Queen Elizabeth Hospital
UH00008015

D1765407

Anesthesiology

Anesthesiology

Second Edition

Edited By

David E. Longnecker, MD, FRCA
Robert D. Dripps Professor Emeritus
Department of Anesthesiology and Critical Care
University of Pennsylvania
Philadelphia, Pennsylvania

David L. Brown, MD
Professor and Chair
Anesthesiology Institute
Cleveland Clinic Lerner College of Medicine
Cleveland, Ohio

Mark F. Newman, MD
Merel H. Harmel Professor and Chairman
Department of Anesthesiology
Duke University Medical Center
Durham, North Carolina

Warren M. Zapol, MD
Reginald Jenney Professor of Anesthesia
Department of Anesthesia
Critical Care and Pain Medicine
Harvard Medical School
Director, Anesthesia Center for Critical Care Research
Massachusetts General Hospital
Boston, Massachusetts

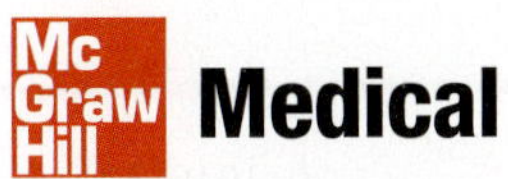

New York Chicago San Francisco Lisbon London Madrid Mexico City
Milan New Delhi San Juan Seoul Singapore Sydney Toronto

The McGraw-Hill Companies

Anesthesiology, Second Edition

1 2 3 4 5 6 7 8 9 0 CTP/CTP 16 15 14 13 12

Set ISBN 978-0-07-178513-6
Set MHID 0-07-178513-2
Book ISBN 978-0-07-166484-4
Book MHID 0-07-166484-X
DVD ISBN 978-0-07-178512-9
DVD MHID 0-07-178512-4

This book was set in Minion Pro by Cenveo Publisher Services.
The editors were Brian Belval and Christie Naglieri.
The production supervisor was Catherine Saggese.
The illustration manager was Armen Ovsepyan.
Project management was provided by Rajni Pisharody, Cenveo Publisher Services.
The designer was Alan Barnett; the cover designer was The Gazillion Group.
China Translation & Printing Services, Ltd. was printer and binder.

Library of Congress Cataloging-in-Publication Data

Anesthesiology / edited by, David E. Longnecker ... [et al.]. — 2nd ed.
p. ; cm.
Includes bibliographical references and index.
ISBN-13: 978-0-07-166484-4 (hardcover : alk. paper)
ISBN-10: 0-07-166484-X (hardcover : alk. paper)
1. Anesthesiology—Textbooks. I. Longnecker, David E., 1939-
[DNLM: 1. Anesthesia. 2. Anesthesiology—methods. 3. Anesthetics.
WO 200]
RD81.P7427 2012
617.9′6—dc23

2011019552

"Life is no brief candle to me; it is a sort of splendid torch which I've got a hold of for the moment and I want to make it burn as brightly as possible before handing it on to future generations."

George Bernard Shaw
Irish playwright (1856–1950)

The editors were fortunate indeed to have outstanding mentors who dedicated their professional lives to the development of our generation in the specialty. Through their guidance, wisdom, and actions, they truly handed the torch to us. As their progeny, we are ever grateful for both their professional guidance and their personal friendship. In recognition of their influence on us individually, and the specialty overall, we dedicate this book to:

Robert M. Epstein,
Harold Carron Professor and Chair
Emeritus of Anesthesiology,
University of Virginia,
on behalf of David E. Longnecker

Daniel C. Moore, Chair Emeritus of Anesthesiology,
Virginia Mason Medical Center, Seattle, Washington,
on behalf of David L. Brown

Jerry Reves, Vice-President for Medical Affairs and Dean,
College of Medicine, Medical University of South Carolina,
Professor of Anesthesiology and Pharmacology
(former Chair, Duke University Department of Anesthesiology),
on behalf of Mark F. Newman

Richard J. Kitz, Henry Isaiah Dorr Distinguished Professor
of Research and Teaching in Anaesthetics and Anaesthesia,
Harvard Medical School and Massachusetts General Hospital,
on behalf of Warren M. Zapol

Edward Lowenstein, Henry Isaiah Dorr Professor of Research
and Teaching in Anaesthetics and Anaesthesia,
Harvard Medical School and Massachusetts General Hospital,
on behalf of Warren M. Zapol

Contents

Contributors

Basem Abdelmalak, MD
Associate Professor of Anesthesiology
Director, Anesthesia for Bronchoscopic Surgery
Departments of General Anesthesiology and Outcomes Research
Director, Center for Sedation and Remote Anesthesia Services
Anesthesiology Institute
Cleveland Clinic
Cleveland, Ohio

Mark Abel MD
Attending Anesthesiologist
Lawrence Hospital
Bronxville, New York

Hassan H. Ali, MD
Professor Emeritus
Harvard Medical School
Boston, Massachusetts

Solomon Aronson, MD, FACC, FACCP, FASE, FAHA
Professor, Duke University Medical Center
Executive Vice Chair, Business Development and Finance
Department of Anesthesiology
Finance Chair, Physicians Diagnostic Clinic
Durham, North Carolina

Edwin G. Avery IV, MD
Chief, Division of Cardiac Anesthesiology
Associate Professor of Anesthesiology
Department of Anesthesiology and Perioperative Medicine
University Hospitals Case Medical Center
Cleveland, Ohio

Michael S. Avidan, MBBCh, FCA SA
Associate Professor, Department of Anesthesiology
Washington University
St. Louis, Missouri

Rafi Avitsian, MD
Associate Professor of Anesthesiology
Section Head, Neurosurgical Anesthesiology
Program Director, Neuroanesthesia Fellowship
Anesthesiology and Neurological Institutes
Cleveland Clinic
Cleveland, Ohio

Douglas R. Bacon, MD, MA
Professor and Chair
Department of Anesthesiology
Wayne State University
Detroit, Michigan

Jane C. Ballantyne, MD, FRCA
Professor, Department of Anesthesiology and Critical Care
University of Pennsylvania School of Medicine
Philadelphia, Pennsylvania

Michael C. Banks, MD
Assistant Professor
Anesthesiology & Critical Care Medicine
Johns Hopkins Hospital
Baltimore, Maryland

Shahar Bar-Yosef, MD
Assistant Consultant Professor
Department of Anesthesiology and Critical Care
Duke University Medical Center
Veterans Affairs Medical Center
Durham, North Carolina

Salvatore J. Basta, MD
Assistant Professor, Department of Anesthesiology
Harvard Medical School/Massachusetts General Hospital
Medical Director, Day Surgery
Department of Anesthesiology, Critical Care and Pain Medicine
Massachusetts General Hospital
Boston, Massachusetts

Loren A. Bauman, MD
Associate Professor, Department of Anesthesiology
Wake Forest University School of Medicine
Winston-Salem, North Carolina

Joseph Bayes, MD
Assistant Professor of Anesthesia
Harvard Medical School
Director of Preoperative Evaluation
Massachusetts Eye & Ear Infirmary
Boston, Massachusetts

David S. Beebe, MD
Professor, Department of Anesthesiology
University of Minnesota Medical School
Minneapolis, Minnesota

Kumar G. Belani, MBBS, MS
Professor Department of Anesthesiology
University of Minnesota Medical School
Adjunct Professor, Medicine & Pediatrics & Environmental Health Sciences
University of Minnesota Schools of Medicine & Public Health
Minneapolis, Minnesota

Patrick E. Benedict, MD
Assistant Professor of Anesthesiology
Director, Preoperative Assessment Clinic
Department of Anesthesiology
University of Michigan Health System
Ann Arbor, Michigan

John R. Benjamin, MD, MS
Assistant Professor, Department of Anesthesiology
The Uniformed Services University of the Health Sciences
Bethesda, Maryland
Anesthesia Critical Care Fellow
Department of Anesthesia, Critical Care, and Pain Management
The Massachusetts General Hospital
Boston, Massachusetts

Claudia Benkwitz, MD, PhD
Instructor, Pediatric Anesthesia
Department of Anesthesia
Stanford University School of Medicine
Stanford, California

Christopher M. Bernards, MD
Anesthesiology Faculty, Department of Anesthesiology
Virginia Mason Medical Center
Clinical Professor of Anesthesiology, Department of Anesthesiology
University of Washington
Seattle, Washington

Sascha Beutler, MD, PhD
Anesthesiologist, Instructor
Harvard Medical School
Department of Anesthesiology
Brigham and Women's Hospital
Boston, Massachusetts

Luca M. Bigatello, MD
Professor of Anesthesiology, Tufts School of Medicine
Director of Surgical Critical Care
Department of Anesthesiology and Pain Medicine
St. Elizabeth's Medical Center
Officer for Critical Care Quality, Steward Healthcare Network
Boston, Massachusetts

Edward A. Bittner, MD, PhD
Assistant Professor, Harvard Medical School
Anesthesiology, Critical Care and Pain Medicine
Massachusetts General Hospital
Boston, Massachusetts

George T. Blike, MD
Quality and Patient Safety Officer
Medical Director of the Patient Safety Training Center
Professor of Anesthesiology and Staff Anesthesiologist
Department of Anesthesiology
Dartmouth College of Medicine
Dartmouth Hitchcock

Cecil O. Borel, MD
Professor, Department of Anesthesiology
Duke University School of Medicine
Durham, North Carolina

Gary J. Brenner, MD, PhD
Director, MGH Pain Medicine Fellowship
Assistant Professor, Harvard Medical School
Department of Anesthesia, Critical Care and Pain Medicine
Massachusetts General Hospital
Boston, Massachusetts

Margaret F. Brock, MD
Assistant Professor, Department of Anesthesiology
Wake Forest University School of Medicine
Winston-Salem, North Carolina

David S. Bronheim, MD
Associate Professor, Department of Anesthesiology
Mount Sinai School of Medicine
New York, New York

David L. Brown, MD
Professor and Chair, Anesthesiology Institute
Cleveland Clinic Lerner College of Medicine
Cleveland, Ohio

Allen W. Burton, MD
Professor and Chairman, Department of Pain Medicine
University of Texas MD Anderson Cancer Center
Houston, Texas

John Capacchione, MD
Assistant Professor, Department of Anesthesiology
Uniformed Services University of the Health Sciences
Bethesda, Maryland

Maurizio Cereda, MD
Assistant Professor, Anesthesiology and Critical Care
University of Pennsylvania School of Medicine
Philadelphia, Pennsylvania

Mark A. Chaney, MD
Professor, Director of Cardiac Anesthesia
Department of Anesthesia and Critical Care
University of Chicago
Chicago, Illinois

Albert T. Cheung, MD
Professor, Department of Anesthesiology and Critical Care
University of Pennsylvania
Philadelphia, Pennsylvania

Ellen P. Convery, MD
Critical Care Fellow, Anesthesia Institute
The Cleveland Clinic
Cleveland, Ohio

Jeffrey B. Cooper, PhD
Professor of Anesthesia, Department of Anesthesia
Harvard Medical School
Biomedical Engineer
Department of Anesthesia, Critical Care and Pain Medicine
Massachusetts General Hospital
Boston, Massachusetts

Mark Dershwitz, MD, PhD
Professor and Vice Chair of Anesthesiology
Professor of Biochemistry & Molecular Pharmacology
University of Massachusetts
Worcester, Massachusetts

Clifford S. Deutschman, MS, MD, FCCM
Professor of Anesthesiology and Critical Care and Surgery
University of Pennsylvania School of Medicine
Philadelphia, Pennsylvania

Teresa E. Dews, MD
Clinical Associate Professor of Anesthesiology
Vice Chair, Department of Pain Management
Anesthesiology Institute Cleveland Clinic
Medical Director, Hillcrest Hospital Pain Management Center
Cleveland Clinic
Cleveland, Ohio

Franklin Dexter, MD, PhD
Professor, Division of Management Consulting
Departments of Anesthesia and Health Management & Policy
University of Iowa
Iowa City, Iowa

Joshua R. Dooley, MD
Assistant Professor, Department of Anesthesiology
Duke University Medical Center
Durham, North Carolina

Adam M. Dryden, MD
Anesthesia Resident
Department of Anesthesiology and Pain Medicine
University of Alberta
Edmonton, Alberta, Canada

Roderic G. Eckenhoff, MD
Austin Lamont Professor
Department of Anesthesiology and Critical Care
University of Pennsylvania
Philadelphia, Pennsylvania

Talmage D. Egan, MD
Professor of Anesthesiology
KC Wong Presidential Chair
University of Utah School of Medicine
Department of Anesthesiology
Salt Lake City, Utah

James B. Eisenkraft, MD
Professor, Department of Anesthesiology
Mount Sinai School of Medicine
New York, New York

Richard H. Epstein, MD, CPHIMS
Professor, Department of Anesthesiology
Jefferson Medical College
Philadelphia, Pennsylvania

Holly C.L. Evans, MD, FRCP(C)
Assistant Professor, Department of Anesthesiology
University of Ottawa
Ottawa, Ontario

Lucinda L. Everett, MD, FAAP
Associate Professor, Anesthesiology
Harvard Medical School
Chief, Pediatric Anesthesia
Department of Anesthesiology, Critical Care, and Pain Medicine
Massachusetts General Hospital
Boston, Massachusetts

Alex S. Evers, MD
Henry Mallinkrodt Professor and Chairman
Department of Anesthesiology
Professor of Internal Medicine and Molecular Biology and Pharmacology
Washington University School of Medicine
Anesthesiologist-in-Chief, Barnes-Jewish Hospital
St. Louis, Missouri

Ehab Farag, MD, FRCA
Associate Professor, Anesthesiology Institute
Cleveland Clinic Lerner College of Medicine
Cleveland, Ohio

Brendan T. Finucane, MBBCh, FRCPC
Professor Emeritus, Anesthesiology and Pain Medicine
University of Alberta
Director Anesthesia Services, Cross Cancer Institute
Edmonton, Alberta, Canada

Michael G. Fitzsimons, MD, FCCP
Assistant Professor, Interim Director Cardiac Anesthesia
Department of Anesthesia, Critical Care, and Pain Medicine
Massachusetts General Hospital
Boston, Massachusetts

Lee A. Fleisher, MD
Robert Dunning Dripps Professor and Chair
Department of Anesthesiology and Critical Care
University of Pennsylvania, School of Medicine
Philadelphia, Pennsylvania

Stuart A. Forman, MD, PhD
Associate Professor of Anesthesia, Harvard Medical School
Associate Anesthetist, Department of Anesthesia
Critical Care and Pain Medicine
Massachusetts General Hospital
Boston, Massachusetts

Robert Gaiser, MD, MSEd
Professor of Anesthesiology and Critical Care, Obstetrics and Gynecology
Department of Anesthesiology and Critical Care
University of Pennsylvania School of Medicine
Philadelphia, Pennsylvania

Rodolfo Gebhardt, MD
Director Acute Pain, Department of Pain
University of Texas MD Anderson Cancer Center
Houston, Texas

Edward George, MD, PhD
Instructor, Harvard Medical School
Assistant Anesthetist, Department of Anesthesia and Critical Care
Massachusetts General Hospital
Boston, Massachusetts

Vijaya Gottumukkala, MB, BS, MD (Anes), FRCA
Professor, Deputy Chairman & Clinical Director
Director, Cancer Anesthesia Fellowship
Department of Anesthesiology and Perioperative Medicine
MD Anderson Cancer Center University of Texas
Houston, Texas

Loretta Grecu, MD
Assistant Professor, Department of Anesthesiology
Yale School of Medicine
Attending Physician, Department of Anesthesiology
Yale New Haven Hospital
New Haven, Connecticut

Katherine Grichnik, MD, MS, FASE
Professor, Department of Anesthesiology
Duke University Medical Center
Durham, North Carolina

Hilary P. Grocott, MD, FRCPC
Professor of Anesthesia and Surgery
University of Manitoba
St. Boniface Hospital
Winnipeg, Manitoba

Judith C. Haas, MD, JD
Director, Department of Anesthesiology
Lakewood Hospital, Cleveland Clinic Health System
Lakewood, Ohio

Basem Hamid, MD
Director, Comprehensive Pain Center of Texas
Memorial Hermann Southeast
Houston, Texas

C. William Hanson III, MD
Professor of Anesthesiology & Critical Care, Surgery and Internal Medicine
Department of Anesthesiology and Critical Care
University of Pennsylvania School of Medicine
Philadelphia, Pennsylvania

James S. Harrington, MD
Instructor, Department of Anesthesiology
Harvard University
Associate in Anesthesia (Cardiac)
Children's Hospital Boston
Boston, Massachusetts

Jessica A. Hathaway, MD
Cardiothoracic Anesthesia Fellow
Department of Anesthesiology
Duke University Medical Center
Durham, North Carolina

James E. Heavner, DVM, PhD
Professor, Anesthesiology and Cell Physiology and Molecular Biophysics
Texas Tech University Health Sciences Center
Lubbock, Texas

Judith Hellman, MD
Associate Professor, Anesthesia and Perioperative Care
University of California, San Francisco
San Francisco, California

Michael R. Hernandez, MD
Assistant Professor, Department of Anesthesia and Critical Care
University of Chicago Biological Sciences Division
Attending Physician
Department of Anesthesia and Critical Care
University of Chicago Hospitals
Chicago, Illinois

Dean R. Hess, PhD, RRT
Associate Professor of Anesthesia
Harvard Medical School
Assistant Director of Respiratory Care
Massachusetts General Hospital
Boston, Massachusetts

Paul R. Hickey, MD
Professor, Department of Anesthesiology
Harvard Medical School
Anesthesiologist-in-Chief
Department of Anesthesiology, Perioperative and Pain Medicine
Children's Hospital Boston
Boston, Massachusetts

Robert S. Holzman, MD, MA (Hon), FAAP
Senior Associate in Perioperative Anesthesia
Department of Anesthesiology, Perioperative & Pain Medicine
Children's Hospital Boston
Professor of Anaesthesia
Harvard Medical School
Boston, Massachusetts

Marc A. Huntoon, MD
Professor, Department of Anesthesiology
Mayo Clinic College of Medicine
Rochester, Minnesota

William E. Hurford, MD
Professor and Chair, Department of Anesthesiology
University of Cincinnati College of Medicine
Cincinnati, Ohio

A. D. John, MD
Assistant Professor, Anesthesia & Critical Care Medicine
Johns Hopkins Medical Institutions
Baltimore, Maryland

Ken B. Johnson, MD
Professor of Anesthesiology
Carter M. Ballinger MD Presidential Chair in Anesthesiology
Department of Anesthesiology
University of Utah
Salt Lake City, Utah

Robert M. Kacmarek, PhD, RRT
Professor, Department of Anesthesia
Harvard Medical School
Director, Department of Respiratory Care
Massachusetts General Hospital
Boston, Massachusetts

John C. Keifer, MD
Associate Professor, Department of Anesthesiology
Duke University
Durham, North Carolina

Max B. Kelz, MD, PhD
Assistant Professor
Department of Anesthesiology and Critical Care
University of Pennsylvania School of Medicine
Philadelphia, Pennsylvania

Sean Kennedy, MD
Associate Professor Emeritus
Department of Anesthesiology and Critical Care
University of Pennsylvania School of Medicine
Philadelphia, Pennsylvania

Miklos D. Kertai, MD, PhD
Assistant Professor of Anesthesiology
Department of Anesthesiology
Division of Cardiothoracic Anesthesia and Critical Care Medicine
Duke University Medical Center
Durham, North Carolina

Sachin Kheterpal, MD, MBA
Assistant Professor
Department of Anesthesiology
University of Michigan
Ann Arbor, Michigan

Stephen M. Klein, MD
Associate Professor, Department of Anesthesiology
Duke University Medical Center
Durham, North Carolina

John C. Klick, MD, FCCP
Assistant Professor of Anesthesiology
Divisions of Cardiac Anesthesia and Intensive Care Medicine
Department of Anesthesiology and Perioperative Medicine
University Hospitals Case Medical Center
Case Western Reserve University School of Medicine
Cleveland, Ohio

P. Allan Klock, Jr, MD
Professor and Vice Chair for Clinical Affairs
Department of Anesthesia and Critical Care
University of Chicago
Chicago, Illinois

W. Andrew Kofke, MD, MBA, FCCM
Professor, Director of Neuroanesthesia
Co-Director Neurocritical Care
Department of Anesthesiology and Critical Care
Department of Neurosurgery
University of Pennsylvania
Philadelphia, Pennsylvania

Benjamin A. Kohl, MD
Assistant Professor
Department of Anesthesiology and Critical Care
University of Pennsylvania School of Medicine
Philadelphia, Pennsylvania

Mojca R. Konia, MD, PhD
Assistant Professor and Program Director
Department of Anesthesiology
University of Minnesota
Minneapolis, Minnesota
Attending Physician
Department of Anesthesiology
Fairview, University of Minnesota
Minneapolis, Minnesota

Jean Kwo, MD
Assistant Professor of Anesthesia, Harvard Medical School
Assistant Anesthetist
Department of Anesthesia, Critical Care, and Pain Medicine
Massachusetts General Hospital
Boston, Massachusetts

Riad Laham, MD
Cleveland Clinic-Hillcrest Hospital Pain Management Center
Cleveland Clinic Lerner College of Medicine
Cleveland, Ohio

Marilyn Green Larach, MD
Senior Research Associate
The North American Malignant Hyperthermia
Registry of MHAUS
Pittsburgh, Pennsylvania

Stephanie L. Lee, MD, PhD, FACE
Associate Professor
Department of Medicine
Boston University School of Medicine
Director, Thyroid Health Center
Section of Endocrinology, Diabetes and Nutrition
Boston Medical Center
Boston, Massachusetts

Frederick W. Lombard, MBChB, FANZCA
Assistant Professor
Department of Anesthesiology
Duke University Medical Center
Durham, North Carolina

David E. Longnecker, MD
Robert D. Dripps Professor Emeritus
Department of Anesthesiology and Critical Care
University of Pennsylvania School of Medicine
Philadelphia, Pennsylvania

G. Burkhard Mackensen, MD, PhD
Associate Professor, Department of Anesthesiology
Duke University Medical Center
Durham, North Carolina

Jonathan B. Mark, MD
Professor and Vice Chair, Department of Anesthesiology
Duke University Medical Center
Chief, Anesthesiology Service
Veterans Affairs Medical Center
Durham, North Carolina

Gavin Martin, MB, FRCA
Associate Professor, Department of Anesthesiology
Duke University Medical Center
Durham, North Carolina

J. A. Jeevendra Martyn, MD, FRCA, FCCM
Director of the Clinical and Biochemical Pharmacology Laboratory
Department of Anesthesia
Massachusetts General Hospital
Anesthetist-in-Chief at the Shriners Hospital for Children
Professor of Anesthesia
Harvard Medical School
Boston, Massachusetts

Joseph P. Mathew, MD, MHSc, FASE
Jerry G. Reves Professor of Anesthesiology
Chief of the Division of Cardiothoracic Anesthesiology
Duke University Medical Center
Durham, North Carolina

Judith A. May, MD
Assistant Professor
Department of Anesthesiology
Medical College of Wisconsin
Milwaukee, Wisconsin

Douglas B. Mayers, MD, PhD
Clinical Associate Professor, Anesthesiology Institute
Cleveland Clinic
Lerner College of Medicine
Cleveland, Ohio

Steve Melton, MD
Assistant Professor, Department of Anesthesiology
Duke University Medical Center
Durham, North Carolina

William T. Merritt, MD, MBA
Department of Anesthesiology and Critical Care Medicine
Johns Hopkins School of Medicine
Department of Surgery
Johns Hopkins School of Medicine
Baltimore, Maryland

Philip J. Mesisca, MBA, CMPE
Chief Operating Officer
Department of Anesthesiology & Critical Care
University of Pennsylvania School of Medicine
Philadelphia, Pennsylvania

Susan Chapman Moss, MPH
Corporate Director
Business Planning & Market Development
Partners Healthcare
Charlestown, Massachusetts

Sheila Muldoon, MD
Professor, Department of Anesthesiology
Uniformed Services University of the Health Sciences
Bethesda, Maryland

Joseph M. Neal, MD
Anesthesiology Faculty
Department of Anesthesiology
Virginia Mason Medical Center
Clinical Professor of Anesthesiology
Department of Anesthesiology
University of Washington
Seattle, Washington

Patrick J. Neligan, MD
Consultant in Anaesthesia and Intensive Care Medicine
Galway University College Hospitals
Honorary Senior Lecturer in Anaesthesia
National University of Ireland
Galway, Ireland

Mark F. Newman, MD
Merel H. Harmel Professor and Chairman
Department of Anesthesiology
Duke University Medical Center
Durham, North Carolina

Alina Nicoara, MD
Assistant Professor of Anesthesiology
Duke University School of Medicine
Durham, North Carolina

Lokesh B. Ningegowda, MD
Staff Physician, Department of Pain Management
Anesthesiology Institute
Cleveland Clinic Lerner College of Medicine
Cleveland, Ohio

E. Andrew Ochroch, MD, MSCE
Associate Professor
Departments of Anesthesiology and Critical Care and Surgery
University of Pennsylvania School of Medicine
Philadelphia, Pennsylvania

Babatunde O. Ogunnaike, MD
Professor, Vice Chairman and Chief of Anesthesia Services, Parkland Health and Hospital System
Department of Anesthesiology and Pain Management
University of Texas Southwestern Medical Center
Dallas, Texas

Ronald P. Olson, MD
Associate Professor, Department of Anesthesiology
Co-director, Preoperative Screening Unit
Duke University Medical Center
Durham, North Carolina

James A. Onigkeit, MD
Department of Anesthesiology
Mayo Clinic College of Medicine
Rochester, Minnesota

Fredrick K. Orkin, MD, MBA, SM
Adjunct Professor of Anesthesiology (proposed)
Yale University School of Medicine
New Haven, Connecticut

Charles W. Otto, MD, FCCM
Professor of Anesthesiology
Associate Professor of Medicine
University of Arizona College of Medicine
Director, Critical Care Medicine
University Medical Center
Tucson, Arizona

Paul S. Pagel, MD, PhD
Staff Anesthesiologist, Anesthesia Service
Clement J. Zablocki Veterans Affairs Medical Center
Professor and Director of Cardiac Anesthesia
Department of Anesthesiology
Medical College of Wisconsin
Milwaukee, Wisconsin

C. Lee Parmley, MD, JD
Executive Medical Director, VUMC Critical Care Units
Director and Professor, Critical Care Anesthesiology
Vanderbilt University Medical Center
Nashville, Tennessee

Michelle C. Parra, MD
Assistant Professor of Anesthesiology
Director Acute Pain Management
Dartmouth Medical School
Dartmouth-Hitchcock Medical Center
Lebanon, New Hampshire

Yash J. Patil, MD, FACS
Assistant Professor, Department of Otolaryngology
Head and Neck Surgery
University of Cincinnati
Cincinnati, Ohio

Robert A. Peterfreund, MD, PhD
Associate Professor, Department of Anesthesia
Harvard Medical School
Anesthetist, Department of Anesthesia,
Critical Care, and Pain Medicine
Massachusetts General Hospital
Boston, Massachusetts

Marc T. Petre, MSc, PhD
Executive Director of Clinical Engineering
Cleveland Clinic Lerner College of Medicine
Cleveland, Ohio

Phillip C. Phan, MD
Assistant Professor, Department of Neurosurgery
Baylor College of Medicine
Director of Pain Management
Interventional Pain Management
Houston Pain Associates
Houston, Texas

James C. Phero, DMD
Professor of Clinical Anesthesia
Clinical Surgery and Clinical Pediatrics Department of Anesthesiology
College of Medicine
University of Cincinnati Academic Health Center
Cincinnati, Ohio

Eric T. Pierce, MD, PhD
Assistant Professor
Department of Anesthesia, Critical Care and Pain Medicine
Massachusetts General Hospital/Harvard Medical School
Boston, Massachusetts

Michael A. Pilla, MD
Associate Professor of Clinical Anesthesiology
Department of Anesthesiology
Vanderbilt University School of Medicine
Nashville, Tennessee

Carlos A. Pino, MD
Director, Center for Pain Medicine
Assistant Professor, Department of Anesthesiology
University of Vermont College of Medicine
Burlington, Vermont

Richard M. Pino, MD, PhD
Associate Anesthetist
Department of Anesthesia, Critical Care, and Pain Medicine
Massachusetts General Hospital
Associate Professor, Harvard Medical School
Boston, Massachusetts

Mihai Podgoreanu, MD, FASE
Associate Professor of Anesthesiology
Department of Anesthesiology
Division of Cardiothoracic Anesthesia and Critical Care Medicine
Duke University Medical Center
Durham, North Carolina

Bil Ragan, MD
Director Residency Education
Associate Anesthesiologist, Department of Anesthesiology
Massachusetts Eye and Ear Infirmary/MGH
Harvard Medical School
Boston, Massachusetts

Douglas E. Raines, MD
Associate Anesthetist
Department of Anesthesia, Critical Care, and Pain Medicine
Massachusetts General Hospital
Associate Professor, Harvard Medical School
Boston, Massachusetts

Atif Raja, MD
Fellow, Duke Adult Cardiothoracic Anesthesiology Fellow
Department of Anesthesiology
Duke University Medical Center
Durham, North Carolina

James P. Rathmell, MD
Professor of Anaesthesia, Harvard Medical School
Chief, Division of Pain Medicine
Department of Anesthesia, Critical Care and Pain Medicine
Massachusetts General Hospital
Boston, Massachusetts

Ron H. Rawlings, MD
Department of Anesthesiology
Duke University Hospital
Durham, North Carolina

Ihab A. Riad, MD
Staff Anesthesiologist, Department of Anesthesia
Fairview Hospital
Cleveland, Ohio

Richard W. Rosenquist, MD
Chairman, Pain Management Department
Cleveland Clinic
Cleveland, Ohio

Mark I. Rossberg, MD
Assistant Professor
Department of Anesthesiology and Critical Care Medicine
The Johns Hopkins Medical Institutions
Baltimore, Maryland

Carl E. Rosow, MD, PhD
Professor of Anesthesia, Harvard Medical School
Department of Anesthesia, Critical Care and Pain Management
Massachusetts General Hospital
Boston, Massachusetts

Raymond C. Roy, MD, PhD
Professor, Department of Anesthesiology
Wake Forest University School of Medicine
Winston-Salem, North Carolina

Robert H. Rubin, MD, FACP, FCCP
Gordan and Marjorie Osborne Professor of
Health Sciences and Technology
Professor of Medicine, Harvard Medical School
Co-director, Division of Infectious Disease
Brigham and Women's Hospital
Boston, Massachusetts

Nyamkhishig Sambuughin, PhD
Research Assistant Professor, Department of Anesthesiology
Uniformed Services University of the Health Sciences
Bethesda, Maryland

Warren S. Sandberg, MD, PhD
Professor and Chair, Department of Anesthesiology
Vanderbilt University School of Medicine
Nashville, Tennessee

Joseph S. Savino, MD
Professor, Department of Anesthesiology and Critical Care
University of Pennsylvania School of Medicine
Philadelphia, Pennsylvania

Rebecca A. Schroeder, MD
Associate Professor, Department of Anesthesiology
Duke University Medical Center
Veterans Affairs Medical Center
Durham, North Carolina

Benjamin K. Scott, MD
Department of Anesthesiology and Critical Care
University of Pennsylvania School of Medicine
Philadelphia, Pennsylvania

John W. Sear, MA, BSc, MBBS, PhD, FFARCS, FANZCA
Emeritus Professor, Nuffield Department of Anesthetics
University of Oxford
Headington, Oxford, UK

Sally P. Seraphin, MD
Assistant Professor, Department of Anesthesia and Critical Care
University of Chicago Pritzker School of Medicine
Attending Physician
Department of Anesthesia and Critical Care
University of Chicago Hospitals
Chicago, Illinois

Nirav J. Shah, MD
Assistant Professor, Tufts Medical Center
Department of Anesthesiology
Boston, Massachusetts

Andrew D. Shaw, MBBS, FRCA, FCCM
Associate Professor of Anesthesiology
Duke University Medical Center
Veteran's Affairs Anesthesiology Service
Durham, North Carolina

Stanton K. Shernan, MD, FAHA, FASE
Professor of Anaesthesia, Director of Cardiac Anesthesia
Brigham and Women's Hospital
Harvard Medical School
Boston, Massachusetts

Avinash C. Shukla, MD
Assistant Professor
Department of Anesthesia
Harvard Medical School
Associate in Anesthesia (Cardiac)
Children's Hospital
Boston, Massachusetts

Nathaniel Sims, MD
Assistant Professor of Anesthesia
Department of Anesthesia and Critical Care
Massachusetts General Hospital
Boston, Massachusetts

Kieran A. Slevin, MD
Chief, Interventional Pain and Spine
Virtua Pain and Spine
Virtua Health System
Voorhees, New Jersey

Martin K. Slodzinski, MD, PhD
Clinical Associate, Anesthesiology and Critical Care Medicine
Johns Hopkins University
Baltimore, Maryland

Brian C. Spence, MD
Assistant Professor, Department of Anesthesiology
Director, Same Day Surgery
Dartmouth-Hitchcock Medical Center
Lebanon, New Hampshire

Mark Stafford-Smith, MD, CM, FRCPC
Professor of Anesthesiology
Director of Fellowship Education
Director, Duke Adult Cardiothoracic Anesthesiology Fellowship
Department of Anesthesiology
Duke University Medical Center
Durham, North Carolina

Madhav Swaminathan, MD, FASE, FAHA
Associate Professor, Anesthesiology
Duke University Health System
Durham, North Carolina

BobbieJean Sweitzer, MD
Professor of Anesthesia and Critical Care
Professor of Medicine
Director of Anesthesia Perioperative Medicine Clinic
Department of Anesthesia and Critical Care
University of Chicago
Chicago, Illinois

Richard S. Teplick, MD
Chief of Staff, University of South Alabama Hospitals (retired)
Professor of Medicine, Surgery and Anesthesiology
University of South Alabama College of Medicine (retired)
Mobile, Alabama

Joseph R. Tobin, MD
Professor and Chairman, Department of Anesthesiology
Wake Forest University School of Medicine
Winston-Salem, North Carolina

Slobodan M. Todorovic, MD, PhD
Professor, Department of Anesthesiology and Neuroscience
University of Virginia School of Medicine
Charlottesville, Virginia

Tony A. Tran, MD
Anesthesia Resident, Department of Anesthesia
University of Manitoba
Winnipeg, Manitoba

Kevin K. Tremper, PhD, MD
Robert B. Sweet Professor and Chairman
Department of Anesthesiology
University of Michigan Health System
Ann Arbor, Michigan

Christopher A. Troianos, MD
Professor and Chair
Department of Anesthesiology
Western Pennsylvania Hospital
West Penn Allegheny Health System
Western Campus of Temple University School of Medicine
Pittsburgh, Pennsylvania

Lawrence C. Tsen, MD
Associate Professor of Anaesthesia, Harvard Medical School
Vice Chair, Faculty Development and Education
Department of Anesthesiology, Perioperative and Pain Medicine
Brigham and Women's Hospital
Boston, Massachusetts

Ban C.H. Tsui, MSc, MD, FRCPC
Professor
Department of Anesthesiology and Pain Medicine
University of Alberta
Edmonton, Alberta, Canada
Director, Regional Anesthesia and Acute Pain Service
Department of Anesthesiology and Pain Medicine
Stollery Children's Hospital/University of Alberta Hospital
Edmonton, Alberta, Canada

Brian S. Uthlaut, MD
Assistant Professor of Medicine
Department of Medicine
University of Virginia Health System
Charlottesville, Virginia

Jean-Louis Vincent, MD, PhD
Professor of Intensive Care Medicine
Head, Department of Intensive Care
Erasme Hospital, Free University of Brussels, Belgium

Maria Voelkel, BA
Contractor, HJF
Comprehensive National Neuroscience Program
Department of Neurology
Uniformed Services University of the Health Sciences
Silver Spring, Maryland

Brian J. Wainger, MD, PhD
Instructor, Harvard Medical School
Department of Anesthesia, Critical Care and Pain Medicine
Massachusetts General Hospital
Boston, Massachusetts

David B. Waisel, MD
Associate Professor of Anaesthesia
Harvard Medical School
Department of Anesthesiology, Perioperative and Pain Medicine
Children's Hospital
Boston, Massachusetts

Binbin Wang, MD
Assistant Clinical Professor
Department of Anesthesia and Critical Care
University of California, San Francisco
San Francisco, California

David O. Warner, MD
Professor of Anesthesiology
Mayo Clinic College of Medicine
Rochester, Minnesota

Daniel T. Warren, MD
Section Head, Director, Anesthesiology Pain Clinic
Program Director, Pain Medicine Fellowship
Department of Anesthesiology
Virginia Mason Medical Center
Seattle, Washington

Stuart J. Weiss, MD, PhD
Associate Professor
Department of Anesthesiology and Critical Care
University of Pennsylvania School of Medicine
Philadelphia, Pennsylvania

Lynda T. Wells, MBBS, FRCA
Associate Professor of Anesthesiology and Pediatrics
University of Virginia Health System
Charlottesville, Virginia

Ian J. Welsby, BSc, MBBS, FRCA
Associate Professor
Department of Anesthesiology and Critical Care
Duke University Medical Center
Durham, North Carolina

Randall C. Wetzel, MBBS, MRCP, LRCS, MBA, FAAP, FCCM
Ann O'Melveny Wilson Professor of Critical Care Medicine
Department of Pediatrics Anesthesiology
University of Southern California
Los Angeles, California

Charles W. Whitten, MD
Professor and Chairman
Margaret Milam McDermott Distinguished Chair in Anesthesiology and Pain Management
Department of Anesthesiology and Pain Management
UT Southwestern Medical Center
Dallas, Texas

Richard A. Wiklund, MD
Associate Clinical Professor, Department of Anesthesia
Harvard Medical School
Honorary Anesthetist
Department of Anesthesia, Critical Care, and Pain Management
Massachusetts General Hospital
Boston, Massachusetts

Jessica L. Willert, MD, MSc
Attending Physician, Active International Cardiovascular Institute
Good Samaritan Hospital
Suffern, New York
Attending Physician, Department of Anesthesiology
St Mary's Hospital
Passaic, New Jersey

Myron Yaster, MD
Richard J Traystman Professor
Departments of Anesthesiology, Critical Care Medicine, and Pediatrics
Johns Hopkins University
Baltimore, Maryland

Warren M. Zapol, MD
Reginald Jenney Professor of Anesthesia,
Department of Anesthesia, Critical Care and Pain Medicine
Harvard Medical School
Director, Anesthesia Center for Critical Care Research
Massachusetts General Hospital
Boston, Massachusetts

David A. Zvara, MD
Professor and Chair, Department of Anesthesiology
The University of North Carolina at Chapel Hill School of Medicine
Chapel Hill, North Carolina

Preface

Anesthesiology, and indeed all of US health care, is influenced currently by two dominant trends. First, the passage of the Patient Protection and Affordable Care Act (PPACA) of 2010 codified the US commitment to broad-based access to health care, and it underscored that such care must be more efficient and cost effective. Second, the emphasis on quality and safety in health care has gained even greater momentum. Together, these trends emphasize the concept of value in health care. These trends are not unique to the United States. Rather, they represent global trends in health care policy and practice. We believe they will be dominant themes for many years to come and thus they are guiding principles in the second edition of this text.

Fortunately, the specialty of anesthesiology is well positioned to lead these initiatives. Anesthesiology is already recognized as the pioneering leader in patient safety and we see no reason why anesthesiologists should not be leaders in efficiency and value in health care as well. Indeed, we believe that continuing to position our specialty at the forefront of these initiatives is a key strategy for both the current and future success of anesthesiology and its practitioners.

In 2000, the Institute of Medicine (IOM) published its landmark analysis of American health care, "To Err is Human," a treatise that emphasized the fallibility of even highly motivated humans, and emphasized that systems of safe care must be constructed to protect patients from potential harm. That report specifically cited anesthesiology as a leader in the patient safety movement and urged other disciplines to follow, which many have done subsequently. A subsequent IOM publication, "Crossing the Quality Chasm; A New Health System for the 21st Century" (2001) described the attributes of a model health care system that is safe, timely, efficient, effective, patient centered and equitable to all. The PPACA legislation underscored these principles and subsequent regulations translated them into operational policies and practices. We agree with these principles and have worked diligently to adopt them in our own practices and departments, for they are guideposts to the professional and ethical practice of medicine and anesthesiology. Further, we have designed this text around the concepts of safe, effective, efficient, and patient-centered care, and we urge others to approach their practice with a similar commitment to these principles.

Our goal is to provide the practitioner with a single resource that captures the essence of the full spectrum of anesthesia practice. There are multiple sources of information about anesthesiology but many ignore the full breadth of the practice. Further, there are numerous focused texts that delve into specific subdisciplines in great detail; often more detail than the trainee or practitioner desires or needs. In this text, we have focused on what is truly important for the clinical practice of anesthesiology in all its dimensions, while being efficient in the presentation of this essential material. Throughout, we have asked "What is important?" "Why is it important?" "When should it be applied?" and "How should it be applied?" Our goal was to write for practitioners, not physician scientists. That said, this is not a users' manual of anesthesia care, but rather a text that constantly builds on the concepts of safe, effective (ie, evidence-based), efficient, and patient-centered care, distilled in a manner that facilitates easy access to the key scientific concepts that underpin the rationale for that practice. Thus one finds Key Points and Key References in each chapter, while an extensive reference list is provided online for those who seek in-depth research-based documentation.

Throughout, we embrace an encompassing view of modern anesthesiology practice, including especially perioperative medicine, critical care medicine, and pain medicine, each of which improves patient care and enhances the value of anesthesia care within the overall health care process. We have emphasized important trends in both the specialty and in health care in general, to ensure that the reader is not required to go elsewhere for additional information to support the mainstream of their practice. These trends include the expanded use of regional anesthesia, the remarkable explosion in pain medicine practice, and the expanded need for practitioners who are skilled in the practice of critical care medicine. No careful observer of the specialty could miss these trends, and no text could be considered "comprehensive" if it did not embrace them as full components of the modern practice of anesthesiology.

Further, we have woven the concepts of quality, safety, cost effectiveness, and value into the text by emphasizing that anesthesia care is one system of care within a larger system of care that focuses on overall patient outcomes, not independent events by individual practitioners working in isolated clinical disciplines.

We have approached these and other key "drivers" of contemporary and future anesthesia practice with care, commitment, and enthusiasm for the future of the specialty. We trust that you share this enthusiasm and hope our efforts will serve you well as you continue to translate your knowledge and skills into safe, effective, efficient, and patient-centered care; our patients want nothing less and our surgical and medical colleagues are looking to anesthesiology to continue to set the example for implementation of these principles. We are honored to serve you through our efforts here.

David E. Longnecker, MD
David L. Brown, MD
Mark F. Newman, MD
Warren M. Zapol, MD

PART 1

The Specialty of Anesthesiology

CHAPTER 1

The Evolution of Anesthesiology as a Clinical Discipline: A Lesson in Developing Professionalism

Douglas R. Bacon

KEY POINTS

1. The history of anesthesiology is an interesting and complicated story of professionals seeking to understand the anesthetic state and to anesthetize patients safely.
2. Shortly after the first public demonstration of ether anesthesia on October 16, 1846, the news spread across the world. At first anesthetics were given based on written accounts, often in the lay press.
3. John Snow, a London physician, worked out the physics of vaporization of volatile agents by observation off ether and chloroform and used this information to design vaporizers and anesthetic techniques that were safer for the patient.
4. The first professional organization devoted to anesthesia was the London Society of Anaesthetists founded on May 30, 1893. The first similar group in the United States was the Long Island Society organized by Adolph Frederick Erdmann in 1905. The Long Island Society eventually became the American Society of Anesthesiologists.
5. Francis Hoffer McMechan organized professional anesthesia. He helped create the first national organization, the Associated Anesthetists of America in 1912, and went on to found several national and international organizations, of which the International Anesthesia Research Society (IARS) remains active. He was the founding editor of the first journal in the world devoted to the specialty, *Current Researches in Anesthesia and Analgesia,* which is currently published as *Anesthesia and Analgesia*.
6. Ralph Water is credited with the first department of anesthesia within an academic setting at the University of Wisconsin in 1927. Much of the current residency structure comes from this seminal department that helped establish the specialty on an equal footing with other medical specialties and created a method to train physicians in the art and science of anesthesia.
7. John Lundy, working at the Mayo Clinic, organized the Anaesthetists Travel Club, whose members were the leading young anesthetists of the United States and Canada. These individuals helped create, by 1938, the American Board of Anesthesiology, which defined what it meant to be an anesthesiologist in the United States.
8. The need for physician specialists in World War II exposed a large number of young men to anesthesiology who would not have otherwise considered the specialty. After the hostilities ceased, these physicians returned and helped create the tremendous growth in the 1950s and 1960s that the specialty enjoyed.
9. In the mid-1950s, the World Federation of Societies of Anesthesiologists (WFSA) was formed. It was the culmination of a dream that dated to the late 1930s. The WFSA made it possible for nations with a long tradition of physician specialization in anesthesia to help train and create the specialty in countries where it did not or does not exist.
10. In the 1980s, the Anesthesia Patient Safety Foundation (APSF) and the Foundation for Anesthesia Education and Research (FAER) were created. They are additional examples of the professionalism demonstrated throughout the history of anesthesiology. These two organizations work to create a safe anesthetic environment. In addition, they support educational and research efforts in the specialty.

The quest for insensibility to the surgeon's knife is a primordial one. Stretching back to antiquity, physicians have sought ways to render a patient pain free while an operation was being performed. Many different regimens were tried, with varying success, until October 16, 1846, when surgical anesthesia was publicly demonstrated at the Massachusetts General Hospital by William Thomas Green Morton. Yet there remained a long road from that fall day in Boston to the current operating room full of electronic machines whose sole purpose is to measure the physiologic parameters of the anesthetized patient. How did anesthesiology evolve from a simple glass globe inhaler to the vast array of machines that makes the modern operating room?

The history of anesthesiology is the history of the men and women who have devoted their career to the administration of anesthetics. Without physicians interested in the anesthetic state and the ability to adapt to new conditions demanded of anesthesiologists by surgeons, there would be neither modern surgery nor the specialty of anesthesiology. Yet each individual was a real human, many displaying professionalism beyond what was required or expected; others seem reprehensible by "modern" standards. Although many of the individuals in this story would not consider themselves specialists in anesthesia, their contributions were critical in moving the specialty forward. The development of anesthesiology can be told as the history of involved physicians who dedicated themselves to providing safer, focused care of the patient, first in the operating room and later in the critical care unit and pain clinic. The story begins in ancient Egypt and continues to evolve in untold ways.

PREHISTORY: THE QUEST FOR SURGICAL ANESTHESIA

Imagine for a moment that there is no surgical anesthesia. The Edwin Smith Papyrus describes 48 surgical cases done between 3000 and 2500 BC. Although there is no specific anesthetic agent, within the papyrus there is evidence of compression anesthesia. In one instance, a surgeon is compressing the antecubital fossa while operating on the hand; in another instance, the patient is compressing his brachial plexus while the surgeon operates on his palm.[1] The ancient Chinese reported the use of an anesthetic for surgery in the 2nd century BC.[2] The use of hemp smoke as an anesthetic was noted in India[3] long before Western medicine developed crude forms of anesthesia.

During the Middle Ages and early Renaissance, a mixture of herbs purported to induce anesthesia was created. Boiled into a sponge, at the time of surgery the sponge was placed in water and the vapors inhaled. Although the vinca alkaloids were a major component of the drugs used in the *spongia somnifera*, the resultant anesthetic was less than satisfactory. Another Renaissance solution was the use of parallel lines of ice, with the incision placed between them. This was effective for simple operations and found use in the Russo-Finnish War of 1939-1940.[4] Alcohol, when drunk in sufficient quantities, was noted to render individuals insensible. Thus the age-old intoxicant was used as a standard against which all anesthetics could be measured.[3]

In the early 1840s, the effects of nitrous oxide and diethyl ether were well known. Both drugs were well known to medical students as intoxicants. Humphry Davy had described the intoxicating effects well in his book, *Researches Chemical and Philosophical: Chiefly Concerning Nitrous Oxide*, published in 1800. Ether, which had been first synthesized in the 1500s, had been observed to lessen the "air hunger" of asthmatics.[5] In January 1842, in Rochester, New York, a medical student, William E. Clark, anesthetized the sister of a classmate for the extraction of a molar using ether. Instructed not to pursue this observation, as it most likely was a "hysterical reaction of women," Clarke continued his training and became a respected physician in the Chicago, Illinois, area.[6]

Two months later, in rural Georgia, a country doctor, Crawford Long, who had hosted parties where ether was used as an intoxicant, used the drug to render James Venable insensitive for the removal of tumors from the back of his neck. Long charged Venable $2 for the anesthetic, thus delineating anesthesia as part of a physician's professional service.

Two years later, in 1844, Horace Wells, a dentist in Hartford, Connecticut, would gain the insight that, during a nitrous oxide (N_2O) show, when an individual was intoxicated by N_2O, pain was abolished. Wells then tried this idea on himself for the removal of one of his teeth by his partner, and it was successful. Soon he was using "painless dentistry" as part of his professional advertisement. Wells even attempted to demonstrate a painless tooth extraction at the Massachusetts General Hospital in 1844, but the patient groaned, although later had no memory of the event, and the demonstration was considered a failure.[7]

Clearly, by the middle of the 19th century, there were sufficient observations about specific agents that could potentially abolish the pain of surgery. On a limited scale in rural Jefferson, Georgia, surgery with ether anesthesia was happening. Yet Long felt he lacked sufficient cases to study the effects of this new agent.[8] Wells's use of N_2O was groundbreaking, yet he lacked the emotional stability to overcome his failed demonstration.[9] Thus the stage was set for another dentist to demonstrate reproducible surgical anesthesia and give birth to what would grow and develop into the specialty of anesthesiology.

DISCOVERY

On October 16, 1846, William Thomas Green Morton, a dentist and medical student, provided surgical anesthesia for Gilbert Abbott for the removal of a tumor of the jaw at Massachusetts General Hospital. The events of that day are well known.[10] Upon completing the operation, the surgeon, John Collins Warren, remarked, "Gentlemen, this is no humbug." The miracle of pain-free surgery so impressed the Boston medical establishment that letters were sent to colleagues across the world. Considerable scholarship has been spent discerning when these letters arrived, where they arrived, and who provided anesthesia first in the new location. For example, the generally accepted view of the spread of anesthesia to the United Kingdom is a letter from Jacob Bigelow to Francis Boot. However, by careful study of the ships sailing between Boston and Liverpool, another letter, written almost 2 weeks before Bigelow's and only 12 days after the public demonstration of ether, arrived in England on November 1, 1846. Interestingly, this letter was to a patent attorney.[11]

Morton wanted to patent the process by which ether was administered, so writing to the foremost patent attorney in England to secure rights to the administration of ether in the United States and the United Kingdom,[9] and perhaps the world, is not surprising. He also tried to patent ether itself, calling his anesthetizing mixture "Letheon." However, the distinctive odor of ether gave away the true nature of the concoction. The Boston medical establishment had convinced Morton to allow Massachusetts General Hospital to use Letheon without charge. With ether a well-known and easy-to-synthesize compound, and its effects reproducible without the "Morton's Inhaler," the patent was unenforceable. Morton would spend the rest of his life attempting to be compensated for patent infringement, fighting with the medical establishment and into the halls of Congress.[8] Morton clearly was not the embodiment of medical professionalism as we currently understand it.

News of Morton's achievement did travel, and quickly, given the nature of communication in the 1840s. On December 16, 1846, ether anesthesia, in the form of a letter, arrived in London. On December 19, the first ether anesthetic was given in the United Kingdom for the removal of a tooth. On December 21, Robert Liston, the famous surgeon, amputated the leg of a butler and uttered the famous words, "This Yankee dodge beats mesmerism hollow." By early 1847, anesthetics were being given across Europe. In June of that year, the news had spread to Australia.[12] Peter Parker, minister and physician missionary in China, gave the first anesthetics there on October 4, 1847.[13]

For the history of the specialty of anesthesiology, what is interesting is how willing physicians and dentists were to use ether to induce insensibility. Consider for a moment that outside of Boston, none of the recipients had actually witnessed surgical anesthesia. Many accounts, especially those reaching South Africa and Australia, were newspaper articles or letters to the editor, often signed by a pseudonym. The hope of these medical professionals, their desperation at their inability to alleviate pain, and their desire to help patients may well have motivated them to try this new technique. Yet when viewed from the perspective of current 21st-century medical practice, this willingness to go on purely written accounts, often in the lay press, without the collaborating voices of the medical profession, seems to be dangerous and without regard for the basic principle of medicine: first do no harm.

And what of the surgeons? Tolerance of the pain of surgery limited operations to those that could be performed quickly. Anesthesia obviated the need for speed, presenting the possibility of operating within the visceral cavities for hours rather than seconds. But as the physician responsible for the patient, long before the specialty of anesthesiology would be defined, why were these professionals willing to risk lives to find an anesthetic? What does this behavior say to the modern student of medical professionalism?

JOHN SNOW, SPECIALIZATION, AND EARLY PROFESSIONALISM

As reprehensible as Morton's actions appear in patenting his "discovery," he was acting within the ethics of his time. The American Medical Association (AMA) was only just beginning to be formed. Meeting for the first time in May 1846, 5 months before the public demonstration, the National Medical Convention adopted a resolution to write a code of medical ethics. A year later, the code was adopted. Morton's actions were covered under section 4: "Equally derogatory to professional character is it, for a physician to hold a patent for any surgical instrument, or medicine, or to dispense a secret nostrum, whether it be the composition or exclusive property of himself or others. For, if such nostrum be of real efficacy, any concealment regarding it is inconsistent with beneficence and professional liberality."[14]

Thus at the time when Morton was trying to patent either ether or the apparatus for its vaporization, medicine was starting to organize and promulgate statements against such behavior.

In contrast, John Snow (**Fig. 1-1**), a London physician, began to study the chemical and physical properties of ether, and by 1847 he had

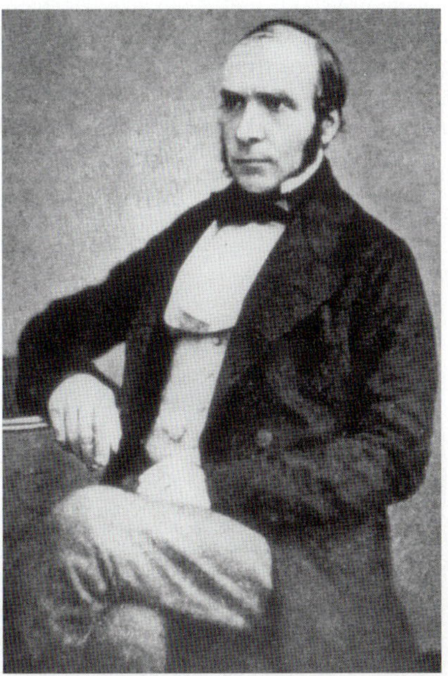

FIGURE 1-1. John Snow. [Photograph courtesy of the Wood Library-Museum of Anesthesiology.]

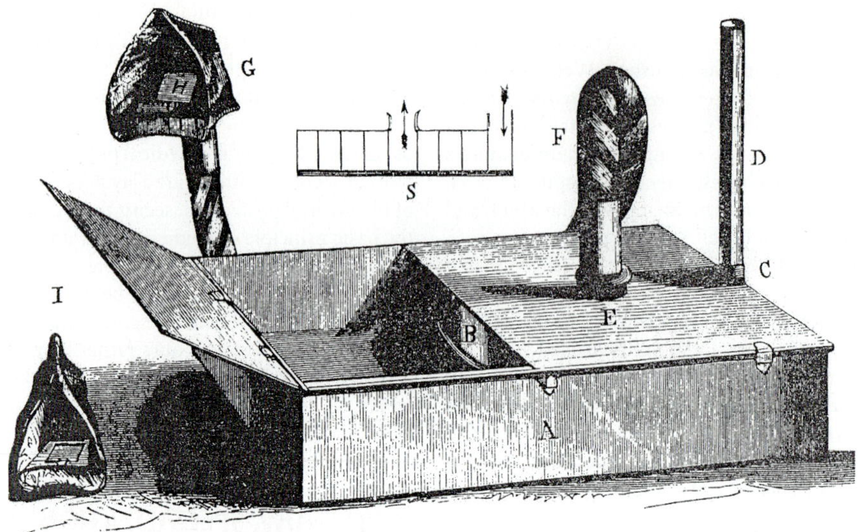

FIGURE 1-2. Snow's vaporizer. [Image courtesy of the Wood Library-Museum of Anesthesiology.]

developed a vaporizer. "Snow never patented any apparatus he designed. On the contrary, he published clear descriptions, including engraved figures, so that others could copy them if they chose."[15] Snow, by careful observation, worked out the vaporization characteristics of ether. His vaporizer (**Fig. 1-2**) was temperature compensated, being made of coiled copper (**Fig. 1-3**), an excellent heat-conducting metal, housed in a water bath to ensure constant temperature of the ether. Thus Snow was able to calculate the amount of ether a patient required for anesthesia within a few years of the discovery of anesthesia.[13]

Following the introduction of chloroform as an anesthetic in 1847 by Edinburgh obstetrician James Young Simpson, Snow began to investigate this second anesthetic agent. Snow used his experience with ether as a guide for investigating the properties of chloroform. He concluded that it was far safer to give this new anesthetic in measured quantities through an inhaler and did not favor the handkerchief method, whereby chloroform was applied to a cloth and held close to the nose and mouth because the anesthetic depth of the patient could not be adequately controlled. His deliberate nature and strong powers of observation allowed Snow to create a calibrated, temperature-compensated vaporizer for chloroform as well.[13]

Snow was unique among his colleagues in the 1850s in London. In a day when operations were still rarely performed, Snow specialized in anesthetics. In some ways, his expert knowledge allowed him entrée into the upper echelons of both social and physician circles, a status he could not have obtained had he not limited his practice. Perhaps this is best illustrated by his attendance on Queen Victoria for the birth of her last two children. Although Snow did not use his inhaler, he also did not induce the full anesthetic state in the queen. Rather, he strove for analgesia with chloroform, and in so doing, he created a form of obstetric analgesia, *chloroform à la reine*, which would persist in various forms over the next century.[13]

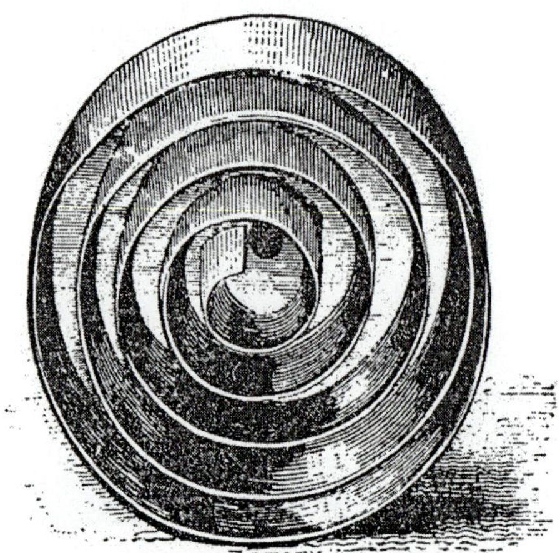

FIGURE 1-3. Coil from Snow's vaporizer. [Image courtesy of the Wood Library-Museum of Anesthesiology.]

Aside from working out the physics of vaporization, Snow was intensely interested in outcome data. He studied every report concerning a death under anesthesia and oftentimes had data in advance of the published reports of death. He commented extensively on the death of Hannah Greener, thought to be the first death under anesthesia in the world.[16] In his posthumous book, *On Chloroform and other Anesthetics,*[17] published in 1858, Snow compiled the first 50 deaths under chloroform, with comments about the pathophysiology present. Snow's spirit of inquiry, which went from the bench top to the pathologic findings at death, helped him understand the nature of the anesthetic process and the agents that produced insensibility, thus the scientific underpinnings for a specialty.[18]

A PROFESSION EMERGES

After Snow's untimely death, anesthesia faded into the medical background again. In larger cities, there were those who made most of their clinical income from providing anesthesia, yet it would not be until the advent of Listerism and the "taming" of infection that operations would become more frequent. As the number of operations increased, so did the need for anesthesia, and, unfortunately, mortality became an issue. Chloroform was responsible for deaths that seemed unexplainable. Ether appeared to be safer, yet the side effects of nausea and vomiting, and the prolonged induction when compared with chloroform, made ether a less-than-ideal agent. Surgeons began to search for alternative methods for the administration of anesthetics.

In 1884, Carl Koller, a resident in ophthalmology in Vienna, was introduced by Sigmund Freud to a new crystalline substance called cocaine. Koller sought a local anesthetic to replace ether anesthesia for operations on the eye; because fine suture material to close the eye wound did not exist, any postoperative retching potentially could cause the loss of vision. Thus when Koller's tongue became numb from droplets of a solution containing cocaine, he made the conceptual leap that this same solution could be applied to the cornea with similar anesthetic effects on the eye. Using the facilities of the laboratory in which he worked, Koller soon numbed the eyes of several animals, a fellow investigator, and himself. He took this new topical anesthetic to the clinic and used it with great success. On September 15, 1884, Koller's paper on the subject was accepted at the German Ophthalmological Society meeting in Heidelberg. Too poor to travel, his colleague, Dr Josef Brettauer, presented the paper for Koller.[19]

While Koller continued his career in ophthalmology, eventually emigrating to the United States, other physicians modified this new form of anesthesia into an alternative to general narcosis. One of the early practitioners was William Halstead, future chair of surgery at Johns Hopkins University, who was in Vienna at the time of Koller's discovery. Using cocaine topically, Halstead dissected down to a nerve and directly anesthetized it. Much of the work he did on himself, becoming addicted to cocaine in the process.[20] Another of the pioneers of regional anesthesia was the German surgeon Carl Ludwig Schleich, who developed the technique of infiltration anesthesia.[21] Combining infiltration techniques with the newly discovered lumbar puncture, August Bier, another academic German surgeon, initiated spinal anesthesia in the late 1890s. Working with his fellow, August Hildebrandt, Bier successfully cannulated the subarachnoid space of Hildebrandt and produced a satisfactory anesthetic state. Hildebrandt was unsuccessful in cannulating Bier's subarachnoid space; however, both men suffered postdural-puncture headaches.[22] Ten years later, Bier described an intravenous regional anesthetic technique that is still referred to as the Bier block.[23]

At the same time when regional anesthesia was being developed in Germany, concern over the safety of chloroform, especially when compared with ether, was developing. In India, then a colony of England, a Chloroform Commission was seated in Hyderabad to attempt to determine which anesthetic agent was safest. Funded by the Nizam of Hyderabad, the 1888 study of anesthetic agents was an effort to find out if there was an intrinsic mortality associated with chloroform. The findings were tainted by the British medical officer in charge, Dr Edward Lawrie, who was a strong chloroform proponent, having trained in Edinburgh, chloroform's birthplace. The findings of the Hyderabad Chloroform Commission were not conclusive, and a second was ordered, which also was inconclusive. But what was important in these commissions is that physicians were studying anesthesia and trying to increase patient safety. For many physicians, the need for a specialty practice of anesthesia was slowly becoming apparent.[24]

Early in the 20th century, the AMA set up a commission to study anesthetics. A preliminary report was issued in 1908.[25] All forms of anesthesia were accounted for, including spinal anesthesia and various combinations of inhalational agents. The conclusions of the report are interesting, for they foreshadow the development of a separate specialty:

> [A]ll the newer methods demand expertness, experience, and special apparatus. They appeal especially to the surgeons who are equipped with the paraphernalia of expensive and highly specialized clinics. They are little suited to physicians in general practice. For the latter great class of practitioners, the old general anesthetics, chloroform and ether, will probably hold their own until increasing experience has enabled us to simplify and to make safe the newer and more novel methods.[25]

The commission had three very interesting recommendations:

1. That for the general practitioner, and for all anesthetists not specially skilled, ether must be the anesthetic of choice—ether administered by the open-drop method.
2. That the use of chloroform, particularly for the minor operations, be discouraged, unless it is given by an expert.
3. That the training of skilled anesthetists be encouraged and that undergraduate students be more generally instructed in the use of anesthetics.[25]

The third suggestion of the commission would take almost the entire 20th century to implement.

THE RISE OF THE SPECIALIST

In 1905 in Brooklyn, New York, a group of 8 physicians and a medical student, led by Adolph Frederick Erdmann (**Fig. 1-4**), gathered to discuss the problem of anesthetics. These young physicians thought, like the AMA commission, that there was more to the giving of an anesthetic than simply dropping ether on a cloth held near the patient's face, and that discussions and a free exchange of scientific and practical information were needed.[26] This was the second specialty group in the world that was created. The first was the London Society of Anesthetists in 1893, and it would become the catalyst for the development and recognition of physicians who were specialists in anesthesia.[27] Thus the Long Island Society of Anesthetists was born. The society met quarterly, in the evening, with a short business meeting followed by the presentation of 2 or 3 papers and perhaps the demonstration of a new anesthetic technique or apparatus. Science aside, the society provided a support group for those seeking to improve their anesthetic skills and a forum at which to exchange ideas and deal with problems beyond the science of anesthesia.[26]

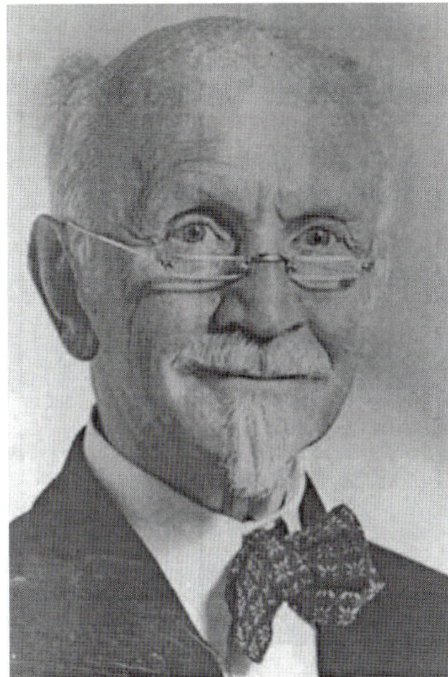

FIGURE 1-4. Adolph Frederick Erdmann. [Photograph courtesy of the Wood Library-Museum of Anesthesiology.]

The group flourished and, in 1912, moved across the river to New York City, changed the organization's name, and became the New York Society of Anesthetists. Over the next 24 years, the society would grow, both in membership and in scope. Starting out as a New York City group, by the mid-1920s, the group encompassed all of the state. By 1936 it had become a national organization.[28] The transformation focused on the recognition of physicians who primarily anesthetized patients as specialists.

The first significant political move of the New York Society was a motion put before the House of Delegates of the AMA asking for a Section on Anesthetics in 1912. The members of the society were concerned about nonphysicians giving anesthetics, and they echoed some of the findings of the AMA's Commission on Anesthetics some 6 years earlier.[28] James Gwathmey (**Fig. 1-5**), the society's president, was developing a new method of anesthesia: rectal ether. Like chloroform, rectal ether could be unpredictable and needed to be administered by someone very familiar with its use and with the effects of anesthesia in general.[29] The quest for a section within the AMA was, in some ways, the beginning of a quest for patient safety in anesthesia, a movement that would take the specialty by storm in the latter half of the 20th century.

The motion was denied by the AMA House of Delegates. However, Gwathmey and Francis Hoeffer McMechan (**Fig. 1-6**) gathered the defeated physician anesthetists and created the American Association of Anesthetists (AAA). This was the first national group of physician anesthetists in the United States who met the following year, 1913, for

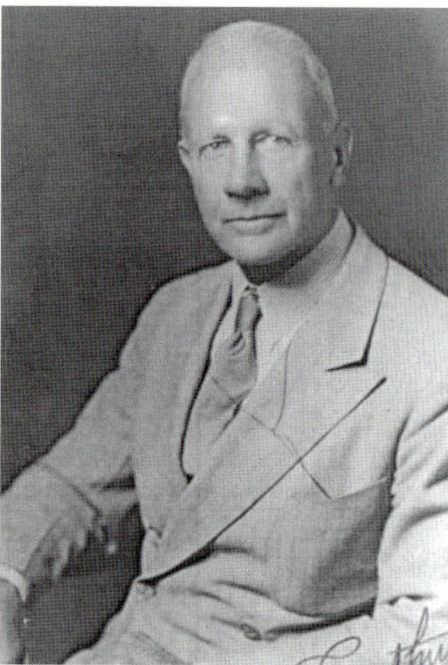

FIGURE 1-5. James Tayloe Gwathmey. [Photograph courtesy of the Wood Library-Museum of Anesthesiology.]

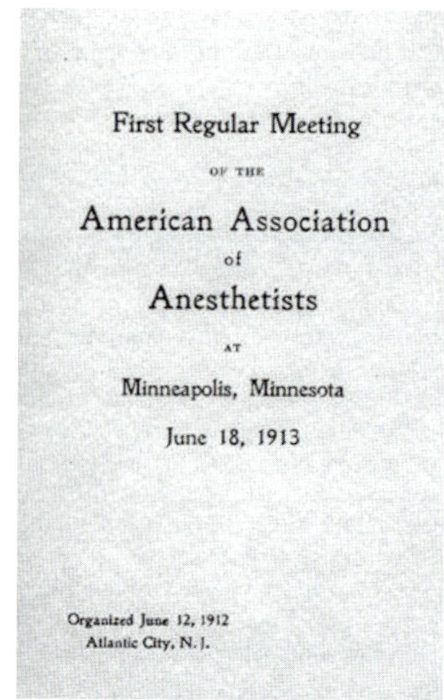
First Regular Meeting

OF THE

American Association

of

Anesthetists

AT

Minneapolis, Minnesota

June 18, 1913

Organized June 12, 1912
Atlantic City, N. J.

FIGURE 1-7. Program of the first meeting of the American Association of Anesthetists, June 18, 1913, Minneapolis, Minnesota. [Image courtesy of the Wood Library-Museum of Anesthesiology.]

a day of papers, mostly clinical in origin, and a dinner, with spouses (**Fig. 1-7**). A day devoted to the science of anesthesia is memorable; the evening meal signified a group, however small, that was willing to be recognized as specialists in anesthetics and by uniting, to move the field forward.[28]

The AAA, and its successor, the Associated Anesthetists of the United States and Canada, were run by Francis Hoeffer McMechan. A third-generation physician who entered anesthesia against the advice of his physician father, McMechan had crippling rheumatoid arthritis and was out of clinical practice by 1911. He was a visionary who hoped to see, on a worldwide scale, the elevation of anesthesia to "stand shoulder to shoulder" with surgery and internal medicine. He realized that without a place to publish papers on the specialty and without a place to gather the news of the various societies and names of physicians practicing anesthesia, the specialty would be doomed. Convincing his friend Joseph McDonald, the editor of the *American Journal of Surgery,* to publish a supplement on anesthesia gave the physician specialty its first US quarterly. McMechan also edited the *Yearbook of Anesthesia* between 1914 and 1919, compiling all the papers published in the specialty in the preceding year into a single volume.[30]

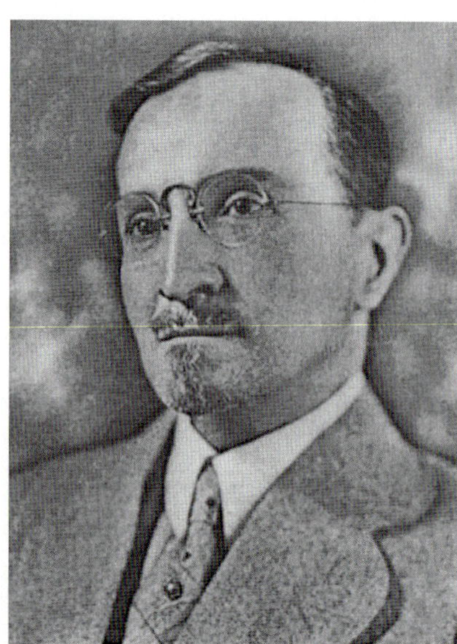

FIGURE 1-6. Francis Hoeffer McMechan. [Photograph courtesy of the Wood Library-Museum of Anesthesiology.]

McMechan also understood that the specialty would never develop as a discipline within medicine without a strong scientific underpinning. To that end, first nationally, and internationally in the mid-1920s, McMechan organized a society devoted to research in anesthesia. The International Anesthesia Research Society (IARS) brought together basic science researchers and the physicians most in need of their talents. Most importantly, the IARS sponsored the first journal in the world devoted to anesthesiology, *Current Researches in Anesthesia and Analgesia.*[31]

The education of physician specialists, especially in the postgraduate period, was another of McMechan's concerns. Partnering with Ralph Waters, an opportunity emerged at the University of Wisconsin in 1926 as the medical school transformed itself from a 2-year institution offering only basic science education into a 4-year curriculum with all the clinical sciences. One addition was a section on anesthesia, headed by Waters, in the Department of Surgery. Waters immediately began to teach anesthesia to medical students and interns. He collaborated with the basic science researchers, at first on problems of carbon dioxide absorbance, and later, through various members of his department, on all aspects of anesthesiology. Perhaps most importantly, Waters established the first residency training program in an academic center. The training was 3 years beyond the intern experience. Years 1 and 3 were clinical, with year 2 devoted to laboratory research. Two weekly conferences were established, one discussing the week's cases in a format similar to current morbidity and mortality conferences, and another devoted to the current literature in anesthesia. By 1933 the teaching program was the envy of the world, and Waters understood that one final step had to be taken. He sent one of his faculty members, and an early graduate of the program, Emery Rovenstine, to Bellevue Hospital and New York University to try to replicate the University of Wisconsin department. Rovenstine was successful beyond any expectation and, in some ways, his graduates would eclipse the contributions of Waters's graduates in the development of academic anesthesiology across the country.[32]

In 1929, the year of the stock market crash and the beginnings of the Great Depression, another pivotal event occurred in anesthesiology. The Anaesthetists Travel Club was organized by John Lundy at the Mayo Clinic. The group was created along the lines of the Society of Clinical Surgery, with members going to other members' institutions to see their anesthetic practice in action. It was a young man's group, with the oldest member Lahey Clinic anesthesiologist Lincoln Sise at 55 years of age and the youngest the Philadelphian and future first editor of *Anesthesiology* Henry Ruth at 30 years of age, and Mayo resident Ralph Tovell at 28 years of age. The average age was just 40 years. These young, influential anesthesiologists were those "standing in line" in the McMechan organization or those who believed that McMechan's international vision of the specialty, although important, would not solve domestic issues. The Travel Club would come to dominate the New York Society and become the nidus of leadership for the effort to create the American Board of Anesthesiology.[33]

THE CREATION OF THE AMERICAN BOARD OF ANESTHESIOLOGY

Once there was an organization in place to address national issues, regular meetings of a society devoted to the specialty, a university presence, ongoing research into clinical problems, and a residency training program to continue to retain and transmit the knowledge already gained, some recognition of a physician practicing the specialty was important. The gains in clinical practice in the 1920s and 1930s are best summed up by Harold Griffith, a leading Canadian physician-anesthetist of the time when he wrote, in 1939, the following:

> Seventeen years ago when I began to give anesthetics, the anesthesia equipment in the small hospital which has ever since been my hospital home, consisted of bottles of ether and chloroform and a few face masks. This was typical of the fairly well-equipped hospitals of that time. Today in that hospital there are eight gas machines of various models, suction equipment in every room, oxygen- and helium-therapy equipment, at least fifteen different anesthetic agents, and much technical equipment for their administration. This transformation has been taking place everywhere in anesthesia.[34]

Economic reasons played a role in the need to define a specialist in anesthesia, for physician anesthetists were not well compensated and faced competition from a number of groups. Surgeons, for example, could hire a nurse to help in the office and give anesthetics. The surgeon could then charge each patient a fee for anesthesia in addition to the fee for surgery. The income generated from the anesthetic fee was in excess of what he paid the nurse, and thus profitable. Likewise, hospitals could hire nurses to give anesthetics, charge a fee that cumulatively was in excess of the salaries, and make a profit. Finally, general practitioners would refer cases to surgeons with the caveat that they could give the anesthetic and collect the anesthetic fee.[35]

McMechan proposed an International College of Anesthetists and certified the first fellows in 1935. There were two serious problems with his certification process. First, and foremost, the clinical criteria were weak. The applicant only had to document 10 anesthetic cases, with lessons learned, to be eligible. In one instance, an intern on the anesthesia service for 1 month wrote up the necessary cases and was certified. In another, a surgeon who occasionally gave an anesthetic completed the necessary paperwork and was certified. With certificate in hand, he attempted to become the head of a hospital division of anesthesia. Second, the college had no standing with the AMA, and the certificate meant nothing "official" in the United States.[36]

Members of the Anaesthetists Travel Club, especially Paul Wood, John Lundy, and Ralph Waters, believed that certification was essential if anesthesiology was going to be recognized as an equal with all other specialty practices. Using AMA criteria, which included documentation of either postgraduate training in the specialty, or 2500 cases where the applicant had administered the anesthetic, Wood and his colleagues at the New York Society created a special classification of members called "fellows." This new form of membership was extremely popular, and the membership of the New York Society skyrocketed. Now national in membership, the society changed its name to the American Society of Anesthetists in February of 1936.[37] In 1945 the American Society of Anesthetists became the American Society of Anesthesiologists (ASA).

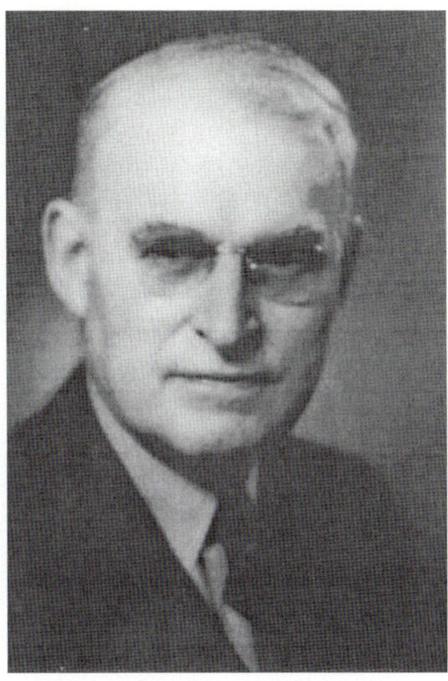

FIGURE 1-8. Erwin Schmidt. [Photograph courtesy of University of Wisconsin Archive Collection, Madison, Wisconsin.]

The AMA took note largely through Lundy's efforts, and Waters, working closely with Erwin Schmidt (**Fig. 1-8**), the chair of surgery at the University of Wisconsin, was able to secure an agreement for the American Board of Anesthesiology (ABA) to be created as a subboard of the American Board of Surgery. Using AMA criteria, which included, in addition to the heavy clinical training, the stipulation that the physician had to be in full-time practice of the specialty, the ABA was created in 1938. The first written examination of the ABA was held in March 1939. It was an essay format, with 5 subject subheadings: pharmacology, anatomy, physics and chemistry, pathology, and physiology. There was an oral examination and a practical one at the candidate's place of practice.[38]

WORLD WAR II AND BEYOND

The New York World's Fair opened on April 30, 1939, the eve of World War II. In the Hall of Man, an anesthesiology exhibit (**Fig. 1-9**) allowed the general public to learn more about the specialty. The exhibit was paid for by the Winthrope Chemical Company at a cost equivalent to several million dollars today. This is important for two reasons: First, it demonstrated that anesthesia had enough of a market impact that industry was willing to spend lavishly to support such a display. Second, the clinical practice of anesthesiology had become both complex and commonplace enough that the lay public would recognize and want to learn about it.[39]

At the same time, Lewis Wright was hired by Squibb Pharmaceuticals to investigate new anesthesia drugs, among them curare. Wright was a self-taught anesthesiologist who, in midcareer, took a leave of absence from his job at Squibb and did a residency with Emery Rovenstine at Bellevue Hospital.[40] It was to Rovenstine and Emmanuel Papper that he gave some of the first commercially prepared curare. Papper felt that the agent was a poor anesthetic because all the test animals stopped breathing when it was administered to them.[41] It was Harold Griffith and Enid Johnson, of Montreal, who discovered the true value of curare in anesthesia.[42]

As the United States plunged into World War II, the anesthesia community was determined not to repeat the mistakes of World War I.

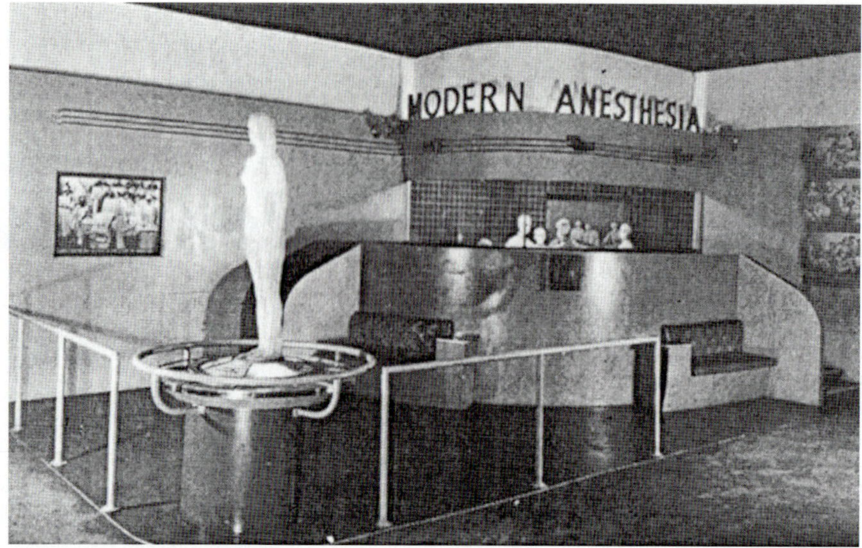

FIGURE 1-9. Postcard image of the anesthesia exhibit at the 1939 World's Fair. [Image courtesy of the Wood Library-Museum of Anesthesiology.]

Physician anesthetists had been in short supply and often ran from unit to unit training corpsmen in the administration of ether by open drop.[43] By the early 1940s, anesthesia had become too complex for this to be successful. The leaders of the ASA worked with the advisers to the armed forces and developed short 90-day courses to train medical officers in the basics of anesthesia. These young physicians managed many horrific clinical situations and, applying what they learned, were able to decrease mortality.[44] The case of Samuel Lieberman, who won the Legion of Merit for his work in the South Pacific, is illustrative. By using continuous spinal anesthesia, he decreased the mortality from abdominal wounds from 46% to 12.5%.[45]

Returning from the war, these physicians had tremendous clinical experience, especially with regional anesthesia. Nerve blocks were invaluable because corpsmen could take vital signs and talk to the soldier while the operation was ongoing, freeing the anesthesiologist to treat others. These military anesthesiologists had extensive experience with transfusion and fluid therapy. Returning to the United States, approximately 40% sought additional formal training. Thus the specialty expanded tremendously, not only because of the returning physicians, but also because surgeons exposed to the field work of the anesthesiologists demanded physician involvement in anesthesia.[44]

THE SECOND HALF OF THE 20TH CENTURY

McMechan's vision of an international community of anesthesiologists came to fruition in the 1950s. The first world meeting of anesthesiologists had been scheduled for Paris in the spring of 1940 but was canceled as the German army took the city. By the early 1950s, Europe was starting to recover from the effects of the war and the original French organizers were still interested in seeing the meeting become a reality. Working within the European community and Canada, and with help from the World Heath Organization, preliminary meetings were organized and the structure of the World Federation of Societies of Anesthesiologists (WFSA) was created. The first World Congress, held at The Hague in the Netherlands in 1955, was a success despite the absence of the ASA. The WFSA wanted to bring the best clinical practice of the specialty to the fore; the World Congress was a way to bring first-, second-, and third-world anesthesiologists together to discuss problems and to seek solutions. The WFSA set up programs to share information with those in need of it.[46]

However, it would not be until the end of the 1950s that the ASA would join the WFSA. The reluctance on the part of the Americans was multifactorial. First, because dues to the WFSA were on a per capita basis, the ASA felt they would be providing most of the finances of the organization without an equal voice in its government. There was also reluctance on the part of some American anesthesiologists to join an organization that had communists among its members. Time, dialogue, and the performance of the WFSA eliminated those fears.[47]

Along with the international concerns, the specialty faced a challenge in the United States as well. There was a significant part of the anesthesiology community that believed no physicians should accept a contract for services and allow a third party, such as a hospital or other employer, to bill in the physician's name. Enforcement of this edict was done by the component societies of the ASA, for an anesthesiologist could not be a member if he or she was not a component society member. Furthermore, to be eligible to take the ABA examination, an anesthesiologist had to be an ASA member.[48] In response to this, the Association of University Anesthesiologists (AUA) was formed. Most academic anesthesiologists were employed by the university for a salary, in violation of the ASA edict. The establishment of the organization is important not only as a protest, but because it underscores how important academics had become to the fledgling field in the 30 years between the creation of the Waters department to the first AUA meeting.[49] It was a rapid expansion and one that continued to delineate the scientific underpinnings of the specialty. The AUA was also the first subspecialty society formed in anesthesiology and worked to promote scientific research and teaching in anesthesiology.

In the 1960s, the US federal government sought to support medical research and created the National Institutes of Health (NIH). Emmanuel Papper (**Fig. 1-10**) was invited to Washington DC, to help organize the new agency. Papper worked tirelessly to see that anesthesiologists were treated fairly by the NIH and were eligible for funding. However, he was unable to secure an independent study section for anesthesia, and the battle to obtain this for the specialty remains a leading agenda item for many.[41]

The 1970s was a decade of crisis for anesthesiology. To ensure billing commensurate with services, the ASA had endorsed a relative value guide that helped place a unit value on work done by the physician. Other specialties, including orthopedics and radiology, had adopted similar guides, but the Federal Trade Commission (FTC) thought this was a monopolistic practice. All of the specialties but anesthesiology agreed to cease and desist; the ASA went to court. After a 2-week trial, the judge ruled that the relative value guide did not represent a monopolistic practice; rather, it was simply a tool that applied monetary value differently in different parts of the country. In one of history's little ironies, 30 years after the verdict, the federal government now

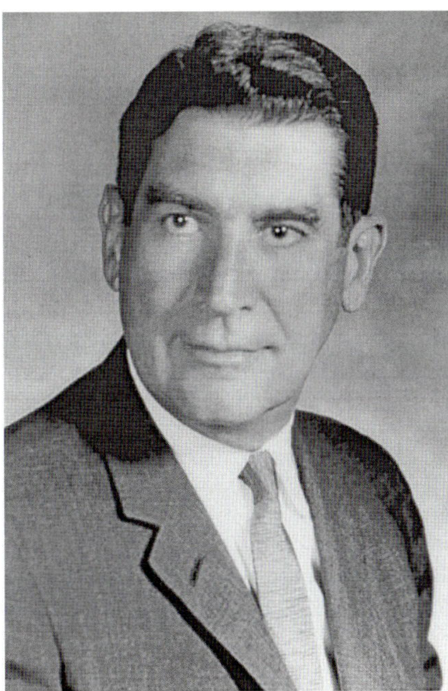

FIGURE 1-10. Emmanuel Papper. [Photograph courtesy of the Wood Library-Museum of Anesthesiology.]

states the relative value guides are the preferred billing methodology. The 1970s also saw another federal government suit against the ASA for the fee-for-service rule. While there was little chance of a successful suit, the federal government, cautious after its defeat, agreed to a cease-and-desist order.[50]

The 1970s also oversaw the beginnings of the subspecialty movement in anesthesiology. Just before the beginning of the decade, the Society for Obstetric Anesthesia and Perinatology was formed in 1968. The group remains diverse with anesthesiologists, obstetricians, and perinatologists all presenting work of interest to the group.[51] Likewise in the early 1970s, Maurice Albin and others interested in neuroanesthesia created the Society of Neurosurgical Anesthesia. John Mitchenfelder was the first president in 1973.[52] Two years later, the American Society of Regional Anesthesia (ASRA) was reformed, although without knowledge of the group formed by Gaston Labat in the 1920s. Dedicated to the promotion of regional anesthesia, which also meant teaching and research, the society has grown and prospered. Publishing the first subspecialty journal, *Regional Anesthesia*, the society provided a place for a peer-reviewed publication in regional anesthesia. Coupled with the annual meeting, where information and demonstrations about the topic were presented, the society also provided a forum for anesthesiologists interested in pain medicine to interact. Eventually the society would change its name to the American Society of Regional Anesthesia and Pain Medicine and the name of journal to *Regional Anesthesia and Pain Medicine* emphasizing the importance of this emerging field in anesthesiology.[53] Mid-decade, the Society of Cardiovascular Anesthesiologists came into being. This group disseminated information about cardiac bypass and the emerging fields of vascular surgery.

The 1980s, by contrast, witnessed the development of two organizations that have served anesthesiology well. The Foundation for Anesthesia Education and Research (FAER) is devoted to the promotion of research within the specialty. The group has a special interest in those just beginning their careers, and it has supported a successful starter grant program. Indeed many of the leaders of academic anesthesiology in the early 21st century began their careers with a FAER grant. At the same time when FAER was being established, the Anesthesia Patient Safety Foundation (APSF) was created. Its mission is simple: No patient should ever be harmed by an anesthetic. APSF has partnered the academic, private practice, and industrial communities to work toward decreasing anesthetic risk. The establishment of the Harvard standards of monitoring, at the beginning of the APSF, was an important step in this direction. APSF and its work is the model for the patient safety movement across the country, and it is used by the AMA as a model for its patient safety foundation.[54]

The subspecialty movement in anesthesiology continued into the 1980s. In 1987 the first meeting of the Society for Pediatric Anesthesia was held. An outgrowth of the anesthesia section of the American Academy of Pediatrics, the society strove to be inclusive of all anesthesiologists interested in the care of children undergoing anesthesia, not simply anesthesiologists in full-time pediatric practice. Another society formed in the mid-1980s was the Society for Ambulatory Anesthesia.[55] In response to the growing trend of day surgery and having patients return home on the day of operation rather than spending a night in the hospital, the society strove and continues to strive for the highest standards in anesthesia care in the ambulatory setting.[56] Likewise the American Society of Critical Care Anesthesiologists was formed to establish a forum where anesthesiologists interested in critical care could meet to exchange ideas and information.[57]

During the 1990s, the ABA recognized the trend toward subspecialization by creating special qualifications that could be added to board certification in anesthesiology in both critical care medicine and pain medicine. This trend continues to the present with added qualifications available in palliative care and pediatrics. One of the greatest challenges before anesthesiology currently remains the proper role for these credentials in the clinical setting and which subspecialties are appropriate to endorse for them.

CONCLUSIONS

By comparison with most other medical specialties, the history of clinical anesthesia is short. Perhaps Francis Hoeffer McMechan summed it best when in 1935 he wrote,

> Anesthesia was the gift of pioneer doctors and dentists to suffering humanity, and every significant advance in its science and practice has been contributed by doctors, dentists, and research workers of similar standing. In contrast, technicians have added nothing of any consequence. Anesthetics are among the most potent and dangerous drugs used in the practice of medicine; they penetrate to every cell and organ of the body and may cause almost instant or delayed death by their toxic effects. The dosage of general inhalation anesthetics cannot be prescribed in advance but must be determined from moment to moment during administration. The dosage of local and other anesthetics must be determined by the risk of the patient, the nature and duration of the operation to be done—certainly a challenge to the knowledge and experience of the keenest doctor. No patient should ever be given an anesthetic whose condition and risk has not been diagnosed in advance of the operation, so that every resource of medical science can be used to lessen the risk and make the recovery more assuring. Certainly in this preoperative evaluation and the selection of the safest anesthetic and best method of administration, the medical anesthetist is more in a position to act as a consultant than a technician. . . .

The safety of the patient demands that the anesthetist be able to treat every complication that may arise from the anesthetic itself by the use of methods of treatment that may be indicated. The medical anesthetist can do this, the technician cannot. More recent developments have extended the field of medical anesthesia to include resuscitation, oxygen therapy, and therapeutic nerve block for intractable pain, and treatment of various conditions of disease, and the rehabilitation of the disabled—all fields of practice quite beyond the capacity of the technician.[58]

McMechan's vision of professionalism, and its 21st-century equivalents, needs to continue to guide the specialty. The history of anesthesia is interesting, filled with fascinating events and people, and replete with the highest examples of professionalism, and the best is yet to come!

KEY REFERENCES

- Bacon DR. The New York Society of Anesthetists: building the foundation. In: Bacon DR, Lema MJ, McGoldrick KE, eds. *The American Society of Anesthesiologists: A Century of Challenges and Progress.* Park Ridge, IL: Wood Library-Museum of Anesthesiology Press; 2005:9-18.
- Bacon DR. The World Federation of Societies of Anesthesiologists (WFSA): McMechan's final legacy? *Anesth Analg.* 1997;84:1130-1135.
- Bacon DR, Lema MJ. To define a specialty: a brief history of the American Board of Anesthesiology's first written examination. *J Clin Anesth.* 1992;4:489-497.
- Fenster J. *Ether Day.* New York, NY: HarperCollins; 2001.
- Goerig M, Agarwal K, Schulte am Esch J. The versatile August Bier (1861-1949), father of spinal anesthesia. *J Clin Anesth.* 2000;12:561-569.
- Griffith HR, Johnson GE. The use of curare in general anesthesia. *Anesthesiology.* 1942;3:418-420.
- Johansen PV, Paneth N, Rachman S, Rip M. *Cholera, Chloroform, and the Science of Medicine: A Life of John Snow.* New York, NY: Oxford University Press; 2003:113.
- Smith HM, Bacon DR. The history of anesthesia. In: Barash P, Cullen B, Stoelting R, eds. *Clinical Anesthesia.* 5th ed. Philadelphia, PA: Lippincott Williams & Wilkins; 2005:3-26.
- Waisel DB. The role of World War II and the European theater of operations in the development of anesthesiology as a physician specialty in the USA. *Anesthesiology.* 2001;94(5):907-914.
- Wells CJ. Francis Hoeffer McMechan. *Curr Res Anesth Analg.* 1948;26(Suppl):1-19

REFERENCES

Complete references available on DVD and online version at www.LongneckerAnesthesiology.com

CHAPTER 2 The Scope and Future of Anesthesia Practice

Michael S. Avidan
Alex S. Evers

KEY POINTS

1. The operating room remains the primary focus for the vast majority of anesthesiologists.
2. The anesthesiologist's primary responsibility is to ensure patients' comfort and safety when they are exposed to the trespass of surgery.
3. The intraoperative conduct of anesthesia has effects on patient safety and comfort in the postoperative period.
4. The provision of safe anesthetic care across geographically dispersed sites and encompassing wide ranges of patient health, in an economically responsible manner, is a challenge that anesthesiologists need to address proactively.
5. It is arithmetically impossible to provide a fully trained individual anesthesiologist for every anesthetic procedure.
6. Meeting the labor, safety, and cost demands of the future will require that we overcome the political infighting between organized anesthesiology and nurse anesthesia.
7. Many believe it is important for the future of the specialty that anesthesiologists increase their commitment to critical care medicine.
8. Recent advances in knowledge and technology create an enormous opportunity for anesthesiologists to address the scientific questions at the core of the specialty as well as a variety of important clinical problems.
9. Apart from traditional areas of involvement, such as operating room anesthesia, critical care, pain medicine, teaching, research, and resuscitation, there will be future opportunities for anesthesiologists in pharmacogenomics, health care systems management, and new technologies.

Anesthesiology arose as a medical specialty because the dangers associated with anesthetic drugs and techniques demanded that they be administered by skilled and knowledgeable physicians. As safer drugs were developed and physiologic monitoring improved, the need for anesthesiologists was propelled by increasing surgical complexity and severity of patient illness, as well as by increasing expectations for patient safety. Whereas the original raison d'être for the specialty remains today, a variety of professional and economic factors have challenged anesthesiology and produced large "swings of fortune" during the past few decades.

During the 1970s and 1980s, the emergence of critical care attracted many talented medical students to American anesthesiology training programs. However, these were halcyon days for anesthesiologists practicing in the operating room, where professional income was high, job opportunities were ample, and increasing surgical complexity demanded an increasing level of medical knowledge and skills. Thus there was little incentive for anesthesiologists to expand their roles beyond the confines of the operating suites, and most of the trainees who were initially attracted by critical care subsequently practiced operating room anesthesia only. In contrast, anesthesiologists in Europe and Canada were consolidating their positions during this same period in the burgeoning subspecialties of pain, intensive care, and resuscitation.

In the mid-1990s, gloom beset anesthesiology in the United States as predictions, widely reported in lay press such as the *Wall Street Journal,* suggested that the need for anesthesiologists would decrease dramatically in an anticipated managed care environment. Medical graduates were discouraged from pursuing careers in anesthesiology, and residency programs contracted dramatically. In the last 10 years, US anesthesiology programs have enjoyed a revival, and many talented medical graduates have chosen to enter the specialty. Another encouraging recent trend has been the marked increase in the proportion of US graduating residents who are choosing to pursue fellowships to bolster their specialist knowledge and refine their clinical skills. All anesthesiology subspecialties (eg, pain medicine, critical care, pediatrics, clinical scientist) are benefiting from this growing cadre of subspecialists. Anesthesiologists in the other parts of the world have also experienced fluctuating fortunes. Currently there is a shortage of doctors, in general, and anesthesiologists, in particular, in many countries. The future of anesthesiology depends on several factors, including changes in surgery and interventional medical practice, technological advances in anesthesiology, the evolving scope of anesthesia practice, and the role of nonphysicians (eg, nurse anesthetists and anesthesia physician assistants) and physicians trained in other specialties, in the provision of anesthesia care; health care financing will also influence trends in anesthesia practice. This chapter briefly reviews the current scope of anesthetic practice and offers some possible scenarios for future directions of the specialty.

OPERATING ROOM ANESTHESIA

The operating room remains the primary focus for the vast majority of anesthesiologists. The anesthesiologist's primary responsibility in this arena is to ensure the patients' comfort and safety when they are exposed to the trespass of surgery; this includes protecting the patient from pain, undesired awareness, and organ system injury, and fostering full recovery from the surgical and anesthetic interventions. Over the past decades it has become increasingly clear that the intraoperative conduct of anesthesia has profound effects on patient safety and comfort in the postoperative period. For example, modest intraoperative hypothermia can either decrease the incidence of wound infection[1] or provide neuroprotection[2] depending on the clinical situation. Anesthesiologists are increasingly sophisticated in their understanding of patient safety, and they are focusing on such issues as appropriate perioperative medications, antibiotic prophylaxis and infection control, multimodal analgesia, maintenance of normothermia and normoglycemia, and appropriate fluid and electrolyte therapy. Recent research shows that an estimated 1.85% of adult patients die within 30 days of undergoing operations across the entire surgical spectrum, with some operations having much higher mortality (eg, vascular surgery: 5.97%) and others having lower mortality (eg, breast surgery: 0.07%).[3] It is likely that, with appropriate interventions, many of these deaths could be prevented. This growing responsibility for overall postoperative outcomes raises new expectations for knowledge and skills of the practicing anesthesiologist and challenges our previously narrower definitions of anesthetic outcome.[4]

Despite the demands imposed by increasing severity of illness in surgical patients, growing surgical complexity and more comprehensive postoperative considerations, anesthesiology is often viewed as a victim of its own perceived success. One widely cited study from the United Kingdom, the Confidential Enquiry Into Perioperative Deaths (CEPOD), reports that patients undergoing general anesthesia have a 1 in 185 000 chance of dying as a consequence of anesthetic misadventure.[5-7] This finding was highlighted in the Institute of Medicine report on medical errors,[8] and anesthesiology was cited as the specialty that had best addressed safety issues (see Chapter 3 for a more comprehensive review of quality and safety in anesthesia practice). Unfortunately, this widely publicized perception that anesthesia is "safe" has encouraged nonphysician anesthesia providers to advocate for independent practice and has suggested to insurers that anesthesia care by an anesthesiologist is needlessly expensive. However, studies from other countries have reported much higher rates of death attributable to anesthesia than those reported in the CEPOD study.[9] In a large French study, the perioperative mortality directly attributable to anesthesia was found to be 1 in 13,000.[10] In studies reported from Australia,[11] Denmark,[12] Finland,[13] and the Netherlands,[14] perioperative death attributable to anesthesia ranged from 1 in 2500[12] to 1 in 67,000.[13] The mortality attributable to anesthesia is probably much greater in underdeveloped countries. For example, a 1992 study from a Zimbabwean teaching hospital reported an alarming incidence of death or coma attributable to anesthesia of 1 in 388.[15] Whereas the bulk of evidence suggests that anesthesia is not nearly as safe as publicized,[16] it is undoubtedly true that advances in anesthetic practice in developed countries have rendered the care of healthy patients undergoing low- or intermediate-risk surgery much safer than in the past (see Chapter 25 for a more detailed review of anesthesia risk).

The challenges to anesthesiology are exacerbated by the massive expansion in demand for anesthesia services for a variety of nonoperative procedures ranging from cerebral aneurysm coiling to general anesthesia for screening colonoscopy, and by the introduction of freestanding ambulatory surgery centers and office-based surgical suites where anesthesia is administered. The demands for safe anesthesia care provided in numerous remote locations present significant challenges to the workforce, financing, and practice of anesthesiology.

Current practice models vary widely both in the United States and worldwide. In the United States, some anesthesiologists (or practice groups) personally provide all anesthetic care regardless of complexity, an approach that is also common in the United Kingdom, Canada, and Australia. In other practices, anesthesiologists supervise ancillary providers (eg, nurse anesthetists, residents, or anesthesia assistants) in more than one operating room, a practice model that is also common in the Netherlands. The provision of safe anesthetic care across geographically dispersed practice sites and encompassing wide ranges of severity of patient illness, in an economically responsible manner, is a major challenge that anesthesiologists need to address proactively.

The expectations for operating room anesthesia can be simply stated: *We will need to provide an ever-increasing quality of perioperative care for a lower cost.* In turn, these expectations and predictions require that the anesthesiology community consider who will, or should provide each component of anesthesia care, what levels of knowledge and skill will be required of each provider, and how the responsibility for care will be organized, managed, and rewarded.

Currently, at least 50% of anesthesia care in the United States involves nurse anesthetists; in several states, physician supervision is not mandatory. Worldwide, anesthesia practice often includes some form of nonphysician provider or physician provider who is not a fully trained anesthesiologist. For example, staff-grade noncertified anesthetists provide a significant proportion of anesthesia care in the United Kingdom. There is one report asserting that nonanesthesiologists can safely provide anesthesia for selected procedures (eg, colonoscopy) and patients.[17] It is also clear that patients with minimal physiologic reserve, those undergoing major interventions, and those with complex medical problems require the direct involvement of a skilled anesthesiologist to enhance patient safety.[18,19] Unfortunately, practitioner skill and experience are often not matched to these factors but determined by the availability of providers or a fixed model of care delivery rather than one tailored to the specific clinical situation. This is a fruitful area for further work by anesthesiologists to ensure proper matching of resources to clinical needs.

It is arithmetically impossible to provide a fully trained individual anesthesiologist for every anesthetic procedure. Further, the increasing demands for anesthesia services (aging population, proliferation of ambulatory surgery centers, escalating demand for nonsurgical anesthesia and sedation) will outstrip even the most aggressive output of anesthesiologists. Medical schools simply do not have the capacity to train sufficient doctors to feed exponentially increasing anesthesia programs. For reasons of both anesthesiologist availability and cost, it is thus apparent that the future of anesthesia practice will involve an increasing role for nonphysician providers. How can this be made compatible with the demands for increasing safety and quality? This can be accomplished by involving skilled anesthesiologists in the cognitive aspects of *every* anesthetic. This will require coordination and cooperation with nonphysician providers, allowing them to perform at the highest levels their training allows while ensuring that a fully trained specialist is involved in planning and managing care for high-risk cases and is readily available for complex diagnostic and therapeutic decision making. Technological developments in monitoring and information systems should facilitate these changes. The development of telemedicine could make this model of care feasible even in communities where an anesthesiologist is not physically present.[20] Meeting the labor, safety, and cost demands of the future will require that we overcome the political infighting between organized anesthesiology and nurse anesthesia. Further, the training of anesthesiologists will increasingly need to encompass the development of skills in supervising other anesthesia providers. It is in the interests of public safety and health care delivery that unity be forged among anesthesia providers under the leadership of specialist anesthesiologists, whose medical training and education is required for complex medical decision making, supplemented by the skills and abilities of nonphysician providers who enhance this team approach.

OUTSIDE THE OPERATING ROOM

PREOPERATIVE CARE

Perioperative morbidity is frequently attributable to poor preoperative patient assessment and optimization. These roles have always been integral to the anesthesiologist's practice. However, as patients increasingly present to the hospital on the day of surgery, it has become necessary to ensure that patients are properly evaluated well before the immediate preoperative interval. Recognizing this need has led to burgeoning preoperative assessment clinics, where problems such as ischemic heart disease, pulmonary disease, or sleep apnea may be evaluated and appropriate perioperative interventions may be planned (see Chapter 4 for a more detailed discussion of the benefits and operation of preoperative clinics). In some practice settings, preoperative assessment of complicated patients has been largely relegated to non–anesthesiology-trained physicians or physician extenders. In other settings, the challenge of same-day surgery admission has left preoperative assessment as a day-of-surgery activity; neither of these approaches is optimal. From the standpoint of continuity of care and so that anesthesiologists can implement best practices that contribute to the continuum of care and long-term outcomes, it is essential that anesthesiologists continue to play an integral role in preoperative assessment clinics. This should also be a key component of anesthesia resident training programs, for it represents an important aspect of future anesthesia practice.

PAIN MEDICINE

Doctors cannot always cure disease, but they should always try to alleviate suffering. Physical pain is among the most unpleasant of human experiences. Anesthesiologists are often involved in the management of severe pain associated with surgery, and the perioperative use of analgesics constitutes an important component of anesthetic care. Anesthesiologists are more comfortable with opiate administration than many other physicians, both because of their knowledge of pharmacology (especially opioid pharmacology) and their skill and experience in managing side effects such as respiratory depression. Anesthesiologists have pioneered regional anesthetic techniques, many of which are applicable to the treatment of chronic intractable pain. Increasing numbers of anesthesiologists are specializing in pain management, and the effective relief of pain will remain an important component of the anesthesiologist's role even for those who do not subspecialize specifically in pain medicine.

CRITICAL CARE MEDICINE

Anesthesiologists pioneered the development of critical care medicine.[21] In many countries, anesthesiologists constitute the bulk of the physician workforce in critical care. In most of Europe, full training in critical care is an integral component of an anesthesia residency, and critical care anesthesiologists are responsible for organizing and staffing most hospital critical care units. In contrast, US anesthesia residents receive only a few months of critical care training, and anesthesiologists constitute a minority of the nation's critical care physicians. Many believe it is important for the future of the specialty that anesthesiologists increase their commitment to critical care medicine. To achieve this, leading academic programs must expand their critical care fellowships and promote critical care as a financially viable and intellectually rewarding subspecialty for talented graduating residents.

CLINICAL SERVICES ADMINISTRATION

The operating suite is a complex environment, one that often has not been efficiently managed. Anesthesiologists are an integral component of this important but unwieldy organization. The need for effective management and administration is being increasingly recognized, and anesthesiologists are often sought for this management function. In many countries, including in Europe and North America, anesthesiologists are acquiring formal training in management and business administration. Today's doctors, even in academic institutions and national health services, cannot afford to isolate themselves from the realities of reimbursement, cost, efficiency, patient satisfaction, and overall system performance. There appears to be a bright future for physician leaders in health care organizations; anesthesiologists are, and will continue to be, an important part of this management evolution.

PATIENT SAFETY

Anesthesiologists have been at the forefront of pioneering patient safety. The improvements have been so dramatic that liability insurance for anesthesia practice has decreased while that for most other specialties has steadily increased (some dramatically). The Anesthesia Patient Safety Foundation was founded in the United States in 1984 with the expressed purpose of ensuring "that no patient shall be harmed by the effects of anesthesia." Since 1985 the Committee on Professional Liability of the American Society of Anesthesiologists (ASA) has been studying records of closed malpractice claims files for anesthesia-related patient injuries.[22] More than 5000 claims have been studied. Subsequently, the Australian Patient Safety Foundation was established in 1987 and the Australian Incident Monitoring Study was initiated.[23] More than 4000 critical incidents have been reported to date. Analysis of these incidents has reinforced the value of technological advances, such as capnography and oximetry, in improving patient safety. The results also confirm the value of structured algorithms in anesthesia care, by documenting favorable outcomes in a range of life-threatening crises during anesthesia. CEPOD was started in the United Kingdom in 1989. Changes in consultant practice, increase in medical audits, improvement in physiologic monitoring, appropriate matching of specialist experience to patient's medical conditions, and increased awareness of the need for critical care services are believed to have been influenced by this inquiry.[24]

Critical events occur within the context of complex system failures, and anesthesiologists have been developing safeguards to decrease the likelihood that human error may result in patient harm. Examples include written "checklists," audible alarm settings, and automated anesthesia machine checks. A seminal study showed how the routine implementation in hospitals around the world of a simple 19-item surgical safety checklist designed to improve team communication and consistency of care markedly reduced 30-day complications (from 11% to 7%) and deaths (from 1.5% to 0.8%) associated with surgery.[25] Expertise in patient safety should be developed and translated into the broader medical context, including application in areas not historically viewed as the purview of anesthesia practice (such as diagnostic and treatment suites, obstetric suites, intensive care units, and intermediate care units).

RESEARCH

Anesthesiology has a vibrant history of research and intellectual contributions to clinical medicine. Historically, anesthesia research has focused on laboratory investigations in physiology and pharmacology and their application to patient care. These contributions have improved the safety of anesthesia and surgery, and they constituted pioneering efforts in the initial application of scientific principles to individual patient care. Until recently many of the scientific questions at the core of anesthesiology have been relatively inaccessible to investigation; this stems from the absence of tools to study the mechanisms of the complex behaviors (eg, consciousness, memory, pain) that anesthesiologists manipulate. Recent advances in cellular physiology (ie, patch clamp recording), molecular biology, genetics, functional imaging, and behavioral sciences have enabled serious investigation of these complex behaviors. It is thus now possible that the fundamental mysteries of anesthesia (including the molecular mechanism of the hypnotic, amnestic, and analgesic effects of anesthetics agents) will be solved. These same new scientific tools also make it feasible to define the mechanisms of hyperalgesia and chronic pain and to design effective treatments. Finally, advances in the understanding and manipulation of inflammation and the immune response provide a new opportunity to delineate how organ system injury occurs in the perioperative period and to identify strategies for protection of the brain, heart, kidneys, and other organs. Collectively, recent advances in knowledge and technology create an enormous opportunity for anesthesiology to address the scientific questions at the core of the specialty, as well as a variety of important clinical problems. Innovative anesthesiology training programs are offering integrated scholarship tracks to the most academically competitive residency applicants, and several graduates are pursuing fellowships in clinical and translational research.

The application of information technology and epidemiologic techniques (often referred to as outcomes research) to the perioperative period has also created new research opportunities for anesthesiology. These approaches quantify and describe perioperative morbidity and mortality, facilitating recognition of patterns and causes of adverse patient outcomes. The broad application of information technology coupled to epidemiologic analysis will provide the opportunity to define and monitor "best practices" and to evaluate systematically the efficacy of new technologies, techniques, and approaches. Recognizing the need for detailed perioperative clinical data, the American Society of Anesthesiologists established the Anesthesia Quality Institute in 2008, which will house the National Anesthesia Clinical Outcomes Registry, a patient data registry that will be combined with other data sources to enable provider benchmarking, quality improvement, research, public reporting, credentialing, and maintenance of certification. The National Anesthesia Clinical Outcomes Registry will contain anesthesia-specific data elements that are essential for comprehensive perioperative clinical research.[26]

Academic anesthesia has been challenged in recent years, with decreased academic funding of some departments, a decreasing share of extramural grant funds,[27] and a contraction in the number of young anesthesiologists embarking on rigorous research training and careers. One of the reasons put forward for reduced funding for anesthesia research is that the current safety of anesthesia implies that anesthesia research is not a pressing public health concern. As noted earlier, this may be a misconception; although intraoperative mortality is rare, postoperative mortality and major morbidity still occur commonly, and anesthesia care has been shown to contribute to this process, both positively and negatively. There is much room for improvement before any field can conclude that we have overcome the hurdles in surgical care that challenge the extremes of age, those with significant comorbidities, or those undergoing extensive surgical procedures. Many of the advances in these areas will come from improved perioperative care, built on evidence-based techniques that are confirmed by careful clinical investigation and innovation. One of the priorities for research, as identified by the National Institutes of Health, is for investigators to embark on more multidisciplinary and multicenter research initiatives. It is also crucial to foster translational research where advances in the basic sciences, including genetics, can lead to progress in the clinical arena. A strong commitment to research will be necessary to ensure the continued advance of the specialty and to ensure that anesthesiology remains a mainstream medical discipline that contributes to the overall good of society.

EDUCATION AND TRAINING

Clearly, the future of the specialty requires a robust commitment to education and training at all levels, from undergraduate medical education through the most advanced subspecialty levels. Strong training programs depend on an excellent teaching faculty, ample and diverse clinical cases, a well-organized teaching program, and an emphasis on the knowledge required for future as well as current practice. Adequate funding for anesthesiology education by the federal government, by teaching hospitals, and by our specialty societies is an imperative if the specialty is to flourish in future decades. The current shortfall in anesthesiologists (particularly in teaching hospitals) creates a temptation to increase training numbers and churn out many more anesthesiologists; this may be particularly true in training programs that need to use residents primarily as the workforce. The danger is that this approach will decrease the selectivity of training programs and downgrade the quality of anesthesiologists. Training must be broadened as well; if the next generation of anesthesiologists is to be prepared for the future, anesthesiology training programs must emphasize preoperative assessment, critical care, pain management, supervision of nonphysician providers, and operating room administration, among others. Also important will be an increased emphasis on fellowship programs, with formal recognition of fellowships in areas such as regional anesthesia, transplant anesthesia, and obstetric anesthesia.

To attract high-caliber applicants to anesthesiology, medical students must continue to receive adequate exposure to the specialty. In addition to perioperative medicine and pain medicine, anesthesiologists are well placed to teach medical students applied respiratory and cardiovascular physiology, several aspects of neuroscience, and numerous aspects of pharmacology, in addition to their more traditional educational roles in resuscitation and emergency airway management. The model of academic anesthesia care facilitates excellent learning, with medical students able to spend high-quality one-on-one time with experienced anesthesiologists.

SIMULATION

The aerospace industry has long appreciated the value of simulation in increasing safety and decreasing errors. Within the medical profession, anesthesiologists have been among the first to recognize the potential role of simulation in improving both education and patient safety. Anesthesiologists established simulation facilities to train anesthesiologists in the management of infrequent but life-threatening problems that arise in the operating room. It rapidly became apparent that simulation might be useful for teaching other topics that are not unique to anesthesia practice (eg, diagnosis and management of pneumothorax, hemorrhagic shock, myocardial infarction, and insertion of central vascular catheters). Computer modeling can be used in research as well. Speculation is rife about a role for simulation in credentialing and recredentialing in various medical specialties. Increasingly, physician and nursing professionals, including those in critical care and emergency medicine, are seeking time in simulation facilities for purposes of training and honing their skills in crisis management. Simulation centers are mushrooming internationally and are also being embraced by medical schools. Anesthesiologists have led this initiative, and it is important that we continue to lead innovation in this field of evolving technology. Maintenance of certification is increasingly emphasized for specialist medical practice and is particularly valued by the public.[28] Simulation offers a practical and potentially objective method to assess anesthesiologists and other practicing clinicians, and to ensure uniform methodological rigor in complementing both initial certification and maintenance of certification programs.[29-31]

PUBLIC PERCEPTION OF ANESTHESIOLOGISTS

Anesthesiology is one of the largest physician-based specialties, but few mainstream medical specialties are as poorly understood by members of the public and by other health professionals.[32] Many patients do not realize that anesthesiologists are doctors or that they have responsibilities outside the operating room.[32] In Swiss and Austrian studies, 93% to 99% of patients knew that anesthesiologists are qualified physicians. In addition, many of the patients were aware that the anesthesiologists are engaged in activities outside the operating room. However, many patients also thought that the anesthesiologists played a subservient role to the surgical team.[33,34] In studies from Singapore, Pakistan, and the West Indies, only 56% to 66% of patients were aware that anesthesiologists are physicians, and most patients had a limited knowledge of the anesthesiologists' roles.[35-37] In contrast to these findings, a Finnish study reported that anesthesiologists were generally recognized as specialist physicians and were held in high esteem.[38] In the United Kingdom, the organizations representing anesthesiologists initiated National Anaesthesia Day in an attempt to increase the profile of anesthesiologists. Clearly there is variation among countries in the way anesthesiologists are perceived. Heightening public awareness and improving public perception about anesthesiologists and their many essential functions may be important to the future of the specialty in several respects, including allocation of research funding, quality of applicants to residencies, and the future role of anesthesiologists within health care in general.

A recent Scandinavian study explored perceptions of the anesthesiologist's role. The study was titled "Professional Artist, Good Samaritan, Servant and Co-coordinator: Four Ways of Understanding the Anaesthetist's Work."[39] According to these authors, the current scope of anesthesia practice encompasses the following:

1. The provision of safe anesthesia while controlling patients' vital functions.
2. Helping patients including the alleviation of pain and anxiety.
3. Providing service to the whole hospital including support to other doctors and nurses who are caring for severely ill patients.
4. Participation in the organization and direction of the operating suites to ensure that lists run smoothly.

Whereas these are essential and important components of the specialty, even collectively they do not encompass the spectrum of anesthesiology as we view it currently or as we look to the future, which seems particularly attractive if we maintain a comprehensive view of the opportunities for our discipline.

THE FUTURE OF ANESTHESIA PRACTICE

The future of the specialty depends on several key drivers: (1) The vision and actions of organized anesthesiology, (2) technological changes in surgery and anesthesiology, and (3) the directions chosen by academic institutions, the trainers of future practitioners. These drivers will influence the attractiveness of anesthesiology as a specialty choice for medical students, the career paths of young anesthesiologists, and the scope and organization of anesthetic practice.

There will be tough choices faced by future anesthesiologists. New drugs and increasingly sophisticated monitoring will facilitate safer anesthesia. Such technological advances will allow more effective remote supervision of anesthesia providers. There is likely to be a steady growth in the demand for anesthesia. Anesthesiologists will have to decide whether to try to expand their ranks at all costs and to defend their turf or whether to refine their training according to future conditions. It is highly unlikely that anesthesiologists alone will be able to meet all the demands for anesthesia.

Anesthesiology faces many challenges in the years ahead. To meet these challenges, perioperative medicine, which includes the spectrum of care from preoperative assessment to postoperative care, may offer the best chance for the specialty to survive and prosper.[40] Although there is a vision that future anesthesiologists will practice as much outside as inside operating rooms,[41] the expansion of anesthesiologists' activities could lead to dilution of the specialty's identity, endangering the vitality of anesthesiology in an era of sweeping changes in health care delivery systems.[42] An expansion of anesthesiology practice into nonoperative domains of perioperative medicine may also be challenged by other specialties. The role of perioperative physician may fall to hospitalists, the role of critical care physicians to intensivists, and the role of pain management to pain specialists. Anesthesia may grow and acquire new tentacles or it may have its subspecialties amputated, leaving it as a restricted operating room–bound specialty (**Fig. 2-1**).

As an academic specialty, anesthesiology evolved out of fundamental contributions to health care, including the prevention of pain from surgery and the development of critical care medicine, cardiopulmonary resuscitation, and pain medicine.[43] In recent years, many advances have occurred in the basic science of anesthesiology; these include mechanisms of pain, receptor physiology, modes of action of anesthetic agents, and cellular responses to sepsis. If anesthesiology is to flourish as an academic specialty, it is crucial that research is pursued and encouraged. Without intellectual advances, anesthesiology is in danger of becoming a sterile technical discipline.[43] University departments of anesthesiology are increasingly experiencing pressure to emphasize clinical delivery at

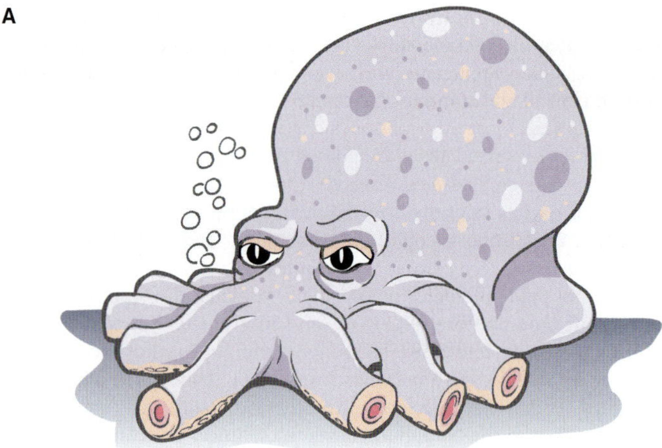

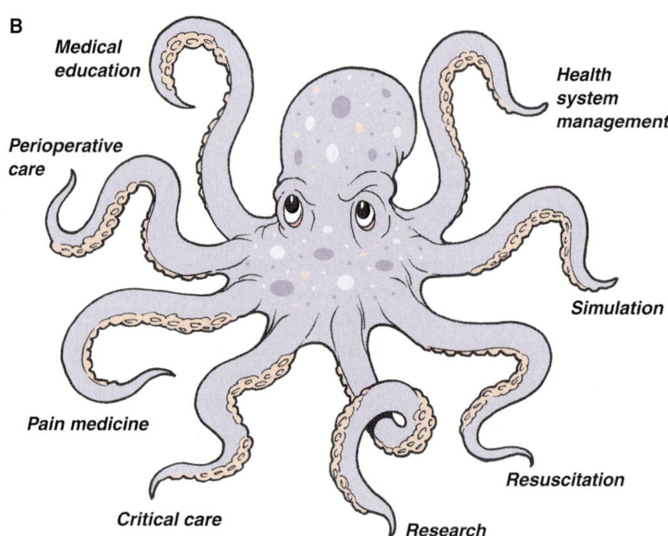

FIGURE 2-1. The future of anesthesiology: two possible outcomes. **A.** The specialty may come to resemble a bloated octopus, based only in the operating room with all its tentacles amputated. **B.** Anesthesiology may retain its integral role in the operating room but expand its tentacles in other areas, such as critical care, pain medicine, medical education, health system management, simulation, resuscitation, and research.

the expense of academic pursuits. If they succumb to these pressures, this will threaten undergraduate perioperative medicine teaching, development of critical appraisal skills among anesthesiologists, and the future of research programs.[44] The irony would be that by immersing themselves entirely in the clinical arena, anesthesiologists would neglect the education of medical students and trainees, thus jeopardizing the future of clinical anesthesiology practice.

Although it is easy to teach others as we were taught, or as we practice today, focus on the future is an essential element of education. Long-term success for the specialty will depend on our efforts in undergraduate and graduate medical education, whereas short-term success will depend on our efforts in the continuing medical education of current practitioners.[45] A different approach may be required to redefine the scope of the practice with broadened training to provide increased expertise in the evolving medical marketplace. This approach could include solid training in business, informatics, data management, and critical thinking on outcomes. This paradigm shift may be challenging, and it requires redirection, reallocation of assets, reeducation, and a new mindset. If successfully applied, however, it presents a means to strengthen the respected position of the specialty and to promote the medical care and practice of perioperative specialists in the rapidly changing landscape of modern medicine.[46]

VISIONS OF THE FUTURE

SCENARIO 1: TO EACH PATIENT A DEDICATED ANESTHESIOLOGIST

This is the current model of anesthesia care in much of the developed world, and many in the United States are adherents to this model. Most American residency programs are structured to train anesthesiologists to practice in this model. As discussed earlier in this chapter, it is unlikely that this model of anesthesia care will be sustainable given the mismatch between surgical demand and the anesthesiology workforce and the inevitable pressure to reduce the cost of anesthesia.

SCENARIO 2: PHYSICIANS FOR THE PERIOPERATIVE PERIOD

Many advocate that anesthesiologists should play a greater role in perioperative care. This is an appealing option but fraught with difficulties. An expansion of anesthesiologists' roles will mean that even more anesthesiologists must be trained. There is simply a limited capacity to achieve this. It is also not clear whether anesthesiologists are prepared to compete financially in many perioperative roles. Anesthesiologists are accustomed to high remuneration for their procedure-driven roles, whereas hospitalists are willing to accept lower compensation. Thus far anesthesiologists have not shown enthusiasm in adopting the mantle of perioperative physicians. Tremendous inertia will have to be overcome for this to become a possibility.

SCENARIO 3: PROCESS MANAGERS AND PERIOPERATIVE CARE DIRECTORS

To achieve this, anesthesiologists will require formal training in business, management, and finance. They will also need to broaden their medical knowledge and experience. Perhaps most importantly, anesthesiologists would have to be trained to supervise others effectively and to use physician extenders throughout the perioperative period. Certified registered nurse anesthetists are also expensive, and other physician extender roles should be explored too. This model runs counter to the current training process. There are anesthesia programs that are offering novel fellowships, such as operating room management. The philosophy behind this model is that anesthesiologists would receive broader training, where operating room anesthesia would be only a component. Fellowships and academic tracks would also increase. If this model is to succeed, residencies will have to undergo major paradigm shifts.

MEETING THE CHALLENGE OF CHANGE

At the ASA's 2005 Rovenstein Lecture, Mark Warner opined that as long as anesthesiologists remain steadfast in their commitment to the specialty's core values, the specialty would continue to develop as a vibrant academic medical specialty.[47] Warner identified two quintessential values of anesthesiology[47]:

1. Commitment to the care of critically ill patients as well as those experiencing acute and chronic pain.
2. Promoting and improving patient safety in the operating room and in the perioperative period.

Change will be driven by several imperatives, including shifting demographics, technological advances, patterns of surgery, and economic realities. There will be an increasing number of elderly people, high-risk obstetric patients, and children with complex medical problems requiring surgery. It is important to further increase the safety of surgical, anesthetic, and perioperative care to minimize both short-term morbidity and long-term deterioration when vulnerable patients undergo surgery and anesthesia.

Improved monitoring, safer drugs, less invasive surgery, and sophisticated communication networks may allow anesthesiologists and other anesthesia providers to extend their roles without compromising patient safety. Intensive care units may serve as a useful model. Typically 1 nurse attends to 1 or 2 critically ill patients. Usually a small number of physicians, with one experienced intensivist, regularly assess all the patients and modify treatment plans over the course of the day. A derivative of this model could be conceptualized for future operating room anesthesia care. As individual patients present with their genetic profiles, it may become possible to tailor anesthetic and analgesic therapy with increased efficacy and decreased side effects. This pharmacogenomics model would represent a major advance in patient safety.

CONCLUSION

Health care systems are evolving at a rapid rate. Anesthesiology as a specialty must adapt to the changes in order that anesthesiologists remain valuable and essential members of the health care team. Anesthesiologists must extend their physician skills and increasingly pursue subspecialty fellowships. Anesthesiologists should have a meaningful presence in all areas of medicine. Apart from traditional areas of involvement, such as operating room anesthesia, critical care, pain medicine, teaching, research and resuscitation, there will be future opportunities for anesthesiologists in pharmacogenomics, health care systems management, and new technologies.

KEY REFERENCES

- Brennan TA, Horwitz RI, Duffy FD, Cassel CK, Goode LD, Lipner RS. The role of physician specialty board certification status in the quality movement. *JAMA.* 2004;292(9):1038-1043.
- Haynes AB, Weiser TG, Berry WR, et al. A surgical safety checklist to reduce morbidity and mortality in a global population. *N Engl J Med.* 2009;360(5):491-499.
- Lagasse RS. Anesthesia safety: model or myth? A review of the published literature and analysis of current original data. *Anesthesiology.* 2002;97(6):1609-1617.
- Larsson J, Holmstrom I, Rosenqvist U. Professional artist, good Samaritan, servant and co-ordinator: four ways of understanding the anaesthetist's work. *Acta Anaesthesiol Scand.* 2003;47(7):787-793.
- Noordzij PG, Poldermans D, Schouten O, Bax JJ, Schreiner FA, Boersma E. Postoperative mortality in the Netherlands: a population-based analysis of surgery-specific risk in adults. *Anesthesiology.* 2010;112(5):1105-1115.
- Schwinn DA, Balser JR. Anesthesiology physician scientists in academic medicine: a wake-up call. *Anesthesiology.* 2006;104(1):170-178.
- Warner MA. Who better than anesthesiologists? The 44th Rovenstine lecture. *Anesthesiology.* 2006;104(5):1094-1101.

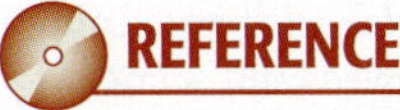

REFERENCES

Complete references available on DVD and online version at www.LongneckerAnesthesiology.com

CHAPTER 3

Safety and Quality: The Guiding Principles of Patient-Centered Care

Jeffrey B. Cooper
David E. Longnecker

KEY POINTS

1. The patient should be the focus of anesthesia care.
2. The goal of anesthesia care must be to ensure that *no* patient is harmed.
3. Preventing harm is challenging because care is complex and serious adverse events are relatively rare and often the result of many causes rather than a single one.
4. Serious adverse events are usually the result of weaknesses in the "system" of anesthesia care, not the fault of incompetent clinicians.
5. To prevent adverse events, a strategy is needed, not simply vigilance.
6. Organizations, departments, and groups must use a top-down approach and a commitment to creating a safe environment and system for safety.
7. Safety must be the number 1 priority to create an organization that operates at the highest level of reliability.
8. Anesthesia professionals must employ a broad array of safety tactics.
9. Teamwork and communication among the perioperative caregivers are critical components of patient safety.

Anesthesia providers develop a comfort with their craft, despite its inherent dangers. Over time, the administration of potentially lethal drugs, the management of apnea, and the control of altered physiologic systems become almost routine. With experience, they may even take for granted the inherently hazardous art and science of rendering patients insensible to pain, unconscious, and paralyzed. Yet patients do not take anesthesia for granted. To the contrary, they fear the possibility of experiencing pain or awareness, as well as the potential for death or other serious complications.[1,2] They also fear what professionals might consider "minor complications"; patients often view postoperative nausea and vomiting as dreaded and prominent complications associated with the procedure.

This chapter focuses on patient safety and quality and is based on the principle that the patient is the center of care. The person or team performing the procedure will have medical requirements that are embedded in the anesthetic plan, but the patient's concerns, fears, values, and expectations also must be addressed. Although that may seem obvious, historically, the design of health care systems, including anesthesia care, has been centered on the needs and convenience of the providers and the facility. The underlying concept was that quality of care alone was enough, whereas quality of service (ie, "patient centeredness") was relatively insignificant in the process. That concept is changing, and this chapter begins by emphasizing that patient perceptions must be considered in the design of a safe, high-quality anesthetic experience.

The patient's most fundamental needs are for high quality and complete safety. Meeting these expectations demands knowledge, skills, and continuous vigilance. Equally important is a system that ensures safe practitioners; provides the appropriate drugs, technologies, policies, and procedures to foster safe practice; monitors performance of the entire process (including both outcomes and patient satisfaction); identifies safety and quality problems; and implements corrections. All of these demand a culture of safety and quality at all levels of the system, a culture that supports these needs not just in words but in deeds and actions.

In 2001, an Institute of Medicine (IOM) committee identified patient safety, quality of care, and patient-centered care (ie, individualized care) as progressively increasing levels of excellence in the overall health care process.[3] This view is consistent with the tenets of other organizations that serve the public while dealing with potentially lethal outcomes (eg, the commercial aviation industry). In short, safety is the foundation on which quality (eg, the application of evidence-based approaches) and then patient-centeredness are built, but all are required to meet the goal of highest-quality care.

The demands for quality and safety start with the patient's needs guided by the needs of the physicians performing the procedure (medical, surgical, or diagnostic) that requires anesthesia care. Sometimes these are competing expectations, requiring thoughtful tradeoffs based on essential priorities. When balancing these tradeoffs, involvement of the patient is a key to positive patient satisfaction with the overall process.

Every subsequent chapter in this text has the delivery of safe and high-quality care as its primary objectives. This chapter defines a strategy and generic principles for achieving these objectives, centering on the patient while also meeting the other demands of modern perioperative care. Subsequent sections in this book provide specific elements of evidence-based anesthesia care that are required to meet these strategic objectives.

DEFINING QUALITY AND SAFETY

The key terms commonly used to discuss quality and patient safety include the following:

- *Patient-centered care* encompasses the qualities of compassion, empathy, open and complete communication, and responsiveness to the needs and preferences of each patient.[3]
- *Quality of care* is the extent to which health services for individuals and populations increase the likelihood of desired health outcomes and are consistent with current professional knowledge.[4]
- *Patient safety* is the avoidance, prevention, and amelioration of adverse outcomes or injuries stemming from the processes of health care. These events include "errors," "deviations," and "accidents." Safety emerges from the interactions among the components of the system; it does not reside in a single person, device, or department. Improving safety depends on learning how safety emerges from the interactions of the components through analysis of "near misses" and adverse outcomes or injuries. Patient safety is a subset of health care quality.[5]
- *Quality improvement.* The US Agency for Healthcare Research and Quality defines high-quality health care as "doing the right thing, at the right time, in the right way."[6] *Quality improvement* is the process used by individuals and organizations to ensure that these goals are met through a system of constant scrutiny, measurement, review, and revision.[7]
- *Adverse event* is an injury caused by medical management that results in measurable disability.[8]
- *Accident* is an unplanned, unexpected, and undesired event, usually with an adverse consequence.[9]
- *Error* is when a planned sequence of mental or physical activities fails to achieve its intended outcome and these failures cannot be attributed to the intervention of some chance agency.[10]
- *Near miss* is an event or situation that could have resulted in an accident, injury or illness but did not, either by chance or through timely intervention.[7] Also known as close call or near hit.
- *Human factors* refers to the scientific discipline concerned with understanding interactions among humans and other elements of a system, and to the profession that applies theory, principles, data, and methods to design so as to optimize human well-being and overall system performance.[11]
- *Risk management* is the clinical and administrative activities undertaken to identify, evaluate, and reduce the risk of injury to patients, staff, and visitors, and to identify, evaluate, and reduce the risk of loss to the organization itself.[12]

The concepts of quality and safety are a continuum. Some view safety as a subset of quality; most agree that quality care must be founded on safe care. One important difference is that quality is generally measured in terms of success in achieving desired outcomes, whereas safety is measured in failures, particularly catastrophic failures. Success in achieving the desired outcomes includes not only a safe experience but also one that incorporates the elements of evidence-based medicine, especially because personal provider experience is almost never adequate to evaluate either the overall positive or negative consequences of a specific drug, technique, or procedure. Because anesthesia is generally not therapeutic, complete safety must be the most important goal of every anesthetic. This means a goal that *no patient is caused any injury or complication from the effects of the overall anesthesia encounter.* This may seem unattainable. But, as described later, adopting such lofty goals and committing to achieve them leads to greater safety and better care.

To the benefit of all, quality and safety have attained increasing importance in modern health care. There is a rich history of attention to the processes of improving care. Those activities can be traced to the work of Donebedian, who developed principles by which quality can be measured and improved for health care in general, but with specific applications to hospital care.[13] It was only in the late 1990s that the concept of patient safety was raised to prominence in the broad health care environment, a result of a landmark study of medical error.[14] Yet, in anesthesia, patient safety has a much richer history. Indeed, the specialty of anesthesiology is often identified as the earliest adopter of patient safety principles, and it is lauded for achieving dramatic improvements in outcomes (see "Anesthesia Risk and Accidents" for the history of patient safety in anesthesia).

The concepts of patient safety, quality improvement, and risk management are related but have important distinctions. Patient safety is focused on prevention of injury. Quality improvement generally deals with the broader spectrum of quality, including the success of treatments. Risk management historically was directed at managing the aftermath of adverse outcomes, especially to manage legal issues, malpractice, and avoidance of financial loss for insurers. But modern risk management is focused on proactive patient safety, based on the principle that prevention of injuries via error reduction and system improvements reduces the adverse events from which malpractice awards arise.

Because safety focuses on preventing rare events, it is much harder to develop an evidence base for actions that create safety. Randomized controlled trials, although possible for testing many types of quality improvement practices, are almost unheard of for trials of safety practices. Many safety initiatives arise from investigation of serious adverse events. More intuitive arguments and judgments guide the implementation of safety principles.

ANESTHESIA RISK AND ACCIDENTS

The roots of safety run deep in anesthesiology. Dating to the first survey of anesthetic deaths,[15,16] there has been a regular and continuous self-examination within the anesthesia profession to understand the causes of harm and how to prevent them. In the modern era of health care, anesthesia was the specialty that coined the term *patient safety,* which is now in the lexicon of health care and broadly applied to all medical disciplines.

HISTORY OF PATIENT SAFETY IN ANESTHESIA

The history of safety in anesthesiology may have begun with the first description and review of an anesthetic death—that of Hannah Greener, who died during administration of chloroform for amputation of her large toe in 1848.[17] Although outcome studies were reported over the years, it was not until the landmark study of Beecher and Todd that a large population was sampled and specific causality suggested.[18] Other studies followed during the 1950s and 1960s, with a focus generally on the morbidity and mortality associated with general or regional anesthesia, and the cause of death or serious injury in surgical patients.[19,20]

Safety interventions in the 1950s and 1960s focused on the development of safety features of anesthesia equipment. Features such as the fail-safe system for protecting against loss of oxygen supply pressure and pin-indexing of gas cylinders to prevent their being interchanged are still in use today.

The concept of "patient" safety arose in the early 1980s, in response to several factors. The first study of the contribution of human error in anesthesia was reported in 1978, followed by larger studies that focused on the sources of errors and strategies for their prevention.[21,22] In these studies, Cooper et al studied "critical incidents" to elucidate the mechanisms of what were then called anesthesia "mishaps" as being multidimensional, resulting from a number of errors and other contributing factors to each event. Other reports described attributes of a specific event, disconnection in the breathing circuit, and a generic contributor to critical events, the relief of one anesthesia provider by another. Several studies replicated the methods and general findings in other settings and countries.[23,24]

A "crisis" of increasing costs for malpractice insurance for anesthesiologists prompted intense interest in tort reform and in reducing the number of adverse events that led to claims. The American Society of Anesthesiologists (ASA), under its then president, Ellison C. Pierce Jr, MD, led this initiative, which resulted in the formation of the Anesthesia Patient Safety Foundation in 1985.[25] Its activities represented the first organized efforts in health care to address patient safety as a single topic. The ASA later sponsored studies of closed malpractice claims, which led to numerous reports about causes of the most severe adverse events and their trends.[26]

Many efforts contributed to what appears to be a substantial reduction in catastrophic adverse anesthesia outcomes among relatively healthy patients.[27] Among these were improvements in educational programs, safer drugs and equipment, more intense patient monitoring (especially oxygen analyzers, pulse oximetry, and capnography), and new technologies for managing difficult airways (a specific contributor to numerous severe adverse outcomes). Standards and guidelines for anesthesia care also played a role in reducing adverse events. The Harvard Medical School Department of Anaesthesia promulgated the first standards for care in 1986[28]; these were later adopted by the ASA as national standards. It is claimed that these standards are associated with a reduction in serious outcomes among ASA physical status (ASA-PS) 1 and 2 patients in the ensuing years.[28] Many other standards and guidelines followed. **Box 3-1** summarizes key milestones in the path to safer anesthesia care.

A national movement in patient safety was catalyzed by the 1999 publication of the IOM report *To Err Is Human: Building a Safer Healthcare System.*[14] It and subsequent reports recommended fundamental changes in the health care system to combat a problem with deep roots in the way patient care is organized (or disorganized), particularly the culture of health care that did not place a high priority on the overall safety of patients relative to the delivery of specific services. Anesthesiology was singled out in the IOM's report, and in other writings, as the one specialty that addressed patient safety early and with positive results.

BOX 3-1

Key Influences Leading to Increasing Patient Safety in Anesthesia

Research in human error, human factors, and closed claims.

Development and routine use of pulse oximetry.

Development and routine use of capnometry.

Enhanced alarms and safety features in anesthesia machines/workstations.

Development of safer anesthetic drugs.

Anesthesia Patient Safety Foundation focus on patient safety.

American Society of Anesthesiologists adoption of standards and guidelines for safe practice.

Development of new airway management tools such as fiberoptic bronchoscopy.

CURRENT STATE OF KNOWLEDGE OF ANESTHESIA RISK AND RELATIONSHIP TO ERROR

There is a general belief that the risk of preventable death or injury from anesthesia is relatively low compared with many other medical and nonmedical risks. Yet there are no accurate estimates of the rate of adverse outcomes in general or for an individual patient presenting with specific risk factors. One reason is that there are no standard methods for assigning causality appropriately among numerous factors that include anesthesia, surgery, the facility (and its systems), and the patient's disease. Particularly in the United States, the fear of malpractice claims hinders reporting and open, candid discussion of errors. Federal legislation, similar to that enacted in Australia in the late 1980s, now protects voluntary reporting.[29] Despite the absence of strong evidence, estimates of the risk of untoward outcome to a relatively healthy patient are believed to be on the order of 1 in 100,000 patients.[30, 31] However, for patients presenting at greater risk, the risk may be on the order of 1 in 10,000, which is not different from early estimates for all patients.[30,32] Thus there remains substantial room for improvement in the overall safety of anesthesia. Chapter 25 has a comprehensive discussion of risk, mortality, and morbidity.

ACCIDENT MODELS

Most people, both in and out of health care, seek to assign blame to specific individuals for specific lapses in performance associated with an adverse event. Yet the evidence demonstrates that most injurious accidents are typically complex events for which there is no single cause.[33-35] Although it would be possible to envision a scenario in which a specific act by one individual led to an accident, assigning such pinpoint causality is not a useful approach to accident prevention. Substantial research is targeted at learning how accidents occur and how humans are involved in that process. The science emerging from that research supports the concept that there are few simple solutions for prevention of accidents. However, it offers possible strategies and tactics for lowering the potential for accidents, by preventing human error and its precursors (ie, the factors that promote and propagate errors), and by creating resilience in systems to respond to those errors that will inevitably occur despite the best of intentions and preventive actions.

The goal of adverse-event-free anesthesia care can be achieved only by applying a broad spectrum of prevention strategies and building resilience throughout the entire system of anesthesia care, for the overall system is no stronger than its weakest links. This section examines several models and issues at the organizational and human levels to inform our thinking about designing for failure.

THE "SYSTEM" OF ANESTHESIA CARE

Whereas anesthesia could be viewed simply as a single provider administering drugs to a single patient, that narrow perspective does not represent the much more intricate and multidimensional processes that characterize care delivery. Rather, the anesthesia encounter consists of several components that comprise the "system of anesthesia care." The anesthesia processes can be thought of broadly in three phases: preanesthetic planning and preparation, provision of anesthesia for the procedure, and postanesthesia care. Within each of these phases, the anesthesia provider(s) performs a set of tasks intended to provide quality care for the patient, surgeon, or other operator, and the health care organization. Achieving safety and quality requires that these anesthesia activities be synchronized with the needs of other providers, allied health professionals, technical staff, support staff, hospital or organization programs, and, especially, with the patient's needs and expectations. The interactions between all of these components comprise a "system" of care that has yet to be fully modeled for the perioperative experience. Further, this "anesthesia system" takes place within a system of systems that includes the overall course of care, and numerous elements of this larger system may interact with anesthesia care at multiple points in the delivery process; such interactions often contribute to a less-than-optimal experience for the patient.

The Accreditation Council for Graduate Medical Education (ACGME) has established a set of 8 competencies that must be met for all medical trainees.[36] One competency is to understand and know how to practice within a system of health care. That requirement arose in recognition of the interdependencies among all the members of the care team and the larger system in which they operate. In the case of anesthesia, that implies having an understanding of the requirements and needs of all other participants in the perioperative system and implementing an anesthesia plan that appropriately meets these various needs, rather than acting individually in an introverted fashion.

MODELS OF ORGANIZATIONAL FAILURE

James T. Reason is perhaps the most widely cited author for overall conceptual thinking about the mechanisms of human error and system failures, although his work is founded on the basic work of Rasmussen. Their thinking derives from research in high-hazard industries, such as nuclear power, aviation, and chemical manufacture. Gaba has offered insightful interpretations of this work and other research as it applies specifically to anesthesia practice.[35] The basic concepts are relatively simple: Accidents are not unidimensional; rather, they are the result of the interaction of several elements; each accident is somewhat unique in the way that elements combine to result in injury. (Note that in the context of "safety," we are addressing only those adverse outcomes that could be prevented given the application of current knowledge; death or injury that appears to be caused primarily by the patient's disease process or the unpredictable influences of drugs or operation likely cannot be altered by safety interventions.) Reason depicted the process of accident evolution in what is widely referred to as the "Swiss cheese" model (**Fig. 3-10**).[10]

The "Swiss cheese" model illustrates that accidents are typically the result of a series of events that include precursors, which trigger or allow the chain of events that result in the final (active) adverse event. Reason termed these precursors *latent errors*. This concept is now widely accepted in understanding health care system failures. Latent factors exist regularly in any work environment. They have the potential for initiating or propagating an evolving accident. Examples are failure to maintain equipment or replace obsolete equipment, selection of low-quality supply items, poor scheduling practices that promote haste or fatigue, and case scheduling and staffing models that allow assignment of relatively inexperienced clinicians to unfamiliar cases or high-risk patients. Cultural influences are an important source of latent failures. Examples include the pressure to proceed with cases in remote locations where the resources are insufficient to meet minimal anesthesia safety requirements, pressures to move rapidly to avoid "turnover delays," pressures to assign an inexperienced provider to a case to "keep the schedule moving," a hostile atmosphere within an operating room that limits communication of concerns about quality and safety, and failure to heed a patient's warnings or concerns. Latent errors rarely lead to an immediate accident. Rather, they can be seen as a lurking enemy, or, as Reason called them, "resident pathogens," awaiting the circumstances that will combine to produce a catastrophic outcome, often in ways that are unusual and what may be called "unpredictable." Avoiding the consequences of latent errors requires broad defenses and resilience throughout the system, to mitigate evolving failure that results from alignment of the "holes in the cheese."

Reason's model highlights the need for broad and varying mechanisms to trap errors and failures during the patient's health care encounter and thus mitigate or prevent the full cascade from unfolding. His work on managing risk begins at the organizational level and offers a spectrum of strategies and tactics for accident prevention. Both the attitude and actions of the organization and each individual in the chain of care can either bolster or undermine those defense mechanisms.

There is a competing theory that postulates that prevention is not always possible or even probable. The normal accident theory (NAT),

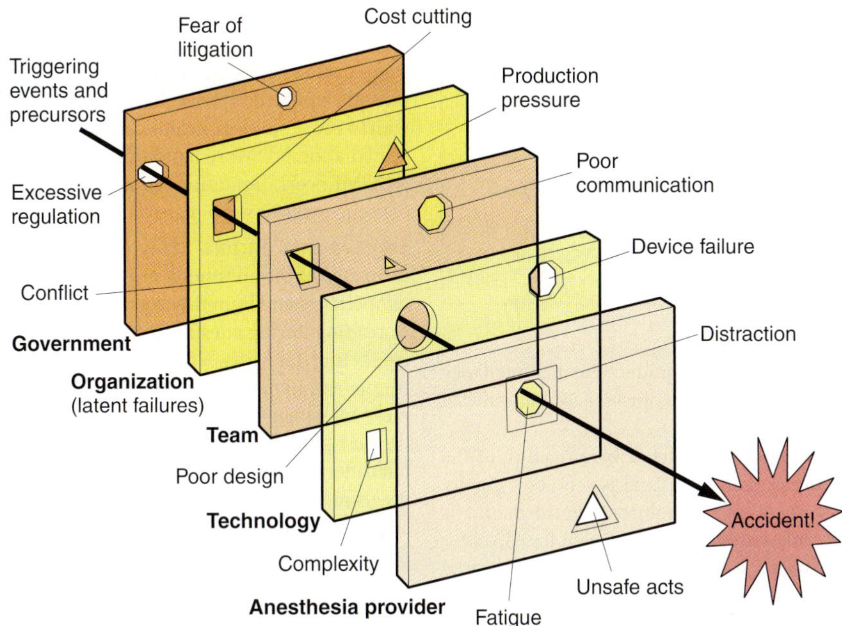

FIGURE 3-1. "Swiss cheese" model of accidents in anesthesia. [Reason J. *Managing the Risk of Organizational Accidents.* Aldershot, Hants, UK: Ashgate Publishing; 1997.]

as described by Perrow,[32] characterizes some industrial systems as particularly resistant to strategies for prevention of catastrophic accidents if the systems are both complex and "tightly coupled"; that is, the connections between processes are such that one quickly affects the other in ways that can evolve into an accident that is not predictable by deterministic analysis. Fortunately, although all the patient and provider processes involved in anesthesia administration may create a "complex" system, they are not usually "tightly coupled" to the extent envisioned in Perrow's model, although it may occur in certain high-risk patients whose disease processes present a less stable condition. Still, Perrow's NAT provides many lessons for anesthesia practice and for constructing resilient systems to minimize the potential for accidents. Of special concern is that some protections and safety features can actually make systems more complex, mask impending problems, and impart a false sense of security. Further, certain prevention or mitigation strategies may affect other parts of the system in unanticipated ways and thus lead to new, unexpected risks. Anesthesia has many examples: Pulse oximetry can lead to practicing closer to the edge of acceptable levels of oxygenation or inappropriate assumptions that a functioning pulse oximeter implies adequate blood flow as well, automated noninvasive blood pressure monitors can fail to cycle and thus continue to present falsely high readings even in the presence of blood loss, or alarms on anesthesia monitors may be turned off to avoid "distraction" during the procedure. Moreover, the relative safety of anesthesia itself has been called an "insidious hazard," for some become complacent about anesthesia care and vigilance and assume that nothing will go wrong, based on prior experience.[22] The development of complacency about safety based on prior experiences has led to major disasters in a variety of organizations; a prime example is the loss of the orbiter ("shuttle") *Columbia* on February 1, 2003. The Columbia Accident Investigation Board identified a number of contributing latent factors that resulted in complacency within the National Aeronautics and Space Administration (NASA), including the acceptance of "normal deviation" and the loss of checks and balances that should have guided NASA safety efforts; many of these latent factors resulted from the lack of serious events in the years immediately preceding the loss of *Columbia*.[37]

Reason's commentary about creating effective defenses against accidents fits well for anesthesia:

> If eternal vigilance is the price of liberty, then chronic unease is the price of safety. Studies of high-reliability organizations—systems that have fewer than their share of accidents—indicate that the people who operate and manage them tend to assume that each day will be a bad day and act accordingly. But this is not an easy state to sustain, particularly when the thing about which one is uneasy has either not happened or has happened a long time ago, and perhaps in another organization. Nor is this Cassandra-like attitude likely to be well received within certain organizational cultures.[34]

MODELS OF HUMAN ERROR/FAILURE

The modern theory of accident causality and safety views the human as a component of a system. Most experts now tend to play down the operator's responsibility for accidents, perhaps because so often the attention and blame has been so heavily directed at those who are at what Cook and Woods term the *sharp end* of the pyramid of accident control.[38] In fact, there is substantial evidence about human error and how humans interact with systems in diverse ways to either help or hinder the accident process. The vast majority of research has been in industry, most notably aviation and nuclear power applications, but there has been substantial investigation in anesthesia, where some of the earliest studies of human error and human factors in health care are found.

The studies of critical incidents mentioned earlier identified the basic issue of human error as a component of what were termed *mishaps.* Factors associated with mishaps, what would now be called *latent factors,* were identified, such as lapses in training, equipment design weaknesses, and the contribution of fatigue. In these and other areas, the science of human performance and human factors has revealed much more about the weaknesses of humans and the many ways in which we can fail, including how system design and other factors can influence our performance and conspire to weaken even the most expert clinician.

There has been a strong reliance on "vigilance" during anesthesia as the primary approach to error prevention, so much that the word is the motto of the ASA. Vigilance means sustaining attention.[39] It has been defined as having 3 components: alertness, selection of information, and conscious effort. It is a much more complex process than is immediately apparent, and vigilance is the subject of much investigation in many fields that require sustained attention to ensure safety and performance. The observant practitioner is aware of some of the many ways that

BOX 3-2

Slips and Mistakes

Slip: The plan is adequate, but the actions fail to go as planned. These are unintended failures of execution, also referred to as lapses, trips, or fumbles. They are further divided into attentional slips of action and lapses of memory.

Mistake: The actions conform to plan, but the plan is inadequate to achieve its intended outcome. Mistakes are divided into rule based (eg, misapplication of normally good rules but not correct for this situation) and knowledge based (eg, incorrectly thinking out a solution for which there is not a prepackaged solution).

vigilance can be thwarted and performance degraded. Further, vigilance is only one of a complex set of elements that comprise safe anesthesia practice.

Human error in general is the subject of intense investigation in the fields of human factors, ergonomics, and industrial psychology. Again, James Reason provided an overview of the subject.[10] Performance is defined at 3 levels: skill based, rule based, and knowledge based. Error is defined as the failure of planned actions to achieve their desired ends without the intervention of some unforeseeable event. Errors are divided into 2 main types: slips and mistakes (**Box 3-2**). The thoughtful practitioner will consider that his or her slips and mistakes vary in type and cause, most of all recognizing that all forms of error require efforts toward prevention, or mitigation of their consequences because errors occur despite the best of efforts.

Many factors influence vigilance and performance (performance-shaping factors), including fatigue and sleep deprivation, environmental influences, production pressures, human-interface design, and teamwork. Other factors associated with adverse events in anesthesia that either may promote errors or foster their propagation have been identified.[21,22] We consider some as examples of the issues that anesthesia providers must address to maintain accident-free performance throughout a professional career. Measures to prevent performance decrement or to help maintain optimal performance are described in "Creating Safety at the Organizational and Department Level."

Fatigue and Sleep Deprivation There is evidence (in trainees) that shows an association between sleep deprivation and human errors, including lack of attention to task, serious auto accidents, and medical errors involving both diagnosis and treatment.[39-41] There are many examples of large-scale industrial accidents where sleep deprivation or fatigue was identified as a major contributing factor.

Howard et al reviewed the literature on sleep and fatigue with particular reference to anesthesia.[42] Among the key findings were the following: (1) Inadequate sleep degrades performance, (2) individuals require different amounts of sleep to feel awake and alert, (3) the failure to obtain adequate sleep results in a sleep "debt" that is cumulative and can only be diminished by sleep to pay back the debt, (4) circadian rhythms have an important influence both on the tendency to sleep and the ability to sleep; the circadian lull associated with degraded performance is between 2 and 6 AM and 2 and 6 PM, and (5) stimulants such as caffeine can aid in maintaining alertness and wakefulness, but side effects must be understood to use these effectively.[43]

Transitions Among Care Providers ("Handoffs" or "Handovers") There are conflicting findings about the impact of handoffs among anesthesia providers to mitigate the effects of fatigue, boredom, hunger, and so forth. Cooper et al examined critical incidents associated with relief of one anesthesia provider by another.[44] They concluded that, overall, relief provided more benefit from detecting undiscovered problems than harm from transferring responsibility to a provider with less serial knowledge of the specific patient and procedure. These conclusions were verified by interpretation of data from a similar study by Short et al.[45] More recently, Arbous et al found that a change of anesthesiologists was associated with a greater incidence of severe morbidity and mortality.[46] Yet routine breaks are generally found to be useful and necessary in anesthesia and in high-hazard industries. Provisions for adequate transfer of critical information and situational awareness are required. Cooper suggested a specific set of guidelines for conduct of handoffs, which was recently updated.[47,48] The hazards of transitions in care are now more widely recognized in health care and receiving increasing attention for remediation.[49,50] More handoffs now occur among trainees as a result of ACGME work-limitation requirements that are intended to mitigate the consequences of sleep deprivation and fatigue.

Environmental Factors Many environmental factors can affect the performance of the anesthesia provider. Among these are noise, extremes of temperature and humidity, lighting, and toxic vapors.[51] Listening to music or reading during anesthesia administration are controversial issues with conflicting tradeoffs.[52,53] There are no robust studies in health care or simple extrapolations from studies in other fields to guide the development of evidence-based standards. Rather, good judgment appears to be the best guideline. Background music can alleviate stress and boredom, but different musical tastes may lead to varying effects among the operating team. Loud music or other noises can obscure verbal communications and be especially disruptive during periods of high workload or management of critical events. Similarly, reading, texting, e-mailing, and so on in the operating room could alleviate boredom during uneventful intervals, but these could also foster a lack of vigilance and alertness. They appear especially problematic intuitively and would be difficult to justify during an accident investigation involving pilots, air traffic controllers, train operators, or anesthesia providers, among others.

Human Factors and Human Interface Design Human factors engineering (HFE) is a broad topic that encompasses all of the different aspects of the ways in which humans interact with systems.[54] The importance of human factors, especially the design of the human–machine interface, is well known in other fields but greatly underappreciated in health care.[11] The goal of HFE is to "design tools, machines, and systems that take into account human capabilities, limitations, and characteristics."[55] Given that anesthesia is technology intensive, human factors play an important role in prevention of errors and adverse outcomes.

Several studies have examined how the design of displays and of anesthesia alarms have an impact on equipment use and errors.[51,56,57] The results indicate that technology is not generally well designed to accommodate the ways people use it. There are numerous examples of how the design of a device interface can be especially dangerous.[58-60] The design of anesthesia monitors is particularly problematic. Anesthesia providers work in facilities that have various models or different suppliers of devices. For example, differences in software design or data displays can cause confusion and distract the provider from other important tasks that should be higher priority. A new standard requiring attention to human factors in the design of medical devices is intended to address these issues, but it will be years until the effects can be felt.[61]

Production Pressure Production pressure refers to "overt or covert pressures and incentives on personnel to place production, not safety, as their primary priority."[62] Based on a survey of anesthesiologists in California, Gaba et al reported that nearly half of the respondents had witnessed instances of what they believed to be unsafe actions by an anesthesiologist because of production pressure.[62] These included internal pressures (eg, to foster good relations with a surgeon, accrue personal income) and external pressures (eg, proceed rather than cancel a case to appease patient or family, accept an unfamiliar patient or procedure to foster facility throughput).

Teamwork The importance of good teamwork and communication is now more widely recognized in health care, especially for surgical teams. A substantial body of literature from high-hazard domains, especially aviation, and in health care demonstrates the value of teamwork for successfully preventing and managing critical situations.[63-65] Gaba et al were the first to develop teamwork and crisis management training techniques for health care, adapting crew resource management (CRM) techniques from aviation for applications in anesthesia.[66] These approaches have since been extended to nearly all health care

BOX 3-3

Some Effective Practices of High-Performance Teams

Introduce all members of the team to each other at the start of each procedure.

Regularly conduct *preoperative briefings* with the entire operative team, which can be done via a specific checklist as described by Lingard et al[67]

Use specific *communication protocols* within the team (SBAR is gaining increasing acceptance. It calls for a specific sequence for describing the patient's status: the Situation, the Background, Assessment, and Recommendations [SBAR]).[65]

Establish communication standards such as "read-back" of all verbal orders (eg, medications).

Conduct *debriefings* with the team following unusual occurrences, near misses, or critical events.

Establish an environment that encourages cross-monitoring and backup behaviors across the entire team.

Create a language that signifies recognition of potential hazards.

Practice for emergency situations (Box 3-4).

settings but are particularly applicable to those where rapid action is required to successfully treat acute complex events, such as dire surgical emergencies.[68]

Box 3-3 lists some characteristics of effective teams.[63,67,69] These definitions and characteristics, derived from other industries, generally apply to health care and to anesthesia practice. Good teamwork can prevent errors or mitigate their impact. Teamwork is vital to the successful management of critical events. The team within which anesthesia providers work varies depending on the setting, but it typically includes at least a surgeon, a circulating nurse, a surgical technician, and other support personnel, including environmental workers, technicians (eg, blood bank, laboratory, or radiology), and clerical personnel. Within the broad system of care, the team can include those who provide care pre- and postoperatively and specialists, such as radiologists, pathologists, and intensivists. The immediate operative team has been given the most attention for training and research.

Surgical teams have several distinguishing features that create obstacles to effective performance. The hierarchy in surgical care places physicians above other workers. It is common for surgeons to be accorded higher status and to assume a self-designated role of "captain of the ship." Whereas leadership is a key feature for team success, the person in that role should vary depending on the situation. Similarly, anesthesia providers may treat other team members as subordinates rather than colleagues. High-reliability organization (HRO) theory (see "The Elements of Safe, High-Quality Anesthesia Care/The High-Reliability Organization Model"), which is based on characteristics of organizations that function at high levels of safety, calls for a nonhierarchal culture in which the leader is the one with the most expertise, not the highest status. Conflict among these roles can complicate the management of acute operative events, especially when the care team does not work together regularly (eg, during nights and weekends when the care team consists of "night call" personnel from various work rosters).

CRM and team-building techniques have been applied for training teamwork skills and performance. There are different approaches to training, but the principles are generally the same. Teamwork needs should be assessed for the specific environment; all team members must be motivated and engaged in accepting the need for teamwork and agree about skills and behaviors they will adopt; those behaviors must be taught and practiced via drills and the behaviors assessed and periodically reinforced via more drills and didactic sessions.[63,70]

In anesthesia, simulation of the patient and environment in which anesthesia is administered has been used, both for motivation and for training of technical and nontechnical (behavioral) teamwork skills.[71,72] There is some evidence that such sessions can effectively instill good team behaviors[74] (see later discussion of simulation). Team training without simulation also is effective, as is the combination of both approaches.[65,75]

SOME SPECIFIC HAZARDS ASSOCIATED WITH ANESTHESIA

There are a seemingly infinite number of case reports of specific hazards and complications of anesthesia that were largely preventable, although a litany of isolated cases is perhaps less helpful than a series of organized observations. Studies of closed malpractice claims, funded by the ASA, have examined many of these events in a more systematic manner, one that assists in developing action plans for reducing risks. These closed claims studies have explored several categories of adverse outcomes, the most notable addressing errors related to airway management, monitoring, sudden cardiac arrest during spinal anesthesia, equipment failures, or nerve injuries.[26,76,77]

The Australian Incident Monitoring project analyzed 4000 critical events and developed an algorithm (COVER ABCD: A Swift Check) that accounts for the most common anesthetic emergencies (**Box 3-4**).[78] Use of the mnemonic will prevent injury in most cases if specific practices are followed. A detailed review of even a substantial subset of these concepts is beyond the scope of this chapter. Rather, we present here examples of the types of failures that establish an argument for having organized principles for general prevention of errors. Analysis of these types of events also suggests tactics that could reduce the likelihood that these would become a trigger or propagator of an accident chain.

ADVERSE RESPIRATORY EVENTS

Events associated with management of respiration are the most serious remaining hazards in anesthesia, as evidenced by data from the ASA closed claims analyses.[77] The three most common causes of death and brain damage are inadequate ventilation, esophageal intubation, and difficult tracheal intubation. The large majority of cases in the first two groups were judged to have been preventable if "better monitoring" had been used. For management of the difficult airway, prevention is more challenging. Peterson et al reported that "Persistent failed attempts at intubation were associated with an outcome of death or brain damage in claims in which a 'cannot ventilate and cannot intubate' emergency situation developed prior to surgical incision."[79] They concluded that this was confirming evidence for limiting conventional ventilation efforts to 3 attempts before using other strategies. Despite substantial

BOX 3-4

Crisis Management Algorithm–Memorize and Practice: An Explanation of Each Cue in the Mnemonic COVER ABCD[78]

C1	Circulation
C2	Color
O1	Oxygen
O2	Oxygen analyzer
V1	Ventilation
V2	Vaporizer
E1	Endotracheal tube
E2	Elimination
R1	Review monitors
R2	Review equipment
A	Airway
B	Breathing
C	Circulation
D	Drugs

advances in technologies that aid endotracheal intubation and some helpful, although far from foolproof, methods of airway assessment, there remain many opportunities for unanticipated difficulties with airway management, tracheal intubation, and effective ventilation (see Chapters 10 and 36). Each is an opportunity for a serious adverse outcome. Although airway management skills are greatly emphasized during training, there is great variance in experience and abilities among anesthesia providers, as are the opportunities to practice emergency skills. Thus periodic retraining and practice in the application of difficult airway management protocols is prudent. (This is an example of the value of simulation as a tool for learning and maintaining skills that may be needed infrequently but are essential for patient safety.)

MONITORING AND ALARMS

Failure to monitor the patient adequately is an important contributor to anesthesia-adverse events. Aside from failures of vigilance, which are often related to performance-shaping factors, monitoring technology design and lack of experience with technology can contribute to adverse outcomes. There are numerous ways in which pulse oximetry, capnometry, and automated noninvasive blood pressure monitors can give false information, leading to missed or incorrect diagnoses. The failure to use alarms has led to a requirement in the relevant standard that when a pulse oximeter is used, the variable pulse pitch tone and low-threshold alarm of the oximeter must always be audible.[80] Similarly, when capnography or capnometry is used, the end-tidal carbon dioxide alarm must be audible.

MEDICATION ERRORS

Medication errors are among the most frequent errors in anesthesia and in health care practice in general.[22] Similarity of drug names, containers, and label colors contribute to the ease by which such errors can be made, especially during periods of high stress. Dosing errors are also common and related to the frequent need for individual numerical calculations when drawing and mixing drugs for bolus administration or intravenous infusion. Choosing the wrong form of drug (eg, among various insulin formulations), flushing a catheter with a solution containing another potent drug, and confusion in the programming of infusion pumps are other examples of ways in which patients can be injured.

An obvious recommendation for prevention of some medication errors is to admonish the provider to read the label carefully.[81] Another tactic is to read each label 3 times. Yet human factors issues are widely recognized as contributing greatly to medication errors, especially because of similarity of drug names, the small or obscure print on vials or ampules, and the failure to organize medication carts optimally to avoid errors. Distractions and production pressure also are likely contributors to medication errors. No universal remedy for prevention has been identified. There is a standard for label colors and grouping by drug type, but some argue that it is unlikely to be effective and, if anything, all drug labels should be in black and white to force careful reading of the drug identity and concentration.[82] Numerous health care organizations are implementing barcode technology to address this hazard in other clinical environments, but this is not in wide use in anesthesia practice.

ERRORS IN DIAGNOSIS

Diagnostic errors are likely underreported because of the difficulty in their identification. Yet it is likely that diagnostic errors occur, especially during the management of critical events. Gaba has described 3 forms of fixation errors, including "this and only this" (fixating on a single diagnostic possibility to the exclusion of others, a form of "tunnel vision"), "everything but this" (searching among many possibilities but not including the real explanation), and "everything's OK" (persistent belief that there is no problem in spite of substantive signs there is a problem).[66]

EQUIPMENT ERRORS AND FAILURES

Current anesthesia machines and associated technology incorporate substantial safety features (see Chapter 39), which have been developed over decades in response to specific series of patient injuries associated with failure or misuse of equipment. Equipment failure is frequent and can occur in many ways, but it rarely causes injury directly.[21,80,81] When there is an equipment-associated injury, it is more likely to be from misuse than from overt failure of a device. Whereas the end user may be at fault, human factors research dictates that causes related to the design of technology and the lack of training and practice are equally, if not more, responsible. Among the legendary failures associated with poor human factors are the failure to turn on a ventilator that was briefly suspended during measurement of cardiac output or performance of radiologic studies, or the accidental, unnoticed disconnection of an intravenous or arterial pressure cannula leading to blood loss or failure of fluid or drug administration. Users can reduce hazards by ensuring they obtain adequate training before using a new device, conducting a systematic pre-use inspection of devices, and using backup monitoring devices as aids to vigilance. Never turning off an alarm is an essential precept to safe care.

ERRORS ASSOCIATED WITH A LACK OF STANDARD PRACTICE AND UNUSUAL SITUATIONS

The complexities of anesthesia create many opportunities for preventable adverse events caused by unusual circumstances or pitfalls. Goldhaber-Feibert and Cooper, taking from a convenient sample of clinician experiences, offer numerous examples[48]:

- A Passy-Muir valve, a form of "talking" tracheotomy tube, left on a tracheostomy when inflating the cuff to deliver positive-pressure ventilation causes repeated inflation of the patient's lungs with no mechanism for exhalation.
- An emergency can arise during transport of the intubated patient if the tracheal tube is accidentally dislodged.
- Administration of undiluted phenytoin (Dilantin) by rapid intravenous infusion can cause refractory hypotension, arrhythmias, and death.
- Administration of undiluted potassium by rapid intravenous infusion can cause ventricular fibrillation and cardiac arrest.
- Neostigmine given without an antimuscarinic drug (eg, glycopyrrolate) can cause asystole/severe bradycardia and atrioventricular block, and can be fatal.
- Inadvertent intravascular injection of local anesthetics during a nerve block can cause neurologic and cardiac toxicity, which can be fatal (especially with bupivacaine).
- Air embolism can occur during the placement or removal of central venous catheters.
- Limb necrosis can develop if the tourniquet used for intravenous placement or blood draw is left on the anesthetized patient for a prolonged period.
- Intracranial pressure (ICP) may be increased if a ventriculostomy drain is connected to a pressurized bag of heparinized saline (in a patient who likely already has a high ICP).

Even though these situations are likely obvious to experienced clinicians, they might occur under periods of stress and might not be obvious to the uninformed neophyte. Learning may arise haphazardly in the absence of a systematic approach to training.

THE DIMENSIONS OF QUALITY

What is quality as applied to health care? "Quality" is an abstract concept, with little intrinsic meaning. Rather, it represents the extent to which the expectations of health care consumers are met by health care providers, whether that consumer is the patient, a professional colleague, the payer, or the facility that provides resources for the care delivery. In this context, the "consumer" of anesthesia services includes not only the patient but the surgeon or other operator who requires anesthesia services to perform a diagnostic or therapeutic procedure.

Numerous definitions of quality exist, but a widely accepted definition is that of the IOM, which we noted earlier: Quality is the "extent to which health services for individuals and populations increase the likelihood of desired health outcomes and are consistent with current professional knowledge."[4] Thus quality represents not a distinct entity or end point but a continuum in the process of meeting the rational expectations of others who interact with the providers of health care services. Two major concepts are inherent in the IOM definition of quality: measurement (ie, "outcomes") and evidence-based care (ie, "current professional knowledge"). Inherent in the definition of quality is the view that safety is the essential foundation for quality and that high-quality practice cannot be achieved in the absence of safe practice. **Figure 3-2** illustrates these concepts. Another definition is that of the Agency for Health Care research, also noted previously: Quality is "doing the right thing, at the right time, in the right way, for the right person—and having the best possible results."

Donabedian, a leader in the genesis of the quality movement, proposed that quality could be evaluated by examining its major components: structure, process, and outcomes.[13] Structure involves the facilities and environment in which care is delivered (eg, governance, policies and procedures, and specific details, such as cleanliness, attractiveness, ease of access, noise levels, privacy); process involves how care is actually delivered, including the interactions between clinicians and patients (eg, the elements of communication including listening, sensitivity, compassion, the development of trust); outcomes involves measures of results of the care provided (eg, mortality, morbidity, speed of recovery). Inherent in these evaluations of quality are the patients' perspectives on each of these areas; thus the role of the consumer (especially the patient) in the evaluation of health care quality has increased considerably in recent years.

The IOM went further in defining quality, by identifying 6 desired characteristics of health care. Thus high-quality care should be safe, timely, effective, efficient, equitable, and patient centered (often abbreviated as STEEEP, for ease of recall). Here, also, the concepts of measurement and current knowledge are apparent throughout.

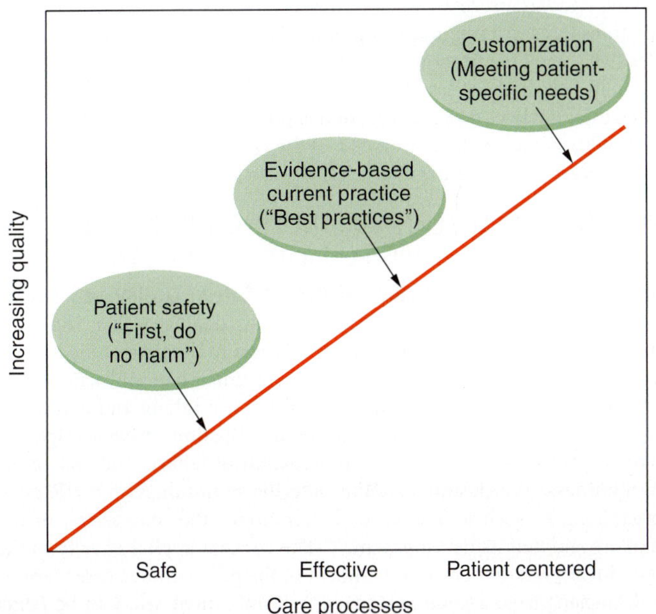

FIGURE 3-2. The relationship between safety and quality and the process of care.

The relationships among providers are key elements in the care process, especially in an era when complex care management is provided by specialists and subspecialists who focus on specific aspects of care. That complexity often leads to communication lapses and fragmentation without subsequent integration into a coordinated system of care that focuses on the patient's needs for understanding, planning, and decision making. Thus patients often rate communication as one of the most important components in the evaluation of quality health care, whereas physicians often rate technical abilities as considerably more important than communication.[85]

Eliminating these lapses in communication is essential for both patient compliance and patient satisfaction; eliminating the lapses benefits both process and outcome in the delivery of care. Further, it minimizes the frustrations that patients and families experience as a result of conflicting or inadequate communications among professionals, leading to mistrust of the provider by the consumer. Finally, the development of relationship-centered care teams, in which all parties have developed a pattern of open communication and mutual respect and trust, increase both safety and quality in multiple industries, including health care.[86]

These concepts apply as much to the discipline of anesthesiology as to other disciplines in health care. Anesthesia providers, as individuals and departments, must institute these principles, including practical measurement of outcomes and the development of relationship-centered clinical teams, if they expect to practice at the higher levels of the quality spectrum (ie, beyond the fundamental level of safe practice).

THE ELEMENTS OF SAFE, HIGH-QUALITY ANESTHESIA CARE

Creating a safe, high-quality practice of anesthesia depends on a combination of broad strategies and effective tactics for day-to-day work. Many models for establishing safe environments and practices and for ensuring quality have been described, but there is no empirical evidence from controlled studies to demonstrate that a specific model is superior to others. Still, there is face validity from qualitative studies in specific industries and organizations to suggest that having an overall systematic approach leads to both safer and higher-quality care. Indeed, a combined report from the National Academy of Engineering and the IOM emphasized that systems approaches to health care delivery were most likely to transform health care to deliver the goals of safe, timely, effective, efficient patient-centered care in the future.[87]

THE HIGH-RELIABILITY ORGANIZATION MODEL

Although several models have been promulgated for managing quality (see Chapter 25), there are fewer directed primarily at safety. For the latter, the concept of the high-reliability organization (HRO) was formulated from observations in highly hazardous industries that, despite operating under conditions of high risk, have many fewer serious accidents than expected.[88,89] Such industries included naval aviation and nuclear power. Weick and Sutcliffe further describe how organizations can be successful if they appropriately "manage uncertainty."[90] Gaba applied these concepts to health care.[35] Weick and Sutcliffe[90] lists the following elements that characterize a typical highly reliable organization:

- *Preoccupation with failure:* Despite its good safety records, an HRO will constantly look for any signs of weak systems or impending failure. An HRO assumes that failure is imminent and plans for the worst. In anesthesia, this extends to organizational and individual planning for potential failures or problems in every procedure.
- *Reluctance to simplify interpretations:* Managers often look for simple answers to problems. In an HRO, interpretations are more nuanced; skepticism about apparent explanations is encouraged. Rather than simply blaming the people who are the proximal agents in a causal chain of events, an HRO seeks to understand the latent failures that led to an individual's failure to perform flawlessly.

- *Sensitivity to operations:* An HRO pays close attention to how work actually gets done on the frontline rather than merely proposing solutions that appear reasonable from a distance. Cook and Woods wrote about the danger of ignoring the ways in which workers must act to do their jobs, often needing to circumvent rules made by managers or regulators who do not understand the complexity and challenges in health care systems.[37]
- *Commitment to resilience:* The HRO understands that regardless of its best efforts, things do go wrong and people do make mistakes. An HRO "develop[s] capabilities to detect, contain, and bounce back from those inevitable errors that are part of an indeterminate world." In the operating room, this translates to ensuring adequate backup of personnel, supplies, and equipment.
- *Deference to expertise:* During a crisis in an HRO, decision making falls to the person most experienced in dealing with that kind of problem (ie, situational leadership), not to the most senior person. A good leader seeks out that expertise rather than squelching disagreement or demanding loyalty.

Another critical feature of an HRO is that safety is the highest priority among all concerns. That is, the interests of production and speed are not allowed to supersede the need to ensure safety.[35] Another element of HROs, one that has direct implications for anesthesia practice, is the need for intensive and regular training, especially with simulation.[87] For high-hazard industries that face rare events requiring expertise to avoid an adverse outcome, frequent training and practice are essential; all of these conditions are met in the practice of anesthesiology.

HROs are also noted for organizational learning, especially from accidents and near misses. Health care recently embraced the process of root cause analysis (RCA).[12] An RCA is applied to unusual, potentially harmful events in an effort to understand the many elements that contribute to an event and use the findings to design and implement corrective interventions (see Chapter 26 for more detail on RCA). Failure mode and effect analysis (FMEA) is one of several industry techniques to study new processes proactively before an adverse event occurs.[92] The FMEA is used to identify potential failure modes and key points where barriers are needed to minimize the potential for failure (see Chapter 26 for a more detailed discussion of RCA and FMEA as risk-reduction strategies).

Vaughan described the concept of "normalization of deviance" that arises when an otherwise safe organization drifts into unsafe conditions.[93] In analyzing the sociologic features of the disintegration of the *Challenger* orbiter ("shuttle") in 1986, Vaughan identified how NASA, under intense financial and political pressures, evolved from an organization that had once highly valued safety to one that gave production a higher priority. This led to what she called a "normalization of deviance" in the way engineers made decisions about safety issues. Rather than demanding that assurance of safety was the highest priority at each step, the "burden of proof" had shifted—to cancel or delay a launch, engineers were asked to prove that conditions were unsafe, where previously, to allow a launch, they were required to prove that each item was safe. This critical shift in emphasis has direct applications to anesthesia and surgery.

To ensure safety, strategies and tactics must be implemented at all levels throughout an organization, from senior management to bedside provider. That process has two major elements of responsibility: the organization and the individual.

CREATING SAFETY AT THE ORGANIZATIONAL AND DEPARTMENT LEVEL

The organization is responsible for creating a safe culture throughout its various levels (Chapter 26 focuses on quality improvement at the department level). Culture is the "shared values and beliefs that interact with an organization's structures and control systems to produce behavioral norms."[34] More simply stated, it is "the way we do things around here." Cultural characteristics are usually deeply ingrained, not immediately visible, and often difficult to modify. Yet it is the culture that defines the overall commitment to safety of an organization. Although highest reliability can likely only be achieved within a consistent culture of safety across an organization, the perioperative subcultures and anesthesia practices and departments can establish strong safety cultures within their sphere of influence. Mohr et al refer to these smaller elements as "microsystem environments" and emphasizes that safety and quality must be applied at these levels, as well as in the more global "macrosystems environments" (ie, it must be brought from the corporate or departmental office to the bedside to be effective).[94] In contrast, the individual practitioner working in various environments (eg, locum tenens practice) may find it difficult to achieve an overall high-quality safe practice in an organization that gives only lip service to safety.

There is a growing literature about *safety culture* (also referred to as *climate*; the terms are similar but not synonymous) in health care.[95,96] One technique to assess the organizational culture is to conduct periodic surveys. Helmreich and Merritt reported on use of one survey instrument, the Operating Room Management Questionnaire, and compared attitudes of surgeons to pilots, whose safety culture is generally believed to be superior to that found in many industries as a result of long-standing attention to safety training and interventions.[97] Although there are many similarities with pilots, surgeons appear to have attitudes that are not aligned with safety science, such as a perception that their performance is not affected by fatigue. Flin et al reported on results of a survey from anesthesia departments in the United Kingdom with a similar finding about the effects of stress and fatigue.[98] Although perceptions of teamwork were generally positive, only 65% of respondents perceived that operating room personnel worked well together as a team. Respondents also reported variable compliance with procedures and policies. Similar findings have been replicated for operating room teams.[98] Notably, physicians and nurses have different perceptions of the quality of teamwork by their colleagues—physicians generally rate themselves as much better team players than do their nursing colleagues.

Extrapolating from the earlier descriptors of an HRO, we can imagine that a safe perioperative culture demonstrably places safety as its priority with regular meetings of the group and teams; organizational learning via reporting systems that are open, fair, and nonpunitive; a formal and active quality improvement process; by implementing corrective actions on learning of unsafe practices; having policies and procedures defining standard operations; have regular training for common emergencies; being nonhierarchical during emergencies; rewarding those who raise safety concerns and have open discussions about those concerns; having processes for briefing and debriefing about near misses and adverse events; having standard processes for communication among providers especially for transitions in care; and using other similar processes and attributes. Relatively few organizations have these attributes, especially those related to multispecialty analyses of the causes of errors and adverse events; too often these analyses take place in parallel processes that result in the allocation of blame rather than resolution of the root causes that are embedded in the larger system, or the interfaces between services or providers.

PRACTICAL ELEMENTS FOR THE PRACTITIONER FOR PRODUCING SAFE, HIGH-QUALITY PATIENT CARE

Importance of Instilling Values of Patient Safety, Quality and Patient Centeredness Safety demands that each individual, as well as the organization, make preventing any injury or harm to the patient the highest priority. For the individual clinician, a continual commitment to safe practice includes avoidance of unnecessary risk taking and avoidance of corner cutting, an almost unending anticipation of what might go wrong, projection of actions in anticipation of failure, and, above all, mindfulness. Weick and Sutcliffe describe mindfulness for HROs as organizing in such a way as to "better notice the unexpected in the making and halt its development."[90] The concept applies equally to the individual practitioners and members of the perioperative care team.

Clinicians have a good reason aside from patient safety to be being eternally mindful: Those who lead, design, and manage local care systems may have an equal or greater responsibility for an adverse event. But when systems fail, blame is usually assigned, fairly or not, to the clinician closest to the last action in the chain. Protecting oneself from the impact of system failures is, if nothing else, an act of self-preservation.

Maintaining Vigilance and Mitigating Performance Decrement Although vigilance cannot be relied on solely to protect the patient from harm, it remains the strongest underpinning of safety in anesthesia. This requires that the anesthesia provider must maintain alertness and be aware of, compensate for, and counteract the forces working against vigilance. This, too, requires mindfulness about the state of one's own vigilance.

Fatigue and sleep deprivation are probably the most common causes of lapses in vigilance. Howard et al have recommended several "fatigue countermeasures,"[42] and a 2009 IOM report has explored this in detail.[100] Such countermeasures include education about the effects of fatigue on vigilance, limiting duty hours to avoid fatigue, using good sleep hygiene (regular bedtime and wakeup time; restricting alcohol, caffeine, and nicotine use; creating good conditions for sleep), rest breaks, strategic napping, and selected medications, if necessary.

There is little evidence to support a specific time between breaks, but awareness of a fatigued state can suggest when a break is needed. Naps are often inconsistent with daily clinical routines but may be appropriate when routines are disrupted or during "on-call" intervals. Optimal nap times are on the order of 45 to 60 minutes to improve alertness while minimizing sleep inertia on awakening. Napping is best done when circadian rhythms are enabling sleep (between 2 and 6 PM and 2 and 6 AM) and is more difficult to do when circadian rhythms are encouraging wakefulness. The evidence that napping improves performance of flight crews is strong enough that appropriate napping is recommended during long duration flights.[102] Caffeine can be used judiciously to compensate for fatigue.[42] Excessive use or inappropriate timing of caffeine use can have the negative consequence of preventing subsequent sleep.

Relief breaks, either during a procedure or at a change of shift, are a double-edged sword, providing an opportunity to identify an undiscovered problem or to create a new problem because of lesser situational awareness by the relieving provider.[44,45] Although it is widely recommended that a preplanned protocol be followed to optimize information transfer during the handoff, the evidence for the effectiveness of such handoffs or how they should be conducted is lacking in anesthesia or elsewhere in health care.[47,48,103] Until such evidence is established, local procedures must suffice. These can be informed by the procedures found to be effective in other high-hazard industries.[49,104]

Teamwork The importance of anesthesiologists integrating into the larger system of team-based care was described earlier. Although teamwork can be seen as a subset of working within a system of care, it also includes specific practices for optimizing safety. Box 3-3 lists some of the recommended practices of high-performance teams in non–health care domains. Various forms of teamwork training have been implemented in health care, and there is evidence to demonstrate its effectiveness at improving teamwork performance and some evidence that it improves outcomes.[104] The preoperative checklist developed by the World Health Organization's Safe Surgery program is specifically intended to promote teamwork and has been demonstrated to be effective in improving surgical outcomes.[106,107] All anesthesia professionals should actively and seriously participate in the preoperative briefing that uses a form of the WHO checklist.[106]

Preparation The failure to prepare adequately for anesthesia administration often contributes to anesthesia critical incidents.[21,22,108] Preparation encompasses a large set of issues, including complete preoperative assessment (see "Preoperative Assessment and Planning"); ensuring availability of emergency drugs, equipment, and supplies; checking out the function of equipment (especially using the recommended procedure for ensuring functionality of the anesthesia machine[109]); and ensuring communication pathways in the event of an emergency.

Preoperative Assessment and Planning Preoperative assessment and planning involves evaluation of the patient and development of the anesthesia plan that includes the anesthetic technique, the requirements for monitoring, and the plans for postoperative care, all of which must be consistent with the wishes of the patient and the needs of the surgeon or other operator (eg, radiologist, cardiologist), and the resources of the facility. (Preoperative evaluation is considered in Chapter 6, and for specific conditions in Chapters 9-24.) Similarly, an anesthetic plan must be developed that is consistent with both patient wishes and operator requirements, and with the plans for postoperative care. Chapter 7 addresses the development of the anesthetic plan in detail.

Monitoring Because failure to monitor is so often associated with adverse outcomes, this issue deserves special attention. The safe practitioner follows the standards promulgated by the ASA except in truly extraordinary situations, and should those occur, he or she documents the reason for noncompliance. Critical alarms should never be disabled.[110]

Human Factors Although the individual anesthesia provider has little control over the design of equipment and local systems, he or she does have substantial control over many of the human factors features that are part of the environment. Attention to the organized arrangement of supplies and drugs, especially adherence to consistent labeling of drugs, and establishing and adhering to local standards are examples. Care to keep arterial and intravenous cannulae and monitoring cables orderly, ensuring reasonable lighting, and reducing clutter, noise, and distractions are general, sound safety practices. Control of noise levels and background music can be contentious issues among staff, surgeons, and anesthesia providers, who sometimes are urged to compromise the principle that patient safety takes preeminence. Reasonable efforts should be made to reach compromise, and music should be discontinued during management of critical events.

Applying Systematic Crisis Management Techniques Anesthesia crisis resource management (ACRM) is an organized set of principles for managing crisis situations in anesthesia. Adapted by Gaba et al from CRM in aviation, it consists of several founding principles for effective management of acute events.[66,74,111,112] Although there is no single adopted standard, the following principles are generally applicable:

- Seek assistance early and quickly—inform others on the surgical team and call for extra assistance as soon as unusual circumstances are recognized.
- Establish clarity of roles for each person involved in management of the event; especially identify who will manage the event (event manager).
- Use effective communication processes, including reading back of instructions, being clear to whom directions are being given.
- Use resources effectively and identify what additional resources (people, supplies, equipment, transportation, etc) are available to manage the situation.
- Maintain situational awareness and avoid fixations, which is perhaps the most challenging task as situational awareness is difficult to retrieve once it is lost. Having one person act as event manager, observing the big picture rather than becoming immersed in the details, is thought to be effective.

The algorithm of ABCD COVER swift check discussed earlier (Box 3-4) should be available for reference. Simulation has been shown to be an effective for learning and maintenance of CRM skills.

Infection Control Care in the safe use and sterility of all anesthesia systems is essential, especially in the modern hospital environment where hospital-acquired infections with resistant organisms (eg, methicillin- or vancomycin-resistant *Staphylococcus aureus* organisms) are increasingly common. Adherence to carefully timed protocols for antibiotic administration in the perioperative interval reduces postoperative wound infection.[113] Surgical wound infection rates are increased 3-fold by hypothermia and reduced by increased perioperative oxygen administration.[114,115] The importance of using strict sterile technique protocols for placing central venous catheters and other venous or arterial access are now well documented.[116] There is simply no excuse for laxity in adherence to following proscribed protocols.

BOX 3-5

Key Standards of Care of the American Society of Anesthesiologists

- Ambulatory Anesthesia and Surgery, Guidelines for (2008)
- Basic Anesthetic Monitoring, Standards for (2005)
- Clinical Privileges in Anesthesiology, Guidelines for Delineation of (2008)
- Critical Care by Anesthesiologists, Guidelines for the Practice of (2009)
- Documentation of Anesthesia Care (2008)
- Ethical Guidelines for the Anesthesia Care of Patients With Do-Not-Resuscitate Orders or Other Directives That Limit Treatment (2008)
- Ethical Practice of Anesthesiology, Guidelines for the (2008)
- Labeling Pharmaceuticals for Use in Anesthesiology, Statement on (2009)
- Nonoperating Room Anesthetizing Locations, Guidelines for (2008)
- Obstetrics, Guidelines for Regional Anesthesia Care in (2007)
- Obstetrics, Optimal Goals for Anesthesia Care in (2008)
- Office-Based Anesthesia, Guidelines for (2009)
- Patient Care in Anesthesiology, Guidelines for (2006)
- Postanesthesia Care, Standards for (2009)
- Preanesthesia Care, Basic Standards for (2005)

Data from American Society of Anesthesiologists.[117]

Following Standards and Practice Guidelines The ASA has established a large set of practice standards and guidelines.[117] Standardizing practices across providers is widely accepted as a critical component for safety and reliability. **Box 3-5** lists common practice standards. Each practitioner is obligated to be familiar with such guidelines and apply them appropriately in his or her practice. Similarly, health care facilities are required to establish local policies and procedures to ensure standardization of basic practices. These, too, must be known and followed.

Periodic Training Because critical events are relatively rare and demand expert and effective treatment, it is important to practice skills periodically. Schwid and O'Donnell demonstrated that advanced cardiac life support skills are generally maintained for only approximately 6 months.[118] Periodic training includes practice in management of the unanticipated difficult airway, generic skills in ACRM, and drills for operating room fires and other specific anesthetic emergencies, such as malignant hyperthermia.

Simulation Simulation is used increasingly throughout health care to address many of the issues in this chapter. Simulation has been applied in many high-hazard industries for years, but its applications in health care arose from pioneering work in anesthesia.[71,119] Simulation is a technique that replicates reality in ways that allow deliberate, repetitive practice for many applications. It can use technologies that represent clinical care with relatively high or low clinical, environmental, or psychological fidelity depending on the training objectives and philosophy.[120] Increasingly sophisticated mannequin and task trainers are now used widely. Yet simpler task trainers suffice for many purposes (eg, for learning basic intubation or difficult airway management skills, skills in placing central venous catheters, regional anesthesia). A variety of computer-based simulators and trainers have been shown to be effective for obtaining knowledge and skills for the management of acute events.[121]

For patient safety, simulation is especially useful for training novices without exposing patients to risk. As well, it can be used for periodic training for the purposes noted previously, particularly for training in the management of critical events using the CRM concepts described earlier. One of several models of computer-controlled mannequin is used to simulate the patient, whose physiology, anatomy, and life signs can be varied to simulate normal or abnormal situations.[71,73] In high-fidelity simulation, props and actors are used to create realism, which is believed to strengthen the engagement of the learners. The early applications were for the anesthesia "crew" of the larger surgical team. More recently, simulations have involved training for entire operative teams. In addition to other skills, these CRM training sessions reinforce the concept that all team members are expected to communicate openly and without hesitation regarding safety-related matters. Examples include confirming a directive (eg, "heparin, *xx* units, has been administered," "I'm confirming that these are Mrs. Jones's radiographs"), to speaking out when a concern for safety exists (eg, "Are you sure you should be prepping the right hand? The consent says left." or "Have you noticed that this patient's blood pressure has been falling over the past several minutes?"). Training sessions use patient care scenarios to elicit treatment and behavioral responses from the individuals or teams being trained. Debriefing using videotapes of the session are conducted to review actions. Simulation training has been demonstrated to be effective across a variety of clinical domains for improving both clinical/technical and behavioral skills.[69,74,122]

Most academic anesthesia training programs now have either their own designated simulation programs or share resources with other departments in their hospitals or communities. Simulators of various types are being deployed in hospitals of essentially all types of sizes. Although there are no data on the actual numbers of simulation programs, there is a growing community of simulation professionals, evidenced by the existence of a society and journal.

Effective in 2010, the American Board of Anesthesiology requires a simulation training experience with both technical and behavioral crisis management practice for maintenance of certification of anesthesia credentials (MOCA).[123] The ASA led a process for endorsing anesthesia simulation programs that are qualified to offer that training. Currently, the simulation requirement is purely formative (ie, skill enhancing). It is likely that the experience of other industries will be repeated and, after sufficient validation, some summative (ie, pass or fail) requirements may well be implemented. The very use of simulation is a sign of a move toward a deeper culture of safety in anesthesia and other clinical disciplines.

INVOLVING THE PATIENT IN SAFETY AND QUALITY

Patients increasingly are being urged to take a role in ensuring the safety of their own care, as well as being involved in patient safety by their health care providers.[124] Anesthesia professionals should encourage and assist in this because it benefits everyone. Providers should also be concerned with the patient's perceptions of the quality of care and consider more than just the needs of the direct surgical process. There are several ways in which these goals can be achieved.

To encourage patient involvement, actions can be taken to foster "patient-centered communication," which has been defined as including the following[125]:

- Eliciting and understanding the patient's perspectives—concerns, ideas, expectations, needs, feelings, and functioning.
- Understanding the patient within his or her unique psychosocial context.
- Reaching a shared understanding of the problem and its treatment with the patient that is concordant with the patient's values.
- Helping patients share power and responsibility by involving them in choices to the degree that they wish to be involved.

What specific things can anesthesia providers do to involve patients in their own care that will not just improve satisfaction but also safety? Consider the following:

- Tell the patient as much as practical (assessing how much the patient can handle knowing) about the process of anesthesia care the patient will experience.
- Provide information preoperatively about the process of anesthesia care and expectations; several references are available on the Internet in addition to books and pamphlets.
- Encourage the patient to speak up if the patient does not understand something or believes something is inappropriate, such as drugs being given, absence of handwashing or glove wearing.

- Involve the patient's family members in care whenever practical.
- Advise the patient to contact you if there are any concerns or possible side effects after the anesthetic.
- In concert with other providers, disclose errors and adverse events (a strategy that enhances trust and decreases skepticism in concerned patients).
- Involve patients on committees that involve the design of anesthetizing locations and in the process of patient flow and family communication in such facilities.

SUMMARY AND CONCLUSIONS

The concepts of quality, safety, and patient-centeredness are prominent themes throughout American health care, and they have been embraced by patients and affirmed by third-party payers, specialty societies, and health care organizations, both governmental and private. Despite the increased focus on these factors, the goals have yet to be met, especially because most initiatives have focused on individual practitioners or within specific disciplines. To achieve the full goals of quality and safety, the processes must include systematic approaches that cross the boundaries of specialties, clinical services, and facilities. In short, the delivery of care must be recognized as a complex matrix of interactions among multiple providers, including both clinicians and facilities, all interacting with one another in a system of systems. The specialty of anesthesiology is a leader in the development of patient safety approaches within its discipline; the next steps involve building safety and quality into this larger system of care. Anesthesia providers can contribute significantly to achieving these goals by participating fully in the system-of-systems approach, as well as by building highly reliable microsystems within their department or group. These approaches are best understood by adopting a patient-centered approach, whereby all providers interpret the integrated care process from the patient's viewpoint and include that viewpoint in the design and delivery of care.

KEY REFERENCES

- Kohn LT, Corrigan JM, Donaldson MSE. *To Err Is Human: Building a Safer Healthcare System.* Washington, DC: National Academy Press; 1999.
- Cooper JB, Newbower RS, Kitz RJ. An analysis of major errors and equipment failures in anesthesia management: considerations for prevention and detection. *Anesthesiology.* 1984;60(1):34-42.
- Reason J. *Managing the Risk of Organizational Accidents.* Aldershot, Hants, UK: Ashgate Publishing; 1997.
- Baker DP, Salas E, King H, et al. The role of teamwork in the professional education of physicians: current status and assessment recommendations. *Jt Comm J Qual Patient Saf.* 2005;31(4):185-202.
- Gaba D, Fish K, Howard S. *Crisis Management in Anesthesiology.* Philadelphia, PA: Churchill Livingstone; 1994.
- Gaba DM, Howard SK, Fish K, et al. Simulation-based training in anesthesia crisis resource management (ACRM): a decade of experience. *Simul Gaming.* 2001;32(2):175-193.
- Two chapters: Impact of duty hours on resident well-being. Strategies to reduce fatigue risk in resident work schedules. In: Ulmer C, Wolman DM, Johns MME, eds. *Resident Duty Hours: Enhancing Sleep, Supervision, and Safety.* Washington, DC: National Academies Press; 2009:159-178 and 217-262, respectively.

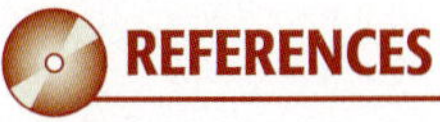

REFERENCES

Complete references available on DVD and online version at www.LongneckerAnesthesiology.com

CHAPTER 4

The Role of Genomics in Anesthesia Practice

Mihai V. Podgoreanu
Miklos D. Kertai

KEY POINTS

1. Hundreds of genome-wide association studies have been performed in recent years to identify common variants that are associated with complex disease. Although there have been some notable success stories, overall common variation has explained little of the high heritability of these traits. It is likely that the use of whole-genome sequencing to extend the study of rare variation in complex diseases will greatly advance our understanding of perioperative biology.
2. Preliminary candidate gene studies suggest that susceptibility to adverse perioperative events, including cardiac (myocardial infarction [MI], ventricular dysfunction, atrial fibrillation), neurologic, and renal, among others, is genetically determined.
3. Potential applications of biomarkers in perioperative medicine and critical care include prognosis, diagnosis, and monitoring of adverse outcomes, as well as informing and refining therapeutic decisions. Very few so far have been rigorously evaluated to demonstrate additive performance to existing risk stratification models (clinical validity) or change therapy (clinical utility). Most promising among those are natriuretic peptides and C-reactive protein for cardiovascular risk prediction, and procalcitonin to assess infection in the critically ill.

SCIENTIFIC FOUNDATIONS OF GENOMIC AND PERSONALIZED MEDICINE

DNA technology has already changed our health care, the food we eat, and our criminal justice system. Underlying these profound societal implications is the process of elucidating the relationship between specific differences encoded in our DNA (ie, *genotypes*) and our interindividual variability in morphology, development, behavior, athletic prowess, physiology, and disease susceptibility (ie, *phenotypes*). Many common diseases like atherosclerosis, coronary artery disease, hypertension, diabetes, cancer, asthma, and our responses to stress, injury, drugs, and nonpharmacologic therapies are genetically complex, characteristically involving interplay of many genetic variations in molecular and biochemical pathways (ie, *polygenic*) and interactions between genes and environment (ie, *multifactorial*). In other words, complex phenotypes can be viewed as the integrated effect of many susceptibility genes and many environmental exposures. The proportion of phenotypic variance explained by genetic factors is referred to as *heritability* and can be estimated by examining the increased similarity of a phenotype in related as compared with unrelated individuals.

In 2003 the 50th anniversary of Watson and Crick's description of the DNA double-helix structure also marked the completion of the Human Genome Project.[1] This major accomplishment has provided the discipline of genomics with basic resources to study the functions of all genes in a systematic fashion, including their interaction with environmental factors, and to translate the findings into clinical and societal benefits. *Functional genomics* uses large-scale experimental methodologies and statistical analyses to investigate the regulation of gene expression in response to physiologic, pharmacologic, and pathologic changes. It also uses genetic information from clinical studies to examine the impact of genetic variability on disease characterization and outcomes. One of the major challenges and ongoing research efforts facing the postgenomic period is to connect the nearly 26,000 protein-coding genes of mammalian organisms to the genetic basis of complex polygenic diseases

TABLE 4-1 Milestones on the Path From Human Genome Project to Genomic Medicine

1. Uncovering human gene function	Sequencing genomes of key model organisms	Enable comparative genomic studies
	The Encyclopedia of DNA Elements (ENCODE) Project[193]	Identify the location of all functional elements in the human genome
	The NIH Roadmap Epigenomics Program[194]	Investigate the patterns that determine whether genes are switched on or off in a given tissue
2. Identifying all human genetic variation	The International HapMap Project	Determine the common points at which human genomes differ
	The 1000 Genomes Project[195]	The most detailed and accurate catalog of human genetic variation
3. Elucidating the genetic basis for human diseases	Genome-wide association studies (GWAS)	Identify genetic variants that point to region of human genome where the disease-causing mutation likely resides.
	NHGRI Office of Population Genomics initiatives	
	• Genome-Wide Association Research Network Into Effects of Treatment (GARNET) • Gene Environment Association Studies (GENEVA) • Electronic Medical Records and Genomics (eMERGE) Network • PhenX	• A series of GWAS of treatment response in randomized clinical trials • Assess the interplay between genetic and nongenetic factors • Combine DNA biorepositories with electronic medical record systems for large-scale genetic research • Develop consensus measures for phenotypes and exposures for use in GWAS

and the integrated function of complex biologic systems. The rapidly evolving field of *genomic medicine* proposes to use genomic information to assist medical decision making and tailor health care to the individual patient.

A breathtaking acceleration on the path from the Human Genome Project to genomic medicine has been paved by landmark "big biology" efforts concentrated on the main themes of uncovering the function of human genes, identifying all human genomic variation, and elucidating the genetic basis for human diseases (**Table 4-1**). Furthermore, dramatic improvements in sequencing technologies and cost reductions have fueled even more ambitious initiatives such as the ongoing Personal Genome Project,[2] which aims to publish the complete genomes and medical records of a number of volunteers to enable personalized medicine research. Nevertheless, it is fair to say a decade after its completion, that although the Human Genome Project has revolutionized the pace and scope of biomedical science, it has failed so far to fulfill the promise and grand vision of "personalized medicine," leaving the scientific community somewhat sobered and divided.

The perioperative period represents a unique and extreme example of gene–environment interaction. As we appreciate in our daily practice in the operating rooms and intensive care units, one hallmark of perioperative physiology is the striking variability in patient responses to the acute, robust, and systemic perturbations induced by surgical injury, hemodynamic challenges, vascular cannulation, extracorporeal circulation, intra-aortic balloon counterpulsation, mechanical ventilation, partial/total organ resection, transient limb/organ ischemia, transfusions, anesthetic agents, and the pharmacopoeia used in the perioperative period. This translates into substantial interindividual variability in the incidence or severity of immediate perioperative adverse events, as well as long-term outcomes (**Table 4-2**). For decades we have attributed this variability to many complexities such as age, nutritional state, comorbidities—what we colloquially call "protoplasm." Now we are beginning to appreciate that genetic variation is also in part responsible for this observed variability in outcomes. Overall, an individual's genetic susceptibility to adverse perioperative events stems not only from genetic contributions to the development of comorbid risk factors (like coronary artery disease [CAD] and reduced preoperative cardiopulmonary reserve) during his or her lifetime but also from genetic variability in specific biologic pathways participating in the host response surgery (**Fig. 4-1**). With increasing evidence suggesting that genetic variation can significantly modulate risk of adverse perioperative events,[3-6] the emerging field of *perioperative genomics* aims to apply functional genomic approaches to discover underlying biologic mechanisms that explain why similar patients have such dramatically different outcomes after surgery. It is justified by a unique combination of environmental insults and postoperative phenotypes that characterize surgical and critically ill patient populations. To take full advantage of the unique opportunities offered by the genomic revolution, the cycle of innovation in perioperative medicine must include a comprehensive and standardized definition of the phenotypes of interest (including short- and long-term adverse outcomes such as organ injury/dysfunction, adverse drug responses, transition to chronic pain), followed by identification of the underlying genes, characterization of the mechanism from DNA

TABLE 4-2 Categories of Perioperative Phenotypes

Immediate Perioperative Outcomes	• In-hospital mortality • Perioperative myocardial infarction • Perioperative low cardiac output syndrome/acute decompensated heart failure/ventricular dysfunction • Perioperative vasoplegic syndrome • Perioperative arrhythmias (atrial fibrillation, QTc prolongation) • Postoperative bleeding • Perioperative venous thrombosis • Acute postoperative stroke • Postoperative delirium • Perioperative acute kidney injury • Acute perioperative lung injury/prolonged postoperative mechanical ventilation • Acute allograft dysfunction/rejection • Postoperative sepsis • Multiple organ dysfunction syndrome • Postoperative nausea and vomiting • Acute postoperative pain • Variability in response to anesthetics, analgesics, and other perioperative drugs • Intermediate phenotypes (plasma biomarker levels)
Long-Term Postoperative Outcomes	• Event-free survival / Major adverse cardiac events • Progression of vein graft disease • Chronic allograft dysfunction/rejection • Postoperative cognitive dysfunction • Postoperative depression • Transition from acute to chronic pain • Cancer progression • Quality of life

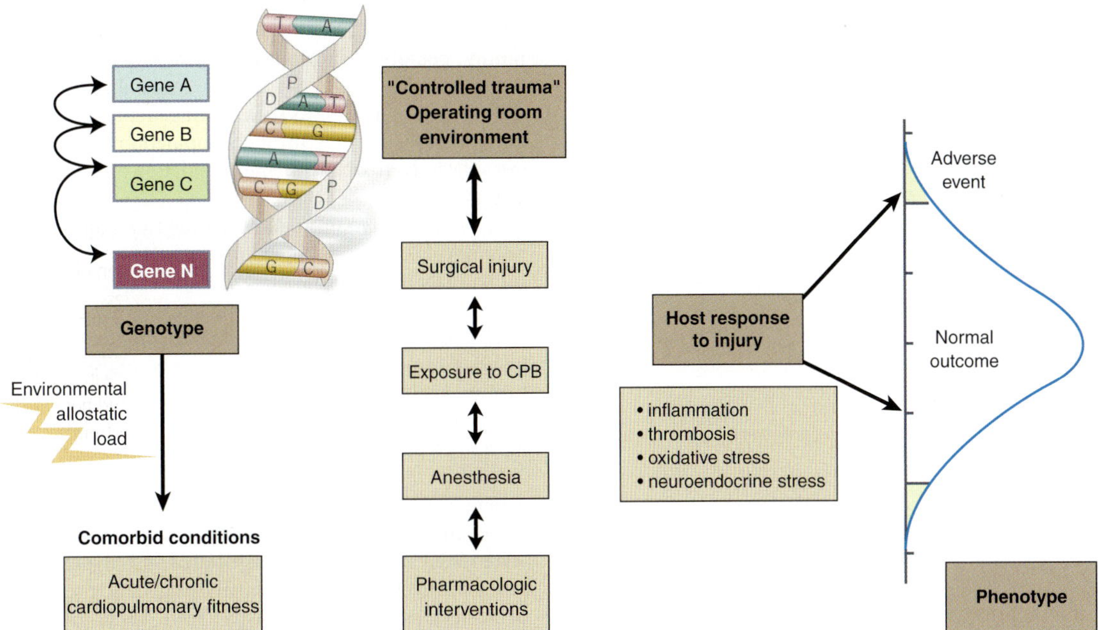

FIGURE 4-1. Perioperative adverse events are complex traits, characteristically involving an interaction between robust operative environmental perturbations (surgical trauma, hemodynamic challenges, exposure to extracorporeal circulation, drug administration) and multiple susceptibility genes. The observed variability in perioperative outcomes can be in part attributed to genetic variability modulating the host response to surgical injury. CPB, cardiopulmonary bypass.

to phenotype, and rigorous development and validation of diagnostic or therapeutic applications ultimately having an impact on our patients and families.

To integrate this new generation of molecular tests into clinical practice, perioperative physicians need to become familiar with several key concepts, including patterns of human genome variation, gene regulation, basic population genetic methodology, gene and protein expression analysis, and, most importantly, the general principles for evaluating biomarker performance. This chapter serves as a primer in genomic medicine by highlighting the rapidly evolving current and future applications of molecular (including genomic) technologies for perioperative risk stratification, outcome prediction, mechanistic understanding of surgical stress responses, as well as identification and validation of novel targets for perioperative organ protection.

HUMAN GENOMIC VARIATION

In elucidating the genetic basis of disease, much of what was investigated before the Human Genome Project era focused on identifying rare genetic variants (*mutations*) responsible for >1500 monogenic disorders such as hypertrophic cardiomyopathy, long-QT syndrome, sickle cell anemia, cystic fibrosis, or familial hypercholesterolemia, which are highly penetrant (carriers of the mutant gene will likely have the disease) and inherited in Mendelian fashion (hence termed *Mendelian diseases*). However, most of the genetic diversity in the population is attributable to more widespread DNA sequence variations (*polymorphisms*), typically single nucleotide base substitutions (*single nucleotide polymorphisms* [SNPs]), or to a broader category of previously overlooked *structural genetic variants* that include short sequence repeats (*microsatellites*), insertion/deletion of one or more nucleotides (*indels*), inversions, and the recently discovered copy number variants (*CNVs;* large segments of DNA that vary in number of copies),[7] all of which may or may not be associated with a specific phenotype (**Fig. 4-2**). The first published drafts of the human genome were of haploid genomes, and they identified only a small amount of variation (0.1%) between individuals. However, with the completion of the first diploid genome sequence of an individual human,[8] it became apparent that the two parental genomes surprisingly differed from each other by 0.5% when insertion and deletions were included along with SNPs. It was subsequently discovered that the genomes of different individuals differ by 1% to 3%.

To be classified as a polymorphism, the DNA sequence alternatives (ie, *alleles*) must exist with a frequency of at least 1% in the population. About 15 million SNPs are estimated to exist in the human genome, approximately once every 300 base pairs, located in genes as well as in the surrounding regions of the genome. Polymorphisms may directly alter the amino acid sequence and therefore potentially alter protein function or alter regulatory DNA sequences that modulate protein expression. Sets of nearby SNPs on a chromosome are inherited in blocks, referred to as *haplotypes*. As shown later, haplotype analysis is a useful way of applying genotype information in disease gene discovery. However, CNVs involve approximately 12% of the human genome, often encompass genes (especially regulating inflammation and brain development), and may influence disease susceptibility through dosage imbalances. In this chapter, we review the common strategies used to incorporate genetic analysis into clinical studies.

BASIC GENETIC EPIDEMIOLOGY

Most ongoing research on complex disorders focuses on identifying genetic variants that alter susceptibility to given conditions. Often the design of such studies is complicated by the presence of multiple risk factors, gene–environment interactions, and a lack of even rough estimates of the number of genes underlying such complex traits. Two broad strategies have been used to identify complex trait loci. The *candidate gene* approach is motivated by what is known about the trait biologically and can be characterized as a hypothesis-testing approach but is intrinsically biased. The second strategy is the *genome-wide scan*, in which thousands of markers uniformly distributed throughout the genome are used to locate regions that may harbor genes influencing phenotypic variability. This is a hypothesis-free and unbiased approach, in the sense that no prior assumptions are being made about the biologic processes involved and no weight is given to known genes, thus allowing the detection of previously unknown trait loci. Both the candidate gene and genome scan approaches can be implemented using one of two fundamental methods of identifying polymorphisms affecting common

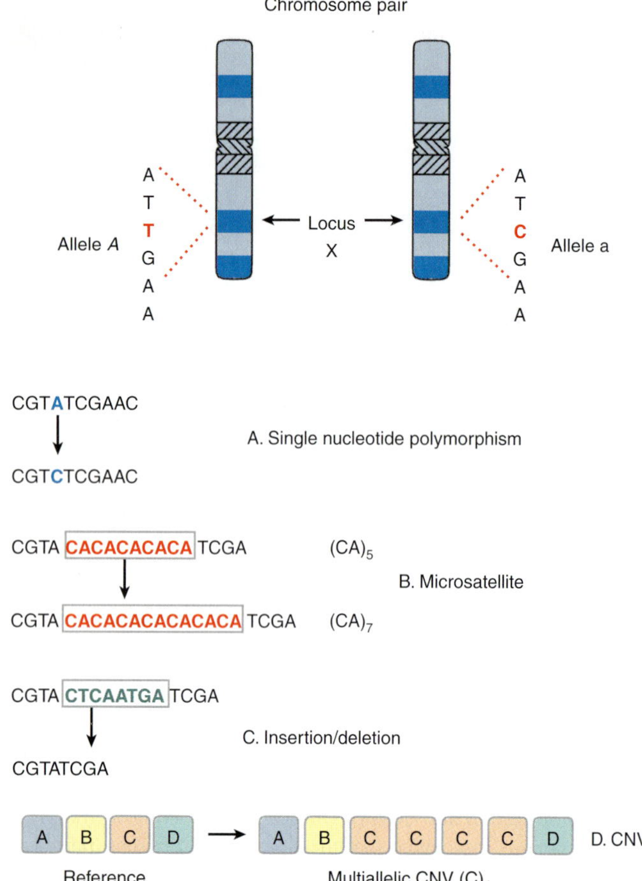

FIGURE 4-2. Categories of common human genetic variation. **A.** *Single nucleotide polymorphisms* (SNPs) can be silent or have functional consequences: changes in amino acid sequence or premature termination of protein synthesis (if they occur in the coding regions of the gene) or alterations in the expression of the gene, resulting in more or less protein (if they occur in regulatory regions of the gene such as the promoter region or the intron/exon boundaries); structural genetic variants include **(B)** Microsatellites with varying number of dinucleotide $(CA)_n$ repeats; **(C)** *Insertions-deletions*; and **(D)** Copy number variation (CNV). A to D are long DNA segments; segment D shows variation in copy number. Glossary: *locus:* the location of a gene/genetic marker in the genome; *alleles:* alternative forms of a gene/genetic marker; *genotype:* the observed alleles for an individual at a genetic locus; *heterozygous:* two different alleles are present at a locus; *homozygous:* two identical alleles are present at a locus. A SNP at position 1691 of a gene with alleles G and A would be written as 1691G>A.

diseases: linkage analysis or association studies in human populations. Importantly, the ability of either one of these mapping strategies to discover genetic susceptibility for complex traits depends on the joint contributions of two independent factors: the *frequency* of the risk allele in the population and the magnitude of its *effect*.

Linkage analysis maps the chromosomal location of gene variants related to a given disease by studying the distribution of disease alleles in affected individuals throughout a pedigree. Traditionally, family-based linkage studies have been successful at identifying rare genetic variants of large effects involved in rare monogenic (ie, classical Mendelian) disorders. The approach is less effective for common complex diseases, however, which are characterized by a multitude of genes with rare and/or common alleles creating an apparently chaotic pattern of heterogeneity within and between families. Nevertheless, a few positive findings have emerged, including susceptibility loci for stroke (chromosome 5q12),[9] myocardial infarction (chromosome 14),[10] and pulse pressure variation, an emerging risk factor for perioperative adverse outcomes (chromosomes 22 and 10).[11] Furthermore, the nature of most complex diseases, in general, and perioperative adverse outcomes in elderly patients, in particular, makes the study of extended multigenerational family pedigrees impractical (with few exceptions, eg, malignant hyperthermia), due to the lack of availability of pedigree information and/or DNA samples. As such, most genetic susceptibility variants have been identified so far through population studies of association and are relatively frequent in the population but have individually small effects.

Genetic association studies examine the frequency of specific genetic polymorphisms in a population-based sample of unrelated diseased individuals and appropriately matched unaffected controls. As previously discussed, the increased statistical power to uncover small clinical effects of multiple genes[12] and the fact that they do not require family-based sample collections are main advantages of this approach over linkage analysis. Until recently, most significant results were gathered from candidate gene association studies, with genes selected because of a priori hypotheses about their potential etiologic role in disease based on current understanding of the disease pathophysiology.[13] For example, genetic variants within the renin-angiotensin system, nitric oxide synthase, and β_2-adrenergic receptors, known to modulate vascular tone, were tested and found to be associated with hypertension. Similarly, the possible effects of polymorphisms on genetic predisposition for CAD[14] or restenosis after angioplasty[15] have been extensively investigated; more recently, two large-scale association studies identified gene variants that might affect susceptibility to myocardial infarction.[16] As presented in more detail later, accumulating evidence from candidate gene association studies also suggests that specific genotypes are associated with a variety of organ-specific perioperative adverse outcomes, including myocardial infarction,[17,18] neurocognitive dysfunction,[19-21] renal compromise,[22-24] vein graft restenosis,[25,26] postoperative thrombosis,[27] vascular reactivity,[28] severe sepsis,[29,30] transplant rejection,[31] and death (for reviews, see [3,6]).

One of the main weaknesses of the genetic association approach is that, unless the marker of interest "travels" (ie, is in *linkage disequilibrium*) with a functional variant or the marker allele *is* the actual functional variant, the power to detect and map complex trait loci will be reduced. Other known limitations of genetic association studies include potential false-positive findings resulting from population stratification (ie, admixture of different ethnic or genetic backgrounds in the case and control groups), and multiple comparison issues when large numbers of candidate genes are being assessed.[32] Replication of findings across different populations or related phenotypes remains the most reliable method of validating a true relationship between genetic polymorphisms and disease,[13] but poor reproducibility in subsequent studies has been one of the main criticisms of the candidate gene association approach.[33] However, a recent meta-analysis suggested that lack of statistical power may be the main contributor to this inconsistent replication, and it proposed more stringent statistical criteria to exclude false-positive results and the design of large collaborative association studies.[34]

At last, after several decades of frustrating limitations in the ability to find genetic variations responsible for common disease risk, with the completion of the International HapMap Project (a high-resolution map of human genetic variation and haplotypes)[35] and advances in high-throughput genotyping technologies, the past 3 years have marked an explosion of adequately powered and successfully replicated *genome-wide association studies* (GWAS) that identified very significant genetic contributors to risk for common polygenic diseases like CAD,[36-38] MI,[39] diabetes (type 1 and 2),[40,41] atrial fibrillation,[42] obesity, asthma, common cancers, rheumatoid arthritis, Crohn disease, and others. At the time of this publication, the NHGRI GWAS catalog included 782 publications and 3902 associations, with the list growing every day.[43] GWAS make use of the known linkage disequilibrium pattern between SNPs from the human HapMap and the new high-density SNP chip technology to interrogate comprehensively and accurately between 65% and 80% of common variation across the genome, with even higher coverage being possible using statistical imputation techniques. One of the most comprehensive GWAS to date was conducted by the Wellcome Trust Case-Control Consortium, investigating the association between 500,000 SNPs and seven common diseases in 2000 cases and 3000 shared controls. It identified 25 independent association signals at stringent levels of significance ($p < 5 \times 10^{-7}$).[36] Interestingly, variants in or near *CDKN2A/B* (cyclin-dependent kinase inhibitor 2 A/B) conferred increased risk for both type 2 diabetes (odds ratio [OR]: 1.2; $p = 7.8 \times 10^{-15}$) and MI (OR: 1.64, $p = 1.2 \times 10^{-20}$), which may lead to a mechanistic explanation for the link between the two disorders. This finding also highlights the power of GWAS to identify variants outside described genes: While one of the signals occurs in the *CDKN2A/B* region, the other much stronger association signal occurs more than 200 kb from these genes, in a gene desert, and thus would not have been picked up by a candidate gene approach. Identifying the mechanism by which this variant may affect *CDKN2A/B* expression will provide new insights into the regulation of these genes. To maximize the power of identifying novel susceptibility loci for CAD and MI, even larger consortia have been assembled, like the Coronary ARtery DIsease Genome-wide Replication And Meta-analysis (CARDIoGRAM),[44] which includes 22,000 cases and 60,000 controls. It has already successfully mapped 27 new loci.

An important theme has emerged from GWAS: Most SNPs associated with common diseases collectively explain only a small proportion of the observed contribution of heredity to the risk of disease (eg, 6% for type 2 diabetes) or other complex traits (eg, 2% for body mass index and 5% for height). This *missing heritability* problem limits substantially the potential application of genomic markers to risk prediction, and it remains an important obstacle to overcome to develop evidence-based guidelines recommending the use of SNPs in clinical care. Two broad explanations have been proposed and considerable resources invested in discovering the unknown sources of heritable risk, which are briefly reviewed here.

First, the underlying rationale for GWAS is the "common disease-common variant" hypothesis, which postulates that common diseases may arise secondary to cumulative effects of common variants. Most genes, however, lack a common functional coding variant with a detectable functional effect, yet they typically contain several rare variants. A counterhypothesis has emerged stating there are additional novel genes harboring such low-frequency variants (possibly with larger effects) that may be the primary drivers of common disease. Currently these variants are poorly detected by genotyping microarrays, but with the advent of sequencing technologies, the potential exists to revolutionize complex traits genetics by identifying and typing rare variants and thus rendering virtually every gene susceptible for genetic analysis.

The second theme emerging from GWAS that may offer clues into the missing heritability problem is that most variants identified so far are located either in intergenic regions or in genes of unknown function. This among other findings has challenged the very concept of the "gene" as the traditional unit of heredity. Discovery of the diverse and ubiquitous roles of new classes of RNA (including *microRNAs* and *short interfering RNAs*) led to an emerging picture of gene regulation as interdependent layers of control consisting of interactions of DNA with regulatory proteins and RNA (**Fig. 4-3**).[45] Furthermore, on top of the DNA sequence lies another (*epigenetic*) code that influences when and what genes should be transcribed or silenced. The epigenome is laid down during prenatal and postnatal development, and it is heritable through cell divisions. Given previous studies implicating changes in DNA methylation patterns or histone modification (the most commonly studied epigenetic marks), for instance as prognostic biomarkers in various cancers, one can assume that epigenetics will soon find a role in the perioperative management of cancer patients.

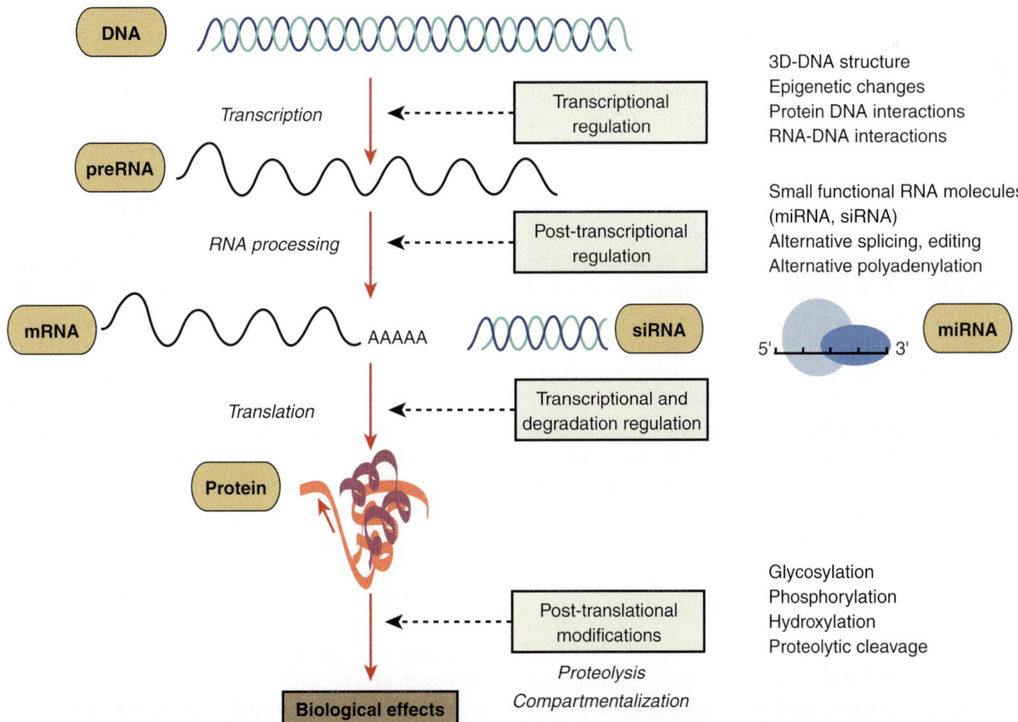

FIGURE 4-3. Increasing complexity of the central dogma of molecular biology. Protein expression involves two main processes, RNA synthesis (*transcription*) and protein synthesis (*translation*), with many intermediate regulatory steps. A single gene can give rise to multiple protein products (isoforms) via processing of preRNA molecules yielding multiple RNA products, including microRNA (miRNA) and small interfering RNA (siRNA) molecules, as well as alternative splicing and RNA editing. Thus functional variability at the protein level, ultimately responsible for biologic effects, is the cumulative result of genetic variability as well as extensive transcriptional, posttranscriptional, translational, and posttranslational modifications.

As discussed previously, both family-based linkage studies and genetic association studies depend fundamentally on the concept of linkage for their practical execution (ie, the identified variant is in linkage disequilibrium with, but not necessarily the, causal variant). Newer ("next-generation") approaches based on direct *whole-genome sequencing* depart from the concept of linkage by attempting to directly identify causal alleles.[46] One particular application of genome-scale sequencing is called *whole-exome sequencing*. The *exome*, defined as the protein-coding portion of the genome, is composed of approximately 30 megabases (1%) split among about 200,000 exons in humans. Aside from the ability to identify rare variants and the obvious substantial cost reduction (~20-fold), this approach has the advantage of focusing on nonsynonymous variants in coding genes for which there are well-established methods of functional validation and interpretation of biologic effects, thus enabling their implication as causal variants. However, it completely misses noncoding and structural variation in the genome. Early results suggest that whole-exome sequencing is an effective approach to identify causal mutations for monogenic disorders but also to distinguish signal (causal rare variants) from noise (background rate of rare mutations) for complex traits. Successful studies so far (eg, early-onset MI) sequenced individuals were informed by the following key observations: The younger the age when developing MI, the greater the heritability; selecting extremes of the phenotype distribution (eg, young with MI versus old without MI as a "hypernormal" control group) is likely to improve power; that genetic discovery may be enhanced by studying multiple ethnicities. These studies have demanded the development of novel statistical methods to associate rare variants with the phenotype. One such promising solution for overcoming the statistical challenges revolving around sequencing low-frequency variants is to combine all nonsynonymous SNPs (by gene or biologic pathway) into a single statistical test. The first integrated analysis of a complete human genome in a clinical context, in a patient with a family history of vascular disease and early sudden death, was reported in the *Lancet* in 2010.[47] The analysis revealed increased genetic risk for CAD, MI, type 2 diabetes, and some cancers, as well as rare variants in three genes clinically associated with sudden cardiac death. Furthermore, the patient had variants associated with clopidogrel resistance, a positive response to lipid-lowering therapies, and a low initial dosing requirement for warfarin, suggesting that routine whole-genome sequencing can yield clinically relevant information for individual patients.

A further advantage of high-quality genome sequence generated by the next-generation sequencing technologies stems from the ability to assemble the sequence data independently and sort it into the two sets of parental chromosomes in a process termed *haplotype phasing*. Establishing the complete set of genetic information that we received from each parent is crucial to understanding the links between heritability, gene function, regulatory sequences, and our predisposition to disease.[48] Several additional next-generation technologies involve sequencing of multiple genomes per person, such as matched tumor and blood DNA samples from 20 common types of cancer in the Cancer Genome Atlas, which enable development of targeted therapeutics based on a detailed molecular understanding of pathogenesis. Equally important for medical progress is the sequencing of genomes of the billions of microorganisms that dwell within us as part of the Human Microbiome Project.

BIOMARKER DISCOVERY: PROFILING GENE/PROTEIN EXPRESSION AND METABOLITES

Genomic approaches are anchored in the "central dogma" of molecular biology, the concept of transcription of messenger RNA (mRNA) from a DNA template, followed by translation of RNA into protein (Fig. 4-3). Because transcription is a key regulatory step that may eventually signal many other cascades of events, the study of RNA levels in a cell or organ (ie, quantifying gene expression) can improve the understanding of a wide variety of biologic systems. Furthermore, although the human genome contains only about 26,000 genes, functional variability at the protein level is far more diverse, resulting from extensive posttranscriptional, translational, and posttranslational modifications. It is believed that there are approximately 200,000 distinct proteins in humans, which are further modified posttranslationally by phosphorylation, glycosylation, oxidation, and disulfide structures. There is increasing evidence that variability in gene expression levels underlies complex disease and is determined by regulatory DNA polymorphisms affecting transcription, splicing, and translation efficiency in a tissue- and stimulus-specific manner.[49] Thus, in addition to the assessment of genetic variability at the DNA sequence level using various genotyping techniques as described in previous sections (*static genomics*), analysis of large-scale variability in the pattern of RNA and protein expression both at baseline and in response to the multidimensional perioperative stimuli (*dynamic genomics*) using microarray and proteomic approaches provides a much needed complementary understanding of the overall regulatory networks involved in the pathophysiology of adverse postoperative outcomes. Such dynamic genomic markers can be incorporated in genomic classifiers and used clinically to improve perioperative risk stratification or monitor postoperative recovery.[50] This concept of *molecular classification* involves the description of informational features in a training data set using changes in relative RNA and protein abundance in the context of genetic predisposition and applying to a test data set to recognize a defined "fingerprint" characteristic of a particular perioperative phenotype (**Table 4-3**). For example, Feezor et al used a combined genomic and proteomic approach to identify expression patterns of 138 genes from peripheral blood leukocytes and the concentrations of 7 circulating plasma proteins that discriminated patients who developed multiple organ dysfunction syndrome (MODS) after thoracoabdominal aortic aneurysm repair from those who did not. Importantly, these patterns of genome-wide gene expression and plasma protein concentration were observed *before* surgical trauma and visceral ischemia-reperfusion injury, suggesting that patients who developed MODS differed in either their genetic predisposition or their preexisting inflammatory state.[51]

Alternatively, dynamic genomic markers can be used to improve mechanistic understanding of perioperative stress, and to evaluate and catalog organ-specific responses to surgical stress and severe systemic stimuli such as cardiopulmonary bypass (CPB) and endotoxemia, which can be subsequently used to identify and validate novel targets for organ-protective strategies.[52] Using a similar integrated approach of transcriptomic and proteomic analyses, Tomic et al[53] characterized the molecular response signatures in peripheral blood to cardiac surgery with and without CPB, a robust trigger of systemic inflammation. The authors demonstrated that, rather than being the primary source of serum cytokines, peripheral blood leukocytes only assume a "primed" phenotype upon contact with the extracorporeal circuit that facilitate their trapping and subsequent tissue-associated inflammatory response. Interestingly, many inflammatory mediators achieved similar systemic levels following off-pump surgery but with delayed kinetics, offering novel insights into the concepts of contact activation and compartmentalization of inflammatory responses to major surgery.

Several studies have profiled myocardial gene expression in the ischemic heart, demonstrating alterations in the expression of immediate-early genes (c-*fos*, *jun*B), as well as genes coding for calcium-handling proteins (calsequestrin, phospholamban), extracellular matrix, and cytoskeletal proteins.[54] Upregulation of transcripts mechanistically involved in cytoprotection (heat shock proteins), resistance to apoptosis, and cell growth has been found in stunned myocardium.[55] Moreover, cardiac gene expression profiling after CPB and cardioplegic arrest has identified the upregulation of inflammatory and transcription activators, apoptotic genes, and stress genes,[56] which appear to be age related.[57] Microarray technology has also been used in the quest for novel cardioprotective genes, with the ultimate goal of designing strategies to activate these genes and prevent myocardial injury. Preconditioning is one of such well-studied models of cardioprotection, which can be induced by various triggers, including intermittent ischemia, osmotic

TABLE 4-3 Summary of Gene Expression Studies With Implications for Perioperative Cardiovascular Outcomes

Tissue (Species)	Stimulus/Method	Genomic Signature: Number/Types of Genes	Reference
Myocardium (rat)	Ischemia/μA	14 (wound-healing, Ca-handling)	54
Myocardium (human)	CPB/circulatory arrest/μA	58 (inflammation, transcription activators, apoptosis, stress response): adults 50 (cardioprotective, antiproliferative, antihypertrophic): neonates	56 57
Myocardium (rat)	IPC vs APC/μA	566 differentially regulated/56 jointly regulated (cell defense)	58
Myocardium (rat)	APC vs ApostC/μA	Opposing genomic profiles, 8 gene clusters, <2% jointly regulated genes	196
Myocardium (human)	APC, OPCAB, postoperative LV function/μA	319 upregulated and 281 downregulated gene sets in response to OPCAB; deregulation of fatty acid oxidation, DNA-damage signaling and G-CSF survival (perioperative) and PGC-1α (constitutive) pathways predict improved LV function in sevoflurane-treated patients	60
PBMC (human)	APC, sevoflurane/μA	Deregulation of late preconditioning, PGC-1α, fatty acid oxidation, and L-selectin pathways	59
Atrial myocardium (pig)	Pacing-induced AF/μA+P	81 (MCL-2 ventricular/atrial isoform shift)	197
Atrial myocardium (human)	AF/μA	1434 (ventricular-like genomic signature)	125
PBMC (human)	Cardiac surgery, PoAF/μA	1302 genes uniquely deregulated in PoAF/401 upregulated (oxidative stress), 902 downregulated	126
PBMC (human)	Cardiac surgery, POCD/μA	1201 genes uniquely deregulated in POCD/531 upregulated, 670 downregulated (inflammation, antigen presentation, cell adhesion, and apoptosis)	148
PBMC (human)	Heart transplant/μA	30 (profile correlated with biopsy-proven rejection; persistent immune activation in response to treatment)	198
PBMC (human)	Heart transplant/ RT-PCR	11 (AlloMap, AlloMap score)	128
Myocardium (human)	Heart transplant/P	2 (increased αB-crystallin and tropomyosin serum levels)	199
PBMC, plasma (human)	TAAA/μA+P	138 genes and 7 plasma proteins predicted MODS	51
PBMC (human)	Obstructive CAD in non-diabetic patients/RT-PCR	23-gene expression signature	200
Ventricular myocardium (human)	End-stage cardiomyopathy on LVAD/μA	Combined signature of 28 microRNAs and 29 mRNAs had superior performance to classify status and predict recovery	130

AF, atrial fibrillation; APC, anesthetic preconditioning; APostC, anesthetic postconditioning; CAD, coronary artery disease; CPB, cardiopulmonary bypass; G-CSF, granulocyte colony stimulating factor; IPC, ischemic preconditioning; LV, left ventricle; LVAD, left ventricular assist device; μA, microarray; MCL-2, myosin light chain 2; MODS, multiple organ dysfunction syndrome; mRNA, messenger RNA; OPCAB, off-pump coronary artery bypass; P, proteomics; PBMC, peripheral blood mononuclear cells; PGC-1α, peroxisome proliferators-activated receptor γ cofactor-1α; PoAF, postoperative atrial fibrillation; POCD, postoperative cognitive decline; RT-PCR, real-time polymerase chain reaction; TAAA, thoracoabdominal aortic aneurysm repair.

or redox stress, heat shock, toxins, and inhaled anesthetics. The main functional categories of genes identified as potentially involved in cardioprotective pathways include a host of transcription factors, heat shock proteins, antioxidant genes (heme-oxygenase, glutathione peroxidase), and growth factors, but different gene programs appear to be activated in ischemic versus anesthetic preconditioning, resulting in two distinct cardioprotective phenotypes.[58] More recently, a transcriptional response pattern consistent with late preconditioning was reported in peripheral blood leukocytes following sevoflurane administration in healthy volunteers, characterized by reduced expression of L-selectin as well as downregulation of genes involved in fatty acid oxidation and the peroxisome activated receptor gamma coactivator (PCG)1α pathway,[59] which mirrors changes observed in the myocardium from patients undergoing off-pump coronary artery bypass grafting (CABG) (Table 4-3).[60] Deregulation of these novel survival pathways thus appears to generalize across tissues, making them important targets for cardioprotection, but further studies are needed to correlate perioperative gene expression response patterns in end organs such as the myocardium to those in readily available surrogate tissues such as peripheral blood leukocytes.

The *transcriptome* (the complete collection of transcribed elements of the genome) is not fully representative of the *proteome* (the complete complement of proteins encoded by the genome) because many transcripts are not targeted for translation, as evidenced recently with the concept of gene silencing by RNA interference. Alternative splicing, a wide variety of posttranslational modifications, and protein–protein interactions responsible for biologic function, would remain therefore undetected by gene expression profiling (Fig. 4-3). This has led to the emergence of a new field, *proteomics*, studying the sequence, modification, and function of many proteins in a biologic system at a given time. Rather than focusing on "static" DNA, proteomic studies examine dynamic protein products, with the goal of identifying proteins that undergo changes in abundance, modification, or localization in response to a particular disease state, trauma, stress, or therapeutic intervention (for a review, see [61]). Thus proteomics offers a more global and integrated view of biology, complementing other functional genomic approaches. Several preclinical proteomic studies relevant to perioperative medicine have characterized the temporal changes in brain protein expression in response to various inhaled anesthetics[62,63] or following cardiac surgery with hypothermic circulatory arrest.[64] This may focus further studies aimed to identify new anesthetic binding sites and the development of neuroprotective strategies. Furthermore, detailed knowledge of the plasma proteome has profound implications in perioperative transfusion medicine,[65] in particular related to peptide and protein changes that occur during storage of blood products. The development of protein arrays and real-time proteomic analysis technologies has the potential to allow the use of these versatile and rigorous high-throughput methods for clinical applications and is the object of intense investigation.

Emerging *metabolomic* tools have created the opportunity to establish metabolic signatures of myocardial injury. In a population of patients undergoing alcohol septal ablation for hypertrophic obstructive cardiomyopathy, a human model of planned (albeit chemical) MI that recapitulates spontaneous myocardial infarction targeted mass spectrometry-based metabolite profiling identified changes in circulating levels of metabolites participating in pyrimidine metabolism, the TCA cycle, and the pentose phosphate pathway as early as 10 minutes after MI in an initial derivation group and were validated in a second, independent group. Coronary sinus sampling distinguished cardiac-derived from peripheral metabolic changes. To assess generalizability, the planned MI-derived metabolic signature (consisting of aconitic acid, hypoxanthine, trimethylamine N-oxide, and threonine) differentiated with high-accuracy patients with spontaneous MI.[66] We applied a similar approach to cardiac surgical patients undergoing planned global myocardial ischemia/reperfusion (I/R) and identified clear differences in metabolic fuel uptake based on the preexisting ventricular state (left ventricular dysfunction, CAD, or neither) as well as altered metabolic signatures predictive of postoperative hemodynamic course and perioperative MI.[67] While simultaneous assessment of coronary sinus effluent in addition to the peripheral blood improves cardiac specificity of the observed signatures, direct measurements of metabolites in myocardial tissue allow marked enrichment and easier detection of potential biomarkers compared with plasma, as well as an assessment of how metabolic substrates are used in the tissue of interest. Such studies are possible in cardiac surgical patients where atrial tissues are routinely removed; for example, one study using high-resolution ^{1}H-NMR spectroscopy identified alterations in myocardial ketone metabolism associated with persistent atrial fibrillation, and the ratio of glycolytic end products to end products of lipid metabolism correlated positively with time of onset of postoperative atrial fibrillation.[68]

GENOMICS AND PERIOPERATIVE RISK PROFILING

More than 40 million patients undergo surgery annually in the United States at a cost of $450 billion. Each year approximately 1 million patients sustain medical complications after surgery, resulting in costs of $25 billion annually. The proportion of the US population older than 65 years is estimated to double in the next 2 decades, leading to a 25% increase in the number of surgeries, a 50% increase in surgery-related costs, and a 100% increase in complications from surgery. Recognizing the significant increase in surgical burden due to accelerated aging of the population and increased reliance on surgery for treatment of disease, the National Heart, Blood and Lung Institute recently convened a working group on perioperative medicine. The group concluded that perioperative complications are significant, costly, variably reported, and often imprecisely detected; and they identified a critical need for accurate comprehensive perioperative outcome databases. Furthermore, presurgical risk profiling is inconsistent and deserves further attention, especially for noncardiac, nonvascular surgery and older patients.[69]

Although many preoperative predictors have been identified and are constantly being refined, risk stratification based on clinical, procedural, and biologic markers explains only a small part of the variability in the incidence of perioperative complications. As mentioned earlier, it is becoming increasingly recognized that perioperative morbidity arises as a direct result of the environmental stress of surgery occurring on a landscape of susceptibility that is determined by an individual's clinical and genetic characteristics, and it may even occur in otherwise healthy individuals. Such adverse outcomes will develop only in patients whose combined burden of genetic and environmental risk factors exceeds a certain threshold, which may vary with age. Identification of such genetic contributions not only explains disease causation and susceptibility but also influences the response to disease and drug therapy; and incorporation of genetic risk information in clinical decision making may lead to improved health outcomes and reduced costs. For instance, understanding the gene–environment interactions involved in atherosclerotic cardiovascular disease and neurologic injury may facilitate preoperative patient optimization and resource utilization. Furthermore, understanding the role of allotypic variation in proinflammatory and prothrombotic pathways, the main pathophysiologic mechanisms responsible for perioperative complications, may contribute to the development of target-specific therapies, thereby limiting the incidence of adverse events in high-risk patients. To increase clinical relevance for the practicing perioperative physician, we summarize the existing evidence by specific outcome while highlighting candidate genes in relevant mechanistic pathways (**Tables 4-through 4-6**).

BIOMARKERS OF ADVERSE PERIOPERATIVE CARDIOVASCULAR OUTCOMES

Perioperative Myocardial Infarction and Ventricular Dysfunction Patients with underlying cardiovascular disease can be at increased risk for perioperative cardiac complications. Over the last few decades, several multifactorial risk indices have been developed and validated for both noncardiac (eg, Lee's Revised Cardiac Risk Index) and cardiac surgical patients (eg, Hannan scores), with the specific aim of stratifying risk for perioperative adverse events. However, these multifactorial risk indices have only limited predictive value for identifying patients at the highest risk of perioperative myocardial infarction (PMI).[70] In this context, it has been proposed that genomic approaches could aid in refining an individual's risk profile. Several reports from animal models, linkage analysis, and family, twin, and population association studies have confirmed the role of genetic factors in the etiology and progression of CAD. Specifically, both deaths from CAD as well as hazardous patterns of angiographic CAD (left main and proximal disease), known to be major risk factors for adverse perioperative events, are highly heritable. Similarly, a number of linkage and association studies,[10,16] including a well-powered and replicated GWAS,[39] have identified genetic susceptibility to MI in ambulatory population-based cohorts. The collective evidence from these studies suggests a strong genetic contribution to the risk of adverse cardiovascular outcomes in general but do not directly address the heritability of adverse perioperative myocardial events.

The incidence of PMI following cardiovascular surgery remains between 7% and 19%,[71,72] despite advances in surgical, cardioprotective, and anesthetic techniques, and it is consistently associated with reduced short- and long-term survival in these patients. The pathophysiology of PMI after cardiac surgery involves systemic and local inflammation, "vulnerable" blood, and neuroendocrine stress.[3] In noncardiac surgery, PMI occurs as a result of two distinct mechanisms: (1) coronary plaque rupture and subsequent thrombosis triggered by a number of perioperative stressors including catecholamine surges, proinflammatory, and prothrombotic states; and (2) myocardial oxygen supply-and-demand imbalance.[73] Interindividual genetic variability in these mechanistic pathways is extensive, which may combine to modulate overall susceptibility to perioperative stress and ultimately the magnitude of myocardial injury. Nevertheless, until recently, only a few studies have explored the role of genetic factors in the development of PMI,[25,74,75] mainly conducted in patients undergoing CABG surgery (Table 4-4).

Inflammatory Biomarkers and Perioperative Myocardial Outcomes Although the role of inflammation in cardiovascular disease biology has long been established, we are just beginning to understand the relationship between genetically controlled variability in inflammatory responses to surgery and PMI pathogenesis. Recently, three inflammatory gene SNPs were described to have an independent predictive value for incident PMI after cardiac surgery performed with CPB.[17] These include the proinflammatory cytokine interleukin-6 (*IL6*-572G>C) and two adhesion molecules: intercellular adhesion molecule-1 (*ICAM1* Lys469Glu) and E-selectin

TABLE 4-4 Representative Genetic Polymorphisms Associated With Altered Susceptibility to Adverse Perioperative Cardiovascular Events

Gene	Polymorphism	Type of Surgery	OR	Reference
Perioperative Myocardial Infarction, Ventricular Dysfunction, Early Vein Graft Failure				
IL6	−572G>C −174G>C	Cardiac/CPB Thoracic	2.47 1.8	17 76
ICAM-1 *SELE*	E469L 98G>T	Cardiac/CPB	1.88 0.16	17 17
MBL2	LYQA secretor haplotype	CABG/CPB	3.97	18
ITGB3	L33P (Pl^{A1}/Pl^{A2})	CABG/CPB Major vascular	2.5[a] 2.4	96 98
GP1BA	T145M	Major vascular	3.4	98
TNFA	−308G>A	Thoracic	2.5	76
TNFB (LTA)	TNFB2	Cardiac/CPB	3.84	81
IL10	−1082G>A	Cardiac/CPB	n.r.	83
F5	R506Q(FVL)	CABG/CPB	3.29	100
CMA1	−1905A>G	CABG/CPB	n.r.	25
ANRIL	rs10116277 G>T (9p21)	CABG	1.7	116
NPR3	rs700923 A>G rs16890196 A>G rs765199 C>T rs700926 A>C	CABG/CPB	4.28 4.09 4.27 3.89	107
NPPA/NPPB	rs632793 T>C rs6668352 G>A rs549596 T>C rs198388 C>T rs198389 A>G	CABG/CPB	0.52 0.44 0.48 0.51 0.54	107
PAI-1	4G/5G	CABG	n.r.	94
Perioperative Vasoplegia, Vascular Reactivity, Coronary Tone				
DDAH II *NOS3* *ACE*	−449G>C E298D In/del	Cardiac/CPB	0.4 n.r. n.r.	114 110,201 28,111
ADRB2	Q27E	Tracheal intubation	11.7[b]	112
GNB3	825C>T	Response to α-AR agonists	n.r.	201
PON1	Q192R	Resting coronary tone	n.r.	201
TNFβ+250	−1082G>A	Hyperdynamic state		202
Postoperative Arrhythmias: Atrial Fibrillation, QTc Prolongation				
IL6	−174G>C	CABG/CPB β-Blocker failure Thoracic	3.25 n.r. 1.8	120,122 203 76
RANTES	−403G>A	β-Blocker failure	n.r.	203
TNFA	−308G>A	Thoracic	2.5	76
ATFB5	rs2200733 C>T rs2220427 T>G	Cardiac/CPB	1.97 1.76	119
IL1B	−511T>C 5810G>A	Cardiac/CPB	1.44 0.66	204
Postoperative MACE, Late Vein Graft Failure				
ADRB1	R389G	Noncardiac with spinal block	1.87[c]	109
ACE *ITGB3*	In/del L33P	CABG/CPB	3.1[d] 4.7	75 97
MTHFR	A222V	PTCA and CABG/CPB	2.8	205

(Continued)

TABLE 4-4 Representative Genetic Polymorphisms Associated With Altered Susceptibility to Adverse Perioperative Cardiovascular Events (*Continued*)

Gene	Polymorphism	Type of Surgery	OR	Reference
ADRB2	R16G Q27E	Cardiac surgery/CPB	1.96 2.82	131
HP	Hp1/Hp2	CABG	n.r.	74
CR1,KDR *MICA* *HLA-DPB1* *VTN*		CABG/CPB	n.r.	26
LPL	HindIII		n.r.	206
THBD	A455V	CABG/CPB	2.78	132
IL6	−174G>C nt565 G>A	Noncardiac vascular surgery	2.14 1.84	84
IL10	−1082 G>A −819 C>T −592 C>A ATA haplotype	Noncardiac vascular surgery	2.16	84
		Cardiac Allograft Rejection		
TNFA *IL10* *ICAM1*	−308G>A −1082G>A K469E	Cardiac transplant	n.r. n.r. n.r.	207 207 208
IL1RN *IL1B*	86-bp VNTR 3953C>T	Thoracic transplant	2.02 20.5[e]	209 209
TGF-β	915G>C	Cardiac transplant	n.r.	210

ACE, angiotensin-converting enzyme; ADRB1, β_1-adrenergic receptor; ADRB2, β_2-adrenergic receptor; ANRIL, antisense noncoding RNA in the INK4 locus; ATFB5, atrial fibrillation, familial 5; CABG, coronary artery bypass grafting; CMA1, heart chymase; CPB, cardiopulmonary bypass; CR1, complement component 3b/4b; DDAH II, dimethylarginine dimethylamino hydrolase II; F5, factor V; GNB3, G-protein β_3 subunit; GP1BA, glycoprotein Ibα; HLA-DPB1, β chain of class II major histocompatibility complex; HP, haptoglobin; ICAM1, intercellular adhesion molecule 1; IL1B, interleukin 1β; IL1RN, interleukin 1 receptor antagonist; IL6, interleukin 6; IL10, interleukin 10; ITGB3, glycoprotein IIIa; KDR, kinase inert domain receptor; LTA, lymphotoxin α; LPL, lipoprotein lipase; MBL2, mannose binding lectin 2; MICA, MHC I polypeptide; MTHFR, methylenetetrahydrofolate reductase; n.r., not reported; NOS3, endothelial nitric oxide synthase; NPPA/NPPB, natriuretic peptide precursor A/B; NPR3, natriuretic peptide receptor 3 precursor; OR, odds ratio; PAI-1, plasminogen activator inhibitor 1; PON1, paraoxonase 1; RANTES, regulated upon activation normally T-expressed and secreted; SELE, E-selectin; SELP, P-selectin; TGF-β, transforming growth factor-β; TNFA, tumor necrosis factor α; TNFB, tumor necrosis factor β; VNTR, variable number tandem repeat; VTN, vitronectin.

[a]Relative risk; [b]F-value; [c]hazard ratio; [d]β-coefficient; [e]in haplotype with IL1RN VNTR.

TABLE 4-5 Representative Genetic Polymorphisms Associated With Altered Susceptibility to Adverse Perioperative Neurologic Events

Gene	Polymorphism	Type of Surgery	OR	Reference
		Perioperative Stroke		
IL6 *CRP*	−174G>C 1846C>T	Cardiac/CPB	3.3	133
	Perioperative Cognitive Dysfunction, Neurodevelopmental Dysfunction			
SELP	E298D	Cardiac/CPB	0.51	21
CRP	1059G>C	Cardiac/CPB	0.37	21
ITGB3	L33P (Pl^{A1}/Pl^{A2})	Cardiac/CPB	n.r.	20
APOE	ε4 ε2	CABG/CPB (adults) Cardiac/CPB (children)	n.r. 7; 11	19 141,142
APOE	ε4	CABG/CPB	1.26	211
		Postoperative Delirium		
APOE	ε4	Major noncardiac Critically ill	3.64 7.32	139 140

APOE, apolipoprotein E; CABG, coronary artery bypass grafting; CPB, cardiopulmonary bypass; CRP, C-reactive protein; IL6, interleukin 6; ITGB3, platelet glycoprotein IIIa; n.r., not reported; OR, odds ratio; SELP, P-selectin.

(*SELE* 98G>T). Furthermore, the predictive ability of a PMI model based only on traditional risk factors was improved by the addition of genotypic information. Similarly, Collard et al identified a combined haplotype in the mannose-binding lectin gene (*MBL2 LYQA* secretor haplotype), an important recognition molecule in the lectin complement pathway, to be independently associated with PMI in a cohort of white patients undergoing first-time CABG with CPB.[18] Genetic variants in *IL6* and *TNFA* have also been described in association with increased incidence of postoperative cardiovascular complications including PMI after lung surgery for cancer.[76] Several polymorphisms in key proinflammatory genes have been associated with robust increases in perioperative inflammatory responses in patients undergoing cardiac surgery with CPB. These include the promoter SNPs in *IL6* (-572G>C and -174G>C),[77] also shown to prolong the hospital length of stay[78]; the apolipoprotein E genotype (the *ε4* allele)[79]; SNPs in the tumor necrosis factor genes (*TNFA*-308G>A, *LTA*+250G>A),[80] also associated with postoperative left ventricular dysfunction[81]; and a functional SNP in the macrophage migration inhibitory factor (MIF).[82] Conversely, a genetic variant modulating the release of the anti-inflammatory cytokine interleukin-10 (*IL10*-1082G>A) in response to CPB has been described, with high levels of *IL-10* surprisingly being associated with postoperative cardiovascular dysfunction.[83] In patients undergoing elective surgical revascularization for peripheral vascular disease, several SNPs in *IL6* (-174 G>C, nt565 G>A) and *IL10* (-1082 G>A, -819 C>T, -592 C>A, and the ATA haplotype) were associated with endothelial dysfunction and an increased risk of a composite end point of acute postoperative cardiovascular events.[84]

TABLE 4-6 Representative Genetic Polymorphisms Associated With Other Adverse Perioperative Outcomes

Gene	Polymorphism	Type of Surgery	OR	Reference
Perioperative Thrombotic Events				
F5	FVL	Noncardiac, cardiac	n.r.	27
Perioperative Bleeding				
F5	R506Q(FVL)	Cardiac/CPB	−1.25[a]	99
PAI-1	4G/5G		10[b]	212
ITGA2	−52C>T, 807C>T	CABG/CPB	−0.15[a]	213
GP1BA	T145M		−0.22[a]	213
TF	−603A>G		−0.03[a]	213
TFPI	−399C>T		−0.05[a]	213
F2	20210G>A		0.38[a]	213
ACE	In/del		0.15[a]	213
ITGB3	L33P (PI[A1]/PI[A2])		n.r.	214
PAI-1	4G/5G	Cardiac/CPB	10[b]	212
TNFA	−238G>A	Brain AVM treatment	3.5[c]	215
APOE	ε2		10.9[c]	215
ELAM-1	98 G/T 561 A/C	CABG/CPB	n.r.	216
Perioperative Acute Kidney Injury				
IL6	−572G>C	CABG/CPB	20.04[d]	22
AGT	M235T		32.19[d]	22
NOS3	E298D		4.29[d]	22
APOE	ε4		−0.13[a]	22,24
Perioperative Severe Sepsis				
APOE	ε3		0.28[e]	30

ACE, angiotensin-converting enzyme; AGT, angiotensinogen; APOE, apolipoprotein E; AVM, arteriovenous malformation; CABG, coronary artery bypass grafting; CPB, cardiopulmonary bypass; CRP, C-reactive protein; ELAM-1, endothelial-leukocyte adhesion molecule-1; F2, prothrombin; F5, factor V; FVL, factor V Leiden; GP1BA, glycoprotein Ibα; IL6, interleukin 6; ITGA2, glycoprotein Ialla; ITGB3, glycoprotein IIIa; NOS3, endothelial nitric oxide synthase; n.r., not reported; OR, odds ratio; PAI-1, plasminogen activator inhibitor 1; TF, tissue factor; TFPI, tissue factor pathway inhibitor; TNFA, tumor necrosis factor α.

[a]β-Coefficient; [b]odds ratio; [c]hazard ratio; [d]F-value; [e]relative risk.

C-reactive protein (CRP) is the prototypical acute-phase reactant and the most extensively studied inflammatory marker in clinical studies, and high-sensitivity CRP (hs-CRP) has emerged as a robust predictor of cardiovascular risk at all stages, from healthy subjects to patients with acute coronary syndromes and acute decompensated heart failure.[85] Whether CRP is merely a marker or also a mediator of inflammatory processes is yet unclear, but several lines of evidence support the latter theory. In perioperative medicine, elevated preoperative CRP levels have been associated with increased short- and long-term morbidity and mortality in patients undergoing primary elective CABG (cut-off >3 mg/L)[86] as well as in higher acuity CABG patients (cut-off >10 mg/L).[87] Interestingly, in a retrospective analysis of patients with elevated baseline hs-CRP levels undergoing off-pump CABG surgery, preoperative statin therapy was associated with reduced postoperative myocardial injury and need for dialysis.[88] In elective major noncardiac surgery patients, preoperative CRP levels (cut-off >3.4 mg/L) independently predicted perioperative major cardiovascular events (composite of MI, pulmonary edema, and cardiovascular death) and significantly improved the predictive power of the Revised Cardiac Risk Index (RCRI) in receiver operating characteristic analysis.[89]

In addition to the already established heritability of elevated baseline plasma CRP levels, recent reports indicate that the acute-phase rise in postoperative plasma CRP levels is also genetically determined. The *CRP*1059G>C polymorphism was associated with lower peak postoperative serum CRP following both elective CABG with CPB,[90] as well as esophagectomy for thoracic esophageal cancer.[91] Furthermore, *CRP*-717C>T polymorphism was associated with stress hyperglycemia in patients undergoing esophagectomy for cancer, leading to increased postoperative infectious complications and intensive care unit length of stay.[92]

Hemostatic Biomarkers and Perioperative Myocardial Outcomes The host response to surgery is also characterized by alterations in the coagulation system, manifested as increased fibrinogen concentration, platelet adhesiveness, and plasminogen activator inhibitor (PAI)-1 production. These changes can be more pronounced after cardiac surgery, where the complex and multifactorial effects of hypothermia, hemodilution, and CPB-induced activation of coagulation, fibrinolytic, and inflammatory pathways are combined. Dysfunction of the coagulation system following cardiac surgery may manifest on a continuum ranging from increased thrombotic complications such as coronary graft thrombosis, PMI, stroke, pulmonary embolism at one end of the spectrum, to excessive bleeding as the other extreme. The balance between normal hemostasis, bleeding, and thrombosis is markedly influenced by the rate of thrombin formation and platelet activation, with genetic variability known to modulate each of these mechanistic pathways,[93] suggesting significant heritability of the prothrombotic state (see Table 4-6 for an overview of genetic variants associated with postoperative bleeding). Several genotypes in hemostatic genes have been associated with increased risk of coronary graft thrombosis and myocardial injury following CABG. A genetic variant in the promoter of the *PAI-1* gene, consisting of an insertion (5G)/deletion (4G) polymorphism at position -675 has been associated with changes in the plasma levels of *PAI-1*. Because PAI-1 is an important negative regulator of fibrinolytic activity, its polymorphism has been associated with increased risk of early graft thrombosis after CABG[94] and, in a meta-analysis, with increased incidence of MI.[95] Similarly, a polymorphism in the platelet glycoprotein IIIa gene (*ITGB3*), resulting in increased platelet aggregation (PI[A2] polymorphism), has been associated with higher levels of postoperative troponin I release following CABG[96] and with increased risk of thrombotic coronary graft occlusion, MI, and death 1 year following CABG.[97] In the setting of noncardiac surgery, two polymorphisms in platelet glycoprotein receptors (*ITGB3* and *GP1BA*) have been shown to be independent risk predictors of PMI in patients undergoing major vascular surgery and resulted in improved discrimination of an ischemia risk assessment tool when added to historic and procedural risk factors.[98] Finally, a point mutation in coagulation factor V (1691G>A), resulting in resistance to activated protein C (factor V Leiden), was also associated with various postoperative thrombotic complications following noncardiac surgery.[27] Conversely, in patients undergoing cardiac surgery, factor V Leiden was associated with significant reductions in postoperative blood loss and overall risk of transfusion.[99] Nevertheless, in a prospective study of CABG patients with routine 3-month postoperative angiographic follow-up, carriers of factor V Leiden had a higher incidence of graft occlusion.[100]

Natriuretic Peptides and Perioperative Myocardial Outcomes Circulating B-type natriuretic peptide (BNP) is a powerful biomarker of cardiovascular outcomes in many circumstances. Produced mainly in the ventricular myocardium, BNP is formed by cleavage of its prohormone by the enzyme corin into the biologically active C-terminal fragment (BNP) and an inactive N-terminal fragment (NT-proBNP). Known stimuli of BNP activation are myocardial mechanical stretch (from volume or pressure overload), acute ischemic injury, and a variety of other proinflammatory and neurohormonal stimuli inducing myocardial stress. Although secreted in a 1:1 ratio, circulating levels of BNP and NT-proBNP differ considerably due to different clearance characteristics.

A large number of studies have reported consistent associations of baseline plasma BNP or NT-proBNP levels with a variety of postoperative short- and long-term morbidity and mortality end points, independent of the traditional risk factors. For noncardiac surgery, these were summarized in two meta-analyses that overall indicate an approximately 20-fold increase in risk of adverse perioperative cardiovascular outcomes.[101,102] Similarly, for cardiac surgery patients, preoperative BNP was a strong independent predictor of in-hospital postoperative ventricular dysfunction, hospital length of stay, and 5-year mortality following primary CABG,[103] performing better than peak postoperative BNP.[104] The current guidelines for preoperative cardiac risk assessment in noncardiac surgery list BNP and NT-proBNP measurements as class IIa/level B indications.[105] However, despite the large number of studies conducted in both cardiac and noncardiac surgery, precise cut-off levels for BNP still need to be determined and adjusted for age, gender, and renal function. Similarly, no BNP-based goal directed therapies have been reported in the perioperative period. However, a role for BNP assays in monitoring aortic valve disease for optimal timing of surgery has been described.[106]

Furthermore, a recent study by Fox et al identified genetic variation in natriuretic peptide precursor genes (*NPPA/NPPB*) to be independently associated with a decreased risk of postoperative ventricular dysfunction following primary CABG, whereas variants in natriuretic peptide receptor *NPR3* were associated with an increased risk (Table 4-4),[107] offering additional clues into the molecular mechanisms underlying postoperative ventricular dysfunction.

The Role of Genetic Variability in Perioperative Vascular Reactivity The perioperative period is characterized by robust activation of the sympathetic nervous system, which plays an important role in the pathophysiology of PMI. Thus patients with CAD who carry specific polymorphisms in adrenergic receptor (AR) genes can be at high risk for catecholamine toxicity and cardiovascular complications. Several functionally important SNPs modulating the AR pathways have been described.[108] One of them is the Arg389Gly polymorphism in β_1-AR gene (*ADRB1*), a SNP associated with increased risk of composite cardiovascular morbidity at 1 year after noncardiac surgery under spinal anesthesia.[109] Of note, perioperative β-blockade had no effect. These findings prompted the investigators to suggest that stratification on AR genotype in future trials may help identify patients likely to benefit from perioperative β-blocker therapy. Significantly increased vascular responsiveness to α-adrenergic stimulation (phenylephrine) has been observed in carriers of the endothelial nitric oxide synthase (NOS3) 894>T polymorphism[110] and angiotensin-converting enzyme (ACE) insertion/deletion (I/D) polymorphism[28,111] undergoing cardiac surgery with CPB. Differences in perioperative vascular reactivity in relation to genetic variants of the β_2-AR (*ADRB2*) have also been noted in patients undergoing noncardiac surgery. In patients with a common functional *ADRB2* SNP (Glu27), increased blood pressure responses to endotracheal intubation were observed in one study.[112] In a different study, in obstetric patients who had spinal anesthesia for cesarean delivery, the incidence and severity of maternal hypotension and response to treatment was affected by ADRB2 genotype (Gly16 and/or Glu27 led to lower vasopressor use for the treatment of hypotension).[113] In patients undergoing cardiac surgery, the frequently observed vasoplegic syndrome and vasopressor requirements have been associated with a common polymorphism in the dimethylarginine dimethyl-aminohydrolase II (DDAH II) gene, an important regulator of nitric oxide synthase activity.[114]

Two recent studies have revealed the association of a common SNP at the 9p21 locus with both perioperative myocardial injury[115] and all-cause mortality after primary CABG.[116] This SNP was previously correlated with a wide array of vascular phenotypes in ambulatory populations (including CAD, MI, carotid atherosclerosis, abdominal aortic aneurysms, intracranial aneurysms) in replicated GWAS analyses. The mechanism of action of this SNP in the development of PMI and mortality is not completely understood, but it involves altered regulation of cell proliferation, senescence, and apoptosis. It seems that cardiac surgery with CPB may trigger the effects of the 9p21 gene variant leading to accumulation of senescent cells or cells that show evidence of necrotic death with cellular edema and lysis.

Perioperative Atrial Fibrillation Perioperative atrial fibrillation (PoAF) remains a significant clinical problem after cardiac and noncardiac thoracic procedures. With an incidence of 27% to 40%, PoAF is associated with increased morbidity, hospital length of stay, rehospitalization, health care costs, and reduced survival. The high incidence of PoAF has prompted several investigators to develop comprehensive risk indices for the prediction of PoAF based on demographic, clinical, electrocardiographic, and procedural risk factors. Nevertheless, the predictive accuracy of these risk indices remains limited,[117] suggesting that genetic variation may play a significant role in the occurrence of PoAF. Heritable forms of AF have been described in the ambulatory nonsurgical population, and it appears both monogenic forms like "lone" AF as well as polygenic predisposition to more common acquired forms like PoAF do exist.[118] A recent GWAS for AF found two polymorphisms on chromosome 4q25 to be significantly associated with AF,[42] findings replicated in other patient groups from Sweden, the United States, and Hong Kong. Recently, this locus was also associated with new-onset PoAF after cardiac surgery with CPB (CABG with or without concurrent valve surgery).[119] The mechanism of action of the genetic locus identified by the 2 noncoding SNPs is unknown, but it lies close to several genes involved in the development of the pulmonary myocardium, or the sleeve of cardiomyocytes extending from the left atrium into the initial portion of the pulmonary veins. Clinical studies have demonstrated that ectopic foci of electric activity arising from within the pulmonary veins and posterior left atrium play a substantial role in initiating and maintaining AF.

Other candidate susceptibility genes for PoAF include those determining the duration of action potential (voltage-gated ion channels, ion transporters), responses to extracellular factors (adrenergic and other hormone receptors, heat shock proteins), remodeling processes, and magnitude of inflammatory and oxidative stress. It has been described that inflammation, reflected by elevated baseline CRP or IL6 levels and exaggerated postoperative leukocytosis, predicts the occurrence of PoAF. A link between inflammation and the development of PoAF is also supported by evidence that postoperative administration of nonsteroidal anti-inflammatory drugs may reduce the incidence of PoAF. Several recent studies have found that a functional SNP in the *IL6* promoter (-174G>C) is associated with higher perioperative plasma IL6 levels and several adverse outcomes after CABG, including PoAF.[120-122] In noncardiac surgery, polymorphisms in *IL6* and *TNFA* genes have been shown to be associated with an increased risk of postoperative morbidity, including new-onset arrhythmias.[76] There is, however, a contradictory lack of association between CRP levels (strongly regulated by IL6) and PoAF in women undergoing cardiac surgery,[123] which may reflect gender-related differences. However, a recent study reported that both pre- and postoperative PAI-1 levels were independently associated with development of PoAF following cardiac surgery.[124]

Several investigations in the transcriptional responses to AF in human atrial appendage myocardium collected at the time of cardiac surgery or in preclinical models (Table 4-3) have identified a ventricular-like genomic signature in fibrillating atria, with increased ratios of ventricular to atrial isoforms, suggesting dedifferentiation.[125] It remains unclear whether this "ventricularization" of atrial gene expression reflects cause or effect of AF, but it likely represents an adaptive energy-saving process to the high metabolic demand of fibrillating atrial myocardium, akin to chronic hibernation. Recently, a different mechanism was proposed as being involved in PoAF; it has been found that patients who exhibit PoAF after cardiac surgery display a differential genomic response to CPB in their peripheral blood leukocytes, characterized by upregulation of oxidative stress genes, which correlated with a significantly larger increase in oxidant stress both systemically (as measured by total peroxide levels) as well as at the myocardial level (as measured in the right atrium).[126]

Cardiac Allograft Rejection Identification of peripheral blood gene- and protein-based biomarkers to noninvasively monitor, diagnose, and predict perioperative cardiac allograft rejection is an area of rapid scientific growth. Although several polymorphisms in genes involved in alloimmune interactions, the renin-angiotensin-aldosterone system, and the transforming growth factor-β superfamily have been associated with cardiac transplant outcomes, their relevance as useful clinical monitoring tools remains uncertain. However, peripheral blood mononuclear cell–based molecular assays have shown much promise for monitoring the dynamic responses of the immune system to the transplanted heart, discriminating immunologic allograft quiescence and predicting future rejection.[127] A noninvasive molecular test to identify patients at risk for acute cellular rejection is commercially available (Allomap, XDx), in which the expression levels of 11 genes are measured by quantitative real-time polymerase chain reaction (qRT-PCR) and translated using a mathematical algorithm into a clinically actionable AlloMap score that enhances the ability to deliver personalized monitoring and treatment to heart transplant patients.[128] Furthermore, several clinically available protein-based biomarkers of alloimmune activation, microvascular injury (troponins), systemic inflammation (CRP), and wall stress and remodeling (BNP) correlate well with allograft failure and vasculopathy and have good negative predictive values, but they require additional studies to guide their clinical use. Similarly, molecular signatures of functional recovery in end-stage heart failure following left ventricular assist device (LVAD) support using gene expression profiling have been reported using only mRNA[129] or combined microRNA and mRNA profiling,[130] and they could be used to monitor patients who received an LVAD as destination therapy or assess the timing of potential device explantation.

GENETIC VARIABILITY AND POSTOPERATIVE EVENT-FREE SURVIVAL

Several large randomized clinical trials examining the benefits of CABG surgery and percutaneous coronary interventions relative to medical therapy and/or to one another have refined our knowledge of early and long-term survival after CABG. These studies have helped define the subgroups of patients who benefit from surgical revascularization, and they also demonstrated a substantial variability in long-term survival after CABG, altered by important demographic and environmental risk factors. Increasing evidence suggests that the *ACE* gene indel polymorphism may influence post-CABG complications, with carriers of the *D* allele having higher mortality and restenosis rates after CABG surgery compared with the *I* allele.[75] As discussed earlier, a prothrombotic amino acid alteration in the β_3-integrin chain of the glycoprotein IIb/IIIa platelet receptor (the Pl^{A2} polymorphism) is associated with an increased risk for major adverse cardiac events (a composite of MI, coronary bypass graft occlusion, or death) following CABG surgery (Table 4-4).[97] We found preliminary evidence for association of two functional SNPs modulating β_2-adrenergic receptor activity (Arg16Gly and Gln27Glu) with incidence of death or major adverse cardiac events following cardiac surgery,[131] and recently identified a functional polymorphism in thrombomodulin (*THBD* Ala455Val; OR: 2.64) gene associated with increased 5-year mortality after CABG independent of EuroSCORE.[132]

GENETIC SUSCEPTIBILITY TO ADVERSE PERIOPERATIVE NEUROLOGIC OUTCOMES

Despite advances in surgical and anesthetic techniques, significant neurologic morbidity continues to occur following cardiac surgery, ranging in severity from coma and focal stroke (incidence: 1%-3%) to more subtle cognitive deficits (incidence up to 69%), with a substantial impact on the risk of perioperative death, quality of life, and resource utilization. Variability in the reported incidence of both early and late neurologic deficits remains poorly explained by procedural risk factors, suggesting that environmental (operative) and genetic factors may interact to determine disease onset, progression, and recovery. The pathophysiology of perioperative neurologic injury is thought to involve complex interactions between primary pathways associated with atherosclerosis and thrombosis, and secondary response pathways like inflammation, vascular reactivity, and direct cellular injury. Many functional genetic variants have been reported in each of these mechanistic pathways involved in modulating the magnitude and the response to neurologic injury, which may have implications in chronic as well as acute perioperative neurocognitive outcomes. For example, Grocott at al examined 26 SNPs in relationship to the incidence of acute postoperative ischemic stroke in 1635 patients undergoing cardiac surgery, and they found that the interaction of minor alleles of the CRP (1846C>T) and IL6 promoter SNP -174G>C significantly increases the risk of acute stroke.[133] Similarly, a recent study suggests that P-selectin and CRP genes both contribute to modulating the susceptibility to postoperative cognitive decline (POCD) following cardiac surgery.[21] Specifically, the loss-of-function minor alleles of *CRP* 1059G>C and *SELP* 1087G>A are independently associated with a *reduction* in the observed incidence of POCD after adjustment for known clinical and demographic covariates (Table 4-5).

Our group has demonstrated a significant association between the apolipoprotein E (*APOE*) E4 genotype and adverse cerebral outcomes in cardiac surgery patients.[19,134] This is consistent with the role of the *APOE* genotype in recovery from acute brain injury, such as intracranial hemorrhage,[135] closed-head injury,[136] and stroke,[137] as well as experimental models of cerebral I/R injury[138]; two subsequent studies in CABG patients, however, have not replicated these initial findings. Furthermore, the incidence of postoperative delirium following major noncardiac surgery in the elderly[139] and in critically ill patients[140] is increased in carriers of the *APOE* ε4 allele. Unlike adult cardiac surgery patients, infants possessing the *APOE* ε2 allele are at increased risk for developing adverse neurodevelopmental sequelae following cardiac surgery.[141,142] The mechanisms by which the *APOE* genotypes might influence neurologic outcomes are yet to be determined, but they do not seem to be related to alterations in global cerebral blood flow of oxygen metabolism during CPB[143]; however, genotypic effects in modulating the inflammatory response,[79] extent of aortic atheroma burden,[144] and risk for premature coronary atherosclerosis[145] may play a role.

Recent studies have suggested a role for platelet activation in the pathophysiology of adverse neurologic sequelae. Genetic variants in surface platelet membrane glycoproteins, important mediators of platelet adhesion and platelet–platelet interactions, have been shown to increase the susceptibility to prothrombotic events. Among these, the Pl^{A2} polymorphism in glycoprotein IIb/IIIa has been related to various adverse thrombotic outcomes, including acute coronary thrombosis[146] and atherothrombotic stroke.[147] We found the Pl^{A2} allele to be associated with more severe neurocognitive decline after CPB,[20] which could represent exacerbation of platelet-dependent thrombotic processes associated with plaque embolism.

Cardiac surgical patients who develop POCD demonstrate inherently different genetic responses to cardiopulmonary bypass from those without POCD, as evidenced by acute deregulation in peripheral blood leukocytes of gene expression pathways involving inflammation, antigen presentation, and cellular adhesion.[148] These findings corroborate with proteomic changes, in which patients with POCD similarly have significantly higher serologic inflammatory indices compared with those patients without POCD[149,150] and add to the increasing level of evidence that CPB does not cause an indiscriminate variation in gene expression but rather distinct patterns in specific pathways that are highly associated with the development of postoperative complications such as POCD. The implications for perioperative medicine include identifying populations at risk who might benefit not only from an improved informed consent, stratification, and resource allocation, but also from targeted anti-inflammatory strategies.

In noncardiac surgery, a study conducted in patients undergoing carotid endarterectomy demonstrated that preoperative plasma levels of fibrinogen and hs-CRP were independently associated with new periprocedural cerebral ischemic lesions caused by microembolic events, as determined by MRI diffusion-weighted imaging.[151]

GENETIC SUSCEPTIBILITY TO ADVERSE PERIOPERATIVE RENAL OUTCOMES

Acute renal dysfunction is a common, serious complication of cardiac surgery; about 8% to 15% of patients develop moderate renal injury (>1.0 mg/dL peak creatinine rise), and up to 5% of them develop renal failure requiring dialysis.[152] Acute renal failure is independently associated with in-hospital mortality rates of greater than 60% in patients requiring dialysis.[152] Several studies have demonstrated that inheritance of genetic polymorphisms in the *APOE* gene (ε4 allele)[24] and in the promoter region of the *IL6* gene (-174C allele)[121] are associated with acute kidney injury following CABG surgery (Table 4-6). Stafford-Smith et al reported that major differences in peak postoperative serum creatinine rise after CABG are predicted by possession of combinations of polymorphisms that interestingly differ by race: the angiotensinogen (*AGT*) 842T>C and *IL6* -572G>C variants in whites and the endothelial nitric oxide synthase (*NOS3*) 894G>T and angiotensin-converting enzyme (*ACE*) insertion/deletion in African Americans are associated with >50% reduction in the postoperative glomerular filtration rate.[22] Further identification of genotypes predictive of adverse perioperative renal outcomes may facilitate individually tailored therapy, risk stratify the patients for interventional trials targeting the gene product itself, and aid in medical decision making (eg, selecting medical over surgical management).

GENETIC VARIANTS AND RISK FOR PROLONGED POSTOPERATIVE MECHANICAL VENTILATION

Prolonged mechanical ventilation (inability to extubate patient by 24 hours postoperatively) is a significant complication following cardiac surgery, occurring in 5.6% and 10.5% of patients undergoing first and repeat CABG surgery, respectively.[153] Several pulmonary and nonpulmonary causes have been identified, and scoring systems based on preoperative and procedural risk factors have been proposed and validated. Recently, genetic variants in the renin-angiotensin pathway and in proinflammatory cytokine genes have been associated with respiratory complications post-CPB. The *D* allele of a common functional insertion/deletion polymorphism in the angiotensin-converting enzyme (*ACE*) gene, accounting for 47% of variance in circulating ACE levels,[154] is associated with prolonged mechanical ventilation following CABG[155] and with susceptibility to and prognosis of acute respiratory disease syndrome (ARDS).[156] Furthermore, a hyposecretor haplotype in the neighboring genes tumor necrosis factor α (*TNFA*) and lymphotoxin α (*LTA*) on chromosome 6 (*TNFA-308G/LTA+250G* haplotype)[157] and a functional polymorphism modulating postoperative IL6 levels (*IL6*-174G>C)[121] are independently associated with higher risk of prolonged mechanical ventilation post-CABG. The association is more dramatic in patients undergoing conventional CABG than in those undergoing off-pump CABG (OPCAB), suggesting that in high-risk patients identified by preoperative genetic screening, OPCAB may be the optimal surgical procedure.

A next crucial step in understanding the complexity of adverse perioperative outcomes is to assess the contribution of variations in many genes simultaneously and their interaction with traditional risk factors to the longitudinal prediction of outcomes in individual patients. The use of such outcome predictive models incorporating genetic information may help stratify mortality and morbidity in surgical patients, improve prognostication, direct medical decision making both intraoperatively and during postoperative follow-up, and even suggest novel targets for therapeutic intervention in the perioperative period.

PHARMACOGENOMICS AND ANESTHESIA

Interindividual variability in response to drug therapy, both in terms of efficacy and safety, is a rule by which anesthesiologists live. In fact, much of the art of anesthesiology is the astute clinician being prepared to deal with outliers. The term *pharmacogenomics* is used to describe how inherited variations in genes modulating drug actions are related to interindividual variability in drug response. Such variability in drug action may be *pharmacokinetic* or *pharmacodynamic* (**Fig. 4-4**). Pharmacokinetic variability refers to variability in a drug's absorption, distribution, metabolism, and excretion that mediates its efficacy and/or toxicity. The molecules involved in these processes include drug-metabolizing enzymes (such as members of the cytochrome P450, or CYP, superfamily) and transport molecules that mediate drug uptake into, and efflux from, intracellular sites. Pharmacodynamic variability refers to variable drug effects despite equivalent drug delivery to molecular sites of action. This may reflect variability in the function of the molecular target of the drug or in the pathophysiologic context in which the drug interacts with its receptor target (eg, affinity, coupling, expression).[158] Thus pharmacogenomics investigates complex, polygenically determined phenotypes of drug efficacy or toxicity, with the goal of identifying novel therapeutic targets and customizing drug therapy.

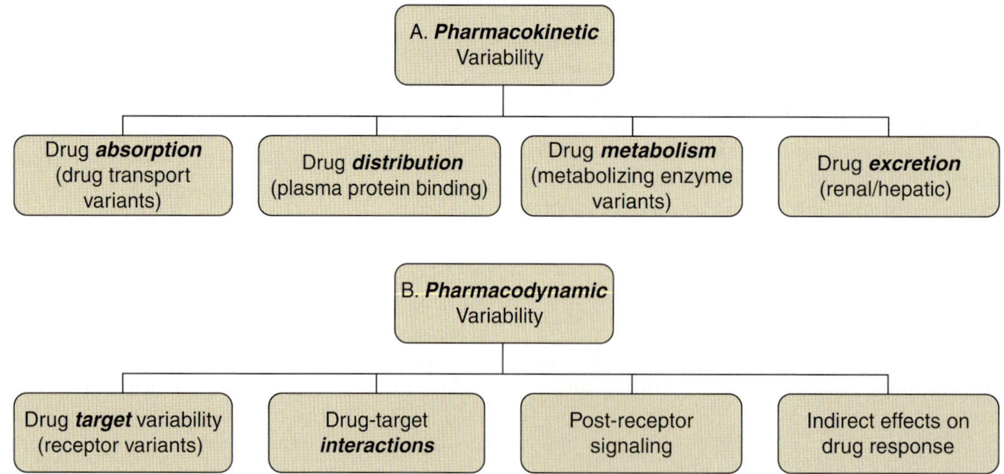

FIGURE 4-4. Pharmacogenomic determinants of individual drug response operate by pharmacokinetic and pharmacodynamic mechanisms. **A.** Genetic variants in *drug transporters* (eg, ATP-binding cassette sub-family B member 1 or *ABCB1* gene) and *drug metabolizing enzymes* (eg, cytochrome P450 2D6 or *CYP2D6* gene, *CYP2C9* gene, N-acetyltransferase or *NAT2* gene, plasma cholinesterase or *BCHE* gene) are responsible for *pharmacokinetic* variability in drug response. **B.** Polymorphisms in *drug targets* (eg, β_1 and β_2-adrenergic receptor *ADRB1*, *ADRB2* genes; angiotensin-I converting enzyme *ACE* gene), *postreceptor signaling molecules* (eg, guanine nucleotide binding protein β3 or *GNB3* gene), or *molecules indirectly affecting drug response* (eg, various ion channel genes involved in drug-induced arrhythmias) are sources of *pharmacodynamic* variability.

PSEUDOCHOLINESTERASE DEFICIENCY

Historically, characterization of the genetic basis for plasma pseudocholinesterase deficiency in 1956 was of fundamental importance to anesthesia and the further development and understanding of genetically determined differences in drug response.[159] Individuals with an atypical form of pseudocholinesterase resulting in a markedly reduced rate of drug metabolism are at risk for excessive neuromuscular blockade and prolonged apnea. More than 20 variants have since been identified in the butyrylcholinesterase gene (*BCHE*), the most common of which are the A-variant (209A>G) and the K-variant (1615G>A), with various and somewhat poorly defined phenotypic consequences on prolonged neuromuscular blockade. Therefore, pharmacogenetic testing is currently not recommended in the population at large but only as an explanation for an adverse event.[160]

GENETICS OF MALIGNANT HYPERTHERMIA

Malignant hyperthermia (MH) is a rare autosomal dominant genetic disease of skeletal muscle calcium metabolism, triggered by administration of general anesthesia with volatile anesthetic agents or succinylcholine in susceptible individuals. The clinical MH syndrome is characterized by skeletal muscle hypermetabolism and manifested as skeletal muscle rigidity, tachycardia, tachypnea, hemodynamic instability, increased oxygen consumption and carbon dioxide production, lactic acidosis and fever, progressing to malignant ventricular arrhythmias, disseminated intravascular coagulation, and myoglobinuric renal failure. MH susceptibility has been initially linked to the ryanodine receptor (*RYRI*) gene locus on chromosome 19q.[161] However, subsequent studies have shown that MH may represent a common severe phenotype that originates not only from point mutations in the *RYRI* gene (Arg614Cys), but also within its functionally and/or structurally associated proteins regulating excitation-contraction coupling (such as *α1DHPR* and *FKBP12*). It is becoming increasingly apparent that MH susceptibility results from a complex interaction between multiple genes and environment (such as environmental toxins), suggested by the heterogeneity observed in the clinical MH syndrome and the variable penetrance of the MH phenotype.[162] Current diagnostic methods (the caffeine-halothane contracture test) are invasive and potentially nonspecific. Unfortunately, because of the polygenic determinism and variable penetrance, direct DNA testing in the general population for susceptibility to MH is currently not recommended; in contrast, testing in individuals from families with affected individuals has the potential to greatly reduce mortality and morbidity.[160] Furthermore, genomic approaches may help elucidate the molecular mechanisms involved in altered RYRI-mediated calcium signaling and identify novel, more specific therapeutic targets.

GENETIC VARIABILITY AND RESPONSE TO ANESTHETIC AGENTS

Anesthetic potency, defined by the minimum alveolar concentration (MAC) of an inhaled anesthetic that abolishes purposeful movement in response to a noxious stimulus, varies among individuals, with a coefficient of variation (the ratio of standard deviation to the mean) of approximately 10%.[163] This observed variability may be explained by interindividual differences in multiple genes that underlie responsiveness to anesthetics, by environmental or physiologic factors (eg, brain temperature, age), or by measurement errors. With growing public concern over intraoperative awareness, understanding the mechanisms responsible for this variability may facilitate implementation of patient-specific preventive strategies. Evidence of a genetic basis for increased anesthetic requirements is beginning to emerge, suggested, for instance, by the observation that desflurane requirements are increased in subjects with red hair versus dark hair,[164] and by recently reported variability in the immobilizing dose of sevoflurane (as much as 24%) in populations with different ethnic (and thus genetic) backgrounds.[165] Several studies evaluating the genetic control of anesthetic responses, coupled with molecular modeling, proteomic, neurophysiology, and pharmacologic approaches have provided important developments in our understanding of general anesthetic mechanisms. Triggered by the seminal work of Franks and Lieb,[166] research shifted from the membrane lipid bilayer to protein receptors (specifically ligand- and voltage-gated ion channels) as potential anesthetic targets, ending a few decades of stagnation that were primarily due to an almost universal acceptance of the dogma of nonspecific anesthetic action (the so-called lipid theory). Some of the genes responsible for phenotypic differences in anesthetic effects have been mapped in various animal models, and following genomic manipulation of plausible candidate receptors to investigate their function in vitro, they were evaluated in genetically engineered animals for their relationship to various anesthetic end points, such as immobility (ie, MAC), hypnosis, amnesia, and analgesia (for reviews, see Sonner et al[167]). Several thousand different strains of knockout mice have been created and are used to investigate specific functions of particular genes and mechanisms of drug action, including the sensitivity to general anesthetic in animals lacking the β_3 subunit[168] or the α_6 subunit[169] of the $GABA_A$ receptor. In contrast, *knock-in* animals express a site-directed mutation in the targeted gene that remains under the control of endogenous regulatory elements, allowing the mutated gene to be expressed in the same amount, at the same time, and in the same tissues as the normal gene. This method has provided remarkable insight into the mechanisms of action of benzodiazepines[170] and IV anesthetics. In a seminal study by Jurd et al, a point mutation in the gene encoding the β_3 subunit of the $GABA_A$ receptor, previously known to render the receptor insensitive to etomidate and propofol in vitro,[171] was validated in vivo by creating a knock-in mouse strain that proved also essentially insensitive to the immobilizing actions of etomidate and propofol.[172] A point mutation in the β_2 subunit of the $GABA_A$ receptor results in a knock-in mouse with reduced sensitivity to the sedative[173] and hypothermic effects[174] of etomidate. Knock-in mice harboring point mutations in the α_{2A}-adrenergic receptor have enabled the elucidation of the role of this receptor in anesthetic-sparing, analgesic, and sedative responses to dexmedetomidine.[175]

The situation is far more complex for inhaled anesthetics, which appear to mediate their effects by acting on several receptor targets. Based on combined pharmacologic and genetic in vivo studies to date, several receptors are unlikely to be direct mediators of MAC, including the $GABA_A$ (despite their compelling role in IV anesthetic-induced immobility), $5\text{-}HT_3$, AMPA, kainate, acetylcholine and α_2-adrenergic receptors, and potassium channels.[176] Glycine, NMDA receptors, and sodium channels remain likely candidates.[167] These conclusions, however, do not apply to other anesthetic end points, such as hypnosis, amnesia, and analgesia. Several preclinical proteomic analyses have identified in a more unbiased way a group of potential anesthetic targets for halothane,[61] desflurane,[62] and sevoflurane,[63] which should provide the basis for more focused studies of anesthetic binding sites. Such "omic" approaches have the potential to evolve into preoperative screening profiles useful in guiding individualized therapeutic decisions, such as prevention of anesthetic awareness in patients with a genetic predisposition to increased anesthetic requirements.

GENETIC VARIABILITY AND RESPONSE TO PAIN

Similar to the observed variability in anesthetic potency, the response to painful stimuli and analgesic manipulations varies among individuals. The sources of variability in the report and experience of pain and analgesia (ie, the so-called pain threshold) are multifactorial, including factors extrinsic to the organism (such as cultural factors or circadian rhythms) and intrinsic factors (such as age, gender, hormonal status, or genetic makeup). Increasing evidence suggests that pain behavior in response to noxious stimuli, its modulation by the central nervous system in response to drug administration or environmental stress, as well as the development of persistent pain conditions through pain amplification are strongly influenced by genetic factors.[177-179]

Results from studies in twins[180] and inbred mouse strains[181] indicate a moderate heritability for chronic pain syndromes and nociceptive sensitivity, which appears to be mediated by multiple genes. Various strains of knockout mice lacking target genes like neurotrophins and their receptors (eg, nerve growth factor), peripheral mediators of nociception, and hyperalgesia (eg, substance P), opioid and nonopioid transmitters and their receptors, and intracellular signaling molecules have significantly contributed to the understanding of pain processing mechanisms.[182] A locus responsible for 28% of phenotypic variance in magnitude of systemic morphine analgesia in mouse has been mapped to chromosome 10, in or near the *OPRM* (μ-opioid receptor) gene. The μ-opioid receptor is also subject to pharmacodynamic variability; polymorphisms in the promoter region of the *OPRM* gene modulating interleukin 4–mediated gene expression have been correlated with morphine antinociception. The much quoted *OPRM* 188A>G polymorphism is associated with decreased responses to morphine-6-glucuronide, resulting in altered analgesic requirements but also reduced incidence of postoperative nausea and vomiting, and reduced risks of toxicity in renal failure patients. Conversely, variants of the melanocortin 1 receptor (*MC1R*) gene, which produce a red hair/fair skin phenotype, are associated with increased analgesic responses to κ-opioid agonists in women but not men, providing evidence for a gene-by-gender interaction in regulating analgesic response (for a review, see Somogyi et al[183]). Very recent reports suggest that peripherally located β2-adrenergic receptors (*ADRB2*) also contribute to basal pain sensitivity, the development of chronic pain states, as well as opioid-induced hyperalgesia.[179] Functionally important haplotypes in the *ADRB2*[178] and catechol-O-methyltransferase (*COMT*)[184] genes are associated with enhanced pain sensitivity in humans.

In addition to the genetic control of peripheral nociceptive pathways, considerable evidence exists for genetic variability in the descending central pain modulatory pathways, further explaining the interindividual variability in analgesic responsiveness. One good example relevant to analgesic efficacy is cytochrome P450D6 (*CYP2D6*), a member of the superfamily of microsomal enzymes that catalyze phase I drug metabolism and are responsible for the metabolism of a large number of therapeutic compounds. The relationship between the *CYP2D6* genotype and the enzyme metabolic rate has been extensively characterized, with at least 12 known mutations leading to a tetramodal distribution CYP2D6 activity: ultrarapid metabolizers (5% to 7% of the population), extensive metabolizers (60%), intermediate metabolizers (25%), and poor metabolizers (10%). Currently, pharmacogenomic screening tests predict CYP2D6 phenotype with more than 95% reliability. The consequences of inheriting an allele that compromises CYP2D6 function include the inability to metabolize codeine (a prodrug) to morphine by O-demethylation, leading to lack of analgesia but increased side effects from the parent drug (eg, fatigue) in poor metabolizers.[160,177]

GENETIC VARIABILITY IN RESPONSE TO OTHER DRUGS USED PERIOPERATIVELY

A wide variety of drugs used in the perioperative period display significant pharmacokinetic or pharmacodynamic variability that is genetically modulated (**Table 4-7**). Although genetic variation in drug-metabolizing enzymes or targets usually results in hypervariable drug response, genetic markers associated with rare but life-threatening side effects have also been described. Of note, the most commonly cited categories of drugs involved in adverse drug reactions include cardiovascular, antibiotic, psychiatric, and analgesic medications, and interestingly, each category has a known genetic basis for an increased risk of adverse reactions.

There are more than 30 families of drug-metabolizing enzymes in humans, most with genetic polymorphisms shown to influence enzymatic activity. Of special importance to the anesthesiologists is the *CYP2D6*, one of the most intensively studied and best understood examples of pharmacogenetic variation, involved in the metabolism of several drugs including analgesics (codeine, dextromethorphan), β-blockers, antiarrhythmics (flecainide, propafenone, quinidine), and diltiazem. Another important pharmacogenetic variation has been

TABLE 4-7 Examples of Genetic Polymorphisms Involved in Variable Responses to Drugs Used in the Perioperative Period

Drug Class	Gene Name (Gene Symbol)	Effect of Polymorphism
	Pharmacokinetic Variability	
β-blockers	Cytochrome P450 2D6 (*CYP2D6*)	Enhanced drug effect
Codeine, dextromethorphan	*CYP2D6*	Decreased drug effect
Calcium channel blockers	Cytochrome P450 3A4 (*CYP3A4*)	Uncertain
Alfentanil	*CYP3A4*	Enhanced drug response
Angiotensin II receptor type 1 blockers	Cytochrome P450 2C9 (*CYP2C9*)	Enhanced blood pressure response
Warfarin	*CYP2C9*	Enhanced anticoagulant effect; risk of bleeding
Phenytoin	*CYP2C9*	Enhanced drug effect
Angiotensin-converting enzyme inhibitors	Angiotensin I converting enzyme (*ACE*)	Blood pressure response
Procainamide	N-acetyltransferase 2 (*NAT2*)	Enhanced drug effect
Succinylcholine	Butyrylcholinesterase (*BCHE*)	Enhanced drug effect
Digoxin	P-glycoprotein (*ABCB1, MDR1*)	Increased bioavailability
	Pharmacodynamic Variability	
β-blockers	β_1 and β_2 adrenergic receptors (*ADRB1, ADRB2*)	Blood pressure and heart rate response' airway responsiveness to β_2-agonists
QT-prolonging drugs (antiarrhythmics, cisapride, erythromycin, etc)	Sodium and potassium ion channels (*SCN5A, KCNH2, KCNE2, KCNQ1*)	Long QT syndrome; risk of torsade de pointes
Aspirin, glycoprotein IIb/IIIa inhibitors	Glycoprotein IIIa subunit of platelet glycoprotein IIb/IIIa (*ITGB3*)	Variability in antiplatelet effects
Phenylephrine	Endothelial nitric oxide synthase (*NOS3*)	Blood pressure response

described in cytochrome P450C9 (*CYP2C9*), involved in metabolizing anticoagulants (warfarin), anticonvulsants (phenytoin), antidiabetic agents (glipizide, tolbutamide), and nonsteroidal anti-inflammatory drugs (celecoxib, ibuprofen), among others. Three known *CYP2C9* variant alleles result in different enzyme activities (extensive, intermediate, and slow metabolizer phenotypes) and have clinical implications in the increased risk of life-threatening bleeding complications in slow metabolizers during standard warfarin therapy. This illustrates the concept of "high-risk pharmacokinetics," which applies to drugs with low therapeutic ratios eliminated by a single pathway (in this case CYP2C9-mediated oxidation); genetic variation in that pathway may lead to large changes in drug clearance, concentrations, and effects.[158] Dose adjustments based on the pharmacogenetic phenotype have been proposed for drugs metabolized via both CYP2D6 and CYP2C9 pathways,[160] and a commercially available approved test by the Food and Drug Administration (FDA) (CYP450 AmpliChip, Roche Molecular Diagnostics) allows clinicians for the first time to test patients for a wide spectrum of genetic variation in drug-metabolizing enzymes. Using this technology, Candiotti et al showed that patients carrying either 3 copies of the CYP2D6 gene, a genotype consistent with ultrarapid metabolism, or both have an increased risk of ondansetron failure for the prevention of postoperative vomiting but not nausea.[185] The strongest evidence to date for use of pharmacogenomic testing is to aid in the determination of warfarin dosage by using genotypes in the *CYP2C9* and vitamin K epoxide reductase complex 1 (*VKORC1*) genes, and at least four FDA-approved tests are now commercially available.

Genetic variation in drug targets (receptors) can have a profound effect on drug efficacy, and more than 25 examples have already been identified. For example, functional polymorphisms in the β_2-AR (Arg16Gly, Gln27Glu) influence the bronchodilator and vascular responses to β-agonists, and β_1-AR variants (Arg389Gly) modulate responses to β-blockers and may have an impact on postoperative cardiovascular-adverse events.[108,109]

Finally, clinically important genetic polymorphisms with indirect effects on drug response have been described. These include variants in candidate genes like sodium (*SCN5A*) and potassium ion channels (*KCNH2, KCNE2, KCNQ1*), which alter susceptibility to drug-induced long-QT syndrome and ventricular arrhythmias (torsade de pointes) associated with the use of drugs like erythromycin, terfenadine, disopyramide, sotalol, cisapride, or quinidine. Carriers of such susceptibility alleles have no manifest QT-interval prolongation or family history of sudden death until QT-prolonging drug challenge is superimposed.[158] Predisposition to QT-interval prolongation (considered a surrogate for risk of life-threatening ventricular arrhythmias) has been responsible for more drug withdrawals from the market than any other category of adverse event in recent times, so understanding genetic predisposing factors constitutes one of the highest priorities of current pharmacogenomic efforts.

Pharmacogenomics is emerging as an additional modifying component to anesthesia along with age, gender, comorbidities, and medication usage. Specific testing and treatment guidelines allowing clinicians to modify drug use appropriately (eg, adjust dose or change drug) already exist for a few compounds[160] and will likely be expanded to all relevant therapeutic compounds, together with identification of novel therapeutic targets.

FUTURE DIRECTIONS

SYSTEMS BIOLOGY APPROACH TO PERIOPERATIVE MEDICINE: THE "PERIOPTOME"

Systems biology is a conceptual framework within which scientists attempt to correlate massive amounts of apparently unrelated data into a single unifying explanation of how biologic processes occur.[186] This evolving discipline that merges experimental and computational approaches to observe, record, and integrate information from the molecular, cellular, tissue, and whole organism level into testable models of a dynamic biologic process can be applied to understand the way patients respond to a multidimensional stimulus such as a surgical procedure and the mechanistic basis of perioperative morbidity. Such an approach involves multiple levels of data integration. First, delineating the composition of the *perioperative phenome* (the representation of all perioperative phenotypes expressed by a given patient) requires standardized definitions, controlled vocabularies, and data dictionaries (a perioperative phenotype ontology), new (molecular) imaging technologies, and the availability of comprehensive data warehousing capabilities that will allow cataloging of individual perioperative phenotypes as well as correlations between combinations of phenotypes (organ cross-talk, multiple organ failure). Second, the orthogonal integration of whole-genome genotypic, transcriptomic, proteomic, and metabolomic data, augmented by more recent functional genomic and proteomic approaches including protein–protein, protein–DNA, or other "component–component" interaction mapping (*interactome*), transcript, or protein three-dimensional localization mapping (*localizome*),[187] and literature data within individual biologic systems involved in perioperative morbidity. This highest level of data integration is the mapping of the integrated high-throughput static and dynamic genomic data into regulatory networks to model interactions of the different components of the system and identify modules of highly interconnected genes and hub points that can be prioritized as therapeutic targets. Ultimately, mathematical models require experimental validation in animal models of disease or tissue culture, in an iterative process that is one of the core characteristics of systems biology.[188] Such integrative approaches to study cardiovascular function (the Cardiome Project), but also perioperative morbidity (the Perioptome)[189] have already been outlined, and they promise to increase the identification of key drivers of perioperative adverse events beyond what could be achieved by genetic associations alone.

TARGETED THERAPEUTIC APPLICATIONS: THE "5 P'S" OF PERIOPERATIVE MEDICINE AND PAIN MANAGEMENT

Genomic and proteomic approaches are rapidly becoming platforms for all aspects of drug discovery and development, from target identification and validation to individualization of drug therapy. As mentioned, the human genome contains about 26,000 genes encoding for approximately 200,000 proteins that represent potential drug targets. However, only about 120 drug targets are currently being marketed, thus making identification of novel therapeutic targets an area of intense research. Following gene identification, its therapeutic potential needs to be validated by defining the sequence function, its role in disease, and demonstrating that the gene product can be manipulated with beneficial effect and no toxic effects. A developing field, *toxicogenomics*, studies the influence of toxic or potentially toxic substances on different model organisms by evaluating the gene expression changes induced by novel drugs in a given tissue. Sponsored by the National Institutes of Health, a nationwide collaborative effort called the Pharmacogenetics Research Network (http://www.nigms.nih.gov/pharmacogenetics/) is aiming to establish a strong pharmacogenomics knowledge base (http://www.pharmgkb.org/) as well as create a shared computational and experimental infrastructure required to connect human sequence variation with drug responses and translate information into novel therapeutics.

The epidemiologic framework for assessing the applicability of previously identified biomarkers of perioperative morbidity and the successful implementation of molecular diagnostics in perioperative medicine is contingent on demonstrating their *clinical validity, analytical validity*, and *clinical utility*.[190] Perioperative genomic investigators are currently conducting replication studies in different surgical patient populations to formally assess the clinical validity of the markers reported so far. For genomic classifiers, the emphasis during external validation is placed on prospectively testing the accuracy of the entire molecular fingerprint in a new patient population rather than corroborating results in individual genes. In perioperative and critical care settings, it is vital to have fast turnaround time (several hours) and easy-to-use testing capabilities, so that meaningful therapeutic interventions can take place. In this regard, new molecular diagnostic systems based on the random access technology such as the GeneXpert (Cepheid), eSensor (Osmetech), and Liat Analyzer (Iquum) are already becoming available. Clinical utility (targeted interventions to reduce perioperative morbidity among patients with a certain genomic profile) remains to be evaluated in future genomically stratified perioperative trials. Indeed, a landmark study on the effects of a 5-lipoxygenase–activating protein (FLAP) inhibitor on biomarkers associated with the risk of MI demonstrates that by defining at-risk patients for two genes in the leukotriene pathway, one can predict who will respond to targeted drug therapy. Specifically, in patients carrying the at-risk variants in FLAP and in the leukotriene A4 hydrolase genes, use of a FLAP inhibitor in a randomized controlled trial resulted in significant and dose-dependent suppression of biomarkers associated with increased risk of MI.[191] It is expected that similar principles of targeted therapeutics could be operational in the perioperative period, thus beginning to fulfill the 5 P's of modern medicine (*p*ersonalized, *p*reventive, *p*redictive, *p*articipatory, and *p*rospective).

ETHICAL CONSIDERATIONS

Although one of the aims of the Human Genome Project is to improve therapy through genome-based prediction, the birth of personal genomics opens up a Pandora's box of ethical issues, including privacy and the risk for discrimination against individuals who are genetically predisposed for a medical disorder. Such discrimination may include barriers to obtaining health, life, or long-term care insurance or obtaining employment. Thus extensive efforts are made to protect patients participating in genetic research from prejudice, discrimination, or uses of genetic information that will adversely affect them. To address the concerns of both biomedical research and health communities, the U.S. Senate approved in 2003 the Genetic Information and Nondiscrimination Act, which provides the strong safeguards required to protect the public participating in human genome research.

Another ethical concern is the transferability of genetic tests across ethnic groups, particularly in the prediction of adverse drug responses. It is known that most polymorphisms associated with variability in drug response show significant differences in allele frequencies among populations and racial groups. Furthermore, the patterns of linkage disequilibrium are markedly different between ethnic groups, which may lead to spurious findings when markers, instead of causal variants, are used in diagnostic tests extrapolated across populations. In exploring racial disparities in health and disease outcomes, considerable debate has focused on whether race and ethnic identity are primarily social or biologic constructs, and the contribution of genetic variability in explaining observed differences in the rates of disease between racial groups. With the goal of personalized medicine the prediction of risk and treatment of disease on the basis of an individual's genetic profile, some have argued that biologic consideration of race will become obsolete. However, in this discovery phase of the postgenome era, continuing to incorporate racial information in genetic studies should improve our understanding of the architecture of the human genome and its implications for novel strategies aiming at identifying variants protecting against, or conferring susceptibility to, common diseases and modulating drug effects.[192]

CONCLUSIONS

The Human Genome Project has revolutionized all aspects of medicine, allowing us to assess the impact of genetic variability on disease taxonomy, characterization, and outcome, and individual responses to various drugs and injuries. Mechanistically, information gleaned through genomic approaches is already unraveling long-standing mysteries behind general anesthetic action and adverse responses to drugs used perioperatively. However, a strong need remains for prospective, well-powered genetic studies in highly phenotyped surgical populations, which require the development of multidimensional perioperative databases. For the anesthesiologist, this may soon translate into prospective risk assessment incorporating genetic profiling of markers important in thrombotic, inflammatory, vascular, and neurologic responses to perioperative stress, with implications ranging from individualized additional preoperative testing and physiologic optimization, to choice of perioperative monitoring strategies and critical care resource utilization. Furthermore, genetic profiling of drug metabolizing enzymes, carrier proteins, and receptors, using currently available high-throughput molecular technologies, will enable personalized choice of drugs and dosage regimens tailored to suit a patient's pharmacogenetic profile. At that point, perioperative physicians will have far more robust information to use in designing the most appropriate and safest anesthetic plan for a given patient.

Future trends and challenges in perioperative genomics are still being defined, but they mainly concern interdisciplinary studies designed to combine an analytical system approach, mathematical modeling, and engineering principles with the multiple molecular and genetic factors and stimuli, and the macroscale interactions that determine the pathophysiologic response to surgery.

Acknowledgments: Supported in part by NIH grants HL075273 and HL092071 (to MVP).

KEY REFERENCES

- Ashley EA, Butte AJ, Wheeler MT, et al. Clinical assessment incorporating a personal genome. *Lancet.* 2010;375:1525-1535.
- Body SC, Collard CD, Shernan SK, et al. Variation in the 4q25 chromosomal locus predicts atrial fibrillation after coronary artery bypass graft surgery. *Circ Cardiovasc Genet.* 2009;2:499-506.
- Diatchenko L, Nackley AG, Tchivileva IE, et al. Genetic architecture of human pain perception. *Trends Genet.* 2007;23:605-613.
- Feero WG, Guttmacher AE, Collins FS. Genomic medicine—an updated primer. *N Engl J Med.* 2010;362:2001-2011.
- Fox AA, Collard CD, Shernan SK, et al. Natriuretic peptide system gene variants are associated with ventricular dysfunction after coronary artery bypass grafting. *Anesthesiology.* 2009;110:738-747.
- Fox AA, Muehlschlegel JD, Body SC, et al. Comparison of the utility of preoperative versus postoperative B-type natriuretic peptide for predicting hospital length of stay and mortality after primary coronary artery bypass grafting. *Anesthesiology.* 2010;112:842-851.
- Mathew JP, Podgoreanu MV, Grocott HP, et al. Genetic variants in P-selectin and C-reactive protein influence susceptibility to cognitive decline after cardiac surgery. *J Am Coll Cardiol.* 2007;49:1934-1942.
- Muehlschlegel JD, Liu KY, Perry TE, et al. Chromosome 9p21 variant predicts mortality after coronary artery bypass graft surgery. *Circulation.* 2010;122:S60-S65.
- Podgoreanu MV, Schwinn DA. New paradigms in cardiovascular medicine: emerging technologies and practices: perioperative genomics. *J Am Coll Cardiol.* 2005;46:1965-1977.
- Podgoreanu MV, White WD, Morris RW, et al. Inflammatory gene polymorphisms and risk of postoperative myocardial infarction after cardiac surgery. *Circulation.* 2006;114:1275-1281.
- Rosenberg S, Elashoff MR, Beineke P, et al. Multicenter validation of the diagnostic accuracy of a blood-based gene expression test for assessing obstructive coronary artery disease in nondiabetic patients. *Ann Intern Med.* 2010;153:425-434.

- Turer AT, Stevens RD, Bain JR, et al. Metabolomic profiling reveals distinct patterns of myocardial substrate use in humans with coronary artery disease or left ventricular dysfunction during surgical ischemia/reperfusion. *Circulation.* 2009;119:1736-1746.
- Zaugg M, Bestmann L, Wacker J, et al. Adrenergic receptor genotype but not perioperative bisoprolol therapy may determine cardiovascular outcome in at-risk patients undergoing surgery with spinal block: the Swiss Beta Blocker in Spinal Anesthesia (BBSA) study: a double-blinded, placebo-controlled, multicenter trial with 1-year follow-up. *Anesthesiology.* 2007;107:33-44.

REFERENCES

Complete references available on DVD and online version at www.LongneckerAnesthesiology.com

CHAPTER 5 Ethics and Conflicts of Interest in Anesthesia Practice

David B. Waisel

KEY POINTS

1. Treat patients and families with the grace and consideration you would want for your family.
2. The goal of informed consent is to maximize the ability of the patient to make substantially informed autonomous decisions.
3. Physicians are obligated to protect patient information from unauthorized and unnecessary disclosure.
4. Patients with limited decision-making capacity should participate in decision making to the extent their capacity permits.
5. Competent patients have a virtually unlimited right to refuse life-sustaining medical treatment.
6. The risk of liability for honoring properly documented do-not-resuscitate (DNR) orders is no more than the risk of not honoring it.
7. Patients opting for goal-directed perioperative DNR orders usually choose to authorize temporary therapeutic interventions to manage easily reversible events.
8. Anesthesiologists face conflicts of interest in daily practice from production pressure, interactions with industry, and safety and quality care initiatives. Anesthesiologists need to recognize potential conflicts, characterize the potential severity of the conflict, and determine the likelihood and resultant harm of the influence or the appearance of influence.
9. The discipline of medical ethics provides expertise in recognizing, analyzing, and managing ethical dilemmas.
10. Anesthesiologists are obligated to "own" the advancement and advocacy of all things anesthesiology.

PATIENT–PHYSICIAN RELATIONSHIP

The goal of informed consent is to enable patients to make substantially autonomous informed decisions.[1,2] The modifier "substantial" emphasizes that the realistic goal for consent is to sufficiently, as compared to fully, inform the patient.

COMPONENTS OF INFORMED CONSENT

Decision-Making Capacity Patients have decision-making capacity when they are capable of making a specific decision at a specific time. Patients show capacity by understanding proposed treatments, alternatives, consequences of proceeding or not proceeding, and the ability to express a preference based on rational, internally consistent reasoning. Decision-making capacity is different than competency. The clinician at the bedside determines decision-making capacity for a specific decision, whereas competency is a legal determination of the global abilities required to provide legal and other authorizations. Adults are presumed competent.

Anesthesiologists should pay particular attention to the decision-making capacity of patients with temporary or more permanent limitations in decision-making capacity.[3] Patients with more permanent limitations in decision-making capacity should be encouraged to participate in decision making to the extent of their abilities. Sedated patients with temporarily limited decision-making capacity should be assessed for decision-making capacity with regard to the specific decision. Decisions with riskier consequences require more comprehensive decision-making capacity. In patients with temporarily insufficient decision-making capacity, anesthesiologists should delay nonemergent care until patients regain sufficient decision-making capacity.

Voluntariness Physicians should only perform procedures on competent patients who participate willingly. Anesthesiologists manipulate patients by distorting, downplaying, or omitting information to influence decision making. Anesthesiologists hinder voluntariness when they chemically or physically restrain patients who have sufficient decision-making capacity.[4] For example, in *Shine v Vega,* Shine, a competent adult, went to the hospital for treatment for an asthma attack.[5] The emergency department attending Vega recommended tracheal intubation. Shine refused. Later, Shine and her sister tried to leave but were forcibly detained. Shine was restrained and Vega intubated her trachea.[6] The Massachusetts Supreme Court stated that the competent patient has a right to refuse potentially life-sustaining treatment, even if her decision is considered unwise.

Disclosure Disclosure is the process of supplying relevant information to the decision maker. Skilled disclosure builds trust and facilitates patient self-determination.

The predominant legal standard in the United States is the reasonable person standard that requires disclosure of information based on what a theoretical reasonable person would consider material for decision making.[7] However, the preferences of the reasonable person are not precisely defined by statute or case law. Further, patients vary in their desire to receive information. For example, one typical study found that 10% of patients did not want to know alternative methods for anesthesia, 7% did not want to know about preoperative medications, 11% did not want to know all possible complications, and 10% did not want to know dangerous complications.[8] Patient preferences for disclosure cannot be wholly predicted from socioeconomic status, age, sex, ethnicity, and history of previous surgery.[9-11] Variation in anesthesiologists' customary practices of risk disclosure indicates the complexity of using the "reasonable person" standard to guide clinical practice.[12,13] For example, in one typical survey, approximately half of the respondents disclosed transient or persistent neuropathy as a risk for central neuraxial blockade.[14]

These data indicate that rather than presenting a standard laundry list of data, anesthesiologists should tailor information to the preferences of the patient. Anesthesiologists do this by highlighting options that affect the perioperative experience, such as regional versus general anesthesia, and by informing patients about significant risks that the anesthesiologist considers relevant to decision making. Anesthesiologists should also prepare patients for common but less severe risks, such as postoperative nausea and vomiting. Patients should be informed whether trainees are participating in care.[15,16]

To customize disclosure, anesthesiologists may then ask patients whether they want more information. For example, if there are no significant risks relevant to decision making, the anesthesiologists can say, "There are significant but very rare risks of receiving anesthesia. Would you like me to tell you about them"? Although the likelihood of being sued based on informed consent malpractice issues is very rare, increasing satisfaction by meeting the patients' needs likely decreases complaints and lawsuits. In any case, disclosure does not prevent medical malpractice liability for adverse events. Liability is based on negligence theory and depends mainly on whether the standard of care was met and if the failure to meet the standard of care was a proximate cause of injury.

The original concept of therapeutic privilege permitted physicians to withhold information if disclosure would prevent patients from making a rational decision. More recently, some suggest a valid use for therapeutic privilege is to give patients time to adjust to jarring events, to prevent stress-impaired decision making, and to preserve hope.[17,18]

Recommendation Anesthesiologists should highlight the advantages and disadvantages of options, and recommend a plan by explaining how well each option suits the patient's preferences.

Understanding It is difficult to determine if a patient substantially understands the risks, benefits, and indications of the proposed procedures.[19-21] Translating population data into data relevant and understandable to the patient is problematic.[22] Numerous biases affect both physician and patient understanding of risks. In addition, patients commonly misunderstand frequently used terms such as *anaphylaxis, antibiotics, aspiration, fasting, local anesthesia, reflux, and sedation.*[23,24]

"Teach-back" has been suggested to assess patient understanding during the informed consent process. Patients are asked to articulate key information about the proposed treatment to help physicians redress gaps or misunderstandings. There is insufficient literature about whether "teach-back" improves the quality of understanding and therefore improves informed consent. Although superficially this seems like a potentially beneficial and harmless technique, how "teach-back" is performed will likely affect whether patients view this as a positive interaction. Perhaps the benefit of "teach-back" simply will be the greater focus on assessing patient understanding.

Most research relating to understanding is based on the less applicable surrogate end points of recall of information or patient satisfaction. Recalling information does not reflect the ability of patients to understand and use information, and lack of recall does not mean inadequate understanding and use of information. Recall is generally poor.[25,26] Even the most successful interventions improve recall only to about 50% of the presented information. Written information for patients to review may improve recall.[27-29] Pain and distress do not seem to compromise the ability to recall risks, particularly among parturients.[10,30-32]

Decision Patients vary in their preferences for participation in decision making. The desire to participate in the decision-making process may be a function of the individual, extent of illness, gender, age, and level of education. Older studies indicate that younger patients and more formally educated patients tended to prefer more significant participation in decision making.[9,33-36,37] These preferences are more likely due to generational differences than absolute age, and therefore it should be assumed that older patients are by now also more likely to prefer greater participation in decision making. It is legally and ethically superior for anesthesiologists to tailor participation in decision making to the patient.[38]

Anesthesiologists should obtain *informed refusal* when patients refuse recommendations or request a relevantly suboptimal technique. The concept underlying informed refusal is that these patients need to be more extensively informed about risks, benefits, and alternatives when they desire inadvisable techniques. Anesthesiologists are not ethically obligated to provide care for these patients in nonemergent situations, although they may wish to assist in finding a willing colleague.

Autonomous Authorization Anesthesiologists should seek the patient's explicit authorization to perform a specific procedure.

ISSUES IN INFORMED CONSENT

Refusing to Provide Care Society's interest in preserving the moral fabric of individual physicians permits anesthesiologists to withdraw from care with which they morally disagree, such as the elective termination of pregnancy. Anesthesiologists may be obligated to make a reasonable effort to find a willing colleague, although some find this recommendation ethically objectionable.[39] There is controversy about whether anesthesiologists should perform emergent care that violates their conscience. Some argue that the altruistic obligation toward patients cannot supersede a physician's most cherished values. Others argue that medicine is first and foremost a service profession, and in extreme circumstances physician are obligated to put patients first. This argument is in part based on the social contract the profession of medicine has with society.[40] Although this situation rarely occurs in clinical practice, the role of the physician vis-à-vis the patient is worthy of consideration.

Although anesthesiologists may refuse to provide care when a patient makes a sufficiently inappropriate request, this determination should be made only after extensive consideration and perhaps consultation with colleagues. Anesthesiologists may not refuse to care for patients based on race, gender, or disease status, such as the patient with an infectious disease.[41] Anesthesiologists should refuse to provide nonemergent care if they do not feel that the environment, including their own and other clinicians' abilities, operating room capabilities, and consultative and postoperative care, provides a sufficient quality of care.

Emergency Situations Anesthesiologists should seek informed consent as practicable in emergency situations. The assumption is that patients want potentially life-sustaining therapy. Reversibility is the key to determining how to intervene when there is incomplete evidence that the patient would prefer not to receive emergency treatment. For example, because tracheal intubation is reversible, it is appropriate to intubate the trachea of the unconscious patient when there is insufficient documentation of preferences, even if a relative declares that the patient's preferences would be to refuse tracheal intubation. Therapy may be withdrawn later if appropriate. In this case, the slight burden of temporary tracheal intubation is traded for improved clarification and certainty of the patient's wishes.

Irreversible interventions do not offer this opportunity. Consider the unconscious Jehovah's Witness patient with a critically low hemoglobin. Transfusion represents irreversible contamination. However, because the standard is an explicit refusal of potentially life-sustaining treatment, anesthesiologists should probably provide transfusion in the absence of unambiguous evidence.

Jehovah's Witness Jehovah's Witnesses interpret biblical scripture to mean that those who take in human blood shall be "cut off" from eternal life.[42] Case law unequivocally supports the rights of adult patients to refuse transfusion therapy.[43] In particular, physicians have not been held liable when honoring a parturient's properly documented refusal of transfusion therapy, even in the face of maternal or fetal death.[44]

Jehovah's Witness patients consider transfusion therapy preferences as a "matter of conscience." Primary concerns center on whether it is blood from another human and whether their own blood has been outside of the body. Thus blood components, autologous blood, and banked blood are generally unacceptable. Some patients will accept blood harvested intraoperatively and returned while being kept in a closed loop, such as with cell salvage of shed blood or presurgical removal of blood. Some patients will accept recombinant erythropoietin, which depending on the brand contains small amounts of human albumin. Acceptable techniques include synthetic colloid solutions, erythropoietin-stimulating protein, and preoperative iron.

Precisely documenting patient preferences forces clarification of acceptable interventions. Nonemergent care should proceed only if all clinicians are wholly certain they can satisfy the patient's requirements.

Confidentiality Physicians are obligated to protect patient information from unauthorized and unnecessary disclosure. For example, anesthesiologists should seek permission from patients before sharing information

TABLE 5-1 Graduated Involvement of Minors in Medical Decision Making

This broad outline should be viewed as a guide. Specific circumstances should be taken into consideration.

Age	Decision-Making Capacity	Techniques
< 6 y	None	Best interest standard
6-12 y	Developing	Informed permission Informed assent
13-18 y	Mostly developed	Informed assent Informed permission
Mature minor	Developed, as legally determined by a judge, for a specific decision	Informed consent
Emancipated minor	Developed, as determined by statutes defining eligible situations (eg, being married, in the military, economically independent)	Informed consent

with family members. Anesthesiologists should be aware of and should seek to comply with public privacy guidelines. In particular, electronic medical and financial records may lead to inappropriate distribution of sensitive personal information.[45] Exceptions to confidentiality rules include when a patient makes a credible threat to harm someone.

Pediatric Ethics Patients, parents, other surrogate decision makers, and physicians use the concepts of best interest, informed assent, and informed permission to guide decision making about health care for minors (**Table 5-1**).[46] The best interest standard is used when the ability to apply self-determination is impossible, such as with an infant or a child with severe developmental delay. The parent or surrogate decision maker should then apply what they believe to be in the best interests of the child, but this decision must be within an acceptable range of decision making. Parents may not opt for grossly inappropriate overtreatment or undertreatment.[47] Whether anesthesiologists should intervene about potentially inappropriate treatment depends primarily on the amount of harm to the child by the therapy or its absence, the likelihood of a successful therapy, and the overall risk-to-benefit ratio. Interventions include ethics consultation, legal consultation, and legal intervention. The term *informed permission* has been suggested to emphasize that only the individual receiving care can provide informed consent and therefore the parent or surrogate decision maker is more accurately providing permission.

Pediatric patients should participate in decision making to the extent their development permits. Anesthesiologists therefore should incorporate informed assent with older children. The extent of participation of children should increase throughout adolescence depending on the patient's maturity and the consequences of the decision. Anesthesiologists should go out of their way to respect the right of adolescents not to assent to a procedure. In those cases, achieving assent may necessitate further discussions with patients, parents, and other clinicians, and such discussions may best take place away from the operating room.

Loss of confidentiality may lead adolescent to curtail or delay seeking medical care, or be less forthright about information, particularly when care involve sexually transmitted infections, contraception, and mental health.[48-50] Anesthesiologists may want to ask sensitive questions privately. Although anesthesiologists should encourage adolescents to be forthright with their parents, anesthesiologists should maintain the confidentiality of adolescents unless prohibited by reporting statues.[51] Of particular relevance, state statutes may limit the anesthesiologist to informing *only* the adolescent about a positive pregnancy test.

Emancipated minors and adolescents declared mature minors are authorized to make their own health care decisions. States statutes may award emancipated minor status to adolescents in the military, who are married, who have children, and who are economically independent. Judges may award mature minor status if the adolescent is capable of giving legal consent in a specific situation.[52] Judges base mature minor decisions on the maturity of the child and the consequences of the decision.

Disclosure and Apology Patients desire appropriate disclosures and apologies about medical errors.[53] On the whole, physicians and administrators agree. But fear, lack of training, and inadequate support limits the ability of physicians to disclose and apologize.[53-56]

More than half the states have laws prohibiting the admission of apology or sympathy as evidence of wrongdoing.[57] Nonetheless, the quality of these laws vary and an apology conceivably may influence whether legal action is sought or is successful.[58,59] But in the long run, sincere disclosures and apologies followed by appropriate post-event actions improve patient satisfaction and trust, possibly forestalling legal action.[38] Consider the alternative: Hiding or dissembling about an event infuriates patients and will likely spur a lawsuit.

When disclosing potential errors, anesthesiologists should be very precise about communicating only what is known. Anesthesiologists should not speculate about what is not known, particularly about fault. Initial disclosure should occur promptly and should focus on the medical implications of the event.[60] A specific permanent contact person should be identified to be the liaison for the patient and family. The contact person should be able to answer questions, arrange meetings, explain the results of the investigation, and describe the plan to prevent comparable events.

The quality of the apology matters. It is very appropriate to apologize for the effects of an event. Although anesthesiologists should generally not assume responsibility for an event during the initial disclosure and apology, it seems bizarre to evade responsibility for a clear error. Dodging responsibility in that situation likely delegitimizes the apology in the patient's eyes.

ETHICAL AND LEGAL ASPECTS OF END-OF-LIFE CARE

The Supreme Court has grounded the virtually unlimited right of a competent patient to refuse treatment in the liberty interest of the Fourteenth Amendment, which states, "No State shall make or enforce any law which shall abridge the privileges or immunities of citizens of the United States; nor shall any State deprive any person of life, liberty or property."[61]

For the incompetent patient, formal written or oral directives are the preferred method of directing end-of-life care.[62] If a patient does not have declared preferences, surrogates direct care by using their judgment of what the patient would have chosen. This is known as *substituted judgment,* and it is presumably based on intimate knowledge of the patient. Nonetheless, making these choices burden surrogates. For the never competent patient, the best interest standard is used.

A *substituted interests* model proposes that clinicians integrate substituted judgment and best interests.[63] Surrogates articulate the patient's values and beliefs, which is less burdensome than declaring the patient's specific preferences. Clinicians and surrogates then work together to determine what would be in the best interest of the specific patient. Physicians familiar with the patient's values may alleviate surrogates' burdens by having knowledgeable people with whom to share the decision making.

PERIOPERATIVE LIMITATIONS ON POTENTIALLY LIFE-SUSTAINING THERAPY

The rights of patients to limit unwanted perioperative therapy is well accepted. Patients implement limitations on cardiopulmonary resuscitation (commonly known as DNR [do-not-resuscitate] orders) because the likely burdens outweigh the potential benefits. Patients with DNR orders reasonably seek invasive therapy to improve their quality of life while rejecting the burdens of perioperative resuscitation. Patients seek interventions to reduce pain, improve vascular access, and treat urgent problems unrelated to the primary disease. But desiring these benefits

TABLE 5-2 Components of a Perioperative Do-Not-Resuscitate Discussion[66,78]

- Planned procedure and anticipated benefit
- Advantages and opportunities of having specific, identified clinicians providing therapy for a defined period
- Likelihood of requiring resuscitation
- Reversibility of likely causes requiring resuscitation
- Description of potential interventions and their consequences
- Chances of successful resuscitation including improved outcomes of witnessed arrests compared with unwitnessed arrests
- Ranges of outcomes with and without resuscitation
- Responses to iatrogenic events
- Intended and possible venues and types of postoperative care
- Postoperative timing and mechanisms for reevaluation of the DNR order
- Establishment of an agreement through a goal-directed approach or revocation of the DNR order for the perioperative period
- Documentation

DNR, do not resuscitate.

does not minimize their desire to avoid potential burdens of resuscitation such as extensive ventilatory support, cognitive deficits, or physical limitations that can follow resuscitation. "Potentially" modifies "life-sustaining therapy" to emphasize the uncertainty that a therapy will be life sustaining. Keeping this doubt in mind may help anesthesiologists communicate more successfully with patients.

The American Society of Anesthesiologists and the American College of Surgeons recommend mandatory reevaluation of preoperative DNR orders before proceeding with invasive interventions.[64,65] Reevaluation should consider the goals for surgery and end-of-life care.[66] In reevaluating the DNR order, anesthesiologists should emphasize pertinent differences between perioperative and ward care (**Table 5-2**). Perioperative clinicians can weigh the etiology of the event, the effects of clinical interventions, and a detailed knowledge of the goals for end-of-life care to tailor the extent of resuscitation to the likelihood of achieving those goals.

Perioperative DNR orders should be clarified and documented using the goal-directed approach.[66] The goal-directed approach permits patients to communicate their goals for surgery and end-of-life care in terms of outcomes. ("I do not want to suffer for my last 3 months in the intensive care unit.") Patients then authorize anesthesiologists to use clinical judgment to determine how specific interventions will affect achieving the goals. Contemporaneous decisions about using and continuing specific interventions are more likely to be consistent with end-of-life goals. The goal-directed approach promotes trials of therapy such as cardioversion that test assumptions about whether a therapy will achieve the patient's goals. Because witnessed arrests receive immediate therapy for a cause that is likely known, outcomes are typically better than unwitnessed ward arrests.[67,68]

The flexibility inherent in goal-directed approaches enables perioperative physicians to honor patients' desires without getting "caught" in a technicality. In contrast, typical ward procedure-directed approaches listing acceptable interventions (eg, tracheal intubation, chest compressions, etc) are too inflexible for use in the operating room. For example, restrictions on resuscitation intended to limit lengthy and burdensome therapy are not intended to prevent a time-limited intervention to reverse a temporary process.

Reevaluation should include determining preferences for postoperative trials of therapy. Anesthesiologists should consult with the physicians responsible for postoperative care to ensure that those physicians have adequate understanding of the goals of end-of-life care. It is also wise to ensure that advance directives are prepared.

Patients opting for goal-directed perioperative DNR orders usually choose to authorize temporary therapeutic interventions to manage easily reversible events, but they reject interventions likely to result in permanent sequelae, such as neurologic impairment or dependence on life-sustaining technology.[64] For example, a dysrhythmia that responds quickly to intravenous therapy and cardioversion would be characterized as a temporary, easily reversible event unlikely to have significant sequelae. But extended therapy would be more likely to result in unacceptable burdens and postoperative decrements in functional status. In that case, it would be appropriate to cease resuscitation. Anesthesiologists should base decisions on continuing resuscitation on the likelihoods of outcomes; absolute certainty is not only *not required* but is also a standard that impairs honoring the patient's goals to avoid end-of-life burdens.

Iatrogenicity should not influence the extent of resuscitation.[69-71] Patients initiate DNR orders to minimize potential burdens. From the patient's perspective, the outcome is relevant, not the cause. Anesthesiologists should base the extent of the resuscitation on achieving the patient's goals.

The "temporary and reversible" goal-directed perioperative DNR order can be documented as "The patient desires resuscitative efforts during surgery and in the PACU only if the adverse events are believed to be both temporary and reversible, in the clinical judgment of the attending anesthesiologists and surgeons."[64] With the patient's permission, anesthesiologists may want to include selected family members in the reevaluation discussion to enable the best communication of the patient's preferences.

BARRIERS TO HONORING LIMITATIONS ON POTENTIALLY LIFE-SUSTAINING THERAPY

Barriers to honoring limitations on potentially life-sustaining therapy center on clinician attitudes and inadequate knowledge about policy, law, and ethics (**Table 5-3**).[72-76] Clinicians tend to honor limitations on resuscitation in patients who are closer to dying and patients seeking palliative therapy. However, patients prioritize functional status when choosing to limit resuscitation.[77]

Clinicians often believe that policy or law requires full resuscitation during the perioperative period. The risk of liability for honoring properly documented DNR orders is no more than the risk of not honoring it.[78] In addition, many states include clinician immunity provisions in statues addressing DNR orders.[78] Immunity provisions tend to protect clinicians from liability as long as they follow statutory requirements

TABLE 5-3 Barriers to Limitations on Potentially Life-Sustaining Therapy[72-76]

Anesthesiologists may care for patients who would appear to benefit from limitations on potentially life-sustaining therapy. Although the choice may be well considered, at times barriers prevent thoughtful assessment of the goals of end-of-life care. Understanding these barriers may be helpful.

Patient and Family Barriers

- Unrealistic expectations about prognosis or effectiveness of treatment
- Inadequate education/guidance from clinicians
- Guilt (often arising from minimal contact with the patient) leading to overtreatment
- Emotional overtones of "causing death"
- Stories about "miraculous" cures
- Mistrust of clinicians, hospitals, or medical system
- Personal beliefs
- Denial of death

Clinician Barriers

- No process in place for addressing end-of-life goals
- Unrealistic expectations about prognosis or effectiveness of treatment
- Inadequate communication with patient or surrogates regarding end-of-life goals
- Inadequate communication among clinicians regarding end-of-life goals
- Disagreement among clinicians about the benefit-to-burden ratio of treatment
- Influence from recent personal, hospital, or national events
- No clearly identified physician coordinating care

and act in good faith. In clinical practice, inadequate time and a lack of standardized procedures impair the reevaluation of the DNR order.

FUTILE THERAPY AND INADVISABLE CARE

Futile therapy is best defined as treatments unable to achieve a specific goal, such as maintaining sinus rhythm. Defining futile therapy as achieving physiologic goals means that dilemmas about implementing futile therapy seldom occur. But dilemmas do occur in therapy that may be inadvisable because of a questionable benefit-to-burden ratio as defined by the patient.

Discussions about inadvisable care begin with a careful evaluation of the goals of the therapies under consideration. Decision makers should understand whether the predicted outcomes are based on intuition, clinical experience, or sufficiently relevant scientific studies. The options and likely outcomes should then be considered in light of the patient's end-of-life goals.

Hospitals should have inadvisable care policies. Good policies are public and explicate procedures for identifying stakeholders, implementing the policy, resolving conflicts, and initiating appellate mechanisms. As with all potentially controversial policies, public policies that reflect the values of the community are more likely to be successful.[79]

In 1999 a modification to the Texas law permitted a due process approach to resolving disputes about appropriate care.[80] Physicians were permitted to request an ethics committee review of potentially nonbeneficial life-sustaining therapy. If the ethics committee agreed that the therapy was nonbeneficial, the treatment was considered inadvisable and could be unilaterally withheld or withdrawn by the physician if the patient could not be transferred within a 10-day waiting period.

Although there is no central repository for these data, effects of this statute were reviewed in a 2004 survey of Texas hospitals.[81] In 70% of cases, the ethics committee concurred with the physician's assessment. Of those cases, 40% of families withdrew therapy upon knowledge of the committee's agreement with the physician, an additional 44% of patients died during the 10-day waiting period, 17% of patients were transferred, and 4% of patient improved (some patients were assigned to more than one category). Resolving conflicts about inadvisable care by due process through an ethics committee instead of honoring patient or surrogate preferences may be the vanguard for future policies or may be a temporary aberration.

MANAGING POTENTIAL CONFLICTS OF INTEREST

Conflict of interest has been defined as "a set of conditions in which professional judgment concerning a primary interest (such as patient's welfare or the validity of research) tends to be unduly influenced by a secondary interest.[82] Although commonly viewed as financial benefits, secondary interests also include personal and professional gains such as prestige, promotion, personal gratification, and respect.[83,84] Conflict of interest is characterized as "potential" because individuals are placed in situations that create the opportunity for conflicts of interest. The goal is to recognize and manage the ever-present potential conflicts of interest.[85] Anesthesiologists need to recognize potential conflicts, characterize the potential severity of the conflicts, and determine the likelihood and resultant harm of the influence or the appearance of influence.[82]

Production Pressure Anesthesiologists face potential conflicts of interest from production pressure. Production pressure is "the internal or external pressure on the anesthesiologist to keep the operating room schedule moving along speedily."[86] Production pressure can influence clinical practice by affecting the extent of preoperative discussions, the postponement of cases, the use of invasive monitoring, and the placement of catheters for postoperative analgesia. Production pressure may encourage anesthesiologists to provide anesthesia outside of their skill set or in inappropriate situations. Secondary gains for anesthesiologists may include increased referrals, positive feedback, heightened reputation, and misplaced internal pride. Anesthesiologists should carefully consider and frequently reassess whether economic and administrative pressures induce inappropriate changes in behavior. Concerns are often best addressed by implementing systems that reduce production pressures.

Interaction with Industry Interaction with industry is widespread and results in potential conflicts of interest for anesthesiologists.[87-91] Overwhelming evidence indicates that intimacy with industry unconsciously affects clinical behavior through unrecognized feelings of gratitude, reciprocity, or obligation.[82,92-95] Physicians may also unconsciously rationalize accepting industry gifts because of sacrifices made in terms of education, time, and compensation.[96] Most physicians claim that interaction with industry does not affect their clinical practice. But in addition to contrary evidence in the literature, consider that a core strategy of advertising is to influence unwitting patrons through familiarity and positive associations.

The claim that industry provides necessary education about the availability and use of medications is belied by the need for physicians to have unbiased information and unaffected decision making.[89,97,98] Although physicians supposedly independently evaluate industry information, busy physicians with insufficient abilities to critically evaluate studies devolve into accepting industry materials "as is." Industry representatives and materials routinely overrepresent the benefits and underrepresent the risks of drugs.[99-105] National guidelines for industry gifts, originally considered draconian, are now considered relatively weak. Academic centers have begun implementing policies more stringent than national guidelines.

Prohibiting relationships between academic health centers and industry is counterproductive. More appropriate goals are greater participation, the use of guidelines, and more rigorous oversight.[106] For example, in clinical trials, academic researchers should participate in trial development, have the right to examine the raw data, and be able to publish data without the company's authorization.[107] Industry relationships with powerful members of the hospital community should be examined to determine if the potential for influence can be minimized.[108]

Research Research has potential financial and nonfinancial conflicts of interest.[109] In 1985 and 1989, published results from a large trial suggested that lumpectomy was preferable to mastectomy for breast cancer. But a principal investigator had falsified records, in large part to be a more prominent author. Although reanalysis still endorsed lumpectomy, the event distressed patients and families. In 2009 an anesthesiologist allegedly fabricated clinically influential data supporting the use of cyclo-oxygenase-2 inhibitors for multimodal pain therapy.[110] The anesthesiologist was a paid speaker for industry and received financial support for research. Supporting the benefits of oversight, irregularities found in a routine audit initiated the revealing comprehensive evaluation. Management of potential conflicts of interest may include disclosure of financial interest, independent review of research, and prohibiting relationships that create the potential for conflicts of interest.[109] Disclosure is an inadequate remedy. Physicians do not accurately disclose payments from industry during presentations of research, and it is unrealistic for clinicians to assume they can properly appreciate the influences of payments or other second gains.[111,112]

Safety and Quality Care Initiatives Participation in safety and quality care initiatives is pointedly placed in the section on conflict of interest. Many perceive participation in safety and quality care initiatives as bothersome, unnecessary, distracting, and inefficient.[113] These policies are then met with resistance and perfunctory performance. But individual physicians need to recognize that they have limited perspective, knowledge, and experience regarding potential medical errors. Patient care obligations require anesthesiologists to incorporate into practice hospital safety and quality care initiatives, even if they do not understand or support them. Anesthesiologists, as frontline clinicians, are also obligated to speak out. If a policy seems harmful, anesthesiologists should inform the appropriate individuals. Routinely bypassing the problem by ignoring the policy prevents policy remediation and hinders the effectiveness of implementing policies in general.[114]

TABLE 5-4 Obligations of Anesthesiologists

Physicians are obligated to their communities. Community may be considered broadly to be a physical location, a type of patient, or groups with whom physicians electively associate. Here is one perspective of communities to which anesthesiologists are obligated. Individual anesthesiologists are not expected to fulfill every obligation. Units of anesthesiologists such as private practice groups, academic departments, and state societies should fulfill these obligations collectively.[133]

Patient Community	Local Community

• **Treat every patient with the grace and consideration you would want for your family**
• Tailor the perioperative experience to the individual
• Respond to problems that may harm patients (eg, impaired colleagues)
• Practice mindfulness and critical self-reflection
• Actively engage in continuing medical education
	• Foster patient safety
	  • Participate in surveillance data collection
	  • Comply with policies intended to improve care
	  • Seek best practices
	  • Participate in collaborative care
	• Participate in hospital governance
	• Build hospital systems that improve patient care (eg, sedation services, preoperative clinics, pain management services)

Society	**Anesthesiology Community**
• Be politically active • Participate in social advocacy of an area of choice (eg, tobacco use, socioeconomic disparities in general and in health care, health care delivery) • Support national and international health care missions	• Teach, do research, or support teaching and research • Participate in professional organizations related and unrelated to anesthesiology • Prepare future generations through mentoring, creating opportunities, and designing practice styles that encourage participation

THE ETHICS CONSULTATION SERVICE

The discipline of medical ethics encompasses recognizing, analyzing, and managing ethical dilemmas. Ethics consultants identify relevant facts, facilitate communication, apply principles of ethical analysis, define precise ethical questions, and discover alternative, more palatable, solutions. The law and medical ethics have different responsibilities. By defining boundaries of behaviors, the law prescribes what must be done. Medical ethics works within these boundaries to help determine what ought to be done, to recognize when to challenge boundaries, and to provide guidance in areas not governed by law.

Ethics consultations are typically performed by an individual, a small group, or the full committee.[115,116] Ethics committees seek to have a heterogeneous membership that spans the hospital and may include physicians, nurses, social workers, chaplains, administrators, and laypeople. Most ethics consultation services permit patients, families, and those participating in the care of the patient to request a consultation. Many require notification (not permission) of the patient, surrogate, and attending physician prior to initiating the consultation and many prepare a written report for the clinical record and the patient. The standard of care is that ethics consultation services have no formal authority and are only advisory. But respected committees often have considerable informal authority.

One large urban hospital reported an incidence of ethics consultation in 0.16% of hospital admissions and 0.64% of intensive care unit admissions.[117] Most of these consultations involved patients with primary diagnoses of neurologic disease, infectious disease, malignancy, and trauma. The most common reasons for consultation were questions regarding the level of care. Anesthesiologists may find ethics consultation helpful with questions about informed consent, decision-making capacity, resuscitation decisions, and resolving disagreements among patients, families, and caregivers.[116,118-120] Ethics committees also provide formal education sessions, ward ethics rounds, policy development, and institutional ethics consultation.[121]

PROFESSIONAL OBLIGATIONS

Anesthesiologists have overlapping professional obligations to patients, the local community, anesthesiology, and societal health (**Table 5-4**).[122-132]

It is fashionable to bemoan the financial and clinical fate of physicians. Among other legitimate and illegitimate complaints, physicians are paid too little, work too hard, are forced to assume untenable loans, and are being treated as technicians. These issues are irrelevant in terms of the physician obligation to fulfill the social contract. Society invested limited resources to develop the medical infrastructure of education, materials, expertise, and opportunities that enables physicians to practice. Despite these concerns, medical practice still provides significant compensation, official authority, unofficial influence, and the exquisite privilege of making a difference in individuals and society. In exchange for these considerable privileges, the implicit social contract calls for physicians to use their professional skills altruistically to better society.[113,130]

Anesthesiologists are obligated to "own" the advancement and advocacy of all things anesthesiology.[131]

KEY REFERENCES

- Berwick DM. What 'patient-centered' should mean: confessions of an extremist. *Health Aff.* 2009;28:w555-w565.
- Churchill LR. The hegemony of money: commercialism and professionalism in American medicine. *Camb Q Healthc Ethics.* 2007;16:407-414; discussion 39-42.
- Dana J, Loewenstein G. A social science perspective on gifts to physicians from industry. *JAMA.* 2003;290:252-255.
- Epstein RM. Mindful practice. *JAMA.* 1999;282:833-839.
- Gallagher TH, Studdert D, Levinson W. Disclosing harmful medical errors to patients. *N Engl J Med.* 2007;356:2713-2719.
- Greene NM. Familiarity as a basis for the practice of anesthesiology. *Anesthesiology.* 1976;44:101-103.
- Greene NM. The 31st Rovenstine Lecture. The changing horizons in anesthesiology. *Anesthesiology.* 1993;79:164-170.
- Truog RD, Waisel DB, Burns JP. DNR in the OR: a goal-directed approach. *Anesthesiology.* 1999;90:289-295.
- Waisel DB. Developing social capital in the operating room: the use of population-based techniques. *Anesthesiology.* 2005;103: 1305-1310.
- Wazana A. Physicians and the pharmaceutical industry: is a gift ever just a gift? *JAMA.* 2000;283:373-380.

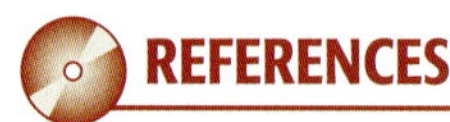

REFERENCES

Complete references available on DVD and online version at www.LongneckerAnesthesiology.com

PART 2

Preparing for Anesthesia

SECTION A

Approach to the Anesthesia Patient

CHAPTER 6

Overview of Preoperative Assessment and Management

Bobbie Jean Sweitzer
Michael Pilla

KEY POINTS

1. Comprehensive preoperative evaluation and management improve patient satisfaction, outcomes, and safety.
2. Inadequate preoperative evaluation and management increase perioperative adverse events and often lead to delays or cancellations of procedures.
3. At a minimum, the preanesthesia visit should include an interview with the patient to review the medical history (including medications, allergies, comorbid conditions, previous operations, and anesthetics), an appropriate physical examination, review of diagnostic data, assignment of an American Society of Anesthesiologists physical status score, and a formulation and discussion with the patient of the anesthetic plan.
4. The medical history is the most important component of preoperative assessment.
5. Findings from the history and physical examination determine the need, if any, for further diagnostic testing.
6. Diagnostic tests should only be ordered if the results will alter the planned anesthetic or procedure or establish an already suspected diagnosis. "Screening" tests are never appropriate.
7. Cardiovascular morbidity and mortality are the leading cause of significant perioperative adverse events.
8. Identification and management of cardiovascular disease is an important goal of preoperative evaluation.
9. Knowledge of risk factors for cardiovascular disease and familiarity with the American College of Cardiology–American Heart Association guidelines for cardiovascular evaluation for noncardiac surgery is essential.
10. A determination of functional capacity or the patient's cardiorespiratory fitness can guide further testing and predict a wide range of complications and outcome.
11. Potentially high-risk patients include those with the following conditions:
    a. Ischemic heart disease
    b. Heart failure
    c. Murmurs
    d. Pacemakers, implantable cardioverter-defibrillators (ICDs)
    e. Vascular stents
    f. Pulmonary disease
    g. Obstructive sleep apnea
    h. Obesity
    i. Diabetes mellitus
    j. Poorly controlled hypertension
    k. Renal disease
    l. Hepatic disease
    m. Substance abuse
    n. Advanced age
    o. Difficult airway
12. Knowledge and management of antiplatelet therapy in patients with coronary stents is imperative in the perioperative period.
13. Poor communication is a common source of medical errors, patient dissatisfaction, and malpractice claims.
14. Practice guidelines can standardize care, decrease delays, and improve outcomes.
15. Anesthesia-directed preoperative evaluation centers can be cost-effective, improve care and safety, and offer services beyond history acquisition, physical examinations, and diagnostic testing.

GOALS AND BENEFITS

As the practice of medicine becomes increasingly outcomes driven and cost conscious, clinicians need to reevaluate and streamline methods of patient care. The role of the anesthesiologist as a consultant is more important than ever. No single clinician is better informed and capable than the anesthesiologist to evaluate patients who require anesthesia. Preoperative assessment and management have evolved as the role of the anesthesiologist has expanded outside of the operating theater and as an increasing number of procedures are performed on patients who are not hospitalized before their anesthetics. Reasons for preoperative assessment may entail some or all of the following:

1. To screen for and properly manage comorbid conditions.
2. To assess the risk of anesthesia and surgery and lower it.
3. To identify patients who may require special anesthetic techniques or postoperative care.
4. To establish baseline results for perioperative decisions.
5. To educate patients and families about the objectives and risks of anesthesia and the anesthesiologist's role in perioperative care.
6. To obtain informed consent.
7. To facilitate timely care and avoid cancellations on the day of operation.
8. To determine the appropriateness of patients to undergo anesthesia in out-of-operating room or ambulatory surgical facilities.
9. To motivate patients to stop smoking, lose weight, or commit to other preventive care.
10. To train personnel in the art and science of preoperative assessment and optimization of a patient's condition.

The Australian Incident Monitoring Study (AIMS) found that 3.1% (197 of the first 6271 reports) of adverse events were unequivocally related to insufficient, and 11% to inadequate, preoperative assessment.[1] More than half of incidents were considered preventable. An analysis of the first 2000 reports to AIMS found a 6-fold increase in mortality in patients who were inadequately assessed preoperatively.[2] Davis concluded that 53 (39%) of 135 deaths attributed to anesthesia involved inadequate preoperative assessment and management.[3] Delays, complications, and unanticipated postoperative admissions are significantly reduced by preoperative screening and patient contact. Others have shown that preoperative health status can predict operative outcomes and resource use. Preoperative preparation and education can facilitate recovery and reduce the incidence of postoperative morbidity. In

France, a preoperative consultation has been mandated since 1994. Although debates continue regarding both the financial implications and convenience to society and patients, this process has been associated with a greater than 10-fold decrease in anesthetic-related complications.[4] Anxiety, postoperative pain, and length of stay have been positively affected by comprehensive preoperative care. Adequate pain management correlates significantly with patients receiving sufficient preoperative information.[5] From the patient's perspective, an opportunity to meet an anesthesiologist (preferably the one providing anesthesia on the day of surgery) is very important. In a study conducted in Canada and Scotland, patients rated meeting the anesthesiologist as the highest priority, above that of information on pain relief, alternative methods of anesthesia, and complications.[6]

Preoperative evaluation must be efficient for both patient and hospital personnel. It can be cost-effective and can reduce turnover times, cancellations, and length of hospital stays. In a retrospective analysis of practices at one major US teaching hospital, significant reductions in case cancellations were observed for same-day surgery patients (8.4% vs 16.2%) and main operating room patients (5.3% vs 13%) when patients had a preoperative evaluation.[7] Preoperative visits should be comprehensive, including plans for postdischarge patient care. Many anesthesiologists perform preoperative evaluations, review diagnostic studies (often chosen and ordered by someone else), discuss anesthetic risks, and obtain informed consent moments before a patient undergoes a major, potentially life-threatening or disfiguring procedure. This choice offers little opportunity to manage comorbid conditions or alter risk. Legally, morally, and psychologically, anesthesiologists and patients are in awkward, and often unpleasant, situations. The effects of extensive disclosure are stressful for patients and families at a time when they may be ill prepared to consider the implications rationally. An increase in preoperative anxiety may adversely affect postoperative outcomes because increased anxiety correlates with increased postoperative analgesic requirements and prolonged recovery and hospital stay. Anxiety impairs retention of information, which could result in legal action because of inadequate communication or discussion of the risks of anesthesia.

At a minimum, the guidelines of the American Society of Anesthesiologists (ASA) indicate that a preanesthesia visit should include the following:[8]

1. Interview with the patient to review medical, anesthesia, and medication history
2. Appropriate physical examination
3. Review of appropriate diagnostic data (laboratory, electrocardiograms, radiographs)
4. Assignment of ASA physical status score
5. Formulation and discussion of the anesthesia plan with the patient or a responsible adult

Table 6-1 outlines the criteria and medical conditions of patients likely to benefit from evaluation in a preanesthetic clinic before the day of surgery.

RISK ASSESSMENT AND REDUCTION

The current ASA risk classification system was developed in 1941 by Meyer Saklad at the request of the ASA (**Table 6-2**). This classification was the first attempt to quantify risk associated with anesthesia and surgery. The type of anesthesia and the operation are not even considered in this classification system. Moreover, this system attempted to estimate the mortality rate based only on the patient's preoperative medical condition. Since then, other studies have corroborated an association of mortality and morbidity with ASA physical status (ASA PS) scores. Studies also have shown a correlation between ASA PS and unanticipated intensive care unit admissions, longer hospital stays for some procedures, and adverse cardiopulmonary outcomes. No correlation was shown between ASA PS class and cancellations, unplanned admissions, and other perioperative complications and cost.[9] Few studies have evaluated the effect of combining the risk of the surgical procedure and the ASA PS score. Among the first was the Johns Hopkins Risk Classification System.[10] Many institutions use a more simplified version of high, intermediate, and low risk.[11] **Figure 6-1** offers one example of such a risk stratification.

Goldman et al further advanced risk assessment by identifying risk factors and cardiac complications in noncardiac surgery. Several studies followed, culminating in the joint guideline publication by the American College of Cardiology and the American Heart Association (ACC/AHA) in 1996, which was most recently updated in 2007.[11] (see "Heart Disease" later and Chapter 9 for more detailed discussions of the ACC/AHA guidelines.) However, there are limited studies or guidelines addressing specific disease states and their effects on perioperative risk. Pulmonary and renal risk and the implications of certain laboratory abnormalities (albumin and hematocrit levels) have been evaluated.[12-15]

Some assessment of risk is important to prepare for the anesthetic and surgical procedure. The need for invasive monitoring, blood salvage and hypothermic techniques, postoperative care in the intensive care unit, and special monitoring must be considered. Patients must be informed during the consent process. Technical terms used in the consent may be misunderstood.[16] Risk assessment is useful to compare outcomes, control costs, allocate compensation, and assist in the difficult decision of canceling or recommending a procedure not be done when the risks are too high. Yet risk assessment, at its best, is hampered by individual patient variability.

TIMING OF ASSESSMENT

The Practice Advisory for Preanesthesia Evaluation commissioned by the ASA determined that the time of the preanesthesia assessment depends on the patient's condition, the type of procedure, the health care system, and the patient's access to care providers.[8] The recommendations, which were based on the opinions of experts and randomly selected ASA members, favor assessments on or before the day of surgery for low to medium invasive procedures and before the day of operation for highly invasive procedures. The consensus is for assessments before the day of surgery for patients with less severe disease if they are scheduled for highly invasive procedures and for patients with severe disease for less invasive procedures. For selected patients, evaluations on the day of surgery can be safe and effective.

The importance of a visit to the preoperative clinic before a surgical procedure cannot be overstated.[17] A Canadian survey found that more than 60% of patients thought it was important to see an anesthesiologist preoperatively, more than 30% thought it was extremely important, and more than half indicated that the visit should be before the day of operation.[18] Anesthesiologists at Massachusetts General Hospital demonstrated that a preoperative visit before the day of surgery was as good as or better than medication in reducing preoperative anxiety and postoperative pain.

DETECTING DISEASE

Several studies have proved the usefulness of the history and physical examination in deciding a diagnosis. A study of patients in a general medical clinic found that 56% of correct diagnoses were made with the history alone and rose to 73% with the physical examination. In patients with cardiovascular disease, the history established the diagnosis 66% of the time, and the physical examination contributed to 25% of diagnoses. Moreover, routine investigations, mainly chest radiography and electrocardiography (ECG), helped with only 3% of diagnoses, and special tests, mainly exercise ECG, assisted with 6%.[19] ECG alone was only 14% predictive in the diagnosis of left ventricular dysfunction in patients with suspected neuromuscular disease.[20] History is also the most important diagnostic method in respiratory, urinary, and neurologic conditions. The skill of performing a clinical examination derives from pattern recognition learned by seeing patients and listening to the stories of their illnesses. The diagnostic acumen of the physician is a result of the ability to assimilate information and develop an overall impression, rather than just reviewing a compilation of facts.

TABLE 6-1 General Criteria and Medical Conditions for Which Preoperative Evaluation Is Recommended Before the Date of Surgery

Medical Condition	Criteria
General	Age
Normal activity inhibited	>75 y, unless surgery is minor (eg, cataract, cystoscopy) and under monitored anesthesia care
Monitoring or medical assistance at home within 2 mo	
Hospital admission within 2 mo	Language
Obesity >140% ideal body weight	Patient or parent/guardian cannot hear, speak, or understand English
Cardiovascular	Anesthesia related
Coronary artery disease	Patient or family has had previous difficult intubation, elevated temperature during anesthesia, is allergic to succinylcholine, has malignant hyperthermia or pseudocholinesterase deficiency or paralysis or nerve damage during anesthesia
Arrhythmias	
Poorly controlled hypertension	
Systolic blood pressure >180 mm Hg or diastolic blood pressure >110 mm Hg	Procedure related
Heart failure	Intraoperative blood transfusion likely
Respiratory	ICU admission likely
Asthma requiring daily medications	High-risk surgery
Chronic obstructive pulmonary disease (COPD) with symptoms	Pregnancy
Exacerbation or progression of COPD within 2 mo	Patient is pregnant (unless the procedure is termination)
Previous airway surgery	
Unusual airway anatomy	
Airway tumor or obstruction	
Home ventilatory assistance or monitoring	
Endocrine	
Diabetes	
Adrenal disorders	
Active thyroid disease	
Neuromuscular	
Seizure disorder	
CNS disease (eg, multiple sclerosis)	
Myopathy or other muscle disorders	
Hepatic	
Active hepatobiliary disease or compromise	
Renal	
Renal insufficiency or failure	
Musculoskeletal	
Kyphosis or scoliosis compromising function	
Temporomandibular joint disorder limiting mouth opening	
Cervical or thoracic spine injury/disease	
Oncology	
Chemo- or radiotherapy within last 2 mo	
Significant physiologic compromise from disease or treatment	

This table has been updated and adapted with permission from Pasternak LR. Preoperative evaluation of the ambulatory surgery patient. Ambulatory surgery. *Anesthesiol Rep.* 1990;3(1):8.

Medical History One common problem is the variability of the medical history. Asking and recording symptoms in ordinary words leads to greater interobserver agreement between practitioners. History taking is not simply asking the questions; history taking includes interpreting and carefully recording the answers. Complete and thorough histories not only assist in planning appropriate and safe anesthesia care, but they also are more accurate and cost-effective in establishing diagnoses than screening laboratory tests.

The patient's medical problems, past operations, previous anesthesia-related complications, allergies, and use of tobacco, alcohol, or illicit

TABLE 6-2 American Society of Anesthesiologists Physical Status Classification

P1	Healthy patient without organic, biochemical, or psychiatric disease.
P2	A patient with mild systemic disease (eg, mild asthma or well-controlled hypertension). No significant impact on daily activity. Unlikely impact on anesthesia and surgery.
P3	Significant or severe systemic disease that limits normal activity (eg, renal failure or dialysis or class 2 heart failure). Significant impact on daily activity. Likely impact on anesthesia and surgery.
P4	Severe disease that is constant threat to life or requires intensive therapy (eg, acute myocardial infarction, respiratory failure requiring mechanical ventilation). Serious limitation of daily activity. Major impact on anesthesia and surgery.
P5	Moribund patient who is equally likely to die in the next 24 h with or without surgery.
P6	Brain-dead organ donor.

"E" added to the above (P1-P5) indicates emergency surgery.
Adapted from American Society of Anesthesiologists. ASA physical status classification system. ASA Web site. www.asahq.org.

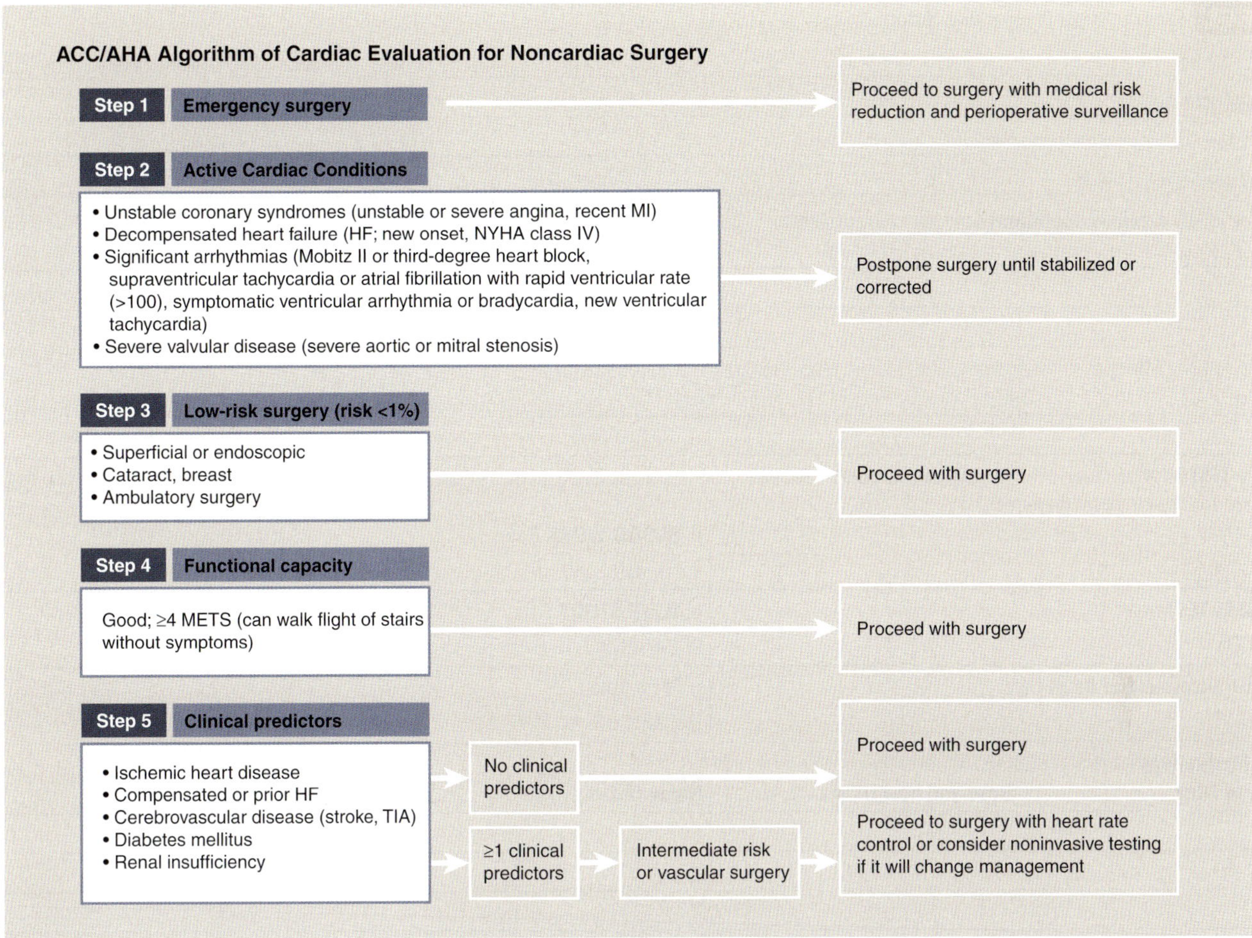

FIGURE 6-1. Simplified cardiac evaluation for noncardiac surgery. ACC, American College of Cardiology; AHA, American Heart Association; METS, metabolic equivalent of task score; MI, myocardial infarction; NYHA, New York Heart Association; TIA, transient ischemic attack.

drugs should be documented. Equally important to identifying the presence of a disease is establishing the severity, the stability, and prior treatment of the condition. A screening review of systems needs special emphasis on airway abnormalities, personal or family history of adverse events related to anesthesia, and cardiovascular, pulmonary, endocrine, or neurologic symptoms.

The patient's medical problems, previous operations, and responses to questions elicit further questions to establish the severity of disease, its stability, current or recent exacerbations, and recent or planned interventions. Rarely is a simple notation of diseases or symptoms such as hypertension (HTN), diabetes mellitus (DM), coronary artery disease (CAD), shortness of breath (SOB), or chest pain sufficient. The severity, extent, degree of control, and the activity-limiting nature of the problems are equally important.

A determination of the patient's cardiorespiratory fitness or functional capacity is useful in guiding additional preanesthetic evaluation and predicting outcome and perioperative complications.[11,21] Exercise or work activity can be quantified in the metabolic equivalent of task score (METS), which refer to the volume of oxygen consumed during an activity.[22] One's ability to exercise is two pronged in that better fitness decreases mortality through improved lipid and glucose profiles and reductions in blood pressure and obesity. An inability to exercise may be a *result* of cardiopulmonary disease. Several studies show that inability to perform average levels of exercise, equivalent to 4 to 5 METS (walking 4 blocks on level ground, climbing 2 flights of stairs or 1 flight of stairs carrying 20 lb), identifies patients at risk of perioperative complications.

Table 6-3 shows the important components of an anesthesia history. The form can be completed by the patient in person (paper or electronic version), via Internet-based programs, via a telephone interview, or by anesthesia staff. A more detailed discussion of important components of the history for specific medical conditions is presented later (see "High-Risk Patients").

Physical Examination At a minimum, the preanesthetic examination should include the airway, a heart and lung examination, vital signs, including oxygen saturation, and height and weight. Increased body mass index (BMI) is one of many factors associated with development of chronic diseases such as heart disease, cancer, and DM, and it can be calculated from an individual's height and weight. The two formulas for calculating the BMI are the English and the metric.

English formula:

$$\text{BMI} = \left(\frac{\text{Weight in pounds}}{(\text{Height in inches}) \times (\text{Height in inches})}\right) \times 703$$

Metric formula:

$$\text{BMI} = \left(\frac{\text{Weight in kilograms}}{(\text{Height in meters}) \times (\text{Height in meters})}\right)$$

or

$$\text{BMI} = \left(\frac{\text{Weight in kilograms}}{(\text{Height in centimeters}) \times (\text{Height in centimeters})}\right) \times 10000$$

TABLE 6-3 Sample Patient Preoperative History

Patient's Name ______ Age____ Sex _____ Date of Surgery ______

Proposed operation ______

Primary care physician name/phone # ______ Height ________ Weight ______

Cardiologist name/phone # ______

1. Please list **all previous operations** (and approximate dates)

a.	d.
b.	e.
c.	f.

2. Please list any **Allergies** to medications, latex, food or other (and your reactions to them)

a.	c.
b.	d.

3. Circle **TESTS** that you have already completed, list where and when you had them. Please bring all existing reports for your visit. We are NOT suggesting that you require (or need to have) these tests.

a. **ECG** Date: LOCATION:	d. **BLOOD WORK** Date: LOCATION:
b. **STRESS TEST** Date: LOCATION:	e. **SLEEP STUDY** Date: LOCATION:
c. **ECHO/ultrasound of heart** Date: LOCATION:	f. Other: Date: LOCATION:

4. List **Medications** taken in the last month (over-the-counter meds, inhalers, herbals, aspirin)

Name of Drug	**Dose and how often**	**Name of Drug**	**Dose and how often**
a.		f.	
b.		g.	
c.		h.	
d.		i.	
e.		j.	

(Please check YES or NO and circle specific problems)	**YES**	**NO**
5. Have you taken steroids (prednisone or cortisone) in the last year?	☐	☐
6. Have you *ever* smoked? (quantify in ___ packs/day for ___ years)	☐	☐
7. Do you still smoke? (quantify in ___ packs/day)	☐	☐
8. Do you drink alcohol? (if so, how much?) ______	☐	☐
9. Do you use or have you ever used any illegal drugs? (we need to know for your safety)	☐	☐
10. Can you walk up one flight of stairs without stopping?	☐	☐
11. Have you had any problems with your heart? **(circle all that apply)**	☐	☐
(chest pain or pressure, heart attack, skipped beats, murmur, palpitations, heart failure)	☐	☐
12. Do you have high blood pressure?	☐	☐
13. Do you have diabetes?	☐	☐
14. Have you had any problems with your lungs or your chest? **(circle all that apply)**	☐	☐
(shortness of breath, emphysema, bronchitis, asthma, TB, abnormal chest x-ray)	☐	☐
15. Are you ill now or were you recently ill with a cold, fever, chills, flu or productive cough? Describe recent changes______	☐	☐
16. Have you or anyone in your family had serious bleeding problems? **(circle all that apply)**	☐	☐
(prolonged bleeding from nose, gums, tooth extractions, or surgery)	☐	☐
17. Have you had any problems with your blood ? **(circle all that apply)**	☐	☐
(anemia, leukemia, lymphoma, sickle cell disease, blood clots, transfusions)	☐	☐

(Continued)

TABLE 6-3 Sample Patient Preoperative History (*Continued*)

18. Have you ever had problems with your: **(circle all that apply)**		
Liver (cirrhosis; hepatitis A, B, C; jaundice)?	☐	☐
Kidney (stones, failure, dialysis)?	☐	☐
Digestive system (frequent heartburn, hiatus hernia, stomach ulcer)?	☐	☐
Back, neck, or jaws (TMJ, rheumatoid arthritis, herniation)?	☐	☐
Thyroid gland (under active or overactive)?	☐	☐
19. Have you ever had: **(circle all that apply)**		
Seizures?	☐	☐
Stroke, facial, leg, or arm weakness, difficulty speaking?	☐	☐
Cramping pain in your legs with walking?	☐	☐
Problems with hearing, vision, or memory?	☐	☐
20. Have you ever been treated with chemotherapy or radiation therapy? **(circle all that apply)**	☐	☐
List indication and dates of treatment: ______		
21. Women: Could you be pregnant? Last menstrual period began: ______	☐	☐
22. Have you ever had problems with anesthesia or surgery? **(circle all that apply)** (severe nausea or vomiting, malignant hyperthermia [in blood relatives or self], breathing difficulties, or problems with placement of a breathing tube)	☐	☐
23. Do you have any chipped or loose teeth, dentures, caps, bridgework, braces, problems opening your mouth or swallowing, or choking while eating? **(circle all that apply)**	☐	☐
24. Do your physical abilities limit your daily activities?	☐	☐
25. Do you snore?	☐	☐
26. Do you have sleep apnea?	☐	☐
27. Please list any medical illnesses not noted above: ______		
28. Additional comments or questions for the anesthesiologist? ______		

See "Obesity" for further discussion and for definitions of BMI categories for adults.

Components of the airway examination should include the following[23]:

- Length of upper incisors
- Condition of the teeth
- Relationship of upper (maxillary) incisors to lower (mandibular) incisors
- Ability to protrude or advance lower (mandibular) incisors in front of upper (maxillary) incisors
- Interincisor or intergum (if edentulous) distance
- Visibility of uvula
- Presence of heavy facial hair
- Compliance of mandibular space
- Thyromental distance
- Length of neck
- Thickness of neck
- Range of motion of head and neck

Because of the relatively frequent incidence of dental injuries during anesthesia, a thorough documentation of preexisting tooth and gum abnormalities is useful. Either a tooth chart (**Fig. 6-2**) or standard nomenclature (eg, right upper central incisor, left lower lateral incisor, or right lower bicuspid) can be helpful.

It is important to discuss potential dental risks, especially in the presence of poor dentition.[24] A good time to discuss with patients variant options of airway management, including possible fiberoptic intubation when necessary, is after examination of the airway. Findings from the airway examination may predict difficult intubations.[25] When challenging airways are identified, advance planning ensures that necessary equipment and skilled personnel are available.

Auscultation of the heart and inspection of the pulses, peripheral veins, and extremities for the presence of edema are important diagnostically and for risk assessment in development of care plans. One should auscultate for murmurs, rhythm disturbances, and signs of volume overload. Murmurs, without a clear etiology (anemia, hyperthyroidism, or pregnancy, with confirmation that the murmur was not present prior to these conditions), warrant further evaluation (see "Heart Disease").

The pulmonary examination includes auscultation for wheezing, decreased or abnormal breath sounds, notation of cyanosis or clubbing, and effort of breathing. Observing whether the patient can walk up 1 to 2 flights of stairs can predict a variety of postoperative complications, including pulmonary and cardiac events and mortality, and aid in decisions regarding the need for further specialized testing such as pulmonary function tests (PFTs) or noninvasive cardiac stress testing.[11,26,27] For selective patients (eg, those with deficits or disease who are undergoing neurologic surgery or regional anesthesia), a neurologic examination is necessary to document preexisting abnormalities that may aid in diagnosis, interfere with positioning, or establish a baseline in defense of potential malpractice claims of adverse events.[28]

Obesity, HTN, and large neck circumference predict an increased incidence of obstructive sleep apnea (OSA). See "Obstructive Sleep Apnea."

PREOPERATIVE TESTING

Preoperative testing is performed to evaluate existing medical conditions and to diagnose asymptomatic conditions based on known risk factors for particular diseases. Diagnostic tests can aid in the assessment of the risk of anesthesia and operation, guide medical intervention to lower this

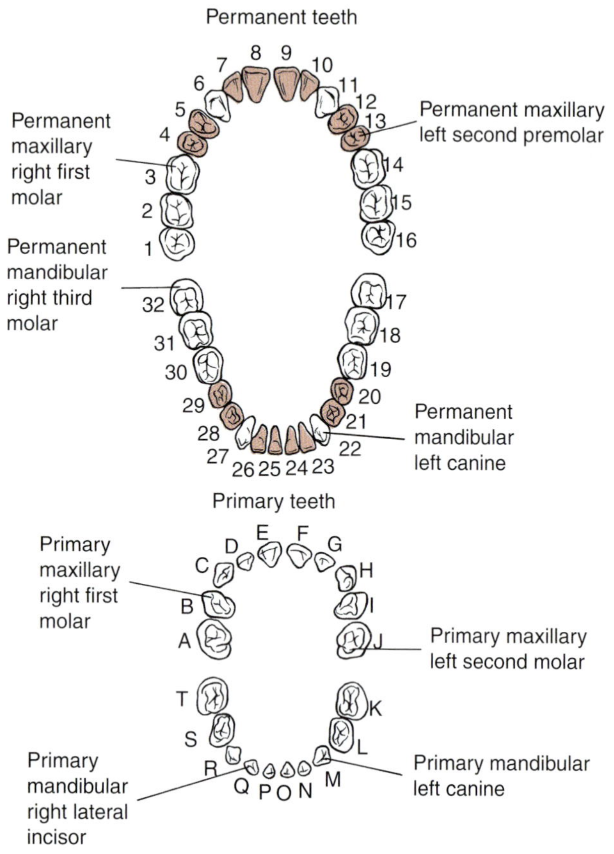

FIGURE 6-2. Dental chart. [From Tintinalli JE, Kelen GD, Stapczynski JS. *Tintinalli's Emergency Medicine: A Comprehensive Study Guide.* 6th ed. New York, NY: McGraw-Hill; 2004.]

risk, and provide baseline results to direct intra- and postoperative decisions. The choices of laboratory tests depend on the probable impact of the test results on the differential diagnosis and on patient management. A test is ordered only if the results will have an impact on the decision to proceed with the planned procedure or alter the care plans, The history and physical examination are used to direct test ordering. **Table 6-4** contains recommendations for testing based on specific medical conditions. Guidelines in this table are not intended for all patients with those conditions but to aid in diagnosing a disease, to optimize the patient if the disease state is out of control, or for high-risk surgeries.

Preoperative tests without specific indications lack clinical usefulness and may actually lead to patient injury because of unnecessary interventions, delay of surgery, anxiety, and even inappropriate therapies. The history is responsible for the diagnosis 75% of the time and is more important than the physical examination and laboratory investigations combined. In addition, the evaluation of abnormal results is costly. Many studies have evaluated the benefits of disease/condition-indicated testing versus screening batteries of tests.[29] Few abnormalities detected by nonspecific testing resulted in changes in management, and rarely have such changes had a beneficial patient effect.[30] At most 1 in 1000 patients has benefited from findings derived from nonindicated testing.[31] Blery et al found that 0.4% of tests without specific indications provided useful clinical information.[30] However, 1 in 2000 preoperative tests resulted in patient harm from pursuit of abnormalities detected by those tests; only 1 in 10 000 was of benefit to the patient.[9] It has been suggested that not following up on an abnormal result is a greater medicolegal risk than not identifying the abnormality to begin with. Several studies have demonstrated that routine preoperative testing in ambulatory surgery patients is not useful and cite disparity in requirements for tests among anesthesia providers.[29,32]

Preoperative ECGs are one of the most frequently ordered and costly noninvasive tests. Occult heart disease is common in the middle-age population and increases with advancing age. Preexisting heart disease increases perioperative risk. Recommendations for age-based testing

TABLE 6-4 Preoperative *Diagnostic* Testing Order Form for Intermediate- to High-Risk Procedures by Disease and Therapy-Based Indications[a]

☐	AST/AlkP	Alcohol abuse; exposure to hepatitis; hepatic disease; history of bleeding
☐	β-hCG	Possible pregnancy
☐	BUN/Cr	Cardiovascular, hepatic, or renal disease; diabetes; poor exercise tolerance; systemic lupus; use of digoxin, diuretics, steroids; procedures with radiographic dye
☐	CBC w/plt	Alcohol abuse, anemia; cardiovascular, pulmonary, or renal disease; malignancy; malnutrition; history of bleeding; procedures with significant blood loss
☐	CXR	Active, acute symptoms especially with cardiovascular or pulmonary disease; rheumatoid arthritis, systemic lupus; smoking >40 pack-years; radiation therapy
☐	ECG	Alcohol abuse; cardiovascular, cerebrovascular, intracranial, peripheral vascular, pulmonary, or renal disease; diabetes; morbid obesity; poor exercise tolerance; rheumatoid arthritis; sleep apnea; smoking >40 pack-years; systemic lupus; radiation therapy to chest or breasts; use of digoxin
☐	Electrolytes	Intracranial, or renal disease; diabetes; malnutrition; use of digoxin, diuretics
☐	Glucose	Intracranial disease; diabetes; morbid obesity; steroid use
☐	PT	Alcohol abuse; hepatic disease; malnutrition; personal history of bleeding; use of anticoagulants
☐	aPTT	Personal or family history of bleeding, heparin use
☐	Thyroid tests	Thyroid disease; use of thyroid medications
☐	T&S	Procedure with significant blood loss potential
☐	Urinalysis	Suspected urinary tract infection

AST/AlkP, aspartate transaminase/alkaline phosphatase; β-hCG, β-human chorionic gonadotropin; BUN/Cr, blood urea nitrogen/creatinine; CBC w/plt, complete blood count with platelets; CXR, chest x-ray; ECG, electrocardiogram; PT, prothrombin time; aPTT, activated partial thromboplastin time; T&S, type and screen.

[a]Guidelines are not for routine testing in all individuals with stated conditions but are only indicated if the medical condition is newly diagnosed, evolving, or unstable or results will alter anesthetic management. Guidelines may not apply for low-risk procedures where testing is rarely indicated except in situations when the patient's medical condition is significantly deranged. With the exception of β-hCG for pregnancy, all tests are valid for 2 months before surgery unless abnormal or patient's condition has changed.

were derived from the high incidence of abnormalities found on ECGs of elderly patients. The Centers for Medicare and Medicaid Services (CMS) do not reimburse for "preoperative" or age-based ECGs; one must provide a supporting diagnosis with an acceptable International Classification of Diseases, Ninth Revision (ICD-9) code. (Centers for Medicare and Medicaid Services. Available at http://www.cms.hhs.org. Accessed May 19, 2010.) Even the ASA Practice Advisory for Preanesthesia Evaluation states, "The Task Force recognizes that age alone may not be an indication for an electrocardiogram."[8] A *resting* ECG is not a reliable screen for CAD and is a poor predictor of heart disease (without a supporting history) in nonsurgical patients. It appears that only some ECG abnormalities are important in the perioperative period (eg, new Q waves and arrhythmias). One study found only 2% of patients had one or both of these abnormalities.[33] The frequency of silent Q-wave infarctions found *only* by ECG in men age 75 years or older (the highest risk group) is approximately 0.5%. Gold et al found that in ambulatory surgical patients, the incidence of abnormal ECGs was 43%. Only 1.6% (12 of 751) of patients had an adverse perioperative cardiac event and in only half (6 of 751) of these was the preoperative ECG of potential value.[34] History is far more important. An abnormal ECG will be found in 62% of patients with known cardiac disease, in 44% of patients with strong risk factors for ischemic heart disease, and in only 7% of patients older than 50 years with no risk factors. Results are abnormal in only 3% of patients between ages 50 and 70 years without risk factors for heart disease.[35]

Some abnormalities may have implications for anesthesia care beyond the detection of CAD. Arrhythmias, such as atrial fibrillation, which can be detected on physical examination and confirmed by ECG, conduction abnormalities, and left ventricular hypertrophy, may alter anesthesia plans. Adjustments may be necessary to avoid hemodynamic instability, ischemia, or pulmonary edema because of drug interactions or the stress of surgery combined with previous, but not necessarily clinically significant, disease. Plans can be made on the day of operation when monitors are placed in the preoperative area or the operating room rather than incurring the expense of a 12-lead ECG beforehand. Many practitioners espouse the need to establish a baseline. However, this approach is misguided and costly. A preoperative 12-lead ECG is rarely comparable with the intraoperative ECG due to varying lead placement. Anesthetic drugs, position, and volume changes affect the ECG. An unchanged ECG does not eliminate the possibility of ischemia; nor does any change on an ECG absolutely establish a diagnosis. A better comparison can be obtained once the patient is in the operating room with the monitoring ECG in place right before induction of anesthesia by printing off rhythm strips of various leads, most importantly leads II, V_4, or V_5.

The ACC/AHA *Guidelines for Perioperative Cardiovascular Evaluation for Noncardiac Surgery* no longer consider ECG abnormalities in deciding on further noninvasive stress testing.[11] A prospective observational study in patients 50 years or older having noncardiac surgery found abnormalities in 45% of the preoperative ECGs, and bundle branch blocks were associated with postoperative myocardial infarction (MI) and death but had no added predictive value over clinical risk factors.[36] The ASA Preoperative Evaluation Practice Advisory recognized that ECG did not improve prediction beyond risk factors identified by patient history.[8] Chung et al showed that elimination of testing did not increase risk as long as patients had a clinical evaluation preoperatively.[29] In a retrospective study of 23 036 patients, patients undergoing low- to intermediate-risk noncardiac surgery with abnormalities on their preoperative ECG had only a 0.5% increase in cardiovascular mortality as compared with cohorts with normal ECGs.[37] In summary, the prevalence of abnormalities on ECG may incur costly evaluation, delaying necessary surgery, and the yield of these workups is quite low. Table 6-4 provides guidance for ECG testing.

Hemoglobin (Hgb) and hematocrit (Hct) levels are frequently abnormal in otherwise healthy patients, but they rarely have an impact on anesthetic care or management unless the planned procedure involves the potential for significant bleeding. Abnormal Hgb levels (both higher and lower than normal) predict postoperative complications and mortality. However, interventions to correct anemia such as transfusion or erythropoietin carry risks of their own. Anemia is often an indication of disease related or unrelated to the planned surgery. If the discovery of anemia will lead to an alteration in surgical plans or prompt further evaluation for disease, such as colonoscopy, and previous laboratory values are unavailable, then testing is warranted.[12,15]

Coagulation studies (platelet count, prothrombin, or activated partial thromboplastin time) are not recommended unless the patient history suggests a coagulation disorder. If a patient has a negative history for a bleeding disorder, the cost of screening coagulation tests before most surgeries outweighs the benefit. Many practitioners mistakenly believe that a *screening* prothrombin time (PT) is more likely to be abnormal because of the numbers of patients with liver disease, malnutrition, or warfarin use, conditions that should be readily identified by history. If "screening" tests (not based on history) are ordered, a platelet count and activated partial thromboplastin time (aPTT) are indicated to detect the uncommon patient with thrombocytopenia, an acquired anticoagulant (eg, lupus anticoagulant), or a reduced level of a contact activation factor (eg, von Willebrand disease or factor VIII, IX, XI, or XII deficiencies). Additionally, a *short* aPTT may be equally as important as a prolonged aPTT. A short aPTT increases the risk of postoperative thromboembolism. The CMS does not reimburse for "routine" or "preoperative" PT/aPTT without an appropriate ICD-9 code.[38]

There are few data to recommend age-based testing. No correlation has been established, independent of coexisting disease, a positive history, or findings on physical examination, between age and abnormalities in Hgb, serum chemistries, radiographs, or PFTs.[31,39,40] Chest radiographs are indicated only in patients with pulmonary signs or symptoms of undetermined cause or severity.[13]

There is much controversy about and no consensus regarding routine pregnancy testing, especially in adolescents.[41] Surveys show that 30% to 50% of practitioners mandate testing in women of childbearing age, primarily because of the unreliability of the history, especially from minors, and the concern over the potential harm to the pregnancy or fetus with anesthesia and surgery, with the attendant medicolegal implications.[42,43] Opponents of mandatory testing cite the false-positive rate, cost, the belief that history is reliable if taken in privacy, and the paucity of data establishing risks of anesthesia in early pregnancy. When minors are pregnant, their privacy is governed by state laws. One must be familiar with local statutes and how unexpected positive pregnancy results will be handled. With the high reliability of urine testing, it is best to delay testing until the day of operation instead of testing in the preoperative clinic, unless the patient suspects pregnancy or the menstrual period is delayed. This delay in testing will obviate a negative test days before surgery that may be positive on the day of surgery. The ASA Preoperative Evaluation Practice Advisory "[r]ecognizes the literature is insufficient to inform patients or physicians on whether anesthesia causes harmful effects on early pregnancy. Pregnancy testing may be offered to female patients of childbearing age and for whom the result would alter the patient's management.[8]

Healthy patients or those with chronic, stable diseases, of any age undergoing low- or intermediate-risk procedures without expected significant blood loss are unlikely to benefit from any tests (Tables 6-4 and 6-5).[29] Exceptions are a procedure with the injection of contrast (creatinine level is indicated) or the possibility of pregnancy (a pregnancy test should be done) as shown in **Table 6-5.** If significant blood loss is expected, Hgb and/or Hct and type and screen are indicated (Table 6-5). Table 6-4 contains the recommendations for *diagnostic* tests for patients who either have poorly managed coexisting diseases or are suspected of having a condition that has not been diagnosed. Even these tests may not be indicated in this same patient population if they are anticipating low-risk operations, especially with sedation only. In general, tests are recommended only if the results may:

TABLE 6-5 Basic Preoperative Testing Guidelines

Procedure/Patient Type	Tests
Injection of contrast dye	Creatinine[a]
Potential for significant blood loss	Hemoglobin/hematocrit[a]
Likelihood of transfusion requirement	Type and screen
Possibility of pregnancy	Pregnancy test[b]
End-stage renal disease	Serum potassium[c]
Diabetes	Blood glucose on day of surgery[c]
Active cardiac condition (eg, decompensated heart failure, arrhythmia, chest pain, murmur)	Electrocardiogram

[a] Results from laboratory tests within 3 months of surgery are acceptable unless major abnormalities are present or a patient's condition has changed.

[b] A routine pregnancy test before surgery is not recommended before the day of surgery. A careful history and local practice determine whether a pregnancy test is indicated.

[c] There is no absolute level of either potassium or glucose that precludes surgery and anesthesia. The benefits of the procedure must be balanced against the risk of proceeding in a patient with abnormal results.

- Change, cancel, or postpone the surgical procedure
- Change anesthetic and medical management
- Change monitoring or intra- or postoperative care
- Establish a diagnosis in a patient who has not been adequately prepared

Many facilities have developed diagnostic testing guidelines to improve patient care, standardize clinical practice, improve efficiency, and reduce costs. With implementation of guidelines, one facility reduced the tests ordered by 60%, improved testing by 81%, and saved almost $80 000 per year. The Mayo Clinic reduced preoperative testing and its costs without a change in outcomes. A cost-to-benefit analysis found that routine urinalysis for all knee replacement surgery in the United States would cost $1.5 million to prevent 1 wound infection.[44] Interestingly, one study found 50% more routine ECGs and 40% more chest radiographs were done in a fee-for-service versus a prepaid practice.[45]

HIGH-RISK PATIENTS

Many of these conditions are discussed in greater detail in other chapters of this text, but here is a brief review of some common diseases that often require perioperative intervention. Identification of patients with these comorbid conditions often presents an opportunity for the anesthesiologist to intervene to lower risk. The following conditions are best managed before the day of surgery, which allows ample time for thoughtful evaluation, consultation, and planning.

HEART DISEASE

Cardiovascular complications are the most common serious adverse event perioperatively. It is estimated that 1% to 5% of unselected noncardiac surgical patients will suffer a cardiac morbidity. Next is a brief discussion of a few high-risk issues that are likely to be encountered in the preoperative clinic. The patient with ischemic heart disease, coronary stent(s), heart failure (HF), a rhythm disturbance, an abnormal ECG, an undiagnosed murmur, or a cardiac rhythm management device is discussed. Chapter 9 provides a comprehensive review of cardiovascular disease.

Ischemic Heart Disease The goals in the preanesthetic encounter are to:

- Identify the risk of heart disease based on comorbid diseases (Fig. 6-1)
- Identify the presence and severity of heart disease from symptoms, physical findings, or diagnostic tests
- Determine the need for preoperative interventions
- Modify the risk of perioperative adverse events

The basis of cardiac assessment is the history, the physical examination, and the ECG. The guidelines for cardiac evaluation before noncardiac surgery published by the ACC/AHA are the national standard of care.[11] Figure 6-1 presents a simplified approach to the evaluation of patients at risk of heart disease before noncardiac surgery. The complete ACC/AHA algorithm is found in Chapter 9. The goal is to identify patients with heart disease who have a significantly high risk of cardiac morbidity and mortality perioperatively, not to simply find patients with mild or stable ischemic coronary artery disease. Clinical predictors, functional or exercise capacity, and level of surgical risk guide further diagnostic and therapeutic interventions. Not included in the ACC/AHA guidelines are conditions such as chronic inflammatory diseases (eg, rheumatoid arthritis, systemic lupus erythematous); chronic steroid use, and chest irradiation, that either alone or associated with more traditional risk factors, identifies patients at risk for CAD and cardiac complications.[46-48]

Anesthesiologists who apply the ACC/AHA recommendations and develop practice guidelines (Fig. 6-1) are well positioned to initiate evaluation with stress tests. Results may obviate the need for a cardiac consultation or be available at the time of consultation. Exercise treadmill testing is indicated for patients with normal ECGs who can exercise. Pharmacologic tests, such as dobutamine echocardiography or nuclear perfusion imaging, are necessary for those unable to exercise or who have significant ECG abnormalities that may interfere with the interpretation of ischemia via ECG.

Currently, the benefits versus risk reduction in coronary revascularization before noncardiac surgery are controversial.[49] Factors to consider are the urgency of the noncardiac surgery (eg, in cancer cases) and the potential long-term benefits of revascularization. Noncardiac surgery soon after revascularization (bypass grafting and percutaneous coronary intervention with or without stents) is associated with high rates of perioperative cardiac morbidity and mortality.[50] Coronary revascularization may offer only moderate protection in patients undergoing elective vascular surgery.[51]

Patients who have had a percutaneous coronary intervention, especially with newer, drug-eluting stents, require several months, if not a lifetime, of antiplatelet therapy to avoid restenosis or acute thromboses (see "Coronary Stents"). These patients must be identified in the preoperative period and managed in collaboration with a cardiologist. Given that up to half of all perioperative MIs and cardiac deaths can be attributed to plaque rupture in noncritical coronary stenoses, intensive medical management in revascularized patients is likely to be helpful and may account for the lack of benefits of revascularization.[49,52] Decisions to revascularize patients before noncardiac surgery should be made only after evaluating the risk of perioperative cardiac-adverse events, the risks and benefits of the various methods of risk reduction, the benefits of the noncardiac surgery, and the patient's preferences. A face-to-face dialogue with all involved parties, similar to "tumor board" discussions, may assist decision making. Because cardiac complications are the leading cause of perioperative morbidity and mortality, anesthesiologists must be current on the latest evidence-based recommendations and be active in decision making and in the management of patients at risk.[52]

Coronary Stents More than 1 million patients receive coronary stents each year in the United States. The number of patients presenting for surgery who have stents continues to rise. Bare metal stents (BMS) were the first devices and are still widely used. However, drug-eluting stent (DES) implantation has steadily risen. DES are less likely to cause neointimal hyperplasia and restenosis of the coronary artery, but they are associated with late thrombosis, with an often catastrophic outcome. Thrombosis of either type of stent is more common if antiplatelet therapy is interrupted. Dual antiplatelet therapy with aspirin and a thienopyridine (typically clopidogrel) should not be interrupted for at least 1 month after BMS placement and 12 months after DES insertion.[53] See **Table 6-6** and **Fig. 6-3.**

In 2009 the ASA published a practice alert warning practitioners of the risk of premature discontinuation of antiplatelet therapy in patients

TABLE 6-6 Recommendations for Perioperative Management of Patients With Coronary Stents Who Are Receiving Antiplatelet Therapy

- Health care providers who perform invasive procedures must be aware of the potentially catastrophic risks of premature discontinuation of thienopyridine (eg, clopidogrel or ticlopidine) therapy. Such professionals should contact the patient's cardiologist to discuss optimal strategies if issues regarding antiplatelet therapy are unclear.
- Elective procedures involving risk of bleeding should be deferred until an appropriate course of thienopyridine therapy (12 mo after drug-eluting stents [DES] and 1 mo after bare-metal stents [BMS]) has been completed.
- Patients with DES who must undergo procedures that mandate discontinuing thienopyridine therapy should continue aspirin if at all possible and have the thienopyridine restarted as soon as possible.

Adapted from Grines CL, Bonow RO, Casey DE Jr, et al. Prevention of premature discontinuation of dual antiplatelet therapy in patients with coronary artery stents: a science advisory from the American Heart Association, American College of Cardiology, Society for Cardiovascular Angiography and Interventions, American College of Surgeons, and American Dental Association, with representation from the American College of Physicians. *J Am Coll Cardiol.* 2007;13;49(6):734-739.

with coronary stents, and it recommended delaying nonemergency surgery for 1 month in patients following BMS placement and 1 year in patients who had received DES.[54] If emergent or urgent surgery is required, it is recommended that aspirin therapy be continued at a minimum through the perioperative period and the thienopyridine restarted as soon as possible after the surgery.[54] See Table 6-6, Fig. 6-3, and Table 6-7.

Heart Failure HF affects 4 to 5 million people in the United States and is a significant risk factor for postoperative adverse events. Asymptomatic left ventricular dysfunction predicts cardiovascular events at 1 month and long term in vascular surgery patients having open procedures.[55] The goal in the preoperative period is to identify and minimize the effects of HF. Recent weight gain, complaints of SOB, fatigue, orthopnea, paroxysmal nocturnal dyspnea, edema, recent hospitalizations, and recent changes in management are all significant. Physical findings focus on examination for third or fourth heart sounds, rales, jugular venous distension, ascites, hepatomegaly, and edema. Classifying the patient's medical status according to the New York Heart Association's (NYHA) categories is useful.[56]

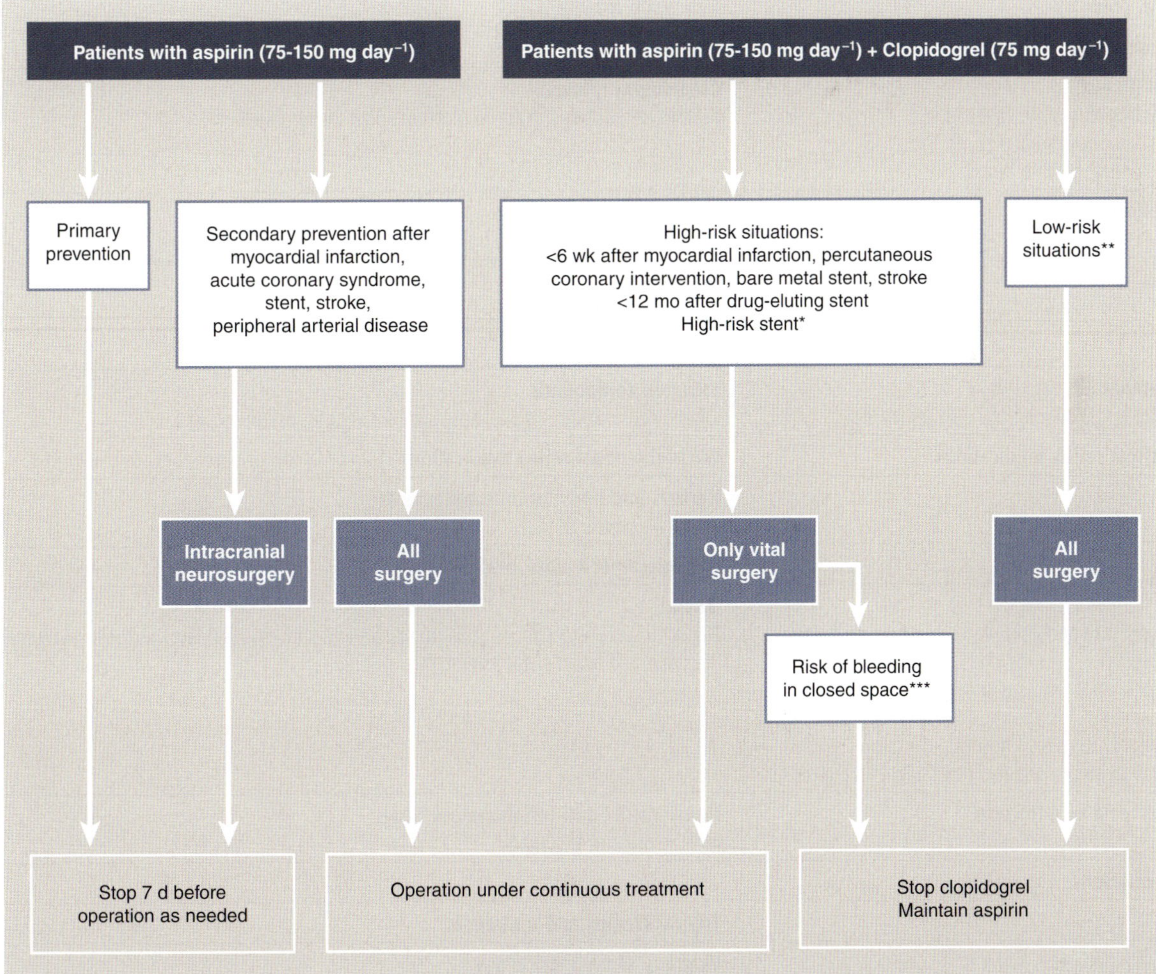

FIGURE 6-3. Algorithm for preoperative management of patients taking antiplatelet therapy. ACS, acute coronary syndrome; BMS, bare metal stent; DES, drug-eluting stent; MI, myocardial infarction; PAD, peripheral arterial disease; PCI, percutaneous coronary intervention. *High-risk stents: long (>36 mm), proximal, overlapping, or multiple stents, stents in chronic total occlusions, or in small vessels or bifurcated lesions. **Examples of low-risk situations: more than 3 months after BMS, stroke, uncomplicated MI, PCI without stenting. ***Risk of bleeding in closed space: intracranial neurosurgery, intramedullary canal surgery, posterior eye chamber ophthalmic surgery. In these situations, the risk-to-benefit ratio of upholding versus withdrawing aspirin must be evaluated for each case individually; in case of aspirin upholding, early postoperative reinstitution is important. [Adapted from Chassot PG, Delabays A, Spahn DR. Perioperative antiplatelet therapy: the case for continuing therapy in patients at risk of myocardial infarction. *Br J Anaesth.* 2007;99:316-328. By permission of Oxford University Press.]

TABLE 6-7 Preoperative Medication Guidelines

Continue on Day of Surgery	Discontinue on Day of Surgery
Antidepressants, antianxiety, and psychiatric medications (including monoamine oxidase inhibitors)[a]	
Antihypertensives Generally to be continued	**Antihypertensives** Consider discontinuing angiotensin-converting enzyme inhibitors or angiotensin receptor blockers 12-24 h before surgery if taken only for hypertension; especially if: Lengthy procedures, significant blood loss or fluid shifts, use of general anesthesia, multiple antihypertensive medications, well-controlled blood pressure; hypotension is particularly dangerous
Aspirin[b] Patients with known vascular disease Patients with vascular stents Before cataract surgery (if no bulbar block) Before vascular surgery Taken for secondary prophylaxis	[*]**Aspirin** Discontinue 5-7 d before surgery: If risk of bleeding > risk of thrombosis For surgeries with serious consequences from bleeding Taken only for primary prophylaxis (no known vascular disease)
Asthma medications	
Autoimmune medications Methotrexate (if no risk of renal failure)	**Autoimmune** Methotrexate (if risk of renal failure) Etanercept (Enbrel), Infliximab (Remicade), Adalimumab (Humira): Check with prescriber
Birth control pills	
Cardiac medications	
Clopidogrel (Plavix) Patients with drug-eluting stents <12 mo Patients with bare metal stents <1 mo Before cataract surgery (if no bulbar block)	**Clopidogrel (Plavix)** Patients not included in group recommended for continuation
Cox-2 inhibitors	**Cox-2 inhibitors** If surgeon concerned about bone healing
Diuretics Triamterene, hydrochlorothiazide	**Diuretics** Potent loop diuretics
Eye drops	
Estrogen compounds When used for birth control or cancer therapy	**Estrogen compounds** When used to control menopause symptoms or for osteoporosis
Gastrointestinal reflux medications	**Gastrointestinal reflux medications** (Tums, Maalox, or other particulate antacids)
	Herbals and nonvitamin supplements 7-14 d before surgery
	Hypoglycemic agents, oral
Insulin Type 1 diabetes: take about a third of intermediate to long-acting (NPH, lente) Type 2 diabetes: up to half long-acting (NPH) or combination (70/30) preparations Glargine (Lantus): decrease if dose is ≥1 unit/kg If insulin pump delivery, continue lowest night time basal rate	**Insulin** Regular insulin (exception: insulin pump, continue lowest basal rate, generally nighttime dose) Discontinue if blood sugar level <100
Narcotics for pain or addiction	**Nonsteroidal anti-inflammatory drugs** 48 h before day of surgery
Seizure medications	
Statins	**Topical creams and ointments**
Steroids (oral or inhaled)	**Viagra** or similar medications Discontinue 24 h before surgery
Thyroid medications	**Vitamins, minerals, iron**
Warfarin Cataract surgery, no bulbar block	**Warfarin**[c] Discontinue 5 d before surgery

[a]Need consultation for planning ahead of day of surgery.

[b]Except when the risk or consequences of bleeding are severe (generally only intracranial, posterior eye procedures).

[c]Bridging may be necessary; check with prescribing physician.

- Class I: no limitation of physical activity; ordinary activity does not cause fatigue, palpitations, or syncope
- Class II: slight limitation of physical activity; ordinary activity results in fatigue, palpitations, or syncope
- Class III: marked limitation of physical activity; less than ordinary activity results in fatigue, palpitations, or syncope; comfortable at rest
- Class IV: inability to do any physical activity without discomfort; symptoms at rest

Diastolic dysfunction may be as common as systolic dysfunction and predicts a poor prognosis outside the perioperative period. The significance of diastolic dysfunction for anesthesia and surgery is less well defined. In a study of patients undergoing major vascular surgery, isolated diastolic dysfunction diagnosed preoperatively by echocardiography was an independent predictor of postoperative HF.[57]

An objective measure of left ventricular ejection fraction (LVEF) and ventricular performance is helpful, especially in patients with NYHA class III or IV HF. Normal LVEF is greater than 50%; mildly diminished, 41% to 49%; moderately diminished, 26% to 40%; and severely diminished, less than 25%. Patients with class III or IV heart failure should be evaluated by a cardiologist before undergoing general anesthesia or any intermediate- or high-risk procedure. Very minor procedures under monitored anesthesia care can proceed as long as the patient's condition is stable.

Rhythm Disturbances and Electrocardiogram Abnormalities Arrhythmias and conduction disturbances are common in the perioperative period. Supraventricular and ventricular arrhythmias are associated with a greater risk of perioperative adverse events because of the arrhythmia itself and because they are markers for cardiopulmonary disease. Because uncontrolled atrial fibrillation (AF) and ventricular tachycardia are high-risk clinical markers, elective surgery is postponed until evaluation and stabilization are complete.[11] Patients with preexisting paroxysmal AF who progress to persistent AF have worse outcomes due to increases in major cardiovascular events.[58]

New-onset AF, recent conversion from paroxysmal to sustained AF, AF with a rate more than 100 beats per minute, symptomatic bradycardia, or high-grade heart block (second or third degree) identified preoperatively warrant postponement of elective procedures and referral to cardiology for further evaluation. Left and right bundle branch blocks on preoperative ECG have been shown to predict major cardiac morbidity and mortality, but they had no added predictive value over the clinical history.[36] Brugada syndrome is a congenital disease characterized by right bundle branch block (RBBB) with ST-segment elevation in the right precordial leads and is associated with a risk of sudden death and lethal arrhythmias. If the history and physical do not suggest significant pulmonary or congenital heart disease, no further evaluation is warranted because of an isolated RBBB. If congenital heart disease or Brugada syndrome is suspected, a cardiology consultation is indicated. RBBB in a patient with pulmonary symptoms is suggestive of severe respiratory compromise that warrants a pulmonary evaluation and echocardiography if an intermediate- or high-risk operation is planned. Prolonged QT intervals prompt an evaluation of electrolytes, magnesium, and calcium and a cardiology referral.

Murmurs The quandary is to determine the cause of cardiac murmurs and to distinguish between significant murmurs and clinically unimportant ones. Diastolic murmurs are always pathologic and require further evaluation. Regurgitant disease is tolerated perioperatively much better than stenotic disease.

Aortic stenosis is the most common valvular lesion in the United States, affecting 2% to 4% of adults older than 65 years of age; severe stenosis is associated with a high risk of perioperative complications.[11] Once considered a degenerative lesion with increasing age or a congenital bicuspid valve, aortic stenosis is now thought to have much in common with CAD and is an independent marker of CAD.[59]

Aortic *sclerosis,* which also causes a systolic ejection murmur similar to that of aortic stenosis, is present in 25% of adults 65 to 74 years of age and almost half of those older than 84 years of age.[59] Aortic sclerosis is associated with a 40% increase in the risk of MI and a 50% increase in the risk of cardiovascular death in patients without a history of CAD.[60] There is no hemodynamic compromise with aortic sclerosis.

The cardinal symptoms of severe aortic stenosis are angina, HF, and syncope, although patients are much more likely to complain of a decrease in exercise tolerance and exertional dyspnea. Aortic stenosis causes a systolic ejection murmur that is best heard in the right upper sternal border, which often radiates to the neck. Any patient with a previously undiagnosed murmur needs an ECG, and any ECG abnormality warrants an echocardiogram. Because of the difficulties noncardiologists have in distinguishing murmurs of aortic stenosis from those of aortic sclerosis, an echocardiogram should be ordered even without ECG abnormalities, especially if general anesthesia or an intermediate- or high-risk procedure is planned. Current guidelines recommend echocardiography annually for patients with severe aortic stenosis, every 1 to 2 years for moderate stenosis, and every 3 to 5 years for mild stenosis.[61]

Mitral stenosis is much less common than aortic stenosis and is usually associated with a history of rheumatic heart disease. Mitral stenosis causes a diastolic murmur and should always be further evaluated with ECG and echocardiography. Patients with hypertrophic obstructive cardiomyopathy are often young and male, and they may be asymptomatic and without murmurs. An ECG and echocardiogram is done if there is a personal or family history of syncope with exertion or sudden death, or if a murmur is detected. LVH and ST-segment and T-wave abnormalities on an ECG in an otherwise healthy nonhypertensive patient need to be further evaluated with echocardiography.

Cardiac Rhythm Management Devices: Pacemakers and Implantable Cardioverter-Defibrillators It is estimated that more than 100 000 new cardiac rhythm-management devices (CRMDs), which include both pacemakers and ICDs, are implanted yearly in the United States. Electromagnetic interference is likely to occur with electrocautery, radiofrequency ablation, magnetic resonance imaging, and radiation therapy, and it can result in malfunction or adverse events.[62] Some patient monitors and ventilators may cause electromagnetic interference in patients with CRMDs with rate-adaptive mechanisms. The type of device and the features (eg, rate-adaptive mechanisms) likely to malfunction with electromagnetic interference need to be determined during the preoperative evaluation.

Magnets cause most pacemakers to pace asynchronously at a preset rate. Although most ICDs suspend tachydysrhythmia detection (and therefore therapy) when a magnet is appropriately placed, many can be programmed to ignore the magnet. Placement of a magnet may deactivate the device permanently, requiring a programmer to reenable it. Magnets do not affect the pacing function of ICDs.

Ideally, patients with CRMDs have these devices interrogated preoperatively. Consultation with the device manufacturer, cardiologist, or the electrophysiology service may be needed. Special features, such as rate adaptive mechanisms and anti-tachyarrhythmia functions, need to be disabled or the device reprogrammed to an asynchronous pacing mode before surgical procedures and anesthesia where electromagnetic interference is anticipated.[62] Newer-generation devices are more complex, and reliance on a magnet, except in emergency situations, is not recommended. ASA guidelines recommend interrogation of the device and disabling the antiarrhythmic function during the procedure. Patients must be in a monitored setting with defibrillation capabilities until the device is reactivated.[62] This requires planning so the appropriate device-specific interrogator and trained personnel are available. This may pose a problem for free-standing ambulatory centers.

PULMONARY DISEASE OR PATIENTS WITH RISK FACTORS FOR POSTOPERATIVE PULMONARY COMPLICATIONS

Postoperative pulmonary complications develop in 5% of patients undergoing nonthoracic surgery, and as many as 1 in 4 deaths occurring within a week of operation are pulmonary related, making it the second most common serious morbidity after cardiovascular-adverse events.[63] Established risk factors for an increased risk of pulmonary complications include the following[13]:

- Advanced age
- Poor general health status
- ASA PS scores >2
- Chronic obstructive pulmonary disease
- Head, neck, thoracic, upper abdominal, aortic, neurologic, vascular, or emergency surgery
- Anticipated prolonged procedures (>2 hours)
- Planned general anesthesia (especially with endotracheal intubation)
- Heart failure

Surprisingly absent predictors in the preceding list are asthma or results from arterial blood gas (ABG) analysis or PFTs. Risk of complications is surprisingly low in well-controlled asthma and in patients treated preoperatively with corticosteroids.[64] Risk is greater in patients with asthma with recent exacerbations, a history of postoperative pulmonary complications, recent hospitalizations, or recent intubations for asthma. ABGs are useful in predicting pulmonary function after lung resection surgery but do not predict risk for complications. The extent of airway obstruction, measured by the forced expiratory volume in 1 second is not predictive of pulmonary complications.[65] The predicted postoperative diffusing capacity of the lungs for carbon monoxide predicts postoperative pulmonary complications following thoracic surgery.[66, 67]

The focus is on identifying patients at risk for postoperative pulmonary complications and on optimizing those patients with preexisting pulmonary disease. Rarely, PFTs may be indicated to diagnose disease (dyspnea caused by lung disease or heart failure?) or assess management (can dyspnea or wheezing be improved further?) but *not* as a risk assessment tool or to deny a beneficial procedure.[65]

The pulmonary status of patients with recent exacerbations or infections needs to be improved whenever possible. Prescriptions for bronchodilators or steroids, referral to pulmonologists or internists, or delay of surgery might be necessary. Training patients preoperatively in lung expansion maneuvers, such as deep-breathing exercises and incentive spirometry, reduces pulmonary complications more than giving the training postoperatively.[68] Additionally, a change in perioperative management, including altering the planned surgical procedure if possible, discussing alternatives to general anesthesia, and educating the patient about the benefits of epidural pain management, may provide effective measures to decrease pulmonary complications.[69]

Patients with pulmonary arterial hypertension have a high rate of perioperative morbidity and mortality. The patient's care should be coordinated with a pulmonologist. An ECG and echocardiogram are useful in patients with more than mild disease. Signs and symptoms of disease severity include the following[70]:

- Dyspnea at rest
- Metabolic acidosis
- Hypoxemia
- Right heart failure (peripheral edema, hepatomegaly, jugular venous distension)
- History of syncope

Traditionally, especially with children, cases scheduled for elective procedures were cancelled for patients with current or recent upper respiratory tract infections. With modern anesthetic practices, cancellation is not routine.[71] In patients with severe symptoms, especially those with underlying conditions that may further compromise a safe anesthetic, elective surgery is postponed for at least 4 weeks. When infection is mild or uncomplicated in healthy patients, there is little risk in proceeding with a procedure to avoid the inconvenience of a cancellation. The dilemma lies with the patients between these extremes. Decisions regarding suitability to proceed should be made on an individual basis. Chapter 20 discusses the pediatric patient with an upper respiratory tract infection in greater detail. Chapter 11 discusses the patient with pulmonary disease in detail.

OBSTRUCTIVE SLEEP APNEA

Sleep-disordered breathing affects up to 9% of middle-age women and 24% of middle-age men; fewer than 15% of these cases have been diagnosed. OSA, the most common serious manifestation of sleep-disordered breathing, is caused by intermittent airway obstruction. OSA is characterized by total collapse of the airway with complete obstruction for more than 10 seconds. Obstructive hypopnea is partial collapse (30% to 99%) associated with at least a 4% arterial oxygen desaturation. OSA severity is measured on the apnea-hypopnea index (AHI), the number of apneic and hypopneic episodes per hour of sleep. Patients with severe OSA have more than 30 episodes per hour.

Cardiovascular disease is common in patients with OSA. These patients have an increased incidence of hypertension, atrial fibrillation, bradyarrhythmias, ventricular ectopy, endothelial damage, stroke, HF dilated cardiomyopathy, and atherosclerotic CAD.[72] Mask ventilation, direct laryngoscopy, endotracheal intubation, and even fiberoptic visualization of the airway are more difficult in patients with OSA than in healthy patients. Patients with OSA are at risk of postoperative oxygen desaturation.[73] There is an association of OSA with obesity.

The STOP-Bang Questionnaire is useful to identify patients with undiagnosed OSA.[74] Preoperative evaluation focuses on identification of patients at risk for OSA and improving associated comorbid conditions. Echocardiography may be indicated if HF or pulmonary hypertension is suspected.[75] Patients should be instructed to bring their continuous positive airway pressure (CPAP) devices to the hospital on the day of operation. Chapter 11 discusses OSA in detail.

OBESITY

An overweight person has a BMI of 25 to 29.9 kg/m^2; obesity is defined as a BMI of 30 to 39.9 kg/m^2. A BMI of 40 kg/m^2 or higher defines extreme obesity. See the formulas for calculating BMI earlier in this chapter. An estimated 64% of adults in the United States are overweight or obese, and 4.7% are extremely obese. Annually 300 000 US adults die of obesity-related issues, and almost 10% of health care expenditures in the United States are associated with obesity and inactivity. Obesity is an independent risk factor for heart disease. Hypertension, stroke, hyperlipidemia, osteoarthritis, DM, cancer, and OSA are more common in obese people.

Extremely obese patients may have challenging airways that require specialized equipment, techniques, and personnel. They may need prophylaxis for deep venous thrombosis (DVT) with advanced techniques such as inferior vena cava filter placements. They require special operating room tables and gurneys to support excessive weight. Venous access and invasive and noninvasive monitoring can be difficult. Preoperative identification and planning for these contingencies will avoid delays on the day of the operation. Preoperative evaluation is directed toward coexisting diseases (Table 6-4). Chapter 23 discusses this in greater detail.

DIABETES

An estimated 18 million US adults have DM, which increases the risk of CAD, is considered a CAD equivalent, and is a risk factor for perioperative cardiac complications on a par with angina or a previous MI.[11,76] Figure 6-1 and Chapter 9 address cardiac evaluation for noncardiac surgery.

Heart failure is twice as common in males and 5 times as common in females with DM as in those without DM. Poor glycemic control is associated with an increased risk for heart failure, and both systolic and diastolic dysfunction may be present. People with diabetes are also at increased risk for renal failure perioperatively (see Chapters 13, 14, and "Renal Disease" later) and for postoperative infections. Patients with poor preoperative management of glucose are likely to be more out of control intra- and postoperatively.[77] Obtaining a glycosylated hemoglobin concentration preoperatively can guide glucose management with intensification of therapy well before the procedure.[77] Aggressive management of hyperglycemia decreases postoperative complications. The American College of Endocrinologists' position statement recommends a target fasting glucose of less than 110 mg/dL in noncritically ill patients.[78]

Preoperatively, the focus is on assessing organ damage and the control of blood sugar. Cardiovascular, renal, and neurologic systems should be evaluated. Ischemic heart disease is often asymptomatic in the person with DM. The goals of perioperative diabetic management include avoidance of hypoglycemia and marked hyperglycemia. Table 6-7 has suggestions for hypoglycemic medication management.

HYPERTENSION

HTN, defined by 2 or more measurements of blood pressure greater than 140/90, affects 1 billion individuals worldwide. The incidence of HTN increases with age. In the United States, 25% of adults and 70% of patients older than 70 years of age have HTN, and fewer than 30% are treated adequately. The degree of end-organ damage and morbidity and mortality correlate with the duration and severity of HTN.

Ischemic heart disease is the most common form of organ damage associated with HTN. The odds ratio for an association between HTN and perioperative cardiac risk is 1.31.[79] There is little evidence of an association between preoperative blood pressures lower than 180/110 mm Hg and perioperative cardiac risk. Heart failure, renal insufficiency, and cerebrovascular disease are more common in hypertensive patients.

It is generally recommended that elective surgery be delayed for severe HTN (diastolic blood pressure > 115 mm Hg; systolic blood pressure > 200 mm Hg) until the blood pressure is lower than 180/110 mm Hg. If severe end-organ damage is present, the goal is to normalize blood pressure *as much as possible* before the operation.[79] There is no evidence to justify cancellation of an operation when blood pressure is lower than 180/110 mm Hg, although interventions preoperatively are appropriate. Severely elevated blood pressure should be lowered over several weeks.

Guidelines suggest that cardioselective β-blocker therapy is the best treatment preoperatively because of a favorable profile in lowering cardiovascular risk.[80] Effective lowering of risk may require 6 to 8 weeks of therapy to allow regression of vascular changes, and too rapid or extreme lowering of blood pressure may increase cerebral and coronary ischemia. The Antihypertensive and Lipid-Lowering Treatment to Prevent Heart Attack Trial (ALLHAT) showed that effective treatment of HTN is not simply a matter of lowering blood pressure.[81] Continuation of antihypertensive treatment preoperatively is critical (Table 6-7). Chapter 9 has more information on the hypertensive patient.

RENAL DISEASE

A normal creatinine level is often not an accurate indicator of renal function. A doubling of serum creatinine from 0.8 to 1.6 mg/dL represents a halving of glomerular filtration rate (GFR). Creatinine does not exceed the normal limits until GFR has fallen below 50 mL/min. GFR decreases with age, and the renal reserve of a healthy 80-year-old is less than half that of a healthy 40-year-old. The focus of the preoperative evaluation of patients with renal insufficiency or failure is on the cardiovascular and cerebrovascular systems, fluid volume, and electrolyte status. Chronic metabolic acidosis is common but usually mild and compensated for by chronic hyperventilation.

Chronic renal disease is a significant risk factor for cardiovascular morbidity and mortality and is an ACC/AHA cardiac risk factor equal to a history of known CAD (Fig. 6-1).[11] The annual incidence of death from CAD in patients with both DM and end-stage renal disease requiring hemodialysis is 8.2%. A creatinine of 2.0 mg/dL or higher triggers an assessment of cardiac risk using the ACC/AHA guidelines (Fig. 6-1).[11] In a study of 23 016 patients undergoing cardiac surgery, those requiring preoperative hemodialysis had an increased 30-day morbidity and mortality equal to patients having urgent surgery, valvular surgery, or an ejection fraction less than 30%.[82]

In elective cases, hemodialysis needs to be performed within 24 hours of the operation, but not immediately before, due to the risk of hypovolemia and electrolyte shifts. Hemodialysis is associated with fluid and electrolyte (sodium, potassium, magnesium, phosphate) imbalance and shifting of electrolytes between intra- and extracellular compartments. Hemodialysis is performed to correct volume overload, hyperkalemia, and acidosis.

Patients at risk for perioperative renal failure include those with preexisting renal insufficiency and DM, especially in combination, and those undergoing procedures with the administration of contrast medium. If all 3 conditions are present, the risk of renal failure may be as high as 50%. Preoperative identification of at-risk patients may change management, such as administration of sodium bicarbonate, hydration, a change in type of contrast medium, and avoidance of hypovolemia or even vigorous hydration. Chapter 14 has a complete discussion of the patient with renal disease.

HEPATIC DISEASE

Predictors of poor perioperative outcome in patients with liver disease include the following[83]:

- Acute hepatitis (viral or alcoholic)
- Chronic active hepatitis with jaundice, encephalopathy, coagulopathy, or elevated liver enzymes
- Child C cirrhosis (bilirubin > 3 mg/dL, albumin < 3 g/dL, PT > 6 seconds more than control, poor nutritional status, large amount of ascites, and moderate encephalopathy)
- Abdominal surgery
- PT longer than 3 seconds; prolongation refractive to vitamin K therapy

Salt and water restriction, diuretic therapy (spironolactone is preferred), enteral nutritional supplements, and oral vitamin K (1-5 mg daily for 3-5 days) are indicated preoperatively to correct deficiencies. Delaying elective surgery until after an acute episode of hepatitis or an exacerbation of chronic disease has resolved is appropriate. Chapter 15 discusses the patient with liver disease in detail.

ANEMIA

The ASA Task Force on Blood Component Therapy concluded that red blood cells should not be transfused solely because of a Hgb level but rather because of risk for complications from inadequate oxygenation.[84] Transfusion is rarely indicated when the Hgb is more than 10 mg/dL and almost always needed when the Hgb is less than 6 mg/dL. Anemia is associated with an increase in postoperative mortality independent of transfusion.[12,15] The goal in the preoperative period is to determine the etiology, duration, and stability of the anemia, and to consider the extent and type of surgery, the anticipated blood loss, and the patient's comorbid conditions that may impact oxygenation, such as pulmonary, cerebrovascular, or cardiovascular disease. Type and screen testing before the day of operation and planning for the availability of blood will avoid delay of the procedure (Table 6-5). This can ease the burden on the blood bank personnel for same-day admission or outpatient surgery. A protocol can be instituted with the department of surgery and the blood bank. Intraoperative blood salvage can be planned, if appropriate. In special circumstances, such as a patient's refusal of perioperative blood transfusions or for elective procedures with expected significant blood loss in anemic patients, postponement of surgery to treat with iron may be warranted.

Sickle cell disease is a hereditary hemoglobinopathy, and vasoocclusion is responsible for most of the associated complications. Preoperative assessment focuses on identification of organ dysfunction and acute exacerbations.[85] Chapter 16 discusses in detail the patient with anemia.

NEUROLOGIC DISEASE

For a patient with neurologic disease (eg, stroke, seizure disorder, multiple sclerosis), a detailed history is required with focus on recent events, exacerbations, or evidence for poor control of the medical condition. A basic neurologic examination documenting deficits in mental status, speech, cranial nerves, gait, and motor and sensory function is important. This baseline enables postoperative comparison and evaluation of new deficits. If a stroke or transient neurologic deficit is not fully evaluated or occurs within 1 month before the operation, elective surgery is typically delayed pending complete evaluation. A carotid bruit requires a careful history of related symptoms. If symptoms are present, carotid Doppler studies are indicated. Significant abnormalities on Doppler studies should prompt a referral to a vascular surgeon or neurologist.

Routinely ordering tests for serum drug levels of antiseizure medications is not warranted unless toxicity is a concern or the patient is having breakthrough seizures. Patients with good control of seizures may have levels outside the therapeutic range and results may be confounded if the timing of the administration of the drugs in relation to when the test is drawn is not considered. Chapter 12 discusses neurologic diseases in detail.

CANCER PATIENTS

Patients with a history of cancer may have complications related to the disease or the treatment. Preoperative evaluation focuses on evaluation of the heart, lungs, and neurologic and hematologic systems. Previous head and neck irradiation may cause carotid artery disease, hypothyroidism, or difficulty with airway management.[86] Auscultation for bruits, thyroid function tests (thyroid-stimulating hormone levels), and carotid Doppler studies may be needed.

Mediastinal, chest wall, and left breast irradiation can cause conduction abnormalities, cardiomyopathy, valvular abnormalities, and premature CAD even without traditional risk factors.[87] Cardiovascular disease is the second most common cause of mortality in survivors of Hodgkin disease. One study found that 88% of patients had echocardiographic abnormalities 5 to 20 years after treatment, most of them asymptomatic. Treatment at a younger age increases risk. These risk factors were not considered in the ACC/AHA *Guidelines for Cardiac Evaluation for Noncardiac Surgery,* but they may be important predictors of CAD.[87] ECG, echocardiography, and stress testing may be indicated.

Patients with cancer may have significant pain associated with their primary illness and take large amounts of narcotics. Consultation with a pain specialist may be necessary in complicated and difficult pain management cases. A discussion with the patient needs to occur preoperatively to help allay patient concerns and fears about inadequate pain control. Similar issues may occur in patients with chronic pain or who abuse substances.

SUBSTANCE ABUSE

Patients who use alcohol to excess or illicit drugs may not give a reliable history. Addicts may be at risk for a myriad of perioperative complications, including withdrawal, acute intoxication, an altered tolerance to anesthetic and opioid medications, infections, and end-organ damage. Preferably, patients with drug or alcohol dependence should be drug free well before an elective operation. Acute preoperative abstinence in alcoholics, however, is associated with a poorer outcome postoperatively than if drinking is continued.[88]

Preanesthesia clinic staff should be prepared to refer patients to addiction specialists or programs or prescribe medications to prevent withdrawal in the preoperative period if patients agree to abstinence. Intravenous drug use prompts an evaluation for cardiovascular, pulmonary, neurologic, and infectious complications. Because intravenous access is often limited in users, interventional radiology may be needed to help with line placement. Alcoholics need assessment of cardiovascular, hepatic, and neurologic alterations. Planning for adequate postoperative analgesia is important because these patients often have a higher requirement from chronic abuse and misuse of substances. Testing depends on symptoms and findings from the history and physical. ECG, echocardiography, chest radiography, and chemistry and hepatic panels may be needed. Table 6-4 and Chapter 24 provide additional information.

PATIENTS WITH OR AT RISK OF THROMBOEMBOLISM AND/OR PULMONARY EMBOLI

Recent arterial or DVT requires postponement of non–lifesaving procedures. Without anticoagulation, the risk of recurrent DVT within 3 months of a proximal DVT is approximately 50%. A month of warfarin treatment reduces the risk to 10%; 3 months of warfarin treatment reduces the risk to 5%. Patients with a hereditary hypercoagulable state, cancer, or multiple episodes of DVT are at higher risk indefinitely. Patients with nonvalvular atrial fibrillation who have had a previous cerebral embolism also are at high risk, as are patients with mechanical heart valves, especially multiple valves. Risk is greater with mitral than with aortic valves. Surgery increases the risk of DVT, but there is no evidence that surgery increases the risk of arterial embolism in patients with atrial fibrillation or mechanical valves.[89]

An elective operation scheduled for the first month after an episode of venous or arterial thromboembolism should be postponed. If postponement is not possible, then the patient should receive preoperative heparin while the international normalized ratio (INR) is below 2.0.[89] Ideally, 3 months of anticoagulation is recommended before an elective operation. In a large cohort study, thromboembolism, excessive bleeding, and death were low when anticoagulation was temporarily suspended for invasive procedures. Patients with cancer had the greatest risk of thrombosis and bleeding as compared with noncancer patients.[90] See the section on medication instructions and Table 6-7 for further discussion of warfarin management preoperatively. Chapter 16 discusses patients with coagulation disorders.

SMOKERS AND THOSE EXPOSED TO SECONDHAND SMOKE

Exposure to tobacco, directly or through "secondhand" smoke, increases the risk of many perioperative complications. Smokers are more likely to experience wound infections, respiratory or airway complications (including oxygen desaturation), and severe coughing.[91] Smoking decreases macrophage function, negatively impacts coronary flow reserve, and causes vascular endothelial dysfunction, hypertension, and ischemia. Smoking causes inflammation and may cause immunosuppression. [92] Smokers require longer hospital stays and more often need postoperative intensive care than do nonsmokers.

The greatest benefit of smoking abstinence is probably only realized after several months of cessation. In studies reporting a greater perioperative risk in recent quitters than in smokers, selection bias may have contributed to the results. The patients who were motivated to stop or advised to quit smoking may have been at greater risk because of health status. Soon after a patient quits smoking, carbon monoxide levels decrease, which improves oxygen delivery and use. Cyanide levels decrease, which benefits mitochondrial oxidative metabolism. Lower nicotine levels improve vasodilatation, and many toxic substances that impair wound healing decrease. Patients without a history of ischemic heart disease who smoked shortly before their operation had significantly more episodes of rate-pressure product-related ST-segment depression than did nonsmokers, former smokers, or chronic smokers who did not smoke in the immediate preoperative period.[93]

A preoperative smoking cessation intervention in patients who underwent knee and hip replacements decreased rates of surgical-site infections from 23% in the conventional group to 4% in those who stopped smoking. The US Public Health Service recommends that "*all* physicians should strongly advise every patient who smokes to quit because evidence shows that physician advice to quit smoking increases abstinence rates."[94] Nearly 70% of smokers want to quit. Patients presenting for surgery are more likely to quit smoking compared with smokers not having surgery.[95]

Effective interventions include medical advice and pharmacotherapy, such as nicotine-replacement therapy, varenicline (Chantix), and bupropion (Wellbutrin), which are safe in the perioperative period. Nicotine patches, gum, and lozenges are available without a prescription; nasal spray, varenicline, and bupropion require prescriptions. Clonidine is also effective. Varenicline, bupropion, or clonidine should be started 1 to 2 weeks before a quit attempt; nicotine replacement therapy is effective immediately.[95] Individual and group counseling may increase rates of long-term abstinence. Many hospitals, insurance companies, and communities offer smoking cessation programs. Excellent resources are available on the Internet and from the US government. Advice and guidelines are available at http://www.surgeongeneral.gov/tobacco/default.htm. Patients can be referred to 1-800-QUITNOW. Tobacco-intervention training during medical school and residency can significantly improve the quality of physician counseling and rates of abstinence.

THE ELDERLY

By the year 2030, almost 70 million persons older than 65 years will be alive in the United States, and a significant portion of these will be 85 years of age or older. The number of patients older than 65 years who will undergo noncardiac surgery will increase from 7 to 14 million by 2025. Chronological age, however, is a less important determinant of operative outcome than are comorbid conditions and physiologic age. Age older than 70 years is an independent predictor of postoperative mortality, cognitive dysfunction, major perioperative complications, and longer hospital stays.[13, 96] Organ function declines in the elderly, who respond differently to medications and have a greater number of comorbid conditions. Among the conditions are arthritis, hypertension, heart disease, and DM. One study found coexisting disease in 95% of geriatric patients scheduled for surgery. Postoperatively 35% of patients had cardiac or pulmonary complications that were associated with comorbid conditions, and many could have been predicted preoperatively.[97] Other studies have found that the rate of perioperative complications among the very elderly (>85 years) is not prohibitive.[96]

Elderly individuals often do not return home immediately after an operation for various reasons. They need rehabilitation, their recovery takes longer, they have a high incidence of postoperative cognitive dysfunction (41.4% prevalence at discharge, 12.7% at 3 months), or support services are lacking.[98] Discharge planning in advance may lessen the costs of perioperative elder care. Preoperative clinics can be designed to offer multidisciplinary care and after-discharge planning that coordinates with surgical, nursing, and social service departments.[99]

Testing in the elderly patient should be based on disease indications rather than age alone (see Table 6-4 and the section in this chapter on age-based testing, "Preoperative Testing"). Chapter 21 presents an expanded discussion of the evaluation of the geriatric patient.

CATARACT PATIENTS

Patients undergoing cataract surgery are often elderly with extensive comorbid disease. The procedure is minor, however, without expected systemic physiologic disturbances or significant postoperative pain. Topical anesthesia is commonly used, and because general anesthesia is rarely required, the risk is lessened. Elective cataract surgery has the enormous benefits of allowing individuals to drive, read, avoid isolation, watch television, and decrease the incidence of falls. The cost of routine medical testing before cataract surgery is estimated at $150 million annually. In a study of more than 18 000 patients randomly allocated to no *routine* testing before cataract surgery or to a battery of tests, including ECG, complete blood count, and electrolytes, blood urea nitrogen, creatinine, and glucose levels, no differences in postoperative adverse events were found between the two groups.[100]

The results of this study do not suggest that patients undergoing cataract surgery require no laboratory testing.[100] The study of cataract patients eliminated routine tests, not tests indicated for a new or worsening medical problem. The group that crossed over from no testing to some testing had significantly more coexisting illness and poor self-reported health status. This finding suggests that the preoperative care provider screen patients to order tests for those who require them. In the study described, exclusion criteria were general anesthesia or an MI within 3 months. *All* patients underwent a *preoperative medical assessment*. More than 85% of enrollees reported good to excellent health status, almost 25% reported no coexisting illnesses (including hypertension, anemia, DM, and heart or lung disease), almost 30% were older than 70 years, and 65% were ASA PS 1 or 2 status, suggesting a fairly healthy group.[100] If patients are comparable with those in the study, are routinely evaluated by primary care physicians, have stable mild disease, and will undergo cataract operation under topical or bulbar block, then no special testing is required because of cataract surgery. Serious, poorly controlled conditions must be normalized before surgery, and selective testing suggested by history and physical examination may be necessary. One center showed a 90% savings in laboratory costs in a 4-month period by eliminating routine testing for cataract patients.[101]

Although testing is rarely necessary *because* of cataract surgery, patients with limited access to health care services may benefit from medical evaluation. The ACC/AHA *Guidelines for Cardiac Evaluation for Noncardiac Surgery* consider cataract surgery to be low risk.[11]

THE DIFFICULT AIRWAY

An important part of preoperative evaluation is assessment of the airway. If a patient with a difficult airway can be identified before the day of operation, special equipment or personnel with advanced training and skills in airway management can be available without delaying or postponing procedures or compromising patient safety.[1] Patients with the following characteristics may have a challenging airway:

- OSA
- Snoring
- Obesity
- Facial and neck deformities from previous operation
- Head and neck radiation
- Head and neck trauma
- Congenital abnormalities
- Rheumatoid arthritis
- Down syndrome
- Scleroderma
- Cervical spine disease or previous operation

The ease or difficulty of laryngoscopy and intubation are discussed extensively in the literature. However, equally, if not more, important is the ability to predict difficulty with mask ventilation.[102] The following patient characteristics independently suggest difficulty with mask ventilation:

- Age older than 55 years
- BMI higher than 26 kg/m^2
- Lack of teeth
- A beard
- Snoring history

Patients with Down syndrome or rheumatoid arthritis may have asymptomatic atlantoaxial subluxation and cervical spine instability. A careful history may elicit neurologic deficits or neck and shoulder pain.

Patients with neurologic deficits or symptoms and rheumatoid arthritis patients with long-standing, severely deforming disease need cervical spine radiographs with special flexion, extension, and open-mouth odontoid views. Patients with oral piercings are counseled to remove all jewelry on the day of surgery and about the potential risks if piercings are not removed.[103]

Chapter 10 discusses the evaluation of the patient with a difficult airway. The goals in the preoperative clinic should be documentation of an airway examination, including size of the oral opening, Mallampati score, status of teeth (Fig. 6-2), range of motion of the neck, thyromental distance, body habitus, presence of facial hair, and pertinent deformities. Previous anesthetic records should be obtained and a discussion of awake fiberoptic intubation with the patient may be appropriate. See "Physical Examination" earlier for components of the airway examination.

ANESTHESIA-SPECIFIC CONCERNS

A personal or family history of pseudocholinesterase deficiency is identified preoperatively. Records from previous anesthetics may clarify an uncertain history. If time allows, a dibucaine number and pseudocholinesterase, chloride, and fluoride levels should be obtained. A history of malignant hyperthermia (MH) or a suggestion of it (hyperthermia, rigidity during anesthesia, or unplanned admission to an ICU following a general anesthetic) either in a patient or family member should be clearly documented and arrangements made before the day of the operation. Chapter 87 provides a comprehensive review of MH, its prevention and management.

AMBULATORY SURGERY

Approximately 60% to 70% of surgical procedures are performed on an outpatient basis, and of these, 5% to 8% are performed in an office setting. A study of ambulatory surgery in Medicare beneficiaries older than 65 years found no deaths on the day of operation when the procedure was performed in a physician's office; 2.3 deaths per 100 000 procedures when performed in a freestanding ambulatory surgical center; and 2.5 deaths per 100 000 when performed at an outpatient hospital. The 7-day mortality was 35 per 100 000, 25 per 100 000, and 50 per 100 000, respectively. Age older than 85 years, significant comorbidity, and type of procedure predicted adverse events.[104]

Almost half of ambulatory surgical procedures are performed in patients 65 years and older. Elderly patients may bring specific problems to the ambulatory setting because they often have multiple chronic conditions and poor eyesight, and they may be unable to perform activities of daily living such as feeding themselves or driving. Some patients have limited support during the stress of recovery from anesthesia and surgery.[99]

Patients with OSA may require skilled and specialized airway management. They are typically sensitive to anesthetic agents (less airway muscle tone than normal, which leads to airway collapse) and narcotics (greater than average respiratory depression). They may require longer postoperative monitoring, and the American Sleep Apnea Association suggests that some patients with sleep apnea might not be candidates for ambulatory surgery. Patients are told to bring their CPAP machines on the day of surgery.

Obese patients may require specialized equipment to accommodate their weight, which might not be readily available in ambulatory facilities. Patients with a history or family history of MH may require prolonged observation in the recovery period, so planning is important. Whether a patient susceptible to MH is a candidate for ambulatory surgery should be decided well before the day of operation. Individuals with pacemakers and ICDs may not be candidates for freestanding ambulatory facilities if electromagnetic interference is likely or sudden patient movement is undesirable, and personnel are not available to reprogram the devices.[62] The ACC/AHA *Guidelines for Cardiac Evaluation for Noncardiac Surgery* consider ambulatory surgery to be low risk.[11]

PATIENT MANAGEMENT

Management of comorbid conditions and interventions to reduce risk is as important as identification and diagnosis of medical disease. If anesthesiologists are not going to intervene to improve new or chronic disease states, then close collaboration with primary care physicians, specialists, and surgeons are essential. Far too many anesthesia practices collect information without having processes in place to follow through to manage patients and risk to improve outcomes and reduce adverse events.

CONSULTATIONS

Collaborative care of patients is often necessary and beneficial. Consultation initiated by the preoperative physician should seek specific advice regarding diagnosis and status of the patient's condition(s). Asking specific questions such as "Does this patient have CAD?" or "Is this patient in the best medical condition for planned thoracotomy with lung resection under general anesthesia?" is the first step. Letters or notes stating "cleared for surgery" are rarely sufficient to design a safe anesthetic. A summary of the patient's medical problems and current status, medical therapy, and results of any recent diagnostic tests is necessary.

Close coordination and good communication among the preoperative anesthesiologist, surgeon, and consultant is vitally important. Miscommunication among care providers was central to most reported incidents in the Australian Incident Monitoring Study (AIMS) whenever preoperative assessment was implicated.[1]

In many practices the cardiology service is most frequently consulted perioperatively. In one survey, however, the usefulness of such consultations was questioned by anesthesiologists. Unfortunately, only 17% of anesthesiologists felt obligated to follow the consulting cardiologist's recommendations. Forty percent of the consultations contained only the recommendation to "proceed with the case," "cleared for surgery," or "continue with current medications." Recommendations regarding intraoperative monitoring or cardiac medications were largely ignored. Part of this responsibility lies with the consulting physicians (be that surgeons or anesthesiologists) and the long-standing practice of asking for or receiving cardiac "clearance." This is a vague request, and a response (often scribbled on a prescription pad) simply stating "low risk" or "cleared for surgery" is meaningless and unhelpful. In general, preoperative consultations are sought for diagnosis, evaluation, and improvement of a new or poorly controlled condition, and for creation of a clinical risk profile that the patient, anesthesiologist, and surgeon use to make management decisions.

Detailed discussions and communication, preferably oral, are essential for the best management of complicated patients. Copies of diagnostic studies that accompany the consultation letter help the anesthesiologist to make an independent decision about patient risk and to plan anesthetic care. Chapter 8 has a detailed discussion of consultations.

PRACTICE GUIDELINES

An important element for a successful preoperative evaluation system is a uniform, consistent method for assessment and management. Even though individual judgment is necessary, guidelines and policies for the group should be developed. Cancellations, delays, or demands for additional diagnostic testing on the day of operation after a patient has been evaluated and deemed acceptable for anesthesia by the preoperative clinic is detrimental to the success of a preoperative assessment program.

Practice guidelines improve the process of preoperative evaluation and management and affect surgical outcomes. Guidelines minimize variation in clinical practice and make good use of resources. They may help to avoid cancellations or delays on the day of operation when the anesthesiologist in the preanesthetic clinic and the one performing the anesthesia have differences in opinion about the patient's fitness for operation. This will prevent patient inconvenience and disappointment and surgeon dissatisfaction. Guidelines synthesized from the best, most current sources help practitioners stay up to date with recommendations and the literature by assimilating treatments and diagnostics into their practices. Guidelines can be as simple as an organization of the type and timing of care delivered to typical, uncomplicated patients or as complex as instructions for dealing with a specific issue expressed by decision trees in branching logic format.[105] Acceptance is more likely when disease-specific algorithms are developed and agreed to by all stakeholders. The intent is not to design inflexible standards but to provide a consistent, straightforward method to evaluate a particular disease such as hypertension or CAD, a finding such as a murmur, or a symptom such as chest pain. Practice guidelines recommend care based on scientific evidence and broad consensus but leave room for justifiable variations in practice.

Practice guidelines typically rely on evidence-based medicine that examines the data from clinical research. Intuition, personal clinical experience, and pathophysiologic rationale are less important. The practice and teaching of evidence-based medicine requires skills that are not part of traditional medical training. Precisely defining a problem and the information required to resolve the problem are important first steps. The pertinent studies from a well-conducted literature search are selected and applied to the treatment of medical conditions found in patients.

Algorithms such as in Figs. 6-1 and 6-3, and guidelines such as in Tables 6-4 through 6-7, are examples.

NOTHING-BY-MOUTH GUIDELINES

Historically, patients have been told to abstain from oral intake (nothing by mouth [NPO]) after midnight regardless of the time of their procedure to reduce the risk of aspiration. Twenty years ago Miller found that a light breakfast (of tea and toast) 2 to 4 hours before an operation did not negatively impact gastric pH or volume. In many European countries today, patients are allowed to eat a "light breakfast" if an operation is scheduled for noon or after. However, this practice has not received widespread adoption in the United States. Because oral fluids have short gastric transit times, many, if not most, departments of anesthesia modified the "nothing after midnight" approach. The ASA recommends that healthy patients who will undergo elective procedures be allowed to drink clear liquids (eg, water, juice without pulp, coffee or tea without cream or milk) until 2 hours before anesthesia; breast milk until 4 hours before anesthesia; and nonhuman milk, infant formula, or a light breakfast until 6 hours before procedures requiring anesthesia (**Table 6-8**).[106] In a prospective cohort study there were no differences in aspiration, and delays or cancellation of cases between groups who followed traditional NPO versus liberalized (clear fluids until 2-3 hours before surgery) guidelines. There were more cases of regurgitation, and rapid-sequence and awake intubations in the NPO after midnight group.[107]

TABLE 6-8 Guidelines for Food and Fluids Before Elective Surgery

Time Before Surgery	Food or Fluid Intake
Up to 8 h	Food and fluids as desired
Up to 6 h[a]	Light meal (eg, toast and clear liquids[b]), infant formula, nonhuman milk
Up to 4 h[a]	Breast milk
Up to 2 h[a]	Clear liquids[b] only; no solids or foods containing fat in any form
During the 2 h	No solids, no liquids

[a]This guideline applies only to patients who are not at risk for delayed gastric emptying. Patients with the following conditions are at risk for delayed gastric emptying: morbid obesity, diabetes mellitus, pregnancy, a history of gastroesophageal reflux, a surgery limiting stomach capacity, a potentially difficult airway, opiate analgesic therapy.

[b]Clear liquids are water, carbonated beverages, sports drinks, and coffee or tea (without milk). The following are *not* clear liquids: juice with pulp, milk, coffee or tea with milk, infant formula, and any beverage with alcohol.

MEDICATION INSTRUCTIONS

Some medications should be continued on the day of operation because of their beneficial effects; others may be harmful or contraindicated.[108] Medications associated with withdrawal effects (eg, β-blockers, centrally acting sympatholytics, benzodiazepines, and opioid analgesics) should be continued through the preoperative period. Table 6-7 and Fig. 6-3 describe in detail drugs to be continued or discontinued before an operation.

Most antihypertensive medications, with the possible exception of angiotensin-converting enzyme inhibitors (ACEIs) and angiotensin receptor–blocking agents (ARBs) should be taken before operation.[109] ACEIs and ARBs may be associated with greater risk for hypotension upon induction of general anesthesia. There is no consensus as to whether these agents should be held before anesthesia. No large studies exist to support any specific recommendation. For high-risk procedures with planned neuraxial blockade or general anesthesia in well-controlled hypertensive patients, it may be beneficial to hold these drugs on the day of operation. In our preoperative clinic patients who will undergo minor procedures with monitored anesthesia care, and those with poorly controlled HTN are advised to continue these drugs on the day of operation to reduce the risk of significantly elevated blood pressure in the pre- and postoperative periods. β-Blockers and centrally acting sympatholytics (eg, clonidine) can be associated with rebound hypertension when withdrawn.

Consensus is lacking on the recommendations to discontinue diuretics preoperatively. Diuretics (eg, hydrochlorothiazide) to treat HTN will likely help to control blood pressure when continued on the day of operation. Withholding potent loop diuretics (eg, furosemide) on the day of operation may decrease the risk of volume depletion and renal insufficiency.[110] Intravenous admission by the anesthesiologists on the day of operation is an option.

Medications used by patients with a history of or who are at risk for heart disease, such as β-blockers, digoxin, antiarrhythmics, and statins, should not be withdrawn before operation. Not only are they beneficial, but risk may be increased when they are not taken.[11]

Aspirin, taken for primary prophylaxis of vascular disease or for pain, and other nonsteroidal anti-inflammatory drugs (NSAIDs) are generally discontinued before the day of operation.[111,112] Circumstances may dictate otherwise to prevent MI or stroke, to improve patency of vascular grafts, and to achieve better pain control. There is increasing evidence supporting continuation of aspirin when taken for secondary prophylaxis (ie, patients with established vascular disease).[111,112] Aspirin is continued for patients scheduled for vascular reconstruction and for those at high risk for cardiovascular and cerebrovascular complications except for intraspinal and intracranial procedures. Aspirin and other NSAIDs do not need to be discontinued for planned neuraxial or regional anesthesia techniques.[113] If the decision to discontinue these agents is made, aspirin is stopped 5 to 7 days and other NSAIDs 48 hours before the operation.[114] Many cold preparations and over-the-counter drugs (eg, Alka-Seltzer and Pepto-Bismol) may contain aspirin.

More potent antiplatelet agents, such as clopidogrel (Plavix) may be associated with a substantial risk of perioperative bleeding. These drugs are discontinued 7 days before the operation if appropriate.[111,112] Patients with DES placed less than 12 months ago, BMS placed less than 4 to 6 weeks previously, or percutaneous coronary interventions without stents less than 2 weeks before surgery should have only lifesaving surgery, preferably while continuing dual antiplatelet therapy (Table 6-6 and Fig. 6-3).

Statins reduce strokes, renal dysfunction, MI, length of hospital stay, and even death.[115-117] Patients having coronary artery bypass grafting who take perioperative statins have a dose-dependent reduction in adverse cardiac events.[118] No study of perioperative statin therapy has reported serious risks with the use of these drugs.[116] Abruptly stopping statins may be associated with an increased risk, including death.[117] Statins are continued in the perioperative period. Serious consideration should be given to starting them in patients with risk factors for or known atherosclerotic disease, especially because these patients have indications independent of surgery. This is an important intervention with long-term benefits.

Pulmonary medications, such as theophylline, inhaled β-agonists, inhaled anticholinergics, and inhaled or oral steroids, should be continued preoperatively. These drugs are prescribed for patients with reactive airways who require optimization.[119]

Oral hypoglycemic agents typically are held the day of operation to avoid hypoglycemia. Taking small amounts of long-acting insulin on the day of operation presents little risk of hypoglycemia but results in improved perioperative control. Patients with types 1 and 2 DM discontinue all short-acting bolus doses of insulin on the day of operation. Patients with type 2 DM take none or up to one-half dose of long-acting (eg, lente or neutral protamine Hagedorn [NPH]) or combination (70/30 preparations) insulins on the day of operation. Ultra–long-acting insulin (eg, glargine) is best continued as scheduled. People with type 1 DM take a small amount (usually a third to a half) of their usual morning long-acting insulin (eg, lente or NPH) on the day of operation to avoid diabetic ketoacidosis. Patients with an insulin pump continue their basal rate only.

Warfarin may be associated with increased bleeding except for minor procedures such as cataract surgery without bulbar blocks. There is no consensus on the optimal perioperative management of patients on warfarin. The usual recommendation is to withhold 4 to 5 doses of warfarin before operation (if the INR is 2.0-3.0) to allow the INR to decrease to less than 1.5, a level considered safe for surgical procedures and neuraxial blockade. [113] If the INR is higher than 3.0, it is necessary to withhold warfarin longer than 4 doses. If the INR is measured the day before the operation and remains higher than 1.8, a small dose of vitamin K (1.0-5.0 mg orally or subcutaneously) can reverse anticoagulation. [90]

Substitution with shorter-acting anticoagulants such as unfractionated or low-molecular-weight heparin, referred to as bridging, is controversial and should be individualized.[89] Kearon recommends preoperative bridging with intravenous heparin only for patients who have had an acute arterial or venous thromboembolism within 1 month before operation if the procedure cannot be postponed.[89]

Most medications for neurologic and psychological problems should be continued on schedule in the preoperative period. Antiepileptics, antiparkinson medications, antidepressants, including monoamine oxidase inhibitors (MAOIs), antipsychotics, benzodiazepines, and drugs to treat myasthenia gravis are best maintained to avoid exacerbations of symptoms. Antianxiety and psychiatric medications should be continued up until the time of the procedure. Communication is crucial to alert the day of operation caregivers because alterations in anesthesia may be necessary when caring for patients on these medications, especially for patients taking MAOIs. Highly active antiretroviral regimens to treat human immunodeficiency virus require regular dosing to prevent drug resistance. It is important to maintain these as scheduled. Antibiotics should be taken to complete a prescribed course of therapy.

Patients taking narcotic pain medications are told to continue these medications as needed, including on the day of operation. Missed doses may result in withdrawal symptoms and significant pain with the associated stress response and hemodynamic perturbations.

Thyroid replacement drugs and antithyroid medications are continued on schedule.[108] Patients taking steroids regularly take their usual dose on the day of operation.[120] Patients who have taken more than the equivalent of 7.5 mg of prednisone a day for at least 3 weeks within the previous year may be at risk for stress-associated adrenal insufficiency.

Postmenopausal hormone replacement therapies containing estrogen increase the risk of perioperative thromboembolic complications and should be discontinued before operation.[121] Estrogens must be stopped approximately 1 month before the operation to return coagulation to baseline. Most modern oral contraceptives have low doses of estrogen that increase thromboembolic risk minimally. The risk of unanticipated pregnancy may outweigh the benefits of discontinuing oral contraceptives.

Herbals and supplements may interact with anesthetic agents, alter the effects of prescription medications, and increase bleeding. Many patients do not consider supplements to be medications and will not report them in a list of their medications unless asked. Gingko biloba, echinacea, garlic, ginseng, kava, St. John wort, and valerian may be associated with increased bleeding, or a resistance or increased sensitivity to anesthetic and sedative agents.[122] Herbals and supplements are discontinued 7 to 14 days before the operation. The exception is valerian, a central nervous system depressant that may cause a benzodiazepine-like withdrawal when discontinued. If time permits, valerian should be tapered before a planned anesthetic.

Patients who are particularly anxious should be offered a prescription for a short course of benzodiazepines, such as lorazepam, to be taken in the days preceding the operation, as well as on the day of operation.

CLINICAL MODELS AND MANAGEMENT

As the practice of surgery has moved into the outpatient arena with most patients presenting to the hospital within minutes to hours of undergoing complex procedures, anesthesiologists have struggled with how best to accomplish their evaluations. Various models exist. Lee originally proposed an anesthesia-based outpatient clinic in 1949. Some clinics do no more than document information provided by the patient, the medical record, or others who have seen the patient. Some anesthesiologists rely on other physicians operating independently to prepare patients for operation, either based on anesthesia-derived guidelines or not. This allows for review of information but little direct oversight of the process. Practices that do not have preanesthesia clinics need to develop guidelines to direct testing and to prepare patients for anesthesia (Fig. 6-1, Tables 6-4 through 6-8, and **6-9**).

Many surgeons and anesthesiologists rely on prior screening of patients or referrals to primary care physicians, internists, or specialists to "clear" patients or to manage comorbid conditions. Although this reliance may be appropriate for a few, very select diseases and patients, the management of conditions for everyday life and for reducing long-term complications is very different from the stresses of a surgical procedure and anesthesia. Proficiency in preoperative care is a prerequisite for board certification in anesthesia; internists who are not specifically trained in preoperative care may feel insecure when called on to evaluate the preoperative patient because this important aspect of medicine is not formally taught in many training programs.[123] Anesthesiologists are best suited to do preoperative assessments because of our comprehensive understanding of surgical procedures, anesthetic techniques, and the pharmacologic and physiologic responses of patients during procedures.

Anesthesiologist-staffed preoperative clinics improve the satisfaction of patients and physicians, reduce operating room cancellations and delays, and decrease unnecessary testing and costs.[7] To expand the anesthesiologist's responsibilities beyond the operating room, an educational system must be developed to train anesthesiologists in preoperative care. Concern has been expressed that current anesthesiology training programs are inadequately preparing practitioners to evaluate and manage patients with complicated medical conditions prior to anesthesia and operation.[124] Previously, during residency training, honing the cognitive aptitude for preoperative medicine had not been emphasized because of the inordinate amount of time anesthesiologists spend in the operating room learning technical and procedural skills. One study found that fewer than half of residency programs have a formal preoperative management curriculum.[124] Recently, the American Board of Anesthesiology mandated a 1-month requirement in preoperative evaluation training for anesthesia residents.

TABLE 6-9 Surgeon's Preoperative Checklist

If the patient has not had an anesthesia consultation before the day of surgery, please adhere to the following guidelines:	
☐	1. Surgical history and results of physical examination are available on the day of the operation.
☐	2. Preoperative Questionnaire (Table 6-3) is given to the patient with instructions to complete and bring it on the day of surgery or fax it beforehand to ________________
☐	3. Appropriate diagnostic tests are completed and are available. You are responsible for follow-up on any tests that you order (Tables 6-4 and 6-5 and Fig. 6-1).
☐	4. Medical information from outside our health care system (diagnostic tests, blood work, cardiac stress tests, echocardiograms, catheterizations, pulmonary function tests, consultations) is available on the day of the operation.
☐	5. Patient has been given preoperative medication instructions (Table 6-7).
☐	6. Patient has been given NPO guidelines (Table 6-8).
☐	7. "Clearance" letters or notes are rarely sufficient to design a safe anesthetic. A letter summarizing the patient's medical problems and condition and verifying that the patient's medical status is optimized is necessary. Surgery may be delayed or postponed for patients with chronic medical conditions if they have not been evaluated in the Anesthesia Preoperative Medicine Clinic (APMC) and necessary information is not available preoperatively, or their medical status is not optimized. The staff of APMC encourage you to use the clinic for complex patients or those undergoing major operations (Table 6-1).

As anesthesiologists assume a greater out-of-operating room presence and take on the tasks of evaluating and managing patients before operation and anesthesia, expert practices using cost-efficient management, outcomes measures, and practice guidelines must be developed. Diagnostic expertise and clinical decision making should be emphasized. It would be unrealistic to expect anesthesiologists to manage the administrative and clinical roles of perioperative medicine without training in these skills during residency.[124] Greater involvement of anesthesiologists in preoperative medicine has potential benefits to patients, institutions, the health care system, and the specialty. Preoperative clinics enable anesthesiologists to be responsible for perioperative care resources, to attract a diverse population of health care providers to the specialty, and to establish an expertise beyond the operating suite. Kluger, from the AIMS study, stated, "Anaesthetists must recognize they are responsible for the overall clinical management of the patient rather than simply providing a technical service.[1]

Preanesthesia clinics vary widely in services offered and the personnel involved in preoperative evaluation. They are staffed by anesthesiologists, internists, or physician extenders, such as nurse practitioners, physician assistants, registered nurses, or some combination.[105] Depending on services that are offered, additional staff might include clerks, phlebotomists, ECG technicians, administrators, social workers, case managers, and physical therapists. When outcomes were compared between patients cared for by nurse practitioners versus primary care physicians, no difference in health status of patients or quality of care was found. In one study, a physician's diagnostic accuracy was improved 20% to 30% after a physician's assistant took a detailed history.[125] Little data from preanesthetic clinics exist to guide staffing.

SCHEDULING

Scheduling is based on the anticipated requirements of the preoperative visit, such as the numbers and types of practitioners (eg, nurses, physicians, physical therapists, phlebotomists) who will be seeing the patient, required diagnostic studies, and the general health of the patient. The general health of the patient is estimated by the ASA PS or a screening mechanism offered by various Internet-based tools, a previsit telephone call, or a patient-completed information form sent from the surgeon's office (Table 6-3). Standardized appointment times for all patients inherently result in delays and long waits. Facilities should consider open-access scheduling that accommodates walk-ins for those patients traveling long distances or who have physical disabilities or unexpected scheduling of operation to prevent inconveniencing them with a return appointment. Reserving a block of time to coordinate appointments with high-volume office visits to surgeons might be useful. Scheduling patients far enough in advance allows time for ordering tests, improving the patient's medical condition, and recruiting social services. Evening and weekend hours afford patients the least disruption from work or family responsibilities.

Because long wait times contribute to patient dissatisfaction, strategies should lessen wait times to improve satisfaction. If patients arrive early or late for an appointment, if practitioners take longer than an appointment time, or if patients without appointments delay the evaluation of other patients, wait times will increase. Scheduling appointments that reflect time needed, using longer appointment intervals, providing necessary clinical information, using a computerized anesthesia record, accepting provider idle time, scheduling breaks, and deliberately expecting many "no-show" patients might decrease wait time.

IMPROVING PATIENT EXPERIENCE WITH PREOPERATIVE EVALUATION

Patients who are scheduled for operation want information, want to have their concerns addressed, and want their questions answered.[126] Patient anxiety is reduced when a patient's coping style is not threatened. Too much information, especially detailed information about the dangers of anesthesia and operation, creates anxiety in patients who prefer to cope by avoidance. Patients without prior anesthetic exposure desire more information than patients who have had previous anesthetics. Patients desire information in layperson language[16] Respecting a patient's feelings, explaining complex issues in a simple manner, and learning effective communication skills can improve patient satisfaction.[127] Nonverbal communication, dress, and avoidance of jargon are important.[16] Videos about anesthesia can be time efficient and well received. Written instructions, especially regarding NPO guidelines, medications, and when and where to go on the day of operation, are essential.

Patient satisfaction questionnaires are used to improve the processes.[128] Some questions that might be asked in such a survey are as follows:

- Did the anesthesiologist explain the planned anesthetic in terms you understood?
- How well did the anesthesiologist answer your questions and address your concerns?
- How well did the anesthesiologist explain what you could expect after your anesthesia?
- Did you have to wait long?
- Was the staff courteous and respectful to you?
- Overall, how satisfied were you with your preanesthetic visit?
- How might we improve our services?

INFORMATICS

Modern, up-to-date information systems streamline acquisition, storage, and transfer of data about patients among primary care providers, the laboratory, consultants, surgeons, and operating room and clinic personnel. Many institutions have developed their own computer-based programs (**Figs. 6-4 through 6-6**), and a variety of commercial products are available. These can be as simple as a questionnaire (Table 6-3) or as advanced

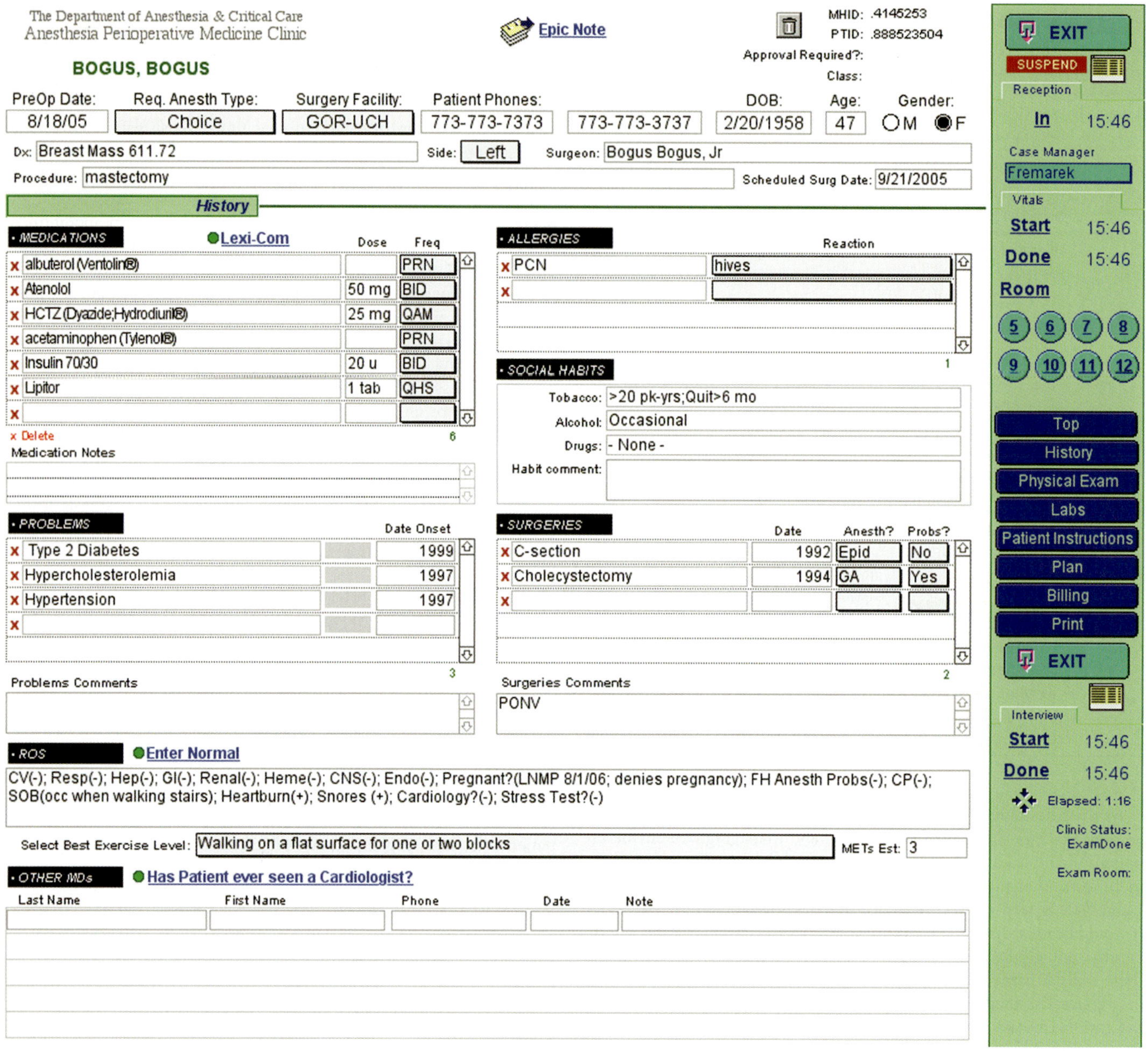

The Department of Anesthesia & Critical Care
Anesthesia Perioperative Medicine Clinic

Epic Note

MHID: .4145253
PTID: .888523504
Approval Required?:
Class:

BOGUS, BOGUS

PreOp Date:	Req. Anesth Type:	Surgery Facility:	Patient Phones:		DOB:	Age:	Gender:
8/18/05	Choice	GOR-UCH	773-773-7373	773-773-3737	2/20/1958	47	○M ●F

Dx: Breast Mass 611.72 Side: Left Surgeon: Bogus Bogus, Jr

Procedure: mastectomy Scheduled Surg Date: 9/21/2005

History

MEDICATIONS Lexi-Com

	Dose	Freq
albuterol (Ventolin®)		PRN
Atenolol	50 mg	BID
HCTZ (Dyazide;Hydrodiuril®)	25 mg	QAM
acetaminophen (Tylenol®)		PRN
Insulin 70/30	20 u	BID
Lipitor	1 tab	QHS

x Delete 6

Medication Notes

ALLERGIES

	Reaction
PCN	hives

1

SOCIAL HABITS

Tobacco: >20 pk-yrs;Quit>6 mo
Alcohol: Occasional
Drugs: - None -
Habit comment:

PROBLEMS

	Date Onset
Type 2 Diabetes	1999
Hypercholesterolemia	1997
Hypertension	1997

3

Problems Comments

SURGERIES

	Date	Anesth?	Probs?
C-section	1992	Epid	No
Cholecystectomy	1994	GA	Yes

2

Surgeries Comments
PONV

ROS Enter Normal

CV(-); Resp(-); Hep(-); GI(-); Renal(-); Heme(-); CNS(-); Endo(-); Pregnant?(LNMP 8/1/06; denies pregnancy); FH Anesth Probs(-); CP(-); SOB(occ when walking stairs); Heartburn(+); Snores (+); Cardiology?(-); Stress Test?(-)

Select Best Exercise Level: Walking on a flat surface for one or two blocks METs Est: 3

OTHER MDs Has Patient ever seen a Cardiologist?

Last Name	First Name	Phone	Date	Note

EXIT
SUSPEND
Reception
In 15:46
Case Manager
Fremarek
Vitals
Start 15:46
Done 15:46
Room
5 6 7 8
9 10 11 12
Top
History
Physical Exam
Labs
Patient Instructions
Plan
Billing
Print
EXIT
Interview
Start 15:46
Done 15:46
Elapsed: 1:16
Clinic Status: ExamDone
Exam Room:

FIGURE 6-4. Computerized patient history.

as complex systems that include decision support tools for diagnostic testing, suggestions for consultations, physician computer order entry, direct links to laboratory databases, and the capability of printing patient preoperative instructions, as well as a summary of the evaluation.

Computerized order-entry, prescription generation, and management programs can improve patient care and reduce costs. Patients can transfer information via e-mail, facsimile machines, and interactive telephone systems. Simple telephone reminders improve appointment keeping, patient satisfaction, patient compliance, use of services, and medication compliance, and they decrease use of alcohol and tobacco (prevention programs).

Computer-program patient interviews save valuable clinician time and may be convenient for the patient. Computer programs that gather information directly from patients allow planning for needed services in advance, and they can provide patient education and instruction. Internet-based sites and telemedicine have been used for preoperative evaluation.[105,129] Airway evaluation is particularly enhanced with telemedicine.[129]

Electronic technology has enhanced the ease and efficiency of data acquisition, and these data can be accessed for patient care simultaneously by multiple providers in diverse locations. Technology can improve management of clinical studies, be used for cost analysis, and used for staffing, resource allocation, and managed care or capitated contract negotiations.

A computerized preanesthetic evaluation system can improve hospital (not just preoperative clinic) reimbursement by improved documentation of diagnosis-related group codes when ICD-9 codes are changed.[130]

MEDICOLEGAL CULPABILITY

As anesthesiologists broaden their scope of practice and responsibilities, concerns over medical liability arise. Professional negligence, or malpractice, is generally characterized as a failure on the part of the physician to possess or exercise reasonable skill or diligence in the diagnosis or treatment of a patient. The essential elements of a medical

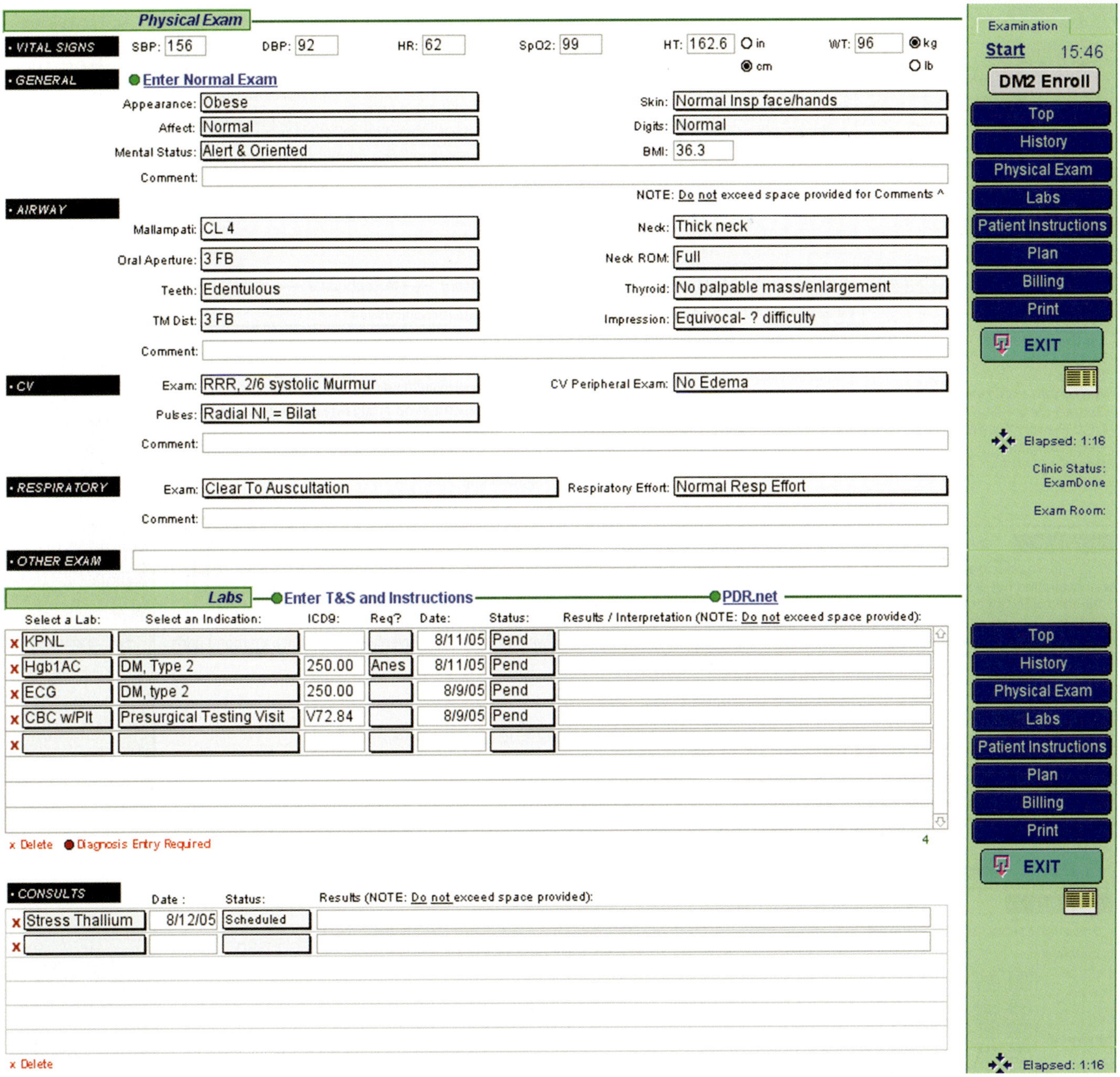

Physical Exam

• VITAL SIGNS — SBP: 156 DBP: 92 HR: 62 SpO2: 99 HT: 162.6 ○ in ◉ cm WT: 96 ◉ kg ○ lb

• GENERAL — ● Enter Normal Exam

Appearance:	Obese	Skin:	Normal Insp face/hands
Affect:	Normal	Digits:	Normal
Mental Status:	Alert & Oriented	BMI:	36.3

Comment:

NOTE: Do not exceed space provided for Comments ^

• AIRWAY

Mallampati:	CL 4	Neck:	Thick neck
Oral Aperture:	3 FB	Neck ROM:	Full
Teeth:	Edentulous	Thyroid:	No palpable mass/enlargement
TM Dist:	3 FB	Impression:	Equivocal- ? difficulty

Comment:

• CV — Exam: RRR, 2/6 systolic Murmur CV Peripheral Exam: No Edema

Pulses: Radial Nl, = Bilat

Comment:

• RESPIRATORY — Exam: Clear To Auscultation Respiratory Effort: Normal Resp Effort

Comment:

• OTHER EXAM

Labs — ● Enter T&S and Instructions ● PDR.net

Select a Lab:	Select an Indication:	ICD9:	Req?	Date:	Status:	Results / Interpretation (NOTE: Do not exceed space provided):
x KPNL				8/11/05	Pend	
x Hgb1AC	DM, Type 2	250.00	Anes	8/11/05	Pend	
x ECG	DM, type 2	250.00		8/9/05	Pend	
x CBC w/Plt	Presurgical Testing Visit	V72.84		8/9/05	Pend	
x						

x Delete ● Diagnosis Entry Required 4

• CONSULTS

	Date :	Status:	Results (NOTE: Do not exceed space provided):
x Stress Thallium	8/12/05	Scheduled	
x			

x Delete

Examination — Start 15:46 — DM2 Enroll — Top — History — Physical Exam — Labs — Patient Instructions — Plan — Billing — Print — EXIT — Elapsed: 1:16 — Clinic Status: ExamDone — Exam Room: — Top — History — Physical Exam — Labs — Patient Instructions — Plan — Billing — Print — EXIT — Elapsed: 1:16

FIGURE 6-5. Computerized patient physical examination and diagnostic test ordering.

malpractice claim include a duty toward the patient, a breach of that duty, and an injury to the patient because of the breach of duty. A physician's responsibility is to act in accordance with *national* standards of care established by the profession, which are defined in terms of care delivered by an average practitioner, not the *best* practitioner.

Duties of the preoperative physician include examination of the patient and referral to a specialist if necessary. Part of the examination requires the use of diagnostic information or techniques that an average, reasonable practitioner would use in similar circumstances.

Often physicians are concerned about failure to diagnose a condition by failing to order a diagnostic screening test. The traditional system of ordering standard preoperative tests evolved from the mistaken belief that more information, no matter how irrelevant or expensive, will improve care, enhance safety, and decrease liability. In reality, nonselective screening may increase legal culpability. Unanticipated significant abnormalities on laboratory test results are uncommon. The relationship between these abnormalities and surgical and anesthetic morbidity is weak at best. More than half of all abnormal test results obtained in routine preoperative screening are ignored or not noted in the medical record, which is the document of interest to the courts. Failure to follow up an abnormal result is, from a legal point of view, probably riskier than failure to order the test in the first place.

Physicians without malpractice claims are more likely than physicians with malpractice claims to encourage patients to talk and give their opinions. The physicians clarify what has been discussed, and they keep patients informed about what to expect during a visit. One study found that communication problems were predominant in most of the reported incidents involving a failure of preoperative preparation.[1] Chapter 94 discusses legal issues in anesthesiology in greater detail.

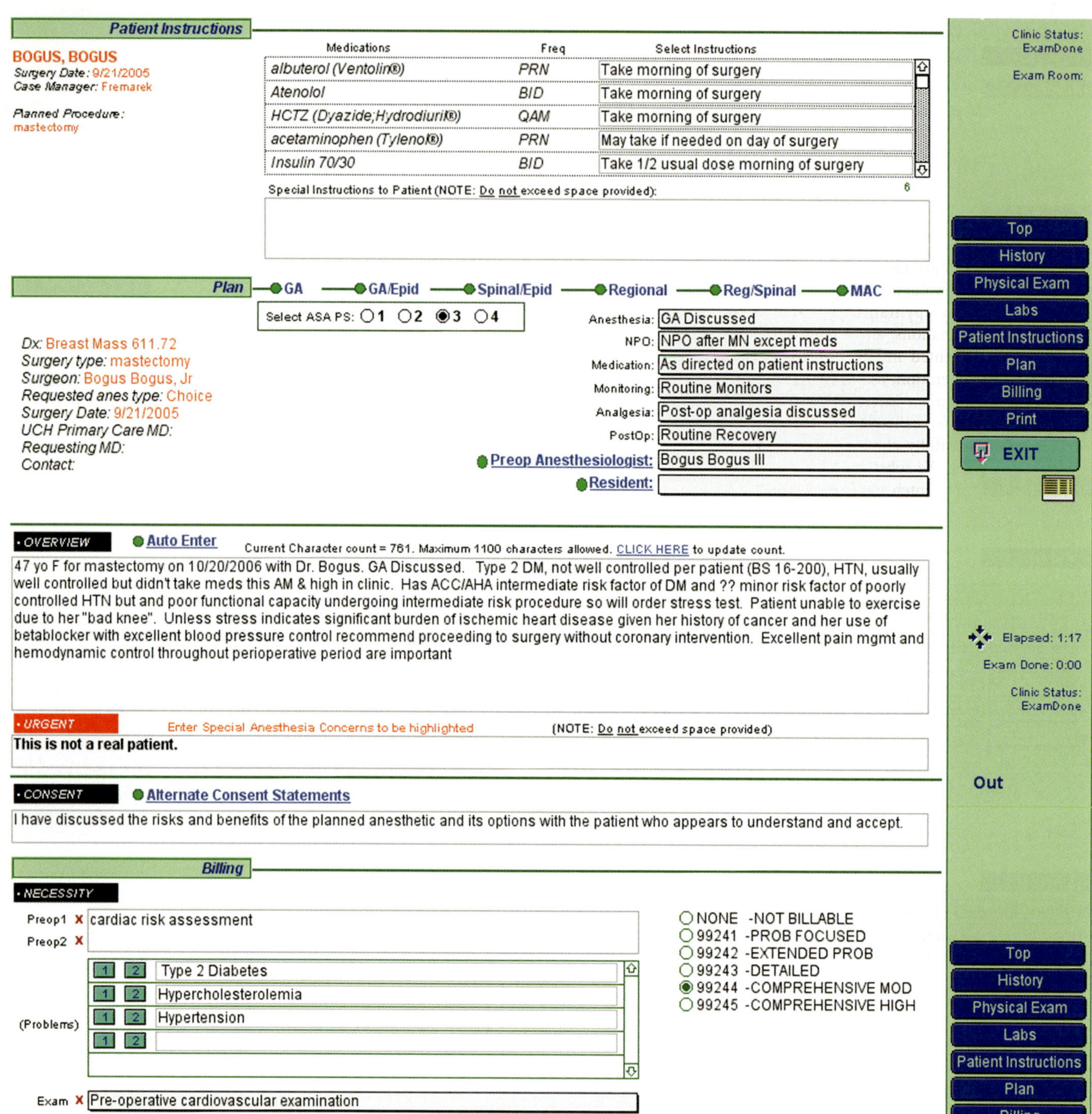

Patient Instructions

BOGUS, BOGUS
Surgery Date: 9/21/2005
Case Manager: Fremarek

Planned Procedure:
mastectomy

Medications	Freq	Select Instructions
albuterol (Ventolin®)	PRN	Take morning of surgery
Atenolol	BID	Take morning of surgery
HCTZ (Dyazide;Hydrodiuril®)	QAM	Take morning of surgery
acetaminophen (Tylenol®)	PRN	May take if needed on day of surgery
Insulin 70/30	BID	Take 1/2 usual dose morning of surgery

Special Instructions to Patient (NOTE: Do not exceed space provided): 6

Plan — GA — GA/Epid — Spinal/Epid — Regional — Reg/Spinal — MAC

Select ASA PS: 1 2 3 4

Dx: Breast Mass 611.72
Surgery type: mastectomy
Surgeon: Bogus Bogus, Jr
Requested anes type: Choice
Surgery Date: 9/21/2005
UCH Primary Care MD:
Requesting MD:
Contact:

Anesthesia: GA Discussed
NPO: NPO after MN except meds
Medication: As directed on patient instructions
Monitoring: Routine Monitors
Analgesia: Post-op analgesia discussed
PostOp: Routine Recovery
Preop Anesthesiologist: Bogus Bogus III
Resident:

• OVERVIEW Auto Enter Current Character count = 761. Maximum 1100 characters allowed. CLICK HERE to update count.

47 yo F for mastectomy on 10/20/2006 with Dr. Bogus. GA Discussed. Type 2 DM, not well controlled per patient (BS 16-200), HTN, usually well controlled but didn't take meds this AM & high in clinic. Has ACC/AHA intermediate risk factor of DM and ?? minor risk factor of poorly controlled HTN but and poor functional capacity undergoing intermediate risk procedure so will order stress test. Patient unable to exercise due to her "bad knee". Unless stress indicates significant burden of ischemic heart disease given her history of cancer and her use of betablocker with excellent blood pressure control recommend proceeding to surgery without coronary intervention. Excellent pain mgmt and hemodynamic control throughout perioperative period are important

• URGENT Enter Special Anesthesia Concerns to be highlighted (NOTE: Do not exceed space provided)
This is not a real patient.

• CONSENT Alternate Consent Statements
I have discussed the risks and benefits of the planned anesthetic and its options with the patient who appears to understand and accept.

Billing
• NECESSITY
Preop1 X cardiac risk assessment
Preop2 X
(Problems) 1 2 Type 2 Diabetes
1 2 Hypercholesterolemia
1 2 Hypertension
1 2
Exam X Pre-operative cardiovascular examination

NONE -NOT BILLABLE
99241 -PROB FOCUSED
99242 -EXTENDED PROB
99243 -DETAILED
99244 -COMPREHENSIVE MOD
99245 -COMPREHENSIVE HIGH

Clinic Status: ExamDone
Exam Room:
Top
History
Physical Exam
Labs
Patient Instructions
Plan
Billing
Print
EXIT
Elapsed: 1:17
Exam Done: 0:00
Clinic Status: ExamDone
Out
Top
History
Physical Exam
Labs
Patient Instructions
Plan
Billing

FIGURE 6-6. Computerized patient assessment and plan, patient medication instructions, and billing documentation.

ECONOMICS

Although anesthesiologists do not regularly receive separate payment for preoperative evaluations, the fee for preoperative assessment is part of the total operating room payment, and preoperative assessment by an anesthesiologist is required by both regulatory bodies and CMS.[40] One study showed that preanesthetic care can reduce delays and cancellations on the day of operation.[7] This can improve revenues by increasing time spent on billable cases rather than incurring personnel costs with an empty operating room. Avoiding delays and cancellations on the day of operation eliminates waste associated with unnecessary setups with disposable products. Preoperative assessment clinics also reduce costs by decreasing unnecessary testing and identifying patients with special needs on the day of operation.

According to CMS, preoperative assessments by anesthesiologists can be billed separately as visits or consultations "if medically necessary" and "beyond a routine preanesthetic assessment."[38] When anesthesiologists perform at the level of a perioperative physician by ordering diagnostic studies such as echocardiograms or stress tests, by identifying problems and requesting consultations with specialists, by prescribing therapies such as β-blockers or bronchodilators, and by coordinating care beyond a simple anesthetic plan, they are offering care "beyond a routine preanesthetic assessment" and should bill for consultative services. Chapter 97 describes the criteria required to bill for preoperative consultations.

Physicians working in or administering preanesthetic clinics must become familiar with the CMS Advance Beneficiary Notice (ABN) billing rules. These rules govern whether physicians and other Medicare Part B providers can bill beneficiaries directly if Medicare does not cover services because of a lack of medical necessity. CMS rules relieve beneficiaries from financial liability if the provider fails to disclose that the service is not reimbursable. Unless the physician or facility has followed the ABN rules, payment may not be sought from the patient. ABN rules apply only to outpatient services. Additional information can be obtained from http://www.cms.hhs.gov.

THE FUTURE OF PREOPERATIVE CLINICS

Preoperative clinics are ideal settings for offering comprehensive care beyond anesthesia evaluation. Advanced care and postdischarge planning, respiratory therapy training, counseling about smoking and substance abuse, vaccinations, and end-of-life care discussions have been effectively implemented in preanesthesia clinics.[96,131] When a patient is scheduled for operation, the patient may be more focused on health issues and improvement interventions may be particularly successful. These times have been called "teachable moments."[95,131]

Warner has rightfully challenged the anesthesia community to do its part in reducing the substantial burden of tobacco abuse.[95] Physical therapists can offer crutch training, social workers can begin postdischarge planning, especially for patients requiring rehabilitation services, and case managers can coordinate care across many disciplines. A 5-minute intervention in a preoperative clinic significantly increased and improved discussions of advance care planning and increased completion of a durable power of attorney to 25%, compared with 10% by controls.[132]

Some day it may be possible to identify patients with genetic polymorphisms linked to adverse outcomes during the preoperative assessments. Then pharmacologic interventions and management can directly alter morbidity and mortality.[133] Molecular biology is rapidly changing our ability to identify genetic variability and its effects on diseases and responses to therapies. This new approach could dramatically alter the way we perform risk assessment and how we design management plans. It would allow us to move away from expectations of results based on population studies to treatments based on individual patient characteristics. Pharmacogenetics may eventually lead to genetic screening tests to identify patients who are at risk for adverse perioperative outcomes, such as patients with pseudocholinesterase deficiency, halothane hepatitis, and susceptibility to malignant hyperthermia, as well as less familiar traits associated with the duration and response to drugs such as benzodiazepines, opioids, anesthetics, and NSAIDs, and pain tolerance.[133]

CONCLUSION

The prevention of complications during and after procedures requiring anesthesia is the most important task for preoperative anesthesiologists. Identification of risk requires fundamentally good medicine, systems of care, clinical and laboratory assessment, and experienced, knowledgeable, and dedicated health care providers. Risk reduction and outcome improvement are the ultimate goals of preoperative assessment and management.

KEY REFERENCES

- American College of Cardiology/American Heart Association Task Force on Practice Guidelines (Writing Committee to Revise the 2002 Guidelines on Perioperative Cardiovascular Evaluation for Noncardiac Surgery), American Society of Echocardiography, American Society of Nuclear Cardiology, et al. ACC/AHA 2007 guidelines on perioperative cardiovascular evaluation and care for noncardiac surgery: executive summary: a report of the American College of Cardiology/American Heart Association Task Force on Practice Guidelines (Writing Committee to Revise the 2002 Guidelines on Perioperative Cardiovascular Evaluation for Noncardiac Surgery). *Anesth Analg.* 2008;106(3):685-712.
- American Society of Anesthesiologists Task Force on Preanesthesia Evaluation. Practice advisory for preanesthesia evaluation: a report by the American Society of Anesthesiologists Task Force on Preanesthesia Evaluation. *Anesthesiology.* 2002;96(2):485-496.
- American Society of Anesthesiologists Task Force on Perioperative Management of Patients With Cardiac Rhythm Management Devices. Practice advisory for the perioperative management of patients with cardiac rhythm management devices: pacemakers and implantable cardioverter-defibrillators: a report by the American Society of Anesthesiologists Task Force on Perioperative Management of Patients With Cardiac Rhythm Management Devices. *Anesthesiology.* 2005;103(1):186-198.
- Bonow RO, Carabello BA, Chatterjee K, et al. 2008 focused update incorporated into the ACC/AHA 2006 guidelines for the management of patients with valvular heart disease. A report of the American College of Cardiology/American Heart Association Task Force on Practice Guidelines (Writing Committee to Revise the 1998 Guidelines for the Management of Patients With Valvular Heart Disease). *J Am Coll Cardiol.* 2008;52(13):e1-142.
- Chassot PG, Delabays A, Spahn DR. Perioperative antiplatelet therapy: the case for continuing therapy in patients at risk of myocardial infarction. *Br J Anaesth.* 2007;99(3):316-328.
- Chung F, Yegneswaran B, Liao P, et al. STOP questionnaire: a tool to screen patients for obstructive sleep apnea. *Anesthesiology.* 2008;108(5):812-821.
- Chung F, Yuan H, Yin L, Vairavanathan S, Wong DT. Elimination of preoperative testing in ambulatory surgery. *Anesth Analg.* 2009;108(2):467-475.
- Ferschl MB, Tung A, Sweitzer B, Huo D, Glick DB. Preoperative clinic visits reduce operating room cancellations and delays. *Anesthesiology.* 2005;103(4):855-859.
- Grines CL, Bonow RO, Casey DE Jr, et al. Prevention of premature discontinuation of dual antiplatelet therapy in patients with coronary artery stents: a science advisory from the American Heart Association, American College of Cardiology, Society for Cardiovascular Angiography and Interventions, American College of Surgeons, and American Dental Association, with representation from the American College of Physicians. *J Am Coll Cardiol.* 2007;49(6):734-739.
- Horlocker TT, Wedel DJ, Rowlingson JC, et al. Regional anesthesia in the patient receiving antithrombotic or thrombolytic therapy: American Society of Regional Anesthesia and Pain Medicine Evidence-Based Guidelines (Third Edition). *Reg Anesth Pain Med.* 2010;35(1):64-101.
- Howell SJ, Sear JW, Foëx P. Hypertension, hypertensive heart disease and perioperative cardiac risk. *Br J Anaesth.* 2004;92(4):570-583.
- Kearon C, Hirsh J. Management of anticoagulation before and after elective surgery. *N Engl J Med.* 1997;336(21):1506-1511.
- Le Manach Y, Coriat P, Collard CD, Riedel B. Statin therapy within the perioperative period. *Anesthesiology.* 2008;108(6):1141-1146.
- Liao P, Yegneswaran B, Vairavanathan S, Zilberman P, Chung F. Postoperative complications in patients with obstructive sleep apnea: a retrospective matched cohort study. *Can J Anaesth.* 2009;56(11):819-828.
- McFalls EO, Ward HB, Moritz TE, et al. Coronary-artery revascularization before elective major vascular surgery. *N Engl J Med.* 2004;351(27):2795-2804.

- Practice guidelines for preoperative fasting and the use of pharmacologic agents to reduce the risk of pulmonary aspiration: application to healthy patients undergoing elective procedures: a report by the American Society of Anesthesiologist Task Force on Preoperative Fasting. *Anesthesiology*. 1999;90(3):896-905.
- Shi Y, Warner DO. Surgery as a teachable moment for smoking cessation. *Anesthesiology*. 2010;112(1):102-107.
- Smetana GW, Lawrence VA, Cornell JE. Preoperative pulmonary risk stratification for noncardiothoracic surgery: systematic review for the American College of Physicians. *Ann Intern Med*. 2006;144(8):581-595.
- Tait AR, Malviya S. Anesthesia for the child with an upper respiratory tract infection: still a dilemma? *Anesth Analg*. 2005;100(1):59-65.

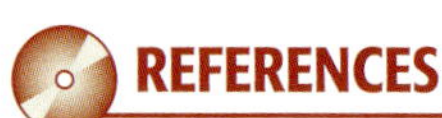

REFERENCES

Complete references available on DVD and online version at www.LongneckerAnesthesiology.com

CHAPTER 7 The Anesthetic Plan for Healthy Patients

Patrick E. Benedict
Kevin K. Tremper

KEY POINTS

1. The main objectives in anesthetizing healthy patients are safety and efficacy.
2. The purpose of the anesthetic history and physical examination in healthy patients is 4-fold:
   - To elucidate the nature of the surgical problem and the specific requirements of the planned operation
   - To ensure that the patient is, in fact, healthy
   - To identify patient features that could complicate the anesthetic
   - To ascertain and document patient expectations and preferences
3. A successful anesthetic plan must take into account the needs of the patient, the surgeon, and the anesthesiologist.
4. Healthy patients can undergo most of their preoperative evaluation and preparation immediately before surgery.
5. Extensive evaluation and testing are rarely necessary in healthy patients undergoing uncomplicated surgical procedures.
6. Anesthetic monitoring has evolved greatly and is believed to prevent complications and improve outcomes.
7. Healthy patients rarely require more than basic, noninvasive monitoring.
8. Healthy patients occasionally undergo complicated surgical procedures that require additional and more invasive monitoring.

INTRODUCTION

Like their medically ill counterparts, healthy patients undergo a variety of surgical procedures. By virtue of their favorable physical status, however, healthy patients generally undergo shorter and simpler operations. This is fortunate because surgical complexity is one contributor to perioperative risk. Healthy patients, by definition, are free of medical comorbidity, which is another contributor to perioperative risk. For purposes of this chapter, "healthy" patients are defined as American Society of Anesthesiologists[1] (ASA) class I or II. Despite the fact that perioperative risk is low in healthy patients, development of an anesthetic plan is largely the same as that for patients with serious comorbidities. Successful development of this plan consists of several important steps. The first is a thorough evaluation of the patient via history and physical examination. In healthy patients, a key component of this evaluation is the history of perioperative, and specifically anesthetic, problems and complications. A successful plan must also take into account any special considerations that may be associated with the proposed surgical procedure. Finally, expectations and needs of both patient and surgeon must be taken into consideration. Of these, safety and efficacy are of utmost importance. This chapter reviews the evaluative phase of the anesthetic plan, with special focus on recognition and avoidance of complications that can occur in healthy patients. Focus is then placed on the derivation of a safe and efficacious anesthetic plan that will meet the needs of both patient and surgeon. Finally, we review the use of routine and special monitors in healthy patients undergoing elective operations.

EVALUATION OF THE HEALTHY PATIENT

HISTORY

Formulating an anesthetic plan begins with a thorough evaluation of the patient. The starting point for this evaluation is the complete history and physical examination. In October 2001, the ASA published a Practice Advisory for Preanesthesia Evaluation.[2] This advisory provides guidelines regarding minimum requirements for the history, physical examination, testing, and timing of the preoperative assessment. Throughout this chapter we invoke principles of this advisory when specific issues relate to the healthy patient.

In the context of the healthy patient, the purpose of the history and physical examination is 4-fold:

- To fully elucidate the nature of the proposed operation and the problem for which the operation is being performed
- To ascertain the presence or absence of comorbidities or conditions that can heighten perioperative risk (to verify that the patient is, in fact, healthy)
- To ascertain whether the patient has a history of perioperative complications
- To educate the patient and then devise a plan that takes into account his or her preferences

The preoperative history and physical examination is typically a joint effort between the surgeon and the anesthesiologist. Following are specific goals and methods for the conduct of such a preoperative history and physical examination, which are well summarized in the ASA Practice Advisory for Preoperative Evaluation.[2]

Type of Surgical Disease and Planned Surgical Procedure In planning an anesthetic, the primary goals of the anesthesiologist are patient safety and satisfaction, and the provision of ideal operating conditions. The starting point for development of this plan is a thorough understanding of the surgical problem. The physical problem that necessitates operation can often have a significant impact on the provision of safe anesthesia. For example, patients presenting for surgical correction of temporomandibular joint disease may have significant issues with airway management. In addition, operations that achieve the same end point are often performed using different approaches and techniques. For example, otherwise healthy men may undergo prostatectomy using either a laparoscopic or an open approach. Surgical technique alone can alter the anesthetic choice.

Much information regarding the surgical condition and planned procedure is obtained from the surgical history and physical examination, which is performed by the surgeon or a clinical "extender" of the surgeon (physician assistant, resident, nurse practitioner). It is critical that effective

TABLE 7-1 American Society of Anesthesiologists Physical Status Classification

Class	Description	Examples
I	No organic, physiologic, biochemical, or psychiatric disturbances	Otherwise healthy patient
II	Mild to moderate systemic disturbance(s)	Hypertension, well-controlled diabetes, mild obesity, age <1 y or >70 y, malignancy without evidence or significant spread or physiologic disturbance
III	Severe systemic disturbance that may or may not be related to the reason for surgery	Angina, poorly controlled diabetes, massive obesity, controlled thyroid dysfunction
IV	Severe systemic disturbance that is life threatening	"Unstable" angina, congestive heart failure, debilitating respiratory disease, hepatorenal failure
V	Moribund patient who has little chance of survival	Septic patient with multiorgan failure, patient in cardiac arrest from major trauma
VI	Brain-dead patient for organ harvesting	
E	Any patient in whom an emergency operation is required	

[a]Reproduced with permission from Classification of Physical Status. ASA Relative Value Guide. 2011. http://www.asahq.org/clinicallphysicalstatus.htm.

communication be maintained between members of the surgical and anesthesia teams to develop an optimal anesthetic plan. Computerized medical records aid greatly in achieving this goal. Most healthy patients do not require an anesthetic evaluation in advance of their operation. However, the surgical team must recognize when an advance visit with an anesthesiologist is appropriate, ensuring that such visits occur when indicated. To this end, preoperative anesthesia assessment clinics have evolved, along with screening criteria to aid surgical teams in deciding who needs this consultation. Preoperative clinics are discussed in subsequent sections.

Defining "Healthy" "Healthy" patients are considered to be ASA physical status classification I and II.[3] By definition, these patients either have no disease or have minor disease processes that are well controlled and cause no physical limitation. Menke and colleagues demonstrated in 1993 that ASA classification independently predicted overall perioperative risk and that this risk was low in ASA I and II patients.[4] Similar findings have been verified by other authors, and the classification is still in common use[5] (**Table 7-1**).

After the surgical condition and the specifics of the operation have been clarified, the next goal of the anesthesia provider is verification that the patient is, in fact, free of disease. This constitutes the bulk of the preoperative history and physical in healthy patients, and it is a joint venture between surgical and anesthetic teams. A comprehensive review of systems is the method of choice for this purpose, which is generally obtained by a member of the surgical team. It is good practice for anesthesiologists to verify and further explore these findings when pertinent for provision of safe anesthesia. Assessment tools and guidelines are helpful for this purpose. The American College of Cardiology/American Heart Association guidelines are useful for patients with suspected cardiovascular disease.[6] Similar guidelines exist for evaluation of the respiratory system. The review of systems is also a valuable tool for careful screening of other organ systems including the coagulation system.

Occasionally, findings from the review of systems (eg, history of gastroesophageal reflux disease, neuropsychiatric disorders, clotting abnormalities) can alter the anesthetic plan in otherwise "healthy" patients. In addition, medical disease (hypertension, diabetes, coronary artery disease, asthma, obstructive pulmonary disease, etc) is occasionally diagnosed in surgical patients previously assumed to be "healthy"; such patients may require further evaluation and treatment before operation. Communication with the referring surgeon is important because this evaluation and treatment can delay the planned procedure.

Identifying Potential Anesthetic Complications Even patients who lack comorbidities may have a spectrum of potential anesthetic complications (**Table 7-2**).

In healthy patients, a primary determinant of the success of an anesthetic is avoidance of these complications. Hence a major focus of the anesthesiologist's medical history in healthy patients is identification of potential complications. Patients may have a personal or a family history of complications, and when such a history is elicited, the patient should always be asked to provide a thorough account of the events and their consequences. In addition, it is important to obtain the medical records if possible. Once the complication has been identified and elucidated, the anesthetic plan should be altered to minimize the risk of that complication recurring. This plan should be clearly documented and the patient informed that steps have been taken for prevention. Next is a discussion of common anesthetic complications and steps that can be taken to minimize or eliminate them.

Postoperative Nausea and Vomiting The most common complication associated with anesthesia is postoperative nausea and vomiting (PONV). This complication is highly distressing yet amenable to prevention.[7] Recognition of this problem, followed by alteration in the anesthetic plan, has resulted in marked improvements in patient outcome and satisfaction.[8] Untreated nausea occurs in as many as 40% of patients undergoing general anesthesia.[9] Golembiewski's excellent review of this subject outlines patient characteristics that heighten risk (**Table 7-3**).

When these characteristics, or a strong history of PONV, are encountered, the anesthetic plan should include use of anesthetics with less likelihood of causing the disorder (eg, total intravenous anesthesia [TIVA] with propofol).[8] In addition, strong consideration should be given to prophylactic use of antiemetic drugs that are highly effective.[8] The PONV algorithms used at the University of Michigan are illustrated in **Figs. 7-1** and **7-2**. Note that, after induction, droperidol (0.625 mg intravenously [IV]) is included as a primary prophylactic agent in high-risk patients. The US Food and Drug Administration (FDA) has placed a "black box" warning on droperidol, given its propensity to prolong the QT interval, which may be associated with serious cardiac rhythm disturbances.[10] Subsequent investigations have challenged this measure, citing remarkable safety at typical dosages used in modern anesthetic practice.[11] It is therefore controversial whether there should be a limit on the use of droperidol, given its track record of safety and efficacy.

TABLE 7-2 Potential Anesthetic Complications in Healthy Patients

Complication	Frequency
Postoperative nausea and vomiting	1:3[7]
Ocular injury	1:600-1:1600[12,13]
Unanticipated difficult airway	1:8-1:1000[14]
Intraoperative awareness	1:100-1:500[15,16]
Malignant hyperthermia	1:30,000[17,18]

TABLE 7-3 Risk Factors for Postoperative Nausea and Vomiting

Patient	Surgical	Anesthetic	Postoperative
Female gender	Longer duration	Nitrous oxide use	Pain
History of postoperative nausea and vomiting or motion sickness	Gynecologic surgeon	Gastric distension	Dizziness
High preoperative anxiety level	Laparoscopic surgery	Reversal of neuromuscular blockade	Early oral intake
Obesity	Middle ear surgery	Opioid use	Opioid use
Delayed gastric emptying			
Nonsmoking patient			
Younger age			

Adapted from Golembiewski JA, O'Brien D. A systematic approach to the management of postoperative nausea and vomiting. *J Perianesth Nurs.* 2002;17(6):364-376 With permission.

Finally, anxiety as a possible causative factor can often be effectively addressed by a frank acknowledgment to the patient that the problem has been recognized and that steps are in place for prevention.

History of Difficult Airway When difficult airway management is known or suspected, a thorough account of the findings and management must be sought from both patient and old medical records. "Difficult airway" usually means that airway anatomy was such that standard laryngoscopy was either difficult or impossible. When this is identified in the preoperative history, subsequent management via an awake technique should be considered. Patients with difficult airways are often otherwise healthy, but this alone presents significant anesthetic risk. The prospect of awake airway management usually provokes anxiety. The possibility of awake intubation is best communicated well in advance of the operative date. Explanation of the plan in a slow,

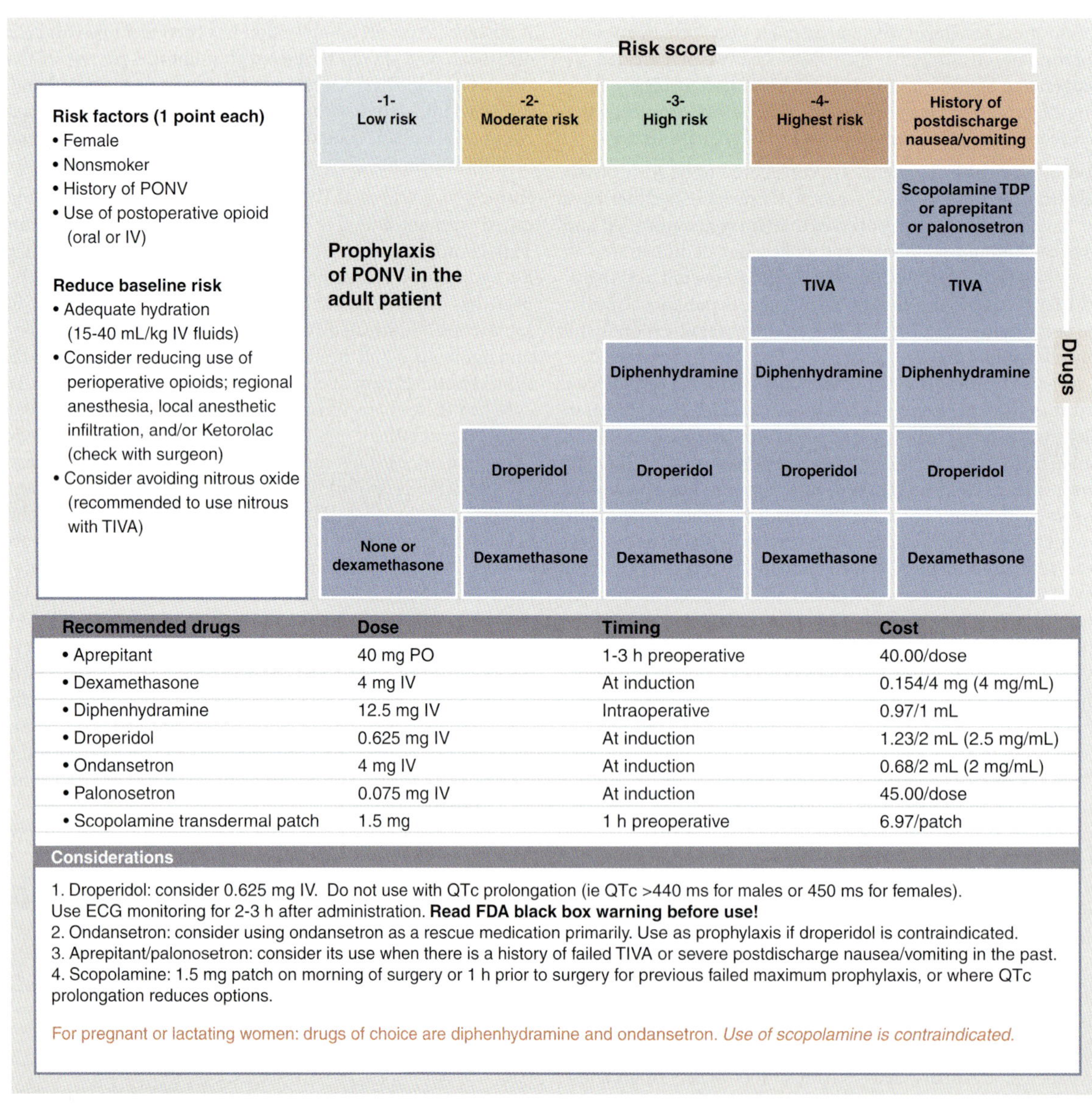

Recommended drugs	Dose	Timing	Cost
• Aprepitant	40 mg PO	1-3 h preoperative	40.00/dose
• Dexamethasone	4 mg IV	At induction	0.154/4 mg (4 mg/mL)
• Diphenhydramine	12.5 mg IV	Intraoperative	0.97/1 mL
• Droperidol	0.625 mg IV	At induction	1.23/2 mL (2.5 mg/mL)
• Ondansetron	4 mg IV	At induction	0.68/2 mL (2 mg/mL)
• Palonosetron	0.075 mg IV	At induction	45.00/dose
• Scopolamine transdermal patch	1.5 mg	1 h preoperative	6.97/patch

Considerations

1. Droperidol: consider 0.625 mg IV. Do not use with QTc prolongation (ie QTc >440 ms for males or 450 ms for females). Use ECG monitoring for 2-3 h after administration. **Read FDA black box warning before use!**
2. Ondansetron: consider using ondansetron as a rescue medication primarily. Use as prophylaxis if droperidol is contraindicated.
3. Aprepitant/palonosetron: consider its use when there is a history of failed TIVA or severe postdischarge nausea/vomiting in the past.
4. Scopolamine: 1.5 mg patch on morning of surgery or 1 h prior to surgery for previous failed maximum prophylaxis, or where QTc prolongation reduces options.

For pregnant or lactating women: drugs of choice are diphenhydramine and ondansetron. *Use of scopolamine is contraindicated.*

FIGURE 7-1. Prophylaxis of postoperative nausea and vomiting (PONV) in the adult patient.

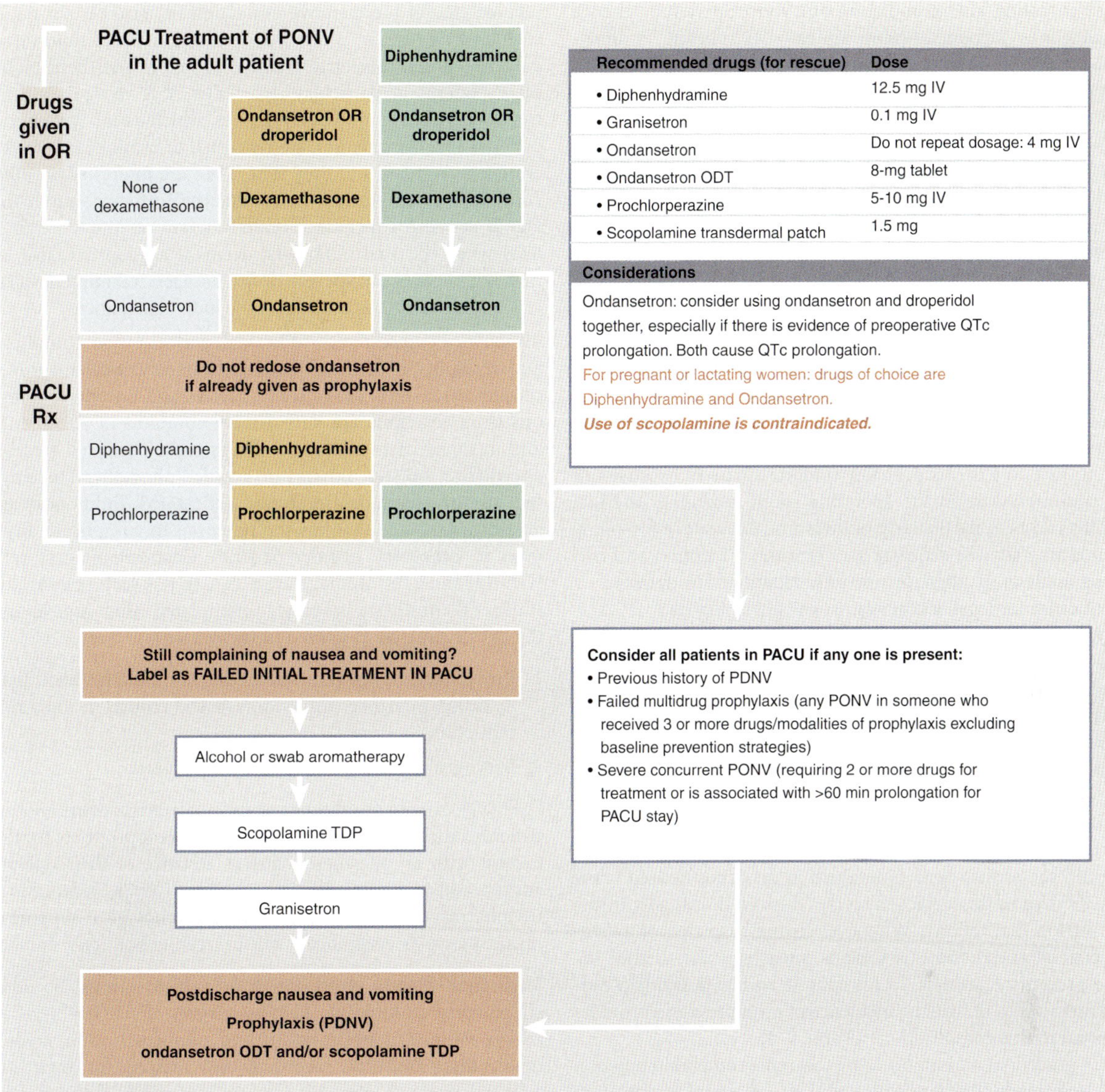

FIGURE 7-2. Postanesthesia care unit (PACU) treatment of postoperative nausea and vomiting (PONV) in the adult patient. OR, operating room; TIVA, total intravenous anesthesia.

reassuring fashion serves to inform and prepare the patient and thus minimize anxiety on the day of operation. A brief overview of airway assessment follows in the physical examination section, but a full review is considered in greater detail in Chapter 36.

Malignant Hyperthermia A rare anesthetic complication that must be recognized and planned for is malignant hyperthermia (MH). Estimates of the incidence of this complication range from 1 in 20 000 to 1 in 70 000.[17] Recognition, prevention, and treatment of MH have been a major success story in anesthesia. (See Chapter 87 for an in-depth review of MH; it is considered only briefly here, but detailed knowledge is required by all anesthesia practitioners.) Patients with potential MH risk must be seen well in advance of operation so that a complete clinical history is obtained and a plan of care can be devised and communicated to the patient and other providers.

Nearly uniformly fatal in the past, this disorder now has a mortality rate of less than 10%.[19] When patients present with either a personal or family history of the disorder, the anesthesiologist is confronted with decisions regarding testing and perioperative management. Muscle biopsy testing for the disorder is available at a diminishing number of centers and is costly, time consuming, and not completely reliable.[20] Although genetic testing appears promising, it is not widely available currently. Many anesthesiologists therefore proceed with the assumption that the patient is at risk and provide a nontriggering anesthetic. In some cases, regional anesthesia or conscious sedation may be appropriate. In others where these are not appropriate, a nontriggering general anesthetic is provided. Bryson et al demonstrated recently that even general anesthesia could be safely provided to MH susceptible outpatients, as long as "triggers" were avoided.[21] "Nontriggering" in this sense means avoidance of the only 2 reliable MH triggers: succinylcholine and potent inhaled anesthetics. This is typically accomplished with TIVA (see Chapter 43), which includes propofol, nondepolarizing neuromuscular blocking agents, and opiates. A minimum of 4 hours of observation are recommended following an uneventful anesthetic.[22]

Pseudocholinesterase Deficiency Pseudocholinesterase (butyrylcholinesterase) is a plasma enzyme with no known physiologic function. Deficiency of this enzyme is attributable to alterations in the gene that codes for it. In 2003 Yen and colleagues estimated the incidence of homozygous (affected) individuals to be approximately 1 in 1800.[23] Deficiency is usually identified when an anesthetized patient has prolonged recovery from the depolarizing neuromuscular blocking agent succinylcholine. Suspicion of this deficiency first arose in 1953 when Nilsson gave a patient succinylcholine, who then failed to resume spontaneous ventilation after completion of a short operation,[24] hence the colloquial name "suxamethonium apnea." Mivacurium, a short-acting nondepolarizing neuromuscular blocking agent, has also been shown to depend on this enzyme for elimination.[25] Despite being far more common than its inherited counterpart MH, pseudocholinesterase deficiency poses far less danger to patients. In addition, testing for the disorder is far simpler and more widely available than that for MH. Once identified, safe management entails ventilatory support combined with sedation until the drug is eliminated via the kidney (after several hours in homozygous recessive patients). Identification of this condition in advance allows for alteration of the anesthetic plan so that use of these drugs can be avoided. (More extensive review of MH is provided in Chapter 87.)

Awareness There has been growing public concern about intraoperative awareness and so-called awake paralysis, leading to increased anxiety in patients undergoing general anesthesia. Unfortunately, the true incidence of intraoperative awareness under general anesthesia, reported to range from 0.2% to 1.0%, is probably underestimated[15] because not all patients who are aware in the operating room remember the fact afterward. This can be a particularly bothersome experience for many patients, and lasting adverse sequelae are common.[26] Domino and colleagues, using analysis of litigation records, identified awareness as a common root cause for legal action against anesthesiologists.[27]

As with other complications, a thorough account of the events from both the patient and their records should be sought. Occasionally, patients misinterpret the goals of conscious sedation and label this as intraoperative awareness. It is important to clarify this distinction to patients preoperatively, so that expectations are realistic. In light of the recent focus on intraoperative awareness, the Bispectral Index Sensor (BIS) monitor has evolved.[28] Although use of BIS monitoring may reduce the incidence of awareness, recent reports by Mychaskiw and Rampersad cast doubt on this technology. Both demonstrated awareness despite BIS values that were maintained in the "anesthetized" (low value) range.[29,30] Use of this device is reviewed more thoroughly in the monitoring section that follows. Whenever strong suspicion of awareness under general anesthesia exists, plans must be made to alter the anesthetic to prevent recurrence. In his concise review, Kazanjian outlines several methods to reduce the incidence of awareness and provides steps to respond to this complication[31] (**Table 7-4**).

Recent ASA guidelines on intraoperative awareness and brain function monitoring also provide clinicians with useful information for evaluation and treatment plans to prevent this worrisome complication.[32] These include careful preoperative evaluation because certain patient features such as drug resistance may be predictive.[27] In addition, various types of surgery (cardiac, obstetric, trauma) as well as anesthetic techniques may place patients at particular risk.[33] The ASA recognizes that processed electroencephalogram (EEG) devices, which assign a numeric value to a patient's level of sedation, are marketed to minimize the risk of intraoperative awareness, and they state, "We are interested in following their continued evolution and in conducting further research in this area." Hence the ASA concludes, "Brain function monitors are an *option* to be used when the anesthesiologist deems it appropriate, just as he or she makes choices about specific drugs, dosages, warming devices, and other types of monitors depending on the individual patient."

Additional Complications Additional perioperative complications exist, and recognition of these complications is critical in preventing their reoccurrence. In a 2004 review, Mertes and Laxenaire found that serious drug reactions are surprisingly common in anesthetic practice,[34] and in many cases alternative drugs can be selected (antibiotics, local anesthetics, opiates, others) or avoided altogether (succinylcholine in the case of pseudocholinesterase deficiency). Pulmonary aspiration of acidic gastric contents has the potential to complicate any anesthetic, even in otherwise healthy patients. Gastroesophageal reflux disease (GERD) and a full stomach are potential risk factors in healthy patients. If general anesthesia is being contemplated when aspiration risk exists, the anesthetic plan is altered in two ways:

1. Prophylactic antiaspiration measures should be taken (gastric motility drugs, pharmacologic stomach acid reduction, and rapid sequence induction).
2. Laryngeal mask airway should not be used.

Finally, even in the absence of anticipated risks or complications, many patients simply have high anxiety levels. It is appropriate for these patients to visit with an anesthesiologist in advance of their operative date to address and ameliorate this anxiety. There is even evidence to suggest that nonpharmacologic strategies, such as psychological support or soothing music, may play a significant role in treating both pain and anxiety.[35]

Medication Review A thorough drug history must be obtained from all patients undergoing elective surgery. Even healthy patients may take a variety of prescription and nonprescription medications. All medications must be recorded, and reasons for their use must be assessed. Patients must also be questioned carefully about drug allergies and intolerances, and clear a distinction between the two must be

TABLE 7-4 Intraoperative Awareness

Prevention	Follow-up
Amnestic premedication (midazolam, scopolamine)	Punctual postoperative checks with queries about awareness
Routine equipment checks (eg, correct placement of vaporizer)	Precise documentation of suspected events, as reported by patient
End-tidal monitoring of volatile anesthetics with low concentration alarm	Attempt to corroborate patient's account with actual events
Adequate dosing of induction agents	Do not trivialize or deny patient's assertion
Use of appropriate volatile anesthetic concentration or propofol dose for maintenance	Provide a full explanation of events
Realize potential for awareness with hypotension/hypovolemia	Offer patient appropriate follow-up (eg, psychological support, if desired)
Judicious use of neuromuscular blocking drugs combined with careful monitoring	Try to determine a cause
Frequent checks of intravenous catheters and pumps when using total intravenous anesthesia	Assure patient that risk of awareness is still low with subsequent anesthetics
Clear labeling of all syringes	Notify hospital risk management
Quiet, professional operating room atmosphere; minimize auditory input	Notify surgeon and primary care physician
Consider use of anesthetic depth monitor (bispectral index)	
Calm reassurance when strong possibility of awareness suspected	

Adapted from the chapter *Anesthesia Complications* by Kazanjian P, in: Mulholland W, Doherty G, eds. *Complications in Surgery*. Philadelphia, PA: Lipincott Williams & Wilkins; 2006.

TABLE 7-5 Pharmacologic Effects and Potential Perioperative Complications of 8 Commonly Used Herbal Remedies

Name of Herb	Common Uses	Pharmacological Effects	Potential Perioperative Complications
Echinacea, purple coneflower, root	Treatment of viral infections	Immune system stimulation	Reduced effectiveness of immunosuppressants. Infection with long-term use. Potential hepatotoxicity
Ephedra, ma huang	Weight loss, athletic performance	Indirectly and directly acting sympathomimetic	Dose-dependent increase in heart rate and blood pressure with potential for perioperative myocardial infarction and stroke. Arrhythmias with halothane. Tachyphylaxis with intraoperative ephedrine
Garlic, ajo	Antihypertensive, antithrombus forming	Inhibits platelet aggregation	Concerns for perioperative bleeding
Ginkgo, maidenhair; fossil tree	Circulatory stimulant	Inhibits platelets	Concerns for perioperative bleeding. May potentiate platelet inhibitors
Ginseng, ajo	General well-being	Poorly understood	Concerns for perioperative bleeding
Kava-kava	Anxiolytic, sedative	Anxiolytic, sedative	Potentiates sedative effects of anesthetic agents
St. John's wort	Depression, anxiety	Inhibition of serotonin, noradrenaline and dopamine. P450 enzyme induction	Decreased effectiveness of multiple medications
Valerian, vandal root, all heal	Anxiolytic and sleep aid	Sedation	Potentiates anesthetic agents

Adapted from Skinner CM, Rangasami J. Preoperative use of herbal medicines: a patient survey. *Br J Anaesth*. 2002;89(5):792-795. With permission.

documented in the medical record. When obtaining a drug history, it is important to ask that *all* regularly ingested exogenous compounds, including over-the-counter medications, herbal preparations, and vitamin supplements, be reported. Several of these compounds have been associated with serious perioperative complications and drug interactions.[36] Planning for a safe anesthetic usually entails discontinuation of many of these preparations well in advance of the planned procedure, which the ASA recommends.[37] **Table 7-5** contains a list of common herbal preparations and adverse interactions that have been associated with them.

Finally, it is important to determine whether patients are using illicit drugs because many of these drugs have also been associated with anesthetic complications.[38] Patients must be advised to abstain from all forms of illicit drugs well in advance of an elective procedure.

PHYSICAL EXAMINATION

The purpose of the physical examination in healthy surgical patients is to corroborate and augment findings from the medical history. Thus the first goal of the physical examination is to rule out disease. The second goal is to identify physical features that may make provision of anesthesia difficult or potentially lead to complications. In actuality, the physical examination begins while the history is being obtained. This direct interaction is a good time to observe the gross physical appearance and mental status of the patient. It is also a good time to look for obvious skin (jaundice, cyanosis, signs of dehydration, rashes) or musculoskeletal abnormalities (especially spine deformities) that may give clues to underlying pathologic conditions. This examination begins with a set of vital signs, including room-air oxygen saturation. Even if previously documented from the surgical history and physical examination, it is important for anesthesiologists to perform baseline examinations of both the cardiovascular and respiratory systems before elective surgery. Finally, a meticulous examination of the airway must be performed to assess for features that predict difficult airway management if the need for general anesthesia should arise.

Vital Signs Even in the presence of a negative medical history, abnormal vital signs can be an important first clue to the presence of underlying disease. In fact, potential medical risks such as hypertension and thyroid disease are occasionally diagnosed during the preoperative history and physical examination. The so-called white coat phenomenon is responsible for hypertension in many preoperative patients.[39] Significant elevations in blood pressure or heart rate, however, especially on repeated measures, warrant further investigation and possible therapy. Rather than simply asking, height and weight should be accurately measured. Arterial blood pressure should be determined either via sphygmomanometry or oscillometry, using an appropriate-size cuff. It is desirable to obtain blood pressure in both arms. We feel strongly that baseline room-air oxygen saturation should be measured via pulse oximetry in every patient.

Cardiorespiratory Examination Examination of cardiovascular and respiratory systems also begins with observation of the patient, which is conveniently accomplished while obtaining the history. Findings such as labored breathing, wheezing, coughing, clubbing of the nails, jugular venous distention, and cyanosis are typically identified while simply conversing with a patient. Obviously, these are signs of potentially serious pathologic conditions and should be investigated further by more in-depth examination. Physical examination of the cardiovascular system aids in ruling out hypertension, valvular heart disease, and heart failure. Palpation and auscultation of the heart should be performed to identify heaves, rubs, extra heart sounds, and murmurs. Peripheral pulses should be assessed for both quality and magnitude. The chest should be examined for wheezes, rales, and rhonchi.

Airway Evaluation Regardless of the anesthetic chosen for a particular operation, it is important that careful examination of the airway be performed in every patient. Although much of the remainder of the physical examination represents a combined or even redundant effort between anesthesiologists, surgeons, and internists, a complete airway evaluation is generally not the purview of other medical specialists. The anesthesiologist is solely responsible for securing the airway and establishing ventilation. Difficulty with these processes may place the patient in great peril. This is borne out by the fact that airway management problems account for a relatively large proportion of anesthesia-related morbidity and mortality. In ASA closed claims analyses, both Caplan et al and Domino et al demonstrated that loss of the airway is a frequent cause of litigation associated with severe injury or death.[40,41] If a patient is known to have a difficult airway, alternative management plans are available (eg, awake fiberoptic intubation). Identifying patients with difficult airways, followed by these alternative induction techniques, should eliminate the "unconscious patient, can't intubate, can't ventilate" scenario. It is therefore a major goal of anesthesiologists to predict the potentially difficult airway in advance of anesthetic induction.

TABLE 7-6 Features Associated With Difficult Laryngoscopy

Feature	Likelihood Ratio (LR) That Laryngoscopy Will Be Difficult
Difficult mask ventilation Body mass index >26 Edentulars Age >55 y History of snoring Facial hair	>2 factors, LR = 2.5[42]
Mouth opening/jaw protrusion	Limited jaw protrusion (class III), LR = 6.5[43]
Mallampati classification	Class III, IV, LR = 1.5-6[44,45]
Mandibular space	Thyromental distance <6 cm, LR = 2[46]
Obesity	BMI >35, LR = 2[47]

Adapted from Pearce A. Evaluation of the airway and preparation for difficulty. *Best Pract Res Clin Anaesthesiol.* 2005;19(4):559-579. With permission.

Tests to Predict Difficult Laryngoscopy Preoperative airway assessment, with the aim of detecting and thus anticipating the difficult airway, has evolved over the years. Currently, a number of strategies exist for systematic evaluation of the airway, and various guidelines endorse the use of such strategies.[48] Key elements of the airway examination include neck anatomy, neck flexion and extension, thyromental distance, mouth opening, Mallampati score, and, more recently, jaw protrusion and the presence of a beard. Excellent reviews are available on the various tests and strategies commonly used by anesthesiologists to assess physical and symptomatic features that may predict difficult laryngoscopy[49] (**Table 7-6**).

Mandibular displacement (upper lip bite test) was correlated with the difficulty of laryngoscopy and may have clinical utility.[43] Although these various tests and maneuvers are simple to perform, they have questionable sensitivity and specificity, and hence unreliable predictive value.[14] This explains the occasional finding of the "unanticipated difficult airway" after seemingly reliable testing preoperatively predicted otherwise.[14] Typically, the goal of these tests is to correlate symptomatic (eg, sleep apnea) and anatomic patient features with difficult laryngoscopy.[49]

Difficult Mask Ventilation Although successful laryngoscopy followed by endotracheal intubation constitutes definitive management for an unconscious and apneic patient, ventilation by mask can be a lifesaving maneuver. Despite this fact, the historical precedent for investigators with an interest in predicting the difficult airway has been to focus on laryngoscopy alone. Given the potentially lifesaving importance of mask ventilation, however, investigators have begun to stress both laryngoscopy and mask ventilation in their predictive strategies. Langeron and colleagues, in 2000, estimated the incidence of difficult mask ventilation and identified several predictive physical features: history of snoring, body mass index (BMI) higher than 26, lack of teeth, age older than 55 years, and beard.[42] In 2004 Han et al devised a scale for categorizing the difficulty of mask ventilation. This 4-point scale elaborates on the work by Langeron, who only noted difficult and impossible ventilation. In contrast, the Han scale describes four degrees of assessment of ventilation, similar to scales used for laryngoscopy (**Table 7-7**).

Han et al found an incidence of difficult mask ventilation of 1.5% in the 3000 patients they studied.[50] More recently, a study of more than 41 000 patients confirmed the incidence of difficult ventilation to be approximately 1.5% and that the incidence of impossible ventilation was 0.5%.[51] This large study by Kheterpal et al found 6 independent predictors (4 of Langeron's) of difficult mask ventilation: history of snoring, age older than 58 years, BMI higher than 30, Mallampati class III or IV, limited jaw protrusion, and the presence of a beard (**Table 7-8**).

Of these, the only modifiable risk factor is the presence of a beard. This suggests that anesthesiologists should consider recommending

TABLE 7-7 Mask Ventilation Scale

Mask Ventilation Scale	
0	Not attempted
1	Easy mask ventilation (with and without neuromuscular block)
2	Ventilated by mask with oral airway or other adjuvant (with or without neuromuscular block)
3	Difficult mask ventilation: inadequate, unstable, or required two practitioners
4	Unable to ventilate

From Han R, Tremper KK, Kheterpal S, O'Reilly M. Grading scale for mask ventilation. *Anesthesiology.* 2004;101(1):267. With permission.

that patients shave prior to elective procedures if they possess other risk factors for difficult mask ventilation. **Table 7-9** illustrates the standard preoperative airway features that we assess and record via electronic data entry at the University of Michigan.

Anticipated Difficult Airway Strategy When a potential difficult airway is identified, it is the anesthesiologist's responsibility to develop a management strategy, in the event that general anesthesia becomes necessary. When a truly difficult airway is known or strongly suspected, and general anesthesia is necessary, the usual management plan entails placement of an oral or nasal endotracheal tube while the patient is awake and spontaneously breathing. Techniques for awake endotracheal intubation are reviewed in Chapter 36. Several important steps in planning and patient preparation, however, are worth mentioning.

The very thought of a potential airway problem can be anxiety provoking. The source of this anxiety often stems from patients' perception that theirs is a rare problem that places them in danger. To allay this anxiety, it is helpful to have a frank discussion with patients to fully inform them about the nature of the problem, and the rationale and plan for safely dealing with it. Patients are reassured knowing that the difficult airway is relatively common and that appropriate management poses no untoward danger. Careful anxiolytic sedation is appropriate preoperatively, to the extent that airway compromise is avoided. Antisialagogue premedication (typically glycopyrrolate 0.4-0.6 mg IV) aids greatly in the ability to anesthetize airway mucosa (typically with

TABLE 7-8 Independent Predictors of Difficult Mask Ventilation and Difficult Mask and Difficult Intubation

Difficult Mask Ventilation	*p* value
Beard	0.0001
History of snoring	0.001
Body mass index >30	0.0001
Mallampati III or IV	0.001
Age >50 y	0.01
Severely limited jaw protrusion	0.03
Difficult Mask[a] and Difficult Intubation[b]	***p* value**
Severely limited jaw protrusion	0.0001
Thick neck/mass	0.02
History of sleep apnea	0.04
Body mass index >30	0.05
History of snoring	0.05

[a]Difficult mask is a grade III or IV mask (see Table 7-7).

[b]Difficult intubation is a grade III or IV laryngoscopic view.

Adapted from Kheterpal S, Han R, Shanks A, et al. Incidence and predictors of difficult and impossible mask ventilation. *Anesthesiology.* 2005;103:A1415. With permission.

TABLE 7-9 Airway Physical Examination Elements

Test	Findings
Dentition	Normal Dentures Edentulous Poor dentition
Beard	Yes/No
Mouth opening	≥3 cm <3 cm Unable to assess
Mallampati	I, II, III, IV, Unable to assess
Hyoid to mentum	≥6 cm <6 cm
Cervical spine	Normal Limited flexion Limited extension Limited flexion and extension Known unstable Possibly unstable Unable to assess
Existing airway	None Tracheostomy Endotracheal tube Unable to assess
Neck anatomy	Normal Laryngeal mobility limited status Postradiation therapy Mass Previous tracheostomy scar Radiation changes Thick, obese Thyroid cartilage not visible Tracheal deviation Unable to assess
Jaw protrusion	A: Normal: lower incisors can protrude past upper B: Limited: lower incisors can only be advanced to meet upper C: Severely limited: lower incisors cannot protrude to meet upper

2%-4% lidocaine). Profound topical anesthesias of upper airway mucosa, combined with judicious sedation, are the key elements in conducting a safe, effective, and comfortable awake intubation.

Special Preoperative Considerations

Preoperative Anesthesia Assessment Clinics Currently, the vast majority of patients presenting for elective surgery present to the hospital on the day of their procedure. Fortunately, most healthy patients can be seen and assessed by the anesthesia team immediately before their operation. The ASA Practice Advisory on Preanesthesia Evaluation recommends that timing of the preoperative evaluation be based not only on the health of the patient but also the invasiveness of the surgical procedure.[52] They recommend that all patients undergoing highly invasive surgical procedures be seen before the day of surgery. These patients require evaluation, counseling, and possibly therapy in advance of their surgical date. An appropriate and convenient place to coordinate this workup is the preoperative anesthesia assessment clinic (PAC). To derive the most benefit from PACs, surgeons need to use them discriminately. We find it helpful to provide screening criteria to our surgeons in the form of a patient self-assessment sheet.[53] This screening questionnaire is filled out by the patient using a series of checkboxes. The boxes are aligned to a back page such that positive answers will check (via carbon copy) the recommended preoperative laboratories and whether a PAC consultation is suggested. For example, if an affirmative answer is recorded for the question "Do you have heart disease?" an electrocardiogram is ordered (if not recently done) and the patient may be referred for further evaluation (**Table 7-10**).

Obesity and Obstructive Sleep Apnea Obesity is a well-established public health problem in developed countries. More specifically, obesity presents a major problem for practitioners who care for patients in the perioperative period. Obese patients have alterations in physiology at baseline that result in major lifestyle limitations, but they also have a well-documented increase in perioperative risk.[54] This would seem to justify an ASA Physical Status classification of at least II, and perhaps III. Multiple physiologic comorbidities exist in obese patients (diabetes mellitus, obstructive sleep apnea [OSA], cardiovascular disease, osteoarthritis, and others).[55] In addition, anatomic alterations of the airway also place these patients at increased risk for difficult mask ventilation and laryngoscopy.[53] IV access can be extremely difficult in obese patients, and in some cases central access must be considered. Some consider obesity a risk factor for gastric aspiration, and preventive measures should be considered. Obesity clearly heightens risk for adverse perioperative respiratory outcomes.[56] Blum et al reviewed the quality assurance events recorded from 25 767 anesthetics. They found a statistically significant increase in failed intubation, reintubation, dental injury, and airway obstruction associated with increasing BMI.[54]

Short of substantial weight loss prior to elective surgery (which has a dismal success rate), the perioperative risks just listed generally are not modifiable. Hence a key element for practitioners to consider in preparation for elective operation in obese patients is counseling, specifically with regard to weight loss (if time permits) and full disclosure of significantly heightened perioperative risks.[57]

It may also be beneficial to prepare obese patients for practical issues such as difficult IV access and the possible need for awake intubation. OSA is a syndrome commonly associated with obesity and is characterized by periodic, partial, or complete airway obstruction during sleep. It is estimated that approximately 9% of women and 24% of men have some degree of OSA; severe symptomatic disease is present in approximately 2% of women and 4% of men.[58] In October 2005 the ASA published a practice guideline, "Perioperative Management of Patients With Obstructive Sleep Apnea." This practice guideline comprehensively reviews the preoperative and postoperative management of patients with this disorder.[59] On occasion, patients who are considered to be healthy may have undiagnosed OSA, and therefore it is important to get a complete history, specifically as it relates to snoring and daytime somnolence. If the patient is indeed suspected of having the syndrome, then they should be evaluated before an elective procedure as recommended by the practice guideline.

Old Age The US population is aging rapidly, and an increasing proportion of surgical procedures are performed in the elderly. In 1986 Tiret et al provided evidence that the elderly have higher perioperative complication rates and higher risk than their younger counterparts, even in the absence of comorbidities.[60] The issue of perioperative risk, as it relates solely to advancing age, however, is far from settled.[61] Some would therefore assert that anesthetizing "healthy" elderly patients poses no significant elevation in perioperative risk. But even "healthy" elderly patients may have marked diminution in the function of major organ systems.[62] This would cause some to assign the ASA classification of II or even III to all such patients. Aside from the universal physiologic changes seen in all elderly patients ("aging"), elderly patients definitely tend to accumulate coexisting disease. Importantly, Kim and colleagues clearly demonstrated that coexisting disease in the elderly is a strong predictor of complications.[63] Elderly patients often have additional and unique perioperative challenges. Many have poor hearing and eyesight, and some suffer from cognitive impairment. This can make communication difficult. Simple issues like transportation home after conscious sedation can become logistical problems in the elderly. Another important effect of aging is altered drug disposition. Elderly patients have diminished volumes of distribution, decreased clearance,

TABLE 7-10 Patient Information Report Sample Questions

Question	Criteria	Answer	Action
Do you have or have you had any of the following heart-related conditions?	a. Heart disease	Yes or no	If yes, send pt. for ECG and preoperative anesthesia visit
	b. Heart attack within the last 6 months?	Yes or no	If yes, send pt. for ECG preoperative anesthesia visit
	c. Angina (chest pain)	Yes or no	If yes, send pt. for ECG preoperative anesthesia visit
	d. Irregular heartbeat	Yes or no	If yes, send pt. for ECG preoperative anesthesia visit
	e. Heart failure	Yes or no	If yes, send pt. for ECG preoperative anesthesia visit
Do you have or have you ever had any of the following?	a. Rheumatoid arthritis	Yes or no	If yes, send pt. for preoperative anesthesia visit
	b. Kidney disease	Yes or no	If yes, send pt. for electrolytes, creatinine, blood urea nitrogen, complete blood count, preoperative anesthesia visit
	c. Liver disease	Yes or no	If yes, send pt. for SGOT/ALK, PT/PTT, preoperative anesthesia visit
	d. Diabetes	Yes or no	If yes, send pt. for ECG preoperative anesthesia visit

ALK, alkaline; ECG, electrocardiogram; PT, prothrombin time; PTT, partial thromboplastin time; SGOT/ALK, serum glutamic-oxaloacetic transaminase/alkaline phosphatase.

Adapted from Tremper KK, Benedict P. Paper "preoperative computer." *Anesthesiology.* 2000;92(4):1212-1213. With permission.

and heightened sensitivity to nearly all medications. This explains why elderly patients are more sensitive to the therapeutic actions of most drugs and markedly more susceptible to side effects. In summary, despite changes attributable to normal aging, there is no strong association between age itself and perioperative risk. Thus chronologic age per se should not be a contraindication to surgery. Finally, to avoid complications and dissatisfaction in the elderly, anesthesia providers need to understand the altered pharmacology, physiology, and special needs that accompany the normal aging process.

Smoking Approximately one in five adult Americans currently smoke, and millions of elective surgical procedures are performed each year on these individuals. This is unfortunate because cigarette smoking is independently responsible for an alarming increase in the rate of perioperative pulmonary complications.[64] Cigarette smoking is an addictive disease that adversely alters the lifestyle of those affected. This fact, coupled with the well-known perioperative risks that smoking confers,[65] should result in otherwise healthy smokers being classified as at least ASA II and, in many cases, ASA III. A 2000 US Public Health Service guideline advised *all* physicians to "strongly advise every patient who smokes to quit because evidence shows that physician advice to quit smoking increases abstinence rates."[66] Further, anesthesiologists are uniquely positioned to give such advice. The preoperative interaction has been described by Warner as a "teachable moment" that not only lowers immediate perioperative risk but is also of great benefit to the long-term health of smokers.[67] Quitting smoking immediately before surgery has not been shown to heighten risk, produce untoward anxiety, or consistently precipitate nicotine withdrawl.[68] Hence patients who smoke should not be considered "healthy." These patients should be advised of the elevation in perioperative risk that is attributable to their habit and be encouraged to quit as soon as possible before their elective surgical procedure.

Preoperative Testing in Healthy Patients Billions of dollars are wasted in the United States each year on unnecessary preoperative testing.[69] In the case of healthy patients, this testing is almost always unnecessary.[70] It is generally accepted that healthy patients undergoing low-risk surgical procedures require no specific laboratory testing unless clinically indicated.[71] Little evidence exists regarding the propriety of such routine testing in healthy patients undergoing more complicated procedures with the potential for major blood loss (eg, major corrective orthopedic procedures, brain aneurysm clipping). Many recommend obtaining a preoperative hematocrit level in menstruating women, but there is little evidence to support this.[72] Women of childbearing age should be given pregnancy tests if it cannot be ascertained for certain whether or not they are pregnant. It is our institutional policy that women 18 years of age and older be asked, "Is it possible that you could be pregnant?" If they answer "no," they are not tested. This is in general agreement with the ASA stance on this issue: "The task force believes that the literature is inadequate to inform patients or physicians on whether anesthesia causes harmful effects on early pregnancy. Pregnancy testing may be offered to female patients of childbearing age and for whom the result would alter the patient's management."[54]

The indiscriminate ordering of batteries of routine tests, even in patients with serious comorbidity, has been the subject of intense recent review and been found to be excessively expensive and ineffective.[31] In fact, batteries of routine tests and their subsequent interpretations were found to predict morbidity more poorly than simple use of either the ASA physical status classification or the ACC/AHA[6] guidelines. The ASA Practice Advisory recommends that "specific tests and their timing should be individualized and based upon information obtained from sources such as the patient's medical record, interview, physical examination, and the types and invasiveness of the planned procedure."[54] These concepts were well summarized by Halaszynski et al, in their 2004 article addressing this issue[31] (see **Table 7-11**).

They suggest that age be used as a basic criterion for testing, with the additional components of surgical complexity and medical illness allowing for layers of flexibility. According to this paradigm, healthy patients younger than 45 years having uncomplicated operations require no testing. As patients deviate from this healthy/uncomplicated baseline, testing may be indicated but in a directed and temporally related fashion (if a test has been done recently, it does not generally need to be repeated). Thus if it can be ascertained from a history and physical examination that a patient is healthy, "routine" testing is rarely indicated in patients having uncomplicated surgical procedures. Age-based thresholds (men >45 years, women >55 years) for obtaining preoperative ECGs were recently called into question due to their arbitrary nature and unsatisfactory yield.[73]

TABLE 7-11 Preoperative Testing in Healthy Patients

	Low-Risk Surgery				High-Risk Surgery					
Test	Age <45 y	Age 45-55 y	Age 55-70 y	Age >70 y	Cardiac/Thoracic	Vascular	Major Abdominal	Major Blood Loss Possible	Intracranial	Major Orthopedic
ECG		M	Y	Y	Y	Y	S	S	S	S
CBC			Y	Y	Y	Y	Y	Y	Y	Y
Electrolytes				Y	Y	Y	Y	Y	Y	Y
Glucose				Y	Y	Y	Y	Y	Y	Y
LFTs							S			
Coagulation factors					Y	Y	S			
Urinalysis										
Pregnancy	S				S	S	S	S	S	S
CXR					Y		S	S		S
BUN/Cr					Y	Y	Y	Y	Y	Y

KEY: M = Male; **Y** = Usually indicated.

S = Sometimes indicated, may be requested by surgeon.

BUN/Cr, blood urea nitrogen/creatinine; CBC, complete blood count; CXR, chest x-ray; ECG, electrocardiogram; LFTs, liver function tests.

Adapted from Halaszynski TM, Juda R, Silverman DG. Optimizing postoperative outcomes with efficient preoperative assessment and management. *Crit Care Med.* 2004;32(4 Suppl):S76-S86. With permission.

IMPLEMENTATION OF THE PLAN

TYPE OF ANESTHESIA: GENERAL, REGIONAL, MONITORED ANESTHESIA CARE

Once the goals of medical evaluation and preoperative preparation have been accomplished, the anesthesiologist and patient must devise an anesthetic plan. This is where surgeon requirements and patient preference directly interface. Surgeon requirements vary widely, but most patients simply want their surgical experience to be safe and comfortable. Surgeons want the best conditions possible to perform their operations. It is advisable that surgeons and anesthesiologists communicate in advance to express their requirements and limitations. Anesthesiologists have direct control over many variables that surgeons require to carry out their operations safely and swiftly: degree of consciousness, blood pressure control, ventilatory control, level of consciousness at the conclusion of surgery, and so on. If other factors are equal (patient has no particular preference, perceived safety is equal), surgeon preference must be taken into consideration. Patient safety is always of paramount importance. At times this issue may outweigh surgeon preference (eg, providing a regional anesthetic for lower extremity surgery in a patient with severe pulmonary disease).

Keeping safety in mind, the anesthetic choice is often influenced by two key patient features: coexisting disease and aging. A completely acceptable technique for a particular operation (eg, a subarachnoid block for a total knee arthroplasty) may be contraindicated in patients presenting with certain disease states (aortic stenosis). Whereas general anesthesia is performed rather indiscriminately in young healthy patients, regional or even local anesthesia with sedation may be the safest option in patients with severe respiratory disease. The same holds true for the elderly patient. Even "healthy" elderly patients have well-documented diminutions in the function of renal, hepatic, cardiorespiratory, and drug-metabolizing systems,[62] and these changes are progressive. Drugs and doses that are innocuous in young healthy patients can have lasting and debilitating effects in the elderly. It is therefore desirable, whenever possible, to consider regional or even local anesthetics with minimal sedation in the elderly.

Type and location of surgery play an important role in planning for anesthesia, but patient preference and the destination of the patient in the postoperative phase also must be considered. Newer, more rapidly eliminated anesthetics have made postoperative destination less of an issue than in times past but one that still must be considered. For example, long-lasting regional blocks and long-acting IV medications may be inappropriate for patients scheduled on an outpatient basis. Following is an overview of common surgical operations and factors that influence the anesthetic plan.

Head and Neck Procedures Head and neck procedures range from minor, superficial operations to complex resections and reconstructions involving nerve monitoring, fluid shifts, and major blood loss. Many simple superficial operations are performed for skin cancer excision, followed by closure of the defect. Unless these lesions are deep or large, the cases can usually be safely and comfortably managed with conscious sedation combined with local anesthetic applied by the surgeon. Unless brief and superficial, ear surgery usually necessitates general anesthesia to achieve suitable patient comfort. It is common for these procedures to be performed on an outpatient basis. Cosmetic facial surgery is often performed with conscious sedation combined with local anesthesia to preserve awake muscle tone. Complex head and neck operations are often performed for invasive (mouth, throat, neck) cancers. These operations can be very complex and involve much fluid shifting and blood loss. In addition, these lesions can compromise the airway, necessitating nonstandard (awake) airway management techniques. Presence of a tracheostomy is common at completion of these operations. Due to the duration and complexity of these procedures, invasive monitoring (eg, intra-arterial catheter) is common. Communication with the patient and family is important in achieving realistic expectations.

On occasion, intracranial neurosurgery is performed in the awake patient, but most craniotomies are performed under general endotracheal anesthesia. Anesthesia for awake craniotomy is beyond the scope of this chapter. Success in these cases depends on an intimate surgeon-patient-anesthesiologist interaction with much preoperative communication. Because operating conditions for intracranial operations depend on, and conversely, can have an impact on vasomotor control, invasive (particularly arterial) monitoring is common. Neurologic function (somatosensory evoked potentials) monitoring is common, and the anesthesiologist must be knowledgeable in the interactions of anesthetic agents and these monitors. Additionally, neurosurgeons often request (if feasible) that a rapid wakeup be accomplished at the conclusion of surgery so that early assessment of neurologic function can be carried out.

Thoracic Procedures Thoracic surgical procedures range from outpatient thoracoscopic procedures (minor pulmonary resections and biopsies, sympathectomy) to major pulmonary and upper gastrointestinal tract procedures involving major body cavity and cardiovascular trespass, blood loss, and fluid shifting. Many of these procedures require single lung ventilation, which must be planned for. Open thoracic procedures are typically associated with a high degree of postoperative pain that is best controlled with epidural analgesia. Because of their proximity to major vascular structures and potential for adverse ventilatory interactions, these procedures often necessitate invasive intravascular lines and monitors that must be discussed with the patient as part of the preoperative plan.

Abdominal Procedures Increasingly, abdominal procedures are being performed laparoscopically. General anesthesia with endotracheal intubation must be used for patients to tolerate this approach safely and comfortably. Regional techniques can be used successfully for open intra-abdominal procedures, but these operations are frequently long and complex, so general anesthesia is often favored. When general anesthesia is used, endotracheal intubation is indicated to provide abdominal muscle relaxation and to protect against gastric aspiration. Epidural is an excellent option for postoperative analgesia in open abdominal operations but is usually not necessary when procedures are performed laparoscopically. Because of the potential for vascular involvement, major blood loss, and fluid shifting, invasive monitors are sometimes indicated, even in otherwise healthy patients.

Urologic Procedures Many urologic procedures are performed through a cystoscope and are of relatively short duration. In these cases, either short-acting regional or general anesthesia is an equally safe and effective option. Patient preference can play a major role in devising a plan for these cases. Both nephrectomy and prostatectomy have typically been performed via large open approaches, but they are increasingly being performed laparoscopically. Open prostatectomy has been performed successfully under both general and regional anesthesia, but the laparoscopic approaches for these procedures necessitate general anesthesia with endotracheal intubation.

Gynecologic Procedures As with abdominal and urologic procedures, gynecologic procedures are being performed increasingly via the laparoscopic approach. The same principles previously mentioned for abdominal and urologic procedures apply. When performed via an open abdominal approach, gynecologic procedures generally require general anesthesia with endotracheal intubation to allow profound muscle relaxation. Vaginal, cervical, and hysteroscopic procedures can be completed safely and comfortably using either general or regional anesthesia. Thus patient preference combined with anesthetist experience must be taken into account when planning for these cases.

Orthopedic Procedures At one extreme, orthopedic operations can be brief and minor peripheral extremity procedures amenable to either regional or local anesthesia with sedation. At the other end of the spectrum are long, complicated procedures involving blood loss, fluid shifting, and intraoperative nerve monitoring. Total knee and hip joint replacement operations are very common and can be carried out with either general or regional anesthesia. Epidural anesthesia is an effective choice and can be continued into the postoperative period to provide excellent analgesia. Some patients are extremely anxious about the prospect of being awake during orthopedic procedures. Consideration must be given to general anesthesia in these patients. Major spine surgery, operations for orthopedic malignancies, and revision hip operations can be long and complex, so general anesthesia with endotracheal intubation and invasive monitoring should be considered. Upper extremity nerve blocks are increasingly common for procedures on the shoulder and arm. Interscalene blocks and catheters are useful for shoulder surgery. Infraclavicular blocks and/or catheters are useful for procedures on the forearm and hand. Use of these techniques is discussed in Chapter 49. Because of the significant pain associated with shoulder reconstructive surgery and the need for postoperative manipulation for rehabilitation, interscalene catheters have become popular. These blocks have proven efficacy in the successful treatment of immediate postoperative pain.[74]

Ocular Procedures Many surgical procedures on the eye can be carried out safely and comfortably using local anesthesia. When formulating the preoperative anesthetic plan, this technique must be fully explained so that the patient has realistic expectations. Some ocular procedures can be very long in duration and hence necessitate use of general anesthesia to provide optimal operating conditions. In these cases plans may need to be devised for "deep" extubation to avoid coughing and elevation of intraocular pressure upon emergence from anesthesia.

Regional Anesthesia versus General Anesthesia The superiority of general anesthesia versus regional anesthesia for major surgical operations is controversial. Both techniques have advocates and detractors from both a safety and efficacy standpoint (see Chapter 46).

Although there is no convincing evidence that morbidity and mortality are decreased with either technique, there is a suggestion of improvement in specific outcomes with use of regional anesthesia.[75] Despite the common perception that regional anesthesia is generally safer than general anesthesia, its principal advantage is in providing analgesia postoperatively. For certain operations, regional anesthesia offers distinct advantages compared with general anesthesia,[76] but some of the perceived benefits of regional anesthesia have recently been called into question.[77] For regional techniques to be successful, the patient must be accepting of the technique, a skilled clinician must be available to perform it, and the block must be effective. If long-lasting blocks or indwelling catheters are to be used, educational efforts must be made regarding the special care that these techniques require. Lastly, patients must be informed of the potential complications that can result from the use of regional anesthesia.

Monitored Anesthesia Care: Potential Pitfalls Superficial operations and "noninvasive" (eg, cardiac electrophysiologic, endoscopic) procedures are commonly performed in healthy patients using the "monitored anesthesia care" (MAC) technique. This entails use of anxiolytic, sedating, and analgesic medications administered by anesthesia personnel, combined with local anesthesia administered by the surgeon. In a recent editorial, Hug describes the attitude of anesthesia providers regarding such cases as "routine, simple, and low-risk."[78,79] In addition these operations are often performed hastily, in remote locations, and involve positioning that provides anesthetists poor access to the airway. This can result in a situation where "diligence is less by both the anesthetist and the surgeon."[78] This, combined with liberal use of sedating respiratory depressant medications, has the potential to result in life-threatening anesthetic-related complications.

Complications attributable to MAC anesthesia have been reported in the literature, and a recent closed claims analysis by Bhanaker et al sheds new light on this devastating, yet uncommon problem. In this study, MAC anesthesia represented a "liability profile similar to claims associated with general anesthesia." This led the author to conclude that "oversedation leading to respiratory depression was an important mechanism of patient injury during MAC. Appropriate use of monitoring, vigilance and early resuscitation could have prevented many of these injuries."[79] Hence anesthesia providers need to be cognizant of the potential for serious complications associated with MAC anesthesia and avoid the pitfall of trivializing this technique to the extent of compromised vigilance and potential serious complications.

PREOPERATIVE INSTRUCTIONS

A clear, concise set of preoperative instructions can contribute greatly to patient safety and operating room efficiency. Provision of these instructions can be carried out in a variety of ways, but we believe a combination of both verbal and written communication is most likely to achieve the desired result. At our institution the verbal communication is carried out in either the preoperative clinic or via a combination of surgical and nursing preoperative "teaching." Our written preoperative instructions are in the form of a folder or packet that is periodically reviewed by perioperative surgical, anesthesia, and nursing teams. The most important elements of preoperative instruction that relate to the provision of safe anesthesia are dietary (nothing by mouth [NPO]) and medication instructions. Fasting guidelines for elective surgery are clearly delineated by the ASA,[80] and we tend to instruct patients conservatively (eg, interpreting "clear liquids" to mean "water").

ASA I and II patients may be taking a variety of prescription and nonprescription medications. To avoid potential complications, clear instructions must be given regarding continuation and avoidance of various medications before elective surgery. Medications that are typically continued include antireflux medications, cardiovascular and antihypertensive medications (with the possible exception of angiotensin-converting enzyme inhibitors and angiotensin receptor blockers),[81] pain medications (with the possible exception of aspirin and nonsteroidal anti-inflammatory medications), psychotropic medications (with the exception of monoamine oxidase inhibitors), asthma medications, and antiseizure medications. Medications taken on the day of surgery should be consumed with as little water as possible. Alternative medications and herbal preparations deserve special consideration. Many patients do not consider these to be medications and hence must be specifically asked about their use. These products are poorly regulated and often contain unknown quantities of substances that can lead to serious perioperative drug interactions and complications.[82] Because of the lack of data on many of these preparations, the ASA recommends that practitioners continually familiarize themselves with alternative medications, and it advises the discontinuation of all such products for at least 2 weeks before elective surgery.[83]

PREMEDICATION

It is difficult to find consensus on what constitutes the best plan for pharmacologic premedication before anesthesia. What is important is that each agent be administered only if there is a clear and specific indication for its use. The most common indications for preoperative administration of medications are anxiolysis, analgesia, gastric aspiration prophylaxis, surgical wound infection prophylaxis, and thromboembolic prophylaxis. None of these classes of medications should be administered on a purely routine basis. Each of these medications has a unique set of potentially dangerous side effects, including allergic reactions, drug–drug interactions, prolonged effects, and added cost. Hence in the absence of clear indications, healthy patients undergoing elective operations should receive little or no pharmacologic premedication.

Anxiety is common in patients undergoing even minor surgery, and it tends to heighten as the surgical event approaches. It is difficult to discern which patients will be anxious before surgery by any other means than a direct interview. Treating preoperative anxiety not only improves patient satisfaction[84] but may have more far-reaching effects such as reduction in surgical stress response and lowering the incidence of PONV.[85] Although the most commonly used agents used for this purpose are benzodiazepines, and particularly midazolam, other agents such as melatonin have proven to be safe and efficacious.[86]

Preoperative analgesia may be considered when painful conditions such as orthopedic fractures are present. If opiates are chosen for this purpose, patients must be monitored for sedative and respiratory depressant side effects. Some studies even support use of "preemptive analgesia" with agents such as ketorolac as a means to lower anesthetic requirements and their attendant side effects. Evaluation for the risk of nausea and vomiting were discussed previously. When this risk is identified, consideration should be given to single, or in select cases, multimodal therapy to prevent this complication. Healthy patients occasionally require thromboembolism prophylaxis in the perioperative period. This is most commonly accomplished with use of either low-dose or low-molecular-weight heparin preparations.

POSTOPERATIVE DESTINATION

The anesthetic plan must take into account the postoperative destination of the patient. Pre- and intraoperative planning must be flexible, so that safe and appropriate medical care is available if ongoing needs of the patient change. For example, many airway procedures can be accomplished on an outpatient basis. There is a relatively high risk with this type of surgery, however, that complications could require admission or even mechanical ventilation in an intensive care unit. This sort of eventuality must be taken into account for two reasons. First, operations with a relatively high likelihood of admission or intensive care unit management (even in otherwise healthy patients) should not be scheduled in facilities that lack the means to provide this care. Second, patients and their families must be advised beforehand of this possibility. Patients and family members must be aware that intraoperative events can change the postoperative destination of the patient, even if the initial plan was for same-day discharge.

Patients have three ultimate postoperative destinations: home, a hospital "floor" or "ward" bed, or the intensive care unit. A stay in the postanesthesia care unit (PACU, or "recovery room") may precede any one of these final destinations. Planning for the eventuality of any of these destinations must occur in both the pre- and intraoperative phases of an anesthetic. In the case of both the PACU and the intensive care unit, advance planning must be carried out so that a bed is available and the unit is appropriately staffed. Both patients and family members need to be made aware of the destination that was initially planned and of any changes that may have been made based on intraoperative (or PACU events). Fortunately, many procedures that are planned on an outpatient basis and are free of complications may entail very short PACU stays or (as is becoming increasingly common) bypass a recovery room altogether. This is generally safe, cost effective, and well received by patients but requires simple but crucial advance planning. For example, it is mandatory that patients who have received sedating medications have safe transportation home, usually in the person of a caregiver who can also assist with medication, surgical dressing issues, and other forms of assistance.

POSTOPERATIVE PAIN

Postoperative pain resulting from surgical procedures performed in healthy patients ranges from none to severe and relatively long lasting. As such, treatment of postoperative pain ranges from no treatment at one extreme (noninvasive endoscopic procedures) to invasive techniques including epidural analgesia and indwelling nerve plexus catheters. This section serves as a simple overview of available pain control options in healthy patients. See the comprehensive section on postoperative pain management in Chapter 72 for a more in-depth review of this subject. It is the anesthesiologist's responsibility to couple analgesia with hypnosis in the intraoperative phase and then continue some form of analgesia postoperatively while minimizing additional drug effects such as sedation and respiratory depression. A key feature in the success of this plan is education and physician-caregiver rapport in the preoperative phase. Although it is important for patients to wake up as pain free as possible, it is also critical that they be informed that they will likely experience some degree of postoperative pain. Realistic expectations regarding postoperative pain are a vital component in patient satisfaction and avoidance of complications related to pharmacologic control of pain.

As stated previously, healthy patients generally undergo short, simple surgical procedures. Occasionally, however, complicated operations are performed that result in severe postoperative pain. Thus the entire array of pain control modalities at the anesthesiologist's disposal must be available in this population. Despite controversy over its efficacy,[87] preemptive analgesia with agents such as acetaminophen and nonsteroidal anti-inflammatory drug (NSAID) compounds should be considered. Use of these compounds is also typically the first line of therapy in patients having minor operations such as carpal tunnel repair or vasectomy. These compounds are generally devoid of side effects, but patients must be cautioned regarding overdose with resultant liver and kidney damage.

Opiates are indicated for moderate to severe pain via either oral or intravenous routes of administration. Patient-controlled analgesia (PCA) represents a major advance in the use of opiates for postoperative analgesia, but success with the technique depends on proper planning and patient instruction. Grass has recently reviewed this subject, including its history, safety, efficacy, and current practice guidelines.[88] Major nerve conduction blockade (nerve blocks, plexus blocks) and epidural analgesia are occasionally necessary in healthy patients undergoing surgical procedures that will result in severe pain (eg, orthopedic procedures, intra-abdominal and pelvic procedures). Liu published an excellent practical review of indwelling catheters for postoperative pain relief.[89] Although highly successful, both techniques are associated with potentially serious complications, and proper planning and consent requires disclosure of both aspects of these techniques. Finally, the issues of aging, opiate dependence, and abuse all have important implications for the successful planning and management of postoperative pain (see Chapter 72).

MONITORING IN HEALTHY PATIENTS

The medical community, the anesthesia community, and patients, to some extent, assume that monitoring during anesthesia and surgery results in fewer preventable mishaps and improved outcomes. Fortunately, since its introduction into modern medicine, anesthesia has become an increasingly safe proposition.[90] As Domino and others continue to point out, however, rare anesthesia mishaps continue to have catastrophic outcomes (death, major morbidity) that are very costly to society.[41] Every year, thousands of cases of death and serious morbidity are attributed solely to the provision of anesthesia.[91] In a large proportion of these cases, the cause of the morbidity or mortality is believed to be preventable.[92] Failure to prevent anesthetic catastrophes usually results from lapses in vigilance or simple human error. Anesthetic monitors are therefore intended to aid in the maintenance of vigilance and to alert providers to the possibility of human error. Following is an overview of monitors commonly used in healthy patients and the rationale for their use in various clinical scenarios. (See Chapters 30-35 for an in-depth review of monitoring.)

Despite the assumption that there is a correlation between monitoring and outcome, there is little in the way of scientific validation to support this assumption. Eichhorn and colleagues, in 1986, suggested that intraoperative monitors may reduce adverse events and therefore improve outcomes.[93] From this body of work arose the ASA guidelines for intraoperative monitoring,[94] which were recently amended (**Table 7-12**).

The assumption that monitoring improves outcome, coupled with anesthesia providers' zeal to gather information, can lead to practitioners erring on the side of more, rather than less monitoring devices. This would be ideal if monitors were cheap, completely accurate, and completely safe. Some modern monitoring devices, however, are expensive and do not always bring value. Some forms of monitoring have the potential to mislead anesthesia providers; others are even capable of causing serious physical harm.[95,96] Therefore, in planning for an anesthetic, anesthesiologists must weigh the perceived advantages with the known potential for complications when choosing a monitoring strategy (**Table 7-13**).

Healthy patients having uncomplicated surgical procedures rarely need more than the ASA basic intraoperative monitors. Before considering machines that monitor the human body, however, it is vital that anesthesiologists maintain basic physical examination skills. These skills can give

TABLE 7-12 American Society of Anesthesiologists Standards for Basic Intraoperative Monitoring

Standards
Standard 1: Qualified anesthesia personnel shall be present in the room throughout the conduct of all general anesthetics, and regional and monitored anesthesia care
Standard 2: Oxygenation, ventilation, circulation, and temperature shall be continually evaluated
Oxygenation
Oxygen analyzer inspired gases
Observation for the patient
Pulse oximetry
Ventilation
Auscultation
Observation of the patient
Observation of reservoir bag
End-tidal carbon dioxide analysis
Circulation
Continuous electrocardiogram display
Heart rate and blood pressure recorded every 5 min
Evaluation of circulation: auscultation of heart sounds, palpation of pulse, pulse plethysmography, pulse oximetry, intra-arterial pressure tracing
Temperature
Core temperature and/or skin temperature

Note: The term *continuously* means prolonged without interruption, whereas *continually* means repeated regularly and frequently.

vital information about patients quickly and reliably. For example, failure of the chest to rise combined with a bubbling sound emanating from the patient's throat may indicate cuff failure or improper placement of an endotracheal tube. Tactile sensation of a bounding pulse, in the presence of a low machine reading, may indicate a problem with mechanical blood pressure measurement. Discoloration of a patient's skin combined with a feeling of warmth could be an early indicator of MH. Smelling a potent anesthetic vapor could be a sign of an airway leak or disconnect. Although it would be crude and unwise to rely solely on sense perception to assess patients, clinicians must maintain vital physical examination skills in addition to their knowledge and skills in the use of mechanical monitoring devices. Analysis of anesthetic mishaps leading to serious morbidity and mortality[41] has consistently revealed one common mechanism as a root cause for catastrophe: failure to deliver oxygen to vital organs. The most common cause of critical end-organ hypoxia is failure to ventilate the lungs, hence the ASA recommendation for continuous evaluation of oxygenation and ventilation, even in healthy patients. The goal of this monitoring is early recognition of ventilatory inadequacy that can be rectified before end-organ damage ensues. Observation is still a vital skill in assessing tissue oxygenation, especially in the case of the awake patient. Signs of hypoxemia in an awake patient include decreased level of consciousness and loss of judgment and disorientation, but these signs are not specific and occur in many other conditions. Cyanosis may be an indicator of hypoxemia, but it occurs late and is generally unreliable. Given the devastating consequences of arterial hypoxemia, however, this cause must be at the top of any differential diagnosis when these physical signs are encountered.

MEASUREMENT OF OXYGENATION

Three methods of assessing oxygen delivery are widely available: arterial blood gas analysis, pulse oximetry, and measurement of inspired oxygen concentration. The need for blood gas analysis in healthy surgical patients is relatively rare. This test is invasive (and therefore has potential complications), relatively expensive, and can only be performed intermittently. Its use in healthy patients should be considered when

TABLE 7-13 Types of Anesthesia Monitors and Their Properties

Type of Monitor	What Is Measured	Invasiveness	Potential for Complications
Physical examination	Heart tones, breath sounds, pulse, color, etc	Noninvasive	–
Pulse oximetry	Arterial oxygen saturation	Noninvasive	–
Arterial blood gas analysis	Ventilatory and acid/base status	Invasive	++
Sphygmomanometry, oscillometry	Blood pressure	Noninvasive	+
Arterial catheterization	Blood pressure	Invasive	++
Electrocardiography	Cardiac rhythm, integrity	Noninvasive	–
Capnography	Ventilatory, circulatory status	Non-semi-invasive	–
Electroencephalogram, bispectral index, entropy, others	Brain function, depth of anesthesia	Noninvasive	+/–
Temperate probes	Body temperature	Non to semi-invasive	+/–
Central venous cannulation, pulmonary artery catheter	Volume status, cardiac function	Invasive	+++

complex surgical procedures are being performed or when perioperative complications necessitate in-depth analysis of ventilation and acid-base status. Pulse oximetry is completely noninvasive, well accepted (despite being a continuous monitor), and is relatively inexpensive. Extensive reviews of the development, theory, and applications of pulse oximetry are available. Pulse oximetry and inspired oxygen analysis should be used in every patient undergoing general anesthesia. Pulse oximetry should be used in all patients anesthetized with sedating IV medications. What follows is a summary of its technical aspects, perioperative uses, and limitations.

Pulse oximetry relies on two principles to continuously measure the degree of arterial blood oxygenation: differential light absorption of oxy- and deoxyhemoglobin, and pulsation of arterial blood. The pulse oximeter displays a number that corresponds to the arterial saturation obtained from an in vivo cooximeter. Also displayed on most units is a plethysmograph, or pulse waveform. Some advantages of pulse oximetry can also be viewed as limitations. First, the pulse oximeter is quite accurate when compared with in vivo oximetry but only under ideal conditions and within a fixed range of arterial saturation. Artifacts that create less than ideal conditions include shivering, cold extremity, intravascular dyes, venous congestion, and electrocautery. In addition, the processor algorithms built in to the device are unable to give meaningful output for oxygen saturations below 70%. Second, users must be familiar with limitations of the plethysmograph feature. It should not be assumed that the plethysmograph accurately reflects the magnitude of the arterial pulsation and hence the adequacy of perfusion. This signal is variably (and sometimes highly) amplified, however, to aid in the measurement of oxygen saturation.[97] Hence the plethysmograph magnitude should not be used to infer information about the adequacy of blood perfusion.

HEMODYNAMIC MONITORS

Hemodynamic monitors are those intended to assess the adequacy of circulatory function. All anesthetized patients must have at least intermittent blood pressure monitoring. For healthy patients having uncomplicated surgical procedures, intermittent cuff measurement is usually sufficient. Cuff measurement of blood pressure can be achieved via either sphygmomanometry or oscillometry. Both methods are accurate, noninvasive, and well tolerated. Clinicians using either of these methods must understand a few guidelines to ensure accurate measurement. First, cuff size must be appropriate for the patient. Too large or too small cuff size can underestimate or overestimate blood pressure, respectively. This is most common in obese patients where cuff size is too small. Second, this method of blood pressure measurement is subject to motion artifact.

Direct intra-arterial blood pressure monitoring involves insertion of a catheter into an artery followed by connection to a pressure transduction system. Arterial cannulae are occasionally necessary in healthy patients, due to procedural length or complexity. This technique is invasive, and serious complications can result from its use. When correctly performed, this method provides continuous measurement of blood pressure that is very accurate. The data obtained from this measurement technique can even be used as an accurate measure of intravascular volume status.[98]

In patients who are intubated and mechanically ventilated, variation in the peak systolic pressure with ventilation has been used as a method to estimate intravascular volume status.[99] This measurement, known as systolic pressure variation (SPV), has been compared with central venous pressure measurements, pulmonary artery occlusion pressure measurements, and transesophageal echocardiographic measurement of left ventricular volume, and it has been found to be more accurate than other pressure measurements for determining adequacy of volume resuscitation.[99] Normal values of SPV are between 5 and 10 mm Hg, with greater values representing possible underresuscitation (hypovolemia) and lesser values implying that the patient may be overresuscitated.[99] This SPV has been described as a "dynamic variable of volume responsiveness."[99,100]

Clinicians must not forget basic physical examination skills that can be valuable when specifically assessing circulatory status. The two most useful of these skills are palpation and auscultation. These tests can be immediately performed and require no mechanical devices. These methods are not sufficient to completely monitor the circulatory status in healthy patients. Regular use of these techniques, however (especially when baseline assessments were performed for comparison), can give anesthesia providers accurate and early information that may guide therapy or aid in selection of more complex assessment techniques. Palpation of a peripheral pulse can give valuable information about the circulatory status of the patient. Two properties of the pulse must be ascertained: magnitude and character. The pulse of a healthy patient at baseline should be strong and regular. Performing a baseline examination is mandatory so that later comparison can be made.

Auscultation is another physical examination skill with usefulness in the modern operating room. Auscultation is simple to perform, even on a continuous basis, and is an excellent qualitative measure of ventilation. Auscultation is most valuable to the clinician when a baseline examination is performed and used for later comparison. Baseline auscultation of heart and lungs should be performed in every anesthetized patient. As with palpation, both the quality and the magnitude of the sounds must be ascertained. Auscultation is never sufficient on its own to make definitive diagnoses or guide therapy, but it can be performed easily, immediately, and without harm and may guide the clinician in planning additional diagnostic steps. An example is development of a third heart sound, combined with new pulmonary rales, raising suspicion of fluid overload and pulmonary edema.

The heart is not only a pump, but a vital end organ, susceptible to hypoxic insult. In addition, even healthy anesthetized patients may be susceptible to cardiac rhythm abnormalities that can compromise circulatory adequacy. Therefore, anesthesiologists routinely monitor the integrity of the heart muscle and heart rhythm during anesthesia. This is accomplished mainly via ECG and, when possible, feedback from an awake patient (angina or anginal equivalent). ECG monitoring is considered the standard of care in modern anesthesia. ECG monitoring is completely noninvasive, relatively inexpensive, and can be assessed continuously. ECG is a crude representation of the heart's electrical activity, but critical information can be inferred from the trace regarding the integrity of the myocardium. Specific patterns of abnormality on ECG tracings can represent cardiac dysrhythmias, cardiac ischemia, and electrolyte imbalances that can compromise the integrity of the heart muscle and its function as a pump.

The most common ECG abnormality found in healthy anesthetized patients is dysrhythmia. Therefore, when using ECG to monitor in healthy patients, it is wise to monitor leads that are best suited for rhythm identification such as lead II or V_1. Common causes of perioperative dysrhythmias are autonomic nervous system overactivity, ventilatory abnormalities such as hypoxemia and hypercarbia, and cardiac effects of anesthetic medications and adjuvants. Perioperative dysrhythmias in otherwise healthy patients are often well tolerated and self-limited. Some, such as severe bradycardia and junctional rhythms, can compromise circulatory status and require intervention. On occasion, the perioperative ECG will identify myocardial ischemia in patients who were previously thought to be healthy.

By definition, healthy patients are free of coronary artery disease. Use of perioperative ECG monitoring, however, will identify possible coronary ischemia in patients who were previously thought to be free of ischemic heart disease. The relationship between perioperative ECG evidence of coronary ischemia and the diagnosis of ischemic heart disease remains unclear. For ECG to function well as a monitor for myocardial ischemia, the correct combinations of leads must be used. Highest sensitivity can be achieved when these combinations include lead V_5. Changes in ST segments and in T-wave configurations are the most universally accepted ECG findings representative of coronary ischemia, but specificity of these findings is far from perfect.[101] Newer monitors use computer-assisted ST segment analysis to assist in early detection of coronary ischemia. Most monitors allow printing or "freezing" of a short ECG trace to compare with later findings. When these are not performed, clinicians should closely observe a preinduction ECG tracing so that comparisons can be made later, if necessary.

CAPNOGRAPHY

Measurement of respiratory carbon dioxide is useful and strongly encouraged in all anesthetized patients. The methodology most commonly used is end-tidal carbon dioxide measurement, or capnography, to measure the carbon dioxide concentration in respiratory gas. Portable colorimetric devices are also available for use at the bedside or in the emergency department and are used to confirm proper placement of an endotracheal tube. Capnographic samples can be obtained from closed or open (eg, near the nose of a patient who is spontaneously breathing room air) breathing circuits. Capnography gives clinicians vital information regarding the pattern and the magnitude of ventilation. It gives useful information regarding cardiopulmonary function. To produce a normal capnogram, the patient must be producing carbon dioxide at the normal rate, blood must be returning it to the pulmonary circulation, and the lungs must be ventilated. Therefore, a continuous capnogram ensures, on a breath-to-breath basis, that all of the following are functioning normally: metabolism, blood flow, and ventilation.

A sudden decrease in end-tidal carbon dioxide may be an early and reliable indicator of pulmonary embolism.[102] Capnography is useful in confirming proper placement of endotracheal tubes, but it is not useful in ruling out endobronchial intubation. End-tidal carbon dioxide concentration can be monitored continuously, the machinery is relatively inexpensive, and the technique is noninvasive.

MENTAL STATUS AND DEPTH OF ANESTHESIA

The best monitor of cerebral function in healthy patients requiring anesthesia is interaction with a conscious patient. This is the rationale for using awake anesthetic techniques in certain settings where feedback regarding brain integrity is critical (carotid endarterectomy, prostatic resection with use of nonionic irrigants). In many surgical settings, however, awake anesthetic techniques are not suitable. A concept intimately related to perioperative cerebral function is the ability of anesthesia providers to assess the efficacy, or "depth" of anesthesia accurately in unconscious patients. The ideal general anesthetic renders a patient unconscious and pain free, facilitates ideal surgical working conditions, is rapidly reversible at the conclusion of surgery, and has no lasting side effects. During anesthesia-induced unconsciousness, however, there is no completely reliable method of assessing whether a patient is aware and possibly perceiving intraoperative events. Anesthesia providers undergo rigorous training in pharmacology and physiology to dose medications and interpret physiologic data correctly so that they can provide assurance on *these grounds that* patients are adequately anesthetized. Unfortunately, correct drug dosing and "normal" physiologic values do not ensure that all patients are unconscious and free from pain.

EEG is used only occasionally for monitoring brain function (and presumably, consciousness). This monitoring technique is cumbersome, expensive, and requires highly trained personnel to interpret the complex data that it generates. Currently, unprocessed EEG is rare in intraoperative settings. A variation of EEG that has gained attention in both the medical community and with the lay media is BIS or "entropy" monitoring. These devices use only select EEG leads and then filter and transform the signals into a single digitized value.[103] BIS or entropy values correlate inversely with depth of anesthesia.[103] Use of the device has been advocated for two reasons: reducing the incidence of intraoperative awareness during general anesthesia and reducing anesthetic drug costs.[104] Although intraoperative awareness is a real problem, the issue has been somewhat sensationalized by the public media, which has led to much public interest in BIS. The ability of BIS to eliminate awareness, however, remains controversial,[105] and some even argue that BIS could actually cause anesthesiologists to underdose their medications, leading to a higher incidence of awareness.[106] This issue remains unsettled and requires further investigation.

TEMPERATURE MONITORING

Temperature must be monitored in some way in all anesthetized patients, especially when general anesthesia is chosen or when MH-triggering agents are used. Multiple investigators have shown improved outcome with maintenance of normothermia during major operations.[107] Hypothermia slows metabolism, inhibits coagulation, can cause cardiovascular lability, and is very uncomfortable in awake patients. Hypothermia is easily and commonly achieved in the operating room, but the best treatment strategy is prevention. Several methods of temperature monitoring are available to anesthesia providers. The simplest and least invasive method is use of a skin temperature probe. These probes are somewhat accurate, but it must be kept in mind that skin temperature is not truly representative of core, or internal, temperature. In addition, skin probes are easily rendered inaccurate by ambient conditions such as warming and cooling mattresses and forced air blowers. Several semi-invasive methods of temperature monitoring are available such as tympanic, nasopharyngeal, esophageal, and rectal. Although these methods are quite safe, accurate, and more reflective of core temperature, complications are possible (ruptured tympanic membrane, nosebleed, irretrievable probe wires). The most accurate monitors of core body temperature are also the most invasive. Temperature probes are present on the tips of pulmonary artery and urinary catheters, but these are generally reserved for major operations in medically ill patients.

CONCLUSION

Safety and efficacy are the primary determinants of a successful anesthetic. Safety in anesthesia is mainly achieved through the avoidance of complications. A main source of complications is patient comorbidity. Healthy patients, by definition, lack comorbidity but may still experience anesthetic complications. The main goals of the anesthetic plan in healthy patients are ensuring the absence of comorbidity and the identification of potential complicating factors. The primary method of accomplishing these goals is the careful performance of a preoperative history and physical examination, which is typically a joint effort between the surgeon and anesthesiologist. In most cases, the anesthetic portion of this evaluation can be performed on the same day as surgery. Once the evaluation of the healthy surgical patient is complete, the plan is formulated, taking into account the needs of both the patient and the surgeon. The patient must be fully informed of the nature of the operation and type of anesthesia involved. Patient instructions and use of premedications are also important steps leading to safe and successful anesthesia. Finally, monitoring devices are believed to be a major contributor to avoidance of complications and overall patient safety. Generally, healthy patients only need basic ASA intraoperative monitoring, but, on occasion, the extent of surgery may dictate a more invasive monitoring scheme.

KEY REFERENCES

- Bryson GL, Chung F, Cox RG, et al. Patient selection in ambulatory anesthesia—an evidence-based review: part II. *Can J Anaesth.* 2004;51(8):782-794.
- Domino KB, Posner KL, Caplan RA, Cheney FW. Awareness during anesthesia: a closed claims analysis. *Anesthesiology.* 1999;90(4):1053-1061.
- Eagle KA, Berger PB, Calkins H, et al. ACC/AHA guideline update for perioperative cardiovascular evaluation for noncardiac surgery—executive summary. A report of the American College of Cardiology/American Heart Association Task Force on Practice Guidelines (Committee to Update the 1996 Guidelines on Perioperative Cardiovascular Evaluation for Noncardiac Surgery). *Anesth Analg.* 2002;94(5):1052-1064.
- Halaszynski TM, Juda R, Silverman DG. Optimizing postoperative outcomes with efficient preoperative assessment and management. *Crit Care Med.* 2004;32(4 Suppl):S76-S86.
- Lagasse RS. Anesthesia safety: model or myth? A review of the published literature and analysis of current original data. *Anesthesiology.* 2002;97(6):1609-1617.
- Pearce A. Evaluation of the airway and preparation for difficulty. *Best Pract Res Clin Anaesthesiol.* 2005;19(4):559-579.
- Warner MA, Saletel RA, Schroeder DR, Warner DO, Offord KP, Gray DT. Outcomes of anesthesia and surgery in people 100 years of age and older. *J Am Geriatr Soc.* 1998;46(8):988-993.

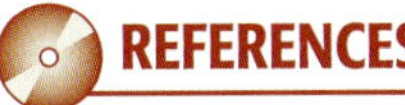

REFERENCES

Complete references available on DVD and online version at www.LongneckerAnesthesiology.com

SECTION B

Preoperative Evaluation of the Anesthesia Patient

Appropriate and Effective Use of Consultants

Lynda T. Wells
Brian Uthlaut

KEY POINTS

1. The increasing complexity of modern medicine requires greater involvement of consultants and coordination of care across medical specialties.
2. Primary physicians and consultants should have clear, direct communication about the reason for consultation and the role of each provider.
3. Consultants should prioritize their recommendations, provide continuity of care perioperatively, and be sensitive to the content and delivery of their recommendations.
4. Preoperative evaluations should be evidence-based, coordinated with all involved physicians, and performed well before surgery to facilitate effective management of comorbidities or complex medical problems.
5. Consultants should facilitate the use of guidelines and consensus statements when recommending therapy and. where necessary, deviate from existing guidelines based on new knowledge.
6. Consultants should actively provide education to the physicians who consult them as well as to the patients on whom they consult (eg, healthy lifestyle interventions).

INTRODUCTION

Recent evolution in the practice of medicine has increased the need for consultants and their role in the perioperative period. These changes arose in response to these situations:

- An aging patient population requiring more medical and surgical care
- The advent of same-day admission and outpatient surgery
- Better outcomes in sicker patients through technological and pharmacologic advances in surgery, anesthesiology, and medicine
- An appreciation that the complexity of care of sick people requires multiple specialties
- Increasing numbers of nonphysician providers who rely on physicians for medical advice
- Market pressures: the need to decrease costs by reducing errors and improving efficiency

The potential for consultation to have a positive impact on patient care and health care indices has never been greater. This chapter addresses the role of the consultant, the consultation process, factors influencing its effectiveness, and medicolegal considerations.

ROLE OF THE CONSULTANT

The consultant enters into a relationship with the patient at the request of the primary physician. The requesting physician should ensure that the patient understands the reason for the consultation prior to the referral and that the patient agrees to this relationship. The consultant should respect the existing professional relationship between the patient and the primary physician. If at any time confusion arises over the requested role of the consultant, this should be clarified with the referring physician. However, once involved with the patient, the consultant's responsibility is to put the patient's interest first.

Consultants should focus their attention on issues pertinent to the clinical question posed in the consult request. They should perform their own history and physical in addition to reviewing the medical record. Providing an estimated quantitative risk of both cardiac and noncardiac perioperative events for that patient and the proposed surgical procedure is ideal (**Table 8-1**), as well as proposing strategies to mitigate these risks. Evaluating medical versus surgical management; anticipating potential intra- and postoperative complications; and outlining a plan for postoperative care to prevent, detect, and treat complications is germane. Findings and recommendations should be clearly and concisely recorded in the chart and discussed directly with the primary physician. Unless the primary physician has given permission to the consultant to do so, the duty to convey important information to the patient remains with the primary physician.[1]

When making an assessment and recommendations, consultants should limit their direct discussion with the patient to their area of expertise (eg, management of diabetes) and should be careful to avoid direct discussion of issues within the domain of the surgeon or the anesthesiologist. The patient should understand that recommendations are simply that. The role of the referring physician is to decide which recommendations they wish to enact. An exception to this arrangement exists in a model of comanagement, in which the medical "consultant" has a set of clearly defined areas in which they may be actively managing as a "primary" physician and should make this role clear to the patient.

Consultants should avoid commenting on areas outside their scope of practice (eg, telling an anesthesiologist how to give an anesthetic or a surgeon how to operate). These comments are not authoritative and can cause animosity within the perioperative care team. Additionally, consultants should be sure to avoid trivial comments, such as "avoid hypotension," that are obvious to any physician and unlikely to improve patient care.[2] When surgeons reviewed a series of medical consultations, 12% of the comments were rated as "insulting."[3]

Conflicts between primary physicians and consultants over medical or surgical decision making can be complex to resolve. A trilateral deliberative model has been proposed to deal with conflicts between the consultant(s) and referring physician. This model describes the ethical duties of the primary physician and consultant.[4] It cautions against attempts to dominate each other and advocates minimizing differences

TABLE 8-1

Key Functions of the Consultant	Key Functions of the Primary Physician
1. Estimate cardiac and noncardiac risks using literature-based guidelines	1. Ultimate decision making for patient
2. Identify ways to minimize risk and manage the patient's comorbidities	2. Identification of problems beyond their expertise
3. Anticipate postoperative complications and challenges	3. Obtaining patient's consent for involving a consultant
4. During the postoperative follow-up, assist in medical management and handoff of care	4. Making a written request for a consultant to address a specific, clearly communicated question
5. Educate primary team and patient	5. Communicating the results and decision making to the patient

of opinion over minor issues. Both the consultant and primary physician are obliged to maintain patient confidentiality separately if requested, except when relevant to immediate health care concerns. This model allows direct discussion between the consultant and patient over a difference of opinion with the referring physician. However, it also assumes that resolution between physicians was attempted and failed before the patient was alarmed by these discussions.

A further role of the consultant is as educator to the physician requesting the consult. This should be done tactfully and sensitively. Opinions should be concise and presented without condescension. Presentation of a differential diagnosis and selected references may help. Brevity is best because long treatises are unlikely to be read and consequently would be of no value.

THE CONSULTATION PROCESS

PREOPERATIVE ASSESSMENT

Preoperative assessment clinics were created to streamline patient assessment and evaluation before surgery, and they appear to be effective. Preoperative evaluation has been shown to enhance management of existing conditions, diagnose new conditions, and help in arranging follow-up care.[5-8] They can reduce costs by facilitating rational use of preoperative testing and consultation. Medical specialties have created consultation services to ensure appropriate physician specialists are available to respond to requests for consultations in a timely manner. Clinical guidelines such as the American College of Cardiology/American Heart Association (ACC/AHA) 2007 guidelines on perioperative cardiovascular evaluation and care for noncardiac surgery have also been helpful in guiding appropriate preoperative evaluation and care.[9]

Consultation is usually performed by an anesthesiologist, internist, medical subspecialist, or a combination. Multiple studies have demonstrated improvement in surgical care from anesthesiologist-staffed preoperative clinics; less evidence has been generated from internist-staffed preoperative clinics.[10-13] The surgical history and physical should be sufficiently detailed to identify the need for further workup. If indicated, the most appropriate specialist(s) should be consulted and specific clinical questions articulated. Internists and medical subspecialists are most appropriate for assessing and managing complex medical problems and for engaging in ongoing medical care. Anesthesiologists are best for assessing anesthetic risks, appropriate location for surgical care based on risk (eg, free-standing outpatient surgery center vs hospital), and whether patients are candidates for nurse sedation, monitored anesthesia care, or another type of anesthesia.

Multiple studies have indicated that the most important factors in effective consultation relate to communication. The reason for the consultation should be stated precisely and confirmed by the consultant with the referring physician. One study showed that 14% of consultants and consultees disagreed on the reason for consultation.[14] Miscommunication such as this at least partially explains compliance rates with consultant recommendations of only 54% to 77%.[3,15] "Please clear for surgery" is not a meaningful consult request.[16] It is unrealistic for any patient to be "cleared" because no patient is *entirely* without *some* medical risk. Additionally, regulations governing consult reimbursements require that a medically appropriate question be asked of a consultant.[1] The physician requesting a consult should be clear as to the type of intervention being sought: consult with recommendations only, consult and treat immediate problems, consult and comanage care, and so on.

Data suggest that in the preoperative period, patients are uniquely receptive to information on health and lifestyle. These educational opportunities should be exploited by all members of the health care team because these interventions can be especially effective for reinforcing other recommendations for a healthy lifestyle. Patients and their families should be counseled to stop smoking,[17,18] limit alcohol intake[19] and drug use, and improve diet and exercise. Referrals and supporting information should be provided whenever appropriate.

As with all types of medical intervention, perioperative consultations are subject to three basic types of medical errors: overuse in patients unlikely to benefit, underuse in patients with clear potential for benefit, and misuse.

TIMING OF THE PREOPERATIVE CONSULTATION

Requests for consultation should ideally be made sufficiently ahead of the scheduled procedure to allow time for necessary investigations and for appropriate medical interventions if warranted. The most commonly diagnosed unexpected morbidities are cardiac related. Allowing sufficient time for evaluation avoids last-minute delays in the event that the patient requires additional evaluation (eg, stress testing or echocardiogram), medication adjustment, or management of abnormal laboratory findings.

If a consultation is requested at the "last minute," the consultant should strive to fulfill their obligation to the patient and referring physician under the circumstances. It is appropriate to use these experiences as "teachable moments" for the referring service and to evaluate system issues that contribute to suboptimal timing.

IMMEDIATE PERIOPERATIVE PERIOD

The surgeon and anesthesiologist comanage patients in the recovery room. Consultation with other services in this setting is unusual. When it occurs, the consultant should be familiar with the normal range of physiologic changes in the recovery period when making their evaluations. More commonly, the consultant is requested de novo, or for follow-up after a preoperative consultation, after the patient returns to the ward or intensive care unit.

A multimodal fast-track surgical care model to promote healing, earlier discharge and return to function, and fewer complications is being advocated.[20,21] This approach requires carefully coordinated team-based care involving surgeons, anesthesiologists, nurses, and other clinicians. Consultants should be aware of this model and facilitate its use as indicated by the clinical situation. Most major postoperative complications occur in the first 72 hours; therefore, the consultant should be available to assist during this interval, and longer if their expertise is indicated in the management of subsequent complications.[22] Further, the primary physician has an obligation to inform the consultant of any subsequent developments that may be relevant to the consultant's expertise.[23,24] Increasingly, surgeons are engaging internists or others to assist or provide perioperative medical care while they focus on surgical management, so such engagement will likely be more common in the future.

POSTOPERATIVE CARE

Increasingly, models of comanagement between surgeons and various medical specialists, including anesthesiologists, have been developed to enable more expedient and skilled medical care to be provided on the wards and to enable surgeons to concentrate their efforts on busier operative workloads. In one study, the frequency of comanagement by medicine-trained physicians for patients undergoing 15 common inpatient operations increased 11.4% annually from 2001 to 2006.[25] Proposed models of comanagement have emphasized more efficient and cost-effective preoperative testing, shorter lengths of stay, and the potential for improved medical outcomes (all these are consistent with the fast-track approach described earlier). To date, studies of comanagement have not clearly demonstrated statistical benefits in outcomes beyond minor medical improvements such as decreased urinary tract infections and electrolyte abnormalities and improved staff satisfaction. Separate studies showed varying results in terms of outcomes such as cost of care, length of stay, time to surgery, and major medical complications.[26-29]

Another role that is increasingly appropriate for consultants involves the need for effective communication at the time of patient transition out of the hospital. Literature focused on effective "handoff of care" and the medical errors occurring at the time of patient transition to home or to rehabilitation settings has shown the need for greater attention to this area.[30] Traditionally, consultants have not always played a major role in this area, but their skills and experience suggest they could be valuable contributors, and the opportunity is consistent with their commitment to strive for the patient's best interests. They should be aware of the service they can provide for the patient by ensuring that issues related to their area of expertise are well communicated to the health care provider who will be responsible for the patient after discharge from the hospital. Checklists and "readback" are effective strategies to enhance transfer of information.[30]

Rapid response systems or rapid response teams have also developed as a strategy for early identification of hospitalized patients with potentially unstable or deteriorating conditions. Depending on the medical center, these systems may or may not involve physicians on the team of emergency providers. If present on this team, internists (often hospitalists), intensivists, or anesthesiologists may practice in either a consultative or comanagement role. Literature to date remains inconsistent regarding the statistical benefits of these systems.[31-34]

FACTORS ASSOCIATED WITH EFFECTIVENESS OF CONSULTATIONS

Consultations can be useful in diagnosis, management of existing conditions, triage to a new service, and in delaying or even cancelling surgery on occasion.[5-7,35] Yet half of all recommendations are ignored.[15] This could reflect lack of relevance of the consultant's comments, failure to communicate reasoning or urgency, or a decision to ignore relevant information.

Communication is essential if a consultation is to be relevant to the requester. The clinical question must be clearly stated and understood. This is achieved by direct and precise communication between requester and provider, both written and orally (**Table 8-2**).[36]

Fewer than 6 recommendations should be made if possible. Data show that compliance decreases with increasing numbers of recommendations.[37,38] This is true regardless of the severity or complexity of the patient's medical condition. Therefore, recommendations should be carefully selected and prioritized. Annotating recommendations as "crucial" may help focus the requesting service on highly important items requiring immediate attention and improve compliance.[36] Recommendations should be written concisely and also communicated to the requesting service directly so that any understanding can be clarified. It is wise to avoid insulting, unhelpful, or redundant advice (eg, avoid hypoxia).

Alternatively, recommendations can be prioritized as preoperative and postoperative courses of action. For example, a patient's medical condition may require many interventions, but only a few may be necessary to prepare a patient for surgery and anesthesia[22]; the remainder can be implemented postoperatively. This information, too, must be clearly stated both in writing and verbally. The presence of the consultant after surgery is important to facilitate the implementation of postoperative recommendations.

Recommendations should be specific and concise. For example, when recommending a drug regimen, the drug name, dose, schedule, duration of therapy, and therapeutic goals should be clearly stated. This precision facilitates compliance and reduces errors in interpretation.[39] Providing reasons for further testing is always helpful and educational to the consultee and others. Continued presence and follow-up by the consultant with visits noted in the medical record and ongoing communication with the requesting service to reiterate recommendations also improves compliance. Nonurgent recommendations that can be pursued as an outpatient should be communicated clearly.

TABLE 8-2 Factors Associated With Compliance With Consultant's Recommendations

- Direct contact between consultant and primary physician[36]
- Continued follow-up of patients[15,38,40]
- Limited number of recommendations[37,38]
- Identification of high-priority recommendations[37]
- Specification of drug dosage, route, and duration[39]

TABLE 8-3 Ten Commandments for Effective Consultations

1. Determine the question
2. Establish urgency
3. Look for yourself
4. Be as brief as appropriate
5. Be specific
6. Provide contingency plans
7. Honor thy turf
8. Teach . . . with tact
9. Talk is cheap . . . and effective
10. Follow up

Goldman L, Lee T, Rudd P. Ten commandments for effective consultations. *Arch Intern Med.* 1983;143:1753.

Many of these principles of consultation are summarized well in Goldman and Lee's Ten Commandments for Effective Consultations (**Table 8-3**).[41] The issue of contingency plans is controversial, as stated by Caplan et al.[42] In general, contingency plans should not be provided in lieu of timely reevaluation of the patient and are best used for non-urgent issues or to clarify what foreseeable scenarios should prompt notification of the consultant.

MEDICOLEGAL ISSUES

Primary providers should seek consultation when a clinical problem is outside their scope of practice or exceeds their level of expertise.[23] Consultants should be used to enhance care, not be used defensively to "cover one's back." The requesting provider should inform the patient why the consultation is requested because the patient must give consent to see the consultant.[24] It is the job of the consultant from a medicolegal perspective to appropriately document his or her independent assessment of the patient's condition and to review and interpret all data independently (ie, laboratory results, diagnostic studies) appropriate to their medical specialty. The consultant should confirm, ideally verbally, that the primary physician receives his or her written assessment and recommendations, comprehends the reason for these recommendations, and has the opportunity to ask questions. In doing so, effectiveness of communication between providers is enhanced, but it is also important from a legal perspective that a consultant ensures that his or her input is understood. The primary physician in a traditional model has ultimate responsibility for medical decision making, which should be made clear to patients when a consultant is involved. This becomes more complicated when "consult and treat" is the model requested or in comanagement scenarios where dual responsibility is involved. Both primary physicians and consultants should avoid informal "curbside consultations" as a general rule, for they can be inadequate medically and convoluted legally.[43] When in doubt, consultants should see the patient formally if he or she feels a complex question is being asked.[44]

Consultants and primary physicians may both be responsible for the adequate and accurate "handoff" of information and plan of care when patients transition between levels of care, such as from the intensive care unit to ward or from hospital to rehabilitation or home.[45]

SUMMARY

The work of the consultant has increased due to shorter planned inpatient treatment, greater numbers of sicker patients able to benefit from surgery and other invasive procedures, and increased use of physician extenders whose supervising service lacks the necessary medical expertise to manage various and complex medical problems. The role of the consultant in many settings has evolved from the traditional information-only model to one of more engagement in care of the patient and education of the consultee.

All parties should ensure effective verbal and written communication. Primary providers should know when consultations are needed and be precise in their clinical requests. Consultants should respond in a timely manner with brief, clear, and focused recommendations. The doctor–patient relationship that exists with the requesting provider should be respected. The consultant should remain engaged throughout the perioperative period and be available for assistance with postoperative care. When comanagement is requested, it is essential that everyone's role be clearly understood, including by the patient. Consultants should facilitate the use of guidelines and consensus statements when recommending therapy but, where necessary, deviate from existing guidelines based on new evidence.[46,47]

KEY REFERENCES

- Emanuel LL, Richter J. The consultant and the patient-physician relationship: a trilateral deliberative model. *Arch Intern Med.* 1994;154:1785.
- Fischer SP. Development and effectiveness of an anesthesia preoperative evaluation clinic in a teaching hospital. *Anesthesiology.* 1996;85:196-206.
- Goldman L, Lee T, Rudd P. Ten commandments for effective consultations. *Arch Intern Med.* 1983;143:1753.
- Kleinman B, Czinn E, Shah K, et al. The value to the anesthesia-surgery care team of the preoperative cardiac consultation. *J Cardiothoracic Anesth.* 1989;3:682.
- Lubarsky D, Candiotti K. Giving anesthesiologists what they want: how to write a useful preoperative consult. *Cleve Clin J Med.* 2009;76:S32-S36.

REFERENCES

Complete references available on DVD and online version at www.LongneckerAnesthesiology.com

CHAPTER 9 Evaluation of the Patient With Cardiovascular Disease

Ronald P. Olson
Ron Rawlings

KEY POINTS

1. Perioperative ischemia results from an imbalance of oxygen supply and demand of the myocardium during perioperative stress, rupture of a vulnerable plaque with subsequent thrombosis of a coronary artery, endothelial dysfunction, or some combination of all of these.
2. The history and physical examination, along with limited indicated tests, are often adequate to determine the general perioperative risk of a patient.
3. Preoperative cardiac testing is usually not needed in patients who have good functional status or are undergoing low-risk procedures. Further testing is unlikely to change management, and these patients may proceed directly to surgery.
4. Many interventions, such as control of diabetes, hypertension, stable coronary artery disease, congestive heart failure, and endothelial function, can be well within the scope of an anesthesiologist's skill set. If anesthesiologists wish to consider themselves perioperative clinicians, they must be active in these well-established aspects of medicine.
5. The attending anesthesiologist of a specific patient, not a consultant, is in the best position to balance the risks and determine the best anesthesia techniques for that case. Other clinicians and consultants are often needed to ensure optimization, although increasingly, the anesthesia team can do at least some of this.

INTRODUCTION

Preoperative evaluation continues to change. In the distant past, the attending anesthesiologist would interview the hospitalized patient and family a day or two before surgery. All resources of the medical systems were mobilized to ensure that all aspects of the patient's health were assessed and treated. Surgery was delayed until any cardiac condition was fully addressed.

Practice changed; it then became common for any potentially complex patient to see a consultant to get "clearance" so surgery could proceed with some nebulous guarantee of acceptable risk, or surgery would be cancelled until such clearance could be provided.

Current practice includes surgery and anesthesia techniques that are numerous and changing. Anesthesiologists are able, if needed, to shepherd high-risk patients through high-risk surgery. Consideration is given to striking a balance between risks at either end of a spectrum, weighing the risk of postponing surgery versus proceeding. At one end, postponing surgery for investigations may be higher than the risk of proceeding. At the other end of the spectrum, some surgical procedures are unlikely to cause more stress than the activities of daily living. In essence, the paradigm of preoperative assessment is shifting from predicting risk to actively managing risk.[1] The issue is less whether to cancel surgery and more whether indicated cardiac tests and management need to be done preoperatively under the supervision of the perioperative physician or postoperatively in a more elective fashion by primary care clinicians.

As medical therapy of cardiovascular disease improves, routine care is sometimes as effective as interventional therapy in reducing cardiac morbidity and mortality.[2] This chapter reviews current understanding of the physiology of perioperative ischemia, followed by examination of how an individual patient's perioperative risk can be assessed. More importantly, it then discusses when and how more detailed risk management should be undertaken.

This chapter focuses on the patient presenting for noncardiac surgery. Many of the studies in this area have been done on patients having vascular or cardiac surgery, but as much as possible, evidence on other surgical populations is presented. Although it will focus on perioperative cardiac complications (PCCs), it is important to remember that the same process is occurring in the rest of the cardiovascular system[3] as well as in other organs such as the brain and kidneys.

FREQUENCY OF PERIOPERATIVE CARDIAC COMPLICATIONS

Gastrointestinal, pulmonary, renal, infectious, wound, and pain control complications are not insignificant in the surgical patient.[4] Approximately 50% of patients with cardiac disease develop other complications perioperatively,[5] but it is cardiovascular complications that garner the most concern. In patients with cardiovascular disease, known or unknown, perioperative cardiac complications occur at a higher rate. An analysis of the 6 studies assessing the incidence of major cardiac complications in patients with some risk factor for coronary artery disease (CAD) revealed an overall rate of 3.9%.[6] Patients with peripheral vascular disease (PVD) are a well-studied group because they are easily identifiable and have a high complication rate. Even vascular patients with no risk factors for CAD have a 5% incidence of PCC.[7] The Coronary Artery Revascularization Prophylaxis (CARP) trial found a PCC rate of 15.6% in vascular patients[8] and a 27% rate in vascular patients with known CAD.[9] Risk of perioperative complications in patients with no evidence of cardiac disease is very low (<1%).[10,11] An analysis of 188, 110 joint-replacement surgeries showed the excess mortality resulting from complications to be only 0.12%.[12]

PREOPERATIVE ASSESSMENT OF CARDIOVASCULAR DISEASES

The main reason for performing preoperative assessments is ultimately to get the surgery done. But additionally, in a sometimes fragmented health care system, the preoperative encounter may be one of the few times a careful assessment of a patient's cardiac status will occur. Following a comprehensive assessment, conditions such as atherosclerotic disease, hypertension, congestive heart failure (CHF), chronic obstructive pulmonary disease (COPD), asthma, and diabetes may be identified and treated so the patient's health will be improved for years to come. Some medications, such as antihypertensives, β-blockers (BBs), statins, and hypoglycemics, can be easily initiated with instructions for follow-up with primary care. Anesthesiologists have traditionally been reluctant to prescribe medications whose effects last past the immediate encounter. But primary care clinicians routinely and safely initiate drug therapy with follow-up done weekly or monthly at best. Because the limitations to successful treatment are usually patient access and compliance, these clinicians will enthusiastically welcome any assistance in drug therapy initiation, and willingly assume follow-up. The risk of initiating recommended medications is minimal, manageable, and a necessary part of ethical medical care. To miss these opportunities to forward improvement in the patient's health would be disappointing (**Table 9-1**).

DANGERS OF TESTING IN LOW-RISK POPULATIONS

In contrast, routine screening investigations of asymptomatic patients should not be undertaken unless a plan for follow-up is in place. Testing a low-prevalence population inevitably produces mild abnormalities that are likely to be either false positives or true positives that have little bearing on the perioperative period. If surgery is delayed even to follow up on just the true positives, the inconvenience and risks of delayed surgery may outweigh the minimal benefits of follow-up. The likelihood of using this data to modify plans is also small.[13] The perioperative period is currently too short and isolated for disease screening. Screening is better done by primary care, where follow-up is conducted over time in the context of addressing overall health and where the few true positives will be sifted out from the many false positives. Case finding—the investigation not of asymptomatic patients but of those who have manifested some indication of possible disease—is sometimes appropriate perioperatively.

Each institution must balance how much intervention can be done without exposing the patient and institution to the dangers of providing inadequate follow-up. Generally, what can be done easily and safely should be done; other investigations or interventions that do not have a direct impact on the perioperative period should be deferred to primary care. Ideally, the perioperative team and the primary care practitioners should share information and resources.

WHO SHOULD DO THE PREOPERATIVE ASSESSMENT?

As mentioned previously, one method of preoperative assessment is to refer any patient with potential cardiac risk to the cardiology or internal medicine service and await "clearance" for surgery by that specialist. Unfortunately, cardiologists may not be in the best position to judge the risk of surgery, the risk of not proceeding with surgery, the risks of various anesthesia techniques, and the skills of a specific anesthesiologist. Thus it is inappropriate for a cardiologist or any other clinician to "clear" the patient for surgery. It is sometimes very important to get a consultant's advice on how to optimize a patient for surgery and an opinion on whether the risk/benefit of surgery is favorable, but the decision on whether a specific patient can undergo a specific procedure with the given resources can only be done by the anesthesiologist responsible for that patient on the day of surgery. Again, this chapter clarifies what information the anesthesiologist needs to make that final decision and to formulate the anesthesia plan. As a side note, many preoperative clinics use nurse practitioners or physician assistants. If these clinicians are educated and supported by anesthesiologists and consultants knowledgeable in anesthesia and surgical issues, they do a comprehensive and meticulous job of focusing on critical issues. However, because the anesthesiologist is the main consumer of the preoperative assessment, it behooves every anesthesiology department to remain intimately involved in the preoperative assessment process.

PHYSIOLOGY OF PERIOPERATIVE CARDIAC ISCHEMIA

Patients with cardiac disease are at increased risk for perioperative morbidity and mortality. The overall rate of perioperative myocardial infarction (MI) in these patients is approximately 5%.[6]

Several cardiac complications can occur perioperatively (**Table 9-2**). Because most of these are either the cause or the result of ischemia,[13] all of which may ultimately lead to infarction, the emphasis in this chapter is on the causes of ischemia.[14]

The etiology of perioperative ischemia is clearly multifactorial and defies simple classification, but understanding the theories on the physiology helps us understand the optimal ways to minimize it.[15] As the theory changes, so does the treatment. Or as different treatments are proven superior, our theories must change. The physiology of ischemia is another area of perioperative medicine that is entering the third swing of the pendulum, back to one of caution.

SUPPLY-DEMAND MISMATCH

Ischemia traditionally was believed to be due to a supply-demand mechanism at a critical stenosis. Infarction from this source probably occurs only after several hours of ischemia.[16] Reduction in the mismatch by reducing heart rate and/or increasing oxygen supply may relieve the ischemia, or a thrombus may form and cause complete coronary occlusion. In that case, thrombolytics, coronary artery bypass grafting (CABG), or percutaneous transluminal coronary angioplasty (PTCA) with stenting is indicated. On this basis, the preoperative treatment of critical stenosis made sense, and early studies such as the Coronary Artery Surgery Study in 1986 showed this was the case.[17] Until recently, surgical intervention appeared superior to medical therapy alone.[18]

TABLE 9-1 Benefits of Preoperative Assessment
Determine if the risk of proceeding to surgery is acceptable
Identify conditions that may be improved
Coordinate optimization
Assist anesthesiologist in reducing and balancing risks
Assist surgeon in choosing procedure with best risk-to-benefit balance
Identify those cases that are inappropriate for ambulatory surgical sites
Assist in informed consent by patient

TABLE 9-2 Perioperative Cardiac Complications
Sudden death
Myocardial infarction
Myocardial ischemia
Systolic heart failure
Diastolic heart failure
Arrhythmias

THROMBOSIS FROM ENDOTHELIAL DYSFUNCTION

Over the last few decades, there has been increasing appreciation of another mechanism of ischemia: erosion and rupture of unstable endothelial plaques, with resultant abrupt occlusion. These episodes result in ST depression as demonstrated on an electrocardiogram (ECG). They may resolve spontaneously but leave the damaged areas vulnerable to further plaque rupture.[19,20] The Task Force on the Redefinition of Myocardial Infarction defines this mechanism as causing type 1 MI and the supply-demand mismatch mechanism as causing type 2 MI.[21]

In the last decade, several new studies have suggested that plaque rupture of noncritical lesions was a more common cause of ischemia, at least in the case of perioperative ischemia.[22] The study by Dawood et al of coronary artery autopsies showed evidence of plaque disruption in 55% of fatal perioperative MIs and in 40% of nonoperative MIs.[23] Ellis et al assessed the preoperative angiograms of vascular patients experiencing a postoperative MI and compared them with the findings in a matched group of nonoperative MIs; they did not find a high-grade stenosis (>70%) in any of the patients who had a PCC.[24] Cohen and Aretz studied the coronary artery autopsies of 26 cases of fatal postoperative MIs. A thrombus occurred on a stenosis of more than 50% in only 33% of cases[25] (**Fig. 9-1**).

Vasoconstriction can be considered as part of endothelial function, although plaque rupture is probably not involved. This may be a fairly common cause of cardiac ischemia, especially in women.[26]

These theories are consistent with accumulating evidence, such as that from the CARP trial,[27] in demonstrating that medical therapy is sometimes as effective as invasive treatment of critical stenosis. In the CARP study, McFalls et al randomized 510 Veterans Administration patients undergoing abdominal aortic aneurysm repair to either coronary artery revascularization before surgery or no revascularization before surgery. Percutaneous coronary intervention was performed in 59% and bypass surgery in 41%. There was no difference in MI in the first 30 days after surgery or in mortality at 2.7 years.[27] A recent post hoc analysis of the high-risk patients in that study came to the same conclusion.[8] A major criticism of this study was the exclusion from randomization of patients with greater than 50% stenosis of the left main coronary artery. But the Clinical Outcomes Utilizing Revascularization and Aggressive Drug Evaluation (COURAGE) trial, which between 1999 and 2004 randomized 2287 patients to either percutaneous coronary intervention and medical therapy or medical therapy alone, did include patients with multiple vessel disease, diabetes, and it likewise showed no difference at 4.6 years of follow-up,[28] even in advanced age patients.[29]

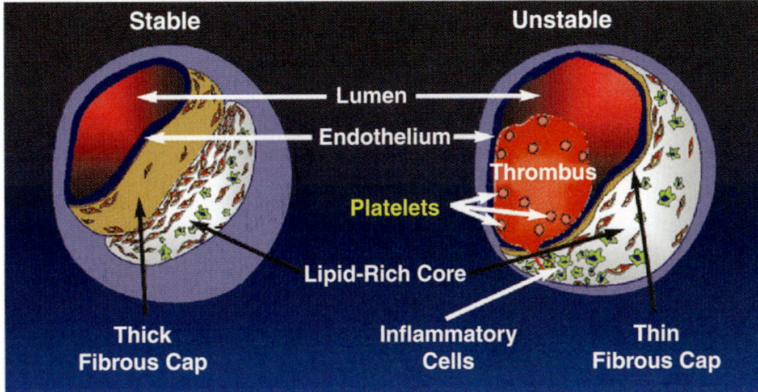

FIGURE 9-1. Characteristics of unstable and stable plaque. Although the stable plaque may be associated with significant luminal narrowing, it tends to have a thick fibrous cap, a small lipid core, and a paucity of inflammatory cells. In contrast, the unstable plaque tends to have a large lipid core and a thin fibrous cap. Inflammatory cells accumulate at the shoulder region and contribute to plaque rupture with subsequent thrombus formation. [From Fuster V, O'Rourke R, Walsh R, et al. *Hurst's The Heart.* 12th ed. New York, NY: McGraw-Hill; 2008.]

Endothelial dysfunction is a result of three broad groups of cardiovascular etiologies: hypercoagulability, inflammation, and sympathomimetic overdrive. These detrimental forces, discussed later, are controlled to some extent by endothelial protective factors (**Fig. 9-2**).

Hypercoagulability Surgery induces a prothrombotic state that may be variable and hopefully measurable.[30] If this state could be measured, it would be valuable for selecting which high-risk patients to treat with anticoagulants. Some patients are probably predisposed to hypercoagulability. The patient group with factor V Leiden is one example where it has not generally been necessary to require perioperative investigation or treatment additional to that which is standard prophylactic practice.[31]

Inflammation Atherosclerosis is largely an inflammatory process,[32] and surgery initiates further inflammatory response. Current research on the usefulness of markers such as C-reactive protein (CRP) in the prediction of perioperative MI from this source is promising.[33] This topic is discussed further later in this chapter.

Sympathetic Stimulation The obvious sympathetic response to the stress of surgery may be attenuated by neuraxial anesthesia,[34,35] clonidine,[36] or BBs.[37] Reduction in anxiety by pharmacologic and interpersonal intervention is important to reduce all three of the factors of endothelial dysfunction: hypercoagulability, inflammation, and sympathomimetic overdrive.

Protective Factors A few short episodes of ischemia may induce preconditioning that results in less damage if later ischemia occurs.[38] One mouse study suggests that the surgical incision induces protective cardiac preconditioning.[39] Nitric oxide induces endothelial stability. The anesthetic nitrous oxide does the opposite. An example of how these factors are interrelated is a study by Zafar et al of the relationship between clinical anxiety, depression, and platelet reactivity measured by optical aggregometry[40] (**Fig. 9-3**).

MULTIFACTORIAL STENOSIS

Countering the evidence that much perioperative ischemia is from noncritical stenosis, a recent ultrasound assessment of culprit lesions[20] and several recent analyses of patients presenting to an angio catheterization lab all showed that most infarcts did occur at high-grade stenosis.[41-43] Some authors still believe that type 2 supply-demand ischemia is the most common cause of perioperative MI.[22] Part of the apparent discrepancy occurs because angiography likely is not the gold standard for detecting sites of critical stenosis. Because atherosclerosis is a systemic disease in which all of the arteries are affected to some degree, but angiography compares the lumen of a segment with the lumen before and after that segment, a severe stenosis in the middle of moderate stenosis will not show up as a critical lesion (**Fig. 9-4**). There is also evidence of a "Glagov" phenomenon of vascular remodeling where the plaque may increase in size, yet the lumen remains unchanged or even enlarges slightly.[44,45] Intravascular ultrasound or cardiac magnetic resonance imaging (MRI) shows promise in more accurately assessing lumens.[46,47]

The other reality is that high-grade critical stenosis probably forms because of repeated plaque rupture. Progression of lesions probably occurs in a phasic fashion, with the perioperative period a time of potential rapid progression.[48] The study by Galal et al with transesophageal echocardiography showed that the high-grade lesions detected preoperatively are not necessarily the sites of perioperative ischemia.[49] Whether ischemia occurs because of either acute plaque rupture or preexisting coronary blockage,[20] endothelial dysfunction likely is common to both mechanisms. Both identifiable high-grade stenoses and numerous smaller vulnerable plaques are amenable to systemic treatment of this endothelial dysfunction as well as interventional procedures where appropriate.[50] BB therapy addresses both mechanisms: from reduced demand and probably more importantly from pleotropic benefits on the endothelium. As medical treatment improves, that treatment is becoming a viable option for treating even high-grade stenosis. This has fairly revolutionary implications in that if medical optimization can be safely and easily applied to any patient at risk, then detailed cardiac

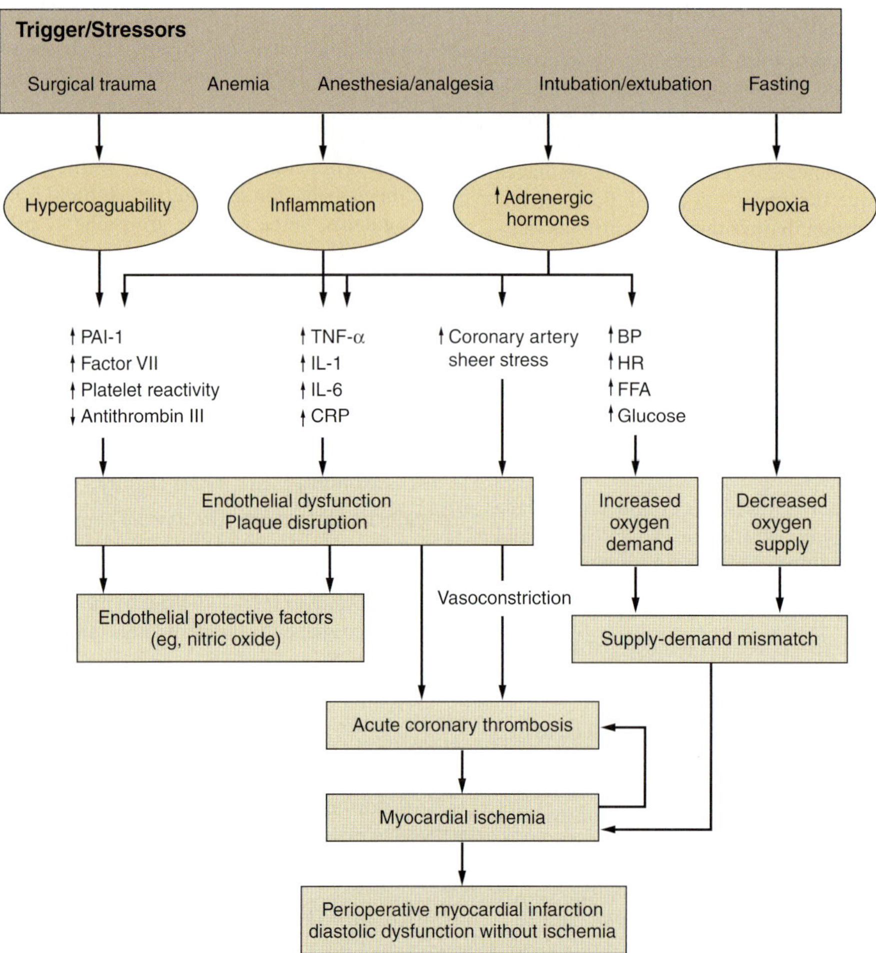

FIGURE 9-2. Etiology of perioperative myocardial infarction. BP, blood pressure; CRP, C-reactive protein; FFA, free fatty acids; HR, heart rate; IL, interleukin; PAI-1, plasma activator inhibitor-1; TNF, tumor necrosis factor. [Adapted from Devereaux PJ, Goldman L, Cook D, et al. Perioperative cardiac events in patients undergoing noncardiac surgery: a review of the magnitude of the problem, the pathophysiology of the events and methods to estimate and communicate risk. *CMAJ*. 2005;173:627-634. Reprinted with permission of the publisher. Copyright 2000, CMA Media Inc.]

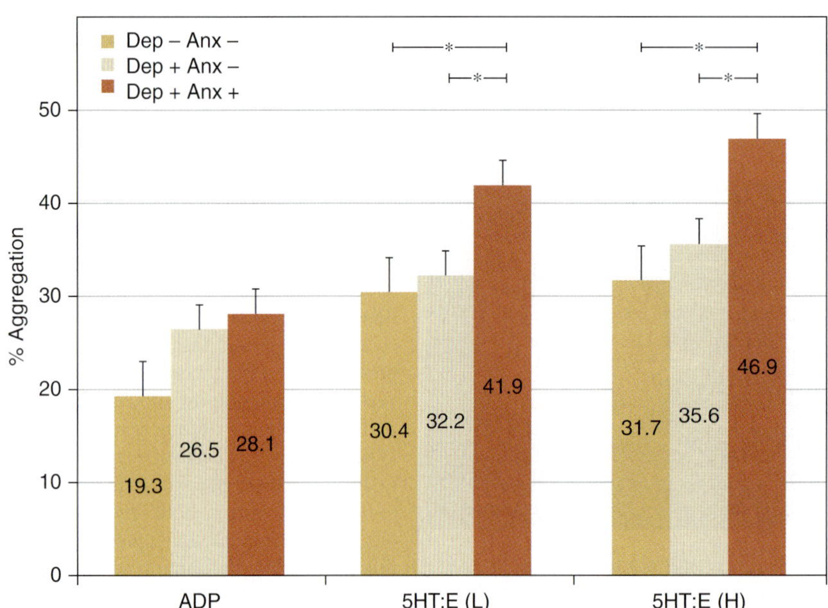

FIGURE 9-3. Platelet aggregation and depression and anxiety. Platelet aggregation result (estimated means plus standard error) in stable CAD patients. Dep–Anx–, nondepressed and nonanxious; Dep+ Anx–, depressed only; Dep+ Anx+, depressed and anxious. ADP, adenosine diphosphate; 5HT:E (L), serotonin with epinephrine; 5HT:E (H), serotonin with epinephrine. [From Zafar M, Paz-Yepes M, Shimbo D, et al. Anxiety is a better predictor of platelet reactivity in coronary artery disease patients than depression. *Eur Heart J.* 2010;31:1573-1582.]

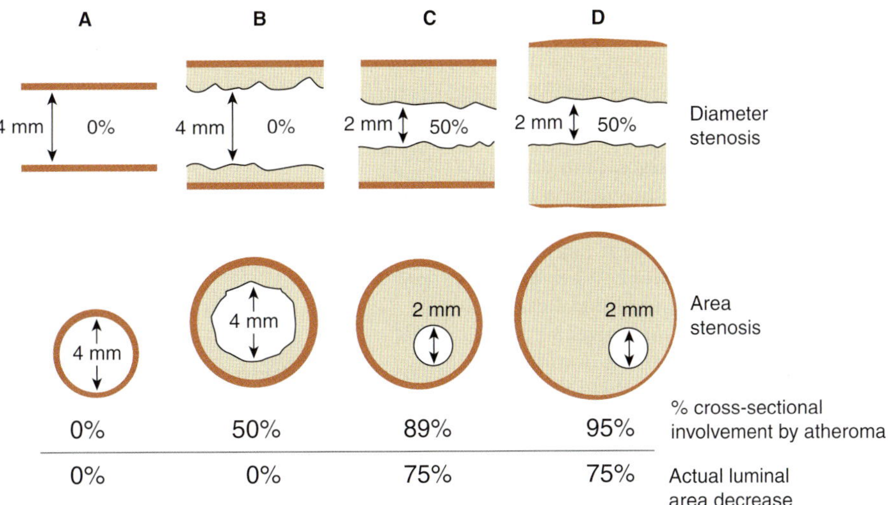

FIGURE 9-4. Angiographic versus pathologic views of stenosis. **Top row:** angiographic views; **bottom row:** pathologic views. **Column A:** normal artery; **column B:** artery with "moderate" atherosclerosis. Because of remodeling, angiography shows a normal lumen with enlargement of the vessel. A pathologic view of the same artery would see the same lumen, but 50% of the cross-sectional area would be occupied by plaque. **Column C:** more involved artery. Angiography shows that the lumen is 50% less in diameter than the adjacent "normal" (**B**) segment. Pathology shows the 2-mm lumen but a larger plaque and measures the stenosis as an 89% narrowing. **Column D:** same situation but with even more remodeling present. Angiography shows a 50% diameter narrowing, even though the plaque is much larger than in column C, and still concludes that this is not severe disease. Because of the greater enlargement of the artery, the pathology now shows the stenosis as a 95% cross-sectional narrowing, even though the lumen size is actually the same as in column C. [Reproduced with permission from Fishbein MC, Siegel RJ. How big are coronary atherosclerotic plaques that rupture? *Circulation*. 1996;94(10):2662-2666.]

investigations or invasive therapies are probably unnecessary, at least in the short term.

POSTOPERATIVE ISCHEMIA

Advances in anesthesia have meant that the intraoperative period is a controlled and safe period. Most ischemia occurs in the immediate postoperative period during emergence from anesthesia, when catecholamines are surging,[51] rather than during anesthesia. Landesberg et al showed that most ischemic events, and most ischemic events that result in infarction, occur immediately postoperatively (**Fig. 9-5**).[52] Several studies have shown that postoperative MIs occur mostly in the first few days after an operation (**Fig. 9-6**), and are often asymptomatic.[3,51,53,54]

Prolonged ischemia is more likely to result in infarct than a shorter duration of ischemia. When the endothelium is damaged, acetylcholine causes muscarinic receptor–mediated vasoconstriction instead of endothelium-dependent vasodilatation.[55] Thus prolonged ischemia may be the cause, as well as the result, of vasoconstriction and subsequent thrombus formation.[22]

Mangano et al showed that the risk from surgery may extend up to 2 years beyond the immediate perioperative period.[56] Although much emphasis is placed on ischemia, postoperative stress may also result in patients reaching their anaerobic threshold. Once this threshold is met, diastolic dysfunction develops, possibly causing later morbidity, even if no ischemia occurs.[57] Cardiac damage is a continuum, not a dichotomy of infarction or no infarction.[58] Even asymptomatic ischemia may lead to long-term complications.[13] Asymptomatic plaque rupture may heal but may leave the plaque more vulnerable to subsequent rupture.[19,20]

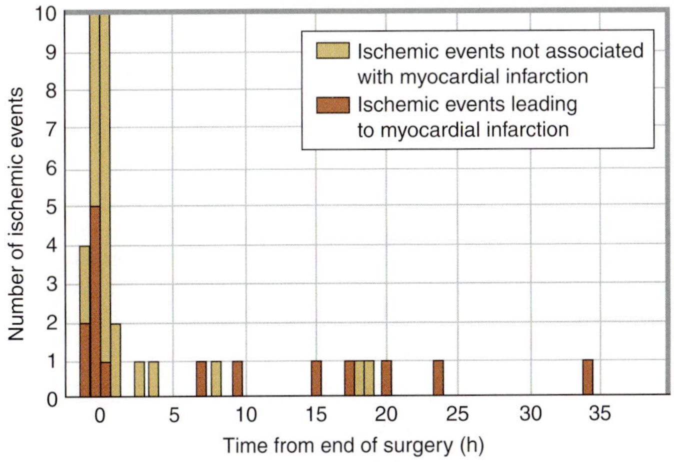

FIGURE 9-5. Timing of postoperative ischemia. The time of onset of longest ischemia relative to the end of surgery (T = 0). *Orange bars* represent the onset time of longest ischemic events of all patients who had ischemia but no myocardial infarction; *blue bars* represent the onset time of longest ischemic events that culminated in myocardial infarction. [Reprinted from Landesberg G, Mosseri M, Zahger D, et al. Myocardial infarction after vascular surgery: the role of prolonged stress-induced, ST depression-type ischemia. *J Am Coll Cardiol*. 2001;37(7):1839-1845, with permission from American College of Cardiology Foundation.]

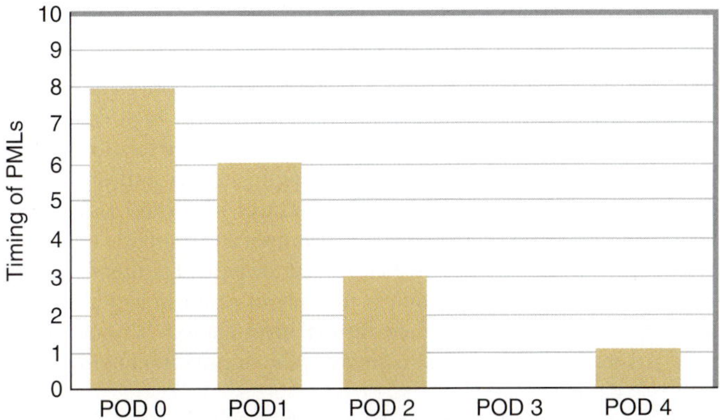

FIGURE 9-6. Timing of postoperative myocardial infarctions (PMLs). [Reproduced with permission from Badner NH, Knill RL, Brown JE, Novick TV, Gelb AW. Myocardial infarction after noncardiac surgery. *Anesthesiology*. 1998;88(3):572-578.]

With these mechanisms in mind, we proceed to an analysis of risk for these events.

GENERAL ASSESSMENT OF PERIOPERATIVE RISK

Preoperative assessment should occur in two stages: first, through a clinical assessment that defines general risk and/or determines that more detailed assessment will be useful. Only after this stage should more selective tests be ordered. The initial assessment can usually be conducted using questions, hands, and a stethoscope. When previous medical records are added, this basic history and physical examination often provide all the information needed for a given anesthesia plan. If further testing will not result in interventions or a change of anesthesia plan, it should at least be deferred to the postoperative period.

This section reviews the initial stage of general overall assessment of factors that affect perioperative risk. The information resulting from this assessment will determine if the next level of investigations are indicated. Risk indices have been a key part of this assessment, and following is a review of the common ones. A discussion of the latest American College of Cardiology/American Heart Association (ACC/AHA) guidelines is followed here by a more detailed review of individual patient risk factors. Particulars of more intensive investigations that may be indicated are covered in the following section, "Rationale for Selective Testing."

COMPARISON OF RISK INDICES

Beginning with Lee Goldman in 1977,[308] a number of collections of risk factors have been proposed to determine which patients are at high risk perioperatively and thus require detailed cardiac investigations. The simple and rather vague American Society of Anesthesiologists (ASA) Physical Classification system may predict risk almost as well as more complex indexes.[59] The most commonly used algorithm for determining the need for assessment of risk for cardiovascular disease is the one created by the ACC/AHA.[72] It is based largely on what is the best studied and validated index for use in predicting PCC: the Revised Cardiac Risk Index proposed and validated by Lee et al.[10,60,61] Risk indices are cost-effective in vascular surgery.[62,63] They are derived from populations and most appropriately applied to them.[58] Although they do not perform well in defining exact risks in individuals, they can help place a patient in a general risk category.[64] A study by Paul et al of four risk factors—history of diabetes, prior angina, previous MI, and history of congestive heart failure (CHF)—in 878 vascular surgery patients showed a good correlation with coronary angiography[65] (**Fig. 9-7**).

Most indices divide patients into one of three risk groups: high, moderate, or low. A patient who has three or more risk factors on the Revised Cardiac Risk Index has a risk for postoperative MI of 11.4%; a patient with no risk factors has a risk of 0.3%.[10] Patients scheduled for vascular surgery with no other cardiac risk factors have a PCC rate of 1.6% versus 23.4% in those with 3 or more risk factors.[8]

High Risk for Perioperative Cardiac Complications Those patients with a greater than 5% risk of developing PCC are termed high risk. These patients occasionally warrant postponement of surgery to allow assessment of the risk-benefit ratio of proceeding to surgery and/or to allow optimization or special perioperative measures to control risk. In the past, it was believed that these patients required an automatic referral to cardiology. However, as described earlier, if the patient is already known to be optimized or investigation is unlikely to result in any change in perioperative management, then further investigation is unnecessary. Standard medical therapy increasingly is the optimal therapy even for high-risk patients.

Moderate or Indeterminate Risk for Perioperative Cardiac Complications This group of patients is not clearly either high risk or low risk, and these are the patients who often warrant further risk analysis. Increasingly, however, if these patients are stable, they may proceed to surgery with relatively simple risk reduction. Even if they turn out to be high-risk patients, the management may be no different, and therefore there is no need to change perioperative management.

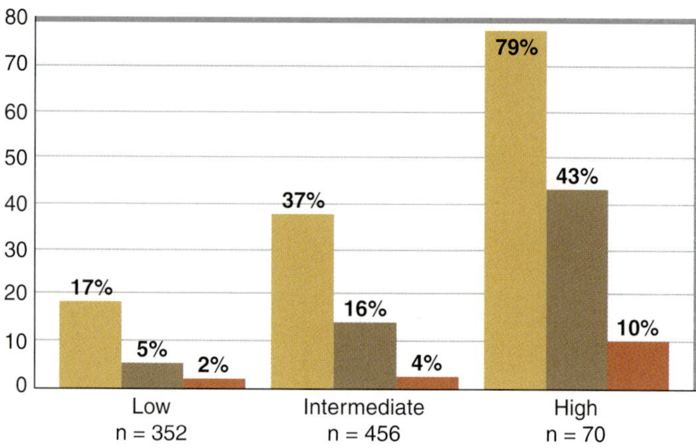

FIGURE 9-7. Concordance of clinical risk score and severity of coronary angiography. Bars represent proportions of patients with severe multivessel disease (*orange*), critical three-vessel and/or left main disease (*green*), and left main stenosis ≥70% (*blue*) within each clinical risk group. [Reproduced with permission from Paul SD, Eagle KA, Kuntz KM, Young JR, Hertzer NR. Concordance of preoperative clinical risk with angiographic severity of coronary artery disease in patients undergoing vascular surgery. *Circulation.* 1996;94(7):1561-1566.]

Low Risk for Perioperative Cardiac Complications These low-risk patients rarely require preoperative testing.[67,68] Tests that might be indicated in routine primary care should not be ordered unless follow-up of results can be arranged. However, the preoperative assessment may be one of the few opportunities in a fragmented health care system to initiate or adjust needed medical care. Each institution must determine the optimal amount of involvement by the perioperative staff in the patient's overall health care. **Table 9-3** compares the contents of the most common risk indices.

RATIONALE FOR SELECTIVE TESTING

Selective testing is cost-effective and safe[62]; indeed, it is statistically and medically inappropriate to test low-risk populations.[69] The Bayesian theorem describes how testing a group with a low prevalence of a given condition results in too many false positives for the information to be useful. The purpose of the clinical assessment is to select patients who have a roughly 5% or greater likelihood of developing PCCs[70] and in whom further testing will yield a useful change of pretest to posttest probabilities. Applying tests to a lower prevalence group is ineffective. For example, the recent Detection of Ischemia in Asymptomatic Diabetics (DIAD) study showed that even routine investigation of diabetics for cardiac disease using myocardial perfusion testing does not result in any significant reduction in morbidity and mortality if it is applied to asymptomatic diabetics.[71] Even angiography is imprecise in a low-risk population.[65] The application of this principle to cardiac testing is discussed later in this chapter.

AMERICAN COLLEGE OF CARDIOLOGY/AMERICAN HEART ASSOCIATION GUIDELINES

The clinical history and examination will uncover any of several risk factors for PCC, which each need to be assessed in a general fashion. However, more detailed investigation and management is not always needed perioperatively. This decision to investigate further is multifactorial, and the ACC/AHA algorithm, based on the Revised Cardiac Risk Index,[10] is a useful aid to determine if such detailed investigation and management are indicated (**Fig. 9-8**). This aid should be used after a standard clinical examination has identified general issues of concern. The first four steps of the algorithm provide for potential

TABLE 9-3 Comparison of Risk Indices

Risk Factor	Cardiac Risk Index Goldman 1977[308]	Points	Modified Cardiac Risk Index Detsky 1986[309]	Points	Revised Cardiac Risk Index Lee 1999[10]	Boersma 2001[104]	ACC/AHA 2007[72]	Chassot 2002[82]	Kertai 2005[105, a]	Points
Ischemic heart disease	MI <6 mo ago	10	MI <6 mo	10	History of MI, or Q waves	Current or prior angina, prior MI	Previous MI by history or Q waves on ECG	Prior MI >6 wk and <3 mo	Prior MI, prior or current angina	13
			MI >6 mo	5	History of + treadmill test		Angina CCS I or II	Angina CCS I or II		
			CCS angina class III; CCS angina class IV	10 20	Use of NTG, current angina			Post CABG/PTCA >6 wk and <3 mo, or >6 y		
			Unstable angina <6 mo	10						
CHF		11	Pulmonary edema <1 wk	10	CHF or History of	History of CHF	Compensated or prior HF	Compensated or prior, EF <0.35	CHF	14
			Pulmonary edema ever	5						
CVD					History of TIA or stroke	History of CVA			History of CVA	10
Arrhythmias	Other than sinus or premature atrial contractions on last preoperative ECG, >5 premature ventricular contractions/min	7	Other than sinus or premature atrial contractions on last pre-operative ECG, >5 premature ventricular contractions/min	5				Ventricular	CHF	
High-risk surgery	Intraperitoneal, Intrathoracic, aortic	3			Vascular, thoracic, abdominal, orthopedic				AAA rupture	43
									Thoracoabdominal	26
									Abdominal aortic	26
									Infrainguinal	15
	Emergency	4	Emergency	10						
Diabetes					Requiring insulin[b]		Diabetes mellitus	Diabetes mellitus		
Renal insufficiency					Creatinine >2 mg/dL[b]		Renal insufficiency		Renal dysfunction	16
Age	>70 y	5	>70 y	5		>70 y		Physiologic >70 y		
Valvular disease	Aortic stenosis	3	Aortic stenosis	20						

(*Continued*)

TABLE 9-3 Comparison of Risk Indices (*Continued*)

Risk Factor	Cardiac Risk Index Goldman 1977[308]	Points	Modified Cardiac Risk Index Detsky 1986[309]	Points	Revised Cardiac Risk Index Lee 1999[10]	Boersma 2001[104]	ACC/AHA 2007[72]	Chassot 2002[82]	Kertai 2005[105, a]	Points
Medical status	Po_2 <60 mm Hg; Pco_2 >50 mm Hg; K <3.0 mmol/L; HCO_3 <20 mmol/L; BUN >50 mg/dL (18 mmol/L); creatinine >3.0 mg/dL (260 μmol/L); abnormal AST; chronic liver disease; bedridden	3	Po_2 <60 mm Hg; Pco_2 >50 mm Hg; K <3.0 mmol/L; HCO_3 <20 mmol/L; BUN >50 mg/dL (18 mmol/L); creatinine >3.0 mg/dl (260 μmol/L); abnormal AST; chronic liver disease; bedridden	5						
Other									Hypertension	7
									COPD	7
									β-Blocker use	−15
									Statin use	−10

[a]Vascular surgery, predictors of all-cause mortality.

[b]Although trending to association, it was not a statistically significant independent predictor.

AAA, abdominal aortic aneurysm; ACC/AHA, American College of Cardiologists/American Heart Association; AST, aspartate aminotransferase; BUN, blood urea nitrogen; CABG, coronary artery bypass grafting; CCS, Canadian Cardiovascular Society; CHF, congestive heart failure; COPD, chronic obstructive pulmonary disease; CVA, cardiovascular accident; CVD, cardiovascular disease; ECG, electrocardiogram; EF, ejection fraction; HCO_3, bicarbonate; HF, heart failure; MI, myocardial infarction; NTG, nitroglycerin; Pco_2, partial pressure of carbon dioxide; Po_2, partial pressure of oxygen; PTCA, percutaneous transluminal coronary angioplasty; TIA, transient ischemic attack.

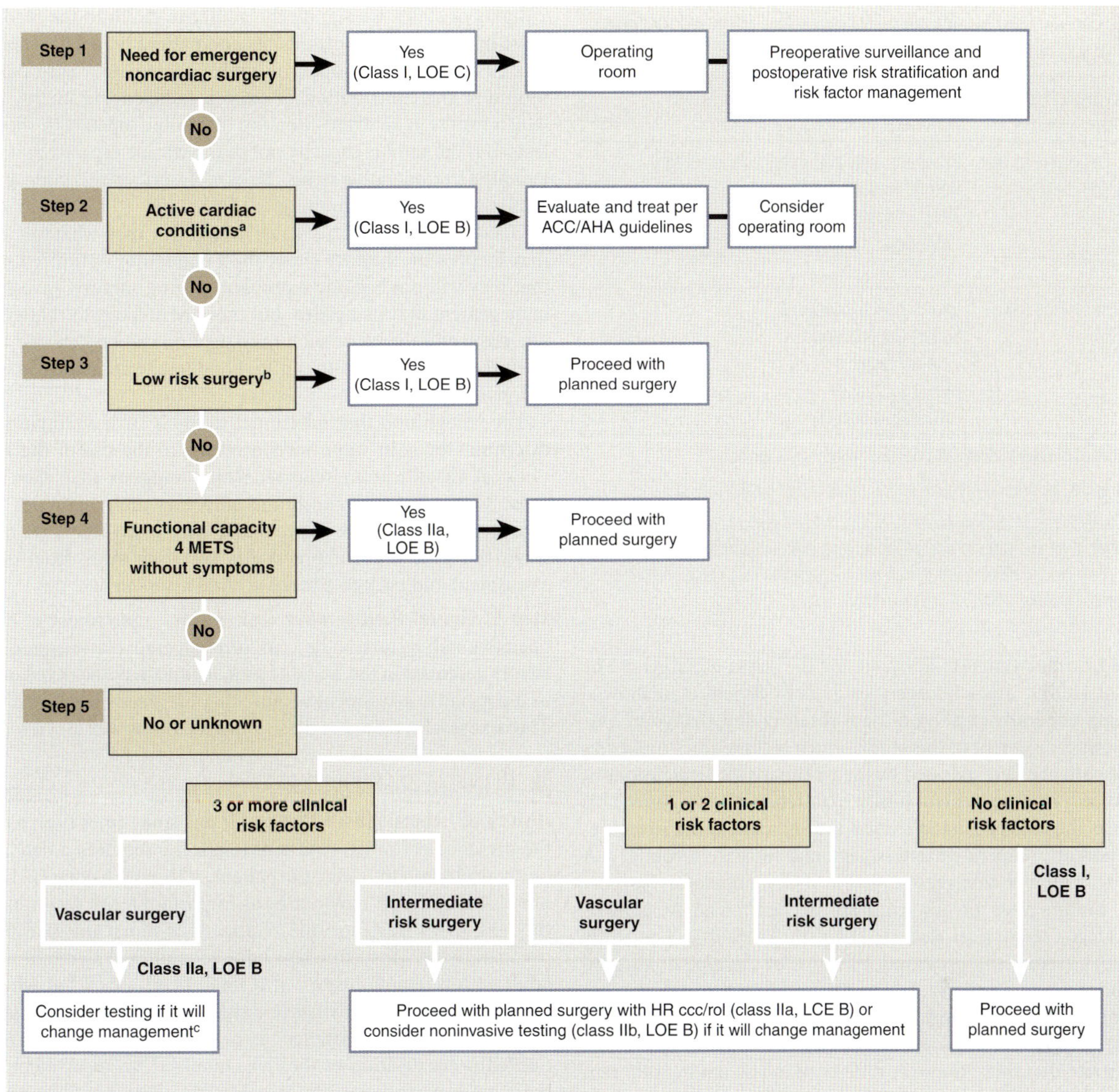

FIGURE 9-8. Clinical determination of need for preoperative cardiac investigation. [a]Active cardiac conditions = Acute coronary syndrome, decompensated heart failure, significant arrhythmias, and severe valvular disease; [b]Clinical risk factors include ischemic heart disease, compensated or prior heart failure, diabetes mellitus, renal insufficiency, and cerebrovascular disease; [c]Consider perioperative beta blockade for populations in which this has been shown to reduce cardiac morbidity/mortality. ACC/AHA, American College of Cardiology/American Heart Association; HR, heart rate; LOE, level of evidence; METS, metabolic equivalent of task score. [From Fleisher LA, Beckman JA, Brown KA, et al. ACC/AHA 2007 guidelines on perioperative cardiovascular evaluation and care for noncardiac surgery: executive summary: a report of the American College of Cardiology/American Heart Association Task Force on Practice Guidelines. *J Am Coll Cardiol.* 2007;50(17):1707-1732.]

"Reasons to Bypass Detailed Preoperative Assessment." If none of these reasons to bypass apply—need for emergency surgery, presence of active cardiac conditions, low-risk surgical procedure, and good functional status of the patient—a more detailed assessment of risk factors is indicated. However, this fifth step remains quite flexible in that the end recommendation—"consider testing if it will change management"—applies to most branches of the algorithm, regardless of the number of risk factors. Thus counting the number of risk factors is less important than assessing each risk factor in light of that question, "Would more investigation change management?" Having said this, presence of two unoptimized risk factors is a reasonable simple threshold for ordering more detailed investigation. The first five steps of the algorithm are described here. The fifth step involves assessment of 5 main risk factors:

Step 1. Emergency Surgery The need to proceed with truly emergent surgery with the information and resources at hand is fairly self-explanatory.

Step 2. Active Cardiac Conditions Acute coronary syndrome, decompensated heart failure, significant arrhythmias, and severe valvular disease generally warrant postponement of surgery and urgent attention by emergency or cardiology clinicians. In earlier versions of the ACC/AHA guidelines, these conditions were grouped as Major Clinical Predictors of PCC. But they are more than risk factors; they are manifestations of actual disease. In the latest guidelines they are termed *Active Cardiac Conditions*,[72] and the algorithm states they must be addressed before proceeding with anything other than emergency surgery. That these patients should have preoperative cardiac investigation is one of the rare class I recommendations in the guidelines. The details of management of these conditions are not discussed here.

Step 3. Is the Surgical Procedure Low Risk? Many low-risk procedures entail risks that do not differ greatly from activities of daily living. If the patient can walk to the surgical suite, he or she has probably

TABLE 9-4 Cardiac Risk[a] Stratification for Noncardiac Surgical Procedures

Risk Stratification	Procedure Examples
High: Vascular (reported cardiac risk often >5%)	Aortic and other major vascular surgery Peripheral vascular surgery
Intermediate (reported cardiac risk generally 1%-5%)	Intraperitoneal and intrathoracic surgery Carotid endarterectomy Head and neck surgery Orthopedic surgery Prostate surgery
Low[b] (reported cardiac risk generally <1%)	Endoscopic procedures Superficial procedure Cataract surgery Breast surgery Ambulatory surgery

[a]Combined incidence of cardiac death and nonfatal myocardial infarction.

[b]These procedures do not generally require further preoperative cardiac testing.

From Fleisher LA, Beckman JA, Brown KA, et al. ACC/AHA 2007 guidelines on perioperative cardiovascular evaluation and care for noncardiac surgery: executive summary: a report of the American College of Cardiology/American Heart Association Task Force on Practice Guidelines. *J Am Coll Cardiol.* 2007;50(17):1707-1732.

demonstrated cardiac function adequate for the stress of surgery. The large study of 18,189 cataract surgery patients by Schein et al showed that forgoing preoperative testing did not result in any change in outcome.[73] The critical element of this study, which is sometimes missed, is that all these patients were assessed by their primary care practitioners, and any tests required for general health maintenance were done. This study supports the concept that a clinical examination is the irreplaceable foundation of preoperative assessment, and tests are secondary. A pilot study by Chung et al suggested that in many ambulatory surgery patients no routine tests of any kind are needed.[68] The ACC/AHA guidelines categorize surgical risk as shown in **Table 9-4**. The study by Kumar et at verifies the profound influence of the type of surgical procedure on perioperative risk.[74] Noordzij et al performed a recent assessment of postoperative mortality in 3.7 million surgical procedures in the Netherlands that shows an overall death rate of 1.42%. These data demonstrate that there is a wide difference in risk among different procedures and suggest that grouping procedures into 3 risk categories is too simplistic. For example, where both gastric surgery and biliary duct surgery are usually considered medium risk, the overall multivariable adjusted mortality for the former is 6.5% but for the latter is 1.6%.[75] The ACC/AHA guidelines no longer make different recommendations for intermediate- versus high-risk surgery.[73] Probably a more important differentiator is elective versus urgently needed surgery.

Step 4. Functional Status Asking about the functional status of the patient is a remarkably simple tool that provides good prediction of risk for PCC, or more specifically, those who are not at risk of PCC. Functional status is a descriptor of how much the previously mentioned risk factors have an impact on the patient. Reilly et al showed that patients who reported they could not climb 2 flights of stairs or walk 4 blocks had twice as many PCCs as those who reported they could.[76] Although patient self-description of exercise capacity correlates well with actual functional capacity,[77] the accuracy of this test can be improved by actually observing the stair climbing. Girish et al observed maximum stair climbing in 83 surgical candidates.[78] The overall rate of postoperative complications, including cardiac events, arrhythmias, reintubation, atelectasis, and pneumonia, was 25%. The rate was 89% in those who could not complete 1 flight of stairs. No patient able to climb seven flights of stairs had a complication.

Climbing 1 flight of stairs suggests having an aerobic capacity of 4 metabolic equivalents[77] and probably represents a capacity to endure postoperative stresses without ischemia. The definition of a "flight of stairs" is quite variable: from 8 to 30 steps. By using a threshold of 2 flights of stairs, we signify the ability to climb to the second story of most houses. It is important that the patient be able to climb 2 flights of stairs without developing dyspnea, chest pain, or leg pain; this will minimize the contribution of oxygen-independent energy generation, which results in an overestimation of aerobic capacity in short-duration tests. It is the aerobic capacity not the anaerobic capacity that is critical in handling perioperative stress. Biccard described this concept and other limitations of a stair-climbing test.[79]

Good functional status usually signifies that whatever risk factors may be present, they are either mild enough or optimized well enough that they will not become a problem during surgery. Investigation and management may be needed, but they are unlikely to change perioperative risks, and therefore such investigation can be deferred to the postoperative period when it can be conducted methodically with careful follow-up.

The recognition that functional status is such a simple yet effective discriminator is in some ways a return to the use of the simple ASA Physical Classification scheme, which suggests that class 3 patients, those whose medical conditions affecting daily activities (as well as those in class 4), are the patients of concern, the others are not. In some ways, the pendulum of practice is swinging away from detailed risk assessment and back to a more general assessment.

Step 5. Clinical Perioperative Risk Factors Assessment of clinical perioperative risk factors is the crux of preoperative assessment. The 5 risk factors described in the ACC/AHA guidelines have achieved unique status in preoperative assessment because they are clearly associated with PCC.[72] The next section discusses those 5 risk factors as well as a few others.

CLINICAL RISK FACTORS

History of Ischemic Heart Disease It has sometimes been assumed that the presence of known CAD automatically required a detailed cardiology consultation to "clear" the patient. Although having CAD is an obvious risk for PCC, it may not be as important a risk factor as previously thought, or at least not one requiring as much invasive intervention preoperatively. Most clinicians have encountered a vibrant middle-aged adult with a remote history of a small heart attack but who now runs marathons and probably has less risk than younger video-gamers.

A cardiologist's "clearance" is of limited usefulness. What is really needed is clarification of the risks involved, an assessment of whether these risks have been minimized as much as possible, as well as an assessment of the stability of the patient. When is CAD considered stable? Certainly either lack of symptoms or optimization and stabilization of symptoms is an important part of this assessment. Left main vessel disease or 3-vessel disease should be carefully assessed even if asymptomatic because progression is more likely to be clinically significant. But as the previous discussion of the physiology of ischemia addressed, even high-grade stenosis may be relatively stable, with preoperative investigation or treatment not adding benefit additional to that provided by routine care such as statin therapy.

Previous Myocardial Infarction A few decades ago, a patient was considered at high risk for PCC for 6 months after an MI, and for some patients at some increased risk forever. But many MIs were treated with bed rest alone. Today, advances in treatment of acute coronary syndrome have improved the prognosis after MI. The angiography study by Van Belle et al of 56 post-MI patients showed that plaques remain unstable and vulnerable to reocclusion for 4 weeks, even after thrombolysis.[80] Cardiac scar tissue heals in 5 to 6 weeks.[21] Therefore, the high-risk period is now 6 weeks, with a period of relative risk from 6 to 12 weeks. In this relative-risk period, cardiac function is more important than time elapsed since the event.

Recent Coronary Artery Bypass Graft In 1997 the Coronary Artery Surgery Study showed that high-risk patients undergoing a variety of noncardiac operations fared better if they had CABG surgery than if they had not. Clinically stable patients who had undergone CABG within the last 5 or 6 years were relatively "protected" from MI complicating noncardiac surgery and thus probably did not warrant routine preoperative stress testing.[81] Then, a study by McFalls et al in vascular patients suggested revascularization may not be necessary preoperatively.[27] Revascularization should be performed if it would have been indicated irrespective of the planned surgery. Which procedure should be done first requires a case-by-case analysis. This topic is discussed in more detail in the section "Managing Risk: What Interventions?"

Recent Percutaneous Transluminal Coronary Angioplasty Recommendations for surgery after PTCA have changed dramatically as the type of intervention has changed, and they continue to be refined. In the 1990s, it appeared that PTCA performed a few weeks before an operation resulted in halving the rate of PCC.[82] However, other studies quickly showed it was advantageous to wait some time after PTCA before undergoing surgery. Posner et al retrospectively studied 686 matched pairs of patients with CAD undergoing noncardiac operations: one set having undergone PTCA preoperatively and one set who did not undergo revascularization of their CAD. These groups were compared with 2155 normal controls. There was no difference in PCC between the 142 patients who had had PTCA less than 90 days before surgery and the matched patients with CAD who were not revascularized. Patients who had PTCA more than 90 days before the operation had a lower risk of PCC than did CAD patients who were not revascularized, although not as low a risk as that of normal controls.[83] On this basis, it is recommended that surgery be delayed until at least 6 weeks after PTCA without stents.

Recent Bare Metal Stent Placement With the advent of stenting during PTCA (**Fig. 9-9**), the vulnerable period initially appeared to be unchanged. In 2002 Kaluza et al studied 40 patients who underwent noncardiac surgery less than 6 weeks after PTCA using stents. Ticlopidine and aspirin were continued postoperatively. There were 8 deaths, all in patients who had operations less than 2 weeks after PTCA. Six deaths were from MI; 2 were from bleeding complications.[84]

A retrospective analysis by Nuttall et al of 899 patients who underwent noncardiac surgery within 1 year of percutaneous intervention (PCI) with bare metal stent placement showed the highest rate of PCC occurred when surgery was performed less than 30 days after PCI and the lowest if done more than 90 days after PCI.[85] Thus the ACC/AHA guideline is to delay surgery to at least 90 days after bare metal stent placement.

Recent Drug-Eluting Stent Placement With the introduction of the drug-eluting stent (DES) in about 2002, evidence quickly emerged to substantiate that although there were clear advantages regarding early stent thrombosis, there was an increase in late stent thrombosis, especially if antiplatelet therapy was discontinued.[86] The late stent thrombosis was due to delayed endothelialization,[87] and although late stent thrombosis was rare at about 1% to 2%, it was fatal half the time. Thus in 2007 the ACC/AHA issued a scientific advisory about the importance of perioperative continuation of antiplatelet therapy for at least 6 months, and preferably 12 months after placement of a DES, including during the entire perioperative period[88] (**Fig. 9-10**).

Further studies show that antiplatelet therapy is more important than time between stent placement and surgery in reducing stent thrombosis.[89] Although dual antiplatelet continuation for 12 months is mandatory, clopidogrel treatment beyond 12 months may not be necessary.[90,91] A new generation of DES using everolimus shows promise of reduced stent thrombosis.[92]

Diabetes The second clinical perioperative risk factor is diabetes. Patients with asymptomatic type 2 diabetics have the same risk of MI as patients with previous MI.[93] Diabetes is considered a risk factor for PCC by most sources[94,75,95] (**Fig. 9-11**), although some studies have not shown evidence in this regard.[10,96,97] Patients with diabetes who do have perioperative MIs have more complications than patients without diabetes.[9] Although diabetes is a risk factor for cardiac disease, screening asymptomatic persons with diabetes for ischemia has not proven beneficial.[66,71] The American Diabetes Association recommends screening asymptomatic persons for diabetes only in high-risk patients.[98] Hyperglycemia is a risk factor for PCC; whether strict control of diabetes reduces risk is discussed in the section "Medications."

Congestive Heart Failure/Cardiomegaly The third clinical perioperative risk factor, CHF, is both a cause and a result of ischemia. Discovery of unknown or decompensated CHF is one of the main purposes of

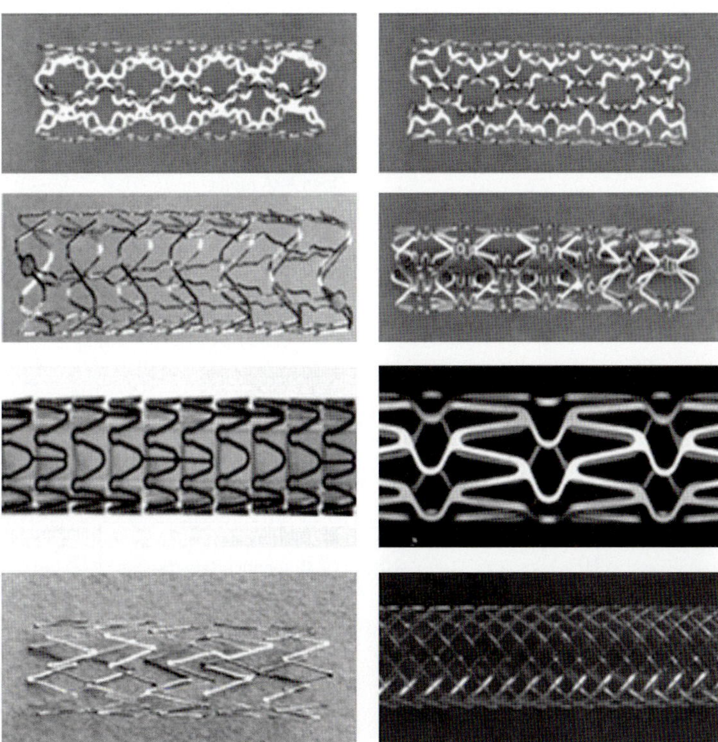

FIGURE 9-9. Coronary stents. Examples of various coronary stent designs. Each design is shown in the expanded state. [Modified from GW Stone. In: Baim D, ed. *Cardiac Catheterization, Angiography and Intervention*. 7th ed. Philadelphia, PA: Lippincott Williams & Wilkins; 2006.]

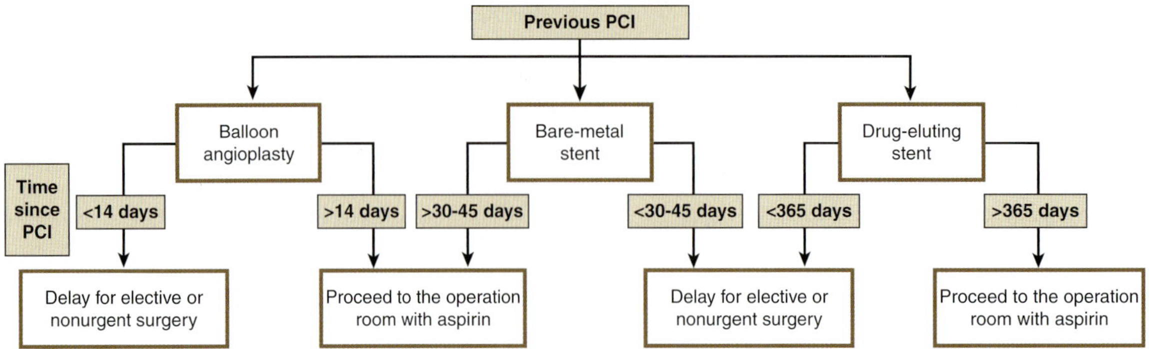

FIGURE 9-10. Perioperative management of patients with percutaneous coronary intervention. Proposed approach to the management of patients with previous percutaneous coronary intervention (PCI) who require noncardiac surgery, based on expert opinion. [From Fleisher LA, Beckman JA, Brown KA, et al. ACC/AHA 2007 guidelines on perioperative cardiovascular evaluation and care for noncardiac surgery: executive summary: a report of the American College of Cardiology/American Heart Association Task Force on Practice Guidelines. *J Am Coll Cardiol.* 2007;50(17):1707-1732.]

conducting preoperative assessment. Decompensated CHF is an unstable cardiac condition that always warrants preoperative optimization, but even stable CHF warrants respect. Hammill et al, in a retrospective multivariate analysis of 159327 Medicare patients undergoing major noncardiac surgery, showed that patients with the diagnosis of CHF have 51% more perioperative morbidity than those with CAD but no CHF[99] (**Fig. 9-12**).

Cardiomegaly is a risk factor for PCC.[100] Routine preoperative assessment of left ventricular function is a IIA recommendation (reasonable, may benefit) in the ACC/AHA guidelines.[72] CHF can usually be detected with a careful history and physical examination, although subclinical levels of cardiomyopathy may develop postoperatively, which lead to late morbidity. In high-risk groups there may be benefit to preoperative echocardiography even in asymptomatic patients.[50] Testing for B-type natriuretic peptide (BNP) may assist in monitoring mild changes.[49,101]

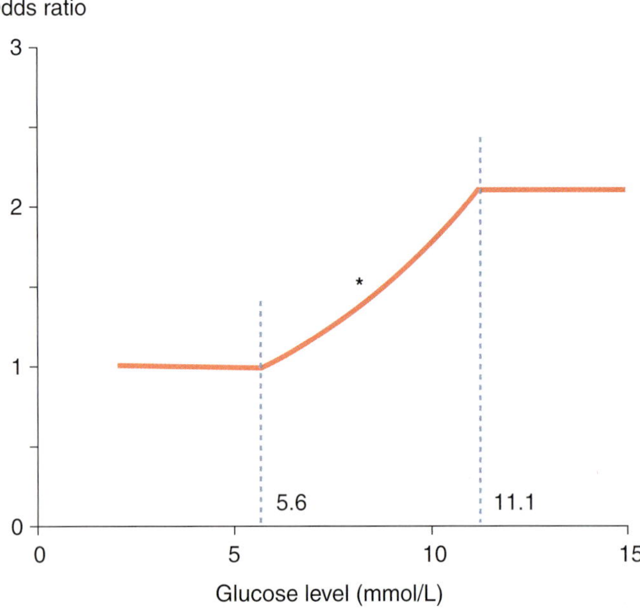

FIGURE 9-11. Glucose level and perioperative mortality. Odds ratios are adjusted for age, sex, medical conditions, type of surgery, family history of coronary artery disease, cardiac interventions, and medications. Odds ratio for perioperative mortality is 1.19 (95% confidence interval, 1.1-1.3) per mmol/L increase in glucose level. [From Noordzij PG, Boersma E, Schreiner F, et al. Increased preoperative glucose levels are associated with perioperative mortality in patients undergoing noncardiac, nonvascular surgery. *Eur J Endocrinol.* 2007;156(1):137-142.]

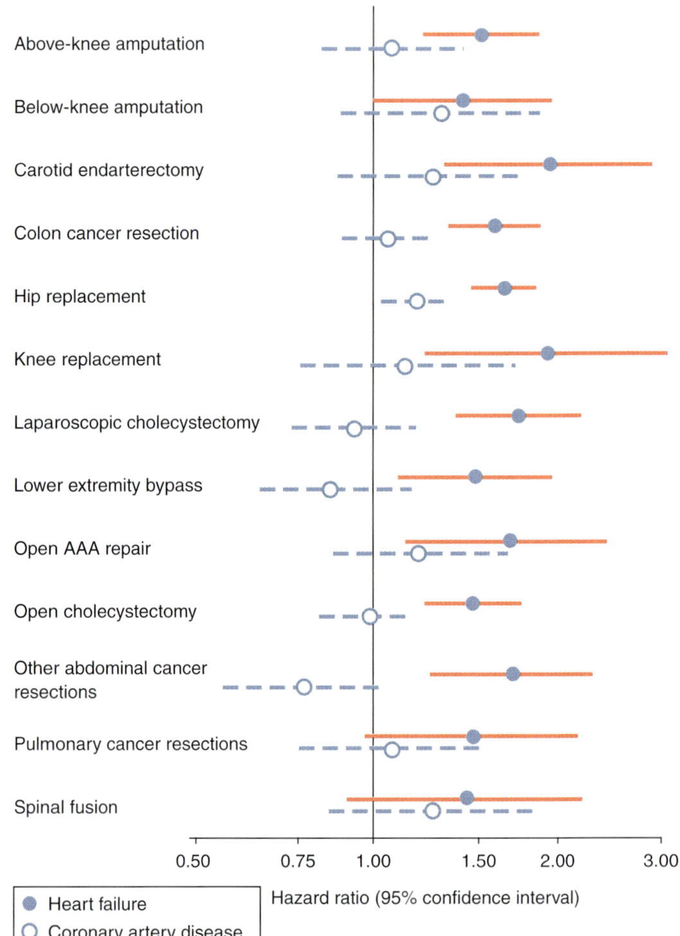

FIGURE 9-12. Effects of congestive heart failure and coronary artery disease on operative mortality. Effects of heart failure and coronary artery disease, compared with neither (hazard ratio: 1), on operative mortality by procedure. Procedure-specific models include indicators for disease group, age, sex, race, admission characteristics, comorbidities, and hospital teaching status. AAA, abdominal aortic aneurysm. [From Hammill BG, Curtis LH, Bennett-Guerrero E, et al. Impact of heart failure on patients undergoing major noncardiac surgery. *Anesthesiology.* 2008;108(4):559-567.]

Renal Insufficiency Renal insufficiency was added to the list of intermediate clinical predictors of PCC by the 2002 update of the ACC/AHA guidelines,[102] and it is the fourth of the clinical perioperative risk factors. An analysis by Lee et al showed increased risk with creatinine more than 2 mg/dL in the derivation cohort but not the validation cohort.[10] A recent validation of the Lee Risk Index by Hoeks et al verified that renal insufficiency along with cerebrovascular disease and insulin-dependent diabetes are the predominant contributors to predicting late mortality.[103] Often, the only optimization that can be done for renal insufficiency is to ensure that a reversible cause such as a drug reaction has not been missed. It is wise to document preoperatively the etiology and level of insufficiency or failure so that the cause of perioperative changes can be appropriately attributed.

Cerebrovascular Disease The fifth clinical perioperative risk factor is a history of cerebrovascular disease. History of stroke or transient ischemic attack (TIA) was an independent correlate of PCC in both the derivation and the validation cohort of the Revised Cardiac Risk Index,[10] as well as in studies conducted by Boersma et al and Kertai et al.[104,105] Optimization includes appropriate anticoagulation.

Carotid stenosis, in addition to being a marker for cardiovascular disease, may predispose a patient to perioperative stroke. Therefore, whether or not carotid surgery should precede other operations has been a dilemma. The risk of serious stroke in patients undergoing a nonvascular operation is less than 1%. It is no higher in patients with bruits than in those without bruits.[106] In 2004 the Asymptomatic Carotid Surgery Trial showed benefit from carotid endarterectomy performed in patients younger than 75 years who had asymptomatic stenosis greater than about 70%, but that was probably achievable only in certain centers.[107,108] There is no evidence to support prophylactic carotid endarterectomy before general surgery.[109] Medical therapies have improved in recent years to provide benefits similar to surgery.[110-112] Thus in asymptomatic carotid stenosis, medical therapy for peripheral vascular disease should be optimized, but no further screening in this low-risk group is needed. Even a carotid bruit is not an indication for screening in asymptomatic patients. The practice guidelines of the American Society of Neuroimaging as well as the Society of Vascular and Interventional Neurology recommend screening for carotid stenosis only in patients undergoing CABG and in symptomatic vascular patients.[113]

Valvular Lesions Asymptomatic valvular conditions are generally of no specific concern perioperatively. Aortic stenosis, however, is of grave concern to the anesthesiologist, and the discovery of this condition is a primary objective of preoperative assessment. The history may give evidence of some recent change in exercise capacity if this lesion is becoming significant. However, where aortic stenosis is a possibility, the threshold for investigation of a heart murmur should be very low because the rate of PCC can be very high.[114] New murmurs and probably any murmurs in an older patient warrant echocardiographic assessment. Physiologic murmurs are common but do not preclude development of aortic stenosis later in life. If aortic stenosis is discovered, the risk can be minimized with advance planning and careful technique.[115,116] Detection of any new diastolic murmur requires further investigation.

Infective endocarditis (IE) prophylaxis was simplified in updated guidelines.[117,118] The risk of IE is so low, the benefit of prophylaxis is so limited, and the concern of developing antibiotic resistance is significant enough that the recommendations have been scaled back considerably. There are no longer any class I recommendations (should be performed) for IE prophylaxis. Basically, the class IIa recommendations (reasonable) are that prophylaxis is recommended for high-risk patients (those with prosthetic valves, repairs with prosthetic material, history of IE, some congenital heart conditions, some heart transplant) undergoing invasive dental procedures. Only severe mitral regurgitation warrants prophylaxis, although this is somewhat controversial.[119] Prophylaxis for these high-risk patients who are undergoing invasive respiratory or infected-skin procedures is a class IIb recommendation (may be considered) with level of evidence C (consensus only). A similar recommendation is made for high-risk patients with established genitourinary (GU) or gastrointestinal (GI) infection undergoing GI or GU tract procedures, but this is mostly to prevent wound infection or sepsis; it is unlikely to prevent IE. The British guidelines include a slightly stronger recommendation for prophylaxis in GU and GI procedures.[120] The European guidelines are slightly more restrictive than those of the ACC/AHA in that no heart transplant patients are considered high risk, and prophylaxis in any procedure except dental is considered class III (not recommended).[121] Most needs for prophylaxis of subacute bacterial endocarditis are satisfied as part of usual surgical prophylaxis.

Peripheral Vascular Disease Peripheral vascular disease is a condition that shows up in 2 locations on most assessments of perioperative risk. Vascular surgery has been repeatedly demonstrated to be high risk because of the comorbidities and risk the patient brings to the procedure,[122,123] as well as those of the procedure itself. But some vascular surgical procedures such as endovascular carotidectomy are proving to be of low to moderate risk. Therefore vascular patients should be individualized according to the specific procedure and almost inevitable comorbidities. As with CAD, if optimal medical treatment is in place, further investigation is probably not needed. However, these are often very complex patients who are not optimized and may need assistance organizing overall care. Aspirin should be continued, although the overall benefit of this is under some debate.[124]

OTHER CORONARY ARTERY DISEASE RISK FACTORS

Several other conditions or markers are associated with CAD, but the association with PCC is still being clarified. With further studies, some of these conditions may become promoted to the previous category of clinical perioperative risk.

Smoking Smoking is a clear risk factor for cardiac disease and poor wound healing. Smoking cessation is one of the most effective ways to reduce cardiovascular risk. The unsolved question is how long before surgery cessation is necessary for there to be some benefit. There is concern that the stress of withdrawal may add to perioperative catecholamine surge. The issue of preoperative cessation is discussed in the section on smoking cessation.

Hyperlipidemia Hyperlipidemia is a major risk factor for CAD, and improving the lipid profile leads to a reduction in risk. Initially it was assumed that because lipid profiles change so slowly, management of lipids was not a practical perioperative issue. However, treatment with statins is proving to have some fairly rapid benefits, although this is probably unrelated to improvement of hyperlipidemia. Perioperative statins are discussed in detail in the next section.

Arrhythmias Arrhythmias are a cause and an effect of ischemia. Significant arrhythmias such as ventricular tachycardia are considered unstable conditions needing preoperative attention, but arrhythmias in and of themselves do not generally precipitate problems unless the heart is already compromised. Therefore, arrhythmias are of more concern if there is other evidence of cardiac disease. In otherwise healthy persons, conditions that may occur which are of perioperative concern are Wolff-Parkinson-White disease and prolonged QT syndrome. These conditions have a bearing on which drugs are selected to treat potential arrhythmias.

Prolonged QT Interval Patients with a long QT interval—a corrected QT interval (QTc) greater than 470 milliseconds for males or 480 milliseconds for females—are at increased risk for perioperative cardiac arrhythmias and morbidity and mortality. Congenital long QT syndrome affects 1 in 5000 people and occurs because of cardiac ion channel abnormalities.[125] Acquired long QT syndrome is more common and usually occurs secondary to medication side effects or electrolyte disturbances. A prolonged QT interval increases the likelihood of torsades de pointes ventricular tachycardia and ventricular fibrillation. In patients with newly identified long QT interval, elective surgery should be delayed for patient optimization or workup. The strategies for management

TABLE 9-5 Drugs Associated With Prolongation of QT Interval and Risk of Torsade de Pointes[b]

Known Risk of Torsades de Pointes[a]
Amiodarone, Arsenic trioxide, Astemizole, Bepridil, Chloroquine, Chlorpromazine, Cisapride, Clarithromycin, Disopyramide, Dofetilide, Domperidone, Droperidol, Erythromycin, Halofantrine, Haloperidol, Ibutilide, Levomethadyl, Mesoridazine, Methadone, Pentamidine, Pimozide, Probucol, Procainamide, Quinidine, Sotalol, Sparfloxacin, Terfenadine, Thioridazine
Possible Risk of Torsades de Pointes[b]
Alfuzosin, Amantadine, Atazanavir, Azithromycin, Chloral hydrate, Clozapine, Dolasetron, Dronedarone, Felbamate, Flecainide, Foscarnet, Fosphenytoin, Gatifloxacin, Gemifloxacin, Granisetron, Indapamide, Isradipine, Lapatinib, Lapatinib, Levofloxacin, Lithium, Moexipril/HCTZ, Moxifloxacin, Nicardipine, Nilotinib, Octreotide, Ofloxacin, Ondansetron, Oxytocin, Paliperidone, Perflutren lipid microspheres, Quetiapine, Ranolazine, Risperidone, Roxithromycin, Sertindole, Sunitinib, Tacrolimus, Tamoxifen, Telithromycin, Tizanidine, Vardenafil, Venlafaxine, Voriconazole, Ziprasidone
Conditional Risk of Torsades de Pointes[c]
Amitriptyline, Ciprofloxacin, Citalopram, Clomipramine, Desipramine, Diphenhydramine, Diphenhydramine, Doxepin, Fluconazole, Fluoxetine, Fluoxetine, Galantamine, Imipramine, Itraconazole, Ketoconazole, Mexiletine, Nortriptyline, Paroxetine, Protriptyline, Ritonavir, Sertraline, Solifenacin, Trazodone, Trimethoprim-Sulfa, Trimethoprim-Sulfa, Trimipramine

[a]Drugs generally accepted to be associated with QT prolongation and torsades de pointes.

[b]Drugs that, in some reports, have been associated with torsades de pointes and/or QT prolongation but at this time lack substantial evidence for causing torsades de pointes.

[c]Drugs that, in some reports, have been weakly associated with torsades de pointes and/or QT prolongation but that are unlikely to be a risk for torsades de pointes when used in usual recommended dosages and in patients without other risk factors (eg, concomitant QT prolonging drugs, bradycardia, electrolyte disturbances, congenital long QT syndrome, concomitant drugs that inhibit metabolism).

This list is continually updated. See http://www.torsades.net for the most up-to-date list.

Data from www.torsades.net. Accessed August 8, 2010.

of patients with long QT syndrome include suppressing sympathetic nervous system activity through establishing β-blockade, avoidance of sympathomimetics, and ensuring adequate pain control and anxiolysis. Drugs that may lengthen the QT interval (typically antiarrhythmics, antibiotics, or antiemetics) should be avoided (**Table 9-5**). Some inhaled anesthetics have been associated with prolongation of QT interval, resulting in recommendations for anesthesia maintenance with isoflurane or propofol infusion. Hypothermia should be avoided. The QT interval should be monitored and a defibrillator should be available during the perioperative period. Table 9-5 and other information on prolonged QT is available at www.torsades.net.[126]

Hypertension Although hypertension has clearly been shown to be a risk factor for cardiovascular disease,[127,128] the evidence that hypertension actually results in increased PCC is limited. A meta-analysis of 30 observational studies demonstrated an odds ratio for the association between hypertension and PCC of 1.35 (range: 1.17-1.56[129]; **Fig. 9-13**). This difference is not clinically significant in the short term. However, even if hypertension in and of itself is not a significant perioperative risk factor, the cardiac conditions that often accompany hypertension are. These include left ventricular hypertrophy, renal failure, and stroke. Uncontrolled hypertension is an unoptimized risk factor that should be addressed preoperatively.

The understanding of the nature of hypertension and its relation to cardiovascular disease is changing. Peripheral arterial pressure, which is what we usually measure, does not reflect large-artery stiffness, pulse wave reflection, and central artery pressure; these are a major part of the hypertension pathology, especially in the elderly.[130,131] The initial pulse wave from systole travels down the vasculature and is reflected back at bifurcation points. If these reflected waves return to the central artery before diastole, there is a summation wave that increases the stress on the heart. Measurements of central aortic pressures, although impractical at this time, are probably better predictors of cardiac morbidity and mortality than peripheral blood pressure. Some medications such as BBs may improve peripheral pressure but actually increase central pressures.[132,133] Part of the atherosclerotic process is a stiffening of the vasculature that results in augmentation of a reflection of the systolic pulse. Angiotensin-converting enzyme inhibitors (ACEIs) may reduce this augmentation.[134]

Even white-coat hypertension is associated with increased cardiovascular risk and endothelial dysfunction,[135] but evidence as to whether this affects overall cardiac risk, let alone perioperative risk, is mixed.[128, 136-139] Hypertension likely has a different pathophysiology in the young, obese, and elderly. Management of preoperative high blood pressure is discussed in the section "Management of Hypertension."

Anemia In addition to disrupting the supply-demand balance, anemia is a marker for other comorbidities. Anemia is associated with increased postoperative morbidity,[140] and measures other than transfusion may be needed to improve outcomes.[141] There is a trend toward greater tolerance of perioperative anemia except in patients with CAD.[142] If significant anemia is identified far enough in advance of the operation,

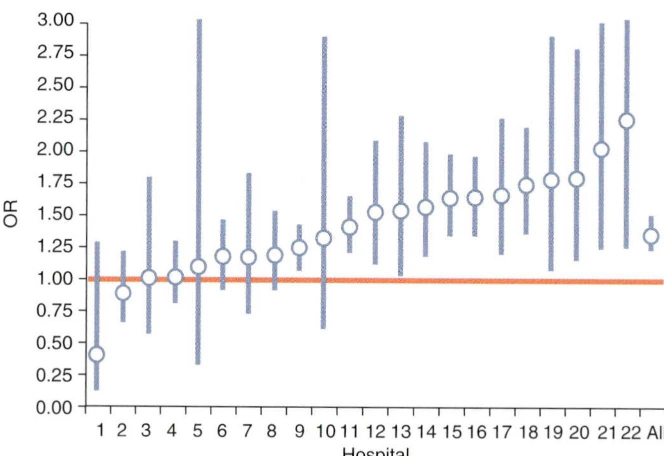

FIGURE 9-13. Association of hypertension and interoperative events in Swiss hospitals. Adjusted odds ratios (ORs) of cardiovascular events associated with hypertension in patients undergoing 124 939 anaesthetic interventions in 22 hospitals. The population averaged value OR of 1.38 is labeled "all." [From Beyer K, Taffe P, Halfon P, et al. Hypertension and intra-operative incidents: a multicentre study of 125,000 surgical procedures in Swiss hospitals. *Anaesthesia.* 2009;64(5):494-502.]

transfusion may still be avoided through the use of preoperative erythropoietin and iron, intraoperative isovolemic hemodilution, and special intensive care unit (ICU) maneuvers.[143]

Age Age older than 70 years was an independent risk factor for PCC in some multivariate analyses[9,59,60,144,145] but not in others.[10,74,105] Age in and of itself is probably not a significant risk factor in the absence of associated comorbidities, but increased age may magnify the impact of other risk factors.[146] For example, if an MI does occur, mortality is higher in older patients.[147] Nevertheless, the COURAGE trial did not show any benefit in adding percutaneous cardiac intervention to optimal medical therapy, even in patients older than 65 years.[148]

Biomarkers B-type natriuretic peptide (BNP) is a biomarker of inflammation and mild myocardial damage that is abnormal in advanced heart failure.[149,150] BNP has a high negative predictive value and might be useful to select out some high-risk patients who do not need echocardiograms to rule out ventricular dysfunction.[151] Recent studies show that preoperative levels may predict myocardial injury[152-154] and hospital length of stay.[155] As we become more aware of the effect of mild cardiac failure, BNP may be a useful marker of perioperative deterioration.[101]

High-sensitivity C-reactive protein (CRP) was shown by the Women's Health Initiative, which analyzed more than 14000 women, to be predictive of adverse cardiovascular events.[156] CRP is particularly predictive of postoperative morbidity in cardiac surgical patients.[157,158] The US Preventive Services Task Force states that CRP is useful in CAD risk stratification.[159] Measurement of CRP was instrumental in the somewhat controversial JUPITER (Justification for the Use of Statins in Primary Prevention: An Intervention Trial Evaluating Rosuvastatin) trial on statin use in healthy patients with normal cholesterol.[160-162]

CRP is probably more than a biomarker in that it is actually part of the inflammation cascade. If so, then decreasing CRP may directly improve endothelial function.[163] Even so, at-risk patients should already have been identified by clinical examination and optimal treatment with statins instituted.[159]

Albumin Low albumin is a marker of overall debilitation and acute-phase reactants, and thus it serves as a very good prognostic test for PCC. Unfortunately, this test result does not offer much guidance in perioperative management, aside from suggesting a longer delay in surgery to allow improved nutrition.

Depression Many studies show a that depression and major affective disorder are predictors of CAD, imposing about a 2-fold increase in risk.[164-166] The relationship is likely multifactorial with mechanisms such as compliance to treatment and antiplatelet activity of antidepressants completing part of the picture.[167,168] Successful treatment of depression is correlated with reduced risk of postoperative death.[169] Again, this serves to remind us of the importance of cooperation with primary care or consultant specialists in treating the whole patient, not just the organs and chemistry.

Genetic Polymorphisms Genetic testing is increasingly commonplace, and there is great interest in how this might be applied to perioperative risk stratification.[170] Factor V Leiden is an example of a common genetic polymorphism. However, with the possible exception of cardiac surgery, routine antithrombotic measures are sufficient to counteract the effects of this condition, and routine preoperative testing for this is not recommended.[31]

Some studies show an association of specific genetic polymorphisms with atherosclerotic complications after CABG,[171,172] whereas other studies have not shown strong associations.[173,174] The Multicenter Study of Perioperative Ischemia Research Group showed that certain polymorphisms for platelet glycoprotein IIIa as well as the degree of platelet activation are related to levels of troponin after CABG, suggesting that this platelet polymorphism contributes to perioperative myocardial injury.[175] Inflammatory response is also altered by genetic variability of key inflammatory genes.[176-178] Genetic variability in β-adrenergic responses may assist in determining who should receive perioperative BBs and who should not.[179-181]

Although not routinely used at this time, genetic testing is a significant frontier in perioperative medicine.

DETAILED PREOPERATIVE INVESTIGATION

As routine medical therapy becomes almost as effective as more invasive interventions, whether a patient has moderate or severe disease is often less critical to short-term management.

WHEN NOT TO START DETAILED PREOPERATIVE INVESTIGATION

If extensive medical investigation would not change perioperative management, it is a poor use of time and resources. It is important to also remember that the patient is an active partner in risk management. For example, if a patient refuses to undergo invasive cardiac intervention, and medical optimization is likely all that will be done, then testing may be a moot point.

This is the main question to be answered in preoperative assessments: "Is the patient as optimized as possible?" Conducting a good functional status assessment often provides evidence that the patient's constellation of medical conditions is adequately optimized for surgery. Thus good functional status is one of the "shortcuts" that precludes the need for preoperative investigation (step 4 of the ACC/AHA guidelines).

A common scenario is a patient with stable cardiac disease for whom it would be "nice" to have more information. A stress echocardiogram is arranged, and the result is indeterminate. The cardiologist, when faced with the possibility that the patient has serious cardiac disease, wants to be sure nothing is missed. This motivation may stem as much from the concern for litigation as from a logical medical indication. Thus an angiogram is scheduled, and it shows a stenosis amenable to stenting. A stent is placed and clopidogrel started, which means that surgery should be delayed for up to 12 months.[88] All this is done for cardiac disease that may have been less hazardous than the indication for an operation. Delay in surgery is inconvenient at least, probably unnecessary, and possibly dangerous. The CARP study[27] and, more recently, the DECREASE (Dutch Echocardiographic Cardiac Risk Evaluation Applying Stress Echocardiography) V study[182] show there is no benefit in preoperative versus postoperative cardiac intervention in vascular surgery (**Fig. 9-14**).

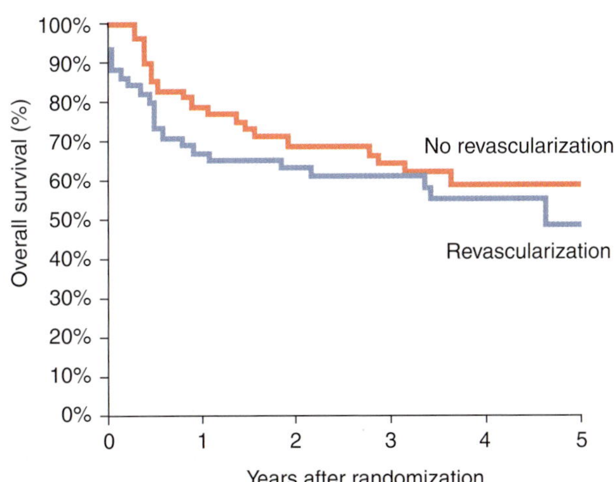

FIGURE 9-14. Survival comparison of preoperative revascularization versus no revascularization. Overall survival in 101 randomly assigned patients with documented extensive stress-induced ischemia in DECREASE V Trial. [From Schouten O, van Kuijk J-P, Flu W-J, et al. Long-term outcome of prophylactic coronary revascularization in cardiac high-risk patients undergoing major vascular surgery (from the randomized DECREASE-V pilot study). *Am J Cardiol.* 2009;103(7):897-901.]

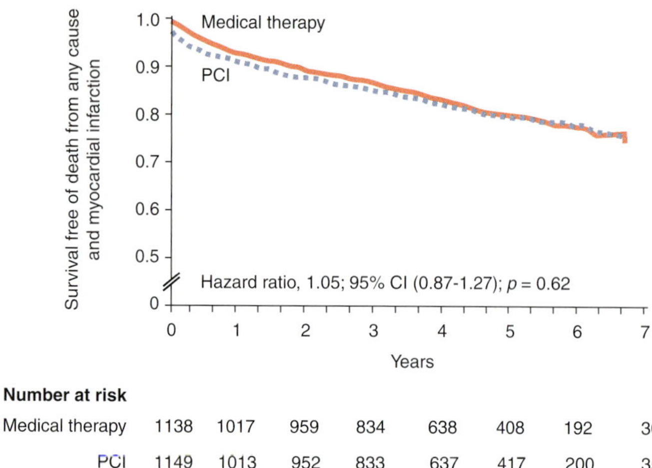

Number at risk								
Medical therapy	1138	1017	959	834	638	408	192	30
PCI	1149	1013	952	833	637	417	200	35

FIGURE 9-15. Survival of patients with coronary artery disease: percutaneous intervention (PCI) versus medical therapy. Estimated 4.6-year rate of the composite primary outcome of death from any cause and nonfatal myocardial infarction was 19.0% in the PCI group and 18.5% in the medical-therapy group. [From Boden WE, O'Rourke RA, Teo KK, et al. Optimal medical therapy with or without PCI for stable coronary disease. *N Engl J Med.* 2007;356(15):1503-1516.]

More recently the COURAGE trial, which randomized 2287 patients with CAD to PCI versus medical therapy, raises further doubt about the benefit of putting stable cardiac patients on the "cardiac train" of progressively increasing investigation and intervention.[183] (**Fig. 9-15**). The results were the same whether the end point was all-cause mortality or only cardiac events.[28]

These findings are consistent with the DECREASE II trial that showed that although the Revised Cardiac Risk Index correlated strongly with postoperative cardiac complications, stress testing did not improve outcome. Median follow-up was 2 years. It must be noted that even the untested subjects received maximal medical therapy including titrated BB therapy.[184] If this result is true for vascular surgery, it is likely even more true for lower-risk operations and lower-risk patients[184] (**Fig. 9-16**).

Thus if a patient is generally stable (good functional status), it is often best to keep a patient off the cardiac train of a stress test, angiogram, angioplasty, and an antiplatelet agent because, once on board, he or she is unavailable for elective surgery until the end of the journey. Before purchasing the "ticket" of a stress test, the clinician and patient must be willing to go the full journey before scheduling the procedure.

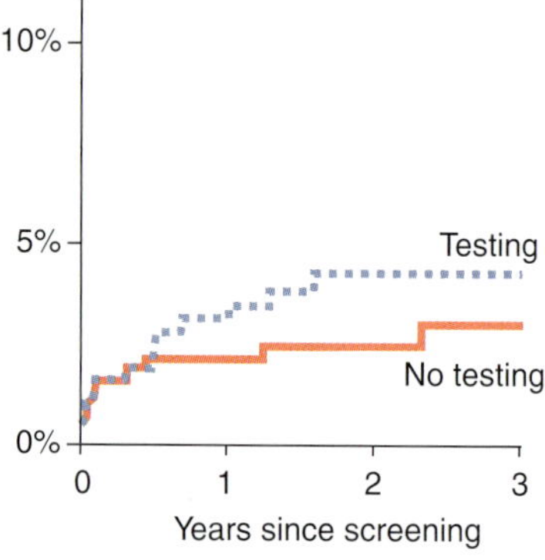

FIGURE 9-16. Relation between preoperative cardiac testing and postoperative cardiac event. Incidence of cardiac death or myocardial infarction (MI) during 3-year follow-up according to the allocated strategy in patients with 1 or 2 cardiac risk factors only. No significant difference (p = 0.30). [From Poldermans D, Bax JJ, Schouten O, et al. Should major vascular surgery be delayed because of preoperative cardiac testing in intermediate-risk patients receiving beta-blocker therapy with tight heart rate control? *J Am Coll Cardiol.* 2006;48(5):964-969.]

WHEN TO UNDERTAKE DETAILED PREOPERATIVE CARDIAC INVESTIGATION

However, there certainly are times when detailed preoperative testing is appropriate. Just as a good surgeon can handle most conditions that might be encountered but still prefers radiologic investigations so as to be as forewarned as possible, so the anesthesiologist may benefit from knowledge of the balance of risks and the range of physiologic reserves.

A simplification of the previously discussed ACC/AHA guidelines is that when there are 2 or more unoptimized clinical risk factors,[105,185] when surgery is assessed as more than low risk, and when good functional status is not present, consideration of further testing is appropriate for optimization. The tests are needed not primarily because the patient falls above a threshold for testing but because the patient's place on the risk continuum and adequacy of optimization are unknown. This testing can sometimes be done by the anesthesia team without cardiac consultation.

The main questions to be answered are these: Can the patient's health be improved? Can the risk of PCC be reduced? Are special perioperative measures needed? Can the procedure be done at an ambulatory surgery center?

WHAT TESTS?

Second-level tests, for purposes of discussion, are divided into resting cardiac tests, cardiac stress tests, and postoperative tests. Invasive tests, such as angiography, or alternatives such as intravascular ultrasonography,[186] coronary artery calcium by electron-beam tomography,[159]cardiac computed tomography,[187,188] or cardiac MRI[47,189] are not discussed. These specialized tests are rarely ordered or interpreted without a cardiology consultation.

Resting Cardiac Tests

Electrocardiogram Routine preoperative electrocardiograms have limited value.[68,190] The specificity of abnormalities is low, resulting in so many false positives requiring further testing and delay of surgery that the ACC/AHA guideline considers routine ECGs a class III recommendation (not recommended because probable harm is greater than benefit).[72] Some of the abnormalities, such as major Q waves, ST-segment alterations, T-wave changes, Mobitz type II or higher blockade, left bundle-branch block, and atrial fibrillation, are associated with increased risk of PCC. But even these abnormalities do not add predictive value to that provided by the clinical examination.[66] A careful clinical history and physical examination is the best screening test. If that assessment shows that the patient was asymptomatic, the optimal preoperative therapy is likely to be medical therapy, which would have been instituted even in the absence of an abnormal ECG. Infarction cannot be diagnosed on the basis of ECG changes unless there is also an elevation in troponin.[21] Troponin levels are rarely drawn in absence of symptoms. A study by Liu et al study suggests that even ECG changes in patients older than age 70 are not predictive of PCCs.[190] Thus most jurisdictions are selective, with overall ECG use rate as low as 13%.[191]

In contrast, selective ECGs in higher-risk patients do have value. The ACC/AHA guidelines recommend preoperative ECGs in patients with at least one clinical risk factor undergoing vascular surgical procedures, or patients with known coronary heart disease, peripheral arterial disease, or cerebrovascular disease undergoing at least intermediate-risk surgery.[72] The recent study by Correll et al adds some evidence-based guidance. Their results showed that age older than 65 years, history of heart failure, high cholesterol, angina, MI, or severe valvular disease are associated with clinically significant abnormalities on ECG.[192] Notice that this list does not include diabetes, which has often been considered an indication for preoperative ECGs, to detect silent MIs. The DIAD study showed that even screening with myocardial perfusion testing did not confer a reduction in cardiac events.[71] The much less precise ECG presumably has even less utility in patients with asymptomatic diabetes.

If the ECG uncovers disease, it is usually in a setting where a careful history has not been taken. If, for whatever reason, a hospital is not able to provide consistent clinical examinations, screening ECG may have some value.

One argument for obtaining preoperative ECGs is to document any baseline abnormality and thereby assist in determining if an abnormality discovered postoperatively represents a perioperative change.[193] No published evidence supports this argument, although it is logical. For such baseline purpose, an ECG less than 12 months old is likely adequate if there have been no clinical changes.

Two-Dimensional Echocardiography Transthoracic (2D) echocardiography is used to detect major wall-motion anomalies, measure ejection fraction, and assess valvular lesions. Certainly identification of severe valvular disease is important. Left ventricular dysfunction is a predictor of future cardiovascular events and increased overall mortality.[194,195] In the case of high-risk surgery and poor exercise tolerance in addition to suspicion of heart failure, knowledge of cardiac capacity will be useful to guide intraoperative management. If there is concern about ischemia, it is preferable to select one of the tests described next.

Cardiac Stress Tests Cardiac stress tests involve two components: a stressor and a test. These can be mixed in any way, but the most common combinations are treadmill ECG, dobutamine echocardiography, and adenosine radionuclide perfusion.

Treadmill Exercise Testing The simplest of the stress tests, treadmill ECG testing is a good first-line test in those patients able to tolerate the exercise.[82,112] It is not useful in patients unable to exercise, with baseline ECG changes (left bundle-branch block, pacemaker, Wolf-Parkinson-White disease, ST elevation at rest), or with a history of revascularization. Treadmill exercise testing produces 30% false positives in women.[196] In practice, if a patient is able to do treadmill testing, he or she probably has already demonstrated adequate functional capacity to preclude the need for preoperative testing. If further testing is needed, a more sensitive test, such as stress echocardiography, is generally preferred.

Older et al showed that cardiorespiratory exercise testing for anaerobic threshold is useful for identifying high-risk patients who are unlikely to develop diastolic heart failure postoperatively and therefore are unlikely to need postoperative ICU admission.[57] Unfortunately, few institutions can logistically arrange these tests preoperatively.

Dobutamine Stress Echocardiography This test has the advantage of requiring relatively little time to complete. It is a functional test in that it shows how cardiac function is affected by underlying pathology. Image quality is variable and usually limited in obese patients. Meta-analyses show that the receiver operating curve of dobutamine stress echocardiography is better than that of other tests.[197] An analysis by Beattie et al, which included 68 studies of 10 049 patients, evaluated stress echocardiography to be superior to radionucleotide imaging because the negative predictive of stress echocardiography was superior.[198] Because accuracy and availability vary between locations, each institution may have a different preferred test.[82]

A common dilemma is whether a dobutamine stress echocardiogram should be postponed in the case of a patient taking BBs. If the test is being done to assess whether CAD is present and whether β-blockade might be indicated, then testing without BBs has theoretical advantage. However, because continuation of BB has no significant effect on sensitivity or specificity,[199] and there is risk with stopping β-blockade, in most cases continuation is a better course. Stopping BBs for the investigation might only prove that the BBs should not have been stopped.

Galal et al compared preoperative dobutamine echocardiography, intraoperative transesophageal echocardiography (TEE), and postoperative cardiac events. Although new wall-motion abnormalities noted on TEE were more predictive of postoperative events, neither of the echocardiographs reliably predicted the anatomic site of the postoperative event.[49] Thus echocardiograms may be mostly markers of more systemic atherosclerosis, with limited ability to predict the specific site of thrombosis.

Radionucleotide Imaging This test may be more sensitive than others in this category because it detects flow anomalies that do not yet cause wall-motion abnormalities; however, the test is also less specific. It does have the advantage of allowing use of vasodilation, which is a gentler stressor of the heart or aneurysms that may be present. Compared with echocardiography, its accuracy is less affected by obesity but is altered by large breasts.

Cardiac Magnetic Resonance Imaging This test can combine flow studies with wall-motion studies in remarkable resolution. It is useful for complex high-risk cases but is time consuming and does not yet have a clear role in preoperative screening.[47]

Tests of Endothelial Dysfunction As described earlier, endothelial dysfunction is one of the unifying mechanisms of PCC. Several new biomarkers and tests for this are showing prognostic value for cardiovascular disease in general and may prove to be useful in the perioperative period. One of these biomarkers is brachial artery flow-mediated dilation. In this "stress test" of the vasculature, nitroglycerin dilation is the "stressor," and ultrasonic observation of the brachial artery is the test.[200-202]

Postoperative Tests Because most ischemia occurs postoperatively and is silent, it makes sense to monitor for it, at least in high-risk patients.[203] Postoperative ECG changes suggesting ischemia may be predictive of postoperative morbidity and mortality even in low-risk patients.[204,205]

Postoperative troponin elevation indicates increased risk of cardiac events.[9,129,206,207] This test has become the gold standard for identifying postoperative ischemia. Le Manach et al studied the postoperative troponin levels of 1136 abdominal aortic aneurysm surgical patients and found that a slightly elevated level was associated with delayed postoperative MI.[16] Discovery of elevated postoperative troponin may represent an opportunity to reduce asymptomatic ischemia.

MANAGING RISK: WHAT INTERVENTIONS?

After general risk level has been determined and more specific risks identified, that information must be used to reduce the perioperative risk where practical. Although consultation and cooperation with cardiology specialists are needed for many aspects of optimization, the anesthesiologist assigned to a case knows best what information is needed or not needed to balance risks, obtain informed consent, and formulate an anesthesia plan.

This section focuses mostly on preoperative and a bit on postoperative interventions. Interoperative management is addressed in other chapters.

Many of the medical interventions for reducing perioperative risk are part of the secondary prevention of cardiac disease. Although the perioperative team must limit itself largely to the management required in the perioperative period, this is an ideal time to institute or reinforce long-term cardiac care, especially the simple proven interventions such as control of hypertension, diabetes, and endothelial dysfunction.

PREOPERATIVE INVASIVE INTERVENTIONS: WHEN SHOULD CORONARY ARTERY BYPASS GRAFTING OR PERCUTANEOUS TRANSLUMINAL CORONARY ANGIOPLASTY BE DONE PREOPERATIVELY?

Glance, in 1999, in a decision tree model, found that proceeding directly to vascular surgery resulted in the poorest 5-year survival (77.4%) compared with 3 screening strategies: (1) nuclear stress test in everyone (86.1% 5-year survival); (2) coronary angiography in everyone (87.9% 5-year survival); and (3) angiography in high-risk patients, nuclear stress in intermediate-risk patients, and no testing in low-risk patients (86.0% 5-year survival). Although the 5-year survival rate was similar in all of the screening strategies, the cost ($/year of life saved) of selective screening was half that of either nonselective strategy. There was no difference in 30-day outcome between any of the 4 strategies.[62]

The CARP trial, published in 2004, showed that preoperative medical therapy is as effective as invasive treatment of vascular surgery patients with moderate disease. Similarly, the COURAGE trial showed that percutaneous coronary intervention added no additional benefit to medical therapy at 4.6 years of follow-up, even in patients with multiple vessel disease or diabetes.[28] The recent retrospective study of 23991 surgical patients undergoing preoperative stress testing in Ontario, Canada, who were propensity matched to a cohort without testing, showed only slight benefit from testing (improved 1-year survival hazard ratio of 0.92; 95% confidence interval [CI], 0.86 to 0.99, $p = 0.03$) and reduced mean hospital stay (difference: −0.24 days, 95% CI, −0.07 to −0.43; $p < 0.001$). The authors conclude that much of the benefit of preoperative stress testing is from the medical management that results.[69] It might be argued that this medical management could and should have been instituted regardless of stress testing.

The DIAD study has shown that even in patients with diabetes, ischemia detected with stress testing often resolves over time with medical therapy alone.[208] Biccard and Rodseth's meta-analysis separating PCTA from CABG suggests there may be benefit to preoperative CABG in some situations.[209]

Coronary interventions should generally be performed as indicated by guidelines used in nonsurgical settings. Whether or not an operation should be delayed depends more on the urgency of the surgery than on the presence of CAD. Because of the evidence previously cited that preoperative surgical intervention is not necessarily needed, and also because of improving medical therapy options, the finding of mild reversible ischemia on stress testing does not necessarily require proceeding to angiography. It is not necessarily predictive of PCC.[210] It may be appropriate to stop the cardiac train at this point if medical therapy is optimal. In essence, the destination has been reached, and it is best to get off the train.

MANAGEMENT OF HYPERTENSION

Hypertension as a risk factor for cardiovascular disease was discussed previously in "Other Coronary Artery Disease Risk Factors." Management is usually elective, and an operation does not need to be delayed unless blood pressure is quite high. There are no evidence-based guidelines on the threshold of hypertension that warrant delay of surgery. The oft-quoted threshold for postponing surgery of 180/110 mm Hg is the result of a recommendation by Goldman and Caldera in their 1979 study that included 5 such patients, none of whom had any complications.[211] Roghi et al did show an increased risk of cardiac complications in vascular surgery patients whose diastolic blood pressure was higher than 110 mm Hg despite taking two or more antihypertensive medications,[63] but evidence to support postponing surgery because of severe hypertension is surprisingly absent.[212]

The important aspect of management of severe hypertension (>180/110 mm Hg) is the search for end-organ damage (cardiac ischemia, renal dysfunction, cerebral impairment). If there is any evidence of end-organ damage, the patient has an active cardiac condition that needs emergency care. This should be managed according to ICU protocols.[213] In the absence of these, the condition is termed a hypertensive urgency, and the treatment goal is to gradually improve blood pressure control. Indeed, rapid reduction in blood pressure has added risks. If these patients are sent to the emergency department, they will be assessed with a clinical examination, ECG, and simple blood tests to rule out end-organ damage. If there is no such damage, oral antihypertensive therapy will be adjusted and the patient will be sent home. The anesthesiologist can often do this as well as the emergency department and at significantly less cost and inconvenience to the patient. There is probably no need to delay an operation if there is no end-organ damage and improvement in long-term management is underway.[129]

Blood pressure control must be continued through and beyond the perioperative period.[214] Hypertension is the classic condition that may present preoperatively and whose treatment will result in long-term health benefits. Treatment of hypertension results in improvement in endothelial function within hours[134] and reduction in cardiovascular events in 6 months.[215] The reasons for treating hypertension may not stem so much from perioperative benefits as from the clear lifelong benefits. Patient compliance is often suboptimal, and perioperative attention to this condition by the anesthesiologist will assist greatly in long-term management. Compared with the potent drugs used daily for anesthesia, antihypertensives have great margins of safety. Anesthesiologists need to learn to write prescriptions where needed for long-term hypertension management. Primary care physicians can assume responsibility for titration of medication initiated perioperatively.

SMOKING CESSATION

Smoking is one of the strongest modifiable risk factors for cardiovascular disease. Whether the stress of smoking cessation outweighs the short-term benefits of preoperative cessation is unclear. An early study by Warner et al showed that it took more than 6 months to see a benefit from preoperative smoking cessation. This study is often quoted as showing that there was actually an increase in pulmonary complications during the first 2 months of cessation efforts.[216] But the CIs for pulmonary complications were much too wide to support this apparent trend. Although sputum production does not decrease for at least 2 months, it is likely that benefits from smoking cessation increase with time.[217] Møller et al studied 120 joint-replacement patients who were randomized to either a 6-week preoperative cessation program that included weekly meetings and free nicotine replacement medication or to standard care.[217A] The overall complication rate was 18% in the smoking intervention group and 52% in controls ($p = 0.0003$). The wound-related complication rate was 5% in the intervention group and 31% in the controls ($p = 0.001$). There were no cardiovascular complications in the intervention group and 10% in the controls ($p = 0.08$).

Results of decision analytical modeling showed that it would be cost-effective to introduce a smoking cessation program even to patients undergoing surgery for lung cancer.[218] It is likely that smoking cessation programs would pay for themselves in the savings from reduced postoperative complications, to say nothing of the long-term benefits of smoking cessation.

MEDICATIONS: WHAT TO START AND WHAT TO STOP

β-BLOCKERS

Recommendations on the use of BBs continue to swing from enthusiasm to caution and back again. Over a decade ago, a few small studies in high-risk patients showed dramatic benefit from the use of perioperative BBs (**Fig. 9-17**). But there were only 83 serious adverse events in all the studies.[219]

These are efficacious medications, but like virtually all drugs, they have significant side effects. Recent studies have shown more adverse effects and probably less benefit than was previously appreciated. Effective use requires appreciation of new understanding in the mechanism and indications of BBs: which agents to use in which patients.

Understanding of the mechanisms of action of BBs continues to evolve. Reductions of heart rate and blood pressure are only two of the actions of BBs, and these may not always be beneficial.[133] The pleiotropic effects such as vasodilatation, reduction in inflammation, and improvement of endothelial function are likely the more useful mechanisms, and these must be maximized while minimizing adverse mechanisms.

Titration of heart rate is important, if not for benefit, at least for prevention of adverse effects.[220,221] Titration to a low heart rate is necessary for benefit after MI,[222,223] whether this is necessary for benefit perioperatively, as shown by Raby et al[37] and Poldermans et al,[184] or for treatment of hypertension is coming under some debate.[224] It is possible that in some patients, lower heart rate may increase central blood pressure.[133]

BBs probably reduce postoperative asymptomatic ischemia and resultant long-term morbidity. Although this may not affect immediate

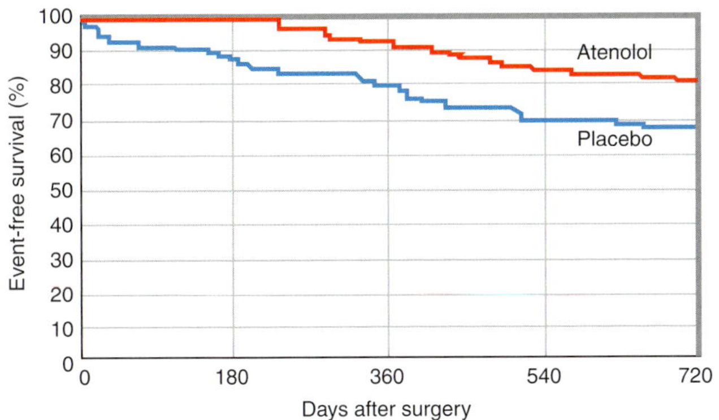

FIGURE 9-17. Event-free survival after surgery: atenolol versus placebo. Event-free survival in the 2 years after noncardiac surgery among 192 patients in the atenolol and placebo groups who survived to hospital discharge. The outcome measure combined the following events: myocardial infarction, unstable angina, the need for coronary artery bypass surgery, and congestive heart failure. The rate of event-free survival at 6 months (180 days) was 100% in the atenolol group and 88% in the placebo group ($p < 0.0001$); at 1 year (360 days), the rates were 92% and 78%, respectively ($p = 0.003$); and at 2 years (720 days), 83% and 68% ($p = 0.008$). Reprinted with permission from Mangano DT, Layug EL, Wallace A, Tateo I; The Multicenter Study of Perioperative Ischemia Research Group. Effect of atenolol on mortality and cardiovascular morbidity after noncardiac surgery. *N Engl J Med.* 1996;335(23):1713-1721. Copyright 1996, Massachusetts Medical Society. All rights reserved.]

PCC,[225,226] it reduces long-term PCC for up to 2 years.[14] BBs also reduce the likelihood of fibrillation with ischemia. Some short-acting BBs augment anesthetic effects.[227,228]

Some contraindications to use of BBs have not turned out to be appropriate. Asthma and COPD are not contraindications to initiation of cardioselective β-blockade unless the patient is having an acute attack.[229,230] In fact, the cardioselective BBs may actually improve pulmonary function.[231] Patients with diabetes benefit from BBs, although other cardiac medications may be preferable.[99]

BBs are no longer recommended for all perioperative patients. Studies such as the POISE (Perioperative Ischemic Evaluation) trial have reminded us that they must be used selectively.[220] They have little or no benefit in low-risk populations.[184,232] In the latest ACC/AHA update on perioperative use, the only class I perioperative recommendation is for continuation in patients who are already receiving BBs for treatment of conditions that have ACC/AHA class I guideline indications for BBs.[233] BB withdrawal has risks and must not be done in the perioperative period. Thus we need to review those indications, which have been or are in the areas of hypertension, CAD, CHF, and diabetes.

Hypertension A few years ago, BBs were given as one of the first-line therapies for all hypertensive patients. When this indication was combined with the apparent perioperative benefits, it was an easy decision to start them preoperatively. However BBs have fallen to as low as fourth-line therapy in hypertension.[133,234] As described in the previous section on hypertension, the treatment of large-artery stiffness, pulse wave reflection, and central artery pressure is more important than just treating peripheral artery pressure. And although BBs reduce peripheral blood pressure, they may change the timing of the reflected pulse wave, resulting in an increase, not a decrease in central pressures.[132] Thus BBs may be largely used for treating blood pressure numbers that are not good indicators of cardiac risk and are not effectively treating important pathology. Hypertension is no longer a reason to start BBs preoperatively, with the following exception.

The latest ACC/AHA update recommends, at a IIa (reasonable) level, the use of perioperative BBs in all patients with CAD or two or more cardiac risk factors undergoing vascular or intermediate-risk surgery.[221]

Coronary Artery Disease β-Blockers continue to be one of the first-line options for treatment of hypertension in patients with CAD.[235] The 2007 ACC/AHA guidelines on treatment of chronic stable angina state that for hypertensive patients with well-established CAD (but no history of MI or acute coronary syndrome), it is useful to add blood pressure medication as tolerated, treating initially with BBs and/or ACEIs. This is a class I recommendation, albeit with level C (very limited) evidence. For those patients who have had an MI or acute coronary syndrome, irrespective of hypertension, it is a class I recommendation to start and continue BB therapy indefinitely. This is supported by level A evidence.[235]

There is evidence that risks may outweigh benefit if BBs are given to an unstable patient.[236] This may be partly because newer cardiac medications and interventions that were not available during previous studies have reduced the additional benefit possible from BBs, whereas the adverse effects persist. Nevertheless, the benefits of BBs in patients with CAD[237] are still unchallenged. Thus if such a patient presents to surgery without β-blockade, it should be started, albeit at a low dose for subsequent titration.

Congestive Heart Failure Use of BB in CHF is another area of changes between enthusiasm and caution. At one time it was considered malpractice to use BBs in someone with CHF, but eventually it was realized they should be first-line agents for this condition.[238] Recently, some dangers have come to light regarding beginning use of BBs in initially unstable heart failure patients and patients with diabetes, and this has resulted in more conservative approaches. But BBs continue to be strongly recommended for most patients with CHF.[239] The ACC/AHA 2009 Guidelines for the Diagnosis and Management of Heart Failure in Adults makes a class I recommendation with level A evidence that bisoprolol, carvedilol, or sustained-release metoprolol succinate be used for all stable patients with current or prior symptoms of heart failure and reduced left ventricular ejection fraction.[240] Contraindications are allergy, major side effects from BBs, or recent use of inotropes for stabilization.

Diabetes Early concerns that BBs should not be used in patients with diabetes because they blocked counterregulatory hormones and masked symptoms changed to general recommendation for use because of the apparent cardioprotective effect in this high-risk group. Recently, however, observations that at least some BBs actually promote the development of diabetes[241-243] as well as increase doubt about the true extent of the cardioprotective effect has led to more cautious use in these patients. Diabetes on its own is not a reason to start BBs preoperatively.

BBs are still useful agents, and we must use them appropriately. All the recent studies showing limited benefits from BB use older medications. Third-generation agents such as carvedilol[244] and nebivolol,[245] which have actions of vasodilatation, reduction in platelet activation, and endothelial function enhancement, as well as fewer side effects, may improve the safety profile.[133] The DECREASE IV study showed significant reduction in PCCs in intermediate-risk patients at 30 days postoperatively with the use of titrated bisoprolol, a β_1 selective agent[246] (**Fig. 9-18**).

Not all individuals respond to BBs equally. Evidence is emerging on which genotypes respond best to β-blockade,[247] although this is not yet a practical option for selecting patients. Most studies showing benefit from perioperative BBs start the medication many days before surgery. At the other end of the continuum, prolonged use after the perioperative period may result in diminishing benefit but mounting risk. Chronic BB use does not seem to provide the same benefit as that of acute perioperative use.[248] There are no studies comparing the different timing of perioperative BB use. More research is clearly needed. The rule of thumb is the sooner the better, so as to allow titration to maximum effect without side effects. But whereas early institution is ideal, encountering this issue shortly before surgery does not justify doing nothing; it does warrant starting with a low dose and arranging follow-up. Above all, BBs must not be discontinued perioperatively.[249,250]

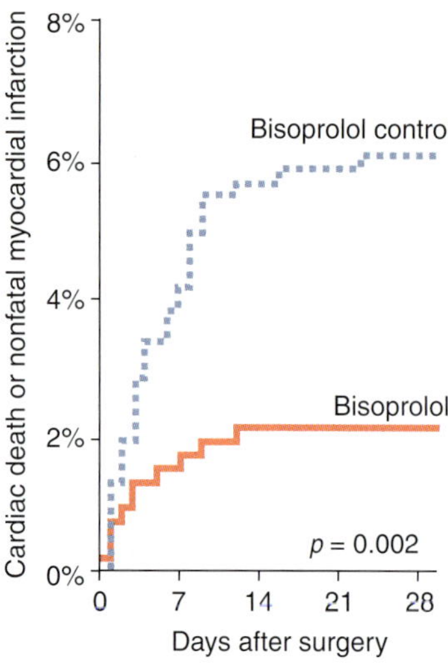

FIGURE 9-18. Association of perioperative bisoprolol and cardiac death or myocardial infarction. Incidence of primary study end point for bisoprolol versus control. [Adapted from Dunkelgrun M, Boersma E, Schouten O, et al. Bisoprolol and fluvastatin for the reduction of perioperative cardiac mortality and myocardial infarction in intermediate-risk patients undergoing noncardiovascular surgery: a randomized controlled trial (DECREASE-IV). *Ann Surg.* 2009;249(6):921-926.]

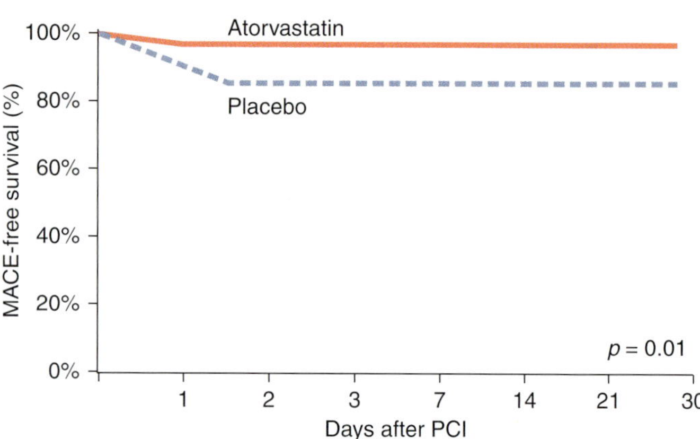

FIGURE 9-19. Effect of preoperative statin on postoperative major adverse cardiac events. Actuarial curves of 30-day major adverse cardiac event (MACE)-free survival in 12-hour preoperative atorvastatin versus placebo (postoperative statin only). PCI, percutaneous coronary intervention. [Adapted from Patti G, Pasceri V, Colonna G, et al. Atorvastatin pretreatment improves outcomes in patients with acute coronary syndromes undergoing early percutaneous coronary intervention: results of the ARMYDA-ACS randomized trial. *J Am Coll Cardiol.* 2007;49(12):1272-1278.]

In summary, perhaps perioperative BBs have not turned out to be quite as wonderful as initially believed, but they are clearly beneficial. Like all medications, there is a risk-benefit ratio that requires some selectivity. BBs that are being used for appropriate indications should not be stopped perioperatively. Patients who present for intermediate- or high-risk surgery, and who have class I indications to be on BBs (such as a history of CAD or CHF), but are not on them, should be started. Initial dose should be low, with plans for follow-up and titration postoperatively if necessary. If the anesthesiologist is uncomfortable with this type of protocol, the hospital system may need to employ a nurse practitioner, physician assistant, or primary care physician who is knowledgeable in these medical practices. In complex or unstable cases, a cardiology consult may be appropriate. Class II recommendations can be addressed more electively after surgery.

STATINS

Inhibitors of 3-hydroxy-3-methylglutaryl coenzyme A reductase (statins) have demonstrated efficacy in decreasing cardiovascular morbidity and overall mortality with chronic therapy and in the perioperative setting. Statins inhibit the rate-limiting step in cholesterol synthesis, decreasing serum cholesterol levels, improving high-density lipoprotein (HDL) to low-density lipoprotein (LDL) cholesterol ratios, and stabilizing vulnerable plaques. Large randomized placebo-controlled studies have shown that statin therapy is effective in the primary and secondary prevention of coronary heart disease and MI and decreases overall mortality in at-risk populations.[251] The Heart Protection Study (2002) also demonstrated a decrease in ischemic stroke from statin use even in patients with normal LDL.[252]

The benefits of statin therapy cannot wholly be explained by, and in fact often appear to be independent of, the lipid-lowering effects of statin therapy. The Prove-It Timi22 (2005) data demonstrate that statin therapy has anti-inflammatory effects that are predictive of cardiac outcomes.[156] It has been shown that statins can improve endothelial function in both coronary and peripheral arteries after just 24 hours of therapy.[253,254] In a small study, 171 patients presenting with non–ST-segment elevation acute coronary syndrome subject were randomized to 2 doses of atorvastatin or placebo within the 12 hours before percutaneous coronary intervention, and then followed by atorvastatin and clopidogrel in both groups. There were significantly improved outcomes in the pre-procedure atorvastatin group[255] (**Fig. 9-19**).

The pleiotropic effects of statin therapy are likely due to downregulation of membrane-bound g-proteins, such as Rho/Rho kinase (ROCK), and suppression of their subsequent pathways, decreasing inflammatory intermediates and increasing nitric oxide availability. Isoprenoids are cholesterol intermediates inhibited by statin therapy that are necessary to translocate and anchor the g-proteins to the cell membranes. It has been demonstrated that statin therapy inhibits ROCK activity in humans but that this effect is smaller when lipids are lowered to a similar level with a combination of a statin and ezetimibe, a cholesterol-absorbing agent.[256,257]

Although the data regarding perioperative statin use are less robust, they do indicate a protective effect. The strongest perioperative data reflect patients undergoing major vascular surgery. Durazzo et al (2004) conducted a small clinical trial in which 100 patients were randomized to receive atorvastatin 20 mg or placebo for 31 days (average) prior to undergoing vascular surgery. Cardiovascular events were 3-fold higher in the placebo group as compared with the statin group at 6 months[258] (**Fig. 9-20**). The DECREASE III trial (2009) randomized 497 patients to fluvastatin extended-release (XL) 80 mg or placebo for 37 days (average) prior to major vascular surgery. Statin therapy resulted in a 43% relative reduction in MI (number needed to treat [NNT] =12), and a 53% relative reduction in death (NNT = 19).[259] Meta-analysis performed in 2006 regarding use of statin therapy in major vascular surgery examined 7 studies, including one randomized controlled trial and one prospective cohort study, and demonstrated postoperative mortality was lower with statin therapy (1.7% vs 6.1%). MI was also reduced with statin therapy (2.9% vs 6.2%).[260]

In this same study, a meta-analysis of statin therapy in patients undergoing cardiac surgery examined 7 studies including one randomized controlled trial. Statin therapy was identified as being associated with decreased postoperative mortality (1.9% vs 3.1%). Postoperative MI, however, was increased with statin therapy (4.6% vs 3.6%).[260] The likely explanation for this increase in postoperative MI is postoperative interruption of statin therapy resulting in a rebound overexpression of ROCK and other g-protein–mediated pathways. Le Manach et al analyzed 669 patients in a prospective cohort in which statin therapy was continued postoperatively (median delay of 1 day until statin continuation) or discontinued (median delay of 4 days until statin

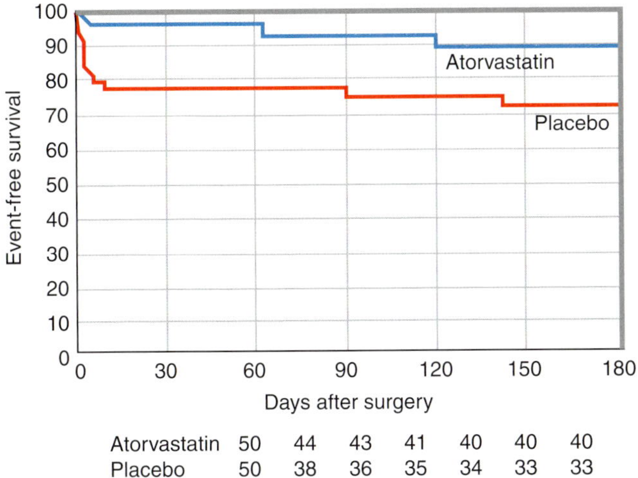

FIGURE 9-20. Event-free survival after vascular surgery—with and without statin. Event-free survival in the 6 months after vascular surgery, according to study group. Outcome measures included death from cardiac causes, nonfatal acute myocardial infarction, ischemic stroke, and unstable angina. Rate of event-free survival at 6 months (180 days) was 91.4% in the atorvastatin group and 73.5% in the placebo group ($p = 0.018$). [Reprinted from Durazzo A, Machado F, Ikeoka D, Caramelli B. Reduction in cardiovascular events after vascular surgery with atorvastatin: a randomized trial. *J Vasc Surg*. 2004;39:967-976, with permission from Society for Vascular Surgery.]

continuation). Continuation of statin therapy was associated with a decrease in MI (odds ratio [OR] = 0.38), whereas discontinuation of statin therapy was associated with an increase in MI (OR = 2.1) compared with controls.[261]

Lindenauer et al retrospectively studied 780 591 patients who underwent a variety of noncardiac surgical procedures, of which fewer than 10% were vascular cases. Of the studied patients, 77 082 received lipid-lowering agents, which included statins in 70 145 (91%) of these patients. Using propensity-matched groups and conditional logistic regression, they showed that treated patients had a risk of mortality with an adjusted OR of 0.62. The lowest quintile of risk did not benefit from lipid-lowering therapy.[15]

The ACC/AHA 2007 Guidelines on Perioperative Cardiovascular Evaluation and Care for Noncardiac Surgery makes the following recommendations for perioperative statin therapy.[72]

1. For patients currently taking statins and scheduled for noncardiac surgery, statins should be continued. (*Class I Recommendation, Level of Evidence: B*)
2. For patients undergoing vascular surgery with or without clinical risk factors, statin use is reasonable. (*Class IIa Recommendation, Level of Evidence: B*)
3. For patients with at least one clinical risk factor who are undergoing intermediate-risk procedures, statins may be considered. (*Class IIb Recommendation, Level of Evidence C*)

Use of extended-release statins during the perioperative period, as was done in the DECREASE III trial is another strategy to minimize disruption of therapy.

ANGIOTENSIN-CONVERTING ENZYME INHIBITORS/ ANGIOTENSIN RECEPTOR BLOCKERS

The cardiovascular benefits of ACEIs have been demonstrated in studies such as the Anglo-Scandinavian Cardiac Outcomes Trial–Blood Pressure Lowering Arm (ASCOT-BPLA).[242] The effects could not be attributed to blood pressure reduction alone[224] and may be due to improvement of arterial function.[134]

Angiotensin receptor blockers (ARBs) have similar benefits.[242,262] Although it would seem that these medications should be continued perioperatively, there have been reports for some time of intractable intraoperative hypertension attributed to ACEIs and ARBs. Some studies have not shown any relation between preoperative ACEIs and intraoperative hypotension,[263] but most do.[264,265] A retrospective study by Comfere et al of 267 hypertensive patients described increased intraoperative hypotension if ACEIs and ARBs are not stopped, but that it is usually easily managed.[265] That study did not show an increase in the incidence of severe hypotension, although other studies have.[266] Shahzamani et al observed a dose-related relation between hemodynamic stability and preoperative ACEIs given to CABG patients.[267]

Angiotensin is important for reversal of hypotension in volume-depleted states, especially during general or epidural anesthesia.[264] Therefore it is advisable to stop ACEIs and ARBs 12 to 24 hours before surgery.

CALCIUM CHANNEL BLOCKERS

Although there is some evidence for perioperative benefit from use of calcium channel blockers,[268,269] they are generally second-line agents that should be continued; routine perioperative addition is not indicated.[270] The dihydropyridine calcium channel blockers tend to cause a reflex tachycardia and should not be used.[271]

DIURETICS

Whether or not to discontinue diuretics should be determined on a case-by-case basis. The benefit of withholding them is a reduction in the dehydration induced by conservative preoperative fluid restrictions. The benefit of continuing them is in the control of heart failure,[272] and they should be continued in patients whose optimization is tenuous.

Use of diuretics is another aspect of medicine that has undergone 3 swings of the pendulum. Initially one of the few medications available for treating hypertension and heart failure, they were replaced by what appeared to be better options. But recent reexamination of studies shows the thiazides to be at least as good as other options.[273] Chlorthalidone is the thiazide most studied, although it is underused in the United States.

CLONIDINE

Clonidine is an old drug with several beneficial perioperative effects. In addition to possessing interesting analgesic properties, it appears to reduce preoperative ischemia[36,274,275] (**Fig. 9-21**). Clonidine may be a good alternative for those patients for whom BBs are not indicated. The European guidelines classify the perioperative use of clonidine as a IIb recommendation for vascular surgery patients.[270]

NITROGLYCERIN

A small prospective study by Dodds et al did not show any benefit to use of preoperative nitroglycerin.[276] A small case-control study by Sear et al suggested slightly increased risk.[226] There are no randomized studies of postoperative benefit of preoperative nitroglycerin.

ANTIPLATELET AND ANTICOAGULANT AGENTS

Balancing antiplatelet cardioprotection in the procoagulant milieu of perioperative stress with the increased risk of surgical bleeding must be done on a case-by-case basis. Aspirin should be stopped 5 days before an operation, and clopidogrel should be stopped 5 to 10 days before.[277] In vascular surgery cases, aspirin is generally continued throughout the perioperative period.[277,278] In some cases, continuation of both aspirin and clopidogrel provides the best balance of risks.[279] Anekstein et al showed that femur fracture repair on patients taking aspirin resulted in the transfusion of an average of 0.5 more units of blood.[280] In many cases this is a small increase in risk compared with the benefit.

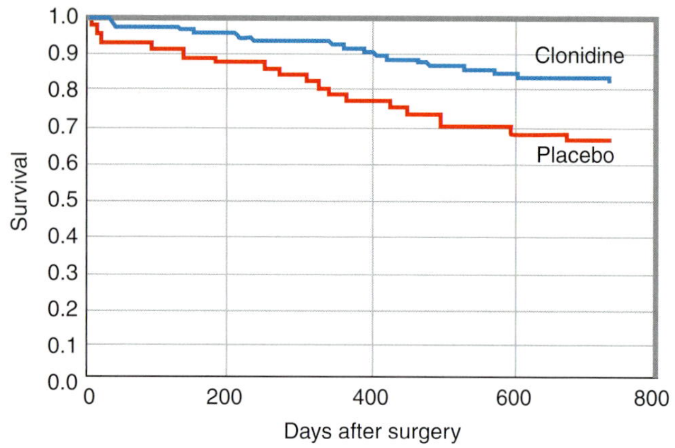

FIGURE 9-21. Postoperative survival: clonidine versus placebo. Survival for clonidine-treated versus placebo-treated patients. Survival curves for 2 years after surgery for patients treated with clonidine (n = 125) and placebo (n = 65). Clonidine reduced the incidence of death ($p = 0.01$ by log-rank test and $p = 0.01$ by Wilcoxon test). [Reproduced with permission from Wallace AW, Galindez D, Salahieh A, et al. Effect of clonidine on cardiovascular morbidity and mortality after noncardiac surgery. *Anesthesiology.* 2004;101(2):284-293.]

TABLE 9-6 CHADS$_2$ Score for Risk of Stroke From Atrial Fibrillation

1 point for each of
- C–recent CHF
- H–hypertension
- A–age ≥75 years
- D–diabetes mellitus

2 points for a history of
- S–stroke or TIA

From Gage BF, Waterman AD, Shannon W, Boechler M, Rich MW, Radford MJ. Validation of clinical classification schemes for predicting stroke: results from the National Registry of Atrial Fibrillation. *JAMA.* 2001;285(22):2864-2870.

Patients with CAD should ideally never stop aspirin.[277,281] There is a rebound phenomenon that results in about a 3-fold increase in the risk of PCC.[282] A cohort analysis of patients presenting with acute coronary syndrome showed that about 20% of those who had ischemic events within 30 days had recently stopped aspirin.[283] An 81-mg dose is as protective as higher doses.[284]

Oscarsson et al, in a small prospective randomized trial in 220 higher-risk patients, showed that preoperative aspirin use resulted in a 7.2 % absolute risk reduction in PCCs and no difference in bleeding complications. The study was not sufficiently powered to allow firm conclusions, but any further trials requiring a planned stoppage of aspirin in high-risk patients would likely be considered unethical.[285] Stopping aspirin in patients with CAD must only be done if the risk is justifiable.

Patients with atrial fibrillation can usually have aspirin and warfarin stopped unless the CHADS$_2$ score is high, about 4 or more (**Table 9-6**). Stroke or TIA within the past year generally warrants either continuation or bridging therapy.

Patients on anticoagulants because of valvular heart disease and prosthetic valves likewise require a balancing of the risk of bleeding from continued anticoagulation versus the increased risk of thromboembolism resulting from a cessation of therapy. Patients who are at high risk for thromboembolism should stop warfarin 5 days before surgery and institute bridging therapy with unfractionated or low molecular weight heparin. Patients who are at moderate risk should likewise stop warfarin 5 days preoperatively and institute bridging therapy, although the evidence for this is less robust. Patients at low risk, for example those with bileaflet mechanical valve and no other risk factors, do not need bridging therapy.[277] The ACC/AHA guidelines suggest that for these patients warfarin can be stopped 48 to 72 hours before surgery, as long as the international normalization ratio (INR) is reduced to below 1.5.[286] Because the evidence defining the perioperative management of anticoagulation in this patient population is so sparse, the specifics of cessation or bridging with heparin of a patient with any of the risk factors in **Table 9-7** must be individualized.[287] A rough guideline is that a patient with two risk factors should have therapeutic doses of intravenous heparin started when the INR has been allowed to fall below 2.0 (typically 48 hours before surgery). Heparin should be adjusted to maintain the activated partial thromboplastin time at 55 to 70 seconds, stopped 4 to 6 hours before the procedure, restarted as early after the operation as possible, and continued until the INR is therapeutic on warfarin.[286] Although there have been some concerns that low-molecular-weight heparin for bridging in patients with mechanical valves does not provide enough protection,[288] its use is becoming common with no reported problems.[289] The European guidelines recommend twice-daily dosing at therapeutic rather than prophylactic levels.[290] Ongoing studies may soon provide guidance in this area.

ANTIPLATELET AGENTS AND RECENT CORONARY STENTS

Generally, dual antiplatelet therapy must be continued for at least 6 weeks after bare metal stent placement[291] and 12 months after placement of DESs. Heparin bridging is of unknown utility; it does not provide

TABLE 9-7 Suggested Patient Risk Stratification for Perioperative Arterial or Venous Thromboembolism

	Indication for VKA Therapy		
Risk Stratum	Mechanical Heart Valve	Atrial Fibrillation	VTE
High	Any mitral valve prosthesis Older (caged-ball or tilting disc) aortic valve prosthesis Recent (within 6 mo) stroke or transient ischemic attack	CHADS$^a_2$ score of 5 or 6 Recent (within 3 mo) stroke or transient ischemic attack Rheumatic valvular heart disease	Recent (within 3 mo) VTE Severe thrombophilia (eg, deficiency of protein C, protein S or antithrombin, antiphospholipid antibodies, or multiple abnormalities)
Moderate	Bileaflet aortic valve prosthesis and one of the following: atrial fibrillation, prior stroke or transient ischemic attack, hypertension, diabetes, congestive heart failure, age > 75 y	CHADS$_2$ score of 3 or 4	VTE within the past 3-12 mo Nonsevere thrombophilic conditions (eg, heterozygous factor V Leiden mutation, heterozygous factor II mutation) Recurrent VTE Active cancer (treated within 6 mo or paliative)
Low	Bileaflet aortic valve prosthesis without atrial fibrillation and no other risk factors for stroke	CHADS$_2$ score of 0-2 (and no prior stroke or transient ischemic attack)	Single VTE occurred > 12 mo ago and no other risk factors

[a]CHADS$_2$ = Congestive heart failure-Hypertension-Age-Diabetes-Stroke.

From Douketis JD, Berger PB, Dunn AS, et al. The perioperative management of antithrombotic therapy: American College of Chest Physicians Evidence-Based Clinical Practice Guidelines (8th Edition). *Chest* 2008;133;299S-339S.

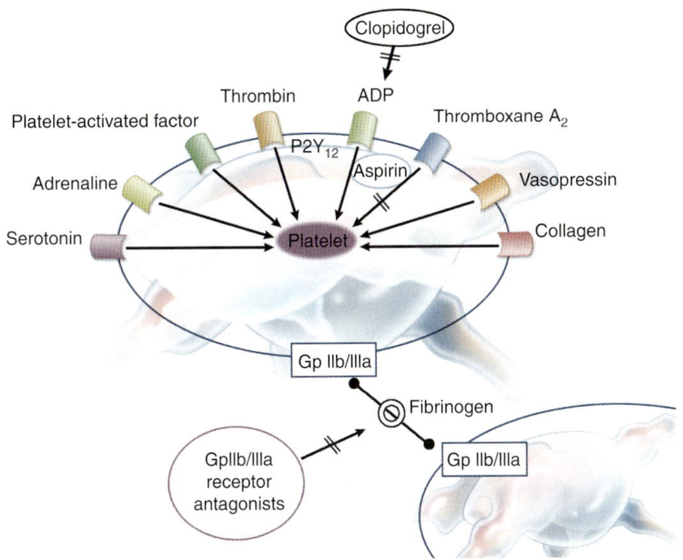

FIGURE 9-22. Antiplatelet agents. Mode of action of the 3 main types of antiplatelet agents (thienopyridines [eg, clopidogrel], aspirin, and glycoprotein [Gp] IIb/IIIa inhibitors) in relation to inhibition of platelet function. ADP, adenosine triphosphate. [From O'Riordan JM, Margey RJ, Blake G, O'Connell PR. Antiplatelet agents in the perioperative period. *Arch Surg.* 2009;144(1):69-76.]

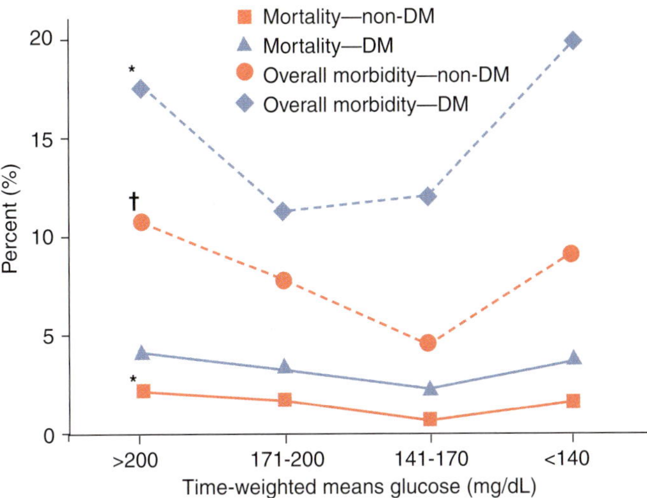

FIGURE 9-23. Intraoperative glucose and morbidity/mortality. Univariate analysis comparing risk of mortality and overall morbidity between patients with and without diabetes related to mean intraoperative glucose levels. $^{*}p < 0.05$ and $^{\dagger}p < 0.001$ overall between levels of mean glucose within patient group. DM, patient with diabetes; non-DM, patient without diabetes. [Adapted from Duncan AE, Abd-Elsayed A, Maheshwari A, Xu M, Soltesz E, Koch CG. Role of intraoperative and postoperative blood glucose concentrations in predicting outcomes after cardiac surgery. *Anesthesiology.* 2010;112(4):860-871.]

the level of antiplatelet activity that must be maintained. In fact, heparin might actually decrease platelet activity.[292] Some initial evidence has shown that bridging with an intravenous glycoprotein (GP)IIb/IIIa receptor blocker such as tirofiban may be beneficial[293, 294] (**Fig. 9-22**).

DIABETES MEDICATIONS

In the past, metformin was stopped up to 1 week preoperatively because of fear of metabolic acidosis and renal insult. A recent Cochrane analysis revealed no cases of fatal or nonfatal lactic acidosis in 70 490 patient-years of metformin use.[295] Metformin is proving to be valuable in improving endothelial function.[296,297] Stopping use of this drug preoperatively is probably counterproductive.

Ideally, no patient should proceed to an elective operation without stable glucose control. Although there is strong evidence that perioperative hyperglycemia increases risk of surgical wound infections in cardiac surgery[298,299] and fairly good evidence that hyperglycemia increases overall risk of CAD,[300] a recent Cochrane review concludes there is no evidence that tight perioperative glucose control is advantageous,[301] and it may actually be detrimental.[302]

A study by Duncan et al of intraoperative glucose levels in 4302 cardiac patients shows a U-shaped curve of morbidity from glucose control; that is, morbidity decreases as glucose levels decrease until they reach near normal, at which point the morbidity becomes as high as with hyperglycemia[303] (**Fig. 9-23**).

ANTIBIOTICS

Clinicians should refer to established guidelines for the use of preoperative antibiotics to prevent surgical infections[304] and to prevent endocarditis.[117] Effective prophylaxis against surgical infections requires that the antibiotic be administered within the hour before incision. Antibiotics for endocarditis prophylaxis are often overused and should be given only when indicated.

NUTRITIONAL SUPPLEMENTS

Many patients take nutritional supplements, herbal medications, and/or well-advertised placebos. Because these are not regulated, it is difficult to know what is really in them. Although most supplements are probably innocuous, some may have detrimental perioperative effects, and so patients are usually asked to stop all of them. However some supplements have beneficial effects or may at least have produced a new homeostasis of coagulation or endothelial function that should not be upset. For example, vitamin D,[305] long-chain n-3 polyunsaturated fatty acids,[306] and isoflavones[163] have positive effects on endothelial function, and benefits of continuing them likely outweigh adverse effects. Recent updated guidelines from the American Society of Regional Anesthesia and Pain Medicine on regional anesthesia in patients receiving antithrombotic or thrombolytic therapy state that "The use of herbal medications does not create a level of risk that will interfere with the performance of neuraxial block. We recommend against mandatory discontinuation of these medications or avoidance of regional anesthetic techniques in patients in whom these medications have been administered (Grade 1C)."[307] Time may prove that some supplements should be actively started in most patients.

CONCLUSION

The patient's perioperative plan can often be created on the basis of good interviewing and examination skills. Specialized tests should only be applied as needed to refine management decisions. Perioperative management now entails more than just identifying high-risk patients and referring them back to other specialists. It is possible for the anesthesiologist to actually reduce perioperative risk through relatively simple medical interventions. The extent and timing of interventions can be tailored to each patient according to specific perioperative risks. Anesthesiologists are well positioned to reduce perioperative risk efficiently and institute simple forms of secondary disease management.

KEY REFERENCES

- Boden WE, O'Rourke RA, Teo KK, et al. Impact of optimal medical therapy with or without percutaneous coronary intervention on long-term cardiovascular end points in patients with stable coronary artery disease (from the COURAGE trial). *Am J Cardiol.* 2009;104(1):1-4.

- Chung F, Yuan H, Yin L, Vairavanathan S, Wong DT. Elimination of preoperative testing in ambulatory surgery. *Anesth Analg.* 2009;108(2):467-475.
- Correll DJ, Hepner DL, Chang C, Tsen L, Hevelone ND, Bader AM. Preoperative electrocardiograms: patient factors predictive of abnormalities. *Anesthesiology.* 2009;110(6):1217-1222.
- Douketis JD, Berger PB, Dunn AS, et al. The perioperative management of antithrombotic therapy: American College of Chest Physicians Evidence-Based Clinical Practice Guidelines (8th Edition). *Chest.* 2008;133(6 Suppl):299S-339S.
- Fleisher LA, Beckman JA, Brown KA, et al. 2009 ACCF/AHA focused update on perioperative beta blockade incorporated into the ACC/AHA 2007 guidelines on perioperative cardiovascular evaluation and care for noncardiac surgery: a report of the American College of Cardiology Foundation/American Heart Association Task Force on Practice Guidelines. *Circulation.* 2009;120(21):e169-276.
- Oscarsson A, Gupta A, Fredrikson M, et al. To continue or discontinue aspirin in the perioperative period: a randomized, controlled clinical trial. *Br J Anaesth.* 2010;104(3):305-312.
- Schouten O, Boersma E, Hoeks SE, et al. Fluvastatin and perioperative events in patients undergoing vascular surgery. *N Engl J Med.* 2009;361:980-989.
- Schouten O, van Kuijk J-P, Flu W-J, et al. Long-term outcome of prophylactic coronary revascularization in cardiac high-risk patients undergoing major vascular surgery (from the randomized DECREASE-V Pilot Study). *Am J Cardiol.* 2009;103(7):897-901.
- Wijeysundera DN, Beattie WS, Austin PC, Hux JE, Laupacis A. Non-invasive cardiac stress testing before elective major non-cardiac surgery: population based cohort study. *BMJ.* 2010;340:b5526.

REFERENCES

Complete references available on DVD and online version at www.LongneckerAnesthesiology.com

CHAPTER 10

Evaluation of the Patient With a Difficult Airway

James C. Phero
Yash J. Patil
William E. Hurford

KEY POINTS

1. A patient with a history of difficult intubation should be treated as having a difficult airway, even though physical appearance and physical examination may be unremarkable.
2. A patient with anatomic variations indicative of possible difficult intubation should receive a careful history and physical examination to define the extent of the potential airway problem.
3. Possible or potentially difficult intubation may be predicted by the Mallampati test, evidence of receding mandible, limited mouth opening as a result of tissue or temporomandibular joint (TMJ) restriction, enlarged teeth, high arched palate, narrow small mouth, or restricted cervical spine movement.
4. All current tests to predict difficulty with airway management are associated with a high incidence of false-positive and false-negative results and have low predictive value. To minimize airway-related complications, it is optimal to accept a high incidence of false-positive predictions by the various tests and treat any patient identified as having a possible difficult intubation accordingly.
5. Unexpected failed ventilation and intubation may result from oropharyngeal, laryngeal, or tracheal pathology that may not be identified by external examination.
6. In pediatrics, infection-related airway compromise and congenital airway malformations are the major airway management problems.
7. In adults, stridor at rest indicates a serious degree of obstruction with a cross-sectional opening less than 4 mm.
8. Upper airway endoscopy with a standard or videolaryngoscope and/or fiberoptic bronchoscope is useful in defining anatomic challenges in patients with upper airway pathology before induction of general anesthesia.

SCOPE OF THE PROBLEM AND INCIDENCE

A challenging airway may present as difficulty with ventilation, difficulty with rigid laryngoscopic tracheal intubation, or both. The American Society of Anesthesiologists' (ASA) *Practice Guidelines for Management of the Difficult Airway* has defined difficult ventilation as a circumstance where "it is not possible for the unassisted anesthesiologist to prevent or reverse signs of inadequate ventilation during positive pressure ventilation."[1]

Difficult rigid laryngoscopy is defined as a situation in which "it is not possible to visualize any portion of the vocal cords with conventional laryngoscopy." A difficult intubation is defined as a circumstance in which "the proper insertion of an endotracheal tube using conventional laryngoscopy requires more than three attempts, or greater than 10 minutes."[1]

The incidence of difficult intubation by rigid laryngoscopy varies from 0.5% to 13.6% in published studies.[2-8] Discrepancies in the reported incidence of difficult intubation are to be expected because most reports are retrospective studies and apply different definitions of what constitutes a difficult intubation.[9] The incidence of failed intubation in the general surgical population has been reported as 1 in every 2230 patients.[4] The incidence of failed intubation in the parturient population has been reported as 1 in 283 to 750 patients.[4,8] This represents a 3- to 10-fold increase compared with the incidence in nonparturient patients. The precise frequency of difficult mask ventilation is unknown, but an Australian study indicated that 15% of difficult intubations were also associated with difficult mask ventilation.[10] In an evaluation of 22 600 attempts at mask ventilation at the University of Michigan, 1.4% (313 cases) were difficult to ventilate, and 0.16% (37 cases) were impossible to ventilate. Of the difficult and impossible to mask ventilate cases, 0.37% (84 cases) were also observed to be a difficult intubation. Of the 37 impossible to ventilate cases, only 1 patient required surgical airway access.[11]

Approximately 30% to 50% of all anesthetic deaths have been attributed to the inability to manage a difficult airway.[12] The ability to predict difficulty with ventilation and intubation accurately would help minimize disasters related to airway management. Unfortunately, the positive identification of all difficult airways is not currently possible. The coexistence of difficult ventilation is even more difficult to predict accurately.

Difficult airway management results from anatomic extremes or diseases affecting the airway. These factors may prevent a good mask fit, adequate positioning of a supraglottic airway, proper positioning of the head and neck, and opening of the mouth. Inability to ventilate the lungs or intubate the trachea may of course also result from poor technique and/or lack of technical expertise.[13]

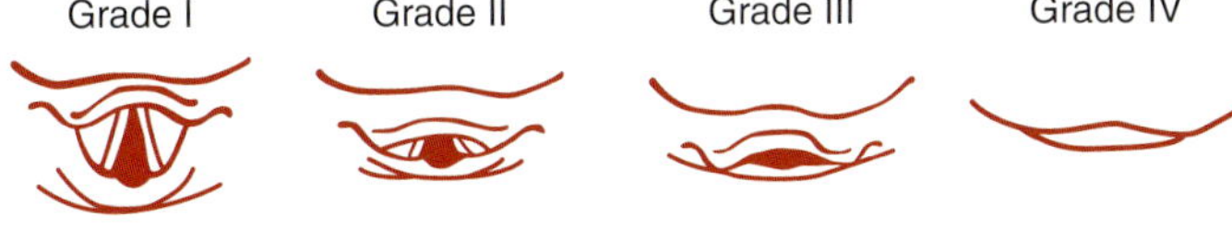

FIGURE 10-1. Laryngoscopic views obtained per Cormack and Lehane.

GRADING THE DIFFICULTY OF TRACHEAL INTUBATION

Cormack and Lehane developed a classification for the view obtained at laryngoscopy.[14] This classification uses four grades as follows: grade I, a full view of glottis; grade II, only the posterior commissure is visible; grade III, only the tip of the epiglottis is visible; grade IV, no glottic structures are visible (**Fig. 10-1**). Use of the original Cormack and Lehane scoring system led Yentis and Lee to develop a modified Cormack and Lehane scoring system in which grade II (only part of the glottis visible) was divided into IIa (part of the cords are visible) and IIb (only the arytenoids or the very posterior origin of the cords are visible) (**Fig. 10-2**).[15] In this system, grade IIb denotes a laryngoscopic view that is relatively common and often associated with difficulty passing a tracheal tube. This system is now frequently used for recording the ease or difficulty in laryngoscopic view in the anesthetic record and in studies of tracheal intubation.

The Intubation Difficulty Scale (IDS) is another tool used in airway research that can be a useful indicator of total intubation difficulty in a prior intubation.[16,17] The IDS is a quantitative measure of the total intubation difficulty encountered during a chosen procedure or sequence of procedures and is calculated after the fact. The score is based on 7 parameters known to be associated with difficult intubation. The 7 parameters are number of supplementary attempts, number of supplementary operators, number and type of alternative techniques used, laryngoscopic grade, subjective lifting force, the use of external laryngeal manipulation, and mobility or position of the vocal cords. The scoring of each individual parameter represents a divergence from ideal, and the total score represents the sum divergence from a zero difficulty, ideal intubation.

Patients with difficult tracheal intubation can be categorized into 3 groups (**Box 10-1**). The first group consists of patients in whom tracheal intubation is known or expected to be difficult. The second group includes patients with external anatomic features indicative of probable airway difficulties. The third group includes patients who present no external anatomic evidence or history of a difficult airway but nonetheless prove to be difficult.

BOX 10-1

Categories of Difficult Airway

- Known or expected difficult airway
  - History of difficult or failed intubation
  - History of difficult or failed mask ventilation
  - Conditions associated with difficult airway
    - Acquired
    - Congenital
- Potentially difficult airway
  - Limited neck extension
  - Limited mouth opening
  - Receding mandible
  - Mallampati class III or IV
  - Short thyromental distance
- Unexpected difficult airway
  - Unknown supraepiglottic mass
    - Hyperplasia of lingual tonsils
    - Supraepiglottic cyst or tumor
  - Missed evidence of difficult airway
    - Poor preoperative evaluation
    - Ignoring presence of evidence

EVALUATION OF THE POTENTIALLY DIFFICULT AIRWAY

These patients have anatomic variations that may interfere with rigid laryngoscopy and tracheal intubation. The failure to identify these patients correctly may lead to an improper anesthetic induction plan and an unexpected failed intubation. If ventilation proves impossible, a life-threatening emergency is created.

To identify patients with potentially difficult-to-manage airways, a careful history regarding patient breathing, sleep position, and voice quality is taken. During physical examination, the patient should be viewed from a frontal and profile view to assess mandibular size. Thyromental distance is measured, and neck rotation, flexion, and extension mobility are evaluated and graded. The neck is palpated for identification of the cricothyroid membrane. Additionally, one should check for TMJ problems, mouth opening, loose or protruding teeth,

Original Cormack and Lehane system	I Full view of the glottis	II Partial view of the glottis or arytenoids		III Only epiglottis visible	IV Neither glottis nor epiglottis visible
View at laryngoscopy	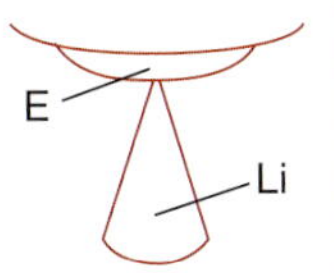 E Li	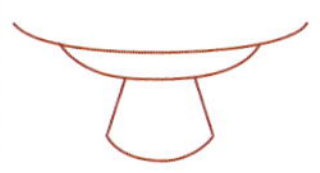	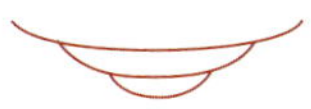	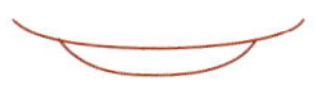	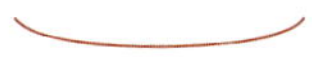
Modified system	I As for original Cormack and Lehane above	IIa Partial view of the glottis	IIb Arytenoids or posterior part of the vocal cords only just visible	III As for original Cormack and Lehane above	IV As for original Cormack and Lehane above

FIGURE 10-2. Original versus modified Cormack and Lehane scoring system: Description of the two scoring systems used for recording laryngoscopy view. E, epiglottis; Li, laryngeal inlet.

BOX 10-2

Tests Applied to Predict Difficult Intubation

External anatomic features

Head and neck movement (atlantooccipital joint)

Jaw movement (temporomandibular joint)

- Mouth opening
- Subluxation of mandible

Receding mandible

Protruding maxillary incisors

Obesity

Thyromental distance

Sternomental distance

Visualization of the oropharyngeal structures

Anterior tilt of larynx

Radiographic assessment

TABLE 10-1 Five Risk Factors of Difficult Intubation

Risk Factor	Level of Risk
Weight	
<90 kg	0
90-110 kg	1
>110 kg	2
Head and neck movement	
>90°	0
~90°	1
<90°	2
Jaw movement	
Interincisor gap (IG) measured with mouth fully open	
Subluxation (SLux) (maximal forward protrusion of the lower incisors beyond the upper incisors)	
IG >5 cm or SLux > 0	0
IG <5 cm or SLux = 0	1
IG <5 cm or SLux < 0	2
Receding mandible	
Normal	0
Moderate	1
Severe	2
Protruding maxillary anterior teeth	
Normal	0
Moderate	1
Severe	2

From Wilson ME, Spiegelhalter D, Robertson JA, et al. Predicting difficult intubation. *Br J Anaesth.* 1988;61:211. The Board of Management and Trustees of the British Journal of Anesthesia. Reproduced by permission of Oxford University Press/British Journal of Anesthesia.

degree of overbite, size of the tongue, visibility of faucial structures, and patency of the nares.

A number of predictive tests have been described that detect potentially difficult intubation (**Box 10-2**). These clinical examinations are straightforward and can be done at the bedside. Although useful in airway evaluation, all these tests are associated with relatively high rates of false-positive and false-negative predictions (**Box 10-3**).

ANATOMIC CONSIDERATIONS

In the early development of rigid laryngoscopy, certain anatomic features were recognized as contributing to the difficulty of intubation.[18] These features included a recessed mandible, limited extension of the head and neck, limited mouth opening, and mandibular depth.

Five physical features were evaluated prospectively by Wilson et al in an attempt to identify potentially difficult intubations (**Table 10-1**).[6] Each risk factor was given three possible scores (0, 1, or 2). A total score of greater than 2 predicted a 75% chance of difficult intubation but with a significant incidence of false-positive results. Changing the prediction criteria to a score of greater than 4 reduced the number of false-positive results but also increased the incidence of false-negative predictions. In this study of 778 patients, 1.5% of rigid laryngoscopies were found to be difficult.

Atlantooccipital Mobility Adequate cervical mobility and mouth opening are essential for alignment of the oral, pharyngeal, and laryngeal axes required for visualization of the glottis during rigid laryngoscopy.[18,19] Decreased neck mobility also limits maneuvers that can be used to keep the airway open, thereby predisposing to difficult mask ventilation.

Evaluation of atlantooccipital extension is performed by having the patient sit straight and extend the head while maintaining the cervical spine in a neutral position.[19] The greater the atlantooccipital distance in the neutral position, the greater the possible degree of head extension. A reduction in atlantooccipital extension by a third or more will contribute to the difficulty of intubation.[19] If the posterior tubercle of the atlas is in contact with the occiput in the neutral position, attempts to extend the head result in anterior bowing of the cervical spine and forward displacement of the larynx.[20] Limitations in head extension may occur secondary to anatomic variations of the atlantooccipital gap in otherwise healthy people or secondary to pathologic conditions such as rheumatoid arthritis.

BOX 10-3

Shortcomings of Tests Predicting Difficult Intubation

High incidence of false-positive results

High incidence of false-negative results

Do not address lower airway problems

Do not address mask ventilation difficulties

Miss lingual tonsil as cause of failed intubation

Mouth Opening, Dentition, Mandibular Space In addition to head and neck extension, other anatomic factors may interfere with the line of vision from the mouth opening to the vocal cords. The hinge movement of the mandible controls mouth opening. A horizontal gliding movement allows for subluxation of the mandible, which allows additional anterior displacement of the tongue during rigid laryngoscopy. A mouth opening (distance between mandibular and maxillary central incisors) limited to 3.5 cm or less tends to make intubation more difficult. TMJ dysfunction, congenital fusion of the joints, trauma, tissue contracture around the mouth, and trismus may limit mouth opening. Trismus secondary to pain associated with infection usually relaxes under general anesthesia, but this cannot be assured if the infection has been long standing or involves the pterygoid space.

In addition, protruding maxillary anterior teeth may interfere with laryngoscope placement and passage of the endotracheal tube during intubation.

During rigid laryngoscopy, the tongue is displaced into the mandibular space, opening the line of vision from mouth to the larynx. A small mandibular space may fail to accommodate tongue displacement adequately, thus interfering with visualization of the larynx.

Thyromental Distance Patil et al reported that rigid laryngoscopy may be impossible in adults if the thyromental distance (TMD) is less than 6.0 cm (3 finger breadths).[21] Practitioners are cautioned that when measuring TMD, the use of a paper ruler is preferred over the traditional thought that 3 finger breadths equal 6.0 cm unless one has checked which distal interphalangeal joint combination equals 6 cm. This distance may be 3 fingers on those with larger hands and 4 fingers on those with narrow fingers.[22] Alignment is more difficult in the patient with a receding mandible where the TMD short, as the laryngeal axis forms a more acute angle with the pharyngeal axis. The TMD is measured between the bony point of the mentum of the mandible and the thyroid notch with the head fully extended. Maximum extension of the head ensures reproducibility of measurements.

Sternomental Distance The sternomental distance is measured with the head fully extended and the mouth closed. This measurement is reported to be more sensitive and specific in predicting difficult rigid laryngoscopy than the Mallampati test, TMD, mouth opening, and mandibular subluxation measurements.[5] The predictive value of sternomental distance regarding difficult intubation has not been studied by other investigators.

VISIBILITY OF OROPHARYNGEAL STRUCTURES

Predicting probability of difficult laryngoscopy by physical evaluation was reported by Skolimowski et al in 1975 when describing a micrognathic patient who could not be intubated: "The anteroposterior dimension of the pharynx was markedly reduced by a large tongue reaching far posteriorly. It was not possible to examine the lower pharynx by means of a laryngoscope mirror because the tongue was situated too far posteriorly to be pulled forward."[23]

Mallampati described the examination signs and related them to intubation difficulty. He correlated the degree of visibility of the oropharyngeal structures with the difficulty of rigid laryngoscopy.[24] In this study, a sitting patient was asked to open his or her mouth as wide as possible and maximally protrude the tongue. The visibility of the faucial pillars, soft palate, and uvula was noted. The airway was classified into 3 categories: class I, soft palate, fauces, uvula, and pillars are visualized; class II, soft palate, fauces, and pillars are visualized, but the uvula is masked by the base of the tongue; and class III, only the soft palate can be visualized. In class III, visualization of the glottis with rigid laryngoscopy is expected to be difficult.[24] Samsoon and Young extended the oropharyngeal exposures to include a fourth class.[4] This four-category system is in common use and classified as follows: class I, soft palate, fauces, uvula, and pillars are visualized; class II, soft palate, fauces, uvula are seen; class III, only the soft palate and base of the uvula are observed; class IV, the soft palate is not visible (**Fig. 10-3**). A further modification of the Mallampati visualization scoring included a class 0 view.[25,26] Class 0 is defined as the ability to see any part of the epiglottis upon mouth opening and tongue protrusion. Ezri et al evaluated 764 patients and reported that 1.18% of patients had a class zero airway.[27] A class 0 airway was noted to be an excellent predictor of uncomplicated laryngoscopy.

In a retrospective study of 13 patients with failed intubations, Samsoon and Young found that in 12 of the patients there was a good correlation between the degree of difficulty of tracheal intubation and the visibility of the oropharyngeal structures.[4] Rocke et al reported the association between Mallampati class and difficulty of intubation to be significant (p <0.001), but only 6.6% of class IV airway cases were associated with difficult tracheal intubation, and all could be intubated.[8] Using the concept of relative risk, they calculated the probability of difficult intubation. The presence of class III airway was associated with a relative risk of 7.58 times greater than class I, and airway class IV had a relative risk of 11.2 times greater than class I. Oates et al compared Mallampati's classification with that of Wilson's 5 risk factors.[28] The predictive value of both tests was found to be similar, but both tests had a high incidence of false-positive and false-negative predictors. Interobserver variability was less with Wilson's scoring system. Other investigators have found Mallampati's classification too subjective and the class III classification not useful as a predictor of difficult intubation when used alone.[29-31]

Phonation during tongue protrusion increases the specificity of the Mallampati test, thus improving its correlation with difficult intubation, but also increases the number of false-negative results.[30] Tham et al reported that phonation created a marked improvement in view.[32] Evaluation of the airway in the supine position produced a small but nonsignificant worsening of the view. Lewis et al recommended that the visibility of oropharyngeal tissues be conducted with the patient in the sitting position, with the head in full extension, the tongue out, and during phonation.[33]

In a retrospective review of failed intubations by Samsoon and Young, 7 of 1980 obstetric patients could not be intubated (incidence of 1 in 280) and 6 of 13380 surgical patients could not be intubated (incidence of 1 in 2230).[4] All patients had a class IV airway except one class II patient who had tracheal stenosis. These authors believed that preanesthetic assessment using the Mallampati classification had merit. Lee et al used the Cormack and Lehane grading system in their systematic meta-analysis review of the accuracy of Mallampati tests to predict the difficult airway.[34] In their review of 42 studies involving 34513 patients, they found that both versions of the Mallampati test had good accuracy for predicting difficult laryngoscopy. The modified Mallampati score had good accuracy, but the original Mallampati had poor accuracy in predicting difficult tracheal intubation. Both versions of Mallampati score were poor at identifying difficult mask ventilation. The authors concluded that to be useful the Mallampati test must be part of a comprehensive evaluation that also includes assessment of dentition, TMD, and neck extension, as recommended by the ASA Task Force on the management of the difficult airway.[1]

In summary, the Mallampati test has been broadly applied, even though its predictive value for difficult intubation is low. As a result, some essential factors, such as suppleness and mobility of the neck or dentition status, may be minimized. No single test is perfect, but this should not discourage practitioners from seeking a more reliable test or combination of tests, especially as most currently used tests require only a minimal amount of time during the physical examination.[35]

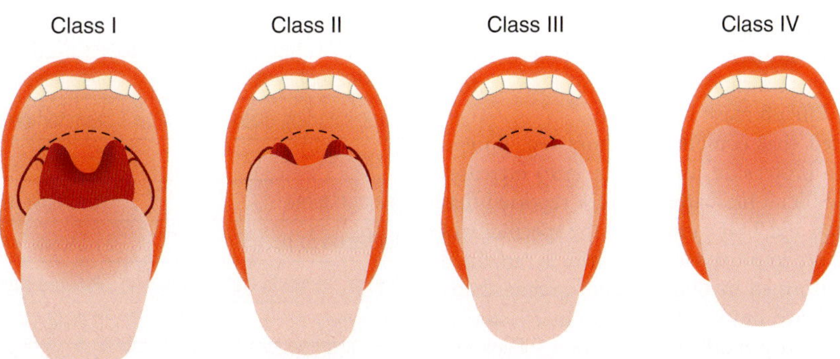

FIGURE 10-3. Classification of pharyngeal structures as proposed by Mallampati and Samsoon. Note: Class III, soft palate visible; class IV, soft palate not visible.

ANTERIORLY TILTED LARYNX

Roberts et al measured the degree of anterior tilt of the thyroid cartilage relative to the horizontal and demonstrated a relationship between degree of the thyroid cartilage tilt and the difficulty of laryngeal exposure using a Macintosh laryngoscope.[36] Laryngeal tilt can be directly measured using a bubble inclinometer. When the tilt of the anterior surface of the thyroid cartilage is greater than 40°, rigid laryngoscopy was predicted to be difficult. The sensitivity of this test was reported to be 70%, with a specificity of 95% and a positive predictive value of 80%. Anterior laryngeal tilt is reduced by depression of the thyroid cartilage but is increased by cricoid pressure.

DIRECT VISUALIZATION ASSESSMENT

Upper airway endoscopy preoperatively using topical anesthesia for patient comfort provides excellent information in defining anatomic challenges in patients with upper airway pathology. The fiberoptic nasopharyngeal scope and the pediatric bronchoscope have been the standard for this evaluation. The classic rigid laryngoscope has not been as useful due to patient discomfort when it is used. However, newer model videolaryngoscopes may be used due to their ability to visualize the oropharyngeal and supraglottic regions more comfortably.

RADIOGRAPHIC ASSESSMENT

Lateral radiographs of the head and neck and the measurement of distances between bony landmarks have been used to identify predictive factors for difficult rigid laryngoscopy.[37] Reduction in the distance between the occiput and the spinous process of C1 (atlantooccipital distance), and to the C1-C2 interspinous gap, has been correlated with the degree of difficulty in intubation. Reduction in the atlantooccipital gap may be found in some otherwise normal cases. Any limitation of cervical extension may interfere with rigid laryngoscopy and glottic exposure. Radiographic assessment is not considered cost-effective for routine airway evaluation.

MULTIPLE FACTORS

Combining several tests for the prediction of difficult laryngoscopy and tracheal intubation improves the accuracy of the assessment. The simplified airway risk index (SARI) was developed to evaluate airway status preoperatively using multiple factors: mouth opening measurement, TMD, ability to protrude the mandible, Mallampati class, head mobility, and body weight.[38] Calculation of the SARI in 136 patients revealed good interobserver agreement in assessing the Mallampati classification, mouth opening, and mandible protrusion. However, because there are more variables in measuring the TMD and evaluating neck mobility, there was not good interobserver agreement with these factors.[39]

Multiple factors often play roles in both difficulty with intubation and difficulty with mask ventilation. In a prospective study of 1502 patients, difficult mask ventilation was reported in 5%, with one occurrence of impossible ventilation.[40] Difficulty with mask ventilation was anticipated by the anesthesiologist in only 17% of the cases in which difficulty occurred. Using multivariate analysis, 5 criteria were recognized as independent factors for difficult mask ventilation: age older than 55 years, body mass index (BMI) greater than 26 kg/m^2, presence of a beard, lack of teeth, and a history of snoring. The presence of two factors suggested a high likelihood of difficult mask ventilation.

Bellhouse and Dore reported that combining factors (eg, limited atlantooccipital extension, chin protrusion, and tongue size) increases the sensitivity of predicting a difficult intubation.[19] Frerk reported that combining two tests, Mallampati and TMD, improved the specificity of the prediction to 97.8% but did not improve sensitivity, which remained at 81.2%.[41] A meta-analysis performed by Shiga et al of preanesthetic airway evaluation test performance on 50760 patients in 35 studies demonstrated a 5.8% overall incidence of difficult intubation.[42] Each test in their analysis, including the Mallampati classification, TMD, sternomental distance, mouth opening, and the Wilson risk score,[6] possessed only poor to moderate sensitivity and moderate to fair specificity. The most useful evaluations were found to be combinations of the Mallampati classification and TMD distance. These authors concluded that the clinical value of airway evaluation tests for predicting difficult intubation remains limited.

A stepwise approach to decision making in the evaluation of the airway is the airway approach algorithm.[43] This algorithm is based on 5 clinical questions: Is airway control necessary? Is there potential for difficult laryngoscopy? Can supralaryngeal ventilation be used? Is there an aspiration risk? Will the patient tolerate an apneic period? Answers to these basic questions can help guide the practitioner in potential use of the ASA difficult airway algorithm.

EVALUATION OF THE COMPLEX AIRWAY

Patients with a history of difficult ventilation or intubation and patients with anatomic or abnormal conditions associated with a complex airway fall into the category of known difficult airway.[44] The causes of the expected difficult airway may be grouped into congenital or acquired conditions and be further classified on the basis of the location of involvement or disease.

Increased frequency of ventilation, chest retractions, increased use of accessory muscles, stridor, voice weakness, or hoarseness, alone or in combination, may indicate a potential airway problem (**Table 10-2**). Stridor is a particularly important sign and may provide evidence of the site and severity of airway obstruction related to severe oropharyngeal, glottic, and/or upper tracheal occlusion. Stridor during inspiration generally indicates obstruction at or above the larynx. Expiratory stridor is most often associated with intrathoracic or subglottic obstructions. Obstruction associated with the larynx or glottic region may produce biphasic stridor, although either inspiratory or expiratory sounds may predominate. In the adult, stridor at rest indicates a serious degree of obstruction with a cross-sectional airway opening of less than 4 mm or an irregularly narrowed airway several centimeters in length.

OBESITY

Airway assessment of the obese patient should be performed with the patient in both the sitting and supine positions. Respiratory function and airway patency can be significantly altered by this change in position.[45] A large neck circumference is associated with obstructive sleep apnea (OSA) in obese patients. In evaluating 123 patients with thick necks for OSA, Katz et al found that the sleep apnea-hypopnea index correlated with external neck circumference, BMI, and the internal circumference of the distal pharynx.[46] Men more commonly have sleep-disordered breathing than women, and the sleep-disordered breathing

TABLE 10-2 History Findings That Suggest Difficult Airway Management

Finding	Implication
Dry cough	Possible tracheobronchial compression
Easy bleeding	Epistaxis risk
Gastroesophageal reflux	Aspiration risk
Long-standing diabetes mellitus	Limited cervical mobility
Loud snoring	Prone to soft tissue obstruction
Major trauma	Unstable neck, limiting safe mobility
Radiation to neck	Fibrosis, immobility
Recent temporal craniotomy	Limited mandibular motility
Smoking	Salivation, cough, laryngospasm
Undigested food returning to mouth	Aspiration risk from pharyngeal pouch

tends to be more severe.[47] In an evaluation of 3942 OSA patients, the frequency and severity of OSA in the sleep clinic population was found to be greater in men than women, with unknown factors other than neck circumference, age, and BMI contributing to the gender differences.[48] In a prospective study of 100 morbidly obese patients (BMI >40 kg/m^2), preoperative measurements of height, weight, neck circumference, width of mouth opening, sternomental distance, TMD, and Mallampati score were recorded.[49] The view during direct laryngoscopy was graded, and the number of attempts at tracheal intubation was recorded. Neither absolute obesity nor BMI was associated with intubation difficulties. Large neck circumference and high Mallampati score were the only predictors of potential intubation problems.

In the supine position, changes in chest compliance and vital capacity may interfere with adequate spontaneous ventilation. The incidence of hiatal hernia, gastric pH of 2.5 or lower, and reduced functional residual capacity found in obese patients places these patients at increased risk for the consequences of aspiration of gastric contents.[50,51] To minimize the risk of aspiration, a rapid sequence induction is commonly performed in obese patients.

There is consensus that airway management is more difficult in the morbidly obese patients. Opinions differ, however, on the difficulty of endotracheal intubation. Wilson and coworkers regarded obesity as a weak predictor of difficult intubation.[6] Buckley et al reported a 13% rate of difficult intubation using a rapid sequence technique in the obese patient.[51] Rocke et al excluded obesity as a risk factor in intubation.[8] Bond found no correlation between BMI and difficulty of laryngoscopy.[50] Juvin et al compared difficulty in tracheal intubation in obese to lean patients using the IDS and patient vital signs.[52] A Mallampati score of III-IV was the only independent risk factor for difficult intubation in obese patients. Difficult tracheal intubation was more frequent in obese (15.5%) than lean (2.2%) patients. The use of the IDS score demonstrated that tracheal intubation, not laryngoscopy, was more difficult in obese than lean patients.

Body weight may not be as critical as the location of excess weight. Massive weight in the lower abdomen and hip area may be less important than when the weight is in the upper body area. A short, thick, immobile neck caused by cervical spine fat pads will interfere with rigid laryngoscopy. Furthermore, the redundancy of soft tissue structures inside the oropharyngeal and supralaryngeal area may also make visualization of the laryngeal structures difficult.

Mask ventilation may prove difficult in the obese patient. When high positive pressure is required to ventilate the patient, the chance of inflating the stomach is increased. Rapid oxygen desaturation during apnea, secondary to reduced functional residual capacity, limits available intubation time. In the case of the cannot intubate, cannot ventilate situation, access to the neck for transtracheal jet ventilation or establishing a surgical airway (eg, emergency tracheostomy or cricothyroidotomy) will also be more complex.

PREGNANCY

The incidence of failed intubation is predicted as 1 in 300 patients undergoing cesarean delivery.[4] Airway-related problems account for a third of all anesthetic-related maternal mortality.[53] During pregnancy, mucosal vascular engorgement, laryngeal edema, immobility of the floor of the mouth related to tongue engorgement, enlarged breasts, and general weight gain contribute to difficult intubation.[53-55]

Airway anatomy may become distorted during prolonged labor or toxemia, leading to edematous soft tissue encroachment of the upper airway.[54,55] Nasal intubation in these patients should be avoided because the mucous membranes become increasingly engorged and friable during late pregnancy. Similar to the obese patient, the obstetric patient should be considered to have a full stomach and at increased risk for gastric aspiration.

The physical changes created by pregnancy may lead to marked alteration in cardiovascular and respiratory function when the patient changes from a sitting to a supine position. Furthermore, in cases of fetal distress or maternal hemorrhage, the emergency nature of the circumstances compounds airway management problems.

RHEUMATOID ARTHRITIS

The airway management of these patients should be based on an understanding of the pathologic changes affecting the airway. In patients with advanced rheumatoid arthritis and spondylosis, airway management may be extremely difficult. Rheumatoid arthritis may involve any joint of the body, including the cervical spine, TMJ, and cricoarytenoid joint. A change in voice, the presence of dysphagia, dysarthria, stridor, or a sense of fullness in the oropharynx may indicate laryngeal involvement. A careful fiberoptic examination of the larynx and glottic structures may be informative when such signs and symptoms are present. An edematous larynx with hyperemic arytenoids and/or mucosa with swollen aryepiglottic folds and false cords may be observed. Changes in phonation may be associated with decreased mobility of the vocal cords. In the case of a narrowed glottic opening, endotracheal intubation frequently requires a smaller sized endotracheal tube. TMJ ankylosis may prevent orotracheal intubation because of limited mouth opening.

Physical examination of the patient with rheumatoid arthritis should include flexion, extension, and rotation of the head with palpation of the larynx and trachea for evidence of deviation and/or limitation. Upper-extremity radiculopathy suggests cervical spine arthritis. Progressive cervical spondylosis associated with rheumatoid arthritis leads to severe flexion deformity of the cervical spine, which complicates airway management.[56] Synovial destruction and vertebral erosion, along with ligamentous changes, lead to instability of the cervical spine.[57] Instability of the atlas and odontoid or of subaxial vertebral alignments may lead to subluxation of the cervical spine and cord compression. Cervical spine flexion and extension radiographs may be required for evaluation of instability and potential spinal cord compression. Although chin lift and jaw thrust are commonly used to improve mask ventilation and oxygenation, these maneuvers may increase the possibility of spinal cord compression and damage.[58] If a head and neck stabilizing device is used by the patient, it generally should be left in place to prevent unintended movement of the cervical spine.[59] Chest wall distortion in patients with rheumatoid arthritis may produce a major decrease in total lung volume and vital capacity. Pulmonary function tests may be helpful in determining a patient's ventilatory status in some cases.

CONGENITAL DISEASE

Anomalies of the cardiovascular, nervous, musculocutaneous, endocrine, or excretory systems may produce abnormalities of the head, neck, or upper airway. Rosenberg and Rosenberg have tabulated the syndromes most often accompanied by aberrations of the upper airway.[44] These include Crouzon, Goldenhar, Pierre Robin, and Treacher Collins syndromes, which are known for their grossly abnormal head and neck anatomy. Patients with congenital malformations associated with micrognathia, retrognathia, and macroglossia have a smaller oropharyngeal cross section and are prone to soft-tissue upper-airway obstruction.[54,60] Children with craniocarpotarsal dysplasia have severe microstomia that becomes more inadequate as they grow older and develop teeth. These children often require repeated anesthetics for correction of their musculoskeletal and soft tissue deformities and can pose a significant problem for the anesthesiologist.

The most significant vascular malformations related to airway compromise are vascular rings, usually of aortic arch origin, encircling the trachea. Tracheomalacia, congenital tracheal stenosis, shortened trachea, and bronchogenic cysts can contribute to difficult airway management (**Fig. 10-4**).[61] Wells et al reported that a significant percentage of infants with congenital malformation syndromes associated with cardiovascular anomalies and skeletal dysplasia have a shortened trachea.[62] These infants may benefit from fiberoptic evaluation of endotracheal tube position to avoid unrecognized bronchial intubation.

Acromegaly, the syndrome that results from the pituitary gland producing excess growth hormone after epiphyseal plate closure at puberty, requires careful airway evaluation. This condition is seldom seen today in the United States due to early diagnosis and management. Most

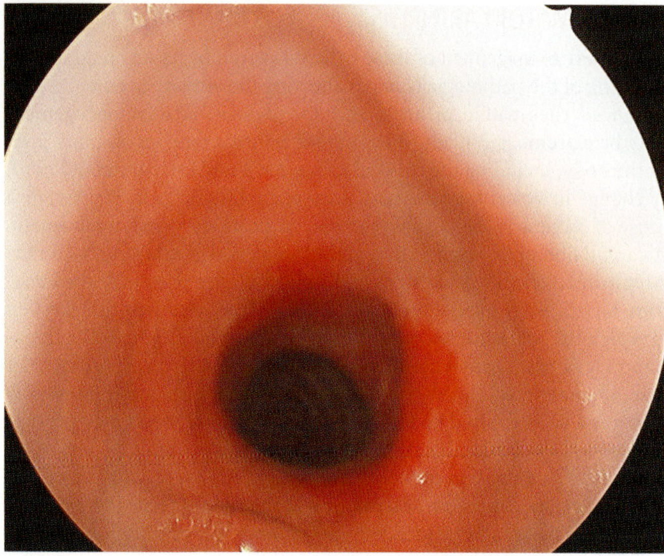

A

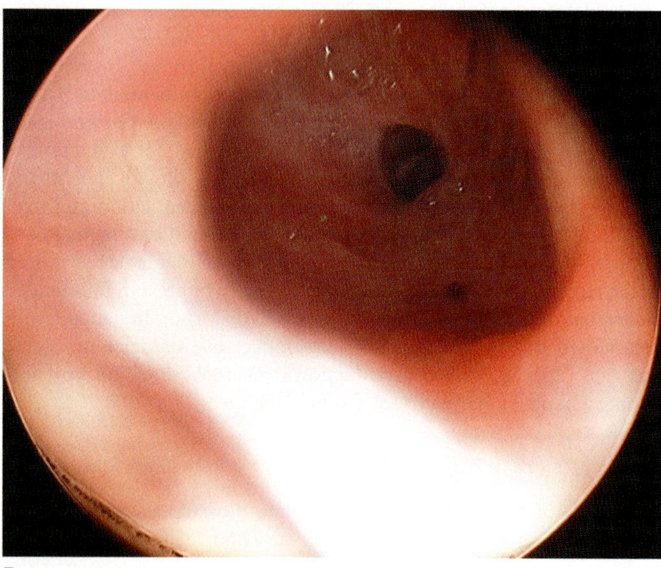

B

FIGURE 10-4. **A, B.** Tracheal stenosis.

patients with acromegaly have poor Mallampati grade due to soft tissue overgrowth and macroglossia. The practitioner may also wish to include evaluation of growth hormone levels and duration of disease symptoms in evaluation of cases with this condition.[63, 64] Congenital malformation syndromes also may be associated with varying degrees of acute, progressive, or chronic airway obstruction. Congenital tumors or cysts may invade or obstruct the airway. Preoperative assessment should include determination of the site of the tumor and the extent of obstruction or distortion of the airway.

AIRWAY INFECTION

Inflammation and edema can distort anatomy, fix soft tissues, and compress the airway, interfering with ventilation and intubation.[65,66] Airway compromise by infection poses a major airway management problem in patients younger than 10 years. Of 90 deaths resulting from upper airway obstruction in children, 36 were related to airway infections (**Fig. 10-5**).[67, 68] Anesthetists are most often involved in the management of urgent conditions such as peritonsillar abscess, retropharyngeal abscess, submandibular abscess, Ludwig angina, croup, and epiglottitis. Each of these infections presents in a specific manner, which then dictates airway management.

Peritonsillar Space Infections The peritonsillar space is a potential space located at the junction of the oral cavity and oropharynx. It is formed by the palatine tonsil, as well as the palatoglossus, palatopharyngeal, and superior pharyngeal constrictor muscles. Clinical findings of peritonsillar abscess include acute onset of fever, pain, dysphagia, and cervical adenopathy. As the infection spreads, it may involve the muscles of mastication, producing trismus secondary to pain and spasm. On examination, there is displacement of the uvula to the contralateral side, tonsillar enlargement, and fetid breath. At times, surgical drainage of the peritonsillar space is indicated. Management of the airway in this subset of patients is generally accomplished with orotracheal intubation. Rapid sequence intubation is generally possible. Reduced interdental distance that may be noted on preoperative evaluation of these patients is due to pain and usually resolves on administering anesthetic agents.

Retropharyngeal Space Infections/Prevertebral Space Infections The retropharyngeal space is a midline compartment located between the middle and deep cervical fascia. The prevertebral space is a bilateral space located posterior to the deep cervical fascia. Infection of the retropharyngeal space most commonly occurs in children and presents with irritability, fever, dysphagia, muffled speech or cry, noisy breathing, stiff neck, and cervical adenopathy.[69] Prevertebral space infection is much less common and is seen after spread of retropharyngeal abscess or more rarely primary infection of the prevertebral space. Airway management in these infections typically uses endotracheal intubation or tracheotomy. During laryngoscopy after induction, the posterior pharyngeal wall appears displaced anteriorly. Care must be taken to avoid lacerating and draining a posterior pharyngeal wall abscess with subsequent aspiration before the airway is controlled.

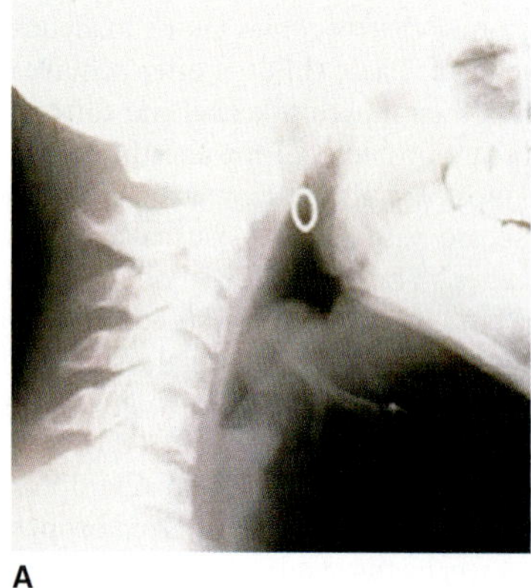

A

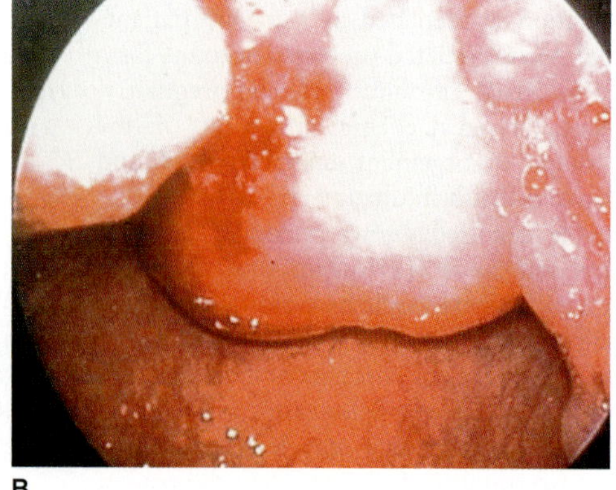

B

FIGURE 10-5. **A:** Epiglottis lateral radiograph. **B:** Afebrile fungal epiglottitis. [Photo courtesy of Dr. Dana M. Thompson, Department of Otolaryngology, Mayo Clinic, Rochester, Minnesota.]

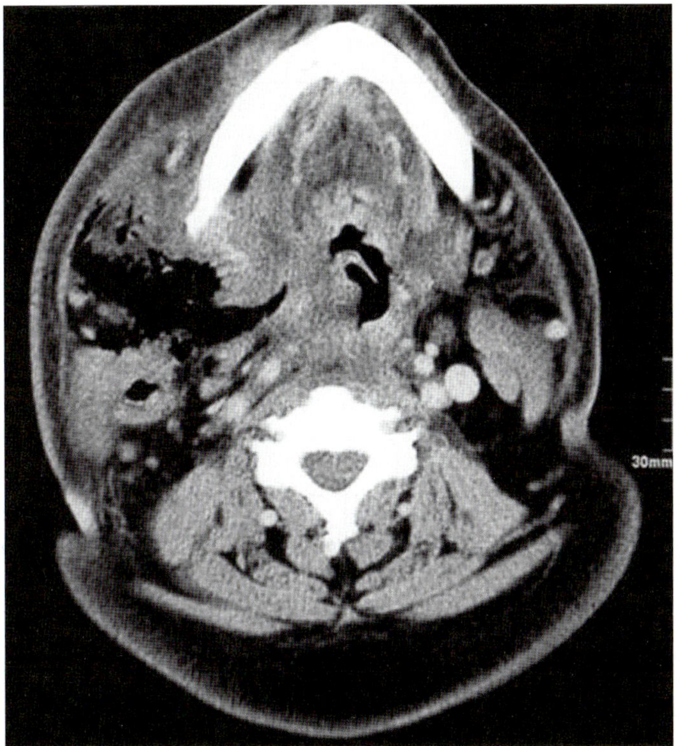

FIGURE 10-6. Computed tomography scan of patient with Ludwig angina.

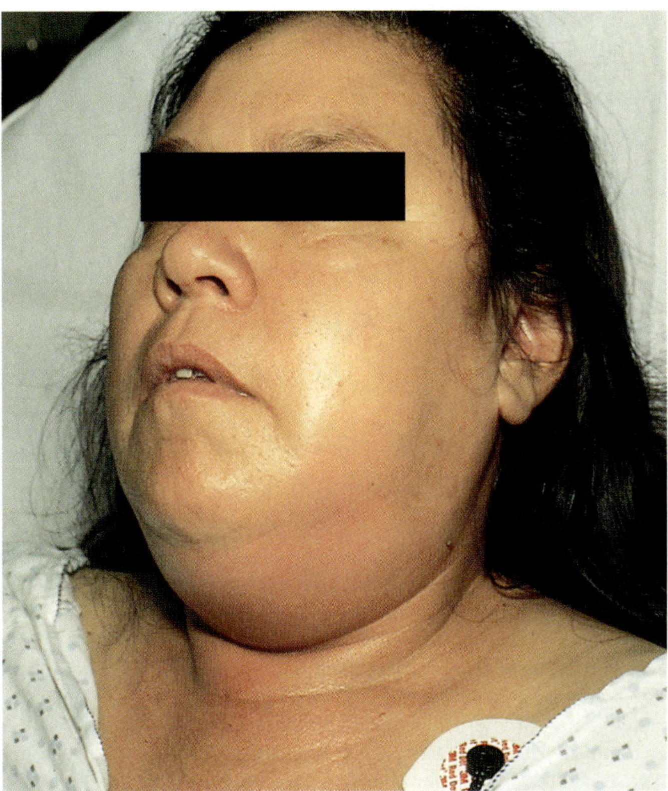

FIGURE 10-7. Ludwig angina. [Courtesy of Jeffrey Finkelstein, MD. From: Knoop KJ, Stack LW, Storrow AB, et al. *The Atlas of Emergency Medicine.* 3rd ed. New York, NY: McGraw-Hill; 2010.]

Ludwig Angina/Submandibular Space Infection that arises in this space may be odontogenic in origin or due to chronic sialadenitis. The submandibular space is divided by the mylohyoid muscle. Infection localized above the mylohyoid muscle creates edema and distortion of the floor of the mouth. Upper airway endoscopy with a standard or videolaryngoscope and/or fiberoptic bronchoscope is useful in defining anatomic challenges in patients with upper airway pathology before induction of general anesthesia.

An infection inferior to the mylohyoid muscle may displace the base of tongue posteriorly. Ludwig angina is typically seen in patient with poor oral hygiene and presents as a bilateral neck cellulitis with displacement and swelling of the tongue base and floor of mouth. (**Figs. 10-6 and 10-7**). Both submandibular space infection and Ludwig angina present with acute onset of fever, dysphagia, pain, and swelling. The airway is best managed in these cases in a collaborative manner with the surgical team.

Epiglottitis With the advent of the haemophilus influenza B vaccine in 1991, the incidence of epiglottitis has precipitously decreased by 90%. Although uncommon today, acute epiglottitis does occasionally present, particularly in the pediatric population, with a rapid onset of high fever, respiratory distress, drooling, and painful swallowing. On examination patients are noted to have tachycardia, tachypnea, and appear toxic. On phonation, a muffled quality may be appreciated.[70] This classic presentation was often seen in the pediatric population before the introduction of the Hib vaccine. In the adult population, acute epiglottitis may be preceded by a viral upper respiratory infection. Noninfectious causes of epiglottitis may also be seen after thermal injury or caustic ingestion. Thermal injury after crack cocaine abuse is not infrequent. Once again, the airway is best managed in these cases in a collaborative manner with the surgical team. Any manipulation of the airway prior to intubation should generally be avoided.

Croup Acute croup, or laryngotracheobronchitis, is often caused by the parainfluenza virus in children between the ages of 1 and 3, particularly in the spring and fall. Children typically present with low-grade fever, increased respiratory rate, barky cough, and hoarseness.[70] Most children can be managed without intubation. When retraction or oxygen desaturation is noted, orotracheal intubation is indicated with an appropriate-size endotracheal tube.

Trauma Trauma to the head and neck may produce major acute or chronic anatomic changes. These changes may affect airway accessibility, making tracheal intubation or mask ventilation difficult. Blunt or penetrating trauma to the larynx, trachea, hyoid structure, and facial bones can result in a complex, difficult-to-manage airway.[71,72] Subcutaneous emphysema, hoarseness, stridor, and tracheal deviation are warning signs of airway injury. Such patients should be observed closely because progression of the condition may lead to airway obstruction.

The signs and symptoms of laryngeal trauma may be quite subtle. Patients with laryngeal trauma are often hoarse or short of breath, although this clinical presentation may not correlate with the severity of injury. Dysphagia is not a common symptom of laryngotracheal injury. Nevertheless, esophageal injury should be strongly considered in patients with laryngotracheal trauma. On physical examination, the presence of hemoptysis may indicate laryngeal or tracheal injury. External palpation of the neck should include evaluation of the hyoid bone, and thyroid and cricoid cartilages (**Fig. 10-8**). The skin should be examined for abrasions and subcutaneous air. Open wounds should not be probed, but entrance and exit wounds should be noted to better understand the trajectory of the injury, particularly with bullet wounds. Cricotracheal separation should be suspected when the mechanism of injury is via a "clothesline" or hanging injury. In these patients, stridor and subcutaneous emphysema should prompt immediate evaluation. Orotracheal intubation is contraindicated because it may cause more harm than good. In these cases, an endotracheal tube can migrate through a perforation into the cervical soft tissues or mediastinum, creating a tenuous and possibly dangerous airway for the patient.[73] Thus awake tracheostomy below the site of injury remains the mainstay of airway management in these cases.

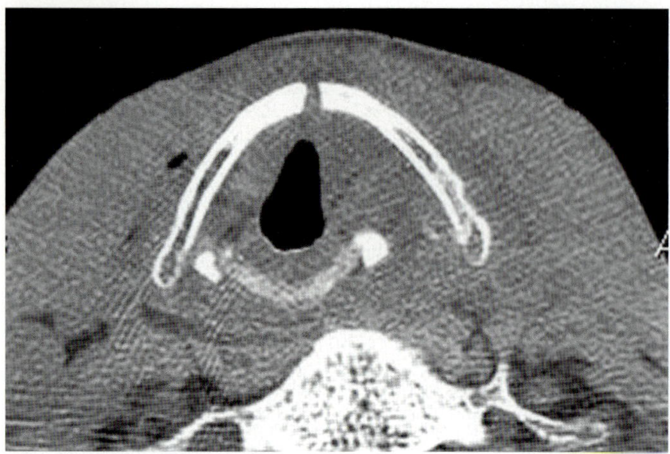

FIGURE 10-8. Computed tomographic scan revealing thyroid cartilage fracture.

The trauma patient should also be examined for cervical spine injuries because movement of the neck during intubation may lead to irreversible paralysis. Maintaining cervical collar placement or applying axial traction may minimize spinal cord injury during intubation.[74] The anesthetist should also be aware that mouth opening may be limited in the patient with facial trauma. Improvement in the ability to open the patient's mouth after induction of anesthesia and paralysis cannot be guaranteed. Therefore, a fiberoptic bronchoscope and a tracheostomy tray should be available for awake management of the airway.

TUMORS

Head and neck tumors, both benign and malignant, may make intubation difficult. Mouth opening and proper positioning of the head and neck for rigid laryngoscopy can be limited by tumors, surgical scars, or radiation fibrosis of head and neck tissues (**Table 10-3**).[2,57]

Tumors of the oral cavity and oropharynx may create trismus due to invasion of the muscles of mastication. This trismus can often be overcome after induction with muscle relaxants. Anesthesiologists should work collaboratively with the otolaryngology service to perform safe laryngoscopy for intubation, diagnosis, and staging biopsies. Care should be taken to avoid trauma of these tumors, which will cause bleeding. This is especially true of friable tumors of the base of tongue and tonsil that, in addition to trismus, prevent proper mask ventilation and preclude the use of a supraglottic airway.

Tumors of the larynx create significant difficulty during orotracheal intubation. Exophytic tumors above the vocal cords may prolapse into and block the airway when even the slightest bit of sedation is administered.[75,76] Once again, consultation with the otolaryngology service is indicated to avoid an emergently obstructed upper airway. In these cases, the airway can be managed with closed laryngoscopes such as a Dedo or anterior commissure (Holinger) laryngoscope (**Fig. 10-9**). Preparation for an awake tracheostomy under local anesthetic may be required in this subset of patients.

The presence of cancerous goiters is also a concern. Difficult tracheal intubation is reported in 17 (5.3%) of 320 patients undergoing thyroidectomy.[77] In this study, multivariate analysis suggests that the presence of a cancerous goiter and Cormack and Lehane grade III or IV laryngoscopic view are independently associated with difficult intubation. However, the same study reported that the size of goiter was not associated with increased difficulty with intubation. In any case, it is important to be aware that a goiter can narrow the airway due to extrinsic compression (**Fig.10-10**). Last, although infrequent, vocal cord paralysis due to malignant thyroid disease or due to surgical trauma may complicate extubation.

Radiologic studies are indicated in the presence of trauma or tumors in or near the airway.[78] Lateral cervical spine films, computed tomography (CT), or magnetic resonance imaging (MRI) may be used to assess the degree of airway compression and the involvement of associated structures. Topical anesthesia with fiberoptic laryngoscopy and bronchoscopy may prove beneficial in airway inspection.[59]

TABLE 10-3 Physical Findings That Suggest Difficult Airway Management

Finding	Implication
Obesity	Easily obstructed airway, aspiration risk, diminished chest wall compliance, difficult laryngoscopy because of macroglossia and immobile head
Pregnancy	All the problems associated with obesity, especially aspiration risk; large breasts impair laryngoscope insertion; swollen mucosa bleed easily
Ascites	Aspiration risk, diminished chest wall compliance
Whiskers, flat nasal bridge, large face	Difficult mask seal
Mouth opens <40 mm	Glottic exposure blocked by maxillary teeth
Cervico-occipital extension limited to an angle at the hyoid <160°	Difficult to align mouth and pharynx for glottic exposure
Short, thick, muscular neck	Prone to soft tissue obstruction, difficult to extend neck for intubation or mask ventilation
Thyromental distance <60 mm, receding chin	Difficult to mobilize tongue for glottic exposure, glottis too anterior to visualize
Maxillary gap from missing incisors with other teeth present to the right	Laryngoscope fits into gap while adjacent teeth, lip, or gums block view of glottis and passage of tracheal tube
Edentulous with atrophic mandible	Small face and furrowed cheeks impair mask fit; tongue and soft palate block exhalation
Prominent or protruding maxillary incisors	Teeth block view of glottis
Advanced caries, loose teeth, caps, bridges	Dentition can be damaged or aspirated; rough edges can tear tube cuff
Stridor, retractions	Risk of insurmountable airway obstruction
Hoarseness	Chance of vocal cord dysfunction or airway masses
"Underwater" voice	Vallecular or epiglottic cysts
Nasogastric tube in situ	Difficult to seal mask
Poorly visualized soft palate and fauces in upright patient with mouth fully open (Mallampati sign)	Difficult to expose glottis with rigid laryngoscopy
Large goiter or immobile tumor displacing trachea	Difficult to expose glottis, airway obstruction, or tracheal collapse
Tracheostomy scar	Possible tracheal stenosis

AIRWAY STENTS

The purpose of an airway stent is to prevent obstruction caused by malacia, stricture, or extrinsic compression that is not suitable for surgical correction either due to location or morbidity (**Figs. 10-11** and **10-12**).[79,80] Conditions treated by stent placement include tracheomalacia, postintubation stricture, stricture related to lobectomy, tuberculosis, traumatic injury or compression secondary to malignancy, multinodular goiter, or an intrathoracic process. Tracheostomy and Montgomery T tubes are used extensively in the management of glottic, subglottic, or tracheal stenosis due to benign or malignant

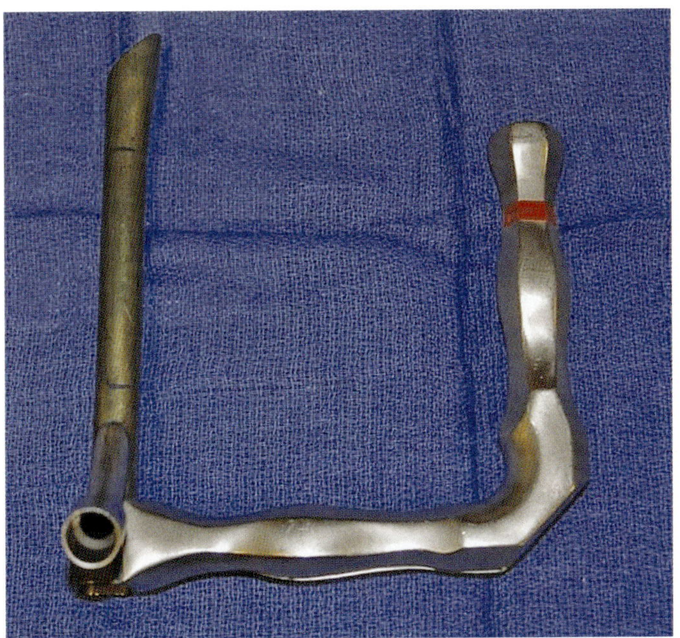

FIGURE 10-9. Anterior commissure laryngoscope.

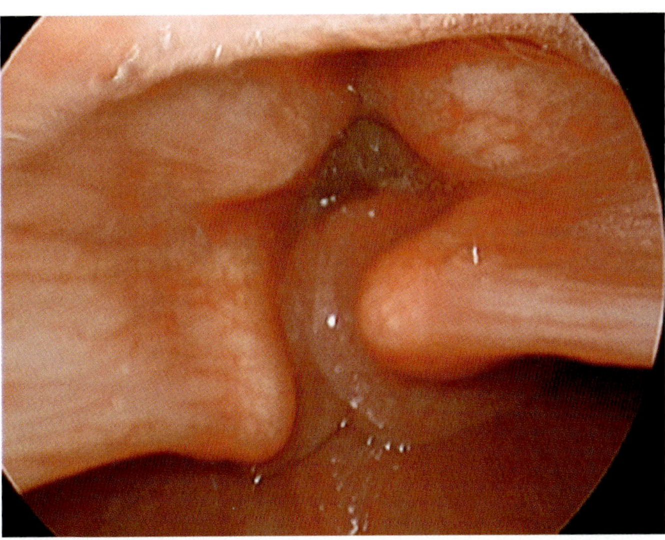

FIGURE 10-11. Relapsing polychondritis. [Photo courtesy of Dr. Dana M. Thompson, Department of Otolaryngology, Mayo Clinic, Rochester, Minnesota.]

disease. More recently, tracheobronchial stents have been developed to help manage malacia, extrinsic compression, and stenosis of the distal airway (**Figs. 10-13** and **10-14**).

Preoperative evaluation requires communication with the otolaryngologist to verify the underlying diagnosis, position of the stent, and the best method of airway management. Presence of a stent may complicate or prevent traditional endotracheal intubation. Also, attempted orotracheal intubation with a stent in place can damage the airway or dislodge the stent. Laryngeal mask airways, however, can often be used to safely manage the airways of such patients.

Frequently, laryngectomy patients wear a silastic stent or a heat-moisture exchange system over the stoma. These "lary" tubes or buttons are uncuffed and often used in conjunction with a speaking valve or prosthesis placed across the tracheoesophageal wall (**Figs. 10-15** through **10-17**). Given that these patients are "neck breathers" with potentially confusing surgically altered anatomy, their airway is best managed by collaborating with an otolaryngologist. Typically direct intubation of the stoma after removal of the laryngectomy tube is the best method of airway management. The speaking valve should not be removed during intubation because this is an indwelling device and will not obstruct placement of a tracheal tube.

INTRATHORACIC LESIONS

Intrathoracic lesions can compromise airway integrity through compression of the tracheobronchial tree or by invasion of the trachea or

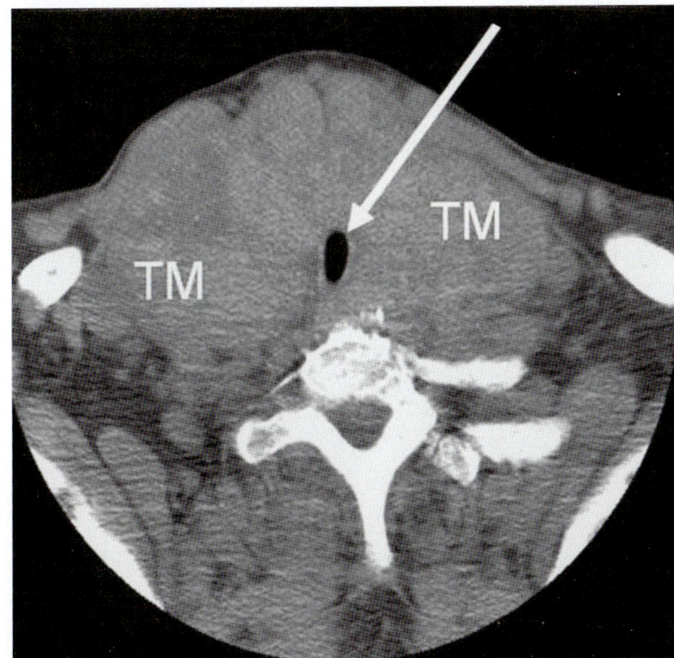

FIGURE 10-10. Thyroid mass (TM).

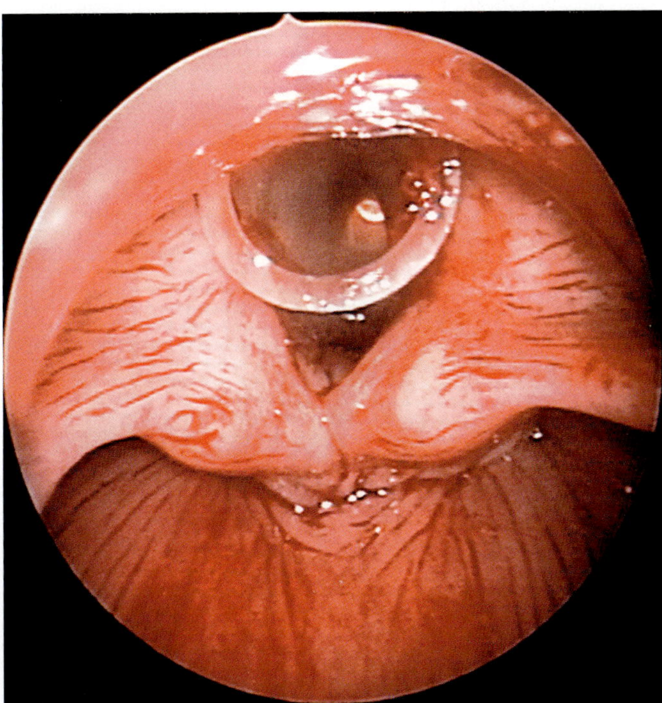

FIGURE 10-12. Suprastomal stent for management of tracheal compromise caused by subglottic and glottic stenosis. [Photo courtesy of Dr. Dana M. Thompson, Department of Otolaryngology, Mayo Clinic, Rochester, Minnesota.]

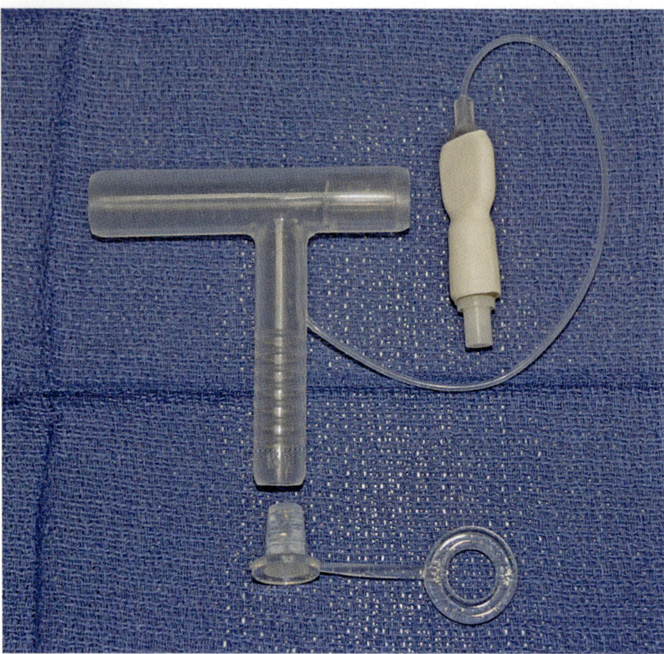

FIGURE 10-13. Montgomery T tube.

bronchi. Mediastinal lesions leading to life-threatening airway obstructions may be found in neonates, infants, children, or adults.[66, 81-84] Congenital tumors or tumors arising in early infancy include hemangiomas, lymphangiomas, cystic hygromas, teratomas, dermoids, rhabdomyosarcomas, neurofibromas, neuromas, and thymic hyperplasia. Adults with mediastinal masses, commonly lymphomas and thymic tumors, appear to be less at risk for perioperative complications than children.[85,86]

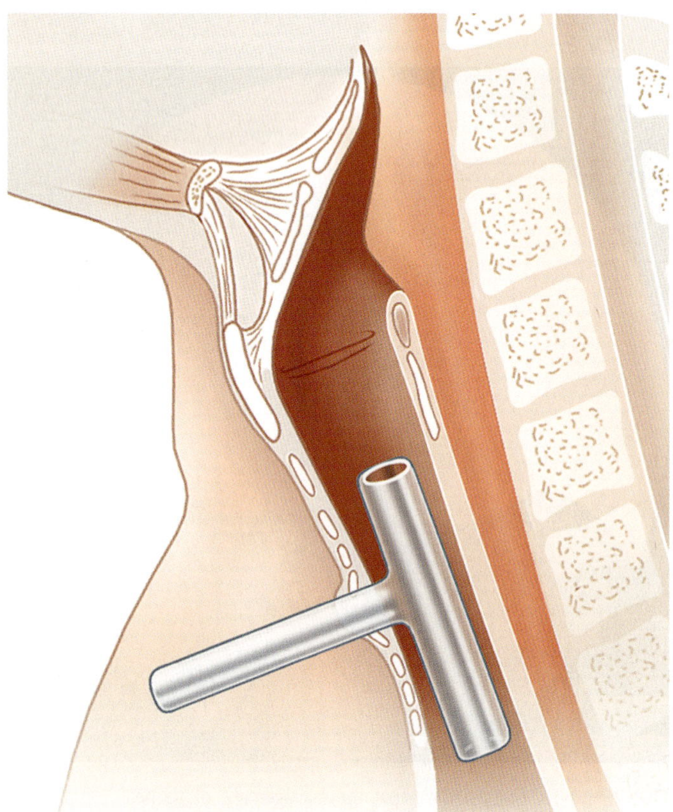

FIGURE 10-14. Montgomery T tube.

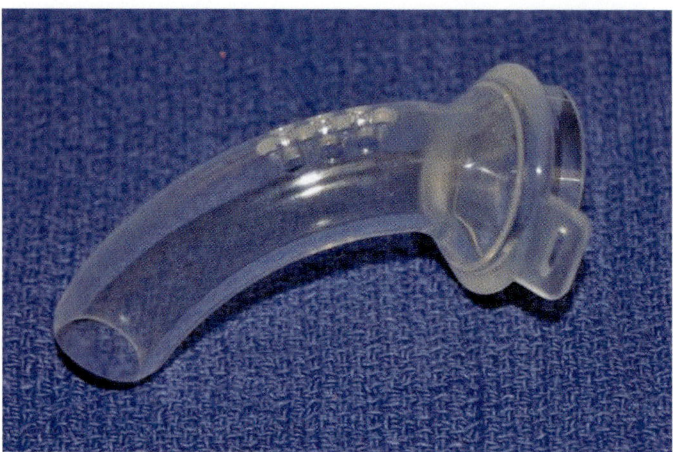

FIGURE 10-15. Laryngectomy tube.

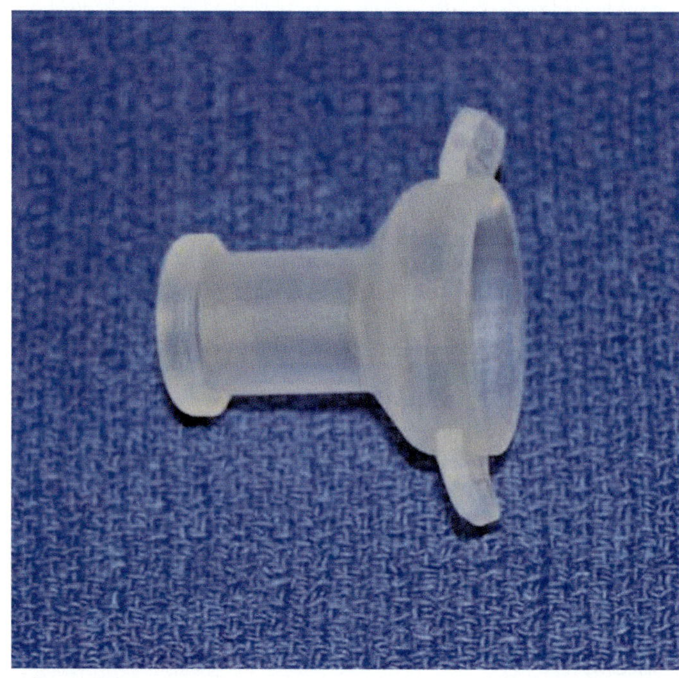

FIGURE 10-16. Laryngectomy button.

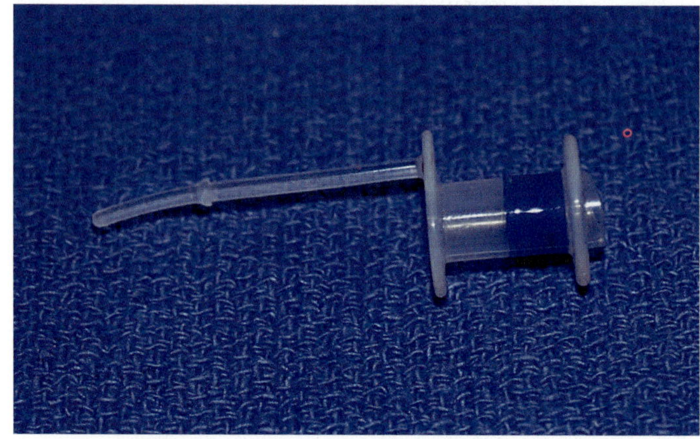

FIGURE 10-17. Tracheoesophageal prosthesis.

By nature of their anatomic location, these lesions may produce compression of the heart, compression of the large vessels, primarily the vena cava, and compression of the trachea and main bronchi. Anterior mediastinal tumors that are undiagnosed or underestimated as to degree of airway obstruction may completely block the airway on induction of anesthesia and induced muscle relaxation.[82,87] Evaluation focuses on an estimate of the presence and degree of obstruction of the tracheobronchial tree and the possibility of avoiding general anesthesia if possible.

Evaluation to assess the patency of the airway at the tracheal and the bronchial level is necessary to formulate an anesthetic plan. By history, symptoms of airway obstruction including dyspnea at rest, on exertion, and in different positions require additional evaluation. The presence of stridor, wheezing, rhonchi, and diminished breath sounds should be reviewed with the patient in different positions. Careful analysis of chest radiographs, CT, and MRI studies may prove essential for planning airway control in the patient with a mediastinal mass. Chest radiographs in the posteroanterior position allow measurement of the tracheal diameter at the level of the clavicles.[88] A lateral chest view shows the degree of compression of the trachea in an anteroposterior position. A CT scan of the chest permits accurate measurements of airway diameters and indicates the exact level and extent of compression of the tracheobronchial tree.

Pericardial effusion on preoperative CT scan was the only variable associated with intraoperative complications in a review of 98 patients with mediastinal mass.[85] In this population, postoperative respiratory complications were related to tracheal compression of greater than 50% on a preoperative CT scan and a finding of mixed restrictive and obstruction disease on pulmonary function testing. A review of 29 pediatric patients with mediastinal masses who were undergoing general anesthesia concluded that CT evidence of superior vena compression along with symptoms and signs of superior vena cava syndrome (SVCS) were associated with potential development of life-threatening situations.[86] In this review, SVCS was the only nonrespiratory sign or symptom that was associated with increased anesthetic risk. All 4 children with SVCS developed acute airway compromise with general anesthesia.

Pulmonary flow volume loop studies performed in the upright and supine positions may sometimes assist in defining the severity of position-related airway compromise. Maximal inspiratory and expiratory flow volume curves may help to quantify the degree of impairment and differentiate extrathoracic from intrathoracic obstruction.[66,82] In an evaluation of 37 patients with anterior mediastinal masses by Hnatiuk and Corcoran, however, the incidence of perioperative surgical complications was found to be low. The results of upright and supine spirometry did not always alter the anesthetic technique, and normal spirometry results did not exclude the occurrence perioperative complications.[89] In a review of 77 mediastinal mass in patients who underwent pulmonary function tests prior to general anesthesia, airway collapse did not occur in any patient.[85] This patient population included 10 cases with a peak expiratory flow rate (PEFR) that was less than 50% of the predicted rate and 6 cases with a PEFR that was 40% or less of the predicted rate. A PEFR of 40% or less of predicted, however, was associated with a more than 10-fold increase in the risk of postoperative respiratory complications.

In general, patients with mediastinal masses are considered at high risk for perioperative complications if they have cardiorespiratory signs and symptoms, tracheal compression more than 50%, pericardial effusion on CT scan, or combined obstructive and restrictive patterns on pulmonary function testing.[85] General anesthesia and the use of neuromuscular blocking agents may reduce lung volume, relax bronchial smooth muscle leading to greater compressibility of the airway from the overlying mass, and reduce the transmural pressure gradient across the airway that helps maintain airway diameter.[82] A conservative management strategy may be necessary in such patients because mask ventilation may not be possible. Tracheostomy may not relieve airway obstruction because the obstruction may occur at or below the level of the carina. Some clinicians have advocated femoral vessel cannulation in high-risk patients so that cardiopulmonary bypass can immediately be initiated in a crisis.[87]

FOREIGN BODY

Foreign bodies in the upper aerodigestive tract are an important cause of morbidity and mortality for patients at both age extremes. Both the elderly and children younger than 3 years are at risk for foreign body ingestion. Impacted food in the upper aerodigestive tract tends to be a problem in the elderly. These patients may have dentures that prevent the detection of a small bone fragments or proper mastication of food. In addition, elderly patients are more likely to suffer from esophageal dysmotility, Zenker diverticulum, malignancy, or stricture, all of which predispose to esophageal foreign bodies. Symptoms of an impacted bone include stabbing pain on swallowing. Typically the bone protrudes from the lingual or palatine tonsil. Generally, when a foreign body is lodged in the upper esophagus, the patient can point to the level of obstruction. Dysphagia, regurgitation of food, bloody secretions, and an inability to tolerate secretions may be noted. Removal of an impacted foreign body may be performed under general anesthesia depending on the patient's age, material that is impacted, and location. In these situations, it is imperative to control the airway to prevent aspiration. Even if the foreign body is noted on laryngoscopy, unless it is obstructing the airway, tracheal intubation should be achieved before removal.

Children, particularly those younger than 3 years, can also present with an upper airway foreign body in addition to the more common esophageal foreign body. Airway foreign bodies may involve the larynx, trachea, or bronchi. Most inhaled foreign bodies enter the right mainstem bronchus, which is larger and has a straighter takeoff from the carina than the left. The symptoms associated with aspiration can include gagging, coughing, spasmodic choking, stridor, wheezing, tachypnea, tachycardia, and decreased breath sounds on auscultation.[90] Removal of an inhaled foreign body may involve a general anesthetic depending on the patient's age, as well as the location and material of the foreign body. Careful control of the airway in these situations is imperative. The anesthetist should work closely with the otolaryngologist to perform laryngoscopy and bronchoscopy for removal of the foreign body.

IMPORTANCE OF PREOPERATIVE AIRWAY EVALUATION

The ASA's Closed Claims Project evaluated adverse anesthetic outcomes obtained from the closed claim files of 35 US liability insurance companies. This database dates from 1985 and accrues about 300 cases per year. One of the first reviews of this data evaluated respiratory events, the most common cause of adverse outcomes. This study found respiratory events to be the single largest class of injury accounting for 34% of all claims, with 85% of these adverse outcomes resulting in death or brain damage. Critical review found that most outcomes could have been prevented. It is not surprising that 30% of the mortalities in these claims were attributable to an anesthetic malpractice and were the result of an inability to manage a difficult airway. More recent examination of the data looked at outcomes from perioperative airway claims from 1985 to 1999. In this series, 57% of claims resulted in brain damage or loss of life with the difficult airway being encountered upon induction. Remarkably, in more than half of the claims the difficult airway was anticipated but still was inadequately managed, and 25% of these patients were patients with head and neck pathology.

In an effort to improve management of the difficult airway, the ASA released an airway algorithm in 1993.[91] The current edition is only slightly revised and includes the use of supraglottic devices such as the laryngeal mask airway. Since its release, the closed claims data reports a 35% decrease in induction-related airway complications resulting in death and brain damage.[1] The study highlights the importance of having in place a plan for airway management as well as the necessary equipment.

RECOMMENDATIONS

A patient with a history of difficult intubation or with conditions associated with difficult airway management should be approached with organized primary and secondary plans for airway management. Often awake intubation, especially if a history of difficult mask intubation is present, is the optimal approach. Patients with physical findings suggestive of a high possibility of difficult intubation may benefit from an awake intubation or the maintenance of spontaneous ventilation during induction of anesthesia. The patient who unexpectedly presents with a difficult or failed intubation history is at most risk because the anesthesiologist may not be prepared.

The hidden cause of a difficult airway (eg, an asymptomatic supraepiglottic cyst) may not be detectable without direct or indirect laryngoscopy. Physicians involved with airway management should be aware of the weaknesses of various tests used to predict difficult airway management and must be prepared to manage an unexpected difficult airway. The ASA's difficult airway algorithm suggests limiting attempts at intubation to avoid trauma. It encourages changing to other techniques to establish ventilation and oxygenation. In a prospective study of 11 257 intubations, this predefined algorithm was effective in solving most problems.[92] Impossible ventilation never occurred during the 18-month study; 100 cases (0.9%) of unexpected difficult intubation were recorded. A preanesthetic diagnosis of difficult intubation remains a task of recognizing subtle signs, with a tendency for the experienced practitioner to err on the side of a conservative diagnosis because of the difficulty associated with managing an unexpected airway problem.

KEY REFERENCES

- American Society of Anesthesiologists Task Force on Management of the Difficult Airway. Practice guidelines for management of the difficult airway: an updated report by the American Society of Anesthesiologist's Task Force on Management of the Difficult Airway. *Anesthesiology*. 2003;98:1269-1277.
- Combes X, Le Roux B, Suen P, et al. Unanticipated difficult airway in anesthetized patients: prospective validation of a management algorithm. *Anesthesiology*. 2004;100:1146-1150.
- Goh MH, Liu XY, Goh YS. Anterior mediastinal masses: an anaesthetic challenge. *Anaesthesia*. 1999;54:670-674.
- Hastings RH, Marks JD. Airway management for trauma patients with potential cervical spine injuries. *Anesth Analg*. 1991;73:471-482.
- Henderson JJ, Popat MT, Latto IP, Pearce AC; Difficult Airway Society. Difficult Airway Society guidelines for management of the unanticipated difficult intubation. *Anaesthesia*. 2004;59:675-694.
- Lee A, Fan LT, Gin T, Karmakar MK, Ngan Kee WD. A systematic review (meta-analysis) of the accuracy of the Mallampati tests to predict the difficult airway. *Anesth Analg*. 2006;102:1867-1878.
- Rosenblatt WH. The airway approach algorithm: a decision tree for organizing preoperative airway information. *J Clin Anesth*. 2004;16:312-316.
- Rosenstock C, Gillesberg I, Gätke MR, Levin D, Kristensen MS, Rasmussen LS. Inter-observer agreement of tests used for prediction of difficult laryngoscopy/tracheal intubation. *Acta Anaesthesiol Scand*. 2005;49:1057-1062.
- Rosenstock C, Hansen EG, Kristensen MS, Rasmussen LS, Skak C, Østergaard D. Qualitative analysis of unanticipated difficult airway management. *Acta Anaesthesiol Scand*. 2006;50:290-297.
- Shiga T, Wajima Z, Inoue T, Sakamoto A. Predicting difficult intubation in apparently normal patients: a meta-analysis of bedside screening test performance. *Anesthesiology*. 2005;103:429-437.

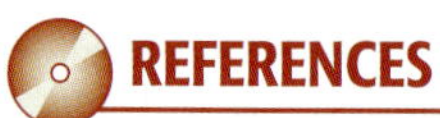

REFERENCES

Complete references available on DVD and online version at www.LongneckerAnesthesiology.com

CHAPTER 11

Evaluation of the Patient With Pulmonary Disease

James A. Onigkeit
David O. Warner

KEY POINTS

1. Postoperative pulmonary complications are a significant source of morbidity, mortality, and excess costs in modern anesthesia practice.
2. Pulmonary disease is the predominant patient-related risk factor for postoperative pulmonary complications, with other factors including age, general health status, and cigarette smoking. The predominant procedural risk factor is the site of surgery, with thoracic and upper abdominal surgery associated with the highest risk.
3. Routine screening or other testing for pulmonary function is not indicated. Rather, testing should be used to make an initial diagnosis in a patient with previously undiagnosed pulmonary disease, to monitor the status of patients with respiratory disease, or to assist with postoperative management.
4. Once pulmonary disease has been identified, it should be optimally treated before surgery. For example, patients with reactive airway disease may require adjustment of bronchodilator and corticosteroid therapy if their airway reactivity is not under optimal control.
5. The perioperative period is an excellent opportunity to provide tobacco interventions in patients who smoke cigarettes.
6. Useful intraoperative techniques to decrease the incidence of postoperative pulmonary complications include prophylaxis to minimize bronchospasm, rational use of neuromuscular blocking agents, and limiting tidal volumes during mechanical ventilation.
7. Postoperatively, therapies that promote lung expansion may reduce the risk of pulmonary complications.

INTRODUCTION

Postoperative pulmonary complications can range from atelectasis to exacerbation of underlying chronic lung disease to respiratory failure. They remain a significant source of morbidity in modern practice, occurring in up to 25% of surgical patients[1] and significantly prolonging the length of hospital stay.[2,3] They are also among the most costly postoperative complications; for example, one study found that the median incremental hospital cost for postoperative pulmonary complications was $52 466 versus $7789 for cardiovascular complications.[4] The goal of this chapter is to provide the anesthesiologist with a framework to (1) identify which patients are at an increased risk for postoperative pulmonary complications, with an emphasis on the role of preexisting pulmonary diseases, (2) understand the underlying pathophysiology of pulmonary diseases that can impact perioperative management, (3) optimize medical management of patients with pulmonary disease prior to surgery, and (4) plan the perioperative management of patients with pulmonary disease to optimize their outcome.

PATIENT RISK FACTORS FOR PULMONARY COMPLICATIONS

The definition of pulmonary complications varies widely. This variation makes comparisons of reported incidences and risk factors problematic among studies. Although nonspecific definitions such as cough or an

TABLE 11-1 Patient Risk Factors for Pulmonary Complications
Chronic obstructive pulmonary disease
Asthma
Interstitial lung disease
Pulmonary hypertension
Heart failure
Functional status
Hypoalbuminemia
Smoking
Age

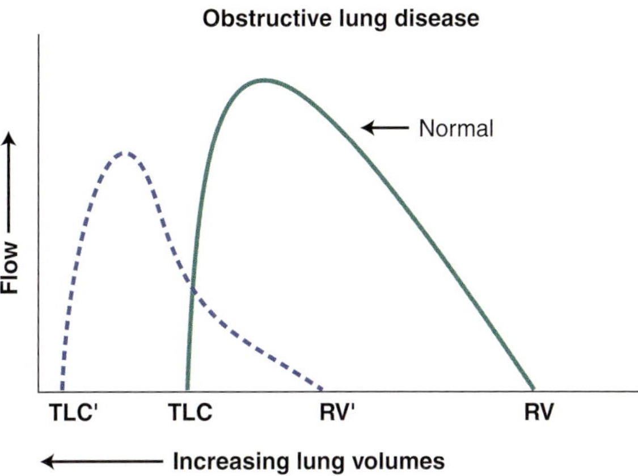

FIGURE 11-1. Spirometry in obstructive lung disease.
RV: residual volume, RV': residual volume in disease, TLC: total lung capacity, TLC': total lung capacity in disease

abnormal lung examination or changes on a chest radiograph[5,6] have been utilized, a more useful definition of a postoperative pulmonary complication is a pulmonary abnormality that significantly affects the clinical course. Examples of clinically relevant pulmonary complications include bronchospasm requiring therapy, pulmonary infections such as pneumonia, and respiratory failure requiring mechanical ventilatory support. Patient risk factors for pulmonary complications are listed in **Table 11-1**.

In patients with pulmonary disease, the effects of anesthesia and surgery on pulmonary physiology interact with underlying disease to determine perioperative pulmonary function. Thus it is important for the anesthesiologist to have a good understanding of those pulmonary diseases commonly encountered in practice that can influence the risk of pulmonary complications. This section reviews patient factors, including pulmonary diseases, that may contribute to the risk of pulmonary complications.

CHRONIC OBSTRUCTIVE PULMONARY DISEASE

Chronic obstructive pulmonary disease (COPD) includes both chronic bronchitis and emphysema. Chronic bronchitis is defined by a chronic productive cough for 2 successive years when other causes for the cough have been ruled out. Emphysema is defined by abnormal and permanent enlargement of airspaces distal to the terminal bronchioles. Both are characterized by chronic airflow limitation that is not fully reversible. Although COPD is often associated with smoking, several other factors, including other noxious particles or gases from occupational exposure, can also contribute to pathophysiology. Patient factors such as α_1-antitrypsin deficiency or a history of childhood respiratory infections can also cause COPD. The final common pathway is inflammation leading to deleterious alterations in the pulmonary vasculature and lung parenchyma.[7]

Patients with COPD usually present with a combination of dyspnea, cough, and wheezing or with an acute chest illness. Physical examination may be normal or demonstrate wheezes and a prolonged expiratory phase. As the disease progresses, the physical examination may show distant breath sounds, hyperinflation, crackles, and an increased anterior-posterior chest diameter. Signs of patients with end-stage COPD may include use of accessory breathing muscles, pursed lip breathing, cyanosis, and an enlarged liver from right heart failure. COPD should be suspected in patients with symptoms and signs compatible with COPD along with a history of exposure or the risk factors described previously. These patients should then undergo pulmonary function testing. The diagnosis is confirmed in patients with a history and symptoms compatible with COPD who also have evidence of airway obstruction (a forced expiratory volume in 1 second [FEV_1]/forced vital capacity [FVC] ratio [FEV_1/FVC] of <0.70 and an FEV_1 of <80% of predicted [**Fig. 11-1**]). Absolute lung volumes, including total lung capacity, residual volume, and total lung capacity are also typically increased.

COPD is an independent risk factor predicting postoperative pulmonary complications.[8-10] However, even in patients with severe airway obstruction the absolute risk is not high, and case series of these patients suggest that most can safely undergo anesthesia and surgery.[11,12] For example, one study found that for patients undergoing major abdominal surgery, severe airway obstruction as measured by spirometry was a significant predictor of perioperative bronchospasm, but did not independently increase the risk of prolonged endotracheal intubation or intensive care unit admission.[11]

ASTHMA

Asthma is an obstructive airway disease characterized by chronic airway inflammation that produces airflow obstruction that is at least in part reversible. The hallmark of asthma is airway hyperreactivity, an exaggerated bronchoconstrictor response to airway irritants (eg, cigarette smoke, allergens, cold air, and airway instrumentation) that produces symptoms of dyspnea, cough, and wheezing. However, the airway inflammation characteristic of asthma may produce persistent symptoms in the absence of obvious triggers. The underlying cause of the airway inflammation is usually unknown. Sequelae of chronic airway inflammation include bronchial smooth muscle hypertrophy and hyperplasia, bronchial wall edema from microvascular leakage, and increased mucus production.[13]

Patients with asthma typically have episodes of airway obstruction characterized by wheezing, dyspnea, cough, and chest tightness, especially at night or early in the morning. Cold, exercise, or airway irritants often trigger these episodes, which are usually associated with airflow limitation. Asthma is classified as intermittent or persistent, with persistent asthma further categorized as mild, moderate, or severe, depending on symptoms, frequency of bronchodilator use, interference with normal activity, and lung function as measured by spirometry.[13] Spirometry may be useful to confirm the diagnosis by demonstrating an increased sensitivity to inhaled bronchoconstrictors such as methacholine. Spirometry may also be a useful tool to follow lung disease status. Optimal treatment of asthma includes (1) patient education, (2) controlling known triggers and contributing conditions, and (3) pharmacologic therapy.[13] Pharmacologic therapy depends on the severity of the asthma (**Fig. 11-2**) and consists of a stepwise approach starting with short-acting inhaled β-agonists and incrementally adding long-acting inhaled β-agonists, inhaled corticosteroids, leukotriene receptor antagonists, and finally oral corticosteroids if needed.

Asthma is clearly associated with an increased incidence of perioperative bronchospasm.[14] However, population-based studies show that the absolute rate of other serious pulmonary complications in patients with asthma is low,[14] and a systematic review of studies looking at predictors

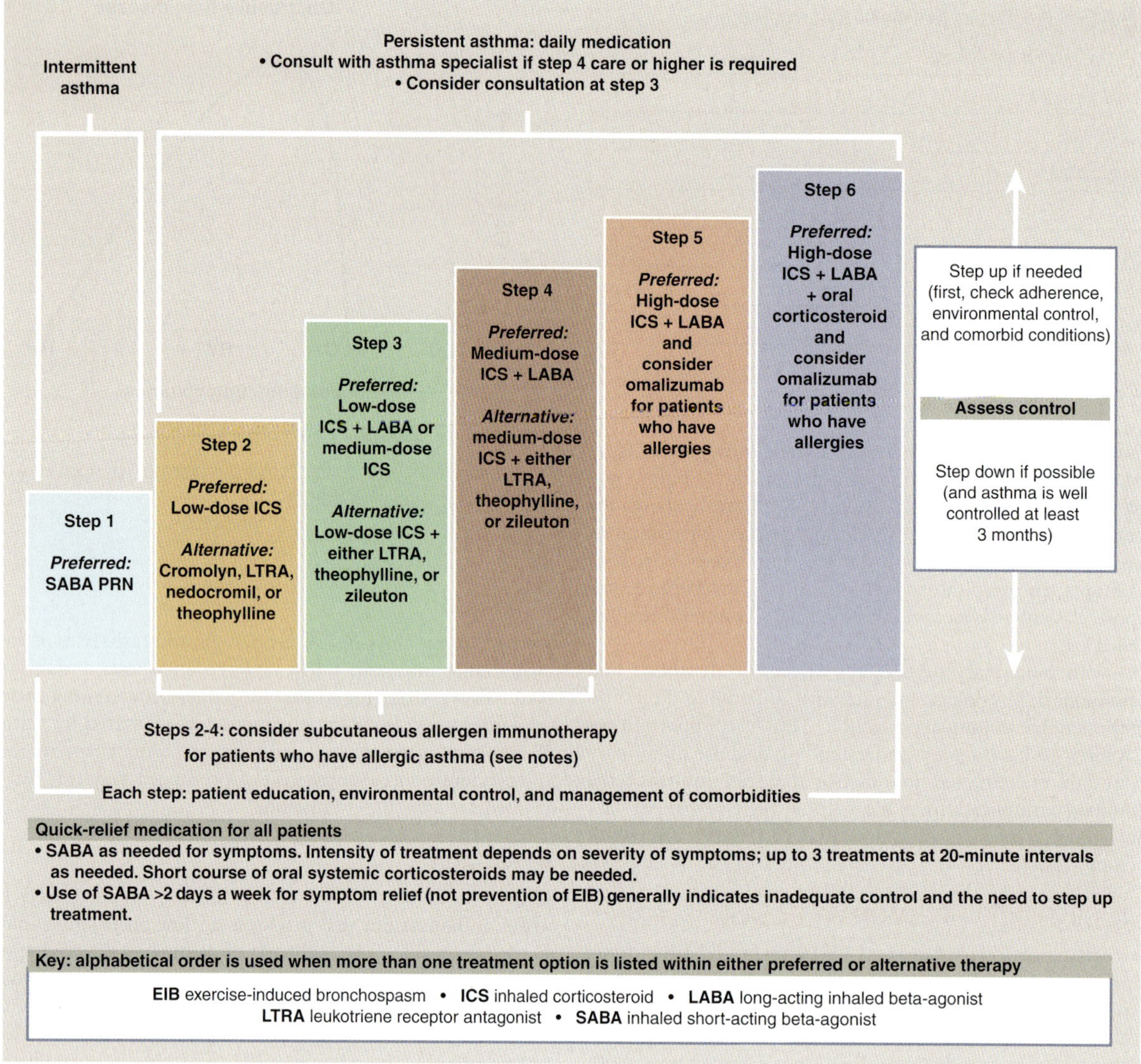

FIGURE 11-2. Stepwise approach to asthma management. [Used with permission from National Heart, Lung, and Blood Institute. Expert Panel Report 3: Guidelines for the Diagnosis and Management of Asthma. NIH Publication no. 08-4051. Bethesda, MD: National Heart, Lung, and Blood Institute; 2007.]

of other postoperative pulmonary complications failed to identify asthma as a risk factor.[9,10]

INTERSTITIAL LUNG DISEASE

Interstitial lung disease (ILD) is a broad collection of diffuse parenchymal lung disorders with unifying clinical, pathophysiologic, and radiologic features (**Table 11-2**). ILD may be associated with exposure to dusts, drugs, toxins, and other airway irritants and connective tissue diseases, although in many cases the cause is unknown. Patients commonly present with progressive dyspnea and a dry, nonproductive cough. The chest radiograph is often abnormal, and high-resolution computed tomography of the chest may show airspace or reticular opacities, consolidation, or cysts, depending on the type of ILD. A resting arterial blood gas tensions may or may not show hypoxemia at rest, and hypercarbia is usually not evident except in end-stage disease. Patients may, however, have significant desaturation with exercise, and evaluating gas exchange with serial arterial blood gas tension measurements during exercise can be useful to follow disease progression and response to therapy. Pulmonary function testing in ILD classically shows a restrictive pattern with decreased residual volume, functional residual capacity, and total lung capacity with decreased flows as evidenced by a low FEV_1 and a low FVC but with a normal or increased FEV_1/FVC ratio (**Fig. 11-3**). The diffusing capacity of carbon monoxide is typically decreased.

There are few data regarding perioperative pulmonary complications in patients with ILD. One study found that in patients with ILD undergoing surgical lung biopsy, the ratio of arterial carbon dioxide tension

TABLE 11-2 Classification of Interstitial Lung Disease (ILD)
Idiopathic pulmonary fibrosis
Respiratory bronchiolitis interstitial lung disease
Cryptogenic organizing pneumonia
Lymphocytic organizing pneumonia
Desquamative interstitial pneumonia
Acute interstitial pneumonia
Nonspecific interstitial pneumonia
ILD secondary to known cause (eg, drugs, collagen vascular disease)
Granulomatous ILD (eg, sarcoidosis)
Other forms of ILD (eg, lymphangioleiomyomatosis, histiocytosis X)

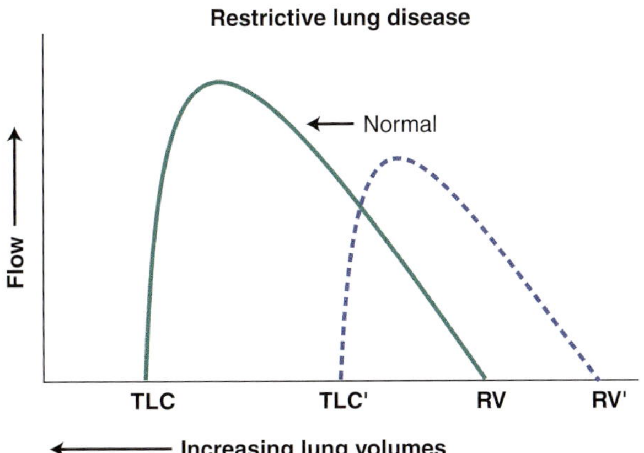

FIGURE 11-3. Spirometry in restrictive lung disease.

RV: residual volume, RV': residual volume in disease, TLC: total lung capacity, TLC': total lung capacity in disease

to arterial oxygen tension and dyspnea as quantified by the American Thoracic Society Shortness-of-Breath Scale predicted mortality.[15] In patients with ILD undergoing lung resection for cancer, an FEV_1 or FVC of less than 60% of predicted or a low diffusing capacity of lung for carbon monoxide identified patients at high risk for postoperative pulmonary complications.[16,17] These 3 studies examined patients with ILD undergoing thoracic procedures, and data for nonthoracic surgical procedures are not available. In addition, ILD can also be associated with other factors such as pulmonary hypertension (see next section, Pulmonary Hypertension) or concomitant airway obstruction (eg, in respiratory bronchiolitis interstitial lung disease) that may increase risk.

PULMONARY HYPERTENSION

Elevated pulmonary artery pressure and subsequent right heart dysfunction characterize pulmonary hypertension, defined as a mean pulmonary artery pressure of greater than 25 mm Hg at rest.[18] There are multiple etiologies of pulmonary hypertension, including COPD, ILD, left heart failure, obstructive sleep apnea, chronic pulmonary thromboembolic disease, connective tissue diseases, drugs, toxins, and genetic and host factors in the case of idiopathic pulmonary artery hypertension.[19] These causes can be grouped into 6 clinical classifications (**Table 11-3**). Symptoms include dyspnea, lethargy, and fatigue and progress to angina, exertional syncope, and peripheral edema. Physical examination findings include an increased pulmonic component of the second heart sound, an elevated jugular venous pressure, a tricuspid regurgitant murmur, hepatomegaly, ascites, and peripheral edema.[20]

Pulmonary hypertension is associated with respiratory as well as other complications postoperatively. All-cause morbidity and mortality is higher in patients with pulmonary hypertension versus matched controls undergoing noncardiac surgery.[21] Another study examining 145 patients with pulmonary hypertension undergoing surgery found that respiratory failure was the most frequent complication, occurring in 28% of patients.[22] However, given that pulmonary hypertension may well be underdiagnosed and is often associated with other conditions that may increase pulmonary risk, the role of pulmonary hypertension as an independent risk factor for pulmonary complications remains to be defined.

TABLE 11-3 Clinical Classification of Pulmonary Hypertension[19]

Group 1: Pulmonary arterial hypertension
Group 1′: Pulmonary veno-occlusive disease and/or pulmonary capillary hemangiomatosis
Group 2: Pulmonary hypertension secondary to left heart disease
Group 3: Pulmonary hypertension secondary to lung disease and/or hypoxia
Group 4: Chronic thromboembolic disease
Group 5: Pulmonary hypertension with unclear multifactorial dimensions

HEART FAILURE

Heart failure (HF) is a risk factor for postoperative pulmonary complications as well as cardiac complications. HF can be either secondary to decreased left ventricular systolic function (systolic heart failure) or due to abnormal left ventricular relaxation causing increased filling pressures (diastolic heart failure).[23] Both forms of HF can lead to postoperative pulmonary complications in the setting of fluid overload, arrhythmias, hypertension, or myocardial ischemia causing pulmonary edema and subsequent respiratory failure.[24] In a systematic review of risk factors for postoperative pulmonary complications from the American College of Physicians, the risk of pulmonary complications in patients with HF was comparable to that of patients with COPD.[25] Likewise, a retrospective study of more than 180,000 patients undergoing general or vascular surgery identified HF as a risk factor for postoperative pulmonary complications.[26]

FUNCTIONAL STATUS

Overall health status and functional capacity predict postoperative pulmonary complications.[25] Various markers of overall health status can be used as a marker of pulmonary risk. A multifactorial risk index for predicting postoperative pulmonary complications after noncardiac surgery included hypoalbuminemia (serum albumin <3.0 g/dL), used as an index of overall metabolic status, as a significant predictor.[1] Another study found that hypoalbuminemia conferred a magnitude of risk similar to that of other patient-related risk factors.[25]

SMOKING

Cigarette smoking continues to be a major public health problem throughout the world. In the United States, approximately 20% of adults smoke cigarettes.[27] Multiple studies identify smoking as a risk factor for postoperative pulmonary complications.[28-31] These complications range from airway events during the induction of anesthesia[32] and pneumonia[30] to respiratory failure and unanticipated intensive care unit admission.[31,33] Even in the absence of overt symptoms, the lung's structure and function are abnormal in smokers.[34,35] Smoking has multiple effects on pulmonary function that can contribute to pulmonary complications,[36] including inducing lung inflammation, depressing alveolar macrophage function, increasing mucus production, and decreasing mucociliary clearance.[36] The net results are structural changes in the airway wall that accelerate the normal age-related decline of the FEV_1 compared with nonsmokers.[37,38] Smoking cessation can attenuate this accelerated decline.

AGE

Older age is an independent risk factor for postoperative pulmonary complications. The risk of pulmonary complications increases with age and approximately doubles for patients 60 to 69 years of age and triples for those 70 to 79 years of age as compared with patients younger than 60 years.[25,39,40] The effects of aging on the respiratory system[41] and the higher prevalence of coexisting disease may in part account for this increased risk.[42] Several age-related factors may contribute to the increased risk of postoperative pulmonary complications.

The chest wall becomes less compliant with age secondary to changes in the geometry of the chest from osteoporosis, stiffening of the intercostal joints, and structural changes in the intercostal muscles.[43,44] Likewise, the shape and muscle mass of the diaphragm change with aging such that peak transdiaphragmatic pressure is reduced.[45,46] When challenged with an increased ventilatory load, these changes predispose the diaphragm to fatigue.[47] Aging also changes the mechanical properties of the lung's parenchyma. In contrast to the decrease in chest wall compliance, lung compliance increases with age[44,46] because of a decrease in static recoil pressure.[48] The loss of elastic recoil can lead to airway obstruction with air trapping and potential dynamic hyperinflation during mechanical ventilation. This age-related loss of elastic recoil also can cause an increase in closing volume (the lung volume at which dependent airways collapse),[49,50] predisposing the patient to developing atelectasis. Finally, the aging lung exhibits increased ventilation/perfusion mismatching and a decreased diffusing capacity.[51]

Altered upper airway patency and changes in the regulation of breathing with aging may also contribute to increased pulmonary risk. Upper airway muscle hypotonia associated with aging predisposes elderly patients to upper airway obstruction.[52-55] This may exaggerate the effects of sedative or anesthetic drugs, which also interfere with normal upper airway muscle function. Impaired upper airway protective reflexes coupled with an inefficient cough attributed to an age-related change of peripheral and central nervous system activity may increase the risk of the elderly for pulmonary aspiration.[56] Along the same lines, elderly patients have dysfunction of central chemoreceptors and peripheral mechanoreceptors, causing an approximately 50% to 60% reduction in the ventilatory response to hypoxia and hypercapnia when compared with younger subjects.[57] This may increase the risk of hypoxia and hypercarbia in the postoperative period.

OBSTRUCTIVE SLEEP APNEA

Obstructive sleep apnea (OSA) is characterized by (1) obstructive apneas, hypopneas, or respiratory effort–related arousals; (2) excessive daytime somnolence leading to fatigue, headaches, or poor concentration; and (3) signs of disturbed sleep, such snorting, snoring, or restlessness. OSA is diagnosed on the basis of the frequency of respiratory events during sleep as measured by polysomnography in the setting of related symptoms. An apnea-hypopnea index (the number of apneas and hypopneas per hour of sleep, with >75% having an obstructive component) of >15 or >5 plus signs or symptoms is diagnostic for OSA.[58] OSA is estimated to be present in 4% of men and 2% of women in the United States, with up to 80% of these not having a formal diagnosis of OSA.[54,58] OSA is found in up to 9% of general surgical patients[59] and is frequently underdiagnosed. For example, one study found that 15% of morbidly obese patients scheduled for bariatric surgery were diagnosed with OSA preoperatively; however, 77% met criteria for OSA according to formal polysomnography.[60] Patients with OSA are suspected to be at risk for respiratory complications such as catastrophic respiratory depression,[61] but data to support this assertion are scarce. A case-control, observational study found that patients with diagnosed OSA had a greater risk for overall complications, but their risk of respiratory complications was not significantly elevated.[62] Another study found that OSA was not a risk factor for unanticipated admissions after ambulatory surgery.[63] Patients with OSA may be at increased risk for difficult mask ventilation and difficult direct laryngoscopy.[64]

OBESITY

Obesity produces multiple changes in pulmonary physiology and mechanics. Lung volumes are reduced and ventilation/perfusion mismatching increases with resultant hypoxemia as compared with normal weight subjects.[62] This has implications in other disease processes such as pulmonary hypertension and may complicate intraoperative management. Despite these effects, obesity per se has not been consistently shown to increase postoperative pulmonary risk. For example, in a prospective study of thoracic surgical patients, body mass index (BMI) had no effect on the incidence of postoperative pulmonary complications.[65] Only 1 study of 8 in a systematic review of predictors of postoperative pulmonary complications found obesity to be an independent predictor of postoperative pulmonary complications.[25] Morbid obesity is not a risk factor for unanticipated admissions after outpatient surgery,[66] suggesting that pulmonary risk does not preclude ambulatory surgery in the obese.

PROCEDURAL RISK FACTORS FOR PULMONARY COMPLICATIONS

In addition to patient factors, other factors related to the planned surgical procedure may modify risk and thus affect the approach to perioperative evaluation and planning. The site of surgery is an important risk factor for developing postoperative pulmonary complications,[1,40] with the incidence of postoperative pulmonary complications increasing the closer that the surgical incision is made to the diaphragm. For example, the rate of postoperative pulmonary complications in upper abdominal surgery ranges from 13% to 33% versus 0% to 16% for lower abdominal surgery.[67] Likewise, a systematic review found complication rates for lower abdominal surgery, upper abdominal surgery, and esophagectomy 8%, 20%, and 19%, respectively.[25] The higher complication rates are likely related to the effects of surgery on diaphragmatic and accessory respiratory muscle function.[68] Other surgical procedures may also pose an increased risk via other mechanisms, including neurosurgery,[69] head and neck surgery,[70] trauma surgery, cardiac surgery requiring cardiopulmonary bypass, esophagectomy, and lung resection.[71-74] A long duration of surgery may also augment pulmonary risk, with a surgical procedure time greater than 3 hours associated with an increased risk of pulmonary complications.[10,33,75-78]

There are limited data to suggest that less invasive surgical techniques such laparoscopy mitigate postoperative pulmonary complications. Proposed benefits of laparoscopic techniques include less postoperative pain, shorter recovery times, and less reduction in postoperative lung volume.[25] Despite this, a systematic review of laparoscopic surgery was found not to provide a decreased incidence of pulmonary complications, despite being associated with lower pain scores and increased postoperative lung volumes.[79] Similarly, a review of laparoscopic versus open colectomy found no difference in postoperative pulmonary complication rates.[25]

PREOPERATIVE EVALUATION OF THE PATIENT WITH PULMONARY DISEASE

The goals of preoperative evaluation are to gather sufficient information to guide the optimization of pulmonary status prior to surgery and to provide some estimation of risk that will allow for obtaining an appropriately informed consent from the patient.

HISTORY AND PHYSICAL EXAMINATION

A history and physical examination focused on the cardiopulmonary system is the single most useful tool in preoperative evaluation and should be the basis for further diagnostic evaluation if needed. Patients who present with new symptoms may require further evaluation for undiagnosed disease. In patients with known respiratory disease, signs and symptoms are important indicators of whether pulmonary function is optimal. For example, in patients with asthma, the recent pattern of medication use and recent symptoms are valuable measures of the state of airway inflammation and important guides to the need for further testing and therapy—and are themselves predictive of perioperative pulmonary complications.[14]

PULMONARY FUNCTION TESTING

The hope would be that preoperative pulmonary function tests (PFTs) could identify patients at high risk for postoperative pulmonary complications who could benefit from aggressive perioperative therapy or would identify patients in whom the risks of surgery outweigh the benefits.[80] Earlier literature proposed spirometric criteria that diagnosed the risk of postoperative pulmonary complications.[81] However, more recent data suggest that in patients undergoing PFTs prior to abdominal surgery, spirometry is not an independent predictor of postoperative pulmonary complications.[25,70] For example, Brooks-Brunn[76] found that abnormal preoperative spirometry in patients with severe COPD

(FEV_1 <50% of predicted) did not predict their postoperative pulmonary complications. Another study compared smokers with severe COPD (FEV_1 <40%) with smokers with a normal FEV_1. Although the patients with more severe airflow obstruction had a higher incidence of bronchospasm, the incidence of other postoperative pulmonary complications was not different between the 2 groups.[11] Based on the available data, the American College of Chest Physicians has recommended against the routine measurement of PFTs in the preoperative pulmonary evaluation,[39] echoing earlier concerns that routine preoperative spirometry wastes health care dollars.[82] Thus, with the possible exception of patients undergoing a lung resection who may benefit from an estimation of pulmonary function before a resection (see Chapter 54), *routine* preoperative pulmonary testing is not indicated. This is not to say that preoperative pulmonary testing should never be performed. Rather, the role of preoperative testing should be to (1) selectively evaluate patients who present with previously undiagnosed pulmonary disease, or (2) function as a tool to optimize patients with known pulmonary disease when prior tests are available that can be used in conjunction with recent testing to objectively assess the current status of disease (eg, serial spirometry in patients with COPD), and (3) guide postoperative care of patients with marginal status who are undergoing high-risk procedures.

ARTERIAL BLOOD GAS ANALYSIS

There are no compelling data to suggest that arterial blood analysis independently predicts the risk of postoperative pulmonary complications.[83-85] A recent review of pulmonary risk stratification for noncardiothoracic surgery[25] was unable to identify a study of sufficient quality to provide data on the predictive value of arterial blood gas tension analysis. As with pulmonary function tests, arterial blood gas tension analysis may play a role in the diagnosis, evaluation, and optimization of pulmonary disease or to provide baseline measurements for those high-risk patients undergoing high-risk surgery that may require postoperative ventilatory support.

CHEST RADIOGRAPHY

Chest radiographs have been a component of routine preoperative evaluation in the past. Despite this practice, there are few data to support routine preoperative chest radiography.[86] Anesthesiologists can largely predict chest radiographic abnormalities from patients' history and physical examination, and chest radiographic findings rarely influence perioperative management.[25,86] Although patients at an increased risk of postoperative pulmonary complications may well have abnormal chest radiographs,[25] this does not provide additional prognostic information beyond the presence of other risk factors already described, such as a history of pulmonary disease.

STRATEGIES TO MINIMIZE PULMONARY COMPLICATIONS IN PATIENTS WITH PULMONARY DISEASE

Strategies to minimize pulmonary complications begin with seeking risk factors and optimizing the treatment of identified pulmonary disease.[79] In general, strategies should be tailored to the particular needs of an individual patient, rather than applied as a part of a routine.

BRONCHODILATORS, CORTICOSTEROIDS, AND ANTIBIOTICS

For patients with reactive airway diseases such as asthma, it is important to minimize hyperresponsiveness to the extent possible. In most patients, this involves achieving optimal control of the underlying airway inflammation. This can be monitored by serial measurements of pulmonary function (eg, peak expiratory flows) or by analyzing patient history according to the persistence and severity of symptoms. Effective therapy can modify risk. For example, patients with reactive airway disease not already treated with corticosteroids and a bronchodilator were found to have less bronchospasm after endotracheal intubation when they received a preoperative 5-day course of albuterol and methylprednisolone.[87] However, the routine application of preoperative corticosteroids to all patients with reactive airway disease is not indicated, as population-based case series show that most patients with asthma do not develop pulmonary complications in the absence of routine treatment.[14] Rather, the decision to initiate or increase preoperative corticosteroid treatment should be individualized and based on the needs of the particular patient.

Although previously included as a part of "pulmonary preparation" regimens,[88,89] there is no indication for routine additional perioperative antibiotics in patients with stable COPD or asthma unless there is a superimposed respiratory infection. In this case, surgery may be delayed until completion of antibiotic therapy and resolution of the acute infection.[90]

SMOKING CESSATION

Because current smokers have an increased risk of postoperative pulmonary complications, patients should be counseled to stop smoking at the preoperative evaluation.[91] Although it appears that more extended preoperative abstinence from smoking (2-6 months) is required to significantly reduce pulmonary risk,[36,92,93] the salutary effects of abstinence to reduce airway hyperreactivity is measurable within a few days.[94] Although extended abstinence may be necessary to reduce pulmonary risk, even a brief perioperative abstinence period may reduce the cardiovascular risk and the risk of wound-related complications. Thus physicians should recommend and assist preoperative smoking abstinence regardless of when the patient is evaluated. Prior reports that a brief abstinence will increase the risk of pulmonary complications by increasing cough and secretions is not supported by the evidence[36,95] and should not be a barrier to recommending smoking abstinence at any time prior to surgery. There are now effective means available by which physicians can support their patients in maintaining abstinence from cigarettes in the perioperative period.[96]

INTRAOPERATIVE MANAGEMENT

It would seem intuitive that avoidance of general anesthesia with airway instrumentation and muscle relaxation would decrease the risk of postoperative pulmonary complications. However, the evidence to support the potential benefits of regional anesthesia techniques is not compelling.[79,97-99] Regional techniques may be indicated for a variety of reasons but have their own pulmonary risks. For example, a level of neuraxial blockade resulting in paralysis of the accessory muscles of respiration[100,101] or interscalene block causing paralysis of the phrenic nerve[102-104] may be poorly tolerated in a patient with marginal pulmonary ventilatory reserve.

Several intraoperative steps can help prevent bronchospasm in patients with reactive airways. Such patients should be pretreated with inhaled β_2-adreneric agonists (eg, albuterol) or anticholinergic agents (eg, ipratropium) preoperatively, especially if endotracheal intubation is planned.[105,106] If possible, endotracheal intubation should be avoided by using a laryngeal mask airway or similar device. Propofol and ketamine are the induction agents of choice.[107,108] Volatile anesthetics have excellent bronchodilating properties, with the exception of desflurane, which, because of its irritant properties, should be avoided in these patients. Other adjuvants such as lidocaine or fentanyl may also be useful to include as part of the induction sequence,[109,110] although intravenous lidocaine may have no effect or may actually exacerbate bronchospasm in some settings.[106,111,112]

The use of neuromuscular blocking drugs may be a valuable adjunct to providing optimal surgical conditions, but inadequate reversal of neuromuscular blockade in the postoperative period can contribute to respiratory complications.[113,114] Longer-acting neuromuscular blockade is associated with a greater risk of postoperative pulmonary complications than shorter-acting neuromuscular blockers,[115-117] likely because of inadequate reversal. Adequate monitoring of neuromuscular blockade, ensuring reversal of neuromuscular blockade prior to extubation, and preferential use of shorter-acting neuromuscular blockers may decrease the incidence of postoperative pulmonary complications.[79,116]

In mechanically ventilated critically ill patients with acute lung injury or acute respiratory distress syndrome,[118] using a lung-protective ventilatory strategy of providing a tidal volume of 6 mL/kg and limiting plateau pressure to less than 30 cm H_2O improves mortality compared with strategies that use higher tidal volumes.[119] There is growing evidence that such a lung-protective ventilatory strategy in surgical patients at high risk for lung injury may be beneficial.[120-123] In addition to limiting tidal volumes in high-risk patients, using a ventilatory strategy to minimize intraoperative atelectasis and subsequent lung trauma from the opening and closing of atelectatic lung parenchyma may be beneficial. An example of this "open lung" ventilatory approach involves using a lung-protective tidal volume strategy of 6 mL/kg, recruitment maneuvers of sequential increases in positive end-expiratory pressure (PEEP) to 20 cm H_2O, and then maintaining the PEEP at 12 cm H_2O.[124] When compared with conventional intraoperative mechanical ventilation, this strategy can increase intraoperative Pao_2 and lung compliance and decrease airway resistance. The effects on oxygenation disappear once the PEEP is removed.[125] It remains to be determined whether such a strategy actually reduces the frequency of pulmonary complications.[124]

POSTOPERATIVE ANALGESIA

Much has been written on the possible pulmonary benefits of neuraxial techniques for postoperative analgesia. The hope is that the excellent analgesia afforded by these techniques can reduce the incidence of postoperative pulmonary complications by improving the patient's ability to cough, breathe deeply, participate in chest physiotherapy, and permit early ambulation. However, other mechanisms in addition to pain contribute to impaired postoperative respiratory function, and even excellent analgesia does not prevent this impairment.[68] Most clinical studies show that postoperative analgesia achieved by neuraxial-blocking techniques is superior to that afforded by parenteral opioids, but any reduction in postoperative pulmonary complications is less clear.[68] Meta-analyses have shown that the addition of neuraxial or regional analgesia can reduce the frequency of selected pulmonary complications.[99,126] However, these are limited by methodologic flaws in some of the included studies as well as limitations inherent to meta-analyses.[127] Two randomized, blinded trials involving patients undergoing major abdominal surgery demonstrated that general anesthesia combined with epidural analgesia did not reduce the incidence of postoperative pulmonary complications when compared with general anesthesia combined with postoperative parenteral analgesia.[128,129] The American College of Physicians (ACP) clinical guidelines and a recent ACP systematic review evaluating strategies to reduce postoperative pulmonary complications found only equivocal evidence that neuraxial techniques can reduce pulmonary complications. Thus neuraxial analgesia should be used because of the benefit of excellent analgesia, but not because it consistently reduces pulmonary risk.

POSTOPERATIVE LUNG EXPANSION THERAPY

Postoperative lung expansion aims to increase the mean lung volume and functional residual capacity, reversing or preventing hypoxemia and postoperative atelectasis with the goal of decreasing the incidence of postoperative pulmonary complications, particularly pneumonia. Multiple techniques can enhance postoperative lung expansion, including incentive spirometry, chest physical therapy, ambulation, chest percussion-vibration, continuous positive airway pressure (CPAP), and effective coughing. In addition, assuming an upright position (eg, with early ambulation) significantly increases the functional residual capacity. Incentive spirometry is the most studied and least labor-intensive of these modalities. These devices encourage slow, deep breathing while providing visual feedback to the patient and can decrease atelectasis and hypoxemia.[90,130,131] However, their impact on other postoperative pulmonary complications is uncertain. Three recent systematic reviews examining the role of incentive spirometry in preventing postoperative pulmonary complications found inconsistent evidence for any efficacy,[132-134] although these analyses are complicated by heterogeneity in the application of incentive spirometry and the varying definitions of pulmonary complications. Interestingly, a single-center study examining the effect of preoperative incentive spirometry and inspiratory muscle training on a group of coronary artery bypass patients at high risk for postoperative pulmonary complications found

TABLE 11-4 Perioperative Management of Patients With Pulmonary Disease

Preoperative	

Evaluation of preexisting pulmonary risk	• Assess pulmonary disease status starting with history and physical examination
	  ◦ Pulmonary function tests used as appropriate to guide treatment
	  ◦ Chest radiograph when necessary to evaluate symptoms
	  ◦ Arterial blood gases as needed to evaluate signs/symptoms
	• Optimize pulmonary function
	  ◦ Quit smoking (for as long as possible before and after surgery)
	  ◦ Treatment of disease as appropriate (eg, antibiotics, bronchodilators, corticosteroids)
	  ◦ Consider postponing elective surgery if additional time is needed to optimize disease state
	• Education regarding postoperative lung expansion maneuvers

Anesthetic/surgical planning	• Consider regional analgesia for excellent pain control, not necessarily to reduce pulmonary risk • Limit duration of surgery as possible
Intraoperative	• Avoid endotracheal intubation as possible, especially in those with reactive airways • Use bronchospasm prophylaxis, especially prior to airway instrumentation • Judicious use of long-acting muscle relaxant (to avoid postoperative muscle weakness) • Limit tidal volumes to 6 mL/kg and consider lung recruitment strategies • Avoid use of 100% oxygen to reduce resorption atelectasis.
Postoperative	• Maintain tracheal intubation until full reversal of neuromuscular drugs is achieved • Optimize postoperative pain management to allow early ambulation and effective use of respiratory therapy • Optimize lung expansion via upright positions and modalities such as incentive spirometry • Consider the use of postoperative continuous positive airway pressure for patients at risk

Modified from Sprung, J, Gajic O, Warner DO. Review article: age-related alterations in respiratory function—anesthetic considerations. *Can J Anesth*. 2006;53:1244-1257.

that postoperative pulmonary complications were reduced in the group receiving preoperative interventions along with usual care.[135] It is uncertain whether this benefit resulted from actual changes in muscle strength or the fact that the group receiving preoperative interventions could more readily perform postoperative expansion maneuvers.

CPAP AND NONINVASIVE POSITIVE PRESSURE VENTILATION

Positive pressure may be applied to the airway of postoperative patients in the form of CPAP or bi-level positive airway pressure (BiPAP), a form of noninvasive positive pressure ventilation. BiPAP involves the delivery of mechanically assisted breaths via a tight-fitting facemask, nasal mask, or helmet, avoiding the need for an endotracheal tube (see Chapter 81). It differs from CPAP in that a higher level of pressure is applied during inspiration in addition to the positive expiratory pressure (as in CPAP).[136] Several recent studies suggest that the application of positive airway pressure may decrease pulmonary complications in high-risk patients. For example, a multicenter trial examined the effect of CPAP given to patients with hypoxemia after major abdominal surgery. Patients who received CPAP had a decreased need for re-intubation (1% vs 10%) and fewer developed pneumonia (2% vs 19%) as compared with the control group.[137] Similar results in cardiac,[138-140] thoracic,[141,142] and bariatric surgery[143,144] have been reported. Patients with OSA may also benefit from CPAP postoperatively, most conveniently applied if patients bring their own CPAP device from home.[61] However, there is no evidence that postoperative CPAP reduces pulmonary risk in OSA patients.

SUMMARY

The goals of the preoperative evaluation of patients with pulmonary disease are to optimize their therapy prior to surgery and facilitate the planning of their intraoperative and postoperative management to minimize the risk of complication (**Table 11-4**). A careful history and physical examination is the best and most important tool for preoperative pulmonary evaluation. Routine tests of pulmonary function are not indicated. Rather, such testing and other diagnostic studies should be individually selected and tailored to the particular needs of each patient with known pulmonary disease or be used to make an initial diagnosis in a patient with previously undiagnosed pulmonary disease.

KEY REFERENCES

- Lawrence VA, Cornell JE, Smetana GW. Strategies to reduce postoperative pulmonary complications after noncardiothoracic surgery: systematic review for the American College of Physicians. *Ann Intern Med.* 2006;144(8):596-608.
- Qaseem A, Snow V, Fitterman N, et al. Risk assessment for and strategies to reduce perioperative pulmonary complications for patients undergoing noncardiothoracic surgery: a guideline from the American College of Physicians. *Ann Intern Med.* 2006;144(8):575-580.
- Ramakrishna G, Sprung J, Ravi BS, Chandrasekaran K, McGoon MD. Impact of pulmonary hypertension on the outcomes of noncardiac surgery: predictors of perioperative morbidity and mortality. *J Am Coll Cardiol.* 2005;45(10):1691-1699.
- Smetana GW, Lawrence VA, Cornell JE. Preoperative pulmonary risk stratification for noncardiothoracic surgery: systematic review for the American College of Physicians. *Ann Intern Med.* 2006;144(8):581-595.
- Warner DO. Perioperative abstinence from cigarettes: physiologic and clinical consequences. *Anesthesiology.* 2006;104(2):356-367.
- Warner DO. Preventing postoperative pulmonary complications: the role of the anesthesiologist. *Anesthesiology.* 2000;92(5):1467-1472.

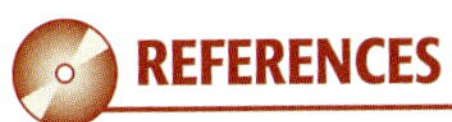

REFERENCES

Complete references available on DVD and online version at www.LongneckerAnesthesiology.com

CHAPTER 12 Evaluation of the Patient With Neuromuscular, Skeletal, or Motion Disorders

Loren A. Bauman
Joseph R. Tobin

KEY POINTS

1. The major cause of death in patients with neuromuscular disorders is respiratory insufficiency. Respiratory involvement varies considerably among the various neuromuscular disorders, and the extent of general muscle weakness does not necessarily correlate with the severity of respiratory muscle involvement.
2. Cardiovascular involvement may manifest as myocardial failure in patients with myopathic disorders and as autonomic dysfunction in patients with neuropathic disorders. Clinical signs of autonomic dysfunction include orthostatic hypotension, resting tachycardia, paralytic ileus, anhidrosis, and constricted pupils. The presence of these clinical signs may indicate profound hemodynamic instability that may manifest during the perioperative period, requiring invasive monitoring to manage intravascular volume status and myocardial contractility.
3. In patients with neuromuscular disorders, the severity of skeletal muscle involvement does not necessarily correlate with the severity of cardiac involvement.
4. Children with asymptomatic, undiagnosed muscular dystrophy are at significant risk for serious, life-threatening anesthetic complications. Specifically, these patients may develop intractable hyperkalemic cardiac arrest after receiving succinylcholine intravenously.
5. Spinal anesthesia has been associated with exacerbation of multiple sclerosis, although the mechanism is unclear. Speculation is that demyelinated areas of the spinal cord are more sensitive to the effects of the local anesthetic, resulting in a relative neurotoxicity.
6. Numerous anesthetics may exacerbate an acute attack of porphyria and should be avoided. Propofol, ketamine, local anesthetics, muscle relaxants, nitrous oxide, isoflurane, and opioids are considered safe.
7. Myasthenic crisis is a rapid deterioration of neuromuscular and respiratory function that may occur at any time perioperatively as a result of infection, stress, or an overdose with anticholinesterase drugs (cholinergic crisis).
8. Patients with myasthenia gravis and myasthenic syndrome are exquisitely sensitive to the effects of nondepolarizing muscle relaxants.
9. Succinylcholine should be avoided in patients with muscular dystrophies; it may further damage the already abnormal muscle membrane and cause the release of intracellular contents.
10. Succinylcholine produces an exaggerated contracture, and its use should be avoided in patients with myotonias. The myotonic response produced by succinylcholine may be so severe that ventilation and tracheal intubation are difficult and may be impossible.
11. Rheumatoid arthritis, osteoarthritis, and ankylosing spondylitis all are associated with possible cervical spine disease and may make airway management difficult.

12. Some musculoskeletal disorders are associated with an abnormal heat dissipation mechanism; central temperature monitoring is essential in these patients.
13. Many etiologies of high creatine kinase concentrations or rhabdomyolysis may be associated with malignant hyperthermia susceptibility.

Perioperative management of patients with neuromuscular disorders is challenging because of the low incidence, diverse etiology, coexisting diseases, and variable responses to anesthetics that often are present. A safe anesthetic plan demands that the anesthesia provider assess the extent of disease and its progression. Despite distinct etiologies, all neuromuscular disorders may adversely affect the respiratory and cardiovascular systems. Unfortunately, the extent of peripheral muscle involvement does not always correlate with the extent of cardiovascular and respiratory system involvement. Indeed, during stressful intervals such as acute illness, anesthesia, or surgery, the patient with a neuromuscular disorder may have his or her reserve easily overwhelmed, resulting in unanticipated complications such as respiratory failure requiring postoperative assisted ventilation, especially when the extent of the underlying neuromuscular disorder is underestimated.

This chapter focuses on the perioperative evaluation of patients with neuromuscular and skeletal diseases, emphasizing the respiratory and cardiovascular systems while highlighting important anesthetic issues. Individual neuromuscular disorders are grouped anatomically in an attempt to delineate specific anesthetic issues and to help predict possible anesthetic complications.

PREOPERATIVE ASSESSMENT

RESPIRATORY SYSTEM

The major cause of death in patients with neuromuscular disorders is respiratory insufficiency.[1] Respiratory involvement often varies considerably among various neuromuscular disorders, and the extent of general muscle weakness does not necessarily correlate with the severity of respiratory muscle involvement.[2] In fact, patients with peripheral neuropathy tend to experience less frequent and less severe respiratory involvement as compared with individuals with myopathy, myelopathy, and neuromuscular junction disease.[3] Significant respiratory muscle involvement may occur early (eg, Guillain-Barré syndrome) in the course of the disease or late (eg, myasthenia gravis), and it may be progressive, reversible, or intermittent. Impaired upper airway function and cranial nerve involvement often result in airflow obstruction and recurrent aspiration. Symptoms of airway involvement may be present preoperatively or after administration of sedation or induction agents, or symptoms may develop early after anesthetic administration, requiring persistent airway control.

Inspiratory muscle disease is frequently observed as a change in respiratory pattern, alternating work between fatiguing muscles and accessory muscles and increasing the respiratory rate to allow more efficient use of weakened muscles early in the course of the disease.[4] In addition, inspiratory time and the ratio of dead space to tidal volume are increased, resulting in decreased ventilatory efficiency, increasing the risk of respiratory embarrassment. More advanced inspiratory muscle disease is characterized by hypoventilation, atelectasis, and hypoxemia. When muscle strength is less than 30% of normal, hypercapnia develops.[5] Ventilatory responses to hypercapnia and hypoxia usually are impaired, especially in the presence of motor neuron and demyelinating disorders.[6] Although central ventilatory drive usually remains intact, it may be diminished in some patients with certain neuromuscular disorders (eg, myotonic dystrophy). Indeed, respiratory drive may reflexively diminish in order to protect against respiratory muscle fatigue, injury, and failure. Chronic hypoventilation or hypoxemia may result in pulmonary hypertension and right ventricular failure, further complicating cardiopulmonary function.

The ability to cough and clear secretions is impaired in patients who have expiratory muscle dysfunction and bulbar palsies, and reductions in forced expiratory capacity after abdominal and thoracic procedures may be exacerbated. When cough is impaired, atelectasis may develop and secretions are retained, predisposing patients to bacterial contamination and pneumonia.

Preoperative evaluation should focus on history, physical examination, and diagnostic studies. Breathlessness on exertion is common; however, many patients who have advanced disease cannot generate sufficient exertion to offer this complaint. Orthopnea is a prominent symptom of diaphragmatic weakness because the abdominal contents limit diaphragmatic movement when a patient is in the supine position. Snoring, morning headaches, and daytime somnolence are indicative of sleep-related breathing disorders that are commonly present in patients with neuromuscular disease. In addition, liquids tend to be harder to swallow than solids in patients who have pharyngeal muscle weakness, and patients often report a perioperative history of aspiration or chest infection after procedures even with minimal sedation. A history of use of nocturnal respiratory assist devices (continuous positive airway pressure [CPAP] or bi-level positive airway pressure [BiPAP]) predicts an increased propensity to postanesthesia airway or respiratory problems and may require advanced monitoring (intensive care unit [ICU] or similar site) for postoperative respiratory/airway complications. Even with a peripheral surgical site not involving the torso, the residual effects of anesthetics may worsen the patient's respiratory status.

Important findings indicative of ventilatory muscle weakness, such as frequent changes in respiratory pattern, tachypnea, use of accessory muscles, and ventilatory muscle incoordination, may be observed during relaxed breathing and auscultation.[7] In addition, paradoxical motion of the abdomen during inspiratory efforts suggests profound weakness of the diaphragm; this is best observed when a patient is supine.

Preoperative laboratory evaluation should focus on the patient's oxygenation and ventilation. Radiographic examination of the chest is useful to exclude pulmonary abnormalities but is not very helpful for diagnosing muscle weakness. Arterial blood gas analysis helps identify patients with hypercapnia and hypoxia. Newer noninvasive technology permits evaluation of preoperative oxygen saturation and hemoglobin estimation; however, these devices do not estimate respiratory reserve. Restrictive patterns typically are demonstrated by classic pulmonary function testing. However, vital capacity is not significantly affected until respiratory muscle strength is 50% below normal. Diaphragmatic weakness is suggested when greater than 25% decrease in vital capacity is observed between upright and supine positions.[8] Total lung capacity decreases in patients with inspiratory muscle weakness, whereas residual volume increases. Flow-volume loop studies commonly reveal truncation of peak inspiratory and expiratory flow rates, a delay in reaching peak expiratory flow rate, and an abrupt decrease in end-expiratory flow rate. Upper airway muscle weakness results in oscillations of forced inspiratory or expiratory flow, as well as plateauing of the inspiratory flow curve.[9] Inspiratory pressure generated by maximal effort against a closed airway can be used to measure the strength of respiratory muscles. Clinically significant ventilatory failure becomes more likely when maximum inspiratory pressure generated is less than 30 cm H_2O.[10]

CARDIOVASCULAR SYSTEM

Cardiovascular involvement in patients with neuromuscular disorders may manifest as myocardial failure in patients with myopathies or as autonomic dysfunction in patients with neuropathic disorders. Patients are at risk for left ventricular thrombi, systemic emboli, pulmonary hypertension, and right ventricular failure. Also, because most patients with neuromuscular disorders are relatively immobile, deep venous thromboses and pulmonary emboli are a concern. With clinically significant symptoms from neuromuscular diseases, patients often cannot demonstrate their cardiorespiratory responses to exercise; therefore, further preoperative testing with echocardiography may be necessary.

Paradoxically, cardiomyopathy can range from subclinical in individuals with advanced neuromuscular disease to severe in patients with mild neuromuscular disorders, such as mildly affected female carriers of Duchenne muscular dystrophy[11] or patients with Friedreich ataxia. Factors influencing the severity of Duchenne muscular dystrophy cardiomyopathy are multifactorial and may not be predicted by the extent of Xp21 (dystrophin) gene deletion.[12]

Heart rate, inotropic state, venous tone, and systemic vascular resistance are regulated by the autonomic nervous system. The most sensitive indicator of autonomic cardiac involvement is loss of beat-to-beat variability.[13] Resting tachycardia and postural hypotension often are observed when autonomic dysfunction is present and has been associated with intraoperative hemodynamic instability. Clinical signs of autonomic dysfunction include orthostatic hypotension, resting tachycardia, paralytic ileus, anhidrosis, and constricted pupils.

The presence of these clinical signs suggests profound hemodynamic instability that may manifest in the perioperative period and require invasive monitoring to manage volume status. Recently, transesophageal echocardiography has been used more commonly to monitor cardiovascular performance and end-diastolic ventricular volume.

Cardiomyopathy is difficult to assess by auscultation in the early stages. Persistent tachycardia usually is the earliest manifestation of cardiomyopathy. Although determination of creatine phosphokinase level is used to detect active systemic myopathy, it may not detect myocardial dystrophy. Both atrial natriuretic peptide and norepinephrine concentrations are useful for detecting and monitoring heart failure. Atrial natriuretic peptide concentrations typically increase in patients with muscular dystrophy when left ventricular ejection fraction is greater than 25%.[14] Preoperative troponin measurement has not been routinely recommended due to chronicity of the cardiomyopathies. Troponin levels are correlated with myocardial damage during acute myocardial injury.

The electrocardiogram (ECG) is a very reliable test for evaluating suspected cardiac involvement in patients with neuromuscular disorders. Characteristics include tall right precordial R and Q waves in leads I, aVL, V_5, and V_6.[15] Fibrous replacement of the myocardium is thought to be responsible for the Q wave often observed on the ECG. Unfortunately, the prognostic value of the ECG is not very good because of very little correlation among the clinical course, ECG alterations, and the level of cardiac enzymes.[16] Chest radiograph may be helpful to determine heart size; however, echocardiography is preferred to determine the size of the cardiac chambers, valvular involvement, and regional wall-motion abnormalities. In addition, serial measurements of fractional shortening and left ventricular ejection fraction are useful to monitor progression of cardiomyopathy and response to therapy.[17]

ANESTHETIC CONSIDERATIONS

In patients with neuromuscular disorders, the severity of disease tends to correlate well with the incidence of perioperative complications. Postoperative respiratory failure can occur, especially in patients with severe restrictive lung disease. The presence of cardiomyopathy can lead to arrhythmias, blood pressure lability, and increased sensitivity to the depressant effects of anesthetics. The risk of aspiration is increased in patients who have a diminished, or absent, gag reflex. Positioning injuries may occur as a result of contractures, skeletal deformity, and lack of subcutaneous adipose tissue. Also, adverse reactions with anesthetics, particularly succinylcholine-induced hyperkalemia, are well documented in patients with neuromuscular disorders.[18–20] The anesthetic concerns for patients with neuromuscular disease are summarized in **Table 12-1**.

Of concern are reports of children with asymptomatic, undiagnosed muscular dystrophy who are at significant risk for serious, life-threatening, anesthetic complications. Specifically, these patients may develop intractable cardiac arrest after receiving succinylcholine intravenously (IV) or after intramuscular injection, with or without the use of halogenated agents.[21,22] In this situation, hyperkalemia, acidosis, and myoglobinuria are common clinical findings. A number of these patients have been found to have abnormal or absent dystrophin, usually indicating myopathy, more specifically Duchenne muscular dystrophy. As a result, the US Food and Drug Administration has determined that succinylcholine should be used in children and adolescent patients only for emergency tracheal intubation or in cases in which immediate securing of the airway is necessary (black box warning).

PERIOPERATIVE ASSESSMENT OF SPECIFIC NEUROMUSCULAR DISEASES

MYELOPATHY

Amyotrophic Lateral Sclerosis Amyotrophic lateral sclerosis (ALS) is a degenerative disease involving the corticospinal tract and anterior horn cells. Loss of motor function is progressive, with development of asymmetric weakness of the limbs (lower motor neurons are affected first), spasticity, and muscle atrophy. Death usually occurs within 3 to 5 years of diagnosis, although approximately 10% of patients may live more than 10 years.[23] The etiology of ALS is unknown, but possible causes include viral or prion infection, glutamate excitotoxicity, free radical stress, autoimmune response, and heavy metal exposures and other undefined mechanisms.[24]

Involvement of the bulbar region typically manifests as respiratory and pharyngeal muscular insufficiency. Pulmonary function tests reveal a decrease in vital capacity, maximal voluntary ventilation, and diminished expiratory muscle function.[25] Ventilatory support will be necessary as the disease progresses because respiratory failure eventually develops in all patients. Indeed, the cause of death in most patients with ALS, as in most patients with neuromuscular disorders, is respiratory failure. Autonomic dysfunction may be present in patients with ALS, as evidenced by resting tachycardia, orthostatic hypotension, and increased concentrations of catecholamines.

The antiglutamate drug riluzole is approved specifically for treatment of ALS. Riluzole has been demonstrated to prolong survival and delay the need for tracheostomy.[26] Anticholinergic agents usually are administered to decrease secretions and facilitate swallowing, whereas dantrolene sodium and benzodiazepines are commonly administered to relieve muscle cramps and spasticity. However, these agents may exacerbate respiratory and skeletal muscle weakness. Anticholinesterase therapy may transiently improve muscle function and therefore is sometimes administered to these patients.

Ventilatory and upper airway muscle impairment significantly affects anesthetic management. Aspiration is an ongoing risk, and the need for postoperative ventilatory support is high because the already decreased respiratory reserve is reduced even further postoperatively. In ALS patients, the response to muscle relaxants, either depolarizing or nondepolarizing, is altered and may be compounded by perioperative administration of anticholinesterase medication. As with other patients with muscle denervation and muscle wasting, ALS patients are susceptible to succinylcholine-induced hyperkalemia and cardiovascular arrest.[27] Therefore, whenever possible, depolarizing and long-acting nondepolarizing muscle relaxants should be avoided. Autonomic dysfunction may produce exaggerated decreases in cardiovascular function in response to anesthesia. No evidence indicates that any one specific anesthetic drug or anesthetic technique is best for patients with ALS. Neuraxial anesthesia has been safely used in patients and can be considered.[28] Concern has been raised regarding neuraxial anesthesia and acute or subacute worsening of symptoms postoperatively, but no scientific evidence has been forthcoming. Multiple novel avenues of investigation are developing new treatments as mechanistic targets are being identified.[29]

Multiple Sclerosis Multiple sclerosis is a chronic disease of the central nervous system (CNS) that is characterized by a demyelinating process of the brain and spinal cord with unpredictable intervals of exacerbations and remissions. The cause of the disease is multifactorial, involving immunologic-mediated events occurring in susceptible individuals.

TABLE 12-1 Anesthetic Considerations in Patients With Neuromuscular Disorders

Disease	Response to Succinylcholine	Response to Nondepolarizing Muscle Relaxants	Other Anesthetic Considerations
Myelopathy			
Amyotrophic lateral sclerosis (ALS)	Hyperkalemia, contracture	Increased sensitivity	Impaired ventilation Aspiration risk Epidural anesthetics have been used successfully
Multiple sclerosis	Hyperkalemia in severe disease	Decreased sensitivity	Avoid stress and hyperthermia Spinal anesthesia may exacerbate disease and cause neurotoxicity Epidural anesthetics have been used successfully
Peripheral Neuropathy			
Guillain-Barré syndrome	Hyperkalemia	Increased/decreased sensitivity depending on phase of disease	Autonomic instability Aspiration risk Postoperative respiratory failure
Porphyrias	Normal response	Normal response	Avoid barbiturates, etomidate Propofol, ketamine, local anesthetics, opioids, nitrous oxide, isoflurane are considered safe
Neuromuscular Junction Disease			
Myasthenia gravis	Decreased sensitivity	Increased sensitivity	Avoid muscle relaxants Postoperative respiratory failure
Myasthenic syndrome	Increased sensitivity	Increased sensitivity	Avoid muscle relaxants
Myopathy			
Dystrophinopathies	Increased sensitivity, hyperkalemic response	Increased sensitivity	Succinylcholine contraindicated Regional anesthesia safe Avoid inhalational agents if possible (membrane destab-lizers) Postoperative respiratory failure Delayed recovery of muscle strength
Myotonias	Induced myotonia	Increased sensitivity if major muscle wasting is present	Avoid factors known to induce perioperative myotonia (cold, succinylcholine, hypothermia, anticholinesterase drugs) Monitor for cardiac dysrhythmias
Periodic Paralyses			
Hyperkalemic	Hyperkalemic response	Increased sensitivity	Avoid factors known to induce myotonia Avoid potassium supplementation Avoid carbohydrate depletion Monitor for dysrhythmias Monitor serum potassium levels Regional anesthetics best avoided
Hypokalemic	Alters serum potassium level	Increased sensitivity	Avoid hypothermia Avoid carbohydrate loading Monitor serum potassium levels Monitor for dysrhythmias Regional anesthetics best avoided

Initially, a virus or other agent triggers an inflammatory response that initiates an autoimmune response to myelin. Plaques in the white matter of the CNS are the fundamental lesions. The ability of the CNS to repair itself during the early phases of the disease accounts for the relapsing nature of the disease. Unfortunately, there is no curative treatment.

The symptoms of multiple sclerosis depend on the site(s) of demyelination. The most common presenting symptoms are sensory losses and ocular disturbances. Limb weakness and paresthesias may occur as a result of demyelination of motor neurons and sensory pathways. The lower extremities are affected more than the upper extremities. Brainstem involvement may produce cranial nerve deficits and abnormal ventilatory drive. Hypotension may reflect the presence of autonomic nervous system involvement. Bowel and bladder irregularities are frequent complaints. The course of multiple sclerosis is characterized by exacerbation of symptoms at unpredictable intervals over a prolonged period. Eventually, residual symptoms persist and lead to progressive disability. However, 10% to 20% of patients have a relatively benign course and trivial disability.[30] Interestingly, pregnancy is associated with an improvement in symptoms, but relapse occurs postpartum.[31]

The diagnosis is based primarily on clinical signs and symptoms. Laboratory confirmation of the diagnosis may be made by analysis of the cerebrospinal fluid (CSF) and magnetic resonance imaging (MRI). The CSF typically reveals increased concentrations of albumin and immunoglobulin G. MRI can detect CNS and spinal cord involvement and can be used as a measure to determine the effectiveness of various treatment modalities.[32,33]

Therapeutic modalities are directed at modulating the immunologic and inflammatory responses that damage myelin. Corticosteroids and interferon are used most commonly. Glatiramer is a polypeptide mixture that mimics the structure of myelin and serves as a distraction for autoantibodies. Mitoxantrone can be used to treat aggressive disease; however, it is cardiotoxic. Dantrolene, baclofen, and benzodiazepines can be used to treat spasticity. Carbamazepine can be used to treat painful dysesthesias, seizures, and paroxysmal symptoms. Antidepressants and anticholinergic drugs can be given for depression and urinary incontinence, respectively. Other promising new therapies are currently under investigation but are not currently approved for routine clinical use.[34] Avoidance of emotional stress, fatigue, and hyperthermia is essential. Indeed, a 0.5°C increase in temperature can block impulse conduction in demyelinated fibers, resulting in an exacerbation or relapse.[35]

Surgery may be required more frequently in patients with multiple sclerosis because of orthopedic, urologic, and neurologic issues. Unfortunately, the effects of surgery and anesthesia on the course of this disease are controversial. Both regional and general anesthesias have been reported to exacerbate multiple sclerosis.[36] However, factors other than anesthesia, such as emotional stress and hyperpyrexia, may increase the risk of an exacerbation as well. The patient should be adequately informed that, despite a well-managed anesthetic, a relapse might occur perioperatively. Patients with multiple sclerosis should undergo a comprehensive, well-documented neurologic examination aimed at identifying any existing deficits before anesthetic management. After surgery, the neurologic examination should be repeated in order to correlate preoperative and postoperative findings. Although patients may reveal no new symptomatology immediately after anesthesia, new symptoms may become present subacutely in the postoperative period.

Spinal anesthesia has been associated with exacerbation of multiple sclerosis, although the mechanism is unclear.[36] Speculation is that lesions may cause the breakdown of the blood–brain barrier, and, in demyelinated areas of the spinal cord, the CNS is more sensitive to the effects of the local anesthetic, causing a relative neurotoxicity. Indeed, higher concentrations of local anesthetics are more likely to cause a relapse than are lower concentrations of local anesthetics. Interestingly, epidural analgesia has been used safely and does not appear to increase the incidence of disease relapse.[31,36] General anesthetics do not appear to have any significant intrinsic adverse effect.

Consideration must be given to the potential interactions of anesthetics with medications patients may be taking for their disease. Patients receiving corticosteroids may require stress doses in the perioperative period. Immunosuppressants may produce subclinical cardiac dysfunction. Anticonvulsants produce resistance to nondepolarizing muscle relaxants,[37-39] whereas baclofen may increase the sensitivity to nondepolarizing agents. Patients with significant muscle denervation or atrophy theoretically have an increased risk of a hyperkalemic response to succinylcholine, so it should be avoided. The hypotensive effects of volatile anesthetics may be exaggerated by autonomic dysfunction, so patients with severe disease may require invasive monitoring, possibly including transesophageal echocardiography. Respiratory dysfunction, when present, increases the likelihood of the need for postoperative mechanical ventilation.

PERIPHERAL NEUROPATHY

Guillain-Barré Syndrome Guillain-Barré syndrome, the most common cause of acute flaccid paralysis, is an autoimmune inflammatory polyneuropathy of motor, sensory, autonomic, and cranial nerves. The syndrome is triggered by an immune response to either a viral or bacterial infection that produces antibodies to an antigen of the infectious agent. The antigen mimics an epitope of the Schwann cell, and affected axons undergo lymphocytic infiltration and demyelination. A respiratory or gastrointestinal infection 3 to 4 weeks earlier usually precedes the onset of this disorder. Usually, the disease evolves over the course of 3 to 4 weeks, with complete recovery eventually occurring in fewer than 80% of patients. Unfortunately, 3% to 10% of patients die, and up to 20% may be permanently disabled.[40]

The clinical course is characterized by an ascending, usually symmetric muscle weakness of the lower extremities that develops over several days, followed by gradual recovery. Paresthesias often precede weakness and paralysis. Difficulty swallowing and impaired ventilation may occur if bulbar and respiratory muscles are involved. Respiratory insufficiency often is characterized by decreased forced exhalation and impaired cough.[41] Rapid shallow breathing indicates inspiratory muscle weakness and usually develops later in the disease. Vital capacity should be measured frequently. When vital capacity is less than 15 to 20 mL/kg, mechanical ventilation often is required.[42] In addition, tracheostomy may be required for management of ventilatory failure and for bulbar muscle weakness even after ventilatory function returns to normal. Autonomic dysfunction may be severe, especially in patients experiencing respiratory failure and quadriparesis. Blood pressure lability, tachycardia, and cardiac conduction abnormalities may be present. Physical stimulation may precipitate hypertension, tachycardia, and cardiac dysrhythmias.[43]

Management is primarily supportive and directed at intensive respiratory care and treatment of autonomic dysfunction. Plasmapheresis and IV immunoglobulin may hasten recovery and may alleviate the harmful effects of the immune response. Corticosteroids and immunosuppressive therapy have not been demonstrated to be effective.[19]

Anesthetic management of the patient with Guillain-Barré syndrome often is dictated by the severity of respiratory and autonomic nervous system dysfunction. Compensatory cardiovascular responses may be absent. Hypotension secondary to hypovolemia, positional changes, and positive-pressure ventilation is possible. Severe autonomic dysfunction may produce exaggerated responses in heart rate and blood pressure; thus invasive monitors may be necessary, and direct-acting vasopressors and antihypertensives must be readily available.

Succinylcholine should be avoided because it can precipitate hyperkalemic arrest.[44] Interestingly, this risk may persist for some time after recovery from the disease. Depending on the phase of the disease, the sensitivity of patients to nondepolarizing muscle relaxants may vary from extreme sensitivity to resistance.[45] Mechanical ventilation should be anticipated postoperatively. Profound sensory disturbance may be present, and patients will need adequate pain control. Although the use of regional anesthesia is limited, the use of epidural opioids has been reported and appears beneficial to patients experiencing intense sensory disturbance.[46] Systemic opioid use must be judicious and closely monitored because these patients may be more sensitive to respiratory weakness or depression secondary to their underlying disease.

Familial Dysautonomia (Riley-Day Syndrome) Familial dysautonomia is an inherited disease thought to be caused by a deficiency of dopamine-hydroxylase with a subsequent decrease in the level of norepinephrine. Patients with this disorder exhibit impaired temperature regulation, denervation supersensitivity, insensitivity to pain, vasomotor instability, and copious pulmonary secretions.

Riley-Day syndrome has numerous anesthetic implications, including excess secretions, pneumonia, decreased responsiveness to hypoxia and hypercarbia, labile blood pressure, intravascular volume depletion, postural hypotension, decreased gag reflex, corneal abrasions, and emetic crisis.[47] Preparation of the patient for surgery includes achieving adequate pulmonary function and correcting fluid and electrolyte imbalance. Opioids should be used sparingly because pain, hypercapnic, and hypoxic responses are blunted. Because of a risk for aspiration, a nonparticulate antacid can be given. Invasive monitoring may be necessary, and vasopressors should be titrated carefully using direct-acting agents as needed.[47] Profound bradycardia and hemodynamic collapse may occur, and the anesthesiologist should be prepared for hemodynamic support and resuscitation.

Porphyrias Porphyrias are a group of inherited disorders of heme synthesis that result in overproduction and accumulation of porphyrin compounds because of a specific enzyme deficiency in the production of heme. Porphyrias are classified as acute (inducible) or nonacute (noninducible) on the basis of clinical presentation. Several reviews contain more detailed discussions of porphyrias.[48,49]

Acute porphyria may affect the CNS and peripheral nervous system via direct neuronal damage, axonal degeneration, and demyelination. Generally, clinical manifestations of acute attacks occur after puberty. Severe abdominal pain, nausea and vomiting, autonomic dysfunction, mental status changes, electrolyte abnormalities, and peripheral neuropathy ranging from paresis to flaccid quadriplegia characterize acute attacks. Death may occur from respiratory muscle paralysis. The cause of neurologic involvement is unknown but may be related to metabolites of heme intermediates or result from deficiency of the heme pigment in the nerve cell. Factors known to precipitate acute porphyric crisis include fasting, dehydration, infection, emotional stress, excessive ethanol intake, and administration of certain drugs.[50] Nonacute porphyrias are not associated with neurologic disorders or acute crisis.

Because the porphyrias are rare disorders, experience with the clinical use of many drugs, particularly anesthetics, is limited. Pharmacologic therapy of acute attacks is aimed at decreasing the activity of aminolevulinic acid synthetase, the rate-limiting step in heme production. Hematin and heme arginate are potent suppressors of aminolevulinic acid synthetase and markedly decrease the pain associated with acute crisis within 48 hours.[51,52] Hydration and correction of electrolyte imbalance, glucose infusion to prevent starvation, and propranolol to control autonomic dysfunction and aminolevulinic acid suppression are several mainstays of treatment. Avoidance of precipitating factors is the foundation of therapy in the latent period.

Commonly used anesthetics rarely precipitate an acute attack during latent porphyria.[53] Numerous anesthetics have been implicated to exacerbate an acute attack of porphyria and should be avoided. Propofol, ketamine, local anesthetics, muscle relaxants, nitrous oxide, isoflurane, and opioids are considered safe (**Table 12-2**). Drugs that induce cytochrome enzyme production may trigger a crisis and should be avoided (eg, barbiturates, ethyl alcohol, etomidate, nonbarbiturate sedatives, hydantoin anticonvulsants, hydralazine, and glucocorticoids).[50] Although regional anesthetic techniques have been described in porphyria, most experts advise against them because of a risk for exacerbating preexisting neuropathy, which could create confusion if neurologic signs develop postoperatively.[54] Perioperative glucose infusion should be administered. Careful positioning is necessary to protect fragile blisters and skin during surgery.

Charcot-Marie-Tooth Disease Charcot-Marie-Tooth disease is the most frequent inherited peripheral neuropathy. Typically, the defect is restricted to the lower third of the legs, causing foot deformities and peroneal muscle atrophy; however, the disease may slowly progress and affect other areas. Patients typically have stocking-glove sensory loss. Sensory deficits usually are milder than are the motor disturbances.[55] Pregnancy has been associated with exacerbations.[56] Despite long-term disability, life expectancy is not decreased, and treatment usually is supportive.

The effects of nondepolarizing neuromuscular blocking agents appear to be predictable. Although succinylcholine has been used without untoward consequences, it seems prudent to avoid using this neuromuscular blocker given theoretical concerns about hyperkalemia and cardiac arrest.[57] Respiratory insufficiency, vocal cord paresis, and cardiac conduction disturbances have been described.[58-60]

TABLE 12-2 Safe Anesthetic Drugs in the Presence of Acute Porphyria

Inhaled Anesthetics
Nitrous oxide: safe
Isoflurane: probably safe
Desflurane: probably safe
Sevoflurane: probably safe
Intravenous Anesthetics
Propofol: safe
Ketamine: probably safe
Analgesics
Morphine: safe
Fentanyl: safe
Sufentanil: safe
Acetaminophen: safe
Neuromuscular Blocking Agents
Succinylcholine: safe
Pancuronium: safe
Cisatracurium: probably safe
Vecuronium: probably safe
Rocuronium: probably safe
Mivacurium: probably safe
Anticholinesterases and Anticholinergics
Neostigmine: safe
Atropine: safe
Glycopyrrolate: safe
Local Anesthetics
Lidocaine: safe
Bupivacaine: safe
Tetracaine: safe
Mepivacaine: safe
Ropivacaine: probably safe
Anxiolytics
Midazolam: probably safe
Antiemetics
Droperidol: safe
Metoclopramide: probably safe
Ondansetron: probably safe

NEUROMUSCULAR JUNCTION

Myasthenia Gravis Myasthenia gravis is an autoimmune disorder involving the neuromuscular junction. Antibodies develop and are directed against postsynaptic acetylcholine receptors and other muscle membrane proteins.[61,62] The thymus is abnormal in 90% of patients with this disorder (ie, thymic hyperplasia, thymoma, or thymic atrophy).[63,64] Autoimmune disorders such as thyroiditis, pernicious anemia, and systemic lupus erythematosus are common in patients with myasthenia gravis.

The hallmark of this disorder is skeletal muscle weakness that is aggravated by exercise and improves with rest. Exacerbations and remissions are common. Any skeletal muscle may be affected, but the most common clinical presentation is ocular muscle weakness. Bulbar involvement may cause difficulty swallowing and respiratory insufficiency. When peripheral muscle groups are involved, ambulation may be difficult. Interestingly, the first manifestation of myasthenia gravis may occur when a patient is administered drugs that stabilize the muscle membrane, such as magnesium sulfate or local anesthetics. Myasthenic crisis occurs in approximately 20% of patients during the course of the disease and usually is precipitated by pulmonary infections.[64]

The diagnosis of myasthenia gravis is suggested by complaints of muscle weakness, particularly ocular and bulbar muscles. In addition to clinical history, the edrophonium tests (or challenge), electromyography, and detection of circulating antiacetylcholine receptor antibodies may confirm the diagnosis. Surprisingly, the extent of the disease is not proportional to the receptor antibody titer.

Treatment aims to improve function by increasing the amount of acetylcholine available at the neuromuscular junction. Cholinesterase inhibitors effectively increase the concentration of acetylcholine available at the neuromuscular junction. Because of its long duration of action, pyridostigmine is the drug of choice. Consistent control of myasthenia gravis with cholinesterase inhibitors may be a challenge. Underdosing results in worsening of the disease, and overdosing may cause cholinergic crisis. Circulating acetylcholine receptor antibodies are reduced by plasmapheresis, immunosuppressants, and corticosteroids. Thymectomy is controversial, but improvement occurs in the majority of patients with myasthenia gravis, especially if performed early in the course of the disease.[65]

Myasthenic crisis is a rapid deterioration of neuromuscular and respiratory function that may occur at any time perioperatively as a result of infection, stress, or an overdose with anticholinesterase drugs (cholinergic crisis). Cholinergic crisis typically presents with respiratory and bulbar muscle weakness, excessive salivation, miosis, bradycardia, and abdominal cramps. The diagnosis usually is made after a small dose of edrophonium is administered and worsening of these symptoms is observed. Control of a cholinergic crisis is achieved with supportive measures and administration of atropine or glycopyrrolate.

Preoperative preparation includes assessment of pulmonary function and optimization of medical therapy. Preoperative plasmapheresis has been shown to decrease ICU stay and the need for mechanical ventilation after thymectomy.[66] Risk factors that have been identified to predict postoperative respiratory failure after transsternal thymectomy are disease duration greater than 6 years, history of chronic respiratory disease, pyridostigmine dose greater than 750 mg/d, and preoperative vital capacity less than 2.9 L.[66] Transcervical thymectomy carries a lower incidence of prolonged postoperative mechanical ventilation than does transsternal thymectomy.[67] Whether anticholinesterase medication should be continued up to and including the day of surgery is controversial.[68]

Volatile anesthetics can be used as the sole anesthetic to provide analgesia, amnesia, and muscle relaxation.[69] Muscle relaxants should generally be avoided in most patients with myasthenia gravis. Anticholinesterase therapy should antagonize nondepolarizing muscle relaxants in theory, but in practice, patients with myasthenia gravis may be up to 100 times more sensitive to nondepolarizing relaxants than are unaffected patients.[70] Increased sensitivity remains in patients who are asymptomatic. The need for careful titration of nondepolarizing neuromuscular blockers via monitoring with a peripheral nerve stimulator in all patients with a history of myasthenia gravis is confirmed by these findings. Also, anticholinesterase therapy prolongs the response to succinylcholine by impairing plasma cholinesterase activity. Phase II block may be seen after administration of low doses of succinylcholine.[71] The decrease in the number of acetylcholine receptors also resists the action of succinylcholine.

Adjuvant drugs such as aminoglycoside antibiotics, magnesium, corticosteroids, loop diuretics, lithium salts, quinidine, and procainamide may exacerbate muscle weakness in myasthenic patients. Central respiratory depression is common in myasthenic patients, and the respiratory depressant effects of opioids and benzodiazepines may be enhanced.[72]

Epidural analgesia and anesthesia have been used in myasthenic patients.[73,74] However, caution is necessary because the muscle relaxation induced by regional anesthesia may accentuate the inherent weakness of myasthenia. Amide local anesthetics are theoretically a better choice than are the ester local anesthetics because cholinesterase activity does not affect amide anesthetic metabolism (see Chapter 45 for a discussion of the local anesthetic structures). Pregnancy has an unpredictable affect on myasthenia, and exacerbations should be anticipated.

Myasthenic Syndrome (Eaton-Lambert Syndrome) Myasthenic syndrome (Eaton-Lambert syndrome) is an acquired autoimmune disorder of the neuromuscular junction, often associated with carcinomas, in which release of acetylcholine from the nerve terminal is impaired despite normal production and processing of acetylcholine by the nerve cell. Onset of this disorder, when present, often precedes discovery of the malignancy by several years. Antibodies are produced against calcium channels, specific to tumor cells, but unfortunately cross-reactivity with calcium channels at the neuromuscular junction results in a decreased release of acetylcholine. Proximal extremity weakness is common, with the bulbar musculature less likely to be involved. In contrast to myasthenia gravis, muscle weakness is not consistently reversed by anticholinesterase administration, and exercise tends to improve muscle function (**Table 12-3**). Diagnosis may be made with electromyography or antibody assay. 3,4-Diaminopyridine is commonly administered and increases the presynaptic release of acetylcholine. Treatment of an underlying neoplasm, if present, usually improves symptoms. Immunosuppression, plasmapheresis, and immunoglobulin may be effective.[75]

TABLE 12-3 Myasthenia Gravis and Myasthenic Syndrome

Myasthenia Gravis	Myasthenic Syndrome
Extraocular, bulbar, facial muscle weakness	Proximal limb (arms > legs) weakness
Fatigue with exercise	Improved strength with exercise
Female > male	Male > female
Thymoma	Carcinoma (small cell of the lung)
Resistant to succinylcholine	Sensitive to succinylcholine
Sensitive to nondepolarizing muscle relaxants	Sensitive to nondepolarizing muscle relaxants
Good response to anticholinesterases	Poor response to anticholinesterases

Adapted from Stoelting RK, Dierdorf SF, eds. *Anesthesia and Co-existing Disease.* 4th ed. New York, NY: Churchill Livingstone; 2002. Copyright Elsevier.

Anesthetic management should focus on interactions with muscle relaxants. Patients with myasthenic syndrome are hypersensitive to the effect of depolarizing and nondepolarizing muscle relaxants. Doses should be reduced and titrated to effect with a peripheral nerve stimulator. Administration of 3,4-diaminopyridine should be continued perioperatively.[76]

MYOPATHIES AND CHANNELOPATHIES

Muscular Dystrophies Muscular dystrophies are disorders associated with abnormalities of the muscle membrane, resulting in variable, and progressive, loss of skeletal muscle function (**Table 12-4**). Dystrophin is a major component of the muscle cell cytoskeleton, which provides structural support to the muscle membrane in normal muscle. Lack of dystrophin results in membrane instability and permeability, eventually leading to intracellular calcium accumulation, cell necrosis, and replacement of degenerated muscle by fibrous and adipose tissue.[77] In addition to skeletal muscle dysfunction, cardiac and smooth muscles are affected. Indeed, in many types of muscular dystrophy, cardiac muscle involvement may be more significant than skeletal muscle involvement.

Duchenne muscular dystrophy is the most common muscular dystrophy (1:3500 male births) and has the most severe clinical course.[78] This disorder is a recessive, sex-linked genetic abnormality that is clinically evident in males, although female carriers may manifest subclinical abnormalities. Duchenne muscular dystrophy is characterized by painless skeletal muscle degeneration and atrophy. Muscle degeneration

TABLE 12-4 Types of Muscular Dystrophies and Myotonias

Muscular Dystrophies
Becker
Congenital
Duchenne
Emery-Dreifuss
Fascioscapulohumeral
Limb-girdle
Oculopharyngeal
Myotonias
Hyperkalemic periodic paralysis
Hypokalemic periodic paralysis
Myotonia congenita
Myotonic dystrophy
Paramyotonia congenita
Proximal myotonic dystrophy
Recessive myotonia

and weakness usually manifest in early childhood (age 2-5 years). Severe limitation in movement with development of contractures and kyphoscoliosis confine the child to a wheelchair by early adolescence. Marked increases in serum creatine kinase levels are present. Death commonly results from congestive heart failure or pneumonia. Although aggressive therapy for cardiopulmonary dysfunction has improved survival, afflicted individuals rarely survive beyond the third decade of life.[79,80]

As the patient ages and the disease progresses, cardiac muscle involvement typically is reflected by a progressive loss of R-wave amplitude in the lateral precordial leads of the ECG. Cardiomyopathy, ventricular dysrhythmias, and mitral regurgitation may develop as cardiac muscle is progressively lost and fibrous tissue replaces myocardial and conducting tissue. Treatment options include administration of angiotensin-converting enzyme inhibitors and β-adrenergic blockers to slow the deterioration of cardiac function.[80] Pulmonary function testing reveals a restrictive pulmonary disease pattern. Ineffective cough, resulting from diminished respiratory muscle strength, causes retention of secretions, pneumonia, and oftentimes death.[81] Many patients and families choose a tracheostomy and assisted ventilation, which may add years of life, but repetitive pulmonary infection contributes to a shortened life span.[82] Intestinal tract hypomotility develops as a result of smooth muscle involvement. Supplemental feedings may slow the process of cachexia, but the disease continues.

Although the cause of Duchenne muscular dystrophy is known, specific genetic therapy is elusive. Therapy is supportive and focuses on improving cardiopulmonary function and better nutrition.

Becker muscular dystrophy is similar to Duchenne muscular dystrophy; however, it has a later onset in life and slower clinical progression. Typically, patients remain ambulatory past the age of 16 years, and cardiac failure caused by occult cardiomyopathy may be the presenting symptom.[83] Any male with a persistent elevation in serum creatine kinase concentration should be evaluated for Becker muscular dystrophy.

Emery-Dreifuss X-linked muscular dystrophy is characterized by humeropectoral muscle weakness and contractures of the spine, elbows, and ankles. The autosomal-dominant type of this disorder is caused by a defect in the protein lamin, whereas the recessive form is caused by a defect in the protein emerin. Clinical manifestations of skeletal muscle weakness usually are mild, but cardiac conduction defects may manifest as sudden death. Patients with this disorder are candidates for implantable defibrillating pacemakers.[84]

Limb-girdle muscular dystrophy patients have weakness of the muscles of the shoulder and pelvic girdles. Most forms of this disorder are inherited in an autosomal-recessive fashion, although autosomal-dominant defects have been discovered. A defect in the sarcoglycan protein is the usual etiology of this abnormality.[85] Cardiomyopathy and cardiac conduction defects may occur.

Fascioscapulohumeral muscular dystrophy is a disease with diverse clinical manifestations that is inherited in an autosomal-dominant fashion. Facial, scapulohumeral, anterior tibial, and pelvic-girdle muscle weakness are common. Cardiac conduction defects as well as deafness and retinal vascular disease may occur.

Oculopharyngeal muscular dystrophy primarily manifests with ptosis and dysphagia late in adulthood. Commonly, weakness of the head and neck develop in addition to dysphagia that is present from pharyngeal muscle weakness and esophageal dysmotility.

Merosin-deficient muscular dystrophy, Fukuyama muscular dystrophy, Walker-Warburg syndrome, Ulrich disease, muscle–eye–brain disease, nemaline myopathy, myotubular myopathy, and rigid spine muscular dystrophy are a group of muscular dystrophies that comprise congenital muscular dystrophy.[85,86] Congenital muscular dystrophies are characterized by early onset of muscle weakness, feeding difficulties, and respiratory dysfunction, frequently with accompanying mental retardation.

Perioperative complications from anesthesia in patients with muscular dystrophies usually result from the effects of anesthetic drugs on myocardial and skeletal muscle. Preexisting myocardial dysfunction makes the patient with muscular dystrophy susceptible to the myocardial depressant effects of anesthetics. The abnormal muscle cell membrane predisposes patients with muscular dystrophy to hyperkalemia and rhabdomyolysis when subjected to volatile anesthetics alone or in combination with succinylcholine, as numerous case reports support. In light of the abnormal muscle membrane, succinylcholine administration may further damage the muscle membrane and cause the release of intracellular contents. Therefore, succinylcholine should be avoided in patients with muscular dystrophies. It has been speculated that volatile anesthetics cause the release of calcium from the sarcoplasmic reticulum and may elicit damage to the muscle cell membrane and cause rhabdomyolysis. Interestingly, sevoflurane appears to be a less potent stimulus for release of calcium from the sarcoplasmic reticulum than are other volatile agents.[87]

Nondepolarizing muscle relaxants may have a prolonged duration of action in patients with muscular dystrophy, although the response to mivacurium appears to be normal.[88] Therefore, close monitoring of neuromuscular function is indicated. Although unpredictable, some patients with muscular dystrophies may be susceptible to developing malignant hyperthermia (MH). Without regard to specific etiology, patients who have chronically increased creatine phosphokinase levels may have a 40% to 45% risk of being MH susceptible.[89] Therefore, careful consideration of anesthetic plan may be to avoid all MH-triggering agents until a patient has been evaluated by the caffeine–halothane contracture test on a muscle biopsy specimen. (A detailed discussion of malignant hyperthermia is provided in Chapter 87.)

Delayed gastric emptying and impaired swallowing increase the risk of perioperative aspiration. Postoperatively, patients with muscular dystrophies must be closely monitored for evidence of pulmonary dysfunction and retained secretions. Vigorous pulmonary toilet and mechanical ventilation are frequently required. Regardless of the need for postoperative mechanical ventilation, these patients should be placed in an advanced monitoring unit (ICU) for appropriate analgesic therapy and respiratory monitoring.

Myotonias The myotonias are a diverse group of hereditary skeletal muscle disorders with a common clinical sign: myotonia (Table 12-1). Myotonia is the persistent contracture and delayed relaxation of skeletal muscle after cessation of voluntary contraction or stimulation of the muscle. One of the typical signs of myotonic dystrophy is the inability to relax the handgrip. Progressive muscle wasting, ptosis, and facial muscle weakness also are common in patients with myotonic dystrophy. Interestingly, in other myotonic syndromes, the most common finding is stiffness that improves with exercise. However, paramyotonia (cold-induced myotonia) is an exception, wherein exercise exacerbates symptoms. Recently, genetic defects in sodium, chloride, and calcium ion channels in the muscle membrane have been identified as the abnormalities responsible for myotonia. Therefore, drugs such as mexiletine, procainamide, tocainide, and quinine may relax myotonic contractures by altering ion channel activity and skeletal muscle membrane excitability.

The most common of the myotonic disorders is myotonic dystrophy (Steinert disease), although proximal myotonic myopathy, myotonic dystrophy type II, and proximal myotonic dystrophy are other myotonic diseases. Myotonic dystrophy is inherited in an autosomal-dominant pattern, and symptoms typically appear in the second or third decade of life. A defect on chromosome 19 produces a decrease in protein kinase that causes degeneration of the sarcoplasmic reticulum.[90] This myotonic dystrophy is the only myotonic disorder to exhibit extramuscular manifestations. Cataracts, premature balding, diabetes mellitus, thyroid dysfunction, adrenal insufficiency, gonadal dysfunction, and cardiac conduction defects are common. Cardiac involvement does not correlate with the severity of skeletal muscle involvement.[91] There is a progressive deterioration of the conduction system resulting in atrioventricular conduction delay. First-degree atrioventricular block, bundle-branch block, and widening of the QRS complex are common. Cardiomyopathy, cardiac failure, and sudden death may occur, and the incidences of septal defects, mitral valve prolapse, and valvular disease are increased.

Recurrent pulmonary infections and aspiration may result when bulbar musculature is affected. Pulmonary function testing demonstrates a restrictive lung disease pattern, mild arterial hypoxemia, and diminished ventilatory responses to hypercapnia and hypoxia. Gastric atony may develop as a result of alterations in smooth muscle function. Exacerbations of myotonic dystrophy often occur during pregnancy as a result of increased concentrations of progesterone. Congestive heart failure is common during pregnancy, and cesarean delivery is indicated because of uterine smooth muscle involvement. Labor typically is prolonged, and the incidence of postpartum hemorrhage is increased. Infants may have congenital myotonic dystrophy, which typically is characterized by hypotonia, respiratory insufficiency, and feeding difficulties.

Therapy for myotonic dystrophy is focused on treating coexisting diseases and cardiac dysrhythmias. Drugs that alter sodium channel function have been the most effective for managing myotonia (eg, mexiletine). Avoiding factors known to precipitate myotonia is important.

Anesthetic considerations for patients with myotonic dystrophy include the presence of coexisting diseases, abnormal responses to drugs, and avoiding factors that are associated with the development of perioperative myotonia. Perioperative myotonia has been precipitated by drugs (propofol and succinylcholine), physical factors (hypothermia), electrocautery, and surgical manipulation. Potassium administration worsens clinical myotonia. Succinylcholine produces an exaggerated contracture, and its use should be avoided. The myotonic response produced by succinylcholine may be so severe that ventilation and tracheal intubation are difficult and may be impossible. The typical presentation of succinylcholine-induced myotonic contracture includes jaw, abdominal, and chest rigidity. Perioperative myotonia may be difficult to differentiate from MH. A recent thorough review of the pathophysiology and clinical experience related to the myotonias concluded that MH is no more common in these patients than in the general population, despite the frequent suggestion of such a relationship (a minor theoretical concern remained for hypokalemic periodic paralysis, but no clinical episodes of MH have been reported in these patients).[92] Nondepolarizing muscle relaxants and peripheral nerve blocks do not abolish myotonic contractures. Induction agents, volatile anesthetics, opioids (systemic and neuraxial), and sedatives may cause profound respiratory depression. Increased sensitivity to nondepolarizing muscle relaxants may occur, especially when there is muscle wasting. Prudence dictates the use of short-acting muscle relaxants when necessary, with careful monitoring of the response. Peripheral nerve stimulation may cause myotonia or be misinterpreted as sustained tetanus, even though significant neuromuscular blockade exists. Reversal of neuromuscular blockade may induce myotonia.

Although no specific anesthetic technique has been determined to be superior for patients with myotonic dystrophy, close monitoring of cardiac and pulmonary function is critical to ensure an optimal perioperative outcome. Mechanical ventilation should be used until muscle strength and function return to baseline.[93] Regional anesthesia has been successfully performed in patients with myotonic dystrophy.[94]

Familial Periodic Paralysis Periodic paralyses are skeletal muscle channelopathies, which include hyperkalemic and hypokalemic periodic paralysis, paramyotonia congenita, and potassium-aggravated myotonia.[95-97] Periodic paralyses are characterized by acute reversible episodes of muscle weakness or paralysis of the extremities, with sparing of the respiratory muscles. Although these disorders are classified by changes in serum potassium concentrations during an acute episode, these changes are relative to the baseline potassium concentration and are not always abnormally increased or decreased (**Table 12-5**).

Hyperkalemic periodic paralysis is inherited in an autosomal-dominant fashion. The dominant trait has been discovered as a mutation in the sodium ion channel on chromosome 17.[90] As a consequence of this dysfunction, when the resting membrane potential becomes slightly more positive, the myofiber can more easily reach threshold and the muscle becomes hyperexcitable, which clinically manifests as myotonia.[98] When the membrane potential becomes even more positive, the myofiber cannot fire an action potential because of the loss of a sufficient membrane potential, and the result is paralysis.[98] Normokalemic periodic paralysis is rare and most likely is a variant of hyperkalemic paralysis in which the potassium concentration does not change during attacks.[99]

TABLE 12-5 Clinical Features of Hypokalemic and Hyperkalemic Familial Periodic Paralysis

Hyperkalemic
Potassium concentration >5.5 mEq/L (or normal) during crisis
Precipitating events
Potassium infusion
Hypothermia
Rest after strenuous exercise
Metabolic acidosis
Duration of paralysis
Minutes to hours (rarely a few days)
Hypokalemic
Potassium concentration <3 mEq/L during crisis
Precipitating events
High glucose intake
Strenuous exercise
Stress (including trauma or surgery)
Hypothermia
Glucose-insulin infusion
Pregnancy
Duration of paralysis
Hours to days

Attacks usually begin during childhood and vary in frequency from several times per week to once in a lifetime. These episodes of myotonia and paralysis may last several hours after exposure to a trigger. Triggering events include eating potassium-rich foods, IV infusion of potassium, fasting, cold exposure, and rest after strenuous exercise. Thiazide diuretics, acetazolamide and a low-potassium diet are the mainstays of preventive treatment. Glucose and insulin infusion, careful catecholamine infusions, and IV calcium administration can be used to manage acute attacks.

Hypokalemic periodic paralysis is usually inherited in an autosomal-dominant pattern. The dominant trait produces a defect in the calcium ion channel on chromosome 1.[100] The dihydropyridine receptor is a voltage-gated ion channel that is responsible for attacks, but the mechanism by which this defect results in attacks of paralysis is under investigation.

Attacks usually begin during childhood or early adulthood and vary in frequency. In contrast to the hyperkalemic form, attacks last longer—from hours to days. Also, cardiac arrhythmias are more common, ventricular dilatation may be seen, myotonia is absent, and permanent muscle weakness eventually develops by the fifth decade of life. Paralysis is commonly triggered by ingestion of carbohydrates, strenuous exercise, glucose and insulin infusion, IV calcium, and exposure to cold. Paralysis often is incomplete, affecting the limbs and trunk but sparing the diaphragm. Rarely are respiratory muscles involved, but asphyxia has been reported. Treatment involves the administration of potassium, acetazolamide, and dichlorphenamide.

Maintenance of normal potassium concentrations and avoidance of events that precipitate weakness are the primary goals of the perioperative management of patients with hyperkalemic and hypokalemic periodic paralysis. Electrolyte abnormalities should be addressed and corrected as best as possible before surgery. Patients may be sensitive to nondepolarizing muscle relaxants; therefore, short-acting relaxants should be administered when necessary. The response should be monitored with a peripheral nerve stimulator. Reversal should be avoided because of concern that reversal agents may precipitate myotonia. However, adequate muscle strength must be assured before extubation.[101] Succinylcholine should be avoided because it alters serum potassium concentrations and therefore may precipitate an attack. Reductions in serum potassium from metabolic changes or medications should be avoided because this situation may initiate an episode of paralysis. Perioperative potassium values should be monitored serially. The ECG should be continuously monitored for evidence of arrhythmia, and normothermia and normocapnia should be maintained. Volatile anesthetics have been administered without complication. Regional anesthesia has been used successfully, although there is concern that regional techniques can create confusion if neurologic signs develop postoperatively.[102] MH has been associated with periodic paralyses.[103]

SKELETAL MUSCLE DISEASES

Central Core Disease Central core disease is a hereditary, nonprogressive, congenital myopathy that typically is characterized by lower extremity muscle weakness. Increased lumbar lordosis, kyphoscoliosis, and hip dislocations may occur. Histologically, type I muscle fibers display amorphous central areas (cores). The underlying defect is thought to be associated with the ryanodine receptor gene, similar to MH.[104] Susceptibility for MH is a great concern when anesthetizing patients with central core disease.[105,106] MH precautions should be taken and nontriggering anesthetics used when anesthetizing patients with central core disease (see Chapter 87 for a thorough discussion of malignant hyperthermia).

Glycogen Storage Diseases Glycogen storage diseases are inherited disorders characterized by a deficiency of enzymes involved in glucose metabolism. An enzyme deficiency results in a lack or excess of precursors and end-products of glycogen formation and breakdown. Type II (Pompe disease) glycogen storage disease is notable for the buildup of glycogen in smooth, skeletal, and cardiac muscle. Cardiac involvement typically leads to congestive heart failure. Anesthetic experience is limited.[107,108] Skeletal muscle involvement predisposes patients to upper airway obstruction secondary to glycogen infiltration of the tongue. Aspiration is common secondary to neurologic involvement and subsequent impairment of cough, gag, and swallowing mechanisms. Volatile anesthetics may precipitate cardiovascular embarrassment or collapse. Administration of succinylcholine to these patients may not be prudent because theoretically it could result in myoglobinuria and perhaps hyperkalemia with subsequent cardiac arrest. Hypoglycemia and acidosis may develop perioperatively, and patients should be hydrated and receive exogenous glucose. Hepatic dysfunction usually is present, so judicious administration of drugs hepatically metabolized should be taken into consideration. Regional anesthesia has been performed in patients with glycogen storage disorders.[109] Patients with type V (McArdle disease) glycogen storage disease are prone to developing myoglobinuria and rhabdomyolysis. Automated blood pressure readings should be performed cautiously, and tourniquets should be avoided to prevent muscle damage.[110]

Mitochondrial Myopathies Mitochondrial myopathies are a group of disorders that affect oxidative phosphorylation, resulting in impaired adenosine triphosphate production. These disorders have many manifestations, including CNS and muscle pathology. Exercise intolerance, fatigue, muscle pain, progressive weakness, and cardiomyopathy may be present. Respiratory depression is common after administration of general anesthesia. There does not appear to be an association with MH with most mitochondrial disorders.[111-114] However, avoidance of succinylcholine seems prudent because of the potential for hyperkalemia.

Kearns-Sayre syndrome and mitochondrial myopathy, encephalopathy, lactic acidosis, and stroke-like episodes (MELAS syndrome) are distinct mitochondrial disorders. The anesthetic concerns are similar to the general concerns previously stated, but, in addition, Kearns-Sayre syndrome is associated with heart block due to involvement of the cardiac conduction system. General anesthesia should be used with caution because it may increase the risk of myocardial depression and cardiac conduction defects.[115] MELAS syndrome is characterized by stroke-like episodes, seizures, dementia, recurrent headaches, vomiting, and lactic acidosis. There is suspicion that MH susceptibility may be increased, and propofol-based anesthesia has been used successfully. Myocardial depression may occur with administration of volatile anesthetics, so they therefore should be used with caution. Additional precautions include maintenance of normothermia, avoidance of lactated solutions or acidosis, and careful attention to blood glucose control. A full discussion of this unusual syndrome is beyond the scope of this chapter, but a recent case report contains a useful review of overall anesthetic considerations.[116]

PERIOPERATIVE ASSESSMENT OF MUSCULOSKELETAL CONDITIONS

Patients with musculoskeletal disease may present varied challenges to the anesthesiologist. A number of more common musculoskeletal conditions are included here for consideration in the evaluation of a patient for anesthesia.

OSTEOARTHRITIS

Osteoarthritis (OA) is a prevalent condition with advancing age.[117] Multiple joints are affected, most commonly weight-bearing joints. Patients with OA may require joint replacement surgery or other intricate orthopedic procedures. In patients with OA, the cervical spine may have a reduced range of motion, and the lumbar spine may be affected with osteal growths such that performing regional anesthesia may be difficult. Determination of what the surgical approach required for patient positioning is important. Whether regional anesthesia will be used intraoperatively or only for postoperative analgesia must be considered. How soon the patient is expected to become ambulatory and require full sensation and motor capabilities may dictate whether long-acting regional anesthetics or techniques can be used.

A careful list of recent nonsteroidal anti-inflammatory drug (NSAID) use should be obtained. With many of the newer, more powerful, and long-lasting NSAIDs, there is concern for possible hematoma formation after regional or neuraxial anesthesia. Most practitioners are willing to perform peripheral blocks in patients who are receiving moderate doses of NSAIDs, provided there is no history of excessive bleeding; however, high-dose NSAID use or a history of bleeding should trigger a note of caution.

OA results in moderate to severe disability that may be relieved by surgical approaches. Of significant concern to the anesthesiologist is cervical spine disease with reduced range of motion and implications of difficulty in visualizing or securing the airway. Neurologic manifestations may occur from development of spinal stenosis at any spinal level. Chronic, subacute, and acute symptoms may be present, and acute neurologic symptoms may require emergency operation. This may require rapid sequence intubation, which may become complicated if the airway is not easily visualized.

Treatment of OA includes salicylates, NSAIDs, local heat, and surgical procedures to ameliorate painful symptoms. There is no effective therapy for slowing the pathogenesis of the disease. Selective cyclooxygenase-2 inhibitors were found to be effective in patients with OA, and their side-effect profile initially was thought to be advantageous compared with that of other nonselective NSAIDs. However, some of these drugs were withdrawn from the market when cardiovascular events associated with use of cyclooxygenase-2 agents were discovered. A careful history of medication use is necessary before considering neuraxial blockade.

RHEUMATOID ARTHRITIS

Rheumatoid arthritis (RA) is an autoimmune disease that attacks numerous joints throughout the body and has some special considerations for the anesthesiologist.[118] Patients with RA may have complications primarily from their disease or secondarily from treatment of the disease, including use of glucocorticoids, NSAIDs, and immunosuppressive drugs.

Patients with advanced stages of RA may have temporomandibular ankylosis that makes direct laryngoscopy for endotracheal intubation very challenging, if not impossible. Fiberoptic intubation may be required, or tracheostomy may be necessary. The cervical spine may be involved, including laxity of the C1-2 ligament, causing instability of the cervical spine. Subluxation of the atlantoaxial joint and instability can progress to spinal cord compression. Long tract signs, including bowel and bladder dysfunction, may occur, and sudden death has occurred from spinal cord laceration by the odontoid process. Recognizing early signs of serious cervical spine instability is critical in planning the approach to the airway. Cricoarytenoid (CA) joint involvement may occur in RA. This condition may make the glottis more rigid and require insertion of a smaller-diameter endotracheal tube. CA joints that are fixed in adduction may be life-threatening and require tracheostomy in order to establish a stable airway.

Awake or fiberoptic intubation may be necessary to permit neurologic examination immediately after placement of an endotracheal tube (see Chapters 10 and 36 regarding airway evaluation and management). Patients with RA often have involvement of multiple digits and may suffer from compression fractures of the vertebral bodies secondary to glucocorticoid use. These presentations in this illness may make anesthesia particularly challenging.

RA afflicts peripheral joints, most often symmetrically. As the disease advances, patients may have severe limitations in movement because of inflammatory contractions, pain with motion, or bone joint fusions due to long-standing inflammation. These patients may present for multiarticular surgical procedures or other surgical procedures secondary to complications of RA.

RA is a systemic disease with pulmonary and cardiac manifestations. Restrictive lung disease occurs from multiple complications. Pulmonary interstitial fibrosis, pulmonary effusions, and parenchymal rheumatoid nodules may lead to crepitations. With advanced disease, ventilation and oxygenation may require attention to small-volume, positive-pressure ventilation during surgery and supplemental oxygen use preoperatively and postoperatively. Consideration for assisted ventilation postoperatively should be discussed with the patient.

RA can be associated with pericardial effusion and pericarditis. Tamponade is rare but well described. Conduction disturbances and valvular dysfunction occurs in advanced stages of RA. Preoperative echocardiographic evaluation and a 12-lead ECG are indicated on the basis of symptomatology or length of duration of the disease.

Treatment of RA includes use of NSAIDs, glucocorticoids, gold salts, penicillin, and immunosuppressive (cytotoxic) drugs.[119] These drugs have multiple serious side effects. Glucocorticoids cause hypertension, cataracts, skin and muscle atrophy, and osteopenia, which may result in vertebral compression fractures. Immunosuppressive therapy may predispose to infections and can be cardiotoxic. NSAIDs and aspirin will result in thrombasthenia or other coagulation disorders, which must be considered before performance of regional neuraxial blockade. Peripheral neural blockade may have less risk of hemorrhagic complications, but the rare complications do not deter some anesthesiologists from careful use of peripheral neural blockade after thorough preoperative assessment of alternatives.

ANKYLOSING SPONDYLITIS

Ankylosing spondylitis is an inflammatory disease of the spine and paraspinal tissue.[120] Ankylosing spondylitis typically affects young men and may become disabling due to chronic pain in less than a decade. Back pain with or without peripheral arthritis occurs. Ankylosis of the hip and sacroiliac joints may occur, and the cervical spine may also be involved. Cauda equina syndrome may occur with devastating consequences.

Anesthetic considerations are similar to those for patients with RA. Cervical fusion (ankylosis) or atlantoaxial subluxation may occur. Cardiopulmonary complications include restrictive pulmonary fibrosis, and possibly cardiac conduction abnormalities and aortic insufficiency.

Pharmacologic therapy includes NSAIDs and glucocorticoids. Side-effect profiles of each of these classes are as discussed previously. Neuroaxial blockade may be contraindicated on the basis of coagulation status and recent use of NSAIDs.

CEREBRAL PALSY

Cerebral palsy (CP) is considered a static encephalopathy. It is included in the discussion of musculoskeletal diseases because of the number of symptoms secondary to loss of upper motor neuron control. Patients have imbalances of flexor/extensor muscle activity resulting in significant contractures. These conditions may make the patient's airway difficult to approach, and the neck may have a reduced range of motion or fixed abnormal position. The usual extremity positions may not be obtainable because of contractures, and IV access may be difficult. Because patients with CP live into adulthood, the anesthesiologist must be aware that multiple procedures for CP are meant to reduce the patient's burden of care by allowing him or her to obtain a more neutral or balanced position. Procedures including osteotomies, botulinum toxin and phenol injections, and other major procedures often are necessary. Patients with CP are one of a group of patients presenting for neuromuscular scoliosis repair. Kyphoscoliosis can be a particularly challenging orthopedic problem requiring extensive instrumentation of the spine posteriorly and sometimes release of multiple ligaments anteriorly. The two-phased approach may be performed in one procedure or may be separated by a number of days or weeks (see Chapter 65 for a discussion of spinal surgery).

Anesthesia considerations include providing a stable airway, appropriate invasive monitoring for anticipated major blood loss, IV access for resuscitative fluid administration, and possible postoperative assisted ventilation. Patients may be limited to nonverbal communication skills, thereby making pain management challenging. Patients with CP may have a seizure disorder from brain injury at birth or traumatic or anoxic brain injury later in life. Anesthesia clinicians should be familiar with the many antiepileptic drugs currently prescribed. If therapeutic monitoring methods are available, optimal serum concentrations should be achieved preoperatively.

OSTEOPOROSIS

Osteoporosis is a generic diagnostic term describing loss of bone mass from one of several disease states. Osteoporosis occurs with advancing age and affects women more frequently than men. Decreased bone density may result in pathologic fractures and kyphosis. Although a systemic disorder, axial spine involvement usually is responsible for acute manifestations, and this is the problem that often presents the most difficulty for the anesthesia practitioner.

Osteoporotic fractures and kyphosis may significantly complicate regional anesthetic neuroaxial procedures. Acute fractures may be severely painful and, in rare circumstances, may result in neurologic compromise necessitating urgent operation. Patients may be unable to assume a sitting or supine position comfortably. With increasing kyphosis, a restrictive lung disease pattern appears. Airway management should include plans to ameliorate the patient's pain, use thorough preoxygenation, and institute assisted ventilation for neurodecompressive procedures with prone positioning. Postoperative respiratory insufficiency should be monitored secondary to underlying respiratory concerns and the moderate-to-heavy opioid requirement for postoperative analgesia.

Most patients with osteoporosis may have an idiopathic etiology. These patients have normal laboratory values for calcium, phosphorus, and alkaline phosphatase. Patients with abnormal laboratory values should be evaluated for coexisting diseases such as hyperparathyroidism or malignancy (hypercalcemia). Paget disease usually is accompanied by a high alkaline phosphatase.

OSTEOGENESIS IMPERFECTA

Osteogenesis imperfecta (OI) is an inherited disorder of connective tissue that usually manifests in 1 of 2 presentations: osteogenesis imperfecta congenita or osteogenesis imperfecta tarda.[121] Newborns and children suffer multiple fractures in the congenital form, whereas the onset of fractures occurs in later childhood, adolescence, and adulthood in the tarda form. In addition to musculoskeletal presentations, these patients may suffer otosclerosis and progressive hearing loss, dental hypoplasia, ligamentous laxity, cardiac valvular insufficiency, and easy bruisability.

Evaluation of a patient with OI includes attention to dental deformities preexisting at the time of anesthesia and echocardiographic evaluation if a murmur is present. Airway management usually is not complicated; however, patient positioning for comfort may be challenging. Regional anesthesia is a reasonable option as in healthy patients, but tourniquet use should be avoided to reduce risk of fracture.

When surgeons may not have the benefit of tourniquet use for a specific procedure, greater than expected blood loss should be anticipated. Although bleeding tendency in patients with OI has been described, this finding does not absolutely contraindicate regional anesthesia.

Patients with OI and many patients with musculoskeletal dysplasias tend to become febrile in the operating room. Ectodermal dysplasia or lack of vasorelaxation may prevent mechanisms of heat loss usually encountered in the operating room or during anesthesia. Special attention should be directed to temperature monitoring and control, even for short procedures. With recent attention to prevention of heat loss during anesthesia, patients often are protected from hypothermia. However, in patients with OI, moderate to severe generalized hyperthermia may occur, and this may be confused with MH. Patients with OI do not have an increased susceptibility for MH.

SCLERODERMA

Scleroderma (progressive systemic sclerosis [PSS]) is a disorder of connective tissue with destruction of small arterioles, leading to fibrosis of the skin and internal organs. It is not specifically a musculoskeletal disease. PSS causes swollen and stiff fingers and Raynaud phenomenon. Pain of the digits and knee joints is common, and a polyarthritis resembling RA may occur. Limited mobility secondary to diffuse fibrosis (scleroderma) becomes a feature that may make patient positioning for surgery difficult.

Visceral involvement in scleroderma includes esophageal (dysphagia and gastroesophageal reflux), gastric atony and dilation, intestinal (abdominal pain), pulmonary fibrosis, and cardiac involvement, including varying degrees of heart block, cardiomyopathy, and pericarditis, which may result in tamponade.[122]

Preoperative evaluation includes a comprehensive history of symptoms related to the airway, pulmonary, and cardiac systems. Airway management may require a rapid sequence or an awake technique. Cardiopulmonary evaluation depends on duration of the disease and symptoms of disability or signs on physical examination. Cardiac rhythm and performance should be thoroughly evaluated before elective anesthesia and operation.

When a patient with PSS presents for emergent surgery, a 12-lead ECG, and possibly echocardiography, should be considered. Electrolytes should be measured. Causes of death in PSS include cardiovascular etiologies and renal failure. Subclinical renal failure (increased blood urea nitrogen and creatinine, hyperkalemia, and hyperphosphatemia) is a relative contraindication to succinylcholine use. Patients may experience amnesia from lack of absorption of nutrients and microangiopathic hemolytic anemia.

Postoperative care should include cardiovascular monitoring, serial electrolytes evaluation, and supplemental oxygen to address the combined effects of pulmonary involvement and opioid use for postoperative analgesia.

CARPEL TUNNEL SYNDROME

Carpal tunnel syndrome is an entrapment neuropathy that may be idiopathic or secondary to a number of illnesses, including RA, tenosynovitis, and amyloidoses, and may occur secondary to edema during pregnancy. The surgical approach to entrapment is decompression by release of the transverse ligaments or removal of a space-occupying lesion compressing the nerve.

The anesthetic approach may include general anesthesia, upper extremity regional blockade, or local intravenous anesthesia (Bier block). These procedures usually are performed in an ambulatory surgical suite, and the anesthesia plan should anticipate the need for rapid recovery. Some surgeons will want to perform a sensorimotor examination immediately postoperatively to establish that no surgical complication occurred, but most are comfortable with regional anesthetic techniques for this procedure.

ACHONDROPLASIA

Achondroplasia is one etiology of dwarfism. A defect in endochondral ossification appears to lead to short tubular bones. Children often are identified at birth by their phenotypic presentation. Relative macrocephaly and hypoplastic midfacial features are common.

The two most concerning issues with achondroplasia are a relative stenotic foramen magnum, which may result in obstructive hydrocephalus, and atlantoaxial instability. These problems may cause acute neurologic presentation of increased intracranial pressure or spinal cord compression, respectively. These problems may present early in infancy and require emergent decompression.

As these children grow, they develop increasing lordosis and require spinal fixation/stabilization.[123] Multiple procedures may be necessary.

Anesthetic implications in patients with achondroplasia include anticipating a difficult seal of a face mask because of midfacial hypoplasia. Tracheal intubation is generally not difficult; however, care should be taken not to hyperextend the neck for visualization of the vocal cords to avoid cervical spinal cord injury. No additional side effects are associated with use of succinylcholine, and there is no association of achondroplasia with susceptibility to MH.

Patients with achondroplasia may have an inability to disseminate heat effectively. Special attention to central temperature monitoring and management should be anticipated. These patients may have an excessive thermal response to anticholinergic agents.

POLYMYOSITIS/DERMATOMYOSITIS

Polymyositis and dermatomyositis are diseases that involve skeletal muscle, connective tissue, and the skin.[124] The etiologies are unknown, but autoimmune phenomena are suspected. Usually slow progressive weakness occurring over months to years affects proximal extremity muscle groups, followed by neck involvement. Pharyngeal and laryngeal muscles also may be involved.

Cardiac involvement may include rhythm disturbances, myocardial necrosis, or inflammation. Pulmonary fibrosis or interstitial pneumonitis may be seen. Treatment of the illness consists of corticosteroids and immunosuppressive drugs. The consequences of these treatments should be considered in the preoperative evaluation (eg, stress doses of corticosteroids may be indicated for major invasive procedures, and meticulous attention to sterile technique is required to prevent risk of infection after vascular access).

Anesthetic implications of these diseases are primarily of pharyngeal muscle activity and the risk for aspiration. No known anesthetic-associated exacerbation of cardiac involvement has been reported. Patients do not routinely experience respiratory weakness after anesthesia or use of neuromuscular blocking agents.

RHABDOMYOLYSIS

Rhabdomyolysis is a condition associated with many inherited disorders,[125] toxin and drug exposure,[126,127] ischemia, crushing, and burn injury.[128] Exercise-induced rhabdomyolysis can occur secondary to inborn errors or secondary to exercise-induced bioenergetic failure at the cellular level. Perioperative rhabdomyolysis has been associated with positioning, cardiopulmonary bypass, an excessive response to succinylcholine, and as a prominent symptom of MH syndrome[129] (see Chapter 87 for details regarding malignant hyperthermia).

A preoperative history of rhabdomyolysis should alert the anesthesiologist to the possibility of inborn genetic errors (carnitine palmitoyltransferase deficiency [not related to MH]) and susceptibility to MH. Exercise-induced rhabdomyolysis patients and patients with chronic hypercreatine kinasemia (hyperCKemia) are considered subgroups at high risk for MH susceptibility.[89,130,131] When in doubt regarding the possibility of susceptibility to MH, the MH hotline consultants are available 24 hours per day (1-800-MH-HYPER) in the United States and Canada (see Chapter 87).

MALIGNANT HYPERTHERMIA

MH is related to very specific muscle disorders as referred (hyperCKemia and exercise-induced rhabdomyolysis, central core disease, and others). MH is covered extensively in Chapter 87.

MOVEMENT DISORDERS: PARKINSON DISEASE

Parkinson disease is the second most common neurodegenerative disease (after Alzheimer disease) and the most common of the movement disorders. This section focuses specifically on Parkinson disease because it is not uncommon in patients requiring anesthetic care for the primary condition (eg, for deep brain stimulation) or for unrelated conditions that occur in the elderly. More than half of persons aged 85 years or older have Parkinson disease or parkinsonian symptoms. The cause of Parkinson disease is unknown, but it involves neuronal destruction in the substantia nigra, locus ceruleus, and other brain centers. The resulting loss of dopamine production produces extrapyramidal signs and symptoms including bradykinesia, festinating (short, jerky, accelerating) gait, tremor, rigidity, and loss of balance. The mainstay of treatment is oral levodopa (L-dopa), a precursor that is converted to dopamine in the brain. Dopamine agonists or type B monoamine oxidase inhibitors (MAOIs) may also be used. The diagnosis of Parkinson disease is made by clinical observation and response to L-dopa; confirmation requires autopsy showing the characteristic Levy bodies in the substantia nigra.

Anesthesia represents a significant hazard for Parkinson disease patients.[132] These patients are susceptible to pulmonary aspiration, laryngospasm, diaphragmatic spasm, and altered function of the ventilatory muscles, resulting in an obstructive breathing pattern.[133-135] Respiratory complications (ie, aspiration) represent the most common cause of death in these patients.[136] Preoperative evaluation should include careful evaluation of the airway and chest, including a chest radiograph if chronic aspiration is suspected.

Perioperative management of multiple medications requires special attention, often among several medical specialists. Withdrawal of Parkinson disease medications in the perioperative period can cause a clinically significant worsening of the respiratory symptoms.[137] Polypharmacy in Parkinson disease patients may also contribute to a greater incidence of orthostatic hypotension.[138] This is further exacerbated by the direct vasodilatory effects of dopamine agonists or tricyclic antidepressants, which are used commonly in this population. The addition of systemic opiates for postoperative analgesia may lead to drug interactions in these patients who are often receiving multiple medications. These factors may contribute to the 8-fold increase in postoperative delirium observed in Parkinson disease patients.[139]

The approach to anesthetic care varies depending on the proposed procedure. Broadly, these patients can be classified as those undergoing deep brain stimulation (ie, primary disease surgery) and those undergoing other procedures (ie, incidental surgery). For the latter, the regularly prescribed medications should be administered immediately preoperatively and resumed as soon as possible postoperatively. Regional anesthesia may offer significant advantages in patients with Parkinson disease by allowing an earlier return to oral intake, eliminating the use of neuromuscular blocking drugs and the risks of general anesthesia.[132,140] Those undergoing deep brain stimulation require a uniquely different approach; their anti-Parkinson medications are withheld before the procedure in order to produce maximum effect during deep brain stimulation, which is performed under local anesthesia[141] (see Chapter 51 for greater discussion of the anesthetic care of patients undergoing deep brain stimulation).

General anesthesia may be required for some procedures, and there are reported problems associated with the use of numerous anesthetics and related medications. Parkinson symptoms were triggered in a patient by general anesthesia who went on to develop the disease.[142] Propofol triggered dyskinetic movements in these patients.[143] Muscle relaxants, including succinylcholine, have been used safely in Parkinson disease patients.[144] Opioids can produce uncommon reactions. Alfentanil has been linked to an acute dystonic reaction in a Parkinson disease patient.[145] Morphine has been reported to reduce dyskinesia at low doses but to induce akinesia at greater doses.[146] The concomitant use of meperidine and selegiline, a selective MAO type B inhibitor, has resulted in agitation, muscle rigidity, sweating, and hyperpyrexia, and their use is not recommended.[147] Ketorolac has been used safely in patients taking MAOIs.[148] Phenothiazines, butyrophenones, and metoclopramide should be used with caution, if at all, in the management of Parkinson disease patients because of their antidopaminergic effects. Finally, the short half-life of oral L-dopa (1-3 hours) can result in symptom exacerbation during long procedures. Although absorption takes place primarily in the duodenum, administration of L-dopa by nasogastric tube has been reported to be effective.[149]

SUMMARY

Patients with neuromuscular or skeletal disease present special problems for anesthetic care. Issues range from physical problems such as airway access or patient positioning to biochemical problems and abnormal thermal regulation. Cardiovascular or respiratory abnormalities accompany several of these diseases and further complicate perioperative anesthetic care. Patients with these differing coexisting comorbidities should be carefully considered for assisted ventilation postoperatively if the effects of residual anesthetics or analgesics remain at the completion of the surgical procedure or if moderate to high doses of opioids will be necessary postoperatively for pain management. Susceptibility to serious anesthetic-related complications, such as rhabdomyolysis or MH, may occur in some patients. Thorough preoperative evaluation, knowledge of the underlying disease, and careful anesthetic planning and management are required to achieve the goals of safe and uneventful anesthetic care.

KEY REFERENCES

- Abel M, Eisenkraft JB. Anesthetic implications of myasthenia gravis. *Mt Sinai J Med.* 2002;69:31-37.
- Briggs ED, Kirsch JR. Anesthetic implications of neuromuscular disease. *J Anesth.* 2003;17:177-185.
- Davies NP, Hanna MG. The skeletal muscle channelopathies: distinct entities and overlapping syndromes. *Curr Opin Neurol.* 2003;16:559-568.
- Dorotta IR, Schubert A. Multiple sclerosis and anesthetic implications. *Curr Opin Anaesthesiol.* 2002;15:365-370.
- Klingler W, Lehmann-Horn F, Jurkat-Rott K. Complications of anaesthesia in neuromuscular disorders. *Neuromuscul Disord.* 2005;15:195-206.
- Rowland LP, Shneider NA. Amyotrophic lateral sclerosis. *N Engl J Med.* 2001;344:1688-1700.

REFERENCES

Complete references available on DVD and online version at www.LongneckerAnesthesiology.com

CHAPTER 13

Evaluation of the Patient With Endocrine Disease or Diabetes

A.D. John

KEY POINTS

1. After diabetes, thyroid disorders are the second most common endocrine disease. The range of presentation is vast, ranging from subclinical hyperthyroidism to life-threatening thyroid storm, and from subclinical hypothyroidism to myxedema coma with high mortality if not appropriately treated.
2. The current thyroid-stimulating hormone (TSH) assays, along with the free thyroxine (FT4) level, often lead to the correct diagnosis of the thyroid disorder. Although the signs and symptoms of hypo- and hyperthyroidism are quite distinct, with aging, the clinical picture may not be quite as clear. A high level of suspicion, the appropriate use of tests, and careful assessment of coexisting conditions will lead to the correct diagnosis.
3. Patients with mild hypo- and hyperthyroidism may safely undergo elective surgery if proper care is exercised, but patients with thyroid storm or myxedema coma may have significant morbidity with elective surgery.
4. Hypercalcemia places a patient at increased risk for hypovolemia, renal dysfunction, and cardiac dysrhythmias. Hypocalcemia may present with decreased myocardial contractility, tetany, dysrhythmias, and altered response to muscle relaxants, leading to increased perioperative patient risk. Prompt recognition and successful treatment can be lifesaving.
5. The complex interplay between the thyroid, adrenal, and pituitary glands must be considered in anesthetizing patients for surgery. Appropriate corticosteroid replacement will often result in a smooth and stable perioperative course.
6. The major goal in preoperative preparation of the patient with pheochromocytoma is to decrease cardiovascular morbidity and mortality resulting from excess catecholamine secretion. However, the optimal drug for preoperative preparation of the patient with pheochromocytoma is controversial.
7. Central diabetes insipidus characterized by decreased vasopressin secretion may have effects on both intravascular volume and electrolytes. Patients with acromegaly have a higher incidence of airway difficulty, as well as diabetes, hypertension, and cardiomegaly.
8. According to the most recent American Diabetes Association guidelines, both hemoglobin A_1C and blood sugar levels can be used to diagnose diabetes mellitus. The most recent consensus conference defines the target hemoglobin A_1C levels and outlines a stepped approach to treatment.
9. Diabetes is a disease with a wide impact. Acute diabetic complications include diabetic ketoacidosis, nonketotic hyperosmolar coma, and infection. Chronic complications from diabetes involve the cardiovascular, neurologic, and immune systems. The confluence of diabetes and other diseases and risk factors are components of the metabolic syndrome.

INTRODUCTION

Disturbances in endocrine function increase the complexity of anesthetic care and the risks to the patient. The anesthesiologist must be aware of endocrine abnormalities and their significance in order to optimize patient care and safety. This chapter focuses on the proper preoperative treatment of patients with specific endocrine abnormalities, emphasizing anesthetic-related issues. Chapter 60 discusses intraoperative care of these patients.

THYROID

PHYSIOLOGY

The synthesis and release of thyroid hormones occurs as a result of the complex interaction between the hypothalamic–pituitary axis, the thyroid gland, and the thyroid hormones. The hypothalamus controls the release of thyrotropin-releasing hormone (TRH), which is secreted by the hypothalamic neurons and is delivered to the adenohypophysis via the hypophyseal portal system. Within the pituitary gland, TRH stimulates the secretion of thyroid-stimulating hormone (TSH), which acts at the thyroid gland. A negative feedback loop is present between the pituitary and the thyroid gland, in which increased levels of thyroid hormone inhibit the secretion of TSH from the pituitary gland. Thyroid hormone levels are the primary determinants of TSH secretion, and increased thyroid hormone levels can override TRH-mediated hypothalamic influences.[1,2]

Thyroid hormones function as important regulators of metabolism and development and have effects on many different organs. Thyroid hormones stimulate calorigenesis and metabolism by increasing metabolic rate and oxygen consumption. In addition to regulating cellular respiration, these hormones are necessary for skeletal maturation in the fetus and for brain development during infancy. They affect multiple processes, including cellular metabolism; the cardiovascular system; bone formation and development, with implications related to osteoporosis; and the nervous system with regard to development, maturation, and maintenance, with implications of neuropsychiatry and dementia in adults. Thyroid hormones exert their effects by binding to nuclear receptors within cells, thereby affecting the synthesis and release of proteins and messengers regulating intracellular processes.[3,4]

The thyroid gland, using the sodium iodide symporter, takes absorbed iodide into the gland and synthesizes the thyroid hormones triiodothyronine (T_3) and thyroxine (T_4). Selenocysteine deiodinases found in tissues, such as the liver, kidney, thyroid, pituitary, central nervous system (CNS), cardiac and skeletal muscle, placenta, and the skin, inactivate both T_4 and T_3 and also convert T_4 into either the more potent T_3 or the physiologically inactive reverse T_3 (rT_3).[1-3] The thyroid gland secretes approximately 80 to 100 μg/d of T_4 with a plasma half-life of 6 to 7 days. Approximately 20% of T_3 is also synthesized and released by the thyroid gland. The remaining T_3 is formed mostly in the liver and kidney by peripheral conversion of T_4 by selenodeiodinases.

Once released into the bloodstream, T_4 and T_3 are tightly protein bound, with T_3 and T_4 being primarily bound to thyroid-binding globulin. Other binding proteins include albumin and transthyretin, with only a very small amount being bound to lipoproteins. T_4 is more tightly bound than T_3, which accounts for the longer half-life of T_4—1 week—as compared with the less than 1 day half-life of T_3. A larger amount of T_3 (0.4%) in comparison with T_4 (0.04%) circulates in a free form. It is the free form that is active and controls the metabolic rate. With stress, the levels of T_3 decrease. Once carrier proteins transport T_4 and T_3 into the cell, cellular nuclear receptors have a far greater affinity for T_3 than T_4, leading to increased protein synthesis and metabolic activity. Thus T_3 is more potent than T_4.[3,4]

THYROID FUNCTION TESTS

When assessing thyroid disease, it is important to combine the clinical picture with laboratory tests of thyroid function. The principal tests currently used include third-generation TSH measurements with a functional sensitivity of 0.02 μU/mL, serum free T_4, serum T_4, serum T_3, resin triiodothyronine uptake (RT_3U), free thyroxine index (FT_4I), serum thyroglobulin, rT_3, and radioactive iodine uptake (RAIU). **Table 13-1** lists the reference ranges for normal values. Even though free thyroxine (FT_4) and free triiodothyronine (FT_3) assays tend to avoid the variation caused by thyroid-binding globulin fluctuations caused by hormones, estrogens, and pregnancy, they may still be affected by artifact and coexisting conditions, such as a severe illness,

TABLE 13-1 Reference Values for Thyroid Function Tests at Johns Hopkins Medical Institutions

Thyroid Function	
Test	**Reference Range**
Thyroid-stimulating hormone	0.5-4.5 μU/L
Thyroxine unbound (FT_4)	0.7-1.6 ng/dL
Triiodothyronine unbound (FT_3)	230-420 pg/dL

heparin therapy, medications, and severe disturbances in binding proteins.[5-7] These circumstances are more likely to occur in the critically ill hospitalized surgical population than in the ambulatory outpatient clinic. The TSH and free T_4 levels can be used to assess common conditions (**Table 13-2**).

With aging, there is an increase in TSH normal values. For patients younger than 50 years of age, the median TSH value is 1.49 μU/mL. After 50 years of age, this value increases to 1.60 μU/mL. After 70 years, it increases to 1.98 μU/mL, and after 80 years it is 2.08 μU/mL in a population without any thyroid disease.[5,8-10]

Other Tests to Assess Thyroid Function The RT_3U does not measure T_3; rather, it is a measure of the binding of thyroid hormone to plasma proteins. RT_3U actually measures the percentage of FT_4 not bound to protein. The FT_4I corrects T_4 for abnormalities caused by protein binding and is calculated by multiplying the T_4 by the RT_3U and dividing the result by 100. rT_3 measures the inactive metabolite of T_4 and may be useful in states of non-thyroidal illness. Serum thyroglobulin levels may be elevated in thyroid cancer and may be useful for differentiating thyrotoxicosis secondary to exogenous administration (low thyroglobulin) from thyroid gland dysfunction (high thyroglobulin). RAIU measures the thyroid's uptake of iodine. This test is helpful in differentiating various entities: iodine deficiency and Graves disease have uniformly increased uptake, whereas a single focus indicates a hyperfunctioning nodule, and multiple foci indicate multiple nodules.

HYPERTHYROIDISM

Hyperthyroidism has a wide clinical spectrum. Laboratory values consistent with hyperthyroidism are a low TSH (<0.05 μU/mL) and a high FT_4 (>1.8 ng/dL). Occasionally the FT_4 may be in the normal range, but the FT_3 may be elevated (>596 pg/dL).[5] In subclinical hyperthyroidism the TSH level is low, but both FT_4 and FT_3 are within the normal range. An elevated TSH with an elevated FT_4 may be suggestive of a TSH-secreting pituitary tumor or thyroid hormone resistance syndrome, both rare entities.[5,6] **Table 13-3** lists the signs and symptoms of hyperthyroidism. Heat intolerance and weight loss despite an increased food intake are two symptoms closely associated with hyperthyroidism.[10-12] Common causes of hyperthyroidism include Graves disease, toxic multinodular goiter, an autonomously functioning thyroid nodule, thyroiditis (subacute, lymphocytic, or postpartum), human chorionic gonadotropin (HCG)–mediated trophoblastic disease, and struma ovarii. Goiter is present in Graves disease and thyrotoxicosis, but may or may not be present in a patient with hyperthyroidism. If a patient has exophthalmos, care must be exercised in protecting the eyes during anesthesia with ointment (lubrication) and protective goggles. In the elderly (>70 years), hyperthyroidism may be difficult to recognize because the hyperkinetic picture is often absent.[12] In the elderly, apathy, tachycardia, weight loss, anorexia, and atrial fibrillation are more frequent, whereas in patients younger than 50 years, heat intolerance, increased appetite, sweating, tremor, hyperreflexia, goiter, and polydipsia are more prevalent.[13,14]

TABLE 13-2 Assessment of Thyroid Function With TSH and FT_4

Condition	TSH	Free T4
Hyperthyroidism	Decreased	Increased
Primary hypothyroidism	Increased	Decreased
Secondary hypothyroidism	Decreased or normal	Decreased
Sick euthyroid		
Mild	Normal to low	Normal
Severe	Decreased	Normal to low
Pregnancy	Normal (may be low in 1st trimester)	Normal; increased total T_4; increased T_3

Adapted with permission from Bigatello LM, ed. *MGH Handbook of Critical Care.* 4th ed. Philadelphia, PA: Lippincott Williams and Wilkins; 2006:496, Table 27-6.

TABLE 13-3 Symptoms and Signs of Hyperthyroidism

Symptoms	Signs
Nervousness	Thyroid enlargement
Increased sweating	Tachycardia
Heat intolerance	Atrial fibrillation
Palpitations	Hyperkinesis
Dyspnea	Tremor
Fatigue and weakness	Hyperreflexia
Insomnia	Eye signs
Weight loss or gain	
Increased appetite	
Hyperdefecation	

Hyperthyroidism affects many systems, including the cardiovascular, respiratory, and neuromuscular systems.[15] The thyroid gland plays a key role in regulating the resting heart rate. Hyperthyroidism causes an increased heart rate when compared with that of healthy individuals. Hyperthyroidism can be associated with an increase in stroke volume, cardiac output, pulse pressure, and ectopy, including premature ventricular contractions and atrial fibrillation. There is a relationship between isolated atrial fibrillation in the elderly and hyperthyroidism. In the elderly hyperthyroid patient, there is also an increase in the incidence of congestive heart failure, with increased chronotropy and decreased lusitropy; a third heart sound may be present. Both increased jugular venous pressure and peripheral edema may occur, even in the absence of heart failure. In hyperthyroidism, cardiovascular events as a result of embolic phenomena or myocardial disease may cause death.[4,17,18] Hypermetabolism caused by hyperthyroidism results in increased CO_2 production and, as a consequence, an increased minute ventilation. Unfortunately, weakness of the respiratory muscles can occur, resulting in reductions of vital capacity and compliance and, ultimately, respiratory collapse. Myopathy is present in more than 50% of patients with hyperthyroidism, with electromyographic (EMG) abnormalities present in more than 90% of hyperthyroid patients.[19] Graves disease may be associated with myasthenia gravis, and an association between hyperthyroidism and familial hypokalemic periodic paralysis has been reported in Asian men.

Treatment of hyperthyroidism[6,18-20] usually consists of antithyroid medications, the thionamides (propylthiouracil or methimazole). Propylthiouracil is given at a dose of 50 to 100 mg 3 times a day, whereas maintenance methimazole is dosed at 5 to 15 mg once a day. These medications are given for weeks, with thyroid function tests being checked to ensure a euthyroid state. Radioactive iodine may be given for recurrent hyperthyroidism or persistent hyperthyroidism. Surgical treatment should be considered after medications have achieved a euthyroid state.

SUBCLINICAL HYPERTHYROIDISM

Subclinical hyperthyroidism is characterized by a low TSH and normal FT_4 and FT_3 levels. The prevalence of subclinical hyperthyroidism is approximately 2%, and it is more common in the elderly, women, and African Americans.[21] Subclinical hyperthyroidism commonly occurs with multinodular goiter, hyperfunctioning solitary thyroid nodule, and excess thyroxine replacement therapy. It is also associated with an increased risk of atrial arrhythmias in patients older than 60 years. There is decreased bone mineral density in postmenopausal women[6] and also an increased risk of mood and affective disorders, with an increased risk of dementia in patients with antithyroid peroxidase antibodies.[22] The consensus panel's (of the American Association of Clinical Endocrinologists, the American Thyroid Association, and Endocrine Society) recommendation is to observe and monitor patients with partial suppression of TSH, but to treat patients who have complete suppression of TSH (<0.1 mU/L).[21]

THYROID STORM

At the other end of the spectrum from subclinical hyperthyroidism is thyroid storm. Thyroid storm is an acute life-threatening form of hyperthyroidism with a significant mortality rate that can exceed 20%.[23,24] The diagnosis of thyroid storm is a clinical one, because serum levels of thyroid hormones are about the same as are encountered in hyperthyroidism. Four clinical features are required for the diagnosis of thyroid storm[23,24]: (1) body temperature elevation with diaphoresis (temperatures above 106°F have been reported); (2) a marked tachycardia that is disproportionate to the temperature elevation—this may manifest as sinus tachycardia, atrial fibrillation, or other supraventricular or ventricular tachycardia; (3) cerebral dysfunction, which may range from agitation, restlessness, and emotional lability to confusion, psychosis, seizures, and coma; and (4) gastrointestinal disturbance ranging from nausea, vomiting, and diarrhea to intestinal obstruction or an acute abdomen. The presence of jaundice is a poor prognostic sign.[23,24] The precipitating event varies and may include (most commonly) infection, surgery, treatment with radioactive iodine or the administration of iodinated contrast dyes, amiodarone, exogenous administration of thyroid hormone, cessation of antithyroid medication, diabetic ketoacidosis, hypoglycemia, congestive heart failure, pulmonary embolism, cerebrovascular accident (CVA), bowel infarction, any acute trauma, toxemia of pregnancy, the postpartum state, dental extraction, and even vigorous palpation of the thyroid.[23,24]

Treatment The approach to treatment of thyroid storm is 4-fold[20,23-25]:

1. Decrease production and secretion of thyroid hormone.
2. Block the peripheral effects of thyroid hormones.
3. Maintain supportive care and aggressively treat fever, acid–base abnormalities, and respiratory and cardiovascular support.
4. Determine the underlying cause.

A more detailed discussion is included in Chapter 60.

Preoperative Care Ideally, before any surgical procedure, the patient should be euthyroid, because of the great risk of precipitating a catastrophic thyroid storm during surgery. Airway compromise by goiters may be present with laryngeal nerve compression, tracheal deviation or displacement, or even erosion of tracheal cartilages by a large goiter. A computed tomographic (CT) scan or magnetic resonance imaging (MRI) of the neck may provide useful information. Because commencing thyroid medications and testing takes a period of weeks to months, 1 to 2 months of treatment with antithyroid medication and a recent TSH and FT_4 level are needed to indicate the levels of effectiveness of treatment before an elective operation. In patients requiring emergency surgery, a combination of antithyroid medication, propranolol, and sodium iodide might be effective. The regimen includes 60 to 120 mg of methimazole or 600 to 1000 mg of propylthiouracil given orally in divided doses in conjunction with intravenous propranolol to control heart rate, followed in 2 to 3 hours by an iodine solution to prevent the release of thyroid hormone.[6,23-25] Corticosteroids should also be administered, both to prevent the release and conversion of thyroid hormones and to avoid the possibility of coexisting adrenal suppression.[6,23-25] Heightened awareness by the anesthesiologist is required to quickly detect manifestations of thyroid storm, even in patients who are well prepared for emergency surgery.

TABLE 13-4 Symptoms and Signs of Hypothyroidism

Symptoms	Signs
Cold intolerance	Bradycardia
Dyspnea	Diastolic hypertension
Decreased appetite	Cardiac rub or soft heart tones caused by pericardial effusion
Weight gain (or loss)	Ileus
Constipation	Oliguria
Decreased libido	Urinary retention
Menorrhagia, amenorrhea	Loss of brow and scalp hair
Galactorrhea	Yellow (carotinemic) skin
Arthralgias	Psychosis
Myalgia, muscle stiffness, and cramps	Coma
Dryness	Carpal tunnel syndrome
Fatigue	
Depression	
Irritability	
Impaired concentration and memory	
Paresthesia	
Pallor	

HYPOTHYROIDISM

Hypothyroidism[5,6,26] is a hypometabolic state with generalized slowing of physical processes and fatigue, lethargy, diminished reflexes, and mental sluggishness. **Table 13-4** lists the signs and symptoms of hypothyroidism. Laboratory values characteristic of hypothyroidism are a high TSH (>10 mU/L) and a low FT_4 level (<0.7 ng/dL). Secondary hypothyroidism, characterized by both a low TSH (<0.5 mU/L) and a low FT_4 (<0.7 ng/dL), is a result of pituitary or hypothalamic dysfunction and is quite rare. The most common cause of hypothyroidism is autoimmune lymphocytic thyroiditis, which is diagnosed with a positive thyroid peroxidase antibody level and may be either atrophic or of the Hashimoto variety. Hypothyroidism may occur after thyroidectomy or after radioactive iodine therapy. In many parts of the world, iodine deficiency is a major cause of hypothyroidism. Hypothyroidism is also inducible by a variety of drugs, including iodine, thionamides, lithium, amiodarone, and interferon, or by impaired intestinal absorption of exogenous thyroid hormone by iron, cholestyramine, and sucralfate. Infiltrative diseases, such as sarcoid, amyloid, and hemochromatosis, are also associated with hypothyroidism. A transient hypothyroidism or sick euthyroid state may be seen in the postpartum period or after illness, trauma, burns, and infections.[5,6,24,26]

Hypothyroid patients can exhibit decreased heart rates, sinus bradycardia, atrioventricular block, and QT prolongation. Pathologically, there is cardiac myofibril swelling, loss of striation, and lipid accumulation in the heart. A widened heart shadow is often caused by a pericardial effusion. There is a decrease in myocardial contractility, with prolonged diastolic relaxation, resulting in decreased myocardial work efficiency.[27,28] Patients with hypothyroidism and heart failure often have underlying cardiac disease. Hyperlipidemia, diastolic hypertension, and increased cardiac risk factors are offset by the decreased metabolic demand and the negative inotropic and chronotropic state of hypothyroidism. The rapid correction of hypothyroidism may precipitate myocardial ischemia.[4]

The pulmonary system may exhibit myxedematous infiltration of the respiratory muscles and possibly depression of respiratory responses to hypoxia and CO_2. Myxedema decreases the maximal breathing capacity and lung diffusion capacity.[29-31] Enlargement of the tongue and changes in the voice may occur with severe hypothyroid myopathy. Even in the absence of muscle symptoms, plasma creatine phosphokinase (CPK) may be elevated.[31] Other abnormalities noted with hypothyroidism include increased bleeding, hyponatremia, hypoglycemia, and hypothermia from a decreased basal metabolic rate.

Subclinical Hypothyroidism Subclinical hypothyroidism in women older than 50 years has a prevalence of almost 20%, whereas the overall prevalence in the population is 4% to 10%.[21] Subclinical hypothyroidism is defined by an elevated TSH (>4.5 mU/L) and normal FT_4 and FT_3 levels. The consensus panel (of the American Association of Clinical Endocrinologists, the American Thyroid Association, and Endocrine Society) recommends that the level of thyroid peroxidase antibody also be measured. If positive, the risk per year of progressing to overt hypothyroidism is almost doubled. There is also an increased risk for other autoimmune diseases such as type 1 diabetes mellitus and adrenal insufficiency. For TSH levels greater than 10 mU/L, the consensus panel recommends treatment to decrease the TSH level in patients with subclinical hypothyroidism.

Treatment In treating hypothyroidism, thyroxine is the preferred agent.[20,24,26,32] Because of its long half-life of approximately 1 week, all that is required is once-daily dosing. Replacement dosing should begin gradually with a starting dose of 25 to 50 μg/d with the possibility that all that is required for replacement is a small dose of 50 μg/d.[20,24,26,32]

MYXEDEMA COMA

Myxedema coma represents an extreme form of hypothyroidism.[23,32,33] In elderly female patients with known hypothyroidism, it has a significant mortality rate (>20%). Three essential components are required for this diagnosis: (1) an altered mental state, which may range from disorientation, lethargy, and confusion to coma; (2) abnormal thermoregulation with temperatures lower than 95°F as a result of impaired hypothalamic temperature regulation (infection may mask the low temperature by causing pseudo-normalization); and (3) a precipitating illness, such as infection, stroke, trauma, heart failure, bleeding, exposure to cold, and medications such as amiodarone and narcotics. Laboratory examination may reveal a markedly elevated TSH with low FT_4 and FT_3 levels, but with concomitant severe illness, glucocorticoid therapy, and pressors, the clinical scenario may not be readily apparent.[23,33]

Preoperative A euthyroid state is desirable before elective surgery. For emergent surgery the treatment of myxedema coma must be based on thyroid hormone replacement and supportive care, with the optimal technique still a matter of debate.[6,20,23,24] It is common to administer 300 to 500 μg of T_4 as an intravenous (IV) bolus and continue with 50 to 100 μg of IV T_4 daily until the patient is able to take oral medications. Glucocorticosteroids are frequently administered to avoid relative adrenal insufficiency as the metabolic rate increases. Supportive care is necessary to address any hypoventilation, hypothermia, hyponatremia, hypoglycemia, hypotension, or sepsis. Hypoventilation often requires mechanical ventilation and the correction of acid–base abnormalities. Hyponatremia needs gradual correction to avoid central pontine myelinolysis. Hypothermia requires gradual correction by ambient warming and warming blankets, because aggressive correction may lead to vasodilatation and subsequent cardiovascular collapse. Hypoglycemia may indicate adrenal suppression, which should be treated with stress-dose steroids. Hypotension should be carefully addressed because of possibly depressed myocardial contractility and the potential for cardiovascular dysfunction from aggressive resuscitation. Appropriate antibiotic coverage for sepsis should be instituted, in addition to volume resuscitation. **Table 13-5** represents a summary of the significance of the various thyroid function tests.

TABLE 13-5 Summary of the Significance of Thyroid Tests

TSH ↑ (increased) and:	
Free T4 ↓	Hypothyroidism
Normal FT_4 and FT_3	Subclinical hypothyroidism
↑ FT_4, ↑ FT_3	Central hyperthyroidism
TSH ↓ (decreased) and:	
Free T_4 ↑	Hyperthyroidism
Normal FT_4 and FT_3	Subclinical hyperthyroidism
↓ FT_4, ↓ FT_3	Central hypothyroidism
When RAIU is used to differentiate thyrotoxicosis	
(1) Increased RAIU	Diffusely (Graves disease)
	Focally (toxic adenoma)
(2) Decreased RAIU	Factitious
	Contrast (IV) or meds (amiodarone)
	Thyroiditis

CALCIUM DISORDERS ASSOCIATED WITH PARATHYROID DISEASE

PHYSIOLOGY

Calcium is a cation that has a vast physiologic impact on processes ranging from subcellular to major organ systems. These include muscular contraction, release of neurotransmitters, coagulation, enzymatic activation, cellular message systems, nuclear and protein function, and cell regulation.[34,42] Most calcium (99%) is found in bone, but it is the ionized calcium that is the most physiologically relevant. The body regulates plasma calcium levels within a narrow range of 8.5 to 10.5 mg/dL. Alterations in serum proteins affect the portion of bound calcium. If plasma albumin is decreased, the total serum calcium concentration should be adjusted upward and vice versa if albumin is increased. The total calcium level is adjusted by 0.8 mg/dL for each 1 g that the serum albumin is below or above 4.0 g/dL. Other processes and acid–base imbalances may also affect the calcium-protein binding.[37,38] For instance, acidosis may provoke hypercalcemia by decreasing calcium binding and increasing the circulating levels of ionized calcium, whereas alkalosis decreases ionized calcium by increasing protein binding.

Three hormones interact to provide calcium homeostasis: parathyroid hormone, vitamin D, and calcitonin. *Parathyroid hormone* (PTH) is secreted by the parathyroid gland and raises serum calcium levels by promoting bone reabsorption, increasing renal calcium resorption, and activating vitamin D through the induction of the 1α hydroxylase gene in renal cells. In the kidney, PTH also increases the excretion of phosphate, bicarbonate, potassium, sodium, and some amino acids. *Vitamin D* and its active metabolites, 25-hydroxycholecalciferol and 1,25-dihydroxycholecalciferol (calcitriol), increase intestinal Ca^{2+} absorption. *Calcitonin* is secreted by the thyroid gland in response to hypercalcemia. Calcitonin decreases bone resorption and promotes renal excretion of phosphate, sodium, and potassium. Several feedback mechanisms serve to regulate the levels of these hormones. PTH release is increased by hypocalcemia, whereas vitamin D inhibits PTH secretion by increasing serum calcium and through direct trophic effects. Hypermagnesemia may inhibit parathyroid hormone release, although severe hypomagnesemia causes paradoxical hypocalcemia by impaired parathyroid hormone secretion and an abnormal end-organ response.[37,38]

HYPERCALCEMIA

Table 13-6 lists the clinical manifestations of hypercalcemia.[37-39] Patients usually are asymptomatic with plasma calcium levels up to 12 mg/dL. At levels between 12 and 14 mg/dL, symptoms vary. Clinical manifestations of hypercalcemia should serve as a guide for the need and speed of treatment. Severe hypercalcemia (serum calcium level >14 mg/dL) may be life-threatening and requires immediate treatment, regardless of symptomatology. The majority of patients presenting with severe hypercalcemia develop this as a complication of malignancy. Hypercalcemia has profound effects on cardiac function, with diverse clinical manifestations. The primary risk in anesthetizing patients with hypercalcemia are cardiac dysrhythmias. Hypercalcemia decreases the refractory period and increases ventricular excitability. These effects depend on the Ca^{2+} level. QT interval changes, however, are not necessarily a reliable indicator of hypercalcemia. Bradyarrhythmias, bundle-branch blocks, and complete heart block are well-documented complications of acute hypercalcemia. Vascular tone increases with hypercalcemia, so the blood pressure often gives an inaccurate assessment of the severity of dehydration and volume status. Other effects of hypercalcemia include renal toxicity, neurologic deficits, and abdominal pain.

TABLE 13-6 Signs and Symptoms of Hypercalcemia

Gastrointestinal
Nausea/vomiting
Anorexia
Constipation
Pancreatitis
Peptic ulcers
Renal
Polyuria
Nephrolithiasis
Free water loss
Oliguric loss
Renal tubular acidosis
Interstitial nephritis
Impaired Na reabsorption
Cardiovascular
Dehydration
Hypertension
ECG abnormalities
Dysrhythmias
Catecholamine resistance
Digitalis sensitivity
CNS disorientation
Obtundation
Confusion
Psychosis
Personality change
Memory impairment
Sedation
Lethargy
Coma
Seizures
Musculoskeletal
Osteopenia/osteoporosis
Weakness/atrophy
Pruritus
Hypomagnesemia

Based on the work of Drs Peterfreund and Lee.

TABLE 13-7 Causes of Hypercalcemia

PTH Dependent
Primary hyperparathyroidism
MEN
Parathyroid Ca
Benign familial hypocalciuric hypercalcemia
Lithium
PTH Independent
Malignancy
Squamous cell cancer
Pancreatic cancer
Myeloma
Breast cancer
Renal cancer
Lymphoma
Leukemia
Drugs
Calcium-containing antacids
Thiazides
Theophylline
Vitamin A
Vitamin D
Iatrogenic
Granulomatous disease
Sarcoidosis
Histoplasmosis
Coccidiomycosis
Tuberculosis
Berylliosis
Endocrine
Hyperthyroidism
Adrenal insufficiency
Acromegaly
Pheochromocytoma
Immobilization
AIDS

Based on the work of Drs Peterfreund and Lee.

Causes **Table 13-7** lists the causes of hypercalcemia. Causes of hypercalcemia are generally divided into PTH-dependent and PTH-independent etiologies. Hypercalcemia secondary to parathyroid disease is a common condition. Laboratory abnormalities in hyperparathyroidism often include hypercalcemia, hypophosphatemia, hypercalciuria, and elevations of serum uric acid and chloride with a decreased serum bicarbonate. The diagnosis of hyperparathyroidism is best supported by an increased PTH level associated with hypercalcemia. The most common cause of hyperparathyroidism is a parathyroid adenoma (80%-90%), followed by parathyroid hyperplasia (15%), with parathyroid carcinoma being uncommon. Hyperparathyroidism also may occur as a manifestation of multiple endocrine neoplasia type I (MEN I; parathyroid hyperplasia, pancreatic islet cell neoplasia, pituitary adenoma) and MEN II (medullary thyroid carcinoma, pheochromocytoma, parathyroid hyperplasia).

Hyperparathyroidism in pregnant women deserves special mention. Maternal hypercalcemia may have profound effects on the fetus and newborn, leading to neonatal hypocalcemia or tetany. The literature suggests that maternal hyperparathyroidism is associated with increased fetal morbidity and mortality rates. Because the primary treatment for symptomatic hyperparathyroidism is surgery, it is not unusual for the anesthesiologist to care for a pregnant woman undergoing parathyroidectomy. Effort should be made to diagnose secondary hyperparathyroidism, a condition characterized by elevated PTH levels but low or normal calcium levels. Secondary hyperparathyroidism is a common factor in vitamin D deficiency and renal disease. It is caused by a physiologic increase in PTH secretion compensating for low calcium or vitamin D levels.

Included among the more common causes of non–PTH-mediated hypercalcemia are malignancy, the milk-alkali syndrome, a granulomatous disorder with excess vitamin D, hyperthyroidism, and immobilization. Hypercalcemia due to malignancy may be caused by the secretion of parathyroid related protein (PTH rP) by the malignant cells, or the local osteolytic effect of malignant cells invasion of bone, or an increase in production of calcitriol (see **Table 13-8**).

Treatment After receiving an elevated plasma calcium value, a repeat calcium level should be checked.[37-39] The basic goals of hypercalcemia therapy include correction of dehydration, enhancing renal calcium excretion, inhibiting bone resorption, and managing the underlying disorder. Saline hydration and furosemide can rapidly decrease the serum calcium level by 2 to 3 mg/dL by correcting the underlying fluid deficit and increasing renal calcium clearance. It is important to correct a fluid deficit before starting loop diuretics. In elderly patients with limited cardiovascular reserve, the rapid correction of a fluid deficit may result in congestive heart failure. Other complications of loop diuretics include hypokalemia and hypomagnesemia.

Specific therapy to inhibit osteoclast-mediated bone resorption should be instituted in patients with persistently elevated calcium levels after aggressive hydration and loop diuretics. Bisphosphonates, calcitonin, and sometimes glucocorticoids are

TABLE 13-8 Mechanism of Malignancy-Induced Hypercalcemia

I. Increased parathyroid-related protein (PTH ↓, Phos ↓)
- Squamous cell carcinoma
- Breast carcinoma
- Renal cell carcinoma
- Islet cell carcinoma
- Ovarian carcinoma
- Transitional cell carcinoma
- T-cell lymphoma

II. Direct invasion of bone (↑ urinary Ca)
- Multiple myeloma
- Adenocarcinoma of the breast
- Lymphomas

III. Increased production of calcitriol
- B-cell lymphoma

Modified from American College of Physicians ©2009 MKSAP 15 Endocrinology, p. 58, Table 28.

used.[37-39] Bisphosphonates bind to hydroxyapatite in bone and inhibit bone resorption. Zoledronate and pamidronate are the bisphosphonates approved by the US Food and Drug Administration. They are given as slow IV infusions and decrease serum calcium within 2 days after the initial dose. Among the drugs used in managing hypercalcemia, calcitonin has a rapid onset. IV calcitonin is given at 4 IU/kg every 12 hours, with the onset of action occurring in 1 to 2 hours and lasting 6 to 12 hours. It is a relatively weak agent and unlikely to normalize the serum calcium alone. Chronic use of calcitonin for hypercalcemia is limited due to the frequent development of tachyphylaxis. Steroids have been used to enhance the effect of calcitonin and are particularly useful in treating hypercalcemia caused by granulomatous disorders.[37-39]

Other agents that have been used to treat hypercalcemia include plicamycin, gallium nitrate, and phosphonates. However, these agents are no longer commonly given because of their side effects. Plicamycin, which acts directly on bone to block calcium resorption, has a relatively fast onset of action. The dosage is 25 μg/kg administered IV over 4 to 6 hours, with effects occurring in 6 to 12 hours. Contraindications to plicamycin therapy include thrombocytopenia, coagulopathy, and overt renal or hepatic dysfunction. Gallium nitrate is administered as a continuous infusion for 5 days and takes 5 days to normalize the calcium level. Nephrotoxicity is a major side effect.[41] Intravenous phosphates have a rapid onset, but are associated with a risk of hypotension, pulmonary edema, hypocalcemia, and metastatic calcification and are contraindicated in renal failure. Oral phosphates chelate calcium in the gastrointestinal tract. Indomethacin, which has a slow onset of action, is used for prostaglandin-associated hypercalcemia.

Preoperative In managing hypercalcemia preoperatively, reversible complications, such as dehydration, mental obtundation, and electrolyte disorders, should be corrected. No intervention other than preoperative hydration is usually necessary for patients with calcium levels of 12 mg/dL or higher. The cause of hypercalcemia, however, should be sought. Patients with more severe hypercalcemia often require management with IV hydration, loop diuretics, and the medications described previously.

HYPOCALCEMIA

Hypocalcemia associated with parathyroid hormone resistance is most commonly caused by hypomagnesemia, whereas decreases in parathyroid hormone are most commonly caused by surgical ablation. There are several other causes of decreased parathyroid hormone levels, such as DiGeorge syndrome and polyglandular autoimmune syndrome type I, but these are far less common. Common causes of hypocalcemia are listed in **Table 13-9**.

TABLE 13-9 Causes of Hypocalcemia

- Hypoparathyroidism
  - Postsurgical
  - Autoimmune
  - Congenital
  - Idiopathic
  - Pseudohypoparathyroidism (PTH resistance)
  - Hemochromatosis
  - Sarcoidosis
  - Amyloidosis
- Vitamin D deficiency
  - Hepatic disease
  - Renal disease
  - Lack of sun exposure
  - Dietary deficiency
  - Malabsorption
- Hyperphosphatemia
  - Rhabdomyolysis
  - Phosphate therapy
  - Renal failure
  - Chemotherapy/tumor lysis
- Critical illness
  - Pancreatitis
  - Burns
  - Toxic shock
  - Fat embolism
  - Sepsis
  - Alkalosis
- Drugs
  - Anticonvulsants
  - INH
  - Rifampin
  - Loop diuretics
  - EDTA
  - Bisphosphonates
- Hypomagnesemia
- Hypoalbuminemia
- Massive transfusion (with calcium chelation)

Based on the work of Drs Peterfreund and Lee.

Table 13-10 lists the signs and symptoms of hypocalcemia. The cardinal sign of hypocalcemia is tetany. The electrocardiogram may exhibit a prolonged QT interval, indicating a predisposition to ventricular dysrhythmias. Primary hypoparathyroidism is often associated with hypocalcemia, hyperphosphatemia, and depressed levels

TABLE 13-10 Symptoms and Signs of Hypocalcemia

Symptoms	Signs
Paresthesias	Dementia
Weakness	Chvostek and Trousseau signs
Anxiety	Bradycardia
Depression	Dysrhythmia
Irritability	QT and ST interval prolongation
Confusion	T-wave inversion
Psychosis	Extrapyramidal manifestations
Hypotension	Coarse, dry, scaly skin
Cardiac insufficiency	Brittle nails
Laryngeal spasm	Thin, brittle hair
Apnea	Cataracts
Bronchospasm	
Tetany	
Muscle spasm	
Seizures	

of parathyroid hormone. When assessing the severity of hypocalcemia, decreased serum calcium levels might not be associated with symptoms if the ionized Ca^{2+} level is normal due to low albumin levels. Alkalosis may predispose patients to hypocalcemia. Magnesium levels should be determined for all patients with hypocalcemia, especially in cases of alcohol abuse, malabsorption, or poor nutrition. Hypomagnesemia can induce hypocalcemia by a reduction in parathyroid hormone secretion, a resistance to the humeral actions of parathyroid hormone, and a direct parathyroid hormone-independent hypocalcemic effect.[37-39,41]

Preoperative The major anesthetic risks of hypocalcemia are cardiac dysrhythmias, decreased contractility, development of tetany (especially with hyperventilation), and an altered response to muscle relaxants. Hypocalcemia patients may be resistant to digitalis therapy.

Clinical signs of hypocalcemia should be controlled before surgical procedures are performed. Hypocalcemia is managed chronically with dietary calcium and vitamin D supplementation. For emergency management of hypocalcemia, 100 to 200 mg of elemental calcium is given as an IV infusion of either 10% calcium gluconate or calcium chloride over 10 minutes and followed by infusion of 0.5 to 2 mg Ca^{2+}/kg/h with monitoring of plasma Ca^{2+} levels. A 10-mL solution of 10% calcium chloride provides three times as much elemental calcium as a 10-mL solution of 10% calcium gluconate. Coexisting hypomagnesemia should be corrected in order to fully correct the hypocalcemia. Magnesium levels can be restored acutely by administering 1 to 2 g of 10% magnesium solution intravenously.[37,38]

ADRENAL DISORDERS

PHYSIOLOGY

Adrenal corticosteroid secretion is controlled via a negative feedback loop with the hypothalamic–pituitary axis.[43-50] Corticotropin-releasing factor from the hypothalamus stimulates the release of corticotropin from the pituitary gland, which, in turn, stimulates the release of adrenal corticosteroids. By a negative feedback loop, elevated corticosteroid levels depress corticotropin secretion. In addition to the influences of corticosteroids, corticotropin release is modulated by stress and exhibits a diurnal variation, with peak secretion occurring in the morning and a nadir in the evening. Random plasma cortisol levels are of marginal benefit in diagnosing the integrity of the adrenal–pituitary axis, and so various stimulation and suppression tests are used. In particular, assessment of adrenal-cortical reserve is done with the corticotropin-stimulation test.

Glucocorticoids have several functions. Steroids increase hepatic gluconeogenesis and decrease fatty acid, nucleic acid, and protein synthesis. They also suppress the inflammatory reaction and reduce calcium absorption from the gut. Steroids antagonize the effects of antidiuretic hormone (ADH) and enhance catecholamine vasoconstriction. High doses of glucocorticoids can exhibit a mineralocorticoid effect, causing sodium and water retention with potassium loss. After surgery the plasma cortisol level increases 5 to 10 times by 6 hours postoperatively, with peak levels decreasing by 24 hours postoperatively, unless the stress continues. Epidural anesthesia delays the cortisol stress response, but does not prevent it.

Aldosterone is secreted by the adrenal cortex in response to hyperkalemia and is inhibited by increases in plasma volume. Aldosterone secretion is also controlled by the renin–angiotensin system and to a lesser extent by the circulating levels of corticotropin. Aldosterone works in the distal convoluted tubules of the kidney to promote sodium retention and potassium excretion. It is a major regulator of potassium balance and extracellular fluid volume.[43,50]

Clinically, disorders of the cortical adrenal gland present as 1 of 3 problems: Cushing syndrome, with an excess secretion of corticosteroids; primary hyperaldosteronism, with excess aldosterone secretion; or Addison disease, with corticosteroid insufficiency.

TABLE 13-11 Symptoms and Signs of Cushing Syndrome

Symptoms	Signs
Weakness/proximal myopathy	Centripetal obesity
Psychiatric changes	Hypertension
Impotence	Skin changes
Oligomenorrhea/amenorrhea	Thin skin/bruising
Backache	Acne, greasy skin
Thirst/polyuria	Hirsutism
Headache	Plethora
Abdominal pain	Abdominal striae
Weight gain	Infection (eg, tinea versicolor)
	Hyperpigmentation (if ACTH dependent)
	Osteoporosis
	Vertebral collapse
	Pathologic fracture
	Glucose intolerance
	Ankle edema
	Renal calculi
	Exophthalmos

CUSHING SYNDROME

Prolonged exposure to excess glucocorticoids-cortisol results in the manifestation of Cushing syndrome (**Table 13-11**). Although the classic features of Cushing syndrome—round faces, supraclavicular fat pad, purple striae, and proximal muscle weakness—are seen in a minority of patients, the nonspecific features—such as obesity, hypertension, glucose intolerance, osteoporosis, osteopenia or fractures, emotional lability, depression, anxiety, easy bruisability, and thick skin—may be attributable to other causes or diseases.[44-46] The most common cause of Cushing syndrome tends to be exposure to exogenous glucocorticoids, such as topical or inhaled corticosteroids. The most common endogenous cause of Cushing syndrome (≈70%) is Cushing disease—the secretion by pituitary tumors of adrenocorticotropic hormone (ACTH). Approximately 15% of endogenous Cushing syndrome is caused by non-pituitary ACTH-producing tumors, and 15% is caused by ACTH-independent secretion of cortisol by adrenal tumors.[44-46] A high level of suspicion should be maintained, especially in patients who are atypical or difficult to control, because many diseases can exhibit similar symptoms.

If Cushing syndrome is suspected, the Endocrine Society recommends that any of 4 initial tests be used to diagnose it.[44-46] They include (1) urine free cortisol on 2 separate occasions, with special care for patients drinking excess fluids and those with a creatinine clearance of less than 60 mL/min; (2) late night salivary cortisol on 2 separate occasions; (3) a 1-mg overnight dexamethasone suppression test; or (4) longer low-dose dexamethasone suppression test (2 mg/d for 48 hours). Once the diagnosis of Cushing syndrome is made, the next step is to determine whether the disease is ACTH dependent or independent. After this is determined, then localization to the pituitary, adrenal, or body is done by CT or MRI, with somatostatin scintigraphy used to detect ectopic sources of corticotropin.

Therapy for Cushing syndrome consists of removing the source of glucocorticoid production. This may mean the removal of exogenously administered medication or the surgical removal of endogenous disease. On occasion, radiotherapy and medication are both used. Ketoconazole and metapyrone are enzyme inhibitors of cortisol synthesis, whereas mitotane is an adrenolytic that may be used to lower cortisol levels. After surgery, steroid replacement will be required until the hypothalamic–pituitary–adrenal axis recovers (see Adrenal Insufficiency section, later).

TABLE 13-12 Symptoms, Signs, and Laboratory Abnormalities in Addison Disease

Symptoms	Signs	Laboratory Abnormalities
Weakness, tiredness, fatigue Weight loss Anorexia Nausea, vomiting Abdominal pain Diarrhea Muscle pain Salt craving Orthostatic hypotension, dizziness, or syncope Lethargy, disorientation	Skin hyperpigmentation Buccal or tongue pigmentation Calcification of the pinnae Vitiligo Hyperthermia or hypothermia Loss of axiliary hair in women Hypotension	Hyponatremia Hyperkalemia Azotemia Fasting or reactive hypoglycemia (infrequent in adults) Hypercalcemia Eosinophilia

PRIMARY HYPERALDOSTERONISM

Primary hyperaldosteronism[44,47,48] is characterized by hypertension, hypokalemic alkalosis, inability to concentrate urine, and skeletal muscle weakness. A plasma aldosterone to plasma renin activity ratio more than 20 and a plasma aldosterone level over 15 mg/dL after IV saline or salt loading is characteristic of the diagnosis. Spironolactone and epleronone are the agents of choice for treatment, with thiazide diuretics being preferred if additional blood pressure control is required. Preoperative preparation focuses on blood pressure control and the correction of fluid and electrolyte imbalance.

ADRENAL INSUFFICIENCY

Adrenocortical insufficiency[43,44,49,50] can be classified as primary, with adrenal gland destruction, or secondary, with hypothalamic–pituitary axis dysfunction. Primary adrenal insufficiency can be iatrogenic, from bilateral adrenalectomy or unilateral adrenalectomy for a hyperfunctioning tumor, or endogenous adrenal gland destruction resulting in Addison disease. Patients with primary adrenal insufficiency usually exhibit hypoaldosteronism. **Table 13-12** lists the signs and symptoms of Addison disease. In patients with secondary adrenal insufficiency related to a suppressed hypothalamic–pituitary axis, aldosterone secretion remains intact, and hyperkalemia does not occur. An additional syndrome of isolated hypoaldosteronism can occur as a result of renin deficiency in patients with normal cortisol secretion but unexplained hyperkalemia. Patients with suspected adrenal insufficiency should undergo further laboratory examinations to assess adrenal function before surgery. Associated laboratory findings include decreased plasma cortisol levels and impaired corticotropin stimulation. Additional provocation testing of the pituitary–adrenal axis might include using metyrapone stimulation. If adrenal insufficiency develops acutely, the symptoms can be severe and dramatic (**Table 13-13**). This may occur in a trauma or intensive care setting in patients with previously unsuspected but inadequate reserve.[43,44,49,50]

Glucocorticoids are given on the basis of the urgency and severity of the clinical situation. Supplementation takes into consideration the type of medical or surgical stress. Minor procedures, such as herniorrhaphy or colonoscopy, are supplemented with 25 mg of hydrocortisone or 5 mg of methylprednisolone IV for the procedure only. Moderately invasive procedures, such as cholecystectomy or hemicolectomy, are supplemented with 50 to 75 mg of hydrocortisone or 10 to 15 mg of methylprednisolone IV on the day of the procedure, followed by a 1- to 2-day taper to the usual dose. A severe stress or procedure, such as cardiac surgery, liver resection, or Whipple surgery, is supplemented with hydrocortisone 100 to 150 mg or methylprednisolone 25 to 30 mg IV followed by a rapid taper over 1 to 2 days.[44-46]

If primary adrenal insufficiency exists, mineralocorticoid replacement should be given. In addition to adequate steroid coverage, preoperative issues again include volume status and electrolyte management, along with the correction of hypotension.

TABLE 13-13 Symptoms and Signs of Acute Adrenal Insufficiency

Symptoms	Signs
Severe clinical deterioration Nausea, vomiting Abdominal or flank pain Lethargy, obtundation	Fever Hypotension Abdominal distension Hyponatremia Hyperkalemia

PHEOCHROMOCYTOMA

Pheochromocytomas are chromaffin cell tumors and are members of the family of amino acid precursor uptake and decarboxylation (APUD) tumors. Massive amounts of catecholamines are released by these tumors, causing their characteristic signs and symptoms. They are rare, occurring in 0.5% of all hypertensive patients.[51-56] Although pheochromocytomas are usually unilateral and intra-adrenal, they may be found in various locations, including the urinary bladder and bilaterally in the chest and abdomen. Extra-adrenal pheochromocytomas are called paragangliomas. Two to three percent of these growths constitute neck or thoracic masses, with most tumors occuring in adults. Children with pheochromocytomas have fewer malignant tumors but tend to have a greater incidence of bilaterality, extra-adrenal location, and associated multiple endocrine neoplasias.

Diagnosis Pheochromocytomas may be either sporadic or hereditary. Most tumors are sporadic, and about 10% of all tumors are hereditary. Pheochromocytoma can be a manifestation of the hereditary disorders of MEN IIA, IIB, neurofibromatosis (NF) type 1, familial paraganglioma syndrome, and von Hippel-Lindau (vHL) disease. A group of susceptibility genes has been identified, including proto-oncogene RET (associated with MEN type II), the tumor-suppressor gene VHL (associated with von Hippel-Lindau disease), and succinate dehydrogenase subunits D and B (which predispose carriers to pheochromocytomas and glomus tumors) (**Table 13-14**). Identification of mutations in

TABLE 13-14 Major Genetic Syndromes Associated With Pheochromocytoma

Syndrome	Clinical Features	Gene
MEN IIA	Medullary thyroid carcinoma Parathyroid hyperplasia Pheochromocytoma	RET
MEN IIB	Medullary thyroid carcinoma Pheochromocytoma Ganglioneuromas Marfanoid habitus	
NF_1	Neurofibromas Café-au-lait spots Lisch nodules Plexiform neurofibromas Sphenoid dysplasia Optic gliomas Axillary and inguinal freckling	NF_1
vHL	Hemangioblastomas (brain, spine, retina) Clear-cell renal cell cancer Pheochromocytoma	vHL

MEN, multiple endocrine neoplasia; NF, neurofibromatosis; vHL, von Hippel-Lindau.

Reprinted and modified with permission from Nathanson KL, Bryant J, Farmer J, Kessler LJ, Townsend RR. Pheochromocytoma: the expanding genetic differential diagnosis. *J Natl Cancer Inst.* 2003;95:1197, Table 1.

TABLE 13-15 Symptoms and Signs of Pheochromocytoma

Symptoms	Signs
Headache (severe)	Blood pressure changes
Excessive sweating (generalized)	Hypertension with wide fluctuations
Palpitations with or without tachycardia	Hypertension induced by physical maneuver such as exercise, postural change, or palpation and massage
Anxiety or nervousness	Orthostatic hypertension
Pain in chest, abdomen, lumbar regions, lower abdomen, groin	Paradoxical blood pressure response to some antihypertensive drugs and marked pressor response with induction of anesthesia
Nausea and vomiting	Hyperhidrosis
Weakness, fatigue, prostration	Tachycardia or reflex bradycardia; very forceful heartbeat, dysrhythmia
Weight loss (severe)	Pallor of face and upper part of body
Dyspnea	Anxious, frightened, troubled appearance
Warmth with or without heat intolerance	Hypertensive retinopathy
Visual disturbances	Leanness or underweight
Dizziness or faintness	Tremor
Constipation	Raynaud phenomenon
Paresthesia or pain in arms	Fever
Bradycardia (noted by patient)	Dilated pupils

these susceptibility genes have been found in 24% of suspected sporadic tumors, suggesting that hereditary syndromes may play a greater role in pheochromocytoma occurrence than previously appreciated.[51-53]

Diagnosis depends on a high index of suspicion and observing for clinical signs and symptoms of this tumor. Signs and symptoms of pheochromocytoma should be sought in hypertensive individuals, and a workup performed in those patients displaying characteristic signs and symptoms (**Table 13-15**). The diagnostic algorithm[55] includes documentation of increased catecholamine breakdown products in plasma and tumor localization by appropriate imaging techniques, including CT, MRI, I-metaiodobenzylguanidine scintigraphy, or positron emission tomography (PET) scanning. The first step in diagnosis is biochemical verification of the presence of a pheochromocytoma. Plasma-free metanephrine levels are the best test to confirm or exclude the tumor. A normal plasma metanephrine level excludes a tumor, and a large elevation confirms its presence. However, the problem comes with marginally elevated values, as there may be a 15% false-positive rate. Patients with marginally elevated plasma metanephrine values should undergo further evaluation via additional biochemical testing (repeat plasma metanephrines or urinary total metanephrine and catecholamines) or pharmacologic testing (eg, clonidine suppression or glucagon stimulation). When interpreting metanephrine and catecholamine levels, physicians should be aware of medical conditions and drugs that can influence the results (**Table 13-16**). Care must be taken to eliminate these confounding factors. After biochemical confirmation, the next step is tumor localization, with adrenal CT and MRI having comparable sensitivity and specificity. Metaiodobenzylguanidine (MIBG) scanning, however, offers superior specificity to MRI and CT and is particularly helpful in localizing extra-adrenal masses. In patients with biochemical evidence of pheochromocytoma, but in whom the presence of the tumor cannot be concluded by CT, MRI, or MIBG, PET scanning may be performed for tumor localization.[51-55]

TABLE 13-16 Potential Causes of False-Positive Results for Catecholamines and Metanephrines

Tricyclic antidepressants and antipsychotics
Levodopa
Drugs containing catecholamines
Ethanol
Withdrawal from clonidine and other drugs
Acetaminophen and phenoxybenzamine (plasma metanephrines)
Major physical stress (ie, surgery, stroke, obstructive sleep apnea)

Preoperative Preparation Preoperative preparation should be a joint venture involving the surgeon, the internist or endocrinologist, and the anesthesiologist. The major goal of preoperative preparation is to decrease cardiovascular morbidity and mortality resulting from excess catecholamine secretion. Pheochromocytomas may secrete norepinephrine, epinephrine, or dopamine.[51-53] The acute effects of catecholamine bursts and their chronic end-organ sequelae may influence postoperative outcome.

The optimal drug for preoperative preparation of the patient with a pheochromocytoma is controversial. A common initial approach has been to use phenoxybenzamine for long-term α-blockade.[51,52,55,58] Preoperative treatment with phenoxybenzamine, an α adrenergic blocker, results in a significantly smoother course than in untreated patients. This drug has a long half-life (approximately 12 hours) and is highly lipid-soluble. However, it has unpredictable absorption from the gut. Its primary side effect is orthostatic hypotension. The starting dosage is 10 to 20 mg daily in 2 doses. Every 3 to 4 days, the dose is increased until either no symptoms of catecholamine excess are evident or the patient complains of side effects from postural hypotension and/or a stuffy nose, with a final dosage range of 40 to 100 mg/d. The adequacy of β-blockade may be assessed by determining whether ongoing symptoms of catecholamine excess are occurring. Signs and symptoms of pheochromocytoma should be specifically sought (see Table 13-15). The preoperative cardiovascular evaluation should seek signs of orthostasis or evidence of heart failure or a cardiomyopathy and determine volume status. Preoperative preparation should include 1 to 2 weeks of α-adrenergic blocker therapy. Volume replacement is important when starting α-blocker therapy, and patients often have a decreased hematocrit after beginning therapy.

There are several disadvantages to the use of phenoxybenzamine.[50,52,55,56] Adequate volume expansion after institution of the drug may take as long as 2 to 3 weeks. Thus patients presenting for surgery who have been on phenoxybenzamine for a shorter time period should have any hypovolemia corrected preoperatively. Total elimination of cardiovascular changes is seldom achieved despite reaching therapeutic end points with phenoxybenzamine. α-Blockade with phenoxybenzamine is irreversible and depends on synthesis of α-adrenergic receptors. Thus there may be continued α-blockade after tumor removal, which can contribute to postoperative hypotension. Phenoxybenzamine causes significant orthostatic hypotension and reflex tachycardia.

Selective α_1-blockers, such as prazosin and doxazosin, have been used with success for preoperative preparation. The rationale behind their selection is a shorter duration of action providing easier dose adjustment and potentially decreasing the postoperative hypotension risk period. Reflex tachycardia is decreased because the presynaptic α-receptors are not blocked.

β-Blockers are administered for a persistent tachycardia and for control of other peripheral β-adrenergic effects of catecholamine excess. These drugs should never be given before α-blockade because serious hypertensive sequelae may result. Both labetalol and atenolol have been suggested as appropriate drug choices.

The drug α-methyltyrosine inhibits the synthesis of norepinephrine. The drug does not produce hypotension and preserves tissue responsiveness to adrenergic agents when a dosage of 500 to 2000 mg is given 4 times daily. Adequate blockade is achieved in 1 or 2 weeks. α-Methyltyrosine without concurrent α-adrenergic–blocking agents does not prevent a hypertensive crisis. α-Methyltyrosine has fallen out of favor, possibly because there is a high incidence of side effects including somnolence, anxiety, agitation, depression, and tremor.

Calcium channel blockers also have been advocated for preoperative and intraoperative blood pressure control in patients with pheochromocytomas. In comparison with the α-adrenergic blockers, calcium channel blockers do not produce orthostatic or overshoot hypotension. In addition, therapy may be started as late as 24 hours before surgery, and optimal cardiovascular effects are still obtained.[56] Several reports suggest that calcium channel blockers may be the drug of choice for antihypertensive therapy during preoperative preparation of the pheochromocytoma patient.[51,52,55,56]

PITUITARY DISORDERS

The pituitary diseases that are of special concern for the anesthesiologist include those associated with secondary metabolic alterations or diabetes insipidus. A much more in depth discussion of the pituitary is included in Chapter 60.

HYPOPITUITARISM

The pituitary gland is composed of an anterior portion (adenohypophysis) and a posterior portion (neurohypophysis).[57-61] The adenohypophysis responds to hypothalamic release factors by secreting corticotropin, TSH, growth hormone, prolactin, and gonadotropins. The neurohypophysis secretes vasopressin (ADH) and oxytocin. Hormone deficiencies leading to hypopituitarism may be caused by lesions in the brain, a pituitary adenoma (especially a macro-adenoma), trauma, irradiation, or granulomatous disease. Gonadotropin deficiency is not of major significance to anesthetic management. Patients with hypopituitary disorders may present with hypothyroidism and inadequate corticotropin secretion. Steroid coverage or thyroid replacement may be required, although mineralocorticoid therapy usually is not necessary in these patients. Central diabetes insipidus (decreased vasopressin secretion) requires special consideration because blood volume status and electrolytes may be affected. Diabetes insipidus is one of several medical conditions characterized by polyuria and may be nephrogenic or central in origin.

Central diabetes insipidus is an uncommon disease and usually is a result of hypothalamic tumors, infiltrative processes, cerebral aneurysm, ischemia, head trauma, or pituitary surgery. The first step in diagnosis of diabetes insipidus is to determine that the patient has polyuria. Polyuria with a 24-hour urine volume of more than 2.5 L is characteristic of diabetes insipidus.[59] Once polyuria is confirmed, then routine blood tests can eliminate alternative diagnoses such as diabetes mellitus, chronic renal failure, hypercalcemia, or hypokalemia. A water deprivation test is the preferred diagnostic maneuver for diagnosing diabetes insipidus. The water deprivation test involves 2 steps: fluid restriction and desmopressin administration. In normal individuals, water deprivation for approximately 8 hours produces an increased plasma osmolality, stimulating the release of vasopressin, with a subsequently increased urine concentration and decreased urine output. Healthy persons will increase their urine osmolality to greater than 700 mOsm/kg after water deprivation,[59] whereas patients with diabetes insipidus are unable to concentrate their urine. After water deprivation, in patients with suspected diabetes insipidus, exogenous ADH (desmopressin) is administered either subcutaneously or intramuscularly. The desmopressin step distinguishes between central and nephrogenic diabetes insipidus. Patients with nephrogenic diabetes insipidus remain unable to concentrate their urine, whereas those persons with central diabetes insipidus will respond to desmopressin by increasing urine osmolality.

In patients with diabetes insipidus, careful preoperative assessment of volume status, renal function, electrolytes, and plasma osmolarity is important. Management of diabetes insipidus is dependent on whether it is vasopressin responsive (central diabetes insipidus) or unresponsive (nephrogenic diabetes insipidus). In both forms, an intact thirst mechanism helps to ensure adequate hydration. Central diabetes is managed with adequate hydration and oral desmopressin 0.05 to 8 mg once or more daily. Nasal and intramuscular are alternate routes of desmopressin administration. The management of nephrogenic diabetes insipidus is often more difficult and includes hydration, decreased sodium intake, thiazide diuretics, amiloride, and prostaglandin synthesis inhibitors such as indomethacin.[57-59]

HYPERPITUITARISM

Hypersecretion by the pituitary gland presents specific problems for the anesthesiologist. Disease states related to excess secretion of TSH or corticotropin are discussed earlier in this chapter. Excess secretion of growth hormone is associated with acromegaly. Macroglossia and prognathism in this condition may be associated with airway management problems and difficulty with intubation. In a retrospective case series of 28 patients, acromegalic patients were more likely to present a difficult intubation, have an enlarged tongue, and present with airway difficulty.[60] In addition, patients with acromegaly had a higher incidence of preoperative hypertension, diabetes, and cardiomegaly.[58,60,61] With this in mind, the anesthetic pre-evaluation should focus on both the airway and cardiovascular system.

SIADH

The syndrome of inappropriate antidiuretic hormone (SIADH) secretion results from abnormal production or sustained release of ADH. SIADH is associated with normovolemic hyponatremia and has numerous causes (**Table 13-17**). Of note, SIADH is most often not the result of an intrinsic pituitary disorder.[58,59] The criteria for SIADH have been well described (**Table 13-18**). The severity of signs and symptoms associated with SIADH are dependent on the degree of hyponatremia and how rapidly the sodium level decreases. The faster the rate of fall of plasma sodium, and the lower the concentration, the more severe the symptoms. The symptoms and signs are primarily neurologic (**Table 13-19**). The first step in treatment is to eliminate the underlying cause. Fluid restriction is the next step in the correction of chronic hyponatremia. For patients with severe neurologic symptoms or hyponatremia, administration of hypertonic saline with or without furosemide may be required. In patients unable to tolerate fluid restriction, demeclocycline, a tetracycline that causes nephrogenic diabetes

TABLE 13-17 Factors Associated With the Syndrome of Inappropriate Secretion of Antidiuretic Hormone

Tumors	Bronchogenic cancer
	Mesothelioma
	Ureteric cancer
	Pancreatic cancer
	Duodenal cancer
	Lymphoma
	Endometrial cancer
	Leukemia
Pulmonary disease	Lung abscess
	Empyema
	Pneumonia
	Tuberculosis
	Aspergillosis
	HIV infections
	Positive-pressure ventilation
Central nervous system disorders	Cerebral tumors
	Cerebral abscess
	Hydrocephalus
	Subdural hematoma
	Subarachnoid hemorrhage
	Meningitis
	Encephalitis
Drugs	Phenothiazines
	Tricyclic antidepressants
	Chlorpropamide
	Ecstasy
	Carbamazepine
	Cyclophosphamide
	Selective serotonin reuptake inhibitors

TABLE 13-18 Criteria of Syndrome of Inappropriate Secretion of Antidiuretic Hormone

Hyponatremia with hypotonicity of plasma
Inappropriately increased urine osmolality
Increased renal sodium excretion
Absence of edema or volume depletion
Normal renal, thyroid, and adrenal function

insipidus, has been given as adjunctive therapy. More recently, vasopressin receptor antagonists have become available to treat SIADH. Correction of serum sodium should be done gradually because of the possibility of neurologic complications. Therefore, the recommendation is for the rate of correction not to exceed 0.5 mmol/L/h.[58,59]

DIABETES

DEFINITION AND CLASSIFICATION

Diabetes is a complex metabolic disease that affects approximately 7% of the population, more than 24 million people, with almost a million and a half new patients annually.[61-63] Classically diabetes is characterized by hyperglycemia with polyphagia, polydipsia, polyuria, weight loss, and an increased susceptibility to infections. Severely uncontrolled patients may present with marked hyperglycemia and diabetic ketoacidosis or with the nonketotic hyperosmolar syndrome. The interrelationship between diabetes and other disease processes is vast and includes the metabolic syndrome, infections, heart disease, neuropathy, nephropathy, peripheral vascular disease, and retinopathy.

Recently the American Diabetes Association[62,63] modified its diagnostic criteria for the definition of diabetes to include measuring hemoglobin A1c (HgbA1c). When evaluating an abnormal glucose test, the recommendation is still to have the test repeated another day, unless the patient presents with classic symptoms of diabetes or is in a hyperglycemic crisis, in which case a random plasma glucose of 200 mg/dL (11.1 mmol/L) or higher may be used in conjunction with the classic symptoms (ie, criterion #4). The 4 glucose test criteria used by the American Diabetes Association for the definition of diabetes are as follows: (1) HgbA1c of 6.5% or higher with the test being performed in a laboratory using a method that is NGSP certified and standardized to the DCCT assay. If the patient has certain hemoglobinopathies and/or anemias from hemolysis or from nutritional deficiencies, then the use of an HgbA1c of 6.5% or higher alone cannot be used, and other criteria must be used. (An updated list of conditions is available at www.ngsp.org/prog/index3html). (2) A fasting plasma glucose of 126 mg/dL (7.0 mmol/L) or higher, where fasting is defined as no caloric intake for at least 8 hours. (3) A 2-hour plasma glucose of 200 mg/dL (11.1 mmol/L) or higher during an oral glucose tolerance test, which is performed in accordance to World Health Organization standards, with a glucose load containing the equivalent of 75 g of glucose dissolved in water.

TABLE 13-19 Symptoms and Signs of Hyponatremia

Serum Sodium[a]	
<120 mmol/L	<110 mmol/L
Lethargy	Drowsiness
Anorexia	Confusion
Nausea, vomiting	Depressed reflexes
Irritability	Extensor plantar responses
Headache	Seizures
Muscle weakness	Coma
Cramps	Death

[a]The severity of the clinical features is determined by the absolute concentration in which serum sodium falls and its rate of fall.

(4) For patients with classic symptoms of hyperglycemia or hyperglycemic crisis, a random plasma glucose of 200 mg/dL (11.1 mmol/L) or higher. For a clinical situation in which the test results are discordant, the test that is positive should be repeated, and, if positive, then the definition of diabetes applies.

CLASSIFICATION

Diabetes is a disease that is characterized by hyperglycemia, with defects of insulin secretion, insulin action, or both. The American Diabetes Association classifies diabetes into the following 4 specific categories: (1) type 1 diabetes, which is caused by β-cell destruction and usually results in insulin deficiency; (2) type 2 diabetes, which encompasses a range from insulin resistance with relative insulin deficiency, to insulin secretory defects with insulin resistance; (3) specific types of diabetes, which include genetic defects of β-cell function, defects in insulin action, diseases of the exocrine pancreas, endocrinopathies, drug-induced, and infections; and (4) gestational diabetes mellitus.[62,63]

Type 1 Diabetes Type 1 diabetes results from β-cell destruction leading to insulin deficiency and accounts for approximately 5% to 10% of patients with diabetes mellitus. Patients with type 1 diabetes have an increased risk of ketoacidosis due to impaired insulin production. Type 1 diabetes is further subdivided into immune-mediated or idiopathic. Immune-mediated type 1 diabetes is characterized by cell-mediated autoimmune destruction of pancreatic β cells with subsequently decreased insulin secretion. The rate of destruction of β cells may vary. Type 1 diabetes often manifests in childhood or adolescence, but may also present at any age, even in elderly patients, including those in their 80s. Markers of autoimmune destruction such as autoantibodies to islet cells, insulin, glutamic acid decarboxylase (GAD65), and tyrosine phosphatases IA-2 and IA-2B are found in approximately 90% of these patients.[63] There is a strong human leukocyte antigen (HLA) association with the HLA-DR/DQ alleles. Some patients who present with autoimmune destruction of β cells may be obese, but most tend to be thin. Patients with immune-mediated type 1 diabetes are prone to other autoimmune disease, such as Graves disease, Hashimoto thyroiditis, Addison disease, autoimmune hepatitis, myasthenia gravis, and pernicious anemia.[62] In contrast, idiopathic diabetes comprises only a minority of type 1 diabetes, usually in patients of African or Asian descent. Although this form is strongly inherited, there is no HLA association or indication of β-cell autoimmunity, and the requirement for insulin may come and go in affected patients.[62-64]

Type 2 Diabetes The principal and most common form of diabetes is type 2 diabetes, which comprises 90% to 95% of patients with diabetes. Although the cause or causes of this form of diabetes may be varied, patients who have type 1 diabetes, gestational diabetes, or specific type diabetes cannot be classified as having type 2 diabetics. Patients with type 2 diabetes are characterized by a range and progression of insulin resistance and relative insulin deficiency, and they have a stronger genetic predisposition than those with type 1, but these genetic relationships are complex and ill defined. With increasing age, obesity, lack of exercise, hypertension, dyslipidemia, and gestational diabetes there is an increased risk of developing type 2 diabetes. Although ketoacidosis is more characteristic of type 1 diabetes, it may occur with type 2 diabetes in association with the stress of acute illness or infection. Because type 2 diabetes tends to go undetected for years, there is an increased risk of developing a variety of complications.

Other Types of Diabetes[62,63] Genetic defects of β-cell function are due to specific monogenetic defects or specific point mutations. Maturity-onset diabetes of the young (MODY) has been associated with at least 6 different abnormal gene products (ie, MODY 1, Chr 20–HNF4α; MODY 2, Chr 7, glucokinase; MODY 3, Chr 12, HNF-1α; MODY 4, Chr 13, IPF-1; MODY 5, Chr 17, HNF–1β; MODY6, Chr 2, neuro D1). Point mutations of mitochondrial DNA may also lead to diabetes. Gene defects in insulin action are found in type A insulin resistance, leprechaunism, Rabson-Mendenhall syndrome, and insulin-resistant lipodystrophy. Diseases of the exocrine pancreas, such as severe pancreatitis, trauma, pancreatectomy, pancreatic carcinoma, cystic fibrosis, hemochromatosis, and fibrocalculous pancreatopathy, can cause diabetes. Endocrinopathies such as acromegaly, Cushing syndrome, glucagonoma, pheochromocytoma, hyperthyroidism, somatostatinoma, and primary hyperaldosteronism cause diabetes, and with the treatment of the primary disease, the diabetes resolves. Certain drugs may precipitate diabetes in patients with underlying insulin resistance and include IV pentamidine, nicotinic acid, glucocorticoids, thyroid hormone, diazoxide, β-adrenergic agents, thiazides, dilantin, and interferon. Certain viruses such as congenital rubella may result in B-cell destruction. Other viruses such as coxsackievirus B, cytomegalovirus, adenovirus, and mumps can cause diabetes. Uncommon forms of immune-mediated diabetes include "stiff man syndrome" with GAD (glutamic acid decarboxylase) autoantibodies and anti-insulin receptor antibodies found in patients with lupus and other autoimmune diseases. Genetic syndromes such as Down syndrome, Klinefelter syndrome, Turner syndrome, Wolfram syndrome, Fredreich ataxia, Huntington disease, Laurence-Moon Biedl syndrome, myotonic dystrophy, porphyria, and Prader-Willi syndrome are associated with diabetes.

Gestational diabetes occurs in at least 200 000 US pregnancies each year and carries with it a host of other risks. Patients with gestational diabetes are at increased risk for fetal macrosomia, maternal hypertension, cesarean section, neonatal hypoglycemia, and neonatal jaundice and hypocalcemia. The American Diabetes Association is currently working with the obstetrical societies to adopt International Association of Diabetes and Pregnancy Study Group (IADPSG) recommendations.[62,63]

TREATMENT

The American Association of Clinical Endocrinologists/American College of Endocrinology (AACE/ACE) has recently established an algorithm for glycemic control (**Fig. 13-1**). The guiding principle is to

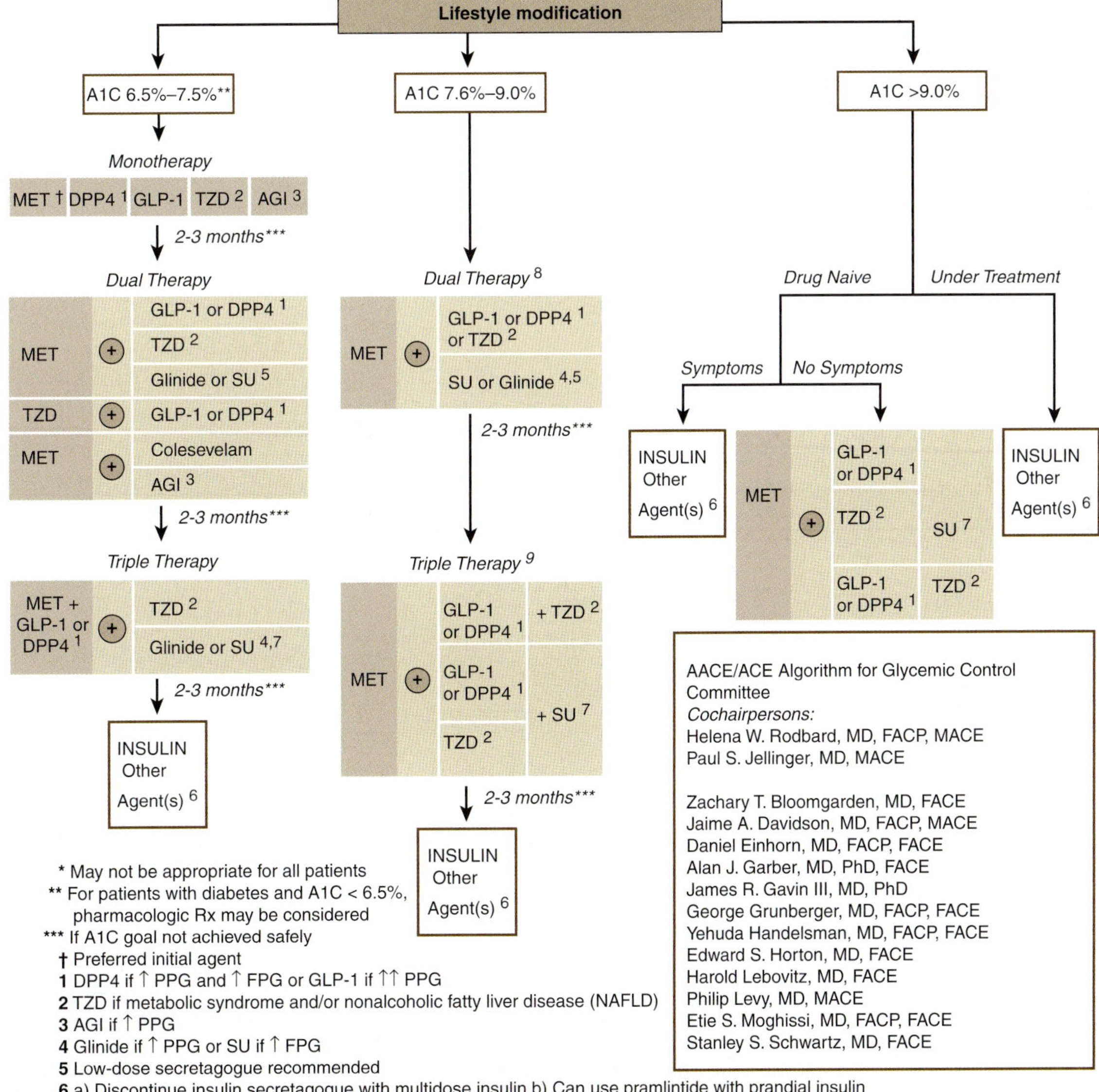

FIGURE 13-1. AACE/ACE diabetes algorithm for glycemic control. [Reproduced with permission from the AACE/ACE Concensus panel.(Rodbard, H.W. and Jellinger, P.S. chairpersons). An algorithm for Glycemic Control. *Endocrin Pract.* 2009;15:546.]

TABLE 13-20 Medications for Glycemic Control

Non-insulin		
Class	**Mechanism**	**Problem**
I. Biguanides Metformin (Glucophage)	Decreases hepatic glucose production	Contraindicated when Cr ≥1.5 or creatine CL <60 mL/min (increased risk of lactic acidosis) Megaloblastic anemia (Impairs vitamin B_{12} absorption)
II. Sulfonylureas Glipizide (Glucotrol) Glyburide (DiaBeta, Micronasis) Glimepiride (Amaryl)	Insulin secretagogue	Hypoglycemia
III. Meglitinides Repaglinide (Prandin) Nateglinide (Starlix)	Insulin secretagogue	Hypoglycemia, weight gain
IV. Thiazolidinediones (TZDs) Rosiglitazone (Avandia) Pioglitazone (Actos)	Insulin-sensitizing agent Edema Heart failure	Weight gain Myocardial infarction
V. α-Glucosidase inhibitors Acarbose (Precose) Miglitol (Glyset)	Inhibits carbohydrate Absorption	GI discomfort Diarrhea
VI. Dipeptidyl peptidose-4 (DPP-4) inhibitors Sitagliptin (Januvia) Saxagliptin (Onglyzia)	Decreases metabolism of incretin hormones	Allergic reactions Renally excreted
VII. Long-acting GLP-1 Analogues Exenatide (Byetta) Liraglutide (Victoza)	Binds to GLP-1 receptor Injection Nausea and vomiting Pancreatitis	Expensive
VIII. Amylin mimetic Pramlintide (Symlin)	Synthetic amylin	Expensive Injection Hypoglycemia
IX. Bili acid sequestrant Colesevelam	Unknown Constipation	Expensive Malabsorption
Insulin		
Name	**Onset/Peak/Duration**	
I. Rapid acting		
Lispro (Humalog)	20 (min)/1 h/3 h	
Aspart (NovoLog)	20 (min)/2 h/3 h	
Glulisine (Apride)	20 (min)/1 h/3 h	
II. Long acting		
Glargine (Lantus)	3 h/no peak/24 h	
Detemir (Levemir)	3 h/no peak/12-24 h (depends on dose)	

use an individualized stepwise approach to achieve an HgbA1c level of 6.5% or less. This should be done with lifestyle modifications, medications including insulin, the use of HgbA1c to guide therapy, and education and compliance on the part of both patients and caregivers.[63,64] **Table 13-20** lists the current classes of medications used for diabetes control.

Non-insulin Medications The *biguanides* suppress hepatic glucose production by decreasing gluconeogenesis and glycogenolysis. There is also decreased absorption of glucose, increased insulin sensitivity, and increased synthesis of GLP-1. Metformin, the principal agent used, is recommended as initial therapy, in combination with other classes of drugs, and may be given in combination with insulin. Nausea and gastrointestinal distress is minimized by a gradual increase in dosage. Metformin is renally excreted and impaired renal function (indicated by a plasma creatinine ≥1.5 or a creatinine clearance of <60 mL/min) may lead to metformin accumulation and lactic acidosis. Metformin therapy is contraindicated in the presence of heart failure, liver disease, alcoholism, sepsis, hypoxemia, and during the administration of intravenous contrast agents. Metformin also decreases the absorption of vitamin B_{12} and may lead to a megaloblastic anemia without vitamin B_{12} supplementation. The insulin secretagogues comprise 2 classes of medicine: the *sulfonylureas* and the *meglitinides*. The sulfonylureas bind to receptors on the β cell to increase insulin secretion. They can have a hypoglycemic effect, which is more pronounced in the elderly, and they can be associated with weight gain and edema. The meglitinides are rapid-acting and short-duration insulin secretagogues. They are tightly bound and metabolized in the liver by cytochrome P450. *Thiazolidinediones* (TZDs) are insulin-sensitizing agents that act on muscle, adipose tissue, and the liver to increase insulin-mediated glucose uptake. Side effects include weight gain and edema, which is not responsive to loop diuretics. TZDs are contraindicated in New York Heart Association functional class III or IV heart failure. TZDs cause patients to be at risk for bone fractures. In addition, a "black box warning" has been issued for rosiglitazone because of its possible association with increased ischemic heart disease. The *α-glucosidase inhibitors* acarbose and miglitol act on the brush border of the intestine to inhibit the breakdown of carbohydrates. Their main side effects are gastrointestinal discomfort, diarrhea, and, in rare instance, cholestatic jaundice. The *dipeptidyl C-peptidase-4 inhibitors* sitagliptin and saxagliptin inhibit DPP-4, an enzyme that metabolizes GLP-1 and gastric inhibitory polypeptide. The incretin hormones cause increased insulin secretion, increased peripheral glucose uptake, and suppression of glucose production in the liver. Allergic reactions may occur. Because these medications are renally excreted, caution must be used in the presence of renal insufficiency. The *GLP-1 agonists*, exenatide and liraglutide, bind to GLP-1 receptors, resulting in increased glucose-dependent insulin secretion and suppression of glucagon secretion. This results in increased satiety, reduced appetite, and weight loss, with the principal side effects being gastrointestinal, although renal insufficiency and pancreatitis have been reported, as well as hypoglycemia when used with sulfonylureas. Pramlintide is a *synthetic amylin* that decreases glucagon secretion, promotes satiety, decreases gastric emptying, and causes weight loss but is associated with nausea and hypoglycemia. Colesevelam is a *bile acid sequestrant* that decreases glucose, but whose precise mechanism of action is unknown.

Insulin The American Association of Clinical Endocrinologists (AACE)/American College of Endocrinology (ACE) consensus panel no longer recommends the use of either regular insulin or NPH insulin for the treatment of type 2 diabetes.[63,64] Regular insulin has an onset of action that is too slow and persists for too long, so that effective glucose control is not achieved, and the risk of delayed hypoglycemia is increased. NPH insulin does not have a consistent absorption pattern from day to day, nor does it persist long enough to provide a basal insulin level, and this increases the risk of hypoglycemia. The AACE/ACE recommends a basal insulin supply, such as provided by glargine or detemir, and treatment with rapid-acting insulins, such as aspart, lispro, or glulisine, to cover postprandial glucose elevations. This more closely mimics normal physiology and minimizes the risk of hypoglycemia.[63,64] The use of continuous insulin infusions requires frequent blood glucose monitoring in order to provide optimal control.

PERIOPERATIVE CHANGES IN GLUCOSE METABOLISM

The surgical stress response[65-71] is characterized by increases in sympathetic tone, glucagon levels, pituitary hormone levels (notably corticotropin and growth hormone), and interleukin-1. During the perioperative period, increases in plasma norepinephrine and epinephrine also occur. Epinephrine and norepinephrine stimulate liver glycogenolysis and gluconeogenesis[68,70] and inhibit glucose uptake by insulin-dependent tissues. The α and β effects of the catecholamines may influence glucose metabolism. For instance, epinephrine increases the metabolic rate through its β effects.[69,70] The α and β effects also have profound influences on pancreatic function. β-Receptor stimulation enhances insulin and glucagon release, whereas α-receptor stimulation inhibits the release of insulin. During the intraoperative and immediate postoperative course, α effects predominate, causing suppression of insulin secretion. Decreased insulin levels coupled with increased gluconeogenesis and insulin resistance cause hyperglycemia and glucose intolerance, prompting the term "the diabetes of injury."

During the convalescent stage after surgery, there is increased gluconeogenesis, and glucose uptake by the peripheral tissues is normal and insulin secretion is increased. The normal pancreas is able to respond normally to the increased glucose loads. A contributing factor to this metabolic change in glucose kinetics is the hormonal shift from α- to β-adrenergic catecholamine effects.[71] Plasma glucagon levels increase after surgery and promote hepatic amino acid uptake, gluconeogenesis, and glycogenolysis.[70,71] Nonetheless, the increase in splanchnic glucose production with glucagon is a transient phenomenon, and it is only with the combined effects of all the stress hormones that hepatic gluconeogenesis is maintained.[70,71] Increased pituitary release of corticotropin leads to increased glucocorticoid levels, which can produce a moderate glycemic response.[67,68] Postoperative increases in growth hormone have an anabolic effect, causing nitrogen retention, protein synthesis, lipolysis, and decreased peripheral glucose uptake.[72] The net effects of the neuroendocrine response on metabolism during the convalescent stage after acute tissue injury include an increased rate of gluconeogenesis, increased blood glucose level, and stimulation of lipolysis.

During surgery, blood glucose concentrations in nondiabetic patients may increase to as much as 60 mg/dL above preoperative levels.[73] The extent of operative stress is the primary determinant of the absolute increase in glucose values. Inadequate insulin secretion, coupled to the stress hormone milieu and the preoperative fasting state, makes the diabetic patient more susceptible to hyperglycemia, osmotic diuresis, hypovolemia, ketosis, and possible changes in acid–base balance. Hyperglycemia may have detrimental effects if it is unmanaged. Osmotic diuresis resulting from the osmotic activity of glucose occurs when the patient's blood glucose level exceeds the renal glucose threshold (approximately 180-250 mg/dL). This osmotic diuresis can result in dehydration, acidosis, and electrolyte abnormalities. Although hyperglycemia per se does not have direct effects on the patient's acid–base status, the ketone bodies that result from inadequate insulin therapy can elicit such effects. Acetoacetic acid and β-hydroxybutyric acid lower serum pH by dissociation of hydrogen ions.

COMPLICATIONS OF DIABETES

Diabetes reduces the overall life span[75] and produces multisystem complications. **Table 13-21** summarizes the principal complications of diabetes.

TABLE 13-21 Diabetic Complications

A. Acute
   1. Diabetic ketoacidosis
   2. Nonketotic hyperglycemic hyperosmolar syndrome
   3. Hypoglycemia
B. Chronic
   1. Cardiovascular
      Coronary heart disease
      Hypertension
      Dyslipidemia
      Prothrombotic state
      Cerebrovascular accident
      Peripheral vascular disease
   2. Diabetic neuropathy
      Small fiber
      Large fiber
      Autonomic
   3. Diabetic nephropathy
      Chronic kidney disease
      Cystopathy
      Infection
   4. Diabetic retinopathy
      Neovascularization
      Blindness
   5. Diabetic foot
      Vascular insufficiency
      Infection
      Ulcer
   6. Immune dysfunction
      Impaired wound healing
      Increased infectious susceptibility
      Periodontal disease
   7. Difficult laryngoscopy and intubation

Cardiovascular Disease and Diabetes The relationship between diabetes and cardiovascular disease is complex. Not only is cardiovascular disease a major complication of diabetes, but diabetes is a major risk factor for cardiovascular disease. Diabetes patients have a higher incidence of cardiovascular disease than the general population.[76-78] Diabetes patients are at increased risk of myocardial infarction and exhibit a greater risk of both pre-hospital and in-hospital mortality after a myocardial infarct.[79] The National Cholesterol Education Program has defined diabetes as a coronary risk equivalent because a higher mortality is associated with diabetes and coronary artery disease.[80] With intensive focus, the risk as a consequence of cardiovascular disease has decreased, but there has not been a decrease in the number of patients with diabetes.[81] Thus risk factor modification assumes greater significance in diabetics.

Similarly, the relationship between diabetes and hypertension is complex and interrelated. Not only should diabetes be aggressively treated, but hypertension should be aggressively treated, as revealed in 2 key studies—the United Kingdom Prospective Diabetes Study (UKPDS) and the Hypertension Optimal Treatment (HOT) trial.[82-84] The UKPDS study found that although intensive glucose therapy was beneficial in reducing cardiovascular risk, there was an even more significant effect of reducing blood pressure, not only for cardiovascular events but also for cerebrovascular events. The HOT study demonstrated that aggressive diastolic blood pressure reduction reduced cardiovascular mortality. These findings have been incorporated into the Joint National Committee on Prevention, Detection, Evaluation, Treatment of High Blood Pressure 7th Report (JNC-7) guidelines.[85] In high-risk cardiovascular patients, angiotensin-converting enzyme (ACE) inhibitors improve cardiovascular morbidity and mortality.[86,87] Despite all the recommendations and the higher prevalence of hypertension among diabetes patients, unfortunately hypertension remains, for many patients, uncontrolled.[88,89]

Dyslipidemias are widely prevalent among diabetes patients and are part of the complex relationship between diabetes and the associated cardiovascular and cerebrovascular events leading to increased morbidity and mortality. Multiple studies—the Heart Protection Study,[89] the Veterans Affairs High-Density Lipoprotein Cholesterol Intervention Trial Study Group,[90] the Scandinavian Simvastatin Survival Study,[91] and the MRC/BHF Heart Protection Study[92]—show a clear benefit of aggressive lipid management. The American Diabetes Association used this information to help set its lipid goal recommendations[63,93]: low-density lipoprotein (LDL) cholesterol in diabetes patients should be less than 100 mg/dL. The National Cholesterol Education Program (NCEP) has set a more aggressive goal in high-risk patients: LDL less than 70 mg/dL, triglycerides less than 150 mg/dL, and high-density lipoprotein greater than 40 mg/dL.[63,93] The Lescol Intervention Prevention Study found a marked reduction of more than 50% in major adverse cardiac events such as death or nonfatal myocardial infarction with the use of statin therapy.[94]

Diabetes is associated with a prothrombotic state that contributes to the increased risk of mortality from cardiovascular disease.[95,96] One of the early studies to show the benefits of aspirin was the Physicians Health Study,[97] which noted a marked reduction in myocardial infarctions among diabetic physicians taking aspirin. Subsequent work, such as the HOT trial, continued to show a significant reduction in cardiovascular events, as well as myocardial infarction for patients taking aspirin. The benefits of aspirin plus clopidogrel, as well as aspirin plus glycoprotein 2b/3a inhibitors, has been noted,[95] although the risk of bleeding is increased with these combinations versus aspirin alone.

Although recent studies[98] indicate that current assessment guidelines may miss patients with silent ischemia, there is still no well-established data in asymptomatic patients demonstrating that advanced testing with nuclear stress tests or stress echocardiography can lead to better outcomes. The emphasis should rather be on risk reduction and adopting proven beneficial therapies—lipid reduction, blood pressure control, smoking cessation, weight reduction, increasing physical activity, and aspirin therapy. A detailed history and physical examination including laboratory and electrocardiogram (ECG) analysis should be done. Exercise capacity should be determined in accordance with the American College of Cardiologists/American Heart Association preoperative assessment guidelines.

Diabetic Neuropathy Diabetic neuropathy is common, varied, and affects between 75% and 90% of all diabetes patients, with the elderly having more pronounced effects. There are many classification systems for diabetic neuropathy.[99,100] The American Diabetes Association[63] classifies neuropathies as (1) sensory neuropathies—acute sensory neuropathy and chronic distal symmetric polyneuropathy; (2) focal and multifocal neuropathies; and (3) autonomic neuropathy. The classification system used by Vinik and Mehrabyan[102,103]—small-fiber neuropathies, large-fiber neuropathies, and autonomic neuropathy—is somewhat more intuitive. A key point emphasized by the American Diabetes Association[63] is that early recognition and treatment of neuropathy is important; it is equally important to determine which neuropathies are not attributable to diabetes and to correctly diagnose and exclude them.

The small-fiber neuropathies[63,102] are characterized by being electrophysiologically silent with preservation of reflexes and motor strength, but with loss of cutaneous nerve fibers on tissue staining. Allodynia with burning superficial pain of the c-fiber type is a characteristic, but later there is hypoalgesia. There is decreased thermal sensation with impaired vasomotor and blood flow and decreased autonomic function, leading to decreased sweating, dry skin, and an increased risk of foot ulceration and gangrene.

The large-fiber neuropathies encompass both sensory and motor nerves and are more amenable to diagnosis with electromyography, nerve conduction velocity studies, and quantitative sensory tests.[99,101,103] Clinical manifestations include changes in perception presenting with impaired vibratory perception and position sense. There is depression of the deep tendon reflexes, sensory ataxia, and a deep-seated, dull, aching pain in the feet. Initially there may be a feeling of warmth in the feet because of increased blood flow. There is a shortening of the Achilles tendon and wasting of the small muscles of the feet, with hammertoes and subsequent weakening of the hands and feet. Distal muscle weakness can been seen as leading to an inability to stand on the heels or toes. Distal symmetric neuropathy, diffuse motor neuropathy, and distal motor neuropathy are part of the large-fiber neuropathy syndrome. It is important to exclude other causes of these types of neuropathies, such as familial B_{12} deficiency, folate deficiency, Lyme disease, heavy-metal poisoning, reaction to cytotoxins, and the neuropathies caused by malignancy. In the elderly, there is an increase in proximal muscle neuropathy. These can present as pain in the buttocks, thighs, and hips that can be either abrupt or gradual in onset. Symptoms can progress to weakness with inability to get up from a sitting position and can coexist with distal symmetric polyneuropathy. Fasciculations may be provoked by percussion or may occur spontaneously with electrophysiologic studies indicating a lumbosacral plexopathy. The elderly are also at greater risk for mononeuropathies. These tend to occur spontaneously, acutely, and with pain. They tend to affect the ulnar, median, peroneal nerves, and cranial nerves III, VI, and VII and are characterized by a spontaneous remission and lack progression. These mononeuropathies must be distinguished from nerve-entrapment syndromes such as carpal tunnel, which are more frequent in diabetes patients but which tend to be gradual in onset and progressive in nature.[63,99,101]

Autonomic neuropathy[99-103] has many clinical manifestations and involves multiple physiologic systems. Cardiovascular manifestations include a resting tachycardia, exercise intolerance, orthostatic hypotension, cardiac degeneration and silent myocardial infarction, alterations in blood flow to skin and extremities, and temperature intolerance. The gastrointestinal system is affected by a variety of changes, including esophageal dysmotility, diarrhea, constipation, incontinence, and diabetic gastroparesis. Genitourinary syndromes include cystopathy, neurogenic bladder, and sexual dysfunction in women and erectile dysfunction in men. Besides temperature intolerance, there are abnormalities of sweating. There is decreased lower-body sweating, with resulting skin dryness and cracking contributing to increased infections and ulcerations of the diabetic foot. Autonomic neuropathy affects the metabolic response to glucose regulation with both a decreased ability to detect and respond to hypoglycemia. Ocular manifestations of autonomic neuropathy include Argyll-Robertson–like pupil and a decreased diameter of a dark-adapted pupil.[102]

As pointed out by Luukinen and Airaksinen,[104] orthostatic hypotension for older diabetes patients portends a higher risk of vascular death. The increase in morbidity and mortality associated with autonomic neuropathy is one of the reasons the American Diabetes Association[63,102] advocates the performance of standard examinations to diagnose autonomic neuropathy. Examination of the resting heart rate is key, because a resting heart rate greater than 100 beats per minute is abnormal. Next, an examination of fasting, nonhypoglycemic heart rate with a study of heart rate variability is done with a patient monitored by an ECG breathing at 6 breaths per minute; the difference in heart rate between resting and supine should be greater than 15 beats per minute, and if the heart rate variability is less than 10 beats per minute, and the R-R interval ratio is not greater than 1.17, then the heart rate variability is considered abnormal.

As noted by Cox et al,[105] hyperglycemia impairs cognitive performance in diabetes patients. Arvanitakis et al[106] notes that diabetes, in addition to aging, contributes to the progression and worsening of rigidity and gait disturbance in the elderly. The DCCT trial[107,108] demonstrated the beneficial effect of tight glucose control on limiting the microvascular complications of diabetes; the goal advocated is an HgbA1c level less than 7%. In addressing the pain and discomfort associated with diabetic neuropathy, the American Diabetes Association[63,102] recommends a stepwise approach starting with exclusion of nondiabetic causes, stabilizing the blood sugar, and then attempting to achieve an HgbA1c level of less than 7%. Tricyclics are the first-line drugs for pain control, then anticonvulsants, and finally opiates. However, Gilron et al[109] recently demonstrated that the lower-dose combination of opiates and anticonvulsants achieves better analgesia than higher doses of either drug alone. The EURODIAB Study Group,[110] in addition to the findings of the UKPDS, emphasizes the importance of addressing all modifiable risk factors to minimize diabetic neuropathy.

Nephropathy and Urologic Complications Diabetic effects on the urologic system encompass diabetic nephropathy, urologic cystopathy, erectile dysfunction, and infection. Diabetic nephropathy affects more than 40% of patients with type 1 diabetes and more than 20% of those with type 2 diabetes.[63,111,112] The National Kidney Foundation[112] defines diabetes as a risk factor for chronic kidney disease and recommends screening and risk factor reduction. The effects of diabetes in leading to end-stage renal disease are worse for certain ethnic groups, namely Native Americans, Hispanics, and African Americans.[63] It appears that aggressive risk-factor reduction and tight blood pressure and glucose control[113] can decrease both the rate of progression to end-stage kidney disease and the renal complications of diabetes. The American Diabetes Association recommends the early diagnosis and treatment of microalbuminuria along with aggressive risk-factor reduction and blood glucose control to prevent the albuminuria, blood pressure elevation, and persistent decline in glomerular filtration rate (GFR) that is characteristic of diabetic nephropathy and which ultimately contributes to increased mortality and morbidity.

Diabetic cystopathy affects almost 50% of diabetes patients and increases with age.[102] In diabetic cystopathy there is impaired sensation of bladder fullness, an increase in bladder capacity, a reduction in bladder contractility, and increased residual urine volume. Residual urine increases the risk for urinary tract infections, urethral reflux, hydronephrosis, pyelonephritis, and urosepsis. A urologic evaluation for cystopathy may include cystometry, sphincter electromyography, uroflowmetry, and urethral pressure profile. Both cystopathy and erectile dysfunction result from microvascular changes of diabetes and the polyneuropathy associated with diabetes.[114]

Diabetic Ketoacidosis and Nonketotic Hyperglycemic Hyperosmolar Syndrome Poorly controlled diabetes may cause severe metabolic abnormalities, including diabetic ketoacidosis or a hyperglycemic hyperosmolar nonketotic state. The hyperosmolar nonketotic state is characterized by marked hyperglycemia, dehydration, and hyperosmolarity, but severe ketosis is absent. Patients unable to compensate for hyperglycemia and dehydration are often elderly type 2 diabetes patients. The presence of diabetic ketoacidosis is suggested strongly by the history and physical examination, along with a high blood sugar level and positive urine ketones, although a definitive diagnosis of diabetic ketoacidosis must be verified with arterial blood gases and consists of (1) hyperglycemia (>250 mg/dL), (2) decreased bicarbonate (<15 mEq/L), and (3) a decreased arterial pH (<7.3) with ketonemia (positive at 1:2 dilution) and moderate ketonuria. The principal therapy includes hydration, IV insulin, and frequent monitoring of electrolytes, glucose, and acid–base status. The details of therapy are addressed in Chapter 60.

DIABETES PREOPERATIVE EVALUATION

Diabetes is a disease with enormous physiologic impact, and the preoperative evaluation should be done in accordance with current American College of Cardiologists/American Heart Association guidelines. The preoperative evaluation should include assessment of the systemic manifestations noted previously. The ECG should be analyzed, bearing in mind the greater incidence of silent myocardial infarctions among diabetes patients. Because diabetic patients tend to receive multiple medications, obtaining a metabolic profile may be worthwhile. The levels of key electrolytes, sodium, and potassium should be determined. Current glucose level both in reference to a patient's baseline and also as a baseline for subsequent comparisons is useful. An HgbA1c level is useful to indicate overall glycemic control, with current American Diabetes Association recommendations being below 7% and values above 10% corresponding to poor glycemic control.[63] A fasting lipid profile provides information regarding concomitant cardiovascular risk. The serum creatinine, along with blood urea nitrogen level, helps to provide information on volume status and renal function. It must be borne in mind that as patients age, their muscle mass diminishes, as does the creatinine that one measures. Because urinary tract infections tend to be common among diabetic patients, a urinalysis can provide insight regarding the presence of infection, ketones, protein, and sediment.

Laryngoscopy and Intubation Diabetes may be associated with a greater incidence of difficult laryngoscopy and intubation. In patients with diabetes, stiff joint syndrome can occur, affecting all joints, including those of the cervical and thoracic spine. The incidence of difficult laryngoscopy in long-term type 1 diabetic patients is reported to be 30% to 40%.[117-119] The diagnosis of stiff-joint syndrome is relatively easy. Besides evaluation of spine mobility, the wrists and elbows should be observed for incomplete extension and flexion. The hands should be assessed for thick, waxy skin and an inability to oppose the interphalangeal joints of the fingers assessed in the "prayer" position.[119]

METABOLIC SYNDROME

Patients with the metabolic syndrome are at an increased risk for cardiovascular disease, cerebrovascular disease, and diabetes. This may be a result of dyslipidemia, vascular dysregulation, a proinflammatory state, prothrombotic state, insulin resistance, or some other mechanism. The recent consensus definition of the metabolic syndrome[120,121] uses in large part the International Diabetes Foundations definition. Currently the consensus conference considers the metabolic syndrome present when any 3 of the following 5 criteria are present: (1) elevated waist circumference that is ethnically and country specific; (2) elevated triglycerides with a value of 150 mg/dL (1.7 mmol/L), or higher, or undergoing drug treatment; (3) reduced high-density lipoprotein cholesterol (<40 mg/dL [1.7 mmol/L] in men and 50 mg/dL [1.3 mmol/L] in women) or undergoing drug treatment; (4) an elevated blood pressure (systolic ≥130, or diastolic ≥85) or undergoing drug treatment; (5) elevated fasting glucose of 100 mg/dL, or higher, or undergoing drug treatment.[121] Whether the metabolic syndrome is a clustering of risk factors or a specific disease itself remains to be determined.

Acknowledgment: The author thanks F.E. Sieber for his work on this chapter in the previous edition.

KEY REFERENCES

- American Diabetes Association. Standards of medical care in diabetes—2010. *Diabetes Care.* 2010;33(Suppl):S11-S61.
- Bondanelli M, Zatelli MC, Ambrosio MR, et al. Systemic illness. *Pituitary.* 2008;11:187-207.
- Drugs for thyroid disorders. *Treat Guidel Med Lett.* 2009;84: 57-64.
- Manger WM. The protean manifestations of pheochromocytoma. *Horm Metab Res.* 2009;41:658-663.
- Michalakis K, Ilias I. Medical management of adrenal disease: a narrative review. *Endocr Regul.* 2009;43:127-135.
- Moe SM. Disorders involving calcium, phosphorous, and magnesium. *Prim Care Clin Office Pract.* 2008;35:215-237.
- Rodbard HW, Jellinger PS, Davidson JA, et al. AACE/ACE Consensus Statement. Statement by an American Association of Clinical Endocrinologists/American College of Endocrinology consensus panel on type 2 diabetes mellitus: an algorithm for glycemic control. *Endocr Pract.* 2009;15:540-559.
- Topliss DJ, Eastman CJ. Diagnosis and management of hyperthyroidism and hypothyroidism. *Med J Aust.* 2004;180:186-193.

REFERENCES

Complete references available on DVD and online version at www.LongneckerAnesthesiology.com

CHAPTER 14 Evaluation of the Patient With Renal Disease

Mark Stafford-Smith
Atif Raja
Andrew D. Shaw

KEY POINTS

1. Kidney functions are centrally involved in whole-body homeostasis and normally keep body fluid volume, osmolarity, electrolyte content and concentration, and acidity within narrow limits.
2. Knowledge of normal kidney function is particularly important to interpret the physiology of the neonate, the parturient, and the elderly patient, where differentiating normal from abnormal may be challenging and even counterintuitive.
3. Although the search continues for a substance with "ideal" properties to assess glomerular filtration (ie, steady production, complete filtration, no secretion or absorption, convenient inexpensive measurement) through its clearance from the circulation, serum creatinine and creatinine clearance are the current clinical standard.
4. Kidney-mediated acid–base, electrolyte, and/or fluid disorders are common preoperatively and may be sufficiently important to require correction before surgery can proceed.
5. Familiarity with the spectrum of acute and chronic renal disorders that may be encountered in the perioperative patient is essential to logically anticipate perioperative problems and design rational therapeutic strategies.
6. Prevention is the most important tool in the approach to perioperative acute kidney injury; this requires knowledge of potential insults, including the renoprotective value of meticulous attention to minimizing hemodilution and transfusion.
7. Major acute kidney injuries significantly impair the kidneys' ability to maintain the internal environment; in these situations adherence to guidelines aimed at preserving volume, electrolyte, acid–base, and nutrition balance within the limits of the remaining renal homeostatic reserve may be sufficiently effective that dialysis can be avoided.
8. Patients with impaired renal filtration have altered responses to normal medication dosing; a simple prescribing approach for water-soluble agents involves a calculated percentage reduction in drug dosage to match the reduction in glomerular filtration. However, drug-level measurement or algorithms for a specific drug dosing may be recommended.

"The composition of blood is determined not by what the mouth ingests but by what the kidneys keep..."[1] This well-known quote of renal physiologist Dr Homer Smith highlights not only the kidneys' domain of influence, but also why even minor renal perturbations have widespread effects. The kidneys play a key role in homeostasis, making review of their function essential for even the most abbreviated perioperative assessment. Although consideration is often limited to issues of filtration and clearance, these tasks comprise only a part of the kidneys' involvement in homeostasis. Normal renal physiology and the consequences of impairment are reviewed here in context of their implications for the perioperative physician.

THE NORMAL KIDNEY: CORRELATES OF STRUCTURE AND FUNCTION

The kidneys are paired mesoderm-derived retroperitoneal organs that weigh approximately 150 g each. Notably, despite the fact that by body weight kidneys make up only 0.4%, they receive 25% of cardiac output; in relative terms, this exceeds muscle blood flow with heavy exercise by 8-fold and makes them the most highly perfused major organ in the body. Partial explanation for this remarkable blood flow comes from unusually high-normal renal vein oxygen levels, which evidence a "luxury perfusion" component to renal blood flow (RBF) that serves plasma filtration at rates as high as 125 to 140 mL/min in adults. Metabolic demands are not the primary determinant of blood flow to the kidney, despite the undisputed major oxygen requirements of tubular active transport. Nonetheless, it is simplistic to assume that kidneys receive excess nutrients and oxygen, because this ignores marked regional differences in perfusion that paradoxically make some kidney "zones," particularly the medulla, highly vulnerable to ischemic injury.

The functions of the kidney are many. Normal "resting" nephrons are continuously processing filtered plasma, involving numerous feedback mechanisms and energy consuming active transport from the tubule to regulate body composition through maintenance of fluid volume, osmolarity, acidity, and the concentration of numerous electrolytes within narrow limits. Every 3 minutes, an amount equivalent to a 12-oz soft drink is filtered, and all but 1%, or 4 mL, is returned to the circulation. Extracellular solutes are tightly regulated, including sodium, potassium, hydrogen ion, bicarbonate, and glucose. The kidneys also generate ammonia and glucose, and eliminate nitrogenous and other metabolic waste, including urea, creatinine, and bilirubin, as well as toxins and many classes of drugs. Finally, circulating kidney hormones

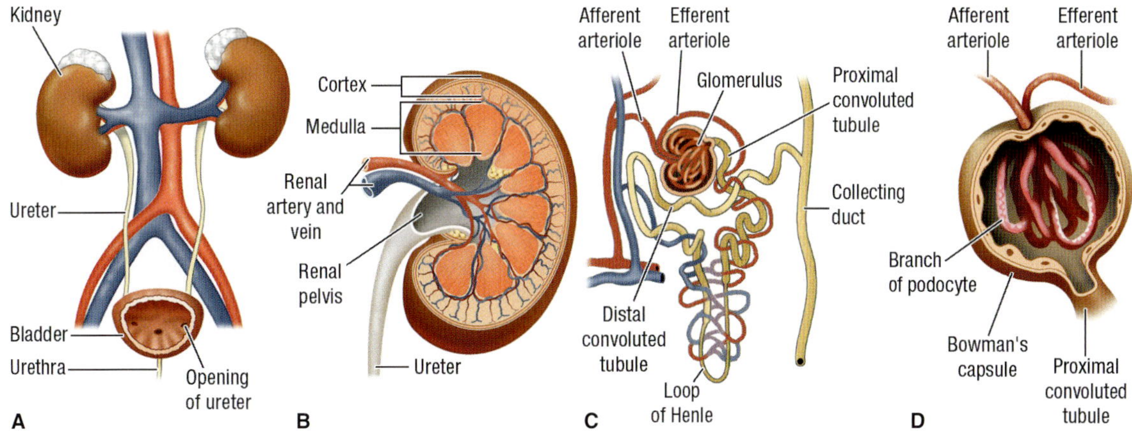

FIGURE 14-1. A. The kidney is part of the genitourinary system. **B.** The internal structure of the kidney includes the vasculature, cortex and medulla regions, and urinary tract structures. **C.** The functional unit of the kidney is the nephron. The glomerulus **(D)** is the site where plasma filtration occurs; approximately 20% of plasma entering the glomerulus will pass through the specialized capillary wall into the Bowman capsule and enter the tubule to be processed and generate urine.

influence erythrocyte generation, calcium homeostasis, and systemic blood pressure.

Detailed descriptions of the anatomy of the kidney are available elsewhere.[2] In summary, each highly internally organized bean-shaped kidney contains a superficial cortical layer, deeper medullary regions, and a network of ducts that feed urine to a renal pelvis and onward to ureter and bladder (**Fig. 14-1**). Each kidney contains approximately 1×10^6 tightly packed nephrons, the functional unit of the kidney. The nephron is a segmented tubular structure made up of specialized elements, including a glomerulus, proximal convoluted tubule, loop of Henle, distal convoluted tubule, and collecting duct (Fig. 14-1). The cortex is the more superficial outer portion of the kidney and contains primarily glomeruli, proximal, and distal convoluted tubules. The medulla is deeper and subdivided into inner and outer (more superficial) layers that contain loops of Henle and collecting ducts. So-called *cortical nephrons* represent the majority (85%) and have glomeruli close to the outer kidney surface, with tubular structures that remain in the cortex, whereas *juxtamedullary nephrons* have glomeruli in the deeper cortex and loops of Henle that pass deep into and out of the medulla forming hairpin curves. The loops of Henle juxtamedullary nephrons participate in *countercurrent exchange*, a mechanism making possible the formation of highly concentrated urine (**Fig. 14-2**).

Like the tubules, the kidney vasculature is highly organized. The *renal artery* enters the kidney at the hilum and divides many times before producing *arcuate arteries* that course the boundary between cortex and outer medulla. *Interlobular arteries* branch from arcuate arteries toward the kidney's exterior capsule, giving rise to numerous *afferent arterioles* that each supply a single *glomerular capillary tuft*. The glomerulus contains the barrier from vascular to tubular space where filtration occurs; this specialized structure includes fenestrated negatively charged capillary endothelial cells and tubular epithelial cells (podocytes) separated by a basement membrane. Selective glomerular permeability typically allows approximately 25% of plasma elements to pass out of the vasculature into the Bowman capsule, preventing large proteins (>60-70 kDa) and cells from escaping. Notably, disease may damage this barrier, evidenced by passage of larger proteins (nephrotic syndrome) and even erythrocytes (glomerulonephritis) into the tubule. Exiting glomerular capillaries merge to form an *efferent arteriole* and subsequently *peritubular capillaries* that nourish the tubules. Peritubular capillaries that accompany loops of Henle are known as *vasa rectae*. The renal vasculature is unusual with its sequence of two capillary beds joined in series by arterioles, and also in its strictly segmental supply, with each nephron provided from only one afferent arteriole and related capillaries. A consequence of this vascular arrangement is that embolic arteriolar obstruction causes infarction in a strict "pizza wedge" distribution from cortex to medulla, involving all related glomeruli and their cortical and medullary elements. Peritubular capillaries perfuse tubular cells and receive reabsorbed fluids, ultimately rejoining to form *venules*. Throughout the kidney, venous tributaries run closely in parallel to their related arterial vasculature, culminating in blood return to the inferior vena cava through *renal veins*.

As a summary of renal plasma processing, the glomerular-filtered fraction enters the Bowman capsule (~120 mL/min) and passes into the proximal convoluted tubule, where active transport processes rapidly reabsorb approximately two-thirds of water and electrolytes. Processing in the loops of Henle and distal convoluted tubules also returns approximately two-thirds of what they receive back into the circulation, with

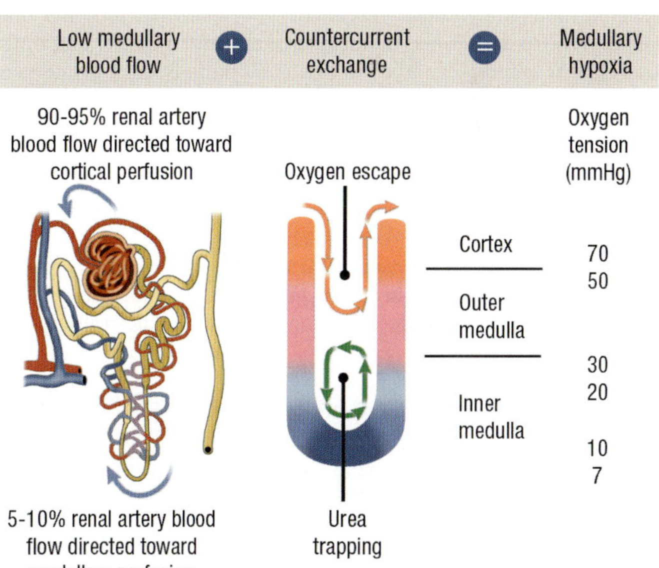

FIGURE 14-2. Medullary hypoxia refers to the physiologically very low Po_2 values (eg, 10-20 mm Hg) in the renal medulla that are present even under normal conditions. Factors contributing to this state include a high rate of oxygen consumption, relatively poor blood supply, and inefficient oxygen delivery related to countercurrent O_2 "escape" due to the parallel arrangement of entering to exiting capillaries. Ironically, this same sluggish perfusion is also essential to create and maintain the urea gradient required to concentrate urine. [From Grocott HP, Stafford-Smith M. Organ protection during cardiopulmonary bypass. In: Kaplan JA, ed., Reich DL, Lake CL, Konstadt SN, assoc. eds. *Cardiac Anesthesia.* 5th ed. Philadelphia, PA: Elsevier; 2006:985-1022.]

generation of highly concentrated urine being a specialized function of medullary loops of Henle. Generally, still more water is reabsorbed as the highly processed effluent enters the collecting duct (5-10 mL/min), with the remnant passing into collecting structures as urine (1-4 mL/min).

Medullary hypoxia is a key concept in understanding the vulnerability of the renal medulla to ischemic insult, even during normal resting conditions. To facilitate the specialized goals of the kidney, an important physiologic compromise appears to have evolved where the ability to form highly concentrated urine comes at the cost of a precariously limited medullary oxygen reserve. Factors necessary to create a urea gradient for medullary countercurrent exchange to occur include a sluggish blood supply and highly "oxygen-expensive" active transport demands; these issues combine with perfusion inefficiency related to "O_2 escape" from entering to exiting vasa rectae capillaries to make normal Po_2 values in the medulla very low (eg, 10-20 mm Hg; Fig. 14-2).[3-5] Much evidence indicates that this precarious arrangement is responsible for the extreme vulnerability of the renal medulla to ischemic injury (see the section Postoperative Renal Disorders).

CLINICAL ASSESSMENT OF THE KIDNEY

There is general agreement that measures such as urine output correlate extremely poorly with the rate of renal filtration[6]; however, much information about the state of the kidneys can be gained by evaluating how effectively they clear circulating substances. Inspection of the urine (ie, urinalysis) can also be informative.

RENAL FUNCTION TESTS

Glomerular filtration is the most clinically evaluated renal function. As a key marker of renal disease, knowledge of limited filtration capacity is useful to guide dosing of drugs cleared by the kidneys but also generally indicates increased perioperative risk. Sudden postoperative declines in filtration indicate acute kidney injury (*AKI*) and consistently predict an even more complicated clinical course.[7] *Glomerular filtration rate* (GFR) refers to the plasma volume filtered by the kidneys per unit time, and normal values range from 90 to 137 mL/min. Normal glomerular filtration rates are proportionate to patient size and body-surface area and decline approximately 10% per decade after age 30 (**Table 14-1**).[8] Generally men have GFR values approximately 10 mL/min higher than those of women. GFR values below 60 mL/min are considered moderately impaired, and individuals with values below 15 mL/min often have uremic symptoms and may require dialysis.

Any substance used to assess GFR through its clearance from the circulation must have certain "ideal" properties; these include a steady supply to the circulation, free filtration by glomeruli, no reabsorption or excretion by the tubules, and, preferably, easy, inexpensive measurement in blood and urine. Unfortunately, the ideal substance has yet to be identified. The most precise and accurate GFR determination tools involve cumbersome "gold standard" methodologies (eg, inulin, ^{51}Cr-EDTA, or ^{99}Tc-DTPA clearance), whereas the role as a clinical tool has been monopolized until recently by a more practical and inexpensive "somewhat ideal" alternate, creatinine. Overall, despite the limitations of creatinine as a marker, its relatively steady supply from muscle breakdown and modest tubular secretion make it the most clinically useful renal filtration marker currently available. Although more ideal substances are being sought as practical clinical tools, candidates currently under evaluation (eg, cystatin C)[9,10] have yet to be generally accepted as superior to creatinine. A notable deficiency of all clearance methods to estimate renal filtration using ideal substances is the requirement for steady-state kinetics, an equilibrium particularly difficult to achieve in the perioperative patient, especially if AKI has occurred.

Estimates of GFR (eGFR) can be made by determining *creatinine clearance* (CrCl) from blood and urine creatinine tests. In stable, critically ill patients, 2-hour urine collections sufficient to determine CrCl[11] are calculated using the following formula:

$$\text{CrCl (mL/min)} = U_{Cr}\ \text{(mg/dL)} \times V\ \text{(mL)}/P_{Cr}\ \text{(mg/dL)} \times \text{time (min)}$$

where U_{Cr} = urine creatinine, V = total volume of urine collected, P_{Cr} = plasma creatinine, and time = collection time.

However, GFR can also be predicted using a single steady-state serum creatinine value if patient characteristics are known. Importantly, as already highlighted previously, predictive formulas from stable nonsurgical populations do not account for perioperative fluid shifts and other sources of "unsteadiness" in the operative patient, reducing the value of serum creatinine as a tool to predict GFR. Nonetheless, serum creatinine is an inexpensive and, thus far, unsurpassed clinical tool (particularly to reflect *trends* and relative changes in renal filtration function) that is useful in predicting outcome, even during the perioperative period.[12-14] Of the many predictive formulas that exist, the Cockroft-Gault equation is one of the most validated and durable.[15] The Cockroft-Gault equation estimates GFR based on patient sex, age (years), weight (kg), and serum creatinine (mg/dL):

$$\text{Cockroft-Gault eGFR (mL/min)} = (140 - \text{age}) \times \text{weight (kg)}/(\text{Cr} \times 72) \times 0.85 \text{ for females)}$$

More recently, an estimating method from the Modification of Diet in Renal Disease (MDRD) study that adds knowledge of ethnicity (black versus nonblack) to standard components of the Cockroft-Gault equation may improve accuracy.[16]

An abbreviated MDRD formula is available that can estimate GFR measured in mL/min/1.73 m^2:

$$\text{GFR} = 186 \times (\text{serum creatinine} - \text{mg/dL})^{-1.154} \times (\text{age})^{-0.203}$$
$$(\times\ 0.742 \text{ for females})$$
$$(\times\ 1.210 \text{ for blacks})$$

In clinical practice, a single preoperative serum creatinine determination can be misleading. Average creatinine values do not increase significantly until GFR rates fall below 50 mL/min, so serum creatinine may be normal, particularly in elderly patients, even with some degree of renal dysfunction. Even the most detailed creatinine-based MDRD eGFR estimation under ideal conditions correlates poorly with GFR by gold standard measures, with more than a 30% error in 10% of patients and 2% deviating more than 50%.[16]

Some consensus definitions for significant perioperative AKI have been published. For example, the RIFLE criteria for AKI require a creatinine increase of 50% risk, 100% injury, or 200% failure.[17] The AKIN criteria are similar to the RIFLE criteria, requiring only a serum creatinine rise of at least 0.3 mg/dL or 50% within a 48-hour period (akinet.org). The Society of Thoracic Surgeon's definition of postoperative AKI includes either a new requirement for dialysis, a rise in serum creatinine

TABLE 14-1 Clinical Correlates of Glomerular Filtration Rate (GFR) Values

GFR Value	Serum Creatinine (mg/dL)	Implication
120 mL/min	1.0	Normal (healthy, 20-year-old)
80 mL/min	1.2	Normal (healthy, 65-year-old)
60 mL/min	1.1	Normal (healthy, 85-year-old)
30-60 mL/min	1.3-2.5	Moderate renal dysfunction Dosage adjustments may be needed
15-29 mL/min	1.7-3.5	Severe decrease in GFR, may reflect chronic disease, prerenal renal failure, or acute tubular necrosis
<15 mL/min	2.0-18.0	Renal failure (acute or chronic) requiring dialysis

Normal kidney filtration keeps serum creatinine levels stable with increasing age due to the roughly matched age-related decline in GFR (creatinine clearance) and reduction in creatinine generation by muscle. Of note, moderate to severe degrees of renal impairment can be associated with only modest rises in serum creatinine in the elderly.

to greater than 2.0 mg/dL, or at least a 50% increase in serum creatinine over baseline values.[18] Another definition requires serum creatinine to rise more than 25% or 0.5 mg/dL (44 µmol/L) within 48 hours.[19] Notably, regardless of definition, the required delay for serum creatinine accumulation to herald renal insult has taken some of the blame for a lack of progress in efforts to intervene early enough in the evolution of perioperative AKI. A search is now on for early biomarker tools that can reflect kidney distress sooner, facilitating timely intervention, much as creatinine kinase and troponin monitoring has advanced myocardial infarction therapies.

Blood urea nitrogen (BUN) remains widely used to assess renal function but possesses few of the characteristics of an ideal substance. Tubular transport of urea changes significantly with some conditions (eg, dehydration), and urea generation can also be highly variable, particularly in the postoperative period (eg, catabolic state). In addition, perioperative hemodilution (eg, CPB) may affect circulating BUN levels.

URINALYSIS AND URINE CHARACTERISTICS

The examination of urine can reveal much information. Standard aspects of urinalysis include gross appearance, specific gravity, chemical tests for abnormal substances, and microscopic examination for cells and formed elements.

Urine inspection can reveal abnormal color, cloudiness, and unexpected odors. There are many available detailed descriptions of examination of the urine[20]; therefore, we provide only a summary here. Color changes reflect increased amounts of dissolved substances; this occurs most commonly with dehydration, but other causes include food colorings, drugs, and liver disease (eg, bilirubin). In contrast, cloudy urine is due to suspended elements, such as crystals and/or white or red blood cells. Lightly centrifuged urine sediment will normally reveal up to 2 red blood cells per high-power field (magnification ×400). In addition, normal urine will contain up to 80 ± 20 mg of protein per day. As noted previously, high levels of protein (eg, > 3.5 g/24 h) or red blood cells reflect abnormal kidney function. Urine protein electrophoresis can trace proteinuria to abnormalities of glomerular (filtering), tubular (reuptake), overflow (supply that saturates the reuptake system), or tissue (eg, kidney inflammation) function.[21] Unusual odors are less common but can also be diagnostic (eg, maple syrup urine disease). Chromogenic "dipstick" chemical tests can determine urine pH and provide a semiquantitative analysis of protein, glucose, ketones, blood, urobilinogen, bilirubin, nitrites, and leukocyte esterase. In addition, urine microscopy can identify bacteria, crystals, cells, and casts from renal tubules.

Urine-specific gravity refers to the weight of urine relative to distilled water; normal values range between 1.001 and 1.035. Specific gravity is often used as a surrogate for osmolarity (normal range, 50-1000 mOsm/kg), with 1.010 reflecting a urine-specific gravity the same as plasma osmolarity. High specific gravity (>1.018) implies a preserved concentrating ability of the kidney, unless substances that raise specific gravity without significantly changing osmolarity are present in large amounts (eg, glucose, protein, contrast dye).

Although poor urine output (eg, <400 mL of urine/24 h) may reflect hypovolemia or impending "prerenal" renal failure, the majority of renal failure episodes develop in the presence of normal urine output.[6] The kidney's typical response to hypovolemia is to retain solute; this produces concentrated urine with a low-sodium content (<20 mEq/L) through fluid and electrolyte retention. In contrast, if renal injury has impaired concentrating ability, urine will approach plasma osmolarity (isosthenuria) and have a higher-sodium content (>40 mEq/L). Calculation of *fractional excretion of sodium* (FE_{Na}) evaluates the kidneys' ability to retain electrolytes by comparing sodium and creatinine excretion from a spot sample of urine and blood; this test can be useful to distinguish hypovolemia and renal injury:

$$FE_{Na} = U_{Na}/P_{Na} \times P_{Cr}/U_{Cr} \times 100$$

where U_{Na} = urine sodium, P_{Na} = plasma sodium, U_{Cr} = urine creatinine, and P_{Cr} = plasma creatinine.

FE_{Na} values less than 1% imply that sodium is being normally conserved by the tubules, whereas values above 1% are consistent with acute tubular necrosis.

THE NORMAL KIDNEY IN SPECIAL CIRCUMSTANCES: MATURATION, AGING, AND PREGNANCY

For additional discussion see Chapters 20 through 23.

THE IMMATURE KIDNEY

Amniotic fluid (fetal urine) through the third trimester amounts to about a cup every hour. At birth, much of the anatomic kidney development has occurred, including growth of approximately 1 million nephrons per kidney. However, nephrons continue to increase in size and steadily gain function, with some activities fully developed a few weeks after birth (eg, urine acidification) but others only attaining adult levels between 1 and 3 years of age (eg, EVF, GFR, urea clearance, tubular excretion, concentrating capacity).[22] In preterm infants, renal maturation relates to conceptual age, with normal kidney function expected but sometimes delayed. Children undergoing heart surgery are vulnerable to postoperative renal dysfunction relative to adults, and renal failure after surgery that requires dialysis carries a particularly grave prognosis.[23]

THE KIDNEY DURING PREGNANCY

Progesterone and relaxin, hormones secreted by the corpus luteum, are believed to mediate most of the renal effects of pregnancy. Rates of EVF, GFR, and clearance of nitrogenous waste rise early in pregnancy and are 50% to 60% increased at term, making typical serum creatinine and urea values 40% lower for pregnant patients (and levels usually considered normal concerningly high). Saturation of tubular uptake mechanisms with increased tubular flow may contribute to some of the aminoaciduria, proteinuria, and glycosuria that are common during pregnancy. Other renally mediated alterations include mild hyponatremia and mild alkalemia with bicarbonate and carbon dioxide tension (P_{CO_2}) values 4 mEq/L and 10 mm Hg below normal, respectively. Maternal blood volume is doubled by 7 months, and at term the pregnant mother is 7.5 L of water and 900 mmol of sodium net positive. Preterm labor can be precipitated by dehydration and sometimes halted by rehydration. The combination of hormonal factors and functional obstruction of the ureters between the pelvic rim and gravid uterus contribute to dilation of all renal collecting structures observed from the first trimester to 3 to 4 months after delivery. The major practical concern of the resulting urine stasis is increased risk for urinary tract infection.

THE AGING KIDNEY

An approximately parallel progressive decline of all renal functions with age starts at approximately 30 to 40 years of age, including EVF, GFR, tubular active transport, urine concentration, dilution, and acidification.[24] In addition, decreased thirst and impaired hormonal functioning of the renin–angiotensin system, vitamin D metabolism, and antidiuretic hormone response are also associated with aging. Creatinine clearance and production of creatinine from muscle decrease at approximately the same rate (1% per year); hence, curiously, serum creatinine values typically do not change with age (Table 14-1).[25,26] However, by the eighth decade, GFR is reduced by one-third to one-half.[27] Practical consequences of these changes include reduced renal reserve to deal with extreme challenges of any kind to the internal environment and changes in the pharmacokinetics of drugs that are cleared by the kidneys. Toxicity of renally excreted drugs is common, and dosage decisions in the elderly should include careful consideration of kidney function. In addition, the aging kidney is more likely to be subject to potentially harmful processes, including chronic illness (eg, hypertension, diabetes, atherosclerosis) and toxic effects (eg, nonsteroidal anti-inflammatory drugs, antibiotics, diuretics).[28]

ACID–BASE, FLUID, AND ELECTROLYTE DISORDERS

For additional discussion see Chapter 43.

Preoperative awareness of kidney-mediated acid–base, electrolyte, and/or fluid disorders can significantly influence selection of intravenous fluids and choice of anesthetic agents and may occasionally require the anesthesiologist to recommend that surgery be delayed to correct abnormalities; therefore, review of these conditions is presented next.

SODIUM DISORDERS

Sodium is the principal electrolyte of the extracellular environment, and derangements of this cation primarily affect normal functioning of excitable cells, including nerve and muscle tissue. Normal serum values are regulated by the kidney between 135 and 145 mmol/L, but test values may be falsely lowered as a result of hyperglycemia, hyperproteinemia, or hyperlipidemia; low serum osmolality will differentiate true hyponatremia from pseudohyponatremia.

Hyponatremia Hyponatremia is the most common electrolyte disorder.[29,30] Symptoms rarely occur unless sodium values are less than 125 mmol/L, and these include a spectrum ranging from anorexia, nausea, and lethargy to convulsions, arrhythmias, coma, and even death from osmotic brain swelling.[31-33] Notably, hyponatremia symptoms resemble those of local anesthetic toxicity, presumably due to similar effects on intracellular sodium levels. Notably, excessively rapid correction of chronic hyponatremia can also produce severe neurologic complications (central pontine myelinolysis) and death.[34] Hyponatremia may occur in the setting of an expanded, normal, or contracted extracellular fluid volume (**Table 14-2**). Volume status and urine sodium concentration are key markers to differentiate the numerous causes of hyponatremia. Dilute urine (sodium >20 mmol/L) suggests water excess, whereas avid sodium conservation (urine sodium <20 mmol/L) accompanies isolated sodium loss.

If hyponatremia is acute, the risk of neurologic complications is high, and treatment may be indicated to prevent cerebral edema and seizures. This should be accomplished with cautious administration of intravenous hypertonic saline and furosemide to enhance water excretion and prevent sodium overload. More conservative management such as water restriction is usually appropriate for chronic hyponatremia, unless the patient is symptomatic.

Hypernatremia Hypernatremia (serum sodium > 145 mmol/L) is generally related to sodium gain or water loss and, most commonly, from a negative water balance, such as occurs when respiratory, sweating, or urinary losses are not replaced. Febrile infants have immature kidneys and, with a high surface area to body mass ratio, are particularly at risk for water losses. Dehydration of brain cells leads to symptoms ranging from confusion to convulsions and coma.

In evaluating the hypernatremic patient, studies often indicate hemoconcentration (high hematocrit and protein levels) and evidence of prerenal failure (elevated BUN and serum creatinine). Urine is usually hyperosmolar (>1000 mOsm) and low in volume (<500 mL/d) and sodium concentration. Occasionally, the urine is not concentrated, suggesting causes such as osmotic diuresis or an intrinsic renal disorder (eg, nephrogenic diabetes insipidus). A primary goal of treatment is restoration of serum tonicity; usually, this is achieved with isotonic or hypotonic parenteral fluids and/or diuretics unless irreversible AKI has required dialysis.

METABOLIC ACID–BASE DISORDERS

The balance between plasma bicarbonate (HCO_3^-) concentration and $P{CO_2}$ in the extracellular space is the primary factor that predicts serum pH. Acid–base homeostasis involves the tight regulation of HCO_3^- and $P{CO_2}$. Extracellular pH derangements due to primary abnormalities in renal bicarbonate reabsorption and proton (H^+) elimination cause most metabolic acidosis or alkalosis, whereas factors affecting respiratory drive affect $P{CO_2}$ tension, leading to respiratory acidosis or alkalosis (**Fig. 14-3**). Because patients presenting with 2 or more coexisting acid–base disorders are common in the perioperative and critically ill setting, an approach to both "pure" and "mixed" acid–base disorders is presented next.

TABLE 14-2 Causes of Hyponatremia

Volume Status	Cause
Hypovolemic	Edema due to burns Sweating Hemorrhage Peritonitis Diuretics GI loss • Vomiting • Diarrhea • Pancreatitis
Euvolemic	SIADH Pseudohyponatremia • Hyperglycemia • Hyperlipidemia • Hyperproteinemia
Hypervolemic	Cirrhosis TURP syndrome CHF Nephrotic syndrome Primary polydipsia Dilute infant formula Hyperthyroidism Glucocorticoid deficiency

CHF, congestive heart failure; GI, gastrointestinal; SIADH, syndrome of inappropriate antidiuretic hormone; TURP, transurethral resection of the prostate.

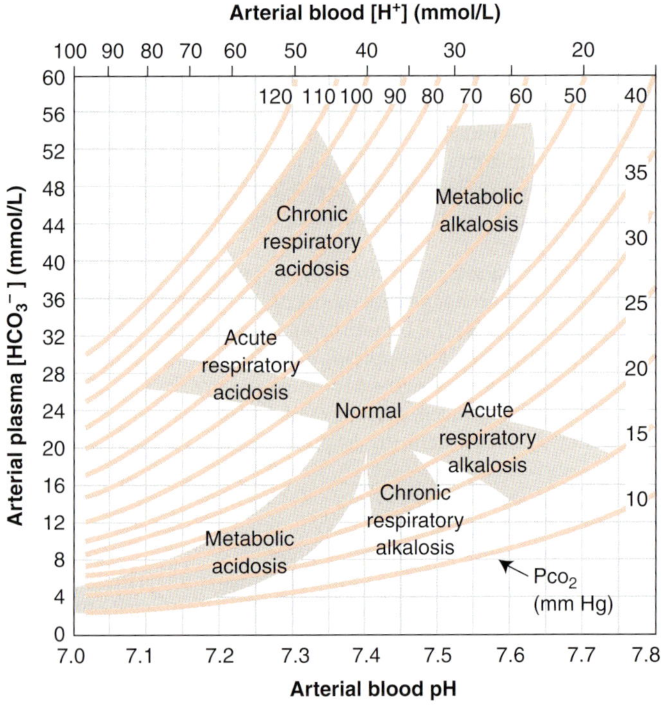

FIGURE 14-3. Acid–base map. Plotting plasma HCO_3^- (from the serum chemistry panel) against the $P{CO_2}$ and H^+ (from the ABG) will fall in the shaded areas in a simple acid–base disorder. Should a mixed disorder exist, the values may fall in the non-shaded areas. [From DuBose TD, Jr. Acid-base disorders. In: Brenner BM, ed. *Brenner and Rector's The Kidney.* 7th ed. Philadelphia, PA: Saunders; 2004:938.]

Metabolic Acidosis Accumulation of nonvolatile acid is the basis for metabolic acidosis and can result from numerous causes. A key tool to differentiate the source of metabolic acidosis is the anion gap (AG; AG = $[Na^+] - ([HCO_3^-] + [Cl^-])$). As calculated from serum electrolyte values, the AG reflects unmeasured anions and differentiates metabolic acidoses into normal AG (8 ± 4) and increased AG types (>16 mmol/L). Normal AG metabolic acidosis is always associated with high chloride levels (*hyperchloremic metabolic acidosis*) and most commonly results from renal or gastrointestinal bicarbonate loss or excess sodium chloride infusion. In contrast, increased AG metabolic acidosis is caused by raised levels of other negatively charged ions (eg, lactate, salicylate). A usual response to all types of metabolic acidosis is compensatory hyperventilation, which partially corrects pH toward normal. *Winter's formula* predicts the Pco_2 response to a metabolic acidosis as follows:

$$Pco_2 = (1.5 \times [HCO_3^-]) + 8 \pm 2$$

Metabolic Alkalosis Metabolic alkalosis is almost always due to an increase in extracellular HCO_3^- related to net loss of H^+ and/or HCO_3^- addition. This disorder is very common, being noted in 51% of patients with an acid–base abnormality in one analysis of more than 13 000 arterial blood gas samples.[35] The biggest single cause is gastrointestinal acid loss due to vomiting or nasogastric suctioning, with any related hypovolemia also contributing through renal retention of HCO_3^-. Diuretics are another common cause of metabolic alkalosis. Thiazides (eg, hydrochlorothiazide) and loop diuretics (eg, furosemide) induce a net loss of chloride and free water, without altering bicarbonate excretion, and can cause a volume "contraction" alkalosis. When metabolic alkalosis is persistent, it usually reflects an inability of the kidney to excrete HCO_3^-. Rare inherited renal causes of metabolic alkalosis exist (eg, Bartter syndrome). A typical response to all types of metabolic alkalosis is hypoventilation and a pH correction toward normal.

RESPIRATORY ACID–BASE DISORDERS

Respiratory Acidosis Respiratory acidosis results from failure to adequately eliminate CO_2. Arterial blood gas values reflect abnormally high Pco_2 levels but can also be used to differentiate acute from chronic conditions. Over several days a renal response mounts to chronic hypoventilation, involving HCO_3^- generation and excretion of acids (eg, ammonium). Thus with *acute respiratory acidosis*, blood gas analysis reveals a normal HCO_3^- level, whereas an increased HCO_3^- level is characteristic of longstanding *chronic respiratory acidosis* with renal compensation. Often the cause(s) of acute respiratory acidosis is obvious from a bedside history and physical examination. For example, in a postoperative patient, respiratory depression from opioid analgesia and residual anesthetic effects may combine with inadequate neuromuscular blockade reversal, acute bronchospasm, or pulmonary edema. In contrast, potential causes of chronic respiratory acidosis include obesity, restrictive and obstructive lung disease, and neuromuscular disease (eg, myasthenia gravis, Guillain-Barré syndrome).

Respiratory Alkalosis Respiratory alkalosis results from excess ventilation. As with respiratory acidosis, blood gas analysis is useful to separate acute from chronic forms. Acute Pco_2 decreases are not associated with the compensatory decreases in plasma HCO_3^- seen with *chronic respiratory alkalosis*. Although pain and anxiety are obvious sources of *acute respiratory alkalosis*, there are many other sources of abnormal respiratory drive that can be acute or chronic, including stimulants and toxins (eg, salicylate, caffeine, nicotine, progesterone), central nervous system abnormalities (eg, anxiety, stroke, increased intracranial pressure), pulmonary abnormalities (eg, pulmonary embolus, pneumonia), mechanical hyperventilation, and systemic conditions such as liver failure and sepsis.

Mixed Acid–Base Disorders The Henderson-Hasselbalch equation ($pH = pK \times \log([HCO_3^-]/(0.03 \times Pco_2))$) predicts that as long as a normal ratio exists between HCO_3^- and $Paco_2$, blood pH will be normal. Combined metabolic and respiratory derangements are common in the perioperative setting, and although a single patient may be suffering from numerous acid–base abnormalities and a state far from normal, the net effect may result in a "normal" blood pH. Hence a superficial preoperative assessment of acid–base status may be inadequate, particularly in the critically ill patient.

A general approach to the diagnosis of mixed acid–base disorder requires a stepwise logical approach that begins with a focused history and physical examination. An arterial blood gas and a simultaneously obtained chemistry panel, which includes Na^+, K^+, Cl^-, and total CO_2 concentrations, should also be obtained, and use of an acid–base map will differentiate simple from mixed disorders (Fig. 14-3).

POTASSIUM DISORDERS

Nearly 98% of all potassium (50 mEq/kg) is intracellular. Although long-term body potassium regulation occurs through renal and gastrointestinal mechanisms, short-term shifts between intra- and extracellular compartments mediated by effects such as hyperventilation, acidosis, insulin, or β_2-adrenergic receptor stimulation can produce dramatic changes in circulating levels. Acute shifts are important because even minor potassium excursions have major effects on serum levels and can lead to symptomatic skeletal muscle weakness, gastrointestinal ileus, rhabdomyolysis, myocardial depression, malignant ventricular arrhythmias, and even sudden death. Dietary potassium approximates 100 mEq/d and is normally balanced by renal (90%-95%) and gut (5%-10%) excretions that maintain extracellular levels between 3.5 and 4.4 mEq/L. In the kidney, 70% of filtered potassium is reabsorbed by the proximal tubule and 15% to 20% by the loop of Henle. Fine tuning of potassium homeostasis can also occur through potassium excretion by the collecting duct under the influence of aldosterone. Renal potassium secretion is influenced by factors such as distal tubule flow rate and acid–base balance. Increased distal tubule flow augments, whereas metabolic and respiratory acidosis attenuates tubular potassium secretion. Metabolic alkalosis has the opposite effect.

Hypokalemia Interpreting serum potassium levels is challenging. Hypokalemia can reflect normal body potassium with an acute intracellular shift or true net deficiency. Equally confusing are conditions such as diabetic ketoacidosis, which are notorious for presenting normal extracellular potassium levels in the setting of net body depletion. In addition to extra- to intracellular potassium shifts as outlined earlier, causes of hypokalemia can be grouped as due to extrarenal loss (eg, vomiting, diarrhea), renal loss (impaired processing due to drugs, hormones, or inherited renal abnormalities), and rarely inadequate intake. Clinical manifestations of hypokalemia include electrocardiogram (ECG) changes (flattened T waves, U waves, proarrhythmic state) and skeletal muscle weakness. Because hypokalemia interferes with the concentrating ability of the kidney, nephrogenic diabetes insipidus may also result. Hypokalemia treatment involves supplementation with intravenous or oral potassium; however, overly rapid intravenous administration of potassium should be strictly avoided due to the potential for lethal arrhythmias.

Hyperkalemia Because a long-standing elevated potassium level is better tolerated than an acute serum elevation, a duration estimate should always accompany the diagnosis of hyperkalemia (>4.4 mEq/L). Beyond laboratory artifact (eg, hemolyzed sample), causes of hyperkalemia group by abnormalities of renal excretion, release from cells, or distribution between intra- and extracellular spaces (**Table 14-3**). Hyperkalemic electrocardiographic changes are well displayed in cardiac surgery procedures when high-potassium cardioplegia is infused immediately after aortic crossclamp application; these include peaked T waves, shortened QT interval, and ST-segment depression with mild elevations, widened QRS complex, increased PR interval, and decreased P-wave amplitude with moderate and absent P waves, sine wave QRS, ventricular fibrillation, and asystole with severe hyperkalemia. Several drugs have acute

TABLE 14-3 Causes of Hyperkalemia

Pseudohyperkalemia	Hemolysis Leukocytosis Thrombocytopenia
Decreased renal potassium excretion	Acute or chronic kidney failure Aldosterone deficiency Diabetic nephropathy Adrenal insufficiency Drugs (eg, potassium-sparing diuretics, some antibiotics, spironolactone, β-blockers) Intrinsic kidney disease
Abnormal potassium distribution	Insulin deficiency Metabolic or respiratory acidosis
Abnormal potassium release from cells	Rhabdomyolysis Tumor lysis syndrome

Adapted from Greenberg A, ed. *Primer on Kidney Diseases.* 4th ed. Philadelphia, PA: Elsevier Saunders; 2005.

effects on potassium levels; in some settings (eg, denervation, insulin therapy), succinylcholine, β-blockers, and certain antibiotics can cause symptomatic hyperkalemia. Fortunately, several interventions are available to counteract symptomatic hyperkalemia by blocking its effects or shifting potassium back into the intracellular space (**Fig. 14-4**).

CALCIUM, MAGNESIUM, AND PHOSPHORUS DISORDERS

Adults contain 1 to 2 kg of calcium. Most calcium is in bone (98%); the remaining 2% exists in either ionized, chelated, or protein-bound forms. Normal serum calcium values range between 8.5 and 10.2 mg/dL, but only the ionized fraction (50%) is biologically active and precisely regulated. Hypocalcemia related to reduced serum protein levels (eg, hypoalbuminemia) is physiologically unimportant. Ionized extracellular calcium concentration (iCa^{++}) is controlled by the combined actions of parathyroid hormone (PTH), calcitonin, and vitamin D and further modulated by dietary and environmental factors. Extracellular magnesium represents only 0.3% of total stores, making normal serum levels (1.6-2.2 mg/dL) a poor reflection of total body (mainly intracellular) magnesium, much as outlined earlier for potassium. Magnesium is an essential cofactor in adenosine triphosphate (ATP) reactions, DNA replication and transcription, and translation of mRNA, and deficits can adversely effect energy production and protein metabolism. Phosphorus is a major intracellular anion involved in regulation of glycolysis, ammoniagenesis, and calcium homeostasis, but is also essential for ATP and red blood cell 2,3-diphosphoglyceric acid synthesis.

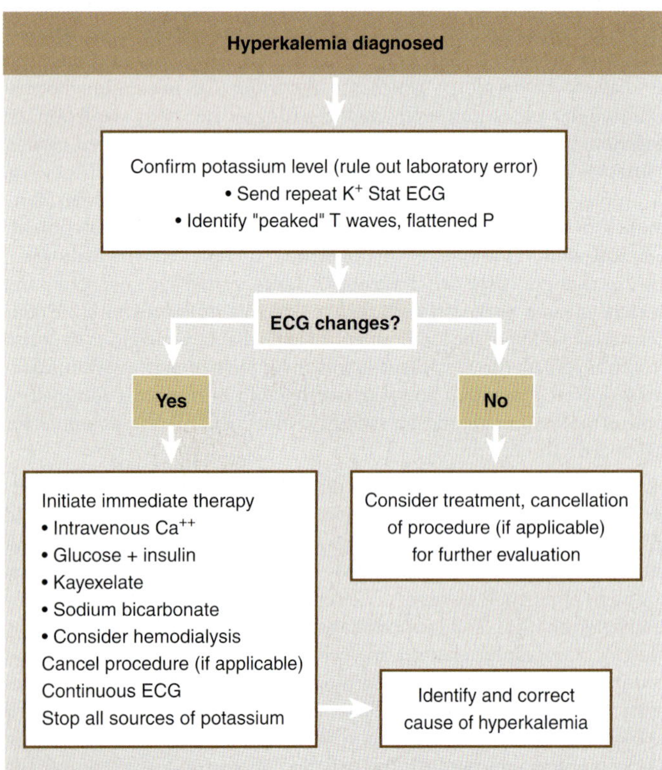

FIGURE 14-4. Treatment algorithm of hyperkalemia.

Hypocalcemia Hypocalcemia symptoms are mainly neurologic and muscular, including cramping, numbness in the digits, laryngeal spasm, carpopedal spasm, bronchospasm, seizures, and even respiratory arrest. Mental status changes including irritability, depression, and impaired cognition may also occur. A positive *Chvostek sign* (facial muscle twitching in response to tapping the facial nerve) and/or *Trousseau sign* (carpal spasm induced by brachial artery occlusion) are classic but often absent. Cardiac manifestations include prolonged QT interval and arrhythmias. Dry skin, coarse hair, alopecia, brittle nails, and evidence of basal ganglia and cerebral cortex calcifications may develop with long-standing hypocalcemia.

Hypocalcemia can be caused by several conditions (**Table 14-4**), including abnormalities of vitamin D or PTH physiology (abnormal hormone secretion, activity, or bone responsiveness) or calcium sequestration. With transfusion, when liver-mediated citrate clearance is unavailable (the anhepatic phase of liver transplantation) or overwhelmed (massive or rapid transfusion), citrate toxicity can cause significant hypocalcemia, clinically manifest as acute hypotension.[36] Although unresponsive to standard vasopressors, hypotension due to acute citrate toxicity quickly responds to 1 to 3 g of calcium gluconate or chloride given intravenously. Citrate for regional anticoagulation with dialysis can also cause hypocalcemia and hypomagnesemia from long-term decreased PTH secretion. The most common source of acquired hypoparathyroidism is deliberate or inadvertent parathyroidectomy during neck surgery.[37] Other explanations for chronic hypocalcemia include hypomagnesemia, renal failure, vitamin D deficiency, and other causes for hypoparathyroidism. Overzealous use of medications to address hypercalcemia (eg, bisphosphonates, mithramycin, and calcitonin) is an obvious source of hypocalcemia. Other drugs associated with hypocalcemia include pentamidine, ketoconazole, asparaginase, cisplatin, and doxorubicin. Oral calcium supplementation is usually sufficient treatment for chronic conditions.

Hypercalcemia Symptomatic hypercalcemia reflects elevation of the ionized fraction of serum calcium. Clinical symptoms correlate with the

TABLE 14-4 Common Causes of Hypocalcemia

Hypoparathyroidism	Altered Ca^{++}/parathyroid hormone set point (calcium receptor mutations) Parathyroid hormone gene defects Post-parathyroidectomy Neck irradiation Infiltrative disease Hypomagnesemia/hypermagnesemia Autoimmune disease
Parathyroid hormone resistance	Hypomagnesemia Pseudohypoparathyroidism Pseudo-pseudohypoparathyroidism
Other	Vitamin D deficiency Altered vitamin D metabolism Drug induced Acute citrate toxicity

acuity of hypercalcemia and include constipation, nausea and vomiting, drowsiness, lethargy, weakness, stupor, and coma. Cardiovascular manifestations include hypertension, shortened QT interval, heart block, and other arrhythmias. Hypercalcemia can also cause polyuria and polydipsia due to its effect on vasopressin-mediated water reabsorption; kidney stones are common. The most frequent causes of hypercalcemia are primary hyperparathyroidism and malignancy. Other causes include thiazide (increase renal calcium reabsorption) or lithium (inhibits PTH release) drug usage and rarer medical conditions, including granulomatous disease, thyrotoxicosis, and multiple endocrine neoplasia types I and II.

Although hypercalcemia is usually chronic and treatment involves addressing the underlying cause, occasionally acute severe hypercalcemia (or acute worsening of chronic hypercalcemia) may require prompt intervention. Because hypercalcemic patients are often volume depleted, intravenous saline can both rehydrate and induce calcium diuresis.[38] Loop diuretics (eg, furosemide) inhibit renal calcium reabsorption and can expedite treatment. In addition, drugs such as bisphosphonates (etidronate pamidronate, clodronate), gallium, and plicamycin (mithramycin) can lower serum calcium concentrations by impairing or inhibiting osteoclast function. In severely hypercalcemic patients, dialysis may be required.

Hypermagnesemia Clinical manifestations of hypermagnesemia (>4-6 mg/dL) are serious and potentially fatal. Minor symptoms include hypotension, nausea, vomiting, facial flushing, urinary retention, and ileus. In more extreme cases, flaccid skeletal muscular paralysis, hyporeflexia, bradycardia and bradyarrhythmias, respiratory depression, coma, and cardiac arrest may occur.

Hypermagnesemia generally occurs in 2 clinical settings: compromised renal function (GFR < 20 mL/min) and excessive magnesium intake (eg, excessive intravenous therapy in preeclamptic patients or oral magnesium containing antacids and cathartics). An abnormally low (or even negative) serum AG may be a clue to hypermagnesemia.[39] Although mild hypermagnesemia in the setting of normal renal function can be treated with supportive care and withdrawal of the cause, in some cases dialysis is necessary.

Hypomagnesemia Although low serum magnesium levels (<1.6 mg/dL) may be asymptomatic, clinically important problems may manifest, including neuromuscular (muscle cramps and weakness, positive Chvostek and Trousseau signs), cardiac (torsades de pointes and other arrhythmias), neurologic (apathy, seizures), and related electrolytic (hypokalemia and hypocalcemia) abnormalities. Causes of hypomagnesemia can be divided into 4 broad categories: decreased intake, gastrointestinal loss, renal loss, and redistribution. Many drugs (eg, loop and thiazide diuretics, cisplatin, aminoglycosides, amphotericin, cyclosporine) induce renal magnesium wasting (24-hour urine magnesium excretion >24 mg in the face of hypomagnesemia).[40] Nutritional deficiency can result from malabsorption syndromes, can occur in patients receiving parenteral nutrition, and is present in 25% of alcoholics.[41-43] Redistribution occurs with acute pancreatitis, administration of catecholamines, and "hungry bone syndrome" after parathyroidectomy.[44] Magnesium can be supplemented orally or via the parenteral route. More than half of hypomagnesemic patients are also hypokalemic, and potassium deficits are usually refractory to repletion, unless magnesium also is supplemented.

Hypophosphatemia Hypophosphatemia has more clinical relevance than hyperphosphatemia to the perioperative physician because it can contribute to muscle weakness, respiratory failure, and even difficulty in weaning critically ill patients from mechanical ventilation when serum levels are less than 0.32 mmol/L. In addition, low phosphate levels may diminish oxygen delivery to tissues and rarely cause hemolysis. Hypophosphatemia can result from intracellular redistribution due to catecholamines, or an anabolic state, inadequate intake, or absorption secondary to alcoholism or malnutrition or increased renal or gastrointestinal losses.[45] Hypophosphatemia is common in alcoholic and poorly controlled diabetic patients, in whom increased urine phosphate excretion can occur. Intravenous and oral supplementation can be used to treat hypophosphatemia.

Hyperphosphatemia Clinical manifestations of hyperphosphatemia (>5 mg/dL) are generally related to the hypocalcemia that often accompanies this disorder, although increased phosphorus levels may also lead to calcium precipitation and decreased intestinal calcium absorption.[46,47] Significantly elevated serum phosphate levels are most commonly due to reduced excretion from renal insufficiency (GFR <25 mL/min) but can also result from excess intake or redistribution of intracellular phosphorus. Treatment of chronic hyperphosphatemia includes dietary phosphate restriction and oral phosphate binders.

DIURETICS AND EDEMA

Fluid overload occurs when salt or water intake exceeds combined renal and extrarenal losses and is generally characterized by increased total body water and sodium. Fluid overload may be evenly distributed among the body compartments (eg, congestive heart failure [CHF]) or unevenly weighted toward the interstitial space, whereas the circulating blood volume may be normal or even decreased (eg, post-traumatic or post-operative increased vascular permeability). Pulmonary edema is a life-threatening complication of fluid overload. Edema results when Starling forces, which regulate fluid transfer between capillaries and interstitium, favor passage of fluid into the interstitial space. A variety of chronic medical conditions (CHF, renal failure, or hepatic cirrhosis) can lead to fluid overload and edema that may even require surgery to be delayed for treatment to reduce operative risk. The first line of therapy for fluid overload that includes all body compartments involves restriction of salt and water ingestion; however, diuretic therapy is often indicated.

Physiologic Basis of Diuretic Action The different classes of diuretic agents have numerous effects that are important for the perioperative physician to consider that extend beyond the common ability of these drugs to increase urine flow. Diuretics are grouped according to their site and mechanism of action (**Fig. 14-5**). Under normal conditions, kidney function ensures that less than 1% of filtered Na^+ load enters the urine (ie, fractional excretion of Na^+ [FE_{Na}] is < 1%) . The Na^+–K^+ ATPase pump on the basolateral surface (blood side) of renal tubular

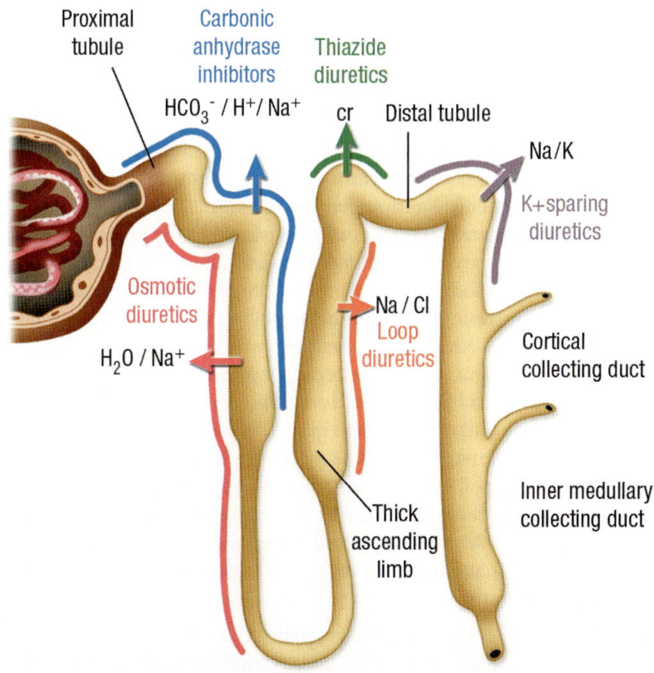

FIGURE 14-5. Site of action of commonly available diuretics.

cells is primarily responsible for active pumping of Na^+ out of cells into blood in exchange for K^+. This pump causes net movement of positive charges out of the cell (2 K^+ in, for every 3 Na^+ out), creating an electrochemical gradient that also causes Na^+ to enter the luminal (urine) side of the cell. Renal tubular cells in different portions of the nephron have different luminal "systems" to allow this Na^+ influx. These systems are the sites of action where the different diuretics work.

Proximal Tubule Diuretics In the proximal tubule, a specialized luminal transporter exchanges protons (H^+) for sodium ions; the result is sodium reabsorption and acidification of the urine. The excreted H^+ combines with bicarbonate HCO_3^- in the tubule to form carbonic acid:

$$H^+ + HCO_3^- \rightarrow H_2CO_3$$

Carbonic acid converts to water (H_2O) and carbon dioxide (CO_2) in a reaction catalyzed by *carbonic anhydrase*:

$$H_2CO_3 \rightarrow H_2O + CO_2$$

The same enzyme, carbonic anhydrase, allows this reaction to occur in reverse within tubular cells, converting H_2CO_3 to HCO_3^- and H^+, generating more H^+ for countertransport with Na^+ and releasing bicarbonate that passes into the circulation.

Carbonic anhydrase inhibitors are drugs that inhibit this enzyme; the net effect of these agents is that sodium and bicarbonate, which would otherwise have been reabsorbed, remain in the urine, resulting in an alkaline diuresis.

Although patients may develop metabolic acidosis when taking these agents, interestingly, compensatory processes in the tubule accommodate to the effects of carbonic anhydrase inhibitors so that their long-term use rarely causes this problem. However, these agents can be useful, for example, with contraction alkalosis from aggressive diuresis with loop diuretics (discussed later); administration of these agents can reduce $Pa{CO_2}$ and improve $Pa{O_2}$ for these patients with little change in blood pH. Specific use for carbonic anhydrase inhibitors includes the treatment of mountain sickness and open-angle glaucoma and to increase respiratory drive in patients with central sleep apnea.[48,49]

Osmotic Diuretics Substances such as mannitol that are freely filtered at the glomerulus but poorly reabsorbed by the renal tubule will cause an osmotic diuresis. In the water-permeable segments of the proximal tubule and loop of Henle, fluid reabsorption occurs, and filtered mannitol is concentrated. Eventually, oncotic pressure in the tubular fluid resists further fluid reabsorption. Mannitol also draws water from cells into the plasma and effectively increases renal blood flow (RBF).

Mannitol has been widely used, especially for the prophylaxis of acute renal failure (ARF). In select patient populations, such as cadaveric kidney transplant recipients, it has been found to be effective.[50] However, in a controlled trial of mannitol prophylaxis in patients with mild chronic renal failure, it was less effective than hydration alone in contrast-associated nephropathy.[51] This trial has reduced enthusiasm for the prophylactic use of mannitol. Although animal studies showed initial promise, apart from ARF prophylaxis in kidney transplantation, there is no clear evidence that mannitol is effective in prevention or treatment of ARF.[52] However, as a therapy for cerebral edema, mannitol therapy is more effective than loop diuretics or hypertonic saline in reducing brain water content.[53]

As mannitol shifts water between fluid compartments, there are effects on plasma and intracellular electrolyte concentrations, including hyponatremia and hypochloremia and intracellular increases in K^+ and H^+. Patients with normal renal function quickly correct these changes, but patients with renal impairment may develop significant circulatory overload with hemodilution and pulmonary edema, hyperkalemic metabolic acidosis, central nervous system depression, and even severe hyponatremia requiring urgent hemodialysis.[54]

Loop Diuretics The electrochemical gradient established by the Na^+–K^+ ATPase in the loop of Henle drives the electroneutral transport of 1 Na^+, 1K^+, and 2 Cl^- ions into the tubule cells from the tubular fluid. Because the thick ascending segment of the loop of Henle is water-impermeable, reabsorption of solute concentrates the interstitium and dilutes the tubule fluid. Loop diuretics, such as furosemide, bumetanide, and torsemide, directly inhibit the electroneutral transporter preventing salt reabsorption from occurring. Because 25% of filtered NaCl is normally reabsorbed in the loop of Henle, loop diuretics cause a large salt load to pass to the distal convoluted tubule beyond the extra reserve of this segment to reabsorb; consequently, large volumes of dilute urine ensue. Other effects of loop diuretics include a weak inhibition of carbonic anhydrase (see earlier discussion) and an increase in the fractional excretion of Ca^{++}.

Interestingly, hormones that stimulate cyclic adenosine monophosphate, such as arginine vasopressin, enhance salt reabsorption by the thick ascending limb of the loop of Henle, making the effect of loop diuretics all the more impressive. Conversely, substances that stimulate cyclic guanosine monophosphate, such as nitric oxide and atrial natriuretic peptide, inhibit thick ascending limb reabsorption and attenuate loop diuretic responsiveness.[55,56]

Loop diuretics are a first-line therapeutic modality for acute treatment of CHF. Although diuretics have no proven mortality benefit, they reduce left ventricular filling pressures and effectively relieve symptoms of congestion, pulmonary edema, extremity swelling, and hepatic congestion.

Adverse loop diuretic effects include hypokalemia, hyponatremia, and acute renal dysfunction. Heart failure patients with atrial fibrillation may also be prescribed digitalis, which, in combination with furosemide, can lead to hypokalemia-induced arrhythmias. Loop diuretics, especially furosemide, may cause ototoxicity, particularly in patients with renal insufficiency.[57]

Distal Convoluted Tubule Diuretics Distal convoluted tubule diuretics, such as thiazides (eg, hydrochlorothiazide) and metolazone, act in the earliest part of this segment to block the NaCl cotransport mechanism across apical plasma membranes. Because the distal tubule is relatively water impermeable, NaCl absorption causes urinary dilution. Distal tubule diuretics also increase magnesium excretion, but, unlike loop diuretics, they inhibit calcium excretion.

Clinically, distal convoluted tubule diuretics are used for the treatment of hypertension (often as sole therapy), volume overload disorders, and to relieve the symptoms of edema in pregnancy.

Adverse reactions associated with distal tubule diuretics include electrolyte disturbances and volume depletion. Hydrochlorothiazide specifically has been associated with a number of other side effects, including pancreatitis, jaundice, diarrhea, aplastic anemia, and anaphylaxis.

Distal (Collecting Duct) Acting Diuretics Unlike in more proximal nephron segments, NaCl absorption in the collecting duct cells (also called principal cells) is electrogenic. That is, a net electrical gradient is maintained both by the Na^+–K^+ ATPase Na^+ ion channels and in the luminal membranes. As a result, the tubule lumen is negatively charged with respect to the blood. This normally causes K^+ secretion into the tubular lumen through K^+-specific ion channels. Distal K^+-sparing diuretics (eg, amiloride and triamterene) directly inhibit luminal Na^+ entry, blocking this mechanism, and resulting in a K^+ "sparing" effect. In addition, H^+ secretion is inhibited.

A second class of distal-acting K^+-sparing diuretics comprises the competitive aldosterone antagonists (eg, spironolactone and eplerenone). Ordinarily, the mineralocorticoid hormone aldosterone is released in response to angiotensin II or hyperkalemia. Aldosterone normally stimulates Na^+ reabsorption and K^+ excretion by the collecting duct. Inhibition of the aldosterone effect by these drugs causes a mild natruresis and K^+ retention. Distal K^+-sparing agents are used primarily for K^+-sparing diuresis (eg, in patients with volume overload receiving digitalis or with hypokalemic alkalosis). In addition, these drugs are especially useful in treating disorders involving secondary hyperaldosteronism, such as cirrhosis with ascites. Spironolactone treatment has been shown to improve survival with volume overload and left ventricular dysfunction or heart failure.[58]

Hyperkalemia and hyperkalemic hyperchloremic metabolic acidosis are significant complications of the injudicious use of spironolactone, triamterene, or amiloride. Metabolic acidosis itself can further contribute to hyperkalemia. These effects are dose-dependent, and the risk of their occurrence increases considerably with renal failure or therapy with K^+ supplements, angiotensin-converting enzyme inhibitors, angiotensin receptor blockers, β-blockers, heparin, or ketoconazole.[59] In addition, amiloride and triamterene accumulate with renal failure, and triamterene also accumulates with liver impairment.[60,61] Spironolactone can cause gastrointestinal distress and antiandrogenic effects (eg, impotence, loss of libido, gynecomastia). Gynecomastia is dose-related.[62]

Other Diuretics

Dopaminergic Agonists Intravenous low-dose infusion of dopamine (1-3 μg/kg/min) is natriuretic owing primarily to a modest increase in the GFR and reduction in proximal Na^+ reabsorption mediated by dopamine type 1 receptors.[63] At higher doses, the pressor response to dopamine, mediated through adrenergic receptors, is beneficial in patients with hypotension but appears to have little or no renal effect in critically ill or septic patients.[63,64] Fenoldopam is more selective than dopamine for the dopamine type 1 receptor with little cardiac stimulation. So-called renal-dose dopamine for the treatment of ARF, although advocated, has not been demonstrated to have significant renoprotective properties in numerous studies[65-67] and can cause worsened splanchnic oxygenation, impaired gastrointestinal function, impaired endocrine and immunologic system function, blunting of ventilatory drive, and increased risk of post–cardiac surgery atrial fibrillation.[68-70]

RENAL DISORDERS ENCOUNTERED IN THE PERIOPERATIVE PATIENT

Acquired disorders of the nephron can be classified by their selective involvement of the glomerulus, the tubule, or both and may reflect localized or systemic disease. Other considerations include inherited conditions and transplanted kidney physiology. These topics are extensively reviewed elsewhere,[20] but an abbreviated summary with focus on features important to the perioperative physician is presented here.

PRERENAL AZOTEMIA

Prerenal azotemia accounts for approximately 70% of hospital-acquired ARF.[71,72] Prerenal azotemia is a normal physiologic response to decreased renal perfusion that produces a hemodynamically mediated reduction in the GFR. No immediate injury occurs to the renal parenchyma, and GFR rapidly returns to normal with reversal of the hemodynamic insult. Overt pathologic changes can occur if the renal hypoperfusion is sustained. The decrease in glomerular ultrafiltration pressure can be secondary to an absolute decrease (eg, hemorrhage, dehydration) or effective decrease in arterial blood volume (eg, CHF, cirrhosis, capillary leak syndromes, sepsis). Progression of this prerenal state can lead to acute tubular necrosis (ATN). Prerenal azotemia and ischemic ATN reflect the spectrum of manifestations of renal hypoperfusion. The severity and duration of insult from prerenal azotemia dictate the likelihood of progression to ischemic tubular damage.

In hypoperfusion states, GFR is maintained by the interplay of several neurohumoral systems. The renin–angiotensin axis increases efferent arteriolar vasomotor tone, whereas afferent arteriolar tone decreases under the influence of nitric oxide, vasodilatory prostaglandins, and the kallikrein-kinin system. The sympathetic nervous system reacts to hypoperfusion with release of norepinephrine and antidiuretic hormone (ADH). With sustained reductions in renal perfusion, the ability of the kidney to maintain glomerular filtration is overwhelmed, and GFR declines, causing first azotemia and then tubular hypoxia with ischemic damage.

Nonsteroidal anti-inflammatory drugs (NSAIDs) can influence renal perfusion. These drugs can be grouped as nonselective inhibitors of both cyclooxygenase-1 (COX-1) and cylcooxygenase-2 (COX-2) or selective inhibitors of COX-2. Both drug classes cause inhibition of various prostaglandins and other substances, including some involved in the paracrine regulation of renal perfusion. Patients at greatest risk for NSAID-induced ARF include those with CHF, advanced liver disease, atherosclerotic vascular disease, or chronic kidney disease.[73,74] Caution should be observed in treating elderly patients with NSAIDs of any type. In a population-based study, the risk of ARF in the elderly increased by 58% with prescription NSAID use.[75] Nonselective NSAIDs inhibit the prostaglandins responsible for vasodilatation in the kidney and can promote prerenal azotemia in susceptible patients. Selective (COX-2) inhibitors cause similar renal vasoconstriction and have the similar consequences. One selective COX-2 inhibitor, rofecoxib, was found to have a higher incidence of renal toxicity than the nonselective inhibitors or celecoxib.[76] The renal toxicity of NSAIDs is increased when they are used in combination with other medications with the potential to alter the kidneys' ability to autoregulate glomerular filtration pressure, such as angiotensin-converting enzyme inhibitors and angiotensin receptor blockers. The renal vascular changes associated with NSAID use are typically reversible, although prolonged use can lead to permanent kidney damage. NSAIDs are also known to cause acute tubulointerstitial nephropathy (see Tubulointerstitial Nephropathies and Disorders of the Urinary Tract), in which case there is often a sudden change in GFR that may persist for days to weeks.

Much like the prostaglandin inhibitors, angiotensin-converting enzyme inhibitors and angiotensin receptor blockers increase the risk of ARF in patients on diuretic therapy; those with volume depletion, CHF, or diabetes; and in the elderly.[77,78] Angiotensin-converting enzyme inhibitors reduce blood pressure by inhibiting the proteolytic cleavage of angiotensin I to angiotensin II. Angiotensin receptor blockers occupy the angiotensin receptor. The renin–angiotensin system contributes to the autoregulation of glomerular perfusion pressure, and inhibition of this system has potential to induce prerenal azotemia. Angiotensin-converting enzyme inhibitors or angiotensin receptor blockers usage in conjunction with NSAIDs, cyclosporine, tacrolimus, and aprotinin may put patients at an even greater risk for ARF.[77,79,80] Furthermore, the incidence of ARF is also higher in patients with chronic kidney disease of any etiology. Patients with chronic kidney disease usually depend on local angiotensin II production to maintain GFR in the face of decreased functional renal mass.[78] Therefore, a 10% to 20% decline in GFR when these patients receive angiotensin-converting enzyme inhibitors is not unusual. More dramatic increases in serum creatinine suggest the presence of underlying renal vascular disease.

GLOMERULAR DISEASES

Glomerular diseases declare in numerous different ways (**Table 14-5**), but the commonest presentations are either as a nephritic or nephrotic syndrome. Nephritic syndrome involves a collection of renal signs and symptoms that predominantly reflect inadequate and/or ineffective glomerular filtration, including accumulation of nitrogenous waste products (azotemia), fluid retention, edema, hypertension, oliguria/anuria, proteinuria, and hematuria. In contrast, nephrotic syndrome

TABLE 14-5 The Spectrum of Clinical Disorders Involving Glomerular Disease

Asymptomatic proteinuria
Nephrotic syndrome
Asymptomatic microscopic hematuria
Recurrent gross hematuria
Acute nephritis
Focal or diffuse proliferative glomerulonephritis
Type I and type II membranoproliferative glomerulonephritis
Fibrillary glomerulonephritis
Rapidly progressive nephritis
Pulmonary-renal vasculitic syndrome
Anti-neutrophilic cytoplasmic antibodies vasculitis
Chronic kidney disease

involves signs and symptoms that predominantly reflect excessively porous filtration and "escape" of substances into the urine that are normally retained in the circulation, including significant proteinuria (>3 g/d/1.73 m^2), hypoproteinemia, edema, lipiduria, and hyperlipidemia. With nephrotic syndrome, characteristic oval fat bodies appear in the urine, and these may help guide diagnosis. The nature and severity of the presentation is determined by the underlying glomerular insult; a definitive diagnosis almost always requires a renal biopsy. The 2 commonest primary diseases causing nephrotic syndrome are minimal change glomerulopathy and membranous glomerulopathy. More commonly, nephrotic syndrome arises in adults as a manifestation of diabetic glomerulosclerosis or systemic amyloidosis.

TUBULOINTERSTITIAL NEPHROPATHIES AND DISORDERS OF THE URINARY TRACT

Tubulointerstitial nephritis (TIN) accounts for 10% of new-onset renal dysfunction in hospitalized cases and primarily involves the renal tubule.[81] The hallmark of TIN is an interstitial mononuclear cell infiltrate on renal biopsy, including T and B lymphocytes, macrophages, and natural killer cells.[82]

Most TIN involves cell-mediated immune responses, although some cases are the direct consequence of infection.[83-87] The clinical features of TIN are variable and depend partly on the initiating process.[88] Disruption of the normal tubulointerstitial compartment is associated with a urinary concentrating defect, hyperchloremic metabolic acidosis, hypo- or hyperkalemia, hypomagnesemia, and typically modest proteinuria. A few triggering medications, such as NSAIDs, interferon-α, and methicillin, are sometimes associated with nephrotic range proteinuria. TIN can progress to ARF requiring dialysis. Notably, TIN triggered by NSAIDs is much more common in women than men, and the onset may be weeks to months after the start of the offending agent. Although recovery usually occurs within days to weeks of drug cessation, up to 20% progress to chronic renal failure.

Drug-Induced Tubulointerstitial Nephritis Drug reactions are a major cause of TIN in hospitalized patients; the most common agents are penicillins,[89] cephalosporins,[88,89] and NSAIDs.[90,91] Other offending agents include proton pump inhibitors, vancomycin, fluoroquinolones,[89,92] sulfonamides,[93] interleukin-2, and α-interferon.[94,95] After exposure, it is often difficult to establish a single nephrotoxic agent with certainty. Additionally, comorbid conditions capable of causing kidney injury may be present, and because renal biopsy is not routine, the diagnosis of TIN is often presumptive. TIN typically occurs within days to a few weeks of drug exposure and is not related to cumulative dose. The commonest presentation is with symptoms of edema, hypertension, diminished urine output, and renal failure. Occasionally, flank pain is prominent. Classic allergic manifestations such as skin rash, arthralgias, fever, eosinophilia, and eosinophiluria are rare; eosinophiluria has only a 40% positive predictive value and 70% negative predictive value.[89,96,97] The diagnosis of TIN requires a high index of suspicion and knowledge of the potential causes.

Primary treatment of drug-induced TIN is cessation of the causative agent. Although some reports indicate clinical response to corticosteroid administration,[88,98,99] there are no large randomized placebo-controlled trials to guide treatment, and steroids are generally restricted to patients with progressive renal failure despite stopping the offending drug. Renal biopsy is often performed in these cases to confirm the diagnosis of TIN.

Infection-Induced Tubulointerstitial Disease Renal biopsy findings of TIN from infection usually have acute interstitial inflammatory cells and microabscesses. There are many causes, including bacterial,[100] fungal (candidiasis, zygomatosis, histoplasmosis), and viral (adenovirus, polyomavirus, Epstein-Barr virus) sources.

Bacterial cases usually present with a history of ascending urinary tract infection superimposed on obstructive nephropathy. Pyelonephritis may cause renal failure due to TIN (direct bacterial effects) or ATN from septic shock. The prognosis in acute bacterial TIN is significantly worse than for ATN. Whereas patients with ATN are expected to make full recovery, bacterial TIN often progresses to severe interstitial scarring and progressive chronic renal failure. Patients require prolonged antibiotic treatment to eradicate the infection and close monitoring to minimize chronic progressive renal damage.

Renal candidiasis is common in patients with a history of prolonged hospitalization, prior exposure to antimicrobial agents, corticosteroid therapy, the postoperative state, surgical wounds, chronic indwelling urinary catheters, and/or underlying malignancy. Renal candidiasis should be considered in vulnerable patients whenever unexplained progressive renal failure occurs, particularly if it is accompanied by flank pain, fever, candiduria, and microscopic hematuria.[101,102] A useful diagnostic test in the catheterized patient with candiduria involves bladder washings with amphotericin B; this will clear the urine of colonization but not renal candidosis.[103] In septic patients, a positive urine culture for candida is considered proof of renal candidiasis.[104]

Most other viral and fungal causes are seen only in immunocompromised patients.[105-110] However, Epstein-Barr virus is associated with TIN and renal failure in both immunocompetent and immunocompromised patients.[111] Other renal lesions associated with Epstein-Barr virus and infectious mononucleosis include acute glomerulonephritis, hemolytic-uremic syndrome, and rhabdomyolysis-induced ARF.[112]

THE KIDNEY IN SYSTEMIC DISEASE

Abnormal kidney function sometimes reflects the impact of a systemic disorder. Some of the more common conditions pertinent to the perioperative period are reviewed next.

Congestive Heart Failure Congestive heart failure is the one cardiovascular disease whose incidence and prevalence is still increasing in the Western world. In fact, the long-term prognosis for CHF is now worse than for many common cancers. Uniquely, the kidneys both suffer from and contribute to the pathophysiology of CHF; this is summarized in **Fig. 14-6**. Despite obvious differences between CHF and hypovolemia, the hormonal response aimed at augmenting a reduced effective arterial volume and cardiac output is common to both. Of course, with CHF the primary cause of reduced perfusion—pump failure—does not improve, but the cycle of volume retention, edema, vasoconstriction, and increased myocardial oxygen consumption continues, leading to

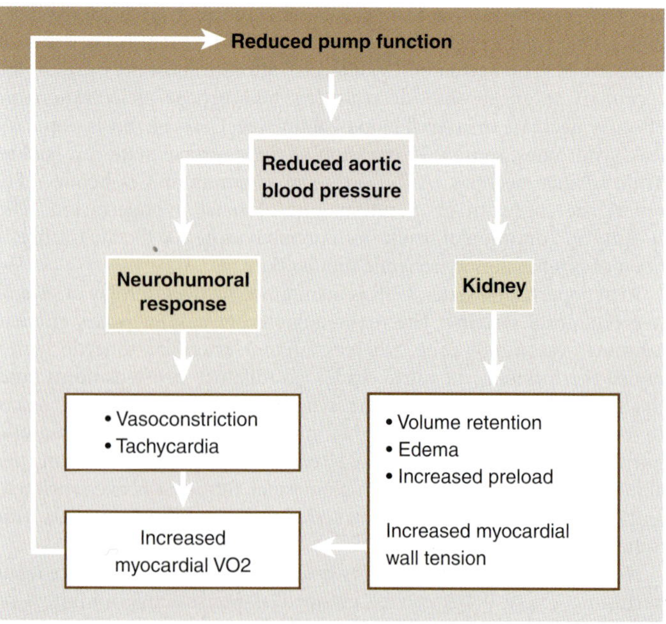

FIGURE 14-6. The pathophysiology of fluid retention that contributes to congestive heart failure.

further reductions in pump function. When CHF or pulmonary edema is diagnosed preoperatively, it is imperative that aggressive treatment occur *prior* to surgery, because uncorrected, this condition is highly predictive of early postoperative mortality.

Diabetes Diabetic nephropathy is the commonest cause of kidney failure in the United States and accounts for more than 40% of all end-stage renal disease. Of these patients, more than 80% suffer from type 2 diabetes. In affected patients, together with better glycemic control, good blood pressure management can postpone but not prevent the onset of end-stage renal disease. Beyond antihypertensive and glycemic therapies, evidence suggests a sizeable portion of unexplained variability in diabetic nephropathy onset, and progression is genetically based. Metformin is a relatively contraindicated treatment once diabetic nephropathy has developed due to the risk of significant lactic acidosis, whereas other hypoglycemic drugs including insulin may require dose reductions to avoid hypoglycemic episodes. Blood pressure control often requires more than one agent and frequently involves drugs that inhibit the renin–angiotensin–aldosterone axis, such as angiotensin-converting enzyme inhibitors and angiotensin receptor blockers.

Liver Failure Hepatorenal syndrome (HRS) is a poorly understood condition of declining renal function related to liver failure that presents as prerenal azotemia with evidence of renal vasoconstriction and decreased GFR, but normal renal histology. A partial explanation for HRS involves liver failure–related decreases in systemic and splanchnic vascular resistance that reduce effective arterial volume and cause renal hypoperfusion. Compensatory renal artery vasoconstriction occurs due to increased renin–angiotensin–aldosterone, ADH, α_1-adrenergic, and endothelin-mediated activity. The kidney also responds by increasing salt and water retention, leading to worsening ascites and edema.[113,114] The diagnosis of HRS is by exclusion, characterized by liver failure and unexplained oliguric ARF with very low urine sodium and bland urine sediment. Other causes for the ARF should be excluded, including alternate explanations for prerenal azotemia, intrinsic renal disease, and obstructive nephropathy. Major and minor criteria have been established for the diagnosis of HRS (**Table 14-6**). Patients who develop HRS before liver transplant have worse graft and overall survival.[115] Potential HRS therapies include vasopressin analogs such as ornipressin and terlipressin, which act as splanchnic vasoconstrictors, although these agents have been associated with mesenteric ischemia.[116-118] Other potential therapies include oral midodrine (a selective α_1-adrenergic agonist) in combination with octreotide,[119] *N*-acetylcysteine,[120] and transjugular intrahepatic portosystemic shunting (TIPS).[116,121] Liver transplant is the only definitive therapy for HRS, and renal failure typically resolves after transplantation. Given the poor prognosis of HRS, patients with the combination of liver failure and renal failure are rarely offered dialysis unless they are candidates for liver transplant or are expected to have hepatic recovery.[113,114,122]

TABLE 14-6 Diagnostic Criteria for Hepatorenal Syndrome

Major Criteria
- Acute or chronic liver disease with advanced hepatic failure and portal hypertension
- Depressed GFR with a serum creatinine > 1.5 mg/dL or a creatinine clearance < 40 mL/min
- Absence of shock, ongoing bacterial infection, fluid loss, and treatment with nephrotoxic medications
- No sustained improvement in renal function after withdrawal of diuretics and fluid resuscitation with 1.5 L of isotonic saline.
- Proteinuria < 500 mg/d and no evidence of obstructive nephropathy on ultrasound

Minor Criteria
- Oliguria
- Urine sodium < 10 mEq/L
- Urine osmolality > plasma osmolality
- Urine red blood cells < 50 per high-power field
- Serum sodium concentration < 130 mEq/L

From Arroyo V, Gines P, Gerbes AL, et al. Definition and diagnostic criteria of refractory ascites and hepatorenal syndrome in cirrhosis. International Ascites Club. *Hepatology.* 1996;23:164-176.

HEREDITARY RENAL DISORDERS

Autosomal-dominant polycystic kidney disease affects 0.1% to 0.25% of live births in the United States and accounts for 5% of all end-stage renal disease. The causative genetic defect is in the polycystin gene on chromosome 16p13.3 (type 1) or chromosome 4q21.2 (type 2). Hypertension is common early in the course of autosomal-dominant polycystic kidney disease, although initial presentation often involves flank or back pain symptoms and sometimes hematuria due to acute cyst hemorrhage. A clinical hallmark of autosomal-dominant polycystic kidney disease is massive cystic enlargement, a diagnosis often made in at-risk individuals by ultrasonography. When kidney volume exceeds 1000 mL (normal 150 mL), it is usually associated with a decline in GFR. Reduced glomerular filtration is related to ischemia from stretching and narrowing of intrarenal vessels and inflammatory cell infiltration and interstitial fibrosis from cytokine release. Renal transplant is the treatment of choice once renal failure develops, and autosomal-dominant polycystic kidney disease patients generally outlive their non-cystic transplant peers. Of note, autosomal-dominant polycystic kidney disease is associated with intracranial aneurysm formation, hepatic cysts, and secondary hypertension.

CONTRAST-INDUCED NEPHROPATHY

Contrast-induced nephropathy occurs in 2% to 7% of patients and constitutes 10% of all in-hospital AKI. The diagnosis is usually made by serum creatinine rise within 5 days after contrast injection.[123,124] Patients with pre-procedure renal impairment are at greatest risk[125]; the pathophysiology involves direct renal tubular cell injury and vasoconstriction. Notably in some patients, renal atheroembolism related to catheter manipulation during interventional procedures may be misdiagnosed as contrast nephropathy. Prehydration with normal saline or sodium bicarbonate (154 mEq/L, 3 mL/kg bolus 1 hour before the procedure, then 1 mL/kg infusion × 6 hours) is useful as prophylaxis for contrast-induced nephropathy.[126] Because some studies indicate that pre-cardiac surgery (<4-8 hours) contrast administration is predictive of postoperative renal complications,[127] avoiding elective procedures soon after contrast injection and/or permitting recovery of contrast-induced nephropathy before surgery would seem prudent.

THE RENAL TRANSPLANT PATIENT

After corneal transplant, kidney transplant is the commonest transplant surgery, with more than 17 000 procedures performed annually in the United States. A variety of anesthetic considerations are pertinent to patients with a previously transplanted kidney presenting for other surgeries. These individuals have a spectrum of GFR values ranging from normal to severely impaired and are receiving immunosuppressant medications that often possess acute and chronic nephrotoxic effects. In addition, renal allograft rejection may be recognized at preoperative assessment, usually heralded by an unexplained rise in serum creatinine. Rejection is a medical emergency, and suspicion obliges referral preoperatively for further investigation; if impending graft loss is overlooked, return to chronic dialysis may be required.

Three types of allograft rejection are recognized: hyperacute, accelerated acute, and acute. Hyperacute rejection occurs within minutes to hours of transplant reperfusion and is related to preexisting human leukocyte antigens and/or ABO blood type antibodies. Antibodies bind to graft endothelium and activate complement, inflammatory, and coagulation pathways, causing widespread thrombosis and subsequent loss of graft function. Hyperacute rejection is now rare due to improved matching of donors and recipients. Accelerated acute rejection occurs in the first 5 days after transplant reperfusion and is due to activation of recipient T and B "memory" lymphocytes. This diagnosis is confirmed by a graft biopsy that demonstrates cells staining positively for C4d. Finally, acute rejection occurs between 5 days and 3 months after reperfusion. It is a cell-mediated process that classically presents as fever, chills, arthralgia, myalgia, and pain over the graft site. Modern immunosuppressive therapy with calcineurin inhibitors (eg, cyclosporine, tacrolimus) has significantly reduced this clinical presentation, and diagnosis is usually made after renal biopsy prompted by a subacute rise in serum creatinine noted on routine testing.

Beyond standard procedure-related infectious risk, renal transplant recipients are vulnerable to specific infections, including *Pneumocystis carinii* pneumonia, urinary tract infections, and sinusitis, and require trimethoprim-sulfamethoxazole therapy for a period after transplant to protect against them. Any post-transplant antibiotics should be continued through subsequent (and unrelated) perioperative periods.

The calcineurin inhibitors tacrolimus and cyclosporine A (CSA) are commonly used immunosuppressants after solid organ and bone marrow transplantation. These agents can cause both AKI and chronic renal disease through direct afferent arteriolar vasoconstriction. Acute effects may require discontinuation, but dose reduction is sometimes sufficient to attenuate drops in glomerular filtration pressure and GFR. Chronic nephrotoxicity can manifest as soon as 6 months after initiation of therapy, including arteriolar damage, interstitial fibrosis, tubular atrophy, and glomerulosclerosis. Common clinical problems associated with prolonged calcineurin inhibitor use include irreversible proteinuria, tubular dysfunction, arterial hypertension, and rising serum creatinine values.[128-130] A less common complication of tacrolimus and CSA therapy is hemolytic uremic syndrome; patients may have partial recovery with drug discontinuation.[131-133] Calcineurin inhibitors have also been associated with hyperkalemia due to tubular resistance to aldosterone.[134]

POSTOPERATIVE RENAL DISORDERS

Acute deterioration of renal function is present in 5% of all hospital patients and 30% of those admitted to intensive care units.[71] Many of these patients sustain their AKI as a consequence of surgery or its complications. Certain surgical procedures are highly associated with postoperative AKI. Significant renal injury complicates up to 30% of trauma, cardiac, vascular, and hepatobiliary procedures.[135] The importance of AKI after surgery lies not only in the resulting physiologic derangements but also in the strong association with in-hospital mortality, even after adjustment for other contributing factors.[7,136,137] Not all surgical procedures are vulnerable to postoperative AKI. Although there is a perception that most noncardiac surgical procedures (eg, thoracotomy) are not associated with important AKI,[138] recent studies indicate that perioperative AKI is more prevalent than previously assumed. Even small perioperative declines in renal function are associated with increased risk of major complications and mortality, possibly due to the effects of AKI on the normal functioning of many other organ systems.[139-141] Preoperative predictive factors include African American race,[142] advanced age,[7,143-147] obesity,[7] hypertension,[148,149] peripheral or carotid atherosclerotic vascular disease,[7,148] elevated preoperative serum glucose and diabetes,[7,146,149,150] obstructive pulmonary disease, and reduced left ventricular function.[7,143,148,151,152] Preoperative genetic testing may be useful in the future[153,154]; however, there are no tests currently available as predictive tools.

The role of preexisting renal disease as an AKI risk factor is complicated. It is undeniable that patients with severe preexisting disease need to only have a small additional insult to lose function sufficient to tip them into renal failure and the need for dialysis. Postoperative patients requiring new dialysis *are* more likely to have preexisting renal dysfunction.[7,144,146-148] However, interestingly patients with preexisting renal dysfunction *are not* more likely to sustain AKI, described as a relative change in renal function perioperatively (eg, 50% rise in serum creatinine).[145,155,156] Patients with preexisting renal disease as a group have more associated comorbidities, and these individuals also have a higher risk for other major postoperative complications.[157-159]

The high metabolic demands and poor oxygen delivery to tubule cells in the outer medulla make this the most vulnerable region of the kidney.[5] As outlined earlier (see The Normal Kidney: Correlates of Structure and Function), the medulla plays an important role in water and solute reabsorption but receives limited perfusion (5%-10% EVF). Normal oxygen extraction in the outer medulla is the highest in the body (79%), exceeding even that of the heart (65%). In the face of hypoperfusion (eg, salt and volume depletion, dehydration), 3 components of renal homeostasis preserve body composition at the expense of further stress on the medulla. First, avid reabsorption of electrolytes by tubular cells increases metabolic requirements. Second, autoregulation preserves glomerular filtration at the "cost" of efferent arteriolar constriction, further reducing medullary perfusion. Finally, the vasa rectae hairpin loops within the medulla allow oxygen to "escape" from vessels entering to those leaving the medulla. As medullary perfusion drops, this *countercurrent exchange* of oxygen increases such that medullary Po_2 may be as low as 10 to 20 mm Hg (Fig. 14-2).[4,5] Outer medullary oxygen supply/demand inequalities are believed to be an important substrate for onset of ARF syndrome.[3] The outer medulla is also vulnerable as the site of concentration for many nephrotoxins. Unfortunately, although "renal angina" is an appealing concept, renal ischemia is a painless and, to date, unmonitorable state.

RENAL FAILURE AND ITS THERAPY

Loss of adequate renal function may have occurred long before surgery and be irreversible or may be acute, in which case, renal recovery usually takes days or weeks; in both cases, the goal is to support the patient through this period.

Patients with serious renal impairment have limitations in their ability to regulate electrolyte, acid–base, and volume homeostasis. Approaches that avoid the complications of exceeding the renal homeostatic reserve with renal failure are outlined next. The most severe cases of renal impairment require rigorous adherence to guidelines aimed at limiting complications. When guidelines are inadequate, generally dialysis is required.

VOLUME HOMEOSTASIS

Free water deficit or excess is normally adjusted for by renal elimination of less or more dilute urine, respectively. When kidneys fail, they usually lose their ability to respond to these challenges and commonly produce a fixed amount of isosmotic urine. If this occurs, the clinician must *maintain euvolemia* without help from the kidneys through fluid management. To achieve this state, meticulous attention must be paid to accurate assessment of volume status and review of fluid status (ins versus outs). A fluids prescription should then be formulated. If an individual is otherwise euvolemic, then the daily fluid volume required should match the daily urine output plus an additional 500 mL (based on a 70-kg adult) for insensible losses. Additional fluid supplementation or restriction should occur if hypo- or hypervolemia are present, respectively.

ELECTROLYTE HOMEOSTASIS

Because a major problem with renal failure is clearance of accumulated substances, fluid should contain supplemental electrolytes (eg, potassium, magnesium, phosphorus) if deficits are identified. Sodium intake should be 2 g or less per day. Excess potassium can be avoided by a restrictive diet and identifying other sources (eg, fluids, parenteral nutrition, potassium penicillin). Hyperkalemia that causes cardiac dysrhythmias should be treated emergently (eg, intravenous calcium chloride or calcium gluconate). Inhaled β agonists and an infusion of sodium bicarbonate or insulin and glucose can also be used to shift potassium intracellularly. Hyperventilation may be used in mechanically ventilated patients as an emergent, temporary, measure to further encourage potassium shift into cells. Although these approaches antagonize the cardiac effects of hyperkalemia, they do not reduce total body potassium. Elimination of excess body potassium in patients with ARF can only be accomplished with resins, continuous gastric suction, or dialysis. Potassium removal with peritoneal dialysis approaches 10 to 15 mEq/h compared with 50 mEq/h for hemodialysis.

Low calcium levels are common with ARF but rarely symptomatic. Hypocalcemia in these settings is often accompanied by hypomagnesemia. Because this state inhibits PTH release, calcium and magnesium should be supplemented accordingly. Functional hypoparathyroidism, together with the decreased vitamin D synthesis by the failing kidney, contributes to the hypocalcemia. Hyperphosphatemia is also common and requires phosphorus restriction and/or administration of calcium salts or aluminum hydroxide gels.

ACID–BASE HOMEOSTASIS

When the inability of failing kidneys to reclaim filtered bicarbonate removes the ability to eliminate all the acid produced by protein breakdown, the result is an anion gap metabolic acidosis. Sometimes restricting protein intake to 0.6 to 0.8 g/kg of body weight is sufficient to treat this problem, but this may not be ideal in the healing phase for postoperative patients. Acidosis that represents lactic or ketoacidosis should always be considered as alternate causes of metabolic acidosis in the critically ill patients.

UREMIA

Uremia results from the accumulation of nitrogenous waste products and is a syndrome characterized by lethargy, fatigue, nausea, anorexia, asterixis, and hiccups. BUN measurement can be used as a marker; values higher than 70 mg/dL are rarely symptomatic, whereas values lower than 100 mg/dL are almost always associated with symptoms. When uremic symptoms develop, dialysis is usually required.

NUTRITION

Adequate nutrition is essential to successful postoperative recovery, and any benefits of avoiding short-term dialysis by protein restriction should be weighed against this. Parenteral or enteral nutrition should provide a daily minimum of 30 to 35 kcal/kg and 1.0 to 1.2 g/kg of protein. Sodium bicarbonate or acetate should be added to buffer the acid generated by protein breakdown (60-80 mEq/d).

DRUG PRESCRIBING IN PATIENTS WITH RENAL IMPAIRMENT

For additional discussion see Chapter 48.

Patients with renal impairment have altered responses to normal dosing of medication. In the case of water-soluble agents, this impairment is often due to changes in rates of drug clearance from the circulation. Other factors such as effects on absorption, distribution, and metabolism related to renal dysfunction may also be important.

If an agent relies solely on the kidney for clearance, then a simple prescribing approach involves a calculated percentage reduction in drug dosage that matches the reduction in GFR. Although GFR can be accurately measured, an estimated clearance derived from serum creatinine is usually adequate for these purposes. Unfortunately, clearance of most medications involves a more complex combination of both hepatic and renal function, and drug-level measurement or algorithms for a specific drug dosing may be recommended.

ARF may affect drug absorption. For example, a reduced first pass effect through the gastrointestinal tract and liver is attributed with the increased serum levels of oral β-blockers and opioids in patients with ARF. Also, an increase in volume of distribution is seen in most patients with chronic renal failure due to increased plasma volume and decreased plasma protein binding. However, plasma protein binding is highly variable, with acidic drugs (eg, warfarin, phenytoin) having reduced binding and basic agents (eg, amide local anesthetics) having increased binding. Importantly, for drugs with less binding, "normal" drug levels may reflect dangerously high active (unbound) drug levels. For example, therapeutic phenytoin levels are 10 to 20 μg/mL normally but 4 to 10 μg/mL with renal failure. Finally, liver metabolism of drugs is difficult to predict in the setting of renal failure; some hepatic enzymes are inhibited, whereas others are induced, and accompanying liver disorders may alter the relationship of drug clearance with GFR.

SUMMARY

Review of kidney function is an essential component of even the most hurried preoperative assessment for surgical candidates. To best manage patients, clinicians must be familiar with the kidney responses to hemodynamic stress and other homeostatic disturbances and with normal states that influence kidney function, such as pregnancy, maturation, and aging. Special considerations are required in caring for surgical patients with kidney disease, and the consequences of kidney injury and postoperative renal dysfunction play importantly into the care of the critically ill patient. The well-being of the kidney throughout the perioperative period is highly associated with good outcomes. Renal insult and injury are predictive of other complications. Thus, in the absence of effective interventions to treat AKI, and limited point-of-care tools to monitor renal stress, perioperative clinicians must act as ambassadors to protect the kidney throughout the perioperative period.

KEY REFERENCES

- Bellomo R, Ronco C, Kellum JA, et al. Acute renal failure—definition, outcome measures, animal models, fluid therapy and information technology needs: the Second International Consensus Conference of the Acute Dialysis Quality Initiative (ADQI) Group. *Crit Care.* 2004;8:R204-R212.
- Chertow GM, Lazarus JM, Christiansen CL, et al. Preoperative renal risk stratification. *Circulation.* 1997;95:878-884.
- Chertow GM, Levy EM, Hammermeister KE, et al. Independent association between acute renal failure and mortality following cardiac surgery. *Am J Med.* 1998;104:343-348.
- Greenberg A, ed. *Primer on Kidney Diseases.* 4th ed. Philadelphia, PA: Elsevier Saunders; 2005.
- Kramer L, Hörl WH. Hepatorenal syndrome. *Semin Nephrol.* 2002;22:290-301.
- Porter GA. Contrast-associated nephropathy: presentation, pathophysiology and management. *Miner Electrolyte Metab.* 1994;20: 232-243.
- Schoolwerth AC, Sica DA, Ballermann BJ, et al. Renal considerations in angiotensin converting enzyme inhibitor therapy: a statement for healthcare professionals from the Council on the Kidney in Cardiovascular Disease and the Council for High Blood Pressure Research of the American Heart Association. *Circulation.* 2001;104:1985-1991.
- Stafford-Smith M. Perioperative renal dysfunction: implications and strategies for protection. In: Newman MF, ed. *Perioperative Organ Protection.* Baltimore, MD: Lippincott Williams & Wilkins; 2003:89-124.
- Swaminathan M, Phillips-Bute BG, Conlon PJ, et al. The association of lowest hematocrit during cardiopulmonary bypass with acute renal injury after coronary bypass surgery. *Ann Thorac Surg.* 2003;76:784-791.
- Verbalis JG. Hyponatremia: epidemiology, pathophysiology, and therapy. *Curr Opin Nephrol Hypertens.* 1993;2:636-652.

REFERENCES

Complete references available on DVD and online version at www.LongneckerAnesthesiology.com

CHAPTER 15 Evaluation of Patients With Hepatic Disease

Eric T. Pierce
Richard A. Wiklund

KEY POINTS

1. The Child-Pugh and MELD scoring systems predict the risk of surgery for patients with liver disease. The Child-Pugh system requires knowledge of the patient's international normalized ratio (INR), plasma bilirubin level, plasma albumin level, degree of encephalopathy, and volume of ascites. The MELD system uses only creatinine, total bilrubin and INR.
2. The leading causes of perioperative death or complications for patients with advanced liver disease include hemorrhage secondary to coagulopathy, elevated intracranial pressure, sepsis secondary to peritonitis or pneumonitis, an ascites fluid leak at the site of surgical incision, and acute renal failure secondary to hemodynamic instability or hepatorenal syndrome.
3. Serious but rare complications of chronic liver disease include the hepatorenal syndrome, the hepatopulmonary syndrome, and portopulmonary hypertension. These may resolve after liver transplantation.
4. Most forms of chronic liver disease lead to cirrhosis, a histologic diagnosis that is characterized by fibronodular hyperplasia leading to compression and obstruction of sinusoidal capillaries and bile canaliculi. These histologic findings account for the development of portal hypertension that is manifested by ascites, esophageal varices, and hypersplenism.
5. Inflammatory cellular mechanisms play a role in the development of most forms of liver disease. Inflammatory mechanisms initiate hepatocellular dysfunction, hepatocyte necrosis, and portal fibrosis.
6. Laboratory testing for the evaluation of liver disease includes tests of synthetic function (INR, serum albumin, and other serum proteins), excretory function (plasma bilirubin levels), and metabolic function (blood glucose, cholesterol, lipoprotein levels), as well as evaluation of bile duct obstruction (plasma alkaline phosphatase) and hepatocellular injury (plasma aspartate aminotransferase and alanine aminotransferase levels). Ultrasonography, computed tomography, and magnetic resonance imaging contribute to establishing an anatomic cause of liver dysfunction.
7. Transmission of viral infection by means of blood product administration has become rare because of routine immunologic and molecular screening of donors for various infectious diseases. Transmission to health care workers continues to be a hazard because of the lack of immunization against hepatitis C. Health care workers who are carriers of hepatitis B or C should limit the risk of transmitting their disease to their patients.
8. Nonalcoholic fatty liver disease is emerging as a leading cause of liver disease in the United States. Its prevalence is tied to the frequency of type 2 diabetes and the increasing problem of morbid obesity.
9. Preoperative attention to the control of ascites, correction of coagulopathy, control of encephalopathy, optimization of renal and pulmonary function, and reduction in the risk of sepsis will decrease the risk of postoperative complications and improve survival rates after surgery in patients with liver disease.
10. Anesthesia-related drugs such as sedatives and vasopressors should be used with increased caution in patients with liver disease. Benzodiazepines may unmask a subclinical encephalopathy. Vasopressors may decrease total hepatic blood flow, inducing ischemia and potential acute liver failure.

The liver is a unique vital organ because it serves multiple, independent functions, each of which is necessary for sustaining life. These include synthesis of proteins required for coagulation (fibrinogen, prothrombin, factor VII) and fluid volume homeostasis (albumin), conjugation and excretion of metabolic products (bilirubin and ammonia), carbohydrate metabolism (glycogen storage and glucose release), drug metabolism (muscle relaxants, local anesthetics, narcotics, many others), and defense from pathogens (reticuloendothelial cells). When the liver fails, these functions are compromised and cause a cascade of effects that results in multiorgan failure. Patients with liver failure can develop abnormal neurologic function (encephalopathy), altered cardiovascular performance and hemodynamics, altered metabolism with accumulation of waste products (jaundice), accumulation of extracellular fluid volume (ascites), and compromised immune and endocrine function. Some patients are at risk for acute renal failure (hepatorenal syndrome) and altered pulmonary physiology (hepatopulmonary syndrome or portopulmonary hypertension).

Despite advances in perioperative care, patients with acute or chronic liver failure continue to experience an increased risk of postoperative complications and death.[1] Identifying and addressing risk factors preoperatively may prevent postoperative morbidity and possibly reduce mortality. This chapter reviews the fundamentals of hepatic anatomy, physiology, and biochemistry and presents an overview of liver disease to provide a foundation for identification of risk (see Key Points).

OVERVIEW OF THE LIVER

The liver is the largest solid organ in the body, typically weighing between 1200 and 1500 g (~2% of body weight). Unlike most organs, the liver is able to regenerate itself after injury. With repeated injury, however, regeneration is limited by surrounding fibrous scar tissue (cirrhosis). Early in the course of many hepatic diseases, the liver becomes enlarged as a consequence of fatty infiltration, cellular infiltration, and fibronodular regeneration. With continued injury, however, it decreases in size, as bridging fibrosis leads to cirrhosis.

FUNCTIONAL ANATOMY OF THE LIVER

The functional anatomy follows the vascular supply and biliary drainage. This anatomy determines the acceptable boundaries for hepatic resection for cancer surgery, as well as living-related liver donor hepatectomy (**Fig. 15-1**). The liver has a dual blood supply consisting of the hepatic artery, which directly supplies arterial blood, and the portal vein, which provides venous blood from the intestines and spleen. Despite being partially desaturated, the portal venous flow typically provides approximately half of the liver's oxygen supply. The branches of the vasculature and bile ducts demarcate the boundaries of the 8 liver segments. The hepatic acinus is the functional unit of the liver. It is elliptical in shape, centering along the vascular anastomoses, connecting 2 portal triads, and extending out toward the central hepatic venules. Portal venule and hepatic arteriolar blood flows from the portal triads to the hepatic venules through the sinusoids (**Fig. 15-2**).[2] Fibrosis leads to portal hypertension from compression of these blood vessels. Hepatocytes are described as being in zone 1, 2, or 3 on the basis of their distance from the center of the acinus with its nutrient and oxygen supply. Those in zone 3 are at greatest risk of ischemic, viral, and toxic injury as they are more remote from their source of oxygen and nutrients.[3] Zone 3 is the area of the hepatic acinus where bridging fibrosis first occurs after ischemic or metabolic injury.

FUNCTIONS OF THE LIVER

Hepatocellular function includes synthesis of proteins, production of bile, clearance of drugs and metabolites, glycogenesis and glycogenolysis, and metabolism of cholesterol and fatty acids (**Table 15-1**). Reticuloendothelial function includes phagocytosis (Kupffer cells), hematopoiesis (stem cells for both red and white blood cells), production of immunoglobulins (lymphoid tissue), and lipid metabolism (lipocytes). All of these functions may be impaired with liver disease.

Synthetic Function Albumin, fibrinogen, prothrombin, other coagulation factors, glycoproteins, transferrin, pseudocholinesterase, and

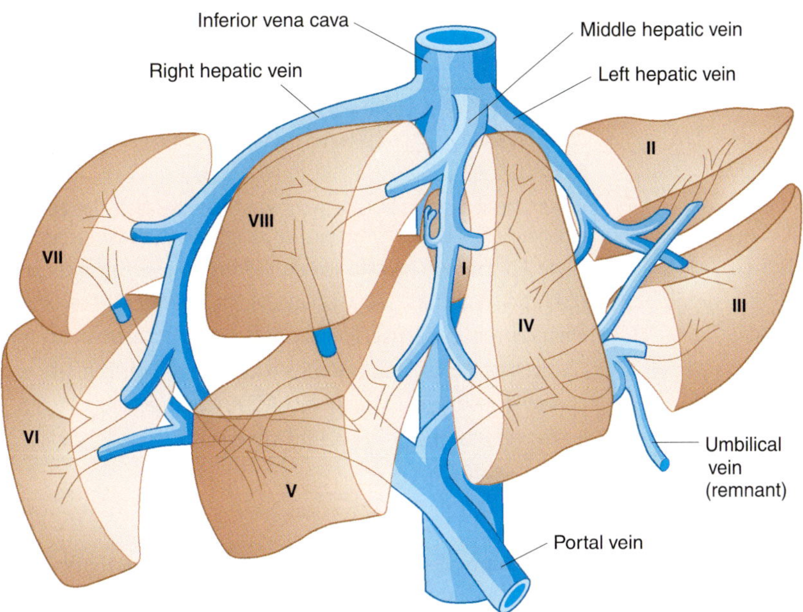

FIGURE 15-1. Segmental anatomy of the liver. The liver is divided into 8 segments based on the branches of the portal and hepatic veins. The left, middle, and right hepatic veins functionally divide the liver into 4 sectors, and these are further subdivided based on the portal inflow into a total of 8 segments. [Adapted with permission from Tanabe KK, Blaszkowsky LS, Chung R T, et al. Case 23–2005: a 57-year-old man with a mass in the liver. *N Engl J Med.* 2005;353:401. Copyright 2005, Massachusetts Medical Society. All Rights Reserved.]

α-globulins (eg, ceruloplasmin) are the major proteins synthesized in the liver. The liver also synthesizes cholesterol and glycogen.

Excretory Function Bile excretion is the final pathway for the hepatic elimination of heme, cholesterol, and drug metabolites cleared from the plasma. The principal mechanism of hepatic excretion is the conversion of nonpolar, lipid-soluble compounds to polar, water-soluble compounds by means of conjugation with glucuronic acid.

Heme molecules are oxidized and eventually conjugated to form direct bilirubin. Approximately 80% of bilirubin is derived from hemoglobin. The remainder comes from other heme molecules, such as those contained by myoglobin and cytochromes. Excretion of conjugated bilirubin at the canaliculi requires energy and is a rate-limited process that occurs against a concentration gradient. Transport failure leads to direct hyperbilirubinemia. Bacteria in the colon convert conjugated

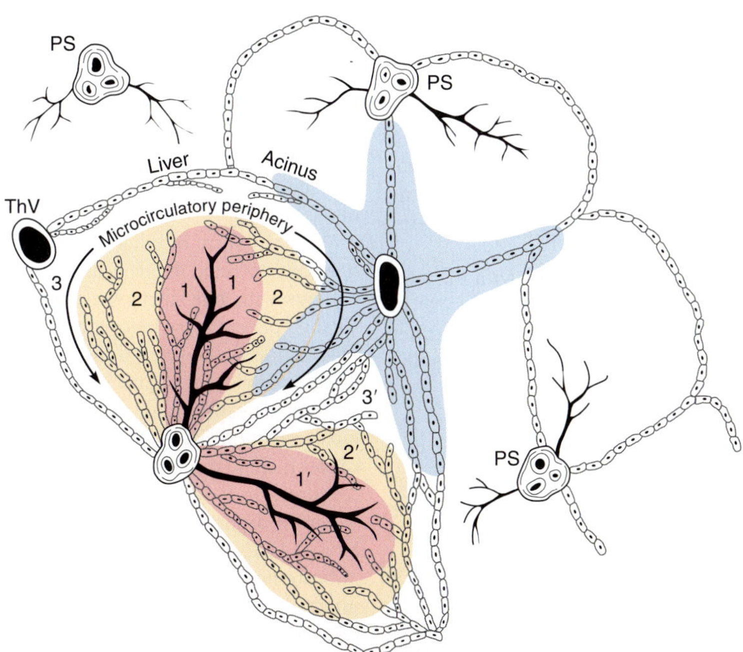

FIGURE 15-2. Anatomy of the hepatic sinusoids. The sinusoids are low-pressure vascular channels that deliver blood from the portal triads at the periphery of the hepatic lobules to the central hepatic venules. Hepatocytes line the sinusoids. The locations of the hepatocytes are divided into zones 1, 2, and 3 based on their proximity to the available oxygen supply. The hepatocytes in zone 3 are most vulnerable to ischemic injury. As such, this is the zone where fibrosis first begins. Kupffer cells and lymphatics are located in the periphery. [Adapted with permission from Sherlock S, Dooley J. Anatomy and function. In: Sherlock S, Dooley J, eds. *Diseases of the Liver and Biliary System.* 9th ed. London, UK: Blackwell Scientific; 1993:9.]

TABLE 15-1 Physiologic and Biochemical Functions of the Liver

Liver Function	Examples
Protein synthesis	Albumin, fibrinogen, γ-globulin, ceruloplasmin, α_1-antitrypsin, α_1-fetoprotien, others
Bilirubin excretion	Active transport and conjugation with glucuronic acid
Coagulation	Factors II, V, VII, IX, X
Drug elimination	Phase I metabolism (oxidation, hydroxylation, dealkylation, demethylation, deamination, desulfuration, sulfoxide formation, dehydrogenation) involving microsomal P450 enzymes
	Phase II metabolism (glucuronidation, sulfonation, acylation, methylation)
	Highly extracted drugs, poorly extracted drugs, enterohepatic circulation, enzyme induction
Waste-product elimination	Ammonia conversion to urea, amino acid elimination, hemoglobin, myoglobin, others
Energy metabolism	Glycogen synthesis, glucose production, cholesterol formation, fatty acid metabolism
Hormone metabolism	Estrogens, androgens, thyroxine, TSH, ACTH, catecholamines
Immune response	Kupffer cell phagocytosis, γ-globulins, complement, protein C and S

ACTH, adrenocorticotropic hormone; TSH, thyroid-stimulating hormone.

bilirubin to urobilinogen, which can be reabsorbed by the ileum but not the colon. The liver normally metabolizes the small amount of urobilinogen reabsorbed in the small bowel (enterohepatic circulation).

Jaundice is more apparent with conjugated hyperbilirubinemia because the conjugated bilirubin is water-soluble and diffuses easily through tissues. Jaundice can be prehepatic (a result of hemolysis), hepatocellular (metabolic, toxic, viral, alcoholic, cirrhotic), or cholestatic (sex hormones, hepatobiliary-pancreatic malignancies, gallstones). Unconjugated (indirect) bilirubin is the primary component of hyperbilirubinemia with prehepatic disease, whereas conjugated (direct) hyperbilirubinemia is present with cholestatic disease. Both may be elevated with hepatic disease. History, physical findings, clinical course (encephalopathy, ascites, steatorrhea, etc), and laboratory testing (plasma albumin and hepatic enzymes) can determine the cause of hyperbilirubinemia.

Metabolic Function The liver, as a target for insulin, plays an important role in glucose metabolism and energy production. Insulin is also a hepatotropic growth factor contributing to hepatocyte regeneration after injury.[4]

Glucagon and β-adrenergic agonists are second-messenger hormones that stimulate the production of cyclic adenosine monophosphate (cAMP) and the release of glucose from hepatocytes. Both glucagon and insulin are secreted into the portal venous blood flowing into the liver. Drainage into the portal venous system is critical for the binding of insulin and glucagon and the release of glucose. Insulin and glucagon are much less effective in stimulating the release of glucose when pancreatic venous blood flow is extraportal (eg, pancreatic transplantation) or when they are administered intravenously.

Insulin is not cleared effectively in cirrhosis.[5] Patients with diabetes and cirrhosis manifest hyperinsulinemia. Hypoglycemia can occur in late acute liver failure but is rare in chronic liver failure. On the other hand, patients may continue to secrete glucose from the liver even in the face of severe hyperglycemia.[6]

ASSESSMENT OF LIVER FUNCTION

The results of liver function tests should provide information about hepatocyte integrity, cholestasis, and liver function (**Table 15-2**). Other tests are valuable in establishing the extent of hepatocellular injury, as well as morphologic and histologic effects of disease.

Hepatic synthetic function is easily assessed by measurement of plasma albumin and fibrinogen and determination of the prothrombin time or the international normalized ratio (INR).* Assay of plasma cholinesterase activity can be used to measure synthetic function, but this test should not be confused with the determination of the dibucaine number.[7] The dibucaine number can remain normal in patients with decreased levels of the normal isoform of pseudocholinesterase.

In acute liver failure, plasma protein levels decrease late in the time course of the disease because of their long half-lives (albumin = 22 days). Factor VII, however, has a short half-life (approximately 4-6 hours)[8] and is a better index of hepatocellular synthetic function in the face of acute hepatocellular injury following transplantation. Serum albumin and the prothrombin time are the standard tests of synthetic function and are used in the algorithm establishing the Child-Pugh score (see later discussion).[9]

The best laboratory tests of hepatic excretion are serum levels of indirect and direct bilirubin (**Table 15-3**). These lab values are also used in the determination of the Child-Pugh score. Although most forms of liver disease will eventually produce an elevation of bilirubin, it is most common with biliary obstruction or secondary autoimmune biliary disease. Plasma levels of hepatocellular enzymes are used to diagnose hepatocellular injury and bile duct obstruction (**Table 15-4**). The pattern of enzyme elevation helps distinguish between hepatocellular injury (ischemic, toxic, inflammatory), biliary obstruction, and alcohol abuse. Beyond that, they are relatively nonspecific and do not provide sufficient information to discriminate among the different liver diseases.[10]

With any form of biliary obstruction, alkaline phosphatase, which is normally excreted in bile, leaks into the systemic circulation. As a result, patients with bile duct obstruction develop elevated plasma levels of alkaline phosphatase before they develop hyperbilirubinemia. Bile duct obstruction at the level of the canaliculi can occur with granulomatous disease, amyloidoses, and infections, as well as with infiltrative disease such as leukemia and metastatic malignancies. Cholelithiasis is the most common cause of extrahepatic bile duct obstruction, but other causes include tumors, strictures, infection, inflammation, and extrinsic compression.

Serum aspartate aminotransferase (AST) and alanine aminotransferase (ALT) are hepatic mitochondrial enzymes. Elevated serum levels indicate hepatocellular injury from a variety of causes, including viral infection, alcohol abuse, and obesity (**Fig. 15-3**). The highest elevations (approximately 50 times normal values) of the transaminases occur with ischemic or toxic liver injury and acute viral hepatitis. γ-Glutamyl transpeptidase (γ-GT) and lactate dehydrogenase are enzymes that can be elevated in both hepatocellular injury and bile duct obstruction.

The serum liver enzyme response to hepatocellular injury can be confusing because elevations occur in the early phase of injury. Decreasing enzyme levels may indicate either recovery or worsening to severe, irretrievable injury. A good example is the fulminant hepatic failure seen

*(INR: INR = [PTpatient/PTmidrange control]ISI, where ISI is the international standardization index and PT is prothrombin time. The ISI shows the relative activity of the reagents used to generate prothrombin. The ISI correction allows the comparison of the INR from one laboratory with that of another laboratory. Most clinical laboratories use reagents with an activity equal to 1.)

TABLE 15-2 Key Biochemical Markers in Hepatic Systems and Function

System or Function	Marker	Site or Significance	Function
Hepatocyte integrity	AST	Liver, heart, skeletal muscle, kidney, brain, red blood cell	
	ALT	Liver	Aminotransferases catabolize amino acids for entry into the citric acid cycle
Cholestasis	Alkaline phosphatase	Bone, intestine, liver, placenta	Canalicular enzyme that plays a role in bile production
	γ-GT	Correlated levels with alkaline phosphatase indicate hepatobiliary origin	Catalyzes transfer of γ-glutamyl group from peptides to other amino acids
	Bilirubin	Elevations may indicate hepatic or extrahepatic disorder	Breakdown product of hemolysis taken up by liver cells and conjugated to water-soluble product excreted in bile
Liver function mass	Serum albumin	Diet or liver	Liver synthesizes albumin
	Prothrombin time	Liver synthesizes vitamin K-dependent clotting factors	Bile salts are necessary for normal vitamin K absorption

ALT, alanine aminotransferase; AST, aspartate aminotransferase; γ-GT, gamma-glucuronyl transpeptidase.

Adapted from Giannini EG, Testa R, Savarino V. Liver enzyme alteration: a guide for clinicians. *CMAJ.* 2005;172:367-379, by permission of the publisher. ©2005 CMA Media Inc.

TABLE 15-3 Causes, Clinical Features, and Biochemical Abnormalities of Hyperbilirubinemia

Type	Cause	Clinical Features and Biochemical Abnormalities
Unconjugated (indirect) hyperbilirubinemia	Hemolysis	Decreased hemoglobin and haptoglobin levels
	Gilbert syndrome	None
	Hematoma absorption	Increased CK and LDH levels
	Ineffective erythropoiesis	Bone marrow abnormalities
Conjugated (direct) hyperbilirubinemia	Bile duct obstruction	Preceded by marked increase in AST/ALT levels
	Hepatitis	Presence of abdominal pain
	Cirrhosis	Increase in AST/ALT levels
	Autoimmune cholestasis	AST/ALT normal or slightly elevated
	Parenteral nutrition	Presence of physical findings of chronic liver disease
	Toxic hepatitis	Marked elevation of ALP with normal AST/ALT levels
	Vanishing bile duct syndrome	Increased ALP and γ-GT
		Concomitant increase in ALP levels
		Associated with drug reactions or liver transplantation

ALP, alkaline phosphatase; ALT, alanine aminotransferase; AST, aspartate aminotransferase; CK, creatine phosphatase; γ-GT, gamma-glucuronyl transpeptidase; LDH, lactate dehydrogenase.

Adapted from Giannini EG, Testa R, Savarino V. Liver enzyme alteration: a guide for clinicians. *CMAJ.* 2005;172:367-379, by permission of the publisher. ©2005 CMA Media Inc.

TABLE 15-4 Biochemical Features of Common Causes of Moderate to Marked Increase in Aminotransferase Levels

Cause	AST/ALT Level Increase (value × reference limit)	Bilirubin Level Increase (value × reference limit)	Comments
Ischemic injury	>10 to >50	<5	AST > ALT; rapid decrease in both after initial peak; ALT:LDH <1; presence of comorbid conditions
Toxic injury	>10	<5	Pattern of enzyme alteration similar to that of ischemic hepatitis History suggestive of toxic injury
Acute viral hepatitis	5-10 to >10	5-10	Slow decrease in AST/ALT levels Presence of risk factors
Acute biliary obstruction	5-10	5-10 to >10	AST/ALT increase precedes cholestasis Presence of typical symptoms
Alcoholic hepatitis	5-10	5-10 to >10	AST:ALT >2 May occur as both acute and acute-on-chronic injury

ALT, alanine aminotransferase; AST, aspartate aminotransferase; LDH, lactate dehydrogenase.

Adapted from Giannini EG, Testa R, Savarino V. Liver enzyme alteration: a guide for clinicians. *CMAJ.* 2005;172:367-379, by permission of the publisher. ©2005 CMA Media Inc.

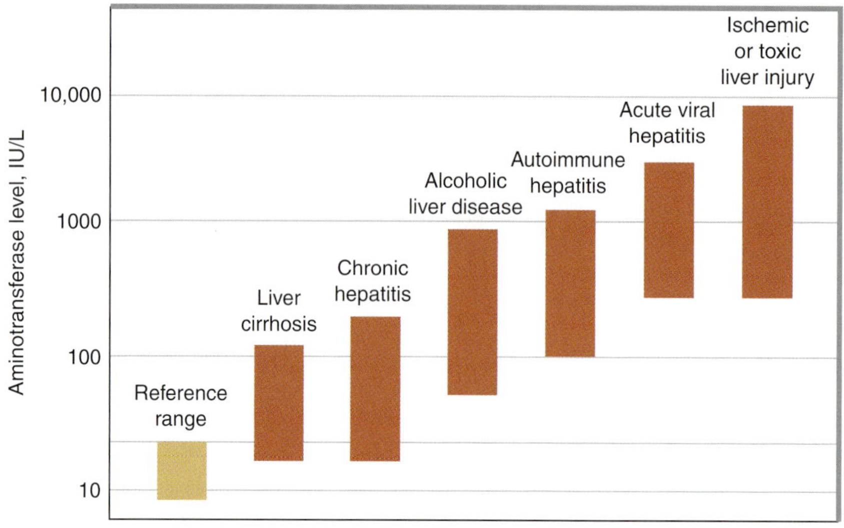

FIGURE 15-3. Serum aminotransferase levels in various liver diseases. The early elevation of the level of aminotransferase corresponds to the extent of inflammatory response in the hepatic sinusoids. [Adapted from Giannini EG, Testa R, Savarino V. Liver enzyme alteration: a guide for clinicians. *CMAJ.* 2005;172:367-379, by permission of the publisher. ©2005 CMA Media Inc.]

with acetaminophen overdose. Falling enzyme levels can lead to a false sense of security and lower the sense of urgency for liver transplantation. In this situation, factor VII levels can be helpful.

Chronic hepatitis is the most common indication for liver biopsy. Serial liver biopsies are helpful in following the progression or resolution of disease, as well as gauging the effects of treatment. Percutaneous imaging and a guided biopsy can establish the diagnosis of hepatocellular carcinoma, metastatic malignancy, or other invasive diseases of the liver.

Needle biopsy helps establish the severity of cirrhosis of the liver by grading the extent of fibrosis in areas of fibronodular hyperplasia.[3] Ishak grade 0 to 2 reflects no or minimal fibrosis, Ishak grade 3 to 4 reflects incomplete bridging fibrosis, and Ishak grade 5 to 6 reflects precomplete and complete cirrhosis (**Fig. 15-4**).

High-resolution ultrasonography and Doppler ultrasonography examinations of the liver are noninvasive, uncomplicated, and simple to perform.[11] Doppler examination can demonstrate the patency or occlusion of the hepatic artery, portal vein, hepatic veins, and inferior vena cava. Lesions as small as 1 cm can be identified with high-resolution ultrasonography, and ultrasonographic imaging can guide needle biopsy with good accuracy. Intraoperatively, ultrasonographic imaging can be used to guide hepatic segmentectomy. Ultrasonography is most

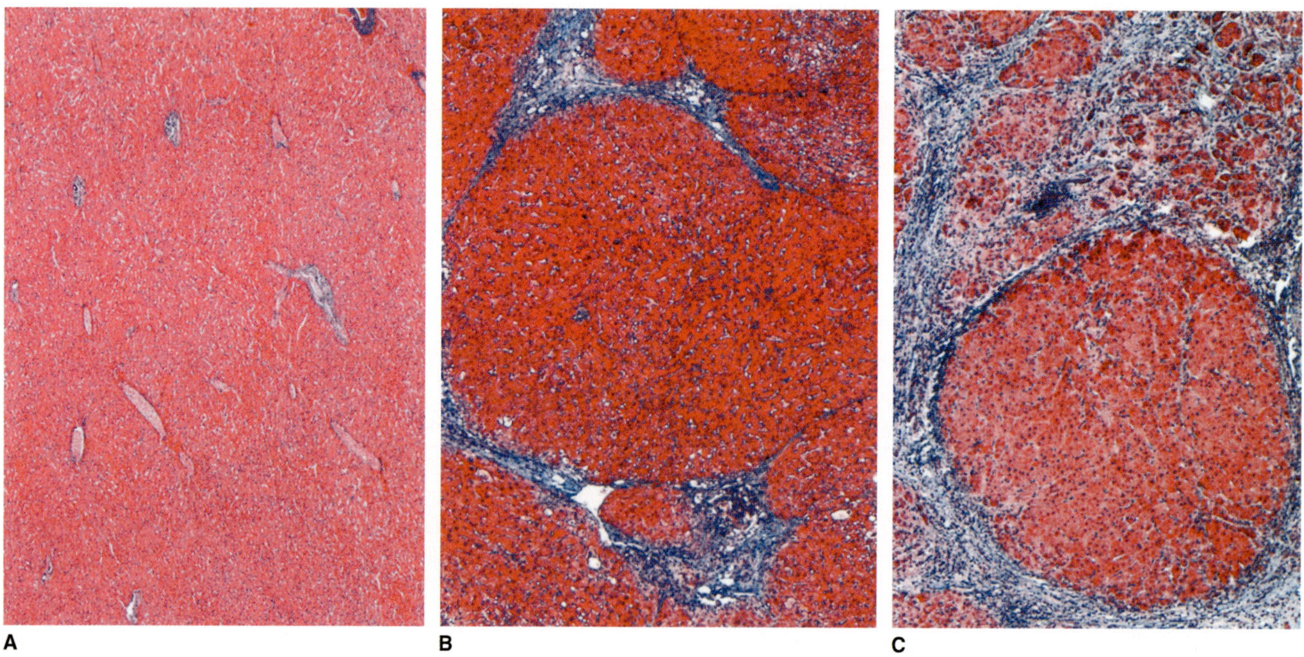

FIGURE 15-4. Ishak classification of cirrhosis. **A.** There is minimal fibrosis and no bridging between areas of fibrosis. Synthetic and excretory functions are maintained. These findings do not cause significant portal hypertension, and they are compatible with Child-Pugh class A. **B.** There is moderate fibrosis with incomplete bridging between segments. Synthetic function is diminished and hyperbilirubinemia may be present. These findings are compatible with Child-Pugh class B, and there may be mild portal hypertension. **C.** There is complete bridging fibrosis and nodular hyperplasia. Patients will have portal hypertension with ascites, varices, and encephalopathy. They meet the criteria for Child-Pugh class C. [Used with the permission of the Department of Pathology, Massachusetts General Hospital, Boston, Massachusetts.]

helpful in determining the cause of cholestatic jaundice and in locating gallstones.[12] It is less helpful in obese patients and in patients with gaseous distension of the stomach or intestines.

Computed tomography (CT) and magnetic resonance imaging (MRI)[11] have advantages over ultrasonography. Hard copy images are produced and can be readily interpreted. The spiral CT has greatly improved liver imaging because a complete scan with high resolution can be obtained during voluntary breath holding, thus eliminating motion artifacts.[13] Blood vessel anatomy is enhanced with oral or intravenous contrast material and CT scanning.[14] CT and MRI studies also provide additional information about surrounding structures, such as the spleen, kidney, collateral circulation, and shunts. CT with blood vessel enhancement provides better definition of liver segments for future resection. High-resolution ultrasonography and serum α-fetoprotein are the most sensitive and specific means of surveillance for patients at risk for hepatocellular carcinoma.[15]

HEPATIC DRUG METABOLISM

HEPATIC METABOLISM OF HIGHLY EXTRACTED DRUGS

Hepatic drug extraction occurs at the level of the hepatocyte with its dual afferent blood flow. Systemically administered drugs arrive at the hepatic sinusoid via the hepatic artery, whereas most orally administered drugs are absorbed in the small intestine and arrive at the liver via the portal vein (**Fig. 15-5**). Drugs can be divided into 2 groups based on the ability of the liver to remove them from the circulation: highly extracted, lipid-soluble (nonpolar) compounds and poorly extracted, water-soluble (polar) compounds. In reality the distinction between these 2 groups is imperfect, but it serves to help understand hepatic drug clearance.

Hepatic clearance is expressed as

$$CL_H = Q_{THBF}\,[(C_{THBF} - C_{HV})/C_{THBF}]$$

where Q_{THBF} is total hepatic blood flow, C_{THBF} is the drug concentration in the mixed portal venous blood and hepatic arterial blood, and C_{HV} is the concentration in hepatic vein blood.

If a drug is highly extracted from either or both the hepatic arterial or portal venous blood, the concentration in the hepatic vein approaches 0, and the value of $[(C_{THBF} - C_{HV})/C_{THBF}]$ approaches 1. Then CL_H is proportional to Q_{THBF}. Thus clearance of highly extracted drugs is proportional to total liver blood flow. Liver disease, abnormal hemodynamics, and drugs can decrease both hepatic artery and portal vein blood flow and exaggerate the systemic effects of a drug that is normally highly cleared by the liver. Also, intra-abdominal surgery and inhalational anesthetics can reduce liver blood flow by more than 80%.[16] Because cirrhosis of the liver markedly decreases total hepatic blood flow as a result of fibrosis at the portal triad, patients with cirrhosis can be expected to have increased sensitivity to highly extracted drugs. For example, propranolol, which also decreases total hepatic blood flow and is commonly prescribed for esophageal varices, increases the sensitivity of patients to highly extracted drugs.

Nitroglycerine, which is highly extracted, undergoes first-pass hepatic clearance when it is administered orally. Consequently, it is most effective when given sublingually or intravenously. Examples of other highly extracted drugs include labetalol, metoprolol, morphine, verapamil, and acetaminophen.

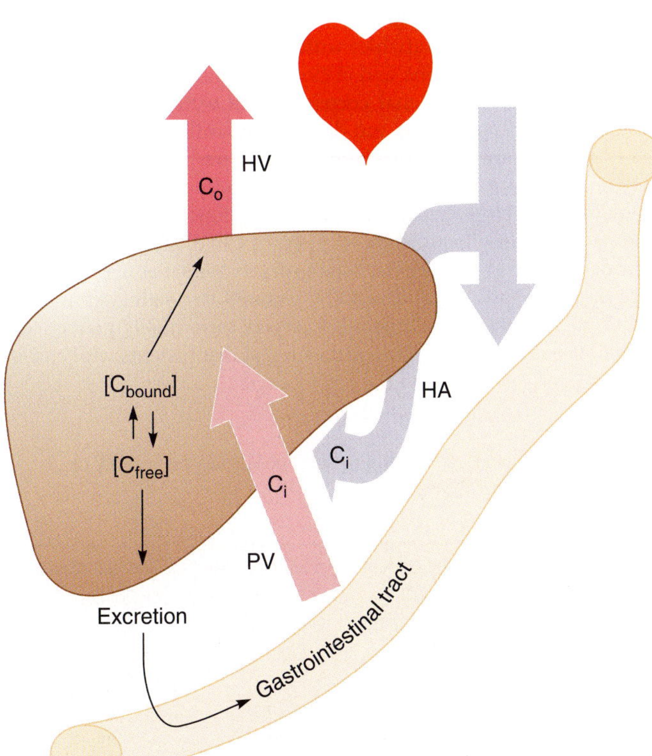

FIGURE 15-5. Hepatic drug metabolism. Drugs are cleared by the liver from blood flow via the hepatic artery (HA) and the portal vein (PV). Drug concentration (C_o) in the hepatic vein (HV) of highly extracted drugs approaches 0. Thus clearance is dependent on the concentration of drug (C_i) in blood from the total hepatic blood flow (HA + PV). Total hepatic blood flow is proportional to cardiac output. Poorly extracted drug blood concentration is dependent on the extraction ration (C_o/C_i). The extraction ratio is decreased with diminished hepatocellular microsomal function. [Courtesy of Richard A. Wiklund, MD.]

PROTEIN BINDING OF DRUGS METABOLIZED BY THE LIVER

Drug binding to plasma proteins will influence liver metabolism. Drugs are typically in equilibrium between bound and free forms. The percentage of free form is determined by the affinity each drug has for the various binding proteins including albumin, α-1 glycoprotein, and lipoproteins. Only the free fraction is available for metabolism, with the bound complex serving a reservoir for additional free drug as it is removed. For drugs that undergo rapid metabolism, such as lidocaine, extraction is nearly complete despite protein binding resulting in "first-pass clearance." Highly extracted drugs are rapidly cleared from blood because the total hepatic blood flow is equivalent to 30% of the cardiac output. However, for drugs with slower metabolism, changes in the free fraction will alter clearance. Variables including total drug concentration, plasma protein concentrations, and other protein-binding drugs will influence the free fraction.

HEPATIC METABOLISM OF POORLY EXTRACTED DRUGS

The clearance expression shown above can also be used to understand the role of the liver in the metabolism of poorly extracted drugs. In this case, however, C_{HV}, the hepatic vein blood concentration, is not zero, and Q_{THBF}, the mixed portal venous and hepatic arterial blood concentration, is not as important as the ability of the liver to extract drugs:

$$C_{HV} = C_{THBF}\,{}^{*}\,ER \sim C_f{:}C_b$$

where ER is the extraction ratio, C_f is the concentration of free drug (unbound), and C_b is the protein bound concentration of the drug. The ER is a hepatocellular microsomal function.

Hepatic microsomal enzymes are responsible for the metabolism of many of the drugs cleared by the liver. Because the activity of microsomal enzymes is dependent on normal hepatocellular function, hepatic metabolism is decreased after hepatocellular injury and in cirrhosis of the liver. The principal hepatic microsomal enzymes include the monooxygenases, cytochrome c reductase, and cytochrome P450. These enzymes convert drugs into polar, water-soluble compounds. Alternatively, alcohols can be converted to acetaldehydes by alcohol dehydrogenase. Once these reactions have occurred, the drugs' metabolites are conjugated with glucuronic acid and undergo active excretion (energy requiring) into the bile. Patients with cirrhosis are more sensitive to these drugs as the process can be saturated because of compromised hepatocellular function. Some examples of drugs that are poorly extracted and are enzyme dependent for their metabolism include certain barbiturates, benzodiazepines, nonsteroidal anti-inflammatory drugs (NSAIDs), diphenylhydantoin, caffeine, theophylline, and warfarin.

The cytochrome P450 system is a complex collection of endoplasmic heme proteins capable of producing toxic drug metabolites. Many of the P450 enzymes are inducible by drugs (ethanol, phenobarbital, omeprazole, isoniazid), and enzyme induction leads to abnormal responses to drugs that undergo hepatic metabolism (acetaminophen, β-blockers, neuroleptics, benzodiazepines). This is important for causing increased sensitivity to acetaminophen-induced acute liver failure and is brought on by chronic alcohol abuse (see Acetaminophen Toxicity) or isoniazid therapy.

OTHER PHARMACOKINETIC ABNORMALITIES IN LIVER DISEASE

Liver disease leads to other intrinsic and extrinsic effects that alter the plasma half-life or pharmacokinetic profile of drugs. Hypoalbuminemia is a characteristic finding in advanced liver disease. The normal liver is capable of producing 10 g of albumin per day. This production may be limited to less than 4 g per day in advanced cirrhosis. Albumin is the principal plasma protein capable of drug binding. Severe hypoalbuminemia increases the unbound concentration of any polar drug.

Hypoalbuminemia and portal hypertension lead to an accumulation of extracellular fluid in the form of peripheral edema, ascites, and pleural effusion. The apparent volume of drug distribution is greatly increased in the patient with a large volume of ascites.

Cirrhosis secondary to chronic alcohol abuse leads to increased sensitivity to drugs that affect the central nervous system, such as benzodiazepines.[17] This effect results from both generalized cerebral cortical atrophy and the accumulation of ammonia in the central nervous system. Benzodiazepine antagonists improve mental function in advanced encephalopathy.[18] Benzodiazepine therapy for agitation should be used with caution in patients with any evidence of hepatic encephalopathy.

The kidney shares the load of drug excretion with the liver, especially of lower-molecular-weight conjugated compounds. Renal blood flow is diminished in advanced liver disease by virtue of the increased abdominal pressure seen with uncontrolled ascites. Acute renal failure (hepatorenal syndrome, see Chronic Liver Failure) can be a complication of severe, usually acute, liver failure.

MUSCLE RELAXANTS

The metabolism of muscle relaxants deserves special attention. Succinylcholine is metabolized by plasma pseudocholinesterase. Patients with advanced liver disease may have decreased plasma levels of pseudocholinesterase, leading to a prolonged duration of neuromuscular blockade after succinylcholine administration. Pseudocholinesterase has a high affinity for its substrate (succinylcholine) and metabolizes it rapidly. Even very low concentrations of plasma pseudocholinesterase will result in only moderately prolonged paralysis. This is an unlikely cause of clinical problems. Purified pseudocholinesterase has been administered to homozygotes for atypical pseudocholinesterase that have received ester muscle relaxants.[19] This resulted in significant acceleration of recovery from neuromuscular blockade.

Aminosteroid nondepolarizing muscle relaxants (pancuronium, vecuronium, rocuronium) are metabolized in the liver, and metabolites are excreted either in bile or urine or both. Active metabolites of vecuronium accumulate in the plasma of patients with advanced liver disease. Although there are theoretical advantages of using benzylisoquinolinium muscle relaxants (atracurium, cisatracurium, mivacurium) that undergo hydrolysis in the plasma, in patients with cirrhosis, the prolonged paralytic effects of repeated doses of vecuronium are not an important clinical problem.

HISTORY OF SURGICAL RISK

CHILD-PUGH STRATIFICATION OF LIVER DISEASE

In 1964, Child and Turcotte[20] described the features of advanced liver disease leading to a high mortality rate in a group of 128 patients undergoing a portocaval shunt. Mortality was increased in patients with jaundice, malnutrition, encephalopathy, elevated serum bilirubin levels, or decreased serum albumin levels. Mortality was proportional to the extent of these abnormalities. All patients had variceal bleeding and had failed conservative treatment. The mortality rate for patients with advanced cirrhosis was 53%; it was only 4.3% for patients with earlier stages of cirrhosis.

Pugh et al modified Child's classification 10 years later.[9] Pugh et al then added the prolonged prothrombin time as an additional laboratory measurement that was predictive of a poor outcome. Estimation of the severity of encephalopathy, malnutrition, ascites, hyperbilirubinemia, hypoalbuminemia, and prolongation of the prothrombin time became the basis for the Child-Pugh score. Each abnormality was graded as minimal (score = 1), moderate (score = 2), or severe (score = 3). Child-Pugh class A patients had an aggregate score of 5 to 6; class B patients, 7 to 9; and class C patients, 10 to 15 (**Table 15-5**). The operative mortality was 77% for patients in class C, 38% in class B, and 29% in class A. None of the patients in class C survived for more than 1 year, and the overall mortality was 68% at 6 months.

Garrison et al[21] reviewed 100 consecutive patients with cirrhosis undergoing non-shunt laparotomies (**Table 15-6**). No patient had variceal hemorrhage. The authors correlated preoperative, intraoperative, and postoperative variables with survival without complications, survival with complications, and in-hospital death. Multivariate analysis showed that the features that correlated well with intraoperative and postoperative complications and death were similar to those factors in the Child-Pugh classification. Poor outcome was associated with malnutrition, uncontrolled ascites, late stages of encephalopathy, perioperative sepsis, coagulopathy, and abnormal liver function tests. Garrison's study added 2 new parameters to those of Child and Pugh that need consideration in evaluating the risk of surgery for patients with chronic liver disease. Sepsis, as evidenced by elevated circulating white blood cell (WBC) counts, and reoperative surgery were highly predictive of complications and death. Their data suggest that patients with chronic

TABLE 15-5 Child-Pugh Scoring System for Staging the Severity of Liver Disease

Child-Pugh Class	A	B	C
Ascites	None evident (1 point)	Adequate control (2 points)	Poorly controlled (3 points)
Encephalopathy	None evident (1 point)	Grade 1-2 (2 points)	Grade 3-4 (3 points)
Albumin	>3.5 g/dL (1 point)	3.0-3.5 g/dL (2 points)	<3.0 g/dL (3 points)
Bilirubin	<2.0 mg/dL (1 point)	2-3 mg/dL (2 points)	>3.0 mg/dL (3 points)
Prothrombin time (INR)	<4 s > control (INR <1.7) (1 point)	4-6 s > control (INR = 1.7-2.2) (2 points)	>6 s > control (INR >2.2) (3 points)
Total score	5-6 points	7-9 points	10-15 points

Adapted from Pugh RN, Murray-Lyon IM, Dawson JL, et al. Transection of the oesophagus for bleeding oesophageal varices. *Br J Surg.* 1973;60:646. Copyright British Journal of Surgery Society Ltd. Reproduced with permission. Permission is granted by John Wiley & Sons Ltd on behalf of the BJSS Lt.

TABLE 15-6 Variables Associated With Morbidity and Mortality After Intra-abdominal Surgery

Preoperative

Preoperative Variable	Survivors Without Complications	Survivors With Complications	Nonsurvivors
Ascites	12.5%	33%	70%
Malnutrition	7.5%	16.7%	43%
Emergency surgery	15%	40%	80%
Infection	7.5%	16.7%	47%
Elevated bilirubin	1.2 mg/dL	2.0 mg/dL	4.1 mg/dL
Decreased albumin	3.7 g/dL	3.3 g/dL	2.5 g/dL
Prolonged PT (> control)	0.3 s	1.5 s	4.5 s
Prolonged PTT (> control)	3.0 s	0.8 s	7.9 s
Child-Pugh class[a]	1.25	1.6	2.4

Operative

Operative Variable	Mortality if Present (%)	Mortality if Absent (%)
Ascites	58	11
Malnutrition	62	22
Emergency surgery	57	10
Infection	64	21
Elevated bilirubin	62	17
Decreased albumin	58	12
Prolonged PT	47	7
Prolonged PTT	54	18
Child-Pugh class A	10	50
Child-Pugh class B	31	30
Child-Pugh class C	76	18

Postoperative

Postoperative Variable	Mortality if Present (%)	Mortality if Absent (%)
Lung failure	100	0
Heart failure	92	8
Renal failure	73	9
Liver failure	66	8
Infected ascites	85	16
Ascitic leak	82	18
Second operation	81	20
Blood >2 units	69	22
FFP	61	19

[a]Average Child-Pugh class calculated assigning a numerical value of 1 for class A, 2 for class B, and 3 for class C.

FFP, fresh-frozen plasma; PT, prothrombin time; PTT, partial thromboplastin time.

Adapted with permission from Garrison RN, Cryer HM, Howard DA, Polk HC Jr. Clarification of risk factors for abdominal operations in patients with hepatic cirrhosis. *Ann Surg.* 1984;199:648.

liver disease are at high risk for sepsis syndrome whenever they develop respiratory, urinary, or intra-abdominal infections in the perioperative period. The mortality rate was 100% for exploratory laparotomy, most likely because these patients had developed spontaneous bacterial peritonitis. Reoperative surgery, for the most part, was performed to control ascites leaking out via the surgical wound, providing another portal of entry for infection.

In 1997, Mansour et al[22] reported results of 92 patients who were undergoing elective and emergency surgery. The mortality rate for Child-Pugh class A was 10%; Child-Pugh class B, 30%; and Child-Pugh class C, 82%. For all 3 groups, mortality rose significantly following emergency surgery (26% overall for elective cases; 50% after emergency surgery). Furthermore, Aranha et al[23] reported an 83% mortality rate associated with cholecystectomy and common duct exploration for patients with liver disease and a prothrombin time more than 2.5 seconds greater than the control. Cholecystostomy and retrograde cholangiography were recommended as options with a much lower mortality (14%).[24]

There are reports of improved outcome after laparoscopic cholecystectomy in patients with cirrhosis. Fernandes et al[25] compared liver disease patients with matched controls. The patients with cirrhosis had greater length of stay, longer duration of surgery, greater need for transfusion, more frequent complications, and a higher rate of conversion of open cholecystectomy. Mortality, however, was not significantly greater. There were no Child-Pugh class C patients in this series. In fact, 80% were Child-Pugh class A.

MODEL OF END-STAGE LIVER DISEASE

The Model for End-Stage Liver Disease (MELD) score was initially developed to assess the short-term prognosis of cirrhotic patients undergoing the transjugular intrahepatic portosystemic shunts (TIPS) procedure.[26] It was later adopted, in modified form and effectively used in assigning priority ranking of patients waiting for a liver transplant.[27] More recently, it has also been shown to be predictive of 30-day postoperative mortality in cirrhotic patients undoing a variety of non-transplant surgical procedures.[28,29]

The MELD score is calculated using 3 objective and routinely obtained laboratory tests: creatinine, total bilirubin, and INR. Calculators for the MELD score can be found on multiple websites, including www.mayoclinic.org/gi-rst/mayomodel5.html. MELD scores of less than 10, 10 to 14, and greater than 14 roughly correspond to Child-Pugh classes A, B, and C, respectively.[28,30] Mortality rates for a given MELD score may vary with different patient populations and the trend in each patient's score.

MELD has undergone more rigorous statistical validation than Childs-Pugh. It should be noted that this validation was performed on cohorts screened for the absence of acute reversible complications. Therefore, the MELD score is more valid when based on the patient's baseline labs in the absence of acute conditions such as infection or azotemia.[31] Unlike MELD, Child-Pugh includes subjective variables such as ascites and encephalopathy. By not including subjective variables, MELD avoids the potential for observer bias. However, because of the potential for postoperative peritoneal leak and fistula formation, ascites may be an important factor in determining outcome for patients undergoing abdominal surgery.

The ability of MELD to predict postoperative mortality and morbidity in cirrhotic patients has been evaluated for a variety of surgical procedures. In a review of 140 cirrhotic patients undergoing surgical procedures including intra-abdominal, musculoskeletal, cardiovascular, and urologic, the overall 30-day mortality rate was 16%. The mean MELD score of the survivors (16.9; 95% confidence interval [CI] 15.6-18.2) was significantly (p=0.0003) lower than that of nonsurvivors. (23.3, 95% CI; 19.6-27.0). For MELD score between 5 and 20, there was approximately a 1% increased risk of mortality with each additional integer in the MELD score, and this increased to 2% for scores greater than 20.[28] MELD also has predictive power for cirrhotic patients undergoing hepatectomy for hepatocellular carcinoma. A review of 82 such patients found that there were no deaths in patients with a MELD score of 8 or less, but there was a 29% mortality rate for those with a MELD score of 9 or more.[32] Similarly, in another study of 154 cirrhotic hepatectomy patients, a MELD score of 8 or less was associated with no liver failure and had a low rate of postoperative mortality (8.1%).[33]

A number of studies have compared the ability of MELD and Child-Pugh to predict postoperative outcomes. One found that for cirrhotic patients undergoing intra-abdominal surgery, a MELD score of 14 or greater was a better predictor of poor outcome than Child-Pugh class C.[34] In cirrhotic patients undergoing cholecystectomy, it was demonstrated that both MELD and Child-Pugh accurately predicted postoperative 90-day morality and that a preoperative MELD score of 8 or greater had sensitivity and specificity of 91% and 77%, respectively, for predicting postoperative mortality.[35] A retrospective review of 44 cirrhotic patients undergoing various cardiac surgery procedures found that both MELD and Child-Pugh scores were significantly associated with postoperative hepatic decompensation and mortality. The receiver operating characteristic curves for mortality for MELD (0.87 ± 0.09) and Child-Pugh (0.84 ± 0.09) were similar.[36]

In summary, MELD is more convenient and objective as well as better validated than Child-Pugh but, on an individual basis, may not be superior for predicting surgical risk in patients with cirrhosis. MELD is increasingly used to predict postoperative mortality and morbidity for cirrhotic patients undergoing a wide variety of surgical procedures.

The risk of complications and death after major surgery for patients with cirrhosis is high (**Table 15-7**), and there has been little reduction in these risks despite the advances in surgery, anesthesia, intensive care, and blood component therapy that have evolved over the past several decades. Intra-abdominal surgery is associated with a high-risk of complications and death in patients with early, moderate, and advanced liver disease. The increased risk is proportional to the extent of liver disease, which is readily estimated by simple clinical and laboratory data. The traditional risk factors of encephalopathy, uncontrolled ascites, malnutrition, abnormal serum albumin and bilirubin, and prolonged prothrombin time should be expanded to include the presence of sepsis and emergency surgery.

TABLE 15-7 Estimated Risk of Major Intra-abdominal Surgery[a] for Patients With Cirrhosis

Child-Pugh Classification	Mortality
A	10%
B	30%
C	80%

[a]Does not include orthotopic liver transplantation.

Data from Child and Turcott[20]; Pugh et al[9]; Garrison et al[21]; and Mansour et al.[22]

BRIEF OVERVIEW OF LIVER DISEASES

CONGENITAL AND INFANTILE LIVER DISEASE

Biliary Atresia Biliary atresia results from destruction of bile ducts in utero. The cause is unknown. Infants do not survive childhood with complete atresia. Surgical correction of a distinct segment of biliary atresia with a choledochojejunostomy or Kasai procedure (hepatic portoenterostomy) may provide relief from severe jaundice and liver failure until liver transplantation can be performed.

Reye Syndrome Reye syndrome is characterized by a severe encephalopathy and a fatty liver. The cause is unknown but it occurs in children with acute viral infection. In the United States, the incidence of Reye syndrome has been tied to aspirin (salicylate) ingestion, and the incidence has fallen as acetaminophen is substituted for salicylates in children with viral illness.

Wilson Disease Wilson disease consists of progressive lenticular degeneration associated with cirrhosis of the liver. Symptoms typically begin between 6 and 20 years of age. It is an autosomal-recessive abnormality of copper metabolism and results in characteristic, greenish Kayser-Fleischer rings in the cornea. The plasma ceruloplasmin level is decreased. However, Wilson disease is not a failure to produce ceruloplasmin; it is a failure of copper transport followed by coupling to ceruloplasmin. Penicillamine therapy chelates copper, leading to improvement of the neurologic symptoms and prevention of cirrhosis. Fulminant hepatic necrosis can occur in 25% of cases and requires urgent liver transplantation. Patients with Wilson disease require uninterrupted penicillamine therapy in the perioperative period.

Hemochromatosis Chronic excessive iron exposure causes hepatic fibrosis (hemochromatosis) irrespective of whether the accumulation is the result of multiple transfusions or abnormal absorption and accumulation of dietary iron. MRI is highly specific and sensitive for iron overload in hemochromatosis and can be used to gauge the effectiveness of iron depletion therapy.[39] Hemochromatosis leads to cirrhosis and hepatocellular carcinoma.

Hereditary hemochromatosis results in macronodular cirrhosis, diabetes from pancreatic fibrosis, and cardiac iron deposition, often with heart failure, conduction abnormalities, and coronary atherosclerosis. This disease is an autosomal-recessive metabolic disorder. Although present from birth, tissue injury does not begin until age 30 to 40 years. Iron toxicity is controlled by aggressive removal of blood. Multiple organ (heart, liver, pancreas) transplantation may be required.

α_1-Antitrypsin Deficiency α_1-Antitrypsin is an enzyme inhibitor produced in the liver that inhibits key proteases (eg, trypsin) and neutrophil elastase. Two genes (Pi or protease inhibitor gene), one received from each parent, control the production of α_1-antitrypsin. There are many alleles, but only 2 are associated with disease. M is the normal allele; S and Z are the 2 alleles that are clinically significant. Liver disease can be associated with the PiMZ and PIZZ genotypes.

Other Inherited Liver Diseases Hereditary tyrosinemia is an autosomal-recessive inborn error of metabolism that results in progressive liver disease and possible acute liver failure early in life.

There are at least 10 defects in glycogen synthesis or storage that affect the liver, skeletal muscle, and red and white blood cells.[40] For the most part all result in excessive amounts of glycogen stored in these tissues.

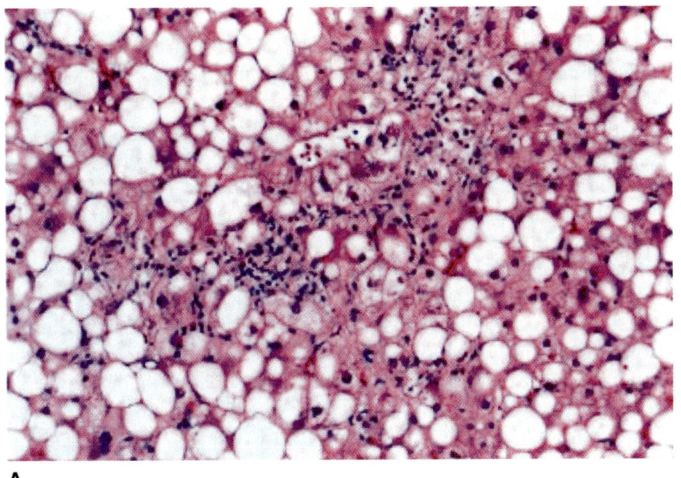
A

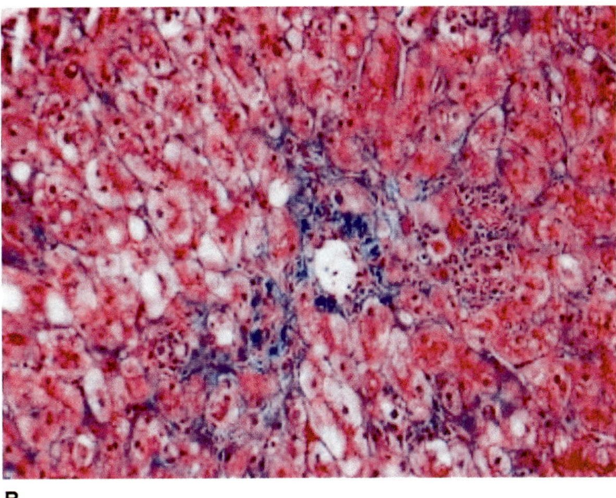
B

FIGURE 15-6. Histologic findings with nonalcoholic fatty liver disease. **A.** Photomicrograph shows macrovesicular fatty infiltration, an inflammatory infiltrate, Mallory hyaline deposits, and hepatocyte ballooning. **B.** This panel shows zone 3 fibrosis in a pattern typical of nonalcoholic liver disease as opposed to that seen in alcoholic liver disease. [Adapted with permission from Angulo P. Nonalcoholic fatty liver disease. *N Engl J Med.* 2002;346:1221. Copyright 2002, Massachusetts Medical Society. All rights reserved.]

The mucopolysaccharide storage disorders are a group of lysosomal storage disorders associated with deficiencies of the lysosomal enzymes required for normal sequential degradation of glycosaminoglycans. Abnormal lysosomal enzymes lead to lysosomal storage diseases such as Hurler syndrome, another autosomal-recessive abnormality.

NUTRITIONAL LIVER DISEASE

Nonalcoholic Fatty Liver Disease Nonalcoholic fatty liver disease (NAFLD) is prevalent in the obese population.[41] In a prospective study of 1124 asymptomatic patients referred for evaluation of abnormal liver function tests, 73 of 81 patients without markers for liver disease (infection, metabolic, autoimmune, hereditary, alcoholic, toxic) were found to have some degree of steatosis on liver biopsy.[42] In its earliest stage, NAFLD is manifested by macrovesicular fatty infiltrate with minimal inflammation, but in more advanced forms, extensive fibrosis in periportal areas is evident (**Fig. 15-6**). NAFLD is believed to be the most common cause of abnormal liver function tests in the United States.[43] It is most prevalent in morbidly obese patients with type 2 diabetes mellitus.[44] Paradoxically, it occurs frequently after bariatric surgery.[45]

It is hypothesized that NAFLD results from an abnormality of lipid uptake, synthesis, degradation, or secretion resulting from insulin resistance.[30] Although NAFLD is an infrequent indication for liver transplantation,[46] it has the potential to be a precipitating cause of postoperative liver dysfunction.

ACQUIRED LIVER DISEASE

Viral Hepatitis Viral hepatitis is a broad collection of illnesses that have hepatic dysfunction as the only common thread. The etiologies, modes of transmission, clinical courses, and late complications are different (**Table 15-8**).[47]

TABLE 15-8 Clinical and Chemical Characteristics of Viral Hepatitis

Disease	Viral Particle	Transmission	Testing	Course	Immunization and Treatment
Hepatitis A	RNA	Fecal–oral contamination of food or water	HVA-AB	Self-limited icteric disease FHF rare	Vaccine HIG
Hepatitis B	DNA	Sexual and familial contact Blood products Intravenous drug abuse Healthcare workplace exposure Immunocompromised patients	HVBsAg HVBeAg HVB-AB HVB-AB HBV DNA	Subclinical anicteric illness, or full recovery in 4-6 mo, or chronic active hepatitis High incidence of FHF	Vaccine HIG Corticosteroids Interferon Antiviral therapy
Hepatitis D	Defective RNA	Intravenous drug abuse Blood products Immunocompromised patients	HVD-AB HVD RNA	Coinfection with hepatitis B Chronic active hepatitis	Protection with hepatitis B vaccination
Hepatitis C	RNA	Blood products Intravenous drug abuse Sexual contact Healthcare workplace exposure	HVC RNA	Subclinical hepatitis Chronic active hepatitis common FHF rare Cirrhosis and hepatocellular carcinoma	HIG and antiviral therapy (exposure) Interferon No vaccine
Hepatitis E	RNA	Fecal–oral contamination of water in tropical climates	HVE-Ag HVE-AB	Self-limited FHF a risk during pregnancy	Vaccine pending
Hepatitis G	RNA	Possibly blood products Unknown		Uncertain May coexist with hepatitis C	None

FHF, fulminant hepatic failure; HIG, human immunoglobulin; HVA, hepatitis A; HVB, hepatitis B; HVC, hepatitis C virus; HVD, hantavirus disease; HVE, hepatitis E.

Data from Hoofnagle JH, di Bisceglie AM. The treatment of chronic viral hepatitis. *N Engl J Med.* 1997;336:347.

All forms of viral hepatitis show diffuse acute inflammation with leukocyte and histiocyte infiltration followed by hepatic necrosis and regeneration with recovery. Zone 3 hepatocytes suffer the greatest injury. Inflammation may be limited to zone 3 in mild forms of viral hepatitis, or it may extend to the entire acinus in fulminant hepatic necrosis. When the entire acinus is involved, the patient will eventually develop postnecrotic scarring with fibrosis (bridging fibrosis).

Hepatitis A is the least severe of the known forms of viral hepatitis. The fecal–oral route, typically by way of consumption of contaminated drinking water or uncooked shellfish, is the mode of transmission of hepatitis A. The incubation period for the disease is approximately equal to or greater than 15 days, and plasma transaminases and bilirubin levels may not rise until several weeks into the course of disease.

Although recovery may take several weeks to months, most patients with hepatitis A have an unpleasant course but uncomplicated recovery. Fulminant hepatic necrosis with liver failure requiring transplantation is extremely rare with hepatitis A infection.

Hepatitis E is a form of viral hepatitis that is very similar to hepatitis A. It occurs in developing countries where there is fecal contamination of the drinking water. Fulminant hepatic failure following hepatitis E infection can be a serious complication in the third trimester of pregnancy.[48]

Although hepatitis B is often an anicteric illness, it can lead to either fulminant hepatic necrosis with acute liver failure or to chronic hepatitis. Hepatitis B is transmitted through sexual contact or exposure to infected blood products. Hepatitis B is a viral infection of the liver caused by a complex virion that contains double-stranded DNA, DNA polymerase, a surface antigen (HBsAg), a core antigen, and the e antigen. The antigens and antibodies found in patients with hepatitis B form the basis for both diagnosis and prognosis. HBsAg is present in the bloodstream during the acute phase of the disease and persists for more than 6 months if the patient becomes a carrier of hepatitis B. HBsAg disappears with recovery and is replaced with the antibody (anti-HB) to HBsAg. Anti–hepatitis-B antibodies (anti-HBs) persist and are evidence of prior hepatitis B infection or exposure. Serum immunoglobulin M (IgM) antibodies to the core antigen (HBcAb) rise during the acute phase of infection and then disappear.

Bodily fluids, including blood, urine, saliva and semen, have been shown to carry hepatitis B virus (HBV) DNA in samples obtained from HBsAg-positive patients. HBsAg is routinely tested by radioimmunoassay in all blood donors in the United States and Europe and is found in approximately 0.1% of potential first-time blood donors. High-risk populations are identified by predonation questionnaires. Testing has contributed significantly to the reduction in the risk of viral hepatitis from the transfusion of blood or blood products (1:75 000). Today, hepatitis B vaccination of health care workers is mandated by institutional regulation, but in the past there were reports of health care workers who had become carriers of hepatitis B and had transmitted the disease to their patients.[49]

Hepatitis D is a severe viral infection of the liver that occurs as a coinfection of a patient with acute hepatitis B or as a superinfection in a patient with chronic hepatitis B, but hepatitis D does not cause hepatitis independently. In Western cultures, it occurs most often in patients with a history of intravenous drug abuse, but health care workers and transfusion recipients are also at risk, as are other patients who have acquired acute or chronic active hepatitis B.

Hepatitis C virus is an enveloped single-stranded RNA virus. Immunologic identification of infection with the hepatitis C virus (HCV) can be difficult. Antibodies against hepatitis C may not be present for long periods after initial infection. However, routine testing of donated blood for HCV and HIV by polymerase chain reaction (PCR) has reduced the incidence of transmission of hepatitis C and HIV to approximately 1:2 000 000 transfusions. Much like hepatitis B, those patients at increased risk of hepatitis C include recipients of blood products, intravenous drug abusers, hemophiliacs, and health care workers after hollow needle sticks. Sexual transmission of hepatitis C is possible.

Hepatitis C rarely causes fulminant hepatic failure; in fact subclinical, chronic, nonicteric infection is fairly common. Unfortunately, approximately half of the patients with acute hepatitis C infection will have evidence of ongoing hepatitis after 1 year. At least 20% of these patients will eventually develop cirrhosis. These patients are also at high risk of developing hepatocellular carcinoma through several possible immunologic and genetic events.[50] There is no vaccine yet to prevent hepatitis C infection.

An RNA virus has been identified in the serum of blood donors and blood recipients that may be responsible for the remaining portion of cases of transfusion hepatitis. This virus has been classified as non-A, non-B, and non-C.[51] However, many of the patients who have received blood products containing this RNA virus did not develop clinical or laboratory signs of hepatocellular injury. In the few cases that have been followed for months to a few years, hepatitis G virus RNA has been present in the serum of some patients, suggesting the possibility of a persistent viral infection, but the target organ may not be the liver.[52] To add to the confusion on this issue, the so-called hepatitis G virus may be an agent that coexists with the hepatitis C virus.

Hepatitis can occur from systemic infections caused by other viruses, such as the Epstein-Barr virus (infectious mononucleosis) and cytomegalovirus. These are important infections of immunocompromised patients.

Chronic Hepatitis The histologic findings on needle biopsy of the liver will define several types of chronic hepatitis, including, in increasing order of severity, chronic persistent, chronic lobular, mild chronic active, and severe chronic active hepatitis. The extent of portal hepatitis, the degree of necrosis, and the presence of fibrosis all indicate increasing severity. Viral hepatitis, autoimmune hepatitis, and drug-induced hepatitis are the most common causes of chronic hepatitis. Of the viral diseases, hepatitis B and hepatitis C are the most important.

When all other causes of hepatitis have been eliminated, there remains a group of patients with cirrhosis with no identifiable etiology. These patients are given the diagnosis of cryptogenic cirrhosis, a diagnosis of exclusion, but one with the features of advanced cirrhosis.

The role of liver transplantation for the treatment of chronic hepatitis is discussed in Chapter 57.

HEPATOTOXICITY

Because the liver plays a central role in drug metabolism and first-pass detoxification of ingested substances, it is susceptible to the toxicity of these substances and their metabolites. This toxicity can be induced by more than a thousand drugs and other compounds, resulting in a wide range of liver dysfunction from mildly elevated liver function tests to acute liver failure. Drug overdose or reactions account for the majority of patients admitted with acute liver failure. Acetaminophen overdose is the most common drug-related cause, accounting for nearly 40% of cases in a large multicenter study.[53]

Alcoholic Liver Disease The excessive daily consumption of alcohol can lead to alcoholic hepatitis, especially in individuals with a low-calorie and low-protein diet. Ingestion of 80 g of alcohol a day places the individual at risk for alcoholic hepatitis, a precirrhotic lesion. Chronic consumption of lower doses of alcohol may lead to fatty infiltration of the liver and, eventually, to cirrhosis of the liver.

Alcohol is metabolized by alcohol dehydrogenase to acetaldehyde. Acetaldehyde dehydrogenase is the rate-limiting step in eliminating acetaldehyde, but it can be overwhelmed when large amounts of alcohol are ingested. Acetaldehyde, when it cannot be rapidly eliminated, is toxic to a number of cellular components and can lead to zone 3 hepatic necrosis. Alcohol can also be metabolized by the microsomal ethanol-oxidizing system, an alcohol-inducible P450 enzyme that also metabolizes acetaminophen.

Severe hepatitis secondary to alcohol ingestion alone is rare; however, a fatty liver and chronic alcoholic hepatitis will lead to cirrhosis. Advanced cirrhosis secondary to long-term alcohol abuse is irreversible, and patients will demonstrate the cardinal features of portal hypertension secondary to the obliteration of portal venules. In the early stages, patients with alcoholic cirrhosis do well compared with those with cirrhosis of other etiologies, provided they abstain from alcohol and correct the nutritional deficiencies (primarily vitamins and protein) that are associated with alcohol abuse. However, the 5-year survival rate in patients with ascites, jaundice, and variceal bleeding who are from higher socioeconomic backgrounds is 50% overall, 40% with continued alcohol abuse, and 60% with abstinence. With patients in lower socioeconomic groups the chance of survival is lower and can be as low as 50% at 33 months. Chronic alcohol abuse of greater than 90 g (6-7 standard drinks) per day for more than 5 years can lead to alcoholic cardiomyopathy in addition to cirrhosis of the liver. Alcohol abuse is the leading cause of nonischemic cardiomyopathy in the United States.[54] Cardiac performance may improve with abstinence from alcohol.

Many patients with alcoholic cirrhosis often have concomitant risk factors for coronary atherosclerosis; others may have cardiac valvular abnormalities requiring valve replacement. Cardiac surgery performed using cardiopulmonary bypass has a high mortality rate, especially in Child-Pugh class B and class C patients.[55]

Acetaminophen Toxicity Suicide attempts are the most common cause of acetaminophen-induced hepatic necrosis and subsequent fulminant hepatic failure. The lethal adult dose of acetaminophen is approximately 10 g, but the lethal dose can be greatly reduced in patients with concomitant alcohol abuse or preexisting liver disease. Acetaminophen is metabolized by the P450 system in the macrosomes of hepatocytes to metabolites (*N*-acetyl-*p*-benzoquinone) (**Fig. 15-7**). Alcohol and drugs that induce the P450 system can therefore increase metabolism of acetaminophen, resulting in increased levels of its toxic metabolites. Glutathione normally binds to and clears the metabolites of acetaminophen, and its depletion may lead to accumulation of toxic acetaminophen metabolites. Acetylcysteine can increase the production of glutathione and may prevent hepatic necrosis.[56] Acetylcysteine is most effective when given intravenously or orally within 24 hours after the ingestion of acetaminophen, but it may be effective even if given up to 72 hours after ingestion.

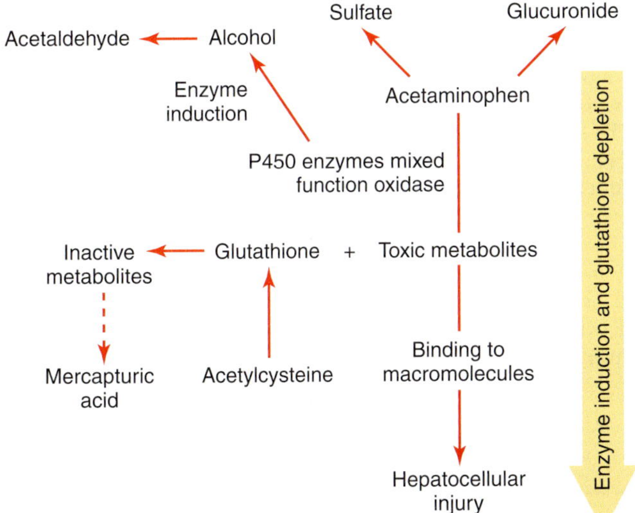

FIGURE 15-7. Mechanism of acetaminophen hepatotoxicity. Acetaminophen can be conjugated to a sulfate or a glucuronide prior to excretion. Alternatively, it can be oxidized to highly reactive compounds by P450 mixed function oxidases. Binding to glutathione inactivates these toxic compounds. When glutathione is depleted, the reactive metabolites bind to hepatocellular macromolecules and cause cell necrosis. P450 enzyme activity is induced by chronic alcohol ingestion. Increased P450 enzyme activity can deplete glutathione and enhance the toxic binding to macromolecules. Acetylcysteine can augment glutathione and prevent hepatic necrosis if given early after the ingestion of a lethal dose of acetaminophen. [Courtesy of Richard A. Wiklund, MD.]

Fulminant hepatic necrosis and acute liver failure can occur 2 to 3 days after an acetaminophen overdose. Plasma transaminases are markedly elevated during the first few days after ingestion. Coagulopathy can become severe when the INR increases. Severe coagulopathy and encephalopathy are signs of a poor prognosis. The outcome of acetaminophen-induced hepatic necrosis can be predicted by measuring the plasma level of acetaminophen 4 hours after ingestion. Blood levels greater than 300 μg/mL predict that hepatic necrosis will occur. Blood levels less than 120 μg/mL usually do not result in hepatic necrosis.

Halothane and Other Halogenated Anesthetics Halothane, a halogenated alkane, was introduced in the late 1950s. It was followed by methoxyflurane, the first of the halogenated methyl-ethyl ethers, which now include enflurane, isoflurane, desflurane, and sevoflurane. A series of case reports describing fulminant hepatic necrosis after surgery led to a review of 850 000 halothane anesthetics and the famous report of the National Halothane Study.[57,58] After other causes of severe acute liver failure were ruled out, 7 cases were identified wherein exposure to halothane was the probable cause. The controversy about the continued use of halogenated anesthetics gradually faded with the subsequent introduction of isoflurane and the replacement of halothane. As much as 17% to 20% of an administered dose of halothane undergoes oxidative and reductive metabolism, mostly in the liver. Reactive metabolites bind to hepatocellular proteins as haptens to produce antigens that can rarely provoke an immune response, evidenced by the appearance of immunoglobulins, an inflammatory response in the liver, eosinophilia, and hepatic necrosis. The immunologic basis of halothane hepatitis has been challenged by other theories suggesting that hepatic oxygen deprivation (decreased supply and increased demand) or direct toxicity of metabolites may be responsible. Massive hepatic necrosis was seen more often in patients with prior or frequent exposures to halothane. Few patients survived massive hepatic necrosis believed to be caused by halothane, which usually occurred before the era of liver transplantation.

OTHER HEPATOTOXINS

Many other drugs are hepatotoxic; their toxicity mimics other liver diseases. Carbon tetrachloride, for one, causes zone 3 hepatocyte necrosis. Valproic acid causes fatty infiltration of the liver. Drugs such as NSAIDs, methyldopa, amiodarone, nifedipine, and isoniazid may mimic acute viral hepatitis and chronic active hepatitis. Methotrexate may cause hepatic fibrosis and portal hypertension. Antibiotics, tranquilizers, and sex hormones may cause cholestasis. Sex hormone therapy may also cause thrombosis of portal and hepatic veins. In most cases of drug-induced hepatic dysfunction, recovery occurs after withdrawal of the drug. Recovery may be prolonged with a drug like amiodarone because of its long half-life and the extremely long time required for elimination of metabolites. Furthermore, some drugs, such as diazepam, can become "locked" in the enterohepatic circulation by the intestinal reabsorption of their potentially toxic metabolites.

AUTOIMMUNE AND INFLAMMATORY LIVER DISEASE

Autoimmune hepatitis, primary biliary cirrhosis, and primary sclerosing cholangitis appear to result from autoimmune mechanisms.[59] At times they are difficult to distinguish from each other or from other inflammatory disease such as viral hepatitis. Patients with these autoimmune diseases often do well after liver transplantation.

Autoimmune Hepatitis Autoimmune hepatitis is a disease characterized by autoantibodies against a variety of liver antigens, including mitochondrial and nuclear antigens. It is most common in young women.[60] Blood testing shows elevated γ-globulins and positive antinuclear antibodies. Early treatment with corticosteroids and anti-inflammatory drugs can slow the progression of this disease and delay or prevent the need for liver transplantation.[61] Azathioprine therapy can be used to decrease the dose and side effects of corticosteroid therapy and may eliminate the need for corticosteroids once remission is achieved.[62] Patients with autoimmune hepatitis may develop cirrhosis and hepatocellular carcinoma if the autoimmune process is not controlled.

Consequently, it is important to distinguish autoimmune hepatitis from other forms of hepatitis with similar histology on liver biopsy.

Primary biliary cirrhosis (PBC) is an inflammatory disease of the intrahepatic bile ducts.[63] Ninety percent of patients are women, with onset occurring between the ages of 30 and 70 years. PBC is characterized by severe jaundice, disproportionate to the other features of liver disease, and thus higher bilirubin levels are used for the Child-Pugh stratification. Serum bilirubin levels rise dramatically as the disease progresses and are predictive of the length of survival. Once serum bilirubin levels exceed 6 mg/dL, expected survival is less than 2 years.[64] Human leukocyte antigens (HLAs) expressed in bile ducts appear to be a target for the lymphocytes. Patients with PBC develop disabling cutaneous xanthomas of their hands and feet and severe pruritus. They may have other autoimmune diseases and can also have interstitial lung disease with giant cell granulomas. However, these patients appear clinically healthier than patients with similar levels of jaundice secondary to alcoholic cirrhosis and can do well after transplantation. It is unclear whether they are at risk of developing recurrent PBC in the transplanted liver.

Primary sclerosing cholangitis (PSC) is another inflammatory disease of the intra- and extrahepatic bile ducts of undetermined etiology affecting more men than women.[65] It may be difficult to distinguish in the early phases from primary biliary cirrhosis. Serum antimitochondrial antibodies are positive in primary biliary cirrhosis and negative in primary sclerosing cholangitis. This inflammatory disease will eventually obliterate the bile ducts, causing jaundice and then liver failure. Cholangiography reveals a characteristic beading and stenosis of the common bile duct. Ulcerative colitis is diagnosed in as many as 70% of patients with primary sclerosing cholangitis.[66] In addition, PSC patients are at increased risk of developing cholangiocarcinoma. The only successful treatment of primary sclerosing cholangitis is liver transplantation.

AMYLOIDOSIS

Amyloidosis is often not a single-organ disease, and its variants can involve single or multiple organs.[67] Each variant involves infiltration of a fibrillar, insoluble protein with a unique pleated structure.[68] The liver is involved in most forms of amyloidosis, but infiltration of the kidneys or heart may produce for most of the clinical symptoms. Treatment includes chemotherapy for primary amyloidosis and treatment of the underlying disease in secondary amyloidosis. The causes of death from the amyloidoses include sepsis from the underlying disease, renal failure, or cardiac failure, but usually not liver failure. In rare cases of slowly progressive primary amyloidosis (multiple myeloma), liver transplantation may be recommended for liver dysfunction.[69]

MALIGNANT LIVER DISEASE

Hepatocellular carcinoma (HCC) is rare in Western countries, but common in Asian and African countries. It can present as a discrete encapsulated mass (most common in Asian countries), as an infiltrative disease, or as a multicentric disease (most common in the United States). Predisposing factors for HCC include chronic active viral hepatitis, hemochromatosis, long-standing heavy alcohol abuse, cigarette smoking, diabetes, and fatty liver.[70,71] α-Fetoprotein is a biochemical marker for HCC. Serial plasma levels correlate with the growth of HCC, as well as with improvement after tumor mass resection. Hepatic resection for HCC in patients with intact synthetic liver function offers a 26% 5-year survival rate.[72] Liver transplantation as a therapy for limited HCC is now an established therapy (see Chapter 57).

Cholangiocarcinoma is a highly malignant disease that is rare in the Western world, but endemic in Asia.[73] It is also associated with primary sclerosing cholangitis and ulcerative colitis. Liver transplantation is contraindicated for patients with advanced cholangiocarcinoma. Patients are often jaundiced but without other signs of liver failure. When the tumor involves the secondary branches of the left and right hepatic ducts, it is not resectable, but palliation can be achieved with stenting of the bile ducts.[74]

VASCULAR DISEASES OF THE LIVER

Hepatic vein thrombosis (Budd-Chiari syndrome) is usually secondary to another systemic disease, often a myeloproliferative disorder.[75] This syndrome can be acute or chronic and can be asymptomatic or lead to chronic liver failure. Treatment options include anticoagulation in the absence of a coagulopathy, thrombectomy, thrombolysis, transjugular intrahepatic portosystemic shunting (TIPS), or liver transplantation.[76,77]

Portal vein thrombosis is most often a complication of orthotopic liver transplantation.

LIVER FAILURE

ACUTE LIVER FAILURE

Acute liver failure, or fulminant hepatic failure (FHF), is a catastrophic illness resulting from many of the liver diseases described in this chapter; it develops within 2 weeks of the onset of disease and carries a poor prognosis without transplantation. It occurs so rapidly that patients may not have developed jaundice. Subfulminant hepatic failure, with onset occurring up to 8 weeks after the onset of jaundice, has a better prognosis, with some chance of complete recovery. Transaminase levels rise rapidly with FHF, but they may fall to normal levels after massive necrosis occurs. Coagulopathy can become progressively more severe.

The common features of fulminant hepatic failure include a severe coagulopathy, metabolic acidosis, hypoglycemia, rapidly progressive encephalopathy, and acute renal failure.[78] Cerebral edema is the usual cause of death, which may occur while the patient awaits a donor liver (**Table 15-9**).

The most common cause of FHF is acute viral hepatitis (A, B, others). FHF in patients with hepatitis B can be precipitated by superinfection with hepatitis D. Immunocompromised patients are at high risk for FHF with acute viral hepatitis, including hepatitis A and B, herpes simplex, cytomegalovirus, Epstein-Barr virus, and varicella.[79]

TABLE 15-9 Grading of Hepatic Encephalopathy

Grade	Consciousness	Cognition	Signs	Electroencephalogram (EEG)
0	Normal	Normal	None	Normal
Subclinical	Normal	Normal	Abnormal on psychometric testing	Normal
1	Restless; abnormal sleep pattern	Forgetful, confused, agitated	Tremor, ataxia, uncoordinated, impaired handwriting	Abnormal
2	Lethargic	Disoriented at times; uninhibited, inappropriate behavior	Asterixis, dysarthria, ataxia, hyporeflexia	Abnormal
3	Somnolent but rousable, confused	Disoriented, aggressive	Asterixis, hyperreflexia, Babinski sign, muscle rigidity	Abnormal
4	Coma	None	Decerebration	Abnormal

Modified with permission from Riordan SM, Williams R. Treatment of hepatic encephalopathy. *N Engl J Med.* 1997;337:473.

There is another cause of FHF that needs to be considered in surgical patients. Alterations of total hepatic blood flow during anesthesia and surgery may precipitate FHF in patients with stable, underlying chronic liver disease. In these patients, acute liver failure is usually noticed on the second or third postoperative day and can be manifested by an unexplained encephalopathy. These patients have adequate hepatocellular function preoperatively but with very little reserve to combat acute stress associated with anesthesia and surgery. Small decreases in hepatic oxygen supply associated with decreased total hepatic blood flow during surgery cause acute hepatocellular ischemic injury and failure. The encephalopathy of FHF is different than that noted with chronic liver failure, and the blood ammonia levels are much higher. In addition, amino acids, which can contribute to the encephalopathy, accumulate in the central nervous system and are excreted in the urine as tyrosine and leucine crystals; FHF with grade 3 or worse encephalopathy is associated with an 80% mortality rate. In contrast, two-thirds of patients survive if encephalopathy does not proceed beyond grade 2.[80] The principal causes of death are cerebral edema, hemorrhage secondary to a severe coagulopathy, and sepsis syndrome secondary to pneumonia.

Metabolic derangements seen in FHF may include severe hypoglycemia, hyperinsulinemia, hyponatremia, hypokalemia, and lactic acidosis. Respiratory alkalosis may be caused by hyperventilation. Acute renal failure (hepatorenal syndrome) is seen in as many as 55% of patients with FHF. Acute respiratory failure may be caused by aspiration pneumonitis or form part of the multiorgan failure associated with sepsis.

Survival is frequent with transplantation, but many patients die while awaiting the availability of a donor organ.

CHRONIC LIVER FAILURE

Chronic liver failure eventually can impair most of the organ systems in the body. Many of the manifestations are caused by the hepatic fibrosis that follows hepatocellular injury. Portal fibrosis produces compression of the portal venules, capillaries, and biliary canaliculi and obliteration of hepatocytes. The result is portal hypertension, obstructive jaundice, coagulopathy, encephalopathy, and metabolic abnormalities. If the underlying cause of fibrosis is treated effectively, fibrosis of the liver may be reversible.[81] In the early stages of chronic liver failure (Child-Pugh class A), ascites is controlled with diuretic therapy. In later stages, ascites is uncontrolled, and patients develop the protuberant abdomen, with a fluid wave on physical examination that is typical of advanced cirrhosis (**Box 15-1**). Portal hypertension leads to abnormal renal function, with marked sodium reabsorption in response to a decreased effective circulating plasma volume. Volume receptor stimulation increases renin secretion and aldosterone production. Urinary excretion of sodium is limited, and total body sodium is greatly increased, yet the patient shows mild hyponatremia. This forms the basis for therapy with loop diuretics, such as furosemide, and aldosterone antagonists, such as spironolactone. Renal blood flow and glomerular filtration rate can be decreased in chronic liver failure because of the increased intra-abdominal pressure caused by ascites, diuretic therapy, and other hemodynamic abnormalities.

BOX 15-1

Physical Findings Suggestive of Advanced Cirrhosis

Scleral icterus
Fetor hepaticus
Asterixis
Neck vein distension
Spider angiomata
Caput medusa
Abdominal distension with demonstrable fluid wave
Palpable liver with appreciable nodular hyperplasia
Splenomegaly

Ascites is associated with spontaneous bacterial peritonitis (SBP), another life-threatening complication of chronic liver failure. An aerobic gram-negative organism is the usual cause of the peritonitis. It may be truly spontaneous and caused by incidental bacteremia but often follows paracentesis to reduce the volume of ascites. The 30-day mortality rate for SBP is approximately 32%; 1-year mortality 78%.[82] Survivors are at high risk of recurrence.

Portal hypertension can lead to the development of collateral circulation, with large veins in the abdominal and chest walls, the mediastinum, stomach, and esophagus. In extreme cases these venous collaterals can anastomose with pulmonary vessels, leading to portopulmonary shunting. This can produce a high-blood volume, high-blood flow state with intrapulmonary shunts, the so-called hepatopulmonary syndrome (HPS). The collateral circulation that occurs with portal hypertension can produce esophageal, gastric, and intestinal varices that are prone to rupture and bleeding.

Obstructive jaundice is a late finding in most forms of cirrhosis and indicates a poor prognosis. Severe jaundice predicts death within a few years. Severe jaundice is usually accompanied by poor synthetic function with coagulopathy, progressive encephalopathy, and severe malnutrition.

There are 2 causes of the coagulopathy associated with chronic liver disease. The first is decreased production of coagulation factors produced in the liver (all except factor VIII); the second is the hypersplenism resulting from portal hypertension. Measuring the INR, plasma fibrinogen level, or direct measurement of coagulation factor activity readily assesses coagulopathy secondary to impaired synthetic function. Hypersplenism with sequestration of platelets is common in advanced liver disease and results in platelet concentration 70 000/μL or less. Bleeding from thrombocytopenia is uncommon unless it is complicated by other causes of thrombocytopenia, such as active bleeding with either a consumption coagulopathy or a dilutional coagulopathy. Metabolic abnormalities include hypoglycemia, hyperinsulinemia, aminoacidemia and aminoaciduria, respiratory alkalosis, lactic acidosis, hyponatremia, and hypokalemia. If patients require rapid multiple transfusions, hypocalcemia secondary to citrate toxicity may become a problem.

Encephalopathy in chronic liver failure is associated with elevation of the plasma ammonia level. However, the cause of hepatic encephalopathy is much more complex than ammonia intoxication. Ammonia is only one of the many potentially neurotoxic compounds that are produced in the intestines and reach the brain by virtue of the collateral portosystemic shunting of chronic liver disease. Other compounds that contribute to encephalopathy include octopamine and the aromatic amino acids, tyrosine, phenylalanine, and tryptophan. Normally, the liver extracts all of these compounds from portal venous blood. Central nervous system γ-aminobutyric acid (GABA), an inhibitory neurotransmitter, is also increased in chronic liver disease, as are GABA and benzodiazepine receptors in the brain.[83]

There are other causes of abnormal neurologic findings in chronic liver disease. There can be generalized cortical atrophy and the increased presence of astrocytes, often associated with Alzheimer disease. The electroencephalogram (EEG) shows generalized slowing. Vitamin deficiencies can lead to Wernicke encephalopathy (inadequate thiamine and B_1), which also contributes to the neurologic findings of chronic liver disease. Portal-systemic encephalopathy is characterized by depressed consciousness, personality changes, slurred speech, apraxia, and a flapping tremor. Severity is graded from minimal confusion through coma (Table 15-9).[84] Grade 4 coma is usually a terminal event.

The circulation in chronic liver disease is hyperdynamic and characterized by a markedly increased cardiac index, a low systemic vascular resistance, mild tachycardia, a normal to increased stroke volume, a high mixed venous oxygen saturation, and a poor oxygen extraction ratio. Patients with a normal cardiac index at cardiac catheterization should be considered to have a cardiomyopathy, and the differential diagnosis should include ischemic cardiomyopathy, alcoholic cardiomyopathy, and cardiomyopathy secondary to hemochromatosis. Systemic precapillary arteriovenous shunting can cause the hemodynamic changes seen in chronic liver disease. Circulating blood volume is reduced, and extracellular fluid volume is often markedly increased.

Coronary artery disease in patients with advanced liver disease may require coronary revascularization. Patients who are Child-Pugh class A may tolerate coronary artery bypass grafting (CABG) with cardiopulmonary bypass without an increased mortality, but patients who are class B or C have an elevated risk of death.[85] Combined CABG and orthotopic liver transplantation has been performed, but there are insufficient data to support this intervention as a standard approach.[86]

Two pulmonary syndromes are noted in patients with advanced liver disease. The first is the HPS; the second is portopulmonary hypertension (PPH).[87] HPS, as described previously, is characterized by pulmonary precapillary and capillary vasodilatation and direct pulmonary arteriovenous communications. This syndrome is associated with 3-fold elevation of exhaled nitric oxide as compared with control subjects.[88] The patients are short of breath and cyanotic and display systemic arterial hypoxemia. Dyspnea with tachypnea and oxygen desaturation is worsened in the upright position, a syndrome described as platypnea and orthodeoxia.[89] This is a high-volume/low-pressure pulmonary blood state with normal right ventricular function and a low pulmonary vascular resistance.[90] PPH, on the other hand, is a high-pressure state similar to primary pulmonary hypertension. The right ventricle is often dilated, cyanosis is absent, right ventricular ejection fraction is low, and systemic hypoxia is rare. These patients may acutely respond to inhaled nitric oxide. Patients with HPS fare better after liver transplantation than do those with PPH.[91]

Hepatorenal syndrome is a form of renal failure associated with liver disease. It is more common in acute liver failure but also occurs in patients with chronic liver failure. Hepatorenal syndrome is the result of intense renal arteriolar vasoconstriction in response to the functional hypovolemia caused by splanchnic vasodilatation and other physical changes of liver failure.[92] Type 1 hepatorenal syndrome typically evolves over less than 1 week and is an indication for urgent liver transplantation.[92] Type 2 hepatorenal syndrome develops over a period of months and is less of an emergency. Standard treatment of hepatorenal syndrome includes intravascular volume expansion with administration of albumin, and the reduction in intra-abdominal pressure by relieving tense ascites. The prognosis of the hepatorenal syndrome is poor. The administration of a vasopressin analogue, terlipressin, may improve renal function by its action as a splanchnic vasoconstrictor.[93] Portal venous pressure reduction by TIPS has been used for hepatorenal syndrome, but it is not recommended on the basis of controlled clinical trials.[94]

APPROACH TO MANAGEMENT

CORRECTION OF COAGULOPATHY

Fresh-frozen plasma infusion and/or cryoprecipitate administration greatly improve the coagulopathy of either acute or chronic liver failure.[95] Recombinant factor VII may also improve the coagulopathy.[96,97] Therapy should be guided by measurement of the INR, plasma fibrinogen levels, and specific coagulation factor analysis when available. Patients may require infusion of large volumes of fresh-frozen plasma, which can itself contribute to circulatory overload. If there is evidence of a consumption coagulopathy, ε-aminocaproic acid can be administered. It is important to avoid the inadvertent administration of small doses of heparin via monitoring lines to patients with a coagulopathy secondary to liver disease. Platelet transfusion is not indicated unless the platelet count is less than 70 000/μL. Platelets can be sequestered in the spleen when the patient has hypersplenism. The coagulopathy can be monitored by the use of the thrombelastogram (TEG).[98,99] Coagulopathy (**Fig. 15-8**) is manifested on the TEG by a delayed onset of coagulation (prolonged R time), decreased or flattened slope (A), and decreased maximum amplitude (MA). A useful technique to rule out inadvertent heparin administration is to perform a dual assay using heparinase in 1 cuvette of the TEG assay. A normal tracing in the presence of heparinase and an abnormal tracing without suggest a significant heparin anticoagulant effect.

VARICES AND VARICEAL HEMORRHAGE

Endoscopic band ligation therapy is the mainstay of treatment to reduce esophageal varices and prevent variceal hemorrhage.[100] Treatment with nonspecific β-adrenergic blockers, particularly propranolol and nadolol,[101,102] may decrease the size of esophageal varices. However, these agents do not reduce the portal hypertension, which caused the development of the varices.

Portal decompression can be accomplished surgically (portocaval shunt, mesocaval shunt, splenorenal shunt) or by means of a transjugular intrahepatic portal vein-to-hepatic vein shunt.[103] TIPS has a high complication rate and a mortality rate that is similar to that reported by centers with extensive experience in surgical shunting.[104] However, recent

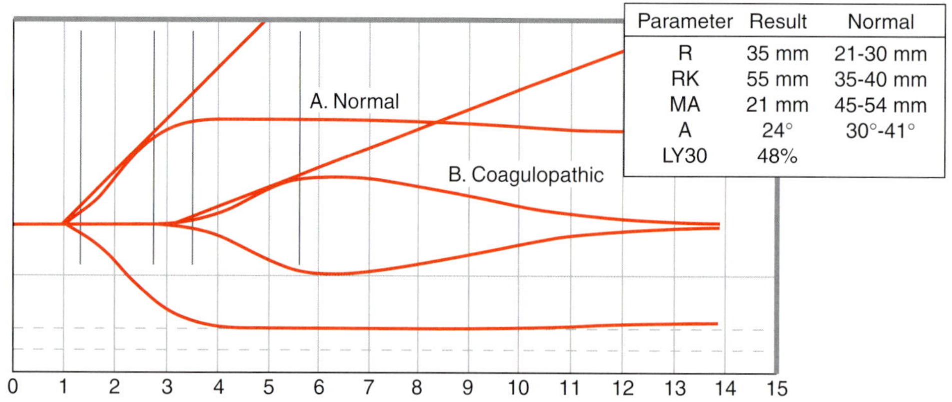

Parameter	Result	Normal
R	35 mm	21-30 mm
RK	55 mm	35-40 mm
MA	21 mm	45-54 mm
A	24°	30°-41°
LY30	48%	

FIGURE 15-8. Thrombelastogram. **A.** Normal onset of coagulation, normal platelet function, no significant fibrinolysis. **B.** Delayed onset of coagulation (prolonged R value and diminished angle A), evidence of decreased platelet function (diminished maximum amplitude [MA]), and early onset of marked fibrinolysis (decreased amplitude at 30 minutes [LY30]). [Courtesy of Richard A. Wiklund, MD.]

evidence suggests that early use of TIPS in patients with cirrhosis and variceal bleeding reduces treatment failure.[105] Preexisting encephalopathy may preclude any form of portal shunting because of the decrease in ammonia extraction that follows the decrease in portal vein blood flow to the liver.[106]

Octreotide is a somatostatin[107] that has been used for control of nonvariceal upper and lower gastrointestinal bleeding secondary to portal hypertension.[9,108] It is administered as a continuous infusion and produces vasoconstriction of the portal circulation vessels.

ASCITES

Ascites is the accumulation of an extracellular colloidal fluid in the abdominal cavity as a result of long-standing portal hypertension. It is a consistent finding in patients with cirrhosis, and it is a poor prognostic finding, as only 50% of patients with ascites will survive for 2 years.[109] The diagnosis of ascites can be made by ultrasonography when it is not apparent on physical examination. Ascites can be controlled by restriction of sodium intake in the diet, by the administration of diuretics, or by abdominal paracentesis. Dietary sodium restriction is often difficult to maintain because of noncompliance. Diuretic therapy includes the use of furosemide and spironolactone or amiloride. Optimal diuretic therapy requires several weeks during which time the balance of sodium intake versus renal excretion of sodium is monitored. Potassium balance is achieved with the use of potassium-wasting diuretics (furosemide) and potassium-sparing diuretics (spironolactone or amiloride). If diuretic therapy is ineffective, invasive procedures may be necessary to relieve tense abdominal swelling. These procedures include large volumes of fluid removal by paracentesis, peritoneovenous shunting (LeVeen shunt), or TIPS. Large-volume paracentesis leads to progressive wasting of protein but not usually to hemodynamic instability. Slow removal of ascites by paracentesis can relieve the symptoms of massive ascites and improve quality of life for these patients.[109]

Currently, peritoneovenous shunting is performed infrequently because of the risks associated with the procedure and the lack of advantages over paracentesis and TIPS.[110] The risks include hepatic failure secondary to a major surgical procedure in patients with marginal hepatocellular function, the risk of bacterial contamination with subsequent peritonitis, and the risk of a postoperative ascites leak. The procedure can be complicated by thrombosis followed by nonfunction of the shunt. Fluid overload is another consideration in patients who may have a concomitant cardiomyopathy.

CONTROL OF ENCEPHALOPATHY

Encephalopathy is present in the majority of patients with cirrhosis, although at times it may only be demonstrated by psychometric testing.[111] Because encephalopathy can progress rapidly from subclinical findings to overt coma, it should be anticipated in any patient with cirrhosis undergoing surgery. Encephalopathy is graded according to the level of consciousness, personality and intellectual features, neurologic signs, and electroencephalographic findings (Table 15-9).[84] Standard therapy for the cerebral edema contributing to grade 3 and grade 4 encephalopathy includes endotracheal intubation, moderate hyperventilation, and monitoring and control of intracranial pressure (ICP). ICP monitoring involves substantial risk of intracranial hemorrhage in coagulopathic patients. Control of ICP may prevent seizures, which may exacerbate elevated ICP.

Encephalopathy can be improved in the short term by limiting protein in the diet. Obviously this counters the objective of improving protein nutrition in chronic liver disease, but limitation of protein in the diet will decrease the amount of nitrogenous waste and ammonia produced in the bowel. Ammonia is an uncharged molecule that readily passes into the blood from the gut. It can be converted to ammonium ion in the presence of excess hydrogen ions; ammonium ion does not cross the gut mucosa. Conversion of ammonia to ammonium ion can be achieved by the oral administration of lactulose, an enzyme that increases the acid content of the colon.[112] Acidification of the stool traps ammonia as ammonium ion in the gut contents. Neomycin can reduce the number of bacteria producing ammonia from protein.

If encephalopathy is life-threatening, charcoal hemoperfusion can be used to eliminate the responsible metabolites from the blood. So can exchange transfusion and extracorporeal organ perfusion.[113,114] However, these are experimental therapies that may worsen the coagulopathy and are used only as a bridge to transplantation.

SUMMARY

The liver is a complex organ that serves multiple functions, including protein synthesis, carbohydrate and lipid metabolism, excretion of waste products, and drug metabolism. Recognizing that each of these vital functions can be impaired with liver disease leads to an understanding of the primary features of liver failure, namely ascites, jaundice, coagulopathy, encephalopathy, altered metabolism, and abnormal fluid balance. Cirrhosis is the final common histologic manifestation of most forms of liver disease.

In the preadmission anesthesia assessment clinic, the severity of liver disease and the risk of surgery can be estimated using the Child-Pugh and MELD scoring systems. The Child-Pugh includes 2 clinical and 3 laboratory assessments. The clinical features are the degree of ascites and the history of encephalopathy; laboratory assessments are determination of the INR and plasma albumin and bilirubin levels. Each of these 5 parameters can be assessed as normal or near normal (class A), moderately abnormal or fairly well controlled (class B), and markedly abnormal or poorly controlled (class C). The surgical mortality rate, particularly for intra-abdominal and other major surgery, is near 10% for patients assessed to be class A, up to 30% for class B, and up to 70% for class C. The MELD uses just 3 laboratory assessments (INR, creatinine, and bilirubin) and is now widely used in surgical risk prediction.

Preoperative preparation includes correction of coagulopathy by the administration of fresh-frozen plasma or cryoprecipitate, control of ascites with diuretic therapy or paracentesis, and correction of encephalopathy by limiting protein intake and the administration of lactulose. Transfusion of packed red blood cells may be necessary to correct blood loss from bleeding esophageal varices. Preoperative platelet transfusion is usually unnecessary unless the platelet count is less than 70 000/μL. Prevention of sepsis by minimizing invasive procedures and use of strict sterile technique for the insertion of lines and surgery is extremely important. These steps may reduce the risk of complications or death for surgical patients with acute or chronic liver disease.

Acute liver failure should be anticipated in the postoperative period in patients presenting with marginal liver function, especially following intra-abdominal procedures, because of the effects of surgery and anesthesia to decrease total hepatic blood flow.

Hepatitis B and C viruses are highly infective after exposure. Immunization against hepatitis B virus is critically important for all health care workers, especially anesthesia providers, because it is effective and safe. Hepatitis B can be a fulminant illness with high mortality. Immunization against hepatitis C virus is not available. Exposure caused by accidental hollow-needle sticks can cause acute hepatitis C infection, which has a high risk of evolving into chronic active hepatitis, cirrhosis, and hepatocellular carcinoma. Most hospitals offer the options for prophylaxis against viral infection after inadvertent needle stick. These include the administration of hyperimmune γ-globulin for prophylaxis against transmission of hepatitis C. Universal precautions are effective in controlling the risk of transmission of hepatitis B and C.

With current testing standards in the United States, viral infection after the administration of blood products is rare, approximately 1:75 000 to 1:2 000 000 transfusions.

KEY REFERENCES

- Bunker JP. Final report of the National Halothane Study. *Anesthesiology.* 1968;29:231.
- Garrison RN, Cryer HM, Howard DA, Polk HC Jr. Clarification of risk factors for abdominal operations in patients with hepatic cirrhosis. *Ann Surg.* 1984;199:648.
- Gelman SI. Disturbances in hepatic blood flow during anesthesia and surgery. *Arch Surg.* 1976;111:881.
- Giannini EG, Testa R, Savarino V. Liver enzyme alteration: a guide for clinicians. *CMAJ.* 2005;172:367.
- Kamath PS, Kim WR. The model for end-stage liver disease (MELD). *Hepatology.* 2007;45(3):797-805.
- Lyew MA, Isaacson IJ. Template for rapid analysis of the thrombelastogram. *Anesth Analg.* 1992;74:782.
- O'Grady JG. Acute liver failure. *Postgrad Med J.* 2005;81:148.
- Piano MR. Alcoholic cardiomyopathy: incidence, clinical characteristics, and pathophysiology. *Chest.* 2002;121:1638.
- Pugh RN, Murray-Lyon IM, Dawson JL, Pietroni MC, Williams R. Transection of the oesophagus for bleeding oesophageal varices. *Br J Surg.* 1973;60:646.
- Riordan SM, Williams R. Treatment of hepatic encephalopathy. *N Engl J Med.* 1997;337:473.
- Shiffman ML, Jeffers L, Hoofnagle JH, Tralka TS. The role of transjugular intrahepatic portosystemic shunt for treatment of portal hypertension and its complications: a conference sponsored by the National Digestive Diseases Advisory Board. *Hepatology.* 1995;22:1591.
- Wiklund RA. Preoperative preparation of patients with advanced liver disease. *Crit Care Med.* 2004;32:S106.

REFERENCES

Complete references available on DVD and online version at www.LongneckerAnesthesiology.com

CHAPTER 16 Anesthetic Considerations for the Patient With Anemia and Coagulation Disorders

John C. Klick
Edwin G. Avery, IV

KEY POINTS

1. Anemia is common in perioperative patients.
2. Hemoglobin (Hb) concentration or hematocrit (HCT) level can be used to rapidly assess the severity of anemia.
3. Treatment of anemia should be based on the physiology and etiology of anemia. Maintenance and restoration of normovolemia and cardiac output (CO) are necessary but insufficient aims in treating anemia.
4. Tachycardia and hypotension are important clinical signs of hypovolemia and anemia, but compensatory increases in heart rate and CO may be impeded by an insufficient cardiac reserve or anesthetic-induced sympathectomy.
5. Consideration of the physiologic signs and laboratory evidence for inadequate tissue oxygen delivery is mandatory before making a decision to transfuse red blood cells (RBCs).
6. Evidence-based outcomes supporting a specific transfusion trigger level of Hb or HCT do not yet exist for perioperative patients; however, the limited present information suggests that Hb levels as low as 7 to 8 g/dL may be as safe as higher levels of Hb in cardiac surgical and critically ill patients without clinical evidence of ischemia. Further clinical investigations are needed to guide transfusion decisions in critically ill patients.
7. Alternatives to transfusion of allogeneic RBCs are available and should be integrated into a blood-conservation strategy for selected surgical patients.
8. Goals of the perioperative management of patients with sickle cell disease are focused on clinical measures to avoid precipitating a vaso-occlusive crisis and include avoiding hypoxia, hypothermia, and dehydration.
9. Implementation of standard or exchange transfusions for sickle cell patients with the goal of reducing Hb S concentration to less than 30% to 40% can be helpful to reduce the incidence of a perioperative vaso-occlusive crisis.

ANEMIA

Anemia is a common blood disorder of perioperative patients.[1] The primary physiologic consequence of severe anemia to the surgical patient is inadequate tissue oxygen delivery, which may lead to tissue hypoxia, biochemical imbalances, organ dysfunction, and ultimately organ damage.[2] Mismanagement of the anemic surgical patient can adversely affect perioperative outcomes.[3] Understanding the laboratory techniques used to assess anemia, the various anemia classifications, and the physiology and appropriate treatment of anemia permits the anesthesiologist to provide better perioperative care for anemic patients.

ANEMIA DEFINED AND MEASURED

Anemia is defined as a reduction in the total red cell mass (RCM). Both hematocrit (HCT) level and hemoglobin (Hb) concentration measurements reflect the body's RCM but do not define it. The HCT level, defined as the fractional volume of sampled blood that erythrocytes occupy, is an indirect measurement of the body's RCM (**Fig. 16-1**). The HCT is a simple, commonly used test to indirectly assess the severity of anemia as well as estimate whole-blood viscosity, oxygen-carrying capacity, and RCM.[4] Hb is the predominant protein component of blood and serves as the major carrier transporting oxygen, carbon dioxide, and some nitric oxide.[4,5] Hb concentration is a directly measured value that is commonly used to indirectly assess RCM. An isotopic dilution assay of tagged red cells can provide a more accurate assessment of RCM, but is not commonly used in clinical medicine because of the complex, costly, and impractical nature of performing a test that can require the use of radioisotopes.[4]

Although measurements of Hb and HCT values generally provide reliable estimates of a patient's RCM, they inaccurately reflect the total circulating RCM under certain conditions.[6,7] The importance of considering the measured HCT and Hb values in the context of overall blood volume cannot be overemphasized. Hb and HCT values are influenced by dynamic changes of plasma volume and thus can be subject to errors. Examples of when Hb or HCT values misrepresent the RCM occur in clinical scenarios involving major, acute blood loss. In this situation the concurrently obtained circulating Hb and HCT values will overestimate the RCM because there has not been sufficient time to redistribute fluid from the interstitial space into the intravascular compartment. The HCT and Hb values will then spuriously indicate an increased RCM. A second example of a failure of the HCT and Hb values to adequately reflect RCM occurs during pregnancy. During normal pregnancy both the RCM and the plasma volume expand. The plasma volume increases more rapidly and to a greater extent than the RCM and creates an apparent anemia termed the *physiologic anemia of pregnancy.*[7]

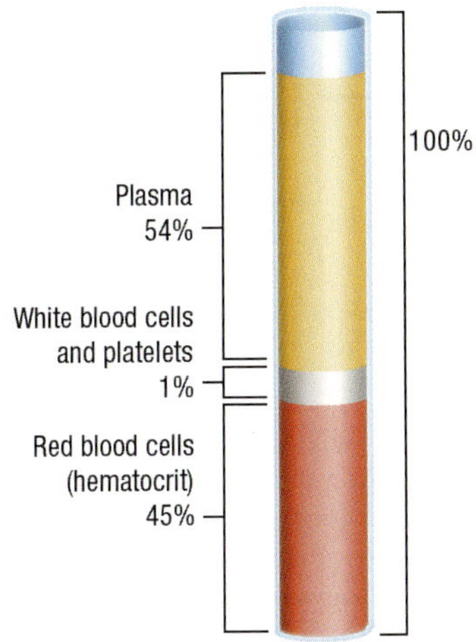

FIGURE 16-1. Graphic representation of a centrifuged sample of whole blood that illustrates its different components.

Beginning in the first trimester of pregnancy, the reduced HCT value does not represent a decreased RCM. Dehydration is a third example of when HCT and Hb values can misrepresent the RCM. In the dehydrated patient, an apparently normal or elevated HCT or Hb value can mislead the clinician to erroneously overestimating the patient's RCM.[6]

There are 2 necessary considerations when attempting to correctly identify anemia in an individual patient. First, the laboratory values of Hb and/or HCT must be compared with standard age/sex normalized reference values (**Table 16-1**).[8] Second, the patient's overall plasma volume status must be assessed to determine whether the patient is significantly plasma volume contracted (ie, dehydration, acute bleeding) or expanded (ie, anemia of pregnancy or volume overload).

PREVALENCE OF ANEMIA IN SURGICAL PATIENTS

Large studies reveal prevalence of anemia in the US population of 4.4% to 5.9%; however, the prevalence of anemia in surgical populations ranges from 5% to 75%.[1,9] Anemia may be produced or exacerbated in the perioperative period.[10]

RED BLOOD CELL MATURATION

Normal red blood cells (RBCs) mature by proliferation and differentiation of bone marrow precursor stem cells (ie, erythropoiesis) (**Fig. 16-2**). A mature RBC will circulate for a period of approximately 100 to 120 days, after which time it is removed from the circulation by the body's reticuloendothelial system. The body replenishes the total RCM with the goal of achieving a steady state depending on the rate at which RBCs are being produced and removed (or lost). The kidney plays a vital role in this process by producing the hormone erythropoietin. This process is up-regulated when the kidney responds to decreased oxygen delivery due to a contracted RCM (**Fig. 16-3**). Optimal erythropoiesis occurs when the body possesses sufficient substrates (eg, folate, iron, vitamin B_{12}, and other nutrients) to produce new erythrocytes.[8]

CLASSIFICATIONS OF ANEMIA

Anemia is classified as either (1) relative or (2) absolute on the basis of determining the total RCM. Relative anemia is characterized by a normal total RCM; this is a condition that does not represent a hematologic disorder but rather a disturbance in plasma volume regulation.[11] The absolute anemias (ie, those characterized by a decreased RCM) are divided into 3 classes: hemorrhage-related, hypoproliferative, and hyperproliferative anemias. Additionally, the anemias are classified as either primary or secondary. Secondary anemias result from a separate disease process that precipitates the decreased RCM. Many RBC-related laboratory parameters may help determine the etiology of anemia, including the reticulocyte count, mean corpuscular volume, and RBC size distribution. Examination of the peripheral smear using light microscopy can also aid in determining etiology. This chapter provides an introduction to various RBC parameters enabling classification of anemia rather than a comprehensive review of all known anemia diagnoses and their associated RBC parameter alterations. The association of these parameters with the various classes of anemia is summarized in **Tables 16-2** through **16-4**.[8]

Hemorrhage-Related Anemia Anemias due to acute or chronic loss of RCM are frequently encountered by the anesthesiologist.[1] The anesthetic implications for the various classes of anemias are discussed in a later section of this chapter (The Decision to Transfuse Red Blood Cells).

TABLE 16-1 Normal Red Blood Cell Values

	Hemoglobin (g/dL)		Hematocrit (%)		Red Cell Count (10^{12}/L)		MCV (fL)		MCH (pg)		MCHC (g/dL)	
Age	Mean	−2SD	Mean	−2SD	Mean	−2SD	Mean	−2SD	Mean	−2SD	Mean	−2SD
Birth (cord blood)	16.5	13.5	51	42	4.7	3.9	108	98	34	31	33	30
1-3 d (capillary)	18.5	14.5	56	45	5.2	4.0	108	95	34	31	33	29
1 wk	17.5	13.5	54	42	3.1	3.9	107	88	34	28	33	28
2 wk	16.5	12.5	51	39	4.9	3.6	105	86	34	28	33	28
1 mo	14.0	10.0	43	31	4.2	3.0	104	85	34	28	33	29
2 mo	11.5	9.0	35	28	3.8	2.7	96	77	30	26	33	29
3-6 mo	11.5	9.5	35	29	3.8	3.1	91	74	30	25	33	30
0.5-2 y	12.0	11.0	36	33	4.5	3.7	78	70	27	23	33	30
2-6 y	12.5	11.5	37	34	4.6	3.9	81	75	27	24	34	31
6-12 y	13.5	11.5	40	35	4.6	4.0	86	77	29	25	34	31
12-18 y												
Female	14.0	12.0	41	36	4.6	4.1	90	78	30	25	34	31
Male	14.5	13.0	43	37	4.9	4.5	88	78	30	25	34	31
18-49 y												
Female	14.0	12.0	41	36	4.6	4.0	90	80	30	26	34	31
Male	15.5	13.5	47	41	5.2	4.5	90	80	30	26	34	31

MCH, mean corpuscular hemoglobin; MCHC, mean corpuscular hemoglobin concentration; MCV, mean corpuscular volume.

Reproduced with permission from Marks PW, Glader B. Approach to anemia in the adult and child. In: Hoffman R, Benz EJ, Shattil SJ, et al. *Hematology: Basic Principles and Practice*. 5th ed. Philadelphia: Churchill Livingstone Elsevier; 2008:Chapter 34 online text.

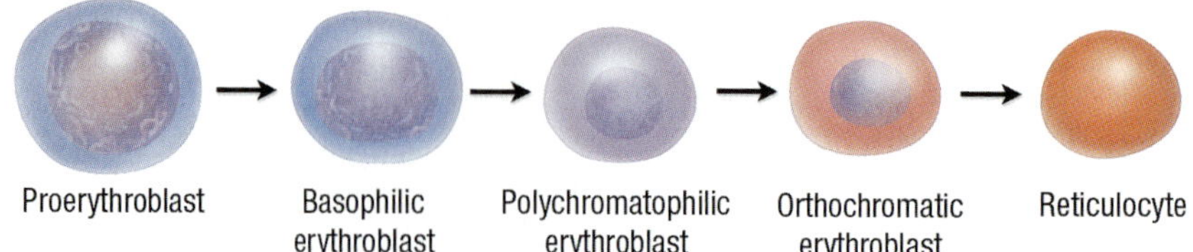

FIGURE 16-2. Illustration of the maturation of a reticulocyte before erythrocyte formation. [Reproduced with permission from Marks PW, Glader B. Approach to anemia in the adult and child. In: Hoffman R, Benz EJ, Shattil SJ, et al, eds. *Hematology: Basic Principles and Practice*. 5th ed. Philadelphia, PA: Churchill Livingstone Elsevier; 2008.]

Hypoproliferative Anemia Hypoproliferative anemias are common in surgical patients and are due to impaired RBC production. These anemias result from an inability to synthesize an adequate number of erythrocytes in response to a physiologic stimulus (eg, increased plasma erythropoietin levels). Hypoproliferative anemias (ie, absolute reticulocyte count <75 000/μL) are commonly due to acquired nutritional deficiencies (eg, iron deficiency anemia) and/or systemic disease (eg, anemia of chronic disease) (Table 16-2).[8]

Hyperproliferative Anemia Hyperproliferative anemias (ie, absolute reticulocyte count >100 000/μL) are commonly termed *hemolytic anemias*. These anemias occur due to premature destruction of RBCs and may be attributable to a host of disorders, either congenital or acquired, such as sickle cell anemia, β-thalassemia major, glucose-6-phosphate dehydrogenase deficiency, autoimmune hemolytic anemia, or microangiopathic hemolytic anemia. Sickle cell anemia has important implications for anesthetic management and is discussed in a later section of this chapter (Table 16-2).[8]

ANESTHESIA AND ANEMIA

The perioperative management of anemia frequently requires a decision of whether to transfuse RBCs or to consider transfusion alternatives (eg, use RBC salvage techniques). Making the best transfusion decision for an individual patient involves considering the balance of risks and advantages of transfusing allogeneic and/or autologous RBCs. We do not have prospective, randomized controlled trials to guide clinicians in making appropriate perioperative transfusion decisions. However, based on retrospective studies, it is likely that transfusing critically ill patients (especially with blood stored >14 days) is independently associated with significantly greater morbidity (ie, increased incidence of infection, multiorgan dysfunction syndrome, acute respiratory distress syndrome) and mortality.[3,12]

Hb concentration and HCT level are important predictors of transfusion risk; therefore, it is prudent to continue using these simple tests in concert with wise clinical judgment to make a transfusion decision for an individual patient.[13] Given the lack of supportive clinical trial data to guide our transfusion decisions, it is of paramount importance to fully understand the physiology of anemia. The subsequent sections of this chapter review the physiology of anemia, present a practical approach to determining an individual patient's transfusion threshold that is supported by the current studies, discuss alternatives to RBC transfusion and risks of RBC transfusion, and describe the special anesthetic considerations for patients with sickle cell disease.

Physiology of Anemia The physiologic response to anemia should be considered from at least 2 vantage points: acute anemia and chronic anemia. The physiologic response to acute anemia, most often due to hemorrhage, will depend on the extent and rate of acute blood loss. There are several normal physiologic responses to acute anemia that are related by the common goal of increasing blood flow and oxygen delivery to the peripheral tissues. Baroreceptor reflexes help to mediate the initial response to acute blood loss; chemoreceptors do not play a significant role.[14] Heart rate and minute alveolar ventilation initially increase after hemorrhage in the absence of volume replacement. Hyperventilation and tachycardia serve to increase cardiac output (CO) that in turn increases blood flow to tissues. The increased heart rate augments CO more directly than hyperventilation, which increases CO by augmenting right heart filling.[15] Acute hyperventilation reduces $Paco_2$,

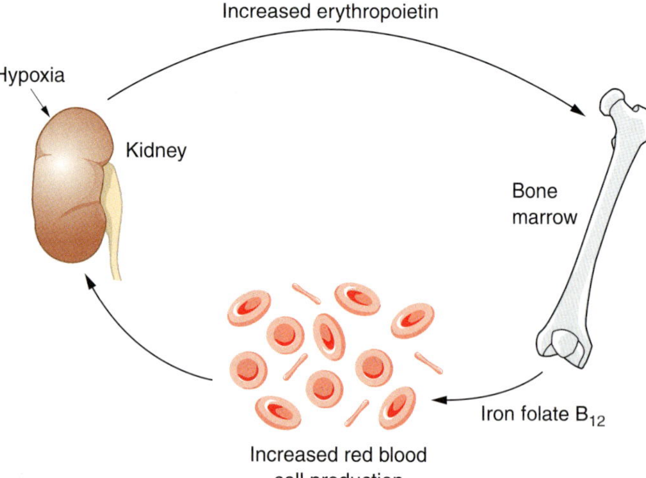

FIGURE 16-3. Regulation of erythropoiesis. [Reproduced with permission from Marks PW, Glader B. Approach to anemia in the adult and child. In: Hoffman R, Benz EJ, Shattil SJ, et al. *Hematology: Basic Principles and Practice*. 5th ed. Philadelphia, PA: Churchill Livingstone Elsevier; 2008:Chapter 34 online]

TABLE 16-2 Usefulness of the Reticulocyte Count in the Diagnosis of Anemia

Diagnosis	Value
Hypoproliferative anemias	Absolute reticulocyte count <75 000/μL
Anemia of chronic disease	
Anemia of renal disease	
Congenital dyserythropoietic anemias	
Effects of drugs or toxins	
Endocrine anemias	
Iron deficiency	
Marrow replacement	
Maturation abnormalities	Absolute reticulocyte count <75 000/μL
Vitamin B_{12} deficiency	
Folate deficiency	
Sideroblastic anemia	
Appropriate response to blood loss or nutritional supplementation	Absolute reticulocyte count >100 000/μL
Hemolytic anemias	
Hemoglobinopathies	
Immune hemolytic anemias	
Infectious causes of hemolysis	
Membrane abnormalities	
Metabolic abnormalities	
Mechanical hemolysis	

Reproduced with permission from Marks PW, Glader B. Approach to anemia in the adult and child. In: Hoffman R, Benz EJ, Shattil SJ, et al. *Hematology: Basic Principles and Practice*. 5th ed. Philadelphia: Churchill Livingstone Elsevier; 2008:Chapter 34 online.

TABLE 16-3 Usefulness of the Mean Corpuscular Value (MCV) and Red Blood Cell Distribution Width (RDW) in the Diagnosis of Anemia

	Low MCV (<80 fL)	Normal MCV (80-99 fL)	High MCV (>100 fL)
Normal RDW	Anemia of chronic disease alpha or beta Thalassemia trait Hemoglobin E trait	Acute blood loss Anemia of chronic disease Anemia of renal disease	Aplastic anemia Chronic liver disease Chemotherapy/antivirals/ alcohol
Elevated RDW	Iron deficiency Sickle cell, β-thalassemia	Early iron, folate, or vitamin B_{12} deficiency Dimorphic anemia (eg, iron + folate deficiency) Sickle cell anemia Sickle cell disease Chronic liver disease Myelodysplasia	Folate or vitamin B_{12} deficiency Immune hemolytic anemia Cytotoxic chemotherapy Chronic liver disease Myelodysplasia

Reproduced with permission from Marks PW, Glader B. Approach to anemia in the adult and child. In: Hoffman R, Benz EJ, Shattil SJ, et al. *Hematology: Basic Principles and Practice*. 5th ed. Philadelphia: Churchill Livingstone Elsevier; 2008:Chapter 34 online.

increasing pH_a, and both of these changes increase the oxygen saturation of arterial Hb via the Bohr effect; these changes favor a higher affinity of oxygen for the Hb molecule and decrease oxygen unloading at the tissues.[14,16] The reduced $Paco_2$ causes a left shift in the oxyhemoglobin dissociation curve, which augments oxygen uptake in the pulmonary capillaries but ultimately may decrease the amount of oxygen unloaded to tissues.[17] (**Fig. 16-4**). The increased CO that accompanies this left shift of the oxyhemoglobin dissociation curve may compensate for the higher affinity of oxygen for the Hb molecule. Insufficient cardiac reserve to increase CO and/or existing vascular dysfunction may worsen tissue hypoxia by interfering with compensatory mechanisms.[5,18]

Recent insights suggest that nitric oxide (NO) works in concert with the lungs and RBCs to provide additional regulation of both pulmonary and tissue blood flow augmenting O_2 delivery. NO is a free radical that is known to be a potent dilator of arterial microvasculature. NO is carried to hypoxic tissue beds by RBCs and nitrite and can serve to increase tissue blood flow.[5]

Concurrent with the rapid baroreceptor-mediated response to acute blood loss is the release of catecholamines, angiotension II, and vasoactive hormones.[14] These biochemical mediators increase systemic vascular resistance and systemic blood pressure. The increase in systemic vascular resistance is selective; blood flow is increased to a lesser extent to gut, skin, muscle, and renal tissue than to the heart and brain, so these vital organs receive preferential blood flow.[18] The increase in catecholamines also confers a positive inotropic and chronotropic effect on the heart that further augments CO.

Decreased intravascular volume stimulates the renin–angiotension–aldosterone axis, contributing to increasing CO and improving tissue oxygen delivery by water retention. Water retention augments cardiac preload.[18] Acute hemorrhage is associated with redistribution of water from the extravascular space into the intravascular space, accompanied by a decreased Hb concentration. As intravascular volume is replenished, Hb concentration and HCT level decline, reducing blood viscosity. Redistribution of water occurs rapidly with severe hemorrhage; a significantly lower Hb concentration is measurable within 2 minutes after an acute loss of 40% of the circulating blood volume. Complete fluid redistribution, however, takes hours. The rapid redistribution of water is attributable to the decreased hydrostatic pressure of the intravascular compartment and an increased plasma oncotic pressure due to acute mobilization of albumin from the interstitial matrix as well as increased hepatic production of glucose and amino acids.[19] The resulting lower blood viscosity serves to reduce resistance to blood flow and increase venous return to the right heart; these changes help to maintain or increase CO. Reduced resistance to blood flow reduces myocardial work and oxygen consumption despite the overall increased CO.[18]

If the rate of blood loss is too severe for these compensatory changes to restore blood flow to tissues, or cardiac performance cannot be increased due to preexisting cardiac pathology (eg, cardiomyopathy), then unmet tissue oxygen needs will result in lactic acid production and decreased pH_a. Under these conditions acidosis reduces the Hb–oxygen affinity augmenting the delivery of oxygen to hypoxic tissues (ie, there is a right shift of the oxyhemoglobin dissociation curve)[20] (Fig. 16-4).

Another compensatory mechanism for acute anemia occurs within the erythrocyte; RBCs can increase their intracellular concentration of 2,3-diphosphoglycerate (2,3-DPG), a product of anaerobic metabolism within RBCs. Increased levels of 2,3-DPG reduce the affinity of Hb for oxygen and result in decreased oxygen uptake in the pulmonary capillaries but result in increased tissue oxygen delivery (Fig. 16-4).[20] Stored allogeneic RBCs have lower 2,3-DPG levels immediately after transfusion (ie, there is a left shift of the oxyhemoglobin curve) and may not readily unload oxygen to tissues. It may take days for 2,3-DPG levels to increase in transfused red cells.

By linking NO and O_2 flux, RBCs effectively couple arterial vessel diameter (ie, resistance) to O_2 availability in the lung and to O_2

TABLE 16-4 Combining the Reticulocyte Count and Red Blood Cell Parameters for Diagnosis

	Corrected Reticulocyte Count <2%	Corrected Reticulocyte Count ≥2%
Low MCV, normal RDW	Anemia of chronic disease	
Normal MCV, normal RDW	Anemia of chronic disease	
High MCV, normal RDW	Chemotherapy/antivirals/alcohol Aplastic anemia	Chronic liver disease
Low MCV, high RDW	Iron deficiency anemia	Sickle cell, β-thalassemia
Normal MCV, high RDW	Early iron, folate, vitamin B_{12} deficiency Myelodysplasia	Sickle cell anemia, sickle cell disease
High MCV, high RDW	Folate or vitamin B_{12} deficiency Myelodysplasia	Immune hemolytic anemia Chronic liver disease

MCV, mean corpuscular volume; RDW, red blood cell distribution width.

Reproduced with permission from Marks PW, Glader B. Approach to anemia in the adult and child. In: Hoffman R, Benz EJ, Shattil SJ, et al. *Hematology: Basic Principles and Practice*. 5th ed. Philadelphia: Churchill Livingstone Elsevier; 2008:Chapter 34 online.

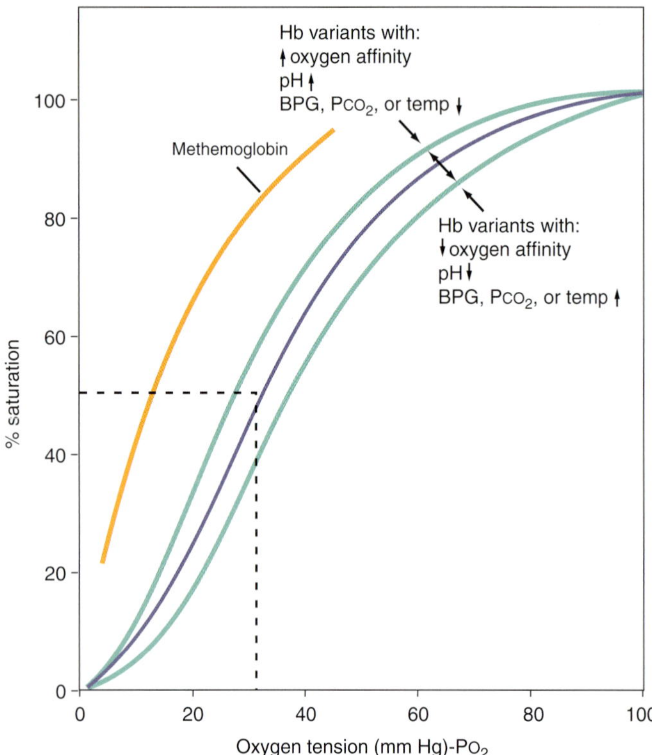

FIGURE 16-4. Oxyhemoglobin dissociation curve. Hb, hemoglobin; BPG, 2,3-bisphosphoglycerate; PCO_2, partial pressure of CO_2; Temp, temperature. [Reproduced with permission from Steinberg MH, Benz EJ, Adeloye AH, et al. Pathobiology of the human erythrocyte and its hemoglobins. In: Hoffman R, Benz EJ, Shattil SJ, et al, eds. *Hematology: Basic Principles and Practice*. 5th ed. Philadelphia, PA: Churchill Livingstone Elsevier; 2008.]

demand in the periphery. The NO is carried from the lungs via RBCs to peripheral tissues, where regional blood flow is regulated by selective release of NO to tissues requiring increased amounts of O_2 (**Fig. 16-5**). RBCs regulate the existing form of NO (eg, NO^+, NO^-, or S-nitroso-hemoglobin [SNO-Hb]), protecting it from degradation during transport to peripheral tissue beds. Specifically, the heme and cysteine thiol portions of Hb within RBCs react with NO free radicals. NO reacts with soluble guanylyl cyclase (sGC) in smooth muscle cells, inducing the rapid production of cyclic guanylate monophosphate (cGMP), which results in vasodilation (ie, increased blood flow). Relevant to transfusion physiology is the fact that stored allogeneic blood with usual blood bank collection methods is completely depleted of SNO-Hb in less than 1 day, raising a concern that the complex storage lesion associated with banked blood causes depletion of SNO-Hb.[5]

Subsequent to these physiologic compensations (eg, hyperventilation, decreased $Pa{CO_2}$, increased 2,3-DPG levels, regulation of selective NO deployment, and ultimately an increased CO), there is increased erythropoiesis (Fig. 16-3). Increased erythropoietin concentration and an increase in the circulating reticulocyte count can be detected as little as 2 days after a hemorrhage event. Blood Hb concentration begins to increase within 7 days after a major hemorrhage. This continuum of physiologic responses occurs in the healthy surgical patient. An individual patient's ability to mount these physiologic responses largely depends on the patient's ability to increase CO and augment tissue oxygen delivery.[18] The compensatory physiologic response to acute, unreplaced volume loss may be reduced during general anesthesia, emphasizing the importance of maintaining intravascular volume.[21] The sympathetic stimulatory response to acute anemia can be impaired during general anesthesia because the heart rate does not increase to the same degree as in unanesthetized patients, and the systemic vascular resistance is lower.[22] The inability to appropriately increase heart rate and augment CO during general anesthesia or due to medications (eg, β-blockers) must also be considered when determining an individual patient's transfusion threshold. Anesthetized patients with a marked impairment of their compensatory responses to anemia may benefit from treatment with more liberal transfusions despite limited data supporting this approach.

Chronic anemia is associated with expansion of plasma volume, hyperventilation, and an increased CO.[23] In deciding whether to perform transfusion on a chronically anemic patient, the clinician should inquire about the signs and symptoms of anemia (eg, fatigue, decreased exercise capacity, and increased frequency of angina in patients with ischemic cardiac disease). For anesthetized patients who are chronically anemic but have been partially volume repleted, electrocardiographic evidence of myocardial ischemia or a systemic acidosis should prompt the clinician to transfuse erythrocytes. However, rapid transfusion of physiologically compensated chronically anemic patients can precipitate congestive heart failure due to intravascular volume overload, even in patients with normal myocardial function.

In forming an understanding of the physiology of anemia, one must consider oxygen delivery (Do_2) to the body, oxygen consumption (Vo_2), and the relationship between them (Vo_2/Do_2, or the oxygen extraction ratio). Do_2 is calculated by the formula:

$$Do_2 = CO \times (\{Sao_2 \times k_1 \times [Hb]\} + \{k_2 \times Pao_2\})$$

where CO is cardiac output, Sao_2 % arterial oxygen saturation, k_1 is the oxygen carrying capacity of Hb and equals 1.34 mL·g^{-1}, [Hb] is the hemoglobin concentration, k_2 is the plasma oxygen solution coefficient at body temperature and equals 0.23 mL·L^{-1}·kPa^{-1}, and Pao_2 the partial pressure of oxygen in arterial blood.[13] Vo_2 is determined by multiplying the oxygen content difference between the arterial and venous blood by CO. Unfortunately all the data required for these calculations are not routinely available to clinicians. When these data are available, they can aid in determining the transfusion trigger point. Additional information on physiologic transfusion triggers will be provided in a later section of this chapter.

CRYSTALLOID VERSUS COLLOID FOR NON-ERYTHROCYTE FLUID REPLACEMENT

Options to replace intravascular fluid loss include crystalloidal and colloidal based solutions. Crystalloidal solutions are composed of solutes with a molecular weight below 30 kDa, whereas colloidal solutions usually contain molecules greater than 30 kDa in size.[24] Crystalloidal solutions (eg, normal saline, lactated Ringer's, hypertonic saline) possess a lower viscosity compared with the more viscous colloidal solutions (eg, blood, 5% albumin, hydroxyethyl starch [HES]), and although the crystalloidal solutions can be delivered more rapidly, contemporary rapid infusion devices make flow rate differences negligible (**Fig. 16-6**). In practice, roughly 2 to 5 times greater volumes of crystalloid are required to obtain the same degree of volume expansion as that obtained with an equivalent volume of colloid, a fact attributed to the greater oncotic pressure of colloids relative to crystalloids.[25]

Crystalloids do not present a risk of infectious disease transmission and are significantly less expensive than colloidal solutions (**Table 16-5**). Although administration of large volumes of crystalloid can produce a dilutional coagulopathy, HES colloidal solutions incur a risk of anaphylactoid reactions, coagulopathy, renal impairment, protracted pruritus, and a trend toward higher mortality rates in patients receiving large doses.[26,27] Human albumin represents an expensive colloidal solution that does not produce coagulopathy and renal failure. Finfer et al[28] established the safety of albumin over normal saline for volume expansion in the critically ill. Subjects in their trial required roughly 1.4 times more total fluid as crystalloid when compared with albumin to reach equal resuscitation endpoints. However, it is possible that albumin-treated patients with traumatic brain injury had a higher mortality, whereas

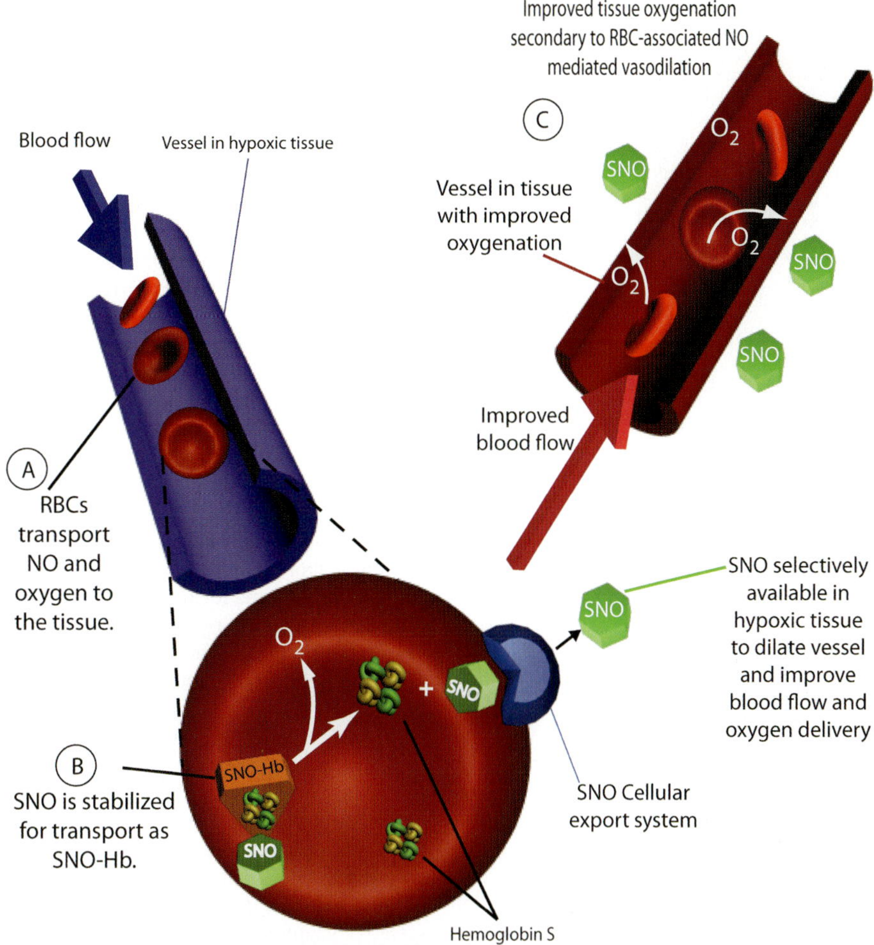

FIGURE 16-5. Red blood cells (RBCs) transduce tissue oxygen gradients to regulate nitric oxide bioactivity in order to improve tissue blood flow and oxygen delivery where metabolic demand is greatest. **A.** RBCs trap nitric oxide (NO) in oxygen-rich tissue (ie, within the pulmonary circulation) as well as bind oxygen, which are ultimately transported to tissues that require oxygen. NO is converted to the S-nitrosothiol (SNO) form, which is highly vasoactive. **B.** SNO is stabilized for transport in the blood by complexing with HbS as SNO-Hb. In tissue with steeper oxygen gradients, the SNO is transported outside of the RBC by specialized cellular export systems. **C.** The SNO vasodilates the local vasculature and improves local blood flow (large red arrow), which in turn improves oxygen delivery.

those subjects with severe sepsis and septic shock suffered a higher mortality rate in the saline group.[28]

Gelatin solutions are known to be associated with a high incidence of anaphylactoid reactions. They are derived from bovine collagen and are not currently available in the United States. Dextran colloidal solutions (eg, dextran-40 and dextran-70, referring to their average molecular weight in kilodaltons) are produced by the hydroxylation of polysaccharides and produce various effects on coagulation. Dextrans decrease platelet adhesion, induce fibrinolysis, decrease fibrinogen levels, and lower blood viscosity. Dextran solutions have been linked to the development of renal failure in hypovolemic patients and are associated with a high incidence of anaphylactoid reactions.[29]

A newly available starch-based colloidal solution is 6% HES 130/0.4 in 0.9% sodium chloride (Voluven). It was expected that this lower-molecular-weight starch would produce fewer adverse effects and provide a more cost-effective alternative to albumin; however, these hopes remain unproven.[27] At present all the synthetic colloids can produce important noxious side effects, and the search continues for a safe and cost-effective alternative to infusing human albumin.

THE DECISION TO TRANSFUSE RED BLOOD CELLS

Clinical Indicators of Organ Ischemia

After establishing normovolemia, the anesthesiologist should review the patient's vital signs and physiologic data and assess the patient's ability to compensate for anemia while weighing the risks (eg, immunosuppression, infection, transfusion-related acute lung injury, transfusion mismatch) and benefits (eg, relieving organ ischemia) of administering a blood transfusion.[3,30] Consideration should be given to the patient's ability to increase cardiac output, given the important role that augmented systemic oxygen delivery plays in compensating for anemia. Physiologic indications of inadequate tissue oxygenation include electrocardiogram (ECG) or echocardiographic evidence of myocardial ischemia (eg, new ST-segment elevation/depression, regional wall motion abnormalities, or spectral Doppler new evidence of significant diastolic dysfunction), systemic acidosis related to enhanced lactate production, an increased calculated oxygen extraction ratio (Vo_2/Do_2) (ie, normal Vo_2/Do_2 is 20%-30%; a Vo_2/Do_2 >50% may indicate inadequate tissue oxygenation), a reduced mixed venous oxygen saturation (Svo_2) (ie, Svo_2 <50%), a low mixed venous oxygen partial pressure (Pvo_2) (ie, Pvo_2 <32 mm Hg), a 25% or greater decrease in baseline regional cerebral oximetry values (rSo_2), a reduced local tissue oxygen saturation (StO_2), or a persistent tachycardia unrelated to hypovolemia and/or inadequate anesthesia (**Table 16-6**).[12] Often these measurements reflecting tissue hypoxia are not available; therefore, clinicians often consider systemic acidemia in the setting of tachycardia and hypotension without other apparent causes to indicate the need to transfuse RBCs.

Clinical Trial Data on Transfusion Triggers To date no appropriately powered, prospective, randomized controlled trials have been reported that definitively compare a liberal versus restrictive RBC transfusion

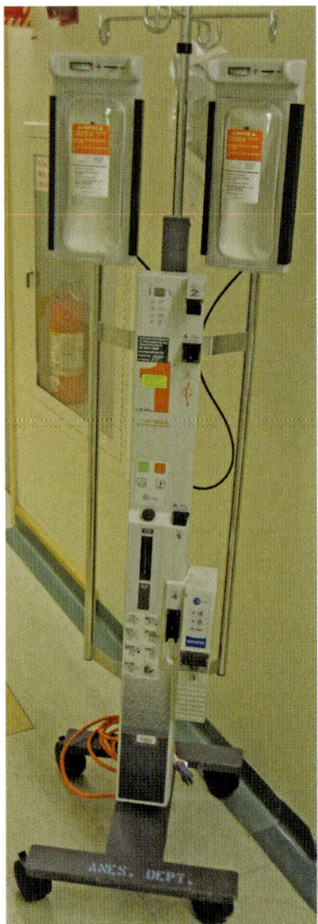

FIGURE 16-6. Level one rapid fluid administration system.

strategy on the morbidity and mortality of critically ill patients. One multicenter, prospective, randomized, controlled study sought to effectively address this question but was stopped for administrative reasons. This study, the Transfusion Requirements in Critical Care (TRICC) trial, enrolled 838 (<20% of projected patient enrollment) intensive care unit (ICU) patients randomized to either a restrictive (ie, [Hb] 7.0-9.0 g/dL) or liberal (ie, [Hb] 10.0-12.0 g/dL) transfusion strategy. The overall 30-day mortality was lower in the restrictive transfusion strategy group (18.7% vs 23.3%), but this difference was not statistically significant ($p = 0.11$). An a priori subgroup analysis of subjects who were less acutely ill and older than 55 years of age demonstrated a significantly lower mortality in the restrictive transfusion group. Although the TRICC trial is the largest study to date, it was stopped prematurely and thus did not answer the question of an appropriate transfusion strategy in ICU patients. The authors concluded that a restrictive approach to RBC transfusion was as effective and potentially superior to a liberal transfusion strategy for ICU patients, with the possible exception of patients with unstable angina and acute myocardial infarction.[31] Unfortunately, the TRICC trial was conducted before leukoreduction of transfused blood became a common practice. A review of the importance of leukoreduction suggests that it may improve the clinical outcomes of patients undergoing transfusion.[32] An additional weakness of the TRICC trial is the fact that it did not include cardiac surgical patients, a group requiring more blood transfusion than any other patient group.

TABLE 16-5 Hospital Acquisition Costs for Intravenous Volume Replacement Solutions

Fluid	Volume (mL)	Cost[a] (US Dollars)
0.9% Sodium chloride	1000	1.03
Lactated Ringers	1000	1.06
Hespan	500	11.23
5% Albumin	250	36.00
25% Albumin	50	36.00

[a]Fluid costs reflect established purchasing through University Hospitals Case Medical Center.

More recently, the results of a single-center, prospective, randomized, controlled non-inferiority trial assessing the effects of 2 transfusion strategies (liberal [HCT ≥ 30%] vs restrictive [HCT ≥ 24%]) in a group (n = 502) of cardiac surgical patients has been completed. The primary outcome measure was the occurrence of the composite end point of all-cause 30-day mortality and severe morbidity. The occurrence of the primary end point was similar in both groups (liberal 10% vs restrictive 11%; $p = 0.85$). Independent of group assignment, the number of RBC units transfused is an independent risk factor for death or clinical complications at 30 days (hazard ratio for each additional RBC unit transfused 1.2 [95% confidence interval, 1.1-1.4]; $p = 0.002$). Unfortunately, blood was not leukoreduced, a common practice in US blood banks, and the median storage time for the transfused RBCs was only 3 days, dramatically shorter than most US centers (ie, average is approximately 14 days). The authors concluded that among cardiac surgical patients, the use of a restrictive perioperative transfusion strategy as compared with a more liberal strategy resulted in non-inferior rates of their composite outcomes.[33]

A third, slightly smaller (n = 428), prospective, randomized, controlled trial of a restrictive (transfused if Hb <8 g/dL) versus liberal (transfused if Hb <9 g/dL) transfusion strategy in cardiac surgical patients was published over a decade ago.[34] The authors did not report any significant differences in morbidity, mortality, or anemia-related fatigue self-assessment scores and concluded that a transfusion threshold of 8 mg/dL did not adversely affect the outcome. Because the conservative group was transfused with significantly less blood (0.9 ± 1.5 vs 1.4 ± 1.8 RBC units, restrictive vs liberal; $p = 0.005$), they concluded that using 8 mg/dL as a transfusion threshold would conserve RBCs without increasing the patient's risk.[34] A number of smaller trials failed to provide any additional insights into the question of determining a transfusion threshold.[3]

Presently, a large, multicenter, National Heart, Lung, and Blood Institute–sponsored, prospective clinical study comparing a liberal transfusion strategy versus a symptom-driven strategy is occurring. Named the FOCUS trial (The Transfusion Trigger Trial for Functional Outcomes in Cardiovascular Patients Undergoing Surgical Hip Fracture Repair), the primary end point is to determine whether a 10 g/dL transfusion strategy is associated with an improved ability to walk 10 ft without assistance at 60 days after hip surgery as compared with a symptom-driven transfusion strategy. The goal of trial enrollment is 2600 subjects, and greater than 2000 subjects are enrolled presently. The FOCUS trial has a number of secondary end points, including assessing the composite outcome of 30-day mortality, myocardial infarction, pneumonia, stroke, and thromboembolism.[35,36]

Several large retrospective studies assessing transfusion-related outcomes in varied patient groups have been completed.[37-39] In a study by Corwin et al,[37] the number of transfused RBC units was found to be an independent risk factor for hospital length of stay, mortality, and a number of complications. In another large study by Vincent et al,[38] mortality was significantly higher in patients with similar levels of organ dysfunction in whom RBCs were transfused. A large (n = 8787) observational study of elderly, orthopedic surgical patients by Carson et al[39] found that postoperative transfusion did not influence 30- or 90-day mortality after adjusting for the transfusion strategy (ie, transfusion trigger between 8 and 10 g/dL^{-1} vs < 8 g/dL^{-1}), cardiovascular disease, and other risk factors.[39] Similar to reported prospective studies, these larger retrospective studies suggest a clear relationship between more RBC transfusions and a worse outcome. However, it

TABLE 16-6 Physiologic Transfusion Trigger Parameters

Situation	Patients	Hb (g/dL)	Circulation	Myocardial Ischemia	Pvo_2 <32 mm Hg, O_2ER >50%, Svo_2 <50%, decrease in Vo_2 >10%
Intraoperative, ICU	All patients	6	Rel. inc. HR/ dec. BP	ST-segment changes	Yes
	>80 y	7	Rel. inc. HR/ dec. BP	ST-segment changes	Yes
	CAD	8	Rel. inc. HR/ dec. BP	ST-segment changes	Yes
	CVD	7	Rel. inc. HR/ dec. BP	ST-segment changes	Yes
	Fever/ hypermetabolism	7	Rel. inc. HR/ dec. BP	ST-segment changes	Yes
Ward	All patients	6	Rel. inc. HR/ dec. BP	Clinical signs	NA[i]
	>80 y	8	Rel. inc. HR/ dec. BP	Clinical signs	NA
	CAD	9	Rel. inc. HR/ dec. BP	Clinical signs	NA
	CVD	8	Rel. inc. HR/ dec. BP	Clinical signs	NA
	Fever/ hypermetabolism	8	Rel. inc. HR/ dec. BP	Clinical signs	NA

Hb-based and physiologic transfusion triggers as a function of patient-related and logistical factors. RBC transfusion is indicated if one of the criteria given in the table is reached: Hb threshold, circulation criterion, myocardial ischemia, or one of the oxygenation variables (Pvo_2, O_2ER, Svo_2, or Vo_2). For all physiologic transfusion triggers, normovolemia, optimization of the anesthesia, and the correction of tachycardia (if present) are assumed, and anemia should be the only probable cause. Includes all patients except the subcategories patients older than 80 years, patients with CAD, patients with CVD, and patients with fever/hypermetabolism. One may choose *not* to transfuse the individual patient without any physiologic transfusion triggers.

CAD, coronary artery disease; CVD, cardiovascular disease; NA, not applicable; O_2ER, oxygen extraction ratio (%); Pvo_2, partial venous pressure of oxygen (mm Hg); Rel. inc. HR, relative increase in heart rate defined as heart rate more than 120% to 130% of baseline or more than 110 to 130 beats/min; Rel. dec., relative decrease in systemic hypotension defined as a mean arterial pressure less than 70% to 80% of baseline or less than 60 mm Hg (<55 mm Hg in young healthy patients, <70-80 mm Hg in patients with CAD or CVD and in hypertensive patients, and even higher in severely hypertensive patients); ST-segment changes, new ST-segment depression more than 0.1 mV or ST-segment elevation more than 0.2 mV. To be confirmed with ECG and/or troponin measurement if possible in a timely fashion; Svo_2, venous oxygen saturation (%); Vo_2, oxygen consumption.

Reproduced with permission from Madjdpour C, Spahn DR: Allogeneic red blood cell transfusions: Efficacy, risks, alternatives and indications. *Br J Anaesth* 95:33, 2005.

remains debatable whether patients who received transfusions were equivalently ill.

Our distillation of peer-reviewed, threshold-related transfusion literature suggests that no critical hemoglobin concentration for moderately anemic patients should be used, but rather clinical signs and symptoms of organ ischemia should be assessed in each patient in whom a transfusion of RBCs is considered. The available literature appears to consistently show independent relationships between the number of RBC units transfused and a worse clinical outcome when other measured variables are taken into account and controlled for, regardless of the transfusion treatment strategy. Furthermore, drawing from the limited body of available evidence, it appears to be just as safe to accept Hb concentrations of 7 or 8 mg/dL in critically ill patients, including those with cardiovascular disease, provided they are not exhibiting signs or symptoms of end organ ischemia. Additional prospective investigations are needed to shed light on these important clinical questions.

UNDESIRABLE EFFECTS OF RED BLOOD CELL TRANSFUSION

Retrospective studies report that transfusion of allogeneic RBCs is associated with increased morbidity and mortality in both cardiac and noncardiac surgical populations.[3] Perioperative transfusion is associated with undesirable outcomes including prolonged hospital length of stay, infections, immunosuppression, and acute transfusion reactions.[40] Presently, human error, or a mistransfusion, accounts for the second highest incidence of adverse transfusion effects, whereas the transfusion-associated viral infectious risk remains remarkably low (**Table 16-7**).[41]

More than 200 cases of transfusion-associated graft-versus-host disease have been reported, with a near 90% fatality rate. Irradiation of blood products can prevent this problem, but irradiation induces detrimental effects on RBCs.[42] Allogeneic blood transfusion is associated with an increased risk of tumor recurrence in patients previously treated for cancer, and this appears to be a dose-dependent effect.[43]

Transfusion-related acute lung injury (TRALI) is the leading cause of transfusion-related mortality Estimated TRALI incidence is once for every 3000 to 70 000 plasma-rich components transfused and 1 per 50 000 units of low plasma volume components transfused.[44,45] Large-scale

TABLE 16-7 Current Risk Estimates of Transfusion-Transmitted Disease in the United States

Pathogen	Average Estimated Risk Per Unit
Hepatitis A	Unknown, presumably <1:1 million
Hepatitis B	1:205 000[a]
Hepatitis C	1:1 935 000[b]
Human immunodeficiency virus-1	1:2 135 000[b]
Human T-lymphotropic virus-I,II	1:2 993 000
Cytomegalovirus	Infrequent with leukocyte-reduced components
Parvovirus B19	Unknown, presumably <1:1 million
West Nile and other Arbo viruses	Regional and seasonal risk, observed incidence of transmissions during 2003 season after implementation of pooled NAT approximately 1:1 million recipients
Bacterial contamination associated with symptomatic sepsis	1:5 million per red blood cell unit; 1:100,000 per apheresis or pooled platelet unit[c]
Malaria	<1:1 million
Babesia	<1:1 million, higher in endemic areas
Chagas disease	Unknown, presumably <1:1 million
Creutzfeldt-Jakob disease (CJD), vCJD	Single probable case reported in the United Kingdom

NAT, nucleic acid testing.

[a]Estimates for hepatitis B virus reflect risk projections before implementation of blood donor screening with NAT.

[b]Estimates for human immunodeficiency virus and hepatitis C virus indicate risk projections after implementation of NAT for these agents in 1999.

[c]Risk estimate reflects the experience of a 2-year US national study from 1998 to 2000, prior to implementation of standards to detect and limit bacterial contamination. Because of likely underreporting, true risks were probably higher.

Reproduced with permission from Fiebig EW, Busch MP. Infectious risks of transfusion. In: Spiess BD, Spence RK, Shander A. *Perioperative Transfusion Medicine*. 2nd ed. Philadelphia: Lippincott Williams & Wilkins; 2006:131-152.

efforts to decrease the risk of TRALI have been initiated.[46] TRALI is an antibody-mediated reaction characterized by the acute onset of respiratory distress within 4 hours of transfusion. Typical manifestations include severe hypoxemia, hypotension, fever, and diffuse pulmonary edema. Patients with TRALI require immediate aggressive respiratory support, with the majority requiring intubation and mechanical ventilation. Despite the severity of symptoms, permanent lung injury does not occur. The majority of patients return to their baseline respiratory function within 48 hours of symptom onset and have total resolution of pulmonary edema within 4 days.[46] Present measures to mitigate against the rising TRALI incidence appear to be reducing the incidence.[45]

Other potentially fatal complications of allogeneic blood transfusion include hemolytic transfusion reactions due to antigen-antibody interactions, transfusion-associated circulatory overload (TACO), anaphylaxis, and post-transfusion purpura due to platelet-specific antigens.[47] Administration of large volumes of stored blood can also lead to hyperkalemia, hypoglycemia, hypothermia, and citrate-induced hypocalcemia.

TRANSFUSION ALTERNATIVES

Acute Normovolemic Hemodilution Acute normovolemic hemodilution (ANH) involves intraoperative removal of a predetermined quantity of the patient's blood (ie, up to 50% of a healthy patient's total circulating RCM can be safely removed) while intravascular volume is concurrently replaced. Because the RCM is decreased before intraoperative bleeding begins, there is a smaller net loss of RCM per unit blood loss by surgical hemorrhage. Additionally, the benefit of transfusing the shed autologous whole blood, including functional platelets and coagulation proteins, is available to the patient at any point during or after the operative procedure.[22] Individuals with religious prohibitions to RBC transfusion (eg, Jehovah's Witnesses) provide a group of patients who can often benefit from ANH if the shed blood is maintained in a parallel circuit connected to the patient.

Red Blood Cell Substitutes Further development and testing of RBC substitute–based transfusion solutions is needed to learn whether they can provide a safe alternative to erythrocyte transfusion. Extensive laboratory and clinical research has been done with Hb-based oxygen-carrying (HBOC) solutions, but despite 50 years of laboratory and clinical research efforts with HBOC solutions, there is presently no US Food and Drug Administration (FDA)–approved product available for clinical use. Recently, the FDA convened a workshop to review the issues affecting the development of blood substitutes. Problems impeding the development of HBOC solutions include renal toxicity, gastrointestinal symptoms, systemic arterial hypertension, coronary vasoconstriction, pulmonary hypertension, short half-life of the transfused molecules, methemoglobin production, and a significant systemic arterial inflammatory response occurring several days after transfusion. The vasoconstrictor effects of these molecules appear to be related to their small size, tendency to migrate into the interstitium, and ability to scavenge nitric oxide produced by vascular endothelium. Perfluorocarbons are a non–Hb-based RBC substitute, but these synthetic solutions are also not available for clinical use in the United States.[48]

Red Blood Cell Salvage Red cell salvage techniques are associated with a significant reduction in allogeneic transfusion requirements and a cost benefit for some patients.[47] Autologous RBC salvage involves the collection of blood from a wound site, processing (eg, centrifugal washing and/or filtering through a 20-μm filter) of scavenged blood, and reinfusion. Centrifugal washing concentrates the salvaged blood to allow the infusion of an autologous product with a high HCT level (eg, 45%-65%) and removes undesirable components of shed blood (eg, free Hb, tissue debris, fibrin split products). Cell salvage requires specialized equipment and disposable devices (**Fig. 16-7**). Processed autologous blood infuses normally biconcave disc-shaped erythrocytes suspended in normal saline. In contrast, allogeneic RBCs develop an abnormal echinocyte shape after 14 days. This conformational change impairs the cells' ability to transit capillary beds[49] (**Fig. 16-8**). Centrifugal washing

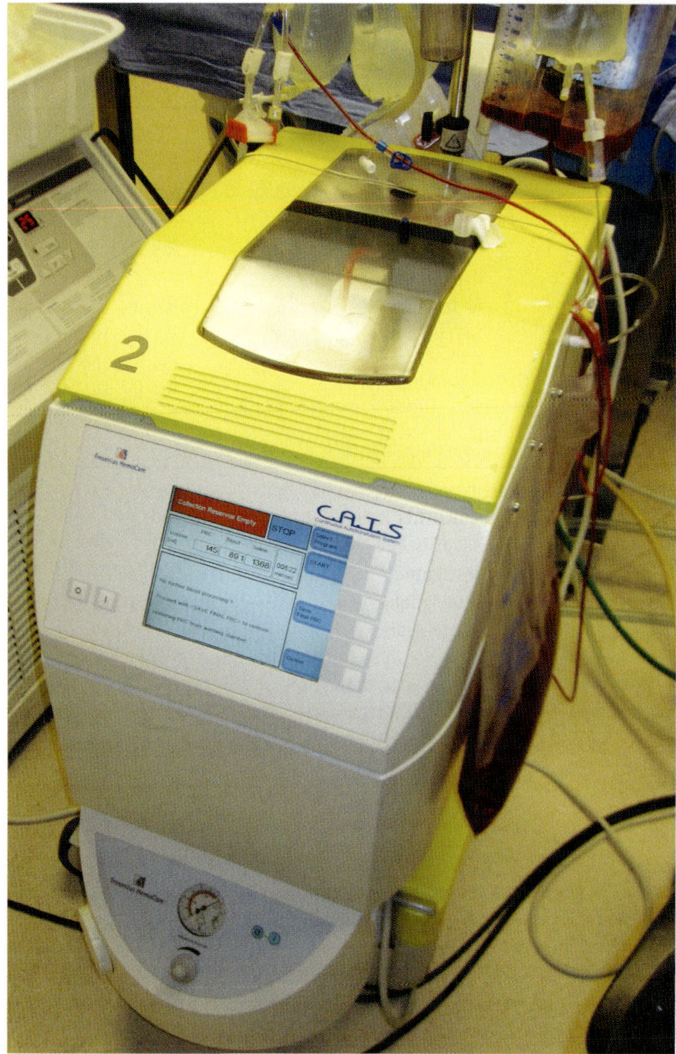

FIGURE 16-7. Red blood cell salvage system.

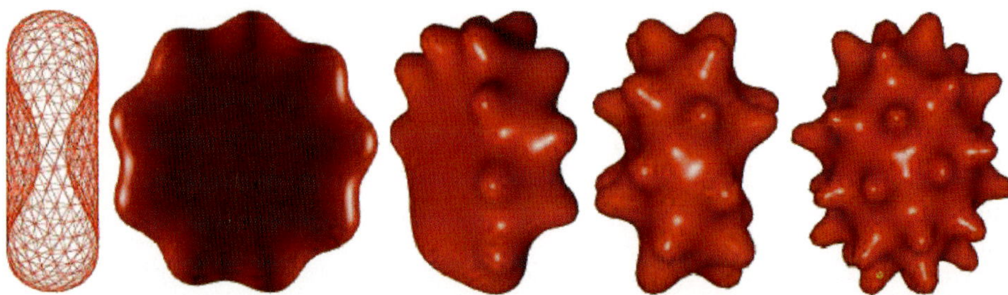
FIGURE 16-8. Graphic depiction of the 3-dimensional shape of echinocytes found in stored allogeneic blood. [Reproduced with permission from Bull BS, Herrmann PC. Morphology of the erythron. In: Lichtman MA, Kipps TJ, Seligsohn U, et al, eds. *Williams Hematology*. 8th ed. New York, NY: McGraw-Hill; 2008.]

removes coagulation proteins, although some leukocytes and platelets are autotransfused.

Alternatively, collected shed autologous blood is passed through a filter with 20-μm pores and re-transfused without centrifugal washing.[47] Red cell salvage with centrifugal washing within certain guidelines has been studied and found to be generally safe; however, current recommendations of The Society of Thoracic Surgeons and the Society of Cardiovascular Anesthesiologists do not allow re-transfusion of shed blood without centrifugal washing.[50] Infection at the operative site or the use of microfibrillar collagen materials are contraindications to using RBC salvage techniques.[47]

Malignancy has been regarded as a contraindication to the use of a cell saver and transfusing autologous blood products. However, recent experience with the cell saver in cases of prostate cancer resection did not show an increased cancer recurrence rate and effectively reduced the need for autologous transfusion. A small prospective observational study of the use of the cell saver for orthotopic liver transplantation for hepatocellular carcinoma has been reported.[43] No large-scale randomized controlled trials have examined the safety of using the cell saver in cases of malignancy; thus this practice is usually avoided.

The use of the cell saver in cases of enteric perforation is avoided. One prospective study investigated the use of the cell saver with a leukocyte depletion filter with the goal of reducing bacterial contamination of salvaged blood.[43] No large-scale randomized controlled trials have been conducted to investigate the safety of using the cell saver in the setting of blood contamination; thus this use should be avoided.

Known risks incurred with the use of cell salvage include nonimmune hemolysis, air embolism, febrile nonhemolytic transfusion reactions, coagulopathy, and contamination with drugs, infectious agents, and cleansing solutions. Incomplete blood washing can lead to administration of activated leukocytes, cytokines, and other microaggregates. Risks of coagulopathy are minimal in patients with blood loss less than 3 L, and technological advances have reduced other risks.[43]

It is currently recommended to use cell saver technology for surgical cases if anticipated blood loss is more than 1 L or more than 20% of estimated blood volume. Other situations of clear benefit are for patients with a low preoperative Hb level at risk for bleeding, patients with multiple antibodies or rare blood types, and patients who object to receiving allogeneic blood.[43,47] A recent systematic review reports that processing cardiotomy blood in cardiac surgery patients through the cell saver can reduce postoperative neurocognitive dysfunction, most likely through the reduction in lipid related microembolization.[47]

Antifibrinolytic Therapy Antifibrinolytic therapy (eg, aprotinin, and the lysine analogues [ε-aminocaproic acid and tranexamic acid]) can reduce blood loss in patients at risk of major hemorrhage (eg, cardiac surgical patients, orthotopic liver transplant patients, selected orthopedic surgery

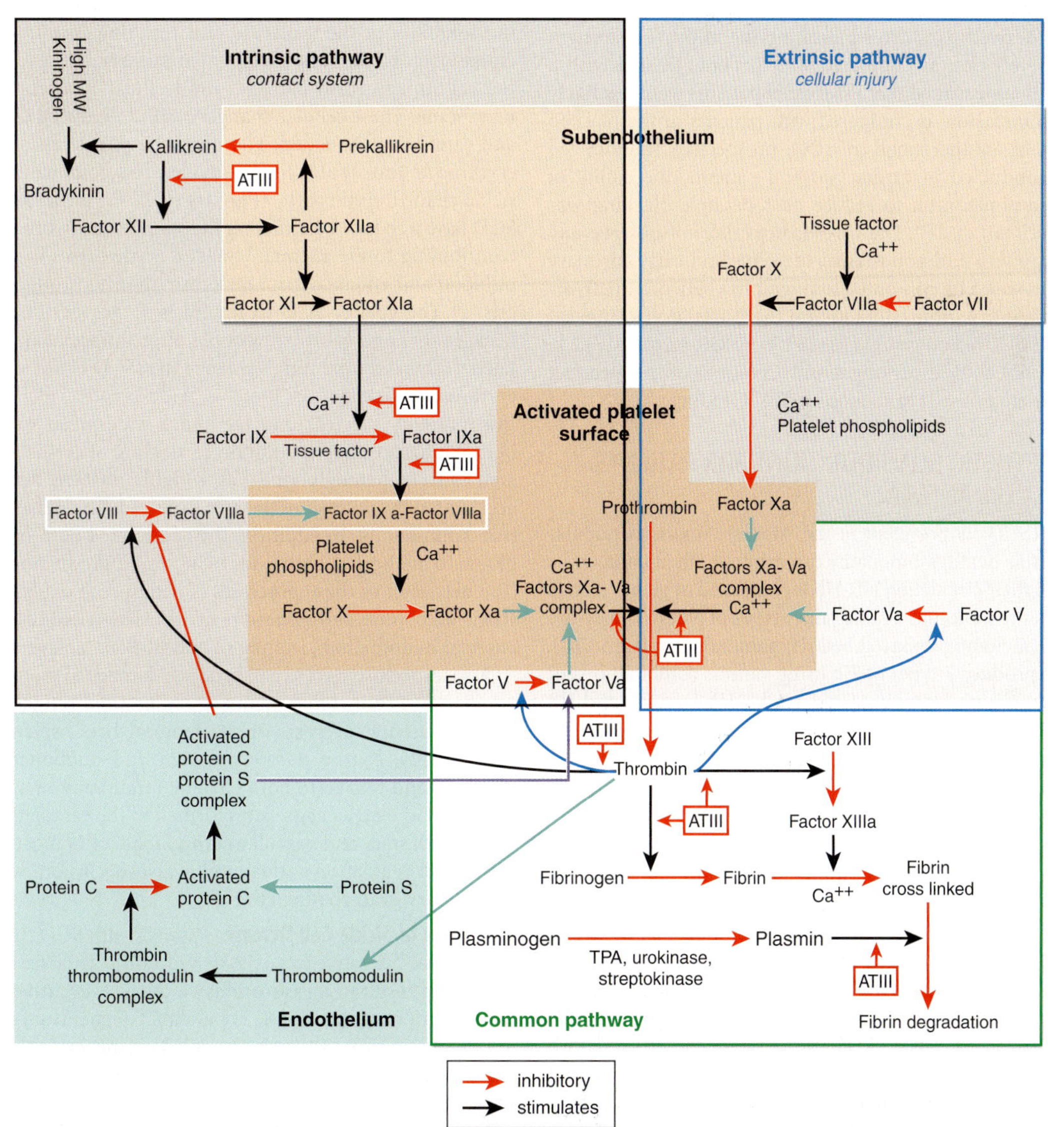

FIGURE 16-9. The coagulation cascade.

patients).[51,52] These agents inhibit fibrinolysis (ie, inhibit conversion of plasminogen to plasmin or directly inhibit the action of plasmin on fibrin) that often accompanies major surgery (**Fig. 16-9**). The results of several prospective, randomized controlled trials indicate that aprotinin therapy can reduce transfusion requirements as well as the incidence of surgical reexploration for hemorrhage. However, recent data report that aprotinin use is associated with a significantly higher morbidity and mortality in high-risk cardiac surgical patients and resulted in the removal of aprotinin in 2007 from the world market.[54-56] Aprotinin is presently only available for investigational use and requires local institutional review board approval as well as individual patient consent before administration. The lysine analogues have been proven effective in blood conservation for selected patient populations.[51,55] Tranexamic acid use has been associated with an increased incidence of perioperative seizures in cardiac surgical patients.[54] The lysine analogues remain in widespread clinical use.

Additional Adjuncts to Promote Blood Conservation There are data suggesting that the administration of a human, pooled fibrinogen concentrate (Riastap) may be beneficial for perioperative patients who develop coagulopathic bleeding. In a prospective, randomized, placebo-controlled study of 20 general surgery patients who developed a hydroxyethyl starch infusion–induced dilutional coagulopathy and were treated with either a fixed dose of fibrinogen concentrate (FC) or a placebo, Fenger-Ericksen et al[57] demonstrated that FC-treated patients exhibited improved maximal clot firmness (MCF), a rotational thromboelastometric (ROTEM)–derived parameter indicating the improved strength and quality of a blood clot, as compared with patients treated with a placebo. They also demonstrated that FC-treated patients were less likely to require blood transfusion as compared with patients in the placebo group ($p = 0.023$). In another small (n = 20), prospective, randomized controlled study conducted in cardiac surgical patients, the ability of prophylactic FC administration to reduce postoperative bleeding was investigated by Karlsson et al.[58] The investigators did not observe any difference in the primary end point (adverse events and early coronary graft occlusion as assessed by computed tomography) between the treatment group and a control group. In addition there was less postoperative bleeding in the FC-treated group (565 ± 150 vs 830 ± 268 mL/12 h; $p = 0.010$). Additional clinical investigation is required of this product before it is appropriate to use it to reduce surgical bleeding.

SPECIAL ANESTHETIC CONSIDERATIONS FOR PATIENTS WITH SICKLE CELL ANEMIA

Sickle cell disease (SCD) is prevalent in the African American population. Patients with this hemoglobinopathy can exhibit both anemia and a functional defect of their circulating Hb. Hb is composed of globin chains combined with a heme molecule. Four distinct types of globin chains are normally produced, including alpha (α), beta (β), gamma (γ), and sigma (σ). Normally humans produce 3 types of Hb using various combinations of the 4 distinct globin chains, including Hb A ($\alpha_2\beta_2$), Hb F ($\alpha_2\gamma_2$), and Hb A_2 ($\alpha_2\sigma_2$). In early infancy, 97% percent of the circulating Hb exists as Hb A. Hemoglobinopathies result from decreased synthesis of normal globin chains (eg, thalassemia syndromes) or, in SCD, a functional defect of the Hb complex involving a qualitative defect in globin synthesis.[59]

Pathophysiology of Sickle Cell Disease The pathophysiology of SCD and sickle cell trait (SCT) is due to a substitution of the amino acid valine for glutamine at the sixth amino acid location of the β-globin chain, resulting in production of Hb S. In humans with both chromosomes directing Hb S synthesis (homozygous SS disease), the normal Hb A is substituted by Hb S. Increased production of Hb A_2 and Hb F is minimally effective in alleviating the pathophysiologic changes of SCD. A major percentage (80%-95%) of the synthesized Hb is Hb S in patients afflicted with homozygous SS disease.[60,61] SCT represents the heterozygous state and is produced by 1 sickle cell gene locus and 1 normal gene locus. SCT results in few clinical problems, despite the Hb S level rising to nearly 40% of circulating Hb.[60] Among African Americans in the United States, approximately 0.4% exhibit homozygous SCD status, with a prevalence of 6% to 8% heterozygotes.[61]

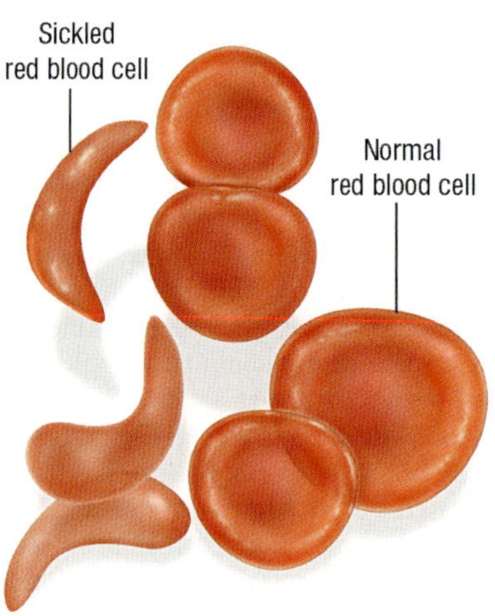

FIGURE 16-10. Diagram art of a normal RBC and a sickled RBC.

There is a spectrum of abnormal tissue oxygen delivery resulting from the pathophysiologic mechanisms of SCD. Patients with SCD exhibit an abnormal conformation of the deoxygenated Hb S molecule, reducing the solubility of the molecule and resulting in intra-erythrocytic precipitation of Hb S.[62] The precipitated intraerythrocytic deoxy-Hb S alters red cell function and damages intracellular RBC contents and the cell membrane. These cellular changes result in reduced capillary blood flow and early cell destruction. The normally pliable, biconcave disc-shaped erythrocyte transmutes into a smaller, less compliant, characteristically sickle-shaped erythrocyte (**Fig. 16-10**).[63] Erythrocytes of patients with SCD have a reduced circulating life span of approximately 10 to 20 days, contributing to the anemia.[64] Sickled erythrocytes increase the viscosity of blood and enhance thrombus formation to produce a vaso-occlusive crisis.[61] The goal of SCD treatment is to prevent initiation of sickling, because this process is irreversible once intracellular Hb S has precipitated.[61] There is mounting evidence that SCD is not simply the result of erythrocyte sickling, as there is widespread evidence of progressive inflammatory vascular damage and a widespread vasculopathy. It has been confirmed that in addition to sickling of erythrocytes, the oxygenated form of hemoglobin S has a highly unstable structure, leading to accelerated breakdown of the molecule and the release of toxic heme and iron compounds. In addition, the accelerated auto-oxidation of hemoglobin to methemoglobin leads to increased production of hemichromes. The net result of these processes is widespread oxidative damage to the RBC membrane and adhesion of iron-laden–oxidized erythrocytes to vascular endothelium, leading to endothelial damage and dysfunction.[61]

A vaso-occlusive crisis can produce damage to many organs (eg, renal papillary necrosis, renal medullary infarction, retinal or vitreous hemorrhage, aseptic necrosis of the femoral head, splenic infarction).[64-66] Additionally, central nervous system and pulmonary infarctions are common and related to both chronic inflammation and emboli of sickled cells and platelet aggregates formed in the vasculature. Alterations of cellular, plasma, and vascular components of hemostasis and impaired vasomotor regulation contribute to vaso-occlusion, with sickling being a secondary exacerbating effect.[64]

Treatment of Sickle Cell Disease Patients with SCD should be treated to prevent perioperative hypoxia, dehydration, acidosis, and hypothermia, which can result in a vaso-occlusive crisis. Preventive measures are the mainstay of treatment for SCD patients.[67] General anesthesia per se does not overtly increase the risk of sickled erythrocytes.[64]

One approach to avoid a perioperative vaso-occlusive crisis is to reduce the percentage of Hb S to less than 30% to 40% before surgery by exchange and standard blood transfusions.[64,67] As with other chronic anemic states, there is physiologic compensation for anemia that results in an increased intravascular volume and augmented CO. The increase in intravascular volume places the anemic SCD patient at risk for volume overload if they are rapidly transfused with allogeneic blood; thus a cautious approach to transfusion is mandated. The benefit of transfusion can persist for weeks after the postoperative period, as evidenced by a reduced incidence of sickling episodes. Perioperative mortality in SCD patients is most commonly caused by a fulminant infection related to immunosuppression associated with prior splenic infarctions.[67]

COAGULATION DISORDERS

KEY POINTS

1. Given the broad range of congenital and acquired disease states as well as the multiple pharmacotherapies producing a hypocoagulable state, serious attention to these pathologies and drugs is warranted to avoid the adverse effects of transfusions, excessive perioperative bleeding, and depletion of community blood bank resources.
2. The management of patients with hypercoagulable disorders is a responsibility of the anesthesiologist because many of these patients require perioperative management of their anticoagulant regimens.
3. Hematology consultation is vital to obtain for the perioperative management of patients with complex hypocoagulable and hypercoagulable disorders in order to avoid unnecessary perioperative morbidity and mortality. After surgery, many of these patients will be managed by a hematologist.

The human coagulation system maintains a delicate balance between hemostasis and the distribution of fluid blood to the tissues. Pathologic changes within the coagulation system may result in either a hypocoagulable state (ie, a tendency to hemorrhage inappropriately) or a hypercoagulable state (ie, a tendency to inappropriately form thrombus). The coagulation system relies on the appropriate level and function of several blood components to allow normal clotting. The process of blood coagulation relies on the interaction of platelets, vascular endothelium, vascular smooth muscle, soluble coagulation proteins, and various local and systemic biochemical mediators to produce a hemostatic clot.[68]

HYPOCOAGULABLE STATES

It is crucial to recognize and treat a preexisting hypocoagulable state to avoid massive hemorrhage and potentially unnecessary blood product transfusion. Optimal treatment of a hypocoagulable disorder is best accomplished by selectively transfusing the blood component(s) that is/are deficient (eg, transfuse factor VIII concentrate into a hemophiliac requiring surgery rather than fresh-frozen plasma). Hypocoagulable states are usually either congenital or acquired; both can occur simultaneously in the same patient. Knowledge of both the coagulation cascade and the biologic half-life of a particular coagulation element are needed to effectively treat many hypocoagulable disorders (Fig. 16-9, **Table 16-8**). It is of paramount importance to combine a history and physical examination with appropriate laboratory testing to discover congenital and/or acquired hypocoagulable/hypercoagulable disorders in surgical patients. After direct questioning of whether a patient has a known coagulation disorder, one must ask specific questions to elicit the presence or absence of these disorders (**Table 16-9**). If a patient answers "yes" to any of these questions, inquire regarding the details and frequency of the problem. Depending on the complexity of the presenting hypocoagulable or hypercoagulable state, a hematology consultation may be indicated.[68]

FACTOR VIII DEFICIENCY (HEMOPHILIA A)

Patients with a factor VIII deficiency, or hemophilia A, can require urgent surgical intervention for bleeding episodes (eg, craniotomy to decompress an intracranial hemorrhage or fasciotomy to relieve a compartment syndrome). Hemophilia A is an X-linked recessive trait that occurs with a frequency of 1 in 5000 male births.[69]

Individuals with hemophilia A manifest a range of bleeding symptoms, with a severity inversely correlated to their plasma activity level of factor VIII. Normally, factor VIII activity ranges from 50% to 150% (or 0.5-1.5 U/mL). Mild hemophilia is present in patients with factor VIII activity levels greater than 5%. Moderate hemophilia is present in patients with factor VIII activity levels from 1% to 5%, and severe hemophilia symptoms manifest at levels less than 1% (or 0.01 U/mL).[69]

Spontaneous hemarthroses are the hallmark of severe hemophilia. Recurrent joint hemorrhage produces painful degeneration of the cartilage (hemophilic arthropathy) that eventually can destroy the joint (**Fig. 16-11**).[70] Hemophiliacs with 1% to 5% of factor VIII activity do not

TABLE 16-8 Summary of Clotting Factor Deficiencies

	Prevalence and Biologic Half-Lives		Screening Abnormalities		
Factor Deficiency	Biologic Half-Life	Estimated Incidence	Type of Bleeding	Abnormal	Normal
I	2-4 d	1:1 million	None to severe	PT, PTT, TCT, BT	None
II	3 d	Very rare	Mild-moderate	PT, PTT	TCT, BT
V	36 h	1:1 million	Moderate	PT, PTT, BT	TCT
VII	3-6 h	1:500,000	Mild-severe	PT	PTT, TCT, BT
X	40 h	1:500,000	Mild-severe	PT, PTT	TCT, BT
XI	80 h	Rare	Mild-moderate	PTT	PT, TCT, BT
XII	50-70 h	Unknown	No bleeding	PTT	PT, TCT, BT
XIII	9 d	1:5 million	Moderate-severe	None	PT, PTT, TCT, BT
PK	35 h	Unknown	None	PTT	PT, TCT, BT
HK	150 h	Very rare	None	PTT	PT, TCT, BT
α_2-Pi	3 d	Unknown	Mild-moderate	None	PT, PTT, TCT, BT
α_1-ATP	--	Very rare	Variable-severe	PT, PTT, TCT, BT	None
Protein Z	2-3 d	Unknown	None	None	PT, PTT, TCT, BT
ZPI	Unknown	Unknown	None	None	PT, PTT, TCT, BT

α_1-ATP, alpha$_1$ antitrypsin Pittsburgh; α_2-Pi, alpha$_2$ plasmin inhibitor; BT, bleeding time; HK, high-molecular-weight kininogen; PK, prekallikrein; PT, prothrombin time; PTT, partial thromboplastin time; TCT, thrombin clotting time; ZPI, protein Z–dependent protease inhibitor.

Reproduced with permission from Kitchens CS. Surgery and hemostasis. In: Kitchens CS, Alving BM, Kessler CM. *Consultative Hemostasis and Thrombosis*. 2nd ed. Philadelphia: Saunders Elsevier; 2007:613-634.

TABLE 16-9 Preanesthetic Assessment Coagulation Disorder Queries

- Is there a family history of making blood clots inappropriately or of excessive bleeding after dental or surgical procedures?
- Do you bleed excessively after having a blood sample drawn?
- Have you ever required a transfusion for any reason? If so, why was the transfusion administered?
- Do you have problems with bleeding gums when you brush your teeth?
- Do you bruise easily?
- Do you have a history of nosebleeds, bloody/red-tinged urine, or tarry, black stools?
- Do experience heavy bleeding with menstruation?
- Are you taking any medications or herbal supplements? If so, which ones?

Modified with permission from Kitchens CS. The consultative process. In: Kitchens CS, Alving BM, Kessler CM. *Consultative Hemostasis and Thrombosis*. 2nd ed. Philadelphia: Saunders Elsevier; 2007:3-15.

generally have spontaneous bleeding events, but trauma and surgery can precipitate a hemorrhage.

Intracranial and intracerebral bleeding are the most common causes of death in hemophiliacs. Approximately half of the intracranial hemorrhages in hemophiliacs occur spontaneously. Gastrointestinal and oropharyngeal bleeding may also occur. Oropharyngeal bleeding is of great importance because it can lead to airway compromise. In severe hemophilia, recurrent hemorrhagic episodes may produce an enlarged pseudotumor that can invade local soft tissue and bone. Operative removal of pseudotumors is associated with a high mortality despite the provision of recommended perioperative therapies.[71]

In the United States, the diagnosis and management of hemophilia A is achieved with an activated partial thromboplastin time (aPTT)–based 1-stage assay. The aPTT is abnormally prolonged in all hemophiliacs. The prothrombin time (PT), thrombin time (TT), bleeding time, platelet count, and platelet function are usually normal in hemophiliacs.[69]

Hemophilia A is usually treated by administration of factor VIII concentrate. The goal of chronic therapy is to maintain the trough level of factor VIII activity at approximately 3% of normal to reduce the incidence of spontaneous intracranial hemorrhage and minimize spontaneous intra-articular hemorrhage.[69] Plasma-derived and recombinant factor VIII concentrates are available, and both provide equally effective treatment (**Table 16-10**). The treatment goal for acute, life-threatening bleeding episodes (eg, intracranial hemorrhage or limb-threatening hemorrhage) is to attain a factor VIII activity of 50% to 100% of normal, as estimated by the aPTT-based 1-stage assay.

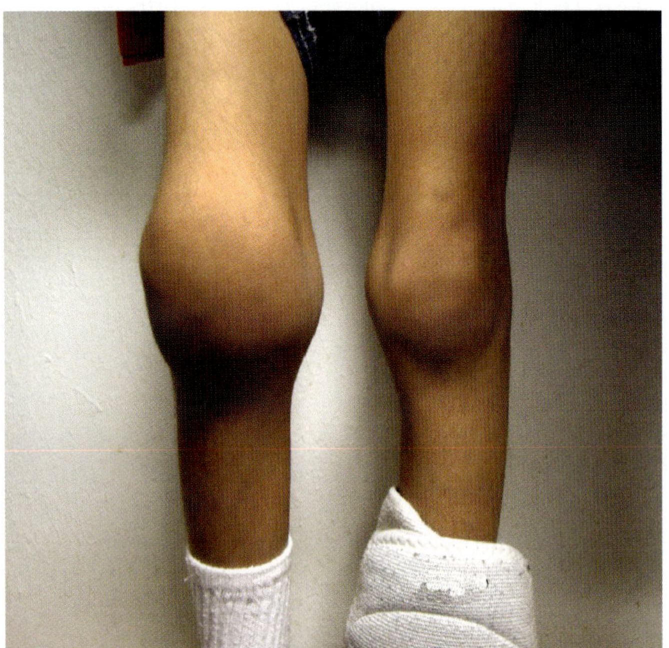

FIGURE 16-11. Image of hemophilic arthropathy in the knee joint. [Reproduced with permission from Roberts HR, Key NS, Escobar MA. Hemophilia A and hemophilia B. In: Lichtman MA, Kipps TJ, Seligsohn U, et al, eds. *Williams Hematology*. 8th ed. New York, NY: McGraw-Hill; 2008.]

TABLE 16-10 Factor VIII Concentrates Licensed in the United States

Type/Product Name	Manufacturer	Specific Activity (IU/mg Protein, Discounting Albumin)
Ultrapure Recombinant		
Recombinate	Baxter Hyland	>3000
Kogenate FS	Bayer	>3000 (albumin-free formulations)
Helixate FS	Aventis-Behring	>3000
Re Facto	Genetics Institute (American Home Products)	11 200-15 500 (albumin-free formulations)
Ultrapure Plasma-Derived		
Monoclate P	Aventis-Behring	>3000
Hemofil M	Baxter Hyland Immuno	>3000
Monarc M	Baxter (using volunteer donor plasma collected by American Red Cross)	>3000
Intermediate-Purity and High-Purity Plasma-Derived		
Alphanate SD	Alpha Therapeutics	8-30
Humate P	Aventis-Behring	1-2
Koate DVI	Bayer	9-22

Reproduced with permission from Boggio LN, Kessler CM. Hemophilia A and B. In: Kitchens CS, Alving BM, Kessler CM. *Consultative Hemostasis and Thrombosis*. 2nd ed. Philadelphia: Saunders Elsevier; 2007: 45-59.

One anesthetic consideration for patients with hemophilia A involves increasing preoperative factor VIII activity levels to approximately 100% of normal. Additionally, it is reasonable to avoid nonsteroidal anti-inflammatory drugs (eg, ibuprofen or ketorolac) because they can precipitate spontaneous, gross hematuria in hemophiliacs. Patients requiring a lumbar puncture should first be restored to approximately 100% of normal factor VIII activity levels; outcome data regarding spinal anesthesia in hemophiliacs are not available, but a similar therapeutic goal appears warranted if the benefits of spinal anesthesia outweigh the risks. Administration of factor VIII concentrates to hemophiliacs with active pharyngeal hemorrhage may not provide acute airway protection; thus elective intubation may be needed to protect against life-threatening airway obstruction.[69] In bleeding hemophiliacs or those requiring prophylaxis who have developed inhibitors to factor VIII treatment, recombinant activated factor VII (NovoSeven) is indicated. Additionally, a complete history and physical examination will reveal whether the hemophiliac has developed narcotic tolerance associated with prior treatment of painful complications related to the disease (eg, hemophilic arthropathy or ureteral blood clots).

FACTOR IX DEFICIENCY (HEMOPHILIA B)

Factor IX deficiency, also termed *hemophilia B*, or Christmas disease, results in a clinical syndrome that is similar to hemophilia A. Hemophilia B is transmitted as an X-linked recessive trait and occurs in 1 of 30 000 male births. The clinical manifestations of hemophilia B are similar to those described for hemophilia A. Mild, moderate, and severe forms of hemophilia B are defined by the same criteria used for hemophilia A (ie, severe hemophilia B is defined by a factor IX activity level of less than 1% [or 0.01 U/mL]). Severity of disease correlates with

TABLE 16-11 Classification of von Willebrand Disease

Type	Inheritance	Frequency of vWD Type	vWf Activity	RIPA	Multimer Pattern
Type 1 (classic)	Autosomal dominant	70%-75%	↓	↓	Uniform ↓ All multimers present
Type 2 (variant)					
2A	Autosomal dominant (and recessive)	10%-15%	↓	↓	↓ Large and intermediate multimers
2B	Autosomal dominant	5%	↓	↑	↓ Large multimers
2M	Autosomal dominant (and recessive)	Infrequent	↓	↓↓	Normal multimers
2N	Autosomal recessive	Infrequent	Normal	Normal	Normal multimers
Type 3 (severe)	Autosomal recessive	Rare	↓↓	↓↓	Undetectable (usually cannot visualize)

RIPA, ristocetin-induced platelet aggregation; vWD, von Willebrand disease; vWf, von Willebrand factor; ↓, decrease; ↑, increase; ↓↓, marked decrease.

Reproduced with permission from Rick ME. von Willebrand Disease. In: Kitchens CS, Alving BM, Kessler CM. *Consultative Hemostasis and Thrombosis*. 2nd ed. Philadelphia: Saunders Elsevier; 2007:97-109.

the factor IX plasma activity; patients with less than 1% activity will exhibit spontaneous hemarthroses, intramuscular hemorrhages, and gross hematuria as symptoms. The diagnosis of hemophilia B is also made with an aPTT-based 1-stage assay. The aPTT will be prolonged in patients with hemophilia B but will correct when the patient's plasma is mixed in equal parts with plasma from a normal individual.[69]

Hemophilia B is treated by administration of concentrated factor IX. Factor IX concentrates are available as either recombinant or plasma-derived preparations. The plasma half-life of transfused or endogenous factor IX is approximately 18 hours. The same levels of factor activity replacement are targeted as described in the preceding section on hemophilia A. Development of inhibitory antibodies can complicate the treatment of both factor VIII and IX deficiency. Antibodies occur more commonly in patients treated with ultra-high-purity factor concentrates (ie, the incidence is approximately 1%-4% in patients with severe factor IX deficiency).[69] Recombinant activated factor VII (rVIIa or NovoSeven) is FDA approved for the treatment of hemophilia B in patients with inhibitors to factor IX.[72] The anesthetic implications for factor IX deficiency are analogous to those of hemophilia A.

VON WILLEBRAND DISEASE

von Willebrand disease (vWD) is a disorder of platelet function caused by a deficiency of normally functioning von Willebrand factor (vWF). vWD can result in a hypocoagulable state that manifests as bleeding episodes.[73] vWD is an autosomal-dominant congenital disorder with an equal male-to-female distribution ratio occurring with an incidence of approximately 1%.

vWF plays 2 major roles in the hemostatic process. First, vWF acts as a bridge between platelet receptors and exposed collagen in disrupted endothelium. Platelet binding to exposed collagen in disrupted endothelium initially occurs via a glycoprotein Ib-vWF and collagen interaction and is followed by firmer adhesion of the platelet to the collagen molecule via a glycoprotein IIb/IIIa-vWF and collagen interaction. vWF enables platelets to create a primary plug in disrupted endothelium and commence the hemostatic process at the site of vessel injury. vWF also acts as a bridge between platelet receptors, specifically between glycoprotein IIb/IIIa receptors, to allow platelet aggregation.[73] Second, vWF circulates in the plasma to create a complex bound to factor VIII and provides protection for factor VIII against proteolytic cleavage.[73,74]

There is a broad range of bleeding severity associated with vWD. Individuals with moderate or severe vWD tend to bleed abnormally in childhood or young adulthood. The majority of affected individuals have only mild to moderate disease. Symptoms of vWD include easy bruising, epistaxis, and bleeding from mucous membranes. Menorrhagia and life-threatening gastrointestinal bleeding occur in vWD. Surgical procedures can also be associated with excessive bleeding in vWD patients.[73]

The diagnosis of vWD is complex and is made with laboratory tests, including vWF antigen, vWF activity, factor VIII activity, and bleeding time. These tests are followed by a second series of assays to determine the classification of vWD and include a ristocetin-induced platelet aggregation assay as well as vWF multimer studies.[73]

The treatment of vWD depends on the type of vWD that is diagnosed (**Tables 16-11** and **16-12**). Use of nonsteroidal anti-inflammatory drugs can further impair preexisting compromised platelet function and thus

TABLE 16-12 von Willebrand Disease Treatment Approaches

Medication	Dose	Comments
DDAVP (desmopressin)	IV: 0.3 mg/kg in 50-mL saline over 20 min (maximum 20 mg) Nasal spray: Weight >50 kg = 300 mg (1 spray in each nostril) Weight <50 kg = 150 mg (1 spray in only 1 nostril)	Useful in most patients with type 1; variable in type 2[a]; not useful in type 3. Patient should have therapeutic trial before invasive procedure. May repeat dose after 12 h and q24h. Tachyphylaxis and hyponatremia may occur: need to monitor patient
vWf concentrates containing all vWf multimers	20-30 IU/kg q12h to keep vWf levels 50%-100% or to control clinical bleeding. Levels should be maintained 3-10 d for major surgery	Dose and duration based on clinical experience
Antifibrinolytic agents:		Use alone or in conjunction with other therapy
ε-Aminocaproic acid	50 mg/kg (maximum 5 g/dose) QID	Especially useful for mucosal bleeding (often for dental procedures)
Tranexamic acid	25 mg/kg TID	
IVIg (for use in immune acquired inhibitors of vWf)	1 g/kg daily for 2 d; infusion over 8-12 h	Use after trial of DDAVP or other measures in patients with acquired vWD, particularly when associated with autoimmune diseases

DDAVP, 1-desamino-8-D-arginine vasopressin; IVIg, intravenous immunoglobulin; vWf, von Willebrand factor.

[b]Type 2, thrombocytopenia may worsen in some type 2B patients.

Reproduced with permission from Rick ME. von Willebrand Disease. In: Kitchens CS, Alving BM, Kessler CM. *Consultative Hemostasis and Thrombosis*. 2nd ed. Philadelphia: Saunders Elsevier; 2007:97-109.

are contraindicated in vWD. The correlation of the degree of diagnostic laboratory test abnormalities in vWD with the bleeding severity is poor, and therefore empirical goals of treatment are pursued. The treatment goal for the perioperative period should be to increase the activity of vWF and factor VIII to 50% to 100% of normal, an analogous goal to the usual treatment of bleeding episodes in vWD.[73]

vWF and factor VIII activity levels are increased in patients with vWD by IV administration of DDAVP (1-desamino-8-D-arginine-vasopressin or desmopressin) and giving vWF-rich plasma-derived blood products. The use of topical hemostatic agents (eg, fibrin glue, Gel-foam, or thrombin-soaked Surgicel) will also promote hemostasis in vWD patients.[73] Alternatively, intravenous (IV) vWF concentrates (eg, Humate P) can be given to patients who do not respond positively to DDAVP therapy. Pregnant patients with vWD merit special considerations. Although evidence-based recommendations for central neuraxial blockade in vWD do not exist, consideration should be given to the fact that causing a spinal or epidural hematoma may be permanently debilitating. vWF levels increase 2 to 3 times above the baseline during the second and third trimesters of a pregnancy and may provide some protection from bleeding complications. The increased levels should be verified by selected assays because an increase in vWF is not universal, and some patients with qualitative vWF defects will not correct their vWF activity during pregnancy. DDAVP can be administered to vWD patients in active labor who are known to have a positive response to this therapy. vWF replacement therapy can be given to patients who are still bleeding after DDAVP administration. Patients who are known nonresponders to DDAVP should be treated with vWF concentrates. Lysine analog antifibrinolytic agents (eg, ε-aminocaproic acid and tranexamic acid) have been successfully used as both adjuncts and monotherapy in some patients with vWD-related hemorrhage.[73]

RARE FACTOR DEFICIENCIES

The individual deficiencies of factors V, VII, X, and XI have all been described and are known to be rare. The reader is referred to in-depth subject matter on these disorders if further information is needed, because covering these hypocoagulable disorders is beyond the scope of this text.[75] Table 16-8 provides some detailed information on these factor deficiencies and their treatment.

CONTACT FACTORS DEFICIENCY

Factor XII, high-molecular-weight kininogen, and prekallikrein constitute the contact factors of the coagulation cascade (Fig. 16-9); definitive diagnosis is made with a specific assay for the deficient contact factor. Contact factor deficiencies are not associated with bleeding, although these individuals demonstrate a prolonged aPTT. No specific perioperative treatment is required for these disorders.[75]

FACTOR XIII DEFICIENCY

Factor XIII is important for the structural stabilization of a fibrin clot; it creates cross-linking peptide bonds between the fibrin strands in a blood clot (Fig. 16-9). Blood clots that lack cross-linked peptide bonds are unstable, permeable to blood, and susceptible to fibrinolysis and provide a poor framework for wound healing. Although 3 different forms of congenital factor XIII deficiency have been described, each is extremely rare. All share the tendency for excessive perioperative bleeding, as well as a lifelong history of bleeding problems when factor XIII activity is less than 1%. Hemorrhage may be seen from birth and throughout life. Although most bleeding episodes are triggered by trauma, spontaneous intracranial bleeding can occur.[75,77]

Definitive diagnosis of factor XIII deficiency is made with a specific clot solubility assay and an assay to quantify the level of factor XIII deficiency. An acquired version of factor XIII deficiency exists that involves the generation of factor XIII autoantibody.[75,77]

The treatment of factor XIII deficiency is accomplished by administration of fresh-frozen plasma or cryoprecipitate. In Europe, factor XIII concentrate (Fibrogammin-P) is available to treat this disorder. Normal hemostasis occurs with factor XIII levels of greater than 5%. Preoperative preparation of individuals with factor XIII activity levels of less than 5% is to give 2 to 3 mL/kg of fresh-frozen plasma or 1 unit of cryoprecipitate per 10 to 20 kg of body weight. The long plasma half-life of factor XIII (9-10 days) usually obviates a need to re-dose. Lifelong supplementation of factor XIII is indicated in individuals with very low levels to prevent intracranial hemorrhage, even when surgery is not planned. The treatment of individuals who have developed inhibitory antibodies to factor XIII is complex and may involve exchange transfusion, administration of platelets (ie, platelets are known to contain factor XIII), or administration of immunosuppressants (eg, intravenous gamma globulin, steroids, and cyclophosphamide).[75,77]

AFIBRINOGENEMIA

Fibrinogen serves as the precursor molecule for the proteinaceous fibrin scaffolding of a blood clot. A congenital or acquired deficiency of fibrinogen can produce clinically important bleeding disorders, especially in the surgical patient. Congenital homozygous afibrinogenemia is a rare disorder that is associated with a varying severity of bleeding problems (eg, easy bruising, mucosal hemorrhage, hematuria, hemarthroses, hemopericardium, hemoperitoneum, menometrorrhagia, obstetrical complications, intracerebral hemorrhage, and spontaneous splenic rupture). These patients have no detectable serum fibrinogen and a markedly prolonged PT, aPTT, and TT; occasional thrombocytopenia; and a plasma fibrinogen assay reveals no detectable fibrinogen.[75]

Preoperative fibrinogen levels must be restored to 50 to 100 mg/dL by infusing cryoprecipitate or human-derived pooled fibrinogen concentrate (Riastap). Five to ten units of cryoprecipitate are needed to increase fibrinogen levels to 50 to 100 mg/dL. A single unit of cryoprecipitate contains approximately 250 to 300 mg of fibrinogen and is expected to raise the plasma fibrinogen level approximately 10 mg/dL. Fibrinogen levels will persist for 2 to 4 days after infusion. The following formula is used to determine the necessary dose of fibrinogen concentrate:

Dose (mg/kg body weight) = (target level [mg/dL] – measured level [mg/dL])/(1.7 [mg/dL per mg/kg body weight])

or, when the fibrinogen level is unknown, administer 70 mg/kg body weight of fibrinogen concentrate.[78] Operations associated with postoperative hemorrhage result in decreased fibrinogen levels so they should be monitored perioperatively on a daily basis. Thrombosis has been reported in patients with fibrinogen levels normalized via cryoprecipitate infusion.[75,79]

DYSFIBRINOGENEMIA

Many variants of congenital dysfibrinogenemia exist. They share the common feature of abnormal conversion of fibrinogen to fibrin. Most individuals with dysfibrinogenemias are heterozygous and usually produce nearly 50% of normal plasma fibrinogen levels, enabling effective hemostasis. Some dysfibrinogenemia variants result in fibrinogen levels well below normal or despite near normal levels of fibrinogen are associated with bleeding problems if the abnormal variant affects the function of the fibrinogen.[75]

Clinical manifestations of dysfibrinogenemia include the following: thrombosis (17%), mild bleeding after trauma (20%), both thrombotic and hemorrhagic manifestations (20%), no hemorrhagic phenomenon, or asymptomatic (43%). Affected patients who demonstrate bleeding problems usually manifest with soft tissue bleeding, easy bruising, menorrhagia, and most commonly perioperative bleeding. Individuals who manifest thromboses can experience either venous (eg, deep venous thrombosis, pulmonary embolism) or arterial involvement (eg, thrombosis of the aorta and carotid arteries). Individuals with thrombotic manifestations can possess concurrent disorders of other portions of the coagulation system (eg, factor V Leiden mutation or other thrombophilias) contributing to their propensity to inappropriately clot. Poor surgical wound healing can be associated with dysfibrinogenemia.[75]

Standard laboratory tests of the coagulation system (eg, PT, aPTT, TT) are usually prolonged despite normal levels of fibrinogen due to a functional defect in the circulating fibrinogen. The reptilase time is often prolonged and fibrinogen immunoelectrophoresis using agarose gels can reveal an abnormal pattern of protein migration. Acquired dysfibrinogenemia associated with hepatic disease can be differentiated from congenital dysfibrinogenemia because it will demonstrate decreased levels of other clotting factors that are synthesized by the liver.

Symptomatic dysfibrinogenemia is treated by administering cryoprecipitate in a manner similar to that described in the Afibrinogenemia section of this chapter (ie, the goal is to restore functional fibrinogen levels to 50-100 mg/dL). Fresh-frozen plasma or fibrinogen concentrates (eg, Riastap) may also be administered to restore functional levels of fibrinogen to normal. The thrombotic variants of dysfibrinogenemia require treatment with intravenous anticoagulation with unfractionated heparin and eventual conversion to oral anticoagulation.[78]

PROTHROMBIN (FACTOR II) DEFICIENCY

Prothrombin deficiency consists of either a quantitative (hypoprothrombinemia) or qualitative (dysprothrombinemia) defect. Prothrombin is normally converted to thrombin (factor IIa) (Fig. 16-9). Thrombin is needed for the conversion of fibrinogen to fibrin, which serves as the protein scaffold of a blood clot. Dysprothrombinemia is an extremely rare disorder that can be either homozygous, heterozygous, or compound heterozygous.[75]

Heterozygous individuals generally have prothrombin activity levels of 50%, normal quantitative levels of prothrombin, and are asymptomatic or have only minor bleeding symptoms (eg, may develop bleeding only after surgical procedures). Homozygous or compound heterozygous individuals demonstrate a lifelong history of bleeding.[75]

Dysprothrombinemia is definitively diagnosed using an assay of functional prothrombin activity. PT and aPTT are prolonged; both will correct when mixed 1:1 with normal plasma. Hepatic function may cause acquired dysprothrombinemia. Acquired dysprothrombinemia is distinct in that multiple hepatic synthetic defects are present in the absence of a history of bleeding problems.[75]

Symptomatic dysprothrombinemia may be treated by administration of fresh-frozen plasma at a loading dose of 15 to 20 mL/kg followed by 3 mL/kg every 12 to 24 hours (ie, an appropriate regimen for individuals with severe bleeding), administration of prothrombin complex concentrates with a loading dose of 20 U/kg prothrombin followed by 5 U/kg every 24 hours, with care not to exceed these doses to avoid the risk of thromboembolism, or plasma exchange transfusion to restore normal levels of prothrombin.[75]

DRUG-INDUCED HYPOCOAGULABLE STATES

Thrombotic complications associated with surgery and percutaneous coronary interventions have stimulated the development of intravenous, subcutaneous, and oral anticoagulant drugs. The 2 general classes of anticoagulant drugs include antiplatelet and antithrombotic agents.[79,80]

Knowing the pharmacodynamic and pharmacokinetic profiles of drugs that affect the coagulation system is necessary to make safe decisions regarding the timing of surgical procedures. Safe conduct of regional anesthesia requires knowledge of how these drugs affect coagulation. An anticoagulant drug's half-life may not predict the duration of its effects on the coagulation system if it irreversibly inhibits one or more aspects of the coagulation system. For example, aspirin has an elimination half-life of 15 to 20 minutes but irreversibly inhibits platelet activation through a selective enzymatic pathway.[81] Consideration of the route of elimination and the individual patient's level of organ function is necessary to predict a drug's effect. For instance, compromised renal function will prolong the elimination half-life of a drug that relies on the kidney to clear its active form. In some instances, suppression or supplementation of components of the coagulation system will be necessary to allow the safe conduct of an invasive procedure (ie, patients who are systemically anticoagulated with unfractionated heparin may require the administration of protamine to neutralize the effects of the heparin-antithrombin complex on factor II and activated factor X).

THE ANTITHROMBOTIC AGENTS

The antithrombotic agents include 5 subcategories of drugs: unfractionated heparin (UFH), low-molecular-weight heparin (LMWH), activated factor X inhibitor, direct thrombin inhibitors, and coumarins. Antithrombotic agents are used to both treat and prophylax against thrombotic events.[79]

UFH, a large molecule that is extracted either from porcine intestine or bovine lung, exerts its antithrombotic effect primarily via an interaction with antithrombin (Fig. 16-9). The heparin-antithrombin complex permits an approximately 1000-fold increase in the ability of heparin to inhibit factor II (prothrombin) activity and activated factor X activity.[82] The result of UFH's action is suppression of the coagulation cascade, as reflected in a dose-dependent prolongation of both the aPTT and the activated clotting time (ACT). The half-life of the anticoagulation effect of UFH as estimated by the aPTT is approximately 1.5 hours irrespective of the heparin dose. In contrast, the functional half-life varies with the magnitude of the administered dose from approximately 40 to 150 minutes, with larger doses yielding a longer duration. UFH's elimination half-life is not affected by renal dysfunction because the drug is cleared from the plasma by transfer to the extravascular space, most likely to the reticuloendothelial system. UFH dosage is calculated according to actual body weight; depending on the anticoagulation goal, different dosing schemes are used (eg, initiation of cardiopulmonary bypass requires a bolus of approximately 300 U/kg, whereas treatment of a venous thrombosis requires an IV bolus of approximately 5000 units plus an infusion).[82] Laboratory monitoring is required (eg, the aPTT, ACT, whole-blood heparin concentration, or anti–factor Xa activity) because some individuals exhibit insensitivity to heparin.[83] An elapsed time of 4 hours after IV heparin therapy cessation may be required to achieve an aPTT of less than 35 seconds, indicating abatement of UFH's anticoagulant effects, before safely initiating an elective surgical procedure or attempting central neuraxial blockade. Alternatively, IV protamine sulfate can be administered to rapidly neutralize UFH's anticoagulant effect. In practice, protamine is given in a range of 0.7 to 1.3 mg: 100 units of UFH administered, or alternatively the protamine dose can be titrated to effect by giving small doses (25-50 mg) and checking the ACT or aPTT to assess whether values have normalized. Protamine is best administered slowly to prevent systemic hypotension and/or pulmonary hypertension. Additional specific recommendations related to UFH treatment can be found in the American Society of Regional Anesthesia and Pain Medicine Practice Guidelines.[84]

LMWH was developed to create an antithrombotic agent that does not require anticoagulant monitoring in the absence of renal insufficiency. LMWH is produced from UFH by a process that decreases the size of the polysaccharide chains of the heparin molecule, resulting in a smaller molecule with potent anti-activated factor X activity. Both UFH and LWMH require antithrombin to exert their effect on activated factor X (Fig. 16-9). A number of LWMH preparations are available for clinical use: enoxaparin (Lovenox), dalteparin (Fragmin), ardeparin (Normiflo), and tinzaparin (Innohep). Patients with renal insufficiency receiving LMWH require dose adjustment and plasma monitoring of anti-activated factor X activity.[85,86] The elimination half-lives of the various preparations of LMWH vary from 3 to 5 hours. Therefore waiting 24 hours after administration is recommended after higher doses (ie, any dose of enoxaparin >1 mg/kg or dalteparin >120 U/kg) of LMWH before an elective surgical procedure or attempting central neuraxial blockade.[84] Although the anticoagulant effects of LMWH can be partially reversed by protamine sulfate, its use has been associated with increased bleeding complications perioperatively, despite protamine reversal.[87]

The activated factor X inhibitor fondaparinux (Arixtra) requires interaction with antithrombin to exert its anticoagulant effect. Once bonded with antithrombin, the fondaparinux-antithrombin complex selectively increases the ability of antithrombin to inhibit activated factor X activity approximately 300-fold. The molecule is smaller than LMWHs and does not elicit formation of or react with the platelet factor 4 (PF4) antibody associated with heparin-induced thrombocytopenia type II. The elimination half-life is 17 to 21 hours. No definite recommendations exist for management of this drug before attempting neuraxial blockade, although it is recommended to use a single-needle atraumatic placement technique and avoid an indwelling catheter if a neuraxial procedure is required. Although no evidence-based recommendations exist, delaying elective surgery for approximately 5 half-lives, or 4 days, is a conservative management strategy for patients treated with this drug.[84] Because there is minimal metabolic breakdown and the primary route of elimination is renal, dose adjustment is required for patients with renal insufficiency. Assays of anti-activated plasma factor X levels are not required in the absence of renal insufficiency.[85]

Direct thrombin inhibitors (DTI) include dabigatran (Pradaxa), lepirudin (Refludan), argatroban, desirudin (Iprivask), and bivalirudin (Angiomax). They exert their effect by interacting with free or clot-bound thrombin to inhibit conversion of fibrinogen to fibrin (Fig. 16-9). DTIs do not rely on the presence of antithrombin to exert their effects. They are given to treat or prevent thrombotic events, including the treatment of patients undergoing percutaneous coronary interventions with or at risk for heparin-induced thrombocytopenia (argatroban) or for PCI (bivalirudin).[88] The half-lives of these drugs vary (**Table 16-13**). Bivalirudin has recently been demonstrated to be a safe and effective anticoagulant for cardiac surgical patients requiring cardiopulmonary bypass.[89,90] Although no evidence-based recommendations exist, conservative management suggests that patients on continuous IV infusions of DTIs should have the drug discontinued 5 elimination half-lives before an operation or neuraxial blockade; no antidote exists for DTI-related bleeding.[84] DTIs do not elicit formation of or cross-react with the PF4 antibody associated with heparin-induced thrombocytopenia type II and are therefore useful to prevent and treat thrombotic events in patients with this syndrome. Clinical effects of DTIs are commonly followed by either the aPTT or the ACT. Dabigatran is the only FDA-cleared oral DTI available in the United States and has a half-life of approximately 17 hours (considerably longer than the half-lives associated with the IV DTIs) in patients with normal renal function, necessitating discontinuation of this drug approximately 4 to 5 days prior to implementing central neuraxial blockade or a regional anesthetic procedure.[84,91]

Coumarins, a subclass of oral antithrombotics, exert their anticoagulant effect by inhibiting the hepatic synthesis of vitamin K–dependent coagulation factors. Coumarins inhibit the synthesis of factors II, VII, IX, and X as well as proteins C and S. Assessing the PT or international normalized ratio (INR) can be used to quantify low levels or activities of these specific coagulation proteins. Vitamin K–dependent factors participate in the extrinsic and common coagulation pathways (Fig. 16-9); therefore, the PT or INR is the best test to assess coumarin effects. PT is reported as the INR to avoid inter-laboratory variation of absolute PT results.[79] Warfarin is the only coumarin approved by the FDA. It is metabolized by the liver and possesses an elimination half-life of 20 to 60 hours. Anticoagulant effects of warfarin take several days to abate depending on the level of warfarin effect at discontinuation. Administration of vitamin K will decrease the time for the effects of warfarin to abate, but may make it difficult to reinstitute a therapeutic warfarin effect, thereby complicating postoperative anticoagulation therapy. Alternatively, administration of fresh-frozen plasma will acutely reverse the anticoagulant effects of warfarin. However, anticoagulation may recur several hours later due to the longer half-life of warfarin than the coagulation factor levels that it inhibits (ie, warfarin's half-life is 20-60 hours; half-life of factor VII is approximately 6 hours). Administration of prothrombin complex concentrates (eg, Beriplex) may offer another option for rapid and effective reversal of warfarin's effects. Excessive operative hemorrhage and neuraxial anesthesia associated with spinal or epidural hematoma may occur if warfarin is not neutralized.[84] Individuals at increased risk for a serious thrombotic event should be anticoagulated with a second intravenous or subcutaneous antithrombotic agent (eg, UFH, LMWH, or a short-acting direct thrombin inhibitor) before warfarin is discontinued or neutralized. Titration of antithrombotic therapy is complex in the presence of more than 1 antithrombotic agent or when a preexisting factor deficiency is present.

Guidelines from the American Society of Regional Anesthesia recommend stopping warfarin 5 days before attempting a central neuraxial blockade or regional anesthesia and verifying that its effects have abated by obtaining an INR value of 1.4 or less.[84]

TABLE 16-13 Direct Thrombin Inhibitor Elimination Half-Lives

Drug	Half-Life
Argatroban	30-51 min
Bivalirudin (Angiomax)	25 min
Lepirudin (Refludan)	48-120 min
Dabigatran (Pradaxa)	11-17 h

Data from Thomson MICROMEDEX 1.0. Direct thrombin inhibitors. New York. http://www.thomsonhc.com/home/dispatch. Accessed January 30, 2011.

ANTIPLATELET AGENTS

The 5 subcategories of antiplatelet agents include nonsteroidal anti-inflammatory drugs, glycoprotein IIb/IIIa receptor inhibitors, platelet adhesion inhibitors, platelet adenosine diphosphate (ADP) receptor antagonists, and platelet production-limiting agents. Platelets can be activated by more than 1 stimulus, and therefore not all antiplatelet agents will place surgical patients at an increased risk for bleeding. Indeed, antiplatelet drugs have proven quite beneficial to patients with cardiovascular disease.[92,93] The increasing use of herbal medications in the United States has drawn attention to the anticoagulant effects of select agents; limited evidence-based data exist describing the interactions of herbal medications with other medications and their effect on the clinical course of surgical patients.[84,94,95]

Nonsteroidal Anti-inflammatory Drugs Aspirin exerts its antiplatelet effects by irreversibly inhibiting the platelet enzyme cyclooxygenase. This prevents the formation of thromboxane A2 from arachidonic acid for the lifetime of the platelet, which in turn blocks platelet activation and aggregation and the release of thromboxane A2, which propagates further platelet activation. Normal platelets have an average circulating life span of approximately 10 days; thus it may take up to 5 days for half-normal platelet function to return after treatment with aspirin, despite measurement of a normal platelet concentration. Aspirin's half-life is 15 to 20 minutes in the plasma, and it undergoes primarily hepatic metabolism as well as plasma esterase metabolism. Other nonsteroidal anti-inflammatory drugs (NSAIDs), such as ibuprofen, ketorolac, and naproxen, produce reversible platelet cyclooxygenase inhibition. Therefore, the return of platelet function correlates with the drug's half-life, and perioperative management with these antiplatelet agents is easily accomplished when one considers that permitting 5 half-lives to elapse after the last dose will completely eliminate the effects of these NSAIDs. For aspirin a distinct perioperative treatment strategy is needed. After aspirin removal, antiplatelet effects of aspirin can only be overcome by platelet transfusion.[81] Doubt exists whether NSAIDs result in significant surgical hemorrhage. If an NSAID is the only inhibitory influence on the coagulation cascade, then later central neuraxial blockade can be safely undertaken.[84] In selected patients with severe peripheral arterial vascular disease, it is advisable to continue perioperative aspirin.[96]

Glycoprotein IIB/IIIA Receptor Inhibitors The glycoprotein IIb/IIIa (GP IIb/IIIa) receptor inhibitors are available only as IV preparations and are among the most potent inhibitors of platelet function. Currently the following GP IIb/IIIa receptor inhibitors are approved for clinical use in the United States: abciximab (ReoPro), eptifibatide (Integrili), and tirofiban (Aggrastat). Platelets are activated by various stimuli, including thromboxane, ADP, epinephrine, serotonin, and mechanical shear stress. The final common pathway of platelet activation involves platelet aggregation via interaction of GP IIb/IIIa receptors and either fibrinogen or vWF as an intermediate molecule. Complete inhibition of this final step of platelet aggregation could render a patient completely thrombasthenic.[97-99]

Abciximab is the Fab portion of the chimeric human/murine monoclonal antibody 7E3 that is directed against the platelet GP IIb/IIIa receptor. In therapeutic doses it creates a marked decrease in the ability of platelets to aggregate. In approximately 1% to 2% of patients, it produces significant thrombocytopenia.[97] Abciximab also inhibits thrombus formation by suppressing tissue factor-induced thrombin generation. It is FDA approved for use as an adjunct in both percutaneous coronary interventions (PCI) and the treatment of refractory angina. Abciximab has a 30-minute plasma half-life. However, once bound to the platelet GP IIb/IIIa receptor, it remains in the circulation for up to 15 days. The putative mechanism for this is migration from platelet to platelet. The anti-aggregation effect lasts 12 to 48 hours. Platelet transfusion may partially restore platelet function if significant bleeding occurs 12 to 48 hours after infusion.[97] Central neuraxial blockade is contraindicated within 24 to 48 hours of abciximab administration.[84] Delaying cardiac surgery in the stable patient treated with abciximab for 12 to 24 hours will allow for some return of platelet function.

Tirofiban, a non-peptide chemical antagonist of the platelet GP IIb/IIIa receptor, produces a greater than 90% reversible reduction in platelet aggregation. Tirofiban is FDA approved for the treatment of acute coronary syndrome (ACS) in patients undergoing angioplasty or being medically managed.[98] The half-life is reported at 90 to 180 minutes; it undergoes renal excretion largely as unchanged drug. Central neuraxial blockade should be delayed for 4 to 8 hours in patients who are receiving tirofiban.[84] It does not appear to confer an increased risk of hemorrhage after emergent or urgent coronary surgery.[100] No specific recommendations are available for general surgical patients at this time.

Eptifibatide is a heptapeptide molecule that inhibits the platelet GP IIb/IIIa receptor and is a potent inhibitor of platelet aggregation, with FDA approval for use in PCI and for the treatment of ACS. The drug is cleared from the circulation by the kidneys with a half-life of 2.5 hours. Approximately 71% of the drug is eliminated unmetabolized.[99] A 4- to 8-hour delay is recommended after discontinuation of this drug before attempting central neuraxial blockade.[84] Data from a large trial suggest that it is safe to perform coronary surgery within 2 hours of the discontinuation of eptifibatide.[99]

ADP Antagonists Clopidogrel (Plavix), ticlopidine (Ticlid), and prasugrel (Effient) are FDA-approved ADP receptor antagonists, selectively and irreversibly inhibiting ADP-induced platelet aggregation by blocking the P2Y12 ADP receptor on the platelet's surface. These oral agents lack effects on prostacyclin and thromboxane synthesis and work by preventing the ADP platelet P2Y12 receptor from transmitting a signal to the platelet to activate GP IIb/IIIa receptor complexes.

Clopidogrel is FDA approved to reduce thrombotic events related to a recent myocardial infarction or stroke and established peripheral arterial disease. Additionally, clopidogrel is approved for both medical management and PCI treatment of acute coronary syndrome. Clopidogrel and ticlopidine both undergo extensive hepatic metabolism. Clopidogrel is excreted in both urine and feces. The half-life of clopidogrel is approximately 8 hours.[101] The irreversible nature of the inhibitory effect of clopidogrel on platelets requires 5 to 7 days before a sufficient population of functional platelets are restored. Seven full days are recommended after treatment with this drug before attempting central neuraxial blockade.[84] Clopidogrel-treated patients exhibit significant bleeding and transfusion requirements after cardiac surgery.[102] Evidence-based recommendations do not exist for general surgery patients at this time.

Ticlopidine is FDA approved for coronary stenting in conjunction with aspirin therapy. Ticlopidine is also FDA approved for the prophylaxis of thromboembolic stroke. At least 1 metabolite of ticlopidine is a potent inhibitor of ADP-induced platelet aggregation. This metabolite is excreted primarily in the urine. Ticlopidine has a reported half-life of 12.6 hours, which increases dramatically to 5 days with repeated dosing. Ticlopidine is used less frequently than clopidogrel because of toxicity (eg, neutropenia, agranulocytosis, and thrombotic thrombocytopenic purpura).[103] A delay of 14 days is recommended after discontinuation of this drug before attempting central neuraxial blockade.[84] Evidence-based recommendations do not exist for general surgery patients at this time.

The recently FDA-approved P2Y12 receptor inhibitor, prasugrel, is metabolized by both intestinal and serum esterases as well as the liver. It is given to reduce thrombotic cardiovascular events (including stent thrombosis) in patients with ACS who are managed with PCI. The effects of prasugrel on platelets are analogous to those of clopidogrel and abate approximately 5 to 9 days after discontinuation. It has a half-life of approximately 7 hours, which is irrelevant because it irreversibly inhibits ADP-mediated platelet aggregation.[104] Perioperative recommendations related to bleeding and regional anesthesia are identical to those of clopidogrel.

Platelet Adhesion Inhibitors Dipyridamole (Persantine, Aggrenox) and cilostazol (Pletal) are drugs classified as platelet adhesion inhibitors. Dipyridamole, available in oral and IV preparations, has a complex mechanism of action that ultimately inhibits platelet aggregation by blocking their activation by ADP, collagen, and platelet-activating factor. Dipyridamole is FDA approved to be used as an adjunct with warfarin for the prophylaxis of thromboembolic complications associated with cardiac valve replacement and for use with thallium in myocardial imaging studies. It is also given to prevent thromboembolic events associated with coronary surgery. Dipyridamole primarily undergoes hepatic metabolism and has a half-life of approximately 9 to 13 hours.[105]

Dipyridamole administration is associated with bleeding. The risk is greater when dipyridamole is combined with aspirin therapy. A combination of dipyridamole and aspirin, Aggrenox, is commercially available. Aggrenox is FDA approved for the prophylaxis of cerebrovascular accidents in patients with a previous history of stroke or transient ischemic attacks.[106] It may be prudent to delay central neuraxial anesthesia for 7 days after Aggrenox therapy to allow the recovery of approximately 50% of normal platelet aggregation. Published literature does not suggest the use of dipyridamole alone to be a direct contraindication to proceeding with elective surgery or neuraxial blockade; however, because dipyridamole works by suppressing platelet aggregation, it may be prudent to avoid elective surgery and neuraxial blockade for 4 days. One reported meta-analysis concludes that among the antiplatelet drugs, dipyridamole was associated with the lowest incidence of bleeding complications.[107] In a large trial of antiplatelet drugs used for the prevention of stroke in medical patients, dipyridamole was indistinguishable from placebo in terms of producing bleeding complications.[108]

Cilostazol increases intracellular cyclic adenosine monophosphate (cAMP) by inhibiting the enzyme phosphodiesterase III. An increase in levels of cAMP results in reversible inhibition of platelet aggregation. It is FDA approved for reduction in the symptoms of intermittent claudication. It is extensively metabolized by the liver into active metabolites that are primarily cleared by the kidneys and has a reported elimination half-life of 11 to 13 hours. Because no evidence-based recommendations exist, a conservative management approach would be to delay elective surgery or central neuraxial blockade for 48 hours after administration.[109]

HERBAL THERAPIES

Self-medication with herbal therapies has been increasing in the United States.[94] Select herbal therapies are now recognized as having deleterious effects on elements of the coagulation cascade, although there is a paucity of research.[95] Garlic, ginkgo, ginseng, ginger, feverfew, fish oil, and dong quai have been implicated as inhibiting normal hemostasis; several of these agents can interfere with platelet aggregation.[84,94,95] Anesthesiologists should routinely inquire during preoperative evaluation whether patients are taking herbal supplements. Patients taking herbal supplements should be advised to discontinue their use preoperatively. The current lack of literature makes it uncertain whether to recommend delaying elective surgical procedures or neuraxial blockade for patients using these supplements. One may expect that individuals taking these herbal therapies along with the concurrent use of other antiplatelet or antithrombotic agents could exhibit synergistic suppressive effects on their coagulation system.

HYPERCOAGULABLE STATES

Thrombophilias, or hypercoagulable states, place surgical patients at increased risk for experiencing a postoperative thrombotic event. Many of these hypercoagulable states are managed with temporary or lifelong systemic anticoagulation therapy. Environmental influences (eg, trauma, surgery, infection, or administration of a drug) will increase the likelihood of a patient with either a congenital or acquired hypercoagulable disorder to develop a thromboembolic event and thus can impact the perioperative management of these patients.[110,111] Several thrombophilias are currently recognized, and anesthesiologists should be familiar with them to aid in the provision of optimal perioperative care. Discontinuation and reinitiation of systemic anticoagulation in the perioperative period is most safely managed in consultation with a hematologist.

ANTITHROMBIN DEFICIENCY

Antithrombin (also termed *antithrombin III*) is a plasma protein produced by the liver that prevents hypercoagulability by binding to and neutralizing thrombin, factors IXa, Xa, XIa, and XIIa (Fig. 16-9). Antithrombin (AT) deficiency is associated with a predilection for thrombosis. AT deficiency is a congenital disorder inherited as an autosomal-dominant trait that is estimated to occur with a prevalence of 1 in 250 to 500 people.[112] Individuals with a history of an unexplained thrombotic event should be evaluated to rule out this disorder.

AT deficiency may be due to decreased synthesis (type I) of this protein or due to decreased protein activity despite normal levels (type II). AT levels are between 75% and 120% in normal individuals. AT levels are measured with a specific assay. Disease states associated with reduced AT activity include sepsis, disseminated intravascular coagulation, burns, acute thrombosis, hepatic disease, severe trauma, and nephritis.[112]

Patients with AT deficiency have a predisposition to develop deep vein thromboses and therefore are often maintained on warfarin. Perioperative management of anticoagulation should be tailored to the invasiveness of the planned intervention or surgical procedure. Surgery induces a prothrombotic state and increases the risk of perioperative thrombosis.[113]

Anticoagulation with UFH is frequently required perioperatively. Importantly, many AT-deficient patients exhibit a relative resistance to UFH because UFH anticoagulation requires coupling with AT to induce an increase in AT's neutralizing effect on the procoagulant factors IIa, IXa, Xa, XIa, and XIIa.[83] ACT or aPTT assays will reveal heparin resistance in patients with an AT deficiency. Heparin resistance in this context is defined as a failure of UFH to produce the expected degree of ACT or aPTT prolongation. Heparin resistance due to AT deficiency is most efficiently treated with plasma-derived, purified AT III concentrate (Thrombate). A bolus of AT III concentrate at 50 IU/kg has been recommended for therapy. If AT III concentrate is not used, heparin resistance can be treated with 2 to 4 units of fresh-frozen plasma with the effect of this therapy assessed by an ACT or aPTT assay.[114]

PROTEIN C DEFICIENCY

Protein C is a hepatically synthesized vitamin K–dependent protein that, when converted to its active form (activated protein C), exerts an anticoagulant effect through interaction with factors Va and VIIIa (Fig. 16-9). Protein C deficiency may be due to either a quantitative or qualitative defect. It is estimated to occur with a prevalence of 1 in 200 to 500.[115]

Many patients with protein C deficiency exhibit a prothrombotic tendency and can require systemic anticoagulation. Protein C deficiency is diagnosed with an aPTT-based clotting assay.[116] The diagnosis of protein C deficiency in patients who have recently been treated with warfarin is complex. Patients with protein C deficiency requiring a surgical intervention require perioperative modification of their anticoagulation therapy.

PROTEIN S DEFICIENCY

Protein S is synthesized primarily in the liver and functions as a cofactor for activated protein C. Quantitative and qualitative congenital protein S deficiencies have been described. Patients with protein S deficiency can have a prothrombotic tendency and may be maintained on systemic oral anticoagulation as outpatients; therefore, this necessitates perioperative modification of their outpatient regimen.[112]

FACTOR V LEIDEN (ACTIVATED PROTEIN C RESISTANCE)

Factor V Leiden, also termed *activated protein C resistance*, is associated with recurrent venous thromboembolic events. It is caused by a single point mutation in the gene that encodes for factor V. This mutation is common among patients who experience thrombotic events. It is commonly diagnosed by an aPTT-based assay. Patients with the factor V Leiden mutation may be on either temporary or lifetime systemic oral anticoagulation.[112]

PROTHROMBIN G20210 MUTATION

Prothrombin, or factor II, is an essential element of the coagulation cascade. A single base pair substitution mutation results in affected individuals expressing higher plasma prothrombin activity associated with the occurrence of thromboembolic disease in these patients. This disorder is the second most common thrombophilia, with a prevalence of 2% in whites, with considerable geographic variation. It is commonly diagnosed using a polymerase chain reaction–based test.[112]

HEPARIN-INDUCED THROMBOCYTOPENIA

Heparin-induced thrombocytopenia (HIT) involves an immune-mediated response to either low-molecular-weight or unfractionated heparin administration that results in pathologic platelet activation causing arterial and/or venous thrombosis with or without associated tissue ischemia and infarction. There are 2 types of HIT. Type I is a non–immune-mediated activation of platelets in heparin-treated patients causing a mild reduction in circulating platelets. HIT type II, or heparin-induced thrombocytopenia with thrombotic syndrome (HITTS), is immune-mediated. It is caused by the interaction of a heparin-dependent immunoglobulin G (IgG) antibody with the molecular complex of platelet factor 4 (PF4) and heparin. The heparin-PF4–bound IgG antibody stimulates platelet activation via the platelet FcγIIa receptor. Once platelets are activated they release internal biochemical mediators that induce platelet aggregation and stimulate other platelets to become activated. The same biochemical mediators that are released from the activated platelets will also stimulate thrombin generation. Heparin-PF4 IgG antibody-induced platelet aggregation along with thrombin contributes to the formation of thrombus. Although venous thrombosis occurs most commonly in HIT type II, arterial thrombosis is also observed, especially at the site of arterial disruption (eg, aortotomy site in cardiac surgery). Thrombi can cause organ ischemia and/or infarction. Loss of limbs and damage to vital organs, such as renal failure or strokes, are recognized complications of this disorder.[117]

Numerous features of HIT type II are poorly understood. Only a portion of patients exposed to heparin develop the IgG antibody directed against heparin and PF4 (commonly termed the *PF4 antibody*). Only a small percentage of patients who develop the PF4 antibody will develop thrombocytopenia and a recognized thrombotic event. At least a 50% decrease in platelet count from the pre–heparin administration baseline is preferred to establish the diagnosis of HIT type II. Using the absolute laboratory criterion of fewer than 150 000 platelets/mm^3 is not completely appropriate to diagnose HIT type II. Patients who are generating the PF4 antibody on initial exposure to heparin characteristically take at least 5 days to develop sufficient amounts of PF4 antibody to cause thrombocytopenia.[117] Patients previously exposed to heparin who have generated PF4 antibody in the past 100 days may develop thrombocytopenia more rapidly. In contrast, the thrombocytopenic response and thrombotic event can occur several days to weeks after the discontinuation of heparin therapy.[118]

HIT type II may be diagnosed using either an antigen assay (ie, highly sensitive) or a platelet activation assay (ie, highly specific); these tests are indicated in patients with a history of thrombocytopenia temporally related to heparin administration or in patients receiving heparin with previously documented HIT type II. The antigen test uses the enzyme-linked immunosorbent assay (ELISA) to detect the presence of the PF4 antibody and has proven to be highly sensitive.[117,119] The activation assays detect PF4 antibodies by detecting their ability to activate platelets in the presence of heparin. The platelet serotonin release assay is an example of an activation assay that detects HIT type II by quantifying the release of ^{14}C-labeled serotonin from platelets activated by heparin in the presence of the PF4 antibody.[117]

Treatment of HIT type II consists of immediate and complete discontinuation of heparin by any routes. Additionally, immediate systemic anticoagulation is indicated in the setting of thrombosis; the current agents of choice are the direct thrombin inhibitors (DTIs). After systemic levels of a DTI are achieved, oral anticoagulation with a coumarin may be established and the DTI discontinued. Oral coumarin therapy must not begin until effective thrombin suppression has been achieved to avoid precipitating warfarin-induced skin necrosis.[120]

Given the widespread use of heparin, HIT type II is an important consideration for anesthesiologists. Heparin should be avoided in patients with HIT type II and an elevated PF4 antibody titer in order to prevent precipitation of a thrombotic event. Patients with a remote history of an elevated PF4 antibody titer should not be treated with heparin if this can be avoided (ie, use a DTI). No reversal agents are available for the DTIs; their suppression of thrombin abates when the drug is cleared from the circulation.

DISSEMINATED INTRAVASCULAR COAGULATION

Disseminated intravascular coagulation (DIC) is a deviation from the normal physiologic balance between the processes of thrombus formation and fibrinolysis. Pathologic hemorrhage, pathologic thrombosis, or both can occur in DIC. Numerous disease processes have been identified as causing DIC (**Table 16-14**). All of these disease states have in common the production of intense, sustained stimulation of the coagulation axis, achieved by inflammatory mediators and resulting in dysregulation of coagulation and/or fibrinolysis. The association of DIC with inflammation explains why this condition can be associated with multiorgan dysfunction syndrome and acute respiratory distress syndrome, 2 disorders that are characterized by insufficient regulation of the inflammatory response. The pathophysiologic mechanisms of DIC are not completely understood. Pathologic thrombosis at the microcirculatory level results in organ malperfusion, ischemia, infarction, and dysfunction as well as pathologic consumption of essential coagulation elements (eg, platelets, fibrinogen, and soluble coagulation proteins). Dysregulation of fibrinolysis can contribute to DIC-associated thrombosis (ie, there is over-suppression of fibrinolysis from excessive plasminogen activator inhibitor-1) or to DIC-associated hemorrhage

TABLE 16-14 Processes That May Induce DIC

Tissue Damage	**Obstetric Conditions**
Trauma	Abruptio placentae
Crush injuries	Placenta previa
CNS injuries	Uterine atony
Heat stroke	Therapeutic abortion
Burns	Toxemia of pregnancy
Hemolytic transfusion reaction	Retained dead fetus syndrome
Acute transplant rejection	Amniotic fluid embolism
Neoplasia	**Miscellaneous**
Cancers	Shock
Leukemias	Cardiac arrest
Cancer chemotherapy	Near drowning
Tumor lysis	Fat embolism
syndrome	Aortic aneurysm
Infections	Giant hemangiomas
Gram-positive bacteria	Snake bites
Gram-negative bacteria	
Spirochetes	
Rickettsia	
Protozoa	
Fungi	
Viruses	

Reproduced with permission from LaBelle C, Kitchens CS. Disseminated intravascular coagulation. In: Kitchens CS, Alving BM, Kessler CM, eds. *Consultative Hemostasis and Thrombosis.* 2nd ed. Philadelphia, PA: Saunders Elsevier; 2007:183-198.

(ie, with overstimulation of fibrinolysis from high levels of inflammatory mediators including interleukin-1, interleukin-6, interleukin-10, and tissue necrosis factor).[121]

The diagnosis of DIC is approached from 2 vantage points. First, because DIC is a manifestation of a primary disease process, one must investigate potential clinical causes that may give rise to DIC (Table 16-14). Second, although DIC is often initially suspected as a clinical diagnosis, central laboratory values may help to establish the diagnosis. Some authorities advocate for more readily available central laboratory tests, including the aPTT, PT, TT, fibrinogen, fibrin degradation products (FDP) level, D-dimer level, and complete blood count. Although an elevation of FDPs or D-dimers, prolonged aPTT, PT, and TT as well as a decreased fibrinogen level and platelet concentration are not universally seen in DIC, they can be useful in making the diagnosis with strong clinical evidence.[121]

The treatment of DIC is most appropriately directed at the underlying cause of the disorder (eg, intra-abdominal abscess drainage and antibiotics in a patient with sepsis). Exhaustive efforts to correct laboratory abnormalities may not be needed in all cases of DIC, especially those in which patients require surgical treatment. Perioperative goals include maintaining the platelet concentration in the range of 25 000 to 50 000/μL and the fibrinogen level greater than 50 mg/dL. However, few studies exist on the most effective management of the patient with DIC. Presently, with the exception of Trousseau syndrome, anticoagulation is not recommended as the treatment of DIC. Administration of antithrombin concentrate, though advocated by some, is also not recommended.[121] Hemorrhaging DIC patients should be volume resuscitated as appropriate to restore intravascular volume to a level consistent with organ perfusion. As previously stated, this coagulopathy is not expected to improve until the underlying cause of DIC has been appropriately treated.

HYPERHOMOCYSTEINEMIA

Hyperhomocysteinemia has been established as an independent risk factor for stroke, myocardial infarction, carotid artery disease, and venous thrombosis. Plasma homocysteine levels are partially genetically determined but are also influenced by environmental factors, specifically by dietary intake of folic acid and vitamins B_{12} and B_6. Hyperhomocysteinemia is present in 10% to 20% of patients who develop venous thrombosis. Hyperhomocysteinemia is diagnosed by measuring plasma levels of homocysteine. No specific recommendations exist for the perioperative management of patients with hyperhomocysteinemia, although vitamin supplementation reduces plasma homocysteine levels in the elderly. Reduction in homocysteine levels by vitamin supplementation has not been demonstrated to decrease the risk of vascular disease. It may be prudent to use postoperative venous thrombosis prophylaxis, especially in patient populations considered at risk for developing postoperative thrombosis (eg, orthopedic surgical patients). However, there are no specific recommendations on the best antithrombotic or antiplatelet treatment regimen.[112]

ANTIPHOSPHOLIPID ANTIBODY SYNDROME

Antiphospholipid antibodies are directed against proteins that bind to phospholipid. They consist of 2 major subgroups: the lupus anticoagulants and the anticardiolipin antibodies. The lupus anticoagulants (LA) are antibodies that prolong phospholipid-dependent coagulation assays (eg, the aPTT). Anticardiolipin antibodies (aCL) target a molecular congener of cardiolipin (a bovine cardiac protein). The aCL antibodies share a common in vitro binding affinity for cardiolipin. Patients with arterial or venous thrombosis (ie, more common in this disorder) in whom these LA and aCL antibodies are detected are said to have the antiphospholipid antibody syndrome (APS). Primary APS occurs alone, whereas secondary APS occurs in association with other disease states, such as systemic lupus erythematosus (SLE).[112]

Treatment of APS is complicated by a lack of laboratory standardization and randomized treatment trials. Depending on the assay, antiphospholipid antibodies are reported in up to 10% of healthy people and in 30% to 50% of patients with known SLE. The antibodies are more common in patients with thrombosis, but a direct causal association remains unproven. The clinical relevance of transient or low titers of antiphospholipid antibodies is uncertain.[122]

The Sapporo criteria define APS as the presence of at least 1 clinical and 1 laboratory criterion. Clinical criteria include confirmed arterial, venous, or small-vessel thrombosis, recurrent fetal loss prior to the 10th week of gestation, or premature birth secondary to placental insufficiency, eclampsia, or preeclampsia. Laboratory criteria include medium or high titers of IgG or IgM aCL antibodies or the presence of LA on 2 or more occasions at least 6 weeks apart.[112,122]

APS patients with arterial thrombosis tend to have recurrence in an artery, whereas those who experience a venous thrombosis tend to redevelop venous thrombosis. Initial treatment consists of UFH or low-molecular-weight heparin for 5 days and then moderate-intensity warfarin (ie, INR 2.0-3.0) is continued for 6 months or longer or even indefinitely.[112,122]

Arterial thrombosis in APS most frequently involves the cerebral circulation. Studies have not demonstrated any difference in the risk of thrombotic events in patients treated with warfarin versus those treated with aspirin. Pregnant women with a history of APS and pregnancy loss are treated with UFH (5000 units subcutaneously twice daily) and aspirin (75-81 mg/d). Consensus opinion is that aspirin 81 mg/d may be considered for asymptomatic individuals who are not pregnant. The optimal treatment of patients with antiphospholipid antibodies who have arterial thrombosis not involving the CNS remains uncertain. Many of these patients are treated empirically with long-term warfarin therapy.[112,122]

THALASSEMIA

Thalassemia is a congenital hemolytic disorder caused by partial or complete deficiency of hemoglobin α- or β-globin chain synthesis. Homozygous carriers of the β-globin gene defect suffer from severe anemia and require chronic blood transfusion, often resulting in iron overload and progressive organ failure. Concurrent with improved care for patients with thalassemias has been a significant prolongation of their life expectancy; recognition of a chronic hypercoagulable state has accompanied this prolonged life span.[123]

Cerebral thromboembolic events, deep venous thrombosis (DVT), pulmonary embolism, and recurrent arterial thromboses have been described in different subtypes of thalassemia. Echocardiographic findings of pulmonary hypertension and right ventricular dysfunction in many patients with thalassemias, along with common autopsy findings of thrombotic lesions in the pulmonary arteries, lend support to a major incidence of recurrent pulmonary thromboembolism.[123]

Thalassemic patients have low levels of proteins C and S, enhanced platelet consumption, and ongoing activation of platelets, monocytes, granulocytes, and endothelium. There is evidence of continuous thrombin generation and enhanced fibrinolysis. Recently it has been suggested that prophylactic antithrombotic therapy should be given to thalassemic patients who are exposed to transient thrombotic risk factors, such as surgery, immobilization, and pregnancy.[123]

NEPHROTIC SYNDROME

The nephrotic syndrome is a condition characterized by loss of plasma protein in urine, leading to profound hypoalbuminemia. These same urinary losses can also result in deficiencies of natural anticoagulants such as antithrombin and protein S. In addition, increased levels of procoagulants including fibrinogen, factor V, and factor VII as well as increased platelet aggregation can occur. Treatment of the syndrome can involve steroids and cyclosporine; both can increase procoagulant activities.[124]

The incidence of thromboembolism in adults with the nephrotic syndrome is reported to be as high as 44%. Both arterial and venous thromboses have been reported. Prophylactic anticoagulation is recommended for adults with nephrotic range proteinuria.[124] No specific perioperative recommendations exist for patients with nephrotic syndrome.

PARANEOPLASTIC HYPERCOAGULATION

Both arterial and venous thromboses are known complications of cancer, with venous thromboembolism being the most common. Thrombosis is currently the second most common cause of death in cancer. The hemostatic system plays an important role in tumor angiogenesis. Tumor cells produce tissue factor, which directly activates factor X, creating a procoagulant microenvironment[125] (Fig. 16-8). The interaction of monocytes and macrophages with malignant cells causes release of tumor necrosis factor, interleukin-1, and interleukin-6. These cytokines produce endothelial damage and sloughing of endothelial cells with exposure of the underlying thrombogenic surface (ie, exposed collagen). The interaction of tumor cells and macrophages also activates platelets, factor XII, and factor X, leading to generation of thrombin and subsequent thrombosis.[126] The administration of chemotherapy agents further increases the risk of thromboembolism. The overall risk of risk of thromboembolism varies depending on tumor type, chemotherapy, use of erythropoietin-stimulating agents, presence of central venous catheters, and surgery. Many cancer patients receive long-term anticoagulation therapy with low-molecular-weight heparin.[126]

THROMBOTIC THROMBOCYTOPENIC PURPURA

Thrombotic thrombocytopenia purpura (TTP) is a disorder of platelet aggregation leading to microvascular occlusion. Both familial and acquired forms of this disorder exist; the mechanism of it remains unknown. Idiopathic TTP seems to strike randomly, whereas certain medications such as ticlopidine, clopidogrel, and various chemotherapy agents are associated with TTP. It is characterized by a severe hemolytic anemia and thrombocytopenia along with various neurologic and psychiatric manifestations. Patients may experience hematuria, proteinuria, and ischemia to the retinal, coronary, and abdominal arteries. Coagulation studies are typically normal during the early stages of a TTP episode, but DIC may develop if significant tissue necrosis occurs. Treatment of the disorder consists of the administration of FFP, glucocorticoids, and plasma exchange with fresh-frozen plasma.[127]

KEY REFERENCES

- Avery EG. Anesthetic considerations in the patient with 1) anemia and 2) coagulopathy. In: Longnecker DE, Brown DL, Newman MF, et al, eds. *Anesthesiology*. New York, NY: McGraw-Hill; 2008: 239-266.
- Doctor A, Stamler JS. Nitric oxide transport in blood: A third gas in the respiratory cycle. *Compr Physiol*. 2011, 1-28. doi: 10.1002/cphy.c090009
- Francis CW. Antithrombotic agents. In: Kitchens CS, Alving BM, Kessler CM, eds. *Consultative Hemostasis and Thrombosis*. 2nd ed. Philadelphia, PA: Saunders Elsevier; 2007:449-460.
- Hébert PC, Van der Linden P, Biro G, et al. Physiologic aspects of anemia. *Crit Care Clin*. 2004;20(2):187-212.
- Horlocker TT, Wedel DJ, Rowlingson JC, et al. Regional anesthesia in the patient receiving antithrombotic or thrombolytic therapy: American society of regional anesthesia and pain medicine evidence based guidelines (3rd edition). *Reg Anesth Pain Med*. 2010;35(1):64-101.
- Marik PE, Corwin HL. Efficacy of blood transfusion in the critically ill: a systematic review of the literature. *Crit Care Med*. 2008;36(9):2667-2674.
- Roberts HR, Escobar MA. Less common congenital disorders of hemostasis. In: Kitchens CS, Alving BM, Kessler CM, eds. *Consultative Hemostasis and Thrombosis*. 2nd ed. Philadelphia, PA: Saunders Elsevier; 2007:61-79.
- Saidenberg S, Petraszko T, Semple E, Branch DR. Transfusion-related acute lung injury (TRALI): a Canadian blood services research and development symposium. *Transfus Med Rev*. 2010;24(4):305-324.
- Society of Thoracic Surgeons Blood Conservation Guideline Task Force, Ferraris VA, Ferraris SP, et al. Perioperative blood transfusion and blood conservation in cardiac surgery: The Society of Thoracic Surgeons and The Society of Cardiovascular Anesthesiologists clinical practice guidelines. *Ann Thorac Surg*. 2007;83:S27-S86.
- Vamvakas EC, Blajchman MA. Transfusion-related mortality: the ongoing risks of allogeneic blood transfusion and the available strategies for their prevention. *Blood*. 2009;113(15):3406-3417.

REFERENCES

Complete references available on DVD and online version at www.LongneckerAnesthesiology.com

CHAPTER 17 Evaluation of the Patient With Perioperative Malnutrition

Benjamin K. Scott
Clifford S. Deutschman

KEY POINTS

1. Numerous studies suggest that malnutrition in the perioperative period is associated with poor postoperative outcomes, including increased rates of infection, poor wound healing and anastomotic integrity, increased intensive care unit and hospital length of stay, increased need for mechanical ventilation, and increased mortality after transplant and major intra-abdominal or cardiothoracic surgery.
2. A lack of standardized definitions and indices has hampered attempts to study the epidemiology and pathophysiology of malnutrition. Nevertheless, the problem appears to be widespread in patients presenting for surgery. In addition, many patients will acquire protein-energy malnutrition (PEM) during hospitalization.
3. Malnutrition is a complex metabolic disorder, involving inflammatory and neurohumoral mediators, that affects virtually every organ system.
4. The metabolic and physiologic changes accompanying malnutrition can significantly alter response to anesthetics.
5. Decreased total circulating albumin has wide implications for drug administration and volume of distribution.
6. As a result of decreased microsomal enzyme activity and altered cytochrome P450/nicotinamide adenine dinucleotide phosphate–dependent transport mechanisms, protein deficiency may reduce drug metabolism. Decreased transformation of compounds that are hepatically detoxified may lead to pathologic responses that require dosage alteration.
7. Uncertainty surrounds the optimal dose, route, and timing of perioperative nutritional support, but there is increasing evidence that reversal of perioperative malnutrition, especially when severe, can reduce complications and improve outcomes.
8. Recent interest has focused on the use of immunonutrient supplementation, preoperative oral carbohydrate loading, and selective elimination of preoperative fasting in an effort to ameliorate postoperative catabolism and insulin resistance.
9. Accurate estimation of the presence and severity of PEM remains problematic for the anesthesiologist, whose evaluation of the patient is often brief. The most useful tool for assessing a patient's nutritional status is a well-performed history and physical examination.
10. Anesthesiologists have an important role to play in perioperative nutrition and should ensure that patients presenting for surgery are in the best possible condition to tolerate the surgical stress and postoperative recovery period. In hospitalized patients, efforts should be made to continue enteral or parenteral nutrition when appropriate. Finally, anesthesiologists should be at the forefront of clinical and basic science research on perioperative nutrition.

In recent years, anesthesiologists, surgeons, and intensivists have gained experience caring for older, more debilitated patients. Surgical intervention is now routinely offered to patients who would once have been considered "too sick for the operating room." Many of these patients suffer from, or will develop, malnutrition during the course of their illness. In order to provide optimal perioperative care, today's anesthesiologist must understand the effects of malnutrition and disease-altered metabolism on organ function, drug metabolism, and patient outcome. This chapter reviews (1) definitions of malnutrition and its prevalence in surgical patients, (2) clinical assessment and diagnosis of malnutrition, (3) effects of malnutrition on organ system function and drug metabolism, (4) the consequences of therapeutic nutrition, and (5) the association between malnutrition (or its reversal) and patient outcomes.

DEFINITION AND SCOPE OF PROTEIN-ENERGY MALNUTRITION

Inadequate intake of macronutrients (carbohydrate, protein, fat) leading to a reduction in lean body cell mass is referred to as *protein-energy malnutrition* (PEM). Historically, studies of malnutrition tended to focus on children in underdeveloped nations and in adult victims of forced starvation or those receiving experimental diets designed to replicate "life-raft" or "European famine" conditions. This literature led to an early focus on malnutrition primarily as a state of undernutrition or depletion. Subsequent work, focusing on medical and surgical patients in developed countries, demonstrated the important relationship between starvation and alterations in normal human metabolism induced by inflammatory processes or diseases. More recently, malnutrition has come to be understood as a complex interplay between derangements in nutrient intake (or uptake) and a more general state of inflammation (acute or chronic).[1]

Although no internationally accepted consensus exists, most current definitions of malnutrition parallel the 1993 European Society of Parenteral and Enteral Nutrition (ESPEN) statement that malnutrition is "a state resulting from lack of uptake or intake of nutrition leading to altered body composition...specifically body cell mass (BCM), and diminished function."[2] Soeters et al[3] have recently urged that this definition be expanded to incorporate both over- and undernutrition as well as inflammation because each alone or in combination can produce changes in body composition and diminished function. In 2010, in recognition of this emerging perspective, the American Society of Parenteral and Enteral Nutrition proposed a new nomenclature that distinguished 3 classes of malnutrition based on etiology and coincident degree of inflammation. According to this classification scheme, starvation-related malnutrition is associated with minimal inflammatory changes, chronic disease-associated malnutrition with long-standing moderate inflammation, and acute disease- or injury-related malnutrition with a high degree of inflammation.[4] However, it is increasingly clear that pure starvation is very unusual, and a wide range of nutritional conditions, even including anorexia nervosa and morbid obesity, are actually chronic inflammatory states. Thus recent work has begun to erase the traditional distinction made between chronic starvation (described in children as marasmus) and stress-hypermetabolism (leading to changes described in protein-malnourished children as kwashiorkor). Nevertheless, it is useful to briefly review these classic paradigms to illustrate the body's response to starvation as well as the metabolic changes that accompany acute stress.

STARVATION

In the initial period of fasting, metabolic rate decreases to conserve endogenous substrate, especially nitrogen. Glucose is the predominant fuel of early starvation and continues to be made available to those tissues that require it (brain, fibroblasts, erythrocytes, leukocytes, renal medullary tissue). Other tissues quickly alter metabolism to adapt to alternative substrate. Glucose is derived initially from glycogen, but following the depletion of stores (approximately 24 hours of fasting), hepatic and renal gluconeogenesis from amino acids supplied by muscle catabolism predominate.[5] Insulin secretion decreases because gluconeogenesis is unable to maintain blood glucose concentration at prestarvation values.[5] Decreased insulin promotes lipolysis (by activation of a hormone-sensitive lipase) and ketonemia. Ketones inhibit pyruvate dehydrogenase and prevent the conversion of pyruvate to acetyl coenzyme A (CoA), thereby blocking use of the end products of glycolysis in the tricarboxylic acid cycle. As a consequence, the primary fuel for most tissues switches to acetyl CoA derived from fat or ketones. This change is reflected in a decrease in the respiratory quotient (carbon dioxide production/oxygen consumption).[5] In addition, the drop in serum glucose levels is associated with secretion of epinephrine, cortisol, and glucagon. The effect of these 3 "counterregulatory" hormones is stimulation of proteolysis, lipolysis, and gluconeogenesis.[5] Muscle-derived gluconeogenesis provides fuel for tissues that are obligate glucose users. If allowed to continue unchecked, such a process would culminate in rapid depletion of endogenous protein, primarily because of the demands of neural tissue. To counter this effect, brain tissue adapts to the use of ketones, permitting a further decrease in glucose demand and some sparing of lean body mass.[6]

In starvation, adaptation to exogenous substrate is effective; when given glucose, a starved individual responds to the increase in serum glucose by increasing insulin secretion and decreasing levels of counterregulatory hormones. This decreases levels of proteolysis, lipolysis, and gluconeogenesis. The resulting reliance on the externally supplied glucose spares endogenous tissues and decreases ketosis (blocked by insulin).[5] Similar patterns are observed when exogenous fuel is supplied as fat or protein. When demand for energy increases, as in exercise, both aerobic and anaerobic metabolism of glucose in skeletal muscle increases. Primary use of branched-chain amino acids by muscle may help meet the new demand.[5] Lactate from anaerobiosis and amino acids derived from proteolysis (that result, in part, from increased catecholamines) are released by exercising muscle and are recycled by the liver via the gluconeogenic pathway. The newly synthesized glucose can return to skeletal muscle and again be metabolized to lactate. These processes make metabolic rate responsive to tissue demand and exogenous substrate availability with only modest neuroendocrine modulation.[7] Prolonged fasting metabolism eventually results in a clinical picture similar to the form of PEM described in children as marasmus. This is characterized by uniform loss of fat and muscle mass in all tissues and a concomitant loss of water in proportion to nonaqueous mass.

STRESS HYPERMETABOLISM

In contrast to starvation, acute stress metabolism involves extensive neurohumoral modulation.[8] Inflammation, surgery, trauma, or infection activates monokines, lymphokines, prostanoids, hormones, neural pathways, complement, and other endogenous mediators that "drive" metabolism and increase energy expenditure. Part of the source for this alteration appears to be derived directly from the energy and substrate demands of hepatic macrophages and the leukocyte infiltrate in wound tissue.[8] After a specific injury, this response follows a regulated time course, with a peak in metabolic rate approximately 2 to 3 days after the insult and a gradual decline to baseline by postinjury day 7.[8,9] The response will persist if a new activating event occurs or if the source of the initial event (eg, an undrained abscess) is not removed.[8,9] The magnitude of the response is proportional to the magnitude of the injury.[8,9]

The liver responds to neurohumoral stimulation by generating substrate for the increased metabolism. Amino acids from proteolysis, lactate from devascularized tissues, and glycerol from lipolysis are directed into gluconeogenic pathways.[9] Amino acids are also used to synthesize enzymes and structural proteins, whereas free fatty acids provide an alternate energy source. Endogenous mediators, stimulated in part by devascularized wound tissue, mediate this process. Because the response is initiated and driven by this internal source, it remains relatively unresponsive to exogenous substrate.[10] The hormonal pattern is characterized by increased glucagon, cortisol, and epinephrine that appear to be driven by demands from damaged tissue and infiltrating leukocytes. As blood glucose levels increase, insulin secretion is stimulated. This pattern of metabolism leads to depletion of visceral protein (in excess of muscle mass) and fat and is associated with an expansion of the extracellular fluid compartment.[11] Physical findings (edema, hypoalbuminemia, fatty liver) are similar to those noted in childhood kwashiorkor.[12]

PREVALENCE OF MALNUTRITION

Without a universally accepted definition, and in the absence of clearly established criteria for the diagnosis or quantification of malnutrition, it is not surprising that estimates of its incidence also vary widely. Nevertheless, it seems clear from available data that the problem is widespread. In widely cited work from the 1970s, Bistrian et al[13] identified abnormalities of anthropometrics or biochemical markers consistent with malnutrition in 50% of general surgical patients[13] and 44% of general medical patients[14] in a large urban hospital. Reviewing studies published since 1990, Norman et al[15] found prevalence estimates ranging from 20% to 50% of hospitalized patients and a weighted mean prevalence derived from all US and European studies of 31.4%. Perhaps of even greater significance is a study noting that 75% of patients admitted to the hospital without PEM developed abnormalities consistent with PEM during hospitalization.[16] Some studies in critically ill patients have demonstrated improvements in indices of malnutrition over time, reflecting either advances in treatment or simply better recognition leading to routine treatment of the problem. On the other hand, the apparent stability of overall prevalence estimates from the 1970s to the present may reflect a balance between improved nutrition and sicker patient populations.[15] In summary, these findings suggest that, although the actual incidence of malnutrition is unclear, the problem exists on a relatively wide scale in hospitalized patients and may develop or worsen over the course of hospitalization. For the anesthesiologist, there are 2 key points. First, PEM represents a real and not uncommon problem that alters normal physiology. Second, PEM acquired over the course of hospitalization may change a patient's response from one anesthetic episode to the next.

ASSESSMENT OF PROTEIN-ENERGY MALNUTRITION

Because PEM can significantly alter perioperative physiology, it would be useful to diagnose this condition during routine preoperative patient evaluation. In practice, however, the detection and quantification of malnutrition have proven challenging. Direct measurement of body cell mass requires multiple isotopic techniques and is not feasible in the clinical setting.[17] Instead, a wide variety of proxies have been proposed. These include anthropometrics and body-composition analysis, estimation of basal energy expenditure, biochemical markers, and tests of muscle, cognitive, or immunologic function. We review each of these methods briefly, noting those that might be used by the perioperative clinician.

Many anthropometric measures were developed for the assessment of malnutrition in childhood starvation.[18] Consequently, parameters that are of key importance in adults but are negligible in children (frame size, build, fat patterning) have been under-analyzed, and 95% confidence intervals have not been determined.[12,18] Furthermore, because edema is a prominent characteristic in inflammation-induced PEM, the interpretation of anthropometric measurements becomes difficult. Despite these limitations, body mass index (BMI), skin-fold thickness, arm muscle circumference, and calculated fat-free mass have shown some promise in the development of screening guidelines and warrant further study.[1]

Bioimpedance analysis (BIA) involves measurement of the body's electrical resistance to estimate total body water (TBW). Because the human body maintains fairly stable ratios between tissue water and tissue solids, this approach assumes that TBW reflects lean body mass. BIA has been validated and appears relatively reliable in healthy or clinically stable populations.[1] Unfortunately, the assumption that TBW reflects lean body mass breaks down in the presence of acute stress as well as in severe malnutrition.

In 1919 Harris and Benedict, based on their study of healthy volunteers, introduced the first predictive equations for resting energy expenditure (REE).[19] In recent decades, numerous modifications and alternatives (eg, "stress-correction factors") have been proposed to address shortcomings arising from the application of these equations to various disease states.[20] Today, indirect calorimetry has made measurement of REE clinically feasible, although it remains labor- and time-intensive. This technique directly measures oxygen consumption and carbon dioxide production and uses these values to calculate resting energy expenditure. In a small trial, use of indirect calorimetry improved nitrogen balance and outcome.[21] As with bioimpedance analysis, indirect calorimetry appears to lose accuracy as illness severity increases. Disease-related accumulations of intermediate metabolites, continuous enteral feeding, bicarbonate loss, and hemodynamic or respiratory instability have all been observed to invalidate this technique.[20]

Conceptualizing malnutrition as an inflammatory condition has focused attention on the potential utility of biomarkers that might aid in diagnosis or quantification of PEM. Despite its clear association with morbidity and mortality from several chronic inflammatory conditions, C-reactive protein has not been demonstrated to be useful in the assessment of individual patients.[22] Several hepatic-derived transport proteins (albumin, transferrin, prealbumin, retinal-binding protein) have also been used to detect PEM. Serum albumin has a half-life of 14 to 20 days, making it insensitive to acute changes in nutritional status. It is also affected by albumin transfusion, dehydration, inflammation, and liver disease. Serum albumin less than 3.5 g/dL is suggestive of malnutrition, and less than 2.5 g/dL is suggestive of severe malnutrition. Serum transferrin is also somewhat useful for evaluating malnutrition. It has a half-life of about 9 days, which is midway between albumin and prealbumin. Unfortunately, unlike albumin and prealbumin, transferrin increases whenever there is bleeding. This decreases its reliability in the perioperative state. Serum prealbumin is most reliable of the hepatic-derived transport proteins to signal acute malnutrition. It has a half-life of 24 to 48 hours. Prealbumin is a negative acute phase reactant and, in the postoperative setting, prealbumin levels decline.

Alterations in these hepatic proteins are common in any inflammatory state and reflect the interplay of decreased synthesis, tissue extravasation, and extracellular fluid expansion from both endogenous and exogenous sources.[23] The relationship between actual depletion of body cell mass and these biochemical markers is unclear. In inflammation, serum proteins will decrease irrespective of the extent of loss of body cell mass.[23] Serum protein concentrations may be only mildly decreased in pure starvation PEM despite significant loss in body cell mass because the loss of mass and water is proportional.[24] Conversely, low serum albumin may primarily reflect dilution of the plasma concentration in the setting of increased extravascular volume and capillary leak rather than decreased synthesis.[25] Despite this, serum proteins are frequently used in the metabolic assessment of the chronically malnourished patient. Irrespective of whether changes represent decreased synthesis or derangements in the distribution of body water, low serum albumin has been consistently associated with increased morbidity and mortality in surgical and chronically ill patients.[25-27] Changes in the serum concentration of the hepatic proteins probably are not direct reflections of nutritional status. More likely they are markers of inflammation, oxidative stress, or illness severity. But as such, they remain important in identifying patients who are at risk for accelerated nutritional depletion and poor outcome.[28]

An alternative strategy has been to focus on more qualitative aspects of malnutrition. Serial 24-hour dietary recall and screening tools such as the Subjective Global Assessment (SGA), Malnutrition Universal Screening Tool (MUST), and Nutritional Risk Screening (NRS 2002) have been advocated as simple and reliable methods for detecting patients at risk.[29] Some authors have proposed that a thorough history and physical examination, coupled with evidence of weight loss or the presence of known "catabolic" disease, is as valid as any sophisticated test or technique.[30] Finally, in the context of recent definitions of malnutrition highlighting functional impairment, there has been a renewed interest in testing of muscle, cognitive, and immunologic function.

Studies of patients with chronic obstructive pulmonary disease (COPD) suggest that malnourished patients are more prone to changes in muscle fiber–type and mitochondrial dysfunction that predispose to fatigue.[31] Skeletal muscle fatigue, maximal inspiratory mouth pressure, and handgrip strength have all been evaluated as markers of malnutrition. Handgrip strength in particular correlates with loss of total body protein,[32] has been associated with postoperative morbidity, and predicts loss of functional status in hospitalized patients.[33,34]

Malnutrition almost certainly has cognitive sequelae, and it has been suggested that cognitive testing might be used as a global measure of function in the nutritionally depleted state. Cognitive function has been shown to correlate well with physical fitness.[35] Conversely, cognitive dysfunction is a well-described feature of chronic malnutrition. Tools such as the mini-mental status examination (MMSE) have been proposed as a screening technique but probably do not have the power to detect subtle changes.[1] Unfortunately, quantification of cognitive function remains exceedingly challenging, limiting the utility of cognitive testing as a measure of malnutrition.

Recent attention to the inflammatory nature of malnutrition has also fostered interest in the role of immune function testing in malnourished patients. Testing of immunologic function via delayed cutaneous hypersensitivity has been in use for decades. Anergy, or the inability to mount a reaction in the face of an antigenic challenge, has been associated with delayed recovery from illness or trauma.[1] Recent work on quantification of T-cell subpopulations, in particular natural killer cells, has shown promise. However, a graded, quantitative measure of immune function has yet to be elucidated.

In short, despite a great deal of research interest and some promising early work, clinical assessment of malnutrition remains problematic. For the anesthesiologist, whose evaluation of the patient before surgery is often necessarily brief, accurate diagnosis and quantification of malnutrition is even more challenging. A focused history and physical with attention to the presence of chronic illnesses suggestive of depletion of body cell mass (eg, aggressive malignancy), chronic conditions that limit intake or absorption (vomiting, diarrhea, upper gastrointestinal obstruction, bariatric surgery), and physical manifestations of weight loss or altered body composition (muscle atrophy, cachexia, edema) probably remains the best available screening method. As detailed in the following sections, malnutrition, in addition to being common, can have profound effects on organ function, physiology, and pharmacokinetics. Consequently, the anesthesiologist should suspect the presence of PEM and recognize its potential for precipitating difficulties in perioperative management.

EFFECTS OF PROTEIN-ENERGY MALNUTRITION AND NUTRITIONAL REPLETION ON INDIVIDUAL ORGAN SYSTEM FUNCTION

The effects of PEM and its correction on individual organ systems are reviewed in this section. When possible, human data are cited; otherwise, appropriate animal studies are presented. An attempt has been made to separate the effects of starvation from inflammation, but the former is disproportionately represented.

Cardiovascular Changes Starvation PEM is associated with morphologic, functional, and electrical abnormalities in the cardiovascular system. Heart size decreases in proportion to loss of body mass,[36] and the left ventricular free wall is thinned.[37] Histologic examination reveals myocardial atrophy and interstitial edema.[38] Left atrial, aortic root, and left ventricular end-systolic and end-diastolic dimensions are decreased relative to normal controls valves,[39] and left ventricular compliance is reduced.[37]

Functionally, resting heart rate, blood pressure, and pulse pressure are reported to decrease in PEM,[40] and a subnormal response is noted in each of these parameters during exercise testing.[39] Cardiac index and ejection fraction remain at prestarvation levels[37] and appear to increase appropriately with exercise[39] or β-adrenergic stimulation.[37]

On electrocardiography (ECG), amplitude is diminished, the axis shows a rightward deviation, PR and QT intervals are prolonged, T waves are inverted to flattened, ST-T segments are depressed, and nodal escape beats and ventricular tachycardia have been reported.[39]

Echocardiographic studies done in anorexic patients reveal decreased ventricular mass with associated ventricular dysfunction.[41] Also common in the anorexic population are prolonged QT and QTc intervals with ventricular arrhythmias.[42] In one study, treatment and weight recovery resulted in normalization of ventricular mass and improvement in ventricular function in adolescents with anorexia.[42]

Stress metabolism in cachectic humans is associated with a somewhat different picture than noted in isolated starvation. Heart rate and indexed ventricular mass (per kilogram of body weight) are increased.[43] This suggests that stressed myocardium is spared from some of the protein-depleting aspects of PEM. It is logical to assume that the heart in stress can respond normally to increased demand for work even when other tissues are being wasted. This may in part occur because the heart can use virtually any fuel (glucose, fat ketones, lactate) to support energy requirements.

Protein and calorie repletion in previously healthy adults subjected to semi-starvation results in a rapid increase in heart size.[39] With refeeding, heart rate, blood pressure, and pulse pressures initially increase to above prestarvation levels and gradually return to baseline. Ejection fraction and cardiac output/index may decrease, and congestive failure has been reported. The cause of these abnormalities is unknown but may reflect mobilization of interstitial fluid coupled with the inability of depleted cardiac muscle to handle the fluid load. ECG amplitude and QT interval abnormalities persist for variable periods despite repletion.[39]

To date, very little research has focused on the effects of correction of stress-induced PEM on cardiac function. In one study, ventricular mass, heart rate, end-diastolic volume, cardiac output, and ejection fraction all increased, but congestive heart failure developed in 3 of 5 patients and pericardial effusion developed in a fourth patient.[43]

Pulmonary Changes Relative cell mass (lung weight/body weight) appears to increase in cases of PEM, but overall wet and dry lung weights decrease with depletion.[44] Morphologic changes similar to those observed in emphysema are characteristic; distances between alveolar walls are increased, the surface area for gas exchange is decreased, and air space is grossly enlarged as a result of disruption of alveolar septae.[45] Peripheral lung tissue is more affected than central mass, and a significant loss of collagen and elastin is noted.[45] The phospholipoprotein content of surfactant is grossly depleted.[46] In the early stages of depletion, pressure-volume relationships are normal,[46] but after prolonged starvation, surfactant concentrations decrease, active surface forces increase, and exposure of alveolar surfaces leads to an altered functional residual capacity.[47]

Diaphragmatic muscle mass decreases in direct proportion to the loss of body weight.[48] As a result, the tension developed in isolated diaphragmatic muscle strips is reduced. Mechanical efficiency appears to be unchanged.[38] Observed changes in the time to achieve 50% tension reduction following 20- or 100-Hz tetanus indicate that diaphragmatic fatigability is reduced.[48] Animal studies indicate a selective depletion of fast (glycolytic) fibers with sparing of the slow oxidative fibers, a finding that supports the notion of decreased fatigability.[48]

After an acute period of mild starvation in otherwise healthy adult women, forced vital capacity, forced expiratory volume, inspiratory pressure, and maximal voluntary ventilation were normal.[49] A prolonged course of severe depletion in both human and animal subjects results in decreases in all lung volumes, maximal pressure generation, and maximal ventilatory effort.[50] Respiratory rate is decreased, perhaps reflecting altered carbon dioxide production; the ventilatory response to carbon dioxide is preserved, but hypoxic ventilatory drive is markedly attenuated.[51] The number of alveolar macrophages and their ability to clear aerosolized *Staphylococcus aureus* is decreased.[52] Refeeding in rats leads to a return to normal lung weight and normal levels of lung hydroxyproline, elastin, and surfactant contents.[44] Parenchymal emphysematous changes are incompletely reversed.[44] Diaphragmatic contractile force is regained as body weight is regained.[50] Respiratory muscle function, maximal inspiratory pressure, and phagocytic capacity improve also, but abnormalities of hypoxic ventilatory drive are not prevented despite the provision of amino acid formulas sufficient to prevent negative nitrogen balance.[53] The effects of repletion on lung volumes and hypoxic ventilatory drive are not well characterized.

Renal Changes During starvation, renal mass is lost in proportion to body mass, and renal protein content is reduced. Clearance of creatinine and free water are decreased, and effective renal plasma flow, glomerular filtration rate, and filtration fraction decrease dramatically, although total renal blood flow is not reduced. The ability to concentrate the urine in response to water restriction is impaired.

Total body water is decreased by starvation PEM, but exchangeable sodium remains normal, implying that cellular mass and exchangeable potassium are decreased.[54] Free water clearance and sodium excretion are increased early in the course of starvation but decline after several days. Renin and aldosterone are increased in this early natriuretic period. Their role in sodium homeostasis during PEM is uncertain. Titratable acid excretion is decreased, whereas serum bicarbonate and urinary ammonia concentrations increase. Refeeding after starvation PEM improves glomerular filtration rate, filtration fraction, concentrating ability, and free water clearance.[55] Sodium and acid excretion increase, as do plasma and extracellular volume. After a period of refeeding accompanied by increasing plasma osmolality, interstitial water moves into the intravascular compartment. This is associated with a diuretic phase.

Surgical or traumatic stress activates renal mechanisms to conserve salt and water[8,17] and thus expand the vasculature to improve substrate delivery. Both antidiuretic hormone and aldosterone are involved in this response, and plasma volume contraction in this setting can produce a metabolic alkalosis. The consequences of prolonged stress remain unclear, and the effects of repletion have not been adequately studied.

Gastrointestinal Changes Intestinal mass, a rapid turnover tissue, is lost at a proportionately greater rate than body weight in starved rats.[56] Small intestine as a whole, and mucosal cells in particular, have decreased contents of DNA, RNA, and nitrogen. Epithelial cell renewal and migration are reduced, and villus size and crypt cell number, size, and mitotic rate are decreased. Gastric ulceration, gastric and intestinal atrophy, and mucosal hemorrhage are all present to a great extent, perhaps reflecting mucosal breakdown either as a result of increased lysosomal acid hydrolase[57] or failure to synthesize mucosal glycoproteins. Gastrin concentrations decrease. Long-term fasting appears to be required for mucosal changes to occur; Knudsen et al[58] found normal histologic conditions after a 7-day fast in obese individuals.

Mucosal transport, reflected in decreased uptake of oral mannitol, may be impaired. Sucrase and maltase (but not lactase) activities are decreased, with these changes most prominent in the proximal gastrointestinal tract. Glucose transfer across the mucosa decreases, but mucosal-to-serosal transport of both glucose and histidine increase. Loss of brush border enzymes impairs absorption and promotes bacterial overgrowth.

Healing of mucosal ulcerations has been reported in depleted patients with Crohn disease who receive parenteral nutrition. Increased nitrogen retention and improved gastric motility in starved individuals have been noted.[59] Cell populations and absorptive capacity improve, activity of brush border enzymes is restored,[57] and lysosomal enzyme activities decrease to normal.

Enteral feeding seems to be more effective than parenteral nutrition in restoring gastrointestinal function postoperatively.[60] Mucosal integrity, brush border enzyme levels, and absorptive capacity all improve rapidly in depleted animals that are refed orally.[61] Use of glutamine is implicated in this improvement; it appears that even parenterally administered glutamine (which is not present in most total parenteral nutrition formulas) is of benefit.[62]

In critically ill patients, there is a concern that bacteria may overgrow and translocate from the intestinal lumen to the systemic circulation, leading to infection. In theory, part of the benefit of early enteral nutrition in the critically ill is to prevent this overgrowth. Although multiple animal studies support this theory, a study by Moore et al[63] failed to find bacteria or endotoxin in the blood from the portal vein in severely injured trauma patients. Indeed, careful examination of most of the work on translocation in animals demonstrates that at least 2 insults (overgrowth of a single bacterial species and some form of injury) are required for translocation, and bacteria translocate to the intestinal lymph nodes and occasionally the liver but rarely beyond.[64] Thus the clinical importance of translocation is unlikely to be great.

Pancreatic Changes Pancreatic mass decreases in direct proportion to body mass, and acinar atrophy, loss of architecture, fibrosis, and exocrine duct dilation are all noted in response to starvation PEM.[5] Rough endoplasmic reticulum and mitochondria are decreased. Amylase and trypsinogen content in the pancreas falls, and lipase is increased.[5] Duodenal aspirates show a sequential decrease in level of lipase, trypsin, and amylase as PEM progresses. Bicarbonate secretion also decreases in adults. Loss of structural integrity is reflected in increased serum amylase levels and indices of amylase production in patients with anorexia nervosa.[65] Following PEM in rats, the exocrine pancreas shows decreased responsiveness to carbachol stimulation, and insulin responsiveness to glucose stimulation is attenuated.[66,67] Insulin secretion, exocrine responses to carbachol, and serum amylase and lipase values return to normal after refeeding.[67]

Hepatic Changes In humans, starvation results in a rapid loss of liver glycogen. Because of defective triglyceride excretion and carnitine-limited uptake, reesterification of free fatty acids in the periportal region occurs.[5] Prolonged PEM will eventually deplete even periportal fat deposits. In chronic protein deficiency in rats, liver mass and rough endoplasmic reticulum are lost.[56] Loss of RNA, water, fat, and protein as well as cellular atrophy have been reported, but it appears that hepatocytes are remarkably resistant to loss of structure or number.[5] Patients with weight loss as great as 55 kg have had histologically normal liver biopsies, although the presence of pigment deposits, fibrosis, and fatty infiltration has also been reported.[5] In pure starvation, hepatic enzymes and bilirubin may be normal or increased[68]; albumin synthesis and total albumin content decrease, but concentrations may be normal. Urinary nitrogen loss decreases reflecting activation of amino acid–conserving enzymes and decreased urea cycle activity.[69]

Protein deficiency often reduces drug metabolism, reflecting decreased microsomal enzyme activity and altered cytochrome P450/nicotinamide adenine dinucleotide phosphate–dependent transport mechanisms.[14] Thus decreased transformation of compounds that are hepatically detoxified may lead to pathologic responses that require dosage alteration. Conversely, compounds that are biotransformed into toxic metabolites are better tolerated.[70]

Many products of hepatic protein synthesis are altered during stress. Messenger ribonucleic acid (mRNA) is increased for acute-phase products, such as fibrinogen or α_1-antiproteases, whereas synthesis of transport proteins such as albumin is decreased.

Liver size and function return to normal with refeeding; gross and ultrastructural morphology are restored after several weeks of repletion. Serum hepatocellular enzymes increase initially with refeeding but then return to normal.[71] Effects of repletion on drug metabolism are unknown.

Immunologic Changes PEM is associated with a reduction in the mass of lymphoid tissue in excess of loss of body mass. Both small lymphocytes and germinal centers are affected. Total circulating polymorphonuclear (PMN) cell counts are reduced, but the fraction of total erythrocytes that are PMNs is increased. Macrophage and PMN chemotaxis, bacterial engulfment, and intracellular killing are impaired. Serum levels and activity of complement components C3 and C5 are normal in stress, but all other components of both the direct and indirect pathways are reduced in stress, and all components are reduced in starvation.[72]

Circulating B-cell numbers are reduced but account for an increased percentage of the total lymphocyte count. Serum immunoglobulin may be low, normal, or high. Impairments of antibody binding and antigen specificity have been reported.[73] Impaired cell-mediated immunity is one characteristic of the malnourished state.[73] Absolute numbers of T cells and the ratio of T cells to total leukocytes are reduced.[73] The proportion of T-helper and T-suppressor cells is normal in starvation but reduced in stress; T-killer cells are reduced in both states.[74]

Lymphoid tissue mass, cell populations, and germinal center populations respond well to nutritional repletion. Phagocytosis and chemotaxis improve, but the effects of refeeding on engulfment and intracellular killing are unknown.[73] Delayed hypersensitivity to skin testing,[75] antibody levels (circulating or fixed),[75,76] and complement levels return to normal with nutritional therapy.[76] Short-term repletion has no effect on T-cell subpopulations in stress or starvation.[74] The effects of longer treatment are unknown.

Nervous System Changes Peripheral nerve conduction velocity is decreased, and associated sensory abnormalities have been reported in PEM.[77] In moderate PEM, nerve biopsies are normal, but severe depletion is associated with segmental demyelination.[77] Chronic malnutrition may lead to lethargy, confusion, and impaired initiative.[78] Cerebral atrophy, ventricular dilatation, and diffuse electroencephalographic slowing have been noted.[8] In adult rats deprived of protein, the phosphatidylglycerol and sphingophospholipid fraction are decreased, but other myelin components are present in normal quantities.[79] Refeeding appears to restore nerve conduction and structure[80] and improve mental status.[78]

Anesthetic Implications of Organ System Dysfunction The dysfunctions caused by PEM have important perioperative implications. Cardiac reserve may compromised, as evidenced by subnormal blood pressure and heart rate responses to stress testing, but appropriate increases in cardiac output in response to exercise or β-adrenergic stimulation argue against this. The potential for myocardial depression caused by volatile anesthetics should be considered in patients with PEM. In addition, the partially repleted patient may be at risk for pulmonary edema when mobilization of fluid occurs because the cardiac response to fluid challenges may be inadequate. Cardiac dysfunction and renal abnormalities make it important to watch fluid balance. Assisting postoperative diuresis may be necessary.

Pulmonary disease resembling emphysema may impair gas exchange, whereas respiratory muscle failure may preclude early extubation, especially with residual paralysis. The selective depletion of fast muscle fibers may alter the ability to respond to acute increases in carbon dioxide. It may be prudent to mechanically ventilate the severely depleted patient for a time postoperatively. In the healthy individual, resistance to pulmonary infection is maintained by bacterial clearance (ciliary action and coughing) and macrophage function. Both are impaired in PEM and further decreased by general anesthesia.

Renal abnormalities may reduce the clearance of both solute and solvent, resulting in retention of water as well as toxic by-products. Thus fluid loads may be poorly tolerated and clearance of drugs and cellular debris impaired. Altered gastric motility increases the risk of aspiration. In addition, because of the loss of brush border enzymes and depletion of gastrointestinal mucosa, oral absorption of drugs may be altered.

Blood sugar values should be monitored perioperatively because of the relatively impaired insulin response to hyperglycemia.

Hepatic drug metabolism may also be altered, but this is unpredictable. Clearance of some drugs (eg, vecuronium) may be impaired, but tolerance for others with toxic metabolites (eg, nitroprusside) might be noted. Metabolism of inhalational anesthetics may be decreased. Perhaps most importantly, decreased total circulating albumin has wide implications for drug administration and volume of distribution. **Table 17-1** is a partial list of commonly used drugs that might be affected by decreased total circulating albumin.

Other effects occur as well. For example, the increased risk of infection mandates the use of careful sterile technique for even routine vascular access. Use of inhalational anesthetics may further depress leukocyte function. Finally, the associated peripheral neuropathy may alter the effects of conduction anesthesia, and mental status changes associated with PEM may impair rapid recovery from general anesthesia.

TABLE 17-1 Commonly Used Drugs That Are Plasma-Protein Bound and Thus Affected by Malnutrition

Narcotics
Morphine
Meperidine
Fentanyl
Sufentanil
Alfentanil
Barbiturates
Thiopental
Phenobarbital
Benzodiazepines
Diazepam
Midazolam
Lorazepam
Nonbarbiturate Induction Agents
Etomidate
Propofol
Local Anesthetics
Tetracaine
Lidocaine
Mepivicaine
Bupivacaine
Etidocaine
Prilocaine
Cardioactive Drugs
Digitalis
Labetalol
Propranolol
Nadolol
Pindolol
Captopril
Others
Phenytoin

EFFECTS OF PERIOPERATIVE PROTEIN-ENERGY MALNUTRITION ON OUTCOME IN SURGICAL PATIENTS

The impact of malnutrition on postoperative outcomes was recognized as early as 1936, when Studley[81] reported that mortality after gastric surgery for peptic ulcer disease was markedly increased in patients whose preoperative weight loss exceeded 20% of their premorbid weight. Subsequent work has reinforced and expanded Studley's conclusions. Evidence is mounting that hospital and intensive care unit (ICU) length of stay, surgical complication rates, and mortality all increase in the setting of perioperative malnutrition.

Effects of Malnutrition on Morbidity Regardless of whether malnutrition is an independent risk factor, it is clear that patients with markers for PEM have increased perioperative morbidity. Patients with anergy, for example, have increased rates of postoperative infections and twice the number of nonseptic postoperative complications.[82] Hypoalbuminemia and other abnormalities of plasma proteins have been associated with a doubling of wound infection rates as well as increased rates of wound dehiscence.[83] Reviewing outcomes in nearly 24 000 surgical wounds, Cruse and Foord linked malnutrition to an 8-fold increase in clean wound infections, from 1.8% to 16.6%.[84] Pressure ulcers also appear to be more common in the setting of PEM.[85] Another group has suggested that recent preoperative intake, and not overall nutritional status, is the most important factor in wound healing.[86] Nevertheless, in both human patients and experimental animals, malnutrition appears to prolong inflammation, impair collagen synthesis and fibroblast proliferation, and retard neoangiogenesis.[87,88]

Despite the absence of standardized criteria for the diagnosis malnutrition, data from selected surgical populations are impressive. Among patients undergoing orthotopic liver transplantation, for example, preoperative malnutrition has been linked to increased ICU length of stay and prolonged mechanical ventilation.[89] In patients undergoing thoracotomy for cancer or lung reduction surgery, preoperative nutritional status correlates with need for re-ventilation as well as overall postoperative morbidity.[90-92] After cardiac surgery, malnutrition is associated with an increased likelihood of acute renal failure, pneumonia, and respiratory failure and postoperative infections.[93] In another study, patients with head and neck cancer who lost more than 10% of their premorbid body weight in the 6 months before resection were 4 times more likely to experience a major postoperative complication, including major wound infection/sepsis, fistula or anastomotic breakdown, or cardiac/respiratory failure.[94] Finally, after major vascular surgery, preoperative nutritional status was found to predict severity of the systemic inflammatory response syndrome (SIRS).[95]

Effects of Malnutrition on Mortality As with morbidity, it appears clear that pathologic changes accompanying malnutrition are also associated with increased mortality in both medical and surgical patients. Reinhardt et al[96] found that serum albumin values less than 3.0 mg/dL were associated with a 30-day mortality of 24% and that levels below 2.0 mg/dL were associated with a mortality of 62% in patients undergoing intra-abdominal surgery. In a study on similar patients, Seltzer et al[97] noted that albumin values less than 3.5 mg/dL were associated with 4-fold increases in mortality and morbidity, whereas lymphocyte counts of less than 1500/μL were associated with a 4-fold increase in mortality alone. Concurrent abnormalities of both albumin and lymphocyte counts were associated with an 18-fold increase in mortality relative to patients with normal indices.

Impaired cell-mediated immunity also appears to be an important marker for increased mortality. Meakins et al[82] noted a perioperative death rate of 3.1% in general surgical patients with normal delayed hypersensitivity (assessed by intradermal injection of a battery of antigens), whereas anergy was associated with a mortality of 35%. The development of anergy after normal initial testing was invariably fatal. A number of studies have confirmed the association of anergy and poor postoperative outcome.

In an attempt to improve specificity, Harvey et al[98] developed a discriminate function that was used to predict the development of sepsis and surgical mortality. This function was based primarily on delayed hypersensitivity testing, transferrin, albumin, and total lymphocyte counts. Prospective evaluation of the index has not been reported. Mullen et al[99] developed a "prognostic nutritional index" (PNI) based on a number of nutritionally relevant variables. Patients identified by this index as high risk had a mortality of nearly 60%; those categorized as low risk had mortalities of only 3%. Prospective evaluation of this index has confirmed its usefulness for identifying high-risk patients, but the true relationship between the variables studied and malnutrition is unclear.

Once again, data from selected surgical populations suggest a clear association between indices of malnutrition and mortality. Liver transplant patients with significantly abnormal resting-energy expenditure or an estimated body cell mass less than 35% of their body weight had significantly reduced 5-year survival after transplant.[100] In lung transplant patients, those with a BMI less than 17 or greater than 25 had an increased risk of 90-day postoperative mortality (odds ratio = 3.7; $p = 0.085$). In addition to increased morbidity, multiple studies of cardiac surgery[93] and thoracotomy for lung reduction or tumor resection[90,92] have demonstrated increased mortality among patients with preoperative malnutrition. Echoing Studley's early work, Ray-Ferro et al[101] found that severely malnourished patients (by nutritional risk index) with gastric cancer suffered 33.3% postoperative mortality versus just 6.5% for those with moderate malnutrition.[101]

Together, the available data strongly support a link between malnutrition and postoperative morbidity and mortality. It is worth remembering, however, that many of the biochemical and clinical markers associated with malnutrition may also be correlated with other risk factors for poor outcome. Anergy, for example, is associated with numerous pathologic processes, all of which may increase perioperative risk independent of malnutrition. In other words, it has yet to be definitively proven that malnutrition is an independent risk factor for poor outcome and not just a marker of disease severity.

Effect of Nutritional Repletion on Outcome Although nutritional repletion may reverse many of the abnormalities that develop in individual organ systems as a result of malnutrition, the overall effect of perioperative alimentation on outcome is unclear. Most studies that address the issue were poorly designed—patients were not randomized, investigators were not blinded, and patient populations lacked uniformity. Most investigations compared different alimentation regimens without an untreated control group. Finally, the end points are not objective measures of outcome. Despite these limitations, some conclusions can be drawn.

First, the effects of perioperative repletion may depend on the severity of preoperative deficit. Patients with mild to moderate preoperative depletion do not appear to benefit from combined preoperative and postoperative alimentation as compared with postoperative support alone. In comparing nonrandomized, mildly depleted patients with gastrointestinal malignancies to undepleted control patients, Thompson et al[102] were unable to demonstrate that combined preoperative and postoperative repletion altered mortality or morbidity.

Outcome appears to be improved when significant malnutrition is corrected before surgery. When comparing combined preoperative and postoperative intravenous alimentation with postoperative support alone, both Mullen et al[99] and Smale et al[103] reported reductions in mortality (9% vs 47%) and morbidity (23% vs 56%). Müller et al[104] confirmed these findings in a randomized study of patients with cancer. Outcome is significantly affected by the duration and efficacy of therapy. Thus Rombeau et al[105] retrospectively studied patients undergoing surgery for inflammatory bowel disease and noted that only 5% of patients who had received hyperalimentation for 5 or more days had postoperative complications, whereas 46% of those receiving fewer than 5 days of therapy had complications.[105] Grimes et al[106] noted similar findings in general surgical patients who were severely depleted. In another study, only 4% of patients who responded to 1 week of repletion had a perioperative complication, whereas 9 of 20 (45%) who did not respond had perioperative morbidity.[107] When therapy in nonresponders was continued for an additional 4 to 6 weeks, until a response consistent with improved nutritional status was noted, the complication rate was 13%. Thus it appears that preoperative repletion of appropriate duration to improve nutritional status also improves perioperative outcome. Questions of methodology in all the studies cited mandate that conclusions be drawn cautiously.

Second, the impact of nutritional repletion strategies probably depends on route. In 2007 Koretz et al[108] published a systematic review of 44 randomized controlled trials of perioperative enteral nutrition. The studies fell into 3 broad categories: enteral feeding compared with no artificial nutrition, enteral versus parenteral feeding, and the use of oral nutritional supplements versus no supplementation. No survival benefit was demonstrated in any of the 3 groups of studies. Compared with those receiving no artificial nutrition, patients who received enteral nutrition had an 11% absolute reduction in the risk of infection (95% confidence interval, –20% to –1%). In this comparison group, enteral nutrition had no impact on length of hospitalization. Compared with total parenteral feeding (TPN), patients receiving enteral nutrition also had fewer infections (11% absolute risk reduction; 95% confidence interval, –15% to –6%), a 6% reduction in major complications (95% confidence interval, –10% to –1%), and a 1.7-day reduction in hospital length of stay (95% confidence interval, –2.65 to –0.75 days). Those trials addressing the use of oral supplements were noted to be of poorer quality, and although several of these studies did report reductions in infections and length of stay, the only high-quality trial in this group did not show a benefit.[108]

Trials of parenteral nutrition have generated conflicting results. The VA Cooperative study, a well-designed, randomized controlled trial, compared patients receiving 7 to 15 days of preoperative TPN followed by 3 days of postoperative TPN, with groups receiving either enteral or no nutrition until postoperative day 3. Patients in the TPN group were found to have increased rates of infection (14.1% vs 6.4%), but a nonsignificant trend toward reduced 30-day mortality (4.9 vs 7.3%) was observed. However, when patients were stratified according to severity of preoperative malnutrition, the TPN group had fewer major postoperative complications (20%-25% vs 40%-50%).[109] A 1997 systematic review by Klein et al[110] included 13 randomized trials of preoperative TPN as well as 8 randomized trials of TPN in the postoperative period. Interestingly, preoperative TPN was associated with a 10% reduction in postoperative complications, whereas postoperative TPN was associated with a 10% increase. In a 2001 meta-analysis of 26 randomized trials, Heyland et al[111] found that TPN appeared to reduce complications in those patients who were malnourished (using varying definitions) and in those receiving lipid-free solutions. The largest meta-analysis to date included 41 trials of TPN in various phases of the perioperative period. Although there were nonsignificant trends favoring TPN over no nutrition, for most outcome measures TPN conferred no statistically significant benefit in mortality, length of stay, or complication rates.[112]

Unfortunately, many of the studies discussed here did not assess the efficacy of enteral or parenteral feeding protocols in normalizing indices of malnutrition prior to surgery, further complicating efforts to interpret their conclusions. In comparing interventions, it would be useful to know the extent to which outcomes reflect a correction of the underlying pathology. Another area of uncertainty surrounds the role of nutritional support in the patient with normal preoperative nutritional status about to undergo a preoperative fast, the physiologic stress of a major operation, and a variable postoperative fasting period. Recent interest in this area has focused on immunonutrition and preoperative hypocaloric feeding.

IMMUNONUTRITION

Attention to the role of nutrition in the maintenance of mucosal barrier integrity, immune system function, and recovery from acute stress has led to a reconsideration of the importance of many nutrients once considered nonessential. These nutrients are depleted or ineffectively synthesized during periods of severe illness or major tissue damage and are therefore probably better thought of as "conditionally essential." Several commercially available formulas have been developed that include a combination of arginine, glutamine, omega-3 fatty acids, and RNA nucleotides. These "immunonutrients" are reviewed in more detail in **Table 17-2**. Several small studies have found benefit using 1 or more of these agents in the perioperative period. To date, no survival benefit has been demonstrated, and it is probably premature to recommend routine use of these compounds. **Table 17-3** reviews the available evidence for use in selected patient populations.

PREOPERATIVE NUTRITIONAL SUPPLEMENTATION AND SHORTENED FASTING

Another area of recent interest surrounds the possible benefits of shortening or otherwise negating the period of preoperative fasting. Several studies have investigated the use of oral carbohydrate solutions designed to limit perioperative catabolism and reduce postoperative insulin resistance. A series of trials have assigned patients to receive 800 mL of a carbohydrate-rich solution on the night before surgery and a 400-mL load 2 hours before their operation. This protocol has been demonstrated to be safe in terms of aspiration risk and, in colorectal and orthopedic surgery patients, reduced postoperative insulin resistance by approximately 50%.[126] Hausel et al[127,128] reported reductions in perioperative discomfort from thirst, hunger, and anxiety as well as decreased postoperative nausea and vomiting following a similar protocol. Alleviation of preoperative hunger and thirst after oral carbohydrate loading was confirmed by Wang et al,[129] who also demonstrated in a randomized controlled trial that use of this technique stimulated the phosphatidyl-inositol 3-kinase (PI3K)/protein kinase B (PKB) pathway, an important component of insulin sensitivity. In another randomized trial enrolling orthopedic surgery patients, assignment to preoperative oral carbohydrate loading was associated with a reduction in postoperative immunosuppression (as measured by monocyte function, and likely a reflection of insulin and glucose handling).[130]

TABLE 17-2 Immunonutrients

Immunonutrient	Physiologic Mechanisms	Potential Benefits	Evidence
Arginine	• Conditionally essential amino acid • An intermediate of the urea cycle and precursor for creatine • The guanidino nitrogen atom of L-arginine provides the nitrogen used to synthesize nitric oxide (NO) • NO modulates cytokine production and white blood cell function • Essential to regulation of vascular tone	• Precursor to substrates for energy metabolism • As a free radical, can kill pathogenic bacteria, may be important in host defense • May have beneficial effects on wound healing	• A relative arginine deficiency state is theoretically produced where induced nitric oxide synthase activity increases; it has been shown that septic patients with low systemic arginine levels have a greater mortality rate[113]
Omega-3 fatty acids	• Omega-3 and -6 fatty acids are long-chain fatty acids that cannot be endogenously produced • Omega-3 fatty acids have immune-suppressive effects • Omega-6 fatty acids have immune-stimulating effects	• Alterations in ratios of omega-3 to omega-6 levels may be beneficial	• In septic rats, substitution of omega-3 for omega-6 fatty acids lowered prostaglandin E_2 production in Kupffer cells, and decreased mortality[114] • Human outcome data are lacking
Glutamine	• A nonessential amino acid • Fuel source in cell lines with rapid turnover • Preferred fuel source in the rat gastrointestinal tract, may have similar role in humans • Precursor to the antioxidant glutathione	• May prevent gut mucosal atrophy • May decrease bacterial translocation • May improve immune function	• Parenteral glutamine reduced mortality and increased jejunal villus height in septic rats[115] • Increases intestinal absorptive capacity in critically ill humans[116] • Showed benefit in a meta-analysis. Reduced infectious complications and hospital length of stay in surgical patients[117]
Nucleotides	• Nonessential • Necessary for gene expression	• May improve type 1 response to antigen challenge[118] • May prevent gut mucosal atrophy[119]	• Mice injected with *Candida albicans* had improved survival if they also received nucleotide supplementation[120] • Human data on nucleotide therapy alone are lacking

TABLE 17-3 Recommendations on -Enhanced Diets (Combinations of Arginine, Glutamine, Omega-3 Fatty Acids, and Nucleotides)

Surgery	Patient Group	Recommendation
Elective gastrointestinal surgery	Esophageal, gastric, pancreatic, hepatobiliary Colonic and rectal surgery	Patients with moderate to severe malnutrition (albumin <3.5 g/dL) benefit from preoperative immunonutrition for 5-7 d[121] Patients with severe malnutrition (albumin <2.8 g/dL) benefit from perioperative immunonutrition
Trauma patients	Blunt and penetrating	ISS >20 or ATI >25 benefit of reduced length of stay and septic morbidity[122]
Burn patients		Theoretically beneficial, lack of sufficient number of studies
Coronary artery	Elderly patients	Small study shows benefit of reduced infection[123]
Critically ill patients	Heterogeneous group	No benefit[124]
Severe sepsis		May harm patient[125]

Many of the benefits attributed to preoperative carbohydrate loading are probably mediated by improved insulin sensitivity. However, the diversity of salutary effects described in recent studies implicates multiple additional metabolic and hormonal pathways. In ASA (American Society of Anesthesiologists) class III and IV patients undergoing elective cardiac surgery (including those with type 2 diabetes mellitus), Breuer et al[131] reported reduced inotropic requirements during weaning from cardiac bypass in patients who received a preoperative oral carbohydrate solution. Two other randomized trials of preoperative oral carbohydrate solutions in colorectal surgery patients have also demonstrated improvements in postoperative skeletal muscle mass[132] and strength.[133] In a sophisticated analysis of the biochemical and genetic effects of a preoperative nutrition protocol, Schricker et al[134] randomly assigned colorectal surgery patients to receive either an intravenous hypocaloric solution of glucose and amino acids starting 20 hours before surgery or preoperative hydration with normal saline. Both groups received the hypocaloric solution from the time of skin incision until the second postoperative day. Patients in the preoperative nutrition group had statistically significant reductions in the breakdown of endogenous proteins, smaller elevations in amino acid oxidation, and a positive perioperative whole-body protein balance. Further, these patients had reduced expression of genes associated with muscle proteolysis and increased hepatic albumin synthesis.

Despite numerous unanswered questions surrounding the optimal timing, duration, amount, and content of perioperative nutrition, evidence supporting early and consistent enteral nutrition is mounting. In critically ill surgical patients, one of the most significant obstacles to maintaining adequate nutrition are the frequent interruptions to enteral feeding that occur when patients must undergo multiple procedures. Many institutions routinely mandate a 6- to 8-hour preoperative fast for patients being fed enterally, and this is often achieved by liberal use of an "NPO after midnight" physician order, regardless of the timing of the next day's procedure. Procedures may be postponed or canceled, leading to further feeding interruptions.

The necessity of prolonged fasting for extra-abdominal surgical procedures in critically ill patients has increasingly been called into question. In burn patients, who have particularly high metabolic demands, continuing enteral feeding during operative procedures has been shown to decrease caloric deficits without increasing infectious complications. Moncure et al[135] prospectively evaluated patients undergoing extra-abdominal procedures with jejunal nutrition and reported no cases of aspiration. Pousman et al[136] implemented a reduced fasting protocol for critically ill patients with a protected airway (defined as a cuffed endotracheal or tracheostomy tube) who were scheduled to undergo selected operative and nonoperative procedures. Intra-abdominal, intrathoracic, and neurosurgical procedures were excluded, as were those requiring prone positioning. Post-pyloric feeding was continued until the time of the procedure, and gastric feedings were continued until 45 minutes before the procedure. In a pre- and postimplementation analysis, the protocol led to nonsignificant trends toward faster attainment of nutritional goals and greater delivery of enteral nutrition. Outcomes including length of stay, ventilator days, and infectious complication rates were similar in both groups. More importantly, there were no cases of aspiration or regurgitation associated with the abbreviated fast.[136] A randomized trial is needed, but many institutions have already begun implementing similar protocols.

INTRAOPERATIVE MANAGEMENT OF THE PATIENT RECEIVING NUTRITIONAL SUPPORT

Three general principles should guide intraoperative nutritional support: (1) Parenteral nutrition should be continued whenever possible; (2) post-pyloric enteral nutrition should be continued with the possible exception of intra-abdominal procedures; and (3) gastric enteral nutrition should be discontinued 6 to 8 hours before procedures requiring general anesthesia and endotracheal intubation.

Total parenteral nutrition should be continued throughout surgery. Most formulas have some form of carbohydrate, putting the patient at risk for hyperglycemia. Careful evaluation of blood glucose should be continued throughout the perioperative period. Post-pyloric feeding probably can be continued safely in the presence of a protected airway, except during intra-abdominal or prone procedures. Patients who will require intubation and general anesthesia should fast for 6 to 8 hours before their procedure.

SUMMARY: IMPLICATIONS OF PERIOPERATIVE NUTRITIONAL SUPPORT FOR THE ANESTHESIOLOGIST

Anesthesiologists have an important role to play in the diagnosis and treatment of perioperative malnutrition. The anesthesiologist should ensure that the patient presenting for nonemergent surgery is in the best possible condition to tolerate the operation and postoperative course. The relatively poor outcome associated with malnutrition, coupled with the apparent benefits of repletion in the severely depleted individual, constitutes one more problem that can be addressed by anesthesiologists in their role as perioperative physicians to improve patient outcomes. An appropriate course of repletion in a highly malnourished individual may well be necessary, and calling attention to this potential problem and relevant therapeutic interventions is part of a comprehensive anesthesia evaluation and plan. Finally, anesthesiologists should be at the forefront of clinical and basic science research efforts to clarify the optimal timing, composition, and indications for perioperative nutrition support.

KEY REFERENCES

- Cerra FB. Hypermetabolism, organ failure, and metabolic support. *Surgery.* 1987;101:1-14.
- Koretz RL, Avenell A, Lipman TO, Braunschweig CL, Milne AC. Does enteral nutrition affect clinical outcome? A systematic review of the randomized trials. *Am J Gastroenterol.* 2007;102:412-429.
- Norman K, Pichard C, Lochs H, Pirlich M. Prognostic impact of disease-related malnutrition. *Clin Nutr.* 2008;27(1):5-15.
- Nygren J. The metabolic effects of fasting and surgery. *Best Pract Res Clin Anaesthesiol.* 2006;20:429-438.
- Schricker T, Meterissian S, Lattermann R, et al. Anticatabolic effects of avoiding preoperative fasting by intravenous hypocaloric nutrition: a randomized clinical trial. *Ann Surg.* 2008;248(6):1051-1059.
- Soeters PB, Schols AM. Advances in understanding and assessing malnutrition. *Curr Opin Clin Nutr Metab Care.* 2009;12(5):487-494.

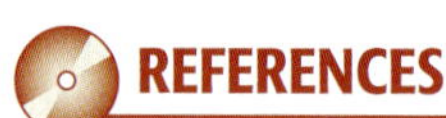

REFERENCES

Complete references available on DVD and online version at www.LongneckerAnesthesiology.com

CHAPTER 18 Principles of Antimicrobial Therapy

Richard Teplick
Robert H. Rubin

KEY POINTS

1. Antibiotic therapy should be based on the infection site, host defenses, antibiotic toxicity, antibiotic pharmacokinetics and pharmacodynamics, and the regional resistance organisms and antibiotic susceptibility patterns.
2. Methicillin-resistant *Staphylococcus aureus,* which is generally spread by contact, has become a major cause of serious hospital-associated infections and ensuing morbidity despite the development of newer effective antibiotics.
3. The term *catheter-associated infection* is used for surveillance and is a diagnosis of exclusion based on the presence of a catheter within 48 hours of a bloodstream infection and no other identifiable source.
4. Ventilator-associated pneumonia typically arises as an extension of upper airway bacteria and is related to duration of intubation. Several "bundles" are recommended for prevention, although their efficacy is controversial.
5. Most guidelines recommend avoiding central venous catheters when possible, removal as soon as it is no longer needed, and placement using full sterile procedures with barrier precautions.
6. Intra-abdominal infections are often associated with mixed flora and generally require anaerobic as well as aerobic antibiotic treatment.
7. Recommended surgical prophylaxis for infective endocarditis is evolving. In contrast with past guidelines, it is currently recommended for only a few conditions.

In general, antimicrobial drugs may be used in 3 different modes: therapeutic, prophylactic, and preemptive. In the therapeutic mode, they are prescribed to treat established clinical infection. This requires prompt diagnosis of clinical infection and a clear understanding of the pharmacologic principles governing treatment of such infections. In the prophylactic mode, antimicrobials are prescribed to all members of a given population before an event (eg, surgery) to prevent infection. Successful prophylactic programs require that the antimicrobial therapy be sufficiently nontoxic, inexpensive, and efficacious to justify the intervention. Finally, in the preemptive mode, antimicrobial therapy is administered to a subgroup of individuals based on either laboratory markers or clinical epidemiologic characteristics that place them at significant risk of a serious clinical infection (eg, patients undergoing organ transplants).[1] Effective preemptive therapy requires the careful delineation of the factors that justify antimicrobial intervention at a point when clinical disease is not yet manifest.[2-4] Clearly, there is some overlap between prophylactic and preemptive modes.

The purpose of this chapter is to present the pharmacologic and clinical principles that underlie all 3 forms of antimicrobial use, distinguishing between what is known, what is suggested by consensus but lacks definitive evidence, and what needs further study. The focus is primarily on antibiotics rather than antifungal and antiviral drugs. Specific information on newer antibiotics such as cyclic lipopeptides, glycylcyclines, ketolides, oxazolidinones, streptogramins, and newer fluoroquinolones can be found in review articles[5-8] and newer textbooks such as Mandell et al.[9] Aside from the specifics of a particular antibiotic, it is important to recognize the different characteristics among the various antibiotic classes. For example, some antibiotic classes such as tetracyclines are bacteriostatic in contrast to bacteriocidal antibiotics which directly kill bacteria, bacteriostatic antibiotics prevent bacteria from growing but generally require leukocytes to kill them. Another important difference among antibiotic classes is their mechanisms of action, especially the distinction between antimicrobials that directly affect cell-wall synthesis and those that affect protein or nucleic acid synthesis. β-Lactams and vancomycin are examples of the former, whereas aminoglycosides, macrolides, glycylcyclines, and fluoroquinolones are examples of the latter. Other important distinctions include the rate of development of resistance, induction of β-lactamases, presence of postantibiotic effect, pharmacokinetics, and pharmacodynamics.

When antimicrobials are used prophylactically for surgical patients, initial therapy is often empirical, directed against the most likely microbes while taking into account their antimicrobial resistance patterns not only in a region, but also in a particular hospital or even an area within the hospital, such as an intensive care unit (ICU). Most commonly, surgical antimicrobial prophylaxis is directed against the organisms most likely associated with a particular type of surgery. Other important considerations in selecting a prophylactic antimicrobial agent are its toxicity, its spectrum, its antimicrobial properties (ie, bacteriostatic or bacteriocidal), post-antibiotic effect, the likely source of bacteria (eg, colon, skin, biliary tract), and the drugs' pharmacokinetics and pharmacodynamics.

It is of great concern that a significant proportion of antimicrobial use, particularly broad-spectrum agents, both in the inpatient and outpatient setting, are often inappropriate, both because they are unnecessary and because they do not cover the infecting organisms.[10-12] Antibiotic use has been clearly associated with the emergence and dissemination of antibiotic-resistant organisms, with this occurring far more commonly in ICUs than in non-ICU inpatient areas and more commonly in inpatient than outpatient settings.

GENERAL PRINCIPLES OF ANTIMICROBIAL THERAPY

MINIMAL INHIBITORY CONCENTRATION AND MINIMAL BACTERICIDAL CONCENTRATION

Antimicrobial therapy designed to treat active infection is predicated on the reliable delivery of the drug to the site of infection at the concentration and duration required to contain or eradicate the infection. The effects of antimicrobials may be either to kill the targeted organisms (*bacteriocidal*) or to inhibit their growth (*bacteriostatic*). Although it would seem likely that bactericidal therapy would be inherently superior to bacteriostatic therapy, in most instances of clinical infection, either form of therapy is effective. There are, however, a few instances in which there is an absolute requirement for a bactericidal regimen, largely because the infection is inaccessible to the body's defenses or the patient is immunocompromised. Predictably, they are as follows:

- Systemic infection in a severely neutropenic patient
- Staphylococcal and, presumably, other forms of osteomyelitis
- Cardiovascular infection (eg, endocarditis)
- Central nervous system (CNS) infection: meningitis, cerebritis, and abscesses
- Infection in the presence of a foreign body, such as a joint prosthesis

If there are no bactericidal regimens for the invading organism, then high-dose and prolonged bacteriostatic therapy in association with aggressive surgery, if possible, becomes the alternative management strategy.

Modern microbiologic techniques not only permit the isolation and identification of the infecting microbe, but also can determine the susceptibility to different antibiotics, thus guiding the choice of antibiotics for a particular patient. When exposed in vitro to possible therapies, bacteria may be killed or their growth may be inhibited without being killed. The lowest concentration required to prevent growth is termed the *minimal inhibitory concentration* (MIC; variants of which are the MIC_{50} and MIC_{90}, which are the concentrations of drug required to inhibit 50% and 90%, respectively, of strains of the same species, in contrast to MIC, which measures inhibition of 1 strain). Similarly, the *minimal bactericidal concentration* (MBC) is the lowest concentration required to kill the bacterial isolate (with the MBC_{90} defining the lowest concentration of drug needed to kill 90% of isolates of the same species). The MBC is technically much more difficult and time-consuming to determine than the MIC; it is subject to multiple potential errors and is generally not important for routine clinical care.[13]

These in vitro results are then interpreted in terms of blood levels that are attainable when appropriate doses of the antimicrobial agent in question are administered. One of the 3 results is usually reported: *susceptible*, *resistant*, or *intermediate*. *Susceptibility* suggests that blood levels attainable with the therapeutic doses of an antibiotic should be effective in the management of infection due to this organism. Whether such efficacy is actually obtained depends on other factors, particularly activity and penetration in the site of infection. For example, blood levels may not provide adequate concentrations at sites such as the eye, the brain, or the prostate gland, and even with adequate concentrations, antibiotics can be inactivated by host factors. For example, daptomycin is inactivated by pulmonary surfactant and aminoglycosides and polymyxins by low pH. Thus in vitro susceptibility is only the first step in choosing the appropriate antimicrobial.

Susceptible sensitivity means the MIC is at or below the concentration achieved with the usual recommended dose of the antibiotic. *Intermediate* sensitivity means that MICs of the organism(s) in question are higher than blood and tissue levels that are achievable without potential toxicity. For the most part, the use of antimicrobial agents to which the bacterial isolate exhibits intermediate susceptibility should be avoided. However, particularly in dealing with a broadly resistant infection in the urinary tract, the issue is not the attainable blood levels, but rather the relationship between the MIC of the isolate and the attainable urine concentration. For example, tetracycline can often be used to treat "resistant" *Pseudomonas aeruginosa* strains isolated from urine because the levels in urine may be 100 times higher than in blood.

Resistant sensitivity generally means the MIC is greater than the concentration achievable in therapeutic or nontoxic doses. However, it can also mean that clinical efficacy has not been reliable or that special resistance mechanisms are likely to develop, such as induction of genes encoding inactivation of the antibiotic.

PHARMACOLOGIC PRINCIPLES IN THE SUCCESSFUL USE OF ANTIMICROBIAL AGENTS

The application of certain pharmacologic principles is important in optimizing the effectiveness of antimicrobial therapy. These principles are particularly important in treating infections, because unlike most anesthetic drugs, a direct measure of efficacy either does not exist or is delayed for long enough that by the time it is determined that the treatment failed, adequate treatment might be much more complex or possibly ineffective.

Pharmacokinetics and Pharmacodynamics The terms *pharmacokinetics* **and** *pharmacodynamics*[14,15] are used to describe the interaction of the drug administered with the individual receiving the therapy. *Pharmacokinetics* (PK) describes the quantitative relations between the administered doses of a drug and the concentrations of that drug in different body compartments. The most common PK models assume that there are only 2 compartments in the body, central and peripheral, which obviously do not correspond exactly to physical locations. Nonetheless, PK takes into account the effects of drug absorption, distribution, metabolism, and excretion. *Pharmacodynamics* (PD) describes the quantitative effects, both toxic and beneficial, of the plasma or tissue concentrations of a drug on the individual.[16,17] PK/PD models quantify the relationships between PK and PD. Perhaps the most useful measure of antimicrobial levels is the area under the time-concentration curve (AUC) divided by the dosing interval. This permits estimation of the average drug concentrations over the dosing interval. However, such data are usually available only for blood (the central compartment) and therefore may not accurately reflect the value at the tissue or site of interest. For example, aminoglycosides are highly concentrated in the kidney. Nonetheless, determining the PK–PD relationship is the foundation of efforts to define the appropriate therapeutic antimicrobial dose.

The *volume of distribution* is the ratio of the drug concentration in blood or plasma, assumed to be in equilibrium with all spaces where it distributes, to the amount of drug administered. For many drugs the volume of distribution vastly exceeds total body water. This large *apparent volume of distribution* may occur because of tissue or protein binding if only free drug is measured. This value is also altered by lipid solubility, the drug's blood–tissue partition coefficient, perfusion, volume status, and pH.

High serum protein binding of a drug can alter the PK behavior of the molecule without significant effects on the PD profile by serving as "buffers" so that there is little change in the concentration of free drug, despite its distribution to extravascular sites. Because albumin is the major binding protein, most binding usually occurs in the plasma, and serum albumin concentration can markedly affect the PK of highly bound drugs. In addition, at sites of active inflammation, there can be leakage of serum proteins, accounting for higher concentrations of drug at these sites.

The nature of the capillary bed at a particular site is also an important factor in the distribution of antimicrobials. At most sites the capillary bed has small pores (fenestrations) that allow for the unencumbered movement of substances with molecular weights of less than 1000 daltons (the great majority of antibiotics are of that size—the so-called small molecules). There are, in addition, specialized sites, such as the retina, the brain, and the prostate gland, where the capillaries are unfenestrated. Because the antimicrobial molecules must pass through these capillaries, diffusion is enhanced by high lipid solubility, small size, and the degree to which they are not ionized. β-Lactams, because they are highly ionized at plasma pH, may exhibit impaired penetration at these sites.[18] A final mechanism affecting the distribution of antimicrobial molecules is active transport pumps. These pumps act on organic anions and are present in the choroid plexus, the retina, the proximal tubules of the kidney, and the biliary ducts. β-Lactam drugs are pumped out by these active transport pumps, with probenecid competitively inhibiting this mechanism.

Pharmacokinetics and the Choice of Antimicrobial Therapy Three PK/PD issues should be considered in the choice of antimicrobial therapy: the ability of the drug to penetrate to the site of presumed infection, the presence of local factors at the site of infection that might modify the efficacy of particular antimicrobial including bacterial resistance and the presence of biofilms and the route of delivery that should be used. Thus if infection of the CNS is suspected, drugs that reach effective concentrations within the CNS should be used in doses adequate to achieve this objective (**Table 18-1**). However, there are exceptions. For example, although not recommended, meningitis due to high-level penicillin-resistant *Streptococcus pneumoniae* has been successfully treated with antibiotics that typically do not penetrate the CNS well. This may be a result of increased penetration resulting from inflammation. Moreover, serum levels may not be indicative of cerebrospinal fluid (CSF) levels. For example, cefotaxime serum levels peak and decline rapidly, whereas CSF levels are much lower but remain elevated much longer than serum levels, probably because the cerebral capillary endothelium is not fenestrated and lacks pinocytotic vesicles.[19]

Local factors that modify the effectiveness of particular antimicrobial agents include the following:

1. Inadequately drained abscesses. For example, aminoglycosides are far less effective in the presence of pus (both aminoglycosides and vancomycin are bound by pus, limiting their antimicrobial activity) and in environments with low pH and low oxygen tension.[20]
2. Low Po_2. Some antibiotics (eg, aminoglycosides) require oxygen-dependent transport to penetrate the outer membranes of susceptible bacteria. This explains why aminoglycosides are generally ineffective against anaerobic bacteria.[21]
3. The presence of β-lactamases. In mixed microbial infections, organisms such as *Bacteroides fragilis* produce β-lactamases, which cause local inactivation of β-lactam antibiotics despite their in vitro sensitivity to other bacteria.[20] Production of β-lactamases may also be induced by certain antibiotics.

TABLE 18-1 Penetration of the Cerebrospinal Fluid by Different Antimicrobial Agents[19]

Penetrate Noninflamed Meninges	Penetrate to Therapeutic Levels in the Presence of Inflammation	Penetrate Poorly or Unreliably Even in the Presence of Inflammation
Chloramphenicol	Penicillin	Cephalothin
Fluoroquinolones	Ampicillin	Cefazolin
Trimethoprim-sulfamethoxazole	Oxacillin	Cephapirin
Isoniazid	Nafcillin	Cefoxitin
Rifampin	Ticarcillin	Cefotetan
Metronidazole	Azlocillin	All aminoglycosides
Pyrazinamide	Mezlocillin	Tetracyclines
Flucytosine	Piperacillin	Ketoconazole
Fluconazole	Cefuroxime	Itraconazole
	Cefotaxime	Amphotericin B
	Ceftriaxone	
	Ceftizoxime	
	Ceftazidime	
	Cefepime	
	Imipenem	
	Meropenem	
	Vancomycin	

4. Binding to hemoglobin. Penicillins and tetracyclines bind to hemoglobin, thus decreasing the efficacy of these drugs for infected hematomas.[22]
5. Presence of foreign bodies. In most instances, the presence of a foreign body at the site of infection will prevent the elimination of the microbial invaders, even with the best antimicrobial regimens.[23]
6. The inoculum effect. High bacterial counts can increase the MIC of some antibiotics.
7. Decreased bioavailability. Oral administration of some antimicrobials (eg, trimethoprim-sulfamethoxazole, fluoroquinolones, fluconazole) can achieve blood levels that are comparable to those obtained with parenteral therapy if gastrointestinal function is adequate. However, absorption of some antimicrobials (eg, levofloxacin) is inhibited by food or substances containing divalent metal ions. A number of other factors can affect bioavailability, including the first-pass effect, in which drugs absorbed in the small intestine are metabolized in the liver; drug-metabolizing enzymes in the gut; and the presence of diseases that interfere with absorption, such as inflammatory bowel disease, parasitic infestation, and diarrhea of any etiology. Nonetheless, even if therapy is initiated intravenously, completion of a course of treatment can be accomplished with a more cost-effective oral regimen once the patient stabilizes.

Postantibiotic Effect Some antibiotics continue to suppress the growth of certain bacteria after the antibiotic is no longer detectable in the media—a phenomenon termed the *postantibiotic effect* (PAE). For example, after a 2-hour exposure of susceptible staphylococcal cultures to penicillin, growth is still inhibited for 1.4 to 1.6 hours after multiple washings removed the penicillin from the culture medium.[24] Although PAE can be demonstrated for virtually all antimicrobials, the bacteria affected and the duration of the effect are highly variable. β-Lactam antibiotics, with the exception of carbapenems such as imipenem and meropenem, have significant PAEs only for some gram-positive bacteria. In contrast, most antibiotics that inhibit protein or nucleic acid synthesis in gram-negative bacteria generally exhibit a PAE for these organisms. For example, for gram-negative bacteria, aminoglycosides and fluoroquinolones produce PAEs for 1 to 4 hours, whereas β-lactams have essentially no PAEs for these bacteria. Importantly, the PAE duration tends to be reduced for aminoglycosides and fluoroquinolones in acidic media, such as encountered in necrotic tissue. A related but poorly understood phenomenon is that during the PAE phase, bacteria are more susceptible to killing by leukocytes, an effect termed *postantibiotic leukocyte enhancement* (PALE).[25,26] In addition, the PAE itself may be prolonged by leukocytes.

Concentration-Dependent and Time-Dependent Killing Agents The distinction between time-dependent and concentration-dependent killing coupled with the presence or absence of a PAE has important clinical ramifications, particularly with respect to dosing intervals. For antimicrobial/bacteria combinations that exhibit time-dependent killing, especially when there is no PAE, the duration that the antimicrobial level is above the lethal range (usually about 4 times the MIC) is important, whereas concentrations above the bacteriocidal levels cause little additional bacterial killing. Vancomycin and β-lactams with the exception of carbapenems typically exhibit time-dependent killing. There is general agreement that for β-lactams to be effective, their concentration must be well above the MIC for most of the dosing interval. This is best achieved using continuous infusions for at least part of the dosing interval or prolonging each bolus administration. This should be especially true for gram-negative bacteria, which usually do not exhibit PAE for β-lactams. Although this concept is supported by animal data, it is puzzling that studies in humans have not generally shown superiority of continuous infusions.[27-29] Nonetheless, for this class of drugs, it seems logical to adjust dosing frequency to maintain levels in a bacteriocidal range for as long as logistically possible.[30]

In contrast, for antibiotic/bacteria combinations that exhibit concentration-dependent killing and significant PAEs, the bacteriocidal rate and the duration of the PAE are dose-dependent (eg, for aminoglycosides, fluoroquinolones, daptomycin, colistin, metronidazole, ketolides, and possibly azithromycin). Therefore, it may be more important to achieve very high peak levels and allow the trough to decrease below the MIC because efficacy will still be maintained by the PAE, whereas toxicity may be minimized. For these drugs, the AUC divided by the MIC is more important than the dosing frequency or the time greater than the MIC. For combinations of antibiotics, the situation is more complicated. The PAEs for gram-positive bacteria are increased either additively or synergistically when aminoglycosides are added to cell-wall active antibiotics. However, this does not occur with gram-negative bacteria, except when imipenem or meropenem is used with an aminoglycoside or for certain bacteria such as the enterococci.[31]

These considerations led to the concept that administering aminoglycosides in larger doses once daily would prove more beneficial and less toxic than the usual standard of 3 times daily.[32] In particular, because aminoglycosides exhibit concentration-dependent killing and have a PAE, concentrations that reach a level 8 to 10 times the MIC will rapidly kill all susceptible bacteria and suppress the survival of higher MIC mutants. Because of the PAE, suppression can be sustained during the period that the concentration drops below the MIC. The maintenance of drug-free intervals for a period before the next dose might also help prevent adaptive resistance, which may occur from decreased aminoglycoside uptake by bacteria exposed to lower levels of the drug. Finally, because renal uptake is saturable, the very high initial levels are not accompanied by proportionally increased renal uptake. Consequently, renal toxicity does not increase. Numerous studies show that in most patients and even in febrile neutropenic patients, these tenets seem to hold; efficacy is at least equal to multiple daily dosing, but surprisingly, renal toxicity is not decreased.[33,34]

A third group consists of antimicrobials that are predominately bacteriostatic and have prolonged PAEs. Because of the prolonged PAE, efficacy is more dependent on an AUC that is greater than the MIC rather than time above the MIC. This group includes macrolides, clindamycin, quinupristin/dalfopristin, tetracyclines, tigecycline, and linezolid.[15]

RESISTANCE

General Concepts Bacteria may be intrinsically resistant to antimicrobials, or they may acquire resistance. *Intrinsic resistance* reflects a natural resistance to an antibiotic. It is demonstrated when bacterial growth is not inhibited or the bacteria are not killed by the antibiotic, even though no new genetic information has been acquired. For example, vancomycin is ineffective against gram-negative bacteria because it cannot penetrate their outer membrane. *Acquired resistance* reflects a genetic alteration in a microorganism that renders a once effective antimicrobial ineffective. The general mechanisms for bacterial resistance to antibiotics are as follows: (1) decreased permeability to the antimicrobial, thus preventing its entry; (2) increased efflux pumps that pump antimicrobials out of gram-positive bacteria or keep the antimicrobial concentrations in the space between the inner and outer membranes of gram-negative bacteria and/or the cytoplasms low; (3) antimicrobial inactivation; (4) modification of the antimicrobial target, interference of binding to the target, or overexpression of the target; (5) binding of the antimicrobial by false binding sites; (6) development of pathways that bypass the target.

The genes encoding these phenotypes may be chromosomal or plasmid/transposon in origin, inducible, or constitutive. Methicillin-resistance in *Staphylococcus*, vancomycin-resistance in *Enterococcus*, and broad-spectrum β-lactam resistance in gram-negative bacteria have important diagnostic and therapeutic implications, particularly in the hospital setting.[35-40]

In gram-negative bacteria, antibiotics usually must penetrate the hydrophobic lipopolysaccharide outer membrane via specialized channels, termed *porins*. Alterations in the permeability of porins to specific antibiotics can either prevent sufficient quantities from entering the bacteria or limit the rate of entry to the extent that even a relatively low inactivation rate is sufficient to render them ineffective. The former is a frequent cause of *P aeruginosa* resistance to aminoglycosides and carbapenems, and the latter allows many gram-negative bacteria to inactivate β-lactams via β-lactamases. Increased active efflux of antimicrobials is a less common mechanism of resistance but can be important for tetracyclines, macrolides, streptogramins, fluoroquinolones, some β-lactams, and possibly meropenem.

Inactivation is the predominant mechanism of resistance for several classes of antibiotics. Aminoglycosides can be inactivated by both gram-positive and gram-negative bacteria, usually by plasmid-mediated enzymes. These enzymes modify specific sites on the aminoglycoside molecule, such that *N*-acetylation, *O*-nucleotidylation, or *O*-phosphorylation takes place. These modified aminoglycoside molecules bind poorly to the ribosome target, rendering them inactive in normally susceptible bacteria. Target modifications in penicillin-binding proteins account for methicillin resistance in staphylococci and penicillin resistance in pneumococci and enterococci. Bypass pathways account for vancomycin resistance in *Enterococcus faecium* and resistance of many bacteria to folate antagonists, such as trimethoprim-sulfamethoxazole.

Specific Mechanisms Perhaps the most comprehensively studied and categorized inactivating enzymes are the β-lactamases. There are at least 890 different β-lactamase protein sequences (www.lahey.com/studies), one or more of which can inactivate virtually any β-lactam, monobactam, or carbapenem-based antimicrobial.[41] They are carried on chromosomal genes, plasmids, transposons, and integrins, the latter often producing multidrug resistance (MDR). The classification schemes for β-lactamases are based on both phenotype and genotype and continue to evolve. One scheme groups them into classes A, B, C, and D based on amino acid motifs. However, it is also common to classify them into the more subjective Bush-Jacoby functional groups 1, 2, and 3 based largely on which β-lactams they hydrolyze and which are blocked by the β-lactamase inhibitors. Certain β-lactam antibiotics induce β-lactamases. For example, clinical failure associated with the emergence of resistance often occurs when serious *Enterobacter* infection is treated with a cephalosporin despite initial cephalosporin susceptibility.[42] Thus cephalosporins should be used carefully in the setting of infection with the previously mentioned gram-negative pathogens.[35]

Although β-lactamases are produced by some gram-positive bacteria, notably staphylococci (but not streptococci) and many anaerobes, the efficacy of these β-lactamases is limited because they are diluted by the extracellular space, in contrast to being confined in the periplasmic space of gram-negative bacteria, where they reach high concentrations.[38,43] Although plasmid-encoded β-lactamases cause staphylococcal resistance to many penicillins, resistance of some staphylococci and other gram-positive bacteria can also occur by completely different mechanisms. For example, methicillin-resistant *Staphylococcus aureus* (MRSA) is caused by the chromosomal presence of the mecA gene, which decreases the binding affinity of methicillin to penicillin-binding protein 2a. Similarly, ampicillin-resistant *E faecium* has an altered penicillin-binding protein 5 that has a greatly reduced affinity for these antibiotics and most β-lactams. In contrast, in the majority of cases, vancomycin resistance in enterococci is related to a multigene plasmid, which is easily spread among enterococci. This plasmid alters a terminal amino acid group in one of the cross-linking amino-acids that prevents vancomycin from binding to the growing cell membrane.[44,45]

It is astonishing that the first time vancomycin-resistant enterococci (VRE) were observed was in 1986,[46] and within 15 years it has come to represent more than 24% of ICU enterococcal isolates in the United States. Unfortunately, there are limited options for the treatment of severe infections related to VRE, which are typically also resistant to ampicillin and aminoglycosides. Several new antibiotics (eg, tigecycline, a glycylcycline; quinupristin/dalfopristin, a streptogramin; and linezolid, an oxazolidinone) that have recently been approved by the US Food and Drug Administration (FDA) have efficacy against VRE and other resistant gram-positive bacteria.[7]

TABLE 18-2 Emergence of Antibiotic Resistance

Resistant to	Bacteria	% Resistance by Year			
		1998	1998-2002[a]	2003	2006-2007[b]
Vancomycin	Enterococci	23.9	25.4	28.5	80.0[c] 6.9[d]
Methicillin	*S aureus*	46.7	53.6	59.5	56.2
Third-generation cephalosporin	*K pneumoniae*	10.7	14.0	20.6	16.8[e]
Third-generation cephalosporin	*Enterobacter* spp.	34.0	33.1	31.1	
Imipenem	*P aeruginosa*	17.1	18.3	21.1	25.3
Quinolones	*P aeruginosa*	23.3	27.1	29.5	

[a]Average percentage resistant from 1998 to 2002. Data from NNIS.[67,191]

[b]Data from NHSN.[66]

[c]*E faecium.*

[d]*E faecalis.*

[e]*K oxytocia.*

There is great concern that *S aureus* will acquire the vancomycin-resistance determinant from enterococci. This was first shown to be possible in the laboratory,[47] and scattered clinical cases have now been reported of MRSA strains with both decreased vancomycin susceptibility (known as vancomycin-intermediate *S aureus* [VISA]) and vancomycin resistance (known as vancomycin-resistant *S aureus* [VRSA]).[48] The mechanism for this diminished susceptibility appears to be due to a thickening of the cell wall leading to decreased antibiotic penetration and sequestration of vancomycin, rather than the transfer of vancomycin resistance genes from *Enterococcus* leading to an altered vancomycin binding target.[49-51]

Emerging Bacterial Resistance In the last decade, there has been a dramatic increase in the development and dissemination of antibiotic-resistant organisms. As shown in **Table 18-2**, resistance of enterococci, especially *E faecium*, to vancomycin has shown the greatest increase, whereas MRSA has remained stable up to 2007, which is the last year when such data were available. Many factors have contributed to the marked increase in resistance; however, indiscriminate broad-spectrum antibiotic use is an important contributor.[52] Other factors that select for resistance include dosing that is too low or given for too short a duration. Thus it is critically important to use antimicrobials judiciously, as overuse facilitates the propagation of pathogens that are difficult or impossible to treat. One example of antimicrobial misuse is in farming, where the widespread deployment of antimicrobials to animals has resulted not only in resistant flora on farms, but also in the spread of such resistant organisms to humans.

COMBINATION ANTIMICROBIAL THERAPY

A common practice in the hospital use of antimicrobial agents is "double coverage" in an effort to improve efficacy and prevent resistance from developing. Indeed, in vitro studies often suggest benefits from such an approach, with at least the following justifications.

Prevention of the Development of Antimicrobial Resistance Combination therapy to prevent development of resistance is most effective when the mechanism for resistance involves chromosomal mutations, with the merits of combination therapy being most easily seen for tuberculosis. The microbial burden in a particular patient and the known rate of mutational resistance to each of the antituberculous drugs are the major determinants of the most effective regimen for a particular patient. Thus, in a nonimmunosuppressed host, the pulmonary microbial burdens are as follows: primary tuberculosis of approximately 10^4 organisms, noncavitary reactivation 10^6 to 10^8 organisms, cavitary disease 10^8 to 10^{10} organisms, and so forth. The rates of mutation to resistance for tuberculosis antimicrobials are approximately 1 in 10^6 for isoniazid and ethambutol, 1 in 10^8 for rifampin, and 1 in 10^5 for streptomycin. Therefore, the treatment for primary tuberculosis typically requires a single drug (usually isoniazid), noncavitary reactivation disease requires 2 drugs, and so on. Although other factors enter into the design of the therapeutic regimen, the approach outlined fits with the efforts to avoid resistance. However, chromosomal mutation is an uncommon mechanism of resistance (the great majority of bacterial resistance is due to the acquisition of a plasmid or transposon that mediates resistance). Thus the prevention of development of resistance is not an adequate reason for combination therapy of pyogenic infection.

Known or Suspected Polymicrobial Infection This can be a valid reason for deploying multiple drugs. For example, a perforation of the distal colon will result in the release of anaerobes (particularly *B fragilis*), gram-negative bacilli, and bowel streptococci (including enterococci) into the peritoneal cavity. This event had traditionally required a 2- or 3-drug regimen (eg, ampicillin, metronidazole, and gentamicin) to deal with the range of aerobic and anaerobic organisms. However, today there are single antibiotics such as carbapenems, β-lactam/β-lactamase combinations, newer fluoroquinolones, and tigecycline with a spectrum of activity that will accomplish the same task.

Initial Therapy When the initial assessment of a patient suggests the possible presence of a therapeutic emergency, broad-spectrum therapy is obligatory, at least until the results of cultures are available. The issue that remains controversial is whether this is best accomplished with a single drug or multiple drugs. Current evidence does not generally support the older concept that a combination of a β-lactam with an aminoglycoside provides a higher probability of success than a single drug, even if *P aeruginosa* is likely to be involved. Nonetheless, commonly therapy is initiated with a broad-spectrum drug or combination of drugs, which may have overlapping spectra with different resistance patterns to ensure the initial coverage is adequate. However, once cultures and sensitivities are available, the regimen should be changed to the drug or drugs with the narrowest spectra that provide sufficient coverage.

Decreased Toxicity A principle of cancer chemotherapy is that in some cases the toxicity can be decreased by using multiple drugs with different mechanisms of action and toxicities at lower doses. Unfortunately, the efficacy of this approach in the treatment of significant infection has not been demonstrated.

Synergistic Therapy In vitro and in animal models of serious infection, enhanced killing with certain antibiotic combinations for some species of both gram-positive and gram-negative bacteria can be demonstrated. This has been most evident with combinations of β-lactams and aminoglycosides. Whether this can be demonstrated in clinical situations is not yet determined. Moreover, whether this truly constitutes synergy is debatable, as the methodology (eg, the checkerboard method) usually does not adhere to standard methods for demonstrating drug synergy. The best evidence of the utility of enhanced efficacy of combination therapy comes from the study of patients with enterococcal endocarditis. Treatment of enterococcal endocarditis with penicillin (or ampicillin) alone results in an inferior clinical outcome compared with that achieved with the addition of streptomycin or gentamicin to the penicillin. Enterococcal strains with high-level aminoglycoside resistance (MIC >2000 μg/mL) do not have the potential for bactericidal therapy and have a distinctly poorer outcome. Although combination of a penicillin and gentamicin may also shorten the requisite duration of therapy for some nonenterococcal gram-positive endocarditis, outcomes are not improved.

Part of the problem with existing studies is the lack of stratification of patients into "therapeutic emergency" versus "a need for parenteral therapy" versus "outpatient management." As a result, even with the lack of definitive evidence, our approach to staphylococcal endocarditis is as follows: stable patients get single-drug therapy with nafcillin; those who are more ill (hemodynamic instability, evidence of emboli, etc) receive potentially synergistic therapy with a minimum of 2 drugs. Although many experienced clinicians use potentially synergistic therapy for other serious gram-negative infections, particularly those occurring in compromised hosts, definitive evidence is lacking and most current data favor monotherapy.

CLINICAL PHARMACOLOGY: GENERAL PRINCIPLES OF THERAPEUTIC ANTIMICROBIAL USE

Effective antimicrobial therapy requires the integration of a sizable body of information regarding the patient, the invading microbe(s), and the antimicrobial agents themselves into an effective antimicrobial prescription. The factors that must be considered include the following.

IDENTITY OF THE ORGANISM

The identity of the infecting organism(s) must be known, or at the very least, it must be possible to make a high-probability assessment of the most likely culprit(s). The initial choice of antimicrobial agents is usually based on probability assessments of the most likely pathogens causing a particular clinical syndrome arising in a particular environment, with subsequent adjustment of the regimen once specific microbiologic information becomes available. Important factors to be weighed in determining the likely infecting organism include the probable source (eg, vascular access device, lung, or urinary tract) and whether the infection is likely to be community-acquired or hospital-associated. Other issues of importance include recent antibiotic use, the presence of such growth factors as iron and elevated blood sugar, and the existence of devitalized tissue.

URGENCY OF TREATMENT

The key question is whether one is dealing with a therapeutic emergency or a diagnostic dilemma. In the former case, the broadest possible regimen should be utilized initially, with later modifications based on precise microbiologic information. This is often termed *front loading* of the antimicrobial regimen. In the latter case, narrower spectrum initial therapy is possible, with fine-tuning of the regimen once specific information is available.

EPIDEMIOLOGY

Epidemiologic considerations must also be factored into antimicrobial decision making. When dealing with primary illnesses acquired in the community, the nature and timing of possible exposures must be considered. Important exposures include the geographically restricted systemic mycoses (*Blastomyces dermatitidis*, *Coccidioides immitis*, and *Histoplasma capsulatum*), *Mycobacterium tuberculosis*, influenza, group A streptococci, *Legionella*, and meningococcus. Even more important is the special epidemiology of the hospital-associated environment, be it a nursing home, a patient with a recent admission to a hospital or recent antibiotic treatment, a hospital, or a specialized area of the hospital such as an ICU. Specifically, the microbiologic flora within a hospital or even a particular ICU within the hospital and their respective resistance patterns are essential information. The rising incidence of infection with difficult to treat organisms such as MRSA, VRE, and multiresistant gram-negative bacilli has a profound influence on the initial choice of antibiotics. For example, vancomycin is usually preferred over nafcillin as initial therapy for suspected staphylococcal infection, and advanced spectrum β-lactam agents such as imipenem rather than cefazolin or gentamicin for gram- negative infections that could be caused by highly resistant *Klebsiella* species.[53,54] It is likely that these problems with antibiotic resistance will increase, not just in terms of these organisms, but also with rising incidences of infections with penicillin-resistant pneumococci[55,56] and ampicillin-, vancomycin-, and gentamicin-resistant enterococci.[56]

These considerations highlight the importance of the reservoir of a given organism and the selective pressure that reservoir is under (eg, *Salmonella* and *Campylobacter* in domestic animals vs *S pneumoniae* in the community at large and multidrug-resistant gram-negative rods in the nosocomial environment).[57,58] By understanding the reservoir, the prevalence of antimicrobial resistance in the reservoir, and the risk of exposure of a patient to a given organism, one can determine appropriate initial antimicrobial therapy.

The implication of these principles is 2-fold. First, every hospital and patient area within the hospital must engage in ongoing surveillance of the most common organisms and antimicrobial susceptibility patterns causing infection in their particular areas. Second, decisions about antimicrobial use should take into consideration such information, particularly for patients who have been subjected to the selection pressures of previous courses of antibiotics or environments that may have rendered them more vulnerable to colonization and/or invasion with resistant flora.

HOST FACTORS

A number of host factors must be considered in formulating an antimicrobial regimen. These can be divided into 3 groups: (1) those that increase a patient's risk for a specific type of infection; (2) those that increase a patient's risk of complications from an infection (eg, the presence of prostheses such as artificial joints, synthetic vascular grafts, or cardiac valves); and (3) those that increase the risks of treating an infection with specific drugs because of patient comorbidities, such as renal insufficiency.

Specific Drug Risks Perhaps the most important consideration is the history of previous adverse reactions to the drugs in question. Great precision is needed in defining the nature of a history of an adverse reaction. For example, nausea, vomiting, and diarrhea, particularly after oral administration, do not preclude the use of an antimicrobial, especially intravenously. In contrast, a history of anaphylaxis, Stevens-Johnson syndrome, toxic epidermal necrolysis, or allergic interstitial nephritis does preclude further use. Commonly, the exact nature of the allergy is unclear. In this circumstance, either the class of drug implicated should be avoided or else skin testing with a subsequent desensitization regimen should be performed.

The presence of renal dysfunction in the patient being treated can also have a profound effect on antimicrobial therapy because many antimicrobials are cleared by the kidney and therefore require adjustment of the dosing regimen. Unless such adjustments are made, toxic side effects may occur, such as injury to the 8th cranial nerve and further renal injury with aminoglycosides,[59] seizures with penicillins and carbapenems,[60] and bleeding due to platelet dysfunction (added to that already caused by a uremic state) induced by ticarcillin, mezlocillin, and piperacillin.[61] Although many antimicrobials are cleared or metabolized by the liver, hepatic dysfunction usually requires less dosage adjustment than renal dysfunction. In general, little dosage adjustment is required until the bilirubin exceeds approximately 5 mg/dL (**Table 18-3**). However, with hepatic dysfunction, chloramphenicol, clindamycin, the tetracyclines, and the antituberculous drugs isoniazid and rifampin should be avoided, if possible (in the case of the antituberculous drugs, if they are required for emergency therapy, then special effort should be made to monitor blood levels in the face of serious hepatic dysfunction).[62] When both renal and hepatic dysfunctions are present, then therapy with essentially all β-lactam antimicrobial agents should be carried out with great care.[63]

Impaired Host Defenses Special considerations need to be extended to those patients who have specific impairments in host defenses. Impairment may be anatomical, such as cutaneous ulcerations or mucosal abnormalities, or it may be secondary to functional host defense defects, such as neutropenia, asplenia, malignancy, immunosuppressive therapy, diabetes mellitus, or human immunodeficiency virus (HIV) infection. Patients with prosthetic heart valves, prosthetic joints, vascular grafts, or other prostheses can suffer dire consequences from metastatic spread of infection if initial therapy is inadequate. Therefore, such patients should be considered for front-loading of the regimen, ideally with a bactericidal drug, even if their initial clinical state would not normally require it.

TABLE 18-3 Use of Antimicrobial Agents in the Presence of Renal or Hepatic Dysfunction

Contraindicated in the Presence of Renal Failure	Require No Dosage Change in the Presence of Renal Failure	Require Dosage Adjustment With Moderate Renal Failure	Require Dosage Adjustment Only With Severe Renal Failure	Avoid or Adjust Dose in the Setting of Significant Hepatic Dysfunction (eg, bilirubin > 5 mg/dL)
Tetracyclines (except doxycycline), nitrofurantoin, cephaloridine, long-acting sulfonamides, methenamine, paraaminosalicylic acid	Erythromycin, azithromycin, clarithromycin, clindamycin, chloramphenicol, doxycycline, cefoperazone, nafcillin, oxacillin, rifampin, amphotericin B, ceftriaxone, metronidazole, grepafloxacin, minocycline, linezolid, quinupristin/dalfopristin	Carbenicillin, ticarcillin, cefazolin, all aminoglycosides, vancomycin, imipenem, flucytosine, penicillin G, 5-fluorocytosine, fluconazole	Ampicillin, cefoxitin, cefotaxime, ceftizoxime, piperacillin, isoniazid, ethambutol, trimethoprim-sulfamethoxazole, cefotetan, ceftazidime, cefuroxime, mezlocillin, meropenem, nalidixic acid, ciprofloxacin, ofloxacin, levofloxacin, norfloxacin, itraconazole	Quinupristin/dalfopristin, chloramphenicol, clindamycin, lincomycin, all the tetracyclines, cefoperazone, ceftriaxone, metronidazole, nafcillin, nitrofurantoin, fusidic acid, isoniazid, rifampin, rifabutin, pyrazinamide, rimantadine, ketoconazole, fluconazole, itraconazole

Modified from Amsden GW. Tables of antimicrobial agent pharmacology. In: Mandell GL, Bennett JE, Dolin R, eds. *Principles and Practice of Infectious Diseases*. 6th ed. Philadelphia, PA: Elsevier; 2005:634-700.

Pregnancy A critically ill patient who is pregnant, and for whom termination of the pregnancy is not an option, represents a particular challenge. First, the pharmacokinetics of many antibiotics are altered in pregnancy due to a larger volume of distribution and increased glomerular filtration rate.[64] Second, the database on the safety of different antibiotics during pregnancy is woefully incomplete. The safety classifications of various antimicrobials during pregnancy are listed in **Table 18-4**. Importantly, this list is constantly updated. Therefore, before using any antimicrobial, current data should be checked. Aminoglycosides and isoniazid should only be prescribed if absolutely necessary because the former may be associated with 8th cranial nerve dysfunction in the infant and the latter with an increased incidence of psychomotor retardation, myoclonus, and seizures.

TABLE 18-4 Safety of Selected Antimicrobials in Pregnancy[a]

Class	Definition	Antimicrobials
A	No adverse effects in human studies	None
B	No adverse effects in human studies with adverse effects in animals *or* no human data but no adverse effects in animal studies	All penicillins All cephalosporins except moxalactam Azithromycin Macrolides Clindamycin Sulfa before third trimester
C	No human data but adverse effects in animals *or* no data in humans or animals	Fluconazole Isoniazid, pyrazinamide, rifampin Imipenem-cilastin All fluoroquinolones Trimethoprim Vancomycin Gentamicin Chloramphenicol
D	Adverse effects in humans but benefit may outweigh risks	Amikacin, tobramycin All tetracyclines
X	Adverse effects in humans. Risk outweighs benefits	None

[a]This list is constantly evolving. Check for current recommendations before use.

Data from Draper JC, Cox KW, Matthews KJ et al. Teratology and drug use during pregnancy. http://emedicine.medscape.com/article/260725-overview#showall. Accessed 10/23/11.

PRACTICAL ASPECTS OF DRUG ADMINISTRATION: ANTIMICROBIAL THERAPY OF PARTICULAR CLINICAL SITUATIONS

GENERAL

When choosing the appropriate antibiotic therapy, it is critical to decide whether the infectious process is nosocomially acquired or present at admission (ie, community-acquired). In 2005, the Centers for Disease Control and Prevention (CDC) published rigorous definitions of nosocomial infections in various body sites.[65] The CDC defines *health care–associated infections* (HAI) as those that develop during hospitalization but are neither present nor incubating upon the patient's admission to the hospital. This generally includes infections that occur more than 48 to 72 hours after admission and within 10 days after hospital discharge. Under the aegis of the CDC, the National Healthcare Safety Network (NHSN), has subsumed the surveillance functions of the National Nosocomial Infections Surveillance system (NNIS) in collecting and analyzing HAI surveillance data. **Figure 18-1** shows the site distribution

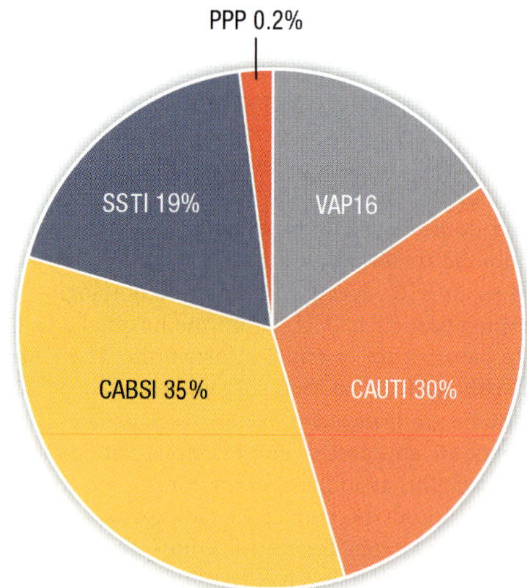

FIGURE 18-1. Site distribution of 28 502 antimicrobial-resistant health care–associated infections in 463 hospitals reporting more than 1 infection to the NHSN.[66] Note that these are derived from surveillance data and are not necessarily proven sources of infection. CABSI, catheter-associated bloodstream infections; CAUTI, catheter-associated urinary tract infections; PPP, post-procedure pneumonia; SSTI, skin and soft tissue infections; VAP, ventilator-associated pneumonia.

TABLE 18-5 Distribution and Rank Order of HAI Pathogens by Site of Infection[66]

	CLABSI	CAUTI	VAP	SSI
Pathogen	% (rank)	% (rank)	% (rank)	% (rank)
Staphylococcus, coag negative	34.1 (1)	2.5 (7)	1.3 (9)	13.7 (2)
S aureus	14.5 (4)	2.2 (8)	24.4 (1)	30.0 (1)
E faecalis	3.5 (2)	3.6 (3)	0.4 (10)	2.8 (3)
E faecium	5.6 (2)	6.0 (3)	0.6 (10)	4.9 (3)
E coli	9.6 (5)	21.4 (1)	4.6 (6)	9.6 (4)
P aeruginosa	7.9 (6)	10.0 (4)	16.3 (2)	5.6 (5)
K pneumoniae	5.8 (7)	7.7 (5)	7.5 (5)	3.0 (7)
K oxytoca	1.1 (10)	0.9 (10)	2.2 (8)	0.7 (9)
Enterobacter spp.	4.8 (8)	4.1 (6)	8.4 (3)	0.6 (9)
A baumannii	2.7 (9)	1.2 (9)	8.4 (3)	4.2 (6)
C albicans	6.8 (4)	14.5 (2)	2.4 (7)	1.6 (8)
C non-albicans	3.9 (4)	6.5 (2)	0.3 (7)	0.4 (8)

CAUTI, catheter-associated urinary tract infection; CLABSI, central line–associated bloodstream infection; SSI, surgical site infection; VAP, ventilator-associated pneumonia. Rank is based on sum of percentages.

of 28 502 antimicrobial-resistant HAIs collected by the NHSN in 463 hospitals from January 2006 until October 2007.[66] These data show that approximately 80% of antimicrobial-resistant HAI pathogens were associated with 3 sources: 35.3% with intravascular catheters, 30.1% with bladder catheterization, and 15.9% with ventilators. This accounts for the enormous regulatory interest in minimizing or eliminating infections in these 3 sites. The primary pathogens associated with these various sites are shown in **Table 18-5**. Note, however, that these are from surveillance data and therefore may overestimate actual infection rates because the former include associations that may lack definitive evidence of the causative device or organism.

It is important to recognize that gram-positive pathogens, particularly *Staphylococcus epidermidis*, *S aureus*, and enterococci are the leading bloodstream pathogens, whereas *S aureus* and gram-negative bacteria, particularly *P aeruginosa*, are the predominant pathogens associated with nosocomial pneumonia. In addition to *S aureus* and *P aeruginosa*, *Escherichia coli* and *Candida albicans* are the primary pathogens found in urinary tract infections, with the great majority of these being associated with urinary tract instrumentation.[67-73] These data are consistent across continents.[73] It is of interest that *Candida* species now account for the fourth most common cause of nosocomial bloodstream infection. Ten years ago, it was 24th, a testimonial to the increasing importance of this organism, particularly in ICU patients and possibly to the overuse of antibiotics.

As indicated in Fig. 18-1, the incidence of nosocomial infections is highly associated with the use of devices such as ventilators, vascular access catheters, and urinary catheters. This is likely a result of the breakdown of normal host defenses and clearance mechanisms. In addition, these devices may support the growth of various microorganisms in different ways. For example, the development of biofilms on urinary and central venous catheters enhances the adherence of certain microorganisms such as *E coli* and may impair the penetration of antimicrobials or alter the resistance patterns, whereas the condensation of water in ventilator circuits is a conducive environment for *Pseudomonas* and *Acinetobacter*.[71] The device-associated infection rates are surprisingly constant for different devices and types of ICUs. For example, from the most recent NHSN data, the maximum and minimum rates per 1000 device days for catheter-associated urinary tract infections was 25.7 in medical–surgical ICUs and 2.4 in burn ICUs; for central line–associated bloodstream infections, the maximum was 20.6 in medical–surgical ICUs, and the minimum was 2.7 in neurosurgical ICUs; and for ventilator-associated pneumonia, the maximum was 25.1 in medical–surgical ICUs and the minimum was 3.5 in cardiac medical ICUs.[67] Surprisingly, these rates are consistently near the lowest in burn ICUs.

MULTIDRUG-RESISTANT BACTERIA

Methicillin-Resistant *Staphylococcus aureus* *S aureus* is the leading cause of hospital-associated infections. The mortality rate for invasive *S aureus* infections approaches 20%, and an increasing percentage of all such infections are resistant to methicillin (MRSA). *S aureus* developed resistance to penicillin in the 1940s due largely to its inducible production of a penicillinase that hydrolyzes penicillin and most other β-lactams. Methicillin and oxacillin, which are resistant to penicillinase, were developed in the late 1960s. *S aureus* resistance to these newer drugs emerged shortly after they were developed. Today, at least 80% of *S aureus* isolates are resistant to methicillin and most β-lactams, including penicillin and cephalosporins. β-Lactams work by inactivating penicillin-binding proteins (PBPs), which are enzymes that are essential to the formation of the cell wall. Resistance to methicillin (and oxacillin) is due to PBP2a, which is encoded by the mecA gene. PBP2a has low affinity for β-lactams and is not present in methicillin-sensitive *S aureus* (MSSA). Aside from multiple mechanisms that impair the efficacy of antimicrobial therapy, *S aureus* can produce a wide variety of substances that promote adherence to cells and artificial materials (eg, catheters), as well as a panoply of exotoxins, all of which enhance its virulence. Because of the virulence of *S aureus* coupled with the resistance of MRSA to most antibiotics, its containment and treatment of infections caused by it are major problems for hospitals and other chronic care facilities.[9]

Currently approximately 60% of *S aureus* infections in hospitalized patients are MRSA, although this varies somewhat regionally.[74] Initially, the hospital-acquired and community-acquired MRSA differed markedly. MRSA are often classified into species by pulsed-field gel electrophoresis of DNA fragments into USA100 to USA700.[75] Initially, hospital-acquired MRSA (HA-MRSA) comprised USA100 and USA 200, which are resistant to all but a few antibiotics (eg, vancomycin). In contrast, the community-acquired variant (CA-MRSA) largely included USA 300 and USA 400 genotypes, which are sensitive to many antibiotics (eg, clindamycin), excepting most β-lactams.[76] However, this distinction has blurred as an increasing number of HA-MRSA are now caused by USA300 CA-MRSA, which evolved independently of HA-MRSA. CA-MRSA usually carries genes that encode Panton-Valentine leukocidin (PVL), a pore-forming exotoxin that is associated with necrotizing pneumonia as well as skin, soft tissue, and leukocyte necrosis. Although it is not clear which strains are most virulent, PVL is thought to be important in the virulence of USA300.

There are several reasons that MRSA has attracted so much attention. First, regardless of the species, MRSA infections are a major cause of morbidity and mortality. Second, until recently, vancomycin was the only antimicrobial that could be used to treat HA-MRSA. Third, MRSA is highly contagious, spread primarily by contact. Fourth, both patients and non-patients frequently carry MRSA in their nares without any signs or symptoms. Consequently, they may inadvertently spread the organism, causing infections among susceptible contacts. Lastly, MRSA causes many types of infection, ranging from furuncles and carbuncles to metastatic infections, necrotizing pneumonia, osteomyelitis, and endocarditis. It is also responsible for a substantial percentage of catheter-associated bloodstream infections. There are many strategies intended to prevent HAIs in hospitalized patients, many of which center around handwashing and contact precautions, and the incidence of MRSA infections seems to be declining.[77-79] Although it is tempting to attribute this to mandatory reporting in some states as well as an emphasis on a variety of measures intended to help prevent MRSA infections, the decrease began before widespread implementation of these measures and may reflect a natural biologic trend.[80] The role of nasal screening and decontamination, usually with topical mupirocin, is controversial and probably not generally cost effective, except possibly in patients with recurrent infections.[81]

Although CA-MRSA and HA-MRSA both are resistant to β-lactams because of PBP2a, CA-MRSA is usually sensitive to clindamycin, trimethoprim-sulfamethoxazole, and doxycycline. Current guidelines recommend empirical treatment with one of these drugs for outpatient treatment of purulent cellulitis, abscesses with constitutional symptoms, or with comorbidities such as diabetes or immunosuppression.[81] Otherwise, drainage alone may suffice. Notably, these antimicrobials are not effective against HA-MRSA. Pending sensitivities, it should be assumed that all staphylococcal infections in hospitalized patients are multidrug resistant. Therefore, initial treatment is limited to vancomycin, linezolid, daptomycin, or tigecycline, with certain caveats as reviewed by Neuner et al.[82] Daptomycin should not be used for MRSA pneumonia because it is inactivated by pulmonary surfactant. Linezolid may be at least as effective as vancomycin for treating MRSA pneumonia and may have an advantage because, at least in vitro, it inhibits the production of several toxins, including PVL. Of concern, however, is its potential for inducing toxicity in combination with drugs that inhibit serotonin uptake because it is weak inhibitor of monoamine oxidase. Unfortunately, strains of *S aureus* that have partial (VISA) or complete (VRSA) resistance to vancomycin are emerging. Fortunately, aside from the previously mentioned antibiotics, several new antibiotics, including the cephalosporins ceftaroline and ceftobiprole, that have activity against MRSA are currently undergoing development.

Multidrug-Resistant Gram-Negative Bacteria The plethora of bacterial resistance mechanisms and the mobility of some of the responsible genes have posed an ongoing problem in the management of both gram-negative and gram-positive infections. However, for gram-negative bacteria, this problem has increased with the emergence of strains that are resistant to 3 or 4 different antibiotic classes. Such *multidrug resistance* (MDR) has been a problem for some strains of *Klebsiella pneumoniae*. More recently, the incidence of infections caused by *Acinetobacter baumannii*, which is intrinsically MDR, has increased. In the past, these organisms were usually sensitive to carbapenems, but lately they have acquired serine and metallo-β-lactamases (carbapenemases), which hydrolyze carbapenems as well as all other β-lactams.[83] As a result, some strains of *A baumannii*, *P aeruginosa*, and other species of Enterobacteriaceae (eg, *E coli*) have exhibited resistance to 4 different antibiotic classes.[84] The genes responsible for production of these carbapenemases usually reside on plasmids that have apparently been transmitted from *K pneumoniae* to other Enterobacteriaceae, including *E coli*. These genetic islands often carry with them resistance mechanisms for multiple classes of non–β-lactam antibiotics. Between 2006 and 2008, approximately 60% of *A baumannii* infections throughout the United States were MDR, in contrast to only 10% of *P aeruginosa* and 15% of *K pneumoniae*.[84]

MDR in *Acinetobacter* species have become particularly problematic. They are usually restricted to hospitals, especially ICUs, and community-acquired infections are uncommon. However, because they are found in soil and water, they may be present in trauma and burn patients on admission. Moreover, for reasons that are not understood, they are also being found with increasing frequency in military personnel injured in the Middle East. *Acinetobacter* species can colonize skin, respiratory tract, and gastrointestinal tract, and because they are transmitted by contact, meticulous handwashing and contact precautions are essential in preventing hospital outbreaks. Furthermore, they can survive desiccation for weeks. Consequently, eradication of outbreaks may require closing the offending area (eg, an ICU) for complete decontamination. *A baumannii* infections occur mostly in ICU patients with ventilator-associated pneumonia and catheter-associated bloodstream infections, whereas *P aeruginosa* and *K pneumoniae* are most prevalent in catheter-associated urinary tract infections.

These MDR bacteria may be resistant to all antibiotics except colistin (polymyxin E). Unfortunately, colistin is nephrotoxic. Because it was approved before the FDA's promulgation of more rigorous standards, the appropriate doses and dosing schedules are not well established. Therefore, minimization of cross contamination is vital to contain these bacteria.

CATHETER-RELATED INFECTIONS

Intravascular access devices are common causes of bacteremia and fungemia. A *primary bloodstream infection* (BSI) is defined as at least 1 positive bacterial or fungal culture drawn from a peripheral site without any known source. Although a BSI is usually central to defining infections attributable to a catheter, the terminology has become somewhat confusing. A *central line–associated bloodstream infection* (CABSI) is defined as a BSI when an arterial or central venous catheter (CVC) was in place within the past 48 hours.[85] Importantly, as noted earlier, this definition is used for surveillance rather than clinical care and has several limitations.[86] First, using the total catheter days as the denominator for CLABSI as per CDC recommendations implies that for a given patient, the probability of getting a CLABSI is constant over the CVC dwell time. Yet, clearly, dwell time does matter, which implies that the probability per day is not constant. Moreover, if this were not true, there would be no infection-control reason to advocate minimizing CVC dwell times. Therefore, in assessing CLABSI rates, a correction should be applied for dwell times rather than normalizing the rate per 100 catheter days. Second, because there are no accepted criteria for when to obtain blood cultures, the incidence of BSI within 48 hours of the presence of CVC may underestimate CLABSI or even central line–related bloodstream infections (CRBSI) unless blood cultures are obtained every time a catheter is removed. Finally, statistical comparisons among rates cannot be made unless the total number of catheter days is known or confidence limits are included in the data. The latter practice was used by the CDC,[87] but not in reporting by individual states.

In contrast, a *suspected* CRBSI is defined as a BSI in a patient with a CVC or arterial catheter in place, whereas a *definite* CRBSI is defined as a BSI with the same organism grown from the catheter tip. If the catheter is still in place, a CRBSI is confirmed if blood sampled through the catheter grows more than 15 colony-forming units (CFU) of the same organism on blood media. Alternatively, if a peripheral blood culture cannot be obtained, a CRBSI may be confirmed if blood is sampled through at least 2 lumens of a multilumen catheter and 1 lumen yields a colony count at least 3 times greater than the other lumen(s).[88] However, this definition is occasionally supplanted with a *laboratory-confirmed bloodstream infection* (LCBSI), which is defined either as a CRBSI or a patient with a CVC and with fever (>38°C) or chills or hypotension not related to an infection at another site and with a common skin contaminant (eg, *Corynebacterium* spp., *Bacillus* spp., *Propionibacterium* spp., coagulase-negative staphylococci including *S epidermidis*, viridans group streptococci, *Aerococcus* spp., or *Micrococcus* spp.) grown from 2 or more blood cultures drawn on separate occasions.[89] The most widely used diagnostic technique to culture a catheter tip is a semiquantitative method, which involves rolling the catheter tip or the introducer tip used with a pulmonary artery catheter across an agar plate and then counting the number of CFUs after overnight incubation. Although a positive culture drawn through a catheter is relatively nonspecific and has a higher rate of false-positive results than peripheral blood cultures, a negative culture generally rules out a catheter-related infection because of the low false-negative rate.[90] It is difficult to find current data on the risk of bacteremia associated with various vascular devices, probably because of the large variation in type of catheter (number of lumens, catheter material, antibiotic coated or not), techniques (skin preparation), care of the site, and barrier precautions between regions of the country and hospitals within a region.

To put this risk in perspective, it is worth noting that 50 000 to 100 000 patients in US hospitals develop nosocomial bloodstream infections each year, with approximately 70% of these infections related to arterial or central venous catheters of various types.[67] Such infections are associated with a mortality rate of 25% to 35% and a 2- to 3-fold increase in attributable mortality. In 2009, The Infectious Diseases Society of America (IDSA) published guidelines revised from 2001 for the management of intravascular catheter-related infections.[88] The guidelines generally divide CRBSI into early (<14 days after placement) or late, and percutaneous or tunneled catheters. The guidelines state that the initial choice of antibiotics depends on the severity of the patient's clinical disease, the risk factors for infection, and the likely organisms associated with the specific intravascular device. Understanding the pathogenesis and virulence of the typical organisms involved permits this problem to be approached rationally.

For nontunneled short-term catheters, the organism usually comes from skin flora that colonizes the external surface of the catheter. The most common of these is *S epidermidis*, followed by *S aureus*, *Candida* species, and enteric gram-negative bacteria. In contrast, long-term and tunneled catheters are typically colonized intraluminally from the catheter hub. The most common microorganism is still *S epidermidis*, but for these catheters, it is followed by enteric gram-negatives and then *S aureus*, with *P aeruginosa* becoming more important. Gram-negative bacteria are more common with femoral catheters, probably because of perineal flora, and are therefore discouraged. They are also more common when there are gram-negative infections of the respiratory tract or surgical wounds or drains because they increase the incidence of gram-negative skin colonization, thereby providing a reservoir of organisms for such infections. This pathogenic mechanism explains the increasing infection rate associated with central line position: femoral > internal jugular > subclavian. Presumably, the incidence of infections is higher for internal jugular catheters than for subclavian catheters because the former is more likely to be exposed to orotracheal secretions. The use of antibiotic-impregnated catheters has been shown to prevent microbial contamination of the catheter and subsequent bacteremia in some but not all studies. In one study, catheter-associated bacteremia decreased from 3.4% to 0.3% with the use of a minocycline- and rifampin-impregnated catheter.[91] However, these results should be interpreted cautiously because these coatings may lead to false-negative catheter cultures.

Initial therapy of suspected CRBSI usually includes vancomycin because of the high prevalence of methicillin-resistant *S aureus* and *S epidermidis* in the hospital environment. However, the latter microorganism poses a particular problem because it is both the most common CRBSI but also the most common contaminant. For this reason, the 2009 IDSA guidelines recommend confirmation via additional blood cultures obtained via the catheter and peripherally before initiation of therapy or catheter removal for *S epidermatitis*-suspected CRBSI. Additional coverage directed at gram-negative organisms should be considered based on local susceptibility data, especially if gram-negative infection is present at other bodily sites or if the patient manifests cardiovascular instability. In the latter case and for immune-compromised patients, therapy should also be directed at multidrug-resistant organisms such as *P aeruginosa*. Empiric therapy directed at vancomycin-resistant enterococci is rarely indicated, as this organism is an unusual cause of acute hemodynamic instability. Antifungal therapy is also not initiated unless the patient has been receiving total parental nutrition, prolonged use of broad-spectrum antibiotics, the catheter is in a femoral artery or vein, the patient is immune-compromised, or there is microbiologic evidence of fungal infection (see later discussion). Fluconazole is acceptable therapy if the patient has not received it within the past 3 months and the risk of *Candida krusei* or *Candida glabrata* is low. Otherwise, an echinocandin is recommended. Once the offending bloodstream pathogen is identified and its resistance profile known, focused antimicrobial therapy should be used. There are no definitive data for duration of therapy, but the catheter should be removed and therapy prolonged (4-8 weeks) for complicated CRBSI such as suppurative thrombophlebitis, endocarditis, osteomyelitis, or metastatic seeding. For uncomplicated CRBSI, generally the catheter should be removed and, if needed, replaced de novo rather than over a guidewire if possible. Therapy is recommended for 7 to 14 days.

There are several important issues to consider in the treatment of the common CRBSI pathogens. As mentioned, *S epidermidis* is often a contaminant. However, when it does cause a BSI, it typically behaves as a relatively avirulent pathogen. Consequently, it usually can be treated with removal of the catheter and a short course of antibiotics. Nonetheless, this organism has a propensity to adhere to prosthetic devices such as cardiac valves and artificial joints. Therefore, when *S epidermidis* bacteremia occurs in such a patient, one must carefully evaluate the prosthetic device for evidence of secondary infection. In light of these considerations, patients with indwelling prostheses should be considered at higher risk for consequences of central catheter placement.

S aureus, on the other hand, is an extremely virulent organism, which in the setting of bacteremia, often disseminates, causing osteomyelitis, endocarditis, and other severe, tissue-destructive infections. Thus when a bacteremia with this organism is confirmed, a careful evaluation for metastatic infection should occur, and prolonged therapy (2 to 4 weeks) is often recommended. Enterococcal BSI behaves in a similar manner as *S epidermidis* and typically responds to removal of the catheter. However, endocarditis may occur, particularly in the setting of prolonged bacteremia. The optimal therapy for this organism is ampicillin plus an aminoglycoside, although single-drug therapy with some of the newer antibiotics such as daptomycin and tigecycline show therapeutic promise. When *C albicans* is cultured from the blood, the patient should be evaluated for metastatic infectious foci (eg, hepatic, ocular, and skin), the catheter should be removed, and antifungal therapy initiated, typically with fluconazole, unless *C glabrata* or *C krusei* is prevalent in the environment or isolated, in which case an echinocandin should be used.[92] If metastatic foci of candidal infection are found, then the optimal management of these complications will determine the duration of therapy.

PROPHYLAXIS

Surgical

Need for Prophylaxis The need for antibiotic prophylaxis for surgery depends on the risk of a *surgical site infection* (SSI), generally defined as purulence within the wound. The occurrences of SSIs are related to the wound classification, patient-related factors such as immunocompetence, the bacterial milieu, hospital infection rate for various procedures, and factors relating to the wound itself.[93] As shown in **Table 18-6**, wounds are usually classified as clean (class I), clean-contaminated (class II), contaminated (class III), and dirty/infected (class IV).[94] The increasing risk of SSI from class I to class IV is related to the wound's bacterial burden, although dirty/infected wounds are often already infected. However, careful microscopic examination shows that even clean wounds are contaminated with skin flora.[95]

Staphylococcal species are the most common wound pathogens in most SSIs. Antibiotic prophylaxis is debatable for some clean procedures such as an inguinal hernia repair or mastectomy. However, for other clean procedures (especially for neurosurgical, cardiothoracic, and vascular surgery; hip or knee arthroplasty; and any procedure in which bone is excised or a prosthesis is inserted), gram-positive coverage, in the past with vancomycin but currently usually with cefazolin, has been recommended. However, because of the increasing incidence of MRSA in both hospitals and in the community, the trend seems to be shifting back toward vancomycin. Trials comparing vancomycin with cefazolin to prevent surgical site infections in cardiac surgical patients have had variable results, but in one study the incidence of SSI in coronary artery bypass surgery was decreased when vancomycin was used for prophylaxis instead of cefuroxime,[96] and The Society of Thoracic Surgeons recommends vancomycin prophylaxis for selected patients.[97]

Prophylactic antibiotics should be administered for all clean contaminated and contaminated wounds, as well as for hysterectomies and most invasive urologic procedures. Sterilization of the urinary tract is recommended before any urologic procedure if possible. Even with successful treatment of a urinary tract infection, deep-seated infection of the prostate gland can be reactivated by manipulation

TABLE 18-6 Surgical Wound Classification[111,193]

Classification	Criteria	Typical Examples	Infection Rate (%)
Clean: Typically skin and environmental bacteria	Atraumatic. No break in sterile technique. Respiratory, alimentary, or genitourinary tracts have not been entered	Exploratory laparotomy Mastectomy Neck dissection Thyroidectomy	<2
Clean Contaminated: Bacteria colonizing epithelial surfaces and lumens	Clean urgent or emergent. Areas known to harbor bacteria such as the biliary, respiratory, alimentary, and genitourinary tracts, when there is no or minimal spillage of contents	Cholecystectomy Appendectomy Small bowel resection Transurethral prostate resection	<10
Contaminated: Site-dependent organisms	Major break in sterile technique. Surgery on a traumatic wound. Gross gastrointestinal spillage. Entrance into an infected biliary or genitourinary tract. Incisions in area of acute nonpurulent inflammation	Appendectomy with inflammation Bile spillage during cholecystectomy Diverticulitis	<20
Dirty/Infected: Preexisting infecting organisms	Purulence or abscess. Old wounds with devitalized tissue. Perforated viscus. Penetrating trauma >4 h old	Abscess excision and drainage Perforated bowel Peritonitis	40

and/or surgery. Prophylaxis is advised for high- and moderate-risk patients undergoing procedures involving infected tissues and should include anti-staphylococcal antibiotics for the prevention of cellulitis and osteomyelitis. Similar coverage is advised for patients receiving prosthetic cardiac valves. Patients with urinary tract infections should receive antibiotics such as fluoroquinolones, third-generation cephalosporins, or an aminoglycoside that are active against gram-negative bacilli. Convincing evidence for prophylactic antimicrobial benefit is also found for patients undergoing endoscopic manipulation of an infected biliary tree or urinary tract. For these conditions, antibiotics such as ampicillin-sulbactam and piperacillin-tazobactam are reasonable choices, although the increasing frequency of *E coli* resistance to the former drug has led to suggestions to avoid it.

Timing of Prophylaxis It is generally accepted that intravenous administration of prophylactic antibiotics should be initiated no sooner than 1 hour before incision. Theoretically, this ensures adequate tissue levels before surgery begins. The major impetus for this practice comes from a study that retrospectively analyzed the timing of prophylactic antibiotic administration for patients for whom a wound infection was reported.[98] These investigators concluded that patients who developed SSIs were more likely to have received prophylaxis between 24 and 2 hours before surgery or after skin incision. Often unnoticed in this study was that the incidence of wound infection was statistically unchanged if the antibiotics were given within 2 hours before incision or within the first 4 hours after incision. When these data were subjected to a multiple logistic regression, the only variables related to wound infection were underlying disease, nursing service, type of surgery, duration of surgery, and time after the start of surgery when the first dose of prophylactic antibiotic was administered. Notably, of the 41 SSIs, 58% were resistant to the antimicrobial drug used. Thus although this study is widely quoted as showing that prophylaxis must be given within 2 hours of the incision, these data do not fully support this conclusion. Moreover, this study was retrospective, so at best it could only detect associations rather than cause and effect. It also did not address when the antibiotic infusions were completed.

Although it seems logical to have adequate tissue levels of prophylactic antimicrobials before skin incision, supporting data are only inferential, and it is likely that the importance depends on the type and size of the inoculum. Nonetheless, administration of prophylactic antibiotics within 1 hour of surgery (2 hours for vancomycin) has become a standard of care that is publicly reported as part of the Surgical Care Improvement Project (SCIP). Moreover, the Centers for Medicare and Medicaid Services (CMS) may reduce hospital reimbursement if it is not reported. CMS also will not pay additional costs associated with mediastinitis after cardiac surgery or SSIs after bariatric surgery or certain orthopedic procedures.

In toto, SCIP has 6 surgical infection prevention measures, but only 3 are core measures: (1) timely administration of prophylactic antibiotics as described previously, (2) administration of antibiotics recommended for a given procedure, and (3) discontinuation of prophylactic antibiotics within 24 hours after surgery (48 hours for cardiac surgery). The latter exception occurred because of a document drafted by The Society of Thoracic Surgeons that made the following points: (1) although prolonged use of antibiotics can lead to the emergence of resistant infections, there are no data that this can occur with administration for under 48 hours; (2) antibiotic prophylaxis for 48 hours is "clinically effective in minimizing infectious complications in cardiac surgery" and is as effective as prophylaxis administered for more than 48 hours; and (3) antibiotic prophylaxis should not be used for indwelling catheters of any type or chest tubes.[99] There is general agreement on this last point for all types of surgery, with the possible exception of transplantation.

Despite the CMS mandate, to date no study has convincingly shown that adherence to the 3 SCIP core measures has reduced the surgical infection rate. A study of vancomycin prophylaxis in 2048 cardiac surgical patients was interpreted as showing that vancomycin initiated from 16 to 60 minutes before incision and administered over 1 hour was associated with the lowest rate of surgical site infections.[100] However, the relative risks were not significantly increased for any time from 16 to more than 180 minutes before surgery. Results were similar for odds ratios calculated using a logistic regression that adjusted for various patient variables. Thus this study actually found that SSI rate was not affected if the vancomycin infusion was completed essentially any time before surgery or as long as 30 minutes after surgery began. A single prospective study[101] and 2 purportedly prospective studies that were actually based on data mined from several databases[102,103] failed to show any relation between postoperative infections and timing of antibiotic prophylaxis. Most recently, the largest retrospective data-based cohort study also failed to show a relation between SSI and any of the 3 SCIP core measures or all 3 combined, although a reduction in SSI rate was associated with meeting any 2 or more of the 6 infection prevention measures.[104] This engendered an editorial view that "The current metrics does not appear to discriminate between effective and noneffective care at the patient or hospital level" and that "investing resources in SCIP reporting is no longer cost-effective."[105] Finally, an animal study widely cited as documenting the need to have the antimicrobial given before the incision lacked statistical testing and used very high inocula and varying doses of antimicrobials.[106]

Other Measures to Prevent Surgical Site Infections Aside from maintaining strict sterile procedures, hair removal on the morning of surgery that does not create microabrasion (eg, using clippers rather than razors) is logical and effective, although there are few data to support hair removal at all. Showering with chlorhexidine has not been shown to be effective, possibly because of the interval between showering and surgery. Successful treatment of distant infections and drain removal as soon as possible is also logical although not carefully studied. Surgical technique such as careful approximation of tissue planes and avoidance of hematomas may be the single most important factor. One important factor that is now part of CMS quality measures is maintenance of normothermia both intraoperatively and postoperatively. Normothermia presumably reduces SSI rates because of increased skin blood flow. A seminal study of 200 patients undergoing colorectal surgery randomized to an intraoperative temperature of 34.5° or 36.5° yielded SSI rates of 19% and 6%, respectively.[107] Postoperative oxygen supplementation has met with mixed results. Controlling blood glucose to less than 200 mg/dL in diabetic cardiac surgical patients reduced the incidence of deep wound infections.[108] However, it is unclear whether these results can be extrapolated to noncardiac surgery, although the concept seems logical.

To compare SSI rates among hospitals or even physicians, adjustment must be made for patient risk. One of the earliest predictors of postoperative SSI was the Study on the Efficacy of Nosocomial Infection Control (SENIC) index.[109] This index gave 1 point to each of the following: operative time greater than 2 hours; abdominal procedures; contaminated or dirty procedures; and at least 3 discharge diagnoses, the latter probably serving as a surrogate for patient health. On the basis of data accrued from 1970 and 1975 to 1976, patients with 4 points had approximately a 30% SSI rate, whereas it was 1% for patients with 0 points. This index was subsequently modified into the National Nosocomial Infection Surveillance (NNIS) index, which gave 1 point for each of the following: an American Society of Anesthesiologists score of 3, 4, or 5; a contaminated or dirty procedure; and length of procedure greater than 75% of that expected for each operation. One point was subtracted for laparoscopic surgery.[110] Interestingly, using this NNIS index, the SSI rates were similar for all surgical classifications except clean operations. Although many factors relating to both the patient and the environment have been identified, they have not been incorporated into risk predictors.[111] In fact, since the NNIS index, there has not been any further development in multivariable risk predictors. Therefore, although publicly available, comparisons of hospital SSI rates are problematic because of inadequate risk stratification.

ICU Comparable successes with prophylactic antimicrobial regimens in ICU patients have been more difficult to prove, as have attempts to prevent infection with selective gut decontamination regimens. The latter involves using either nonabsorbable antimicrobial agents or fluoroquinolones to eliminate the aerobic gram-negative flora while leaving the anaerobic flora intact, which provides some protection against colonization with a variety of potential pathogens, which is termed *colonization resistance*. Similarly, aerosolized antibiotics, particularly polymyxin or aminoglycosides, have not been shown to prevent pneumonia. Topical antibiotic ointments also have not been shown to decrease the incidence of intravenous access–related bloodstream infection.

Preemptive Therapy Recently the concept of *preemptive therapy* has come to the fore. Preemptive therapy was initially defined in transplant patients, where the initiation of ganciclovir therapy in bone marrow transplant patients with evidence of cytomegalovirus (CMV) replication either in the blood or in the respiratory secretions, at a time when they were asymptomatic, prevented the development of otherwise life-threatening CMV pneumonia. In organ transplant patients, the initiation of preemptive ganciclovir during intensive antirejection therapy markedly decreases the incidence of systemic CMV infection normally associated with such therapy.[2,3]

The efficacy of preemptive therapy for fungal infection in, for example, abdominal fecal contamination has not been well established. Data for fungal prophylaxis suggest that fluconazole may be effective prophylaxis for certain high-risk patients, such as those undergoing bone marrow transplants or reoperation for gastric or upper small bowel perforations, anatomic sites where large numbers of *Candida* species are normally found. Nevertheless, there is no evidence that this reduces mortality.[112,113] However, such studies are difficult to interpret because the diagnosis of invasive fungal infection is often challenging, and distinguishing between candidal colonization and invasion is problematic. Several studies have shown that when a patient is colonized with a fungus at 3 or more sites, there is a 30% to 60% incidence of invasive disease, with a high associated mortality. There is some agreement that preemptive therapy should be initiated only after recent abdominal surgery with recurrent gastrointestinal perforations or anastomotic leaks and is not necessary for the initial surgery, even if there is fecal soilage, so long as it has not been present for a relatively long period.[114] However, this issue is further complicated by the emergence of fluconazole-resistant *C albicans* and the change in common fungal species to more resistant species such as *C krusei* and *C glabrata*, which are not sensitive to fluconazole but can be treated with echinocandins..

Bacterial Endocarditis The guidelines for prophylaxis for endocarditis have changed markedly since first published in 1955 and continue to evolve, including the most recent update published in 2008,[115] which supplanted those published in the preceding year.[116] Although these guidelines are generally agreed on, they are not supported by any Class I evidence (benefit >>> risk) that definitively show that antibiotic prophylaxis prevents bacterial endocarditis during procedures that can produce a bacteremia. Nonetheless, given the consequences of endocarditis and the minimal risk associated with prophylaxis, the use of antibiotics to prevent cardiac infection is sensible for high-risk procedures. The most recent guidelines (2008) modify recommended prophylaxis for dental procedures. They are based on 4 rationales: (1) endocarditis is more likely to result from random bacteremias associated with daily activities than dental, gastrointestinal, or genitourinary procedures; (2) prophylaxis would prevent few if any cases of endocarditis; (3) the risk of prophylaxis exceeds the potential benefit; and (4) maintenance of oral health is more important than prophylaxis.

The major changes in these recommendations are that prophylaxis for dental procedures is reasonable only for cardiac conditions associated with the highest risk of an adverse outcome from endocarditis. This includes patients with prosthetic valves, patients with a history of infective endocarditis, patients with unrepaired complex cyanotic congenital heart disease or repaired with prosthetic material within the past 6 months, and cardiac transplant patients with regurgitation from a structurally abnormal valve. Prophylaxis is recommended for these patients only for procedures that involve manipulation of gingival tissue or the periapical region of teeth or perforation of the oral mucosa. Prophylaxis is not recommended for genitourinary or esophageal procedures or colonoscopy. Interestingly, in contrast to older guidelines, these new guidelines no longer recommend prophylaxis for patients with mitral valve prolapse, even those with audible murmurs or thickened valve leaflets. However, this recommendation is not universally accepted and is an enlightening controversy for several reasons.[117] First, prolapse can occur in normal mitral valves under conditions that reduce the end-diastolic volume of the left ventricle, such as hypovolemia or enhanced contractility, especially in young adults. Second, prolapse without regurgitation is not thought to increase the risk of bacterial endocarditis because the regurgitant jet seems to cause the abnormalities that increase bacterial adherence to the valve. Thus it was thought that only patients with mitral valve prolapse who also have mitral regurgitation should receive antibiotic prophylaxis, although this is no longer recommended.

Procedures such as central catheter placement through skin that is otherwise normal and has been cleansed with povidone-iodine or chlorhexidine are not associated with significant bacteremias and therefore do not warrant prophylaxis. Regardless of the source, viridans streptococci (α-hemolytic streptococci) are the most common cause of endocarditis, followed by *S aureus* and enterococci. If prophylaxis is used, a single oral dose of 2 g of amoxicillin given 1 hour before the procedure or intravenous ampicillin or penicillin is recommended. Clindamycin or azithromycin is alternative for penicillin-allergic patients. Endocarditis prophylaxis is recommended for some clean procedures, such as abdominal and lower extremity vascular procedures, craniotomies, orthopedic procedures with hardware insertion, and any procedure that includes implantation of permanent prosthetic material. In contrast, the need for prophylactic antibiotics for orthopedic procedures such as laminectomies and spinal fusions is controversial.

The rate of endocarditis-causing bacteremia with genitourinary tract surgery or instrumentation is high in patients with urinary tract infections and prostatitis and in prostatic surgery. *E faecalis* is the most common bacterial species, but *Klebsiella* species are also common. The recommended prophylaxis for these high-risk patients undergoing such procedures is ampicillin. Vancomycin may be substituted for ampicillin in penicillin-allergic patients. Gentamicin may be added in high-risk patients. Attempted sterilization of the urinary tract before any procedure is also thought to be beneficial. Prophylaxis is not recommended for uncomplicated vaginal delivery, cervical biopsy, or manipulation of an intrauterine device in the absence of infection.

PNEUMONIA

Patients with pneumonia had been divided into 2 general categories: those with community-acquired pneumonia (CAP) and those with hospital-acquired (ie, nosocomial) pneumonia (HAP). However, much of health care is now delivered in nonhospital settings such as nursing homes, where bacterial infections have a risk of being caused by MDR organisms similar to that of hospitalized patients, as is the severity of such infections. Recognition of this led to classifying pneumonia in patients exposed to such environments as health care–associated pneumonia (HCAP). Accordingly, in 2005 pneumonias were categorized into the following 3 groups:[118] (1) hospital-acquired pneumonia (HAP), which occurs at least 48 hours after admission; (2) ventilator-associated pneumonia (VAP), which occurs at least 48 hours after endotracheal intubation; and (3) HCAP, which occurs in patients who were hospitalized in an acute care hospital within the past 90 days or who within the past 30 days resided in a nursing home or a long-term care facility or received intravenous antibiotic therapy, wound care, hemodialysis, or chemotherapy. These patients either present with pneumonia or develop it within 48 hours of admission.

Whether HCAP should be considered a single entity or should be subdivided into subcategories by, for example, host, environment, hospital exposure, and immunosuppression is controversial.[119,120]

To facilitate the study of pneumonia in hospitalized patients, the NHSN published detailed diagnostic criteria.[65] Despite this, caution must be exercised in interpreting studies on pneumonia because defining criteria may vary from those used by NHSN.[121] Nonetheless, there are clear differences in the microbiology of CAP and HCAP, whereas that of HCAP, HAP, and VAP is similar.

Community-Acquired Pneumonia It is useful to consider CAP in 3 different categories. First are the typical pneumonias of conventional bacterial origin, which are characterized by the abrupt onset (within <24 hours) of fever, chills, systemic toxicity, cough, purulent sputum production, and dyspnea, often after a preceding viral illness. Second are the atypical pneumonias, characterized by a subacute onset of fever, nonproductive cough, and malaise, with a gradual progression over a several days. Legionnaire disease, which combines features of both, has an abrupt onset of fever, rigors, nonproductive cough, systemic toxicity, and increasing dyspnea, often after a several day prodrome of gastrointestinal upset, headache, malaise, and encephalopathy. Although there is considerable overlap among these presentations, initial therapy can be guided by such categorization and by considering the different etiologies within each category.

The bacterial species or virus causing CAP is never identified in approximately 40% to 60% of patients. **Table 18-7** shows the frequencies of the most common bacterial pathogens subdivided into typical and atypical pneumonias. *S pneumoniae* is the most common cause, accounting for approximately 40% of bacteremic pneumonias. Other relatively common typical bacteria are *Haemophilus influenzae*, *S aureus* (with an increasing frequency of methicillin-resistant strains), *K pneumoniae*, and *Moraxella catarrhalis*. The atypical bacteria are *Chlamydia pneumoniae*, *Mycoplasma pneumoniae*, and *Legionella pneumophila*. The most common viruses are influenza A and B, depending on the season, respiratory syncytial virus, and respiratory syncytial virus and human metapneumovirus.[122] The choice of appropriate antimicrobial therapy is helped by Gram stain of sputum, which cannot detect atypical bacteria of viruses. For detection of atypical bacteria, urinary *Legionella* antigen assay detects more than 80% of cases of pneumonia due to *L pneumophila* type I, which accounts for approximately 70% of all cases, but not other *Legionella* species or types; a polymerase chain reaction test detects mycoplasma; and immunoglobulin M titers detect *Chlamydia*. Respiratory viruses can be detected by the appropriate antigen or nucleic acid amplification tests. However, for most patients, antimicrobial therapy needs to be initiated in the absence of clear-cut microbiologic information.

TABLE 18-7 Etiologies of Community-Acquired Pneumonia[194]

Etiology	Incidence (%)
Typical (acute onset or abrupt deterioration after viral prodrome, with productive cough, systemic toxicity, and a lobar infiltrate)	
S pneumoniae	42
H influenzae	9
S aureus	6
K pneumoniae	3
E coli	2
M catarrhalis	2
Total	64
Atypical (subacute onset, nonproductive cough, interstitial infiltrate)	
M pneumoniae	19
C pneumoniae	10
L pneumophila	4
Total	33

In patients with respiratory failure for whom a typical pneumonia is suspected and who do not have a predisposing immunologic defect or a history of a gross aspirational episode, initial therapy should be directed against *S pneumoniae*, *H influenzae*, and possibly *S aureus*, particularly if they also have influenza. Recommended empirical therapy for such inpatients is a β-lactam plus a macrolide, usually azithromycin, or a fluoroquinolone, such as levofloxacin, alone.[123] For patients with CAP who require an ICU, the recommended empiric therapy is a β-lactam plus a fluoroquinolone or a β-lactam plus a macrolide, although the supporting data are very limited. If *S aureus* is suspected and the incidence of MRSA in the community is high, adding vancomycin or linezolid may be appropriate until the organism and its sensitivities are confirmed. If an atypical pneumonia is suspected, a fluoroquinolone such as levofloxacin or erythromycin or one of the newer macrolides, azithromycin or clarithromycin, with or without trimethoprim-sulfamethoxazole, would constitute reasonable initial therapy. For patients with a *Legionella*-like presentation, high-dose erythromycin has been the traditional therapy of choice. However, azithromycin or levofloxacin may be preferable, combined with of one of the regimens used for the treatment of typical bacterial pneumonia (eg, ampicillin-sulbactam or ceftriaxone), if resistant pathogens are a concern. It is also important to consider viral pathogens because they are a common cause of CAP; rapid diagnostic tests are available, and the possibility of antiviral therapy exists. Although the initiation of empiric therapy is often obligatory, invasive diagnostic techniques such as bronchoalveolar lavage or lung biopsy should be considered for any patient with respiratory failure in whom the etiologic diagnosis is not quickly apparent or fails to respond to therapy. This is especially important for individuals with underlying conditions that predispose them to a broader range of pathogens, such as alcoholics and the immunocompromised.

Nosocomial Pneumonia Nosocomial pneumonia includes both HAP, defined as occurring more than 48 hours after admission, and HCAP. It can be divided further into early onset, which occurs within the first 4 days of hospitalization, and late onset, occurring 5 or more days after hospitalization. The term *nosocomial pneumonia* will therefore refer to all HCAP and late-onset HAP because early onset non-HCAP nosocomial pneumonia is similar to CAP. It is less likely to result from MDR bacteria and has a better prognosis than late-onset pneumonia. The common organisms are essentially the same as those found in CAP. MRSA that is often sensitive to clindamycin is also increasingly common in non-HCAP or CAP pneumonia.

The etiology of nosocomial pneumonia, especially when acquired within the ICU, is vastly different from the etiology of non-HCAP CAP. The pathogenesis is typically an extension of a tracheobronchitis. Relatively antibiotic-resistant, aerobic, gram-negative bacilli had been the most frequent invading pathogens, but recently this has been surpassed by gram-positive bacteria. This is thought to be due to the increased rate of oropharyngeal and gastric colonization with these organisms. This colonization serves as a reservoir for the introduction of this flora into the lower respiratory tract, usually due to aspiration and impaired clearance. This is especially true among intubated patients, those with previous lung injury, significant atelectasis, or immunocompromised patients.

Simple measures to help prevent VAP have been promulgated by the Institute for Healthcare Improvement (IHI) (www.IHI.org) as a ventilator bundle that includes elevation of the head of the bed to 30 to 45 degrees, daily trials of spontaneous breathing without sedation, daily "sedation vacation," prophylaxis for both peptic ulcer disease and deep venous thrombosis, and daily oral care with chlorhexidine. Notably, only 2 IHI recommendations, elevation of the head of the bed and oral care, directly relate to VAP. Although these recommendations seem logical, there are no convincing data that they have resulted in a decrease in the incidence of VAP.[124,125] Other recommendations for preventing VAP include using enteral rather than parenteral nutrition, orotracheal intubation, orogastric tubes, and subglottic secretion drainage and, obviously, minimizing the duration of intubation. Some studies have also demonstrated a reduction in VAP using silver-coated endotracheal tubes. However, this remains controversial, largely because of study design and incremental expense.[126]

Figure 18-2 shows the bacterial etiologies of HAP and VAP. Although gram-negative bacillary pneumonia had been the major problem, gram-positive bacteria, especially MRSA, have overtaken gram negatives. Regardless, the bacteria causing infection and their antibiotic sensitivity patterns vary widely in different hospitals and even in different areas within a hospital. Thus precise antibiotic recommendations for initiating therapy must be based on ongoing surveillance of the resident bacterial flora and antibiotic sensitivities in the particular hospital area.

Initial therapy should be modified based on sputum examinations including Gram stains, which provide important information about the relative importance of a particular organism found on culture. Initial therapy should be based on a single advanced-spectrum antibiotic with broad gram-negative protection, possibly with an aminoglycoside for patients with more severe illness, although this practice is less common than when these guidelines were published.[127] As noted previously, clear-cut evidence in humans that 2-drug, potentially synergistic therapy is more effective than a single drug is controversial, but such therapy is used by many clinicians in the face of rapidly progressive *Pseudomonas* or *Klebsiella* infection.[128] Because of the increasing prevalence of MRSA, vancomycin or linezolid is often appropriate pending more definitive bacterial identification.

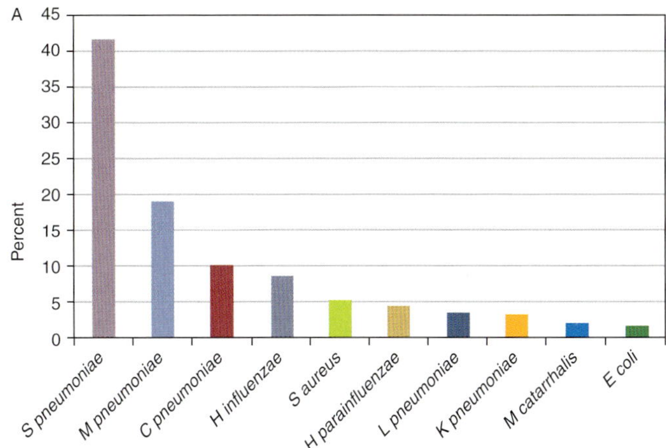

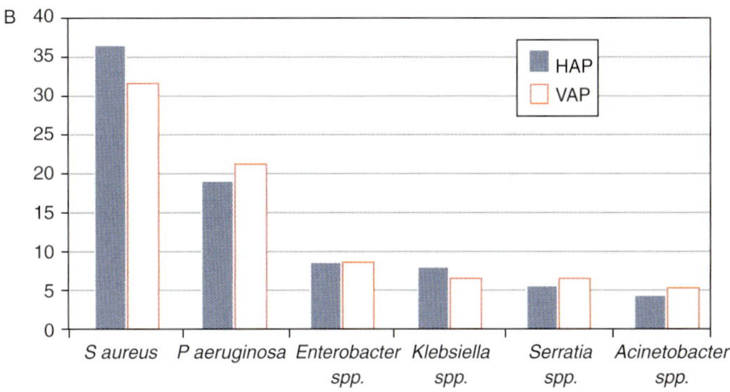

FIGURE 18-2. A. Bacteria recovered from community-acquired pneumonia (CAP). **B.** bacteria recovered from both hospital-acquired pneumonia (HAP) and ventilator-associated pneumonia (VAP). Note that the bacteriology of HAP and VAP are similar but differ markedly from that in CAP. [Adapted from Jones, Ronald N. Microbial etiologies of hospital-acquired bacterial pneumonia and ventilator-associated bacterial pneumonia. *Clin Infect Dis.* 2010;51:S81-S87.]

In immunocompromised patients, pneumonia is the most common life-threatening infection. Although a detailed discussion of the approach to pulmonary infection in these patients is beyond the scope of this chapter, certain antimicrobial strategies are worth noting. As outlined in **Table 18-8**, particular host defense defects are associated with specific infections, and initial therapy should reflect these associations. Even more than other ICU patients, these immunocompromised individuals are especially susceptible to nosocomial infection, both with the resident gram-negative flora and with *Aspergillus* species. Because of the importance of such infections in these patients, precise diagnosis is essential, using invasive techniques if necessary.

BACTEREMIA

Bacteremias occurring in hospitalized patients can be considered as arising from 2 separate pathogenic routes. One is a consequence of definable infection at an anatomic site such as the lung, biliary and urinary tracts, pancreas, and gut, as discussed later. The incidence of bacteremia with pneumonia varies according to which organism is causing the infection. Bacteremia occurs in 30% to 50% of patients with pneumococcal pneumonia, whereas this occurs in fewer than 10% with gram-negative or aspiration pneumonia. In pneumococcal infection, the bacteremia is typically caused by hematogenous seeding from the pulmonary infection, whereas in gram-negative VAP the bacteremia is likely related to heavy oropharyngeal colonization leading to skin contamination with consequent seeding of a central venous catheter. Thus,

TABLE 18-8 Frequent Causes of Pneumonia in Patients With Various Defects in Host Defenses and Initial Antimicrobial Therapy

Host Defense Defect	Pulmonary Infection	Initial Therapy
Impaired antibody formation or splenectomized	*S pneumoniae*, *H influenzae* type B	Levofloxacin, azithromycin or ampicillin + β-lactamase inhibitor
Depressed cell-mediated immunity	*P jiroveci*, *Mycobacterium* species, fungi, *Nocardia*, *Legionella*, herpes group viruses, *Strongyloides stercoralis*	Trimethoprim-sulfamethoxazole
Decrease in the number and/or function of granulocytes	Oral bacterial flora, Enterobacteriaceae, *P aeruginosa*, *Aspergillus*	Ceftazidime, carbapenem, ± an aminoglycoside
Oral and tracheobronchial ulcerations	Oral bacterial flora, Enterobacteriaceae	Ceftazidime, carbapenem

in the setting of VAP, all vascular access devices should be carefully evaluated, especially for duration of implantation, exit site erythema and drainage, and by blood cultures. The initial antimicrobial therapy of bacteremia secondary to invasive tissue infection is identical to that which would be prescribed in the absence of bacteremia.

URINARY TRACT INFECTION

Urosepsis is relatively uncommon unless complicating factors are present, such as obstruction to urine flow, diabetes, advanced age, spinal cord injury, or bladder catheterization. The likely bacteria are also different from those in uncomplicated urinary tract infections (UTI) or asymptomatic UTIs. In these 2 instances, the likely organisms are *E coli* or other Enterobacteriaceae, which can be treated with a fluoroquinolone or trimethoprim-sulfamethoxazole. In patients with complicating factors, gram-positive and antibiotic-resistant gram-negative bacteria, including *P aeruginosa*, are more common.[129] Consequently, therapy should be initiated with broader-spectrum antibiotics, usually fluoroquinolones or advanced-spectrum β-lactam agents such as ceftazidime, ampicillin-sulbactam, ticarcillin-clavulanate, aztreonam, or imipenem. As with all infections, antimicrobial therapy should be adjusted so that the spectrum is as narrow as possible.

A more common problem in hospitalized patients, especially those with urinary catheters, is nosocomial bacteriuria. The literature on UTI in patients with urinary catheters is confusing because definitions vary in different studies. For patients with indwelling urinary catheters, the Infectious Disease Society of America defines catheter-associated asymptomatic bacteriuria (CA-ASB) as greater than 10^5 CFU/mL of 1 or more bacteria collected from the catheter in patients without symptoms compatible with a UTI. A catheter-associated UTI (CA-UTI) is a CA-ASB with symptoms and signs (eg, a new-onset fever, altered mental status, lethargy, flank pain, and acute hematuria) that occur without another identified cause.[130] The etiology of such infections is far different from that observed in community-acquired infections. Whereas *E coli* accounts for more than 85% of community-acquired urinary tract infections, it is responsible for only one-third of nosocomial UTIs. Enterococci, *P aeruginosa*, relatively antibiotic-resistant Enterobacteriaceae such as *Klebsiella*, *Proteus*, *Enterobacter*, *S epidermidis*, and *Serratia*, and *Candida* species now account for the majority of these infections.[129,130] Antibiotic therapy can delay the appearance of bacteriuria, but the price to be paid if catheterization is maintained is that when infection does occur, it will be relatively resistant.

The incidence of bacteria in patients with urinary catheters is estimated to be 5% to 10% per day. Thus duration of catheterization is the most important risk factor for CA-ASB and CA-UTI. Moreover, approximately 15% of nosocomial bacteremias are attributable to bacteriuria. Thus catheters should be placed for well-defined reasons and removed as soon as possible. Moreover, Medicare will no longer reimburse a hospital for additional length of stay related to a CA-UTI that was not present on admission (http://www.cms.gov/HospitalAcqCond/06_Hospital-Acquired_Conditions.asp). Aside from minimizing the duration of catheterization, for short-term use (<30 days), studies suggest that the use of silver alloy or antibiotic-coated catheters may reduce the incidence of bacteriuria, although this is not generally recommended.[131]

Treatment of asymptomatic positive cultures when the catheter is still present is generally not indicated because this usually represents colonization rather than invasive infection, and long-term benefits of such therapy are unlikely. However, when to treat critically ill patients may be problematic because they may not be able to relate symptoms. Usually a quantitative colony count of more than 10^5 CFU is used as a criterion for treatment, with the choice of antibiotic guided by the culture and the urinary excretion of the antimicrobial.[132] However, colony counts can be misleading because of the formation of biofilms and encrustations on the catheter surfaces, particularly from *Proteus* species, *P aeruginosa*, *K pneumoniae*, and *Providencia* species.[130] Treatment is clearly indicated if symptoms develop and/or instrumentation of the urinary tract is to be carried out.

CLOSTRIDIUM DIFFICILE

Clostridium difficile is the leading cause of gastrointestinal infection in the nosocomial environment. This pathogen is an important cause of fever and leukocytosis, which may precede the diarrheal phase. The spectrum of *C difficile* infection (CDI) may vary from mild and resolving without treatment to toxic megacolon or perforation and associated life-threatening septic shock. The latter requires emergency surgery, which is associated with a high mortality. Surgery should also be considered for any patient who does not respond to medical therapy within 24 to 48 hours. The most common etiology is prolonged antibiotic therapy, not necessarily recent, especially with clindamycin, fluoroquinolones, second- or third-generation cephalosporins, and broad-spectrum penicillins, with the exception of those that are β-lactamase-stable. Patients receiving immunosuppressive therapy appear to be at particularly high risk for severe CDI.

The pathogenesis of this disease is typically mediated by enterotoxin A or cytotoxin B, and bacteremia is extremely rare. The diagnosis is usually confirmed by an enzyme immunoassay for the aforementioned toxins. Recently, a hyper-virulent *C difficile* strain has emerged, which, although still sensitive to metronidazole and vancomycin, produces much more toxin and is associated with an increased mortality rate. The spores from *C difficile* are extremely hearty and impervious to antimicrobial therapy, which explains reports of relapse rates varying from 8% to 50% within 2 weeks to several months in successfully treated patients.[133] Although oral metronidazole had been the therapy of choice even for relapsing cases, recent studies showed a higher rate of recovery from diarrheal symptoms and a lower rate of recurrence with oral vancomycin, which is now considered the drug of choice for severe infection.[9,134] This may be related to metronidazole's complete absorption in the small intestine, reaching the colon via enterohepatic circulation and leakage from the bowel wall, which may also account for the undetectable colonic levels after resolution of diarrhea.

For patients being treated with other antibiotics for an ongoing pyogenic process, the treatment of *C difficile* is particularly vexing. In this setting, where continued broad-spectrum antibiotic use is required, we recommend continuing the CDI therapy in parallel with the other antimicrobial agents and extending the course of therapy for *C difficile* after completion of the other antibiotics typically for 5 to 10 days. The extended *C difficile* course of therapy is required because of the role of antibiotic therapy in provoking CDI by altering the normal bowel flora, which takes days to reconstitute. Patients with a history of CDI are more likely to have a recurrence with subsequent antibiotic therapy, probably because of the presence of latent spores. Patients who are severely ill from CDI may benefit from several adjuvant approaches, including minimization of other antimicrobial therapy, toxin-binding resins such as cholestyramine, fecal enemas, and, in severe cases, surgical resection of the colon (eg, in the setting of toxic megacolon). For a patient who undergoes a colectomy for *C difficile* toxic megacolon, the rectal stump, if it is left behind, may be a source of residual disease.

INTRA-ABDOMINAL INFECTIONS

There are many sources for intra-abdominal infections, and there are substantial differences in presentation and therapy, but treatments share 2 common elements: source control and antimicrobial administration. Source control is defined as any procedure or series of procedures that eliminate infectious foci and correct any anatomic defects contributing to the foci (eg, colonic perforation).[114] In addition, in concert with pneumonias, intra-abdominal infections are frequently divided into community-acquired and hospital-associated. As noted previously, hospital-associated infections are thought to be microbiologically similar to true hospital-acquired (ie, nosocomial) intra-abdominal infections. Tigecycline, a relatively new glycylcycline antibiotic that is FDA-approved for complicated intra-abdominal infections, has a spectrum that covers gram-positive, gram-negative, and anaerobic bacteria. Because it covers MRD bacteria including MRSA, *S epidermidis*, and enterococci (including those that are vancomycin resistant) and is not inactivated by Amp C β-lactamases, it appears to be an excellent single drug for complicated intra-abdominal infections. However, it does not cover *P aeruginosa*.[135] Unfortunately, because of a paucity of prospective studies, guidelines and recommendations are usually based on expert opinion. This section only considers 4 relatively common acute sources of intra-abdominal infections: cholangitis and acalculous cholecystitis, diverticulitis, appendicitis, and pancreatitis.

Cholangitis and Acalculous Cholecystitis Cholangitis and cholecystitis, though technically an inflammation of the common bile duct and gallbladder, respectively, usually refer to their infection. Cholangitis may result from bile stasis and increased ductal pressure from an obstruction, from bacteria ascending from the small intestine, and possibly via the portal system or lymphatics. Biliary obstruction may also lead to cholecystitis, which usually begins as a sterile inflammatory process causing gallbladder distention and mural ischemia and ultimately leading to infection. Cholecystitis also occurs without obstruction in conjunction with total parenteral nutrition and serious illnesses, including trauma and burns. This entity, termed acalculous cholecystitis, is probably precipitated by factors that reduce gallbladder microcirculation, leading to ischemia. Regardless of etiology, if left untreated, the gallbladder may become gangrenous and ultimately perforate. Because symptoms and signs of both cholangitis and cholecystitis may be masked in the perioperative period, a high index of suspicion is required. Source control via percutaneous cholecystostomy for a critically ill patient may circumvent the need for a cholecystectomy. Nonoperative procedures are also available to decompress the biliary ducts. Once stabilized, procedures that are more definitive may be required.

Bacteria isolated from patients with infected cholecystitis and cholangitis usually reflect normal gut bacterial flora, most commonly *E coli*, followed by *Klebsiella* and *Enterobacter* species. Anaerobes, particularly *Clostridium* and *Bacteroides*, are found in approximately 5% to 10% of patients, as is *E faecalis*, which is usually found in association with other bacteria.[136] Although there are no evidence-based guidelines for antibiotic treatment of either entity, by consensus, therapy should include those drugs that are active against these organisms, taking into account local resistance patterns.[114] If either entity meets criteria for being health care–associated, as recommended for all such infections, antimicrobial therapy should be broadened to account for higher resistance rates and less common bacteria (eg, *P aeruginosa*), guided by local epidemiology and sensitivities.

Diverticulitis Diverticulitis is usually caused by a sigmoid perforation resulting from continued mucus secretion in a diverticulum that has become obstructed at its neck. Management depends on severity, usually defined by the Hinchey classification[137]: stage 1, localized perforation with pericolic phlegmon; stage 2, perforation with abscess; stage 3, purulent peritonitis; and stage 4, free perforation with fecal peritonitis. Stages 1 and 2 are associated with less than a 5% mortality rate, whereas mortality rates for stages 3 and 4 are approximately 13% and 43%, respectively.[138] Stage 1 can be treated initially with antibiotics alone, whereas stages 3 and 4 usually require early operative intervention. Stage 2 is often managed with antibiotics and percutaneous drainage. The bacteriology, as expected, generally reflects that of the colon and is usually polymicrobial. As many as 5 different organisms may be recovered. Anaerobic organisms, especially *B fragilis* because it outnumbers other bacteria in the colon by roughly 100:1, are common, but aerobic gram-negative bacteria, especially *E coli*, are also usually present. Thus antibiotic therapy should be directed against both anaerobic and gram-negative bacteria. However, there is only 1 randomized study of different antibiotic regimens, cefoxitin alone or gentamicin plus clindamycin, with the former having a higher clinical success rate. Although enterococci are present in approximately 10% of cultures, the need to cover these organisms is controversial but recommended for health care–associated diverticulitis.[114]

Appendicitis The pathophysiology and management of acute appendicitis in many ways resembles that of diverticulitis. Appendiceal obstruction is likely the precipitating event, and the course can range from mild, resolving without any treatment, to gangrene and perforation with abscess formation or peritonitis. Culture data are also similar to those found in diverticulitis, and as many as 14 different bacteria have been recovered from cultures. In addition, as with diverticulitis, although controversial, it is likely that some patients can be managed with antibiotics alone, whereas those with gangrene or perforation require prompt surgery. There are very few studies defining these populations, but there are advocates of a trial of antibiotics without surgery for patients without perforation or gangrene. Generally, if the patient is improving, surgery may be unnecessary, although recurrence rates without surgery are approximately 14% within a year.[139] For patients without gangrene, perforation, or abscesses, some advocate that antibiotics be given preoperatively and for a maximum of 24 hours postoperatively, whereas treatment for those with such complications should be continued for approximately 7 days or until signs and symptoms of infection have resolved.[114]

Acute Pancreatitis Antibiotic management in acute pancreatitis is challenging because the severity of illness often indicates a therapeutic emergency, yet the traditional markers of infection may not be present and there may be limited supporting clinical data. Patients with severe pancreatitis without infection may present with septic pathophysiology including hypotension, tachycardia, hypoxemia, tachypnea, metabolic acidosis, leukocytosis with a left shift, thrombocytopenia, elevated lactate, and coagulopathy. These findings are all consistent with the pathogenesis of this disease, where an inciting event such as alcohol, gallstones, or trauma leads to pancreatic injury and inflammation, which in turn leads to autodigestion, liquefaction, and necrosis with associated inflammatory cytokine release. If the necrotic pancreatic tissue becomes infected by, for example, biliary reflux, colonic bacterial translocation, or hematogenous seeding, there is an associated increased morbidity and mortality.[140] It is important to note that infection is rarely the inciting event but rather a sequel of pancreatic necrosis and often occurs weeks into the hospital course. Abdominal imaging, with a contrast CT scan, has enabled stratification of those patients at risk for developing superimposed infection by an increasing degree of pancreatic necrosis. Unfortunately, imaging, like the physical examination and laboratory evaluation, cannot reliably distinguish an infection from sterile inflammation. Therefore, the time to initiate antibiotic therapy in the presence of documented pancreatic necrosis remains largely based on the patient's clinical state, with deterioration often used as the trigger. Logically, a fine-needle aspirate of necrotic areas should be diagnostic of infection. However, there is a relatively high false-negative rate, and the trend seems to be moving away from its use.[141] Although an infected necrotic pancreas has been thought to require source control with surgical debridement or percutaneous drainage in addition to antibiotic therapy and supportive care, there is a trend toward delaying intervention so that the necrotic area can consolidate. However, no studies conclusively support such delays.

It would seem logical to administer antibiotics preemptively, to prevent infection of necrotic pancreatic tissue. However, multiple randomized studies and meta-analyses have failed to find support for this concept, and there are risks of selecting for resistant organisms if the necrotic tissue becomes infected.[142] For these reasons, this practice is no longer recommended. Nonetheless, in the critically ill patient for whom it is too risky to delay antimicrobial therapy, targeting the typical infecting organisms, which includes aerobic enteric gram-negative rods and gram-positive cocci, is appropriate. A variety of antibiotics, such as fluoroquinolones, imipenem, ceftazidime, cefepime, metronidazole, clindamycin, chloramphenicol, doxycycline, and fluconazole, have been shown to achieve pancreatic levels above the MIC for the commonly encountered bacteria, but either imipenem or a fluoroquinolone plus metronidazole are commonly recommended. However, because resistant organisms such as *S aureus* species (which usually are not sensitive to these antibiotics) and *Candida* species (including *C glabrata*, which is generally not susceptible to fluconazole) are emerging as significant pathogens in severe acute pancreatitis, it is likely that these recommendations will be modified. Interestingly, multiple studies have indicated that enteral, as opposed to parenteral nutrition, initiated as soon as tolerated may decrease the infection rate and complications in severe acute pancreatitis with no difference between gastric and jejunal routes.[143]

HIV INFECTION AND AIDS

A remarkable body of information regarding the treatment of HIV infection has emerged since 1981, when acquired immune deficiency syndrome (AIDS) was first recognized. The occurrence of oral thrush, *Pneumocystis jiroveci* pneumonia, *Toxoplasma* encephalitis, and other opportunistic infections in apparently healthy gay males was quickly recognized as something unusual; that is, the net state of immunosuppression should not have been great enough to allow such infections to occur. Very quickly, the characteristics of this epidemic emerged: profound and progressive immune compromise and efficient transmission from infected individuals by intimate contact, blood transfusion and organ transplantation, intravenous drug abuse, and perinatal route. In 1984 the identification of the cause of these events, infection with a unique retrovirus now known as the human immunodeficiency virus (HIV), was reported. HIV is now recognized as the cause of a worldwide pandemic of infection, particularly those due to opportunistic organisms, as well as Kaposi sarcoma and other malignancies. More than 30 million individuals are believed to have been infected by HIV since 1981, with devastating consequences.[144-146] **Table 18-9** lists the CDC definitions of the stages of HIV infection, including AIDS. The long list of AIDS-defining conditions is similar to those found in severely immunocompromised patients.[147]

Three different phases of disease have been recognized once HIV has been acquired[148,149]:

Primary HIV Infection A mononucleosis-like illness is observed in ~50% of individuals 2 to 6 weeks after infection. Primary infection is associated with a marked increase in plasma viremia, which can exceed 1 000 000 copies per milliliter; a significant decrease in the CD4 T-lymphocyte count; and a large increase in the blood CD8 T-lymphocyte count.

Chronic Asymptomatic Stage An extended phase of clinical latency occurs, persisting for 10 to 12 years in the majority of individuals. An estimated 20% of individuals, the so-called rapid progressors, have an accelerated course, having full-blown AIDS in less than 5 years; conversely, approximately10%, the so-called slow progressors or non-progressors, remain free of AIDS for 7 to 12 or more years. At the end of this period, the level of viremia rises rapidly and there is a significant decrease in the CD4 T-lymphocyte count. AIDS-defining opportunistic infections begin to appear.

AIDS In the absence of effective therapy, there is a progressive decrease in CD4-positive lymphocytes and an increase in viral load. These events are correlated with recurrent opportunistic infection, the occurrence of certain malignancies, and death in 2 to 3 years.

The specifics of anti-HIV therapy are constantly evolving, although certain principles remain constant: HIV replication remains at a very high level throughout the stages of illness. This high rate of replication is coupled with a remarkable amount of errors in the function of the reverse transcriptase (the daily production of ~10^8 to 10^{10} virions and a mutation rate of 3×10^{-3}). The frequency of these events virtually guarantees the presence and the rapid development of mutants that are responsible for drug resistance. Resistant clones of HIV may be present even before the initiation of any therapy. Such findings mandate that multiple drugs will be needed to treat this infection effectively.

The general principle that applies to HIV therapy is "hit early and hit hard," with multiple drugs being started simultaneously.[149-151] Although the precise point when therapy should be instituted is still being studied, at present it is recommended that highly active anti-retroviral therapy (HAART) or ART, which consists of multidrug regimens, be initiated

TABLE 18-9 Surveillance Definitions of HIV Stages[171]

Stage	Laboratory Criteria[a]	Clinical Criteria
1–HIV infection	$CD4^+$ T-lymphocyte count of >500 cells/μL or $CD4^+$ T-lymphocyte percentage of total lymphocytes of >29	No AIDS-defining condition
2–HIV infection	$CD4^+$ T-lymphocyte count of 200-499 cells/μL or $CD4^+$ T-lymphocyte percentage of total lymphocytes of 14-28	No AIDS-defining condition
3–AIDS	$CD4^+$ T-lymphocyte count of <200 cells/μL or $CD4^+$ T-lymphocyte percentage of total lymphocytes of <14	*Or* laboratory confirmation of HIV infection with documentation of an AIDS-defining condition[b]
4–Unknown	No information	No information

[a]All laboratory criteria require laboratory documentation of HIV infection, which requires a positive Western blot or indirect immunofluorescence or a positive test for HIV virus.

[b]The long list of AIDS-defining conditions is available in Stamm et al.[147]

TABLE 18-10 Classes of Antiviral Drugs Used to Treat HIV

Class	Mechanism	Side Effects
Nucleoside and nucleotide reverse transcriptase inhibitors (NRTI)	Prevent proviral synthesis by blocking reverse transcriptase from synthesizing viral cDNA from HIV RNA	Hyperlactatemia, lactic acidosis, hepatic steatosis, peripheral neuropathy, myopathy, lipoatrophy
Non-nucleoside reverse transcriptase inhibitors (NNRTI)	Inhibit proviral synthesis by binding to reverse transcriptase away from active site, reducing its activity	CNS toxicity, rash, hepatotoxicity, sleep disorders, teratogenicity, induction of cytochrome P450
Protease inhibitors	Cleave HIV proteins	CYP3A4 inhibition, dyslipidemia, hyperbilirubinemia, elevated transaminases
Fusion and entry inhibitors	Interfere with HIV binding to cells, preventing entry	Gastrointestinal upset, cough, fever
Integrase strand transfer inhibitors	Inhibit incorporation into cellular genome	Fatigue, nasopharyngitis, rash, herpes zoster infection, elevations of alanine aminotransferase and aspartate aminotransferase, increased triglycerides, increases in creatine kinase

in asymptomatic patients who have circulating CD4 T-lymphocyte counts fewer than 500 cells/mL and/or an HIV RNA load of 5000 to 10 000 copies/mL. Initiation of treatment is also recommended regardless of CD4 count if the viral load exceeds 100 000 copies/mL or if the CD4 count declines by more than 100 per year. It is also recommended for all patients older than 60 years and all pregnant women and when there is coinfection with hepatitis B or C. Further details may be found in Thompson et al.[152]

Treatment of HIV is very complex, both in terms of drug therapy and because HIV can impair virtually any organ system. Moreover, the antiviral regimens are constantly evolving and may require changes during the course of the disease. There are now a large number of drugs available for HAART regimens, which generally fall into 1 of 5 classes based on mechanism of action (**Table 18-10**). Aside from the development of resistance, 2 key issues must be considered for all of these drugs: side effects (eg, pancreatitis, hepatotoxicity, and a lipodystrophy syndrome) and drug–drug interactions, including changes in drug metabolism by the hepatic cytochrome P450 enzymes (Table 18-10). This is made even more complex because to help with compliance, combinations of antiviral drugs supplied in a single pill are often appropriate. For these reasons, specialists in HIV should always be involved.

The goal of HAART therapy is to lower and maintain the HIV viral load to undetectable levels. Such an approach has been quite effective, but drug resistance remains an important impediment in treatment. Clinically important resistance is particularly likely when the level of mutations and the ability of these mutant strains to replicate is relatively high.[151,153-155]

INVASIVE FUNGAL INFECTION

Advances in therapy for invasive fungal diseases have improved survival of immunocompromised patients (eg, HIV, transplant, and cancer patients and patients with autoimmune diseases). The most common cause of invasive fungal infection has long been *Candida* species, and this is still true, but there has been an increase in the range of fungal species causing serious infection, as well as an increase in antimicrobial resistance. In addition, new sites of infection are being seen. For example, the ICU use of invasive vascular access devices is becoming an important source for candidemia, whereas this was uncommon in the past. Today, *Candida* species are the sixth most common nosocomial isolate and fourth most common cause of nosocomial bloodstream infections. As this has occurred, the range of candidal species has changed from azole susceptible *C albicans* to more resistant non-albicans infections.[156-158]

The risk of invasive fungal infection is largely determined by the interaction of the following 4 factors[156]:

1. The environmental exposure to which a patient is subjected is an important factor in the occurrence of many fungal infections. The density of organisms that are aerosolized and then inhaled is the critical first step in the initiation of many fungal infections. These exposures can occur in the community or within the hospital. In the hospital, the patient is vulnerable to organisms that are aerosolized and inhaled on the ward where the patient resides (ie, domiciliary exposure) or to exposure to aerosols while being transported through the hospital for studies or procedures. In both instances, ongoing construction is the most common activity resulting in aerosolization of infectious organisms, particularly *Aspergillus* species that have resided in the building interstices. In addition, person-to-person spread via the hands of medical personnel is a relatively common event, with the spread of antimicrobial-resistant *Candida* species being a particular problem.[156-160]
2. Also important is the patient's net state of immunosuppression, which is a complex function determined by deficits in innate host defenses that may occur in conjunction with many conditions such as underlying diseases and their therapy; infection with immunomodulating viruses including HIV, cytomegalovirus, and the hepatitis viruses; and the presence of protein-calorie malnutrition.[156]
3. The presence of foreign bodies such as orthopedic prostheses, devitalized tissues, undrained fluid collections, and invasive vascular and urinary catheters contributes significantly to the pathogenesis of invasive *Candida* infection. Whether one is dealing with candidemia associated with vascular access catheters, peritonitis in association with peritoneal dialysis catheters, or orthopedic prosthesis infection, the chances of successful therapy are greatly enhanced by the removal of the foreign body in association with effective antifungal therapy.[156,161,162]
4. Darwinian factors can play an important role as well. Thus prolonged therapy with broad-spectrum antibacterial drugs will create an ecologic niche easily occupied by *Candida* species. The presence of excess growth factors such as glucose and iron can significantly increase the occurrence of mucocutaneous candidiasis, invasive mucormycosis, and other types of invasive fungal infections. Unless the ecologic niche is eliminated, recurrent fungal infections may occur. For example, therapy with the newer azoles can be associated with the development of mucormycosis.[156,158,160,161]

The fungal species capable of causing invasive infection can be divided into 3 general categories:

1. The geographically restricted systemic mycoses, blastomycosis, coccidioidomycosis, and histoplasmosis are important in North America. In addition, paracoccidioidomycosis in Latin America and penicilliosis in Southeast Asia exhibit similar clinical and epidemiologic patterns. These are dimorphic fungi that grow as molds in soil and as yeast-like forms in tissue. Invasive infection with one of these is greatly amplified by the presence of immunocompromise. Treatment of these infections at present has 2 parts: induction therapy with amphotericin to gain control of the disease and then prolonged oral therapy with an azole to consolidate the antifungal effects.

At present, itraconazole is the therapy of choice for this purpose, with the exception of fluconazole for treating coccidioidomycosis.[156,161-165]

2. The opportunistic fungi are ubiquitous in the environment, where they are nonpathogenic, particularly for normal hosts, but they can cause invasive infection when the inhaled inoculum harbors a high microbial burden and when the host is immunocompromised. These organisms include *Aspergillus* species, *Cryptococcus neoformans*, and *Sporothrix schenckii*. Voriconazole is currently the treatment of choice for *Aspergillus* infection and fluconazole for cryptococcal infection, often after induction therapy with amphotericin plus flucytosine and saturated potassium iodide or itraconazole for sporo trichosis.[156,161,162,166,167]
3. The newly emerging fungi now account for approximately 10% of invasive fungal infections, with the major species involved, including *Mucorales*, *Fusarium*, and *Trichosporon*. These species tend to be more resistant to fluconazole, echinocandins, and even amphotericin. Drugs such as voriconazole and posaconazole should be considered as the first choices for therapy. Posaconazole is the first really effective agent for mucormycosis, particularly when combined with surgery.[156,161,162]

Several types of exposure are important in the development of invasive fungal infections, with the effects of both being amplified if immunocompromise is present. Candidal infections frequently result from contaminated vascular access devices. Less commonly, infections may occur when the mucocutaneous surfaces are compromised. In this case, not only is candidal infection a concern, but invasion by *Aspergillus*, *Mucorales*, and other fungal species can also occur.[157,158,162,168] The respiratory tract can also be an important portal for fungal infections. Inhalation of the organisms can result in invasive fungal infection of the nasal sinuses and the lungs, with *Aspergillus* species being the most common invader. The first host response to these organisms is the migration of polymorphonuclear leukocytes, which can kill the inhaled inoculum. If the inhaled organisms escape this first defense, bloodstream invasion with the potential for metastatic spread may occur, as may tissue invasion both at the primary site of infection and metastatic sites. Cell-mediated immunity including alveolar macrophages is then mobilized. With histoplasmosis, persistent infection of macrophages is established, making lipid-associated amphotericin B particularly effective by targeting the macrophages with the lipid moiety. Thus an increased risk of invasive aspergillosis and other such infections (eg, fusariosis) is to be expected in patients with neutropenia and/or impaired cell-mediated immunity.[159,160,162,168-170]

Drugs that are available for the treatment of invasive fungal infection are as follows:

1. Amphotericin B is a broad-spectrum polyene that acts by binding to fungal cell membranes, specifically ergosterol (for which it has a >500-fold increase in affinity when compared with binding to cholesterol in mammalian cell membranes). Binding to ergosterol results in increased membrane permeability and cytolysis, which are the probable mechanisms of fungal injury and death. Amphotericin B remains the broadest-spectrum antifungal known, producing fungicidal effects against the majority of pathologic fungi, including those that are resistant to other antifungal compounds. The dose-limiting toxicity is to the kidneys, which is particularly important when such nephrotoxic drugs such as gentamicin or cyclosporine are administered to a patient receiving amphotericin. In addition, the administration of amphotericin B usually produces a "cytokine storm," which can include not only fever and chills, but also hypotension. These storms are usually not a problem after the first several days of therapy. Lipid-associated amphotericin appears to decrease but not eliminate both the febrile reactions and the renal toxicity. However, as with all the amphotericin products, the optimal dosing regimen is not known, but the recommended doses are 3 to 5 mg/kg/d for a lipid-associated drug and 0.1 to 1.5 mg/kg/d for the standard amphotericin. The optimal duration of therapy also is unclear. Our practice is to treat until all overt disease is gone and then add a buffer for safety. The duration of this buffer is a clinical decision usually determined by the nature of the original infection and the speed with which the patient responded.
2. Flucytosine is synergistic with amphotericin for the treatment of cryptococcosis. This regimen protects against a single step mutation to flucytosine resistance. Dose-related hepatic and bone marrow toxicity can occur with the use of flucytosine. A common approach is to administer amphotericin and flucytosine for 7 to 10 days to gain control of the process and then complete the course of therapy with oral fluconazole.[171,172]
3. The azoles act by blocking the cytochrome P450-associated enzyme lanosterol synthetase, which results in the inhibition of ergosterol synthesis. The effect is fungistatic. There are 5 azoles that have been approved for the treatment of systemic fungal invasion. However, ketoconazole and miconazole are essentially of historical interest only and are rarely prescribed today.

   Itraconazole has an appealing spectrum of activity, including *Aspergillus* and other fungal species. The problem has been poor and unreliable drug delivery. With substitution of an oral suspension, more reliable bioavailability has been achieved, and the utility of the drug should be reassessed. Up to now, the major use of this drug has been in oral "wrap-up" therapy after amphotericin had gained control of the infection.[172]

   The advent of fluconazole, in contrast, was a major advance in antifungal therapy. Its only weakness is a rather narrow spectrum of activity limited mostly to *Candida* species and *C neoformans*. Most *C krusei* are resistant to fluconazole, as are approximately 10% to 20% of *Candida tropicalis*.[173] Pharmacokinetically, fluconazole penetrates into the urinary tract, the eye, and the brain, as well as the spleen, liver, and other sites. The bioavailability when given by mouth is complete, and thus the dose given by mouth is the same as the parenteral dose. Side effects are relatively uncommon or minor and include a measles-like rash, hepatocellular dysfunction, and minimal gastrointestinal complaints. Fluconazole does interact with cytochrome P450 enzymes, as do all the azoles, and thus can increase the blood levels of such important therapies as cyclosporine and tacrolimus.[172]

   Voriconazole, a newer azole, can be administered either orally or parenterally.[174] Its candidal spectrum is broader than that of fluconazole, with only about 5% of *C krusei* resistant.[173] Voriconazole is fungicidal for *Aspergillus* and is the most effective of the current anti-*Aspergillus* drugs, including amphotericin, as well as having efficacy for other resistant molds. Side effects are similar to those of other azoles (rash, hepatocellular dysfunction, nausea, etc.). Voriconazole does have a unique side effect: the occurrence of visual effects, including bright colors, lights, and so forth, akin to that seen with digitalis toxicity. Such symptoms appear to be most common with high doses and appear to be due to retinal dysfunction. All such symptoms disappear when the drug is stopped, and extensive study has failed to reveal any persistent visual or structural consequences. Voriconazole appears to be the drug of choice for invasive aspergillosis. Treatment with voriconazole, however, carries a small risk of selecting for *Mucorales* infection (mucormycosis).[172,175]

   Posaconazole is the newest azole and is available only in oral formulation.[176,180] Although its antifungal spectrum includes most candidal species and many molds including aspergillosis, clinical data are still limited. It is, however, approved for prophylaxis of candidal infections and aspergillus in immunocompromised patients.
4. The echinocandins are large lipopeptide molecules that damage fungal cell walls by inhibiting the synthesis of 1,3-β-D-glucan, a fungal cell wall component. In vitro, these compounds are fungicidal for *Candida* and fungistatic for *Aspergillus* species. These molecules appear to have activity against candidal strains that are amphotericin, fluconazole, and itraconazole resistant. On the other hand, species such as *C neoformans* and the *Mucorales* are inherently resistant to echinocandin therapy, presumably because they do not possess significant β-glucan in their cell walls.[177]

Three echinocandins—caspofungin, micafungin, and anidulafungin—have been approved by the FDA. All 3 must be administered intravenously and have similar antifungal spectra and pharmacodynamics. They all exhibit a post-antifungal effect, which is analogous to the post-antibiotic effect, with durations that vary among different fungi. Interestingly, there is in vitro evidence that they also exhibit the so-called eagle effect, which is an increase in fungal growth at concentrations well above their MIC, but it is unclear if this occurs in vivo.[178] The echinocandins seem to be equivalent to fluconazole for the treatment of invasive candidiasis and theoretically should be superior for treatment of *Candida* normally resistant to fluconazole to be useful in the treatment of both drug-resistant candidiasis and invasive aspergillosis. The results thus far suggest comparable efficacy to that achieved with amphotericin and the licensed azoles. The possibility of achieving better results with combination therapy that includes an echinocandin is particularly intriguing. The cell wall damage that is caused by echinocandins is reminiscent of synergistic therapy of enterococcal infection with ampicillin and gentamicin, with the echinocandin playing the role of a cell wall active agent that potentiates the penetration of additional drugs. Indeed, the echinocandins have been called "the antifungal penicillins."[177,179]

THE FUTURE OF ANTIFUNGAL THERAPY

Since the advent of new drugs for the treatment of fungal disease, great progress has been made in terms of efficacy and adverse events. What we need now is a new generation of diagnostic tests that will inform us regarding the appropriate drugs to use, how long to treat, whether multiple drugs should be deployed, and a determination to define microbial load objectively, which will allow us to treat preemptively rather than empirically. The present data on the use of (1-3)-β-D-glucan testing in defining the presence or absence of invasive fungal infection suggest that we are getting closer to that possibility.

NEW DIAGNOSTICS

One of the greatest frustrations when caring for a potentially septic patient is having to wait 1 to 2 days for culture results to find out if the patient is infected and then to wait another day or 2 to discover the identity and later the susceptibility profile of the infecting organism. With the molecular biologic revolution, new tests have emerged, typically polymerase chain reaction–based technology, enabling the rapid identification of specific pathogens directly from the infected body site. Nonetheless, this technology is prone to many of the same interpretation challenges. For example, does a positive result represent colonization or disease? To help both diagnostically and prognostically, the development of new assays are focusing on the levels (or presence) of mediators in the inflammatory cascade or on circulating bacterial moieties, such as endotoxin or nuclear factor kappa B, to improve our ability to risk stratify patients or determine the infecting pathogen.[181-184]

A broad array of pathogens can now be identified by molecular techniques, including viruses (HIV, CMV), fungi (*Candida*, *Aspergillus*), and bacteria (VRE, *E coli*, *M tuberculosis*, *Bacteroides*).[185-190] As learned for HIV-positive patients, monitoring the HIV viral load has become an important parameter in gauging the success of therapy. The development of technology may allow us to provide pathogen-directed therapy earlier in a patient's illness, enabling more focused narrow-spectrum antimicrobial use. This would diminish the selective pressure, which leads to the emergence and dissemination of resistance, as well as yielding novel markers to gauge the duration and intensity of therapy.

SUMMARY

Antimicrobial therapy is complicated by the increasing incidence of bacterial, fungal, and viral resistance. As a result, a broader range of antimicrobial agents has come into use, with the basic approach to antimicrobial therapy in these patients being front-loading broad-spectrum antimicrobials. This therapy is then modified to relatively narrow spectrum-specific therapy. The regimens chosen and the doses prescribed are based on the principle that effective therapy is dependent on the delivery of a level of antimicrobial agent to the site of infection that significantly exceeds the MIC of the invading organism. Bactericidal therapy is essential when dealing with cardiovascular infection, CNS infection, prosthesis-associated infection, osteomyelitis, and infection in the neutropenic patient. Combination therapy may be important when dealing with life-threatening enterococcal, *P aeruginosa*, and perhaps other gram-negative infections, but the definition of synergy varies and the clinical efficacy is not firmly established. Finally, it is hoped that a better definition of high-risk patients will permit the more effective use of preemptive antimicrobial regimens. It is clear that many questions remain unanswered and that many therapeutic decisions must be based on a thorough understanding of the properties of antimicrobials and the pathogenesis of infections, rather than efficacy demonstrated in clinical studies.

KEY REFERENCES

- Bonten MJ, Chastre J, Craig WA, et al. Guidelines for the management of adults with hospital-acquired, ventilator-associated, and healthcare-associated pneumonia. *Am J Resp Crit Care Med.* 2005;171:388-416.
- Craig WA. Pharmacokinetic/pharmacodynamic parameters: rationale for antibacterial dosing of mice and men. *Clin Infect Dis.* 1998;26:1-10.
- Hooton TM, Bradley SF, Cardenas DD, et al. Diagnosis, prevention, and treatment of catheter-associated urinary tract infection in adults: 2009 International Clinical Practice Guidelines from the Infectious Diseases Society of America. *Clin Infect Dis.* 2010;50:625-663.
- Liu C, Bayer A, Cosgrove SE, et al. Clinical practice guidelines by the Infectious Diseases Society of America for the treatment of methicillin-resistant *Staphylococcus aureus* infections in adults and children. *Clin Infect Dis.* 2011;52:285-292.
- Mermel LA, Allon M, Bouza E, et al. Clinical practice guidelines for the diagnosis and management of intravascular catheter–related infection: 2009 Update by the Infectious Diseases Society of America. *Clin Infect Dis.* 2009;49:1-45.
- Nishimura RA, Carabello BA, Faxon DP, et al. ACC/AHA 2008 guideline update on valvular heart disease: focused update on infective endocarditis: a report of the American College of Cardiology/American Heart Association Task Force on Practice Guidelines: endorsed by the Society of Cardiovascular Anesthesiologists, Society for Cardiovascular Angiography and Interventions, and Society of Thoracic Surgeons. *Circulation.* 2008;118:887-896.
- Rubin RH. *Clinical Approach to Infection in the Compromised Host.* 4th ed. New York, NY: Kluwer/Academic Press; 2003.
- Rubin RH. Surgical wound infection: epidemiology, pathogenesis, diagnosis and management. *BMC Infect Dis.* 2006;6:171.
- Solomkin JS, Mazuski JE, Bradley JS, et al. Diagnosis and management of complicated intra-abdominal infection in adults and children: guidelines by the Surgical Infection Society and the Infectious Diseases Society of America. *Clin Infect Dis.* 2010;50:133-164.
- Teplick R. Caveats for comparing catheter-associated bloodstream infection rates. *Crit Care Med.* 2011;39:392-394.

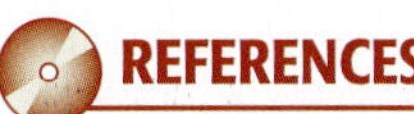

REFERENCES

Complete references available on DVD and online version at www.LongneckerAnesthesiology.com

CHAPTER 19

Preoperative Assessment of the Newborn

Myron Yaster
Mark I. Rossberg

KEY POINTS

1. It is our belief that, except for extraordinary circumstances, all newborns require anesthesia for surgery.
2. Maternal factors associated with increased perinatal risk include hypertension, diabetes, prolonged rupture of membranes, drug abuse (tobacco, alcohol, opioids, amphetamines) and use (antipsychotics, antidepressants, anticonvulsants), collagen vascular disease, and maternal infection (prolonged rupture of membranes) or inflammation.
3. Small for gestational age and large for gestational age babies often have glucose homeostatic instability and require 10% glucose infusions to maintain normoglycemia (45-100 mg/dL).
4. The definition of prematurity is an infant born at less than 37 weeks of gestation.
5. The younger the infant, the more fragile the neurologic, pulmonary, and gastrointestinal systems and the more likely the severity of complications.
6. The presence of 1 congenital anomaly should always alert the anesthesiologist to the potential for others.
7. It is always a good idea to check this site (http://www.ncbi.nlm.nih.gov/omim) before the induction of anesthesia, particularly if you are unfamiliar with the syndrome, defect, or malformation and/or its anesthetic implications.
8. A good rule of thumb to remember is that the presence of any midline defect is almost *always* associated with another defect.
9. The newborn is an obligate nose breather.
10. The narrowest part of the infant's airway is at the level of the cricoid ring and not the vocal cords.
11. The weight in kilograms + 6 is where the endotracheal tube in centimeters should be taped at the lip.
12. Increasingly, cuffed endotracheal tubes are being used even in the newborn, particularly in situations in which aspiration of gastric content or poor lung compliance makes ventilation with an uncuffed endotracheal tube difficult.
13. Oxygen consumption in the newborn is 2 to 3 times that of older children and adults.
14. A history of prematurity (ie, <37 weeks postconceptual age) or apnea must alert the anesthesiologist to possible respiratory compromise in the postoperative period, particularly if an opioid, vapor, or ketamine are used during anesthesia. Indeed, premature infants are at risk of developing postanesthetic apnea for weeks after birth (48-60 weeks postconceptual age) and require overnight admission to a high-surveillance in-hospital care unit regardless of the surgical procedure performed.
15. Arterial hypoxemia, hypercarbia, hypothermia, pain, or acidosis will reverse this transitional circulation and restore the fetal circulatory pattern and is referred to as *persistent fetal circulation* or *persistent pulmonary hypertension* of the newborn.
16. An intravenous infusion of prostaglandin E_1 to maintain the patency of the ductus arteriosus may be life-sustaining in these ductal-dependent patients.
17. The newborn's myocardium is less compliant than that of the adult or older child, and cardiac output is primarily heart rate dependent.
18. The most common cause of bradycardia in the newborn is hypoxia, and in the operating room, unexplained bradycardia should always be considered to be due to hypoxia until proven otherwise.
19. The central nervous system is the least mature major organ system at birth. This structural immaturity predisposes the newborn to certain risks, including intraventricular hemorrhages, seizures, respiratory depression, hypoxic–ischemic injury, and retinopathy of the premature.
20. Intraventricular hemorrhage, in which subependymal hemorrhage occurs, is now the leading cause of death and morbidity in premature infants.
21. Evaporative heat loss is the major source of heat loss in the perioperative period.
22. The newborn's ability to concentrate urine is also significantly reduced.
23. Hypoglycemia is common in infants born to diabetic mothers and in infants who required resuscitation, are premature, or who are small for gestational age.
24. Neonatal hypocalcemia is common in the first few days of life. Infants at particular risk are those born prematurely or to diabetic mothers, who are small for gestational age, or who have received large volumes of citrated blood products or sodium bicarbonate.

The newborn presenting for surgery is among the most daunting and challenging patients facing the anesthesiologist. Critically ill and hemodynamically unstable, these tiny and fragile patients demand a level of specialized knowledge, skill, and attention to detail that is inversely proportional to their size and gestational age. Providing safe anesthesia is only possible when the specialized equipment and techniques necessary to conduct an anesthetic are in the hands of individuals who understand the anatomic, physiologic, and pathologic differences that characterize these patients during their transition from intra- to extrauterine life.

With rare exception (eg, circumcision), newborn surgery is always emergent and never elective. The types of surgical procedures in the newborn span a wide variety of life-threatening congenital anomalies, each with its own set of unique management strategies. Nevertheless, there are many aspects of preoperative and intraoperative anesthetic management common to all neonates. This chapter focuses on neonatal physiology and its impact on anesthetic and surgical techniques. Emphasis is placed on those aspects of preoperative assessment, monitoring, and supportive care that are pertinent to newborn patients in general, with special attention to disease states, anesthetic agents, and surgical interventions that can influence the infant's transition from fetal to newborn existence.

Historically, the newborn has been undertreated for pain and for painful experiences, including surgery. Who but the newborn would undergo a surgical procedure with physical restraints and without the benefits of anesthesia? Unfortunately, in North America this remains commonplace (circumcision) even in 2011, albeit not in the operating room. It is our belief that, except for extraordinary circumstances, all newborns require anesthesia for surgery.[1-3] Why this even remains an issue in the 21st century is discussed in detail in Chapter 63.

FAMILY INTERACTIONS AND PREPARATION

The parents of critically ill children require substantial support and reassurance that their newborn child will perceive no pain during surgery and will be as safe as possible. Parents experience an acute emotional crisis when their newborns face surgery. Aside from the deprivation of contact with their child, parents experience anticipatory grief and a profound sense of failure.[4,5] When confronted with surgery and anesthesia, many parents undergo a period of mourning for the loss of the perfect infant or anticipate their infant's death or mutilation. The overwhelming nature of the situation may deafen parents to explanations during the preoperative interview, and repetition may be necessary. The child's parents should be counseled that the overwhelming majority of children not only survive their surgery, but grow up to live healthy and productive lives. Without being inappropriately optimistic or avoiding the issues of informed consent, it is important to emphasize the normal, healthy aspects of the baby and give positive affirmation regarding the correction that will be achieved by surgery. Failure at this may significantly impact the parents' future interactions and bonding with their child.

The newborn undergoing surgery must be optimally prepared within the constraints of performing an emergent procedure. Essential to this process is a thorough history and physical examination. This evaluation must focus on maternal and peripartum history, neonatal physiology and its relation to anesthesia, and the presence of coexisting anomalies present in the child.

MATERNAL AND PERIPARTUM HISTORY

A thorough review of maternal past medical history and prenatal assessments is essential for the preoperative evaluation of the neonate. Maternal medical history may indicate diseases, complications of pregnancy, or behaviors that result in fetal anomalies (**Table 19-1**). Maternal factors associated with increased perinatal risk include hypertension, diabetes, prolonged rupture of membranes, drug abuse (tobacco, alcohol, opioids, amphetamines) and use (antipsychotics, antidepressants, anticonvulsants), collagen vascular disease, and maternal infection (prolonged rupture of membranes) or inflammation. Maternal exposures to teratogens such as thalidomide, phenytoin, or ethanol are well described and are associated with specific anomalies. Less dramatic are the effects of tobacco, alcohol, and opioids, which may affect brain development or somatic size. Additionally, maternal intravenous drug addiction, particularly to opioids, may result in acute withdrawal and seizures in the neonate or to infection with HIV. Finally, some perinatal conditions provide insight into potential future problems. For example, polyhydramnios is associated with high intestinal obstruction and oligohydramnios with renal and lung hypoplasia (Tables 19-1 and **19-2**).

TABLE 19-1 Maternal History

Pregnancy
- Polyhydramnios
  - High intestinal obstruction (eg, duodenal atresia, congenital diaphragmatic hernia, omphalocele)
  - Central nervous anomalies (eg, hydrocephalus, spina bifida)
  - Respiratory abnormalities (eg, pulmonary hypoplasia, pleural effusions)
  - Genitourinary tract abnormalities (eg, posterior urethral valves, urethral stricture)
  - Maternal diabetes
  - Rh-isoimmunization
  - Multiple pregnancy
- Oligohydramnios
  - Renal failure
  - Hypoplastic lungs
  - Marked crowding of fetal limbs, causing multiple skeletal contractures
  - Neonatal infection (chorioamnionitis)
- Toxemia of pregnancy
  - Frequently associated with decreased placental perfusion and premature separation of the placenta; associated problems include small for gestational age infants, hypoglycemia, and anemia; magnesium used in blood pressure control produces neonatal hypotonia and apnea
- Diabetes: large for gestational age infants; hypoglycemia despite enormous glucose loading, prematurity (yet >2500-g birth weight); congenital heart disease; anencephaly; sacral agenesis
- Maternal seizures: 2 to 3× greater incidence of congenital malformations
- Intrauterine infection: prematurity; fetal infection, particularly pneumonia; persistent fetal circulation; heart defects (rubella)
- Medication: teratogens (eg, anticonvulsants, warfarin, antimetabolites); hypoglycemia, floppy infant
- Drug abuse
  - Fetal alcohol syndrome: growth retardation, mental deficiency, heart defects, flexion contractures
  - Opioid withdrawal: seizures; jittery, irritable infants; hypoglycemia; diarrhea
  - Amphetamines: congenital heart disease
- Maternal age: trisomy 13, 18, 21
- Single umbilical artery: renal malformations

TABLE 19-2 Peripartum History

- Prolonged labor
  - Abnormal fetus (eg, hydrocephalus, abdominal wall defect, breech presentation)
- Premature rupture of membranes
  - Prematurity
  - Infection, pneumonia
  - Oligo- or polyhydramnios
- Traumatic delivery
  - Intracranial hemorrhage, skull fracture, vocal cord paralysis, brachial plexus injury
- General anesthesia
  - Hypotonia, respiratory distress
- Prematurity (<37 wk postconceptual age or birth weight <2500 g)
  - Hyaline lung disease
  - Hypocalcemia, hypoglycemia, hypomagnesemia
  - Infection
  - Necrotizing enterocolitis
  - Patent ductus arteriosus
  - Hyperbilirubinemia
  - Increased risk of oxygen toxicity to the eyes (retinopathy of prematurity or "retrolental fibroplasia")
- Postmaturity (>41 wk postconceptual age)

The peripartum history is of equal importance for the evaluation of the neonate (Table 19-2). Prolonged labor and premature rupture of membranes are indicators for potential infectious complications in the neonate. Moreover, a traumatic delivery or abnormal fetal presentation may imply fractures or nerve injury. Other factors that may imply coexisting disorders include an abnormal umbilical cord or placenta, as well as the child's age, birth weight, and Apgar score.

Infants who are asphyxiated at birth must be identified before surgery. These newborns have depressed myocardial function and decreased perfusion to the brain and gastrointestinal system. Additionally, a variety of metabolic derangements, such as hypoglycemia, hypocalcemia, and hyperkalemia, occur in asphyxiated newborns. Other problems seen in these infants are clotting abnormalities, pulmonary aspiration of meconium-stained amniotic fluid, and intracranial hemorrhage. The latter is particularly devastating and may be due to impaired autoregulation of the cerebral circulation and/or large swings in blood pressure, cardiac output, and arterial blood gasses.

MECONIUM-STAINED AMNIOTIC FLUID

Under normal circumstances, the passage of meconium from the fetus into the amniotic fluid is prevented by the lack of intestinal peristalsis. Meconium-stained amniotic fluid may be a natural phenomenon that neither indicates nor causes fetal distress but simply reflects a postterm fetus with a mature gastrointestinal tract. Vagal stimulation produced by cord or head compression also may be associated with the passage of meconium in the absence of fetal distress. In contrast, meconium passage may occur secondary to an in utero stress, with resultant fetal hypoxia and acidosis producing relaxation of the anal sphincter. Term and postterm neonates are more likely to pass meconium in response to such a stress than preterm neonates. Perinatal conditions associated with an increased risk of meconium staining are listed in **Table 19-3**.[6]

GESTATIONAL AGE

Babies born at term, 37 to 42 weeks after conceptual age, can either be normal in size, small (<10th percentile) for gestational age (SGA), or large (>90th percentile) for gestational age (LGA). SGA and LGA babies often

TABLE 19-3 Risk Factors for Meconium-Stained Amniotic Fluid[6]

Maternal hypertension
Maternal diabetes mellitus
Maternal heavy cigarette smoking
Maternal chronic respiratory or cardiovascular disease
Postterm pregnancy
Pre-eclampsia/eclampsia
Oligohydramnios
Intrauterine growth retardation
Poor biophysical profile
Abnormal fetal heart rate patterns

have glucose homeostatic instability and require 10% glucose infusions to maintain normoglycemia (45-100 mg/dL).[7] Additionally, calcium homeostasis may be abnormal in these infants. The well-accepted definition of prematurity is an infant born at less than 37 weeks of gestation. Like the full-term infant, they too can be SGA or LGA. The physiologic variability between 24 and 36 weeks of gestation is enormous, and it is probably best to subdivide this group into infants on the edge of survivability (<26 weeks of gestation), fragile infants between 27 and 30 weeks of gestation, and more robust infants between 31 and 35 weeks of gestation. The younger the infant, the more fragile the neurologic, pulmonary, and gastrointestinal systems and the more likely the severity of complications.

PATIENT HISTORY–CONGENITAL ANOMALIES

The presence of 1 congenital anomaly should always alert the anesthesiologist to the potential for others. Currently, approximately 2% of liveborn infants have a congenital anomaly recognized at birth.[8,9] Congenital anomalies fall into 4 broad categories. The first is known as a *congenital malformation*. This is a primary structural defect that results from a localized error of morphogenesis, such as a cleft lip or a ventricular septal defect. The second category is a *malformation syndrome*. This is a recognized pattern of malformations believed to have the same etiology, but not the result of a single error of morphogenesis, such as trisomy 21. The third category is known as an *anomalad*. It is described as a single localized error of morphogenesis, as in Pierre Robin syndrome. Finally, patterns of recognized malformations that occur in a nonrandomized fashion are called an *association*. The VATER (vertebral defects, imperforate anus, tracheoesophageal fistula, and renal defects), which is currently also known as the VACTERL (vertebral defects, imperforate anus, congenital heart disease, tracheoesophageal fistula, renal and limb defects) association, is a classic example.

Table 19-4 provides a concise list of the more common congenital anomalies, syndromes, and associations. **Table 19-5** represents a more detailed account of the anesthetic implications of the more common syndromes and malformations. An excellent Internet resource can be found at the website of the National Center for Biotechnology Information (NCBI) Online Mendelian Inheritance in Man (OMIM) (http://www.ncbi.nlm.nih.gov/omim). It is always a good idea to check this site before anesthetic care, particularly if you are unfamiliar with the syndrome, defect, or malformation or its anesthetic implications (if you do not, you can be sure your patient's family will!). The presence of an anomaly or an associated defect can often be inferred from a detailed history and physical examination, as well as from the child's parents, neonatologist, and referring physician. Finally, a good rule of thumb to remember is that the presence of any midline defect is almost *always* associated with another defect.

REVIEW OF SYSTEMS AND DEVELOPMENTAL PHYSIOLOGY

HEAD AND NECK

The newborn is an obligate nose breather. If both nostrils are obstructed, respiratory distress will occur. Choanal atresia, an anomaly in which there is absence or complete obstruction of the nasopharynx bilaterally, is diagnosed by respiratory distress in the delivery room that is easily treated by oral intubation and by an inability to pass a catheter through the nostrils. A subset of patients with choanal atresia have the CHARGE syndrome: colobomas of the eye, congenital heart disease, atresia choanae, retardation, genital hypoplasia, and ear abnormalities. Occasionally, respiratory distress is caused by obstruction of the nasopharynx by a nasogastric tube and overzealous taping that occludes the opposite nostril. The airway must be evaluated for any abnormality that may result in a difficult intubation, such as a small or receding jaw (micrognathia) (Pierre Robin syndrome, Treacher Collins syndrome) or a large tongue (Beckwith syndrome, glycogen storage diseases, hypothyroidism, and Down syndrome). In many of these patients, intubation with conventional laryngoscopy is extremely difficult, if not impossible, and alternative methods (eg, laryngeal mask airways, light wands, fiberoptic bronchoscopy) and surgical backup should always be available. Additional lesions that make intubation difficult or impossible are airway hemangiomas, lymphangiomas, cystic hygromas, and laryngeal webs and cysts. The presence of a hemangioma should always raise a "red flag"; some of these lesions trap and consume platelets and may produce a bleeding diathesis. When an impossible airway situation arises and the patient's condition is known in utero, the EXIT (ex utero intrapartum treatment) procedure may be lifesaving.[10,11] In the EXIT procedure, which was originally designed for fetal surgery, the infant is partially delivered via a cesarean section and intubated in a controlled manner, prior to delivery of the placenta. The placenta acts as a "heart lung machine," and the procedure avoids a "crash" intubation or tracheostomy at birth in the delivery room. On the other end of the spectrum, cleft lips and palates do not usually present intubation problems.

TABLE 19-4 Commonly Encountered Lesions in the Neonate

Airway lesions
Choanal atresia
Pierre Robin syndrome
Upper airway obstruction
Cystic hygroma
Cleft lip and/or palate
Upper airway cysts and webs
Thoracic lesions
Tracheoesophageal fistula (TEF) or atresia
Congenital diaphragmatic hernia
Congenital heart disease
Pneumothorax, pneumomediastinum, pneumopericardium
Lobar emphysema, cystic adenomatoid malformation
Mediastinal masses
Abdominal lesions
Omphalocele
Gastroschisis
Intestinal obstruction
Malrotation and volvulus
Imperforate anus
Exstrophy of the bladder or cloaca
Hirshsprung disease
Biliary atresia
Incarcerated hernia
Necrotizing enterocolitis
Neurosurgical lesions
Myelomeningocele
Encephalocele
Craniosynostosis
Intracranial masses
Arteriovenous malformations (vein of Galen)
Skull fractures
Hydrocephalus
Subdural hemorrhage
Spinal tumors

TABLE 19-5 Anesthetic Implications of Syndromes and Unusual Disorders (http://www.ncbi.nlm.nih.gov/omim)

Name	Description	Anesthetic Implications
Arthrogryposis multiplex	Multiple congenital contractures; congenital heart disease	Possible airway problems due to limitations of mandibular movement
Asplenia syndrome	Absent spleen; complex congenital heart disease; malrotation of abdominal organs	Cyanotic heart disease very common; echocardiography essential preoperatively
Beckwith syndrome	Birth weight > 4000 g; macroglossia, visceromegaly	Airway problems due to large tongue; hypoglycemia common
Cherubism	Fibrous dysplasia of the mandible and maxilla	Intubation may be extremely difficult; tracheostomy may be the only way to secure the airway
Congenital hypothyroidism	Goiter; large tongue; respiratory depression; hypoglycemia; hypotension	Airway obstruction secondary to large tongue, particularly in supine position; slow to awaken at the completion of surgery
Crouzon disease	Craniosynostosis, hypertelorism, hypoplastic mandible	Intubation may be difficult
Dandy-Walker syndrome	Hydrocephalus	Increased intracranial pressure rare in the newborn period; head may be enormously enlarged
DiGeorge syndrome	Thymus and parathyroids absent; hypocalcemia, immune deficiency; aortic arch abnormalities	Irradiate all blood products to prevent graft-versus-host disease; stridor may be due to hypocalcemia
Down syndrome (trisomy 21)	Large tongue, unstable cervical spine, small mouth; high incidence of congenital heart disease, particularly AV canal; intestinal obstruction	Intubation may be difficult; ? inline traction during intubation, ? cervical spine films prior to intubation in older children; echocardiography required prior to surgery in the newborn
Ehlers-Danlos syndrome	Collagen abnormality-hyperelasticity and fragile tissue; dissecting aneurysm of aorta; bleeding diathesis; heart, lung, GI problems	Poor tissue and clotting defects may lead to hemorrhage; spontaneous pneumothorax
Ellis-van Creveld syndrome	Ectodermal and skeletal defects; congenital heart disease; cleft lip and palate, mandibular hypoplasia; hepatosplenomegaly	Airway problems, intubation may be difficult; chest wall anomalies cause poor lung function
Epidermolysis bullosa	Skin cleavage at dermal–epidermal junction, minor trauma denudes skin	Do not use adhesive tape of any sort; avoid instrumentation of the airway if possible; use a well-padded mask or apply ointment to rim; secure IV, monitoring devices with Kerlix; sterile technique
Familial dysautonomia (Riley-Day syndrome)	Poor suck and swallow; hyper- and hypotension; insensitivity to pain; absent sweating and lacrimation	Recurrent aspiration and pneumonia; respiratory center insensitive to CO_2; labile intraoperative blood pressure
Fetal alcohol syndrome	Growth retardation; microcephaly, craniofacial abnormalities; congenital heart disease; renal abnormalities	Intubation is usually not difficult, ventricular septal defects are common and require prophylaxis for subacute bacterial endocarditis
Glucose-6-phosphate deficiency	Hemolytic anemia caused by drugs and infection	Aspirin, sulfa, methylene blue cause anemia
Goldenhar syndrome	Hemifacial microsomia, congenital heart disease	Very difficult intubation, vertebral instability
Hemangioma with thrombocytopenia	May involve the airway; bleeding, anemia	Airway involvement may require radiation therapy; transfuse components as necessary
Jeune syndrome (asphyxiating thoracic dystrophy)	Severe thoracic malformations, renal failure	Respiratory failure, prolonged mechanical ventilation; care with drugs excreted by kidneys
Klippel-Feil syndrome	Hemi- or fused vertebra	Intubation may be difficult
Maple syrup urine disease	Inability to metabolize leucine, isoleucine, and valine	Acid–base imbalance; avoid preoperative fasting, start glucose early and check frequently
Mucopolysaccharidoses (Hurler, Hunter, Morquio syndrome)	Bony abnormalities, dwarfism, kyphoscoliosis, abnormal facies, congenital heart disease	Very difficult intubations, unstable necks, respiratory failure perioperatively
Myasthenia congenita	Similar to adult form	Avoid muscle relaxants and narcotics
Osteogenesis imperfecta	Pathologic fractures; abnormal platelets, vascular fragility	Extreme caution when positioning and during intubation; blood pressure cuff may cause fractures
Pierre-Robin syndrome	Cleft palate, micrognathia, glossoptosis, congenital heart disease	Very difficult intubation, may require tongue suture or awake tracheostomy; best nursed in prone position
Prader-Willi syndrome	Hypotonia, obesity	Hypoglycemia common; assisted ventilation may be required postop
Prune-Belly syndrome	Agenesis of the abdominal musculature, renal failure	Respiratory failure common, postoperative ventilation, avoid respiratory depressants; avoid drugs excreted by the kidneys

(*Continued*)

TABLE 19-5 Anesthetic Implications of Syndromes and Unusual Disorders (http://www.ncbi.nlm.nih.gov/omim) (*Continued*)

Name	Description	Anesthetic Implications
Treacher Collins syndrome	Micrognathia, mid-face hypoplasia, congenital heart disease	Very difficult intubation, may require tongue suture or awake tracheostomy; best nursed in prone position
Thrombocytopenia with absent radius syndrome	Episodic thrombocytopenia precipitated by stress, infection, surgery; congenital heart disease	Platelet transfusions prior to surgery; prophylaxis for subacute bacterial endocarditis
Trisomy 18	Congenital heart disease; micrognathia; renal malformations; most die in infancy	Ethical considerations concerning surgery in a patient with a fatal anomaly; assess cardiac status carefully
Trisomy 21 (see Down syndrome)		
VATER syndrome	Vertebral, anal, tracheal esophageal fistula, renal, cardiac	Examine carefully for associated anomalies

Indeed, the cleft may provide more room for the laryngoscope blade and facilitate endotracheal intubation.

Infants with a history of endotracheal intubation who are stridorous or who have a weak cry may have developed subglottic stenosis or subglottic granulomas. Unlike the adult, the narrowest part of the infant's airway is at the level of the cricoid ring and not the vocal cords.[12] Furthermore, the infant's trachea may be only 4 to 5 cm in total length, making endobronchial intubation extremely easy to accomplish, even by very experienced practitioners. To minimize this risk, we use the "1-2-3...7-8-9" rule to assist in correct endotracheal tube positioning. The "1-2-3" refers to the patient's weight in kilograms, and the "7-8-9" refers to the position of the endotracheal in centimeters at the patient's lip. An alternative reminder is the weight in kilograms + 6, which identifies the depth in centimeters where the endotracheal tube should be taped at the lip. Thus a 1-kg infant would have the tip of the endotracheal tube taped at the 7-cm mark at the lip. The trachea is very easily injured and explains in part the use of noncuffed endotracheal tubes in this age group.[13] However, the recent development of low-pressure, thin-walled, cuffed endotracheal tubes has challenged this decades-long held convention. Increasingly, cuffed endotracheal tubes are being used even in the newborn, particularly in situations in which aspiration of gastric contents is likely or poor lung compliance makes ventilation with an uncuffed endotracheal tube difficult.[14,15] In our practice we continue to use uncuffed endotracheally tubes primarily. Typically the trachea of most infants can be intubated with a 3.0-mm endotracheal tube. Premature infants occasionally require smaller, 2.5-mm tubes. In infants in whom subglottic narrowing is anticipated or who require intubation with tubes smaller than 2.5 mm, tracheostomy and/or bronchoscopy should be considered and discussed with the parents before surgery.

GAS EXCHANGE AND OXYGEN CONSUMPTION

During fetal life, respiratory gas exchange occurs at the placenta. The first breath after birth generates a negative intrapleural pressure of 80 cm of H_2O, expands the lungs, establishes the residual volume and the functional residual capacity, increases alveolar oxygen content, and causes pulmonary arterial vasodilation.[16] Gas exchange in the lungs is maintained with successful removal of the lung fluid from the airways and alveoli. This is achieved by drainage and increased pulmonary lymphatic flow for several hours after birth and by the presence of surface active phospholipids (surfactant).[17-19] The increase in arterial oxygen content that occurs with the successful transition to extrauterine life decreases pulmonary vascular resistance and leads to the functional closure of the ductus arteriosus and atrial septum.[16,20-22]

Oxygen consumption in the newborn is 2 to 3 times that of older children and adults. Unfortunately, the newborn responds to hypercarbia and hypoxia paradoxically as compared with the adult or older child.[23-29] Unlike the adult, the newborn's response to hypoxia during the first 3 weeks of life is biphasic and paradoxical; that is, rather than maintaining an increased minute ventilation, they rapidly develop apnea.[23,24,30,31] Further, hypoxia, which normally increases the respiratory response to hypercapnia, paradoxically depresses the newborn's ventilatory response to carbon dioxide. Indeed, apnea may also occur in response to hypothermia or when energy reserves are limited (eg, in the premature infant).[32] Thus a devastating cascade of events may be set in motion. Increased oxygen consumption, depressed respiratory function, and limited reserves lead to hypoxemia. Hypoxemia results in apnea and cardiovascular collapse. Other disadvantages of the newborn include a very compliant rib cage, which tends to collapse the chest wall; inefficient diaphragmatic contraction, and a low percentage of fatigue resistant type I muscle fibers in the diaphragm.[33,34] The combination of high work of breathing, increased oxygen consumption, and less resistance to muscle fatigue can produce abnormal breathing patterns, such as periodic breathing and apneic episodes, and respiratory failure.

The respiratory depressant effects of opioids and inhalational agents are also profound and long-lasting. Morphine penetrates the newborn's brain more easily than that of the adult and achieves levels that are 2 to 4 times higher.[35,36] Furthermore, the mu opioid receptor is exquisitely sensitive to respiratory depression in the newborn when compared with the adult.[37,38] Thus a history of prematurity and/or apnea must alert the anesthesiologist to possible respiratory compromise in the postoperative period, particularly if an opioid-based anesthetic is used. Indeed, premature infants are at risk of developing postanesthetic apnea for weeks after birth (48-60 weeks postconceptual age) whenever a potent vapor, opoid, or ketamine is used.[39-42]

Neonates suffering from respiratory distress syndrome (hyaline membrane disease) have low lung compliance, a diminished functional residual capacity, and diffuse microatelectasis. These infants are often hypoxemic and hypercarbic and exhibit tachypnea, expiratory grunting, and inspiratory retractions. They are often intubated and either positively pressure ventilated or spontaneously ventilating on continuous positive airway pressure. Maintaining normal gas exchange in these infants requires careful monitoring and respiratory support. Increased peak inspiratory pressures and positive end-expired pressures may be needed to maintain adequate oxygenation. Unfortunately this may lead to pneumothorax, pneumomediastinum, and interstitial emphysema. Indeed, the perioperative development of pulmonary barotrauma should alert the anesthesiologist to the possibility of intraoperative pneumothorax, which will manifest itself by catastrophic and sudden cardiovascular collapse.

CARDIAC PHYSIOLOGY

The fetal circulation is characterized by the preferential shunting of "arterialized" placental ("right-sided") blood across the foramen ovale and ductus arteriosus into the systemic ("left-sided") circulation.[43,44] This right-to-left shunting of blood is caused by the increased pulmonary vascular resistance and decreased systemic vascular resistance that characterizes the fetal circulation. The combination of breathing room air and clamping the umbilical cord reverses these resistances and results in the functional closure of the foramen ovale and the ductus arteriosus. Bidirectional shunting through the ductus arteriosus or an incompletely closed foramen ovale may normally persist for 24 to 72 hours and underscores the potential for paradoxical air embolus and the need to meticulously debubble all intravenous (IV) tubing. Unfortunately, arterial hypoxemia, hypercarbia, or acidosis will reverse this transitional circulation and restore the fetal circulatory pattern and is referred to as *persistent fetal circulation* or *persistent pulmonary hypertension of the newborn*.[45-47] It has catastrophic consequences. The increased pulmonary artery hypertension caused by arterial hypoxemia reduces pulmonary blood flow and reopens the foramen ovale and ductus arteriosus. This further exacerbates the hypoxemia and acidosis. It can occur with sepsis, hypotension, meconium aspiration, diaphragmatic hernia, and inefficient ventilation. Treatment with some combination of inhaled nitric oxide, oscillatory ventilation, and/or extra corporeal membrane oxygenation is increasingly successful.[46,48]

On the other hand, closure of the foramen ovale and ductus arteriosus may be detrimental in patients with certain types of congenital heart disease. Patients with transposition of the great vessels, complete or partial tricuspid or pulmonary valvular obstruction or atresia, and hypoplastic left heart syndrome are critically dependent for their very survival on continued flow across these shunts. An intravenous infusion of prostaglandin E_1 (PGE_1) to maintain the patency of the ductus arteriosus may be life-sustaining in these patients. Indeed, any newborn with refractory shock or hypoxemia should receive PGE_1 until a ductal-dependent lesion can be ruled out with echocardiogram. The usual dose of PGE1 is 0.01 to 0.4 µg/kg/min as a continuous IV infusion.[49] The starting dose is typically 0.05 µg/kg/min. Side effects include apnea, fever, hypotension, cutaneous vasodilation, and seizures.

The newborn's myocardium is less compliant than that of the adult or older child, and cardiac output is primarily heart rate dependent.[50-52] The heart has incomplete or decreased sympathetic innervation, with reduced catecholamine stores.[53] Studies performed in newborns during exchange transfusions have revealed that the newborn has reduced capacity for peripheral vasoconstriction during hypovolemia.

Several powerful reflexes control the cardiovascular system of the neonate. The arterial baroreceptor is the most powerful of these and consists of the carotid sinus and aortic arch baroreceptors. These receptors are stretch receptors stimulated by pressure deformation of the vessel wall tissue in which they reside. An increase in transmural pressure stretches these receptors and increases the rate of baroreceptor firing. Afferent nerves carry these signals to the vasomotor centers of the medulla and parasympathetic and sympathetic efferent fibers slow the heart rate, strengthen contraction, and reduce venous and arterial resistance. A reduction in arterial blood pressure has the opposite effect, causing a central afferent sympathoadrenal discharge that increases systolic and diastolic blood pressure. The arterial baroreceptor reflex is intact in healthy full-term newborns but may be significantly depressed in stressed or premature infants. Anesthetics, particularly halothane, may also significantly depress this response.[54,55]

The arterial chemoreceptors form a second powerful cardiovascular reflex arc. The carotid and aortic chemoreceptor bodies are responsible for the cardiovascular response to acute hypoxia. The primary central response to hypoxia is bradycardia.[56] The peripheral chemoreceptors, once stimulated, cause tachypnea and increased sympathetic discharge to the heart and peripheral tissues. These receptors are stimulated by hypoxic hypoxia (low PaO_2) and decreased cardiac output, but not by reduced oxygen content due to anemia. Once again, the stressed or premature infant or the full-term infant anesthetized with halothane may have a blunted or absent sympathetically mediated response to hypoxia. Indeed, the most common cause of bradycardia in the newborn is hypoxia, and in the operating room, unexplained bradycardia should always be considered to be due to hypoxia until proven otherwise.

Thus it may be dangerous to anesthetize a stressed neonate who is either hypovolemic or dehydrated, particularly with the potent inhalational anesthetic vapors. Hypovolemia or dehydration should be assumed in septic patients (necrotizing enterocolitis), ventilated patients who are being treated with diuretics and fluid restriction (hyaline membrane disease, patent ductus arteriosus), and, in the operating room, when hemorrhage occurs.

CENTRAL NERVOUS SYSTEM

The central nervous system is the least mature major organ system at birth. This structural immaturity predisposes the newborn to certain risks, including intraventricular hemorrhages, seizures, respiratory depression, hypoxic–ischemic injury, and retinopathy of the premature.[57-60] Hypoxia, hypercarbia, hypotension, acidosis, and pain may produce any and all of these complications. Further, hypoxia–ischemia in the perinatal period may be an important cause of cerebral palsy and associated disabilities in children. The stressed premature infant is particularly at risk. Indeed, intraventricular hemorrhage, in which subependymal hemorrhage occurs, is now the leading cause of death and morbidity in these infants, particularly among the premature born at less than 28 weeks of gestation, and has an incidence as high as 50%.[57,58,61-64]

Hydrocephalus also occurs frequently either as noncommunicating hydrocephalus, in which the flow of cerebral spinal fluid is obstructed (aqueductal stenosis, spina bifida) or as communicating hydrocephalus, in which the flow of cerebral spinal fluid is unimpeded, but resorption is affected (intraventricular hemorrhage). Increased intracranial pressure secondary to hydrocephalus may or may not be present because the newborn's cranial sutures are open at birth and allow for intracranial decompression. On the other hand, the resulting large head may present very difficult airway management problems. Furthermore, the stretching of cranial nerves that may occur with hydrocephalus or with other intracranial pathology, such as the Arnold-Chiari malformation, may cause vocal cord paralysis and/or stridor.[65] Finally, autoregulation may be disrupted during hypoxia, acidosis, seizures, or in the presence of a patent ductus arteriosus. Thus rapid increases in blood pressure may produce intracerebral bleeding, and rapid decreases may produce ischemia.[66-69]

THERMOREGULATION

The newborn infant, even the premature, is quite capable of maintaining a stable core temperature in the face of modestly changing ambient temperatures. This is accomplished by balancing heat production with skin blood flow, sweat production and changing minute ventilation. However, when exposed to cold, neonatal compensatory mechanisms operate only within a narrow temperature range. For adults, the lower range of thermoregulation is 0°C, whereas for full-term newborns it is 22°C. Premature infants require even higher ambient temperature to ensure thermal homeostasis. Indeed, at ambient temperatures of less than 32° to 34°, the premature infant must significantly increase its oxygen consumption to stay warm.[70] The ambient temperature at which a state of thermal equilibrium exists, that is, in which heat loss and heat production are equal and occur without an increase in oxygen consumption, is called the *neutral thermic state*.[71,72]

After delivery, the newborn infant rapidly loses heat as a result of its large surface area relative to its body mass and its lack of heat-insulating subcutaneous tissue (fat). The infant loses heat by evaporation, convection, conduction, and radiation. Evaporative heat loss is the major source of heat loss in the perioperative period.[73,74] Physical factors that govern evaporative losses include relative humidity, velocity of air flow, and minute ventilation. The driving force for evaporative heat loss is the difference between vapor pressure on the surface of the skin and vapor pressure in the environment. Physiologic factors that affect evaporative loss relate to the infant's ability to sweat and to increase minute ventilation. Premature infants less than 30 postconceptual weeks of age have underdeveloped sweat glands and do not perspire. Preventing or minimizing evaporative heat loss is the primary means of heat control in the perioperative period. Wrapping newborns inside plastic bags is one of the easiest ways of minimizing evaporative heat losses and should be used not only in the operating room during surgery, but in transport as well.[75,76]

Heat production is achieved by voluntary muscle activity, shivering, and nonshivering thermogenesis. Shivering is rarely observed in the newborn and, with the small muscle mass present, would not be very effective. Nonshivering thermogenesis is a heat-producing and oxygen-consuming mechanism stimulated by cold, in which there is a generalized increase in metabolism and a marked increase in the metabolic activity in certain specialized tissues, most notably in the brown adipose tissue ("fat").[77] This tissue is principally located in the interscapular region, mediastinum, and the tissues surrounding the kidneys and adrenal glands. Unlike white fat, it has a rich blood supply and very high oxygen consumption when metabolically active. Morphologically, brown fat contains multiloculated cells with numerous mitochondria. The mitochondria appear densely packed with cristae and have increased respiratory chain components. It is also abundantly enervated by the sympathetic nervous system. In fact, the metabolism of brown fat is stimulated by the local release of catecholamines, particularly norepinephrine.[70,77]

Thus the control of heat-producing mechanisms depends on skin (not central) thermoreceptors. When skin temperature decreases, central control mechanisms trigger increased metabolic activity in brown adipose tissue. This is mediated by the sympathetic nervous system. Unfortunately, vapor anesthetics may paralyze these systems and convert the infant into a poikilotherm. Alternatively, hypoxia may interfere with thermoregulation. Hypoxia impairs heat production and impairs heat conservation by producing peripheral vasodilation.

The infant can be protected from unnecessary heat loss quite easily. Aside from wrapping the infant in plastic bags and humidifying the anesthetic vapors, heat can be conserved by warming the operating room to 25°C (85°F), using a forced air heating blanket, warming intravenous fluids, blood, and irrigation solutions, and using a radiant heater with a servo control mechanism.[78]

RENAL PHYSIOLOGY AND METABOLISM

The glomerular filtration rate in newborns is less than a quarter of the adult's. Further, the newborn's ability to concentrate urine is also significantly reduced. In fact, the maximum concentrating ability of the newborn's kidney does not exceed 700 mOsm/kg as compared with 1400 mOsm/kg in the older child.[79] Thus the newborn requires sodium-containing fluids intraoperatively.[80] Not only will these infants lose salt intraoperatively through third space and hemorrhagic losses, but they also continue to lose sodium through obligate urinary losses because of tubular inability to increase sodium reabsorption.

GLUCOSE METABOLISM

Another physiologic transition that must occur at birth involves glucose and energy homeostasis. Before birth, all of the newborn's nutritional needs are continuously provided by the maternal circulation. After birth, major physiologic and metabolic changes are required to adjust to intermittent enteral feeding. Glucose is the substrate used for the energy production necessary for maintenance of body temperature, respiration, and muscular activity.[81-83] Blood glucose concentration is normally maintained at a relatively constant level by a fine balance between hepatic glucose output and peripheral glucose uptake. Hepatic glucose output depends on adequate glycogen stores, sufficient supplies of endogenous gluconeogenic substrate, a normally functioning gluconeogenic and glycogenolytic system, and a normal endocrine system for modulating these processes. The newborn has limited glycogen stores that may be rapidly depleted. On the other hand, endogenous gluconeogenic substrate availability is not a limiting factor, nor is the liver's gluconeogenic and glycogenolytic systems.

Hypoglycemia is common in infants born to diabetic mothers and in infants who required resuscitation, are premature, or who are small for gestational age.[82-84] By definition, hypoglycemia is a blood glucose level less than 45 mg/dL in the infant during the first 3 days of life.[7,82-84] After 3 days of age, glucose values should be greater than 75 to 90 mg/dL. The clinical manifestations of hypoglycemia include tremors or jitteriness, apnea, cyanotic spells, convulsions, limpness or lethargy, hypothermia, sweating, refusal to feed, and cardiac failure or arrest. These are nonspecific signs and symptoms and must be differentiated from birth asphyxia, central nervous system abnormalities such as hemorrhage or cerebral edema, congenital heart disease, sepsis, drug withdrawal, apnea, and other metabolic abnormalities such as hypocalcemia, hypomagnesemia, and hyponatremia.

Symptomatic babies must be treated rapidly to prevent neurologic damage. Treatment should be started with a 250- to 500-mg/kg bolus of glucose (25% dextrose-containing solution, D25), followed by an infusion of 4 to 6 mg/kg/min (65-100 mL/kg/h) of a 10% dextrose-containing solution. Failure of this regimen to produce blood glucose concentration of 80 to 120 mg/dL should alert the physician to the possibility of hyperinsulinism. Hyperinsulinism and hypoglycemia occur in maternal diabetes, erythroblastosis, Beckwith-Wiedemann syndrome, SGA and LGA infants, polycythemia, and insulin-secreting tumors (nesidioblastosis).

CALCIUM

Calcium in the blood circulates as 3 fractions, protein bound, complexed, and ionized, and is tightly regulated by the intricate interplay of parathyroid, renal, and skeletal factors.[85,86] Ionized calcium is the only physiologically active fraction, whereas the protein-bound calcium provides a reserve of available calcium should a need for increased ionized calcium arise acutely.[85,86] In fact, if total calcium levels in the blood are reduced as a result of low plasma protein and if the ionized fraction remains normal, there may be no physiologic changes. On the other hand, if total calcium levels are normal, but the ionized levels are low, as may occur when chelating agents are used (eg, as with citrated blood products), significant physiologic effects occur.

During pregnancy, there is rapid transfer of calcium from mother to fetus, via an active placenta pump.[87] At birth there is an abrupt termination of maternal to fetal calcium supply. Further, dietary calcium in the first few days of life is significantly less than the amount normally received from the mother. A decrease in serum calcium is expected to occur. In the sick newborn, even greater deprivation of calcium is common because of the conventional withholding of milk feeding and the substitution of calcium-free intravenous feeding.

Neonatal hypocalcemia is therefore common in the first few days of life. Definitions vary regarding the level of serum calcium required for the diagnosis, but most agree that in infants up to 3 months of age, hypocalcaemia is defined as a serum total calcium level of less than 8.8 mg/dL or ionized calcium less than 4.9 mg/dL (1.22-1.4 mM).[86] Infants at particular risk are those born prematurely or to diabetic mothers, SGA infants, or those who have received large volumes of citrated blood products or sodium bicarbonate. Additionally, infants who are alkalotic secondary to hyperventilation, who experienced birth asphyxia, or who are hypoparathyroid or born with the DiGeorge syndrome present with hypocalcemia as well.

The classic clinical signs and symptoms of hypocalcemia, namely Chvostek sign (facial muscle twitching when stimulated) and Trousseau sign (carpal spasm after constriction of the upper arm), are of little value in the newborn. Rather, nonspecific symptoms occur, namely, jitteriness, twitching, convulsions, and, occasionally, hypotension. An electrocardiogram will reveal prolonged QT intervals. The treatment of symptomatic hypocalcemia is the administration of calcium salts. Acute intravenous administration of 1 to 2 mL/kg of either 10% calcium gluconate or chloride should be administered while the heart rate is monitored continuously. In the newborn the acute administration of calcium can produce significant bradycardia. The other important complication of this therapy relates to extravasation of calcium into the soft tissues when a peripheral intravenous catheter is utilized. This can cause skin sloughing and necrosis.

SUMMARY

Except for extraordinary circumstances, all newborns require anesthesia and analgesia for surgery. During the first month of life, the newborn must function independently and adapt to extrauterine life. This involves anatomic, physiologic, and pharmacologic changes to maintain homeostasis and to ensure the infant's survival. Disease, congenital anomalies, surgery, and anesthesia may interfere with these adaptations and threaten survival. In this chapter we have attempted to provide an in-depth review of developmental physiology and pathophysiology that are essential in the provision of safe anesthesia to the newborn.

KEY REFERENCES

- Anand KJ, Hickey PR. Pain and its effects in the human neonate and fetus. *N Engl J Med.* 1987;317:1321-1329.
- Berde CB, Jaksic T, Lynn AM, Maxwell LG, Soriano SG, Tibboel D. Anesthesia and analgesia during and after surgery in neonates. *Clin Ther.* 2005;27:900-921.
- Coté CJ, Zaslavsky A, Downes JJ, et al. Postoperative apnea in former preterm infants after inguinal herniorrhaphy. A combined analysis. *Anesthesiology.* 1995;82:809-822.
- Cramer K, Wiebe N, Hartling L, Crumley E, Vohra S. Heat loss prevention: a systematic review of occlusive skin wrap for premature neonates. *J Perinatol.* 2005;25:763-769.
- Gregory GA. The baroresponses of preterm infants during halothane anaesthesia. *Can Anaesth Soc J.* 1982;29:105-107.
- Hirose S, Farmer DL, Lee H, Nobuhara KK, Harrison MR. The ex utero intrapartum treatment procedure: looking back at the EXIT. *J Pediatr Surg.* 2004;39:375-380.
- Hsu SC, Levine MA. Perinatal calcium metabolism: physiology and pathophysiology. *Semin Neonatol.* 2004;9:23-36.
- Kalhan S, Peter-Wohl S. Hypoglycemia: What is it for the neonate? *Am J Perinatol.* 2000;17:11-18.
- Kiserud T. Physiology of the fetal circulation. *Semin Fetal Neonatal Med.* 2005;10:493-503.
- Maze A, Bloch E. Stridor in pediatric patients. *Anesthesiology.* 1979;50:132-145.
- McCrea HJ, Ment LR. The diagnosis, management, and postnatal prevention of intraventricular hemorrhage in the preterm neonate. *Clin Perinatol.* 2008;35:777-792, vii.
- Konduri GG. New approaches for persistent pulmonary hypertension of newborn. *Clin Perinatol.* 2004;31:591-611.
- Pang LM, Mellins RB. Neonatal cardiorespiratory physiology. *Anesthesiology.* 1975;43:171-196.
- Tálosi G, Katona M, Rácz K, Kertész E, Onozó B, Túri S. Prostaglandin E1 treatment in patent ductus arteriosus dependent congenital heart defects. *J Perinat Med.* 2004;32:368-374.
- Volpe JJ. Brain injury in the premature infant: overview of clinical aspects, neuropathology, and pathogenesis. *Semin Pediatr Neurol.* 1998;5:135-151.
- Weber T, Salvi N, Orliaguet G, Wolf A. Cuffed vs non-cuffed endotracheal tubes for pediatric anesthesia. *Paediatr Anaesth.* 2009;19(Suppl 1):46-54.

REFERENCES

Complete references available on DVD and online version at www.LongneckerAnesthesiology.com

CHAPTER 20

Evaluation of Children

Randall C. Wetzel

KEY POINTS

1. Children have significantly different physiology and psychology and behavior to necessitate a comprehensive pediatric approach for the child and the family based on their requirements.
2. The percentage of total body composition that is water decreases with age; intracellular fluid increases, whereas extracellular fluid decreases.
3. Fat and muscle mass increase from 13% to 22% and 20% to 50%, respectively, with age.
4. The distribution of blood flow varies, with a decreased percentage of flow going to the vessel-rich groups with increased age.
5. Infants have a large tongue and relatively small jaw. Infants usually are described as having an anterior and cephalad displacement of the airway, with the narrowest segment at the level of the cricoid. The epiglottis generally is large and floppy compared with that of adults.
6. Younger children tend to experience airway closure and alveolar collapse with atelectasis because the end-expiratory lung volume from which tidal breathing occurs is close to closing capacity.
7. Although the functional residual capacity in milliliters per kilogram is smaller in infants compared with adults (30 vs 34), increased oxygen consumption is the major factor in the rapid desaturation of infants.
8. The perioperative risk of reversion to a transitional circulation is related to pulmonary hypertension triggered by hypoxemia, hypercarbia, hypothermia, acidosis, and increased catecholamines.
9. Cardiac output depends on heart rate in infants and young children. Infants have parasympathetic hypertonia, decreased sympathetic innervation, and a ventricle with less muscle and more noncontractile mass per unit volume. These all lead to a myocardium that is less able to generate adequate force than in adults.
10. A hematocrit nadir of approximately 35 at approximately age 3 months is the so-called physiologic anemia of infancy.
11. The glomerular filtration rate/1.73 m^2 increases from 40 to 130 mL/min with age. Ability to concentrate urine is limited, and maximal osmolarity may be only 700 mOsm.
12. Slack lower esophageal sphincter tone with reflux is common in infants younger than 6 months, but the maintenance of low gastric volumes by nothing-by-mouth (NPO) regulations should be balanced by awareness of the risk of hypoglycemia.
13. The liver is functionally immature in children, affecting synthetic and metabolic function.
14. Defending the thermoneutrality of infants is a cornerstone of pediatric anesthesia.
15. Cold stress in neonates can increase oxygen consumption and decrease oxygen delivery, leading to increased hydrogen ion concentration and decreased glycogen and glucose. This may result in respiratory distress, disseminated intravascular coagulation, shock, and persistent fetal circulation.
16. The large surface-area-to-mass ratio in children and decreased subcutaneous tissue mass lead to increased heat loss via conduction, convection, radiation, and evaporation.
17. The large volume of distribution noted in neonates is related to decreased protein binding and a greater proportion of extracellular water.
18. In preoperative evaluation, the anesthesiologist should prepare himself or herself, the family, and the child for the procedure. The primary objective is to ensure that the child is in optimal condition. Developmental milestones

and growth charts should be reviewed to assist in the general assessment of well-being. Optimal drug levels (eg, anticonvulsants and theophylline) should be ensured.

19. Many congenital anomalies are associated with airway and cardiac abnormalities.
20. In children with known cardiopulmonary disease, it is imperative that the anesthesiologist be completely familiar with the child's current status and be assured that therapy has been optimized preoperatively.
21. In infants, feeding is the major exercise, and failure to thrive may indicate compromised cardiovascular function.
22. The "runny nose" remains a controversial area, but whenever possible, surgery and anesthesia should be delayed at least 2 weeks when the child has a runny nose associated with lower respiratory or systemic symptoms.
23. Routine laboratory testing for healthy children remains controversial and should be dictated by clinical situation.
24. The trend of NPO status is toward a more liberal NPO restriction for clear liquids.
25. Rigorous, compulsive, and systematic evaluation of critically ill children is essential.

The preanesthetic evaluation of the child requires not only an understanding of the different surgical procedures children undergo, but also an understanding of the unique psychology, development, and physiology of children. There are many obvious differences between adults and children that affect anesthetic management. Apart from the differences of size, communication skills, and issues involving parents, there also are multiple, less obvious differences in the physiology, psychology, anatomy, and pharmacology of children. The most characteristic and important feature of childhood is development. Not only does children's responsiveness to other people follow recognized patterns of psychological development that require appropriate responses from the anesthesiologist, but virtually every organ system undergoes distinct, well-described development that is relevant to the anesthetic management of children. The key to understanding pediatric anesthesiology is to recognize the dynamic processes that occur at the various developmental stages of childhood. The mindset required is not that of understanding anesthesia that is appropriate for adult physiology and adapting this approach to children, but rather to flexibly approach the child as the child grows from fetus to adult. A specific anesthetic plan appropriate to developmental stages should be designed for each child. Because the developmental characteristics of children determine anesthetic management, this chapter focuses on those changes that occur after the neonatal period. Chapter 19 discusses neonatal physiology. This chapter familiarizes the anesthesiologist with the anesthetic implications of development from neonates to adults.

DEVELOPMENTAL IMPLICATIONS

Growth is not solely a process of proportional enlargement. Total body composition, including proportional fluid content, the relationship of head-to-body size, and cardiorespiratory function, all change disproportionately during development. For example, the head becomes proportionately smaller, with relatively little change in the size of the cranial vault after 2 years of age. At the same time, major changes in facial configuration occur. Most striking is the development of the mandible, which develops from being small and obliquely set to the skull of infants to becoming proportionately larger, less obliquely set, and more mobile in adults.

The development of body composition is important because it is an essential determinant of developmental pharmacology. In the fetus, 90% of total body composition is water; at full term, 75% of total body composition is water, but by age 1 year, 60% of total body content is water.[1] Adult water composition is attained by age 1 year. There is also a change in the relative proportion of extracellular water over the first years of life. Extracellular water volume demonstrates a greater decrease than intracellular volume, which undergoes a complementary increase. Intracellular fluid increases from approximately 20% in premature infants to 30% in term infants and to 40% in adults, whereas extracellular fluid falls from 60% in premature infants to 45% in term infants and 20% in adults.[2] The percentage of body composition that is muscle in premature infants is less than 20% and increases to more than 20% at term, and attains 50% in adults.[1] Fat likewise increases with age, from 13% in term infants to 22% of total body weight in adults.[1] There also is an age-dependent change in the relative proportion of blood flow to the various organs. Distribution of blood flow to various organ groups defined by their vascularity (vessel-rich group [VRG], muscle group [MG], and vessel-poor group [VPG]) also demonstrates major developmental change (**Table 20-1**).[3] For example, there is a decreased percentage of flow going to VRGs with increasing age. The VRG in neonates accounts for 22% of total body volume, whereas in adults, it only accounts for 10%. Thus an anesthetic caregiver would expect a smaller portion of blood flow to VPGs in infants and a more rapid attainment of the plateau phase of the alveolar end-tidal concentration (FA)-to-inspired concentration (FI) ratio with use of inhalational anesthetics. This has clear implications for the induction of inhalational anesthesia in children, and, not surprisingly, the uptake and distribution of inhalational anesthetics in children.[3]

TABLE 20-1 Tissue Type Volume as Percent of Body Volume

Age	Vessel-Rich Group	Muscle Group	Vessel-Poor Group
Neonate	22	39	13
1 year	17	39	25
4 years	17	41	23
8 years	13	45	21
Adult	10	50	22

From Eger EL II, Gahlman SH, Munson ES: The effect of age on the rate of increase of alveolar anesthetic concentration. *Anesthesiology*. 35;365, 1971.

RESPIRATORY SYSTEM

The major features of the respiratory system that undergo important developmental changes are (1) the upper airway, (2) airway caliber, (3) respiratory system (chest wall and lung) mechanics, (4) central control of breathing, and (5) respiratory muscle characteristics. Each is described in the following material.[4]

The upper airway undergoes major development (**Fig. 20-1**). The first developmental difference is that an infant's tongue is relatively large compared with the rest of the airway. Intubation may be hampered by the overlarge tongue situated in the relatively small jaw. Infants usually are described as having an anterior, cephalad-displaced glottis, with the airway forming an inverse cone (**Fig. 20-2**). The narrowest segment of the airway is at the cricoid cartilage and remains so until puberty. These factors are important for intubation. An endotracheal tube that will be admitted to the glottis may be too tight for the subglottic area. The presence of an air leak below 30 cm H_2O airway pressure always should be ensured for routine anesthesia.

In infants, the glottis is located at C2, 2 to 3 vertebral bodies higher than in adults, in whom the glottis is located at C4-C5. The cricoid cartilage is found at C4 in children and at C6-C7 in adults. The obliquity of the vocal cords also changes with age. In infants, these are slanted down and anteriorly compared with adults. This makes the angle for intubation more acute and more difficult in children, and makes blind nasal intubation difficult. Another difference in the child's airway is the nature of the epiglottis. The epiglottis in small children is relatively larger, longer, more curved (omega [Ω] shaped), and floppy compared with that in adults. Maturation begins to occur at age 2 years, and the adult configuration is achieved sometime near puberty, when the epiglottis is shorter,

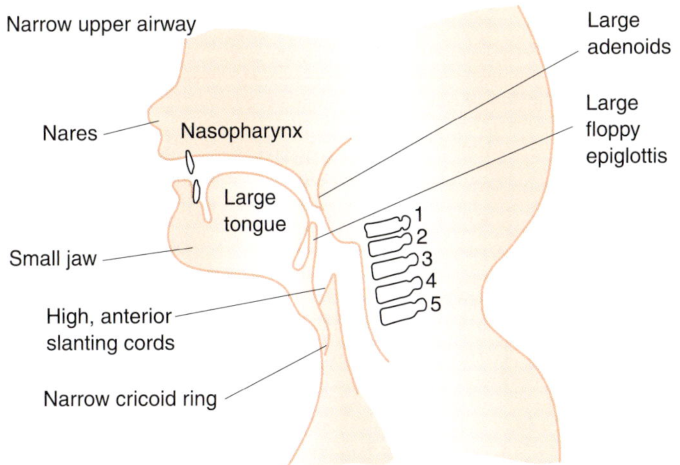

FIGURE 20-1. Diagram of a coronal section through the airway of an infant. Areas where there are important differences from adults are highlighted. [Reproduced with permission from Wetzel RC. Anesthesia for pediatric trauma. In: Stene JK, ed. *Pediatric Trauma*. Baltimore, MD: Williams & Wilkins, 1989;312-329.]

smaller, blunter, and less curved rather than Ω shaped. These anatomic differences in the airway have a major effect on which intubation techniques will be useful in children. For example, a straight laryngoscope blade (eg, Miller blades) that can lift directly the epiglottis out of the larynx during glottic visualization is useful in children.

Airway caliber undergoes continuous developmental change from the nares to the small airways. Although airway branching has been completed by birth, the caliber of the airways continues to increase. Airway resistance is inversely proportional to the fourth power of the radius, as seen in the Poiseuille equation:

$$\text{Resistance} = 8\,Ln/r^4$$

where L is the airway length, n is the viscosity of the fluid, and r is the radius of the airway. It should be noted that total airway resistance is affected by consideration of caliber from the nares to the alveoli. Small airways have high resistance. The consideration of size also makes the seriousness of airway edema greater in younger children. A proportional

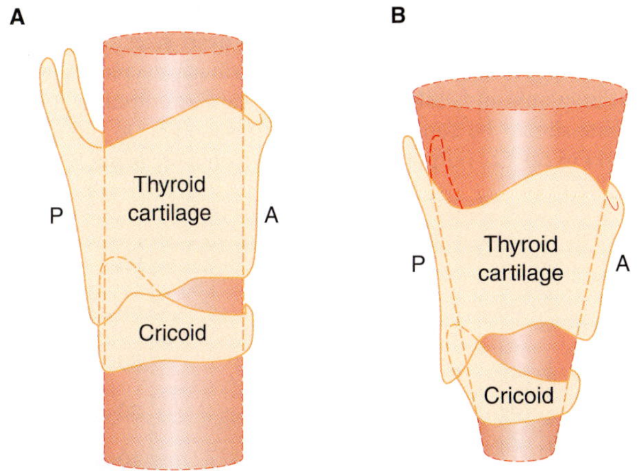

FIGURE 20-2. Schematic of an adult (**A**) and infant (**B**) airway. Note the comparison between the cylindrically shaped airway with uniform diameters in the adult and the conically shaped airway of the child with the narrowest region at the cricoid. A, anterior; P, posterior. [Reprinted from Cote CJ, Todres ID. The pediatric airway. In: Ryan JF, Todres ID, Cote CJ, et al, eds. *A Practice of Anesthesia for Infants and Children*. Philadelphia, PA: WB Saunders; 1986;35-58, with permission from Elsevier.]

increase in mucosal thickness in children increases resistance to a greater extent than it does in adults because equal mucosal thickening proportionately decreases caliber more in children. Airway resistance decreases approximately 15 times from infancy to adulthood, with a dramatic change occurring near age 8 years.[5] This decrease in resistance with increasing age largely results from an increase in diameter of the small airways.[6] Infants are obligate nose breathers, and nasal obstruction can cause severe respiratory embarrassment, which is more severe in premature infants.[7]

Respiratory mechanics change dramatically from birth to adulthood. These changes result from increased alveolarization, increased airway size, and changes in the chest wall. Only as the rib cage ossifies does its configuration change and become more rigid. In infants, the chest wall is soft and pliable because of its largely cartilaginous structure, which makes the chest wall highly compliant. This compliance promotes chest wall collapse when increased work of breathing requires more negative intrathoracic pressure. The clinical consequences associated with these chest wall factors are seen in infants with respiratory distress as marked sternal and subcostal retractions. In infants, the chest wall is at a mechanical disadvantage during breathing because greater pressure is required per unit of tidal volume moved. In addition to the compliance of the chest wall, there is also a decrease in elastic recoil of the total respiratory system and chest wall. This low elastic recoil tends to alter the relationship between closing volume, functional residual capacity (FRC), and residual volume.

The respiratory system undergoes significant and dramatic neuromuscular development. Central respiratory control, muscle fiber makeup (type I vs type II), and neural innervation of the chest wall show distinct developmental changes in infants and small children.[8] The central respiratory control undergoes dramatic developmental changes. For example, full and preterm neonates demonstrate depression of the CO_2 response curve and secondary apnea with hypoxia.[9,10] This contrasts with the characteristic adult response, which is increased CO_2 responsiveness in the presence of hypoxia, resulting in tachypnea. The impact of hypoxia in the presence of this paradoxic, immature response can be catastrophic in neonates.[9] This infantile pattern of respiratory control is related to the risk of postanesthetic apnea in neonates.[11] Anesthetic effects on the CO_2 response curve are similar in infants and adults. The CO_2 response curve undergoes depression by potent inhalational anesthetic agents and narcotics in children as it does in adults.[12]

Respiratory muscle type reaches the adult pattern of distribution at approximately age 2 years. This predisposes the infant to fatigue. Type II muscle fibers predominate and do not have the ability to perform repeated exercise against increased workloads as do type I fibers.[8] Type I fibers become predominant at approximately age 2 years. Regarding neural innervation, reflex responses and spindle innervation of the thoracic cage also undergo developmental changes. For example, the Hering-Breuer response is accentuated in preterm infants compared with full-term infants and leads to apnea with lung inflation in preterm infants.[13] These characteristics have a major impact on cyclic respiration, as can be seen from the immature respiratory pattern of periodic breathing. In addition, sleep state–dependent respiratory patterns show distinct developmental differences.[14]

These changes in chest wall recoil, elasticity, compliance, and neural control have a major effect on lung volumes (**Fig. 20-3**). One of the most important factors is the tendency in younger children for airway closure and alveolar collapse with atelectasis to occur. Children breathe from an end-expiratory lung volume (EELV) close to closing capacity (CC). Their FRC is actually below CC in premature infants and term neonates, increasing with age. Airway closure may occur even during normal tidal respiration in small infants.[15] Induction of anesthesia is associated with decreased elastic recoil and airway tone and decreased respiratory muscle tone. Thus an expected lung volume decrease occurs with tidal respiration falling below closing volumes. These factors and those responsible for the decrease in EELV to less than FRC on induction of anesthesia in part account for the rapid occurrence of hypoxemia in apneic infants during induction of anesthesia. The other major factor related to the

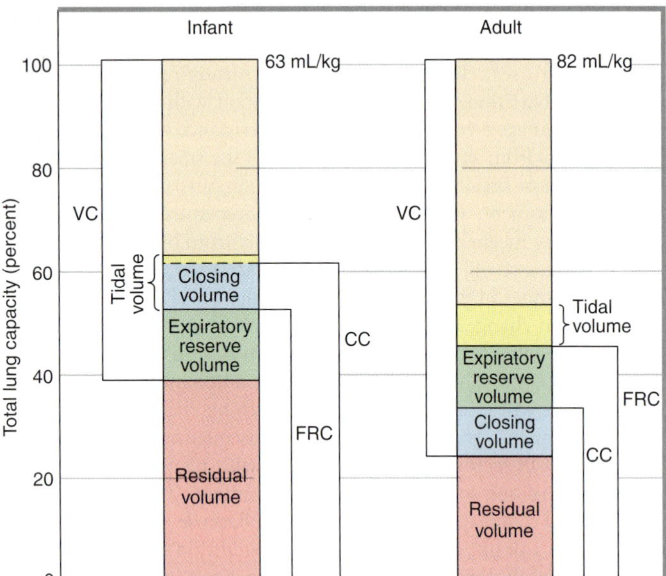

FIGURE 20-3. Bar graphs representing proportional lung volumes in infants and adults. Note the relationship of functional residual capacity (FRC) to closing volume and how this changes with age. CC, closing capacity; VC, vital capacity. [Smith CA, Nelson NM. *The Physiology of the Newborn Infant*. Springfield, IL: Charles C Thomas; 1976. Courtesy of Charles C Thomas Publisher, Ltd., Springfield.]

TABLE 20-2 Respiratory Mechanics

	Infant	Adult
Respiratory frequency (breaths/min)	30-40	12-16
Inspiratory time (s)	0.4-0.5	1.2-1.4
I:E ratio	1:1.5-1:2	1:2-1:3
Inspiratory flow (L/min)	2-3	24
Tidal volume		
mL	18-24	500
mL/kg	6-8	6-8
Functional respiratory capacity (FRC)		
mL	100	2200
mL/kg	30	34
Vital capacity		
mL	120	3500
mL/kg	33-40	52
Total lung capacity		
mL	200	6000
mL/kg	63	86
Total respiratory compliance		
mL/cm H_2O	2.6-4.9	100
mL/cm H_2O/mL FRC	0.004-0.06	0.04-0.07
Lung compliance		
mL/cm H_2O	4.8-6.2	170-200
mL/cm H_2O/mL FRC	0.04-0.07	0.04-0.07
Specific airway conductance		
mL/s/cm H_2O/mL FRC	0.24	0.28
Respiratory insensible water loss		
mL/24 h	45-55	300

Data from Powell FL, Heldt GP, Haddad G. Respiratory physiology. In: Nichols DG, ed. *Roger's Textbook of Pediatric Intensive Care*. Philadelphia, PA: Lippincott Williams & Wilkins; 2008:631-661.

rapid occurrence of hypoxemia in apneic infants is their relatively increased oxygen consumption. In neonates, oxygen consumption is approximately 7 mL/kg/min.[16] On a consumption-to-weight basis, this is approximately double that seen in adults, in whom oxygen consumption undergoes a gradual decrease with age. Although FRC/kg is less (30 vs 34 mL) in infants than adults, increased oxygen consumption is the major cause of the rapidity of desaturation in infants and small children who are apneic. **Table 20-2** summarizes the developmental differences in respiratory physiology between infants and adults.

In addition to oxygenation issues, development of the respiratory system also affects ventilation. For example, V_{DS}/V_T, the ratio of dead space gas volume to tidal gas volume ventilation, is approximately 33% in neonates and adults.[16] Thus an infant would be expected to have a 7-mL dead space gas volume with a 20-mL tidal gas volume. The addition of a few milliliters of dead space gas volume by the superimposition of anesthetic equipment may increase dead space gas volume from 7 to 12 mL and have a serious effect on V_{DS}/V_T and CO_2 clearance in neonates. The dead space gas volume of all ventilatory equipment, endotracheal tubes, and especially face masks and anesthesia circuitry should be minimized.

CARDIOVASCULAR SYSTEM

The cardiovascular system also undergoes dramatic developmental changes.[17-19] The most obvious and dramatic changes occur perinatally, and these are detailed in the section on perinatal physiology. Even in full-term infants, there is a perioperative risk of complications related to the transitional circulation. Any factor that contributes to pulmonary hypertension (eg, infection, acidosis, hypoxia, hypercarbia, hypothermia, and aspiration) may lead to a serious decrease in cardiac output, hypoxemia, and hypotension. These factors should be avoided in the anesthetic plan for infants.

Multiple developmental changes occur in myocardial function. Changes in the proportion of muscle to connective tissue with development lead to an alteration in myocardial compliance.[18] Developing left ventricular dominance also alters ventricular characteristics. Nearly every determinant of cardiac output (heart rate,[19] contractility,[20] afterload,[21] and preload relationships[22]) undergoes distinct developmental changes (**Fig. 20-4**).[17,23] Although myocardial ischemia only rarely plays a role in the anesthetic management of children, these factors and the varying responses to pharmacologic agents can lead to rapid, and occasionally catastrophic, hemodynamic decompensation in children undergoing anesthesia.[23,24]

In neonates and infants, heart rate is the predominant determinant of cardiac output.[25] The infant's heart is able to sustain greater rates than that of the adult while maintaining preload, contractility, and myocardial oxygenation before there is a decrease in cardiac output (**Fig. 20-5**). **Figure 20-6** shows the normal heart rates for infants and children. Bradycardia can drastically and seriously decrease the cardiac output in infants and children. Increasing cardiac output by increasing heart rate should be considered early in responding to intraoperative decreases in cardiac output as represented by hypotension. Bradycardia

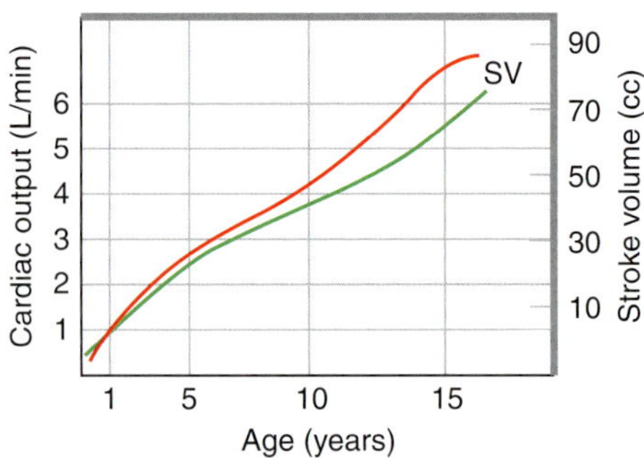

FIGURE 20-4. Stroke volume and cardiac output increase with age. Data from Wetzel RC, Rogers MC. Pediatric hemodynamic monitoring. In: Shoemaker WC, Thompson WL, eds. *Critical Care–State of the Art*. Fullerton, CA: The Society of Critical Care Medicine; 1983.

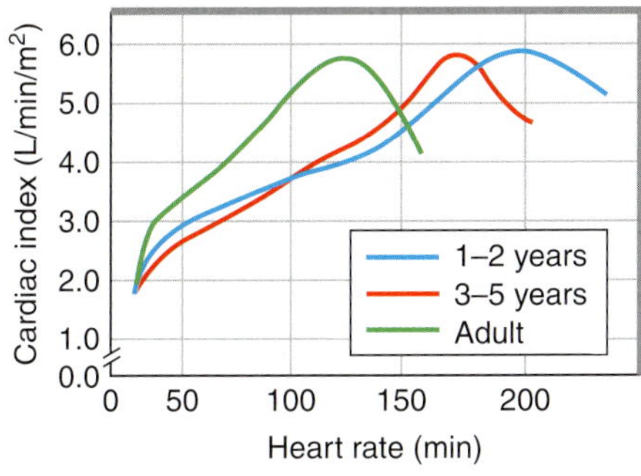

FIGURE 20-5. Cardiac output is shown as it relates to heart rate in healthy children and adults. [Data from Wetzel RC, Rogers MC. Pediatric hemodynamic monitoring. In: Shoemaker WC, Thompson WL, eds. *Critical Care–State of the Art*. Fullerton, CA: The Society of Critical Care Medicine; 1983.]

results from a predisposition to parasympathetic hypertonia, which is common in young children and can be induced by painful stimuli or hypoxia. Laryngoscopy, intubation, eye surgery, airway surgery, abdominal traction, and herniorrhaphy frequently are associated with marked increases in vagal tone and profound bradycardia. Under these circumstances, the cardiac output of the heart rate–dependent infant heart can decrease dramatically. That children adapt to changes in cardiac output by changes in heart rate accounts for the wide ranges in heart rate seen in healthy children. Anesthetic suppression of atrial conduction and loss of P waves on the electrocardiograph with nodal escape rhythms are seen in children during anesthesia, and the resultant bradycardia can be dramatic. Heart-rate depression during anesthesia is readily treated with atropine and is the reason many anesthesiologists make atropine part of any inhalational anesthetic plan in infants and small children. Sinus dysrhythmia, a variation in the heart rate with respirations, is so common in children that it is considered normal, although it can be confused with extra systoles or sinus arrest during anesthesia.

As Friedman originally reported in 1973, the myocardial length–tension relationships vary between the hearts of children and adults, and developmental differences in contractility are clearly seen.[18] These differences are explained by changes in muscle mechanics, innervation, myocardial blood flow, and histologic structure, all of which have been implicated in children's relative inability to increase contractility. Fetal myocardial muscle sarcomeres are active and have about the same contractile power as the adult sarcomere.[18] The fact that neonatal ventricular tissue contains less muscle mass and more noncontractile mass per unit volume than adult tissue accounts for the fact that the neonatal myocardium is less able than the adult myocardium to generate adequate force.[26] The neonatal heart is only innervated partially by the autonomic nervous system (this innervation increases until mid childhood). Therefore, not only is the myocardium less able to develop inotropic force, but sympathetic innervation also is decreased. The Frank-Starling preload relationship also appears to be altered by differences in

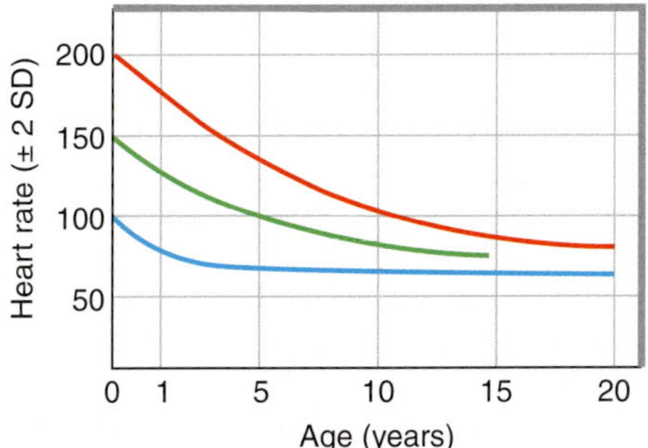

FIGURE 20-6. Normal heart rates +2 standard deviations (SD) shown in relation to age.

TABLE 20-3 Normal Range of Blood Pressures

Age	Mean Systolic/Diastolic
Premature neonates	Systolic 40-60
Full-term neonates	75/50
1-6 months	80/50
6-12 months	90/65
12-24 months	95/65
2-6 years	100/60
6-12 years	110/60
12-16 years	110/65
16-18 years	120/65
Adult	125/75

Approximate ranges: pressure ± 20% = 95% confidence limits. Levels for females are approximately 5% lower than these levels.

Data from Lowry GA. *Growth and Development of Children*. 6th ed. Chicago, IL: Year Book Medical Publishers; 1975; and Report of the Task Force on Blood Pressure Control in Children, National Heart, Lung, and Blood Institute. *Pediatrics*. 1977;59(Suppl):803.

the fiber makeup of the infant myocardium and by the relationship of the right and left ventricles.[18] These changes in compliance characteristics frequently make the infant heart preload insensitive. Volume load may generate higher filling pressures over a narrower proportional range in infants and small children than in adults.[27] Normal adult contractility and compliance is reached between 1 and 2 years of age.

The final determinant of cardiac output—afterload—also changes with age. At birth, systemic resistance greatly increases with removal of the placenta, whereas afterload in the pulmonary circuit decreases dramatically.[26,27] Adjustment to this massively increased afterload in the systemic circulation occurs rapidly, but further increases in afterload may be poorly tolerated in the first year of life. Right and left ventricular mass and wall thickness are relatively equal in neonates. During the next year or so of life, the left ventricle becomes markedly dominant. As a result of the factors mentioned previously, optimal cardiac output occurs at lower filling pressures in neonates compared with adults.[27]

All of these factors lead to optimal cardiovascular function at higher heart rates and lower blood pressures in infants than in adults (Fig. 20-5). Familiarity with the normal range of blood pressures (**Table 20-3**) is essential to guide appropriate intraoperative management.

Congenital heart defects can affect the determinants of cardiac output: heart rate, contractility, preload, afterload, and oxygenation. Left-to-right intracardiac shunting alters preload, potentially alters contractility, and even alters right ventricular afterload as pulmonary vascular resistance increases. Right-to-left shunting affects systemic oxygenation. Valvular disease can increase preload (regurgitant lesions), decrease preload (mitral and tricuspid stenosis), or increase afterload (aortic and pulmonic stenosis). Congenital and surgically acquired lesions can alter conduction and give rise to cardiac dysrhythmias. Thus careful evaluation of all aspects of cardiac function is necessary in assessing children with congenital heart disease. The specific anatomic diagnosis, the presence of intracardiac shunts, and myocardial function all have a bearing on the conduct of the anesthetic in children.

Hemoglobin content and oxygen affinity also vary with age.[28] In the infant born at term, the normal hemoglobin concentration falls dramatically during the first year of life, reaching a nadir at approximately age 2 to 3 months, the so-called physiologic anemia of infancy.[28] Although a physiologic hematocrit at this age could dip below 29%, a hemoglobin of less than 10 g/dL is rare. In the preterm infant, the hemoglobin concentration may fall to between 6 and 8 g/dL within the first 6 to 8 weeks of life.[29] Although not unusual, this should not be considered "physiologic," and the same concern regarding a hematocrit of less than 25% in older children is appropriate. The hematocrit slowly increases to adult levels after puberty. Knowledge of these normal levels is necessary to guide blood transfusion and the timing of elective surgery that may be associated with significant blood loss.

TABLE 20-4 Intravascular Blood Volume

Age	Blood Volume/Kilogram Body Weight (mL/kg)
Infants	
Premature	90-100
Full-term	80-90
<1 y	75-80
1-6 y	70-75
>6 y and adult	65-70

From Wetzel RC. Evaluation of Children. In Longnecker DE, Tinker JH, Morgan GE, et al, eds. *Principles and Practice of Anesthesiology.* Vol I, 2nd ed. St. Louis, MO: Mosby; 1998.

TABLE 20-5 Development of Renal Function

Age	Kidney Weight (g)	GFR/1.73 m² mean ± SD mL/min
Infants		
Term	27	20 ± 4
6 mo	32	77 ± 18
1 y	71	115 ± 25
Children		
2 y	93	127 ± 19
8 y	149	127 ± 19
12 y	191	127 ± 19
Adults	290	131 ± 21

Modified from Chantler C. The kidney. In: Godfrey S, Baum JD, eds. *Clinical Paediatric Physiology.* Oxford, United Kingdom: Blackwell Scientific; 1979.

Circulating blood volume is greater in neonates than in adults on the basis of body weight. Intravascular volume for neonates generally is 80 to 90 mL/kg (**Table 20-4**). Understanding this relative change in total estimated blood volume (EBV) (body weight × estimated blood volume/kg) is necessary when determining allowable blood loss (ABL) in children. The following formula is useful for estimating how much blood children can lose before the hematocrit is unacceptably low (ABL):

$$\text{ABL} = \text{EBV} \times \frac{\text{Hct}_1 - \text{Hct}_2}{\text{Mean Hct}}$$

where Hct_1 is the starting hematocrit, Hct_2 is the minimum desired or allowable hematocrit, and the mean hematocrit is the simple arithmetic mean of $\text{Hct}_1 - \text{Hct}_2$. Thus, in a 12-kg, 1-year-old child with an initial hematocrit of 37% in whom a final hematocrit of 25% is acceptable, the ABL is:

$$\text{ABL} = 12\text{ kg} \times \frac{75\text{ mL}}{\text{kg}} \times \frac{0.37 - 0.25}{0.5(0.25 + 0.37)} = 348\text{ mL}$$

A comparison of the estimate of expected intraoperative loss with the estimate of allowable loss should be made before surgery. If possible, preoperative therapy should be designed to decrease the need for blood transfusion. Iron and nutritional supplements may be beneficial. Erythropoietin should be considered in some children to increase the preoperative hemoglobin concentration when the child is chronically anemic, where there are religious reasons to refuse transfusion, or if the child is erythropoietin deficient (eg, renal disease). Preoperative treatment with erythropoietin has been advocated to increase the hematocrit in children to facilitate autotransfusion, either in directed autotransfusion with preoperative blood collection, or to facilitate intraoperative autotransfusion.[30]

RENAL FUNCTION

Renal function changes dramatically with age.[31] For example, glomerular filtration rate (GFR)/1.73 m² changes from less than 40 mL/min at birth to 100 mL/min in the first year of life, which compares with 130 mL/min in adults (**Table 20-5**). These changes in renal function and GFR are accompanied by changes in the ability to regulate salt and water metabolism and by responses to changes in antidiuretic hormone (ADH) that occur during anesthesia.[32] Although the factors regulating neonatal kidney function are complex in the transitional phase, the net result is that water is excreted in excess of sodium. The neonatal kidney wastes sodium, and there is a tendency toward hyponatremia in the premature and full-term neonate.[33] The kidney of the full-term infant is able to conserve sodium.[33,34] The ability of the kidney to concentrate urine is limited, and maximal osmolarity may be only 700 mOsm/L in infants.[31,32] Thus infants are less able to defend intravascular volume against water deprivation.

Complete maturation of renal function usually occurs by approximately age 2 years. These developmental aspects of renal function have an effect on pharmacology. The effects of these changes are most prominent in the first few months of life and require careful fluid management in neonates and attention to sodium and potassium balance.[34] Blood pressure regulation and the characteristics of hypertensive renal disease also show distinct differences in children.[35] In children with renal disease, hypertension should be looked for because intraoperative blood pressure regulation may be difficult.

DENTITION

Although teeth occasionally are present at birth, they may not erupt until nearly 1 year of age. The mean age for the development of the first tooth, usually a lower incisor, is around 6 months. By 1 year, children usually have upper and lower teeth present. By age 6 years, permanent teeth begin to appear, and the average 6-year-old has an intubation gap between the front incisors. The importance of deciduous teeth is that they fall out, and they should not fall out during anesthesia. Children younger than 12 years of age, especially those with loose incisors at around age 6 years, should be questioned and examined for the presence of loose teeth. Loose and carious teeth are at increased risk for dislodgment by the placement of oral airways, laryngoscope blades, and endotracheal tubes. A history of endotracheal intubation in the neonatal period is associated with subsequent development of abnormal dentition in neonates.[36] Whether this is a result of direct trauma from the laryngoscope or from long-term placement of an endotracheal tube is not clear.[37] Attention to children's oropharynx and condition of dentition is an essential part of the anesthetic evaluation.

GASTROINTESTINAL SYSTEM

Developmental changes in the gastrointestinal (GI) tract also have important anesthetic implications. At birth, gastric pH is alkalotic; however, by the second day of life, the normal physiologic range of gastric pH is achieved. The secretion and amount of gastric contents in full-term infants is similar to that of adults. Although fasting gastric contents and pH in children are similar to those in adults, the reflex coordination of swallowing and lower esophageal sphincter (LES) function is not fully mature until age 6 months.[38-40] Slack LES tone with reflux is common in this age group. This is relevant to the question of preoperative fasting. The maintenance of low residual gastric volumes by nothing-by-mouth (NPO) regulations (a questionable assumption) should be balanced against the propensity of fasting children to develop hypoglycemia.[38,39] This especially is true if the infants or children are born prematurely, small for gestational age (SGA), nutritionally deprived, or with increased metabolic needs because of conditions such as fever, sepsis, increased respiratory effort, or the condition that requires surgery. To ensure a suitable period of fasting, especially in small, ill children, preoperative intravenous (IV) supplementation with dextrose-containing solutions is indicated.

Development of the GI tract generally is complete at birth. Problems caused by congenital malformations or developmental anomalies generally are obvious within the first few days after birth.[38] Upper GI obstruction (eg, duodenal atresia, malrotation) is indicated by bilious vomiting and regurgitation within the first few days of life. Lower intestinal anomalies (eg, volvulus or atresia of the small or large bowel) are manifested by failure to pass stools and by abdominal distension. Pyloric stenosis, another major cause of GI dysfunction in the first year of life, usually presents between ages 3 and 6 weeks. Its major symptoms are failure to gain weight and projectile vomiting.

The liver in neonates and young infants is functionally immature. This functional immaturity generally is a result of 2 main causes: (1) the development and growth of enzyme systems that, although present at birth, are not fully induced, and (2) relatively decreased hepatic blood flow.[41] The ability of the liver to conjugate and catabolize circulating substrate and pharmacologic substances is diminished at birth. For this reason, drugs tend to have longer half-lives in neonates compared with older children. This functional immaturity of the liver is reflected by decreased concentrations of products of hepatic synthesis, such as albumin, in neonates.[42] These decreased concentrations lead to decreased protein binding of many pharmacologic agents, which alters pharmacokinetics and pharmacodynamics.[43,44] Hepatic function usually reaches adult levels within the first few months of life.

THERMOREGULATION

Perhaps no area is of greater concern to the pediatric anesthesiologist than the need to maintain normal body temperature perioperatively. The need for thermoregulatory control is underemphasized in adults but is critical in the treatment of children. Defending the thermoneutrality of infants has been a cornerstone of pediatrics since the 19th century. In 1900, Pierre-Constant Boudin demonstrated that there were striking differences in the survival of infants weighing less than 2000 g that depended solely on their rectal temperatures.[45] The mortality rate for infants with core temperatures less than 95°F (35°C) was greater than 90% and for those with temperatures greater than 95°F (35°C) was only 23%. Boudin designed an incubator that provided heated air and humidity and then conclusively demonstrated that its use could dramatically improve the survival of neonates.[45] This observation found its way to Julius Hays Hess, who is considered the founder of premature care in North America.[46] He recognized the importance of these observations and, in 1922, opened the first premature infant center at the Michael Reese Hospital in Chicago.

Thermoregulation is a complex process involving peripheral and central thermoreceptors, the central nervous system (CNS), and hypothalamic integration with central thermoreceptors.[47] A complex integration of responses leads to alterations in cutaneous blood flow and thermogenesis from shivering and nonshivering sources.[48] This complex system is necessary to maintain mammalian core temperature within a normal range. Sources of heat production include basal metabolism, movement, shivering thermogenesis, and nonshivering thermogenesis. Basal metabolism is responsible for the greatest amount of baseline heat production. Shivering thermogenesis is the uncontrolled, rapid contraction of skeletal muscles and is common on emergence from anesthesia in older patients. Nonshivering thermogenesis is under direct control of the autonomic nervous system and produces heat by mobilizing fat from muscles, liver, and brain.[49] Although neonates metabolize both white and brown fat, brown fat is used by neonates to a greater extent than by adults. This is important because neonates cannot respond to cold stress with shivering thermogenesis until age 6 months to 1 year. Brown fat is distributed around the back of the neck, mediastinum, and interscapular regions, and around the kidneys and adrenals. Brown fat owes its color to a high content of mitochondria and rich blood supply, which mirror its metabolic capability. Brown fat metabolism increases heat production when stimulated by autonomic catecholamine release.[49] Cold stress also leads to norepinephrine secretion, which causes adipocytes to release glycerol and fatty acids from brown fat depots. Brown fat metabolism provides the only possibility of increasing body temperature in the immobile, anesthetized infant with decreased metabolic rate. Cardiac output is diverted from other organs to brown fat depots. Vasoconstriction of the systemic and pulmonary circulations occurs as a result of norepinephrine release. Consequently, cold stress can lead to peripheral vasoconstriction, pulmonary vasoconstriction, decreased cardiac output, and shunting of cardiac output away from other organ systems to brown fat depots, all of which may pose a serious threat to neonates. Importantly, inhalational anesthetics inhibit brown fat-dependent thermogenesis, which explains the propensity of neonates to become hypothermic during inhalational anesthesia.[50] This complex system can compensate for heat loss, but at a high cost. Avoiding cold stress is preferred.

During anesthesia, environmental challenges to thermal integrity should be minimized, especially as inhalational anesthetics inhibit brown fat thermogenesis.[50] Hypothermia increases cardiorespiratory demand because of increased oxygen demand and the need for thermogenesis and alters every basic enzyme system. Environmental cold stress in neonates leads to increased oxygen consumption, hypoxia, acidosis, respiratory distress, depletion of glycogen stores, hypoglycemia, pulmonary vasoconstriction, pulmonary hypertension with persistence of the fetal circulation, shock, and even disseminated intravascular coagulation. Altered drug metabolism, delayed emergence, prolongation of the effects of neuromuscular blocking agents, and other pharmacologic effects accent the need for intraoperative thermoregulatory control in children.[46]

Heat loss occurs through 4 basic mechanisms: conduction, convection, radiation, and evaporation. Each of these, under certain circumstances, can be the major cause of heat loss. Conductive heat losses can be eliminated by minimizing the direct contact of children with surfaces colder than themselves. The use of a warming pad or heating blanket in the operating room can eliminate heat loss to the cold operating room table. Warming of the operating room greatly reduces conductive heat loss. Convective heat losses can be further limited by the use of an incubator, by surgical drapes, and warm blankets for the child. Radiant heat losses also should be minimized. Heat is radiated to objects of lower temperature. Warming objects in the patient's environment will lead to decreased radiant losses. This is the principle that underlies "radiant" neonatal warmers.[51] The use of double-walled incubators decreases radiant losses. Transportation of neonates to the operating room in double-walled isolettes probably is optimal, but the use of radiant warmers that minimize convective loss also is acceptable. Finally, evaporative losses intraoperatively should be curtailed to minimize heat loss.

The use of warmed solutions for skin preparation and irrigation is important. The use of heated humidified air for ventilation also contributes to the thermoregulatory control of children. It is the Children's Hospital of Los Angeles' routine practice to use humidifiers in all pediatric circuits, maintain warm operating rooms with a high humidity, and use heating pads for all children who are anesthetized. For newborns and small neonates, the operating room should be maintained at 80°F (26.7°C), for infants ages 0 to 6 months at 78°F (25.6°C), and for children age 6 months to 2 years at 76°F (24.4°C), always maintaining a minimum of 80% humidity. Warming of intravascular fluids and rapidly transfused blood also is necessary. Factors that contribute to infants becoming cold are basically related to their large surface-area-to-mass ratio. In addition, areas richly supplied with blood, such as the head and cranial vault, are proportionally larger in infants, giving rise to heat loss. In premature neonates, this situation is aggravated by their decreased subcutaneous tissue. Some method should be used to eliminate heat loss from the skin surface, especially the head, such as the use of plastic wraps and blankets. Convective warming with forced warm air devices is probably more effective than conductive (heat pad) warming and appears to decrease postoperative thermal stress when used in the recovery area.[52,53]

GENERAL PRINCIPLES OF PEDIATRIC PHARMACOLOGY

The developmental differences among neonates, infants, and adults impact pediatric pharmacology. Until recently, our understanding of pediatric pharmacology was at best sketchy and at worst incorrect. Pharmacokinetic principles that govern the distribution and metabolism of anesthetic agents in adults are not directly applicable to children. Pediatric drug dosages initially were determined by calculating the proportionate amount of an adult dose on a weight basis. Some assumptions about converting adult dosages to children's dosages on a per kilogram, surface area, or age basis have been proven incorrect.[43] Perhaps no other area demonstrates more clearly that children are not small adults. There are many reasons why merely scaling down dosages on a per-kilogram basis does not yield equivalent drug concentrations or pharmacologic effects. During the development from fetus to adult, factors that affect drug uptake, distribution, metabolism, and sensitivity to drugs change. Volume of distribution, elimination half-lives, drug sensitivity, side effects, organ function, protein binding, and clearance undergo major changes with age.

Complex issues of clinical investigation contribute to the poor knowledge of pharmacokinetics in children. Medicolegal and ethical issues affect the ability to obtain data directly applicable to children. These factors have resulted in a largely empiric approach to pediatric anesthesia. This empiricism is yielding to better-designed, better-informed studies in small children, aided by the advent of microassay techniques that require smaller volumes of blood sampling. There are now several excellent studies of the pharmacokinetics of many agents, including local anesthetics, narcotics, and sedatives, and of the uptake and distribution of inhalational agents in children.

DRUG ADMINISTRATION

Anesthetic agents may be delivered orally, rectally, transnasally, percutaneously, conjunctivally, intramuscularly, intravenously, or by inhalation. Administration of drugs across mucous membranes requires passive diffusion, which depends on the concentration and the chemical properties of the agents used and on the amount of surface area exposed. The fact that agents are absorbed across the mucous membrane in the rectum has made this route of administration popular for numerous sedatives and induction agents, such as fentanyl, methohexital, midazolam, thiopental, and ketamine.[54] Because the degree of ionization generally depends on pH and surface area, formulation is particularly important. Rectal absorption is generally slow and uneven, but can be enhanced by large volumes of dilute solutions, which come in contact with a greater surface area.[55] Analgesic agents also can be administered by this route, allowing mild analgesia without the need for oral administration perioperatively. This route is acceptable for most children younger than 5 years old.

Intranasal and transconjunctival administration of benzodiazepines, ketamine, and narcotics has been reported.[56-58] Formulation, solubility characteristics, desired end points, and concentration affect the rapidity, duration, and depth of sedation and define an agent's suitability to induce anesthesia. Novel formulations, such as oral transmucosal fentanyl citrate, have yet to find a place in routine clinical practice.[54,59]

Intramuscular administration is not recommended in children because of pain on injection and pain after injection, which may last for several days.[60] Induction, neuromuscular blocking, and analgesic agents may be administered intramuscularly. When no other route of administration of an induction agent is possible, intramuscular ketamine (5-10 mg/kg) might achieve anesthetic induction in agitated, uncooperative children within 5 to 7 minutes. Although intramuscular administration of narcotics is time-honored, it is generally avoided. Administration of diazepam is associated with burning and muscle pain; however, water-soluble midazolam appears to be less irritating. Pain on injection and its variable duration make intramuscular administration rarely used in children.[60]

The distribution of drugs administered intravenously depends on many factors, most of which are affected by developmental changes. Degree of binding to circulating blood elements, such as proteins and erythrocytes, blood–tissue partition coefficients, distribution of blood flow to various tissue beds, and changes in tissue volumes, affect the distribution of intravenously administered agents.

DRUG DISTRIBUTION

The existence of the free, nonbound, water-soluble moiety in the circulation is required for a drug to cross the endothelium and other cell membranes (where its effect is achieved) and for plasma clearance. The bulk of protein binding is by albumin; however, α_1-acid glycoprotein also is a significant circulating protein to which drugs bind. The concentration of the latter and its contribution to protein binding appear to be greater in older children than in adults. In contrast, infants have low concentrations of α_1-acid glycoprotein, therefore, they may have a larger, unbound, circulating concentration of certain drugs.[61] Curare, metocurine, propranolol, lidocaine, bupivacaine, digoxin, barbiturates, and narcotics demonstrate protein binding. Their protein affinities have a major effect on the pharmacokinetics of drugs in infants and children. Because the protein-bound fraction acts as a reservoir for the drug to maintain tissue and plasma concentrations, concomitant presence of substances that displace drugs from binding sites, such as bilirubin in the neonate, will alter the pharmacology of highly protein-bound agents. Substances that reduce protein binding include free fatty acids, maternal steroids, and sulfonamides. Protein binding affects a drug's volume of distribution. Agents that are poorly protein bound have a larger apparent volume of distribution because the free drug penetrates tissues more easily. Thus a reduction in plasma protein binding causes an increase in the apparent volume of distribution, which partially explains the large volume of distribution frequently found in neonates. Nearly twice as much barbiturate and morphine is bound in the neonatal CNS as compared with what is bound in adults and older children, at least partly as a result of reduced plasma protein binding in neonates.[62] Plasma protein binding also may have a major effect on determination of blood–gas and blood–tissue partition coefficients and leads to developmental differences in uptake and distribution of anesthetics.[63]

The developmental changes of blood flow to various tissue compartments and body fluid composition cause differences in drug distribution with increasing age.[43] Distribution is altered by the relatively small muscle mass and fat stores in neonates, which results in greater flow to the central organs, such as the liver, brain, blood, heart, and kidneys. A water-soluble drug may require a larger initial dosage to achieve a desired blood level. This is relevant for most antibiotics and, most notably, for succinylcholine. The increased volume of distribution also has an effect on clearance, causing delayed excretion and metabolism and prolonged half-lives. A further effect of change in body composition is seen with fat-soluble drugs. Drugs that rely on redistribution into fat for the termination of their therapeutic effects, such as thiopental, may have a more prolonged clinical effect in younger children. Those that redistribute into muscle, such as narcotics, also have a prolonged effect.[64]

Other factors may alter the uptake and distribution of anesthetic agents. First is the change in the blood–brain barrier that occurs perinatally.[15,43] The integrity of the blood–brain barrier is immature at birth. Because many anesthetic drugs are lipid-soluble, this leads to a more rapid uptake of anesthetic agents by the neonatal CNS than occurs in adults. The proportion of blood flow to the brain is higher in neonates than in adults, and for highly lipid-soluble drugs, diffusion across the blood–brain barrier leads to higher brain concentrations and a larger apparent volume of distribution in neonates compared with adults. A second factor that may affect uptake of anesthetic agents arises from differences in dose–response relationships, which may result from receptor affinities, changes in receptor density, or sensitivity with age. With uptake and distribution considered, the minimum alveolar concentration (MAC) of inhalational anesthetics, the hypnotic dose of thiopental, and the sensitivity to succinylcholine have age-related differences that can be explained by potential differences in receptor sensitivity to these agents.

The termination of a drug's effect depends on distribution, metabolism, and excretion. Distribution, as shown previously, varies dramatically with age. Drug metabolism and the enzyme systems responsible, especially cytochrome P450 and hepatic conjugation, also undergo distinct developmental changes.[15,62] Finally, the developmental differences in renal function also have an effect on the clearance and termination of drug effects.

Myriad developmental differences and multiple factors varying dramatically with age determine the uptake, distribution, metabolism, and excretion of anesthetic agents. Thus it is not surprising that there is no simple relationship between age and a dosage calculated on a milligrams per kilogram basis.

PREOPERATIVE EVALUATION AND PREPARATION

Examining and preparing children for anesthesia and surgery require a specialized approach because of the unique physiologic and psychological needs of children and their families. The same basic goals of preoperative examination that should be achieved in adults also are applicable to children, but in addition, the emotional and psychological needs of not only the child but the child's family should be addressed. Familiarity with the specific perioperative needs of children and their families is necessary for the anesthesiologist to obtain an appropriate history, physical examination, and thorough preoperative evaluation from a wailing infant, a hyperactive child, or a shy, frightened 5-year-old, without undue trauma for all concerned. In these situations, although it may be difficult, it is necessary to thoroughly examine children. Understanding the physiology and psychology of children is necessary.[65,66]

PURPOSE

The two goals of preoperative evaluation are (1) for the anesthesiologist to obtain, through interview history and physical examination of the patient, information pertinent to the child's physiologic and emotional preparedness for surgery; and (2) for the patient, to allay the anxieties of the child and parent and prepare them for surgery. Both of these goals are important and should be viewed as necessarily compatible in the anesthetic treatment of children. From the outset, both goals should be constantly kept in mind (**Box 20-1**).

The anesthesiologist's first contact with the child and family necessarily sets the stage for the remainder of the anesthesia management. The information obtained and the interactions that occur during the preoperative evaluation will determine the quality of the intraoperative management and the postoperative recovery. Although this is obvious when examining the physiologic status of the child, which is used to guide the choice of preoperative medication, induction agent, and anesthetic maintenance, as well as the postoperative requirements, it likewise is true for addressing the emotional and psychological needs of the child and family. Not only should the preoperative evaluation familiarize the anesthesiologist with the child and the parents, it also should provide an excellent and critical opportunity for the child and family to become comfortable with the anesthesiologist and to understand the anesthesiologist's responsibilities. The preconceived notions of children and their families about the events that will occur in the perioperative period and the personnel with whom they will interact form the background for the preoperative interview. The skilled and experienced anesthesiologist is aware of these preconceptions and addresses them whether or not they are mentioned by the child or the family. This anticipatory approach to the child's needs frequently smoothes the path for induction and emergence from anesthesia for the child, the family, and, not unimportantly, the anesthesiologist.

The key to smooth anesthetic management is not only the complete familiarity of the anesthesiologist with the child's medical and psychoemotional background, but also of the child's and family's understanding of the procedures associated with anesthesia and surgery. A comfortable and competent anesthesiologist, familiar with all aspects of the perioperative course of surgery in children, is able to optimize this experience for all concerned. This approach applies to infants or older children, as well as to inpatients and outpatients. The exact setting and the child's unique characteristics determine the specific technique for dealing with each circumstance. Whereas it may be necessary in one case to separate the child from the family early and use preoperative sedation, in another case, parental presence during induction and emergence may be the optimal approach. The knowledge and experience of the anesthesiologist are important in determining which approach is best for which child.

The first objective of preoperative examination and preparation is to ensure that the child is in his or her optimal status for the procedure planned. The question of whether or not the child can tolerate the anesthetic and surgery is less relevant than in the past. Pediatric anesthesiologists are capable of providing the most advanced physiologic support for children who require complex surgery. It almost always is possible to provide monitored critical care and analgesia for any surgical procedure. What does vary from patient to patient is not the ability of the anesthesiologist to deliver anesthesia care and ensure survival, but the risk to the child for each set of circumstances. The all-important question of whether the anesthetic and surgical risk to the child is greater than the benefits of the procedure should be addressed. Concerns of survival largely are replaced by a precise, accurate, and clear evaluation of the risks of anesthesia for each child, which then can be realistically compared with the child's surgical needs. The underlying goal is that for each child, given the circumstances, the best possible preoperative status will be attained for the procedure. This varies tremendously if the child is undergoing decompression of an epidural hematoma after a traffic accident in which the child has sustained bilateral femoral fractures, a ruptured spleen, pulmonary contusion, and intracranial injury with little time for preoperative assessment compared with myringotomy in a child with Down syndrome and a recently diagnosed atrioventricular canal defect who also happens to be wheezing. Both of these children can be anesthetized and are likely to survive the anesthetic; however, the wisdom of immediately proceeding varies considerably based on the results of an analysis of the specific risk-to-benefit relationship.

It is the anesthesiologist's responsibility to ensure that an accurate assessment of the risks and benefits of the anesthetic is as clear as possible to the child, the parents, the surgeon, where necessary the operating room (OR) team, and the pediatrician. Careful attention to these details is essential in evaluating and preparing children for anesthesia. Questions of preoperative preparation, timing of surgery, specific surgical procedure, and anesthetic plan are within the anesthesiologist's purview. These should be addressed by the anesthesiologist in the preoperative evaluation. A thorough and adequate examination of the child is essential for identifying and predicting physiologic as well as psychological and emotional problems that the child might encounter intraoperatively and postoperatively.[65,67] The anesthesiologist, armed with this extensive background information, can provide the best intraoperative care and advise on postoperative treatment (**Box 20-2**).

BOX 20-1

Purposes of Preoperative Evaluation

Prepare the anesthesiologist

Prepare the child and family

Prepare the OR team

BOX 20-2

Preparation for Surgery

Goal

- Optimal physical and mental status for surgery

Contingencies

- Medical judgment
- Optimization of medical therapy
- Timing
- Psychoprophylaxis of child and family

BOX 20-3

Sources of Parental Anxiety

- Anesthesia complications
  - Brain damage
  - Death
- Results of surgery
  - Disfigurement
  - Dismemberment
  - Death
- Separation, loss of control
- Hostility generated by
  - Poor information and communication
  - Apparent lack of due concern by caregivers and physicians

GENERAL APPROACH

Preconceptions It is essential to understand some of the preconceived notions that the child and family may have acquired from society and the surgeon. Most parents think that anesthesia is a source of some risk to their child; the spectrum may vary from fear of postoperative nausea, vomiting, headaches, and behavioral disturbances, to fear of a serious threat to the child's life. It is important to recognize, inquire about, and address these issues because these preconceptions frequently differ from the anesthesiologist's view.

Whereas the anesthesiologist may view a child whose American Society of Anesthesiologists physical status (ASA PS) score is P1 for a unilateral myringotomy as being at extremely low risk and very low on the anxiety scale, parents do not necessarily always appreciate this (**Box 20-3**). They frequently may demonstrate a parental "Moro response" to any perceived threat to their child, no matter how trivial the threat. Any threat to their child naturally may trigger defensive and protective responses, as well as high levels of anxiety in families. The underlying concerns and anxieties experienced by parents of children undergoing what to anesthesia caregivers may be a routine procedure frequently do not qualitatively differ from those of parents whose children have been admitted to the pediatric intensive care unit. For parents of former premature infants and critically ill children, the perception of vulnerability, not surprisingly, heightens anxiety.[68] Although anesthesia caregivers may consider this parental response inappropriate, it is important to recognize that the parents of a child undergoing a routine procedure may be terribly concerned for their child's well-being. A sympathetic and understanding approach to this parental response is a crucial ingredient of expert management. Ensuring calm, informed, confident parents is frequently the most essential aspect of ensuring calm, cooperative children. Terrified, nervous, defensive, angry, ill-informed parents are incapable of allaying their child's anxieties for the upcoming procedure.[69] Time taken to explain, answer questions, anticipate and allay anxieties, and demonstrate care and concern for the child is time well spent.

Areas of Childhood Anxiety Childhood anxieties in the perioperative period center on 5 areas (**Box 20-4**).[66] The first, fear of injury is universal; fear of death (even for minor procedures) often is present. Fear of pain and the potential for resulting body disfigurement is common. Second, fear of parental separation (separation anxiety) is common in children age 6 months or older and can be a concern in adolescents. Common sense dictates that the less time the conscious child is separated from the parents the better for all concerned. Apart from obvious humanitarian concerns, a calm, comfortable, nonscreaming child is more aesthetic physiologically and is better able to tolerate anesthesia and surgery than a distraught child.[69] The third area of anxiety that correlates with the developmental stage of separation—individuation—concerns fears centered on the loss of individuality and autonomy, which may be a source of considerable stress in children. Taking a child who has spent several years learning to walk, who is comfortable away from his or her parents only for short times, and who has independent control of major functions, and suddenly reducing the child to lying on his or her back, surrounded by what appear to be giants, with no control of the situation, certainly provokes anxiety. Along with the loss of autonomy is the threatened loss of function and loss of control that were won so recently. Anything that can be done to encourage and enhance the child's autonomy and control of the situation, such as allowing choices (eg, position [sitting, lying, standing], method of induction, which stuffed animal to bring to the operating room, or color of gown) can help calm the child's fears.

BOX 20-4

Sources of Childhood Anxiety

- Fear of pain, injury, and death
- Fear of parental separation
- Fear of loss of autonomy
- Fear of the unknown
- Fear of punishment

The fourth issue is fear of the unknown. Children often are intimidated by the new. Most children will not have undergone either anesthesia or surgery in the past, and this generates anxiety. Recognition of this issue, followed by frank, honest, and as complete a disclosure as possible of the procedures and occurrences that the child will experience is necessary. The child's knowledge reduces the dark, mysterious areas of ignorance and uncertainty. The phrases "it won't hurt" or "you have nothing to worry about" can be some of the most anxiety-provoking words an anesthesiologist can utter. The child knows it is not true and suspects a coverup.

The fifth area, and perhaps the least obvious, is the child's fear of breaching behavioral standards and eliciting from authority figures, including parents, a reprimand. The fear of transgression and punishment is a characteristic underlying anxiety of childhood (and frequently extends into adulthood) and may be a major source of concern to the child. Explaining the permissibility of crying appropriately, of expressing anxiety and fear about the procedure, and of having a negative attitude toward the procedure, thus validating the child's emotions, decreases the anxiety associated with this childhood concern.

These areas should be always remembered and addressed consciously by the anesthesiologist in his or her approach to the child.[65,66] Openness, honesty, and cheerful confidence are the main tools for allaying child and family anxieties and in producing a setting that is most conducive to obtaining information by history and by physical examination. Children are capable of seeing through fraud and spotting lack of confidence. Once their trust is lost, the ability to provide them with the best anesthesia care also is lost. Honestly telling a child that an IV start might be unsuccessful and will be painful is preferable to saying "it won't hurt" and then repeating this painful procedure unsuccessfully several times. Spending the extra time to gently talk a child through a mask inhalational induction frequently may be more rewarding (although more time consuming) for the child, the parent, and the anesthesiologist than walking into the room and, with little preparation, jabbing a needle in the child's thigh. Developing the skills necessary to approach children and their families increases the facility with which the anesthesiologist provides the best anesthesia care and increases the rewards of anesthesia practice.[70,71]

Developmental Stage Just as an adult approach is inappropriate for the child, so is an approach that does not consider the developmental stage of the child. The anesthesiologist's approach to a 6-month-old infant is different from the approach taken with a 14-year-old pubertal adolescent. Developmental stage determines approach (**Table 20-6**).

TABLE 20-6 Developmental Behavior

Age	Stage	Characteristics
0-6 mo	Infantile	No expression Passivity Dependence
9 mo-5 y		Separation–individuation Communicative Separation anxiety Poor reality perception Developing independence
5 y-adolescent	Childhood	Imaginative rationale Self-focused Fearful Limited expressiveness

From Wetzel RC. Evaluation of children. In: Longnecker DE, Tinker JH, Morgan GE, et al, eds. *Principles and Practice of Anesthesiology.* Vol I, 2nd ed. St. Louis, MO: Mosby; 1998.

Neonates and Infants Younger Than 6 Months Probably because infants and neonates are unable to express themselves, it is assumed that the psychological ramifications of separation and surgery are minimal. This assumption may be as erroneous as the assumption by earlier medical practitioners that infants were unable to feel pain. Although infants do not have the apparent adverse responses to strangers that are seen in older children (older than 6 months of age) and can be comforted by a nurse or physician, they unquestionably recognize their mother and are comforted by her presence.[72] Consequently, it is judicious to minimize the time children are separated from their parents. For this age group, although direct psychological preparation of children is not possible, parental preparation can form the basis of the approach to neonates and young infants. Experience indicates that fretful, anxious, uptight parents frequently convey this attitude to their young infants. Psychological preparation should be directed toward the child's family. Parents know that anesthesia and surgery present a threat to adults and reason that this threat is much greater for frail infants. Specifically addressing this frequent, although false, assumption and pointing out that a robust infant undergoing routine surgery is more likely to recover rapidly from the stress of surgery and anesthesia than a grandparent or a parent is important. Such information can alleviate anxiety and remarkably calm the parents, who, in turn, calm the infant.

Nine Months to 5 Years Older infants and preschool children ages approximately 9 months to 5 years are in a difficult stage. They are aware of their environment and surroundings, are able to perceive a threat, and can remember painful experiences. Unfortunately, this is combined with an inability to reason and a poor perception of reality. Although these children are able to recognize stressful situations, they are unable to express their fears by modes of communication other than crying, regressive behaviors, sullen withdrawal, or other nonspecific responses to stressful situations.[73] Even though it may not be possible to determine exactly what is most disturbing to a child, attention to the areas mentioned previously and a specific explanation can alleviate their concerns. There is value in explaining what is going to happen and in familiarizing the child with the procedure, even though the child might not appear to be receptive. If this has no benefit other than to demonstrate the anesthesiologist's concern for the child's well-being to the parents, it is worthwhile.

Five Years to Adolescence This developmental stage of childhood is characterized by an increasing capability of expression and reasoning. Gaining control over behavioral and emotional responses is one of the major tasks of this period. The ability to understand and trust adults, even strangers, generally develops during this time. Disclosure of anesthetic procedures and careful, honest, and compassionate explanation of the events that surround surgery generally is rewarded in this age group. Explaining to the child and parents the anesthesiologist's role and what happens during the perioperative period decreases anxiety. In this age group, and throughout adolescence, children's imaginations are well developed. Frequently, this imagination, aided and abetted by exposure to the hyperkinetic modern media (eg, television), can lead to vivid and distorted anticipation of what actually goes on inside an operating room. As much realistic exposure to personnel, equipment, and methods of dress as possible before the procedure may drive some of these vivid, preconceived, and frequently terrifying notions from the child's (and parents') mind.[66,70] It often is informative to ask the child what he or she anticipates, and, if one is fortunate to have a communicative child, this can be worthwhile and permit the practitioner to directly assess and address the child's concerns.

In older children and adolescents, an underlying fear is that of death. This fear may be reinforced by well-meaning parents, friends, and adults, as well as by medical personnel. Saying that the child "will be put to sleep" or the anesthesiologist's reference to "getting him down" may be counterproductive. Unfortunately, these statements may remind a child of what happened to a pet. In adolescents, the fear of death can be strong, and this, coupled with the loss of control and autonomy that accompanies anesthesia, frequently worries children and teenagers. Talking expectantly and openly about the postoperative period is worthwhile. Discussing how the child will feel and what steps will be taken to awaken him or her and to relieve pain will confidently lead the child away from any notion that he or she will not awaken after surgery.

A "macho" attitude in teenagers may lead them to be trapped in silence with their fears. In dealing with adolescents, it is worthwhile to specifically ask if they have any fears and specifically ask if there is concern about pain and dying. The frequency with which these questions are answered affirmatively is revealing. Understanding these underlying anxieties and specifically, honestly, and openly addressing them is valuable and certainly rewards the time required to do it. This is true even if the adolescent bravely denies such fears.

PREOPERATIVE PSYCHOLOGIC PREPARATION

Psychologic preoperative preparation begins for children before coming to the hospital. Informing the parents that they should explain openly and honestly to the child what is about to occur can begin the child's psychological preparation at home.[74] Honesty and an open demeanor cannot be overemphasized as the cornerstones of this reassurance.[69-71] Many hospitals have programs for inpatients and outpatients designed to introduce children and their families to the hospital and operative setting in an enjoyable manner. There are many alternatives for accomplishing these goals, including a preoperative film, a puppet show, a coloring book, a tour of the hospital, and a friendly meeting with doctors and nurses.[71,72] Selecting from these options is not as important as implementing a program to ensure that the child's association with the hospital or surgical center begins on a positive note. This provides a major contribution to the preoperative preparation of children. Younger children, and occasionally older children, should be encouraged to bring familiar things to the hospital. They should bring their stuffed animals and their own pajamas, arrive in their own clothes, and be allowed to retain them as long as possible. Comforting, familiar books and toys certainly should be encouraged. Parents should be reminded of the importance of this. Encouraging older children to be involved in the planning of the surgery also can be beneficial. Allowing them to select the time of surgery and participate in the planning process can raise the young adult's spirits and reassure the child.

During the preoperative evaluation, it should be remembered that the evaluation is a 2-way process. Not only does the medical establishment (whether it is a nurse, nurse practitioner, or anesthesiologist) gain information pertinent to the anesthetic management of the child, but also the child and family gain information that is useful for building confidence and anxiolysis about the anesthesiologist and hospital setting. It is useful to remember that throughout the interview with the family, the child is the center of attention.[71] The battle may be lost with the parent and child if the anesthesiologist interacts only with the parent to obtain information about the child, tells the parent the procedure, and leaves the room. The initial contact should be made with the child with a cheerful greeting and an attempt made to win the child's confidence before beginning the medical interview. Assuring the child that the main intent is not to inflict injury but to get to know him or her is crucial. No one will appreciate this more than the parents. Making it clear to the child and family that the anesthesiologist takes the child's procedure as seriously as the child does and is there to help, not only during the painful times but also during the anxiety-provoking times, is beneficial. Explanations of how the child will awaken and what will be done to manage pain are worthwhile.

Many parents will expect to be with their child during the induction of anesthesia. This may frequently be a pleasant experience for the child, parent, and practitioner. The benefit for the child has been greatly debated recently.[71] Parents seem to prefer to be present, whereas practitioners prefer they are not. The focus should be on the child and, after much study, parental presence does not appear to provide a significant benefit over preoperative medication. Clearly, tearing a terrified child away from the comforting arms of a parent is difficult for the child, the parent, and the caregivers. If this parental separation cannot be achieved comfortably with preoperative psychoprophylaxis and behavioral modification as described previously, or with pharmacologic means, such as preoperative medications including benzodiazepine and barbiturates, then there may be a need to defer parent–child separation until general anesthesia has been induced. Medicating the child preoperatively with an oral benzodiazepine more frequently provides smooth, calm conditions for induction than does parental presence without medication.[65] A confident, competent anesthesia practitioner may be able to reduce the need for preoperative medication. Parental presence appears neither to decrease emergence phenomena nor the incidence of postoperative behavioral changes and does not add an advantage over that provided by preoperative sedative medication, such as oral midazolam.

PREOPERATIVE EVALUATION

Just as psycho-emotional preoperative preparation of the child should begin before the anesthesiologist meets the child, the anesthesiologist also should have prepared before the meeting. The anesthesiologist should be familiar with the surgery that the child requires, the surgeon's needs, and the anesthetic implications of the surgical procedure. The anesthesiologist should be as familiar as possible with the child's medical background as documented in the medical records. Communication with the pediatrician and surgeon before meeting the child and family will reveal areas of particular interest to the anesthesiologist before the interview.[74] An anesthesiologist who is aware of the child's name, age, general background, medical problems, and surgical procedure and who has communicated with the child's pediatrician and surgeon is in a strong position to win the confidence of the child and family. When a child has an extensive previous medical history, it is worthwhile reviewing old records. Specific attention should be directed to the presence of congenital anomalies and pediatric syndromes that may be associated with anomalies that are unrelated to the surgery but that could complicate the anesthetic management. A review of the drug and allergy history may provide information critically important to the anesthetic management.

Finally, if there were any previous anesthetic procedures, careful review of these records may provide an opportunity to improve anesthetic management. Specifically noting whether premedication was necessary, its effect when given, the response to various anesthetic agents, airway management, and emergence particularly may be useful. There may be information in this record that the anesthesiologist wishes to have before speaking to the parents. If the child, after what appeared to be a minor procedure, was intubated and ventilated in the intensive care unit for 3 days, the parents would be, not surprisingly, somewhat skeptical should the anesthesiologist be unaware of this occurrence. In children who have had several operations, consideration of latex allergy is important. A review of the previous anesthetic records for unexplained hypotension or wheezing should raise the consideration of latex allergy and the need for latex precautions.[75]

It may be worthwhile to discuss areas of concern with the surgeon and the child's physicians before meeting the family so the family can have the most complete information possible at the preoperative assessment. When meeting with the family, the anesthesiologist can determine the child's general health, level of activity, interests, favorite toys, background, and mental and medical condition. Knowledge of the parents' nickname for the child might be useful during emergence. Finding out which fingers or thumb the child sucks as a guide to IV placement may make the difference between a calm patient and an inconsolable patient postoperatively.

A systems review of appropriate depth always is indicated. A history of current and recent drugs and a history of allergies should be completed in all patients. Specific questioning about previous anesthetics and any history of siblings or family members who have had prolonged awakening, canceled surgery while in the operating room, intraoperative cardiorespiratory catastrophes, or unexplained fevers specifically should be sought in each case. Frequently, no one else will have asked questions concerning potential drug allergies, malignant hyperthermia, or adverse anesthetic reactions.

PHYSICAL EXAMINATION

The examination of the child should begin as soon as the physician enters the room. During the time spent obtaining the history from the parents and, when appropriate, from the child, important observations can be made. This period is invaluable for establishing rapport with the child and family. Constant efforts to gain the child's confidence (eg, by getting down to the child's level [sitting down is necessary], offering a toy, or interacting with the child) are of tremendous help. While discussing the child with the family, attempting to interact with the child and desensitizing the child to the close presence of the anesthesiologist is critical. Briskly walking into the room, interrogating the mother or father, and turning to the child will not yield optimal information from the physical examination. Interacting with, humoring, reassuring, and playing with the child during the interview not only calms the child, but can also provide valuable information regarding the child's general health status, developmental status,[76] respiratory condition, level of activity, state of hydration and perfusion, and level of anxiety concerning hospitalization.

The examination of the child falls into 3 areas: (1) general health and systems examination, (2) areas specifically related to the provision of anesthesia, and (3) areas related to surgery. The physical examination is guided by the findings in the history and interview and the needs of the surgical procedure. As mentioned previously, the examination begins when the anesthesiologist first meets the child. A great deal can be learned about the patient's perfusion, hemodynamic status, and respiratory status by general observation. Determining the child's growth and weight (eg, short stature, failure to thrive) is essential because they guide anesthetic management and may indicate the necessity for closer evaluation (**Figs. 20-7** through **20-10**).[76]

The airway can be assessed by observing phonation, inspiratory sounds, and respiratory rate; evidence of respiratory distress, such as retractions or tachypnea, are readily noted without interfering with the child. Coughs, runny noses, and upper respiratory tract infections can be detected without hands-on examination of the child. With specific regard to airway evaluation, determining the presence of airway anomalies, such as cleft lip or palate, large tonsils, the state of the child's dentition, loose teeth, or absent teeth is essential. A small jaw or a skeletal anomaly that may indicate a difficult intubation should be noted. It is possible to obtain a fairly comprehensive impression of the child's overall status without actually having to physically examine the child.

Familiarity with the surgical procedure also is necessary. The anesthesiologist should have a fair idea of how extensive the surgery is, whether it will affect airway management, what sort of blood loss to

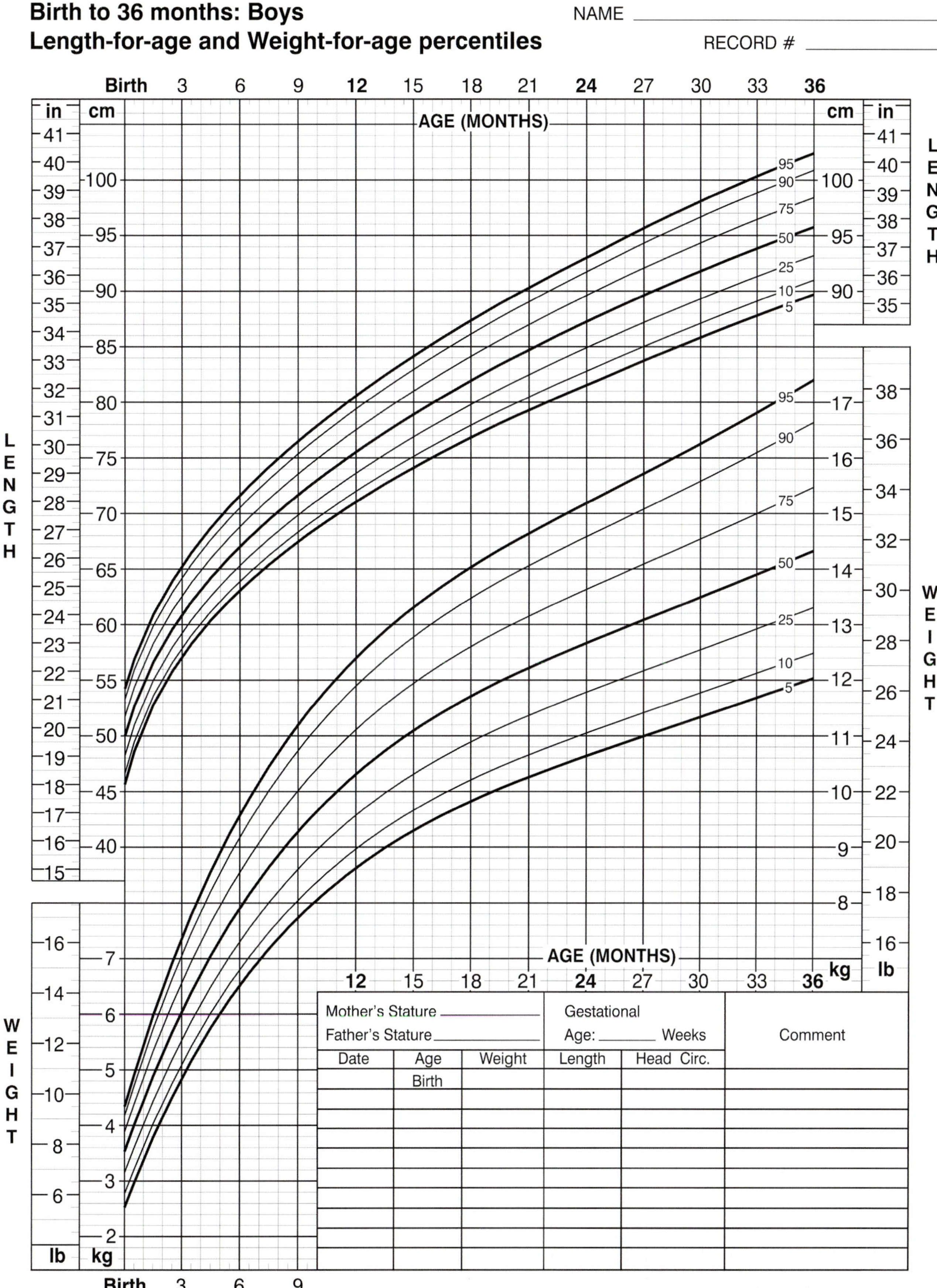

FIGURE 20-7. Standard growth curves for length and weight for newborn to 36-month-old boys. [Developed by the National Center for Health Statistics in collaboration with the National Center for Chronic Disease Prevention and Health Promotion (2000). Available at: http://www.cdc.gov/growthcharts/clinical_charts.htm Last accessed February 2011.]

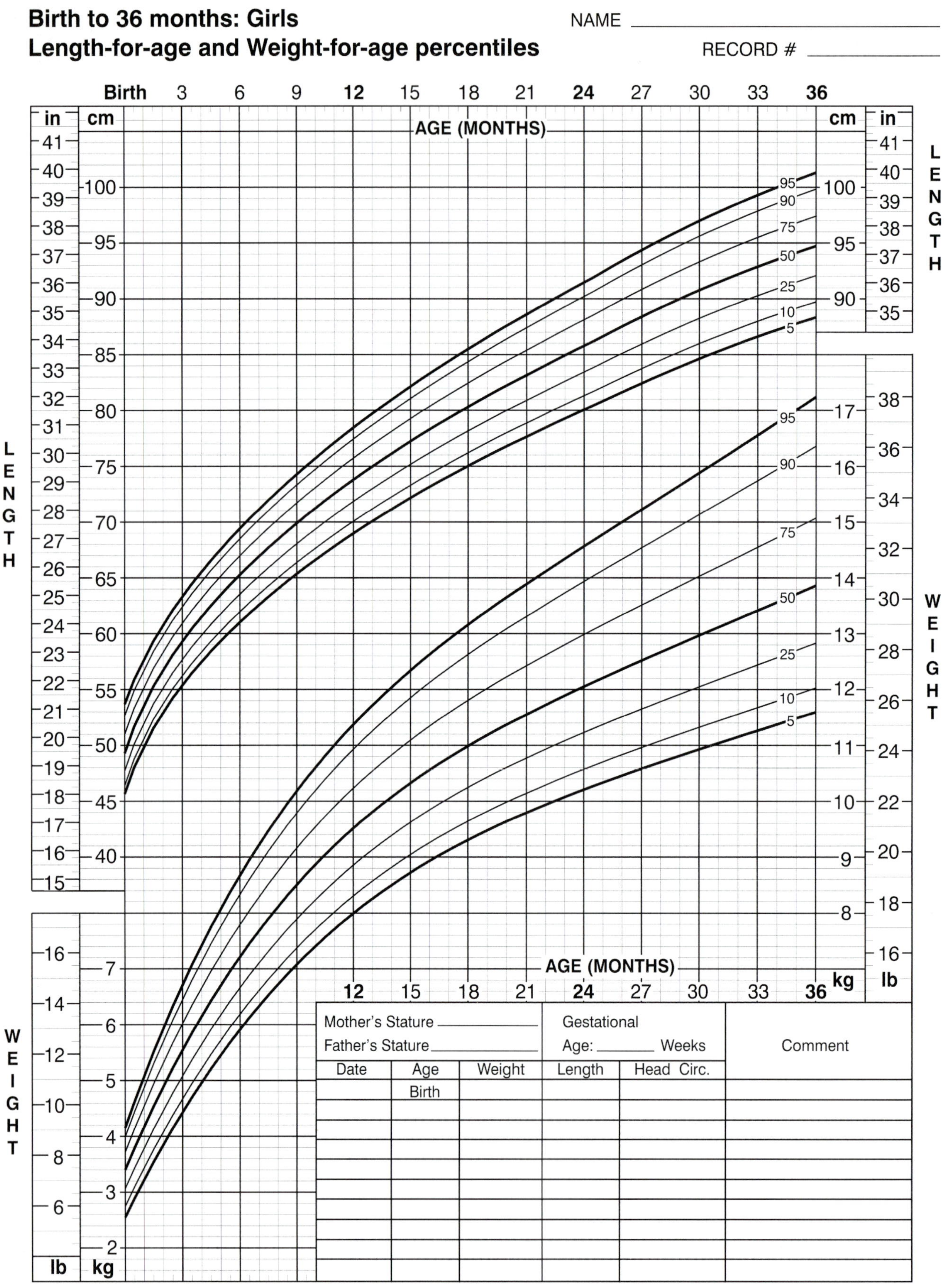

FIGURE 20-8. Standard growth curves for length and weight for newborn to 36-month-old girls. [Developed by the National Center for Health Statistics in collaboration with the National Center for Chronic Disease Prevention and Health Promotion (2000). Available at: http://www.cdc.gov/growthcharts/clinical_charts.htm Last accessed February 2011.]

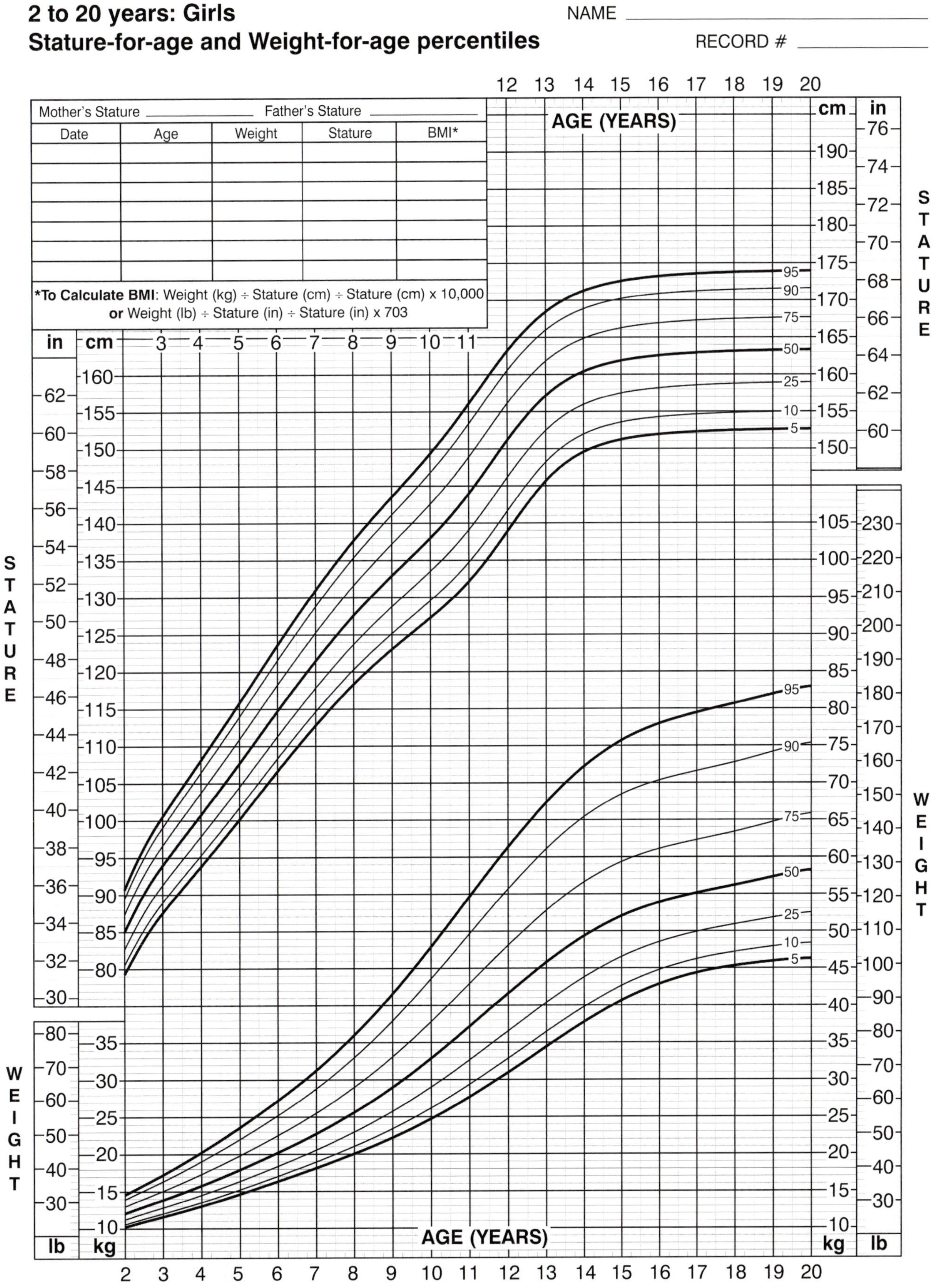
2 to 20 years: Girls
Stature-for-age and Weight-for-age percentiles
NAME
RECORD #
Mother's Stature
Father's Stature
Date
Age
Weight
Stature
BMI*
*To Calculate BMI: Weight (kg) ÷ Stature (cm) ÷ Stature (cm) x 10,000
or Weight (lb) ÷ Stature (in) ÷ Stature (in) x 703
AGE (YEARS)
STATURE
WEIGHT
in
cm
kg
lb
95
90
75
50
25
10
5

FIGURE 20-9. Standard growth curves for height and weight for girls aged 2 to 20 years. [Developed by the National Center for Health Statistics in collaboration with the National Center for Chronic Disease Prevention and Health Promotion (2000). Available at: http://www.cdc.gov/growthcharts/clinical_charts.htm Last accessed February 2011.]

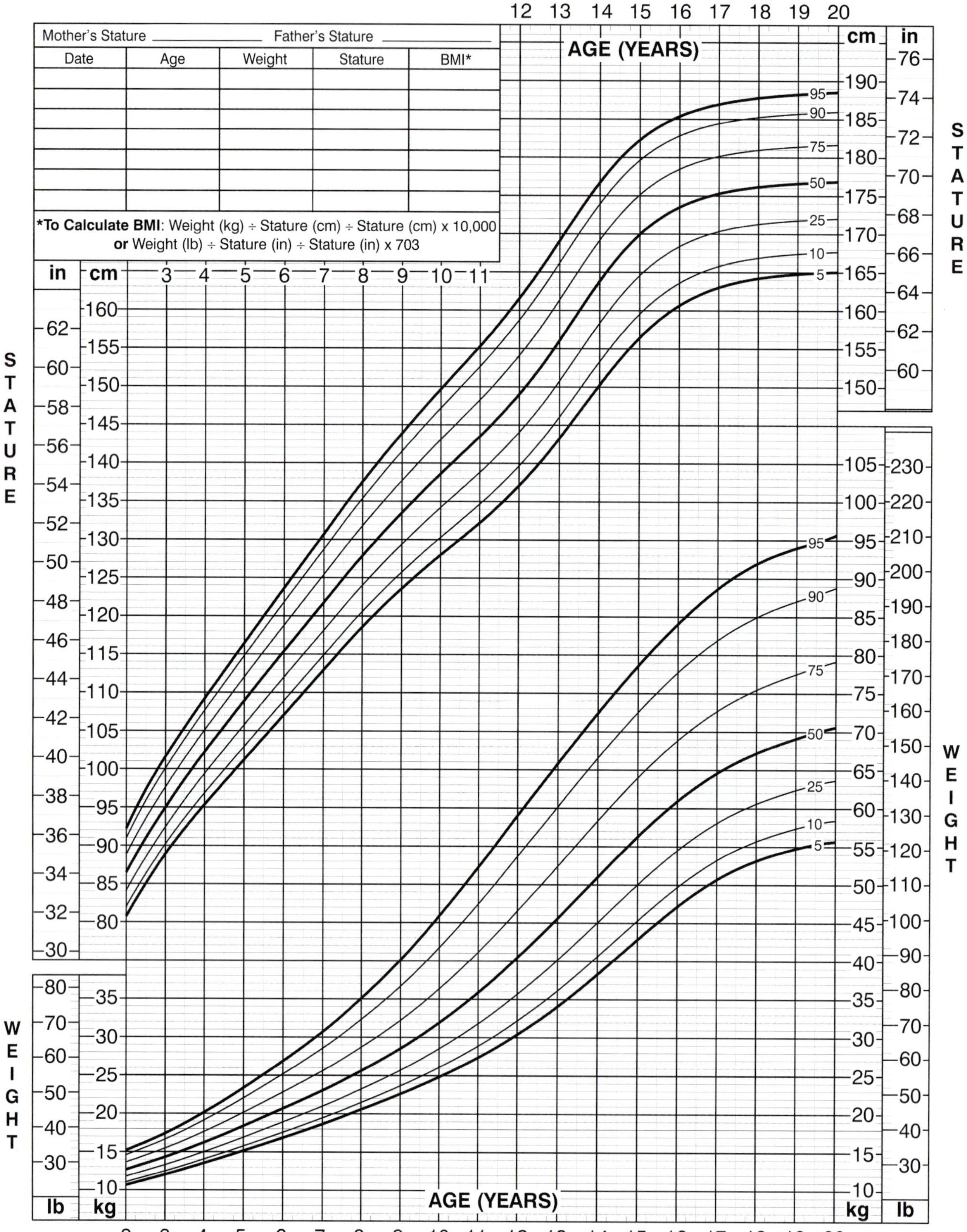

FIGURE 20-10. Standard growth curves for height and weight for boys aged 2 to 20 years. [Developed by the National Center for Health Statistics in collaboration with the National Center for Chronic Disease Prevention and Health Promotion (2000). Available at: http://www.cdc.gov/growthcharts/clinical_charts.htm Last accessed February 2011.]

expect, and if there are any particular factors complicating anesthesia management. Concerns about positioning and duration of surgery should be addressed. The presence of a cystic hygroma, for example, should dictate meticulous examination of the airway, auscultation for upper airway sounds, and determination of whether any airway involvement may have occurred. Discovery of capillary hemangiomas also may indicate the need to rule out airway involvement.

SYSTEMS REVIEW

Neuromuscular System Much will be apparent about the developmental stage of the child's CNS during the initial contact. Conversely, assessment of anesthetically relevant neurologic conditions will depend on the child's age and developmental status. Familiarity with the development of children gives the anesthesiologist a background by which to assess the child (**Fig. 20-11**). A wide spectrum of neuromuscular disorders that are important to the anesthesiologist accompanies various childhood conditions. In all children, information concerning mental and developmental stage, gestational age, gross motor function, presence of a seizure disorder, and any preexisting neurologic sensory deficits should be sought.

Cerebral Palsy and Mental Retardation A common problem in children who present for surgery for either multiple congenital anomalies or complications after prematurity is mental retardation or cerebral palsy. It should be stressed that not all children with cerebral palsy, even those with severe neuromuscular involvement, are mentally retarded. Incapacitating hypertonicity and spasticity, which may render a child unable to readily express himself or herself, do not necessarily interfere with the ability of the child to understand or the anesthesiologist's responsibility to inform the child about the course of the perioperative period. The anesthetic implications of mental retardation and cerebral palsy are legion. The response to a host of anesthetic drugs, including muscle relaxants, sedatives, analgesics, and hypnotics, varies and is less predictable in these children compared with healthy children. Older children with mental retardation and cerebral palsy also may have significant pulmonary complications that arise from musculoskeletal anomalies caused by imbalance of muscle groups, resulting in scoliosis and kyphosis and leading to restrictive lung pathology. Pharyngeal discoordination, difficulty with handling secretions, and the not infrequent association of gastroesophageal reflux in children with mental retardation and cerebral palsy can lead to recurrent, chronic, pulmonary parenchymal injury, which may complicate the anesthetic management. The presence of gastroesophageal reflux should be sought because it is frequent in this patient population. This may have particular relevance to NPO precautions and may indicate the need for histamine receptor (H_2) antagonism, antacids, agents that hasten gastric emptying, and rapid sequence intubation. Specific questioning about gastroesophageal reflux, recurrent aspiration, recurrent pneumonias, and wheezing should be directed toward the parents, and the anesthetic should be altered accordingly.[40]

Seizure Disorders Children with a history of epilepsy or seizure disorders also are of concern perioperatively. In the past, problems have resulted from a failure to maintain adequate anticonvulsant levels perioperatively. Most oral anticonvulsants can be given on the morning of surgery and have a sufficiently long half-life to ensure adequate levels intraoperatively. Sodium valproate and carbamazepine may be exceptions. The anesthesiologist should ensure that the optimal serum levels of anticonvulsants are achieved preoperatively and that these are maintained perioperatively. If a prolonged NPO status postoperatively is anticipated, alteration of anticonvulsant therapy preoperatively may be indicated to include agents that can be given parenterally. A consultation with the child's pediatrician or pediatric neurologist may be required. Preoperative awareness of the child's epilepsy should lead to avoiding epileptogenic anesthetic agents, such as methohexital and possibly etomidate.

Intracranial Hypertension The management of anesthesia for children with intracranial hypertension requires special care. Recognition of the classic triad of hypertension, bradycardia, and apnea in children who may require neurosurgical procedures, or ventricular peritoneal shunts, or who have suffered acute head injury is crucial in determining the anesthetic management of these children. In younger children with chronically elevated intracranial hypertension, the need for perioperative management of intracranial pressure is indicated by complaints of nausea, vomiting, headache, irritability, lethargy, and finding on physical examination of the sunsetting sign. Careful questioning for an acute change in the child's status may indicate the need preoperatively for measures directed at decreasing intracranial pressure, such as diuresis and osmolar therapy. Intraoperative provision of deep anesthesia and controlled ventilation to maintain normocapnia would be wise.

If the child has an existing decompressive shunt, the anesthesiologist should be aware of it. If it contains a valve and pump mechanism, its function should be evaluated. Perioperative fluid shifts may alter cerebrospinal fluid (CSF) function and upset the balance of CSF production and drainage, leading to elevated intracranial pressure and perioperative catastrophe, especially in the anesthetized child. Assurance of shunt patency and functional history is necessary.

Muscular Dystrophy Congenital neuromuscular disease, such as muscular dystrophy, myotonic dystrophy, and acquired diseases, such as myositis, dermatomyositis, and collagen vascular diseases, raise questions concerning the use of muscle relaxants. In patients with myotonic dystrophy, the use of succinylcholine should be avoided.[77] Although this is less clear in patients with some of the muscular dystrophies, the occurrence of rhabdomyolysis and the suspicion of an increased incidence of malignant hyperthermia in patients with Duchenne muscular dystrophy suggests caution in the use of depolarizing muscle relaxants and inhalational anesthetics.[78] The use of nondepolarizing muscle relaxants in children who have muscle weakness and neuromuscular impairment should be guided by meticulous perioperative monitoring and perhaps are best avoided when possible (**Box 20-5**).

The majority of neurologic deficits and impairments will be obvious from a review of the patient's records, the parents' interview, and observation of the child. If detailed neurologic examination and documentation are required, or if the presence of serious CNS disease is suspected, a pediatric neurologist should be consulted. With the increasing use of regional anesthesia, it is wise for the anesthesiologist to search for and document existing neurologic deficits before performing nerve blocks.

Respiratory System A host of illnesses and congenital abnormalities affect respiratory function in children. Many congenital anomalies are associated with small, difficult-to-visualize airways, upper airway obstruction, and difficult intubation. All of these conditions should specifically be sought and investigated whenever the suspicion arises (**Table 20-7**). The relatively small diameter of a child's airway, a child's different anatomic makeup, and high oxygen consumption relative to FRC put children at increased risk for developing hypoxia, decreasing the margin for error.

Specific questioning about airway obstruction (eg, snoring), recurring episodes of croup, tonsil or adenoid hypertrophy, and any history of apnea is part of routine history taking in pediatric anesthesia. Noticing characteristic facies, such as those associated with Treacher Collins syndrome, Pierre Robin syndrome, or Hunter and Hurler mucopolysaccharidosis, is an essential skill of the pediatric anesthesiologist in detecting the potential for difficulty with intubation and upper airway obstruction perioperatively. Careful examination of the nares, of the oropharynx for loose teeth, and for the presence of respiratory distress indicating airway obstruction should be part of every examination. Routine attention to these airway issues may prevent potentially lethal complications in the operating room.

Assessment of children with chronic respiratory disease also is necessary. The high frequency of chronic lung disease (bronchopulmonary dysplasia [BPD]) in former premature infants who required ventilatory support in the neonatal period should be remembered.[79] Evidence should be sought for this in the patient's record and by questioning the parents. BPD may range from mild recurrent wheezing to a chronic

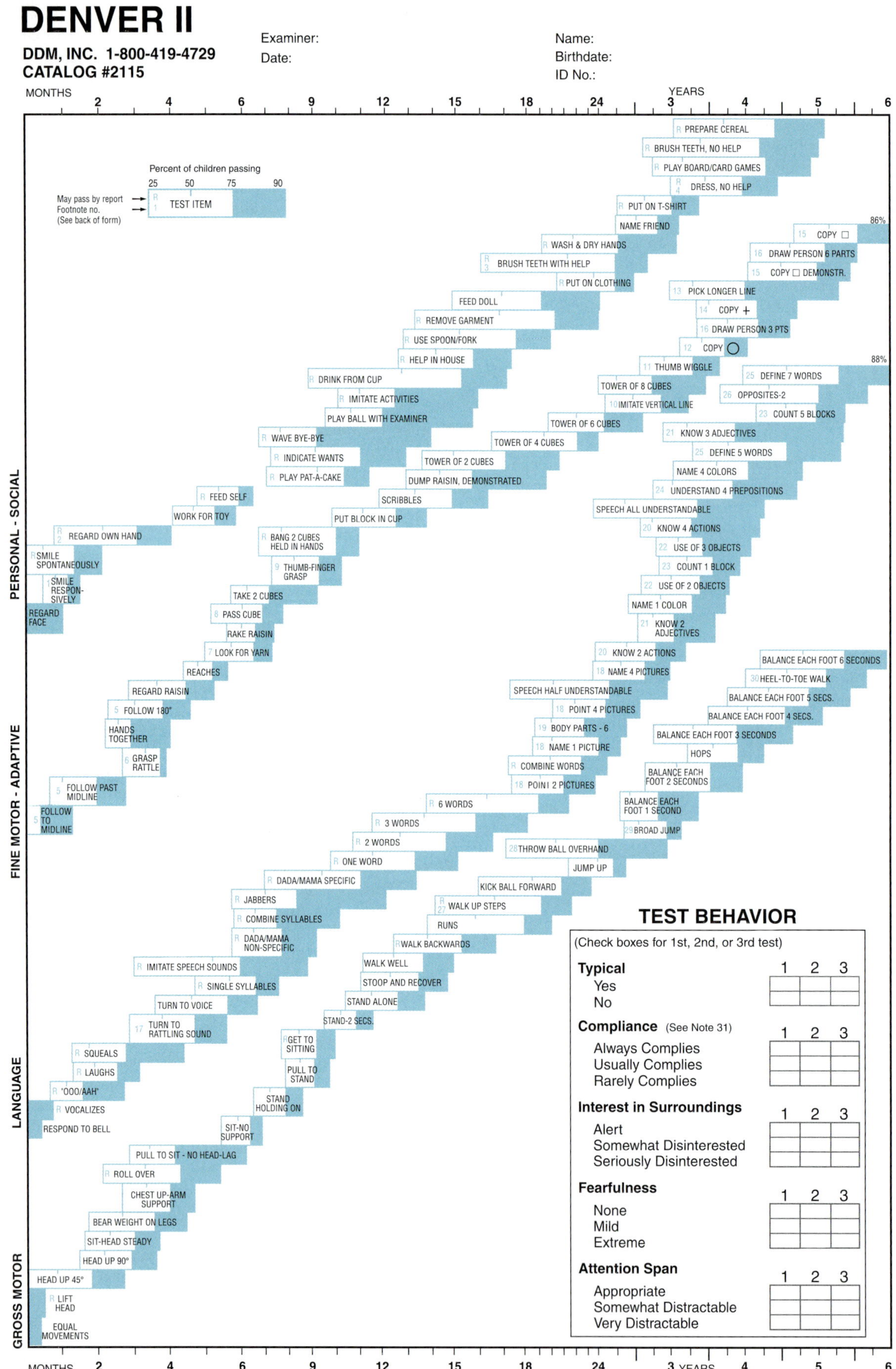

FIGURE 20-11. Denver Developmental Screening Test serves as a guide to the development of language, motor, and social skills of children aged from 1 month to 6 years. [©1969, 1989, 1990 W.K. Frankenburg and J.B. Dodds ©1978 W.K. Frankenburg ©2009 Wilhelmine R. Frankenburg–Contact DDM, Inc. 1-800-419-4729 or Sales@denverii.com.]

BOX 20-5

Neuromuscular Diseases in Which Neuromuscular Agents Should Be Used With Caution

- Muscular dystrophy
  - Facioscapulohumeral
  - Duchenne
- Myasthenia gravis
  - Eaton-Lambert (very rare)
- Cerebral palsy
- Myotonias
  - Myotonia congenita
- Spinal muscle atrophy
- Spina bifida (thoracic level)

oxygen requirement—even mechanical ventilation at home. In children with BPD and asthma, the anesthesiologist should be completely familiar with the child's respiratory status and ensure that therapy has been optimized preoperatively. The child's exact therapy should be ascertained, and when possible, an effort should be made to ensure that appropriate doses of bronchodilator therapy have been achieved. A history of recent steroid use should be sought, and consideration should be given to initiating steroid therapy preoperatively.

Particular attention should be directed to the history of exercise tolerance in children with or suspected of having chronic lung disease. In patients with musculoskeletal disease, especially kyphosis or scoliosis, one should seek evidence of restrictive lung abnormalities. Preoperative investigations in children with chronic lung disease may include determination of blood gases and pulmonary function tests. A cardiac examination with electrocardiography and possibly echocardiography may be necessary to discover and define the severity of pulmonary hypertension and cor pulmonale.

Acute lung disease is an indication for canceling elective surgery. Pneumonia, croup, and acute asthma pose serious perioperative threats, both acutely as well as after apparent resolution. Airway reactivity is increased for several weeks after an acute asthmatic attack.[80,81] Deteriorating pulmonary status caused by viral or bacterial infection, superimposed on BPD, cystic fibrosis, or asthma may cause serious intraoperative hypoxia, increased secretions with the risk of endotracheal tube obstruction, and difficulty in maintaining airway patency. Postoperative atelectasis and pneumonia can be serious complications after surgery. Specific questioning about episodes of apnea should be included because these may be associated with fatal postoperative respiratory difficulties.[82]

TABLE 20-7 Common Syndromes Associated With Difficult Intubation

Syndrome	Airway	Associated Anomalies
Achondroplasia	Small nares and mouth Midface hypoplasia Megacephaly	Hydrocephalus Atlantoaxial instability Atropine sensitivity
Apert	Narrow, occasionally cleft palate Small maxilla Craniosynostosis Flat facies	Mental retardation Cardiac anomalies Renal abnormalities Syndactyly, often severe
Arthrogryposis, congenital	Small mandible Cleft palate Torticollis, contracture Klippel-Feil syndrome	Scoliosis Ventricular septal defect
Beckwith-Wiedemann	Large tongue Prognathism	Retardation Hypoglycemia Exomphalos Gigantism
Cornelia de Lange	Micrognathia Short neck Cleft palate Mandibular spurs	Cardiac abnormalities Retardation
Crouzon	Small maxilla Large tongue Craniosynostosis	Proptosis
Down	Large tongue Small mouth Small mandible	Cardiac abnormalities Atlantoaxial instability Hypotonia
Goldenhar	Small mandible and zygoma Cleft palate Macrostomia	Cervical spine defects
Congenital hypothyroidism	Large tongue	Hypothermia Retardation, if untreated Umbilical hernia
Freeman-Sheldon (whistling face)	Very small mouth High palate	Scoliosis
Klippel-Feil	Short neck, limited extension	Deafness Ventricular septal defect
Marfan	Narrow face Narrow palate	Cardiac anomalies Scoliosis Restrictive lung disease
Möbius	Small mandible Small mouth Aspiration	Talipes equinovarus Ptosis Cranial nerve palsies
Mucopolysaccharidosis	Large tongue Narrow airway Limited opening	Cardiac abnormalities
Pierre-Robin	Micrognathia	
Robinow	Small mouth Micrognathia Crowded teeth Large tongue	Hemivertebra Hypertelorism Atrial septal defect
Rubinstein-Taybi	Small maxilla Narrow palate	Retardation Cardiac anomalies Cervical instability
Russel-Silver	Small stature Small mandible	Hypoglycemia
Treacher-Collins	Facial hypoplasia Mandible, maxilla Cleft palate Choanal atresia	Cardiac disease Cervical vertebral anomalies
Turner	Small narrow maxilla, mandible Short neck	Coarctation Hypertension
Zellweger	Small mandible Short neck	Cardiac anomalies Contractures

Data from Smith DW. *Recognizable Patterns of Human Malformation: Genetic, Embryologic and Clinical Aspects*. 5th ed. Philadelphia, PA: WB Saunders; 1997.

Runny Nose Problem Frequently, the problem of the child with a runny nose arises. Rhinorrhea can be caused by an acute viral or bacterial upper respiratory tract infection (URI), allergic rhinitis, or foreign object. There is evidence that recent URIs increase airway hyperreactivity for 6 to 8 weeks after infection.[80] Anecdotally, most anesthesiologists believe that URIs are associated with increased secretions, incidence of laryngospasm and bronchospasm, endotracheal tube obstruction, and intraoperative respiratory difficulties.[83] An increased incidence of postintubation stridor and other postoperative respiratory complications also has been reported.[84] Experience in recent years has failed to substantiate an increased risk of complications in patients with simple URIs.

When is it appropriate to cancel elective surgery on the basis of rhinorrhea? The patient should be in optimal condition before induction of anesthesia. The recent onset of mucopurulent rhinorrhea, especially if accompanied by pharyngitis and fever, is an indication for cancellation of elective surgery. The child who always has clear rhinorrhea on the basis of allergic rhinitis probably is at no increased anesthetic risk. Multiple considerations, such as the inconvenience to the family because of long travel or arranged time off work, the potential of complications from delaying surgery, and the risks of proceeding, need to be weighed when deciding whether to proceed. With healthy children who are afebrile and have clear rhinorrhea, we proceed with elective surgery. Anesthesia caregivers are more cautious with other respiratory diseases, especially asthma and BPD.[80,81] Although this topic remains controversial, whenever possible, surgery and anesthesia should be delayed for at least 2 weeks.[85]

Cardiovascular System Because of the multiple cardiovascular effects of anesthetics in children and the frequency with which cardiac anomalies accompany other congenital malformations, particular attention to the cardiovascular system is necessary (**Table 20-8**). Recognition of the setting in which congenital heart disease may occur, coupled with careful attention to the previous history and questioning of the family, help define the type and severity of the defect. Examination of the child may lead to discovery of hitherto undiagnosed cardiac defects or to the presence of a cardiac murmur and demonstrate the need to alter the anesthetic plan and perhaps to seek further pediatric cardiology consultation. The cardiovascular system undergoes significant developmental changes, and reference to normal age-related values is essential in assessing children (see Figs. 20-4 through 20-6).[86,87]

Poor exercise tolerance, as in adults, is a hallmark of inadequate cardiovascular function. Children who tire easily, become tachypneic, have dyspnea on exertion, or have orthopnea must be evaluated carefully. In infants, the major exercise is feeding. An irritable child with a history of poor feeding accompanied by diaphoresis and tachypnea may have borderline cardiac function. Failure to thrive may indicate compromised cardiac function. In younger infants, clubbing is never present, and cyanosis may be difficult to detect. Palpation and auscultation remain the cornerstones of the cardiology examination. Particular attention should be paid to the presence of a brachial–femoral delay, indicating coarctation, and for left and right ventricular heaves. Detection of a new murmur frequently raises the question of whether it is benign or significant. Differentiating between a venous hum or ventricular outflow murmur and more serious murmurs requires specific examination (**Table 20-9**). When in doubt, consultation with a pediatric cardiologist is indicated. The child with a murmur who is asymptomatic, acyanotic, healthy, and gaining weight along appropriate percentiles and who has a normal S_1 and S_2 almost certainly will tolerate routine anesthesia without serious complications. Questions arise regarding the need for further cardiology follow-up, evaluation- and infective endocarditis (IE) prophylaxis (**Table 20-10** and **Box 20-6**). When the history and physical examination indicate possible serious cardiac disease, a hematocrit, electrocardiogram (ECG), chest radiograph, and oxygen saturation (pulse oximetry) form the basis of the laboratory workup. In patients with known serious heart disease, the anesthesiologist should understand the anatomy and physiology of the defect. A hemodynamically inconsequential atrial septal defect, ventricular septal defect, mitral valve prolapse, or the presence of a bicuspid aortic valve may predispose the child to an untoward intraoperative event, and consultation with a pediatric cardiologist may be indicated. For most children with heart disease, it is prudent to obtain a recent consultation with the child's pediatric cardiologist.

Renal System Asymptomatic renal disease, apart from bacteriuria, is rare in children. The likelihood of discovering a new renal lesion during routine physical examination done for the preanesthetic evaluation is almost nonexistent. The presence of hypertension (see Table 20-3) should indicate the need for urinalysis and electrolyte analysis.[35] The unexpected presence of anemia also may indicate chronic renal disease. The anesthetic implications of renal disease in the presence of normal electrolytes, normal growth and development, and normotension are minimal. In infants, there may be the inability to concentrate urine or to handle a large fluid load, both of which dictate cautious fluid management perioperatively.

In the presence of serious preexisting renal disease, careful attention should be paid to the child's preoperative preparation. If the child requires dialysis (peritoneal dialysis or hemodialysis) to maintain optimal electrolyte levels and growth, consideration of dialysis on the day before surgery is indicated. Antihypertensive therapy, if required, should be optimized. Electrolytes should be monitored carefully. Particular

TABLE 20-8 Syndromes Associated With Congenital Heart Disease

Syndrome	Associated Disease
Apert	Pulmonic stenosis, VSD
Asplenia or polysplenia	ASD, VSD
Cornelia de Lange	VSD
DiGeorge	Aortic arch, truncus, VSD, PDA, tetralogy
Down	AV canal, ASD, VSD
Ellis–van Creveld	ASD
Fetal alcohol	VSD, cardiomyopathy
Holt-Oram	ASD, VSD
Kartagener's	ASD, VSD
Marfan	Aortic and mitral valve diseases, dilated aortic root
Noonan	Pulmonic stenosis, ASD
Opitz	ASD
Robinow	ASD
VATER	VSD
Williams	Pulmonic stenosis

ASD, atrial septal defect; AV, atrioventricular; PDA, patent ductus arteriosus; VSD, ventricular septal defect.

Data from Smith DW. *Recognizable Patterns of Human Malformation: Genetic Embryologic, and Clinical Aspects.* 5th ed. Philadelphia, PA: WB Saunders; 1997.

TABLE 20-9 Innocent Asymptomatic Murmurs

	Venous Hum	Vibratory Murmur
Area	Aortic area into neck Pulmonary	Apex to sternum Basal (occasionally mitral) Not transmitted to axilla
Timing	Continuous (ductus murmur)	Systolic Diastolic accentuation
Character	Increased with inspiration Loudest in sitting position Jugular pressure diminishes intensity S_1 and S_2 normal	Coarse, low-pitched, scratchy, twang Short, limited area Decreased with inspiration S_1 may be softened; S_2 normal Very common

From Wetzel RC. Evaluation of children. In: Longnecker DE, Tinker JH, Morgan GE, et al, eds. *Principles and Practice of Anesthesiology*. Vol I, 2nd ed. St. Louis, MO: Mosby; 1998.

TABLE 20-10 Infective Endocarditis Prophylaxis Regimens

	Time	Dosage
Dental and routine prophylaxis only in high-risk patients		
Routine		
Amoxicillin PO	1 h before procedure	50 mg/kg (max 3 g)
Or if NPO		
Ampicillin IV	Within 30 min of procedure	50 mg/kg
Or cefazolin IV		
Or ceftriaxone IV		
For maximal protection		
Ampicillin IV	Within 30 min of start of procedure	50 mg/kg
And		
Gentamicin IV	Within 30 min of start	1.5 mg/kg
Followed by:		
Ampicillin IV		25 mg/kg
Or		
Amoxicillin PO	6 h after initial dose	50 mg/kg
PCN-allergic patients		
Cephalexin PO		20 mg/Kg
Azithromycin PO		15 mg/kg
Or		
Clindamycin PO/IV	1 h before start	20 mg/kg
Or		
Cefazolin IV	Within 30 min of start	25 mg/kg
Minor or repetitive in low-risk children		
Amoxicillin PO	1 h before procedure	50 mg/kg (max 3 g)

Data from AHA Guidelines: Prevention of Infective Endocarditis. *Circulation.* 2007:1736-1754; and Gerber MA. New AHA guidelines for prevention of infective endocarditis. *Pediatr Infect Dis.* 2008;27:647-649.

BOX 20-6

Infective Endocarditis Prophylaxis

Indications

Moderate risk (routine)

- Congenital or acquired valvular heart disease (rheumatic heart disease)
- Hypertrophic cardiomyopathy
- Mitral valve prolapse with regurgitation
- Subaortic stenosis
- Recently corrected congenital heart disease (within 6 mo)

High risk (maximal)

- Surgically constructed shunts (Waterston, Blalock-Taussig, Potts, etc)
- Uncorrected or palliated complex cyanotic heart disease (single ventricle, transposition of the great arteries, tetralogy)
- Prosthetic valve or other material
- Previous bacterial endocarditis
- Cardiac transplant patient with valvulopathy

Procedures

- Tonsillectomy/adenoidectomy
- Endoscopic retrograde cholangiopancreatography, stricture dilation, biliary tract surgery
- Dental extractions, implants, where gingival bleeding is anticipated, endodontics, periodontal surgery, mucosal perforation
- Incision and drainage procedures
- Airway surgery or rigid bronchoscopy

Prophylaxis not necessary for secundum atrial septal defect or patent ductus arteriosus repaired >6 mo ago, endotracheal intubation, tympanostomies

BOX 20-7

Conditions Associated With Gastroesophageal Reflux

- Apnea
- Prematurity
- Recurrent pneumonia syndromes
- Cerebral palsy or mental retardation
- Gross obesity
- Tracheoesophageal fistula
- Bronchopulmonary dysplasia
- Pregnancy
- Recurrent, persistent vomiting

attention is necessary concerning the serum potassium concentration. Serum potassium greater than 5.5 mEq/L is worrisome in children with renal disease. The propensity of succinylcholine to induce hyperkalemia in patients who may have a concurrent metabolic acidosis puts these patients at particular risk. Elective surgery should be canceled in the presence of a potassium level higher than the acceptable upper level of normal for the individual hospital's laboratory (5.5 mEq/L, generally). Regarding hematocrit in patients with chronic renal failure, there is some controversy. It is usual practice to accept a lower hematocrit (20%) in these children than would be normally tolerated. This is based on the assumption of chronic adaptation, which includes increased blood volume and increased cardiac output. These may be compromised during anesthesia. Although the child may be chronically adapted, it should be remembered that the reserve necessary to tolerate the stresses that may accompany anesthesia and surgery is markedly decreased. Preoperative erythropoietin therapy and transfusion before surgery may be administered if time allows.

Gastrointestinal System The major anesthetic issues concerning the GI system center on a predisposition to aspiration pneumonitis. Children with increased gastric residual volumes and gastroesophageal reflux should be identified preoperatively. Those children who have a history of tracheoesophageal fistula, mental retardation, cerebral palsy, apnea, and recurrent aspiration pneumonia always should be suspected of having gastroesophageal reflux (**Box 20-7**).[40,88] Careful scrutiny of medical records and questioning of the parents may indicate that gastroesophageal reflux has been evaluated in the past. If not, consultation with pediatricians might prove worthwhile. The history of recurrent aspiration pneumonia in a child with a predisposing condition raises the likelihood of aspiration during anesthesia, and a rapid sequence induction is indicated. The treatment of children with gastroesophageal reflux includes administration of antacids, histamine (H_2) receptor antagonists, agents that encourage gastric emptying (metoclopramide), and the Sellick maneuver during induction and intubation.[89] Consider awake intubation in young infants.

Halothane hepatitis developing de novo in children appears to be exceedingly rare, occurring in perhaps less than 1 in 50|000 to 250|000 anesthetic inductions.[90] The relationship between the occurrence of halothane toxicity in patients with previous liver damage and resulting hepatitis is unclear. Many premature infants have abnormal liver function tests and elevated bilirubins. Some children also may have hyperbilirubinemia and elevated transaminases. Although the advisability of using halothane under these circumstances is not clear, it probably is best avoided because suitable alternatives are available. Currently, sevoflurane has almost entirely replaced halothane in practice, and reports of hepatitis after sevoflurane are extremely rare.

LABORATORY INVESTIGATIONS

It may seem surprising that the American Society of Anesthesiologists, the American College of Surgeons, and the American Academy of

Pediatrics do not make any specific recommendations for preoperative testing in children.[91] Specific laboratory testing that is indicated by information obtained from the chart review, history, and examination of the child is straightforward. Routine testing for healthy children remains controversial. In the past, guidelines that had been developed for adults were applied to children. These tests included a complete blood count, urinalysis, and chest radiograph. With the streamlining influence prevalent in health care systems today, critical appraisal of the need for these examinations has been undertaken. All aspects of the preoperative laboratory investigation have been questioned. The standard that required a routine chest radiograph in healthy children without symptoms or signs was abandoned.[92] Recent experience with large numbers of outpatient anesthetics has raised serious questions about the need for routine performance of other laboratory tests. In general, preoperative laboratory testing should be dictated by the child's condition and status, rather than merely by the need for an anesthetic.[66]

Hematology It generally is accepted that a preoperative hematocrit is unnecessary in most healthy children for operations in which significant blood loss is not expected. The value of a complete blood count and whether there is a role for determination of platelets and coagulation studies are also unclear. These decisions should be guided by patient considerations. There are developmental differences in the standard level of hematocrit (**Table 20-11**).[93] For years, "normal" hematocrits were required for elective surgery. Later, the lower limit of normal (ie, hematocrit of 30% or a hemoglobin of >10 g/dL) became the requirement. Elective surgery probably should await attaining this level, short of transfusion. Iron and nutritional support are indicated. In the emergent situation, transfusion therapy may be indicated as directed by patient need, such as anticipated blood loss and cardiorespiratory status. Transfusion should not rely on arbitrary and unsupported boundary of "normal" hemoglobin.[94]

What are the essential considerations? In a healthy child with normal cardiorespiratory function, a fully saturated hemoglobin of 10 g/dL would require a cardiac index of 3.4 L/min/m^2 to provide an oxygen delivery 3 times the average oxygen consumption. If the child's hemoglobin were 7 g/dL (hematocrit approximately 20%), a cardiac index of 4.8 L/min/m^2 is required to maintain the same level of oxygen delivery. This is well within a healthy child's cardiac reserve and should represent no major difficulty. The assumptions underlying this are that the child remains 100% saturated, receives no cardiac-depressant drugs, and loses little blood. These circumstances frequently cannot be guaranteed during surgery and anesthesia, and this lack of guarantee is the key issue. The major concern is not for healthy children having minor surgery, but when surgery will result in blood loss and lower this margin of reserve further. A child whose hemoglobin drops to 5 g/dL from 10 g/dL should double cardiac output to around 6.6 L/min/m^2 to maintain oxygen delivery. This remains well within the average child's cardiac reserve. If a child's hemoglobin drops to 2 g/dL from 7 g/dL intraoperatively, the child requires a cardiac index of nearly 17 L/min/m^2 to maintain a marginal oxygen delivery, which is beyond the ability of even the healthy child's cardiovascular system to compensate for, especially when anesthetized.

A third issue that frequently is raised is adaptation. The classic teaching is that children with renal disease tolerate lower hematocrits because they have had time to adapt. There is little evidence to demonstrate this is so; 2,3-diphosphoglyceric acid may not be increased in children with renal disease, and there is no reason to suggest that they have a shift in the oxyhemoglobin dissociation curve. The concept that they can adapt to lower levels of oxygen delivery or consumption is unsupported. If serious blood loss is expected perioperatively, the margin of safety is considerably less in patients who begin with low hematocrit.

As mentioned previously, there are no absolute guidelines for preoperative hematocrit, and at present, each anesthesiologist should decide on a standard for each child. Motoyama[95] found that a hemoglobin of 7.5 to 8.5 g/dL will deliver oxygen to the tissues of children equivalent to what a hemoglobin of 10 g/dL will in adults. In neonates, 12 to 13 g/dL is necessary. This is largely related to shifts in the P50 (partial pressure of oxygen at which hemoglobin is 50% saturated).[95] It seems reasonable that a hemoglobin of 8 g/dL in an ASA PS P1 child may be acceptable if no major perioperative blood loss is expected. A child who has chronic restrictive lung disease and is about to undergo scoliosis repair probably should have a hemoglobin higher than 10 g/dL (at least initially).

Many abnormalities can be discovered during preoperative laboratory screening.[96] These abnormalities fall into 2 categories: those that are relevant to the anesthetic management of the child and those that are relevant to the child's general health. The degree to which a preanesthesia screening clinic wishes to be responsible for the general health care of children needs to be determined by each facility. There is a responsibility to ensure follow-up evaluation for abnormal laboratory tests that may be discovered coincidentally with preoperative assessment. O'Connor and Drasner[97] reported that 17% of children who had a complete blood count (CBC) were anemic or had a microcytosis. Only 2 of these children had surgery canceled because of anemia (hemoglobins <10 g/dL).[97] A mechanism to arrange follow-up evaluation with the pediatric clinic should be available, and communication should be assured.

Sickle Cell Disease The American Academy of Pediatrics recommends that a sickle preparation or other screening test be performed in all children of African descent.[98] Is it reasonable for the anesthesiologist to insist on receiving the results of a sickle cell preparation in all children of African descent requiring anesthesia and surgery?[99] Is anesthetic management different for those who have sickle trait than for those who do not? Is it necessary to have a sickle cell preparation in nonanemic at-risk children? Anesthetizing a child with sickle cell disease who is anemic and with 95% sickle hemoglobin poses a major threat to that child and should never be undertaken without good reason. The likelihood of a child older than age 2 years with a normal hemoglobin having sickle cell disease is extremely low. If all children with hemoglobins less than 10 g/dL require further investigation, among the factors to be investigated, in addition to iron deficiency, is sickle hemoglobin status in at-risk children. This might not apply to neonates or infants who may have hemoglobin concentration greater than 10 g/dL and have sickle cell disease and high levels of sickle hemoglobin. Unless a sickle hemoglobin preparation is performed, cases might be missed in this population which is at risk for hypoxia and low cardiac output during anesthesia. Common practice is to perform a sickle cell preparation on all children of African descent unless their status is known and to screen for anemia in all other children. In those with positive sickle screen, hemoglobin electrophoresis is required.[100,101] It should be noted that infants younger than age 4 months have maternal antibodies that interfere with performing a quick sickle index preparation. These children require hemoglobin electrophoresis to determine their sickle cell disease status.

TABLE 20-11 Mean Hematocrit and Hemoglobin Versus Age

Age	Hct (SD) %	Hgb (SD) g/dL
1-3 d	56 ± 5	18.5 ± 2.0
2 wk	53 ± 4	16.6 ± 1.6
1 mo	44 ± 5	13.9 ± 1.6
2 mo	35 ± 4	11.2 ± 0.9
6 mo	36 ± 3	12.6 ± 0.7
6-24 mo	36 ± 2	12.0 ± 0.8
2-6 y	37 ± 2	12.5 ± 0.5
6-12 y	40 ± 3	13.5 ± 1.0
12-18 y	43 ± 4	14.5 ± 0.7
Adult	41 ± 2	14.0 ± 1.0

From Rowe PC. Laboratory values. In: Oski FA, De Angelis CD, Feigin RD, et al, eds. *Principles and Practice of Pediatrics*. Philadelphia, PA: 1990; JB Lippincott.

Does sickle trait pose a threat to older children who may not be anemic but who have some amount of sickle hemoglobin? Although there are some anecdotal stories of sickling and rare vasoocclusive phenomena in children with sickle cell trait during anesthesia with resulting hypothermia, ischemia, and hypoxia, sickle cell trait generally is associated with less than 40% of hemoglobin S in the circulating blood.[101] This is the target level that is obtained with transfusion protocols for sickle cell disease. Prudent avoidance of tourniquets that cause blood stasis and hypoxia in the affected limb probably is wise in patients with sickle cell trait. Anesthetic management will not vary because the routine goals of anesthesia (avoidance of hypoxia, hypothermia, hypovolemia, and hypotension) are as important in routine anesthetic management as they are for patients with sickle cell trait.[101,102]

In patients with sickle cell disease, preoperative treatment is directed at reducing sickle hemoglobin to less than 40%. Chronic transfusion, exchange transfusion, and acute blood transfusion are reported to be useful in achieving this goal.[98,103]

Leukocyte Counts In one study, leukocyte counts were abnormal only in patients who were ill or otherwise suspected of having an infection.[66,93] No occult leukocytosis was discovered in 463 preoperative screening evaluations.[97] When indicated by suspicion of sepsis, infection, fever, or respiratory tract infection, a CBC might be useful in arriving at the diagnosis; however, routine leukocyte determination does not appear to be warranted.

Urinalysis Routine urinalysis is part of preoperative recommendations in children. Apart from providing a possible contribution to routine health screening, the relevance to anesthetic management is unclear.[66,104] In children who are febrile, have congenital anomalies of the urinary tract, or have suspected renal function anomalies, urinalysis might be beneficial. In otherwise healthy children in whom urinalysis can be difficult to obtain and unreliable, abnormal results appear to occur in 15% of children and usually are asymptomatic bacteriuria.[97] The majority of these are either false-positive results, clinically insignificant, or previously known. In only 2 of 453 cases was surgery canceled, and both of these were canceled because of suspected colonization or asymptomatic bacteriuria, which was of no anesthetic relevance. In afebrile, ASA PS P1 children with no history of renal disease, most centers have abandoned routine urinalysis.

Screening for pregnancy varies widely from center to center. The evidence that anesthesia, per se, is deleterious to the continued pregnancy or the fetus is extremely sparse. On the other hand, the logistic, behavioral, privacy, and social implications of testing all female children of child-bearing age for pregnancy, with or without consent, are quite complex. Each institution must resolve these issues for itself.

Drug Levels In children who are receiving therapeutic drugs, it frequently is worthwhile to know whether the therapeutic level has been achieved. The 2 major areas in which this is of concern are in children with epilepsy and asthma. Obtaining routine blood levels of theophylline (although now only rarely used) and anticonvulsants to ensure compliance with therapy and adequate levels for the perioperative management appears to be a wise precaution. It is not so clear what should be done when an abnormal result is found. Does an asymptomatic healthy child with a nontherapeutic drug level require therapy? Should therapeutic levels of indicated drugs be achieved before elective surgery? These decisions may require input from the child's primary care physician and perhaps a pediatric neurologist in children with epilepsy. Frequently, it is worthwhile to inform the primary caregiver that the level is subtherapeutic so that the drug can be discontinued before surgery. There is a caveat. Discontinuing anticonvulsants may lead to withdrawal seizures, which is not a pleasant prospect perioperatively. Asymptomatic children with low theophylline levels may not be wheezing on the day of examination but may develop wheezing on the day of surgery and may have serious underlying bronchial hyperreactivity, which may pose difficulties intraoperatively. Our current practice is if a child requires theophylline to suppress wheezing episodes, the child requires therapeutic theophylline levels perioperatively. If this is not possible, knowing the level will allow the anesthesiologist to specifically direct therapy intraoperatively if required. Further testing is guided by the patient's underlying medical condition.

Preoperative assessment for elective surgery should be done early enough to allow all special investigations to be performed before surgery. Consultation with other services and the performance of other investigative procedures, such as computed tomography (CT) scans, ECGs, and echocardiograms, should be timed so that the results will be available to the anesthesiologist before induction of anesthesia. Deciding that such information is important preoperatively but acting before it is obtained or reported sets the stage for medical or legal misadventures.

NPO STATUS AND PREOPERATIVE FASTING

Of all the shibboleths of pediatric anesthesia, perhaps the one most time honored and most frequently under attack is the duration of preoperative fasting. The days of NPO after midnight for all children who require surgery is over. For years, we have realized that small infants, with their unique glucose and fluid requirements, do not benefit by being NPO for 12 hours before surgery. Serious hypovolemia with intraoperative hypotension and hypoglycemia is the result.[66,105] Concerns have been raised about hypoglycemia occurring in older children after a prolonged fast.[105-107] There also are concerns about comfort and the need for the imposition of starvation on children preoperatively. The goal is to reduce gastric volume and minimize the risk of aspiration pneumonia perioperatively. There are many studies looking at factors predisposing to gastric acid aspiration and lung injury and their relationship to gastric residual volumes. The fact remains that perioperative aspiration pneumonia is remarkably rare (a fact that may attest to the success of severe NPO restrictions).

There is little evidence that in a healthy child prolonged fasts are required to ensure minimal gastric volumes. NPO for solid foods and large meals for 8 hours before surgery should be maintained because gastric volumes may be increased for up to 6 hours. The question becomes less clear with fluids. Several studies demonstrate that ad lib clear liquids up until 2 hours before surgery are associated with lower gastric volumes and higher pHs than those found in fasting patients.[108,109] If this is the case, the recommendation ought to be to encourage oral clear fluids preoperatively rather than to limit them. Studies demonstrate that not only is there no major burden of hypoglycemia placed on the healthy child by fasting, but that feeding the child clear liquids is not associated with increased gastric volumes.[110]

The final factor that needs to be considered is whether one should change an age-old guideline for a more liberal approach that may be confusing and lead to unintended changes in other requirements. The guideline of NPO after midnight perhaps is draconian, but it is clear to all concerned. No solids after midnight and clear liquids up to 1 hour before surgery ad lib, if the patient is healthy, without gastroesophageal reflux, or other significant GI disease, certainly is less clear. These liberal rules are bound to be applied in inappropriate situations, potentially leading to catastrophe. Some major institutions allow clear liquids until 1 to 2 hours before surgery in their outpatients, and a large series reported from the Children's Hospital of Philadelphia reports no incidence of gastric aspiration after years of this approach.[109] ASA guidelines indicate fasting for clear liquids from 2 hours preinduction. Communication, education, monitoring current protocols, and flexibility in approach, based on known facts, should form the guidelines for anesthesia practice. This is no less true regarding preoperative fasting rules. The trend is toward more liberal fasting requirements for clear liquids (**Table 20-12**).[111,112]

One final question: What are clear liquids? Water, glucose water, and commercially available pediatric electrolyte solutions are clear. Some institutions consider breast milk a clear liquid and cow's milk a solid food. Breast milk is not emptied as rapidly as clear liquids from the stomach, and the ASA guidelines state breast milk should not be

TABLE 20-12 Fasting Guidelines at Children's Hospital Los Angeles: The 2-4-6-8 Rule

Time Before Anesthetic	All Age Groups	Example
Up to 8 h	Full diet	
Up to 6 h	Liquid diet, infant formula, milk	Formula, Jello
Up to 4 h	Breast milk, clear liquids	
Up to 2 h	Clear liquids only	Electrolyte, glucose, water solutions, apple juice
From 2 h before	NPO	

given within 4 hours of induction. Some institutions encourage gelatin (no additives) and fruit juices, including pulp-free orange juice, as perfectly allowable. It is unlikely that there will be hard scientific data to aid the anesthesiologist in these decisions. The application of common sense and the provision of clear instructions for families are essential. Simplicity is best. Adhering to local protocols is important to avoid confusion and ignoring stated regulations is detrimental to the organized anesthetic care of children.

EVALUATION OF THE CRITICALLY ILL CHILD

Intraoperative treatment of critically ill children can present the anesthesiologist with great challenges. The use of cardiovascularly active anesthetic agents in critically ill children can demand the most meticulous anesthesia care. Thorough preoperative evaluation and preparation is essential to ensure optimal intraoperative management. A rigorous, compulsive systematic evaluation of critically ill children is essential, and although it follows the basic outline of systems review, the underlying assumption is that the severity of illness in each system is much worse than in the patient for elective surgery.

Establishing rapport with a child in an intensive care unit can range from difficult to impossible. An unconscious, heavily sedated, paralyzed child requiring mechanical ventilation and neuroresuscitation will not be communicative. Discussing the anesthesia care with the child's family often may be awkward because survival is the parents' primary concern. Before contacting the family, it is essential that the anesthesiologist be completely familiar with the child's problems so that the parents can be confident that all physicians who are caring for their child are knowledgeable and concerned. Many parents have bonded with the intensive care unit staff and transferring their child's care to other physicians can provoke anxiety. The anesthesiologist needs to demonstrate concern and state that the intraoperative care and management will be as meticulous as that provided for the child in the intensive care unit. Although it is natural to focus entirely on the child's immediate surgical needs or indication for admission to the intensive care unit, other problems that may have anesthetic importance should be sought as they would be in a routine evaluation. A systems review, previous drug and allergy history, and family history should not be neglected.

NEUROLOGIC STATUS

The level of consciousness, presence of CNS injury, intracranial pressure, and neurologic deficits specifically should be determined. Psychotropic drugs, sedatives, and other obtunding agents that may supplement, augment, or interact with anesthetic agents should be identified. Some children in the intensive care unit will be essentially anesthetized at transfer to the operating room, whereas others may have received little medication. Complete review of current neurologic status and psychotropic drugs is mandatory.

RESPIRATORY STATUS

Respiratory evaluation should be meticulous. The level of oxygen required, respiratory rate, ventilatory rate, tidal volume, airway pressures, and arterial blood gases form the basis of this information. If the child requires a ventilator, it is necessary to be familiar with the degree of ventilatory support the child requires, including the fraction of inspired oxygen (FiO_2), mean airway pressure, peak end-expiratory pressure, and respiratory rate. A blood gas just before transfer to the operating room may provide critical information. Anesthesia machine ventilators, although more than adequate for patients with normal pulmonary function, may be inadequate in those with advanced stages of lung disease. The anesthesiologist should be able to organize sophisticated ventilatory support in the operating room when indicated. This should be done before transfer of the child to the operating room in conjunction with respiratory therapy.

CARDIOVASCULAR SYSTEM

Complete familiarity with the child's hemodynamic function is essential. All patients in the critical care unit should be suspected of having compromised cardiovascular function and borderline oxygen delivery. Complete evaluation of perfusion status, temperature, and hemodynamic information as obtained from invasive monitor catheterization should be reviewed and optimized. Optimization of intravascular volume and the hematocrit and availability of blood products should be ensured. A review and optimization of cardiovascular drugs the child is receiving should be undertaken. It is necessary to ensure that constant, uninterrupted delivery of cardiovascular drugs and infusions be continued during transportation. Finally, an ECG and review of the child's rhythm history for the presence of cardiac dysrhythmias should be conducted.

RENAL STATUS

Recent urine output, fluid requirements, creatinine, and blood urea nitrogen (BUN) should be reviewed. Renal function should be assessed and may have an important bearing on the use of neuromuscular relaxants, intraoperative fluid requirements, and electrolyte status. Electrolyte abnormalities are common in those with critical illness and may lead to cardiorespiratory failure and cardiac dysrhythmias intraoperatively. These, in general, should be corrected preoperatively.

GASTROENTEROLOGY

All patients who are ill enough to require admission to an intensive care unit should be suspected of having full stomachs. Acute, critical, and chronic illnesses delay gastric emptying. Even though the child may have been NPO for a prolonged period, hypersecretion and high gastric acid content may predispose the child to aspiration on induction. Patients who have suffered trauma and for whom no NPO history is available should, as a precaution, be treated as having full stomachs.

LABORATORY TESTS

Laboratory investigation should be reviewed thoroughly. At a minimum, baseline CBCs, electrolyte profiles, calcium, and blood gases are essential. Therapeutic levels of drugs, such as theophylline and anticonvulsants, are indicated, if the child is receiving them. A final check to ensure cross-matched blood is available, when indicated, is prudent.

KEY REFERENCES

- Allen EC, Manuel JC, Legault C, et al. Perception of child vulnerability among mothers of former premature infants. *Pediatrics.* 2004;113:267-273.
- American Academy of Pediatrics, Section on Anesthesiology. Evaluation and preparation of pediatric patients undergoing anesthesia. *Pediatrics.* 1996;98:502-508.

- Anderson BJ, McKee AD, Holford NH. Size, myths and the clinical pharmacokinetics of analgesia in paediatric patients. *Clin Pharmacokinet.* 1997;33:313-327.
- Buisson P, Bach V, Elabbassi EB, et al. Assessment of the efficiency of warming devices during neonatal surgery. *Eur J Appl Physiol.* 2004;92:694-697.
- Jacoby DB, Hirshman CA. General anesthesia in patients with viral respiratory infections—an unsound sleep? *Anesthesiology.* 1991;74:969.
- Kain ZN, Caldwell-Andrews AA. Preoperative psychological preparation of the child for surgery: an update. *Anesthesiol Clin North America.* 2005;23:597-614.
- Lehrman J. Inhalational anaesthetics. *Paediatr Anaesthesiol.* 2004;14:380-383.
- Marchant WA, Walker I. Anaesthetic management of the child with sickle cell disease. *Paediatr Anaesth.* 2003;13:473-489.
- Maxwell LG, Deshpande JK, Wetzel RC. Preoperative evaluation of children. *Pediatr Clin North Am.* 1994;41:93-110.
- Maxwell LG, Wetzel RC. Induction techniques in pediatric anesthesia. *Anesth Rep.* 1988;1:110.
- O'Connor ME, Drasner K. Preoperative laboratory testing of children undergoing elective surgery. *Anesth Analg.* 1990;70:176.
- Wetzel RC. Gastro-oesophageal reflux: theory over experience? *Paediatr Anaesth.* 1998;8:101-104.
- Zuckerberg AL. Perioperative approach to children. *Pediatr Clin North Am.* 1994;41(1):15-29.

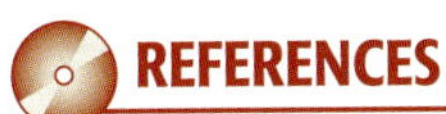

REFERENCES

Complete references available on DVD and online version at www.LongneckerAnesthesiology.com

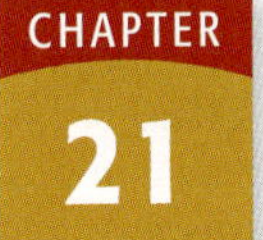

CHAPTER 21 Evaluation of the Geriatric Patient

Frederick W. Lombard
Katherine Grichnik

KEY POINTS

1. The elderly are the fastest growing segment of the population.
2. A healthy elderly patient may have normal organ function but less reserve.
3. There are normal organ and overall functional changes of aging that do not imply disease but must be considered when planning an anesthetic.
4. Elderly patients have a high incidence of chronic disease states.
5. Elderly patients do not require a "special" anesthetic but rather require strict attention to meticulous preoperative assessment, detailed management of intraoperative variables and concurrent disease states, and cautious titration of drug administration and dosages.

In developed countries the elderly population is growing at a remarkable rate, with considerable implications for perioperative health care. Elderly patients now account for more than half of all hospital care days in the United States. In addition, almost a third of all surgical patients are 65 years or older, with an even larger fraction anticipated in the next 2 decades. Virtually every nonpediatric hospital provides a wide range of surgical services for elderly adults; consequently, almost every anesthesiologist in contemporary practice is expected to have expertise in geriatric medicine as it relates to anesthetic practice.[1]

As they age, adults exhibit an increasingly varied array of physical responses to lifelong exposure to environmental and socioeconomic conditions and to the accumulated stigmata of prior traumatic injuries and medical therapies. Prolonged longevity also reveals all intrinsic physiologic strengths and weaknesses and full expression of genetic differences that might not be fully apparent over shorter life-span intervals. The terms *elderly* and *geriatric* are used synonymously in this chapter to describe patients who are 65 years or older. The term *aged* is used to describe individuals older than 80 years.

Neither elderly nor aged surgical patients require a "special" anesthetic. A well-conducted anesthetic of any type can be both safe and appropriate for an elderly patient if the anesthesiologist (1) adheres to high standards of preoperative assessment, (2) closely controls and monitors preexisting disease, and (3) pays meticulous attention to drug dosage and to the details of pain management and postoperative care.[2] The sections that follow describe some of the current concepts of human aging that are relevant to contemporary anesthetic practice, examine common disease states, and review common surgical procedures in the elderly.

CONCEPTS AND THEORIES OF AGING

The exact mechanisms that control the aging process remain unknown. However, it is very clear that aging is not simply the result of accumulated disease. Aging is a physiologic phenomenon that manifests itself in mammalian species as universal and progressive degenerative changes in both the structure and the functional capacity of organs and tissues. The implied consequence of aging in all species is an increasing probability of death as a function of time. Currently, there is no consensus as to when the geriatric era begins in human subjects or whether any single physiologic marker can identify an elderly or an aged patient.

Theories proposed to explain aging broadly fall into 3 categories: *genetic theories*, in which gene-controlled programmed biologic clocks such as telomeres regulate growth, maturity and old age; *neuroendocrine theories*, where changes in neural function and hormones cause age related physiologic changes by interfering with cooperation between organs and impairing the response to external stimuli; and *damage-accumulation theories*, where damage to molecular structures progressively accumulates because repair and maintenance are always less than those required for immortalization. All these mechanisms are important and interrelated.

THE MITOCHONDRIAL FREE RADICAL THEORY OF AGING

Among all the single-cause theories that have been proposed, the mitochondrial free radical theory of aging is without doubt the most studied and the most widely recognized.[3] It is thought that throughout adulthood, increasing levels of oxygen-derived free radicals, or reactive oxygen species (ROS), create oxidative stress within the mitochondria and disrupt the structural and enzymatic machinery of oxidative phosphorylation.[4] Investigations of oxidative phosphorylation in aging mitochondria suggest that aging is associated with progressive impairment of bioenergetic efficiency and increases in the incidence of defects in DNA, primarily mitochondrial DNA (mtDNA), presumably because of increasing levels of ROS.[5] As the ability of the cell to scavenge these by-products of aerobic metabolism declines, ROS may create a self-perpetuating "cycle of aging" within the mitochondria (**Fig. 21-1**).[6] Many gerontologists have concluded that changes in mitochondrial bioenergetics largely explain much of normal human aging and that these appear to play a central role in the diffuse deterioration of cellular and organ function that characterizes human senescence.[7]

However, although it is clear that oxidative damage increases during aging,[8] and it is difficult to doubt that mitochondria play a key role

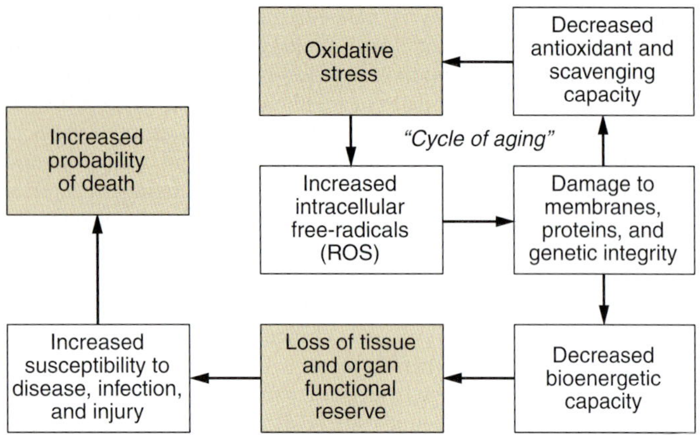

FIGURE 21-1. There may be a self-sustaining "cycle of aging" in which accumulated oxidative stress as a result of aerobic metabolism eventually damages the metabolic machinery and the genetic integrity of mitochondria. ROS, reactive oxygen species.

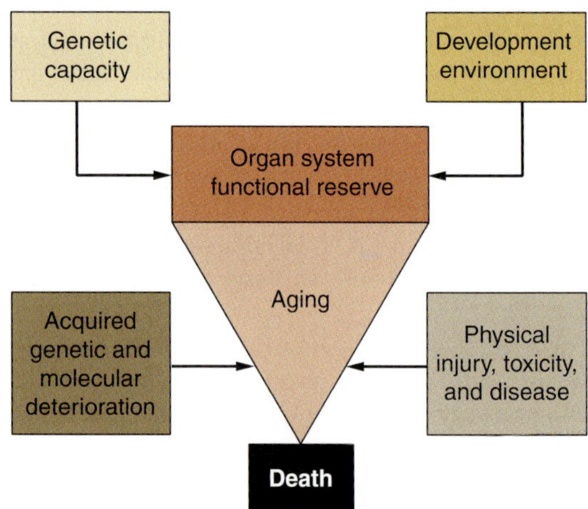

FIGURE 21-3. One concept of organ system functional reserve describes a "wedge" that is broadest at birth but then declines progressively after maturity. Genetically determined organ system functional reserve may determine life *span*, but life *expectancy* reflects "real-world" estimates of human longevity given extrinsic environmental factors. Actual observed life expectancy for a population of individuals is a measure of typical or average longevity and includes those with a "poor" genetic profile as well as those individuals who die of external nongenetic causes. [Reprinted with permission from Jazwinski SM. Longevity, genes, and aging. *Science.* 1996;273:54-59. Copyright, 1996 AAAS.]

in the aging process,[9] the fundamental question regarding whether mitochondrial oxidative stress is causal to the aging process remains unresolved. In fact, a number of studies on long-lived vertebrate species, mutants, and transgenic animals indicate that the concept that aging is triggered by the detrimental action of ROS, produced during normal metabolism, may not be accurate.[10]

ORGAN SYSTEM SENESCENCE

Age-related physiologic change was classically represented as a linear decline of maximal organ system function. The physiologic decline was believed to begin early in young adulthood and continue inexorably downward thereafter. However, contemporary analysis suggests that there is a more complex relationship, with relatively minor decrements in maximal organ function first becoming apparent just after peak of somatic maturation, in the fourth decade of human life. Additional decrements of average maximal function or functional capacity during the middle adult years also appear to be relatively subtle but subsequently become more obvious during the seventh decade of life and beyond (**Fig. 21-2**).

Nevertheless, although some decline of maximal function is inevitable, the competence of integrated organ system function varies greatly from one elderly patient to the next, even in the absence of disease. Functional capacity is significantly altered by differences in physical and mental activity level, comorbidities, social habits, diet, and genetic background. Those elderly patients who maintain greater than average functional capacities are considered "physiologically young." However, when organ function declines at an earlier age than usual, or at a more rapid rate, elderly patients are often described as "physiologically old."

In fact, the extreme variability of signs, symptoms, and physical presentation common among older patients is an essential characteristic of geriatric medicine.[11] This is not surprising, given that human aging represents the interaction of many factors, some universal and some idiosyncratic (**Fig. 21-3**). In all healthy geriatric patients, however, maximal organ system function remains greater than basal demand at all ages. The difference between maximal organ system capacity and basal function defines organ system "functional reserve." Aging is also inevitably associated with a decrease in functional reserve, which also is considered a defining physiologic characteristic of human aging (**Fig. 21-4**).

Clinically, decreased functional reserve implies a universal and predictable increase in the susceptibility of elderly patients to stress- and disease-induced organ system dysfunction. Organ system functional reserve is the "safety margin" that is available to meet, for example, the

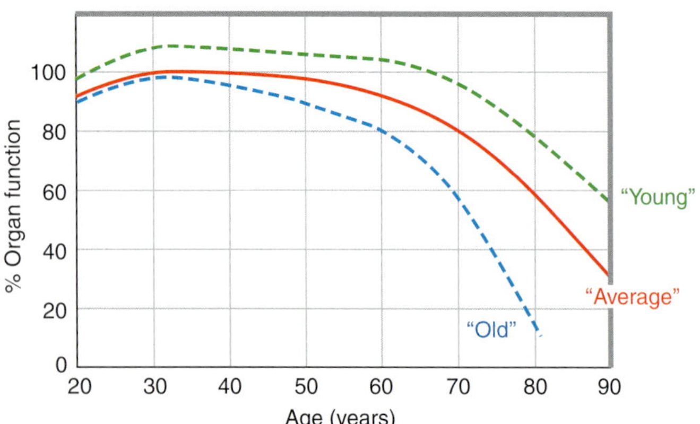

FIGURE 21-2. Differences in the rate at which maximal organ system functions decline with increasing age and differences in initial functional levels explain the inevitable variability seen in geriatric patients, clinically recognized as physiologically "younger" or "older" than average.

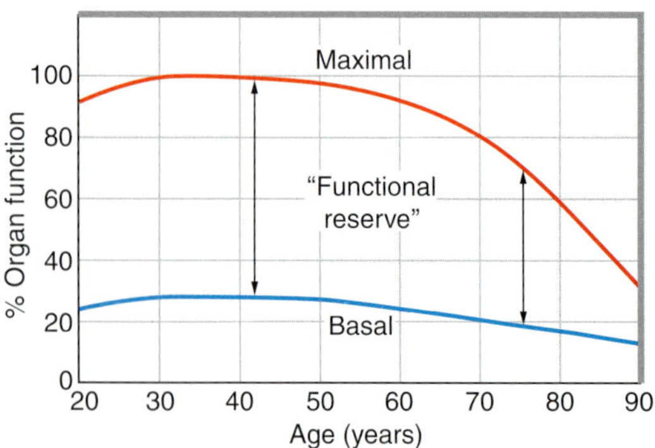

FIGURE 21-4. For any organ system, "functional reserve" represents the difference between basal (minimal) and maximal organ system function. The age-related decline in functional reserve may not be clinically apparent until demands made on the organ system are increased by stress, disease, polypharmacy, or surgical intervention.

additional demands for cardiac output, carbon dioxide excretion, or protein synthesis imposed on the patient by trauma or disease or by surgery, healing, and convalescence. It is therefore of great importance to the anesthesiologist, and preoperative testing in the elderly patient is most effective when it provides the anesthesiologist with a quantifiable assessment of functional reserve. Testing should be clinically directed according to symptoms and complaints referable to age-related disease or to functional decline suggesting erosion of physiologic homeostasis.[12] However, although cardiopulmonary functional reserve can be assessed clinically using various exercise or aerobic stress tests, there are no comparable techniques for assessment of hepatic, immune, or nervous system functional reserve, at least at the present time. These require subjective clinical assessment and detailed clinical history and physical examination, with particular focus on activity levels and the ability to participate fully in the normal activities of daily life.

AGING, METABOLISM, AND BODY COMPOSITION

Older adults of both sexes undergo significant atrophy of most metabolically active tissues, especially brain, liver, and kidney. In addition, normal aging, particularly in men, is associated with a progressive loss of skeletal muscle mass. In aged men, continuing loss of muscle and central organ atrophy eventually produces a significant decline in total body weight, often to levels less than those of young adulthood. In women, however, muscle and bone loss due to osteoporosis are largely offset by increasing body fat, and therefore total body weight usually returns toward, but rarely falls below, young adult values (**Fig. 21-5**).

Skeletal muscle and large well-perfused organs comprise the lean tissue mass (LTM) component of total body weight. Age-related loss of LTM plays a powerful role in altering perioperative metabolism, cardiopulmonary function, and the pharmacokinetics of anesthetic agents. The linear correlation between basal metabolic rate (BMR) and creatinine excretion suggests that decreased muscle mass is largely responsible for the age-related decline in BMR,[13] although middle-age subjects have a slightly lower BMR than younger subjects even when they are comparable in body size, body composition, or activity.[14] BMR decreases in parallel with the contraction of total body water (TBW) throughout most of adulthood, but a more accelerated decline in energy expenditure at rest occurs later in senescence, with kcal/d in the 10th decade only half that of young adults. There do not appear to be any gender-specific differences in the effects of age on BMR that are not related to body composition or activity. Nevertheless, because BMR for both men and women eventually decreases somewhat faster than can be explained from the decrease in LTM, lessened thyroid hormone activity may eventually limit the level of metabolic activity, as well as the mass, of lean tissue components.[15]

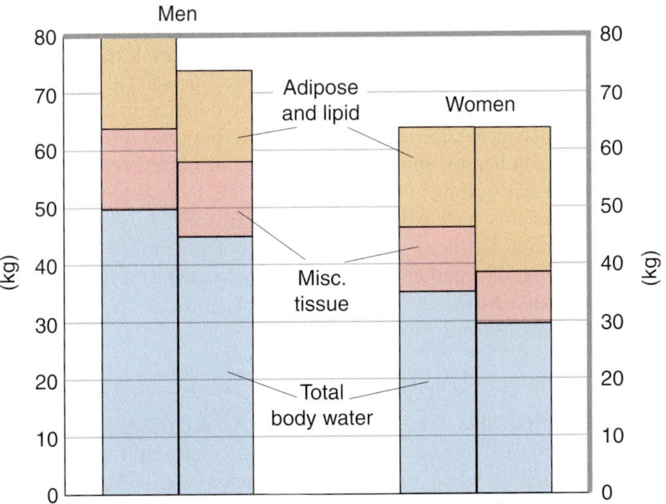

FIGURE 21-5. Age-related changes in body composition are gender specific. In women, total body mass remains constant because increases in body fat (*upper shaded segment*) offset bone loss (*middle segment*) and intracellular dehydration (*lower shaded segment*). In men, body mass decreases despite maintenance of body lipid and skeletal tissue elements because accelerating loss of skeletal muscle and other components of lean tissue mass produces marked contraction of intracellular water (*lower shaded segment*).

After the young adult years, TBW falls 10% to 20%. Virtually all of the age-related changes in body water content are limited to the intracellular compartments. Decreases in circulating blood volume, once believed to be inevitable, actually reflect deconditioning and dehydration and are typical only in bedridden elderly or those with essential hypertension.[16] Plasma volume, red cell mass, and extracellular fluid volumes are well maintained in nonhypertensive elderly individuals who maintain reasonable levels of daily physical activity.

Decreasing LTM reduces the capacity for body heat production, and impairment of thermoregulatory vasoconstriction places elderly surgical patients at increased risk for inadvertent intraoperative hypothermia.[17] In fact, intraoperative core temperature decreases at a rate twice as great as that observed in young adults under comparable conditions, and the time needed for spontaneous postoperative rewarming increases in direct proportion to patient age.[18,19] Because muscle, liver, and other components of LTM provide storage for carbohydrates, aging limits the ability to handle a glucose challenge, even though the timing and the magnitude of insulin release is normal in the elderly. Consequently, aging may be associated with a loss of pancreatic islet cell sensitivity to hyperglycemia, the so-called glucoreceptor defect.[20] Alternatively, age-related glucose intolerance may reflect antagonism of insulin's effect on target tissues.[21] Thus fluid replacement with glucose-containing solutions should be limited to environments that permit frequent measurement of blood sugar levels in elderly patients.

NUTRITION

Malnutrition, also known as undernutrition, is commonly encountered in the geriatric population. The prevalence of undernutrition in hospitalized geriatric medical and surgical patients is particularly high and often unrecognized, unless sought specifically.[22,23] Furthermore, if left untreated, nutritional status continues to deteriorate during the inpatient stay.[24] Moreover, mortality is considerably higher in the malnourished elderly medical patient, compared with those who are nutritionally replete.[25] The etiology of undernutrition in elderly patients is multifactorial and includes (1) functional decline and social isolation from support systems, (2) anorexia associated with older age or chronic illness, (3) anatomic or gustatory impediments to mastication or swallowing, (4) neglect or abuse, and (5) insufficient financial resources.[22]

The postoperative effects of malnutrition are multisystemic with consequences such as poor wound healing, impaired immunity, and poor respiratory function.[26,27] In postoperative patients, food intake may be suboptimal at a time when metabolic requirements are increased. Indeed, it is well established that malnutrition on admission may adversely influence clinical outcome in elderly patients with femoral neck fractures.[28]

CARDIOVASCULAR FUNCTION

Myocardial Stiffening and Diastolic Dysfunction The heart, unlike other major organs, does not atrophy with age. The aging left ventricle is actually thicker and less elastic than its younger counterpart, exhibiting the physical characteristics of *presbycardia*.[29] This is caused by, at least in part, an increase in collagen cross-linking in the myocardial cytoskeleton to which the myocytes are attached.[30] Cross-linking may reflect the buildup of advanced glycation end products produced by the chemical transformation of sugar moieties normally found in tissues.[31] Mitochondrial dysfunction has also been invoked as an explanation for the age-related changes in ventricular dynamics.[32]

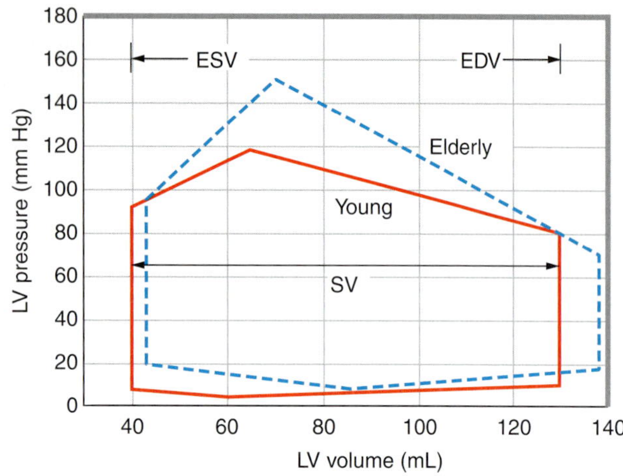

FIGURE 21-6. Left ventricular (LV) cardiac pressure-volume loops for fit young (*solid line*) and elderly (*broken line*) subjects. Older subjects have a slightly higher end-diastolic ventricular volume (EDV) and larger stroke volume (SV), as well as elevated pressures throughout the cardiac cycle, because of increased myocardial stiffness and delayed active relaxation during diastole, delaying the passive phase of ventricular filling. Consequently, aging alters ventricular hemodynamics by increasing dependence on atrial contraction for the maintenance of normal stroke volume.

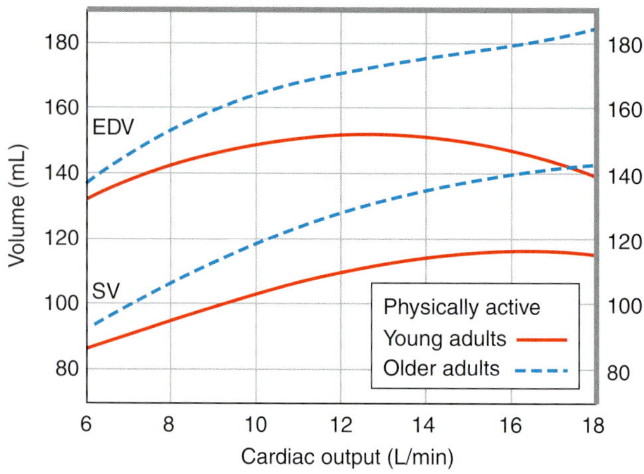

FIGURE 21-7. In healthy older adults (*broken lines*), maximal heart rate is less than that can be achieved by young adults (*solid lines*). Consequently, increases in cardiac output during aerobic metabolic stress are achieved by augmentation of stroke volume (SV) caused by generalized ventricular dilation and increased end-diastolic volume (EDV), with ejection fraction maintained at constant levels.

Whatever the precise mechanism, the stiffer ventricle and atrium do not permit complete chamber relaxation until relatively late in diastole. Consequently, passive ventricular filling, which occurs during the early phase of diastole, is significantly reduced in older adults, producing a form of diastolic dysfunction (**Fig. 21-6**). As a result, the elderly are particularly dependent on the synchronous atrial contraction of sinus rhythm for complete ventricular filling and may experience significant increases in pulmonary blood volume during exercise.[33,34] Small decreases in venous return, such as those produced by positive pressure ventilation, surgical hemorrhage, or venodilator drugs, can significantly compromise stroke volume if even minor cardiac dysrhythmias are present.

Cardiac Output Resting cardiac index in healthy elderly subjects decreases slightly throughout adulthood and into senescence, but this is not evidence of degenerative cardiovascular change.[35,36] To the contrary, reduced cardiac output at rest is an appropriate integrated cardiovascular response to the reduced metabolic activity that occurs because of age-related loss of LTM. Normal aging simply produces a smaller "aerobic machine" with reduced perfusion requirements. Under conditions of submaximal demand, myocardial contractility is well maintained, at least until the eighth decade of life.[37] Short-term demands for increased cardiac output are first met by moderate increases in heart rate and then by increasing left ventricular end-diastolic volumes and pressures.

During vigorous aerobic exercise, the aging, but well-conditioned, heart can increase cardiac output to levels near those of younger adults by generating progressively larger stroke volumes through the Starling mechanism, a nonpathologic adaptation unique to older adults (**Fig. 21-7**).[38] Nevertheless, although many aged individuals compete successfully in a variety of strenuous athletic events, aging does ultimately impose significant limitations of maximal aerobic power generation (maximal oxygen consumption: Vo_2max) by reducing both the inotropic and chronotropic responses to β-agonists and to autonomic reflex pathways.[39,40] In general, however, peripheral factors, such as lactate production and musculoskeletal stiffness, and not cardiac reserve actually limit Vo_2max during strenuous physical exercise in older adults.[35]

Vascular Stiffening and Systolic Hypertension Systolic hypertension with widening of arterial pulse pressure is a major cardiovascular risk factor.[41] It is common in the geriatric population and reflects a gradual increase in large artery stiffness caused by fibrotic replacement of elastic tissues during the adult years.[42] This reduces the ability of the aorta and large arteries to store hydraulic energy and increases vascular impedance to ejection of stroke volume. The end result of these changes is a progressive and sustained increase in left ventricular wall tension and myocardial workload that produces symmetrical ventricular hypertrophy and increased ventricular mass. Impedance to the ejection of stroke volume increases in older adults, even when systemic vascular resistance is unchanged.[43] Increased vascular stiffness and loss of arterial cross-sectional area also increase the reflection of arterial pressure waves that produces the familiar "ringing" characteristics of radial artery waveform tracings in geriatric patients.

Autonomic Control Aging affects the autonomic cardiovascular control mechanisms nonuniformly. Although the parasympathetic component of the arterial baroreflex is diminished, the baroreflex control of sympathetic outflow and the vascular response to sympathetic stimulation are maintained.[44]

Basal levels of catecholamines and sympathetic nerve activity are known to increase with age. Plasma norepinephrine levels gradually increase 10% to 15% per decade.[45] However, in isolated ventricular myocytes the EC50 for isoprenaline is nearly doubled in the elderly.[45] A consequence of the decreased contractile response to catecholamines is that the aging heart is more dependent on the Starling mechanism to maintain cardiac output.[46]

Elderly patients have a lower resting vagal tone, fewer muscarinic receptors, and a decline in muscarinic receptor function.[45] This results in the lower parasympathetic activity observed in the elderly, which has been implicated in the diminished heart rate increase in response to atropine compared with young patients.[47]

PULMONARY FUNCTION

Pulmonary Mechanics Loss of tissue elasticity occurs in the lungs as well as in the cardiovascular system, and all elderly individuals eventually demonstrate some degree of emphysema-like increases in lung compliance. However, calcification and stiffening of the costochondral joints of the thorax reduce chest wall compliance, so net pulmonary compliance does not increase but is usually unchanged.[48] Within the lung parenchyma, fibrous connective tissue proliferates, and there is degeneration and cross-linking of lung elastin.[49] Breakdown of alveolar septae also reduces total alveolar surface area, increasing both anatomic and alveolar dead space.

Loss of lung elastic recoil is the primary anatomic mechanism by which aging degrades the efficiency of pulmonary gas exchange.[50] Small

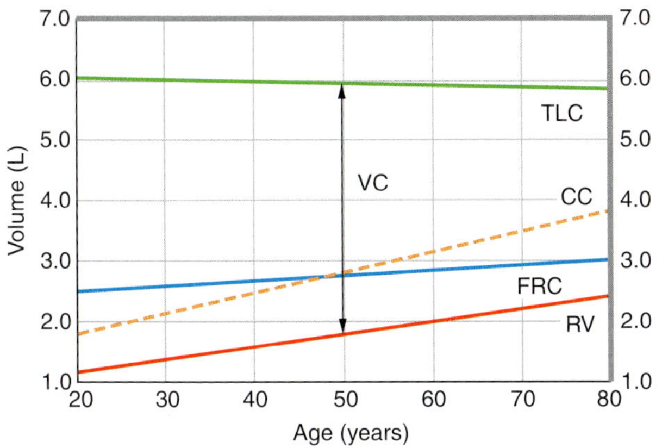

FIGURE 21-8. Total lung capacity (TLC)—the sum of vital capacity (VC) and residual volume (RV)—decreases slowly in older adults of either gender. However, VC, which represents exchangeable intrathoracic gas volume, is markedly compromised by increases in thoracic rigidity and loss of ventilatory muscle power. RV increases because intrinsic lung elastic recoil is progressively reduced. Closing capacity (CC, *dotted line*) increases to a value greater than that of functional residual capacity (FRC). CC greater than FRC implies there is persistent closure of small airways when the lung is at rest in the neutral state.

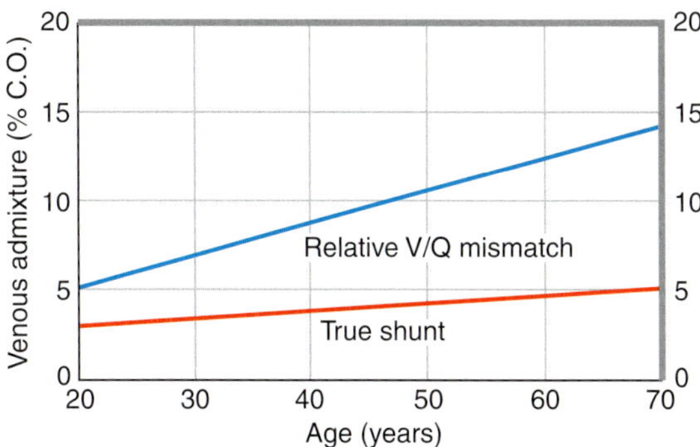

FIGURE 21-9. During anesthesia, total venous admixture (expressed as percentage of cardiac output [CO]) increases with increasing age largely because of a progressively greater amount of diffuse ventilation-perfusion (V/Q) mismatching, with only minimal increases in true intrapulmonary shunting.

airway patency, normally maintained by elastic recoil, is compromised, and closing capacity increases to the point at which it becomes greater than the volume of the lung at rest.[51] The elderly individual probably experiences closure of some small airways even before the end of exhalation, and chronic airway obstruction, detectable as "expiratory scooping" on flow volume loops, is increasingly common but often undiagnosed in senescence.[52] Vital capacity is significantly and progressively compromised because residual lung volume increases at the expense of inspiratory and expiratory reserve volumes (**Fig. 21-8**).[53] Because the changes in elasticity are nonuniform, they severely disrupt the normal matching of ventilation and perfusion within the lungs, increasing both shunting and physiologic dead space.

Informal but clinically valuable assessment of pulmonary function may be possible by questioning the elderly with regard to ability to climb stairs, provided that other causes for stopping, such as claudication, can be excluded. Inability to climb 2 flights of stairs correlates with a forced expiratory volume (FEV) that is less than 70% of predicted value, and failure to achieve 3 flights of stairs may predict severe pulmonary complications after thoracic surgery.[54,55]

Control of Respiration The cardiovascular and ventilatory responses to imposed hypoxia or hypercarbia are delayed in onset and are of smaller magnitude in geriatric patients.[56] However, the moment-to-moment neural control of ventilation and the responses to changes in pH and respiratory gases appear to be essentially unchanged.

Gas Exchange Overall, pulmonary function in older adults during general anesthesia is best characterized as decreased efficiency of gas exchange as a consequence of significant ventilation-perfusion mismatch, primarily because of the deterioration of intrinsic recoil, disruption of alveolar architecture, and increased sensitivity to anesthetic-induced depression of active hypoxic pulmonary vasoconstriction.[57] As a result, total venous admixture during anesthesia increases steadily with advancing age (**Fig. 21-9**).[58] Although the strength and endurance of the ventilatory apparatus remain adequate to meet moderate demands, skeletal calcification and rising airway resistance increase the work of breathing in elderly subjects, predisposing them to acute postoperative ventilatory failure.[59,60]

CENTRAL NERVOUS SYSTEM

With aging, independent of comorbid processes, the brain undergoes a series of deleterious changes. These include gray and white matter atrophy (resulting in reduced brain size and expansion of cerebral ventricles and sulci), synaptic degeneration, blood flow reductions, and neurochemical alterations. These changes are complex and associated with large interindividual variability. There is, however, a pattern of selective loss and preservation.

Brain Atrophy Longitudinal structural magnetic resonance imaging studies have demonstrated a gradual decline in gray matter volume with advancing age.[61,62] In general, these studies suggest that although age is associated with generalized reduction in brain volume, the prefrontal cortical regions are more significantly affected than the rest of the neocortex, with the primary visual cortices maintaining their integrity.[62] The mechanisms of differential brain atrophy are unclear, but vascular risk factors, even at moderate levels, may significantly accelerate its pace.[62] Hippocampal volume is thought to remain relatively stable with age in healthy elderly adults without concurrent hypertension. The relative resilience of hippocampal volume to aging makes hippocampal deviations from normal size a sensitive indicator of pathology, such as vascular or Alzheimer dementia.[62] The loss of brain volume appears not to result from cell death but rather from lower synaptic densities in older adults.[63] Compared with gray matter decline, the decline in white matter volume begins later in life and continues at a more accelerated rate.[61] Diffusion tensor imaging indicates white matter decline in healthy older adults most likely reflects myelin deterioration.[64]

Neurochemical Alterations In addition to the structural effects of aging, there are prominent differences in brain neurochemistry between young and older adults. Progressive, although regionally variable, decrements in dopaminergic and cholinergic signal transduction mechanisms are well described.[65] These are thought to be the result of both pre- and postsynaptic mechanisms. Decreases in the elderly brain neurotransmitter reserves are manifested by decreases in functional activities of daily living and increased sensitivity to anesthetic medications, in particular drugs that might precipitate extrapyramidal symptoms or anticholinergic syndrome. Decreased levels of acetylcholine and dopamine have been implicated in age-related cognitive and behavioral deficits, and they may therefore potentially contribute to postoperative cognitive dysfunction.[66,67]

Cerebral Blood Flow Throughout the adult life span, healthy aging is associated with a 5% per decade reduction in positron emission tomography measures of cerebral blood flow, cerebral blood volume, and cerebral metabolic rate of oxygen in cortical and subcortical regions.[68,69] These reductions can largely be accounted for by the reduction in brain volume associated with aging; flow-metabolism coupling, oxygen extraction ratio, and cerebral autoregulation remain intact.[70,71]

HEPATIC, ENDOCRINE, AND IMMUNE SYSTEMS

The age-related changes in hepatosplanchnic function are predominantly quantitative rather than qualitative.[72] Liver tissue mass decreases approximately 40% by age 80 years, and hepatic blood flow is proportionally reduced, primarily because of decreasing portal perfusion.[73] Hepatic enzyme activities are comparable with those of young adults, but there is great variability of metabolic function that may reflect loss of hepatocyte density.[74] Plasma concentrations of transaminase and other hepatocyte-derived enzymes are similar to those of young adults, but the bromsulfophthalein retention test is prolonged with increasing age, approaching the upper limit of normal in the seventh decade of life.[75] Functional capacity for nitrogen clearance is also progressively reduced in aging adults, as is galactose elimination—both to an extent somewhat greater than can be accounted for based on changes in liver blood flow alone.[76,77] As a result, hepatic biotransformation and protein synthesis, although adequate to meet modest increases in metabolic demand, may easily be overwhelmed by the metabolic demands of trauma, disease, or surgical intervention, especially if associated with arterial hypotension, low cardiac output, hypothermia, or direct hepatic injury.[78] Loss of hepatic functional reserve also explains the reduced rates of plasma clearance and prolonged clinical effects of narcotics and many other xenobiotics in geriatric subjects.[79] Overt hepatic dysfunction and failure appear in approximately 4% of elderly surgical patients, but more subtle degrees of hepatic compromise and limited hepatic functional reserve produce many postoperative complications and may require supportive therapy and intensive care.[80]

Aging appears to have little effect on macrophage and other aspects of phagocytic activity, but even fit elderly subjects exhibit subtle evidence of decreased immune responsiveness and specificity. As people age, the ability of the immune system to distinguish "self" from "nonself" antigens is reduced, increasing the prevalence of autoimmune phenomena and decreasing resistance to infection.[81,82] The effects of aging on mitochondrial function and control of apoptosis may play an important role in this process.[83] Thymic involution at sexual maturity is associated with marked changes in lymphocytic balance that progresses through senescence. Older adults have decreased B- and T-cell lymphocyte activity and depressed serum titers of immunoglobulin E, depressed skin response to exogenous allergens, and impaired delayed hypersensitivity.[84] Older adults are particularly predisposed to streptococcal pneumonia, meningitis, and septicemia. Sepsis is second only to respiratory failure as a cause of morbidity and mortality in elderly trauma patients.[85]

Adrenal tissues also show evidence of age-related atrophy, and cortisol secretion declines at least 15% by 80 years of age, although plasma levels of cortisol remain similar to those of younger adults because of reduced rates of degradation. Similarly, in the pituitary-thyroid axis, thyroxine levels are relatively unchanged, but there is a damped pituitary response to thyrotropin-releasing factor and decline of thyroid-stimulating hormone (TSH) levels, although the end-organ cellular response to TSH is not affected by age.[20,86] However, plasma concentrations of norepinephrine are 2- to 4-fold higher in elderly subjects than in younger adults during sleep, at rest, and even in response to exercise-induced physical stress.[87] These are rarely apparent clinically in elderly patients because aging markedly and progressively depresses β-adrenergic end-organ responsiveness, producing, in effect, endogenous β-blockade.[88] In contrast, there appears to be little change in α-adrenoceptor or cholinoreceptor activity.[89]

RENAL SYSTEM

As people age, there is a progressive reduction in renal tissue mass and renal blood flow (**Fig. 21-10**). Renal plasma flow, glomerular filtration rate (GFR), and, most important, creatinine clearance decline significantly.[90] These deficits are further exacerbated by decreased perfusion caused by cardiovascular system aging and superimposed disease.[91] One must be wary of perioperative fluid balance, potential electrolyte imbalance, and the potential for impaired renal metabolism of perioperatively administered medications. Of note, a "normal" plasma creatinine concentration may not indicate normal renal functional reserve in the elderly patient because creatinine load is greatly reduced by atrophy of skeletal muscle mass. Calculated creatinine clearance remains the most sensitive marker of renal function in the elderly.[90]

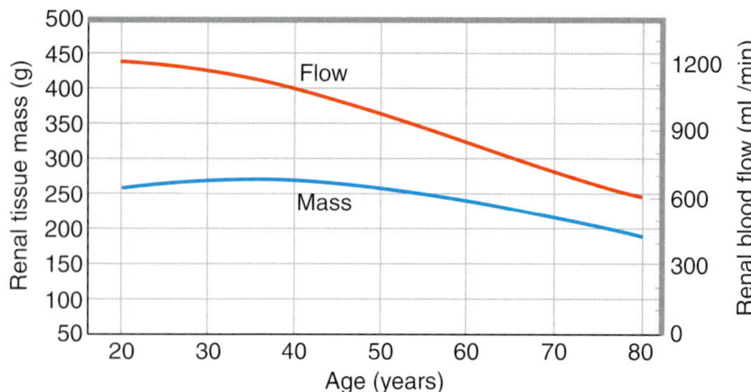

FIGURE 21-10. Renal blood flow decreases more rapidly than does renal tissue mass with increasing age. Glomerular filtration rate (not shown) decreases somewhat more slowly than plasma flow because filtration fraction actually increases in some elderly individuals.

PHARMACOLOGY OF AGING

POLYPHARMACY

The high prevalence of disease in an elderly surgical patient population exposes them not only to the stigmata of the disorders themselves, but also to the risks of polypharmacy from the drugs used for medical therapy.[92] Recent surveys reveal that more than 90% of persons older than 65 years use at least 1 drug per week, 40% take 5 or more drugs, and 12% to 19% use 10 or more medications in a week.[93] Elderly patients account for 30% of all drug prescriptions, approximately twice the rate expected from their representation in the general population, and they consume 40% of all over-the-counter medications.[94] Adverse drug interactions occur more often in older than in younger patients because polypharmacy is more common in older adults, and the reduced hepatic and renal functional reserve of the elderly patient prolongs both the desired and the unwanted effects of their medications.

A detailed medication history is an important part of the geriatric patient's preoperative evaluation. However, inaccurate reporting is common, and it may be necessary to request that patients bring all their medications or a complete list for review by the anesthesiologist.[95] All medications should be carefully reviewed with the specific aim to identify potential interactions.[96] Although it is appropriate to maintain elderly patients perioperatively on all medications needed to effectively control the symptoms of their disorders, especially cardiovascular, neurologic, and metabolic disease, some drug interactions may complicate perioperative management or make the pharmacokinetics of drugs used perioperatively less predictable.[97]

VOLATILE ANESTHETIC AGENTS

The effect of nervous system aging on requirements for general anesthesia is well established.[98] Between young adulthood and the geriatric era, relative minimum alveolar concentration values for the newer inhalational agents decline by approximately 30%, the same decrement seen with older anesthetics such as cyclopropane (**Fig. 21-11**).[99,100] However, the mechanisms producing this age-related increase in pharmacodynamic sensitivity to anesthetic agents remain unknown. Declining neuronal bioenergetics as a consequence of mitochondrial genetic mutation or because of age-related oxidative stress reduce anesthetic requirement, but it is not yet established that this, in fact, explains the reduced anesthetic requirement in the elderly.[101,102] Given this empirical phenomenon, however, agedness itself may be an indication for additional monitoring of anesthetic depth using a processed electroencephalogram or similar device.[103]

INTRAVENOUS ANESTHETIC AGENTS AND OPIOIDS

Clinical experience suggests that there are significant age-related reductions in the dose requirements for virtually all anesthetic agents that

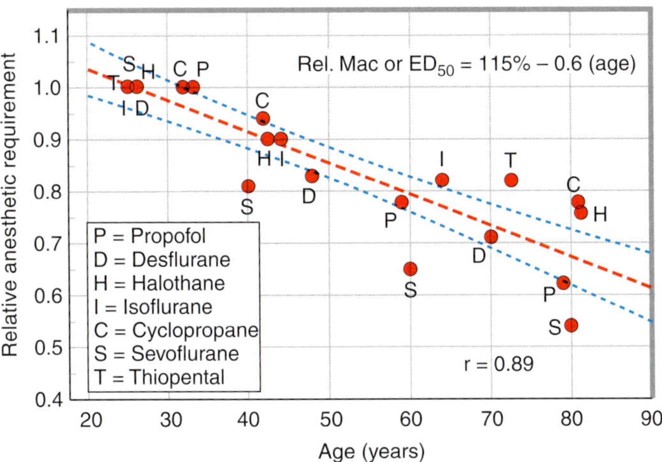

FIGURE 21-11. The age-related decline in relative anesthetic requirement (relative minimum alveolar concentration [MAC] or median effective dose [ED_{50}]) in unsedated human subjects is a consistent characteristic reported for a wide variety of inhaled and injected anesthetic agents.

depress consciousness.[104,105] However, pharmacologic data for the effect of aging on the dose requirements for opioids, barbiturates, and benzodiazepines are less consistent than those for inhalational anesthetics. Most studies suggest that aging increases brain sensitivity to narcotics, but the effects of aging on the pharmacodynamics of barbiturates or etomidate are less impressive.[106-109] Plasma drug concentrations immediately after intravenous injection are usually higher in elderly than in young adults.[110] Consequently, there remains considerable controversy as to whether the clinically apparent age-related increase in the potency of these drugs is truly a pharmacodynamic phenomenon or whether it simply reflects age-related changes in the "alpha" or early phase redistribution pharmacokinetics of injected agents.

In any case, the concentrations of short-acting intravenous (IV) agents in plasma change so rapidly and in such a complex manner that the 2-compartment pharmacokinetic model used in traditional pharmacokinetic studies may be of little value for studying the early or "alpha-phase" behavior of these drugs and their subsequent redistribution in elderly subjects.[111] Because the interaction between subtle changes in both pharmacodynamics and redistribution pharmacokinetics is sufficiently complex and unpredictable, some researchers believe that it must be characterized for each drug to predict the implications of aging on IV drug dosage.[112]

The net effect of age-related structural and functional changes within the nervous system on pain-related neurologic function remains controversial. The study of the amplification, modulation, and selectivity of afferent input within the spinal cord, thalamus, and other locations within the aging nervous system does not yet permit broad generalizations regarding aging and perception of pain.[113,114] In addition, optimizing postoperative pain management in older adults may be further complicated by cognitive impairment and by unrealistic fear of opioid side effects.[115] Perceived intensity of perioperative pain also appears to depend far more on anxiety, personality, and the prospect of long-term debility or disfigurement than on age itself.[116] Nevertheless, the classic observation that opiate requirements are inversely related to patient age and essentially independent of body weight remains a useful and valid general guideline.[117]

NEUROMUSCULAR BLOCKING AGENTS

Although the elderly have reduced skeletal muscle mass, disseminated neurogenic atrophy at the neuromuscular junction allows proliferation of extrajunctional cholinoreceptors. An increased density of cholinoreceptors at the muscle end plate implies that increased concentrations of neuromuscular blocking drugs are needed to produce competitive blockade. In fact, the median effective dose and steady-state plasma concentration required for half-maximal neuromuscular blocking effect (median effective concentration) remain virtually unchanged, or may actually increase slightly, in the elderly patient.[118] Maximal relaxant effect is delayed in onset relative to that produced in young adults, and duration of blockade is prolonged for relaxants with hepatic or renal elimination because plasma clearance declines with increasing age.[119-122] Significant interindividual variability in the duration of neuromuscular blockade has been described with rocuronium and vecuronium in elderly patients.[123,124] This unpredictability may be an important contributor to residual neuromuscular blockade in elderly patients. Relaxants, such as cisatracurium, that do not require organ-based elimination may provide more consistent duration of clinical effects.[123,124] In elderly patients with limited functional reserves, it is therefore mandatory that quantitative neuromuscular monitoring be used to guide maintenance dosing, determine the optimum time for antagonism (train-of = four count = 4), and document the full return of neuromuscular function (train-of-four ratio >0.9) before extubation.[125] Solely relying on expectations of the pharmacokinetics of relaxant elimination and clinical signs such as sustained head lift cannot be justified.[125,126]

Antagonism of neuromuscular blockade with an anticholinesterase or sugammadex should be routine in all geriatric patients.[126] The cardiac muscarinic effects of anticholinesterases, such as bradycardia and conduction defects, are more pronounced with neostigmine (35%) than with pyridostigmine (14%) in elderly patients.[127] Although studies in elderly patients are still lacking, sugammadex has been shown to be safe in clinical trials and free from any significant cardiovascular effects.[128] It does not interfere with acetylcholine metabolism and there should therefore be no effect on the cardiovascular system or smooth muscles and no increase in secretions. There is no requirement to add an anticholinergic drug when giving sugammadex, thereby avoiding any possible side effects due to anticholinergic drugs.

COMMON COMORBID DISEASE STATES

The functional capacity of organs reduces with age, resulting in decreased reserve, decreased compensation for stress, and increased incidence of coexisting diseases. Coexisting diseases further depress organ function, leading to even greater risk with surgical procedures. It is useful to review the common diseases encountered in the elderly.

CARDIOVASCULAR DISEASE

The elderly patient is likely to suffer from altered cardiovascular function. Common disease states include coronary artery disease, cardiac valvular disease, congestive heart failure (CHF) and diastolic dysfunction, abnormal heart rhythm, systolic hypertension, and peripheral vascular disease.

Coronary Artery Disease The presence of coronary artery disease (CAD) increases with age. Anatomic CAD can be detected in more than 50% of people older than 70 years (**Fig. 21-12**).[129] CAD in the aged is more severe and diffuse than in younger patients.[130,131] There are differences in prevalence by gender: At 65 years of age, CAD is more prevalent in men than in women; by age 80, the prevalence of symptomatic congestive heart disease is nearly equivalent in men and women.[131] Despite the high prevalence of anatomic CAD, only 10% to 20% of people older than 65 years carry a diagnosis of active CAD.[131] This may be a result of misdiagnosis, lack of clinical symptoms because of inactivity, or lack of recognition of risk factors leading to diagnosis. One study reported that 37% of elderly patients had subclinical CAD, making it as common as clinically overt CAD in older adults.[132] Furthermore, in this study, the presence of subclinical CAD was significant because it strongly predicted overt CAD, stroke, and mortality, even after adjustment for traditional cardiovascular risk factors.[132] Despite the high prevalence of CAD, over the last 30 years in the United States, the CAD mortality rate has decreased significantly. This includes reduced recurrent myocardial infarction and increased postmyocardial infarction survival.

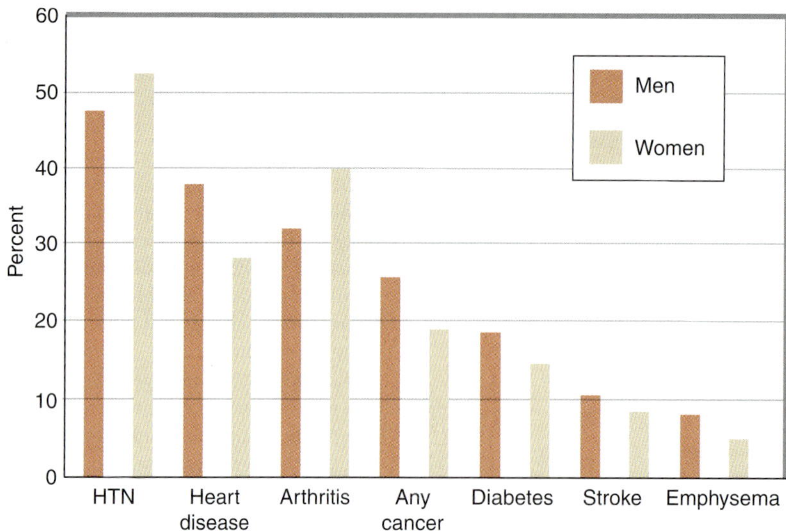

FIGURE 21-12. The percentage of chronic disease in a noninstitutionalized adult population older than 65 years (data averaged from 2000 to 2002). HTN, hypertension. [Adapted from Centers for Disease Control and Prevention, National Center for Health Statistics, National Health Interview Survey. http://www.agingstats.gov/chartbook2004/healthstatus.html. Accessed June 19, 2006.]

Cardiac Valvular Disease

Aortic Valve The mitral and aortic valves may undergo significant age-related dysfunction. Common causes of valvular heart disease in the elderly are degenerative calcification, myxomatous degeneration, papillary muscle dysfunction, and infective endocarditis.[133]

The most frequent valvular lesion in the elderly is degenerative calcified aortic stenosis, with a prevalence of 2.5% at the age of 75 years and of almost 8% at 85 years.[34]Aortic regurgitation, mostly mild, was found in 29% of the entire study cohort. The severity of aortic stenosis in the elderly is often underestimated because its progression is so gradual and because symptoms may be attributed to normal aging, but stenosis severity may progress rapidly after age 80.[135] Common causes of aortic valve stenosis are calcification of a congenital bicuspid aortic valve, degenerative aortic stenosis, and rheumatic heart disease (which may coexist with mitral valve disease).

Mitral Valve Mitral valve disorders are common in the elderly, but the symptoms of mitral valve disease may be masked or exacerbated by coexistent CAD, pulmonary disease, hypertension, and other systemic disorders that commonly occur in older adults.[136] Chronic mitral regurgitation is the most common type of mitral valve disease in the elderly. Rarely, isolated chronic mitral regurgitation occurs as a consequence of papillary muscle dysfunction after myocardial infarction. Chronic mitral regurgitation may also be a result of mitral annular calcification, myxomatous valve degeneration (with mitral valve prolapse), chordal rupture, and rheumatic heart disease. Mitral annular calcification occurs in approximately 6% of people older than 60 years, predominantly in women. The incidence of myxomatous valvular degeneration increases with age.

Mitral stenosis is a disease of younger patients because severe mitral stenosis usually leads to surgery or death before 65 years of age.[136] If present, mitral stenosis is usually a result of rheumatic heart disease, a common condition when the current elderly population was young. Less commonly, mitral stenosis develops because of progressive mitral annular calcification.

Tricuspid Valve Tricuspid regurgitation is usually a result of annular dilation caused by right ventricular failure (usually resulting from left-sided heart failure) or pulmonary hypertension. Unlike in younger patients, infective endocarditis is a less common cause of tricuspid valve dysfunction. Tricuspid stenosis is rare in the elderly.

Pulmonic Valve Pulmonic valve disease as a consequence of primary valve dysfunction is rare but is usually secondary to pulmonary hypertension.

Concurrent Valvular Disease Concomitant mitral and aortic valve disease is common in the elderly. About half of patients with rheumatic mitral regurgitation have associated aortic valve disease, usually aortic regurgitation. In one study, concurrent mitral regurgitation found in elderly patients undergoing isolated aortic valve replacement (AVR) was found to be an independent risk factor for long-term survival.[137]

Systolic Hypertension, Diastolic Dysfunction, and Congestive Heart Failure As reviewed earlier, diastolic dysfunction and systolic hypertension are common and increase with aging. Ninety percent of Americans who have a healthy blood pressure at 55 years of age will have hypertension when they reach 75 years of age.[138] Another common problem in the elderly is chronic heart failure, which can be divided into 2 broad categories: systolic heart failure and diastolic heart failure.[139] Diastolic heart failure occurs more frequently in the elderly, in women, and in those with systolic hypertension, but it is less associated with concurrent CAD than systolic heart failure.[139]

Peripheral Vascular Disease Peripheral vascular disease is not a normal consequence of aging but is associated with systemic atherosclerosis and other risk factors for CAD, many of which are commonly found in the aging patient. The prevalence of peripheral arterial disease increases with age and has a variable presentation: asymptomatic, associated with intermittent claudication, or associated with critical limb ischemia.[140]

Abnormal Heart Rhythm Age-related changes in atrial chamber size and pressure, in left ventricular mass, and in catecholamine levels, in addition to increased incidence of CAD, contribute to a higher incidence of arrhythmias and conduction disturbances in the elderly. Common arrhythmias are atrial fibrillation, ectopic beats, and heart block.

Atrial Fibrillation Atrial fibrillation (AF) is among the most common arrhythmias seen in the general population.[141] The prevalence of this condition is increasing and increases with age; it occurs in approximately 6% of people older than 65 years as compared with approximately 2% of people between 40 and 65 years of age.[142] In all age groups, men are more affected than women. It is believed that by 2050, more than 5.6 million people will have AF and that more than 50% of those older than 85 years will have this condition.[143] Multiple conditions predispose to AF, including structural heart disease, hypertension, CAD, heart failure thyrotoxicosis, sick sinus syndrome, and amyloidosis. Further, AF is common after certain procedures such as cardiac surgery with a perioperative incidence up to approximately 35%. AF is not a trivial rhythm because it increases morbidity and mortality, usually due to stroke.

Heart Block There is a striking increase in the incidence of bradydysrhythmias and conduction abnormalities associated with progressive fibrosis in both the sinus node and atrioventricular conduction system in the elderly; sinoatrial pacemaker cells decrease progressively from 60 years of age such that approximately 10% of the cells are still present at age 75, while fat can also accumulate, serving to separate nodal tissue from the atria musculature.[144] Bradydysrhythmias may be present preoperatively but can initially present as unexpected heart block under general anesthesia.[145]

PULMONARY DISEASE

Emphysema and chronic pulmonary obstructive disease are not associated with normal aging but are the consequences of exposure to environmental toxins, such as tobacco, which may vary among populations. One study from Norway estimated that in people older than 70 years, 11% reported having at least one current obstructive pulmonary disease, 8% reported daily wheezing, and 12% reported significant dyspnea.[146] However, they noted that the only respiratory symptom or disorder to show any clear age-related pattern was dyspnea, which increased through 89 years of age before decreasing.

As noted, because of declines in immunologic function, the elderly person is more prone to pneumonia than a younger person. Furthermore, there may be an increased risk of aspiration pneumonia as a result of other conditions such as gastrointestinal sphincter malfunction or altered mental status.

As is expected in an aging population, the absolute number of patients with lung cancer is increasing. Historically, there has been a reluctance to treat elderly lung cancer patients aggressively because of a lack of supportive data and concern for potential toxicity. However, the bulk of evidence suggests that healthy elderly patients can benefit from therapy in all stages of non–small cell lung cancer and that the decision to offer therapy should be based on comorbidities and performance status rather than age.[147]

GASTROINTESTINAL DISEASE

Although most gastroenterologic disorders that develop in younger people may also develop in the elderly, the presentation, treatment, and prognosis may be different.[148] Disorders that may have a higher incidence in the elderly include peptic ulcer, ischemic complications of vascular abnormalities, drug-induced disorders, malignancies, and passive reflux. Competent upper and lower esophageal sphincters should not be assumed, leading to the increased risk of silent aspiration. Also important to consider in the perioperative patient is the high likelihood of a gastrointestinal side effect of a medication such as a nonsteroidal anti-inflammatory agent.[149] Furthermore, there may be an increased risk of constipation and bowel obstruction with opioids in the elderly.

RENAL DISEASE

Known decreases in renal function and GFR lead to a high incidence of mild chronic renal insufficiency. Progression to chronic kidney disease is associated with a high risk of renal failure, cardiovascular disease, and death.[150] Many common comorbid disease states contribute to the increased incidence of renal dysfunction, including systemic hypertension, systemic arteriosclerotic disease, and chronic CHF. Regardless of the cause, the severity of chronic kidney disease can be classified by GFR (**Table 21-1**). Albuminuria is also used for diagnosis of renal dysfunction. This is a common problem because 18% of people older than 60 years have albuminuria, and 7% have an estimated GFR less than 60 mL/min per 1.73 m^2.[151] In people 70 years or older, those percentages increase to 30% and 26%, respectively.[151]

The diagnosis of renal dysfunction is indirect as GFR is estimated from the serum creatinine concentration or with creatinine-based estimations. One should not rely on creatinine alone; equations for GFR estimation should incorporate additional demographic and clinical variables.

TABLE 21-1 The Severity of Kidney Disease Classified by Glomerular Filtration Rate

Stage	GFR mL/min per 1.73 m^2
1	Normal or mild decrease
2	60-100
3	30-59
4	15-29
5	<15

GFR, glomerular filtration rate.

From National Kidney Foundation. K/DOQI clinical practice guidelines for chronic kidney disease: evaluation, classification, and stratification. *Am J Kidney Dis.* 2002;39:(Suppl 1): S1-S266.

Other problems to consider include urinary tract obstruction, common in elderly patients with an increased rate of benign prostatic hypertrophy, urinary incontinence, and a high incidence of silent urinary tract infections that may lead to perioperative infections or even urosepsis if left untreated.

MUSCULOSKELETAL DISEASE

The known changes in the musculoskeletal system lead to predictable disorders, including tendon and ligament tears, especially in the rotator cuff, the biceps tendon, the quadriceps tendon insertion to the patella, the Achilles tendon, and the posterior tibial tendon. A large study in the United Kingdom identified the odds ratio of an Achilles tendon rupture to be 6.4% in patients ages 60 to 70 years and 20.4% in patients age 80 years or older.[152] There is also an increased incidence of osteoarthritis with age. Less clearly associated with aging but with a high incidence in the elderly patient is rheumatoid arthritis.[153] These conditions are associated with known problems with airway manipulation and positioning. Spinal column intervertebral disk degeneration with disk herniation and osteophyte formation is progressive in the elderly and may lead to cauda equina or nerve root impingement and symptoms of spinal stenosis. Other conditions include polymyalgia rheumatica, gout, and pseudogout.

ENDOCRINE DISEASE

Several endocrine disorders occur frequently in the elderly, including thyroid disorders, diabetes, and androgen deficiency.[154] Glucose intolerance is especially important to assess, and thyroid disease is an underappreciated cause of morbidity in the elderly patient. A study of 3 233 individuals age 65 years or older showed an association between subclinical hyperthyroidism and development of atrial fibrillation.[155] However, this study did not support the hypothesis that unrecognized subclinical hyperthyroidism or subclinical hypothyroidism is associated with other cardiovascular disorders or mortality.

NEUROLOGIC AND MENTAL STATUS DISEASE

Starting with middle age, there is a progressive decrease in learning and memory, a factor to consider when assessing the ability of an elderly person to cooperate with perioperative care. An interesting hypothesis is that this is not caused by loss of the ability to generate new neurons but rather to a reduction in the decline of growth factors (fibroblast growth factor-2, insulin-like growth factor-1, and vascular endothelial growth factor) necessary for new neuron growth.[156] There is also an increased occurrence of all forms of dementia, including Alzheimer dementia and neurologic disorders such as Parkinson disease.[157]

The risk of suffering a stroke increases linearly with age and is associated with other forms of cardiovascular disease, especially atrial fibrillation. For example, the proportion of strokes with AF in the United States is 6.2% for patients who are 50 to 59 years of age, 7.3% for patients 60 to 69 years of age, 16.5% for patients 70 to 79 years of age, and 30.8% for patients 80 to 89 years of age.[158,159] Other causes of stroke are hypertension, cerebrovascular disease, myocardial infarction, structural heart disease, and cardiomyopathy. A history of neurologic dysfunction before a procedure may predict persistent increased cognitive dysfunction.[160]

Depression is very common in the elderly, with fewer reported symptoms than in younger people.[161] It is estimated that more than a third of hospitalized elderly patients may suffer from depression.[162] Not only does depression lead to increased symptoms from medical illness and increased use of health care resources, but it may affect the patient's ability to cooperate with preoperative conditioning and postoperative rehabilitative care. Interestingly, depression may be related to disturbances in other systems, such as the hypothalamic–pituitary–adrenal axis, cerebrovascular disease, inflammatory conditions, and nutrient deficiencies.[163] Another condition to be aware of in the elderly is alcoholism, with implications for perioperative withdrawal and malnutrition.[164]

OPHTHALMOLOGIC DISEASE

Visual impairment is common in elderly and aged patients. The most common causes include presbyopia, macular degeneration, cataract formation, diabetic retinopathy, and glaucoma. Untreated, visual impairment leads to physical handicap, increased incidence of falls, depression, social isolation, and dependency.[165] Visual diseases and the medications used to treat them must be considered with the choice of anesthetic agents. Furthermore, perioperative disorientation or delirium may be in partly a result of declines in visual stimuli.

HEARING IMPAIRMENT

Hearing loss occurs linearly with age, but the variation in hearing thresholds is large. Possible explanations include precipitating medical conditions, coexisting diseases, prior environmental exposure (especially occupational), and undefined genetic contributions.[166] Hearing impairment may also contribute to postoperative delirium.

ONCOLOGIC DISORDERS

Worldwide, the incidence of cancer in the elderly continues to rise with more than 50% of all cancers and approximately 70% of cancer deaths occurring in patients age 70 years and older in developed countries.[167] However, the use of combined modality therapy may improve survival in a variety of malignancies in the elderly, despite the known risks of chemotherapy. Although the elderly are less well studied in clinical trials, age itself should not be used as a criterion for denial of cancer therapy. Rather patients should be carefully selected and evaluated for life expectancy, performance and nutritional status, social support, and presence of medical or social conditions that may impede therapy.[168] Decisions should also be made with respect to the anticipated benefit in quality or quantity of life.

COMMON PROCEDURES IN THE ELDERLY

Currently, more than 20% of people older than 60 years undergo surgery and anesthesia as compared with fewer than 15% of those ages 45 to 60 years. These proportions are expected to increase in the future. Despite the higher numbers of elderly patients having surgery, mortality and morbidity rates have been declining.[169]

Because all types of surgical operations are being offered to increasingly older people, it is important to differentiate the effects of aging from the pathology of individual disease processes and to control for comorbid conditions. In general, preoperative testing is not determined on the basis of age but in consideration of the procedure, the coexistent disease states, and the overall condition of the patient.[170] However, it is reasonable to search for common, but perhaps asymptomatic, comorbid problems, such as subclinical cardiac disease or glucose intolerance. Common procedures in the elderly are briefly reviewed next.

CARDIAC SURGERY

All types of cardiac procedures, including coronary artery bypass grafting (CABG), valvular repair or replacement, and ventricular assist device placement, are being offered to older patients, even those patients older than 80 years. The morbidity and mortality of these procedures increase with age, but the benefits are a greater life expectancy as well as a better quality of life.

In-hospital mortality for CABG is approximately 8% for patients older than 80 years and is similar in highly selected patients older than 90 years.[171] Although there are limited studies, the data appear to suggest that elderly patients at higher risk have better outcomes with revascularization than with medical therapy alone.[171,172]

AVR-combined procedures (AVR and CABG) and, to a lesser extent, mitral valve surgery are increasingly offered to the elderly. The risk appears to be similar to CABG alone; 2 authors reported in-hospital mortality rates of 7.9% and 8.5% for mitral and aortic valve surgery, respectively.[173,174,] Certainly age and comorbid disease states play a role both in morbidity and mortality but also in the choice of valve repair versus the type of prosthetic valve use.[175]

Heart failure is an increasingly common problem, which affects more than 5 million Americans and 15 million Europeans.[176] Left ventricular assist devices have evolved as destination therapy for advanced heart failure patients who are not candidates for heart transplant, leading to a significant increase in use in elderly patients with this condition.[177] This surgical procedure is likely to increase over time as the population ages and patients reach the limit of effective medical management for advanced heart failure.

VASCULAR SURGERY

Vascular disease is prevalent in the elderly population, with major vascular procedures most commonly performed to treat the effects of peripheral vascular disease and carotid artery atherosclerosis. Therefore many elderly patients undergo aortic repair (open and endovascular), femoral-to-popliteal bypass grafting, and carotid endarterectomy. In general, the morbidity and mortality of many vascular operations are not different between a *healthy* elderly patient and a younger patient, but the elderly are often not diagnosed until late in the disease process, leading to higher risk procedures with higher mortality rates.[178] Endovascular interventions have made vascular surgery less invasive; one comparison of aortic endovascular repair to open repair revealed a reduced incidence of perioperative complications compared with open vascular surgery.[179] However, long-term follow-up determined that the incidence of cardiac mortality and myocardial infarction was similar.

CARDIAC CONDUCTION PROCEDURES

With the significant increase in conduction abnormalities, CAD, and CHF in the elderly, it is logical to anticipate an increased incidence of procedures to treat these abnormalities. In fact, half of all pacemakers implanted in the United States are for patients age 75 years and older.[180] Additionally, biventricular pacing for heart failure and cardioverter-defibrillator implantation are also being increasingly used in the care of the elderly, although efficacy and benefit in the elderly are less than those in younger patients.[181,182]

THORACIC PROCEDURES

The choice to undertake thoracic procedures must be carefully weighed against the risks and benefits in an elderly population. For example, an oncologic indication for a procedure may carry more weight than a quality-of-life indication (eg, surgery for emphysema) in this higher-risk population. A study of 356 patients older than 70 years after lung resection found a 33% to 48% 30-day morbidity and a 4% to 69% 30-day mortality rate.[183] Independent predictors for postoperative complications included a low predicted postoperative forced expiratory volume in 1 second (FEV_1), concurrent CAD, and extended resection. Others have found that post–lung resection morbidity is predicted by a reduction in the ability to carry out activities of daily living, decreased cognition, and length of surgery.[184] Brunelli et al suggested that a simple screening test for surgical fitness is the ability to climb stairs because it was determined that concomitant cardiac disease and a low stair height climbed preoperatively predicted cardiopulmonary complications in the elderly after lung resection.[185] The type of procedure contemplated may also affect the decision to offer a surgical intervention, in that a minimally invasive procedure may lead to less immediate morbidity, although the overall long-term mortality may be similar. Esophageal resection has a particularly high morbidity and mortality at baseline, but age as a sole criterion has only a minor influence on overall outcome.[186] There appear to be fewer age-related concerns for other types of smaller thoracic procedures such as bronchoscopies, mediastinoscopies, and esophagoscopies.

TRANSPLANT PROCEDURES

Organ transplant is also becoming increasingly common among the elderly as the contraindications for transplant with respect to age are being relaxed. An especially interesting program is the Eurotransplant Senior Program that allocates kidneys within a narrow geographic area from donors age 65 years or older to recipients 65 years or older regardless of human leukocyte antigen. Graft and patient survival were not adversely affected, but a 5% to 10% higher rejection rate was noted as compared with younger recipients or younger donors.[187] In contrast, survival of elderly heart transplant patients is significantly lower than in young recipients with increased risk of renal failure and malignancy among elderly patients.[188] As above, destination a ventricular assist device may be used to complement heart transplant to treat advanced heart failure. Similarly, lung transplants are being offered to patients up to 70 years but must be cautiously allocated to those most likely to benefit.[189] One group found that the risk of death increased dramatically after age 70 and concluded that lung transplant should be very limited for those older than 70 years.[189]

ORTHOPEDIC PROCEDURES

As osteoarthritis and rheumatoid arthritis increase with age, so do the procedures to treat these conditions, primarily knee and hip replacements. Furthermore, the high prevalence of skeletal disease, combined with an increased predisposition to fall, leads to a high incidence of fractures (especially of the hips, the vertebrae, and the wrists) in older people who then present for treatment on an emergency basis (**Fig. 21-13**).

Hip Replacement Hip replacement and repair of hip fracture are exceedingly common operations in the elderly and aged populations. Unfortunately, hip fracture also carries a very high mortality rate of 20% in the first year after fracture.[190]A Cochrane review of the treatment of evidence-based best practices for elderly hip fracture patients revealed that spinal anesthesia, pressure-relieving mattresses, perioperative antibiotics, and deep venous thromboses prophylaxis were beneficial, whereas preoperative traction was not beneficial, and types of surgical management, postoperative wound drainage, and even "multidisciplinary" care lacked sufficient evidence to determine either benefit or harm.[191] A large study of 2390 patients older than 60 years with hip fracture found a 9.6% 30-day mortality and a 33% 1-year mortality after hip fracture surgery; preoperative variables that predicted mortality included 3 or more comorbid conditions, preexisting chest infection, and concurrent malignancy.[192]

Knee Replacement Total knee replacement (TKR) is primarily a surgery for the elderly, with younger patients less likely to be referred for surgery than older patients.[193] As the population ages, TKR is now almost as common as total hip replacement. Long-term results in patients older than 70 years are excellent, but infection and loosening and malpositioning of the implants are common complications.[194]

GENITOURINARY TREATMENT

Elderly men are subject to abnormalities of the urethra primarily related to benign prostatic hypertrophy and prostate cancer; commonly leading to a transurethral prostrate procedure. In contrast, elderly women are prone to bladder and vaginal relaxation with urinary incontinence and prolapse symptoms. Thus many urethral and urethrovaginal procedures are performed on patients older than 65 years. In one study, preexisting cardiovascular disease increased the risk of perioperative complications in elderly women undergoing urogynecologic surgery, but the overall perioperative morbidity rate was low.[195] Procedures to treat benign prostatic hypertrophy are commonly performed and usually well tolerated in the elderly. Although age is a prognostic factor for bladder cancer resection, this surgical procedure is also being performed frequently in the elderly patient.[196]

ABDOMINAL SURGERY

Abdominal procedures are undertaken in the elderly for a variety of reasons. As surgical and anesthesia techniques have developed, age is no longer considered a contraindication to an intra-abdominal procedure, in part due to increased use of minimally invasive approaches.[197]

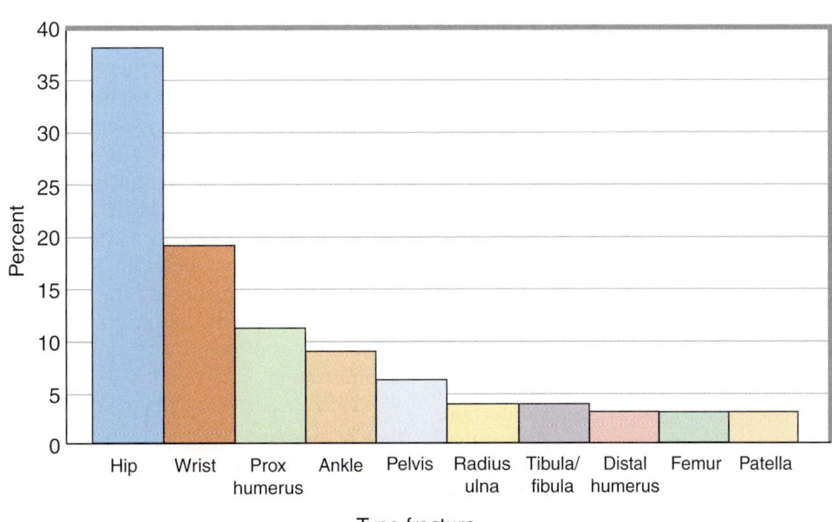

FIGURE 21-13. The most common types of fractures found in Medicare beneficiaries for the 1 year between July 1991 and June 1992. [Data from Grecula MJ, Caban ME. Common orthopaedic problems in the elderly patient. *J Am Coll Surg.* 2005;200:774-783.]

However, one should be aware of mesenteric ischemia as the cause for abdominal surgery in combination with vascular procedures. This condition typically presents in patients older than 70 years and carries a high incidence of morbidity and mortality due to both the predisposing factors of arteriosclerosis, hypertension, CAD, CHF, diabetes, and obesity but also due to the range and inconsistency of presenting symptoms leading to confusion with other abdominal processes.[198]

EYE SURGERY

Visual impairment conditions increase with age, as do corrective surgical procedures to restore sight; elderly patients represent the majority of the surgical population scheduled for ophthalmologic surgery.[199] Eye surgery is usually minimally invasive and performed as day-case surgery despite the high comorbidity of these patients.

OVERALL SURGICAL RISK

Overall surgical risk is related to physiologic organ system age, comorbid diseases, and the risks of the procedure to be undertaken. In general, an otherwise healthy elderly patient can expect a good outcome with continued quality of life. However, there are known overall risks for surgery in the elderly. Emergency procedures have especially high mortality in the elderly, in part because they take longer to exhibit symptoms and thus present with more advanced diseases, such as perforation or necrosis.[200]An example is a study of 48-hour emergency surgery mortality rates in 795 patients in which patients older than 90 years had a mortality of 7.8% as compared with a 0.6% for age-matched patients undergoing elective surgery.[201]

The type and number of coexisting diseases are exceedingly important because it has been proposed that the effects from coexisting disease outweigh the effects of age alone on anesthesia outcome.[169] When age and severity of illness are compared, the number of coexisting diseases is more significant. Additionally, the albumin level may serve as a marker for preoperative health status of the elderly patient because albumin level has been linked to perioperative mortality.[202]

Of elderly patients undergoing surgery, 10% to 40% develop a postoperative complication that can lead to serious adverse events.[203] According to a recent study, even seemingly mild initial complications may profoundly alter postoperative prognosis, beginning a cascade of other complications that result in death.[203] Silber et al examined Pennsylvania Medicare claims and determined that the odds of an elderly patient dying within 60 days after surgery increased 3.4-fold in patients with complications compared with those without complications.[203] Certain complications increased the risk substantially, such as respiratory compromise, associated with a 7.2-fold increase in the risk of dying, and CHF, resulting in a 5-fold risk in the odds of dying compared with patients without any perioperative complications.

One must consider, however, that advances in surgical and anesthetic techniques may allow the stabilization of an elderly patient with an emergent condition. For example, a minimally invasive emergency procedure performed with a regional anesthetic may allow stabilization of an elderly patient, thus affording the opportunity for full resuscitation and optimization before a definitive surgical procedure.[204]

Altered Perioperative Mental Status and Cognitive Dysfunction Perioperative delirium is common in high-risk surgery and associated with age, education, preoperative cognitive functioning, preexisting medical conditions, and postoperative complications. However, the pathophysiology is poorly understood. As well as being linked to narcotics, sedatives, and anticholinergics, delirium is associated with urinary tract infection, pneumonia, hypoxia or hypercarbia, fever, blood loss, and electrolyte disturbances. For example, 102 patients between 41 and 88 years of age underwent elective open abdominal aortic aneurysm surgery. Delirium occurred in 33% of the patients during the first 6 days after surgery. With multivariate analysis, the most powerful preoperative predictors of delirium *were number of pack-years smoked*, mental status scores, and number of perioperative psychoactive medications.[205] Longer duration of delirium was related to lower education, preoperative depression, and greater preoperative psychoactive medication use. Unrelated variables were characteristics of the surgery and hospital stay.

Persistent postoperative cognitive dysfunction is also a common problem after surgical procedures, estimated by some to be as high as 14% in patients older than 70 years.[206] Monk et al further evaluated 1064 patients before, just after, and 3 months after noncardiac surgery.[160] They found at 3 months, young and middle-age patients had similar incidences of cognitive dysfunction (5.7%) but that elderly patients still had significantly more dysfunction at 12%. The risk factors identified were similar to those for postoperative delirium and included increased age, lower educational level, and a history of a prior cerebrovascular accident without residual impairment. Persistent postoperative cognitive dysfunction is important because patients were both more likely to die within 3 months of surgery and in the first year after surgery ($p = 0.02$).[160]

Given the devastating consequences of postoperative cognitive dysfunction in the elderly, the role of anesthetic choice has been investigated. Forty-seven patients older than 60 years who were undergoing major surgery were randomly allocated to receive either regional or general anesthesia. Overall, elderly patients subjected to general anesthesia displayed more frequent cognitive impairment during the immediate postoperative period in comparison with those who received a regional technique.[207]

However, several studies have failed to demonstrate any long-term differences in postoperative cognitive function between general and regional anesthesia. Williams-Russo et al examined 262 patients older than 40 who were undergoing total knee arthroplasty, randomly assigned to either epidural or general anesthesia.[208] No differences were found between the patients for either cognitive or cardiovascular outcome. Rather, at 1 week postoperatively, both anesthetic groups had significant decreases from their preoperative neurocognitive test scores. At 6 months postoperatively, both groups improved, but the incidence of long-term postoperative cognitive deficit remained at 5% regardless of anesthesia group. Rasmussen and colleagues also examined patients older than 60 years randomly allocated to general or regional anesthesia for major noncardiac surgery.[209] They demonstrated that a substantial proportion of patients experienced postoperative cognitive dysfunction at 1 week and 3 months postsurgery (incidence: 10%-20%). There was no significant difference in the incidence of postoperative cognitive dysfunction between the groups at 3 months after surgery. The authors concluded that the choice of anesthesia should be based on an open discussion of patients' preferences, general postoperative complications, and the experience of the anesthetist.

Pain Management It is generally supported in the literature that the elderly have unique needs for analgesia compared with younger patients, including the problem of increased sensitivity to opioids.[210] However, this should not be interpreted to mean that elderly patients do not need pain medication because some have withheld analgesics for fear of prolonged action or increased side effects.[211] To care for the elderly patient in pain, one must also consider the coexisting diseases and their effects on the distribution of analgesics, elimination of analgesics, and the potential for exacerbated or unique side effects from analgesic medications in the elderly. Furthermore, the high incidence of postoperative confusion, delirium, or altered mental status may complicate the assessment and communication of postoperative pain. Consideration should be given to the use of nonopioid analgesics, reduced doses of opioid analgesics, and alternative routes of analgesic administration. One solution is to use regional anesthetic techniques with local anesthetics so that opioids are avoided.

Type of Anesthetic Multiple studies have demonstrated that the type of anesthesia (general vs regional anesthesia) has no substantial effect on perioperative morbidity, but some claim differences in perioperative morbidity.[212,213] However, it intuitively makes sense that elderly patients benefit from an anesthesia technique that allows for minimal cognitive depression with excellent postoperative pain control. It is essential to recognize that many factors influence the outcome; the quality of the anesthetic administered rather than the type of anesthetic is most important.[212]

Quality of Care We know that improved quality of care (QOC) received by patients is strongly associated with better survival among community-dwelling vulnerable older adults.[214] QOC begins with adequate information being obtained from a patient and related to a patient about proposed surgical interventions. An interesting challenge, however, is the finding that there is a strong negative correlation with patient's age and the desire for extensive information about medical care.[215] This may mean that QOC must include family members as well as the elderly individual both for obtaining and relating medical information. Perioperative QOC in elderly patients is also of great importance because of the increasing number of older adults undergoing operations.[216] QOC indicators have been developed in 7 domains: comorbidity assessment (cardiopulmonary disease), elderly issues (cognition), medication use (polypharmacy), patient-to-provider discussions (life-sustaining preferences), intraoperative care (preventing hypothermia), postoperative management (preventing delirium), and discharge planning (home health care), with most indicators rated addressing processes of care not routinely performed in younger surgical populations.[216] However, to address these varied goals, interdisciplinary team care has been applied successfully in hospital, outpatient, home, and nursing home settings.[217] Optimal outcomes are achieved in the elderly patient when clinical care is multidisciplinary and integrated beginning from preoperative assessment to supportive care after discharge.[218]

SUMMARY

The elderly are the fastest-growing segment of the world's population and have unique medical and surgical needs. Decrements in organ function decline combined with increases in organ system disease lead to challenges in surgical and anesthetic care. Assessment of comorbid conditions, nutritional status, and physiologic reserve when planning the most efficacious approach to surgical care can lead to excellent outcomes from a variety of procedures in most elderly and aged patients.

Acknowledgment: Many thanks to Terri Monk, MD, Professor of Anesthesiology at the Durham Veteran's Administration Medical Center in North Carolina, for manuscript review, collaborations, guidance, and her excellent work in geriatric medicine.

KEY REFERENCES

- Barnett CR. Polypharmacy and perioperative medications in the elderly. *Anesthesiol Clin.* 2009;27:377-389.
- Beliveau MM, Multach M. Perioperative care for the elderly patient. *Med Clin North Am.* 2003;87:273-289.
- Brody JA, Grant MD. Age associated diseases and conditions: implications for decreasing late life morbidity. *Aging.* 2001;13:1364.
- Loran DB, Hyde BR, Zwischenberger JB. Perioperative management of special populations: the geriatric patient. *Surg Clin North Am.* 2005;85:1259-1266.
- Monk T, Weldon BC, Garvan CW, et al. Predictors of cognitive dysfunction after major noncardiac surgery. *Anesthesiology.* 2008;108:18-30.
- Papaioannou A, Fraidakis O, Michaloudis D, et al. The impact of the type of anaesthesia on cognitive status and delirium during the first postoperative days in elderly patients. *Eur J Anaesth.* 2005;22:492-499.
- Rosenthal RA, Kavic SM. Assessment and management of the geriatric patient. *Crit Care Med.* 2004;32:S92-S105.
- Sieber JA. Age associated issues. *Geriatr Anesth Clin North Am.* 2004;22:45-58.
- Silber, JH, Rosenbaum PR, Trudeau ME, et al. Changes in prognosis after the first postoperative complication. *Med Care.* 2005;43(2):122-131.
- Stevens LA, Levey AS. Chronic kidney disease in the elderly—how to assess risk. *N Engl J Med.* 2005;352:2122-2124.

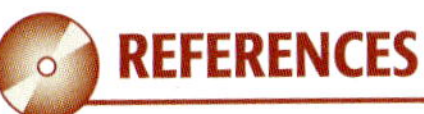

REFERENCES

Complete references available on DVD and online version at www.LongneckerAnesthesiology.com

CHAPTER 22 Evaluation of the Pregnant Patient

Robert Gaiser

KEY POINTS

1. Unlike other operations in which the patient is primarily concerned with himself or herself, the pregnant woman is usually concerned for her infant's welfare.
2. The anesthesia provider must be aware of the various physiologic changes of pregnancy and incorporate them into the anesthetic plan. These changes may affect various concurrent diseases if present.
3. The central nervous system effects of pregnancy include a reduced local anesthetic requirement when these agents are administered intrathecally or epidurally.
4. Pregnant patients in the third trimester and symptomatic patients in the first/second trimester should be considered at risk for aspiration during general anesthesia.
5. There is extremely weak evidence that surgery during the first trimester is linked to central nervous system defects in the fetus.
6. Fetal heart rate monitoring is possible during some surgical procedures, but it is not universally applied in the United States.
7. Preterm labor and delivery remain the leading cause of perinatal morbidity and mortality in the United States. Preterm labor is difficult to control with medication, with the most promising being the calcium channel blocking drugs. Magnesium sulfate is frequently used for neuroprotection in the preterm neonate.
8. The etiology of preeclampsia remains to be elucidated, but it is believed to be triggered by a paternal antigen in a susceptible mother.
9. Magnesium sulfate is the most effective medication for the prevention of seizures in those with preeclampsia.
10. Labetalol is the preferred drug for the control of blood pressure in mothers with preeclampsia. Antihypertensive medication does not treat the disease process; rather it is used to prevent intracerebral hemorrhage.
11. The 2 causes of antepartum hemorrhage are placenta previa and placental abruption. With the increase in cesarean deliveries, there is a high risk of placenta accreta in patients with previous cesarean delivery and placenta previa.
12. The perinatal transmission of human immunodeficiency virus (HIV) is low if the viral load is less than 1000 copies/mL and these patients do not require cesarean delivery. If the viral load is greater, cesarean delivery may decrease the risk of perinatal transmission.
13. Aggressive treatment of gestational diabetes mellitus, even mild gestational diabetes, with diet modification, oral agents, and insulin, is associated with improved maternal and neonatal outcome.

One of the most rewarding as well as challenging aspects of anesthesia is caring for the parturient because it involves 2 patients, the mother and the fetus. When formulating an anesthetic plan, the outcomes for both patients must be considered, although usually the ultimate welfare of the mother guides final management decisions. Fortunately, in most circumstances, optimal care of the mother provides good care of the fetus. Both preoperative evaluation and formulation of the anesthetic plan require an understanding of the physiologic changes that accompany pregnancy. These physiologic changes result from alterations in the hormonal milieu (accounts for the changes early in pregnancy) and from the mechanical factors of the enlarging uterus (accounts for most of the changes later in pregnancy).

PHYSIOLOGIC CHANGES OF PREGNANCY

CARDIOVASCULAR SYSTEM

Pregnancy causes an increase in maternal cardiac output, in response to the increased oxygen consumption associated with the developing fetus. Increases in cardiac output begin during the first trimester, resulting initially from an increase in maternal heart rate (typically 10-20 beats/min).[1,2] As the pregnancy progresses, there is an increase in stroke volume caused by a reduction in systemic vascular resistance. Cardiac output increases progressively, beginning as early as 10 weeks of gestation and continuing until it is 40% over baseline during the second trimester.[3] The increase results in a 10- to 20-fold increase in uterine blood flow. Despite the increase in cardiac output, blood pressure decreases in early pregnancy, reaching a minimum in midpregnancy, and remains low until around 32 weeks of gestation, and then it returns to baseline levels at term. Although systemic vascular resistance decreases during pregnancy, the central venous and pulmonary artery pressures remain similar to the nonpregnant state.

Maternal blood volume increases by 35% during pregnancy. This increase begins in early pregnancy and continues throughout the gestation. The increase in blood volume results from an increment in both extracellular and intravascular volume. Several theories attempt to explain this increase in blood volume. The "underfill" hypothesis proposes that blood volume expands as a result of systemic vasodilation and an attempt to accommodate the increased intravascular space. In contrast, the "overfill" hypothesis suggests that the increase results from the greater levels of salt-retaining steroids that accompany gestation, with the intravascular space expanding to accommodate the increase in volume.[4] Most likely, the increase results from a combination of the 2 theories: there is an initial "underfilling" very early in gestation, and the increase in mineral corticoid levels occurs later in gestation. Whatever the mechanism, the increased blood volume during pregnancy allows parturients to tolerate normal blood loss of delivery (approximately 400 mL during vaginal delivery and 700 mL during cesarean delivery).[5] Further, the uterus contracts at delivery, resulting in autotransfusion of approximately 500 mL. Blood volume returns to prepregnancy levels within 7 to 14 days after delivery.

Vascular responsiveness is altered during pregnancy: Normal parturients are less responsive to vasopressors and chronotropic agents.[6,7] In animals, both the carotid and uterine arteries responded less to norepinephrine.[8] This decreased response may be related to down-regulation of α and β receptors. The clinical implications of decreased vascular responsiveness are 2-fold. First, treatment of hypotension may require an increased amount of vasopressor to treat hypotension as compared with that required in the nonpregnant individual. Second, the response to an intravenous test dose of epinephrine will not increase the heart rate to the same extent as in the nonpregnant individual.[9]

Pregnant patients are particularly susceptible to cardiovascular alterations induced by changes in body position. In the supine position, up to 15% of pregnant patients develop nausea, hypotension, and vomiting (supine hypotension syndrome).[10] The supine position allows the gravid uterus to compress the inferior vena cava and aorta. Caval compression results in decreased venous return to the right atrium and hence decreased cardiac output. Anesthetic drugs or techniques that

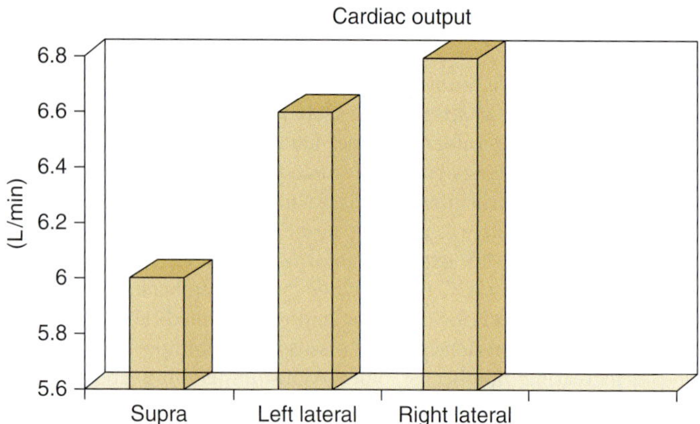

FIGURE 22-1. By tilting the patient to the left, compression of the vena cava by the aorta is relieved, improving cardiac output. [Data from Uleland K, Novy MJ, Peterson EN, et al. Maternal cardiovascular dynamics. IV. The influence of gestational age on the maternal cardiovascular response to posture and exercise. *Am J Obstet Gynecol.* 1969;104:856.]

cause venodilation further decrease venous return accompanying caval obstruction. This hypotension decreases uterine perfusion. Uterine blood flow may be further compromised if the uterus compresses the aorta because the uterine artery is a branch of the hypogastric artery, which emerges distal to the level of aortic compression. Studies performed with pregnant women in the lateral position have not noted major decreases in cardiac output.[11,12] By tilting the patient to the left, the uterus is displaced off the vena cava and aorta (**Fig. 22-1**). As such, pregnant women should not lie supine after 20 weeks of gestation, especially if anesthesia is being provided. Whenever the supine position is required, the uterus should be tilted to the left by placing a wedge underneath the right hip, and this principle applies not only at the time of delivery but throughout pregnancy. For example, during cardiopulmonary resuscitation, effective chest compressions may only be accomplished with the parturient in left uterine displacement.[13]

Physical examination of pregnant women typically reveals a point of maximal cardiac impulse that is displaced cephalad and leftward from its location prepregnancy. Diaphragmatic elevation displaces the heart leftward so that it may appear enlarged on chest radiographs. The electrocardiogram shows left axis deviation. A small pericardial effusion may develop in healthy asymptomatic women during the third trimester of pregnancy.[14]

RESPIRATORY SYSTEM

Various changes occur in the maternal airway during gestation. There is vascular engorgement of the airway, resulting in edema of the oral and nasal pharynx, larynx, and trachea.[15] When parturients were examined at 12 weeks of gestation and then again at 36 weeks of gestation, the percentage of patients with a Mallampati class IV airway had doubled.[16] This airway edema may render intubation of the trachea difficult. This supposition is confirmed by examining maternal deaths from anesthesia in the United States, with approximately half occurring because of failed intubation.[17] For oral tracheal intubation, the likelihood of edema in the false cords mandates the use of smaller endotracheal tubes. A 6.0 cuffed endotracheal tube should be ready and available for every case. Exacerbation of these changes may occur in patients with upper respiratory tract infections or preeclampsia. The mucous membranes are also very friable. Manipulation, such as nasal intubation or the insertion of a nasogastric tube, may result in excessive bleeding.

The gravid uterus results in a 4-cm elevation of the diaphragm; the circumference of the thorax is increased 5 to 7 cm. Despite this elevation, there is little change in total lung capacity as the chest expands in both anterior-posterior and transverse diameters to compensate. The diaphragmatic elevation does cause a 20% decrease in functional residual capacity (FRC) at term. This decrease is a result of decreases in both residual volume and expiratory reserve volume. Oxygen consumption increases by 20% due to increased metabolism and increased work of breathing.[18] The parturient compensates for this increased oxygen consumption in 2 ways: (1) increased alveolar ventilation, and (2) shifting the oxyhemoglobin dissociation curve to the right, thus facilitating unloading of oxygen at the cellular level. The P50 increases from 26 to 30 mm Hg. This shift is caused by an increase in 2,3-diphosphoglycerate.

The decrease in FRC and increased oxygen consumption make parturients very vulnerable to hypoxia. After complete denitrogenation by breathing 100% oxygen, nonpregnant patients tolerate up to 9 minutes of apnea before oxygen saturation is less than 90%, whereas parturients can only tolerate 2 to 3 minutes. The decrease in FRC allows for the rapid denitrogenation, with 4 deep breaths of 100% oxygen equivalent to 3 minutes of tidal volume breathing of 100% oxygen.[19]

Minute ventilation increases by 3 to 4 L/min.[20] This increase results primarily from increased tidal volume and secondarily from a small increase in respiratory rate. Alveolar ventilation also increases by 70%. Hormone-mediated increases in the neural drive contribute to the hyperventilation of pregnancy. The $Paco_2$ decreases to 32 mm Hg as a result of increased ventilation and Pao_2 increases 5 to 10 mm Hg. The respiratory alkalosis is only partially compensated by a lowering of plasma concentrations of bicarbonate from 26 to 22 mm Hg.

Approximately 60% to 70% of healthy pregnant women have mild, intermittent dyspnea. The cause is not clear but may be related to alterations in chest wall proprioreceptors or progesterone-induced hyperventilation.[21] Diaphragmatic elevation may result in increased lung markings, mimicking mild congestive heart failure, on the chest radiographs of healthy pregnant women.

GASTROINTESTINAL CHANGES

Parturients should be considered to be at risk for pulmonary aspiration due to the physiologic changes of pregnancy. The enlarged gravid uterus displaces the stomach cephalad. This displacement alters the angle of the gastroesophageal junction, decreasing competence of the gastroesophageal sphincter. The uterus also displaces the pylorus upward and posteriorly, resulting in delayed gastric emptying. Elevated concentrations of progesterone decrease gastrointestinal motility and food absorption. These changes facilitate the occurrence of gastric reflux and heartburn in as many as 70% of pregnant women.[22] Recent studies question the delayed gastric emptying and increased gastrin concentration. Eleven women had gastric emptying times measured during the first trimester, third trimester, and postpartum.[23] There was no difference between first trimester and postpartum. Gastrointestinal transit time was significantly longer in the third trimester. Thus, despite hormonal changes, it seems that gastric emptying is only affected in the third trimester and during labor. This supposition was further confirmed when the gastric contents were aspirated via a nasogastric tube prior to cesarean delivery.[24] The stomach contents of 100 term parturients were compared with those from 100 nonpregnant women scheduled for gynecologic surgery. The gastric volume in the pregnant patients was greater than that in the nonpregnant group. Unlike previously believed, serum gastrin levels did not differ between the groups (**Fig. 22-2**).

These findings affect approaches to the care of the pregnant patient who presents for nonobstetric anesthesia care. Gastric emptying is not delayed until the third trimester. Greater gastric volume occurs but not early in the pregnancy, and serum levels of gastrin are not elevated. From the perspective of pulmonary aspiration of gastric contents, parturients during the first and second trimesters should be treated like nonpregnant individuals. If the patient has symptomatic reflux, rapid sequence induction and intubation should be done. If asymptomatic, rapid sequence induction and intubation are not required. During the third trimester, it may be prudent to perform rapid sequence induction and intubation, although the literature does not strongly support this contention. Clinical judgment is important here, weighing the risks of rapid sequence induction (failed intubation, tachycardia, hypertension) versus the risks of aspiration in an asymptomatic parturient.

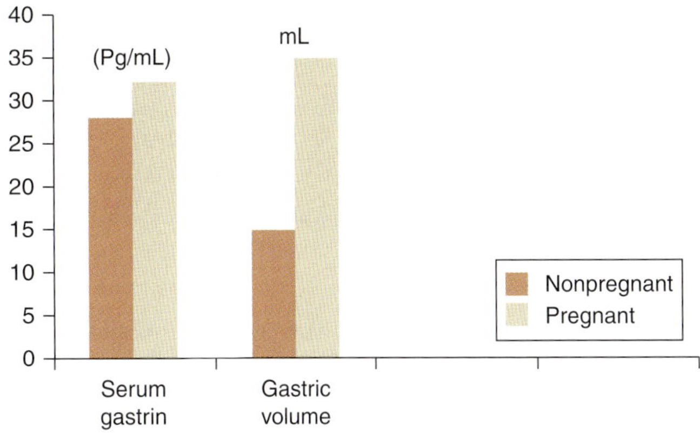

FIGURE 22-2. Although there is a difference in residual gastric volume between parturients at 40 weeks of gestation and nonpregnant patients, there is no difference in serum gastrin levels. Clear, nonpregnant; darkened, 40 weeks of gestation. [Data from Hong JY, Park JW, Oh JI. Comparison of preoperative gastric contents and serum gastrin concentrations in pregnant and nonpregnant women. *J Clin Anesth.* 2005;17:451.]

HEPATIC CHANGES

There is little or no change in hepatic blood flow during normal pregnancy. Healthy pregnant women frequently have an increase in serum aspartate aminotransferase, lactic dehydrogenase, alkaline phosphatase, or cholesterol. Colloid oncotic pressure decreases as a result of decreased total protein and a decreased albumin-to-globulin ratio. Colloid oncotic pressure decreases further after delivery, regardless of method of delivery or anesthesia administered.[25]

Pseudocholinesterase activity is decreased 24% before delivery and by 33% on the third postpartum day.[25,26] It returns to normal 2 to 6 weeks postpartum. The decreased cholinesterase activity is usually not sufficient to result in clinically relevant prolonged paralysis after a single dose of succinylcholine.

HEMATOLOGIC CHANGES

Plasma volume increases 45% (increasing approximately 1000 mL from onset of pregnancy to 36 weeks of gestation), but the red cell mass increases only 20%, leading to the physiologic (dilutional) anemia of pregnancy. Hemoglobin concentration typically decreases by 2.4 g/dL from prepregnancy to 36 weeks of gestation; hematocrit typically decreases 6.5%.[27] A maternal hemoglobin concentration less than 11 g/dL is abnormal. The most common cause of anemia during pregnancy is iron deficiency.

Platelet count is usually elevated, but one can see a modest decrease without any other hematologic pathology. It is believed that gestational thrombocytopenia is an exaggerated normal response in which platelets are consumed.[28] Pregnancy produces a hypercoagulable state. All coagulation factors, except factors XI and XIII, increase in concentration. Fibrinolytic activity decreases during the third trimester as a result of decreased plasminogen activator concentrations. These changes combined with rapid contraction of the uterus after placental separation help protect women from major hemorrhage. Unfortunately, this hypercoagulability also predisposes pregnant women to thromboembolic complications. Thromboembolism is the leading cause of maternal mortality.[29] Parturients are at greatest risk for deep venous thrombosis and pulmonary embolism immediately after delivery.

ENDOCRINE

Mean blood glucose concentration remains within the normal range, although glucose concentration may be lower in some women than those before pregnancy. Parturients become insulin resistant due to human placental lactogen, causing an increased release of insulin.[30]

TABLE 22-1 Recommendations for Total Weight Gain During Pregnancy

Prepregnancy BMI	Total Weight Gain	Rate of Weight Gain
Underweight <18.5 kg/m^2	28-40 lbs	1 lb/wk
Normal weight 18.5-24 kg/m^2	25-35 lbs	1 lb/wk
Overweight 25-29.9 kg/m^2	15-25 lbs	0.6 lb/wk
Obese >30 kg/m^2	11-20 lbs	0.5 lb/wk

BMI, body mass index.

Recommendations for weight gain have changed, as documented by the Institute of Medicine. Current guidelines are based on the World Health Organization cutoff points for body mass index. The recommended weight gain during pregnancy is presented in **Table 22-1**.[31] The greatest change is the narrow range of weight gain for obese parturients.

The thyroid gland enlarges 50% to 70% during pregnancy. Concentrations of thyroid-binding globulin and total thyroxine increase, but concentrations of free thyroxine and tri-iodothyronine do not change.

RENAL

Renal plasma flow and glomerular filtration rate (GFR) increase during the first trimester to 50% above normal by the fourth month. The increase in renal plasma flow and GFR result in an increased creatinine clearance, with a decreased blood urea nitrogen (BUN) and creatinine.[32] BUN decreases 40% to 8 to 9 g/dL; creatinine decreases to 0.4 to 0.5 mg/dL. A BUN of 15 mg/dL, a serum creatinine of 1.0 mg/dL, or a creatinine clearance of 100 mL/min suggest abnormal renal function in pregnant women who are near term. Glucosuria may occur in healthy pregnant women because tubular glucose reabsorption may not keep up with increased GFR. Proteinuria, up to 300 mg/d, is common.

Maternal progesterone, which is a smooth muscle relaxant, causes dilation of renal calyces, pelves, and ureters. After midpregnancy, the enlarged uterus compresses the ureters of the pelvic brim, exacerbating ureteral dilation. Urinary stasis predisposes pregnant women to urinary tract infections.

DERMATOLOGIC

Hyperpigmentation is the most common dermatologic change in pregnancy; it occurs in approximately 90% of pregnancies.[33] It is usually more evident in women of darker complexion. This hyperpigmentation occurs in the areolar area and also in the clinical appearance of preexisting freckles and nevi. Thickening of scalp hair occurs, and the nails of fingers and toes become softer.

CENTRAL NERVOUS SYSTEM

The pituitary gland increases in size during pregnancy, but, in contrast, the brain decreases in size.[34] The decrease in brain size begins after placental implantation and is maximal at term, reversing slowly after delivery. The precise mechanism and physiologic importance of these changes is not known.

The minimum alveolar concentration for inhaled anesthetics is decreased up to 40% in pregnancy.[35] This decrease occurs with all of the inhalation agents. The mechanism is unclear, although it may be related to progesterone (which has sedative activity) and endorphins. A concentration of an inhalation agent that may not produce loss of consciousness in nonpregnant patients may render pregnant women unconscious, placing the parturient at risk for aspiration. For this reason, inhalation agents for labor analgesia are not desirable.

Pregnant women require less total dose of local anesthetic to produce the same level of epidural or spinal block.[36] In the epidural space, it may be partly due to epidural vein engorgement, thus decreasing the volume of the epidural space. However, this decreased requirement is seen in the first trimester, well before significant mechanical changes have occurred. Acid base changes in cerebrospinal fluid or hormonal changes of pregnancy may cause increased sensitivity to local anesthetics.[37]

REPRODUCTIVE TRACT

The uterus weighs 50 to 70 g in the nonpregnant state and increases to 1.0 to 1.5 kg in pregnant women at term. Total uterine blood flow increases from 50 mL/min in nonpregnant women to 700 mL/min in pregnant women at term, representing approximately 10% of the cardiac output. Most of the uterine blood flow perfuses the intervillous space; the remainder of the blood flow perfuses the enlarged myometrium.

The uterine vasculature appears maximally dilated in healthy pregnant women; therefore, uterine blood flow decreases parallel with maternal arterial pressure. There is little or no autoregulation of uterine blood flow during pregnancy. Any factor that decreases venous return and cardiac output will decrease uterine blood flow. Uterine contractions also decrease uterine blood flow. No known drug specifically or directly increases uterine blood flow.

MONITORING THE FETUS

The use of electronic fetal monitoring to assess fetal well-being has become universal, used by both physicians and nurses.[38] The American College of Obstetricians and Gynecologists has stated that the goal of fetal surveillance is the prevention of fetal death.[39] However, the problem with the current testing methods relates to their predictive value. The negative predictive value is high, meaning that the chance of death within 1 week of a reassuring test is rare. The same does not apply to positive predictive value. A nonreassuring (ie, "positive") test does not imply that the fetus is at risk of death. The obstetrician considers the gestational age of the fetus, other fetal indices, and judgment to arrive at a decision regarding the management of a nonreassuring test.

Monitoring the fetal heart rate is used to determine adequate cerebral oxygenation of the fetus. As the brain modulates the heart, a decrease in fetal heart rate is believed to reflect inadequate fetal cerebral oxygenation. External fetal heart rate monitors use a Doppler detective device with computerized logic to interpret and count the Doppler signals, whereas internal fetal heart rate monitors involve the placement of an electrode on the fetal scalp. The presence of fetal heart tones as well as its rate and rhythm are used to interpret the status of the fetus. The baseline fetal heart rate (FHR) is determined by approximating the mean FHR rounded to increments of 5 beats/min during a 10-minute interval. A normal baseline heart rate is within 110 to 160 beats/min.[40] Baseline FHR variability is defined as fluctuations that are irregular in amplitude and frequency. A normal FHR should have moderate variability defined as an amplitude range of 6 to 25 beats/min. Several characteristics of the FHR depend on fetal gestational age. A preterm fetus is expected to have a more rapid rate with little or no beat-to-beat variability.[41]

Fetal movement is the easiest means to document fetal well-being. The mother perceives fetal movements, which serves as a basis for assessment. A diminution in the perception of fetal movement often precedes fetal death.[42] Perception of 10 distinct movements in a period of up to 2 hours is considered reassuring. The first perception of fetal movement occurs around 20 weeks of gestation. As the pregnancy progresses, the movements are felt on a more regular basis.

Heart rate reactivity is thought to be a good indicator of normal fetal autonomic function. Loss of reactivity is associated most commonly with fetal sleep but also may result from any central nervous system depression. The fetal heart rate typically increases in response to fetal movement. This premise serves as the basis for the nonstress test, in which the mother has the FHR monitored for 20 to 40 minutes and also records the time of fetal movement. A reactive (normal) nonstress test is the presence of 2 accelerations (an increase in fetal heart rate by 15 beats/min lasting for at least 15 seconds) in a 20-minute period. A nonreactive nonstress test is one that lacks accelerations over a 40-minute period.[43] The ability of the fetus to accelerate its heart rate depends on the age of the fetus. As such, the nonstress test is usually not used prior to 32 weeks of gestation.

The contraction stress test is based on the response of the fetal heart rate to uterine contractions. During a uterine contraction, fetal oxygenation worsens due to uterine artery compression. In the suboptimally

TABLE 22-2 Ultrasound Components of the Biophysical Profile

Fetal breathing movements (≥1 episodes of rhythmic fetal breathing movement of ≥30 s within 30 min)
Fetal movement (≥3 discrete body or limb movements within 30 min)
Fetal tone (≥1 episodes of extension of a fetal extremity with return to flexion, or opening or closing of a hand)
Determination of the amniotic fluid volume (a single vertical pocket of amniotic fluid >2 cm)

oxygenated fetus, this further decrease in oxygenation is not tolerated, leading to the fetal heart rate pattern of late decelerations. A contraction stress test requires 3 contractions in a 10-minute period. Contractions may be produced by oxytocin infusion.[44] The contraction stress test is interpreted according to the presence or absence of late fetal heart rate decelerations, which are defined as decelerations that reach the nadir after the peak of the contraction and persist beyond the end of the contraction.[45] The presence of late decelerations suggests that the fetus is compromised and should be delivered, usually by cesarean delivery. The results of the contraction stress test are negative if there are no late decelerations. The test is complex and contraindicated in preterm gestations, parturients with bleeding, and parturients with previous uterine surgery. If the test demonstrates no late decelerations, the incidence of fetal death occurring within 1 week of the negative test results is extremely unlikely. The contraction stress test is rarely used today because of ease of the nonstress test and the biophysical profile.

The biophysical profile (**Table 22-2**) was developed as a method of integrating real-time observations of the fetus directly in its environment. It is used as an assessment tool for both acute and chronic fetal conditions in the antepartum period. The biophysical profile consists of a nonstress test combined with 4 observations made by ultrasonography.[46] The biophysical profile is a reflection of a fetus that can accelerate its heart rate, move appropriately, and is surrounded by a normal amount of amniotic fluid. Each of 5 components is assigned a score of either 2 (normal) or 0 (abnormal). A composite score of 8 to 10 is normal, a score of 6 is considered equivocal, and a score of 4 or less is abnormal. The biophysical profile is frequently performed in the labor suite, necessitating a basic understanding by the anesthesiologist. A score of 8 or 10 has the chance for fetal death within 1 week of the test in normal pregnancies as less than 1 in 1000. A biophysical profile of 6 or less is highly predictive of the need for admission to the neonatal intensive care unit.[47]

Umbilical artery Doppler flow velocimetry is based on the hemodynamic components of vascular impedance and on the observation that flow velocity waveforms in the umbilical artery of normally growing fetuses differ from those of growth-restricted fetuses.[48] Various blood vessels have been investigated, including the maternal uterine artery, fetal middle cerebral artery, and umbilical artery. Commonly measured flow velocities include peak systolic-flow velocity and the diastolic flow velocity occurring at the end of the cardiac cycle. The umbilical flow velocity waveform of normally growing fetuses is characterized by high-velocity diastolic flow, whereas with intrauterine growth restriction, there is a diminution of umbilical artery diastolic flow. Commonly measured flow indices are based on peak systolic frequency shift (S) and end diastolic frequency shift (D). The poor predictive value of Doppler velocimetry limits its use to the setting of fetal growth restriction. A S/D ratio of less than 3 is normal, even in the setting of growth restriction, and supports continuing the pregnancy.

Future monitors may include the transabdominal fetal pulse oximeter. The depth of the fetal head from the maternal abdomen is determined on ultrasound; the distance between the optodes needs to be twice the depth of the fetus. Using this device, oxygen saturations between 50% and 74% have been obtained and are similar to those obtained transvaginally.[49] The monitor provides measures of both the fetal heart rate and the oxygen saturation of the fetal blood. The value of this monitor is evident because not all cases of decreased fetal heart rate variability are due to decreased oxygenation. The transabdominal fetal pulse oximeter allows for the differentiation between normal fetal sleep and decreased oxygen content.

PRETERM LABOR

Preterm birth resulting in a premature neonate is a major health problem in the United States. The overall rate of preterm birth in the United States in 2006 was 12.8%; black (18.4%) and American Indian/Alaska Native (14.1%) women have the highest risk of preterm delivery as compared with white (11.7%), Asian/Pacific Islanders (10.9%), and Hispanic women (12.2%).[50] The concern with preterm labor and birth is its outcome: it accounts for approximately 70% of all neonatal deaths and half of long-term neurologic disabilities.[51] Almost a fifth of all very preterm infants do not survive the first year of life. Of the smallest infants, disabilities occur in about half of survivors.[52] Health care costs resulting from preterm birth are staggering. The financial burden of preterm birth was estimated to be $26 billion in 2005 or approximately $52 000 per preterm infant.[53] **Table 22-3** lists the risk factors for preterm labor and delivery.

The pathophysiology of preterm labor is multifactorial and not well understood. Preterm birth may result from early activation of the mechanisms of normal term labor or from pathophysiologic mechanisms that trigger labor by distinct means. Poverty, maternal race, limited maternal education, young maternal age, and inadequate prenatal care increase the risk of preterm labor and delivery. Infection also has a prominent role in preterm birth. It has been estimated that 80% of preterm births are associated with chorioamnionitis or organisms in the placental membrane.[54] Finally, there is a genetic predisposition. A strong risk factor for preterm birth is a maternal history of preterm birth. However, the association between polymorphisms in certain genes and the risk of preterm birth has been modest. Given the association between preterm labor and bacterial vaginosis, evidence supports its treatment with metronidazole, which decreases the risk of preterm birth by 25% to 75%.[55,56] The other major advance in the prediction of preterm birth comes from genomics, the study of gene expression at the messenger RNA level to provide an integrated view of the relationship between the host genome, gene expression, and disease outcome. Several studies have demonstrated a link between nucleotide polymorphisms and preterm birth.[57,58]

Tocolysis has been a prominent component of efforts to prevent preterm labor and delivery. The premise behind tocolysis is that, by administering medication, uterine contractility will be reduced, thus retaining the fetus in utero. There is increasing consensus among obstetricians that only a minority of patients benefit from tocolysis. Literally hundreds of trials have evaluated medications for the prevention of preterm birth. Acute tocolysis occurs at the initial presentation for preterm labor, which differs from maintenance after successful tocolysis.

The β-mimetic agents, such as terbutaline or ritodrine, have been increasingly falling from favor as tocolytic agents due to the high incidence of maternal adverse effects, such as hypokalemia, hyperglycemia,

TABLE 22-3 Risk Factors for Preterm Labor and Birth

- History of preterm birth
- Current multifetal pregnancy
- Infection
- Diabetes mellitus
- Hypertension
- Asthma
- Lack of prenatal care
- Smoking
- Alcohol
- Cocaine
- Stress
- Long work hours with long periods of standing

tachycardia, decreased systemic vascular resistance, and increased risk of pulmonary edema.[59] These drugs have been linked to at least 25 maternal deaths from pulmonary edema. The β-mimetics act by binding to β_2-adrenergic receptors on the myometrial cell and by increasing the levels of cyclic adenosine monophosphate, resulting in inactivation of the myosin light chain kinase. In a meta-analysis comparing tocolytic agents, only 1 trial found an increase in the length of pregnancy with β-mimetic agents.[60] The American College of Obstetricians and Gynecologists concluded, "It would appear, on the basis of currently available evidence, very difficult to support the use of beta-mimetics, which have a high incidence of side effects. Although these drugs do delay delivery in the short term, there is no demonstrable benefit for the newborn."[61] However, these drugs are frequently used to relax the uterus during uterine tetany, which is a sustained, prolonged uterine contraction.

The use of magnesium sulphate for the treatment of preterm labor has undergone several revisions. Although used frequently in the United States, its reason for use has changed. A meta-analysis of magnesium sulphate for tocolysis concluded that it does not reduce the frequency of delivery within 48 hours, 7 days, or preterm birth.[62] The effect of magnesium sulfate on the fetus and neonate is controversial. Although some data suggested increased adverse neonatal outcomes or fetal death, some evidence suggests a neuroprotective effect.[63] In a systematic review of 5 eligible randomized clinical trials, there was a reduced risk of cerebral palsy with the number needed to treat to prevent 1 case of cerebral palsy being 63. For the mother, magnesium sulfate results in blurry vision and maternal weakness. It potentiates the nondepolarizing muscle relaxants, necessitating a major reduction in dose of these medications.

Calcium channel blockers relax the myometrium by inhibiting the reuptake of calcium in the myometrial wall. The most commonly studied calcium channel blocker for tocolysis is nifedipine which may be administered either orally or sublingually. Maternal side effects include headache and rarely hypotension. A Cochrane review found nifedipine to be superior to β-mimetics in general, with a reduction in the number of women giving birth within 7 days and prior to 34 weeks of gestation.[64] These drugs should not be used in women with cardiovascular disease or those who are hemodynamically unstable.

Prostaglandins play a role in the initiation of labor, and, as such, prostaglandin synthetase inhibitors may treat preterm labor and prevent preterm birth.[65] The most commonly used prostaglandin synthetase inhibitor is indomethacin, which reduces birth before 37 weeks of gestation. Side effects are primarily fetal and include constriction of the ductus arteriosus and fetal oliguria.

Oxytocin receptor antagonists have been developed in response to the observation that labor is accompanied by an increase in oxytocin receptors. Atosiban is the only oxytocin receptor antagonist that has undergone significant study.[66] In regard to its effect on preterm labor, the results have been disappointing. It has no benefit over placebo in regard to increasing the length of labor or infant outcome. No oxytocin-receptor antagonists are yet approved by the Food and Drug Administration for use in the United States.

All tocolytic medications have side effects. The decision of which medication to use depends on the desired outcome. All seem to be effective for short-term tocolysis with only indomethacin and nifedipine demonstrating long-term benefits. In an analysis of 19 trials, the probability for an adverse event from a tocolytic agent was 58% for terbutaline, 27% for nifedipine, 22% for magnesium, and 11% for indomethacin.[67] Both nifedipine and indomethacin are inexpensive compared with magnesium sulfate and terbutaline, suggesting that these 2 agents are the better choices for a patient in preterm labor. Magnesium sulfate is used not for tocolysis but rather for the prevention of cerebral palsy.

PREECLAMPSIA

Preeclampsia is a multisystem disorder unique to human pregnancy. It is characterized by an abnormal vascular response to the placenta that is associated with increased systemic vascular resistance, enhanced platelet aggregation, activation of the coagulation system, and endothelial cell dysfunction. Parturients with preeclampsia develop edema, raised blood pressure, and proteinuria. Preeclampsia occurs typically after the 20th week of gestation, except when associated with a hydatidiform mole, but rarely occurs before the 24th week of gestation.[68] The American College of Obstetricians and Gynecologists has defined preeclampsia as a blood pressure of at least 140 mm Hg (systolic) or at least 90 mm Hg (diastolic) on at least 2 occasions at least 4 to 6 hours apart.[69] **Table 22-4** lists the possible abnormal laboratory values in preeclampsia. In general, maternal and perinatal outcomes are good in patients with mild preeclampsia developing after 36 weeks of gestation. If preeclampsia develops before 33 weeks of gestation or in those patients with preexisting medical disorders, the outcome is less favorable.[70] Preeclampsia usually abates within 48 hours of termination of the pregnancy. Eclampsia is preeclampsia with central nervous system involvement leading to seizures or grand mal convulsions not related to other cerebral conditions. The diagnosis of severe preeclampsia requires the presence of end-organ disease (**Table 22-5**).

TABLE 22-4 Laboratory Abnormalities in Preeclampsia

- Proteinuria
- Elevated hemoglobin
- Elevated creatinine
- Elevated blood urea nitrogen
- Thrombocytopenia
- Elevated uric acid
- Elevated prothrombin time and partial thromboplastin time
- Elevated liver enzymes
- Microangiopathic hemolytic anemia

The incidence of preeclampsia ranges from 2% to 7% of nulliparous patients.[71] It is the third leading cause of maternal mortality in the United States and accounts for 20% of maternal deaths.[72] Several risk factors for preeclampsia have been identified (**Table 22-6**). Preeclampsia tends to occur at both extremes of reproductive age. The greatest risk is a first pregnancy. The importance of the father in the etiology of preeclampsia was highlighted in a study examining the Medical Birth Registry of Norway. If a woman becomes pregnant by a man who has already fathered a pregnancy complicated by preeclampsia in a different woman, her risk of developing preeclampsia is increased 1.8 (95% confidence interval [CI], 1.2-2.6).[73] There is also a genetic component. Using the same birth registry, the authors demonstrated that daughters of women who had preeclampsia during pregnancy had doubled the risk of developing preeclampsia themselves. The same did not apply to the sons who fathered children.[74]

During pregnancy, the placenta exerts a significant influence on maternal blood pressure because of the interaction of its various hormones, vasoactive substances, and structure. In a normal pregnancy, peripheral vascular resistance decreases resulting in a lower blood pressure. Maternal blood pressure decreases as early as 7 weeks of gestation.

TABLE 22-5 Factors That Define Severe Preeclampsia

One of the following will diagnose a preeclamptic parturient with severe preeclampsia necessitating delivery:

- Systolic blood pressure ≥160 mm Hg
- Diastolic blood pressure ≥110 mm Hg
- Proteinuria ≥5 g/24 h
- Oliguria ≤400 mL/24 h
- Cerebral visual disturbances
- Headache
- Pulmonary edema
- Hemolysis, elevated liver enzymes, low platelets (HELLP)
- Epigastric pain

TABLE 22-6 Risk Factors for Preeclampsia

- Maternal age (<20 y or >40 y)
- Multiple births
- Hypertension before pregnancy
- First pregnancy
- Previous pregnancy with preeclampsia
- Diabetes mellitus
- Asthma
- Kidney disease
- Lupus
- Scleroderma
- Obesity

After 28 weeks of gestation, the blood pressure increases, reaching nonpregnant values toward the end of the third trimester. Also, in a normal pregnancy, all fluid compartments expand. In patients with preeclampsia, the opposite occurs, with an increase in blood pressure and a decrease in the fluid compartments.

The cause of preeclampsia is still unknown, but the disease seems to begin at implantation, well before the clinical manifestations allow the diagnosis to be made. The likely culprit in preeclampsia is the placenta. Preeclampsia is seen in patients with molar pregnancies (thus it cannot be a result of the fetus) and also in patients with abdominal pregnancies (thus it cannot be a result of the uterus). Although the etiology remains unknown, current data suggest that various proteins that control angiogenesis are released from the placenta in women who develop preeclampsia. In a susceptible individual, various angiogenic proteins respond differently from the usual. These proteins are important for normal placental development. Because of this varied response, an imbalance in concentrations occurs, causing abnormal placentation. Angiogenic proteins promote the development of a healthy vasculature; antiangiogenic proteins do the opposite. At 20 to 24 weeks, sFlt-1 (soluble fms-like tyrosine kinase 1) was greater in those women who subsequently developed preeclampsia.[75] sFlt-1 is an antiangiogenic factor. It binds placental growth factor (PlGF) and vascular endothelial growth factor (VEGF), 2 factors that promote angiogenesis. The link of sFlt-1 to preeclampsia has been well established. Serum concentrations of this factor are increased in preeclampsia and correlate with the severity of the disease. sFlt-1 does not have a direct effect. It exerts its effect by binding to the angiogenic factors PlGF and VEGF. Although abnormal placentation occurs with the onset of the pregnancy, sFlt-1 levels do not change until the second trimester. Samples analyzed at 10 to 14 weeks of gestation (at least 10 weeks before the onset of disease) were not predictive of preeclampsia. The levels of sFlt-1 in the first trimester in preeclamptic parturients do not differ from those in normal parturients.[76] As such, using sFlt-1 and PlGF is not useful early in the pregnancy. The predictive value of these blood tests did not manifest until the second trimester. Another antiangiogenic factor, endoglin, was examined; it is highly expressed on cell membranes of the vascular endothelium and syncytiotrophoblasts of the placenta.[77] Placental endoglin is upregulated in preeclampsia, releasing soluble endoglin into the maternal circulation. It is an antiangiogenic protein that inhibits VEGF in the vasculature. Unlike sFlt-1, which increases 5 weeks before the onset of disease, circulating soluble endoglin levels increase 2 to 3 months before the onset of disease. Beginning as early as 17 weeks of gestation, levels of soluble endoglin were higher in women who developed preeclampsia. The combination of measuring both endoglin and sFlt-1 should improve the predictive ability of such tests.[78]

If preeclampsia is a state of antiangiogenesis, one would predict that the subsequent health of the mother should be affected. Heart disease, an antiangiogenic state, should be increased in women with preeclampsia. Using a meta-analysis involving 3 488 160 women, of which 198 252 had preeclampsia, the relative risks of hypertension (3.70; 95% CI, 2.70-5.05), ischemic heart disease (2.16; 95% CI, 1.86-2.52), and for stroke (1.81; 95% CI, 1.45-2.27) were all increased.[79] It seems that the occurrence of preeclampsia has significant implications for the mother's future health, despite the apparent resolution of the acute disease process. A review of systems for women should include a history of preeclampsia.

Anticonvulsants were introduced for women with preeclampsia in the belief that they would prevent eclampsia and improve outcome. Predicting who is at risk for eclampsia is difficult, and only 1% to 2% of those with preeclampsia develop eclampsia. However, prophylactic anticonvulsants are used in all parturients with preeclampsia. A variety of anticonvulsants have been proposed and evaluated, but the most widely used drug is magnesium sulfate. Other agents used include diazepam and phenytoin. Evidence continues to support the use of magnesium sulfate for the prevention of seizures, and it appears to be superior to other agents. The largest study that examined magnesium sulfate was a multicenter trial that included centers from the United Kingdom, South America, and South Africa.[80] A total of 10 110 patients were randomized to receive magnesium sulfate (5055 patients) or placebo (5055 patients). There was a greater incidence of side effects in the magnesium sulfate group such as flushing, hot flashes, and blurry vision. The magnesium sulfate group also had a 58% lower risk of eclampsia; this lower risk did not affect maternal mortality. Magnesium does not prevent the progression of the disease to severe preeclampsia. In 222 women with mild preeclampsia, 109 patients received intravenous magnesium. There was no difference in the groups in the progression to severe disease.[81] Magnesium sulfate does relax the uterus. The use of magnesium sulfate in parturients with preeclampsia does not slow labor, but there is a greater need for oxytocin.[82]

It was hoped that low-dose aspirin would be beneficial in preventing preeclampsia. Low-dose aspirin reduces thromboxane production by selective inhibition of platelet thromboxane production without affecting prostacyclin production by the vascular endothelium. The largest study randomized 2539 women to receive either low-dose aspirin (60 mg) or placebo.[83] The use of small-dose aspirin did not affect the incidence of preeclampsia. A meta-analysis of aspirin studies identified 14 trials that met specific criteria. Aspirin was only effective in women with known risk factors. It was not beneficial for the general population.[84]

Treatment of acute hypertension is intended to prevent potential cerebrovascular complications (the most common cause of morbidity in patients with preeclampsia). Antihypertensive medications prevent cerebrovascular problems; they do not alter the course of the disease. Intravenous hydralazine and intravenous labetalol are the most commonly used medications. Originally, it was believed that hydralazine was the drug of choice because it preserves uterine blood flow. In a meta-analysis comparing hydralazine to labetalol, hydralazine was associated with more maternal hypotension, more cesarean deliveries, more adverse effects on the fetal heart rate, and lower 1-minute Apgar scores.[85] It was also associated with less maternal bradycardia as compared with labetalol. Labetalol is used more frequently for the treatment of hypertension of preeclampsia.

In a review of hypertension in pregnant women, Lindheimer and Katz concluded, "Epidural block should be avoided, since in preeclampsia it is associated with sudden falls of blood pressure and on occasion with vascular collapse."[86] The literature does not support this stance.[87,88] Studies have demonstrated the stability of maternal cardiac output after administration of epidural anesthesia in patients with severe preeclampsia. Also, spinal anesthesia is not contraindicated in severe preeclamptic patients.[89] Although it does result in a higher incidence of hypotension, these episodes are not more severe than during epidural anesthesia and are also easily treated. In regard to epidural anesthesia, it provides excellent analgesia during labor and allows patients to remain awake and alert during vaginal and cesarean delivery. Epidural anesthesia has at least 3 specific advantages in parturients with preeclampsia who require cesarean delivery. It reduces circulating concentrations of catecholamines in laboring women, facilitating control of blood pressure and improving intervillous blood flow.[90,91] It also allows for better control of systemic and pulmonary arterial pressures.[92] Finally, epidural anesthesia does not require laryngoscopy and intubation, which might be hazardous or difficult because of pharyngeal edema.[93]

Platelet turnover and function is often altered in preeclampsia. Normal platelets are disk-shaped cells, 2 to 4 μm in diameter, that lack a nucleus. Platelets are formed in the bone marrow from giant cells called megakaryocytes. At any moment, approximately 80% of the platelets are circulating and 20% are localized in the spleen. Platelets participate in coagulation factor reactions leading to thrombin formation by providing a lipoprotein surface on which coagulation enzymes and substrates interact. The bone marrow does not contain a reserve of platelets. If circulating platelets are rapidly destroyed or lost, thrombocytopenia persists for several days until enough platelets are formed to correct it.

Pitkin and Witte measured platelet counts every 4 weeks in 23 pregnant women and found that platelet counts dropped from 322 000/μL in the first trimester to 278 000/μL in the third trimester.[94] This decrease is caused by increased destruction.[95] Preeclampsia is accompanied by endothelial injury, leading to increased platelet activation with consumption in the microvasculature. Platelet consumption is a late finding in preeclampsia, but increased platelet turnover may be an early marker of preeclampsia. Thrombocytopenia is the most common hematologic abnormality in patients with preeclampsia. Its incidence depends on the severity of the disease and the presence or absence of abruption placenta. A platelet count less than 150 000/μL was found in 50% of the women and a count of less than 100 000/μL in 36% of women with preeclampsia.[96] Roberts et al retrospectively studied 292 patients with low platelets.[97] Patients were divided into 2 groups: those with platelet counts less than 50 000/μL and those with platelet counts of 50 000-100 000/μL. Bleeding was only likely if the platelet count was less than 40 000/μL. There is no therapy for the thrombocytopenia of preeclampsia other than delivery. Epidural analgesia has been successfully placed in individuals with platelet counts less than 100 000/μL if there is no other existing coagulopathy.

ANTEPARTUM HEMORRHAGE

The 2 major causes of antepartum hemorrhage are placenta previa and placental abruption. Hemorrhage is the second leading cause of maternal mortality in the United States, and its incidence is expected to increase as the number of cesarean deliveries increase.[97] Hemorrhage can be quite severe because uterine blood flow at term is 500 to 700 mL/min.

Placenta previa is present when the placenta overlies the cervical os. Placenta previa varies in degree and may be complete (in 37% of cases, the placenta completely covers the internal cervical os), partial (in 27% the placenta partially covers the os), or low lying (in 46% the placenta is in the lower segment but does not reach the internal os). Parturients with either complete or partial placenta previa are at an increased risk of antepartum bleeding, are more likely to have placenta accreta, and are more likely to require hysterectomy and to have postoperative complications than women with low-lying placenta previa.[98] Whereas women with complete or partial placenta previa require cesarean delivery, not all parturients with low-lying placenta previa require cesarean delivery. With transvaginal ultrasonography, the location of the placenta may be determined. If the placental edge is greater than 10 mm from the cervical os, the parturient may safely undergo vaginal delivery without increased risk of hemorrhage.[99] Risk factors for placenta previa include uterine fibroids and a history of multiple pregnancies (**Table 22-7**). Placenta previa is more likely to be affected by conditions existing prior to pregnancy, such as maternal age, race, parity, and previous cesarean delivery.[100] The main sign of placenta previa is painless vaginal bleeding. The bleeding usually stops spontaneously but may recur suddenly at any time. Recurrent bleeding is usually more severe. If the diagnosis of placenta previa is suspected, ultrasonography is performed. The accuracy of this technique is 95% and has replaced the double setup technique in which a cervical examination is performed in the operating room with preparation to do an immediate cesarean delivery.[101,102] Before term gestation, the patient with placenta previa is usually managed conservatively with bed rest if the patient is not actively bleeding. If bleeding does occur, emergency cesarean delivery is required. Occasionally, the placenta may implant directly to the myometrium giving rise to 3 situations: placenta accreta (the placenta attaches to the myometrium), placenta increta (the placenta invades the myometrium but does not penetrate it fully), or placenta percreta (the placenta penetrates the entire thickness of the myometrium and may attach to other structures in the pelvis). In the general obstetric population, the incidence of placenta accreta is 1 in 2500. In patients with placenta previa and no prior cesarean delivery, the incidence is 3%. The risk of placenta accreta in patients with placenta previa and who have had a prior cesarean delivery increases with each prior cesarean delivery. With 1 prior uterine incision, the incidence of placenta accreta has been reported to be 11%; 2 prior uterine incisions, 40%; and 3 prior uterine incisions, 61%.[102] In patients with placenta previa and prior cesarean delivery, the anesthesia provider should be prepared for massive hemorrhage. Large-bore intravenous access and the immediate availability of blood products are mandatory.

TABLE 22-7 Risk Factors for Placenta Previa

- Uterine fibroids
- Multiple pregnancies
- Previous cesarean delivery
- Smoking
- Older age
- Previous uterine surgery

Placental abruption refers to separation of the placenta after 20 weeks of gestation but before the birth of the fetus. The incidence ranges from 0.2% to 2.4%, depending on the population studied. From 1979 to 2001, the rate of placental abruption increased 92% among black women and 15% among white women.[103,104] A high infant mortality is associated with placental abruption. Unlike risk factors for placenta previa, placental abruption is more likely to be affected by conditions occurring during pregnancy, such as maternal cigarette smoking, alcohol consumption, and prenatal care. Risk factors for placental abruption are presented in **Table 22-8**. The primary etiology of placental abruption is unknown. It begins with hemorrhage into the deciduas basalis, causing a split in the deciduas and subsequent hematoma formation. This expanding hematoma causes additional separation, compression, and ultimately destruction of the adjacent placental tissue. The classic signs of placental abruption are vaginal bleeding, abdominal pain, uterine tenderness, and contractions. Bleeding is either through the vagina or concealed in the uterus. If the blood is concealed, underestimating blood loss is common. Unlike placenta previa, abruption may not be ruled out by a negative ultrasound examination, as ultrasound evidence of hemorrhage is present in only 50% of patients.[105] Anesthetic management of the parturient with placental abruption requires volume resuscitation. The anesthesia provider must also be prepared to manage a coagulopathic patient because placental abruption is associated with disseminated intravascular coagulation.

TABLE 22-8 Risk Factors for Placenta Abruption

- History of placenta abruption
- High blood pressure
- Preeclampsia
- Trauma
- Cocaine
- Diabetes mellitus
- Advanced maternal age
- Multiple pregnancies
- Smoking

SURGERY DURING PREGNANCY

For surgery during pregnancy, the anesthesia provider must consider possible fetal effects of the maternal disease process. The most common cause of the nonobstetric acute abdomen is appendicitis, occurring in 1 in 500 pregnancies and accounting for approximately 25% of surgeries during pregnancy.[107] The incidence of acute cholecystitis requiring surgery is 1 in 1600 pregnancies. Approximately 3% of parturients have stones in their gallbladder. For surgery during pregnancy, protection of the mother is paramount, but other goals of anesthetic management include maintenance of uterine blood flow and fetal oxygenation, avoidance of teratogenic drugs, and prevention of preterm labor.

Perhaps the greatest concern of pregnant women is whether anesthetics or anesthesia may increase the risk of congenital anomalies. Shnider and Webster were the first to study this possibility when they evaluated the medical records of 9073 women who delivered infants between July 1959 and August 1964.[108] Of these women, 147 (1.6%) had surgery during pregnancy. There was no increased incidence of congenital anomalies in the surgical group, but the authors noted that most of these patients received anesthetics during the second or third trimester (after the period of organogenesis, which is the first trimester). Brodsky et al mailed questionnaires to 287 women who had surgery during pregnancy.[109] Among the women, 187 had surgery during the first trimester. There was no major increase in congenital anomalies in infants born to women who had surgery during pregnancy compared with a control group of pregnant women who did not have surgery. Duncan et al, used health insurance data from 1971 to 1978.[110] They matched 2565 women undergoing surgery during pregnancy to those of similar height and weight who did not. There was no difference in the rate of congenital anomalies. There was an increased risk of spontaneous abortion in those undergoing surgery with general anesthesia in the first or second trimester, especially in those undergoing gynecologic surgery. Mazze and Kallen obtained data from 3 Swedish health care registries to evaluate the risk of adverse reproductive outcomes after anesthesia administration and surgery in pregnant women between 1973 and 1981.[111] They identified 2252 women who underwent surgery during the first trimester. Among these women, 65% received general anesthesia; 35% received regional anesthesia or local infiltration. There was no increase in congenital anomalies among the parturients who had surgery.[112] Another approach to this question is to examine anomalies and determine if there is a link to anesthesia or surgery. Of the 20 830 pregnant women who had a child with a congenital anomaly, 31 patients had surgery with anesthesia. This fraction did not differ from the 35 727 women who had infants without congenital anomalies and 73 of them having surgery during pregnancy. There was no higher rate of surgery or anesthesia in any of the congenital anomaly groups.

The lack of link between anesthesia and surgery during pregnancy and congenital anomalies has not been universal. Kallen and Mazze reexamined their database and noted 6 infants with neural tube defects (an overall incidence in the general population is 1 in 1000).[113] Of these 6 infants, the mothers of 5 of the infants had surgery during gestational weeks 4 to 5, the period of neural tube formation. This group was not the only one to hypothesize a possible link. Infants born with central nervous system defects in Atlanta between 1968 and 1980 were matched to controls by race, birth hospital, and period of birth.[114] Of the 694 mothers of infants with central nervous system defects, 12 reported first-trimester anesthesia exposure (34 of 2984 control mothers reported such exposure). There was an increased risk for hydrocephalus (odds ratio [OR]: 9.6; 95% CI, 3.8-24.6). The strongest association was for hydrocephalus and eye defects (OR: 39.6; 95% CI, 7.5-209.2). These data are influenced by a rare event and by small sample size. In the past, anesthesia providers informed patients that there was a theoretically risk that exposure to anesthesia in the first trimester increased the risk of teratogenesis. These 2 studies raise the possibility of such an existence. When discussing the risk of anesthesia with pregnant women scheduled for surgery, the anesthesia care provider should remind the patient that there is a 3% baseline incidence of fetal anomalies among all pregnant women regardless of exposure.

The use of fetal monitoring during maternal surgery is a debated subject. After 18 to 20 weeks of gestation, the fetal heart rate may be monitored. The argument in favor of intraoperative fetal monitoring is that it may improve fetal outcome. Changes in the fetal heart rate may signal fetal compromise allowing the anesthesia care provider to take steps to improve uteroplacental perfusion and fetal oxygenation. These may include increasing left uterine displacement, higher inspired concentration of oxygen, adjustment of maternal ventilation, augmentation of maternal circulating blood volume, or pharmacologic management of hypotension. Despite these benefits, the use of fetal monitoring during surgery is not universally applied. Hospitals in the United States were surveyed regarding monitoring.[115] Of the 184 respondents, 60% routinely used fetal monitors; 40% did not. The American College of Obstetricians and Gynecologists recognized that there are no data regarding monitoring during surgery and stated

> It is important for physicians to obtain obstetric consultation before performing nonobstetric surgery because obstetricians are uniquely qualified to discuss aspects of maternal physiology and anatomy that may affect intraoperative maternal-fetal well-being. The decision to use fetal monitoring should be individualized and if used, may be based on gestational age, type of surgery, and facilities available. Ultimately, each case warrants a team approach for optimal safety of the woman and her baby.[116]

EVALUATING THE PARTURIENT WITH COEXISTING DISEASE

CARDIAC DISEASE

The cardiovascular changes of pregnancy place a major stress on the maternal heart and circulatory system. The changes may even result in death of the mother if she has cardiovascular disease. In an attempt to quantify this risk, 562 pregnant women with cardiac disease (either congenital or acquired) were followed prospectively in 13 Canadian hospitals.[117] The study followed these women through pregnancy and for 6 months after delivery. Neonatal morbidity, preterm labor, and small for gestational age births occurred in 20% of these patients. Maternal complications included pulmonary edema, stroke, and tachyarrhythmia. The most significant predictor of morbidity and mortality was the presence of left ventricular dysfunction prior to the pregnancy, with an OR of 11 (95% CI, 4-34). The best predictor of maternal outcome is the New York Heart Association functional class (**Table 22-9**). In a study of 482 pregnancies, cardiovascular morbidity was less in mothers with class I as compared with others.[118] The higher the functional class, the greater the incidence of morbidity and mortality.[119] Neonatal complications were seen in 20% and were associated with poor functional class, left heart obstruction, or smoking.

Valvular lesions in pregnant patients are decreasing due to the decrease in rheumatic heart disease. In general, the parturient with valvular incompetence does better than the parturient with stenotic

TABLE 22-9 New York Heart Association Functional Classification of Cardiovascular Disease

Class I: No limitation of physical activity. Ordinary activity does not precipitate cardiovascular symptoms.
Class II: Slight limitation of physical activity. Ordinary physical activity will precipitate cardiovascular symptoms.
Class III: Less than ordinary physical activity precipitates symptoms that markedly limit activity. Patients are comfortable at rest.
Class IV: Patients are unable to carry on any physical activity without discomfort. Cardiovascular symptoms may be present at rest.

lesions. The reduced systemic vascular resistance of pregnancy improves forward flow, thus limiting the effects of regurgitation. In contrast, stenotic valvular lesions create a fixed impediment to the required increase in cardiac output of pregnancy, precipitating heart failure. Mitral stenosis is the most common valvular lesion encountered in the parturient.[120] There is an increased incidence of atrial fibrillation, leading to heart failure. Balloon mitral commissurotomy has been described during pregnancy and is a therapeutic option.[121] Aortic stenosis is infrequently encountered and is usually due to a congenitally abnormal valve. Hypertrophic cardiomyopathy is a genetically transmitted cardiac disease characterized by left ventricular hypertrophy and reduced left ventricular size and compliance. Reduction in preload and afterload results in an increase in the outflow gradient and in a reduction in left ventricular filling. One hundred parturients with hypertrophic cardiomyopathy were compared with the general population.[122] There were 2 pregnancy-related deaths, both in women with severe disease. If the patient were in a stable condition, the progression of symptoms, atrial fibrillation, and syncope were uncommon.

Congenital heart disease is increasingly prevalent in women of childbearing age due to the advances in diagnosis and treatment of these conditions. Approximately 25% of cardiac disease in the parturient is due to congenital heart disease.[123] In pregnant patients with congenital heart disease, both cardiac and neonatal complications are increased. Right subpulmonary ventricular systolic dysfunction and severe pulmonary regurgitation were predictors of an adverse fetal outcome. Congenital heart disease may be divided into 2 groups: those with acyanotic lesions and those with cyanotic lesions. Patients with cyanotic lesions developed significantly more congestive heart failure and deteriorated more often than those with acyanotic lesions. Women with obstructive lesions had a higher incidence of pregnancy-induced hypertension, whereas in the cyanotic group, the mean birthweight was approximately 1 kg less than that the acyanotic group. Acyanotic conditions include atrial or ventricular septal defects or persistent ductus arteriosus with small or moderate left to right shunts.[124] Cyanotic lesions include tetralogy of Fallot and transposition of the great vessels with subsequent Fontan procedure. In cyanotic lesions, the increase in cardiac output and decrease in systemic vascular resistance lead to greater right-to-left shunting, worsening the cyanosis and hypoxemia.

Peripartum cardiomyopathy is a rare form of heart failure with no identifiable cause that occurs within the last month of pregnancy or within 5 months after delivery. The incidence is 1 in 4000. Risk factors include advanced maternal age, multiparity, multiple gestation, black population, obesity, and preeclampsia. There is a high morbidity and mortality with approximately 20% of those developing the condition dying.[125] The remainder of those affected recovers partially or completely. The largest series of women who had the disorder and a subsequent pregnancy involved 44 women.[126] Twenty-eight pregnancies occurred in women who recovered completely; 16 pregnancies occurred in women who had persistent left ventricular dysfunction. All deaths occurred in the patients with persistent left ventricular dysfunction and they were also twice as likely to present with congestive heart failure. These patients also had a greater frequency of premature deliveries.

Acute myocardial infarction during pregnancy is rare, with an incidence of 1 in 10 000 pregnancies. However, the incidence is increasing, most likely reflecting the trend toward an older maternal age.[127] Mortality is approximately 40%, with the greatest risk occurring if the infarction occurs late in the pregnancy. Cardiac troponin is unaffected by pregnancy, allowing for the diagnosis of ischemic infarction.

Pulmonary hypertension is defined as a mean pulmonary artery pressure greater than 25 mm Hg associated with pulmonary capillary wedge pressure less than 12 mm Hg. Primary pulmonary hypertension is a rare disease that affects young women of childbearing age. Pulmonary hypertension may also be secondary to other causes such as congenital heart disease, thromboembolic disease, and connective tissue disorders. The most common cause of pulmonary hypertension in the parturient involves the late consequences of a large cardiac shunt (eg, Eisenmenger syndrome). Pulmonary hypertension is tolerated poorly during pregnancy due to insufficient adaptation of the right heart to increases in cardiac output and a poorly compliant pulmonary vasculature. In a series of 14 parturients with severe pulmonary hypertension (4 primary and 10 secondary), 2 patients died before delivery and 3 died postpartum.[128] It was not possible to determine whether parturients with primary pulmonary hypertension fared better than patients with secondary pulmonary hypertension.

TABLE 22-10 Classification for Severity of Asthma

	Medication Use	Symptoms	FEV_1
Intermittent	No daily medications	≤2 times/wk	≥80%
	Bronchodilator as needed		
Mild persistent	One medication	>2 times/wk but <1 time/d	≥80%
Moderate persistent (no nocturnal symptoms)	Two medications	Daily	>60%
Severe (nocturnal symptoms)	Three medications	Daily	≤60%

FEV_1, forced capacity expiratory volume in 1 second.

ASTHMA

Asthma is a disease of chronic airway inflammation with acute episodes of bronchospasm. Asthma severity is classified according to its clinical features (**Table 22-10**). Approximately 7% of pregnant women are affected by asthma.[129] A number of physiologic changes of pregnancy affect the course of asthma in the parturient. Airway closure that results from decreased functional residual capacity during tidal breathing might lead to exacerbation of the disease.[130] To determine the effect of pregnancy and stage of pregnancy on asthma, 6 electronic databases were searched for prospective studies of asthmatic women during pregnancy. This review demonstrated that asthma improves in 70% of parturients and worsens in the remaining 30%. This improvement peaked in the second trimester and reverted to baseline after delivery. Peak expiratory flow rate declines significantly throughout gestation, returning to normal at 6 weeks postpartum.[131]

Parturients with asthma are at a higher risk of developing complications during pregnancy. Parturients with poorly controlled asthma had a doubling of risk for spontaneous preterm labor.[133] If the asthma is controlled, there is no increased risk of preterm delivery, although there is an increased risk of stillbirth for the male fetus.[134] Frequency of asthmatic symptoms during pregnancy was strongly associated with preeclampsia. Fetal hypoxia has been suggested as the mechanism for the association between asthma and preeclampsia as well as between asthma and intrauterine growth retardation.[135] Parturients with asthma have a greater risk of developing chorioamnionitis, most likely due to premature rupture of membranes coupled with immunosuppressive therapy of asthma.[136]

The treatment of asthma combines allergen avoidance, smoking cessation, pharmacotherapy, and education. The value of smoking cessation was reinforced in a study of 2210 women. Active smoking in women with asthma had a strong association with increased asthma symptoms and fetal growth abnormalities; passive smoke exposure did not exacerbate the disease process.[137] The management of pregnant women with asthma should follow the same guidelines as for nonpregnant patients, with inhaled steroids as the first line of therapy.[138] Inhaled steroids, even in high doses, is not associated with congenital malformations in the neonate.[139] Parturients are not treated with systemic glucocorticoids due to its teratogenetic effect (the risk of orofacial cleft increases by 3).[140] Treatment with inhaled steroids as compared with theophylline results in a greater improvement in FEV_1 in the parturient.[141] The mainstay for treatment of an acute attack is inhaled albuterol. Albuterol is a relatively selective β_2-adrenergic bronchodilator. It has been shown to have no effect on maternal and fetal circulations.[142]

BACK PAIN

Back pain during pregnancy is a frequent problem. A cohort of 200 consecutive women was followed throughout their pregnancy.[143] Of these participants, none reported back pain at the beginning of the study. However, at 12 weeks of gestation, 19% of the study population complained of back pain. The incidence increased to 47% at 24 weeks of gestation and peaked at 49% at 36 weeks of gestation. After delivery, the prevalence of back pain declined to 9.4%. Despite a relatively high prevalence, only 32% of women with low back pain during pregnancy report this problem to their physician, and only 25% of providers recommend a specific therapy.[144] If patients receive osteopathic manipulation during the third trimester, the progression of back pain may be halted.[145]

The etiology of the back pain is multimodal. One popular theory is that the exaggerated lumbar lordosis to compensate for the enlarging uterus places significant mechanical strain on the lower back. There is also a hormonal component. Relaxin is a polypeptide hormone of ovarian origin of the insulin-like growth factor family. Relaxin is associated with remodeling of collagen fibers and pelvic connective tissue. The primary source of circulating relaxin is the corpus luteum. The placenta is also a major source of relaxin. When serum levels of relaxin were measured in parturients with and without back pain, these levels best explained differences in back pain.[146]

Patients who develop low back pain during pregnancy may avoid subsequent pregnancy to prevent recurrence of the back pain. Women with low back pain during pregnancy have an extremely high risk for experiencing a new episode during a subsequent pregnancy.[147]

Most patients with low back pain during pregnancy respond to activity and postural modification. Exercise to increase the strength of the abdominal and back muscles is helpful. Scheduled rest periods with elevation of the feet to flex the hips and decrease the lumbar lordosis help to relieve muscle spasm and pain.[148]

DIABETES MELLITUS

Diabetes mellitus complicates 4% to 7% of pregnancies in the United States, although the incidence is expected to increase with the increase in frequency of gestational diabetes mellitus.[149] Gestational diabetes mellitus is defined as glucose intolerance that first occurs during pregnancy. The reason for the increase is the increase in maternal weight. A large weight gain during the first trimester of pregnancy, especially in overweight or obese women, increases a woman's risk of gestational diabetes mellitus.[150] Type 1 diabetes results from primary failure of endogenous insulin production, whereas type 2 diabetes represents a relative insulin deficiency. The precise etiology of type 1 diabetes is unknown; it appears that to develop type 1 diabetes mellitus, one must have genetic susceptibility and an environmental insult, which leads to an autoimmune attack against the insulin-producing pancreatic islet β cells. (See Chapter 13 for a detailed discussion of endocrine disease.)

During normal pregnancy, the parturient develops an insulin resistance that begins near midpregnancy and progresses through the third trimester. The insulin resistance appears to be a result from a combination of increased maternal adiposity and of hormones excreted by the placenta, such as human placental lactogen and progesterone. The fact that insulin resistance rapidly abates following delivery (important to remember when managing diabetic parturients in the labor suite) suggests that the major contributor to this insulin resistance is placental hormones.

Glucose control is important for both maternal and fetal well-being during pregnancy. Studies have consistently shown a significant positive correlation between ambient serum glucose concentration during organogenesis and the incidence of spontaneous abortion.[151] When glycosylated hemoglobin levels were less than 8.5%, the fetal malformation rate (cardiac defects, sacral agenesis, renal agenesis, polycystic kidneys, anencephaly, meningomyelocele) was 3.4%, but when the glycosylated hemoglobin level was greater than 9.5%, the rate of fetal malformations approached 22%.[152] Glucose crosses the placenta; fetal levels reflect maternal levels. Insulin does not cross the placenta. Maternal hyperglycemia produces fetal hyperglycemia causing stimulation of the fetal β cells and fetal hyperinsulinemia. Insulin is the major fetal growth hormone and produces excessive fetal growth, especially in the fat. The fetus of a poorly controlled diabetic mother is likely to be large, especially in the shoulders and chest, increasing the risk of shoulder dystocia at delivery. Given this risk, there is a higher incidence of cesarean delivery as compared with the general population, with 45% to 73% of parturients with type 1 diabetes mellitus having cesarean delivery. A weight gain of 15 kg and suspected macrosomia are risk factors associated for cesarean delivery without labor.[153] Increased insulin levels in the fetus delays fetal lung maturity. Diabetic parturients also have an increased risk of developing preeclampsia.[154] In 1949, White proposed a system for classifying diabetes in obstetric patients[155] (**Table 22-11**). The White classification is still used today as a means of conveying to others the severity of the disease process.

TABLE 22-11 White Classification of Diabetes in Pregnancy

Class	Age at Onset	Duration	Complications	Insulin Requirement
Gestational Diabetes				
A1	Any	Any	–	No
A2	Any	Any	–	Yes
Pregestational Diabetes				
B	>20 y	<10 y	–	Yes
C	10-19 y	10-19 y	–	Yes
D	<10 y	>20 y	Benign retinopathy	Yes
F	Any	Any	Nephropathy	Yes
R	Any	Any	Proliferative retinopathy	Yes
T	Any	Any	Renal transplant	Yes
H	Any	Any	Cardiac	Yes

The management of diabetes in pregnancy includes a careful combination of diet, exercise, and insulin. An aggressive approach to mild gestational diabetes including dietary intervention and self-monitoring of blood glucose with insulin if necessary was associated with a significant reduction in fetal overgrowth, shoulder dystocia, cesarean delivery, and preeclampsia.[156] Any abnormality of blood glucose should be aggressively managed to improve outcome for mother and fetus. Fasting blood glucose should be maintained near 90 mg/dL and the 1-hour postprandial glucose below 140 mg/dL. During the night, glucose levels should not fall below 60 mg/dL. Glycosylated hemoglobin levels should be no higher than 6%.[157]

Gestational diabetes mellitus is defined as glucose tolerance during pregnancy. Risk factors include advanced maternal age, family history of diabetes, and obesity.[158,159] Long-term follow-up of patients with gestational diabetes indicates that most progress to diabetes after pregnancy.[160] Very few have diabetes soon after delivery; the incidence appears to increase 10 or more years after delivery. The focus of treatment antepartum is to return glucose levels to normal. After pregnancy, the main focus of clinical care should be reducing the risk of diabetes and treating it if it develops.

Much debate has focused on the role of oral hypoglycemic agents for the management of diabetes during pregnancy. These drugs are routinely used in nonpregnant adults with type 2 diabetes. They are also effective in parturients with gestational diabetes. The most commonly used agent is glyburide, the second-generation sulfonylurea. It does not cross the placenta, thus avoiding possible teratogenicity. It has an onset of action of 4 hours and duration of 10 hours. In a study of 404 women, glyburide was similar to insulin in regard to glucose control, with a lower incidence of hypoglycemia in the glyburide group.[161] When compared with glyburide in 149 parturients with gestational diabetes, the failure rate of metformin was 2.1 times higher than the failure rate of glyburide.[162]

THYROID DISEASE

Thyroid disease is more common in women, with a female-to-male ratio of 12:1. (See Chapter 13 for details regarding endocrine disease.) Thyroid autoimmunity is by far the most frequent cause of hypothyroidism in women of reproductive age.[163] The prevalence of hypothyroidism in the general population of reproductive age is 2%. The incidence of hyperthyroidism in pregnant women is estimated at 0.2%, with the most common cause being Graves disease (autoimmune-induced thyroxine overproduction). During pregnancy, normal thyroid activity undergoes significant changes, including a 2- to 3-fold increase in thyroxine-binding globulin concentrations, increased serum thyroglobulin, and increased renal iodide clearance. In addition, human chorionic gonadotropin has mild thyroid stimulating activity.[164]

Hypothyroidism in women may cause infertility. This cause is not surprising because thyroid hormones have direct effects on granulose cells, luteal cells, and oocytes. With mild hypothyroidism, pregnancy may occur, but the resulting pregnancies are often associated with abortion, stillbirth, or prematurity.[165] For the fetus, maternal thyroid hormones are transferred across the placenta. This transfer is important in early gestation because the fetal thyroid gland becomes operational only after midgestation. During pregnancy, the parturient requires a greater iodine intake. Before pregnancy, a woman requires approximately 100 μg/d, which increases to 200 to 250 μg/d to maintain free thyroxine during pregnancy.[166] This higher iodine requirement is a result of the increase in thyroxine production by the mother, a transfer of iodine to the fetus, and an increased renal iodine clearance. In the United States, approximately 11% of parturients do not receive sufficient iodine. Maternal hypothyroidism is associated with neurologic disorders in the newborn because thyroid hormonal levels are important for fetal brain development.[167] In 2007, the Endocrine Society Clinical Practice Guideline on the Management of Thyroid Dysfunction During Pregnancy and Postpartum was published. In a study of 4562 parturients, universal screening reduced the incidence of adverse obstetrical and neonatal outcomes in a low-risk population.[168]

Hyperthyroidism during pregnancy is less common than hypothyroidism. Hyperthyroidism may lead to miscarriage, neonatal death, preterm delivery, and intrauterine growth retardation. Two pregnancy-specific conditions, hyperemesis gravidarum and trophoblastic disease, may cause hyperthyroidism in the mother.[169,170] Hyperemesis gravidarum is characterized by severe vomiting that begins around 6 weeks of gestation and usually resolves by 20 weeks of gestation. The etiology of transient hyperthyroidism in hyperemesis gravidarum is unclear. In trophoblastic disease, there is an increase in human chorionic gonadotropin, which increases thyroid function. In select cases, propylthiouracil may be required.

HUMAN IMMUNODEFICIENCY VIRUS

Acquired immunodeficiency syndrome (AIDS) was first reported in women in 1981 with the percentage of AIDS cases in women increasing thereafter. For AIDS among children younger than 3 years, perinatal transmission accounts for 92% of the cases.[171] Of the women with HIV, 31% were of childbearing age. Pregnancy does not affect HIV or disease progression; levels of virus are not increased by pregnancy.[172] As such, the challenge with HIV in pregnant patients is the prevention of transmission of HIV to the child.

The first major discovery in the prevention of transmission of the virus to the neonate was the demonstration that treatment of the mother with zidovudine during pregnancy and labor and of the neonate during the first 6 weeks of life reduces the transmission rate from 25% to 8%.[173] The introduction of this practice had a dramatic effect on perinatal transmission.[174] However, the use of a single agent is considered obsolete, and patients now receive a combination therapy. Combination therapy consists of 2 nucleoside reverse transcriptase inhibitors and 1 nonnucleoside reverse transcriptase inhibitor or protease inhibitor. Combination antiretroviral therapy has been proven effective in reducing maternal HIV-1 RNA levels to less than 500 copies/mL, which minimizes the risk of perinatal transmission from a baseline of 26% to 1% to 2%.[175] Given that an effective therapy exists, the Centers for Disease Control and the American College of Obstetricians and Gynecologists have recommended that all pregnant women be screened for HIV. HIV-negative infants born to HIV-positive mothers frequently exhibit a range of immunologic abnormalities.[176]

Early studies suggested an association between vaginal delivery and fetal transmission of the virus, with a decreased likelihood of transmission with cesarean delivery.[177,178] In 1999, the International Perinatal HIV Group published a meta-analysis that included only those studies of at least 100 mother-child pairs and defined elective cesarean delivery as that performed before the onset of labor.[179] The number of patients in the final analysis was 7800 mother-child pairs. The study concluded that the likelihood of transmission from the mother to the child decreased by approximately 50% with elective cesarean delivery as compared with other modes of delivery. The addition of antiretroviral therapy during prenatal, intrapartum, and neonatal periods reduced the risk further. The problem with this analysis was that most studies were performed prior to the use of highly active antiretroviral therapy and also without any data concerning maternal viral load. Given these concerns, the American College of Obstetricians and Gynecologists published a committee opinion, which may be summarized as follows:

1. In patients with HIV who did not take antiretroviral therapy, the risk of vertical transmission is 25%.
2. The addition of zidovudine decreases the risk to 5% to 8%.
3. If a cesarean delivery is performed, the risk is approximately 2%.
4. A similar risk of 2% or less is seen among women with viral loads of less than 1000 copies/mL. Women whose viral loads are greater than 1000 copies/mL should be counseled regarding the potential benefit of scheduled cesarean delivery.
5. Viral load should be measured to assist the obstetrician in planning the route of delivery.[180]

COCAINE ABUSE

The consequences of acute and chronic cocaine abuse must be considered in the obstetric population, due to the prevalence of abuse in women of childbearing age. Overall approaches to the perioperative management of substance abuse are provided in Chapter 24; this brief review focuses on the special concerns that affect the parturient and her child. Cocaine is derived from the *Erythroxylum coca* plant. It is taken intravenously, intranasally, or orally. Crack is a form of cocaine that is smoked. Cocaine produces sympathetic stimulation by blocking the presynaptic reuptake of norepinephrine, dopamine, and serotonin. This pathophysiology explains the hypertension and tachycardia frequently seen following acute use. In fact, it is difficult to differentiate preeclampsia from acute cocaine toxicity based on physiologic variables.[181] Urine testing for protein differentiates between the 2.[182] Almost 90% of drug-abusing women are of reproductive age, with an estimated 4.6 million female users of cocaine in the United States and 750 000 drug-exposed births annually.[183] In addition to its cardiovascular effects, maternal ingestion of cocaine is associated with premature labor, placental abruption, nonreassuring fetal heart rate, and uterine rupture. Cocaine rapidly crosses the placenta resulting in a high incidence of fetal anomalies. In children who were exposed in utero to cocaine, performance on tasks that assess sustained attention and behavioral self-regulation are compromised.[184] Evidence indicates that this deficiency is a result of disruption of neuronal pathways associated with attention and behavioral self-regulation. In the mother, cocaine is associated with thrombocytopenia. Propanol is contraindicated in patients with hypertension from acute cocaine use due to unopposed α-adrenergic stimulation.

Labetalol or hydralazine is acceptable. The American Heart Association recommends nitroglycerine and benzodiazepines as first-line agents for patients experiencing cocaine-related myocardial ischemia. For hypotension, ephedrine may not be effective due to a depletion of catecholamines. Phenylephrine would be effective.[185]

PUTTING IT ALL TOGETHER

Unlike other patients, the evaluation of the parturient involves 2 patients, the mother and fetus. Optimal care of the mother provides the best care for the fetus. The parturient undergoes various physiologic changes that vary depending on gestation. These changes must be considered when devising an anesthetic plan. These changes also must be considered when the parturient has an underlying disease. These diseases and conditions typically worsen during pregnancy, ultimately resulting in deterioration of the mother's condition. These changes also have implications in the pharmacologic management. Preterm labor does not entail increased risk to the mother; rather, it carries significant risk to the fetus. However, the use of tocolytic agents places the mother at risk. Magnesium sulfate is typically administered during preterm labor, not necessarily for tocolysis but rather for the neuroprotective effects in the neonate. Magnesium sulfate also remains the cornerstone for seizure prophylaxis in patients with preeclampsia. Magnesium sulfate potentiates both nondepolarizing (significantly) and depolarizing muscle relaxants. Although one of the most challenging aspects of anesthesia is the care of the parturient, it also is one of the most rewarding.

KEY REFERENCES

- Berkman ND, Thorp JM Jr, Lohr KN, et al. Tocolytic treatment for the management of preterm labor: a review of the evidence. *Am J Obstet Gynecol.* 2002;186:587.
- Bonnin M, Mercier FJ, Sitbon O, et al. Severe pulmonary hypertension during pregnancy. *Anesthesiology.* 2005;102:1133.
- Cohen SE, Andes LC, Carvalho B. Assessment of knowledge regarding cardiopulmonary resuscitation of pregnant women. *Int J Obstet Anesth.* 2008;17:20.
- Czeizel AE, Pataki T, Rockenbauer M. Reproductive outcome after exposure to surgery under anesthesia during pregnancy. *Arch Gynecol Obstet.* 1998;261:193.
- Doyle LW, Crowther CA, Middleton P, Marret S. Antenatal magnesium sulfate and neurologic outcome in preterm infants: a systematic review. *Obstet Gynecol.* 2009;113:1327.
- Hong JY, Park JW, Oh JI. Comparison of preoperative gastric contents and serum gastrin concentrations in pregnant and nonpregnant women. *J Clin Anesth.* 2005;17:451.
- Jensen D, Webb KA, O'Donnell DE. Chemical and mechanical adaptations of the respiratory system at rest and during exercise in human pregnancy. *Appl Physiol Nutr Metab.* 2007;32:1239.
- Kain ZN, Mayes LC, Ferris CA, Pakes J, Schottenfeld R. Cocaine-abusing parturients undergoing cesarean section: a cohort study. *Anesthesiology.* 1996;85:1028.
- Kwon H, Belanger K, Bracken B. Effect of pregnancy and stage of pregnancy on asthma severity: a systematic review. *Am J Obstet Gynecol.* 2004;190:1201.
- Landon MB, Spong CY, Thom E, et al. A multicenter, randomized trial of treatment for mild gestational diabetes. *N Engl J Med.* 2009;361:1339.
- Macones GA, Hankins GDV, Spong CY, Hauth J, Moore T. The 2008 National Institute of Child Health and Human Development Workshop Report on Electronic Fetal Monitoring: Update on Definitions, Interpretation, and Research Guidelines. *J Obstet Gynecol Neonatal Nurs.* 2008;37:510.
- Macones GA, Parry S, Elsousy M, et al. A polymorphism in the promoter region of TNF and bacterial vaginosis: preliminary evidence of gene-environment interaction in the etiology of spontaneous preterm birth. *Am J Obstet Gynecol.* 2004;190:1504.
- Negro R, Schwartz A, Gismondi R, Tinelli A, Mangieri T, Stagnaro-Green A. Universal screening versus case finding for detection and treatment of thyroid hormonal dysfunction during pregnancy. *J Clin Endocrinol Metab.* 2010;95:1699.
- Oatridge A, Holdcroft A, Saeed N, et al. Change in brain size during and after pregnancy: study in healthy women and women with preeclampsia. *AJNR Am J Neuroradiol.* 2002;23:19.
- Pilkington S, Carli F, Dakin MJ, et al. Increase in Mallampati score during pregnancy. *Br J Anaesth.* 1995;74:638.
- Silver RM, Landon MB, Rouse DJ, et al. Maternal morbidity associated with multiple repeat cesarean deliveries. *Obstet Gynecol.* 2006;107:1226.
- Siu SC, Sermer M, Colam JM, et al. Prospective multicenter study of pregnancy outcomes in women with heart disease. *Circulation.* 2001;104:515.
- Strathearn L, Mayes LC. Cocaine addiction in mothers: potential effects on maternal care and infant development. *Ann NY Acad Sci.* 2010;1187:172.
- Wang SM, Dexinno P, Maranets I, et al. Low back pain during pregnancy: prevalence, risk factors, and outcomes. *Obstet Gynecol.* 2004;104:65.
- Whittaker PG, Macphail S, Lind T. Serial hematologic changes and pregnancy outcome. *Obstet Gynecol.* 1996;88:33.

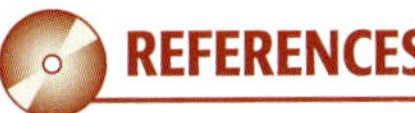

REFERENCES

Complete references available on DVD and online version at www.LongneckerAnesthesiology.com

CHAPTER 23 Evaluation of the Obese Patient

Babatunde O. Ogunnaike
Charles W. Whitten

KEY POINTS

1. Expiratory reserve volume (ERV) is the most sensitive indicator of the effect of obesity on pulmonary function testing.
2. Plasminogen activator inhibitor-1 (PAI-1), secreted by the endothelium, vascular smooth muscle cells, hepatocytes, and adipocytes, is associated with visceral obesity and inhibits the fibrinolytic system. PAI-1 decreases fibrinolysis and increases the risk of coronary artery disease.
3. Gastric emptying may be delayed in obese patients because of increased abdominal mass causing antral distension, gastrin release, and a decrease in pH with parietal cell hypersecretion. However, emptying has been documented to be faster, with high energy content intake such as fat emulsions, but residual volume (RV) is increased because of their larger gastric volume (up to 75% larger). They should follow the same fasting guidelines as nonobese patients.
4. Rhabdomyolysis has been documented in morbidly obese patients undergoing prolonged procedures. Elevations in serum creatinine and creatine phosphokinase (CPK) levels unexplained by other reasons and complaints

of buttock, hip, or shoulder pain in the postoperative period should raise the suspicion of rhabdomyolysis.

5. Difficult laryngoscopy and intubation correlates well with increased age, male sex, temporomandibular joint (TMJ) pathology, Mallampati classes 3 and 4, history of obstructive sleep apnea (OSA), and abnormal upper teeth, not the magnitude of body mass index (BMI).
6. Neck circumference has been identified as the single biggest predictor of problematic intubation in morbidly obese patients.
7. Preoxygenation in the head-up or sitting position is more effective and provides the longest safe apnea period (SAP) during induction of anesthesia in obese patients.
8. The head-elevated laryngoscopy position (HELP) position significantly elevates the obese patient's head, neck, upper body, and shoulders above the chest to a point where an imaginary horizontal line can be drawn from the sternal notch to the external ear to better improve laryngoscopy and intubation.
9. Positive end-expiratory pressure (PEEP) is the only ventilatory parameter that has consistently been shown to improve respiratory function in obese subjects, but it decreases venous return, cardiac output, and subsequent oxygen delivery.
10. Postoperative continuous positive airway pressure (CPAP) does not increase the incidence of major anastomotic leakage after gastric bypass surgery despite the theoretical risk of anastomotic injury from pressurized air delivered by CPAP.

The worldwide epidemic status of obesity is a key factor in the increased incidence of type 2 diabetes mellitus and cardiovascular diseases such as high blood pressure, and stroke.[1] Obesity is defined as an abnormally high percentage of body weight as fat. Overweight is an increase in weight relative to a standard. Approximately 65%, or 2 of every 3 adults, in the United States are overweight or obese.[2]

Approximately 85% of the economic burden of obesity can be accounted for by obesity-related diseases (coronary artery disease, stroke, type 2 diabetes mellitus, hypertension, hyperlipidemia) and prescription drugs.[3] The anatomic distribution of body fat is associated with varying pathophysiologic consequences. Android (central) obesity is commonly seen in men and associated with increased oxygen consumption and increased incidence of cardiovascular disease with a truncal or upper body distribution of the adipose tissue. Visceral fat is particularly associated with cardiovascular disease and ventricular dysfunction. Alcohol encourages deposition of central (android pattern) body fat. Gynecoid (peripheral) obesity, typically seen in women, locates adipose tissue predominantly in the hips, buttocks, and thighs and is less closely associated with cardiovascular disease because it is less metabolically active. Waist circumference (WC), waist-to-stature ratio (WSR), and waist-to-hip ratio (WHR) are body circumference (anthropometric) indices that identify patterns of obesity and correlate strongly with mortality and the development of obesity-related diseases. WC generally represents abdominal fat and is an independent predictor of disease. A WHR greater than 0.9 in women and greater than 1.0 in men is associated with a higher risk of morbidity and mortality than is a more peripheral pattern of body fat distribution (WHR <0.75 in women and <0.85 in men). A WC greater than 102 cm (40 in) in men and 88 cm (35 in) in women increases the risk of obesity-related diseases, including cardiovascular diseases, diabetes mellitus, and dyslipidemia (**Table 23-1**). WSR is the best simple anthropometric index in predicting a wide range of cardiovascular risk factors and related health conditions. It is recommended that a person's WC not exceed half the stature to minimize the incidence of these diseases.[4]

Ideal body weight (IBW) is the weight associated with the lowest mortality rate for a given height and gender. It is estimated using the Broca's index: IBW (kg) = height (cm) – x; where x is 100 for adult males and 105 for adult females. BMI is more appropriate for clinical use. It estimates the degree of obesity using this equation:

TABLE 23-1 Disease Risk According to Waist Circumference

BMI (kg/m²)	Risk/Waist Circumference	
	Male: <102 cm Female: <88 cm	Male: ≥102 cm Female: ≥88 cm
18.5-24.9	Average	Average
25.0-29.9	Increased	High
30.0-34.9	High	Very high
35.0-39.9	Very high	Very high
>40	Extremely high	Extremely high

BMI, body mass index.

$$\text{BMI} = \text{weight (kg) divided by height (m)} \times \text{height (m)}$$

or

$$\text{BMI} = \text{weight (lb) divided by height (in)} \times \text{height (in)} \times 703$$

A BMI of 18.5 to 24.9 is within normal weight range; 25.0 to 29.9 is overweight, and BMIs more than 30 and more than 40 kg/m^2 are considered obesity and extreme obesity, respectively (**Table 23-2**). BMI reliably measures body fat, but it cannot distinguish overweight from overfat because heavily muscled people can be easily classified as overweight using BMI.

Lean body weight (LBW) is the total body weight (TBW) minus the adipose tissue. It is a combination of body cell mass, extracellular water, and nonfat connective tissue. It approximates 80% of TBW in males and 75% in females. In morbidly obese subjects, decreasing the TBW by 20% to 30% gives an estimate of LBW. In nonobese and not overtly muscular individuals, TBW approximates IBW.[5,6]

A simple reversal of the BMI equation can be used to estimate IBW by relating "normal" BMI average of 22 (normal = 18.5-24.9) to a known height so that when the equation is rearranged, it reads: IBW = 22 × height^2. This equation yields weights that fall midway within the range of values obtained with other IBW formulas.[7]

PATHOPHYSIOLOGY OF OBESITY (TABLE 23-3)

RESPIRATORY SYSTEM

Morbidly obese patients have an increased work of breathing due to reduced chest wall compliance associated with the accumulation of fat on the chest wall, diaphragm, and abdomen. There is some contribution from obesity-related respiratory muscle dysfunction. Decreases in functional residual capacity (FRC) and ERV are the most commonly reported abnormalities of pulmonary function in obese subjects.[8] Decreased respiratory compliance leads to decreased FRC, vital capacity (VC), and TLC. These parameters are significantly lower in individuals with upper body fat distribution (central obesity). The reduction in FRC is due to

TABLE 23-2 Classification of Obesity

BMI (kg/m²)	Description	Obesity Class
<18.5	Underweight	
18.5-24.9	Normal	
25.0-29.9	Overweight	
30.0-34.9	Obesity	I
35.0-39.9	Obesity	II
>40	Extreme obesity	III

BMI, body mass index.

TABLE 23-3 Medical Consequences of Obesity

System	Pathology
Respiratory	Obstructive sleep apnea, obesity-hypoventilation syndrome, asthma, pulmonary hypertension
Cardiovascular	Arrhythmias, atherosclerosis, cardiac failure, coronary artery disease, peripheral vascular disease, sudden cardiac death, systemic hypertension, thromboembolism, varicose veins
Gastrointestinal	Colon cancer, gallbladder disease, gastroesophageal reflux disease, hernias, nonalcoholic fatty liver disease, nonalcoholic steatohepatitis
Endocrine/metabolic	Diabetes mellitus, dyslipidemia, hyperinsulinemia, hypothyroidism, insulin resistance, metabolic syndrome
Genitourinary	End-stage renal disease, macrosomia, menorrhagia, preeclampsia and eclampsia, prostate cancer, urinary incontinence
Neurological	Carpal tunnel syndrome, pseudotumor cerebri, stroke
Hematology	Hypercoagulability, polycythemia
Musculoskeletal	Acanthosis nigricans, gout, osteoarthritis, rheumatoid arthritis
Psychology/Psychiatry	Depression, reduced self-esteem, social stigma

decreased ERV. Reduction in ERV is due to encroachment of abdominal contents on the diaphragm, decrease in respiratory system compliance by chest wall fat, and impairment of respiratory muscle strength. ERV is the most sensitive indicator of the effect of obesity on pulmonary function testing. Each kilogram of weight gained results in approximately a 26 mL reduction in VC.[9] RV remains normal. Decreased FRC can result in lung volumes below closing capacity during normal tidal ventilation leading to small airway closure, V/Q mismatch, right-to-left shunting, and hypoxemia (**Fig. 23-1**). Anesthesia worsens the situation such that up to a 50% reduction in FRC occurs in the obese anesthetized patient compared with 20% in the nonobese. Reduction in FRC impairs the ability of the obese patient to tolerate even minimal periods of apnea; hence the rapid desaturation after induction of anesthesia despite adequate preoxygenation.

Obesity increases total oxygen consumption and carbon dioxide production even at rest. This is due to the metabolic activity of excess body fat and increased workload on supportive tissues. Basal metabolic activity in relation to body surface area is usually within normal limits, and an increase in minute ventilation usually maintains normocapnia. The increase in minute ventilation requires an increase in oxygen consumption because most obese patients retain their normal response to hypoxemia and hypercapnia. Morbidly obese patients do extra work to maintain their augmented ventilation; therefore they have to dedicate a high percentage of their total oxygen utilization to perform respiratory work even during regular respiration.[10] Dynamic lung volumes, including the forced expiratory volume in 1 second (FEV_1) and the forced vital capacity (FVC) both, decline with increasing body mass, resulting in an unchanged ratio of FEV_1 to FVC. Significant hypoxemia is attributed in part to the closure of dependent airways within the range of normal tidal ventilation. Substantial weight loss results in gas exchange improvement as evidenced by an increase in Pao_2. Morbid obesity is associated with a reduction in forced expiratory flow during midexpiratory phase and maximum voluntary ventilation (MVV) while the diffusing capacity remains normal.[11] MVV, an index of respiratory muscle strength, is decreased in extreme obesity. Respiratory muscle efficiency is suboptimal in obese patients. Inefficiency is suggested by a sharper increase in oxygen consumption during exercise when compared with nonobese patients. Supine position reduces FRC due to cephalad displacement of the diaphragm. This effect is exaggerated in the obese, leading to a further reduction in FRC, further small airway closure, and increased work of breathing. Clinically significant increases in intrapulmonary shunting and oxygen consumption have been documented in obese patients while changing from a sitting to a supine position. Chest wall and lung compliance are both decreased by fat accumulation on the thorax and abdomen. Increased pulmonary blood volume, which is part of an overall increase in total blood volume, partially explains the decreased lung compliance. Chronic hypoxemia causes polycythemia, which contributes to the increased blood volume. Morbidly obese patients breathing room air have lower arterial oxygen tensions (Pao_2) than that predicted for similar-age nonobese subjects in both sitting and supine positions. Chronic hypoxemia can eventually lead to pulmonary hypertension and cor pulmonale.

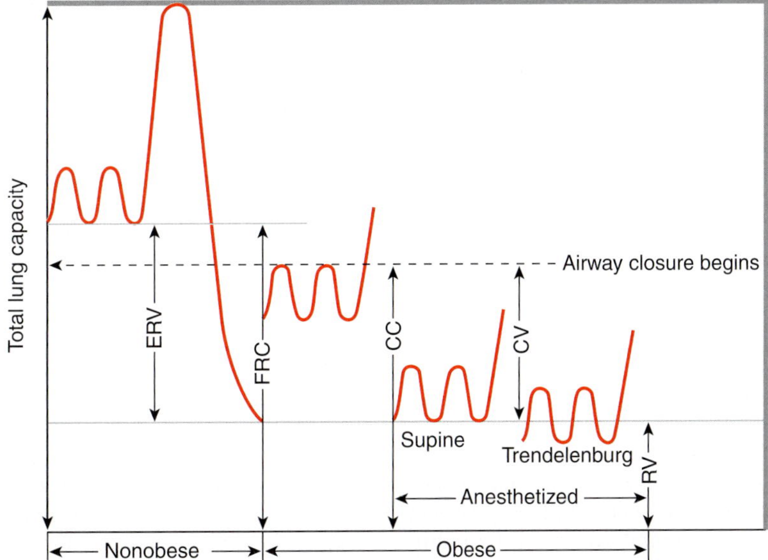

FIGURE 23-1. Effects of obesity, positioning, and anesthesia on lung volumes. CC, closing capacity; CV, closing volume; FRC, functional residual capacity; RV, residual volume. [Reprinted with permission from Ogunnaike BO, Whitten CW. Anesthesia and obesity. In: Barash PG, Cullen BF, Stoelting RK, et al., eds. *Clinical Anesthesia*. 6th ed. Philadelphia, PA: Lippincott, Williams, & Wilkins, 2009:1232].

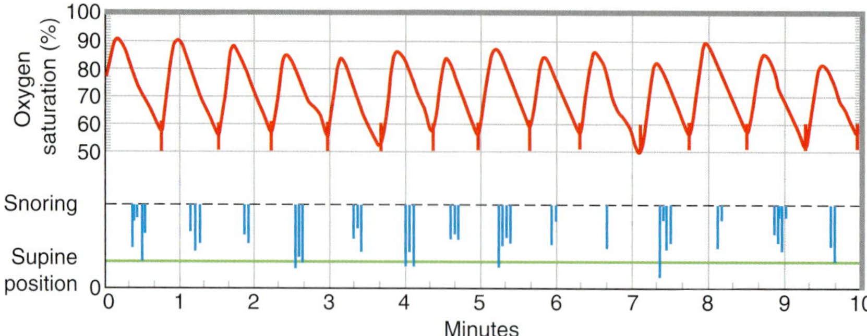

FIGURE 23-2. Pattern of oxygen saturation in a patient with severe sleep apnea. The vertical lines below the oxygen saturation values indicate respiratory disturbances. Episodes of snoring are shown. Patient is in supine position. [Reprinted with permission from Flemons WW. Obstructive sleep apnea. *N Engl J Med.* 2002;347:498.]

OBSTRUCTIVE SLEEP APNEA

Obstructive sleep apnea (OSA) is defined as a cessation of airflow for more than 10 seconds 5 or more times per hour of sleep despite continuous respiratory effort against a closed glottis in combination with a decrease in arterial oxygen saturation of greater than 4% (**Fig. 23-2**). Obstructive sleep hypopnea is a decrease in airflow of more than 50% for more than 10 seconds, 15 or more times per hour of sleep; it is usually associated with snoring and arterial oxygen desaturation greater than 4%. The upper airway resistance syndrome is characterized by arousal in response to increased upper airway resistance without an elevated apnea-hypopnea index (AHI). AHI is the total number of apneas and hypopneas per hour and used to quantify the severity of OSA.[12] The AHI is the total number of apneas and hypopneas per hour. An AHI index higher than 30 signifies severe OSA; values of 5 to 15 and 16 to 30 define mild and moderate OSA, respectively. The total arousal index (AI) is the total number of arousals per hour. The sum of the AHI and total AI is known as the respiratory disturbance index.[13]

Predisposing factors to OSA include male gender, middle age, and obesity. Alcohol consumption or night sedation worsens the situation. BMI higher than 30 kg/m^2 and collar size more than 16.5 in correlate with severe OSA. Resulting physiologic abnormalities include hypoxemia, hypercapnia, and generalized (pulmonary and systemic) vasoconstriction. Secondary polycythemia due to recurrent hypoxemia increases the risk of cerebrovascular and ischemic heart disease. Right ventricular failure is a potential consequence of chronic hypoxic pulmonary vasoconstriction. Electrocardiogram (ECG) pattern of right ventricular hypertrophy or echocardiographic evidence of hypofunction may be seen. Initially, respiratory acidosis occurs only during sleep with return to normal homeostasis when awake. Hypoxemia during apnea can lead to bradycardia, long sinus pauses, second-degree heart block, and ventricular dysrhythmias with markedly increased severity if arterial oxygenation decreases below 60%. The higher incidence of nocturnal angina and myocardial infarction in OSA patients may be explained by the increased incidence of arrhythmias in these patients. Activation of the sympathetic nervous system occurs in response to hypoxemia due to apneic and hypopneic events, which may explain the increased incidence of hypertension in obese OSA patients. As obesity worsens, pharyngeal area decreases due to adipose tissue deposition into pharyngeal tissues including the uvula, tonsils, tonsillar pillars, tongue, aryepiglottic folds, and the lateral pharyngeal walls where it is most pronounced, correlating well with the severity of OSA (**Fig. 23-3**). Weight loss improves the pharyngeal and glottic function of patients with OSA.[14] The upper airway can be compressed externally by superficially located fat masses that increase the pharyngeal extraluminal pressure. This situation is evidenced by a significantly larger neck in the obese patient with OSA when compared to those without OSA and the fact that the severity of OSA correlates better with larger neck circumference than with general obesity.

Central depressant anesthetic drugs (benzodiazepines, opioids, and induction agents such as thiopental and propofol) reduce the action of pharyngeal dilator muscles in obese OSA patients causing pharyngeal collapse. Precurarizing doses of muscle relaxants and nitrous oxide also reduce their action. Addition of opioids will depress ventilation and result in poor response to the ensuing hypoxemia and hypercapnia. OSA is associated with difficult mask ventilation and difficult laryngoscopy, which when combined with decreased FRC and reduced oxygen stores requires anticipation and preparation for an airway emergency.

A significant number of patients with OSA are undiagnosed, which poses various perioperative challenges for the anesthesiologist. The STOP questionnaire, the initial portion of the STOP-BANG scoring model (**Table 23-4**), is a concise and easy-to-use screening tool for OSA. Incorporating BMI, age, neck size, and gender with the STOP questionnaire (STOP-BANG scoring model) significantly increases screening sensitivity especially for patients with moderate to severe OSA.[15]

OBESITY-HYPOVENTILATION SYNDROME

Obesity-hypoventilation syndrome (OHS) is a combination of obesity and chronic hypoventilation that ultimately results in pulmonary hypertension and cor pulmonale.[14] It can also be defined as a combination of obesity (BMI >30 kg/m^2) and awake arterial hypoxemia ($Paco_2$ >45 mm Hg) in the absence of known causes of hypoventilation. OHS is seen in up to 10% of morbidly obese patients. Clinical features are similar to those seen with OSA including excessive daytime somnolence, fatigue, and morning headaches. In addition, there is daytime hypercapnia and hypoxemia that are associated with pulmonary hypertension and right-sided congestive heart failure (cor pulmonale), resulting in substantial morbidity and mortality.[16]

OHS patients have an increased sensitivity to the respiratory depressant effects of general anesthetics. Episodes of central apnea from progressive desensitization of respiratory centers to hypercapnia are initially limited to sleep but eventually leads to a progressive reliance on hypoxic drive for ventilation. Pickwickian syndrome,[17] characterized by obesity, hypersomnolence, hypoxia, hypercapnia, right ventricular failure, and polycythemia, is the end result of OHS. Chronic daytime hypoxemia may be a better predictor of pulmonary hypertension and cor pulmonale than the presence and severity of OSA.[18] There is a strong correlation between increasing BMI (>40 kg/m^2) and the likelihood of developing OHS.[19] Many obese patients with OHS also have OSA, but the reverse is not always true, suggesting that OHS is an autonomous disease.[20]

Arterial blood gas (ABG) analysis should be obtained in any morbidly obese patient with unexplained hypoxemia or features of cor pulmonale because pulse oximetry detects oxyhemoglobin desaturation without consideration for the presence of hypercapnia. This results in inappropriate treatment with supplemental oxygen alone that does not reverse the hypoventilation.[15] ABG confirms the presence of daytime hypercapnia and usually reveals compensated respiratory acidosis and hypoxemia. Elevated bicarbonate level is consistent with chronic hypercapnia.

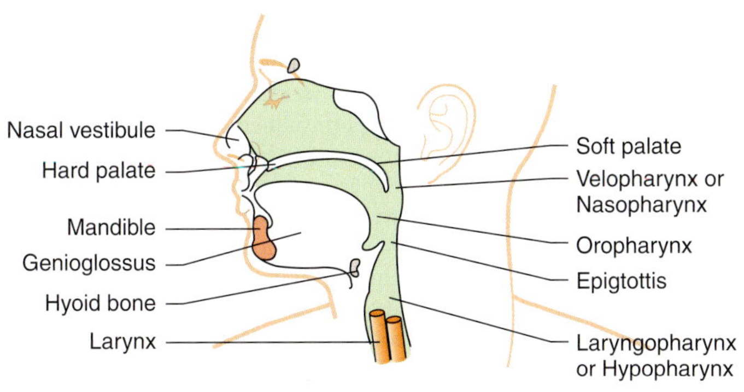

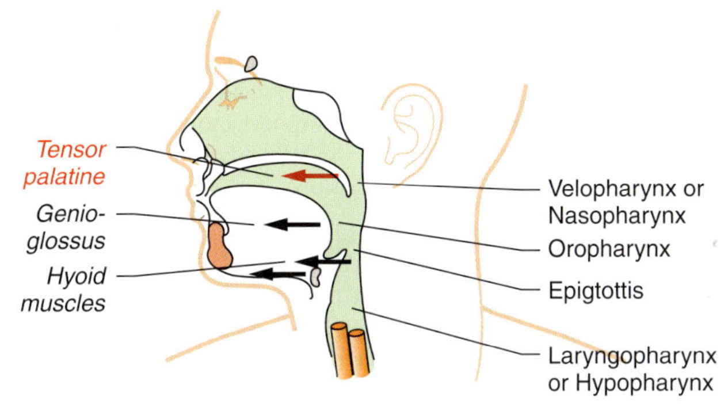

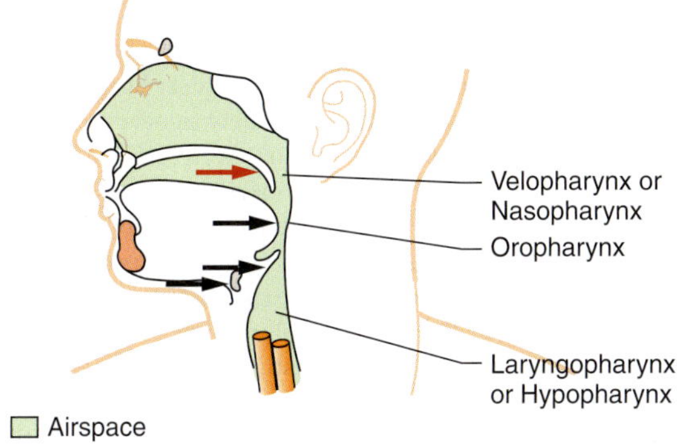

FIGURE 23-3. Airway obstruction during sleep apnea. [Reprinted with permission from Benumof JL. Obstructive sleep apnea in the adult obese patient: implications for airway management. *J Clin Anesth*. 2001;13:144.]

Treatment of OHS with weight reduction, tracheostomy, or nocturnal positive-pressure support improves daytime hypercapnia and hypoxia without changing the abnormal ventilatory responses.

CARDIOVASCULAR SYSTEM

The increased morbidity and mortality of obesity is largely due to cardiovascular problems, including hypertension, ischemic heart disease, cardiac failure, cardiomyopathy, arrhythmias, dyslipidemia, and sudden cardiac death.[21] Total blood volume is increased in the obese, but it is less than that in nonobese individuals when compared on a volume-to-weight basis (50 mL/kg compared with 70 mL/kg). Most of the extra blood volume supplies adipose tissue. Excess adiposity requires an increase in cardiac output to parallel the increase in oxygen consumption,

TABLE 23-4 STOP-BANG Scoring Mode

		Question	Yes	No
1.	**S**noring	Do you **s**nore loudly (louder than talking or loud enough to be heard through closed doors)?		
2.	**T**ired	Do you often feel **t**ired, fatigued, or sleepy during the daytime?		
3.	**O**bserved	Has anyone **o**bserved you stop breathing during sleep?		
4.	Blood **P**ressure	Do you have or are you being treated for high blood **p**ressure?		
5.	**B**MI	**B**MI more than 35 kg/m^2?		
6.	**A**ge	**A**ge >50 y?		
7.	**N**eck Circumference	**N**eck circumference >40 cm?		
8.	**G**ender	**G**ender male?		

Questions 1-4 represent the STOP questionnaire
High risk of OSA: answering yes to 2 or more questions
Low risk of OSA: answering yes to fewer than 2 questions
Questions 1-8 together make up the STOP-BANG Scoring Model
High risk of OSA: answering yes to 3 or more items
Low risk of OSA: answering yes to fewer than 3 three items

Adapted and modified from Chung F, Yegneswaran B, Liao P, et al. STOP questionnaire: a tool to screen patients for obstructive sleep apnea. *Anesthesiology*. 2008;108: 812.

leading to a systemic arteriovenous oxygen difference that remains normal or slightly above normal. Cardiac output increases with increasing weight (20-30 mL/kg of excess adipose tissue) because of ventricular dilatation and an increase in stroke volume. Left ventricular dilatation results in increased left ventricular wall stress leading to eccentric hypertrophy that leads to reduced left ventricular compliance, impairment of left ventricular filling (diastolic dysfunction) elevation of left ventricular end diastolic pressure (LVEDP), and eventual pulmonary edema. The dilated left ventricle has a limited capacity to hypertrophy, so when left ventricular wall thickening fails to keep pace with dilatation, systolic dysfunction ("obesity cardiomyopathy") results with eventual biventricular failure (**Fig. 23-4**). Obese subjects compensate by using cardiac reserve, especially in the presence of hypertension. Systemic vascular resistance (SVR) is usually within normal limits in morbidly obese patients, suggesting that hypertension and obesity can coexist with a normal SVR.

Obesity accelerates atherosclerosis; however, because of reduced mobility, morbidly obese patients appear asymptomatic in the face of significant cardiovascular disease; symptoms such as angina or exertional dyspnea only occur during periods of significant physical activity.[22] Cardiac output rises faster in response to exercise in the morbidly obese and is often associated with a rise in left ventricular end-diastolic pressure and pulmonary capillary wedge pressure. Increase in cardiac output during exercise is achieved by increases in heart rate without a concomitant increase in stroke volume or ejection fraction but with an increase in filling pressures. Similar changes occur during the perioperative period. With the exception of renal and splanchnic blood flows that increase with obesity, organ blood flow does not change significantly because the additional cardiac output is diverted to perfuse excess fat. Blood volume and cardiac output are approximately twice the values predicted for those with ideal body weight, but when it is normalized for body surface area, it is within normal limits or slightly below normal. Chronically increased cardiac output and blood volume may cause the SVR to increase over time. A high SVR and high preload combination may lead to an early left ventricular dysfunction and congestive heart failure.

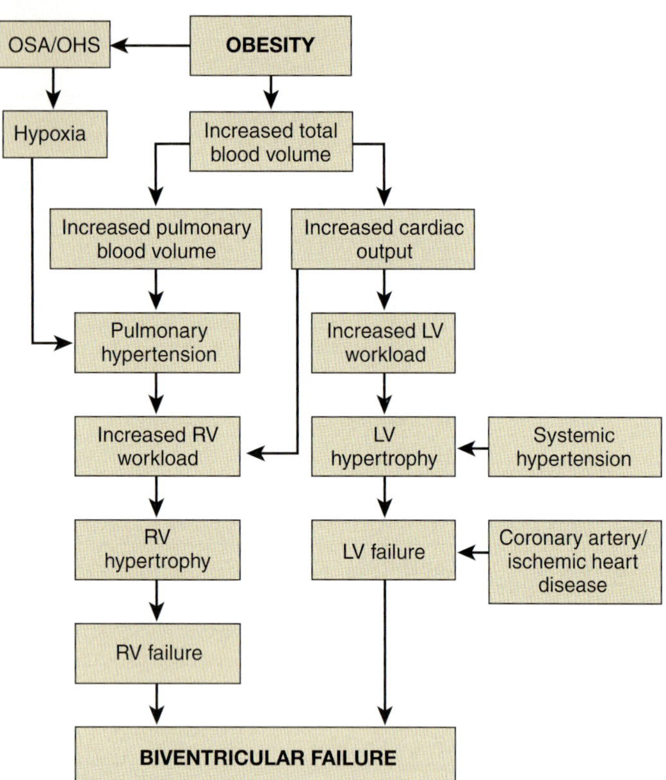

FIGURE 23-4. Interrelationship of cardiovascular and pulmonary sequelae of obesity. LV, left ventricle; OHS, obesity hypoventilation syndrome; OSA, obstructive sleep apnea; RV, right ventricle. [Reprinted with permission from Ogunnaike BO, Whitten CW. Anesthesia and obesity. In: Barash PG, Cullen BF, Stoelting RK, et al, eds. *Clinical Anesthesia.* 6th ed. Philadelphia, PA: Lippincott, Williams, & Wilkins; 2009:1234.]

Obesity is an independent risk factor for ischemic heart disease and eventual heart failure and is strongly associated with central (android) distribution of fat. Angina may actually be a direct symptom of obesity because a significant number of obese patients with angina do not have demonstrable coronary artery disease.[23] The risk of heart failure increases by 5% for men and 7% for women for every increment of 1 kg/m^2 in BMI.[24] Coronary blood flow reserve in obese patients is limited because of ventricular mass and metabolic demands of the myocardium. Intraoperative cardiac failure can occur from rapid intravenous fluid administration (indicating left ventricular diastolic dysfunction), negative inotropy of anesthetic agents, or pulmonary hypertension precipitated by hypoxia or hypercapnia.

Cardiac arrhythmias can be precipitated by fatty infiltration of the conduction system, hypoxia, hypercapnia, electrolyte imbalance, coronary artery disease, increased circulating catecholamines, OSA, and myocardial hypertrophy. ECG findings frequently seen in morbidly obese patients include low QRS voltage, multiple criteria for left ventricular hypertrophy (LVH) and left atrial enlargement, and T-wave flattening in the inferior and lateral leads.[25] In addition, there is a leftward shift of the P-wave, QRS complex, and T-wave axes, lengthening of the corrected QT interval, and prolonged QT interval duration. Echocardiography usually shows an increased cardiac output, increased LVEDP, and LVH in otherwise healthy obese subjects.

Mild to moderate hypertension is common in obese patients. There is a 3 to 4 mm Hg increase in systolic and a 2 mm Hg increase in diastolic arterial pressure for every 10 kg of weight gained. SVR is usually within normal limits, suggesting that hypertension and obesity can coexist with a normal SVR. Their expanded blood volume causes an increased cardiac output with a lower calculated SVR for the same level of arterial blood pressure. The renin-angiotensin system has been implicated in the hypertension of obesity. Increases in circulating levels of angiotensinogen, aldosterone, and angiotensin-converting enzyme occur. With obesity, most tissues have normal to increased level of sympathetic nervous system activity. An increased basal level of sympathetic activity predisposes to insulin resistance, dyslipidemia, and hypertension.[26] Obesity-induced insulin resistance enhances the pressor activity of norepinephrine and angiotensin II.[27] Hyperinsulinemia further activates the sympathetic nervous system causing sodium retention and contributing to the hypertension of obesity.[28] Hypertension causes concentric hypertrophy of the ventricle in normal weight individuals but causes eccentric dilatation in obese subjects.[29] The combination of obesity and hypertension causes left ventricular wall thickening and a larger heart volume and therefore increased likelihood of cardiac failure (**Fig. 23-5**).

A hypofibrinolytic and hypercoagulable state predisposes the obese patient to cardiovascular disease. Obese patients have higher levels of fibrinogen (a marker for the inflammatory process of atherosclerosis) factor VII, factor VIII, von Willebrand factor, and PAI-1 produced by adipose tissue.[30] Increased fibrinogen, factor VII, factor VIII, and hypofibrinolysis due to increased PAI-1 levels are associated with hypercoagulability and an increased risk of coronary artery disease. High factor VIII coagulant activity levels are associated with increased cardiovascular mortality. Visceral (abdominal) fat is associated with increased levels of PAI-1, factor VIII, and von Willebrand factor. Endothelial dysfunction induced by insulin increases von Willebrand factor and factor VIII levels, predisposing to fibrin formation.

GASTROINTESTINAL/HEPATIC SYSTEM

Gastric volume and acidity are increased, hepatic function altered, and drug metabolism adversely affected by obesity. A significant number of fasted morbidly obese patients have gastric volumes in excess of 25 mL and gastric pH less than 2.5, which are the generally accepted volume and pH indicative of high risk for pneumonitis in the event of regurgitation and aspiration. Gastric emptying can be delayed in obese patients because of increased abdominal mass that causes antral distension, gastrin release, and a decrease in pH with parietal cell hypersecretion. However, emptying may be faster, with high-energy content intake such as fat emulsions, but RV is increased because of their larger gastric volume (up to 75% larger). Accelerated gastric emptying induces hunger and frequent eating by reducing the negative feedback satiety signal produced by the presence of nutrients inside the stomach, thus precipitating a feeling of hunger and shortening the interval between consecutive meals.[31]

An increased incidence of hiatal hernia and gastroesophageal reflux (GERD) increases aspiration risk. Fasting nonpremedicated, nondiabetic obese surgical patients who have no significant gastroesophageal pathology are not more likely to have high-volume, low pH gastric contents than lean patients at the time of general anesthetic induction after routine preoperative fasting.[32] They should follow the same guidelines as nonobese patients and be allowed to drink clear liquids (up to 300 mL) until 2 hours before elective surgery, a quantity that has been shown not to affect gastric pH and volume at induction of anesthesia adversely.[33] One mechanism of increased risk of GERD is via mechanical factors whereby abdominal obesity increases intragastric pressure, increasing the frequency of transient lower esophageal sphincter relaxation and/or formation of hiatal hernia. A greater than 3.5 kg/m^2 increase in BMI is associated with a 2.7-fold increase in risk for developing new reflux symptoms.[34] The combination of hiatus hernia, GERD, and delayed gastric emptying, coupled with increased intra-abdominal pressure and a high volume-low pH gastric content, increases the incidence of severe pneumonitis should aspiration occur.

Peculiar morphologic and biochemical abnormalities of the liver associated with obesity include fatty infiltration, inflammation, focal necrosis, and cirrhosis. Fatty infiltration reflects the duration rather than the degree of obesity. Histologic and liver function test abnormalities are relatively common in the obese, but clearance is usually not reduced. Abnormal liver function tests are seen in up to a third of obese patients who have no evidence of concomitant liver disease; increased alanine aminotransferase is most frequently seen. Despite these histologic and

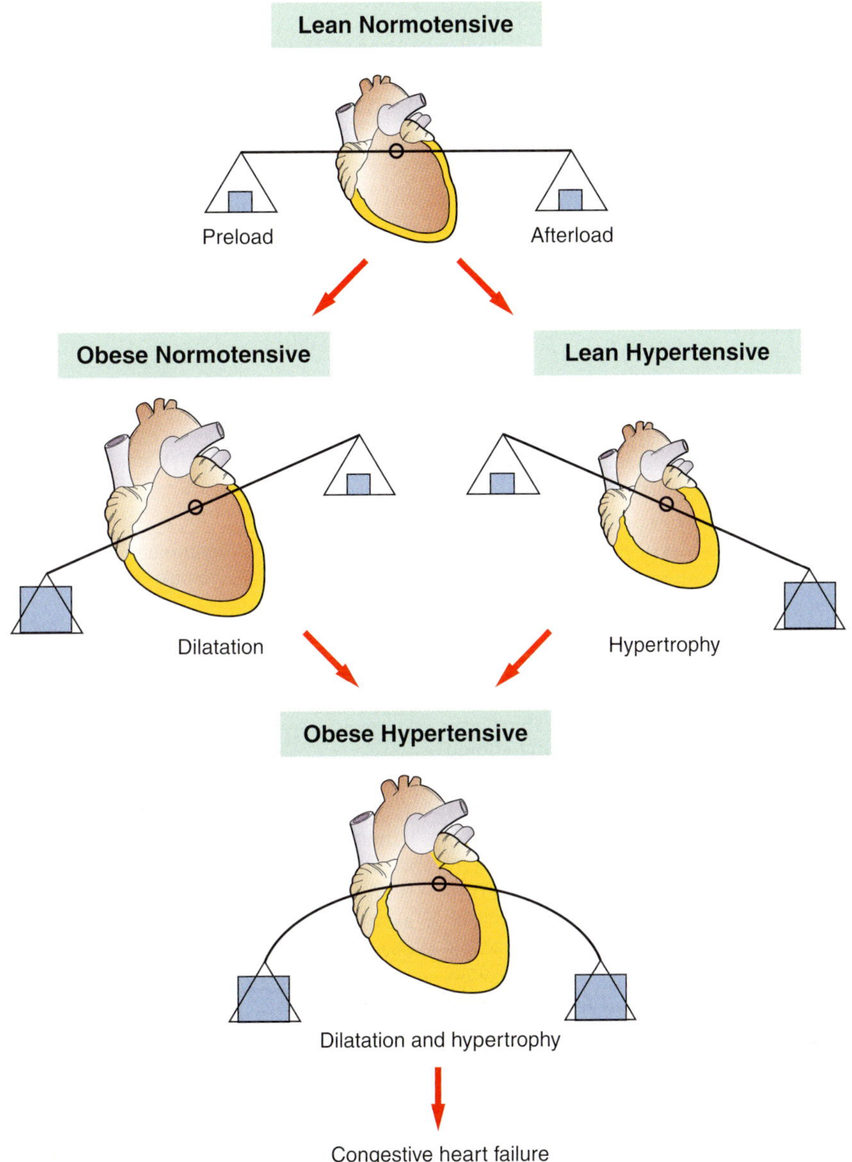

FIGURE 23-5. Adaptation of the heart to obesity and hypertension. [Reprinted with permission from Messerli FH. Cardiovascular effects of obesity and hypertension. *Lancet*. 1982;1:1165.]

enzymatic changes, no clear correlation exists between routine liver function tests and the capacity of the liver to metabolize drugs.[35] Hepatic decompensation can occur after Roux-en-Y gastric bypass (RYGB), which necessitates careful assessment for preexisting liver disease in candidates scheduled to undergo this procedure because of a high prevalence (63%) of nonalcoholic fatty liver disease (NAFLD) and cirrhosis.[36] NAFLD is a group of liver abnormalities associated with obesity and insulin resistance. Hepatomegaly, elevated liver enzymes, and abnormal liver histology (including steatosis, steatohepatitis, fibrosis, and cirrhosis) are an intrinsic part of this disease.[37] Up to 95% of morbidly obese patients have nonalcoholic steatohepatitis (NASH).[38] NASH is an aggressive form of NAFLD that can progress to cirrhosis or hepatocellular carcinoma. The incidence of gallbladder disease, including cholelithiasis, is significantly increased in morbidly obese subjects; the relative risk appears to be positively correlated with increasing BMI.[39] Abnormal cholesterol metabolism is partially to blame.

RENAL, ENDOCRINE, AND METABOLIC SYSTEMS

Impaired glucose tolerance in the morbidly obese is reflected by a high prevalence of type 2 diabetes mellitus due to the resistance of peripheral fatty tissues to insulin. A significant number of obese patients have an abnormal glucose tolerance test that predisposes them to wound infection and an increased risk of myocardial infarction.[40] Exogenous insulin may be required perioperatively, to oppose the catabolic response to the stress of surgery, even in obese patients on oral hypoglycemic agents. Gastric bypass surgery improves or even cures type 2 diabetes mellitus by substantially improving insulin resistance through an unknown mechanism.[41] Subclinical hypothyroidism occurs in about 25% of all morbidly obese patients.[42] Thyroid stimulating hormone levels are frequently elevated, suggesting the possibility that obesity leads to a state of thyroid hormone resistance in peripheral tissues.[43,44] Hypothyroidism should be considered in any obese patient who displays perioperative cardiovascular or respiratory instability. Hypoglycemia, hyponatremia, and impaired hepatic drug metabolism are other adverse consequences of hypothyroidism. Reduction in thyroxine requirements is seen with a decrease in BMI.[45]

Obesity is a major risk factor for end-stage renal disease and essential hypertension. It induces high blood pressure through increased renal tubular sodium reabsorption, impaired pressure natriuresis, and volume expansion due to the activation of the sympathetic nervous system and renin-angiotensin system, and by physical compression of the kidneys especially when visceral obesity is present. Chronic obesity results in increasing urinary protein excretion and gradual loss of nephron function that worsens with time and exacerbates hypertension. Obesity-related glomerular hyperfiltration decreases after weight loss, which decreases the incidence of overt glomerulopathy.[46] Obesity-related glomerulopathy is defined as focal segmental glomerulosclerosis and glomerulopathy or glomerulopathy alone.

THE METABOLIC SYNDROME

According to the International Diabetes Federation, diagnostic criteria for metabolic syndrome include central obesity (defined as WC >94 cm for men and >80 cm for women); plus any 2 of the following 4 factors: raised serum triglyceride, low serum high-density lipoprotein-cholesterol level, high blood pressure or treatment of previously diagnosed hypertension, and abnormal fasting plasma glucose or previously diagnosed type 2 diabetes mellitus.[47] It is a cluster of metabolic abnormalities including diabetes (or prediabetes), abdominal obesity, and changes in cholesterol and high blood pressure. People with this syndrome have up to a 5-fold greater risk of developing type 2 diabetes mellitus (if not already present) and are also twice as likely to die from and 3 times more likely to have a heart attack or stroke compared with people without the syndrome.

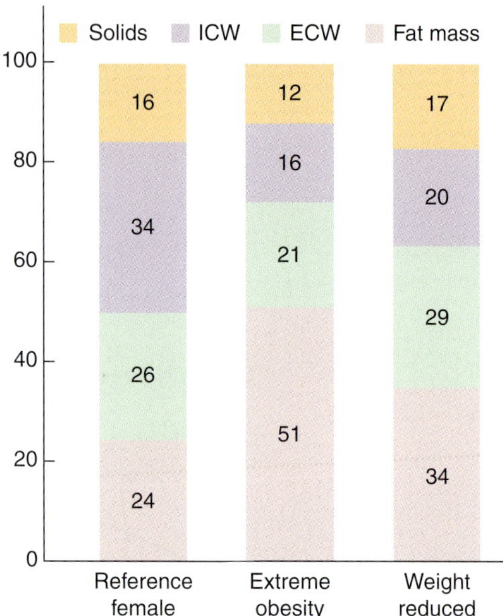

FIGURE 23-6. Body composition in extremely obese and weight-reduced states compared with reference female values. ECW, extracellular water; ICW, intracellular water. [Reprinted with permission from Das SK, Roberts SB, Kehayias JJ, et al. Body composition methods in extreme obesity. *Am J Physiol Endocrinol Metab*. 2003;284: E1080.]

PHARMACOLOGY

General pharmacokinetic principles dictate that drug dosing should take into consideration the volume of distribution (V_D) for administration of the loading dose and or the clearance for the maintenance dose.[48] A drug that is mainly distributed to lean tissues should have the loading dose calculated based on LBW, whereas dosing should be calculated based on TBW if the drug is equally distributed between adipose and lean tissues. For maintenance, a drug with similar clearance values in both obese and nonobese individuals should have the maintenance dose calculated based on LBW; a drug whose clearance increases with obesity should have the maintenance dose calculated according to TBW.

The volume of the central compartment in which drugs are first distributed remains unchanged in obese patients, but absolute body water content is decreased and lean body adipose tissue mass is increased, affecting lipophilic and polar drug distribution (**Fig. 23-6**). The V_D in obese patients is affected by reduced total body water, increased total body fat, increased LBM, altered protein binding, increased blood volume, increased cardiac output, increased serum concentrations of free fatty acids, triglycerides, cholesterol, and α_1-acid glycoprotein, lipophilicity of the drug, and organomegaly.[49] Lipophilic compounds are associated with increases in V_D with some exceptions such as digoxin, procainamide, and cyclosporine that are highly lipophilic substances but have comparable volumes of distribution in obese and nonobese subjects.[49]

The major plasma proteins are albumin (primarily responsible for binding acidic drugs), α_1-acid glycoprotein (primarily responsible for binding basic drugs) and lipoproteins. Plasma protein binding of acidic drugs may decrease because of the obesity-associated decrease in albumin levels and an increase in concentration of α_1-acid glycoprotein. Hyperlipidemia and an increased concentration of α_1-acid glycoprotein affect protein binding and lead to a reduction in free drug concentration. Drugs that are primarily bound to albumin (eg, thiopentone, phenytoin) show no significant changes in protein binding in obese individuals, whereas binding of drugs to α_1-acid glycoprotein increases. Lipoprotein levels may be elevated in obese individuals due to higher triglyceride and cholesterol levels. Histologic and liver function abnormalities are common in the obese with concomitant deranged liver function tests; metabolism and clearance, however, are usually not adversely affected. Drugs that depend on the kidneys for elimination face consistently higher clearance rate in obese patients.[50] Orally administered medications are expected to have decreased bioavailability in obese patients because of increased splanchnic blood flow, but there is no evidence to suggest a significant difference in the absorption and bioavailability of orally administered drugs when compared with nonobese subjects.

Increased blood volume in the obese patient decreases the plasma concentrations of rapidly injected intravenous drugs. Fat, however, has poor blood flow; therefore doses calculated on actual body weight could lead to excessive plasma concentrations. A reasonable approach is to calculate the initial doses based on LBW and subsequent doses determined by pharmacologic response to the initial dose. Repeated injections accumulate in fat leading to prolonged response due to subsequent release from this large fat depot.

SPECIFIC INTRAVENOUS AGENTS (TABLE 23-5)

THIOPENTAL

Thiopental is highly lipophilic and has a larger V_D in obese patients; prolonged somnolence is expected. Increased blood volume and cardiac output and increased muscle mass necessitate an increase in the initial induction dose. The volume of distribution is larger in obese than in nonobese patients; elimination half-life is significantly longer. They are more sensitive to the effects of thiopental dosed according to TBW.[51] Continuous infusion results in longer elimination half-life due to a larger V_D; clearance, however, remains unaltered.

PROPOFOL

Both the V_D and clearance of propofol in obese and nonobese subjects correlate well with TBW without signs of accumulation and prolongation of action because the half-life is similar in obese and nonobese subjects due to the increase in both V_D and clearance.[52] Induction and maintenance dosing for propofol in both obese and nonobese individuals may be based on TBW, but the negative cardiovascular effects of large doses of propofol combined with the negative physiologic effects of obesity on the cardiovascular system should prompt a somewhat reduced total dose.

TABLE 23-5 Intravenous Drug Dosing in Obesity

Drug	Dosing	Comments
Thiopental	LBW (somewhat increased)	Increased V_D, increased blood volume, cardiac output, and muscle mass. Increased absolute dose. Prolonged duration of action. Elimination half-life longer. Adjust loading/induction dose accordingly.
Propofol	Induction: LBW suggested (somewhat increased) Maintenance infusion: TBW	Highly lipophilic. Total clearance and V_D at steady state correlate well with TBW. Keep in mind negative cardiovascular effects that suggest induction dosing based on LBW may be better. High affinity for well-perfused organs. Titrate to effect.
Succinylcholine	TBW	Larger extracellular fluid compartment in obese. Pseudocholinesterase activity increases with increasing weight.
Rocuronium	LBW	Faster onset and longer duration when dosed according to TBW. Pharmacokinetics and pharmacodynamics not altered in obese subjects.
Vecuronium	LBW	Prolonged action when dosed according to TBW. Obesity does not alter distribution or elimination of the drug.
Atracurium	LBW	V_D, absolute clearance, and elimination half-life unchanged by obesity. Unchanged dose per unit body weight without prolongation of recovery because of organ-independent elimination.
Cis-atracurium	LBW	Pharmacokinetics similar to atracurium but prolonged duration of action when dosed according to TBW.
Fentanyl	Derived "pharmacokinetic (PK) mass"	Measured total body clearance has a nonlinear relationship to TBW. Fentanyl dosing based on a derived "pharmacokinetic mass" correlates better with clearance. Dosing based on TBW overestimates dose requirements in the obese.
Sufentanil	LBW	Increased V_D and prolonged elimination half-life that correlates with degree of obesity. Clearance similar in obese and nonobese. Overestimation of plasma concentration occurs in the morbidly obese range (BMI >40 kg/m^2).
Remifentanil	LBW	Pharmacokinetics similar in obese and nonobese subjects. Systemic clearance and V_D corrected per kg of TBW is significantly smaller in the obese. Consider age and lean body mass for dosing.
Dexmedetomidine	TBW	Lacks significant effect on respiration. Ideally suitable as an analgesic adjuvant in morbidly obese subjects.

LBW, lean body weight; TBW, total body weight; VD, volume of distribution.

MIDAZOLAM

There is a significant increase in both V_D and elimination half-life in obese patients. Midazolam is relatively shorter acting compared with other benzodiazepines; therefore the intensity and duration of its sedative side effects after a single intravenous dose correlate better with the extent of distribution of the drug than on the rate of elimination and clearance.[53] The total V_D and elimination half-life of midazolam in the obese are up to 3 times larger and 3 times more prolonged than those in nonobese subjects with no difference in the clearance rates. A single intravenous dose of midazolam should be administered based on TBW, but continuous infusion dosing should be adjusted according to LBW rather than TBW. Even though midazolam is considered short acting, it has the potential to accumulate and cause prolonged sedation in obese patients because larger initial doses are required to achieve adequate serum concentrations.

NEUROMUSCULAR BLOCKING AGENTS

Muscle relaxants are polar and hydrophilic drugs that are distributed poorly into excess adipose tissue. Obese individuals have a larger absolute lean body mass in conjunction with extra adipose tissue and a decreased proportion of muscle mass and body water when compared with nonobese subjects.[35] Therefore drugs with weak or moderate lipophilicity have fairly predictable effects in obese patients due to their distribution mainly into lean tissues; they should therefore be dosed based on LBW rather than TBW.[54]

Succinylcholine Succinylcholine should be dosed based on TBW. Larger extracellular fluid compartment and a linear increase in pseudocholinesterase activity with weight gain necessitate an increase in dosage of succinylcholine in obese patients. The potency estimates for succinylcholine in obese adolescents with BMI more than 30 kg/m^2 are similar to those of nonobese adolescents in the same age group when calculated based on TBW.[55]

Nondepolarizing Muscle Relaxants Nondepolarizing muscle relaxants should be administered according to lean body mass to prevent delayed recovery due to increased V_D and impaired hepatic clearance. There is no alteration in the pharmacokinetics and pharmacodynamics of rocuronium in obese female patients when compared with normal weight patients. The duration of action of rocuronium in obese patients is significantly longer when dosed according to TBW; therefore, rocuronium should be dosed according to LBW.[56] Vecuronium pharmacokinetics and pharmacodynamics in obese patients is consistent with dosing on the basis of LBW because the V_D, plasma clearance, and elimination half-life of vecuronium are not different between obese and nonobese patients.[57] Vecuronium action is prolonged, however, when dosed according to TBW because of the excess dose administered. The V_D, absolute clearance, and elimination half-life of atracurium are unchanged by obesity. However, if dosed according to TBW, atracurium concentrations are higher in obese patients than in the nonobese with no increase in recovery times. The median effective dose is higher; therefore dosing can be based on TBW with some reduction in the total dose.[58] The duration of action of cisatracurium is prolonged in the morbidly obese when dosed according to TBW, suggesting that dosing based on LBW is optimal in this group of patients.[59]

Prompt early reversal but slow full recovery has been documented in overweight and obese patients during neostigmine-induced reversal of vecuronium dosed according to TBW.[60] Sugammadex, a modified γ-cyclodextrin compound that encapsulates rocuronium, and other steroid-based neuromuscular blockers to a lesser extent, may prove invaluable for more rapid and complete neuromuscular blockade reversal in obese patients.[61]

OPIOIDS

All synthetic opioids are highly lipophilic drugs. Application of non-weight-based pharmacokinetic models for fentanyl derived from normal weight patients overestimates the plasma concentration of fentanyl as body weight increases from normal to morbid obesity. Fentanyl dosing based a derived "pharmacokinetic mass" (derived pharmacokinetic body weight for dosing that reflects the influence of TBW on clearance) is clinically more useful than that based on TBW because of the strong linear correlation between this derived mass and total body clearance and also a strong correlation with dosing for postoperative analgesia.[62,63]

Administration of fentanyl according to TBW overestimates fentanyl dose requirements in obese patients. Sufentanil, a highly lipid soluble opioid, distributes extensively in body fat as well as in lean tissues, and it has an increased V_D and a prolonged elimination half-life that correlates positively with the degree of obesity. Plasma clearance, however, is similar in obese and nonobese patients; therefore loading dose should account for TBW while maintenance and infusion dosing should be reduced and dosed according to LBW. Pharmacokinetic parameters derived from nonobese subjects accurately predict plasma sufentanil concentrations in morbidly obese subjects, but at the morbidly obese range (BMI >40 kg/m^2), overestimation of plasma sufentanil concentration rises.[64] Remifentanil, a fentanyl congener, is hydrolyzed by blood and tissue esterases leading to rapid metabolism and inactive products. There is no difference in V_D estimate of remifentanil between obese and nonobese subjects, and remifentanil pharmacokinetics is more closely related to LBW than to TBW; therefore, dosing should be based on LBW.[65]

DEXMEDETOMIDINE

Dexmedetomidine is a highly selective α_2-adrenergic agonist with sedative-hypnotic, anesthetic-sparing, analgesic, and sympatholytic properties but lacks significant effects on respiration, making it ideally suitable as an analgesic adjuvant in morbidly obese subjects in whom opioid-induced respiratory depression may be a risk.[66] At infusion rates of 0.2 to 0.7 µg/kg per hour, dexmedetomidine produces clinically effective sedation with decreased analgesic and anesthetic requirements.

MEDICAL AND SURGICAL THERAPY FOR OBESITY

Antiobesity medications are formulated to reduce energy intake, increase energy utilization, or decrease absorption of nutrients. Indications for drug treatment include a BMI 30 kg/m^2 or higher or a BMI between 27 and 29.9 kg/m^2 in conjunction with an obesity-related medical complication. The combination of phentermine and fenfluramine (Phen-Fen) was previously popular for obesity treatment until evidence indicated its association with valvular heart disease and pulmonary hypertension. Sibutramine and orlistat are antiobesity medications for long-term use that have not yet been associated with such detrimental side effects. Sibutramine inhibits the reuptake of both serotonin and norepinephrine to increase satiety after the onset of eating rather than reduce appetite; it does not promote the release of serotonin, unlike fenfluramine and dexfenfluramine that primarily increase the release of serotonin in brain synapses and also inhibit reuptake to produce anorexia. Sibutramine does not deplete the neural synapses of catecholamines; therefore, dangerous hypotension that is unresponsive to indirectly acting vasopressors, seen with fenfluramine and dexfenfluramine, does not occur. Orlistat blocks the absorption and digestion of dietary fat by binding lipases in the gastrointestinal tract. It improves cardiovascular risk factors associated with obesity such as hypertension, WC, fasting blood glucose levels, and lipid profile.[67] Low-density lipoprotein and total cholesterol levels also decrease. An increase in warfarin's anticoagulant effect is seen with chronic dosing of orlistat because of its side effect of decreasing absorption of fat-soluble vitamins, including vitamin K.[68] This results in an abnormal plasma thromboplastin time due to deficiency of clotting factors II, VII, IX, and X. Rimonabant, a selective cannabinoid-1 receptor antagonist, induces weight loss, reduces WC, and improves lipid profile and glucose management by decreasing appetite, with a concomitant reduced incidence of the metabolic syndrome.[69] Significant side effects that should be considered during the perioperative period include psychiatric disorders, anxiety, and depression. Nausea, dizziness, diarrhea, arthralgia, and back pain are also seen.

Obesity (bariatric) surgery is generally classified into malabsorptive, restrictive, or combined. Malabsorptive procedures that include jejunoileal bypass and biliopancreatic diversion are rarely used presently. Restrictive procedures include the vertical banded gastroplasty and the adjustable gastric banding (ABG). The RYGB combines gastric restriction with a minimal degree of malabsorption. RYGB is the most commonly performed and the most effective bariatric procedure in the United States today. It involves anastomoses of the proximal gastric pouch to a segment of the proximal jejunum, bypassing most of the stomach and the entire duodenum. RYGB patients lose an average of 50% to 60% excess body weight and decrease their BMI by approximately 10 kg/m^2 during the first 12 to 24 postoperative months. Type 2 diabetes mellitus resolves in more than 90% of post-RYGB patients.[70] AGB requires that an adjustable inflatable band be placed around the proximal stomach to limit the stomach capacity. Adjustments can be made to meet a patient's individual needs by adding to or removing saline from the silicone band, making it tighter or less so.

Rhabdomyolysis has been documented in morbidly obese patients undergoing prolonged procedures such as laparoscopic bariatric surgery; the main risk factor is prolonged duration of surgery. Elevations in serum creatinine and CPK levels unexplained by other reasons and complaints of buttock, hip, or shoulder pain in the postoperative period should raise the suspicion of rhabdomyolysis. Measurement of serum CPK pre- and postoperatively aids in early diagnosis and treatment. Myoglobinuric acute renal failure can be as high as 30% when serum CPK is higher than 5000 IU/L.[71] Efforts to determine whether liberal intraoperative intravenous fluid administration used to treat rhabdomyolysis can also be used to prevent it did not show favorable results. Both conservative (15 mL/kg) and liberal (40 mL/kg) fluid administration did not affect the incidence of rhabdomyolysis in obese patients undergoing laparoscopic bariatric surgery.[72]

PREOPERATIVE EVALUATION

Previous experiences as detailed by the patient and anesthetic records are useful sources of information. Obese patients should be evaluated for systemic and pulmonary hypertension, signs of right and/or left ventricular or congestive cardiac failure, and ischemic heart disease. Excess adiposity may make signs of congestive cardiac failure difficult to elucidate. The chronicity of pulmonary impairment including OSA and OHS makes pulmonary hypertension common in morbidly obese patients. Tricuspid regurgitation on echocardiography is the most useful confirmatory test of pulmonary hypertension but should be combined with clinical features such as exertional dyspnea, fatigue, and syncope that reflect the inability to increase cardiac output in response to activity.[73] Features of right ventricular hypertrophy such as tall precordial R waves, right axis deviation, and right ventricular strain pattern may be seen on ECG. Sensitivity of the ECG features correlates well with the degree of pulmonary hypertension. Chest radiographs may show evidence of underlying lung disease and prominent pulmonary arteries. In patients with significant cardiopulmonary disease or abnormal ECG, preoperative echocardiography, spirometry, and arterial blood gas analysis are strongly recommended.[74]

Patients who have previously undergone bariatric surgery should be investigated for long-term metabolic and nutritional abnormalities during the preoperative visit. Common deficiencies include vitamin B_{12}, iron, calcium, and folic acid. A collective form of postoperative polyneuropathy known as acute postgastric reduction surgery (APGARS) neuropathy could result from these deficiencies.[75] Patients with APGARS neuropathy present with protracted postoperative vomiting, hyporeflexia, and muscular weakness. Differential diagnoses of this disorder include thiamine deficiency (Wernicke encephalopathy, beriberi), vitamin B_{12} deficiency, and Guillain-Barré syndrome. Because of the associated hyporeflexia and muscular weakness, close attention should be paid to dosing and monitoring of neuromuscular blocking agents.[76] Electrolyte and coagulation indices should be checked before surgery, particularly in patients on chronic diuretics treatment and weight loss medications and also in the acutely ill or those poorly compliant with vitamin and nutritional supplements. Chronic vitamin K deficiency can result in coagulation abnormalities requiring vitamin K analog or fresh-frozen plasma.

OSA and OHS are frequently associated with difficult laryngoscopy and intubation. Inquiry should be made about the signs and symptoms during preoperative evaluation. History of hypertension or neck circumference greater than 40 cm correlates with an increased probability of OSA. OSA is a legitimate reason to delay surgery to get a proper workup.[13] A formal sleep study helps quantify its severity. Those requiring general anesthesia should be treated as having severe OSA. Regional anesthesia should be considered if it is technically feasible. OSA patients should generally be treated as inpatients; however, outpatient surgery can be considered in the following circumstances: mild OSA, local or regional anesthesia with minimal or no sedation, 23-hour observation postanesthesia care unit following surgery, and patients on oral medication at the time of discharge. Patients on a CPAP device at home should be encouraged to bring them to the hospital for postoperative use. The possibility of invasive monitoring, prolonged endotracheal intubation, and postoperative mechanical ventilation at preoperative evaluation should be discussed. Specialized tests such as pulmonary function tests and liver function tests need not be routinely obtained because they are not cost-effective in the asymptomatic morbidly obese patient. Blood glucose abnormalities should be corrected if present.

PREOPERATIVE MEDICATIONS

All current medications should be continued until the time of surgery; with the possible exception of insulin and oral hypoglycemic agents. Antibiotic prophylaxis is important because of an increased incidence of wound infection in obese patients partly due to a decrease in tissue oxygenation.[77] Oral benzodiazepines are reliable for anxiolysis and mild sedation; intravenous midazolam can be titrated in small doses during the immediate preoperative period. Prophylaxis against both aspiration pneumonitis and deep vein thrombosis (DVT) should be addressed during the preoperative period. H_2 receptor antagonists, nonparticulate antacids, and proton pump inhibitors all reduce gastric volume, acidity, or both, reducing the risk and severity of aspiration pneumonitis.

Obesity is a major independent risk factor for deep vein thrombosis (DVT) and subsequent morbidity and mortality from postoperative pulmonary embolism (PE).[78,79] Minidose subcutaneous heparin 5000 IU administered before surgery and repeated every 8 to 12 hours until the patient is fully mobile reduces this risk. The incidence of clinically evident DVT after laparoscopic RYGB is low when the procedure is accomplished in a relatively short time, with the initiation of calf-length pneumatic compression hose before induction of anesthesia and with routine early ambulation.[80] Prophylactic inferior vena caval (IVC) filter placement is recommended for bariatric surgery patients with prior pulmonary embolus, prior DVT, evidence of venous stasis, or a hypercoagulable state.[81] Four important risk factors that may necessitate prophylactic IVC filter placement include venous stasis disease, BMI 60 or higher, truncal obesity, and obesity hypoventilation/sleep apnea syndrome (OHS/SAS).[82] Many bariatric surgeons prefer low-dose unfractionated heparin as their primary method of thromboprophylaxis.[83] The use of a protocol for heparin dosing in gastric bypass patients as opposed to a fixed dose is the preferred method. Dose calculations based initially on height and weight that is later adjusted according to peak anti–factor Xa activity results in better thromboprophylaxis and few side effects.[84] Low-molecular-weight heparins have better bioavailability when injected subcutaneously.

AIRWAY

Anatomic changes of obesity that contribute to a potentially difficult airway include limitation of movement of the atlantoaxial joint and cervical spine by upper thoracic and low cervical fat pads, excessive tissue folds in the mouth and pharynx, short thick neck, suprasternal, presternal, and posterior cervical fat, and a very thick submental fat pad. Obese patients with OSA are significantly more difficult to intubate than those without OSA; however there is no relationship between the severity of sleep apnea and the occurrence of difficult intubation.[85] A short thick neck is significantly more related to difficult intubation, whereas obesity and a short thick neck are significantly related to each other, in addition to both being related to OSA. Patients with OSA have excess adipose tissue deposited in their pharyngeal area, including the tonsils, tonsillar pillars, uvula, tongue, aryepiglottic folds, and the lateral pharyngeal walls.[13] This fat deposition is most pronounced in the lateral pharyngeal walls, and it may not be noticed during routine airway examination. Even with the presence of these anatomic changes and pathology, the magnitude of BMI does not have much influence on the difficulty of laryngoscopy. Such difficulty correlates better with increased age, male sex, TMJ pathology, Mallampati classes 3 and 4, history of OSA, and abnormal upper teeth.[86] Neck circumference has been identified as the single biggest predictor of problematic intubation in morbidly obese patients.[87] A larger neck circumference is associated with the male sex, higher Mallampati score, grade 3 views at laryngoscopy, and OSA. The probability of a problematic intubation is approximately 5% with a 40-cm neck circumference compared with a 35% probability at a 60-cm neck circumference.[87]

OBESITY AND AMBULATORY ANESTHESIA

The Royal College of Surgeons of England issued guidelines in 1992 that deemed patients with BMI 30 kg/m^2 or higher unsuitable for ambulatory surgery.[88] Subsequent evaluation of adherence to these guidelines discovered that greater than 85% of ambulatory surgery units in England and a significant number in other countries continued routinely to anesthetize patients with BMI higher than 30 kg/m^2.[89,90] Many anesthesiologists believe that morbidly obese patients with comorbidities and no patient escort are unsuitable for ambulatory anesthesia because many of them are in suboptimal health. The presence of cardiovascular or respiratory comorbidity significantly reduces the willingness of anesthesiologists to provide ambulatory care to the obese.[91,92] An excess of adverse perioperative cardiovascular events has not been found in obese patients undergoing ambulatory surgery despite a prevalence of cardiovascular disease in this patient population; however, adverse intraoperative and postoperative respiratory events, including arterial oxygen desaturation and bronchospasm, are quite common.[93] Individual evaluation should dictate which obese patients can undergo ambulatory anesthesia and surgery. Proper equipment and procedures for positioning and monitoring should be readily available, including difficult airway and resuscitation equipment. Arrangements for transfer to a 24-hour observation unit or full admission unit should be in place. Ambulatory anesthesia for morbidly obese patients without significant comorbidities is safe. Obese patients do not have a higher incidence of contact with health care professionals after discharge from the ambulatory surgery unit, neither do they have a higher postambulatory surgery unplanned hospital admission rate than the general population.[94] Obesity is associated with a higher regional block failure and complication rates during ambulatory regional anesthesia. The rate of successful blocks and overall satisfaction, however, is high; therefore, obese patients should not be excluded from ambulatory regional anesthesia procedures.[95]

INTRAOPERATIVE CONSIDERATIONS

POSITIONING

Obese patients may require specially designed tables or 2 regular operating tables for safe anesthesia and surgery. Regular operating tables have a maximum weight limit of approximately 205 kg, but wider and higher-capacity operating tables are also available that can hold up to 450-kg patients and accommodate the extra girth. Electrically operated or motorized tables facilitate maneuvering into various surgically favorable positions. The use of belts and straps and malleable bean bags helps keep obese patients from falling off the operating table. Pressure areas on the body should be protected with care to avoid neural injuries and possible pressure necrosis. Brachial plexus and lower extremity nerve injuries are frequent. A documented association between ulnar neuropathy and increasing BMI quoted a greater than 30% incidence of ulnar neuropathy in patients with a BMI 38 kg/m^2 or higher compared with only 1% in the control group.[96] Peripheral neuropathy occurs more frequently after bariatric surgery than after other abdominal surgery. Intraoperative neural compression or stretching from improper positioning is one of the most common etiologies. Malnutrition may be an important contributing factor; inflammation and altered immunity also play some role.[97] Other associated risk factors include greater absolute weight loss, a faster rate of weight loss, lower serum albumin and transferrin concentrations, prolonged postoperative gastrointestinal symptoms (nausea and vomiting, diarrhea, and dumping syndrome), and reduced vitamin and calcium supplementation.[97] Attention to patient positioning and duration of immobility during surgery helps reduce the incidence of compression injuries and rhabdomyolysis during bariatric surgery. Micronutrient deficiencies such as vitamins B_6, B_{12}, D, E, folate, and minerals such as calcium, magnesium, phosphorus, selenium, and copper contribute to nonmechanical peripheral neuropathies, especially in nutritionally noncompliant patients undergoing postbariatric surgery procedures.[98]

Supine positioning of the obese patient causes aortic and IVC compression and also leads to ventilatory impairment with further decrease in FRC and oxygenation. Trendelenburg positioning, when required, further worsens FRC and should be avoided whenever possible. A simple change from the supine to sitting position in the obese patient causes a significant increase in cardiac output, oxygen consumption, and pulmonary artery pressure. The head-up (semirecumbent) or reverse Trendelenburg (semi-Fowler) position unloads the weight of the intra-abdominal contents from the diaphragm leading to increased pulmonary compliance and better values for FRC and oxygenation. Both intraoperative PEEP and reverse Trendelenburg positions significantly decrease alveolar-arterial oxygen tension difference and increase total respiratory compliance to a similar degree in the obese, but reverse Trendelenburg position results in lower airway pressures. Both maneuvers decrease cardiac output significantly, however, which partially counteracts their beneficial effects on oxygenation.[99] Prone positioning in the obese patient should be correctly performed with freedom of abdominal movement to prevent detrimental effects on lung compliance, ventilation, and arterial oxygenation. Prone positioning increases intra-abdominal pressure, worsening IVC and aortic compression and further decreasing FRC. Lateral decubitus positioning allows for good diaphragmatic excursion during mechanical ventilation because the panniculus is displaced off the abdomen reducing intra-abdominal pressure.[100] Changing from a sitting to a lateral decubitus position after placing an epidural catheter may cause catheter dislodgment, resulting in inadequate analgesia because movement from sitting to lateral position increases the distance from the skin to the epidural space.[101]

MONITORING

Noninvasive blood pressure measurements can be falsely elevated if a cuff is too small for the limb. The blood pressure cuff bladder should encircle a minimum of 75% of the upper arm circumference or, preferably, the entire arm. Forearm blood pressure is a fairly good predictor of upper arm blood pressure in most patients; however, forearm measurements with a standard cuff may overestimate both systolic and diastolic blood pressures in obese patients.[102] Invasive arterial pressure monitoring may be indicated for the morbidly obese with severe cardiopulmonary disease and for those with poor fit of the noninvasive blood pressure cuff. Central venous and pulmonary artery catheters may be indicated for extensive surgery and in patients with significant cardiopulmonary impairment. Difficult intravenous access is an indication for central venous catheterization. A central venous line need not be routinely inserted in obese patients because insertion of peripheral lines is almost always successful.[103]

INDUCTION, INTUBATION AND MAINTENANCE

Obese patients desaturate very rapidly after loss of consciousness because of increased oxygen consumption and decreased FRC; therefore, adequate preoxygenation is vital before the induction of anesthesia. Application of positive pressure ventilation during preoxygenation decreases atelectasis formation and improves oxygenation.[104] Four VC breaths with 100% oxygen within 30 seconds have been suggested as superior to the usually recommended 3 minutes of 100% preoxygenation in obese patients.[105] Preoxygenation in the head-up or sitting position provides the longest SAP and is more effective and significantly extends the tolerance to apnea in obese patients when compared with the supine position.[106-108]

Obese patients may require larger doses of induction agents because blood volume, muscle mass, and cardiac output increase linearly with the degree of obesity. Cardiovascular and respiratory depression may result from larger doses, however. An increased dose of succinylcholine is indicated because of an increase in pseudocholinesterase activity. Myalgia following succinylcholine is not frequently seen in morbidly obese patients so it is highly recommended for tracheal intubation.[109] If difficult intubation is anticipated, awake intubation under topical or regional anesthesia is a prudent approach. During awake intubation, sedative-hypnotic medications should be reduced to a minimum, to prevent cardiorespiratory depression. An immediately available experienced colleague is invaluable during induction and airway management. If endotracheal intubation under general anesthesia is selected, hypoxia and aspiration of gastric contents should be prevented at all costs. Preparation should be made for the possibility of difficult intubation, and a surgeon capable of rapidly surgically accessing the airway should be readily available. Towels or folded blankets under the shoulders and head can compensate for the exaggerated flexed position of posterior cervical fat (**Fig. 23-7**). The object of this maneuver, known as "stacking," is to position the patient so that the tip of the chin is at a higher level than the chest to facilitate laryngoscopy and intubation. The HELP, or "ramped" position,[110,111] is a step beyond stacking. It significantly elevates the obese patient's head, neck, upper body, and shoulders above the chest to a point where an imaginary horizontal line can be drawn from the sternal notch to the external ear to better improve laryngoscopy and intubation. To facilitate proper HELP placement, the preformed Troop Head Elevation Pillow (C&R Enterprises, Frisco, TX, USA) in combination with a standard intubation pillow can be used in place of folded towels or blankets (**Fig. 23-8A-C**). The advantage of the preformed pillow is that it can be prepositioned, inserted, and removed much faster with less effort than that required to build and dismantle a ramp made from blankets and towels.[112] The need for additional lifting can be eliminated by using an inflatable multichambered pillow to facilitate HELP placement more easily[113] (**Fig. 23-9**).

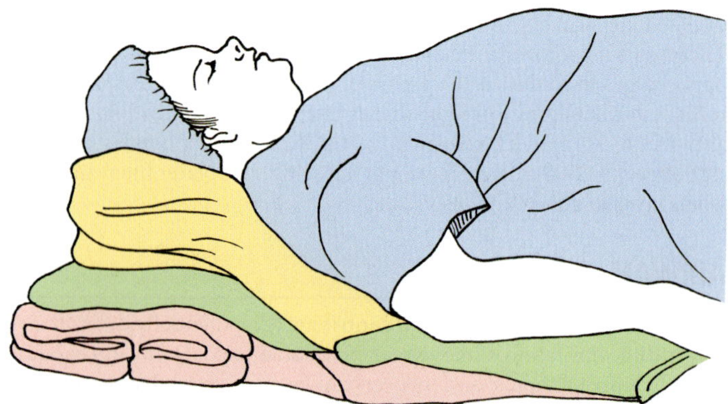

FIGURE 23-7. "Stacking" using towels and blankets. [Reprinted with permission from Ogunnaike BO, Whitten CW. Anesthesia and obesity. In: Barash PG, Cullen BF, Stoelting RK, et al., eds. *Clinical Anesthesia*. 6th ed. Philadelphia, PA: Lippincott, Williams, & Wilkins, 2009:1242).

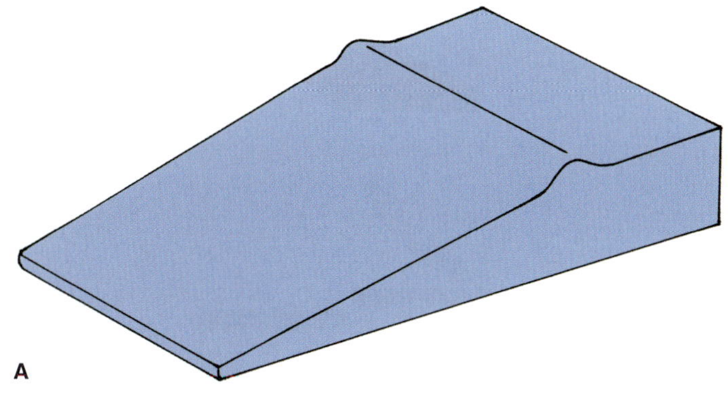

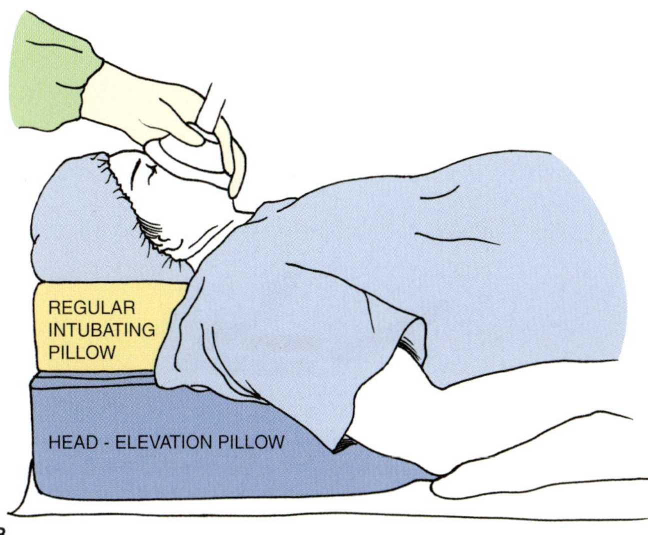

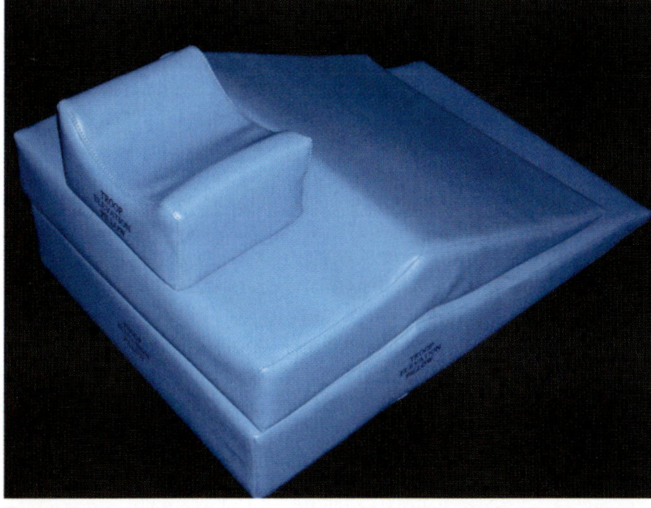

FIGURE 23-8. **A.** The preformed Troop head elevation pillow. **B**. Proper head-elevated laryngoscopy position placement with the head elevation pillow combined with a standard intubating pillow. **C.** Photograph of the Troop elevation pillow with additional layer (for extralarge patients) and preattached intubating pillow. [Reprinted with permission from Ogunnaike BO, Whitten CW. Anesthesia and obesity. In: Barash PG, Cullen BF, Stoelting RK, eds. *Clinical Anesthesia*. 6th ed. Philadelphia, PA: Lippincott, Williams, & Wilkins; 2009:1243.]

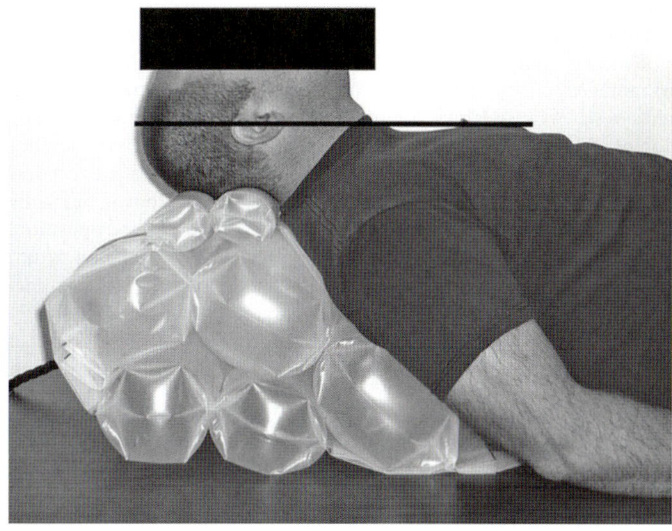

FIGURE 23-9. Prototype of the inflatable multichambered pillow for proper head-elevated laryngoscopy position placement of the obese patient. [Reprinted with permission from Nissen MD, Gayes JM. An inflatable multi-chambered upper body support for the placement of the obese patient in the head-elevated laryngoscopy position. *Anesth Analg.* 2007;104:1305.]

Continuous infusion of a short-acting intravenous agent such as propofol or any of the inhalational agents or a combination may be used to maintain anesthesia. Desflurane, sevoflurane, and isoflurane are minimally metabolized and are therefore useful choices in obese patients. Desflurane may provide better hemodynamic stability.[114] Sevoflurane provides rapid recovery, good hemodynamic control, prompt regaining of psychological and physical functioning, and infrequent incidence of nausea and vomiting when compared with isoflurane.[115] An insignificant difference exists between sevoflurane and desflurane with respect to emergence and cognitive psychomotor recovery characteristics when careful anesthetic titration is used.[116] Morbidly obese patients awake and regain protective airway reflexes significantly faster after desflurane than after sevoflurane anesthesia and also record higher oxygen saturation on arrival in the postanesthesia care unit (PACU).[117-119] Propofol-nitrous oxide anesthesia adjusted to a Bispectral Index Sensor level of approximately 60 combined with thoracic epidural analgesia provides intraoperative hemodynamic stability and prompts recovery during laparotomy for gastric bypass surgery.[120] Metabolism of volatile anesthetics is greater in obese than in normal weight patients, which is reflected by a greater increase in serum inorganic fluoride, including during anesthesia with sevoflurane, whose biotransformation has not been shown to result in significant differences in plasma fluoride levels or differences in pre- and postoperative liver function and renal function tests between obese and nonobese patients.[121] A potentially hepatotoxic reductive pathway metabolizes halothane in obese patients, resulting in an increased incidence of "halothane hepatitis." Fortunately, halothane is rarely needed in modern-day practice. Rapid elimination and analgesic properties make nitrous oxide an attractive choice for anesthesia in obese patients, but high oxygen demand in this patient population limits its use. Short-acting opioids such as remifentanil at the lowest possible dose, combined with a low-solubility inhalation anesthetic, facilitates a more rapid emergence without increasing opioid-related side effects.[122] Cisatracurium possesses an organ-independent elimination profile and is a favorable nondepolarizing muscle relaxant for maintenance of anesthesia in the obese patient with a high prevalence of renal and hepatic compromise. Vecuronium and rocuronium are also useful choices. Dexmedetomidine, an α_2 agonist with sedative and analgesic properties, provides hemodynamic stability without myocardial depression; it has no clinically significant adverse effects on respiration, which makes it an attractive agent for use as an anesthetic adjunct in obese patients.

Furthermore, it reduces the postoperative opioid analgesic requirements and their subsequent detrimental respiratory depressant effects.[66,123.]

Ventilatory tidal volumes greater than 13 mL/kg offer no added advantages during ventilation of morbidly obese patients during anesthesia because larger volumes increase airway pressures and lung compliance without significantly improving arterial oxygen tension but results in severe hypocarbia that increases shunt fraction at a $Paco_2$ less than 30 mm Hg.[124] Arterial oxygenation during laparoscopy in morbidly obese patients is affected mainly by body weight and not body position, pneumoperitoneum, or mode of ventilation, and oxygenation is not significantly improved by increasing either the respiratory rate or tidal volume.[125] PEEP is the only ventilatory parameter that has consistently been shown to improve respiratory function in obese subjects, but it may decrease venous return, cardiac output, and subsequent oxygen delivery.[126]

Blood loss is usually greater in the obese than in the nonobese for the same type of surgery because technical difficulties of accessing the surgical site requires larger incisions and more extensive dissection. Early infusion of colloids and blood products may be necessary because obese patients are less able to compensate for small volumes lost, but rapid infusion of excessive amounts should be avoided because of high prevalence of preexisting congestive cardiac failure.

REGIONAL ANESTHESIA

A regional technique is a useful alternative or adjunct to general anesthesia in the morbidly obese because it may help avoid potential intubation difficulties and assist with postoperative pain control and physical therapy. It can be technically difficult, however, because of the inability to easily identify usual bony landmarks. A peripheral nerve stimulator with or without ultrasound guidance helps with the success of regional anesthesia. Central neuraxial block is easier in the lumbar region because the midline in this area has a thinner layer of fat than other areas of the spinal column. Longer needles and the sitting position are other useful tools that facilitate induction of central neuraxial anesthesia. Ultrasound[127] and fluoroscopy[128,129] can be used to guide a needle or continuous infusion catheter into the spinal or epidural space. Low-current electrical stimulation through an epidural catheter, to achieve trunk or limb movement, can also be used for confirmation of epidural catheter placement.[130] Epidural vascular engorgement and fatty infiltration reduce the volume of the space, making dose requirements of local anesthetics for epidural anesthesia 20% to 25% less in obese patients. Subarachnoid blocks are not technically as difficult as epidural blocks, but the height of a subarachnoid block in obese patients can be unpredictable because it may spread considerably upward within a short time causing cardiovascular and respiratory embarrassment. tContinuous catheter subarachnoid block allows titration of the local anesthetic to the desired effect and level.[131] Combined epidural and balanced general anesthesia allows for better titration of anesthetic drugs, use of larger oxygen concentration, and optimal muscle relaxation. It also allows for continuation of postoperative analgesia through the same catheter used to provide surgical anesthesia, thereby facilitating early postoperative mobilization.

POSTOPERATIVE CONSIDERATIONS

EMERGENCE

Prompt extubation prevents the morbidly obese patient from becoming ventilator dependent. Tracheal extubation should be considered only when there is complete reversal of neuromuscular blockade and full recovery from the effects of anesthetics. The patient should be preferably extubated in the semirecumbent position, which has less adverse effect on the respiratory system. Supplemental oxygen should be administered after extubation. Lifting devices such as the HoverMatt (Patient Handling Technologies; Allentown, PA, USA) and the Patient Transfer Device (PTD; AliMed; Dedham, MA, USA) are useful for transporting morbidly obese patients onto or off the operating table. The PTD can be combined with the Walter Henderson Maneuver (**Fig. 23-10**) to transfer obese patients safely and gently onto their postoperative beds.[132]

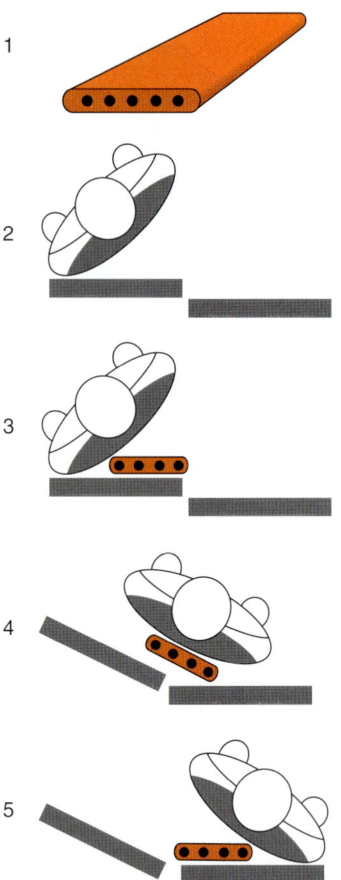

FIGURE 23-10. Illustration of the Walter Henderson maneuver. 1, Patient Transfer Device PTD (also known as patient roller); 2, patient tilted to slip roller under; 3, roller slipped under patient; 4, table tilted to roll patient downhill onto bed; 5, patient rolled onto bed. [Reprinted with permission from Ogunnaike BO, Whitten CW: In response to Rosenblatt MA, Reich DL, Roth R, et al [Letter]. *Anesth Analg.* 2004;98:1809.]

Risk of airway obstruction at extubation is increased in the obese OSA patient; up to 5% incidence of life-threatening postextubation obstruction is seen. Negative pressure pulmonary edema can occur from postextubation obstruction and is best treated by reintubation, which can be difficult in a patient with OSA. Extubation in the fully awake state is advocated. Any regional technique, if instituted for postoperative analgesia, should be operative at the time of extubation.

Patients on preoperative CPAP should continue on it postoperatively. CPAP should not be immediately applied to obese OSA patients upon arrival in the PACU because it impairs access to suctioning and dealing with postoperative nausea and vomiting; it also impairs communication between patient and caregiver, and interferes with monitoring of facial color. Furthermore, intraoperative and postoperative events such as facial edema may change mask fit, and also CPAP requirements may change significantly because it is meant to be used for natural, not drug-induced sleep.[13] Another indication for CPAP is an increased incidence of postoperative atelectasis in morbidly obese patients after general anesthesia.[133] Postoperative CPAP does not increase the incidence of major anastomotic leakage after gastric bypass surgery despite the theoretical risk of anastomotic injury from pressurized air delivered by CPAP.[134] The obese patient may avoid taking deep breaths due to pain after abdominal surgery. Adequate analgesia and a properly fitted elastic binder for abdominal support may encourage them to cooperate with early ambulation and deep breathing exercises with the aid of incentive spirometry. Pulse oximetry and arterial blood gases should be monitored appropriately.

POSTOPERATIVE ANALGESIA

Perioperative use of regional anesthesia and analgesia reduces the incidence of postoperative respiratory complications. Epidural analgesia with local anesthetics, opioids, or both, or intrathecal opioid are viable options. Potential advantages of epidural analgesia in obese patients include prevention of DVT, improved analgesia, and earlier recovery of intestinal motility. Lesser oxygen consumption and decreased left ventricular stroke work are other benefits. Patient-controlled analgesia (PCA) with morphine may be equivalent to low thoracic/high lumbar continuous infusions of bupivacaine/fentanyl epidural analgesia in morbidly obese patients undergoing gastric bypass surgery with regard to the quality of pain control at rest, the frequency of nausea and pruritus, the time to ambulation, time to return of gastrointestinal function, and the length of hospital stay.[135] Incisional local anesthetic infiltration plus PCA produces lower pain scores when compared with epidural anesthesia and analgesia and postoperative PCA for gastric bypass surgery. In addition, infiltration analgesia as part of a multimodal regimen offers a simple, safe, and inexpensive alternative to epidural analgesia alone.[136,137] A combination of intraoperative nonopioid analgesics and anesthetic adjuvants (ketorolac, clonidine, ketamine, lidocaine, magnesium sulfate, and methylprednisolone) decreases sedation during recovery from anesthesia and reduces postoperative morphine requirements when compared with intraoperative fentanyl anesthesia in morbidly obese patients.[138] Delayed respiratory depression from neuraxial opioids coupled with a potentially difficult airway in the obese patient necessitates closer monitoring in a stepdown or intensive care unit. Increased analgesic requirements during the first 3 postoperative days increase the danger of life-threatening apnea during drug-induced sleep. The first postoperative week is a period of increased risk of prolonged apnea during sleep for the postoperative obese patient, especially those with OSA.[13]

RESUSCITATION

Chest compressions may not be effective when improperly performed. Mechanical compression devices may be required. The maximum 400 J of energy on regular defibrillators is sufficient for the morbidly obese because their chest wall is usually not much thicker, but the higher trans-thoracic impedance from fat may obligate several attempts.[139] Mask ventilation is more difficult because of poor mask fit, redundant oropharyngeal tissues, and reduced chest wall compliance. Intubation may be difficult. The gum-elastic bougie may help facilitate successful intubation in emergency situations. The intubating and ProSeal laryngeal mask airways and the esophageal tracheal Combitube are useful temporary supraglottic airway devices. Transtracheal jet ventilation and retrograde wire intubation may be difficult to establish due to difficulty in palpating anatomic landmarks. Tracheostomy and percutaneous cricothyrotomy should be reserved as final options and should be performed by experienced practitioners.[140] Pulse oximetry may be unreliable because of increased finger thickness; the earlobe may be a better choice.

KEY REFERENCES

- Adams JP, Murphy PG. Obesity in anaesthesia and intensive care. *Br J Anaesth*. 2000;85:91.
- Benumof JL. Obesity, sleep apnea, the airway and anesthesia. *Curr Opin Anaesthesiol.* 2004;17:21.
- Brodsky JB, Lemmens HJ, Brock-Utne JG, et al. Morbid obesity and tracheal intubation. *Anesth Analg*. 2002;94:732.
- Chung F, Yegneswaran B, Liao P, et al. STOP questionnaire: a tool to screen patients for obstructive sleep apnea. *Anesthesiology*. 2008;108:812.
- Fraley MA, Bircham JA, Senkottaiyan N, et al. Obesity and the electrocardiogram. *Obes Rev*. 2005;6:275.
- Ogunnaike BO, Jones SB, Jones DB, et al. Anesthetic considerations for bariatric surgery. *Anesth Analg*. 2002;95:1793.
- Schumann R, Jones SB, Cooper B, et al. Update on best practice recommendations for anesthetic perioperative care and pain management in weight loss surgery, 2004-2007. *Obesity*. 2009;17:889.
- Servin F. Ambulatory anesthesia for the obese patient. *Curr Opin Anaesthesiol.* 2006;19:597.
- Wool DB, Lemmens HJM, Brodsky JB, et al. Intraoperative fluid replacement and postoperative creatine phosphokinase levels in laparoscopic bariatric patients. *Obes Surg*. 2010;20:698.
- Xing J, Chen JD. Alterations in gastrointestinal motility in obesity. *Obes Res*. 2004;12:1723.

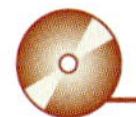

REFERENCES

Complete references available on DVD and online version at www.LongneckerAnesthesiology.com

CHAPTER 24 Evaluation of the Patient With Alcohol or Drug Addiction

Paul S. Pagel
Judith A. May

KEY POINTS

1. Addiction is a very common medical illness. It is characterized by loss of control over an abusable substance, including an inability to voluntarily self-regulate drug use, compulsive preoccupation with obtaining or using a drug, and continued use despite adverse consequences.
2. Addiction may be managed successfully as a chronic disease, and many patients respond positively to treatment with long periods of abstinence.
3. Consultation with an addiction medicine specialist is encouraged when providing care for active or recovering alcohol or drug abusers during the perioperative period.
4. Preoperative assessment of all patients presenting for surgery should include a routine evaluation for alcohol or drug abuse.
5. Establishing a supportive, nonjudgmental but firm approach to the patient with active alcoholism or drug addiction is vital for successful care.
6. Preoperative history, physical examination, and laboratory testing should be guided by the known medical consequences of alcohol and drug addiction.
7. A blood alcohol concentration and a urine drug screen should be obtained in all active and most recovering alcohol or drug abusers.
8. Polysubstance abuse is common among alcohol or drug users.
9. Infectious diseases are epidemic in injection drug users.
10. Alcohol abuse has extensive medical consequences that impact every major organ system and is a major risk factor for perioperative morbidity and mortality.

11. Abuse of sedative–hypnotics, opioids, cocaine, amphetamines, hallucinogens, and inhalants is associated with a wide variety of drug specific medical complications.
12. Withdrawal is commonly encountered during the perioperative period in alcohol or drug abusers, and prophylaxis against withdrawal should be instituted before surgery.
13. Recovery involves abstinence in combination with a series of personal changes to maintain sobriety.

INTRODUCTION

Addiction is a major public health problem. The lifetime prevalence of alcohol or drug addiction in the United States is estimated to be approximately 14% and 7%, respectively.[1] The literature describing the evaluation and treatment of patients with addiction is exhaustive. This chapter focuses on what the anesthesiologist needs to know to effectively manage the perioperative care of the addicted patient.

ADDICTION: DEFINITIONS AND NEUROBIOLOGY

Addiction is defined by loss of control over a drug or substance of abuse. The inability to voluntarily self-regulate drug use, compulsive preoccupation with obtaining or using a drug, and continued use despite adverse consequences are central features of this multifaceted disease.[2] Initial drug use is usually voluntary, and most users do not develop drug dependence, but repetitive drug exposure in a susceptible individual appears to cause fundamental changes in central nervous system function that produce the disease. Evidence suggests that genetic predisposition to addiction may be related to alterations in neurocircuitry that enhance sensitivity to the reinforcing effects of drugs of abuse, thereby overwhelming cognitive control of behavior.[3] Thus addiction is a chronic disease; once present, it is regarded as permanent. However, it may be managed successfully, and many patients respond positively to treatment with long periods of abstinence.[4]

The neurobiology of addiction has been well documented and is not discussed in detail here.[3,5] Three major concepts pertain to the perioperative care of the patient with addiction: drug reward and reinforcement, cross-addiction, and disease permanence. The mesocorticolimbic dopamine system is central to the pathophysiology of addiction.[5] This neurocircuitry involves the ventral tegmental area of the midbrain where dopaminergic neurons originate and the basal forebrain, the nucleus accumbens, and the amygdala to which these neurons project. All drugs of abuse interact with this system to produce reinforcement.[3] Different drugs of abuse, including many of those routinely used by anesthesiologists, may activate sites in this reinforcement cascade, but all lead to reward stimulation.[5] Thus exposure to one drug may mimic the reinforcing effects of another ("cross-addiction"). Alterations in reinforcement neurocircuitry may persist despite long-term abstinence. This observation supports the notion that addiction is a chronic disease[4] and may be particularly important in the recovering addict because drugs commonly used during the perioperative period may inadvertently reactivate addiction independent of the relative duration of abstinence.

APPROACH TO PREOPERATIVE EVALUATION

Medical and psychiatric diseases are very common in patients with addiction. Drugs of abuse produce direct toxic effects on a variety of organ systems or they may exacerbate preexisting medical conditions. Addictive behaviors (eg, sharing injection equipment, high-risk sexual activity) can markedly increase the risk of infectious diseases such as endocarditis, hepatitis, and acquired immunodeficiency virus (AIDS). Depressed socioeconomic conditions (eg, unemployment, reliance on housing in shelters, homelessness) also increase the risk of other infectious diseases such as community-acquired pneumonia and tuberculosis. Routine and preventive health care may be inadequate or nonexistent. Despite these, there is clear evidence that patients with addiction benefit from routine health care, particularly when it is linked to substance abuse treatment.[6] Such an integration of services improves patient outcome and should be an important goal during the perioperative period.

Previously undiagnosed alcohol abuse occurs in many hospitalized patients,[7] and physicians often fail to detect it[8]; thus the preoperative assessment of surgical patients should include an evaluation for alcohol or drug abuse. The CAGE and Michigan Alcohol Screening Test (MAST) questionnaires are brief but extensively validated screening instruments that are useful for the detection of a substance abuse disorder.[9] The simple 4-question CAGE test is particularly helpful for the anesthesiologist because of its brevity and predictive value:

C Have you ever felt you ought to Cut down on your drinking (drug use)?

A Have people *A*nnoyed you by criticizing your drinking (drug use)?

G Have you ever felt bad or Guilty about your drinking (drug use)?

E Have you ever had a drink (or used a drug) first thing in the morning ("*E*ye opener") to steady your nerves or get rid of a hangover?

Two or more positive responses to the CAGE questionnaire indicate that addiction is most likely present, whereas a single affirmative answer suggests that further assessment may be necessary. Corroborating history including evidence of alcohol- or drug-related amnesia ("blackouts"), multiple detoxifications or previous rehabilitation attempts, recurrent unemployment, and habitual criminal activity also suggest the diagnosis of a substance abuse disorder.[10] A blood alcohol concentration and a urine drug screen should be obtained in the patient with a known history of addiction, a positive preoperative screening evaluation, or when indicated by other clinical conditions (eg, trauma, altered mental status, obtunded state). The results identify the class(es) of drugs abused by the patient, alert the anesthesiologist to the possibility of withdrawal or potential drug interactions, and provide the opportunity to challenge denial and initiate a discussion about treatment alternatives, including consultation with an addiction medicine specialist.

A nonjudgmental but firm approach to the patient with addiction is essential for successful care. Unfortunately, patients with addiction may encounter physicians whose attitudes about and treatment may be prejudicial.[11] For example, general surgeons possessed the weakest educational background and the least desire to learn about resources for addiction management compared with psychiatrists and internists.[12] Anesthesiologists displayed more negative attitudes about patients with addiction than primary care physicians[13] (**Fig. 24-1**). A positive rapport also allows the anesthesiologist to strongly encourage the active alcohol or drug abuser to seek or reenter treatment.

Providing reassurance about prompt, effective management of pain to the patient with addiction deserves special emphasis during the preoperative evaluation. Chronic pain resulting from a variety of alcohol- or drug abuse-related medical illnesses was previously identified in many patients enrolled in methadone maintenance programs or residential treatment facilities[14] (**Fig. 24-2**). Chronic opioid abusers frequently display hyperalgesia, in part as a result of drug tolerance.[15] However, even well-intentioned, informed physicians may be hesitant to provide adequate doses of opioid analgesics to such patients because of fears about contributing to the disease process. Some physicians may intentionally withhold or restrict opioid analgesics because they are anxious about adverse consequences imposed by federal or state regulatory agencies,[15] are concerned that patient requests for these drugs may represent manipulative "drug-seeking" behavior,[16] or hold negative attitudes about addiction. These factors contribute to inadequate treatment of pain in patients with addiction,[17] and as a result, these patients often harbor suspicions that they will be deliberately abused by physicians

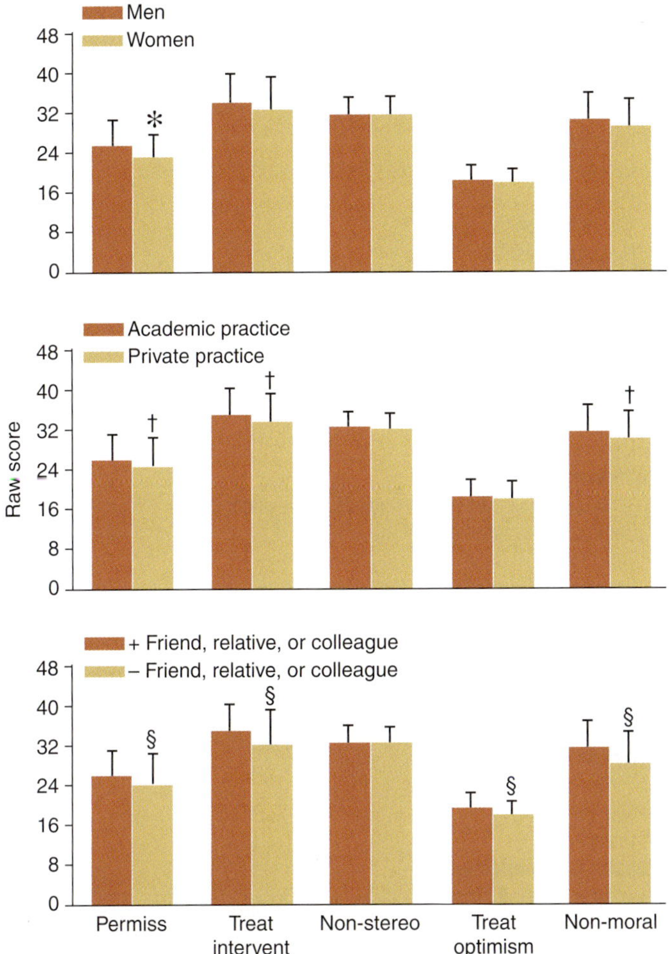

FIGURE 24-1. Histograms illustrating the raw scores for permissiveness, treatment interventions, nonstereotypes, treatment optimism, and nonmoralism factors observed in male (solid bar; top panel) and female (light bar; top panel) anesthesiologists in academic (solid bar; middle panel) or private practice (light bar; middle panel) and anesthesiologists who have (+; solid bar; bottom panel) or do not have (–; light bar; bottom panel) a friend, relative, or colleague with addiction. *Significantly (p <0.05) different from male anesthesiologists; † significantly (p <0.05) different from anesthesiologists in academic practice; § significantly (p <0.05) different from anesthesiologists who have a friend, relative, or colleague with addiction. [Reproduced with permission from May JA, Waltier DC, Pagel PS. Attitudes of anesthesiologists about addiction and its treatment: a survey of Illinois and Wisconsin members of the American Society of Anesthesiologists. *J Clin Anesth.* 2002;14:284-289.]

or nursing staff. Recognition that patients with addiction self-medicate or manipulate prescribed drugs to treat pain may further complicate this situation and thereby create "mutual mistrust."[16] The potential for such a conflict should be honestly addressed during the preoperative evaluation. Guidelines for pain management in patients with addiction encourage early consultation with an addictionologist, meticulous observation of compliance with and clinical response to prescribed opioids, and continuous assessment of function.[18]

HISTORY, PHYSICAL EXAMINATION, AND DIAGNOSTIC TESTING

In addition to the chief complaint that led to the original surgical referral and other relevant past medical history, the known medical consequences of alcohol and drug abuse, the common occurrence of polysubstance abuse, and the presence of other coexisting diseases should guide the preoperative history and physical examination. A thorough

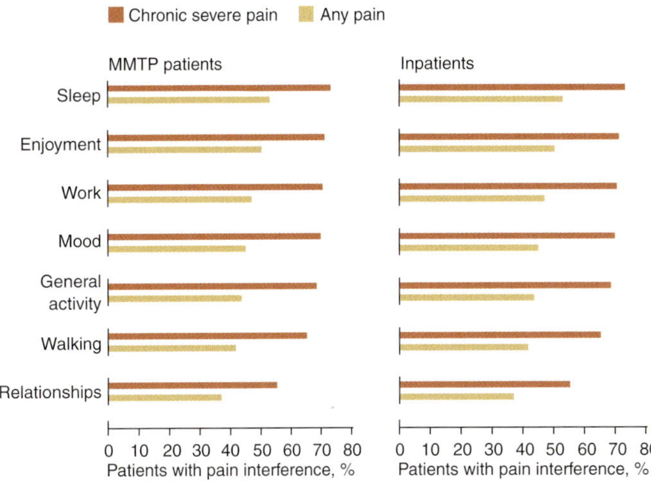

FIGURE 24-2. Histograms demonstrating the percentage of patients in methadone maintenance treatment programs (MMTPs) experiencing chronic severe (dark bars) or any (light bars) pain that interferes with daily activities compared with a cohort of hospital inpatients. Data are patients reporting a score of 5 or higher on the Brief Pain Inventory "interference" item, scored from 0 (does not interfere) to 10 (interferes completely). The data suggest that patients in methadone maintenance treatment programs have higher levels of pain that interfere with their daily activities compared with hospital inpatients. [Reproduced with permission from Rosenblum A, Joseph H, Fong C, Kipnis S, Cleland C, Portenoy RK. Prevalence and characteristics of chronic pain among chemically dependent patients in methadone maintenance and residential treatment facilities. *JAMA.* 2003;289:2370-2378.]

review of systems is required if the interview or laboratory results (blood alcohol concentration, urine drug screen) suggest substance abuse. Importantly, the recognition that constitutional complaints or new presenting symptoms may or may not indicate drug use or withdrawal is a critical feature of the history and physical examination. For example, fever, myalgias, tachycardia, and gastrointestinal symptoms typically characterize alcohol or opioid withdrawal, but such generic complaints may also indicate the presence of an underlying infectious disease. Weight loss due to malnutrition is a very common finding in drug abusers, but infectious diseases including human immunodeficiency virus (HIV) and occult malignancy must also be considered in the differential diagnosis. Similarly, a seizure certainly suggests the presence of alcohol or opioid withdrawal in the patient with a recent history of heavy abuse, but other causes cannot be immediately excluded.

The physical examination of the patient with addiction is directed toward the medical ramifications of specific drugs of abuse, but routine investigation of other coexisting diseases and the potential for complications arising from polysubstance abuse should not be overlooked. Examination of the skin may reveal evidence of acute or chronic infection (eg, cellulitis, abscess), repetitive drug injection ("track" marks), or peripheral venous thrombosis and will help anticipate difficulty inserting intravenous or intra-arterial catheters. Skin examination may also reveal the stigmata of advanced liver disease. Diffuse lymphadenopathy strongly suggests the presence of systemic infection, tuberculosis, or HIV. Poor dentition, oral-pharyngeal carcinoma, or nasal septum damage may be detected during examination of the airway. Such findings may have potentially important implications for airway management. Wheezing, rhonchi, rales, or evidence of pulmonary consolidation detected during the lung examination suggests the presence of reactive airway disease, acute or chronic bronchitis, heart failure, or pneumonia that may be related to alcohol or drug abuse and merit further investigation. A cardiac murmur strongly suggests that active or healed endocarditis may be present. The abdominal examination should be directed specifically toward the liver because most drugs of abuse are associated with the development of hepatic disease. Last, the neurologic examination may reveal evidence of altered mental status, cerebrovascular accident, head trauma, central nervous system infection, or peripheral neuropathy.

Standard recommendations for obtaining preoperative laboratory and diagnostic tests in healthy subjects are often inadequate in patients with a history of alcohol or drug abuse. As in healthy patients, the preoperative laboratory and diagnostic evaluation of alcohol or drug abusers should be guided by the results of the history and physical examination, but a high index of suspicion is required about the possible existence of other subclinical medical complications of alcohol or drug abuse and their potential impact on perioperative management. For example, hepatic dysfunction resulting from drug toxicity or infection is very common in alcohol and injection drug abusers, and obtaining liver function tests, a coagulation panel, and viral hepatitis testing is warranted even if patients are supposedly asymptomatic. Similarly, a tuberculin skin test and a chest radiograph should be performed because subclinical tuberculosis may be present. Serum electrolyte, blood urea nitrogen, and creatinine concentrations and a urinalysis should also be obtained because renal insufficiency resulting from viral hepatitis or HIV infection commonly occurs. Routine screening for HIV should be performed, especially in alcohol or drug abusers who acknowledge high-risk behavior. A positive HIV screen facilitates further testing to confirm the infection, allows early initiation of medical treatment, and alerts the surgical team to the potential for viral transmission.

INFECTIOUS DISEASE IN INJECTION DRUG USERS

Infectious diseases are epidemic in injection drug users,[19] and most hospital admissions of injection users are related to acute infection; the presence of chronic infectious diseases frequently complicates the perioperative management of these patients as well. This section focuses on infectious diseases that are of most immediate relevance to the anesthesiologist (**Table 24-1**).

TABLE 24-1 Infectious Complications of Alcohol and Drug Abuse

Skin and Muscle
Cellulitis
Abscess
Ulcer
Cutaneous or muscular necrosis (cocaine or amphetamines)
Pyomyositis
Thrombophlebitis
Necrotizing fascitis
Cardiovascular
Endocarditis (right > left)
Septic embolization
Hematoma
Ischemic vasculitis (cocaine or amphetamines)
Vascular thrombosis
Mycotic aneurysm
Pulmonary
Septic pulmonary embolism (tricuspid valve endocarditis)
Community-acquired pneumonia
Tuberculosis
Pneumocystis pneumonia (HIV)
Neurologic
Brain or spinal cord abscesses
Cerebral infarction
Cerebral mycotic aneurysm
Meningitis
Encephalopathy
Vertebral osteomyelitis
Botulism
Tetanus
Hepatic/Gastrointestinal
Viral hepatitis (all forms)
Hepatic abscess
Hepatic granulomatosis (talc)
Spontaneous bacterial peritonitis
Renal
Nephrotic syndrome (hepatitis B, HIV)
Nephritic syndrome (hepatitis C)
Rhabdomyolysis
Immunologic
HIV/AIDS

SKIN AND SOFT TISSUE

Skin and soft tissue infections (eg, cellulitis, abscess, ulcer) are frequently responsible for hospital admission of injection drug users, and they may also be initially recognized during the preoperative evaluation. Skin and soft tissue infections with or without necrotizing fasciitis may be present in as many as a third of all active users.[20] *Staphylococcus aureus* and β-hemolytic streptococci are the most frequently identified pathogens responsible for cutaneous and soft tissue infections,[19] but geographic variations in organism identity are regularly reported.[21] The route of administration and frequency of injection, the presence of HIV, and the combined use of heroin and cocaine (known as a "speedball") are known risk factors for abscess development. Ranked in descending order of occurrence, the arms, legs, buttocks, deltoids, and neck are the most common locations for abscess formation and correlate with typically used injection sites.[22] Vasoactive drugs (eg, cocaine) may produce cutaneous or muscular ischemic necrosis at the injection site and contribute to ulcer formation. Infections of large skeletal muscles (pyomyositis) occur more commonly in injection drug users with HIV. Necrotizing fasciitis is associated with substantial morbidity and mortality; aggressive surgical intervention is required to manage this devastating complication.

CARDIOVASCULAR SYSTEM

Endocarditis is one of the most common complications of injection drug abuse.[23] The frequency of injection and the presence of HIV are major risk factors for the development of endocarditis. Mortality in injection drug users with endocarditis may exceed 35%[24] and is undoubtedly higher in those who are immunocompromised. Endocarditis may affect any heart valve, but infection of right compared with left heart valves is more frequent and less likely to prove fatal.[25,26] In contrast to other forms of endocarditis, injection drug use more commonly produces infection of structurally normal right heart valves (tricuspid more than pulmonic). *Streptococcus viridans* and *Enterococcus* are typically identified as responsible for endocarditis in patients without a history of substance abuse, but more virulent species, most notably *S. aureus* (with or without methicillin resistance), are most often implicated in injection drug abusers.

Persistent bacteremia is the major feature of active endocarditis. The diagnosis of the disease is established using standard criteria.[27] The clinical presentation of endocarditis is typified by persistent fever, cardiac abnormalities (eg, new murmur, valvular insufficiency, congestive heart failure, intraventricular conduction defects), septic embolization with bacterial seeding of other structures (eg, meningitis, brain abscess, osteomyelitis), and immune complex–related complications (eg, glomerulonephritis, Roth spots, Osler nodes). Patients often present with cough, pleuritic chest pain, and bilateral pulmonary infiltrates because of septic embolization from the tricuspid valve. Hemoptysis, bronchopleural fistulae, pneumothorax, empyema, or infection of a major bronchial structure complicates necrotizing or cavitary pulmonary defects produced by septic thromboemboli. Echocardiography often provides direct visual evidence of vegetation (consisting of platelets, fibrin, and sequestered bacteria) located on the leaflet surface, but a normal echocardiogram alone does not definitively exclude the diagnosis. Primary treatment of endocarditis with organism-specific antibiotics or antifungal drugs often requires simultaneous surgical intervention to cardiovascular or neurologic sequelae.

Vascular infections also frequently occur in injection drug users. Contaminated injection equipment, hematoma surrounding a direct vascular injury, local ischemic damage from vasoactive drug injection, or thrombosis may cause thrombophlebitis, arteriovenous fistulas, or septic embolization. When septic emboli lodge in the vasa vasorum of an arterial wall, a mycotic aneurysm may result. Right or left heart valve endocarditis-induced septic embolization is the most common cause of pulmonary or brain mycotic aneurysm formation, respectively. Most of these arterial defects resolve with intravenous antibiotic treatment, but some patients with mycotic aneurysms may develop signs and symptoms despite appropriate antibiotic treatment. The clinical presentation of a mycotic aneurysm is typified by the presence of a painful pulsatile mass accompanied by a bruit, thrill, surrounding cellulitis or abscess formation, or frank rupture. Surgical excision is required for definitive treatment of the infection or to prevent rupture in a minority of cases.

PULMONARY SYSTEM

Community-acquired pneumonia is a major cause of hospital admission in injection drug users. Aspiration risk resulting from drug-induced depression of airway-protective mechanisms, poor nutritional status, immunosuppression, and compromised mucociliary and phagocytic function associated with tobacco smoking contribute to increased susceptibility to pneumonia.[28] Injection drug users with HIV are approximately 5 times more likely to develop community-acquired pneumonia than those without HIV.[29] *Streptococcus pneumoniae* and *Haemophilus influenzae* are the most commonly identified pathogens responsible for pneumonia in injection drug users with or without HIV infection, but other bacteria may also be encountered. HIV-positive drug abusers are especially susceptible to opportunistic pulmonary infection with *Pneumocystis jirovecii (formerly Pneumocystis carinii), Mycobacterium tuberculosis, Mycobacterium avium intracellulare*, and cytomegalovirus.

Tuberculosis is also common in injection drug users, especially in those coinfected with HIV.[30] Injection drug users have a prevalence of latent tuberculosis infection that is 3- to 5-fold greater than that observed in healthy subjects. Standard treatment of tuberculosis usually involves therapy with isoniazid, rifampin, ethambutol, and pyrazinamide.[31] Rifampin stimulates methadone metabolism, and chronic opioid abusers in methadone maintenance programs often require dosing adjustments to avoid withdrawal.[32] This drug interaction has potentially important ramifications perioperatively when using opioids for postoperative analgesia. Rifampin and pyrazinamide may also exacerbate preexisting hepatitis leading to severe liver dysfunction in users with tuberculosis.

CENTRAL AND PERIPHERAL NERVOUS SYSTEM

Signs and symptoms of acute drug intoxication or withdrawal often complicate the diagnosis of neurologic infection. Meningitis, brain abscess resulting from septic embolization, cerebral infarction, or rupture of a mycotic aneurysm may occur in as many as 40% of injection drug users with endocarditis. Bacteremia-induced vertebral osteomyelitis with extension into the epidural space may accompany endocarditis, thereby potentially compromising spinal cord integrity. Bacterial invasion from ear, sinus, or mastoid infections, bacteremia resulting from another infectious source, or traumatic injury may also cause infection in the injection drug user. Immunosuppressed injection drug users with HIV are particularly vulnerable to central nervous system infections produced by unusual pathogens such as tuberculosis, *Cryptococcus, Aspergillus*, and *Toxoplasma gondii*. Viral hepatitis may also produce encephalopathy independent of liver dysfunction.

Injection drug users are also susceptible to neurotoxin-mediated infectious diseases. Subcutaneous or intramuscular injection sites infected with *Clostridium botulinum* releases botulinum toxin. The toxin produces blurred vision, dysphagia, descending bilateral flaccid paralysis, and respiratory failure as a result of irreversible inhibition of acetylcholine release. The anaerobic bacterium *Clostridium tetani* produces tetanus toxin (tetanolysin) that irreversibly blocks inhibitory neurotransmitter release in spinal motor neurons, thereby causing spastic paralysis characterized by trismus, dysphagia, hydrophobia, and profound, unrelenting muscle contraction in the upper and lower extremities. Neutralization of circulating tetanus toxin with hyperimmune globulin precedes surgical debridement to avoid additional tetanolysin release from the infected site.

HEPATITIS

Injection drug abuse is strongly associated with all known forms of viral hepatitis. Collectively, these diseases have potentially devastating consequences and pose substantial risks of transmission to anesthesiologists and other health professionals who are responsible for their care. Hepatitis A virus (HAV) is the most common form of viral hepatitis in the United States, and drug abuse is a major risk factor for its transmission. Hepatitis A is often a self-limited disease characterized by fever, fatigue, gastrointestinal symptoms, jaundice, hepatosplenomegaly, and abnormal liver function tests concomitant with sequential appearance of immunoglobulin (Ig)E and IgG anti-HAV antibodies that confer immunity against subsequent infection. In contrast to hepatitis B virus (HBV) infection, a carrier state does not occur with HAV infection, extrahepatic manifestations of the disease are unusual, and most cases require only supportive care. However, acute HAV infection may cause fulminant hepatic failure and mortality in patients who are coinfected with hepatitis C virus (HCV) or those affected by chronic hepatic pathology.[33]

Transmission of HBV among drug abusers most often occurs as a result of sharing contaminated injection supplies or high-risk sexual activity. Drug abuse is responsible for a fifth of new HBV cases reported annually in the United States. Acute infection with HBV has a widely variable clinical course. Many patients infected with HBV remain completely asymptomatic, and fewer than half develop jaundice, hepatosplenomegaly, and elevated serum transaminases. Most patients require only supportive care, but a few (<0.1%) develop fulminant hepatic failure. The presence of antibodies directed against HBV surface and core antigens that occur with the resolution of acute infection confer protection against subsequent infection in most patients. Unlike HAV, a chronic HBV infection occurs in a small percentage of patients (5%–10%) characterized by the continued presence of HBV surface or e antigen, variable extent of hepatic inflammation and dysfunction, and persistent infectivity; cirrhosis or hepatocellular carcinoma may follow. Treatment with interferon-α and lamivudine (3-TC) may reduce the occurrence of these complications. Membranous nephropathy and renal insufficiency may also occur.

As many as 80% of injection drug users chronically infected with HBV are coinfected with the hepatitis D virus, which requires the presence of HBV for activity. Coinfection has a substantially greater incidence of fulminant hepatic failure compared with HBV alone.

Injection drug use is the primary route of transmission of HCV in the United States. The vast majority of injection drug users demonstrate evidence of HCV exposure. Most injection drug users develop the HCV shortly after beginning injection activity. The initial presentation of HCV infection is usually subclinical, but as many as 85% develop a long-term infection. Recent estimates suggest that more than 4 million Americans are chronically infected with HCV.[34] Serum antibodies directed against the virus and the presence of HCV RNA establish the diagnosis of chronic infection. Ominously, as many as 20% of patients with chronic HCV develop cirrhosis, and hepatic failure resulting from this complication is currently the most common indication for liver transplantation in this country. Older patients with chronic HCV who abuse alcohol or those coinfected with HIV appear to be particularly vulnerable to more rapid progression of end-stage liver disease.[35] The combination of peginterferon (interferon with a polyethylene side chain) and ribavirin is currently the most efficacious drug regimen for the treatment of chronic HCV infection and appears to reduce the incidence of cirrhosis and hepatic failure.[36] Chronic HCV is also associated with membranoproliferative glomerulonephritis with or without cryoglobulinemia. Proteinuria, hematuria, hypertension, and renal insufficiency are prominent features of this mixed nephrotic-nephritic syndrome. A membranous glomerulonephropathy produced by the deposition of virus core protein has also been described in injection drug users with chronic HCV. Last, injection drug users with HCV- or HBV-induced cirrhosis are susceptible to bacterial hepatic infections and spontaneous bacterial peritonitis. Enteric gram-negative bacilli are the most common cause of these frequently fatal complications.

HUMAN IMMUNODEFICIENCY VIRUS

Injection drug use is a major risk factor for HIV transmission; the Centers for Disease Control and Prevention identified injection drug use as the presumed route of transmission in 31% of adults with newly diagnosed HIV infection.[37] Injection drug use was also implicated as the primary cause of 39% of reported cases of maternal–fetal transmission of the virus. The use of highly active antiretroviral therapy (HAART) combined with intensive public health emphasis has transformed HIV infection from a "death sentence" diagnosis into a manageable chronic illness. HIV treatment is complex and not reviewed in detail here.

DRUG-SPECIFIC MEDICAL COMPLICATIONS OF ABUSE (TABLE 24-2)

ALCOHOL

Heavy alcohol use (defined as at least 5 drinks per day on >5 days of the week) has been documented in 7% of the US population and is even more common in patients presenting for surgery. Alcohol abuse is a major risk factor for perioperative morbidity and mortality,[41] yet many clinicians often fail to recognize it. Achieving preoperative abstinence before elective surgery substantially reduces postoperative complications.[42] Blood alcohol concentrations as low as 0.05 mg/dL produce acute hemodynamic effects that may have important consequences for patients with heart disease. Mildly intoxicating doses of alcohol reduce myocardial contractility in vitro and cause left ventricular dysfunction in vivo. Such actions cause further reductions in global cardiac performance in patients with preexisting cardiomyopathy. The mechanism responsible for alcohol-induced myocardial depression is unclear. The ingestion of alcohol increases cardiac output in healthy individuals because systemic vascular resistance declines. Conversely, alcohol and its metabolites also indirectly enhance sympathetic nervous system activity, thereby producing tachycardia, arterial vasoconstriction, and attenuation of baroreceptor reflex control of the circulation.[43] These actions combine to increase myocardial oxygen consumption and may contribute to the development of myocardial ischemia or infarction in heavy drinkers with coronary artery disease. Myocardial ischemia or infarction may also occur during alcohol withdrawal in patients with coronary artery disease as a result of elevated sympathetic nervous system tone or coronary vasospasm.

A strong causal relationship between alcohol abuse and hypertension has been established.[44] The combination of chronic alcohol use and withdrawal enhances centrally mediated sympathetic nervous system activity and produces hypertension by overwhelming the direct, but transient, vasodilatory effects of the drug and its metabolites.[43] Heavy alcohol use is linked to the development of coronary atherosclerosis and is associated with increased morbidity and mortality resulting from coronary artery disease.[45] Conversely, consumption of modest amounts of alcohol produces cardioprotection against ischemic injury.[46] Several large-scale epidemiologic studies provided compelling evidence that chronic consumption of small amounts of alcohol reduces cardiovascular mortality, decreases the incidence of coronary artery disease, and improves survival during acute myocardial infarction. Despite these convincing data, substantial individual variability exists, and "rebound" phenomena that theoretically increase the risk of cardiovascular complications are also known to occur with abrupt cessation of alcohol intake. This latter caveat may be of particular importance because temporary abstinence from alcohol consumption is required during the perioperative period.

Chronic alcohol abuse produces a dilated cardiomyopathy characterized by myocardial hypertrophy, chamber dilatation, interstitial fibrosis, disruption of myocyte organelle structure, and severe contractile dysfunction (ie, alcoholic cardiomyopathy). These alterations cause irreversible congestive heart failure.[47] Advanced cirrhosis produces changes in systemic hemodynamics that may obscure the presence of alcoholic cardiomyopathy. Increases in cardiac output occur in response to declines in systemic vascular resistance in patients with decompensated cirrhosis.[48] There is correlation between the extent of hepatic dysfunction and the magnitude of reduction in systemic vascular resistance.[48] Abnormal arterial-venous shunting that accompanies chronic hepatic dysfunction does not appear to be responsible for the decrease in afterload. Instead, enhanced production of nitric oxide is a major cause of cirrhosis-induced declines in peripheral resistance.[49] Notably, the presence of ascites (and the consequent reduction in left ventricular preload) may stimulate compensatory sympathetic nervous system–mediated vasoconstriction that attenuates this vasodilation.

Atrial or ventricular arrhythmias are frequently observed in alcohol abusers, most often after a binge-drinking episode. This "holiday heart" effect usually develops in otherwise healthy subjects without heart disease or abnormal serum electrolytes. An increased risk of sudden cardiac death was also reported in alcohol abusers with or without coronary artery disease, presumably because of malignant ventricular arrhythmias.[50]

Alcohol abuse produces many pulmonary complications that are related to the acute and chronic effects of the drug.[51] Alcohol is a potent depressant of respiratory drive, and intoxication may produce hypoxemia, hypercarbia, acidosis, atelectasis, and respiratory failure. These complications may be more pronounced in patients with preexisting pulmonary or airway pathology (eg, chronic obstructive or restrictive lung disease, obstructive sleep apnea, upper airway neoplasm). An altered level of consciousness and compromise of airway protective reflexes during acute intoxication predisposes to aspiration pneumonitis and adult respiratory distress syndrome. Alcohol ingestion exacerbates bronchospastic lung disease, especially in the presence of histamine-sensitive asthma. Acetaldehyde-induced mast cell degranulation with the release of histamine, leukotrienes, and other inflammatory mediators appears to be a major mechanism for alcohol-induced bronchospasm. Conversely, other patients with asthma report symptomatic improvement with alcohol ingestion. Thus the acute effects of alcohol on airway reactivity may be unpredictable and patient specific. Chronic alcohol abuse also causes several important pulmonary complications in patients with cirrhosis. Large quantities of ascitic fluid reduce vital and functional residual capacities, thereby producing atelectasis, tachypnea, dyspnea, and rapid arterial oxygen desaturation during anesthetic induction. Movement of ascitic fluid across the diaphragm to the pleural space may worsen this clinical picture. Abnormal pulmonary arterial-venous shunts produce hypoxemia in patients with alcoholic cirrhosis. This "hepatopulmonary syndrome" is observed in as many as 15% of patients with cirrhosis and occurs as a result of reduced pulmonary vascular resistance.[52] Enhanced nitric oxide production and altered hepatic metabolism of estrogen and progesterone are possible etiologies of hepatopulmonary syndrome. Conversely, a small minority of patients with alcoholic cirrhosis develops pulmonary hypertension, most likely because the liver fails to metabolize circulating vasoactive substances. The diagnosis of this "portal" pulmonary hypertension may be overlooked because many of the signs and symptoms of right ventricular failure mimic those of chronic hepatic dysfunction. Depression of immunologic function, concomitant tobacco abuse, and malnutrition probably contribute to this increased incidence of pneumonia.

Seizures and cerebrovascular accidents are common in alcohol abusers. Anticonvulsant medications are usually unnecessary for the treatment of alcohol withdrawal seizures because these events are usually self-limited. Seizures occur less frequently during active alcohol consumption. Similar

TABLE 24-2 Medical Complications of Alcohol and Drug Abuse

Drug	Cardiovascular	Pulmonary	Neurological	Hepatic/GI	Renal	Other
Alcohol	LV dysfunction Myocardial ischemia or infarction Coronary artery disease Hypertension Cardioprotection (modest doses) Cardiomyopathy Reduced systemic vascular resistance (hepatic cirrhosis) Atrial and ventricular arrhythmias ("holiday heart") Sudden cardiac death	Respiratory depression/failure Aspiration Exacerbation of asthma Reduced functional vital capacity (ascites) Hypoxemia Hepatopulmonary syndrome Pulmonary hypertension Community-acquired pneumonia	Seizures during use or withdrawal Ischemic or hemorrhagic stroke Cerebral protection against ischemia (modest doses) Impaired cognition Compression neuropathy Peripheral polyneuropathy	Alcoholic fatty liver Alcoholic hepatitis Cirrhosis GERD Upper GI bleeding Pancreatitis (acute or chronic)	Renal tubular dysfunction Renal tubular acidosis Hepatorenal syndrome	Myelopathy Alcoholic ketoacidosis ↓ Potassium ↓ Magnesium ↓ Phosphate ↓ Vitamin K-dependent coagulation factors Pancytopenia Malnutrition Immunosuppression
Sedative-Hypnotics		Respiratory depression Atelectasis Aspiration	Sedation, obtundation, and coma			
Opioids	Reduced LV preload Bradycardia Cardioprotection Endocarditis	Talc granulomatosis Septic pulmonary emboli Mycotic pulmonary aneurysm Pulmonary hypertension/RV failure Pneumo-, hemo-, chylothorax Empyema Mucosal damage Bronchospasm Barotrauma Emphysema Respiratory depression/failure Aspiration pneumonitis Noncardiogenic pulmonary edema Pneumonia Hypersensitivity pneumonitis	Seizures (meperidine, pentazocine) Ischemic or hemorrhagic stroke Myelopathy Guillain-Barré syndrome Encephalopathy	Ileus Intestinal pseudo-obstruction Hepatic granulomatosis	Heroin nephropathy (?) Nephropathy related to infectious disease	Malnutrition Immunosuppression
Cocaine	Sympathetic nervous system activation Myocardial ischemia/infarction Coronary vasospasm Accelerated atherosclerosis Hypertension Ventricular arrhythmias Sudden cardiac death Dilated cardiomyopathy Pulmonary edema Aortic or coronary dissection Peripheral vascular insufficiency	Pulmonary vasoconstriction Reduced diffusion capacity Alveolar hemorrhage Noncardiogenic pulmonary edema eosinophilic hypersensitivity pneumonitis ("crack lung") Mucosal injury Sinusitis Burns ("freebasing")	Ischemic stroke Hemorrhagic stroke Cognitive dysfunction Seizures	Bowel ischemia/infarction Bowel obstruction or drug toxicity (body "packing" or "stuffing") Cocaine hepatitis	Infectious disease-related nephropathies Renal ischemia/infarction Renal insufficiency due to hypertension Rhabdomyolysis Thrombotic microangiopathy	Malnutrition Immunosuppression
Amphetamines	Similar to cocaine Necrotizing vasculitis	Similar to cocaine Pulmonary hypertension	Ischemic and hemorrhagic strokes Seizures associated with drug toxicity Paranoia/psychosis	Hepatic failure (MDMA) Hepatitis A (methamphet-amine)	Accelerated hypertensive renal disease Necrotizing vasculitis Rhabdomyolysis	Iatrogenic hyponatremia Malnutrition Immunosuppression

(*Continued*)

TABLE 24-2 Medical Complications of Alcohol and Drug Abuse (*Continued*)

Drug	Cardiovascular	Pulmonary	Neurological	Hepatic/GI	Renal	Other
Marijuana	Myocardial ischemia/infarction (patients with CAD) Ventricular ectopy	Chronic bronchitis Emphysema CO-hemoglobinemia Fungal pneumonia Hypersensitivity pneumonitis				
Hallucinogens	Similar to cocaine and amphetamines		Hallucinations, delusions, paranoia Seizures Myoclonus Ischemic or hemorrhagic stroke	Hepatic necrosis	Rhabdomyolysis	Profound hyperthermia
Inhalants		Respiratory depression Bronchospasm Hemoptysis Aspiration Barotrauma Asphyxiation Methemoglobinemia (amyl nitrate)	Dementia (toluene) Lead encephalopathy (gasoline) Polyneuropathy (hexane)			Metabolic acidosis (toluene)

CAD, coronary artery disease; CO, carbon monoxide; GI, gastrointestinal; GERD, gastroesophageal reflux disease; LV and RV, left and right ventricular, respectively; MDMA, 3,4-methylene-dioxymethamphetamine.

to previously reported reductions in cardiovascular risk associated with moderate alcohol consumption, several epidemiologic studies have suggested that daily ingestion of small quantities of alcohol may reduce the risk of cerebrovascular accidents (**Fig. 24-3**).[53] In contrast, chronic alcohol abuse is strongly associated with stroke.

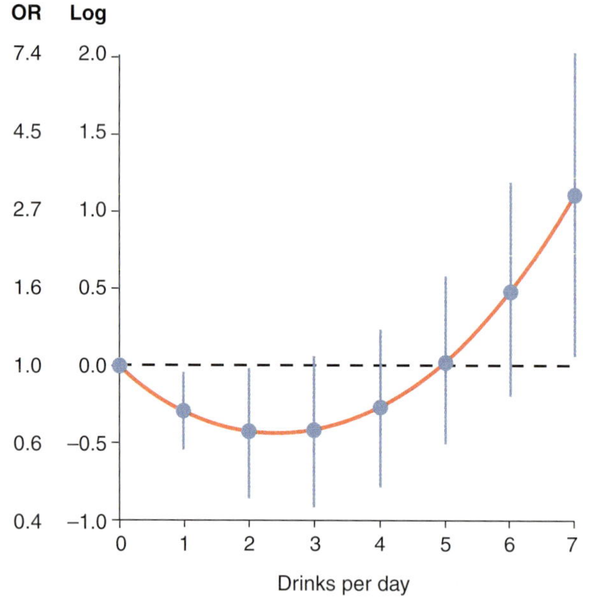

FIGURE 24-3. This illustration depicts the relationship between alcohol consumption (number of drinks per day) and the risk of ischemic stroke (represented as the odds ratio [OR]). Consumption of 2 or 3 drinks per day was associated with a decrease in the risk of ischemic stroke. The reference group used in this study did not consume alcohol for at least 1 year. Analysis was matched for age, gender, race, and ethnicity and was adjusted for hypertension, diabetes mellitus, cardiac disease, tobacco use, and education. [Reproduced with permission from Sacco RL, Elkind M, Boden-Albala B, et al. The protective effect of moderate alcohol consumption on ischemic stroke. *JAMA.* 1999;281:53-60.]

Sustained impairment of cognitive function or frank dementia frequently occurs in chronic alcohol abuse. Severe alterations in cognitive function may jeopardize the ability to obtain informed consent and may also undermine compliance with perioperative treatment. Thiamine deficiency accompanies alcohol-induced malnutrition and produces Wernicke encephalopathy. Confusion, memory and attention deficits, nystagmus, and ataxia characterize Wernicke encephalopathy, which is initially fully reversible with appropriate thiamine replacement. Irreversible memory deficits, amnesia, inability to recall new information, and confabulation are major features of Korsakoff syndrome. Peripheral compression nerve palsies ("Saturday night palsy"), rhabdomyolysis, and compartment syndromes commonly occur because alcohol abusers may lose consciousness and remain immobile for prolonged periods. Alcohol-induced myelopathy and polyneuropathy probably occur as a direct result of drug toxicity, but malnutrition most likely also plays an important contributing role.

Alcoholic liver disease is the most well-recognized complication of alcohol abuse. Hepatic failure resulting from alcohol abuse is responsible for over 25 000 deaths annually in the United States.[54] Until it was recently surpassed by chronic HCV infection, alcohol-induced hepatic cirrhosis was the most common indication for liver transplantation in this country. Fatty liver may be observed in chronic alcohol abusers, but this change may also occur after several days of binge drinking in otherwise healthy subjects. Clinical signs and symptoms of alcohol-induced fatty liver include nausea, vomiting, anorexia, and right upper quadrant pain, whereas liver function tests remained preserved or only modestly elevated. The relative perioperative risk associated with alcoholic fatty liver has not been formally studied, but it may be prudent to delay elective surgery until abstinence is achieved and clinical symptoms resolve. Fever, jaundice, abnormal liver function tests, and right upper quadrant pain characterize the presentation of alcoholic hepatitis. Severe alcoholic hepatitis is associated with high mortality, is often accompanied by ascites, encephalopathy, and coagulopathy, and is a contraindication to elective surgery.[55] Portal hypertension, ascites, esophageal varices, hepatic encephalopathy, spontaneous bacterial peritonitis, and coagulopathy resulting from decreased synthesis of coagulation factors and thrombocytopenia typify end-stage liver disease resulting from cirrhosis. A history of sustained alcohol abuse and characteristic abnormalities in liver function tests establishes the diagnosis of alcoholic liver disease, in addition to clinical signs and symptoms. Markedly increased blood γ-glutamyl transferase concentrations are accompanied by elevations in aspartate aminotransferase (AST) that usually exceed those of alanine aminotransferase (ALT), hyperbilirubinemia, hypoalbuminemia, and prolonged prothrombin time. The severity of alcoholic cirrhosis determines surgical risk; mortality rates for alcohol abusers with Child's classification A, B, and C hepatic disease undergoing abdominal surgery were identified as 10%, 31%, and 76%, respectively.[56]

Alcohol abuse is associated with gastrointestinal complications that are significant for anesthesia care. For example, alcohol abusers are predisposed to acid aspiration. Gastroesophageal reflux occurs frequently during alcohol ingestion because of reductions in lower esophageal sphincter tone. Chronic alcohol use also reduces maximal lower esophageal sphincter pressure. Upper gastrointestinal hemorrhage also increases aspiration risk during anesthetic induction and may occur as a result of esophageal, gastric, or duodenal mucosal injury, esophageal varices, or vomiting-induced tears of the gastroesophageal junction (Mallory-Weiss syndrome). Severe upper gastrointestinal bleeding may cause profound hypovolemia requiring aggressive volume replacement and often compels urgent endoscopic or surgical intervention. Active upper gastrointestinal hemorrhage with or without esophageal varices is a relative contraindication to transesophageal echocardiography. Alcohol abuse is also a major risk factor for acute and chronic pancreatitis.

Hepatorenal syndrome is the most devastating renal complication of chronic alcohol abuse: It is almost always fatal without liver transplantation. Profound hepatic dysfunction, splanchnic vasodilation, and intense renal arterial vasoconstriction are characteristic features of hepatorenal syndrome.[57] Progressive oliguric renal failure and reduced glomerular filtration rate that are unresponsive to volume administration, a gradual increase in serum creatinine concentration, and a markedly reduced urine sodium concentration established the diagnosis of hepatorenal syndrome in the absence of other causes of nephrotoxicity. Hepatorenal syndrome may occur in conjunction with a major complication of alcohol-induced end-stage liver disease (eg, sepsis, upper gastrointestinal hemorrhage) but may also develop insidiously without any apparent underlying cause.

Alcohol abuse produces several acid–base and electrolyte abnormalities because of gastrointestinal losses and malnutrition. Perhaps the most frequent severe metabolic complication is alcoholic ketoacidosis, an anion gap acidosis that usually occurs in alcohol abusers after binge drinking. Hypokalemia is common in alcohol abusers; it occurs as a result of gastrointestinal tract losses combined with secondary hyperaldosteronism and may worsen preexisting hepatic encephalopathy or precipitate rhabdomyolysis. Other common electrolyte abnormalities are hypomagnesemia and hypophosphatemia. Gastrointestinal loss, malnutrition, and alcohol-induced renal tubular dysfunction combine to produce these deficiencies.

Alcohol causes direct bone marrow toxicity and pancytopenia. Iron and folate deficiency with or without acute or chronic blood loss and hemolysis resulting from red blood cell fragility contribute to anemia. Leukopenia and neutrophil dysfunction increase the risk for infection. Thrombocytopenia may be especially profound, and, when combined with reduced coagulation factor synthesis, it substantially increases the risk of bleeding from gastrointestinal causes, trauma, or surgery.

SEDATIVE-HYPNOTICS

The clinical pharmacology of barbiturates and benzodiazepines is discussed in Chapter 42. Briefly, barbiturates, benzodiazepines (including the ultra–short-acting agent flunitrazepam, known as the "date rape" drug), and the gamma-aminobutyric acid (GABA) derivative γ-hydroxybutyrate (GHB, termed "liquid ecstasy") act through GABA receptors to exert anxiolytic, anticonvulsant, amnestic, and sedative effects.[58] The major complications of barbiturate or benzodiazepine abuse are respiratory depression and overdose, especially in the presence of alcohol or opioids. Barbiturate or benzodiazepine abuse produces sedation, obtundation, or coma with eventual loss of airway protective reflexes. Progressive alveolar hypoventilation, hypoxemia, respiratory acidosis, and death subsequently occur. Mortality from barbiturate-induced respiratory depression was previously not uncommon, but the clinical use of these drugs for the treatment of anxiety disorders has been largely supplanted by benzodiazepines or specific serotonin reuptake inhibitors, which have a greater margin of safety. Nevertheless, death resulting from benzodiazepine overdose has been reported, most often in conjunction with the abuse of other drugs.

OPIOIDS

Heroin is the most commonly abused opioid in the United States. The Office of National Drug Control Policy estimates that more than 900 000 individuals in this country suffer from heroin addiction.[59] Heroin and other opioid abusers are at substantially increased risk for a wide variety of devastating medical complications. The clinical pharmacology of opioids is reviewed in detail in Chapter 42. This section focuses on the relevant pathology specifically associated with opioid abuse. Cardiovascular stability is a hallmark of administration of opioids, and even large quantities of opioids (such as those previously used during cardiac anesthesia) usually produce relatively small changes in systemic hemodynamics. Most naturally occurring and synthetic opioids dilate venous capacitance and splanchnic arteriolar vessels. These actions cause modest reductions in arterial pressure independent of histamine release (eg, heroin, morphine). Opioids also modestly reduce heart rate but do not affect left ventricular function or cardiac output under most conditions. Opioids exert cardioprotective effects against infarction[60] and may also produce antiarrhythmic actions in ischemic myocardium. As a result, opioid abuse usually produces few, if any, direct cardiovascular consequences, in sharp contrast to stimulants such as cocaine or amphetamines. As mentioned previously, endocarditis is the most important cardiovascular complication of opioid abuse.

Pulmonary complications are more common; they are responsible for as many as 20% of hospital admissions for opioid abuse. Substances that contaminate the drug or those related to the route of administration cause acute or chronic respiratory consequences. For example, magnesium silicate (talc) is frequently used in oral pharmaceutical preparations or those mixed with an illicit opioid to dilute the drug. Injection or inhalation of magnesium silicate or other contaminants may cause pulmonary granulomatosis, a form of diffuse micronodular interstitial fibrosis characterized by cough, dyspnea on exertion, and diminished diffusion capacity. This "talc granulomatosis" is similar to the presentation of sarcoidosis and may be complicated by direct occlusion of pulmonary arterial branches by granulomas. In addition to this vascular occlusion, chronic hypoxemia and reactive pulmonary arterial vasoconstriction resulting from interstitial fibrosis also contribute to the development of pulmonary hypertension and right ventricular failure. Bullous emphysema is another complication of talc granulomatosis. Septic pulmonary embolization is a frequent complication of injection opioid abuse, as a result of thrombophlebitis or endocarditis. Mycotic aneurysms also occur because of pulmonary vascular seeding with septic emboli. Rupture of a pulmonary mycotic aneurysm may cause life-threatening hemoptysis. Attempted opioid injection into the internal jugular or subclavian vein ("pocket shooting") may cause pneumothorax, hemothorax, chylothorax, and empyema. Smoking or nasal inhalation of opioids produces particulate substances that are distributed throughout the bronchial tree and contribute to mucosal irritation, inflammation, fibrosis, or granulomatosis. Chemical compounds produced by ignition of drugs or solvents also produce mucosal damage. Thus patients who use inhaled opioids are susceptible to the development of bronchospasm, bronchitis, airway injury, or hemoptysis. Barotrauma may occur during inhaled opioid abuse as a result of intense inhalation and breath holding performed to maximize drug uptake. Smoke forcefully exhaled from one user into the lungs of another ("shotgunning") may also cause barotrauma. Finally, chronic abuse of inhaled opioids is associated with the development of emphysema.

The direct actions of opioids on control of respiration, airway reactivity, pulmonary arterial vascular tone, and immunologic response to infectious agents produce several other pulmonary consequences. Opioids bind to mu_2 receptors in the pons and medulla, thereby attenuating respiratory automaticity, inhibiting airway protective reflexes, and reducing the influence of carbon dioxide on respiratory drive in a dose and route of administration-dependent manner. These actions produce respiratory depression, a major cause of mortality associated with opioid overdose.[61] Loss of airway reflexes combined with a diminished level of consciousness further predisposes the opioid abuser to aspiration pneumonitis and its associated complications. Heroin-induced histamine release from mast cells may cause bronchospasm in drug abusers with asthma. This histamine release may occur because of direct activation of mu opioid receptors or through an IgE-mediated mechanism. Noncardiogenic pulmonary edema occurs in as many as half of patients presenting with intravenous or inhalational opioid overdose and is associated with substantial mortality. Opioids may directly increase pulmonary capillary permeability, thereby facilitating accumulation of protein and fluid in the alveoli by hydrostatic forces. A neurogenic mechanism may also cause pulmonary venoconstriction, thereby increasing pulmonary capillary permeability.[62] Histamine release by some opioids also contributes to constriction of pulmonary veins and enhances permeability of pulmonary capillary membranes. Aspiration pneumonitis and pneumonia often complicate the management of patients with opioid-induced pulmonary edema. A hypersensitivity pneumonitis, characterized by cough, dyspnea, and bilateral pulmonary infiltrates, may present several days after nasal heroin inhalation. Opioid abuse attenuates neutrophil and macrophage phagocytosis, reduces T- cell and killer cell activity, decreases CD4 cell count, promotes leukocyte apoptosis (programmed cell death), depresses white blood cell chemotaxis, and inhibits delayed hypersensitivity reactions.[63] These immunologic effects markedly increase the risk and severity of pulmonary infection in the chronic opioid abuser.

Opioid abuse is associated with neurologic consequences. Seizures are a rare side effect of heroin or morphine abuse or withdrawal, and the occurrence of seizures in patients who have abused these opioids should prompt investigation of other potential etiologies. In contrast to the findings with heroin or morphine, seizures may occur with meperidine abuse because of the epileptogenic properties of normeperidine, a major meperidine metabolite.[64] Seizures have also been reported after intravenous abuse of the combination of the mixed opioid agonist-antagonist pentazocine and the antihistamine tripelennamine ("T's and Blues") may also cause seizures. Infectious disease-related complications or renal failure account for most of the hemorrhagic strokes in opioid abusers. A myelopathy distinguished by sensory deficits, paraparesis, and urinary retention has been described in heroin abusers that may be related to spinal cord infarction or vasculitis. Immunologically mediated Guillain-Barré syndrome and brachial or lumbar plexopathies have been reported in heroin abusers. Last, inhalation of heroin vapors produced by heating the drug on metal foil ("chasing the dragon") rarely causes a crippling, often fatal leukoencephalopathy.

Heroin use is associated with the development of focal and segmental glomerulosclerosis. This so-called heroin nephropathy is probably a manifestation of coincident HIV or HCV infection and is not an independent disease process.

COCAINE

More than 3.6 million Americans are chronic cocaine users.[66] Most of the medical consequences of cocaine abuse are related to the pharmacologic properties of the drug[67] or infectious disease implications of its use. In addition to its well-known local anesthetic effects, cocaine produces intense vasoconstriction in nearly all vascular beds. Cocaine inhibits presynaptic reuptake of norepinephrine, enhances actions of circulating endogenous catecholamines, and augments centrally mediated sympathetic nervous system activity. These actions produce tachycardia and hypertension, thereby increasing myocardial oxygen consumption. Cocaine also causes direct epicardial coronary artery vasoconstriction, coronary vasospasm, and prothrombotic effects (eg, increased platelet adhesion and aggregation). These combined actions may produce myocardial ischemia and infarction.[68] Indeed, Mittelman et al reported that the risk of myocardial infarction was increased by greater than 20-fold during the first hour after cocaine use compared with other times.[69] Cocaine use may be responsible for as many as 25% of acute myocardial infarctions in subjects between 18 and 45 years of age[70] independent of route or frequency of administration, drug quantity, or plasma concentration. With the exception of smoking, risk factors for coronary artery disease are most often absent. Angiographically documented coronary stenoses are present in only 50% of these patients.[68] Cocaine inhibits sarcolemmal Na^+, voltage-dependent Ca^{2+}, and K^+ channel conductance attenuates Ca^{2+}-induced Ca^{2+} release from the sarcoplasmic reticulum and reduces myofilament Ca^{2+} sensitivity.[71] When combined with the sympathomimetic and vagolytic actions of the drug, these electrophysiological effects may produce ventricular arrhythmias and sudden cardiac death independent of ischemia or preexisting heart disease. Accelerated coronary atherosclerosis occurs in chronic cocaine abusers and contributes to the risk of myocardial ischemia and infarction.[72] Release of inflammatory cytokines, repeated exposure to elevated circulating catecholamines, enhanced vascular endothelial permeability permitting intimal diffusion of atherogenic lipoproteins, and chronic vasospasm are postulated mechanisms for this accelerated atherosclerosis. Cocaine abuse causes focal myocarditis and necrosis. These pathologic findings are very similar to those observed in disease states in which serum catecholamine concentrations are chronically increased (eg, pheochromocytoma). Cocaine-induced hypertension contributes to the development of left ventricular hypertrophy, dilated cardiomyopathy, and congestive heart failure, especially in patients with preexisting essential or alcohol-induced hypertension. Cocaine abuse is a major risk factor for acute aortic or coronary dissection, peripheral vascular insufficiency, and limb ischemia. A greater risk of aortic or mitral valve endocarditis may occur in intravenous cocaine compared with heroin or amphetamine abusers.[68]

The pulmonary complications of cocaine abuse occur as a result of drug inhalation and are exacerbated by habitual tobacco or marijuana smoking. Like other inhaled drugs of abuse, inhalation of cocaine may cause bronchospasm, chronic bronchitis, barotrauma, hemoptysis, or pulmonary fibrosis.[73] Inhaled cocaine produces intense pulmonary vasoconstriction and increases vascular permeability because of its sympathomimetic properties. These actions contribute to limited diffusion capacity similar to that observed in chronic tobacco smokers. More ominously, inhaled cocaine may cause diffuse alveolar hemorrhage or noncardiogenic pulmonary edema resulting from increased pulmonary capillary permeability.[73] Cocaine-induced pulmonary edema may also occur because of high negative intrathoracic pressures during inhalation or increases in sympathetic nervous system activity in the pulmonary circulation.[73] Despite the acute pulmonary vascular effects of cocaine use, pulmonary infarction has been rare. Irreversible pulmonary hypertension may occur in cocaine abusers resulting from pulmonary arterial medial hypertrophy and the frequent development of interstitial fibrosis mediated by the deposition of talc, silica, or other substances used to "cut" the drug.[73] Inhaled cocaine suppresses B- and T-lymphocyte function and impairs the activity of alveolar macrophages, thereby predisposing the abuser to pulmonary infection. A delayed eosinophilic hypersensitivity pneumonitis that bears many similarities to Loeffler disease has also been described after cocaine inhalation. Pleuritic chest pain, hemoptysis, diffuse infiltrates, hypoxemia, fever, and eosinophilia are characteristic features of this "crack lung" syndrome that usually occurs within hours after binge abuse.[74] Upper airway complications, including mucosal irritation and burns, are common among cocaine abusers. Vasoconstriction produced by nasal cocaine inhalation may cause septal perforation, acute or chronic sinusitis, epiglottis, airway obstruction, or an upper airway vasculitis that resembles Wegener granulomatosis.[73] Severe upper airway burns may also occur as result of freebasing, a potentially explosive chemical process in which a flammable solvent is used to transform cocaine from a salt to a base, thereby increasing the drug's potency. Drugs users who smoke crack cocaine also have a higher incidence of tuberculosis compared with those who inhale other drugs of abuse.

Cerebrovascular accident and seizure are 2 primary acute neurologic complications associated with cocaine abuse. Ischemic strokes, including transient ischemic attacks and cerebral infarction, constitute approximately half of all cocaine-induced cerebrovascular accidents and may be attributed to the combination of cerebral vasoconstriction and a prothrombotic state. Indeed, direct cerebral vasoconstriction was observed using magnetic resonance angiography during administration of cocaine to healthy volunteers.[75] Cocaine-induced hypertension is responsible for most hemorrhagic strokes. Chronic cocaine abusers may suffer from cognitive dysfunction as a result of multi-infarct dementia. Cocaine-induced seizures are usually single grand mal events that most often resolve without the need for therapeutic intervention. Notably, such seizure activity may be observed without signs or symptoms of systemic drug toxicity. Seizures occur more frequently with an inhalational or intravenous compared with an intranasal route of administration. Interestingly, seizures may also develop several hours after cocaine abuse, presumably because benzoylecgonine (a cocaine metabolite) has epileptogenic effects.

Cocaine abuse has several gastrointestinal and hepatic consequences. Mesenteric vasoconstriction and the direct toxic effects of cocaine on intestinal mucosa cause large or small intestinal ischemia, infarction, or perforation. Bowel obstruction or acute drug toxicity has been reported with the intentional ingestion of wrapped packages of cocaine ("stuffing" or "packing") that is performed to smuggle the drug or avoid imminent arrest when in its possession.[76] These complications often require immediate surgical intervention. Cocaine hepatitis is a relatively rare disorder caused by hepatic vasoconstriction combined with toxic oxidative metabolites generated through cytochrome P450 3A1, a secondary route of cocaine metabolism. Cocaine hepatitis develops shortly after drug use and is most often associated with evidence of systemic toxicity. Simultaneous alcohol abuse induces P450 enzymatic activity and facilitates the development of cocaine hepatitis. Cocaine hepatotoxicity also occurs in patients with reduced plasma pseudocholinesterase activity (the major route of cocaine metabolism) because the P450 3A1 pathway assumes a greater role for drug metabolism. Centri- or panlobular hepatic necrosis and marked elevations in serum aminotransferase concentrations are characteristic findings in patients with cocaine hepatitis.

Other acute and chronic renal diseases are quite common in patients who abuse cocaine and are often related to infectious diseases, especially in intravenous users. A nephrotic syndrome characterizes HIV or hepatitis nephropathy, whereas glomerulonephritis results from bacterial endocarditis or sepsis. A mixed nephritic-nephrotic syndrome is most often observed with chronic HCV infection. Renal infarction, accelerated hypertension, rhabdomyolysis, or thrombotic microangiopathy contributes to cocaine-induced renal insufficiency.[77] The pronounced sympathomimetic actions of cocaine and its prothrombotic effects cause direct renal arterial vasoconstriction and thrombosis. These actions produce acute renal ischemia and infarction. Cocaine-induced hypertension clearly worsens preexisting renal insufficiency. Cocaine abuse also causes rhabdomyolysis and acute tubular necrosis. A final cause of acute renal insufficiency in cocaine abusers is thrombotic microangiopathy, a syndrome that may occur and accompany hemolytic uremic syndrome or renal infarction.[78]

AMPHETAMINES

Amphetamines, including *d,l*-amphetamine, methylphenidate, methamphetamine, and 3,4-methylenedioxymethamphetamine (MDMA, "ecstasy"), cause a wide variety of acute and chronic medical consequences. In recent years, abuse of MDMA and methamphetamine has increased dramatically, attracting the attention of federal regulatory agencies and the national media. Similar to the actions of cocaine, amphetamines produce sympathetic nervous system activation, inhibit the presynaptic reuptake of biogenic amines, and exert direct agonist actions on peripheral α- and β-adrenoreceptors to varying degrees depending on minor structural variations in their β-phenylethylamine chemistry. Amphetamines cause dose-related hypertension that may be sustained for several hours depending on each drug's pharmacokinetics. Tachycardia is also observed with methylphenidate and MDMA ingestion because these drugs produce relatively greater β_1-adrenoceptor stimulation than other amphetamines. These hemodynamic effects increase myocardial oxygen consumption and may produce acute myocardial ischemia and infarction, malignant ventricular arrhythmias, and sudden cardiac death. Notably, the cardiovascular effects of amphetamines are potentiated by strenuous physical activity, and deaths attributed to MDMA at nightclubs or dance parties ("raves") may be related to this additive effect.[79] Pathological examination of hearts from amphetamine abusers often demonstrates focal necrosis and myocarditis consistent with chronic catecholamine exposure. Amphetamines produce arterial vasospasm and promote thrombosis as a result of their sympathomimetic effects, and these actions further contribute to myocardial injury. Methamphetamine abuse also causes necrotizing angiitis, a vascular disease of the intima and media that is very similar to polyarteritis nodosa.

Similar to the findings with inhaled opioids and cocaine, inhalation of amphetamines may cause barotrauma, mucosal irritation and hemoptysis, and cardiogenic or noncardiogenic pulmonary edema.[73] Amphetamine overdose may produce central nervous system depression or seizures. Aspiration is quite common under these conditions. In contrast to cocaine, amphetamines are sequestered within pulmonary parenchyma. When combined with pulmonary arterial vasoconstriction, this pulmonary sequestration contributes to the well-known relationship between chronic methamphetamine or methylphenidate abuse and pulmonary hypertension. Epidemiology studies indicated a strong link between the amphetamine derivative fenfluramine and pulmonary hypertension in many patients who had been prescribed the drug as an appetite suppressant.[80] Amphetamines also reduce immune function and increase the risk of bacterial, viral, or fungal pneumonia. For example, inhaled amphetamine increases immunosuppressive cytokine expression and reduces CD4 cell number. These actions may predispose the HIV patient to pulmonary infection.

Cerebrovascular accidents in amphetamine abusers may be ischemic or hemorrhagic in origin. Similar to cocaine, amphetamine-induced ischemic strokes may occur because of cerebral vasoconstriction.[81] Hypertension is the most common cause of amphetamine-induced hemorrhagic stroke. In contrast to seizures produced by cocaine, clinical signs and symptoms of drug toxicity often accompany seizures occurring as a result of amphetamine abuse. Psychological effects are also prevalent with amphetamine abuse. Exaggerated paranoia is a characteristic feature of active drug use, whereas withdrawal may cause prolonged clinical depression as a result of the absence of a stimulant effect.

Fulminant hepatic failure requiring urgent liver transplantation was reported in MDMA abusers.[82] Such hepatic failure may occur acutely independent of drug dose or may develop days or even weeks after abuse. Delayed drug metabolism by cytochrome P450 2D6 in susceptible patients with reduced enzymatic activity or an immunologically mediated cause are proposed mechanisms by which this delayed hepatoxicity occurs. Jaundice, pruritus, severe hyperbilirubinemia, elevated transaminases (AST more than ALT), hypovolemia, hyperthermia, and rhabdomyolysis concomitant with drug abuse are prominent features of MDMA-induced hepatic failure. Methamphetamine use is also associated with the development of HAV. Amphetamine abuse alters kidney perfusion, and accelerated hypertension and acute renal failure are well-known complications of methamphetamine and MDMA abuse. Necrotizing vasculitis with microaneurysm formation and thrombosis may also occur, leading to renal ischemia and chronic renal insufficiency. Rhabdomyolysis and acute tubular necrosis often accompany MDMA abuse, especially during exercise-induced hyperthermia and hypovolemia. Interestingly, many MDMA abusers recognize the risk of developing acute hypernatremia under these conditions and attempt to prevent this complication by ingesting large quantities of water, thereby inadvertently causing neurologically significant hyponatremia.

MARIJUANA

Marijuana or hashish abuse increases heart rate and cardiac output and reduces systemic vascular resistance. As a result, arterial blood pressure is maintained. These hemodynamic effects mirror serum Δ-9-tetrahydrocannabinol (the psychoactive drug in marijuana and hashish) concentration, are more pronounced following inhalation compared with other routes of administration, and are often accompanied by ventricular ectopy. The cardiovascular actions of marijuana are usually well tolerated by healthy subjects but may have important consequences for patients with heart disease. Marijuana-induced tachycardia increases myocardial oxygen consumption. Elevated carboxyhemoglobin levels resulting from smoking the drug reduce myocardial oxygen supply. Thus patients with coronary artery disease who abuse marijuana are at risk of developing myocardial ischemia or infarction.[83] The pulmonary complications of marijuana smoking are similar to those produced by tobacco smoking. Chronic bronchitis and emphysema occur in marijuana smokers, and the additional use of tobacco clearly exacerbates these diseases. Marijuana smoking causes more tar deposition and higher carboxyhemoglobin concentrations than tobacco smoking.[84] These effects are related, at least in part, to sustained inhalation and breath holding, which are performed to maximize drug uptake. Like tobacco smoking, marijuana smoking weakens pulmonary defenses, including alveolar macrophage function, cytokine formation, and ability to combat oxidative stress against pathologic organisms. Chronic, heavy marijuana smoking may also contribute to the development of lung or oropharyngeal cancer. Marijuana is often contaminated with fungi or actinomycetes, inhalation of which may cause an infection or a hypersensitivity reaction. Immunosuppressed marijuana users, including those with HIV, are particularly vulnerable to pulmonary aspergillosis.

HALLUCINOGENS

Similar to cocaine and amphetamines, phencyclidine and lysergic acid diethylamide (LSD) are potent sympathomimetics. Phencyclidine or LSD ingestion causes tachycardia and hypertension, increases myocardial oxygen consumption, produces coronary artery vasoconstriction or vasospasm, and creates a prothrombotic effect. These actions may combine to cause acute myocardial ischemia or infarction. Severe hypertension, left ventricular hypertrophy, and malignant ventricular arrhythmias also occur in chronic phencyclidine and LSD abusers. Notably, the mechanisms by which phencyclidine and LSD stimulate the sympathetic nervous system are somewhat different than cocaine or amphetamines. As a result, cardiovascular cross-tolerance between phencyclidine or LSD and other stimulants may not occur. In addition to cardiovascular consequences, phencyclidine and LSD abuse produce neurologic effects. Like ketamine, phencyclidine causes an acute dissociative state that bears a striking resemblance to schizophrenia. The phencyclidine abuser may be highly agitated and experience delusions, hallucination, and paranoia. Paradoxically, frank catatonia may be present. LSD also produces hallucinations that limit compliance with treatment. LSD users often report "flashbacks" (hallucination recurrence that is temporally remote from drug abuse itself). Abuse of large quantities of phencyclidine, LSD, or other hallucinogens (such as mescaline) may produce seizures, myoclonus, and coma. Phencyclidine or LSD abuse may cause ischemic or hemorrhagic stroke through direct cerebral vasoconstriction or hypertension, respectively. Hyperthermia and acute liver necrosis resembling malignant hyperthermia has been reported in phencyclidine abusers.[85] Rhabdomyolysis and acute tubular necrosis may also occur with the abuse of hallucinogens.

INHALANTS

Inhalants include volatile hydrocarbons (eg, hexane, xylene, toluene) contained in paints, solvents, and adhesives. Teenagers frequently abuse inhalants because they are inexpensive and readily available. These drugs may be directly sniffed or forcefully inhaled using an airtight container ("huffing") to produce rapid intoxication. Inhalant abuse causes many respiratory complications, including asphyxiation resulting from respiratory depression, bronchospasm in the presence or absence of preexisting asthma, airway mucosal irritation, hemoptysis, hypersensitivity pneumonitis, aspiration, and barotrauma.[86] Methemoglobinemia and resultant cyanosis may occur with abuse of amyl nitrate or related compounds ("poppers"). Suffocation by a plastic bag used as an inhalant container has also been reported. Toluene inhalation may cause a white matter dementia in which extrapyramidal signs and symptoms, cerebellar ataxia, and oculomotor effects are present. Inhaled toluene also causes a nonanion gap metabolic acidosis and hypokalemia resulting from formation of the metabolite hippuric acid. Lead encephalopathy has been described in individuals who inhale gasoline. Inhalation of hexane-containing adhesives produces a progressive sensory-motor polyneuropathy ("glue sniffer's neuropathy").

ALCOHOL AND DRUG WITHDRAWAL

Withdrawal commonly occurs during the perioperative period in alcohol or drug abusers, and prophylaxis against withdrawal should be initiated before surgery in patients with a history of recent heavy use. Alcohol withdrawal causes substantial increases in morbidity and mortality.[87] Alcohol withdrawal usually begins within 24 hours after ingestion ceases. The severity of alcohol withdrawal does not appear to be correlated with the total quantity of alcohol ingested or the duration of consumption. Headache, anxiety, nausea, vomiting, diarrhea, and sleep disturbances characterize early alcohol withdrawal (**Table 24-3**). Fever, diaphoresis, tachycardia, hypertension, hyperreflexia, and tremor often accompany these symptoms. Visual, auditory, or tactile hallucinations may also be present, but the alcohol abuser initially recognizes that these hallucinations are not real. Alcohol withdrawal resolves spontaneously in most abusers without progressing to seizures or delirium tremens (DTs). An alcohol withdrawal seizure is usually a single grand mal event, correlates closely with maximal increases in electroencephalographic activity, and occurs in a minority (10%-33%) of alcohol abusers without benzodiazepine prophylaxis.[88] Status epilepticus occurs in fewer than 3% of alcohol abusers who develop withdrawal seizures.[89] Patients who have experienced multiple episodes of abuse and withdrawal are at greater risk of alcohol withdrawal seizures. DTs usually occur 3 to 4 days after alcohol consumption stops. Exaggerated signs and symptoms of withdrawal, vivid hallucinations that are indistinguishable from reality, profound confusion, disorientation, and marked agitation are common. This delirium usually resolves within 72 hours, is more frequent in older patients, and continues to carry a mortality rate of approximately 1% because of delayed or insufficient treatment and the presence of coexisting diseases.

Full discussion of the pathophysiology and treatment of alcohol withdrawal is beyond the scope of this chapter. Briefly, alcohol abuse is assumed to chronically stimulate inhibitory GABA-mediated neurotransmission and attenuate autonomic nervous system sensitivity. In response, an upregulation of GABAergic and central and peripheral adrenergic receptors occurs. Thus anxiety, tremor, hyperreflexia, and a reduction in seizure threshold are observed during alcohol withdrawal because GABA receptors are no longer stimulated and central nervous system excitatory neurotransmission is relatively unopposed. Sudden abstinence from alcohol consumption also causes a rebound activation of the sympathetic nervous system, thereby producing the characteristic findings of fever, diaphoresis, tachycardia, and hypertension during withdrawal. Benzodiazepines are used to treat alcohol withdrawal because these drugs activate GABA receptors and facilitate inhibitory neurotransmission. β_1-or α_2-adrenoceptor agonists may also

TABLE 24-3 Common Signs and Symptoms of Alcohol or Drug Withdrawal

General
Fever
Chills
Headache
Diaphoresis
Myalgias
Fatigue
Piloerection (opioids)
Cardiovascular
Tachycardia
Hypertension
Gastrointestinal
Nausea
Anorexia
Vomiting
Diarrhea
Ophthalmologic
Lacrimation (opioids)
Pupillary dilatation (opioids)
Otolaryngologic
Rhinorrhea (opioids)
Neurologic
Anxiety, irritability, and agitation
Mood disorders
Depression (cocaine, amphetamines)
Drug craving
Sleep disturbances
Insomnia (alcohol, sedative-hypnotics, marijuana)
Hypersomnolence (cocaine, amphetamines, hallucinogens)
Hyperreflexia
Tremor
Disorientation (alcohol, sedative-hypnotics)
Delusion (alcohol, sedative-hypnotics)
Hallucination (alcohol, sedative-hypnotics)
Seizure (alcohol, sedative-hypnotics)
Delirium (alcohol, sedative-hypnotics)
Coma and death (alcohol, sedative-hypnotics)

blunt increases in sympathetic nervous system tone. Close monitoring for developing signs and symptoms of alcohol withdrawal using established guidelines (eg, Clinical Institute Withdrawal Assessment Scale for Alcohol) should be used to direct pharmacologic management and supportive care.

The clinical ramifications of benzodiazepine or barbiturate withdrawal are similar to alcohol withdrawal, largely because the primary site of action of the sedative-hypnotic drugs is also the GABA receptor. Fever, tachycardia, hypertension, gastrointestinal symptoms, and evidence of neurologic excitability occur after abrupt discontinuation of chronic benzodiazepine or barbiturate abuse. More severe withdrawal from these drugs causes hallucinations, seizures, delirium, and death. The elimination half-life of the abused drug determines the onset, whereas the type, dose, potency, and duration of sedative-hypnotic abuse are the major factors that establish the severity of withdrawal. In contrast to the findings during alcohol withdrawal, the duration of benzodiazepine or barbiturate withdrawal may be very prolonged, often extending from several weeks to months. Patients who abuse alcohol or other substances also frequently use benzodiazepines or barbiturates, and withdrawal from other drugs of abuse worsens the symptoms of simultaneous sedative-hypnotic withdrawal. Other factors that contribute to the severity of sedative-hypnotic withdrawal include coexisting psychiatric conditions (particularly anxiety disorders and depression), family history of alcohol abuse, age, and female gender. The addition of an acute surgical stress response may also increase the severity of benzodiazepine or barbiturate withdrawal. As a result, initiation of a cross-tolerant alterative sedative-hypnotic is recommended during the perioperative period to avoid withdrawal.

Prompt recognition and appropriate treatment of withdrawal are also essential in the opioid abuser during the perioperative period. Unlike alcohol or sedative-hypnotic withdrawal, mortality rarely occurs during opioid withdrawal unless significant coexisting diseases are present. Nevertheless, opioid withdrawal is so intensely uncomfortable that untreated abusers often leave the hospital against medical advice. Many opioid abusers report that continued drug use is motivated, in large part, by a desire to avoid withdrawal symptoms. Fever, anxiety, irritability, intense drug ideation, altered thermoregulation, rhinorrhea, piloerection, pupillary dilatation, and gastrointestinal symptoms are prominent features of acute opioid withdrawal. Hypertension and tachycardia also occur in response to sympathetic nervous system activation. The onset of acute opioid withdrawal depends on the elimination half-life of the abused drug. For example, opioid withdrawal usually occurs within 6 hours after heroin abuse, but the onset of withdrawal is delayed if methadone or a sustained-release opioid (eg, oxycodone, morphine) is the drug of abuse. The pharmacokinetics of the abused opioid are also responsible for the duration of the withdrawal symptoms. The duration of abuse, the dose of drug, and the route of administration (intravenous more than inhaled) are also determinants of the severity of opioid withdrawal.

The easiest strategy for managing opioid withdrawal during the perioperative period is methadone substitution therapy.[90] A validated withdrawal evaluation tool to should be used to guide treatment. Using this method, an oral or intravenous loading dose of methadone is administered before the onset of withdrawal. Subsequent doses are titrated until symptoms are controlled and a stable daily dose is established. Methadone may be continued at this constant dose throughout the hospital course or the dose may be gradually reduced as opioid withdrawal symptoms improve. It is essential to recognize that methadone substitution therapy for opioid withdrawal should not be confused with acute or chronic pain management. Perioperative opioid withdrawal may also be treated independent of substitution therapy using a benzodiazepine and an α_2-adrenoceptor agonist administered on a scheduled basis to control anxiety and sympathetic nervous system responses, respectively. Consultation with an addictionologist is recommended to guide perioperative therapy and arrange postoperative substance abuse treatment.

Drug ideation, depression, anhedonia, and hypersomnolence characterize cocaine or amphetamine withdrawal.[91] These symptoms are usually self-limited but may initially be quite pronounced (known as a "crash"). Stimulant withdrawal is usually treated with supportive care alone and most often does not require pharmacologic intervention. Notably, the appearance of cocaine or amphetamine withdrawal symptoms (particularly hypersomnolence) during the perioperative period may be confused with a new neurologic event. Anxiety, irritability, insomnia, and gastrointestinal complaints may occur after abrupt cessation of marijuana use in a minority of patients. Treatment of these symptoms is primarily supportive, but antidepressants may benefit some patients. Specific phencyclidine or hallucinogen withdrawal syndromes have not been described, but some patients report constitutional complaints, including anxiety, fatigue, hypersomnolence, depression, and anhedonia. These acute symptoms and the delayed "flashbacks" of phencyclidine or hallucinogen abuse most often respond to supportive care, but some patients with severe manifestations may benefit from benzodiazepines or antidepressant medications.

GENERAL PRINCIPLES OF PERIOPERATIVE MANAGEMENT

A detailed description of the perioperative management each of the scenarios that might occur in active alcohol or drug abusers is beyond the scope of this chapter. However, the pharmacologic diversity of drugs of abuse combined with the wide range of complications that

TABLE 24-4 General Recommendations for Perioperative Management

Preoperative
- Supportive, nonjudgmental but firm approach
- Obtain a urine drug screen and blood ethanol concentration
- Achieve abstinence and stability of medical comorbidity before elective surgery
- Anticipate and treat alcohol or drug withdrawal, especially in alcohol or drug abusers undergoing urgent or emergent surgery
- Consult an addiction medicine specialist
- Ensure that anxiety and pain are appropriately treated

Intraoperative
- Consider regional or local anesthesia or nerve blocks if possible
- Anticipate hyperalgesia, especially in opioid abusers
- Use general anesthesia or opioids as clinically indicated

Postoperative
- Plan postoperative analgesia including alternative approaches before surgery
- Use continuous local anesthesia, nonopioid analgesics, or alternative pain approaches if possible, but do not avoid opioids if clinically indicated
- Use scheduled but not "as needed" administration of opioids
- Frequently assess behavioral and functional responses to pain therapy
- Integrate initiation of treatment for addiction into the discharge plan

accompany substance abuse requires that the anesthesiologist has a clear understanding of the ramifications of substance abuse and applies this knowledge to the specifics of each patient. The perioperative approach to the patient with addiction varies depending on the type, location, and duration of the anticipated surgical procedure and the presence, severity, and relative stability of alcohol- or drug-related comorbidities. Several general principles should guide the perioperative care of the patient with an active substance abuse disorder (**Table 24-4**). Historical evidence of abstinence from alcohol and other drugs of abuse, confirmed by appropriate laboratory analysis, is strongly recommended before the patient undergoes elective surgery (**Fig. 24-4**) because of the well-recognized increase in the incidence and severity of perioperative complications and the potentially life-threatening consequences of withdrawal. Cessation of drug use before elective surgery also promotes stabilization of many abuse-related medical complications and may increase the probability that the patient will comply with postoperative instructions upon discharge (eg, follow-up appointments, wound care, physical therapy). In some patients, abstinence before elective surgery may be facilitated by frank discussions with the anesthesiologist and surgeon regarding the consequences of continued abuse. Other patients may require the assistance of an addiction medicine specialist to achieve abstinence before an elective procedure. Unfortunately, attaining preoperative abstinence is often an unrealistic goal for many alcohol or drug abusers undergoing urgent or emergent surgery. Under such circumstances, alcohol or drug withdrawal must be anticipated, and appropriate measures (eg, drug prophylaxis guided by history and laboratory tests, anticipated admission to an intensive care unit) should be instituted well before the expected onset of withdrawal signs and symptoms. Vigilance about the potential for drug withdrawal is essential for all patients with a history of recent substance abuse, and the benefits of proactive intervention cannot be overemphasized.

Physicians and nurses should take a straightforward, nonjudgmental approach to the patient. Such a strategy often encourages the alcohol or drug abuser to cooperate with the treatment plan. Patients should be assured repeatedly that withdrawal symptoms, anxiety, and pain will be appropriated addressed. A clear plan for postoperative pain management should be discussed before surgery. Use of continuous local anesthesia, nerve blocks, nonopioid analgesics, neuraxial techniques, or alternative pain modalities may be used for postoperative pain management, but opioids administered on a scheduled basis should be used as clinically indicated. It is critically important that pain be promptly and adequately treated to avoid the development of a "mutual mistrust" relationship between the patient and health care providers.[16] Hyperalgesia is very common in patients with substance abuse disorders, and the

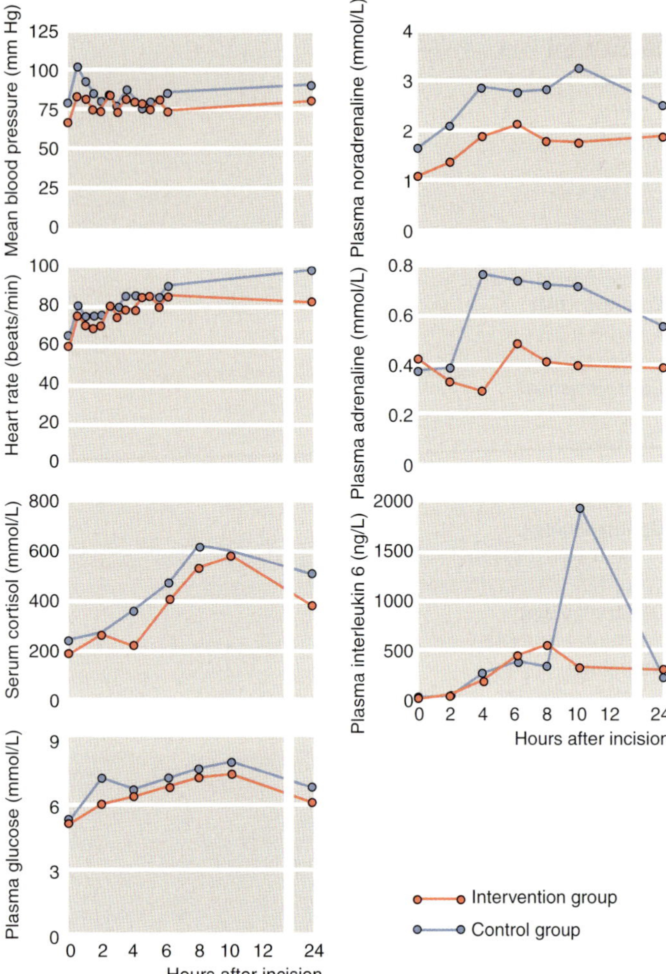

FIGURE 24-4. This illustration demonstrates the effects of a 1-month period of preoperative abstinence in alcohol abusers to surgical stress responses in patients undergoing colorectal surgery. Abstinent patients (intervention group; red lines) had attenuated cardiovascular, endocrine, and inflammatory responses to surgical stress compared with those who were continuously drinking (control group; blue lines) before surgery. [Reproduced with permission from Tonnesen H, Rosenberg J, Nielsen HJ, et al. Effect of preoperative abstinence on poor postoperative outcome in alcohol misusers: randomized controlled trial. *BMJ.* 1999;318:1311-1316.]

anesthesiologist and other clinicians should be prepared to manage pain accordingly. A continuous evaluation of the efficacy of pain management, based on the behavioral and functional responses of the patient, should be conducted throughout the perioperative period.

Active participation of an addiction medicine specialist throughout the entire hospital course is advised. An addictionologist may contribute substantially to the evaluation and treatment of alcohol- or drug-related coexisting diseases, provide guidance about the management of perioperative alcohol or drug withdrawal, and serve as additional resource for pain management strategies. Perhaps most importantly, the addiction medicine specialist also facilitates the transition to substance abuse treatment during postoperative discharge planning. The anesthesiologist and surgeon should recognize that the perioperative experience provides a unique opportunity to intervene in cases of substance abuse.

THE RECOVERING PATIENT

Recovery is a complex process requiring intense, continuous effort that requires abstinence and a series of personal changes to maintain sobriety (**Table 24-5**). Acquisition of knowledge about substance abuse

TABLE 24-5 Therapeutic Objectives in Addiction Management

Affective
- Manage anxiety, depression, shame, and guilt
- Increase coping skills
- Increase emotional awareness of negative consequences of use

Behavioral
- Eliminate drug use behaviors
- Expand healthy behaviors

Cognitive
- Reduce denial
- Enhance personal awareness of addictive disease in self and others
- Increase recognition of negative consequences of use

Physiologic
- Treat withdrawal symptoms and medical consequences of alcohol or drug abuse
- Encourage healthy activities
- Reestablish personal responsibility for health

Social
- Increase personal responsibility
- Increase honesty, reliability, and trustworthiness
- Establish sober social network
- Increase social coping skills

Spiritual
- Increase self-esteem and reduce self-loathing
- Reestablish personal values
- Increase appreciation of transcendence

Adapted with permission from May JA, White HC, Leonard-White A, et al. The patient recovering from alcohol or drug addiction: special issue for the anesthesiologist. *Anesth Analg.* 2001;92:1604, Table 1.

disorders, renewal of self-esteem and personal responsibility, development of sober living abilities and social interactions, identification with sources of inspiration, and a unified approach to guide these changes are essential components of recovery.[92] The terms *cured, former, recovered,* and *ex*-alcoholic or addict are not appropriate to describe the recovering patient. The incidence of relapse may be inversely related to the duration of recovery, but return to use may occur despite many years of recovery. Abstinence alone is not recovery because effective skills for coping with stress independent of drug ideation or use may not be in place. Whether an abstinent individual has more difficulty coping with the perioperative experience than a patient in a well-established recovery program is unknown. Mutual-help organizations including Alcoholics Anonymous (AA) and other Twelve Step programs, individual psychotherapy, behavioral modification, and pharmacologic therapy may all be effective in the management of addiction. The US standard of care in addiction treatment is the Minnesota Model,[93] a multidisciplinary approach that includes participation in a Twelve Step program, individual and group psychotherapy, patient and family education, vocational rehabilitation, and spiritual renewal. The experience of other recovering patients is the key element of the Minnesota Model. AA and related groups are fellowships of recovering patients who help each other maintain sobriety. The Twelve Steps are the central tenet of the AA program that serve as guidelines for recovery. Other components of recovery within AA include regular meeting attendance and sponsorship that increase the likelihood of maintaining sobriety.

Several medications used in sobriety maintenance therapy may have important implications for the anesthesiologist (**Table 24-6**). Alteration of a drug's metabolic consequences (eg, disulfiram in alcoholism), reduction in drug reward (eg, acamprosate in alcoholism), receptor antagonism (eg, naltrexone in opioid addiction), and drug substitution therapy (eg, methadone in refractory opioid addiction) are the major pharmacologic approaches. Several drugs have documented utility in alcohol or opioid addiction, but effective medications for treatment of addiction to other drugs of abuse have yet to be documented. A more frequent incidence of anxiety, psychotic, and affective disorders is also observed in recovering patients. Psychoactive drugs used to treat these disorders reduce the incidence of relapse by limiting self-medication of psychiatric symptoms.

Disulfiram is an alcohol-sensitizing drug that is still occasionally used in the treatment of chronic alcohol abuse. Disulfiram inhibits aldehyde dehydrogenase; acetaldehyde accumulates and a severe aversive reaction occurs when alcohol is ingested. Disulfiram also irreversibly inhibits other sulfhydryl-based enzymes responsible for drug metabolism. For example, disulfiram inhibits dopamine β-hydroxylase, thereby reducing presynaptic neuronal synthesis of norepinephrine. This action may attenuate the cardiovascular response to indirect-acting sympathomimetic amines.

TABLE 24-6 Pharmacologic Therapy in Relapse Prevention

Medication	Drug of Abuse	Pharmacology	Mechanism of Action	Anesthetic Implications
Disulfiram **Calcium carbimide**	Alcohol	Enzyme inhibition	Adverse side effects	Altered response to sympathomimetics; alerted drug metabolism; discontinue disulfiram 10 d before surgery
Naltrexone	Alcohol	Modulation of drug reward	Decreases drug ideation	Altered response to opioid agonists; discontinue 3 d before surgery
Nalmefene	Opioids	Direct receptor antagonist	Decreases euphoric threshold to opioids	
Acamprosate	Alcohol	Modulation of drug reward	Decreases drug ideation	Unknown
SSRIs	Alcohol? Benzodiazepines? Barbiturates?	Modulation of drug reward	Decrease drug ideation; decrease consumption in active users	Rare; may cause hypotension and bradycardia
Antiepileptics	Alcohol; opioids	Reduce neuronal excitability	Decrease drug ideation	Prolonged duration of neuromuscular blockers
Methadone **LAAM** **Buprenorphine**	Opioids	Direct receptor agonist	Decreases drug ideation, positive reward, and withdrawal symptoms	Continue maintenance dose

LAAM, levo-alpha acetyl methadyl; SSRIs, selective serotonin reuptake inhibitors.

Reproduced with permission from May JA, White HC, Leonard-White A, et al. The patient recovering from alcohol or drug addictions; special issue for the anesthesiologist. *Anesth Analg.* 2001;92:1604, Table 3.

Disulfiram also reduces the clearance of benzodiazepines and interferes with the metabolism of barbiturates, tricyclic antidepressants, phenytoin, and warfarin through inhibition of hepatic microsomal enzymes. Calcium carbimide is another alcohol-sensitizing drug used clinically in Europe and Canada that reversibly inhibits alcohol dehydrogenase and may cause less pronounced drug interactions. Naltrexone and nalmefene are mu opioid receptor antagonists that reduce ideation and decrease the incidence of relapse in recovering alcohol abusers.[94] Experience with naltrexone and nalmefene has been less successful in opioid addiction, but either of these drugs may be used as "insurance" in abstinence-based recovery because the threshold dose of opioid required to produce euphoria is increased. The recovering patient who continues to receive an opioid antagonist during the perioperative period will have an increased requirement for opioid analgesics. Conversely, the mu receptor is upregulated during chronic opioid antagonist treatment, and perioperative withdrawal of naltrexone or nalmefene is associated with increased sensitivity to opioid agonists.

Acamprosate is an amino acid derivative that substantially reduces ideation[95] and improves treatment retention in recovering alcohol abusers. Acamprosate decreases neuronal hyperexcitability caused by chronic alcohol abuse by altering GABA- and glutamate-mediated neurotransmission. These actions reduce drug ideation, a major cause of relapse in recovering alcohol abusers. The anesthetic implications of acamprosate are unknown. Antiepileptics (eg, carbamazepine, valproate, gabapentin) also attenuate alcohol- or opioid-mediated drug ideation.[96] Carbamazepine and other antiepileptics hasten recovery from nondepolarizing muscle relaxants by enhancing the drug clearance, increasing serum α_1-acid glycoprotein concentration, and causing postsynaptic acetylcholine receptor proliferation. Selective serotonin reuptake inhibitors reduce alcohol use in chronic alcohol abusers with depression and may also prevent relapse in recovering patients with anxiety or affective disorders.[97] Profound bradycardia and severe hypotension during anesthesia may rarely occur in patients receiving these drugs.

Methadone, the long-acting mu agonist levo-alpha acetyl methadyl (LAAM), and the partial agonist buprenorphine are used successfully as substitution pharmacotherapy in chronic opioid abusers. Methadone, LAAM, and buprenorphine decrease withdrawal symptoms, inhibit drug ideation, and attenuate the opioid-induced positive reward. Patients chronically treated with methadone, LAAM, or buprenorphine remain physically dependent on opioids despite attenuation of the behavioral aspects of addiction. Verification of the dose of methadone, LAAM, or buprenorphine with an addiction medicine specialist before surgery and unconditional administration of the drug throughout the perioperative period are required to prevent withdrawal. Patients receiving opioid substitution therapy may experience exaggerated pain responses to nociceptive stimuli because of drug tolerance.[15] These patients often require inordinately large quantities of additional opioids for postoperative analgesia, and they may benefit from alterative pain control techniques. Substituting a new opioid for methadone, LAAM, or buprenorphine for maintenance therapy during the perioperative period is not recommended. Similarly, increasing the dose or frequency of methadone, LAAM, or buprenorphine administration to provide analgesia should be avoided because the boundaries between treatment of addiction and pain will be obscured.

Anesthesia and surgery may expose the recovering patient to several possible obstacles that increase the risk of relapse. Numerous anecdotal descriptions of drug ideation or relapse after brief perioperative exposure to sedatives or opioids have been reported in recovering patients with years of sobriety, but the precise incidence of such phenomena has not been formally studied. Anxiety about the perioperative experience may be heightened because of concerns about the possibility for relapse and the fear that pain will be inadequately treated. Anxiety and pain are important causes of relapse, and inadequate analgesia produces drug ideation.[98] Recovering patients may also display abnormal behavioral responses to stress that increase the risk of relapse.[99] Similar to the active alcohol or drug abuser, the recovering patient may encounter surgeons or anesthesiologists during the perioperative period who remain cynical about the sincerity or success of the recovery process. Conversely, other apparently well-intentioned physicians may withhold or restrict pain analgesics because they are afraid to contribute inadvertently to relapse. As a result, the recovering patient may be inadequately managed, a situation that may be further complicated if justified requests for additional analgesics are misinterpreted as "addictive behavior."

The preoperative evaluation allows the anesthesia provider to obtain a detailed history of addiction and recovery, and it also provides ample opportunity to allay anxiety. Many patients openly disclose their addiction and recovery, but others may be somewhat reticent to acknowledge this history because of the stigma that remains attached to the disease. Under these circumstances, the history of addiction and recovery may be elicited by tactfully asking direct questions in response to negative answers to routine inquiries about alcohol or drug use. The history of alcohol or drug abuse, type and quality of and compliance with a recovery program, and participation in mutual-help groups are important components of the past medical history. Involvement of an addictionologist, rehabilitation counselor, and sponsor in the patient's recovery should be noted, the duration and relative success of recovery explored, and the history of and apparent factors responsible for triggering relapse episodes identified. Encouraging the patient to intensify the practices of his or her recovery program is strongly recommended because the patient's support system is an essential defense against relapse during periods of stress.[98]

Much of the end-organ damage that occurs as a result of chronic substance abuse is reversible with long-term abstinence, but some permanent pathology may remain that requires further evaluation or stabilization before surgery. A urine drug screen is indicated to exclude drug use and identify the need for further referral. Most recovering patients are aware that drugs used for premedication have abuse potential and may refuse premedication on these grounds. Patients familiar with biofeedback, guided imagery, or meditation may want to use these relaxation techniques instead of drug therapy. Euphoria-associated premedication before surgery may theoretically stimulate drug ideation, but use of anxiolytics to control anxiety may be more important because apprehension and exaggerated stress responses are common in the recovering patient. Twelve Step meetings and increased sponsor contact may also be useful anxiolytics.

Clear strategies for the conduct of anesthesia and the management of postoperative pain should be established with the recovering patient before surgery. Reassurance that the history of addiction will not be an obstacle to anesthetic technique and adequate postoperative analgesia should be provided. The anesthesiologist's broad expertise in pain management also deserves strong emphasis. The anesthesiologist should also discuss evaluation of the recovering patient's possible behavioral responses to pain with the nursing staff before surgery because abnormal attitudes or conduct that may signify drug ideation or loss of control over pain medication need to be identified and promptly reported. Notably, unusual behavior specifically related to pain therapy may also indicate the "pseudoaddiction" (drug-seeking behavior related to inadequate analgesia). In contrast to addiction, extinction of aberrant behavior with adequate analgesia characterizes pseudoaddiction.

Analgesics without abuse potential may initially be proposed for the relief of postoperative pain. These drugs may be used with or without continuous regional anesthesia or selective nerve blocks in some recovering patients to provide adequate pain control and reduce or eliminate the use of opioids (see Chapter 72 for detailed approaches to acute postoperative pain management). Alternative pain techniques may also be considered. Importantly, the potential benefits of these methods must be weighed against the risk of inadequate analgesia, a crucial factor in precipitating relapse. Opioids remain the most efficacious analgesics for treatment of surgical pain, and their use should be guided by specific clinical indications. The selection of the type of opioid and the route of administration may be less important than the scheduling of administration. Mixed opioid agonist-antagonists may have less abuse potential than pure mu agonists, but these drugs are not completely devoid of risk and are often inferior to mu agonists for postoperative analgesia. Neuraxial opioids may be beneficial because of reduced euphoria and drug ideation, but this hypothesis has not been formally tested. Scheduled administration of opioids or patient-controlled analgesia (PCA; administered by intravenous or epidural routes) provides benefits over intermittent dosing by simplifying the pain management plan for nursing staff, reducing delays in drug administration that contribute to inadequate analgesia, and eliminating patient requests for opioids that may be misinterpreted as "addictive behavior." Nevertheless, the use of PCA in recovering patients is somewhat controversial because of the dynamics of self-administration. Prescription of opioids solely on a *pro re nata* basis is not recommended to avoid an association between pain symptoms and administration of the analgesic.

KEY REFERENCES

- Albertson TE, Walby WF, Derlet RW. Stimulant-induced pulmonary toxicity. *Chest.* 1995;108:1140-1149.
- Cherubin CE, Sapira JD. The medical complications of drug addiction and the medical assessment of the intravenous drug user: 25 years later. *Ann Intern Med.* 1993;119:1017-1028.
- Havlir DV, Barnes PF. Tuberculosis in patients with human immunodeficiency virus infection. *N Engl J Med.* 1999;340: 367-373.
- Kitchens JM. Does this patient have an alcohol problem? *JAMA.* 1994;272:1782-1787.
- Linden CH. Volatile substances of abuse. *Emerg Med Clin North Am.* 1990;8:559-578.
- McLellan AT, Lewis DC, O'Brien CP, Kleber HD. Drug dependence, a chronic medical illness. Implications for treatment, insurance, and outcomes evaluation. *JAMA.* 2000;284:1689-1695.
- Qureshi AI, Suri MF, Guterman LR, Hopkins LN. Cocaine use and the likelihood of nonfatal myocardial infarction and stroke: data from the Third National Health and Nutrition Examination Survey. *Circulation.* 2001;103:502-506.
- Rosenblum A, Joseph H, Fong C, Kipnis S, Cleland C, Portenoy RK. Prevalence and characteristics of chronic pain among chemically dependent patients in methadone maintenance and residential treatment facilities. *JAMA.* 2003;289:2370-2378.
- Spies C, Tonnesen H, Andreasson S, Helander A, Conigrave K. Perioperative morbidity and mortality in chronic alcoholic patients. *Alcohol Clin Exp Res.* 2001;25:164S-170S.

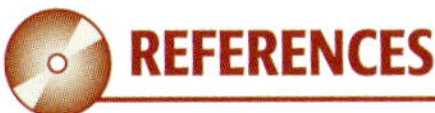

REFERENCES

Complete references available on DVD and online version at www.LongneckerAnesthesiology.com

PART 3

Safety and Risk Reduction in Anesthesia

CHAPTER 25 Anesthesia Risk

Fredrick K. Orkin
David E. Longnecker

KEY POINTS

1. Anesthesia risk estimates are influenced by the circumstances in which they are generated; estimates developed in one clinical setting or selected population may not be relevant to other settings or specific patients.
2. The risk of death related primarily to anesthesia is estimated to be as low as approximately 1 in 200 000 anesthetics in some large populations and reflects improvement of perhaps 2 orders of magnitude over more than 60 years.
3. Despite the very low anesthesia-attributable mortality rate, the very large and increasing number of anesthetics engenders a substantial burden of mortality and morbidity, much of which may be preventable.
4. The very low anesthesia-attributable overall mortality should not be a cause for complacency but rather an impetus toward a greater emphasis on improving anesthesia-related morbidity in selected subpopulations of high-risk patients or high-risk procedures.
5. Approximately 75% of risk actually relates directly to patient-specific characteristics, including age, gender, and comorbidity; 20% to surgical issues, such as experience and judgment; and the remaining 5% to anesthesia factors, including experience, board certification, pharmacologic issues, and overall management of care.
6. The American Society of Anesthesiologists physical status classification correlates with risk for mortality and morbidity, but it is somewhat subjective and, without additional clinical information, is alone not as strong a predictor of poor outcomes as other, morbidity-specific measures.
7. Although randomized clinical trials have rightly become the gold standard for establishing efficacy in clinical research, randomized clinical trials have a limited role in studying anesthesia risk, particularly because they cannot efficiently and at reasonable cost identify the confounding clinically relevant variables.
8. Well-conducted observational studies reveal that anesthesia risk is influenced much more by *how* the anesthesiologist provides care rather than specifically *what* methods are used. Thus careful attention to such factors as blood pressure, perfusion, oxygenation, body temperature, and depth of anesthesia, for example, are often more beneficial than the specific anesthetic drug or technique that is selected.

"What is the risk of anesthesia," patients often wonder. Their concern really is multipart. First, how likely is something to go wrong; then, what "bad things" could happen; and, finally, what can be done to reduce the risk to me and to others following me in the future?

Anesthesia care providers try to allay patients' concerns by citing statistics based on large populations or reassuring that common anesthesia side effects, however annoying, are fortunately transient. Serious, life-threatening complications now are uncommon, if not rare. Such comments may offer comfort, but they do little to specify the magnitude and types of risks that a given individual faces, nor do they indicate that we know how to reduce the risks. The current national focus on patient safety leads to expectations that we provide more to our patients, and this chapter will provide such information.

The concern for enhanced safety has special import for anesthesia care because anesthesia care usually confers no therapeutic benefit but rather facilitates other therapeutic or diagnostic interventions. The potential for harm is expressed quantitatively by a variety of risk metrics, most commonly as the incidence rate for an adverse event. Such metrics enable us to estimate the contributions of various aspects of anesthesia care (eg, anesthesia methods and drugs, clinical care sites, temporal periods) to overall anesthetic risk, allow clinicians to formulate care strategies that are evidence based, and form the basis for comparative effectiveness studies that evaluate new drugs, anesthetic methods, and specific procedures. These diverse efforts have included inquests and closed malpractice-liability claims, case reports and series, study commissions, registries, cohort studies (some with multi-institutional and geographically diverse data), clinical trials, clinical practice guidelines and standards, establishment of the multidisciplinary Anesthesia Patient Safety Foundation, and use of simulation for clinical training, among other initiatives (see Chapter 3).

The intensity of these myriad efforts documents the specialty's commitment to decreasing the occurrence of adverse events and thereby improving anesthesia safety. An almost 100-fold decrease in estimates of anesthesia-attributable mortality among studies over the past 6 decades[1] demonstrates the specialty's high level of professionalism and leadership toward ever-greater patient safety, which has been cited by the Institute of Medicine as a model for the rest of health care.[2]

The risk of death related primarily to anesthesia has been estimated to be as low as approximately 1 in 200000 anesthetics in large populations.[1,3,4] (This chapter emphasizes that such estimates vary greatly depending on circumstances of the given study, and that no rate can be considered representative of all clinical settings.) Yet such figures should not engender complacency among providers; as we will show, the death rate is still 20 to 30 times greater than that of air transportation or working in the construction industry, for example. An estimated 39 to 48 million surgical procedures[5-7] in the United States, plus an uncertain number of diagnostic procedures undertaken with anesthesia, results in several hundred anesthesia-associated deaths each year. Many more—perhaps 10 to 15 times as many—perioperative deaths occur in circumstances where perioperative anesthesia management, surgical care factors, and/or patient-specific characteristics jointly contribute to poor outcomes. Moreover, an even greater prevalence of anesthesia-associated morbidity poses a substantial burden of individual suffering and societal costs. Thus, despite substantial improvement in anesthesia safety, potentially preventable anesthesia-associated mortality and morbidity remain "of sufficient magnitude to constitute a public health problem," as Beecher and Todd[8] noted almost 60 years ago.

This chapter surveys the factors that the practitioner needs to understand both to gain a greater understanding of anesthesia risk and to interpret the literature on anesthesia risk appropriately.

WHAT IS ANESTHESIA RISK?

The concepts risk and hazard are sometimes confused: A *hazard* has the potential to cause harm; examples include stairs, automobiles, motorcycles, hospitals, hypertension, and anesthesia. In contrast, *risk* refers to the *likelihood* of harm resulting from a hazard: Risk is *the probability of an event within a population during a specified period of time.*[9] Although risk is ubiquitous and a natural part of life, it is not uncontrollable; it can be mitigated by knowledge, attitudes, and behaviors. Typically, risk is influenced by a variety of "risk factors," including especially human behavior, equipment, colleagues, fatigue, location, and experience. In common usage, *anesthesia risk* connotes negative occurrence, such as death or injury.

Risk quantifies the occurrence of a *specific* outcome within a *specified* population that is exposed to a *specific* hazard (eg, anesthesia, air travel) under *specific* conditions. For example, the population receiving general anesthesia might share exposure to a hazard (eg, loss of protective airway reflexes) during the period of observation; however, only some among the population develop an adverse outcome (eg, aspiration pneumonitis) that is associated with this hazard. Although the definition of risk is precise, risk estimates can vary widely to the casual observer. Such variation usually results from differences in study design, not from differing definitions of risk. Careful reading of a report often reveals possible sources of the differences (**Box 25-1**).

Although the bulk of the anesthesia risk literature relates to estimates of risk (including identification of risk factors), an important

BOX 25-1

Common Sources of Differences in Anesthesia Risk Estimates Among Studies

Characteristics of study population (eg, age, gender, comorbidities, genomics)

Magnitude or duration of the exposure

Definition of the outcome

Surveillance interval following exposure

Sensitivity and specificity of the diagnostic methods used to identify the outcome

Method of attributing outcome to anesthesia management

Characteristics of the health care setting

Sampling variation (especially with small sample size)

Other factors that might affect the likelihood of the occurrence of the outcome

subset of our risk literature relates to the other, less common usage of *risk*: descriptions of specific adverse outcomes. Examples include case reports, case series (eg, critical incident studies[10]), and registries such as the American Society of Anesthesiologists (ASA) Closed Claims Project.[11] Because such reports do not include information on the "at-risk" or "exposed" population, incidence rates cannot be estimated and risk factors for the occurrence of the outcomes cannot be identified. Yet such reports are widely used to alert us to possible, but still unquantified, risks, and they have been especially useful in developing initiatives to improve safety (see Chapter 3 and this chapter).

HOW DOES ANESTHESIA RISK DIFFER FROM ANESTHESIA SAFETY?

Risk and *safety* often are discussed colloquially as if they were closely related, yet they are not. Whereas *risk* is an objective, probabilistic term, *safety* connotes personal and/or social value judgment about the acceptability of a given level of risk.[12,13] We generally regard as safe that which poses an acceptable level of risk, given that nothing is risk free.[13,14] The acceptability of a given risk level is a function of each individual's *risk tolerance,* which, in turn, is influenced by factors characterizing the adverse outcome, exposure, and perceptions of the individual evaluating the risk (**Box 25-2**).[12,15] The tolerance for risk varies considerably among individuals. Not surprisingly, parents are generally much more concerned about the safety of anesthesia for their children than for themselves, even though the risk of injury is generally similar.

HOW IS ANESTHESIA RISK MEASURED?

MODELS FOR STUDYING ANESTHESIA RISK

Approaches to studying anesthesia risk have evolved over time. Most investigators who published before the late 1980s were guided by a restrictive model that focused almost exclusively on serious clinical outcomes (deaths, adverse events; see **Fig. 25-1**). In this approach, a population of patients is "exposed" to the dual "hazards" of anesthesia and surgery, and the model counts clinical outcomes that result from this experience.

A newer model (**Fig. 25-2**), consistent with studies of anesthesia risk undertaken since the latter 1980s, recognizes that anesthesia care and surgery occur in a complex matrix of administrative, cultural, and clinical processes, all of which can add hazards to the system. This model also includes a broader array of outcomes that include cost, functional status, and patient satisfaction (**Box 25-3**). These assume greater importance now with the growing call throughout medicine for greater patient-centered care (see Chapter 3).

QUANTIFYING ANESTHESIA RISK

If exposure to a "hazard" increases the likelihood of an adverse outcome, then duration of exposure should be a better predictor of a negative outcome than just occurrence of exposure. Indeed, this intuitive notion is the basis for the investigative approach in toxicologic and epidemiologic studies of health hazards. Time-related exposure risks (eg, 1-year odds) of real-world health hazards have been tabulated.[15] Runciman and Moller[17] applied this notion to quantify the mortality risk of anesthesia and complex surgery in relation to a variety of real-world hazards (**Box 25-4**). Although the mortality rates are only approximations, the relative risks are informative for both providers and patients, who can more clearly understand that anesthesia is 20 times more hazardous than commercial flight but 10 times safer than parachute jumping!

Unfortunately, there are few anesthesia risk studies examining time-related hazards. Many studies note an association between greater

BOX 25-2

Factors Associated With Decreased Tolerance for Risk

A. Features of the adverse outcome
   1. Greater versus lesser severity
   2. Permanence versus reversibility
   3. High versus low frequency
   4. "Dread disease," especially social and economic implications
   5. Immediate versus delayed onset
   6. Occurrence in all people versus only in sensitive people
   7. Relationship to intervention known with certainty versus not well established

B. Characteristics of exposure (intervention)
   1. Optional (eg, cosmetic services, treatment for self-limited disease) versus essential (eg, therapy for life-threatening disease)
   2. Related to exposure versus its absence
   3. Alternatives available versus only available intervention
   4. Imposed versus voluntarily assumed
   5. Misuse is likely versus unlikely

C. Perceptions of evaluator (regarding circumstances of exposure)
   1. New versus established
   2. Synthetic or imposed versus natural
   3. Greater uncertainty versus highly predictable result
   4. Less knowledge of situation
   5. Less personal control versus more control
   6. Less trust in the circumstances versus greater trust
   7. Relates to one's child versus oneself versus a stranger

Modified from Strom BL, Kimmel SE, eds. *Textbook of Pharmacoepidemiology.* Copyright © 2007, John Wiley & Sons Ltd. Reproduced with permission;

Ropeik D, Gray G. *Risk: A Practical Guide to Deciding What's Really Safe and What's Really Dangerous in the World Around You.* Boston: Houghton Mifflin; 2002:16-18, 421-428.[15]

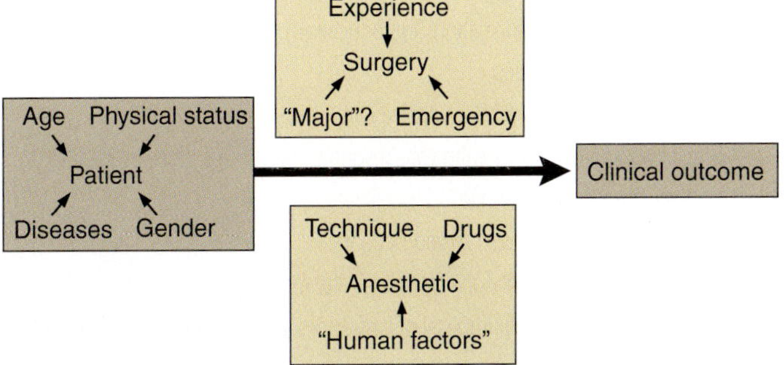

FIGURE 25-1. Traditional model of the determinants of the patient's clinical outcome after surgery and anesthesia care. [Modified from Orkin FK. Patient outcome following anesthesia care: role of the provider. *Probl Anesth.* 1992;6(2):212-227.][16]

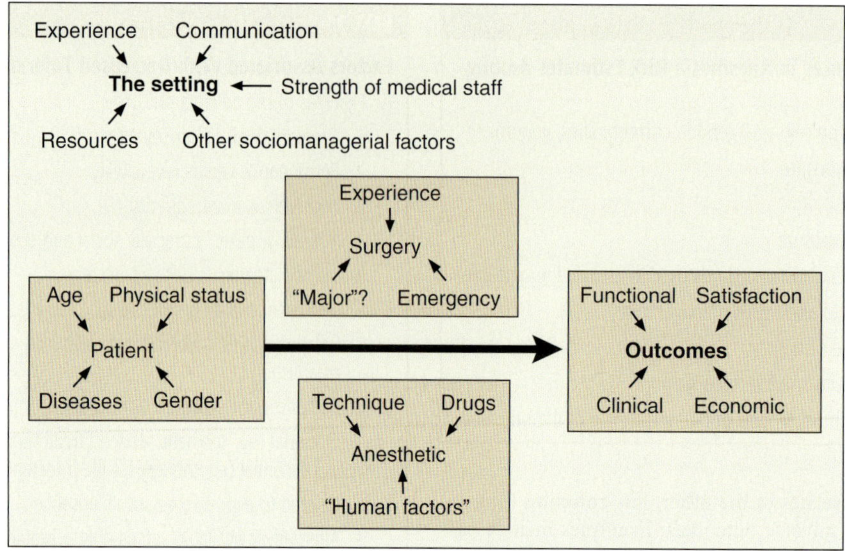

FIGURE 25-2. Revisionist model of the determinants of the patient's outcomes after surgery and anesthesia care. This model acknowledges that the outcomes are far broader than purely clinical and that the care setting has diverse influences on the care and its results. [Modified from Orkin FK. Patient outcome following anesthesia care: role of the provider. *Probl Anesth.* 1992;6(2):212-227.][16]

duration of anesthesia (or surgery) and poorer outcome, but longer anesthesia also reflects longer and/or more complicated surgery, making it difficult to separate the independent role of anesthesia. However, recent research documents that anesthetic depth—or cumulative deep hypnotic time, estimated as the cumulative duration of low Bispectral Index Sensor (BIS <45)—is an independent predictor of postoperative[18-22] and criticalcare mortality,[22] particularly in combination with patient comorbidity and intraoperative hypotension.

In the absence of time-related risk data, anesthesia risk is commonly summarized as an incidence rate computed as the quotient of the number of cases and the overall population:

$$\text{Risk} = \text{Incidence rate} = \frac{\text{Persons with outcome}}{\text{Population exposed to hazard}}$$

BOX 25-3

Taxonomy of Outcomes

I. Clinical outcomes
   A. Clinical end points
      1. Symptoms (eg, nausea, cough)
      2. Laboratory values (especially abnormal values)
   B. Complications and adverse events (eg, dental injury, pulmonary aspiration, arrhythmia, cardiac arrest)
   C. Death
II. Functional health status (health-related quality of life)
   A. Physical
   B. Mental (including psychological and well-being)
   C. Social
   D. Role
III. Patient satisfaction
   A. Patient-based assessment of care
      1. Quality (eg, satisfaction with pain control)
      2. Convenience
      3. Access to care
      4. Adequacy of information (eg, education)
IV. Economic consequences
   A. Length of stay (hospital, intensive care unit)
   B. Utilization of specific health care resources (eg, drugs, tests, procedures)
   C. Institutional performance
      1. Readmission of discharged patients
      2. Unplanned admissions from ambulatory surgery
      3. Other institutional implications of errors and complications ("rework")
   D. Costs
      1. Direct costs
      2. Indirect costs (eg, lost wages, lost productivity, disability)

BOX 25-4

Average Fatal Accident Incidence Rates (Deaths per 100 Million Hours of Exposure)

Being pregnant	1
Traveling by train	5
Working at home	8
Working in agriculture	10
Testing positive for human immunodeficiency virus after receiving a transfusion of 1 unit of blood	10
Being in traffic (overall, in any capacity)	50
Working in the construction industry	67
Flying in a commercial aircraft	100
Being a patient in an Australian hospital	2000
Being anesthetized	2000
Parachute jumping	20 000
Having elective abdominal aortic surgery	200 000
Having emergent abdominal aortic surgery	2 000 000

Modified from Runciman WB, Moller JJ. *Iatrogenic Injury in Australia*. Adelaide, Australia: Australian Patient Safety Foundation: 2001: Table 1. http://www.apsf.net.au. Accessed June 15, 2010.

Four important features of this simple relationship are apparent. First, a risk cannot be estimated without knowing the size of the population from which the cases (ie, those with the outcome) arose. Thus the absence of the denominator precludes estimating risk in studies using case series and registry data, and imprecision in estimating the size of the population influences the computed risk.

Second, risk estimates can range from 0 (ie, no one experiences the outcome) to 1 (ie, everyone suffers the outcome). Depending on the outcome studied, anesthesia risk estimates span much of this range, from death primarily related to anesthesia care in large unselected populations (eg, as low as 0.000005) to postoperative nausea in especially susceptible individuals under specific circumstances (eg, as high as 0.8). Because decimal values can be unwieldy and awkward in conversation, we commonly refer to risks as percentages (eg, the risk of perioperative death in relation to cardiac surgery is "3.0%" rather than "0.03"). For smaller risk values, we often express the risk in either the scientific notation (eg, 5×10^{-6} rather than 0.000005) or, more commonly, the ratio of 1 to the smallest number of individuals whose exposure to the hazard would result in one case (eg, risk of death primarily related to anesthesia is "1 in 200 000" or "1:200 000" rather than "0.000005").

Third, by definition, the calculated risk is the risk faced by the population under study, whereas we are often interested in the risk faced by a particular individual or perhaps a specific group of individuals who were not part of the study population and may have special characteristics that might place them at greater or lesser risk. Thus risk estimates in the literature, especially some very low mortality rates widely touted in public media, may not relate well to the person(s) about whom we are concerned. Again, risk estimates are very much the products of the circumstances in which they are generated (Box 25-1).

Fourth, this simple and common risk calculation is but one approach to expressing the magnitude of risk. The magnitude of risk can be expressed in alternative ways, some of which are particularly useful in understanding clinical trial results and comparing treatment benefit or harm across studies (**Table 25-1**).[23] Such risk metrics are easily computed from summary results presented in the literature (**Box 25-5**).

TABLE 25-1 Risk Metrics Developed With the Epidemiologist's 2 × 2 Table

		Outcome		
		Present	Absent	
Exposure	Present	a	b	
	Absent	c	d	
Risk Metric	**Definition**			**Calculation**
Relative risk (RR)	Proportion of original risk present with new intervention			$\frac{a/(a+b)}{a/(c+b)}$
Relative risk reduction (RRR)	Proportion of outcome risk removed by intervention			$\frac{c/(c+d) - a/(a+b)}{c/(c+d)}$
Absolute risk reduction (ARR)	Proportion of persons spared outcome by intervention			$\frac{c}{c+d} - \frac{a}{a+b}$
Number needed to treat (NNT)	Number of persons treated with intervention to save one			$\frac{1}{ARR}$
Odds ratio (OR)	Ratio of proportion of persons with outcome to those without outcome			$\frac{a/b}{c/d}$

Modified from Table 7-1 by Jaeschke R, Guyatt G, Barratt A, et al. Does treatment lower risk? Understanding the results. In: Guyatt G, Rennie D, eds. *Users' Guides to the Medical Literature: A Manual for Evidence-Based Clinical Practice*. 2nd ed. New York, NY: McGraw-Hill, 2008:88.

BOX 25-5

Calculating Risk Metrics

We can often extract greater risk-related information from studies, particularly clinical trials, by calculating a set of risk metrics (Table 25-1).[23] The first step is to express the study results in an epidemiologist's "2 × 2 table" and then compute a set of risk metrics.

Example 1: How effective is intensive insulin therapy in intensive care?

Van den Berghe et al[24] reported that an intensive insulin regimen was associated with a 48% decrease ($p = 0.005$) in mortality among those receiving more than 5 days of intensive care. Such a decrease certainly appears very meaningful, yet a small *p* value is not a measure of *clinical* significance and is influenced by sample size. Creating a 2 × 2 table from their results (a = 22, b = 208, c = 49, d = 243), we can calculate the number needed to treat (NNT) of 13.6. Such a relatively very low NNT value indicates that the intensive insulin regimen is a very potent intervention.

Example 2: Reconciling perioperative prophylactic atenolol recommendations.

Mangano et al[25] recommended prophylactic perioperative atenolol for all patients at risk for coronary artery disease, but later Lindenauer et al[26] suggested that β-blocker use be reserved only for patients at high risk because lower-risk patients may be harmed. Can we reconcile the 2 recommendations? One hypothesis is that Mangano et al studied higher-risk patients. From a 2 × 2 table constructed from Mangano's principal results (a = 9, b = 90, c = 12, d = 89), we calculate risk metrics, including a NNT of 36 and odds ratio of 0.74. These risk metrics approximate those for the highest-risk patients studied by Lindenauer et al, thus supporting our hypothesis and suggesting that only the high-risk patients should receive prophylactic β-blocker drugs.

RISK VALUES ARE ESTIMATES

Risk values are estimates, and estimates from small samples can vary greatly. For this reason, randomized clinical trials usually involve thousands of patients and, even then, we may learn of new risks in subsequent postmarketing surveillance. Small trials that report "no complications" or similar are especially suspect, and unfortunately small trials are all too common in the medical literature, especially for new procedures (new drugs tend to be evaluated more fully). Thus our personal confidence in small trials or case series should be suspect,[27] and this is expressed mathematically as the *confidence interval* (CI).

As the sample size increases, the CI for the estimated rate narrows, enhancing the precision of that estimate (**Fig. 25-3** and **Box 25-6**).[28] Thus, other things being equal, we regard rates calculated from larger cohorts as more reliable than those from smaller studies, and the statistics support our intuition.

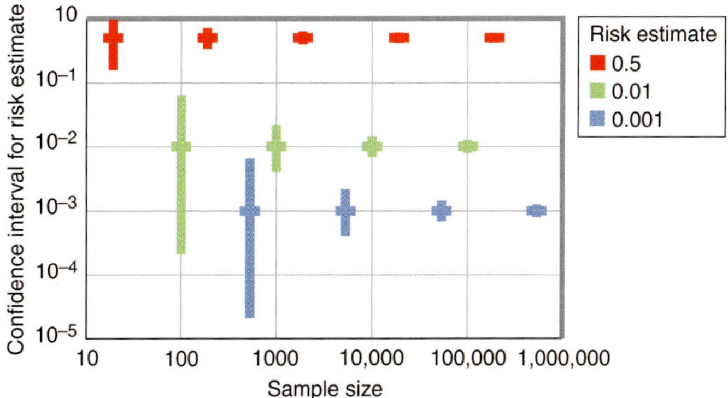

FIGURE 25-3. Span of 95% confidence interval (*vertical bar*) as a function of risk estimate (*horizontal line in vertical bar*) and sample size. Smaller risk estimates require sharply increasing sample size for precision.

BOX 25-6

Calculating Confidence Intervals

When perusing medical literature, physicians hone in on *p* values, looking specifically for values (eg, "<0.05") that are commonly accepted to denote "statistical significance." The latter is not a measure of *clinical* significance, and a smaller *p* value does not indicate a stronger basis for clinical decision making. Indeed, the *p* value tells whether the study result could have happened by chance (not necessarily of great relevance to the clinician); also, the size of the *p* value is sensitive to the study's sample size (ie, smaller *p* value for same "effect size" with larger sample size).

Instead, recognizing that study results vary, the clinician is most interested in knowing the range in which the study result is likely to lie, were the study to be repeated. The 95% *confidence interval* (CI) is the range in which the result would lie in 95 of the next 100 repeat studies.[28]

A special situation arises when an outcome of interest (eg, a complication) does not occur, in which case the rate obviously is 0. But we can have little confidence that the true rate is 0%. Clearly, the lower limit of the confidence interval is 0%, but what is the upper limit? Although we can resort to statistical software or tables, a handy "rule of 3" computes an estimate of the upper limit of the 95% CI: the quotient of 3 divided by the sample size in which no event was observed.[27] (Similarly, there is a "rule of 5" for estimating the upper limit of the 99% CI.)

Example 1: Among 9152 gastroenterologic endoscopies in an ambulatory surgery center where nurses administer propofol sedation, using an anesthesiologist-furnished protocol, there were 7 cases (0.08%) of "respiratory compromise" (3 prolonged apnea, 3 laryngospasm, 1 aspiration requiring hospitalization).[29] What is the likely variation about this rate? Using statistical software, we compute the 95% CI to be 0.03%-0.16%, suggesting that these important complications are likely to continue to be rare.

Example 2: A clinical trial of gastroenterologist-administered sedation for advanced upper endoscopy compared propofol in 38 patients with meperidine/midazolam in 37 patients.[30] Apart from brief, transient respiratory depression monitored by capnography, no major complications occurred. How confident can we be about the risk of major complications? Using the rule of 3, we compute the upper limit of the 95% CI as approximately 8% (statistical software: 9.5% and 9.3%, respectively). Thus, with the risk of a severe complication as high as 1:11, this small trial does not instill a sense of safety.

WHAT ARE THE CHALLENGES IN ESTIMATING ANESTHESIA RISK?

GENERIC CHALLENGES IN STUDYING ANESTHESIA RISK

Identifying the Outcomes of Interest

Diagnostic Problems Diagnosing or identifying an adverse event is critical to the assessment of risk and not a trivial problem. Identifying the occurrence of death might seem inordinately simple, but postanesthesia death may not be recognized if the defined surveillance interval is brief, such as the first 48 hours postoperatively or only during hospitalization. This *ascertainment bias* results in underestimation of the true mortality rate. Even greater challenges are posed by adverse events that present in a graded fashion, from barely detectable to life threatening. Thus differences in incidence rates can be influenced greatly by the prevalent diagnostic methods or definitions. For example, the observed rate of myocardial ischemia is greater if the diagnosis is made by continuous Holter monitoring than by clinical symptoms such as angina. Such imprecision constitutes an important source of systematic error (ascertainment bias, information bias) that can lead to failure to recognize outcome occurrences (misclassification bias) and inaccurate risk estimates.

Diagnostic challenges often are compounded by problems with the definitions and classifications inherent in clinical information systems and administrative databases. Institutional clinical information systems may use nonstandard definitions for data elements, such as adverse events, diagnoses, surgical procedures, and thresholds for abnormalities among laboratory values. Administrative databases, which classify the diagnoses, complications, and surgical procedures relating to care in a standard procedure coding system, are subject to institutional variation in coding practices and typically have few anesthesia-specific categories (eg, "E" codes in the *International Classification of Diseases, Ninth Revision, Clinical Modification [ICD-9-CM]* system), and some can be quite arcane (eg, ICD-9-CM code 968.3: poisoning by intravenous anesthetics).

Surrogate End Points Even if the outcome of interest (eg, death, specific adverse event) can be identified accurately, it may occur so infrequently that a proposed study may not be feasible. Thus investigators have opted for alternative end points that are surrogates or intermediate variables—symptoms, signs, clinical events, laboratory values, and even process variables—which occur more often and are believed to be linked to that outcome. Elevated blood pressure is used as an end point in clinical trials because high blood pressure is a known risk factor for stroke and myocardial infarction (MI); similarly, myocardial ischemia is commonly used as a surrogate for MI.

Such approaches are appropriate only if the surrogate end point truly predicts the occurrence of the outcome. However, this requirement is often not met, possibly because the outcome may occur via some pathway(s) not mediated by the surrogate.[31] Among recent examples is use of ventricular ectopy as the surrogate end point in the evaluation of drugs to prevent sudden death. Food and Drug Administration approval of a new class of antiarrhythmic drugs followed clinical trials demonstrating efficacy of such drugs in treating ventricular ectopy, but a subsequent trial revealed a *greater* risk for sudden death among those receiving the new drugs, and the drugs were withdrawn.[32] Problematic surrogate end points in anesthesia have included the interval to eye opening after general anesthesia, which does not correlate well with earlier discharge after ambulatory surgery, lower rate of unplanned hospital admission after ambulatory surgery, greater patient satisfaction, or overall lower cost of care.[33]

Broadened Array of Outcomes End points of interest have expanded from "clinical outcome" to a more comprehensive set of "outcomes" that reflect many facets of the care process, particularly factors that are important from the patient's perspective, or administrative end points such as the cost of services (Box 25-3). Studies of anesthesia risk already include some nonclinical outcomes, such as unplanned hospital admission after ambulatory surgery[34,35] and poorer quality of immediate postoperative recovery.[36] Patient-reported outcome measures[37] include health-related quality-of-life[38,39] scales (eg, Medical Outcome Study's SF-36 Health Survey[40]) and disease- and condition-specific specific scales (eg, Visual Analog Scale for Pain,[41] McGill Pain Questionnaire[42]). Such instruments have been validated in large populations, typically with chronic disease, for use in longitudinal and cross-sectional studies,[43] and they have been used in chronic pain clinics.

Patient-Specific Descriptive Data Risks are not distributed randomly. Some individuals are more likely to experience health problems as a result of diverse factors, including genetics, coexisting disease, personal health behaviors (eg, smoking, poor diet, sedentary living), socioeconomic status, and environmental setting. Thus estimating anesthesia risk requires accurate information to characterize each patient, including nonclinical information. Such information enables categorizing patients by likelihood of poor outcome (risk stratification) and "risk adjusting" their data for outcome comparisons.[44]

The ASA physical status classification originally was advanced to standardize terminology and group patients[45-47] but subsequently was found to correlate with clinical outcomes.[34,48-51] In addition, the Charlson Comorbidity Score,[52] a disease-specific classification system, is increasingly used in anesthesia risk studies. With growing interest in health care disparities, noting the patient's race and ethnicity accurately is important, typically using categories from the US Census Bureau (white, black or African American, Hispanic or Latino, Asian or Pacific Islander, or American Indian or Alaskan Native).[53] Differential selection for surgical procedures is associated with race: Blacks are more likely to receive nonoperative care for hip fracture, and they experience increased survival compared with whites who receive operative care.[54]

Duration of the Surveillance Interval Intuitively, we know that too short a surveillance interval may miss some occurrences, leading to systematically underestimating risk. Yet, as the time between the "exposure" (eg, administration of anesthesia) and event increases, the greater the chance that the occurrence may be associated with circumstances partially or totally independent of the exposure. These other circumstances might include even chance patient-specific factors (eg, MI that might have occurred 2 weeks preoperatively while walking the dog). This dualism of comprehensiveness versus precision plagues most cohort studies in the anesthesia risk literature.

Variation in the surveillance interval is especially apparent in the early studies of anesthetic-associated mortality. Some considered a death "anesthesia related" only if it occurred during or within 24 hours of administration of the anesthetic or after failure of the patient to regain consciousness after anesthesia.[55-58] Others extended the surveillance interval progressively to 48 hours, 3 days, 6 days, 7 days, 30 days, 1 year, and 2 years.[18,59,25,60-63] Beecher and Todd[8] adopted an empirical approach, using the duration of the surgical hospitalization.

Warner et al[64] found that 39% of major morbidity occurred more than 2 days but within 30 days after ambulatory surgery among 45 090 adults, including 2 of 5 cases of respiratory failure, 5 of 14 cases of MI, and 3 of 5 cases of pulmonary embolism. Although results could not be shown to be statistically different from those of the general population due to sample size, it is clear that substantial numbers of events would have been missed had the surveillance interval been limited to the immediate postoperative period.

There are no formal guidelines on duration of the surveillance interval, yet 30-day duration was adopted by the Veterans Affairs (VA) National Surgical Quality Improvement Project (NSQIP),[65] and this duration is commonly used with Medicare data. For most procedures, this represents a reasonable compromise between too short an interval, which misses adverse events, and too long an interval, which introduces extraneous events.

Assessing the Relationship With Anesthesia Care

Problem of Attribution Attributing causation is inherently problematic. Most studies of anesthesia-associated mortality have included a panel of blinded case reviewers who were asked to attribute the death to one of several possible causes: Was anesthesia care the *primary cause* of death? Or was anesthesia management a *contributory cause* (along with patient- and surgery-related factors)? Or was the poor outcome unrelated to anesthesia care? Panels were often composed mostly or wholly of anesthesiologists, but some have been more inclusive, including surgeons, obstetricians, referring physicians, and others.[66] The latter seem more appropriate, especially given the current emphasis on team-based care.

Unmasking Biases The mere occurrence of a poor outcome that *may* be related to anesthesia management can bias our judgments regarding quality and appropriateness of care.[67] The belief that a poor outcome is presumptive evidence of error on the part of anesthesia providers is a bias that pervades much of the early anesthesia-risk literature.[68] Notably, high interrater reliability in peer review does not ensure that judgments are accurate, for review panel determinations are necessarily products of their collective current knowledge of practice at the particular time, as well as numerous other biases that result from inadequate study designs, limited statistical capabilities, and the complexity of phenomena being studied.

Characterizing the Population Our discussion thus far has focused largely on patients experiencing an outcome of interest (becoming "cases") after exposure to a "hazard." However, if we do not give due consideration to the larger "at-risk" population from which these cases emerge, we have only a set of cases and cannot quantify the risk.[66]

Ecology of Care A large population is not homogeneous with regard to health status or the need for health care services.[69] Rather, there is a hierarchy in the need for health services and, by implication, poorer health status or greater acuity of illness increases sequentially from the unselected general population to outpatient care settings to community hospital settings, and finally to the academic medical center (**Fig. 25-4A**).[70] Surgical care is delivered in a similar spatial hierarchy (**Fig. 25-4B**). Thus risk estimates derived in one setting may differ from those in another environment (Berkson fallacy[71]). Recognizing these relationships can help reconcile seemingly disparate risk estimates from studies undertaken in widely differing clinical settings.

STATISTICAL PROBLEMS IN STUDYING ANESTHESIA RISK

Dealing With Low-Incidence Phenomena Although some anesthesia-related adverse events may occur frequently (eg, postoperative nausea), most severe events do not. The incidence rates may be so low that estimating rates of occurrence with acceptable precision (ie, narrow CI) or demonstrating meaningful differences in occurrence (eg, comparisons of drug regimens or sites of care) can be problematic (**Fig. 25-5** and **Box 25-7**).

The most obvious remedy is merely using a larger sample size. Yet, even when feasible, a larger sample usually connotes higher cost and a longer patient accrual period, during which other countervailing circumstances may arise (eg, deterioration in quality of data collection because of study team turnover or loss of enthusiasm, emergence of better technology that obviates study, information that alters or invalidates earlier results, changes in concurrent care processes that affect the event being studied). Other options include using a more sensitive end point, repeated measurements, matched cases and controls, multiple controls, lower statistical certainty ("power"), a higher-risk population, or concurrent multicenter trials, or some combination of such designs.

Multi-institutional studies, such as the 10-hospital Beecher-Todd study,[8] 34-hospital National Halothane Study,[73] or the 460-hospital study by Tiret et al[57] in France, offer the added benefit of enhancing the external validity (applicability of the results to other settings, termed *generalizability* in epidemiology) of the results because cooperating institutions may have different patient populations, surgical case mixes, clinical care processes, and/or administrative characteristics. Yet multi-institutional designs may introduce additional challenges, such as adherence to study design and definitions. Alternatively, investigators may opt to use a more frequent surrogate end point (eg, myocardial ischemia) that is associated with the outcome of interest (eg, MI), but, as noted earlier, the relationship between the occurrence of the surrogate and outcome may not be sufficiently close for valid results.[31,33]

One especially productive multi-institutional approach involves a consortium jointly collecting large amounts of data prospectively for a series of studies. An example was the Multicenter Study of Perioperative Ischemia Group that began in the late 1980s and comprised as many as almost 200 hospitals worldwide during its 20-year life, each contributing the same data elements to a database on patients having cardiac and noncardiac surgery. This group studied important perioperative risk topics, including the long-term risk of cardiovascular events,[74] atrial fibrillation after cardiac surgery,[75] mortality reduction with prophylactic use of β-adrenergic blocking agents,[25] aspirin-related mortality from cardiac surgery,[76] and risks related to use of aprotinin in cardiac surgery.[77]

Similarly, in the early 1990s, the dozen US Department of Veterans Affairs hospitals that performed cardiac surgery joined to create a common database[78] that became the model for an expanded project covering all major surgery in more than 120 VA hospitals, the VA NSQIP.[79] Using project-specific, trained medical-record abstractors in each hospital, NSQIP collected prospectively defined clinical data that have contributed greatly to measuring risk, outcomes, and quality of care.[65,79,80]

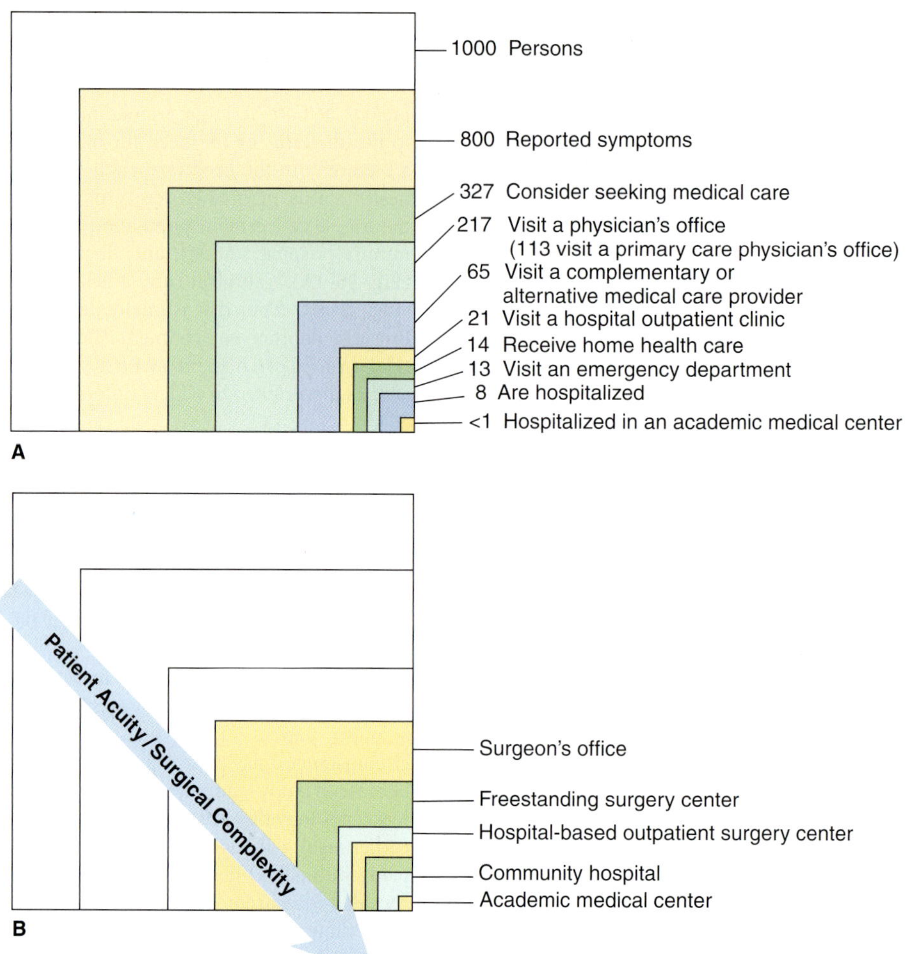

FIGURE 25-4. **A.** Ecology of care, with the site of US health care utilization for each 1000 persons in the year 2001. [Adapted with permission from Green LA, Fryer GE Jr, Yawn BP, et al. The ecology of medical care revisited. *N Engl J Med.* 344:2021, 2001. Copyright ©2001 Massachusetts Medical Society. All rights reserved.] **B.** Analogous spatial distribution of surgical care, with different types of surgical sites reflecting different strata of patient acuity and surgical complexity.

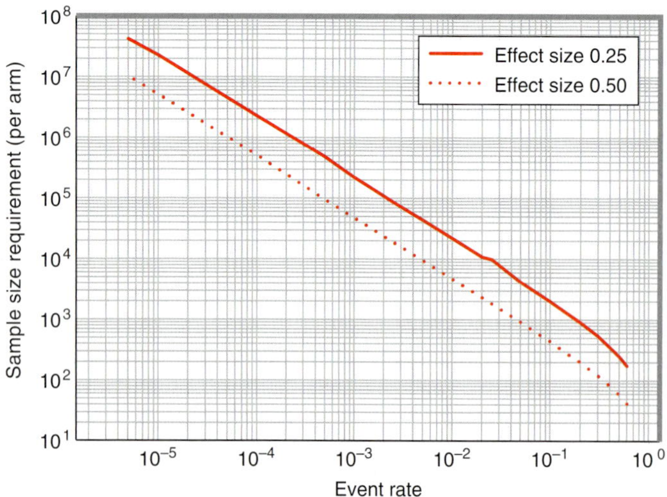

FIGURE 25-5. Sample size requirement for clinical studies comparing risk estimates as a function of adverse-event rate and magnitude of outcome difference ("effect size") sought, with a probability of finding such a difference ("power") of 0.80 and of falsely concluding that no difference exists ("type I error") of 0.05.

Recently, it was adopted by the American College of Surgeons (ACS), as the ACS-NSQIP, a collaboration of more than 200 academic health centers and large community hospitals. Although anesthesia-specific data elements comprise little more than the principal anesthesia method, the VA/ACS NSQIP database includes comorbidities and postoperative complications for thousands of patients having each surgical procedure and is beginning to enhance our understanding of preoperative risk assessment and choice of anesthesia method.[81-84] Similar comprehensive clinical databases relating to cardiac surgery have been established by the Society of Thoracic Surgeons[85] and the New England Cardiovascular Disease Study Group.[86]

As clinical information systems become ubiquitous, other clinical databases will arise from customary clinical care. In turn, vast institutional databases will result, creating innumerable opportunities for observational studies not even imagined by the early pioneers who first used computers to develop crude estimates of anesthesia risk.[63] Examples include the various databases maintained by the University HealthSystem Consortium, a collaboration of 107 academic health centers and 232 affiliated hospitals; member institutions can benchmark their clinical results for performance improvement and enhanced patient safety. Challenges awaiting those exploiting such clinical treasure troves include ensuring that information systems use standard terminology for diagnoses, surgical procedures, complications, and other clinical information; adequate software to merge data from different databases in real time; availability of sufficiently robust risk-adjustment methods

BOX 25-7

Estimating Sample Size Requirements for Risk Studies

Among important steps in planning a study comparing interventions is estimating the minimum sample size needed to demonstrate a true difference, if it exists. Studying too many subjects takes more time, wastes other resources, and potentially puts individuals at unnecessary risk. Studying too few may result in not finding a statistically significant difference–and not knowing whether that reflects an inadequate sample size or a true lack of benefit.[72] Thus institutional review boards now require an explicit sample-size determination in study protocols; proceeding in its absence may be construed to be unethical.

Generically, the estimate is obtained by considering the smallest difference that the investigator believes is *clinically* important or beneficial ("effect size"), the desired level of certainty about the result ("statistical power" or "power"), the risk of accepting a false result ($\alpha = 0.05$), and numerical value(s) with which the intervention is compared (mean and standard deviation as a measure of variation, for continuous variables; proportion, for binary data). Using a statistical table, a formula, or statistical computing software, one can determine the minimal sample size to detect a given effect size (eg, "small" = "0.25" for 25% change, "moderate" = "0.50" for 50% change) at a specified statistical certainty or "power" (eg, minimum = 0.80, with more conservative power being 0.85 or 0.90). The smaller the effect size and/or the smaller the event rate, the greater the sample size needed to demonstrate a meaningful difference with a given power. The sample-size requirement rises in an accelerating fashion as the event rate decreases (Fig. 25-5), placing a severe burden on investigators studying low-incidence events.

Example 1: A new antiemetic drug is being tested to reduce the risk of nausea associated with laparoscopic cholecystectomy. Half of patients have emetic symptoms (rate = 0.5); the investigator believes that a clinically beneficial drug would halve that rate (ie, effect size = 0.5). The comparison involves a "2-sided test" of statistical significance, to identify the possibility that the intervention raises rather than lowers the rate. Assuming minimal power (0.80), the sample-size requirement is 58 patients in each arm of the clinical trial.

Example 2: Another investigator studying the same drug, under the same clinical circumstances, believes that nausea is so distressing that a meaningful clinical effect would be a 25% decrease in symptoms (ie, effect size = 0.25). Assuming minimal power (0.80), the sample size needed is 247 patients in each arm.

Example 3: Recent studies suggest that the anesthesia-attributable death rate associated with anesthesia care may be as low as 1 in 200 000 (rate = 0.000005). An investigator wishes to study a new patient-monitoring configuration and believes that a meaningful clinical benefit would be a 50% decrease in this rate (effect size = 0.50). Assuming minimal power (0.80), the sample size needed is 10 202 941 patients in each arm of the trial!

for meaningful and valid comparisons; user-friendly software to facilitate use of such databases without reliance on computer technicians; and uncertainty whether results generated in large and academic health centers can be generalized to smaller and rural hospitals that often lack resources to participate or invest as fully in required technology.

An alternative source of multi-institutional data has developed as a by-product of the payment system for health care: the Medicare Provider Analysis and Review inpatient ("Part A") file and the federal Healthcare Cost and Utilization Project's all-payer Nationwide Inpatient Sample. Although offering the benefit of millions of patient encounters at much lower cost than clinical databases, claims or administrative data have very limited clinical information. Moreover, challenges in merging this hospital file with other files (eg, physician or "Part B" file) and numerous coding issues, including inconsistency and imprecision (eg, is a given coded disorder a comorbidity or complication?), plague efforts to risk adjust outcomes data.[44] Nonetheless, claims data have been used to explore risk in relation to medical direction of anesthesia care,[87] board certification of the anesthesiologist,[88] and location of surgical care.[35,89] Such data have also enabled identification of patient and hospital characteristics that influence anesthesia time for common major operations.[90] Recently, investigators have developed robust 30-day postoperative mortality and morbidity risk predictors based on readily available claims data—the surgical procedure code, patient age, and ASA Physical Status category—that rival the accuracy of NSQIP risk models.[91] Similar risk indices based solely on procedure and diagnosis codes from claims data perform almost as well as those developed with added patient demographic information.[92]

Hybrid data collection combining claims and clinical data sources are also developing: ASA has recently established the Anesthesia Quality Institute to foster the development and use of a National Anesthesia Clinical Outcomes Registry based on claims and other data volunteered by anesthesia practitioners.

Finally, public health data provide another opportunity to study low-incidence events: The occurrence of death and the chain of events leading to death, including anesthesia-related complications and comorbidity, are entered on multiple cause-of-death certificates, whose information is coded, using the newer, more detailed ICD-10 classification system, and entered into the National Center for Health Statistics' National Vital Statistics System. Using its anesthesia-related ICD-10 codes, with estimates from NCHS's National Hospital Discharge Survey, Li et al in 2009 obtained estimates of anesthesia-related mortality risk similar to those derived in recent studies.[1]

Dealing With Covariates and Confounding Clearly, anesthesia care occurs in a multifactorial setting. The outcome of each episode of anesthesia care—whether administration of anesthesia in the operating room, critical care in an intensive care unit, pain management, or other care—ultimately reflects the interaction of various patient characteristics ("covariates"), including age, gender, and health status (eg, ASA physical status, other metrics, presence of specific comorbidities), as well as factors relating to the particular situation (eg, surgery, obstetric delivery).

When complications occur among elderly men, are the poor outcomes related to the age or gender of the patients as well as the care? Might advanced age merely be common in the study sample? Or perhaps advanced age is a proxy for some underlying severe comorbidity (eg, coronary artery disease) that happens to be more common in older men? Only by disentangling these myriad relationships can we truly understand anesthesia risk and begin to target remedial efforts to the appropriate factor(s) (see Chapter 26).

Underlying this complexity is the reality that covariates may be *confounding variables* that share 2 properties: They may be associated with the exposure (the care) because an older or sicker person is more likely to have the care, *and* they also may be independent risk factors for poor outcome (ie, morbidity begets a poor outcome by itself unrelated to the care). Thus covariates may "confound" the relationship between the exposure and outcome, resulting in an anesthesia risk estimate that mixes the risk due to anesthesia care with that due to the confounding variable.

Such *confounding* can be controlled in the study design by randomization and inclusion criteria in a clinical trial or by matching (eg, ensuring that a specified covariate is present in the study sample in the same proportion as the population).

Stratification If confounding has not been controlled in the study design, as would be the case in an observational design, *stratification* can be used. An anesthesia risk estimate can be calculated for men and women separately, then compared with the rate for the combined study sample, thereby revealing the influence, if any, of gender. Almost all cohort studies of anesthesia-associated death attempted stratification, even if they did not use the term.

Multivariable Modeling When more than a few confounding variables are present, multivariable modeling is used to both control confounding and determine the independent contributions of different factors.

(Strictly defined, *multivariate modeling* refers to simultaneously predicting multiple outcomes, whereas *multivariable modeling* involves predicting a single outcome at a time.)

In developing the "model," the outcome is viewed as a numerical result of a mathematical function composed of risk factors identified by prior research on the selected outcome, candidate variables of special interest to the investigators, and any variables that may potentially confound the relationships between risk factors and outcome. The particular mathematical form of the model is set by the type of outcome. Most commonly, binary outcomes (eg, death vs survival) are modeled using logistic regression analysis, yielding a set of odds ratios (ORs). As in dichotomous circumstances (eg, survival vs death), the OR is the ratio of the probability (odds) of the outcome in the "exposed" group to that in the nonexposed group (Table 25-1); however, the multivariable modeling yields a set of "adjusted" ORs that reflect the independent effect of each variable (covariate) with the influence of other variables held constant. If time to event is believed important in genesis of the outcome, the relationship is modeled with a proportional hazards model, yielding equivalent hazards ratios; the study by Monk et al[18] identifying cumulative deep hypnotic time as a predictor of 1-year mortality is an example.

Although intuitive as one's "chance" of experiencing the outcome, ORs often are less useful in estimating the risk faced by a given individual because several predictors (eg, male gender *and* advanced age) may be relevant for many individuals. Alternatively, Sinclair et al,[93] among others, demonstrated the usefulness of the logistic regression equation, a part of the analytic output not typically presented in study reports, in estimating patient-specific risk of postoperative nausea by substituting into the equation the patient's particular numerical values for the independent predictors.

Propensity-Score Matching Generally, modeling controls confounding adequately; however, confounding and related bias is ever present and often undetected.[94] One type of confounding that is an especially problematic source of bias is *confounding by indication*, where clinical features prompt use of a given intervention that is also related to the patient's outcome. An example is the historical predilection of anesthesia providers to administer spinal anesthesia preferentially to "poor-risk" patients, believing that this method poses a lesser physiologic trespass. Not surprisingly, many early outcome comparisons noted that spinal anesthesia, sick patients, and higher mortality were associated! Because conscientious physicians will naturally opt to "do what's right" for their patients, confounding by indication is a frequent problem with observational data (selection bias).

A special approach for dealing with selection bias is propensity-score matching. This method uses logistic regression first to identify from the observational data matched patient pairs that, based on their covariates, are equally likely to receive the intervention.[95,96] Then, using the matched-pairs subgroup, logistic regression analysis identifies independent predictors for the outcome. This approach has been applied to diverse risk-related topics, including pulmonary artery catheter use in critical care,[97] anesthesia choice for hip fracture repair,[98] medical direction of anesthesia care,[87] and anesthesiologist's board certification.[88] The method is commonly used with observational data because a clinical trial is either logistically difficult or not feasible. As with modeling generally, the propensity-score approach cannot control for confounding by covariates that are unknown or overlooked in the analysis; such oversight itself is unlikely to be detected.[99]

Recursive Partitioning An alternative approach for studying risk amid confounding avoids fitting data to a mathematical regression equation and instead uses the covariates to repetitively partition the study population into "high-risk" and "low-risk" subgroups with regard to the outcome. *Recursive partitioning* (also termed *data mining*) exploits lack of homogeneity among the study population to yield a treelike graphic that depicts how each subject fared with regard to the outcome. This classification approach has been used to identify MI risk among emergency department patients presenting with chest pain,[100] poor credit risks for financial services, and genotypes in genomic analysis, but it is only beginning to find use in studying anesthesia risk.[101] Recently, this method enabled exploration of the relationships between severity and duration of intraoperative hypotension and 1-year postoperative mortality in a sample population that was inadequate for multivariate modeling.[102]

HOW DOES THE CLINICIAN INTERPRET ANESTHESIA RISK STUDIES?

STUDY DESIGNS FOR ANESTHESIA RISK

Taxonomy of Study Designs

Interpreting anesthesia risk literature does not require extensive knowledge of statistics, but it does require an appreciation of the strengths and limitations of study designs. **Box 25-8** presents a taxonomy of study designs used in anesthesia risk studies. It categorizes these studies as randomized controlled trials, cohort studies, or case-control studies and further describes their purpose and design as experimental (eg, clinical trial) or observational; in the latter, the investigator observes what is often a natural or unplanned experiment, hence the alternative name, *observational design*. It also distinguishes between prospective and retrospective studies, with the former denoting explicit definition of study variables and outcomes before data collection begins. Most anesthesia risk reports have been retrospective, although prospective designs have been more prevalent in recent studies.

Ranked in order of reliability of results, the clinical trial is first, followed by well-conducted prospective cohort studies, other cohort studies, case-control studies, and case aggregations.[103] When similar results are obtained from studies using different designs, we gain confidence in those results. The salient features of the 3 principal designs used in anesthesia risk studies are compared in **Table 25-2** as an aid to surveying examples that inform us about anesthesia risk.

MORTALITY AS A RISK OF ANESTHESIA

Early "Anesthesia Deaths" In 1848, only 15 months after William Morton's successful demonstration of clinical anesthesia in Boston, an Edinburgh medical journal reported the death of Hannah Greener, a 15-year-old British girl who had a toenail removed under chloroform anesthesia, some 4 months after she had a similar procedure performed with diethyl ether anesthesia.[104] This first report of an anesthesia-related death initiated a decades-long debate over the relative safety of ether versus chloroform and also indicated that surgical anesthesia could be fatal. Similar case reports followed.

Were these "anesthesia deaths" rare, occasional, or perhaps common? Although case reports and subsequent case series provided descriptions of the fatal events and even clues to possible etiologies, they could not quantitate the frequency of these catastrophes and allow an estimate of

BOX 25-8

Taxonomy of Study Designs for Studying Anesthesia Risk

- I. Experimental designs
  - A. Randomized clinical trial (RCT)
  - B. Nonrandomized clinical trial
- II. Nonexperimental (observational) designs
  - A. Person-level observation
    - 1. Longitudinal measurements
      - a. Cohort study
      - b. Case-control study
    - 2. Cross-sectional measurements
    - 3. Case aggregations (case series, registry)
  - B. Aggregate-level observation (ecology)

TABLE 25-2 Comparison of Common Study Designs for Studying Anesthesia Risk

	Study Design		
Design Attribute	**Randomized Clinical Trial**	**Cohort Study**	**Case-Control Study**
Purpose	Establish efficacy of an intervention or study effects of an exposure	Study ≥1 outcome(s) after an exposure	Study ≥1 exposure(s) resulting in an outcome
Basic design	Experimental	Observational	Observational
Study perspective	Prospective	Prospective	Retrospective
Clinical setting	Ideal clinical practice	Customary clinical practice	Customary clinical practice
Role of subjects	Allocated to exposure groups usually via randomized process	Classified in groups based on exposure status	Sampled from source population based on outcome status
Measurement perspective	Prospective	Prospective or retrospective	Retrospective (for measurements); retrospective or prospective (for disease)
Risk metrics	Incidence, and absolute and relative risks	Incidence, and absolute and relative risks	Odds ratio (which can yield relative risk)
Benefit	Minimizes bias	External validity (generalizability)	External validity (generalizability)
Disadvantage	Possibly limited external validity (generalizability)	Possibly unknown biases	Possibly unknown biases

the risk in undergoing anesthesia. Anesthesia risk measurement benefited from the early epidemiologic work of anesthesiologist John Snow, who applied to an analysis of 50 deaths during chloroform anesthesia the epidemiologic logic that enabled him to identify the mode of transmission of cholera related to colonization of the Broad Street water pump.[105]

Cohort Studies of Anesthesia-Associated Mortality **Table 25-3** presents the principal results of international studies in which the mortality risk of surgical anesthesia was studied. These studies were major, often pioneering efforts, with most performed before the advent of modern information technology that facilitates aggregating and analyzing vast data and well before epidemiology and biostatistics had reached their current level of sophistication. Despite these limitations, their reports provide estimates for surgery-related, anesthesia-attributable mortality and, in many, morbidity.

In surveying the unadjusted or crude mortality estimates listed in Table 25-3, we are immediately impressed by a wide variation in rates. Undoubtedly much of the variation is due to different study designs and other factors listed in Box 25-1. Yet there is a suggestion of improved outcome over time, especially in well-developed countries.

Holland[66,114] documented a 5-fold decrease in anesthesia-attributable mortality in 1 Australian region over 25 years, much of which he attributed to enhanced risk management education of practitioners. Ever greater progress in Australia was documented by Mackay[129] and Gibbs and Borton.[4] Similarly, Lienhart et al[128] noted an 11-fold decrease in anesthesia mortality over 15 years in France when repeating (albeit with different methodology) the study by Tiret et al,[57] which noted poor outcomes in relation to lack of postanesthesia care units.

Moreover, although we might regard the study results listed in Table 25-3 akin to a collection of mixed fruit, a plot of the primary-cause mortality estimates in those studies span almost 2 orders of magnitude (or a near 100-fold decrease) over 6 decades,[1] and the putative improvement trend predates the vigorous US patient safety initiatives of the mid-1980s (**Fig. 25-6**), even if we might be uncomfortable concluding that any specific amount of "improvement" has occurred.

However, even if an apparent trend is wholly an artifact of differing methodologies, as some argue,[126] the clinical terrain has changed dramatically over the past half century. Concerned in 1959 that mortality statistics were unchanged from those decades earlier, the National Academy of Sciences' Committee on Anesthesia invited Chauncey Starr from the National Academy of Engineering to comment. "Well, that is exactly the way it is in farming," he related as he began to discuss the tractor principle[132]: The rate of farming accidents remained high despite many safety improvements in tractors (eg, wider wheel base, roll bars, seat belts). Seeking an understanding, Starr made site visits during which he learned that improved tractor design enabled farmers to plow on steeper inclines! The same is true in medicine, where we now routinely perform major "high-risk" operations on patients who as recently as 35 years ago were "too sick" for surgery. Thus even stable mortality rates in the face of increasing severity of illness reflects improved clinical outcome.

SOURCES OF MORTALITY AND MORBIDITY RISK

Our literature abounds with attempts to allocate overall perioperative mortality and morbidity risk to specific characteristics of the patient, anesthetic, operation, or clinical setting. An important reference point is the perioperative mortality rate that was estimated to be 1.43% (or 1 in 70) for US hospital–based surgery in 2004[133] and has been relatively stable over several decades. Comparable mortality estimates based on individual cohort studies have ranged from 1 in 256 to 1 in 53,[8,59,51,46,63,134] without any apparent temporal trend.

The earliest attempt to identify specific sources of mortality risk appeared in Beecher and Todd's mid–20th-century study,[8] which noted a perioperative mortality rate of 1 in 75 and ascribed 78% of deaths (1 in 95) to the patient's disease, 18% (1 in 420) to surgical management, and 3% (1 in 2680) solely to anesthesia management. They attributed approximately 5% (1 in 1560) to anesthesia when considering it as both a contributing and a primary cause. Subsequent studies attributed somewhat greater proportions of mortality to surgical and anesthesia causes, as understanding of the pathophysiology of disease and the physiologic effects of anesthesia and surgical intervention increased.[3,59,51,46]

However, substantial confounding underlies such simple categorizations. Being male, elderly, and in poorer condition (ie, ASA physical status ≥3), each individually augments the risk of a given surgical procedure. An early (and still valid) effort to model perioperative mortality is that of Cohen et al,[59] who identified the relative importance of patient characteristics (advanced age and ASA physical status, male gender), surgery-related factors (invasiveness, whether emergent), and anesthesia management (method and drug choice; **Table 25-4**).

Although definitive allocation of perioperative risk, and specifically of anesthesia risk, is lacking, what follows is an attempt to dissect some of these relationships, with the goal of offering guidance to practitioners as well as identifying improvement opportunities.

The Patient

Importance of Comorbidity Intuition tells us that sick patients tend to do poorly. Among the many studies[8,34,46,48-50,52,57,59,62,63,65,74,75,78-81,89] documenting

TABLE 25-3 Estimates of Mortality Attributable to Surgical Anesthesia Care

Investigator(s)	Time Period	Location	No. of Hospitals	No. of Anesthetics	Primary Cause	Primary and Associated Causes
Dornette and Orth[58]	1943-1954	Madison, Wisconsin	1	63 105	1:2427	1:1343
Beecher and Todd[8]	1948-1952	United States	10	599 548	1:2680	1:1560
Dripps et al[46]	1949-1957	Philadelphia	1	33 224	1:852	1:415
Minuck[106]	1949-1965	Canada	1	121 786	1:6766	1:3291
Schapira et al[107]	1952-1956	New York, New York	1	22 177	1:1232	1:821
Phillips et al[108]	1953-1959	Baltimore, Maryland	Multiple	Unstated	(1:7692)	(1:2500)
Clifton and Hotten[109]	1952-1962	Australia	1	205 640	1:6048	1:3955
Greene et al[110]	1956-1959	Connecticut	Multiple	120 935	1:3901	1:3183
Memery[111]	1955-1964	Springfield, Massachusetts	1	69 291	1:3139	1:1082
Gebbie[112]	1958-1964	Canada	1	129 336	–	1:6158
Harrison[113]	1956-1960 1963-1966	Cape Town, South Africa	1	177 928		1:3068
Holland[66,114]	1960-1968	New South Wales, Australia	Multiple	(300 000)	(1:5500)	–
Marx et al[63]	1965-1969	New York, New York	1	34 145	–	1:1265
Bodlander[55]	1963-1972	Sydney, Australia	1	211 130	1:14,075	1:1703
Harrison[56]	1967-1976	Cape Town, South Africa	1	240 483	–	1:4537
Holland[114]	1970-1979	New South Wales, Australia	Multiple	(400 000)	(1:10 250)	–
Hovi-Viander[61]	1975	Finland	100	338 934	1:5059	1:1412
Turnbull et al[60]	1973-1977	Vancouver, Canada	1	195 232	1:5138	–
Tiret et al[57]	1978-1982	France	460	198 103	1:13,207	1:3810
Pitt-Miller[115]	1976-1987	Port-of-Spain, Trinidad	1	129 107	1:6795	1:1956
Eichhorn[116]	1976-1985	Boston, Massachusetts	9	757 000[a]	1:151 400	–
	1985-1988	Boston, Massachusetts	9	244 000[a]	0	–
Chopra et al[117]	1978-1987	Leiden, The Netherlands	1	113 074	–	1:16 250
Pausawasdi[118]	1981-1984	Bangkok, Thailand	1	45 362	–	1:1296
Holland[114]	1983-1985	New South Wales, Australia	Multiple	(550 000)	(1:26 000)	–
Tan and Delilkan[119]	1980-1992	Malaysia	1	155 000	–	1:25 833
Lunn and Devlin[3]	1987	United Kingdom	100	485 850	1:185 056	1:1351
Tikkanen and Hovi-Viander[120]	1987	Finland	69	325 585	1:66,700	1:16 279
Pedersen et al[121]	1986-1987	Herlev, Denmark	1	7306	–	1:2500
Cohen et al[122]	1988-1989	Toronto Canada	4	27 184	0	0
Warden et al[123]	1984-1990	New South Wales, Australia	Multiple	(493 000)	–	(1:20 000)
Coetzee[124]	1988-1992	Stellenbosch, South Africa	1	94 945	1:9090	1:2941
Eagle and Davis[125]	1990-1995	Western Australia	Multiple	(84 000)	–	(1:40 000)
Lagasse[126]	1992-1994	New York, New York	1[b]	37 924	–	1:12 641
	1995-1999	New York, New York	1[c]	146 548	–	1:13 322
Arbous et al[127]	1995-1997	Netherlands	Multiple	869 483	–	1:7307
Lienhart et al[128]	1999	France	Multiple	(7 756 121)	(1:145 500)	(1:18 500)
Mackay[129]	1997-1999	Australia	Multiple	(10 336 000)	(1:219 919)	(1:79 509)
Li et al[1]	1999-2005	United States	Multiple	(105 700 000)	(1:121 952)	–
Noordzij et al[130]	1991-2005	Netherlands	102	3 667 875	–	1:54
Gibbs and Borton[4]	2000-2002	Australia	Multiple	(7 650 000)	(1:182,143)	(1:56 000)
Charuluxananan et al[131]	2003-2005	Thailand	Multiple	163 403	1:5882	1:2500

"Multiple" indicates that the study involved many hospitals, but the actual number is unspecified.

Parenthetical values reflect circumstances in which the number of anesthetics was estimated.

[a]ASA physical status 1 and 2 patients only.

[b]Suburban community hospital.

[c]Urban teaching hospital.

this truism is Pedersen's prospective cohort study[51] of 6307 patients, in which the extent of comorbidity was associated with greater complication and mortality rates (**Table 25-5**).

Modeling Outcome With Patient Characteristics Although the general principle is now well established, capturing the precise quantitative relationship between comorbidity and clinical outcome remains an active focus of research. The venerable ASA physical status classification, never designed as a risk metric, has long been known to correlate with perioperative outcome,[49,59,63,126,134] with mortality rising sharply with advanced physical status (Table 25-4 and **Table 25-6**). ASA physical status interacts with age, becoming a much more potent predictor of major complications beyond middle age (**Fig. 25-7**).

Yet there is substantial subjectivity and variability in use of middle ASA physical status categories, even in settings where payment for services is unrelated to this classification.[135-138] Prediction improves when this metric is used in combinations in multivariable modeling

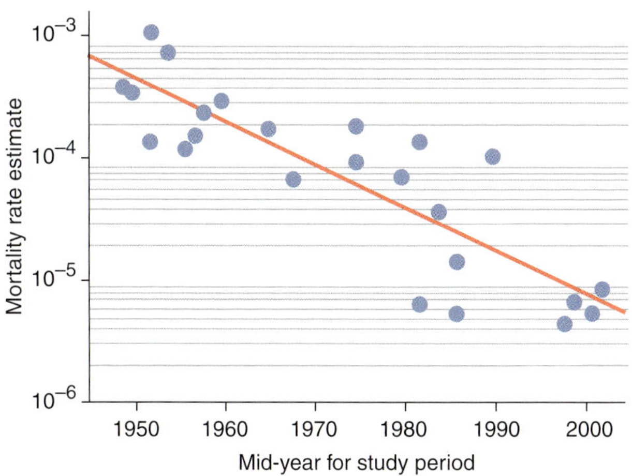

FIGURE 25-6. Rate of perioperative mortality primarily attributable to anesthesia care by the midpoint year of various studies undertaken in developed countries, from 1948 to 2005, as listed in Table 25-3.

with other covariates, such as age and/or the presence of specific morbidities.[18,25,34,48-51,59,65,74,80-83,89,122,139,140] Concerns about subjectivity of the ASA physical status metric may also be addressed in risk modeling studies by including the Charlson Comorbidity Score,[52] a morbidity-specific metric that has been at least as good an outcome predictor in several studies[18,98,141-143]; the Acute Physiology Score (APS) of the Acute Physiology and Chronic Health Evaluation (APACHE) II score, a metric commonly used in critical care[144]; or perhaps the Sickness at Admission Scale Score.[145]

Alternatively, there have been embryonic efforts to reduce the subjectivity in ASA physical status scoring by enhancing its specificity, thereby enhancing its precision and predictive power: Barbeito et al[138] suggested adding a "G" to the scoring of parturients (eg, "2-G" to indicate the gravid status), and Holt and Silverman[146] proposed a superscripted notion to indicate specific morbidity (eg, "3[RESP]" to indicate the affected organ system). Emphasizing the confounding of physical status by surgical complexity, Pasternak[147] suggested a preoperative assessment scale that includes both. These await further development and validation. The Charlson Comorbidity Score was developed to predict 1-year mortality among hospitalized *medical* patients,[52] and, although it has taken several decades, similar morbidity-specific scoring systems for predicting surgical mortality are emerging. For example, Sessler's group has developed a risk metric using age and Medicare comorbidity and surgical procedure codes to predict duration of hospitalization 30-day postoperative mortality and morbidity.[92]

Several simple scoring systems for organ- or operation-specific complications are available. The Cardiac Risk Index of Goldman et al[48]provided an early model that was improved by Detsky et al,[148] by adding angina to the risk factors. Lee et al[149] developed and validated a Revised Cardiac Index that specified 6 independent predictors: history of ischemic heart disease, history of congestive heart failure, history of cerebrovascular disease, preoperative treatment with insulin, preoperative serum creatinine more than 2.0 mg/dL, and high-risk surgical procedure. Similar clinical prediction rules have been developed for early outcome after coronary artery bypass surgery.[150] Glance et al[151] have studied the substantially enhanced postoperative mortality risk associated with the metabolic syndrome (obesity, hypertension, and diabetes).

Even in the absence of simple, comprehensive risk scoring systems, multivariable modeling of several large cohorts has identified a common set of independent risk factors for severe complications and death (Tables 25-4 and **25-5**, and **Box 25-9**). Differences in the risk associated with specific morbidities among studies probably are explained, in part, by differences in how disorder-specific acuity of illness is measured.[152]

TABLE 25-4 Factors Associated With Mortality Within 7 Days of Surgery

Factor[a]		Odds Ratio[b]	95% Confidence Interval
Patient related			
	Age, 60-79 vs <60 y	2.32	1.70-3.17
	Age, ≥80 vs <60 y	3.29	2.18-4.96
	Gender, female vs male	0.77	0.59-1.00
	ASA physical status score, 3-4 vs. 1-2	10.65	7.59-14.85
Surgery related			
	Major vs minor procedure	3.82	2.50-5.93
	Intermediate vs minor procedure	1.76	1.24-2.50
	Length of anesthesia, ≥2 vs <2 h	1.08	0.77-1.50
	Emergent vs elective procedure	4.44	3.38-5.83
Other factors			
	Years of operation, 1975-1979 vs 1980-1984	1.75	1.32-2.31
	Complication in operating room vs none	1.42	1.06-1.89
Anesthesia related			
	Experience of anesthesia-provider, >600 cases for ≥8 y vs <600 procedures for <8 y	1.06	0.82-1.37
	Inhalation agent with narcotic vs inhalation alone	0.76	0.51-1.55
	Narcotic anesthesia alone vs inhalation alone	1.41	1.01-2.00
	Narcotic with inhalation vs inhalation alone	0.79	0.47-1.32
	Spinal anesthesia vs inhalation alone	0.53	0.29-0.98
	Number of anesthetic drugs, 1-2 vs ≥3	2.94	2.20-3.84

[a]Factors were evaluated in logistic regression analysis of data from 100 007 patients performed the 5 most frequently used anesthesia methods (inhalation alone, inhalation with narcotic, narcotic anesthesia alone, narcotic anesthesia with inhalation, spinal anesthesia).

[b]All odds ratios whose 95% confidence intervals do not include the value 1.0 are statistically significant.

Modified from Cohen MM, Duncan PG, Tate RB. Does anesthesia contribute to operative mortality? *JAMA*. 1988;260:2859.

TABLE 25-5 Factors Associated With Perioperative Complications and Death

	Cardiovascular Complications		Pulmonary Complications		In-hospital Mortality	
Factor	%	OR	%	OR	%	OR
Gender						
Female	4.9		3.7		0.7	
Male	8.8[a]	1.8	6.6[a]	1.8	2.2[a]	3.2
Age (y)						
<50	2.6		2.3		0.3	
50-69	8.2		6.7		1.8	
70-79	14.3[a]		8.9		2.9[a]	
≥80	16.7[a]		10.2[a]		5.8[a]	
Ischemic heart disease	29.1[a]	6.5	8.7	1.9	2.9	2.5
Myocardial infection						
>1 y since	20.8[a]		7.7		4.0[a]	
≤1 y since	38.5[a]		10.4[a]		7.7[a]	
Chronic heart failure	35.2[a]		15.1[a]	3.8	9.0[a]	9.9
Hypertension	11.8[a]	2.1	7.1[a]	1.6	1.3	1.1
Hypotension (SBP ≤90 mm Hg)	16.5[a]	2.5	17.3[a]	4.0	9.4[a]	9.8
Chronic obstructive lung disease	12.4[a]	2.1	12.4	3.0	5.0[a]	4.7
Renal failure	14.4[a]	2.2	11.8[a]	2.4	5.9[a]	5.2
Diabetes mellitus	9.2	1.5	7.1	1.5	2.1[a]	1.8
Neurologic disease	5.9	1.0	8.8[a]	1.9	2.9	2.4
Cancer	7.0	1.1	5.5	1.2	1.1	1.0
Cancer, abdominal	19.8[a]	3.2	19.4[a]	4.3	5.0[a]	5.4
Emergent surgery	7.4[a]	1.3	6.3[a]	3.0	2.8	3.2
Duration of anesthesia (min)						
<30	1.2		0.6		0.1	
30-179	6.8		4.5		1.3	
180-299	17.9[a]		13.4[a]		3.2[a]	
≥300	20.4[a]		30.2[a]		4.9[a]	
Minor surgery	3.2		1.8		0.3	
Major surgery	13.0[a]	4.1	10.6	5.8	3.1[a]	4.9
Total study population	6.3		4.8		1.2	

OR, odds ratio; SBP, systolic blood pressure.

[a]Statistically significantly higher rate compared with total study population.

From Pedersen T. Complications and death following anaesthesia: a prospective study with special reference to the influence of patient-, anaesthesia-, and surgery-related risk factors. *Dan Med Bull.* 1994;41(3):319-331.

Racial and socioeconomic characteristics, possibly proxies for unadjusted underlying comorbidity and/or problems with access to care, also influence outcome.[89,153,154]

Failure to Rescue Building on the relationship between health status and clinical outcome, Silber et al[155,156] developed a novel outcome metric, *failure to rescue*. Using multivariable modeling, they showed that patient characteristics (eg, age, gender, comorbidities) predict complications better than they predict death; whether a complication turns into a death reflects the capability of the facility to rescue the patient. The rescue capability itself depends on hospital characteristics that include proportion of board-certified anesthesiologists and ratios of nurses to patients.[88,155,157] Subsequently validated in many studies,

TABLE 25-6 Relationship of ASA Physical Status Classification to Perioperative Mortality

		Perioperative Mortality				
	Author(s)	Vacanti et al[134]	Marx et al[63]	Cohen et al[59]	Lagasse[126]	
	Study Period	1964-1966	1965-1969	1975-1984	1992-1994	1995-1999
	Surveillance Period	48 h	7 d	7 d	48 h	48 h
ASA Physical Status Class	1	1:1179	1:1665	1:1389	0	1:8756
	2	1:371	1:212	1:508	1:7813	1:3084
	3	1:55	1:23	1:87	1:1360	1:644
	4	1:13	1:4	1:13	1:86	1:136
	5	1:11	1:2	1:3	1:4	1:5
Overall		1:256	1:53	1:140	1:332	1:632

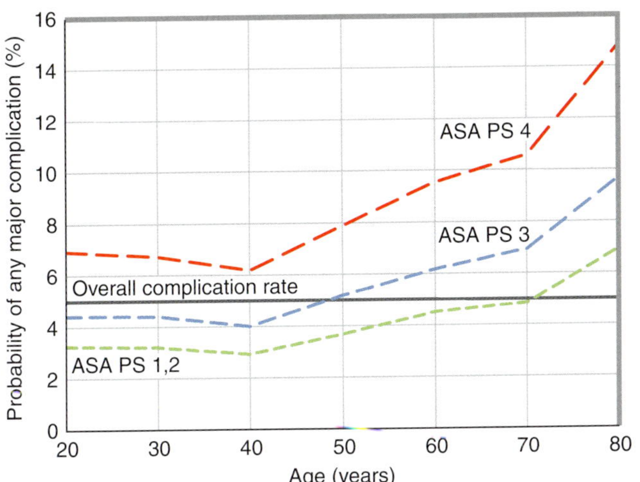

FIGURE 25-7. Probability of a severe perioperative respiratory or cardiovascular complication as a function of both American Society of Anesthesiologists physical status class and patient age, computed from the logistic regression equation developed in the clinical trial of inhalation anesthesia drugs conducted among 17 201 patients by Forrest et al.[50] [From Muravchick S. Anesthesia for the elderly. In: Healy TEJ, Knight PR, eds. *Wylie and Churchill-Davidson's A Practice of Anesthesia*. 7th ed. London, UK: Arnold; 2003:990. Reproduced with permission of Edward Arnold, Ltd.]

this metric is included among quality indicators used by the Agency for Healthcare Quality and Research, National Quality Forum, University HealthSystem Consortium, and independent health care researchers.

The Health Care Setting

Unexplained Variation in Outcome Long before investigators had tools to identify the source of risk differences, they began to document variations in patient outcome for ostensibly similar surgery.[16] Buried in the mid 20th-century Beecher-Todd study[8] is an unexplained 3-fold difference in mortality across the 10 participating university hospitals. A decade later, the mortality variation was so great in the mid-1960s 34-hospital National Halothane Study (0.27%-6.40%) that its statisticians concluded, "Such variation in so important an outcome of surgery compels attention."[158] Even after adjusting their data for age, ASA physical status, and surgical procedure, an unexplained, 3-fold variation remained.

Emergence of an Ill-Defined "Provider" Intrigued by unexplained mortality variation in the National Halothane Study, one of its investigators joined with sociologists and statisticians to explore nonclinical factors, including structural characteristics of hospitals, as potential explanatory variables for the postoperative mortality variation among 1224 hospitals using a chart abstracting service in the early 1970s.[159,160] Despite case-mix adjustments, 3- to 4-fold outcome variations remained for the 15 major surgical procedures studied in this Institutional Differences Study. Probing deeper in a 17-hospital subset with more detailed institutional data, they explored the influence of the individual surgeon's experience, anesthesia-provider type, and various measures of hospital structure and medical staff organization.[161,162] Although such factors were weak predictors of outcome, the mere presence of such relationships heralded the beginning of our understanding of the multifaceted role of an ill-defined "provider" in surgical outcomes. (*Provider* here is a comprehensive term indicating not only the clinicians but also the facility, its associated staff, organizational structure, and policies.)

BOX 25-9

Independent Risk Factors for Severe Complications and Death

Male gender[51,59,89]

Advanced age[48,50,51,59,89,148]

Advanced American Society of Anesthesiologists physical status class[48,50,51,59,65,80]

Moderate and severe specific comorbidity[25,48,50,51,65,80,148,149]

Role of Sociomanagerial Factors The Institutional Differences Study[160,162] identified diverse sociomanagerial factors that are associated with better surgical outcomes, including teaching hospital status, greater number of residency programs, higher hospital expense per day, stringent medical staff admission requirements, power over senior surgeons, higher proportion of surgeons' practices at the study hospital, and board certification of physicians. Subsequent studies have validated the influence of teaching hospital status and board certification,[155,163-165] although research has not explored the full array of care.[166,167] Silber et al[155] specifically identified a low proportion of board-certified anesthesiologists on the anesthesia staff as an important hospital characteristic associated with "failure to rescue" the surgical patient who experiences a complication. Generally, hospital characteristics are stronger predictors of clinical outcome than are surgeon's characteristics.[161,162]

As a natural extension, investigators have explored whether mortality after high-risk surgery is influenced by provider experience. Studying procedures of varying complexity in the mid-1970s in 1498 hospitals using a chart abstracting service, Luft et al[168] found an inverse relationship between mortality and procedure volume for high-risk procedures; a volume–outcome relationship existed for lesser risk surgery but was weaker at low volumes. What underlies this phenomenon, a team effect in the hospital, expertise of individual surgeons, or regional referral patterns? Research has been more equivocal, in part, because of technical issues, such as low statistical power in comparisons of lower total case volume and a statistical association (collinearity) affecting hospital and surgeon-specific volumes.[169,170] Yet accruing literature documents better outcomes for high-risk surgery performed at high-volume sites and suggests that a more experienced team may underlie the phenomenon.[171-173] As a result, performing high-risk surgery at high-volume sites has become a principle that guides contracting for services of some organizations (eg, the Leapfrog Group) and third-party payers.

Certain aspects of critical care medicine are also associated with better surgical outcomes. Pronovost et al[174,175] showed that the presence of a dedicated intensive care physician making daily rounds, a nurse-to-patient ratio of at least 1.2, a monthly case conference, and tracheal extubation in the critical care unit rather than the operating room are associated with better outcomes after abdominal aortic surgery. The implications of not having a dedicated critical care physician are so grave (OR for in-hospital mortality: 3.0; 95% CI, 1.9-4.9) that this has also become a Leapfrog Group standard. The contribution of nurse staffing ratios for good outcomes echoes the studies of general hospital nurse staffing by Aiken et al.[157]

Delivering good outcomes in complex settings also requires effective team functioning, an essential part of an effective patient safety climate.[2] Higher scores on the Safety Attitudes Questionnaire are associated with fewer medication errors, lower ventilator-associated pneumonia rates, and decreased risk-adjusted mortality.[176] Makary et al[177] developed a "teamwork culture" metric that is sensitive to operating room caregivers' perceptions and beginning to be used in improvement work. Awad et al[178] showed that a preprocedural operating room briefing improves teamwork climate, including coordination among caregivers, and Haynes et al have demonstrated a 44% reduction in surgical mortality in association with use of an immediate presurgical checklist that fosters enhanced communication among team members.[179] (See Chapter 3 for a more thorough discussion of team performance.)

Mortality risk appears to be influenced also by the facility in which the procedure is performed (ie, a "provider" effect). Fleisher et al[89] studied outcomes of Medicare patients having surgery in a hospital outpatient unit, freestanding surgery center, or surgeon's office. Although death rates on the day of operation were not different, there were differences among the rates for 7-day mortality (1 in 2000, 1 in 4000, and

1 in 2856, respectively) and 7-day hospital admission (1 in 48, 1 in 119, and 1 in 110, respectively). The readmission rates resembled those in other studies, but the authors could not exclude the likelihood that the differences across sites in both readmission and mortality rates reflected patient referral patterns (selection bias), with sicker patients treated in the more intensive settings (Fig. 25-4B).

The Surgeon and the Operation

The Surgeon's Characteristics The surgeon's board certification,[155,162,164] experience,[3,162,164] and case volume[162, 164,169,171,172] is each associated with clinical outcome when comparing different hospitals, although these relationships may be weak when comparing individual surgeons at the same site. However, outcome variation has been demonstrated among individual surgeons for complex procures.[180] Lunn and Devlin[3] called attention to the association of poor outcomes from surgery and anesthesia care provided by unsupervised and undersupervised trainees at night, particularly in emergent care and sicker patients, as have others more recently.[4,127,129]

Outcomes associated with individual surgeons are confounded by diverse hospital characteristics, such as teaching-hospital status,[162,166,167] total hospital expenditures,[162] total case volume,[162,169,172,173] team culture,[176,177] critical care organizational characteristics,[174,175] and general nurse-to-patient ratio.[157]

The Operation The surgeon's influence on outcome is confounded by important characteristics of the operation. In most cohort studies, invasiveness of the surgical procedure (ie, "major" vs "minor" surgery) and whether the operation is undertaken emergently are potent independent determinants of both mortality and morbidity (Tables 25-4 and 25-5). [34,48,51,59,148] Underlying these relationships undoubtedly are the implications of the extent of physiologic derangement and the limited preparatory care before emergent surgery. Procedure invasiveness interacts with age, becoming a much more potent predictor of major complications beyond middle age, particularly for the more invasive procedures (**Fig. 25-8**).[50] Invasiveness (or complexity) of operation is so potent a predictor of outcome that it has been included in several proposals for modifications of the ASA physical status classification or new approaches to preoperative patient assessment.[82,147]

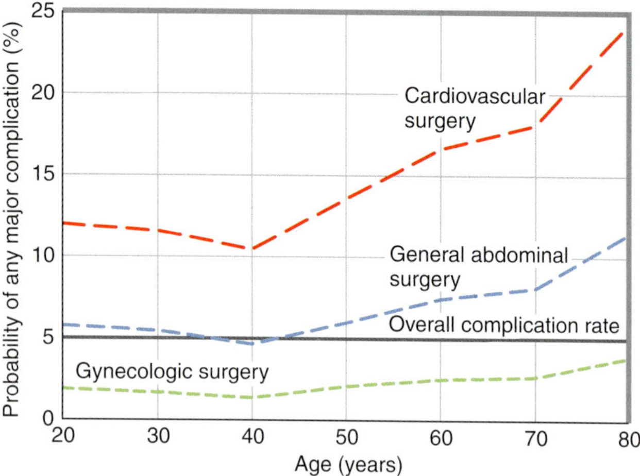

FIGURE 25-8. Probability of a severe perioperative respiratory or cardiovascular complication as a function of both type of surgical procedure and patient age, computed from the logistic regression equation developed in the clinical trial of inhalation anesthesia drugs conducted among 17 201 patients by Forrest et al.[50] ASA PS, American Society of Anesthesiologists physical score. [From Muravchick S. Anesthesia for the elderly. In: Healy TEJ, Knight PR, eds. *Wylie and Churchill-Davidson's A Practice of Anesthesia*. 7th ed. London, UK: Arnold; 2003:990. Reproduced with permission of Edward Arnold, Ltd.]

An especially problematic procedure-related factor is duration of operation (or anesthesia). Consistent with the notion that increasing exposure to a potentially hazardous intervention risks a poorer outcome, duration of operation (or anesthesia) is associated with increased mortality and morbidity[35,51,59] (Tables 25-4 and 25-5) and hospital admission after ambulatory surgery.[34,35] Greater procedure duration may be a proxy for more extensive (perhaps unrecognized) surgical disease, lesser surgical skill, or the occurrence of intraoperative anesthesia and surgical complications, any of which may independently determine the postoperative outcome. Cohen et al[59] specifically included occurrence of intraoperative complications among candidate predictor variables and found that such complications, rather than procedure duration, was an independent predictor of outcome (Table 25-4). Thus, unless the study has included occurrence of intraoperative complications in the outcome modeling, procedure duration alone should be regarded as a possibly "tainted" variable.

The Anesthesia Provider and the Anesthesia Care

The Anesthesiologist's Characteristics Board certification seems an even more important predictor of outcome with the anesthesiologist than with the surgeon.[88,155] Using sophisticated modeling, Silber et al[155,156] showed that a lesser proportion of board-certified anesthesiologists on the anesthesia staff is associated with a greater likelihood of "failure to rescue." In a direct comparison of mortality among Medicare patients treated by midcareer anesthesiologists with and without board certification, Silber et al[88] showed that absence of board certification is associated with greater likelihood of "failure to rescue" (OR: 1.13, 95% CI, 1.01-1.27) and higher mortality (OR: 1.13; 95% CI, 1.00-1.26). So confounded are the outcome predictors, however, that they noted that the poorer outcomes of noncertified practitioners may reflect hospital characteristics as well.

Apart from board certification, the effect of the anesthesiologist's experience on outcome is less clear. In a comparison of anesthesia providers at the Massachusetts General Hospital in the mid-1970s, Gilbert[181] detected slightly better outcomes when anesthesia was administered directly by a senior anesthesiologist. However, Cohen et al[59] were unable to detect an outcome difference among anesthesiologists with greater time in the specialty and greater case volumes (Table 25-4). Lunn and Devlin[3] noted the association between poor outcomes of surgery and anesthesia care and unsupervised and undersupervised trainees at night, as have others.[4,129] Exploring the linkage between myocardial ischemia and MI in anesthesia for coronary bypass, Slogoff and Keats[182] famously identified Anesthesiologist 7, whose cases had a greater proportion of intraoperative ischemia and much greater postoperative infarction than did others in the group practice. They implied this was due to individual skill factors, but analysis was superficial and without risk adjustment of the clinical data.

Anesthesia Provider Type More extensive efforts to explore outcome differences by type of anesthesia provider also have been indeterminant because of design flaws, principally failure to adequately address patient selection bias and/or unmeasured, potentially important clinical confounding variables.

Gilbert[181] found no outcome differences when comparing anesthesiologists providing direct care, anesthesiology residents medically directed by faculty anesthesiologists, and nurse anesthetists similarly medically directed. Yet a fully trained anesthesiologist was involved in every case, the data were only partially risk adjusted, and patients were not randomly allocated to providers (*Note:* The physicians likely received the more difficult cases). Similar flaws are present in an analysis based on the Institutional Differences Study: In one portion of that study, clinical outcomes in "[9] hospitals in which anesthesiologists primarily were the providers" were compared with those in "[7] hospitals in which nurse anesthetists were primarily the providers."[183] Outcomes were the same in both groups, yet anesthesiologists were involved in all care.

Multiple design flaws also plague an analysis of postoperative deaths in North Carolina during the period 1969-1976, in which half of the anesthetics were administered by nurse anesthetists medically directed by the surgeon and the other half by anesthesiologists working alone or a team of a nurse anesthetist and an anesthesiologist.[184] Anesthesia-related death rates were similar across the 3 provider types; yet, unlike the studies by Gilbert[181] and Forrest,[183] there was no attempt to adjust the data for case-mix differences (eg, age, ASA physical status) and type of operation (eg, emergent vs elective, major vs minor). Because nurse anesthetists working without anesthesiologists (then and now) are located typically in smaller, often rural hospitals, the 2 other provider types (with anesthesiologists) likely were treating sicker patients having more complex procedures. Also, as with the other studies, there had been no random allocation of patients to provider type, resulting in likely selection bias.

A more recent provider-type comparison, although much more sophisticated, still suffers from serious design flaws: Pine et al[185] compared mortality of 404 194 Medicare patients having 1 of 8 common surgical procedures, whose anesthesia was provided by nurse anesthetists working without anesthesiologists, anesthesiologists providing direct care, or an anesthesia care team of a nurse anesthetist medically directed by an anesthesiologist. After stratification by procedure and adjustment for patient, institutional, and geographic factors, the mortality rates were similar across the 3 provider types. However, 80% of the cases in which nurse anesthetists worked without anesthesiologists were performed in rural hospitals, most assuredly caring for a lower-risk population (severe selection bias). Direct comparison of outcomes in this circumstance is likely to be misleading because patients in the 3 groups would be expected to differ markedly in measured *and unmeasured* risk factors and thus their likelihood of poor outcome. Just as Silber et al[88] noted that the poorer outcomes of noncertified anesthesiologists may also reflect residual confounding by hospital characteristics, there is likely to be similar, unresolved facility-related confounding in the study by Pine et al,[185] particularly without a propensity-score analysis.

In another study, Silber et al[87] demonstrated in a matched-pair, propensity-score analysis (addressing selection bias) that lack of medical direction by an anesthesiologist is associated with a higher failure-to-rescue rate (OR: 1.10; 95% CI, 1.01-1.18) and higher 30-day postoperative mortality (OR: 1.08; 95% CI, 1.00-1.15). They estimated that the higher mortality rate engenders 2.5 excess deaths per 1000 patients, which represents a number needed to treat (NNT) of 400 (Table 25-1). Although a NNT of 400 reflects a modest effect, anesthesiologist's medical direction gains enormous importance because of the tens of millions of anesthetics administered each year.

Several recent comparisons of clinical outcomes associated with different anesthesia provider types undertaken with less analytical sophistication—principally the absence of a propensity-score analysis—undoubtedly were flawed by selection bias and/or unmeasured confounding variables. For example, a comparison of maternal outcomes following obstetric anesthesia care by the 3 anesthesia provider types for 1 141 641 patients in 369 hospitals in 6 states during the period 1999-2001 found no statistically significant differences[186]: Among sources of selection bias was excluding tertiary hospitals expected to receive referrals of high-risk patients (eg, level 3 obstetric units, facilities having neonatal intensive care, Council of Teaching Hospital membership) and patient populations with low prevalence of important chronic illnesses (eg, diabetes).

Another recent example, with particularly subtle flaws, is a study of *surgery*-related complications and deaths associated with the 3 anesthesia-provider types during the period 1999-2005 in the 14 states that opted out of the Medicare requirement that a physician oversee delivery of anesthesia care by a nurse anesthetist compared with those in states that had not opted out[187]: They specifically chose to focus on *surgery*-related adverse outcomes, given that those specifically related to anesthesia care are generally believed to occur at very low rates. Present is the previously mentioned selection bias (particularly in the absence of a propensity-score analysis) related to comparing outcomes from small, often rural hospitals in which nurse anesthetists treat healthier patients having simpler procedures with those from tertiary care centers where anesthesiologists alone or working with nurse anesthetists in an anesthesia care team provide complex care for patients with the highest acuity. In addition, opting out of the physician-supervision requirement had a minimal impact on anesthesia delivery in the 14 affected states because the opt-out provision does not mandate any change but rather gives each hospital the discretion to permit nurse anesthetists to function without physician oversight. Under this circumstance, anesthesia provider change (to unsupervised nurse anesthetists) would probably occur predominantly in the small rural hospitals where anesthesiologists are often not present. Although the presentation of their analysis is not sufficiently detailed to identify personnel shifts by hospital size, case complexity (as measured by mean ASA Relative Value base units) was noted to be significantly lower for solo nurse anesthetists than for either solo anesthesiologists or the anesthesia care team in both opt-out and non–opt-out states. The multivariate analyses, however seemingly exhaustive, did not include a propensity-score analysis or even variables characterizing the site of care. Finally, anesthesia risk (unmeasured here) is but a very small component of overall surgery risk. Hence the inability to demonstrate statewise outcome differences in relation to states opting out should not be unexpected.

The Anesthesia Care Outcome comparisons of specific anesthesia drugs and methods have not identified a single ideal approach to anesthesia but rather have emphasized characteristics, typically pharmacologic, that can be regarded as tradeoffs among different options. Keats[68] suggested that anesthesia agents are "inherently toxic" and that, as our knowledge grows, anesthesia risk diminishes. Past controversies about specific drugs were resolved by either learning how to use them safely or discarding those that were problematic, usually on a pharmacologic basis (eg, methoxyflurane due to dose-related nephrotoxicity). Thus Beecher and Todd[8] attributed "intrinsic toxicity" to curare (a generic term applied to muscle relaxants) before it was appreciated that post-anesthesia residual paralysis could be both hazardous and avoided with pharmacologic antagonism. That drug class now is a mainstay of anesthesia practice (see Chapter 34).

Perhaps expectedly, well-conducted studies have failed to identify important risk differences among anesthesia options. Regional anesthesia (eg, epidural analgesia) may pose lower risk than general anesthesia for graft thrombosis and deep venous thrombosis, among other morbidity, in vascular, lower extremity, and pelvic surgery (see Chapter 55); however, the magnitude of such benefit is uncertain, and whether it results from neuraxial blockade or avoiding general anesthesia is also unknown.[188] Cohen et al[59] noted that anesthesia-related factors (eg, principal anesthesia method) added negligibly to the contributions of patient- and surgery-related factors in accounting for mortality risk (Table 25-4). However, they did find markedly greater mortality if a single-agent anesthetic rather than "balanced anesthesia" with multiple drugs was used (OR: 4.85; 95% CI, 1.97-11.96). Although their inability to identify benefits of specific anesthesia methods arguably could result from selection bias (confounding by indication), Forrest et al[50] were unable to detect meaningful morbidity differences among inhalation agents in a clinical trial that would minimize biased selection.

However, in support of a long-held belief that it is more important *how* rather than specifically *what* one does, Arbous et al[189] have shown that there are multiple opportunities to decrease anesthesia risk by adopting a set of good practices in the management of anesthesia care (**Table 25-7**). Although the efficacy of most of the practices identified by Arbous et al is well documented in the literature (eg, epidural opiates for postoperative pain management rather than intramuscular or intravenous narcotic administration; antagonism of nonmetabolized muscle relaxants at conclusion of anesthesia), these practices continue to require support and encouragement toward full adoption.

TABLE 25-7 Anesthesia Management Factors Associated With 24-Hour Mortality and Coma

Factor[a]	Odds Ratio[b]	95% Confidence Interval
Preoperative Period		
Equipment check with protocol and checklist (vs none or incomplete)	0.640	0.432-0.948
Documentation of equipment check (vs none)	0.607	0.399-0.923
Intraoperative period		
Availability of and access to attending anesthesiologist (direct vs indirect)	0.455	0.313-0.662
No intraoperative change of anesthesiologist (vs change)	0.444	0.199-0.990
Presence of full-time anesthesia nurse (vs part time)	0.408	0.236-0.704
Presence of attending anesthesiologist at emergence and termination of anesthesia (2 practitioners vs 1)	0.687	0.474-0.996
Reversal of opiates (vs none)	0.636	0.100-4.027
Reversal of muscle relaxants (vs none)	0.101	0.032-0.314
Reversal of opiates and muscle relaxants (vs none)	0.290	0.175-0.482
Postoperative period		
Postoperative pain medication: opiate (vs none)	0.165	0.108-0.254
Postoperative pain medication: local anesthetics (vs none)	0.061	0.009-0.400
Postoperative pain medication: combination (vs none)	0.324	0.140-0.752
Postoperative opiate route: epidural (vs IV)	0.226	0.057-0.887
Postoperative opiate route: intramuscular (vs IV)	0.130	0.074-0.335

IV, intravenous route of administration.

[a]All factors adjusted for characteristics of patient (age, gender, ASA physical status classification); surgical procedure (time, duration, whether emergent, type, complexity); principal anesthetia method (inhalation, total intravenous, combined technique; regional [type]; or combination); and hospital (type, size).

[b]All odds ratios whose 95% confidence intervals do not include the value 1.0 are statistically significant.

Modified from Arbous MS, Meursing AEE, van Kleef JW, et al. Impact of anesthesia management characteristics on severe morbidity and mortality. *Anesthesiology.* 2005;102(2):257-268.

More recently, investigators have begun to probe deeper into specific aspects of anesthetic management to gain insights into additional ways to enhance patient outcome and safety: The identification of a relationship between cumulative deep hypnotic time (BIS <45) and greater 1-year mortality[18-21] has been followed recently by recognition that outcomes worsen when low mean arterial pressure (MAP <75 mm Hg) and low anesthetic concentration (minimal anesthetic concentration <0.7) are also present.[190] Moreover, the duration of such a "triple low" predicts worsening outcomes,[190] and the promptness with which a vasopressor is administered attenuates the potential harm of the "triple low."[191] These findings from Sessler's group, based on observational data from one large academic medical center, require validation in a prospective study; however, other evidence demonstrates that intraoperative parameters influence patient outcome: a surgical Apgar score—a composite reflecting intraoperative blood loss, lowest pulse rate, and lowest MAP—predicts 30-day complications and mortality rates.[192,193]

These results emphasize the inadequacy of viewing anesthesia care as merely the presence of certain drugs, anesthetic methods, and devices. We may infer that anesthesia risk studies that consider patient characteristics and their clinical outcomes—but omit intraoperative detail relating to the anesthesiologist's clinical practices—provide an incomplete and possibly misleading perspective. We also might speculate that the beneficial practices identified are likely to be among those that underlie the anesthesiologist's beneficial influence detected by the failure-to-rescue metric.

HOW DO WE INTERPRET ANESTHESIA RISK TO PATIENTS?

As if the evolving story of anesthesia risk were not sufficiently complex, communicating effectively with patients about anesthesia risk is even more challenging. Basic concepts of risk are confusing, if not foreign, to patients, and they are likely to be wary of risk-related statements, given the many prominent public reversals about the benefits and safety of common drugs (eg, hormone replacement therapy, cyclo-oxygenase-2 analgesics).

CREATING AN EFFECTIVE MESSAGE

Because the hallmark of effective communication is understanding the audience, we should tailor risk-related discussions to the specific patient's needs and knowledge, recognizing that a brief targeted disclosure is likely to be mutually satisfying. We can allay their general concerns by noting that anesthesia care has never been safer, that it may be among the least hazardous parts of overall patient care, that common postanesthesia problems tend to be transient, that serious complications have become very uncommon, and that our expanding perspective on anesthesia care (eg, postoperative pain management) means that they are also likely to be more comfortable and satisfied with their care. We can convey to patients that as a result of myriad improvements, anesthesia methods are more similar than different with regard to risk, and often their anesthesia preferences can be honored.

Problems With Risk Numeracy We should avoid placing undue emphasis on specific risk estimates, in part because they are based on the experiences of large populations and may not predict well a given individual's clinical outcome in a given situation (Box 25-1). Although patient-specific risks can be estimated from regression equations and patients often want to know their "chances" (even if they do not ask), the more problematic issue is that quantitative information about risk is meaningful only to the small minority having facility with probabilities and numerical concepts.[194-196] Rather than regarding an outcome occurring 1 in 10 as "common," 1 in 100 as "uncommon," and 1 in 1000 as "rare," patients tend to focus on the numerator almost to the exclusion of the denominator (ie, odds are less important than the possibility that an event can occur). Framing is also a barrier to communicating risk, with "90% survival" perceived as better than "10% mortality."

Evolving guidance for enhancing effective risk communication includes understanding the patient's experience and expectations, presenting *relative* risks of competing options rather than risk estimates in isolation, using graphics ("decision aids") to help the presentation, encouraging a balanced discussion of options and uncertainties, developing recommendations informed by clinical judgment and patient preferences, and continually checking for understanding and agreement.[197,198] For some patients, comparing the risks of anesthesia to other well-known events, such as parachute jumping or flying in commercial aircraft, may be helpful (Box 25-4), but both the clinician and the patient must recognize that these broad generalities may not apply to a given patient.

HOW DO WE ACHIEVE FURTHER REDUCTION IN ANESTHESIA RISK?

The foregoing dissection of sources of risk emphasizes the need to move beyond the former narrow definition of anesthesia care as the use of drugs, methods, and devices, to embrace a far broader perspective of the overall anesthesia care process, from preoperative assessment to postoperative care, and its role in the overall system of care (see Chapter 3 for a discussion of the system of anesthesia care, within a larger system of overall care). A real benefit of adopting a more comprehensive view of anesthesia care has already been demonstrated by the mortality and morbidity risk reduction achieved by modulating the sympathetic nervous system by administering β-adrenergic blockers to high-risk patients when appropriate[26,199] and preventing hypothermia,[100,101] decreasing surgical wound infections by administering perioperative supplemental oxygen,[200] decreasing perioperative mortality by adopting optimal clinical practice patterns[189] and immediate presurgical checklists,[179] and by having an anesthesiologist directing the anesthesia care.[87] The identification of an association between higher cancer recurrence and metastasis-free survival rates and use of anesthesia approaches known to reduce stress[201] suggests that perhaps only our formerly narrow notions of "anesthesia" risk are preventing further reduction in anesthesia risk.

KEY REFERENCES

- Arbous MS, Meursing AEE, van Kleef JW, et al. Impact of anesthesia management characteristics on severe morbidity and mortality. *Anesthesiology.* 2005;102(2):257-268.
- Gold BS, Kitz DS, Lecky JH, Neuhaus JM. Unanticipated admission to the hospital following ambulatory surgery. *JAMA.* 1989;262(21):3008-3010.
- Li G, Warner M, Lang BH, Huang L, Sun LS. Epidemiology of anesthesia-related mortality in the United States, 1999-2005. *Anesthesiology.* 2009;110(4):759-765.
- Lindenauer PK, Pekow P, Wang K, et al. Perioperative beta-blocker therapy and mortality after major noncardiac surgery. *N Engl J Med.* 2005;353(4):349-361.
- Lunn JN, Devlin HB. Lessons from the confidential enquiry into perioperative deaths in three NHS regions. *Lancet.* 1987;2(8572):1384-1386.
- Pronovost PJ, Jenckes MW, Dorman T, et al. Organizational characteristics of intensive care units related to outcomes of abdominal aortic surgery. *JAMA.* 1999;281(14):1310-1317.
- Rodgers A, Walker N, Schug S, et al. Reduction of postoperative mortality and morbidity with epidural or spinal anesthesia: results from overview of randomized trials. *BMJ.* 2000;321(7275):1493-1505.
- Sessler DI, Sigl J, Manberg PJ, et al. A broadly applicable risk stratification system for predicting duration of hospitalization and mortality. *Anesthesiology.* 2010;113(5):1026-1037.
- Silber JH, Kennedy SK, Even-Shoshan O, et al. Anesthesiologist direction and patient outcomes. *Anesthesiology.* 2000;93(1):152-163.
- Silber JH, Williams SV, Krakauer H, Schwartz JS. Hospital and patient characteristics associated with death after surgery: a study of adverse occurrence and failure to rescue. *Med Care.* 1992;30(7):615-629.

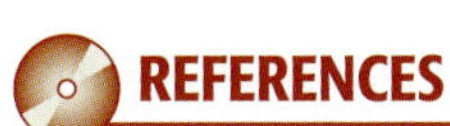

REFERENCES

Complete references available on DVD and online version at www.LongneckerAnesthesiology.com

CHAPTER 26

Approaches to Quality Improvement in Anesthesia Care

George T. Blike
Lee A. Fleisher

KEY POINTS

1. In the United States there is significant public dissatisfaction with the level of safety associated with medical care. This issue has been taken up by many legislative and governmental regulatory bodies at both the federal and state level.
2. The demand for greater patient safety (ie, error reduction) has created multiple new levels of regulation and demands for accountability that go well beyond the traditional.
3. The traditional approach of practitioner accountability is giving way to approaches that additionally emphasize systems redesign and group-managed processes.
4. The demands for accountability require that individual practitioners, groups of practitioners, hospitals, and entire health systems implement methods that allow documentation of outcome and process.
5. The reliance of review systems such as case conference and focus on the individual patient is not adequate for the level of error remediation demanded. New approaches that allow examination of aggregate performance across a hospital or health system need to be developed and implemented. This is particularly challenging for perioperative anesthesia care, considering the already low level of adverse outcome.
6. For many practitioners, reimbursement will be linked to both outcome and the demonstrated compliance with process variables such as perioperative antibiotic administration. Systems that allow documentation at the individual patient level need to be developed or reimbursement and accreditation may be compromised.
7. The level of sophistication with respect to outcome and process evaluation in the intensive care unit has undergone much greater development than that for the operating room. A significant body of work exists to guide the improvement of care and to decrease the error rate in this area of anesthesia practice.
8. Safety and evaluation of outcome for acute pain therapy lags. Part of this may be related to the fact that decisions about acute pain therapy are often split between multiple groups. In addition, there is little definition of what adequate levels of acute pain relief are, how to accurately measure adequacy of pain relief, or how to monitor to prevent the complications of opioid-based pain therapy.

Since the publication of the Institute of Medicine monograph *To Err Is Human* in 1999, there has been a dramatic increase in the public's concern about the quality of patient care and the determination of the extent with which errors occur during the provision of that care.[1] This concept of quality includes ensuring that the care is both beneficial and cost-effective and has placed unprecedented demands on all health care providers to prove the safety and value of the care they deliver.

Until recently, the autonomy of the individual practitioner to provide care in a manner in which they deemed best was paramount. In the hospital setting, the quality of care was ensured by preemployment credentialing with casual periodic renewal and episodic case conferences with the primary reliance on the individual professionalism of each practitioner. This no longer suffices. Groups, regardless of specialty, are being asked to identify potential sources of error both within their practices and the entire health care system. It is now assumed by hospital chief executives and medical officers that groups will establish

TABLE 26-1 Organizations With an Interest in the Quality of Medical Care and Patient Safety

American Society of Anesthesiologists (ASA)
Anesthesia Patient Safety Foundation (APSF)
American Medical Association (AMA)
The Joint Commission
Joint Commission International Center For Patient Safety
Centers for Medicare and Medicaid Services (CMS, part of the US Department of Health and Human Services)
Agency for Healthcare Research and Quality (AHRQ; part of the US Department of Health and Human Services)
Food and Drug Administration (FDA; part of the US Department of Health and Human Services)
National Quality Forum (NQF)
Institute of Medicine of the National Academies (IOM)
Legislative bodies both state and federal
State boards of medicine
Local law enforcement organizations
Purchasers of health care
Consumers of health care
World Health Organization (WHO)

procedures and protocols to minimize risk and to collaborate with other professional groups within a health system. For example, it is expected that anesthesiologists will collaborate with surgeons and nurses to cross-check and confirm correctness at certain critical points in a patient's care (eg, time-out before incision or checking transplant organ compatibility). As part of the continued support of a group, they are expected to document the approaches being used to evaluate and improve the quality and safety of the care provided.

These concerns about patient safety are being driven at many levels (**Table 26-1**). In addition to traditional accrediting agencies, hospital boards of directors and credentialing committees, state boards of medicine, legislatures, the federal government including Congress, and even the courts are increasingly involved. Patient safety and quality improvement is an area that is rapidly changing, the terminology often cryptic and the sources of information outside that usually consulted by anesthesiologists. The key goal of this chapter is to demystify the processes related to quality improvement and discuss several toolsets that are available to provide quality assurance including the approach in use at the University of Pennsylvania Health System. Questions to be addressed include: How does one determine the quality of care provided by a group of anesthesiologists? How does one identify errors in care? What is meant by a critical incident? How does one establish a process to improve the quality and safety of care provided? How should this process be documented?

TERMINOLOGY

A variety of terms are used to define aspects of patient safety, risk reduction, and quality of care. Some of these terms are duplicative. For a number of terms the meaning has changed over time. The following are terms and their definitions used by the Institute of Medicine (IOM) and the Joint Commission in their recent standards and reporting documentation.

HEALTH CARE QUALITY

In *Crossing the Quality Chasm,* the Institute of Medicine (IOM) provided a 6-part definition of health care quality that many view as the emerging standard. According to the IOM, health care should be safe, avoiding injuries to patients from the care that is intended to help them; effective, providing services based on scientific knowledge to all who could benefit and refraining from providing services to those not likely to benefit (avoiding underuse and overuse, respectively); patient centered, providing care that is respectful of and responsive to individual patient preferences, needs, and values and ensuring that patient values guide all clinical decisions; timely, reducing waits and sometimes harmful delays for both those who receive and those who give care; efficient, avoiding waste, including waste of equipment, supplies, ideas, and energy; and equitable, providing care that does not vary in quality because of personal characteristics such as gender, ethnicity, geographic location, and socioeconomic status.[2]

PATIENT SAFETY CULTURE

Lucien Leape, at the Inaugural Gala of the Leape Institute in 2008, said, "A just culture and transparent culture, where no one is punished for making or reporting errors, while at the same time everyone is held accountable. A culture of mindfulness and vigilance where every individual feels personally responsible for practicing safely and for reducing hazards. A culture where everyone feels valued and respected, but processes are standardized and simplified, teamwork trumps autonomy, and safety takes precedence over productivity" (used with permission).

Medical Error Medical error has been defined as the failure of a planned action to be completed as intended (failure of execution) or use of a wrong plan to achieve an aim (error of planning).[3] This is clearly a very broad definition. With regard to unintended acts, it is important to recognize that activities once considered appropriate care may now be considered a medical error and vice versa.

Sentinel Events As defined by the Joint Commission, a sentinel event is "an unexpected occurrence involving death or serious physical or psychological injury, or the risk thereof. Serious injury specifically includes loss of limb or function. The phrase "risk thereof" includes any process variation for which a recurrence would carry a significant change of a serious event outcome." The Joint Commission notes the term *sentinel* reflects an event that requires immediate investigation and response. At a leadership level, the Joint Commission requires an integrated patient safety program that includes in part (1) A definition of the types of occurrences to be addressed, (2) a mechanism to ensure that all relevant areas of the health care organization participate and that their activities are integrated, (3) a procedure of immediate response including care of the affected patient, containment of the risk to others, and preservation of information for future review, (4) clear system for internal and external reporting, (5) a defined mechanism for responding to various types of occurrences, and (6) reporting at least yearly on occurrence of errors and efforts to improve patient safety both proactively and in response to actual occurrences. Thus reporting, categorizing, and review of serious events are required and mechanisms need to be established to accomplish this goal (**Table 26-2**).

In addition to the Joint Commission, other organizations have begun to require the documentation and reporting the equivalent of the Joint Commission sentinel event. Currently in the United States (2010), about 39 states require some form of reporting. Although the specific events and terminology may vary, there are common concepts that tend to follow the Joint Commission descriptions and more recently National Quality Forum Definitions. For example, New Hampshire's Adverse Event Reporting law (HB 592) was passed in 2009 and took effect January 1, 2010. The law requires hospitals to report certain adverse events to the NH Department of Health and Human Services (DHHS) by filing the following via a secure e-mail to DHHS: (1) An Initial Report, due within 15 days of the discovery of an adverse event, and (2) the hospital's Root Cause Analysis (RCA) and Corrective Action Plan (CAP) or a no corrective action taken statement, due within 60 days of the discovery of an adverse event.

The state's objectives with the new reporting are to improve safety by encouraging systematic, open, and transparent reporting of serious adverse events and to improve knowledge and understanding of why serious adverse events occur and how they can be prevented by identifying common underlying causes. HB 592 identifies 28 reportable events in the categories of surgical, product or device related, patient protection, care management, environmental, and criminal. (National Quality Forum: Serious Reportable Events in Healthcare Update 2010,

TABLE 26-2 Joint Commission Sentinel Events That Might Be Related to Anesthesia Care

Events that result in an unanticipated death or major permanent loss of function and are unrelated to the natural course of the patient's illness or underlying condition
Surgery on the wrong patient or body part regardless of magnitude of procedure
Unintended retention of a foreign body after surgery or other procedure
Hemolytic transfusion reactions because of major blood group incompatibilities
Unanticipated death of a full-term infant
Prolonged fluoroscopy with a cumulative dose >1500 rads to a single field
Discharge of an infant to the wrong family
Severe neonatal hyperbilirubinemia
Abduction
Rape
Suicide during treatment or within 72 h of discharge
Delivery of radiotherapy to the wrong body region or >25% above the planned radiotherapy dose
Some of these events may seem remote from the experiences of anesthesiologists whose practices are confined to the operating room. Those doing interventional pain therapy, block placement with fluoroscopic guidance, or intensive care need to be concerned with the broader range of these events.

Source: The Joint Commission: Sentinel event policy and procedures, updated June 2005.

A Consensus Report; www.qualityforum.org). The events are significant and result in either death or a permanent change in function or ability. Not all states have comparable reporting requirements to New Hampshire. However, most states publish an annual report of the number of reportable events that allow a certain level of comparison on this issue.

In some states such as New Jersey, specifically delineated events that might be associated with perioperative anesthetic care include hemolytic reactions from administration of ABO incompatible blood or blood products, electric shock, burns, injuries from the use of restraints, malfunction of ventilators or infusion pumps, surgery on the wrong body part, wrong patient, and wrong surgical procedure. They also include intraoperative or postoperative (within 12 hours) coma, death, or other serious preventable adverse event for any American Society of Anesthesiologists (ASA) class 1 inpatient or any same-day surgery patient regardless of ASA class. Other states such as Pennsylvania are less prescriptive. The Pennsylvania statute, Medical Care Availability and Reduction of Error (MCARE) Act (Act 13 of 2002), does not use the "sentinel event" terminology but rather defines a "serious event" as an event, occurrence, or situation involving the clinical care of a patient in a medical facility that results in death or compromises patient safety and results in an unanticipated injury required the delivery of additional health care services to the patient. The act further defines the term *incident* as an event that could have produced unexpected injury to a patient in a way similar to that defined under serious event. Several investigators have begun using state databases of reported events to determine the safety of different practices such as office-based anesthesia care.

Near Miss This is defined as a "process variation" that did not affect the outcome but for which recurrence carries a significant chance of a serious adverse outcome. These events are not subject to review by the Joint Commission but need to be appropriately reviewed and changes made to decrease the risk of the event happening again.

Hazardous Conditions These are defined as circumstances (not including the disease or condition for which the patient is being treated) that significantly increase the likelihood of a serious adverse outcome. A wet floor, for example, presents a hazardous condition that might increase the risk of a patient fall. The Joint Commission has now made prevention of patient falls a national patient safety goal, and therefore identification of both those at risk and hazardous conditions in those at risk is a national priority.

Sentinel Event Alerts This is a mechanism introduced by the Joint Commission to bring attention to situations that might lead to sentinel events. Among the many are a number that appear potentially to involve the practice of anesthesia or intensive care, including high concentrations of potassium chloride, wrong surgery (wrong side, wrong patient, wrong procedure, etc), restraint deaths, high-alert medications (ie, anticoagulants, hypoglycemics, sedative/analgesics, paralytics, cardio- and vasoactive medications), operative and postoperative complications, infusion pump malfunction, look-alike sound-alike drugs, medical gas mixups, needles and sharps injuries, dangerous abbreviations, ventilator-related events, delays in treatment, nosocomial infections, surgical fires, anesthesia awareness, and patient-controlled analgesia. Once an alert occurs, it is important that it is disseminated throughout the organization.

The specialty of anesthesiology has recently addressed one of these sentinel alerts more formally. On October 6, 2004, the Joint Commission issued an alert, *Preventing, and Managing the Impact of, Anesthesia Awareness.* The alert went on to state:

> To overcome the limitations of current methods to detect anesthesia awareness, new methods are being developed that are less affected by the drugs typically used during general anesthesia. These devices measure brain activity rather than physiological responses. These electroencephalography (EEG) devices (also called level-of-consciousness, sedation-level and anesthesia-depth monitors) include the Bispectral Index® (BIS), spectral edge frequency (SEF) and median frequency (MF) monitors. These devices may have a role in preventing and detecting anesthesia awareness in patients with the highest risk, thereby ameliorating the impact of anesthesia awareness. A body of evidence has not yet accumulated to definitely define the role of these devices in detecting and preventing anesthesia awareness; the Joint Commission expects additional studies on these subjects to emerge. In its review of the Bispectral Index (BIS) ® monitor, the Food and Drug Administration determined that "Use of BIS monitoring to help guide anesthetic administration may be associated with the reduction of the incidence of awareness with recall in adults during general anesthesia and sedation."

The Joint Commission recommended that health care organizations that perform procedures under general anesthesia develop and implement an anesthesia awareness policy. Because many practitioners were concerned that a particular monitoring device was being endorsed, they developed a sample departmental policy on intraoperative awareness that is available to members. It is important to recognize that resources are available to help address some of these alerts.

QUALITY-OF-CARE INDICATORS

A broad definition for reportable events such as those found for sentinel events or serious events presented earlier may be difficult for practitioners to use on a day-to-day basis to decide what should or should not be reported. Without detracting from the need to report at a broad level, defining specific reporting indicators provides operational definitions that speeds this decision making. In 2009, the ASA established the Anesthesia Quality Institute (AQI). Multiple data sources are now flowing into AQI's central repository (**Fig. 26-1**). The *mission* of the AQI is to develop and maintain an ongoing registry of case data that helps anesthesiologists assess and improve patient care. The eventual *goal* of the AQI is to provide a resource for anesthesiologists to obtain patient safety and quality management data and to meet regulatory requirements designed to improve patient care. A key component of the AQI is the National Anesthesia Clinical Outcomes Registry (NACOR), which includes a group of key quality indicators developed by the Committee on Performance and Outcome Measures of the ASA. (**Table 26-3**). There are important process indicators also, such as on-time antibiotic administration or time-out documentation.

Reporting of adverse events needs to be encouraged. The aviation industry has used self-reporting for a number of years to detect situations at risk for serious events (for an overview, see Helmreich and

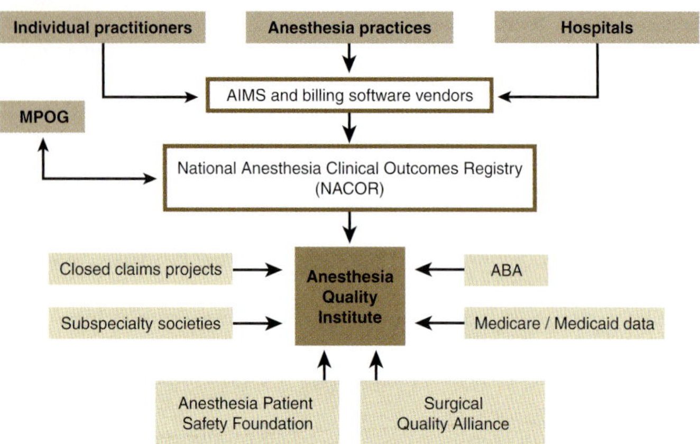

FIGURE 26-1. Map of the multiple sources of process and outcome data being linked to the Anesthesia Quality Institute's central data repository. AIMS, anesthesia information management systems.

Merritt.[4] This reporting is nonpunitive, whereas failure to report may compromise one's employment position. An environment in which reporting is encouraged can only be created if the act of reporting does not create negative repercussions. Anonymous reporting may be helpful but compromises the ability to follow up and determine events at the level of detail that might be required. There has been debate about whether or not voluntary reporting is adequate, and a number of institutions have reported their experiences with scanning of anesthesia records for vital sign excursions beyond predefined boundaries. Others have used chart review by sampling a portion of the anesthetics performed. Given the relative rarity of many of the most serious anesthesia-related incidents and events, sampled chart reviews may miss critical cases. Chart scanning for acceptable vital sign boundaries might generate more false positives than can be reasonably reviewed, depending on the patient population of a particular institution. "Buy-in" for voluntary reporting provides the ability to identify the uncommon but serious events. (As mentioned, in some states, there is also mandatory reporting of medical errors.) Voluntary reporting need not be limited to members of an anesthesia department. We have found that observations by others, such as nurses, surgical house staff, and so on, can be valuable additions to the quality improvement process.

TABLE 26-3 Quality Improvement Indicators Related to Anesthesia From the Committee on Performance and Outcome Measures of the American Society of Anesthesiologists[a]

1. Death
2. Cardiac arrest
3. Perioperative myocardial infarction
4. Anaphylaxis
5. Malignant hyperthermia
6. Transfusion reaction
7. Stroke, cerebral vascular accident, or coma following anesthesia
8. Visual loss
9. Operation on incorrect site
10. Operation on incorrect patient
11. Medication error
12. Unplanned ICU admission
13. Intraoperative awareness
14. Unrecognized difficult airway
15. Reintubation
16. Dental trauma
17. Perioperative aspiration
18. Vascular access complication, including vascular injury or pneumothorax
19. Pneumothorax following attempted vascular access or regional anesthesia
20. Infection following epidural or spinal anesthesia
21. Epidural hematoma following spinal or epidural anesthesia
22. High spinal
23. Postdural puncture headache
24. Major systemic local anesthetic toxicity
25. Peripheral neurologic deficit following regional anesthesia
26. Infection following peripheral nerve block

[a]For full definitions, see http://aqihq.org/CPOM%20Registry%20Data%20Set.pdf).

ASSESSMENT OF PATIENT QUALITY-OF-CARE INFORMATION

PEER REVIEW

Peer review has been a part of anesthesia practice for over 70 years. One of the earliest documented uses of peer review for anesthesia-related mortality was by Ruth in 1935 when he helped establish the first anesthesia study commission to analyze perioperative deaths.[5] The commission relied on voluntary submission of cases and determined the cause of death by majority vote. The peer review process actually approaches the analysis of care in a much more systematic way today, but clearly there is a long tradition in the field of trying to identify those cases in which the actions of the anesthesiologist contribute to mortality and morbidity. The magnitude of iatrogenic morbidity and mortality was not quantified across the spectrum of health care until the Harvard Practice Study, published in 1991.[6] This seminal study used a structured peer review methodology to estimate that iatrogenic failures occur in approximately 4% of all hospitalizations. Specific categories of surgical adverse events have been identified in subsequent review of over 14 700 hospitalizations in Colorado and Utah.[7] The nature of surgical adverse events was categorized by type of injury and by preventability (**Table 26-4**).

It is also common today for many of these categories of complications to be reviewed in a quality assurance (QA) process by multiple individuals who were not directly responsible for the care of the patient. For example, it may include a QA officer in the anesthesia department but may also include individuals in surgery, nursing, and pharmacy.

MORTALITY AND MORBIDITY CONFERENCES (TABLE 26-5)

The "M&M" conference has a long history of reviewing negative outcomes in medicine. The goal of this traditional conference is to learn

TABLE 26-4 Surgical Adverse Events by Type of Injury and by Preventability

Type of Event	% of Adverse Events	% Preventable
Technique-related complication	24	68
Wound infection	11	23
Postoperative bleeding	11	85
Postpartum/neonatal related	8	67
Other infection	7	38
Drug-related injury	7	46
Wound problem (noninfectious)	4	53
Deep venous thrombosis	4	18
Nonsurgical procedure injury	3	59
Diagnostic error/delay	3	100
Pulmonary embolus	2	14
Acute myocardial infarction	2	0
Inappropriate therapy	2	100
Anesthesia injury	2	45
Congestive heart failure	1	33
Stroke	1	0
Pneumonia	1	65
Fall	.5	50
Other	5.5	32

Adapted from Gawande AA, Thomas EJ, Zinner MJ, Brennan TA. The incidence and nature of surgical adverse events in Colorado and Utah in 1992. *Surgery.* 1999;126:66-75.

TABLE 26-5 Comparing Traditional Mortality and Morbidity Conferences With Systems-Oriented Conferences

Absolute individual practitioner responsibility	Examines the role of the "system" in contributing to error without diminishing the need for individual responsibility
Focuses on individual cases	Allows for examination across larger patient groups often beyond individual practitioner
Does not adequately recognize the role of groups and group interaction	Emphasizes group contributions toward common goal of patient safety and error reduction
Exhortation to "do better" key route for problem solution	Explores possible changes in the "system" to reduce probability of error
High rate of medical error despite long history of this approach improving patient care	Too new to know if there will be a significant reduction in error
"Shame" and "blame" may make discussions less than forthcoming	Emphasis on totality of risk may allow better discussion

Adapted from Pierluissi E, Fischer MA, Campbell AR, Landefeld CS. Discussion of medical errors in morbidity and mortality conferences. JAMA. 2003;290:2838-2842.

how to prevent future patients from suffering similar harm and thus incrementally improve care. However, frank discussion of error is often limited in M&M conferences. Also, the actual review practices fail to support deep learning regarding systemic vulnerabilities; indeed, because M&M conferences do not explicitly require medical errors to be reviewed, errors are rarely addressed. One prospective investigation of 4 US academic hospitals found that a resident vigilantly attending weekly internal medicine M&M conferences for an entire year would discuss errors only once. The surgical version of the M&M conference was better with error discussion. However, although surgeons discussed adverse events associated with error 77% of the time, individual provider error was the focus of the discussion and cited as causative of the negative outcome in 8 of 10 conference discussions.[8] Surgical conference discussions rarely identified structural defects, resource constraints, team communication, or other system problems. Further limiting its usefulness, the M&M conference is reactive by nature and highly subject to hindsight bias. This is the basis for most clinical outcome reviews, focusing solely on medical providers and their decision making.[9] In their report, "Nine Steps to Move Forward From Error," in medicine, human factors experts Woods and Cook challenged the medical community to resist the temptation to simplify the complexities practitioners face when reviewing accidents post hoc. Premature closure by blaming the closest clinician hides the deeper patterns and multiple contributors associated with failure and ultimately leads to naive "solutions" that are weak or even counterproductive.[10] The IOM has also cautioned against blaming an individual and recommending training as the sole outcome of case review.[1] Although the culture within medicine is to learn from failure, the M&M conference does not typically achieve this aim.

The single-case approach slights trends and risks that can only be detected by grouping events and performing various types of data analyses. Although this type of conference still has a place as a tool to improve patient safety, it has been less than optimal, and other approaches need to be implemented as well.

One approach to using the morbidity and mortality conferences more effectively is to conduct them in an interdisciplinary manner. At the University of Pennsylvania, cases are periodically presented to a joint group of surgeons and anesthesiologists. There is a focus on cases in which more effective teamwork or communication could have led to better outcomes. These conferences have proven to be a very effective method for obtaining more widespread buy-in to quality assurance processes. Senior faculty members and the respective departmental leaders have been very willing to participate. The concept has expanded from joint conferences with general surgery and anesthesia to conferences with other surgical specialties and even with our colleagues in perioperative nursing. At Dartmouth-Hitchcock Medical Center the Department of Anesthesiology has used a variant of the M&M conference called Quality and Patient Safety Conference. It is multidisciplinary and presents all adverse events reviewed by the departmental Quality Assurance and Quality improvement Committee. The method of review identifies contributing factors and priority corrective actions. Hundreds of problems have been identified and improvements implemented using this approach over the 10 years it has existed.

ROOT CAUSE ANALYSIS

Root cause analysis is a more structured process than traditional peer review for identifying the causal or contributing factors that lead to major morbidity or mortality (see www.patientsafety.gov/rca.html). A root cause analysis must include the following:

1. Determination of human and other factors
2. Determination of related processes and systems
3. Analysis of underlying cause and effect systems through a series of *why?* questions
4. Identification of risks and their potential contributions
5. Determination of potential improvement in processes or systems

The approach demands that bad outcomes not be attributed to the first error discovered, but rather it is important to review all of the potential sources of error or systems problems that led to the adverse event. Analysis depends on a robust model of accident causation. Reason's model is widely respected in high hazardous industries including health care.[11] This model recognized that a combination of triggering factors, unsafe acts by individuals, latent conditions, and faulty defenses, allow a minor incident to progress until harm results (**Fig. 26-2**).

A systems approach allows one to discover all of the potential areas that can lead to an adverse event. We routinely use an approach that systematically investigates for contributory factors.[12,13]

Reason[14] popularized the concept of latent conditions, that is, the "accidents waiting to happen," in a system or process. For example, an anesthesiologist may give the wrong medication, but contributing factors may be containers with similar size and lettering, low light levels in an operating room, a distressingly high level of music, and a malfunctioning

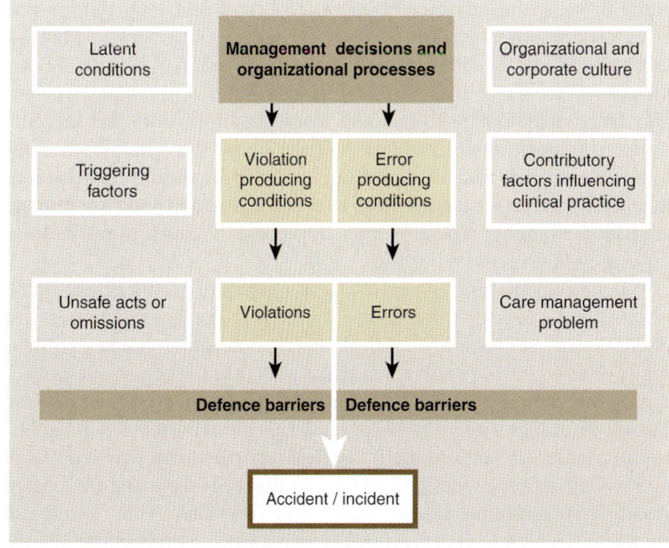

FIGURE 26-2. Model of organizational causes of accidents. Triggering events propagate when a combination of cultural factors, unsafe acts, and multiple gaps in safety defense systems align to cause an accident Vincent C, Taylor-Adams S, Chapman EJ, et al. How to investigate and analyse clinical incidents: clinical risk unit and association of litigation and risk management protocol. *BMJ*. 2000;320:777-781.[13]

inspiratory valve whose correction has created distraction. Typically these factors do not all occur at once, and the patient receives the correct medication. Focusing only on the last error (the giving of the wrong medication) will not correct the underlying cause of the error, nor will it decrease the probability of avoiding a similar error in the future.

FAILURE MODES AND EFFECTS ANALYSIS

Failure modes and effects analysis (FMEA) is a systematic method of evaluating a process to identify where and how it may fail. Whereas root cause analysis assesses cause after an event has occurred, the goal of FMEA is to anticipate risks, alter processes, and thus avoid adverse events. According to the Institute for Healthcare Improvement, FMEA includes review of the following:

- Steps in the process
- Failure modes (what could go wrong?)
- Failure causes (why would the failure happen?)
- Failure effects (what would be the consequences of each failure?)

Tools have been developed to perform a FMEA (http://www.patientsafety.gov/safetytopics.html). Each failure mode gets a numeric score that quantifies (1) likelihood that the failure will occur, (2) likelihood that the failure will be detected, and (3) the amount of harm or damage the failure mode may cause to a person or to equipment. The product of these 3 scores is the risk priority number (RPN) for that failure mode. The sum of the RPNs for the failure modes is the overall RPN for the process.

For example, FMEA can be used to look at blood bank processes even if no adverse event occurred. It can also be used by groups of clinicians to test or simulate a process before it is incorporated into routine clinical care. This may lead to improvements in the process. Paradoxically, a proposed "improvement in care" may be found to increase the RPN rather than decrease it and therefore should not be implemented. The RPN can also be used to determine if implemented process changes actually resulted in lower potential risk.

AN APPROACH TO QUALITY-OF-CARE IMPROVEMENT

DATA ACQUISITION

Observer Reporting Acquiring information about patient outcomes, adverse events, and incidents that might have led to adverse events is the first step for any quality review process. Event reporting by the caregivers or observers has been contrasted to chart review. Manual chart review can be labor intensive, and the yield may be low for the infrequent events of most interest to anesthesiologists. Chart review may be complementary to incident reporting and may in fact identify different populations of patients.[15] Reporting by those involved needs to be encouraged. Ease of reporting,[16] comfort providing reports, and the feeling that reporting may lead to useful evaluation and change may contribute to higher reporting rates. A process that leads to retribution for error will decrease reporting.

Whether or not caregiver incident reporting produces adequate response rates is a topic for debate. Sanborn et al suggested that in his institution there was a low level of compliance with voluntary reporting of defined intraoperative incidents.[17] In contrast, Lagasse described a program claiming a near 100% response rate with a nonthreatening quality assurance system.[18,19] Katz and Lagasse reported on incidents captured after 37 924 anesthetics by self-reporting, chart reviews, and an incident report process.[20] They found that self- reporting for events resulting in disabling patient injury was very high. They found no significant benefit to chart review compared with self reporting.

Automated Data Acquisition Over the past 15 years there has been a marked acceleration of the implementation of hospital information systems and continuing refinement of intraoperative data record keepers or anesthesia information management systems (AIMS). The AIMS have the ability to capture and identify multiple outcomes of interest and intraoperative events (eg, blood pressure changes, drugs). Data from individual patients can be aggregated and linked to predefined clinical and/or resource utilization outcomes. Although there is concern about the accuracy of the information obtained from the AIMS related to the potential "smoothing" of intraoperative data, studies in this area have reported a higher degree of accuracy than data obtained from a traditional "handwritten" record or self-reporting.[21,22] Of greatest concern in the potential use of these large databases is the potential for "data mining." It is important to recognize that the associations that might be found from these types of analyses are just associations, and when a large number of variables are available there is a good statistical probability that these associations will be found. It is therefore important to recognize that these are hypothesis generating, rather than hypothesis confirming or disproving. Nonetheless, the increasing implementation of AIMS should lead to an improved ability to identify morbidity and mortality and to reconstruct the potential factors that led to the complications.

Computer-Assisted Data Acquisition Computers can assist in the acquisition of incident and event information. In 2002, the University of Pennsylvania Medical Center went online with a computerized report entry system. Embedded within the system are the quality improvement indicators that we had been following for anesthesia-related events. The system is accessible from any computer within the medical center's domain that includes computers in every operating room, in strategic locations outside the operating room, postanesthesia care units, intensive care units, and all faculty offices. Prior to this system going online, we would typically receive about 50 to 100 patient-related event reports per year. Most of these came from anesthesia faculty and residents. The year after the computer system went online, 250 events were logged in with at least half coming from nonanesthesia observers. Currently we are receiving about 300 reports per year of events or incidents that might be related to the activities of anesthesiologists. The system has greatly improved our capture of potential issues. In addition there is faster access to these reports than was possible when a paper-based system was in use.

Data Verification The medical record is the ultimate source of data verification. With respect to serious events, discussions with those involved before memory fades, review of the anesthesia record, and other associated records are critical. We have found that single reports may be inaccurate or the reporter not aware of the entire clinical situation. Thus reports are a start, and depending on the nature of the event, more investigation may be required. In some situations we undertake these reviews internally. When there appears to be significant multidisciplinary issues, we have asked our medical center risk management group to conduct a formal root cause analysis.

Database Entry The data obtained often contain patient identifiers and information of a sensitive nature. Clearly basic precautions to avoid theft of this data or its publication need to be taken. Password protection of computer files using strong passwords and possibly encryption appear necessary. Paper records should be kept in locked offices or filing cabinets. We do not store any of our patient safety data on portable computers. We store the data on medical center servers that are routinely backed up and maintained behind a firewall. Patient records are not removed from the medical center because records of this nature have been stolen from automobiles; briefcases have been mislaid in restaurants, and so on. We attempt to maintain all of our patient safety/quality improvement data within the peer review system to decrease the risk of discoverability during any medical legal processes.

Consideration must also be given to the personnel entrusted with database entry. Diversion of records from their intended purposes by clerks and others has occurred. We also make sure that the records are not left out on desks when those doing data entry leave the area.

Review of Data

Moving Beyond the Assessment of a Single Case The single case unless intensively studied may provide little information. Aggregating the data will provide information about trends and special risks depending on the frequency of event occurrence and the time over which the data is accumulated. Particularly for rare events such as anesthesia-related deaths, occurrence and cause may not at all be evident without some sort of data accumulation. However, the key first step is to review the incident to determine its relevance to the anesthetic care provided.

Database Management and Incident Analysis Programs Systematic data review can be done reasonably well using a computerized spreadsheet. Data entry and simple analysis such as frequency, changes over time, or events based on practitioner, type of surgery, or other variables of interest can be relatively easily obtained. The ASA has made available a program from Quality Assurance Research called QA/PDX. Members can apply and then download it from the ASA Web site (for information, see www.asahq.org/qmdaform.htm). According to the information provided by the developers, the program is a relational database that can be used on virtually any computer that uses a Microsoft operating system, including DOS legacy machines. The program has a defined data entry format as well as preconfigured reports.

Computer-Assisted Reporting Programs Many large centers have developed their own reporting systems. However, a number of reporting systems can be purchased. The advantages of using a computer-based (as opposed to a paper-based) system for the entire institution (in contrast to a single department) have been mentioned earlier. Although we have not had personal experience with any of these programs, each has been installed and recommended in general way by a current user. These include Risk MonitorPro; WEBagent by Peminic; Quantros Occurrence report management system; International Developers Healthcare Management System, which includes modules for incident and complaint management, quality, and peer review management, as well as other process management programs.

Feedback Obtaining and analyzing data is a QA function. However, quality improvement requires mechanisms to feed back this information to the involved practitioners and to other stakeholders. Because quality improvement involves system and behavior change, this part of the patient safety process is the most difficult and critically dependent on feedback mechanisms. In teaching departments, the normal turnover of residents and in many cases junior faculty means that the "institutional" memory is short. The intervals required to review or reteach this information may be difficult to determine, as is maintaining an up-to-date list of "what needs to be relearned." Change management in complex sociotechnical systems like health care is not simply common sense. One will quickly find that the major barriers to designing and implementing behavioral change are cultural, and with regard to systems and process, it involves managing the uncertainty found in health care. Interestingly, at both Dartmouth Hitchcock and University of Pennsylvania, we have very similar experiences with managing change to improve quality and patient safety. At both institutions, many reacted to new requirements for universal precautions during central line insertion by viewing them as an impediment rather than a process to be embraced and reliably practiced. We find communication to be critical and that a variety of approaches are needed to reach most of those who need to receive such specific patient safety messages. We regularly use conferences, e-mail both in the form of a periodic "newsletter" and individual e-mail, individual conversation, and policy development. We find that developing policies that can alter processes at the level of the operating nurse or those who prepare the operating room between cases can often effect change faster then working through physicians. We have also found that residents are more receptive than faculty to implementing change rapidly. The need for repetition and follow-up suggests that in larger departments, resources are needed to be devoted to the education component of the patient safety, quality improvement process. Several examples may be helpful. Intraoperative cardiac arrest related to potassium was not finally eliminated until concentrated potassium solutions were removed from the operating room. We achieved virtual 100% compliance with operating room central line placement guidelines when a sterile gown, drape, and towel pack specifically for central line placement was provided with every request for a central line kit. In addition, the circulating nurse and scrub nurse have become actively involved as a double check to ensure compliance.

AGGREGATED PATIENT OUTCOME AND SAFETY DATA IMPROVES ANESTHESIA CARE

One of the first reports in which anesthesia-related patient care data was aggregated was by Beecher and Todd, who studied anesthetic death in 10 institutions and published their work in 1954.[23] Their study included 599 548 anesthetics. The cause of mortality was determined at the local institution by consensus of a surgeon and the chief anesthetist of the institution. Each death was characterized as having one primary cause and may also have had multiple secondary causes. This approach allowed a more thorough analysis of the causes of mortality beyond a primary one.

Dripps and colleagues at the University of Pennsylvania surveyed their experience during the 10-year period from 1947 to 1957.[24] They noted 1285 operative deaths (death within 30 days) in approximately 120 000 anesthetics, for a gross mortality rate of 1.1%. This definition includes late deaths, as opposed to many studies that focus on the intraoperative period or the first 48 postoperative hours. After review of the hospital records, they determined if anesthesia was definitely or possibly contributory to death. This approach allowed the authors to identify systematic issues that could be addressed.

Clifton and Hotten reported on 162 deaths associated with anesthesia in 205 640 operations performed in the Royal Prince Alfred Hospital in Sydney, Australia, between 1952 and 1962.[25] One cause of postoperative mortality was respiratory insufficiency. These authors argued that many of these complications would have been prevented by the use of a recovery unit. The potential safety advantage of a postanesthesia care unit (PACU) was a general theme in these reports from the 1960s, and this quality assurance process led to the routine availability of a PACU.

Numerous other groups have examined the incidence and etiology of perioperative morbidity and mortality over the years. For example, Tiret and colleagues carried out a prospective survey of complications associated with anesthesia in France from 1978 to 1982 in a representative sample of 198 103 anesthetics chosen at random from hospitals throughout the country in a study under the direction of the French Ministry of Health.[26] The investigators evaluated either deaths or coma within 24 hours of surgery. The French survey confirmed previous findings that major complications occurred more frequently in older patients, those undergoing emergent operations, and those with more extensive comorbidity, as measured by the ASA Physical Status Classification.

One of the most important findings of the survey was that postanesthesia respiratory depression was the largest cause of death and coma that was totally attributable to anesthesia. Almost all of the patients with respiratory depression leading to a major complication had received narcotics and muscle relaxants that had not been reversed. They also reported a high incidence of "anaphylactoid shock." The authors contended that this was primarily due to Althesin and succinylcholine. Importantly, there was no category of drug overdose, which may have been a more appropriate label for some of these cases.

The need to look into perioperative morbidity and mortality on a national level was recognized in England. The pioneering work of Lunn and others led to the development of the Confidential Enquiry into Perioperative Deaths (CEPOD), which assessed nearly a million cases of anesthesia during a 1-year period in 1987 in 3 large regions of the United Kingdom.[27,28] Unique to this study was the establishment of "crown privilege" by the government to allow total confidentiality: "The Secretary of State is satisfied that the disclosure of documents about individual cases prepared for the Enquiry into Perioperative Deaths would be against the public interest and would undermine the whole basis of a confidential study. Therefore, the data/information sent to the confidential Enquiry intro perioperative deaths is protected from subpoena."

Deaths within 30 days of surgery were included in the study. Anesthesia was considered the sole cause of death in only 3 individuals, for a rate of 1 in 185 000 cases, and anesthesia was contributory in 410 deaths, for a rate of 7 in 10 000. An important aspect of the CEPOD study was that it established both anesthesia- and surgical-related factors that contributed to mortality. Of the 410 perioperative deaths, there were 9 cases of aspiration or vomit and 18 cases of cardiac arrest.

There remains some debate as to whether anesthetic mortality has actually decreased or, if it has not, what factors (such as increasingly complex procedures or extension of surgical care into the extremes of age) may influence the data. Lagasse reviewed perioperative deaths in the 1990s and concluded that the anesthesia-related mortality rate had remained stable at approximately 1 death per 13 000 procedures, with wide variation making it impossible to detect trends in anesthesia safety. (See Chapter 25 for an extensive discussion of anesthesia risk and mortality.)[29]

Although some uncertainty remains, these types of publications add greatly to understanding the cause of rare outcomes and provide individual clinicians with areas to focus their attention.

AMERICAN SOCIETY OF ANESTHESIOLOGISTS CLOSED CLAIMS STUDY

Studies similar to the CEPOD study have not been performed in United States, most likely because of the legal system. Therefore, potential causes (and treatments) of perioperative mortality had to be obtained from other sources. This led the Professional Liability Committee of the ASA to conduct a nationwide survey of closed insurance claims for major anesthetic mishaps, which has resulted in a series of publications over the past several decades. The Closed Claims Study allowed analysis of very rare events and potential treatments.

One example involved unexpected cardiac arrest during spinal anesthesia, which was observed in 14 healthy patients from the initial 900 claims.[30] The cases were analyzed to identify patterns of management that may have led to the event. Two patterns were identified: oversedation leading to respiratory insufficiency and inappropriate resuscitation of high spinal sympathetic blockade. In another example, Caplan et al reviewed the closed claims study for respiratory events.[31] They identified inadequate ventilation, esophageal intubation, and difficult tracheal intubation as the primary causes of respiratory events. Most of the outcomes were deemed to be preventable with better monitoring. Much of this work formed part of the basis for the ASA Difficult Airway Guidelines and algorithm.[32] More recently, they have evaluated complications that occur in remote locations.[33] Investigators in England have also used this approach to review claims from the National Health Services.[34]

VETERANS ADMINISTRATION HEALTH SYSTEM'S APPROACH TO QUALITY AND THE NATIONAL SURGICAL QUALITY IMPROVEMENT PROGRAM

Based on concern about quality of care within the US Veterans Administration, Congress mandated the development of the National VA Surgical Risk Study (NVASRS) in 1986. Between October 1991 and December 31, 1993, the NVASRS was conducted in 44 VA Medical Centers and developed a risk-adjustment model for predicting 30-day outcome. Based on the NVASRS, the National VA Surgical Quality Improvement Program (NSQIP) was established in January 1994.[35,36] NSQIP collected data on 40 preoperative clinical risk factors (eg, diabetes and heart disease), 20 categories of 30-day postoperative morbidity (eg, venous thrombosis, wound infections, and pneumonia), and 30-day postoperative mortality on patients having major operations under general, spinal, or epidural anesthesia. This VA-led initiative has published numerous articles demonstrating the factors associated with poor outcome and medical errors.[37] As of 2002, the 30-day postoperative mortality after major surgery in the VA had decreased by 27% and the 30-day morbidity by 45%. By 2004, the private sector piloted and then the American College of Surgeons implemented a NSQIP program. Currently, more than 211 independent sites participate and contribute to the shared data and costs of data management and administration. The previously described ASA Anesthesia Quality Institute, although still in its early stages of development, is expected to accelerate identification of factors associated with poor outcomes specific to anesthesia practice.

INVOLVEMENT OF THE PATIENT AND FAMILY

As part of some of the national patient safety initiatives, a critical component has been the involvement of the patient and family. For example, the Joint Commission and the Institute for Healthcare Improvement (IHI) have both advocated informing the patients to ask their physicians and other health care providers to wash their hands. This may seem like a simple request, but multiple observations have suggested that hand washing is not a routine activity between patient encounters. Similarly, the Surgical Care Improvement Project (SCIP) has developed patient "tip sheets" to advise patients about appropriate questions and best practices that should be adopted at the individual hospital. For example, patients are informed to ask about the use of protocols to maintain perioperative β-blockade in those patients already taking the medication and other protocols to prevent deep vein thromboses. It is the authors' belief that this is becoming common practice and that clinicians should be prepared for an educated public who questions their practices.

NATIONAL PATIENT SAFETY GOALS AS THEY RELATE TO ANESTHESIA PRACTICE (TABLE 26-6)

Over the past several years, a series of national patient safety goals have been advanced by The Joint Commission based on sentinel events and other sources of medical errors that occurred in the past. Table 26-6

TABLE 26-6 Joint Commission Patient Safety Goals as They Apply to the Perioperative Period (2003-2006)

Standards and goals vary depending on the health care setting. The ones in this list apply to Hospital and Critical Access Hospital programs.
Goal 1: Improve accuracy of patient identification. 1A: Use at least 2 patient identifiers prior to giving medication or blood products, providing treatment or procedures
Goal 2: Improve effectiveness of communication among caregivers. 2A: "read-back" verbal orders or verbal test results; 2B: Standardize a list of abbreviations that are not to be used; 2E: Implement a standardized approach to "hand-off" communications including an opportunity to ask and respond to questions.
Goal 3: Improve the safety of using medications. 3A: Remove concentrated electrolytes from patient care units (includes potassium chloride and sodium chloride >0.9%); 3B: Standardize and limit the number of drug concentrations available within the organization; 3C: Identify a list of look-alike/sound-alike drugs used in the organization, and take action to prevent errors involving the interchange of these drugs; 3D: Label all medications, medication containers, or other solutions on and off the sterile field in perioperative and other procedural settings.
Goal 4: Eliminate wrong-site, wrong patient, wrong procedure surgery. Protocol-driven preoperative verification process; mark the operative site; conduct a "time-out" before starting the procedure.
Goal 5: Improve safety of using infusion pumps.
Goal 6: Improve effectiveness of clinical alarm systems. Ensure that alarms are activated with appropriate settings; ensure adequate level of audibility.
Goal 7: Reduce risk of health care–associated infections. 7A: Comply with Centers for Disease Control and Prevention's hygiene guidelines; 7B: Manage as sentinel events all identified cases of unanticipated death or major permanent loss of function associated with a health care–associated infection.
Goal 8: Medication reconciliation. 8A: Develop a process for obtaining a complete list of patient's current medications; 8B: Develop a process for communicating the complete medication list to the next provider outside or within an organization.

Adapted from various sources including the Joint Commission Web site.

TABLE 26-7 Draft Candidate 2007 Joint Commission National Patient Safety Goals as They Apply to the Perioperative Period

These are proposed standards and may be modified prior to adoption. Some may not be adopted. This list is based on material released November 2005.

Goal 3E: Reduce the likelihood of patient harm associated with the use of anticoagulant therapy. Strategies include the use of premixed heparin solutions, use of programmable pumps and independent double checks for IV anticoagulants, dosing protocols based on patient weight, elimination of heparin flush in peripheral intravenous lines.

Requirement 15B: Prevent health care–associated pressure ulcers. Assess and periodically reassess each patient's risk for developing a pressure ulcer and take action to address any identified risks. Strategies include maintaining and improving tissue tolerance to pressure, protecting against the adverse effects of external mechanical forces by reducing skin injury from friction and shear forces, repositioning, or mechanical loading and support surfaces.

Goal 16: Discourage disruptive behavior. Implementation strategies include developing a code of behavior, identifying unacceptable behaviors, staff reporting using a nonretributive process, education, programs to manage unacceptable behavior, and develop programs to manage stresses associated with the health care work environment.

Goal 18: Improve recognition and response to changes in patient's condition. Key strategy involves development of an early response team whose composition will vary depending on the needs of the organization. The goal is to provide a route for health care staff members to obtain direct assistance when a patient's condition appears to be worsening.

represents a list of those currently being assessed during unannounced site inspections. The evidence-based goals are updated by The Joint Commission annually (**Table 26-7**), and links to the most current National Patient Safety Goals (NPSGs) and related literature are available at their Web site (http://www.jointcommission.org/patientsafety/nationalpatientsafetygoals/). Because the operating room is a high-risk health care setting, adoption of systems to reduce this risk is deemed critical and adherence to this collection of patient safety best practices is scrutinized.

EVIDENCE-BASED PRACTICES

On a national level, the ability to disseminate best practices has taken the form of standards and guidelines produced by national associations and the federal government. Practice policies or guidelines are the summation by clinicians of the available evidence about the benefits and risks of a treatment plan. Guidelines are a method of codifying recommendations regarding the use of a given technology or practice. Several types of recommendations fall into the general category of a practice parameter. A standard implies that a therapy or practice should be performed on patients with a particular condition. Standards are only approved if an assessment of the probabilities and utilities of the group indicate that the decision to choose the treatment or a strategy would be virtually unanimous. If a particular therapy or strategy is considered a standard, it is cost-effective for those for whom it is recommended. Standards are intended to be applied rigidly. The ASA first adopted Standards for Intraoperative Monitoring in 1986, which were developed from safety guidelines adopted at the Harvard hospital system. Guidelines are intended to be more flexible than standards, but they should be followed in most cases. Depending on the patient, setting, and other factors, guidelines can and should be tailored to fit individual needs. Like standards, guidelines should be cost-effective. The ASA has developed a series of guidelines that they term *practice parameters* or *practice guidelines* on a number of issues such as pulmonary artery catheter use and blood transfusions.[38-40] Similarly, the American Heart Association/American College of Cardiology has established *Guidelines for Perioperative Cardiovascular Evaluation for Noncardiac Surgery*.[41] Local practices can then be benchmarked against these national norms and local performance improvement initiatives can be developed. One example is the development of β-blocker protocols for patients who present to the hospital currently taking β-blockers. As more high-quality studies of best practices become available, practice guidelines will be used to disseminate these practices.

In the absence of strong evidence to support a given practice, expert opinion can help define best practice. For example, there is little high-quality randomized data to support the decision to perform a routine laboratory test before surgery. After reviewing the data, the ASA Task Force on Preoperative Evaluation chose to develop a practice advisory.[42] Practice advisory uses expert opinions and survey of practice results to help inform clinicians.

PROCESS MEASUREMENT AS PART OF THE QUALITY IMPROVEMENT PROCESS

Most of the discussion has focused on outcome measurements, death, or myocardial infarction, for example. However, because anesthesia-related complications are rare, observing outcome changes requires fairly large sample size and may be hard to separate from other factors such as underlying disease or the surgical intervention. For this reason, quality improvement methods typically implement and measure process-based indicators such as antibiotic administration, β-blocker administration, or other processes that have been demonstrated to lead to improved outcome.[43,44] The key issue here is the relationship between the process being measured and outcome. Unfortunately, high compliance with process measures alone may not guarantee an acceptable outcome. Thus the previously discussed patient safety and quality improvement activities cannot be abandoned. Of concern is the use of process variables to institute "pay for performance" financial incentive paradigms and whether or not the processes mandated will in fact be correlated with improved patient care.

PATIENT SAFETY AND QUALITY IMPROVEMENT IN INTENSIVE CARE UNITS

As summarized by Wu et al, in the United States, intensive care units (ICUs) account for about 10% of inpatient acute care beds.[45] ICU mortality has been estimated to be between 8% and 10%, accounting for about 400 000 to 500 000 deaths each year.[46] Errors and adverse events appear to be common in ICUs and may be on the order of 1.7 errors per patient per day.[47] Consequently many believe that ICUs present an ideal area to study the effects of patient safety initiatives on outcome.[48] The National Quality Forum has recently evaluated for endorsement a composite measure of ICU length of stay coupled with mortality. It is important to recognize that shorter ICU lengths of stay are beneficial if and only if they are not associated with increased mortality or readmission rates.

Communication errors may contribute to as many as 67% of adverse events in the intensive care setting.[49] Pronovost and colleagues have described several tools, "the morning briefing" and the concept of "daily goals," that have improved certain measured outcomes.[49,50] The morning briefing approach highlights those patients with the most critical issues; it helps determine the order of rounds and provides focus for the day's activity. The morning briefing form asks 3 questions: "What happened overnight that I need to be aware of? Where should I begin rounds? What are your concerns regarding potential problems for today?" The authors note that this approach provides an immediate overview of the totality of care requirements in the ICU and allows a more rational allocation of resources. They also note anecdotally enhanced teamwork, better identification of defects, and an improved admissions/discharge process.

The "daily goals" is a second form. It is "low tech" but has decreased ICU length of stay in the studied ICU from a mean of 2.2 to 1.1 days and allowed an additional 670 patients to be cared for during the year.[50] According to the authors, this approach allows explicit delineation of the goals for each patient and improved communication with nurses, house staff, and families.

The frequency of ICU-based incidents and their deleterious effect on patient outcome has led to considerable effort to define relevant variables that alter outcome. Berenholtz et al described outcome variables such as ICU mortality rate, average days on mechanical ventilation, suboptimal management of pain; process variables such as appropriate use of blood transfusion, appropriate peptic ulcer disease prophylaxis; access variables such as delayed admissions and rate of delayed discharges; and complication variables such as rate of unplanned ICU readmission and the rate of resistant infections as a starting point to determine which factors seemed the most relevant to improving patient outcomes in the ICU.[51] There is increasing awareness that postoperative pulmonary complications may be an important determinant of outcome.

Others have described various processes for data collection of adverse events, including collaborative, multi-institutional Web-based reporting systems.[46,52] Approaches to encourage reporting within institutions include the trigger tool described by Resar et al, which is a mix of process and outcome variables that led to further review.[53] Triggers in this series include chest tube insertion, positive blood cultures, death, renal failure, and a number of others. The selection was empirical. However, the authors determined a prevalence of 11.3 adverse events per 100 ICU days. Schuerer et al describe an error reporting system involving the use of preprepared cards listing various reporting indicators.[54] They noted that reporting increased with this system compared with the previous online system. This was attributed mostly to ease of reporting, although the attention paid to reporting including inservice sessions may have been a factor.

Other types of data acquisition besides reporting have been attempted. Beckmann et al compared incident reporting to a medical card review.[55] Although the incident reporting and medical chart review often found similar events, medical chart review seemed to detect infections, pain management problems, and myocardial infarction that were missed by the incident reporting system. The authors felt that the 2 systems were complementary, but that the medical chart review required a greater investment of resources.

Adverse events also occur while patients are being moved from other areas of the hospital to the ICU. Gillman et al, for example, determined that during a 6-month period, 22% of 290 patients transferred from the emergency department to the ICU experienced some type of adverse event during the transfer process. These ranged from incorrect identification bands to hypertension, hypotension, hypothermia, and transport equipment problems.[56] Thus any program developed for ICU-related patient care quality needs also to account for patients coming into and leaving the unit.

Despite great efforts by a number of institutions, monitoring for patient safety and improving outcomes in the ICU setting is still in the developmental stage. For efficacy, Pronovost and Holzmueller note that quality improvement and patient safety within the ICU setting is multidisciplinary.[57] They emphasize the need to develop a culture that emphasizes these aspects of patient care. They note that developing work processes that reduce complexity, standardize, and automate may be most helpful for reducing error.

ACUTE PAIN MANAGEMENT

Quality and safety standards with respect to acute pain appear have been especially difficult to develop. Part of the problem relates to the fragmentation of acute pain care between surgeons, nurses, and anesthesiologists that occurs in most institutions. Part is also related to philosophical differences toward the treatment of acute pain and the lack of a quantitative measure outside of patient observation. Practice guidelines from the ASA emphasize that a single approach to pain management may not be appropriate for all types of patients and that multimodality approaches tailored to the patient's clinical conditions and therapeutic requirements have the greatest probability of producing adequate pain relief with the least risk of undesirable side effects.[58] The Joint Commission has published specific pain management standards that may help increase the resources devoted to this often ignored aspect of patient care.[59] The requirement that patient pain needs to have appropriate assessment and management provides the basic underpinning of determining the efficacy and safety of pain control efforts. There are 2 problems. The first is that many institutions have not yet implemented appropriate pain assessment and control programs. The American Pain Society guidelines, now close to 11 years old, provide a very precise approach to instituting an effective approach to acute pain care.[60] The second problem is the focus of this section: Specifically, once an acute pain care plan is in place, how does one go about monitoring for safety and efficacy?

Garnerin et al discuss a single event related to a pump error and the process of root cause analysis related to that error.[61] Karlsten et al found that over a 3-year period the assessment of pain according to the set protocols improved with repeated staff training, meetings, and audits.[62] Bardiau et al reported improved pain relief as indicated by visual analog scale (VAS) scores with the implementation of a multimodal pain therapy approach, routine VAS measurement, and nurse training.[63] Sartain and Barry reported improved pain control with the institution of an acute pain service.[64] Miaskowski et al described the results of a prospective multisite study involving 5837 patients of whom 49% were cared for by an anesthesia-based pain service.[65] Patients cared for by the acute pain service had significantly lower pain scores; they also had a lower level of complications. Meissner et al described an ongoing benchmarking protocol for quality assessment.[66] This approach used a specialized pain nurse who interviewed patients on the surgical wards for quality of pain relief. Benchmarks included pain at rest, pain with ambulation, and maximal pain intensity since surgery. Specific side effects such as nausea, vomiting, and sedation were also determined. Other potential quality indicators might include the documentation of VAS, the frequency of VAS documentation, the appropriateness of pain medication for the expected level of pain, efficiency of transition for one pain modality to another, and complications.[67] The large number of patients being treated for pain allows the construction of control charts based on type of surgery, pain therapy modality, and physical condition of the patient. This might allow determination of the success of pain control efforts and better determination of which approaches are the most effective in a particular patient population.

Postoperative sedation/analgesia care has been associated with preventable deaths, leading to calls for increased monitoring in the postsurgical care setting. Multiple studies have shown that failure to rescue due to sedative/analgesic-induced respiratory depression is relatively common given the millions of patients having surgery annually. Although there is debate as to the effectiveness of rescue teams and methods for deploying them, recent focus on early detection supports expanded monitoring for unexpected respiratory depression.[68-72]

At Dartmouth Hitchcock, surveillance monitoring of all postsurgical patients was associated with significant reductions of rescue activations and the need for ICU transfer when compared with units without this monitoring practice.

IMPEDIMENTS TO REVIEW OF QUALITY-OF-CARE ISSUES

Many physicians are concerned about the confidentiality and discoverability of discussions of patient outcome. Most states provide protection for discussions held within the purview of peer review committees. The degree of protection may vary but tends to protect the members of the committee, those who testify to the committee, and the written work product of these committees. Original patient records are of course discoverable even if taken into the "protected" environment of the peer review committee. Discussions outside the committee environment may be discoverable in legal proceedings. In general, case conferences and mortality and morbidity conferences avoid many of these issues by avoiding the use of specific patient identifiers.

THE FUTURE

CHANGING PATIENT EXPECTATIONS

Patient expectations are changing. Many want greater involvement in the care process. Some demand input into the exact drugs used and evidence significant dissatisfaction with the care provided when their desires are not met. Many also want a near risk-free experience and have little tolerance for what many of us view as relatively minor events such as small degrees of hematoma or bruising, intravenous infiltration, delays in start of surgery, and so on. "Service recovery," measures taken to satisfy the patient or their family when care expectations are not met, has long been used to compensate patients for dental injury. It is now being expanded at our institution to reimburse the copay or uninsured portions of postoperative consultations related to certain aspects of anesthesia care such as ophthalmology consults in the case of eye irritation, plastic surgery consultation for intravenous infiltration, or otorhinolaryngologic consultation for voice changes or persistent sore throat. Patients are also more willing to "complain" to hospital leadership when their expectations are not met.

CHANGING PAYER EXPECTATIONS

Payers for medical care expect better outcomes and are willing to pay for these better outcomes through the use of incentives (ie, pay-for-performance, or P4P). There are 2 different philosophical approaches to P4P: (1) focusing on the outcomes themselves or (2) on care processes that have been associated with the improved outcomes. An example of an outcome-oriented program is the NSQIP. As described previously, the American College of Surgeons has recently adapted NSQIP (ACS-NSQIP) to the private sector and allowed private hospitals to send a standard set of data to a national center and obtain observed versus expected mortality.

The process variable approach is best exemplified by the Surgical Care Improvement Project (SCIP). SCIP represents a partnership that was formed in 2003 and included representatives from the American Hospital Association, the American College of Surgeons, the ASA, the Association of Perioperative Registered Nurses, the Joint Commission on Accreditation of Healthcare Organizations, the IHI, the Department of Veterans Affairs (VA), the Agency for Healthcare Research and Quality (AHRQ), the Centers for Medicare and Medicaid Services (CMS), and the Centers for Disease Control and Prevention (CDC) (see www.medqic.org/scip). In 2005, the group set the goal of reducing surgical complications by 25% by the year 2010. Four major areas of surgical complications were identified: prevention of surgical site infections, perioperative myocardial infarction, postoperative pneumonia, and venous thromboembolism (pulmonary embolism and deep vein thrombosis).

The partnership has used expert panels that included members from the steering committee and from more than 20 additional organizations. The goals are to identify best practices supported by the literature or preferably identified as class I recommendations in guidelines developed by the appropriate societies. For example, the recommendations for perioperative β-blockade were restricted to class I recommendations by the *American College of Cardiology/American Heart Association Guidelines for Perioperative Cardiovascular Evaluation.* In fact, the *Focused Update on Perioperative Beta Blockade* was published in part to ensure that the SCIP measures would be consistent with the most current evidence. The measures for venous thromboembolism are based on recommendations from the American College of Chest Physicians. The most well-described measures are those related to the prevention of surgical site infections. Both timing and appropriateness of perioperative antibiotics were incorporated from the previously commissioned Surgical Infection Project (SIP). Additional measures such as perioperative normothermia in colon surgery and perioperative glucose control in cardiac surgery were also part of this "module." At this time, the SCIP measures are voluntary. Hospitals can report on any one of the 4 major areas, but they must report on all of the measures in that area. The IHI has also included the SCIP project in their national agenda. However, the antibiotic measures of SCIP that were incorporated in SIP are part of the new P4R, or pay-for-reporting, initiative incorporated into the Medicare reimbursement policy. Many private insurers and states are also incorporating this measure, and eventually the overall performance on this measure may affect payment (pay-for-performance, often called "P4P") rather than just reporting. Although the US Congress has clearly identified P4P as an important approach to controlling health care costs and improving quality, there are several investigators who are concerned that better performance on process variables (ie, antibiotic timing) may not lead to improved outcome. Werner and Bradlow found that hospital performance measures only predict small differences in hospital risk-adjusted mortality rates.[73] In a recent study of hospitals in the Premier Inc Perspective Database reporting SCIP performance, adherence measured through a global all-or-none composite infection-prevention score was associated with a lower probability of developing a postoperative infection. However, adherence reported on individual SCIP measures, which is the only form in which performance is publicly reported, was not associated with a significantly lower probability of infection. Importantly, when performance measurement was evaluated over time (2004-2006), hospital process performance improved and was associated with better patient and quality outcomes. For acute myocardial infarction, performance improvements were associated with declines in mortality rates, lengths of stay, and readmission rates. As part of health care reform, an increasing number of measures are being developed for physicians through the American Medical Association Physician Consortium for Performance Improvement. The Consortium is composed of more than 100 national medical specialties and state medical societies; the Council of Medical Specialty Societies; American Board of Medical Specialties and its member boards; experts in methodology and data collection; the Agency for Healthcare Research and Quality; and Centers for Medicare & Medicaid Services. It is committed to the development, testing, and maintenance of evidence-based clinical performance measures and measurement resources for physicians. The measures are then proposed to the National Quality Forum (NQF) and will become those measured included in the P4P measures for CMS.

CHANGING HOSPITAL EXPECTATIONS

Medical centers increasingly are expecting members of their clinical staff to actively participate in programs to improve patient outcomes and safety. The active participation of anesthesiologists in the patient safety time-out process and in the proper identification of organ transplant blood types are just 2 of many. Requests to participate in multidisciplinary process planning groups are increasing. There is an increasing concern with patient satisfaction, and clinician groups are being increasingly asked to review processes that produce less than optimal outcomes, significant patient dissatisfaction, or have higher costs. This will only increase, and a good understanding of the sources of patient dissatisfaction and poorer outcomes within the context of a specific practice will become increasingly necessary.

SUMMARY AND CONCLUSIONS

A robust quality improvement system is essential to ensure that we provide our patients with the highest quality of care. The history of the specialty of anesthesiology has been marked by a focus on patient safety and assessment of outcomes. Anesthesiology has been lauded as the specialty that has focused on achieving a Six Sigma approach to quality. Numerous national projects have attempted to identify factors that contribute to perioperative morbidity and mortality and proposed systems to reduce complications through the publications of guidelines. These guidelines are now being converted into P4P initiatives to ensure that all practitioners practice according to the best evidence. Despite these national efforts, individual providers and groups of providers should develop their own systems to both identify the causes of complications and disseminate practices to reduce these same complications. As an example, participation in the Anesthesia Quality Institute will allow anesthesiologists to benchmark their performance versus peers in an effort to continue to improve.

KEY REFERENCES

- Miaskowski C, Crews J, Ready LB, Paul SM, Ginsberg B. Anesthesia-based pain services improve the quality of postoperative pain management. *Pain.* 1999;80:23-29.
- O'Neil AC, Petersen LA, Cook EF, Bates DW, Lee TH, Brennan TA. Physician reporting compared with medical-record review to identify adverse medical events. *Ann Intern Med.* 1993;119: 370-376.
- Quality improvement guidelines for the treatment of acute pain and cancer pain. American Pain Society Quality of Care Committee. *JAMA.* 1995;274:1874-1880.
- Reason JT. *Human Error.* Cambridge, UK: Cambridge University Press; 1990.
- Rubin HR, Pronovost P, Diette GB. The advantages and disadvantages of process-based measures of health care quality. *Int J Qual Health Care.* 2001;13:469-474.
- Sanborn KV, Castro J, Kuroda M, Thys DM. Detection of intraoperative incidents by electronic scanning of computerized anesthesia records. Comparison with voluntary reporting [see comments]. *Anesthesiology.* 1996;85:977-987.
- Wu AW, Pronovost P, Morlock L. ICU incident reporting systems. *J Crit Care.* 2002;17:86-94.

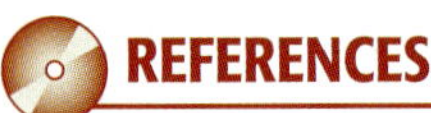

REFERENCES

Complete references available on DVD and online version at www.LongneckerAnesthesiology.com

CHAPTER 27

Positioning of Patients for Operation

Vijaya Gottumukkala

KEY POINTS

1. Proper positioning of the patient during the operative period is important for optimal surgical exposure and outcome.
2. Understanding the pathophysiologic changes and special considerations associated with each position helps reduce positioning-related morbidity.
3. Improper positioning during surgery can lead to spinal cord ischemia, postoperative peripheral neuropathies, muscular sprain injuries, ischemic injury to skin and muscles, and visual loss.
4. Perioperative peripheral nerve injuries are the second most common cause of professional liability among anesthesiologists.
5. New and advanced surgical procedures (robotic) may involve unconventional and extreme positioning techniques, necessitating better understanding of the physiologic consequences of positioning and enhanced vigilance to prevent injury to the patient.
6. Male gender, extremes of body habitus, and prolonged hospitalization are risk factors for postoperative peripheral neuropathies.
7. A thorough assessment of risk factors for complications related to positioning should be an integral part of the preoperative evaluation.
8. As part of the informed consent, risks and benefits associated with positioning should be discussed with the patient.
9. Description of intraoperative positioning techniques and measures taken to prevent injury should be documented in the anesthetic record.
10. Familiarity and understanding of the American Society of Anesthesiologists (ASA) Task Force on Prevention of Perioperative Peripheral Neuropathies may help with minimizing the problems associated with positioning during the perioperative period.
11. Special attention needs to be paid to minimize the potential for visual injuries in high-risk patients during the perioperative period.
12. A report by the ASA Task Force on perioperative blindness is an excellent source of current information and consensus expert opinion on this devastating problem.

The term *surgical posture* or positioning in the perioperative context denotes the body position in which a patient is placed for the surgical procedure. The main purpose of "positioning" is to maximize anatomic exposure for the surgical procedure. In *Epidemics, Book I, Second Constitution,* Hippocrates advised *primum non nocere,* "to first do no harm." Thus intraoperative positioning should make surgical exposure ideal while optimizing patient safety. In spite of anesthesia-related morbidity secondary to inadequate ventilation and oxygenation improving as a result of better physiologic monitoring and ASA standards on minimum monitoring, complications secondary to positioning are on the rise. Many problems arising from positioning such as peripheral nerve injuries fall under the legal doctrine of *Res ipsa loquitur*. This Latin phrase literally means "the thing speaks for itself" and implies that the injury sustained is so evident that it would not have occurred without negligence from someone else. Thus the plaintiff needs only to prove the injury. In cases of *res ipsa loquitur,* the burden of proof falls on health care providers to prove their innocence (ie, the care provided was not negligent). Therefore, safe intraoperative patient positioning is crucial, and a clear protocol must be in place and followed by all members of the perioperative team.

This chapter discusses the positions that are commonly used during surgical procedures (supine, lithotomy, sitting, head down, prone, and lateral decubitus). The rationale and technique for safe establishment of each of these positions are described, followed by the associated pathophysiologic changes, and finally the potential complications particular to each position. With advances in technology and the advent of new surgical therapeutic options, various modifications of the standard positions are continuously being added. It is still possible to minimize positioning-related injury to the patient even in these challenging situations by adhering to the basic principles.

SUPINE (HORIZONTAL DORSAL DECUBITUS POSITION)

Because most surgical procedures involve patients in the supine position, a clear understanding of the pathophysiologic effects of this position is necessary for the perioperative team. A significant portion of our life is spent in the supine position, and this position is not usually considered to pose significant physiologic stress on the body. However, patients with morbid obesity, mediastinal masses, poor cardiac functional status, and term parturients prone to aortocaval compression do not easily tolerate this position.

In the traditional supine position, the patients are placed on their back with some degree of neck flexion. The arms are either padded and restrained in a neutral position alongside the body or abducted on padded arm boards. A pillow is usually placed under the knees to reduce the degree of lumbar lordosis and prevent excessive strain on the lumbar spine. This is a very important consideration in the elderly and those with mechanical low back pain.

PATHOPHYSIOLOGY OF THE SUPINE POSITION

Cardiovascular Moving from erect posture to the supine position increases central blood volume considerably. As a result of this increased blood volume, compensatory stretch and baroreceptors in the central circulation initiate reflex responses that usually maintain blood pressure within narrow limits in healthy adults. Ward et al[1] studied the hemodynamic changes during supine positioning and noted that the mean arterial pressure (MAP), heart rate, and peripheral vascular resistance decrease, whereas cardiac output (CO) and stroke volume (SV) increase in healthy adults. Although these changes are well tolerated in healthy subjects, an increase in myocardial oxygen consumption is noted in patients with coronary artery disease and poor myocardial function.

Pulmonary In the erect position, breathing normally is a function of muscles of the rib cage. In the supine position, however, muscles of the abdominal wall and diaphragm assume the predominant role. Significant changes in the anatomy of the upper airway and abdominal-thoracic areas occur in the supine position. These changes affect the cross-sectional area of the upper airway, ventilatory mechanics, and blood flow to the lungs, contributing to significant alterations in lung volumes and ventilation-perfusion matching.[2]

Cephalad displacement of the posterior diaphragm occurs in the supine position, and in the awake state this allows for improved ventilation in basal portions of the lungs. Because the vertical distance of the capillaries from the pulmonary hilum determines regional blood flow in the lungs, there is corresponding increased perfusion in the basal segments in the supine position. Froese and Bryan[3] studied regional ventilation in awake spontaneously breathing patients as well as in those who are anesthetized (spontaneously breathing or paralyzed) and concluded that a more uniform ventilation per unit lung volume and an overall improvement of ventilation to perfusion matching occurs in the supine position in healthy patients.

Functional residual capacity (FRC) decreases under anesthesia, with most of the reduction occurring immediately after induction of general anesthesia.[4] The relationship between closing volume (CV) and FRC reflects the degree of atelectasis, and therefore hypoxemia, during tidal ventilation. CV is defined as the fraction of the total lung capacity below which airway closure occurs when external pressures overcome natural elastic recoil.[5] The relationship between CV and FRC in erect and supine patients can be divided into 4 groups (**Fig. 27-1**). Craig et al[6] showed that a conscious patient between the ages of 30 and 40 years can have basilar atelectasis on assuming the supine position because CV exceeds FRC. Induction of anesthesia exaggerates these changes, which are further pronounced in obese patients and during procedures involving head-down positioning.

COMPLICATIONS

Excluding peripheral neuropathies, the main complications in the supine position are backache and ischemic pressure injuries. Pressure point changes and alopecia result from ischemia to the tissues overlying bony prominences and the hair follicles, respectively. These complications can be minimized by maintaining tissue perfusion pressure and adequate padding of pressure points in the dependent regions of the body.

Backache in patients under the supine position for long periods results from loss of normal lordotic curvature of the lumbar spine because of reduced tone of paraspinal muscles and ligaments. This problem may be exacerbated in the elderly and in patients with preexisting lower back pain problems or lumbar spinal stenosis. Using the lawn chair position or placing a pillow under the knees in the standard supine position may reduce the incidence of backache.

LAWN CHAIR POSITION

This is a modification of the standard supine position in which the lower and upper half of the body are slightly elevated in relationship to the hips. This position results in an improved tissue perfusion and hemodynamic status because of the better balance between the venous return from the lower half of the body and the perfusion pressure gradient to major organs. An additional advantage of this position is the greater degree of abdominal musculature relaxation, which is facilitated by the shortened distance from the xiphoid process to the symphysis pubis.[7]

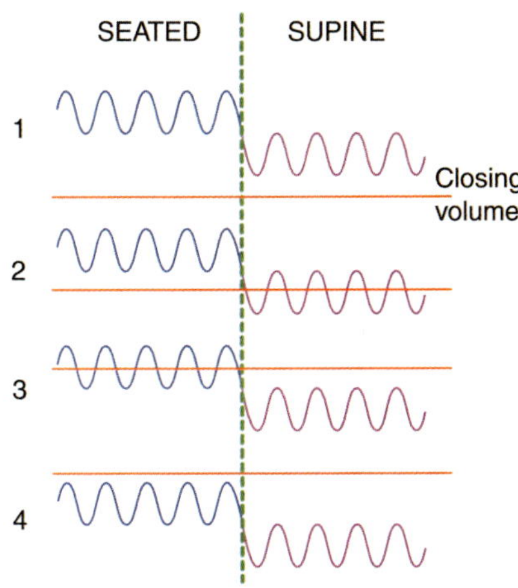

FIGURE 27-1. Classification of subjects into groups (1-4) according to the relationship of closing volume (CV) to functional residual capacity (FRC) in the seated and supine positions. Group 1: FRC > CV in both positions; group 2: FRC > CV in seated position only; group 3: CV in the breathing range in seated position and exceeded in supine position; group 4: CV above breathing range in both positions. [From Craig DB, Wahba WM, Don HF, et al. "Closing volume" and its relationship to gas exchange in seated and supine positions. *J Appl Physiol.* 1971;31(5):717-721. With permission.]

LITHOTOMY POSITION

This position is most often used for genitourinary, gynecologic, and colorectal procedures. The standard lithotomy position is achieved when the patient's legs are abducted from the midline and the hips and knees are flexed so that the lower legs are parallel to the floor. It is prudent that both lower extremities be raised and lowered simultaneously while using this position to avoid rotational stress on the lumbar spine. To minimize the risk of injury to the patient, it is important to understand the advantages and limitations of the various supporting devices (candy cane, knee crutch, calf support, cushioned dorsal boot, adjustable knee, and foot support) for the lower extremities. Improper uses of these devices can lead to postoperative neuropathies, musculoskeletal strain to the lower spine, and ischemic injuries to the skin and muscles. Because many variations of the lithotomy position are currently used, Martin has proposed a standardized classification (low, standard, high, hemi, exaggerated, and tilted) to prevent miscommunication between members of the operating team (**Figs. 27-2** through **27-7**).[7]

PATHOPHYSIOLOGY OF THE LITHOTOMY POSITION

The physiology of a patient in the lithotomy position is not different from that of a supine patient except for the physiologic consequences of

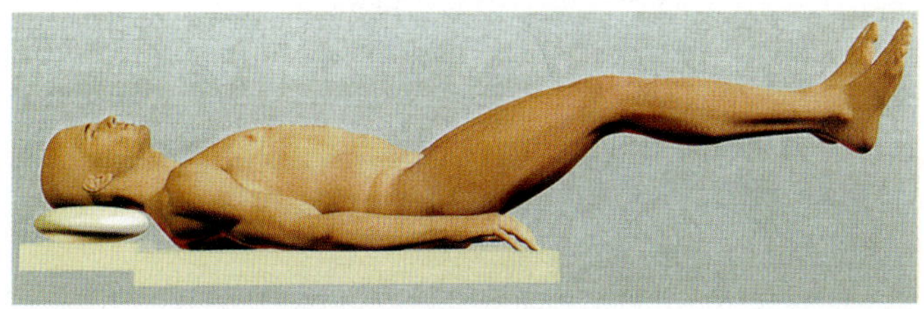

FIGURE 27-2. Low lithotomy position. [Redrawn from Martin JT. *Positioning in Anesthesia and Surgery*. Philadelphia, PA: WB Saunders; 1997. With permission.]

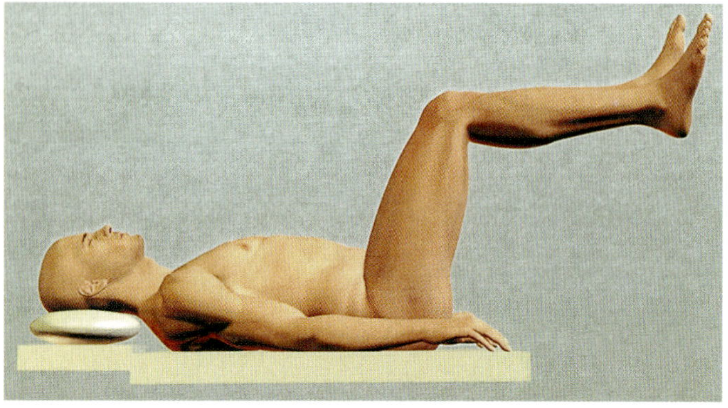

FIGURE 27–3. Standard lithotomy position. [Redrawn from Martin JT. *Positioning in Anesthesia and Surgery*. Philadelphia, PA: WB Saunders; 1997. With permission.]

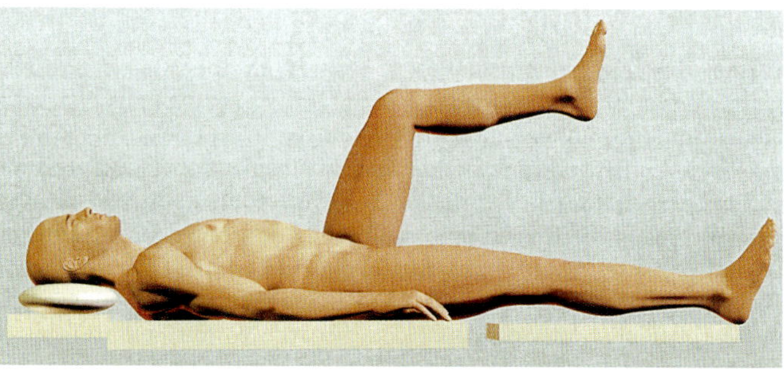

FIGURE 27–5. Hemilithotomy position. [Redrawn from Martin JT. *Positioning in Anesthesia and Surgery*. Philadelphia, PA: WB Saunders; 1997. With permission.]

leg elevation on the central blood volume, the effects of antigravity on tissue perfusion in elevated legs, and the deleterious ventilatory effects of excessive flexion at the hip joints.

Because the legs are elevated, a significant amount of intravascular volume is added to the central circulation. Normal vascular compensatory reflexes tend to compensate for these transient increases in atrial filling pressures, increased intracranial blood volume, and internal carotid blood flow. In disease states, however, these changes may cause significant alterations to the cerebral and cardiac function. Kopman and Sandza[8] have shown that patients with coronary artery disease poorly tolerate head-down tilts greater than 10 degrees and lithotomy position. Because lithotomy position is frequently combined with head-down tilt for improved surgical access, the cardiopulmonary status of the patient has to be taken into consideration to minimize cardiac decompensation.

The MAP at a measurement site varies by 2 mm Hg with each vertical inch above or below the atrium. Enderby[9] clearly demonstrated the variations in MAP with positional changes (**Fig. 27-8**). This is particularly important in older patients (with peripheral vascular disease, diabetes, and hypertension) when compressive stockings are used and the patient is situated in lithotomy position for a prolonged period of time. Inadequate perfusion pressure to the lower extremities in such a situation can lead to ischemic complications of the skin and muscles resulting in skin necrosis and myoglobinuria.

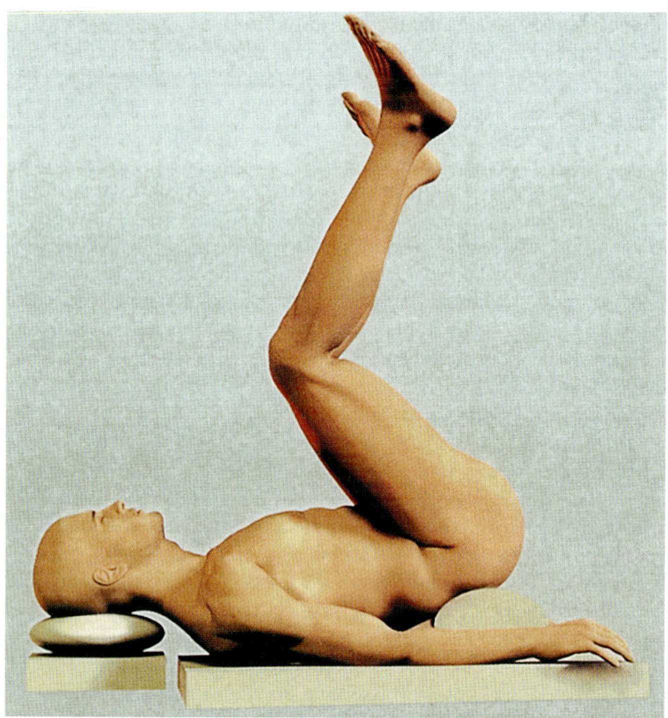

FIGURE 27–6. Exaggerated lithotomy position. [Redrawn from Martin JT. *Positioning in Anesthesia and Surgery*. Philadelphia, PA: WB Saunders; 1997. With permission.]

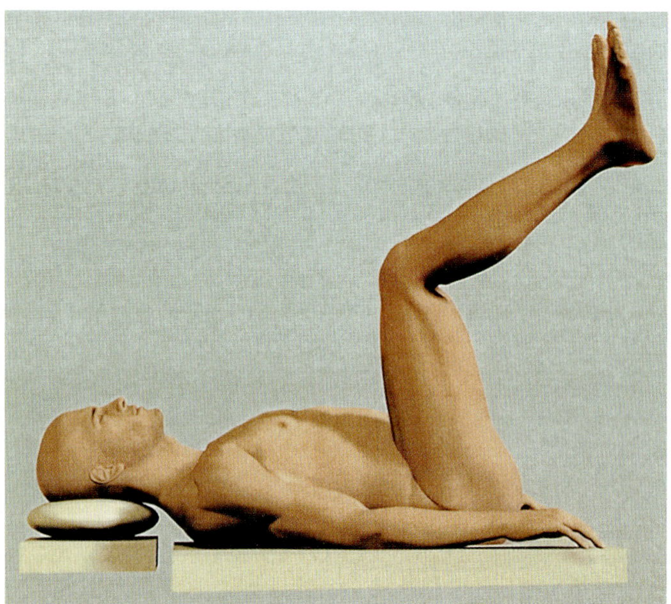

FIGURE 27–4. High lithotomy position. [Redrawn from Martin JT. *Positioning in Anesthesia and Surgery*. Philadelphia, PA: WB Saunders; 1997. With permission.]

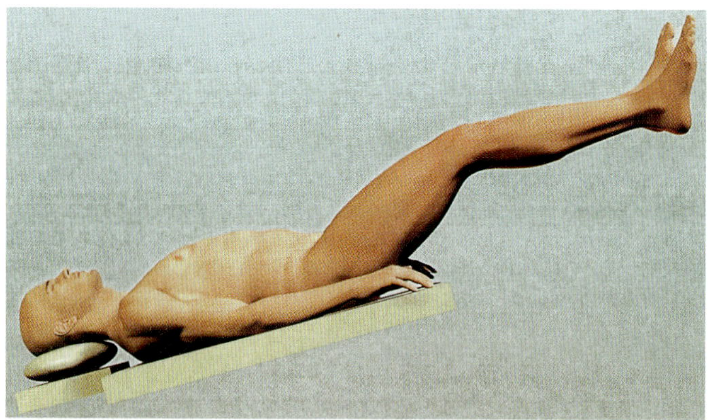

FIGURE 27–7. Tilted lithotomy position. [Redrawn from Martin JT. *Positioning in Anesthesia and Surgery*. Philadelphia, PA: WB Saunders; 1997. With permission.]

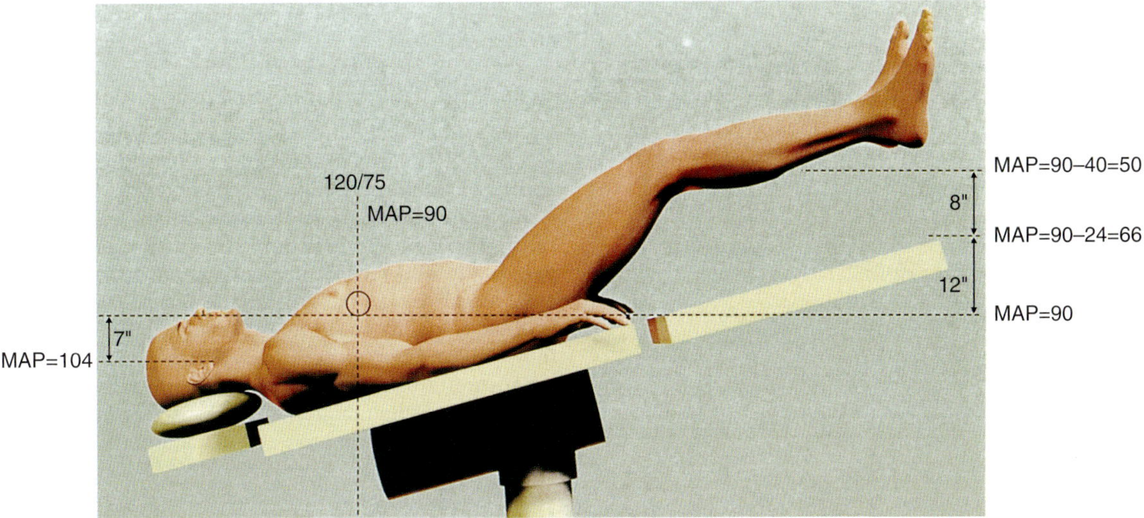

FIGURE 27-8. Effects of gravity on perfusion pressure in the lower extremities in the lithotomy position. MAP, mean arterial pressure. [Redrawn from Martin JT. *Positioning in Anesthesia and Surgery*. Philadelphia, PA: WB Saunders; 1997. With permission.]

Under general anesthesia, with the assumption of the lithotomy position the tidal volume decreases by 3%. With a 10 degrees head-down tilt, tidal volume decreases another 14%.[10] Although conscious patients can usually compensate and tolerate this change in tidal volume because of improved resting position of the diaphragm, anesthetized patients breathing spontaneously may develop basilar atelectasis and hypoxia. Patients with obesity, hiatal hernia, and gastroesophageal reflux disease may have decreased lower esophageal sphincter tone and barrier pressure, increasing the risk for regurgitation and aspiration of gastric contents in the lithotomy position.

Compartment syndromes have been associated with use of the lithotomy position lasting greater than 5 hours.[11] Anatomic compartments are relatively rigid osseofascial partitions in the extremities composed of muscles, nerves, blood vessels, and connective and adipose tissues. A certain amount of perfusion pressure, 9 to 15 mm Hg in the lower extremity,[12] is required for normal perfusion of tissues in these compartments. If the pressure in the compartment rises as a result of external forces (dependent pressure, casts, stockings, tight dressings) or internally by edema/bleeding, the vascular driving pressure (MAP) must increase concurrently to prevent ischemic complications. Inadequate tissue perfusion and ischemia of the contents of these compartments lead to varying degree of injury (endothelial injury, tissue necrosis, and myoglobinuria) that could potentially result in death. Because pain is the most specific symptom for diagnosis of compartment syndromes, a high index of suspicion should be maintained for patients at risk while receiving regional analgesia.

The respiratory complications of the lithotomy position are similar to those of the supine position. The lithotomy position can be an additional factor when diaphragmatic excursion is restricted as a result of excessively flexed thighs or a steep head-down tilt. The duration of the use of the lithotomy position and the body mass index of the patient are reliable predictors for complications pertaining to nerve injuries, respiratory problems, and the compartment syndromes.[11]

SITTING POSITION

An operative surgical site is intentionally elevated above the level of the heart to decrease bleeding in the operative field and to provide better surgical conditions in the sitting position. Although popular in the 1980s and early 1990s for posterior fossa neurosurgical procedures, the sitting position is now commonly used for surgical procedures on the shoulder. Advantages of the sitting position to the anesthesiologist include easier ventilation because of unimpeded diaphragmatic excursion, easier access to the endotracheal tube and airway, unimpeded access to the chest wall for resuscitative measures, and unobstructed view of the face for monitoring cranial nerve function. Disadvantages include the need for a coordinated effort from the operating team (nursing, surgical, and anesthesia) to establish this position safely, hypotension, venous air embolism, consequences of excessive neck flexion (kinking of endotracheal tube and swelling of face and tongue), nerve injuries, pneumocephalus, and blindness.

PATHOPHYSIOLOGY OF SITTING POSITION

Gravity and anesthetic agents have significant effects on the cardiovascular function in the sitting position. In a healthy adult patient, SV and CO are decreased by about 12% to 20%, and cerebral perfusion pressure (CPP) reduces by 15% without much change in the heart rate (HR).[13]

There is an overall increase in ventilation with increased vital capacity (VC) and FRC. However, with positive pressure ventilation and relative hypovolemia, there is reduced perfusion in the nondependent lung fields leading to an increase in physiologic dead space.

During neurosurgical procedures, upon opening of the arachnoid membrane there is loss of cerebrospinal fluid (CSF) allowing air to enter the intracranial CSF pathway leading to pneumocephalus and downward displacement of the brain. Although this gravitation of the brain may be tolerated in most patients, those with thin cerebral mantles may suffer from subdural hematoma.[6]

While positioning the patient, care should be exercised with the following basic principles: maintaining normal body alignment, protecting and padding all pressure points, avoiding placement of rigid oropharyngeal airways and excessive flexion of the neck, exercising care with extremities so their limits of passive range of motion are not exceeded, establishing final position slowly allowing time for hemodynamic compensation, and exercising extreme caution with a horseshoe frame if used for support of the head (**Fig. 27-9**).

Complications The frequent and most common complications are related to the hemodynamic and ventilatory effects as described in the previous section. Neurologic complications pertaining to neuropathies and blindness are detailed at the end of the chapter.

Venous Air Embolism The incidence of venous air embolism (VAE) in posterior fossa surgery in the sitting position is reported to be 41% to 45% with routine monitoring.[14] However, with the use of Doppler ultrasound, the reported incidence is as high as 42% to 85%.[15] VAE is often clinically undetected and frequently not of serious concern in a healthy patient if the volume and rate of air entrainment are minimal.

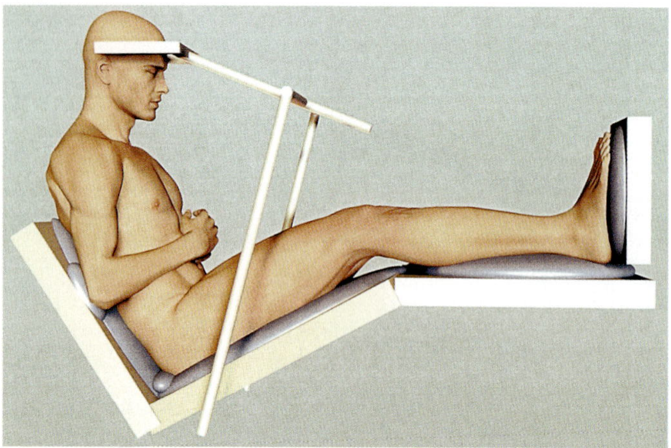

FIGURE 27–9. Sitting position. [Redrawn from Martin JT. *Positioning in Anesthesia and Surgery*. Philadelphia, PA: WB Saunders; 1997. With permission.]

The amount of entrained air that is reported to be lethal in humans is approximately 300 mL.[16] Children generally have greater clinically significant hemodynamic derangement from VAE than adults.

Significant morbidity and mortality from VAE is now less than 1%,[17] predominantly as a result of better monitoring techniques, early detection, and prompt intervention. VAE has significant effects on the cardiopulmonary system, resulting in elevated pulmonary artery pressures, decreased CO, systemic hypotension, and increased dead space ventilation. These physiologic changes are due to the results of mechanical effects of obstructed pulmonary blood flow from the air pocket in cardiac chambers and chemical mediator release from the air–blood interface. The appearance of dysrhythmias can signal the presence of intracardiac air, and therefore a high index of suspicion is warranted.

Paradoxical air embolus occurs whenever there is a communication between the right and the left sides of the heart. Although left-sided pressures are generally higher than the right, right-sided pressures can exceed the left in pathologic conditions (pulmonary hypertension, pulmonic stenosis) and also in healthy subjects during certain phases of the cardiac cycle. Thus increased right-sided cardiac pressures could result in the appearance of the entrained air in the arterial circulation with its associated complications. Therefore, the sitting position is contraindicated in patients with documented intracardiac defects or arteriovenous malformations. Patent foramen ovale (PFO) is the most common congenital defect associated with a paradoxical air embolus.

HEAD-DOWN TILT POSITION

The head-down position as introduced by Trendelenburg in the mid-19th century is still routinely used in genitourinary and colorectal procedures. Anesthesiologists also use this position for cannulation of central veins in the upper half of the body. Head-down tilt is usually combined with lithotomy to get optimal surgical conditions for genitourinary and colorectal procedures, but this combination has special physiologic consequences that anesthesia providers need to be aware of. Steep head-down tilt is frequently used for laparoscopic gynecologic and urologic procedures.

A steep head-down position has significant deleterious effects on the cardiovascular, respiratory, and nervous systems. Although young healthy patients may tolerate this position for short period of time without major sequelae, those with obesity, cardiovascular dysfunction, obstructive airway disease, and intracranial pathology may decompensate when placed in this position. Abdominal insufflation exaggerates and adds to the deleterious physiologic effects of this position. Therefore, special attention is needed for laparoscopic procedures in the steep head-down tilt position. The earlier custom of the head-down position to treat "shock" or hypotension has been disputed by Weil et al[18] and Sibbald et al.[19]

PATHOPHYSIOLOGY OF HEAD-DOWN TILT

Upon instituting the head-down position, the central blood volume increases by roughly 1000 mL in an adult patient, increasing CO and systolic blood pressure. However, there is immediate systemic vasodilatation secondary to reflex barostimulation leading to decreased SV, reduced CO, and diminished perfusion of vital organs. The brain is particularly vulnerable to decreased perfusion (reduced CPP) because of increased venous and CSF pressure. Shenkin et al[20] studied the effects of head-down tilt on cerebral hemodynamics in healthy adults and showed a consistent decrease in cerebral blood flow in spite of increased mean carotid pressure. Increased cerebral venous pressure from the head-down position can result in increased intraocular tension leading to ocular venous thrombosis and retinal detachment. These effects are particularly significant in patients with glaucoma. The occurrence of these complications can be minimized by using a less steep tilt and by decreasing the mean airway pressure.

Sing et al[21] studied the effects of head-down tilt on hemodynamic indices in hypovolemic postoperative patients in an intensive care unit. All hemodynamic variables and indices were measured supine and at 10 minutes after the head-down tilt position. MAP, pulmonary capillary wedge pressure, and systemic vascular resistance (SVR) increased, whereas cardiac index (CI), oxygen delivery, and consumption remained unchanged. They concluded that the immediate increase in blood pressure was not accompanied by a similar improvement in tissue oxygenation.

Johannsen et al[22] studied the cardiorespiratory effects of the head-down position and intraperitoneal insufflation in healthy women undergoing elective diagnostic laparoscopies. They reported about 42% reduction in stroke index and CI, a 50% increase in SVR, and no significant changes in HR or MAP. These changes in cardiovascular variables remained abnormal until the patient was returned to the supine position and the abdomen was deflated. The critical factors that determine the cardiovascular effects of intraperitoneal insufflation are the increase in intra-abdominal pressure and patient position.[23] Transesophageal echocardiographic studies have also shown an increase in SV and CO with the Trendelenburg position. However, with pneumoinsufflation there was a reduction in SV and CO associated with increased left ventricular end systolic wall stress and decreased left ventricular end diastolic volume and aortic diameter.[24,25]

Current evidence does not support the use of head-down tilt to treat hypovolemic shock. Lawn chair position is ideal in such a situation because it gently elevates the head as well as the legs on the torso. The advantage of this position is that cerebral congestion is minimized and peripheral venous return is augmented, thereby augmenting CO and cerebral oxygenation.

Atelectasis occurs when an anesthetized patient is placed in this position. The main reason for atelectasis and hypoxemia is decreased FRC (with induction of anesthesia, increased central blood volume, cephalad displacement of the diaphragm, and the weight of the abdominal contents impeding diaphragmatic excursion). This results in increased impedance to chest wall and lung inflation leading to decreased total compliance and increased work of breathing (if the patient is breathing spontaneously). The cardiopulmonary effects of these changes can be minimized by maintaining intravascular volume, minimizing the time spent in this position, ventilating the patient with larger tidal volumes, and adding positive end-expiratory pressure (PEEP). However, the effects of these ventilatory adjustments on cardiovascular indices and cerebral circulation must be taken into consideration so that oxygen delivery to the brain and vital organs is optimized. Position of the endotracheal tube has to be frequently checked when the patient is placed in the head-down tilt position. Cephalad movement of the diaphragm and compression of the lung bases can shift the carina relative to the fixed endotracheal tube resulting in endobronchial intubation. These changes are exaggerated with abdominal insufflation.

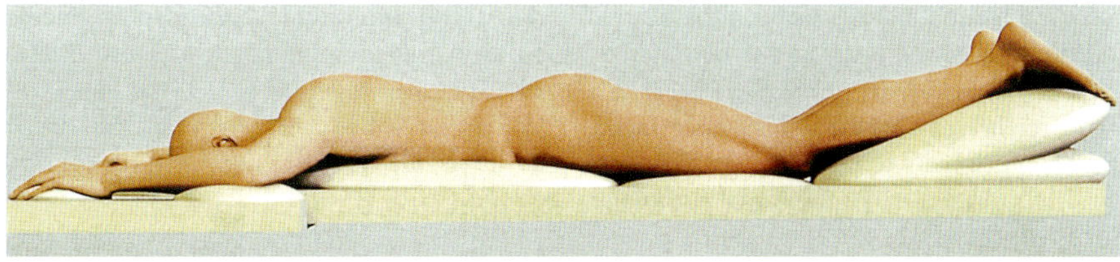

FIGURE 27-10. Prone position. [Redrawn from Martin JT. *Positioning in Anesthesia and Surgery*. Philadelphia, PA: WB Saunders; 1997. With permission.]

PRONE POSITION

Prone, ventral decubitus, or ventral recumbent position is a posture in which the patient is resting "face down" on the operating table. The prone position may be comfortable and even common for some individuals during normal sleep. However, when anesthetized in this position, there are potential complications that result from the loss of active reflexes that normally protect from atelectasis, compressive ischemia, and skeletal stress (**Figs. 27-10** and **27-11**).

In the classic or horizontal prone position, the patient lies face down resting on the ventral aspects of the torso with legs extended and arms raised beside the head or tucked alongside the body. Care should be exercised during positioning of the arms to avoid stretch injury to the neurovascular structures. In the former position (arms raised beside the head), shoulders and the forearms should be ventral to the horizontal axis of the torso. In the latter situation (arms tucked beside the torso), excessive elevation or drooping of the shoulders should be avoided. In all variations of this position, pressure points (such as nipples and genitalia) should be carefully padded and care exercised to avoid any compressive ischemic injury. The patient's torso is usually bolstered or supported to avoid abdominal compression (to minimize undesirable effects on ventilation, venous return, and engorgement of epidural venous plexus) and to allow unimpeded chest wall expansion with ventilation. It is vital that the patient's face (eyes, tip of the nose), mouth, and the endotracheal tube be visualized and accessible at all times.

The operating room table is generally angled or varied (crouching or kneeling) from the classic prone position when used to straighten the spine or decrease the lumbar lordosis for procedures on the dorsal lumbar spine. Numerous devices like the Tarlov seat, Andrews frame, and Hastings frame are also used to help position the patient for surgical procedures on the dorsal spine. Each of these devices has the potential to cause further injury if care is not exercised during positioning and securing the patient. Coordinated team effort during positioning and constant vigilance throughout the procedure is vital to minimize the risk of injury. It is extremely important to be diligent in supporting the head and to minimize injury to the face during prolonged spine procedures. Various devices are commercially available for head support. Some have a mirror attached to the base allowing visualization of the face at all times. Irrespective of the device used, it is the constant vigilance and monitoring of dependent areas and pressure points that may prevent any potential ischemic injury. It is widely believed that the most stable holder for the prone head is the 3-pin C-shaped skull fixation frame. Patients with an unstable cervical spine must be managed in a manner that allows for spinal cord function monitoring during and after the positioning process.

The prone jackknife position is often used for anorectal surgery. The patient is first placed prone and all pressure points are padded. The patient is situated on the table such that when the table is anteflexed the apex of the inverted "V" is at the patient's inguinal region. The final position should be achieved in graded steps to avoid sudden hypotension from venous pooling in dependent lower extremities and venous compression in the groin. A supportive pad is usually placed beneath the pelvis to avoid direct compression to the neurovascular bundle in the inguinal region. Care should be exercised in securing the patient after the desired position is achieved.

The anesthesia team should have a plan to manage the ventilation, invasive monitoring catheters and cables, intravenous lines, ostomy bags, and the urinary catheter during the positioning process.

PATHOPHYSIOLOGY OF THE PRONE POSITION

It is unusual for a healthy adult patient to have significant hemodynamic disturbances during the positioning process if major venous compression is avoided. However, if pressure is exerted on the major vessels (aortocaval and iliac compression), decreased venous return leads to decreased CO. In the presence of abdominal compression (compression of inferior vena cava), blood from the lower half of the body is diverted through other (perivertebral, intercostal, and lumbar veins) low-pressure venous systems to the right atrium, leading to congestion of vertebral venous plexuses. Engorgement of venous plexuses can lead to increased blood loss during surgical procedures on the spine if positioning is not optimized. Various authors have studied the hemodynamic effects of the commonly used supporting devices in the prone position. The single most important factor consistently shown to have a deleterious effect on hemodynamic function is the impact of the device on abdominal and thoracic compression.

Douglas and associates[26] showed an increase in FRC and arterial oxygen partial pressures with no change in respiratory mechanics after the patients were placed prone and properly positioned. The relationship between transpulmonary and airway opening pressures is an important factor in determining the degree of atelectasis. In the supine position, transpulmonary pressures are less than airway opening pressures, leading to atelectasis in the dorsal lung units. Lamm et al[27] showed that in the prone position, the transpulmonary pressure generated in the dorsal lung units exceeded the airway closing pressures in dogs subjected to oleic acid–induced acute lung injury. This may explain the transient improvement in oxygenation in the prone position by increased homogeneity in the gravity-dependent ventilation-perfusion ratios in the dorsal lung regions without adversely affecting ventral lung regions.

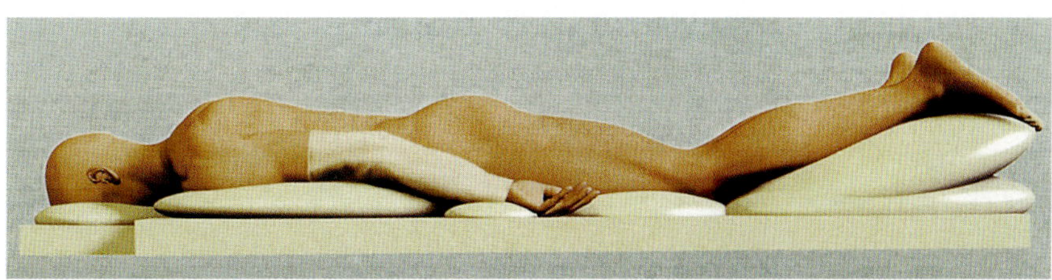

FIGURE 27-11. Prone position. [Redrawn from Martin JT. *Positioning in Anesthesia and Surgery*. Philadelphia, PA: WB Saunders; 1997. With permission.]

No significant changes in cerebral hemodynamics occur if the head of the healthy prone patient is at the level of the heart and is not laterally flexed or rotated. If head is positioned below the level of the heart in a healthy patient, cerebral blood pressure and vascular resistance in the carotid arterial system increase proportionally to maintain constant perfusion pressure and blood flow. In the presence of intracranial pathology, cerebral autoregulation is impaired; therefore, the head of the patient should not be positioned below the level of the heart to prevent pressure-dependent (gravity-induced) increase in cerebral blood flow. Severe rotation (>60 degrees) of the head and neck can have significant deleterious effects on the flow patterns in cerebral circulation. Complete obstruction of the contralateral vertebral blood flow with rotation of the head greater than 80 degrees in humans has been reported.[28] Care must be exercised during rotation of the head because patients can have significant asymptomatic occlusive cerebral vascular disease and/or congenital variations in cerebral vascular anatomy (circle of Willis). Exaggerated rotational movements in such situations can compromise blood flow in the region of the vertebrobasilar systems, leading to neurologic dysfunction.

Other complications related to prone positioning include injury to the eyes, ocular edema and blindness, compressive ischemic injuries to facial structures, compartment syndrome, VAE, breast and genital injuries, thoracic outlet syndrome, neuropathies, ostomy injuries, and hypothermia.

LATERAL DECUBITUS POSITION

Lateral decubitus positions are described as right or left, based on the dependent side of the body. For example, patients are said to be positioned in right lateral decubitus position when they lie with their right side down.

In the classic lateral decubitus position, the patient is positioned on the side with his or her back perpendicular to the surface of the table. The head is supported so the cervical spine is properly aligned with the rest of the body, and a supportive device (axillary roll or chest pad) is placed under the dependent thorax just caudad to the axilla to prevent compression and injury to the axillary neurovascular bundle. The dependent lower extremity is flexed at the hip and knee joints, and the nondependent leg is straightened in such a manner that the pelvis is stabilized and ventral tilt (forward roll) of the torso is avoided. Adequate padding is ensured to protect all the pressure points (pillow between the legs, foam for the dependent greater trochanter, fibular head and lateral malleolus) of the lower extremities. The dependent arm is flexed and supported on a padded arm board; the nondependent arm is slightly abducted and flexed at the shoulder and elbow joints so the scapula is drawn away from the thorax (**Fig. 27-12**). Once the patient is positioned optimally, care should be exercised to avoid injuries related to restraint devices (bean bag, Velcro straps).

The "kidney position" is a variation of the lateral decubitus position that is commonly used for renal procedures. In this version of the lateral decubitus position, the patient's dependent ilium is placed over the flexion point between the torso and thigh sections of the table. The table is then flexed, and the transverse elevating bar of the table (kidney bar) is raised until the lateral flexion has caused the muscles of the upper flank to become tight. During and immediately after the final position, all measures must be taken to avoid inferior venacaval and dependent rib cage compression.

PATHOPHYSIOLOGY OF THE LATERAL DECUBITUS POSITION

For the most part, the lateral decubitus position has minimal effects on major organ function when the patient is carefully positioned. Sudden postural changes are poorly tolerated in deeply anesthetized and hypovolemic patients because there is a dose-dependent depression of the carotid and baroreceptor function under general anesthesia. A gentle change in position with frequent monitoring of blood pressure is indicated in elderly, hypovolemic, and hypertensive patients. Mediastinal shift to the dependent hemithorax and rotation of the heart on its longitudinal axis in the lateral position could impair venous return and decrease CO. Impediment of venous return is usually not a problem except in the lateral jackknife (venous pooling in lower extremities) or kidney positions (caval compression). The right lateral decubitus position appears to have greater propensity for caval compression and reduced venous return with kidney rest because of the closer proximity of the vena cava to the right flank.

Vital capacity in normal awake subjects decreases by a comparable 10% in the lateral and supine positions compared with the erect posture. The kidney position can decrease the VC by another 5% to 10%. Most of this decrease is thought to result from reduced movement of the ribs and diaphragm. Although VC and FRC are reduced, better ventilation-perfusion matching results from increased perfusion in the dependent lung and corresponding increase in ventilation from the stretched dependent hemidiaphragm. However, general anesthesia with or without spontaneous ventilation in the lateral decubitus position causes an increased mismatch in ventilation-perfusion ratios compared with that in awake subjects. This is further complicated by the institution of paralysis and mechanical ventilation, addition of PEEP, opening of the pleura in thoracic procedures, pathologic processes in the dependent and nondependent lung, and use of medications (vasodilators) that affect hypoxic pulmonary vasoconstriction.

Complications from the lateral decubitus position include pressure injuries (ischemic), muscular and ligamentous strain, whiplash-like injury to the cervical spine, neurologic injuries, and ocular complications (corneal abrasions, pressure effects, dependent edema, and blindness).

NERVE INJURIES ASSOCIATED WITH POSITIONING

Perioperative peripheral nerve injuries are a significant source of morbidity for the patient and unfortunately will be encountered by even the most conscientious anesthesia provider. It is the second most common cause (after death) of professional liability among anesthesiologists, accounting for 16% of claims in the ASA closed claims database.[29] The claims secondary to nerve injuries have steadily increased in the last decade, and unfortunately the relationship between current conventional perioperative care with positioning and development of postoperative nerve injury is poorly understood.

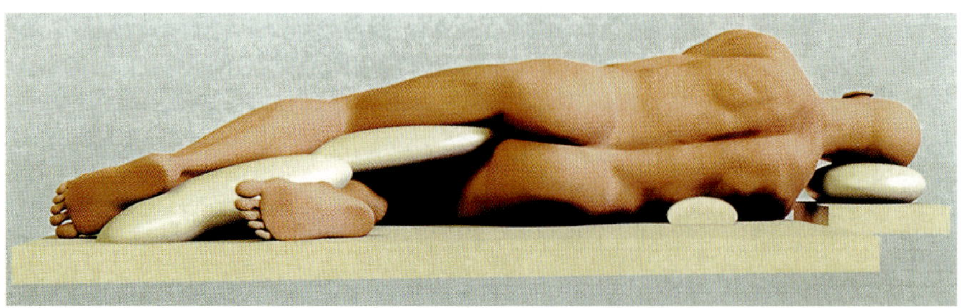

FIGURE 27–12. Lateral decubitus position. [Redrawn from Martin JT. *Positioning in Anesthesia and Surgery*. Philadelphia, PA: WB Saunders; 1997. With permission.]

Injuries to the ulnar nerve, brachial plexus, and the lumbosacral roots account for most of the claims, with the ulnar the most commonly reported nerve injury during the perioperative period. Cited mechanisms for nerve injury during the perioperative period include compression, stretch, ischemia, direct trauma, and laceration. Although injuries to the brachial plexus and lumbosacral roots may be secondary to stretch or compression with malpositioning of the patient, those to the ulnar nerve are usually unexplained and often puzzling. Ulnar nerve injury may occur despite protective padding and careful positioning. In fact, 27% of cases of ulnar nerve injury in the ASA closed claims database occurred despite the documentation of adequate padding at the elbow.[29]

A retrospective review from the Mayo Clinic reported a 0.04% incidence of persistent ulnar neuropathy in noncardiac surgery, with 9% of the reported injuries in this report bilateral.[30] Initial symptoms in most cases were noted only after a 24-hour period, and the distribution of sensory-only and mixed sensory and motor loss injuries were equal. More recent prospective data from the same authors reports a higher incidence (approximately 0.5%) of perioperative ulnar neuropathies.[31] The incidence may be even higher in patients undergoing cardiac surgery. The most consistent risk factors appear to be male gender, prolonged hospitalization, and extremes of body habitus.[30] Prielipp and colleagues reported significant changes in ulnar nerve sensory thresholds with elbow flexion in human volunteers. In the flexed position, nearly all volunteers reported ulnar nerve paresthesias. All the volunteers reporting paresthesias had a significant increase in C-fiber sensory threshold without any change in either Aα or Aβ fiber function. It could be that most hospitalized patients spend a considerably greater time with their elbows flexed, accounting for the finding that prolonged hospitalization is an independent risk factor for nerve injuries. Prielipp et al[32] studied the effects of arm positioning on the pressure exerted at the elbow. They showed that the pressure exerted over the ulnar nerve was greatest when the forearm was pronated. It was also noted that up to 50% of male volunteers who experienced pressure on the ulnar nerve sufficient to impair electrophysiologic function did not perceive concurrent paraesthesia in that nerve distribution. Thus a significant number of male patients could be at increased risk for failure to respond to potentially damaging compression injury over the ulnar nerve during the perioperative period. An additional risk factor may be the sedated state of the patients in the immediate postoperative period from the residual effects of anesthetics and narcotic medications.

Injury to the brachial plexus is the second most common perioperative nerve injury with an estimated incidence of 0.2% to 0.6%.[33] The anatomy of the brachial plexus long and mobile course of its components through the limited space between the first rib and the clavicle—makes it susceptible to stretch and compressive injury. Careful attention to arm positioning during supine position (abduction <90 degrees), steep head-down tilt (avoiding shoulder braces for support), prone positioning (avoiding improper placement of chest roll and positioning of arms), and lateral decubitus position (properly placed axillary roll) can help minimize the risk of injury.

Perioperative lower extremity neuropathies have a clearer relationship with positioning when compared with upper extremity nerve injuries. Warner et al[34] reported an overall 1.5% incidence of all patients undergoing surgery in the lithotomy position. The risk increases with the duration (>2 hours) in the lithotomy position, and almost all of the reported injuries were sensory in nature. Paraesthesia in the affected nerve distribution was the most common complaint. Symptoms in all of their patients were noted within 4 hours. The obturator was the most commonly affected nerve, with lateral femoral cutaneous, sciatic, and peroneal nerve injuries following in order. Sciatic nerve injury is most common after lithotomy positioning or some variant of it. Hyperflexion of the hip with extension at the knee along with external rotation of the thigh during positioning of the legs can produce excessive stretch of the sciatic nerve and result in injury. The common peroneal nerve is particularly vulnerable to compression injury because it wraps around the head of the fibula. Femoral neuropathy is more commonly associated with surgical factors, although ischemic injury could result from extreme abduction and external rotation of the thighs during lithotomy positioning.

Anesthesiologists should be familiar with and follow the recommendations of the ASA practice advisory for prevention of perioperative neuropathies (**Box 27-1**). For particularly long procedures, consideration should be given to minimizing the time spent in a position that amplifies physiologic perturbations or injury to the patient. It may be

BOX 27-1

Summary of ASA Task Force Consensus on Prevention of Perioperative Peripheral Neuropathies

Preoperative assessment

- When judged appropriate, it is helpful to ascertain that patients can comfortably tolerate the anticipated operative position.

Upper-extremity positioning

- Arm abduction should be limited to 90 degrees in supine patients; patients who are positioned prone may comfortably tolerate arm abduction >90 degrees.
- Arms should be positioned to decrease pressure on the postcondylar groove of the humerus (ulnar groove). When arms are tucked at the side, a neutral forearm position is recommended. When arms are abducted on arm boards, either supination or a neutral forearm position is acceptable.
- Prolonged pressure on the radial nerve in the spiral groove of the humerus should be avoided.
- Extension of the elbow beyond a comfortable range may stretch the median nerve.

Lower-extremity positioning

- Lithotomy positions that stretch the hamstring muscle group beyond a comfortable range may stretch the sciatic nerve.
- Prolonged pressure on the peroneal nerve at the fibular head should be avoided.
- Neither extension nor flexion of the hip increases the risk of femoral neuropathy.

Protective padding

- Padded arm boards may decrease the risk of upper-extremity neuropathy.
- Use of chest rolls in laterally positioned patients may decrease the risk of upper-extremity neuropathies.
- Padding at the elbow and at the fibular head may decrease the risk of upper- and lower-extremity neuropathies, respectively.

Equipment

- Properly functioning automated blood pressure cuffs on the upper arms do not affect the risk of upper-extremity neuropathies.
- Shoulder braces in steep head-down positions may increase the risk of brachial plexus neuropathies.

Postoperative assessment

- Simple postoperative assessment of extremity nerve function may lead to early recognition of peripheral neuropathies.

Documentation

- Charting specific positioning actions during the care of patients may result in improvements of care by (1) helping practitioners focus attention on relevant aspects of patient positioning, and (2) providing information that continuous improvement processes use can lead to refinements in patient care.

From Practice advisory for the prevention of perioperative peripheral neuropathies: a report by the American Society of Anesthesiologists Task Force on Prevention of Perioperative Peripheral Neuropathies. *Anesthesiology.* 2000;92:1168-1182. Reprinted with permission of the publisher.

advisable to look for and document symptoms of nerve dysfunction preoperatively in high-risk patients (those with risk factors for perioperative neuropathies or those coming for high-risk surgery, ie, long procedures or surgical positions at risk for injury). A description of the intraoperative positioning and measures taken to prevent injury should be documented in the anesthetic record at the beginning of the procedure and thereafter on a regular basis.

VISUAL INJURY

Postoperative visual complications constitute a broad group ranging from temporary loss of visual acuity to devastating permanent loss of visual function. Corneal abrasions, periorbital and conjunctival edema, ocular hemorrhage, vitreous loss, retinal detachment, central retinal artery occlusion, and ischemic optic neuropathy are the range of complications encountered in the perioperative period.

The reported incidence of perioperative visual injury varies widely (<0.06%-25.6%). The American Association of Nurse Anesthetists Foundation closed malpractice claims study[35] reports an incidence of 3.3%, and the ASA closed claims analysis[36] reports a similar 3.47% for all types of eye injury. In both closed claims projects, corneal abrasions are the most common complications encountered. Patient movement, chemical irritation from preparation solutions, direct trauma from the face mask, pressure from the laryngoscopic blade, pressure effects on the globe from lateral and prone positioning, prolonged procedures on the spine in the prone position, intraoperative hypotension, and anemia have all been implicated as the reasons.

The lateral, prone, and Trendelenburg positions increase the risk for visual complications during the perioperative period. In all these positions, venous pressure in the eye can increase from direct pressure, edema, and/or stasis, leading to decreased choroidal perfusion and increased risk for ischemic optic neuropathy. Other associated factors for visual complications during the perioperative period include prolonged operations on the spine, large-volume blood loss, significant decreases in hemoglobin levels, and intraoperative hypotension. Contributing patient comorbid conditions include hypertension, diabetes, obesity, smoking history, hypercholesterolemia, alcohol abuse, atherosclerosis, anemia, Graves disease, and renal transplantation.[37] Shaw et al[38] reported that 40 of their 312 patients scheduled for coronary artery bypass grafting procedures had preexisting ophthalmologic abnormalities on examination. Currently, preoperative screening ophthalmologic examination of surgical patients to predict postoperative visual complications is not a common practice. Therefore, it is imperative for anesthesia providers to be highly cognizant of the potential for visual complications in high-risk patients. Anesthesia providers should pay special attention to avoid pressure effects on the globe and to maintain adequate oxygen delivery to the optic disc and retinal structures. A report by the ASA Task Force on perioperative blindness is an excellent source of current information and consensus expert opinion on this devastating problem (approved by the ASA house of delegates October 2005).[39]

SPECIAL CONSIDERATIONS OF ROBOTIC SURGERY

Although surgical endoscopy started in the early 1990s, the technology and practice has evolved greatly in the last few decades. Commonly used initially for short diagnostic and sterilization procedures in gynecologic practice, it has now evolved to an alternative and viable option in the youngest and oldest patients alike and in patients with multiple comorbidities who are at increased risk for open procedures. One of the revolutionary advancements in surgical practice has been the adoption of computer-assisted robots in laparoscopic procedures.[40] Robotic surgery has the combined advantages of better surgical precision than the human hand and the minimal invasive benefits of laparoscopic procedures; however, it does have special implications for anesthesia providers.

Robotic procedures typically take a longer time than the open positions and are frequently performed in a nondorsal decubitus position. They commonly involve use of a gas to distend the surgical site and therefore are prone to the adverse effects of the combined mechanical and systemic sequelae of the gas used to create pneumoperitoneum and the physiologic perturbations associated with each individual position for a particular procedure. Because carbon dioxide is commonly used to create the pneumoperitoneum, the systemic cardiovascular effects depend on the raise in intra-abdominal pressure with the creation of pneumoperitoneum, duration of surgery, hypercarbia induced secondary to the pneumoperitoneum, degree of respiratory acidosis, sympathetic tone of the patient, preoperative volume status, preoperative cardiovascular function, and the surgical position used.

Robotic surgery involves complex bulky equipment that makes it difficult for unimpeded access to the patient in an emergency after the system is docked into position. In addition, the bed may be turned away from the anesthesia machine. Therefore, it is vital that the patient be properly positioned, taking appropriate measures to secure the patient to the bed and have unimpeded fluid flow to vascular access sites and pressure tubing of the arterial catheter. The patient has to be covered appropriately to avoid trauma from misplaced or loose equipment and to avoid hypothermia.

Fluid management needs to be based on a goal-directed therapy regimen to maintain adequate perfusion to vital organs. It is prudent to be aware that over the course of a prolonged procedure in steep head-down position there is a risk for increased intracranial pressure, raised intraocular pressure, orbital and laryngeal edema leading to serious intracranial, visual, and upper airway problems with excessive fluid therapy.

Some evidence indicates that retroperitoneal carbon dioxide insufflation for prostate procedures may be associated with lower cardiovascular and respiratory changes compared with intraperitoneal insufflation.[41]

EVALUATION OF POSITIONING RELATED NERVE INJURIES

Although rare, positioning-related nerve injuries (neuropathy) can last for weeks. Pure sensory deficits (numbness and/or tingling only) typically resolve within 5 to 7 days. Assurance to the patient and continued vigilance to avoid stretching of the involved nerve or external pressure may be all that is needed. However, an evaluation by a neurologist may be indicated if the deficit lasts longer than 7 days or is worsening.

If there is a motor component to the deficit, an immediate neurologic evaluation is warranted. Electromyographic studies may be helpful in pinpointing the acuity (relationship to surgery) and location of the lesion. This study may also help in identifying subclinical and/or chronic abnormalities in the contralateral nerve, hence identifying a high-risk patient.

KEY REFERENCES

- *A Report by the American Society of Anesthesiologists Task Force on Perioperative Blindness.* Chicago, IL: American Society of Anesthesiologists; October 2005.
- Cheney FW, Domino KB, Caplan RA et al. Nerve injury associated with anesthesia: a closed claims analysis. *Anesthesiology.* 1999;90(4):1062-1069.
- Lumb AB, Nunn JF. Respiratory function and ribcage contribution to ventilation in body positions commonly used during anesthesia. *Anesth Analg.* 1991;73(4):422-426.
- Martin JT. *Positioning in Anesthesia and Surgery.* Philadelphia, PA: WB Saunders; 1997.

- Prielipp RC, Morell RC, Walker FO, et al. Ulnar nerve pressure: influence of arm position and relationship to somatosensory evoked potentials. *Anesthesiology*. 1999;91(2):345-354.
- Rupp-Montpetit K, Moody ML. Visual loss as a complication of nonophthalmologic surgery: a review of the literature. *AANA J*. 2004;72(4):285-292.
- Warner MA, Warner DO, Harper CM, et al. Lower extremity neuropathies associated with lithotomy positions. *Anesthesiology*. 2000;93(4):938-942.
- Warner MA, Warner ME, Martin JT. Ulnar neuropathy. Incidence, outcome, and risk factors in sedated or anesthetized patients. *Anesthesiology*. 1994;81(6):1332-1340.

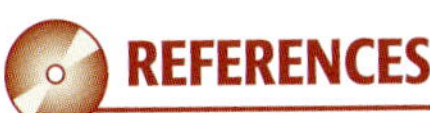

REFERENCES

Complete references available on DVD and online version at www.LongneckerAnesthesiology.com

CHAPTER 28 Environmental Safety

Marc Petre

KEY POINTS

1. Environmental risk factors for anesthesia include electrical, fire, radiation, and chemotherapeutic considerations.
2. Anesthesia providers must have a general understanding of these risks, preventive measures, and reactive procedures to serve as effective advocates for their patients.
3. Many regulatory bodies, professional societies, and standards organizations provide guidelines for environmental safety in anesthetizing locations.

INTRODUCTION

Health care providers recognize patient safety as a primary area of concern. Anesthesia providers must take this responsibility especially seriously because they practice in an environment of increased patient risk, and do so with the intent of reducing the patient's ability to respond to stimulus on his or her own. The anesthesia team must act as the patient's steward in both risk avoidance and crisis management. In addition to the patient's safety, the anesthesia provider must also consider the safety of operating room colleagues and himself or herself. Many decisions as simple as draping technique, electrical outlet connection, supply selection, and equipment positioning can have serious implications for all persons in the vicinity of care.

As minimally invasive interventions increase in popularity, anesthesia care is more frequently pulled out of the relatively highly regulated operating room and into procedure rooms, intensive care unit (ICU) bed spaces, and physician offices. To provide safe and effective care in these areas, it is important that anesthesia providers understand the origins of operating room (OR) safety requirements so that they can apply them as needed during remote anesthetics.

Although much attention has been given to electrical safety in health care, environmental safety in anesthesia also includes consideration of fire, chemical, and radiation risks. A general knowledge of the potential environmental safety hazards associated with anesthesia and its related equipment will help providers protect themselves, their clinical colleagues, and act as effective advocates for their patients. This chapter reviews several common environmental risk factors associated with anesthesia care and discusses infrastructure, equipment, and procedures used to prevent and react to critical events. Safety and prevention of physical accidents such as needle sticks and cuts from broken medication vials are not discussed, although studies have shown that physical accidents may be more prevalent than critical fire and electrical events.[1]

Many regulatory bodies provide guidance on environmental safety. They serve as additional resources for the safe design, construction, and maintenance of anesthetizing locations and are also reviewed for reference and to familiarize providers with the bodies that encourage safety in their clinical space.

ELECTRICAL SAFETY

As electronic and, more recently, computerized equipment becomes more prevalent in anesthetizing locations, it has become increasingly important for providers to understand the specific risks posed by such equipment. This section focuses on the direct risks including temporary physiologic disruption and tissue damage. Ignition of fire or explosion is one of many *indirect* risks associated with electrical equipment and is discussed in the section on fire safety.

ELECTRICITY FOR HEALTH CARE PROVIDERS

Although it is not necessary for health care providers to master electrical circuit theory, they should have an understanding of common electrical concepts and terms in the context of the clinical care they provide.

Coulomb A coulomb (C) is the International System of Units (SI) unit of electric charge equivalent to 6.242×10^{18} electrons. In the case of electrons, each electron carries one charge. In the case of ions, each ion may carry more than one charge. For example, 3.121×10^{18} Ca^{2+} ions = 1 C of charge.

Current The flow of electric charge per unit of time, measured in amperes (1 A = 1 C/s), is called the current. In the case of electrical distribution systems and devices using metallic conductors, the electrical charges in motion are electrons. Biologic currents are often ionic in nature. For example, electrically active cells use Ca^{2+}, Na^+, and K^+ currents for action potential propagation.

Voltage Voltage is the electrical representation of potential energy and expressed in energy per unit charge measured in volts (1 V = 1 joule [J] of energy per coulomb of charge). Just as 1 L of blood may have a different pressure under different circumstances, 1 C of charge may have a different voltage depending on its circumstances. Just as blood flows toward the ground to reduce pressure due to gravitational potential energy, whenever possible, voltage will be eliminated through current flow from a point of higher voltage (potential) to one of lower voltage.

Ground Ground is a point of reference from which all voltages in a circuit are measured. The earth represents a relatively reliable reference point because it is large enough to be viewed as an infinite source or sink for electrons. Because of this fact, earth ground is capable of accepting or producing large currents without a change in its voltage (often designated as zero volt).

Circuit A complete closed-loop path through which current may flow. From a safety standpoint, we are most concerned with electrical circuits that include pathways for current flow through the human body.

Direct Current Direct current (DC) is a type of electrical circuit where charge flows exclusively in one direction (**Fig. 28-1**). Batteries are voltage stores that generate DC current. DC current may be pulsed to create a regular pattern, but charges always flow in a single direction.

Alternating Current Alternating current (AC) is a type of electrical circuit where the direction of charge flow alternates in a regular fashion (**Fig. 28-2**). Electrical power is widely generated and distributed as

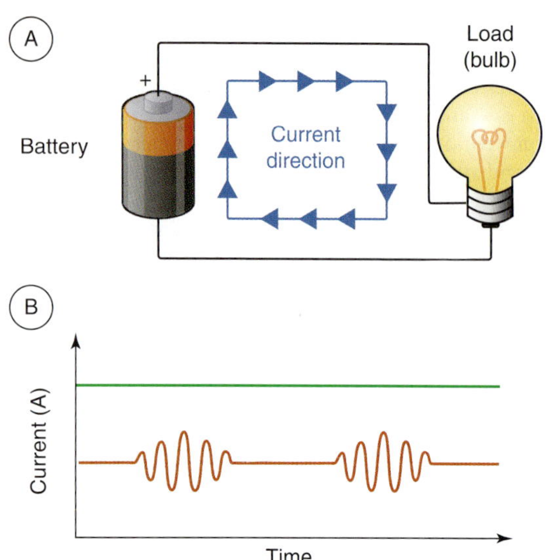

FIGURE 28-1. A. A simple direct current circuit showing the unidirectional flow of current. **B.** Direct current (DC) always flows in one direction but need not be static. DC may be pulsed to generate cyclic waveforms.

AC. Despite being somewhat more dangerous than DC current of the same voltage, AC power has the advantage of being more efficient for transmission across long distances due to the ability to easily transform high AC transmission voltages into lower consumer voltages. Many consumer and medical devices use a power transformer to convert AC into DC near the AC power outlet (known as AC rectification; **Fig. 28-3**).

Electrical Power The rate at which electrical energy is transferred, measured in watts (1 W = 1 VA = 1 J/s), is electrical power.

Resistance Opposition to the flow of electrical charge (DC), measured in ohms (1 Ω = 1 V/A), is called resistance. A resistor is an electrical circuit component designed to provide a known opposition to the flow of charge. Resistors are used to guide and manage current as it moves through engineered circuits. Dry intact human skin and myelin are both examples of biologic insulators with high resistance to electrical current.

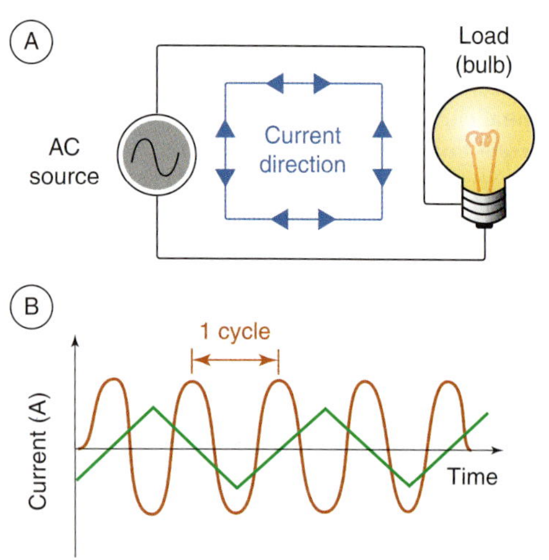

FIGURE 28-2. A. A simple alternating current (AC) circuit showing bidirectional current flow. **B.** AC switches between positive and negative values in a cyclic fashion but is not necessarily sinusoidal (red) in nature and may have other waveforms such as a sawtooth (green). AC current may also be pulsed as in burst-modulated alternating current used in transcutaneous electrical nerve stimulation.

Capacitance The storage of electrical energy by collecting charges on separated conductors, measured in farads (1 F = 1 C/V), is known as capacitance. A capacitor is created, intentionally or accidentally, whenever an insulator separates 2 conductors. No current flows through a capacitor, but the capacitor affects currents elsewhere in the circuit by accumulating and releasing charge(s). Insulating human skin, lipid bilayers, and myelin also create capacitors by separating charges (**Fig. 28-4**).

Inductance The storage and release of electrical energy resulting from conversion of current to a magnetic field and vice versa as measured in henries (1 L = 1 V·s/A) is inductance. The magnetic field created by current passing through a wire is maximized by arranging the wire in a coil and filling the core of the coil with a material of high magnetic permeability, often iron (**Fig. 28-5**). Changes in electrical current must change the electromagnetic field in the core, either building it up or collapsing it, and there is a time delay associated with this change. Inductors are electrical components with a single coil that may be used in a circuit to store current or to resist rapid changes in current.

Transformer When 2 electrically separate coils are placed around the same core, a transformer is created using mutual inductance. Alternating current passing through one coil results in a cyclic magnetic field in the core. The cyclic magnetic field in turn induces an alternating current in the second coil. The ratio of voltages in the 2 coils V_1/V_2 is equal to the ratio of the number of wraps of wire each coil has around the shared core N_1/N_2 (**Fig. 28-6**). Transformers are often used in medical devices to step up or down voltages or to transfer voltage from one circuit to another while maintaining physical separation or isolation of the circuits.

Reactance Opposition to the flow of electrical charge (AC) due to the accumulation of electrical or magnetic fields, measured in ohms (1 Ω = 1 V/A). Reactance is a combination of capacitance and inductance.

Impedance Impedance is essentially a frequency-dependent opposition to the flow of electrical charge (AC) that extends the DC concept of resistance to AC systems. Impedance = resistance + reactance. As the AC frequency approaches zero, the current becomes more DC-like, and impedance is dominated by resistance. At higher frequencies, resistance is less significant, and insulators for DC currents can become conductors. Human skin is an example of a material with high DC resistance but low impedance at higher AC frequencies. Current always flows through a circuit in the direction of least impedance.

Ohm's Law A simple electrical rule relating voltage, impedance, and current is known as Ohm's law. V = IR or I = V/R. The current through a circuit, or section of a circuit, I, increases if the driving force, V, is increased and decreases if the circuit resistance, R, increases.

Leakage Current Leakage current is the current that does not follow an expected path through a circuit but rather escapes along another route and may or may not rejoin the circuit (**Fig. 28-7**). If the leakage current flows through an alternative path to ground, it is often referred to as *ground fault current.* Leakage currents are difficult to avoid in electrical devices and may occur through direct contact with current-carrying components or inductive or capacitive coupling of equipment to grounded objects or people. These currents, although generally small in magnitude, represent a risk for patients undergoing invasive procedures, especially procedures with direct access to the heart.

HUMAN BODY THRESHOLDS

Electricity, like other energy sources such as radiant heat, has the ability to produce burns and tissue damage at high levels. Electricity also has the ability to disrupt the body at much lower energy levels due to interaction with electrically active tissues such as nerves, skeletal muscle, and cardiac muscle. Although the neurons and myocytes that make up these tissues use ions and electrolytes as their source of electrical potential, they are susceptible to modulation by the flow of electrons commonly used for electrical power.

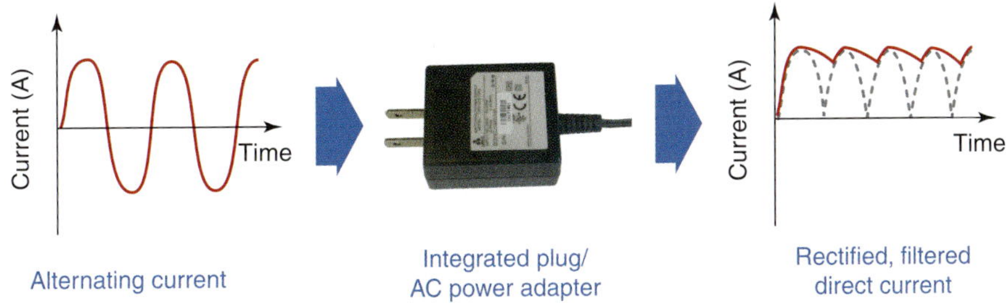

FIGURE 28-3. Medical devices often operate on direct current (DC) for safety and simplicity. Alternating (AC) power from the electrical distribution system is often converted into DC at the outlet using a full-wave rectifier and power transformer (sometimes referred to as a power adapter).

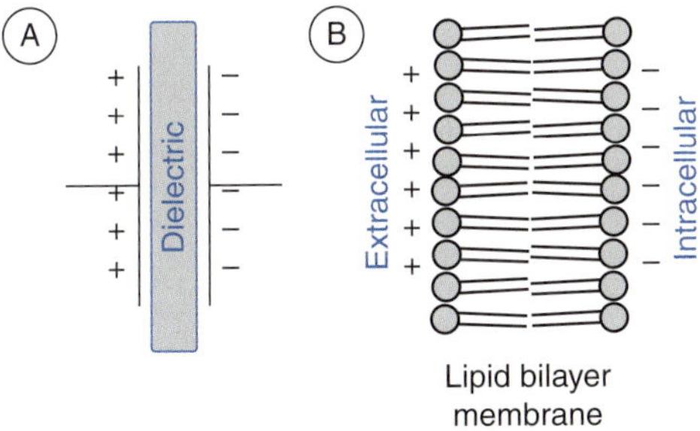

FIGURE 28-4. A. Schematic representation of a capacitor. **B.** The cell membrane as an example of a biologic capacitor. Human skin also acts as a capacitor, separating charge on its inner and outer surfaces.

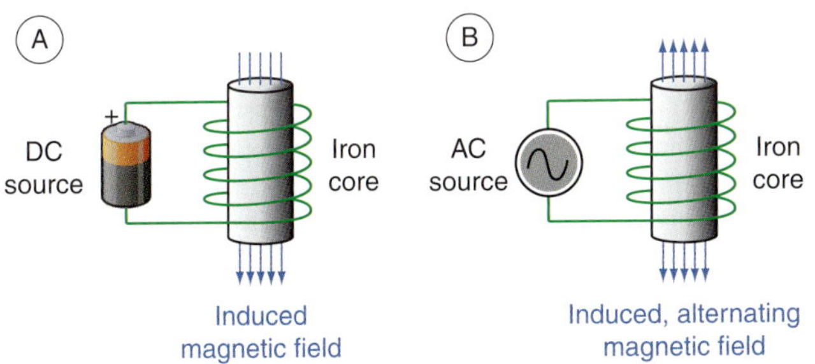

FIGURE 28-5. An inductor is created by wrapping a wire coil around a core. A magnetic field is induced in the core and either built up or collapsed with changes in the coil current. **A.** In the case of direct current (DC), the magnetic field is fixed creating an electromagnet. **B.** In the case of alternating current (AC), the magnetic field varies with time. Maximum inductance is achieved by using a core material that is highly magnetically permeable, such as iron.

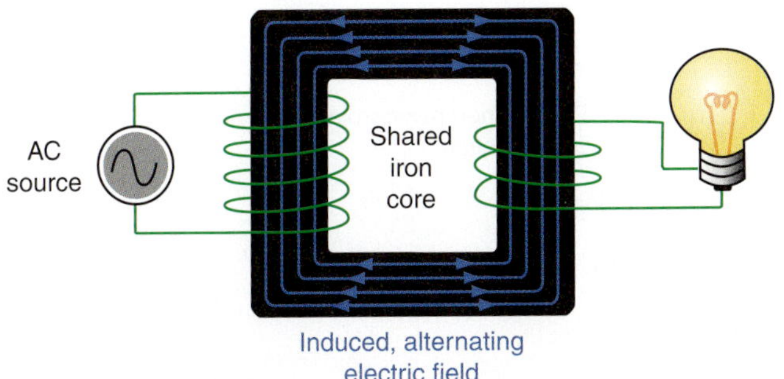

FIGURE 28-6. A schematic of a simple transformer. Wires connected to the light bulb are physically disconnected from the power source. The source, or primary, coil has 5 wraps around the shared core, and the load, or secondary, coil has 3 wraps, so this transformer steps the source voltage down to three-fifths of its original value.

Anesthesia and pain management providers take advantage of this phenomenon when using nerve stimulators to evaluate the quality of pharmacologic paralysis, confirm placement of regional anesthesia needles, or treat chronic pain as in transcutaneous electrical nerve stimulation. Medicine has also harnessed electrical current for use in defibrillators, electrotherapy, and electrosurgery. These intentional exposures to electricity produce a safe and useful response, yet it is obvious that some exposures to electricity do not. It is important for the anesthesia provider to have an understanding of common thresholds for electrical stimulus and their modifiers to use these technologies appropriately and safely.

When examining human thresholds for electricity, the therapeutic effect, interaction, or danger lies in the motion of charge through the body. As such, thresholds are expressed in terms of currents rather than voltages. Ohm's law links voltage and current through impedance (current = voltage/impedance) demonstrating that the danger of high voltage is really in the possibility of generating high currents through a circuit of sufficiently low impedance. **Figure 28-8** shows common responses to varying magnitudes of 60 Hz alternating current. It should be noted that these thresholds are representative of one group of potential users (male, about 70 kg) and one combination of stimulation duration (1-3 seconds pulse), frequency (60 Hz), and current path (hand-to-hand). Any one of these variables, or a combination of them, can be the difference between a tingling sensation and a tissue burn or ventricular fibrillation.

INDIVIDUAL VARIABILITY

Thresholds to electrical stimulation vary between men and women and even within these groups.[2] Men tend to have higher thresholds, possibly due to higher average muscle content leading to higher resistivity. As arm/leg thickness increases, resistance of the limb decreases. The human response to electrical stimulation is also modified by increased resistance in obesity and decreased neuronal response from both advancing age and the presence of chronic illnesses. The threshold for electrical interaction may also be altered by the administration of medications.[3]

INTERACTIONS WITH ELECTRICALLY ACTIVE TISSUES

For all currents with insufficient energy to cause burns and other physical damage, the safety focus is on interaction with electrically active cells and tissues, specifically the ability of the applied current to trigger action potentials artificially in these tissues.

- **Sensory and nociceptive neurons.** The firing of sensory and nociceptive neurons may create sensations of tingling, heat, or pain. The threshold of perception is determined by first activation of these pathways.
- **Skeletal muscle and motor neurons.** Activation of skeletal muscle, either directly or through activation of its innervating motor neuron, may lead to involuntary contraction that prevents victims from removing themselves from the circuit. The current level at which this occurs is known as the "let go" current. If the current passes through the thoracoabdominal region, sustained contraction in the muscles of

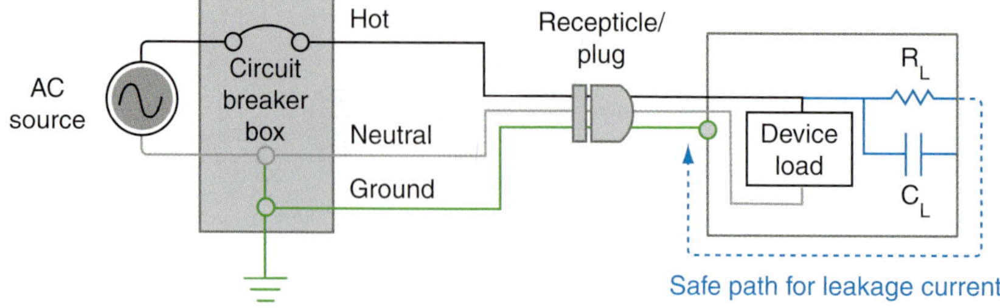

FIGURE 28-7. Current flows through the medical device load, as intended, but may also leak to the device chassis through resistive (R_L) or capacitive (C_L) paths. Leakage current should flow through the low-impedance path to ground created by the ground wire. If the ground wire continuity is broken anywhere between the device and the breaker box, leakage current (and any fault current) will energize the device case creating a potentially dangerous situation. AC, alternating current.

the diaphragm may result in life-threatening paralysis of the breathing mechanism.

- **Cardiac muscle.** Just as sustained contraction of the diaphragm prevents lung function, sustained contraction of the myocardium prevents pumping of the heart. In addition to this transient risk during the application of electrical current, disruption of the carefully coordinated cardiac cycle may reduce the effectiveness of pumping long after the current is removed. This includes the possibly of leaving the heart in life-threatening ventricular fibrillation.
- **Central nervous system.** Although rare in general surgery, it is possible for fault currents to pass through the brain or spinal cord and activate the neurons and ganglia of the central nervous system. This risk is more prevalent in neurosurgery where direct electrical access to the brain may lead fault currents through the patient's vertical axis.

Electrically active cells do not respond instantaneously to external electrical stimulus, but rather have time constants associated with changes in their membrane potential. Membrane time dependence results in tissue-specific sensitivity to the frequency of applied electrical stimulation (**Table 28-1**). This sensitivity depends on at least 3 factors:

1. **Excitability.** The likelihood that a cell will be activated by a given excitation depends on cell membrane properties such as resting potential, threshold potential, and capacitance. Activation follows a magnitude-duration relationship. For example, a large myelinated nerve fiber will be activated in less than 0.05 millisecond with a 4 V excitation but will require 0.35 millisecond if the excitation is decreased to 0.5 V.[4] The chronaxie time, or time to activation when the excitation potential is twice the threshold potential, is commonly used to compare the excitability of different cell types. A longer chronaxie time implies lower excitability.
2. **Stimulation.** The magnitude and duration of the stimulation determine whether or not enough charge will be delivered in a given time to cross the cell's activation threshold and elicit an action potential. The stimulation waveform has no effect on the ability to elicit an action potential[5] but may have effects on efficiency of stimulation, charge accumulation at electrodes, and/or summation of repetitive stimulus.
3. **Refractory period.** Once a cell has been depolarized, its sodium channels enter a deactivated state where ion transport is impossible.[4] During the absolute refractory period, no magnitude of excitation can elicit a response from the cell. This length of this absolute refractory period may be pharmacologically altered (usually lengthened) by medications including antiarrhythmics (**Box 28-1**).

The combination of cell excitability and refractory period result in a cell-type dependent optimal range of stimulation frequencies (Table 28-1). All important electrically active tissues are susceptible to modulation in the 50 to 60 Hz range used in North America and Europe for AC power distribution. For example, the muscle-dependent let-go current is highly frequency dependent with the lowest current threshold, about 16 mA, occurring at a frequency of about 60 Hz.[2] At high frequencies, above about 10 kHz, electrically active cells cannot respond quickly enough to the rapidly alternating electric field and there is little biologic interaction other than heating and desiccation at high current densities (**Box 28-2**).

AC power generally represents a higher risk than DC power at the same voltage due to the alternating nature of the current. When static direct current is applied to the human body, it acts to depolarize cell membranes and hold them in such a state until the current is removed. The effect on the heart, for example, disappears after the stimulus is removed. AC power, in contrast, has a greater probability of leaving the heart in an uncoordinated state such as flutter or fibrillation upon

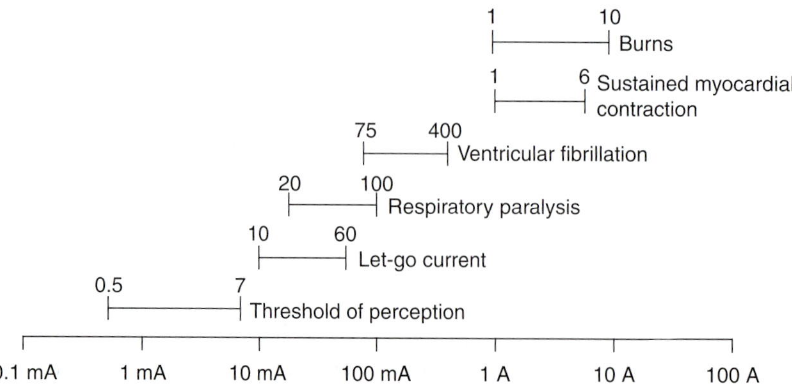

FIGURE 28-8. Threshold ranges for the interaction between 60-Hz alternating current (AC) and the human body when current is applied from hand to hand through intact skin.

TABLE 28-1 Time-Dependent Activation Properties for Selected Electrically Active Tissues[4,52]

Tissue	Chronaxie Time (ms)	Absolute Refractory Time (ms)	Optimal Stimulation Frequency (Hz)
Nerve fiber: large, myelinated type A	0.1-0.2	0.4	10-50
Nerve fiber: small, myelinated type A	0.3	1-2	90-100
Nerve fiber: unmyelinated type C	0.5	1-2	90-150
Muscle: skeletal	0.25-1	1-3	10-100
Muscle: cardiac	1-3	0.1-15	0-30

The chronaxie time represents the time required to activate the fiber when the stimulation magnitude is twice the threshold value. The chronaxie time provides a means to compare cell excitability with longer chronaxie times indicating lower excitability.

removal. If direct current is pulsed to generate a regular waveform, its effects may be similar to those of alternating current.

LOCAL CURRENT MAGNITUDE

The magnitude of the current reaching important structures such as the diaphragm, skeletal muscles, and heart depends on the integrity of the skin barrier and the path and distribution of current flow through the body.

Skin as a Current Barrier The human body can be viewed as a pool of electrolytes inside of a skin envelope of varying impedance. Skin impedance results from a combination of resistance and capacitance, both of which are in large part due to the dense outer layer of dead cells known as the stratum corneum.[2,8] Skin resistance can be lowered by abrasion of the stratum corneum and/or the application of electrolyte gels or fluids, which hydrate the skin. Clinicians take advantage of this reduced resistance when applying external electrodes for monitoring the electrocardiogram (ECG), electroencephalogram, and other low-magnitude biopotentials. A typical resistance value for intact skin is 1 to 10 kΩ. This resistance drops about 35% when skin is moist due to sweating or the application of electrolytic gel and to as little as 1 kΩ when the stratum corneum is mechanically removed.[9] As electrical excitation frequency increases, skin capacitance falls resulting in decreased overall resistivity.[10]

Penetration of the protective skin barrier is common in anesthesia practice not only due to invasive surgical procedures, but also due to invasive pressure monitoring, endoscopy, and venous access. Cardiac surgery often uses postsurgical pacing wires, which also provide a direct path to cardiac tissue. Any procedure that penetrates or bypasses the protective skin layers potentially provides a low-impedance (electrolyte/blood) connection or circuit to the heart. Direct access greatly reduces the required current for adverse events, and in these cases, the patient is at risk for microshocks. Limited data on human microshocks via cardiac catheter have implied that currents between 80 and 600 μA can result in fibrillation, and designers of indwelling devices often use 10 μA as an upper limit for allowable leakage current[2] (**Box 28-3**).

Path and Distribution of Current Electrical shocks that transverse intact skin are often referred to as *macroshocks*. Current that traverses or entirely bypasses the skin travels through the path of least impedance to a lower potential, often ground (**Fig. 28-9**). The internal resistivity of the body is related to the water content and structure of individual tissues with a range from about 10^8 Ω cm in bone to 10^2 Ω cm in blood.[10] The overall resistance of a human limb is approximately 200 Ω; the resistance of the trunk is about 100 Ω.[2] If a wire was held in each hand, a current passing between them would pass through the skin on the right hand, the right arm, the trunk, the left arm, and the skin on the left hand (1000 + 200 + 100 + 200 + 1000 = 2.5 kΩ). By inserting metallic probes into each hand, the skin layers are bypassed and the overall resistance is significantly reduced to 500 Ω. At this reduced impedance, even a 9-V battery would generate a current of 18 mA through the trunk of the body.

The effect of current is also determined by the local magnitude, or distribution of current over an area. Any current passing through the body will be distributed throughout the conductive tissues of the trunk or limb (Fig. 28-9). For currents applied arm to arm in experimental animals, only approximately 3% of the current traversed the heart.[11] In this case, 3% of 18 mA = 540 μA passing directly through the myocardium may still be sufficient to cause cardiac depolarization and induce an arrhythmia (**Box 28-4**).

PROTECTIVE INFRASTRUCTURE

Electrical power arrives at health care facilities from a utility provider via one or more high-voltage supply lines. The hospital power distribution system is responsible for making this power available at user end points (receptacles) at a safe and useful level and providing emergency backup power should the main utility source fail. Power distribution

BOX 28-1

Applied Theory: Cell Excitability and the TASER X26

TASER-brand X26 stun guns are designed to incapacitate suspects by artificially stimulating both sensory and motor neurons. These devices are capable of generating pain and subtetanic involuntary muscle contraction using a high-voltage (50 000 V), low-magnitude pulsed DC (about 3 mA, 19 Hz). Safety advocates have raised questions about the possibility of cardiac injury or incapacitation, but TASER has successfully defended the safety record of their product.[6,7] The waveform used by the device is tuned to activate nerves and avoid cardiac activation using principles of cell excitability:

1. The magnitude and duration of the pulse are just above the threshold for activation of large type A neurons but below the threshold for cardiac muscle activation
2. The current delivery is superficial and therefore the current that reaches the heart is even lower than the surface magnitude.

BOX 28-2

What Were They Thinking?: AC Power Distribution Frequency

AC power is distributed at 60 Hz in the United States and a mixture of 50 and 60 Hz elsewhere in the world. Although it may seem like a bad idea today, these distribution frequencies were originally selected to be high enough to avoid perceptible flicker in incandescent light bulbs (>30 Hz) and low enough to simplify the design of electrical devices. Much more is now known about the biologic consequences of this choice, but power grids are well established, and it is up to device designers and users to work within existing guidelines.

BOX 28-3

Applied Theory: Controlled Macroshock for Defibrillation

The goal of defibrillation is to stimulate all cardiomyocytes simultaneously and send them into a refractory state. The stimulation pulse does not need to be long in duration, and when the current is removed, a fresh substrate will be available for the reestablishment of sinus rhythm. Modern external defibrillators apply about 1000 V through 2 large paddles or disposable electrodes placed against the chest wall such that the current flowing between them passes close to or through the patient's heart. A conductive gel is often used to lower the resistance of the skin. Using external paddles, users may apply up to 360 J to depolarize the myocardium. When internal paddles are applied directly to the myocardium, devices limit energy to about 50 J (Philips HeartStart XL).

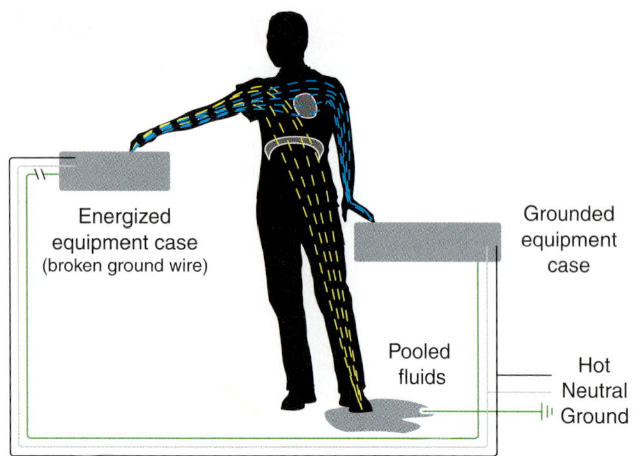

FIGURE 28-9. Two possible current paths to ground for a macroshock condition and their approximate distribution throughout the body. A broken ground conductor and internal fault in the medical device on the left leads to an energized case. Yellow path: Current flows from operator's right hand through diaphragm to the left foot, which is grounded through contact with a puddle of fluids on the operating room floor. Blue path: Current flows from the operator's right hand through the trunk and heart and out of the left hand, which is in contact with a grounded surface. Note that because current is distributed throughout the volume conductor of the body, not all hand-to-hand current will pass through the heart.

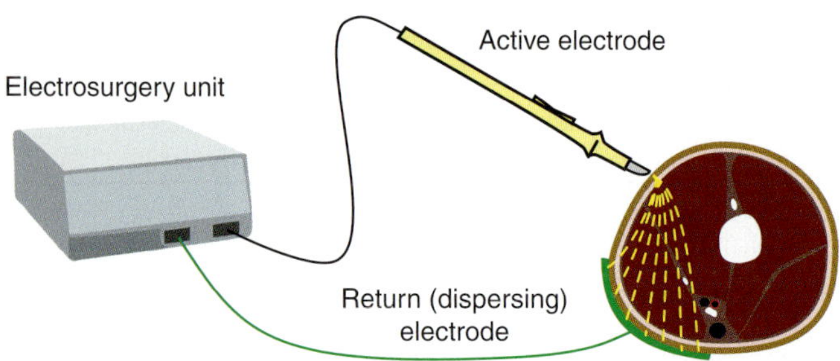

FIGURE 28-10. Monopolar electrosurgery uses high current density at the active electrode tip to cut and coagulate tissue. Current density is then lowered by dispersion at the return electrode to avoid tissue damage from exiting current. Problems may arise if exiting current is refocused by poor return electrode contact or an alternative return pathway such as an electrocardiogram electrode.

systems include all receptacles, wires, fuses, transformers, generators, and circuit breakers within a facility.

Typically, metallic piping, structural beams, and other conductive components of modern buildings are physically and electrically tied to earth ground and can provide a path for current to flow to or from this infinite source and sink for electrons. Humans may become a part of this path (circuit) to ground through direct contact with, or capacitive coupling to, conductive building structures or fluids in contact with building structure or plumbing. Currents flowing to ground through paths other than the expected electrical circuits are often referred to as ground fault currents. A major safety goal of electrical distribution systems is to minimize ground fault currents by limiting maximum currents and providing alternative low-impedance paths to ground. Power distribution systems may contain a variety of safety equipment to manage the flow of stray currents to ground and provide over-current protection.

MANAGEMENT OF CURRENT FLOW TO GROUND

The simplest power distribution system would supply 2 wires with a consistent voltage difference between them to each electrical outlet. Electrons could not flow from either wire to earth ground because it is not part of the circuit unless it contacts both wires simultaneously. Devices connected to these 2 conductors, known as line 1 and line 2, would form a complete circuit and draw current limited only by the supply capacity and the size of the wires carrying the current (**Fig. 28-11A**). A human coming in contact with only one of the conductors could be completely grounded and still have no current flow through his or her body because current can only leave line 1 if it has a path back to line 2. This is a convenient safety feature of isolated 2-wire systems.

> **BOX 28-4**
>
> **Applied Theory: Current Density and Electrosurgery**
>
> Monopolar electrosurgery is a great example of the engineering of current density. A pencil or cutting electrode with a small tip is used to focus radiofrequency current through a small area of tissue resulting in desiccation and/or coagulation. The same current must flow out of the patient's body through the return electrode but with no ill effects. This is accomplished by using a return electrode with a large surface area that disperses the current and decreases the current density to a safe level (**Fig. 28-10**).[12]

Unfortunately, 2-wire distribution systems are susceptible to the conductors being elevated to a high voltage relative to ground by a lightning strike, transformer failure, or a buildup of static electricity. Difficulty maintaining a reference intensifies as the distribution network grows in size and complexity. These drifting voltages may be detrimental or damaging to attached equipment and lead to the potential for large ground fault currents if one of the conductors becomes connected to ground, for example, a wire with damaged insulation in contact with a water pipe.

This limitation of 2-wire systems is commonly addressed by connecting one of the 2 conductors to ground to maintain a consistent reference to Earth and provide a path for fault currents to flow safely (**Fig. 28-11B**). The grounded wire is referred to as the *neutral wire* and the conductor maintained at an elevated voltage is referred to as the *hot wire*. This configuration works well as long as all devices and components function as designed and currents flow only within the designed circuits. The major drawback to a ground-referenced 2-wire system is that building plumbing, structure, and potential occupants represent possible return paths for current that normally would travel to ground down the neutral conductor.

An internal fault in a device that breaks the hot wire → device → neutral wire circuit leaves the high-voltage electrons in the hot wire looking for a means to flow to ground. If the hot wire is in contact with a metallic device case or supporting bracket, the next object to touch the high potential surface may become part of the ground fault current's path to ground. To protect users from providing a path to ground through their bodies, a third conductor was added to the power distribution system, the ground wire (**Fig. 28-11C**). The ground wire provides a very low-impedance path to ground for fault currents, presumably a path of lower impedance than through a person in contact with the device. Thus most of the current would pass through the ground wire rather than through someone in contact with the case and some other ground path. Although both the neutral and the ground wires are maintained at the same voltage (Earth), they serve separate functions. The neutral wire is intended to be the return path for current, and, under normal circumstances, the ground wire carries no current.

For small power distribution systems, such as a single operating room, drift associated with a 2-wire distribution system is manageable, and the benefits of avoiding reference to ground can be exploited. An isolation transformer can be used to convert the ground-referenced power in a hospital's distribution system into nonground-referenced power with the same differential voltage (**Fig. 28-12**). The 2 conductors are supplemented with a ground wire to maintain safety if there is a fault between one of the two isolated lines and ground. When this fault occurs, the isolated system diverts back to a conventional ground-referenced system. The intentionally decoupled, unreferenced, system

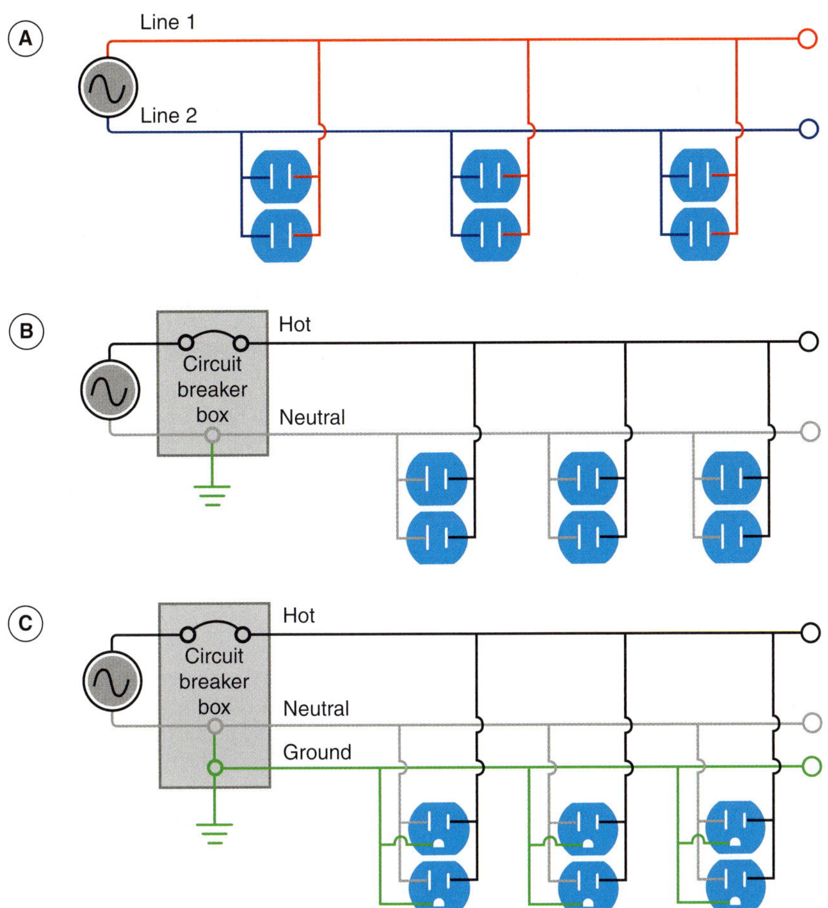

FIGURE 28-11. A. The simplest possible electrical distribution system providing no protection for over-current or lightning strikes. Neither line is referenced to ground. **B.** Ground-referenced power distribution with one of the power lines tied to earth ground at the breaker box. **C.** A 3-wire grounded power distribution system. Although both the neutral and ground wires are tied to earth ground, the neutral wire is intended to carry current during normal operation; the ground wire is only intended to carry current in a fault situation.

is known as line-isolated power. These are some of the benefits of line-isolated power:

1. **Reduced likelihood of arc/spark generation.** In a ground-referenced distribution system, charge buildup on a conductive surface may lead to a high enough potential to a grounded object (building infrastructure, person, etc) to create an arc/spark across the air gap separating the surface from ground. If flammable anesthetic agents or alcohol vapors are present, this could lead to an explosion or fire.
2. **Reduced risk of fault currents flowing through a human.** In an intact state, any current leaving line 1 must flow back into line 2, so for a human to become part of the current path, he or she must be touching both lines at the same time. This is true whether or not the human is grounded. This is especially useful in wet locations

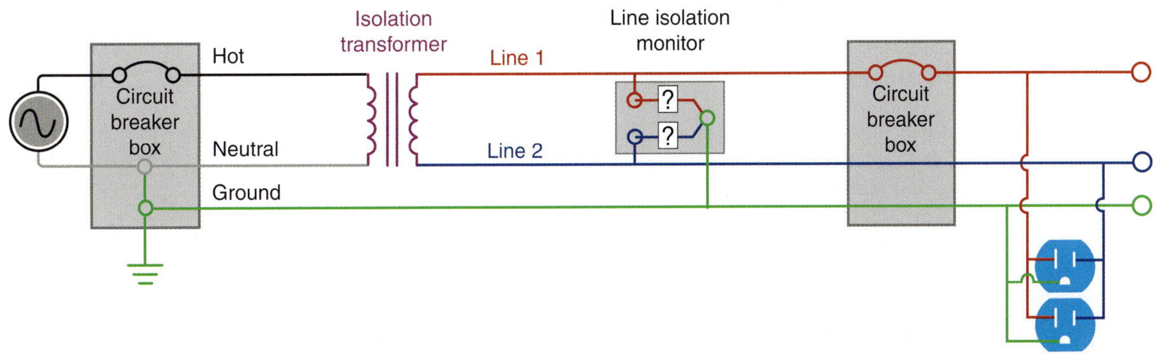

FIGURE 28-12. An isolated power distribution system. Because neither line is referenced to ground (no connection in the circuit breaker box on the isolated side), the lines are referred to as 1 and 2 rather than hot and neutral. It is important to note that the third ground wire is still used to keep equipment cases, and so on, at a safe potential. The line isolation monitor continuously determines the hazard current that would flow to ground should one of the conductors become grounded, converting the system to a traditional ground-referenced distribution.

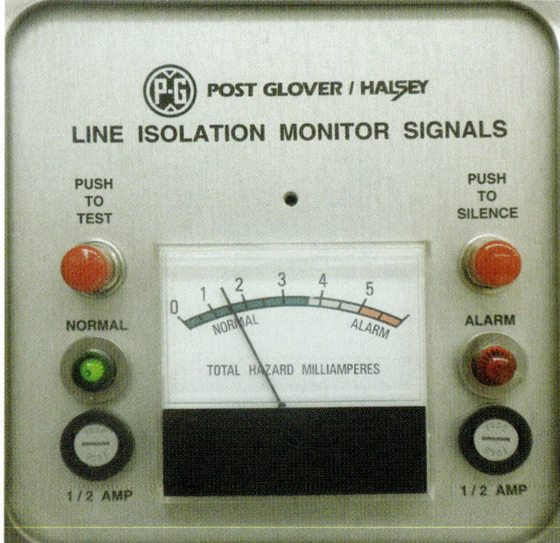

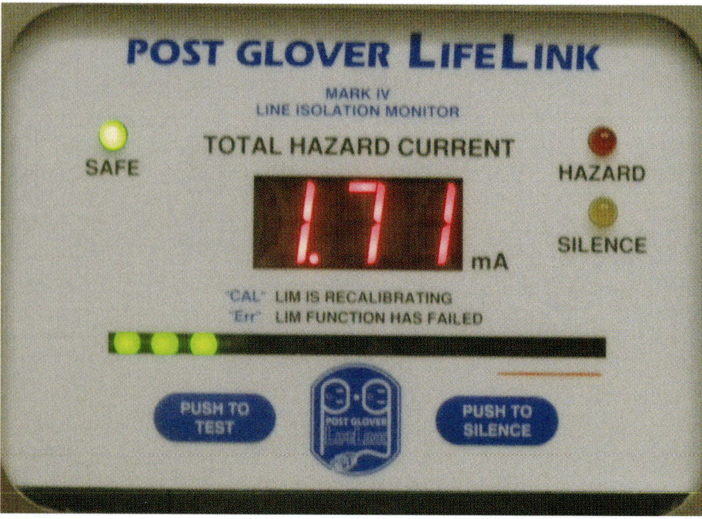

FIGURE 28-13. Examples of line isolation monitor panels: **A.** analog; **B.** digital. Most modern isolation monitors alarm when the potential hazard current reaches 5 mA. Because the line isolation monitor and other devices and wiring are electrically nonideal, they all contribute leakage current to the circuit and result in a nonzero line isolation monitor reading even when no devices are connected to the outlets.

where the presence of conductive fluids makes it much more likely occupants will become part of an electrical circuit to ground. A fault between one line and ground results in the return to standard, ground-referenced power distribution with a third wire still providing grounding of the instrument case. For an adverse event to occur, a second fault must be present.

Initially, the National Fire Protection Association (NFPA) required isolated power in operating rooms to reduce the risk of arc-initiated OR fires. The NFPA Standards for Healthcare Facilities required isolated power in all operating rooms until 1970 and the release of NFPA 56, which recognized differences between sites using flammable anesthetic agents and those without. As flammable agents were phased out in the United States, the main task of line-isolated systems turned to protecting OR occupants from ground fault currents. Isolated power is no longer an NFPA requirement for operating rooms unless they are designated as wet locations by the facility management. The freedom to designate an OR as a dry location has recently been questioned by patient safety advocates from the anesthesiology community.[13] Facilities choosing to include both isolated and nonisolated power in the same room must provide labels on each receptacle indicating whether or not the power source is isolated.[14]

Line-isolated power systems commonly contain a line isolation monitor, or LIM, which monitors the current that *could* flow if one of the 2 isolated lines became electrically connected to ground (**Fig. 28-13**). This potential leakage current is displayed prominently on the front of the line isolation panel within the isolated room. Each piece of equipment attached to the isolated system, including the built-in LIM, contributes to the cumulative potential leakage current. If the predicted leakage current rises to a set level (commonly 5 mA), the LIM sounds an audible alarm to indicate that a potentially unsafe state has been detected. It is important to note that a LIM alarm does not indicate that leakage current is actually flowing, but rather the potential for unsafe current to flow if an occupant came in contact with either line 1 or line 2. LIMs also have no automated mechanism for disconnecting power, which is convenient when critical monitoring or life support equipment is plugged into the distribution system. Operating room and ICU personnel should be familiar with the location of LIMs in their ORs and bed spaces and basic LIM troubleshooting procedures (**Fig. 28-14**).

CURRENT-LIMITING DEVICES

Conductors in a power distribution system are sized according to the expected current that will be carried. Passing too high of a current through a wire can result in resistive heating, insulation breakdown, and electrical fires. Because wires are hidden within the walls and ceilings of buildings, incremental damage would go unnoticed until a critical failure occurred. Unexpectedly high currents also pose risks to humans that, intentionally or unintentionally, become part of an electrical circuit.

One of the earliest and simplest approaches to over-current protection is the fuse. Fuses are current limiting devices, which are strategically placed within electrical circuits to protect segments of the circuit from drawing too much current either through a short circuit or extreme

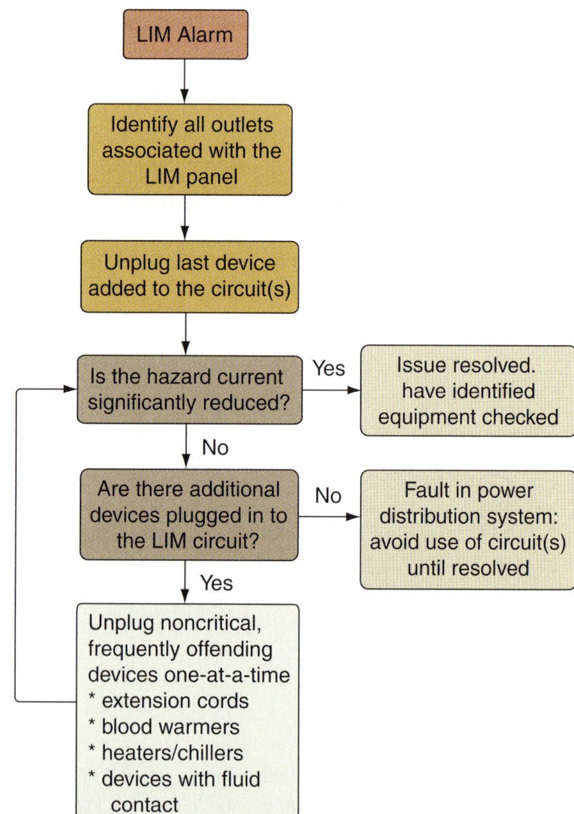

FIGURE 28-14. Line isolation monitor (LIM) troubleshooting flow diagram.

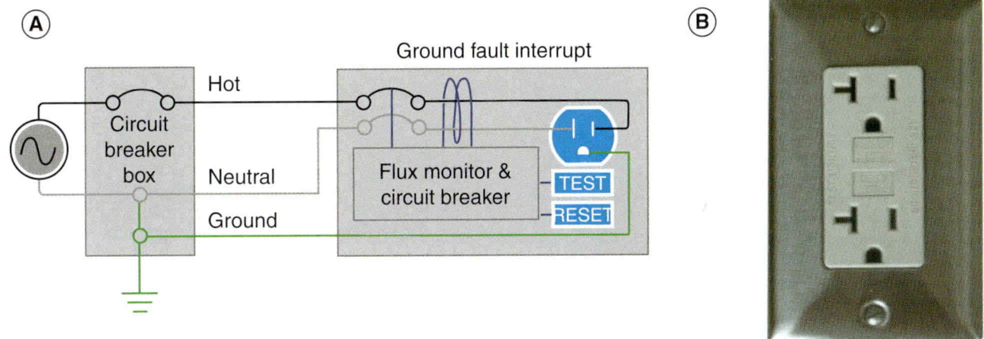

FIGURE 28-15. A. Schematic explanation of ground fault interrupt (GFI) technology. The outlet itself contains a net-current flux monitor and fast-acting breaker that can cut off the flow of current in response to unbalanced currents in the hot and neutral wires. A single GFI outlet may be wired with multiple regular outlets in series so that it monitors and breaks the flow of current to all. **B.** GFI outlet installed.

leakage to ground. Fuses contain a material that fails in a controlled manner at a known current, causing the circuit to open and breaking the path for current flow. Once a fuse has failed, it must be replaced for the circuit to resume function. Fuses respond quickly (within nanoseconds) to increasing currents, are relatively inexpensive, and incredibly reliable (even after years of sitting idle). Fuses are now uncommon in hospital infrastructures but can still be found in biomedical equipment.

Fuses require the inconvenience and cost of replacing a physical component to recover from a fault and therefore have been replaced in many applications with circuit breakers. Circuit breakers also create an opening in an electrical circuit once a specified current is reached, but in the case of a circuit breaker, the fault may be cleared by resetting the breaker via a physical switch or button. This is accomplished using a current-sensitive electromagnet or bimetallic strip. Circuit breakers are relatively slow to respond (on the order of milliseconds) and generally operate in the 5 to 100 A current range. They are common in hospital settings and, in many cases, operating rooms have dedicated electrical panels with a breaker for each electrical circuit in the room. Over-current protection in the form of circuit breakers is also standard in isolated-power systems and is included on the isolated side of the isolation transformer.

Each circuit breaker in a breaker box defines an electrical circuit in an OR or procedure room, and each circuit serves one or more electrical outlets. Outlets are commonly engraved or labeled with the name of the circuit to which they are connected. These names correspond to circuit breaker labels in the room's circuit breaker box. The number of devices that are connected to a given circuit is determined by adding the maximal current draw of each device (usually printed near the power cord connection on the device) and comparing it with the rating on the circuit's breaker (commonly 20 A). When working in an area without a dedicated circuit breaker box, such as a procedure room or physician's office, it can be helpful to determine the location of the corresponding breaker before the onset of any clinical or electrical complications.

Equipment that contains pumping, heating, and cooling features tends to have high current draws. Cardiopulmonary bypass pumps and other motor-driven devices often draw a surge of current on startup and then decrease their steady-state draw while running. For this reason it is important to consider not just the operational current draw, but also the peak current draw from each connected device. Outlets sharing a circuit breaker are often distributed over the walls of the room so that areas with high equipment concentration do not overwhelm any one circuit. The anesthesia machine and patient monitoring is often given its own dedicated circuit to ensure that no devices plugged in across the room can overwhelm a shared circuit and unexpectedly cut off power to the life support and monitoring equipment.

Circuit breakers and fuses provide minimal protection against small leakage currents (5-100 mA) that may pose a risk to patients with compromised skin barriers. A LIM is capable of monitoring the potential for these small currents but does not provide a means to open the circuit and avoid them. In the 1980s, a device called a ground fault interrupter (GFI) became common in commercial and residential buildings as a means of opening circuits in response to even small leakage currents. GFI devices rely on the fact that a conductor passing through the center of a coil of wire induces a current in the coil that is proportional to the magnitude and direction of the current flow. If 2 wires are placed within the same coil, then the net current in the coil is proportional to the sum of the directional currents in the 2 wires (**Fig. 28-15**). In a closed circuit, it would be expected that the same number of electrons flowing out through the hot wire would return through the neutral wire. If both wires are placed within the same loop, the net flux would be zero. If some electrons escape the circuit, say through a short to ground (possibly through a human body), the net flux becomes nonzero. When a GFI device senses a difference between outgoing and incoming currents greater than 20 mA, it reversibly breaks the circuit. In this regard, a GFI acts as a highly sensitive circuit breaker. Underwriters Laboratories (UL), a US government–backed standards and testing organization, requires that GFI devices respond within 25 milliseconds at a leakage current of 250 mA.

The drawback to using GFI devices in acute care areas is that they disconnect power to all devices attached to the affected circuit. This may include OR lighting, patient monitoring, or a patient ventilator. In many cases, disconnection of the circuit is not a viable option, and designers opt for line-isolated power that identifies potential leakage currents and requires 2 faults for an adverse event but places the responsibility for issue resolution on the provider.

EMERGENCY POWER

A complication of the increasing number of electrical and computerized devices in the OR is the increased dependence on a reliable, consistent power source. Equipment downtime can be minimized by supplementing the utility provider's power supply in a variety of ways, each with its own response time and capacity for load and duration of emergency support.

NFPA 99 calls for the installation of an emergency backup power system capable of sensing the absence of power from the utility provider and providing supplemental power within 10 seconds of service loss.[14] This is most often accomplished using large diesel or gasoline generators on the facility grounds. The less-than-for instantaneous response of emergency backup systems is directly associated with the startup time required for internal combustion generators. Generators are able to provide limited power for an extended period of time as long as generator fuel is available.

Facility generators are not sized to replace service to all powered devices but rather to power life safety equipment (alarms, exit signs, egress lighting, communication systems, etc) and selected critical equipment and procedure lighting. Receptacles attached to the emergency

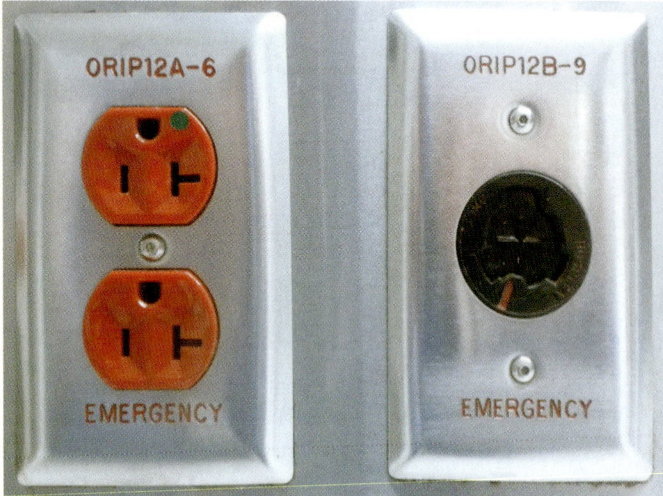

FIGURE 28-16. Emergency power outlets. Note the engraving on the faceplate with circuit identifiers that can be traced back to circuit breakers in the breaker box. The outlet on the right is a Legacy Twist-Lock, or HUBBELLOCK, outlet that prevents arcs during plug insertion and removal and accidental plug removal.

power system are color coded to indicate their special status. In many facilities the faces of receptacles connected to emergency power are colored red (**Fig. 28-16**). Patient monitoring equipment, balloon pumps, infusion pumps, and ventilators are often connected to the emergency power system. Nonessential items, such as personal computers and copy machines, should not be connected to red outlets if it can be avoided to conserve the limited capacity of the generators for critical needs.

For some critical equipment, like OR lighting and patient ventilators, the 10 seconds between loss of utility service and start of backup power can feel like a lifetime. One way to avoid this time delay is to supplement generator backup with a relatively fast-acting battery backup. Batteries have both a finite limit on power delivery and duration of emergency support. Fortunately, if the device is connected to the emergency power system, batteries only have to be capable of transitioning from utility-provided to facility-generated power (about 10 seconds). Most critical care devices, including anesthesia machines and ventilators, are designed to run for several minutes or more from internal batteries. High acuity fixed patient monitoring does not often have extended battery backup, but monitors designed for dual use (wall mounting and transport) often have the ability to monitor vital signs continuously during a transient or extended power outage. Operating and procedure room lighting often have battery backup in place. It is not required that the surgical lights themselves are on emergency power, only that there is sufficient lighting in the room to terminate a procedure safely in the event of an emergency.

Preparation for loss-of-power events includes the following:

- Keep a flashlight with working batteries in the drawer of every anesthesia machine. Change the batteries yearly as part of the anesthesia machine preventive maintenance.
- Know where to get battery-operated equipment in a critical situation. For example, paramedics may have a battery-powered suction device that can be borrowed to complete a case in the OR.
- Maintain the equipment and know-how to observe patient status without a patient monitor.
  - Manual noninvasive blood pressure cuff
  - Stethoscope
  - Lighting that allows for observation of skin color (no blue, red, or green flashlights)
- Know what to expect from your hospital infrastructure.
  - Approximate delays in generator startup
  - Plug equipment into the appropriate outlets
  - Will OR temperature and humidity be maintained?
- Understand how your equipment behaves when power is cut off.
  - Safely test loss-of-power behavior by connecting a patient simulator to the anesthesia machine and patient monitor and switching off the circuit breaker.
  - Does it have battery backup? How long is the battery expected to last?
  - Will the auxiliary oxygen source, or better yet ventilator, operate using only local compressed gas tanks?
  - Bypass pumps often have supplemental hand cranks, but operators may need to be relieved often to avoid exhaustion.
- Create and follow an institutional disaster plan.
  - Who will decide when it is time to evacuate the OR?
  - Where will patients be taken and how?
    - Will elevators be powered and hallways lit?

Much can be learned from simulated disasters and it has been recommended that facilities make the time to physically walk through disaster plans with all personnel.[15,16] The actual role playing of an event may lead to discoveries such as OR tables with casters that cannot clear a building expansion joint or balloon pumps and other crucial equipment that do not fit into elevators. The more prepared that clinicians and facilities are for emergencies, the better the outcome when a real situation arises.

DEVICE SAFETY

Like hospital infrastructure, medical devices play an important role in preventing electricity-related injuries. Medical devices are generally designed to be single-fault safe, meaning that they require 2 faults to present a hazard to the patient or operator. For example, accidentally dropping a device may break an internal wire and expose the metal device case to an electrified wire. Without additional safety features, this single fault would cause the device to pose a risk to patients, visitors, and users. If the device has a second safety feature such as a built-in fuse or a grounded case, the user will not be at risk until a second fault occurs.

LEAKAGE CURRENT

Leakage current is impossible to avoid in electronic devices but needs to be managed to protect patients at risk for microshock (see section on human body thresholds). Unfortunately, the functionality of even the best engineered circuits can be modified by faulty components, accumulated dust, and/or user error that contribute to their overall leakage current. Equipment preventive maintenance usually includes verification that device and power cord leakage current is within the manufacturer's limits when tested in a variety of states (OFF/ON, unenergized, etc).

INTERFERENCE

Biopotentials captured by patient monitoring devices are low-magnitude signals that can be masked or altered by electrical noise. In some cases, this noise will be minor and/or easily identified, but in others, the source of the noise may be difficult to pinpoint and eliminate.

Typical Sources of Artifact Coupling of one signal to another is the most common cause of artifact in medical devices. The signal coupling to the biologic signal may be another biologic signal (respiration modulation of ECG) or a device in proximity to the patient (fluorescent lighting, electrosurgical unit, etc). There are at least 3 types of signal measurement coupling:

1. **Capacitive coupling:** This type of noise occurs from the noncontact coupling of AC signals from 1 conductor to another. Capacitive coupling is more prevalent at higher frequencies, and electrosurgery units are notorious for generating artifact on ECG, temperature, and other patient signals.
2. **Resistive coupling:** This type of coupling requires direct contact of 2 signal sources or transmission wires. Resistive coupling occurs through imperfect or damaged wire insulation.

3. **Inductive coupling:** When wire coils unintentionally share a common core, even if it is air, inductive coupling may occur. This type of coupling is rare and cannot be eliminated through shielding of wires.

Motion is also a possible source of artifact. It is uncommon in the anesthetized patient but can occur wherever electrodes are used to obtain a signal. Motion artifact results from the alteration of the electrode/skin electrochemical equilibrium. This equilibrium is a consequence of the use of polarizing electrodes.

Ways to minimize artifact include the following:

- Whenever possible, amplify and or process signals in close proximity to the patient (source). When amplification is performed 5 to 10 ft away at the medical device, noise picked up on the cable is amplified with the signal.
- When artifact is present and an older cable is being used, consider replacing the cable with one that has shielding that is known to be intact.
- Verify that electrical connections are intact all the way from the patient electrodes (which commonly dry out) to the medical device.
- Regularly inspect equipment in accordance with a hospital equipment management program.
- It can be difficult to identify artifact from postprocessed parameters such as heart rate. Whenever possible, verify data by directly observing the corresponding waveform.

EQUIPMENT MANAGEMENT

The goal of an equipment management program is, first and foremost, to ensure the safety of patients, families, and staff who may come in contact with medical equipment. The US Centers for Medicare and Medicaid Services (CMS) specifies in its conditions for participation that "Facilities, supplies, and equipment must be maintained to ensure an acceptable level of safety and quality."[17] Although this statute is relatively vague, it is often interpreted more specifically by hospital accreditation boards such as the Joint Commission.[18] Hospital equipment management programs may be overseen by a dedicated clinical engineering department or an outside contractor, but in either case patient safety remains the responsibility of the health care institution.

The core of an equipment management program is the documented inspection of medical equipment. Inspection first occurs at initial purchase, lease/rental, or loan and should continue at regular intervals as long as the device remains in service. Although commonly overlooked, this incoming and regular inspection must also apply to trial devices, even if they have been cleared by the Food and Drug Administration (FDA). Inspection criteria generally begin with the manufacturer recommendations but should be modified by hospital experience and the experience and recommendations of independent knowledge bases such as the FDA and ECRI institute. These modifications may include the addition or subtraction of test procedures or alteration of the test frequency. Equipment is categorized based on the likelihood of failure, the possible outcome of a failure, and the ability to prevent failures. For example, the failure of a life-supporting ICU ventilator is unusual but would have serious implications for patient care and may be preventable if seals are routinely replaced and the internal electronics are kept dust free.

Regular inspections are often referred to as preventive maintenance (PM), and medical devices often carry stickers with unique ID numbers (serial numbers may not be unique across all devices) and an indication of when they are due for inspection. Health care providers should contact their local clinical or biomedical engineering department if they encounter a device that is overdue for inspection. Clinical engineering departments are often challenged to locate mobile devices for inspection and will appreciate any help from their clinical partners.

In addition to a regular PM process, anesthesia machines should be subjected to a daily checkout before use. Clinicians maintain the overall responsibility for completing this checkout and verifying function, although in some sites the clinical engineering or anesthesia technicians assist with machine checkouts. Many guidelines have been published for machine checkout,[12] and some modern machines contain software that leads users through a step-by-step machine checkout procedure before a normal case can be started.

FIRE SAFETY

INCIDENCE AND REPORTING

Operating room fires are infrequent occurrences with the potential to cause serious harm to the anesthetized patient and operating staff. The incidence of OR fire is difficult to gauge because few countries have an effective central-reporting agency, and it is generally believed that compliance with fire reporting, even within facilities, is low. Estimates of fire incidence in the United States have ranged from 20 in 1997[19] to 650 fires per year in 2009.[20] It is likely that this is a conservative estimate. Most fires are minor or quickly extinguished by OR staff and cause no permanent harm to the patient. At a minimum, even minor events should be reported within an organization. Only through consistent and thorough reporting can trends be observed and systematic improvements in fire prevention made.

It is also important for providers to recognize that even with the removal of flammable anesthetic agents in the United States, the rate of OR fire appears to have remained relatively steady.[21] This is due to a shift in fire caused from minor ignition sources in highly flammable environments to high-powered ignition sources in oxygen-enriched environments. Three major contributing factors are as follows:

1. **Increased use of electrosurgical units and lasers.** High-powered surgical devices are capable of igniting less reactive and obvious fuel sources.
2. **A shift toward minimally invasive procedures under conscious sedation.** These procedures often use masks and nasal cannula to deliver supplemental oxygen and monitor expired CO_2. Inefficiency in these delivery mechanisms often leads to oxygen enrichment of the surgical environment.
3. **Ubiquity of pulse oximetry.** Continuous measurement of oxygenation encourages the use of high supplemental oxygen concentrations.

CAUSES AND PREVENTION OF SURGICAL FIRES

Fire requires fuel, an oxidizer, and a source of ignition, all of which are readily available in the surgical environment (**Table 28-2**). Fuel sources and oxygen are necessary to provide anesthetics, and ignition sources are necessary for modern surgical techniques, but the interaction of these necessary components may be systematically managed to reduce the risk of fire. This is primarily performed through the elimination of unnecessary risks and separation of necessary fire elements over space and/or time.[55]

Fuel Historically, the largest liability in terms of operating room fires was the highly flammable agents, such as diethyl ether, used to anesthetize patients. These agents made the OR environment sensitive to

TABLE 28-2 Current and Past Fuel, Oxidizer, and Ignition Sources in Anesthetizing Locations

Fuel	Plastics, drapes, flammable anesthetics (fluroxene, cyclopropane, divinyl ether, diethyl ether, ethyl chloride), patient hair, prep solutions containing alcohol, abdominal gas, gauze, sponges, endotracheal tubes, and other supplies
Oxidizer	Oxygen, nitrous oxide
Igniter	Electrical arc, laser, electrosurgery, heated probes, high-intensity light sources, drills and burrs, static electricity

even minor ignition sources such as arcs produced by static electricity buildup. A myriad of safety systems were put in place to avoid sparks, including Twist-Lock (HUBBELLOCK) electrical outlets and plugs, conductive flooring (to avoid static buildup), and line-isolated power.[14] Although flammable anesthetic agents were phased out in the United States around 1985, much of this protective infrastructure remains in place due to either cost of removal (conductive flooring) or the presence of alternative benefits (twist-lock plugs and line-isolated power). It is possible that anesthesia providers traveling to developing countries may still encounter flammable anesthetic agents. The NFPA *Health Care Facilities Handbook* contains an appendix that describes some of the challenges and safety measures associated with these agents.

More recently, high alcohol-content (70% alcohol) surgical site preparation agents have been identified as unnecessary potential fuel sources. The danger surrounding these products comes from inadequate drying time and evaporation of the alcohol diluents. If prep solution is allowed to pool on or under drapes, flammable vapors will continue to be released and possibly trapped by drapes for an extended period of time. The American Society of Anesthesiologists has suggested that all prep solutions should be completely dry before draping to avoid the accumulation of flammable vapors.[22] These items are being steadily removed from use for primary surgical site preparation but in some cases maintained for anesthesia use such as line insertion preparation, regional anesthesia, and pain management procedures. These procedures are generally distant from ignition sources, such as electrosurgery devices and lasers, in both time and distance. If these prep agents are removed from use, they may be replaced with versions containing the same active ingredient, such as 2% chlorhexidine, but lower or no alcohol content.

Published surgical fire case studies often include dry drapes, gauze, and/or sponges in the list of involved fuels. Gauze and/or sponges may be soaked with saline to increase fire resistance, but they must be checked regularly throughout procedures to avoid drying out. Other supplies such as endotracheal tubes, nasal cannula, and nasopharyngeal airways can also contribute to surgical fires. The patient may also be a source of fuel with reports of ignition of body hair, lanugo, gastrointestinal gases (mainly methane), and tissue. The bowel should be evacuated before entry or risk of accidental entry with an electrosurgery unit or laser. Even more preferential is the use of cold cutting devices (scalpels, harmonic scalpels) whenever flammable gas, vapor, or high oxygen concentration may be present including emergency tracheal surgery and incision in the presence of a recently applied alcohol-based containing prep solution.[22] The risk of body hair ignition can be minimized by avoiding contact with alcohol-containing prep solutions and coating with water-based lubricants to increase fire resistance.

Oxidizer Oxygen does not burn in a fire but rather supports combustion of fuel sources by providing a needed element of the exothermic oxidation reaction. Room air contains about 78% inert nitrogen and about 21% oxygen. Any supplemental oxygen supply with more than 21% oxygen provided to the patient creates an oxygen-enriched local environment. Given the same fuel and ignition sources, increasing the oxygen content of the atmosphere increases the risk of fire and rate of fire growth.[22,23] Unlike ignition and fuel sources, the management of oxygen enrichment is entirely under the control of the anesthesia team. The American Society of Anesthesiologists recommends that special attention be paid to this issue in all anesthesiology-directed fire prevention training.[22]

During general anesthesia, the oxygen-enriched environment is restricted to the breathing circuit, patient's airway, and lungs. This environment is only exposed to ignition sources through accidental access to one of these compartments. Leaks in an airway device such as an endotracheal tube or laryngeal mask airway may create a locally oxygen-enriched environment near the site of neck or throat surgery. Thoracic surgery may open the lung compartment intentionally or unintentionally, spilling oxygen into the surgical field.

During monitored anesthesia care (MAC) cases, where supplemental oxygen is provided through loose-fitting masks or nasal cannulae, an oxygen-enriched environment may be created around the patient's face, especially if drapes form a tent around the patient's head or face.[21] Several methods for reducing this risk have been proposed, including the following:

1. Ceasing supplemental oxygen supply with enough time for oxygen dispersion before each use of the electrosurgery unit. This solution limits the possible depth of anesthesia and requires flawless communication between the surgeon and anesthesia team.
2. Modification of the anesthesia machine and/or supply line to allow for delivery of supplemental gas with less than 100% oxygen concentration.[24] Again, this solution may limit the possible depth of anesthesia and requires specially configured equipment.
3. Use of waste anesthesia gas suction to evacuate the excess oxygen from the surrounding area or beneath the drapes.[25] For this approach the waste anesthesia gas vacuum must be used rather than the surgical vacuum due to limitations on the oxygen capacity of surgical vacuum systems (see section on air quality).
4. Administration of supplemental oxygen directly to the nasopharynx through a nasopharyngeal airway rather than to the nostrils using nasal cannula.[26] This method allows for deeper anesthetics while greatly reducing the oxygen content around the patient's face.

At elevated temperatures above about 650°C (candles burn at about 750°C), nitrous oxide decomposes into nitrogen and oxygen. Once started, the decomposition is exothermic and can be self-sustaining. As nitrous oxide (N_2O) decomposes, it contributes nitrogen (62% by weight) and oxygen (38% by weight) to the immediate atmosphere, which results in an oxygen-enriched environment.[27] For this reason, N_2O should be treated as a fire accelerant and avoided whenever possible in cases where ignition sources are close to the airway such as head and neck procedures.[22]

Ignition Source Electrosurgery and lasers are currently the 2 most common initiators of OR fire with the relative percentage of each type of fire varying with surgical specialty and prevalence of laser use. In head and neck surgery the estimated ignition rates are 59% and 32% for electrosurgery and lasers, respectively.[28] In an evaluation of closed claims related to MAC cases, electrosurgery ignited all 20 intraoperative fires.[29] Estimates for surgery in general are 70% electrosurgery and 10% laser ignition.[30] Both techniques represent effective ignition sources, and the higher number of electrosurgery events is probably an indicator of the relative ubiquity of this device. Other possible ignition sources include high-power fiberoptic light sources, damaged electrical equipment or cords, drills, burrs, and other equipment that produce heat during use.[22]

To decrease the risk of fire when using electrosurgery, the probe tip should be kept as clean as possible and the probe should be holstered when not in use. When lasers are used in the head or neck area, laser-resistant endotracheal tubes should be used to prevent airway fires. These specialty tubes often include a reflective coating and/or an outer sheath that can be soaked with saline to reduce flammability. Endotracheal tube cuffs should be inflated with colored saline rather than air to reduce the oxidizer content and provide a visual indication of accidental cuff puncture.[22]

If a laser or electrosurgery unit must be used to enter an oxygen-enriched or flammable gas-containing compartment, the surgeon should communicate in advance so that the anesthesia team can temporarily reduce oxygenation if possible. The convenience of hand and foot controls for lasers and electrosurgery devices leads to an increased likelihood of accidental activation. Electrosurgery pencils, lasers, and even fiberoptic light source cables should be holstered or otherwise managed when not in use.

When sevoflurane vapor is passed through desiccated, high alkali content, CO_2 absorbent, the reaction may produce high heat (in excess of 200°C after 100 minutes at 1.5 MAC), and even flames.[56] Although sevoflurane/absorbent fires have been reported, they are believed to be extremely rare. No such fires have been reported using desflurane or isoflurane, which reach a maximum absorbent temperature of about 100°C at 30 and 75 minutes of 1.5 MAC delivery, respectively. Premium absorbents with decreased alkali content may reduce the (already low) risk of sevoflurane fire. Avoidance of absorbent desiccation by shutting off fresh gas flow when not in use and replacing canisters on infrequently used machines just before use will also greatly reduce the risk of absorbent fire.

MANAGEMENT OF OPERATING ROOM FIRE

An OR fire may be recognized by any member of the operational team by an unusual noise (popping sounds, etc), odor, feeling of warmth, or visual confirmation of smoke and/or flame. When a fire is suspected, the surgical procedure should pause immediately until the fire is extinguished or the possibility of fire is ruled out, even if the fire is not initially near the patient.

OR fires can be categorized into 3 increasingly specific types based on the required response: fires in the operating suite, fires on or in the patient, and airway fires. The American Society of Anesthesiologists has published recommended procedures for managing all types of surgical fires,[22] and many of the procedures are closely mirrored by publications for the surgeon audience.[30]

FIRES DURING ANESTHETICS

Surgical fires are generally small events that begin in the immediate vicinity of the patient and are extinguished quickly by the operating staff without a need for escalation. Modern anesthetizing locations have many systems in place that can help with the management of larger scale fires, including the following devices:

- **Fire extinguishers.** Fire extinguishers may contain different fire suppressants for different types of fires.[12] CO_2 extinguishers are common in health care facilities because they may be used for household, flammable liquid, and electrical fires. CO_2 extinguishers leave no residue and may be used directly on expensive medical equipment or even patients.
- **Sprinklers in the OR.** Operating rooms are required to have sprinkler systems for fire suppression.[14] These systems feed central alarms but are usually locally activated by heat at the sprinkler head level (as opposed to the whole room being activated). Most surgical teams are never aware of sprinklers in the OR due to the low heat generated by surgical fires and in testimony to the rapid response of surgical teams to intraoperative fires.
- **Medical gas zone valves.** Medical gas zone valves provide an accessible means to shut off pipeline gases to a room or zone for construction or emergency purposes. Providers should know where to locate, how to operate, and the scope of these valves (**Fig. 28-17**).
- **Compartmentalized construction.** Unlike other high-occupancy facilities such as schools, arenas, and hotels, health care facilities cannot be expected to protect occupants through evacuation.[14] As such, they are constructed as a grouping of individual compartments separated by fire-resistant barriers, sealed walls, and fire doors (**Fig. 28-18**).

In the event of a fire in the OR suite, policies and procedures laid out by the health care facility should be followed. In general, fires should be extinguished as soon as possible by smothering or patting out the source when directly visible and still small. If this is not immediately successful, CO_2 fire extinguishers should be used to control and extinguish the fire. If the fire still persists, the OR team should activate the central fire alarm and make a decision about the relative risks associated with continuing to fight the fire or moving the patient. If the patient can be evacuated, all staff should leave the room with the patient, shut the door, and deactivate the medical gas supply using applicable zone valves. Wet blankets or towels may be used to prevent smoke from affecting other operating suites.

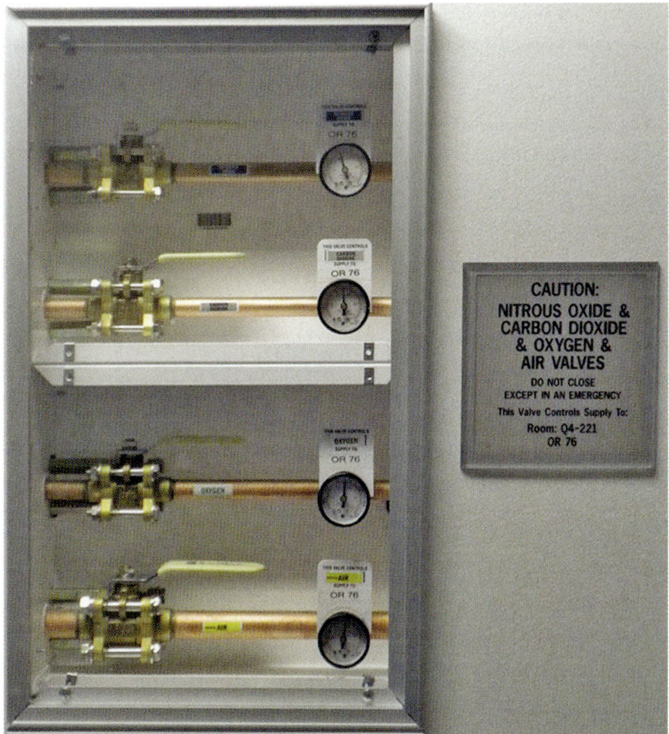

FIGURE 28-17. Medical gas zone valves located in the exterior corridor just outside of an operating room (OR). The zone valves are clearly labeled as to what areas they control. Zone valves may be used to cut off the flow of oxidizer if an OR fire grows out of control and also allow for construction/renovation of an OR without shutting down service to a whole building.

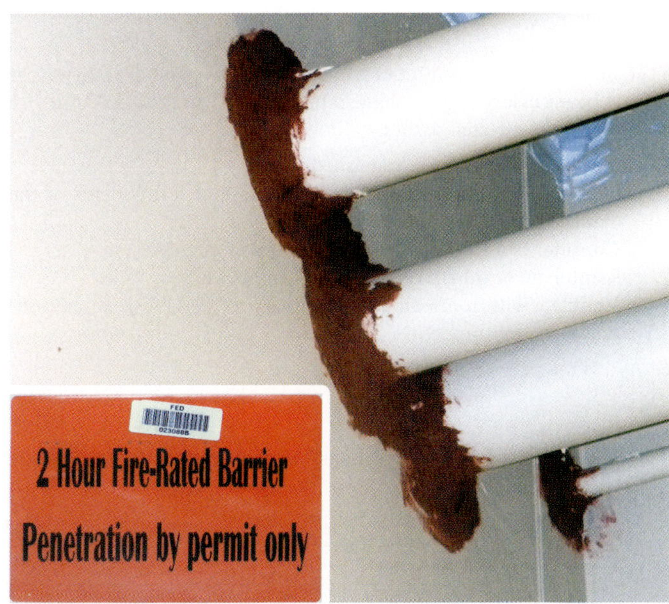

FIGURE 28-18. Rated fire barrier with wall notification. Compartmentalized construction using fire barriers is common in hospitals where mass evacuation is not always a feasible fire response. The red putty surrounding the plumbing that passes through the barrier is known as "fire-stop." Any penetration of the fire barrier must be appropriately sealed to prevent the flow of smoke or heat between compartments.

When anesthetics are being performed outside of the OR, there will likely be a different infrastructure available. Zone valves should still be present but may serve multiple beds, bays, or units. The anesthesia team should inquire as to the location and scope of zone valves in remote areas. Fire extinguishers may not be present in every room or may not be the type of fire extinguishers that can be used directly on a patient (CO_2). Again, it is the anesthesia team's responsibility to check equipment ahead of time and verify that it meets the needs and is functional.

FIRE ON OR IN THE PATIENT

If the fire is on the patient, or inside the patient's body or surgical wound:

1. Immediately stop the flow of airway gases to reduce oxidizer availability. Disconnection of the breathing circuit at the anesthesia machine is a simple way to accomplish this.
2. Extinguish existing flames by pouring saline on top or manually patting out with wet sponges or drapes.
   a. If the fire cannot be put out with saline, use a CO_2 fire extinguisher to suppress the fire by eliminating oxygen (CO_2 extinguishers may be used directly on patients).
3. Remove all possible fuel from the patient (drapes, sponges, etc).
4. Continue to ventilate with room air until it is safe and necessary to recreate an oxygen-enriched environment.
5. Assess the patient.

AIRWAY FIRE

Airway fires are associated with significant morbidity due to the potential for permanent lung damage. Once the lumen of an endotracheal tube is on fire in an oxygen-enriched environment, it will act as a flamethrower spouting flames down into the lungs with every breath. When an airway fire has been identified:

1. Discontinue use of electrosurgery or lasers (remove ignition potential).
2. Disconnect the breathing equipment from the anesthesia machine or supplemental oxygen source (remove O_2).
3. Quickly but carefully remove the endotracheal tube from the patient. Douse the tube in water or saline to extinguish any flames or embers.
4. If smoke or flame continues from the surgical wound or airway, it may be necessary to pour saline into the airway to extinguish the fire and cool the affected tissues.
5. Once the fire has been extinguished:
   a. Examine the endotracheal tube for signs that components of the damaged tube may remain in the airway.
   b. Consider bronchoscopy to evaluate airway damage.
   c. Reintubate or otherwise secure the patient's airway.
   d. Ventilate with room air until necessary to reestablish an oxygen-enriched environment.
6. Assess the patient.

OCCUPATIONAL SAFETY

AIR QUALITY

Heating, Ventilating, Air Conditioning Systems The American Institute of Architects (AIA) guidelines for OR design specify that the air handling system in an operating room should provide 15 to 21 full exchanges of room air every hour with at least 3 of these exchanges infusing filtered outside air.[32] Modern heating, ventilating, air conditioning (HVAC) systems recirculate air rather than bringing fresh air in each cycle, to increase efficiency in temperature and humidity management. Recirculated air is passed through a high-efficiency particulate air filter to remove contaminants. Air generally enters the room from the middle of the ceiling and is returned through wall ducts located near the floor to control the flow of dust particulates and potential contaminants. These design guidelines are intended to facilitate the maintenance of a sterile surgical field, remove toxic fumes produced by electrosurgery and other sources, and clear escaped anesthetic agent from the room.

Electrosurgical and laser cutting and coagulation of tissue result in a noxious-smelling, mutagenic smoke plume. The National Institute for Occupational Safety and Health (NIOSH) and the Association of Perioperative Registered Nurses recommend the use of supplemental suction to remove surgical smoke from the operating room.[33] If electrosurgery devices are used in remote anesthetizing locations, it may be necessary to have a portable suction source available to collect surgical smoke.

ANESTHETIC AGENT EXPOSURE

Much attention has been given to the possible link between occupational exposure to trace inhalational anesthetic agents and spontaneous abortion, vitamin B_{12} metabolism, and other health hazards.[34] The American Society of Anesthesiologists, among others, believes that the evidence remains inconclusive, but that even in the presence of inconclusive evidence, it makes sense to take reasonable measures to limit the exposure of surgical staff to N_2O and other agents.[35] The Occupational Safety and Health Administration (OSHA) has recommended maximum exposure levels, but no levels are known to be safe (**Table 28-3**).[36]

- When filling vaporizers:
  - Use a well-ventilated area
  - Minimize spillage
  - Clean up spills promptly
- Minimize contact with agent when pregnant or trying to conceive.
- Use sealed airway equipment such as cuffed endotracheal tubes and laryngeal mask airway devices whenever appropriate and possible.
- Check equipment daily for leaks, damaged hoses, etc.
- Use active waste anesthesia gas scavenging systems.

Anesthesia gas scavenging systems may either passively or actively exhaust gases to the outside atmosphere. Passive systems are more common in old or renovated construction where the addition of wall gas

TABLE 28-3 Guidelines for Maximal Exposure to Trace Anesthetic Agents From Some Countries With Defined Standards[53]

Volatile Anesthetic Agent	US/NIOSH Limit (ppm)	United Kingdom Limit (ppm)	Netherlands Limit (ppm)	Italy, Norway, Sweden, Denmark Limit (ppm)
Nitrous oxide	25	100	25	100
Halogenated volatile agents	2 (0.5 when used with nitrous oxide)	N/A	N/A	N/A
Enflurane, isoflurane	N/A	50	N/A	N/A
Halothane	N/A	10	N/A	N/A

All values represent maximal time-weighted averages over an 8-hour period except for the US limit for halogenated agents, which is based on a 1-hour sampling period.

outlets would be prohibitively expensive. In a passive system, the waste gas line from the anesthesia machine or breathing circuit is connected to the return side of the HVAC system. The slight positive pressure in the waste gas hose causes its contents to flow into the return air duct and away from the operating or procedure room. Passive systems may also use dedicated exhaust fans to slowly draw waste gas out of a dedicated duct. To avoid recontamination of the surgical area or another area of the hospital with inhalational anesthetic, passive scavenging cannot be used with a recirculating HVAC system.[37]

Both medical vacuum and active waste anesthetic gas disposal (WAGD or sometimes labeled EVAC) systems provide pump-generated suction at anesthetizing locations. Medical vacuum is readily available at most high-acuity bed spaces, making it an attractive alternative for anesthesia gas scavenging where WAGD connections are not present. The NFPA permits the use of medical vacuum plumbing and pumps for WAGD disposal if the plumbing is sized to accommodate the additional flow from the anesthesia equipment and the pumps are of a variety known as "O_2 assured."[14] O_2-assured pumps do not contain lubricating oil that may become saturated with oxygen when oxygen-enriched gas mixtures are moved through the pump. Pumps that are not O_2 assured run the risk of fire or explosion as internal heat builds around fuel (pump lubricant) and oxygen. These fires are rare but have been reported.[38] National or local standards may require completely separate systems (outlets, plumbing, and pumps) for WAGD and surgical vacuum. For example, European and International Organization for Standardization (ISO) standards mandate separate plumbing and pump systems for WAGD and surgical vacuum, limiting the ability to take inhalational anesthetics to areas of the hospital with no dedicated WAGD connections (EN 737-2, ISO 9170).

The postanesthesia care unit (PACU) is seldom equipped for waste gas scavenging on postsurgical patients, although patients may continue to outgas anesthetic agent well after the surgery. HVAC circulation of air within the PACU may help dissipate trace volatile anesthetics. The AIA requires 6 exchanges of PACU room air per hour, 2 of which should be fresh outside air.[32] Even with this management of air flow, studies have detected trace amounts of N_2O and halogenated agents on the breath of PACU nursing staff.[34]

RADIATION

Interventional radiology, endovascular surgery, cardiac catheterization, and pain management all present opportunities for anesthesia staff to be exposed to ionizing radiation, with cardiac catheterization often leading to the highest exposure of these 3.[39] Exposure to ionizing radiation may cause changes in the provider's body by directly damaging cells or leading to cumulative mutations, DNA damage, and associated long-term changes in cell function and reproduction.[40]

The SI unit for radiation exposure is the sievert (1 Sv = 1 J/kg), but it is still often expressed in the historical units of roentgen equivalent human (1 rem = 0.01 Sv). The average human is exposed to about 3 to 3.6 mSv of unavoidable background radiation annually.[41,42] Of this total, about 55% is due to naturally occurring radon gas and about 15% is due to intentional medical exposure. Anesthesia providers who work around x-ray equipment experience an additional occupational exposure that is regulated in the United States by OSHA (**Table 28-4**).[43] As a point of reference, the typical chest computed tomography (CT) scan delivers about 8 mSv to the patient. Radiation exposure of the anesthesia care team is modified by a number of factors, including the following:

- **Source magnitude.** The source magnitude is often manipulated by the surgical and imaging team.
- **Duration.** Fluoroscopy and CT represent significantly higher radiation exposure than traditional 2-dimensional radiographs because they both require the continuous activation of the x-ray source over an extended period. The cancer-inducing and mutagenic effects of radiation are cumulative over not just a case, but a lifetime.
- **Distance.** Radiation levels are proportional to the inverse of the distance from the source squared ($1/d^2$). Doubling the distance between the provider and the source decreases the magnitude of the exposure by a factor of 4. Patient care needs often dictate the maximum distance of the anesthesia provider.
- **Barrier use.** When proximity to the source cannot be avoided, as is the case in many anesthetics, anesthesia providers may protect themselves using radiation-shielding barriers. Whenever present in an imaging suite, staff should wear protective lead vests, aprons, and thyroid guards. Protective equipment should also be available for support staff such as anesthesia technicians and clinical engineers who may need to enter the room briefly during a case. Additional portable barriers such as portable lead-impregnated panels may be positioned to provide extra protection for anesthesia staff standing at the anesthesia machine or monitoring equipment. It is the responsibility of the anesthesia staff to take full advantage of barrier protection because they have little control over the other elements of exposure.

These modifiers also apply to patient exposure and should be exploited to minimize procedural radiation, especially in pain management practice where the anesthesiology staff may have more control over the imaging decisions.[42]

TABLE 28-4 US Occupational Safety and Health Administration Maximums for Radiation Exposure in the General Public and Workers With Regular Exposure to Radiation at Work[54]

	Maximum General Public Exposure (mSv/y)	Occupational Exposure (mSv/y)
Lens of eye	15	150
Skin	50	500
Hands and feet	N/A	500

CHEMOTHERAPEUTICS

Anesthesiologists are often called on to provide sedation for intravenous chemotherapy in children and are more and more frequently getting involved in surgical procedures involving cytotoxic agents such as hyperthermic intraoperative intraperitoneal chemotherapy (HIPEC or HIIC). Although physical contact between the anesthesia team and the chemotherapeutic agent is rare, it is important that anesthesia providers are aware of the unique risks posed by these agents and how to manage them. Chemotherapeutic agents may cause irritation of the skin, decreased fertility, spontaneous abortion, congenital malformations, leukemia, and other cancers.[44] The long-term effects of repeated exposures are currently unknown, but studies have demonstrated that when proper precautions are taken, no detectable exposure occurs.[45]

HIPEC and other intraoperative procedures have the goal of maximum effectiveness in a short period of time and thus use the strongest antineoplastic agents available at elevated temperatures to increase their activity. For example, mitomycin C is 10 to 15 times as cytotoxic when its temperature is raised from 37°C to 43°C.[46] The surgical team can be at risk for exposure to both liquid and vapor forms of the agent. Exposure to aerosolized chemotherapeutic agents should be minimized by covering the open abdomen, leaving only enough access for the surgeon to manipulate the viscera during the mitomycin C soak. All operating personnel should wear appropriate personal protective equipment including protective eyewear and/or facemasks, N-95 masks, impermeable gowns, and double gloves. Masks should be changed every 2 hours and outer gloves exchanged every 30 minutes or whenever there is a possibility that they have come into contact with the chemotherapeutic agent.[47] All used protective equipment should be discarded in biohazard receptacles. With these safety mechanisms in place, studies have shown that there is no detectable exposure of the surgical team to cytotoxic agents.[45] Even with low-risk, pregnant, or breast-feeding women and staff with compromised immune systems should be considered for alternative duty.

The risk of staff exposure is elevated with the necessity of sharing operating rooms and equipment between HIPEC procedures and general surgery procedures. After every case involving cytotoxic agents, the equipment and rooms must be thoroughly cleaned to allow for a return to lower vigilance. Antibacterial agents should not be used in cleanup because they may react with cytotoxic agents; 70% isopropyl alcohol is recommended for cleaning of any equipment that may be contaminated with chemotherapeutic agents.[46]

REGULATORY BODIES

This section briefly describes the structure of bodies regulating environmental safety, their jurisdiction or coverage, and their source of influence on health care organizations. Many of these bodies reference each other or, even more frustratingly, contradict one another. In the case of a contradiction, the more stringent guideline should be followed whenever possible.

It should also be noted that although guidelines are often static for a number of years, it is possible for the *interpretation* of a guideline to change substantially throughout its active life. In addition to a basic understanding of regulation, constant awareness of code alterations and interpretations is important for the maintenance of compliance and safety.

US DEPARTMENT OF HEALTH AND HUMAN SERVICES

The Department of Health and Human Services (HHS) is the branch of the US government with primary responsibility for the health and well-being of its citizens. HHS includes several components well known to health care professionals including the Centers for Medicare and Medicaid Services (CMS), the Food and Drug Administration (FDA), and the National Institutes of Health (NIH) (**Fig. 28-19**). HHS is responsible for the implementation of laws protecting patient rights such as the Health Insurance Portability and Accountability Act (HIPAA) privacy policy and for the prevention and management of infectious disease through the Centers for Disease Control and Prevention (CDC). The power of HHS extends outside US borders through influence over reimbursement, medical devices, and international research.

National Institutes of Health 8 The NIH is the primary government sponsor and regulator of medical research. When NIH-sponsored research involves a new medical device, the NIH requires that an Investigational Device Exemption (IDE) be obtained. The IDE process is handled by the FDA and evaluates the safety of the investigational device.

Food and Drug Administration In the United States, the FDA regulates medication and device safety. FDA regulations also often carry weight with international drug and device manufacturers because the US represents such a large potential market for their products. FDA approval is the first step toward reimbursement and clinical acceptance. For a device or medication to be approved by the FDA, it must either (1) prove that it is substantially equivalent to a previously approved product (510k submission) or (2) prove through extensive scientific testing that it is both safe and effective (premarket submission).

The FDA keeps online public records of device complaints and failures.[48] When patterns are recognized, the FDA requires manufacturers to make formal device corrections or recalls. It is the responsibility of the manufacturer to notify known accounts of device corrections.

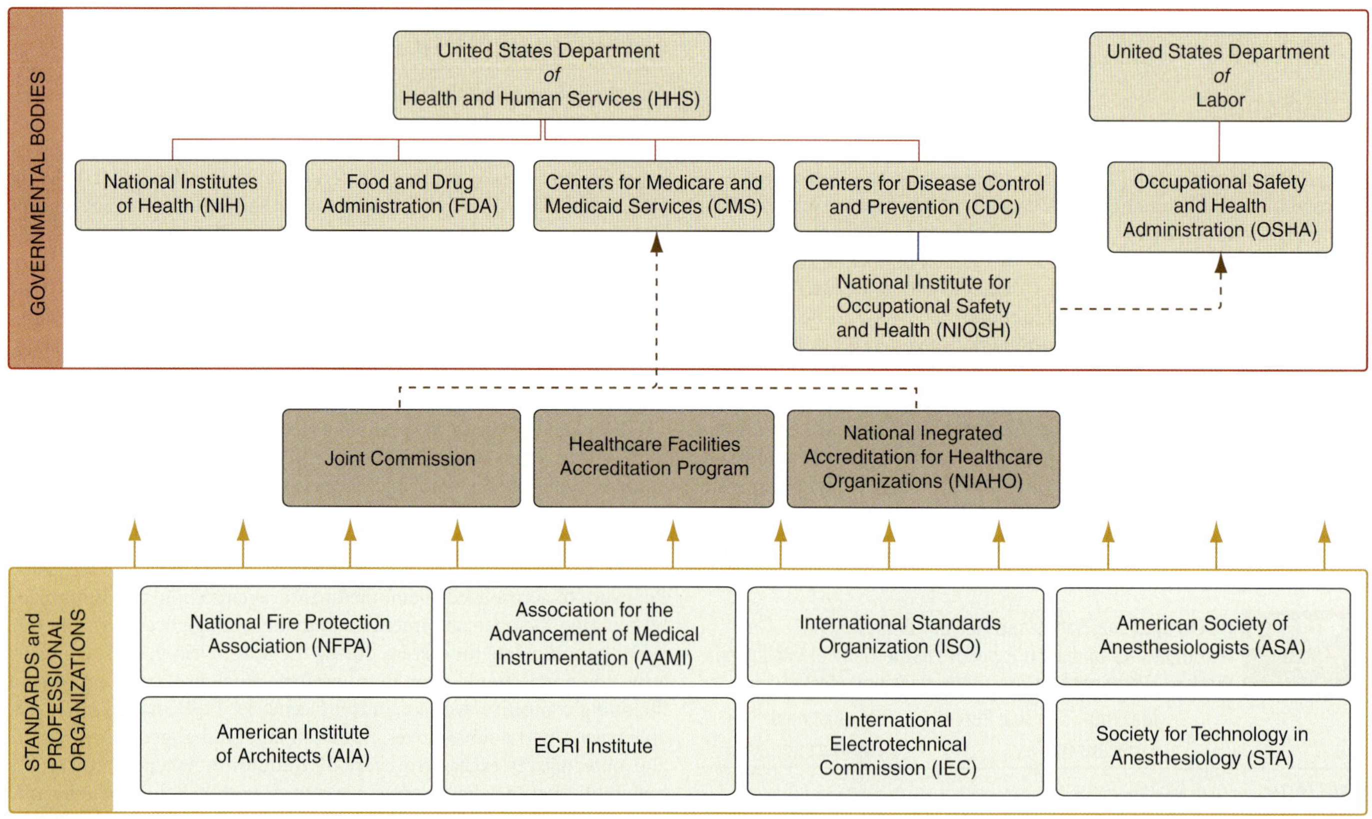

FIGURE 28-19. Interrelationships between regulatory agencies in the United States. Standards and professional organizations do not have legal authority but provide expert recommendations often adopted by the appropriate governmental body.

National Institute for Occupational Safety and Health and the Occupational Safety and Health Administration NIOSH and OSHA were both created in 1970 to improve the safety of the American workplace. NIOSH is a branch of the CDC that performs research into occupational safety, produces training materials, and generates recommendations for formal regulation to OSHA. NIOSH guidance documents are not legally binding. OSHA, a division of the US Department of Labor, is responsible for creating and enforcing workplace safety and health regulations based on recommendations from NIOSH. For example, NIOSH published a guidance document on workplace exposure to inhalational anesthetic agents,[49] and OSHA created a mandate for maximal occupational exposure to anesthetic agents.[37]

Centers for Medicare and Medicaid Services CMS is an important regulator of health care because it defines the standards of care, procedures, and environmental conditions for which the government will provide reimbursement. In 2009, Medicare and Medicaid covered 45.9 (Medicare) + 51.1 (Medicaid) = 97 million people, and this number is expected to grow as the population ages and the Health Care Reform Act of 2010 is phased into practice.[50] Many private insurers also follow the lead of CMS in defining their own reimbursement policies.

CMS accredits hospitals and certifies independent parties to accredit hospitals. Health care organizations must meet CMS Conditions for Participation (CfP) and Conditions for Coverage (CfC) to qualify for, and continue to receive, payments from the government for health care services to beneficiaries of Medicare and Medicaid.[51] As Medicare also funds residency-training programs, CMS also has significant power over teaching institutions. CfP and CfC include references to standards generated by other bodies; for example, CMS adopts the fire safety code of the NFPA.

HOSPITAL ACCREDITATION BOARDS

Independent boards of accreditation are approved by CMS to "deem" health care organizations compliant with Medicare Conditions of Participation and Conditions for Coverage. These boards gain their power through CMS approval and adoption by large numbers of health care institutions. It is possible for a hospital to seek accreditation by more than one independent body or directly by CMS alone.

Joint Commission The Joint Commission (JC), formerly known as the Joint Commission for the Accreditation of Hospital Organizations (JCAHO), was founded in 1951 as a nonprofit validator of health care facilities. It has since become one of the most recognized CMS accreditors of health care facilities. To maintain JC approval, a health care organization must undergo an inspection at least every 3 years.

Healthcare Facilities Accreditation Program The Healthcare Facilities Accreditation Program (HFAP) program of the American Osteopathic Medicine Association is the only osteopathic-driven surveyor with CMS deeming authority. The HFAP may also be used by allopathic or mixed facilities to obtain CMS accreditation.

National Integrated Accreditation for Healthcare Organizations The Swiss-owned DNV Healthcare, Inc. has combined Medicare CfP standards with ISO 9001 quality practices, usually reserved for the manufacturing environment, to create the National Integrated Accreditation for Healthcare Organizations (NIAHO) accreditation program. NIAHO was approved to deem hospitals by CMS in 2008.

NATIONAL FIRE PROTECTION ASSOCIATION

The NFPA is an international nonprofit organization founded in the United States in 1896 to provide standards for fire safety. Since its founding, the NFPA has grown to provide consensus-based standards for electrical safety, ventilation systems, and medical gases. Because NFPA codes are based on the consensus of experts in the field, they are often delayed by debate over controversial issues. The last released guideline for health care facilities was *NFPA 99: Standard for Healthcare Facilities 2002.*[14] NFPA guidelines often reference each other for more detailed information. For example, NFPA 99 heavily references *NFPA 70: The National Electric Code (NEC)*. NFPA guidelines are not legally binding until adopted by a government agency (which is often the case).

ECRI INSTITUTE

The ECRI Institute, formerly known as the Emergency Care Research Institute, is a nonprofit organization dedicated to the evidence-based advancement of patient care. It provides systematic reviews, purchasing guidelines, maintenance recommendations, and safety notifications to hospitals, patients, device manufacturers, payers, and other members of the health care community. The ECRI is respected for its health care expertise and science-based approach to guidance, which does the work of compiling data from many sources into concise practice recommendations.

ASSOCIATION FOR THE ADVANCEMENT OF MEDICAL INSTRUMENTATION

The Association for the Advancement of Medical Instrumentation (AAMI) is a nonprofit organization founded in 1967 to promote the understanding, development, and appropriate use of medical equipment. AAMI generates standards on equipment selection, processing, and maintenance through member and expert consensus.

ARCHITECTURE ORGANIZATIONS

The AIA is a professional group for architects and developer of design standards. AIA most notably produces the *Guidelines for Design and Construction of Healthcare Facilities*, which describes best practices for medical facility design and is referenced by the JC and other standards agencies when inspecting health care facilities. State boards of architecture or building code compliance may also provide additional guidance on local rules and regulations, which may be stricter than federal guidelines.

STANDARDS ORGANIZATIONS

International Organization for Standardization ISO is an independent consortium of high-influence standards organizations from around the world. The ISO member representing the United States is the American National Standards Institute. ISO generates consensus standards on industrial and commercial issues that are often adopted as regulations by national or local governments.

International Electrotechnical Commission Much the same as the ISO, the International Electrotechnical Commission (IEC) represents an international consortium of standards organizations, in this case dedicated to standards for electrotechnical devices and equipment. The IEC works closely with ISO in the definition of standards for overlapping territory such as IT equipment and energy efficiency.

American National Standards Institute The American National Standards Institute (ANSI) is a nonprofit, nongovernmental organization that organizes voluntary consensus in the United States but does not write standards itself. It is a voting member of both the ISO and IEC and thus participates in the global propagation of standards.

ASTM International Formerly known as the American Society for Testing and Materials, ASTM International is one of many standards-generating organizations in the United States that is managed by the ANSI. ASTM International is a prolific generator of consensus standards on subjects ranging from construction to medical devices.

TABLE 28-5 Examples of Certification Marks Commonly Used to Indicate Compliance of a Medical Device With a Specific Set of Standards

Certification Mark(s)	Testing Laboratory	Accepted by
UL ®	Underwriters Laboratory	United States, Canada (in some cases)
MET C US	MET Laboratories	United States, Canada
SP ® SP ® US	Canadian Standards Association	Canada, United States
ETL ® C ETL ®	Intertek Testing Services	United States, Canada
BEAB Approved	British Electrotechnical Approvals Board	Great Britain
CE	Conformance European	European Union countries
CCC	China Compulsory Certification	China

Note: It is not uncommon for a device to carry several markings of conformance.

Testing Laboratories Before sale, medical devices are subject to testing for conformance to safety and operability standards acceptable in the target market. This testing is usually performed by a for-profit independent but government-certified test laboratory. In the United States, OSHA defines acceptable marks of conformance. In Canada, the acceptability of conformance stamps is determined by the Standards Council of Canada. For electrotechnical products, especially those marketed internationally, the manufacturer may pursue marks of compliance from more than one certified laboratory (**Table 28-5**).

KEY REFERENCES

- ASA Taskforce on Operating Room Fires. Practice advisory for the prevention and management of operating room fires. *Anesthesiology*. 2008;108:786-801.
- Dorsch JA, Dorsch SE. *Understanding Anesthesia Equipment*. 5th ed. Philadelphia, PA: Lippincott Williams & Wilkins; 2008.
- Fishman S, Smith H, Meleger A, Seibert JA. Radiation safety in pain medicine. *Reg Anesth Pain Med*. 2002;27(3):296-305.
- National Fire Protection Association. *Health Care Facilities Handbook*. 7th ed. Quincy, MA: NFPA; 2002.
- Webster JG, ed. *Medical Instrumentation: Application and Design*. 3rd ed. New York, NY: John Wiley; 1998.

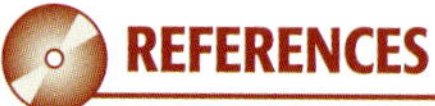

REFERENCES

Complete references available on DVD and online version at www.LongneckerAnesthesiology.com

PART 4

Managing Anesthesia Care

SECTION A
Monitoring the Anesthesia Patient

CHAPTER 29

Perioperative Information Management Systems

Nirav J. Shah
Kevin Tremper
Sachin Kheterpal

KEY POINTS

1. Perioperative information management systems (PIMS) are software systems that manage the documentation, workflow, and charge capture of the operating room (OR) environment. PIMS are composed of two main components: anesthesia information management systems (AIMS) and operating room management information systems (ORMIS).
2. AIMS have been shown to improve processes of care. However, the expense and effort of implementing these systems has prevented widespread adoption.
3. Point-of-care software and hardware are available in many different forms. Each has its advantages and disadvantages. Ultimately, the institutional leaders need to decide on the best fit for its users.
4. Functional components of AIMS include automated device interfaces, user-entered documentation, decision support capabilities, charge capture, and reporting capabilities.
5. Functional components of ORMIS include clinical documentation, process reporting, OR scheduling, resource management, and patient tracking.
6. AIMS and ORMIS need to be configurable systems to account for changes in practice patterns, new regulatory requirements, and updates in medical technology.
7. AIMS need to integrate with hospital-wide electronic medical records (EMRs). The anesthetic record needs to be available for viewing as part of the medical record, and anesthesiologists need to view enterprise patient information in the perioperative environment while using the AIMS.
8. Institutions need to have disaster preparedness strategies including data redundancy plans to account for failure at each level of software and hardware architecture.
9. PIMS vendors will continue to add new features and functionality to their systems. Exciting opportunities lie in the standardization of content and ability to aggregate and analyze large amounts of clinical data.

INTRODUCTION

Information technology is rapidly altering clinical practice. Health care providers interact with, and depend on, electronic medical information every day. From humble beginnings as extensions of billing and registration systems, newer clinical information systems are designed to allow management of clinical workflow, and in best cases, improve the quality of care delivered to our patients. There is ample evidence that perioperative information management systems (PIMS) can improve documentation accuracy, clinical compliance, process-of-care measures, and even improve operational efficiency. However, there are still detractors who feel these systems hamper the clinician's ability to focus on the patient. Although the adoption of PIMS has been slower than expected, the number of successful implementations is clearly increasing, and many departments that do not have systems are in the process of implementing. More than just documenting care, AIMS customers are using the immense amount of data generated to better understand perioperative medicine and develop practices that improve the quality of care. They are also providing feedback to the commercial vendors of these systems that are resulting in improvements in usability and functionality. PIMS have 2 major components: anesthesia information management systems (AIMS) and OR management information systems (ORMIS). AIMS are software that anesthesiologists use to document perioperative care of the patient. OR personnel use ORMIS to schedule surgical procedures, track resources, and document clinical care and billable items. This chapter introduces the functional components of PIMS. It also explains how these components work together and why they are important to the practice of perioperative medicine.

HISTORY OF PERIOPERATIVE INFORMATION MANAGEMENT SYSTEMS

An automated intraoperative anesthesia recording machine was described by McKesson in 1934.[1] This device recorded tidal volume, fraction of inspired oxygen (FIO_2), and blood pressure and represented one of the first attempts to reduce the manual transcription of physiologic parameters. Later, Piepenbrink et al described the use of video recorders to document all the information available to the anesthesiologist as the intraoperative record.[2] Despite these bold yet unsuccessful attempts, paper has endured as the medium of choice to document the perioperative experience. Modern anesthesia information systems initially attempted to replace the paper record primarily by functioning as intraoperative record keepers. They captured physiologic data from the clinical monitors and recorded them in the anesthetic record. These electronically captured data were supplemented by manually entered information to complete the intraoperative record. Over time, these systems have grown from merely intraoperative record keepers to perioperative information management systems (PIMS). These systems now enable electronic documentation of the entire perioperative clinical experience: preoperative, intraoperative, and postoperative care. They also allow users to view historical patient records and help users track patients throughout their perioperative stay. As these systems have moved from functioning as intraoperative record keepers to workflow managers, departments have started to appreciate benefits in billing, compliance, quality assurance documentation, as well the expected benefits in legibility, availability, and clinical research. The impetus to increase the breadth and depth of functionality in PIMS came from several sources. First, more sophisticated hardware and software allowed electronic capture of more parameters from medical devices. This in turn allowed for less manual transcription of information and greater user acceptance of PIMS. As data interfacing became more secure and prevalent, users developed more confidence in the reliability of transmitted variables. Second, as the anesthesiology departments started to understand gaps in the systems, they worked with the PIMS vendors to develop features that allowed for comprehensive workflow management. For example, preoperative clinic, quality assurance, and postoperative care modules were integrated with the intraoperative record keepers. Finally, hospitals began recognizing the important fiscal role of the OR. ORs generate a significant proportion of the health care enterprise's overall profits, and small changes in perioperative anesthesia processes may lead to large changes in revenue collection. As a result, PIMS began to incorporate more billing functionality.

As AIMS have become more prevalent, users have begun to use them as agents of process improvement. Examples of process improvement features include required documentation elements and case documentation templates that allows users to deliver more consistent care for similar patients and procedures. As PIMS have become integrated with

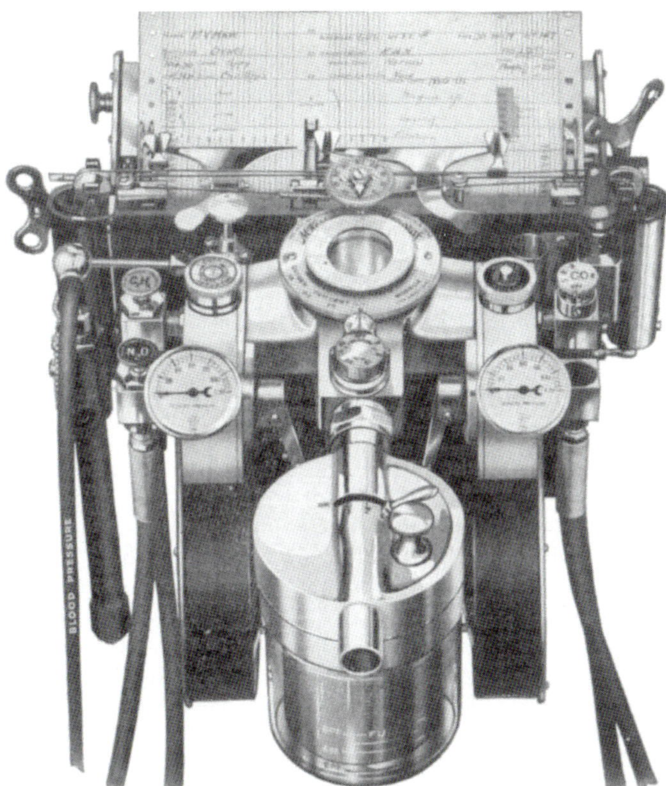

FIGURE 29-1. Close-up view of recording device from early 20th century. [From McKesson EI. The technique of recording the effects of gas-oxygen mixtures, pressures, rebreathing and carbon-dioxide, with a summary of the effects. *Curr Res Anesth Analg.* 1934;13(1):1-14.]

other hospital systems, redundant documentation has been reduced, clinical efficiency has been improved, and documentation accuracy has increased. The integration of preoperative and postoperative care documentation with the intraoperative record keeper has created a comprehensive perioperative record. This has not only allowed for a longitudinal view of the patient's perioperative course but also enabled information to flow more seamlessly.

Billing processes have also demonstrated enormous improvements with the implementation of PIMS. The creation of a legible record, requiring important billing elements to be completed, and electronically transmitting the record to billing departments has streamlined billing processes. Adverse events documentation, long underreported with paper systems, has become more closely integrated with clinical workflow when included with a PIMS. In the most comprehensive implementations, PIMS have become workflow management tools, allowing clinicians to document their entire experience with the patients while improving processes for critical ancillary functions such as billing and quality assurance. Other implementations are much more limited, suggesting that although PIMS have great potential, much improvement in the software, ease of implementation, and affordability needs to be realized (**Fig. 29-1**).

POINT-OF-CARE SOFTWARE

Software systems used in the perioperative environment come from a variety of commercial vendors. However, they can be grouped into 3 broad architectural categories: medical devices, client/server, and Web based.[3] AIMS that are part of the anesthesia machine or physiologic monitor are labeled as medical devices. The software user interface is incorporated into the device. For example, the AIMS may be accessed through the physiologic monitor screen or a monitor on the anesthesia machine. Advantages of this model include reduced probability of error with the recording of hemodynamic parameters. Also, because the user interface of the device is familiar to the clinician, adoption of AIMS may be easier. However, medical devices are more rigorously regulated than medical software. Although this may improve the reliability of the software, new features may take much longer to develop and incorporate.

The second category is the traditional client/server. In this model, software files are installed on the local workstation. These files provide instructions on how the software should interact with the user. The files on the workstation (also known as the client) primarily interact with a central computer housing patient data (the server) by exchanging patient data and user requests. Client/server software is developed in one of two ways: "thick" or "thin" client. A thick client typically provides significant functionality independently of the central server. The name is contrasted to thin client, which describes a computer heavily dependent on a server's applications. A thick client still requires at least periodic connection to a network or central server but is often characterized by the ability to perform many functions without that connection. In contrast, a thin client generally does as little processing as possible and relies on accessing the server each time input data need to be processed or validated.[4] Client/server software maintenance can be very resource intensive for hospital information technology (IT) staff because of the need to update all individual workstations every time there is an update in the client software. In addition, files loaded on the workstation are susceptible to interactions with files from other programs with unintended consequences. Fortunately, advanced system management and automation tools can allow for quick distribution and installation of upgrades to workstations. Although a dichotomy between "thick" and "thin" client has been described here, the implementation reality is a continuum with systems being identified as close to one extreme or the other.

The advantages of thick clients are as follows:

- **Fewer server requirements.** Because the point-of-care computer is doing much of the application processing, the thick client server does not need the level of performance of a thin client server. This allows for less expensive servers to be used.
- **Offline or downtime working.** If the central server is down, clinical care can still be documented on the point-of-care computer. When the central server goes back up, the data can be synchronized.
- **Better user experience.** Thick clients typically allow for a richer user experience because many of the features are in the point-of-care software (and not on the server) and therefore not dependent on network bandwidth, which can be variable.

The advantages of thin clients are as follows:

- **Data not stored on local workstation.** Because the server contains all of the data, possibility of loss of data becomes confined to relatively few servers, instead of the many computers located at the point of care.
- **Less expensive point-of-care hardware.** Although the server needs to be powerful to handle the processing load, the point-of-care computer typically needs to be much less powerful than for a thick client. Less expensive hardware in the ORs, where computing equipment may be easily broken or stolen, could lower overall system costs.

Web-based software uses Web browsers to display the user interface, and it stores the application instructions in a central computer known as the Web server. Software upgrades are limited to only the Web servers. The workstations are spared because it is only used to house the Web browser. This model is extremely advantageous for large workstation deployments in multiple locations or when the software needs to be accessed remotely. However, user interface development tools and capabilities are currently less mature for Web-based software than client/server, so the interaction between the clinician and software is less robust. In addition, the software may be optimized for a particular Web browser (ie, Microsoft Internet Explorer) and be incompatible with others (ie, Mozilla Firefox). The reality is that currently the lines are blurring between client/server and Web-based models. In addition, combinations of all 3 categories of point-of-care software are possible

TABLE 29-1 Commonly Available Commercial Anesthesia Software Vendors

Cerner: Millennium Anesthesia
Draeger Medical: Innovian Anesthesia
General Electric: Centricity Perioperative Anesthesia
McKesson: McKesson Anesthesia Care
Merge Healthcare: Frontiers Anesthesia
Merge Healthcare: DocuSys AIMS
Philips: CompuRecord
Picis: Anesthesia Manager
Surgical Information Systems: SIS Anesthesia
Epic: Anesthesia Information Management System
iMDsoft: MetaVision (MV-OR)
Plexus: Anesthesia Touch
Acuitec: GasChart

Data from http://www.klasresearch.com.

TABLE 29-2 Examples of Hardware and Software Specifications for Perioperative Information Management Systems

- Servers: Operating system and version, processors, RAM, storage, storage redundancy
- Clients: Operating system and version, processor, RAM, storage
- Database type and query capability
- Physiologic device interface architecture
- Network type: Wired and wireless bandwidth requirements
- High availability and disaster recovery implementation
- Programming language
- Software release methodology (major and minor) and timing
- Single logon capability
- Interfaces types
- Custom functionality: Barcoding, image capability, voice recognition, Web enabled
- Handheld devices: Supported models

and may be used to optimize the user's experience and resource requirements of hospital IT staff[3] (**Table 29-1**).

POINT-OF-CARE HARDWARE

Point-of-care hardware the workstation or medical device that the application is accessed from, including the keyboard and monitor, and also the mounting equipment used to house the hardware. Several considerations go into choosing the appropriate hardware for each clinical setting where the software is being used.

1. The hardware should be ergonomic. Mounting equipment should have adequate range of motion to allow the user to interact with the software and simultaneously take care of the patient. Keyboard should be adjustable.
2. The hardware should be compliant with hospital infection control guidelines. Typically, the hospital's infection control team will review all the equipment.
3. The hardware should be durable. It should be resistant to water and other spills, and usable in a variety of temperature settings. The hardware should also withstand the usual "bumps and bruises" of the OR.
4. The hardware should be procured in an economical manner. Workstation prices are continually dropping, and typically the hardware purchase is one of the last purchases in an implementation to take advantage of the downward price trajectory of computing equipment.
5. The hardware should be usable in multiple environments, or the hospital should be able to buy equipment specific to each area that the software will be used.

A few vendors require vendor-specific hardware, either workstations or special keyboards, bar code scanners, or even syringe pumps. Hospitals should evaluate the usefulness of each of the specialized hardware against cost, support, and training issues (**Table 29-2**).

ANESTHESIA INFORMATION MANAGEMENT SYSTEMS

Although each of the commercially available systems has its own set of features and functionality, the most successful systems have enough breadth of functionality to serve the needs of clinicians, billing staff, and quality improvement groups. The core functional components include:

- Automated physiologic device interfaces
- User-entered documentation
- Staff and billing documentation
- Alerts and reminders
- Anesthesia history and physical
- Reporting for quality improvement, compliance, or research purposes

AUTOMATED PHYSIOLOGIC DEVICE INTERFACES

Among the most critical feature of AIMS is its ability to interface data automatically from the medical devices into the intraoperative record. Interfaces are software and hardware that allow one system to communicate with another. Without device interfaces, the user would be required to manually type in all of the physiologic data into the system to create the anesthetic record. User acceptance would be limited. In addition, intraoperative records generated by AIMS with device interfaces have been shown to be more accurate that handwritten records and therefore more useful for review, research, and quality improvement purposes.[5]

In terms of the physiologic parameters that are interfaced from the monitors to the AIMS, a "more is better" philosophy predominates. Although not always possible for technical reasons, every device that records physiologic information should be able to send the information to the intraoperative record electronically. Devices commonly interfaced to the AIMS include physiologic monitors, anesthesia machines, ventilators, bispectral index sensor (BIS), and continuous cardiac output monitors. Less commonly interfaced devices include heart/lung bypass machines and infusion pumps. **Table 29-3** lists many of the commonly recorded parameters by devices found in the anesthesia cockpit. Basic hemodynamic variables such as blood pressure, heart rate, and pulse oximetry must absolutely be interfaced. Other useful parameters include gas analyzer data, such as inspired and expired inhalational anesthetic concentrations, FIO_2, and end-tidal carbon dioxide. Ventilator data such as tidal volume, respiratory rate, and peak pressures should also be sent to the AIMS.

Physiologic device interface implementations typically leverage existing monitoring networks that were created to provide a central viewing area for waveforms (such as ECG) and vital signs from multiple locations. The physiologic device interface server copies information from the monitoring server and places it into the AIMS database. If the physiologic monitors also display information from other devices (such as BIS) and that information is transmitted over the monitoring network, then the interface server can copy information from these other devices as well. If there are devices that are not connected to the monitoring network, the data from those devices must be copied into a local processing device (usually a workstation). This workstation then sends the patient information to a central database server, which then copies it into the AIMS. If there is no monitoring network at all, then all devices must interface to the AIMS at the point of care. Then, all patient information is sent from the client to the server.

Each device may have its own communication protocol with the network. With new devices arriving with increasing frequency to the health care market, the ability for an AIMS vendor to create interfaces with every device can be extremely difficult and expensive, and many have chosen to outsource this work to specialized interface vendors.

TABLE 29-3 Interfaced Physiologic Variables

- Heart rate (ECG monitoring and Spo_2)
- Noninvasive blood pressure (systolic, diastolic, mean)
- Arterial blood pressure (systolic, diastolic, mean)
- $ETCO_2$
- Level of consciousness monitors (BIS, Entropy, SedLine)
- Temperature (all sources)
- Fio_2
- Peak inspiratory pressure
- Tidal volume
- Minute volume
- Respiratory rate (ventilator and $ETCO_2$)
- PEEP
- PA pressures (systolic, diastolic, mean)
- CVP
- Cardiac output
- Cardiac index
- Spo_2
- Svo_2
- Systemic vascular resistance
- Nitrous (inspired and expired concentrations)
- Oxygen (inspired and expired concentrations)
- Inhalational agents measured (inspired and expired concentrations)
- Intracranial pressure
- Flows: oxygen, air, nitrous oxide
- Acceleromyography

BIS, bispectral index sensor; CVP, central venous pressure; ECG, electrocardiogram; Spo_2, pulse oximetry saturation; $ETCO_2$, end-tidal carbon dioxide; Fio_2, fraction of inspired oxygen; PA, pulmonary artery; PEEP, peak end-expiratory pressure; Spo_2, pulse oximetry saturation.

DATA INTERFACED FROM PHYSIOLOGIC DEVICES

Data recorded in the physiological monitors can be either intermittent (eg, noninvasive blood pressure readings) or continuous (eg, pulse oximetry saturation [Spo_2] or invasive arterial blood pressure). For both intermittent and continuous data, there needs to be clear understanding between the user and vendor on how information is captured by the AIMS. For example, if noninvasive blood pressure is set to cycle at 3-minute intervals, then the expectation is that the AIMS will capture each noninvasive blood pressure reading. In contrast, continuous parameters are interfaced at defined intervals that allow an accurate representation of the patient's clinical condition but do not overwhelm the AIMS with data. For example, sampling the Spo_2 every minute may be appropriate; however sampling every second may be information overload. Currently, no standards have been defined for the frequency of data capture. Each AIMS typically has its own algorithm for data capture from physiologic monitors, and institutions should be aware of the data capture interval and algorithm for its system.

PITFALLS OF DEVICE INTEGRATION

Artifact Data artifact can come from a variety of sources such as manipulation of the device (movement of a noninvasive blood pressure cuff), electrocautery, and flushing of an arterial line. Clinicians using paper documentation account for these occurrences when noting vital signs and typically filter out the spurious values. Most AIMS allow the user to annotate the spurious data and remove it from the AIMS display. Although programs with algorithms designed to recognize artifact and annotate clinical records have been described in the literature, they are not in widespread use.[6,7] Institutions with AIMS have found that users manually edit interfaced data (especially pulse rate, pulse oximetry, and blood pressure) in a significant number of cases.[8] Whether this is due to data artifact or other reasons is not entirely clear. However, clinicians using paper documentation have a tendency to artificially smooth out real variations in hemodynamic parameters. AIMS makes this tendency more difficult to carry out, but it does not completely eliminate the ability to artificially reduce variation.

Data Loss When devices are interfaced to the AIMS, the expectation is that the interface will work 100% of the time. In reality, there may be cases when the interfaces are down due to network failure, maintenance, or some other reason. For these instances, AIMS and hospital IT departments typically have a warning system (alert on the screen or automatic page that immediately notifies users of this (hopefully) rare occurrence. In addition to inciting user frustration, failure to recognize loss of data may increase medical liability.[9] Manual input of data or temporary reversion to paper documentation is the most common backup plan.

Complexity Ideally, interfacing between devices and AIMS would be as simple as plugging in all the necessary cables and clicking Start. Unfortunately, medical devices use a range of communication technologies protocols (RS232, RS485, 802.11, IrDA). As updated models are released, they may have slightly different software loaded on them. Each of these models has to be interfaced to the AIMS. Moreover, clinical information requires a completely safe and secure exchange of data. Safeguards to ensure that the interfaces are reliable to health care standards add a considerable amount of cost and complexity to interfacing projects.[10] The device industry and health care professionals have realized the need to improve communication between devices and systems. Integrating the Healthcare Enterprise (IHE) is an initiative that promotes the use of established standards. IHE has created protocols so that systems developed using IHE guidelines communicate better with each other and are easier to implement. Increasing use of these interoperability guidelines should help reduce the cost of interfacing and increase adoption (Table 29-3).

TECHNICAL INFRASTRUCTURE FOR PHYSIOLOGIC DEVICE INTERFACES

The network used to transmit all the information gathered from the devices must be robust, reliable, and secure. Each hospital must perform an accurate analysis of its network before implementing an AIMS. Networks with relatively poor reliability may need a system that supports storage of clinical information locally. Other institutions that have a more reliable network may not need such redundancy. Hospitals and vendors also need to agree on how clinical data streams will be separated from other applications on the network. Options include a separate physical network or a virtual private network.[3]

USER ENTERED DOCUMENTATION

Preoperative Record A thorough history and physical completed in a timely manner allows for optimal care of the patient and minimizes delays in starting cases. In most instances, the preoperative process starts at the surgeon's office, where the initial history and physical is completed and testing is ordered. Then the patient is evaluated in advance (phone triage, preoperative testing clinic) or the morning of surgery, where the anesthesiologist first views the patient's health information. Well-designed preoperative modules of AIMS are able to manage the multiple scenarios in which preoperative information in collected. In comprehensive implementations, much of the information for the history and physical is collected from other sources including previous anesthesia history and physicals, and it is presented to the anesthesiologist for review. The anesthesiologist can then spend less time collecting information and more time analyzing it to produce a safe anesthetic plan (**Fig. 29-2**).

Preoperative documentation can be divided into several categories:

1. Patient demographics: examples include name, gender, and date of birth. This information is usually interfaced from hospital registration systems or OR scheduling systems and rarely entered manually
2. Preoperative testing: laboratory results, ECG, x-ray, echocardiography. Interfacing of preoperative testing data is highly variable among implementations and depends on a number of factors, including the technical ability of the testing systems to interface with AIMS and vice versa. More important is the model of patient care. If the preoperative testing is done at a facility completely unrelated to the OR facility, then it may not be possible to exchange information electronically because systems in unrelated facilities rarely communicate with each other.

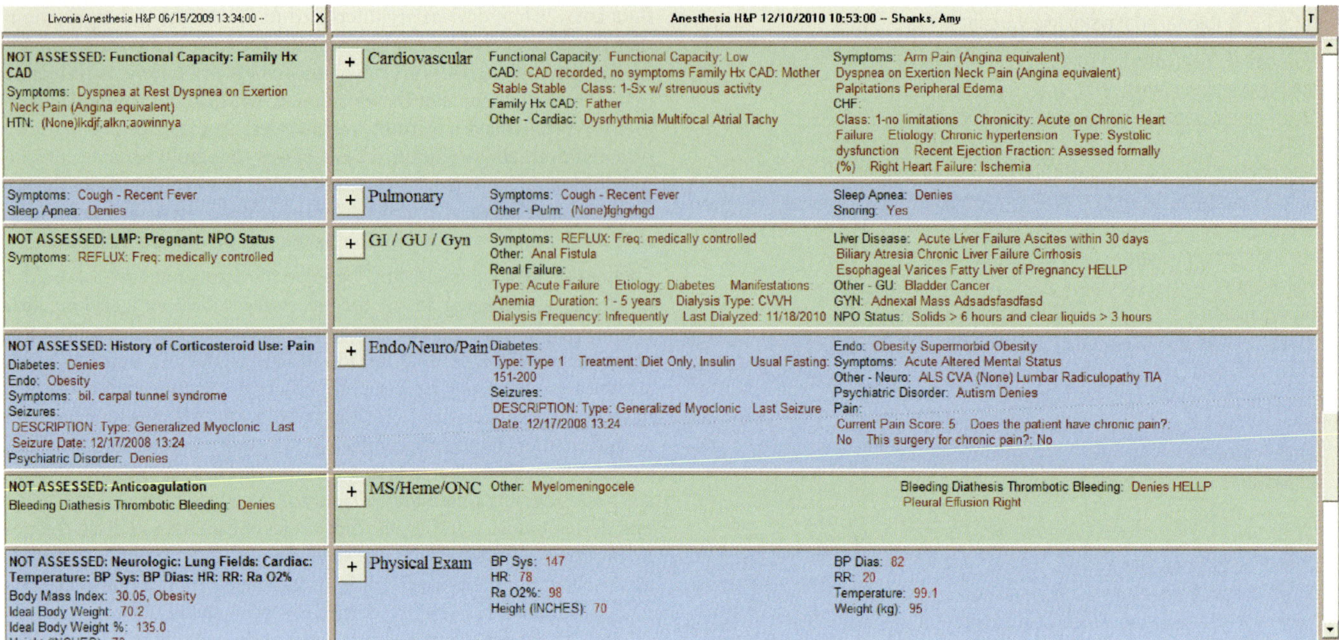

FIGURE 29-2. Preoperative anesthesia assessment, with view of previously documented assessment.

3. Allergies and medications: includes reactions of each allergy and last time that each medication was taken. This information is typically collected by nursing staff or is available from previous visits. If the information is automatically captured from other sources, then the anesthesiologist must verify before completing the history and physical. If not, then the system should be designed to easily input allergies and medications.
4. Past medical history and review of systems: includes previous surgeries and problems with anesthesia. Usually follows a systems approach. If manually entered, then systems typically provide multiple methods to input the information, selecting from a list of choices, typing information into a text box, or choosing a default option (eg, "within normal limits"). If the AIMS has the ability to capture information automatically that was previously entered, then the information must be verified before becoming part of the final medical record.
5. Physical examination: vital signs, height, weight, heart sounds, lung fields, and airway assessment. This information can be interfaced from the physiologic monitor and/or captured from the initial nursing assessment. In addition, AIMS can provide useful tools to take information automatically from the history and physical and calculate derived values such as body mass index or risk prediction scores.
6. Procedure information: includes surgeon and proposed operation. This information should be automatically captured from the OR scheduling system. If not, AIMS typically allow users to select from a list of choices.
7. Anesthetic assessment and plan: includes American Society of Anesthesiologists physical status, airway management plan, monitoring, and patient discussion acknowledgment.

The preoperative components of AIMS help improve the quality of care of patients by helping collect all of the relevant information to perform a safe anesthetic. They can prevent information from being missed or overlooked and automatically provide guidance to prevent adverse events. For example, preoperative information collected in an AIMS can help to predict patients needing antiemetic rescue.[11] They can save clinicians time by eliminating the need to search for information or manually enter information that has already been collected by someone else. Conversely, poorly integrated and designed systems may reduce the satisfaction of providers and patient focus. Preimplementation planning is of utmost importance.

Intraoperative Record The intraoperative component of the AIMS must allow for quick and accurate documentation. Screen layout must be well thought out, methodology of data input should be intuitive, and the overall ergonomics should be conducive to the multitasking that occurs in the OR environment.[12]

Although much of the clinical information is automatically captured from the physiologic monitors or other medical devices into the intraoperative record, there are observations that need to be manually entered because of either the type of information captured or hardware/software limitations. For example, train-of-four information may need to be entered manually because the nerve stimulator does not record the number of twitches. Specific items are required for quality assurance or billing reasons and must be documented by the user in the anesthetic record. AIMS can be used to increase the documentation compliance rate.[13] However, there are also instances where despite the implementation of an AIMS, incomplete documentation persisted in the anesthesia record[14] (**Table 29-4**).

After the case is complete and all the data have been entered in the system, the record is closed, typically triggered by an event (such as anesthesia end). Alternatively, AIMS have a separate action to close the record. After the record is closed, any additional items documented should be highlighted as addendum information (**Fig. 29-3**).

STAFF AND BILLING INFORMATION

AIMS can be extremely useful to billing and compliance teams by ensuring all items required for billing are accurately recorded and that all compliance measures are accounted for. Many institutions that use AIMS have been able to improve billing significantly. Spring et al were able to reduce their percentage of unbillable records from 1.31% to 0.04% and increase annual revenue by $400 000.[15]

Staff Concurrency Checks Many anesthesia care models have a number of anesthetic caregivers involved in a single case. Anesthesiologists

TABLE 29-4 Categories of User-Entered Documentation With Selected Examples

Required Documentation for Billing or Regulatory Guidelines
- Anesthesia and surgical times
- Machine check
- Confirmation of case, history and physical review, and NPO status
- "Time-out" confirming patient, case, side with surgical and nursing colleagues
- Timing of antibiotic dosing
- Patient disposition such as transport to PACU or SICU

Routine and Nonroutine Clinical Events That Occur During the Surgical Case
- Induction events such as laryngoscopic view
- Patient positioning
- Intravenous lines placed
- Adverse events: bronchospasm, laryngospasm

Notes or Forms Completed by the Anesthesiologist During the Case (Fig. 29-4)
- Documentation for procedures such as arterial lines or central venous lines
- Difficult airway letters for patients
- Acute Pain Service consults for PCA management or chronic pain patients

Clinical or Physiologic Data That May Not Be Captured by the Physiologic Monitors
- Train-of-four neuromuscular blockade monitoring
- Fresh gas flows
- Eyes and pressure points checked
- Systolic pressure variation

Medications/Fluids/Infusions/Blood Products
- Bolus medications
- Fluids, with amounts given and rates
- Drug infusions such as vasopressors or narcotics
- Blood products

NPO, nothing by mouth; PACU, postanesthesia care unit; PCA, patient-controlled analgesia; SICU, surgical intensive care unit.

may be supervising multiple nurses or residents, breaks are given, and responsibility of care is transferred from one anesthesiologist to another. Anesthesiologists are expected to sign in and out of cases accurately and reliably as they are associated or disassociated with them. However, in a typically busy day in an OR, time-related documentation mistakes commonly occur. This can have multiple adverse ramifications. Specific institutions, as well as insurance companies, have guidelines on the number of cases that an anesthesiologist can supervise simultaneously. AIMS can keep track of the cases that each anesthesiologist is associated with and perform real-time concurrency checks, so no caregiver is associated with more cases than is allowed at any given time. This saves the billing team a time-consuming task and reduces the possibility of rejected bills; furthermore, it allows anesthesia departments to be compliant with institutional policies.

Automatic Charge Capture Anesthesia charge capture is a complex process, involving not only the complexity of the procedure but the patient's clinical condition and the time spent with the patient. Every single anesthetic is a unique charge. AIMS can provide significant revenue optimization by ensuring that all billable clinical activities are captured and reducing the time spent by the billing staff in generating a charge.

Acute care anesthesia professional services fees include 4 main categories:

1. Base units: refers to the complexity of the case (lower units assigned for monitored anesthesia care [MAC] ophthalmology cases and higher units for cardiac bypass cases).
2. Time units: how long the anesthesiologist was directly responsible for the patient.
3. Qualifying circumstances unit: a variety of special situations such as use of induced hypotension or extremes of patient age
4. Flat-fee procedure charges: non–time-based charges involving invasive procedures such as preoperative placement of arterial lines, use of peripheral nerve blocks for postoperative pain relief, or emergent nonoperative airway management

These categories are then compiled to create a bill. AIMS can help this process by abstracting the necessary billing information from the anesthetic record. This information includes:

- Patient indentifying information (such as medical record number). Medical record numbers are usually interfaced from hospital registration systems or OR scheduling systems.
- Provider information (all anesthesiologists and attending surgeons involved in the case). AIMS allow users to sign in and out of a case. This information is then recorded as part of the anesthetic record. The documentation of surgeons involved in case is either captured from the ORMIS or manually entered by the user into the AIMS.
- Anesthesia times (anesthesia start and end).
- Procedure information (complete procedure and accompanying diagnosis). The billing team requires comprehensive procedural information to generate an accurate bill. For example, it is important that the billing staff know that a spinal procedure was a multilevel fusion with instrumentation to assign the appropriate base unit. Procedures listed in the scheduling system can be used as a starting point for the documented procedure in the anesthetic record, but many times it needs to be modified to reflect the procedure actually performed.[16]
- Anesthesia type and procedures: MAC, general anesthesia, regional block, lines placed.

DECISION SUPPORT

Decision support is any aid that reduces the possibility of error or increases the probability of making the correct decision. Decision support functionality in AIMS can help standardize clinical practices, reduce errors of omission, and prevent anesthesiologists from delivering harmful medication or medication doses.[17]

Case Templates Cardiac anesthesia cases are managed differently from routine hysterectomies. Cataracts are managed different from craniotomies. Intraoperative templates take these into account and enable best practices to be followed. Templates can significantly help institutions follow practice guidelines. Placing antibiotic dosing on case templates, in addition to physician-specific reminders, increased compliance with antibiotic administration from 69% to 92% in one study.[18]

Alerts and Reminders Alerts and reminders are important tools that help ensure the completeness of documentation and adherence to standard of care. When used judiciously, they guide the user to perform the right action without interfering with the speed of documentation. When used excessively, they slow the user down and decrease user acceptance. Alerts and reminders fall under the broader category of decision support. Within the context of the AIMS, they can take several forms, including:

- Pop-up windows in the AIMS
- Pager or e-mail messages
- Highlighting or bolding of certain items within the AIMS

These features have been used in AIMS to address institutional compliance issues. There have been many examples of improved administration of prophylactic antibiotics with AIMS using alerts and reminders.[18-20] Wax et al studied the administration of antibiotic prophylaxis in patients before and after the implementation of a visual reminder. They found that compliance increased from 82.4% to 89.1%

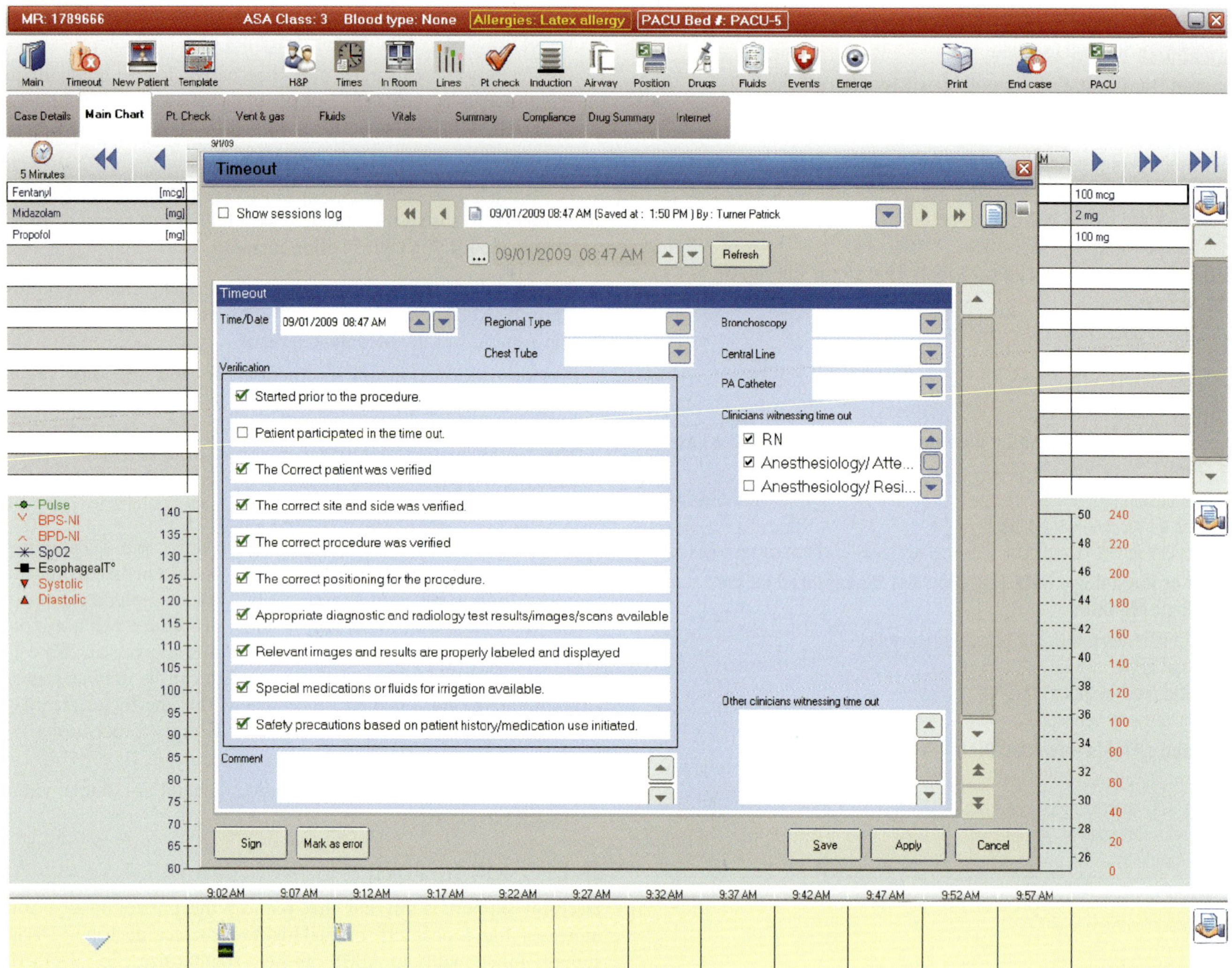

FIGURE 29-3. **A.** Intraoperative case template displaying time out documentation.

with the reminder.[19] Sandberg et al used automated text messaging to reduce missing allergy documentation from 30% to 8%.[21] Kheterpal et al developed an automated reminder system for peripheral arterial catheter documentation in the ORs. The experimental group received pager alerts when the arterial line documentation was not completed in a timely fashion. During the 2-month trial, the group that received pager reminders had a significantly higher documentation rate (88% vs 75%; p <0.001). Interestingly, when all users were sent reminders, the documentation rate increased to 99%. This resulted in a net increase in reimbursement of $40 500 annually.[22] Despite the potential advantages, one must be cautious when implementing alerts. As stated earlier, when too many alerts are activated in a system, "alert fatigue" sets in and effectiveness of all alerts is decreased (**Fig. 29-5**).

Workflow Engine Workflow engines are the tools that allow users to complete their task more efficiently. They work in the background of AIMS as the behind-the-scenes functionality that powers decision support. They can create pending work lists to remind anesthesiologists of documents that need to be signed or patients that need to be evaluated. They can send automatic pages to users informing them of critical labs or test results for upcoming patients. They can also work in conjunction with patient tracking systems to inform users of the status of patients (ready in preoperative holding, OR ready for patient, postoperative care area slot assigned for patient, etc). Workflow engines deliver their output through multiple modalities: on a dedicated screen, via e-mail or pager, or an alert or reminder within the AIMS. They are part of the AIMS toolkit that can improve the quality of care. Kooij et al used a decision support (or workflow) engine to study adherence to postoperative nausea and vomiting (PONV) guidelines. When automated reminders were sent to users, adherence to PONV guidelines jumped from 38% to 73%. When the automated reminders were removed, adherence dropped back down to 37%.[23]

REPORTING FOR QUALITY IMPROVEMENT, COMPLIANCE, OR RESEARCH PURPOSES

Institutions implement AIMS for many reasons: increased operational efficiency, adoption of best practices, and reduced liability. They also implement AIMS to comply with local and national regulatory requirements. The Centers for Medicare and Medicaid Services (CMS) has implemented pay for reporting efforts and is now exploring the implementation of value-based purchasing. Initially, CMS asked for voluntary reporting on a number of quality measures. For anesthesiologists, these included timely administration of prophylactic antibiotics and maintenance of perioperative normothermia.[24] Robust reporting functionality is crucial to meeting or validating all of these objectives. Analyzing clinical, financial, and operational metrics across patients provide data-driven justification for process changes. The resulting cost savings and improvement in charge capture and patient outcomes can provide justification for the cost of implementing AIMS.

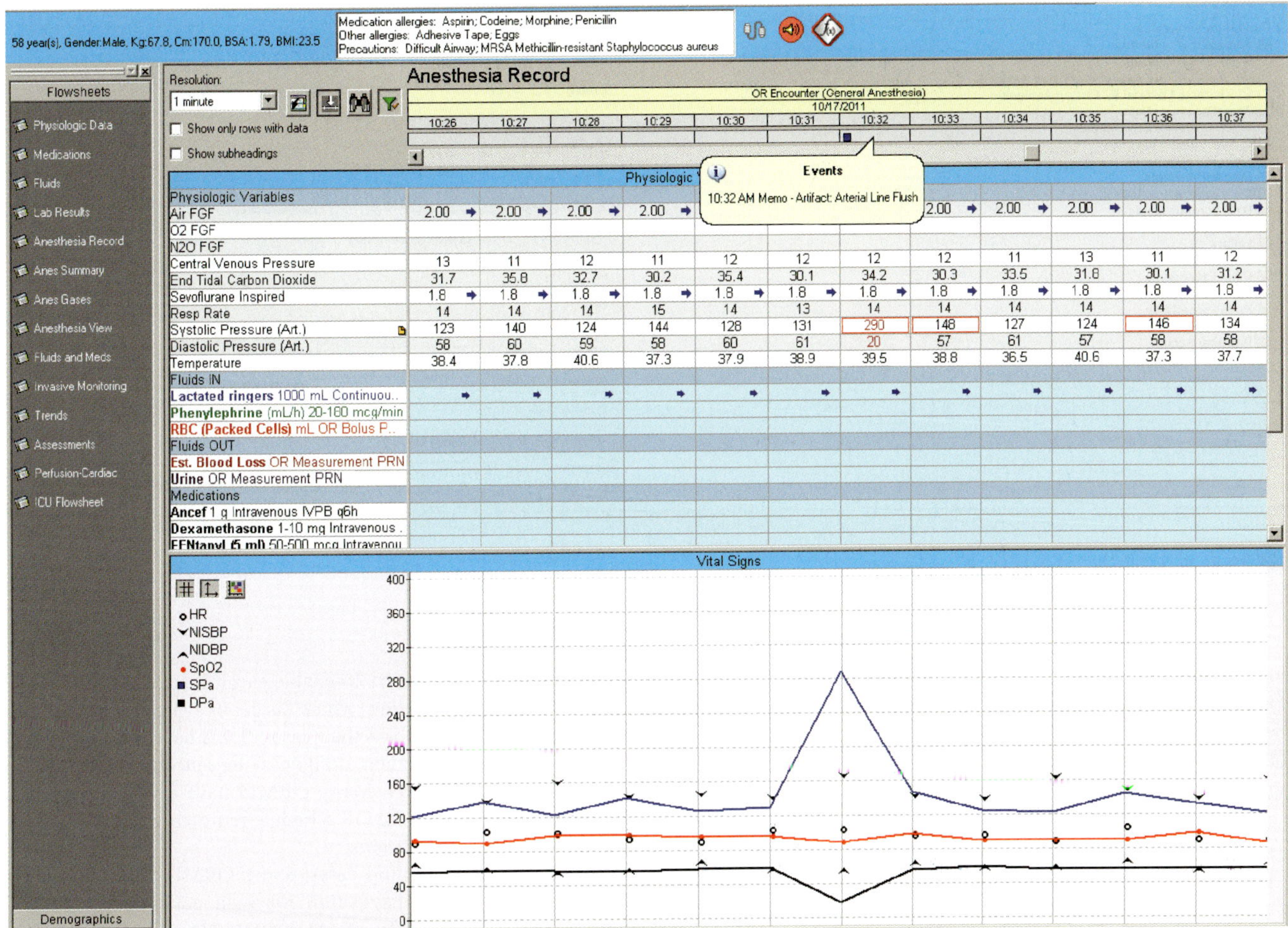

FIGURE 29-3. B. Intraoperative graph showing artifactual data.

Reports can be categorized as standardized or ad hoc. Standardized reports are usually provided by the vendor when an AIMS is purchased. They are commonly used across institutions and include reports such as cases per anesthesia provider, cases by anesthesia type, and total anesthesia time per case type. These reports are either automatically generated or easily obtained from the system. They might be available from the ORMIS as well. In general, OR management software tends to have more standard reports than AIMS due to its increased product maturity. As the number of AIMS implementations continues to increase, we expect more standard reports to be available. Ad hoc reports are unique database queries that answer specific clinical, operational, and financial questions at a given institution. They typically require a deep level of understanding of the system database and querying tools used to access it. Institutions and vendors need to have clear discussions on the availability of standard reports and the limitations of ad hoc reporting tools. Some institutions with large reporting requirements have a separate reporting database. Patient data are transferred from the application database to this reporting database, which is optimized for querying. Then commercially available off-the-shelf reporting tools such as Crystal Reports or SAS can be used to create ad hoc reports.[3]

Limitations A major limitation of the ability to create usable reports is the method of data collection. For example, if difficult airway documentation is a free text box where the clinician types in details about the situation, then creating a report to describe difficult airways may be difficult because of the variability in user input. If the clinician had to select among a several choices in a list specifically built for difficult airways, then the report may be easier to create and much more usable. In addition, reporting tools may assume specific content and data nomenclature. This may limit configurability of the system. Tradeoffs between the ease of report creation and clinician ease of use occur constantly. Institutions must ascertain their reporting needs and configure their systems so they can create the necessary reports but not burden the user with lengthy lists and rarely used choices. Ultimately, a well-defined content development philosophy that balances reporting versus ease of use is of utmost importance to institutions with large reporting requirements (**Table 29-5**).

OPERATING ROOM MANAGEMENT INFORMATION SYSTEMS

ORMIS is a software application or a suite of applications that contains the ability to schedule a case, document all the materials and supplies used, create a bill for those materials and supplies, organize staffing for rooms and cases, and document clinical nursing care in all perioperative areas.[25] An ORMIS may interface with an AIMS, may contain an AIMS as one of its modules, or may be completely unrelated to an AIMS that is being used in the same health care facility (usually not the best workflow). There is usually some overlap in functionality between the ORMIS and AIMS, and deciding which application to use for a specific task is an important decision each facility must make as part of the implementation process (**Table 29-6**).

All commercially available ORMIS use standard off-the-shelf personal computer workstations with keyboards to enter information. Most documentation is entered manually, but some systems have device interfaces and barcode reading technology available as well.

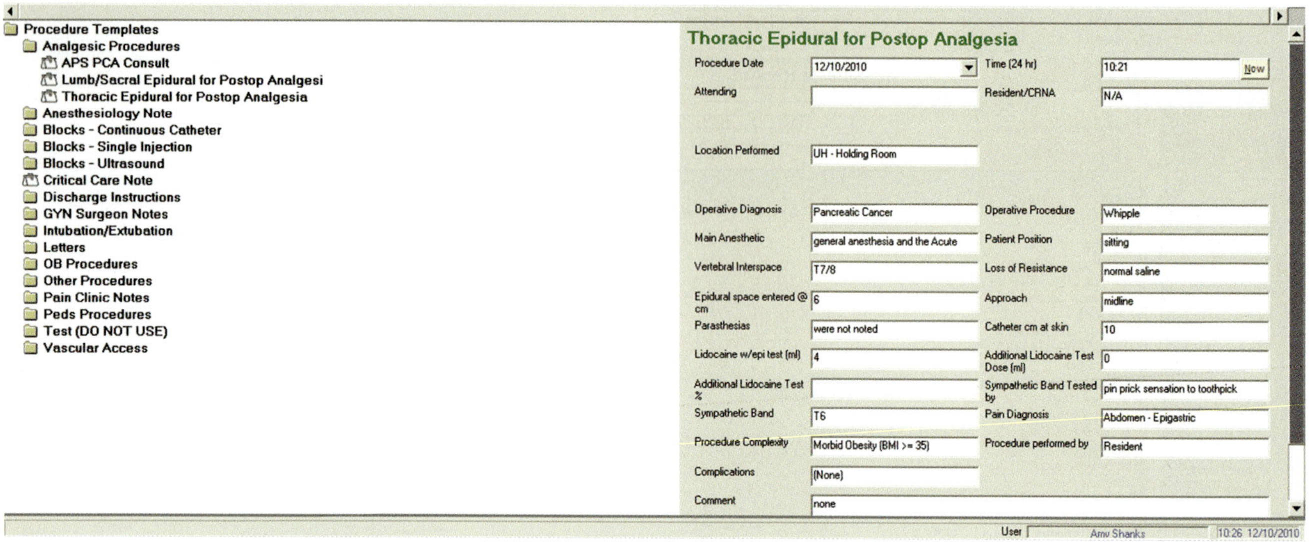

Procedure Templates
- Analgesic Procedures
  - APS PCA Consult
  - Lumb/Sacral Epidural for Postop Analgesi
  - Thoracic Epidural for Postop Analgesia
- Anesthesiology Note
- Blocks - Continuous Catheter
- Blocks - Single Injection
- Blocks - Ultrasound
- Critical Care Note
- Discharge Instructions
- GYN Surgeon Notes
- Intubation/Extubation
- Letters
- OB Procedures
- Other Procedures
- Pain Clinic Notes
- Peds Procedures
- Test (DO NOT USE)
- Vascular Access

Thoracic Epidural for Postop Analgesia

Procedure Date	12/10/2010	Time (24 hr)	10:21 Now
Attending		Resident/CRNA	N/A
Location Performed	UH - Holding Room		
Operative Diagnosis	Pancreatic Cancer	Operative Procedure	Whipple
Main Anesthetic	general anesthesia and the Acute	Patient Position	sitting
Vertebral Interspace	T7/8	Loss of Resistance	normal saline
Epidural space entered @ cm	6	Approach	midline
Parasthesias	were not noted	Catheter cm at skin	10
Lidocaine w/epi test (ml)	4	Additional Lidocaine Test Dose (ml)	0
Additional Lidocaine Test %		Sympathetic Band Tested by	pin prick sensation to toothpick
Sympathetic Band	T6	Pain Diagnosis	Abdomen - Epigastric
Procedure Complexity	Morbid Obesity (BMI >= 35)	Procedure performed by	Resident
Complications	(None)		
Comment	none		

User Amy Shanks 10:26 12/10/2010

FIGURE 29-4. A. Screenshot of epidural procedure note.

Radiofrequency identification (RFID) technology is being increasingly used to track materials, equipment, and sometimes staff and patients.[26]

OPERATING ROOM SCHEDULING

A core component of the ORMIS is the ability to schedule a case. Primary information needed by the application include the surgeon(s), patient, procedure(s), date of procedure, location, and duration of surgery. Additional information collected includes basic patient demographic and medical history, special equipment needed, and preferred type of anesthesia. ORMIS are able to assign anesthesiologists and nursing staff to specific cases and rooms. When cases are scheduled, the ORMIS is able to retrieve the list of required surgical equipment, trays, and supplies from its database automatically and associate those items with the case. It also allows for special equipment or instructions to be added to a specific case.

ORMIS have functionality to enable surgical schedulers to maintain a block model of scheduling, where surgeons typically have dedicated slots during a day to perform their cases. Some have the ability to allow end users (surgeons or their designees) to schedule their own cases within defined parameters. Many ORMIS have a viewing application that allows users to view the OR schedule remotely through the Web or through other hospital systems.

In addition to scheduling cases, some ORMIS have the ability to schedule the proposed disposition for each patient. This allows for more efficient coordination of enterprise-wide resources and patient throughput[25] (**Fig. 29-6**).

MATERIALS MANAGEMENT

The materials management functionality for ORMIS ensures that the correct supplies are present for each case and maintains inventory to keep track

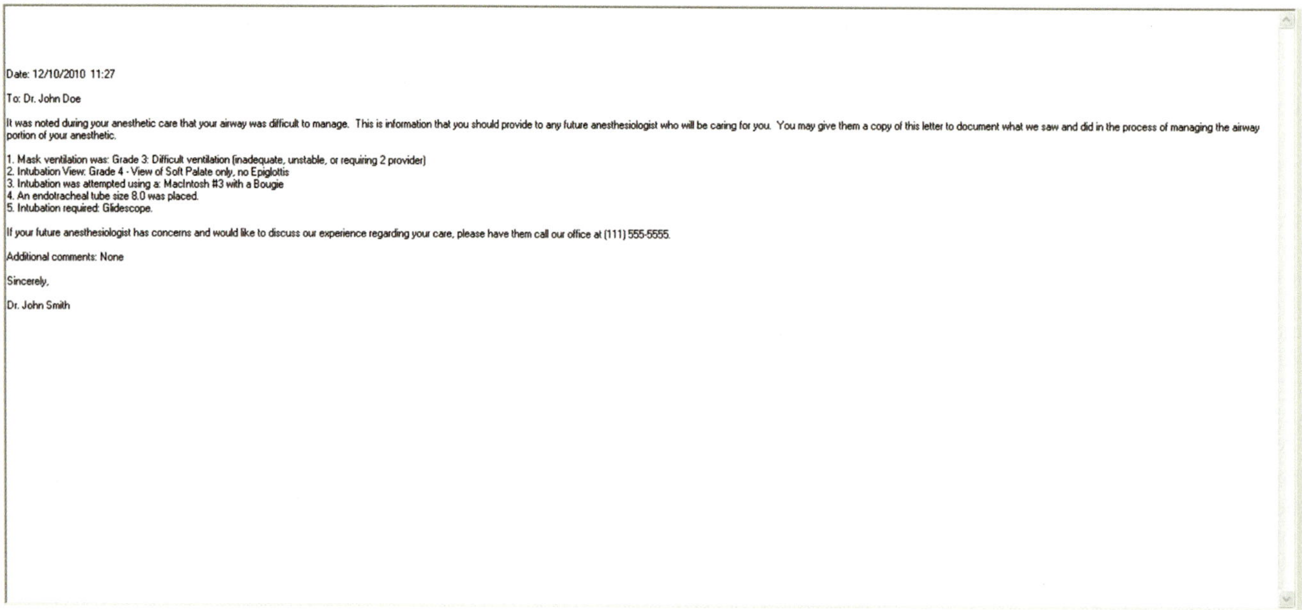

Date: 12/10/2010 11:27

To: Dr. John Doe

It was noted during your anesthetic care that your airway was difficult to manage. This is information that you should provide to any future anesthesiologist who will be caring for you. You may give them a copy of this letter to document what we saw and did in the process of managing the airway portion of your anesthetic.

1. Mask ventilation was: Grade 3: Difficult ventilation (inadequate, unstable, or requiring 2 provider)
2. Intubation View: Grade 4 - View of Soft Palate only, no Epiglottis
3. Intubation was attempted using a: MacIntosh #3 with a Bougie
4. An endotracheal tube size 8.0 was placed.
5. Intubation required: Glidescope.

If your future anesthesiologist has concerns and would like to discuss our experience regarding your care, please have them call our office at (111) 555-5555.

Additional comments: None

Sincerely,

Dr. John Smith

FIGURE 29-4. B. Screen shot of difficult airway letter.

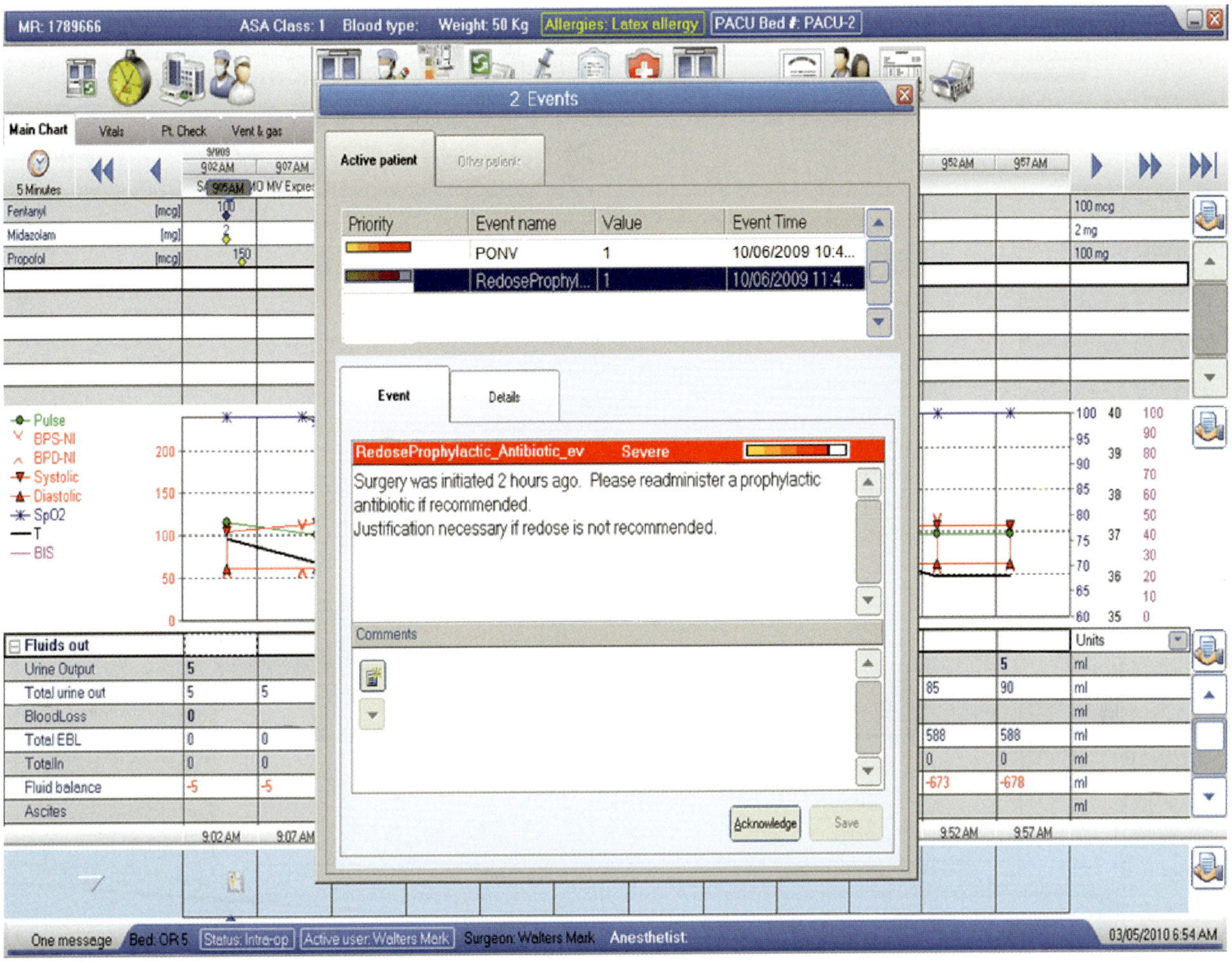

FIGURE 29-5. **A.** Example of antibiotic reminder.

of each item's availability. It can also interface with hospital-wide material management systems so that a facility can keep track of all supplies and equipment that are used and order additional supplies as needed. ORMIS have functionality to manage all the equipment that an OR contains: track location of equipment, servicing information, and maintenance schedules.

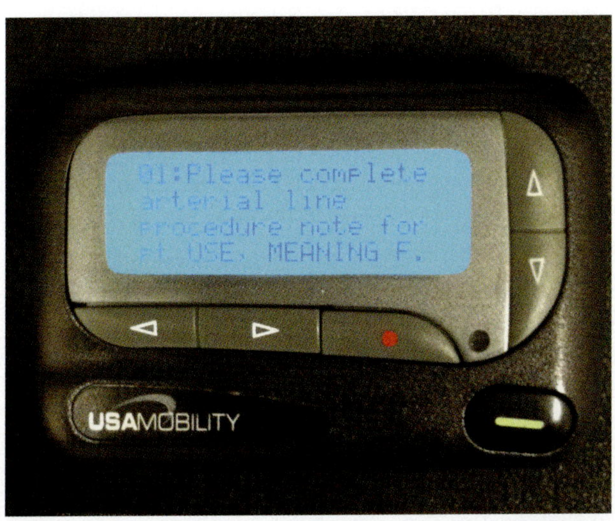

FIGURE 29-5. **B.** Example of pager reminder.

BILLING AND CHARGE CAPTURE

During a case, the circulating nurse is typically responsible for documenting all items that are used during the case (with some exceptions, such as medications given to the patient by the anesthesiologist) in the ORMIS. This information is entered manually, or newer/updated systems allow the use of barcode technology for documentation. All items that are billable are sent to the billing system to generate a charge for the patient.

CLINICAL DOCUMENTATION

ORMIS contain modules to document the perioperative nursing care of the patient. Because there is some overlap between nursing and anesthesia documentation, ideally AIMS and ORMIS interface with each other to reduce redundant documentation.

Intraoperative Documentation Circulating nurses are responsible for the documentation in the OR. In addition to all the billable items, they document certain clinically focused elements as well. Since resource documentation is a significant proportion of the documentation, intraoperative nursing documentation typically resides in the ORMIS. Clinical documentation elements may include:

- Patient position and positioning aids
- Medications administered on surgical field
- Implant information
- Laser use and settings
- Bed types and accessories
- Staff names and roles, with in and out times

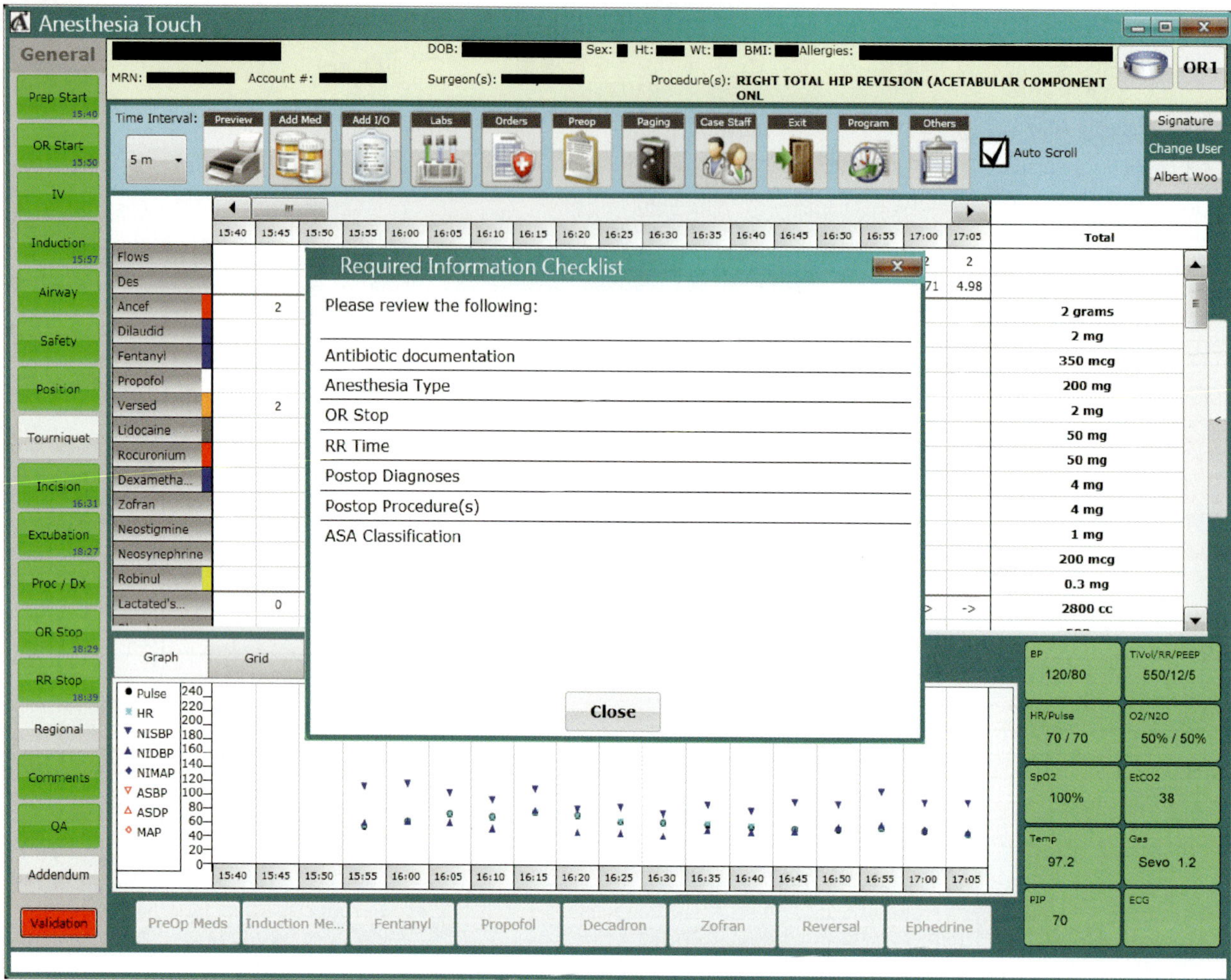

FIGURE 29-5. C. Example of AIMS helping facilitate documentation of required information.

- Actual procedure completed
- Time information (room setup/cleanup, room start/stop, case start/stop, anesthesia start/stop, time out, incision/dressing times)
- Tourniquet on and off times
- Drains, tubes, catheters
- Estimated blood loss

Systems that have templates and easy-to-use lists based on the type of case can significantly ease the burden of data entry.

Preoperative Documentation The main preoperative documentation functionality is the preoperative nursing assessment. Because this is a largely clinical assessment, it often resides in the enterprise clinical information system or the AIMS. Typical elements include:

- Verification of allergies and reactions to allergies
- Medications taken or held
- Brief medical history
- Vital signs and physical assessment.
- Presence of family members
- Mobility issues, activity limitations
- Language/interpreter requirements
- Pain score
- Results of point-of-care testing such as blood glucose and urine pregnancy tests
- Intravenous access obtained
- Medications dispensed

Postoperative Documentation Postoperative documentation is completed by postoperative anesthesia care unit (PACU) nurses. PACUs are high acuity clinical environments and systems that automatically capture vital signs decrease manual documentation for the nurses and allow them to focus on the patients. Because of this physiologic monitoring focus, PACU documentation often resides in the AIMS or hospital EMR. PACU documentation modules allow nurses to document the flow sheet and patient assessment including:

- Pain score
- Level of consciousness
- Wound assessment
- Drain and tube assessment
- Bowel and bladder function
- Aldrete score

PROCESS REPORTING

All the information that is interfaced or painstakingly entered into the ORMIS can be queried to help the perioperative areas provide

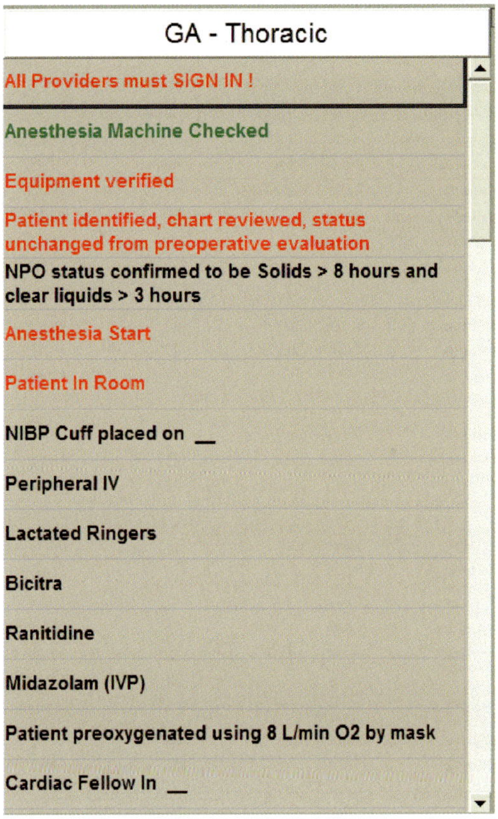

GA - Thoracic

All Providers must SIGN IN !

Anesthesia Machine Checked

Equipment verified

Patient identified, chart reviewed, status unchanged from preoperative evaluation

NPO status confirmed to be Solids > 8 hours and clear liquids > 3 hours

Anesthesia Start

Patient In Room

NIBP Cuff placed on __

Peripheral IV

Lactated Ringers

Bicitra

Ranitidine

Midazolam (IVP)

Patient preoxygenated using 8 L/min O2 by mask

Cardiac Fellow In __

FIGURE 29-5. D. Intraoperative case template facilitating best practice.

better and more efficient care. These reports can be categorized into several different categories: administrative, operational, financial, or clinical.

ORMIS have built-in standard reports, and some also contain functionality that allows creation of ad hoc reports by individual facilities, based on the institution's unique characteristics. ORMIS may also use third-party tools to access the database to create custom reports (**Table 29-7**). Commonly used reports include:

- Daily OR schedule
- Block and room use
- Equipment use
- Number of procedures by location or service or surgeon
- Scheduled case time versus actual case time with reason for delay
- Time per procedure per surgeon

TABLE 29-5 Examples of Reports by Type

Operational
- Cases types by anesthesia provider
- Cases by anesthesia type
- Total anesthesia time by case

Quality Improvement
- Number of patients with postoperative neuropathy
- Number of patients with medication errors
- Number of patients with unplanned intraoperative hypothermia

Compliance
- Percentage of "time-out" documented before incision
- Percentage of antibiotics given before incision
- Number of patients with unverified allergies

TABLE 29-6 Commonly Available Commercial Operating Room Management Information Systems

- Unibased USA ORMS
- Epic OpTime
- Surgical Information Systems SIS Surgery, SISCom (OR Tracking)
- MEDITECH C/S OR Management
- McKesson Horizon Surgical Manager, ORSOS Next Gen
- Picis OR Manager, SmarTrack
- Cerner Millennium SurgiNet
- GE Centricity Perioperative Manager

Data from http://www.klasresearch.com.

PATIENT TRACKING

Patient tracking components of ORMIS take all the scheduling information and clinical documentation entered to create a real-time view showing the progress of the day's cases. The initial starting point is the OR schedule of the day. The progress of each case is shown by a visual cue triggered by a documentation event in the perioperative area. For example, selecting "In Room" in the intraoperative component of the ORMIS when a patient is taken to the operating automatically changes the color of the case as seen on the patient tracker. In this way, the progress of cases becomes readily transparent and changes can be made to facilitate patient throughput as the situation of cases changes during the course of a day. Schedule adjustments, such as room changes or case cancellations, are automatically updated on the patient tracker. If the AIMS is part of the ORMIS or interfaced to it, important information such as anesthesia personnel and anesthesia times can be reflected on the patient tracker. Many ORs currently have large dry-erase boards used as patient trackers. The electronic patient tracker automates this whiteboard, enhances it by adding information provided from the OR in real time, and distributes the information to any workstation that is able to view the tracker. This distribution of information allows all users to participate in enhancing patient throughput (**Fig. 29-7**).

Key features of tracking systems include:

- *Access*
  - Secure, widespread availability
  - Patient information confidentiality functionality
  - View/Edit modes depending on user accessing system
  - Real-time updates
- *Preoperative related*
  - Graphic display of preoperative holding area
  - View of patient's location within preoperative holding area
  - Visual cue that patient is ready/not ready for transport to OR
  - View of pending items if patient is not ready for OR
  - Ability to notify staff with patient's readiness status for OR
- *Intraoperative related*
  - Graphic display the operating rooms
  - View of patient location within OR
  - Ability to see anesthesia providers assigned to the room
  - Ability to see surgeons assigned to the room
  - Ability to see procedure being performed
  - Ability to see stage of case (induction, incision, closing, etc)
  - Ability to see if a room is open/ready for patient, closed, dirty, or in use
  - Visual cue that case is running over allotted time.
  - Ability to notify staff of patient's readiness status for PACU
- *Postoperative Related*
  - Graphic display of postoperative care area
  - View of patient's location within the postoperative care area.
  - Ability to see if a PACU slot is open/ready for patient, closed, dirty, or in use
  - Ability to notify staff with patient's readiness status for PACU discharge

2 Anesthesia - Message: *****Life Flight en route- MCA******

Anesthesia | Tomorrow

Today

✓	Sch Time	Patient Name	Age	Procedure	Surgeon	Anes Type	ASA	Current Checkpoint	Next Checkpoint	Exp End Time
EV_01				**ANES: carlosn ANESRES: kulka j**						
	07:15		42	Amputation Toe	Birdie	Regional Anesthesia	I	Surgery Start	-101	07:45
	08:15			Arthroplasty Total Hip	Aarons	General Anesthesia	I	Patient ready	-87	10:45
	11:15			Grafting, Skin	Dolcen	General Anesthesia	II	Pre-Op	77	12:15
	12:45		31	Arthroplasty Total Hip	Gansh	General Anesthesia	I	Registration	137	15:15
	15:45		18	*Bunionectomy	Ford				287	17:00
EV_02				**CRNA: kdoub ANES: carlosn ANESRES: mazur a**						
	07:15		70	Abdominal Aortic Aneurysm	Almona	General Anesthesia	II	Surgery Start	-41	08:45
	09:15		39	AICD Insertion	Borns	General Anesthesia	II	Patient ready	-27	10:45
	11:15		9M 9D	*Repair Patent Ductus Arteriosus	Miner				17	12:45
EV_03				**ANES: hansb ANESRES: gilbey h**						
	07:15		42	Sinus Endoscopy and Septoplasty	Bordette	General Anesthesia	I	Surgery Complete	-32	08:45
	09:15		35	Arthroscopy TMJ	Bordette	General Anesthesia	I	Patient ready	-27	10:00
	10:30		51	Gastric Bypass	Blocker				-28	12:30
EV_04				**CRNA: kdoub ANES: hansb**						
	07:15		73	Arthroplasty Total Hip	Krafts	General Anesthesia	II	Surgery Start	19	09:45
	10:15		53	Arthroscopy Shoulder	Adison	General Anesthesia	I	In OR	137	11:45
EV_05										
	07:15		21	Arthroplasty Total Hip	Rosen	General Anesthesia	II	PACU	88	09:45
	10:15		58	Cholecystectomy, Laparoscopic w,	Bennigan	General Anesthesia	I	In OR	122	11:30
	12:00		65	Cholecystectomy, Laparoscopic w,	Bennigan				62	13:15
EV_07										
	07:15		71	Replacement Aortic/Mitral Valve	Randall	General Anesthesia	II	Surgery Start	199	12:45
	13:15		71	Incision & Drainage	Kacella	General Anesthesia	I		137	13:45

FIGURE 29-6. Operating room schedule in operating room management information systems (ORMIS).

INTERFACING WITH ANESTHESIA INFORMATION MANAGEMENT SYSTEMS

OR management systems and anesthesia information management systems can be part of the same suite of applications integrated by a single database. More commonly, they are separate systems build specifically for their own end users. Because certain clinical and administrative information overlaps between the 2 systems (eg, allergies and scheduling information), an interface between the 2 systems can be a vital part of any implementation.

Key Considerations for AIMS and ORMIS Interfacing Once it is clear which system will be used for each specific part of the perioperative process, then users must determine the documentation elements common to both systems. There must be consistency in the naming and defining of terms between systems to avoid confusion. Ideally, the systems should be able to both send and receive information to and from each other depending on the item documented and facility-specific workflow. Sources of truth must be defined for vital information such as allergies. Data elements that are typically interfaced include scheduling information and allergies. However, common elements of the nursing assessment and anesthesia history and physical, surgical, and anesthetic time stamps, and key intraoperative patient data such as fluids could also be shared, ensuring consistency between systems and a decrease in redundant documentation.

Scheduling Information The OR schedule is generated from the ORMIS, but the end users of AIMS depend on the schedule as well to access and create the anesthetic record. Updates to the OR schedule should be sent to the AIMS in real time and include relevant procedural and patient demographic information.

Nursing Assessment Preoperative nurses are typically first to see the patient the day of surgery. Information collected by these clinicians that is useful for anesthetics includes allergies, medications, medical history, review of systems, and vital signs. In the best designed implementations, elements in the nursing assessment that can be incorporated into the anesthesia history and physical are sent to the AIMS. This can significantly reduce the time to complete documentation and improves user satisfaction but does not obviate the need for the anesthesiologist to verify and assume responsibility for the information contained in the anesthesia preoperative history and physical.

Surgical and Anesthetic Time Stamps OR facility fees and anesthesia professional services fees both depend on time elements for billing. Therefore, both ORMIS and AIMS users document time stamps. When interfacing time stamps, users must decide which system primarily documents a specific time element and then if the information should be sent to the other system. For example, anesthesiologists should always document the anesthesia start and end times. However, many ORMIS include the ability to document surgeon in-room times. The anesthesiologist would not necessarily require this information for the anesthetic record; therefore, it would not need to be sent to the AIMS. Time stamps that are used in common and should be exchanged include:

- Patient in/out room
- Anesthesia start/stop
- Surgery start/complete

Key Intraoperative Patient Data The documentation of fluids in/out, blood loss, urine output, and other important intraoperative measures is primarily the responsibility of the anesthesiologist but can also be part of the nursing intraoperative record and initial postoperative assessment. As such, data exchange from the AIMS to the ORMIS can reduce redundant manual data entry.

CONFIGURABILITY

PIMS bought from vendors are not ready for use immediately after procurement. They need to be customized for the specific needs of a

TABLE 29-7 Key Features of an Operating Room Management Information System

Scheduling
- Operating room (OR) scheduling, rescheduling, case canceling
- Schedule conflict checking (patient/physician/equipment)
- Ability to keep patient confidentiality on OR schedule
- OR schedule interface to other systems

Materials Management
- Doctor preference cards
- Supplies management
- Equipment tracking
- Instrument counts

Clinical Documentation
- Implant tracking
- Documentation of nursing quality measures
- Data from physiologic monitor interface

Reporting
- Audit trail maintenance
- Average times per procedure per surgeon
- Adverse event reporting
- Utilization reporting
- Custom reporting capability

Administrative and Financial
- Charge capture for staff time, procedures, operating times, supplies, and equipment
- Billing interface
- Registration system interface

facility. Moreover, the system must allow for changes in standards of care and regulatory requirements and advances in medical technology. As facilities grow and mature, processes change, clinical practice evolves, and improvements in workflow are proposed and need to be incorporated by the information system. This adaptability, or configurability, is crucial to the success of the PIMS implementation. Each system has a different level of configurability. Some changes to the application may require the vendor approval or assistance. In other cases, the facility may be able to make the changes. The vendor typically supplies tools that allow the facility to make content changes stored in the database. A few examples of these content changes include:

- Adding or changing names of surgical or anesthesia personnel who use the system
- Adding, removing, or editing elements of the clinical documentation forms
- Adding or removing interfaced devices as the facility changes devices
- Adding or removing locations as new facilities grow or shrink

Facilities need to be aware of the configurability of their system. They should know the aspects that need involvement from the vendor and that can be changed by the facility IT staff.

INTEGRATION WITH INSTITUTIONAL MEDICAL RECORD SYSTEMS

AIMS are just one of many software systems used in an institution. These multitudes of systems were typically implemented over long periods of time and have varying levels of interoperability. They include the hospital EMR, computerized provider order entry systems, laboratory information systems, radiology systems, document imaging systems, and many others. The anesthetic record needs to become part of the EMR so that other providers can view it when necessary. Given that AIMS are not typically fully integrated parts of the hospital EMR, there has to be an interface built between them. Most EMRs and document imaging systems are able to

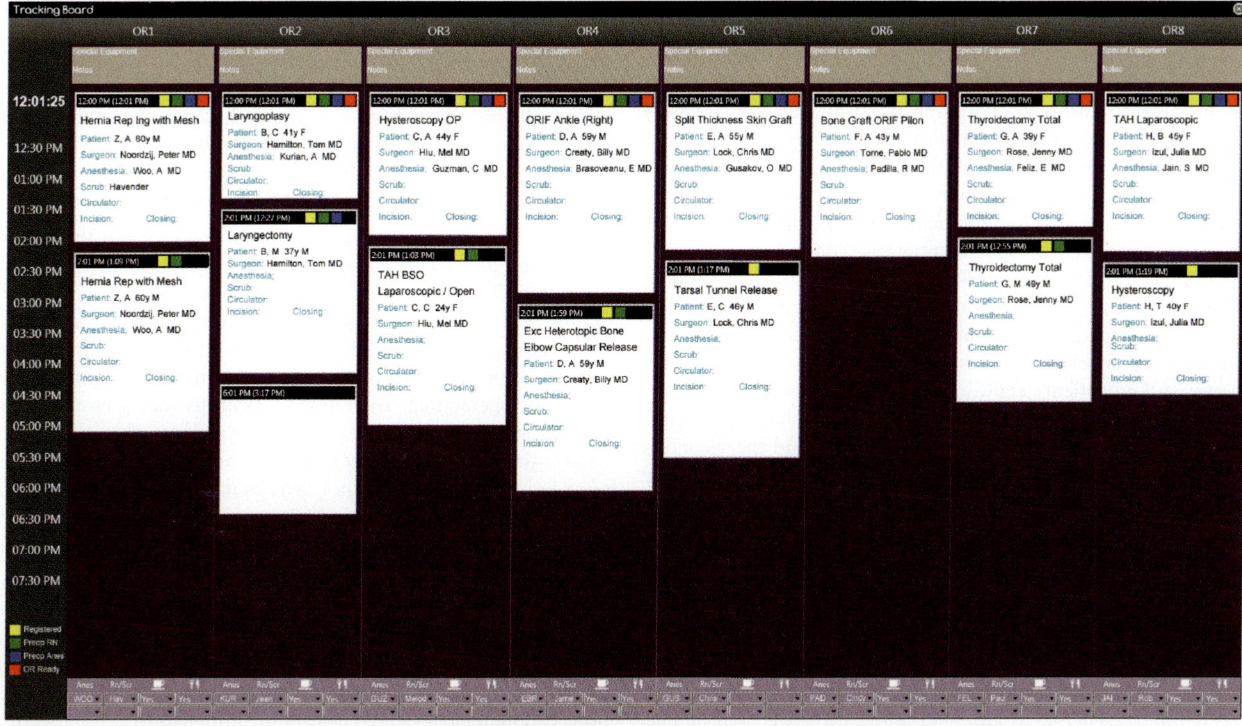

FIGURE 29-7. Patient tracker in an anesthesia information management system.

accept an exported image of the anesthetic record as long as it is in a supported format (PDF, TIFF, etc). AIMS should be able to send a document or image of the anesthetic record to the EMR. The EMR then provides a method for other providers to access and view the record from sites other than the OR where the AIMS are installed. Ideally, documentation of medications given or fluids in/out and other important clinical information would automatically populate an institutions electronic nursing flow sheet and medication administration record. This level of integration is rarely seen today but is certainly a goal for an integrated EMR.

Equally important as accessing the anesthetic record from the EMR is accessing patient information while the anesthesiologist is using the AIMS. There are several ways this can be accomplished, and the methodology depends on many factors: the interfacing capability of the AIMS and institutional software systems, institutional philosophy regarding access of its systems, and breadth of deployment of other systems within an institution. One method is to interface the AIMS with key clinical information systems needed by users. In this scenario, laboratory, pathology, and departmental testing information; dictated notes such as history and physical and discharge summaries; radiology images; medication administration; and electronic orders would be interfaced to the AIMS for viewing by the anesthesiologist. A second scenario is using single logon architecture with patient context to automatically launch other hospital systems such as the hospital EMR with the same patient displayed to avoid having to search for the patient again. This scenario has the advantage of requiring less interfacing work but requires the user to be familiar with each of the applications that are opened. A third scenario is that the user has to open each system manually, including the paper chart, separately to find the necessary clinical information. The reality is that because the transition to EMRs is a long journey, clinicians use combinations of all 3 scenarios to retrieve clinical information in many institutions and a find a way to balance efficiency with retrieving all the necessary information to take care of the patient.

ANESTHESIA INFORMATION MANAGEMENT SYSTEM REDUNDANCY

The information stored in AIMS needs to be available in real time and also be safe and secure. A data redundancy plan as part of an overall disaster preparation strategy is essential to any AIMS architecture. Disaster preparedness strategies look at several different levels of failure and develop a plan for each case. For example, if the network goes down in one or a few ORs, the plan would be different than if the network went out in the entire hospital. A well-designed disaster preparedness plan includes redundancy and automatic failover at important points of failures such as data storage areas, storage network, network switches and routers, and servers. The institution, with input from the clinicians, medical records, and IT staff, should include with this plan a trigger of when to revert to paper charting, also known as "code white."[3]

Data redundancy starts at the workstation level. Some AIMS vendors store patient data locally. In the event of network or central server failure, the clinician would simply continue using the local workstation. When the network or server resumes operation, the data would be sent to the server, and no patient data would be lost. Database servers can be clustered (ie, grouped so that identical servers serve as backup for each other). One server is the designated primary server, and the second is continuously making sure that primary server is working properly. If any significant problems are detected, the backup server automatically takes over and alerts the appropriate personnel. IT staff can usually acquire this backup capability when purchasing the AIMS. They can also manually start up a backup server when problems are detected; however, this method typically causes a short period of downtime for the application.

Backups are also available for the hard drives where the data are stored. A redundant array of independent drives (RAID) system stores the same data on multiple drives. The failure of one drive does not cause the loss of patient data. If a drive fails, it can simply be replaced by the IT staff, and the simultaneous backup continues. Storage area networks (SANs) expand the simple concept of RAID into enterprise storage solutions. Large arrays of redundant hard drives are shared across database servers. The SAN itself can be replicated to a remote backup SAN. In the case of natural disaster such as fire or flood, patient information can simply be retrieved from the mobile SAN. Multilevel and secure data redundancy is complex and expensive. However, no AIMS should be installed without one. The clinical and medicolegal ramifications for unrecoverable data may be far worse.

ANESTHESIA INFORMATION MANAGEMENT SYSTEMS IMPLEMENTATIONS

The decision to implement an AIMS, although offering significant possibilities of improvement on many fronts, is not one to make lightly. The initial cost and maintenance of these systems can consume a significant proportion of a department's annual capital budget. In addition, the implementation process provides not only the excitement of technological advancement but also the frustrations of health care process change. The net result is usually a system that, although not perfect, is superior to the paper record it replaced. After the initial implementation phase, the vast majority of users prefer the AIMS to the paper anesthetic record. AIMS implementations require dedicated personnel from both the vendor and institution. Clinician champions of the system need to come forward or be recruited, and protected time needs to be allotted to the implementation. Once the due diligence has been complete, and the system has been selected and purchased, the real work begins.[27]

PHASES OF THE IMPLEMENTATION PROCESS

Design This is the planning stage. Clinicians and users envision in detail how the system will be used. Workflow is mapped out, screens are reviewed and designed, and use cases are discussed so that the system can be configured appropriately. Vendor implementation teams and institutional IT staff typically help in this stage by mocking up screens, providing guidance on the limits and best use of the features and preventing deviation from initial project scope. In this stage, clinicians test different hardware combinations and decide on the best choice for their facility.

Build This is the configuration stage. Vendor or institution application specialists build out each of the screens. History and physical screens, anesthesia intraoperative templates, nursing assessment modules, and every other screen that needs configuration are built or modified to specification. Specialists upload or input all additional and institution-specific data needed to operate the system. These include locations, users, equipment, supplies, charges, medications, allergies, and many others. In this stage, hardware is purchased and installed, including point-of-care workstations if needed, central servers, and backup equipment. This process can be time consuming and tedious but ultimately makes the system usable for a specific institution.

Test Once the build is complete, it needs to be thoroughly tested. Typically, systems are initially tested by the vendor implementation team and the institution IT staff, and then detailed screen testing and use case testing is performed by selected end users of the system. The testing should cover as many use cases and workflow scenarios as possible to uncover bugs in the system and prevent surprises when the system is live and running in a real clinical or operational environment. Rigorous testing ensures that every data element on every screen is tested in as many combinations as possible. Load testing is done to ensure that when multiple users are performing the same task, the system does not deteriorate. Performance testing ensures that response times are to specifications. Disaster preparedness plans are tested to ensure that backup systems are functioning properly.

Train After adequate testing, the all end users of the system must be trained on the system. Training should be concise, focusing on broad concepts of navigating and documenting. Well-designed systems do not take an overwhelming amount of training for users to grasp basic concepts and be able to function within the system. Many specific questions can then be answered during the initial go-live.

Go-Live Go-live is the culmination of all the hard work put in by the implementation team. The hope is that the effort expended during the previous phases makes for a smooth go-live with satisfied end users. The reality is that issues always arise, minor malfunctions are discovered, and some features do not work as planned. A go-live team that is flexible and responsive to end-users is invaluable to making the initial days successful. For inexperienced institutions, vendor implementation teams can provide valuable expertise during these times.

Maintenance and Upgrade The go-live is just the start of the journey. During the life of the software product, maintenance will be required; changes will be made to both the content and features of the system. Newer releases will come out that provide exciting new functionality but may break existing features that users depended on. As the institution becomes familiar with, then inextricably linked to the product, clinicians will start to forget the time when the product was not around.[28]

FUTURE OF ANESTHESIA INFORMATION MANAGEMENT SYSTEMS

AIMS continue to evolve in features and functionality. As software development technology improves, regulatory requirements change, and users continue to work in partnership with vendors on improving the systems, AIMS vendors are incrementally providing better user experiences and more robust software.

VENDOR ENVIRONMENT

Our expectation is that the vendor environment will continue to consolidate. Although this has the potential to stifle innovation and increase bureaucracy, it can also lead to substantially greater investment in a product. The ultimate outcome of vendor consolidation for clinicians and institutions remains to be seen.

DECISION SUPPORT AND INTEGRATION WITH PHYSIOLOGIC MONITORS

A major opportunity for innovation involves the use of advances decision support in AIMS. Currently, vendors provide relatively straightforward decision support functionality with case templates, simple alerts, and reminders. We expect further integration with medication libraries and drug checking to allow systems to provide timely drug interaction warnings, including:

1. Dose range checking
2. Default drug doses based on patient weight
3. Drug/allergy checking
4. Drug/drug reaction checking

In addition, smart alarms that collect information from multiple devices to help alert the user regarding catastrophic emergencies have developed as research tools and may be on the horizon for commercial products as well. Links to evidence are currently found on many Computerized Physician Order Entry products and should start to be seen in AIMS products as well.

STANDARDIZATION OF CONTENT AND DATA EXTRACTS

The information entered and stored in AIMS is valuable for many reasons, one of which is the opportunity to aggregate and analyze the information to improve the quality of care. Data entered into a system may reflect similar clinical concepts but be entered differently. For example, one user may enter the term *sleep apnea* and the other *OSA*. Content standardization efforts aim to create consistency in data to allow large-scale aggregation and analysis of data. Terminology standards like SNOMED CT already exist.[29] We expect upcoming versions of AIMS to have functionality that allows institutions to map their existing clinical terms to terminology standards like SNOMED CT. This will allow for enhanced interoperability of systems. Benefits include:

1. Ability to conduct large-scale population studies of adverse events using data from multiple institutions.
2. Ability to share quality improvement or other reports between institutions.
3. Ability to interface with other systems in less time with lower expense.

FEATURES AND FUNCTIONALITY

Continued advancement is general features and functionality can be expected. More widespread use of touchscreen and multitouch navigation can be incorporated with current technology. Voice recognition technology is being used in research settings and will hopefully move to commercial availability.[30] Greater use of biometric authentication, barcode technology, and RFID will enhance the user experience. Greater focus on screen layout ergonomics will make the information easier to process. Better search technology will allow quicker documentation of data that references libraries, such as medications and allergies. Finally, more robust networking and processing hardware should allow for faster screen changes and increased speed of documentation.

SUMMARY

PIMS have 2 main components: AIMS and ORMIS. They are available from commercial vendors as (1) part of an enterprise EMR, (2) packaged together as part of a PIMS, or (3) as separate systems with varying levels of integration. They are used to help manage both the documentation and the workflow that OR personnel encounter every day. AIMS have been used for more than 30 years, first as rudimentary record keepers, now as active assistants to anesthesiologists, researchers, and billing staff. The complexity of implementations of these systems has increased as the complexities of the systems have increased. Although the core functionality of AIMS and ORMIS continues to evolve and be updated, the greatest opportunity lies in the standardization of content and resultant large-scale aggregation and analysis of data. Most anesthesiologists still document the anesthetic record on paper, but the day when paper will be the exception and not the norm is approaching. How quickly and with what type of response from the anesthesiology community will largely be determined by carefully applying the lessons learned from those using the systems today.

KEY REFERENCES

- Kheterpal S. Architecture. In: Stonemetz J, Ruskin K, eds. *Anesthesia Informatics.* London, UK: Springer; 2008:147-165.
- Reeves C, Stonemetz, J. Automated charge capture. In: Stonemetz J, Ruskin K, eds. *Anesthesia Informatics.* London, UK: Springer; 2008: 269-294.
- Reynolds, M. Device interfaces. In: Stonemetz J, Ruskin K, eds. *Anesthesia Informatics.* London, UK: Springer; 2008:109-143.
- Ritchie G, Robinson ST. Implementation of an AIMS. In: Stonemetz J, Ruskin K, eds. *Anesthesia Informatics.* London, UK: Springer; 2008:49-66.
- Shah, N, O'Reilly M. Intraoperative charting requirements. In: Stonemetz J, Ruskin K, eds. *Anesthesia Informatics.* London, UK: Springer; 2008:191-208.
- Vigoda MM, O'Reilly M, Gencorelli FJ, Lubarsky DA. Decision support. In: Stonemetz J, Ruskin K, eds. *Anesthesia Informatics.* London, UK: Springer; 2008:295-310.
- Wilson M. Components of an ORMS. In: Stonemetz J, Ruskin K, eds. *Anesthesia Informatics.* London, UK: Springer; 2008:333-344.

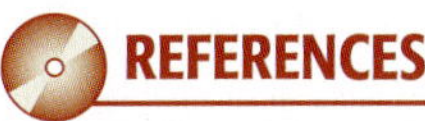

REFERENCES

Complete references available on DVD and online version at www.LongneckerAnesthesiology.com

CHAPTER 30

Hemodynamic Monitoring

Shahar Bar-Yosef
Rebecca A. Schroeder
Jonathan B. Mark

KEY POINTS

1. When interpreting invasive hemodynamic pressures, consideration should be given to technical aspects including the zero reference level, dynamic response of the monitoring system, and effects of changes in intrathoracic pressures.
2. Much diagnostic information can be gleaned from the analog waveform of directly measured pressures, both arterial blood pressure and cardiac filling pressures.
3. Interpretation of filling pressures like central venous pressure (CVP) and pulmonary artery occlusion pressure (PAOP) is confounded by many variables, notably changes in ventricular compliance, valvular abnormalities, and positive pressure ventilation.
4. Pulmonary artery catheter monitoring without a structured therapeutic intervention protocol has generally not been found to be beneficial in most perioperative and critical care settings. It might still be justified in very high-risk patients or in critically ill patients who do not respond to empiric therapy.
5. There are no accepted gold standards for cardiac output measurement. It is more clinically useful to follow trends in cardiac output rather than considering absolute values.
6. Functional indices based on respiratory variation in hemodynamic parameters are better predictors of fluid responsiveness compared with static filling pressures or volumetric indices.
7. Metabolic indices like lactate, base excess, and venous oxygen saturation should be included in the hemodynamic assessment of the critically ill patient.
8. Preemptive goal directed therapy, aimed at optimization of hemodynamic goals before and during surgery, has been found to decrease mortality in high-risk surgical patients and decrease morbidity in moderate-risk patients.

INTRODUCTION

One can ascribe the birth of hemodynamic monitoring to the British anesthesiologist Joseph T. Clover (1825-1882), who emphasized the need to have one's finger on the pulse while giving chloroform anesthesia (**Fig. 30-1**).[1] The word "monitor" originated in the Latin word *monere*, meaning "to warn." Indeed, one of the more commonly associated roles of monitoring devices is to alert the anesthetist of changes in patient condition. However, an additional goal of "monitoring" relates to regulation and control: The anesthetist uses information gleaned from the monitors to modify therapeutic interventions and then uses the monitors again to gauge the effect of these interventions, and so on, in a continual feedback-control loop.[2] For the patient to gain benefit from the monitor used, several conditions must be fulfilled. First, monitoring data need to be correctly interpreted; both the technical and physiologic aspects of the monitor need to be perfectly understood by the physician-user. Second, effective clinical interventions should exist to treat the underlying problem. Third, risks associated with the monitor itself should be recognized and minimized. Monitor information not followed by effective interventions will not benefit the patient, and information that is mistakenly interpreted can even lead to patient harm by prompting wrong interventions.[3]

This chapter describes the technical and physiologic principles behind the more commonly used perioperative hemodynamic monitors, present existing data regarding their accuracy and usefulness, and it then suggests a cognitive framework for using these monitors to answer specific clinical questions.

ARTERIAL BLOOD PRESSURE MONITORING

BACKGROUND

Blood pressure is the vital sign that describes the driving force for perfusion and is the major determinant of left ventricular afterload. Accurate, reliable, and timely measurement of arterial blood pressure (ABP) is crucial for the care of critically ill patients and those undergoing surgical procedures. ABP can be measured accurately with invasive and noninvasive methods, but both are subject to artifacts that could result in inappropriate therapy and patient injury.

NONINVASIVE ARTERIAL BLOOD PRESSURE MEASUREMENT

The auscultatory method for measuring ABP is based on the work of Korotkoff, who described the series of distinct sounds produced by the return of blood flow through the artery during cuff deflation. This method has a variety of limitations, including reliance on pulsatile blood flow and inaccuracy in conditions of extreme vasodilatation or vasoconstriction.[4] Accurate noninvasive blood pressure (NIBP) measurement requires appropriate placement and sizing of the cuff. The bladder midpoint should be positioned over the relevant artery and the cuff wrapped snugly enough to allow only 2 fingers to fit comfortably underneath.[5]

Automated NIBP measurement has been based on the oscillotonometric technique, in which the point of maximal cuff pressure fluctuation corresponds to mean arterial pressure (MAP).[6] The algorithms by which systolic and diastolic pressures are determined vary among device manufacturers, but in general, these correspond to points of rapidly increasing and decreasing oscillations, respectively (**Fig. 30-2**). The time required for a complete cycle makes NIBP monitoring unsuitable for most critically ill patients. However, rapidly cycling "STAT" modes that provide only MAP values have been shown to have good discriminative power in identifying hypotensive patients.[7]

INVASIVE ARTERIAL BLOOD PRESSURE MEASUREMENT

Theory and Background Direct ABP measurement from a catheterized peripheral artery remains the gold standard for care of hemodynamically unstable patients. The dynamic response of the catheter-transducer system is best characterized by 2 physical properties: natural frequency and damping coefficient. Natural frequency describes how rapidly a system oscillates following a stimulus, and the damping coefficient describes how quickly it returns to rest. When the pressure monitoring system has too low a natural frequency, it will resonate and cause overestimation ("overshoot") of true ABP. Underdamped systems further exaggerate high- and low-pressure values and produce artifactual peaks and troughs in the displayed waveform. In contrast, overdamped systems display waveforms devoid of detail with artifactually attenuated peaks and troughs.

The dynamic response of the monitoring system can be assessed quickly with the "fast-flush test," which allows quantitative determination of the natural frequency and damping coefficient (**Fig. 30-3**).[8] In most clinical circumstances, satisfactory system dynamic response exists when the rapid flush results in one large and one small oscillation followed by a return to baseline. Based on the fast-flush test, one can determine whether changes in the monitoring system (eg, reducing the length of extension tubing, removing stopcocks, removing clots or air bubbles) would likely improve natural frequency and decrease resonance of the system. For all invasive pressure monitoring systems, a zero reference value must be established, usually at the upper border of the heart and best estimated in a supine patient at a point approximately 5 cm below the sternal border in the fourth intercostal space.[9]

The Arterial Blood Pressure Waveform The systemic arterial pressure waveform results from forceful ejection of blood from the left ventricle during systole, runoff into the peripheral vessels during diastole,

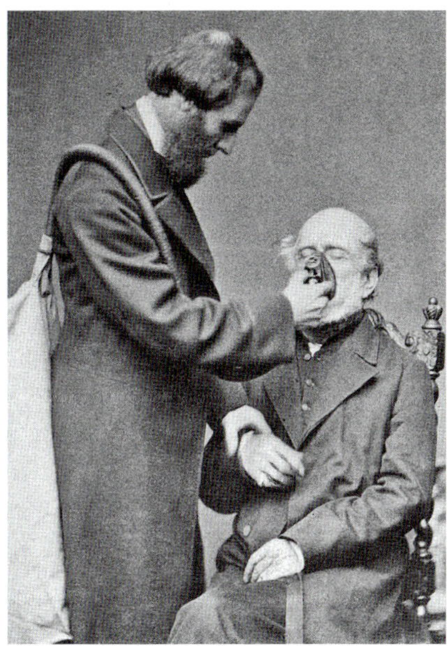

FIGURE 30-1. Joseph T. Clover (1825-1882), a pioneer of monitoring during anesthesia. [Reproduced with permission from the Wellcome Library, London.]

and reflectance of waveform energy from the peripheral circulation (**Fig. 30-4**).[10] As a consequence, ABP waveform morphology differs as the monitoring site moves distally, a phenomenon known as distal pulse amplification. Distal ABP tracings have a wider pulse pressure, delayed upstroke, delayed and slurred dicrotic notch, and a more prominent diastolic wave. Beyond these normal physiologic variations, large pressure gradients may exist between central and peripheral sites in patients in shock and following cardiopulmonary bypass.[11,12]

Specific waveform morphologic patterns have been described that may provide useful diagnostic information in pathologic states (**Fig. 30-5**). Other uses of the ABP waveform include noninvasive measures of cardiac output as well as systolic pressure variation and its derived indices (described later).

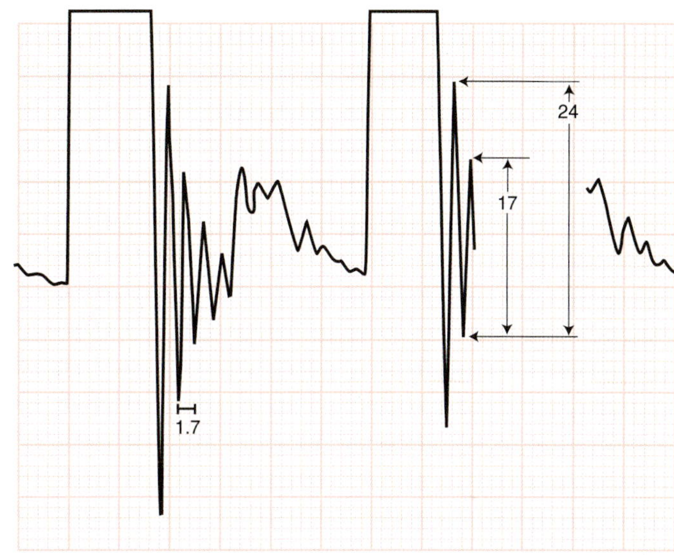

FIGURE 30-3. The "flush test" used to estimate natural frequency and damping coefficient of an invasive pressure monitoring system. A square-wave artifact is created by temporarily opening the flush system, then allowing the monitoring system to return to "resting" state. Natural frequency is calculated as the recording paper speed (25 mm/s) divided by the length of 1 cycle between 2 adjacent pressure oscillation peaks (1.7 mm in this example, resulting in a natural frequency of 14.7 Hz). The damping coefficient is inversely related to the amplitude ratio of 2 adjacent oscillation peaks. [Modified with permission from Gardner RM. Direct blood pressure measurement-dynamic response requirements. *Anesthesiology*. 1981;54(3):227-236.]

Insertion Technique The most common site for monitoring ABP is the radial artery due to its ease of access and low complication rate, although the arterial catheterization procedure is similar regardless of the target vessel. For radial artery cannulation, the wrist should be in the neutral or slightly dorsiflexed position to prevent median nerve or vessel compression. The skin is cleansed with chlorhexidine, and a local anesthetic

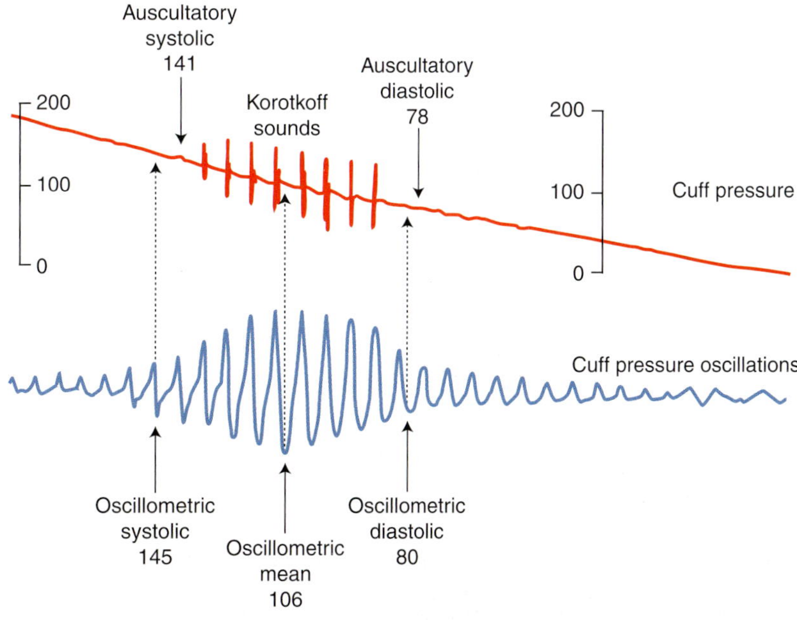

FIGURE 30-2. Noninvasive measurement of blood pressure. In the auscultatory method, systolic and diastolic pressures are determined by the beginning and end of Korotkoff sounds. In the oscillometric technique, the mean blood pressure is the primary measured variable, determined as the point of maximal oscillations in cuff pressure. The exact algorithm used to determine systolic and diastolic pressures varies. [Reproduced with permission of the author from Geddes LA. *Cardiovascular Devices and Their Applications.* New York, NY: John Wiley; 1984:Fig. 3-6).

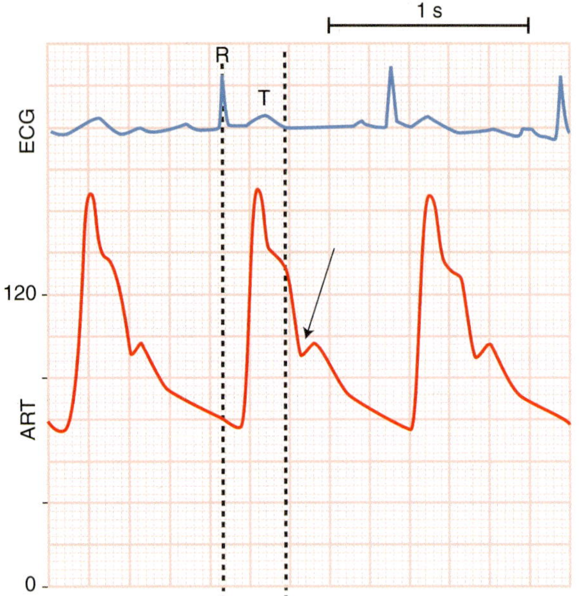

FIGURE 30-4. Normal arterial pressure waveform with sharp systolic upstroke, a peak, and a well-defined dicrotic notch (arrow). Note that the upstroke follows the R wave on the electrocardiogram trace due to the short delay between electrical and mechanical systole.

is injected into the skin and around the artery to anesthetize the site and reduce the risk of arterial spasm. Integrated needle-guide wire-catheter assemblies are frequently used in adults. The angle of needle entry should be shallow and in line with the course of the artery. When blood flows into the reservoir, the wire is advanced into the artery, and the catheter then passed over the wire. The wire should thread without resistance, and the catheter should pass smoothly and painlessly. Some practitioners prefer to place arterial lines without use of a guidewire, threading the catheter directly into the vessel upon appearance of the blood "flash" through the needle hub.[13] If smooth passage into the vessel lumen does not occur, a through-and-through method may salvage the procedure. The needle/catheter assembly is advanced through the back wall of the vessel, the needle removed, and the catheter pulled back slowly until brisk pulsatile flow is obtained through the catheter. At this point, the catheter may be advanced into the artery or a guidewire inserted and the catheter advanced over the wire.

If the radial artery cannot be cannulated successfully, an alternative site must be sought. One should be cautious using the ipsilateral ulnar artery. Many have raised concerns about cannulation of the brachial artery owing to the lack of collateral circulation at this location, but large clinical studies have confirmed its safety.[14] Other possible targets include the dorsalis pedis, axillary, and femoral arteries.

Indications for Invasive Arterial Blood Pressure Monitoring Current standards for intraoperative monitoring require measurement of the blood pressure at least every 5 minutes.[15] Despite traditional teaching that intraoperative blood pressure liability does not result in worse

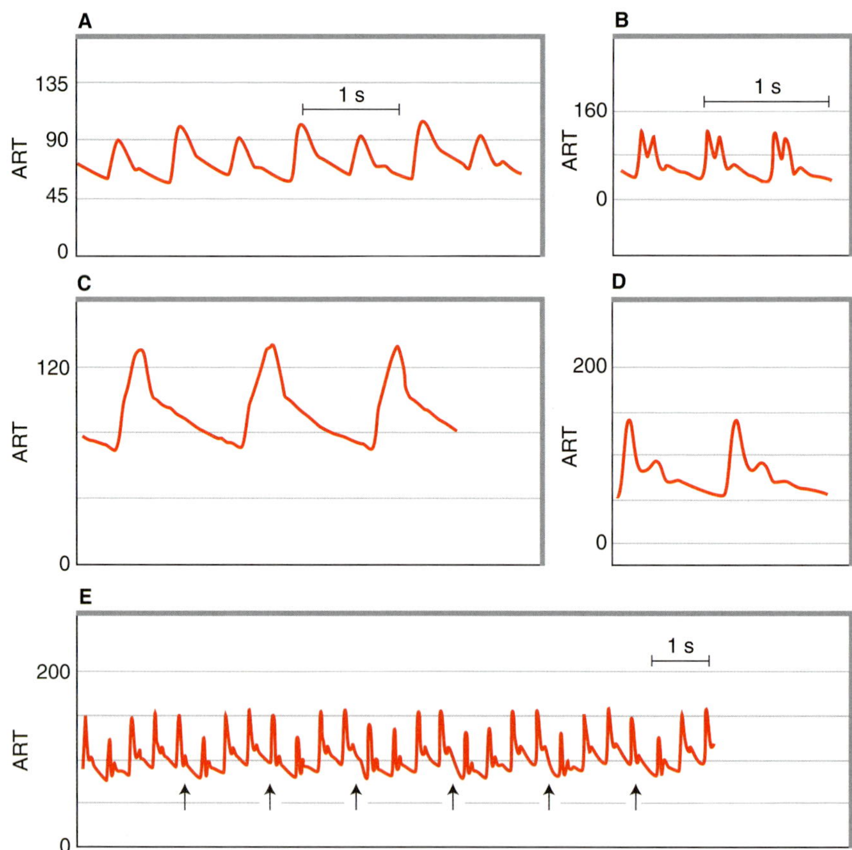

FIGURE 30-5. Pathologic arterial waveforms. **A.** Pulsus alternans: alternating higher and lower systolic peaks, most often associated with severely depressed ventricular function. **B.** Pulsus bisferiens: characterized by a double systolic peak, low diastolic pressure, and a wide pulse pressure, usually indicating severe aortic regurgitation. **C.** Pulsus parvus and tardus: slurred upstroke with a delayed systolic peak, characteristic of severe aortic stenosis. **D.** Spike-and-dome configuration characteristic of hypertrophic obstructive cardiomyopathy, with a normal systolic upstroke but wide delayed dicrotic notch and prolonged ejection phase. **E.** Pulsus paradoxus: cycles of increasing and decreasing systolic blood pressure related to the respiratory cycle (arrows point to onset of inspiration during spontaneous ventilation). In this example, the degree of variation is approximately 35-40 mm Hg. [Reproduced with permission from Mark JB. *Atlas of Cardiovascular Monitoring*. New York, NY: Churchill Livingstone; 1998:Figs. 17.22, 17.24, and 18.10.]

outcome following elective surgery, some clinical evidence indicates that, especially in elderly patients, intraoperative blood pressure variability or large changes from preoperative values are indeed associated with postoperative complications.[16-18]

Direct invasive monitoring of ABP is indicated in cases when large moment-to-moment blood pressure changes are anticipated or when coexisting medical conditions, abrupt blood loss, or large fluid shifts are likely to cause sudden cardiovascular changes. Occasionally, invasive ABP monitoring is performed when noninvasive methods are unreliable or technically difficult. These situations include morbid obesity, burn or trauma patients who have no suitable site for cuff placement, or a patient whose dysrhythmias preclude adequate function of automated noninvasive blood pressure devices. A frequent need to measure arterial blood gases is another indication for invasive arterial cannulation.

Complications of Blood Pressure Monitoring Even a monitoring modality as seemingly innocuous as NIBP measurement is not without risk, although reported complications are rare. Most have followed high-frequency or prolonged periods of cuff inflation, or they have occurred in patients receiving anticoagulation and have resulted in either local trauma or impaired perfusion to the distal extremity.[19] Likewise, peripheral arterial cannulation has been shown to be relatively safe, with a risk of ischemic complications of less than 0.1%.[20] The Allen test, which purports to examine the integrity of the ulnar collateral circulation, is not considered a reliable predictor of ischemic complications following arterial cannulation.[21] Other complications include air or catheter embolism, thrombosis, hematoma formation, vessel injury, blood loss from tubing disconnection, unintentional arterial injection of drugs, and contamination of samples drawn from the arterial line.[20,22] Of note, arterial thrombosis and limb ischemia following femoral or brachial arterial cannulation have been reported predominantly in infants.[20]

CENTRAL VENOUS PRESSURE MONITORING

THE NORMAL CENTRAL VENOUS PRESSURE

Central venous pressure (CVP), or right atrial pressure (RAP), is ideally measured at the junction of the superior vena cava (SVC) and the right atrium (RA), and it reflects the balance between intravascular volume, venous capacitance, and right ventricular (RV) function. In a healthy, spontaneously breathing subject, normal mean CVP ranges between 1 and 7 mm Hg. A normal CVP waveform is displayed in **Fig. 30-6**. It is composed of 3 waves and 2 descents: the *c* wave, *x* descent, and *v* wave occur during ventricular systole, and the *y* descent and *a* wave occur during ventricular diastole (**Table 30-1**). Identification of each wave is easiest when the CVP trace is aligned with the electrocardiogram (ECG) and the ECG R wave is marked to indicate end-diastole. Use of the ABP trace to identify the CVP waves may lead to confusion due to the delay between electrical depolarization and onset of the ABP systolic upstroke. Note that flow from the vena cavae into the RA is greatest when RAP is the lowest (ie, during the *x* and *y* descents). This relationship is responsible for the pattern seen when the hepatic veins are examined with spectral Doppler echocardiography. A similar relationship between left atrial pressure and pulmonary venous flow velocity exists on the left side of the heart.

THE ABNORMAL CVP

Analysis of the CVP waveform can assist in making a variety of clinical diagnoses.[23] Specific dysrhythmias cause unique patterns that are easily interpreted when the underlying physiologic disturbance is kept in mind (**Fig. 30-7**). Atrial fibrillation is recognizable by the absence of the *a* wave and a prominent *c-v* wave. Atrioventricular (AV) nodal rhythms can result in cannon *a* waves that result from retrograde conduction of the cardiac impulse from the AV node to the atrium, producing atrial contraction against a closed tricuspid valve during ventricular systole. Similar cannon waves may be detected during any form of AV

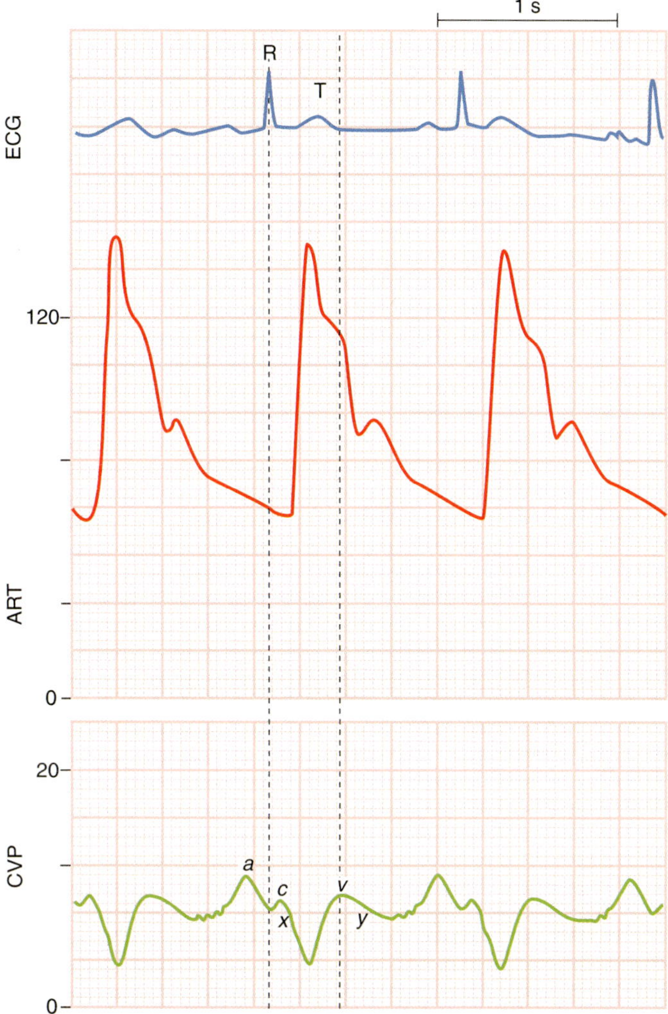

FIGURE 30-6. Normal central venous pressure (CVP) and arterial pressure (ART) waveforms. The diastolic (*a* wave, *y* descent) and systolic (*c* and *v* waves, *x* descent) components of the CVP waveform are noted. Clear identification of venous waveform components is aided by the electrocardiogram (ECG) waveform timing. [Reproduced with permission from Mark JB. *Atlas of Cardiovascular Monitoring*. New York, NY: Churchill Livingstone; 1998:Fig. 2.5.]

dissociation, including ventricular pacing. Effective restoration of AV synchrony with atrial or AV pacing can be confirmed by reappearance of a normal CVP trace.

Disorders of the tricuspid valve can also affect the CVP waveform (**Fig. 30-8**). Severe tricuspid regurgitation results in a broad, tall systolic *c-v* wave (often termed a regurgitant *v* wave), resembling a RV pressure

TABLE 30-1 Components of the Normal Central Venous Pressure Waveform

Waveform Component	Cardiac Cycle Phase	Causative Mechanical Event
a wave	End diastole	Atrial contraction
c wave	Early systole	Isovolumic ventricular contraction
x descent	Mid systole	Atrial relaxation and descent of the base of the heart
v wave	Late systole	Systolic filling of the atrium
y descent	Early diastole	Opening of the atrioventricular valve

Modified with permission from Mark JB. *Atlas of Cardiovascular Monitoring*. New York, NY: Churchill Livingstone; 1998:Table 2.2

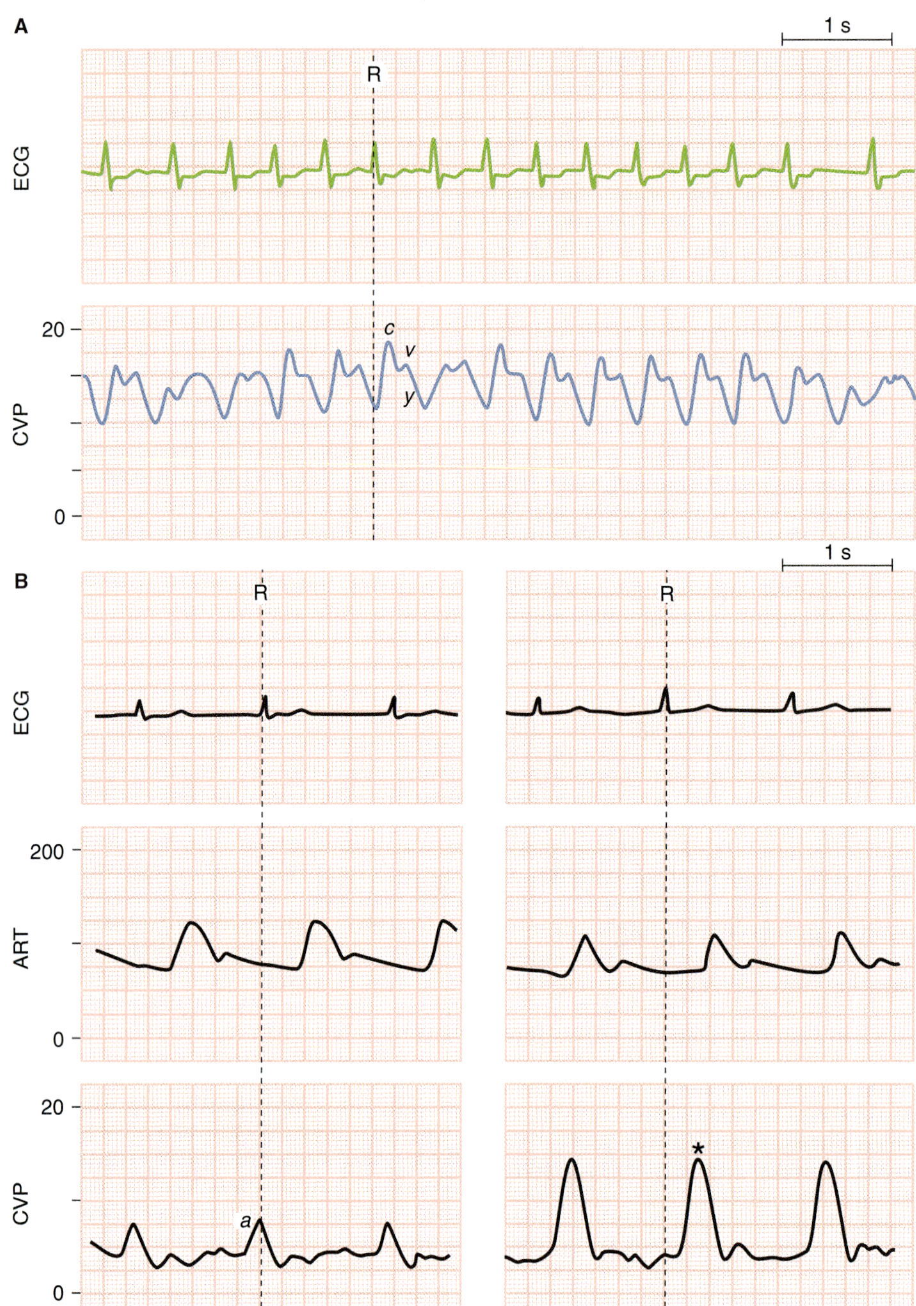

FIGURE 30-7. Effect of dysrhythmias on the central venous pressure (CVP) waveforms. **A.** Atrial fibrillation: Irregular R-R interval leads to an inconsistent CVP waveform, absent *a* wave, and prominent *c-v* wave complex. **B.** Atrioventricular dissociation: Early systolic cannon *a* waves (marked by *) result from atrial contraction against a closed tricuspid valve. ART, arterial pressure; ECG, electrocardiogram. [Reproduced with permission from Mark JB. *Atlas of Cardiovascular Monitoring*. New York, NY: Churchill Livingstone; 1998:Figs. 14.1 and 14.5.]

waveform. In contrast, tricuspid stenosis produces a tall end-diastolic *a* wave and an attenuated early diastolic *y* descent.

In combination with data from the pulmonary artery catheter, the CVP waveform is also useful for diagnosis of other conditions, including right ventricular ischemia, cardiac tamponade, and constrictive pericarditis (see Fig. 30-13).

INSERTION TECHNIQUE

Cannulation of a central vein is necessary for measurement of CVP and for placement of a pulmonary artery catheter or transvenous pacing wire. A variety of sites are available, including femoral, subclavian, internal and external jugular, and even the large antecubital veins. Among anesthesiologists, the internal jugular (IJ) vein approach is the most common due to its ease of access in the operating room and its optimal location for placement of a pulmonary artery catheter. In contrast, the subclavian vein approach is often preferred for long-term access or in the intensive care unit (ICU) due to increased patient comfort and lower infection rate.[24]

During IJ cannulation, one must rely on either superficial anatomic landmarks or imaging techniques to locate the vessel, which usually lies lateral and slightly superficial to the carotid artery (CA). To approach the right IJ, the patient is positioned supine, with mild head-down tilt, and with the head turned slightly to the left. Ultrasound studies have shown that rotation of the head greater than 40° increases overlap of IJ and CA, increasing the risk of arterial puncture.[25] Appropriate aseptic technique is important and includes chlorhexidine-alcohol skin preparation and

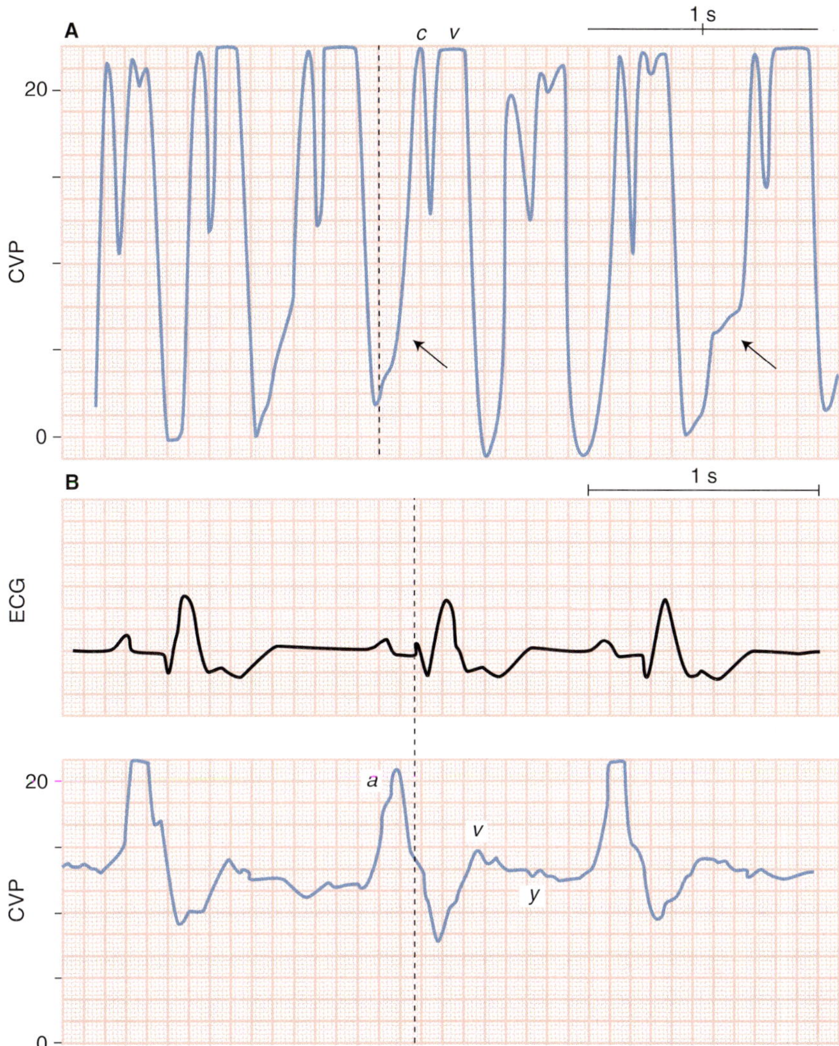

FIGURE 30-8. Effect of tricuspid valve pathology on the central venous pressure (CVP) waveform. **A.** Tricuspid regurgitation: high mean CVP with tall *c-v* wave complex and minimal *x* descent. End-diastolic CVP (arrow) is a better indicator of right ventricle filling than mean CVP. **B.** Tricuspid stenosis: high mean CVP with prominent *a* wave, deep *x* descent, and minimal *v* wave and *y* descent. ECG, electrocardiogram. [Reproduced with permission from Mark JB. *Atlas of Cardiovascular Monitoring.* New York, NY: Churchill Livingstone; 1998:Figs. 17.3 and 17.5.]

full body drape for the patient, and handwashing, mask, gown, gloves, and cap for the operator.[24]

There are a variety of approaches to catheterizing the IJ vein using landmark-based techniques, with the anterior approach the most common and reliable.[26] The CA is palpated with the fingertips of the left hand, the skin is anesthetized near the apex of the triangle formed by the 2 heads of the sternocleidomastoid muscle, and a small-gauge finder needle is then used to locate the vessel. It is common to get the "flash" of blood on withdrawal of the needle rather than on needle insertion, which often compresses the IJ vein as it is advanced.

After location of the vein with the finder needle, an 18-gauge thin-walled needle attached to a syringe is inserted with constant aspiration. On entering the vessel, the syringe is removed, a guidewire is inserted through the needle, and the needle removed. The ECG should be monitored for dysrhythmias during wire manipulation that may cause atrial or ventricular irritation. As an alternative to the thin-walled needle, a 2-in 18-gauge catheter may be used to enter the vessel. With this technique, the catheter is threaded into the vessel, the needle removed, and the guidewire inserted through the catheter. Confirmation of venous rather than arterial cannulation may be accomplished in one of several ways. Detection of pulsatile blood through the thin-walled needle identifies unintended cannulation of an artery but is unreliable as the sole mean of confirming venous location of the needle tip. In addition, when using the 18-gauge catheter to cannulate the IJ vein, attachment of a length of intravenous tubing to measure the intravascular pressure before placement of the guidewire is a common and effective safety check.[27] After confirmation of venous cannulation, the skin, subcutaneous tissues, and vessel opening are dilated, and the catheter is placed. A small skin incision facilitates insertion of the catheter and prevents damage to its leading edge. However, care should be taken with passage of the vessel dilator because it is large, stiff, and capable of perforating or tearing the vessel.

The development of portable ultrasound devices has revolutionized the process of central line placement, and in many institutions, it is now standard of care to use dynamic ultrasound guidance during these procedures.[28] Advantages are many, and include the ability to directly visualize the target vessel as well as the surrounding anatomy and confirm the presence of the guidewire in that vessel.[29,30] In addition, use of ultrasound guidance has been shown to decrease the time required for IJ catheterization, the number of attempts required, and the overall complication rate.[31-33] It is important to note, however, that use of ultrasound has not completely prevented arterial injury.[34-36] Focused training, educational efforts, and equipment investment are required for results to be realized.

BOX 30-1

Indications for Central Venous Line Placement

Monitoring

- Central venous pressure monitoring
- Pulmonary artery catheterization
- Frequent blood sampling

Therapeutic Intervention

- Hemodialysis
- Temporary transvenous pacing
- Aspiration of air emboli (eg, sitting position craniotomy)
- Infusion of vasoactive drugs or total parenteral nutrition
- Cannulae placement (eg, venovenous bypass, portosystemic shunt)
- Inadequate peripheral venous access (obesity, burns, postchemotherapy)

INDICATIONS FOR CENTRAL VENOUS CATHETERIZATION

Box 30-1 lists the indications for central venous catheterization. The main indication for monitoring CVP is as a guide for volume status assessment and fluid resuscitation. Once in place, it may be used for additional purposes such as for obtaining repeated blood samples.

COMPLICATIONS OF CENTRAL VENOUS CATHETERIZATION

Complications arising from a central venous catheter can generally be separated into those arising from the placement of the catheter itself and those that develop while the catheter is in place and in use (**Box 30-2**). However, for all central vein cannulation sites, vascular injury is the most common complication and can result in a wide range of clinical sequelae, from undetectable hematoma to life-threatening cardiac tamponade. Risk for cardiac perforation and tamponade can be minimized by ensuring the catheter tip is located at the level of the carina or higher on a chest radiograph.[37] Unintentional placement of a large-bore catheter into a central artery should prompt consultation with a vascular surgeon. Respiratory compromise can develop from several sources, including embolism of air or clot, pneumothorax, direct airway injury from the needle, or airway compression from arterial bleeding or expanding hematoma. Catheter-related infections range from local skin infection to life-threatening sepsis or endocarditis. In an attempt to decrease infectious complications, specific recommendations have been published by the Centers for Disease Control and Prevention (**Box 30-3**).[24] Furthermore, evidence from large clinical trials have demonstrated the power of bundling several interventions to reduce catheter-related bloodstream infections: handwashing, full barrier precautions, avoiding the femoral site, chlorhexidine skin preparation, and removing unnecessary catheters.[38]

BOX 30-2

Complications of Central Venous Catheterization

Secondary to catheter placement:

- Airway or lung injury (pneumothorax, subcutaneous or mediastinal emphysema)
- Bleeding (subcutaneous/retroperitoneal hematoma, hemothorax)
- Chylothorax
- Arterial injury/cannulation
- Air embolism
- Nerve injury
- Catheter shearing/embolism
- Dysrhythmias

Secondary to in situ catheter:

- Dysrhythmias
- Hydrothorax/hydromediastinum
- Thromboembolism (superior vena cava syndrome, pulmonary embolism)
- Infections (cellulitis, bacteremia, sepsis, endocarditis)
- Vascular/cardiac perforation (arteriovenous or venobronchial fistula, cardiac tamponade)

BOX 30-3

Recommended Measures to Decrease Catheter-Related Infections

- Adequate training of physicians and nurses
- Avoiding femoral vein catheterization
- Use of full sterile technique for catheter insertion (including cap, mask, gown, sterile gloves, and drapes)
- Chlorhexidine rather then povidone-iodine for skin preparation
- Use of heparin-bonded catheters
- Removal of catheters as early as possible

THE PULMONARY ARTERY CATHETER

BACKGROUND

A landmark article in 1970 described the clinical use of a balloon-tipped, flow-directed pulmonary artery catheter (PAC) for treatment of patients with acute myocardial infarction.[39] Since then, use of the PAC rapidly spread as an important monitoring tool for treatment of high-risk surgical and critically ill patients. Numerous studies have shown that standard clinical measurements such as heart rate, blood pressure, and urine output do not always allow early identification of inadequate perfusion states, and experienced clinicians are often wrong in their assessment of the circulatory profile of critically ill patients.[40] Therefore, monitoring using the PAC often reveals new information that should be helpful in diagnosis and management of various hemodynamic disturbances, and guiding fluid and vasoactive drug therapy. However, studies have demonstrated widespread deficiencies both in interpretation of the hemodynamic waveforms[41] as well as in choosing appropriate therapeutic interventions.[3,42]

These studies have led to increasing emphasis on training requirements by the American Society of Anesthesiologists (ASA), Society of Critical Care Medicine, and the National Institute of Health.[43-45] Widespread difficulties with interpretation and application of PAC data confounds evaluation of PAC clinical outcome studies and might explain in part the discrepant results and failure to show benefit in many trials.[46] Correct insertion technique, awareness of indications and complications, and understanding of the physiologic principles involved are all prerequisites for gaining any clinical benefit from use of the PAC.

INSERTION TECHNIQUE

The current PAC for use in adults is 110 cm in length, contains 3 or 4 lumens, and has an embedded thermistor and a 1.5-mL balloon at the tip. The catheter is inserted through a 1-way valve on a large-bore introducer placed into a central vein.

The right IJ vein affords the most direct path for inserting the PAC into the right heart chambers. The left subclavian vein is an alternative choice because the catheter follows the natural curve of the brachiocephalic vein into the superior vena cava. Other routes, including more peripheral sites such as the femoral vein or even a large arm vein, can be used, but catheter positioning might be more difficult, and limited intraoperative access will hinder needed adjustments. Once the catheter is inserted through the introducer to a depth of 20 cm, the balloon at the tip is filled with 1.5 mL air to help float the catheter into the pulmonary

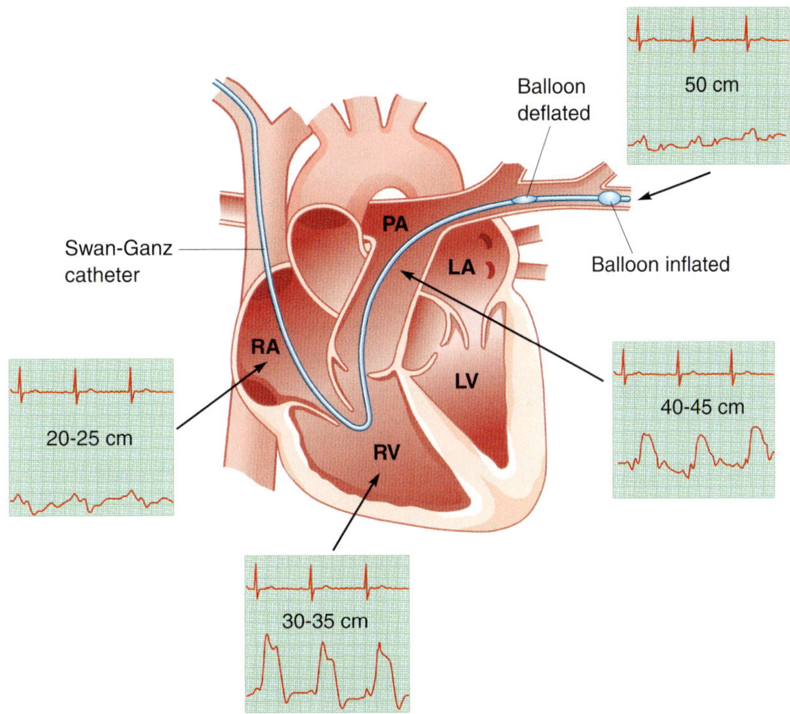

FIGURE 30-9. Pressure waveforms recorded by the pulmonary artery catheter. As the catheter is advanced from the venous cannulation site, the first waveform recorded will be the central venous pressure trace. Passage of the catheter from the right atrium (RA) into the right ventricle (RV) is accompanied by a marked increase in "systolic" pressure. As the catheter tip enters the pulmonary artery (PA), a dicrotic notch may appear in the systolic wave and the diastolic pressure will increase in magnitude and will be downsloping in contrast to the upsloping diastolic pressure in the right ventricle (RV). With further advancement of the catheter, the balloon will occlude blood flow and the tip will record the pulmonary artery occlusion pressure, characterized by disappearance of the "systolic" pressure wave and reappearance of venous *a, c,* and *v* waves. Numbers show the approximate depth when inserting the PAC from the right internal jugular vein. [Modified with permission from Mark JB. *Atlas of Cardiovascular Monitoring*. New York, NY: Churchill Livingstone; 1998:Fig. 3.1.]

artery. Although catheter guidance depends both on balloon flotation as well as blood flow direction, the former is by far the more important.[47] Therefore, patient positioning can influence the ease with which the catheter passes through the heart: A combination of head elevation with patient tilt to the right will place the right ventricular infundibulum and pulmonary valve in a nondependent position and aids flotation into the pulmonary artery.[48]

Identification of correct catheter positioning depends primarily on monitoring changes in the pressure transduced from the distal port of the PAC (**Fig. 30-9**).

The PAC balloon should not be kept inflated for more than a few seconds at a time because of the risks of pulmonary infarction or pulmonary artery rupture. If the pulmonary artery occlusion pressure (PAOP) waveform appears when less than 1 mL air is added to the balloon, the PAC tip has migrated into a small pulmonary artery branch, and the catheter should be withdrawn immediately to a point where this does not occur.

When PAC insertion proves difficult, or when using the femoral or arm veins as entry sites, either fluoroscopy or transesophageal echocardiography (TEE) can help with visualizing the catheter during insertion (**Fig. 30-10**).[49]

PAC-DERIVED PRESSURE MEASUREMENTS

Once the PAC is in place, several physiologic parameters can be measured, calculated, and derived (**Tables 30-2 and 30-3**). The most important measurements are cardiac output (CO), an index of global perfusion, and PAOP, an index of left ventricular (LV) preload. Additional useful pressure recordings are measured from the right atrium and pulmonary artery. Right ventricular pressure can be measured as the catheter tip is advanced or retracted into the right ventricle. To measure PAOP, the balloon is slowly inflated so that pulmonary blood flow carries the catheter to a "wedged" position. At this point, the balloon obstructs forward blood flow through a medium-size pulmonary artery branch, and a static column of blood is created, connecting the catheter tip to a junction point where flow resumes in the pulmonary veins near the left atrium.[50] Because resistance to flow in the large pulmonary veins is low, the PAOP should provide an accurate estimate of left atrial pressure (LAP). Similar in morphology to the CVP trace,

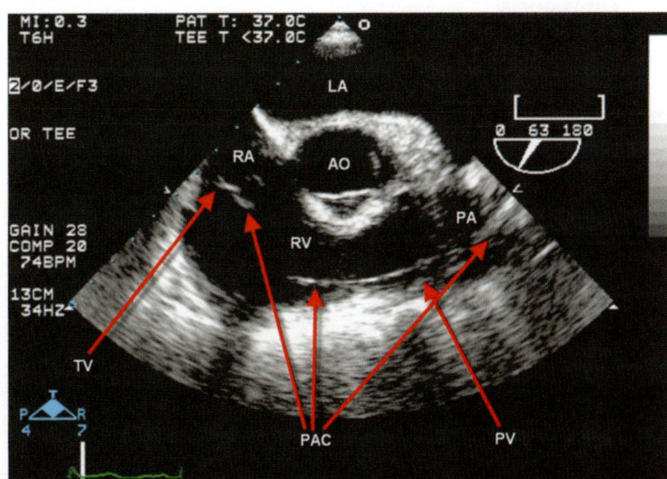

FIGURE 30-10. Midesophageal right ventricle inflow-outflow transesophageal echocardiogram view demonstrating the pulmonary artery catheter (PAC) in the right atrium (RA), right ventricle (RV), and pulmonary artery (PA), traversing the tricuspid valve (TV) and pulmonary valve (PV). Also shown are the left atrium (LA) and aorta (AO).

TABLE 30-2 Hemodynamic Parameters Measured by the Pulmonary Artery Catheter

Measured Parameter	Normal Values	Normal Values Indexed to Body Surface Area
Cardiac output	4-6 L/min	2.8-4.2 L/min per m^2
Central venous pressure	2-7 mm Hg	N/A
Pulmonary artery pressure (systolic/diastolic)	15-30/ 6-15 mm Hg	N/A
Pulmonary artery occlusion pressure	5-12 mm Hg	N/A
Right ventricular ejection fraction	40%-60%	N/A
Mixed venous oxygen saturation	70%-75%	N/A

the PAOP waveform has both *a* and *v* waves that reflect a somewhat delayed and damped LAP waveform. The PAOP is usually reported as a single mean value, whereas the PAOP *a* wave, which just follows the ECG R wave, better reflects preload, which is left ventricular end-diastolic pressure (LVEDP), particularly in patients with left ventricular dysfunction.[51] The mean PAOP, however, is a better estimate of the hydrostatic back pressure that influences pulmonary edema formation. Although the terms *PAOP* and *pulmonary capillary pressure (PCP)* are sometimes used interchangeably, these pressures do not reflect the same physiologic measurement. Because direction of blood flow is from the pulmonary capillaries to the pulmonary veins and thence to the left atrium, true PCP is slightly higher than PAOP and may be significantly higher when either pulmonary venous resistance is elevated, as in acute respiratory distress syndrome (ARDS), or when blood flow is increased.[50]

Factors Affecting Data Validity and Interpretation One of the primary reasons for PAC monitoring is to provide an estimate of left ventricular preload. Physiologically, true preload is the length of the ventricular muscle sarcomere at end-diastole. In the 3-dimensional heart, left ventricular end-diastolic volume (LVEDV) can be considered a global measure of LV preload; however, measurement of this parameter is not readily available clinically. LVEDP can be measured by left heart catheterization, although its relationship to LVEDV depends on left ventricular compliance. Under normal physiologic conditions, upstream pressure measurements of LAP, PAOP, and PA diastolic pressure (PADP), can provide accurate surrogates for LVEDP. However, there are many pathophysiologic conditions in which these surrogate measures of left ventricular preload are subject to error. These are discussed below and are summarized in **Table 30-4.**[50,52]

Artifacts Motion of the PAC tip from ventricular contraction or valve leaflet movements can produce artifactual spikes or troughs in the pressure waveform, termed *catheter whip*. *Overwedging* appears when balloon inflation produces a gradually rising, nonpulsatile pressure that results from the catheter tip being forced against the arterial wall, occluding the distal lumen of the PAC.

Ventricular Compliance Because the pressure-volume relationship of the left ventricle is curvilinear, the same change in ventricular volume can produce either a small or large change in LVEDP, depending on the position on the compliance curve over which the left ventricle is operating. Also, conditions causing a marked shift in the compliance curve may result in pressure and volume changing in opposite directions (**Fig. 30-11**). In the perioperative period, myocardial ischemia, right ventricular failure causing interventricular septal shift, and inotropic drug effects can all induce rapid changes in ventricular compliance.

Catheter Tip Position West et al divided the lung into 3 zones according to gravity-dependent differences in perfusion and ventilation that affect the relationship of pulmonary arterial pressure (P_a), alveolar pressure (P_{alv}), and pulmonary venous pressure (P_v).[53] The PAC tip needs to reside in zone 3 ($P_a > P_v > P_{alv}$) so that a continuous column of blood exists and the pressure measured by the catheter tip will reflect vascular rather than alveolar pressure. In a supine, spontaneously breathing subject, this is rarely a problem. However, with hypovolemia (low P_v) or positive pressure ventilation (high P_{alv}), zone 2 or zone 1 conditions might develop. This may be suspected when the PAOP trace demonstrates excessive respiratory variation in the pressure waveform (**Fig. 30-12**).[54]

Changes in body position also influence the distribution of lung blood flow and the anatomic locations of the different lung zones. This may be an important consideration in a patient who has a PAC inserted while supine but later is positioned in the lateral, prone, or steep head-up or head-down positions.

Ventilatory Pressure Influences With large cyclic variations in intrathoracic pressure, as occurs during labored respiration, coughing, Valsalva maneuver or positive pressure ventilation, both intracardiac and intrapericardial pressures are affected. The PAC will reflect the increased intracardiac pressures, although the true transmural pressure that

TABLE 30-3 Hemodynamic Calculations Derived From Pulmonary Artery Catheter Measurements

Parameter	Formula	Normal Values	Normal Values Indexed to BSA
Stroke volume	Cardiac output/heart rate	60-90 mL	40-60 mL/m^2
Systemic vascular resistance	$\frac{(\text{MAP} - \text{CVP}) \times 80}{\text{Cardiac output}}$	900-1500 dyne·s/cm^5	1600-2400 dyne·s·m^2/cm^5
Pulmonary vascular resistance	$\frac{(\text{mPAP} - \text{PAOP}) \times 80}{\text{Cardiac output}}$	150-200 dyne·s/cm^5	225-320 dyne·s·m^2/cm^5
Left ventricular stroke work	(MAP − PAOP) × stroke volume × 0.0136	60-110 g·m	50-68 g/m
Right ventricular Stroke work	(mPAP − CVP) × stroke volume × 0.0136	8-16 g·m	5-10 g/m
Right ventricular end-diastolic volume	Stroke volume/right ventricular ejection fraction	100-160 mL	60-100 mL/m^2
Oxygen delivery	Cardiac output × Cao_2 × 10	850-1050 mL/min	500-600 mL/min per m^2
Oxygen consumption	Cardiac output × (Cao_2 − Cvo_2) × 10	200-250 mL/min	120-160 mL/min per m^2
Pulmonary shunt fraction	(Pulmonary capillary oxygen content − Cao_2)/ (Pulmonary capillary oxygen content − Cvo_2)	<5%	N/A

BSA, body surface area; MAP, mean arterial pressure; CVP, central venous pressure; mPAP, mean pulmonary artery pressure; PAOP, pulmonary artery occlusion pressure; Cao_2, arterial oxygen content; Cvo_2, mixed venous oxygen content.

TABLE 30-4 Factors Causing Under- and Overestimation of Left Ventricular Preload

Condition	Site of Discrepancy	Cause of Discrepancy
Underestimation		
Aortic regurgitation	LAP < LVEDP	Ventricular filling continues after mitral valve closure
Decreased pulmonary vascular bed	PAOP < LAP	Balloon inflation significantly decreases right ventricular blood flow
Pulmonic regurgitation	PADP < PAOP	Bidirectional runoff for pulmonary artery blood flow
Right bundle branch block	PADP < PAOP	Delayed pulmonary valve opening allows continued fall of PADP
Overestimation		
Decreased left ventricular compliance	LVEDV < LVEDP	Change in pressure-volume relation
Positive pressure ventilation	LVEDP > transmural EDP	
Mitral stenosis/Left atrial myxoma	LAP > LVEDP	Obstruction to flow across mitral valve
Mitral regurgitation	Mean LAP > LVEDP	Retrograde systolic *v* wave
Ventricular septal defect	Mean LAP > LVEDP	Antegrade systolic *v* wave
Tachycardia	PADP > PAOP = LAP > LVEDP	Short diastole creates pressure gradients
Positive end-expiratory pressure	PAOP > LAP	Expansion of West's lung zones 1 or 2
Overwedging	PAOP > LAP	Occlusion of distal catheter lumen
Pulmonary arterial hypertension	PADP > PAOP	Increased pressure gradient over pulmonary circulation

The table lists conditions where PAC-derived estimates for LV preload, such as PADP or PAOP, either overestimate or underestimate LVEDP, and common conditions in which all filling pressures (including LVEDP) provide inaccurate estimates for filling volume or true preload. LAP, left atrial pressure; LVEDP, left ventricular end-diastolic pressure; PAOP, pulmonary artery occlusion pressure; PADP, pulmonary artery diastolic pressure; EDP, end-diastolic pressure.

Modified with permission from Mark JB. *Atlas of Cardiovascular Monitoring*. New York, NY: Churchill Livingstone; 1998:Tables 6.1 and 6.2.

determines cardiac preload has not been changed.[55] Therefore, the PAOP should be measured at end expiration, when intrathoracic pressure approximates atmospheric pressure, whether the patient is breathing spontaneously or is mechanically ventilated. Visual inspection of the waveform display is more accurate than reliance on digital display for identifying end-expiratory pressures. During spontaneous breathing, inspiratory pressures are negative and the end-expiration point corresponds to the higher vascular pressure values. The opposite is true under positive pressure ventilation.

Application of positive end-expiratory pressure (PEEP) also alters intrathoracic pressure and hence PAOP values at end expiration. The magnitude of these effects will depend on the level of PEEP used and the pulmonary and chest wall compliance.[50] As a simple rule of thumb, the increase in measured PAOP is usually less than half the value of the PEEP applied. As lung compliance deteriorates, however, the transmission of airway pressure to the pleural space is attenuated. Therefore the effect of high PEEP, commonly used in these situations, is minimized.[56]

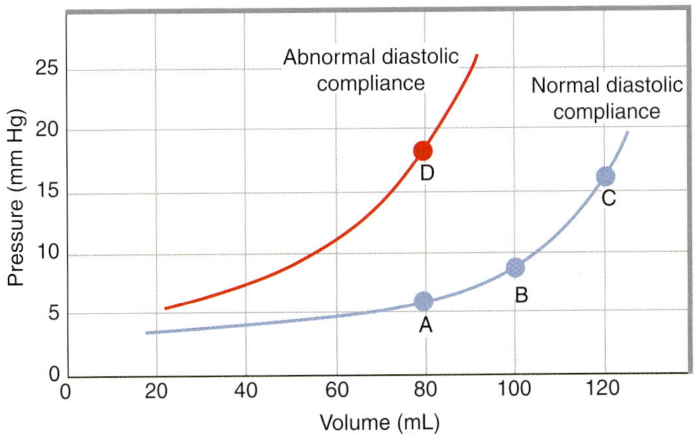

FIGURE 30-11. The effect of change in left ventricular compliance on the pressure-volume relationship. The normal relationship (light blue curve) is curvilinear. Depending on the starting point, the same change in the true preload (ie, end-diastolic volume) will cause a markedly different change in left ventricular end-diastolic pressure and hence in the pulmonary artery occlusion pressure (A-B vs B-C). When ventricular compliance decreases (red curve), an increase in filling pressures (from A-D) does not necessarily reflect increased end-diastolic volume. [Modified with permission from Mark JB. *Atlas of Cardiovascular Monitoring.* New York, NY: Churchill Livingstone; 1998:Figs. 15.1 and 15.2.]

DIAGNOSTIC USE OF THE PAC-DERIVED PRESSURE WAVEFORM

In addition to the quantitative hemodynamic data provided by pressure measurements and cardiac output, the analog pressure waveform can be diagnostic of several pathologic cardiovascular conditions. Although echocardiography has mostly supplanted the PAC for clinical diagnosis of most of these disorders, initial clinical clues can be provided by PAC monitoring (**Fig. 30-13**).[57]

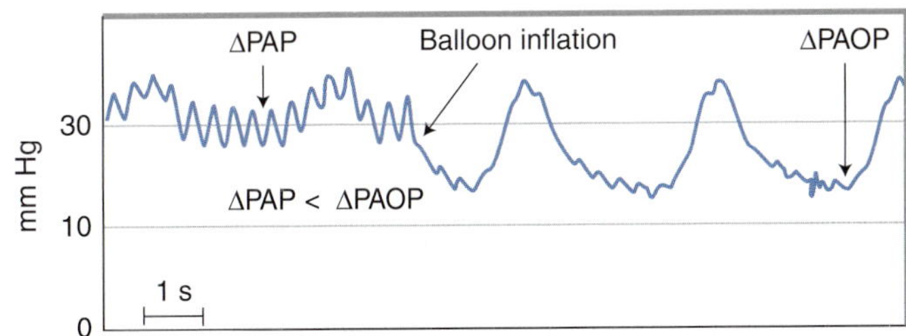

FIGURE 30-12. Pressure trace recorded during positive pressure mechanical ventilation from a pulmonary artery catheter located in West's lung zone 1. Pressure swings in the pulmonary artery occlusion pressure (ΔPAOP) reflect changes in airway pressure and are significantly higher than swings in pulmonary artery pressure (ΔPAP), which result from changes in pleural pressure. [Modified with permission from Teboul JL, Pinsky MR, Mercat A, et al. Estimating cardiac filling pressure in mechanically ventilated patients with hyperinflation. *Crit Care Med.* 2000;28(11):3631-3636.]

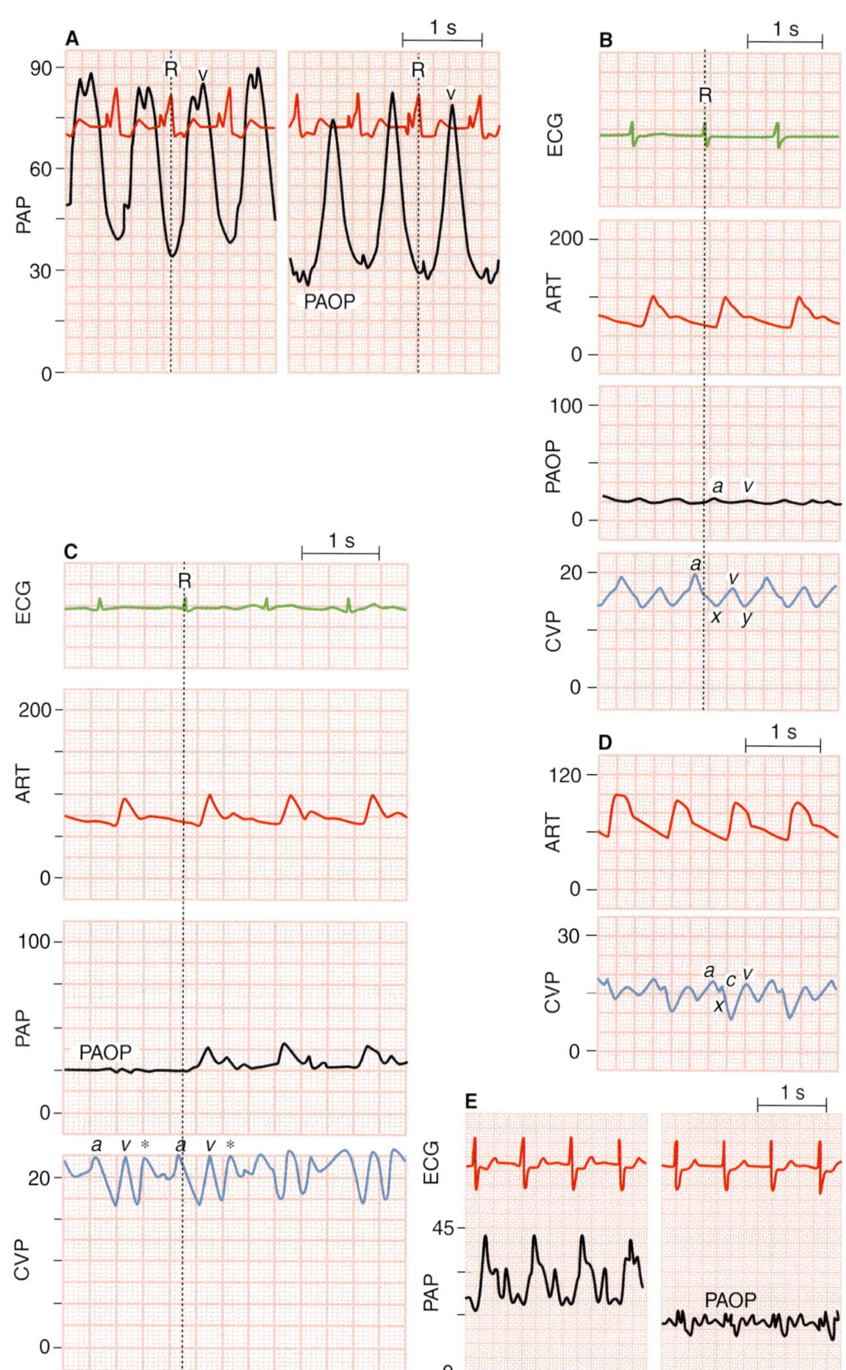

FIGURE 30-13. Pressure waveforms in various clinical situations. **A.** Acute mitral regurgitation: Giant *v* waves are seen in the pulmonary artery occlusion pressure (PAOP) trace, as well as distorting the non-wedged pulmonary artery pressure (PAP) trace. The PAOP pressure can be mistaken as a PAP trace, but the delayed timing of the main pressure wave relative to the electrocardiographic T wave can help correct identification. **B.** Right ventricular infarction: Note prominent central venous pressure (CVP) waves and increased mean CVP (16 mm Hg) almost equal to PAOP (18 mm Hg). **C.** Constrictive pericarditis: Equilibration of end-diastolic pressures across the heart; PAOP, diastolic PAP, and CVP *a* wave, all about 20 mm Hg. Also note the W-shaped CVP trace with the middiastolic plateau wave (marked by *). **D.** Cardiac tamponade: Relatively low blood pressure (84/55 mm Hg) and elevated CVP with dominant *x* descent but attenuated *y* descent. **E.** Pulmonary hypertension: Increased pulmonary pressure (42/20 mm Hg) with markedly lower PAOP (13 mm Hg), caused by increased pulmonary vascular resistance. ART, arterial pressure; ECG, electrocardiogram. [Reproduced with permission from Mark JB. *Atlas of Cardiovascular Monitoring.* New York, NY: Churchill Livingstone; 1998:Figs. 17.11, 12.15, 18.1, 18.5, and 6.11.]

COMPLICATIONS OF PAC MONITORING

Complications associated with the PAC arise from central venous cannulation (Box 30-2), initial PAC placement and positioning, and from continued presence and use of the catheter within the body. Frequency varies greatly between various reports, and most complications have been described only in case reports or small case series.[43] Although minor complications occur in up to 50% of cases, recent practice guidelines concluded that the incidence of serious life-threatening complications is much lower, estimated to be 0.1% to 0.5%.[43] Two large prospective registries of PAC complications in surgical patients support this estimated risk, showing major morbidity in 0.12% to 0.16% and mortality of 0.016%.[58,59] Factors suggested as important to minimize complications include the expertise and experience of the attending physician, close supervision of trainees, and attention to detail during pulmonary artery catheter insertion and use.

Dysrhythmias Transient dysrhythmias, most commonly premature ventricular contractions (PVCs), accompany passage of the PAC through the heart in up to 70% of patients.[58] Clinically significant dysrhythmias, such as complete heart block, ventricular tachycardia, and ventricular fibrillation, are much rarer—about 3% of patients.[58,60]

Transient right bundle branch block occurs in up to 5% of patients during PAC insertion.[61] Therefore, patients with preexisting left bundle branch block are at risk for developing complete heart block.[62] In these patients, a margin of safety can be provided by using a PAC with a pacing port, having transcutaneous pacing readily available, or, rarely, a prophylactic placement of a transvenous pacing wire.

In patients with severe aortic stenosis and other conditions associated with severe left ventricular hypertrophy, effective external cardiac massage is hard to achieve. When cardiac surgery is performed in these patients, many anesthesiologists delay floatation of the PAC until after sternotomy, which enables open cardiac massage to be performed in the event of a life-threatening dysrhythmia.

Catheter Knotting Possible risk factors for looping and knotting of catheters within the heart include low cardiac output states, right heart dilatation, and excessive length of catheter inside the heart.[63] The PAC might also become entangled with intracardiac pacing wires or anatomic structures such as chordae tendineae.[64,65] If knots occur, they can usually be untangled under fluoroscopic guidance. Alternatively, the knot may be pulled tight and the catheter removed with its sheath.[66]

Thromboembolism and Pulmonary Infarction Minor thrombi associated with the PAC were almost universal in the past but became uncommon with the use of heparin-coated catheters.[67] Major pulmonary embolism associated with PAC use has recently been reported in 0.9% of patients receiving PAC versus none in the control group.[68] Pulmonary infarction following PAC can also result from prolonged balloon inflation or distal catheter migration.[69]

Catheter-Related Infections For central venous catheters and PACs alike, catheter-related infections usually result from skin organisms colonizing the introducer sheath.[24] Heparin-coated PACs and regular central venous catheters carry a similar risk of infectious complications (2.6 infections per 1000 catheter days); non-heparin-coated PACs carry a 2-fold increased risk.[24] Leaving the PAC in place for more than 5-7 days also increases the risk of infection.

Valvular Damage and Endocarditis Case reports have described PAC-associated injury of the tricuspid valve[70] and the pulmonary valve,[71] but these injuries appear to be very rare events. The PAC balloon must be completely deflated before catheter withdrawal to avoid valvular injury. Even with proper catheter management, endocarditis, either septic or thrombotic, has been described in autopsy studies, probably representing occult endocardial injury.[72]

Pulmonary Vascular Injury Pulmonary vascular injury and pulmonary artery rupture are rare but life-threatening complications of pulmonary artery catheterization. Pulmonary artery rupture has an incidence of 0.02% to 2.0% but carries a mortality of 40% to 70%.[68,73,74] Risk factors for this catastrophic complication include patient characteristics (advanced age, female gender, hypothermia, anticoagulation therapy, and pulmonary hypertension) as well as operator errors (overdistention of the balloon, unrecognized distal migration of the catheter, and balloon inflation when the catheter tip is wedged).[73,74] In patients with risk factors, consideration should be given to using the PADP as an estimate for PAOP and avoiding repeated balloon inflation.

Sudden hemoptysis is the most common presentation of pulmonary artery rupture. Other signs include hemothorax, hypoxemia, and cardiovascular collapse.[73,74] Maintaining oxygenation and achieving rapid control of bleeding are initial therapeutic goals. Endobronchial intubation with a double-lumen tube or intentional main stem intubation allows selective lung ventilation and isolation of the bleeding segment.[75] Ancillary treatments include lowering the pulmonary artery pressure, reversing anticoagulation, performing bronchoscopy for endobronchial toilet, and identifying the bleeding site. Definitive control of bleeding may be achieved by transcatheter selective pulmonary artery embolization,[76] but surgical lung resection is required when more conservative treatments fail or if life-threatening bleeding develops.[73,74]

INDICATIONS FOR USE AND THE CONTROVERSY SURROUNDING PULMONARY ARTERY CATHETERIZATION

Box 30-4 summarizes the common indications for the PAC. However, studies have shown that factors other than medical indications affect the decision to use the PAC, including institutional, geographic, organizational, demographic, and individual preferences.[77,78]

In a retrospective study published in 1996, Connors et al concluded that PAC use was associated with a 20% increased mortality in critically in patients.[79] This study ignited a major controversy regarding the role of the PAC in clinical medicine.[46,80] Early studies shared problems of inadequate methodology, unequal case mix, and small sample size,[43,44] but several large well-designed clinical trials have been published more recently and have helped to better define the role of the PAC in perioperative medicine. In patients undergoing major noncardiac surgery, a large observational study showed that PAC use was associated with a 2.2-fold increased risk of cardiac complications,[81] and a large randomized study found no benefit for PAC-guided goal-directed therapy compared with standard care without PAC.[68] In moderate-risk vascular surgery, both randomized controlled studies[82] and a meta-analysis[83] demonstrated no benefit associated with routine use of the PAC. And lastly, a large prospective randomized trial in patients undergoing coronary artery bypass surgery compared routine use of PAC versus CVP monitoring and showed no difference in outcome.[84]

Several large randomized studies have also been performed recently in nonsurgical populations, including patients with severe congestive heart failure,[85] patients with acute lung injury,[86] and ICU patients with early shock or multiorgan failure.[60,87,88] All found no therapeutic advantage for use of the PAC.

However, most randomized studies have looked at the routine use of the PAC in large sequential cohorts of patients with relatively moderate risk of death.[89] In most of these clinical trials, specific therapeutic protocols were not mandated and management was left to the physician's discretion. Patients whose physicians considered being too sick to avoid PAC placed were also usually excluded.[90] In contrast, several recent large nonrandomized studies suggest that PAC use may benefit especially high-risk patients characterized by old age, significant physiologic disturbances (ie, large base deficit), and a high level of disease acuity or injury severity.[91-93] In addition, use of the PAC as a rescue monitor in patients who remain hemodynamically unstable despite empirical therapy has received little investigation.

Several expert panels have been convened to provide guidelines to help standardize clinical practice.[43-45] Specifically focused on the perioperative period, the ASA task force practice guidelines suggest that the use of the PAC is considered necessary only in high-risk patients undergoing high-risk surgery, and even then it is contingent on a

BOX 30-4

Common Indications for Pulmonary Artery Catheterization

- Hemodynamic monitoring in high-risk patients undergoing major surgery, including preoperative optimization
- Differential diagnosis and management of shock (hypovolemic, septic, cardiogenic)
- Diagnostic evaluation of major cardiopulmonary disorders (eg, myocardial ischemia, pulmonary hypertension, intracardiac shunt, pulmonary edema)
- Titration of therapy in unstable hemodynamic conditions (eg, hypervolemic therapy in subarachnoid hemorrhage, management of eclampsia)
- Optimization of ventilatory support (positive end-expiratory pressure titration)

favorable practice environment (ie, knowledgeable and experienced physicians and ICU nurses). The term *high-risk patient* generally refers to an ASA class 4 or 5 patient with significant cardiovascular disease, pulmonary dysfunction, renal insufficiency, sepsis, or trauma. High-risk surgery includes procedures commonly associated with large fluid shifts or hemodynamic derangements and high predicted mortality. As new monitoring modalities become clinically available, the need for PAC is expected to decrease even further.

SPECIAL TYPES OF PULMONARY ARTERY CATHETER

Pacing Pulmonary Artery Catheter Two types of PAC have pacing capability. One has 5 electrodes incorporated in the catheter that allow bipolar atrial, ventricular, or atrioventricular sequential pacing. A second type has an extra lumen through which a pacing wire can be placed into the right ventricle. An obvious target population for these catheters includes patients undergoing cardiac surgery using cardiopulmonary bypass, where pacing is frequently required postoperatively for a short period. Other candidates are patients with left bundle branch block, in whom placing a PAC puts them at risk of developing complete heart block. Successful pacing with these catheters is usually achieved intraoperatively in anesthetized patients,[94] but capture becomes less reliable when patients start to move postoperatively. As a result, these catheters are not widely used.

Continuous Mixed Venous Oximetry Measurement of mixed venous oxygen content in the pulmonary artery blood provides an assessment of the balance between total body oxygen supply and consumption.[95] Assuming the contribution of dissolved oxygen is negligible, the mixed venous oxygen saturation can be expressed by rearrangement of the Fick equation (**Box 30-5**). Hence under conditions where oxygen consumption, hemoglobin concentration, and arterial oxygenation remain stable, mixed venous oxygen saturation continuously reflects changes in cardiac output.

Mixed venous oxygen saturation can be measured intermittently using a PAC by sampling blood from the distal pulmonary artery lumen. Co-oximetry should be used to directly measure saturation rather than calculate it from the blood oxygen partial pressure owing to the steep hemoglobin-oxygen saturation curve at partial pressures normally seen in venous blood. Continuous measurement of mixed venous saturation can be achieved using oximetric PACs that use "reflectance spectrophotometry": transmitting light through a fiberoptic bundle, measuring the light reflected from the blood, and calculating the amount of light absorbed by the hemoglobin. Similar to plethysmography, this technique is based on the differential absorption of various wavelengths of light by oxyhemoglobin and deoxyhemoglobin. Oximetric PACs have several technical limitations that should be recognized. They may show a drift artifact, requiring recalibration every 24 hours with a pulmonary artery blood sample, and they may be inaccurate at venous oxygen saturations below 50%. Other technical problems include thrombus formation on the catheter tip or excessive proximity to the vessel wall that may result in inaccurate readings. Most systems warn of a reduction in light signal quality under these conditions. Last, if the catheter is wedged, arterialized blood with high oxygen saturation will be sampled rather than mixed venous blood.

BOX 30-5

Mixed Venous Oxygen Saturation

$$Sv_{O_2} = Sa_{O_2} - \left(\frac{\dot{V}O_2}{CO \cdot 1.36 \cdot Hb}\right) \times 100$$

Where Sv_{O_2} = mixed venous oxygen saturation (%)

Sa_{O_2} = arterial oxygen saturation (%)

$\dot{V}_{O_2}$ = oxygen consumption (mL O_2/min)

Hb = hemoglobin concentration (g/dL)

CO = cardiac output (mL/min)

1.36 = the amount of oxygen carried by hemoglobin (mL/g)

Although continuously monitoring venous oximetry can reliably reflect changes in cardiac output during cardiac surgery,[96] this is not the case in situations associated with rapid changes in oxygen consumption, like graft reperfusion during liver transplantation,[97] aortic cross clamp removal,[98] and high-dose therapy with catecholamines.[99]

Several recent studies, performed in patients with early sepsis,[100] or undergoing either cardiac or noncardiac surgery,[101,102] demonstrated that therapeutic interventions aimed at achieving venous oxygen saturation above 70% result in improved outcome. This contrasts with negative results of an older study performed in critically ill patients,[103] suggesting that early monitoring and prompt therapy are important for achieving benefit.

Recently developed oximetric central venous catheters allow continuous measurement of central venous oxygen saturation in the superior vena cava. Normally, the brain is the major oxygen consumer; therefore, central venous oxygen saturation (70%-75%) is usually slightly lower than mixed venous oxygen saturation (75%).[95] With hypoperfusion, splanchnic blood flow suffers before cerebral blood flow, and oxygen saturation in the inferior vena cava decreases first. Under these situations, central venous saturation in the superior vena cava will be higher than mixed oxygen saturation by 5% to 8%.[104] Despite these complicated relationships, low central venous saturation has been found to be associated with a more severe injury and increased blood loss in trauma patients with otherwise stable hemodynamic parameters[105] and with increased incidence of complications after major surgery.[106] Central venous oximetry has been used successfully to guide therapy in early sepsis[100] and for goal-directed management in both cardiac and noncardiac surgery.[102,107]

Right Ventricular Ejection Fraction PAC This modification of the PAC allows measurement of right ventricular ejection fraction (RVEF) using a fast-response thermistor that measures beat-to-beat changes in pulmonary artery blood temperature.[108] The RVEF PAC incorporates a heating filament that delivers a thermal bolus into the bloodstream. Distal temperature is measured in the pulmonary artery, and from the beat-to-beat temperature decay curve and successive diastolic temperature plateaus, RVEF is computed. Right ventricular end-diastolic volume (RVEDV) can be calculated from RVEF and stroke volume, and this derived variable has been used as an index of cardiac preload. Studies have demonstrated acceptable accuracy of the thermal technique for RVEF measurement compared with radionuclide ventriculography.[109]

Right ventricular dysfunction may result from right ventricular ischemia or acute pulmonary hypertension. These events are not rare during cardiac surgery, especially after weaning from cardiopulmonary bypass (CPB). Indeed, RVEF monitoring in patients following CPB can identify patients with significant right ventricular dysfunction.[110] In patients with septic shock, depressed RVEF has been shown to better predict prognosis compared with cardiac output or cardiac filling pressures,[111] as well as to indicate when inotropic support is needed, rather than fluid resuscitation alone.[112]

CARDIAC OUTPUT MONITORING

BACKGROUND

CO is determined by cardiac preload, afterload, contractility, and heart rate. As such, CO is a global index of circulatory status. Using CO and other hemodynamic measurements, a variety of useful parameters can be derived, including vascular resistances, oxygen delivery to the tissues, and oxygen consumption (Table 30-3). Measurement of CO and its response to therapeutic interventions are commonly used therapeutic protocols in critically ill patients. Although thermodilution CO (TDCO) using the PAC is generally considered the gold standard in both clinical medicine and research, studies comparing it with the Fick method have not shown good agreement.[113] For clinical purposes, though, the absolute CO might be less important than changes in CO and assessing its adequacy in terms of oxygen supply and demand.[114] This section will describe in detail the TDCO technique as well as other less invasive CO measurement techniques.[115]

THE THERMODILUTION TECHNIQUE

TDCO measurement is based on the indicator dilution principle, in which a known amount of indicator is injected into the circulation and its concentration measured over time at a downstream site.[116] For TDCO, a thermal bolus is used as the indicator, and a thermistor incorporated into the catheter 4 cm proximal to the tip measures the change in pulmonary artery blood temperature. Based on these measurements, CO is calculated using the modified Stewart-Hamilton equation (**Box 30-6**). TDCO, therefore, measures right ventricular output, which, at steady state conditions and in the absence of intracardiac shunts, equals left ventricular output.

In clinical practice, 10 mL of room temperature saline or D_5W (0.15 mL/kg in children[117]) is injected rapidly and uniformly through the proximal port of the PAC into the SVC or right atrium. The injectate temperature should be measured at the point of injection, to obviate the influence of injectate rewarming in the syringe. The results from 2 to 3 consecutive measurements are usually averaged, deleting measurements varying more than 10%. The reproducibility of the TDCO technique is not high; therefore at least a 15% change in CO between 2 time points is required to be considered clinically significant.[118]

Right and left ventricular loading conditions as well as pulmonary artery blood temperature all vary considerably during the respiratory cycle.[119] Although synchronizing CO measurement to end inspiration or end expiration might decrease measurement variation and increase reproducibility, a more truly representative mean value for CO is obtained by averaging multiple measurements performed throughout the respiratory cycle.[120]

Technical errors during TDCO measurement are common and may go unrecognized. A real-time display of the pulmonary artery blood temperature curve is an important aid to identify spurious measurements (**Fig. 30-14**).[118] Fluid boluses, given either peripherally or through the PAC introducer sheath, behave as additional positive or negative thermal sources and affect TDCO measurement accuracy.[121] In the immediate post-CPB period, both a rapid drift and an exaggerated respiratory variation of pulmonary artery blood temperature can introduce clinically significant errors in TDCO measurement.[122,123] Right-sided valvular regurgitation, especially tricuspid regurgitation, can have a significant and unpredictable effect on the accuracy of TDCO measurement by causing recirculation of the thermal bolus.[124] Because positive pressure ventilation with high levels of PEEP can either induce or exacerbate tricuspid regurgitation,[125] this may limit the accuracy of TDCO measurement in a large group of critically ill patients. It is also important to remember that intracardiac shunts invalidate TDCO as a measure of systemic CO because under these conditions right and left ventricular outputs are not equal. Additionally, either recirculation (in left-to-right shunts) or injectate bypassing the thermistor (in right-to-left shunts) will introduce errors in the calculation of CO. Last, at low flow states, TDCO might overestimate true CO owing to excessive heat loss from slow transit of the injectate.[126]

Notwithstanding its limitations, the TDCO technique is simple to perform repeatedly and quickly, does not require blood sampling, and uses a nontoxic, nonrecirculating, and nonaccumulating indicator. For these reasons, TDCO is extensively used as the preferred method in a variety of clinical settings. However, because TDCO measurement requires pulmonary artery catheterization, it is a highly invasive monitoring technique.

BOX 30-6

The Modified Stewart-Hamilton Equation for Calculation of Cardiac Output

$$CO = \frac{V_I \times (T_B - T_I) \times K}{\int_0^\infty \Delta T_B(t)dt}$$

Where CO = cardiac output (L/min)

V_I = injected volume (mL)

T_B = blood temperature

T_I = injectate temperature

K = computation constant

$\int_0^\infty \Delta T_B(t)\,dt$ = integral of temperature change over time

The computation constant adjusts for characteristics of the injectate (volume, specific heat capacity, and density) and catheter (specific heat capacity, dead space).

TRANSPULMONARY THERMODILUTION CARDIAC OUTPUT MEASUREMENT

As an alternative to TDCO using a PAC, the transpulmonary thermodilution technique uses a special thermistor-tipped arterial catheter that measures blood temperature change in the systemic circulation (either femoral or axillary artery) following bolus administration of ice-cold injectate through a central venous line.[127] Unlike standard TDCO measurement, this technique requires iced injectate owing to higher thermal noise and greater thermal loss from the longer path that the thermal bolus must traverse from venous injection to systemic arterial detection. Compared with TDCO, this measurement is made over a longer time period, which eliminates the problem of respiratory variation in CO.[128] Both in patients after cardiac surgery and in critically ill patients, transpulmonary thermodilution CO agreed well with standard TDCO, although the transpulmonary values tended to be about 0.3-0.5 L/min higher, possibly reflecting loss of the thermal indicator during passage through the lungs.[129,130] In addition to measuring CO, this method allows calculation of global end-diastolic volume (GEDV) as a measure of preload, extravascular lung water (EVLW) as a measure of pulmonary edema, and cardiac function index (CFI) as a measure of contractility.

LITHIUM DILUTION CARDIAC OUTPUT MEASUREMENT

Another indicator dilution technique uses intravenously injected ionized lithium as the indicator. The dilution curve is built by drawing blood from a standard arterial line over a lithium-sensitive electrode.[131] Similar to transpulmonary thermodilution, respiratory influences are eliminated with this method because CO is measured over several respiratory cycles. Another advantage of this technique is that the injection of the lithium indicator can be done through a peripheral vein, removing even the requirement for central venous catheterization.[132] In small children, lithium dilution CO has been shown to compare favorably with transpulmonary thermodilution CO.[133] In several studies that compared lithium dilution cardiac output with TDCO in postoperative patients in the critical care unit, a good agreement was found, although the lithium dilution technique tends to underestimate TDCO by 0.2-0.5 L/min.[131,132]

The lithium dilution technique has several limitations. It cannot be used in patients who are allergic to or receiving lithium. Nondepolarizing neuromuscular blocking agents can interfere with the lithium electrode, which requires a 15- to 30-minute wait period following use of these drugs before CO can be measured. Also, frequent repetition of the measurement is limited by the risk of lithium accumulation and toxicity.

PARTIAL CO_2 REBREATHING CARDIAC OUTPUT MEASUREMENT

This noninvasive method uses a modification of the Fick principle to measure CO in mechanically ventilated patients. In the partial rebreathing method, CO_2 production and end-tidal CO_2 are measured at baseline and during brief periods of rebreathing, which allows calculation of pulmonary capillary blood flow.[134] The rebreathing is achieved by intermittently diverting exhaled gas through a loop connected to the ventilatory circuit. Although this technique does not involve invasive vascular catheterization, it generally requires a tracheally intubated, mechanically ventilated patient. It provides a semicontinuous CO

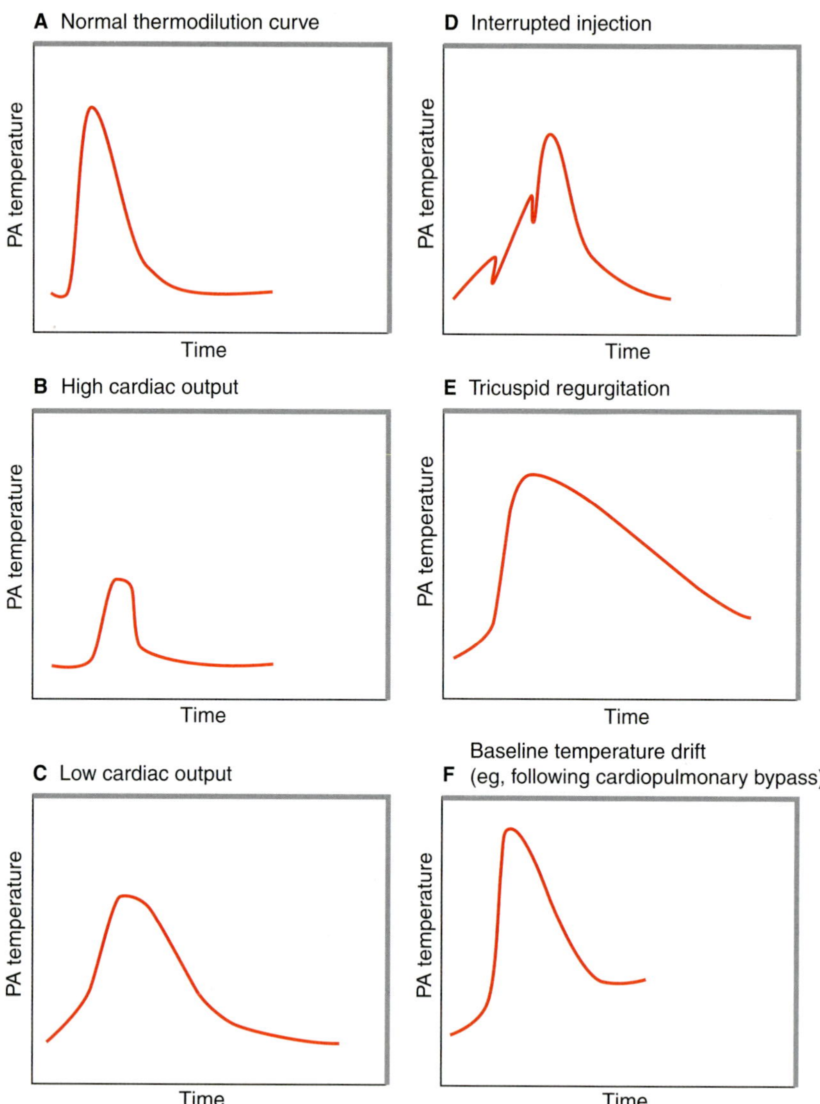

FIGURE 30-14. Thermodilution curves recorded from the thermistor at the tip of the pulmonary artery catheter after injection of cold saline. Because the injectate temperature is usually colder than body temperature, the temperature along the *y* axis is decreasing. The cardiac output is inversely related to the area under the curve, as demonstrated by curves A-C. Curve D shows the effect of a nonsmooth injection. In tricuspid regurgitation (curve E), incomplete mixing of the indicator within the right ventricle and subsequent recirculation between the right atrium and right ventricle will distort the descending limb of the thermodilution curve, usually leading to an increased area under the curve and underestimation of cardiac output. After discontinuation of cardiopulmonary bypass (curve F), blood temperature gradually decreases as blood flow resumes to body parts that are cold (eg, the lungs). The drift in baseline temperature will decrease the area under the curve and lead to an overestimation of cardiac output.

measurement because the rebreathing period can be automatically repeated. A major theoretical drawback of the technique is that it only measures blood that participates in gas exchange, ignoring shunted blood. To account for this, the CO_2 rebreathing measurements can be adjusted by estimating shunt fraction based on FIO_2 and either arterial oxygen partial pressure or saturation.

Clinical studies of the partial rebreathing method in surgical patients have been mainly limited to patients undergoing or recovering from coronary artery bypass grafting (CABG). These small trials have generally shown acceptable measurement bias and precision compared with TDCO,[135] although accuracy at higher CO is reduced.[136] Newer software versions allow use of the partial rebreathing method in modes of ventilation that allow spontaneous breathing and might improve its performance in patients in the ICU.

Because arterial PCO_2 increases 2 to 5 mm Hg during each rebreathing measurement period, the use of the CO_2 rebreathing technique is relatively contraindicated in neurosurgical patients who have increased intracranial pressure.

CONTINUOUS THERMODILUTION CARDIAC OUTPUT MEASUREMENT

The continuous thermodilution PAC incorporates a thermal filament around the right ventricular portion of the catheter, approximately 20 cm from the tip. This filament is intermittently warmed to 44°C, and a thermodilution curve is recorded by the thermistor at the tip of the PAC in the pulmonary artery. Because this warm thermal signal is much smaller than the cold thermal signal of standard TDCO measurement, a stochastic system controls filament heating, switching it on and off with pseudorandom timing, thereby enhancing the signal-to-noise ratio.[137] The displayed CO is updated every 30 seconds and represents the averaged measurement over the previous 3 to 6 minutes, eliminating respiratory variation in CO. Current commercial systems have a "fast" mode that displays the result of each measurement cycle as it is performed, allowing earlier detection of acute changes but at the price of accentuated random variations and errors. Because of the very small thermal signal involved, this method is more susceptible to interference by other sources of heat, such as rapid intravenous fluid infusion or the temperature changes that occur immediately following CPB.[138]

Continuous thermodilution has been quite extensively validated against standard TDCO, mainly in patients undergoing cardiac surgery.[130,139] Although this method is termed *continuous thermodilution*, current devices only provide semicontinuous measurement that is averaged over a several minute interval, and therefore they have an obligate delay of approximately 10 minutes in identifying acute hemodynamic changes.[140] However, compared with TDCO measurements performed every several hours, continuous thermodilution should allow earlier recognition of hemodynamic problems.[141] Thus far, no studies have demonstrated that patient outcome is improved by using these more expensive continuous CO catheters.

PULSE CONTOUR-DERIVED CARDIAC OUTPUT MEASUREMENT

Pulse contour methods calculate stroke volume from the area under the arterial pressure waveform. The pressure waveform as measured in the large arteries is a combination of a forward pressure wave produced by the contraction of the heart and a backward pressure wave reflected from arterial branch points and arterial-arteriolar junctions. The magnitude of wave reflection is affected by changes in arterial resistance and compliance and needs to be taken into account in the calculation algorithm.[142,143] Available commercial devices are based on different models of the circulation and generally require intermittent (every 4-8 h) calibration with a CO reference to establish accurate monitoring in an individual patient, accounting for differences in vascular resistance, compliance, impedance, and wave reflectance.[144] Although the pulse contour method only requires an arterial line for monitoring, the needed calibration methods might require additional invasive procedures. Recently, devices have been developed that replace external calibration with a more sophisticated arterial pressure waveform analysis combined with a scaling parameter derived from patient demographic data. However, their accuracy is still questionable, especially in situations where mean blood pressure and cardiac output change in different directions.[145]

Reliable pulse contour measurement requires a well-defined arterial pressure waveform, in part because the dicrotic notch is often used to identify end-systole. On the other hand, it appears that pulse contour CO monitoring remains accurate across arterial pressure monitoring systems that have a wide range of dynamic response characteristics.[146] This method is also unreliable in the presence of dysrhythmias or severe tachycardias, which lead to a variable or low stroke volume, respectively. Some investigators have shown that large fluctuations in systemic vascular resistance affect vessel compliance and wave reflectance and require recalibration to maintain accuracy of the pulse contour measurements[146]; other studies have shown preserved accuracy despite acute changes in systemic vascular resistance.[147]

Notwithstanding these shortcomings, the pulse contour method provides a true continuous beat-to-beat measurement of stroke volume and CO and has an acceptable agreement with TDCO, with a small mean bias of 0.1-0.3 L/min.[130,143,146] In addition, pulse contour methods can calculate the beat-to-beat variation in stroke volume induced by positive pressure ventilation, which can be used to evaluate volume status.

ESOPHAGEAL DOPPLER CARDIAC OUTPUT MEASUREMENT

Ultrasound waves reflected from a moving target change their frequency, which allows calculation of the direction and velocity of target movement using the Doppler equation (**Box 30-7**). For CO calculation, circulating red blood cells are used as the moving target.

The current Doppler CO technique uses an esophageal probe, similar in size to a standard orogastric tube, which is inserted into the lower esophagus, approximately 35 to 40 cm from the incisor teeth.[148] This position provides a suitable acoustic window to interrogate the descending thoracic aorta because the aorta and esophagus are almost parallel at this anatomic location. With this method, descending thoracic aorta blood flow is calculated from the area under the velocity-time curve and the aortic cross-sectional area. The latter is either derived from a nomogram or continuously measured during the cardiac cycle with a dedicated M-mode echo transducer incorporated into the probe to measure aortic diameter.[149] Because the flow in the descending aorta is only a portion of total CO, some devices report an estimate of total CO that is derived by multiplying descending thoracic aortic flow by an empirical constant of 1.4.[148] In addition to providing a minimally invasive, continuous beat-to-beat estimate of CO, Doppler CO monitors can provide valuable information regarding cardiac preload, contractility, and afterload, all derived from the shape of the velocity-time spectral Doppler waveform (**Fig. 30-15**).[148] The respiratory variation in aortic blood flow velocity can also be used to evaluate preload, similar to systolic blood pressure variation.[150]

BOX 30-7

The Doppler Equation

$$V = \frac{\Delta f \cdot c}{2f_0 \cdot \cos\theta}$$

Where V = blood velocity

Δf = change of ultrasound frequency

f_0 = transmitted ultrasound frequency

θ = angle between the ultrasound beam and velocity vector

c = velocity of ultrasound in blood (1540 m/s)

One shortcoming of the esophageal Doppler monitor is its restriction to tracheally intubated, deeply sedated patients. Relative contraindications include patients with esophageal pathology or severe coagulopathy. In addition, frequent repositioning of the Doppler probe is needed, particularly in ICU patients who are not paralyzed, anesthetized, and immobile. Additional concerns involve the underlying assumptions on which the technique is based: a fixed ratio between descending aortic blood flow and total CO, a constant thoracic aortic cross-sectional area during systole, a uniform flow profile across the aorta, and absence of significant diastolic antegrade aortic flow. It is not surprising that esophageal Doppler CO measurements tend to underestimate total CO measured by other methods, although in some trials, the bias was small enough to be clinically insignificant and changes in cardiac output over time were reliably tracked.[151]

Despite all the theoretical concerns regarding the accuracy of the technique, Doppler-derived CO monitoring is one of the few monitoring modalities that has been tested and found to be clinically effective for resuscitating critically ill and surgical patients. Several studies, both in cardiac and noncardiac surgery, have used esophageal Doppler monitoring to guide fluid therapy for maximizing CO and have shown a reduced incidence of perioperative complications and a shorter hospital length of stay.[152]

GASTRIC TONOMETRY

Gastric tonometry is a unique monitoring modality. Instead of directly measuring total CO, it measures gastric P_{CO_2} and thereby serves as a surrogate measure of regional blood flow and tissue perfusion. As gastric mucosal blood flow decreases, CO_2 clearance is reduced. With further reduction in blood flow and oxygen delivery, CO_2 production increases from titration of H^+ ions generated by anaerobic metabolism.[153] Increased mucosal tissue levels are reflected by increased CO_2 levels in the gastric lumen because CO_2 diffuses freely across membranes. The gastric tonometer consists of a modified gastric tube with a balloon at the tip that is filled with either saline or air. CO_2 in the balloon equilibrates over time with the gas in the gastric lumen, and samples are intermittently aspirated for measurement using either an ABG machine (for saline tonometry) or infrared spectroscopy (for air tonometry).[154] Calculating the gap between gastric P_{CO_2} and arterial

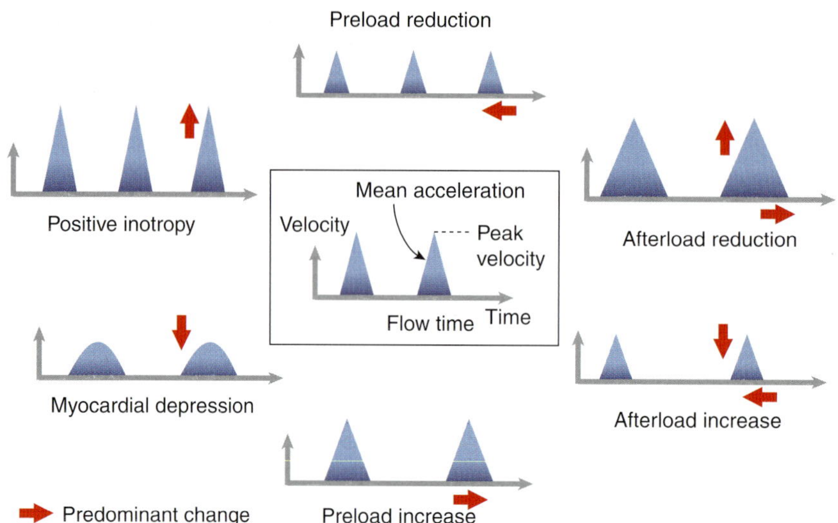

FIGURE 30-15. Spectral Doppler tracings of descending aorta blood flow recorded using esophageal Doppler cardiac output monitoring. Changes in the velocity-time waveform shape result from alterations in contractility (mainly affect peak velocity and mean acceleration), preload (mainly affect systolic flow time corrected for heart rate [FT_c]), and afterload (which affect FT_c, mean acceleration and peak flow velocity). [Modified with permission from Singer M. Esophageal Doppler monitoring of aortic blood flow: beat-by-beat cardiac output monitoring. *Int Anesthesiol Clin.* 1993;31(3):99-125.]

P_{CO_2} controls for the effect of respiratory acidosis on gastric CO_2. Most devices can also calculate gastric pH (pH_i) when the arterial bicarbonate level is measured and entered into the monitor. A pH_i value below 7.32 is considered abnormal, but the P_{CO_2} gap (gastric P_{CO_2}–arterial P_{CO_2}) is currently considered to be a better measure of tissue perfusion.[155]

During low perfusion states, splanchnic blood flow is the first to be compromised as the body diverts blood flow to the brain, heart, and kidneys.[156] Therefore, gastric P_{CO_2} has been considered to be an early monitor of hypoperfusion. Studies of experimental graded hemorrhage[157] as well as clinical studies in trauma patients[158] support this concept. The effects of gut ischemia may be protean because it can contribute to bacterial translocation, inflammatory response, and the development of multiorgan failure, independent of the mechanism that caused the ischemia in the first place.[159] Indeed, intraoperative gastric hypercarbia was shown to correlate with increased complications, length of stay, and mortality after both cardiac and noncardiac surgery.[160,161] Several studies in ICU patients and in patients undergoing noncardiac surgery suggest that therapy guided by gastric P_{CO_2} can reduce morbidity and mortality.[162,163]

Gastric tonometry is contraindicated in patients with esophageal abnormalities, and the measurements might be affected by feeding, gastric insufflation or suctioning, and the use of H_2 blockers. Finally, not all studies have found gastric tonometry to be useful.[164,165]

PROBLEM-ORIENTED HEMODYNAMIC MONITORING

For clinicians, monitoring choices should always stem from a clinical diagnostic or therapeutic question. It is therefore essential to discuss and compare the various existing monitoring modalities in terms of their usefulness to answer specific clinical questions.

ASSESSMENT OF ACUTE MYOCARDIAL ISCHEMIA

Several studies have confirmed the association of perioperative myocardial ischemia with postoperative cardiac complications, mainly myocardial infarction and cardiac death.[166,167] This highlights the importance of early diagnosis of ischemia in the surgical patient. The most commonly used methods to diagnose ischemia perioperatively are ECG monitoring and echocardiography.

Some authors have advocated use of the PAC to monitor for ischemia.[168] Myocardial ischemia typically impairs diastolic relaxation, which leads to decreased ventricular compliance and increased ventricular end-diastolic pressure.[169] This will lead to an increased amplitude of the a wave of the PAOP, reflecting left atrial contraction against an incompletely relaxed ventricle. Less prominent increases in mean PAOP and PADP can also be seen. When systolic dysfunction occurs, reduced stroke volume, left ventricular stroke work, and arterial blood pressure may ensue. If acute mitral regurgitation develops, either due to ischemia-induced geometric changes in the left ventricle or due to papillary muscle dysfunction, a tall *c-v* wave can be observed in the PAOP trace.

The main limitation of using PAC monitoring for diagnosis of ischemia is that no threshold values have been set as diagnostic criteria. In a study where ischemia was defined as wall motion abnormalities seen on TEE, mean PAOP increased by 3.5 ± 4.8 mm Hg.[170] However, a threshold of 3 mm Hg had only 25% sensitivity and only 15% positive predictive value for ischemia. Another study in patients undergoing CABG used myocardial lactate production to diagnose ischemia and found that a 5 mm Hg increase in mean PAOP had almost 100% specificity but only 1.6% sensitivity.[171] Interestingly, ECG monitoring had only 17.5% sensitivity, demonstrating the lack of a clinically reliable and useful ischemia monitor. Given the numerous factors that can affect PAC pressure measurements, these results are not surprising. Also, ischemia in small areas of the myocardium might not induce a large enough change in global myocardial compliance to be detected by the PAC. Lastly, the PAOP cannot be continuously monitored due to the risk of pulmonary infarction.

To summarize, PAC monitoring should probably not be used for the sole purpose of diagnosing perioperative ischemia. However, other currently available monitors, namely ECG and TEE, are also limited in their diagnostic usefulness. Information collected from the PAC can help to corroborate the diagnosis of ischemia, evaluate its hemodynamic significance, and guide therapy.

ASSESSMENT OF PULMONARY EDEMA

Pulmonary edema results from the interplay of 2 different processes: increased pulmonary capillary hydrostatic pressure and increased pulmonary capillary permeability. The critical forces driving edema formation are described by Starling's equation (**Box 30-8**). Pulmonary edema formation will be reduced as pulmonary capillary hydrostatic pressure is lowered (eg, by diuresis), but at a certain point, left ventricular preload reduction will reduce cardiac output without any further benefit in terms of pulmonary edema. In normal alveolar-capillary permeability states, a pulmonary capillary pressure of 18 to 20 mm Hg is considered to be the threshold beyond which alveolar flooding is promoted.[172]

BOX 30-8

Starling's Equation for Fluid Flux Across Membranes

Fluid flux $= K_{fc} \times (P_{capillary} - P_{interstitium}) - K_d \times (\pi_{capillary} - \pi_{interstitium})$

Where P = hydrostatic pressure

π = oncotic pressure

K_{fc} = capillary filtration coefficient

K_d = reflection coefficient

Accordingly, pulmonary edema in the presence of a PAOP below 18 mm Hg has traditionally been classified as noncardiogenic or "permeability" pulmonary edema.[173]

The Usefulness of PAOP Clinical reliance on absolute PAOP values such as 18 mm Hg can be misleading. First, increased hydrostatic pressure might be transient, as in acute ischemic left ventricular dysfunction or acute neurogenic pulmonary edema. Following such an event, by the time the PAOP is measured, it might already be significantly lower. Second, PAOP is used as a surrogate for pulmonary capillary pressure, assuming negligible pulmonary venous resistance. However, in conditions of increased cardiac output or increased pulmonary venous resistance (eg, pulmonary fibrosis, late-stage ARDS, high-altitude pulmonary edema, vasopressor therapy), true pulmonary capillary pressure might be significantly higher than the measured PAOP.[174] In these patients, pulmonary vasodilators might be beneficial for treating pulmonary edema. Third, positive pressure ventilation may increase the PAOP while simultaneously increasing the interstitial tissue pressure, resulting in no net increase in the filtration pressure gradient. Last, in patients with acute lung injury and increased capillary permeability, Starling's equation indicates that pulmonary capillary pressure might play an even greater role in edema formation because as K_d decreases, protein concentration in the interstitium increases and the oncotic pressure gradient decreases (Box 30-8). Under these conditions, pulmonary capillary pressures less than 18 mm Hg might still promote formation of pulmonary edema. Indeed, pulmonary capillary pressure is a major determinant of fluid flux across the alveolar capillary membrane regardless of the degree of capillary permeability. The so-called safe level of PAOP in patients with increased alveolar capillary permeability remains elusive.[175] A recent large randomized study in patients with acute lung injury has shown clinical advantage to a restrictive fluid therapy aiming at PAOP less than 8 mm Hg or CVP less than 4 mm Hg compared with liberal fluid management.[176]

Measuring Extravascular Lung Water A different approach to assess pulmonary edema involves quantification of EVLW, which can be measured using transpulmonary thermodilution.[177] Studies conducted in critically ill patients have demonstrated that the level of EVLW has prognostic value.[178] Also, the ratio of EVLW to another parameter derived using transpulmonary thermodilution, intrathoracic blood volume, has been shown to differentiate between hydrostatic and permeability pulmonary edema.[177]

Of clinical importance, trials in patients with acute lung injury have found that compared with care guided by PAOP monitoring, therapy guided by EVLW monitoring results not only in a reduction in the amount of administered fluid, but also in an improvement in clinically significant end points such as ventilator days, ICU length of stay, and mortality.[175] A more recent study suggests that monitoring EVLW can be used to guide fluid challenges in septic patients at risk for pulmonary edema.[179] Limited data, however, exist regarding EVLW monitoring during the perioperative period, and its usefulness in the operating room remains uncertain.

ASSESSMENT OF VENTRICULAR CONTRACTILITY

Contractility, the force of muscle contraction, can be defined as the velocity of myocardial fiber shortening during systole. Together with the preload, afterload, and heart rate, these are the four determinants of cardiac output. Direct assessment of intrinsic ventricular contractility, independent of loading conditions, is possible under laboratory or research conditions but is not easily available clinically. Instead, several indices of integrative "pump" function can be used, attempting to take into consideration the effects of loading conditions. Under a range of loading conditions, these indices can still give reasonably accurate estimate of ventricular contractility.[180]

Cardiac Function Curve A classical study on the use of the PAC in the setting of myocardial infarction defined cardiogenic shock as the combination of low cardiac index (<2.2 L/min per m^2) and high PAOP (>18 mm Hg).[181] As a rough guide, this combination is commonly used clinically to decide on the need for inotropic support (eg, following weaning from cardiopulmonary bypass). However, significant ventricular dysfunction may be present in a variety of clinical conditions when measured CO is in the normal range, yet inadequate for the bodily needs. Also, CO might be preserved despite low stroke volume due to increased heart rate, or stroke volume might be preserved despite reduced contractility due to reduced afterload. Similarly, PAOP can be abnormally increased from a variety of other causes besides systolic left ventricular dysfunction. Rather than focusing clinically on absolute values for PAOP or stroke volume, "fluid responsiveness" might serve as a better indicator of ventricular function. When a fluid bolus does not lead to a significant increase in stroke volume, while at the same time the PAOP does rise significantly, this can be construed as a sign of a failing left ventricle that is operating on the "flat portion" of its Starling curve (**Fig. 30-16**).[182] Obviously, a flat portion also exists in a normal ventricle, however at a relatively very high stroke volume.

Ventricular Stroke Work Another measure of pump function is ventricular stroke work, which is the energy consumed by the ventricle while transferring the stroke volume from the atrium to the pulmonary artery (RV) or aorta (LV).[183] The higher the pressure differential between the filling pressure and the mean arterial blood pressure (pulmonary or systemic), the higher the ventricular work. A failing ventricle, due to a contractility-afterload mismatch, will display a smaller stroke work index.[184]

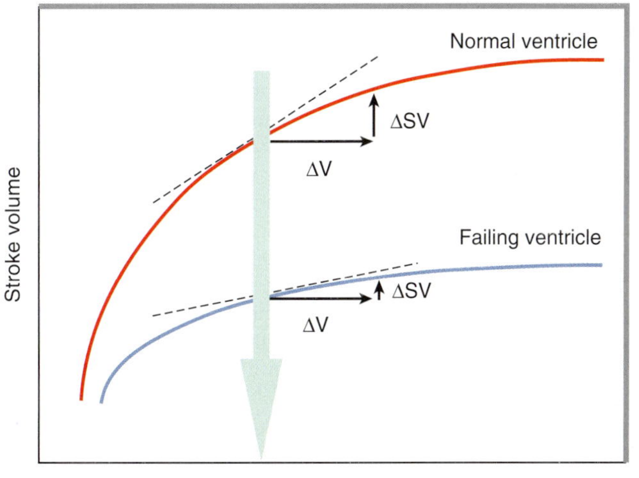

FIGURE 30-16. Lack of fluid responsiveness as a marker of ventricular dysfunction. Starting from the same left ventricular end-diastolic volume (LVEDV, turquoise arrow), a similar preload augmentation (ΔV) leads to a much smaller increase in stroke volume (ΔSV) in the failing ventricle, operating on a much flatter Starling curve (the slope is marked by the dotted line). Therefore, assessment of baseline preload, whether in pressure terms (eg, pulmonary artery occlusion pressure) or in volume terms (LVEDV) cannot predict the cardiac output response to preload augmentation. [Modified with permission from Michard F, Reuter DA. Assessing cardiac preload or fluid responsiveness? It depends on the question we want to answer. *Intensive Care Med*. 2003;29(8):1396.]

Echocardiography Echocardiography has become a widely used monitor to evaluate ventricular function.[185] The most widely used index for assessing left ventricular function is the ejection fraction, although it is both preload and afterload dependent. It is usually estimated from the observed change in ventricular 2-dimensional cross-sectional area, although techniques do exist for more accurate calculation. Because of the nongeometric shape of the right ventricle, calculation of right ventricular ejection fraction is usually abandoned in favor of a more qualitative evaluation of contractility, based mainly on inward movement of the ventricular wall during systole.

The rate of pressure rise during systole, dP/dT, is classically measured using intraventricular pressure manometers. In patients with mitral regurgitation, a similar parameter can be measured using echocardiography from the mitral regurgitation jet Doppler envelope. Because this index is measured during the isovolumic contraction phase, it is afterload independent, although it is still preload dependent.

Newer Monitors Newer monitoring modalities offer additional indices of contractility. From the esophageal Doppler time-velocity waveform, the peak flow velocity as well as the slope of the velocity-time envelope (ie, mean acceleration) can be calculated (Fig. 30-15).[186] These are analogous to the dP/dT index mentioned previously.

Transpulmonary thermodilution provides a measurement termed the *cardiac function index* (CFI), defined as the cardiac index divided by the global end-diastolic volume index (which is a measure of preload). The resulting quotient is proposed to be a preload-independent index of contractility.[187]

Right ventricular ejection fraction can be directly measured using the RVEF PAC. In the presence of right ventricular dysfunction, as a result of either ischemia[110] or sepsis,[112] fluid loading may cause further hemodynamic deterioration by increasing right ventricular end-diastolic volume, inducing leftward shift of the interventricular septum and thereby decreasing left ventricular compliance and preload.[188] This might be diagnosed by RVEF PAC monitoring, prompting inotropic support of the right ventricle.

ASSESSMENT OF VOLUME STATUS

Goals for fluid administration are maintenance of effective intravascular volume and optimization of tissue perfusion and cellular oxygenation. Inadequate intravascular volume resuscitation initially impairs nonvital organ perfusion but eventually leads to shock and inadequate oxygen delivery to all tissues. Although volume expansion is expected to increase stroke volume and cardiac output and ameliorate tissue hypoperfusion, excessive volume administration can result in pulmonary and intestinal edema, exacerbation of cor pulmonale, hemodilution and functional anemia, hyperchloremic acidosis from saline administration, and coagulation abnormalities, all of which may increase morbidity and mortality.[189]

The inflammatory response to surgical trauma, ischemia/reperfusion injury, or sepsis increases vascular permeability, greatly increasing fluid losses from the vascular space.[190] Even without additional pathology, general anesthesia alone has been shown to increase interstitial fluid 3-fold compared with conscious controls.[191] Hence perioperative and critically ill patients are often relatively hypovolemic. Unfortunately, volume expansion alone may not improve organ perfusion; several investigators have shown that up to half of critically ill patients fail to respond to fluid administration.[192,193] The challenge for resuscitation of critically ill patients is to identify individuals who are hypovolemic and who will respond favorably to volume expansion.

Clinical Evaluation In the absence of invasive monitors, standard clinical signs and symptoms are used to guide fluid administration in the operating room. Formulas for calculating volume deficits are based on the length of fasting period, estimates of insensible losses during the operation, blood loss, and third spacing of fluid. The most commonly mentioned signs of hypovolemia are tachycardia and hypotension. Clinical indicators of peripheral perfusion include capillary refill and tactile warmth of the extremities. Laboratory findings consistent with hypovolemia include inappropriately high hematocrit, hypernatremia, high levels of blood urea nitrogen (BUN), increased ratio of BUN to creatinine, hyperlactatemia, or metabolic acidosis. In patients with normal renal function, urine output and composition (osmolarity, fractional excretion of sodium) may provide supplementary clues to intravascular volume status. However, many of these measures indicate perfusion rather than overall volume status, and they are further confounded in pathologic states such as severe vasoconstriction or cardiogenic shock. Other complicating factors are common during the perioperative period, including hypothermia, anxiety, increased antidiuretic hormone, or hyperchloremic metabolic acidosis. Several studies have shown the lack of sensitivity or specificity of the clinical examination and laboratory indices to assess volume status.[194,195]

One of the best and simplest methods to determine the adequacy of volume resuscitation is to administer a fluid challenge and assess the desired physiologic response. A 250 to 500 mL of crystalloid or colloid solution may be infused over 10 to 20 minutes,[196] or, even simpler, passive leg raising can induce transient autotransfusion and increase blood pressure in patients that are volume responsive.[197] In contrast to respiratory variation-based dynamic indices (see later), the passive leg raising test is also useful in patients who are breathing spontaneously or who have significant dysrhythmias.[198] In patients who fail to respond to these simple measures or in whom a fluid challenge carries greater risk, more sophisticated assessment requires additional hemodynamic monitoring.

The Usefulness of Filling Pressures Static pressure measurements, mainly CVP and PAOP, have been traditionally used as preload indicators to guide fluid administration. However, the relationships between intravascular blood volume, end-diastolic ventricular volumes, and cardiac filling pressures are complex and affected by a variety of factors. In particular, the nonlinear nature of ventricular diastolic compliance (Fig. 30-11) confounds the direct pressure-volume relationship, as do variations in pulmonary vascular resistance, chest wall or abdominal compliance, pericardial pressure, intrathoracic pressure, and use of vasoactive drugs. Indeed, no predictable relationship between CVP or PAOP and volumetric measures of preload or cardiac performance could be demonstrated even in healthy volunteers.[199] In a critical review of 12 studies, neither CVP nor PAOP measurements were able to identify patients who would respond to volume expansion with improvements in cardiac output.[192] It should be noted that monitoring PAOP during fluid resuscitation might still be important for high-risk patients because PAOP indicates the hydrostatic force responsible for development of pulmonary edema.[179]

Given the poor predictive ability of static measures, a different approach to evaluate volume status focuses on using changes in filling pressures following administration of a fluid challenge. In one investigation of goal-directed therapy in patients with femoral neck fractures, volume was infused to achieve sustained increases in CVP of more than 3 mm Hg above baseline value, which was associated with improvements in postoperative outcomes.[200]

Volumetric Indices Volumetric indices have been proposed as an alternative to static pressures. Fast-response RV ejection fraction PACs are able to calculate RV end-diastolic volume (RVEDV). As a direct measure of RV preload, RVEDV appears to be a better index of fluid responsiveness than PAOP in some studies[201,202] but not others.[203] RVEDV monitoring might be especially useful in patients requiring mechanical ventilation, where elevated intrathoracic pressures confound interpretation of cardiac filling pressures.[204] Transpulmonary thermodilution techniques allow measurement of global end-diastolic volume (GEDV), representing the volume of blood inside both right and left heart chambers at end-diastole. Several small studies in septic patients[205] and those undergoing cardiac[206] or lung transplant surgery[207] have found GEDV to be a better indicator of volume status compared with static pressure measurements. However, a recent meta-analysis concluded it is no better than the CVP to predict fluid responsiveness.[208]

Echocardiography can be used to measure and derive a number of cardiac volumes and parameters that can help to evaluate preload. Not surprisingly, ventricular end-diastolic area has been found to be a better index of preload compared to filling pressures.[209] In healthy volunteers, echocardiographic volume indices also correlated with response to volume expansion,[199] although threshold values that differentiate responders from nonresponders could not be identified.[192,193] Another echocardiographic measure, the degree of superior or inferior vena cava collapsibility during inspiration, was found to predict fluid responsiveness in mechanically ventilated septic patients.[210,211] Unfortunately, the time, training, cost, and equipment involved in the use of bedside echocardiography limit the applicability of these techniques.

Respiratory Variation-Based Dynamic Indices As an alternative to static preload measurements, a variety of dynamic measures have been proposed to identify hypovolemic patients who will respond to volume expansion with an increase in CO. The physiologic basis for these dynamic indices depends on cardiopulmonary interactions, in which cyclic changes in left ventricular preload are induced by changes in intrathoracic pressure and volume that occur during positive pressure mechanical ventilation. In fluid-responsive (ie, preload dependent) patients, cyclic changes in stroke volume and blood pressure are more pronounced.[212]

Systolic Pressure Variation Systolic pressure variation (SPV) is defined as the greatest measured difference between systolic pressure peaks during a single positive pressure breath. Increased SPV more than 10 mm Hg has been found to reflect blood loss, indicate hypovolemia, and predict a beneficial response to volume infusion.[213,214] SPV has 2 distinct components. An early systolic increase of 2 to 4 mm Hg (Δ Up) immediately follows onset of positive pressure inspiration and results from both a displacement of pulmonary venous blood into the left heart[215] and from increased intrathoracic pressure that decreases left ventricular afterload.[216] The second component of SPV (Δ Down) is a pressure decrease of approximately 5 to 6 mm Hg that reflects a decrease in venous return to the right heart caused by positive intrathoracic pressure, which results in reduced LV filling several beats later.[217] The Δ Down component may be a more sensitive indicator of volume responsiveness compared with total SPV, especially in patients with poor LV function: In those patients the decrease in LV afterload induced by positive intrathoracic pressure might lead to a more pronounced Δ Up and a larger total SPV (**Fig. 30-17**).[193] To easily identify and measure SPV and its components, a printout of the arterial pressure waveform is beneficial, including a short period of recording during apnea to serve as the baseline pressure for Δ Up and Δ Down. In clinical studies, Δ Down 5 mm Hg or more identified patients who were likely to respond to fluid administration. In these "responder" patients, the greater the Δ Down, the greater the resulting increase in end-diastolic area or stroke volume following fluid challenge.[193]

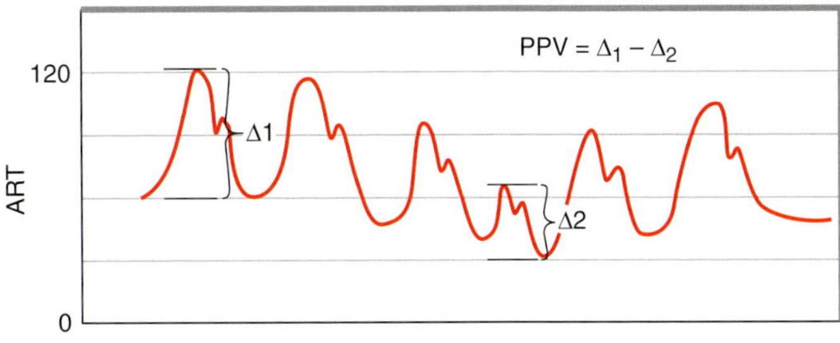

FIGURE 30-18. An example of pulse pressure variation (PPV). Maximal pulse pressure is approximately 62 mm Hg; minimal pulse pressure is 36 mm Hg. The resulting PPV (26 mm Hg/49 mm Hg = 57%) is more than 12% of the mean of the 2 values (49 mm Hg), indicating a high likelihood of hypovolemia and fluid responsiveness.

Pulse Pressure Variation Pulse pressure variation (PPV) is defined as the difference between the maximal and the minimal pulse pressure values during a single mechanical breath, divided by the mean of these 2 values (**Fig. 30-18**). A PPV more than 12% was able to predict fluid responsiveness in patients with ARDS, sepsis, or cardiac surgery, and there was good correlation between the magnitude of PPV and the response to fluid administration.[218,219] Although PPV, like SPV, is affected by both Δ Up and Δ Down and may be misleading in conditions of hypervolemia or cardiac failure, a recent meta-analysis has shown PPV>12.5% to have the best discriminative power for fluid responsiveness among all dynamic indices.[208]

Stroke Volume Variation Stroke volume variation (SVV) can be calculated from arterial pulse contour cardiac output monitors and is defined as the difference between the maximal and minimal stroke volumes during a single mechanical breath divided by the mean stroke volume, and expressed as a percentage. SVV greater than 10% has been found to be a good predictor of fluid responsiveness in patients undergoing neurosurgical or cardiac procedures.[220,221]

A related dynamic index of fluid responsiveness is the respiratory variation in peak blood flow velocity in the descending aorta, which can be measured using esophageal Doppler. Respiratory variation in excess of 18% identified those patients who would benefit from volume infusion.[150]

Plethysmography-Derived Indices A noninvasive dynamic volume index has been described that is based on respiratory variation in the amplitude of the pulse oximetry plethysmography signal. The plethysmogram measures the sum total of volume changes within all vessels contained in tissue below the sensor, with arterial pulsations responsible for the largest portion of these changes. The plethysmogram waveform has a similar morphology to an ABP waveform, although it is important to

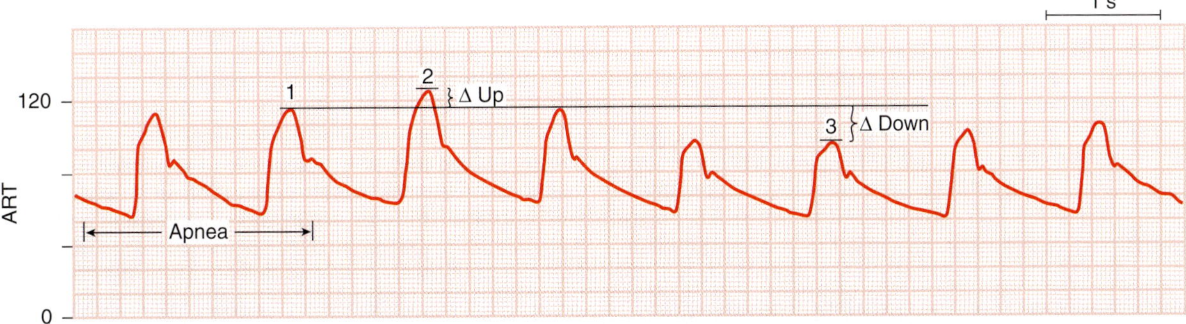

FIGURE 30-17. Systolic pressure variation visible on an arterial pressure trace. Note that Δ Up and Δ Down are measured from an apneic baseline. In this example, Δ Up is approximately 9 mm Hg, whereas Δ Down is approximately 18 mm Hg for a total systolic pressure variation of 27 mm Hg.

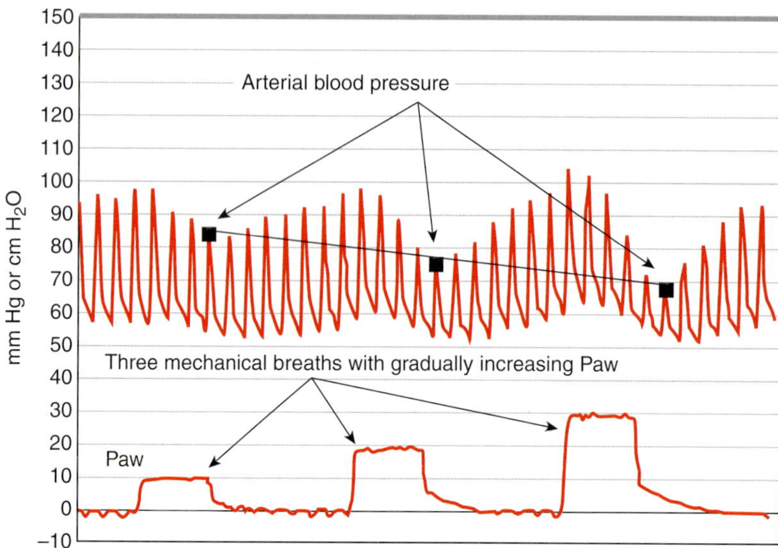

FIGURE 30-19. Respiratory systolic variation test: The steeper the slope of the line created by plotting minimal systolic blood pressures during the standardized protocol, the greater the predicted response to fluid resuscitation. Paw, mean airway pressure. [Reproduced with permission from Preisman S, Kogan S, Berkenstadt H, Perel A. Predicting fluid responsiveness in patients undergoing cardiac surgery: functional haemodynamic parameters including the Respiratory Systolic Variation Test and static preload indicators. *Br J Anaesth.* 2005;95(6):746-755.]

remember that whereas ABP waveforms reflect changes in *pressure*, plethysmography waveforms reflect changes in blood flow or *volume*. Use of plethysmography has generally been shown to correlate with other dynamic indices of volume assessment, although there is some conflicting evidence.[222-226] Whenever plethysmography is used to assess volume responsiveness, it is important to disable the autogain and autocentering functions that are integrated into clinical monitoring systems to allow detection of the respiratory variation in these signals.

Limitations of Dynamic Indices Dynamic preload indices are simple to use, minimally invasive, and accurately reflect the cardiac output response to fluid loading in many clinical conditions. However, they require the patient to be tracheally intubated and mechanically ventilated using a controlled mode of ventilation to ensure uniform tidal volume, generally larger than 8 mL/kg.[227,228] Dynamic indices cannot be used in patients with significant dysrhythmias, notably atrial fibrillation, because nonuniform diastolic filling time will induce its own beat-to-beat variation.

The respiratory systolic variation test has been suggested to eliminate the effects of tidal volume variation on SPV (**Fig. 30-19**).[229] Three or four consecutive pressure-controlled breaths are administered at increasing pressure settings in a stepwise fashion. A plot is then constructed of the lowest systolic pressure value versus peak inspiratory pressure, and a slope is calculated. A slope greater than 0.5 mm Hg/cm H_2O was found to have the best predictive power for fluid responsiveness.[229] The usefulness of this test in patients with abnormal lung compliance has not yet been addressed.

Summary Dynamic measures of volume responsiveness have been shown to be superior to static measures in identifying patients who will respond favorably to volume expansion. However, two important issues must be considered. First is that the dynamic variables previously described are a measure of fluid responsiveness, related to the subject's position on the cardiac function curve and not to an absolute preload (Fig. 30-16). Hypovolemic patients might fail to respond to volume expansion for a host of reasons including but not limited to right or left ventricular failure or increased venous or arterial compliance. Similarly, a change in contractility might induce a change in fluid responsiveness (and in PPV or SVV) without a change in preload, due to a switch to a steeper or flatter cardiac function curve.[230] Last, fluid administration might increase stroke volume due to an associated hemodilution-induced reduction in afterload, with minimal change in end-diastolic ventricular volume.[231]

A second important issue is identification of the clinical goal. Simply being fluid responsive does not necessarily equate with a clinical need for fluid administration. Indeed, fluid responsiveness is a normal characteristic of cardiovascular physiology.[199] The critical question is whether hypoperfusion exists, and only if the answer to this question is affirmative should evaluation of fluid responsiveness proceed.[232]

ASSESSMENT OF PERFUSION

Ensuring adequate perfusion of body organs is the main hemodynamic goal of the anesthesiologist in the perioperative period. Tissue hypoperfusion is the defining characteristic of circulatory shock but can occur long before other signs and symptoms become apparent. Unfortunately, most currently used monitoring modalities provide only indirect measures of organ perfusion. Regional perfusion variability adds to the monitoring challenge because some organs, like the splanchnic bed, might be hypoperfused, whereas vital organs like the brain and heart remain adequately perfused.[233]

Clinical Evaluation A variety of traditional clinical indices have been used to judge the adequacy of tissue perfusion. These clinical signs and symptoms include level of consciousness, urine output, heart rate, capillary refill, and skin temperature and color. All, however, may be unreliable in the perioperative period owing to the many confounding effects encountered during this time, and as a result, hemodynamic monitors have been developed to fill this patient care need.

Pressure-Based Indices The simplest of these monitors are pressure-based measurements, mainly systemic blood pressure and cardiac filling pressures. However, owing to autoregulation, perfusion of major body organs is pressure independent over a wide range of pressures. In addition, compensatory mechanisms help defend blood pressure, so that in many circumstances, arterial hypotension is a late sign of hypovolemia or shock.[157] Indeed, studies in different patient populations have demonstrated the coexistence of normal vital signs despite occult shock as demonstrated by continuing anaerobic metabolism.[234]

TABLE 30-5 Positive Randomized Controlled Studies of Goal-Directed Therapy in the Perioperative Period

Study	Patient Population	*N*	Monitoring Modality	Therapeutic Goals	Interventions	Outcome (Control vs Treatment Group)*
Boyd, 1993[267]	High-risk noncardiac surgery	107	PAC	DO_2 >600 mL/min per m²	Dopexamine	Mortality 22.7% vs 5.7%
Wilson, 1999[268]	Major elective noncardiac surgery	138	PAC	PAOP >12 mm Hg Hb >11 g/dL Sao_2 >94% DO_2 >600 mL/min per m²	Albumin, blood, oxygen, Adrenaline/Dopexamine	Mortality 17% vs 3%
Polonen, 2000[101]	Cardiac surgery	403	PAC	Svo_2 >70% Lactate <2 mmol/L	Dobutamine, fluids	LOS 7 vs 6, organ dysfunction on discharge 5.6% vs 1%
Pearse, 2005[269]	High-risk non-cardiac surgery	122	Lithium dilution	Maximize stroke volume DO_2 >600 mL/min per m²	Colloid boluses, dopexamine	LOS 14 vs 11, postop comp 68% vs 44%
Mythen, 1995[270]	Cardiac surgery	60	Esophageal Doppler	Maximize stroke volume	Colloid boluses	LOS 10.1 vs 6.4, postop comp 6 vs 0
Gan, 2002[271]	Noncardiac surgery with estimated blood loss >500 mL	100	Esophageal Doppler	Maximize stroke volume	Colloid boluses	LOS 7 vs 5
Wakeling, 2005[272]	Colorectal surgery	128	Esophageal Doppler	Maximize stroke volume	Colloid boluses	LOS 11.5 vs 10, GI morbidity 45.3% vs 14.11%
Donati, 2007[102]	Major abdominal surgery	135	Central venous catheter	Oxygen extraction ratio <27%	Colloid boluses, dobutamine, blood	LOS 13.4 vs 11.3, organ failures 27 vs 9
Lopes, 2007[273]	High risk noncardiac surgery	33	Arterial line	Pulse pressure variability <10%	Colloid boluses	LOS 17 vs 7, postop comp (per patient) 3.9 vs 1.4
Mayer, 2010[274]	Major abdominal surgery	60	Autocalibrated pulse-contour cardiac output	CI>2.5 L/min per m²	Fluid boluses, dobutamine	LOS 19 vs 15, postop comp 50% vs 20%

* For all results, *p* is significant at 0.05 unless stated otherwise.

PAC, pulmonary artery catheter; CI, cardiac index; DO_2, oxygen delivery; Vo_2, oxygen consumption; PAOP, pulmonary artery occlusion pressure; Hb, hemoglobin concentration; Sao_2 arterial oxygen saturation; SVR, systemic vascular resistance; Svo_2 mixed venous oxygen saturation; LOS, length of hospital stay (days); Postop comp, postoperative complications incidence.

Flow-Based Indices The next level of hemodynamic monitoring involves flow-based measurements, namely CO, stroke volume, and oxygen delivery. Several studies have suggested that these indices have prognostic value,[235] and many studies of goal-directed therapy have demonstrated their clinical utility (**Table 30-5**). However, these studies also demonstrate that the "optimal" level of cardiac output or oxygen delivery in the perioperative period is not necessarily the "normal" level. With the changes in oxygen requirements resulting from anesthesia on the one hand, or the systemic inflammatory response on the other, the same oxygen delivery might be too high, too low, or just right. The development of "oxygen debt" after major surgery has been found to be associated with both reduced survival and increased complications.[236]

Metabolic Indices Considering the shortcomings of flow-based monitoring methods, metabolic indices might supply the required information about the adequacy of oxygen delivery or cardiac output. These metabolic markers include either global measures, such as base excess, blood lactate level, and venous oxygen saturation, or regional perfusion measures, such as cerebral oximetry and gastric tonometry.

Lactic Acidosis Elevated blood lactate and metabolic acidosis indicate anaerobic metabolism, presumably related to hypoperfusion leading to tissue ischemia. Indeed, various studies have confirmed the prognostic significance of serial lactate and base deficit measurements,[237,238] and the potential of using lactate level as a guide for directing therapy.[101,239] Several pitfalls need to be recognized, however. Lactate levels may increase due to isolated organ damage such as limb ischemia or mesenteric thrombosis, where surgical intervention rather than medical therapy to increase oxygen delivery is warranted. Also, because there are various other etiologies for both hyperlactatemia and metabolic acidosis, lactic acidosis is probably a more specific index for hypoperfusion than either measure alone.[240]

Venous Oximetry Because increased oxygen extraction can initially compensate for reduced oxygen delivery, anaerobic metabolism usually does not occur before venous oxygen saturation has decreased to 30% to 40%.[241] Therefore, monitoring venous oxygen saturation, in either mixed venous (pulmonary artery) or central venous blood, might allow early detection of relative hypoperfusion and developing oxygen debt before tissue ischemia develops. Reduced venous oxygen saturation (<60%-65%) has been shown to predict adverse outcome after both cardiac and noncardiac surgery.[106, 242] In contrast, treating low CO in patients with a normal venous oxygen saturation might be counterproductive.[243] Indeed, venous oxygen saturation may be one of the more important monitors for judging the adequacy of hemodynamic status and determining whether the measured pressure- and flow-based indices are appropriate in the context of the individual patient's oxygen requirements.[244] In several clinical studies, venous oxygen saturation was successfully used to guide therapeutic interventions like blood transfusion and inotropic support, as part of a multidimensional goal-directed therapy.[100-102,107] **Figure 30-20** shows a sample algorithm.

Regional Versus Global Perfusion A major drawback of lactate, base deficit, and venous oxygen saturation is their global nature. Lactate production and increased oxygen extraction induced by ischemia in an isolated organ might be diluted and therefore masked when whole body lactate or mixed venous oximetry are measured. Therefore, monitoring regional perfusion may be advantageous. The best example is gastric

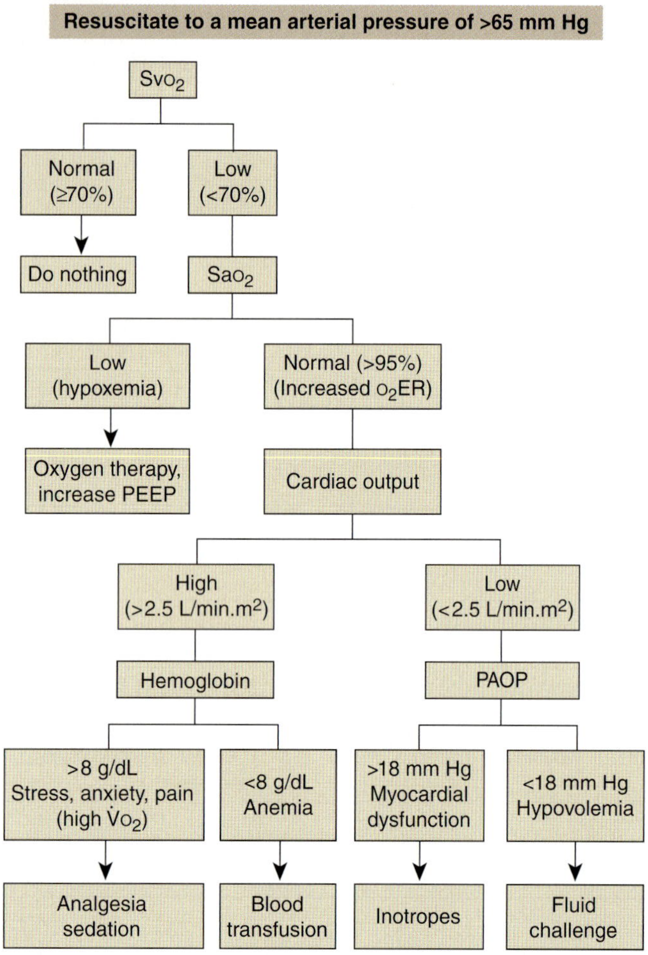

Resuscitate to a mean arterial pressure of >65 mm Hg

Svo_2

Normal (≥70%) → Do nothing

Low (<70%) → Sao_2

Low (hypoxemia) → Oxygen therapy, increase PEEP

Normal (>95%) (Increased O_2ER) → Cardiac output

High (>2.5 L/min.m^2) → Hemoglobin

>8 g/dL Stress, anxiety, pain (high $\dot{V}o_2$) → Analgesia sedation

<8 g/dL Anemia → Blood transfusion

Low (<2.5 L/min.m^2) → PAOP

>18 mm Hg Myocardial dysfunction → Inotropes

<18 mm Hg Hypovolemia → Fluid challenge

FIGURE 30-20. A systematic approach to assessment and treatment of hypoperfusion. Perfusion assessment by measuring mixed venous oxygen saturation (Svo_2) starts after restoration of perfusion pressure (which can be done using fluids and vasopressors). PAOP, pulmonary artery occlusion pressure; PEEP, positive end-expiratory pressure; Sao_2, arterial oxygen saturation; O_2ER, oxygen extraction ratio; $\dot{V}o_2$, systemic oxygen consumption. [Reproduced with permission from Pinsky MR, Vincent JL. Let us use the pulmonary artery catheter correctly and only when we need it. *Crit Care Med.* 2005;33(5):1119-1122.]

tonometry. Other regional monitors include jugular bulb oximetry, sublingual capnography, near-infrared light spectroscopy, tissue oxygen electrodes, and CytoScan imaging.[245,246]

To summarize, a systematic approach to hemodynamic monitoring that combines relatively easily measured metabolic indices with classical hemodynamic measurements might allow early detection of tissue hypoperfusion and appropriate corrective measures.

PREEMPTIVE GOAL-DIRECTED THERAPY

Monitoring alone cannot influence patient outcome unless it is used to guide effective therapeutic interventions. Usually, these interventions are ill defined and highly variable between practitioners, contributing to the difficulty in assessing the usefulness of various monitoring modalities, most notably the PAC.[3,46] "Goal-directed therapy," in contrast, defines a priori set of interventions aimed at achieving specific values for monitored physiologic parameters.[247] In an early retrospective trial in high-risk surgical patients, mostly trauma victims, survivors were found to achieve higher levels of cardiac output (>4.5 L/min per m^2), oxygen delivery (>600 mL/min per m^2) and oxygen consumption (>170 mL/min per m^2) compared with nonsurvivors.[235] This was followed by a successful prospective interventional trial aimed at treating patients to achieve these "supranormal" values preoperatively through use of fluids, blood transfusion, and vasoactive drugs.[248] Many similar trials followed, and most of them confirmed a significantly decreased morbidity and mortality in the goal-directed treatment group (Table 30-5). Meta-analyses of these optimization studies have confirmed a decrease in mortality, reduced length of hospital stay, earlier return of gastrointestinal function, reduced incidence of renal failure, and a decrease in overall postoperative complications.[249,250] In contrast, goal-directed therapy has been less successful when applied to critically ill medical and surgical patients who have an established systemic inflammatory response syndrome, sepsis, or multiorgan failure.[251] The main early pathophysiologic disturbance in trauma and perioperative patients is occult hypovolemia, which can often be ameliorated with fluids alone[252] or fluids plus a moderate inotropic support.[253] In contrast, the pathophysiologic disturbances in critically ill septic patients with multiorgan failure may be much more profound and involve abnormalities at the level of the microcirculation and mitochondria. These critically ill patients might not be able to increase oxygen use regardless of oxygen delivery.[254,255]

Goal-directed therapy is associated with several risks. Retrospective studies suggest that the large fluid volume required for increasing cardiac index and oxygen delivery to supranormal values might result in congestive heart failure[81] and increased abdominal pressure leading to gastric hypoperfusion and acute renal failure.[256] Positive inotropic agents might increase systemic oxygen consumption owing to their thermogenic effect, hence paradoxically decreasing venous oxygen saturation despite increased cardiac output.[99] Increasing myocardial oxygen consumption might also trigger acute ischemic events.[81]

Several recent studies have demonstrated some advantages to "restrictive" versus "liberal" fluid administration, especially during intra-abdominal operations.[257,258] Although "restrictive" management might seem to contradict the goal-directed approach, one should note that in the goal-directed approach patients usually receive more fluid only in the early stages of surgery but not later. Indeed, intraoperatively they usually receive only several hundred milliliters more fluid compared with control patients, and over the whole perioperative period they might actually receive less fluid compared with the control group.[259] Also, most goal-directed therapy studies used colloids whereas most "restrictive" versus "liberal" studies used crystalloid fluids. Although this controversial issue is beyond the scope of this chapter, recent studies suggest that this difference might affect perioperative outcome.[260]

For perioperative goal-directed therapy to have a beneficial effect on mortality, treated patients need to be very high risk (at least 15% to 20% predicted mortality, according to a recent meta-analysis).[261] Older patients with coexisting cardiorespiratory diseases may be one such group.[262] A low anaerobic threshold on preoperative cardiopulmonary exercise testing or a clinical assessment of the ability to climb 2 flights of stairs might help identify patients who will not be able to increase oxygen delivery perioperatively without aggressive therapeutic interventions.[263,264] Patients with lower mortality risk might still benefit from goal-directed therapy by having a reduced complication rate or shortened hospital length of stay, especially when undergoing extensive abdominal or vascular surgery.[247]

To provide any benefit, hemodynamic goals should be achieved early, either pre- or intraoperatively. In most patients, optimization of volume status is all that is required. Patients with known cardiac dysfunction may require inotropic therapy in addition to fluid resuscitation, guided either by cardiac output or venous oxygen saturation. Clinical attention to development of fluid overload and increased oxygen consumption may reduce potential complications of goal-directed therapy. In most studies, goal-directed therapeutic interventions were stopped at the end of surgery or at most a few hours later. When performed properly and applied to appropriate patient cohorts, perioperative hemodynamic optimization may not only improve outcome but also prove to be a cost-effective intervention as the reduction

BOX 30-9

Standard Steps for Troubleshooting Unexpected Monitored Values

- Recognize clinical urgency
- Address technical considerations
- Confirm digital values with accompanying waveforms
- Confirm measurements using another technique
- Cross-validate measurements with another monitored variable
- Consider physiologic and pathophysiologic explanations
- Consider iatrogenic causes

in complications compensates for the increased costs of monitoring and use of the ICU.[265]

DISCREPANT CLINICAL DATA AND TROUBLESHOOTING MONITORING PROBLEMS

One of the more important roles played by the anesthesiologist in the care of the critically ill patient is to determine that the monitored data are accurate. A common challenge arises when monitoring results provide discrepant data or are otherwise inconsistent with the clinical condition of the patient and the working clinical diagnosis. In these circumstances, a methodical approach is helpful, one that is based on a good understanding of monitoring equipment and patient physiology. **Box 30-9** summarizes the recommended steps in the evaluation of discrepant data. These steps can be performed rapidly and some even simultaneously. Although less common, there are certainly clinical situations in which apparently normal monitored values are in fact spurious. Recognition of these problems begins with knowledge of the clinical condition of the patient and the clinical context in which the monitored value is observed.

KEY REFERENCES

- Bloos F, Reinhart K. Venous oximetry. *Intensive Care Med.* 2005;31(7):911-913.
- Lees N, Hamilton M, Rhodes A. Clinical review: goal-directed therapy in high risk surgical patients. *Crit Care.* 2009;13(5):231.
- Mark JB. Central venous pressure monitoring: clinical insights beyond the numbers. *J Cardiothorac Vasc Anesth.* 1991;5:163-173.
- Michard F. Changes in arterial pressure during mechanical ventilation. *Anesthesiology.* 2005;103(2):419-428.
- O'Quin R, Marini JJ. Pulmonary artery occlusion pressure: clinical physiology, measurement, and interpretation. *Am Rev Respir Dis.* 1983;128(2):319-326.
- Pinsky MR. Pulmonary artery occlusion pressure. *Intensive Care Med.* 2003;29(1):19-22.
- Reuter DA, Huang C, Edrich T, et al. Cardiac output monitoring using indicator-dilution techniques: basics, limits, and perspectives. *Anesth Analg.* 2010;110(3):799-811.
- Siegemund M, van Bommel J, Ince C. Assessment of regional tissue oxygenation. *Intensive Care Med.* 1999;25(10):1044.

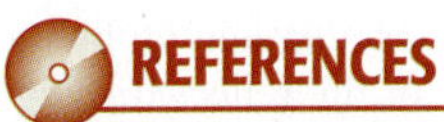

REFERENCES

Complete references available on DVD and online version at www.LongneckerAnesthesiology.com

CHAPTER 31

Intraoperative Transesophageal Echocardiography: A Systematic Approach

G. Burkhard Mackensen
Solomon Aronson

KEY POINTS

1. Transesophageal echocardiography (TEE) is an essential component of anesthesia care for modern cardiac and thoracic aortic surgery.
2. A complete diagnostic examination should include the standard set of views (at a minimum) suggested by guidelines from the American Society of Echocardiography and the Society of Cardiovascular Anesthesiologists.
3. Intraoperative evaluation of acute persistent and life-threatening hemodynamic disturbances in which ventricular function is uncertain and unresponsive to treatment is a Category I indication for TEE.
4. Real-time 3-dimensional echocardiography represents a breakthrough technology that fundamentally transforms intraoperative imaging.

Intraoperative echocardiography now is considered an essential part of modern cardiac and thoracic aortic surgery and is routinely used during other major surgical procedures such as liver and lung transplantations. It can be performed using transesophageal, epicardial, epiaortic, intravascular, and transthoracic approaches. Available imaging modalities include 2-dimensional (2D) and 3-dimensional (3D) imaging; pulsed-wave, continuous-wave, color-flow, and tissue Doppler; M-mode; speckle tracking. The echocardiographic data are obtained in real time (RT) and interpreted by a physician in a timely manner to direct the clinical treatment of surgical patients. The clinical applications of intraoperative echocardiography are numerous, including assessment of left ventricular (LV) and right ventricular (RV) function, assessment of preload, measurement of cardiac output, detection of myocardial ischemia, assessment of valvular function and pathology, detection and assessment of various congenital heart diseases, and evaluation of aortic atheromatous disease before manipulation of the aorta. Intraoperative echocardiography serves as both an important diagnostic tool and a monitor for cardiac surgical patients. With an emphasis on 2D and 3D transesophageal echocardiography (TEE), this chapter combines practical recommendations for a comprehensive 2D TEE examination with some of the key features of the emerging 3D TEE technology.

INDICATIONS FOR PERIOPERATIVE TRANSESOPHAGEAL ECHOCARDIOGRAPHY

Perioperative TEE has evolved as an important clinical tool that aids the hemodynamic management and improves outcome in patients undergoing cardiac surgery for valve repairs, coronary artery bypass grafting (CABG), thoracic aortic surgery, and repair of complex congenital lesions. Perioperative TEE involves the use of cardiac ultrasonography in surgical patients immediately before, during, or after their operations. In the perioperative setting, TEE not only facilitates diagnoses and optimizes the surgical approach during cardiac operations but also guides the institution of specific treatments and helps monitoring interventions throughout the operative course without disrupting the surgical workflow.[1-5]

Since 1996, when evidence-based practice guidelines for perioperative TEE initially were published (**Fig. 31-1**), support for the superiority of intraoperative TEE over other cardiovascular monitoring techniques (eg, electrocardiograms [ECGs] or pulmonary artery catheters) has steadily increased.[6,7] Recently updated guidelines recommend the use of

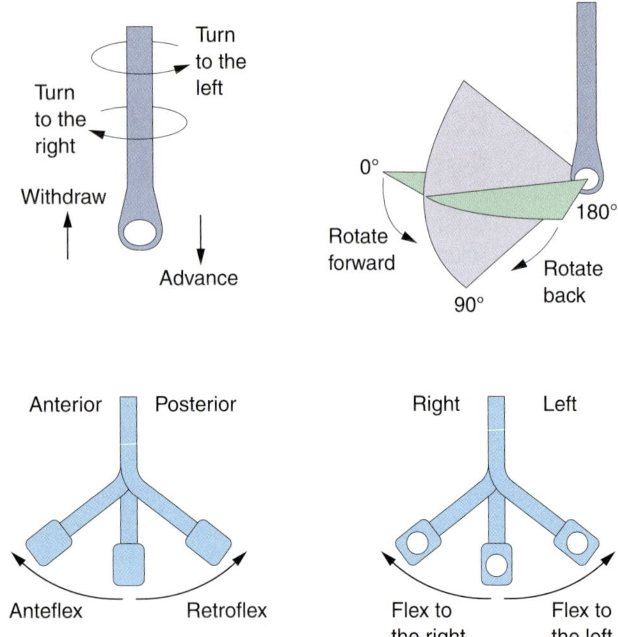

FIGURE 31-1. Probe manipulation of guidelines. [Modified from Shanewise JS, Cheung AT, Aronson S, et al. ASE/SCA guidelines for performing a comprehensive intraoperative multiplane transesophageal echocardiography examination: recommendations of the American Society of Echocardiography Council for Intraoperative Echocardiography and the Society of Cardiovascular Anesthesiologists Task Force for Certification in Perioperative Transesophageal Echocardiography. *Anesth Analg.* 1999;89(4):870-884.]

TEE in all adult patients without contraindications undergoing open-heart (eg, valvular procedures) and thoracic aortic surgical procedures and to consider its use in CABG surgeries to confirm and refine the preoperative diagnosis, detect new or unsuspected pathology, amend the anesthetic and surgical plan accordingly, and evaluate the results of the surgical procedure. In younger patients, the use of TEE should be considered on a case-by-case basis because of risks unique to these patients.[8] In addition, the dynamics of each case should dictate when a TEE examination may reduce critical diagnostic work or distract from it. **Table 31-1** provides some published recommendations.

LIMITATIONS TO AND CONTRAINDICATIONS FOR TRANSESOPHAGEAL ECHOCARDIOGRAPHY

One of the most important limitations to performing an intraoperative TEE examination relates to the skills and expertise of the echocardiographer, now often a TEE-trained anesthesiologist.[9] Recent guidelines published by the American Society of Echocardiography (ASE) and the Society of Cardiovascular Anesthesiologists (SCA) seek to establish recommendations and guidelines for a continuous quality improvement program specific to the perioperative environment.[10] However, substantial patient harm can also result from inappropriate fixation of the anesthesiologist's attention on the TEE examination rather than on the patient. Although performing a useful TEE examination while simultaneously caring for the patient often is possible, a more appropriate practice would be having a colleague perform the TEE examination while the primary anesthesiologist focuses on caring for the patient (especially if a more comprehensive TEE examination is desired or the patient is unstable).

Absolute contraindications to performing a TEE examination in an anesthetized patient include esophageal stricture, tracheoesophageal fistula, recent esophageal surgery, and esophageal trauma. A history of dysphagia, esophageal varices, severe gastroesophageal reflux disease, odynophagia, unstable cervical spine injuries, prior mediastinal radiation, and upper airway pathology should be sought before probe insertion and are considered relative contraindications. Although TEE is considered safe and a relatively noninvasive, severe and life-threatening complications have been reported.[11] Proper insertion of the TEE probe requires skill and judgment. In anesthetized patients, the probe can be inserted blindly or with laryngoscopic visualization. The latter has been shown to reduces the incidence of oropharyngeal mucosal injury, odynophagia, and the number of insertion attempts.[12] It is helpful to have an assistant support the probe during insertion. A bite guard should always be used to protect the patient as well as the probe. Major complications of TEE are rare (0.2%-0.6% of insertion attempts in prospective studies),[13-15] and most examples are based on published case reports.[11] The transducer should never be forced through resistance upon entry into or during passage through the esophagus. Insertion and manipulation of the TEE probe can result in oral, esophageal, or pharyngeal trauma and arrhythmias. Another important risk of performing a TEE examination is misrepresenting a finding as abnormal when it is actually a normal variant or an artifact (**Table 31-2**). Understanding the normal variants enables better diagnostic accuracy when detecting abnormal structures. Significant clinical experience is required for the echocardiographer to be able to confidently make this distinction.

TERMINOLOGY

Table 31-3 lists the terminology used to describe probe manipulation with the patient lying supine with reference to the heart.

BASIC PRINCIPLES OF ECHOCARDIOGRAPHY

Two-dimensional echocardiography displays the intensity of reflected ultrasound waves as brightness along the axis of the scan plane to reconstruct a representative 2D image. Although this 2D qualitative assessment includes the description of cardiac structures, chamber sizes, and shapes, it does not allow for a quantitative hemodynamic approach to determine blood flow and volumes, pressure gradients, valve areas, and intracardiac pressures.

Hemodynamic evaluation with echocardiography consists of both qualitative and quantitative assessment using Doppler ultrasonography. The Austrian physicist Christian Doppler first described the "Doppler effect" in 1843. The Doppler effect is defined as the change in frequency of a sound or light wave that is caused by the motion of the source or the observer. If the sound source (eg, red blood cells) moves toward the observer (eg, ultrasound transducer), the sound frequency increases; when the sound source moves away from the observer, the sound frequency decreases. The term *frequency shift* (or *Doppler shift*) describes the change in frequency between the transmitted sound and the reflected sound. The Doppler shift depends on the velocity of the moving target and the intercept angle θ between the direction of the moving target and the ultrasound beam, all described in the Doppler equation:

$$\text{Doppler equation: } \Delta f = 2\ Ft \times V \times \cos\theta / c$$

Δf = Doppler shift
Ft = frequency transmitted
V = velocity (m/s)
$\cos\theta$ = cosine of the angle between blood flow and ultrasound beam
c = speed of sound (1560 m/s)

Solving for velocity leads to the following equation:

$$V = c \times \Delta f / 2\ Ft \times \cos\theta$$

Clinically, the frequency transmitted and the speed of sound through tissue remains constant. This reduces the determination of blood flow velocity to only 2 variables: the frequency of the reflected signal and the cosine of the angle between the direction of blood flow and the ultrasound beam. It is important to know that the intercept angle between the ultrasound beam and the blood flow needs to be as small

TABLE 31-1 Recommended Indications for Transesophageal Echocardiography

Category I Indications: Supported by the strongest evidence or expert opinion: TEE is frequently useful in improving clinical outcomes in these settings and is often indicated, depending on individual circumstances (eg, patient risk and practice setting).	Category II Indications: Supported by weaker evidence and expert consensus; TEE may be useful in improving clinical outcomes in these settings, depending on individual circumstances, but appropriate indications are less certain.	Category III Indications: Little current scientific or expert support; TEE is infrequently useful in improving clinical outcomes in these settings, and appropriate indications are uncertain.
• Intraoperative evaluation of acute, persistent, and life-threatening hemodynamic disturbances in which ventricular function and its determinants are uncertain and have not responded to treatment • Intraoperative use in valve repair • Intraoperative use in congenital heart surgery for most lesions requiring cardiopulmonary bypass • Intraoperative use in repair of hypertrophic obstructive cardiomyopathy • Intraoperative use for endocarditis when preoperative testing was inadequate or extension of infection to perivalvular tissue is suspected • Preoperative use in unstable patients with suspected thoracic aortic aneurysms, dissections, or disruption who need to be evaluated quickly • Intraoperative assessment of aortic valve function in repair of aortic dissections with possible aortic valve involvement • Intraoperative evaluation of pericardial window procedures • Use in intensive care unit for unstable patients with unexplained hemodynamic disturbances, suspected valve disease, or thromboembolic problems (if other tests or monitoring techniques have not confirmed the diagnosis or patients are too unstable to undergo other tests)	• Perioperative use in patients with increased risk of myocardial ischemia or infarction • Perioperative use in patients with increased risk of hemodynamic disturbances • Intraoperative assessment of valve replacement • Intraoperative assessment of repair of cardiac aneurysms • Intraoperative evaluation of removal of cardiac tumors • Intraoperative detection of foreign bodies • Intraoperative detection of air emboli during cardiotomy, heart transplant operations, and upright neurosurgical procedures • Intraoperative use during intracardiac thrombectomy • Intraoperative use during pulmonary embolectomy • Intraoperative use for suspected cardiac trauma • Preoperative assessment of patients with suspected acute thoracic aortic dissections, aneurysms, or disruption • Intraoperative use during repair of thoracic aortic dissections without suspected aortic valve involvement • Intraoperative detection of aortic atheromatous disease or other sources of aortic emboli • Intraoperative evaluation of pericardiectomy, pericardial effusions, or evaluation of pericardial surgery • Intraoperative evaluation of anastomotic sites during heart or lung transplantation • Monitoring placement and function of assist devices	• Intraoperative evaluation of myocardial perfusion, coronary artery anatomy, or graft patency • Intraoperative use during repair of cardiomyopathies other than hypertrophic obstructive cardiomyopathy • Intraoperative use for uncomplicated endocarditis during noncardiac surgery • Intraoperative monitoring for emboli during orthopedic procedures • Intraoperative assessment of repair of thoracic aortic injuries • Intraoperative use for uncomplicated pericarditis • Intraoperative evaluation of pleuropulmonary diseases • Monitoring placement of intraaortic balloon pumps, automatic implantable cardiac defibrillators, or pulmonary artery catheters • Intraoperative monitoring of cardioplegia administration

TEE, transesophageal echocardiography.

Modified from Daniel MT, Martin A, Bruce AB, et al. Practice guidelines for perioperative transesophageal echocardiography. A report by the American Society of Anesthesiologists and the Society of Cardiovascular Anesthesiologists Task Force on Transesophageal Echocardiography. *Anesthesiology.* 1996;84(4):986-1006.

TABLE 31-2 Normal Structures That May Be Mistaken for Abnormal Cardiac Masses

Left atrium	Tissue ridge between the superior pulmonary vein and left atrial appendage ("Coumadin ridge")
	Atrial suture line after cardiac transplant
Left ventricle	Papillary muscle
	Chordae variant (redundancy)
	Prominent apical trabeculation
Right atrium	Chiari network
	Eustachian valve
	Crista terminalis
	Lipomatous hypertrophy of interatrial septum or lateral tricuspid valve annulus
	Right atrial appendage trabeculations
	Pulmonary artery catheter, pacer wire
Right ventricle	Moderator band
	Pulmonary artery catheter, pacer wire
Aortic valve	Nodules of Arantius
	Lambl excrescences
Mitral valve	Myxomatous mitral valve tissue
	Lambl excrescences
Pericardium	Epicardial adipose tissue

TABLE 31-3 Transesophageal Echocardiography Probe Manipulation

Terminology	Definition
Superior	Toward the head
Inferior	Toward the feet
Anterior	Toward the sternum
Right and left	Patient's right and left sides
Advancing the transducer	Pushing the tip of the probe deeper into the esophagus or the stomach
Withdrawing the transducer	Pulling the tip of the probe up the esophagus toward the head
Turning to the right	Moving the tip of the probe clockwise within the esophagus (scan plane moving toward the patient's right if the transducer is oriented anteriorly)
Turning to the left	Moving the tip of the probe counterclockwise
Rotating forward	Rotation of the multiplane angle from 0 degree toward 180 degrees (using the electronic toggle switch)
Rotating back	Rotation of the multiplane angle in the opposite direction toward 0 degree
Anteflexing	Flexing the tip of the probe anteriorly (clockwise rotation of the large control wheel when oriented anteriorly)
Retroflexing	Flexing the tip posteriorly (counterclockwise rotation)
Flexing to the right	Laterally flexing the tip of the probe to the patient's right (clockwise rotation of the small control wheel). (Fig. 31-1)
Flexing to the left	Flexing the tip to the patient's left (Fig. 31-1)

as possible to prevent underestimation of peak velocity. If the angle is 0, the true peak velocity can be measured because the cosine of 0 is 1. Conventionally, an intercept angle between 0 and 20 degrees is accepted because this will keep the resulting error in the range of 0% to 6%. Clinically, this can be achieved by interrogation of the peak velocity from multiple views to obtain an angle of insonation between 0 and 20 degrees. This necessitates using specific views to obtain accurate measurements, as will be described.

Pulsed-wave Doppler (PWD) uses a single transducer that sends and receives ultrasound beams. The ultrasound crystal sends short bursts of ultrasound beams with a given frequency (pulse repetition frequency [PRF]). These beams are reflected by the moving red blood cells and received by the emitting crystal. PWD displays the mean velocity of a small sample area versus time, resulting in velocity waveforms of that sample. This allows more accurate measurement of velocity waveforms in specific areas (eg, depth) with a high sampling rate but without the 2D structural information (range resolution). Because of the pulsed nature of this Doppler, it can measure velocities only within a given range determined by how long the transducer listens for ultrasound reflections before repeating the pulses. Velocities outside this given range are assigned incorrect velocities, termed *aliasing*. The aliasing velocity (the highest velocity accurately displayed) often can be increased by decreasing the pulse repetition frequency, but this degrades the temporal resolution.

Color-flow Doppler (CFD) uses multiple sampling sites along the ultrasound beams and is based on PWD principles. The frequency shift at each sampling site is measured and expressed in a preset color according to a color flow map. By definition, flow toward the transducer (positive Doppler shift) is expressed in red color; flow away from the transducer (negative Doppler shift) is expressed in blue. Turbulent flow or high-velocity flow (above the Nyquist limit) with changing directions is displayed in bright, mixed, and speckled colors of yellow, green, and orange. This velocity information is overlaid on top of the 2D image, allowing the echocardiographer to visualize the velocity flow patterns of blood through the various structures. The velocity data for the CFD sample area consist of many PWD areas, which reduces the frame rate of the image displayed. Decreasing the lateral area covered by CFD results in less PWD sampling and a higher frame rate. Because PWD is used to construct CFD images, CFD suffers from the same velocity and temporal resolution limitations.

Continuous-wave Doppler (CWD) displays all the blood velocities along a beam of ultrasound rather than at a particular location. The continuous nature of this mode allows for display of the complete range of velocities at the highest temporal resolution. However, this mode cannot determine where along the ultrasound beam the particular velocities originated. This limitation of CWD is termed *range ambiguity*. Often, the echocardiographer will be able to assume where the peak velocities should be originating (eg, a narrowed valve orifice).

Using PWD or CWD, blood flow velocities in cardiac chambers or great vessels can be measured. With the use of the modified Bernoulli equation, these velocities can be converted into pressure gradients (in mm Hg) across a given orifice (eg, across a stenotic valve):

$$\text{Modified Bernoulli equation: } \Delta P = 4(V_2^2 - V_1^2).$$

Simplified Bernoulli equation: $\Delta P = 4V_2^2$ (assuming $V_1 < 1.5$ m/s).

Over the past decade, the introduction of the concepts of strain and strain rate and the development of novel imaging technologies have allowed for the objective quantification of myocardial deformation during the cardiac cycle. These techniques are grouped under the name **myocardial deformation imaging** and comprise tissue Doppler strain, 2D and 3D speckle tracking, and velocity vector imaging.

Strain is a measure of deformation, which means that is measures lengthening and shortening. Strain rate represents the rate of change of that deformation.[16] Strain and strain rate have been shown to provide complementary information when assessing cardiac function.[17-19] Regional assessment of the LV can be accomplished by using tissue Doppler imaging (TDI). Velocity vectors obtained with TDI allow calculating strain as a change in unit length relative to the initial length. Two-dimensional speckle tracking is a new echocardiographic technique developed to measure myocardial strain and strain rate independent of the insonation angle. This is possible because the acoustic markers (speckles) used can be followed in any direction.

Although advances in myocardial deformation imaging have made the intraoperative evaluation of these techniques quite feasible, they have been incompletely studied.

The history of **3D echocardiography** goes back to 1974, when Dekker et al[20] described the first 3D reconstruction of 2D images and the first 3D TEE was performed in 1992.[21] For years, the image quality using reconstructive techniques has been shown to depend critically on the quality of the original 2D images in which minor patient movements (during ventilation) or movement of the heart (during arrhythmia) may result in artifacts.[22,23] Because of cumbersome and time-consuming acquisition and reconstruction processes (15-30 minutes[23]), reconstructive 3D echocardiography remained primarily a research tool. More recent advances in technology have allowed improvements in the acquisition of multiple, gated image planes using ECG and respiratory gating that limits the amount of motion artifacts. Postprocessing of acquired images results in 3D images that can be further optimized. One significant drawback of reconstructive approaches to 3D echocardiography is that live, RT imaging cannot be achieved because the different imaging planes are required sequentially. In the late 1980s, a sparse array matrix transducer containing 256 elements was designed to develop a new approach to 3D echocardiography and to overcome some of these issues. Although this transducer allowed generating different cut planes from a 3D volume online, it was not capable of displaying RT-rendered 3D images.[24-26] Further advances in crystal and computer technology allowed for the introduction of matrix-array transducers for the use in transthoracic echocardiography (TTE). Matrix-array transducers use a greater number of imaging elements (>2500), which are capable of generating RT-rendered 3D images.[27,28] More recently, the reduction in the size of the transducer footprint in addition to other technical developments led to the introduction of a RT 3D TEE transducer and a RT-capable ultrasound system that is available to the operative environment.[29,30]

To date, the only clinical available RT 3D TEE transducer is the X7-2t TEE (Philips Medical Systems, Andover, MA) transducer, which combines xMATRIX technology and PureWave crystal technology. This technology allows creation of live biplane (termed Xplane) imaging with 2 full-resolution planes created simultaneously and therefore enables the parallel acquisition of diagnostic data without moving the probe. Importantly, the system permits live volume imaging with unlimited planes in all directions, allowing the acquisition and rendering of true RT 3D full-volume data. Of note, 3D TEE systems provide all conventional modalities such as 2D multiplane imaging, M-mode, PWD and CWD as well as color Doppler imaging. The following 4 3D imaging modes are possible.

LIVE 3D

This RT mode displays a narrow fixed pyramidal data set of approximately 50 by 30 degrees by the depth of the initial 2D image that conveniently can be used to visualize any cardiac structure located in the near field (**Fig. 31-2**A). Movement of the TEE probe results in a live (RT) change of the 3D image. Live 3D permits for quick 3D imaging and immediate return to a 2D mode. Live 3D achieves frame rates up to 30 Hz and is suitable to guide interventional procedures in RT. Using Live 3D, a thick slice (90 degrees × 1 degree) representing an enhanced 2D image may also be displayed and rotated in space.

LIVE 3D ZOOM

This mode displays a magnified but truncated pyramidal data set of variable size. Live 3D Zoom can be focused on a specific region of interest that should be minimized to optimize frame rate and image quality

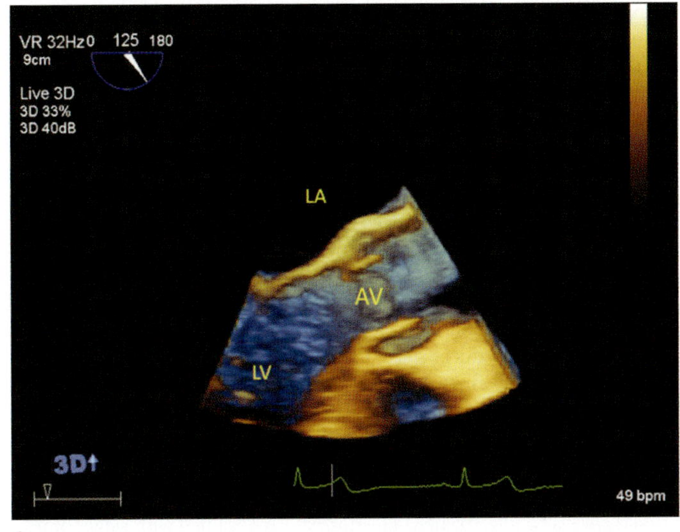

A

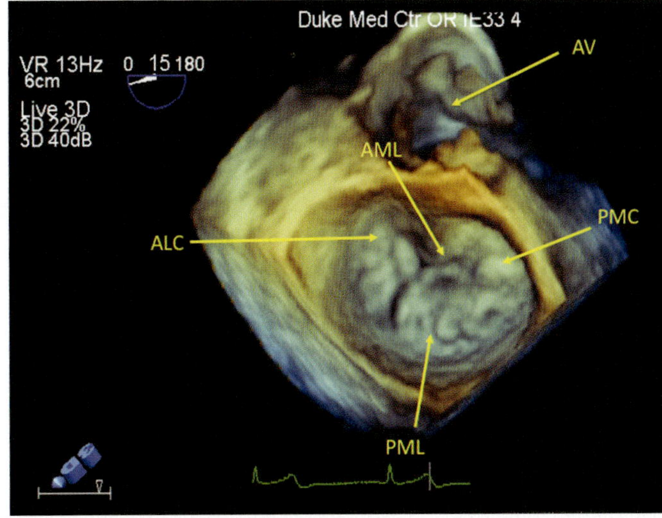

B

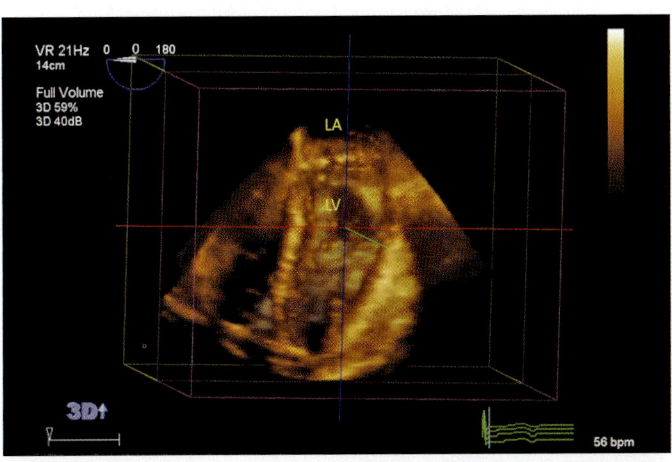

C

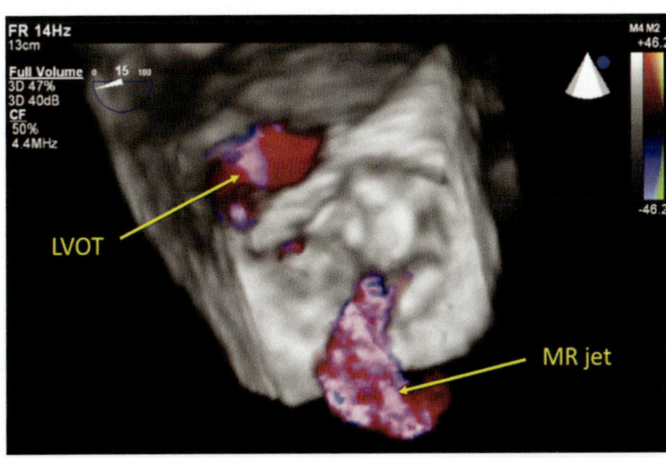

D

FIGURE 31-2. A. Midesophageal live three-dimensional (3D) transesophageal echocardiography (TEE) image of a normal aortic valve in long axis. Live 3D obtains a fixed pyramidal data set of approximately 50 x 30 degrees. **B.** 3D TEE zoom *en face* view of a normal mitral valve with the anterior mitral leaflet (AML) on the top and the posterior mitral leaflet (PML) on the bottom. The orientation of the image is similar to the surgeon's view. **C.** 3D TEE full volume of the left ventricle presented as an auto cropped image revealing only 50% of the larger full-volume data set. **D.** 3D TEE color full volume demonstrating central mitral regurgitation and flow in the left ventricular outflow tract (LVOT). ALC, anterolateral commissure; AV, aortic valve; LA, left atrium; LV, left ventricle; MR, mitral regurgitation; PMC, posteromedial commissure.

(Fig. 31-2B). Live 3D Zoom is preferentially used to display the mitral valve (MV), the tricuspid valve (TV), the left atrial appendage (LAA), or the intra-atrial septum.

3D FULL VOLUME

This mode allows the gated acquisition of a pyramidal data set (~65 degrees × 60 degrees up to 100 degrees × 100 degrees) that includes a larger cardiac volume (Fig. 31-2C). This wide-angle data set is composed by merging 4 to 7 narrower RT 3D pyramidal wedges obtained over 4 to 7 heartbeats. Although artifacts cannot be totally avoided in patients with arrhythmias, they can be minimized in anesthetized patients by holding ventilation and acquiring full-volume loops while electrocautery is not used. With the goal of minimizing artifacts, it is recommended to acquire full-volume loops at the beginning of the comprehensive TEE examination in the operating room before the start of surgery.

3D COLOR FULL VOLUMES

These are acquired similar to the acquisition of a full-volume data set. Again, the wide-angle data set is compiled by merging 7 to 14 narrower RT-3D pyramidal wedges and is similarly prone to artifacts introduced by arrhythmias, movement, or electrocautery. It is essential to place the area of interest (eg, the regurgitant jet) in the center of the sector (Fig. 31-2D).

Postprocessing involves the appropriate orientation and cropping of acquired 3D data and requires a whole new set of skills. Any stored 3D image can be manipulated by rotation so that easily recognized structures such as the aortic valve (AV) become visible to orient the image in space. Cropping of 3D images can be performed by either using 1 of 6 available cropping planes selected from a 3D cropping box (along the 3 axes, X, Y, and Z, using 6 orthogonal planes) or by using a freely adjustable cropping plane. Approximate measurements can be performed in an easy way by using the 3D grid with a specified dot-to-dot distance allowing the estimation of dimensions of cardiac structures (eg, the MV annulus). More sophisticated and accurate measurements require the use of built-in software (QLAB 7.0, Philips Medical Systems, Andover, MA). This software contains several programs, including the MV Quantification (MVQ), the 3D Quantification Advanced (3DQAV) for assessment of LV volumes and function, and the simpler 3D Quantification (3DQ) program. Offline analysis can also be performed using commercially available software such as 4D LV-Analysis,

4D Cardio-view, 4D RV-Function, or 4D MV assessment 2.0 (TomTec Imaging Systems, Unterschleissheim, Munich, Germany).

SYSTEMATIC APPROACH TO A TRANSESOPHAGEAL ECHOCARDIOGRAPHY EXAMINATION

The ASE and the SCA have suggested a set of standard views and the nomenclature for those views.[7] This nomenclature should be followed whenever possible to minimize confusion. Generally, a combination of these views allows for a complete diagnostic examination. However, deviation from these standard views may be necessary to obtain images appropriate to the individual patient. It is beneficial to be flexible about the order in which the views are obtained to allow focusing on a specific clinical question in a timely manner. Each echocardiographer should develop a systematic order for routine diagnostic TEE. This not only allows for increased speed and efficiency but also ensures that an important finding will not be missed simply because a view was forgotten.

Many echocardiographers prefer to order the examination such that they collect multiple views focusing on many different structures from each probe position or depth before moving to the next probe location. This allows for increased efficiency and decreases the total probe manipulation necessary for a complete examination. Alternatively, the echocardiographer may focus on 1 structure or chamber at a time. This results in duplicated views because many structures usually can be seen within single views and increased probe manipulation because each structure is interrogated from different vantage points and angles.

LEFT ATRIUM

Because the left atrium (LA) lies just anterior to the esophagus in most patients, the LA can be seen in the near field (ie, at the top) of most midesophageal (ME) images of the heart (probe tip is approximately 35 cm from the teeth and anteriorly oriented). Evaluation of the LA usually starts from an ME 4-chamber view (**Fig. 31-3**A; multiplane angle at 0 to 20 degrees with transducer slightly retroflexed from the neutral position). It can be evaluated further as the multiplane angle sweeps from 0 to 120 degrees. Within the LA, a tissue ridge ("Coumadin ridge") separates the LAA and left upper pulmonary vein (Fig. 31-3B, 31-3C, and 31-3D). This atrial tissue can accumulate fat, creating a mass-like appearance. Because the majority of LA thrombi are located within the LAA, this structure should always be interrogated. The normal LAA is lined with ridges of pectinate muscle, which may be difficult to differentiate from small thrombi. Thrombi are generally more rounded and often fill the appendage.

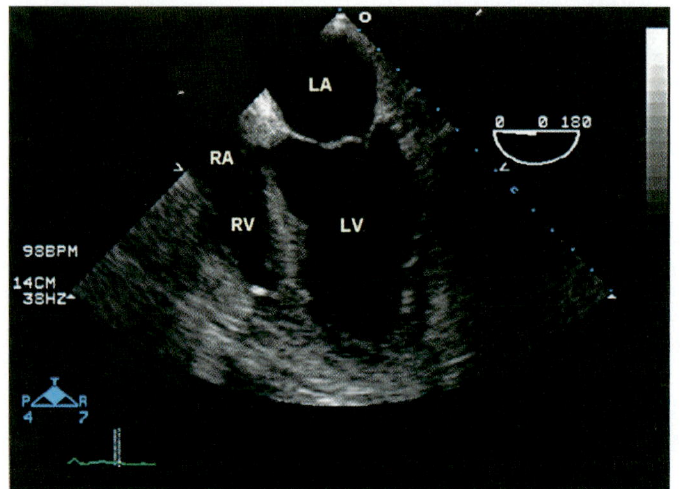

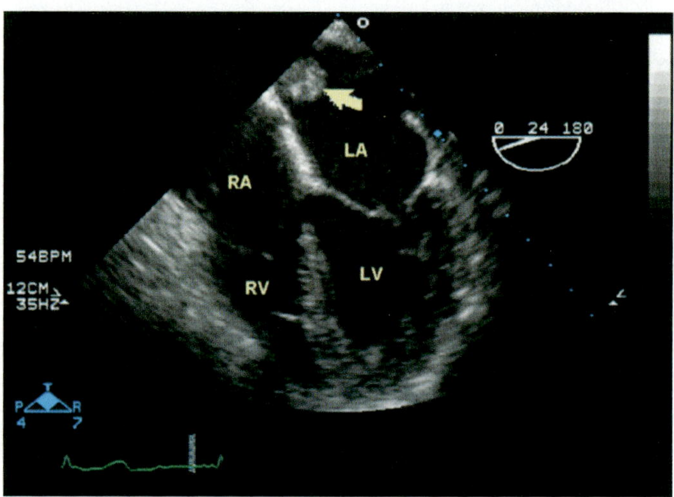

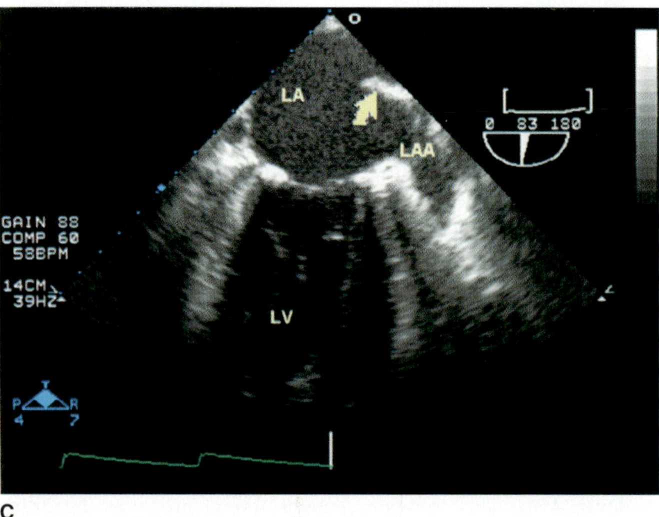

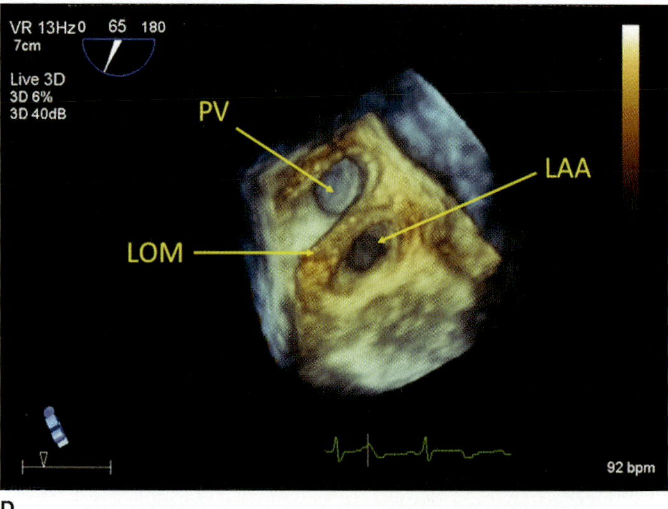

FIGURE 31-3. A. Standard midesophageal 4-chamber view. **B.** Midesophageal 4-chamber view with an atrial myxoma (*arrow*). **C.** Midesophageal 2-chamber view with left atrial appendage (LAA) and Coumadin ridge (*arrow*). **D.** Three-dimensional transesophageal echocardiography zoom of the LAA adjacent to the ligamentum of Marshall and the left superior pulmonary vein (LSPV). LA, left atrium; LV, left ventricle; RA, right atrium; RV, right ventricle.

LA thrombus usually is associated with high-risk structural and functional heart disease, most commonly atrial fibrillation, mitral stenosis, MV prosthesis, or LA enlargement resulting from LV dysfunction. These structural and functional cardiac abnormalities tend to be associated with blood stasis within the LA, which facilitates thrombus formation. Mitral regurgitation (MR) may decrease LA stasis and protect against LA thrombus formation. Aortic stenosis (AS) or an AV prosthesis usually does not result in significant LA stasis unless accompanied by LV dysfunction. Thrombus usually is homogeneous in appearance, more echogenic than the underlying myocardium, appears in multiple imaging planes, and moves in concert with the underlying myocardium.

TEE is considered the gold standard imaging modality for detection of LA and LAA thrombi. This is partly because of the large percentage of LA thrombi that are found in the LAA, which can be well delineated by TEE. The LAA can be evaluated by keeping the LAA centered in the image and rotating the multiplane angle from 0 to 180 degrees. Spontaneous echo contrast (SEC), seen as a slowly swirling "smoke" pattern, indicates low-flow velocities that are strongly associated with LA thrombus. Doppler interrogation of the LA appendage also may be helpful because lower blood flow velocities identify patients at higher risk. Despite a relatively high specificity, 2D TEE imaging may overestimate the incidence of thrombi partly because of the complex 3D morphology of multilobed LAA.[31] This complex structure of the LAA lends itself well to 3D assessment. Recent reports using RT 3D TTE or reconstruction 3D TEE showed that 3D assessment enables excellent visualization of the LAA anatomy and function.[32-34] Furthermore, RT 3D TEE provides excellent visualization of the LAA orifice, which may optimize the guidance for the placement of LAA occlusion devices.[35] Successful application of RT 3D TEE to confirm stable catheter position along the entire length of the ligament of Marshall during LA catheter ablation for atrial fibrillation has also been described. RT 3D TEE could potentially enhance lesion delivery during LA catheter ablation for atrial fibrillation to improve efficacy and safety.[36] Furthermore, RT 3D TEE might become the method of choice to more accurately evaluate the LAA, especially to distinguish thrombi from anatomical variants and might alter the course of therapy in patients with atrial fibrillation, including the placement of a LAA occlusion device.[37] The LAA can be best visualized by using the 3D zoom mode, obtaining the *en face* view of the LAA with the adjacent ligament of Marshall (Fig. 31-3D).

RIGHT ATRIUM

Evaluation of the right atrium (RA) can be approached from the ME 4-chamber view, ME bicaval view (**Fig. 31-4**A; probe turned to the patient's right with a multiplane angle of 110-120 degrees), ME RV inflow–outflow view (Fig. 31-4B; 40-60 degrees), and transgastric (TG) RV inflow view (rotating the angle to 90 degrees and turning the probe to the right from the TG short-axis [SAX] view). The RA is a thin-walled structure. The superior vena cava (SVC) and inferior vena cava (IVC) enter the RA posteriorly and medially, respectively. The coronary sinus (CS) can be imaged echocardiographically as a small tubular sonolucency in the posterior atrioventricular (AV) groove. Remnant embryonic structures should be distinguished from thrombi and other masses. The eustachian valve is an elongated, membranous projection at the junction of the RA and IVC. The Chiari network, a delicate, mobile structure often arising from the eustachian valve and stretching to the interatrial septum (IAS), may be misdiagnosed as an atrial mass. The crista terminalis is a vertical ridge of muscle originating at the junction of the RA and SVC. It runs toward the IVC and has also been misinterpreted as an intracardiac mass. Central venous catheters, pulmonary artery catheters, and pacing wires often can be seen as they course through the right heart and should not be confused as pathologic masses. RA thrombi typically are associated with indwelling catheters or pacemaker leads.

INTERATRIAL SEPTUM

The IAS consists of the thin fossa ovalis centrally and thicker limbus regions anteriorly and posteriorly. The IAS should be examined with both 2D and CFD, which adds to the detection of interatrial shunts. Three-dimensional TEE imaging provides excellent RT images of the IAS and atrial septum defects and aids in guiding percutaneous placement of IAS closure devices (**Fig. 31-5**A).[38]

Structural atrial septal defects (ASDs) can be divided anatomically into defects at the fossa ovalis (ostium secundum type), defects occurring inferior to the fossa ovalis (ostium primum type), and defects occurring superior to the fossa ovalis (sinus venosus type). The most common defect is the ostium secundum type, in which the posterior atrial wall may be totally absent (Fig. 31-5B). The ostium primum type usually can be seen inferior to the fossa ovalis in the ME 4-chamber view. It is associated with other endocardial cushion defects, such as ventricular septal defects, AV canal defects, and TV or MV abnormalities. The sinus

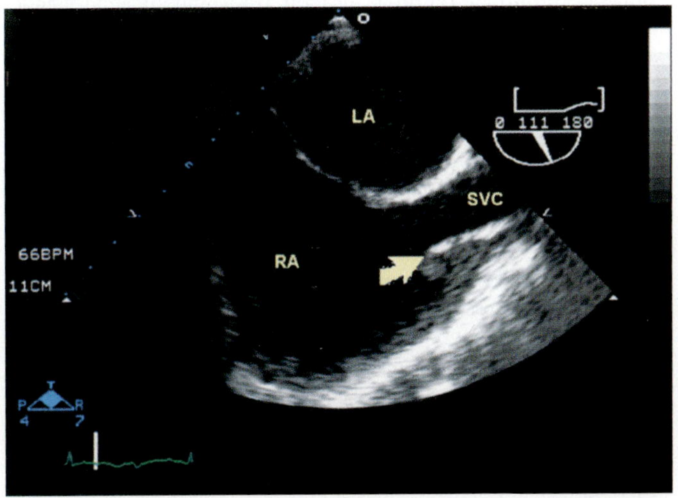

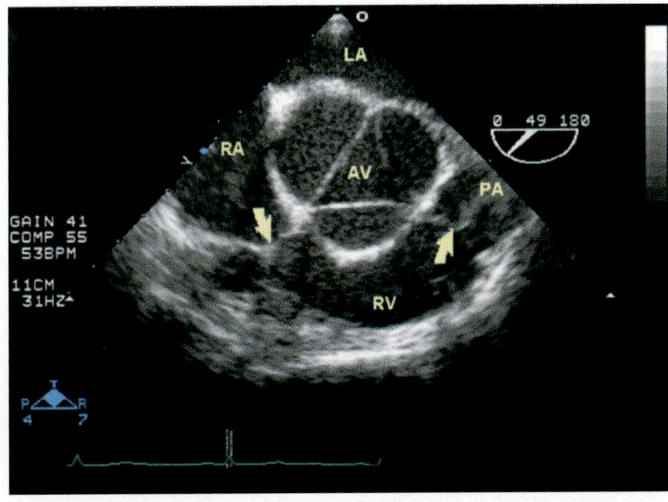

FIGURE 31-4. A. Standard midesophageal bicaval view with crista terminalis (*arrow*) visualized. **B.** Standard midesophageal right ventricular inflow–outflow view in a patient with a large aortic valve. *Down arrow* indicates tricuspid valve; *up arrow* indicates pulmonic valve. AV, aortic valve; LA, left atrium; PA, pulmonary artery; RA, right atrium; RV, right ventricle; SVC, superior vena cava.

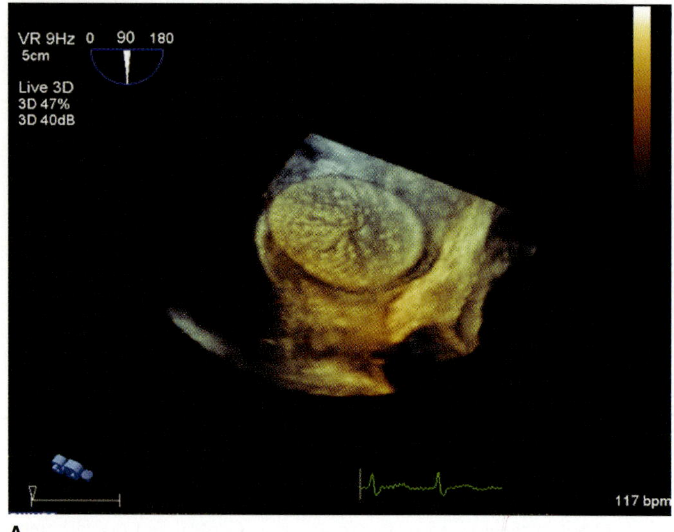

A

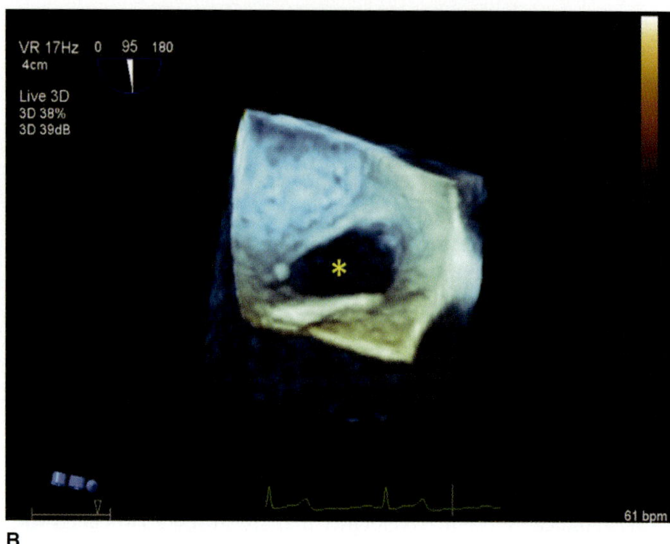

B

FIGURE 31-5. A. Three-dimensional (3D) transesophageal echocardiography (TEE) image of the left atrial disk of an Amplatzer atrial septal defect (ASD) occluder. **B.** Rims of a secundum ASD as image with 3D TEE from the left atrial aspect of a secundum ASD (*asterisk*).

venous type of ASD lies superior to the fossa ovalis close to the opening of the SVC. It may be best seen from an ME bicaval view.

A patent foramen ovale (PFO) is a flaplike opening between the atrial septa primum and secundum at the location of the fossa ovalis that persists after age 1 year. In utero, the foramen ovale serves as a physiologic conduit for right-to-left shunting. PFO is a common functional secundum ASD that results from failure of the septa primum and secundum to completely fuse (**Fig. 31-6**A), allowing an interatrial shunt to occur under certain hemodynamic conditions. TEE is the diagnostic standard for detecting PFO, which is present in approximately 20% of adults. The ME bicaval view often is best for detecting this lesion. CFD interrogations of the IAS and contrast echocardiography both have high sensitivity and specificity for detecting PFO. Intravenous injection of agitated saline often is used intraoperatively to produce a contrast effect (Fig. 31-6C), a maneuver that can be monitored with either 2D or 3D TEE. Simultaneous release of a breath-holding maneuver will increase RA pressures relative to LA pressures and may open a functionally closed PFO.

In the presence of an ASD with left-to-right shunting, the LA usually appears normal, and the RA and RV enlarge from volume overload. As pulmonary hypertension occurs, the RV wall becomes hypertrophied. With an ASD, the pulmonary vasculature dilates and can be as wide as the aorta.

Lipomatous hypertrophy of the atrial septum is a peripherally thickened septum surrounding the thin fossa ovalis (Fig. 31-6B). It results from fat deposits in the atrial septum and should not be confused with intra-atrial masses such as myxomas.

An atrial septal aneurysm is an outpouching of thin, mobile, redundant tissue in the region of the fossa ovalis. The atrial septum is considered to be aneurysmal when a portion at least 15 mm wide has an interatrial excursion of at least 15 mm. Atrial septal aneurysm formation may be secondary to increased interatrial pressure gradients, producing a bulging septal shift toward the low-pressure side, and has been associated with the occurrence of a PFO.[39] An atrial septum aneurysm must be considered in the differential diagnosis of atrial cysts and tumors and has been related to atrial arrhythmias, systemic and pulmonary embolism, MV prolapse, and ASD.

CARDIAC TUMORS

Metastatic cardiac tumors are more common than primary cardiac tumors. Metastatic disease may result from contiguous extension, lymphangitic spread, or hematogenous spread from the primary tumor. It tends to involve the pericardium and myocardium rather than the valves and endocardium. Extension of tumor thrombus via the IVC into the RA is a well-recognized complication of advanced renal cell carcinoma.

Myxomas, the most common primary cardiac tumors, account for approximately 50% of all primary cardiac tumors. Myxomas can cause obstruction and embolization, making prompt surgical removal mandatory. Myxomas usually are solitary and are found most commonly within the LA (Figs. 31-3B and 31-6D), originating from the IAS (often the fossa ovalis). Myxomas characteristically have hemorrhagic cystic spaces and possibly areas of calcification.

LEFT VENTRICLE

Systolic Function Assessment of regional and global systolic LV function often is the primary indication for perioperative echocardiography. TEE is well suited to providing accurate evaluation and monitoring of ventricular filling and systolic function during hemodynamic instability. For purposes of identifying wall motion abnormalities, the ASE divides the LV into 17 segments (**Fig. 31-7**).[40] The basal and midlevels of the LV each have inferior, inferolateral (formerly termed posterior), anterolateral, anterior, anteroseptal, and inferoseptal segments. The apical level has inferior, lateral, anterior, and septal segments. The apical cap is the final segment. All segments (except the apical cap) can be visualized from either an ME or TG probe location. If wall motion abnormalities are observed, the typical blood supply patterns (or actual blood supply patterns from a previous angiogram) to these segments can help identify the compromised coronary artery or graft.

A wall motion description should be assigned for each segment. *Mild hypokinesis* refers to a decrease in inward wall movement and a 10% to 30% increase in endocardial systolic thickening (normal is >30%). *Severe hypokinesis* refers to only slight wall movement and less than 10% thickening. *Akinesis* refers to lack of both movement and endocardial thickening (indicating severe ischemia or infarct). *Dyskinesis* refers to outward wall movement and endocardial thinning during systole (indicating old infarct). Movement may be passive because of contraction of adjacent segments or translational movement of the heart, so thickening is believed to be more reliable than wall movement in determining wall motion abnormalities. If scaled scores are assigned to each type of wall motion abnormality, the average of those scores from each segment provides a semiquantitative assessment of global ventricular function, termed the *wall motion index*. The wall motion index can be converted to estimate ejection fraction (EF) and results in good agreement with other measures of EF.[41]

Many other measures of global ventricular function can be made; only the most common are discussed here. Fractional area change (FAC) can be obtained from the TG SAX view ("donut view"). It is simply the proportion of diastolic area of the LV chamber in the midpapillary SAX view (**Fig. 31-8**A and 31-8B) that is reduced during systole:

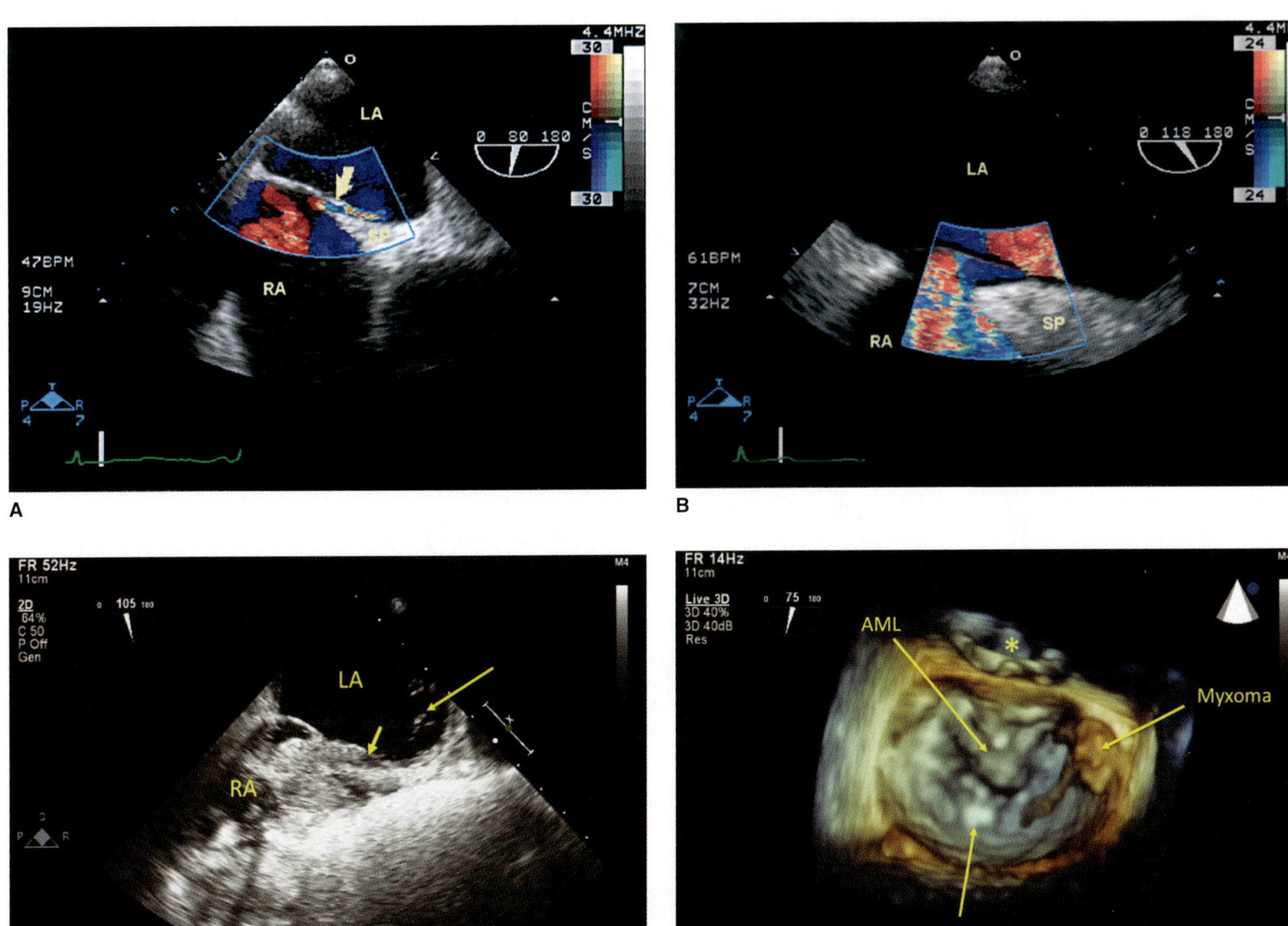

FIGURE 31-6. **A.** Turbulent flow through a patent foramen ovale between the septum primum (SP) and septum secundum portion of the interatrial septum (*arrow*). **B.** Midesophageal bicaval view (with imaging depth reduced) with color-flow Doppler interrogation of the interatrial septum in a patient with a patent foramen ovale (not clearly demonstrated in this frame) and lipomatous hypertrophy of the SP portion of the interatrial septum. **C.** Contrast echocardiography ("bubble study") showing bubbles (*long yellow arrow*) that have crossed through a patent foramen ovale (*short yellow arrow*). **D.** Three-dimensional transesophageal echocardiography zoom *en face* view demonstrating a left atrial myxoma attached to the interatrial septum above the mitral valve with the anterior mitral leaflet (AML) on the top and the posterior mitral leaflet (PML) on the bottom (*asterisk* denotes the aortic valve). LA, left atrium; RA, right atrium.

$$\text{FAC\%} = (\text{End-diastolic area} - \text{End-systolic area}) / \text{End-diastolic area} \times 100$$

Although FAC often is estimated visually, the chamber circumference can be traced in both systole and diastole to provide the areas for more accurate calculation. Because FAC is measured in only 1 plane, it may miss significant wall motion abnormalities outside that plane and therefore has limited accuracy in the assessment of overall ventricular function. Oblique planes of view also may reduce accuracy.

The LV EF, which includes the volume change of the whole ventricle rather than the area change of a change.

$$\text{EF\%} = (\text{End-diastolic volume} - \text{End-systolic volume}) / \text{End-diastolic volume} \times 100$$

Normal EF is 55% to 75%.

Generating accurate 3D volumes from 2D echocardiography can be a source of error. Multiple geometric methods have been developed that assume that the ventricle fits a stereotypical ellipsoidal shape. They include the single-plane ellipsoid method, cylinder–hemi-ellipsoid method, and area–length method; all of these methods estimate volume from diameter and length measurements in 1 or 2 planes. These geometric assumptions limit the accuracy of EF estimation when segmental wall motion abnormalities or unusual ventricular shapes are present. If the plane of measurement does not include the true apex, termed a *foreshortened view*, then the volumes and EF will be unreliable.

The modified Simpson method, also known as the *disk summation method*, is considered the best method for deriving ventricular volumes and EF from 2D echocardiography. For this method, the endocardial border is traced in 2 orthogonal planes (eg, ME 4-chamber and 2-chamber views). Computer software then models the ventricle as a series of 20 or more stacked elliptical disks (**Fig. 31-9**). The volume of each disk then is calculated from the thickness of the disk and the diameters of each ellipsoid disk (Fig. 31-9C), and all of the individual disk volumes are summed to yield the total volume of the ventricle. Similar cylindrical disks or rotating ellipsoid models can be generated from a single tomographic view but with reduced accuracy. This biplane disk summation method allows for variably shaped ventricles. It also can account for significant regional wall motion abnormalities but still may be limited by image quality or foreshortened views. To reduce foreshortening errors, the 2 orthogonal views should not be combined if the chamber lengths appear to differ by more than 20%.

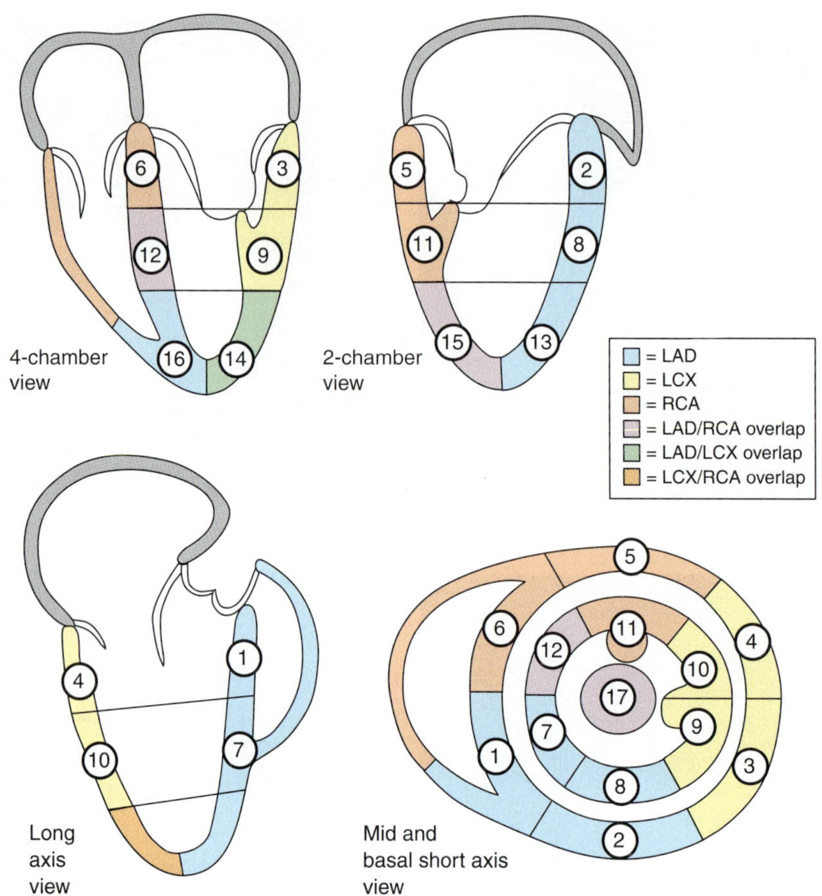

FIGURE 31-7. Depiction of the American Society of Echocardiography's 17 left ventricular wall segments, with color coding according to normal variations of coronary blood flow. 1, Basal anteroseptal; 2, basal anterior; 3, basal anterolateral; 4, basal inferolateral; 5, basal inferior; 6, basal inferoseptal; 7, mid anteroseptal; 8, mid anterior; 9, mid anterolateral; 10, mid inferolateral; 11, mid inferior; 12, mid inferoseptal; 13, apical anterior; 14, apical lateral; 15, apical inferior; 16, apical septal; 17, apical cap (apex). LAD, left anterior descending coronary artery; LCX, left circumflex artery; RCA, right coronary artery.

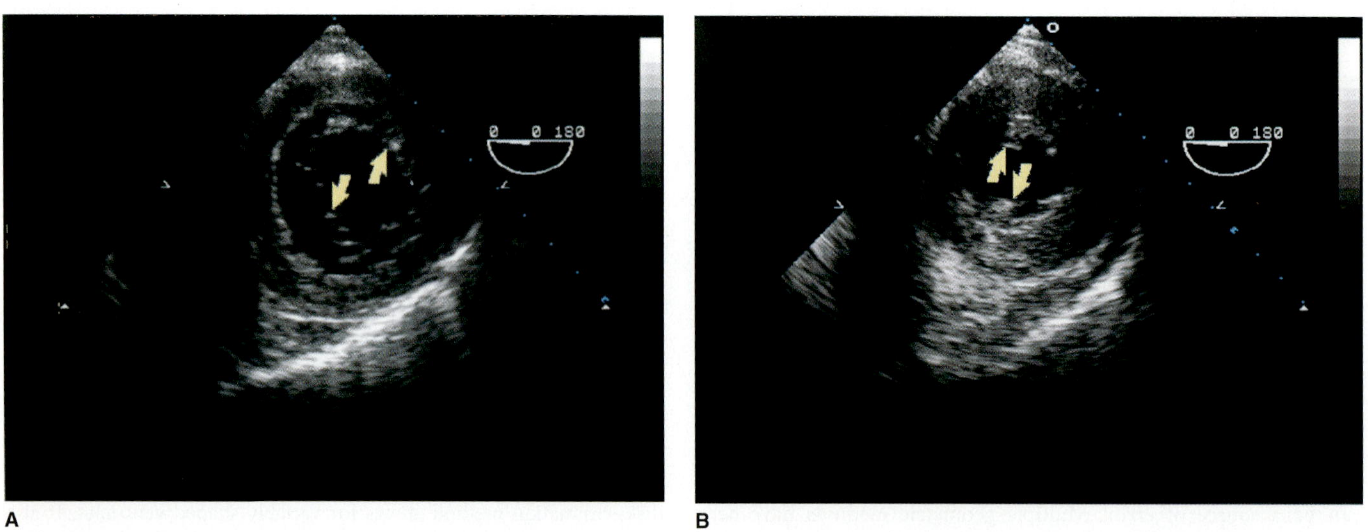

FIGURE 31-8. **A.** Basal transgastric short-axis view showing open mitral valve. Posterior (*up arrow*) and anterior (*down arrow*) mitral leaflets. **B.** Midpapillary transgastric short-axis view. Posteromedial papillary muscle (*up arrow*) and anterolateral papillary muscle (*down arrow*).

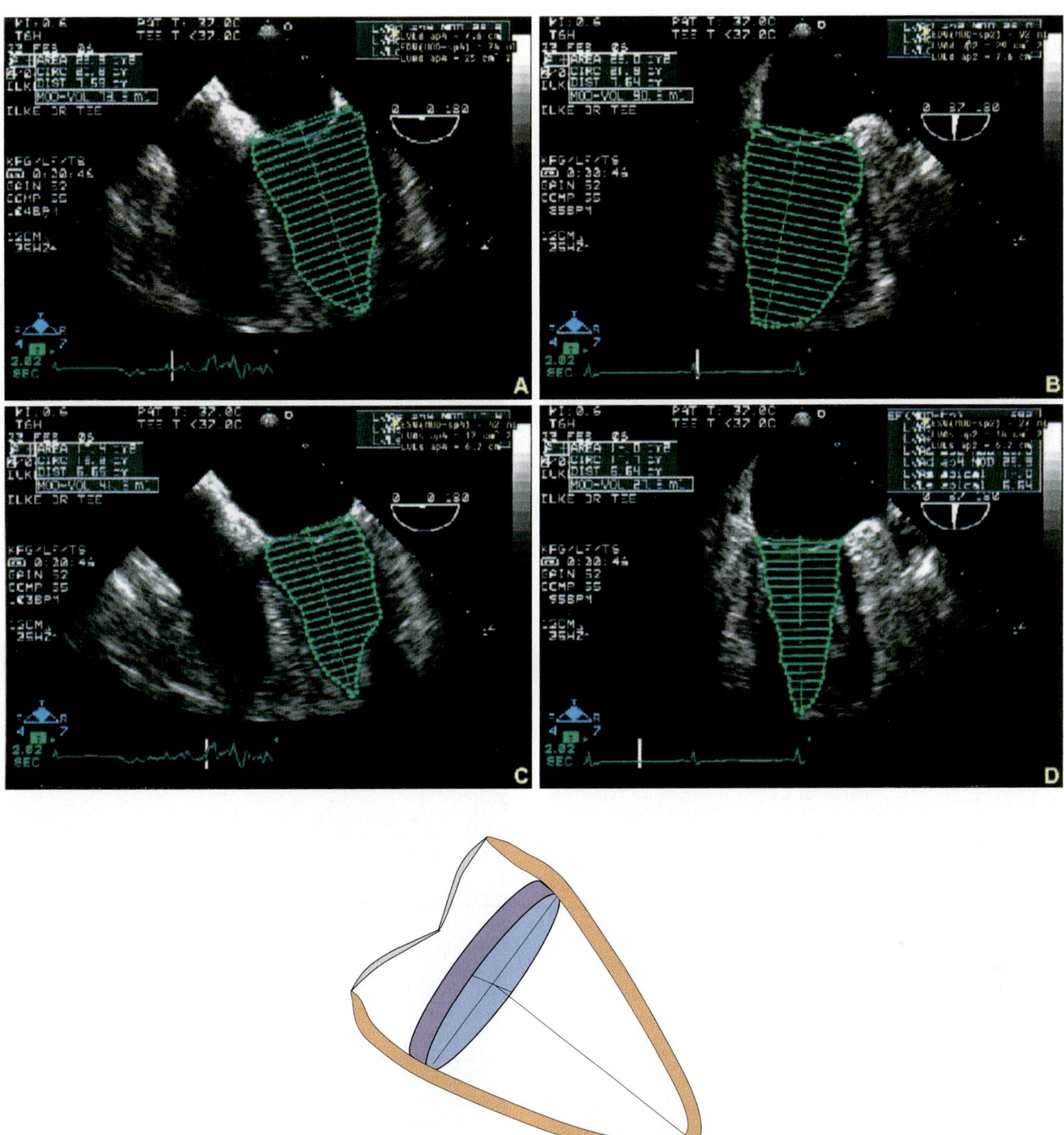

FIGURE 31-9. Ejection fraction calculated using the disk summation method from 4-chamber end diastole (**A**), 2-chamber end diastole (**B**), 4-chamber end-systole (**C**), and 2-chamber end systole (**D**) tracings. **E.** Depiction of a single Simpson disk with elliptical diameters measured from midesophageal 4-chamber and 2-chamber views. Using the software package of the transesophageal echocardiography machines, the volume of each theoretical disk is automatically calculated separately in this way and then summed together to obtain the left ventricular volume in both end diastole and end systole, allowing for calculation of ejection fraction.

In clinical practice, the assessment of the LVEF is routinely performed by "eye-balling," which relies on the echocardiographer's experience and ability to visually integrate spatial information. Further limitations of 2D TEE assessment of the LVEF are attributed to the use of foreshortened views of the LV and the reliance on geometric assumptions to calculate volumetric parameters. However, the reliability of visual estimation of EF by an experienced echocardiographer appears to be similar to wall motion index and EF calculations using the Simpson rule.[41]

The advent of 3D echocardiography along with built-in quantification software, which is based on semiautomated endocardial border detection, allows obtaining fast and accurate measurements of global and regional LV function.[42-44] Studies comparing magnetic resonance imaging (MRI) with 3D echocardiography for the assessment of LV mass and function show very good correlation and agreement that is superior to 2D echocardiography.[45] This also holds true for RT 3D TTE assessment of patients with cardiomyopathies or regional wall motion abnormalities secondary to myocardial infarction (MI) with abnormal LV geometry.[46-48] A recent study suggests that LV function assessment based on 3D-TEE data offers a more reliable perioperative quantification, especially for less experienced users.[49] However, further research comparing 3D TEE with a gold standard such as MRI is required to assess if 3D TEE is superior to 2D TEE in assessing the LV function.

The best mode to assess global and regional LV function by 3D TEE is the full-volume mode, which is acquired based on the ME 4-chamber view. Using built-in software, data for both global LV function as well as regional wall motion abnormalities are obtained in a semiautomatic fashion. The software relies on automatic endocardial border detection and border-tracking algorithms, which can be edited manually. Global LV function is assessed by analysis of end-systolic and end-diastolic volumes, stroke volumes, and EF. Upon completion of the analysis, as many as 17 regional waveforms are displayed simultaneously, thus enabling objective wall motion comparisons. This requires a manually performed definition of the septal, lateral, anterior, inferior, and apical endocardial borders of the LV in the end-systolic and the end-diastolic frames followed by an

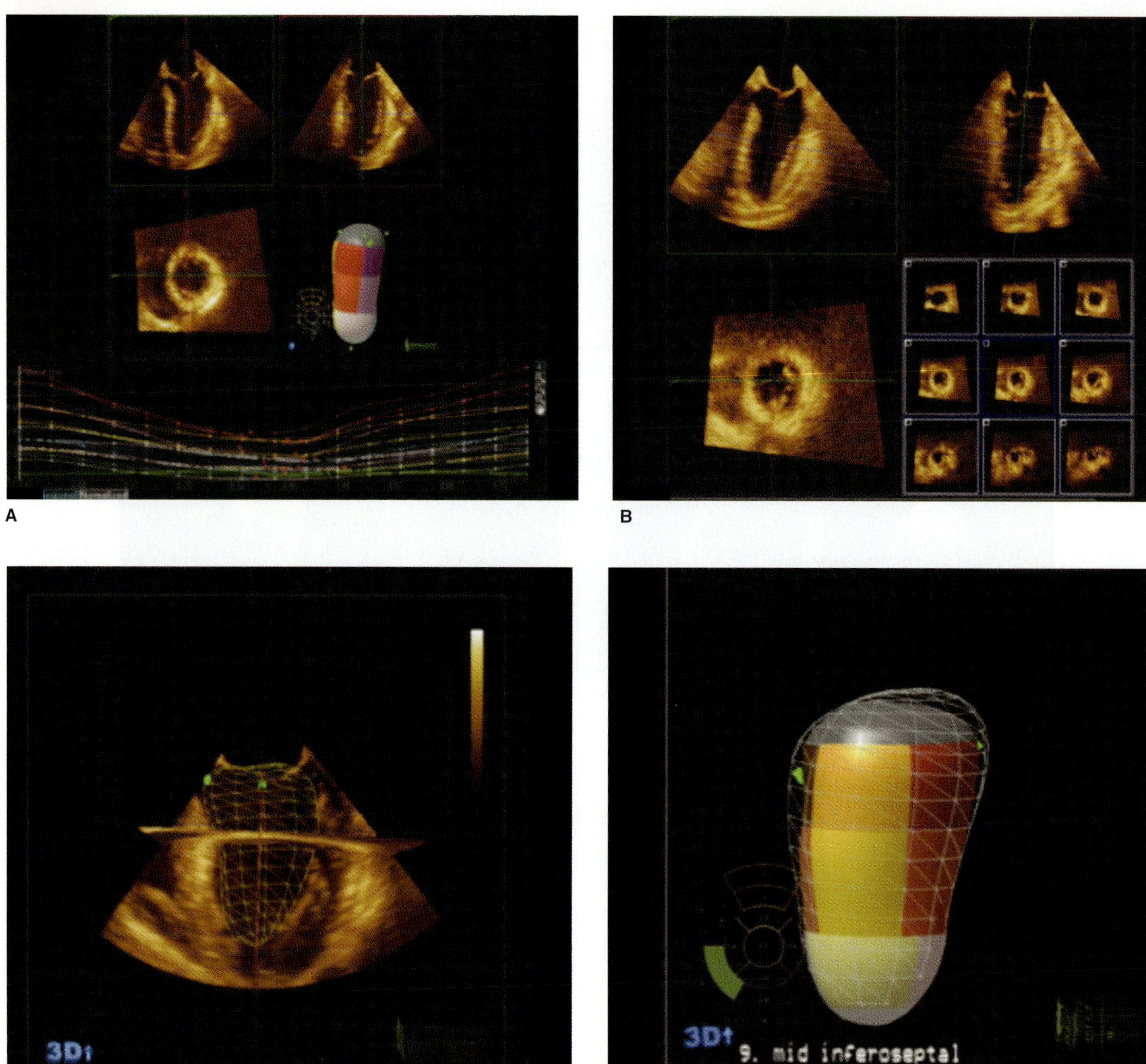

FIGURE 31-10. A. Three-dimensional (3D) transesophageal echocardiography (TEE) full volume of the entire heart displayed in 3 multiplanar reconstruction planes (MPRs, green = 4-chamber view; red = 2-chamber view; and blue = midpapillary short axis view). Manual definition of septal, lateral, anterior, inferior, and apical endocardial border points of the left ventricle (LV) in end systole and end diastole followed by an automatic border-tracking algorithm and segmental analysis will display the LV shell in 17 segments (*right lower quadrant*) along with the corresponding segmental time-volume waveforms. The iSlice view (13C) (**B**). the slice plane view with end-diastolic reference mesh (**C**), and the LV shell views (**D**) are alternative options for display of the data.

automatic border-tracking algorithm (**Fig. 31-10**A). The system will then calculate end-systolic as well as the end-diastolic volumes by summation of the voxels enclosed by the endocardial borders. Thereafter, global stroke volume and EF are derived. The obtained shell view (Fig. 31-10D) is subdivided into 17 regions, which are analyzed separately by performing the "segment analysis," and 17 segmental time-volume waveforms are displayed simultaneously offering the possibility for objective wall motion comparisons (Fig. 31-10A). Activation of "show reference mesh" displays the end-diastolic surface mesh as a diastolic reference point (Fig. 31-10C). Other viewing modes include the "iSlice" view (Fig. 31-10B), which displays 4 and up to 16 simultaneously moving SAX views of the LV and allows verifying appropriate endocardial border detection as well as the "Slice Plane" view, which shows a moving LV surface mesh within 3 orthogonal axis planes (Fig. 31-10C).

Neither FAC nor EF is a pure index of myocardial contractility because both depend on loading conditions, especially at the extremes of preload and afterload. Attempts have been made to measure load-independent indices of ventricular function. Generation of pressure–volume loops at different loading conditions results in a linear end-systolic relationship, the slope of which is termed *end-systolic elastance.* The area within pressure–volume loops is *stroke work,* which can be plotted against the corresponding end-diastolic volumes to obtain preload-recruitable work. These measures are much more complex and include measuring intraventricular pressures or their surrogates and thus are principally used for research purposes at this time.

Less load-dependent measures that are easier to obtain, although rarely reported, include the peak systolic pressure-end systolic volume ratio and cardiac power. *Mean cardiac power* is the product of stroke volume, mean arterial pressure, and heart rate. Peak instantaneous power also can be calculated. These measures can be corrected for end-diastolic volume to make them load independent. If MR is present, dP/dt of the MR jet is a relatively load-independent measure of contractility, which is otherwise difficult to assess when ventricular work is lost into the lower-pressure LA. The *myocardial performance index* is the sum of isovolumic contraction time and isovolumic relaxation time divided by ejection time. It combines systolic and diastolic function into one easily obtainable and reproducible index that has good prognostic value.[50] All of these measures have the benefit of being independent of ventricular geometry and the subjective determination of endocardial borders.

Diastolic Function Diastole is divided into 4 distinct phases: isovolumic relaxation, early rapid filling, diastasis, and atrial contraction (**Fig. 31-11**). Isovolumic relaxation begins with closure of the AV. The LV chamber relaxes, and the pressure within the LV decreases. When the pressure falls below the pressure in the LA, the MV opens, ending the period of isovolumic relaxation. Isovolumic relaxation is an active, energy-dependent process; therefore, abnormalities in systolic function usually are accompanied by abnormalities in isovolumic relaxation. Blood flowing through the MV initiates the early rapid filling phase. The rapid filling of the chamber (early diastole) depends on both LV relaxation (an active process) and chamber compliance (a passive property). As volume fills the ventricle, the pressures between the atrium and the ventricle equalize and the flow begins to slow. This period is referred to as *diastasis* because there is little blood flow between the chambers. The MV leaflets remain in an open position, and the duration of diastasis depends on heart rate and chamber compliance. With the onset of atrial contraction, atrial pressures become greater than ventricular pressures, so again there is a net flow of blood into the ventricle. In normal individuals, atrial contraction contributes approximately 20% to the end-diastolic ventricular volume. The atrial contraction phase depends on the chamber compliance, LA function, and the electrical conduction system.

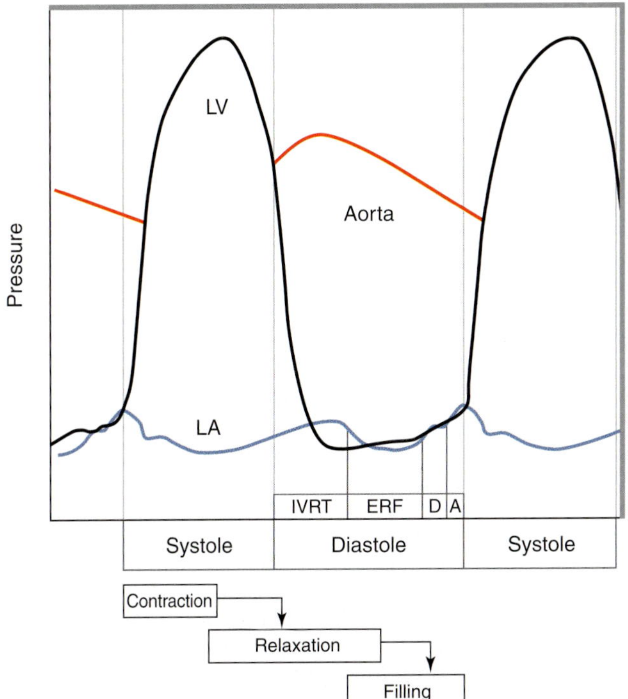

FIGURE 31-11. Pressure tracings from a normal cardiac cycle. Pressure differences (which cannot be measured directly by transesophageal echocardiography [TEE]) between chambers drive the corresponding flow velocities (which are measured with TEE to calculate pressure differences). A, atrial contraction; D, diastasis; ERF, early rapid filling; IVRT, isovolumic relaxation time; LA, left atrium; LV, left ventricle.

From the preceding discussion, one can conclude that flow is driven primarily by pressure gradients between the atrium and the ventricle. For a given pressure, if LV relaxation is brisk, the result is a large, early pressure gradient (often even a suction effect) that drives filling during early diastole. This results in less filling in late diastole. On the other hand, if ventricular relaxation is sluggish, early diastolic filling declines and a greater proportion of diastolic filling is seen in late diastole. In the latter situation, there is a greater dependence on atrial contraction for filling.

It follows then that a decrease in LV relaxation or compliance will lead to a compensatory increase in LA pressures to maintain end-diastolic ventricular volume. Because the rate of LV relaxation and increase in LA pressures is a continuum, many different transmitral pressure gradients and LV filling patterns are possible. This leads to a challenge in quantifying diastolic dysfunction over the continuum of varying patient conditions.

Doppler echocardiography, by virtue of its ability to evaluate flow patterns across valves and in large blood vessels, allows the clinician to diagnose diastolic dysfunction. Two-dimensional echocardiographic inspection of the ventricular systolic function may provide an alternative cause for a patient's heart failure or suggest that diastolic dysfunction is likely. For example, if a patient with the clinical picture of heart failure is found to have normal ventricular systolic function and volumes but LV hypertrophy (end-diastolic wall thickness >1.1 cm) is present, diastolic heart failure is likely. Combined systolic and diastolic failure may be present or a patient may have ventricular hypertrophy without measurable diastolic abnormalities. Therefore, 2D findings are neither sensitive nor specific for diastolic dysfunction, and further investigation is warranted. Therefore, two-dimensional echocardiography is most useful in helping to quantify systolic function and to differentiate isolated diastolic dysfunction from combined systolic–diastolic dysfunction. To fully assess diastolic function, use of Doppler echocardiography techniques is necessary.

The period required for isovolumic relaxation (first phase of diastole) is the isovolumic relaxation time (IVRT). IVRT is measured as the time interval from closure of the AV to opening of the MV. IVRT can be obtained from the deep TG long-axis (LAX) view (multiplane angle at 90 degrees) with a PWD sample at (or CWD through) the junction of the MV inflow and the LV outflow tract (LVOT). Normally, IVRT lasts 60 to 90 milliseconds and reflects the rate of myocardial relaxation. Impaired relaxation delays the decrease in ventricular pressure below that of the atrium, resulting in prolonged IVRT. It probably is the most sensitive Doppler index for detecting impaired relaxation because it is the first to become abnormal, but it is dependent on afterload and heart rate.

If a PWD sample is acquired near the coaptation point of the MV leaflets, transmitral flow velocities can be mapped and measured, corresponding to early diastolic filling. Flow at this time is directed away from the transducer (below the baseline). This wave is the *early* or *E wave.* The time required for the flow velocity to return to zero (from the peak of the E wave back to the baseline) is the *deceleration time.* For a brief time, there is no flow across the MV, and the velocities remain zero (diastasis). Soon after, the LA contracts, and flow again begins. Plotting these velocities versus time will yield the *atrial* or *A wave.* The total duration of the A wave (from the end of diastasis to the return of zero flow) is termed *A-wave duration* (A_{dur}).

Normally, most diastolic filling occurs in early diastole so that the E/A ratio is greater than 1 (**Fig. 31-12**A). However, mitral flow velocity curves vary with loading conditions, age, and heart rate. In healthy young patients, the E/A ratio may be as high as 2. As people get older, LV relaxation slows; there is a gradual decrease in the peak E-wave velocity and an increase in the A-wave component. In most individuals, E and A become approximately equal in the sixth decade of life. Because relaxation is impaired beyond what is "normal" for age, early diastolic filling decreases.

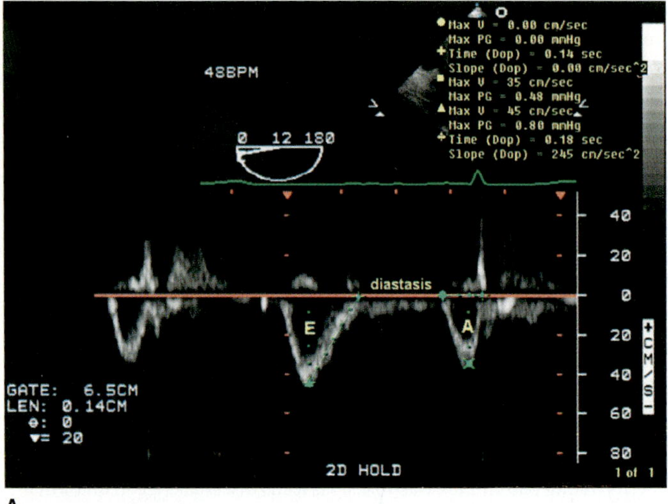

A

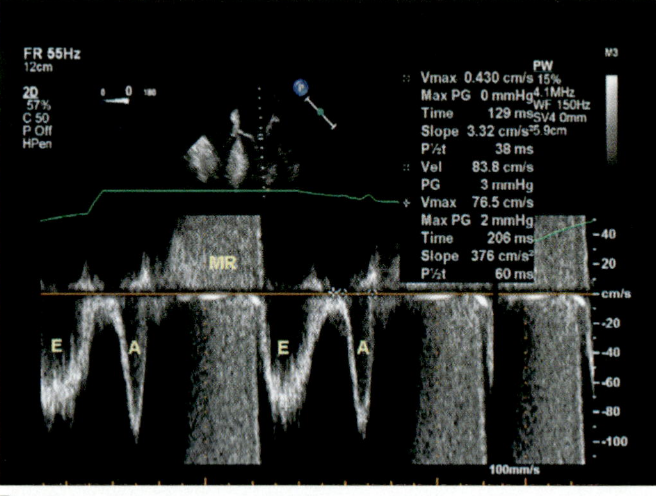

B

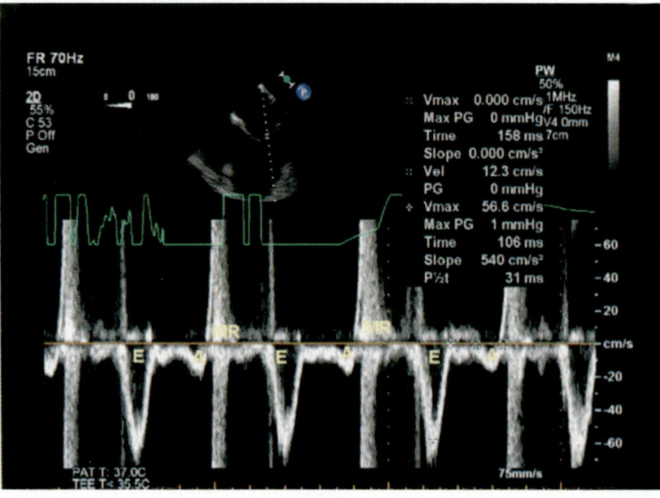

C

FIGURE 31-12. **A.** Normal transmitral flow velocities. **B.** Pseudonormal transmitral flow velocities in a patient with regurgitant mitral flow. **C.** Restrictive diastolic dysfunction in a patient with mitral regurgitation. A, A wave of atrial contraction; E, E wave of early diastolic filling; MR, regurgitant mitral flow velocities (aliasing, a limitation of pulsed-wave Doppler, is also demonstrated, with some mitral regurgitation velocities incorrectly displayed below the baseline as forward velocity).

With diastolic dysfunction, the volume that remains in the atrium at the end of the early filling phase increases, and a progressively vigorous compensatory atrial contraction ("atrial kick") occurs. This results in a reversed E/A ratio (E/A <0.75; delayed relaxation pattern). In this case, the deceleration time is increased (>220 milliseconds) and IVRT is increased (>100 milliseconds).

With further diastolic dysfunction, LV compliance is even lower, and filling pressures begin to increase. This leads to a compensatory increase in LA atrial pressure, resulting in increased early filling velocities despite impaired relaxation. The filling pattern appears relatively normal (termed *pseudonormalization*), and the E/A ratio returns to approximately 1 (Fig. 31-12B). Pseudonormalization represents abnormalities of both relaxation and compliance and can be distinguished from normal filling by a shortened deceleration time.

In patients with severely decreased LV compliance, LA pressure is markedly elevated and drives vigorous early diastolic filling velocities despite impaired relaxation. This restrictive filling pattern (E/A >1.5) is consistent with an abnormal increase in LV diastolic pressure and an abrupt deceleration of early diastolic flow (deceleration time <150 milliseconds) with little additional filling during mid-diastole and atrial contraction (Fig. 31-12C). In the extreme case, the change in pressure in the ventricle exceeds LA pressure so that MR in mid-diastole may occur.

Analysis of pulmonary venous filling patterns provides additional information about LV diastolic function. PWD is used to sample pulmonary venous flow approximately 1.5 to 2.0 cm within the left upper pulmonary vein (or alternatively the right upper pulmonary vein). Flow from the pulmonary veins into the LA occurs in 3 phases: systolic phase (S wave), diastolic phase (D wave), and retrograde flow with atrial contraction (A wave). Under normal conditions (LA pressure is normal and the MV is competent), most of the flow into the atrium occurs during ventricular systole (S-wave velocity > D-wave velocity) as the MV annulus is pulled downward (**Fig. 31-13**A). During diastole, additional blood flows from the pulmonary veins into the LA, which is simultaneously emptying into the LV. During atrial contraction, blood is ejected into the LV, with a small amount of retrograde flow into the pulmonary veins. The smaller A wave is in the opposite direction to the S and D waves.

As pressure in the LA increases (compensating for advancing diastolic dysfunction), systolic flow decreases (decreased S-wave velocity) and flow occurs predominantly in diastole (increased D-wave velocity; Fig. 31-13B). The absolute values of the S and D waves do not necessarily provide any additional information. Because they depend on the volume status of the patient, the absolute values of the S and D waves can vary significantly even under normal conditions.

Pulmonary venous flow patterns help to differentiate normal transmitral filling patterns from pseudonormal patterns. In the pseudonormal pattern, the atrium contracts against an increased afterload in the LV because of an elevated diastolic filling pressure and a stiff LV. More blood is ejected along the "path of least resistance" back into the pulmonary veins. As a result, the A wave in pseudonormal diastolic dysfunction is tall (often >0.35 milliseconds) and prolonged.

Both transmitral and pulmonary venous flow patterns are affected by the patient's volume status. Color M-mode Doppler echocardiography is a relatively new modality that can be used to assess diastolic function in a preload-independent manner. When using color M-mode, an "ice pick" scan line is used to display color Doppler velocity information versus time. By placing the scan line through the mitral inflow jet of the LV, 2 distinct flow profiles are obtained. The displayed profiles correspond to the E and A waves from PWD. The slope of the first (E) wave's aliasing velocity is the propagation velocity (Vp), which is an indication of the velocity at which blood travels from the mitral annulus to the apex during early ventricular filling (**Fig. 31-14**). Vp correlates to the degree of diastolic dysfunction and is independent of preload and heart rate. Another advantage of color M-mode Doppler echocardiography is that it provides a superior combination of temporal, spatial, and velocity resolution. Propagation velocities less than 45 cm/s are consistent

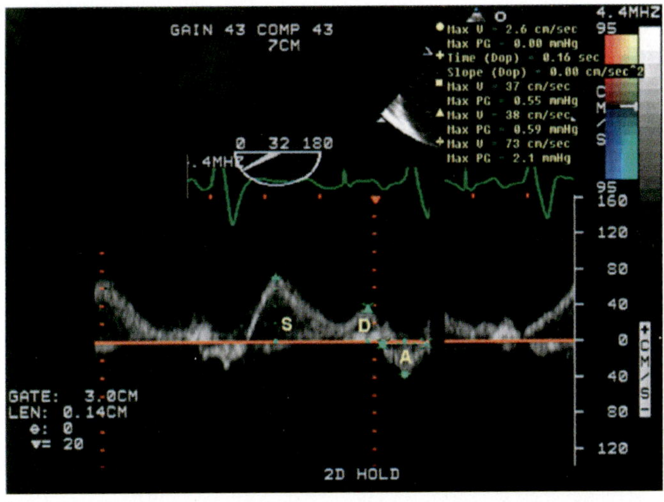

A

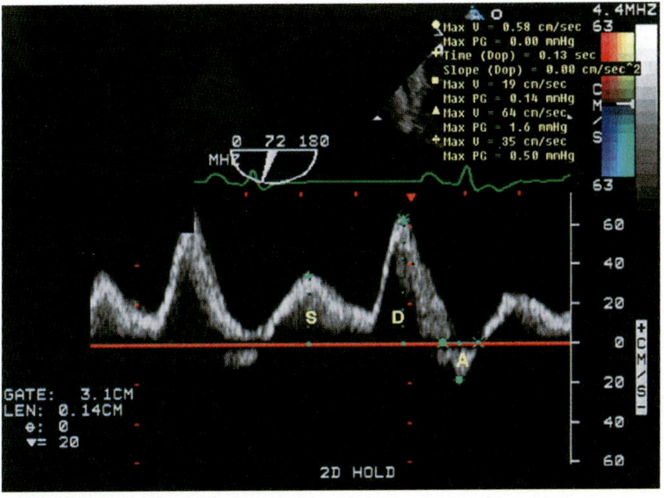

B

FIGURE 31-13. **A.** Normal pulmonary venous flow velocities (S wave > D wave). **B.** Abnormal pulmonary venous flow velocities (D wave > S wave) from diastolic dysfunction. A, retrograde atrial flow wave; D, diastolic phase wave; S, systolic phase wave.

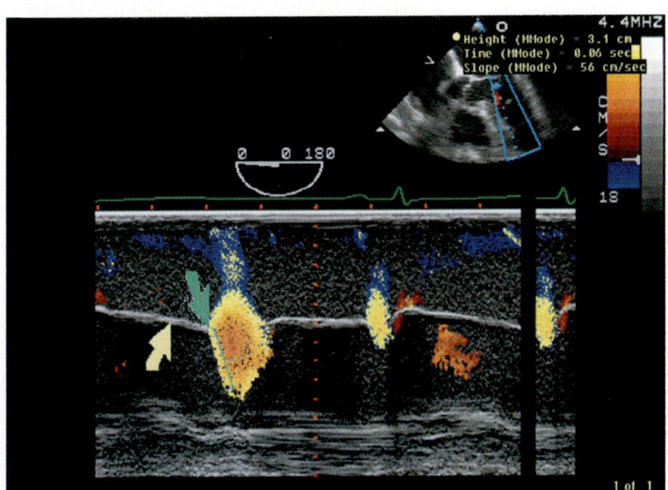

FIGURE 31-14. Normal propagation velocity measured using color M-mode Doppler. *Yellow arrow* indicates closed mitral valve. *Green arrow* indicates the beginning of transmitral early diastolic flow as the mitral valve opens.

with diastolic dysfunction in people who are older than 30 years of age, but Vp less than 55 cm/s is abnormal in younger patients.

Doppler tissue imaging is another relatively new ultrasound imaging modality that measures the velocity of the actual myocardium during the cardiac cycle. Myocardial tissue Doppler shifts typically are higher in amplitude and lower in frequency than the traditional blood flow measurements. PWD tissue imaging provides the capability of recording the low velocities of a moving wall structure with a relatively high sampling rate. A PWD sample is taken at the lateral MV annulus, and the peak early diastolic myocardial velocity (E') is measured. In contrast to blood flow velocity profiles that are below the baseline (away from the TEE transducer), Doppler tissue imaging profiles are above the baseline as the MV annulus recoils toward the transducer in diastole.

During diastole, motion of the mitral annulus shows 2 distinct movements toward the atrial side in patients with sinus rhythm (**Fig. 31-15**A). During the early diastolic period, the onset of E coincides with the beginning of mitral inflow. The E' peak velocity precedes the peak velocity of the transmitral E wave. Unlike transmitral inflow velocities, in which measured parameters are preload dependent, E' is a good index of LV relaxation and appears to be less sensitive to alterations in preload.

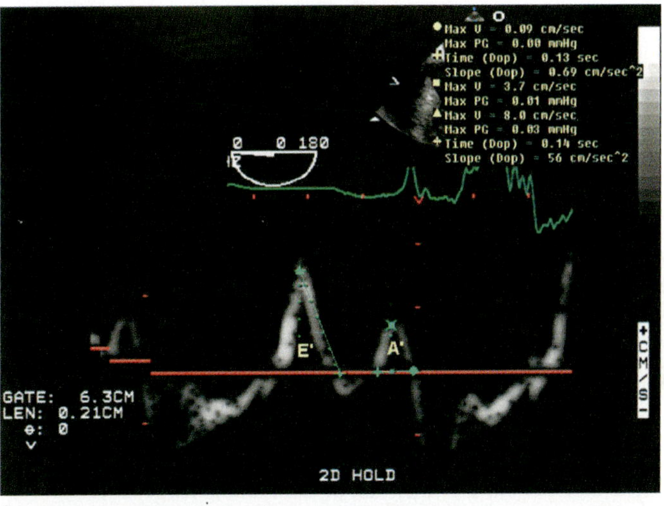

A

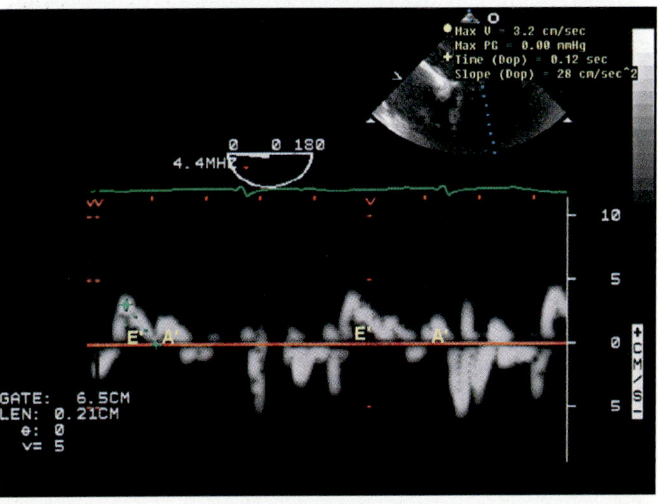

B

FIGURE 31-15. **A.** Normal mitral valve annulus tissue Doppler velocities. A', atrial contraction myocardial velocity; E', early diastolic myocardial velocity. **B.** Mitral valve tissue Doppler showing restrictive diastolic dysfunction. A', atrial contraction (late diastolic) myocardial velocity; E', early diastolic myocardial velocity.

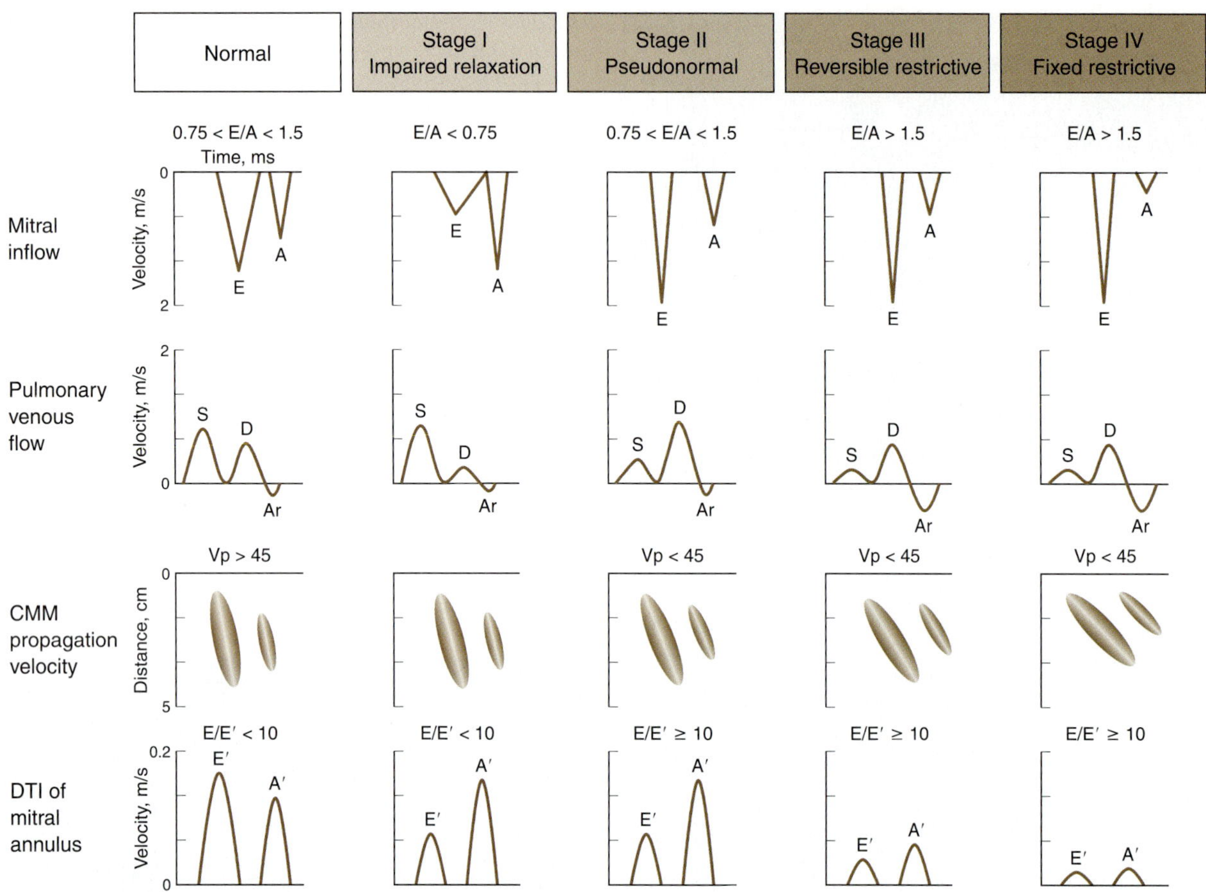

FIGURE 31-16. Transesophageal evaluation of diastolic dysfunction. A, peak late diastolic transmitral flow velocity; A′, peak late diastolic tissue velocity; Ar, peak pulmonary venous (PV) atrial reversal flow velocity; D, peak diastolic PV flow velocity; E, peak early diastolic transmitral flow velocity; E′, peak early diastolic myocardial velocity; S, peak systolic PV flow velocity; Vp, flow propagation velocity.

E' below 8 cm/s is consistent with diastolic dysfunction (Fig. 31-15B). In addition, a peak early transmitral inflow velocity to peak early diastolic myocardial velocity ratio (E/E') greater than 10 is consistent with diastolic dysfunction. E/E' then can be used to differentiate normal from pseudonormal transmitral flow pattern. Whereas E/E' greater than 15 has been shown to be highly specific for elevated LA pressures, E/E' less than 8 is highly sensitive for normal LA pressures (**Fig. 31-16** and **Table 31-4**).

MITRAL VALVE

The MV with its complex saddle-shaped configuration presents one of the most challenging structures to be assessed with 2D TEE. Two-dimensional TEE imaging of the MV requires a mental integration of several views for accurate assessment and therefore depends on observer experience and expertise. Its complex structure and interrelationship of the MV to chordae, papillary muscles, and myocardial walls make it particularly suited to 3D assessment. The MV is attached to a fibrous ring and consists of 2 leaflets, 1 anterior and 1 posterior. Although morphologically different, the surface areas of the anterior and posterior MV leaflets are nearly identical and together exceed the area of the mitral annulus in a greater than 2:1 relationship.[51] The mitral annulus is a 3D, saddle-shaped, ellipsoid structure that changes shape and decreases in area as it descends during systole (**Fig. 31-17**). Coaptation of the 2 leaflets is curvilinear, and both leaflets join at the anterolateral and posteromedial commissures (Fig. 31-2B and **31-18**).

The subvalvular apparatus consists of 2 papillary muscles and chordae tendineae. The anterolateral papillary muscle supplies chordae to the anterior aspect of both the anterior and posterior mitral leaflets; the posteromedial papillary muscle supplies chordae to the posterior aspect of both valve leaflets. Three groups of chordae exist, named in accordance with their insertion points on the MV leaflets (**Figs. 31-19** and **31-20**). *First-order chordae* attach to the free edge of the leaflets, *second-order chordae* attach to the body of the leaflets, and *third-order*

TABLE 31-4 Normal Doppler Values

Parameters	Adults Younger Than 41 Years of Age	Adults Older Than 55 Years of Age
Peak mitral flow velocity (E) (cm/s)	76 ± 13	63 ± 11
Peak mitral filling rate (A) (cm/s)	38 ± 8	52 ± 9
Mitral E/A	2.1 ± 0.6	1.3 ± 0.3
Mitral E deceleration time	184 ± 24	
Isovolumetric relaxation time (ms)	74 ± 26	
Peak pulmonary venous AR wave (cm/s)	18 ± 3	25 ± 5
Peak pulmonary venous S wave (cm/s)	41 ± 10	60 ± 10
Peak pulmonary venous D wave (cm/s)	53 ± 10	38 ± 10

E/A, E wave/A wave ratio.

Reprinted from Rakowski H, Appleton C, Chan, KL, et al. Canadian consensus recommendations for the measurement and reporting of diastolic dysfunction by echocardiography: from the Investigators of Consensus on Diastolic Dysfunction in Echocardiography. *J Am Soc Echocardiogr.* 1996;9:736-760, with permission from Elsevier.

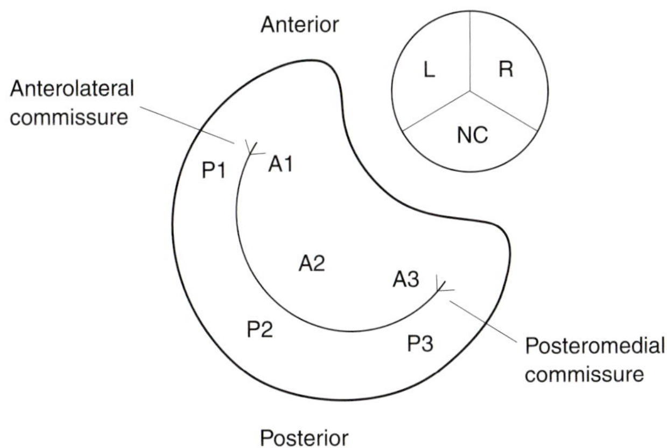

FIGURE 31-17. Anatomic view of the mitral valve viewed from the base of the heart looking toward the left ventricular apex. Orientation of the leaflets and commissures is shown using the Carpentier naming system for mitral segments. The left (L), right (R), and noncoronary (NC) aortic valve leaflets are shown.

chordae attach near the base of the posterior leaflet only.[52] More than 120 chordal tendons subdivide as they project from each papillary muscle to attach to the free edge and body of both MV leaflets.[8] The subvalvular apparatus is responsible for maintaining valve integrity during systole and plays a crucial role in preserving the overall structure–function relationship of the LV.

The MV shares a close anatomic, and at times pathophysiologic, relationship with the AV. In particular, the fibrous skeleton of the heart that gives rise to the anterior MV annulus is intimately associated with both the left and noncoronary cusps of the AV.

Recent advances in 3D echocardiography provide clinicians with spectacular images of complex MV pathology. RT 3D TEE permits an accurate identification of the etiology and mechanism of MR and is more sensitive than 2D TEE in identifying the location of the pathology leading to MR, especially in patients with bileaflet and commissural defects using both reconstruction 3D TEE and RT 3D TEE.[22,53,54] In addition, the severity of MR can be more accurately determined using 3D color Doppler echocardiography,[55] and specific geometric shapes for different MR-pathologies can be identified.[56-58] Ongoing development of dynamic analysis techniques for 3D echocardiography images allows a quantitative and systematic analysis of the MV and demonstrates increasing value of 3D imaging.

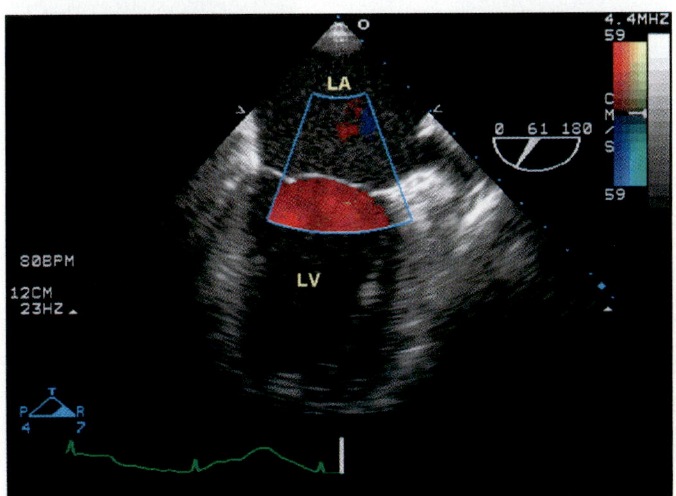

FIGURE 31-18. Midesophageal commissural view of a normal mitral valve. A2 segment of anterior leaflet is seen between the commissures with P1 and P3 segments lateral to commissures. LA, left atrium; LV, left ventricle.

RT 3D TEE provides excellent visualization of prosthetic MVs and annuloplasty rings.[59,60] Thus, it might help in identifying the location of a paravalvular leak (**Fig. 31-21**A and 31-21B).[61] 3D TEE has been shown to provide complementary information in patients with an Alfieri stitch and may aid in long-term follow-up.[62] 3D TEE provides additional information in patients with a postoperative MV dehiscence and thus may help planning an optimal surgical intervention.[60] Prosthetic valve endocarditis remains a challenging diagnosis, especially for TEE. However, initial experiences suggest that 3D TTE might improve the sensitivity of detecting endocarditis.[63]

A comprehensive 3D assessment of the MV involves the acquisition of an *en face* view, a full-volume, and a 3D color full-volume image. The *en face* view refers to a view of the MV with the patient in the supine position through a surgical left atriotomy. The anatomical identification of structures is based on Carpentier's classification. This view is routinely generated using the live 3D zoom mode based on the ME 4-chamber view and by rotating the obtained image to display the AV at the 12 o' clock position as the midpoint of the anterior annulus and the posterior leaflet at the bottom of the image (Fig 31-2B). Three-dimensional zoom MV images may then be manipulated such that the MV may be viewed from either atrial or ventricular perspectives, which is another unique feature of 3D imaging. The full-volume data set allows assessing the intimate interrelationship among the MV, the papillary muscles, the myocardial walls, and the LV outflow tract. Using 3D color, the size and geometry of regurgitant jets can be visualized, and exact quantification of effective regurgitant orifice areas (EROA) can be obtained (**Fig. 31-22**A). These images can be supplemented by 3D quantitative assessment of the MV using built-in software (MVQ). The MVQ offers a semiautomated analysis package for accurate modeling of the mitral annulus, valve commissures, leaflet coaptation, leaflet topography, aortic orifice to MV angle, and so on (Fig. 31-22B). Reconstructive approaches to assess the MV with 3D TEE (Siemens, Mountainview, CA) paired with offline computer software (TomTec Imaging Systems, Unterschleissheim, Munich, Germany) allow for similar quantification of the MV.[64]

To accurately diagnose MV pathology, it is crucial to be able to relate TEE images of this valve to specific anatomic regions. Three approaches to 2D examination of the MV by TEE have been published. Although these approaches all have strengths and limitations, they all emphasize the importance of concise, systematic 2D evaluation of the MV in multiple scan planes and from multiple points of view.

Mitral Regurgitation In the early 1980s, Carpentier introduced a functional classification of mitral insufficiency (Fig. 31-19).[65] Type I MR has normal motion of the leaflets with MR caused by leaflet perforation, usually from endocarditis, or annular dilation, often accompanying LV dysfunction. Type II MR has increased leaflet motion, typically from myxomatous change, leading to either leaflet prolapse or a flail leaflet. Leaflet prolapse, a result of leaflet redundancy and chordal elongation, is defined as doming of the leaflet body above the level of the mitral annulus in systole with the leaflet tip still directed toward the LV. With myxomatous change, the annulus often is significantly dilated in addition to the defect in leaflet tip coaptation. This regurgitant lesion usually evolves slowly and ranges in scale from trivial to severe. A flail leaflet has a leaflet tip directed toward the LA throughout systole. This regurgitant lesion usually is severe with an abrupt onset and is poorly tolerated by the patient. Type III MR is characterized by restricted leaflet motion. Type IIIa dysfunction involves restricted leaflet motion during diastole and systole because of rheumatic changes. Type IIIb dysfunction correlates to restricted leaflet motion during systole secondary to papillary muscle displacement in ischemic or dilated cardiomyopathy.

Mitral insufficiency caused by global LV dysfunction appears to result from a distorted geometric relationship between the MV leaflets and the papillary muscles. At the gross level, the LV is seen to transform from its usual ellipsoid shape into that of a sphere, causing widening of the interpapillary angle and restriction or tethering of leaflet motion.[66] The

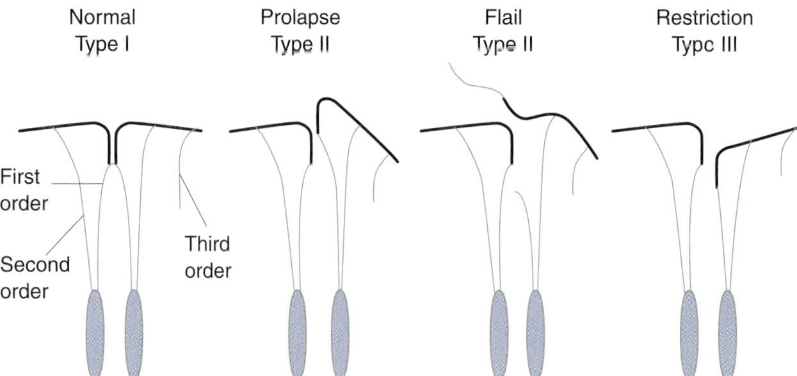

FIGURE 31-19. Carpentier classification of mitral regurgitation with normal, prolapsed, flail, and restricted mitral leaflets. The classification of chordae tendineae is also shown.

valve may appear morphologically normal on 2D imaging but with loss of the usual systolic leaflet overlap or with a visible coaptation defect. With dilated cardiomyopathy, the regurgitant jet usually is central (**Fig. 31-23**). Dilation of the annulus may contribute to regurgitation, most notably in the region of the P2 segment, but in most cases is not the major mechanism of regurgitation.

With ischemic MR, dilation of specific areas of myocardium may lead to asymmetric tethering and an eccentric regurgitant jet. Papillary muscle rupture, which most frequently affects the posteromedial muscle, is an occasional complication of MI and can result in severe bileaflet regurgitation. The papillary muscle and chordae tips can often be seen flinging into and out of the LA. In hypertrophic obstructive cardiomyopathy, the MR jet usually occurs in mid to late systole and is directed posteriorly as the anterior leaflet is pulled into the LVOT (systolic anterior motion of the anterior leaflet), resulting in a coaptation defect (**Fig. 31-24**).

MV endocarditis can affect native valves and result in regurgitation because of perforation or deformation of the valve leaflets (**Fig. 31-25**). Vegetations commonly arise on the upstream side of a valve, which are generally areas of slower flow and therefore are usually seen in the LA. The finding of MV endocarditis mandates careful inspection of the other heart valves to rule out their involvement. Leaflet perforation is identified by the appearance of 1 or more regurgitant jets that do not seem to arise from the coaptation line. A clue to this particular pathology is the presence of multiple convergence zones on color Doppler.

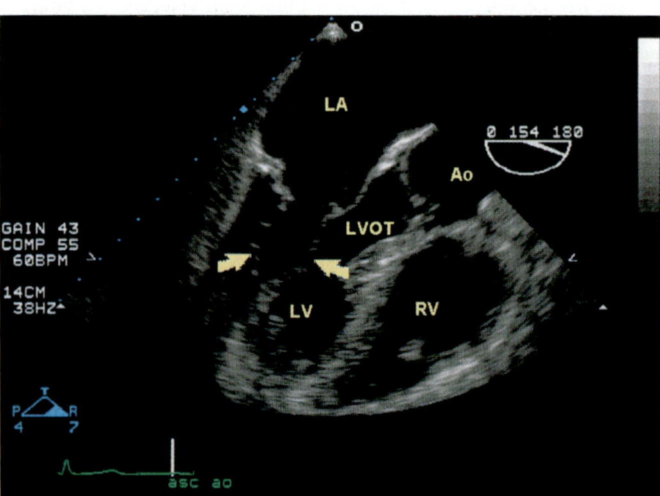

FIGURE 31-20. Midesophageal long-axis view showing subvalvular chordae (*arrows*). Ao, aorta; LA, left atrium; LV, left ventricle; LVOT, left ventricular outflow tract; RV, right ventricle.

A recent study showed that 3D TTE may improve the sensitivity of TTE in detecting endocarditis involving prosthetic valves.[63] 3D imaging may also be useful for assessing complications associated with endocarditis.[67] Studies using 3D-TEE in the diagnosis of IE are very limited but suggest an incremental benefit when used in addition to 2D TEE.[68,69]

Echocardiographic examination of the insufficient MV should involve inspection of other structures in the heart that may be altered as a result

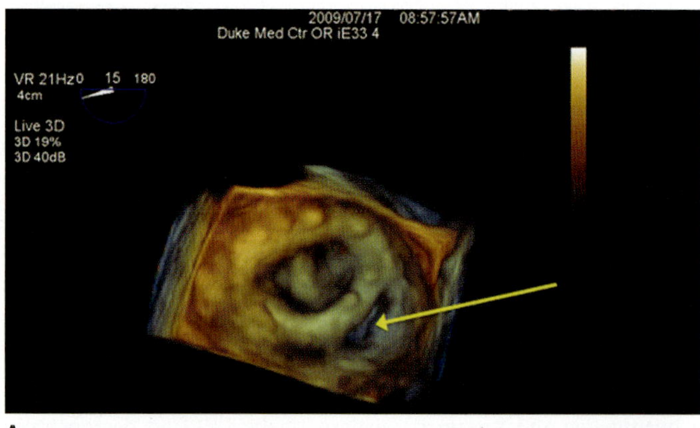

A

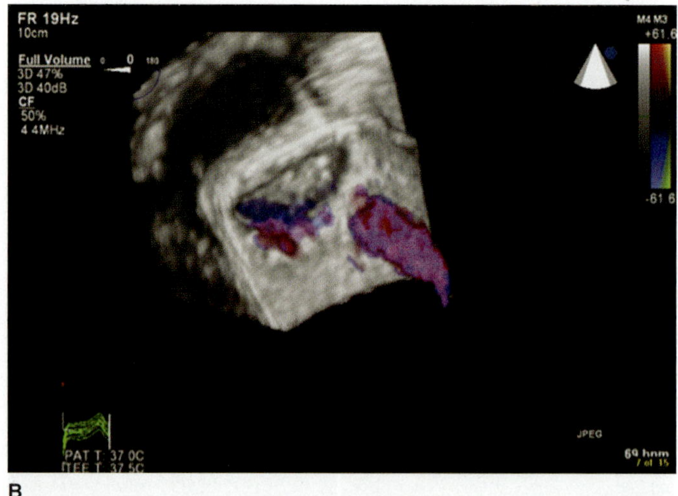

B

FIGURE 31-21. A. Live three-dimensional (3D) image of a repaired mitral valve demonstrating a posterior-medial defect outside the annuloplasty ring (*yellow arrow*). **B.** Corresponding 3D color imaging nicely illustrating the paravalvular leak outside the ring structure.

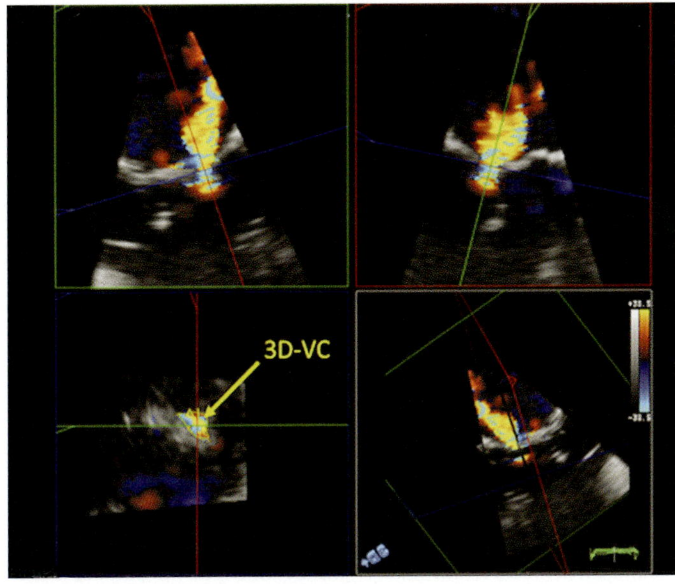

A

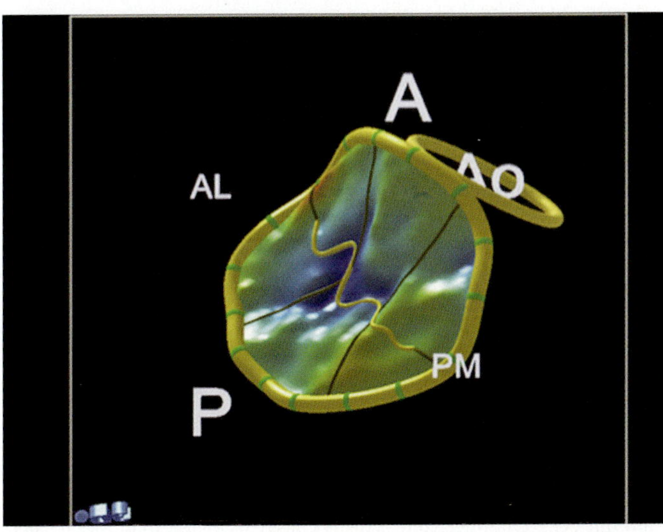

B

FIGURE 31-22. A. Three-dimensional (3D) transesophageal echocardiography color full volume of a mitral valve (MV) with severe mitral regurgitation displayed in 3 multiplanar reconstruction planes (green, red, and blue MPRs). The *left lower quadrant* (blue MPR) depicts the 3D vena contracta (3D-VC) and reflects the effective regurgitant orifice area. This was achieved by carefully cutting the MV at the annular plane. **B.** 3D model of a MV demonstrating the options for quantitative assessment of the MV using built-in software (MV Quantification, QLAB 7.0, Philips Medical Systems, Andover, MA). A, anterior; AL, anterolateral commissure; P, posterior; PM, posteromedial commissure.

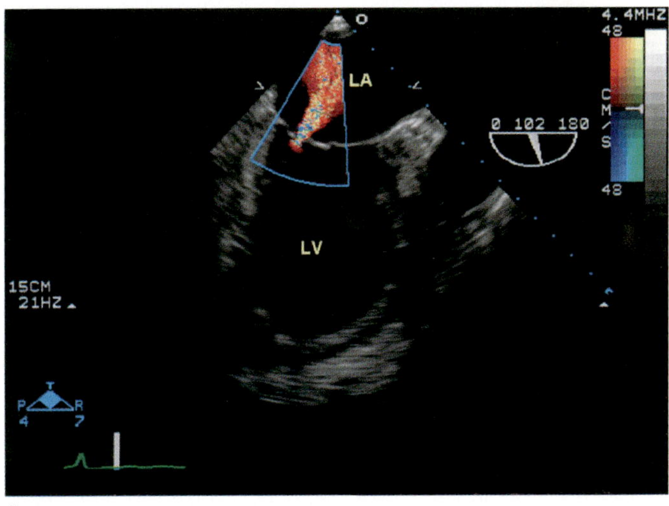

A

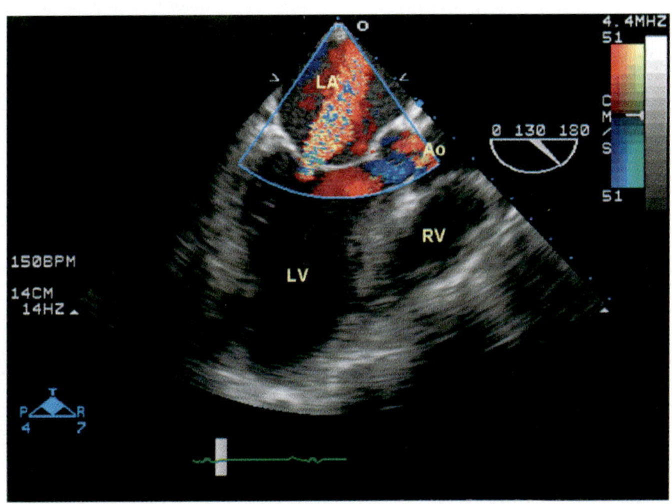

B

FIGURE 31-23. A. Midesophageal 2-chamber view with color-flow Doppler (CFD) showing mild mitral regurgitation from left ventricular dilation. **B.** Midesophageal long-axis view with CFD showing moderate mitral regurgitation. Ao, aorta; LA, left atrium; LV, left ventricle; RV, right ventricle.

of the regurgitant process. LA dilation is commonly found in chronic MR of at least moderate severity but is not a feature of acute MR. Left-to-right bowing of the IAS caused by elevated LA pressure often can be appreciated in the ME 4-chamber or ME bicaval view. Signs of pulmonary hypertension, such as RV and RA enlargement, often accompany progressive MR.

Because a significant portion of the systolic volume is unloaded into the LA with severe MR, normal systolic function should appear like a hypercontractile LV. Therefore, an LV with apparently normal systolic function may actually have significant systolic dysfunction. Spherical enlargement of the LV with eccentric hypertrophy signifies long-standing MR in which the compensatory processes of the ventricle are failing.

Echocardiographic grading of MR severity is based on a number of qualitative and quantitative parameters.[70] Among these, the width of the 2D vena contracta (VC) as visualized by color Doppler has been widely considered to accurately reflect MR severity.[71] However, although this may be true for simple MR orifices, there is a significant overlap between of 2D VC measurements and angiographic severity grades because orifices are multiple and asymmetric. A VC of 6 mm or larger identifies angiographically severe MR with a sensitivity of 95% and a specificity 98%. Eccentric regurgitant jets imaged by CFD commonly appear to occupy less overall area than jets of similar flow rates directed centrally within the LA.[72] An eccentric jet has a different observed morphology compared with free jets secondary to limited expansion because of impingement of the jet along the atrial wall. Consideration of jet morphology in the CFD assessment is important to avoid underestimating the degree of regurgitation. Illustrating variable MV pathology with 3D color imaging and using the additional information to obtain an EROA by cropping into the 3D MR jet takes advantage of the new 3D technology.

A proximal isovelocity surface area (PISA) may be seen on the LV side of the MV during systole as blood flow accelerates toward the regurgitant orifice, causing aliasing with CFD. The product of PISA and

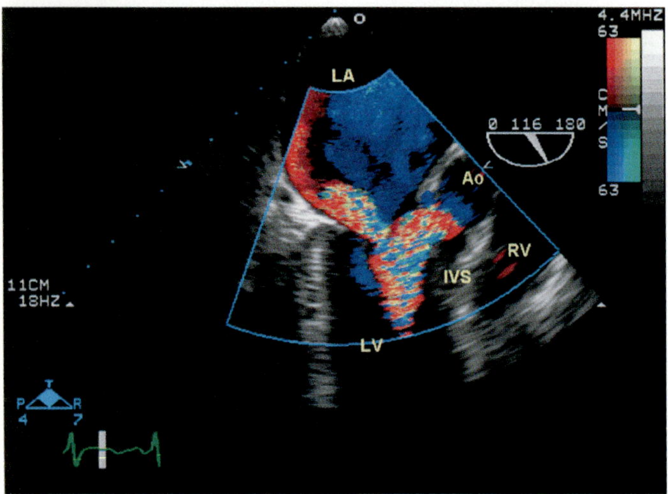

FIGURE 31-24. Midesophageal long-axis view with color-flow Doppler revealing mitral regurgitation caused by hypertrophic obstructive cardiomyopathy. Ao, aorta; IVS, interventricular septum (hypertrophied); LA, left atrium; LV, left ventricle; RV, right ventricle.

the aliasing velocity provides the flow rate through the valve during the measurement. According to the continuity principle, dividing the peak flow rate by the peak regurgitant velocity, as measured by CWD, provides quantitative assessment of the effective regurgitant orifice (ERO):

$$ERO = PISA_{MR} * (Aliasing\ velocity)/(Peak\ regurgitant\ velocity)$$

where $PISA_{MR} = 2Pi*r^2$, and r = radius of semicircular shell of color change at the set Nyquist limit.

The continuity principle also can be used to derive regurgitant fractions by determining stroke volumes through various other sites in the heart (notably the LVOT, AV, and pulmonic valve). Stroke volume is calculated as the product of the velocity–time integral (VTI) through an orifice and the calculated orifice area at the same location.

Alterations in the pulmonary venous Doppler profile are useful in quantifying the severity of MR. Trivial or mild regurgitation is generally associated with a normal flow velocity pattern (Peak S wave > Peak D wave), moderate regurgitation is associated with systolic blunting (Peak S wave < Peak D wave), and severe regurgitation is associated with S-wave reversal (S wave directed away from transducer as regurgitant blood flows retrograde into the pulmonary vein).[73] It is advisable to interrogate at least 1 pulmonary vein from each side of the LA because regurgitant jets may preferentially affect the pulmonary venous profile of one side over the other.

Peak E-wave velocity is another parameter that can be used to qualitatively assess the degree of MR. When the degree of MR increases, the added regurgitant volume across the MV increases the pressure gradient between the LA and the LV. This increase in pressure gradient subsequently increases early mitral inflow velocity. E-wave velocity greater than 1.2 milliseconds identifies patients with severe MR with a sensitivity of 86%, specificity of 86%, positive predictive value of 75%, and negative predictive value of 92%.

One caveat that must be emphasized is that MR severity often can be difficult to interpret in the intraoperative period because of the relatively deranged hemodynamic profile of the patient undergoing general anesthesia. Altered loading conditions and cardiac contractility can lead to varying degrees of MR that may be different from those seen in the awake, physiologically normal state. Furthermore, application of severity estimation methods depends on the technical expertise of the imaging staff, the complexity involved with the measurement technique, associated limitations with the individual method, and time constraints.

Mitral Stenosis Most cases of hemodynamically significant native MV stenoses are caused by rheumatic heart disease. Uncommon causes include severe mitral annular calcification, obstructing lesions such as LA tumors and endocarditis vegetations (**Fig. 31-26**), and congenital deformities such as parachute MV or cor triatriatum. Surgical correction can involve either open commissurotomy or valve replacement. In addition to confirming the severity of the stenosis, it is equally if not more important to evaluate the heart for evidence of LA thrombus (particularly within the LA appendage), RV and LV function, presence and severity of tricuspid regurgitation (TR), and degree of residual stenosis or regurgitation after valve repair or replacement.

Common echocardiographic findings of rheumatic MV stenosis (**Fig. 31-27**A) include leaflet thickening and calcification, leaflet restriction, and subvalvular involvement (shortening, tethering, and calcification of the chordae). The resulting failure of leaflet coaptation causes a regurgitant jet that is directed toward the side of the lesion (Fig. 31-27B). These leaflet changes are best seen in the ME 4-chamber and LAX views. Subvalvular involvement usually is best visualized from the TG 2-chamber view. The TG basal SAX view may reveal calcification in the region of the commissures. Rheumatic heart disease also may involve the pericardium, myocardium, and other heart valves.

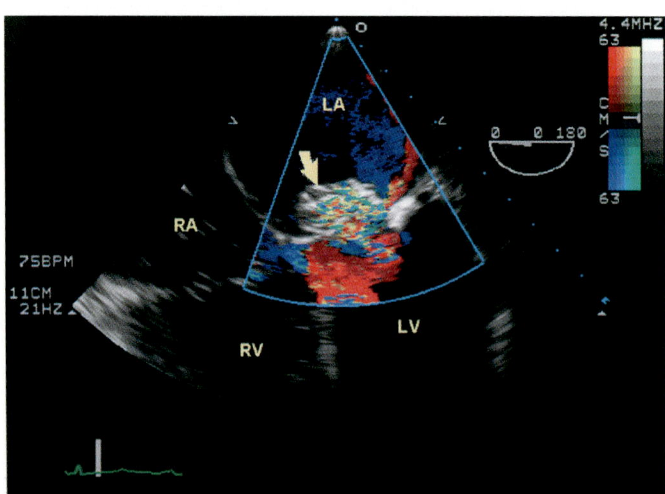

FIGURE 31-25. Midesophageal 4-chamber view with color-flow Doppler demonstrating mitral regurgitation caused by mitral valve endocarditis (*arrow*). LA, left atrium; LV, left ventricle; RA, right atrium; RV, right ventricle.

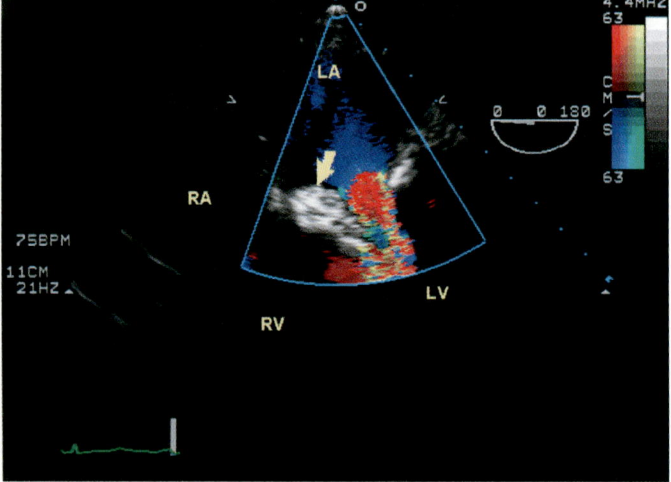

FIGURE 31-26. Midesophageal 4-chamber view with color-flow Doppler demonstrating mitral stenosis from mitral valve endocarditis (*arrow*). LA, left atrium; LV, left ventricle; RA, right atrium; RV, right ventricle.

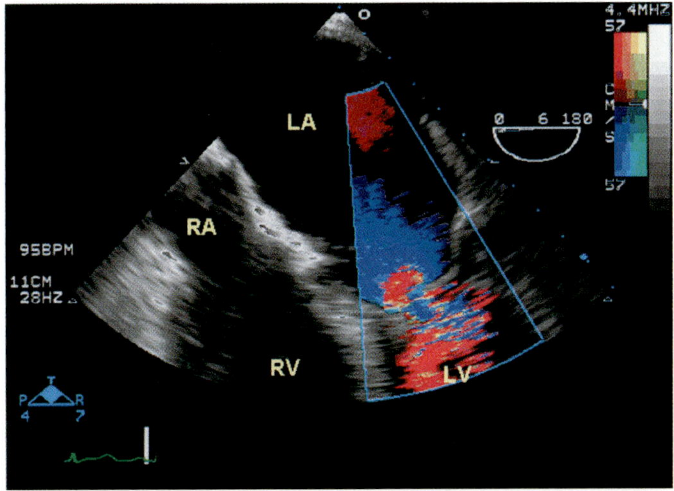

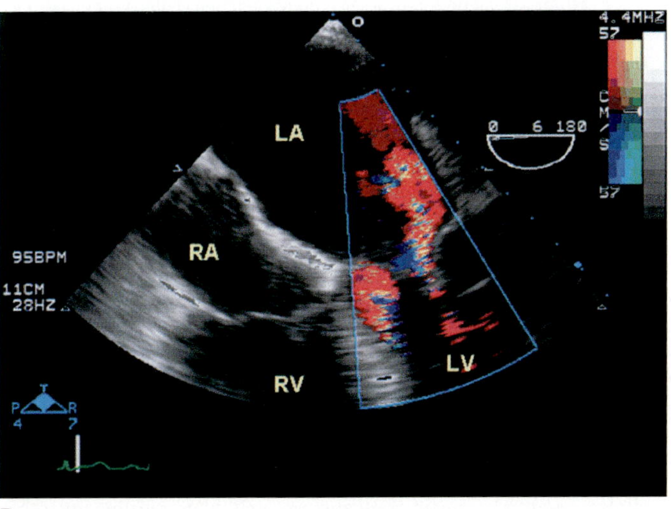

FIGURE 31-27. A. Midesophageal 4-chamber view with turbulent flow through a stenotic rheumatic mitral valve. **B.** Midesophageal 4-chamber view with color-flow Doppler demonstrating mitral regurgitation in a patient with rheumatic heart disease. LA, left atrium; LV, left ventricle; RA, right atrium; RV, right ventricle.

Associated findings in mitral stenosis include atrial dilation, pronounced left-to-right bowing of the IAS, SEC in the LA (with or without atrial thrombus), and signs of pulmonary hypertension (right-heart dysfunction).

A number of methods are available to echocardiographers for assessing the severity of mitral stenosis. Mean transmitral pressure gradients are easily estimated from the transmitral CWD profiles using the simplified Bernoulli equation:

$$\text{Mean pressure difference} = 4(\text{Mean transmitral velocity})^2$$

Severe MV stenosis is associated with mean transvalvular gradients greater than 12 mm Hg.

The pressure halftime (PHT) denotes the rate of diastolic pressure decline across the MV, specifically the time required to reach 50% of the peak pressure gradient. Normally, the diastolic E wave undergoes rapid deceleration because of the abrupt decrease in transmitral pressure gradient as the LV fills during early systole. However, in mitral stenosis, the pressure gradient is sustained much later in diastole, giving rise to a greatly prolonged E-wave deceleration and thus longer PHT. Angiographic experiments have shown that an MV area of 1 cm^2 corresponds to a PHT of 220 milliseconds; thus, the area of the stenotic orifice can be estimated by dividing 220 by the PHT in milliseconds.[74]

The continuity equation can be used in conjunction with the peak transmitral E-wave velocity and PISA measurements to estimate the stenotic orifice area. Providing there is no significant aortic or pulmonary regurgitation or interventricular shunts, the continuity equation also can use stroke volumes of the LVOT, AV or pulmonary valve, and the measured VTI of transmitral inflow to estimate the area of the stenotic mitral orifice.

Assessment of the MV area with 3D planimetry is an alternative approach to grading MS severity and correlates well with catheter-based techniques.[75] RT 3D TEE helps identifying MV commissural fusion and limited MV opening. Furthermore, RT 3D TEE has successfully been used for guidance during percutaneous mitral valvuloplasty and has been shown to be a suitable technique for monitoring its efficacy and complications.[76,77]

AORTIC VALVE

High-resolution images of the AV are provided by TEE because the valve and probe are separated by the LA, which acts as an excellent acoustic window. The AV is composed of 3 leaflets or cusps that are suspended from the aortic wall along 3 crescent-shaped lines. The junctions of the free edges of the cusps are called the *aortic commissures*. Behind each leaflet is the respective sinus of Valsalva, a pouchlike dilation of the aortic root. The leaflets and sinuses are named according to the adjacent coronary artery (ie, left, right, and noncoronary cusps and sinuses).

Four standard views allow examination of the AV and LVOT. Beginning with the imaging depth set at 10 to 12 cm, the ME AV SAX view is obtained by advancing or withdrawing the probe with a multiplane angle of 30 to 50 degrees until the AV appears in the center of the screen (**Fig. 31-28**). All 3 cusps should be seen symmetrically by rotating the multiplane angle and slightly anteflexing the probe. The general morphology of the AV (bicuspid, tricuspid) is noted as well as the thickness and mobility of the leaflets. CFD is applied to detect flow disturbances indicating aortic regurgitation or stenosis. The AV orifice may be traced to measure valve area.

The ME AV LAX view is obtained by rotating the multiplane angle forward 90 degrees from the ME AV SAX to visualize the LVOT, AV, and proximal ascending aorta in the LAX view (**Fig. 31-29**). The AV leaflets appear as 2 thin lines opening parallel to the aortic walls. The right coronary cusp, being farthest from the probe, is visualized toward the bottom of the display. The left or noncoronary cusp (depending on the imaging plane), located closer to the probe, is seen toward the top of the display. The diameters of the LVOT, aortic annulus, sinotubular junction, and ascending aorta can be measured in this view. The annulus is measured where the leaflets insert into the aorta. The proximal ascending aorta should be evaluated for calcification, atheroma, intimal flap or dissection, and aneurysmal dilation. CFD is again applied to detect the flow pattern through the LVOT, AV, and ascending aorta. Turbulent LVOT flow in this view should prompt further evaluation for hypertrophic obstructive cardiomyopathy or another obstruction to LVOT flow. Systolic anterior motion of the MV (often a fluttering motion into the LVOT but sometimes apparently occluding the LVOT), associated MR, premature AV closure or fluttering of the AV cusps, and thickened interventricular septum (>1.4 cm, disproportionate from the free wall) confirm hypertrophic obstructive cardiomyopathy.

The deep TG LAX view can be obtained by advancing the probe tip deep into the stomach and then anteflexing to create an imaging plane originating from the LV apex with the AV appearing in the far field. Alternatively, the TG LAX view is obtained from the TG midpapillary SAX view by rotating the angle forward to 90 to 110 degrees until the AV comes into view in the far field to the right side of the image. Both of these TG views allow for parallel alignment of the ultrasound beam through the AV, making them most useful for measuring Doppler flow velocities through the LVOT and AV rather than visualizing anatomy.

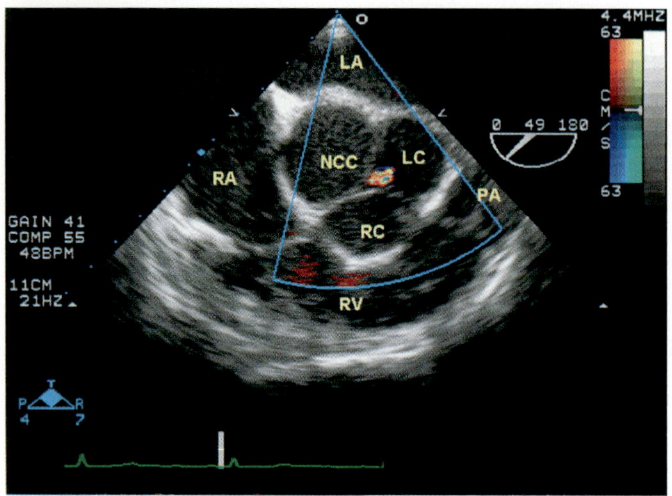

A

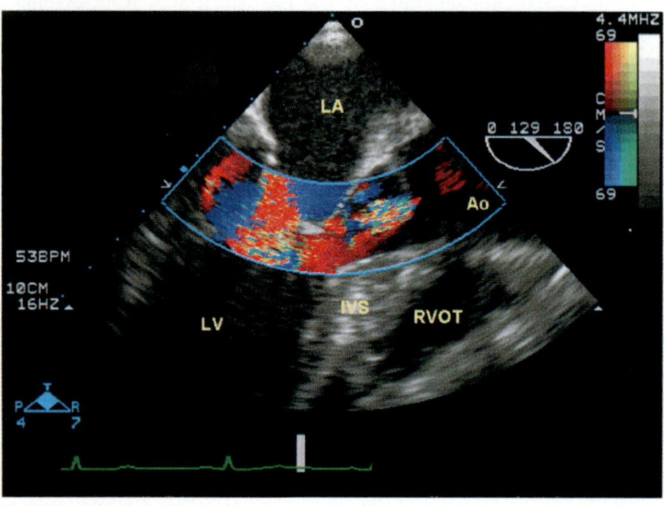

B

FIGURE 31-28. **A.** Midesophageal aortic valve short-axis view with color-flow Doppler (CFD) showing central aortic insufficiency in a dilated aortic valve. **B.** Midesophageal aortic valve long-axis view with CFD demonstrating aortic insufficiency. Ao, aorta; IVS, hypertrophied interventricular septum; LA, left atrium, LC, left aortic valve cusp; LV, left ventricle, NCC, noncoronary aortic valve cusp, PA, pulmonary artery, RA, right atrium, RC, right aortic valve cusp, RV, right ventricle, RVOT, right ventricular outflow tract.

Positioning the PWD sample volume in the center of the LVOT allows Doppler flow measurement in the outflow tract. Flow velocity through the AV is measured with CWD. Either or both of these TG views may be difficult to obtain in some patients, and a severely stenotic AV may make Doppler interrogation difficult. CFD may be helpful in detecting flow through the stenotic orifice, facilitating appropriate placement of the Doppler beam.

The 3D assessment of the native AV is more difficult compared with 3D imaging of the MV. The AV can be optimally visualized only in 18% when using RT 3D TEE, most likely because the AV is an anterior structure with a longer distance to the transducer, is associated with a less favorable angle of insonation and has thin pliable cusps compared with the MV leafets.[59]

Three-dimensional echocardiographic imaging of the AV appears to be most successful when using the live 3D mode (**Fig. 31-30**A and 31-30B). Occasionally, the 3D full-volume mode might offer more detailed information based on higher frame rates, and this mode also permits assessing both AV valves and the AV simultaneously.

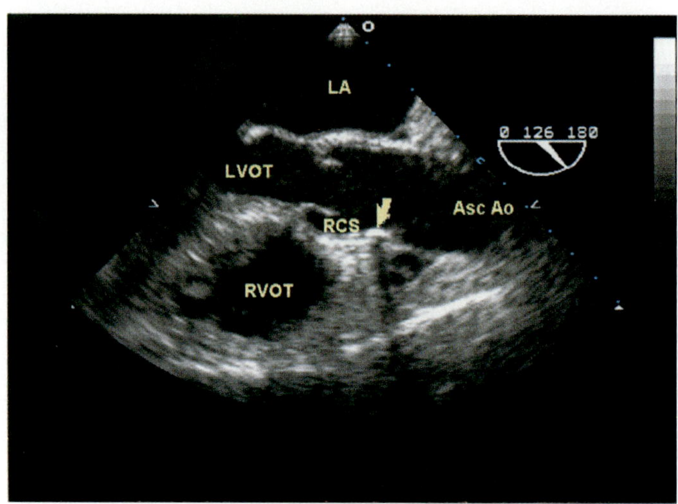

FIGURE 31-29. Midesophageal aortic valve long-axis view. *Arrow* indicates sinotubular junction. Asc Ao, ascending aorta; LA, left atrium; LVOT, left ventricular outflow tract; RCS, right coronary sinus behind right cusp of aortic valve; RVOT, right ventricular outflow tract.

Thickening and calcification of the AV cusps mostly facilitates RT 3D TEE imaging of the AV, but significant calcification results in similar drop-out (shadowing) as seen with 2D TEE. Cropping of a 3D TEE image assists in the planimetric assessment of the AV area, and RT 3D TEE potentially helps differentiating bicuspid from tricuspid anatomy of the AV and helps identify the exact location of an aortic dissection (Fig. 31-30C and 31-30D).

Aortic Insufficiency Acute or chronic regurgitation may result from abnormalities of the AV and the aortic root. Aging, rheumatic heart disease, endocarditis, and congenital bicuspid or unicuspid AV all may lead to aortic regurgitation. Dilation of the aorta resulting from connective tissue diseases (Marfan syndrome, Ehlers-Danlos syndrome), sinus Valsalva aneurysm, aortic root abscess, and hypertension are other causes of aortic insufficiency (AI).

Two-dimensional TEE imaging should be applied in the ME AV SAX and LAX views to detect congenital abnormalities or acquired defects such as myxomatous degeneration and vegetations. The aortic root should be assessed for dilation, and measurements of the LVOT, AV annulus, sinotubular junction, and ascending aorta should be obtained. The area of the end-diastolic gap between the aortic cusps, measured by planimetry, correlates with the severity of AI (mild, <0.2 cm^2; moderate, 0.2-0.4 cm^2; severe, >0.4 cm^2).

The VC should be measured by CFD in the ME LAX view with the imaging depth reduced. A VC less than 0.3 cm indicates mild AI, and a value greater than 0.6 cm signifies severe AI. The ratio of the regurgitant jet area to the LVOT area also can be measured by CFD in the ME LAX view. Similarly, the width of the regurgitant jet can be compared with the width of the LVOT. Values greater than 60% for area and greater than 65% for width indicate severe AI.

The PHT, described previously to grade mitral stenosis, can be applied to grade the severity of AI. The more severe the AI, the shorter the PHT because the aortic diastolic pressure gradient declines more rapidly. Whereas PHT is best obtained in the TG LAX or deep TG LAX views with CWD. PHT greater than 500 milliseconds indicates mild AI, PHT less than 200 milliseconds is compatible with severe AI. PHT measurements can be misleading in patients with elevated LV end-diastolic pressure (diastolic dysfunction). In these instances, the gradient will dissipate rapidly, and the true severity of regurgitation may be overestimated.

Early diastolic flow reversal in the descending aorta, measured with PWD, may be a normal finding. However, holodiastolic flow reversal in the proximal abdominal aorta or distal thoracic aorta indicates severe AI.

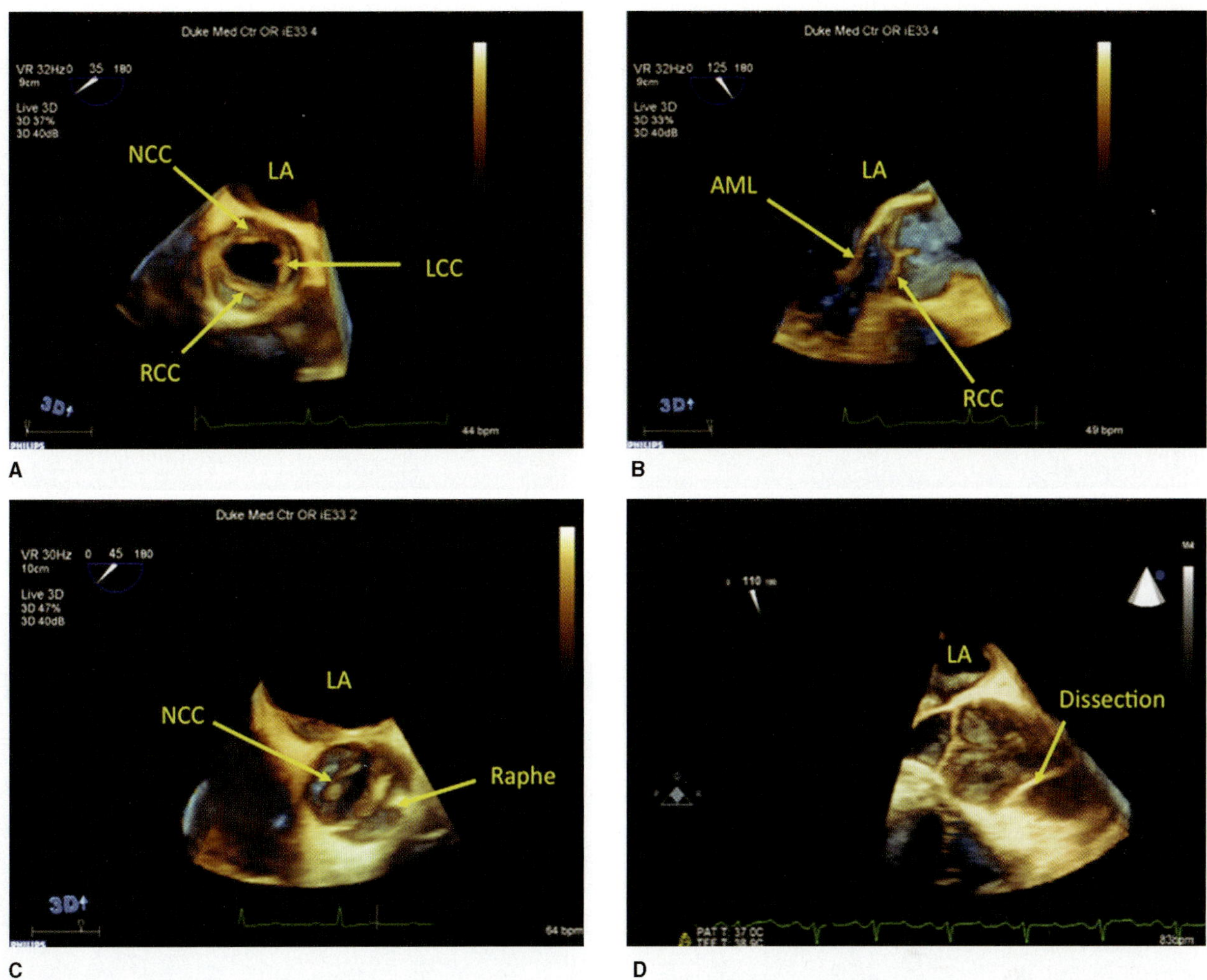

FIGURE 31-30. **A.** Midesophageal live three-dimensional (3D) transesophageal echocardiography (TEE) image of a normal open aortic valve acquired in short axis. **B.** Midesophageal live 3D TEE image of a normal closed aortic valve orientated in long axis. **C.** 3D image showing the elliptical opening of a bicuspid aortic valve. *Arrow* indicates calcification along raphe where right and left aortic valve cusps appear fused into a single cusp. **D.** Type A dissection of the ascending aorta originating very close to the AV, obtained in AV long-axis orientation. AML, anterior mitral valve leaflet; LA, left atrium; LCC, left coronary cusp; NCC, noncoronary cusp; RCC, right coronary cusp.

Aortic Stenosis The echocardiographic assessment of AS is based on a detailed description of cusp morphology, AV function, and the grading of AS severity. Calcific degeneration of the AV, the most common cause of AS, is characterized by restricted leaflet motion and calcification along the free edges of the leaflets. Patients with calcific degeneration usually become symptomatic in their sixth to seventh decades of life.

Rheumatic AS typically is seen in middle-aged immigrants. The tips of the leaflets are thickened and calcified, and the commissures are fused, producing a characteristic "doming" during systole. The orifice may become circular instead of the normal triangular shape. Rheumatic AS almost always is associated with rheumatic involvement of the MV.

Congenital abnormalities of the AV may lead to AS. Bicuspid AV is the most common form, occurring in approximately 2% of the normal population, and symptoms usually occur in the fourth to sixth decades of life. The bicuspid AV orifice is elliptical, and a calcified raphe is often present on one of the leaflets, giving the false impression of a trileaflet valve (Figs. 31-30C and **31-31**).

TEE interrogation should start with 2D imaging in the ME AV SAX and LAX views. Thin and mobile AV leaflets without calcification usually exclude severe AS. Thickening, calcification, and restricted leaflet motion are seen in all cases of AS. Commissural fusion is seen in rheumatic valvulitis. Poststenotic dilation of the aortic root and the proximal ascending aorta may be present. The AV area can be measured by planimetry in the ME AV SAX view using the zoom mode to magnify the frozen image. The inner edges of the distal leaflets should be traced in systole during their greatest excursion. Severe thickening and calcification of the leaflets, shadowing, accentuated cardiac motion, and the inability to obtain a true SAX view near the leaflet tips all may make planimetry difficult and inaccurate. In the ME AV LAX view, leaflet morphology, mobility, calcification, and thickening also can be evaluated. The LVOT can be examined for subaortic pathology.

Turbulent, high-velocity flow can be seen in the proximal ascending aorta with severe AS. Pressure gradients and transvalvular velocity should be measured. To accomplish this, the CWD beam is positioned across the AV in the TG LAX or deep TG LAX views (**Fig. 31-32**), and the edge of the spectrum is traced to obtain the peak and mean pressure gradients and flow velocities. Severe AS corresponds to a peak velocity greater than 4 milliseconds (**Fig. 31-33**A). The VTI of the traced spectrum is calculated and corresponds to the distance traveled by a column of blood during the stroke cycle. This allows use of the continuity principle to calculate the effective AV cross-sectional area (CSA_{AV}). The continuity principle is based on the conservation of flow over time between 2 conduits within a closed circuit (AV and LVOT in this example).

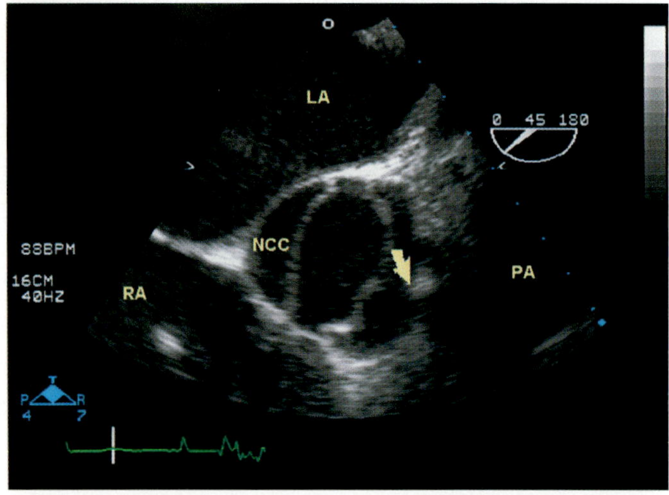

A

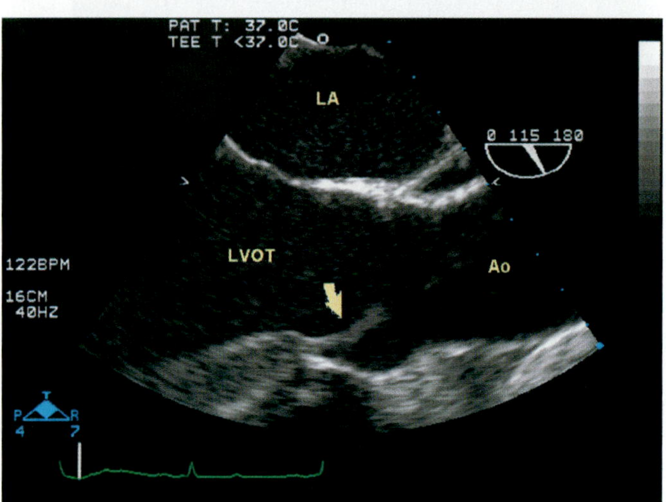

B

FIGURE 31-31. A. Midesophageal aortic valve short-axis view showing the elliptical opening of a bicuspid aortic valve. *Arrow* indicates calcification along the raphe, where the right and left aortic valve cusps appear fused into a single cusp. **B.** Midesophageal aortic valve long-axis view showing bowing of the restricted bicuspid aortic valve leaflet (*arrow*). Ao, aorta; LA, left atrium; LVOT, left ventricular outflow tract; NCC, noncoronary aortic valve cusp; PA, pulmonary artery; RA, right atrium.

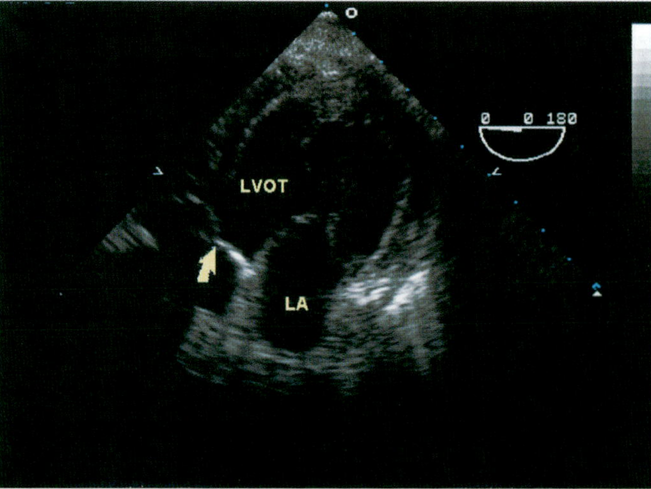

FIGURE 31-32. Deep transgastric long-axis view with aortic valve leaflets (*arrow*) seen on the *left*. LA, left atrium; LVOT, left ventricular outflow tract.

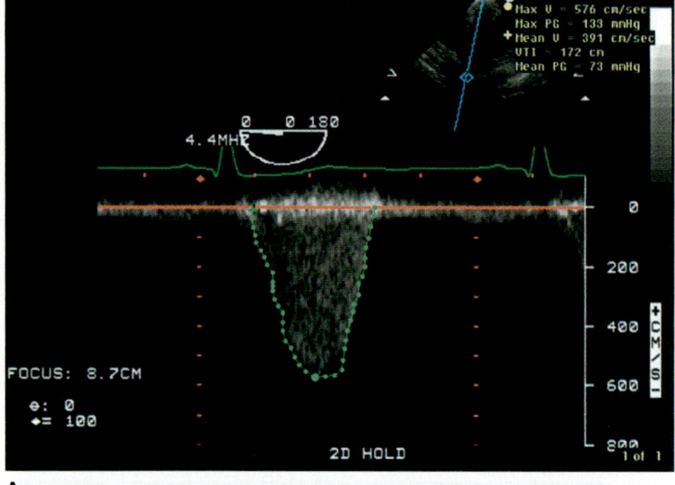

A

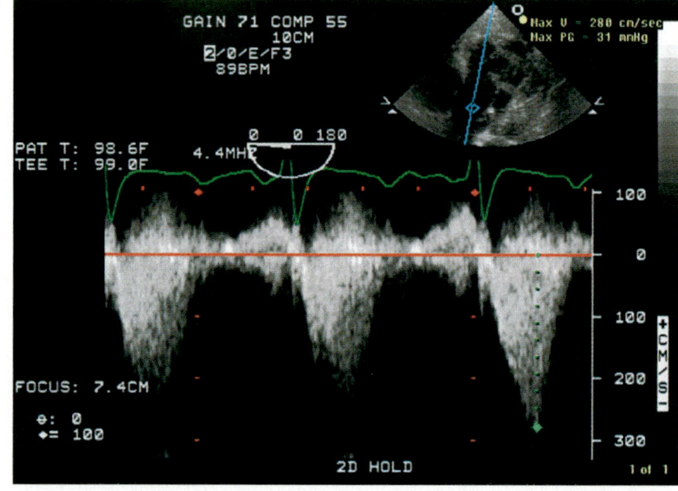

B

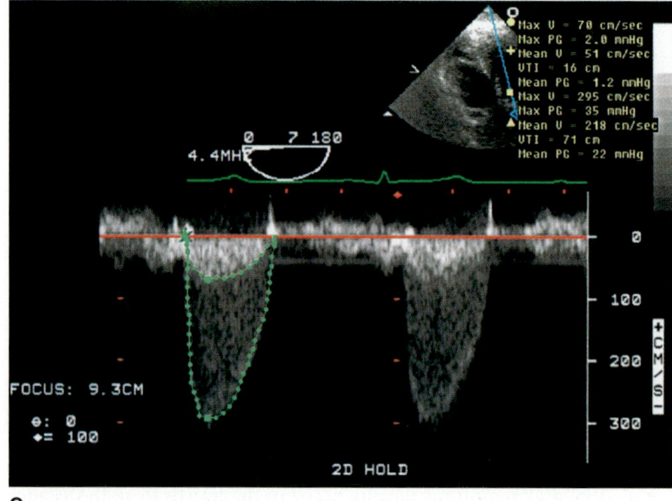

C

FIGURE 31-33. A. Continuous-wave Doppler through deep transgastric long-axis view of the aortic valve showing severe aortic stenosis (velocity >4 milliseconds). **B.** Continuous-wave Doppler through deep transgastric long-axis view of the aortic valve in a patient with hypertrophic obstructive cardiomyopathy (note the sharp "ice pick" contour). **C.** Continuous-wave Doppler through the aortic valve with velocity–time interval measured at the left ventricular outflow tract (inside tracing) and aortic valve (outside tracing) simultaneously.

Because flow is the product of the cross-sectional area of the conduit and the VTI through the conduit:

$$CSA_{LVOT} \times VTI_{LVOT} = CSA_{AV} \times VTI_{AV}$$

where CSA = πr^2, and r = radius of the respective conduit.

The radius or diameter of the LVOT can be measured in the ME LAX view. VTI_{LVOT} can be obtained in the TG LAX or deep TG LAX views using PWD. VTI_{AV} can be directly measured with CWD from the deep TG view. Alternatively, a "double-envelope" technique can be used to simultaneously measure LVOT and AV VTIs by CWD in the TG LAX or deep TG LAX views (Fig. 31-33C). Because the velocity of flow through the smaller AV must accelerate from that of the larger diameter LVOT, the larger envelope must correspond to the VTI of the AV, and the smaller but denser envelope represents the VTI of the LVOT. Demonstration of the noncircular shape of the LVOT by RT 3D TEE has raised questions of the accuracy of this method. However, accuracy in the AV area calculation can be improved by direct volumetric measurement of the LV stroke volume using a 3D full-volume data set.[78]

The role of intraoperative TEE in guiding percutaneous AV implantation for patients with symptomatic AS is evolving. TEE can help to confirm the diagnosis, provides accurate measurements of the AV annulus for appropriate sizing, guides the transcatheter positioning of the prosthetic valve, and permits immediate evaluation of the deployed prothesis.[79] RT 3D TEE modes and biplane imaging provide valuable complementary information to fluoroscopy in guiding these procedures.[80]

AORTA

The aorta is the largest artery in the body with a normal diameter up to 3.5 cm. It is divided anatomically into 4 segments: the ascending aorta, transverse aortic arch, descending thoracic aorta, and abdominal aorta. The ascending aorta begins at the level of the aortic annulus and the AV. Just distal to the aortic annulus, the ascending aorta dilates to form a segment known as the *aortic sinus of Valsalva,* which includes the respective left coronary, right coronary, and noncoronary sinuses. Distal to the aortic sinuses, the aorta has a brief segment with a reduced diameter called the *sinotubular junction.*

In adults, the ascending aorta is approximately 5 cm in length. After originating from the AV annulus, the ascending aorta extends rightward around the main pulmonary trunk and crosses the right pulmonary artery anteriorly. It then ascends rightward and anteriorly until it meets the aortic arch at the origin of the innominate artery (at the level of the second intercostal space). The proximal or near aortic arch is poorly visualized with TEE because of the anatomic interposition of the trachea between the esophagus and the aorta at this level. Whereas the innominate and left common carotid arteries are in close proximity to the trachea, the left subclavian artery lies to the left of the trachea and can be visualized more easily with TEE.

The descending thoracic aorta begins distal to the left subclavian artery at the level of the ligamentum arteriosus. This is an area of narrowing referred to as the *aortic isthmus.* The ligamentum arteriosus is a fibrous connection between the pulmonary artery and the aorta, a remnant of the ductus arteriosus during fetal life. Inferior to the isthmus, the descending aorta courses to the left lateral side of the body of the fourth thoracic vertebrae. The descending aorta is relatively transfixed to the vertebral column here. Therefore, deceleration injuries often occur at the level of the isthmus. The descending aorta continues along a slightly anterior and rightward path as it approaches the diaphragm, where it lies directly posterior to the esophagus. Therefore, at the level of the lower esophageal sphincter, the heart and the aorta are on opposite sides of the esophagus.

The SCA and the ASE have defined 6 2D views for interrogating the thoracic aorta by TEE.[7] Multiple imaging planes from within similar views may be necessary to accurately define aortic pathology.

The ME ascending aorta SAX view is obtained in the 0- to 30-degree imaging plane with the probe approximately 25 cm from the lips. In this view, a SAX view of the ascending aorta along with the main pulmonary artery, right pulmonary artery, and SVC is obtained. Qualitative analysis of the aortic anatomy and wall thickness can be obtained in this view.

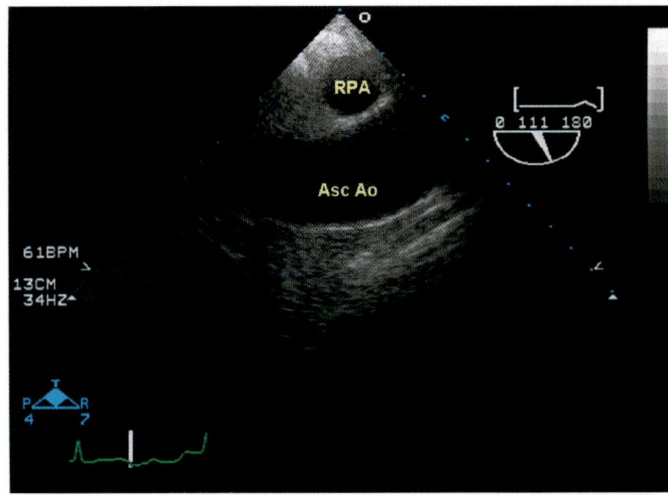

FIGURE 31-34. Midesophageal ascending aorta long-axis view. Asc Ao, ascending aorta; RPA, right pulmonary artery.

The ME ascending aorta LAX view is obtained between 110 and 140 degrees. This view is easily obtained after starting with the ME AV SAX view ("Mercedes Benz" view), which is easily recognized at the ME level with the multiplane angle at 20 to 50 degrees. After the "Mercedes Benz" view has been obtained, rotating the imaging plane forward an additional 90 degrees and withdrawing the probe slightly yields the ME ascending aorta LAX view (**Fig. 31-34**). This view is useful in defining wall thickness, aortic dimensions, and blood flow patterns in the ascending aorta.

From the ME ascending aorta views, turning the probe to the left with a multiplane angle of 0 degree produces a SAX image through the descending aorta. After the aorta has been visualized, the depth of the image should be optimized so the aorta is in the center of the screen. Inserting the probe to the level of the diaphragm (where the image disappears) and then slowly withdrawing the probe allows scanning of the entire descending thoracic aorta. The SAX view is useful for defining wall thickness, determining atherosclerotic severity, and measuring aortic dimensions (**Fig. 31-35**A).

From the SAX view, rotating the plane to 90 degrees produces a LAX view of the descending aorta, or alternatively, both view can be demonstrated with biplane imaging (Fig. 31-35A). These views are useful for defining spatial relationships of SAX findings, interrogating aortic flow patterns, and identifying branch vessels. Three-dimensional TEE may help to communicate the extent of atheromatous disease to the surgeon Fig. 31-35B.

With the scan plane at 0 degree, withdrawal of the probe following the aorta to an upper esophageal window with a rightward rotation produces a LAX view of the aortic arch. This view is used to define aortic dimensions, wall contour, and branch vessels. Advancing the multiplane angle to 90 degrees in the upper esophagus produces a SAX view of the arch. At the proximal arch, the main pulmonary artery and right pulmonary artery may be seen if the depth is sufficient. At the distal arch, multiple views of the arch and its branch vessels may be obtained.

Even using all of these views, TEE does not image the entire thoracic aorta. A "blind spot" in the distal ascending or proximal arch is created by the trachea. The aorta also is subject to echocardiographic artifacts and dropout caused by calcifications. With every image, the examiner should describe the morphology, dimensions, and integrity of the aortic wall. Evaluation for spontaneous echocardiographic contrast or turbulent flow also is recommended. Any fluid collection should be noted.

The aorta is a significant source of atheromatous material that can embolize to the brain, and atherosclerosis of the proximal thoracic aorta is established as an independent risk factor for cognitive dysfunction and stroke after cardiac surgery.[81-83] Multiple strategies can be used to minimize embolization of atheromatous material liberated from the

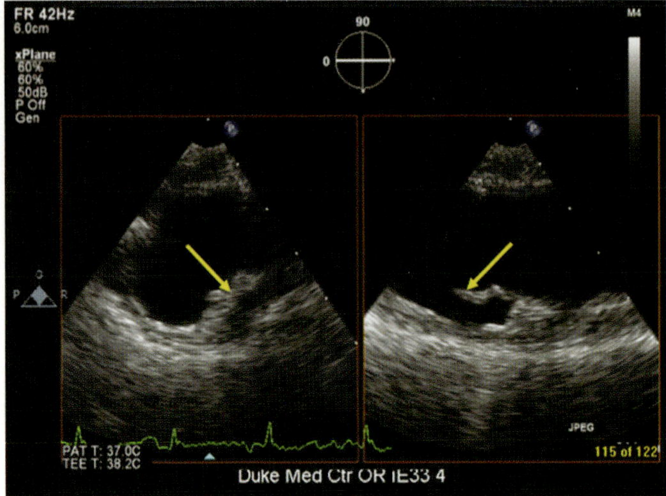

A

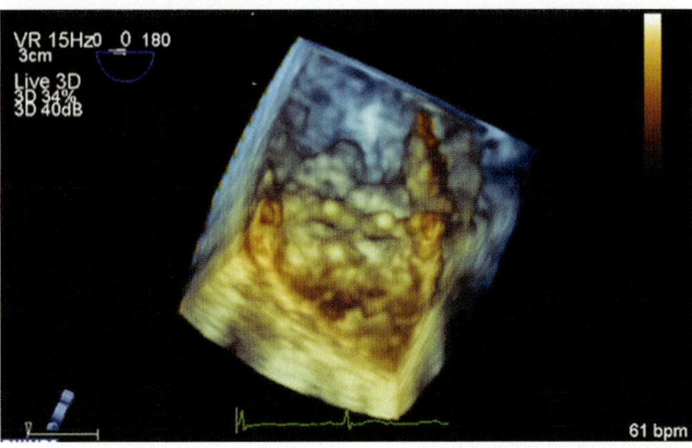

B

FIGURE 31-35. **A.** Biplane view of the descending aorta illustrating a mobile atheroma (*arrow*) short-axis (*left*) and long-axis (*right*) views. **B.** Live three-dimensional image of a descending aorta with significant atheromatous disease.

aortic wall to the cerebral circulation. The use of TEE and epiaortic scanning facilitates a "knowledgeable avoidance" of the atheromatous ascending aorta with respect to cannulation, clamping, and anastomosis placement.[84] Hammon et al[85] have recently demonstrated that avoiding manipulation of the aorta by using only a single-clamp application can significantly reduce postoperative cognitive loss. Optimal placement of the aortic cannula in an area relatively devoid of plaque, and the use of specialized cannulae with optimal hydrodynamics and less "sandblasting" effects[86] can also decrease the embolization of plaque.

Most of the thoracic aorta can be routinely imaged with multiplane TEE because it is adjacent to the esophagus while moving vertically through the mediastinum. TEE offers an advantage over epiaortic ultrasound (EAU) imaging in allowing continuous monitoring without interruption of the surgical procedure. However, because the air-filled trachea is interposed between the esophagus and the distal ascending aorta and proximal aortic arch, these regions usually cannot be visualized with TEE. EAU imaging can be used to examine these areas through a median sternotomy by covering a high-frequency transducer with a sterile sheath and placing it directly on the ascending aorta in the surgical field. Recently published guidelines state that EAU imaging is a superior technique compared with TEE for the detection and localization of ascending aortic atherosclerosis compared with manual palpation and TEE.[84] A comprehensive EAU examination is based on a minimum of 5 views for the evaluation of the ascending aorta from the sinotubular junction to the origin of the innominate artery and the aortic arch. An EAU examination can be performed rapidly and provides valuable information for the management of atheroma burden in patients with cardiac surgical conditions who require aortic manipulation. Further studies are warranted to determine the optimal atheroma grading scale and to delineate management strategies directed toward plaque avoidance and improving patient outcomes.

A case series using RT 3D epiaortic echocardiography showed that 3D was better in displaying diffusely dispersed plaques. Another advantage of 3D epiaortic scans might be the inclusion of discernable landmarks within the aorta like the AV to clarify the relative position of the plaque.[87]

Many different classification systems for aortic atheroma severity have been proposed. The most widely used system was proposed by Katz et al, consisting of a 5-grade classification system. A grade I atheroma has minimal or no intimal thickening. A grade II atheroma has severe intimal thickening without a protruding element. A grade III atheroma has intimal thickening protruding less than 5 mm into the lumen. A grade IV atheroma protrudes more than 5 mm into the lumen. A grade V lesion is any atheroma with a mobile component. Although currently there is no consensus as to the size of plaque that should warrant alteration of the surgical procedure, large atheromas and atheromas with mobile elements should warrant discussion with the surgeon.

TEE is useful for diagnosis and classification of thoracic and abdominal aneurysms (**Fig. 31-36**). An aneurysm of the aorta involves an increase in

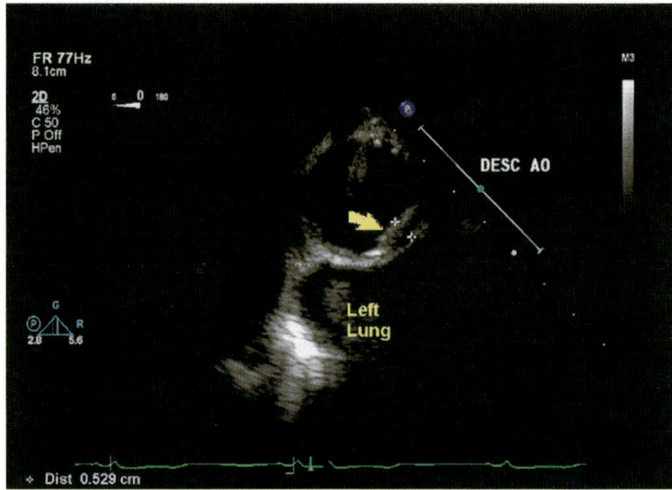

A

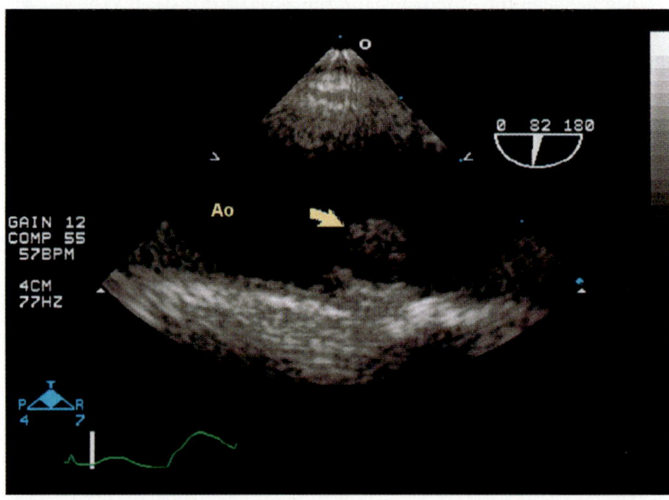

B

FIGURE 31-36. Short-axis (**A**) and long-axis (**B**) views of a descending thoracic aorta aneurysm with ulcerated atheroma.

the luminal diameter of all 3 layers of the aorta. A pseudoaneurysm involves an interruption of the intima and media at the level of the aneurysmal sac and its communication with the native aorta. An ascending aortic diameter larger than 4 cm, descending thoracic aneurysm larger than 6 cm, or abdominal aortic aneurysm larger than 5 cm in diameter is considered an indication for surgical intervention.

Dissection of the aorta is a process in which the intima separates from the adventitial layer. It is characterized by the presence of an intimal flap and resulting false and true lumens. Aortic dissection can result from intimal rupture followed by cleavage formation and propagation of the dissection into the media. Additionally, aortic dissection can result from intramural hemorrhage and hematoma formation in the media followed by perforation of the intima. The presence of an intimal flap is the most characteristic feature of aortic dissection. The pathogenesis of dissection is complex. Medial degeneration tends to be more extensive in older individuals and in patients with hypertension, Marfan syndrome, and bicuspid AVs.[88] The true lumen diameter typically is smaller than the false lumen diameter (**Fig. 31-37**A), and spontaneous contrast can often be seen in the false lumen. However, PWD should be used to confirm forward flow in the presumed true lumen during systole (Fig. 31-37B).

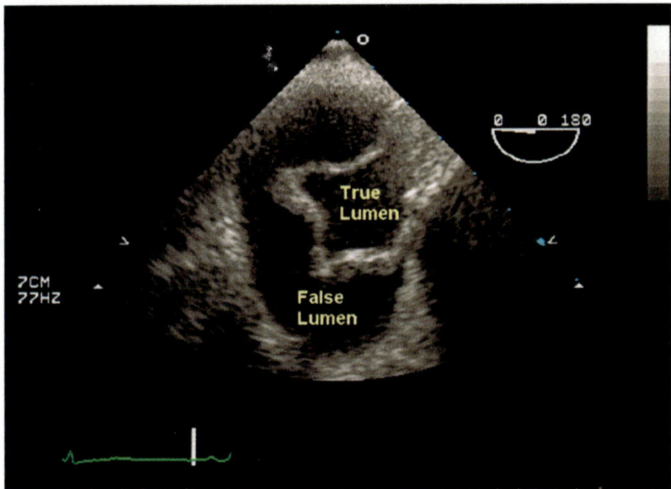

A

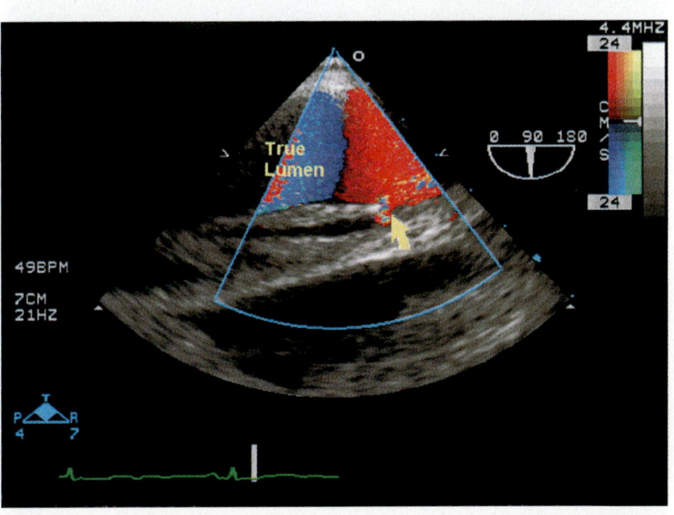

B

FIGURE 31-37. A. Descending aorta short-axis view of an aortic dissection. **B.** Descending aorta long-axis view of an aortic dissection at the level of an intimal tear (*arrow*).

Aortic dissection is divided into acute and chronic types, depending on the duration of symptoms. Acute aortic dissection is present when the diagnosis is made within 2 weeks after the initial onset of symptoms. Approximately one-third of patients with aortic dissection fall into the chronic category in which symptom duration is longer than 2 weeks. The most common site of initiation of aortic dissection is the ascending aorta (50%) followed by aortic regions in the vicinity of the ligamentum arteriosum.

Anatomically, aortic dissection has been classified by 2 schemes. The DeBakey classification consists of the 3 types: type I includes both the ascending and the descending aorta, type II includes only the ascending aorta, and type III includes only the descending aorta. The Stanford classification consists of 2 types: type A involves the ascending aorta regardless of the entry site location, and type B involves the aorta distal to the origin of the left subclavian artery. Whereas any dissection involving the ascending aorta (DeBakey types I and II or Stanford type A) is an indication for repair, dissections confined to the descending aorta can be medically managed, at least initially.

Two-dimensional TEE is one of the most frequently used imaging modalities to diagnose aortic dissection and showed a sensitivity comparable to CT scan and MRI with a lower specificity due to false-positive findings in the ascending aorta.[89,90] Several case reports have demonstrated that 3D TTE might add value to 2D TTE in identifying aortic dissection. Color Doppler 3D TEE allowed detecting an extension of the dissection into the innominate artery.[91-93] The main advantage of RT 3D TEE may be the determination of the interrelationship of the dissection flap to adjacent structures (eg, if the coronary arteries are involved in the dissection) (see Fig. 31-30D). This can be best addressed by using the 3D zoom mode.

Endovascular repair of the aorta has gained popularity as a reliable alternative to conventional repair. TEE is used to supplement intraoperative angiography in guiding placement of thoracic endografts. During endovascular repair, TEE is the most sensitive imaging modality currently available for diagnosing endoleaks immediately after graft deployment. The ability to use intraoperative TEE for visualizing the thoracic and abdominal aorta and monitoring cardiac function makes it an invaluable tool during these procedures.[94]

RIGHT VENTRICLE

The RV is often described as a crescent-shaped, thin walled, and compliant chamber. It is less contractile than the LV, and its oxygen requirements are lessened by its reduced muscle mass and lower afterload. The right coronary artery (RCA) supplies the RV free wall, the posterior descending artery supplies the inferior RV wall, and the anterior RV wall has a dual blood supply from the conus branch from the RCA and the moderator branch from the left anterior descending artery.[95] The RV is a low-pressure system, with an average pressure of 20/5 mm Hg. Therefore, coronary flow to the RV from the aorta follows this favorable pressure gradient, resulting in perfusion during both diastole and systole, unlike the high-pressure LV, which is perfused mainly during diastole.[96,97] RV contraction resembles peristaltic motion, which functions to prolong ejection time by ejecting blood even as proximal RV pressures decline, thus minimizing end-diastolic pressure and promoting venous return.[98] RV ejection results primarily from RV free wall inward motion, with a smaller contribution from descent of the base of the heart.

The RV is highly sensitive to changes in afterload and susceptible to coronary air embolism because of the anterior location of the RCA takeoff. Furthermore, RV myocardial protection during cardiac surgery is more difficult than for the LV. Evaluation of the RV is a necessary part of a comprehensive TEE examination because RV dysfunction in cardiac surgery correlates with mortality.[99] However, because of its anterior position far from the TEE probe and its geometric complexity because of its crescent shape and twisting contraction of its thin free walls, assessment of the RV with TEE is more challenging than that of the LV.

TEE examination of the RV is primarily performed qualitatively by assessing the RV in LAX with the ME 4-chamber (see Figs. 31-3B

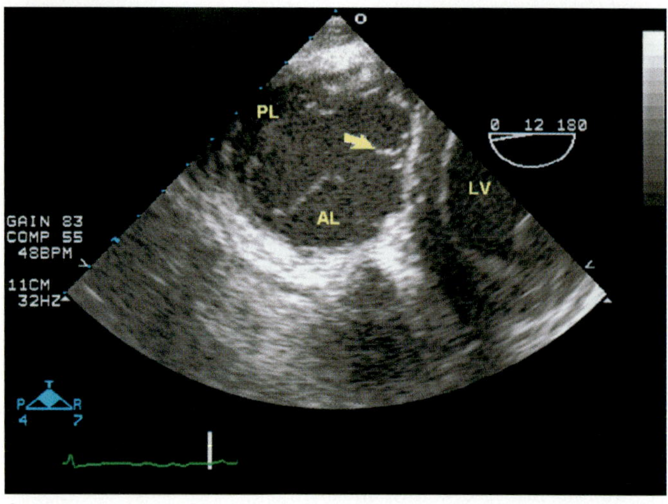

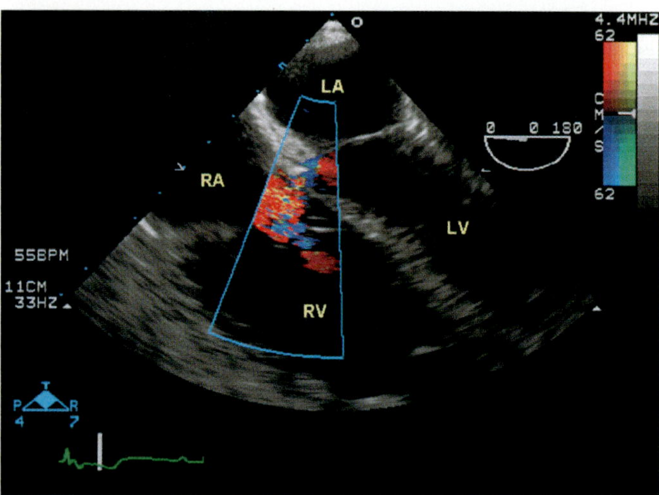

FIGURE 31-38. A. Transgastric short-axis view with rightward rotation at the level of the tricuspid valve leaflets. *Arrow* indicates septal tricuspid leaflet poorly visualized in this plane. **B.** Midesophageal 4-chamber view showing severe right ventricular dilation and associated tricuspid regurgitation. AL, anterior tricuspid leaflet; LA, left atrium; LV, left ventricle; PL, posterior tricuspid leaflet; RA, right atrium; RV, right ventricle.

and **31-38**B) and TG RV inflow views, as well as in SAX with TG mid-SAX (Fig. 31-41) and ME RV inflow–outflow views (Fig. 31-4B). The RV free wall is best viewed from the ME 4-chamber and TG mid-SAX views. When assessing RV function, RV dilation, the presence of interatrial or interventricular septal shift to the left, RV wall motion abnormalities, significant tricuspid insufficiency, and IVC engorgement indicate dysfunction.[100-102] *RV hypertrophy* is defined as end-diastolic free wall thickness larger than 0.5 cm (or greater than half the thickness of the LV).

RV dilation is indicated by an RV diastolic diameter that exceeds the LV diastolic diameter in the TG mid-SAX view. RV dilation also can be graded from the ME 4-chamber view. The normal-sized RV will not form part of the heart apex. If the apex of the heart includes the RV apex, then moderate RV dilation is present; if the apex is entirely formed by the RV, then severe dilation is present.[6]

Semiquantitative assessment of RV systolic function is described by the RV fractional area of contraction in the ME 4-chamber view and the tricuspid annular plane systolic excursion (descent of the tricuspid annulus) in the ME 4-chamber view. In a retrospective study, RV fractional area of contraction below 35% was associated with poorer outcomes.[103] Tricuspid annular plane systolic excursion greater than 25 mm correlates with normal RV EF.[104] However, because of the complexity of the RV anatomy, these measurements may be inaccurate, so a comprehensive qualitative assessment must be performed.

In high-risk cardiac procedures, dynamic analysis of RV performance is important but has been hampered by the inability to reliably image the geometric complexity of the RV. Therefore, all 2D echocardiographic approaches to RV volumes and function are inadequate because they rely on visual estimation and geometric assumptions. With the introduction of RT 3D TTE imaging, dedicated RV quantification software has been introduced and validated in comparison with cardiac magnetic resonance and radionuclide ventriculography as gold standards.[105,106] Recent work suggests that 3D echocardiography is useful for dynamic RV assessment. Three-dimensional echocardiography may be able to overcome the limitations of 2D echocardiography and has been shown to improve the accuracy and reliability of RV quantification compared with 2D.[107,108] Free-standing software (TomTec Imaging software, Unterschleissheim, Munich, Germany) dedicated to RV quantification facilitates the analysis of RV volume and function and can be performed both with 3D TTE as well as 3D TEE data (**Fig. 31-39**).[109]

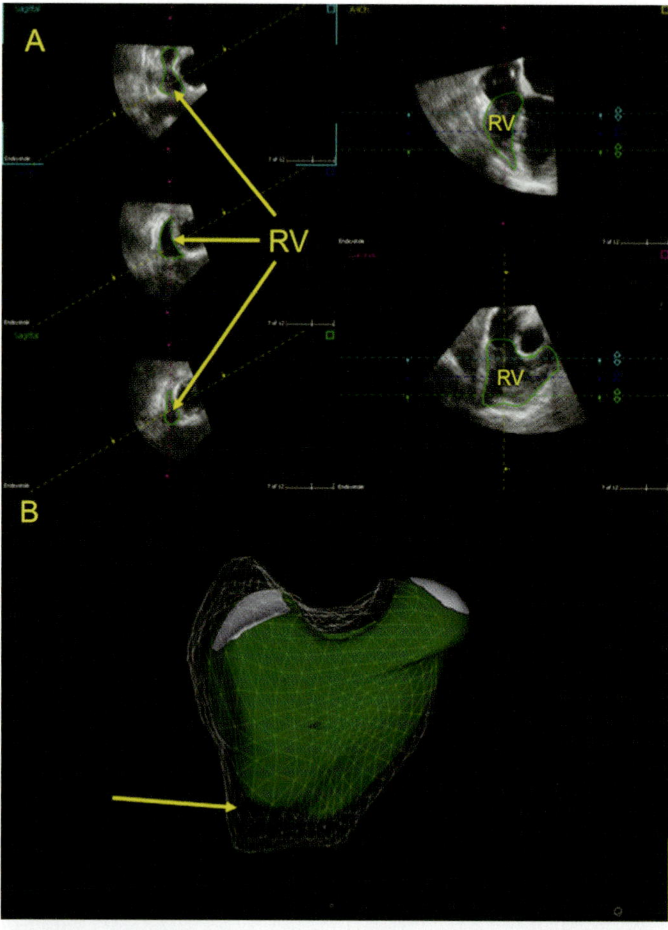

FIGURE 31-39. A. Three-dimensional (3D) transesophageal echocardiography (TEE) full volume of the right ventricle displayed in 3 short-axis and 2 long-axis reconstruction planes. **B.** Offline reconstruction of the right ventricular cavity using TomTec analytical software (4D RV-Function application, TomTec Imaging Systems GmbH, Unterschleissheim, Munich, Germany). Manual definition of several endocardial border points of the right ventricle in end systole and end diastole followed by an automatic border-tracking algorithm and segmental analysis will display the right ventricular shell along with an end-diastolic reference mesh (*arrow*) and volumetric quantification.

TRICUSPID VALVE

The TV consists of anterior, posterior, and septal leaflets; the largest is the septal leaflet (Fig. 31-32A). In the presence of normal leaflets, TR is termed *functional* and is commonly attributable to RV dilation or dysfunction. In contrast, TR caused by abnormalities is rare.

Similar to the RV, the TV lies in the far field, making 2D and 3D imaging difficult. In the ME 4-chamber view, the anterior (or sometimes posterior) and septal leaflets are seen. In the ME RV inflow–outflow view, the posterior and anterior leaflets are seen on the left and right of the image screen, respectively (Fig. 31-4B). In the TG RV inflow view, the posterior leaflet is in the near field, and the anterior leaflet is in the far field. Optimal visualization of the TV using RT 3D TEE is achieved only in a small percentage of patients.[59] It remains to be seen if RT 3D TEE will improve the accuracy in the assessment of valvular dysfunction similar to what has been described for the MV. Early reports using 3D TTE suggest that assessment of tricuspid regurgitation is feasible in most patients and that the shape of the VC is more ovoid than that of MR regurgitant jets.[110] Grading TR should consider many factors, including RA and RV size, hepatic flow patterns, VC, and jet area. Severe TR correlates well with systolic flow reversal in the hepatic veins, a VC measuring larger than 6.5 mm in the apical 4-chamber view, and TR jet area more than two-thirds of RA area.[111,112] In addition, TV annulus larger than 4 cm and tricuspid inflow velocity longer than 1 millisecond by CWD is associated with severe TR.[113]

In the absence of pulmonic stenosis, the pulmonary artery systolic pressure can be estimated if TR is present. To accomplish this, the peak pressure gradient is calculated and added to the measured central venous pressure. To obtain the peak pressure gradient across the TV, the modified Bernoulli equation is applied to the peak TR jet velocity measured by CWD.

With regard to tricuspid stenosis, a mean inflow pressure gradient less than 2 mm Hg is considered mild, 2 to 6 mm Hg is moderate, and greater than 6 mm Hg is severe. CWD is used to measure TV inflow velocities, which are used to determine pressure gradients. Multiple views should be interrogated to obtain the best alignment with diastolic inflow and therefore more accurate measurements.

PULMONIC VALVE

The pulmonic valve is trileaflet, consisting of anterior, left, and right leaflets. Significant pulmonic disease in an adult without congenital heart disease is rare. As with the other right-sided structures, the pulmonic valve is anterior and difficult to image with TEE. The best views for visualizing the pulmonic valve are the ME RV inflow–outflow view (Fig. 31-4B) and upper esophageal aortic arch SAX view (**Fig. 31-40**A).

In adults, pulmonic regurgitation usually is caused by pulmonary hypertension and annular dilation. The examination should include the regurgitant jet VC, jet length, RV size, and degree of CWD flow deceleration. Holodiastolic flow reversal in the main pulmonary artery (measured with PWD in the upper esophageal aortic arch SAX view) is indicative of significant pulmonic insufficiency.

Pulmonic stenosis is rare in adults and is classified as valvular, subvalvular, or supravalvular. CWD is used in the upper esophageal aortic arch SAX view to obtain a peak pressure gradient (mild stenosis, <30 mm Hg; moderate, 30-64 mm Hg; severe, >64 mm Hg).

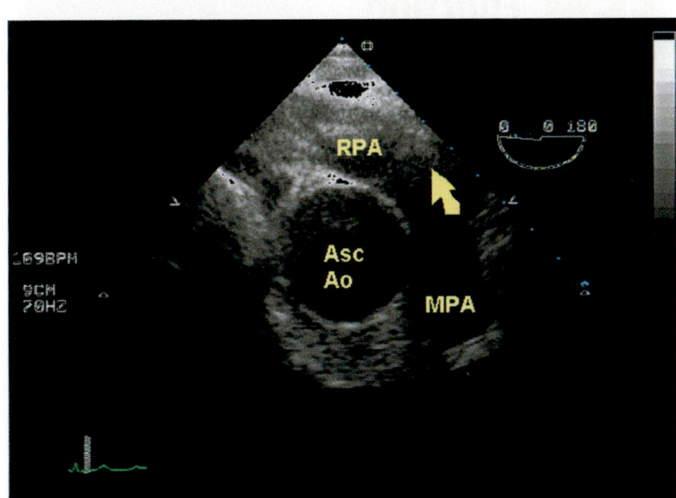

FIGURE 31-40. **A.** Upper esophageal aortic arch short-axis view with pulmonary artery and pulmonary valve in the far field. *Leftward arrow* indicates pulmonic valve. The left pulmonary artery and branch point are not within this two-dimensional ultrasound plane. Ao, aorta with branch vessel (*downward arrow*); PA, main pulmonary artery. **B.** Upper esophageal ascending aorta short-axis view at level of the pulmonary artery branch point. Asc Ao, ascending aorta; IV, innominate vein; MPA, main pulmonary artery; RPA, right pulmonary artery; RVOT, right ventricular outflow tract.

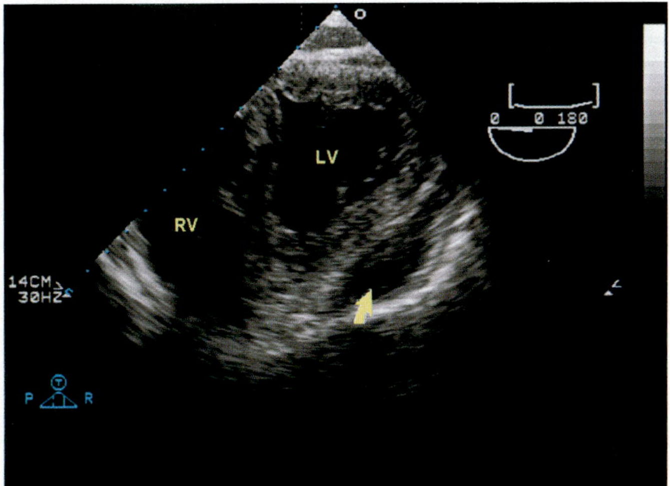

FIGURE 31-41. Transgastric short-axis view revealing a significant pericardial effusion (*arrow*). The right ventricle (RV) is enlarged, and the D-shaped left ventricle (LV) indicates elevated right ventricular pressures.

PULMONARY ARTERY

Evaluation of the main and right pulmonary arteries is performed from the upper esophageal ascending aorta SAX view. The left pulmonary artery is difficult to image because it usually is obscured by air in the left mainstem bronchus. In adults, the main pulmonary artery is approximately 5 cm in length. The normal main and right pulmonary artery dimensions are 0.9 to 2.9 cm and 1.2 to 2.2 cm, respectively. TEE has 80% sensitivity and 100% specificity for the diagnosis of pulmonary embolus, but its low negative predictive value of 53% makes this modality unsuitable for ruling out pulmonary embolus.[114]

PERICARDIUM

The pericardial sac is a potential space between visceral and parietal pericardium. Pericardial effusion is a syndrome in which fluid accumulates in the pericardial sac. A wide variety of disease processes can lead to pericardial effusion. Depending on the size and speed of accumulation, a pericardial effusion can compromise venous return and lead to low cardiac output. Tamponade occurs when pericardial pressure exceeds the distending pressure of the cardiac chambers, resulting in impaired diastolic cardiac filling. Echocardiography is helpful for diagnosing pericardial effusion and cardiac tamponade, but cardiac tamponade ultimately is a clinical diagnosis.

Pericardial effusions can be visualized as an echolucent space surrounding the echogenic external border of the heart chambers (**Fig. 31-41**). A thorough TEE examination, including ME 4-chamber, ME 2-chamber, ME LAX, and TG basal SAX views, should be performed for evaluation of pericardial cavity and surrounding structures. Effusions that separate the visceral pericardium from the parietal pericardium by less than 0.5 cm are small, and those with more than 2-cm separation are large. Three-dimensional imaging may also add to the diagnostic ability of echocardiography.[115]

Characteristic echocardiographic findings of cardiac tamponade are RA systolic collapse, RV diastolic collapse, abnormal ventricular septal motion, and reciprocal respiratory variation in ventricular volumes. RA systolic collapse usually develops before RV diastolic collapse. Because of the tethering effect of the pulmonary veins, LA collapse is rare and implies the presence of a large effusion. PWD of mitral inflow velocity and pulmonary vein flow velocity also shows a pronounced respiratory variation pattern in cardiac tamponade.

CONCLUSION

Intraoperative echocardiography has become a standard of practice for cardiac anesthesia care, reflecting the ever-expanding complexity of surgical techniques and cardiovascular pathology. In addition, it now holds a place as an important and increasingly routine adjunct to noncardiac anesthesia practice. Recent advances in 3D echocardiography provide intraoperative echocardiographers with spectacular images and enhanced diagnostic accuracy and facilitate communication with surgeons. The trend to smaller imaging systems that are less expensive, portable, and user friendly has enabled the expansion of intraoperative echocardiography to a greater variety of settings. Today, handheld as well as portable systems allow for use of ultrasonography in preoperative clinics, postanesthesia care units, and intensive care units and have stimulated a new generation of ultrasound uses. Recent advances of tissue Doppler-derived strain and speckle tracking and 2D-strain imaging make these attractive new tools for the quantification of intraoperative changes in myocardial function.

It is our hope that this chapter with its systematic approach to the perioperative use of 2D and 3D TEE will help grow and stimulate further use of these unique and important imaging modalities.

Acknowledgments: The authors thank Larry C. Field, MD, George D. Lappas, MD, Angus A. Christie, MD, Andrew Green, MD, Steven T. Morozowich, MD, Tamas Szabo, MD, PhD, Qin Zhang, MD, Stephen P. Murphy, MD, and Ravi Bissessar, MD, for their work on the version of this chapter that appeared in the previous edition.

KEY REFERENCES

- Daniel MT, Martin A, Bruce AB, et al. Practice guidelines for perioperative transesophageal echocardiography. A report by the American Society of Anesthesiologists and the Society of Cardiovascular Anesthesiologists Task Force on Transesophageal Echocardiography. *Anesthesiology.* 1996;84(4):986-1006.
- Daniel WG, Erbel R, Kasper W, et al. Safety of transesophageal echocardiography. A multicenter survey of 10,419 examinations. *Circulation.* 1991;83(3):817-821.
- Shanewise JS, Cheung AT, Aronson S, et al. ASE/SCA guidelines for performing a comprehensive intraoperative multiplane transesophageal echocardiography examination: recommendations of the American Society of Echocardiography Council for Intraoperative Echocardiography and the Society of Cardiovascular Anesthesiologists Task Force for Certification in Perioperative Transesophageal Echocardiography. *J Am Soc Echocardiogr.* 1999;12(10):884-900.
- Swaminathan M, Lineberger CK, McCann RL, Mathew JP. The importance of intraoperative transesophageal echocardiography in endovascular repair of thoracic aortic aneurysms. *Anesth Analg.* 2003;97(6):1566-1572.
- Vegas A, Meineri M. Core review: three-dimensional transesophageal echocardiography is a major advance for intraoperative clinical management of patients undergoing cardiac surgery: a core review. *Anesth Analg.* 2010;110(6):1548-1573.

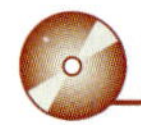

REFERENCES

Complete references available on DVD and online version at www.LongneckerAnesthesiology.com

CHAPTER 32 Monitoring Respiratory Function

Dean R. Hess
Robert M. Kacmarek

KEY POINTS

1. Arterial blood gases are used to assess oxygenation, ventilation, and acid–base balance.
2. The right-to-left shunt fraction is the gold standard index of oxygenation efficiency in the lungs.
3. Dead space is that portion of the minute ventilation that does not participate in gas exchange.
4. Acid–base balance is explained by the Henderson-Hasselbalch equation or the strong ion difference.
5. Whereas arterial blood gases primarily reflect lung function, venous blood gases reflect the adequacy of tissue oxygenation and tissue carbon dioxide clearance.
6. Pulse oximeters pass 2 or more wavelengths of light through a pulsating vascular bed to measure arterial oxygen saturation, carboxyhemoglobin, and methemoglobin.
7. The role of monitoring cerebral oxygenation in patients with traumatic brain injury is unclear.
8. Capnometry is the measurement of CO_2 at the airway opening during the ventilatory cycle.

9. The use of capnometry to monitor procedural sedation is controversial.
10. Current standards recommend the use of capnography to assess the quality of cardiopulmonary resuscitation.
11. Transcutaneous Po_2 is measured with a Clark electrode and transcutaneous Pco_2 is measured using a Severinghaus electrode.
12. Pulmonary mechanics is the expression of lung function through measurements of pressure and flow; from these measurements, a variety of derived indices can be determined, such as volume, compliance, resistance, and work of breathing.

Monitoring is the continuous, or nearly continuous, evaluation of the physiologic function of a patient in real time to guide diagnosis and management decisions, including when to make therapeutic interventions and assessment of those interventions.[1] Many physiologic parameters can be monitored during mechanical ventilation, including both invasive and noninvasive monitoring. Respiratory monitoring is an integral part of the care of mechanically ventilated patients in operating rooms and intensive care units (ICUs). Arterial blood gases are also commonly used to assess respiratory function. This chapter reviews the use of blood gases and monitors for assessment of respiratory function.

ARTERIAL BLOOD GASES

Arterial blood gases refers to measurements of Pco_2 and Po_2. The measurement of pH is also included with blood gases. Measured hemoglobin saturation with oxygen (O_2Hgb), carboxyhemoglobin (COHb), and methemoglobin (metHb) may be included. Many laboratories also report calculated values of oxygen saturation, bicarbonate concentration, and base excess. These measurements assess oxygenation, ventilation, and acid–base status.

OXYGENATION

Hypoxemia results from decreased delivery of oxygen from the atmosphere to the arterial blood, and *hypoxia* refers to decreased delivery of oxygen to the tissues (**Table 32-1**). Oxygen content is a combination of dissolved oxygen and that bound to hemoglobin. The amount dissolved in plasma is small and directly related to Po_2. The normal range of arterial Po_2 (Pao_2) is 80 to 100 mm Hg in healthy young adults breathing air at sea level. Pao_2 normally decreases with increasing age and increasing altitude. Hypoxemia occurs when the lungs fail to adequately oxygenate arterial blood. Pao_2 is often a reflection of lung function and not of hypoxia per se. Hypoxia can occur without hypoxemia and vice versa. Adequate Pao_2 in acutely ill patients is unknown, but most clinicians agree that Pao_2 above 60 mm Hg usually is acceptable.

TABLE 32-1 Causes of Hypoxemia and Hypoxia

Hypoxemia
- Decreased inspired oxygen: altitude
- Hypoventilation: respiratory center depression, neuromuscular disease, respiratory failure
- Shunt: pulmonary (eg, atelectasis, pneumonia, pulmonary edema, acute respiratory distress syndrome) or cardiac (patent foramen ovale)
- $\dot{V}/\dot{Q}$ mismatch: airway secretions, bronchospasm
- Diffusion defect: pulmonary fibrosis, emphysema, pulmonary resection

Hypoxia
- Hypoxemic hypoxia: lower than normal Pao_2 (hypoxemia)
- Anemic hypoxia: decreased red blood cell count, carboxyhemoglobin, methemoglobin, hemoglobinopathy
- Circulatory hypoxia: decreased cardiac output, decreased local perfusion
- Affinity hypoxia: decreased release of oxygen from hemoglobin to the tissues
- Histotoxic hypoxia: cyanide poisoning

Pao_2, partial pressure of oxygen in arterial blood; $\dot{V}/\dot{Q}$, ventilation/perfusion.

ALVEOLAR GAS EQUATION

The alveolar Po_2 (P_{AO_2}) is calculated from the alveolar gas equation:

$$P_{AO_2} = (F_{IO_2} \times EBP) - (Paco_2 \times [F_{IO_2} + (1 - F_{IO_2})/R]) \qquad (32\text{-}1)$$

where F_{IO_2} = fraction of inspired oxygen, EBP = effective barometric pressure (barometric pressure minus water vapor pressure), and R = respiratory quotient. For calculation of Pao_2, R = 0.8 is commonly chosen. For F_{IO_2} 0.6 or greater, the effect of R on the alveolar gas equation becomes the following:

$$P_{AO_2} = (F_{IO_2} \times EBP) - (Paco_2) \qquad (32\text{-}2)$$

For F_{IO_2} <0.6, the alveolar gas equation becomes the following:

$$P_{AO_2} = (F_{IO_2} \times EBP) - (1.2 \times Paco_2) \qquad (32\text{-}3)$$

An increased difference between P_{AO_2} and Pao_2, the $P(A\text{-}a)O_2$ gradient, can be caused by shunt, $\dot{V}/\dot{Q}$ mismatch, or a diffusion defect. $P(A\text{-}a)O_2$ normally is 10 mm Hg or below breathing air and 50 mm Hg or below breathing 100% oxygen. The ratio of Pao_2 to P_{AO_2} (PaO_2/P_{AO_2}) also can be calculated as an index of lung function and normally is greater than 0.75 at any F_{IO_2}. Pao_2/F_{IO_2} is the easiest of the indices of oxygenation to calculate. The acute respiratory distress syndrome (ARDS) is associated with Pao_2/F_{IO_2} less than 200, and acute lung injury (ALI) is associated with Pao_2/F_{IO_2} less than 300.

The oxygenation index (OI) is calculated from F_{IO_2}, mean airway pressure ($\overline{P}aw$), and Pao_2:

$$OI = (F_{IO_2} \times \overline{P}aw \times 100)/Pao_2 \qquad (32\text{-}4)$$

OI is commonly calculated for neonates but is seldom used in the care of adults. In neonates, OI above 40 with maximal therapy is often used as a criterion for severe hypoxemia requiring extracorporeal life support.

OXYHEMOGLOBIN DISSOCIATION CURVE

The oxygen saturation of hemoglobin is determined by the oxyhemoglobin dissociation curve (**Fig. 32-1**), where oxygen saturation is a function of Po_2. The affinity of hemoglobin for oxygen is high at high saturations and less at lower saturations. This effect facilitates oxygen loading in the lungs (where Po_2 is high) and oxygen unloading to the tissues (where Po_2 is low). The position of the oxyhemoglobin dissociation curve is not fixed. Factors that shift the curve to the left increase the affinity of hemoglobin for oxygen, and factors that shift the curve to the right decrease the affinity of hemoglobin for oxygen. The oxygen saturation of hemoglobin is also altered by conditions such as COHb and metHb. Carbon monoxide attaches to the oxygen binding sites of hemoglobin with a high affinity and decreases the ability of hemoglobin to carry oxygen. Thus, the hemoglobin oxygen saturation cannot be above 70% if the COHgb level is 30%. Methemoglobin is produced when the iron in the hemoglobin molecule is converted from its common reduced state (Fe^{++}) to its oxidized state (Fe^{+++}). Hemoglobin can carry oxygen only if the iron is in the reduced state. Thus, metHb decreases the ability of hemoglobin to transport oxygen.

SHUNT

The right-to-left shunt fraction is the gold standard index of oxygenation efficiency in the lungs. It is calculated from the shunt equation:

$$Q_S/Q_T = (C\bar{c}o_2 - Cao_2)/(C\bar{c}o_2 - C\bar{v}o_2) \qquad (32\text{-}5)$$

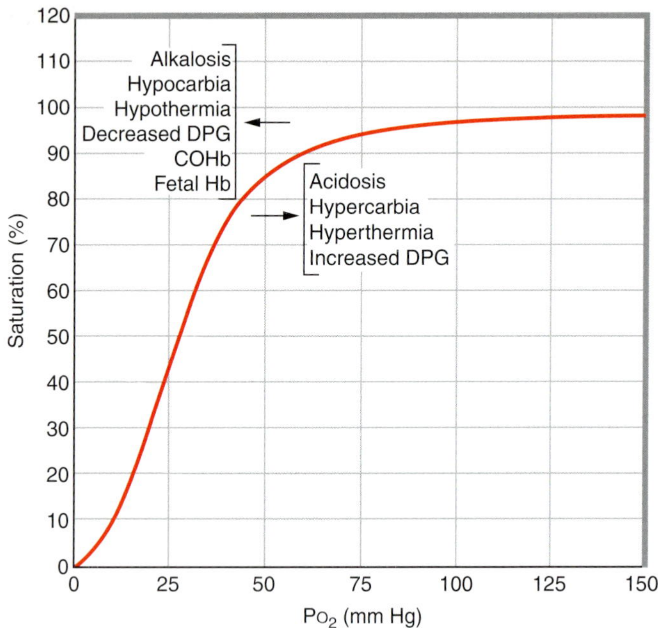

FIGURE 32-1. Oxyhemoglobin dissociation curve. Physiologic conditions that shift the curve to the left and to the right are indicated. Note that a shift to the left increases oxygen saturation for a given Po_2 (increased affinity), and a shift to the right decreases oxygen saturation for a given Po_2 (decreased affinity).

where $C\bar{c}o_2$ = pulmonary capillary oxygen content (mL/dL), Cao_2 = arterial oxygen content, and $C\bar{v}O_2$ = mixed venous oxygen content. Oxygen content is calculated as follows:

$$Co_2 = (1.34 \times Hgb \times HgbO_2) + (0.003 \times Po_2) \qquad (32\text{-}6)$$

To calculate $C\bar{v}O_2$, the pulmonary capillary Po_2 is assumed to equal the alveolar Po_2, and the pulmonary capillary hemoglobin oxygen saturation is assumed to be 100%. If measured when the patient is breathing 100% oxygen, Q_S/Q_T represents shunt (ie, blood that flows from the right heart to the left heart without passing gas-exchanging alveoli). If measured at $F{\small IO}_2$ less than 1.0, then Q_S/Q_T represents both shunt fraction and $\dot{V}/\dot{Q}$ mismatch. Whereas a shunt greater than 50% represents severe respiratory failure, 5% approximates the normal value.

VENTILATION

Arterial Pco_2 ($Paco_2$) reflects the balance between carbon dioxide production $\dot{V}co_2$ and alveolar ventilation ($\dot{V}_A$):

$$Paco_2 = \dot{V}co_2/\dot{V}_A \qquad (32\text{-}7)$$

Thus, $Paco_2$ varies directly with carbon dioxide production and inversely with alveolar ventilation. Note that $Paco_2$ is determined by alveolar ventilation and not total minute ventilation per se. Minute ventilation affects $Paco_2$ only to the extent that it affects alveolar ventilation. Clinical causes of hypoventilation (increased $Paco_2$) and hyperventilation (decreased $Paco_2$) are listed in **Table 32-2**. Because alveolar ventilation is determined by minute ventilation ($\dot{V}_E$) and the ratio of dead space to total ventilation (V_D/V_T), the relationship can be derived as follows:

$$Paco_2 = \dot{V}co_2/[\dot{V}_E \times (1 - V_D/V_T])] \qquad (32\text{-}8)$$

$Paco_2$ increases with an increase in V_D/V_T, an increase in $\dot{V}co_2$, and a decrease in $\dot{V}_E$ (**Fig. 32-2**). Although a goal of mechanical ventilation traditionally has been to normalize $Paco_2$, at times an elevated $Paco_2$ (permissive hypercapnia) may be more desirable than the high alveolar pressure required to normalize $Paco_2$ in patients with acute respiratory failure.

TABLE 32-2 Clinical Causes of Hypoventilation and Hyperventilation

Hypoventilation
- Respiratory center depression: pathologic, iatrogenic
- Disruption of neural pathways affecting respiratory muscles: neuropathy, trauma
- Neuromuscular blockade: disease, paralyzing agents
- Respiratory muscle weakness: fatigue, disease

Hyperventilation
- Respiratory center stimulation: hypoxia, anxiety, central nervous system pathology
- Metabolic acidosis
- Iatrogenic: mechanical ventilation

DEAD SPACE VENTILATION

Dead space is that portion of the minute ventilation that does not participate in gas exchange.[2-4] It consists of anatomic dead space and alveolar dead space. Dead space is calculated using the Bohr equation:

$$V_D/V_T = (Paco_2 - P\bar{E}co_2)/Paco_2 \qquad (32\text{-}9)$$

where V_D/V_T = fraction of total ventilation that is dead space, and $P\bar{E}co_2$ is the partial pressure of CO_2 in mixed exhaled gas. The normal value of V_D/V_T ranges from 0.2 to 0.4. Causes of an increased V_D/V_T include pulmonary embolism, positive-pressure ventilation, pulmonary hypoperfusion, and high-rate, low-tidal-volume ventilation. Increased V_D/V_T has been associated with a high mortality rate in patients with ARDS in a dose-response manner.[5-9] Increased V_D/V_T also has been associated with a lower rate of weaning from mechanical ventilation.[10]

The traditional method for determining $P\bar{E}co_2$ was to collect mixed exhaled gas in a large bag for 5 to 15 minutes. During the gas collection, the patient is undisturbed, with a stable $\dot{V}_E$, and an arterial blood sample is obtained to assess $Paco_2$ during this time. Many current-generation mechanical ventilators have a constant bias gas flow through the circuit, which complicates the collection of mixed exhaled gas to calculate V_D/V_T. In this case, $P\bar{E}co_2$ can be calculated from $\dot{V}co_2$ and $\dot{V}_E$:

$$P\bar{E}co_2 = (\dot{V}co_2/\dot{V}_E) \times P_B \qquad (32\text{-}10)$$

Because dead space determinations require a leak-free system, they cannot be measured in patients with a bronchopleural fistula or with

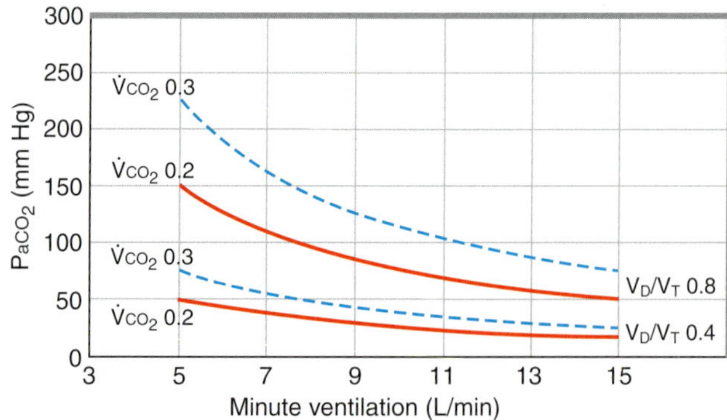

FIGURE 32-2. Relationship between $Paco_2$, minute ventilation, V_D/V_T, and $\dot{V}co_2$. $Paco_2$, partial pressure of oxygen in arterial blood; V_D/V_T, dead space to tidal volume ratio; $\dot{V}co_2$, carbon dioxide production.

TABLE 32-3 Clinical Causes of Metabolic Acidosis and Metabolic Alkalosis

Metabolic acidosis
- Lactic acidosis (eg, hypoxia)
- Ketoacidosis (eg, uncontrolled diabetes)
- Uremic acidosis (eg, renal failure)
- Loss of base from the lower gastrointestinal tract (eg, diarrhea)
- Loss of base from the kidneys (eg, acetazolamide, renal tubular acidosis)
- Poisons (eg, methanol, ethylene glycol, aspirin)

Metabolic alkalosis
- Hypokalemia
- Loss of acid from upper gastrointestinal tract (eg, vomiting, gastric suction)
- Bicarbonate administration

a leaking uncuffed tracheostomy tube. From the exhaled CO_2, $\dot{V}_E$, and barometric pressure (P_B), $\dot{V}_A$ can be calculated as follows:

$$\dot{V}_A = \dot{V}_E \times P\bar{E}CO_2/P_B \quad (32\text{-}11)$$

$\dot{V}_A$ also can be calculated from V_D/V_T as follows:

$$\dot{V}_A = \dot{V}_E - (\dot{V}_E \times V_D/V_T) \quad (32\text{-}12)$$

ACID–BASE BALANCE

Acid–base balance is explained by the Henderson-Hasselbach equation:

$$pH = 6.1 + \log[HCO_3^-]/(0.03 \times PCO_2) \quad (32\text{-}13)$$

Metabolic acid–base disturbances are those that affect the numerator of the Henderson-Hasselbach equation, and respiratory acid–base disturbances are disturbances that affect the denominator. The pH is normal (7.40) whenever the ratio $[HCO_3^-]/(0.03 \times PaCO_2)$ is 20:1. The metabolic component of acid–base interpretation usually is given as $[HCO_3^-]$. The metabolic component also can be expressed as base excess (BE). BE can be estimated as BE = $[HCO_3^-]$ – 24. In other words, $[HCO_3^-]$ less than 24 mmol/L corresponds with a negative BE, and $[HCO_3^-]$ greater than 24 mmol/L corresponds with a positive BE. Clinical causes of metabolic acid–base disturbances are listed in **Table 32-3**, and the degree of compensation for acid–base disturbances is given in **Table 32-4**.

The strong ion difference (SID) is a method of evaluating acid–base disturbances based on the Stewart physiochemical approach to acid–base chemistry.[11] Using this approach, the only variables that affect pH are PCO_2, SID, and the concentration of unmeasured strong ions. The normal value for SID is 40 mmol/L and is calculated as follows:

$$SID = [HCO_3^-] + 0.28 \times [\text{Albumin (g/L)} + \text{Inorganic phosphate (mmol/L)}] \quad (32\text{-}14)$$

Metabolic acidosis is associated with a decreased SID, and metabolic alkalosis is associated with an increased SID (**Table 32-5**).

TABLE 32-4 Expected Compensation for Acid–Base Disturbances[a]

Respiratory acidosis	$\Delta HCO_3^- = 0.10 \times \Delta PaCO_2$ (acute) $\Delta HCO_3^- = 0.35 \times \Delta PaCO_2$ (chronic)
Respiratory alkalosis	$\Delta HCO_3^- = 0.2 \times \Delta PaCO_2$ (acute) $\Delta HCO_3^- = 0.5 \times \Delta PaCO_2$ (chronic)
Metabolic acidosis	$PaCO_2 = 1.5 \times HCO_3^- + 8$
Metabolic alkalosis	$PaCO_2 = 0.9 \times HCO_3^- + 15$

$PaCO_2$, partial pressure of carbon dioxide in arterial blood.

[a]If the acid–base status exceeds the expected level of compensation, a mixed acid–base disturbance is present.

TABLE 32-5 Classification of Acid–Base Disturbances Using the Steward Approach

	Acidosis	Alkalosis
Respiratory	↑$PaCO_2$	↓$PaCO_2$
Metabolic		
Water excess or deficit	↓SID, ↓Na^+	↑SID, ↑Na^+
Chloride excess or deficit	↓SID, ↑Cl^-	↑SID, ↓Cl^-
Unmeasured strong ion excess	↓SID, ↑ unmeasured ions	

PCO_2, partial pressure of oxygen in arterial blood; SID, strong ion difference.

The anion gap is useful to differentiate causes of metabolic acidosis. Metabolic acidosis can be associated with a normal anion gap (hyperchloremic acidosis) or with an increased anion gap (normochloremic acidosis). The anion gap is calculated as follows:

$$\text{Anion gap} = [Na^+] - ([Cl^-] + [HCO_3^-]) \quad (32\text{-}15)$$

A normal anion gap is 8 to 12 mmol/L. Causes of metabolic acidosis with an increased anion gap include lactic acidosis, diabetic ketoacidosis, and azotemic (renal) acidosis. Causes of metabolic acidosis with a normal anion gap include loss of bicarbonate from the gastrointestinal tract (eg, diarrhea), acetazolamide (Diamox) therapy, and excessive chloride administration (eg, HCl, NH_4Cl). The osmolality (osmol gap) is the difference between the measured osmolality of the plasma and that is calculated as follows:

$$\text{Osmolality} = 2[Na^+] + [\text{Glucose}]/18 + [\text{Bun}]/2.8 + [\text{Ethanol}]/4.6 \quad (32\text{-}16)$$

where BUN = blood urea nitrogen. If the measured osmolality is greater than 10 mOsm/L above the calculated value (osmol gap >10 mOsm/L), osmotically active particles whose metabolites may be organic acid may present. Metabolic acidosis with an osmol gap is consistent with the presence of the toxins methanol, ethanol, and ethylene glycol.

TEMPERATURE ADJUSTMENT OF BLOOD GASES

Blood gases and pH are measured in the laboratory at 37°C. If the patient's temperature is abnormal, the in vivo blood gas and pH values differ from those measured and reported by the blood gas laboratory. Using empiric equations, the blood gas analyzer can adjust the measured values to the patient's body temperature. Two ventilation strategies for hypothermic acid–base management have been suggested (usually during cardiopulmonary bypass).[12-17] During α-stat management, $PaCO_2$ is maintained at 40 mm Hg when measured at 37°C. Thus, whereas the dissociation fraction of the imidazole moiety of histidine is constant, pH changes parallel to the neutral pH point of water. During pH-stat management, $PaCO_2$ is corrected to the patient's actual body temperature. Because of increased gas solubility during hypothermia, the α-stat strategy results in relative hyperventilation. This issue is becoming increasingly important with the use of induced hypothermia after cardiac arrest and in the treatment of focal cerebral ischemia. Animal studies suggest that pH-stat management, compared with α-stat management, results in improved cerebral blood flow and neurologic outcomes. The pH-stat approach allows differentiation of temperature-related changes from physiologic changes. Temperature-adjusted values should be used to compare blood gas levels with exhaled gas values (eg, end-tidal PCO_2 [$P_{ET}CO_2$]) and to calculate oxygen content indices (eg, right-to-left shunt) or tension indices [eg, $P(A\text{-}a)O_2$].

POINT-OF-CARE MEASUREMENT OF BLOOD GASES

Point-of-care blood gas monitoring is performed near the site of patient care (eg, operating room, ICU). Point-of-care analyzers are available to measure blood gases and pH. These analyzers also can make other important useful measurements at the bedside, including levels of electrolytes, glucose, lactate, urea nitrogen, and hematocrit, and clotting studies (activated clotting time, prothrombin time, and partial thromboplastin time). Point-of-care analyzers are small and portable (some are handheld), they require minute blood volumes (several drops), and they provide rapid reporting of results (a few minutes). They are relatively easy to use (eg, self-calibrating) and typically incorporate a disposable cartridge that contains the appropriate biosensors. The cost–benefit of these devices is unclear. Furthermore, appropriate documentation for compliance with hospital standards is necessary. This requires appropriate quality control checks and instrument maintenance.

VENOUS BLOOD GASES

Whereas arterial blood gases primarily reflect lung function, venous blood gases reflect the adequacy of tissue oxygenation and tissue carbon dioxide clearance. A low mixed venous Po_2 ($P\bar{v}o_2$) level (<35 mm Hg) reflects tissue hypoxia and may be the result of decreased oxygen delivery or increased tissue oxygen uptake. $P\bar{v}o_2$ typically is much lower than Pao_2, and there is often little relationship between the two. For example, the $P\bar{v}o_2$ may be low and the Pao_2 may be high when cardiac output is reduced, lung function is normal, and Fio_2 is high. Normally, the mixed venous Pco_2 $P\bar{v}co_2$ is only slightly greater than the $Paco_2$. However, the $P\bar{v}co_2$ depends on blood flow (cardiac output), and in cases of low blood flow (eg, cardiac arrest), the $P\bar{v}co_2$ may be high despite a normal or decreased $Paco_2$. When venous blood gases are used to assess acid–base balance, mixed venous or central venous blood samples are preferable to peripheral venous samples. Interest in central venous oxygen saturation has increased with the use of goal-directed treatment of sepsis, in which $S\bar{v}o_2$ greater than 70% was reported to be associated with a survival benefit.[18]

PULSE OXIMETRY

Pulse oximetry, a technology unavailable until the mid-1980s, is now in widespread use. Continuous pulse oximetry is the standard of care in the operating room and for treatment of critically ill patients. A probe passes 2 wavelengths of light (660 and 940 nm) through a pulsating vascular bed. Although most pulse oximeters commonly use transmission oximetry (ie, the light emitted from the light-emitting diodes [LEDs] is transmitted through the tissue and a photodetector is opposite the LEDs), other designs use reflectance oximetry (ie, the light from the LEDs is reflected from the tissue, and the photodetector is on the same side of the tissue as the LEDs). The pulse oximeter probe can be placed on a number of sites, including the finger, toe, earlobe, nose, and forehead. In infants, the probe can be placed on the hand or foot (**Fig. 32-3**).

A number of limitations of pulse oximetry should be recognized, appreciated, and understood by everyone who uses pulse oximetry data.

- *Accuracy*: Most pulse oximeter errors can be explained by too little signal (eg, low tissue perfusion levels, improper probe placement) or too much noise (eg, motion, high levels of ambient light). Pulse oximeters use empirical calibration curves developed from studies of healthy volunteers. At saturations above 80%, the accuracy of pulse oximetry is approximately ±4% to 5%. Below 80%, their accuracy is far worse, but the clinical importance of this is questionable. To appreciate the implications of the limits of accuracy of pulse oximetry, one must consider the oxyhemoglobin dissociation curve. If the pulse oximeter displays an Spo_2 (oxygen saturation measured by pulse oximetry) of 95%, the true saturation could be as low as 90% or as high as 100%. If the true saturation is 90%, the Pao_2 will be approximately 60 mm Hg. If the true saturation is 100%, however, one does not know how high the Pao_2 might be. Also, a shift of the oxyhemoglobin dissociation curve can change the Spo_2, although no change in Pao_2 has occurred.
- *Misunderstanding by those who use pulse oximetry:* It has been reported that many clinicians lacked knowledge and made serious errors in the interpretation of Spo_2.[19-21]
- *Differences between devices and probes:* The pulse oximeter is unique in that it requires no user calibration. However, manufacturer-derived calibration curves programmed into the software vary from manufacturer to manufacturer and can vary among pulse oximeters from a given manufacturer. Moreover, the output of the LEDs can vary from probe to probe.
- *Penumbra effect:* If the finger pulse oximeter probe does not fit correctly, light can be shunted from the LEDs directly to the photodetector. This will cause a falsely low Spo_2 if Sao_2 is greater than 85% and a falsely elevated Spo_2 if Sao_2 is less than 85%.
- *Dyshemoglobinemias:* Because traditionally available pulse oximeters use only 2 wavelengths of light, they are only able to evaluate oxyhemoglobin (O_2Hb) and deoxyhemoglobin (Hb). Abnormal elevations of COHb[22] and metHb[23] both result in significant inaccuracy in pulse oximetry, and pulse oximetry should not be used when elevated levels of these abnormal hemoglobins are present. Fetal hemoglobin[24] and sickle cell anemia[25] do not affect the accuracy of pulse oximetry.
- *Endogenous and exogenous dyes and pigments:* Intravascular dye administration can affect the accuracy of pulse oximetry, with methylene blue having the greatest effect.[26] Nail polish also can affect the accuracy of pulse oximetry.[27] Although this has recently been challenged,[28] nail polish should be removed before pulse oximetry is begun. Hyperbilirubinemia does not appear to affect the accuracy of pulse oximetry.[29]

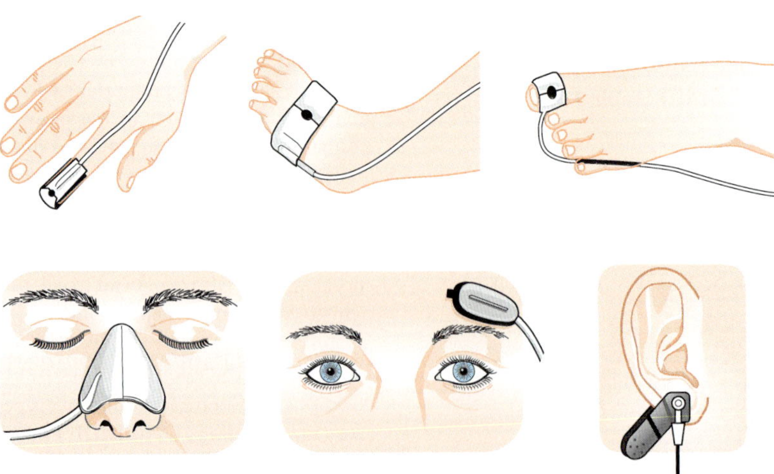

FIGURE 32-3. Examples of pulse oximetry probes. [Adapted from materials provided by Nellcor (Covidien, Mansfield, MA)].

- *Skin pigmentation:* Several studies have found that the accuracy and performance of pulse oximeters are affected by deeply pigmented skin.[30-32]
- *Perfusion:* Pulse oximeters require a pulsating vascular bed to function correctly. Under conditions of low flow (eg, cardiac arrest or severe peripheral vasoconstriction), pulse oximetry becomes unreliable. Under these conditions, an ear probe may be more reliable than a finger probe.
- *Anemia:* Although pulse oximeters are generally reliable over a wide range of hemoglobin levels, they become less accurate and reliable with conditions of severe anemia (hematocrit <24 g/dL at low saturations and hematocrit <10% at all saturations).[33]
- *Motion:* Motion of the probe can produce considerable artifact and unreliable and inaccurate pulse oximetry readings. This problem can sometimes be corrected by using a more stable probe site (eg, the ear or toe rather than the finger).
- *High-intensity ambient light:* Because the photodetector of the pulse oximeter is nonspecific, high-intensity ambient light can produce interference. This problem can be corrected by wrapping the probe with a light barrier.
- *Abnormal pulses:* Venous pulses and a large dicrotic notch may affect the accuracy of pulse oximetry.
- *Safety:* Pulse oximetry is generally considered safe. However, burns as the result of defective probes and pressure necrosis can rarely occur.

Jubran and Tobin[32] evaluated the use of pulse oximetry in titrating supplemental oxygen in 54 critically ill ventilator-dependent patients (**Fig. 32-4**). In white patients, they found that an Spo_2 of 92% was reliable

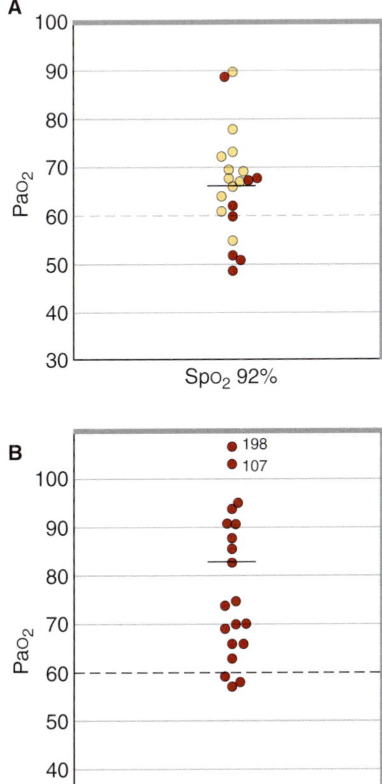

FIGURE 32-4. Top. In white patients (*yellow circles*), Spo_2 of 92% or greater is reliable in predicting Pao_2 of 60 mm Hg or greater. **Bottom.** In black patients (red circles), Spo_2 of 95% or greater was required to reliably predict Pao_2 of 60 mm Hg or greater. Pao_2, partial pressure of oxygen in arterial blood; Spo_2, oxygen saturation measured by pulse oximetry.

in predicting Pao_2 60 mm Hg or greater. In black patients, however, a Spo_2 of 95% was required. Although this method is useful for titrating a level of arterial oxygenation that does not produce hypoxemia, it does not eliminate the need for periodic arterial blood gas measurements. When pulse oximetry is used to titrate the Fio_2, the final Fio_2 setting should be confirmed by an arterial blood gas measurement.

If pulse oximetry is to be clinically useful, it must have a low failure rate. Intraoperative pulse oximeter failure was evaluated by Freund et al.[34] Overall, they found a failure rate below 5%. Pulse oximetry failures tended to be greater in older patients, sicker patients, and during longer surgical procedures. Failure of pulse oximetry in other settings has not been reported. Perhaps the most frequent cause of pulse oximetry failure in ICUs is accidental disconnection or misplacement of the probe.

Motion artifact and low perfusion are common causes of pulse oximetry errors.[35-42] Manufacturers of pulse oximeters have developed improved software algorithms to calculate Spo_2 in an attempt to eliminate motion artifacts from the pulse signal. Three such devices on the market are the FAST (Fourier Artifact-Suppression Technology, Philips Medical Systems, Andover, MA), SET (Signal-Extraction Technology, Masimo, Irvine, CA), and Oxismart N-3000 (Nellcor, Pleasanton, CA). A comprehensive review concluded that the clinical performance of all of the new-generation pulse oximeters was better than that of earlier devices.[36] Although several studies have evaluated the performance of these new designs,[38-42] there was no strong and convincing evidence that the performance of any single new-generation device was superior to that of any other new-generation device.

New pulse oximetry technology (Masimo Rainbow Technology, Massimo Corp, Irvine, CA) uses 8 wavelengths of light to measure Spco (oximetric estimate of COHb), SpMet (oximetric estimate of metHb), and SpHb (oximetric estimate of hemoglobin concentration).[43] Acceptable accuracy has been reported for these devices, but this requires further confirmation.[44-46] However, because it uses conventional 2-wavelength red and infrared signals to determine Spo_2, when there are significant levels of either COHb or MetHb, the Spo_2 will be subject to the same errors described previously. Another limitation is the crosstalk between the metHb and COHb measurement channels. In the presence of significant metHb levels, the device will display a falsely elevated Spco but a correct SpMet. If this occurs, the device displays an error message indicating that the Spco may not be accurate.

Although it allows early detection of hypoxemia and related events, the impact of pulse oximetry on patient outcomes is unclear.[47] A large study (>20,000 patients) of pulse oximetry use during anesthesia and postanesthesia care found no difference in outcome.[48,49] Pulse oximetry is indicated in unstable patients likely to desaturate, in patients receiving a therapeutic intervention that is likely to produce hypoxemia (eg, bronchoscopy), and in patients having interventions likely to produce changes in arterial oxygenation (ie, changes in Fio_2 or positive end-expiratory pressure [PEEP]).

There may be important non-oxygenation monitoring applications for pulse oximetry. For example, Hartert et al[50] reported the effect of pulsus paradoxus, and therefore the severity of air trapping in obstructive airway disease, on the pulse oximetry plethysmographic (POP) waveform (**Fig. 32-5**). They reported that in patients with obstructive lung disease and elevated pulsus paradoxus, an altered pulse oximetry baseline tracing manifested as the respiratory waveform variation. Pulsus paradoxus was significantly correlated with the degree of respiratory waveform variation of the pulse oximetry tracing and the amount of auto-PEEP.

Respiratory variations in POP waveform amplitude has been shown to be useful in predicting fluid responsiveness. POP waveform amplitude is measured on a beat-to-beat basis as the vertical distance between peak and preceding valley trough in the waveform (**Fig. 32-6**). Maximal POP (POP_{max}) and minimal POP (POP_{min}) are determined over the same respiratory cycle. ΔPOP is calculated using the following formula:

$$\Delta POP(\%) = 100 \times ([POP_{max} - POP_{min}]/[POP_{max} + POP_{min})/2]) \quad (32\text{-}17)$$

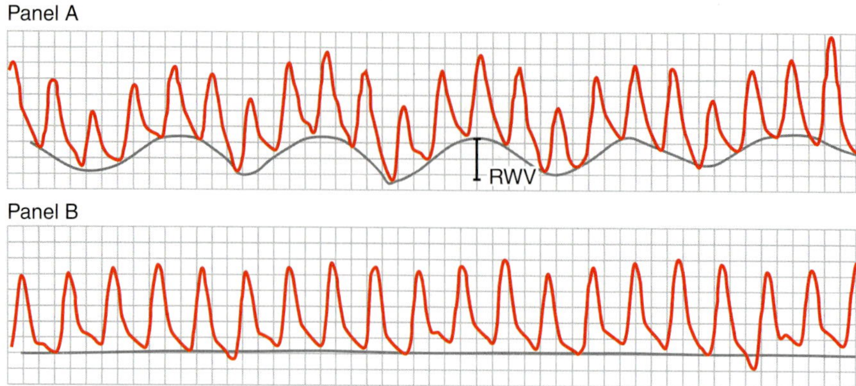

FIGURE 32-5. Pulse oximeter tracings from a 60-year-old woman with exacerbation of chronic obstructive pulmonary disease who was admitted to the intensive care unit in ventilatory failure. **A.** The patient's pulse oximetry tracing at the time of admission reveals respiratory variability in the pulse oximeter plethysmography tracing. Measured pulsus paradoxus at this time was 16 mm Hg. **B.** The patient's pulse oximetry tracing after 12 hours of aggressive therapy. Pulsus paradoxus at this time was 8 mm Hg. Note the absence of respiratory waveform variation (RWV) in the baseline of the oximeter tracing after clinical improvement in airflow and resolution of elevated pulsus paradoxus. [Reproduced from Hartert TV, Wheeler AP, Sheller JR. Use of pulse oximetry to recognize severity of airflow obstruction in obstructive airway disease: correlation with pulsus paradoxus. *Chest.* 1999;115:475-481, with permission.]

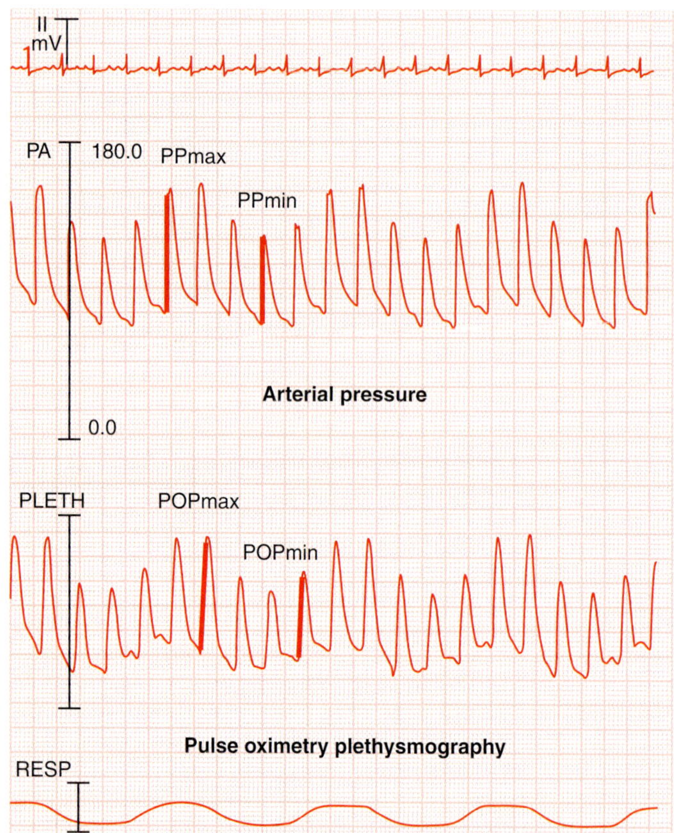

FIGURE 32-6. Comparison between invasive arterial pressure and pulse oximeter plethysmography recordings. Simultaneous recording of electrocardiographic lead (II), systemic arterial pressure (PA), pulse oximetry plethysmography (PLETH), and respiratory signal (RESP) in one illustrative patient. POP, pulse oximetry plethysmographic; PP, pulse pressure. [From Cannesson M, Besnard C, Durand PG, et al. Relation between respiratory variations in pulse oximetry plethysmographic waveform amplitude and arterial pulse pressure in ventilated patients. *Crit Care.* 2005;9:R562-R568.]

The results of one study suggest that ΔPOP greater than 15% is predictive of fluid responsiveness in mechanically ventilated patients with circulatory failure.[51]

Some pulse oximeters display the plethysmogram variability index (PVI) as a reflection of POP. Perfusion index (PI) is the ratio of the pulsatile blood flow to the nonpulsatile blood in peripheral tissue. PVI is a measure of the dynamic changes in the PI that occur during the respiratory cycle:

$$PVI\ (\%) = (PI_{Max} - PI_{Min})/PI_{Max} \tag{32-18}$$

The lower the PVI, the less variability there is in the PI over a respiratory cycle.

CEREBRAL OXYGENATION

Monitoring of cerebral perfusion pressure (difference between mean arterial pressure and intracranial pressure [ICP]) is standard practice in the medical treatment of patients with traumatic brain injury.[52] More recently, monitoring of cerebral oxygenation has become possible either by jugular oximetry (Sjo_2) or measurement of brain tissue oxygen pressure via a parenchymal probe. Whereas jugular oximetry provides a more global estimate of oxygen extraction by the brain, brain tissue oxygen monitoring represents a local measurement of Po_2 (Pbo_2) in a relatively small volume of tissue. Sjo_2 is dependent predominantly on arterial oxygen saturation, cerebral blood flow, and cerebral oxygen uptake. The normal range for Sjo_2 is 50% to 75%. The Licox brain tissue oxygen system is a triple-lumen catheter inserted through an intracranial bolt that measures Pbo_2, brain tissue temperature, and ICP. Normal PbO_2 is 20 to 35 mm Hg. Changes in Pbo_2 reflect a shift in the balance between arterial oxygen delivery and the brain's oxygen consumption. A common threshold for altering treatment is a Pbo_2 less than 20 mm Hg.

The INVOS Cerebral Oximeter (Somanetics Corp, Troy, MI) uses near-infrared spectroscopy (NIRS) to monitor cerebral oxygenation via sensors placed on both sides of the patient's forehead.[53] It measures regional oxygen saturation (rSo_2), the cortical O_2 saturation within an area beneath the sensors, by passing infrared light through the forehead and skull into the brain. Light at specific wavelengths is transmitted through the scalp into the brain, and changes in the light attenuation at the receiving end of the reflected (or transmitted) light are converted into changes in chromophore concentration. Because light within the visible spectrum does not penetrate tissue more than approximately 1 cm, wavelengths in the near-infrared region between 650 and 900 nm are used, which allows deeper penetration. Unlike pulse oximetry, in which only the arterial component is measure, NIRS captures an average of the arterial, capillary, and venous compartments. Various assumptions are made in the calculation algorithm of cerebral oxygen saturation with NIRS, which may not always be valid, and uncertainty exists regarding whether NIRS, as claimed, mainly measures the intracranial compartment or also the extracranial compartment. Translation of NIRS systems and methods into the clinical field requires an understanding of the physiologic basis of the measured NIRS signals, and unfortunately, some uncertainly remains. Changes of rSo_2 reflect a shift in the balance between arterial oxygen delivery and the brain's oxygen consumption. rSo_2 can be measured as either an absolute level or as percent change from the patient's baseline rSo_2. Normal rSo_2 is 58 to 82 points.

Whether monitoring of cerebral oxygenation improves outcome is controversial.[52] One study suggests that the diagnostic accuracy of rSo_2 is limited, and the authors suggest that rSo_2 should not be considered as a substitute for Pbo_2 monitoring.[53] However, the role of Pbo_2 monitoring is equally unclear. A study of 629 patients reported that the mortality in patients with traumatic brain injury whose clinical management was guided by Pbo_2 monitoring was not reduced in comparison with that of patients who received ICP monitoring alone.[54]

CAPNOGRAPHY

Capnometry is the measurement of CO_2 at the airway opening during the ventilatory cycle.[55] Most capnometers measure CO_2 by infrared absorption, analyzing the absorption peak of CO_2 at 4.26 µm. Mass spectrometry and Raman spectrometry can also be used. A portable nonelectronic single-patient-use device is commonly used to produce a color change (colorimetric end-tidal CO_2 detection) in the presence of exhaled CO_2 (ie, tracheal intubation). The color changes from purple with a low CO_2 concentration to yellow with CO_2 concentration of 2.0% to 5.0%.

Capnometers can be configured as mainstream or sidestream devices. With the mainstream capnometer, the measurement chamber is placed directly at the airway. With the sidestream capnometer, gas from the airway is aspirated through fine-bore tubing to the measurement chamber inside the device. Some devices (eg, colorimetric capnometers) can only be used as mainstream devices, and other devices (eg, mass and Raman spectrometers) can only be used as sidestream devices. Infrared capnometers can be configured as either mainstream or sidestream devices. Each approach has advantages and disadvantages (**Table 32-6**). A new capnography technology, microstream, has been introduced, which uses molecular correlation spectroscopy that operates at room temperature and emits only CO_2-specific radiation.[56] It features low flow rates, reduced dead space, and lack of moisture-associated occlusion problems.

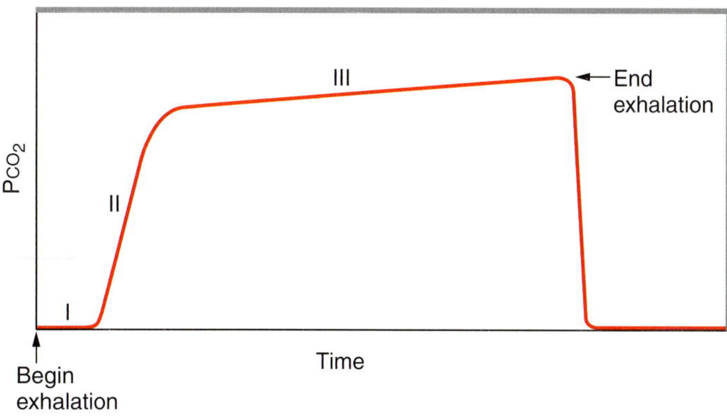

FIGURE 32-7. Time-based capnogram. I, anatomic dead space; II, transition from anatomic dead space to alveolar plateau; III, alveolar plateau.

TIME-BASED CAPNOGRAPHY

For applications in the operating room and critical care unit, the time-based capnogram is often displayed (**Fig. 32-7**). Unlike the volume-based capnogram, the time-based capnogram has an inspiratory segment and an expiratory segment. Pco_2 usually is zero during the inspiratory phase. At the beginning of exhalation, Pco_2 remains zero as gas from the anatomic dead space leaves the airway (phase I). The capnogram then increases sharply as alveolar gas mixes with dead space gas (phase II). The curve then forms an alveolar plateau during most of exhalation (phase III). Pco_2 at the end of the alveolar plateau is the $P{\small ETCO}_2$. The capnogram with airflow obstruction is characterized by an increased slope of phase III (**Fig. 32-8**). This occurs because of the $\dot{V}/\dot{Q}$ heterogeneities that result from airflow obstruction.[57] In patients with asthma with acute bronchospasm, the slope of phase III has been shown to correlate with peak expiratory flow rate, and this slope normalizes with β-agonist therapy.[58,59]

Carbon dioxide homeostasis is affected by $\dot{V}co_2$, CO_2 transport from the tissues to the lungs, and $\dot{V}_A$. Conditions that increase $\dot{V}co_2$ include fever, activity, sepsis, hyperthyroidism, trauma, burn injuries, and a high-carbohydrate diet. Conditions that decrease $\dot{V}co_2$ include hypothyroidism, hypothermia (when shivering is blocked), sedation, and paralysis. Carbon dioxide from tissue metabolism diffuses into the circulation, producing a mixed venous Pco_2 ($P\bar{v}co_2$) of approximately 45 mm Hg. The Pco_2 of an individual lung unit depends on the $\dot{V}/\dot{Q}$ (**Fig. 32-9**). Without perfusion (pure dead space; $\dot{V}/\dot{Q} = \infty$), $Paco_2$ is similar to inspired Pco_2 (ie, zero). With a normal $\dot{V}/\dot{Q}$ unit, $Paco_2$ is the same as arterial Pco_2 (ie, 40 mm Hg). With a low $\dot{V}/\dot{Q}$ unit, $Paco_2$ increases toward $P\bar{v}co_2$ (ie, 45 mm Hg). $Paco_2$, and thus $P{\small ETCO}_2$, must always remain between zero and $P\bar{v}co_2$. $P{\small ETCO}_2$ normally is several millimeters

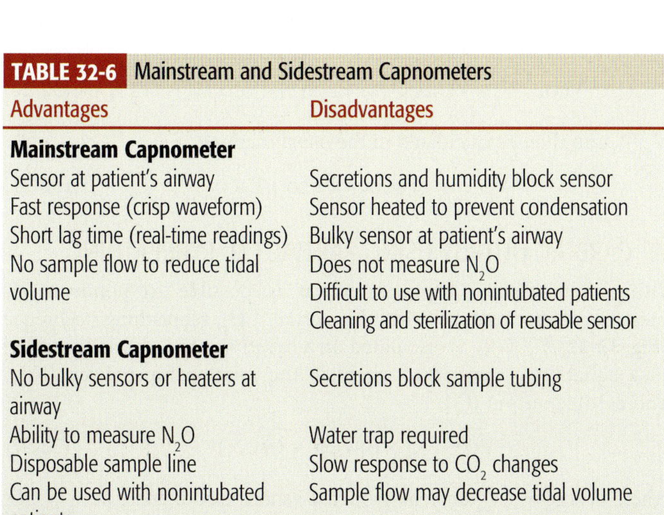

TABLE 32-6 Mainstream and Sidestream Capnometers

Advantages	Disadvantages
Mainstream Capnometer	
Sensor at patient's airway	Secretions and humidity block sensor
Fast response (crisp waveform)	Sensor heated to prevent condensation
Short lag time (real-time readings)	Bulky sensor at patient's airway
No sample flow to reduce tidal volume	Does not measure N_2O
	Difficult to use with nonintubated patients
	Cleaning and sterilization of reusable sensor
Sidestream Capnometer	
No bulky sensors or heaters at airway	Secretions block sample tubing
Ability to measure N_2O	Water trap required
Disposable sample line	Slow response to CO_2 changes
Can be used with nonintubated patients	Sample flow may decrease tidal volume

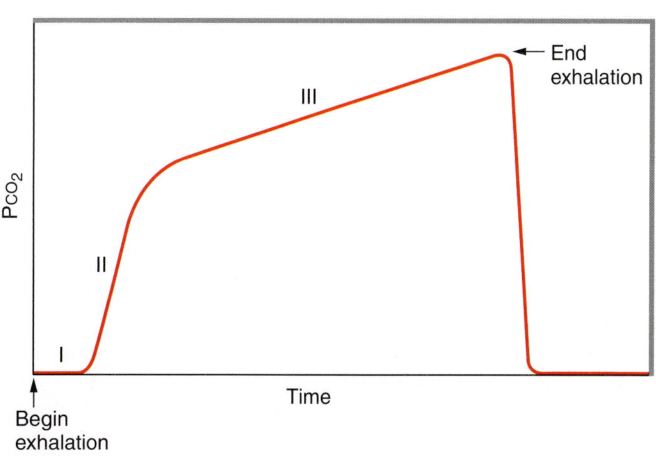

FIGURE 32-8. Capnogram produced with airflow obstruction.

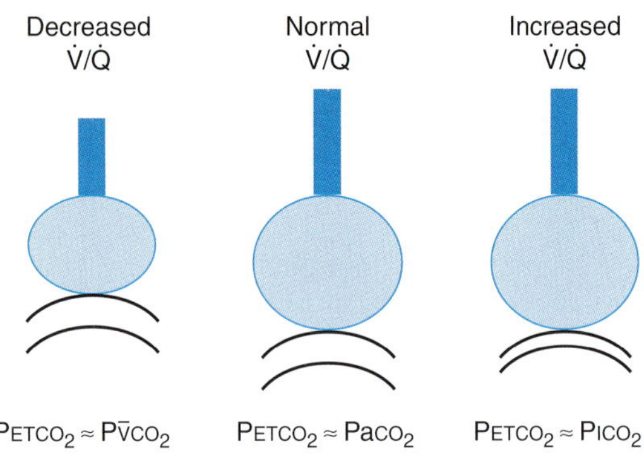

FIGURE 32-9. P_{ETCO_2} with low $\dot{V}/\dot{Q}$, normal $\dot{V}/\dot{Q}$, and high $\dot{V}/\dot{Q}$. P_{ETCO_2}, end-tidal PCO_2; $P\bar{v}CO_2$, mixed venous PCO_2; $PaCO_2$, PCO_2 in arterial blood; $PICO_2$, PCO_2 in inspired gas; $\dot{V}/\dot{Q}$, ventilation to perfusion ratio.

of mercury less than $PaCO_2$. However, the relationship between the $PaCO_2$ and P_{ETCO_2} varies depending on the relative contributions of various $\dot{V}/\dot{Q}$ units comprising the lungs.[57]

Theoretically, P_{ETCO_2} could be as low as inspired PCO_2 (zero) or as high as $P\bar{v}CO_2$ (but not higher than this value). An increased or decreased P_{ETCO_2} can result from changes in $\dot{V}CO_2$ and carbon dioxide delivery to the lungs, changes in alveolar ventilation, or equipment malfunction (**Table 32-7**). However, because of homeostasis, compensatory changes may occur so that P_{ETCO_2} does not change despite some of these changes. For example, if $\dot{V}CO_2$ increases (such as with fever) and alveolar ventilation increases proportionately (the normal homeostatic response), then P_{ETCO_2} may not change. Thus, P_{ETCO_2} is a nonspecific indicator of cardiopulmonary homeostasis and often does not indicate the presence of any specific problem or abnormality.

If $PaCO_2$ is measured, the gradient between $PaCO_2$ and P_{ETCO_2} [$P(a\text{-}ET)CO_2$] can be calculated. This gradient normally is small, usually less than 5 mm Hg. With dead space–producing disease (high $\dot{V}/\dot{Q}$), P_{ETCO_2} may be considerably less than $PaCO_2$ (**Table 32-8**).[60-65] Although right-to-left blood shunting may result in a large gradient between PaO_2 and PaO_2, it will have only a small effect on $P(a\text{-}ET)CO_2$. On occasion, P_{ETCO_2} may be greater than $PaCO_2$. The reason for P_{ETCO_2} greater than $PaCO_2$ is not well understood and may be related to low (but finite) $\dot{V}/\dot{Q}$ regions within the lung that empty at end-exhalation. $P(a\text{-}ET)CO_2$ may decrease when measured at maximal exhalation in patients with airway obstruction.[66]

Perioperative measurement of P_{ETCO_2} is a standard of care to determine proper endotracheal tube position.[67-73] Lack of exhaled CO_2 is consistent with an esophageal intubation. Capnography has also been reported useful for verifying feeding tube placement.[74,75] In the case of tracheal placement of the feeding tube, CO_2 is detected in the gas aspirated from the feeding tube. P_{ETCO_2} may also be useful for assessing the adequacy of cardiopulmonary resuscitation (CPR). The onset of cardiac arrest results in a decrease of P_{ETCO_2} to zero. With the initiation of CPR, P_{ETCO_2} increases and has been reported to increase immediately with return of spontaneous circulation.[76-79] Capnography during CPR is recommended in the guidelines of the American Heart Association; a low P_{ETCO_2} should prompt assessment of the quality of CPR. In one study, patients successfully resuscitated after cardiac arrest had a P_{ETCO_2} of 15 ± 4 mm Hg during CPR, but patients who could not be resuscitated had a P_{ETCO_2} of only 7 ± 5 mm Hg.[80,81]

TABLE 32-7 Causes of Increased and Decreased P_{ETCO_2}

Increased P_{ETCO_2}	Decreased P_{ETCO_2}
Increased CO_2 production and delivery to the lungs: fever, sepsis, bicarbonate administration, increased metabolic rate, seizures	Decreased CO_2 production and delivery to the lungs: hypothermia, pulmonary hypoperfusion, cardiac arrest, pulmonary embolism, hemorrhage, hypotension
Decreased alveolar ventilation: respiratory center depression, muscular paralysis, hypoventilation, chronic obstructive pulmonary disease	Increased alveolar ventilation: hyperventilation
Equipment malfunction: rebreathing, exhausted CO_2 absorber, leak in ventilator circuit	Equipment malfunction: ventilator disconnect, esophageal intubation, complete airway obstruction, poor sampling, leak around endotracheal tube cuff

P_{ETCO_2}, end-tidal PCO_2

TABLE 32-8 Causes of Increased $P(a\text{-}ET)CO_2$

Pulmonary hypoperfusion
Pulmonary embolism
Cardiac arrest
Positive-pressure ventilation (especially positive end-expiratory pressure)
High-rate, low-tidal volume ventilation

$P(a\text{-}ET)CO_2$, difference between $PaCO_2$ and P_{ETCO_2}.

A common clinical cause of increased dead space is pulmonary embolism, and there has been interest in the use of capnography in this setting.[82-84] $P(a\text{-}ET)CO_2$ usually is increased when pulmonary embolism is present, but the gradient also is increased for a variety of other causes when pulmonary embolism is not present (eg, any dead space–producing disease). Extrapolation of phase III of the volumetric capnogram to determine PCO_2 at 15% of the predicted total lung capacity has been reported to be useful in the diagnosis of pulmonary embolism (**Fig. 32-10**). With maximal exhalation, the gradient approaches zero in patients with obstructive lung disease but remains high in patients with pulmonary embolism.[84]

VOLUME-BASED CAPNOGRAPHY

The volume-based capnogram is displayed with PCO_2 on the ordinate and volume on the abscissa. Airway dead space volume (anatomic dead space), physiologic dead space fraction (V_D/V_T), and the volume of exhaled CO_2 ($\dot{V}CO_2$) can be determined from the volume-based capnogram (**Fig. 32-11**). If $\dot{V}CO_2$ is known, it is possible to calculate the metabolic rate:

$$REE = \dot{V}CO_2 \times 5.52 \times 1440 \qquad (32\text{-}19)$$

where REE = resting energy expenditure (kcal/d), $\dot{V}CO_2$ is given in L/min, 5.52 = caloric equivalent for CO_2, and 1440 = number of minutes in a day.

Volumetric capnography can also be used to measure V_D/V_T[85-88] because $P\bar{E}CO_2$ can be calculated from $\dot{V}CO_2$ and $\dot{V}_E$:

$$\dot{V}CO_2 = \dot{V}_E \times P\bar{E}CO_2/P_B \text{ or } P\bar{E}CO_2 = (\dot{V}CO_2/\dot{V}_E) \times P_B \qquad (32\text{-}20)$$

V_D/V_T can then be calculated in the usual manner:

$$V_D/V_T = (PaCO_2 - P\bar{E}CO_2)/PaCO_2 \qquad (32\text{-}21)$$

CARDIAC OUTPUT USING PARTIAL CO_2 REBREATHING

Using volume-based capnography, it is possible to noninvasively measure cardiac output with the partial CO_2 rebreathing technique (**Fig. 32-12**).[89-99] $\dot{V}CO_2$ is calculated on a breath-by-breath basis, and the Fick equation is applied to establish the relationship between $\dot{V}CO_2$ and cardiac output ($\dot{Q}$):

$$\dot{V}CO_2 = \dot{Q} \times (C\bar{v}CO_2 - CaCO_2) \qquad (32\text{-}22)$$

where $C\bar{v}CO_2$ = CO_2 content of mixed venous blood, and $CaCO_2$ = CO_2 content of arterial blood. CO_2 rebreathing is performed for 35 seconds every

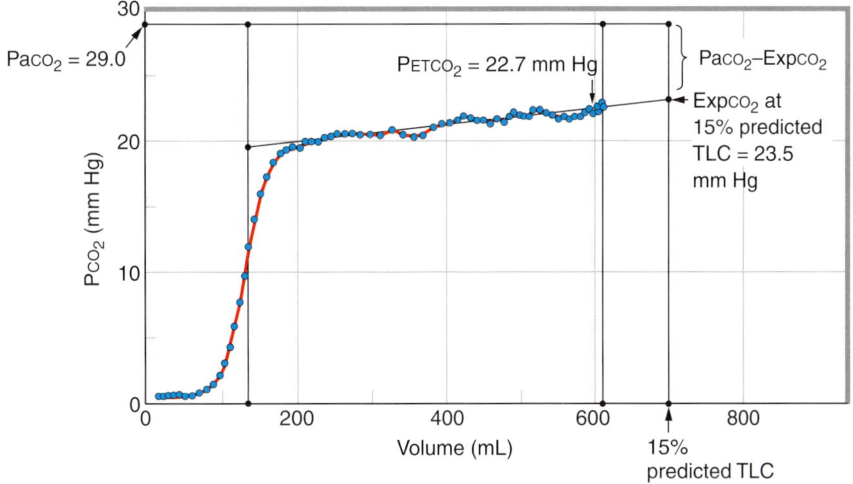

FIGURE 32-10. Capnogram in a patient diagnosed with pulmonary embolism. This patient had V_T of 612 mL. $Paco_2$ was 29 mm Hg, P_{ETCO_2} was 22.7 mm Hg, and 15% of the predicted total lung capacity (TLC) was calculated to be 699 mL. P_{ETCO_2} at this volume was 23.5 mm Hg after extrapolation of phase III. This relatively high percentage theoretically separates a patient with pulmonary embolism from a healthy patient and a patient with chronic obstructive pulmonary disease. P_{ETCO_2} end-tidal Pco_2; $Expco_2$, extrapolated Pco_2 at 15% of predicted TLC. [From Verschuren F, Liistro G, Coffeng R, et al. Volumetric capnography as a screening test for pulmonary embolism in the emergency department. *Chest.* 2004;125:841-850.]

3 minutes. Assuming that $\dot{Q}$ remains constant during the rebreathing procedure yields the following:

$$\Delta\dot{V}CO_2 = \dot{Q} \times (\Delta C\bar{v}CO_2 - \Delta CaCO_2) \quad (32\text{-}23)$$

where $\Delta\dot{V}CO_2$ = change in $\dot{V}CO_2$ between normal breathing and rebreathing, $\Delta C\bar{v}CO$ = change in mixed venous carbon dioxide content, and $\Delta CaCO_2$ = change in arterial carbon dioxide content. If $\Delta C\bar{v}CO_2$ remains constant during rebreathing, the following equation is used:

$$\Delta\dot{V}CO_2 = \dot{Q} \times (-\Delta CaCO_2) \quad (32\text{-}24)$$

When end-capillary content ($CcCO_2$) is used in place of $CaCO_2$, pulmonary capillary blood flow (PCBF), the blood flow that participates in alveolar gas exchange, is measured rather than $\dot{Q}$, and the following equation is used:

$$\Delta\dot{V}CO_2 = PCBF \times (-CcCO_2) \quad (32\text{-}25)$$

Assuming that $-CcCO_2$ is proportional to ΔP_{ETCO_2}, the following equation can be used:

$$PCBF = \Delta\dot{V}CO_2/(S \times \Delta P_{ETCO_2}) \quad (32\text{-}26)$$

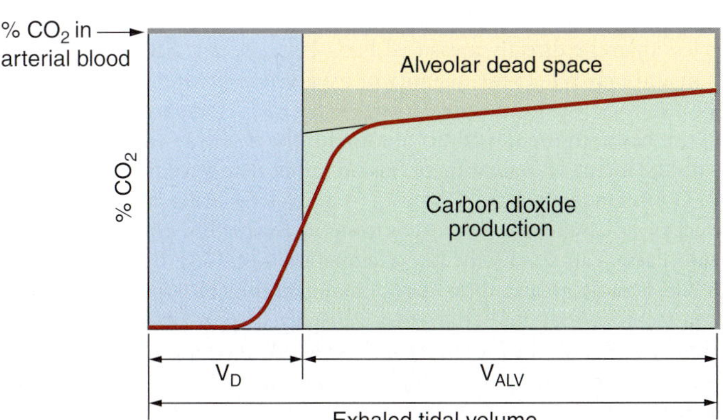

FIGURE 32-11. Components of volume-based capnogram. V_D, anatomic dead space; V_{ALV}, alveolar gas volume.

where ΔP_{ETCO_2} = change in P_{ETCO_2} between normal breathing and rebreathing, and S = slope of the carbon dioxide dissociation curve from hemoglobin. Because cardiac output is the sum of PCBF and intrapulmonary shunt flow:

$$\dot{Q} = PCBF/(1 - \dot{Q}_S/\dot{Q}_T) \quad (32\text{-}27)$$

The noninvasive method for estimating Q_S/Q_T is adapted from Nunn's iso-shunt plots, which are a series of continuous curves indicating the relation between arterial oxygen pressure (Pao_2) and FIO_2 at different levels of right-to-left shunt. Pao_2 is noninvasively estimated using a pulse oximeter.

There are several potential limitations of partial rebreathing for the measurement of cardiac output. In nonparalyzed patients, rebreathing increases the respiratory rate, which reduces the magnitude of the signal and limits the ability to detect changes in P_{ETCO_2} and $\dot{V}CO_2$. Noise is increased by respiratory pattern irregularities that produce an unstable P_{ETCO_2} and $\dot{V}CO_2$, and these may impair accuracy. Additional cardiac output not calculated because shunt fraction is estimated from Spo_2 and FIO_2, and these also may introduce errors.

CAPNOMETRY DURING SPONTANEOUS VENTILATION

Although capnometry is most often used with intubated and mechanically ventilated patients, techniques are available to measure P_{ETCO_2} during spontaneous breathing. Nasal cannulae are commercially available for capnometry (**Fig. 32-13**). When a capnometer is used with a nasal cannula, it is important that the sample is not contaminated with room air or oxygen flow, which will result in significant underestimation of P_{ETCO_2}. Although it can be technically difficult to accurately perform capnometry in nonintubated patients, $P(A\text{-}ET)CO_2$ values that are similar during both spontaneous breathing and intubation have been reported.[100-105]

CAPNOMETRY FOR PROCEDURAL SEDATION

During moderate and deep sedation, pulse rate and rhythm, respiratory rate, blood pressure, and pulse oximetry are commonly monitored. Recently, there has been interest in the use of capnometry during procedural sedation to enhance safety, with the hope that capnometry will identify respiratory depression before the onset of hypoxemia.[106-108]

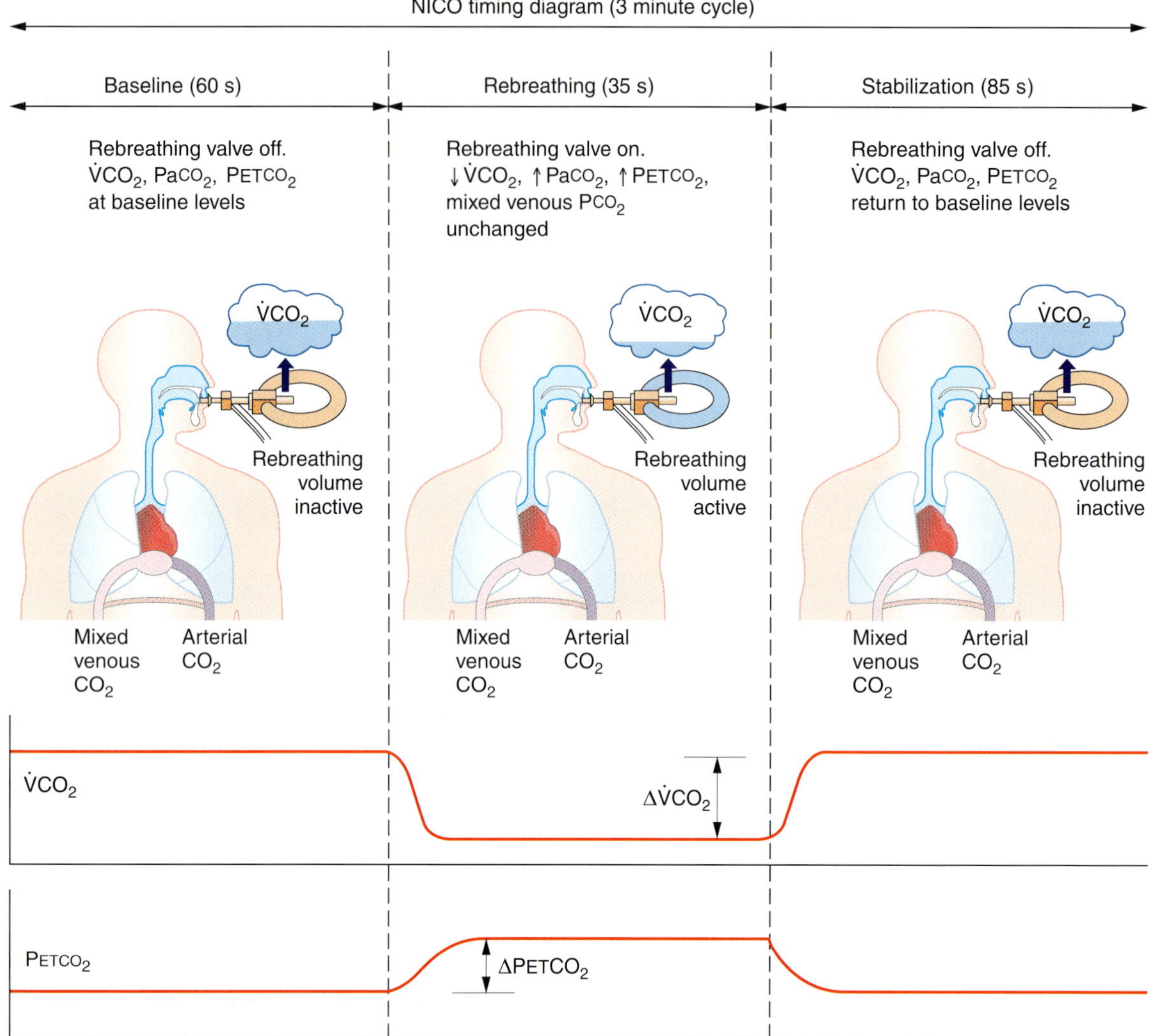

FIGURE 32-12. Rebreathing cycle used by Respironics Noninvasive Cardiac Output (NICO) monitor to measure cardiac output using the partial rebreathing technique. $Paco_2$, partial pressure of CO_2 in arterial blood; P_{ETCO_2}, end-tidal P_{CO_2}; $\dot{V}co_2$, carbon dioxide production.

In a study of adults receiving propofol sedation in an emergency department, the addition of capnography to standard monitoring reduced hypoxemia and provided advance warning for all hypoxic events.[106] Whether capnometry should be used during procedural sedation in nonintubated patients remains controversial.[107]

Bradypneic hypoventilation during procedural sedation and analgesia is characterized by an increased P_{ETCO_2} and an increased $Paco_2$. In this case, respiratory rate is depressed proportionally more than tidal volume, resulting in an increased P_{ETCO_2}. Hypopneic hypoventilation is characterized by a normal or decreased P_{ETCO_2} and an increased $Paco_2$, in which airway dead space is constant and tidal volume is decreased. Thus, there is an increased V_D/V_T. The $P(A\text{-}ET)co_2$ increases with the increase in V_D/V_T. Even though $Paco_2$ is increasing, P_{ETCO_2} may remain normal or may be decreased. If capnometry is used for monitoring of procedural sedation, it is important to appreciate that a decrease in P_{ETCO_2} may be associated with hypoventilation.[108] In one study, many patients (63%) who had respiratory depression during procedural sedation had a decrease in P_{ETCO_2} greater than 10%.[106]

TRANSCUTANEOUS Po_2 AND Pco_2

The transcutaneous Po_2 (P_{TCO_2}) electrode uses the polarographic principle (Clark electrode). To produce a P_{TCO_2} approximating the Pao_2, the electrode must be heated to approximately 44°C. The relationship between Pao_2 and P_{TCO_2} is the result of a complex set of physiologic events. Simply stated, the increase in Po_2 caused by heating roughly balances the decrease in Po_2 caused by skin oxygen consumption and the diffusion of oxygen across the skin. It should be recognized that the close relationship between Pao_2 and P_{TCO_2} that occurs in neonates probably is more coincidental than physiologic. In adults, the P_{TCO_2} value frequently is less than the directly measured Pao_2. P_{TCO_2} is also affected by perfusion and may reflect the quantity of oxygen delivered to the skin under the electrode (the product of cardiac output and arterial oxygen content). P_{TCO_2} has been used in adults to monitor the results of vascular surgery with the intent of evaluating perfusion rather than Pao_2 per se.

Transcutaneous Pco_2 (P_{TCCO_2}) is measured using a Severinghaus electrode. Unlike the P_{TCO_2} electrode, a reasonably good correlation with $Paco_2$ can be obtained at a temperature of 37°C. Because P_{TCCO_2} is consistently greater than $Paco_2$, manufacturers incorporate a correction factor so that the P_{TCCO_2} that is displayed approximates the $Paco_2$. Similar to P_{TCO_2}, the proximity with which P_{TCCO_2} approximates $Paco_2$ is the result of a complex set of physiologic events; thus, it is incorrect to believe that P_{TCCO_2} is the $Paco_2$. For example, decreased tissue perfusion causes P_{TCCO_2} to increase.

A miniaturized single sensor combining the measurement of pulse oximetry (Spo_2) and P_{TCCO_2} (TOSCA, Linde Medical Sensors) has

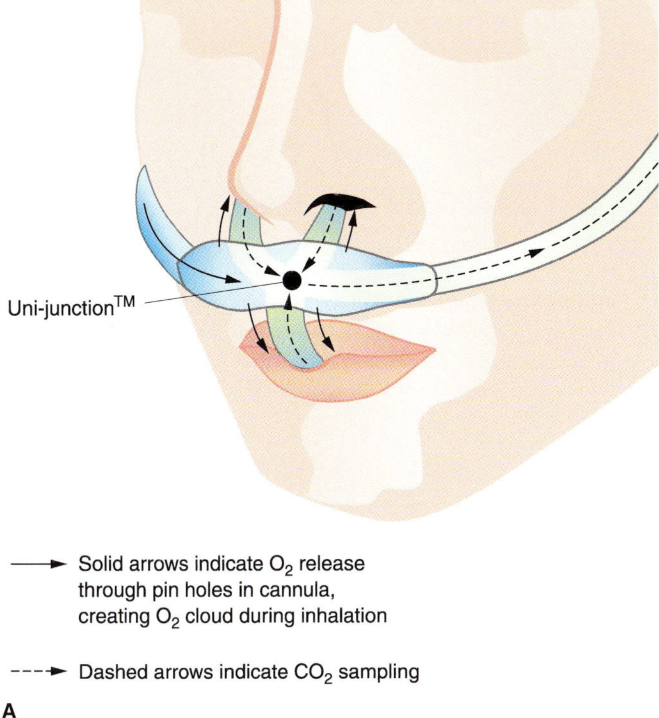

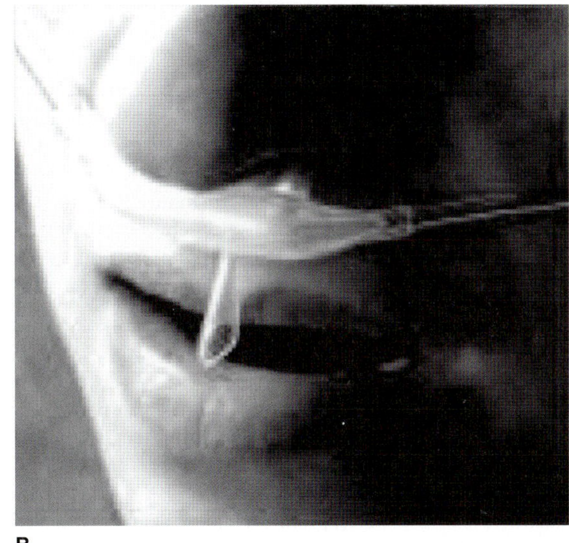

FIGURE 32-13. Nasal cannula designed for CO_2 sampling and oxygen administration (Smart CapnoLine, Oridion [Needham, MA]). The cannula samples CO_2 from both the nares and the mouth while oxygen is delivered through pinholes directed toward both the nose and mouth.

recently become available (**Fig. 32-14**). The TOSCA measurement system is based on a heated Severinghaus electrode combined with a pulse oximetry sensor and is attached to the earlobe with an attachment clip. The pressure exerted by the attachment clip to the skin is approximately 12 mm Hg. According to the manufacturer's data, the in vitro 90% response time for Pco_2 is less than 50 seconds. The sensor is calibrated in vitro using a 1-point dry gas calibration with 7% CO_2 when the sensor is placed in its calibration chamber. The calibration takes 2 minutes, allowing rapid repositioning every 8 hours. The sensor is heated to 42°C to induce local vasodilatation and enhance skin permeability for CO_2 to improve gas diffusion at the site of measurement. The sensor is cleaned with alcohol and dried before each application. One drop of contact gel is applied on the skin in the center of the attachment clip before the sensor is applied. The sensor is removed after 8 hours, recalibrated, and fixed on the other earlobe. Several studies have reported the accuracy of this device compared with $Paco_2$.[109-113]

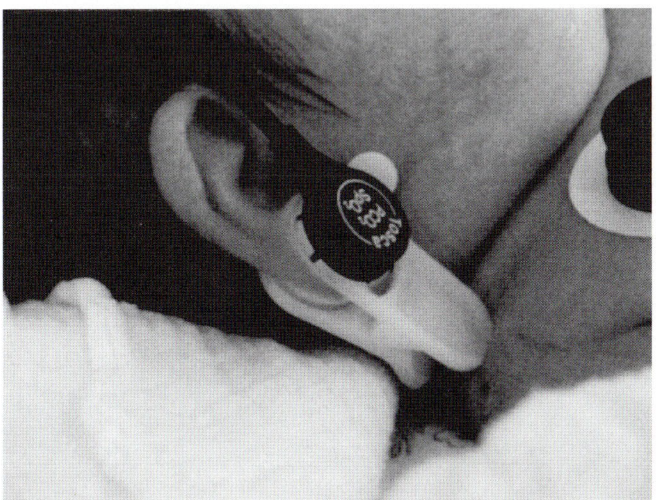

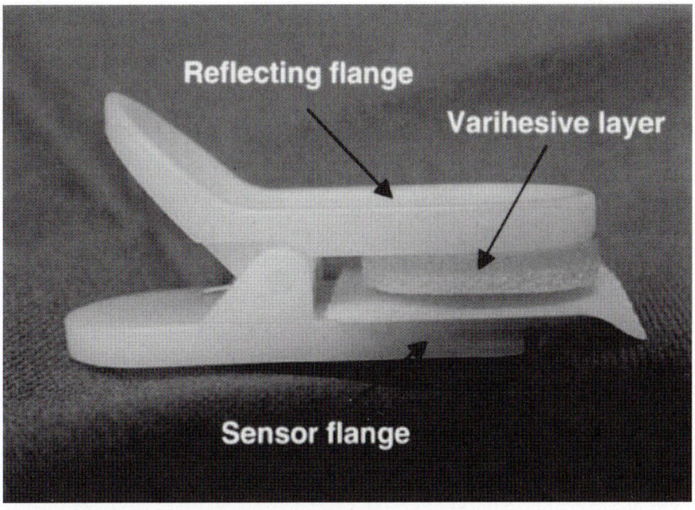

FIGURE 32-14. A and **B.** Disposable low-pressure adhesive attachment clip for transcutaneous sensor placement at the earlobe. The clip consists of 2 clip jaws connected by a coil spring. One of the jaws to be placed at the outside of the earlobe provides a retainer ring for inserting the sensor. This jaw also has a hole in the middle, in which a drop of contact gel must be applied before inserting the sensor. The sensor can be rotated in the retainer ring for finding a position in which the sensor cable is not stretched or twisted. [From Bernet-Buettiker V, Ugarte MJ, Frey B, et al. Evaluation of a new combined transcutaneous measurement of PCO_2/pulse oximetry oxygen saturation ear sensor in newborn patients. *Pediatrics.* 2005;115:e64-e68, with permission.]

LUNG MECHANICS AND GRAPHICS

Pulmonary mechanics is the expression of lung function through measurements of pressure and flow.[114-116] From these measurements, a variety of derived indices can be determined, such as volume, compliance, resistance, and work of breathing. Pulmonary graphics are derived when one of the parameters of pulmonary mechanics is plotted as a function of time or as a function of one of the other parameters. This produces scalar pressure–time, flow–time, and volume–time graphics as well as flow–volume and pressure–volume loops. Current-generation critical care and anesthesia ventilators provide monitoring of pulmonary mechanics and graphics in real time.

Airway pressure is universally measured during mechanical ventilation. Peak airway pressure is predicted mathematically by the equation of motion, which describes the relationship between proximal airway pressure (Paw), the pressure generated by the respiratory muscles (Pmus), respiratory system compliance (C), tidal volume (V_T), airways resistance (R), flow ($\dot{V}$), and the level of PEEP:

$$\text{Paw} + \text{Pmus} = V_T/C + R \times \dot{V} + \text{PEEP} \qquad (32\text{-}28)$$

The equation of motion predicts that proximal airway pressure will increase with a higher tidal volume, lower respiratory system compliance, higher airway resistance, higher inspiratory flow, higher PEEP, and presence of auto-PEEP.

Because of airway resistance, proximal airway pressure will always be greater than alveolar pressure during inspiration when flow is present. During volume-controlled ventilation, plateau pressure (P_{plat}) is measured by applying an end-inspiratory breathhold for 0.5 to 2 seconds, during which pressure equilibrates throughout the respiratory system so that the pressure measured at the proximal airway approximates the peak alveolar pressure (**Fig. 32-15**). P_{plat} cannot be accurately measured during active breathing and thus cannot be measured with ventilator modes such as pressure support ventilation. During pressure-controlled ventilation, the flow may decrease to zero before the end of the inspiratory phase, in which case peak inspiratory pressure (PIP) and P_{plat} are equal. Breath-to-breath variability of airway pressure occurs with patient–ventilator dyssynchrony (**Fig. 32-16**).[117,118]

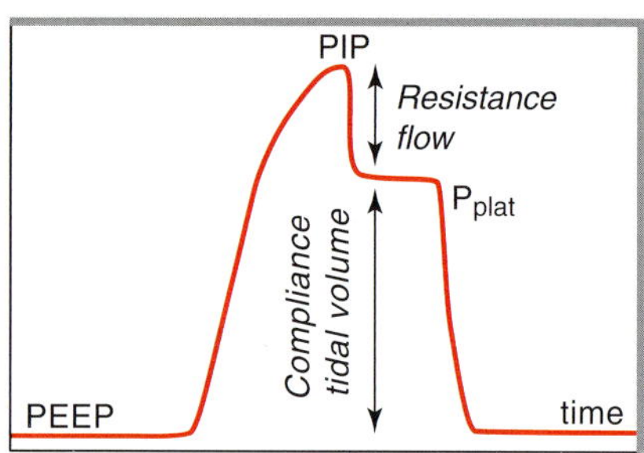

FIGURE 32-15. Schematic representation of a pressure waveform during volume-controlled ventilation. The difference between peak inspiratory pressure (PIP) and plateau pressure (P_{plat}) is determined primarily by airway resistance and flow. The difference between P_{plat} and the level of PEEP is determined by compliance and tidal volume.

P_{plat} is determined by tidal volume and respiratory system compliance:

$$P_{plat} = V_T/C + \text{PEEP} \qquad (32\text{-}29)$$

P_{plat} indicates the risk of alveolar overdistension during mechanical ventilation and should be maintained at 30 cm H_2O[119] or less and as low as possible.[119] The lower the P_{plat}, the lower is the risk of ventilator-induced lung injury.[120,121] However, a higher P_{plat} may be safe (and necessary) if intrapleural pressure is elevated (eg, abdominal distension, decreased chest wall compliance).

Incomplete emptying of the lungs occurs if the expiratory phase is terminated prematurely. When this occurs, alveolar pressure does not equilibrate with proximal airway pressure at end-exhalation and gas trapping results. The pressure produced by this trapped gas is called auto-PEEP or intrinsic PEEP. Auto-PEEP increases the end-expiratory lung volume (hyperinflation). It is measured by applying an end-expiratory pause for 0.5 to 2 seconds (**Fig. 32-17**). The pressure measured at the end of this maneuver that is in excess of the PEEP set on the ventilator is auto-PEEP.[122-126] For a valid measurement, the patient must be

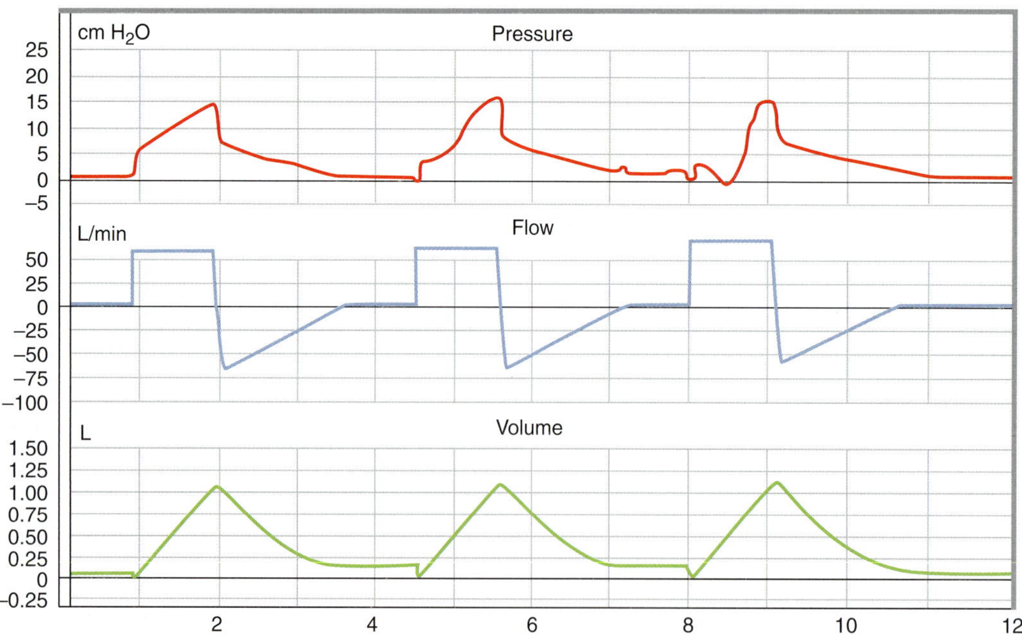

FIGURE 32-16. Example of patient–ventilator dyssynchrony in a patient on volume-controlled ventilation. Note the breath-to-breath changes in airway pressure waveform. [From Nilsestuen JO, Hargett KD. Using ventilator graphics to identify patient-ventilator asynchrony. *Respir Care.* 2005;50:202-234, with permission.]

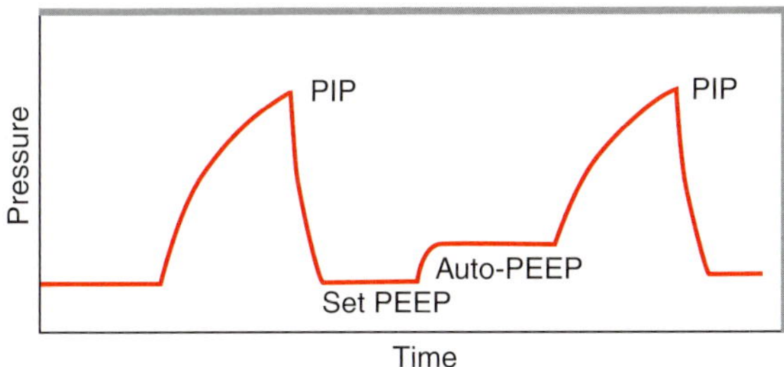

FIGURE 32-17. Measurement of auto-positive end-expiratory pressure (PEEP) with an end-expiratory pause maneuver. The difference between the pause pressure and the set PEEP level is the amount of auto-PEEP. PIP, peak inspiratory pressure.

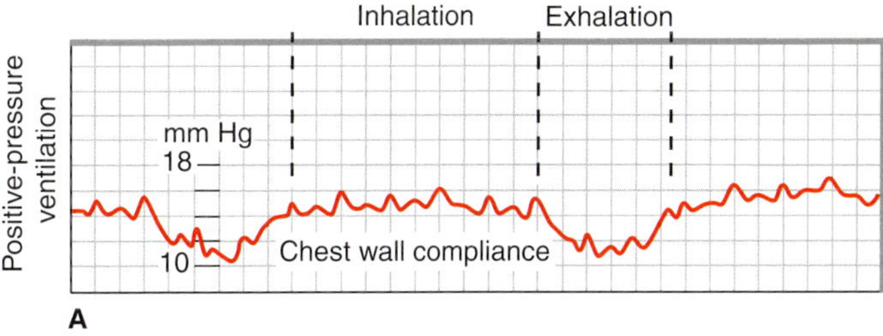

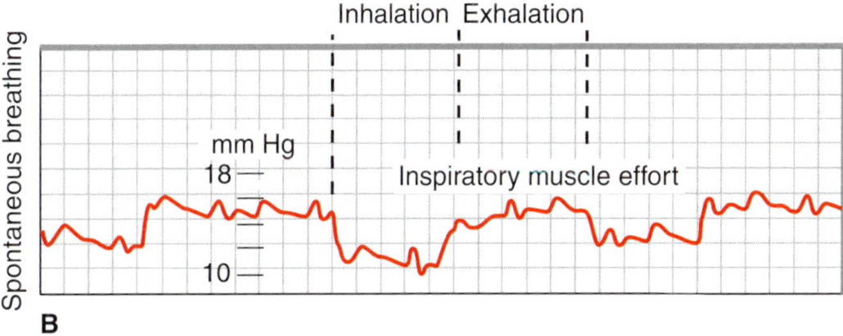

FIGURE 32-18. A. During positive-pressure ventilation in a relaxed patient, the increase in central venous pressure (CVP) during the inspiratory phase is determined by chest wall compliance. **B.** During spontaneous breathing, the decrease in CVP during the inspiratory phase is determined by inspiratory muscle effort.

relaxed and breathing in synchrony with the ventilator. Many patients with chronic obstructive pulmonary disease contract their abdominal muscles during exhalation. This is an important determinant of auto-PEEP for these patients but does not produce hyperinflation. It has also been shown that the end-expiratory pause method can underestimate auto-PEEP with complete airway closure during exhalation, as may occur during mechanical ventilation of patients with severe asthma.[126] The risk of auto-PEEP is greater with increased resistance and compliance (eg, chronic obstructive lung disease), increased respiratory rate or increased inspiratory time (both decrease expiratory time), and increased tidal volume. It follows that auto-PEEP can be reduced by decreasing minute ventilation (rate or tidal volume), increasing expiratory time, or decreasing the airways resistance (eg, bronchodilator administration). During mechanical ventilation, set-PEEP may counterbalance auto-PEEP in patients with flow limitation, and thus auto-PEEP should be measured at PEEP = 0.

Esophageal pressure is measured with a balloon inflated with a small volume of air (<1 mL) that is placed into the lower esophagus.[127,128] Esophageal pressure changes reflect changes in pleural pressure. However, the absolute esophageal pressure does not reflect the absolute pleural pressure. Changes in esophageal pressure can be used to assess respiratory effort and work of breathing during spontaneous breathing, to assess chest wall compliance during full ventilatory support, and to assess auto-PEEP during spontaneous breathing. If an esophageal balloon is not present, changes in pleural pressure can be estimated by observing the respiratory variability of the central venous pressure (**Fig. 32-18**).[128,129]

In critically ill mechanically ventilated patients, a stiff chest wall may increase intrapleural pressure, which may have a collapsing effect on alveoli.[130] This can result in atelectasis, intrapulmonary shunting, and hypoxemia. It might be argued that mechanical ventilation should provide a sufficient transalveolar pressure (the difference between alveolar and pleural pressure) to minimize alveolar collapse. Talmor et al[131] tested the hypothesis that oxygenation in patients can be improved by adjusting PEEP to maintain positive transalveolar pressures. They reported that a ventilatory strategy using esophageal pressures to estimate the transalveolar pressure significantly improved oxygenation and compliance. Whether this might improve outcomes in patients with ARDS is yet to be determined. There are concerns about the accuracy of esophageal pressure measurements in patients with ARDS.[128,132] However, using esophageal pressure measurements from 48 mechanically ventilated patients with ARDS, Loring et al[133] suggest that esophageal pressure can be used to estimate transalveolar pressure that is consistent with known physiology and can provide meaningful information that is otherwise unavailable in critically ill patients.

Gastric pressure can be measured with a balloon inserted into the stomach. Gastric pressure reflects intra-abdominal pressure. Measures of phasic gastric pressure during spontaneous breathing usually reflect diaphragmatic function. Normally, gastric pressure (intra-abdominal pressure) should increase during inhalation. If the gastric pressure decreases during a spontaneous inhalation, this is consistent with diaphragmatic paralysis (**Fig. 32-19**).[134] In the absence of a gastric balloon, respiratory variation of bladder pressure can be used.

If exhalation is passive, the change in esophageal pressure required to reverse flow at the proximal airway (ie, trigger the ventilator) reflects the amount of auto-PEEP. Negative esophageal pressure changes that produce no flow at the airway indicate failed respiratory triggering efforts (Fig. 32-17). Clinically, this is recognized as a patient respiratory rate that is greater than the trigger rate on the ventilator (readily observed by inspecting chest wall movement).[135]

A useful application of the airway flow waveform is for detection of auto-PEEP. If the expiratory flow does not return to baseline, this indicates the presence of auto-PEEP. Although the flow waveform is useful for detecting auto-PEEP, it does not quantitatively indicate the amount of auto-PEEP. Upward swings in expiratory flow indicate trigger efforts in which the patient's inspiratory effort was insufficient to overcome auto-PEEP and trigger the ventilator (**Fig. 32-20**).

Respiratory system compliance (C_{rs}) is assessed in mechanically ventilated patients as the tidal volume divided by the pressure required to deliver that volume:

$$C_{rs} = \Delta V/\Delta P = V_T/(P_{plat} - PEEP) \qquad (32\text{-}30)$$

Normal respiratory system compliance is 50 to 100 mL/cm H_2O in mechanically ventilated patients and is determined by the compliance of the lungs and chest wall. Chest wall compliance is calculated from the change in esophageal pressure (pleural pressure) during passive inflation. Chest wall compliance normally is 200 mL/cm H_2O and can be decreased by abdominal distension, chest wall edema, chest wall burns, thoracic deformities (eg, kyphoscoliosis), and an increase in muscle tone (eg, a patient who is bucking the ventilator). Chest wall compliance is increased with flail chest and paralysis. Lung compliance is calculated using the transpulmonary pressure, or the difference between alveolar pressure (P_{plat}) and pleural pressure (esophageal). Normal lung compliance is 100 mL/cm H_2O and is decreased by pulmonary edema (cardiogenic or noncardiogenic), pneumothorax, lung consolidation, atelectasis, pulmonary fibrosis, pneumonectomy or lung resection, mainstream intubation, and hyperinflation. Lung compliance is increased with emphysema and flail chest.

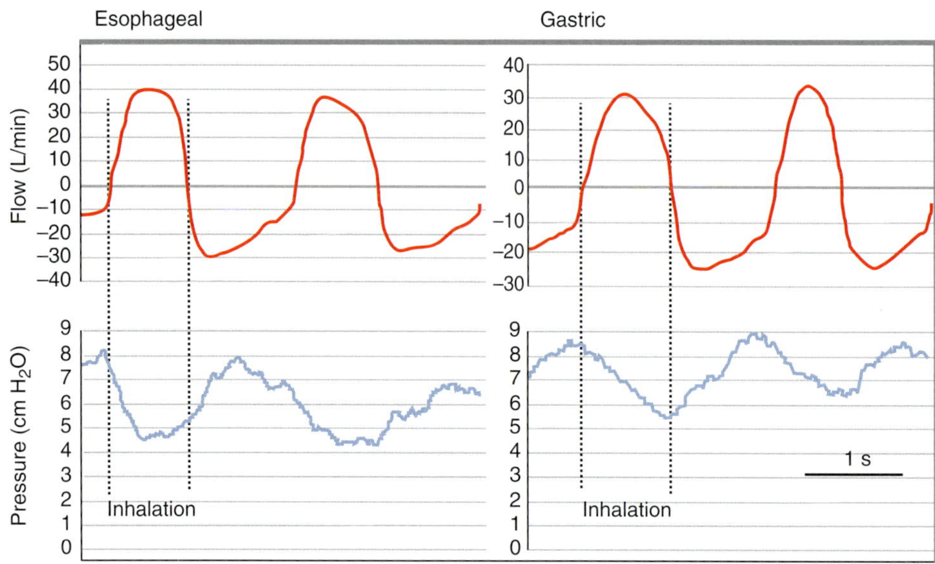

FIGURE 32-19. Esophageal and gastric pressure changes in a patient with diaphragmatic paralysis. Note that both esophageal and gastric pressures have negative deflections during the inspiratory phase. [From Lecamwasam HS, Hess D, Brown R, et al. Diaphragmatic paralysis after endovascular stent grafting of a thoracoabdominal aortic aneurysm. *Anesthesiology.* 2005;102:690-692, with permission.]

During volume-controlled ventilation, inspiratory airways resistance can be estimated:

$$R_I = (PIP - P_{plat})/\dot{V}_I \quad (32\text{-}31)$$

where $\dot{V}_I$ = end-inspiratory flow. A simple way to make this measurement is to set the ventilator for a constant inspiratory flow of 60 L/min (1 L/s). Using this approach, the inspiratory airways resistance is PIP – P_{plat}. Common causes of increased airway resistance are bronchospasm, secretions, a small inner-diameter endotracheal tube, and low lung volume. For intubated and mechanically ventilated patients, airways resistance should be less than 10 cm H_2O/L/s at a flow of 1 L/s. Expiratory airway resistance typically is greater than inspiratory airway resistance.

The pressure–volume curve represents the static relationship between pressure and volume of the respiratory system (lungs, abdomen, rib cage, and respiratory muscles). It can be constructed using a number of techniques that measure pressure as the lungs are inflated or deflated.[136] This requires a completely relaxed chest wall; thus, the patient must be paralyzed for the best results. The respiratory system pressure–volume curve can be separated into the lung and chest wall curves by estimating pleural pressure with an esophageal balloon. In the normal respiratory system, the shape of the pressure–volume curve is nearly linear above the resting volume. The inflation and deflation curves demonstrate differences in their shape and pressure for a given volume (hysteresis). The inflation curve with ALI and ARDS begins with a flat portion

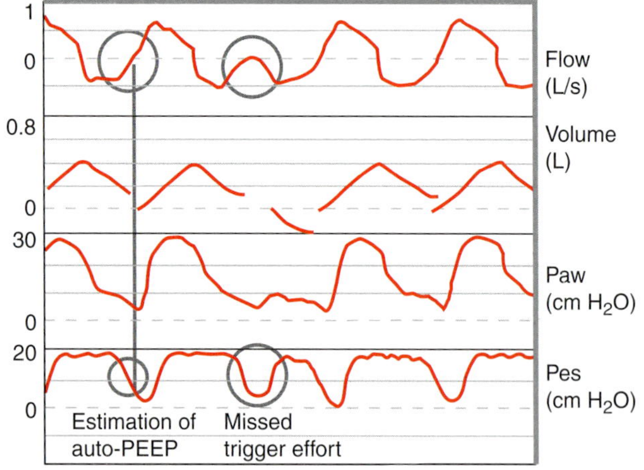

FIGURE 32-20. Esophageal pressure measurements in a patient with auto-positive end-expiratory pressure (auto-PEEP). Note that an esophageal pressure decrease of approximately 10 cm H_2O is necessary to trigger the ventilator. This represents an auto-PEEP level of approximately 10 cm H_2O. Also note an inspiratory effort that is not great enough to overcome auto-PEEP and trigger the ventilator. Expiratory pressure does not return to zero before the subsequent breath is initiated. Paw, airway pressure: Pes, esophageal pressure.

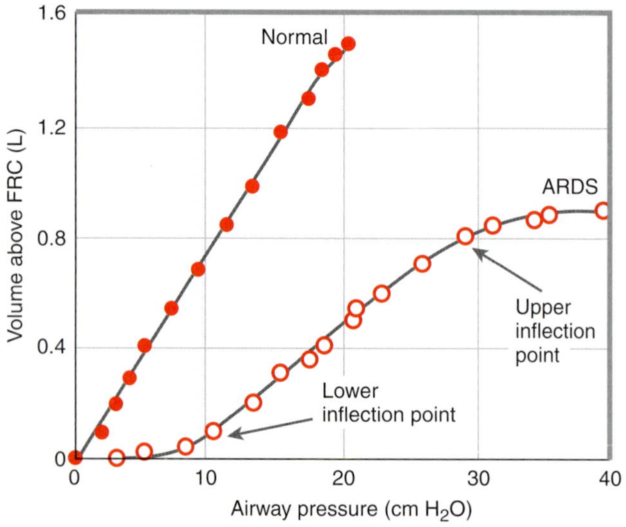

FIGURE 32-21. Pressure–volume curve during mechanical ventilation. Note that the curve is nearly linear in the normal condition. In acute respiratory distress syndrome (ARDS), the curve demonstrates a lower inflection point and an upper inflection point. FRC, functional residual capacity.

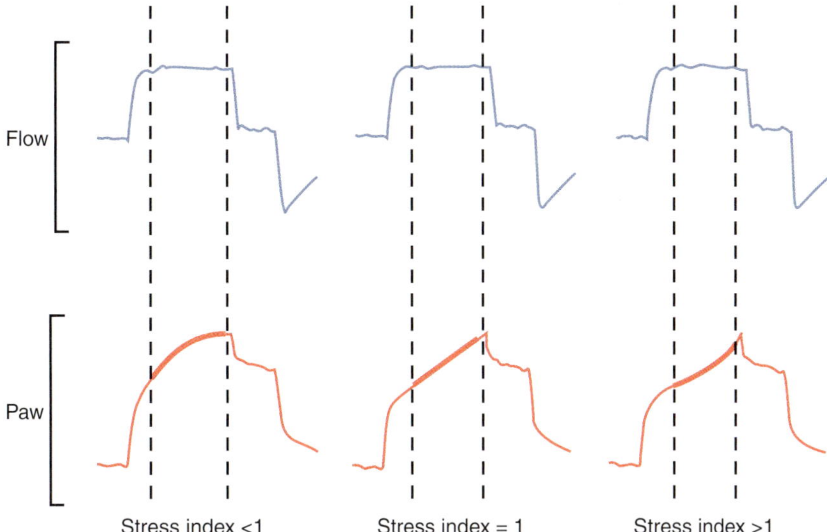

FIGURE 32-22. Graphic representation of the stress index derived from the period of constant-flow inflation (*dotted lines*), during constant-flow, volume-controlled mechanical ventilation. For stress index values of less than 1, the airway pressure curve presents a downward concavity, suggesting an increase in compliance. This is consistent with tidal recruitment. For stress index values higher than 1, the curve has an upward concavity, suggesting a decrease in compliance. This is consistent with overdistension. For a stress index of 1, the curve is straight, suggesting the absence of tidal variations in compliance. Paw, airway pressure. [From Grasso S, Stripoli T, De Michele M, et al. ARDSnet ventilatory protocol and alveolar hyperinflation: role of positive end-expiratory pressure. *Am J Respir Crit Care Med.* 2007;176:761-7677.]

followed by a transition to a steeper more compliant region (**Fig. 32-21**). This transition has been called the lower inflection point (P_{Flex}). The curve continues with a linear progression and at its upper end undergoes another transition to a flat region. This transition has been called the upper inflection point. On deflation, a similar shape is achieved but at a lower pressure than the inflation curve. The lower P_{Flex} has been equated with the closing volume, and the upper P_{Flex} has been equated with overdistension. Determination of inflection points often is arbitrary and inaccurate. Methods have ranged from eyeball approximation to graphical curve-fitting methods. Interobserver variability in the determination of P_{Flex} has been reported.[137] Methods based on curve-fitting equations may provide more accurate estimates of the inflection points.

There has been enthusiasm for use of pressure–volume curves to optimize ventilator settings by setting PEEP above P_{Flex} and keeping P_{plat} below the upper P_{Flex}. Recent observations and analysis of the pressure–volume curve in ARDS have changed its interpretation and implications for management. The chest wall affects P_{Flex} and determination of the upper inflection point.[138-140] These observations imply that the pressure–volume curve should be measured with an esophageal balloon to determine the inflection points for the lung alone. Because the pressure–volume curve represents the sum behavior of all ventilated lung units and given the heterogeneity of lung injury, it might not be possible to determine ideal points of recruitment or overdistension. Mathematical modeling suggests that PEEP settings based on P_{Flex} may not be adequate to ensure an open lung.[141,142]

The stress index has been proposed to assess the level of PEEP avoiding overdistension.[143] This approach uses the shape of the pressure–time curve during tidal volume delivery. If compliance is worsening as the lungs are inflated (upward concavity; stress index >1), this suggests overdistension and the recommendation is to decrease PEEP or tidal volume (**Fig. 32-22**). If compliance is improving as the lungs are inflated (downward concavity; stress index <1), this suggests tidal recruitment and a potential for additional recruitment, thus giving a recommendation to increase PEEP.

MONITORING IN PERSPECTIVE

How much monitoring is needed? This is an important question for both clinicians and administrators. Clinicians often want to monitor everything possible, with a more is better attitude. On the other hand, administrators and managed care providers become concerned with the costs and complexity associated with monitoring.

The presence of many monitors at the bedside can be distracting to clinicians. Many monitoring systems tend to beep, buzz, and blink constantly, attracting attention excessively. Bentt et al[144] found that a pulse oximeter alarm was present up to 47% of the time (28 min/h) in a 10-bed surgical ICU and that many of these were false alarms that required no intervention. During anesthesia monitoring, Kestin et al[145] found that 75% of all alarms that sounded were spurious, and only 3% indicated a risk to the patient. In an adult ICU, monitor alarms were present 20% of the time, with an average peak sound level of nearly 80 dBA (decibels measured using the A weighting filter); the Environmental Protection Agency recommends that noise levels in hospitals not exceed 45 dBA.[146] Monitoring is often useful in patient care. However, monitoring should not be done just because it is technically feasible. Technical capability must be balanced against clinical usefulness, cost effectiveness, and safety. The decision to monitor, like any other clinical decision, should be based on achieving therapeutic objectives in a safe and cost-effective manner.

KEY REFERENCES

- Blanch L, Romero PV, Lucangelo U. Volumetric capnography in the mechanically ventilated patient. *Minerva Anestesiol.* 2006;72:577-585.
- Grasso S, Stripoli T, De Michele M, et al. ARDSnet ventilatory protocol and alveolar hyperinflation: role of positive end-expiratory pressure. *Am J Respir Crit Care Med.* 2007;176:761-7677.
- Fencl V, Jabor A, Kazda A, Figge J. Diagnosis of metabolic acid-base disturbances in critically ill patients. *Am J Respir Crit Care Med.* 2000;162:2246-2251.
- Hess DR. Monitoring during mechanical ventilation. In Mosenifar Z, Soo Hoo GW, eds. *Practical Pulmonary and Critical Care Medicine. Respiratory Failure. Lung Biology in Health and Disease.* Vol 213. New York, NY: Taylor & Francis; 2006.

- Kiziltan HT, Baltali M, Bilen A, et al. Comparison of alpha-stat and pH-stat cardiopulmonary bypass in relation to jugular venous oxygen saturation and cerebral glucose-oxygen utilization. *Anesth Analg.* 2003;96:644-650.
- Lucangelo U, Blanch L. Dead space. *Intensive Care Med.* 2004; 30:576-579.
- Martini RP, Deem S, Yanez ND, et al. Management guided by brain tissue oxygen monitoring and outcome following severe traumatic brain injury. *J Neurosurg.* 2009;111:644-649.
- Pedersen T, Møller AM, Pedersen BD. Pulse oximetry for perioperative monitoring: systematic review of randomized, controlled trials. *Anesth Analg.* 2003;96:426-431.
- Rodriguez P, Lellouche F, Aboab J, et al. Transcutaneous arterial carbon dioxide pressure monitoring in critically ill adult patients. *Intensive Care Med.* 2006;32:309-312.
- Talmor D, Sarge T, Malhotra A, et al. Mechanical ventilation guided by esophageal pressure in acute lung injury.*N Engl J Med.* 2008;359:2095-2104.

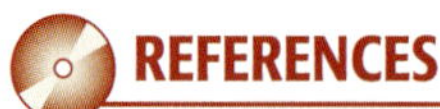

REFERENCES

Complete references available on DVD and online version at www.LongneckerAnesthesiology.com

CHAPTER 33

Intraoperative Neurologic Monitoring

John C. Keifer
Cecil O. Borel

KEY POINTS

1. Anesthetic strategies to enhance intraoperative monitoring of the nervous system include techniques that minimize interference with neurophysiologic monitoring as well as techniques that preserve neurocognitive function during the structure and function mapping in the awake patient.
2. The cellular basis of normal electroencephalography (EEG) reveals a variety of pathways to produce alterations of electrical and neurocognitive function.
3. Synchronous EEG is seen with sleep, sedation and anesthesia, and cerebral ischemia.
4. Processed EEG algorithms can aid the objective assessment of EEG changes. As long as there is an understanding of the EEG features analyzed by these algorithms, pitfalls leading to inaccurate assessment can be avoided.
5. Achieving reliability with evoked potential monitoring depends on minimizing anesthetic effect, maintaining a constant anesthetic level, and ensuring adequate nervous tissue perfusion.
6. Intraoperative wakefulness for cortical mapping has been achieved by a variety of techniques. For a successful procedure, all techniques must address maintenance of effective ventilation during craniotomy and a balance of clear sensorium and sufficient analgesia to enable effective patient participation during cortical mapping.
7. Subarachnoid block for placement of epidural stimulating electrodes allows for maintained patient perception of electrode stimulation while providing effective anesthesia for laminotomy.

Intraoperative neurologic monitoring is based on detecting changes in neurologic function that reflect injury to the nervous system. Neurologic function can be assessed intraoperatively either by repeated neurologic physical examinations or by inducing observable responses through electrical or magnetic stimulation of the nervous system. Because much of intraoperative neurophysiologic monitoring depends on some measurement of the electroencephalogram (EEG), this chapter starts with a brief overview of the cellular mechanisms responsible for the genesis of the EEG. Phenomena that modify electrical brain function and electrical activity are considered so readers can appreciate the possibilities and limitations of electrical monitoring in guiding anesthetic administration and safeguarding the integrity of the nervous system. The use of anesthetic techniques that minimize interference with monitored neurophysiologic function are presented as are techniques that allow for rapid emergence enabling intraoperative neurologic testing, immediate postoperative assessment, and continuous postoperative assessment in the intensive care unit.

ELECTRICAL METHODS

ELECTROENCEPHALOGRAPHY

Electrical activity in the brain, which is what an EEG records, was first measured in 1875 by Richard Caton, who noted the electrical oscillations on the exposed cortical surface of animals. The physiologic mechanisms and cortical morphology responsible for generating the EEG are presented by Martin,[1] and some essential features are summarized here.

Neural Basis of Electroencephalography The EEG is derived from postsynaptic potentials on pyramidal cells. There are 2 major classes of cortical neurons, pyramidal and nonpyramidal. Pyramidal cells derive their name from their distinctive shape and are notable as the only neuron that projects axons out of the cerebral cortex and locally as well. Their apical dendritic spines are oriented perpendicularly to the cortical surface and extend through the lamina of the cortex, enabling connection with all of the nonpyramidal cortical cells. These nonpyramidal cells serve to modulate pyramidal cell output through stimulation (glutamate alteration of postsynaptic potential) or inhibition (GABA [γ-aminobutyric acid] alteration of postsynaptic potentials) (**Fig. 33-1** and **Table 33-1**).

Collective voltage of cortical neuron ensembles is measurable at the scalp. The parallel orientation of the pyramidal cells enables the constructive addition of polarity from each cell to be measured at the surface of the cerebral cortex (**Fig. 33-2**).

Because the postsynaptic potentials last for a relatively long period of time and are geometrically aligned, it is possible for the potentials to summate to a sufficiently large magnitude to be measurable by electrodes placed on the scalp. Action potentials, which are of a much larger magnitude than the postsynaptic potential, are too brief to enable summation and therefore do not contribute to the EEG. Similar mechanisms for the generation of the EEG are presented by Rampil,[2] Lukatch and Greenwald,[3] and McPherson.[4] The EEG is an electrical potential versus time measurement that measures cortical voltages at the scalp resulting from the collective postsynaptic potentials of ensembles of cortical pyramidal cells.

Synchronous Versus Desynchronous Electroencephalographic Patterns This cellular mechanism forms the conceptual basis of 2 basic patterns of EEG, synchronous and desynchronous EEG. A synchronous EEG is composed of large-amplitude peaks with slow-frequency oscillations. Referring to the basic mechanism presented previously, a synchronous EEG results when an ensemble of many cortical dendrites are polarized in synchrony. The voltage amplitude is large because the individual depolarizations are additive. The thalamus serves as the orchestrator of pyramidal cell depolarization during EEG synchrony, and the frequency of thalamic stimulation determines the slow rate of cortical polarization or depolarization.[5] A desynchronous EEG results when cortical

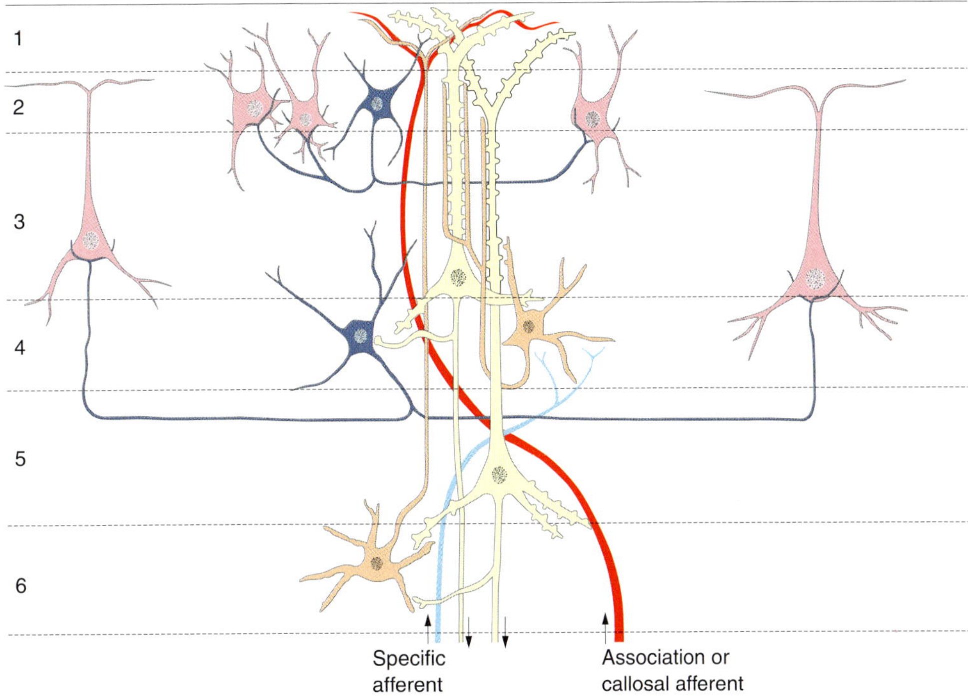

FIGURE 33-1. Schematic of cortical pyramidal, basket, and inter neurons. [From Martin JH. The collective electrical behavior of cortical neurons: The electroencephalogram and the mechanisms of epilepsy. In: Kandel ER, Schwartz JH, Jessel TM, eds. *Principles of Neural Science*. 3rd ed. New York, Amsterdam, London, Tokyo: Elsevier; 1991:777-791.]

dendrites are polarized by a less circumscribed group of afferent nerves. The consequence of diverse sources of polarizations is a faster frequency of oscillation. The polarizations are not additive and therefore are of lower amplitude. Drawing from this conceptual framework, certain patterns are evident in the normal waking and sleeping EEG (**Fig. 33-3**). A normal EEG from an awake, alert person is characterized by irregular EEG oscillations with a variable frequency greater than 12 cycles/s and relatively small amplitude. Low-amplitude, high-frequency EEG activity, the hallmark of desynchronous EEG, is the typical EEG pattern of the awake and dreaming brain (the consciously perceiving brain). Departures from normal waking consciousness during sleep are characterized by a slowing of the oscillation frequency and an increase in amplitude of the voltage oscillation. Neuronal discharge is no longer subject to the ambient environmental stimuli–responses characteristics of wakefulness. Orchestration of neuronal discharge is now directed by central pattern generators (presumably located in the thalamus).[5] The constructive interference of these waves is evidenced by large-amplitude and slow-frequency EEG traces, the hallmark of the synchronized EEG of the sleeping brain.

Desynchronous Electroencephalography: Wakefulness and REM Sleep One of the early findings in sleep research was that the EEG reverted from a synchronous pattern (low frequency, large amplitude) to a desynchronous pattern when a subject passed from non–rapid eye movement (NREM) sleep to rapid eye movement (REM) sleep. Because subjects were able to report dreams (cognitive activity) at the conclusion of these episodes and because awake patients also demonstrated desynchronous EEGs, the notion that EEG desynchrony was the electrical correlate of a cognitively functioning brain. Conversely, EEG synchrony was the hallmark of the unconscious brain. The transition from desynchronous EEG to synchronous EEG during sleep onset is characterized by the gradual appearance of slow oscillations in the EEG. The tendency for an EEG to develop a synchronous pattern is also known as slowing.

Synchronous Electroencephalography: Natural Sleep, Drug-Induced Sedation, "Light" Anesthesia, and Cerebral Ischemia All of these states are usually marked by an alteration of consciousness. But all of these states are not equivalent in terms of the degree of altered wakefulness or in terms of the likelihood of return to normal consciousness. However, for all of

TABLE 33-1 Cortical Neurons Contributing to Generation of the Electroencephalogram

Neuron	Cytologic Features	Synapses With	Neurotransmitter	Stimulates or Inhibits Target Neuron
Pyramidal cell	Spiny dendrites	Only output neurons of the cortex	Glutamate	Stimulates
Interneuron	Stellate shape No dendritic spines	Pyramidal cell dendrites	Glutamate	Stimulates
Basket cell	Envelops the soma of postsynaptic cell bodies, hence the name basket	Pyramidal cell bodies, hence the name basket	GABA	Inhibits Pericolumnar inhibition enabling neurons in a given cortical column to function in relative isolation from neighboring columns

From Martin JH. The collective electrical behavior of cortical neurons: the electroencephalogram and the mechanisms of epilepsy. In: Kandel ER, Schwartz JH, Jessel TM, eds. *Principles of Neural Science*. 3rd ed. New York, Amsterdam, London, Tokyo: Elsevier; 1991:777-791.

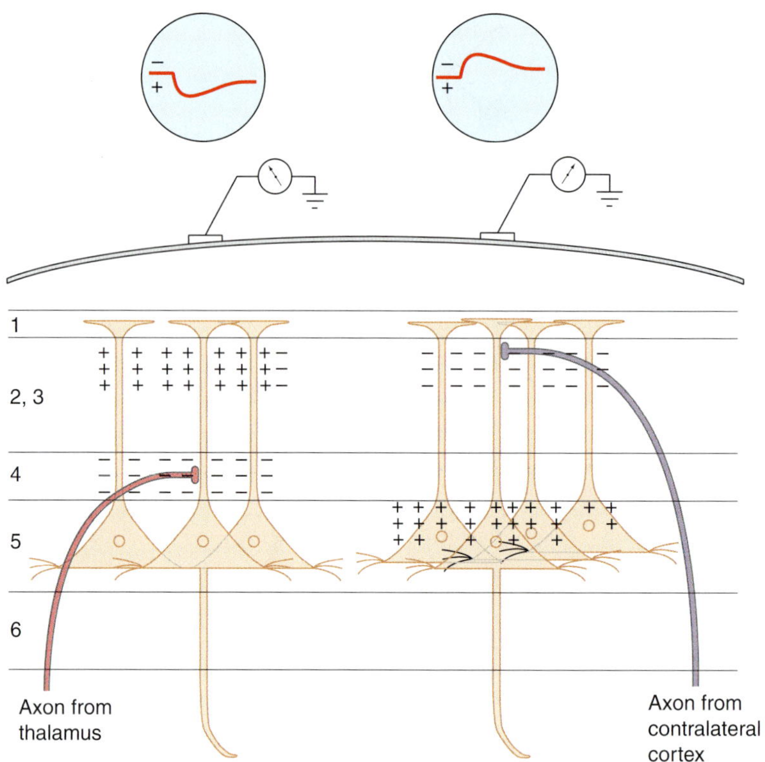

FIGURE 33-2. Scalp voltage potential depends on perpendicular orientation of pyramidal cells and the polarity of the apical dendrites. [From Martin JH. The collective electrical behavior of cortical neurons: The electroencephalogram and the mechanisms of epilepsy. In: Kandel ER, Schwartz JH, Jessel TM, eds. *Principles of Neural Science*. 3rd ed. New York, Amsterdam, London, Tokyo: Elsevier; 1991:777-791.]

these states, a return to normal waking consciousness is associated with a return of a desynchronized EEG pattern. In summary, the synchronous EEG does not specifically identify the cause of the EEG synchrony (and its associated alteration of consciousness). Therefore, synchronous EEG will be less than specific in predicting the consequences.[6]

The following 4 points, although highly simplified, represent key concepts in EEG generation: (1) EEG signals recorded at the skull surface represent the summated postsynaptic potential of hundreds of thousands to millions of pyramidal neurons. (2) Although EEG rhythms recorded at the skull surface are generated by neocortical neurons, these rhythms may originate either in the neocortex itself, or they may be "imposed on" the neocortex by subcortical structures that "pace" the activity of neocortical neurons. (3) Multiple neurotransmitter systems can be involved in generating different types of EEG activity. (4) EEG activity within individual frequency bands (ie, delta, theta, alpha, beta, or gamma) likely represents more than 1 phenomenon."[3]

Studies Suggesting the Cellular Mechanisms for Electroencephalographic Synchrony: How Sleep, Anesthesia, and Cerebral Lesions Slow the Electroencephalogram Amzica and Steriade[5] have reviewed the evidence for the cellular mechanisms of slow wave generation during natural sleep. Their summary describes 3 different oscillations that "coalesce into the polymorphic wave of slow wave EEG sleep" (**Fig. 33-4**). Salient points from their review include

1. Cellular discharge data are obtained from cats anesthetized with ketamine and xylazine. Therefore, there is a leap of faith that the mechanism of slowing from sleep versus anesthesia is the same.
2. Human data during natural sleep are not obtained from single-cell but from scalp EEG. Therefore, there is an assumption that cellular data from anesthetized cats can be extrapolated to unmeasured cellular phenomena of sleeping humans because of a similarity of the EEGs from both groups.
3. Deafferented cortex (cortex disconnected from thalamic input by surgical prep or tumor) tends to reveal a slow wave pattern.

The EPITIDE (enhanced phasic inhibition, tonic inhibition, and depressed excitation) theory of anesthetic action on patterned brain activity proposes that anesthetic-induced prolongation of inhibitory currents may slow EEG activity by limiting neuronal discharge frequencies of EEG-generating neurons. Lukatch and Greenwald[3] propose that the origin of the EEG rhythms arise in neocortical neurons and may also be "imposed" on neocortical neurons by subcortical structures that "pace" the cortex. Multiple neurotransmitter systems are involved, and EEG activity within individual frequency bands likely represents more than 1 phenomenon. The anesthetic effect on EEG is not a simple transition from the desynchronized EEG to the synchronous but rather involves an initial EEG activation at subanesthetic concentrations (perhaps an EEG correlate of the clinical excitement phase of subanesthetic levels during induction and emergence). At greater anesthetic exposure, the EEG evolves into a synchronous pattern of slowing followed at even greater exposure by isoelectric EEG with bursts of oscillation. It is hypothesized that at the network level, this cellular effect could produce a state in which low-frequency EEG oscillations (eg, delta activity) are supported by the network but higher-frequency oscillations are filtered out (much like the activity of a low-pass filter in an electronics circuit). Lukatch and Greenwald[3] state that the theory relies on anesthetic effect on the cortical networks to explain the EEG effect. The theory does not address the role of subcortical networks of cortical slowing proposed for the mechanism of natural sleep-related EEG slowing. Further observations are required for confirmation.

Electroencephalographic changes induced by a variety of insults include EEG slowing, burst suppression, and isoelectric activity. Neuronal electrophysiologic changes responsible for these EEG changes were explored by Rabinovici et al[7] This study used an in vitro rat brain slice model that enabled the measurement of single-cell discharge and

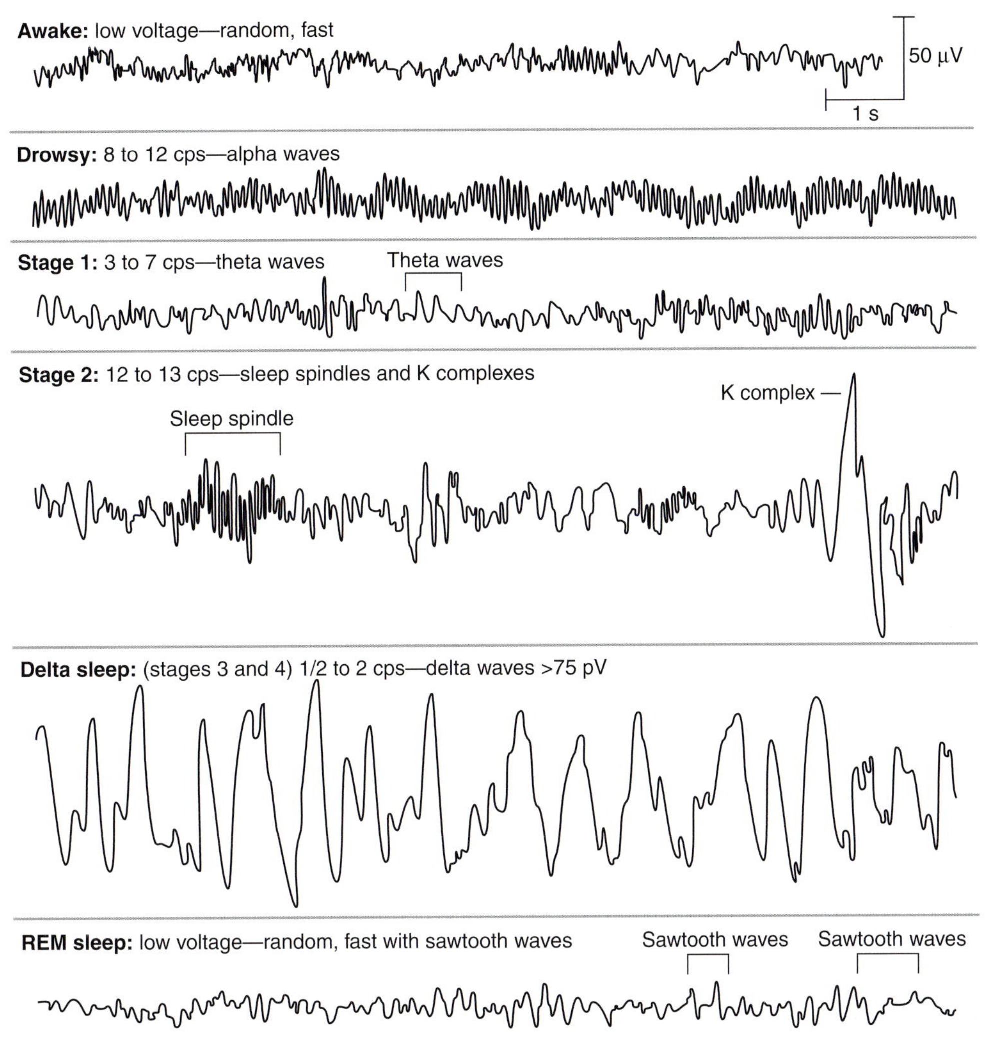

FIGURE 33-3. Electroencephalographic patterns from wakefulness (desynchrony) to sleep (synchrony) to dreaming (desynchrony). [From PowerPoint presentation: Sleep and Epilepsy in Childhood by Lawrence W. Brown, MD Co-Director, Pediatric Neuropsychiatry Program Co-Director, Pediatric Regional Epilepsy Program, The Children's Hospital of Philadelphia. www.aesnet.org/visitors/ProfessionalDevelopment/ Educational/documents/Sleep_Epilepsy.ppt Website for the American Epilepsy Society.]

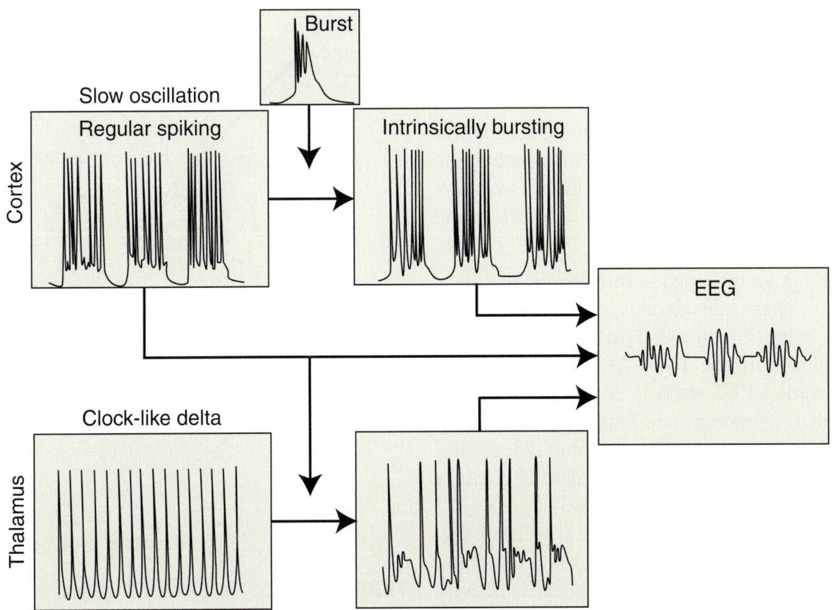

FIGURE 33-4. Cortical and thalamic depolarization leading to delta slow waves. EEG, electroencephalogram. [From Amzica F, Steriade M. Electrophysiological correlates of sleep delta waves. *Electroencephalogr Clin Neurophysiol.* 1998;107:69-83.]

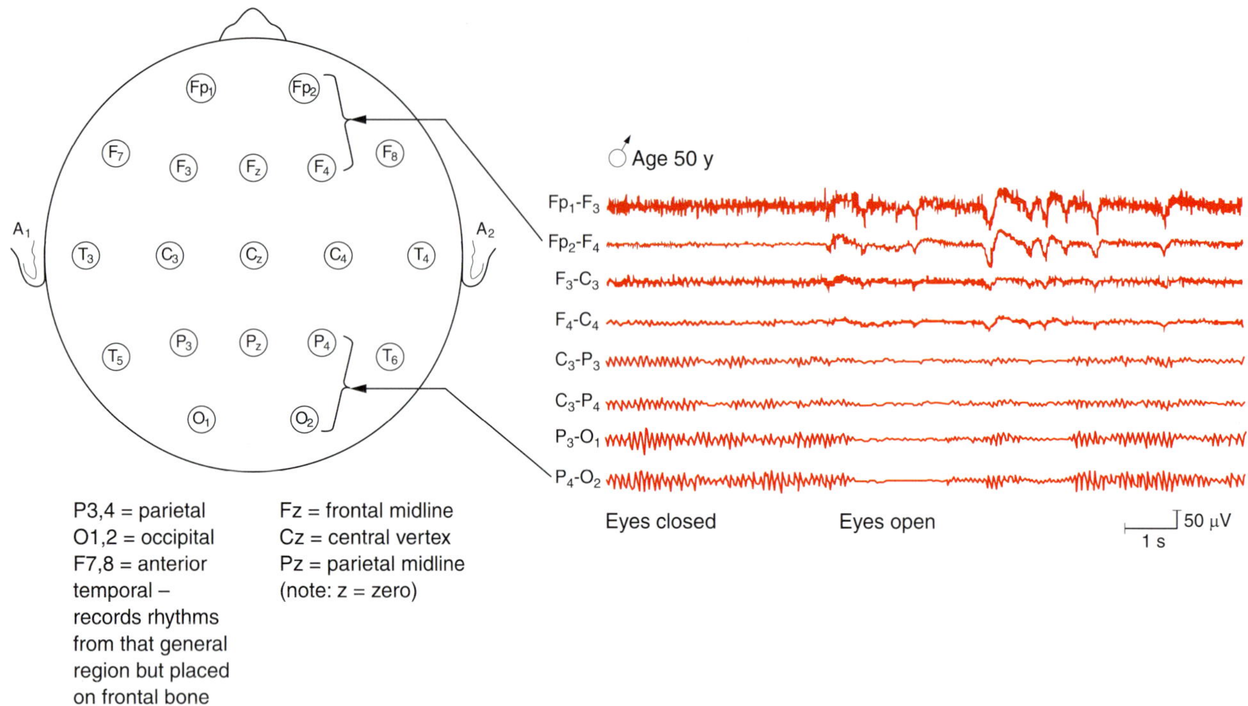

FIGURE 33-5. Heterogeneous appearance of electroencephalograms obtained simultaneously from many sites on the scalp. [Modified from Mahla M, Black S, Cucchira R. *Neurologic Monitoring Miller's Anesthesia*. 6th ed. Philadelphia, PA Churchill Livingstone; 2005:1511-1550.]

simultaneous cortical field potential (analogous to EEG) resulting from exposure to the brain slice to hypoxia, ischemia, and hypoglycemia. The findings show that EEG slowing, burst suppression, and isoelectric EEG occur with varying patterns depending on the lesion and that some patterns of damage occur with recovery from the insult. This study did not specifically address the role of subcortical structures (ie, thalamus) in the generation of slowed EEG, suggesting that thalamic mechanisms may not be necessary for the genesis of a slowed EEG in response to cerebral insult.

The work of Amzica and Steriade[5], Lukatch and Greenwald,[3] and Rabinovici et al[7] illustrates that ischemia, hypoxia, hypoglycemia, and anesthesia produce cortical EEG slowing by a variety cellular electrophysiologic mechanisms that may not be distinguishable from the macroscopic EEG.

Intraoperative Electroencephalography Uses The foregoing discussion indicates that a variety of "natural," pharmacologic, and pathologic causes alter conscious brain function and the associated EEG. This overlap points to the necessity of obtaining confirmatory data to determine the cause and treatment of such EEG changes.

Ischemia Monitor The EEG is not homogeneous throughout the skull (**Fig. 33-5**). The EEG activity varies considerably depending on the location of the electrode pair being monitored. Therefore, a standardized scheme of electrode application, the 10-20-20 system, has been developed to more reliably position EEG sensing electrodes using surface landmarks of the head for reference points. This reference system enables electrode to be placed at positions that are likely to detect EEG changes because of alteration of local perfusion evoked EEG changes because of stimulation of a particular extremity (**Fig. 33-6**).

Doubt has been cast[8] on the standard 10-20-20 system to have sufficient spatial sensitivity to determine small areas of cerebral ischemia. The EEG, however, is symmetric about the midline with EEG activity on 1 hemisphere generating a "mirror image" of the same area on the other side of the midline. This feature adds a benefit of internal control when assessing changes in an area of EEG activity. If the mirror image area of 1 hemisphere does not mimic the change on the other side, then the change is focal and likely attributable to a change in the activity of the area under monitoring. Symmetric changes in the EEGs of both hemispheres' activity suggest a global source of altered neural activity and therefore more likely attributable to global changes (ie, blood pressure,

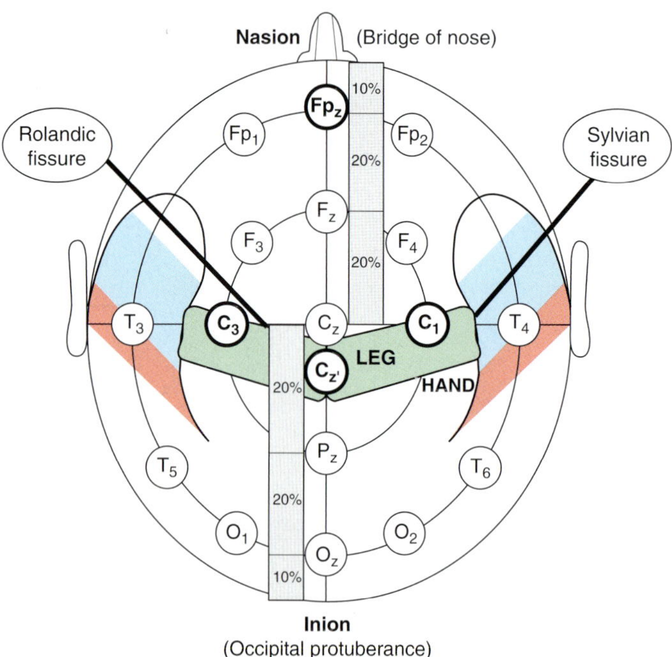

FIGURE 33-6. 10-20-20 system highlighting the position of electrodes to underline cortical anatomy. [From Keifer JC. Somatosensory evoked potentials. In: Russel GB, Rodichok LD, eds. *Intraoperative Neurophysiologic Monitoring.* Boston, MA: Butterworth-Heineman; 1995:125-333.]

TABLE 33-2 Summary of Electroencephalographic Changes in 36 of 367 (9.8%) Human Endarterectomy Patients

Group	Decreased Voltage	Decreased Frequency	Ipsilateral	Bilateral	Immediate	Delayed
I	X		X		X	
II	X			X	X	
III		X	X		X	
IV	X	X	X		X	
V	X	X		X	X	
VI						X

Reproduced with permission from Chiappa KH, Burke SR, Young RR. Results of electroencephalographic monitoring during 367 carotid endarterectomies. Use of a dedicated minicomputer. *Stroke.* 1979;10:381-388.

oxygenation, anesthetic depth). The converse is also true. Focal changes in EEG activity over 1 portion of the brain may not be detected over another portion of the same brain. This fact has consequence when one tries to describe a global change in cerebral activity from 1 focal electrode pair. At least 2 electrode pairs from mirror image sites on either cortex are necessary to conclude that a particular EEG change reflects a "global" change in activity.

The ischemic effect of carotid cross-clamping was reported by Chiappa et al in 1970[9] (**Table 33-2**). There was a variety of postclamping patterns. The changes were not global but reflected local changes in activity, underscoring the importance of a symmetric array of electrodes to detect changes over 1 hemisphere versus the other. EEG changes were sometimes observed over the cerebral hemisphere opposite to the clamped side, suggesting an interruption of collateral circulation.

A Cochrane meta-analysis[10] reviewed 2 prospective randomized studies (composed of 590 patients) that compared routine selective shunting strategy with a no shunt strategy for carotid endarterectomy (CEA). The analysis reviewed a third study that explored the potential benefit of intraoperative EEG monitoring to identify CEA patients who would benefit from shunting. The authors concluded: "There is still insufficient evidence from randomized controlled trials to support or refute the use of routine or selective shunting during CEA. Furthermore, there is little evidence to support the use of one form of monitoring over another in selecting patients requiring a shunt."[10]

As regards the method of monitoring in selective shunting, until the efficacy of shunting has been demonstrated, further trials of the method of monitoring are probably not merited."[10] This Cochrane analysis does not address the use of other potential strategies for brain protection during endarterectomy such as hypothermia, burst suppression, or induced hypertension or techniques performed on an awake patient (either endovascular carotid angioplasty or transcutaneous endarterectomy performed under local anesthesia).

After one has made the decision to monitor EEG for cerebral ischemic changes during any surgery, one is then confronted with the problem of determining if a change in EEG is attributable to focal hypoperfusion, generalized hypoperfusion (from low systemic blood pressure), or anesthetic effect. These possibilities guide anesthesiologists toward a strategy of anesthetic management during procedures that may result in ischemia.

1. Rely on anesthetic agents that have the least effect on EEG activity (short-acting narcotics, benzodiazepine) (**Table 33-3**).
2. Maintain a constant anesthetic level throughout procedure, especially at critical periods.
3. Be prepared to raise and lower blood pressure with nonanesthetic agents (inotropes, chronotropes, vasoactive drugs, and volume).
4. Be prepared to use alternative ischemia monitors (ie, somatosensory evoked potential [SSEP] if burst suppression is to be used for "cerebral protection").
5. Perform the carotid surgery with the patient awake.

Using Electroencephalography to Monitor Burst Suppression The human data regarding burst suppression as a guide to administration of anesthetics for cerebral protection are mixed. Patients in whom focal iatrogenic ischemia is induced during middle cerebral artery (MCA) aneurysm clip ligation have a significant advantage over those receiving isoflurane when they are given pentobarbital as the primary neuroprotective agent or when they receive propofol or etomidate titrated to achieve EEG burst suppression.[11] Melgar et al[12] propose the use of EEG to identify CEA patients who develop ischemic changes following carotid cross clamp that are refractory to induced hypertension. To these patients, these authors administer etomidate to achieve burst suppression and proceed with endarterectomy without shunting. Bush et al[13] conclude: "Percutaneous carotid stenting with neuroprotection provides comparable clinical success to CEA performed under local anesthetic."

However, a multicenter study of the protective effects of propofol-induced burst suppression during cardiac valve replacement showed no effect.[14] Burst suppression achieved through various means (barbiturate or isoflurane) resulted in different effects on cerebral blood flow and calculated cerebral requirement for oxygen,[15] demonstrating that the balance of oxygen delivery to consumption is altered differently by these 2 agents at equivalent degrees of burst suppression. Therefore, the use of burst suppression as a guide to anesthetic administration during procedures that place the cortex at risk must take account of the anesthetic agent used for the burst suppression, the surgical procedure for which it is intended, and the other hemodynamic and ventilatory parameters effecting oxygen delivery to the cortex.

STATE OF ANESTHESIA MONITORS

WHY PROCESS AN ELECTROENCEPHALOGRAM?

The characteristics of the EEG associated with consciousness and unconsciousness are EEG synchrony and desynchrony. Synchronous EEG is obtained in natural sleep, sedation, anesthesia, and cerebral ischemia. Desynchronous EEG is observed during wakefulness and REM sleep (associated with dreaming). The degree of synchrony and desynchrony of the EEG varies. It is difficult for the human observer to reliably measure this feature by an inspection of the unprocessed EEG. Therefore, methods to objectively quantify the frequency and amplitude characteristics of the EEG have been developed.[2,16] Two methods currently in clinical use are the bispectral index (BIS) and entropy.[17,18]

THE PROCESSED ELECTROENCEPHALOGRAM

EEG voltage oscillation is sufficiently irregular so that the voltage measured at one instant does not enable an exact prediction of voltage for the next instant. However, EEG voltage oscillation is not completely random. Knowing the voltage at a particular instant allows for prediction of the next voltage with some probability of certainty. The EEG signal is stochastic (from the Greek, *stokhos*, meaning "to aim"), meaning that it may be analyzed statistically but may not be predicted precisely. The stochastic nature of the EEG requires that the signal be described in terms of probability .The Fourier transformation of the EEG has been used to provide this summary and is the initial step used in both the bispectral and the entropy methods of EEG signal processing.

Bispectral Array The three-pronged strategy underlying the analysis of "raw" EEG to derive a BIS is described by Sigl and Chamoun[16] and Rampil[2] (**Fig. 33-7**). This strategy includes (1) a determination of the slow wave content of the signal (beta ratio), (2) a determination of the bicoherence of all frequency pairs derived from a Fourier transformation (synch slow), and (3) quantifying the amount of burst suppression

TABLE 33-3 Table of Intravenous and Inhalational Anesthetic Effect on Somatosensory Evoked Potential and Electroencephalography*

Drug/Dose	Early Cortical Waveform§ Latency	Early Cortical Waveform§ Amplitude	Subcortical Waveform
Thiopental			
2.5-5.0 mg/kg	<10% ↑	5%-30% ↓	Negligible
75 mg/kg	15% ↑	60% ↓	Negligible
Pentobarbital			
Up to 20 mg/kg	~10% ↑	45% ↓	None (latency) 20% ↓ (amplitude)
Ketamine			
0.5 mg/kg	No effect	No effect	No effect
2-3 mg/kg + 2 mg · kg^{-1} · h^{-1}	No effect	0%-30% ↑	Negligible
Etomidate			
0.3-0.4 mg/kg + 2 mg · kg^{-1} · h^{-1}	<10% ↑	40%-180% ↑	None (latency) 50% ↓ (amplitude)
1 mg/kg	10% ↑	150% ↑	Negligible
Propofol			
2.5 mg/kg	10% ↑	No change	Negligible
Propofol			
2.5 mg/kg, then 10 mg · kg^{-1} · h^{-1} + sufentanil 0.5 μg/kg, then 0.25 μg · kg^{-1} · h^{-1}	10%-105% ↑	50%	NA
Midazolam			
0.1-0.3 mg/kg*	<5% ↑	25%-40% ↓	Negligible
Diazepam			
0.1-0.25 mg/kg	Minimal	↓	NA
Morphine[72]			
0.25 mg/kg	<10% ↑	~20% ↓	NA
Lidocaine			
1.5 mg/kg, then 3 mg · kg^{-1} · h^{-1}	5% ↑	25%-30% ↓†	Negligible
Fentanyl			
2.5 μg/kg + N_2O	5%-10% ↑	Variable‡	No change
25-100 μg/kg	<10% ↑	10%-30% ↓	Negligible
Sufentanil			
Sufentanil + N_2O + 0.5 % Isoflurane/ 1 μg/kg + infusion	5%-10% ↑	~50% ↓	No change
5 μg/kg sufentanil (alone)	~5% ↑	~40% ↓	No change (latency) amplitude: 40% ↓
1 μg/kg + sufentanil propofol	5%-10% ↑	No change	NA
Remifentanil (with 0.4 MAC isoflurane)			
1 μg/kg + 0.2 μg · kg^{-1} · min^{-1}	NA	15%-30% ↓	NA
2.5 μg/kg + 0.5 μg · kg^{-1} · min^{-1}		30%-40% ↓	
5.0 μg/kg + 1.0 μg · kg^{-1} · min^{-1}		~40% ↓	
Clonidine			
2-10 μg/kg	No effect	No effect	10% Amplitude ↓ No effect (latency)
Alfentanil			
10 μg/kg alone	NA	50% ↓	NA
100 μg/kg + 2 with N_2O	No effect	40% ↓	NA
Dexmedetomidine[67]			
Low sedative dose	NA	~10% ↓	~20% Amplitude ↓
High sedative dose	NA	~30% ↓	~10% Amplitude ↓
Halothane			
0.5 MAC + 60% N_2O	<10% ↑	~60% ↓	Negligible
1.0 MAC + 60% N_2O	<10% ↑	~70% ↓	Negligible
1.5 MAC + 60% N_2O	10%-15% ↑	~80% ↓	Negligible
1.5 MAC (alone)	10%-15% ↑	~70% ↓	Negligible

(Continued)

TABLE 33-3 Table of Intravenous and Inhalational Anesthetic Effect on Somatosensory Evoked Potential and Electroencephalography* (*Continued*)

Drug/Dose	Early Cortical Waveform[§] Latency	Early Cortical Waveform[§] Amplitude	Subcortical Waveform
Isoflurane			
0.5 MAC + 60% N_2O	<10% ↑	50%-70% ↓	Negligible
0.5 MAC (alone)	<15% ↑	<30% ↑	Negligible
1.0 MAC + 60% N_2O	10%-15% ↑	50%-75% ↓	Negligible
1.0 MAC (alone)	15% ↑	~50% ↓	Negligible
1.5 MAC + 60% N_2O*	>15% ↑	>75% ↓	5% ↑ in latency
1.6 MAC (alone)*	15%-20% ↑	60%-70% ↓	5% ↑ in latency 20% ↓ in amplitude
Enflurane			
0.5 MAC + 60% N_2O	<10% ↑	~50% ↓	Negligible
0.2-0.6 MAC (alone)	<10% ↑	<20% ↓	NA
1.0 MAC + 60% N_2O*	20% ↑	~85% ↓	Negligible
1.5 MAC + 60% N_2O	Not recordable	Not recordable	Negligible
1.5 MAC (alone)*	>25% ↑	~85% ↓	Negligible
Sevoflurane			
0.5 MAC + 66% N_2O	<5% ↑	38% ↓	Negligible
1.0 MAC + 66% N_2O	<10% ↑	~45% ↓	Negligible
1.5 MAC + 66% N_2O	<10% ↑	~50% ↓	Negligible
1.7-2.5 MAC	10%-15% ↑	~100% ↑[§]	NA
Desflurane			
0.5 MAC	<5% ↑	<20% ↓	Negligible
1.0 MAC	3%-8% ↑	30%-40% ↓	Negligible
1.5 MAC	≤10% ↑	<50% ↓	Negligible
Any with 65% N_2O†	≥15% ↑	>60% ↓	Negligible
Nitrous oxide			
60%-65%	No effect	50%-55% ↓	Negligible

*In several studies, <10 μg/kg fentanyl was added. †In isolated cases, bolus administration of 1-1.5 mg/kg resulted in loss of severe attenuation of the cortical somatosensory evoked potential (SSEP) with preservation of subcortical components.[240] ‡At times, amplitude depression was severe.[76] §For example, N-20 for median nerve SSEPs.

MAC, minimum alveolar concentration; NA, data not available; N_2O, nitrous oxide; ↑, Increase; ↓, decrease.

All data are from humans; percent changes are synthesized from multiple sources and based on reported changes in mean values.

*In a substantial fraction of patients, wave from more not attainable at this concentration. †Complete loss of waveform observed only with 1.5 minimum alveolar concentration (MAC) desflurane plus 65% nitrous oxide (N_2O). ‡Up to 15% in children.[220] §Fusion to a single early cortical high-amplitude wave with abolition of all later wave components. Not proven reliable for intra operative monitoring. ||For example N-20 for median nerve somatosensory evoked potentials (SSEPs) and P-40 for posterior tibial nerve SSEPs.

From Banoub M, Tetzlaff JE, Schubert A. Pharmacologic and physiologic influences affecting sensory evoked potentials: implications for perioperative monitoring. *Anesthesiology*. 2003;99:716-737.

present in the EEG (burst suppression ratio). These 3 features are combined in an unspecified, weighted fashion to derive the BIS.

Because the synchronous activity of EEG (slow, large-amplitude oscillations) occurs during progression from wakefulness to natural sleep, does the BIS identify this as well? Sleigh answered this question in a study of human volunteers undergoing natural sleep (**Fig. 33-8**).[19] The results, summarized in the accompanying figure and table, show that the BIS algorithm assigns low BIS numbers to EEG from naturally sleeping volunteers. A return of desynchronous EEG (ie, dreaming) is also identified by an increase in BIS number. The BIS shows a low number during physiologic sleep based on the prevalence of slow EEG activity during that time. The BIS assumption is that this slow EEG activity also corresponds to a deep state of anesthesia. The BIS algorithm does not uniquely identify an anesthetized EEG.

Phase coupling, which is measured by the bicoherence portion of the algorithm, may be the least useful component of the algorithm.[20] In a study of processed EEG obtained from human subjects undergoing induction of anesthesia, Miller et al[19] conclude that although the power content of slow-frequency EEG increases as subjects progress from wakefulness to anesthesia, the degree of phase coupling remains unchanged (**Fig. 33-9**).

These results show that the bispectral analysis did not give any more information than power spectral-based analysis and that most of the changes in the bispectral values result from decrease in the relative high-frequency content of the EEG caused by anesthesia.[20]

Entropy Monitors Entropy is a concept related to the amount of "disorder" within a system[18] and has been applied to thermodynamics and information theory by Shannon and Weaver[21] and to power spectrums by Johnson and Shore[22] in 1984. There are a variety of ways to compute the entropy of a signal in the time domain or frequency domain. The algorithm implemented by Datex-Ohmeda uses a combination of time and frequency domain approaches (**Fig. 33-10**). This approach allows for the contributions to entropy from any frequency to be explicitly separated. The computations are constructed in such a way that the length of the time window for each individual frequency is individually chosen in order to optimize response times. To summarize the algorithm, the

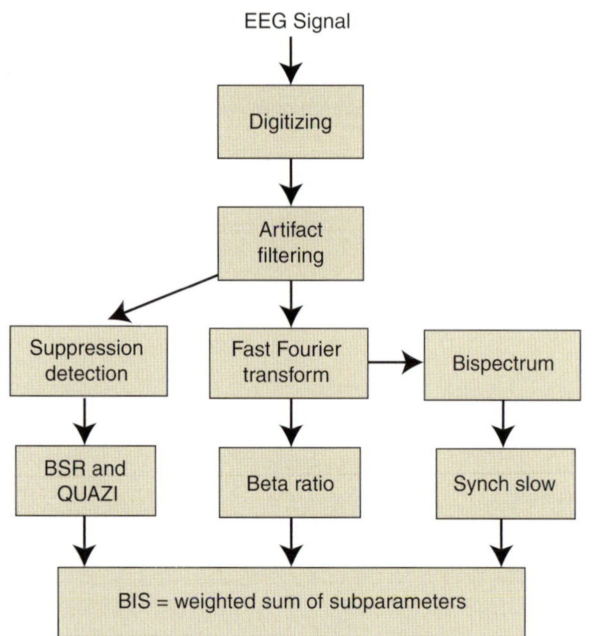

FIGURE 33-7. Three-pronged strategy to generate the bispectral index (BIS). EEG, electroencephalogram. [From Rampil IJ. A primer for EEG signal processing in anesthesia. *Anesthesiology.* 1998;89:980-1002.]

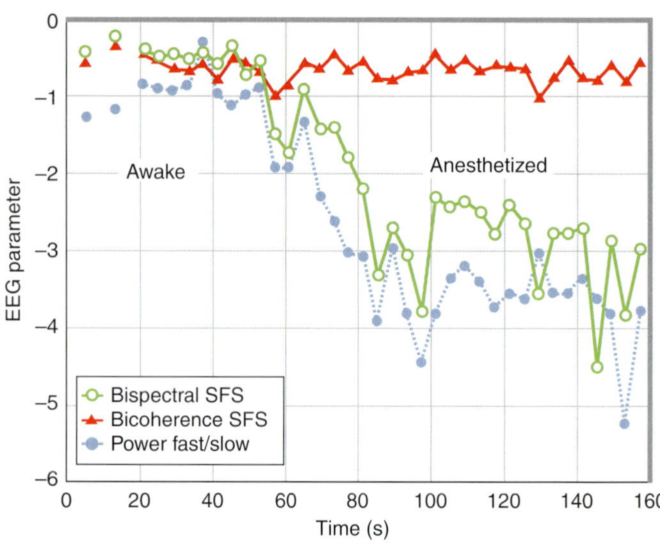

FIGURE 33-9. Wakefulness to anesthesia: comparative change in slow wave content and bicoherence of the electroencephalogram (EEG). SFS, SynchFastSlow. [From Miller A, Sleigh JW, Barnard J, Steyn-Ross DA. Does bispectral analysis of the electroencephalogram add anything but complexity? *Br J Anaesth.* 2004;92:8-13.]

raw EEG (signal) is transformed to a power spectrum by fast Fourier transformation (Fig. 33-10, step 1). A Shannon function is performed on each integer frequency to determine the contribution of each frequency to the overall entropy (Fig. 33-10, step 2). The total amount of entropy is determined by summing all the entropy contributions from each integer frequency (Fig. 33-10, step 3**)**. Entropy ranges from 0 (order) to 1 (complete randomness).

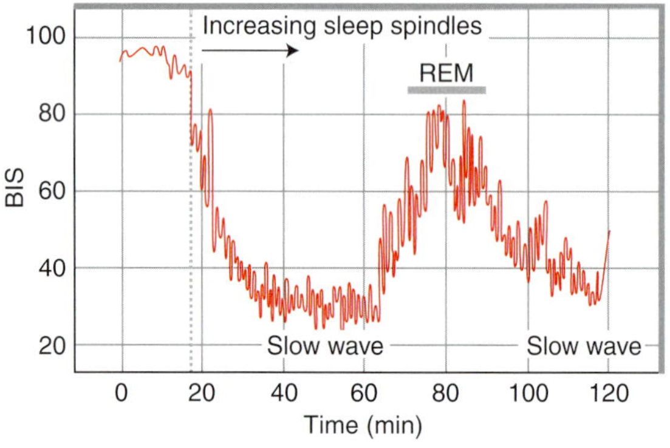

Values of EEG indices at the start of each sleep stage

	BIS	SEF*	EMG	Delta	Alpha
Awake	92 ± 3	21 ± 3	85 ± 12	50 ± 5	52 ± 8
Light sleep	81 ± 9	17 ± 2	88 ± 6	50 ± 5	49 ± 6
Slow wave sleep	59 ± 10	12 ± 2	94 ± 5	50 ± 4	46 ± 7
REM	83 ± 6	14 ± 4	66 ± 14	59 ± 4	44 ± 3

Values are mean + SD.
Data are from 28 sleep stage transitions in 5 subjects.
BIS = bispectral index, SEF = spectral edge frequency, EMG = power in the low EMG waveband (70-110 Hz), EEG = electroencephalogram.
*The units of spectral power are decibels.

FIGURE 33-8. Bispectral index obtained from human volunteers during natural non–rapid eye movement and rapid eye movement sleep. [From Sleigh JW, Andrzejowski J, Steyn-Ross A, Steyn-Ross M. The bispectral index: a measure of depth of sleep? *Anesth Analg.* 1999;88:659-661.]

State Entropy and Response Entropy State entropy (SE) is computed over the frequency range from 0.8 to 32 Hz. It includes the EEG-dominant part of the spectrum and therefore primarily reflects the cortical state of the patient. The time windows for SE are chosen optimally for each particular frequency component and range from 6 to 15 seconds. Response entropy (RE) is computed over a frequency range from 0.8 to 47 Hz. It includes both the EEG-dominant and electromyography (EMG)-dominant part of the spectrum. The time windows for RE are chosen optimally for each frequency.[18] White et al's study[23] of 30 patients undergoing laparoscopy compared the entropy monitor and BIS and showed that both the BIS and RE parameters increased after reversal of cisatracurium paralysis. However, the study was not designed to determine the ability of the RE monitor to function as an early predictor of emergence in a muscle-relaxed patient.

Wheeler et al[24] studied the RE in patients who were induced and paralyzed and found that the RE increased in a portion of patients undergoing arterial catheter placement or head pin placement before recovery from paralysis. They concluded that "increased RE during painful stimulation was not dependent on recovery from paralysis but was seen more often in patients anesthetized with 0.8% compared with 1.4% isoflurane. This suggests that RE reflects FEMG and may be useful to identify inadequate anesthesia and patient arousal during painful stimuli."[24]

Entropy: Clinical Studies Anesthesia Versus Sedation White et al's study[23] concluded "the changes in SE and RE values followed a similar pattern to the BIS values during the perioperative period. Analogous to the BIS, the entropy indices display a high degree of sensitivity and specificity in assessing consciousness during the induction of and emergence from anesthesia and were able to detect changes associated with administration of IV (propofol) and volatile (desflurane) anesthetics during the maintenance period. Finally, the Entropy module experienced less interference with the displayed indices during use of the electrocautery unit than the BIS monitor."

How Does an Entropy Monitor Handle Burst Suppression? Periods of zero EEG voltage have zero entropy because the EEG value is constant. Burst

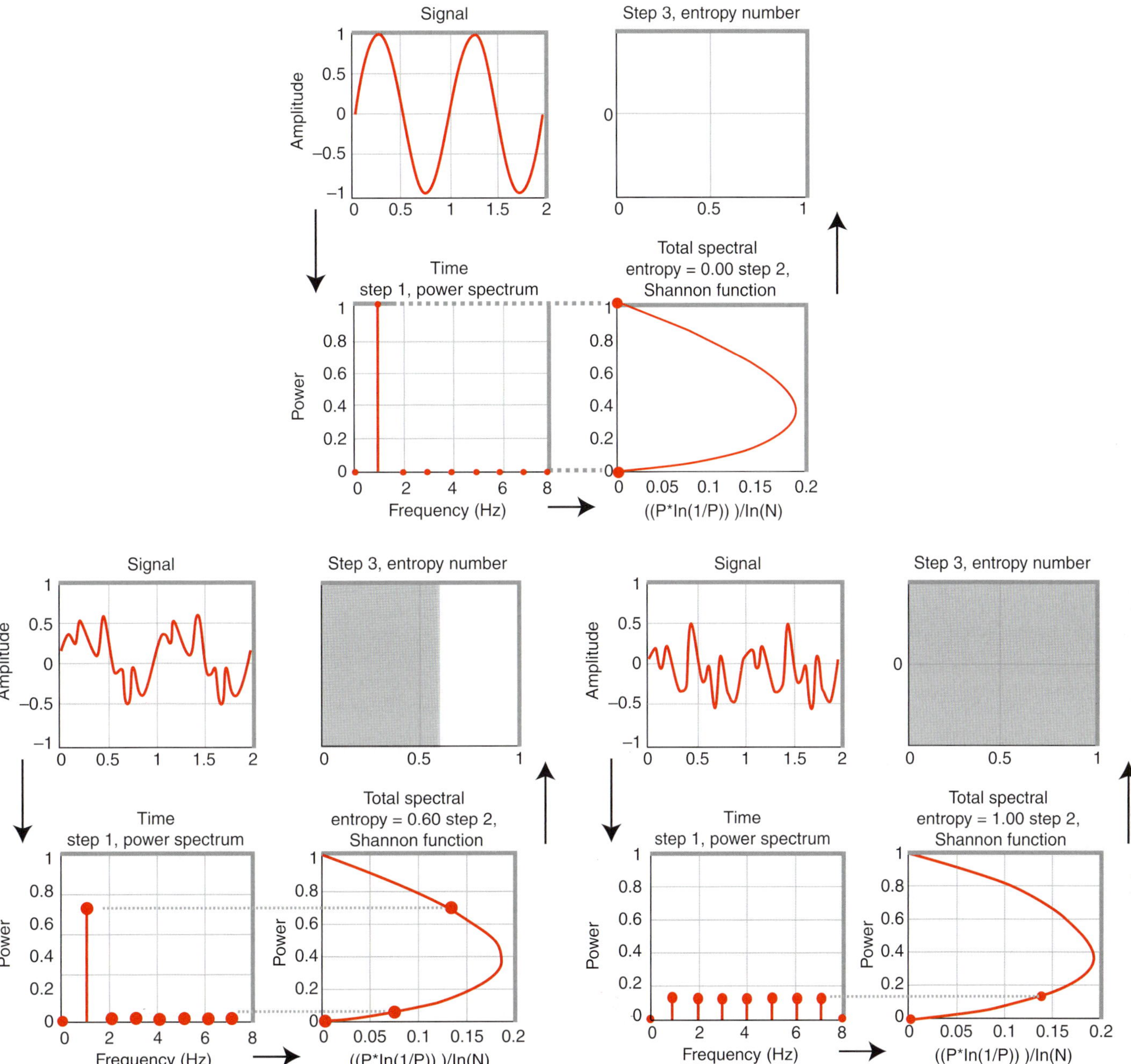

FIGURE 33-10. Schematic representation of the determination of entropy within an electroencephalography signal. [From Viertio-Oja H, Maja V, Sarkela M, et al. Description of the entropy algorithm as applied in the Datex-Ohmeda S/5 Entropy Module. *Acta Anaesthesiol Scand.* 2004;48:154-161.]

suppression patterns contain variable amounts of entropy because a variable amount of the signal is composed of bursts of oscillations. Therefore, the entropy algorithm has been successful in identifying and quantifying the degree of burst suppression.

Conclusion: Bispectral and Entropy Processing of the Raw Electroencephalogram Whatever method is used, bispectral analysis or entropy, the strategy still seems to address the issue of identifying a synchronous versus a desynchronous EEG. The entropy methods use electrical frequencies in the EMG range in an attempt to use muscle activity as a gauge to anesthetic depth. Those strategies are useful if one holds a number of dictums in mind:

1. There are multiple ways to generate a synchronous EEG, including ischemia, natural sleep, and anesthetic. Therefore, a synchronous EEG may not be predictive of the patient's response to stimulation nor for the time for change from a synchronous to desynchronous EEG.
2. Although a synchronous EEG may imply a nonperceiving brain, it does not guarantee that state and it does not define absolute cutoffs for achieving a nonperceiving state.
3. The use of synchrony or desynchrony evaluation of EEG is effectively done when one looks for a change in the EEG pattern in response to stimulus. An absence of change during noxious stimulation may add confidence that cerebral arousal did not occur (retrospective), but it does not add confidence that noxious-induced activation will not occur (prospective). However, if noxious event-related changes in synchrony to desynchrony do occur, the patient might be at risk for a more overt response to noxious stimulus (in the form of gross movement or recollection of the event).

EVOKED ELECTROENCEPHALOGRAM AND EVOKED MUSCLE RESPONSE

Intraoperative evoked potential monitors have received the greatest clinical usage in monitoring the integrity of the spinal cord during surgery to correct spinal column deformities, remove spinal cord tumors and vascular malformations, and correct vascular lesions that jeopardize the spinal cord vascular supply. The decision to use this monitoring is based on the risk and the magnitude of possible deficit versus the predictive value (positive or negative) of the monitor in a given operative setting. Except for a few exceptions, (ie, facial nerve monitoring during acoustic neuroma resection),[25] there are no mandatory uses of this monitoring even though a body of evidence supports its use in a variety of circumstances, including the following: (1) peripheral nerve or plexus surgery, (2) spinal cord surgery (deformity correction, traumatic spinal fracture repair, tumor removal), (3) brainstem surgery (posterior fossa tumor removal), (4) cerebrovascular surgery (CEA, aneurysm repair), or (5) identification of the sensory portion of the sensorimotor cortex (central sulcus identification or cortical mapping).[26]

HOW TO EVOKE A CORTICAL RESPONSE: ANATOMY

Site of Stimulation SSEPs are elicited by stimulation of a peripheral nerve at a distal site, typically the median or ulnar nerves at the wrist for acquiring SSEPs from the upper extremities and the posterior tibial nerve at the ankle or the peroneal nerve at the fibular head for acquiring lower extremity SSEPs. Stimulation is typically delivered by adhesive electrodes or fine-needle electrodes.

Pathway of the Response Through the Spinal Cord The SSEP signal enters the spinal cord through dorsal nerve roots and ascends the spinal cord via multiple pathways.[27,28] The posterior column spinal pathways, which decussate at the cervicomedullary junction, primarily mediate the SSEPs. Other pathways such as the dorsal spinocerebellar tracts and the anterolateral columns, which decussate near the nerve root entry level, may contribute to the early SSEP responses that are used for monitoring purposes.[26]

Implications of Vascular Supply to the Spinal Cord The blood supply for nourishing the posterior column pathways that mediate SSEPs is generally thought to be the posterior spinal arteries (**Fig. 33-11**). The anterior spinal artery is generally believed to provide the primary blood supply to the anterior and anterolateral portions of the spinal cord, which make up the remaining two-thirds of the spinal cord. Motor pathway function is mediated by spinal cord pathways, which receive their blood supply from the anterior spinal artery. Therefore, loss of motor function because of compromise of the blood supply to the anterior spinal artery may be associated with little or no loss of the sensory function that is mediated by the dorsal column pathways (anterior cord syndrome).

Global Cerebral Blood Flow When cerebral perfusion decreases to about 18 cc/min/100 g of tissue, electrical activity of the brain decreases and SSEPs begin to diminish in amplitude. When perfusion decreases to 15 cc/min/100 g of tissue, electrical activity of the brain decreases still further and SSEPs are generally not recordable. Further decreases in blood flow to the brain, particularly if they are sustained, will result in cellular damage and irreversible changes in electrical activity.[26] These responses depend on the blood supply to the brain and brainstem and the specific arterial branches that provide this supply. Perforating branches of the basilar artery and the vertebral artery supply the brainstem. The middle cerebral artery provides the blood supply to the area of the cortex, which mediates the upper-extremity SSEPs, whereas the anterior cerebral artery provides the blood supply to the area of the brain which mediates the lower-extremity SSEPs.

What Is the Response, and How Is It Quantified? Banoub et al[29] conclude: "The single cortical sensory evoked response has a low amplitude (1-2 microV) compared with the much larger electroencephalogram waves (50-100 microV). Therefore, the EP (evoked potential) wave has to be extracted from concurrent spontaneous electroencephalogram activity by repetitive stimulation and computer-signal averaging techniques" (**Fig. 33-12**). They also write: "The EP waveform consists of a series of peaks and valleys presented as a graph of voltage over time and described in terms of amplitude, latency, and morphology. Amplitude is commonly measured as the waves' peak-to-peak voltage difference. Latency is the time from stimulus to the peak of the response. Interpeak latency is the interval between the peaks of interest"[29](**Fig. 33-13**).

ANESTHETIC EFFECT ON SOMATOSENSORY EVOKED POTENTIAL: IMPLICATION OF SYNAPSES BETWEEN PERIPHERAL NERVE SITES, BRAINSTEM, AND CORTEX

General anesthetics do not affect ascending SSEP responses up to the level of the medullary nuclei (nucleus cuneatus and nucleus gracilis). These early subcortical responses are predominantly a reflection of the integrity of spinal cord white matter and provide little direct information about the condition of spinal cord gray matter. The short latency evoked responses from these "subcortical" structures are useful to determine the integrity of the monitoring system (ie, Is the stimulator working? Is electrode impedance sufficiently low to enable peripheral nerve stimulation?) and to distinguish "real problems" in spinal cord integrity from "false-positive problems" caused by anesthetic-induced decrement of cortical SSEPs. Anesthetic effects on sensory responses are more pronounced in regions where synaptic transmission is prominent. Therefore, the effects are more pronounced in the EEG and cortically generated SSEP peaks. Responses of the brainstem, spinal cord, and peripheral nerve are markedly less affected because fewer synapses occur in these pathways. Anesthetic effects are clearly dose related. However, many agents have a disproportionate effect at low doses. Therefore, during periods of acute neural risk, a steady state of anesthesia is important.[30]

Choosing an Anesthetic Plan for Somatosensory Evoked Potential Monitoring[29]

1. Criteria for significant changes are difficult to establish and therefore are empiric. A significant change in SSEP, reflecting loss of integrity of peripheral nerve or spinal cord, is usually taken as a 50% decrease in peak amplitude and a 10% increase in peak latency provided these changes are not caused by anesthetic or temperature.
2. "General anesthesia has an inhibitory effect on neurotransmission and therefore on the EP. The effect of anesthetics is greater on synaptic transmission than on axonal conduction. For this reason, responses recorded from polysynaptic pathways (eg, cortical recordings) are affected by anesthesia to a much greater extent than those recorded from oligosynaptic pathways (eg, spinal cord and subcortical recordings).
3. "All volatile anesthetics produce a dose-dependent increase in SSEP latency and a decrease in amplitude. All volatile anesthetics, even at concentrations above 1.0 MAC [minimum alveolar concentration], only minimally affect the subcortical waveform, resulting in high recordability and reliability."[29]
4. The effect of volatile anesthetics on cortical SSEP amplitude is compounded by nitrous oxide.
5. Intravenous anesthetics generally affect SSEPs less than inhaled anesthetics (Table 33-3).
6. Etomidate and ketamine increase SSEP amplitude.
7. Propofol, midazolam. and barbiturates have a moderate depressant effect on SSEP amplitude. In a normothermic individual, SSEP monitoring can detect cerebral ischemia during barbiturate anesthesia at doses that induce burst suppression.[30-32]
8. Most authors report minimal to no effect of opioids on SSEP amplitude.
9. Clonidine can be used as an anesthetic adjuvant without compromising SSEP monitoring. Dexmedetomidine affects SSEP amplitude minimally at sedative doses. During isoflurane anesthesia, dexmedetomidine blunts isoflurane's effect on SSEP amplitude.

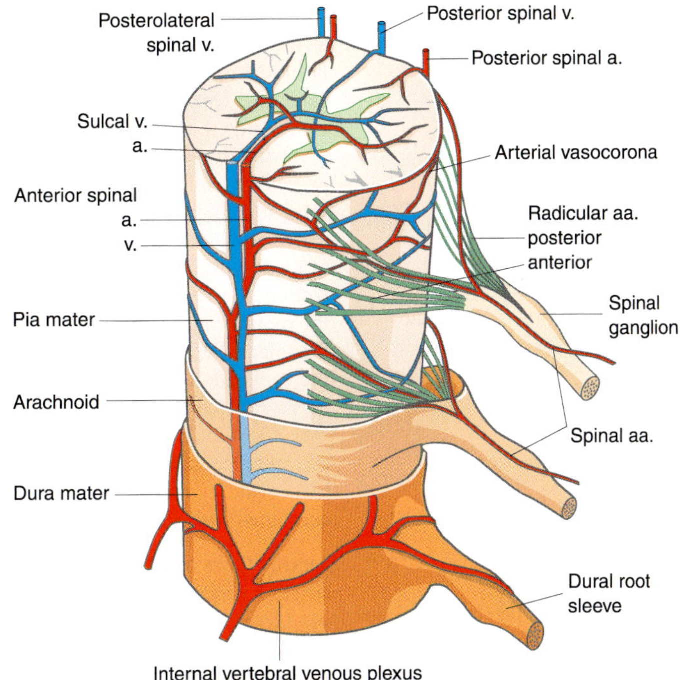

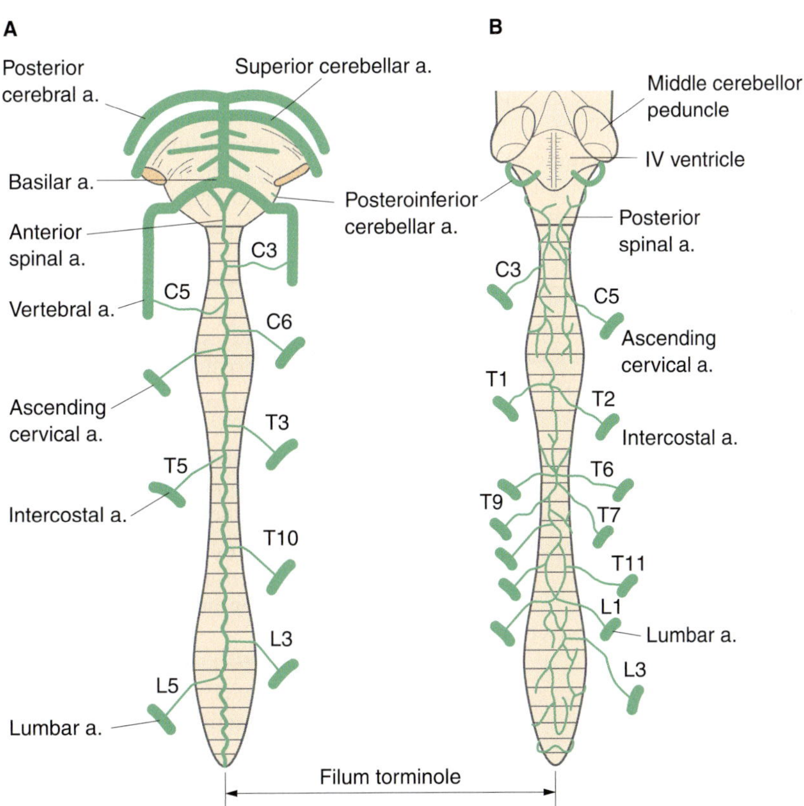

FIGURE 33-11. Vascular supply of the spinal cord. a, artery; v, vein. [From Marshal WK, Mostrom JL. Neurosurgical diseases of the spine and spinal cord: anesthetic considerations. In: Cottrell JE, Smith DS, eds. *Anesthesia and Neurosurgery*. 3rd ed. St. Louis, Baltimore, Boston, Chicago, London, Madrid, Philadelphia, Sydney, Toronto: Mosby; 1994:569-603.]

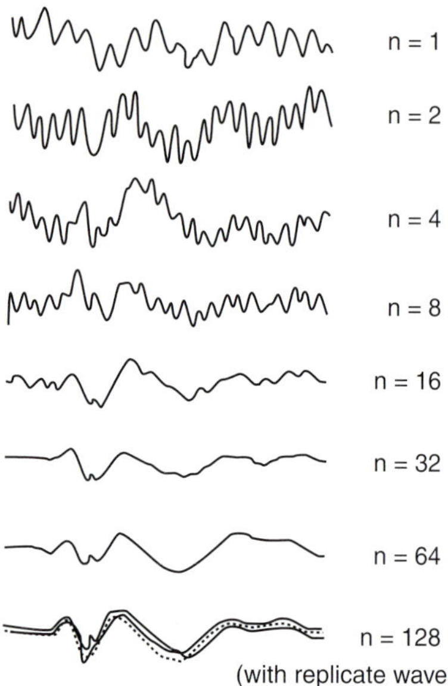

FIGURE 33-12. Evolution of the somatosensory evoked potential from the electroencephalogram (EEG) after repetitive peripheral nerve stimulations and signal averaging of EEG epochs synchronized to each stimulus. [From McPherson R. Intraoperative neurologic monitoring. In: Longnecker D, Tinker J, Morgan E, eds. *Principles and Practice of Anesthesiology*. St. Louis: Mosby; 1998:883-906.]

Application of Evoked Potentials SSEP monitoring is generally used to assess intraoperative spinal cord, brainstem, or regional cortical function. In the spinal cord, SSEP monitoring is used during spinal cord manipulation (eg, spinal distraction and rod placement, intramedullary tumor and vascular malformation removal). In the brainstem, SSEPs are useful for monitoring lesions at the cervicomedullary junction, particularly below the entrance of the eighth cranial nerve to the brainstem, such as clivus cordoma resection. In the cortex, SSEPs are used for monitoring function in the anterior cerebral artery or middle cerebral artery distributions during procedures that place those areas at risk for ischemic damage (eg, vascular surgery or tumor resection).

The brainstem auditory evoked response (BAER) is derived in similar fashion to the SSEP, but in this application, the stimulus is an audible click delivered to the tympanic membrane through earphones. The evoked stimulus traverses the auditory nerve and brainstem tracts and arrives at the auditory cortex. The response of the EEG is summed in similar fashion to the SSEP, and a characteristic pattern of evoked peaks is generated (**Fig. 33-14**) corresponding to synapses that occur between eighth nerve and cortex. BAERs are typically used during surgeries involving the eighth nerve (especially removal of acoustic neuromas) or procedures involving the brainstem or posterior cranial fossa to ensure integrity of neural structures in this area.

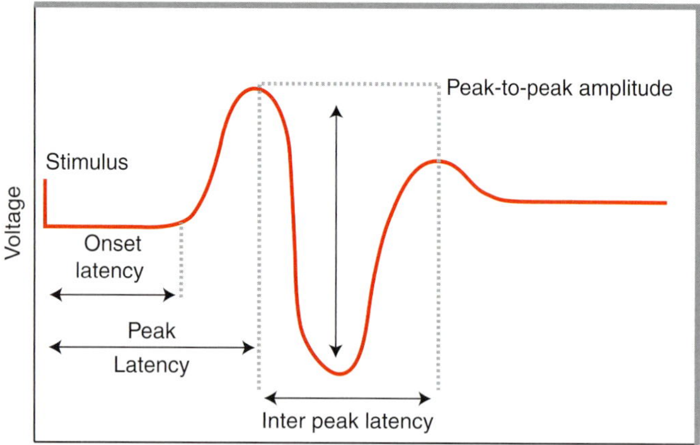

FIGURE 33-13. Amplitude and latency of the somatosensory evoked potential. [From Banoub M, Tetzlaff JE, Schubert A. Pharmacologic and physiologic influences affecting sensory evoked potentials: implications for perioperative monitoring. *Anesthesiology*. 2003;99:716-737.]

The use of mechanically evoked motor potentials has taken the form of identifying muscles that may be rendered paralyzed during the dissection of a tethered spinal cord or meningomyelocele. Other uses are the monitoring of facial nerve function during head and neck surgeries that place the facial nerve at risk. Another method is to determine that the application of a pedicle screw has not come in close contact to the nerve root contained in a neural foramen. Motor evoked potentials (MEPs), stimulated over the motor cortex and measured at the peripheral muscle, enable a monitor of motor tract integrity and are thought to provide a more comprehensive scrutiny of the spinal cord when combined with SSEP monitoring.

Specific Cases and Use of Electrophysiologic Monitoring The variety of surgical procedures and monitoring modalities that have been used productively are listed in **Table 33-4**.[26]

1. Before starting the case, consult with both the surgeon and the neurophysiologist. What is the procedure? What is the tissue at risk (eg, tissue perfusion, mechanical injury)? How is it at risk? When is it at risk (beginning, middle, end, postoperative)? What modality will be used to monitor tissue at risk? Are baseline measurements required preoperatively? Is there anything to be done with the anesthetic plan that enhances the predictive value of the monitor? Usually this takes the form of limiting potent agent and nitrous oxide, but above all keeping these exposure levels as constant as is consistent with an effective anesthetic. Is the monitoring enhanced through use of muscle relaxants or does the use of relaxants impede the detection of an evoked motor response? Monitoring techniques that require an unparalyzed but immobile patient rely on rapidly reversible deep narcotics and/or neuroleptic adjuncts such as dexmedetomidine. Are there alternatives in case of monitor failure (ie, planned intraoperative emergence to perform awake neurologic exam)?
2. There must be constant communication between anesthesiologist, neurophysiologist, and surgeon as to any significant changes in vital signs or administered anesthetic. The neurophysiologist must relay assessment as to the adequacy of monitoring and any change in the monitoring parameters so the cause-and-effect relationship can be identified.
3. Tailor the anesthetic plan to maximize a reliably timed and clear wake-up to enable rapid postoperative assessment of tissue at risk, which enables timely corrective action.

What Is the Effect of Anesthetic Agents on Spontaneous and Evoked EEG? Banoub et al[29] present is a succinct summary of anesthetic effect on SSEP.[29] To summarize

1. All potent inhaled agents prolong SSEP latency in a dose-dependent fashion.
2. All potent inhaled agents diminish SSEP amplitudes in a dose-dependent fashion.
3. Sole use of 60% nitrous oxide decreases SSEP amplitude but does not effect latency
4. Additive use of nitrous oxide with potent agent further decreases SSEP amplitude but does not increase latency more than that seen with the potent agent alone.

Troubleshooting a Change in Somatosensory Evoked Potential Because evoked potential monitoring is highly sensitive and relatively less specific, one can anticipate a fair frequency of "false-positive" changes in

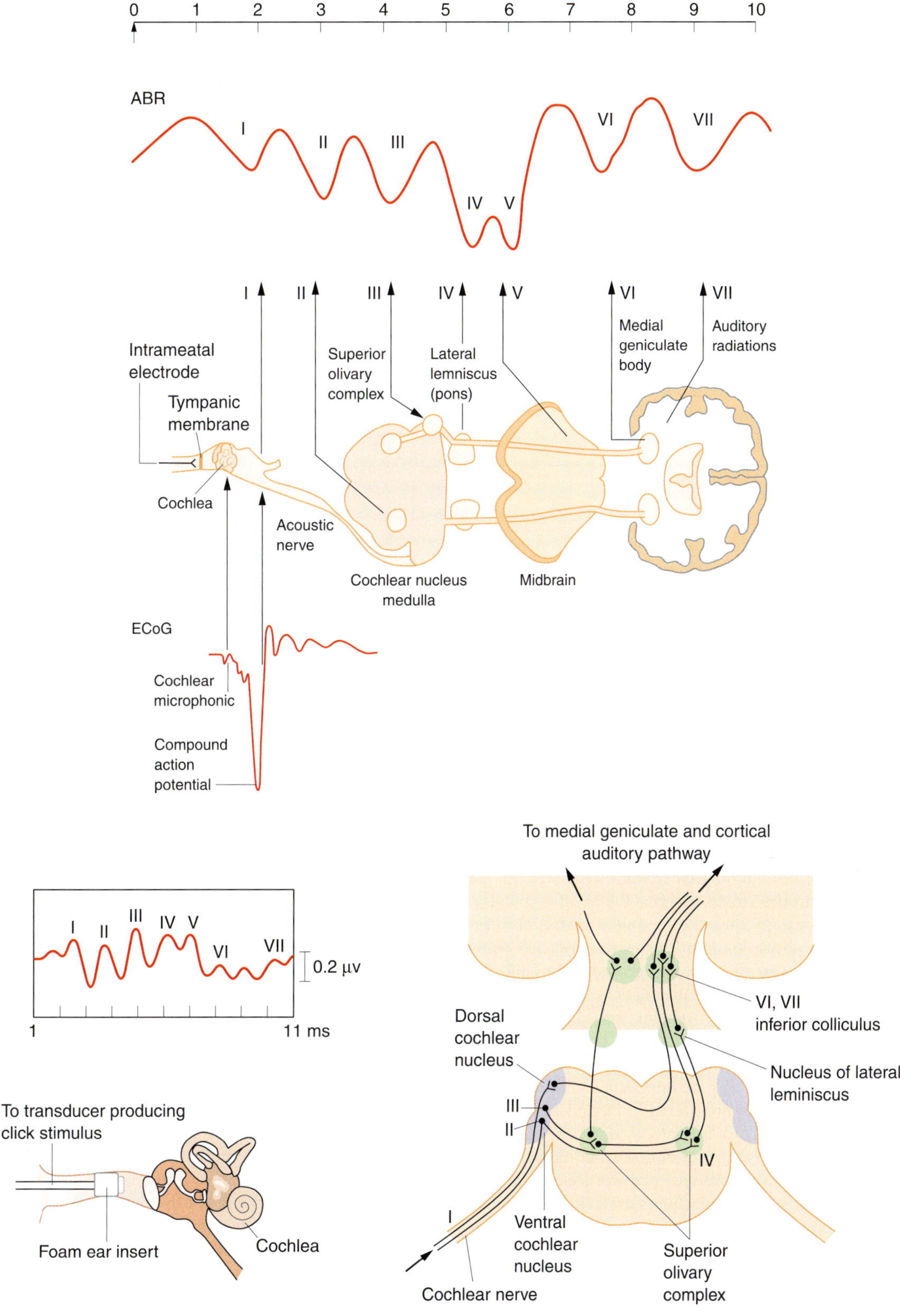

FIGURE 33-14. Schematics of auditory neural pathways. [From Mullatti N, Coakham HB, Maw AR, et al. Intraoperative monitoring during surgery for acoustic neuroma: benefits of an extratympanic intrameatal electrode. *J Neurol Neurosurg Psychiatry.* 1999;66:591-599.]

TABLE 33-4 Specific Procedures for Evoked Potential Monitoring

Procedure	Monitoring	Comments	Reference
Spinal decompression and fusion	EMG	EMG for transpedicle screw placement	
Scoliosis surgery	SSEP MEP or NMEP	Patient prepared for intraoperative wake-up for motor testing	
Acoustic neuroma excision	BAER Facial EMG		
Facial nerve decompression For tic doloreaux	BAER Facial nerve decompression		
Aortic cross-clamping Coarctation and aneurysm	SSEP MEP or NMEP		Weigang et al and Jacobs and Mess
Spinal tumor excision	SSEP MEP or NMEP		
Brachial plexus exploration	EMG		Belzberg et al, Xu et al, and Balakrishnan and Kadadi
Acetabular osteotomy			Pring et al
Pelvic fracture			Arrington et al
Tethered spinal cord	EMG		Sala et al
Intracranial aneurysm clipping	Raw EEG SSEP	EEG for ischemia monitor and burst suppression SSEP for ischemia monitor after burst Suppression Multilobar electrocorticography and scalp EEG Transcranial MEPs	Quinones-Hinojosa et al, Debatisse et al, and Young et al
Carotid endarterectomy	Raw EEG SSEP	EEG for ischemia monitor and burst suppression SSEP for ischemia monitor after burst suppression	

BAER, brainstem auditory evoked response; EEG, electroencephalography; EMG, electromyography; MEP, motor evoked potential; NMEP, neurogenic motor evoked potential; SSEP, somatosensory evoked potential.

the amplitude or latency of evoked responses during surgical procedures. All 3 participants in the monitoring process (neurophysiologist, surgeon, and anesthesiologist) should have a consistent strategy for dealing with these events to determine whether the SSEP is a "false-positive" result (eg, SSEP changes caused by monitor artifact or anesthetic effect impeding the ability to monitor the nervous system). Some preliminary points to consider are the use of preprocedural monitoring in an already damaged nerve tract. If preanesthetic testing results are abnormal, then the likelihood of improvement with anesthesia and surgery is low and monitoring of that tract should not be attempted. The neurophysiologist will be adept at determining false-positive signs to faulty electrode application by way of impedance checks and by determining if the elicited responses are altered in redundant locations along the peripheral nerve–spinal cord–brainstem–cortex circuit. Global changes in SSEP will be explored to determine whether there is a problem with generalized electrical interference from electrocautery or other electrical monitors. While these causes are being eliminated, the anesthesiologist can ensure that the 2 main features of anesthesia-controllable effects—anesthetic depth and tissue perfusion—are optimal. If all of these maneuvers do not improve the SSEP, then plan for rapid wake-up and testing. This part of the plan involves patient preparation for responding to commands to move appropriate extremities.[26]

AUDITORY EVOKED RESPONSES

The genesis of auditory evoked responses (AEPs) shares similarities with the SSEP. They are electrical cortical potentials, evoked through repetitive stimulation of a peripheral nerve, and identified and measured by summating numerous, brief (millisecond) stimulus synchronized EEG epochs recorded from electrodes placed on the vertex and ear lobe. Cranial nerve VIII is stimulated by presenting audible clicks to the cochlea by earphones placed within the auditory canal. The AEPs are grouped based on their respective latencies. Brainstem auditory evoked potentials (BAEP), also called auditory brain stem responses (ABR), are composed of the short-latency waves (~2-10 milliseconds) and are numbered I through VII. The purported neural structures[33] that serve as the substrate for these short-latency waves are noted in Figure 33-14. Procedures that have been monitored effectively include resection of acoustic neuromas, decompression of the facial nerve for hemifacial spasm (which carries a large risk of hearing loss), posterior fossa work in which the brainstem is at risk, clipping of basilar artery aneurysms, and sectioning of cranial nerve VIII for intractable tinnitus.

Midlatency AEPs (MLAEPs) have a poststimulus latency on the order of 20 to 100 milliseconds and are generated from the medial geniculate and primary auditory cortex.[34] Although the amplitude is correlated with increasing indicators of anesthetic depth, this is not a perfect monitoring modality because of poor agreement among experts as to what determines a good peak necessary for analysis.[35] Also, by determining the P_K^{33} of the midlatency BAER, Alpiger et al[37] showed that end-expiratory sevoflurane concentration was a better predictor and may turn out to be more useful in the clinical setting. Long-latency AEPs (also called the auditory late response ALR) have a latency of 50 milliseconds [38] and are generated from the frontal cortex and association areas.[34]

The early-latency BAEPs appear to be exquisitely sensitive monitors for pathologic events during surgery. Because anesthetics and mild hypothermia have minimal effects, they are specific monitors as well. The MLAEPs show promise as evoked responses for monitoring awareness or depth of anesthesia. When the concentration of anesthetics is increased, the amplitudes of the MLAEPs' peaks are decreased and their latencies are elongated. Further testing will determine if these AEP-based monitors may be superior to processed EEG in detecting the transition from unconsciousness to consciousness.[34]

MOTOR EVOKED POTENTIALS

A MEP is an electrical potential evoked from a muscle (myogenic response) or from a motor nerve (neurogenic response) by stimulating the motor cortex, spinal cord, or peripheral nerve. The source of stimulation can be either electrical or magnetic. MEP monitoring is primarily used to ensure integrity of the motor tracts of the spinal cord during spinal cord or spinal column surgery. MEPs are also used to determine the positioning of epidural motor strip electrodes for chronic pain treatment.[39-42]

Why Obtain a Motor Evoked Potential? The review by Sala et al[43] contains an extensive list for surgeries that may be monitored with MEPs:

1. Monitor the anterior cord for spinal tumor removal, spinal vascular surgery (ie, arteriovenous malformation), and spinal column distraction (scoliosis surgery).
2. Identify motor strip for analgesic electrode placement.[39-42,44]
3. Monitor the brainstem and thalamus for ischemia during basilar artery aneurysm surgery.[45]
4. Facial nerve EMG during posterior fossa surgery.[25,46]
5. Upper arm EMG for surgery within the brachial plexus.[47-49]
6. Lower extremity EMG for myelomeningocele repair and release of tethered cord.[43]
7. EMG during acetabular surgery in which epidural was used for the surgery with use of passive EMG.[50]

Why Spinal Cord Stimulation Differs From Transcranial Stimulation Toleikis et al[51]and Rose[52] show that neurogenic monitoring after direct spinal cord stimulation may not specifically evaluate anterior spinal cord function. Measured impulses over the peripheral motor nerve may be attributable to antidromic stimulation of α_1 spindle afferents that stimulate motor neurons. These authors believe that similar "contamination" may occur with transcranial stimulation. They offer a "collision" method of stimulation to circumvent this problem.[51,52]

Motor Evoked Potential Monitoring During Anesthesia The effect of a variety of anesthetic agents, including alfentanil, sufentanil, fentanyl, remifentanil, thiopental, midazolam, etomidate, ketamine, and propofol, on neurogenic and myogenic MEPs was evaluated in a study combining clinical data obtained in 40 patients and experimental investigations conducted in 140 animals. Opioids, propofol, and thiopental suppressed myogenic but not neurogenic MEPs in a dose-dependent fashion; remifentanil exerted the least suppressive effects. Etomidate and midazolam did not suppress myogenic MEP even at plasma concentrations sufficient for anesthesia. Ketamine induced moderate reduction in compound muscle action potential (CMAP) amplitudes only at high doses. Remifentanil and propofol administered via TCI (target controlled infusion) systems allowed recording of myogenic potentials within a defined target plasma concentration range.[53]

The effect of various anesthetics on transcranial MEPs was reported in a review of 20 published studies comprising 537 patients: "Although propofol does demonstrate a dose-dependent reduction in MEP amplitude without effect on latency, it has repeatedly been shown to produce a more stable neurophysiologic environment for monitoring, when compared with inhalational anesthetics."[54] Dexmedetomidine has been used as a supplement to total intravenous anesthetic (TIVA) to reduce the dose of propofol without evidence of detriment. Neuromuscular blockade is known to suppress MEP signal recording. Partial paralysis has been used on rare occasions but is generally too unpredictable to use regularly.

The anesthetics decrement of transcranial MEPs is likely caused by inhibition of the motor neuron because motor potentials evoked from direct stimulation of the spinal cord are maintained even at 1.5 MAC.[55,56] Intraoperative transcranial motor stimulation can be evoked through the use of a TIVA with propofol and remifentanil. Multiple stimulation techniques may improve the quality of weak responses.[56-59]

Direct comparison of an inhaled anesthetic with desflurane and nitrous oxide with a TIVA technique showed successful motor evoked monitoring with both techniques.[60] Tanaka et al[61] propose a method of compensation of transcranial MEP that is an easy and accurate method for removing the effects of muscle relaxants.

The advent of MEP monitoring represents a landmark in this recent progress. MEP monitoring is the most appropriate technique to assess the functional integrity of descending motor pathways in the brainstem and foremost in the spinal cord. Mapping of the corticospinal tract at the level of the cerebral peduncle as well as mapping of the VII, IX–X, and XII cranial nerve motor nuclei on the floor of the fourth ventricle is of great value with which to identify "safe entry zones" into the brainstem[62] (**Figs. 33-15** to **33-17**).

Electromyography Elicited responses to motor nerve stimulation are measured as CMAPs from intramuscular needle electrodes or surface-adherent electrodes placed over the muscle of interest. Stimulation of these responses can be either passive or active. Passive stimulation is used to alert surgeons that a dissection has trespassed on a peripheral nerve by mechanically stimulating a motor fiber resulting in a muscle twitch. Active stimulation is used to electrically stimulate tissue of interest to determine which muscles are innervated by the nerve of interest. This strategy is used for brachial plexus exploration or for identifying nerve roots during meningomyelocele repair or release of tethered spinal cord. The National Institutes of Health Consensus Conference on Acoustic Neuroma recommended that facial nerve monitoring[46] should be used in all patients undergoing surgical resection of an acoustic neuroma.[25]

Intraoperative Wake-up Test Historically, before the use of electrophysiologic spinal cord monitoring, the functional integrity of the complete motor system (upper and lower motor neurons and peripheral musculature) was confirmed after spinal distraction for scoliosis by means of intraoperative emergence from anesthesia and demonstration of voluntary leg movement. This technique, the Stagnara wake-up test (named after one of its originators), was introduced in 1973 by Vauzelle et al[63]and is described by Owens.[64] Careful preoperative patient preparation is necessary to determine that the patient understands what is required and is able to comply. Intraoperatively muscle relaxation and anesthesia are reversed while the narcotic level is maintained. The patient emerges to a level of consciousness at which point he or she is asked to follow commands. The commands include hand grip and movement of the feet. Use of the upper extremities ensures that the patient is sufficiently awake to follow commands. If quadriplegia is a possibility, the patient can be asked to open the mouth or grimace to determine that he or she is sufficiently awake.

The Stagnara wake-up test has a number of limitations. It is a test of gross motor function and cannot precisely assess specific muscle group or nerve root function. It is not a test of sensory function; therefore, a patient could have a significant sensory deficit in the presence of grossly normal motor tract function. The test is time consuming, requires the reversal of anesthetic agents, and poses some risks to the patient, including aggressive patient movement resulting in trauma or extubation. Test administration can be difficult in patients with reduced capacities (eg, mental retardation, deafness, inadequate language skills, insufficient emotional capacity). Repeated administration is difficult and not often undertaken. In most cases, the test is administered at the completion of all corrective maneuvers. This single administration can reduce its sensitivity to the onset of a neurologic injury and the subsequent efficacy of intervention. However, the wake-up test can be useful to further evaluate the veracity of a change in neurophysiologic monitoring parameters in a patient under general anesthesia.

CONSCIOUS INTRAOPERATIVE NEUROLOGIC TESTING

AWAKE CRANIOTOMY

The "silent cortex" is so named because lesions of these cortical regions are not evident by simple neurologic testing. In distinction, lesions in the "eloquent cortex" are identified by alterations in normal neurologic function, including speech and motor and sensory function. Intraoperative

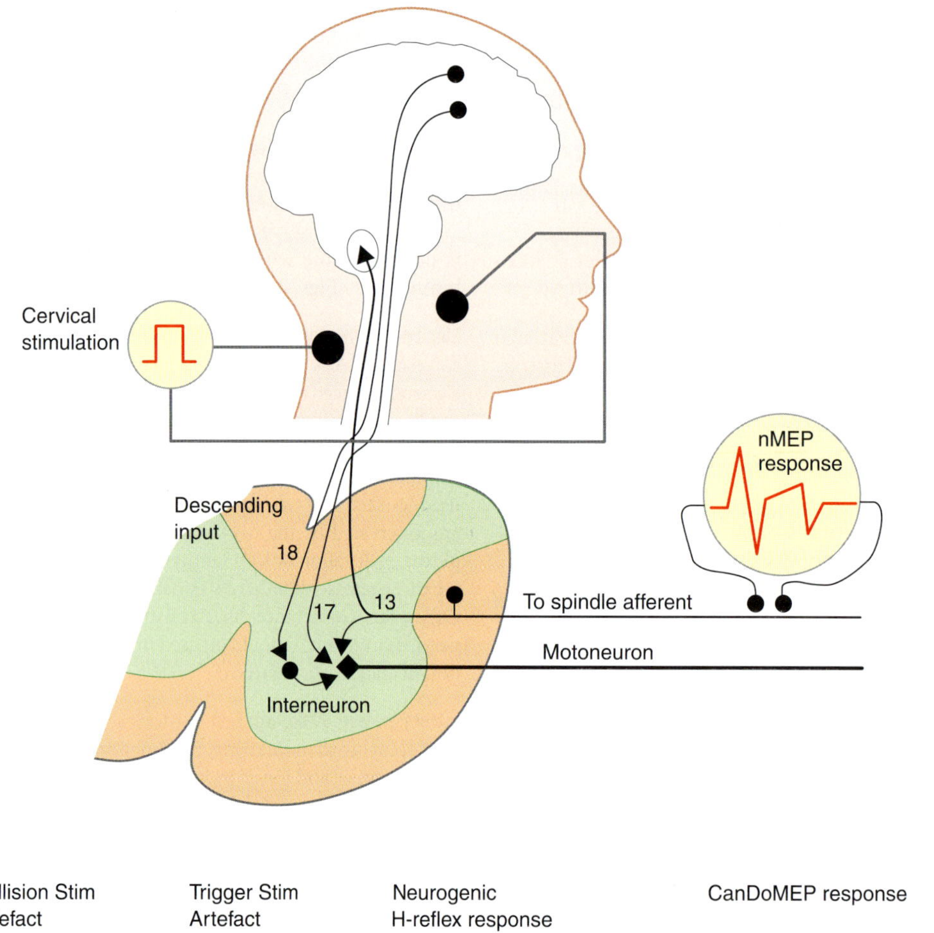

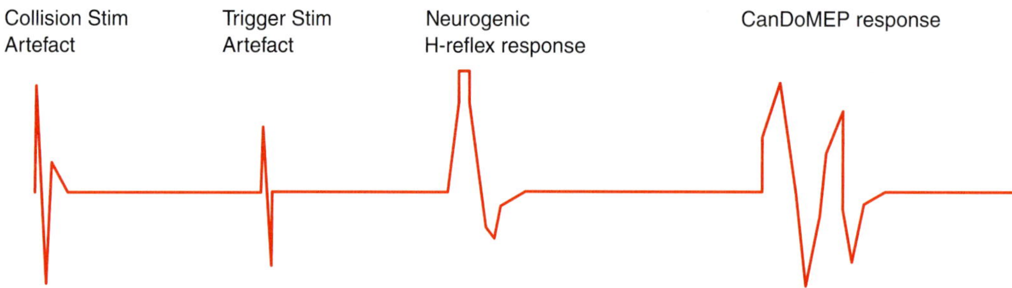

FIGURE 33-15. Schematic of neural circuit responsible for motor evoked potential wave form H reflex. [From Rose RD. Removing the antidromically driven sensory component from cervically evoked motor potentials. *Med Hypotheses.* 1998;50:147-154.]

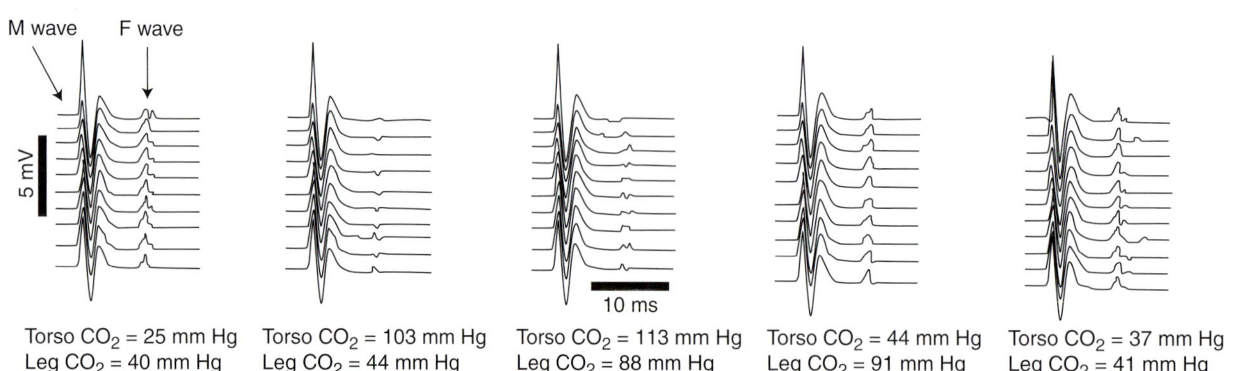

FIGURE 33-16. F wave and M wave. [From Dominguez C, Carstens E, Antognini JF. Carbon dioxide depresses the F wave by a central, not peripheral, mechanism during isoflurane anesthesia. *Anesth Analg.* 2005;100:398-403.]

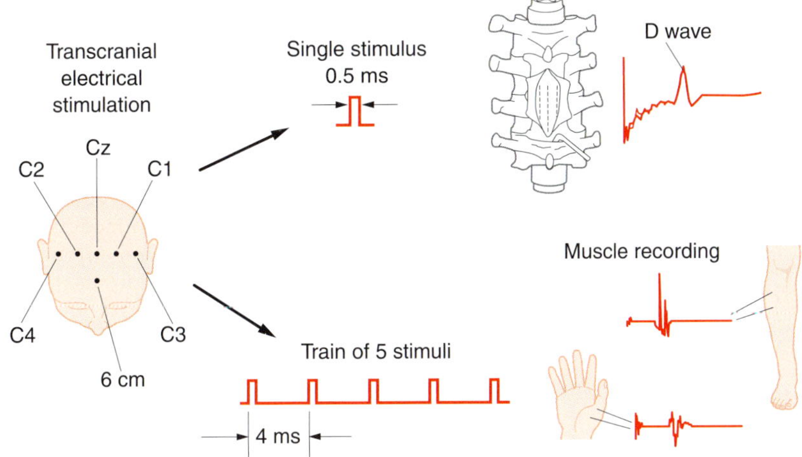

FIGURE 33-17. Obtaining a D wave. [From Sala F, Krzan MJ, Deletis V. Intraoperative neurophysiological monitoring in pediatric neurosurgery: why, when, how? *Childs Nerv Syst.* 2002;18:264-287.]

monitoring of eloquent cortical function can be effectively performed through use of cortical mapping. Mapping is performed intraoperatively by transiently inducing functional ablation of small portions of the cortex with stimulating electrodes. Correlation of structure and function requires an awake patient who is capable of performing the neurologic function under surveillance (ie, speech or directed movement) so a cortical stimulation of a particular portion of cortex can be linked with an interruption of that function (ie, aphasia or uncontrolled contraction of a muscle group). Anesthetic techniques enabling this testing vary from an "awake craniotomy," which relies on local anesthetic blocks of scalp, periosteum, and dura supplemented by a "neurolept anesthetic."[65] More recently, general anesthetic for craniotomy followed by an intraoperative emergence for cortical testing followed by reinduction of general anesthesia (the so called asleep–awake–asleep technique) has gained wide acceptance. Challenges of any method include the issue of airway control (ensuring sufficient airway patency and ventilatory drive to maintain acceptable oxygenation and carbon dioxide level) as well as minimizing coughing and the Valsalva maneuver in a patient with an open cranium. These challenges are met through use of various airway adjuncts, including nasal trumpets and laryngeal mask airways. Significant reflux risk can be addressed by endotracheal intubation followed by extubation at the time of emergence for intraoperative testing. Another challenge is maintaining sufficient balanced analgesia and anxiolysis during the awake portion of the case to enable patient participation. A variety of intravenous anesthetic techniques have been used and tend to rely on quickly titratable and reversible narcotic (eg, remifentanil) and anesthesia provided by an infusion of propofol or infusion of dexmedetomidine.[66] A drawback to propofol is the respiratory depression associated with concomitant narcotic use. A relatively brief exposure to a propofol infusion is associated with a brief predictable emergence time. However, because of context sensitivity, a more prolonged exposure is associated with longer less predictable emergence. Dexmedetomidine infusion used with a narcotic infusion provides dose-related deep sedation as well as maintenance of ventilatory drive during craniotomy. However, airway patency is not ensured at the higher doses, and emergence times are not as brisk. However, a low dose of α_2 agonist may be beneficial as a "rescue" medication for patients after emerging who demonstrate significant anxiety and hypertension that may preclude cortical testing.

SPINAL ANESTHESIA FOR EPIDURAL PLACEMENT OF SPINAL CORD–STIMULATING ELECTRODES

The accurate placement of spinal cord–stimulating electrodes to treat chronic pain requires patient responsiveness to determine that the patient perceives the stimulating current in the same region as the perceived pain. Because the electrode placement may also require a laminotomy to introduce the electrode into the epidural space, the anesthetic challenge is to provide sufficient anesthesia for laminotomy and electrode placement while the patient is in a lateral or prone position. A combination of local anesthetic and conscious sedation is feasible. However, this technique runs the risk of airway loss. Additionally, prolonged deep sedation can impair patient response, which may hinder optimal electrode placement. A technique has recently been described that involves the use of subarachnoid bupivacaine. The spinal block is performed in the prone position, and hypobaric bupivacaine is introduced. Through blockade of the spinal nerve roots, there is complete dermatomal anesthesia, which enables a painless laminotomy to be performed. However, because spinal anesthetic does not completely block sensory tracts within the spinal cord, there is a maintenance of patient perception of stimulation from the epidural electrodes.[67]

SUMMARY

Surgery on and around the nervous system is safer when the functional integrity of the nervous system can be ensured. Anesthetic agents, by definition and design, decrease neurologic function. Therefore, monitoring nervous system function during anesthesia can be challenging. The techniques presented in this chapter offer a standardized approach to assessing intraoperative neurologic function. Much work needs to be done to improve the impact of anesthetics on intraoperative neurologic monitoring, and these techniques will surely evolve.

KEY REFERENCES

- Lind G, Meyerson BA, Winter J, Linderoth B. Implantation of laminotomy electrodes for spinal cord stimulation in spinal anesthesia with intraoperative dorsal column activation. *Neurosurgery.* 2003;53:1150-1153; discussion 1153-1154.
- Martin JH. the collective electrical behavior of cortical neurons: the electroencephalogram and the mechanisms of epilepsy. In: Kandel ER, Schwartz JH, Jessel TM, eds. *Principles of Neural Science.* 3rd ed. New York, NY: Elsevier; 1991:777-791.
- Owen JH. The application of intraoperative monitoring during surgery for spinal deformity. *Spine.* 1999;24:2649-2662.

- Rampil IJ. A primer for EEG signal processing in anesthesia. *Anesthesiology.* 1998;89:980-1002.
- Sala F, Krzan MJ, Deletis V. Intraoperative neurophysiological monitoring in pediatric neurosurgery: why, when, how? *Childs Nerv Syst.* 2002;18:264-287.
- Toleikis JR. Intraoperative monitoring using somatosensory evoked potentials. A position statement by the American Society of Neurophysiological Monitoring. *J Clin Monit Comput.* 2005;19:241-258.

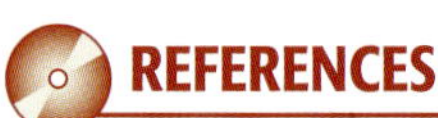

REFERENCES

Complete references available on DVD and online version at www.LongneckerAnesthesiology.com

CHAPTER 34

Monitoring and Managing Neuromuscular Blockade

Richard M. Pino
Hassan H. Ali

KEY POINTS

1. Muscle response to stimulation can be measured by mechanomyography, electromyography, acceleromyography, and direct palpation.
2. Commonly used patterns of stimulation are a single twitch, train of four, double burst, tetanic, and posttetanic count.
3. Succinylcholine, a depolarizing neuromuscular blocking drug (NMBD), is metabolized by plasma cholinesterase. Atypical pseudocholinesterases cannot metabolize pseudocholinesterase at a normal rate, and prolonged neuromuscular blockade may result.
4. Immobility, prolonged use of NMBDs, and upper and lower motor neuron disease may cause a proliferation of extrajunctional receptors. These receptors affect severe hyperkalemia when stimulated with succinylcholine.
5. Nondepolarizing NMBDs are benzylisoquinoline (mivacurium, atracurium, cisatracurium) and steroidal molecules (vecuronium, rocuronium, pancuronium).
6. The degradation of atracurium, cisatracurium, and mivacurium is independent of organ-specific elimination.
7. Pancuronium and vecuronium are metabolized in the liver to derivatives that are cleared by the kidney and that exhibit neuromuscular blocking activities. These derivatives accumulate with prolonged administration and renal insufficiency.
8. Reversal agents increase the concentration of acetylcholine in the junctional clefts to compete with the NMBDs to restore muscle activity.
9. Clinical criteria, in addition to evoked responses, should be used to assess the recovery of neuromuscular blockade.
10. Residual neuromuscular blockade is a persistent and common clinical problem.

Muscle relaxation can be achieved by direct central nervous system depression with volatile inhalation anesthetics or by neural blockade either at the peripheral nerve or with drugs that act at the neuromuscular junction. Neuromuscular blocking drugs (NMBD) are essential in anesthetic practice to facilitate tracheal intubation and provide optimum surgical conditions for a variety of procedures. The use of NMBDs is to significantly reduce the concentration of volatile anesthetics required to provide adequate analgesia. NMBDs have no inherent analgesic or amnestic properties, and their use is contraindicated if artificial ventilation is not possible.

HISTORICAL PERSPECTIVE

In 1850, Pelouze and Bernard demonstrated that curare, the arrow poison used by certain South American Indian tribes, abolished the effect of nerve stimulation on muscle but did not affect the excitability of either nerve or muscle. Curare and nicotine were thought to act directly on muscle through "receptive substances" rather than by action on axonal endings until stimulation of the vagus nerve was demonstrated to produce a substance, later identified as acetylcholine (ACh), as transmitter at the myoneural junction of voluntary muscle.

CELL BIOLOGY OF MUSCLE CONTRACTION

BASIC MYONEURAL STRUCTURE

A motor unit is a series of muscle fibers that is innervated by the same motor nerve.[1] This nerve enters skeletal muscle and ramifies to an extent that depends on the function of the specific muscle. For example, each muscle fiber of an extraocular eye muscle is innervated by a single neuron. In contrast, muscles that contract for more coarse activities (eg, maintenance of posture) have multiple fascicles that are innervated by a single nerve fiber.

Stimulation of a single motor nerve leads to contraction of all the muscle fibers contained within the particular motor unit. As the axons terminate in troughs on the surface of the muscle fibers, their myelin sheaths are lost. The neuromuscular junction is the synapse that is formed at the endplate region of the muscle membrane and bare terminal of the motor nerve (**Figs. 34-1** and **34-2**). The synaptic cleft is a 50-nm-wide extracellular space that spans the short distance between the neuronal and muscle cell membranes.

SYNTHESIS OF ACETYLCHOLINE

Neuromuscular transmission begins with synthesis of the enzyme choline acetyltransferase in the organelle-rich cell body of the axon followed by distal intracellular transport to the nerve terminal where it is concentrated (Fig. 34-1). The choline acetyltransferase catalyzes the synthesis of ACh from acetyl-coenzyme A (acetyl-CoA) and choline. Hydrolysis of ACh in the junctional cleft is the primary source of choline. Most of the ACh (~60%) is stored in thousands of synaptic vesicles of the nerve terminal. These are arranged in a triangular pattern with the apex of each triangle close to a thickened area of the prejunctional membrane (Figs. 34-1 and 34-2). This so-called active zone may be part of a system that orients and controls the site of release of ACh from the synaptic vesicles. The remainder of neural ACh is free in the cytoplasm. In the absence of nerve impulses, spontaneous release of small amounts of ACh depolarizes the postjunctional membrane to a small extent. These 0.5- to 1.5-mV depolarizations, called *miniature endplate potentials*, are approximately 0.01 the magnitude of a standard endplate potential and are not significant enough to trigger muscle contraction. According to the quantum theory,[2] calcium-mediated fusion of synaptic vesicles with the presynaptic membrane simultaneously releases approximately 200 to 400 quanta of ACh into the synaptic cleft. Each quantum contains 500 to 25 000 molecules of ACh. Motor neuron action potentials propagate via voltage-responsive ion channels that, in turn, open channels in the nerve terminal that serve as pathways for the influx of ionized calcium at the active zone.

ACETYLCHOLINE RECEPTORS

The postsynaptic membrane is highly folded, increasing its surface area to allow a high concentration of nicotinic postjunctional receptors (Figs. 34-1 and 34-2). Each receptor is composed of 5 integral linear protein subunits arranged as a rosette in the membrane: 2 α and 1 each

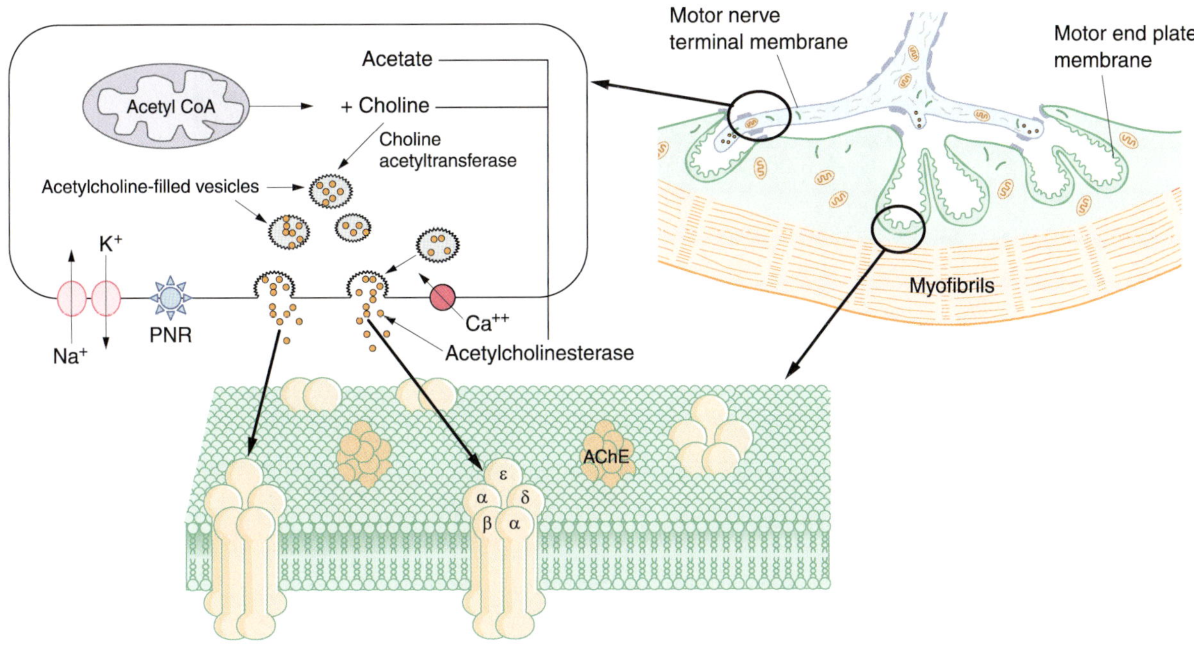

FIGURE 34-1. Schematic representation of the nerve terminal and myoneural junction. See text for details. PNR, prejunctional nicotinic receptor.

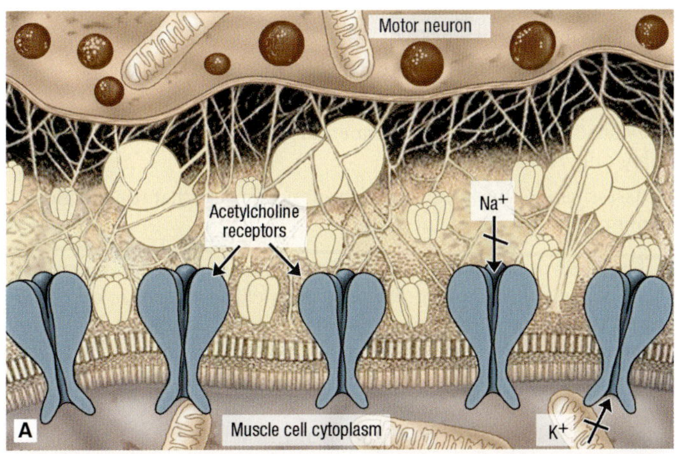

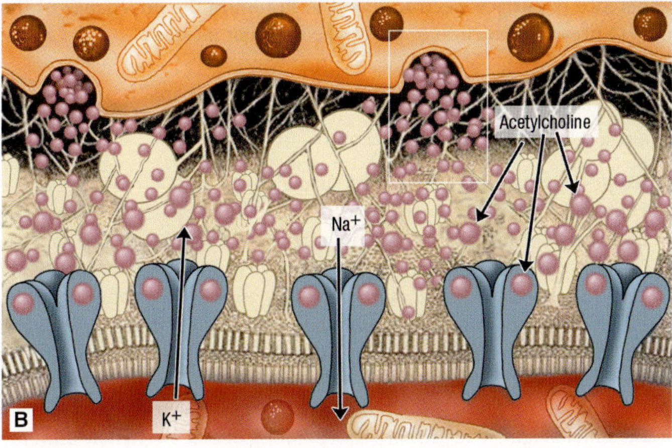

FIGURE 34-2. The myoneural junction. **A.** In the absence of acetylcholine (ACh), receptors of the muscle cell membrane are closed. The transmembrane movement of sodium (Na^+) and potassium (K^+) is blocked, and the muscle does not contract. **B.** A quantum of ACh molecules (outlined in *square*) released from the motor neuron binds to receptors. When these bind to the active site of both α-subunits, the receptor undergoes a conformational change, opening a central channel for the passage of ions, resulting in depolarization and muscle contraction.

of β, δ, and ε. Each subunit contains 4 helical domains. The sites of binding for ACh and NMBD are on the extracellular α-subunits, although the receptors span the entire muscle cell membrane contacting both extracellular and intracellular spaces. The binding sites for ACh on the 2 α-subunits are not identical and can be characterized into high- and low-affinity sites based on their binding of competitive antagonists. Both sites must be occupied by ACh to propagate a muscle cell depolarization (Fig. 34-2). After ACh binds to the active site of both α-subunits, the receptor undergoes a conformational change, opening a central channel within the 5 subunits. The structure of this channel permits the transit of sodium, potassium, and calcium ions while blocking anions and larger cations. When nondepolarizing NMBDs bind to either α-subunit, the channels cannot open and a neuromuscular blockade occurs (**Fig. 34-3**A).

DEPOLARIZATION AND MUSCLE CONTRACTION

Most of the released ACh molecules cross the synaptic clefts, bind to postjunctional receptors, and induce depolarization of the muscle cell. Depolarizations are created by the influx of sodium through specific channels, decreasing the membrane potential from –90 to +50 mV. During depolarization, as the membrane potential approximates 0 mV, potassium channels open, and sodium channels close to limit the voltage flux to +10 mV. The action potential is self-propagating after a threshold has been reached through a decrease in the adjacent membrane potential of approximately 15 mV, which opens sodium channels and depolarizes the membrane.

Depolarization is an all-or-none process. After it has begun, it continues until the entire membrane has depolarized. The strengths of individual contractions are independent of the individual action potential amplitudes. They depend on the sum of repetitive, additive, and fused contractions of different motor units. Calcium is released from the sarcoplasmic reticulum of the muscle upon depolarization to activate actin–myosin coupling within myofibrils resulting in contraction. Upon completion of depolarization, the ionic gradient is restored via an Na^+/K^+-dependent adenosine triphosphate (ATPase) to repolarize the membrane, and a refractory period follows during which time depolarization is not possible. After depolarization is completed, the concentration of ACh markedly decreases in the synaptic cleft by diffusion through the postjunctional receptor. ACh is further reduced by degradation into

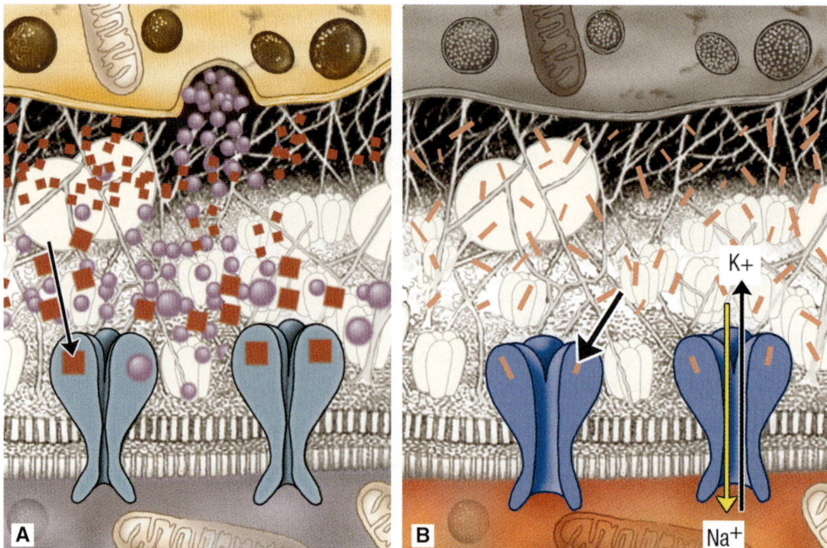

FIGURE 34-3. Comparison of neuromuscular blockade between nondepolarizing blockers and succinylcholine. With nondepolarizing blockade (**A**), a single molecule (*arrow*) bound to an acetylcholine (Ach) receptor channel keeps the channel closed, preventing muscle contraction. In contrast, when succinylcholine is bound to the receptor (**B**), the channel is open, allowing for the movement of potassium and sodium to depolarize the membrane. This depolarized state prevents further muscle contraction by Ach until the succinylcholine diffuses away from the receptor.

acetate and choline by acetylcholinesterase, a key enzyme that is concentrated in the basal lamina of the muscle cell.

PREJUNCTIONAL RECEPTORS

The response of muscle contraction is also modulated by prejunctional receptors of the motor neuron. It is theorized that released ACh interacts with prejunctional nicotinic, and possibly muscarinic, receptors to further augment transmitter release. These receptors are believed to control a sodium-specific ion channel in contrast to the nonspecific cation channels of the postjunctional receptors. Sodium is essential for the synthesis and mobilization of ACh, but it is not directly involved in the release process. Therefore, nondepolarizing NMBD can bind to these ion channels, decrease the mobilization of ACh, and reduce its release from nerves that are stimulated with high-frequency stimuli. The clinical equivalent is seen in the fade to tetanic and train-of-four (TOF) stimulation.

EXTRAJUNCTIONAL RECEPTORS

Muscle cells can also exhibit a variable number of extrajunctional receptors that are embryologic remnants of the muscle cell membrane. In fetuses, these receptors are found throughout the muscle cell membrane. With maturation, extrajunctional receptors become markedly reduced while junctional receptors predominate. In addition to differences in their location, extrajunctional receptors have γ-subunits substituted for the ε-subunit of the junctional receptor. Extrajunctional receptors also have short half-lives of less than 1 day compared with the longer than 1-week half-lives of junctional receptors. Compared with junctional receptors, they are less sensitive to stimulation by ACh but have channels that remain open approximately 4 times longer than the postjunctional receptors. The clinical significance of extrajunctional receptors becomes evident when they proliferate in response to upper and lower neuron damage, muscular injury and disease (some muscular dystrophies, disuse atrophy, and even cast immobilization), and trauma associated with major burns.[3]

TECHNIQUES USED TO MONITOR NEUROMUSCULAR BLOCKADE

We have described the basic mechanisms controlling the contraction of a single muscle fiber. This knowledge must be extrapolated to the bedside analysis of the contraction of anatomically distinct muscles to assess the patient's degree of neuromuscular blockade.

Objectives of clinical monitoring are as follows:

- Titration of NMBD doses to the desired level of paralysis
- Detection of unusual sensitivity, resistance, or altered clearance of a relaxant in the course of the anesthetic
- Evaluation of whether neuromuscular blockade can be pharmacologically reversed
- Assessment of the adequacy of reversal to ensure that residual neuromuscular blockade is not present

The depth of neuromuscular blockade often is assessed by a measurement of the contraction of the adductor pollicis muscle as elicited by stimulation of the ulnar nerve at the wrist with surface electrodes.[4] When the ulnar nerve is not accessible, stimulation of several other peripheral nerves is useful (**Fig. 34-4**). The stimulus used to evoke muscle contraction usually is a rectangular waveform of 0.2-millisecond duration.[4,5] It is important to adequately clean and lightly abrade the skin for optimum adherence of surface electrodes and to minimize the impedance of the skin to prevent reduction in the applied current intensity.

PATTERNS OF STIMULATION

There are 5 patterns of stimulation.

1. *Single-twitch stimulus* (**Fig. 34-5**) usually is given at a frequency of 0.1 Hz, that is, 1 stimulus every 10 seconds.[4,6] The current is incrementally increased until a maximum twitch height is obtained. A current that is slightly greater than that used to achieve maximum twitch height is called the *supramaximal stimulus*. After an NMBD is administered, the decrements in twitch height are compared as percentages of the control twitch. This stimulus pattern is most often used to establish the basic pharmacodynamic properties of an NMBD. For example, the ED_{95} is the dose at which the twitch height is depressed by 95% of maximal height. The primary shortcoming of a single-twitch stimulus is the requirement for a control response before the administration of the NMBD.
2. *TOF stimulation* (TOF; **Fig. 34-6**) is the most commonly used stimulus.[4,7,8] Each train consists of 4 stimuli at 2 Hz (4 stimuli in 2 seconds) that are again repeated every 10 to 12 seconds. In the absence of neuromuscular blockade, the TOF evokes 4 twitches of equal strength when the abducted thumb is palpated after stimulation of the

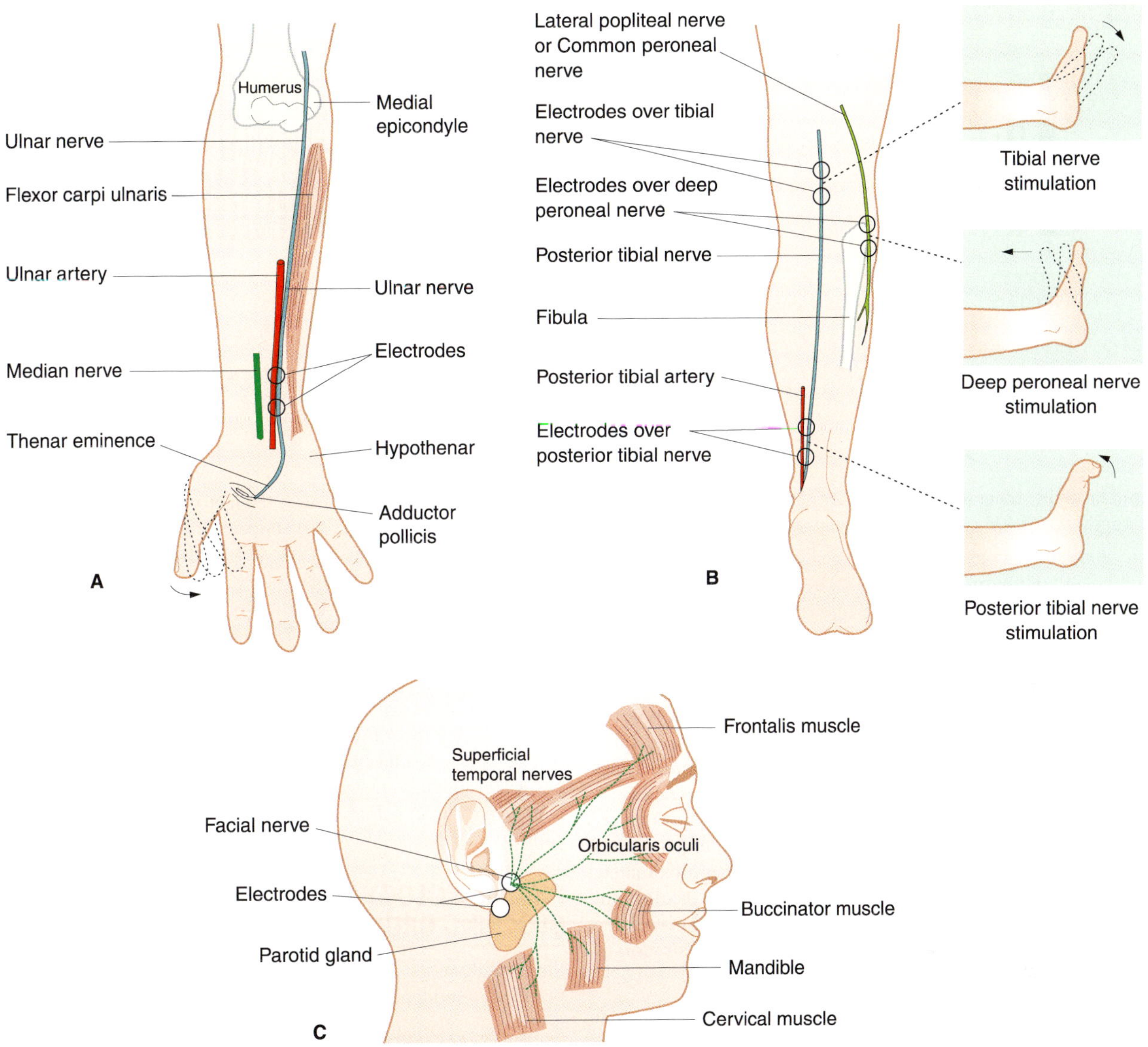

FIGURE 34-4. Diagram of sites suitable for nerve stimulation. **A.** Ulnar nerve. **B.** Tibial, deep peroneal, and posterior tibial nerves. **C.** Facial nerve. [Reprinted and modified from Ali HH. Monitoring neuromuscular function. *Semin Anesth.* 1989;8:158, with permission from Elsevier.]

ulnar nerve. Because the strength of the first twitch (T_1) is compared with the second, third, and fourth twitches, control twitches are not required. With the onset of neuromuscular blockade, release of ACh by the first stimulus often evokes an adequate contraction. However, the ability of neurons to replenish and release ACh progressively diminishes with each stimulus of the TOF in the successive train. This can be manifested in 2 ways. First, with the onset of neuromuscular blockade, the amplitude of the fourth twitch (T_4) decreases with successive stimuli. Second, within each TOF, there is a clear decrement between T_4 and T_1. The ratio of T_4 to T_1 can be easily compared if it is objectively measured. In clinical practice, when the strength of the first twitch is reduced to 75% of the maximal height, only 3 twitches will be demonstrable. With increased neuromuscular blockade to a T_1 of 20%, 2 twitches will be observed. At 90% suppression of T_1, only 1 twitch will be perceptible. These patterns are reversed as muscle activity returns and can be used with other clinical criteria to help determine the patient's suitability for extubation. Initial studies demonstrated that at T_4/T_1 = 0.75, awake patients can sustain a

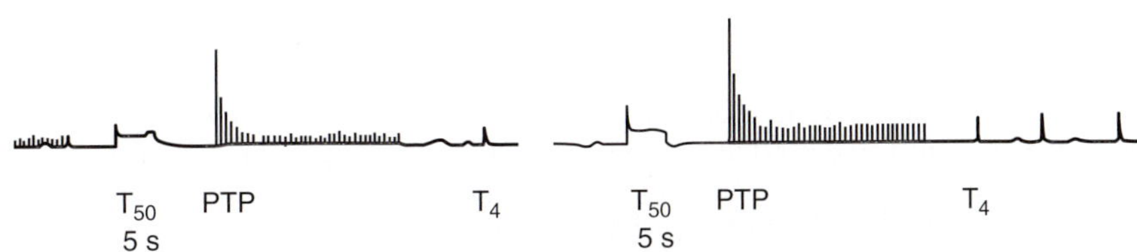

FIGURE 34-5. Evoked thumb adduction in response to single-twitch stimulation of 0.1 Hz before and after tetanic stimulation at 50 Hz for 5 seconds. Note the tetanic fade and posttetanic potentiation (PTP).

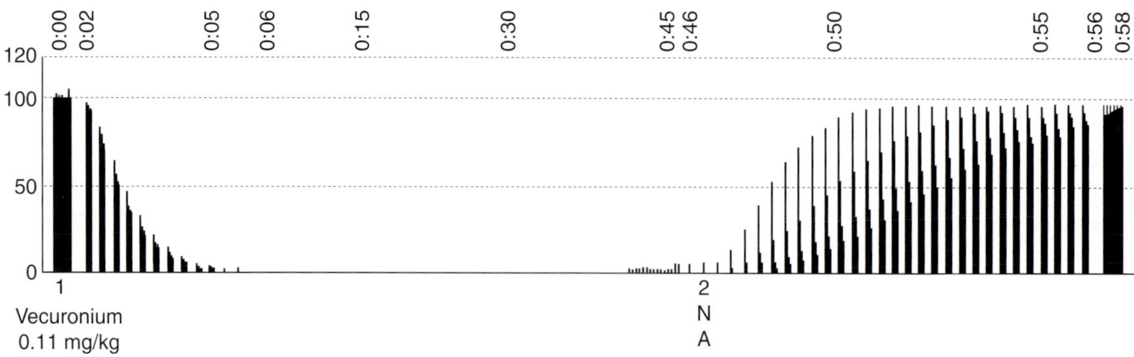

FIGURE 34-6. Integrated evoked electromyographic response to train-of-four (TOF) stimulation shows the response to vecuronium 0.11 mg/kg. At 47 minutes, the first response to TOF recovered spontaneously to 10% of control. Note that during the onset, there is minimal fade compared with that during recovery. Neostigmine (N) 4.0 mg and atropine (A) 1.5 mg were administered. Note the development of T_2, T_3, and T_4 and the progressive increase in the TOF ratio, which reached 0.8 after 11 minutes of reversal.

5-second head lift, generate a vital capacity of 15 to 20 mL/kg with an inspiratory force of −25 cm H_2O, and cough effectively.[9]

3. *Tetanic stimulation* is used in conjunction with the TOF. When a profound depth of neuromuscular blockade has been established, the twitch response to TOF stimulation is abolished.[4,6] With stimulation at a tetanic frequency of 50 Hz for 5 seconds, increased quanta of ACh are released into the synaptic cleft. The increased ACh causes a sustained muscle contraction during the stimulus and also augments its own subsequent release if a single TOF stimulus follows. This enhanced response after tetanic stimulation is called *posttetanic potentiation* (Fig. 34-5). A *posttetanic count* can be obtained when a stimulation of 1 Hz is can be applied 3 seconds after tetanus. A posttetanic count of 10 has been found to coincide with the appearance of the first twitch of the TOF. A posttetanic count of 1 indicates that the first twitch of the TOF should appear in approximately 30 minutes when pancuronium is used or 8 minutes with vecuronium and atracurium.[10] In the absence of a posttetanic twitch, the blockade is sufficiently profound to suggest that immediate administration of reversal agents will not be effective.

4. *Double-burst stimulation* (DBS) was devised to increase the manual perception of fade.[4,11,12] DBS consists of 2 short bursts of 3 stimuli at 50 Hz separated by 750 milliseconds. The responses to each burst are close enough to be palpated as a strong single muscle contraction. Any fade that is manifested with a partial blockade may be easier to detect between the sets of stimuli with DBS than with TOF. In the absence of fade to DBS, there is a 90% chance that TOF is 0.6 or greater, and a 75% chance that TOF is less than 0.6 when fade is present.

METHODS USED TO QUANTIFY MUSCLE RESPONSES[4,13] (FIG. 34-7)

Mechanomyography is an extremely accurate method that has been used for research on the basic pharmacodynamics properties of NMBDs. An isometric tension of a known preload is placed on the thumb. The thumb is attached to a transducer that measures the force of contraction of the adductor pollicis brevis muscle.

Electromyography (EMG) monitors compound motor unit action potentials that are generated a few milliseconds after the stimulus is delivered to a nerve. Two sensing electrodes are placed over a specific muscle and a ground electrode applied between the stimulating and sensing electrodes. The thenar, hypothenar, and first dorsal interosseous muscles of the hand are usually studied. Although each muscle cell responds in an all-or-none fashion, the amplitude of the EMG signal is proportional to the number of individual action potentials. In principle, the advantage of EMG is that it is closest to direct assessment of function of the neuromuscular junction.

Acceleromyography measures the isotonic acceleration across a joint with a small piezoelectric transducer.[14] This technique considers that the acceleration of a muscle is directly proportional to the force of contraction (assuming the muscle mass is constant). Acceleromyography is simple to perform and is clinically useful. One disadvantage is the inconsistency of the response.

Direct palpation of an abducted thumb during contractions evoked by ulnar nerve stimulation is the most common method used to assess neuromuscular blockade. With palpation, the clinician measures both the force of isometric contraction and the force of acceleration. Although it is a subjective assessment of neuromuscular blockade and has a considerable margin of error even in the hands of experienced clinicians,[15] direct palpation with TOF remains the standard in routine clinical practice.

PHARMACOLOGY OF NEUROMUSCULAR BLOCKING DRUGS

Pharmacokinetics and pharmacodynamics are 2 important concepts pertinent to understanding the pharmacology of NMBD.

PHARMACOKINETICS

Pharmacokinetics is the mathematical description of the plasma concentration of the drug over time. The plasma concentration of a drug is initially high after an intravenous (IV) bolus and is followed by a rapid decline toward equilibrium during the distribution phase as a result of transfer between blood and tissue compartments. The initial volume of distribution (V_I) is the distribution space of the vessel-rich organs in contrast to the volume of distribution at steady state (Vd_{ss}), which is the apparent volume needed to explain the drug concentration after equilibrium between blood and the various tissues. The distribution half-life ($t_{1/2}\alpha$) defines the time needed for the blood concentration to decline by 50% and occurs before the elimination phase begins. This is quantified from the slope of the natural log of the blood concentration–time curve in the distribution phase. The $t_{1/2}\alpha$ is 2 to 10 minutes for the nondepolarizing NMBD. During the elimination phase, plasma levels of a relaxant decline at a slower rate than during the distribution phase because of excretion of the drug or its metabolite via the kidneys or the liver, spontaneous degradation, or a combination of both. The elimination half-life ($t_{1/2}\beta$) is computed from the slope of the natural log of the blood concentration–time curve for the elimination phase and is the time required for the plasma drug concentration to decrease by 50%. The $t_{1/2}\beta$ is sensitive to changes in either the volume of distribution at steady state or the clearance (C_L). The latter is defined as the volume of blood that is completely cleared of the drug per unit time. Whereas the $t_{1/2}\beta$ can range from 2.5 minutes (mivacurium) to approximately 2 hours (pancuronium), C_L can vary from 2 to 100 mL/kg/min.

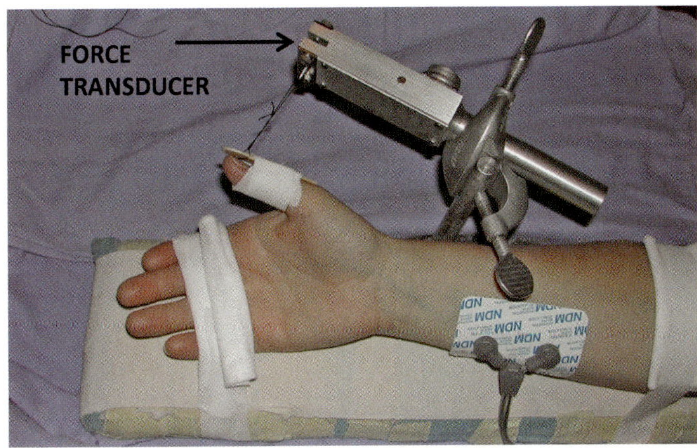

A

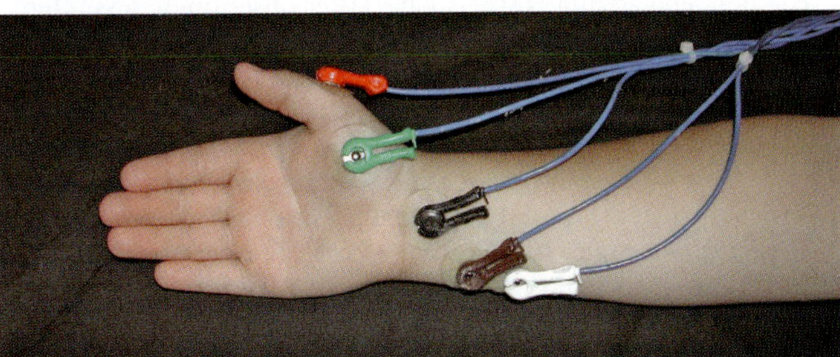

B

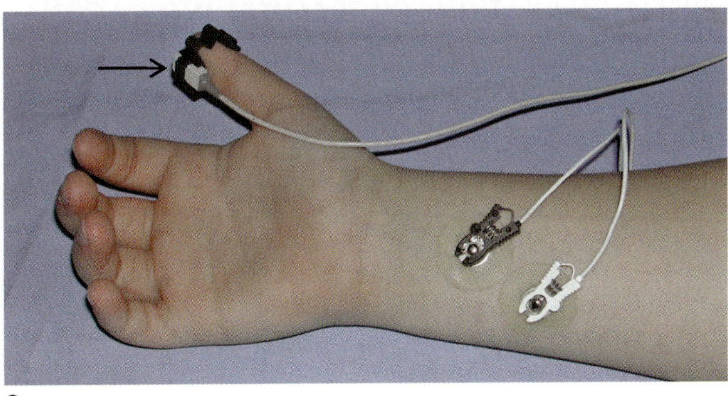

C

FIGURE 34-7. Methods used to quantify muscle responses to stimulation. **A.** Mechanomyography. After stimulation of the ulnar nerve at the wrist with surface electrodes (*arrow*), a transducer measures the force of contraction of the adductor pollicis brevis muscle. This force is recorded as depicted in Fig. 34-16 as an example. **B.** Electromyography. After stimulation of the ulnar nerve (brown and white electrodes), electrical activity of the adductor pollicis brevis is obtained through the green and red electrodes (black electrode is ground). The amplitude of the signal is proportional to the number of individual action potentials (ie, the degree of neuromuscular blockade). **C.** Acceleromyography. The *arrow* indicates a piezoelectric transducer that measures the acceleration of the adductor pollicis brevis muscle as a direct proportion of the force of contraction.

Figures 34-11 to 34-13 and Table 34-6 compare the Vd_{ss}, C_L, and $t_{1/2}\beta$ of the currently used neuromuscular blockers in adults and children.

PHARMACODYNAMICS

Pharmacodynamics is the principle of pharmacology that is most applicable to the clinical use of NMBDs. Pharmacodynamics includes the characterization of the therapeutic, pharmacologic, and toxic effects of the drug as well as the mechanism of drug action at the receptor. Dose–response studies of NMBD have established the relationship between increasing doses of a drug and the extent of neuromuscular blockade. When a dose is simply plotted against response, comparisons of 1 NMBD with another become difficult. The ED_{95} of an NMBD is the dose that blocks neuromuscular transmission to the point of reducing the height of single controlled twitches by 95%. To estimate the ED_{95} of a relaxant and determine appropriate doses for intubation, a straight-line dose–response curve is needed. A log-dose probit analysis assigns an arbitrary number (probit) to each level of blockade (including 0% response and 100% response) to generate a straight line and facilitate the determination of the extent of block versus dose (**Fig. 34-8**). The potency of different NMBD then can be compared by examining the slope and parallelism of these straight lines. Different slopes and the absence of parallelism may indicate different mechanisms of blockade.

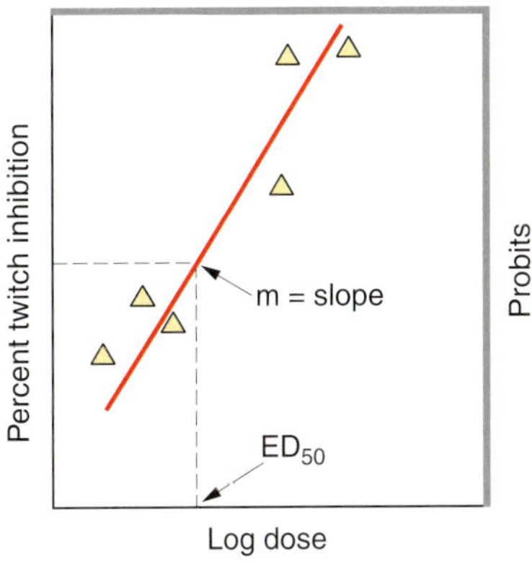

FIGURE 34-8. Log dose-probit transformation allows calculation of dose–response relationship (ED_{50}), estimation of ED_{95}, and comparison of potencies and mechanisms among different neuromuscular blocking drugs.

Although it is desirable to know the concentration–response relationships at the site of drug action, it usually is not possible to do so. An assumption is that a close relationship exists between the concentration of the drug in the plasma and the concentration at postjunctional receptors. This type of relationship for NMBDs is determined during continuous infusions at steady-state conditions, and comparisons between relaxants are noted by concentration in plasma at steady state and 50% paralysis ($Cpss_{50}$). Dose–response relationships (ED_{50}) and concentration–response relationships ($Cpss_{50}$) are altered by disease states, normal differences in physiology, and drug interactions and are reflected in differing dose requirements or plasma levels required to achieve the desired degree of blockade.

ONSET AND RECOVERY OF NEUROMUSCULAR BLOCKADE

The onset time of an NMBD is the time to the maximum neuromuscular blockade. It is inversely related to potency.[16,17] Rapid plasma clearance contributes to a fast onset because the maximum drug effect occurs when the concentrations in the plasma and at the neuromuscular junction are equal. As the plasma concentration is decreasing, the effective concentration at the neuromuscular junction is increasing. Recovery from neuromuscular blockade begins immediately after both the plasma and junctional concentrations of the NMBD decrease. Therefore, when NMBDs have both equal potencies and equilibration rates, the drug with the faster clearance will cause a neuromuscular blockade more rapidly and of lesser magnitude than the NMBD with the slower clearance. A rapid onset and greater peak effect can be obtained by increasing the dose of the more rapidly cleared NMBD as long as there are no side effects with the increased dose. Thus, whereas high-potency, low-clearance drugs have slow onsets, low-potency, rapid-clearance drugs have fast onsets. Succinylcholine (SCh) has the fastest onset time to maximum effect (**Table 34-1**; **Fig. 34-9**). Recovery of NMBD is the spontaneous return to a percentage of activity, for example, the time to 25% of the original twitch height (also called the recovery index). The onset and recovery times for NMBDs are compared in **Figs. 34-9** and **34-10**.

TABLE 34-1 Pharmacodynamics of Succinylcholine

	Dose (mg/kg)	Onset	Time to 25% Recovery (min)	Time to 95% Recovery
ED_{95}	0.2-0.25	1 min	8	12
Routine intubation	0.5-1.0	45 sec	10	12-15
Rapid intubation	1.0	4 sec	10	12-15
Pretreated intubation	1.5	1.5 min	10	12-15
D-Tubocurarine (3 mg)				
Pancuronium (1 mg)				
Vecuronium (1 mg)				
Infusion (mg/kg/min)	60-100	–	6[a]	15-30[a]

[a]After infusion stopped.

[b]The ED_{95} is the dose that blocks the height of single controlled twitches by 95%.

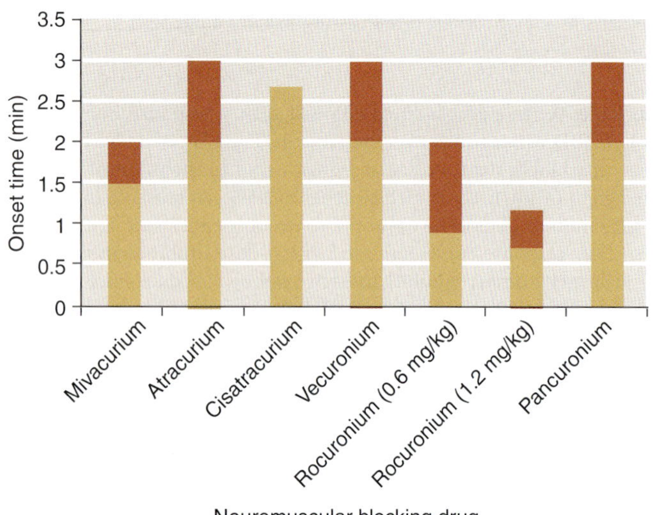

FIGURE 34-9. The onset times of nondepolarizing neuromuscular blockers are compared. In this figure and Figures 34-10 to 34-13, the *blue bars* indicate means, and the *red bars* show the ranges. The chart demonstrates that the onset times are between 2 and 3 minutes with the exception of the higher dose of rocuronium, which has an onset of approximately 1 minute.

The nondepolarizing NMBDs have faster onset times, less intense effects, and more rapid recoveries at the diaphragm and intrinsic muscles of the larynx than at the adductor pollicis.[18,19] This characteristic allows tracheal intubation at lesser degrees of neuromuscular blockade than evidenced at the adductor pollicis under adequate anesthesia. This is especially important for mivacurium because it is possible to have sufficient relaxation of laryngeal muscles while the adductor pollicis and other muscles still have activity. Furthermore, when the adductor pollicis twitch is abolished using small doses of mivacurium (≤0.15 mg/kg), the laryngeal muscles may already be recovering and intubation may be difficult.

MUSCLE RELAXATION FOR TRACHEAL INTUBATION

The most common use for NMDBs is to facilitate endotracheal intubation during general anesthesia. This is especially important during a rapid sequence induction to swiftly intubate the trachea to protect the lungs from gastric contents. The standard drug for such rapid intubation remains SCh (Table 34-1). When SCh is contraindicated, either an awake intubation can be performed or nondepolarizing relaxants can be administered. Conditions appropriate for intubation can be achieved within 2 minutes after administration of large doses of rocuronium, pancuronium, and cisatracurium, although the duration of neuromuscular blockade will be prolonged. To minimize unwanted cardiovascular side effects that may be produced with high doses of

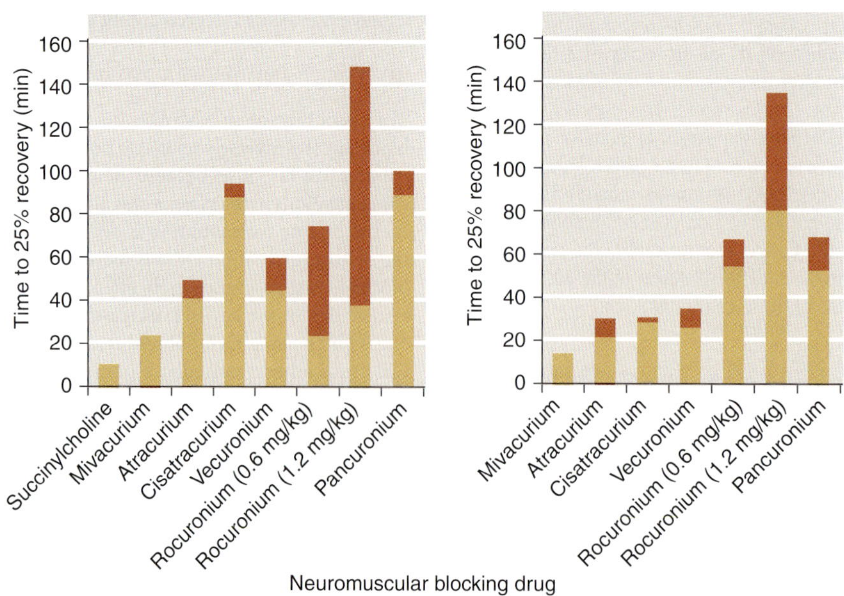

FIGURE 34-10. Times to 25% and 95% recovery. Although rocuronium had the shortest onset time (see Fig. 34-9), it has the widest range of recovery times to both 25% and 95%.

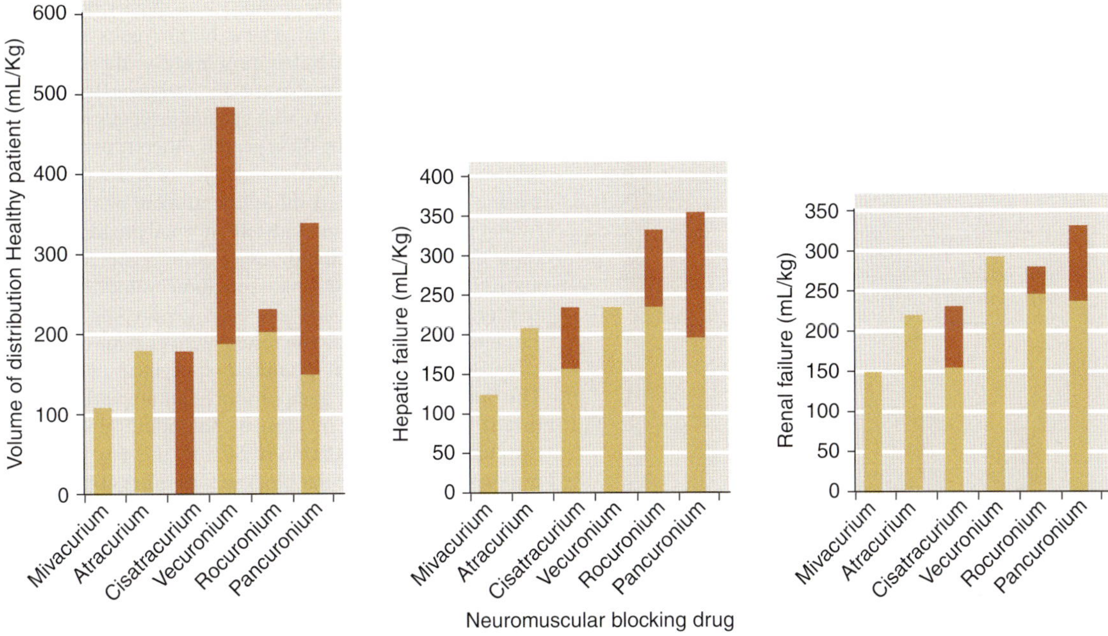

FIGURE 34-11. Volume of distribution of neuromuscular blocking drugs in normal patients and those with liver and kidney disease. The overall trend is the increase in volume of distribution of the steroidal neuromuscular blocking drug compared with the benzylisoquinolines.

pancuronium, atracurium, or mivacurium, a divided dose technique may be used. The rationale for the divided dose technique is the initial binding of a large number of postjunctional receptors by a subparalytic dose of a nondepolarizing relaxant, called the "priming dose," which is insufficient to produce cardiovascular side effects. The balance of receptors subsequently is blocked to facilitate intubation within a short time after administration of the second dose of the NMBD.[20] For example, using the divided dose technique for mivacurium,[21] excellent intubation conditions were achieved by 90 seconds and were identical to those obtained after rocuronium was administered at 3 (0.9 mg/kg) and 4 (1.2 mg/kg) times the ED_{95}.[22]

There are several caveats for the priming principle.[23] In some studies, the priming and intubating doses were determined after induction of anesthesia[24-26] and may not be appropriate for an urgent anesthetic when the patient has a full stomach. Individual patients differ in their sensitivity and response to relaxants. Some patients are not adequately relaxed after 90 seconds, and during light anesthesia, they may cough, jerk, vomit, or have laryngospasm. Many patients have diplopia from the priming dose, and in some patients, more troublesome effects of neuromuscular blockade develop, such as difficulty swallowing, airway obstruction, or inadequate ventilation. Without exception, after a priming dose is given, constant monitoring for these adverse effects is mandatory. Any comorbidity that impairs muscle blood flow (eg, decreased blood volume or decreased cardiac output) will delay delivery of the NMBD to the neuromuscular junction and slow the onset of neuromuscular blockade.[27]

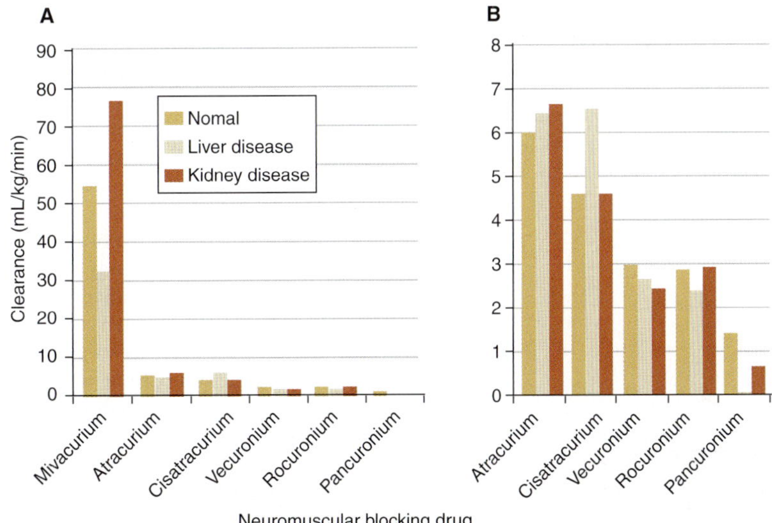

FIGURE 34-12. Clearance of neuromuscular blocking drugs (NMBDs) in normal patients and those with liver and kidney disease. Because of the high rate of clearance of mivacurium shown in **A, B** is provided to better compare the clearance of the intermediate and long-acting NMBD. The benzylisoquinolines have the highest rate of clearance because they do not depend on organ elimination and do not have active metabolites as do the steroidal NMBDs.

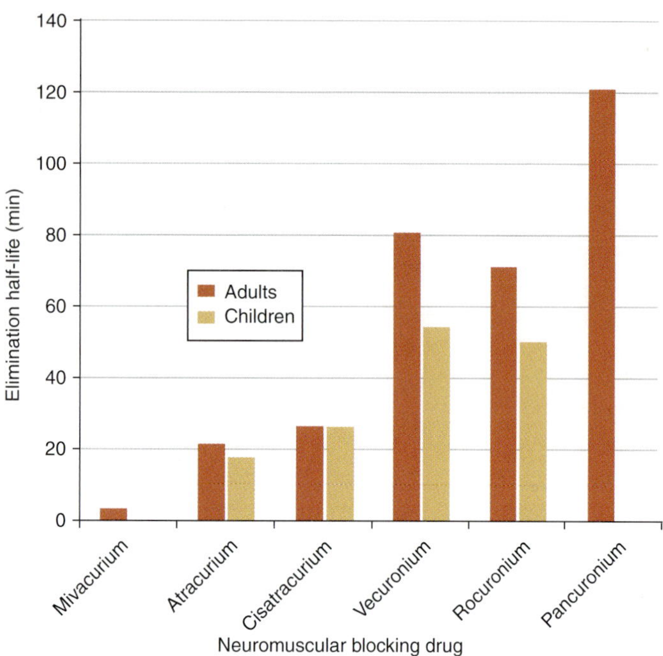

FIGURE 34-13. Elimination half-life of neuromuscular blocking drugs in adults and children. It has been reported that there are no differences between adults and children for mivacurium and pancuronium.

SUCCINYLCHOLINE

SCh is the only depolarizing NMBD in current use (Table 34-1 and Fig. 34-3B).[3] Because it is structurally 2 molecules of Ach linked together via the acetyl moieties (**Fig. 34-14**), SCh reacts with nicotinic receptors at the neuromuscular junction and in autonomic ganglia. Additional SCh binding to muscarinic postganglionic receptors in the heart, secretory glands, and smooth muscle is responsible for many of this drug's side effects. The customary dose for intubation is 1.0 mg/kg (Table 34-1). It has been suggested that a dose of 0.6 mg/kg is efficacious while the time to a return to spontaneous ventilation is decreased.[28]

The rapid onset and brief duration of action of SCh are this drug's major advantages. They result from rapid metabolism of SCh in plasma to succinylmonocholine (a metabolite of minimal potency). The enzyme responsible for this activity is butyrylcholinesterase, usually referred to as *plasma cholinesterase.* The rapid metabolism of SCh by plasma cholinesterase is responsible for its brief duration of action because relatively few of the injected molecules survive intact to reach the motor endplate (Fig. 34-3B). However, SCh molecules that reach the endplate are very resistant to metabolism by acetylcholinesterase, and neuromuscular blockade ends as SCh diffuses away from the neuromuscular junction.

Acetylcholine

$$CH_3\overset{O}{\overset{\|}{C}}OCH_2CH_2{}^{+}\underset{CH_3}{\overset{CH_3}{N}}{-}CH_3$$

Succinylcholine (diacetylcholine)

$$CH_3{-}\underset{CH_3}{\overset{CH_3}{N^+}}CH_2CH_2O\overset{O}{\overset{\|}{C}}CH_2 \vdots CH_2\overset{O}{\overset{\|}{C}}OCH_2{}^{+}\underset{CH_3}{\overset{CH_3}{N}}{-}CH_3$$

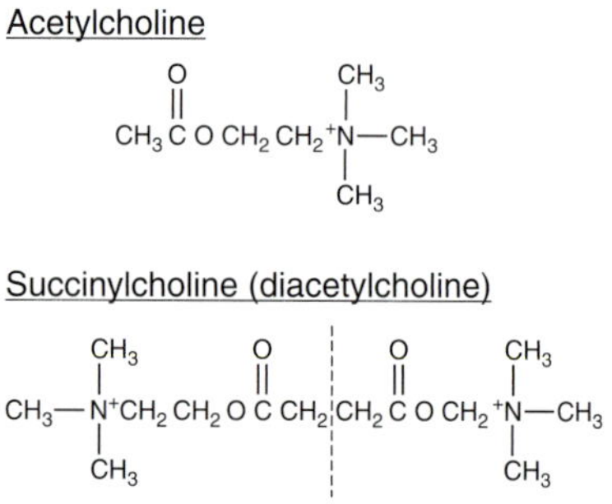

FIGURE 34-14. Chemical structures of acetylcholine and succinylcholine.

Two alleles control the quantity and quality of plasma cholinesterase (**Table 34-2**). The normal gene is homozygous in 96% of patients. The activity of SCh is moderately prolonged in the 4% of patients who are heterozygous with normal and 1 atypical gene. It is greatly prolonged in the remainder of patients who are homozygous for the atypical gene. A clinical test for assessing these genetic differences uses the local anesthetic dibucaine, which inhibits the activity of normal, but not the atypical, plasma cholinesterase. A dibucaine number above 80 (showing marked inhibition of the enzyme) indicates normal pseudocholinesterase, a dibucaine number below 30 indicates a homozygote for the atypical enzyme, and dibucaine numbers between these values indicate heterozygotes. A more recent approach has been genotyping plasma cholinesterase variants and correlating the results with enzyme activity.[29]

Rare genes code for 2 additional atypical plasma cholinesterases.[30] The fluoride-resistant gene produces an atypical plasma cholinesterase that is not inhibited in vitro by the addition of a fluoride ion. The extremely poor degradation of SCh by this enzyme results in a greatly prolonged neuromuscular blockade. Another atypical enzyme produced by the "silent gene" is incapable of metabolizing SCh.

Decreased amounts of plasma cholinesterase that cause prolonged responses to SCh occasionally are problematic in patients with severe liver disease and in peripartum patients. Inhibition of plasma cholinesterase by echothiophate eyedrops, anticholinesterases, organophosphate insecticides, hexafluorenium, phenelzine, and some cytotoxic tumor agents also prolong the duration of SCh's neuromuscular blockade. In the absence or inhibition of SCh metabolism, the drug is eliminated from plasma by redistribution and slow renal elimination.

PHASE I AND PHASE II BLOCKADE (TABLE 34-3)

Because of its structural similarity to ACh, SCh's interaction with the postjunctional receptors (Fig. 34-3B) creates an initial depolarization that spreads to adjacent membranes, causing disorganized contractions of motor units called *fasciculations.* Because SCh is not metabolized in the junctional cleft, the receptors and membranes remain depolarized and unresponsive to further stimuli, and paralysis ensues. After SCh diffuses away from the receptors, the membranes repolarize and again become responsive to normal neuromuscular transmission. This sequence of events is known as *depolarization blockade* or *phase I blockade.* It is characterized by (1) fasciculations, (2) decreased response to single nerve stimuli, (3) absence of fade to tetanus, (4) minimal fade to TOF, (5) no posttetanic facilitations, (6) enhancement of block by anticholinesterase agents, and (7) rapid recovery. However, given prolonged exposure of the neuromuscular junction to SCh, there is a conformational change at the receptors. The block that results, termed *phase II block,* resembles that obtained with nondepolarizing NMBD. This level of paralysis is characterized by (1) marked fade of tetanus and TOF (>50% fade), (2) posttetanic potentiation, (3) a tendency toward prolonged recovery in at least 50% of patients, and (4) the ability to reverse with anticholinesterases after plasma levels of SCh have been allowed to decrease (after waiting at least 10 minutes).

The establishment of a phase II blockade depends on the dose of SCh and the duration of SCh exposure. When inhalation agents are used to maintain anesthesia, a phase II block usually is heralded by a tachyphylaxis to SCh over a cumulative dose range between 10 and 12 mg/kg. The identification of greater than 50% fade on the TOF alerts the practitioner to the presence of phase II block, allows recovery to be followed over time, and permits the assessment of reversal after a plateau in recovery has been reached in patients in whom phase II blockade is prolonged.

SIDE EFFECTS

Hyperkalemia In normal patients, the depolarization induced by SCh administration causes an increase in serum potassium level of 0.5 to 1.0 mEq/L. In some patients with elevated baseline serum potassium levels, this modest increase in potassium level after SCh administration

TABLE 34-2 Plasma Cholinesterase Genotypes and Expected Response to Succinylcholine

Genotype	Incidence	Esterase Activity	Dibucaine Number	Fluoride Number	Response
N : N	96%	Normal	80	60	Normal
N : A	1:25	Moderately low	40-70	45	S_1 prolongation
N : F	1:200	S_1 low	75	50	S_1 prolongation
N : S	1:190	Moderately low	80	60	S_1 prolongation
A : F	1:20 000	Moderately low	45	35	Moderate prolongation
F : S	1:150 000	Very low	60	35	Moderate prolongation
F : F	1:150 000	Moderately low	70	30	Moderate prolongation
A : A	1:2500	Very low	20	20	Very prolonged
A : S	1:29 000	Very low	20	35	Very prolonged
S : S	1:100 000	None	None	None	Very prolonged

A, atypical gene; F, fluoride-resistant gene; N, normal gene; S, silent gene.

Modified from Whittaker M. Plasma cholinesterase variants and the anaesthetist. *Anaesthesia.* 1980;35:174.

will not cause a cardiac dysrhythmia.[31] However, the rapid increase in potassium from normal levels after SCh administration can be life threatening in patients with burns, massive tissue trauma, disuse atrophy, hemiparesis, spinal cord trauma, and neuromuscular disorders (eg, Guillain-Barré disease, amyotrophic lateral sclerosis, Friedreich ataxia).[3] Possible mechanisms for SCh-induced hyperkalemia are (1) loss of motor nerve control over motor endplates that results in a proliferation of extrajunctional receptors, (2) damaged muscle membranes, and (3) defective muscle membranes in certain muscle diseases. In the acutely injured state, the critically dangerous period begins after a grace period of 48 to 72 hours. With burns and trauma, this period of SCh susceptibility can persist until recovery is well under way, even for months. Patients with neuronal injuries, such as spinal cord trauma, can have exaggerated responses for more than 6 months. The use of SCh in children is justified only for rapid sequence inductions. It is not warranted for routine pediatric use based on the increased risk of hyperkalemia in children with as yet undiagnosed congenital myopathies.

Increased Intraocular Pressure SCh can increase the intraocular pressure (IOP). Increased IOP reaches a maximum approximately 2 minutes after SCh is administered and disappears in approximately 6 minutes. This increased IOP traditionally has been considered important for the patient with an open-eye injury wherein an increased IOP may cause irreversible loss of vitreous or global contents. However, studies from institutions with great experience with acute eye injuries have not shown adverse effects from use of SCh.[32-34] Pretreatment with a nondepolarizing relaxant, followed by deep anesthetic induction and SCh for intubation, may prevent an increase in IOP. Alternatively, conditions for rapid endotracheal intubation can be obtained using large doses of nondepolarizing NMBD (2 or 3 times ED_{95}), with the understanding that neuromuscular blockade will be greatly prolonged.

TABLE 34-3 Characteristics of Neuromuscular Blockade With Succinylcholine

Depolarizing (Phase I) Block

- Muscle fasciculation preceding the onset of neuromuscular blockade
- Absence of posttetanic potentiation
- Lack of fade to frequent stimulation (eg, tetanus, train of four, or double burst)
- Block antagonized by nondepolarizing drugs
- Block potentiated by acetylcholinesterase inhibitors

Nondepolarizing and Phase II Block

- Absence of muscle fasciculation
- Presence of posttetanic potentiation
- Fade with frequent stimulation
- Possible synergism between various groups of nondepolarizing relaxants
- Phase II block and nondepolarizing block potentiate each other
- Block may be reversed by acetylcholinesterase inhibitors

Increased Intragastric Pressure Increased intragastric pressure of approximately 40 cm H_2O occurs after SCh administration. This is blunted by pretreatment using a nondepolarizing drug followed by a larger dose of SCh (1.5 mg/kg) to achieve good intubating conditions. However, this increased gastric pressure is not believed to be clinically relevant because it is counterbalanced by an even greater increase in lower esophageal sphincter tone. Therefore, SCh is the most widely used drug for rapid sequence induction of patients with a suspected full stomach.

Increased Intracranial Pressure Increased intracranial pressure can occur via muscle fasciculations, creating a venous pressure elevation in epidural and jugular veins, and through increased cerebral blood flow. Pretreatment with a nondepolarizing relaxant prevents this increase. However, an insufficient depth of anesthesia and hypercapnia are even more significant factors increasing intracranial pressure than the minor effects of SCh.

SCh produces muscle contraction rather than relaxation in patients with myotonia congenita or myotonia dystrophica that can be severe enough to prevent intubation and ventilation. These contractures usually are self-limited and are not inhibited by nondepolarizing agents. Rhabdomyolysis and myoglobinuria can occur with SCh administration in some susceptible patients (eg, those with myopathies or glycogen storage diseases). Finally, SCh is a triggering agent to be avoided in patients susceptible to malignant hyperthermia.

NONDEPOLARIZING NEUROMUSCULAR BLOCKING DRUGS

CLASSIFICATION

Nondepolarizing NMBDs are classified by their duration of action and their chemical composition. The approximate duration of neuromuscular blockade provided by a single dose of these drugs may be short (<20 minutes), intermediate (45-60 minutes), or long (>1 hour). The currently available NMBDs are either benzylisoquinolines (**Fig. 34-15**) or steroidal molecules (Fig. 34-17). The benzylisoquinolines are based on the structure of D-tubocurarine (curare [dTC]), a naturally occurring substance obtained from the vine *Chondodendron tomentosum* found in the Amazon jungle. Curare is no longer commercially available. Pancuronium, the parent chemical of the steroidal NMBD, was formulated from the compound malouetine used by African tribesmen as arrowhead poison. Pancuronium is still used in clinical practice.

A brief discussion of the clinical pharmacology of commonly used nondepolarizing NMBDs is provided, beginning with the benzylisoquinolines in order of the duration of their neuromuscular blockade. Factors associated with either increased resistance and increased sensitivity to

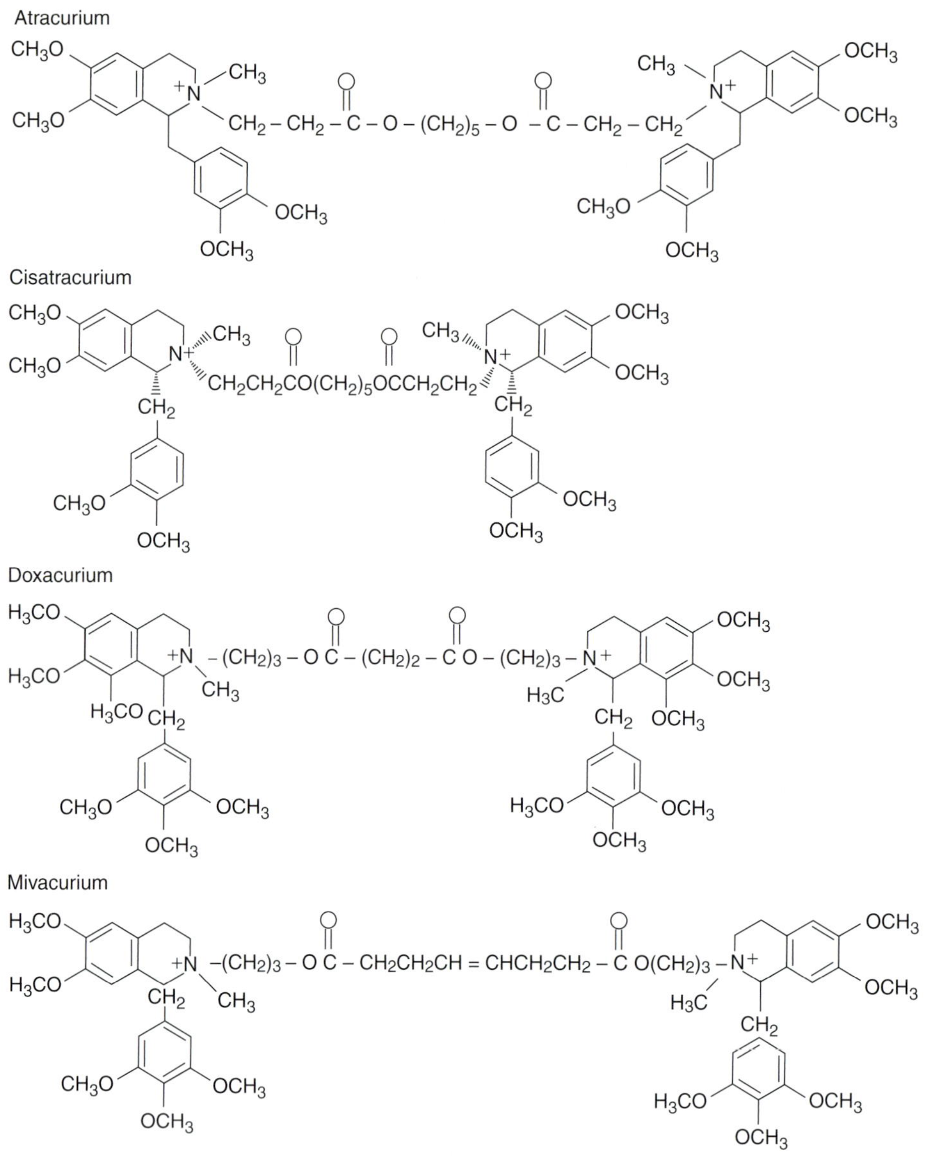

Atracurium

Cisatracurium

Doxacurium

Mivacurium

FIGURE 34-15. Chemical structures of the benzylisoquinoline neuromuscular blocking drugs.

nondepolarizing relaxants are summarized in **Tables 34-4** and **34-5**, respectively. **Table 34-6** lists the characteristics of non-depolarizing NMBDs in normal adults.

BENZYLISOQUINOLINES (FIG. 34-15)

Mivacurium (Short Acting) Mivacurium is a bisquaternary benzylisoquinoline diester with ED_{95} = 0.08 mg/kg, onset of 3.5 minutes (Fig. 34-9), recovery time to 25% of baseline twitch of 15 minutes, and total duration of approximately 25 minutes (Fig. 34-10).[35,36] It is no longer marketed in the United States but is still widely used in other countries. It is a relaxant with both a high potency and a high clearance rate. Although mivacurium is assumed to have an intermediate potency, its high potency is demonstrable in patients with atypical plasma cholinesterase, and its rapid clearance is partly based on destruction of the compound as well as its distribution. Because these characteristics are antagonistic, mivacurium has a slower onset than expected.

At comparable doses, mivacurium has twice the duration of SCh and half the duration of intermediate drugs such as atracurium and vecuronium (Fig. 34-10). The onset time can be shortened to 2 minutes by increasing the dose threefold. This increases the duration of the block by 20%.[35] Mivacurium can cause histamine release when large doses are given by IV bolus.[37] In approximately 50% of patients, histamine is released when 3 times the ED_{95} of mivacurium (0.25 mg/kg) is given within less than 30 seconds. However, when mivacurium was administered in a divided dose regimen of 0.15 mg/kg followed by 0.1 mg/kg

TABLE 34-4 Factors Associated With Resistance to Nondepolarizing Neuromuscular Blocking Drugs
Presence of extrajunctional receptors
Burns
Trauma (massive)
Upper motor neuron lesions
Lower motor neuron lesions
Demyelinating lesions (end-stage lesions may be very sensitive)
Prolonged immobilization
Aminophylline
Theophylline
Corticosteroids
Phenytoin

TABLE 34-5 Factors Associated With the Potentiation of Nondepolarizing Neuromuscular Blocking Drugs

Neuromuscular diseases
Myasthenia gravis
Muscular dystrophies
Inhalation anesthetics
Respiratory acidosis
Neonatal state
Hypokalemia
Hypocalcemia
Hypernatremia
Hypermagnesemia
Antibiotics
Local anesthetics
Calcium channel blockers
Steroids
Diuretics
Immunosuppressants
Antineoplastic agents

30 seconds later, histamine release did not occur, and good-to-excellent intubation conditions were achieved 90 seconds after the initial dose.[21,22] Mivacurium-induced blockade can be maintained by continuous infusion without alteration in its recovery characteristics.

The short duration of block produced by mivacurium (Fig. 34-10) is the result of rapid metabolism by plasma cholinesterase[35,38] at approximately 70% to 80% the rate of SCh hydrolysis.[38] Biochemical genetic analysis has shown that the K variant of the plasma cholinesterase gene prolongs recovery from mivacurium.[39] As a nondepolarizing agent, it is competitively reversed by anticholinesterases by augmenting the concentration of ACh at the neuromuscular junction.[35] However, recovery may be slowed after reversal with neostigmine in the presence of a dense block (the absence of a twitch or 1 twitch on TOF stimulation). This delayed recovery is the result of a concomitant inhibition of plasma cholinesterase slowing the hydrolysis of mivacurium by 20 to 60 minutes and markedly prolonging neuromuscular block in patients with low baseline levels of plasma cholinesterase. Therefore, before attempting reversal of mivacurium with anticholinesterases, there should be evidence of recovery manifested by the appearance of at least 2 twitches in response to TOF stimulation. Edrophonium may be a better choice of anticholinesterase to reverse the action of mivacurium because it inhibits its plasma cholinesterase to a lesser degree than does neostigmine. The recovery after a mivacurium infusion has been compared to recovery after infusions of atracurium, vecuronium, and SCh. Mivacurium blockade recovers from 5% to 95% approximately 15 minutes after stopping an infusion regardless of the duration of infusion.[35] It has half the duration of recovery of atracurium and vecuronium[40] and equals the best of phase II–type recoveries of SCh[41] given by infusion. Because mivacurium does not depend on organ metabolism for elimination, there is no tendency toward accumulation. It behaves consistently across age groups and in patients with comorbid disease states with normal plasma cholinesterase activity and hepatic synthetic function (Figs. 34-11 to 34-13).

Atracurium and Cisatracurium Atracurium and cisatracurium (Fig. 34-15) are bisquaternary benzylisoquinoline diesters with similar intermediate durations of action (Figs. 34-9 and 34-10) that produce 95% blockade.[42,43] They are unique nondepolarizing blocking drugs that were specifically synthesized to degrade spontaneously and are independent of organ elimination. At physiologic temperature and pH, the Hofmann elimination reaction breaks down both drugs to produce a tertiary amine, laudanosine, and a monoacrylate compound.[43,44] Laudanosine at high plasma levels can cause cerebral excitation and seizure activity in animals, but this has not been a clinical problem in humans. Atracurium is additionally metabolized by nonspecific plasma esterases to a quaternary alcohol and acid.[45]

Atracurium has an elimination half-life of approximately 20 minutes, and its plasma clearance rate is 5 to 6 mL/kg/min[46] (Figs. 34-11 to 34-13) This elimination half-life is approximately 7 times shorter than that of long-acting relaxants, with a clearance rate approximately 4 times faster. The pharmacodynamics and pharmacokinetics of atracurium are relatively unaltered in patients with renal failure[47] or hepatic failure,[46] in infants and children,[45,48] in elderly adults,[49] and when given by continuous infusion[50] (Figs. 34-10 to 34-13). Repeated administration or infusion shows no tendency for accumulation as evidenced by increased recovery times[42] (**Fig. 34-16**). Atracurium causes release of histamine and hypotension when administered at doses greater than 2.5 times its ED_{95}, especially when given as a rapid bolus (<15 seconds). When doses below 0.5 mg/kg are given or when a large dose of atracurium (>0.6 mg/kg) is given slowly over 15 to 75 seconds, few patients elicit histamine release and hypotension (Fig. 34-9).[51]

Cisatracurium is one of the 1R-*cis*,1'R-*cis* configurations of one of the 10 isomers of atracurium and is approximately 4 times as potent as atracurium. The ED_{95} is 0.05 mg/kg, with an onset time of 7.5 minutes to complete blockade (2 minutes longer than atracurium), a clinical duration of 45 minutes, and a time to greater than 70% TOF ratio of 67 minutes (Figs. 34-9 to 34-13).[44] Cisatracurium recovery indices are unaffected by the total dose of relaxant or method of administration. In contrast to atracurium, doses of cisatracurium as great as 8 times the

TABLE 34-6 Characteristics of Non-depolarizing Neuromuscular Blocking Drugs in Normal Adults

Drug	ED_{95} (mg/kg)	Onset Time (min)	Time to 25% Recovery (min)	Time to 95% Recovery (min)	Volume of Distribution (ml/kg)	Clearance (mL/kg/min)	Elimination Half-Life (min)
Mivacurium	0.08	1.5-2.0[a]	13	21	112	55	2.3
Atracurium	0.2	3-5[b]	30-40	45-60	182	6.1	21
Cisatracurium	0.05	2.7[c]	66-70	86-71	100-145	4-5.4	21-30
Vecuronium	0.05	2-3[b]	45-60	60-80	190	3.0	80
Rocuronium (0.6 mg/kg)	0.30	1-2[b]	14-28	23-75	193-221	2.9	66-76
Rocuronium (1.2 mg/kg)	0.30	0.7-1.2[c]	38-150	38-150	193-221	2.9	66-76
Pancuronium	0.07	3-5[d]	80-90	120	150-340	1.0-1.9	100-132

[a]Initial dose of 0.15 mg/kg followed by a second dose of 0.1 mg/kg at 30 seconds.

[b]After 2 × ED_{95}.

[c]After 4 × ED_{95}.

[d]After 1 × ED_{95}.

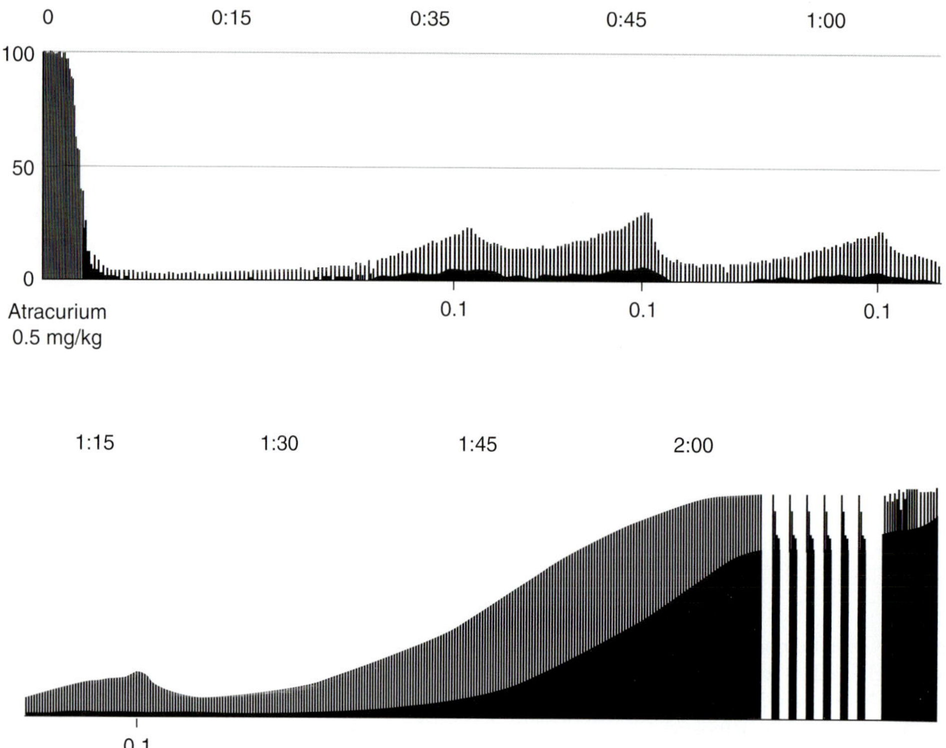

FIGURE 34-16. Initial dose of atracurium was 0.5 mg/kg, followed by four increments of 0.1 mg/kg every 15 minutes. Note when T_1 spontaneously recovered to control height and train-of-four ratio was 0.74 and increased to 0.85 in the next 4 minutes. [From Ali HH, Miller RD. Monitoring of neuromuscular function. In: Miller RD, ed. *Anesthesia*, vol. 2. 2nd ed. New York, NY: Churchill-Livingstone, 1986, with permission from Elsevier. Copyright 1996.]

ED_{95} have been administered rapidly without any evidence of histamine release.

STEROIDAL MUSCLE RELAXANTS (FIG. 34-17)

Vecuronium is the monoquaternary analog of the steroidal relaxant pancuronium.[52] Vecuronium is a more potent NMBD than pancuronium,[53] with half to one-third of its duration of action (Fig. 34-10) by demethylation at the 2 position of the D ring, the position of the steroid nucleus that is responsible for its potency. It is a lipophilic compound that is easily absorbed by the liver and excreted into the bile mostly as the unchanged drug, the predominant method of elimination.[53] The action of this drug can be prolonged in patients with liver disease.[54] Vecuronium is metabolized in the liver to 3-desacetylvecuronium, 17-desacetylvecuronium, and 3,17-desacetylvecuronium.[55] The 3-desacetylvecuronium has neuromuscular blocking properties at approximately half the potency of vecuronium. This metabolite is eliminated by the kidneys (Fig. 34-12), which may account for the prolonged block when vecuronium is given as a continuous infusion to facilitate mechanical ventilation of patients in the intensive care unit (ICU) who have compromised renal function.[56,57] Recovery times are increased in infants younger than 1 year of age based on their increased sensitivity to vecuronium and larger volume of distribution and decreased clearance rate.[58]

Vecuronium does not have effects on heart rate and blood pressure through modification of the A ring of the steroidal nucleus.[59] At doses above 0.1 mg/kg, it may inhibit the enzyme histamine-*N*-methyltransferase,[60] which may contribute to occasional reports of histamine-like reactions to vecuronium.[61,62] This may be a concern, especially when other drugs that release histamine (eg, the antibiotic vancomycin) are administered or when histamine-rich organs are manipulated during a surgical procedure.[60]

Rocuronium is the 2-morpholino, 3-desacetyl 16-*N*-allylpyrrolidino derivative of vecuronium.[63] It was developed specifically to have a rapid onset of action (Fig. 34-9). It achieves this effect partly by being approximately 6 times less potent than vecuronium and by having a similar molecular weight.[16] This results in a larger number of molecules reaching the neuromuscular junction per circulation time and may contribute to the more rapid development of its neuromuscular blockade. Rocuronium undergoes rapid uptake by the liver because of its relative lipophilicity. Unchanged rocuronium has been found in the urine (8.7%) and in the bile (>50%), indicating dual pathways for its elimination.[64] The rapid redistribution of rocuronium from the neuromuscular junction contributes to its intermediate duration of action at lower doses (Fig. 34-10). The pharmacokinetics of this drug have been reported to be altered in patients with major renal[65] and hepatic[66] disease (Figs. 34-11 to 34-13). In both infants and elderly patients, the changes in the pharmacokinetics of rocuronium increases the duration of action.[67] Rocuronium does not produce alterations in heart rate and blood pressure.[68]

The ED_{95} of rocuronium is 0.3 mg/kg, with a recovery index of 8 minutes and a clinical duration of less than 20 minutes. Mean onset times at $2\times ED_{95}$ (0.6 mg/kg), $3\times ED_{95}$ (0.9 mg/kg), and $4\times ED_{95}$ (1.2 mg/kg) are approximately 90, 75, and 55 seconds, respectively, with ranges of 48 to 156, 48 to 144, and 36 to 84 seconds, respectively.[69] These are the most rapid onset times at equipotent doses of any nondepolarizing relaxant currently available. It has been suggested that appropriate doses, this drug in may be useful as an alternative to SCh for rapid intubation of the trachea.[69] Because rocuronium depends on organs of elimination for its termination of action,[70] it has a dose-related escalation of clinical duration. At 2, 3, and 4 times the ED_{95} dose, expected durations to 25% recovery are 37 (range, 23-75), 53 (range, 25-88), and 73 (range, 38-150) minutes, respectively (Fig. 34-10).[69] In addition, recovery from lengthy rocuronium infusions is markedly slower than from single doses of moderate quantity (eg, 0.6 mg/kg).

Pancuronium (Figs. 34-9 and 34-10) is predominantly eliminated by the kidneys and has a prolonged duration of neuromuscular blockade in patients with renal insufficiency (Fig. 34-12). Whereas clearance of pancuronium is minimally altered in patients with obstructive hepatic

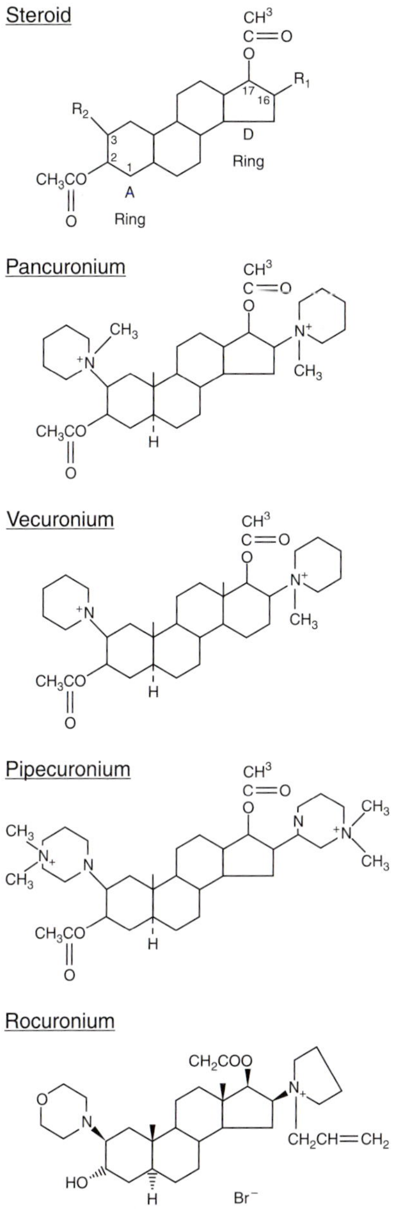

Steroid

Pancuronium

Vecuronium

Pipecuronium

Rocuronium

FIGURE 34-17. Chemical structure of steroidal class neuromuscular blocking drugs.

disease, the volume of distribution at steady state is increased (Figs. 34-11 and 34-12).[71] This implies that in patients with hepatic disease, greater doses may be needed to establish neuromuscular blockade that might be prolonged. In elderly patients, the duration of action is prolonged secondary to compromised clearance of the drug. Approximately 10% to 20% of the injected dose of pancuronium is metabolized in the liver to 3 metabolites: 3-hydroxypancuronium, 17-hydroxypancuronium, and 3,17-dihydroxypancuronium. The 3-hydroxy metabolite is about half as potent as the parent compound and is cleared by the kidneys.

Pancuronium has a tendency to increase heart rate, blood pressure, and cardiac output through a vagolytic action at muscarinic receptors in the autonomic nervous system and via inhibition of catecholamine reuptake at sympathetic nerve terminals.

MAINTENANCE OF NEUROMUSCULAR BLOCKADE BY INFUSION

Intermittent IV bolus doses of nondepolarizing NMBDs to maintain adequate levels of surgical paralysis are readily accomplished by giving one-fifth to one-third the original dose titrated against some objective criteria (eg, number of twitches in the TOF, clinical evaluation of abdominal relaxation). This process usually is necessary every 40 to 60 minutes, although more frequent supplemental doses are needed with the short- and intermediate-acting agents. An appropriate option for maintaining more constant and prolonged neuromuscular blockade is a continuous infusion to achieve steady-state plasma levels of drug within a therapeutic window. The infusion of NMBD can be titrated to achieve a stable depth of neuromuscular blockade (usually 1 or 2 responses to TOF) permitting a rapid reversal when needed, for example, for daily assessment of a patient's neurologic status.

SCh has been given in the past by IV infusion for maintenance of neuromuscular blockade but is no longer routinely used for this purpose. During infusion of SCh, neuromuscular blockade can change from phase I to phase II block in approximately two-thirds of patients receiving a nitrous–narcotic anesthetic, with an extremely variable time of onset. Approximately half of these patients recover rapidly (5%-95% recovery in 15 minutes). The remaining half recover to approximately 75% in roughly 30 minutes and require reversal with an anticholinesterase drug.[72] Inhalational anesthetics hasten the onset of phase II block, which usually is heralded by tachyphylaxis. The key to successful use of SCh as a continuous infusion is to recognize the presence of phase II block (TOF fade >50%) and to not attempt to reverse until a plateau of recovery has been reached.

Vecuronium and rocuronium by infusion have been used with considerable success. After maintaining steady-state paralysis of approximately 95% and then discontinuing the infusion, mean recovery time to 25% is approximately 13 minutes, and mean 5% to 95% recovery times are approximately 32 minutes.[73] However, there is an age-dependent decrease in the steady-state drug infusion requirement and an increased recovery time required for patients older than 60 years of age.[58] These and other findings suggest that disease states or age that alters organ elimination generally decrease maintenance drug infusion requirements and slow the speed of recovery to some extent with vecuronium. This is especially true for long-term infusions in patients with renal failure because the 3-desacetyl metabolite of vecuronium, which is a potent neuromuscular blocking compound, is eliminated by the kidney.[59,74]

Atracurium and cisatracurium have similar recovery characteristics after infusions in healthy patients. The 25% recovery time after infusion is approximately 12.5 minutes, and the 5% to 95% mean recovery time is 26.6 minutes during oxygen, nitrous oxide, and narcotic anesthesia. Unlike vecuronium, atracurium and cisatracurium show no tendency toward prolonged recovery in disease states, such as renal failure, cirrhosis, and hepatic failure, or at the extremes of age because of its spontaneous degradation by the Hofmann elimination reaction and metabolism by nonspecific plasma cholinesterases.

Mivacurium, because of its metabolism by human plasma cholinesterase at 70% the rate of SCh, has significant clinical potential for maintenance of blockade by continuous infusion. During balanced anesthesia, the time from discontinuing the infusion of mivacurium to 25% recovery was 5.7 minutes, with a 5% to 95% recovery time of 13.6 minutes.[40] Its recovery characteristics are much shorter than those of atracurium, cisatracurium, vecuronium, and rocuronium and compare favorably with the short recovery times achieved with SCh.

NEUROMUSCULAR BLOCKADE IN THE INTENSIVE CARE UNIT

NMBDs in the ICU can be valuable adjuncts for managing intubated and mechanically ventilated patients.[75-77] Neuromuscular blockade may be helpful for diminishing the risk of barotrauma by reducing peak airway pressures, minimizing oxygen consumption in hypothermic patients by preventing shivering, decreasing intraabdominal pressure, and stopping respiratory activity that is asynchronous with the ventilatory cycle when all other treatments have failed. NMBD also can be given to help mechanically ventilated patients with unusual problems (status epilepticus, tetanus, botulism) who are resistant to conventional methods of treatment. The administration of cisatracurium for 48 hours during the early stages of severe acute respiratory distress syndrome improved the 90-day survival[76] from potentially several mechanisms, including allowing for better lung-protective ventilation, improvement in oxygenation through a reduction in oxygen consumption of muscle, and improving ventilation/perfusion matching.[77] The use of NMBD in critically ill patients must be balanced with the most serious side effect of severe myopathy.[59,75-82] This critical illness myopathy is characterized by marked atrophy of type I and type II muscle fibers, little evidence of inflammation, and sparing of the motor and sensory nerves.[81] Although the steroidal muscle relaxants have been implicated because the myopathy associated with their use is similar to the myopathy caused by exogenous corticosteroid administration,[59,82] all classes of NMBD may contribute to myopathy. In the ICU, the underlying complex systemic disease processes (including sepsis and burns), prolonged immobility, ventilator dependence, use of various drugs that may affect the neuromuscular system,[75] and the initial more frequent use of the steroidal muscle relaxants compared with the benzylisoquinolines in ICU patients have confounded studies of myopathy caused by prolonged neuromuscular blockade.[77]

Atracurium and *cisatracurium* can be given to critically ill patients with renal failure.[81] The epileptogenic effects of laudanosine, a metabolite of the Hofmann degradation, have not been reported in patients receiving atracurium infusions. The highest plasma concentrations of laudanosine measured in human plasma during continuous infusions in the ICU are below 6 mcg/mL, far lower than the 17 mcg/mL needed to produce seizures in animals.[84]

Pancuronium, because it is the NMBD in longest use, frequently was given to ICU patients before the availability of the benzylisoquinoline NMBD and sedatives, such as propofol, to facilitate mechanical ventilation. Because of its cardiovascular effects, pancuronium may be a poor

TABLE 34-7 Criteria for Adequate Recovery

Criteria used depend on whether the patient is awake or somnolent
Patient is awake
Opens eyes widely to command and denies diplopia
Sustains tongue protrusion
Swallows effectively
Sustains a head lift for 5 s
Sustains a firm hand grip
Has an effective cough
Has a vital capacity of at least 15 mL/kg
Can generate an inspiratory force of at least 30 cm H_2O
Patient is somnolent
Can generate an inspiratory force of at least 30 cm H_2O
Responds to nerve stimulator appropriately, including sustained tetanic response to 50 Hz for 5 s
Train-of-four or double-burst stimulus yields ratio of 0.9 using quantitative methods

choice for patients in whom dysrhythmias and tachycardia would be detrimental. Furthermore, because pancuronium is primarily excreted by the kidneys, patients with compromised renal function may experience a prolonged duration of effect, causing confusion over the patient's neurologic status.[83]

Vecuronium is eliminated primarily by biliary clearance and only minimally by renal clearance. When vecuronium was administered as an infusion to maintain approximately 80% blockade in patients with renal and respiratory failure, recovery to control twitch height after stopping the infusion took from 6 to 37 hours compared with an approximately 1-hour recovery for cisatracurium.[59] A prolonged recovery may occur secondary to accumulation of the 3-desacetyl metabolite

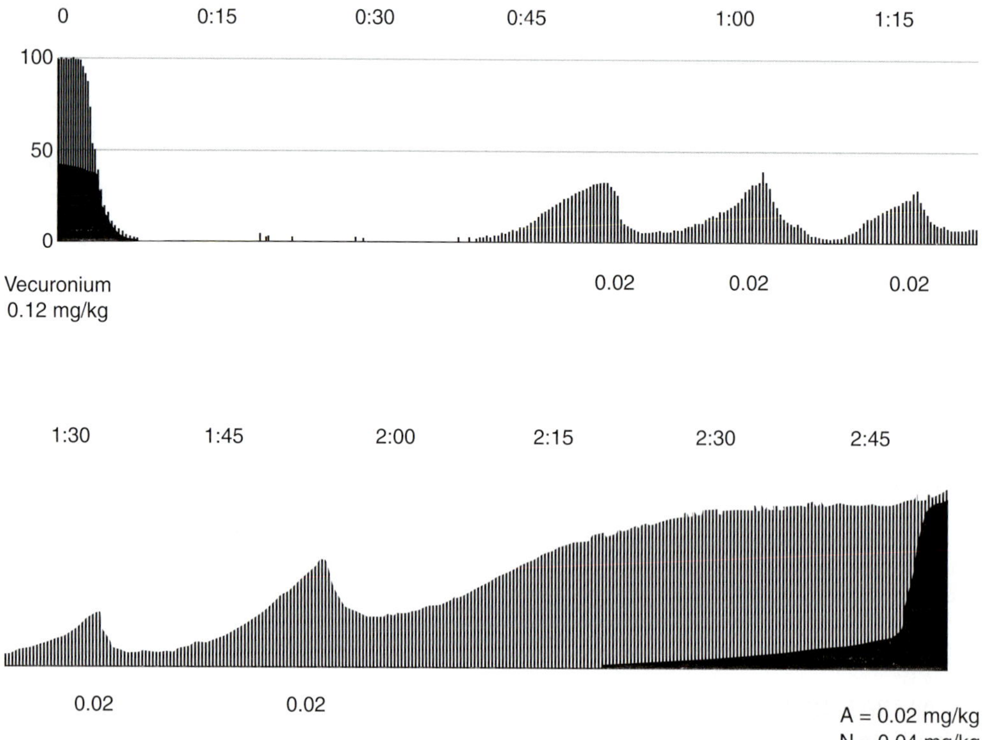

FIGURE 34-18. Tracing of an evoked thenar electromyography after administration of vecuronium. After the initial dose, supplemental vecuronium was given in 15-minute increments. Spontaneous recovery of the first train-of-four (TOF) response to control height took approximately 30 minutes. The fourth response to the TOF occurred 15 minutes later (*dark shadow*) and required reversal with neostigmine and atropine to achieve a ratio of 0.9.

of vecuronium that has approximately 50% of the parent compound's neuromuscular blocking activity and is cleared by the kidney.[57]

RESIDUAL NEUROMUSCULAR BLOCKADE

Residual neuromuscular blockade (RNMB) in patients admitted to the postanesthesia care unit (PACU) is a persistent problem.[85-89] RNMB is associated with impaired pharyngeal function, weakness of upper airway muscles, some attenuation of the hypoxic ventilator response, and the unpleasantness of feeling muscle weakness.[90] *Recurarization* is the term that initially was coined for patients who were re-paralyzed after seemingly adequate reversal of neuromuscular blockade in the operating room. This term is a misnomer because it is realistically a failure to adequately reverse neuromuscular blockade.

One long-standing guide for clinicians has been a return to TOF ratio = 0.7 as an indicator for the return of sufficient muscular function to permit endotracheal extubation[6,91] in concert with the sum total of multiple clinical observations such as respiratory function and the ability to follow commands (**Table 34-7**). If adequate recovery is based on the level of pharyngeal function, recovery to TOF ratios above 0.9 has been advocated.[92] Even with a recovery of the TOF to 0.9, upper airway integrity in some patient may continue to be compromised.[93] However, this ratio is based on quantitative evaluation (eg, with acceleromyography) instead of qualitative observations.[90] The use of intermediate-acting NMBDs can reduce the risk of RNMB but does not completely eliminate this possibility. Interestingly, although patients treated with rocuronium had longer returns to TOF 0.9 compared with those treated with cisatracurium, the number of patients with RNMB was higher with cisatracurium.[94] It is believed that clinicians have compensated for the longer action of rocuronium by stopping its administration sooner.[94]

Reversal of neuromuscular blockade by the administration of an anticholinesterase (eg, neostigmine or edrophonium) (**Fig. 34-18**) is routinely needed in the operating room or PACU. Through inhibition of acetylcholinesterase activity, the concentration of ACh will increase and be available to compete with the nondepolarizing NMBD. A muscarinic antagonist is simultaneously administered to limit any untoward effects of ACh (bradycardia, bronchospasm, or gastrointestinal hyperactivity). Because the anticholinesterase and muscarinic antagonist should have similar durations, the usual drug pairs that are commonly given are neostigmine and glycopyrrolate or edrophonium and atropine. The timing of the administration of anticholinesterases is important. Profound neuromuscular blockade with NMBD that is dependent on organ elimination may require up to 80 minutes for full recovery.[95-97] In routine clinical practice, upon return of the TOF to a single twitch, adequate recovery from neuromuscular blockade to allow successful extubation usually requires at least 15 to 20 minutes.[89]

In lieu of acetylcholinesterase inhibitors,[98] drug-specific reversal agents may provide rapid reversal of neuromuscular blockade. A γ-cyclodextrin, sugammadex, has been synthesized to reverse a profound neuromuscular blockade after rocuronium[99] or vecuronium[100] administration. Sugammadex encapsulates the steroidal NMBD, decreases its free concentration in the plasma, and thereby removes the NMBD from the neuromuscular junction. The sugammadex–NMBD complex is cleared by the kidneys. Although available in Europe, sugammadex has not been approved for use in the United States because of the risks of hypersensitivity and allergic reactions.

NEW NEUROMUSCULAR BLOCKING DRUGS

Gantacurium is an ultra–short-acting nondepolarizing NMBD.[101] It is an asymmetrical isoquiolinium diester of chlorofumaric acid. Its brief duration of action is attributable to a rapid combination with L-cysteine, forming an inactive compound. The duration of action for a dose 5 times the ED_{95} is 7 to 13 minutes. Analogs of gantacurium that have intermediate durations of action have been synthesized. Gantacurium and its analogs can be reversed rapidly by IV administration of L-cysteine.

KEY REFERENCES

- Ali HH. Criteria of adequate clinical recovery from neuromuscular block. *Anesthesiology*. 2003;98:1278.
- Ali HH, Savarese JJ. Monitoring of neuromuscular blockade. *Anesthesiology*. 1976;45:216.
- Brull SJ, Murphy GS. Residual neuromuscular block: lessons unlearned. Part II: methods to reduce the risk of residual weakness. *Anesth Analg*. 2010;111:129.
- Eikermann M, Blobner MM, Groeben H, et al. Postoperative upper airway obstruction after recovery of the train of four ratio of the adductor pollicis muscle from neuromuscular blockade. *Anesth Analg*. 2006;102:937.
- Martyn JA, Richtsfeld M. Succinylcholine-induced hyperkalemia in acquired pathologic states. Etiologic factors and molecular mechanisms. *Anesthesiology*. 2006;104:158.
- Murphy GS, Brull SJ. Residual neuromuscular block: lessons unlearned. Part I: definitions, incidence, and adverse physiologic effects of residual neuromuscular block. *Anesth Analg*. 2010;111:120.
- Naguib M, Flood P, McArdle JJ, et al. Advances in neurobiology of the neuromuscular junction: implications for the anesthesiologist. *Anesthesiology*. 2002;96:202.
- Papazian L, Forel J-M, Gacouin A, et al. Neuromuscular blockers in early acute respiratory distress syndrome. *N Engl J Med*. 2010;363:1007.
- Pino RM. Residual neuromuscular blockade: a persistent clinical problem. *Int Anesthesiol Clin*. 2006;44:77.
- Segredo V, Caldwell JE, Matthay MA, et al. Persistent paralysis in critically ill patients after long-term administration of vecuronium. *N Engl J Med*. 1992;327:524.

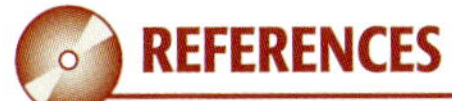

REFERENCES

Complete references available on DVD and online version at www.LongneckerAnesthesiology.com

CHAPTER 35 Monitoring and Managing Perioperative Electrolyte Abnormalities, Acid–Base Disorders, and Fluid Replacement

Patrick J. Neligan

KEY POINTS

1. Water is the single most abundant compound in the body, constituting approximately 50% to 70% of body weight. One-third of body water is extracellular; of this, one-third is located within the intravascular compartment, and two-thirds is extravascular or interstitial.
2. Electrolytes are characterized by their extent of dissociation (strong or weak ions), the number of particles present (millimoles), the number of electrical charges per unit (milliequivalents), and the number of active molecules per unit volume (milliosmoles).

3. Osmolality is uniform through each of the body's compartments, but electrolyte composition varies. Sodium and chloride are principally extracellular. Potassium, phosphate, magnesium, and calcium are principally intracellular.
4. The perioperative stress response elicits significant fluid and electrolyte flux. The magnitude and timing of these changes are key to management strategies.
5. Changes in extracellular sodium concentrations often, but not always, reflect body water composition. Hyponatremia is indicative of free water overload. Hypernatremia is indicative of dehydration.
6. Depletion of serum concentration of principally intracellular ions (potassium, phosphate, magnesium, and calcium) reflects significant total body electrolyte depletion.
7. All acid–base abnormalities can be explained in terms of strong ion difference (SID), weak acid concentration, $Paco_2$, and extracellular free water.
8. The 6 primary acid–base abnormalities are acidosis caused by increased $Paco_2$, acidosis caused by reduced SID, acidosis caused by increased acid-buffering system (A_{TOT}), alkalosis associated with reduced $Paco_2$, alkalosis caused by increased SID, and alkalosis caused by reduced A_{TOT}.
9. A variety of tools are available for interpreting acid–base abnormalities. These include the base deficit (BD) excess, corrected anion gap (AG), strong ion gap (SIG), and the base deficit or excess (BDE) gap.
10. Upper gastrointestinal (GI) losses should be replaced with isotonic saline. Lower GI and extracellular fluid (ECF) losses should be replaced with balanced salt solutions (BSS). Blood loss can initially be replaced with crystalloid in a 1:3 to 1:5 ratio, but as blood loss increases, the volume of crystalloid required increases geometrically.
11. Overresuscitation with crystalloid may lead to poor perioperative outcomes. "Normal saline" solution, given in significant volume, causes metabolic acidosis, and hyperchloremia may reduce splanchnic blood flow.
12. Colloid solutions restore circulating volume more rapidly than crystalloid with less tissue edema, but their use remains controversial.
13. Volume replacement strategies for major surgery should not be formula based but dynamic and goal directed using volume and flow monitoring devices.
14. Postoperative fluid restriction may be appropriate for some patients, especially those undergoing lower intestinal resection.

INTRODUCTION

The human body is an aqueous soup containing carbohydrates, protein, fat, ions, and trace elements bundled into and around cellular structures built on an exoskeleton. Fundamental to the structure and function of the body are the chemical properties of water. Patients undergoing surgery or experiencing critical illness undergo dramatic changes in the volume, distribution, and composition of body water. Patients undergoing the most minor of procedures undertake a period of fasting, rehydration with intravenous (IV) fluids, and neurohormonal changes in fluid distribution. To understand strategies and implications of perioperative fluid administration, it is important that one understands the homeostatic mechanisms by which the body maintains its internal milieu.

Homeostasis refers to the capacity of the human body to maintain a stable constant condition by means of constant dynamic equilibrium adjustments controlled by a medley of interconnected regulatory mechanisms. The concept dates from the foundations of scientific medicine, specifically the work of Claude Bernard (1813–1878). Multiple systems exist in the body to test and control deviations from the normal range in vital functions. These include the autonomic nervous system, the renin–angiotensin–aldosterone–vasopressin axis, and the hypothalamopituitary adrenal axis. The body thus self-regulates to maintain a variety of physiologic and metabolic variables in the state of equilibrium despite a staggering range of variations in the level of human activities and externalities. A key part of homeostasis is maintenance of body water in terms of circulating volume, volume distribution, and composition. The systems involved are dedicated to maintaining the delicate balance of homeostatic function despite externalities such as tissue trauma and surgery. Anesthesiologists are in a unique position to manipulate these systems for the good of the patient.

Key to the understanding of homeostasis is the role of water and ions in body fluids. Changes in water and electrolyte distribution lead to significant physiologic upset, often manifesting as acid–base abnormalities. Acid–base abnormalities result from changes in carbon dioxide tension, water and electrolyte distribution, and extracellular protein concentration. IV fluids, which are administered to the majority of perioperative patients, have significant effects on water and electrolyte distribution and impact the patient's acid–base balance. Initial perioperative or emergency fluid resuscitation strategies involve crystalloid resuscitation to replace insensible loss and restore interstitial volume. Overresuscitation with crystalloid may lead to poor perioperative outcomes. "Normal saline" solution causes metabolic acidosis, and the associated hyperchloremia may reduce splanchnic blood flow.

A careful dynamic or goal-directed approach to fluid administration is supplanting traditional formulaic approaches. Furthermore, widely established practices such as fluid administration to replace third-space losses and postoperative maintenance fluid administration are undergoing rigorous evaluation. This chapter sequentially reviews these concepts.

WATER AND IONS

PHYSICAL CHEMISTRY OF WATER

The human body is composed principally of water. Water is a simple triatomic molecule composed of 2 molecules of oxygen and 1 molecule of hydrogen, bound covalently. There is an unequal charge distribution; oxygen nuclei have a particularly strong attraction for electrons. This results in a H-O-H bond angle of 10 degrees. Thus, water behaves like a charged molecule, a dipole, with a negative oxygen and positive hydrogen end. This polarity (molecules clump together) is responsible for important chemical properties of water. Water has a high surface tension, low vapor pressure, high specific heat capacity, high heat of vaporization, and high boiling point. These factors have enabled life on this planet. Water is a powerful ionizing solvent; substances dissolved in water separate into component parts. Water is slightly ionized: When molecules collide, enough energy is produced to transfer a proton from 1 water molecule to another. Thus, water slightly dissociates in to a negatively charged hydroxylated (OH^-) ion and positively charged protonated (H_nO^+) ion.[1] All metabolic activity in the body occurs in this aqueous medium. Thus compounds ingested or administered to the body are impacted by the chemical properties of water.

WATER DISTRIBUTION IN BODY COMPARTMENTS

Water is the single most abundant compound in the body, constituting approximately 50% to 70% of body weight. Males contain relatively more water (on average, 60%) than do females (on average, 50%). There is an inverse relationship between total body fat and total body water (TBW). Females have less skeletal muscle and have more subcutaneous fat and thus lower TBW. TBW varies dramatically depending on the age of the individual. Neonates have very high TBW (70%–80%). Conversely, elderly patients have relatively lower TBW (52% for men; 45% for women). Body water is neither liquid nor easily accessible. It is divided up into 2 separate compartments, the intracellular and the extracellular compartments (or spaces). Two-thirds of body water is intracellular, principally in skeletal muscle. One-third of body water is extracellular, representing approximately 20% of body weight. Of this, one-third is located within the intravascular compartment, and

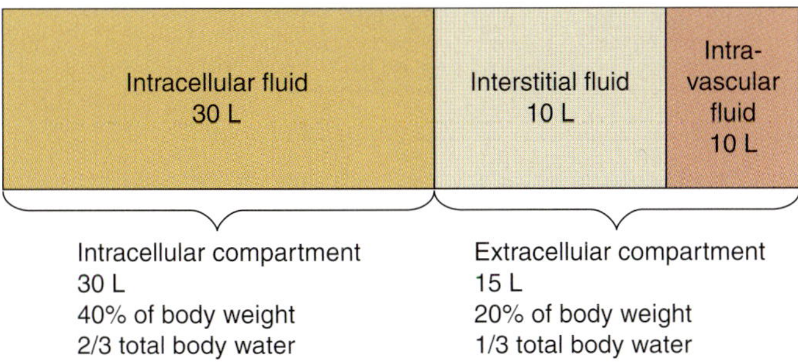

FIGURE 35-1. Body fluid compartments.

two-thirds is extravascular or interstitial. To place this in context, a 75-kg man has a TBW of 45 L, 15 L of which is extracellular, 5 L of which is intravascular (**Fig. 35-1**). The interstitial fluid contains ultrafiltrated plasma (intravascular water), transudated plasma, and fluid and electrolytes actively pumped out of cells (transcellular fluids). Water freely moves from the intracellular to the extracellular space, but dissolved ions cannot do so. Hence, clinicians should be aware that administration of electrolyte-rich solutions may have a dramatic impact on extracellular ionic composition and, indeed, acid–base chemistry.[2,3]

Most of the fluid in the interstitium is derived from filtration and diffusion from the capillaries. The extracellular space is a matrix made up of collagen fiber bundles and proteoglycan filaments. Fluid is entrapped in the minute spaces between the filaments, taking the form of a gel ("tissue gel"). Fluid does not flow easily through this gel. Indeed, fluid diffuses through the gel, molecule by molecule. There is little "free fluid" in the interstitium. Free fluid exists only as small rivulets that course along the collagen fibers or cells. When there is significant extravascular fluid expansion, such as in volume overload or congestive heart failure (CHF), these rivulets turn into pockets and then rivers of free-flowing water. As a consequence, tissues feel boggy or edematous.

IONIC CONSTITUENTS OF BODY COMPARTMENTS

Charge Compounds introduced into aqueous solutions dissociate into their component parts, depending on the ion dissociation constant or pKa.[4] This describes the tendency of the molecule or ion to keep a proton at its ionization center. Strong ions, characterized by low pKa, rapidly split into their component parts. Examples of strong ions include sodium (Na^+), chloride (Cl^-), potassium (K^+), magnesium (Mg2$^+$), and lactate.

The physiologic and chemical activity and thus the importance of electrolytes depend on several variables. These include the number of particles present per unit volume (in terms of moles or millimoles), the number of electrical charges per unit volume (in equivalents or milliequivalents), and the number of osmotically active molecules per unit volume (in osmoles or milliosmoles). It is important that clinicians be aware of these properties and distinguish them when managing and monitoring fluids and electrolytes in perioperative care. It is also important to be aware of the physiologic functions of the most important ions.

The chemical composition of the body's various fluids is described in terms of chemical combining activity or chemical "equivalents." When the concentrations of different ions within each fluid compartment are expressed in this way, the sum of all positive ions (cations) exactly equals the sum of all negative ions (anions). This is the law of electrical neutrality.

The atomic weight of an element is approximately the sum of protons and electrons in the nucleus; the weight of 1 atom of oxygen is 16. The weight of 1 atom of hydrogen is 1. The molecular weight of a compound can be determined by the chemical formula of the compound and then adding together the atomic weights of all the elements constituting that compound.

One mole (1 M) of any substance is its molecular weight expressed in grams (ie, gram-molecular weight) and contains 6.023×10^{23} molecules (Avogadro's number). A millimole of a substance is 1/1000 of a mole, or the substance's weight expressed in milligrams. In addition, 1 M of any *gas* (eg, oxygen, carbon dioxide) under standard conditions occupies a constant volume of 22.4L, and 1 mM of gas occupies 22.4 mL. Regardless of whether a substance is ionized or nonionized, organic or inorganic, the terms *mole* and *millimole* are applicable.

Electrolytes combine with each other strictly in proportion to their ionic valencies. Originally, oxygen was chosen as the standard of reference; 8 g of oxygen combines with 1 g atomic weight of hydrogen. By convention, the chemical standard of reference for combining power is the electric charge (+) of 1 atomic weight (1 g) of hydrogen. Thus, 1 equivalent (1 Eq) of an ion is that amount that can combine with 1 g of hydrogen and is therefore chemically equivalent to 1 g of hydrogen.

One equivalent of hydrogen consists of 6.023×10^{23} particles, weighs 1 g, and carries a positive charge. This quantity of hydrogen ions neutralizes or balances 1 Eq of hydroxyl ions, which consists of 6.023×10^{23} particles, weighs 17 g, and carries a negative electric charge. The result of this neutralization is the formation of 1 M of water weighing 18 g. Such ions are termed *univalent* and balance each other in a 1:1 ratio. For all univalent ions, 1 Eq equals 1 M.

Certain ions (eg, calcium [Ca^{2+}], magnesium [Mg^{2+}], sulfate [SO_4^{2-}]) are divalent and carry either 2 positive charges (divalent cations) or 2 negative charges (divalent anions). These multivalent ions have greater chemical-combining power than do univalent ions. Because electrochemical neutrality must be maintained in all reactions, 1 divalent cation (eg, Ca^{2+}) will react with 2 univalent anions (eg, $2 \times Cl^-$). In other words, 1 M of divalent cation (6.023×10^{23} particles) supplies 2 Eq and will offset 2 M (1 Eq each) of univalent anion.

The ionic concentrations present in body fluids are relatively small and are expressed in terms of milliequivalents (mEq) rather than equivalents. In the case of univalent ions, 1 mEq is equal to 1/1000 of the gram-atomic weight (ie, atomic weight expressed in milligrams), is the same as 1 mM of the ion in question, and consists of 6.023×10^{20} particles. For divalent ions, 1 mEq consists of 3.012×10^{20} particles and weighs 1/2000 of the gram-atomic weight. One mM of divalent ions equals 2 mEq. An equivalent (or milliequivalent) of any ion is its atomic weight expressed in grams (or milligrams) divided by the valence. Electrolytes do not combine gram for gram or milligram for milligram; they combine equivalent for equivalent or milliequivalent for milliequivalent of opposite polarity. Therefore, in any given fluid compartment or IV solution, the number of milliequivalents of cations is balanced by precisely the same number of milliequivalents of anions.

Distribution There are different electrolyte concentrations in each body fluid compartment and the average values are listed in **Table 35-1**. In the extracellular compartment, the major cation is sodium, and the principal anions are chloride and bicarbonate. Sodium and chloride are free in solution, but appreciable fractions of calcium and magnesium are bound to protein. Interstitial fluid represents a partial ultrafiltrate of plasma devoid of platelets and erythrocytes and with a lower concentration of protein. The principal plasma protein, albumin, carries a significant a negative charge at a pH of 7.4, and its diffusion across capillary endothelium is restricted. Consequently, because of the greater protein content (ie, organic anions) in plasma, the total plasma concentration of cations is greater, and the concentration of inorganic anions is less than in the interstitial fluid. Electroneutrality is maintained within each fluid compartment, but because of protein distribution, there is an asymmetry of ion distribution between plasma and the interstitium. Within each fluid compartment, the total cations must equal the total anions, but a greater number of diffusible ions reside in the compartment containing the most organic anions. As a result, a slight osmotic pressure gradient is established, which (under normal conditions) is counterbalanced by capillary hydrostatic forces. This is an example of the Gibbs-Donnan principle, which describes the unequal distribution of diffusible ions on either side of the cell membranes bordering these fluid compartments.

TABLE 35-1 Ion Distribution in Different Compartments

Electrolyte	Plasma (mEq/L)	Plasma Water (mEq/L)	Interstitial Fluid (mEq/L)	Intracellular Fluid (mEq/kg H_2O)
Cations				
Sodium	142	152	145	10
Potassium	4	4	4	156
Calcium	5	5	3	3
Magnesium	3	3	1	26
Total	154	164	153	195
Anions				
Chloride	103	109	114	2
Bicarbonate	27	29	30	10
Phosphate	2	2	2	108
Sulfate	1	1	1	20
Organic acids	5	6	5	
Protein	16	17	1	55
Total	154	164	153	195

The ionic concentrations for plasma water differ from those of plasma because of the exclusion of solids, notably lipids and large proteins, which total approximately 7%. Plasma proteins occupy a volume far out of proportion to the few milliequivalents of anion they represent. One liter of plasma contains about 940 mL of water. The remaining volume is occupied, for the most part, by protein. Ions are generally dissolved in the aqueous phase of plasma so that concentrations in plasma water exceed those in whole plasma by a factor of 1000 to 940. Clinical laboratories usually report electrolyte values as the ionic concentration in a given volume of whole plasma or serum, and although slightly inaccurate, this is generally accepted. However, if the lipid or protein content of plasma is significantly increased, there will be a corresponding decrease in the reported concentration of ions per liter of plasma (eg, pseudohyponatremia). The volume of water in the sample may be significantly less than the total volume; therefore, the ionic concentrations will be underestimated.

Within the intracellular compartment, potassium and magnesium are the predominant cations, and phosphate, sulfate, and protein are the most abundant anions. There is a marked difference between intracellular and extracellular water in terms of ionic concentrations. The ratio of intracellular to extracellular potassium is almost 30 to 1. Likewise, sodium and chloride are portioned along a steep concentration gradient in the opposite direction. There are more ions in the intracellular compartment than the extracellular compartment. Significant proportions of intracellular ions are bound to protein or cellular constituents and are osmotically inactive.

Many biologic processes depend on the presence of transcellular impediments to ion transport. Large polyvalent protein and organic phosphate anions are confined intracellularly because of their absolute membrane impermeability. For smaller ions, maintaining different ionic concentrations across cell membranes partly depends on the active accumulation and extrusion of certain ions from within cells. Active, energy-dependent "ion pumps" (contained within cell membranes) generate the ionic concentration gradients observed among the various fluid compartments. For example, the tendency for sodium ions to diffuse from ECF (high concentration) into cells (low concentration) is opposed by the active transport of sodium ions out of cells. Similarly, the tendency for potassium ions to diffuse along a concentration gradient from the intracellular fluid (ICF; high concentration) to the ECF (low concentration) is opposed by an active accumulation process. For anesthesiologists, this means that when fluids are administered perioperatively, sodium and chloride remain in the extracellular space.

Ionic distribution results in electrical polarization across cells. Sodium is predominantly extracellular, and cells are far more permeable to potassium than to sodium. Thus, potassium ions tend to diffuse down a concentration gradient and out of a cell. The result is an increasing negative charge within the cell that tends to counteract this diffusion, restraining further potassium movement. Membrane polarization is largely a function of the difference in potassium concentration on either side of the membrane. For most cells under normal conditions, the resting transmembrane potential difference is –60 to –90 mV. Alterations in the distribution of ions, particularly in the extracellular space, can result in a change in this resting potential and cellular dysfunction. Hypoxia in particular destroys this delicate charge balance and leads to unopposed diffusion of ions along concentration gradients. This results in cellular swelling caused by sodium and water entering cells and hyperkalemia caused by outward leakage of potassium.

Concentration of Ions By convention, the concentrations of most IV solutions are expressed as percentages (usually weight in grams or milligrams per 100 mL of solution). For example, 0.9% saline solution (normal saline) represents 0.9 g sodium chloride/100 mL water. In the United States, laboratory measurements of glucose, albumin, creatinine, and so on continue to be expressed as milligrams percent (ie, mg/100 mL of blood, serum, or plasma). The major limitation of this measurement technique is the impact of temperature on substance volume.

Internationally, molality and molarity are widely used to describe concentration. Molality is the number of moles of solute per 1000 g of solvent. It is independent of temperature. A mol*al* solution of saline contains 58.5 g of sodium chloride dissolved in 1000 g of water. The mol*ar* concentration is the number of moles of solute per 1000 mL of solution (usually water) at a specified temperature. In clinical practice, millimoles are used. Thus, we use millimoles per kilogram of solution (millimolal or mm) and millimoles per liter of solution (millimolar, or mM).

WATER DISTRIBUTION AND MOVEMENT

Cell membranes are permeable to water. Water molecules continuously move between fluid compartments in the body. Water movement is governed by hydrostatic and osmotic pressures. Hydrostatic pressure is dynamic and results from pulsatile blood flow. This pressure gradually reduces from a mean in the aorta of 90 to 95 mm Hg to a mean of 30 to 40 mm Hg in the capillaries. Hydrostatic pressure is higher in the lower limbs in an erect patient. The capillary network is fenestrated, and the hydrostatic pressure within the capillary is sufficient to push fluid through these fenestrations into the interstitium. In the capillary system, however, osmotic forces are more important than hydrostatic forces. Osmosis is the movement of water through a semipermeable membrane from a location in which solute is in low concentration to a location in which solute is in high concentration. The membrane is permeable to solvent, not solute, resulting in a pressure gradient. Osmotic pressure is the hydrostatic pressure that must be applied to the solution of greater concentration to prevent water movement across the membrane.

Osmotic pressure depends on the number of osmotically active molecules in solution and not their molecular weight, electric charge, or valence number. Small numbers of large molecules are less osmotically active than large numbers of small molecules. One gram molecular weight (ie, 1 M) of a nondissociating compound (eg, glucose, urea) consists of 6.023×10^{23} molecules and is termed 1 osmole (osmol, Osm). For non-dissociating compounds, 1 mM is equivalent to 1 mOsm. One mOsm of any solute dissolved in 1 kg of water will decrease the activity of water by 17 mm Hg. Ionized substances tend to dissociate in solution and thereby generate more osmotically active particles. For example, 1 gram-molecular weight of sodium chloride (NaCl)—consisting of 6.023×10^{23} molecules—dissociates into twice this number of ions in solution and exerts an osmotic effect of approximately 2 Osm. One mole of sodium sulfate (Na_2SO_4) results in 4 Eq (2 Na+, SOa^-) but dissociates so as to exert an osmotic effect approaching 3 Osm (Na, Na, SO_4).

Osmolarity is the number of osmoles of solute per liter of solvent plus solute. Osmolality, on the other hand, is the solute concentration per kilogram of solvent (water). Osmolality is more widely used in clinical practice because its value is unaffected by the presence of fat and protein in plasma. Osmolality is generally measured with a freezing point osmometer.

Extracellular osmolality is approximately 290 ± 10 mOsm/kg H_2O, and presumably, the intracellular osmolality level is identical. Because 1 mOsm/kg H_2O exerts an osmotic effect equivalent to 17 mm Hg, the osmotic pressure of most body fluids is approximately 300 × 17, or 5100 mm Hg.

Quantitatively, osmotic pressures greatly exceed any hydrostatic pressure in the body. The magnitude of these osmotic forces can be appreciated when one realizes that an osmotic pressure difference of only 6 mOsm/L across a semipermeable membrane can move as much water as the entire hydrostatic pressure generated by the heart.

Osmotic forces throughout the body (with the exception of the renal medulla) are equal because water can readily cross cell membranes. Thus, the osmolality of the intracellular and extracellular spaces equalize despite differing compositions. This has significant impact in health and disease. Loss of ECF volume leads to increased ECF osmolality and subsequent cellular dehydration.

Sodium, chloride, and bicarbonate account for 90% to 95% of the osmotic activity present in plasma and interstitial fluid. Other ions and organic compounds (eg, glucose, urea, amino acids) account for most of the remainder. Plasma proteins provide a negligible osmotic effect. The major intracellular osmotic solutes are potassium, magnesium phosphate, and protein. Total-body osmotic solute is portioned such that two-thirds is contained within the ICF compartment and one-third resides in the ECF compartment. This localization of total body solute in turn explains the overall distribution of body water.

In most situations, the concentrations of certain osmotically active substances can be combined to provide a remarkably accurate (within 10%) estimate of serum osmolality (S_{osm}):

$$S_{osm}\ (\text{mOsm/kg H}_2\text{O}) = (2 \times [\text{Na}] + [\text{K}]) + ([\text{glucose}]/18) + ([\text{BUN}]/2.8)$$

where glucose and blood urea nitrogen (BUN) concentrations are expressed in mg/dL and sodium concentration [Na+] is in mEq/L. The calculations for BUN and glucose resolve the results into mmol/L.

Occasionally, osmotically active compounds are present in the ECFs that are not accounted for by the above calculation. When osmolality is measured and then calculated, a gap between the 2 figures becomes evident (osmolal gap). This gap is normally less than 10 mOsm/kg H_2O. Pharmacologically, the gap is increased by the administration of mannitol or alcohol. Pathologically, the gap may be widened by poisoning with ethylene glycol, propylene glycol, or isopropyl alcohol.

Tonicity describes the relative osmolality of solutions. A solution is said to be isotonic when it is iso-osmotic (ie, the same osmotic pressure) with the body fluids. IV fluids that are formulated as BSS (Normosol-R or Plasmalyte) are isotonic with respect to plasma. Normal saline (0.9% NaCl) is slightly hypertonic to plasma. Lactated Ringer solution (LRS) is slightly hypotonic. However, functionally, these fluids act as iso-osmotic solutions and do not impact the size of erythrocytes. Administration of hypertonic fluids (eg, 3% or 7.5% NaCI, 7.5% sodium bicarbonate, 10% mannitol) leads to a dramatic increase in ECF osmolality and cellular dehydration. Often this is intentional, such as the administration of mannitol or hypertonic saline (HS) to patients with head injuries. Occasionally, hyperosmolality occurs pathologically, as in diabetes insipidus, diabetic ketoacidosis (caused by ketones and glucose), or nonketotic hyperosmolar syndrome (caused by glucose) and acute renal failure (caused by urea and other nitrogenous waste products).

Hypotonic solutions (eg, 0.45% NaCl) have fewer osmotically active particles per volume than the reference solution and tend to produce cellular swelling.

Finally, although the terms *tonicity* and *osmolality* are frequently used interchangeably, an alteration in one does not necessarily lead to an alteration in the other. The classic example of this is urea. Urea is freely permeable throughout the body water. It does not affect tonicity but does cause increase extracellular osmolality.

ALTERATIONS IN FLUID AND ELECTROLYTE DISTRIBUTION

IMPACT OF SURGICAL STRESS RESPONSE ON PERIOPERATIVE FLUID DISTRIBUTION INSENSIBLE LOSSES

Perioperative care is characterized by dramatic changes in fluid and electrolyte content and distribution in the various fluid spaces in the body. These changes are predictable and follow a characteristic pattern described by Cuthbertson and Tilstone[5] and Moore,[6,7] widely known as the "stress response." An understanding of this process is central to understanding the dynamics of fluid and electrolyte flux in the perioperative period and is helpful in guiding therapy.

The stress response has traditionally been considered a biphasic "ebb and flow" phenomenon. Initially after an injury or surgical incision, there is significant peripheral vasoconstriction, shunting of blood from the periphery to the midline (to preserve vital organs), and a decrease in body temperature. Simultaneously, there is a decrease in capillary hydrostatic pressure, promoting a rapid shift of protein-free fluid from the interstitium into the capillaries.[8] This is known as "transcapillary refill," and it includes mobilization of fluid from the splanchnic circulation, particularly the splanchnic veins.[9] This induces a state of absolute hypovolemia in the extracellular space. There is a dramatic increase in the release of vasopressin (antidiuretic hormone) and activation of the renin–angiotensin–aldosterone axis to conserve salt and water.

The second phase, the hypermetabolic or "flow" phase, occurs within hours, characterized by a dramatic increase in cardiac output, driven by catecholamines, vasodilatation, increased capillary permeability, and an increase in temperature. A generalized catabolic state ensues characterized by insulin resistance, hypercortisolism, and protein breakdown. Thus, the patient develops tachycardia, leucocytosis, hyperthermia, hyperglycemia, and tissue edema. The magnitude of this response is proportionate to the degree of injury or extent of surgery. Significant ICF deficit may be incurred to maintain circulating volume. A period of fluid sequestration occurs caused by extravasation of fluid consequent of widespread capillary leak, urinary output decreases, and tissue edema may become evident. Vasodilatation and relative intravascular hypovolemia occur. During this period, patients typically require administration of resuscitation fluids to maintain blood pressure and circulating volume. Weight gain ensues.

Eventually, a state of equilibrium arrives, usually day 2 after surgery, when active sequestration stops. This is followed by a phase of diuresis during which the patient mobilizes fluid and recovers. Initially, there is a precipitous decrease in serum albumin. Restoration of albumin levels is associated with recovery. Moreover, ICF volume returns to normal. An inward shift of fluid from the extracellular to the intracellular space is associated with intracellular movement of ions such as potassium, magnesium, and phosphate. Hence, hypophosphatemia, hypomagnesemia, and, in particular, hypokalemia are usually evident on a serum chemistry panel at this time.

The practicing clinician must be aware of the stages of the stress response when deciding whether to administer fluid and electrolytes. For example, early in the flow phase, significant intracellular and interstitial fluid depletion may exist despite the appearance of "normal" cardiovascular measurements (blood pressure, cardiac output, stroke volume). This requires repletion with free water and isotonic crystalloid. During the vasodilatory, hypermetabolic phase, the circulating volume requires support, taking into account the large volume of distribution of administered crystalloid. During the equilibrium phase, the administration of IV fluid depends on the objective of the clinician. The clinician may choose to continue fluid administration to keep organs well hydrated or to stop administering fluid, preventing the formation of further tissue edema. During the diuretic phase, the major objective of the clinician is to allow the patient to return to baseline body weight and to aggressively replete electrolytes.

It can be argued that the administration of anesthesia significantly reduces the ebb or shock phase. Nevertheless, patients undergoing surgery are usually dehydrated secondary to fasting, bowel lavage, or their primary disease (eg, esophageal cancer). Consequently, the perioperative period should be viewed as follows: (1) dehydration phase, (2) shock phase, (3) relative and absolute hypovolemic phase (caused by vasodilatation, fluid sequestration, and blood loss), (4) equilibrium phase, and (5) diuresis phase. Certain operations are associated with greater blood loss because of overt or microvascular bleeding (vascular surgery); other operations are associated with greater tissue injury caused, for example, by bowel handling. Thus, within this paradigm, a "one formula fits all" approach is neither scientific nor effective. Where extensive fluid shifts are to be expected in the perioperative period, it is worthwhile to obtain a preoperative weight to have a baseline goal for the patient's postoperative diuresis.

HYPOVOLEMIA

There is little excess water storage capacity in the human body. With the exception of CHF, perioperative patients are more than likely to present in a state of relative or absolute hypovolemia. This may be mild dehydration caused by fasting or severe dehydration caused by the administration of purgatives (for bowel lavage), persistent diarrhea, nasogastric suctioning, fistula drainage, or the inability to consume water and electrolytes. Clinical findings that may alert the clinician to dehydration include confusion, loss of skin turgor, longitudinal furrowing of the tongue, dry mucus membranes, sunken eyes, collapsed veins, cold extremities, and highly concentrated urine. A 15% to 30% loss of intravascular volume leads to resting tachycardia. Blood pressure is usually maintained despite up to 40% volume loss because of intense vasoconstriction and transcapillary refill. In addition cardiac output and cardiac index remain within normal limits, and the only hemodynamic indication of hypovolemia is a reduction in stroke volume.[10]

On evaluation of the patients' chemistry panel, the clinician will be alerted by a high ratio of urea to creatinine (>10:1), hypernatremia, and metabolic (contraction) alkalosis (caused by increased SID, consequent of free water deficit). A urine specimen (assuming normal renal function) that is significantly concentrated (eg, 500-1400 mOsm/kg H_2O) with a high specific gravity and low sodium content (<20 mEq/L) can confirm an ECF volume deficit.

Of particular importance is the problem of relative hypovolemia. This occurs typically in patients who are being treated with vasodilator drugs such as angiotensin-converting enzyme (ACE) inhibitors, angiotensin receptor blockers, α_1-receptor antagonists (phenoxybenzamine), and α_2-adrenergic agonists (clonidine). Administration of anesthetic agents typically causes widespread vasodilatation and relative hypovolemia; in patients treated with these drugs, severe hypotension may ensue. Likewise, in patients who present with acute shock caused by volume loss or vasoplegia (such as occurs with sepsis), the administration of anesthesia induction agents (propofol or thiopental) followed by the application of positive-pressure ventilation may result in life-threatening hypotension (**Fig. 35-2**).

The decision to rehydrate patients before and during induction of anesthesia must be guided by the clinical assessment, quantification of preoperative fluid deficits, and the nature of the surgery. Preoperative fasting of 12 hours or more may result in a fluid deficit of more than 1 L, consisting principally of free water. Ambulatory patients administered up to 30 mL/kg per have significantly less dizziness and postoperative nausea and vomiting (PONV) that those given less fluid or none at all.[11-13] It is unclear whether prehydration should involve hypotonic crystalloid or BSS. The administration of dextrose-containing fluids is associated with increased pain, thirst, and blood glucose compared with patients given dextrose-free BSS.[14] For patients who have preexisting GI fluid losses, significant electrolyte depletion is to be anticipated. For upper GI losses, for example, secondary to nasogastric suctioning, vomiting, or gastroparesis, hypochloremia is to be anticipated; "normal" saline is the replacement fluid of choice. For patients with

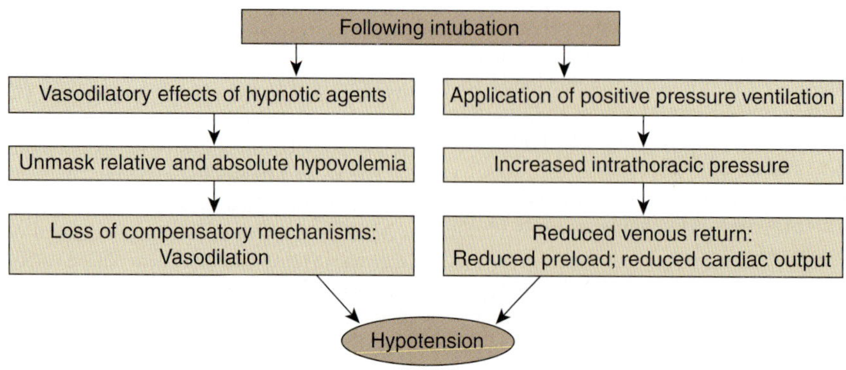

FIGURE 35-2. Hemodynamic consequences of induction, intubation, and positive-pressure ventilation.

lower GI system losses, significant loss of sodium and potassium are to be anticipated, and BSS should be administered. Subsequent to surgical incision, administered fluids should be isotonic because of the 50- to 100-fold increase in antidiuretic hormone (ADH) activity that persists for the duration of the stress response. Large-volume resuscitation with hypotonic fluid may result in acute severe hyponatremia, cerebral edema, and seizures.

HYPERVOLEMIA

Signs of preoperative hypervolemia include a cardiac gallop rhythm, jugular venous distension, ankle or sacral edema, an enlarged liver, and pulmonary edema. There are no pathognomonic laboratory signs of hypervolemia; however, hyponatremia, below normal values of urea and creatinine, and low serum osmolality may be indicative of free water overload.

Postoperative hypervolemia is an inevitable consequence of current fluid administration strategies that has generally been considered benign. Traditionally, generous volumes of IV fluid are administered in the operating room to replete fasting deficits, maintenance requirements and third-space fluid losses. The consequence is an inevitable weight gain of 4 to 6 kg for major surgery.[15] This approach has been challenged, because of emerging evidence of adverse outcomes associated with perioperative fluid overload.[16]

The concept of "third-space" fluid loss or functional ECF deficit derived originally from work by Shires et al[17] The hypothesis behind third spacing is that as a consequence of trauma, hemorrhage, tissue injury, or tissue handling, ECF becomes sequestered in nonfunctional tissue spaces, presumably the injured tissue, the bowel lumen, and other potential spaces such as the pleura and peritoneum. This fluid serves no physiologic purpose and may lead to organ hypoperfusion and, in particular, acute renal failure. Proponents point to the dramatic difference in the incidence of acute renal failure during the Vietnam War, during which liberal fluid management strategies were used, versus the Korean War, when fluid restriction was the norm. A small body of subsequent work investigated ECF volume in the perioperative period with a series of radiolabeled tracers. Brandstrup and colleagues[18] have systematically evaluated this literature and found significant flaws in the methodology. Indeed, there is little or no published evidence that significant third-space fluid loss occurs in clinical practice. Fluid resuscitation strategies based on this premise are associated with an elevated incidence of acute lung injury, abdominal compartment syndrome, prolonged ileus, myocardial ischemia, extensive tissue edema, impaired wound healing, and delayed discharge from the hospital.[16,19,20]

Large-volume fluid resuscitation leads to significant sequestration of fluid in lax tissues in the splanchnic veins and peritoneum. After resolution of the stress response, this fluid is mobilized into the intravascular space, and the patient usually undergoes rapid diuresis. However, in cases of diastolic dysfunction or CHF, the patient may develop acute pulmonary edema ("flash pulmonary edema") or acute myocardial ischemia. This process has been termed *deresuscitation*. Gentle preemptive administration of furosemide may increase venous capacitance and induce earlier diuresis.

SODIUM PHYSIOLOGY

Sodium is the most abundant extracellular ion, responsible for maintenance of the extracellular volume.

There is a dynamic relationship between TBW and extracellular sodium concentration. This water balance is influenced by intakes and outputs, ADH, renin–angiotensin–aldosterone, and serum osmolality. Because sodium ion is excluded from the intracellular space and is the predominant osmotically active substance in the ECF, isolated changes in water volume are generally reflected by inverse changes in the serum sodium concentration and serum osmolality. Hyponatremia generally indicates and expansion in free water volume compared with normal. Hypernatremia generally indicates a reduction in free water concentration.

Total body sodium concentration averages 60 mEq/kg of body weight in a healthy man (ie, 4200 mEq in a 70-kg man). Approximately 2000 to 2200 mEq is dissolved in the ECF. Another 1800 mEq resides within the skeletal system, which constitutes 15% to 16% of body weight. Thus, total body sodium is proportioned as follows: approximately 50% is extracellular, 40% is in bone, and 10% or less is intracellular.

Body sodium is often considered in terms of exchangeable and nonexchangeable moieties. Nonexchangeable sodium is that fraction adsorbed on hydroxyapatite crystals contained deep within the long bones of the skeleton. It amounts to approximately 18 mEq/kg of the total body sodium concentration. Clinically more important is the exchangeable sodium, which represents 42 mEq/kg of total body sodium. This exchangeable fraction includes all sodium within the ECF and ICF and about half of the bone sodium. Exchangeable sodium is in diffusion equilibrium with plasma (serum) sodium and is reflected in the normal ECF concentration of sodium (ie, 136-145 mEq/1). This exchangeable reservoir serves to mitigate concentration changes when sodium is either lost (eg, sweat, diarrhea) or retained (eg, cirrhosis, CHF). As a result, the concentration of sodium may provide little useful information about the total body sodium content.

The daily adult requirement for sodium averages 1 to 2 mEq/kg/d. Normal dietary intake ranges between 100 and 200 mEq/d. The kidney is the principal site of sodium regulation through changes in the rates of glomerular filtration and tubular resorption. Approximately 24 000 mEq of sodium are filtered and resorbed by the kidneys each day. This is modulated by the interaction of a variety of neurohormonal modulators, including the sympathetic nervous system, the renin–angiotensin–aldosterone system, atrial natriuretic peptide, and ADH. Diseases or drugs that impact normal renal function or neuroendocrine function also impact normal sodium–water homeostasis. For example, CHF is characterized by adrenergic activation, release of renin–angiotensin–aldosterone, retention of both salt and water in the renal tubules, and hypervolemia. The administration of ACE inhibitors results in vasodilatation, lowering the blood pressure, diuresis, and natriuresis.

Hyponatremia Hyponatremia exists when the serum (or plasma) sodium is below 135 mEq/L. It may occur in an isotonic, hypertonic, or hypotonic state (**Fig. 35-3**). If the blood is hypo-osmolar in relation to the brain, water enters the brain and can cause acute cerebral edema, particularly in patients who are euvolemic. This may occur with large-volume administration of hypotonic fluids or in patients who develop transurethral resection of the prostate (TURP) syndrome caused by intravasation of hypotonic fluid during TURP. This may lead to a spectrum of neurologic upsets ranging from confusion to seizures to coma to brainstem herniation. Rapid correction of low sodium can lead to osmotic demyelination of the brain or brainstem because of rapid shrinkage of the brain.

Serum osmolality is governed by contributions from all molecules in the body that cannot easily move between the intracellular and extracellular space. Sodium is the most abundant electrolyte, but glucose, urea, plasma proteins, and lipids are also important. A patient with diabetic ketoacidosis may have hyponatremia but normal osmolality because of hyperglycemia, hypertriglyceridemia, and increased plasma ketones. Each of these compounds is osmotically active. Patients with acute renal failure may have hyponatremia caused by uremia characterized by the accumulation of urea and other nitrogenous waste products.

If a patient has hyponatremia, with low measured and calculated serum osmolality, it is called *hypotonic hyponatremia*. If serum osmolality is normal or high, it is isotonic or hypertonic hyponatremia or pseudohyponatremia.

Serum osmolality is calculated from

$$2(\text{Na} + \text{K}) + \text{BUN}/2.8 + \text{Glucose}/16 \text{ (in mEq/L)}$$

or in SI units (mmol/L)

$$2(\text{Na} + \text{K}) + \text{Urea} + \text{Glucose}$$

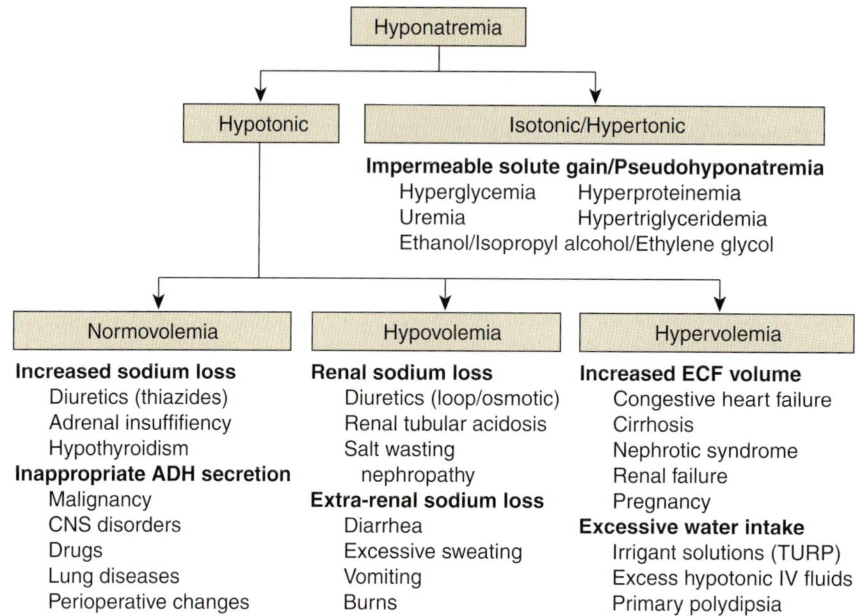

FIGURE 35-3. Hyponatremia. ADH, antidiuretic hormone; CNS, central nervous system; ECF, extracellular fluid; IV, intravenous; TURP, transurethral resection of the prostate.

Classically, pseudohyponatremia is divided into conditions in which the measured and calculated serum osmolalities are the same—hyperglycemia or uremia—and those in which there is an osmolar gap; some osmoles are clearly present as measured by serum osmolality but not identified by standard blood tests. The source of unmeasured osmoles may be endogenous (lipids or proteins) or exogenous (alcohols, including ethanol, ethylene glycol, methanol, or isopropyl alcohol). The recognition of pseudohyponatremia is important because therapy for the decreased serum sodium concentration is not indicated.

Hypertonic hyponatremia occurs when a decreased serum sodium concentration coexists with an increased serum osmolality. An increase in concentration of any osmotically active substance, which is confined predominately to the ECF (eg, glucose, glycerol, mannitol), results in water movement out of cells along the osmolar gradient. The osmolar load usually evokes an osmotic diuresis, leading to urinary loss of both sodium and water. These losses may, in turn, potentiate both the hypertonicity and the hyponatremia. Clinically, the most frequent cause of this water and electrolyte disturbance is the occurrence of significant hyperglycemia in uncontrolled or poorly controlled diabetes mellitus. The measured serum sodium concentration decreases approximately 1.6 mEq/L for each 100-mg/dL increment of blood glucose.

True hyponatremia may result from increased TBW associated with edema (liver failure, CHF, renal failure, or nephrotic syndrome), hypotonic fluid overload, or sodium loss in excess of free water. Total-body sodium concentration is increased, and there is a concomitant defect in the excretion of solute-free water. Water retention is proportionately greater than sodium retention, resulting in hypervolemic hyponatremia. This may be associated with extensive tissue edema. Despite the dramatic increase in ECF volume, there is a tendency toward venous pooling and accumulation of fluid in lax tissues and in the peritoneum. Consequently, the plasma volume and stroke volume may be reduced, leading to renal hypoperfusion and activation of volume defense mechanisms by way of the juxtaglomerular apparatus and renin–angiotensin–aldosterone axis. This leads to a vicious cycle of hypervolemia, characteristically associated with CHF.

Dehydration associated with hyponatremia (hypovolemic hyponatremia) may be of renal or extrarenal origin. Renal losses are identified by a urinary sodium greater than 40 mEq/L and are characterized by the inability of the body to retain sodium. This may be caused by loop, thiazide, or osmotic diuretics; carbonic anhydrase inhibitors; primary aldosterone deficiency (Addison disease or adrenal insufficiency); or cerebral salt wasting (CWS; associated with subarachnoid hemorrhage). If the urinary sodium is less than 20 mEq/L, then the site of sodium loss is outside the kidney, usually the lower GI tract, and associated with diarrhea. The mechanism of hyponatremia is the in-built priority of preservation of volume over osmolality. Hence, in this situation, there is a dramatic increase in plasma ADH levels.

A number of diseases and drugs cause abnormal release of ADH, either caused by ectopic production of ADH (ADH-secreting tumors) or increased release of this compound from the posterior pituitary gland (**Table 35-2**). The result is a paradoxically concentrated urine with dilute blood (the urinary osmolality is higher [>300 mOsm] than the serum osmolality [<300 mOsm]). The result is a state of hypervolemic or euvolemic hyponatremia. The syndrome of inappropriate secretion of ADH (SIADH) is easily confused with CSW; whereas SIADH improves with fluid restriction, CWS does not.

Several factors in perioperative medicine can contribute to functional SIADH. These include emotional stress, anxiety, nausea, pain, the administration of opiates, and mechanical ventilation. Obstetric patients frequently receive oxytocin to increase uterine contractility. Indeed, the acute stress response should be seen as a state of free water retention, and for that reason, large-volume resuscitation hypotonic fluids should be avoided. Conversely, SIADH from other causes (Table 32-1) is treated initially with water restriction (**Table 35-3**). Patients with chronic SIADH may be treated by inducing a state of nephrogenic diabetes insipidus, for example, by administering drugs such as lithium and demeclocycline.

A potentially fatal cause of hyponatremia, particular to perioperative medicine, is TURP syndrome. This procedure requires continuous irrigation of the operative field to improve visibility and distend the bladder or prostatic urethra. The systemic absorption of these irrigating solutions can produce acute and sometimes dramatic hyponatremia. The irrigating fluids cannot contain electrolytes to prevent current dispersion from the resectoscope; hence, distilled water solutions containing isotonic glycine, mannitol, or sorbitol are usually used. During TURP, systemic absorption of the irrigating solutions is influenced by the duration of exposure, the number and size of venous sinuses opened, extravasation of the fluid into tissues outside the bladder or prostatic capsule, and the hydrostatic pressure of the fluid. The majority of patients undergoing TURP probably intravasate some hypotonic

TABLE 35-2 Syndrome of Inappropriate Antidiuretic Hormone (ADH) Secretion

Increased Hypothalamic Production of Antidiuretic Hormone

1. Neuropsychiatric disorders
   Infections: meningitis, encephalitis, brain abscess
   Vascular: thrombosis, subarachnoid or subdural hemorrhage, temporal arteritis, cavernous sinus thrombosis, stroke
   Neoplasm: primary or metastatic
   Skull fracture, traumatic brain injury
   Psychosis, delirium tremens
   Other: Guillain-Barré syndrome, acute intermittent porphyria, autonomic neuropathy, postpituitary surgery, multiple sclerosis, epilepsy, hydrocephalus, lupus erythematosus
2. Drugs
   Intravenous cyclophosphamide
   Carbamazepine
   Vincristine or vinblastine
   Thiothixene
   Thioridazine, other phenothiazines
   Haloperidol
   Amitriptyline, other tricyclic antidepressants or serotonin reuptake inhibitors
   Monoamine oxidase inhibitors
   Bromocriptine
   Lorcainide
   Clofibrate
   General anesthesia
   Narcotics, opiate derivatives
   Nicotine
3. Lung diseases and interventions
   Pneumonia
   Tuberculosis
   Lung abscess, empyema
   Acute respiratory failure
   Positive pressure ventilation
4. Perioperative period: associated with the stress response to injury and pain

Ectopic (Nonhypothalamic) Production of Antidiuretic hormone

1. Cancer
   Small cell carcinoma of the lung (two-thirds of patients with small cell carcinoma have impaired water excretion), bronchogenic, duodenum, pancreas, thymus, olfactory neuroblastoma, bladder, prostate, uterus
   Lymphosarcoma, reticulum cell sarcoma, mesothelioma, Ewing sarcoma
   Hodgkin disease, leukemia
   Pulmonary tuberculosis

fluid, and there are few sequelae. However, when large volumes are absorbed, severe hyponatremia leading to cerebral edema may ensue. Consequently, urologists routinely administer furosemide when resection is complete. On occasion, it is necessary to administer hypertonic fluids to replete a sodium deficit.

TABLE 35-3 Management of Hyponatremia

If Na >125, the treatment is water restriction, 500-1000 mL/d
If Na <125, or water restriction is not possible, furosemide 40-80 mg IV repeated as necessary with replacement of electrolyte losses
If this strategy is unsuccessful at raising serum sodium, treatment with hypertonic saline may be necessary: NaCl 0.9% contains 1 mEq of Na in 6.5 mL (ie, 0.154 mmol/mL), NaCl 1.8% contains ~1 mEq Na per 3.25 mL, and 3% NaCl contains ~1 mEq Na per 2 mL
If the cause is SIADH and the patient does not respond to fluid restriction, then loop diuretics may be helpful. An alternative treatment is to cause a nephrogenic diabetes insipidus by administering demeclocycline 300-600 mg BID

BID, twice a day; IV, intravenous; SIADH, syndrome of inappropriate secretion of antidiuretic hormone.

If HS is to be use, the sodium deficit must be calculated (the normal serum sodium is 140 mEq/L):

Step 1: Find out the patient's weight is kilograms before illness.

Step 2: Calculate the sodium deficit.

It is usual to correct only half the sodium deficit (NaD) (hence the deficit/2)

$$\text{NaD} = (\text{Desired sodium} - \text{Patient's sodium}/2)$$

If the patient's weight is 70 kg and the serum sodium is 120 mEq/L, then the desired change is 10 mEq/L

Total body deficit of sodium is the sodium deficit × TBW

$$\text{NaD} \times (\text{weight in Kg} \times 0.6) = \text{Total deficit (TD)}$$

Using the formula: $10 \times (70 \times 0.6) = 420$ mEq

Step 3: Calculate the rate of replacement.

Most physicians replace the deficit at no more than 0.5 mEq/h. The patient has a deficit of 10 mEq, so at this rate, it will be replaced over 20 hours (10/0.5).

$$\text{Rate of replacement (RoR) in hours} = \text{NaD}/0.5$$

Step 4: Replace the sodium deficit with the fluid of your choice.

The amount of fluid required depends on the sodium content of that fluid (**Table 35-4**):

So,

$$\text{TD}/[\text{Na Fluid/mL}]/\text{RoR} = \text{Per hour fluid replacement}$$

If one is using 3% saline in this 70-kg male patient with a serum sodium of 120 mEq/L:

$$(420/0.513) / 20 = 41 \text{ mL/h}$$

That is, after 20 hours, assuming no other fluids are given, the patient's serum sodium will increase to 130 mEq/L. If 0.9% saline is given:

$$(420/0.13)/20 = 160 \text{ mL/h}$$

Care must be taken when repleting sodium deficits to avoid the problem of osmotic demyelination (central pontine myelinolysis). Rapid correction of hyponatremia may trigger demyelination of pontine or extrapontine neurons, leading to neurologic dysfunction that may include quadriplegia, pseudobulbar palsy, seizures, coma, and even death.[21] For this reason, serum sodium is increased slowly, and only 50% of the deficit is corrected.

Hypernatremia A serum sodium of greater than 145 mEq represents a hypertonic and hyperosmolar state. There is a net deficit of water in relation to sodium. This implies neither an increase in total body sodium nor a deficit in TBW. Hypernatremia is rarely encountered in routine perioperative patients; however, it is a common finding in the intensive care unit (ICU) and consequently in patients traveling to the operating room from the ICU for subsequent procedures. When the

TABLE 35-4 Sodium Content of Various Intravenous Fluids

Fluid (Infusate)	Na Content (mEq/L)	Sodium Concentration per mL
Lactated Ringer solution	130	0.130
0.9% NaCl	154	0.154 mEq/mL
1.8%	308	0.380 mEq/L
3% NaCl	513	0.513 mEq/mL
5% NaCl	855	0.855 mEq/mL

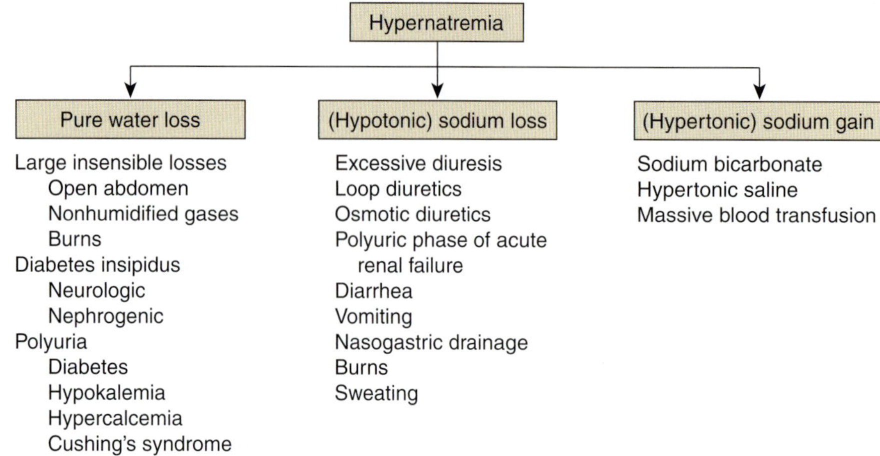

FIGURE 35-4. Hypernatremia.

serum osmolality exceeds 305 to 310 mOsm/kg H_2O, ADH secretion is stimulated, and the urine becomes severely concentrated (ie, osmolality >800-1000 mOsm/kg H_2O). The thirst response is activated in an attempt to stem cellular dehydration. Hypertonicity and hypernatremia rarely develop in the presence of an intact thirst mechanism and access to water. However, critically ill patients are often too sedated to express thirst or unable to drink water.

The imbalance between TBW and sodium that occurs in hypernatremia may develop from either water loss or sodium gain (**Fig. 35-4** and **Table 35-5**).[22] This may result from pure dehydration, the presence of a free water deficit (hypovolemic hypernatremia) such as occurs with administration of loop or osmotic diuretics, excessive evaporative losses (nonhumidified breathing systems), or diabetes insipidus (either cranial or nephrogenic). Patients with diabetes insipidus may present to the operating room in 3 circumstances. First, patients with traumatic brain injury (TBI) complicated by diabetes insipidus may present for neurosurgery, such as for decompressive craniectomy. Second, a patient who has undergone devastating brain injury, either traumatic or hemorrhagic, complicated by diabetes insipidus, may present for organ harvest after brain death. Finally, a patient who has been chronically treated with lithium for bipolar disorder complicated by diabetes insipidus, may present for routine surgery. In each of these situations, the major risk to the patient (or his or her organs) is not hypernatremia but hypovolemia, and the anesthesiologist must be careful to replenish perioperative urinary losses.

TABLE 35-5 Causes of Hypernatremia

Pure water loss
Large insensible losses: no humidifier on mechanical ventilator
Diabetes insipidus
Neurologic: associated with head injury, brain hemorrhage, or meningitis
Nephrogenic: caused by lithium, demeclocycline, amphotericin B, heavy metal poisoning, hypokalemia, and hypercalcemia
Hypotonic fluid loss
Excessive diuresis with loop of osmotic diuretics
Polyuric phase of acute renal failure
Diarrhea
Vomiting
Nasogastric drainage
Burns
Sweating
Hypertonic sodium gain
Sodium bicarbonate infusion
Hypertonic saline administration

Hypernatremic hypernatremia is associated with sodium gain in the presence of either euvolemia or hypervolemia. This may result from administration of HS, sodium bicarbonate, blood transfusion (sodium citrate), or parenteral nutrition (sodium acetate). Hypernatremia may be accompanied by metabolic alkalosis associated with an increase in the SID from either dehydration of sodium gain (see below).

Hypernatremia can be associated with significant neurologic sequelae: Initially, the brain shrinks because of volume depletion, which makes the blood vessels vulnerable to rupture. The brain adapts to dehydration by expressing more solute, which may lead to cerebral edema, a neurologic deficit, or convulsions.

The clinical approach to the management of patients with hypernatremia is to identify and treat the source and replace the free water deficit. To correct hypernatremia, fluid and electrolyte losses must be restored. The rate of correction depends on the duration of hypernatremia: In general, for critically ill patients, correction at a rate of 1 mEq Na/L/h is appropriate; if hypernatremia is prolonged, 0.5 mEq Na/L/h is more advisable (to reduce the risk of rebound cerebral edema).

Calculation of the free water deficit:

$$0.6 \times \text{patient's weight in kg} \times (\text{patient's sodium}/140 - 1)$$

where 0.6 × weight* = Estimated body water and 140 = Desired sodium.

So, for a 70-kg man with a serum sodium of 150 mEq/L = 3 L.

Any fluid can be used to replace the free water loss, either isotonic or hypotonic. However, the more hypotonic the fluid administered, the more rapidly the deficit will be replaced.

In the example above, one wished to reduce the patient's serum sodium by 10 mEq/L, how much of what fluid does one use? This depends on the amount of sodium in the chosen fluid and then applying this figure to the formula below (**Table 35-6**):

$$\text{Change in serum Na per liter} = \text{Infusate Na} - \text{Serum Na/Weight in kilograms} \times (0.6 - 1)$$

If one chose D5% (dextrose 5% in water) and planned to correct this patient's sodium at a rate of 1 mEq/L/h: Because each liter will correct 3.5mEq, the rate of fluid infusion would be 1000 mL/3.5 = 285 mL/h.

Clearly, for simple hypernatremia, the choice of fluid determines the volume required to correct the sodium abnormality (a much larger volume of LRS is required compared with D5%). The administration of free water, for example, via the enteral route, is probably the most effective method replenishing extracellular water deficit.

*This represents TBW for young men; for women and elderly men, multiply the weight in kilograms by 0.5.

TABLE 35-6 Sodium Content of Fluids Used to Treat Hypernatremia

Fluid (Infusate)	Na Content (mEq/L)	Change per Liter in a 70-kg Man With Na 150 mEq/L
Dextrose 5% in water	0	−3.5 mEq Na/L
0.2% NaCl in D5%	34	−2.7 mEq Na/L
0.45% NaCl	77	−1.7 mEq Na/L
Lactated Ringer solution	130	−0.5 mEq Na/L

POTASSIUM PHYSIOLOGY

Potassium is the major intracellular cation in the body and has several roles, the most important being the generation of the resting cell membrane potential and the action potential, as well as protein synthesis, acid–base balance, and maintenance of intracellular osmolality.

The total body potassium content ranges from 50 to 55 mEq per kg of body weight. Potassium is an intracellular cation, and approximately 98% of the body stores are located within the ICF compartment (ie, only a total of 60-70 mEq exists in the ECF). A huge concentration gradient exists between the ICF and ECF compartments (150 mEq/L and 3.5 to 5.5 mEq/L, respectively). The primary mechanism for establishing and maintaining this concentration gradient is the sodium-potassium–activated ATPase "pump" that is located in the plasma membrane of all body cells. These membrane-bound ionic transport pumps and the selective permeability characteristics of cell membranes are responsible for the transmembrane electrical potential difference found in all living cells. Potassium is the ion responsible for generating cellular electrical activity. Hence, hypo- and hyperkalemia result in significant neuromuscular dysfunction.

The total amount of potassium present in the body is approximately 3200 mEq, 90% of which is intracellular, and this is regulated by a variety of homeostatic mechanisms. Of total body potassium, approximately 135 to 150 mEq/L is intracellular compared with plasma levels of 3.5 to 5.5 mEq/L. The daily requirement is about 1 mEq/kg/d absorbed from the small intestine. Potassium excretion exactly matches intake, and body stores are quantitatively stable. Potassium balance is predominately governed by urinary loss. The kidney can adjust urinary potassium excretion from less than 1 mEq/L to greater than 100 mEq/L. In addition, there is some secretion of potassium in the colon.

Two factors impact renal handling of potassium, renal tubular fluid flow and aldosterone. The majority of filtered potassium is reabsorbed in the proximal tubule. The distal tubules then secrete potassium. This is influenced by the intracellular potassium concentration, the rate of urinary flow, and the anionic charge of the urine. As the rate of flow increases, there is a significant increase in potassium excretion. This explains hypokalemia associated with diuresis. Conditions that increase distal tubular sodium delivery promote potassium excretion and sodium reabsorption, particularly in the presence of aldosterone.

One of the most important roles of potassium is the resting membrane potential and in the repolarization phase of action potentials. The normal cell membrane is relatively permeable to potassium ions and impermeable to sodium and anions. The anions generate a negative intracellular potential. Potassium is held intracellularly against the electrochemical gradient by the action of the Na^+/K^+ ATPase pump that maintains the resting membrane potential. The relative ratio for intracellular to extracellular potassium is responsible for electrochemical activity. Hence, abnormalities of potassium concentration directly impact neuromuscular activity.

Hyperkalemia Hyperkalemia is generally defined as a serum potassium concentration of greater than 5.5 mEq/L. Numerous conditions, diseases, and drugs produce hyperkalemia by disrupting the normal external or internal potassium balance (**Table 35-7**) (or both). Factitious hyperkalemia is associated with hemolysis of the blood sample.

TABLE 35-7 Causes of Hyperkalemia

Causes of Hyperkalemia
Increased exogenous potassium load
Potassium supplements, including TPN
Enteral potassium administration
Red blood cell transfusion
Penicillin G administration
Increased endogenous potassium load
Rhabdomyolysis
Impaired excretion
Acute or chronic renal failure
ACE inhibitors
Potassium-sparing diuretics
Congestive heart failure
Heparin
Tacrolimus of cyclosporine
Trimethoprim
Amphotericin
Heparin
Intracellular-to-extracellular exchange
Hyperglycemia
Metabolic acidosis
β-Blockers
Succinylcholine
Digoxin

ACE, angiotensin-converting enzyme; TPN, total parenteral nutrition.

Several factors may produce a transient increase in serum potassium concentration caused by a transcellular shift. This includes administration of succinylcholine (0.3-0.5 mEq/L in normal subjects), burns, diabetes, metabolic acidosis, and nonselective β-blockers.

Succinylcholine may be associated with significant hyperkalemia is certain circumstances. These include conditions with muscle membrane degeneration (eg, trauma, burns, primary muscle disorders) or neural denervation (eg, stroke, multiple sclerosis, Guillain-Barre syndrome, spinal cord injuries). Impaired potassium excretion is associated with acute and chronic renal failure, adrenal insufficiency, hypoaldosteronism (for any reason), and the use of ACE inhibitors.

In hyperkalemia, the resting membrane potential is decreased toward the threshold potential (**Fig. 35-5**). With mild hyperkalemia (ie, serum

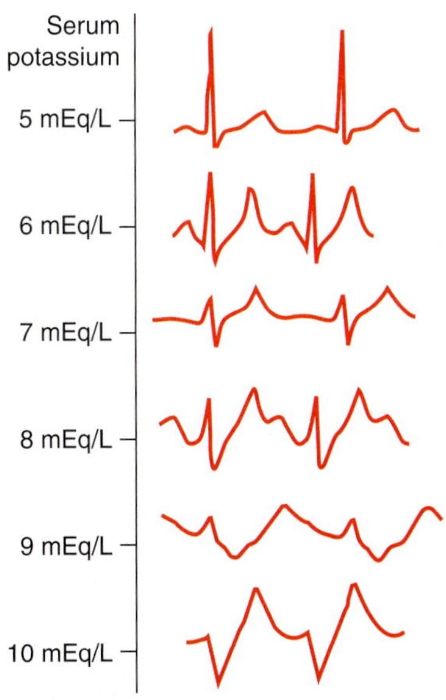

FIGURE 35-5. Electrocardiographic changes associated with progressive hyperkalemia.

potassium concentration of <6-7 mEq/L), there is increased automaticity as reflected by atrial or ventricular ectopy. Progressive hyperkalemia enhances rapid repolarization (phase 3), which causes shortening of the T-wave interval and symmetrical peaking of the T wave. If the serum potassium concentration continues to increase, the inward movement of sodium (phase 0) and calcium (phase 2) diminishes, the PR interval becomes prolonged and eventually the P waves (atrial phase 0) disappear. Within the ventricular muscle mass, both conduction velocity and the height of the action potential are reduced. The net result is a widened QRS complex and reduced contractility. If the hyperkalemia progresses, the QRS complex become smooth, wide, and sinusoidal as it merges with the T wave (serum potassium concentration of >10 mEq/L). Without treatment, ventricular fibrillation will ensue.

Emergency treatment is aimed at quickly stabilizing the myocardium and restoring normal transmembrane electrical potentials. A total of 10 to 30 mL of 10% calcium gluconate can be administered over 3 to 5 minutes (or 5-10 mL calcium chloride may be substituted). Calcium reduces both the threshold potential and the excitability of cell membranes. The duration of action is roughly 30 to 60 minutes; a second dose may be necessary. Alternative temporizing measures include administration of sodium bicarbonate, nebulized albuterol, or insulin and dextrose in combination. Both have the impact of sending potassium into cells, the former by increasing SID and the latter by a direct effect. One unit of regular insulin is recommended for each 2 g of dextrose. For example, 1 ampule of D50 (ie, 50 mL of 50% dextrose) would be immediately followed by 12 units of regular insulin.

More definitive treatment of hyperkalemia can be achieved by administering exchange resins administered orally or rectally. These include calcium or sodium polystyrene sulfonate in combination with sorbitol, which facilitates potassium excretion through colonic exchange of calcium or sodium for potassium. If this approach fails, hemodialysis may be required.

Hypokalemia Hypokalemia is typically considered a potassium level of less than 3.5 mmol/L, although patients may be asymptomatic until the level is less than 2.5 mmol/L. Although the relative decrease in extracellular potassium may appear small (1-2 mEq/L), this represents a significant total body deficit of potassium, up to 500 mEq. On average, plasma potassium decreases by 0.3mmol/L for each 100-mmol reduction in total body stores.

Acute hypokalemia is associated with either inadequate intake or absolute loss of potassium from the body, governed by the law of mass conservation, or transcellular movement (**Fig. 35-6** and **Table 35-8**). Causes of absolute loss include vomiting, diarrhea, bowel fistulae, loop and osmotic diuretics, and the diuretic phase of acute renal failure. Causes of intracellular potassium shifting include metabolic alkalosis, use of β_2-adrenergic agonists, hyperadrenergic states (including the acute stress response), administration of insulin, and hypothermia. Chronic causes of hypokalemia include malnutrition, malabsorption, diuretic usage, corticosteroid administration, and Conn syndrome (hyperaldosteronism).

TABLE 35-8 Causes of Hypokalemia

Altered transcellular (internal) balance
Metabolic alkalosis
Insulin
β_2-Adrenergic agonists
After resolution of the stress response
Anabolism
Periodic Paralysis
Altered external balance
Decreased intake
Inadequate content in intravenous fluids
Malabsorption
Malnutrition
Increased renal excretion
Diuretics
Polyuria
Hyperaldosteronism
Hypomagnesemia
Renal tubular acidosis
High dose penicillins
Increased gastrointestinal loss
Vomiting
Nasogastric suctioning
Diarrhea

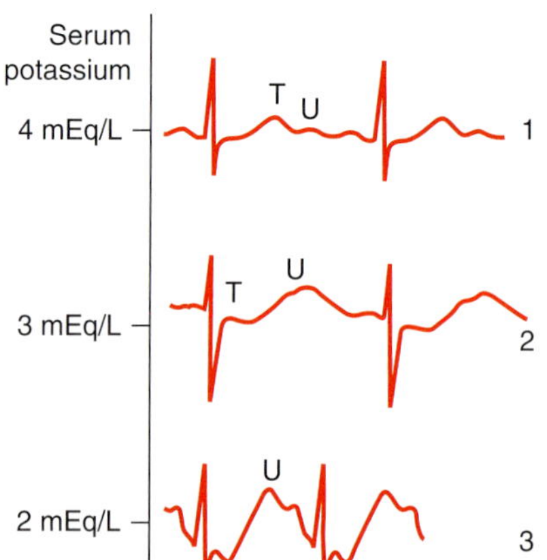

FIGURE 35-6. Electrocardiographic (ECG) changes associated with progressive hypokalemia. Strip 1, normal ECG. Strip 2, flattened T wave, prominent U wave. Strip 3, Prolonged PR interval, prolonged QRS, ST segment depression, heightened U waves, and prolonged QU interval.

Potassium depletion causes muscle weakness. The ratio of intracellular to extracellular potassium increases, thereby reducing the resting potential (phase 4) and creating a state of hyperpolarization. When the action potential is initiated (phase 0), it is of super-normal magnitude. The time allotted for calcium entry (phase 2) is shortened, and repolarization (phase 3) is prolonged, leading to a greater relative refractory period. The diminished calcium entry affects skeletal muscle and may lead to myalgia, cramps, and weakness. The smooth muscle components of the bladder, GI tract, and the peripheral vasculature are also affected, leading to urinary retention, ileus, and postural hypotension. The ensuing vasoplegia may be catecholamine insensitive.

Hypokalemia impacts cardiac conduction and contractility. Progressive electrocardiographic (ECG) changes are typical (**Fig. 35-7**): T-wave amplitude decreases, QT interval lengthens, the U wave appears or becomes broader and taller, the ST segment sags, and P-wave amplitude and QRS duration increase. Cardiac arrhythmias are relatively common. The most common dysrhythmias are atrial fibrillation and premature ventricular systoles, but supraventricular tachycardia, junctional tachycardia, and Mobitz type I second-degree atrioventricular block may also occur. Hypokalemia may induce digitalis toxicity.

It is probably unnecessary to administer potassium supplements to patients with mild hypokalemia. If moderate to severe hypokalemia (<3.0 mEq/L) is present, IV potassium chloride or potassium phosphate is usually administered. The maximal recommended rate of infusion is 0.5 to 0.7 mEq/kg/h. The repletion of total body potassium stores requires approximately 200 mEq for each 1-mEq/L reduction in the serum potassium concentration. Magnesium is an essential cofactor for transcellular sodium–potassium ion pumps. If hypomagnesemia coexists, magnesium supplements should be administered to ensure intracellular potassium repletion.

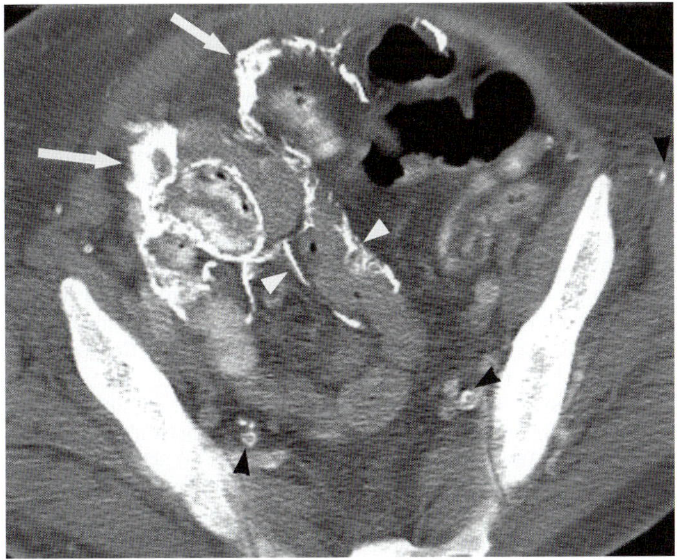

FIGURE 35-7. Sclerosing peritonitis. A 77-year-old woman with chronic renal failure, secondary hypercalcemia, and on chronic peritoneal dialysis with abdominal pain. An axial noncontrast computed tomographic image through the pelvis demonstrates thick calcification of the peritoneum (*arrows*) and of the serosa of small bowel loops (*white arrowheads*). Note also extensive vascular calcification (*black arrowheads*). [Courtesy of Diane Bergin MD, Thomas Jefferson University Hospital, Philadelphia, PA]

Calcium Physiology Calcium is an essential inorganic element that plays a crucial role in many biologic functions. It is the single most abundant electrolyte in the human body. A normal adult contains between 1000 and 1400 g of calcium, of which 99% is located in bone, where it is the primary structural component. Approximately 1% of the total calcium pool resides in the soft tissues and the ECF compartment. Circulating calcium exists in 3 forms, a free ionized fraction (50%); a fraction bound to protein (mostly albumin) (40%); and a diffusible, nonionized fraction (10%) in which calcium is chelated with circulating anions (eg, bicarbonate, phosphate, citrate). The ionized fraction is the calcium that is physiologically active, and it is the concentration of this fraction that is closely regulated by parathyroid hormone (PTH), vitamin E, and calcitonin. These substances alter the resorption of calcium from various target organs, including the skeletal system, GI tract, and kidneys.

A measurement of total serum calcium (the analysis most often performed when a calcium level is requested) reflects the quantitative contribution of all 3 forms of circulating calcium. The normal value varies depending on the particular laboratory but is generally in the range of 8.5 to 10.5 mg/dL (4.5-5.5 mEq/L or 0.96-1.27 mmol/L). The reported quantity may be misleading because of albumin binding, and calcium concentration measured in this way must be corrected for albumin concentration. Modern laboratories have the capability of directly measuring ionized calcium. The normal values for this measurement usually range from 4 to 5 mg/dL (2.1-2.6 mEq/L or 1.17-1.29 mmol/L).

Calcium has a number of important physiologic functions. As an essential component in neuromuscular transmission, calcium is involved in myocardial contractility by way of voltage-sensitive calcium channels in the myocardium. Calcium is involved in both depolarization and the magnitude of muscle contraction. Calcium is stored in the sarcoplasmic reticulum. Neurochemical activation leads to an increase in cytoplasmic calcium concentration. Calcium binds to troponin C, and this complex binds to tropomycin, which facilitates the interaction between actin and myosin, resulting in cardiac muscular contraction. Increased intracellular calcium is associated with increased contractility, inotropy, and cardiac output. Calcium is removed by reuptake into the sarcoplasmic reticulum and by extrusion via the Ca^{2+}-Na^{+} pump located in the plasma membrane. This results in relaxation. Calcium is also an essential component in both skeletal muscle and smooth muscle contractility.

Calcium is an important cofactor for blood coagulation. The cytoplasm of platelets contains contractile filaments of actin and myosin that enable activated platelets to change their shape and release the contents of their granules. This process is driven by intracellular calcium. Calcium is important in the activation of thrombin, acting as a cofactor with factors VII, IX, and X.

Calcium is absorbed by the small intestine under the influence of calcitriol, a derivative of vitamin D. Calcitriol also facilitates absorption of phosphate from the intestine and absorption of calcium from the nephron and influences bone formation and osteoclastic activity. The major control hormone for calcium metabolism is PTH. This hormone causes release of calcium and phosphate from bone. It also enables renal calcium reabsorption and renal phosphate excretion and activates calcitriol. Calcitonin has the opposite impact on serum calcium to PTH. It inhibits renal reabsorption of calcium and osteoclastic bone formation.

Hypercalcemia Hypercalcemia is associated with numerous conditions and disorders, including hyperparathyroidism, immobilization, chronic renal failure, adrenal insufficiency, thyrotoxicosis, sarcoidosis, and various drugs (**Table 35-9**).

The commonest cause of hypercalcemia is hyperparathyroidism. Anesthesiologists encounter these patients because they are frequently scheduled for parathyroidectomy. The second most common cause of acute hypercalcemia is malignancy secondary to bone destruction by metastases or caused by secretion of calcemic factors by the tumor. This problem is most frequently encountered in patients with breast cancer, myeloma, bronchogenic, and renal cell carcinoma.

A wide variety of clinical symptoms are characteristic of hypercalcemia, often described as "bones, stones, groans, and moans." Patients develop bony pain, renal calculi, abdominal symptoms, and neuropsychiatric problems. Abdominal problems include nausea and vomiting, constipation, and acute and chronic pancreatitis. Hypercalcemia may impact cardiac electrical conduction by progressive shortening of the QT interval, leading to arrhythmias and possible cardiac arrest. Hypertension caused by contraction of vascular smooth muscle is common. Hypercalcemia has varying effects on the kidneys. It may cause polyuria and polydipsia (mimicking diabetes mellitus) by interfering with ADH activity on the collecting ducts. It may reduce renal blood flow and glomerular filtration. It may cause nephrocalcinosis, interstitial nephritis, and urolithiasis. In the central nervous system, hypercalcemia may cause anxiety, depression, irritability, lethargy, confusion, and psychosis.

The mainstay of therapy is hydration, either with or without the use of loop diuretics such as furosemide. Renal clearances of sodium and chloride are closely linked, so the co-administration of salt solutions and diuretics allows rehydration and naturesis. Other alternative therapies include chelators (eg, phosphates and EDTA), osteoclast inhibitors (eg, mithramycin, glucocorticoids, calcitonin, diphosphonates), and calcium channel blockers (verapamil).

Hypocalcemia Ionized hypocalcemia develops when there is significant calcium loss from the body. In perioperative medicine, this may be associated with massive blood transfusion, massive crystalloid resuscitation,

TABLE 35-9 Causes of Hypercalcemia

Hyperparathyroidism
Malignancy
Adrenal insufficiency
Sarcoidosis
Thyrotoxicosis
Immobilization
Drugs
Thiazide diuretics
Exogenous calcium or vitamin D
Furosemide
Tamoxifen
β-Adrenergic agonists

TABLE 35-10 Causes of Hypocalcemia

Overhydration with calcium-free intravenous fluids
Massive blood transfusion
Hypoparathyroidism
After parathyroid surgery
Hypomagnesemia
Metabolic alkalosis
Chronic renal failure
Vitamin D deficiency
Osteomalacia
Sepsis or other critical illness
Burns
Anticonvulsant therapy

or after parathyroidectomy (**Table 35-10**). Other causes include acute and chronic renal failure, vitamin D deficiency, hypomagnesemia, rhabdomyolysis, malnutrition, burns, sepsis, and acute pancreatitis. Critically ill patients frequently have hypocalcemia. During massive transfusion, the presence of citrate in the blood may result in significant hypocalcemia. The hallmark of hypocalcemia is neuromuscular irritability, with symptoms ranging from paresthesia to tetany and seizures. In addition, hypocalcemia may augment the neuromuscular blockade caused by nondepolarizing muscle relaxants. Mild hypocalcemia (ionized calcium levels of 3.2-3.9 mg/dL), even in critically ill patients, usually does not evoke symptoms. Patients undergoing parathyroidectomy may develop acute postoperative hypocalcemia, requiring supplementation.

The clinical features of acute hypocalcemia are listed in **Table 35-11**. Acute hypocalcemia is associated with increased neuromuscular irritability. In mild hypocalcemia, the patient may complain of paraesthesia of the fingers and toes and numbness (and burning) around the lips and mouth. With more severe hypocalcemia (ionized Ca <1.0 mmol/L), the patient may complain of painful muscles spasms, particularly of the fingers and thumb (carpal spasm). The term *tetany* has been used to describe this process, whereby there is repetitive neuromuscular discharge after a single stimulus. Tetany can be elicited by tapping over the facial nerve proximal to the auricle; this leads to twitching of the ipsilateral facial muscles, particularly around the eyes and mouth (Chvostek sign). Carpal spasm can be elicited by inflating a blood pressure cuff around the arm for several minutes, presumably causing mild ischemia and provoking muscle contraction (Trousseau sign). Pain, anxiety, and hyperventilation may precipitate muscular spasms in postoperative patients, potentially causing stridor or laryngospasm.

TABLE 35-11 Clinical Features of Hypocalcemia

Neurologic
Paraesthesia
Muscle cramps
Tetany
Muscle weakness
Hyperactive reflexes
Convulsions
Respiratory
Laryngeal spasm
Bronchospasm
Cardiovascular
Hypotension
Impaired contractility
Bradycardia
Arrhythmias
Digitalis insensitivity
Cardiac arrest
ECG changes: QT and ST prolongation, T-wave inversion
Psychiatric
Anxiety
Confusion
Irritability
Depression
Psychosis
Dementia

Acute symptomatic hypocalcemia is a medical emergency that warrants the IV administration of calcium. Therapy should not be withheld even if the cause of the hypocalcemia is unclear. In adults, the recommended treatment is a 100-mg bolus of elemental calcium (over 5-10 minutes) followed by a continuous infusion administered at a rate of 0.5 to 2 mg/kg/h. Note that a bolus dose of calcium will only increase the ionized calcium concentration for 1 to 2 hours. Consequently, repeated boluses or an infusion is required.

Two different calcium salt preparations are readily available for IV administration, calcium chloride and calcium gluconate. Calcium chloride 10% contains 27.2 mg of elemental calcium in 10 mL. Calcium gluconate contains 9.3 mg of elemental calcium per 10 mL. Calcium chloride is very irritating to the peripheral vasculature and should be administered directly into the central venous circulation, if at all possible. In addition, the chloride salt is acidifying and theoretically should not be used when acidemia coincides with hypocalcemia. Thus, in the presence of significant metabolic acidosis, calcium gluconate should be used.

MAGNESIUM PHYSIOLOGY

Magnesium is the fourth most abundant cation within the body and is the second most prevalent intracellular cation next to potassium. Within the body, magnesium is distributed such that 50% to 60% resides in the skeletal system and another 20% is located within muscle tissue. The ICF-to-ECF concentration ratio is about 15:1. At any one time, less than 1% of total body magnesium circulates within the intravascular fluid compartment, and thus serum levels do not reflect total body stores.

Depending on the particular laboratory, the normal total serum magnesium concentration ranges from 1.5 to 2.0 mEq/L. Similar to calcium, the circulating magnesium consists of 3 components: a chelated fraction (5%); a protein-bound fraction (33%); and an ionized, diffusible fraction (62%). It is this that is physiologically active and carefully regulated to maintain homeostasis. Currently, laboratories cannot report ionized magnesium, hence total magnesium is used.

Magnesium is a cofactor for more than 300 enzymatic reactions involving energy metabolism and nucleic acid synthesis. It is also involved with hormone receptor binding, calcium channel gating, transmembrane ion flux, regulation of adenylate cyclase, muscle contraction, neuronal activity, vasomotor tone, cardiac excitability, and neurotransmitter release.[23] From many perspectives, magnesium can be viewed as a physiological calcium antagonist.

Both PTH and vitamin D have regulatory influences on renal and GI magnesium absorption. In turn, the ionized magnesium concentration influences PTH secretion. The circulating ionized magnesium is primarily regulated by the kidneys; the majority of filtered magnesium is conserved through proximal tubular resorption. Renal magnesium wasting occurs with hypermagnesemia, hypercalcemia, hypophosphatemia, hypercalciuria, loop diuretics, ACE inhibitors, aminoglycosides, amphotericin, cyclosporine, and cisplatin. Hypomagnesemia is almost universal in patients undergoing major surgery. Hypomagnesemia may also result from malnutrition, malabsorption, inadequate administration (including ECF dilution), diarrhea, laxatives, vomiting, and diabetes (**Table 35-12**).

Hypomagnesemia is associated with a variety of clinical manifestations that involve the neuromuscular and cardiovascular systems (**Table 35-13**). One interesting manifestation of hypomagnesemia is a cardiac arrhythmia known as torsade de pointes. This is derived from a French ballet expression for "twisting of the points." It refers to a specific polymorphous ventricular tachyarrhythmia in which the morphology of the QRS complexes varies from beat to beat. The ventricular rate

TABLE 35-12 Causes of Hypomagnesemia

Perioperative
Overhydration with calcium-free intravenous fluids
Massive blood transfusion
Recovery phase of the stress response
Administration of epinephrine
Acute respiratory alkalosis
Cardiopulmonary bypass
Gastrointestinal
Diarrhea
Malabsorption
Gastrointestinal fistulae
Malnutrition
Alcoholism
Endocrine
Hyperaldosteronism
Hyperparathyroidism
SIADH
Diabetes
Ketoacidosis (diabetic, alcoholic, starvation)
Drugs
Loop diuretics
Laxatives
Digitalis
Aminoglycosides
Amphotericin
Cyclosporin
Cisplatin

SIADH, syndrome of inappropriate secretion of antidiuretic hormone.

varies from 150 to 250 beats/min. The arrhythmia is effectively treated with potassium and magnesium boluses.

In cases of hypomagnesemia, the total deficit is often greater than anticipated because this is primarily an intracellular cation. The deficit of magnesium is often 1 to 2 mEq/kg, and effective repletion may require a total dose of elemental magnesium in the range of 2 to 4 mEq/kg (given over several days). For mild acute hypomagnesemia, 4 to 6 g of magnesium can be added into IV fluids and infused over 30 minutes. Rapid infusion is associated with an unpleasant hot flash and may induce acute hypotension. A continuous maintenance infusion of magnesium sulfate should then be administered for 4 to 7 days. This maintenance fluid should contain a total daily dose of 600 to 900 mg of elemental magnesium. In emergency situations, the loading dose can be infused more rapidly as long as continuous ECG monitoring is performed, and the rate of administration does not exceed 15 mg/min of elemental magnesium. For the duration of IV magnesium therapy, patients should be carefully monitored for evidence of magnesium toxicity, and frequent assessment of the total serum magnesium concentration is mandatory.

TABLE 35-13 Clinical Manifestations of Hypomagnesemia (<1.2 mg/dL, 0.5 mmol/L)

Neuromuscular (symptoms and signs similar to hypocalcemia)
Muscle weakness
Difficult to reverse from neuromuscular blockade
Tetany
Positive Chvostek and Trousseau signs
Muscle cramps
Muscle fasciculations and tremor
Neurologic
Nystagmus
Apathy
Delirium
Convulsions
Coma
Cardiovascular
Supraventricular arrhythmias
Ventricular arrhythmias
Torsade de pointes
Digitalis toxicity
Electrolyte disturbances
Hypokalemia
Hypocalcemia

Hypermagnesemia results from magnesium-containing antacids, enemas, total parenteral nutrition, acute renal failure, adrenal insufficiency, hypothyroidism, and nephrogenic diabetes insipidus.

Hypermagnesemia impairs neuromuscular function and produces progressive neuromuscular blockade. There is a heightened sensitivity to both depolarizing and nondepolarizing muscle relaxants. Magnesium has significant cardiac and hemodynamic effects. As a functional calcium channel blocker, magnesium may cause vasodilatation and hypotension.

Magnesium has been used in a variety of clinical situations, including perioperative care (**Table 35-14**). Magnesium has been used to control blood pressure and prevent seizures in preeclampsia. Magnesium may be used to control heart rate in ventricular and supraventricular arrhythmias, particularly when hypokalemia coexists. It has been used to treat torsade de pointes and digitalis toxicity. Magnesium has been used to reduce the adrenergic response to induction of anesthesia and intubation.[24] It has been used therapeutically as a smooth muscle relaxant in patients with acute severe asthma.[25] Other therapeutic roles for magnesium in perioperative medicine and critical illness include perioperative analgesia, treatment of myocardial infarction, and treatment of tetanus.[26] The analgesic properties of magnesium appear to be associated with its antagonistic properties on neuromuscular depolarizing receptors and calcium channel blockade. Calcium channel blockers are antinociceptive and potentiate the effects of morphine.[26]

The clinical manifestations of hypermagnesemia correlate well with the total serum magnesium concentration. These include somnolence, hypoventilation, postural hypotension, and, at higher doses, respiratory and cardiac arrest. In patients treated with high-dose magnesium, (eg, in obstetric patients with preeclampsia and eclampsia), careful monitoring of neuromuscular function must be performed to avoid devastating neuromuscular blockade, leading to respiratory arrest.

Treatment for hypermagnesemia includes enhancing urinary excretion, principally by combining saline infusion and furosemide. Direct antagonism of toxic effects can be provided by IV calcium, although the

TABLE 35-14 Therapeutic Uses of Magnesium

Cardiovascular
Supraventricular arrhythmias (associated with hypokalemia)
Torsade de pointes
Digitalis toxicity
Acute myocardial infarction (reperfusion, antiarrhythmia, coronary vasodilatation)
Pulmonary
Acute severe asthma
Obstetrics
Blood pressure control in preeclampsia
Anticonvulsant in preeclampsia
Anesthesia
Anti-adrenergic therapy for intubation
Prevention of succinylcholine induced muscular pain
Reduction in postoperative pain (NMDA antagonism)
Neuromuscular blockade (including treatment of tetanus)

NMDA, *N*-methyl-D-aspartate.

duration of action is relatively short. In circumstance in which reversal of effect is not possible because of acute renal failure, hemodialysis is required.

PHOSPHATE PHYSIOLOGY

Phosphorous is the most abundant intracellular anion; its concentration is approximately 100 mmol/L. One hundredth of the body's mass is made up of phosphate. Most of this is stored as hydroxyapatite crystals in the bone matrix. Only 15% is metabolically active, and 1% is present in the blood. The average diet provides 800 to 1400 mg of phosphorous daily. Of this, 70% is absorbed through the gut, mainly by passive transport, but there is also some active transport stimulated by vitamin D metabolites. Normal plasma range is between 2.8 and 4.5 mg/dL. The main organ of regulation of phosphate is the kidney. Phosphorous is filtered by the nephron, and mostly reabsorbed in the proximal tubule in co-transport with sodium. This co-transport is regulated by phosphorous intake (ie, serum phosphorous levels) and PTH. PTH inhibits the co-transport mechanism and increases urinary excretion of phosphorous. In the blood, phosphate is present in multiple forms as phospholipids, $PO4^{3-}$, $H_2PO_4^-$, and HOP_4^{2-}.

Every metabolic action in the body requires chemical energy, principally in the form of adenosine triphosphate (ATP). The high-energy bonds in ATP are derived from phosphate. This is essential for muscle contractility, neuronal transmission, and electrolyte transport. Phosphate is a key building block for many essential intracellular compounds, including nucleic acids, phospholipids, enzymes, and nucleoproteins. Many of the intracellular messenger chemicals employ phosphate, these include cyclic AMP and cyclic GMP. Phosphate has an essential role in both aerobic and anaerobic metabolism and in 2,3-DPG (2,3-diphosphoglycerate), which is involved with hemoglobin–oxygen interactions at the tissue level. Phosphate is involved in cascades within the coagulation and immune systems. Finally, phosphate is the main intracellular buffer in the body and is a component of the extracellular weak acid buffering system (A_{TOT}).

Hypophosphatemia is caused by inadequate intake, excessive loss, or redistribution within the body (**Table 35-15**). Inadequate intake may result from malnutrition or malabsorption (short bowel syndrome, tropical sprue, celiac and Crohn disease, radiation enteritis). Agents that bind with phosphate may reduce its absorption. These include magnesium and aluminium antacids and sucralfate (which contains aluminium).

Excessive loss of phosphate is associated with diuresis and dialysis. Osmotic diuretics and hyperglycemia cause increase urinary loss, as does theophylline and acetaminophen in overdose. The most phosphaturic diuretics are carbonic anhydrase inhibitors. Hypophosphatemia may rapidly occur during intermittent and continuous renal replacement therapies.

Hypophosphatemia may result from intracellular redistribution, during administration of catecholamines or beta-adrenergic agonists, insulin surges (hyperglycemia), and alkalosis for any reason.

In general, muscles do not function well in hypophosphatemic states (**Table 35-16**). This relates to the importance of phosphate as the body's source of chemical energy. Hypophosphatemic causes weakness of respiratory muscles, particularly the diaphragm, and causes a leftward shift of the oxyhemoglobin dissociation curve (increasing the tendency for hemoglobin to cling onto oxygen). Patients who are hypophosphatemic may be slow to wean from mechanical ventilation.[27,28] As one would expect, hypophosphatemia causes skeletal muscle weakness, which may mimic myopathy. In addition, low serum phosphate may interfere with blood cell function and cause increased red blood cell (RBC) fragility.

Hypophosphatemia may cause myocardial dysfunction[29] and may make the myocytes less sensitive to the stimulatory effects of catecholamines. This effect is reversible. Other complications of hypophosphatemia are listed in table below.

A particularly important cause of hypophosphatemia is the "refeeding syndrome." Severely malnourished individuals develop a total-body

TABLE 35-15 Causes of Hypophosphatemia

Decreased absorption
- Malnutrition
- Phosphate-binding antacids
- Malabsorption syndromes
  - Crohn disease
  - Celiac disease
  - Gastrointestinal fistulae
- Phosphate-binding agents
- Magnesium and aluminum antacids
- Sucralfate
- Vitamin E deficiency

Increased loss
- Volume expansion
- Diuretics
- Dialysis
- Steroids
- Alcoholism
- Renal transplantation
- Hyperparathyroidism
- Metabolic acidosis
- Pancreatitis
- Burns

Redistribution

Shifts from serum into cells
- Recovery from the stress response
- Carbohydrate infusions
- Hyperglycemia
- Hormonal effects
  - Catecholamines (epinephrine, dopamine, terbutaline, albuterol)
  - Insulin
  - Glucagon
  - Calcitonin
- Respiratory alkalosis
- Refeeding syndrome
- Leukemic blast cell crises
- Hungry bone syndrome

TABLE 35-16 Clinical Manifestations of Hypophosphatemia

Musculoskeletal
- Chronic myopathy
- Rhabdomyolysis
- Osteopenia
- Osteomalacia

Cardiovascular
- Cardiomyopathy
- Arrhythmias (ventricular)

Pulmonary
- Respiratory failure
- Failure to wean

Neurologic
- Delirium
- Seizures
- Encephalopathy
- Hallucinations
- Peripheral neuropathy

Hematologic
- Impaired oxygen release
- Hemolysis
- Leucocyte dysfunction

Metabolic
- Metabolic acidosis
- Glucose intolerance

depletion of phosphorous; serum phosphorous levels are maintained by redistribution from the intracellular space. The body uses endogenous fuel stores as its main source of energy. Fat and protein (from muscle) are metabolized. Glucose delivery, either enterally or parenterally, as part of a feeding strategy leads to a dramatic increase in circulating insulin levels. This results in rapid uptake of glucose, potassium, phosphate, and magnesium into cells. The serum concentration of these species decreases dramatically. Simultaneously, there is a dramatic increase in ECF volume. There is an increase in cardiac workload, with increased stroke work, heart rate, and oxygen consumption. This sudden increase in demand for nutrients and oxygen may outstrip supply. Moreover, in patients with cardiovascular disease, the sudden increase in cardiac work and circulating fluid can precipitate acute heart failure. The sudden administration of carbohydrates exerts a considerable strain on the respiratory system, whose musculature may well be atrophied because of starvation. There is an increase in CO_2 production and O_2 consumption and a resultant increase in the respiratory quotient. The consequence of this is an increase in minute ventilation, leading to dyspnea and tachypnea and potentially acute respiratory failure.

The serum phosphorous level decreases precipitously with refeeding because of a shift of phosphate from the extracellular to the intracellular compartment. This results from increased intracellular demand for the synthesis of phosphorylated compounds. This may result in respiratory failure, cardiac failure, cardiac arrhythmias, rhabdomyolysis, seizures, coma, and RBC and leukocyte dysfunction.

Perioperative patients are vulnerable to hypophosphatemia, because of the catecholamine surge associated with the stress response. If severe malnutrition is suspected, the anesthesiologist should be careful to avoid the administration of glucose-containing IV fluids and aggressively supplement intracellular ions, potassium, magnesium, calcium, and phosphate (**Table 35-17**).

Hyperphosphatemia is caused by increased administration or absorption, decreased loss, or increased production (**Table 35-18**). Increased intake can occur as a result of excessive IV administration or oral supplementation or vitamin D intoxication. Occasionally, hyperphosphatemia results from recurrent administration of phosphate-containing enemas. There is reduced excretion in renal failure, hypoparathyroidism, and hypomagnesemia. Increased serum phosphate levels may result from diseases that cause widespread cell destruction, including tumor lysis syndrome, rhabdomyolysis, bowel ischemia, hemolysis, and malignant hyperthermia. Pseudohyperphosphatemia may occur because of hypertriglyceridemia.

Acute hyperphosphatemia is associated with hypocalcemia, muscle weakness, and tetany. In chronic hyperphosphatemia, as occurs in chronic renal failure, calcium may be deposited in the tissues (ectopic or metastatic calcification). The treatment for acute hyperphosphatemia is administration of phosphate-binding salts (ie, calcium, magnesium, and aluminum).

CHLORIDE PHYSIOLOGY

Chloride is the second most abundant extracellular ion and the most important extracellular anion. Chloride is absorbed in roughly equimolar concentrations with sodium in the small bowel. In addition, chloride is actively secreted into the gastric lumen with potassium that is subsequently pumped back into the parietal cell. The consequence is a significant decrease in pH (gastric acidity). Chloride has a wide variety of other functions in the body. It represents one-third of extracellular osmoles and is involved in volume homeostasis; regulation of pH in the kidneys; organic solute transport; and cell migration, proliferation, and differentiation.

Chloride channels are abundant in the body.[30] These are involved in a variety of functional roles in diverse processes, such as blood pressure regulation, cell cycle and apoptosis, muscle tone, volume regulation, synaptic transmission, and cellular excitability.[31] The benzodiazepine receptor gates a chloride channel, a key element in anesthesia pharmacology. A significant number of diseases appear to result from chloride channel abnormalities (**Table 35-19**). Mutations that result in a loss of function of the voltage-gated chloride channel, CLC-5, are associated with Dent disease, which is characterized by low-molecular-weight proteinuria, hypercalciuria, nephrolithiasis, and renal failure.[32] Mutations of another voltage-gated chloride channel, CLC-Kb, are associated with a form of Bartter syndrome; other forms of Bartter syndrome are caused by mutations in the bumetanide-sensitive sodium–potassium–chloride cotransporter (NKCC2) and the renal outer medullary potassium channel (ROMK). Mutations of the thiazide-sensitive sodium-chloride cotransporter (NCCT) are associated with Gitelman syndrome.[32] Mutations

TABLE 35-17 Preparations Available for Phosphate Repletion

Intravenous Preparations	Phosphate Concentration (mmol/mL)	Sodium Concentration (mEq/mL)	Potassium Concentration (mEq/mL)
Neutral sodium potassium PO_4	1.1	0.2	0.02
Neutral sodium PO_4	0.09	0.2	0
Sodium PO_4	3.0	4.0	0
Potassium PO_4	3.0	0	4.4

TABLE 35-18 Causes of Hyperphosphatemia

- Increased intake
  - Intravenous infusion
  - Oral supplementation
  - Vitamin D intoxication
  - Phosphate-containing enemas
  - Acute phosphorus poisoning
- Increased production or release
  - Tumor-lysis syndrome
  - Rhabdomyolysis
  - Bowel infarction
  - Malignant hyperthermia
  - Hemolysis
  - Acid–base disorders (lactic acidosis, diabetic ketoacidosis, respiratory acidosis)
- Reduced loss
  - Renal failure
  - Hypoparathyroidism
  - Acromegaly
  - Tumoral calcinosis
  - Vitamin D intoxication
  - Bisphosphonate therapy
  - Magnesium deficiency
  - Pseudohyperphosphatemia
  - Multiple myeloma
  - Hemolysis in vitro
  - Hypertriglyceridemia

TABLE 35-19 Known Disorders That Result From Chloride Channel Abnormalities

- Myotonia congenita
- Myotonic dystrophy
- Bartter syndrome
- Renal tubular acidosis
- Dent disease (hypercalciuria)
- Gitelman syndrome
- Nephrogenic diabetes insipidus (in mice)
- Cystic fibrosis
- Epilepsy
- Osteopetrosis

of chloride transport proteins are responsible for cystic fibrosis, renal tubular acidosis, neuromuscular disorders, and some forms of epilepsy.

The role of chloride in acid–base chemistry is discussed in that section below. Essentially, hyperchloremia is associated with metabolic acidosis; hypochloremia is associated with metabolic alkalosis. Chloride has an important role in renal function.[32] Thiazide diuretics may modulate blood pressure by controlling serum chloride concentration by way of a sodium–chloride cotransporter. Hyperchloremia produces progressive renal vasoconstriction and a decrease in glomerular filtration.[33] In addition, hyperchloremia results in splanchnic hypoperfusion.[34] Administration of chloride-rich solutions such as 0.9% saline may result in hyperchloremia, renal dysfunction, nausea and vomiting, and hyperventilation.

PHYSIOLOGY OF ALBUMIN

Albumin is the most abundant extracellular protein. It is a single polypeptide with 585 amino acids and a molecular weight range of 65 000 to 69000 D. It is thus a medium-sized compound (IgG is 150 000) which, in addition to being highly soluble, is small enough to pass through fenestrated endothelium, such as in the nephron. Proteinuria does not occur in normal individuals because of the strong negative charge (−17 mEq) carried by albumin, which rebuts the protein in the glomerulus. Albumin is a weak acid whose concentration significantly impacts extracellular buffering capacity.

Albumin is manufactured in the liver at a rate of 9 to 12 g/d. The normal serum albumin level is 30 to 50 g/L (3-5 g/dL). There are no storage and no reserve. Being the major source of oncotic pressure in health, the rate of production of albumin is controlled by changes in osmotic pressure and the osmolality of the extravascular perihepatic space. There is limited capacity to increase production. Increased synthesis is driven by the neuroendocrine system, chiefly by insulin, thyroid hormones, and cortisol.

Albumin is catabolized at a rate of 9 to 12 g/d (the same rate as it is produced) by pinocytosis in cells adjacent to the vascular endothelium. Albumin is not catabolized in starvation; under these circumstances, protein is derived from muscle after exhaustion of fat stores.

Although albumin is perceived as intravascular protein, the total extravascular albumin actually exceeds the total intravascular amount by 30%.[35] The ratio of albumin to water is, however, higher in the intravascular space (the ECF is two-thirds interstitial and one-third intravascular), hence the colloidal effect. Albumin cyclically leaves the circulation through the endothelial barrier at the level of the capillaries, passes into the interstitium, and returns to the bloodstream through the lymph system via thoracic duct. The circulation half-time for this process is 16 to18 hours. A total of 4% to 5% of total intravascular albumin extravasates in this way per hour; this rate of movement is known as the transcapillary escape rate, and this is determined by capillary and interstitial free albumin concentration, capillary permeability to albumin, and movements of solvent or solute and the electrical charges across the capillary wall. The concentration of albumin in lymph protein content is approximately 80% that of plasma.

Albumin has a variety of physiologic and pharmacologic roles (**Table 35-20**). Albumin binds drugs and ligands and reduces the serum concentration of these compounds (Table 35-20). An example is the serum calcium, the free (ionized) concentration of which needs to be corrected for albumin. There are actually 4 binding sites on albumin, and these have varying specificity for different substances. Competitive binding of drugs may occur at the same site or at different sites (conformational changes; eg, warfarin and diazepam). The drugs that have important albumin binding are warfarin, digoxin, nonsteroidal anti-inflammatory drugs, midazolam, and thiopental. The relevance of a low albumin and drug binding is unknown.

Albumin is a major source of sulfhydryl groups; these "thiols" scavenge free radicals (nitrogen and oxygen species). Albumin has anticoagulant and antithrombotic effects that are poorly understood.

Low serum albumin is a nonspecific marker of disease. A decrease in the albumin concentration appears to reflect deterioration; an increase reflects recovery. Very low levels of albumin appear to reflect a poor outcome. The relevance of low albumin on ligand binding is unknown.

TABLE 35-20 Physiologic Roles of Albumin

Maintenance of the COP
Binding and transport
Drugs
Benzodiazepines (including midazolam)
Thiopental
Nonsteroidal anti-inflammatory drugs
Warfarin
Tacrolimus
Indomethacin
Digitalis
Furosemide
Chlorpropamide
Penicillins
Thyroxine
Calcium
Magnesium
Free radical scavenging.
Acid–base balance
Pro- and anticoagulant effects
Inhibits platelet aggregation
Enhances the inhibition of factor Xa by antithrombin III
Effects on vascular permeability

COP, colloid osmotic pressure.

In critical illness, there is a reduction in the production of albumin because of favored hepatic production of acute-phase proteins such as globulins, fibrinogen, and haptoglobin. Other proteins whose levels decease in this situation include prealbumin, retinal-binding protein, transferrin, and somatomedin C. This process is known as "hepatic reprioritization." During conditions of stress or tissue injury, such as major surgery, trauma, or critical illness, a generalized increase in vascular permeability develops associated with release of cytokines and cytotoxic material. This leads to leakage of protein-rich fluid into the interstitium (capillary leak). Aggressive volume resuscitation with crystalloid, gelatins, or hydroxyethyl starch (HES) significantly reduces the albumin concentration by a dilutional effect. Hence, hypoalbuminemia during the stress and systemic inflammatory response is caused by hemodilution, redistribution, and hepatic reprioritization. Low serum albumin (and prealbumin) represents a negative acute-phase response.

In critical illness, there is a stronger correlation between colloid oncotic pressure (COP) and total protein than with albumin. In these patients, the decreased albumin is compensated for by an increase in acute-phase proteins.[36] Nonetheless, there is increased leakage of albumin, and this drags fluid into the extravascular space. The overall fluid flux is less than would be predicted if albumin was the only protein responsible for oncotic pressure in the Starling equation. Thus, low serum albumin does not necessarily mean low plasma oncotic pressure and does not always cause edema.

Hypoalbuminemia has been associated with various disease states (**Table 35-21**). These include liver dysfunction, nephropathies (particularly nephrotic syndrome), preeclampsia and eclampsia, and burns. Hypoalbuminemia in preoperative patients is indicative of severe malnutrition and is a known indicator of poor surgical outcomes. Preoperative nutrition targeting an increase in albumin has been shown to improve outcomes.[37] In critically ill patients, there is a strong relationship between the dynamic decrease in serum albumin concentration and patient outcomes.[38] The lower the serum albumin plunges, the greater the mortality, morbidity, length of stay, and complication rate. Blunt and colleagues[39] have shown that nonsurvivors in the ICU had lower mean albumin concentrations than survivors, and there was, significantly, no difference between the COPs of the 2 groups. Finally, changes in albumin concentration have significant impact on acid–base balance, which is discussed in detail in the following section.

TABLE 35-21 Causes of Decreased Plasma Albumin

Decreased synthesis
Increased catabolism (very slow)
Increased loss
- Nephrotic syndrome
- Exudative loss in burns
- Haemorrhage
- Gut loss

Redistribution
- Haemodilution
- Increased capillary permeability (leakage into the interstitium)

Decreased lymph clearance

ACID–BASE CHEMISTRY

PRIMARY PRINCIPLES

Acid–base chemistry refers to the study of the relative ratio of hydrogen to hydroxyl ions in ECF, particularly arterial blood. Intracellular hydrogen ion concentration, or pH (its negative logarithm), is equivalent to the pH of water at body temperature and varies little despite significant changes in extracellular pH. The body carefully controls the relative concentrations of hydrogen and hydroxyl ions in the extracellular and intracellular spaces. Alterations in this "balance" lead to significant cardiovascular problems caused by dysfunction of transcellular ion pumps. Anesthesiologists are expected to identify changes in acid–base chemistry, determine their origins, and treat them. However, the tools available heretofore, based on traditional methods derived from epidemiologic studies of patients with chronic lung disease and extrapolation of the Henderson-Hasselbalch equation, are often unhelpful in perioperative medicine. These approaches, the "Boston" approach of Schwartz and Brackett and the "Copenhagen" approach of Siggaard-Anderson, frequently fail to identify perioperative acid–base abnormalities, particularly when multiple abnormalities are present simultaneously. Moreover, these approaches do not provide guidance with regard to the source of the anomaly.[40] In general, the cause of acid–base disturbances is more clinically relevant than the acid–base anomaly itself. The majority of causes of such perturbations are easily explained, but some, such as dilutional and hyperchloremic acidosis, have traditionally eluded description.

The "modern" physical-chemical approach, originally introduced by Stewart[41] and subsequently refined by several investigators,[42-44] has significantly enhanced our understanding of these problems and simplified the clinical application.[4,45] This approach has gained widespread acceptance in perioperative medicine and critical care and is the basis of this segment of the chapter.[46]

Acids, Bases, and Water As we have seen, water is a highly ionizing solvent that autodissociates into a negatively charged hydroxylated (OH) ion and positively charged protonated (H_nO^+) ion.[47] Conventionally, this self-ionization of water is written as follows:

$$H_2O \leftrightarrow H^+ + OH^-$$

The symbol H^+ is convenient because, although protons dissociating from water have many aliases (eg, H_3O^+, $H_5O_2^+$ and $H_9O_4^+$), most physicians and chemists refer to them as hydrogen ions. Indeed, the concept of "free hydrogen ions" referred to in texts is metaphorical. Water dissociation is constant (K_w) and is governed by changes in temperature, dissolved electrolytes, and cellular components:

$$K_{w'} = [H^+][OH^-]$$

In other words, if $[H^+]$ increases, then $[OH^-]$ decreases by the same magnitude. The self-ionization of water is miniscule. In pure water at 25°C, the $[H^+]$ and $[OH^-]$ are 1.0×10^{-7} mEq/L.[48] Using the Sorenson negative logarithmic pH scale, this is a pH of 7.0. Physiologic pH, that at which the body resides, differs between the intracellular (pH, 6.9) compartment (pH, 7.4) and between venous (pH, 7.5) and arterial (pH, 7.4) blood. Conventionally, acid–base balance refers to changes in hydrogen ion concentration in ECF from 7.4. This is reasonable because cells are relatively impervious to ionic materials, and the ECF is rapidly influenced by changes in fluids, electrolytes, and carbon dioxide tension. Thus, acidosis (an increase in hydrogen ion concentration) occurs when the pH is less than 7.3, and alkalosis (a decrease in hydrogen ion concentration) occurs when pH is greater than 7.5.

All acid-base reactions in the body are associated with water dissociation.[49] Water is an amphiprotic molecule – simply it can be an acid or a base – a proton donor or a proton acceptor.

$$H_2O\ (acid) + H_2O\ (base) \leftrightarrow H_3O^+ + OH^-$$

Whether water acts as an acid or a base depends on compounds dissolved in it. For example, if HCl is dissolved in water:

$$HCl + H_2O \leftrightarrow H_3O^+ + Cl^-$$

In this situation water acts as a conjugate base – a proton acceptor. Note that there is no net generation of OH^- as the proton donor was Chloride. Chloride, in this situation is a Brønsted–Lowry acid. Likewise, as Chloride delivers a hydrogen ion into water, it is also an Arrhenius acid.

Likewise, NaOH is dissolved into water:

$$NaOH + H_2O \leftrightarrow Na^+ + H_2O + OH^-$$

So water, in this situation, acts a conjugate acid, a proton donor – the conjugate acid of a strong base. Sodium, in this situation, is a Brønsted–Lowry base.[4,50] Likewise, as Sodium delivers a hydroxyl ion into water, it is also an Arrhenius base.

ECF, as we have seen, is an ionic soup containing uncharged cells and particles, dissolved gases (oxygen and carbon dioxide), and fully and partially dissociated ions. Many of these factors influence water dissociation, dependent on chemical charge, quantity, and degree of dissociation.[51] In addition, ionized particles, particularly sodium and chloride, exert a significant osmotic effect. Thus, physical chemistry and ECF volume are interconnected. These particles obey 3 distinct laws[45]: (1) electrical neutrality (the net positive charge must equal the net negative charge), (2) mass conservation (the total quantity of a substance in the extracellular space is constant unless added, removed, generated, or destroyed), and (3) dissociation equilibria for all incompletely dissociated substances (albumin, phosphate, and carbonate) must be obeyed at all times. Thus, to determine the acid–base status of a fluid, all substances to which these rules might be applied must be accounted for. These include fully dissociated ("strong") ions, partially dissociated ("weak") acids, and volatile acid species.

Stewart explained that the relative concentration of hydrogen and hydroxyl ions in health and disease is determined by 3 independent variables, the SID, the total concentration of weak acids (A_{TOT}), and the partial pressure of carbon dioxide (Pco_2) (**Table 35-22**).[4,41] Hydrogen, hydroxyl ions, and bicarbonate are dependent variables. Their concentrations are entirely dependent on independent variables. Hence, isolated loss of hydrogen ions or bicarbonate from the gut or kidney cannot induce a change in acid–base balance.

Strong Ions Strong ions are completely dissociated at physiologic pH. The most abundant strong ions in the extracellular space are sodium (Na^+) and chloride (Cl^-). Other important strong ions include K^+, SO_4^{2-}, Mg^{2+}, and Ca^{2+}. Each applies a direct electrochemical and osmotic effect.

In the extracellular space, the difference between the charge carried on strong cations and strong anions is calculated by:

$$SID = ([Na^+] + [K^+] + [Ca^{2+}] + [Mg^{2+}]) - ([Cl^-] + [\text{Other strong anions: } A^-]) = 40 \text{ to } 44 \text{ mEq}$$

This excess of positive charge, called the *strong ion difference* by Stewart,[41] is always positive and is balanced by an equal amount of "buffer base" (BB), principally in the form of phosphate, albumin, and bicarbonate.[52]

TABLE 35-22 What Determines pH?

Using a physiochemical approach, it is possible to determine the effect of carbon dioxide, completely dissociated ions, and partially dissociated ions on water dissociation and hence hydrogen ion concentration. Six simultaneous equations can be constructed and solved for $[H^+]$[4,40]:

1. Water dissociation equilibrium: $[H^+] \times [OH^-] = K_w$
2. Weak acid dissociation equilibrium: $[H^+] \times [A^-] = K_A \times [HA]$
3. Conservation of mass for weak acids: $[HA] + [A^-] = [A_{TOT}]$
4. Bicarbonate ion formation equilibrium: $[H^+] \times [HCO_3^-] = K_C \times Pco_2$
5. Carbonate ion formation equilibrium: $[H^+] \times [CO_3^{2-}] = K_3 \times [HCO_3^-]$
6. Electrical neutrality: $[SID] + [H^+] - [HCO_3^-] - [A^-] - [CO_3^{2-}] - [OH^-] = 0$

Interestingly, there are 6 independent simultaneous equations and just 6 unknown dependent variables determined by them: [HA], $[A^-]$, $[HCO_3^-]$, $[CO_3^{2-}]$, $[OH^-]$, and $[H^+]$. There are 3 known independent variables: [SID], $[A_{TOT}]$, and Pco_2. Although the above equations look relatively simple, fourth-order polynomials are required for resolution.

Solving the equations for $[H^+]$:

$$[SID] + [H^+] - K_C \times P_C/[H^+] - K_A \times [A_{TOT}]/(K_A + [H^+]) - K_3 \times K_C P_C / [H^+]^2 - K_W / [H^+] = 0$$

In other words, $[H^+]$ is a function of SID, A_{TOT}, Pco_2, and a number of constants. All other variables, most notably $[H^+]$, $[OH^-]$, and $[HCO_3^-]$ are dependent and thus cannot independently influence acid–base balance. Hence, it is possible to resolve all acid–base abnormalities into a problem of 1 or more of these 3 variables.

A_{TOT}, acid-buffering system; SID, strong ion difference.

SID independently influences water dissociation, determined by electrical neutrality and mass conservation. If all other factors (Pco_2, albumin, and phosphate) are kept constant, an increase in SID will decrease hydrogen ion concentration (and increase hydroxyl ion concentration), causing alkalosis (**Fig. 35-8**). A decrease in SID is associated with increased hydrogen ion concentration and results in acidosis.

The chief determinant of SID is the relationship between the relative concentration of sodium, chloride, and free water in ECF. The normal ratio of sodium to chloride is approximately 1.4:1. Any process that reduces that ratio reduces SID and leads to acidosis (sodium loss, chloride gain, or free water gain). Any process that increases that ratio increases SID and leads to alkalosis (sodium gain, chloride loss, or free water gain).

Weak Acids Albumin and phosphate are weak acids whose degree of dissociation is related to temperature and pH. Weak acids, represented by the symbol A_{TOT}, independently influence acid–base balance, depending on absolute quantity and dissociation equilibria.[41,53]

The principal limitation of traditional approaches to acid–base balance has been the limited attention paid to changes in A_{TOT}.[54] Although this may be valid in otherwise healthy patients, perioperative care and critical illness cause hypoalbuminemia because of crystalloid administration, hepatic prioritization, and capillary leak.[55] A reduction in serum albumin or phosphate leads to metabolic alkalosis.[43] Hypophosphatemia is associated with malnutrition, refeeding, diuresis, and hemodilution.

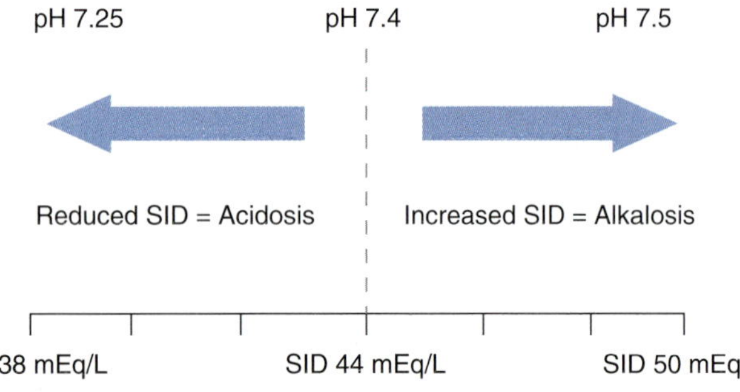

FIGURE 35-8. Impact of changes in strong ion difference (SID) on pH. Increased SID causes metabolic alkalosis. Decreased SID causes metabolic acidosis.

Hyperphosphatemia occurs in renal failure. Hyperphosphatemia leads to metabolic acidosis.

Carbon Dioxide Aerobic metabolism results in the production of large quantities of carbon dioxide. Carbon dioxide is hydrated by carbonic anhydrase in erythrocytes to carbonic acid. This liberates the equivalent of 12 500 mEq of H^+ per day. Hemoglobin is the major extracellular buffer of CO_2. Hydrogen ions bind to histidine residues on deoxyhemoglobin, and bicarbonate is actively pumped out of the cell. Carbon dioxide exists in 4 forms: carbon dioxide [denoted CO_2(d)], carbonic acid (H_2CO_3), bicarbonate ions (HCO_3^-), and carbonate ions CO_3^{2-}. The principal mechanism of excretion is through alveolar ventilation, although some CO_2 is excreted from the kidneys as bicarbonate as part of a sodium–chloride co-transporter.

Chronic respiratory acidosis is associated with increase in total body CO_2 content, reflected principally by an increase in serum bicarbonate. Mathematically, $\Delta HCO_3^- = 0.5\ \Delta Paco_2$.[40] It is important that this is not confused with "metabolic compensation for hypercarbia," a relatively slow process that reduces SID by increased urinary chloride excretion.[56]

ACID–BASE DISTURBANCES

Overview Acid–base disturbances are an important part of clinical and laboratory investigation of perioperative and critically ill patients. There are 6 primary acid–base abnormalities (**Table 35-23**):

1. Acidosis caused by increased $Paco_2$
2. Acidosis caused by decreased SID: Increased chloride (hyperchloremic), reduced sodium (dilutional), increased free water
3. Acidosis caused by increased A_{TOT}: Hyperphosphatemia, hyperproteinemia
4. Alkalosis caused by decreased $Paco_2$
5. Alkalosis caused by increased SID: Decreased chloride (hypochloremic), increased sodium, decreased free water (contractional)
6. Alkalosis caused by decreased A_{TOT}: Hypophosphatemia, hypoalbuminemia

Acute Respiratory Acidosis and Alkalosis Acute respiratory acidosis results from hypoventilation caused by a loss of respiratory drive, neuromuscular or chest wall disorders, or rapid-shallow breathing, which increases the fraction of dead space ventilation. Acute respiratory acidosis is often associated with a precipitous reduction in pH caused by the absence of a rapid buffering system for large quantities of carbon

TABLE 35-23 Classification of Acid–Base Abnormalities

	Acidosis	Alkalosis
Respiratory	Increased Pco_2	Decreased Pco_2 ↑ SID^+ + ↓ $[Cl^-]$
Metabolic		
1. Abnormal SID^+		
a. Caused by water	Water excess = dilution ↓ SID^+ ↓ [Na +]	Water deficit = contraction ↑ SID^+ ↑ [Na +]
b. Caused by electrolytes Chloride (measured)	Chloride excess ↓ SID^+ ↑ $[Cl^-]$	Chloride deficit ↑ SID^+ + ↓ $[Cl^-]$
Others (unmeasured anions) eg, Lactate, ketoacids	↓ SID^+ ↑ $[A^-]$	–
2. Abnormal A_{TOT}		
a. Albumin [Alb]	↑ $[Alb^-]$ (IV albumin)	↓ $[Alb^-]$
b. Phosphate [Pi]	↑ $[Pi^-]$	↓ $[Pi^-]$

A_{TOT}, acid-buffering system; IV, intravenous; SID, strong ion difference.

dioxide (see below). Acute respiratory alkalosis (pH >7.5) is caused by hyperventilation, caused by anxiety, central respiratory stimulation (as occurs early in salicylate poisoning), or excessive artificial ventilation. Acute respiratory alkalosis usually accompanies acute metabolic acidosis (pH <7.35), in which case the reduction in Pco_2 from baseline (usually 40 mm Hg) is equal to the magnitude of the BD (see below). For example, in a patient with lactic acidosis with a lactate level of 10 mEq/L, the BD should be −10 and the Pco_2 30 mm Hg. If the Pco_2 is higher than expected, then there is a problem with the respiratory apparatus. This is seen, for example, in multi-trauma patients with massive blood loss, causing lactic acidosis, plus a flail chest, causing respiratory acidosis.

Acute Metabolic Acidosis Acute metabolic acidosis is caused by an alteration in the relative concentrations of extracellular electrolytes (SID) or proteins (A_{TOT}). SID is changed by an alteration in the relative quantity of strong anions to strong cations. This can be caused by anion gain, as occurs with lactic-, renal-, keto-, and hyperchloremic acidosis, or cation loss, as occurs with severe diarrhea. Acidosis also results from increased free water relative to strong ions, or "dilutional acidosis." This results from excessive hypotonic fluid intake, certain poisonings (methanol, ethylene glycol, or isopropyl alcohol) or hyperglycemia (**Fig. 35-9**).

In acute metabolic acidosis, 3 diagnoses should be immediately investigated, lactic acidosis (the serum lactate concentration should be obtained; it should mirror the magnitude of BD), ketoacidosis caused by diabetes (the patient should have hyperglycemia and have positive urinary ketones), and acute renal failure demonstrated by high serum urea and creatinine and low total CO_2. The latter is a diagnosis of exclusion. The presence of a low serum sodium concentration (<135 mEq/L) should alert the clinician to the possibility of a dilutional acidosis caused by alcohol poisoning. Alcohols such as ethanol, methanol, isopropyl alcohol, and ethylene glycol are osmotically active molecules that expand extracellular water. (Glucose and mannitol have the same effect but also promote diuresis because the molecules are small enough to be filtered by the kidneys.) Alcohol poisoning is suspected by the presence of an osmolar gap: A difference between the measured and calculated serum osmolality of greater than 12 mOsm demonstrates the presence of unmeasured osmoles. Toxicology laboratories can investigate for the presence of various toxic alcohols.

Renal acidosis is caused by accumulation of strong ion products of metabolism excreted exclusively by the kidneys. These include sulphate and formate. In addition, there is accumulation of a weak acid, phosphate.

The administration of IV fluids to patients has significant impact on acid–base balance. Changes occur in free water volume, SID, and A_{TOT} (principally albumin). "Dilutional acidosis" results from administration of pure water to ECF (which is alkaline). This can occur with large-volume administration of any fluid whose SID is 0, including 5% dextrose, 0.9% saline (contains 154 mEq of both Na^+ and Cl^+), or other hypotonic saline infusions. Dilutional acidosis thus results from a reduction in serum sodium or an increase in chloride relative to sodium. This "hyperchloremic acidosis" is frequently seen in the operating suite after large-volume administration of 0.9% saline solution or 6% hetastarch (both formulated in normal saline) (**Fig. 35-10**).[57,58] Kellum[59] has shown in an experimental model of sepsis that dogs treated with lactated Ringer solution and 5% HES diluted in LRS (Hextend) (both with a SID of 20) had less acidosis and longer survival than those treated with normal saline.

Hyperchloremic acidosis as a consequence of isotonic saline administration is common in perioperative care and is probably clinically significant. IV infusion of 1000 mL of 0.9% NaCl results in the administration of 154 mEq/L of NaOH and 154 mEq/L of HCl. Functionally, this results in the accumulation of 50 mEq/L of HCl or more accurately 50 mEq/L of Cl^- and 50 mEq/L of H^+.

It is known that acidosis caused by hyperchloremia is associated with better outcomes than with lactic or ketoacidosis; in these situations, the acid–base abnormality is a manifestation of disease rather than iatrogenic electrolyte imbalance.[60] Nonetheless, acidosis per se is not benign and is associated with cardiovascular dysfunction that includes negative

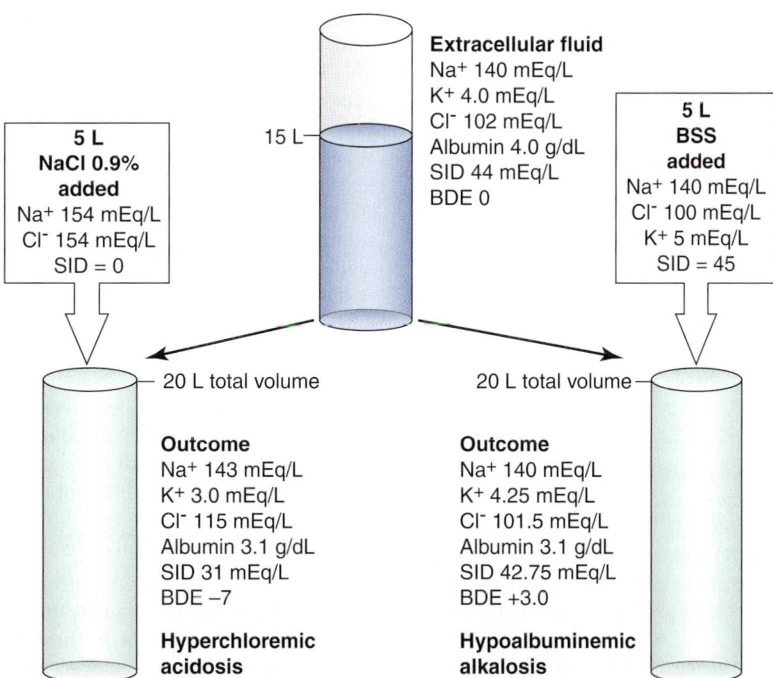

FIGURE 35-9. Impact of loss and gain of free water on acid–base chemistry. In the left-sided example, removal of 3 L of water leads to increased strong ion difference (SID) and increased albumin. The former is alkalinizing, the latter acidifying: the result is a contraction alkalosis. In the *left panel*, the ECF is diluted with 3 L of dextrose 5% (SID 0, a physiologic method of delivering free water). Note the impact of the fluid on both SID and on albumin concentration (A_{TOT}). The main impact of hemodilution with free water is reduced SID; this is dilutional acidosis. BDE, base deficit or excess; BSS, balanced salt solution.

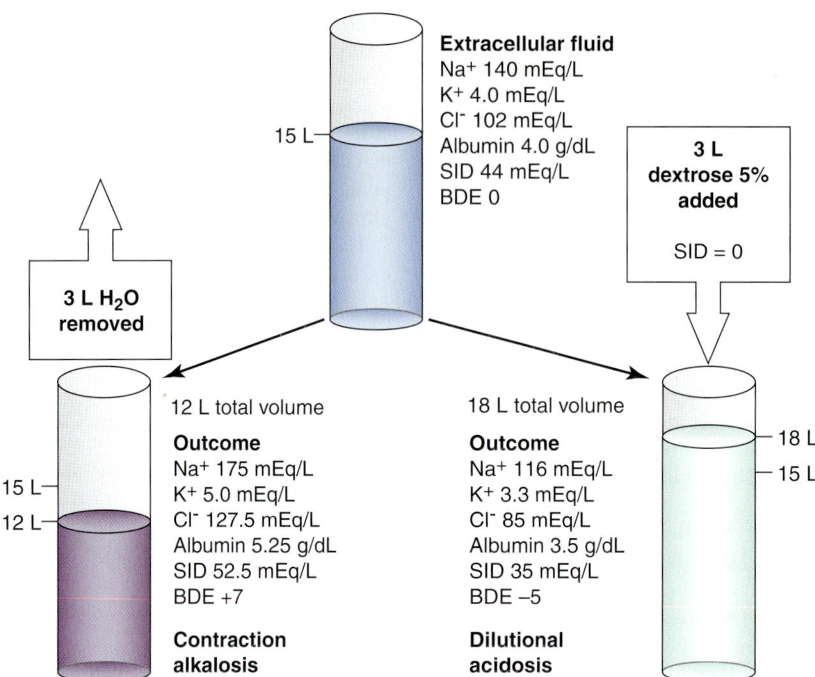

FIGURE 35-10. Impact of extracellular fluid (ECF) expansion with NaCl 0.9% versus an idealized balanced salt solution (BSS) on acid–base chemistry. Note the impact of the fluid on both SID and on albumin concentration (A_{TOT}). In both of these examples, the contribution of albumin dilution to base deficit excess is approximately 3 mEq/L. ECF expansion with NaCl with a SID of 0 leads to hyperchloremic acidosis; the magnitude of acidosis is less than would be predicted by the change in SID. ECF expansion with the idealized BSS is alkalizing because of albumin dilution. BDE, base deficit or excess.

inotropy, vasoplegia, and microcirculatory dysregulation. Acidosis inactivates membrane calcium channels and inhibits the release of norepinephrine from sympathetic nerve fibers, leading to vasodilatation and maldistribution of blood flow. In clinical practice, this appears to affect splanchnic blood flow.[34] For example, metabolic acidosis is associated with an increased incidence of PONV.[61] Hyperchloremia can reduce renal blood flow and the glomerular filtration rate (GFR).[62] Plasma chloride levels affect afferent arteriolar tone through calcium-activated chloride channels and modulate the release of renin.[63] In a study of healthy volunteers, normal saline was associated with reduced urinary output compared with LRS.[64] Two studies have provided circumstantial evidence that saline versus sodium bicarbonate may be associated with adverse renal outcomes in high-risk patients. Merten and colleagues,[65] in study of fluid prehydration to prevent contrast nephropathy, demonstrated that the use of sodium bicarbonate was associated with an 11.9% absolute reduction in the risk of renal injury (defined as a 25% increase in creatinine). Haase and colleagues[66] compared perioperative isotonic sodium bicarbonate with isotonic saline (4 mmol/kg over 24 hours) in patients undergoing cardiac surgery. There was a 20% absolute risk increase in renal dysfunction in the patients receiving saline (odds ratio 0.43 [95% confidence interval 0.19-0.98]); $p = 0.043$).

Acute Metabolic Alkalosis Perioperative metabolic alkalosis is usually of iatrogenic origin. Hyperventilation of patients with chronic respiratory failure results in acute metabolic alkalosis caused by chronic compensatory alkalosis associated with chloride loss in urine. More frequently, metabolic alkalosis is associated with increased SID caused by sodium gain. This occurs because of administration of fluids in which sodium is "buffered" by weak ions, citrate (in blood products), acetate (in parenteral nutrition), and bicarbonate.

The most frequent single disturbance in acid–base chemistry in perioperative and critically ill patients is hypoalbuminemia.[67] This is ubiquitous and causes an unpredictable metabolic alkalosis. This may mask significant alterations in SID, such as lactic acidemia. All IV fluids that do not contain albumin are alkalizing (Fig. 35-10). Thus, all patients who receive significant volumes of IV fluid in the operating room develop hypoalbuminemic alkalosis. It is unknown whether this anomaly has any clinical significance.

Critically ill patients are vulnerable to significant changes in SID and free water. Nasogastric suctioning causes chloride loss; diarrhea leads to sodium and potassium loss. Surgical drains placed in tissue beds may remove fluids with varying electrolyte concentrations (eg, the pancreatic bed secretes fluid rich in sodium). Fever, sweating, oozing tissues, and inadequately humidified ventilator circuits lead to large-volume insensible loss and contraction alkalosis. Loop diuretics and polyuric renal failure may be associated with significant contraction alkalosis caused by loss of chloride and free water.

Parenteral infusions may be responsible for stealth alterations in serum chemistry. Many antibiotics, such as piperacillin–tazobactam, are diluted in sodium rich solutions. Others, such as vancomycin, are administered in large volumes of free water (5% dextrose). Lorazepam is diluted in propylene glycol, large volumes of which will cause metabolic acidosis similar to that seen with ethylene glycol.[68]

Continuous renal replacement therapy (CRRT) is widely used in critical care to hemofiltrate and hemodialyze patients who are hemodynamically unstable. It has a complex effect on acid–base status: CRRT resolves the acidosis of acute renal failure by removing strong ions and phosphate[69]; however, metabolic alkalosis ensued because of the unmasking of metabolic alkalosis caused by hypoalbuminemia. Serum lactate increases, but this does not result in acidosis.[70]

REGULATION OF ACID–BASE BALANCE

Carbon dioxide tension is controlled principally by chemoreceptors in the medulla and peripherally in the carotid body and aortic arch. An increase in the P_{CO_2} or in the acidity of cerebrospinal fluid (CSF) stimulates the breathing center to increase alveolar ventilation. Hence, acidosis, regardless of cause, results in increased respiratory effort. When respiratory failure occurs, the principal CO_2 buffering system, hemoglobin, becomes overwhelmed, leading to the rapid development of acidosis. In response, the kidney excretes an increased chloride load, using $NH4^+$, a weak cation, for electrochemical balance. Thus, ECF osmolality is maintained, but the process is slow and may take weeks or months to restore normal range pH.

"Metabolic" acid is controlled principally by increased alveolar ventilation (resulting ion respiratory alkalosis) and buffered extracellular weak acids. Strong acids (strong ions) characteristically have low pKa (the acid dissociation constant); the farther the pKa is from extracellular pH, the greater the degree of dissociation—lactate has a pKa of 3.6 (fully dissociated). Functionally weak acids, which have relatively high pKa (6-7) buffer strong acids, which have low pKa (≤5); because weak acids are not fully dissociated, and as pH decreases, the capacity to bind hydrogen ions increases (the pH-to-pKa range narrows). Weak acid buffers include plasma proteins, hemoglobin, phosphate, and bicarbonate. The bicarbonate buffering system (92% of plasma buffering and 13% overall) is the most important extracellular buffer. The pKa of bicarbonate is 6.1. In all clinical situations in which hydrogen ions are liberated from water as a result of the addition of anions or loss of cations, bicarbonate binds the majority of free hydrogen ions and forms carbon dioxide. It is important to understand that this merely represents a change in the nature of the acid: An *acid* (for example lactate) is buffered by an *acid* (bicarbonate), and this produces a different *acid* (carbon dioxide). A change in CSF acidity stimulates respiration, and increasing amounts of CO_2 are excreted through the lungs. Under conditions in which respiratory failure accompanies metabolic failure (eg, multi-trauma associated with lung injuries, diabetic ketoacidosis precipitated by pneumonia, or renal failure associated with acute respiratory distress syndrome [ARDS]), the body cannot compensate, and devastating acidosis results.

In metabolic acidosis, chloride is preferentially excreted by the kidneys. Indeed, this is the resting state of renal physiology because sodium and chloride are absorbed in the diet in relatively equal quantities.[71] In metabolic alkalosis, chloride is retained, and sodium and potassium are excreted.

Abnormalities in the renal handling of chloride may be responsible for several inherited acid–base disturbances. In renal tubular acidosis, there is an inability to excrete Cl^- in proportion to Na^+.[72] Similarly, pseudohypoaldosteronism appears to be caused by high reabsorption of chloride.[73] Bartter syndrome is caused by a mutation in the gene encoding encoding the chloride channel, *CLCNKB*, which regulates the Na-K-2Cl cotransporter (NKCC2).[74]

ANALYTIC TOOLS USED IN ACID–BASE CHEMISTRY

Abnormalities of acid–base balance provide valuable information regarding changes in respiratory function, electrolyte chemistry and underlying disease processes. Although blood gas analysis is ubiquitous, it provides only partial information regarding acid–base chemistry. Abnormalities of pH, BDE, or bicarbonate concentration reflect effect (and not always accurately) but not always cause. Measurement of each of the strong and weak ions that influence water dissociation, although cumbersome, is essential.[42]

This section considers some of the tools have evolved over the past 50 years to assist our interpretation of acid–base conundrums. None are entirely accurate, and each has a dedicated group of followers.[75] Clinicians often confuse mechanisms of interpretation with the underlying causes of acid–base abnormalities. For example, a decrease in serum bicarbonate during metabolic acidosis reflects hyperventilation and the consumption of bicarbonate as a buffer (producing CO_2). The acidosis is not caused by depletion or dilution of bicarbonate rather by decreased SID (usually by unmeasured anions [UMAs]) or increased A_{TOT}. Nevertheless, the decrease in the quantity of bicarbonate from its resting concentration, in simple situations, mirrors the quantity of acid produced. We will deal with each of these approaches chronologically and discuss the merits and demerits.

The CO_2-Bicarbonate (Boston) Approach The decrease in serum bicarbonate concentration associated with metabolic acidosis has long been a core principle in acid–base interpretation. This was formalized by a group at Tufts University in Boston and widely disseminated over the past half century. This approach to acid–base chemistry uses acid–base maps and the mathematical relationship between carbon dioxide tension and serum bicarbonate (or total CO_2) derived from the Henderson-Hasselbalch equation to predict the nature of acid–base disturbances.[76] The maps were derived from a large number of patient observations with known acid–base disturbances at steady states of compensation. The term *compensation* was used to describe the change in $[HCO_3^-]$ relative to $Paco_2$ and normal levels, and this was calculated for each disease state. The investigators were able to describe 6 primary states of acid–base imbalance using the linear equations and maps they had developed (**Table 35-24**). For any given acid-base disturbance, an expected HCO_3^- concentration was determined.

TABLE 35-24 Changes in Pco_2 and $[HCO_3^-]$ in Response to Acute and Chronic Acid–Base Disturbances

Disturbance	HCO_3^- Versus $Paco_2$
Acute respiratory acidosis	$\Delta HCO_3^- = 0.2\ \Delta Paco_2$
Acute respiratory alkalosis	$\Delta HCO_3^- = 0.2\ \Delta Paco_2$
Chronic respiratory acidosis	$\Delta HCO_3^- = 0.5\ \Delta Paco_2$
Metabolic acidosis	$\Delta Paco_2 = 1.3\ \Delta HCO_3^-$
Metabolic alkalosis	$\Delta Paco_2 = 0.75\ \Delta HCO_3^-$

Modified from Narins RB, Emmett M. Simple and mixed acid-base disorders: a practical approach. *Medicine.* 1980;59:161-187.

This approach has remained robust; however, its major drawback is that it treats HCO_3^- and CO_2 as independent rather than interdependent variables. This has resulted in a "bicarbonate-centered" culture in which bicarbonate has been considered a leading player in acid–base chemistry rather than a passive factor, hence the concept of "bicarbonate deficit" and the elevation (among clinicians) in importance of bicarbonate over the truly more important ion, chloride. The bicarbonate approach is entirely consistent with the physical chemistry model as proposed by Stewart. Hence, the limitation of the Boston approach is not in the underlying science but in the way clinicians have sought to understand it. For example, the administration of "bicarbonate" to replace a perceived deficit of this compound actually involves the co-administration of Na^+, a strong ion that obeys the laws of mass conservation.

The Base Deficit or Excess (Copenhagen) Approach An early version of the electrical neutrality approach to metabolic disturbances was proposed by Singer and Hastings in 1948.[52] They proposed the concept of whole-blood BB as a counterbalance to metabolic acid. The BB represented sum of the bicarbonate and the nonvolatile buffer ions (essentially the serum albumin, phosphate, and hemoglobin). Applying the law of electrical neutrality, the BB was forced to equal the electrical charge difference between strong (fully dissociated) ions. Thus, normally, BB = $[Na^+] + [K^+] - [Cl^-]$. Alterations in BB represented changes, essentially in strong ion concentrations (which could not be easily measured in 1948). BB increases in metabolic alkalosis and decreases in metabolic acidosis. The major drawback of the use of BB measurements is the potential for changes in buffering capacity associated with alterations in hemoglobin concentration.

In 1958, Siggard-Anderson developed a simpler measure of metabolic acid–base activity, the BDE.[77] This, they defined, is the amount of strong acid or base required to return the pH of 1 L of blood to 7.4, assuming a Pco_2 of 40 mm Hg and temperature of 38°C. The initial use of whole-blood BE was criticized because of the dynamic activity of RBCs within the acid–base paradigm—gas and electrolyte exchange. This approach was modified in the 1960s to use only serum BE, and the calculation became the *standardized* base excess. Current algorithms for computing the SBDE are derived from the Van Slyke equation (1977).[78] This approach has the advantage of being simpler to apply in clinical practice than the Boston (bicarbonate) approach; a negative number

TABLE 35-25 Changes in Standardized Base Deficit or Excess (BDE) in Response to Acute and Chronic Acid–Base Disturbances

Disturbance	BDE Versus $Paco_2$
Acute respiratory acidosis	$\Delta BDE = 0$
Acute respiratory alkalosis	$\Delta BDE = 0$
Chronic respiratory acidosis	$\Delta BDE = 0.4\ \Delta Paco_2$
Metabolic acidosis	$\Delta Paco_2 = \Delta BDE$
Metabolic alkalosis	$\Delta Paco_2 = 0.6\ \Delta BDE$

Modified from Narins RB, Emmett M. Simple and mixed acid-base disorders: a practical approach. *Medicine.* 1980;59:161-187.

(BD) quantifies the degree of acidosis, and a positive number quantifies the degree of alkalosis (base excess). The BDE approach to acid–base chemistry has been successfully validated.[79,80] However, functionally, the bicarbonate and the BD approaches are really 2 sides of the same coin; both use serum bicarbonate as the primary variable.

Simple mathematical rules can be applied using the BDE in each of the common acid–base disturbances (**Table 35-25**). For example, in acute respiratory acidosis or alkalosis, BDE does not change. Conversely, in acute metabolic acidosis, the magnitude of change of the Pco_2 (in mm Hg) is the same as that of the BDE (in mEq/L), and the change in BDE represents the overall sum total of all acidifying and alkalinizing effects. This makes interpretation of acid–base abnormalities simple but misleading.

The BD approach has 2 significant limitations. First, it does not account for changes in acid–base chemistry associated with hypoproteinemia; indeed, the Van Slyke equation assumes normal serum proteins, which is not the case in critical illness. The second limitation is that this approach does not distinguish between metabolic acidosis associated with hyperchloremia and that associated with UMAs.

Anion Gap Approach The AG approach is a continuation of the electrochemical balance approach of Singer and Hastings and is consistent with all of the other approaches (Boston, Copenhagen, and Stewart). It was developed by Emmett and Narins in 1975,[81] and its function is to determine whether the cause of acidosis is chloride or (unspecified) UMAs. This is based on the law of electrical neutrality. The sum of the difference in charge of the common extracellular ions reveals an unaccounted for "gap" of −12 to −16 mEq/L (AG = (Na^+) − [(CL^- + HCO_3^-]) (**Fig. 35-11**). The "gap" represents A_{TOT} or the charge carried by albumin and phosphate. If the patient develops metabolic acidosis and the gap "widens" to, for example, −20 mEq/L, then the acidosis is caused by UMAs (lactate or ketones). The widening of the gap represents the reduction in serum bicarbonate concentration associated with buffering the acidosis. If the gap does not widen, then the anions *are* being measured, and the acidosis has been caused by hyperchloremia (bicarbonate cannot independently influence acid–base status). Although this is a useful tool, it is weakened by the assumption of what is or is not a "normal gap."[82] The majority of critically ill patients have hypoalbuminemia, and many also have hypophosphatemia.[44] Consequently, the gap may be normal in the presence of UMAs. Figge et al[83] have provided us with a variant known as the "corrected AG":

$$\text{AG corrected (for albumin)} = \text{Calculated AG} + 2.5(\text{Normal albumin g/dL} - \text{Observed albumin g/dL}).$$

The great value of the AG is its simplicity, which is also its greatest weakness. The BD and AG frequently underestimate the extent of the metabolic disturbance.[42]

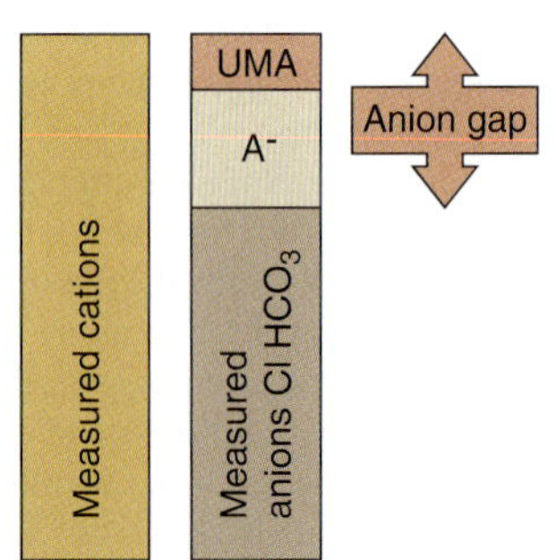

FIGURE 35-11. The anion gap. A^- represents phosphate and albumin. UMA, unmeasured anions.

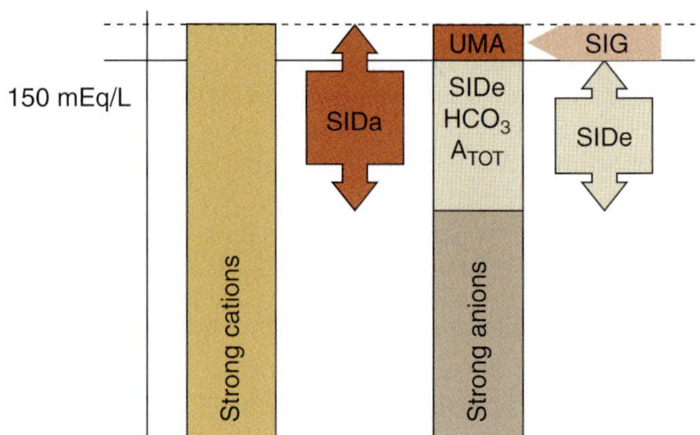

FIGURE 35-12. The strong ion gap. SIDa, apparent strong ion difference; SIDe, effective strong ion difference; SIG, strong ion gap; UMA, unmeasured anions.

Stewart-Fencl Approach A more accurate reflection of true acid–base status can be derived using the Stewart-Fencl approach.[4,45] Similar to the AG, the Stewart-Fencl approach is based on the concept of electrical neutrality. There exists in plasma a SID [(Na^+ + Mg^{2+} + Ca^{2+} = K^+) − (Cl^- + A^-)] of 40 to 44 mEq/L balanced by the negative charge on bicarbonate and A_{TOT} (the BB). There is a small difference between SIDa (apparent SID) and weak acid buffers (SIDe, or effective SID). This represents an SIG, which quantifies the amount of UMA present (**Fig. 24-12**).

$$\text{The SIDa (apparent SID)} = ([Na^+] + [K^+] + [Mg^{2+}] + [Ca^{2+}]) - [Cl^-]$$

The SIDe (effective) is $[HCO3^-]$ + [Charge on albumin] + [Charge on Pi] (in mmol/L)

Weak acids' degree of ionization is pH dependent, so one must calculate for this:

$$[\text{alb}-] = [\text{alb g/L}] \times (0.123 \times \text{pH} - 0.631)$$
$$[\text{Pi}]\ (\text{in mg/dL}) = [\text{Pi}]/10 \times \text{pH} - 0.47$$
$$\text{SIG} = \text{SIDa} - \text{SIDe}$$

The BDE and SIG approaches are consistent with each other and can be derived from a master equation.[84] The Stewart approach,[45] refined by Figge,[43,85] Fencl,[4,42] and others, more accurately measures the contribution of charge from weak acids, which change with temperature and pH.

The weakness of this system is that the SIG does not necessarily represent unmeasured strong anions, merely all anions that are unmeasured. Furthermore, SID changes quantitatively in absolute and relative terms when there are changes in plasma water concentration. Fencl et al[42] have addressed this by correcting the chloride concentration for free water (Cl^- *corr*) using the following equation:

$$[Cl^-]corr = [Cl^-]\text{observed} \times ([Na^+]\ \text{normal}/[Na^+]\ \text{observed}$$

This corrected chloride concentration may be then inserted into the SIDa equation above. Likewise, the derived value for UMAs should also be corrected for free water using UMA instead of Cl^- in the above equation.[42] In a series of 9 normal subjects, Fencl et al[42] estimated the "normal" SIG as 8 +/− 2 mEq/L.

The SIG is a useful tool in clinical medicine. Lactic acidosis upon admission to the emergency department is a marker of severity of illness.

The magnitude of acidosis and the degree of elevation of serum lactate correlate well with patient outcomes.[86-88] Also, the speed of clearance of lactate from the circulation is another known prognostic indicator.[88-91] This probably reflects the status of lactate as an acute-phase compound rather than quantitative evidence of tissue hypoperfusion.[92] BD does not reliably reflect lactate in the emergency setting.[93-95] Kaplan and Kellum[96] looked at a variety of acid–base measurements in the acute trauma setting. SIG was superior at predicting outcome versus all other measures. Only 1 (2%) survivor had an SIG greater than 5 mEq/L, and only 2 (7%) nonsurvivors had an SIG less than 5 mEq/L. Admission pH, HCO_3^-, and lactate were poor predictors of hospital mortality after trauma. Similar data have been reported by a variety of groups in emergency settings.[97-99]

To date, studies of critically ill patients have failed to demonstrate that SIG predicts outcomes.[100,101] This may be attributable to the magnitude of acid–base disturbances that occur simultaneously. Moviat and colleagues[102] found that unmeasured strong anions were present in 98%, hyperchloremia was present in 80%, and elevated lactate levels were present in 62% of patients. Not all UMAs are harmful; for example, succinylated gelatin, when administered as part of a resuscitation strategy, will increase the SIG.[103]

Although accurate, the SIG is cumbersome and expensive, requiring measurement of multiple ions and albumin. An alternative approach, used by Gilfix and colleagues,[104] and subsequently by Balasubramanyan et al[105] and Story et al,[106] is to calculate the BDE gap (BEG). This allows recalculation of BDE using strong ions, free water, and albumin. The resulting BEG should mirror the SIG and indeed AG.

The simplified calculation of Story et al is most useful. They use 2 equations to calculate the BDE for sodium, chloride, and free water (BDE_{NaCl}) and for albumin (**Table 35-26**). A unified approach to solving acid–base problems is presented in **Fig. 35-13**.

TABLE 35-26 Calculation of Base Deficit or Excess (BDE) of Sodium-Chloride–Free Water and Albumin[a]

BDE_{NaCl} = ([Na+]-[Cl-]) – 38
BDE_{Alb} = 0.25 (42 – Albumin g/L)
BDE_{NaCl} - BDE_{Alb} = BDE_{calc}
BDE – BDE_{calc} = BDE gap = The effect of unmeasured anions or cations
These calculations simplify the framework for "eyeballing" a chemistry series:
Normal Na = 140:
- For every 1-mEq/L increase in Na from 140, base excess increases by +1 (Na 150 = BDE +10 = Contraction alkalosis)
- For every 1-mEq/L decrease in Na from 140, base deficit increases by –1 (Na 130 = BDE – 10 = Dilutional acidosis)

Normal Cl = 102
- For every 1-mEq/L increase in Cl from 102, base deficit increases by +1 (Cl 110 = BDE – 8 = Hyperchloremic acidosis)
- For every 1-mEq/L decrease in Cl from 102, base excess increases by +1 (Cl 90 = BDE +12 = Hypochloremic, chloride-sensitive alkalosis)

Normal albumin = 42 g/L or 4.2 g/dL
- For every 0.4-g/dL decrement in albumin from 4.0, there is a 1.0-mEq/L increase in the base excess

[a]This approach involves calculating the BDE for sodium, chloride, and free water (BDE_{NaCl}) and that for albumin (BDE_{Alb}). The result is the calculated BDE (BDE_{calc}). This is subtracted from the measured BDE to find the BDE gap.

TREATING ACID–BASE DISTURBANCES

Although acid–base disturbances are associated with adverse outcomes, correcting the pH has never been demonstrated to improve outcomes. Moreover, the use of therapeutic sodium bicarbonate to treat patients with lactic acidosis is particularly controversial.[107] Therapeutic sodium bicarbonate has 3 effects: (1) volume expansion because the 7.5% and 8.4% solutions are hypertonic (hence the often remarked improvement in cardiovascular performance); (2) increased SID caused by to the administration of sodium without accompanying strong anion[108]; and (3) increased CO_2 generation. Much discussion has focused on bicarbonate inducing intracellular acidosis,[109] but this is probably

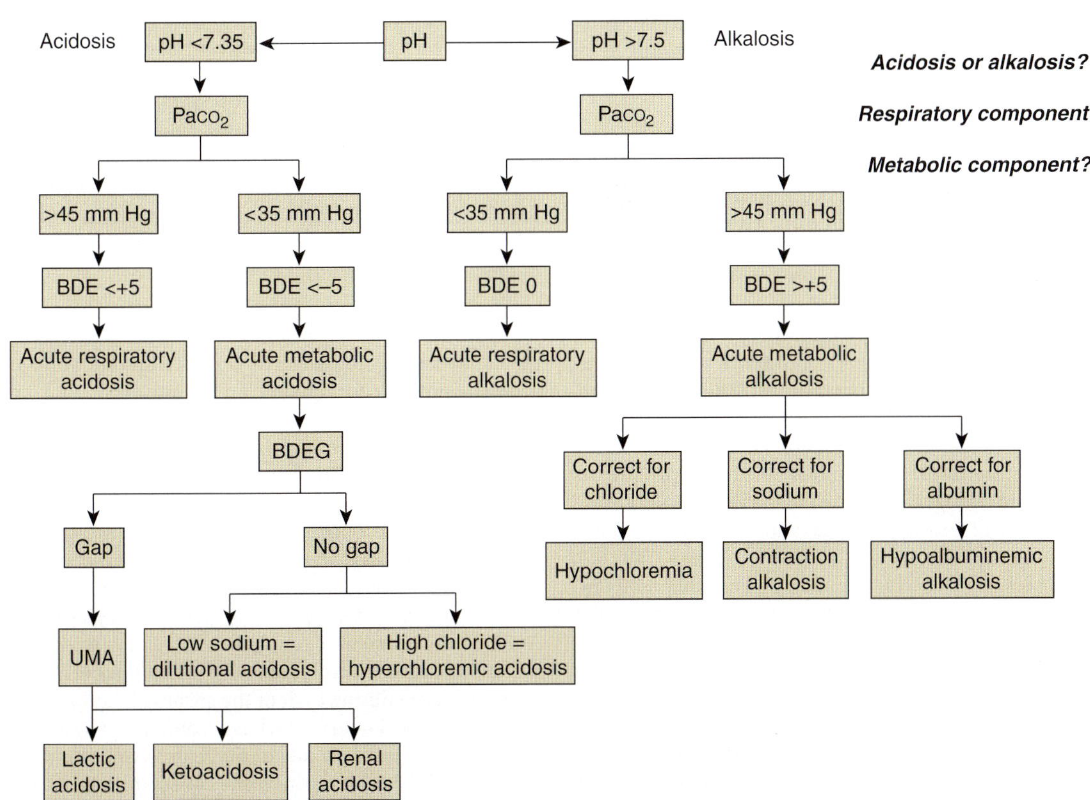

FIGURE 35-13. Mechanism for solving an acid–base problem. BDE, base deficit or excess; BDEG, base deficit or excess gap; UMA, unmeasured anions.

clinically insignificant.[107,110] Patients with lactic acidosis are treated volume resuscitation and source control. Those with diabetic ketoacidosis are treated with volume resuscitation and insulin.

Patients with hyperchloremic or dilutional acidosis can be treated by increasing the SID of infused fluids, for example, by infusing sodium without chloride (isotonic sodium bicarbonate and sodium acetate solutions).

Hypernatremic alkalosis is "chloride sensitive" and can be treated by administration 0.9% NaCl or potassium chloride and calcium chloride. It is probably worthwhile for the clinician to treat chloride-sensitive alkalosis. The normal compensatory measure for alkalosis is hypoventilation, increasing $Paco_2$ that may lead to CO_2 narcosis, or failure to liberate from mechanical ventilation. There is no specific treatment for patients with hypoalbuminemic alkalosis; it resolves with recovery from perioperative stress or critical illness.

Patients with renal acidosis are treated with dialysis, resulting in the removal of a variety of UMA compounds. Both sodium bicarbonate and sodium citrate have been used to increase SID in patients awaiting dialysis; there are little or no published data regarding the utility of this approach.

It is unclear whether or not hypercapneic acidosis is harmful or beneficial for patients, particularly those with lung injuries. Permissive hypercapnia is now a central tenet in mechanical ventilation of critically ill patients with ARDS; the goal is to prevent ventilator-associated lung injury.[111] Accumulating evidence indicates that hypercapnia has a lung-protective effect and that reversing the acidosis[112,113] may have adverse effects.[114] Severe hypercarbia in the setting of limiting mechanical ventilation is extremely difficult to treat and strategies include hypocaloric feeding, neuromuscular blockade, cooling, extracorporeal CO_2 removal, and THAM[115] (*tris*-hydroxymethyl-amino-methane). THAM titrates hydrogen ions (eg, lactic acid, CO_2) according to the following reaction:

$$R\text{-}NH_2 + HA <\!\!-\!\!> R - NH_3^{\ +} + A^-$$

THAM is a proton acceptor that generates NH_3^+/HCO_3^- without generating CO_2, and the protonated $R\text{-}NH_3^{\ +}$ is eliminated by the kidneys along with chloride. THAM has the significant advantage of buffering acidosis without increasing serum sodium or generating more carbon dioxide.

MONITORING BLOOD GASES: ALPHA STAT VERSUS pH STAT

Water dissociation is temperature dependent. Thus, extracellular pH varies with body temperature, becoming more alkalotic with progressive hypothermia and more acidotic with hyperthermia. Hence, patients presenting in a state of hypothermia or induced hypothermia (for cardiac surgery) would be expected to exhibit significant alkalosis on a blood gas. Blood gas machines heat the blood sample to an idealized 37°C. Thus, the clinician is able to make inferences regarding the presence or absence of respiratory or metabolic abnormalities from a constant perspective. This "alpha-stat" approach is widely used in perioperative medicine. An unfortunate drawback of this consensus is that many clinicians are unaware of the impact of temperature on pH. Incumbent in this hypothesis is that despite temperature changes, the body is capable of maintaining homeostatic function, and intracellular enzymes and transcellular ion pumps continue to function.

Intracellular pH is 6.8 at 37°C, which is neutral pH at that temperature. Extensive animal investigation has established that intracellular pH remains neutral across a wide array of body temperatures. The reason that this occurs appears to relate to the constant buffering capacity of intracellular histidine moieties across a spectrum of pH values.[116] This has the effect of maintaining intracellular enzymatic activity.

Carbon dioxide becomes more soluble in blood as temperature decreases. Moreover, hypothermia is associated with reduced metabolic activity. Consequently, hypothermia results in respiratory alkalosis and reduced cerebral blood flow.

Poikilothermic animals (reptiles) use an alpha-stat system of pH control and can function over a broad range of temperatures.[118] Hibernating animals, however, use a pH stat strategy induced by hypoventilation. The consequent increase in intracellular CO_2 content reduces cellular metabolism and, indeed, may have a protective effect.[118]

Some clinicians believe that pH should be kept constant despite changes in temperature (the pH-stat hypothesis). Thus, when measuring a blood gas, the patient's current body temperature is entered into the machine, and a series of calculations corrects the blood gas values to the entered body temperature. For example, if a patient has a temperature of 28°C with otherwise normal metabolic and respiratory function, the specimen is heated in a blood gas machine, and the pH is reported at 37°C; the pH will be 7.40 and the Pco_2 40 mm Hg. In the pH-stat approach, the result will be corrected to the current patient temperature, and the pH will be reported at 7.65 and the Pco_2 at 22 mm Hg. The clinician may then elect to actively correct the pH to the physiologically normal range of 7.4. This is achieved, for example, by adding carbon dioxide during cardiopulmonary bypass (CPB). The resulting respiratory acidosis is thought to improve neurologic outcomes in cardiac surgery. For example, CBF (cerebral blood flow) decreases 40% during CPB at 26°C using alpha-stat management but remains similar to baseline with pH-stat management.[120]

The higher Pco_2 in the pH-stat approach is thought to improve neurologic outcomes by inducing a rightward shift of the oxyhemoglobin dissociation curve, promoting O_2 unloading to tissues; reducing $CMRO_2$ (cerebral metabolic rate of oxygen) and increased neuronal tolerance to ischemia; and modulating the *N*-methyl-D-aspartate receptor that limits the neurotoxic effects of excitatory amino acids.[121] There are few data to support the use of the pH-stat approach in adults, and the benefit, if it exists at all, is probably confined to infants undergoing cardiac surgery.[121] The author does not recommend the adoption of the pH stat approach for the majority of perioperative patients.

ESTIMATING PERIOPERATIVE FLUID REQUIREMENTS

Traditional approaches to perioperative fluid management have focused on rigorous calculation of fluid deficits, the administration of "maintenance" fluids (calculated on body weight and metabolic activity), repletion of insensible losses and third-space losses (depending on the anatomical region of surgery), and replacement of blood loss with crystalloid (in a 1:3 ratio) or colloid (in a 1:1 ratio). There are many limitations to this approach; chief among them is the potential for significant weight gain and fluid overload. Additionally, as previously described, the actual presence of third-space fluid loss has been questioned. Nevertheless, these approaches continue to be widely advocated in practice; a short description follows.

PREOPERATIVE DEFICITS

In adults undergoing elective surgery, despite guidelines that water is permissible up to 2 hours preoperatively,[121] oral intake is usually restricted for up to 12 hours before the procedure. This period of restricted oral intake may be considerably longer when surgery is scheduled late in the day. The resulting fluid deficit is primarily because of water loss.

The traditional approach involves calculating the hourly maintenance fluid rate and multiplying that by the time of restricted fluid intake. The maintenance fluid is calculated using a 4:2:1 system (4 mL/kg for the first 10 kg, 2 mL/kg for the next 10 kg, and 1 mL/kg beyond that per hour). An alternative system is to administer 1.5 mL/kg. Of this total, 50% of this deficit volume is replaced over the first hour of IV fluid therapy, and 25% is replaced during each of the ensuing 2 hours. The entire deficit is then replaced in 3 hours, which is accomplished by adding the fluid deficit to the basal infusion rate of the maintenance fluids. Simultaneously, account must be taken for insensible losses during and after surgery. This is associated with evaporation at the site of surgery, hyperventilation, fever, sweating, denuded skin, burns, the use of nonhumidified oxygen

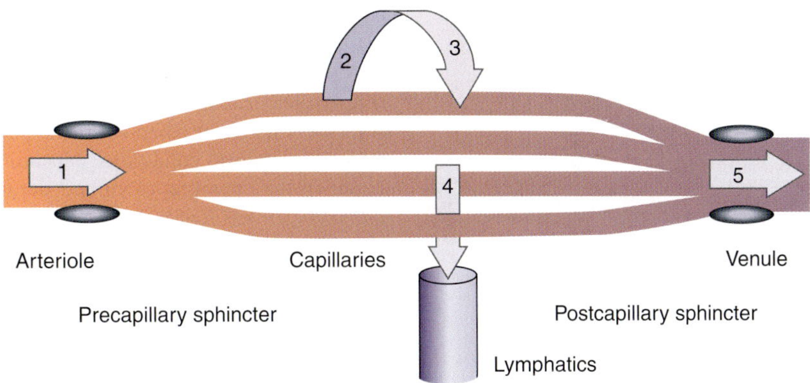

FIGURE 35-14. The normal microcirculation.

therapy administered at high flow rates, and so on. Again, much of this loss is in water, not ECF.

Additional preoperative deficits may also occur. The most common is volume loss through the bowel as a consequence of preoperative administration of purgatives ("bowel preparations"). This leads to an absolute deficit of water and electrolytes, principally sodium and potassium, but also chloride because of renal compensatory loss. This requires replacement with BSS. There is no clear published guideline for the absolute volume that must be replaced to overcome bowel prep losses, but the majority of anesthesiologists estimate this at 1000 to 2000 mL. Other preoperative causes of absolute hypovolemia with associated electrolyte loss include vomiting, gastric suction, diarrhea, and ostomy output. Upper GI losses should be repleted with chloride-rich solutions, preferably 0.9% saline. Lower GI losses should be repleted with BSS.

Internal losses are volume deficits that cannot be easily quantified because they represent redistribution of fluid within the body. Traditionally, these are considered "relocation" losses into cavities and third spaces, but they also represent expansion of the ECF space secondary to capillary leak. The cavitary losses (eg, pleural, ascitic, and pericardial fluid) are simple transudates of plasma that often require a relatively prolonged period to accumulate in significant quantities. The impact on the ECF volume is therefore generally minor because there is usually some degree of compensation for this redistribution of vascular fluid. Although significant cavitary fluid accumulation does occur in hypervolemic states, the most important variant of this is ascites. Ascitic fluid secondary to cirrhosis ovarian cancer, or carcinomatosis, after it has been drained, inevitably reaccumulates, leading to massive fluid shifts and the potential for significant intravascular dehydration.

There are many other causes of fluid redistribution losses in perioperative medicine. These usually involve significant edema in conjunction with injured tissue (as may occur with obstructed, ischemic, or dead bowel), particularly when compartment syndromes occur and when secretory fluid becomes trapped in obstructed bowel. These "third-space" and cavitary losses create a new ECF pool that is sequestered and essentially nonfunctional.

Internal blood loss also diminishes the ECF volume. Such losses may be significant when associated with retroperitoneal hematoma, leaking aneurysm, pseudoaneurysm or vascular anastomosis, pelvic or femoral fracture, or splenic rupture. Depending on the acuteness of the hemorrhage, some degree of compensation may have occurred. Typically, this involves transcapillary refill (**Figs. 35-14** and **35-15**), the movement of ECF into the vascular space to maintain perfusion of fight-or-flight organs (midline structures and skeletal muscle). Although this may lead to a small decrease in the hemoglobin concentration, it is essential

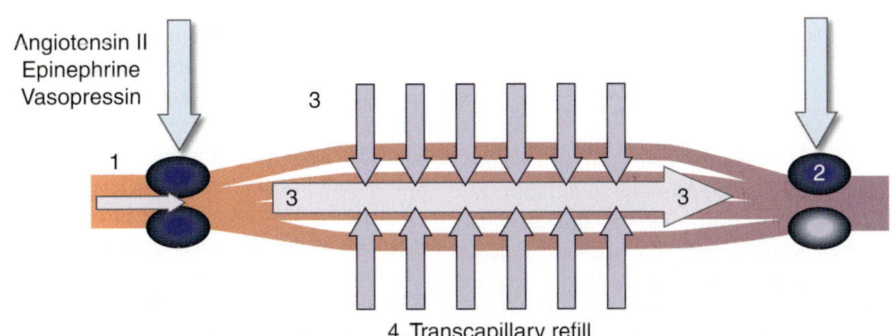

FIGURE 35-15. Compensation for hypovolemia.

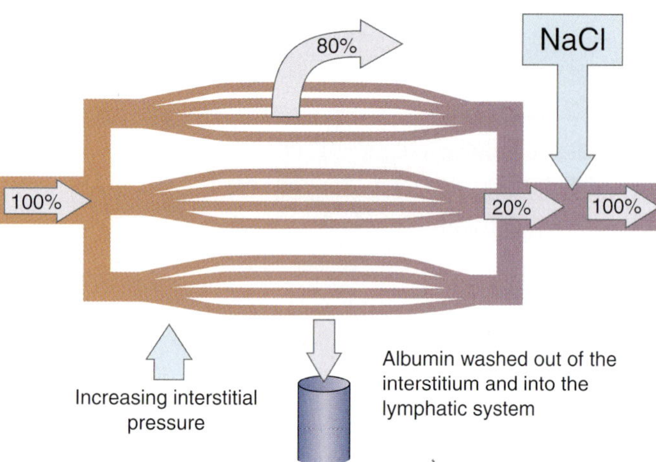

FIGURE 35-16. Crystalloid extravasation. When isotonic crystalloid fluids are administered to a perioperative patient, up to 80% of the infused volume extravasates into the interstitium.

to understand that in situations of acute isovolemic blood loss, hemoglobin remains essentially unchanged despite massive blood loss. This may lead to false reassurance, particularly in young patients, who have tremendous compensatory capacity through tachycardia and intense vasoconstriction.

Clearly, estimation of fluid deficits and ongoing fluid losses is different depending on the nature of the patients and the type of surgery. Emergency procedures are often associated with significant fluid shifts that must be accounted for.

Fluid used to replace pure volume losses should be nearly isotonic with respect to plasma and should also contain sodium and chloride. In general, a polyvalent, BSS (eg, mildly hypotonic LRS) is used. Ideally, both internal and external preoperative fluid deficits should undergo total correction before the administration of an anesthetic. However, an urgent need for surgery may preclude replacement of the entire deficit. Relatively small-volume deficits (ie, <20% of the blood volume) can often be replaced with an isotonic or BSS administered over a period of 15 minutes or less. Most patients will tolerate this amount of acute intravascular volume expansion, but care must be taken in patients with a history of hypertension or diastolic dysfunction. In these cases, rapid volume administration may precipitate acute pulmonary edema. Importantly, 40% to 60% of the infused solution will redistribute to the extracellular compartment within 15 to 30 minutes, and 80% will redistribute by 1 hour (**Fig. 35-16**). If the patient has significant ECF deficit, as we will see, then this is an effective method of resuscitating that space. However, if blood loss is the problem, significant tissue edema will result from large-volume crystalloid resuscitation to maintain hemodynamic goals.

INTRAOPERATIVE FLUID LOSSES

Intraoperative fluid losses (similar to preoperative losses) can be categorized as either internal or external. Traditional approaches to intraoperative fluid management involve estimation of distribution volume deficits and repletion of this apparent ECF volume loss with isotonic fluids. Significant volume is lost or sequestered into "third" spaces. It is assumed that the volume of fluid sequestered is proportional to the amount of surgical trauma. Thus, major orthopedic procedures, surgery within the chest cavity, bowel resections, and hysterectomies are examples in which a significant quantity of third spacing occurs (ie, perhaps 4%-5% of body weight). The exact quantity of sequestered fluid is impossible to ascertain, and replacement of these third-space losses is an approximation.

Conservative approaches to third-space fluid replacement, based on the amount of tissue exposure and degree of tissue trauma are 2 to 4 mL/kg/h for minimal trauma, 4 to 6 mL/kg/h for moderate trauma, and 6 to 12 mL/kg/h for extensive trauma. This volume replacement is in addition to maintenance fluids and repletion of preoperative losses.

External fluid losses during surgery are predominantly attributable to insensible or evaporative losses and blood loss. Significant evaporative losses may occur when either the peritoneal or pleural surfaces are exposed to ambient conditions, depending on the relative humidity of the air in the operating room and the rate of exchange of air within the room. This is free water loss, that is, again, almost impossible to quantify. Traditional approaches involve the administration of 1 to 4 mL/kg/h fluid to replete these losses with higher volumes administered depending on the cavity or tissue surface exposed. Patients with extensive burns have massive insensible volume losses, and volume repletion is formula driven based on the surface area burned.

Intraoperative blood loss may lead to significant tissue hypoperfusion and organ injury. It is, however, difficult to quantify as a result of accumulation in drains, drapes, suction canisters, administration of lavage fluid, and so on. The estimated blood loss almost always underestimates true blood loss. Administration of crystalloid or colloid to fixed hemodynamic goals will progressively deplete the hemoglobin concentration, providing a useful index of blood loss. However, underresuscitation of the patient is often associated with a falsely reassuring hemoglobin concentration.

Traditional approaches to blood replacement have identified a 3:1 ratio of crystalloid to blood loss. This is incorrect.[122] With increasing volumes of crystalloid administration, the extracellular space becomes progressively more compliant, with the result that transcapillary leakage of fluid increases geometrically, and volume replacement for blood loss parallels this.[123] This process is known as *cytopempsis* and reflects, principally, progressive hypoalbuminemia associated with volume replacement.[10] In his original animal study, Moss[10] described a 5:1 ratio of crystalloid replacement to blood loss when losses reached 35% of blood volume, reaching an inflection point at this level, with subsequent ratios increasing geometrically. At 75% blood loss, the ratio reaches 16:1.[10] Consequently, consideration should be given to repleting blood losses with colloid solutions or blood component therapy.

POSTOPERATIVE FLUID LOSSES

Both internal and external fluid losses continue into the postoperative period. Depending on the patient's preoperative status, intraoperative management, and surgical procedure, combinations of volume, concentration, and composition disturbances are not infrequent. Over the first 24 to 36 hours postoperatively, fluid continues to be sequestered into the extracellular space, principally because of capillary leakage (**Fig. 35-17**).[124] Evidence of end-organ hypoperfusion, particularly oliguria, may become apparent. Recurrent boluses of fluid may be required to restore organ function. On day 2 after surgery, a steady state appears to be reached followed by fluid mobilization and diuresis. Patients lose up to 1000 mL of water per day in insensible losses, but they also gain water from metabolic activity. Although traditional teaching emphasizes the administration of hypotonic glucose containing IV fluids to prevent dehydration and ketosis, there is very little support for this position in the literature. Indeed, the controversy of "dry" versus "wet" has existed for as long as IV fluid therapy has been available.[125] Furthermore, as we shall see, postoperative clear fluid administration may be associated with worse outcomes, and dextrose administration is associated with undesirable hyperglycemia.

External losses may persist into the postoperative period as a result of continued bleeding, nasogastric suctioning, surgical drains, diarrhea, evaporative losses, and so on. It is imperative that the clinician quantify these losses and replenish them with fluids appropriate for the site of loss (eg, BSS for ECF loss, normal saline for upper GI losses).

FLUID REPLACEMENT CRYSTALLOIDS

NATURE AND MAKEUP OF CRYSTALLOID SOLUTIONS

Crystalloid solutions are IV fluids that involve electrolytes or dextrose dissolved in sterile water (**Table 35-27**). Crystalloid solutions may be hypotonic, isotonic, or hypertonic. They may have a SID of 0 (dextrose

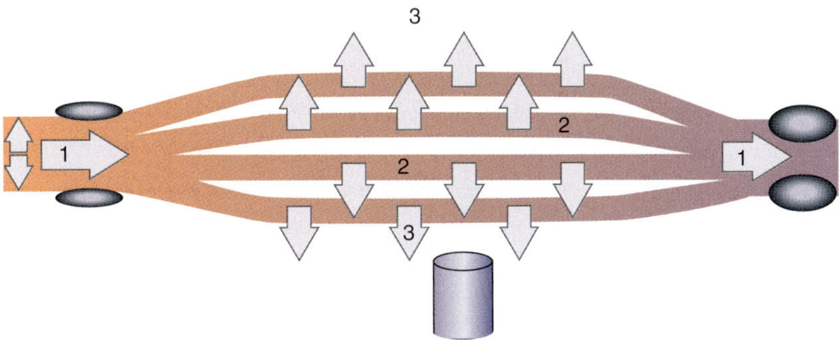

FIGURE 35-17. Extravasation of fluid into the extracellular space caused by capillary leak.

solutions or NaCl 0.9%) or may have a SID that approximates plasma (BSS, including LRS, Normosol, Plasmalyte). Dextrose-based fluids distribute evenly across TBW. Hypotonic fluids distribute across body water in proportion to electrolyte content. Isotonic fluids, being electrolyte based, distribute evenly through the ECF but remain extracellular (**Fig. 35-18**). Hypertonic fluids remain in the compartment into which they are injected (eg, the bloodstream) and expand that compartment by dragging fluid from the intracellular and extracellular space along the osmotic gradient.[126] The choice of IV fluids, used therapeutically, is determined by the clinical indication and prevailing conditions. For example, hypotonic fluids are typically used to replace free water deficits. Isotonic fluids are used to replace ECF losses. Slightly hypotonic BSS, such as LRS, replace free water and ECF losses. Hypertonic fluids are typically used as plasma expanders used in acute resuscitation but may reduce edema volume. HS is typically used in TBI. A comprehensive set of crystalloid solutions is listed in Table 35-27. The following section addresses the most commonly administered formulations.

DEXTROSE 5%

Water cannot be administered into the intravascular space because RBC lysis results. Dextrose as a 5% solution is isosmotic with plasma but rapidly becomes free water as the glucose content is metabolized. Hence, free water therapy has traditionally taken the form of dextrose solutions. Alternative "hypotonic fluids" include 0.45% NaCl + dextrose 5% and 0.25% NaCl. Water, administered as dextrose, distributes to the TBW. Consequently, when 1000 mL of dextrose is delivered, two-thirds enters the intracellular space and a tiny fraction remains intravascular. Consequently, dextrose and all hypotonic fluids should be avoided when intravascular volume expansion is desired. Dextrose has been used traditionally to treat dehydration losses before and after surgery. However, the caloric content of dextrose is problematic (200 kcal/L). Glucose cannot be used as fuel in perioperative patients. Administration of glucose results in hyperglycemia because of stress catecholamine release and insulin resistance during the stress response. Perioperative hyperglycemia has been associated with an increased risk of death, myocardial ischemia, and stroke.[127-129] Thus, traditional postoperative fluid regimens that emphasize the use of glucose to prevent ketosis and replenish free water deficits require reevaluation.

"NORMAL" SALINE

"Normal saline" consists of an equimolar solution of sodium (154 mEq/L) and chloride (154 mEq/L). The solution has an osmolality

TABLE 35-27 Composition of Commonly Used Crystalloid Solutions

Solution	Osmolarity (mOsm/L)	Na^+ (mEq/L)	Cl^- (mEq/L)	K^+ (mEq/L)	Ca2+ (mEq/L)	Mg^{2+} (mEq/L	Glucose (g/L)	Lactate (mEq/L)	Gluconate (mEq/L)	Acetate (mEq/L)
NaCl 0.45% Dextrose 5%	406[a]	77	77				50			
NaCl 0.9% Dextrose 5%	560[a]	154	154				50			
NaCl 0.9%	308	154	154							
Lactated Ringer solution	273	130	109	4	3			28		
Lactated Ringer solution and dextrose 5%	525[a]	130	109	4	3		50			
Dextrose 5%	252						50			
Dextrose 50%	2520						500			
Plasmalyte 148	294	140	98	5		3			23	27
Normosol	294	140	98	5		3			23	27

[a]This is the apparent osmolarity. However, dextrose is rapidly metabolized, so the effective osmolarity is approximately 50% lower.

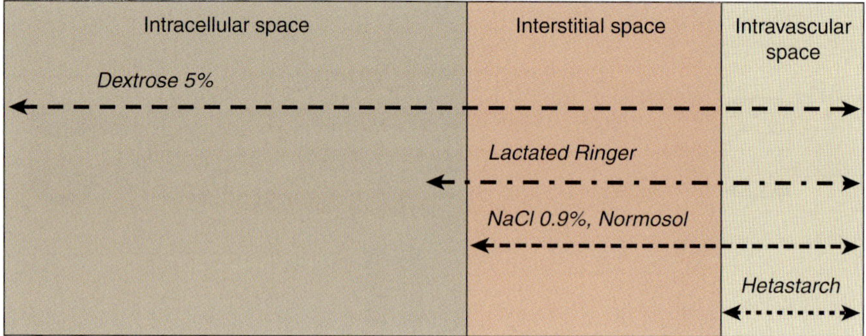

FIGURE 35-18. Volume of distribution of crystalloid solutions.

of 308 mOsm, slightly hypertonic to plasma, and a SID of 0. Consequently, administration of moderate to large quantities of this fluid is associated with mild hypernatremia, progressive hyperchloremia, and metabolic acidosis (Fig. 35-10).

Saline continues to be widely used in hospital practice, particularly in neurosurgery, in which it is used as a component of osmotic therapy. The widely accepted use of this solution in patients with renal failure has been questioned. Traditionally, BSS were avoided in this patient population because of concerns regarding accumulation of potassium in renal failure. However, a study by O'Malley and colleagues[131] demonstrated a 20% absolute risk increase (NNT [number needed to treat] 5) for hyperkalemia, in patients undergoing renal transplantation who were administered saline rather than LRS. Moreover, there was a 30% incidence of metabolic acidosis, requiring treatment, in the saline group versus 0% in the LRS group. A similar study by Hadimioglu and colleagues[131] looked at 0.9% NaCl, LRS, and Plasmalyte in the same setting. Saline was associated with hyperchloremic acidosis, and LRS was associated with elevated serum lactate; potassium levels were unchanged among the groups. Plasmalyte was associated with the best metabolic profile.

Although not widely recognized, chloride ion excretion is one of the primary roles of the kidneys because sodium and chloride are absorbed in roughly equimolar concentrations in the diet; a net excretion of chloride over sodium is necessary. Chloride is involved with regulation of renal vascular tone.[132] Hansen et al[132] have demonstrated that K^+-induced contraction of smooth muscle cells in the afferent arteriole is highly sensitive to chloride. Thus, chloride is a functional renal vasoconstrictor. Hyperchloremia has been shown to produce dose-dependent renal vasoconstriction and a reduction in GFR.[133,134] In addition, hyperchloremia may be associated with an increased risk of acute renal failure in vulnerable patients, such as those receiving radiographic contrast dye.[66,135]

Wilkes and colleagues[34] demonstrated that, compared with BSS, patients receiving intraoperative saline-based solutions had significantly reduced splanchnic blood flow, as estimated using gastric tonometry. Williams et al[64] randomized healthy volunteers to 0.9% saline versus an equal volume of LRS. Saline administration was associated with lower pH and longer time to first urination. This tendency toward fluid retention may result from the higher chloride content or the higher osmolality of the solution that induces inappropriate ADH secretion by "fooling" the midbrain that the patient is dehydrated.[64]

Crystalloid solutions of any type enhance coagulation as measured by thrombelastography (TEG) analysis and routine coagulation studies.[136-138] Saline and LRS produce a hypercoagulable state at 20% and 40% dilutions, respectively.[139] Saline produces a hypocoagulable state at 60% dilution.[141] BSS cause fewer coagulation abnormalities. The most likely mechanism is an imbalance between the naturally occurring anticoagulants and activated procoagulants, with a reduction in antithrombin III probably being the most important.[140] This effect lowers the threshold above which positive feedback into the intrinsic coagulation pathway occurs, leading to the enhanced coagulation. Although it has been suggested that resuscitation with 0.9% normal saline is associated with increased risk of bleeding versus BSS,[143] there are limited human data to support this claim.[139] One study of 0.9% saline versus LRS in aortic aneurysm surgery showed no difference in outcome variables but a higher perioperative blood loss in the saline group.[142]

LACTATED RINGER SOLUTION

Lactated Ringer solution is the most widely used BSS and is recommended as part of advanced trauma life support. Although balanced, it does not fully reflect the electrolyte distribution of the ECF. The sodium component is relatively low (130 mEq/L) and the chloride level high (109 mEq/L). Thus, SID is significantly lower than plasma. Nevertheless, perioperative patients tend to lose more water than sodium because insensible losses, and because all IV fluids dilute albumin, a slightly hyperchloremic solution is favored (**Fig. 35-19**). Hence, studies looking at the acid–base changes associated with LRS have reported few abnormalities.[34,64] The slight hypotonicity may worsen

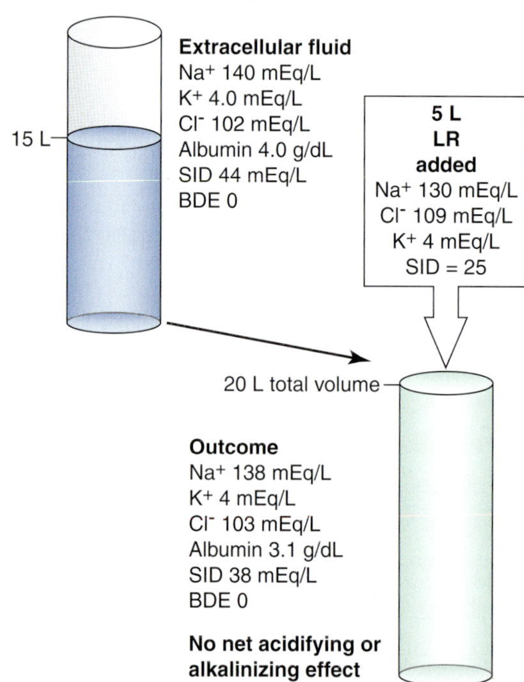

FIGURE 35-19. Extracellular fluid dilution with lactated Ringer solution (LRS). Although moderate volumes of this fluid have both acidifying effects (low strong ion difference [SID]) and alkalinizing effects (dilution of albumin), these effects offset each other and the net acid–base change is negligible. BDE, base deficit or excess.

cerebral edema in patients with TBI, although this has never been proven. In these circumstances, LRS is generally avoided. Because bicarbonate is unstable in electrolyte solutions, LRS is buffered in lactate. Lactate is metabolized by the liver to carbon dioxide and water. Care must be taken with this fluid in end-stage liver disease because these patients cannot metabolize lactate, which then functions as a strong ion, leading to metabolic acidosis. In addition, lactate may be converted to glucose, leading to hyperglycemia; consequently, this solution is rarely administered during diabetic crises. There is little published evidence to support this contention.

An important issue with the use of LRS concerns its interaction with packed RBCs for transfusion. LRS contains calcium, which may lead to clotting of the blood before it enters the bloodstream. Secondly, there is the theoretical concern that mixing this hypotonic fluid with blood will lead to hemolysis.

BALANCED SALT SOLUTIONS

A variety of BSS are available that attempt to mimic ECF content. The solutions available in North America are Normosol-R and Plasmalyte 148, which are essentially identical. Although attractive in conception, there are few published data to suggest that any of these fluids are superior to LRS. Plasmalyte comes in a number of different formulations and different buffering solutions. Normosol is buffered in acetate and gluconate, both weak anion buffers; this suggests a better acid–base profile in liver failure. Both Normosol and Plasmalyte 148 contain 140 mEq/L of Na, 98 mEq/L of Cl, and 5 mEq/L of K, with a SID of 47. Administration of either of these solutions leads to progressive metabolic alkalosis (Fig. 35-10). Because calcium is not a component of either of these solutions, Normosol and Plasmalyte can be safely administered alongside blood.

In choosing a crystalloid solution to administer to a patient, the clinician must take into account the patient's hydration status, the anticipated volume of crystalloid to be administered, and the potential side effects. For the majority of patients, a BSS such as LRS (Hartmann's) solution should be administered. This has the advantages of relative isotonicity, an electrolyte composition similar to ECF, minimal impact on acid–base chemistry, universal familiarity, low cost, and a strong safety profile. Concerns about hyperkalemia and renal failure are probably overstated. LRS is an excellent choice for both resuscitation and rehydration, resulting in neither hypernatremia nor hyperchloremia. Isotonic saline solutions should not be administered in large volume.[143] If blood is to be administered through the same IV line as the crystalloid, Normosol-R or Plasmalyte 148 should be substituted for LRS.

HYPERTONIC SALINE

Normal plasma osmolality, as we have seen, is 280 to 295 mOsm/L. Any solution whose osmolality exceeds 310 mOsm/L is a hypertonic fluid. In practical terms, this refers to HS and sodium bicarbonate solutions (**Table 35-28**). A variety of different HS solutions are commercially available, the most commonly used are 1.8%, 3%, 7.5%, and 23.4% HS. The latter is not generally used as an IV fluid, but is, for example, injected into hydatid cysts.

There are 2 well-defined uses of hypertonic fluids. The first is intravascular volume expansion in patients in hypovolemic shock as a means of low-volume, high-impact resuscitation. The second is a corollary, intracellular volume depletion. This approach is widely used in neurosurgery and neurocritical care to reduce cerebral volume and intracranial pressure (ICP).

Hypertonic saline dramatically increases the osmotic pressure in the compartment into which it is injected. Water flows along the osmotic gradient into the compartment, expanding its volume for several hours. In the intravascular space, HS causes endothelial cell shrinkage, arteriolar dilatation, and reduced viscosity, thus increasing flow.[144] It may also increase myocardial contractility, although there are conflicting data on this issue. The metabolic consequences of HS are hypernatremia, hyperosmolality, and hyperchloremic acidosis.[145] The degree of hypernatremia and hyperosmolality is lower than one would expect because of the relatively low volume administered.[146]

TABLE 35-28 Characteristics of Hypertonic Solutions

Fluid	Sodium Concentration (mEq/L)	Chloride Concentration (mEq/L)	Bicarbonate Concentration (mEq/L)	Osmolality (mOsm/L)
0.9% NaCl	154	154	–	308
1.7% NaCl	291	291	–	582
3% NaCl	513	513	–	1026
7.5% NaCl	1283	1283	–	2566
10% NaCl	1712	1713	–	3424
23.4% NaCl	4004	4004	–	8008
Mannitol	–	–	–	1098
7.5% $NaHCO_3$	900	–	900	1600
8.4% $NaHCO_3$	1000	–	1000	2000

The logic behind the use of HS in shocked states is based on 2 observations: (1) isotonic crystalloids are very inefficient plasma volume expanders and result in significant tissue edema, and (2) hypertonic solutions expand the plasma volume by a significantly greater amount than the volume administered. Consequently, significant hemodynamic benefit accrues from relatively low volumes of fluid administered. This may be of particular use in combat situations, during which the weight and size of medical supplies are of great importance.

Numerous small studies and case reports suggest that patients have better hemodynamic profiles when given HS than if administered isotonic crystalloid.[147] No study of prehospital administration of HS has shown an overall statistically significant benefit. Indeed, published benefits accrue in statistically weaker subgroup analysis. For example Mattox and colleagues[148] studied 422 patients in a randomized, double-blind, multicenter trial of prehospital HS plus dextran (HSD) versus an equal volume of isotonic crystalloid. Patients who had been administered HSD and required surgery had improved survival. Wade and colleagues[149] reported improved survival in patients with penetrating trauma who were administered HS. A meta-analysis by the same group failed to demonstrate benefit using HS in trauma patients.[150] A more recent large clinical trial failed to demonstrate improved clinical outcomes at 6 months.[153] Currently, HS is not used in this setting. The major controversy in trauma is not the utility of HS but the timing of use.

Hypertonic saline has been used in the perioperative care of cardiac surgical patients. To date, data have revealed only that HS reduces perioperative weight gain and has a diuretic effect.[152] HS may be an effective component of a goal-directed approach to fluid resuscitation, but this has yet to be studied.

The most frequent indication for HS use has been in TBI.[153] Death from brain injury is primary, as a direct result of the event, or secondary, caused by ischemic brain injury, cerebral edema, and brain herniation. Intracranial hypertension is the clinical manifestation of secondary brain injury. Under normal conditions, the blood–brain barrier (BBB) limits bulk flow of fluid from cerebral capillaries into brain parenchyma by forming a semipermeable membrane, which is moderately permeable to water and relatively impermeable to small solutes and proteins. The balance of Starling forces (the transcapillary hydrostatic pressure gradient that is counterbalanced by an osmotic pressure gradient) determines the magnitude of flow into the brain substance.[152] In areas where the BBB is disrupted, this balance disappears, facilitating the flow of proteins and electrolytes across the membrane.[153] Hydrostatic pressure becomes the dominant driving force for fluid movement from the intravascular space to brain tissue. This leads to brain swelling with an increase in ICP, a decrease in CPP, cerebral hypoxia, and secondary brain injury. Interruption of this continuing cycle of injury is the basis of treatment in TBI.[154] Osmotherapy using mannitol has been the therapy of choice in TBI for a generation. However, mannitol has several limitations. These include hyperosmolality, osmotic diuresis leading to hypotension, accumulation in brain tissue leading to reverse osmotic effects, and so on.

Hypertonic saline has reemerged over the past decade as an alternative to mannitol. The permeability of the BBB to sodium is low. HS produces a significant osmotic gradient, leading to shrinkage of brain tissue (assuming that the BBB is intact), and reduces ICP. HS, as we have seen, improves overall systemic perfusion and presumably oxygen delivery and may modulate the inflammatory response.[155]

FLUID REPLACEMENT COLLOIDS

COLLOIDS AND COLLOID ONCOTIC PRESSURE

For the majority of patients undergoing surgery and anesthesia, gentle hydration with crystalloid repletes dehydration losses and mild blood losses. However, significant tissue injury (including major surgery) leads to a slightly different paradigm that involves classic inflammatory stress response associated with increased capillary permeability. This facilitates the extravasation of intravascular fluid into the extracellular space (Fig. 35-17). Fluid sequestered in this way does not remobilize until the stress response resolves. In these circumstances, up to 80% of crystalloid solutions used as volume replacement collect in extravascular tissues (Fig. 35-16). This leads to weight gain and tissue edema, particularly in lax tissues and in the abdomen. Oxygen delivery is reduced, and the cumulative effect may be worsened perioperative outcomes.[16] In addition to increased capillary permeability, there is a reduction in plasma oncotic pressure in surgery, trauma, and critical illness; this is attributable to reduced circulating albumin concentrations caused by dilution, extravasation, and reduced hepatic production (negative acute-phase response).

High-molecular-weight solutions are used widely as plasma substitutes. These have the purported advantages of remaining in the intravascular space, plugging leaky capillaries, and increasing COP, thus expanding intravascular volume. Compared with crystalloid solutions, lower volumes are required to achieve hemodynamic goals.[16]

Colloids are homogenous noncrystalline substances, consisting of large molecules or ultramicroscopic particles of 1 substance dispersed through a second substance.[156] Colloid solutions remain in the intravascular space because of their large molecular size, which leads to relative membrane impermeability (**Fig. 35-20**). The principal biologic colloids are plasma proteins, principally albumin and globulin. These proteins impart 2 distinct forces: an osmotic pressure and a Gibbs-Donnan effect. The latter refers to an electrochemical effect of the protein: the protein is negatively charged, and positively charged cations are held in plasma. The combined effect is a pressure that draws water out of the interstitium and into the plasma—the COP. The COP is about 50% greater than that would be expected from the plasma proteins alone.

Albumin, with a molecular weight of 69 000 kD and a significant negative charge, normally accounts for nearly two-thirds of the plasma COP. Serum albumin decreases in the perioperative period and during inflammation from tissue injury or sepsis. Many clinicians mistakenly ascribe hypoalbuminemia as the cause of the edema of critical illness. However, edema occurs secondary to increased capillary permeability and fluid overload. In addition, albumin production decreases as a consequence of "hepatic reprioritization" toward inflammatory proteins. The result is maintenance of COP despite low levels of albumin.[157] Thus, the serum or plasma protein concentration is an unreliable predictor of COP. Globulins are larger molecules than albumin, and they impart significantly fewer osmotic effects. COP can be measured in a laboratory using a colloid osmometer (ie, oncometer); however, this is rarely measured in modern clinical practice.

It is important to note that although colloids have an important role in maintaining intravascular volume, the oncotic effect is significantly less important vis-à-vis extracellular volume than the osmotic effect of electrolytes, such as sodium or chloride. This is because of the significantly lower total number of osmotically active particles involved. The COP is only one of several factors that determine the fluid flux across a vascular membrane. The Starling equation describes the movement of fluid across the capillary endothelium:

$$Qf = k1[(P_c - P_i) - \sigma(\pi_c - \pi_i)]$$

where Qf indicates transcapillary fluid flux, k1 is the fluid filtration coefficient, P_c indicates capillary hydrostatic pressure, P_i indicates interstitial hydrostatic pressure, π_c indicates intravascular oncotic pressure, π_i indicates interstitial oncotic pressure, and σ is the reflection coefficient.

The reflection coefficient in the Starling equation is a function of the permeability and surface area of the capillary bed. The numeric value varies from 0 to 1. For example, the reflection coefficient of the pulmonary endothelium is normally 0.7, but it may decrease to 0.3 or 0.4 in conditions that increase microvascular permeability.

INCREASED CAPILLARY PERMEABILITY

The forces responsible for normal or abnormal fluid flux are the net colloid and hydrostatic pressures on either side of the capillary membrane (**Fig. 35-21**). The capillary hydrostatic pressure is the driving force for fluid moving out of the intravascular compartment. Because the interstitial hydrostatic pressure is usually negative or zero, the plasma COP is the force primarily responsible for counterbalancing the capillary hydrostatic pressure. Any increment in the forces that enhance filtration may induce changes that then retard further transcapillary fluid loss (eg, increased tissue hydrostatic pressure, increased plasma COP, and decreased tissue COP). In addition, the lymphatic system provides a means for returning filtered capillary water and protein back to the intravascular compartment. The rate of lymphatic flow appears

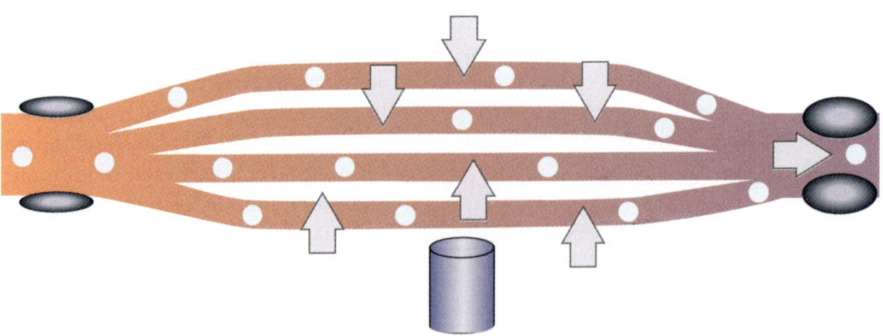

FIGURE 35-20. Colloid therapy. Colloids are hypothesized to remain intravascular despite the presence of widespread capillary leak. Fluid (represented by *white arrows*) is drawn back into the circulation because of increased colloid oncotic pressure.

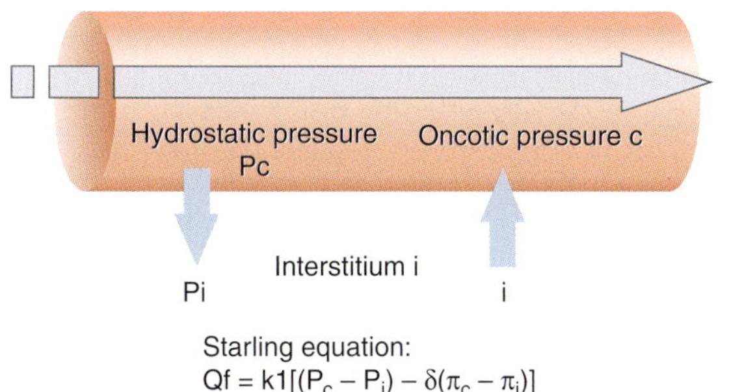

FIGURE 35-21. The Starling hypothesis. Hydrostatic pressure: Pc in capillaries, Pi in the interstitium.

linked to the filtration characteristics of the capillary wall and interstitium and the net flow of transcapillary fluid. When these protective adaptations are overwhelmed, the rate of interstitial fluid accumulation may surpass the rate of lymphatic drainage, and edema will result.

During tissue injury, sepsis, or surgery, there is a significant increase in capillary permeability, with leakage of protein rich fluid into the interstitial space (Fig. 35-17). Thus, the reflection coefficient of the Starling equation changes, and fluid accumulates in lax tissues, leading to edema. The rate of edema formation varies linearly with the volume of crystalloid administered. Colloidal solutions (**Table 35-29**) are purported to remain intravascular in conditions of widespread capillary leak (Fig. 35-20).[158] There is some evidence to support this contention.[159,160] This leads to more rapid achievement of hemodynamic goals, volume expansion equal of greater than the volume administered, and reduction in tissue edema.

Despite these logical arguments, there is a strong counter argument that colloid solutions are expensive, probably leak into the extracellular space, and impact blood coagulation. Three influential meta-analyses were published in the late 1990s that suggested that colloid solutions may actually worsen patient outcomes.[161-163] There is reason to be skeptical of the results of these reviews. A myriad of compounds labelled "colloid" were included, many no longer administered. The studies accrued data over a 30-year period during which fundamental changes occurred in the practices of anesthesia, trauma, and critical care. Moreover, the endpoints listed in the reviews (principally mortality) were not necessarily endpoints measured in the studies. The majority of these studies were not carried out in the controlled operating room environment, did not use specific goals for resuscitation, and tended to compare isolated crystalloid resuscitation with isolated colloid resuscitation, not in combination. Most studies of colloids have compared one agent against another rather than against crystalloid solutions.

There is an emerging body of evidence to support the limited use of colloid solutions in perioperative medicine. These data are discussed in the final section of this chapter. The following sections review the most frequently prescribed colloid solutions.

INTRAVENOUS ALBUMIN

Albumin is commercially available in concentrations of 5% (250- and 500-mL vials) and 25% (50- and 100-mL vials). These monodisperse solutions are derived from pooled human blood, serum, or plasma and have been pasteurized at 60°C for 10 hours. In addition, these preparations contain no clinically important antibodies and may be administered without regard to the recipient's blood group or Rh factor. Whereas the more frequently used 5% solution contains 50 mg of albumin per milliliter of physiologic salt solution, the 25% solution has an albumin concentration of 250 mg/mL. All commercial albumin products contain 130 to 160 mEq of sodium per liter of solution. The 5% solution is isooncotic with respect to human plasma; the 25% solution is 4 to 5 times more oncotically active than is an equivalent volume of normal plasma. Albumin has a very low incidence of allergic reactions (0.5%-1%), and these are usually mild (rash, fever, chills, nausea). Albumin solutions do not appear to directly alter blood coagulation.

Albumin administration is associated with a rapid but unpredictable expansion of the plasma volume. In profoundly hypovolemic patients, the interstitial compartment should be resuscitated first, so the use of albumin should follow initial administration of crystalloid. Albumin has been widely used to minimize weight gain, prevent pulmonary edema, diminish ascites, and reduce tissue edema. There is some evidence that this agent may have some impact on improving organ function and facilitating enteral nutrition.[164] Beyond this, there is no evidence that albumin reduces mortality. Previous concerns that albumin may increase mortality[165] appear to be unfounded. The Saline Versus Albumin Fluid Evaluation (SAFE) study, an Australian randomized, controlled trial that recruited more than 7000 patients, showed no differences in outcome between patients treated with 4% albumin as their resuscitation fluid and those receiving saline.[166] Currently, there is no clear clinical indication for the use of albumin in perioperative medicine.[167] In particular, low-molecular-weight HES appears to have significant therapeutic physiologic and economic advantages over human albumin solutions.[168]

DEXTRANS

Dextrans are high-molecular-weight D-glucose polymers joined largely by α-1,6 bonds into linear-branched macromolecules. They are biosynthesized commercially from sucrose by the B512 strain of Leuconostoc mesenteroides using the enzyme dextran sucrase. For clinical purposes, dextrans are designated by their weight-average molecular weights because these solutions are polydisperse colloids containing both large and small molecules. Dextran 40, with an average molecular weight of 40 000 D (range, 10 000-90 000 D), is available in 0.9% sodium chloride

TABLE 35-29 Properties of Colloid Solutions

Fluid	Weight Average Molecular Weight (D)	Number Average Molecular Weight (D)	Colloid Osmotic Pressure (mm Hg)
5% Albumin	69 000	69 000	19
25% Albumin	69 000	69 000	78
Plasma	119 000	88 000	21
6% Hetastarch	450 000	70 000	30
10% Pentastarch	264 000	63 000	40
6% Pentafraction	280 000	120 000	28
10% Dextran 40	40 000	26 000	148
6% Dextran 70	70 000	41 000	60

or 5% dextrose, as is dextran 70, which has an average molecular weight of 70 000 D (range, 20 000–200 000 D). Dextrans have a strong colloidal osmotic effect: 1 g of dextran 40 retains 30 mL of fluid.

After administration, the lower-molecular-weight particles are rapidly cleared by the kidney. The threshold for the renal excretion of dextran is a molecular weight of roughly 50 000 D. Particles less than 15 000 D are rapidly filtered and not reabsorbed. The remainder is excreted through the gut or phagocytosed by cells of the reticuloendothelial system. Within 24 hours after infusion, approximately 70% of dextran 40 and 50% of dextran 70 is excreted unchanged in the urine. Severe renal dysfunction (creatinine clearance <30 mL/min) prolongs the intravascular half-life and causes an accumulation of the smaller dextran molecules.

In most instances, the dextran preparations produce an expansion of plasma volume that is approximately equal to the volume of solution infused. Acutely, dextran 40 produces a greater increment in plasma volume compared with dextran 70 because of the greater number of molecules and the more powerful osmotic effect. Intravascular volume expansion is generally more prolonged with dextran 70.

Dextrans are known to have a significant impact on coagulation. When more than 1.5% g/kg is administered, bleeding time is prolonged. The observed hemostatic abnormality is similar to that seen in von Willebrand syndrome. Dextran also impairs the polymerization of fibrin. Dextrans have been traditionally used for postoperative thromboembolic prophylaxis in vascular and plastic and reconstructive surgery.

Dextran 40 may interfere with the cross-matching of blood if a proteolytic enzyme technique is used. Dextran 70 can induce erythrocyte aggregation and rouleaux formation that may also impede cross-matching. Both solutions can produce a factitious hyperglycemia, and the lower-molecular-weight dextran solution can increase serum transaminase (aspartate aminotransferase and alanine aminotransferase) levels. Dextran 40 can produce highly viscous urine that may actually obstruct the renal tubules and cause acute renal failure.

Dextrans have been associated with a relatively high incidence of anaphylactoid and anaphylactic reactions. Anaphylactoid reactions are caused by dextran-reactive immunoglobulin G antibodies.[169] The best available data suggest that the risk of a major anaphylactoid reaction is 13 of 100 000 doses sold for dextran 40 and 25 of 100 000 doses sold for dextran 70.[170] Severe anaphylactoid reactions can nearly always prevented by preinfusing dextran 1 (Promit, Meda AB Pharmaceuticals, Solna, Sweden), a low-molecular-weight (1000) dextran moiety.[172] Dextran 1 acts to prevent severe anaphylactoid reactions by competitively inhibiting dextran from binding to IgG antibodies.

HYDROXYETHYL STARCHES

Hydroxyethyl starches (hetastarch) are modified natural polysaccharides, derived from amylopectin, that structurally resemble glycogen. Solutions of starch are unstable as they are rapidly hydrolyzed by alpha-amylase. The solution is stabilized by hydroxyl-ethylation. This results in hydroxyethyl substitutions predominantly at carbon 2 (c2), but also at c3 and c6, in the glucose ring (**Fig. 35-22**). The pharmacokinetics of these starches is determined by the degree and type of hydroxylation. A higher c2/6 substitution ratio results in slower enzymatic degradation. The molecular weight of the compound impacts its side effects. The main route of elimination is urinary. A fraction is taken up by the reticuloendothelial system from whence it is slowly eliminated. Hetastarches contain molecules of variable molecular weights, the average weight is usually that listed. After infusion of HES, the dispersion of molecular weights changes: first the small molecules are rapidly eliminated, the large molecules are partially hydrolysed to middle sized molecules.

Hydroxyl-ethyl starch products can be divided into 3 classes by their weight-averaged MW: high-molecular-weight (450-480 kDa), medium-molecular-weight (~200 kDa), and low-molecular-weight (70-130 kDa). Examples of commercially available starches are 6% high-molecular-weight hetastarch in saline (Hespan), 6% high-molecular-weight hetastarch in balanced electrolytes (Hextend), medium-molecular-weight pentastarch in saline (Pentaspan, EloHAES, HAES-steril), and low-molecular-weight tetrastarch in saline (Voluven) or balanced salt (Volulyte).

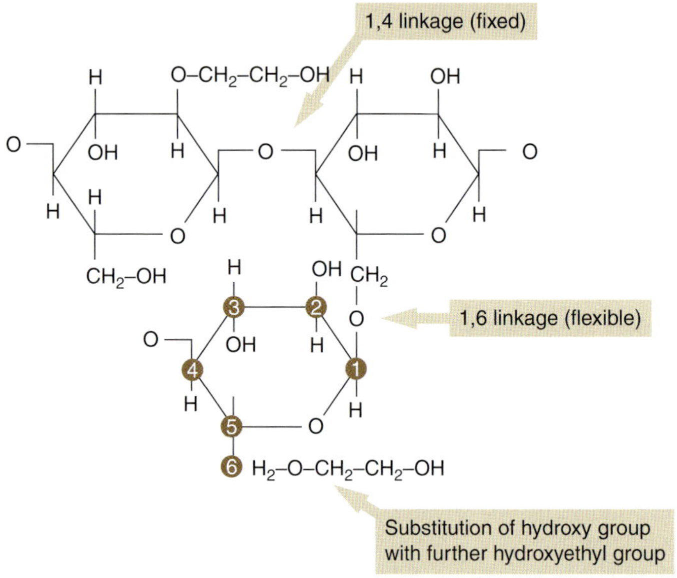

FIGURE 35-22. Hydroxyethyl starch structure.

The most commonly used HES in the United States, Hespan, is a high-molecular-weight HES (480/0.7), with an average molecular weight of 450 000 D and a number-average molecular weight of 70 000 D; 80% of the polymers fall in the range of 30 000 to 2 400 000 D. This HES is usually formulated in 0.9% sodium chloride. The COP of this solution is approximately 30 mm Hg, and each gram of hetastarch has a water-binding capacity of 20 mL. On the average, 46% and 64% of the dose is excreted in the urine within 2 and 8 days, respectively. The average terminal half-life is 17 days. Plasma volume expansion persists for at least 48 hours,[171] with 40% of the peak effect persisting after 24 hours. Hetastarch produces a significantly greater increase in plasma COP compared with an equal volume of 5% albumin. In addition, HES significantly reduces capillary leakage compared with albumin.[172]

Serum amylase may increase significantly after infusion of HES because of the formation of a stable hetastarch–amylase complex that retards amylase excretion. Allergic reactions to HES are uncommon.

HES solutions have varying effects on coagulation that depend on the molecular weight of the polypeptide molecule. This appears to occur principally with high-molecular-weight HES that dilutes coagulation factors and induces abnormalities on TEG but not standard coagulation tests. HES appears to induce an abnormality of platelet function by impairing von Willebrand factor and factor VIIIc. The effect on hemostasis appears to be dose related. Large volumes of hetastarch in vitro and in vivo produce progressive abnormalities in TEG studies. However, it is unclear if this translates into increased risk of perioperative bleeding. Many clinicians assert that the dose of hetastarch be limited to 20 mL/kg/d. Lower-molecular-weight HES and pentastarch solutions appear to be associated with reduced risk of coagulopathy[173] as does formulation in BSS rather than saline.[174] Roche and colleagues[139] have elegantly described changes in coagulation associated with crystalloid and colloid administration. Hetastarch in saline, pentastarch in saline, tetrastarch in saline, and human albumin solutions all produce a hypocoagulable state at 60% dilution. Hetastarch in saline also produces a hypocoagulable state at 40% dilution. The larger-molecular-weight starches produce more intense coagulation abnormalities than the medium-molecular-weight compounds formulated similarly (ie, suspended in saline or BSS). The balanced salt solutions caused fewer coagulation abnormalities, especially pentastarch in balanced salt solution. This balanced salt pentastarch preparation produced the least derangement of coagulation of the colloid solutions at all dilutions, causing hypercoagulability at the lower dilutions and minimal coagulation derangement at 60% dilution.

The VISEP (Efficacy of Volume Substitution and Insulin Therapy in Severe Sepsis) study[39] was a multicenter two-by-two study that randomized patients with severe sepsis to tight glycemic control or conventional therapy and fluid resuscitation with 10% pentastarch, middle-molecular-weight HES 200/0.5, or LRS. The author looked at 28-day mortality and organ failure as primary endpoints, and the study was stopped early after 537 patients had been enrolled (at the first planned interim analysis) for safety reasons. Glycemic control made no difference to outcomes at 28 days, although there were some adverse events in the tight glycemic control group. Patients in the HES group had a lower median platelet count (179 600/mm^3; interquartile range, 122 000-260 000/mm^3) than did those in the LRS group (224 000/mm^3; interquartile range, 149 800-314 800/mm^3; p <.001) and received more units of packed RBCs than did patients in the LRS (lactated Ringer solution) group. In addition, HES was associated with increased 90-day mortality (57.6% vs 30.9%; ARI 26.7%; NNT 4 in patients [with high-dose HES alone] increased renal failure ARI 12%; p <.05) and a 9.1% increase in length of dialysis.

There were significant issues with this study. Older starches than are currently promoted were used.[175] The patients were administered higher than recommended dose (>20 mL/kg) for a long period, 21 days. One of the colloids was hyperoncotic (10%; COP 68) with respect to plasma. Finally, there are known adverse outcomes associated with primary colloid resuscitation.[176] There was no difference between mortality levels at 28 days or indeed at 90 days. Hence, the published 90-day mortality difference may represent pharmacologic poisoning caused by HES accumulation rather than failure of therapy, conflicting with decades of positive HES data.[40]

GELATINS

Gelatin solutions are widely used in Europe, particularly in the British Isles. Currently, no gelatin is licensed for administration in the United States. The colloidal compounds are derived from hydrolysis of bovine collagen. Gelatins are medium-sized compounds, with molecular weights of 30 000 to 40 000 D. The 2 most common preparations are succinylated gelatin (Gelofusin), presented in a carrier solution of Na 154 mmol and Cl 120 mmol, and urea-linked gelatin (Hemaccel), presented in a carrier solution of isotonic saline plus K 5.1 mmol and Ca 6.25 mmol/L. Care should be used when administering the latter product in patients requiring blood transfusions. The presence of calcium in the fluid giving set may cause blood coagulation. Administration of gelatin is followed by intravascular volume expansion of an equivalent volume, although after 4 hours, up to 50% of the volume expansion will have been lost. Thus, use of gelatins is limited to cases in which rapid volume expansion is required, but the source of the problem is rapidly reversible. An example of this situation is acute vasoplegia associated with epidural analgesia.

The pharmacokinetics of gelatins are not well understood. Gelatins are cleared principally by glomerular filtration but may also be broken down by proteases in the reticuloendothelial system. The impact of these compounds of coagulation is unclear; however, urea-bridge gelatins may result in a reduction of platelet aggregation. The incidence of allergic reactions is relatively high compared with HES. The bovine origin of these products has led to so significant discussion about the risk of transmission of bovine spongiform encephalopathy to humans.[177] However, there have been no reported cases of new variant Creutzfeldt-Jakob disease associated with pharmaceutical-grade gelatins to date.

MONITORING FLUID REPLACEMENT

LIMITATIONS OF CRYSTALLOID RESUSCITATION

Traditional approaches to perioperative fluid management had emphasized the use of careful calculation of fasting fluid deficits, insensible losses, third-space loss, blood loss, and maintenance requirements. Fluid replacement regimens have been formulaic, centered on crystalloid resuscitation in the belief that dehydration and excessive third-space loss will lead to adverse outcomes. However, there is an emerging movement that questions these assumptions.[16,178] For example, the human body evolved many processes to sustain itself in the face of inadequate hydration. Hence, the renin–angiotensin–aldosterone–vasopressin axis developed to maintain homeostasis until a source of water became available. Conversely, the human body does not appear to be able to store water. Consequently, few mechanisms appear to be in place to deal with significant hypervolemia. Moreover, advocates of aggressive crystalloid resuscitation have tended to ignore the impact of this fluid on tissue compartments (a dramatic increase in interstitial fluid volume), water dissociation (acid–base balance), electrolyte composition, colloid balance, and coagulation. Proponents of an alternative system for perioperative fluid balance, goal-directed resuscitation, use dynamic flow-directed physiologic endpoints that emphasize timing rather than total volume for fluid administration.

Resuscitation with crystalloid fluids may actually reduce oxygen delivery and tissue perfusion. Funk and Baldinger[179] undertook a laboratory experiment of isovolemic hemodilution of awake Syrian golden hamsters. The hamsters were given either LRS or dextran 60 to replace blood loss. Four times the volume of blood loss was replaced with LRS to maintain mean arterial pressure, central venous pressure (CVP), and heart rate. Tissue perfusion and Pao_2 were unchanged in the colloid group but reduced by 62% and 58%, respectively, in the crystalloid group. Lang et al[180] investigated the impact of colloid fluid replacement versus crystalloid therapy on tissue oxygen tension in major abdominal surgery. A total of 42 patients were randomized to receive 6% HES plus LRS alone for 24 hours targeted to a CVP of 8 to 12 mm Hg. The investigators measured tissue oxygen tension in the deltoid muscle; a Licox CMP monitoring device was placed after induction of anesthesia. Patients in the crystalloid group had received significantly more fluid by the end of surgery (5940 mL +/− 1910 mL vs 3920 mL +/− 1350 mL; p <.05) and at the end of 24 hours (11 740 +/− 2630 mL vs 5950 mL +/− 800 mL; p <.05). The patients in the combined crystalloid–colloid group had significantly greater tissue perfusion (oxygen tension increased from baseline) compared with the crystalloid only group (oxygen tension reduced from baseline).

An ideal resuscitative fluid would maintain intravascular volume without expanding the interstitial space. Ernest et al[181] investigated the volume of distribution of NaCl 0.9% versus albumin 55 in cardiac surgical patients. Plasma and ECF volumes were measured by dilution of radiolabeled albumin and sodium. Administration of isotonic saline increased plasma volume by 9% +/− 23% of the volume infused. Administration of 5% albumin increased plasma volume by 52 +/− 84% of the volume infused. Albumin increased cardiac index significantly more than saline and had an equal impact of hemoglobin dilution. In the saline treatment group, the mean net fluid balance (Fluid infusion + Fluid losses) was approximately double the mean increase in ECF volume, which on average was distributed equally between the plasma volume and interstitial fluid volume. In contrast, in the albumin treatment group, the net fluid balance approximated the mean increase in ECF volume, which approximated the mean increase in plasma volume.

The tendency for crystalloids to extravasate may lead to relative hypoperfusion.[182] Wilkes and colleagues[34] studied saline-based IV fluids (crystalloid and HES) versus BSS-based fluids (crystalloid and HES) on acid–base status and gut perfusion, estimated using gastric tonometry. Patients who received saline were significantly more acidotic and had a lower gastric mucosal pH (indicative of gut perfusion) compared with the patients receiving BSS. This was strongly related to increases in serum chloride.

PRO- AND ANTI-INFLAMMATORY EFFECTS OF INTRAVENOUS FLUIDS

Conventional wisdom holds that IV fluids impart adverse effects consequent of increases in hydrostatic pressure, leading to pulmonary edema, tissue edema, and interference with oxygen perfusion into tissues. However, emerging evidence indicates that IV fluids may have indigenous pro- and anti-inflammatory properties. In a pig model of volume-controlled hemorrhagic shock, Rhee and colleagues[183] demonstrated a significant increase in neutrophil activation and oxidative burst activity associated with the administration of LRS. This solution activated inflammation regardless of whether blood was shed or not. This did not occur when volume was replaced with whole blood or 7.5% HS. Similar findings were reported with isotonic saline, dextran, and HES but not with albumin (5% or 25%), blood, or anesthesia.[184]

LRS administration was associated with expression of adhesion molecules that were increased in the lungs and spleen whether or not hemorrhage took place. This was not seen if animal was not resuscitated or resuscitated with fresh blood.[185] However, when preceded by shock, LRS resuscitation was associated with histologic evidence of pulmonary edema and inflammation.[186]

Ketone-buffered IV fluids, such as ethyl pyruvate, may have opposite anti-inflammatory effects. In a rat model, the use of ethyl pyruvate versus LRS resulted in significantly less pulmonary cellular apoptosis.[187] To date, no commercially available product has confirmed this hypothesis in humans.

FLOW- AND GOAL-DIRECTED VOLUME RESUSCITATION

Because of significant limitations regarding formulaic approaches to fluid resuscitation, concerns about overresuscitation, and the need for a scientific approach based on the dynamics of the stress response, an emerging body of evidence supports the use of goal-directed volume resuscitation (GDVR) that combines crystalloid and colloid in perioperative medicine and critical illness.[179,191,192] The modern approach to GDVR involves the use of specific "normal" endpoints of blood flow and tissue perfusion.[189]

The goal-directed approach involves the use of specific monitors that measure input (fluid loading), tissue blood flow, and response (**Fig. 35-23**). Arterial and central lines are placed, and goals for resuscitation are set; these include a CVP of 8 to 12 cm H_2O; a mean arterial pressure (MAP) of greater than 65 mm Hg; and if the appropriate device(s) is placed, a mixed venous oxygen saturation of greater than 70% and a stroke volume of between 0.7 and 1.0 mL/kg (ideal body weight). The purpose of stroke volume monitoring is to construct Starling curves using one of a variety of surrogates of end-diastolic volume as an index of cardiac preload. These include CVP, pulmonary artery occlusion pressure, or pulmonary artery diastolic pressure (**Fig. 35-24**). Changes in stroke volume are more sensitive to changes in circulating volume than changes in cardiac output or cardiac index.[10] In and of itself, CVP is probably an inadequate measure of volume responsiveness.

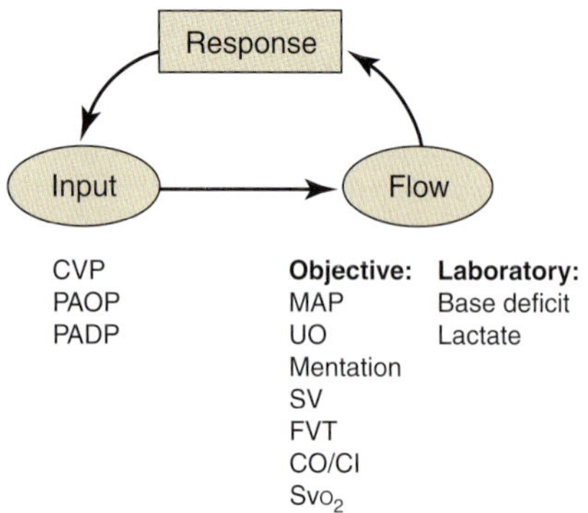

FIGURE 35-23. Principles of goal-directed resuscitation. CI, cardiac index; CO, cardiac output; CVP, central venous pressure; FVT, flow velocity time; MAP, mean arterial pressure; PADP, pulmonary artery diastolic pressure; PAOP, pulmonary artery occlusion pressure; SV, stroke volume; Svo_2, mixed venous oxygen saturation; UO, urinary output.

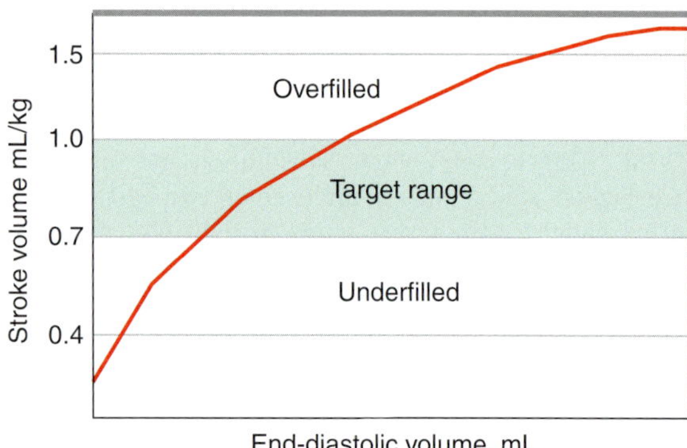

FIGURE 35-24. Stroke volume monitoring.

A variety of other devices that measure surrogates of stroke volume or cardiac output are available. These include esophageal Doppler monitors (EDMs), lithium dilution cardiac output, pulse-pressure variability stroke volume variability pulse contour analysis devices (peripherally inserted cardiac output, and Flotrac-Vigileo), Fick principle CO_2 rebreathing cardiac output (noninvasive cardiac output), bioimpedance cardiac output, and echocardiography. An alternative approach is to directly measure tissue perfusion or surrogates of blood flow. These include gastric tonometry and tissue oxygen monitoring probes, such as Licox.

Central venous pressure has been used to ensure precise perioperative hydration. Moretti et al[190] randomized 90 patients undergoing major elective (noncardiac surgery) to receive 6% hetastarch (in normal saline), 6% hetastarch (in balanced salt solution), or LRS on the basis of a resuscitation algorithm. CVP was used for therapeutic goals (**Fig. 35-25**). Patients who received colloid received significantly less fluid than those receiving crystalloid alone and had significantly lower incidence of PONV, requirement for rescue antiemetics, severe pain, periorbital edema, and double vision.

A number of studies have used EDM stroke volume to guide perioperative fluid administration. Mythen and Webb[191] studied 60 patients undergoing cardiac surgery randomly assigned to a protocol that included 200-mL boluses of colloid throughout to specified stroke volume using EDM or control. The volume administration approach in the control group was at the anesthesiologist's discretion. Patients in the EDM group had higher splanchnic perfusion at the end of surgery, fewer major complications, and shorter intensive care and hospital stays.

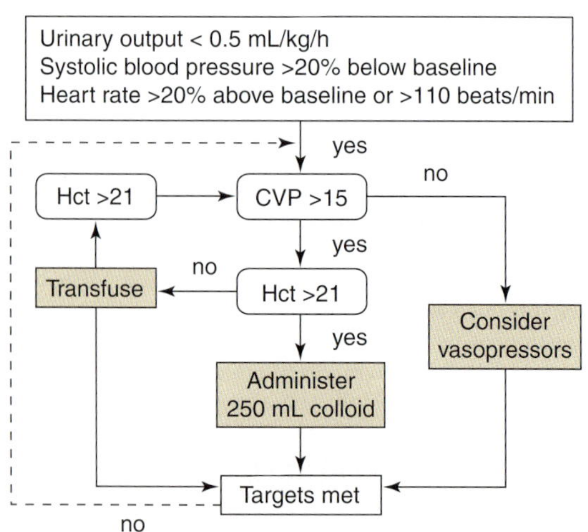

FIGURE 35-25. Use of central venous pressure (CVP) as part of goal-directed volume resuscitation. Hct, hematocrit.

Gan and colleagues[192] studied 100 patients undergoing major elective surgery with anticipated blood losses of greater than 500 mL randomly assigned to a control or protocol group. The protocol included EDM-guided plasma volume expansion (with colloid) to maximize stroke volume. The protocol group had a significantly shorter duration of hospital stay, tolerated solid oral food earlier, and had significantly less PONV.

Venn and colleagues[193] randomized 90 patients into 3 groups: one that received conventional fluid management (CVM; based on formulae), one that received colloid fluid challenges with a CVP line, and a third that received colloid fluid challenges with EDM. Patients were deemed medically fit for discharge more rapidly in the EDM group versus the CVP group and in the CVP group versus the CVM group.

Sinclair et al[194] randomized 40 patients who were undergoing repair of proximal femoral fracture to receive CVM versus EDM and colloid fluid challenges, again, to a specific stroke volume goal. Patients in the EDM group were deemed medically fit for discharge earlier than in the conventional therapy group. Wakeling et al[195] randomized 128 consecutive patients who were undergoing colorectal surgery to EDM-guided or CVP-based (conventional) intraoperative fluid management. The CVP-guided protocol aimed at a CVP of 12 to 15 mm Hg. There was a significant reduction in postoperative stay, shorter time to resuming full diet, and lower incidence of GI morbidity in the patients randomized to EDM-guided therapy.

Noblett et al[196] recruited 108 patients undergoing elective colorectal resection and inserted EDMs into all. The patients were randomized into fluid therapy that was at the discretion of the anesthesiologist versus protocolized fluid therapy that included colloid boluses. The intervention group had a reduced postoperative hospital stay, had fewer intermediate or major postoperative complications, and tolerated diet earlier. In addition, there was a reduced increase in perioperative level of the cytokine interleukin-6 in the intervention group.

An alternative approach to flow monitoring derived from the seminal work of Shoemaker et al[197] is to use oxygen consumption (or its surrogate, mixed venous oxygen saturation [Svo_2]) to determine tissue oxygen flow. Low Svo_2 is indicative of excessive extraction per unit volume, strongly suggestive of hypovolemia. Rivers et al[198] studied early goal-directed therapy in sepsis in 263 patients randomized to "standard" therapy versus aggressive goal-directed therapy that included the use of an oximetric CVP line. They measured Svo_2 in the superior vena cava distribution. The patients in the study group received significantly more fluid than the control group in the first 6 hours, more RBC transfusions overall, and an equivalent volume of IV fluid over the first 72 hours. There was a 16% decrease in 28-day mortality (number needed to treat, 6). The implication of this study is early aggressive volume resuscitation ensures tissue blood flow. After goals are met, further resuscitation is not helpful and may be harmful.

Taking these data together, it appears that perioperative patients undergoing major nonvascular surgery require early aggressive goal targeted volume resuscitation. Stroke volume monitoring appears to be more effective than CVP, which appears to be more effective than the use of standard formulaic approaches. Patients appear to do better if resuscitated on the day of surgery and if colloids are administered to achieve volume goals.

FLUID RESTRICTION

One of the questions that arise from these data is whether the convention of administering postoperative maintenance fluids to patients who have undergone major abdominal surgery is helpful or hurtful. Brandstrup and colleagues[199] performed a randomized, observer-blinded, multicenter trial (8 Danish hospitals) that included 172 patients randomized to a restrictive or standard perioperative fluid regimen. All of the patients underwent colorectal surgery. The patients receiving restrictive therapy received no volume preloading, no adjustment for third-space loss, and hetastarch or blood to replace blood losses. Postoperative fluid management was adjusted to prevent weight gain of more than 1 kg. The standard therapy group received formula-driven volume replacement. There was a significant reduction in postoperative (including cardiopulmonary and wound healing) complications in the restrictive therapy group.

In another study, 152 patients with an American Society of Anesthesiologists (ASA) physical status of I to III who were undergoing elective intra-abdominal surgery were randomized to receive intraoperatively either liberal or restrictive amounts of LRS.[200] The liberal protocol group received 10 mL/kg followed by 12 mL/kg/h. The restrictive protocol group received 4 mL/kg/h and no bolus. The majority of patients underwent lower GI surgery. The median volume of fluid administered to the restrictive group was 1230 mL versus 3670 mL in the liberal group. The number of complications was lower in the restrictive protocol group. Return of bowel function was later in that group and their hospital stay was longer.

Another group randomized 10 patients undergoing surgery for colonic cancer to receive liberal postoperative fluids (≥3 L water and 154 mmol sodium per day) and 10 to receive a restricted intake (≤2 L water and 77 mmol sodium per day).[201] Patients in the fluid restriction group (ie, weight gain of <3 kg) had an earlier return of GI function and shorter duration of hospital stay. A similar study by Tambyraja and colleagues[202] demonstrated a significant relationship between postoperative sodium and water gain and complications, again after colonic surgery.

SUMMARY

Perioperative fluid management is a complex process that must take into account the patient's preexisting disease, preoperative volume status, physiologic reserve, degree of perioperative stress, and perioperative fluid losses.

For the majority of patients, prehydration with 2 mL/kg/h fasting or 30 mL/kg crystalloid, before or at the time of induction, will reduce postoperative nausea, vomiting, pain, and light-headedness. For patients undergoing minor surgery or ambulatory surgery without appreciable blood loss, this is all the IV fluid that is required. There are few data available with respect to youthful patients with low ASA physical status scores. A formula-based approach to perioperative

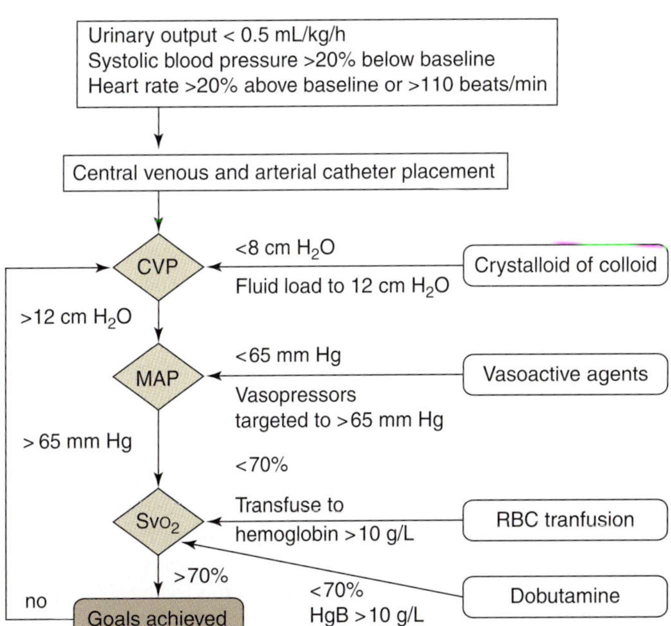

FIGURE 35-26. Use of SVO_2 (mixed venous oxygen saturation) as part of goal-directed resuscitation. CVP, central venous pressure; HgB, hemoglobin; MAP, mean arterial pressure; RBC, red blood cell.

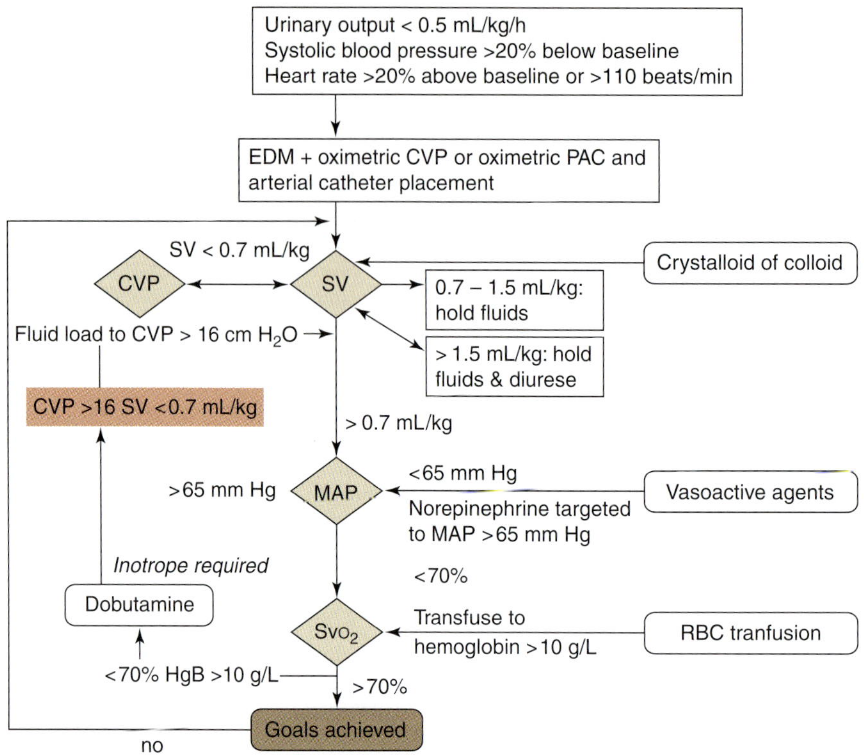

FIGURE 35-27. Use of stroke volume (SV) and Svo_2 (mixed venous oxygen saturation) as part of goal-directed resuscitation. CVP, central venous pressure; EDM, esophageal Doppler monitor; HgB, hemoglobin; MAP, mean arterial pressure; PAC, pulmonary artery catheter; RBC, red blood cell.

fluid management appears reasonable for low-risk patients undergoing moderately traumatic surgery (eg, laparoscopic operations, peripheral vascular surgery, neurosurgery). However, the management of patients undergoing extensive or high-risk surgery requires a more elegant approach. Patients undergoing bowel resection appear to have worse outcomes when overresuscitated with crystalloid. Patients undergoing major vascular surgery, hip surgery, or extensive upper abdominal surgeries appear to benefit from a dynamic flow-based, goal-directed approach to volume resuscitation. This can be achieved (in increasing order of invasiveness) using CVP (volume responsiveness; Fig. 35-25); CVP and mixed venous oxygen saturation (volume responsiveness and tissue flow; **Fig. 35-26**) or stroke volume and mixed venous oxygen saturation (dynamic volume responsiveness and tissue flow; **Fig. 35-27**). In the latter approach, stroke volume is targeted to 0.7 to 1 mL/kg of ideal body weight. A stroke volume in excess of 1.0 mL/kg is indicative of overresuscitation and fluids are withheld until the stroke volume drifts back into normal range. If the stroke volume exceeds 1.5 mL/kg, serious consideration is given to the administration of diuretics. Respiratory pulse pressure variation is gaining popularity and may emerge as a simple surrogate for stroke volume.[203] Intraoperative blood loss should be replaced 1:1 with blood or colloid or with 4:1 with crystalloid; crystalloid requirements to replace blood increase geometrically as blood loss continues. Patient outcomes appear to be optimal when the patient is resuscitated fully on the day of surgery or injury and resuscitation efforts rapidly decelerate.

Postoperative fluid management remains a controversial area. Although transcompartmental fluid sequestration continues for 1 or 2 days after surgery or injury (longer if a septic source remains uncontrolled), continued administration of crystalloid leads to increasing tissue edema and weight gain. Conversely, intravascular dehydration may lead to hypoperfusion organ injury, particularly to the kidney. A prudent approach to postoperative fluid administration is recommended. Maintenance fluids are probably unnecessary unless the period of fasting is prolonged. Patients with evidence of tissue hypoperfusion, as evidenced by low urinary output, low Svo_2, or low stroke volume, should be treated with fluid boluses, keeping in mind that lower volumes of colloid are required to achieve the same hemodynamic goals. After spontaneous diuresis commences, continuous fluid infusions should be discontinued and attention directed toward repletion of intracellular ions, potassium, magnesium, and phosphate. A reasonable goal for perioperative fluid management is restoration of normal body weight by day 7 postoperatively.

KEY REFERENCES

- Alfaro V, Torras R, Ibanez J, Palacios L. A physical-chemical analysis of the acid-base response to chronic obstructive pulmonary disease. *Can J Physiol Pharmacol.* 1996;11(74):1229-1235.
- Boldt J. Use of albumin: an update. *Br J Anaesth.* 2010;104:276-284.
- Brandstrup B, Tonnesen H, Beier-Holgersen R, et al. Effects of intravenous fluid restriction on postoperative complications: comparison of two perioperative fluid regimens: a randomized assessor-blinded multicenter trial. *Ann Surg.* 2003;238:641-648.
- Chappell D, Jacob M, Hofmann-Kiefer K, et al. A rational approach to perioperative fluid management. *Anesthesiology.* 2008;109:723-740.
- Corey HE. Stewart and beyond: new models of acid-base balance. *Kidney Int.* 2003;64:777-787.
- Curley G, Laffey J, Kavanagh B. Bench-to-bedside review: carbon dioxide. *Crit Care.* 2010;14:220.
- Fencl V, Jabor A, Kazda A, Figge J. Diagnosis of metabolic acid-base disturbances in critically ill patients. *Am J Respir Crit Care Med.* 2000;162:2246-2251.
- Fencl V, Leith DE. Stewart's quantitative acid-base chemistry: applications in biology and medicine. *Respir Physiol.* 1993;91:1-16.

- Fisher M. Postoperative intravenous therapy. *Anaesth Intensive Care.* 1977;5:339-346.
- Grocott MPW, Mythen MG, Gan TJ. Perioperative fluid management and clinical outcomes in adults. *Anesth Analg.* 2005;100:1093-1106.
- Holte K, Sharrock NE, Kehlet H. Pathophysiology and clinical implications of perioperative fluid excess. *Br J Anaesth.* 2002;89:622-632.
- Narins R, Emmett M. Simple and mixed acid-base disorders: a practical approach. *Medicine (Baltimore).* 1980;59:161-187.
- Nicholson JP, Wolmarans MR, Park GR. The role of albumin in critical illness. *Br J Anaesth.* 2000;85:599-610.
- Nisanevich V, Felsenstein I, Almogy G, et al. Effect of intraoperative fluid management on outcome after intraabdominal surgery. *Anesthesiology.* 2005;103:25-32.
- Perioperative total parenteral nutrition in surgical patients. The Veterans Affairs Total Parenteral Nutrition Cooperative Study Group. *N Engl J Med.* 1991;325:525-532.
- Rivers E, Nguyen B, Havstad S, et al. Early goal-directed therapy in the treatment of severe sepsis and septic shock. *N Engl J Med.* 2001;345:1368-1377.
- Roche AM, James MFM, Nett-Guerrero E, Mythen MG. A head-to-head comparison of the in vitro coagulation effects of saline-based and balanced electrolyte crystalloid and colloid intravenous fluids. *Anesth Analg.* 2006;102:1274-1279.
- The SAFE Investigators. A comparison of albumin and saline for fluid resuscitation in the intensive care unit. *N Engl J Med.* 2004;350:2247-2256.
- Shoemaker WC, Montgomery ES, Kaplan E, Elwyn DH. Physiologic patterns in surviving and nonsurviving shock patients. Use of sequential cardiorespiratory variables in defining criteria for therapeutic goals and early warning of death. *Arch Surg.* 1973;106:630-636.
- Siggaard-Anderson O. *The Acid Base Status of the Blood.* Copenhagen, Denmark: Munksgard; 1963:134.
- Stewart PA. Modern quantitative acid-base chemistry. *Can J Physiol Pharmacol.* 1983;61:1444-1461.

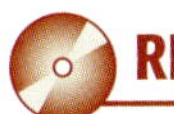

REFERENCES

Complete references available on DVD and online version at www.LongneckerAnesthesiology.com

SECTION B

Managing the Airway

CHAPTER 36 Airway Management

P. Allan Klock, Jr
Michael Hernandez
Sally Seraphin

KEY POINTS

1. Tracheal intubation can be accomplished using several techniques, including direct visual (rigid) laryngoscopy, video laryngoscopy, indirect visual (fiberoptic) laryngoscopy, guided blind (retrograde), and complete blind (eg, intubation through supraglottic airway [SGA] or blind nasal) intubation. Each technique has its preferred indication, risks, and benefits.
2. Soft tissue upper airway obstruction is common after induction of anesthesia. Insertion of an oropharyngeal airway or an SGA or application of a jaw thrust often is successful for overcoming soft tissue airway obstruction.
3. General anesthesia and muscle relaxants facilitate tracheal intubation. A rapid-acting muscle relaxant is used during rapid-sequence induction and intubation.
4. During general anesthesia, airway management without tracheal intubation has become well-accepted common practice since the introduction of SGA devices. As with any technique, it is incumbent upon the physician to determine what technique is most appropriate given the clinical scenario.
5. Securing the airway under topical anesthesia with or without sedation (an "awake intubation") provides the optimal approach for a patient with a severely compromised or difficult airway.
6. Awake intubation should be encouraged, taught, and practiced regularly to help maintain comfort and skill with the technique.
7. The availability of a difficult airway cart should be assured for every anesthetizing location.
8. Many major anesthetic complications are frequently associated with airway mismanagement, including inadequate ventilation or oxygenation and unrecognized esophageal intubation.
9. Laryngospasm is common with airway stimulation during light anesthesia. Stridor indicates partial blockade of the airway. Lack of stridor may indicate complete closure of the larynx with no air exchange.
10. For patients in whom the upper airway is obstructed, establishing emergency ventilation with a supraglottic device (eg, laryngeal mask airway), esophageal device (eg, Combitube), cricothyrotomy, or transtracheal jet ventilation is a must and should be applied as soon as possible to prevent brain injury and death.
11. Trauma to laryngeal structures can leave patients with vocal cord paralysis and serious voice dysfunction.
12. Many airway disasters have been reported after patient extubation. A well-planned and prepared extubation is a must for high-risk patients to minimize airway-related complications.

In the anesthetic environment, an artificial airway conducts gases between the anesthesia machine's breathing system and the alveoli. Effective management requires keeping the airway free of secretions, contamination, and obstruction while minimizing complications. Critical illness often causes weakness and obtundation sufficient to impair gas exchange. The sedative, narcotic, anesthetic, and relaxant drugs that facilitate surgery predictably compromise airway patency and protection. The Closed Claims Study of the American Society of Anesthesiologists Committee on Professional Liability has shown that tragic and costly complications of anesthesia frequently have resulted from problematic airway management.[1] Some of the obligations of the anesthesiologist include ensuring that the patient is adequately oxygenated, the lungs are ventilated, and airway patency is maintained. Essential attributes of the expert airway manager include knowledge, sound judgment, skills for a range of techniques, and a plan for all conceivable contingencies.[2,3]

APPLIED ANATOMY OF THE AIRWAY

Mastery of the airway demands familiarity with normal and variant anatomy and the alterations caused by sedation, anesthesia, and abnormal states.

THE PHARYNX

The pharynx, extending from the sphenoid bone to the sixth cervical vertebrae (C6), parallels the vertebrae. The retropharyngeal space lies between the more superficial buccopharyngeal fascia and the prevertebral fascia. Abscesses may form in this space and infiltrate the superior mediastinum.

The anterior communications of the pharynx take place in the nasopharynx, oropharynx, and laryngopharynx (**Fig. 36-1**). The nasopharynx extends from the skull base to the soft palate at the level of the first cervical vertebrae (C1). From there to the bottom of C3 lies the oropharynx. The laryngopharynx extends from C3 to C6, where it merges with the esophagus (**Fig. 36-2**). There, the cricopharyngeus muscle, originating on the cricoid cartilage, encircles the esophagus to form the upper esophageal sphincter. In anesthetized patients, pressing the cricoid ring against C6 (Sellick maneuver) mimics esophageal sphincter constriction and reduces the risk of passive regurgitation of gastric contents.[4]

NASOPHARYNX AND NOSE

The pharyngobasilar fascia anchors the pharynx superiorly to the occipital and the sphenoid bones. In the presence of basilar skull fractures, attempted passage of nasotracheal and nasogastric tubes has resulted in their entry into the cranium. Superficial to the bones that roof the pharynx and C1 lies the pharyngeal tonsil (called *adenoids* when hypertrophied), a site of potential obstruction or hemorrhage during nasal intubation. In patients whose tongue is large enough to fill the oral cavity, gas enters through the nasopharynx into the lungs with face mask ventilation, but the soft palate, posterior pharyngeal wall, and tongue often form a unidirectional valve that blocks exhalation. Gas trapping is prevented by periodic release of the mandible or by insertion of an artificial airway.

Anteriorly, the nasopharynx opens through the choanae, nasal passages, and nostrils. The filtration and humidification functions of the nose are well served by the convoluted surfaces of the 3 turbinates on each lateral wall (**Fig. 36-3**). Their fragility can lead to epistaxis after nasal intubation attempts unless the tube is guided parallel and adjacent to the hard palate, and perpendicular to the face through the channel beneath the inferior turbinate.

OROPHARYNX AND MOUTH

The oropharynx opens to the oral cavity at the palatoglossal folds, marking the division between the anterior two-thirds and posterior one-third

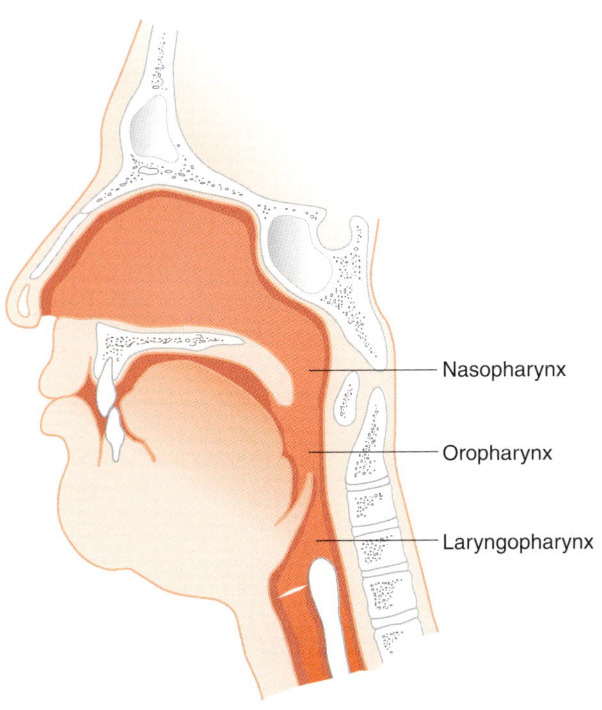

FIGURE 36-1. Diagram of a sagittal section of the pharynx illustrating the 3 subdivisions of the pharynx.

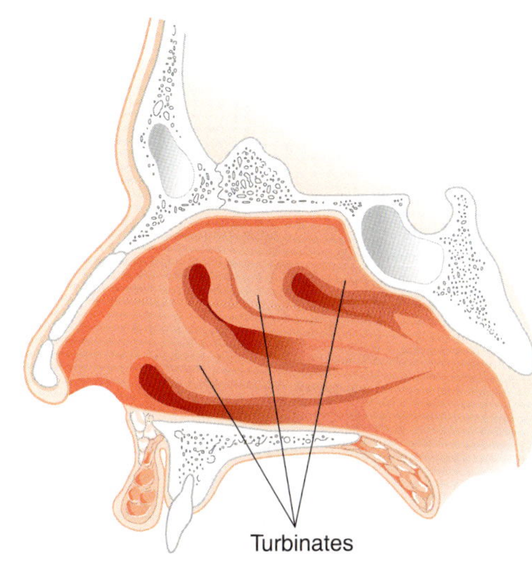

FIGURE 36-3. Lateral wall of the nasal cavity demonstrating the superior, middle, and inferior conchae (turbinate bones). [Reprinted from Finucane BT, Tsui BCH, Santora AH. *Principles of Airway Management*. 4th ed. New York, NY: Springer; 2010, with permission from Springer.]

of the tongue. The posterior third of the tongue forms the anterior wall of the oropharynx. In a sleeping or anesthetized patient in the supine position, muscle relaxation combined with gravity approximates the base of the tongue to the posterior oropharyngeal wall, causing varying degrees of airway obstruction. Partial airway obstruction is aggravated by negative inspiratory pressure collapsing the loose pharyngeal walls inward.

In the absence of an artificial airway, airway patency may be improved by extending the neck or subluxing the mandible anteriorly. This anterior displacement, through stretching of the mylohyoid, geniohyoid, and genioglossus muscles, indirectly relieves oropharyngeal obstructions (**Fig. 36-4**). Mandibular mobility depends in turn on the hinging

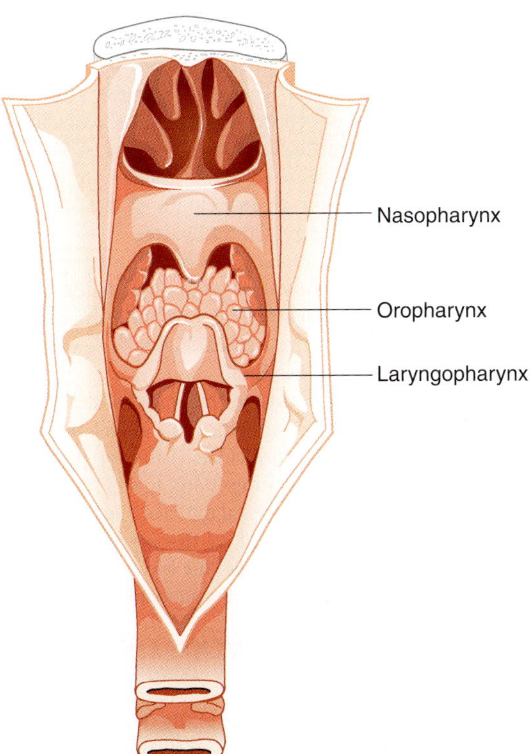

FIGURE 36-2. Posterior view of the pharynx showing subdivisions of the pharynx.

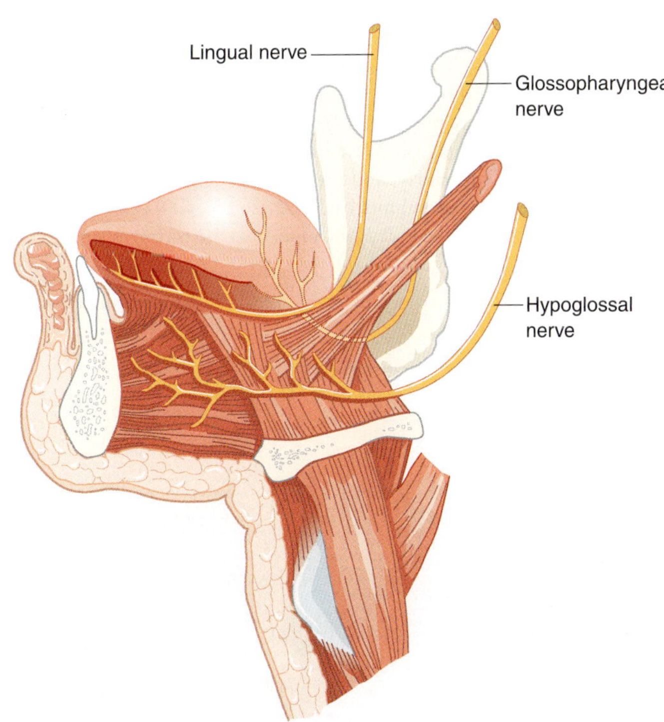

FIGURE 36-4. Sagittal section of the mouth to illustrate the tongue and its innervation.

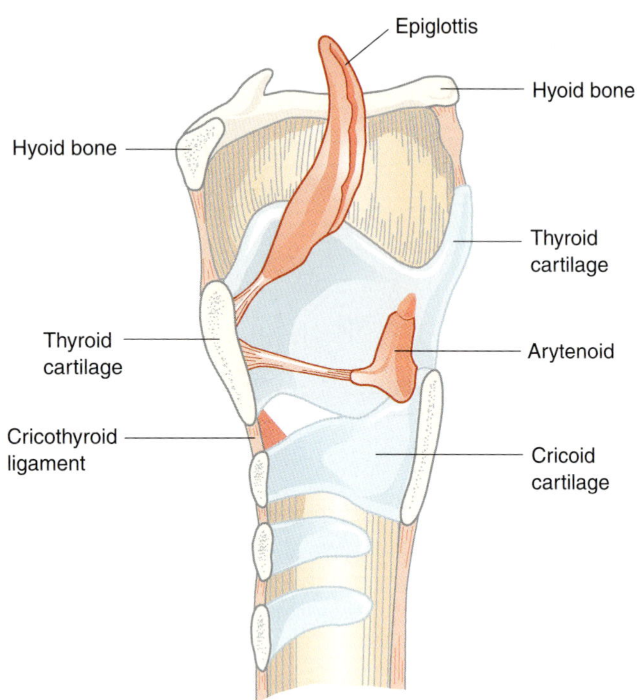

FIGURE 36-5. Diagrammatic illustration of sagittal section of the larynx. The epiglottis, thyroid, cricoid, and arytenoid cartilages and the position of the vocal cord ligaments are demonstrated.

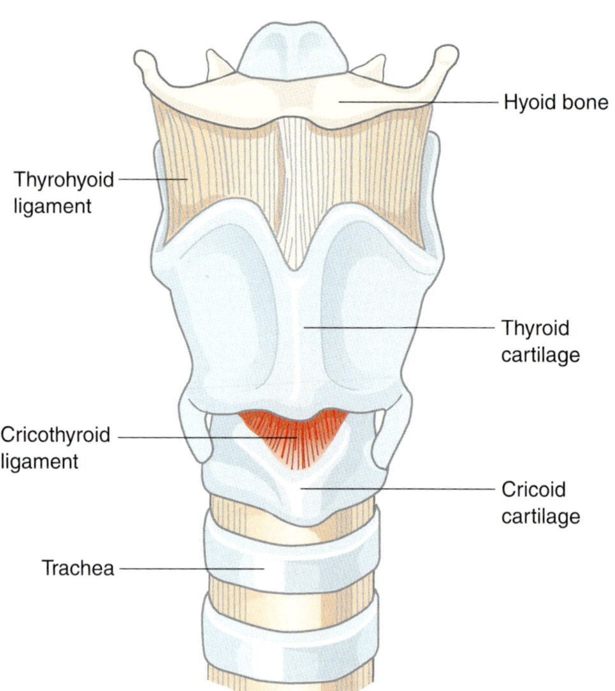

FIGURE 36-7. Diagrammatic illustration of the anterior view of the larynx. The larynx is suspended from the hyoid bone by the thyrohyoid ligament. The cricothyroid ligament provides easy and fast access to the larynx. Translaryngeal injection of local anesthetics and transtracheal jet ventilation are performed through this ligament.

and gliding motions of the temporomandibular joint. For successful rigid laryngoscopy, the tongue is displaced anteriorly for visualization of the larynx.

LARYNGOPHARYNX AND LARYNX

The epiglottis, thyroid, and cricoid cartilages and 6 smaller, paired cartilages (arytenoid, corniculate, cuneiform) shape the larynx (**Fig. 36-5**). To each side of the larynx and inferior to the aryepiglottic folds are the piriform recesses, which are separated by a prominence in the anterior laryngopharyngeal wall created by the lamina of the cricoid cartilage (**Fig. 36-6**).[3] A properly positioned laryngeal mask airway (LMA) seals against the cricoid cartilage and cricopharyngeus muscle inferiorly, the base of the tongue superiorly, and the piriform recesses laterally.[5] The superior laryngeal nerves, submucosal in these recesses, can be blocked with local anesthetic-soaked pledgets applied to the piriform sinuses.

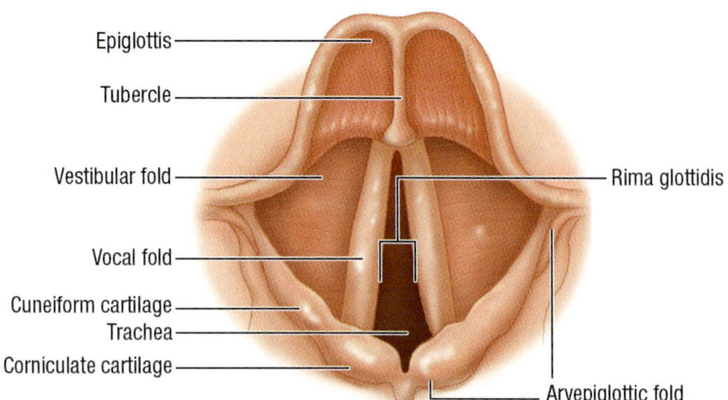

FIGURE 36-6. Diagrammatic illustration of the superior view of the larynx simulating the structures seen during direct laryngoscopy.

The hyoid (Greek: "U-shaped") bone at C4 suspends the thyroid cartilage by the thyrohyoid membrane, which is penetrated when performing superior laryngeal nerve blocks (**Fig. 36-7**). At C5, atop the 3-cm long thyroid cartilage, is the thyroid notch and laryngeal prominence (Adam's apple), an important landmark that may be subtle in women. The thyroid (Greek: "shield") cartilage sends superior cornua cephalad toward the hyoid bone and its inferior cornua to articulate with the cricoid (Greek for "ring") cartilage. In the midline at C6, the cricothyroid membrane is an easily palpated and avascular site for emergency cricothyrotomy or cannulation for instillation of local anesthetics, jet ventilation, or retrograde wire-guided intubation.

The upper edge of the epiglottis blends with the aryepiglottic folds. The tip of a curved (Macintosh) laryngoscope blade fits into the glossoepiglottic reflection. Two lateral valleculae in this reflection are created by the hyoepiglottic ligament, which keeps the resting epiglottis out of the laryngeal vestibule.

Atop the posterior cricoid lamina sit the paired arytenoid (Greek for "ladle") cartilages with superior, anterior, and lateral projections. The superior projections support the corniculate (Latin for "little horn") cartilages, and the anterior and lateral projections attach, respectively, to the vocal cords and various intrinsic laryngeal muscles (Fig. 36-5). Corniculate and cuneiform cartilages embedded in the aryepiglottic fold form 2 prominences, commonly referred to as "the arytenoids," which serve as important landmarks for intubation during suboptimal laryngoscopy.

NORMAL VOCAL CORD MOVEMENTS AND LARYNGEAL NERVE PALSIES

Normal vocal cord movements include abduction during inspiration, partial adduction during exhalation, and full adduction during phonation. All intrinsic muscles of the larynx are adductors or tensors, with the exception of the posterior cricoarytenoid muscles, which are the sole abductors. All intrinsic muscles of the larynx are innervated by

TABLE 36-1 Comparison of Infant and Adult Airways

Feature	Infant (Birth to 1 Year Old)	Adult (Older Than 8 Years)
Cricoid–carina distance (cm)	5-6	10-20
Angle: trachea–right bronchus (degrees)	30	20
Angle: trachea–left bronchus (degrees)	45	45
Narrowest portion of airway	Cricoid cartilage	Glottis
Level of glottis	C3-C4 interspace	C5
Inclination of vocal cords	Anteroinferior	Horizontal
Protrusion of corniculate and cuneiform tubercles into laryngeal aditus	Prominent	Minimal
Epiglottic cross-section	Omega shaped	Crescent shaped or flat
Glottic–epiglottic angle	Small	Large
Ease of mobilizing epiglottis to expose cords	Generally awkward, especially with curved blade	Usually easy with curved or straight blade
Height of thyrohyoid and cricothyroid ligaments	Almost nonexistent	Several millimeters
Preferred breathing route	Nasal	Nasal or oral
Prominence of occiput	Large (no headrest needed to attain the "sniff" position)	Small (headrest needed)

the recurrent laryngeal nerve, with the exception of the cricothyroid, a tensor innervated by the external branch of the superior laryngeal nerve. Laryngeal nerve palsies are classified as central or peripheral and unilateral or bilateral.[6-9] Simultaneous malfunction of the superior and recurrent laryngeal branches implies a central lesion or a high interruption of the vagus nerve. Brain infarction or a complete vagus nerve interruption causes the cord to assume a flaccid, wavy, partially abducted, or "cadaveric" position more commonly seen as a result of administering muscle relaxants. Central causes include posterior fossa surgery or brainstem infarctions. Peripheral lesions are more commonly caused by neck or cardiothoracic surgery than by endotracheal tube (ETT) cuff pressure on the larynx. Damage to the superior laryngeal nerve or its external branch results in an inability to sound a high-pitched "C" note, which improves over time as the contralateral muscle compensates. During phonation, the aryepiglottic folds and glottis are asymmetric. A complete unilateral recurrent laryngeal nerve injury causes hoarseness and a motionless cord that is joined during phonation by the contralateral cord crossing the midline.

Incomplete bilateral recurrent laryngeal nerve palsies result in a glottic opening so small that an emergency surgical airway may be needed. Bilateral complete recurrent laryngeal nerve palsies result in severe hoarseness, but, because the cords neither adduct nor abduct, a safe glottic opening may remain.

GLOTTIC AND LARYNGEAL CLOSURE

Three forms of laryngeal airway closure can be distinguished. First, during light anesthesia or phonation, the intrinsic laryngeal muscles approximate the vocal cords during exhalation, causing expiratory stridor or moaning. Second, if the vocal cords are edematous or are resting close together, the Bernoulli effect draws the cords together during rapid inhalation, resulting in inspiratory stridor.[10] The third kind of closure involves the entire larynx instead of simply the glottis; the thyrohyoid and other strap muscles contract in a forceful, longitudinal compression of the larynx.[11] During deglutition, the Valsalva maneuver, or laryngeal spasm, the thyroid cartilage and hyoid bone approximate, bulging the epiglottis down into the vestibule against the false cords in a ball-valve fashion. Muscle relaxants and maneuvers to elongate the larynx (application of the sniff position, neck extension, and jaw thrust) tend to counteract such closure; in contrast, face mask positive pressure may expand the piriform recesses and compress the aryepiglottic folds, compounding laryngeal closure.

THE LOWER AIRWAY

The lower airway includes the subglottic larynx, trachea, and bronchi. The subglottic larynx is 2 cm in length and extends from the true vocal folds to the lower border of the cricoid ring. The trachea extends from the lower border of the cricoid ring at the level of C6 to the carina at the level of the fifth thoracic vertebrae (T5) posterior to the angle of Louis (manubriosternal junction).[12]

Neck flexion can advance an ETT in a caudad direction; the Trendelenburg position or laparoscopic pneumoperitoneum can move the carina in a cephalad direction. These maneuvers can move a properly placed ETT into a bronchus.[13,14] False reassurance that a tube tip is not in a bronchus often is given by a radiograph taken with the head transiently thrown into extension by removing the pillow while supporting the chest with a film cassette.

During fiberoptic examination, the trachea is distinguished from bronchi by its flat, muscular posterior wall, creating a "D"-shaped cross-section. The right mainstem bronchus is roughly half as long as the 5-cm left mainstem bronchus. Being wider and almost parallel to the trachea, the right mainstem bronchus is more likely than the left bronchus to be accidentally intubated. Also, foreign bodies, aspirated material, and suction catheters preferentially end up in the right bronchus. Tracheobronchial anatomy and other features of the airway differ between infants and adults (**Table 36-1**).[12,14]

EVALUATION OF THE AIRWAY

A difficult airway can present as difficult mask ventilation, difficult rigid laryngoscopic intubation, or both. The major task during preoperative airway evaluation is to identify patients at risk for a "cannot intubate, cannot ventilate" situation, which is caused by congenital or acquired anatomic variations or by abnormal afflictions of the upper and lower airway (**Box 36-1**).[15-17] The variations or abnormalities are found by reviewing old records, taking an anesthetic and airway-focused history, examining the patient with reference to the normal and desired mobility of airway structures, and reviewing relevant laboratory and radiologic studies.An inability to ventilate presents a more urgent problem than

BOX 36-1

Some Causes of Difficult Airway Management

Anatomic features

Short, muscular neck

Limited neck mobility

Prominent maxillary incisors

Awkwardly placed, incomplete dentition

Long, highly arched palate with narrow mouth

Small mouth opening

Receding chin

Abnormal states

Anaphylactic airway edema

Arthritis and ankylosis

- Cervical spine
- Temporomandibular joint
- Larynx

Congenital syndromes

- Klippel-Feil (short, fused neck)
- Pierre Robin (micrognathia, cleft palate, glossoptosis)
- Treacher Collins (mandibulofacial dysostosis)

Endocrinopathies

- Obesity
- Acromegaly
- Hypothyroid macroglossia
- Goiter

Infections

- Ludwig angina (floor of the mouth abscess)
- Peritonsillar abscess
- Retropharyngeal abscess
- Epiglottitis

Mediastinal masses

Myopathies demonstrating myotonia or trismus

Scarring from burns or radiation

Trauma and hematomas

Tumors and cysts

Technical and mechanical factors

Body cast

Halo fixation or cervical collar

Airway foreign bodies

Leaks around a face mask

- Edentulous
- Flat bridge of nose
- Large face and head
- Whiskers, beard
- Nasogastric tube

Poor technique, inexperience, or haste

inability to intubate with adequate mask ventilation. Independent risk factors for difficult mask ventilation include age older than 55 years, body mass index greater than 30 kg/m^2, facial hair, missing teeth, limited mandibular protrusion, abnormal neck anatomy, sleep apnea, and a history of snoring.[18,19] Special attention should be paid to syndromes associated with a problematic airway. Details of the airway evaluation appear in Chapter 10.

Part of developing an airway management plan is to determine whether or not the patient is best served by a supraglottic airway (SGA) or an ETT. One also needs to determine if the airway should be instrumented while the patient is awake or after induction of the anesthetic. Despite a thorough evaluation of the airway, anatomic variants such as supraepiglottic cysts[20] or lingual tonsillar hypertrophy[21,22] can lead to unexpected difficult ventilation or intubation. The ever-present possibility of instrument failure requires backup plans and familiarity with algorithms for handling unanticipated challenges.

VENTILATION DURING ANESTHESIA

Alveolar ventilation delivers the oxygen (O_2) consumed by tissues and removes metabolic carbon dioxide (Co_2). An average anesthetized adult consumes about 250 mL/min of O_2 and produces 200 mL/min of Co_2. Because the normal alveolar effluent contains 5% (1/20) Co_2, removing 200 mL Co_2 each minute requires 4 L/min (20 × 200 mL/min = 4000 mL/min) of alveolar ventilation. Since one-third of minute ventilation is dead space (ie, does not participate in gas exchange), the required total minute ventilation to maintain normocapnia is 6000 mL/min, or roughly 90 mL/kg/min. Unless the metabolic rate is reduced, alveolar hypoventilation results in hypercapnia. Arterial oxygenation can be sustained during hypoventilation by increasing the fraction of inspired oxygen (Fio_2).

In the presence of narcotics, sedatives, and inhaled anesthetics, the brain's normal compensatory responses to hypercapnia and hypoxemia are blunted. Thus, the spontaneously breathing patient during general anesthesia will become hypercapnic, although surgical stimuli offset ventilatory depression and tend to return $Paco_2$ toward normal. Spontaneous ventilation is acceptable during general anesthesia when muscle relaxants are not administered and airway patency is properly maintained.

The anesthesiologist may assist ventilation by timing the compression of the reservoir bag to the patient's spontaneously initiated breaths, a task requiring considerable practice.[23] Assisted ventilation can test the quality of a face mask or laryngeal mask seal, minimize atelectasis, and offset the increased work of breathing caused by partial airway obstruction. In an anesthetized patient, apnea may result either from hyperventilation until the $Paco_2$ decreases below the apneic threshold or from a series of breaths large enough to elicit the Hering-Breuer inspiratory reflex. Assisting breathing enough to lower the $Paco_2$ by 5 mm Hg reduces it below the apneic threshold. For this reason, assisted ventilation cannot generally reverse hypercapnia to a meaningful extent without becoming controlled ventilation. In the presence of muscle relaxants, an unfavorable position, critical illness, or a requirement for hyperventilation, the anesthesiologist may choose to initiate controlled ventilation (mechanical ventilation if the work is performed by a machine).

An inhalation induction is performed by letting a patient breathe a volatile anesthetic, starting with a concentration low enough to avoid airway irritation and gradually increasing as the central effects of the vapors begin to depress the cough reflex. As alveolar ventilation decreases, breaths are assisted with increasing intensity until ventilation is manually controlled. Inhalation inductions, popular for children, have some merit in adults when the ability to ventilate the patient's lungs after induction of anesthesia is uncertain.[23] If worsening of airway obstruction is encountered during inhalation induction, the anesthetic can be turned off with the hope that the patient will awaken.

HYPOVENTILATION

Hypoventilation, consequent to depressed ventilatory drive, laryngeal spasm, or most commonly supraglottic soft tissue airway obstruction, results in hypercapnia and hypoxemia. Normally, although room air is 21% O_2, alveolar gas has an O_2 concentration of 16% because of the presence of water vapor and Co_2. Arterial O_2 desaturation in hypoventilating patients breathing room air results in part because increasing alveolar Co_2 displaces alveolar O_2. Small increases in FIO_2 elevate alveolar O_2 enough to maintain an acceptable arterial O_2 saturation during hypoventilation; large increments in FIO_2 can maintain close to normal arterial O_2 saturation despite profound hypoventilation (**Fig. 36-8**).

During apnea, arterial oxygenation can be sustained by apneic oxygenation.[24] In this technique, the patient breathes pure O_2 long enough to wash nitrogen from the alveoli, leaving only O_2, CO_2, and 6% water vapor (47-mm Hg vapor pressure at 37°C). If 100% O_2 continues to be available to a patent airway, it will be drawn into the alveoli during apnea. Without exhalation, the alveolar Co_2 concentration increases 5 or 6 mm Hg the first minute (equilibration between venous and alveolar Pco_2) and 3 to 6 mm Hg/min thereafter (metabolic production). Ten minutes into apneic oxygenation that begins with normocapnia, the alveolar composition of gases is 47 mm Hg of water vapor, 72 mm Hg of Co_2, and 641 mm Hg of O_2. In the absence of metabolic acidosis, the pH is approximately 7.24.

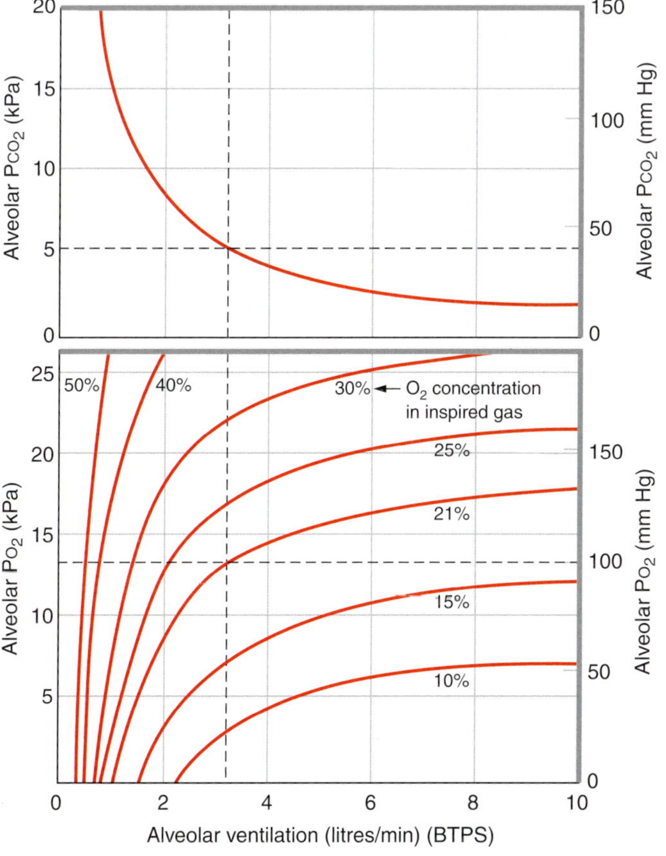

FIGURE 36-8. Dependency of alveolar oxygenation on alveolar ventilation at low fraction of inspired oxygen (FIO_2) values. Supplemental O_2 largely frees the Pao_2 of its dependency on alveolar ventilation. For example, the *broken vertical line* shows that a patient breathing room air with an alveolar ventilation of 3.2 L/min has a Pao_2 of 100 mm Hg, which would decrease to 50 mm Hg if the alveolar ventilation decreases by 50%. Yet even at the lower alveolar ventilation, increasing the FIO_2 to 0.4 elevates the Pao_2 to 200 mm Hg. BTPS, body temperature, standard pressure, saturated (with water vapor). [Modified from Lumb AB. *Nunn's Applied Respiratory Physiology*. 6th ed. Italy: Elsevier; 2005, with permission from Elsevier, NY.]

BOX 36-2

Conditions Aggravated by Hypercapnia

- Preexisting metabolic acidosis (eg, lactic acidosis, uremia)
- Hyperkalemia
- Elevated intracranial pressure
- Pulmonary hypertension
- Right-to-left cardiac shunts
- Cardiac dysrhythmia
- Poor myocardial contractility

In general, it is the risk of hypoxia that threatens to permanently harm the hypoventilating patient. This realization justifies the popularity of supplemental O_2 to lessen the likelihood of hypoxemia during hypoventilation. Except under certain conditions, the consequences of hypercapnia are well tolerated or reversible (**Box 36-2**).

DENITROGENATION

Because it is impossible to ensure the ability to ventilate the lungs of a patient about to receive general anesthesia, proper preanesthetic denitrogenation is recommended. Eighty percent of the average 2.5-L adult functional residual capacity (FRC) that starts out as N_2 is replaced with O_2.[25] If ventilation becomes impossible, the extra 2 L of O_2 may sustain vital organs for up to 8 minutes, enough time to establish other means of oxygenation.

Because it may make the difference between life and death for the patient, proper denitrogenation (**Box 36-3**) should be a top priority for an anesthesiologist preparing to induce a general anesthetic.[25,26]

MONITORING THE ADEQUACY OF VENTILATION AND OXYGENATION

The gold standard for assessing the adequacy of ventilation and oxygenation is the measurement of the partial pressures of CO_2 and O_2 in sampled blood (ie, arterial blood gases). Because of cost and delay, a number of alternative technologies have become popular since 1980. Clinical observations remain invaluable to anesthesiologists, who should constantly evaluate the validity of pulse oximetric and capnographic data.

CLINICAL OBSERVATION

Airway management demands constant awareness of the patient's physiologic status, obtained through observations of skin color, vital signs, chest and abdominal movements, and use of accessory muscles.

BOX 36-3

Proper Denitrogenation

Technique

- High flow of oxygen
- Fully open pop-off valve
- Leak-free mask fit to prevent entraining room air
- Tidal breathing for 2 or 3 minutes or a series of 4 vital capacity breaths

Confirmatory observations

- Reservoir bags empty and refill
- End-tidal CO_2 approaches 40 mm Hg
- End-tidal O_2 approaches 85%

TABLE 36-2 Reassuring and Worrisome Signs and Their Implications During Airway Management

Reassuring	Worrisome	Implication of Worrisome Sign
Concurrent pectoral and subcostal rising alternating with concurrent falling	Stepwise expansion of subcostal region	Stomach filling with gas or unidirectional expiratory obstruction
No retractions	Subcostal expansion with concurrent pectoral collapse	Partial upper airway obstruction, or intercostal weakness
No tug	Subcostal rocking with no chest expansion	Complete airway obstruction
Breathing without accessory muscles	Submandibular, intercostal, or supraclavicular retractions	Partial or complete upper airway obstruction
Sequential fogging and clearing of plastic mask	Inspiratory tracheal tug	Intercostal weakness with preserved diaphragmatic strength
Normal vital signs	Use of sternocleidomastoid and trapezius muscles	Respiratory muscle fatigue or weakness
Rebreathing bag quickly refills during exhalation	Stertor (snoring)	Soft tissue obstruction
Volumeter indicates appropriate tidal volumes	Stridor (harsh, high pitched)	Laryngeal obstruction
Normal breath sounds heard with pretracheal auscultation	Audible phonation or palpable purring	Light anesthesia or partial airway obstruction

Even before arterial blood gases deteriorate, anesthesiologists usually are able to detect problems and make adjustments to maintain airway patency and gas exchange (**Table 36-2**).[12,23]

PULSE OXIMETRY

In the majority of patients, pulse oximetry affords reliable but noninvasive measurement of the arterial O_2 saturation. Provided that hemoglobin concentration and organ perfusion are acceptable, satisfactory arterial O_2 saturation makes organ hypoxia unlikely. The reassurance offered by pulse oximetry lets the anesthesiologist proceed carefully during intubation.[27] Pulse oximetry is not sensitive to hypoventilation if F_{IO_2} is high and it gives late notification of esophageal intubation after denitrogenation.[28]

Most failures of pulse oximetry (eg, movement artifact, vasoconstriction) are obvious. The anesthesiologist may incorrectly assume adequate oxygenation during carbon monoxide poisoning or illumination of the pulse oximeter's probe by lights of unusual wavelength.

CAPNOMETRY

Capnometry, using one of several detection methods, continuously displays the waveform of $P_{ET}CO_2$ sampled at the patient end of the breathing circuit. When the tidal volume is large enough, alveolar gas reaches the CO_2 sampling site and the displayed $P_{ET}CO_2$ closely approximates Pa_{CO_2}, affording a noninvasive, breath-by-breath method to judge the adequacy of ventilation. In patients with normal cardiopulmonary physiology, expiratory gas has a P_{CO_2} that is 2 to 5 mm Hg less than the arterial P_{CO_2}.

Significant and common clinical events create P_{CO_2} gradients (arterial to alveolar to sampled to measured) so that the Pa_{CO_2} is normally higher than that displayed on the capnometer (**Box 36-4**). In most patients, $ETCO_2$ suggests better alveolar ventilation than actually exists because significant amounts of CO_2-free inspired gas dilute the sample. For example, during spontaneous face mask ventilation of a patient with elevated intracranial pressure, the peak measured P_{CO_2} displayed by the capnometer may be only 18 mm Hg, but the first few breaths after tracheal intubation may show a P_{CO_2} of 30 mm Hg. The rapid, shallow ventilatory pattern before intubation prevents transport of undiluted alveolar gas to the capnometer.

An important application of capnometry is confirmation of the position of an intratracheal tube by the appearance of stable CO_2 concentrations in sequential breaths immediately after intubation. This application is mandated by the American Society of Anesthesiologists (ASA) Standards for Basic Anesthetic Monitoring.[29,30] Despite tracheal intubation, the expected levels of CO_2 may fail to appear if the delivery of CO_2 to the lungs is limited by low cardiac output, hypovolemia, gas or thrombotic embolization, or cardiac arrest.

AIRWAY MANAGEMENT WITHOUT TRACHEAL INTUBATION

The majority of airway-related deaths and severe neurologic morbidity result not from a failure to intubate the trachea but rather from a failure to ventilate and oxygenate.[1] Resourceful anesthesiologists command an array of techniques for ventilation without tracheal intubation when the

BOX 36-4

Increased Gradient Between Pa_{CO_2} and $P_{ET}CO_2$

Arterial-to-alveolar gradients

Pa_{CO_2} increases and $P_{ET}CO_2$ decreases (decreased perfusion relative to ventilation)

Decreased perfusion

- Embolization
- Pulmonary thromboembolism
- Air embolism
- CO_2 embolism (laparoscopic insufflation)

Hypovolemic shock

Right-to-left intracardiac shunting

Sudden increase in ventilation-to-perfusion ratio

- Bronchial intubation

Alveolar-to-sampled gradient

Anatomic or apparatus dead space

- Rapid, shallow breaths
- Apparatus dead space (face mask)

Dilution at the sampling site of exhaled gas by fresh gas (eg, loose connection, cracked sampling line)

Low velocity in sampling tubing, causing laminar rather than preferred turbulent flow

Sampled-to-measured gradients

Calibration errors

Slow capnometer response time with rapid breaths

latter is not indicated or has failed. These ventilation techniques may use a face mask with or without an oral or nasal airway or supraglottic devices such as LMAs, or esophageal devices.[12,23,31]

FACE MASK VENTILATION

Positioning to Facilitate Face Mask Ventilation In the supine position, gravity draws the relaxed tongue and epiglottis into configurations that can obstruct the airway. Patients recovering from anesthesia or obtunded, intoxicated emergency room patients may be safest in a semi-lateral position with the dependent leg straight and the other one bent, the dependent arm flexed, and the dependent cheek on the bed (the tonsillar position). Gravity will draw the tongue away from the posterior pharyngeal wall, and blood or vomitus can drain out the mouth more easily.

If the anesthesiologist suspects that gastric contents have entered the pharynx, the patient's head is turned to the side and the table is quickly positioned head down to maximize drainage while the pharynx is cleared with a Yankauer suction catheter.

Students of basic life support are taught to overcome upper airway obstruction by extending the head and neck and by displacing the mandible anteriorly with jaw thrust. Although these maneuvers move the hyoid and attached structures anteriorly, their effectiveness can be limited by 2 factors. Some vertebral columns can bow anteriorly and impinge on pharyngeal patency. More commonly, the forceful cervico-occipital extension tightens the strap muscles sufficiently to limit the anterior mobility of the larynx and the mandible. For these reasons, anesthesiologists often favor the sniffing position, in which the occiput rests on a firm pad about 10 cm anterior to the scapula. Atlanto-occipital extension and jaw thrust maneuvers then are superimposed. The anterior displacement of the head shrinks the sternomental distance, so the hyoid and its attached structures can be pulled out of the pharynx without tightening the strap muscles. Greater comfort for the awake patient and preparedness for laryngoscopy are additional advantages of the sniffing position. The position is natural in infants and small children because of a large occiput, obviating the need for a pad.

In some patients, best airway patency is achieved by rotating the head to either side. Airway visualization and manipulation are easier when the operating room table is elevated so the patient's forehead is brought to the level of the anesthesiologist's xiphoid.

Achieving a Seal The skill of sealing a mask to the face develops only after months of hands-on training. Although masks are of a few basic designs (**Fig. 36-9**), facial contours assume an endless variety. Clear plastic masks with large-volume, low-pressure cushions seal easily to most faces (including the faces of patients with a flat nasal bridge) while affording a view of ventilatory condensation and evaporation cycles and early detection of regurgitated gastric contents.

A mask strap can be used to affix hooks around connectors where the mask attaches to the circuit. When used with the mask, the strap makes a better seal and minimizes hand fatigue for the anesthesia provider. (**Box 36-5**) Concern about excessive apparatus dead space in patients with tiny tidal volumes led Rendel-Baker and Soucek to develop pediatric masks without a cushion and made from molds of infants' faces. In contrast with the racial and ethnic variability displayed in later life, infants share impressive uniformity of facial contours. Their full cheeks can be pulled up and around the rims of these masks. Undue submandibular pressure by the anesthesiologist's fingers tends to worsen airway obstruction. When using mask ventilation for children, the anesthesiologist's third through fifth fingers must engage only the mandible and not compress the soft tissues overlying the tongue.

Beards or broad mustaches may hinder a good mask seal to make controlled ventilation simply impossible. For edentulous patients who are too alert to tolerate an airway, the lower margin of the mask can be placed against the mucosal reflection in the vestibule of the mouth while the lower lip is drawn over the mask. By inserting an oropharyngeal airway an anesthesiologist can minimize the furrows in the cheeks of edentulous patients. Inserting an oral airway lengthens the distance between the supramental depression and the nasal bridge, occasionally necessitating substitution for the next larger mask size. For this reason, it is essential to have small, medium, and large masks available.[12,23]

BOX 36-5

Achieving a Seal With a Face Mask

1. Place the mask strap beneath the occiput.
2. Apply the mask's nasal groove to the low point of the nasal bridge to avoid pressure on the eyes.
3. Grip the left mandible with third, fourth, and fifth fingers of the left hand.
4. Lower the mask so its inferior rim contacts the face between the lower lip and the mental prominence.
5. If there is a leak between the mask and the cheeks, consolidate the seal by dragging mobile tissue of the left cheek toward and under the mask cushion, stabilizing the tissue with the ulnar margin of the left hand.
6. Bracing the mentum against the mask, pull the mandible up and forward with the third through fifth fingers while the thumb and index finger grip the mask above and below the connector.
7. Maintaining the left-sided seal, tilt the mask toward the right cheek, consolidating the seal by dragging the mobile tissue forward to the cushion and by keeping it there with 1 limb of the mask strap.
8. The other limbs of the mask strap may improve the seal, especially for anesthesiologists with small hands. Crossing the lower limbs of the mask strap prevents the mask from riding up the face.

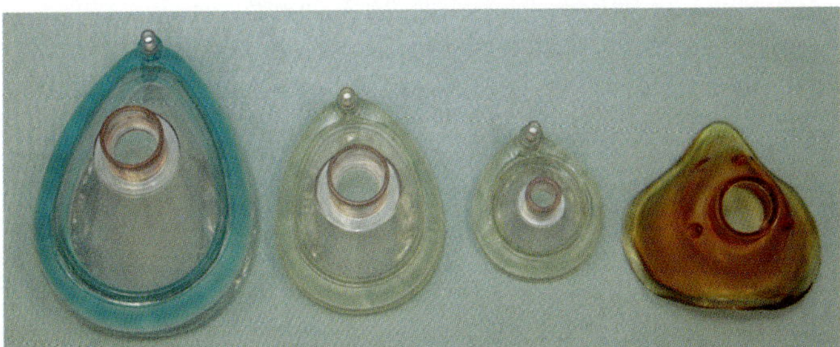

FIGURE 36-9. Face masks. Three universal masks are on the left. The Rendell-Baker pediatric mask is shown on the far right.

APPLYING POSITIVE PRESSURE

Essential for applying positive airway pressure are a functioning breathing system (a backup self-inflating resuscitation bag is needed at all anesthetizing locations) and a leak-free mask seal. The anesthesiologist learns to adjust the pop-off valve and speed of reservoir bag compression to keep airway pressures below the 20 cm H_2O associated with gastric inflation. Most patients can be ventilated well with peak airway pressures of 15 cm H_2O or lower, providing a margin of safety against gastric insufflation.

Fit patients can tolerate generous doses of intravenous (IV) induction drugs without hypotension. A combination of an opioid, a benzodiazepine, and a hypnotic agent acts synergistically and generally renders the airway nonreactive for several minutes, during which inhaled anesthetics may be introduced. Large vigorous breaths and rapid escalations in inspired anesthetic concentrations may precipitate hiccups, coughing, breath holding, and laryngospasm, thereby delaying induction. Increasing sevoflurane or desflurane vaporizer settings by 0.5% increments every 5 breaths depresses airway reflexes before irritating inspired concentrations are reached. Intubating doses of neuromuscular blockers eliminate coughing or hiccups in minutes.

Positive pressure not only ventilates the patient's lungs but also may overcome minor degrees of soft tissue obstruction of the airway. In a spontaneously breathing patient who is too lightly anesthetized to accept insertion of an airway, 5 to 15 cm H_2O of continuous positive airway pressure achieved by partially closing the "pop-off" valve may relieve airway obstruction and increase the minute ventilation. Well-synchronized intermittent positive-pressure breaths can achieve the same end. Inflation of the stomach with respiratory gases should be avoided because it decreases thoracic compliance and increases the risk of regurgitation.

PHARYNGEAL AIRWAYS

An inability to ventilate with a face mask despite proper positioning, jaw thrusts, and a good mask seal may be caused by laryngeal spasm in response to light anesthesia or by soft tissue upper airway obstruction resulting from deepening anesthesia and the onset of muscle relaxation (**Box 36-6**).[2,3] If a careful assessment suggests simple supraglottic obstruction, insertion of pharyngeal airway to separate soft tissues from the posterior pharyngeal wall is a logical next step (**Fig. 36-10**). Success confirms that the soft tissue had been obstructing the airway, but persisting or worsening obstruction is often indicative of active closure of the larynx. Active closure may be relieved by administering muscle relaxants or deepening anesthesia with IV agents. The anesthesiologist should sidestep the trap created by the pathologic causes of catastrophic obstruction that may be worsened by the loss of muscle tone.

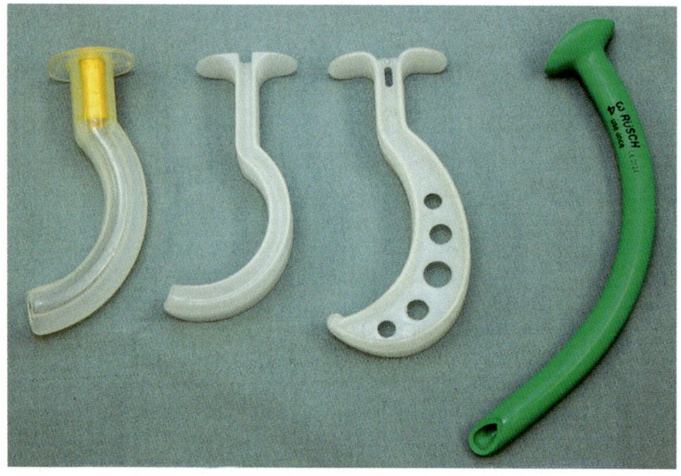

FIGURE 36-10. Artificial oropharyngeal and nasopharyngeal airways.

Until the arrival of the LMA and esophageal devices, oropharyngeal or nasopharyngeal airways were the best ways to relieve simple supraglottic obstructions. They remain inexpensive, safe, and generally effective.[23,31] Trial and error often are necessary for even the experienced anesthesiologist to select an oropharyngeal airway long enough to anteriorly displace the base of the tongue without pushing the epiglottis into the laryngeal inlet. The forward portion of the oropharyngeal airway separates the teeth or gums; its flange keeps the device from dropping into the hypopharynx. Displacing the tongue into the hypopharynx is avoided by drawing it anteriorly with a tongue blade held in the left hand while the right hand opens the mouth and inserts the oropharyngeal airway.

The onset of soft tissue relaxation and airway obstruction usually heralds depression of cough and gag reflexes sufficient to tolerate pharyngeal stimulation. Swallowing or gagging triggered by a tongue blade or airway touching the base of the tongue suggests waiting until the patient is more deeply anesthetized; the stimulus itself often restores airway patency. Coughing and breath holding after uneventful placement of an oropharyngeal airway suggests airway irritation by anesthetic vapors. Approaches to coughing and breath holding include turning down the vaporizer and temporarily abandoning attempts at positive-pressure ventilation or deepening the depth of anesthesia with IV agents.

A nasopharyngeal airway can be inserted before extubation in a patient with a clenched jaw who has an obstructed airway. Unfortunately, unless precautions are taken (**Box 36-7**), epistaxis may complicate the

BOX 36-6

Causes of an Inability to Ventilate

- Light anesthesia
- Laryngeal spasm or vocal cord adduction
- Supraglottic soft tissue relaxation (obstruction)
    - Soft palate and pharyngeal walls
    - Tongue
    - Epiglottis
- Chest wall rigidity
    - Breath holding
    - Narcotic induced
- Pathologic, glottic, and subglottic
    - Foreign body
    - Enlarged lingual tonsil
    - Edema
    - Infection
    - Tumor or hematoma
    - Congenital
    - Superior vena caval syndrome
    - Bilateral vocal cord palsy
    - Tracheal stenosis
    - Tracheal or bronchial compression
        - Great vessel anomalies
        - Mediastinal mass
- Equipment failure
    - Selector valve accidentally in the "ventilator" position
    - CO_2 absorbent canister preventing gas flow (eg, plastic overwrap not removed)

BOX 36-7

Precautions for Introducing Nasopharyngeal Airways

- Prepare the larger nasal passage with a vasoconstrictor.
- Choose a soft, blunt-tipped nasopharyngeal airway.
- Soften it by warming (not applicable for some materials).
- Lubricate the airway.
- To protect the turbinates, point the bevel medially.
- Direct the device directly posteriorly parallel to the hard palate and beneath the inferior turbinate.
- If resistance is encountered, withdraw, rotate 90 degrees medially, and readvance with gentle, steady pressure.
- Ease difficult passage by using a soft suction catheter as an introducer.

hasty introduction of an airway through the nasal passages. Because of alignment with the glottic opening, blind tracheal suctioning may be possible by passing a catheter through a nasopharyngeal airway. The need for and tolerance of repeated tracheal suctioning usually are indications for intubation.

SUPRAGLOTTIC AIRWAYS

The first modern SGA device was the LMA developed in the early 1980s by Dr Archie Brain.[5] The LMA corporation manufactures several varieties based on the original LMA classic (cLMA) (**Fig. 36-11**). These and other supraglottic devices have achieved great popularity for addressing simple, SGA obstruction in a variety of contexts.[32,33] Their unique capabilities (**Boxes 36-8** and **36-9**), relative ease of use, and low incidence of serious complications enssure SGAs a place in the anesthesiologist's armamentarium.[34-41] Several studies have indicated that trained but inexperienced resuscitators are more likely to be successful ventilating with an LMA than intubating the trachea with direct laryngoscopy.[42]

Becoming adept at proper SGA insertion requires consideration of a patient's anatomy, patience, and practice.[43] Even when using suboptimal insertion techniques, success rates with SGAs are high, leading some practitioners to adopt unconventional techniques. Adherence to proper technique maximizes success and reduces complications. An LMA should be deflated with finger pressure on the dorsal aspect of the cuff so that the totally flattened cuff curves away from the aperture (**Fig. 36-12**). A water-soluble lubricant should be applied to the dorsal surface of the cuff and kept from drying. The recommended technique for LMA placement is summarized in **Fig. 36-13**.[44] When the epiglottis is dragged downward, the aperture bars of the LMA prevent impaction of epiglottis into the LMA and possible obstruction (Fig. 36-11).

During insertion, the SGA must navigate past the soft palate, uvula, tonsillar fauces, oral-pharyngeal angle, tongue, and epiglottis. Placing the patient in the sniffing position with marked cervico-occipital extension aligns laryngeal structures to help accommodate the mask.

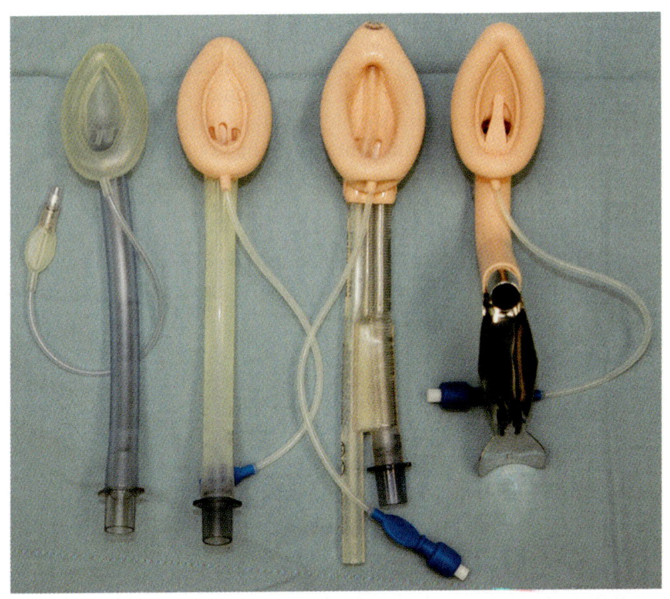
A

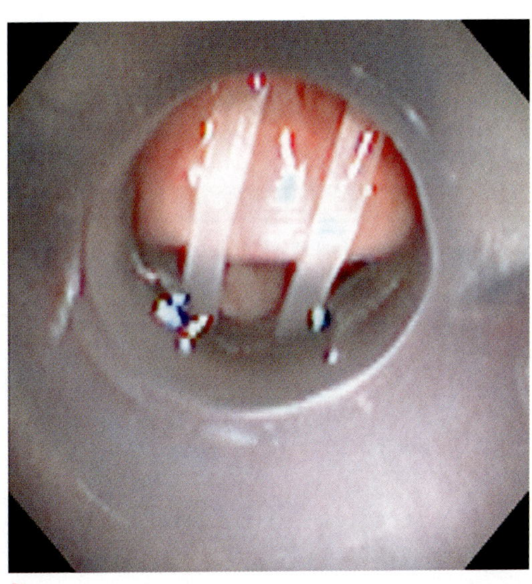
B

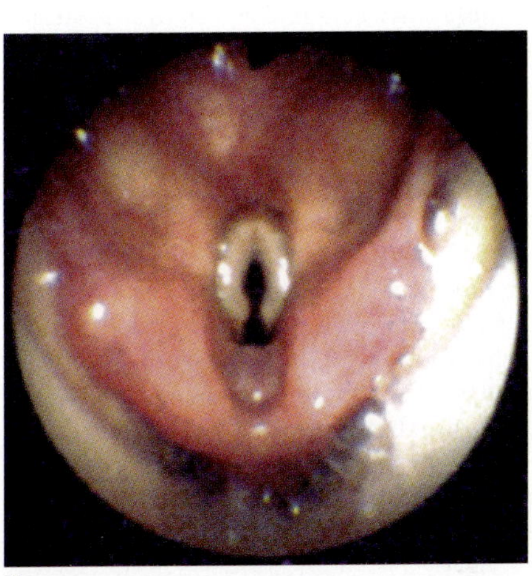
C

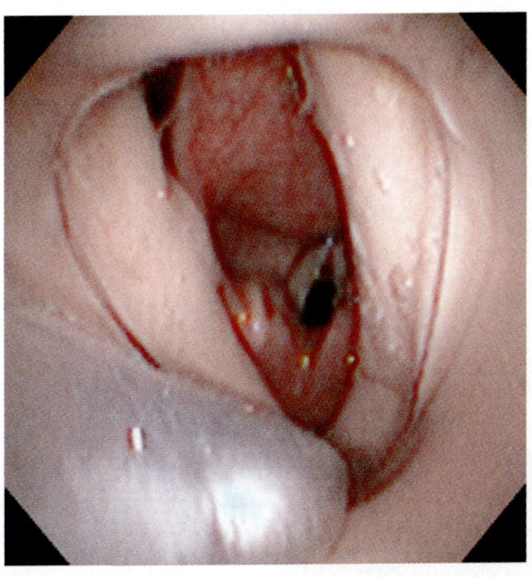
D

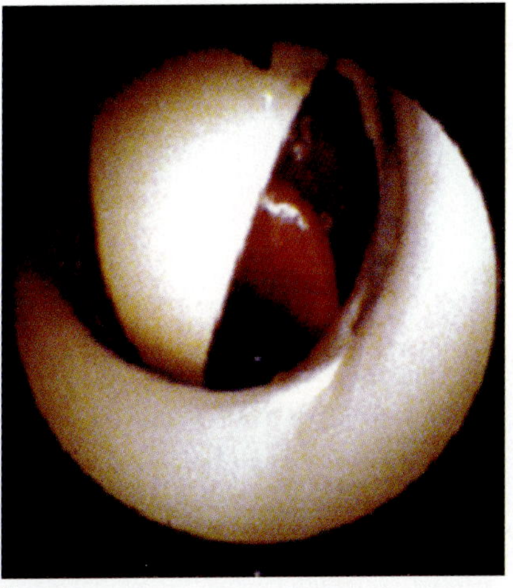
E

FIGURE 36-11. Various laryngeal mask airways (LMAs) and endoscopic views of them. **A.** Shown from left to right are the LMA Unique, Classic, ProSeal, and Fastrach. **B.** The 2 epiglottic bars of the LMA Unique and Classic prevent entry of epiglottis inside the lumen of LMA. **C, D.** The LMA ProSeal does not have epiglottic bars, but the drain tube supports the epiglottis and prevents it from impacting inside the LMA tube. In the LMA Fastrach. **E.** The epiglottis bar elevates the epiglottis as the endotracheal tube passes into the trachea.

BOX 36-8

Clinical Use of a Laryngeal Mask Airway

Indications

Surgical anesthesia without intubation

Airway management without neuromuscular blocking agent

Repeated anesthetics

Emergency ventilation when intubation has failed

Improving airway seal without tracheal intubation

- Patient with facial hair
- Edentulous patient

Assisting tracheal intubation

Providing a patent airway with minimal changes in blood pressure, heart rate, intraocular or intracranial pressure, or bronchial tone

Contraindications

High risk of aspiration (relative contraindication)

Glottic or subglottic obstruction

Supraglottic pathology interfering with placement

Extremely limited mouth opening or neck extension

Prone position (relative contraindication)

Need for high airway pressure ventilation

BOX 36-9

Benefits and Limitations of a Laryngeal Mask Airway (LMA)

Benefits

Permits ventilation when face mask and intubation have failed

Permits lighter anesthesia and faster emergence

Facilitates blind or fiberoptic tracheal intubation

Provides a good airway for fiberoptic bronchoscopy

Easier to learn than tracheal intubation

Limitations

Proper position of the LMA may be difficult to achieve

Probable gas leak with LMA classic when airway pressure >20 cm H_2O

Limited protection against aspiration

No protection against laryngospasm

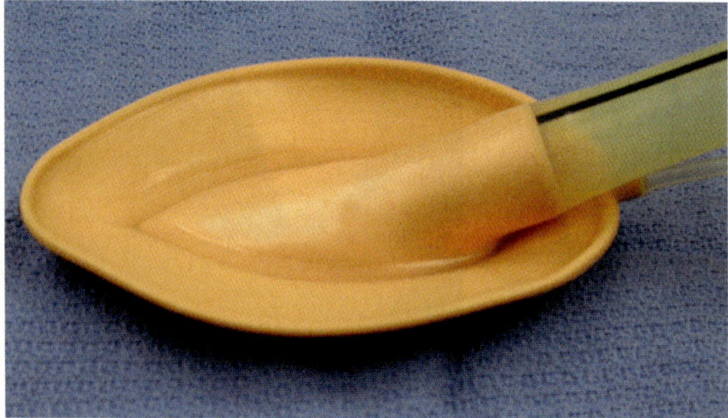

FIGURE 36-12. Diagram of a deflated laryngeal mask airway. The cuff of the laryngeal mask airway is deflated before its insertion. The rim of the cuff should evenly face away from mask aperture with no folds near the tip.

A gloved hand flattens the tip of the mask against the hard palate to start it on a path that will not engage the epiglottis. The patient must be at a sufficiently deep plane of general anesthesia if SGA is to be inserted easily and function properly. Alternatively, the SGA can be inserted in an awake or sedated patient after proper topical anesthesia has been established.

Although careful placement, cuff inflation, and adaptation time improve the seal, leakage often occurs at 20 cm H_2O airway pressure with the classic LMA. Obesity, a head-down tilt, abdominal insufflation, airway obstruction, or any other conditions necessitating ventilation with high airway pressures increase the risk of hypoventilation, gastric insufflation, and regurgitation.

SGAs are particularly well suited for the lightly anesthetized, spontaneously breathing ambulatory surgery patient. Compared with face mask or endotracheal anesthesia, there seems to be less need for an anesthetic plane deeper than that required for the surgery itself.[45] Patients instrumented with an SGA tolerate a lighter depth of anesthesia with less chance of coughing, breath holding, stridor, or laryngeal spasm compared with patients whose tracheas have been intubated.[46] Increasing anesthetic depth usually manages episodes of movement, tachypnea, or hyperpnea. Finally, patients tolerate a return to consciousness and can follow commands while an inflated SGA is still in place. Positive-pressure ventilation can be applied through the LMA[36]; however, the tidal volume, respiratory rate, and inspiratory:expiratory ratio should be adjusted to avoid high airway pressures. Newer anesthesia ventilators that synchronize breaths or provide support ventilators are practical for the patient with an SGA in place.

Using an SGA in an unfavorable setting increases the likelihood of unfortunate results. The devices do not protect as effectively as an ETT against pulmonary aspiration of gastric contents.[47-49] In low-risk populations, the incidence of aspiration with the laryngeal mask is reported to be similar to that of mask anesthesia and very close to that of endotracheal intubation.[50] Application of cricoid pressure impedes placement of the LMA.[51] Reported but rare complications include 12th cranial nerve paralysis,[52] unilateral hypoglossal nerve paralysis,[53] and transient bilateral vocal cord paralysis.[54]

Laryngeal Mask Airway ProSeal Pulmonary aspiration of regurgitant gastric material has long been a concern with the use of devices such as the LMA. Modifications were made to the cLMA design in 2000 to produce the LMA ProSeal (pLMA). The pLMA is a reusable, cuffed laryngeal mask with an integrated gastric drainage tube and posterior doral cuff. The gastric drainage tube exits the tip of the mask cuff and is designed to lie over the esophageal inlet. In addition to the gastric drainage tube, the pLMA also makes use of a posterior dorsal cuff for sizes 3 and above. The posterior cuff of the pLMA is designed for greater seal pressure than the cLMA. Greater seal pressure makes the pLMA attractive for applications that require high-pressure ventilation such as laparoscopic procedures or the care of obese patients.[55]

The pLMA can be inserted using a special introducer or in a manner similar to a classic LMA. A very reliable technique for pLMA insertion uses a gastric drainage tube such as a Salem Sump as a guide to ensure proper positioning while minimizing the risk of the pLMA's folding. First, the gastric tube is advanced through the pLMA drainage tube, and the gastric tube is inserted into the patient's esophagus, either blindly or under direct visualization with a laryngoscope. The pLMA is then advanced over the gastric tube and into the patient's hypopharynx.[56] In a similar technique, a gum elastic bougie is inserted in the esophagus with the pLMA drainage tube advanced over its proximal end.[57]

After the pLMA has been inserted, proper positioning is confirmed with a 4-step process. First, ventilation is confirmed by appropriate chest rise and CO_2 presence on the capnograph. Second, the leak pressure is measured by closing the automatic pressure-limiting valve

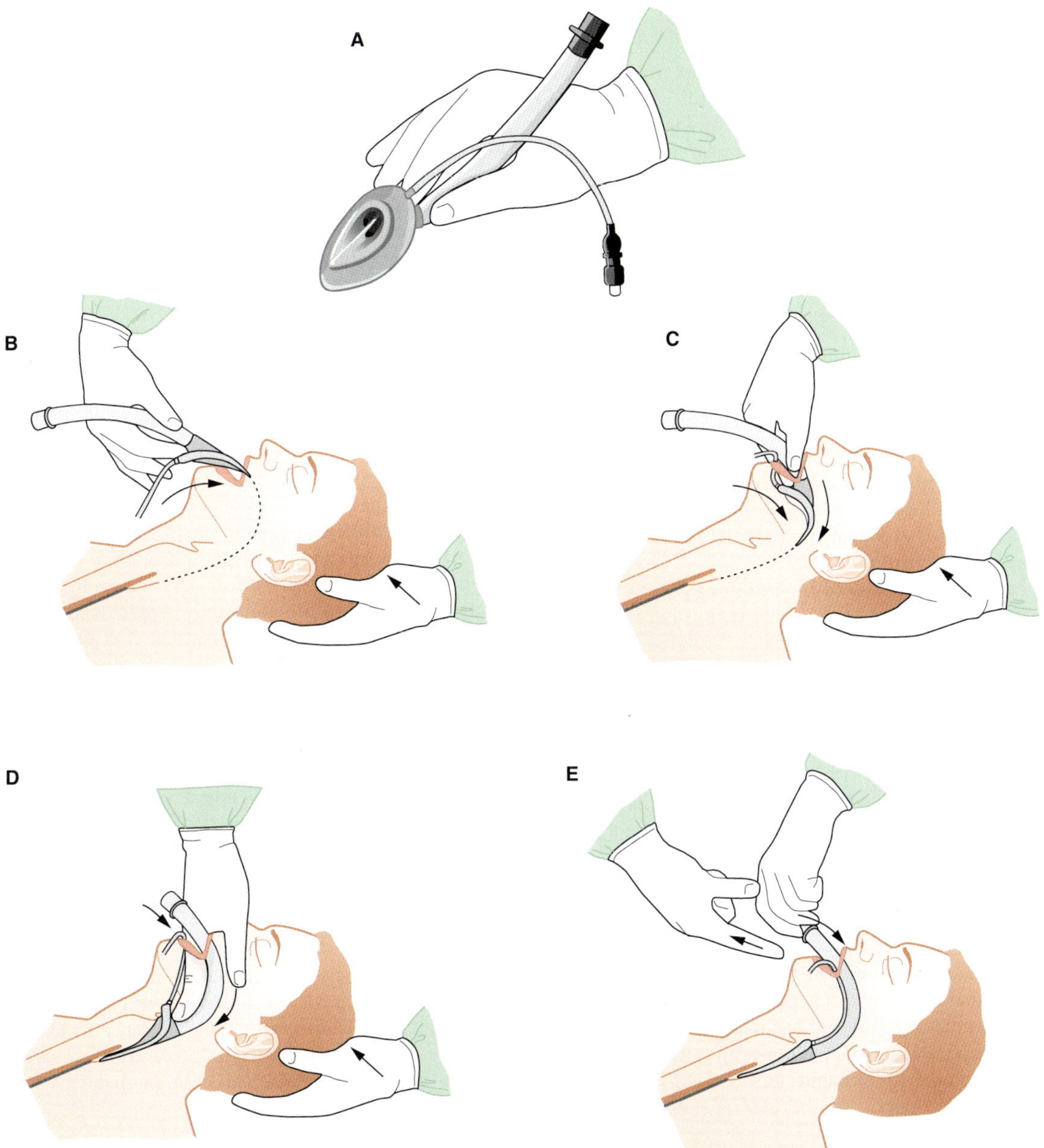

FIGURE 36-13. Technique for placing a laryngeal mask airway (LMA). **A.** The LMA is held by the index finger and the thumb facing the bowl of LMA caudally toward the larynx. The index finger is positioned between the shaft of the LMA and the deflated cuff. The occiput is stabilized with the left hand. **B.** The deflated and lubricated LMA is placed into the open mouth pressed against the hard palate. **C.** The LMA is advanced behind the tongue and into the oropharynx using the index finger. **D.** The LMA is pushed farther down deep into the hypopharynx using the tip of the index finger. **E.** The index finger is removed. The LMA is pushed farther down to its final position by holding the tube of the LMA with the left hand. Without holding the tube of the LMA, the cuff is inflated with the recommended volume of air. The LMA may protrude slightly on inflation of the cuff. [Modified from *LMA Airway Instruction Manual*. San Diego, CA: LMA North America, 2005. Courtesy of LMA North America, San Diego.]

and slowly increasing the pressure in the breathing circuit until a leak is heard or 25 cm H_2O pressure is reached. Third, a small amount of water-soluble lubricant or a thin film of soap is applied to the proximal end of the drainage tube.[58,59] When properly positioned, the meniscus will move slightly during respiration, reflecting normal variation in esophageal pressure. A kinked or folded device will have a motionless meniscus. If the tip of the device is not positioned properly in the proximal esophagus, gas will travel from the respiratory part of the device up the gastric drainage tube, displacing the lubricant proximally or causing the soap film to form a visible bubble. The fourth and final step involves passage of a lubricated suction catheter or gastric drainage tube, 14 Fr or smaller, through the gastric drainage lumen of the device. Easy passage through the gastric drainage port demonstrates that the device is not folded and that the gastric drainage port is patent.

The suprasternal notch test is also assessed for drainage tube patency.[60,61] In the suprasternal notch test, the patient's airway is palpated at the suprasternal notch while observing for a corresponding movement of the lubricant placed in the proximal drainage tube. The lubricant should be displaced slightly by the pressure transmitted from the suprasternal notch to a patent drainage tube. No movement might indicate an obstructed, and therefore nonfunctional, drainage lumen.

Alternatively, the smooth passage of an orogastric tube through the drainage tube past the level of the pLMA mask also confirms patency.

Flexible Laryngeal Mask Airway The Flexible LMA (fMLA; LMA Company North America, San Diego, CA) is helpful when access to intraoral structures is desired or space is limited by the patient's face. The fLMA has enjoyed use in dental surgery, otolaryngologic procedures such as tonsillectomy, and even ophthalmologic procedures.[62]

Intubating LMA (Fastrach iLMA) The Fastrach intubating LMA (iLMA; LMA North America, San Diego, CA) is designed to assist with ventilation and intubation. In 1 series of 254 patients with difficult-to-manage airways, 96.5% of patients had successful blind intubation via the iLMA. The remaining patients were intubated using a fiberoptic scope placed through the iLMA.[63] Patients have been intubated through the iLMA using a variety of ETTs.[64-66] Please refer to the section on tracheal intubation for a discussion of intubation through the iLMA.

Laryngeal Mask Airway Supreme The LMA Supreme (sLMA), a single-use supraglottic device with features of the pLMA (gastric port and integrated bite block) and of the LMA Fastrach (curved shaft), was introduced in 2007. Limited studies of the sLMA appear to show ease of use and function similar to that of the pLMA.[67,68]

As the LMA has grown in popularity and its design has been modified, there has been no shortage of novel SGAs introduced by other manufacturers.

Laryngeal Tube The Laryngeal Tube (LT) uses a double-cuff system fed by a single inflation line. The larger proximal cuff is a pharyngeal cuff; the second and smaller distal cuff is designed to rest in the proximal esophagus. Ventilation is provided by a shaft that terminates between the 2 cuffs near the laryngeal inlet. The original LT has a single lumen, but the Laryngeal Tube Suction (LTS) adds access to a second esophageal lumen and drainage tube. The newest addition to the LT family is the Gastro-Laryngeal Tube. Upper endoscopy is possible via its large esophageal lumen while ventilation is maintained with the ventilating lumen.

Cobra PLA The Cobra Perilaryngeal Airway (PLA) is another device that makes use of a pharyngeal cuff. The Cobra PLA has a soft plastic, wedge-shaped mask that lies distal to a large pharyngeal cuff. The mask does not contain an inflatable cuff and has many small, flexible bars covering its distal orifice. A Cobra PLA Plus measures temperature with an integrated probe, and there is a channel for distal gas sampling.

i-gel The i-gel airway is unique in that it does not have inflatable cuffs. The i-gel relies on a soft thermoplastic elastomer material for its mask. The i-gel mask becomes pliable when warmed by a patient's body temperature and forms a seal. The i-gel's broad ventilating shaft prevents rotation of the device, and there is an integrated drainage tube for gastric venting.

Air Q/Intubating Laryngeal Airway The air Q (single use) and Intubating Laryngeal Airway (ILA, reusable) are SGAs designed to facilitate endotracheal intubation. Both devices use a cuffed mask bowl attached to a ventilating shaft. Both have removable 15-mm adapters for introduction of an ETT introduction and predate the eLMA in this design feature. The air Q and the ILA lack aperture or epiglottic elevating bars.

ESOPHAGEAL–TRACHEAL AIRWAY

The esophageal–tracheal Combitube (**Fig. 36-14**) is intended for establishing emergency ventilation when there is simple, supraglottic obstruction or when the operator cannot ventilate with a face mask or intubate the trachea.[69-73] This device differs from the earlier esophageal obturator airway because the lungs can be ventilated whether the device enters the esophagus or the trachea.

When the lubricated Combitube is passed through the pharynx of a comatose or anesthetized patient, a neutral position or slight flexion of the neck generally directs the device to follow the posterior pharyngeal wall into the esophagus. Approximately 4% to 6 % of the time, the Combitube enters the trachea. A large 100-mL balloon seals the oropharynx, and a smaller one seals the esophagus. Two lumens protrude from the end of the Combitube. The one continuous with the inserted tip is used to ventilate if the tip has entered the trachea. More commonly, the other lumen that opens into multiple pharyngeal fenestration is used to ventilate the patient's lungs. Lifesaving ventilation has been provided by this device.[74] Rusch has introduced the Easytube (Teleflex Medical, Research Triangle Park, NC), a latex-free alternative to the Combitube.

COMPLICATIONS OF NONINTUBATED AIRWAY MANAGEMENT

Improperly conducted or monitored airway management can result in hypercapnia, hypoxic organ damage, or both, although supplemental oxygen and pulse oximetry reduce the incidence of the latter.[1] Hypercapnia is nearly always well tolerated; however, there are rare situations (Box 36-2) in which hypercapnia causes morbidity.

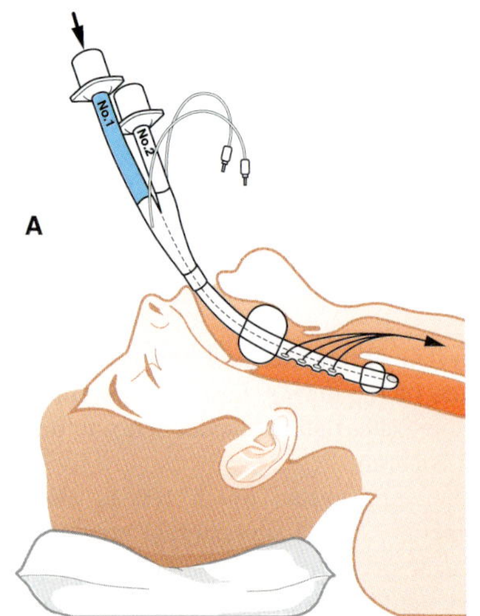

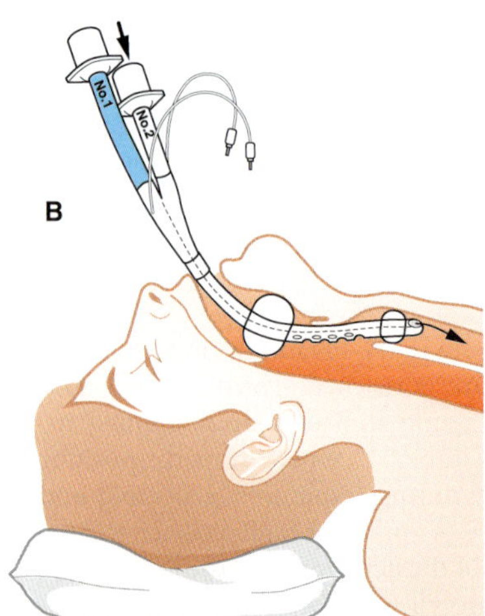

FIGURE 36-14. Combitube. **A.** Combitube positioned in the esophagus. Ventilation is performed via the blue lumen, marked No. 1. **B.** Combitube positioned in the trachea. Ventilation is performed via the clear lumen, marked No. 2. [Modified from Hagberg CA. *Benumof's Airway Management*. 2nd ed. Philadelphia, PA: Elsevier; 2007, with permission from Elsevier.]

BOX 36-10

Progression of Steps to Manage Difficulty in Ventilating a Patient

Confirm that the machine's selector valve is set to "bag" and that the reservoir bag is not twisted.

Deliver 100% oxygen.

Without exceeding 25 cm H_2O, increase airway pressure while intensifying jaw thrust and observing for ventilation or gastric distension.

If blood pressure is adequate and if awakening the patient is unnecessary, deepen anesthesia with a rapidly acting IV drug (eg, thiopental, propofol).

If depth of anesthesia is judged adequate, insert an oro- or nasopharyngeal airway or an SGA such as an LMA.

Consider whether it would be safest to awaken the patient.

Administer 5 to 20 mg of IV succinylcholine.

Consider the wisdom of a full dose of relaxant to facilitate tracheal intubation.

Consider using an alternative extraglottic airway such as a Combitube.

Consider establishing a transcricothyroid or surgical airway.

IV, intravenous; LMA, laryngeal mask airway; SGA, supraglottic airway.

Laryngeal spasm is an abnormal airway reflex of a sustained, disinhibited glottic closure precipitated by instrumentation, fluid irritation, or ill-timed stimulation of the larynx or other body parts (eg, moving or examining the patient in a light plane of anesthesia) in the setting of insufficient anesthetic depth. The anesthesiologist should consider a wide variety of causes (Box 36-6) when treating a patient whose lungs are difficult to ventilate (**Box 36-10**).

Aspiration of regurgitant material is a rare but serious complication of deep sedation and general anesthesia. Although anesthesia deep enough to obliterate airway reflexes eliminates active vomiting, passive regurgitation is possible at any time during the care of an anesthetized or critically ill patient. Repeated inspiratory efforts against an obstructed airway and gastric distension with fluid, food, or air or other gasses are predisposing factors to regurgitation.[75,76] During regurgitation, liquids should be removed from the pharynx by rapidly lowering the patient's head, turning it to the side, and suctioning with a rigid-tipped (eg, Yankauer) catheter. Subsequent pulmonary aspiration of fluid, solid, or acid may result in bronchospasm and oxygen desaturation, tracheobronchial obstruction, or chemical pneumonitis. Although the ASA closed claims studies indicate that aspiration is rare in modern anesthetic practice, the consequences are dire enough to consider the possibility of aspiration in every patient and to plan and prepare for it.[1]

Using a face mask with straps presents the risk of traumatic pressure to the eyes or branches of the facial nerve. Upper airway laceration may precipitate mucosal bleeding sufficiently severe to render laryngoscopy impossible.

AIRWAY MANAGEMENT WITH TRACHEAL INTUBATION

Tracheal intubation is undertaken for reasons of physiology, pathology, or convenience (**Box 36-11**). Reflecting an appreciation for the consequences of hypoventilation, hypoxia, and aspiration or because of a desire to free the anesthesiologist's hands for other tasks, the prevalence of tracheal intubation during anesthesia increased until the introduction of the LMA in the 1980s, after which the proportion of anesthetics with endotracheal intubation was reduced.

Visualization of the pharyngeal and glottic structures ensures the greatest likelihood of successful tracheal intubation. Tracheal intubation is optimally undertaken after careful setup in an operating room or critical care area with an appropriately stocked cart

BOX 36-11

Indications for Tracheal Intubation

Anesthesia

Provides maximal control of the airway

Provides an unobstructed leak-free airway for prolonged ventilation

Minimizes aspiration risk

Facilitates resuscitation of a moribund patient

Permits attention to complex diagnostic and therapeutic matters

Has preemptive utility if it is feared that ventilation and intubation may later become impossible

Allows ventilation during thoracoabdominal surgery

Permits flexible positioning

Allows the anesthesiologist to be distant from the head

Allows full range of positions (eg, prone, sitting, lateral, head down)

Keeps blood and secretions out of the trachea during airway surgery

Critical care

Establishes airway patency

Protects against pulmonary aspiration

Facilitates tracheobronchial toilet

Provides a route for airway positive-pressure ventilation modes

(**Box 36-12**). Alternative techniques of intubation and ventilation may be lifesaving when suboptimal circumstances prevent visualized tracheal intubation.

ENDOTRACHEAL TUBES

Most ETTs are disposable and made of clear, bioinert polyvinyl chloride (PVC) that molds to the contour of the airway after softening at body temperature. Lengths are marked in centimeters, and internal diameters are indicated in millimeters. Implantation testing in animals has shown these materials to be nonirritating by the standards of the American Society for Testing and Materials' Committee F-29 on Anesthetic and Respiratory Equipment. During laser surgery in the airway, PVC tubes can burn rapidly, producing hydrochloric acid and other pulmonary toxins. To minimize the risk of an airway fire during laser surgery, the use of tubes made of metal, metal-wrapped red rubber, or silicone is recommended.[77]

Although the resistance of a small ETT can impair the ventilatory weaning of a critically ill patient, it generally is not necessary in the operating room to use the largest possible tube. In many cases, a 7.0- or 7.5-mm internal diameter ETT is chosen for female patients, and an 8.0-mm ETT is used for men. Good judgment dictates even smaller tubes for patients with airway edema (eg, preeclamptic) or for nasal or blind intubation. Pediatric ETT sizes can be selected by an age-related formula and tested for leaks in situ. Cuffs often are not traditionally used until children have reached the age of 8 or 9 years, when the cricoid ring ceases to be the narrowest, edema-prone portion of the airway. Cutting ETTs renders them less obtrusive and easier to handle, but 26 cm of length should be sufficient for adult oral tubes, allowing 3 cm more for nasal tubes. One can firmly affix the 15-mm adapter by wiping it with alcohol and twisting it firmly into place in the ETT.

High-volume cuffs contact the trachea over a broad area, minimizing the pressure on the mucosa and improving the seal, which helps minimize aspiration risk. The pressure in the cuff is estimated by squeezing the pilot balloon, or it is set to be less than 25 cm H_2O when measured by a manometer. With longer periods of intubation, cuff overinflation is prevented by periodically measuring pressure or by injecting an additional 1 cc of air after an audible air leak has been sealed. A cuff initially inflated with air merits periodic checks to detect

BOX 36-12

Preparation for Tracheal Intubation

Assemble and confirm functionality of:

Skilled assistance

- Equipment for face mask ventilation
- Source of positive-pressure oxygen
  - Anesthesia machine
  - Self-inflating bag
- Tongue blade and oro- or nasopharyngeal airways

Bright laryngoscope

- Straight blade(s)
- Curved blade(s)

Intubating stylet or introducers

Stiff (tonsil-style) suction device

Position and environment

- Access to patient's head
- Elevate bed so the patient's forehead is at the level of the anesthesiologist's xiphoid
- Occipital elevation (sniffing position)
- Adequate light
- Monitors

Local anesthetics

  - Injectable
  - Nerve blocks
  - Laryngotracheal spray
  - Transcricothyroid spray
- Topical
  - Spray
  - Ointment for tongue
  - Viscous
  - Atomized

Intravenous access for

- Sedation or anesthetic induction
- Neuromuscular blockers
- Volume administration
- Cardioactive drugs (eg, antiarrhythmic)

Intubating (Magill) forceps

Backup equipment for unanticipated difficult intubation or ventilation (difficult airway cart)

overinflation when nitrous oxide is used during an anesthetic because if nitrous oxide enters the cuff, high pressures may result, injuring the tracheal mucosa.

The standard ETT has a bevel that opens toward the patient's left when the concavity of the tube's curve faces anteriorly. The Murphy eye is a fenestration in the tip of the tube opposite the bevel that is added to protect against obstruction. A variety of ETTs are available for specific applications (**Table 36-3**; **Figs. 36-15** and **36-16**).

LARYNGOSCOPES

These instruments are designed to create a line of sight for passage of the ETT by displacing the tongue and epiglottis anteriorly.[77] A battery-operated bulb may sit near the tip of the blade or in the handle itself,

TABLE 36-3 Special Tracheal Tubes and Their Applications

Description	Use
Embedded wire (armored or anode)	Minimizes chance of kinking
Endotrol with an intrinsic cable to flex the tip	Facilitates entry into the glottis
J-shaped laryngectomy	Fits into a tracheal stoma without entering a bronchus
Laser adapted	Minimizes chance of ignition
Lumen-containing	Sample airway gas or medicate the airway (eg, with lidocaine)
Microlaryngeal 4- to 6-mm ID with adult length and cuff (MLT)	Traverse a narrowed stretch of the airway
Preformed oral or nasal (Ring-Adair-Elvyn or RAE)	Avoid the surgical field during head and neck procedures
Uncuffed	Prevent subcricoid edema in patients younger than 8 years
Double lumen	Lung separation
Univent bronchial blocker	Lung separation

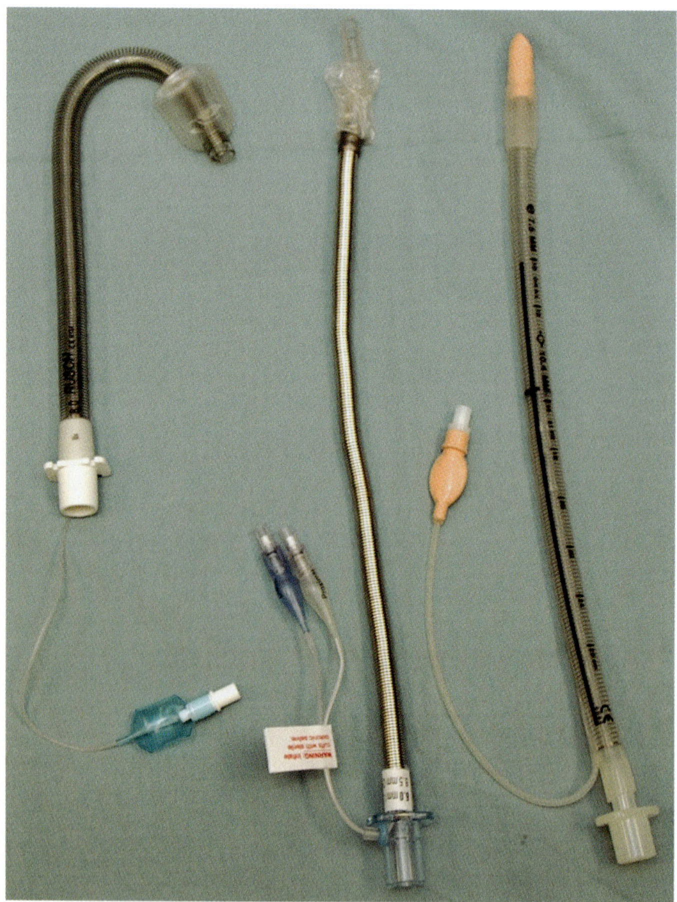

FIGURE 36-15. Varieties of tracheal tubes. Shown from *left* to *right* are the armored laryngectomy tube, laser tube, and laryngeal mask airway flexible nondisposable tube used for Fastrach intubation.

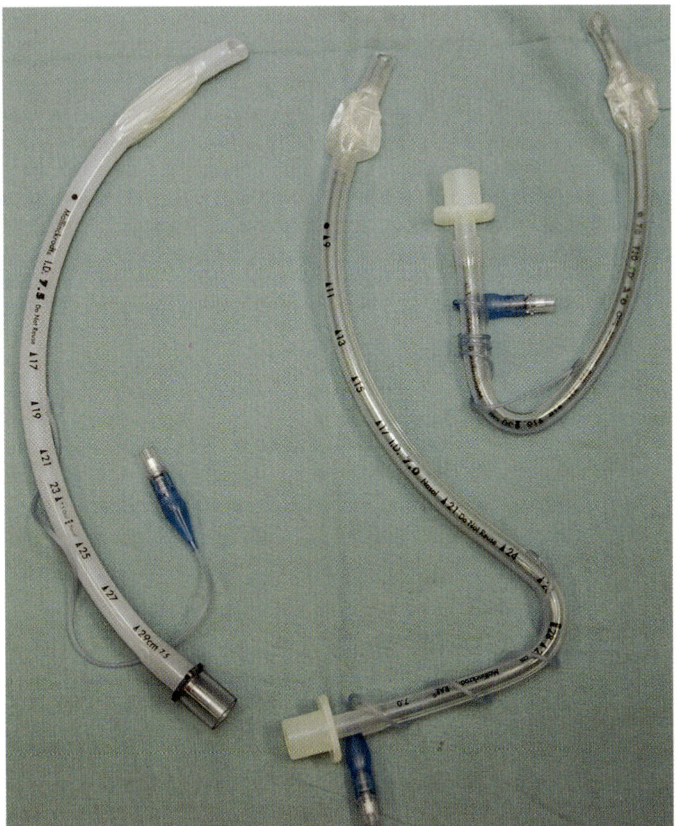

FIGURE 36-16. Varieties of tracheal tubes. From *left* to *right* are a standard tube for oral or nasal intubation, a preformed tube for nasotracheal use (Ring-Adair-Elwyn [RAE]; Mallinckrodt Inc, Boulder, CO.), a preformed tube for orotracheal use (Mallinckrodt Inc, Boulder, CO.).

in which case illumination is directed by a fiberoptic bundle to the laryngeal structures. Blade-mounted bulbs operate erratically if their contacts are not corrosion free.

Laryngoscope blades require a high level of disinfection to kill vegetative organisms but do not necessarily need to be sterilized. They should be soaked and brushed clean in an enzyme detergent before disinfection. Autoclaving or soaking in glutaraldehyde will corrode the contact between the bulb and blade over time. Gas sterilization is effective but time consuming. Disposable plastic covers keep handles and blades free of saliva and blood and minimize cross-contamination.

Although innumerable laryngoscope blade designs have been developed, the 2 remain the most popular: the straight Miller, which lifts the epiglottis directly, and the curved Macintosh, which does so with traction on the glossoepiglottic and hyoepiglottic ligaments (**Fig. 36-17**).

STYLETS

Because of the position of the tongue and epiglottis, a glottic opening not exposed by routine laryngoscopy seems to hide anteriorly. Stylets are blunt-tipped, flexible tools used to give a different shape to the ETT to facilitate tracheal intubation. Stylets are lubricated and inserted in the ETT but are not intended to protrude from the tube (the distal tip of the stylet is positioned inside the ETT). The tip of the ETT and stylet are bent about 5 cm from the end to achieve a "hockey stick" shape. The ETT is passed beneath the epiglottis, and an assistant removes the stylet as the ETT enters the trachea. Excessively stiff, carelessly placed, or improperly used stylets can cause life-threatening complications. A stylet that is used repeatedly may fracture during intubation.

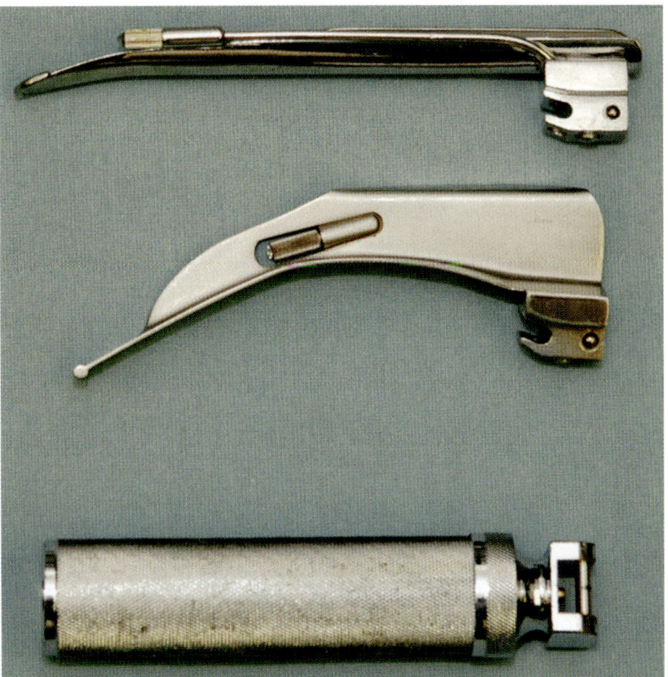

FIGURE 36-17. From *top* to *bottom*: Straight blade (Miller), curved (Macintosh) blade, laryngoscope battery handle.

INTRODUCERS

Introducers exemplified by the angle-tipped Eschmann gum elastic bougie can guide an ETT into the trachea. Longer and less rigid than stylets, introducers facilitate difficult intubation. Passed through the tracheal tube, the tip is guided into the trachea, and the ETT is threaded over it.

A soft, flexible introducer can serve as tracheal tube exchanger and guide the blind insertion of a new tube if an exchange of tubes is necessary. Dedicated tube changers include models with a Luer lock or 15-mm male adapters at the proximal end for oxygenating with jet ventilation until a new tube can be placed. Even if the glottic opening cannot be visualized, it may be helpful to use a rigid laryngoscope to create open space in the hypopharynx, thereby facilitating the passage of the ETT over the tube changer or stylet into the trachea. An ETT is least likely to get stuck on the epiglottis or aryepiglottic folds if its internal diameter is not much larger than the introducer.

TRACHEAL INTUBATION

Tracheal intubation usually is performed after induction of anesthesia and muscle paralysis but is also easily accomplished in conscious patients. In some patients, muscle relaxants are avoided, and intubation is done during general anesthesia with the patient breathing spontaneously.

An ETT can be passed orotracheally, nasotracheally, or through a tracheostomy. Although passage of an ETT through a mature tracheostomy requires no special instruments, intubating through the mouth or nose can be extremely difficult or impossible.

Many techniques exist to assist routine and difficult tracheal intubation (**Box 36-13**).[3,12,75] They vary in their level of sophistication, invasiveness, tendency for blood and secretions to obviate visualization, and potential for major complications. In selecting a technique, the anesthesiologist weighs risks against the likelihood of success, keeping in mind a backup plan to deal with unexpected failure. Expertise may vary depending on when the anesthesiologist trained. For example, whereas recent American trainees may not have extensive experience

BOX 36-13

Techniques of Tracheal Intubation

Visualized

- Rigid laryngoscope (direct)
- Flexible fiberoptic laryngoscope (indirect)
- Video laryngoscope (indirect)

Guided blind

- Laryngeal mask
- Bougie
- Retrograde wire

Blind nasal

Combination of techniques

Surgical

- Cricothyrotomy
- Tracheostomy

in blind nasal intubation, those of an earlier vintage may be less comfortable with fiberoptic techniques. The ideals against which a technique may be judged are summarized in **Box 36-14**. Fiberoptic bronchoscopy scores high as a technique to manage difficult airways. Its shortcomings include its size, cost, relatively fragile nature, and susceptibility to obliteration of the view by blood and secretions. Compact, battery-powered light sources for bronchoscopes have proven advantageous when portability, compact size, and low weight are important.

Disposable, single-use bronchoscope availability removes the concerns of high per-unit expense, allowing the devices to be strategically deployed throughout the hospital in areas such as intensive care units and emergency departments. These areas may not previously have been candidates for expensive but rarely used capital equipment. In addition, concerns about device breakage, sterilization, and reprocessing costs are removed with disposable devices.

BOX 36-14

Desired Features of an Intubation Technique

Primary

- High success rate in those with difficult airways
- Useful for upper and lower airway problems
- Useful for oral and nasal intubations
- Allows ventilation during intubation
- Performed with visual guidance
- Allows application of topical anesthesia
- Devoid of technique-specific complications
- Head and neck manipulations are not crucial for success
- Useful in combination with other techniques
- Blood and secretions do not interfere with its use

Secondary

- Avoids dental trauma
- Equipment is easily cleaned and stored
- Portable
- Easily learned and mastered
- Cost-effective

TECHNIQUES OF INTUBATION

RIGID DIRECT LARYNGOSCOPY

Rigid laryngoscopy retains its popularity because of its simplicity, high success rate, and good visualization.[12,23,75] In adults, it is critical to elevate the occiput on a pad to flex the neck so that the atlanto-occipital extension will align the pharynx with the mouth and larynx (**Fig. 36-18**). If the patient has been given muscle relaxants, a neuromuscular blockade monitor is the best way to ensure complete neuromuscular blockade. Although succinylcholine provides the most rapid onset of relaxation, the effect of nondepolarizing relaxants can be hastened by using either large doses or the priming principle.

The left hand grasps the open laryngoscope with the fifth finger just above the blade. Although simply extending the neck adequately opens some mouths, the best access is achieved by pushing on the right mandibular premolar with the right thumb while stabilizing the maxillary teeth with the third finger. With barrel-chested or obese patients, extra elevation of the head and shoulders or directing the laryngoscope handle to the left (rather than keeping it in a sagittal plane) prevents

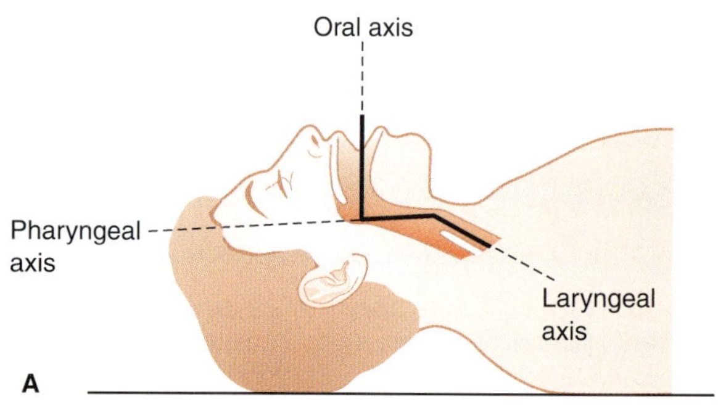

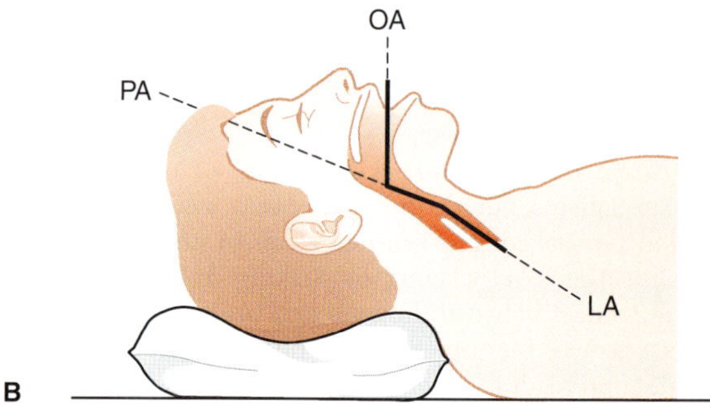

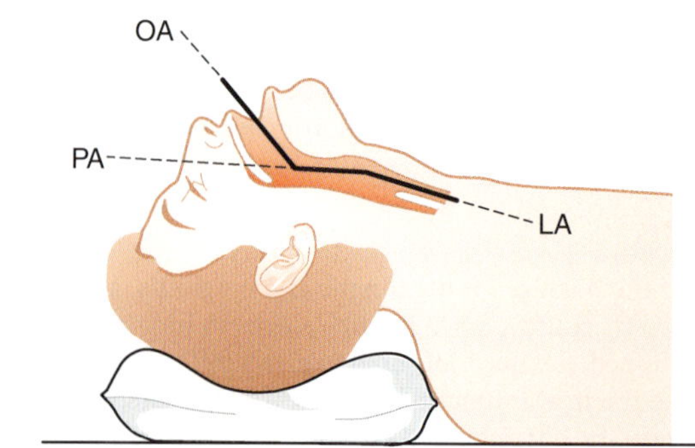

FIGURE 36-18. Intubating position during rigid laryngoscopy. **A.** Supine patient without a headrest. **B.** Head elevation and neck flexion bring the pharyngeal and laryngeal axes into line. **C.** Extension of head at atlantooccipital joint aligns the oral axis with the other 2 axes. [Reprinted from Ovassapian A, Meyer R. Airway management. In: Longnecker DE, Murphy FL, eds. *Introduction to Anesthesia*. 9th ed. Philadelphia, PA: WB Saunders; 1996, with permission from Elsevier.]

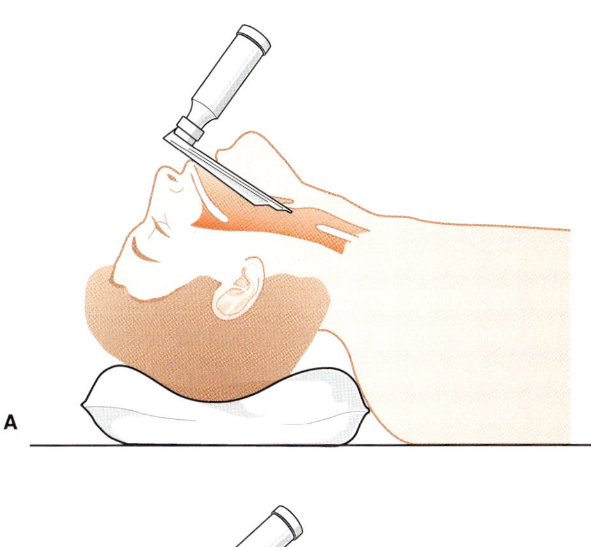

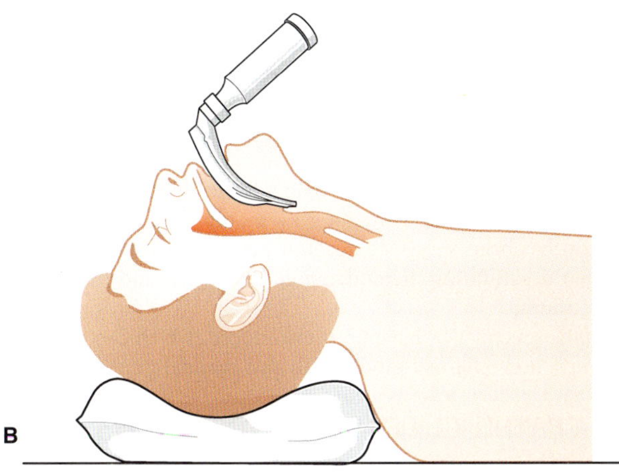

FIGURE 36-19. A. The straight blade is placed under the epiglottis to lift the epiglottis up to expose the glottis. **B.** The curved blade is positioned in the vallecula during rigid laryngoscopy. [Reprinted from Ovassapian A, Meyer R. Airway management. In: Longnecker DE, Murphy FL, eds. *Introduction to Anesthesia*. 9th ed. Philadelphia, PA: WB Saunders; 1996, with permission from Elsevier.]

interference from the sternum while inserting the blade in the mouth. The laryngoscope blade can then be slid along the right side of the tongue so that its flange displaces the tongue leftward. When it passes the right fauces, the blade is directed medially to the epiglottis, a key landmark. The tip of a curved blade, placed in the midline of the glossoepiglottic reflection, will maximally lift the epiglottis to expose the glottis. Straight blades are slid beneath the epiglottis to lift it directly (**Fig. 36-19**). Elevation of the tongue and epiglottis is accomplished with the left hand pulling up and away from the anesthesiologist, keeping the left elbow close to the anesthesiologist's side. Rotating the laryngoscope or "levering" the device is to be avoided as the maxillary teeth can easily be injured. The view of the glottis may be improved by applying the right thumb and index finger to the thyroid cartilage for lateral or backward, upward, and rightward pressure (the BURP maneuver).[75] Initiated by the laryngoscopist, laryngeal pressure can be maintained by an assistant during intubation. In small children, the relatively large occiput eliminates the need for a pad, and the more cephalad glottis increases the importance of laryngeal pressure.[14]

Common avoidable causes of difficult laryngoscopy include improper positioning of the head, inadequate opening of the mouth, selecting the wrong blade, allowing the tongue to hang over the right side of the blade, applying leverage rather than traction, and obscuring the line of vision with the ETT during its insertion. If the epiglottis is not seen, the blade may have been inserted too far, placing the esophagus at the end of the laryngoscope. Slowly backing out the laryngoscope may bring the epiglottis into view. Conversely, selecting too short a blade prevents the tip from reaching the glossoepiglottic reflection.

Particular situations may call for either a straight or curved blade. With its effective flange and its panoramic exposure of the anatomic features, the Macintosh curved blade is recommended for those learning intubation. It retracts large tongues and the prominent lips of edentulous patients. Because a curved blade avoids contact with the sensitive laryngeal surface of the epiglottis, it is well suited for intubation in conscious patients. In patients with micrognathia, a floppy epiglottis, or an anteriorly hidden glottis, the straight blade can lift the epiglottis for a superior view of the larynx. The Miller straight blade, with its small cross-section, is especially useful in the right corner of the mouth in patients with prominent maxillary teeth or limited temporomandibular mobility.

Nasotracheal intubation guided by rigid laryngoscopy may be used in oral and maxillofacial surgery and in the intensive care setting. Introduced through the right corner of the mouth so as not to block laryngoscopic visualization, a Magill intubating forceps directs the ETT tip to the glottis while an assistant advances the tube on command.[75,78] The nasally inserted tube may hang up on the anterior laryngeal structures, requiring rotation of the tube or flexion of the neck or occipitocervical junction to facilitate the ETT entering the trachea.

Intubation in the Conscious Patient In patients with a difficult airway or at high risk of aspiration, serious consideration should be given to securing the airway before inducing anesthesia.[2,3] Intubation in a conscious patient is the choice when both risk of aspiration and difficult airway factors coexist. To ensure maximum cooperation, preanesthetic preparation includes an explanation of the procedure to the patient before premedication.

Sedation to an extent that may cause apnea or airway obstruction is contraindicated. Opioid-induced analgesia and depression of airway reflexes increase the risk of aspirating gastric contents but facilitate oropharyngeal instrumentation while providing a patient who is cooperative enough to follow commands. Protective reflexes remain more active when a benzodiazepine is used, but the patient may be less cooperative, reacting more vigorously to instrumentation. A combination of fentanyl and midazolam (≤1.5 mcg/kg and 30 mcg/kg in divided doses) has been used successfully.[79] In ensuring that these synergistic drugs have reached their peak effect, 3 to 5 minutes should elapse between doses. Continually asking the patient to take deep breaths helps assess the patient's responsiveness, avoiding oversedation and hypoxemia.

Glycopyrrolate, 0.2 to 0.3 mg IV, minimizes secretions and improves the effectiveness of topical anesthetics.[80] Patients may benefit from medications that increase gastric fluid pH or enhance gastric emptying.

Topical anesthesia is achieved by an oropharyngeal spray of 4% lidocaine and translaryngeal injection of 3 mL of 4% lidocaine. Topical anesthesia with lidocaine begins to work within 30 seconds after its application and is fully effective within 2 minutes but lasts only 20 to 30 minutes. For nasotracheal intubation, 4% cocaine or a 3-mL mixture of 4% lidocaine with 1 mL of 1% phenylephrine provides anesthesia while shrinking mucosae.[81] Use of lidocaine jelly before application of other anesthetics to normal mucosa increases patient satisfaction.[82]

During rigid laryngoscopy in a conscious patient, the anesthesiologist continually instructs and reassures the patient while proceeding gently. Time may be required to spray more topical anesthetic on the tongue base or epiglottis. Laryngeal pressure by an assistant is particularly helpful, and lingual nerve block may decrease refractory gagging.

Rapid-Sequence Induction and Intubation Preoxygenation, avoidance of mask ventilation, and compression of the cricoid cartilage (Sellick maneuver; **Fig. 36-20**) to resist passive regurgitation of gastric contents into the oropharynx are elements of a traditional rapid-sequence induction.[4,23,75] Anesthesia begins with a rapid-sequence injection of propofol or thiopental followed by succinylcholine and intubation as soon as muscle relaxation is confirmed. An assistant maintains cricoid

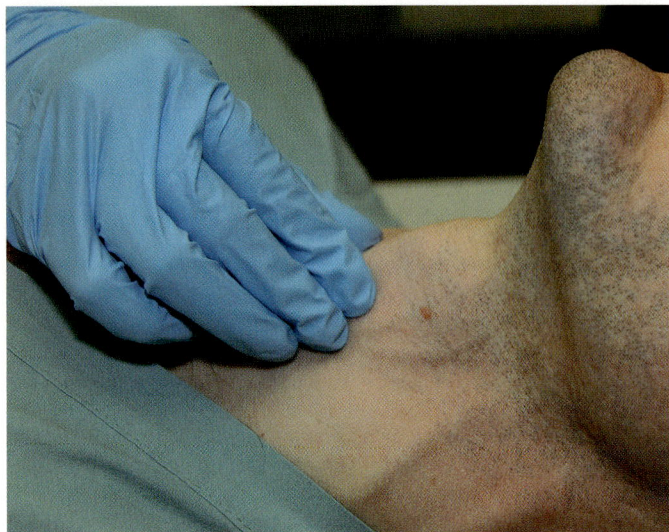

FIGURE 36-20. Proper application of cricoid pressure during rapid-sequence induction and intubation to prevent passive regurgitation of gastric contents.

pressure from the onset of hypnosis until tracheal intubation is confirmed, and the cuff is inflated. Other induction agents and nondepolarizing muscle relaxants are alternatives for induction.

Cricoid pressure, as described by Sellick, should be firm enough to prevent the esophagus from slipping laterally but not so firm as to obstruct ventilation.[4,83,84] This pressure may be difficult to attain as described because the 30-Newton force currently recommended may obstruct the view of the larynx.[85] Application of cricoid pressure is a safe and effective maneuver, with only 1 reported case of esophageal rupture after vomiting. Complete anesthesia and paralysis, confirmed with a blockade monitor, eliminates any chance of active vomiting. With this knowledge, the anesthesiologist can be confident in having the assistant maintain cricoid pressure until position of the tube in the trachea is certain.

If intubation fails, the risk of asphyxia may exceed the risk of aspiration. Mask ventilation with maintained cricoid pressure was described by Sellick in 1961.[4] If mask ventilation proves difficult, the patient may be placed in a 5-degree head-down tilt or kept in a flat supine position while cricoid pressure is slowly decreased until it is released. If mask ventilation is improved, the possibility of airway obstruction caused by improperly applied cricoid pressure[28,83] should be considered, and intubation may proceed without cricoid pressure. If mask ventilation is impossible, previously unsuspected pathology (eg, hypertrophic lingual tonsils) should be considered. If an LMA or other supraglottic or extraglottic airway is needed for rescue breathing, it is important to remember that cricoid pressure may prevent proper positioning of these devices. Cricoid pressure should be released if the rescue breathing device is not working properly.

Anything that increases the intragastric-to-esophageal pressure gradient increases the risk of regurgitation of stomach contents. Factors that elevate this pressure gradient include inflation of the stomach with air, a steep head-down position, high intra-abdominal pressure, and spontaneous respiratory efforts against a fully or partially obstructed airway (this lowers the intraesophageal pressure). Airway pressures below 15 cm H_2O during mask ventilation rarely inflate the stomach, but in adults not subjected to cricoid pressure, the minimum airway pressure required to push air into the stomach is reported to be 20 cm H_2O.

In infants and children, appropriate application of cricoid pressure prevents gastric gas insufflation during mask ventilation with an airway pressure up to 40 cm H_2O.[86] Complete airway obstruction is one of the complications of improperly applied cricoid pressure. This is more likely in infants and children because of their more pliable trachea and laryngeal cartilages.

VIDEOLARYNGOSCOPY

Rigid video laryngoscopes (VLs) are devices that have a small video camera and light source incorporated into a rigid metal or plastic blade. The real-time image from the camera is displayed on a video screen and can be recorded for later viewing, teaching, or research. VLs are designed to improve the view of the larynx to ease tracheal intubation. Because they do not rely on a straight line of sight, the user can "see around the corner" of the natural airway, obviating the need for alignment of the oral, pharyngeal, and laryngeal axes.[87] This facilitates visualization of the glottic opening with minimal force against the airway structures.

A viewing angle of up to 80 degrees is possible compared with the 15-degree viewing angle of direct laryngoscopy.[88] This extended viewing angle may be helpful in difficult intubations secondary to limited neck mobility, cervical spine immobilization, retrognathia, or reduced thyromental or interincisor distance.[89] In addition to facilitating laryngoscopy and orotracheal intubation, VLs can be used for awake, nasotracheal or fiberoptic intubation, confirmation of proper tracheal tube placement, and placement of a transesophageal echocardiography probe.

Views of the glottis are generally better with VLs than with direct laryngoscopy. A better view, however, does not always translate into an easy tracheal intubation. Tracheal intubation is difficult when the glottic view is obstructed by secretions, blood, gastric contents, fogging of the lens, or most commonly, the inability to advance the ETT through the larynx or into the trachea. Difficult ETT manipulation under *indirect* visualization has been shown to account for increased time to intubation, oxygen desaturation, hemodynamic instability, and the potential for airway trauma.[90]

Since 2001, several VLs have been introduced, which can be divided into 2 groups: non–channel-guided VLs and channel-guided VLs.

NON–CHANNEL-GUIDED VIDEOLARYNGOSCOPES

Non–channel-guided VLs include the GlideScope (Verathon Inc, Bothell, WA), the McGrath Series 5 (Aircraft Medical, Edinburgh, UK), and the Storz C-MAC (Karl Storz, Tuttlingen, Germany). These devices are similar to a Macintosh blade in shape and in use; a view of the glottis is obtained before the introduction of the ETT (**Figs. 36-21** to **36-23**).

To perform videolaryngoscopy with a non–channel-guided VL, the blade is inserted into the midline of the oropharynx under *direct*

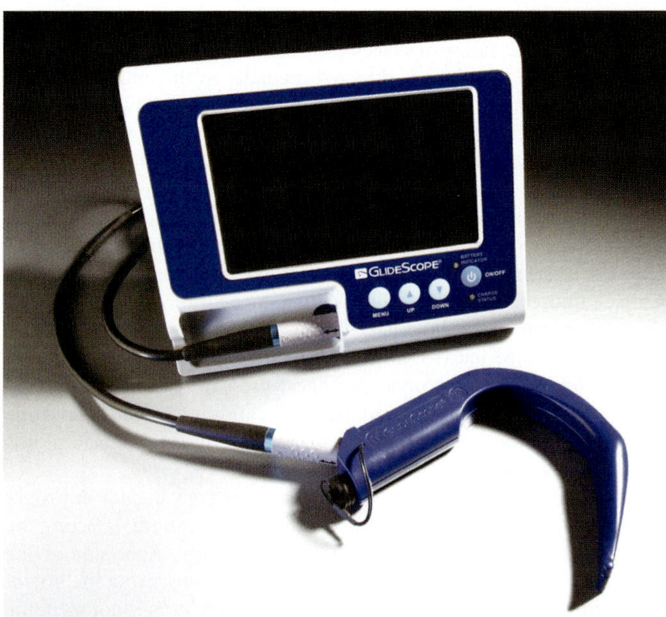

FIGURE 36-21. GlideScope. [Courtesy of Verathon Inc., Bothell, WA.]

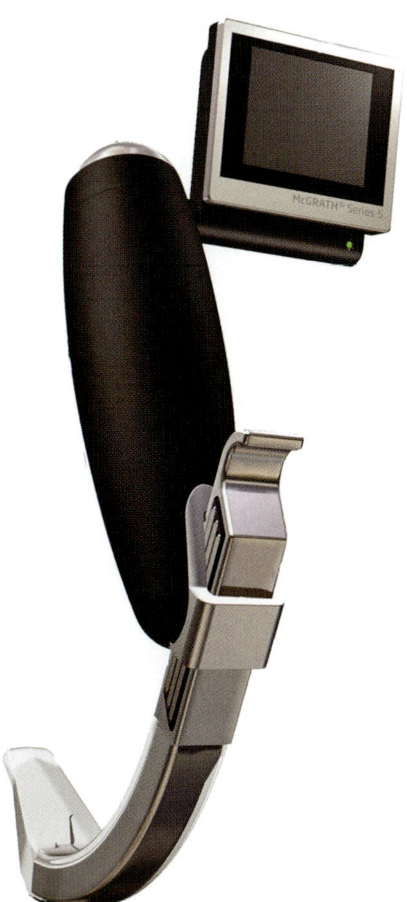

FIGURE 36-22. McGrath Series 5. [Courtesy of LMA North America, Inc., San Diego, CA.]

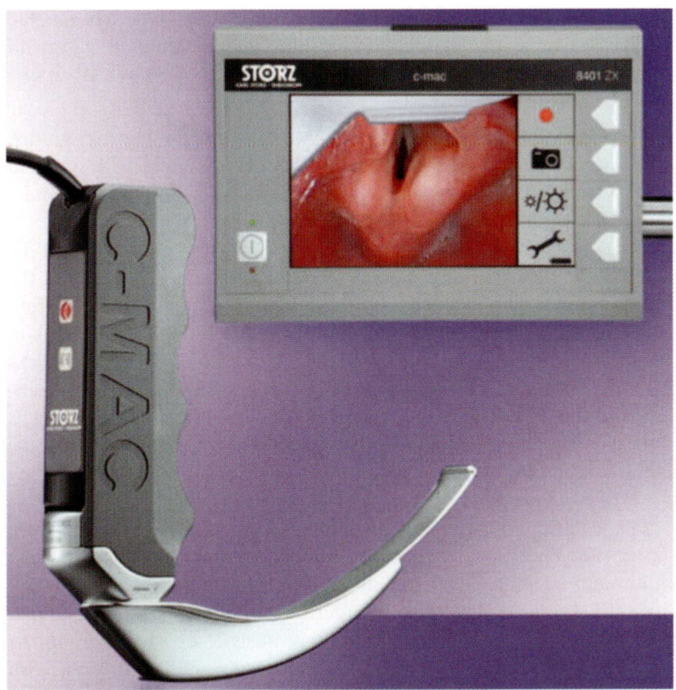

FIGURE 36-23. STORZ c-mac. [©2011 Photo Courtesy of Karl Storz Endoscopy-America, Inc., El Segundo, CA.]

visualization until the tip of the blade is past the posterior tongue. Performing this under direct vision helps prevent damage to the soft palate or palatoglossal arch.[91] When the device is past the tongue, attention is directed to the video screen and the blade is advanced midline until a Cormack-Lehane grade II view is achieved. A grade II glottic view is acceptable because if additional anterior force is applied to the blade, the larynx may be directed further anterior, impeding passage of the ETT into the trachea.[91] After the glottis is visualized, the operator's attention is directed away from the video screen to the oropharynx, and the ETT is inserted under direct visualization until its tip is past the posterior tongue, paying careful attention not to injure the soft palate or palatoglossal arch with the ETT. The operator then looks at the video monitor while directing the tip of the ETT into the vestibule of the larynx and then advancing the tube over the stylet, through the vocal cords, and into the trachea.

As the ETT passes over the stylet, its trajectory becomes less parallel to the axis of the trachea, occasionally causing the tip of the ETT to impact the anterior tracheal wall. This problem can be addressed in 3 ways. The ETT may be loaded on the stylet with "reverse camber" orienting the natural curve of the tube posteriorly. This allows the tube to pass off the stylet in direction parallel to the axis of the trachea. The operator may also spin or "corkscrew" the ETT as it passes off the stylet to minimize the impact of the ETT with the anterior tracheal wall. Finally, an ETT with no curve such as the Parker Tube (Parker Medical, Highlands Ranch, CO) or the Verathon Glideright tube may be used.

GlideScope The GlideScope was introduced in 2001. The blade, available in 3 sizes, has a steep 60-degree curvature, which improves the view of the glottis because the tongue is not displaced anteriorly. (Fig. 36-21) The maximum thickness of the largest blade is less than 15 mm, allowing use in a patient with an interincisor distance of 2 cm.[91] The camera lens, heated to prevent fogging, requires no other preparation before use.

Tracheal intubation with the GlideScope generally requires use of a preloaded, specially curved stylet.[92] The GlideRite Rigid Stylet, curved to follow the 60-degree angulation of the blade, or a standard stylet can be used. If a standard stylet is used, the ETT and stylet should be bent to approximate the angle of the convex side of the GlideScope blade to facilitate advancement of the ETT into the trachea.[91]

The primary advantage of the GlideScope over direct laryngoscopy is an equal or improved glottic view in both normal and difficult airways. In patients with anticipated difficult airways, the GlideScope increased the percentage of Cormack-Lehane grade I to II views compared with views with direct laryngoscopy.[89,93]

Because the improved views are attained without aligning the oral, pharyngeal, and laryngeal axes, less cervical manipulation is required. Cervical spine motion was reduced 50% during GlideScope intubation compared with cervical spine motion during direct laryngoscopy.[94] The GlideScope can accommodate any size and type of ETT, and ratings for time to intubation and "ease of use" were better with both experienced and inexperienced users in simulated difficult airways.[95]

Although the GlideScope may offer improved glottic views, advancement of the ETT into the trachea still can be difficult. Difficult advancement may prolong intubation times; increase the number of intubation attempts; and lead to failed intubation, oxygen desaturation, hemodynamic instability, and trauma to the soft palate and palatoglossal arch.[87,89,92,93,96,97] If difficult intubation is encountered, the blade can be withdrawn 2 to 3 cm and the stylet 3 to 5 cm to lessen the anterior displacement of the larynx. Withdrawal improves the alignment of the axes of the larynx, trachea, and ETT.[91,92]

McGrath Laryngoscope The McGrath Series 5 (Aircraft Medical, Edinburgh, UK) was introduced in January 2006 (Fig. 36-22). This VL has a reusable CameraStick handle, which incorporates a small camera and light source. A sterile, transparent, single-use blade with a 60-degree angle covers the CameraStick. The camera image is displayed on a screen that tilts for viewing and is located on the handle.

Within the handle is a single AA battery, which provides 60 minutes of operating time.

Similar to other VLs, the McGrath Series 5 has been shown to improve glottic views in both routine and difficult airways. Compared with direct laryngoscopy with a Macintosh blade, the McGrath improved Cormack-Lehane views by 2 to 3 grades in more than 90% of patients.[90] Similar to the GlideScope, the McGrath Series 5 requires a stylet to facilitate intubation. This requirement may pose difficulties with ETT manipulation, leading to multiple intubation attempts, airway trauma, or failed tracheal intubation. As with the GlideScope, the blade and stylet can be withdrawn slightly, and the handle can be rotated caudally to advance the tube through the vocal cords without abutting the anterior tracheal wall.

Storz C-Mac The C-MAC was introduced in 2003. It has a Macintosh-shaped steel blade with a slim 14-mm profile, can be equipped with a suction catheter, and is available in 3 sizes[98] (Fig. 36-23). The C-MAC incorporates a digital video camera and a high-power light-emitting diode located laterally in the distal third of the blade. The image from the camera is displayed on a lightweight, portable, color LCD monitor and can be recorded as a single image or a video stream. The monitor houses a rechargeable lithium ion battery for approximately 2 working hours.[98]

The C-MAC differs from other VLs because it can be used as a direct or indirect laryngoscope. As with a Macintosh blade, advancement of the ETT into the trachea does not routinely require a stylet. The C-MAC improved glottic views and facilitated successful tracheal intubation when attempts with direct laryngoscopy failed.[98] Compared with the GlideScope, Airtraq, and Macintosh blade in airway simulations, the C-MAC had the highest ratings for ease of use, provided the best glottic view (along with the Airtraq), and needed the shortest time for intubation.[87] The Storz D-blade has a unique shape and works with the C-MAC platform. More curved than other C-MAC blades, the D-blade lets the user "see around the corner" of the tongue. Although this blade improves visualization of the larynx in some settings, it may require intubation techniques similar to those for the Glidescope system.

CHANNEL-GUIDED VIDEOLARYNGOSCOPES

The channel-guided VLs include the Pentax AWS-100 (Pentax Medical Company, Montvale NJ) and the Airtraq (Prodol Meditec, SA, Guecho Vizcaya, Spain) (**Figs. 36-24** and **36-25**). These VLs have highly curved blades with a channel to hold the ETT during laryngoscopy and guide it during intubation.

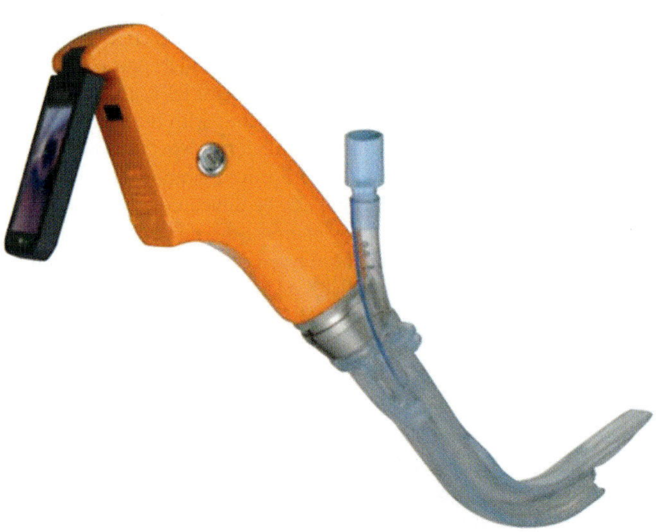

FIGURE 36-24. Pentax AWS. [Courtesy of Pentax, Ballerup, Denmark.]

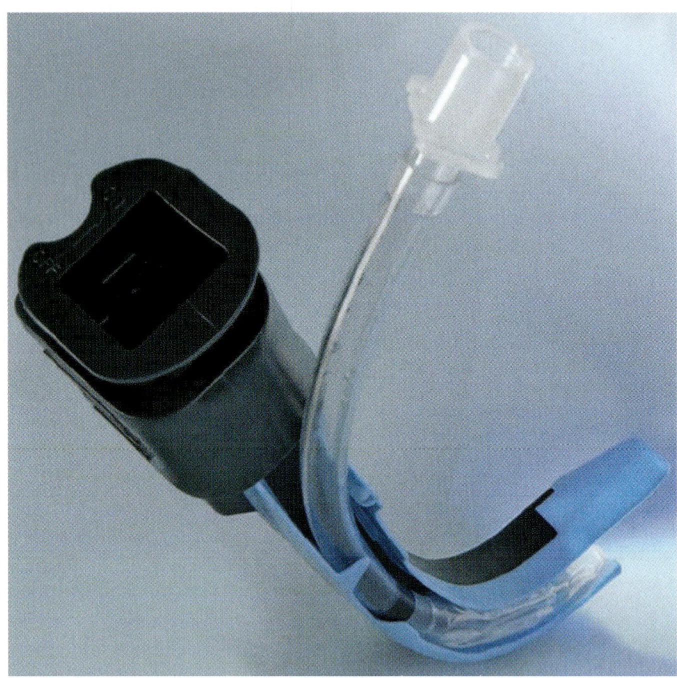

FIGURE 36-25. Airtraq. [Courtesy of Airtraq, LLC. Fenton, MO.]

With channel-guided VLs, view of the glottis is indirect, obviating the need for alignment of the oral, pharyngeal, and laryngeal axes.[87] A well-lubricated ETT is positioned in the tube channel of the blade, with only the tip visible on the LCD screen. The blade is inserted midline into the oropharynx under direct visualization until its tip is past the posterior tongue, preventing damage to the soft palate and palatoglossal arch. When it is past the tongue, the blade is kept midline and attention is turned to the video display. The Pentax AWS PBlade is inserted under the epiglottis and used like a Miller blade. The Airtraq blade may be placed in either the vallecula (Macintosh style) or under the epiglottis (Miller style). After the glottic opening is observed on the monitor, the device is lifted up, and the ETT is advanced into the trachea. If the ETT abuts the epiglottis or arytenoids, the manufacturers recommend rotating the devices back (ie, out of the mouth) and lifting them anteriorly before readvancing the ETT.

Pentax AWS The Pentax AWS, a battery-operated, channel-guided VL, was introduced in Japan in 2006. It has a handle with a 2.4-in LDC screen; a 12-cm image tube with a camera and light source; and a disposable rigid blade, the PBlade[99] (Fig. 36-24).

The tube channel can accommodate an ETT with a 6.0 to 8.5 mm ID. The PBlade comes in only 1 size (18 mm thick) and is larger than the blades of other VLs. It is used only if a patient's mouth opening is larger than 2.5 cm. A distinct feature of the Pentax AWS is a target symbol on the monitor that highlights the intended path of the ETT as it advances from the tube channel. This target mark is aligned with the glottic opening, and the ETT is advanced into the trachea. Because the monitor is attached to the handle and the ETT is preloaded and directed toward the target symbol, the operator does not have to look away while advancing the ETT, which may lower risk for airway trauma.

Studies comparing the AWS with direct laryngoscopy show improved glottic visualization and tracheal intubation and less cervical spine motion in routine and difficult airways with the AWS.[94,99] Novice operators using the AWS have a high success rate visualizing the larynx. Tracheal intubation was faster and more likely to be successful on the first attempt for novices using the AWS compared with Macintosh direct laryngoscopy.[95]

The Pentax AWS has been used for awake intubation of the trachea. When the glottic view is obtained on the monitor, lidocaine can be injected through the suction channel to anesthetize the airway, and the ETT can be advanced through the tube channel.[100]

As with other VLs, advancement of the ETT into the trachea may be problematic after the glottic view is obtained on the monitor. The ETT may impinge on the epiglottis or arytenoids, in which case a gum elastic bougie is used. The bougie is inserted through the ETT and directed into the glottic opening. When the bougie is in the trachea, the ETT can be advanced over the bougie through the glottis. The bougie also has proved useful when the PBlade is too short to reach the epiglottis or larynx.[101]

Airtraq The Airtraq is a single-use, channel-guided VL with a viewfinder and disposable blade (Fig. 36-25). The blade has 2 separate tracks, the optical channel and the tube channel. The optical channel contains a series of lenses, a prism, and a viewfinder at the proximal portion of the device. There is an optional video camera, which can be attached to the viewfinder to transmit the image to a monitor, and a rechargeable battery-operated LED at the tip of the blade for illumination up to 90 minutes. The antifog system for the lenses is activated by the LED for 30 to 60 seconds before use to warm the lens. The Airtraq comes in 4 sizes for orotracheal intubation with ETTs from 2.5 to 8.5 mm ID. The Airtraq has special blades for nasotracheal and endobronchial intubation and can accommodate double-lumen tubes from 35 to 41 Fr.

The Airtraq blade containing the ETT is inserted midline into the oropharynx while the airway structures are visualized through the viewfinder. The blade tip is directed either into the vallecula (Macintosh style) or to the epiglottis (Miller style). The blade is manipulated in all planes until the vocal cords are in the center of the viewfinder at which time the ETT is advanced through the channel into the trachea. If advancement is difficult, the Airtraq is rotated slightly out of the airway and lifted anteriorly. If these maneuvers fail, the operator can try reducing cervical extension.[102] When ETT placement in the trachea is confirmed, the Airtraq blade is tilted laterally away from the ETT and removed.

The Airtraq has advantages in routine and difficult laryngoscopy. Compared with direct laryngoscopy, it improves glottic views; facilitates first-attempt tracheal intubations; and lowers the incidence of oxygen desaturation, airway trauma, and hemodynamic instability. The Airtraq is easy to master for both novice and experienced anesthetists. It reduces cervical spine motion but causes less dental compression than other VLs and the Macintosh blade.[103,104]

Hemodynamic stability with use of the Airtraq versus the Macintosh blade may be attributed to less force needed to elevate the mandible during laryngoscopy. Constant visualization of the glottis and alignment of the preloaded ETT with the trachea cause less trauma to the vocal cords.[104]

The introduction of VL has significantly changed difficult and routine airway management. All of the commercially available devices improve glottic visualization even in the hands of novice operators. The user should understand the fundamental differences between direct and VL. Direct laryngoscopy requires a straight line of sight from the operator's eye to the vocal cords. The line of sight may be difficult to establish, but once the vocal cords are seen, tracheal intubation is usually easily achieved. On the other hand, VLs make viewing the larynx easy even when the airway maintains its normal, highly curved architecture. Thus, viewing the cords is often easier with a VL than with direct laryngoscopy, but passage of the tube through the cords may be harder. As with any tool, its proper use and unique strengths and weaknesses must be understood.

Fiberoptic Intubation A flexible fiberoptic bronchoscope (ie, a fiberscope) (**Fig. 36-26**) can be used for routine or challenging intubations in patients with airway tumors, infections, or cervical spine fractures or fixation (**Fig. 36-27**).[3,105-110] Indications for fiberoptic tracheal intubation are summarized in **Box 36-15**.

Because normal airway architecture is maintained, fiberoptic intubation is easier in conscious patients: The tongue and epiglottis are less likely to obscure the vocal cords, and patients can assist by phonating or protruding the tongue. Haste is unnecessary in a breathing patient. The patient with a history of failed intubation, upper airway abnormality, or expected difficult intubation may benefit from an awake fiberoptic intubation. Proper topical anesthesia and sedation ease the task. With experience, topical anesthesia of the larynx and trachea may be achieved by spraying local anesthetic through the working channel of the fiberscope. Inhalation of nebulized lidocaine may minimize coughing.

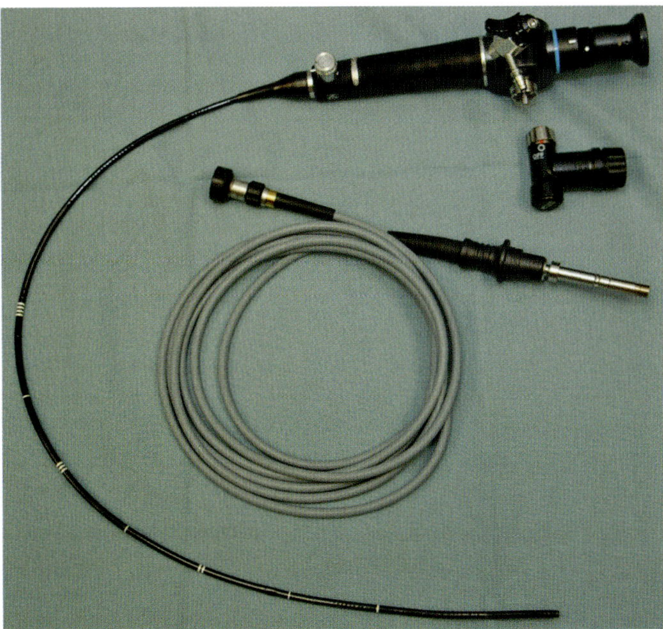

FIGURE 36-26. Olympus LF-GP bronchoscope. This bronchoscope can use a battery-powered, self-contained, or standard halogen light source.

Oral Fiberoptic Approach After applying topical anesthetic to the tongue and oropharynx, a special oropharyngeal airway is inserted to prevent biting on the fiberscope, to keep the instrument in the midline, and to restrain the tongue (**Fig. 36-28**).[3] The oropharynx is suctioned, and the lubricated ETT is placed 4 or 5 cm inside the airway. The fourth and fifth fingers of the right hand stabilize the ETT while the index finger and thumb feed the fiberscope through it (**Fig. 36-29**). If the fiberscope is accidentally passed through the Murphy eye of the ETT, intubation will not be successful even after the fiberscope is guided into the trachea.

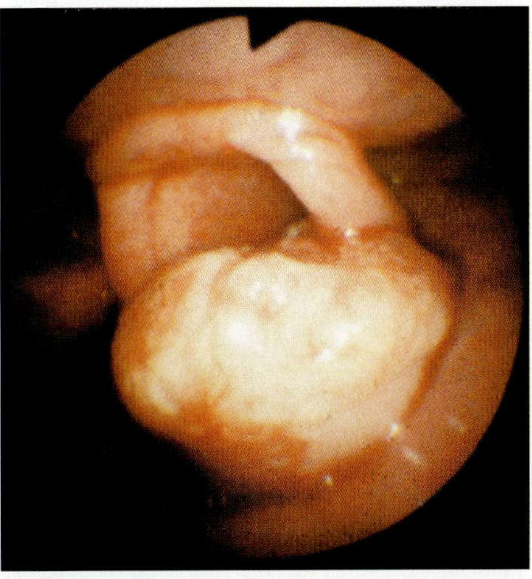

FIGURE 36-27. Advanced carcinoma of the larynx.

BOX 36-15

Indications for Fiberoptic Intubation

- Routine intubation (teaching and learning)
- Difficult intubation
  - Anticipated
    - History of previous difficult intubation
    - Physical evidence of difficult intubation
  - Unanticipated
- Compromised airway
  - Upper airway abnormality
  - Tracheal stenosis or compression
- Minimization of neck movement
  - Unstable cervical spine
  - Vertebral artery insufficiency
- High risk of dental damage
  - Poor, loose, or fragile teeth
  - Extensive dental restoration
- Awake or sedated intubation

As the fiberscope is advanced toward the oropharynx, the soft palate and uvula come into view (**Fig. 36-30**). With entry into the oropharynx, the tip is deflected anteriorly to expose the epiglottis and vocal cords. To separate a floppy epiglottis from the posterior pharyngeal wall, the head is extended at the atlanto-occipital joint and tongue traction or jaw thrust are applied. In an obese patient or one with a difficult airway, the sitting position will improve airway patency and pulmonary physiology.

After the glottis is exposed, it is maintained in the center of the field of view by fine manipulations of the control lever. The fiberscope is advanced into the midtrachea, as confirmed by a view of the carina and flat posterior wall. The ETT is slipped over the fiberscope and advanced with a twisting motion into the trachea, positioning the tip 3 to 4 cm above the carina.

In many patients, even though the fiberscope has entered the trachea, the ETT catches on laryngeal structures and cannot pass. In such a case, the ETT is pulled back and rotated 90 degrees counterclockwise until the leading edge of the bevel is oriented anteriorly. The patient is instructed to inspire deeply, abducting the vocal cords, and the tube is readvanced over the fiberscope. In some patients, this maneuver may have to be repeated 2 or 3 times, particularly when a large discrepancy exists between the size of the fiberscope and the ETT. Passage of the tube over the fiberscope into the larynx can be facilitated by using a larger fiberscope,[111] a special tube with tapered tip[112] such as the tube used to intubate through the Fastrach LMA (**Fig. 36-31**), or a Parker tube (Parker Medical, Highlands Ranch, CO). Laryngospasm also may prevent ETT advancement. Additional topical anesthesia applied through the fiberscope usually remedies this problem.

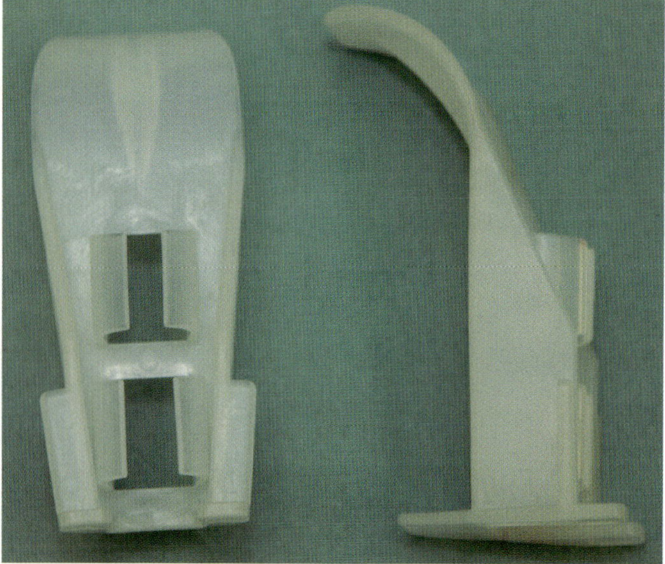

FIGURE 36-28. Ovassapian fiberoptic intubating airway. [Courtesy of Hudson RCI, Research Triangle Park, NC.]

Nasal Approach In the conscious patient, fiberoptic nasotracheal intubation often is easier than an oral approach.[3] Minimal pressure on the base of the tongue causes less gagging, and the patient cannot bite the tube. By creating a "straight shot," passing the fiberscope through the nose facilitates locating the glottis and advancing the fiberscope and tube into the larynx. A warmed, softened, lubricated tube advanced into the pharynx through a nasal passage prepared with anesthetic with or without a vasoconstrictor serves as a channel to suction the pharynx and to find the glottis with a fiberscope. Laryngeal anesthesia and intubation proceed as described for the oral approach. The gag reflex is minimized or eliminated during nasal intubation, so minimal or no oropharyngeal topical anesthesia is needed. If the tube does not easily pass from the nasopharynx to the posterior oropharynx, it is pulled back, rotated 90 degrees, and reintroduced. If this maneuver fails, the ETT is withdrawn and a lubricated fiberscope is advanced from the nasopharynx to the posterior oropharynx. The ETT is then gently advanced over the fiberscope into the oropharynx.

Passing the tube too far into the oropharynx may direct the fiberscope into the esophagus or away from the midline, preventing laryngeal exposure. The oropharynx is suctioned thoroughly through the ETT before the lubricated fiberscope is inserted through it. In most patients, the epiglottis and vocal cords are seen immediately with minimal manipulation of the fiberscope tip. In heavily sedated or edentulous patients, the tongue and pharyngeal tissues may block exposure of the glottis, necessitating head extension, jaw thrust, or tongue traction. The fiberscope is advanced into the mid trachea followed by the ETT.

Asleep Fiberoptic Intubation Fiberoptic oral and nasal intubation in an anesthetized patient requires an assistant to monitor the patient and apply jaw thrust.[3] Intubation attempts are interrupted to ventilate the patient's lungs as needed. With oral and nasal approaches, the ETT is loaded on the fiberscope before intubation is attempted. The fiberscope is then passed through the nostril or intubating airway into the mouth and advanced through the glottis into the trachea. The ETT then is advanced over the fiberscope into the trachea (**Fig. 36-32**).

Failed direct rigid laryngoscopic intubation during a rapid-sequence induction leaves the patient vulnerable to aspiration. If the patient's lungs can be ventilated via face mask, oral fiberoptic intubation with cricoid pressure is an effective technique that should be seriously considered. The ability to perform rapid fiberoptic intubation may prevent airway catastrophes. Repeated unsuccessful attempts at blind nasal intubation or rigid laryngoscopy traumatize the airway, converting a manageable airway into one that is impossible to ventilate.

In a rapid-sequence induction incorporating fiberoptic intubation, 1 assistant maintains cricoid pressure while another applies jaw thrust (**Fig. 36-33**). Excessive cricoid compression may block the endoscopist's view of the glottis by folding the epiglottis posteriorly. In this setting, it may be appropriate to gradually release cricoid pressure until the larynx is visualized.

RETROGRADE INTUBATION

In retrograde intubation, a guidewire is passed through a needle that has been percutaneously inserted into the larynx. The wire is delivered

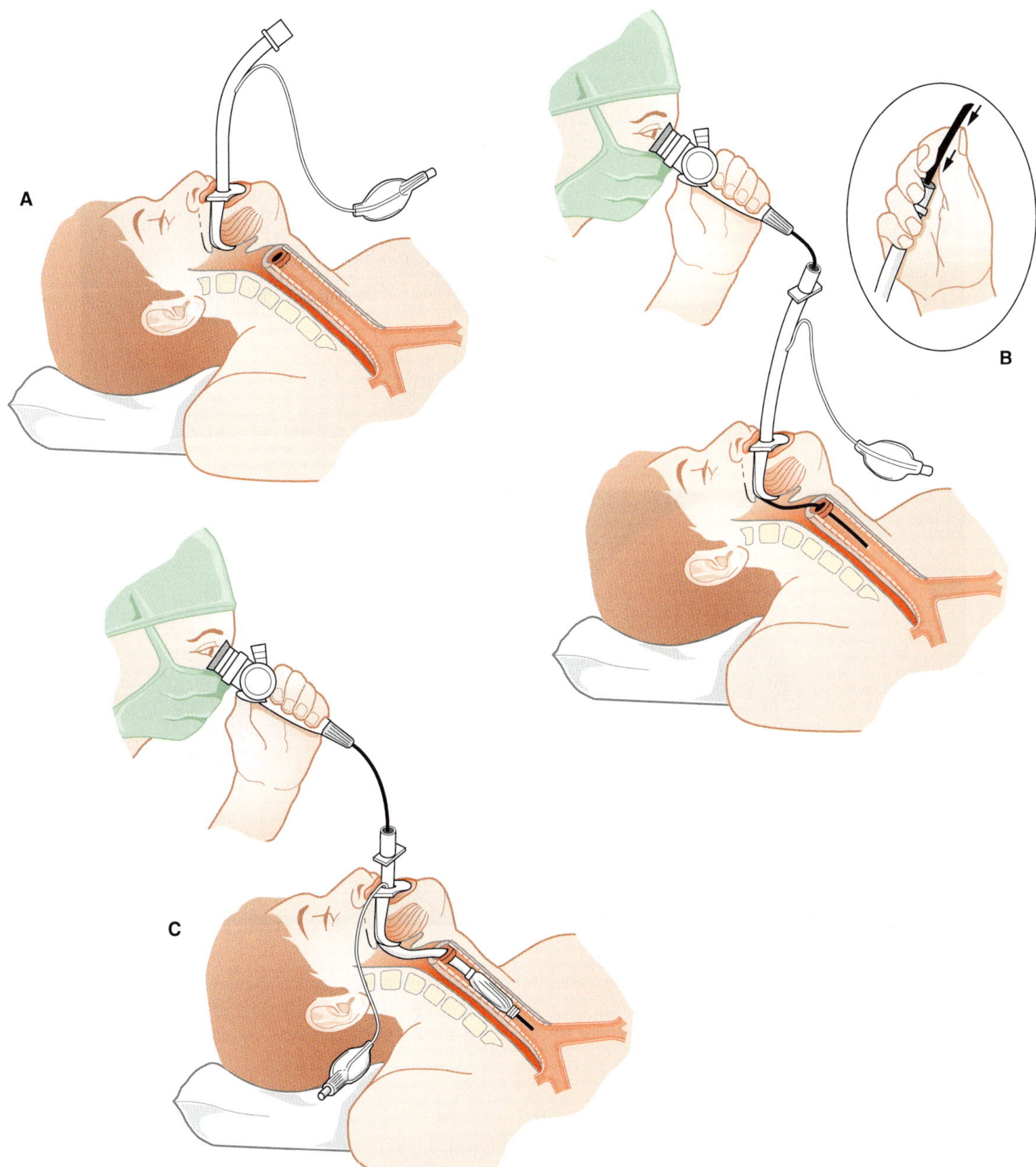

FIGURE 36-29. Fiberoptic orotracheal intubation during sedation and topical anesthesia. **A.** After sedation and application of topical anesthesia, an Ovassapian intubating airway is placed, and the oropharynx is suctioned. **B.** The endotracheal tube is removed from a warm water bath, lubricated, and placed inside the airway. The fiberscope is advanced through the endotracheal tube into the oropharynx, under the epiglottis, and inside the trachea. Care should be exercised to avoid passing the fiberscope through the Murphy eye. **C.** The endotracheal tube is passed over the fiberscope into the trachea. The distance between carina and tip of the endotracheal tube is measured using the fiberscope before it is removed. [From Ovassapian A. *Fiberoptic Endoscopy and the Difficult Airway*. 2nd ed. New York, NY: Lippincott-Raven; 1996, with permission.]

through the mouth or nose to serve as a guide for the ETT.[113-119] Dedicated kits (Cook Retrograde Intubation Set, Bloomington, IN) are available for pediatric and adult use.

The supine patient is placed in the sniffing position. Then the oropharynx, larynx, and trachea are topically anesthetized. A Touhy or other 18-gauge needle attached to a syringe containing 2 mL of lidocaine 4% is inserted into the larynx through the cricothyroid membrane in a slightly cephalad direction. Aspiration of air confirms correct placement of the needle, and the local anesthetic is injected into the larynx. The guidewire is threaded through the needle into the pharynx, and the tip is delivered through the mouth. A guide is passed over the wire, through the mouth, through the vocal cords, and into the trachea. Before the wire is removed, the ETT is advanced over the guide into the trachea (**Fig. 36-34**).

A fiberscope loaded with an ETT may be advanced over the guidewire or next to the guidewire to assist retrograde intubation.[113,115,117] A technique that involves passing the guidewire through the suction channel of the fiberscope has greatly improved the success rate of retrograde intubation.

If the larynx is entered through the cricotracheal membrane rather than the cricothyroid membrane, the ETT can be advanced farther into the larynx.[119] In this method, the cricothyroid arteries that cross the cricothyroid membrane at its proximal section are avoided.

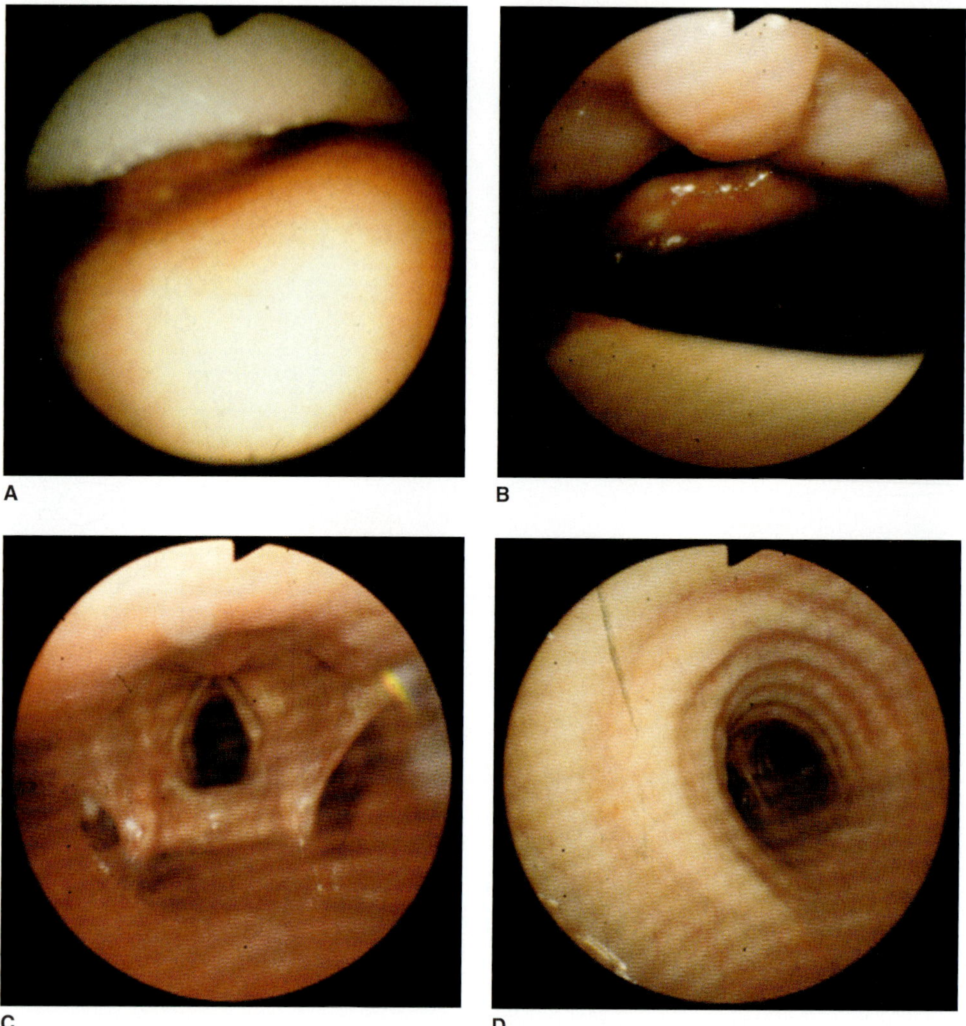

FIGURE 36-30. Endoscopic view during orotracheal intubation. **A.** As the fiberscope enters the intubating airway, the white laryngeal surface of the Ovassapian airway is seen at the top of the circle. The soft palate is visualized in the lower half of the image. **B.** When the tip of the fiberscope is advanced to the oropharynx, the epiglottis is in the center of the view. **C.** With the tip of the fiberscope passed beneath the tip of the epiglottis, the glottic opening is visualized. **D.** The tip of the fiberscope is located in the lower third of the trachea, revealing the carina.

The most common complication in the retrograde technique is bleeding in and around the airway. Bleeding usually is minor and does not require special treatment. Other complications are trauma to the airway, pneumomediastinum, and failed intubation.[120]

BLIND NASAL INTUBATION

Blind nasal intubation is a valuable technique in patients who are uncooperative, unable to open the mouth, or have a fair amount of secretions or blood in the airway.[75,121-123] The nasal mucosa is prepared with cocaine or a mixture of vasoconstrictor and local anesthetic. If sedation is needed, ketamine has been used for sedation with spontaneous ventilation or to induce general anesthesia for blind nasal intubation.[121]

The head is placed in the sniffing position, and a lubricated ETT is advanced gently into the oropharynx. If resistance is encountered at the oropharynx, the tube is pulled back about 2 cm, rotated 90 degrees, and readvanced. If the maneuver is unsuccessful, a suction catheter or a nasogastric tube passed through the ETT into the oropharynx serves as a guide. The intensity of breath sounds and bulging in the neck guide maneuvers.[122] As the tube is advanced toward the larynx, the breath sounds become louder. To help pass through the cords, the patient is encouraged to breathe deeply and rapidly, and the tube is advanced swiftly during inspiration. Successful intubation is confirmed by continued breath sounds through the tube and the patient's inability to phonate. Coughing is common when topical anesthesia is omitted.

If breath sounds stop being transmitted through the tube, the tube has not entered the trachea. It may be in the esophagus, vallecula, or one of the piriform recesses. A loss of breath sounds without resistance to passage indicates esophageal placement. In this case, the tube should be withdrawn and readvanced after further elevating and extending the patient's head. Inflating the tracheal tube cuff with 15 mL of air may accomplish the identical end.[123] The tube is advanced 1 to 3 cm before the cuff is deflated and advanced farther into the trachea. Entry into a piriform recess is corrected by withdrawal and rotation. Obstruction by the epiglottis necessitates neck flexion and jaw thrust or application of traction on the tongue.

Success rates between 86% and 97% have been reported for blind nasal intubation. Success rates in emergency room patients are approximately 90%.[124] Blind nasal intubation is less successful when the larynx is distorted by a mass, edema, or scarring from previous surgery. Contraindications to blind nasal intubation include nasal pathology, coagulopathy, thrombocytopenia, severe midface trauma, or prior transsphenoidal surgery after which an ETT may pass into the cranium.

Complications of blind nasal intubation include trauma to the nasopharyngeal mucosa, entry into the submucosal plane of the pharynx,

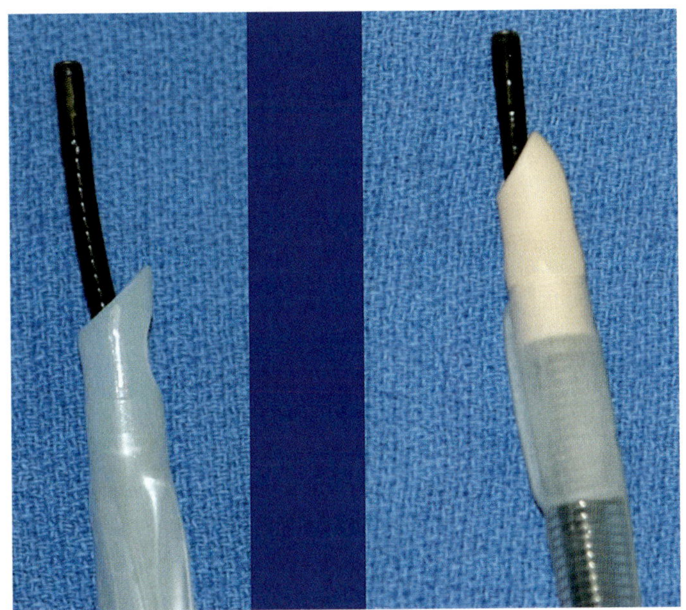

FIGURE 36-31. Endotracheal tubes over a 4.0-mm flexible bronchoscope. The tube designed for intubation through the Fastrach LMA (*right*) has a curved tip, which eases passage of the tube into the trachea.

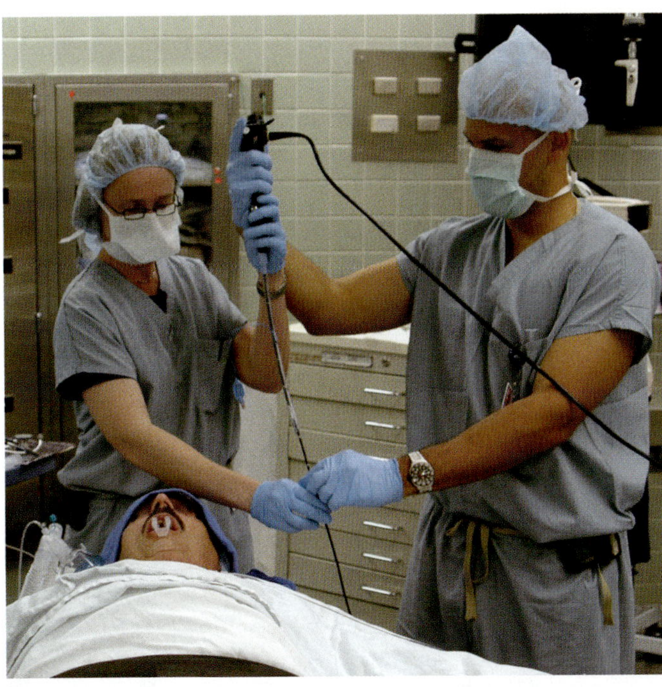

A

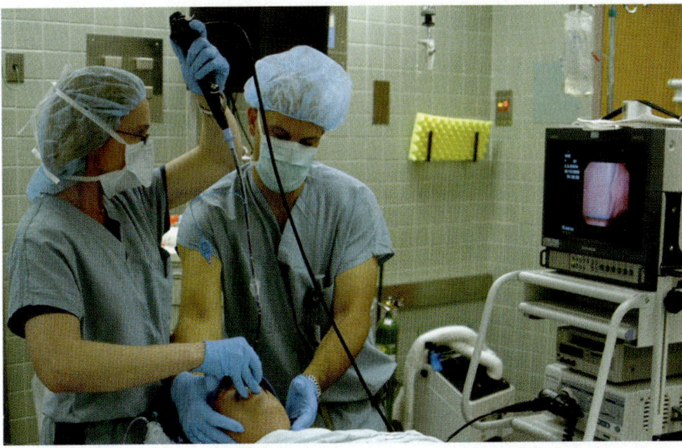

B

FIGURE 36-32. Fiberoptic orotracheal intubation during general anesthesia. **A.** The patient is paralyzed, the intubating airway is in place, and the oropharynx has been suctioned. The operator receives the fiberscope from an assistant and inserts the tip of the fiberscope inside the intubating airway. **B.** The assistant applies a jaw thrust as soon as the fiberscope has been passed to the operator. The operator looks at the monitor and advances the insertion cord through the airway and vocal cords into the trachea. The tube is rotated 45 to 90 degrees counterclockwise if resistance is encountered during advancement through the vocal cords. Note the position of the endoscopist's right hand.

dislodging nasal polyps, pushing foreign bodies into the larynx, and nasal bleeding.[122,124] Difficulty advancing the tracheal tube into the oropharynx may be the result of a deviated septum, a turbinate spur, hypertrophied inferior turbinates, or nasopharyngeal lymph nodes. A smaller tube or use of the other nostril may remedy these problems.

INTUBATION THROUGH A LARYNGEAL MASK AIRWAY

The LMA can be used to manage a "cannot intubate, cannot ventilate" situation or to facilitate tracheal intubation.[125-132] There are 3 distinct techniques for tracheal intubation through a classic or unique LMA: blind passage of a 6.0-mm inner diameter or smaller ETT,[131] blind insertion of a guide to facilitate the threading of a large ETT after LMA removal,[130] or fiberoptic-assisted tracheal intubation through the LMA.[63,129,132] With perfect LMA position, the aperture lies opposite the glottic inlet for blind insertion of an ETT or guide. When the epiglottis partially blocks the laryngeal inlet, fiberoptic assistance is needed. The Aintree intubation catheter (Cook Critical Care, Bloomington, IN), which is 56 cm long with a 4.7 mm internal diameter, is specifically designed to facilitate intubation when an LMA is in place. A fiberoptic bronchoscope is placed through the catheter. The fiberscope and catheter are then directed through the LMA into the trachea. Leaving the Aintree catheter in place, the fiberoptic scope is removed, and then the LMA is removed over the catheter. The trachea is intubated over the catheter.

If rescue intubation is attempted by passing an ETT blindly through a classic LMA, it is important to remember that the distance from LMA aperture bars to the vocal cords is 3.5 cm.[133] If the length of a 6-mm ETT is limited to 26 cm, the cuff of the ETT will be positioned inside the larynx just millimeters beyond the vocal cords, which increases the possibility of a laryngeal nerve palsy.

The LMA Fastrach is an SGA device designed to aid endotracheal intubation. It can serve as a primary airway, but its primary purpose is to serve as a conduit for endotracheal intubation. Blind endotracheal intubation with the LMA Fastrach is successful 96.5% of the time. One study of high-risk airway patients showed that using a flexible fiberoptic bronchoscope in conjunction with an intubating LMA produced a 100% success rate for tracheal intubation.[63]

Properly positioning the LMA Fastrach facilitates introduction of an ETT into the trachea, but suboptimal positioning can result in failure. The Chandy maneuver is a 2-step technique used to improve position of the Fastrach before using it for blind intubation.[63] The first step of the Chandy maneuver uses the device's metal handle for rotation in the sagittal plane until ventilation is optimized. In the second part of the Chandy maneuver, the Fastrach is lifted to displace it anteriorly away from the posterior pharyngeal wall. The second part of the Chandy maneuver is applied as the ETT is advanced through the device.[63]

Correct position is important for success during LMA Fastrach–assisted endotracheal intubation, but the type of ETT is also a consideration. The manufacturer produces a reusable, reinforced ETT for use

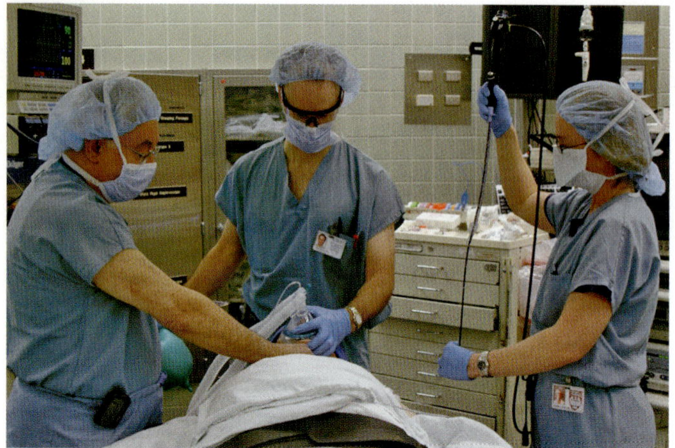

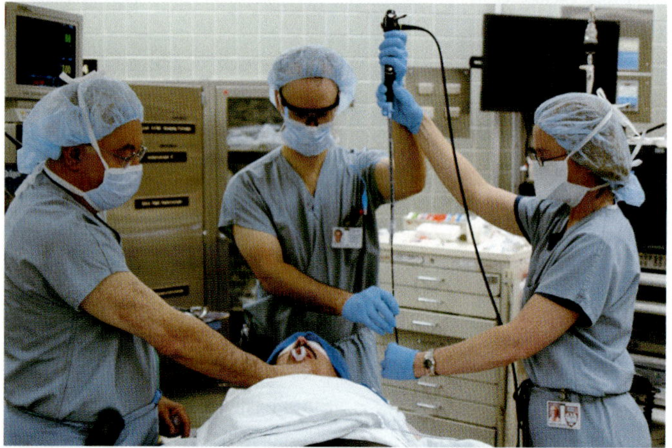

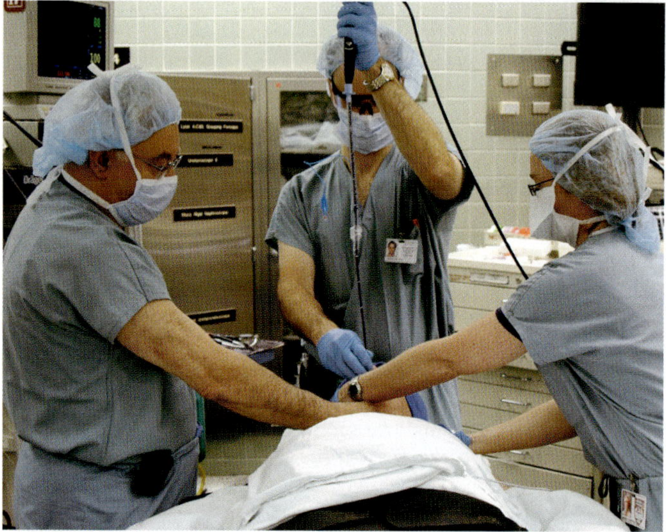

FIGURE 36-33. Fiberoptically aided rapid sequence induction and intubation. The first assistant on the right side of the operator applies cricoid pressure before induction of anesthesia. The second assistant on the left of the operator administers the induction agents, passes the fiberscope to the operator, and then applies jaw thrust.

with the LMA Fastrach. The Fastrach ETT is made of silicone with a blunted tip, features that help with its smooth introduction into the trachea. Standard PVC ETTs can be used with the LMA Fastrach, but their rigid design and sharper bevel increase the risk of resistance or injury during blind intubation. A comparison of the manufacturer's ETTs and standard PVC ETTs during blind intubation via the Fastrach showed better success with the silicone Fastrach ETT even when the standard ETTs were rotated on advancement to avoid bevel impact on glottic structures.[64] Another study evaluating Fastrach-assisted blind endotracheal intubation found similar success rates with the manufacturer's silicone ETT and a warmed PVC ETT.[65] Reverse loading of a standard ETT, so that the curve of the tube points posteriorly, has been reported to increase first attempt success at blind intubation with the LMA Fastrach, although overall success was the same with a traditionally loaded standard ETT.[66] The unique ability to establish ventilation in an unanticipated difficult mask ventilation, coupled with a mechanism to definitively secure the airway, makes the LMA Fastrach a strong addition to the airway management arsenal.

CRICOTHYROTOMY AND TRACHEOSTOMY

Surgical airway access through the anterior neck is indicated in patients with severe upper airway obstruction or failed tracheal intubation combined with impossible ventilation. Cricothyrotomy involves entering the larynx through the cricothyroid membrane to pass a small ETT or a special cricothyrotomy tube into the trachea. Cricothyrotomy is preferred to tracheostomy when an airway must be established promptly. Cricothyrotomy is faster, easier to perform, and is farther away from the mediastinum than a tracheostomy. Several kits are available for percutaneous cricothyrotomy, including the Melker cricothyrotomy system, (Cook Critical Care, Bloomington, IN). Applying the Seldinger technique for cricothyrotomy is familiar for nonsurgeons treating a patient with a difficult airway.[134] Cricothyrotomy usually is performed during emergency situations and under less-than-optimal conditions, which increases the chances for laryngeal injury. After the patient's condition is stabilized, the wound and the larynx should be examined.

PERCUTANEOUS TRANSTRACHEAL VENTILATION

Placement of a large-bore catheter through the cricothyroid membrane (needle cricothyrotomy) into the trachea gives rapid access to the airway and can be lifesaving when mask ventilation and tracheal intubation have failed.[135-137] Percutaneous transtracheal jet ventilation is also an interim means of oxygenation during difficult intubation.[136]

The incidence of malfunctioning of thin-walled 16- or 14-gauge IV catheters caused by kinking or dislodgement is high and can cause major complications. This problem is more likely to happen with an awake, struggling patient. The Arndt emergency cricothyrotomy catheter set (Cook Critical Care, Bloomingdale, IN) may minimize these problems. The set features a 3-mm kink-resistant catheter with a 15-mm connector coaxially positioned over a Luer lock connector. A hollow, tapered-tip dilator assists the placement of the catheter into the trachea. After it is in place, the airway catheter and its 15-mm connector may be attached to the common gas outlet of the anesthesia machine, self-inflating resuscitating breathing bag (Ambu bag) or directly to a jet ventilator through the Luer lock connector. The relatively large tracheal catheter is effective for high-pressure jet ventilation. Bag-valve manual ventilation delivers oxygen but is ineffective for ventilation with a progressive increase in CO_2 concentration.

Rupture of the lungs may produce a pneumomediastinum, pneumothorax, or other serious complications. In the event of total upper airway obstruction, percutaneous transtracheal jet ventilation requires that an exit airway be established. The technique can cause barotrauma, including pneumothorax; pneumomediastinum; or injury to the larynx, trachea, and esophagus. Inadequate time for exhalation or inability of gas to escape can lead to "breath stacking" or pulmonary tamponade. The resultant impairment of venous return can lead to hypotension and even pulseless electrical activity similar to that seen with a tension

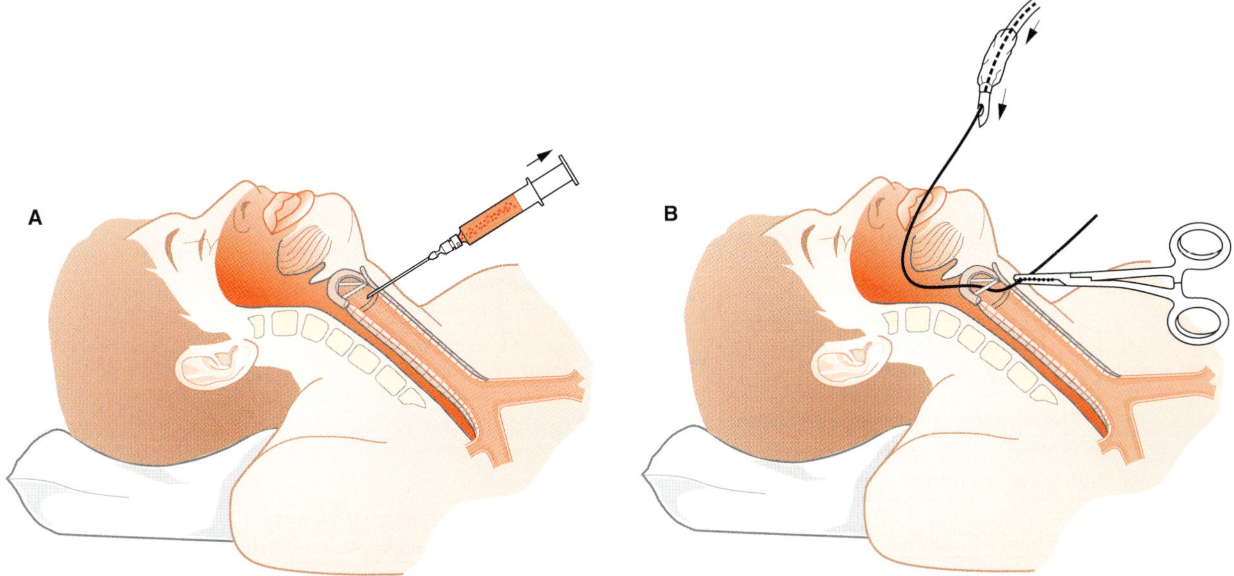

FIGURE 36-34. Retrograde intubation. **A.** A needle attached to a syringe filled with lidocaine is passed through the cricothyroid membrane into the larynx. Free aspiration of air confirms correct placement of the needle. Lidocaine is injected to provide topical anesthesia of the airway. **B.** The guidewire is passed into the needle, retrograde through the larynx, and up into the oropharynx. The guidewire is retrieved through the mouth using a hook or forceps. The endotracheal tube is advanced over the guidewire into the trachea. [From Ovassapian A. *Fiberoptic Endoscopy and the Difficult Airway*. 2nd ed. New York, NY: Lippincott-Raven; 1996, with permission.]

pneumothorax. It is prudent to practice the technique first on a mannequin and then during controlled patient care conditions before applying it to emergency situations.

CARE AFTER TRACHEAL INTUBATION

CONFIRMATION OF TRACHEAL INTUBATION

While visually observing the position of the ETT between the vocal cords after passage is a reliable indicator of tracheal intubation, it is not sufficient to meet the standard of care. Immediately after intubation, the cuff is inflated, and the anesthesiologist should observe the sequential rise and fall of the chest while auscultating over each mid-axillary line and the epigastrium for assurance that the trachea, not the esophagus or bronchi, has been intubated.[138] Because breath sounds have misled even skilled clinicians, the intraoperative monitoring standards of the ASA mandate that tracheal intubation be confirmed by detecting consistent levels of exhaled CO_2 in successive breaths.[29,30] CO_2 can be sampled while the esophagus is ventilated, but its exhaled concentration declines after a few breaths (**Fig. 36-35**).[30] During circulatory shock, exhaled CO_2 levels may be low despite proper tracheal tube position. If there is no sustained CO_2 and the patient has a perfusing rhythm, the tracheal tube is removed, and the lungs are ventilated by mask, particularly if the risk of aspirating gastric contents is low.

The self-inflating bulb (Ambu TubeChek B, Ambu Inc., Glen Burnie, MD) relies on anatomy rather than the physiology of CO_2 in exhaled gases. The device is similar to a "turkey baster" used in many kitchens. The bulb is collapsed and applied to the end of the ETT. The device will reinflate within 5 seconds if the tube is in the trachea but should remain collapsed if the tube is in the esophagus. (**Fig. 36-36**).[139,140]

The ideal position for the tip of an ETT is 3 to 4 cm above the carina. For an average-sized woman, the ETT should be taped with the teeth at the 21-cm mark. For most men, 23 cm at the upper incisors is the appropriate depth. Nasotracheal tubes should be inserted 3 cm deeper.

MAINTAINING THE TRACHEAL TUBE

To avoid tracheal mucosal ischemia, many clinicians inflate the cuff until there is a small audible leak at peak airway pressure. During prolonged intubation, regular checks are conducted to prevent overinflation. Tracheal tubes usually are secured with adhesive tape. Tincture of benzoin, Mastisol (Ferndale Pharma Group, Ferndale, MI), or other

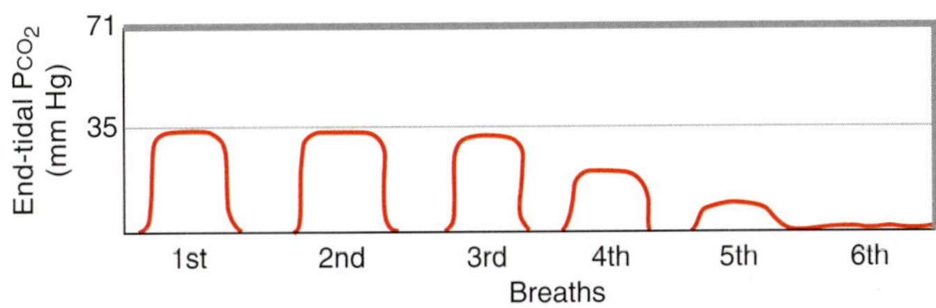

FIGURE 36-35. CO_2 waveform after esophageal intubation. The first 3 breaths may look like normal waves but will decrease in amplitude quickly. With tracheal intubation, the CO_2 level remains constant. [From Sum Ping ST. Esophageal intubation [letter]. *Anesth Analg.* 1987;66:483, with permission.]

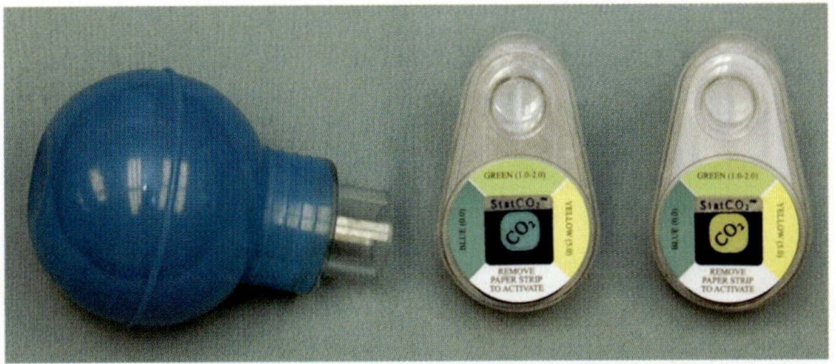

FIGURE 36-36. Left, self-inflating bulb fitted with a standard 15-mm adapter used as an esophageal detector device. Middle, disposable CO_2 detector showing the green color change to yellow color (*right*) with CO_2 exposure.

DIFFICULT AIRWAY INTUBATION

1. Assess the likelihood and clinical impact of basic management problems:
   - A. Difficult Ventilation
   - B. Diffcult Intubation
   - C. Difficulty With Patient Cooperation or Consent
   - D. Difficult Tracheostomy
2. Actively pursue opportunities to deliver supplemental oxygen throughout the process of difficult airway management
3. Consider the relative merits and feasibility of basic management choices:

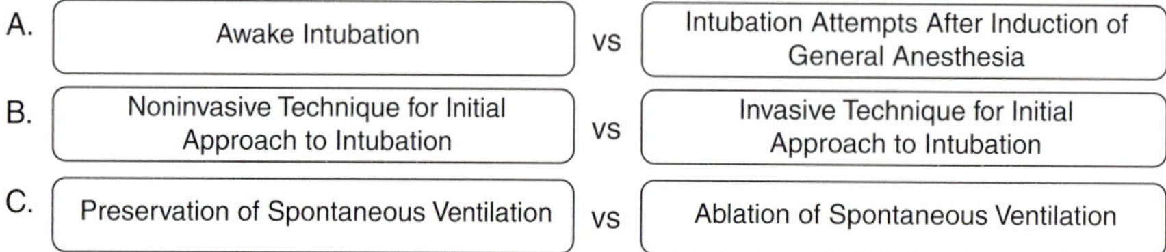

4. Develop primary and alternative strategies:

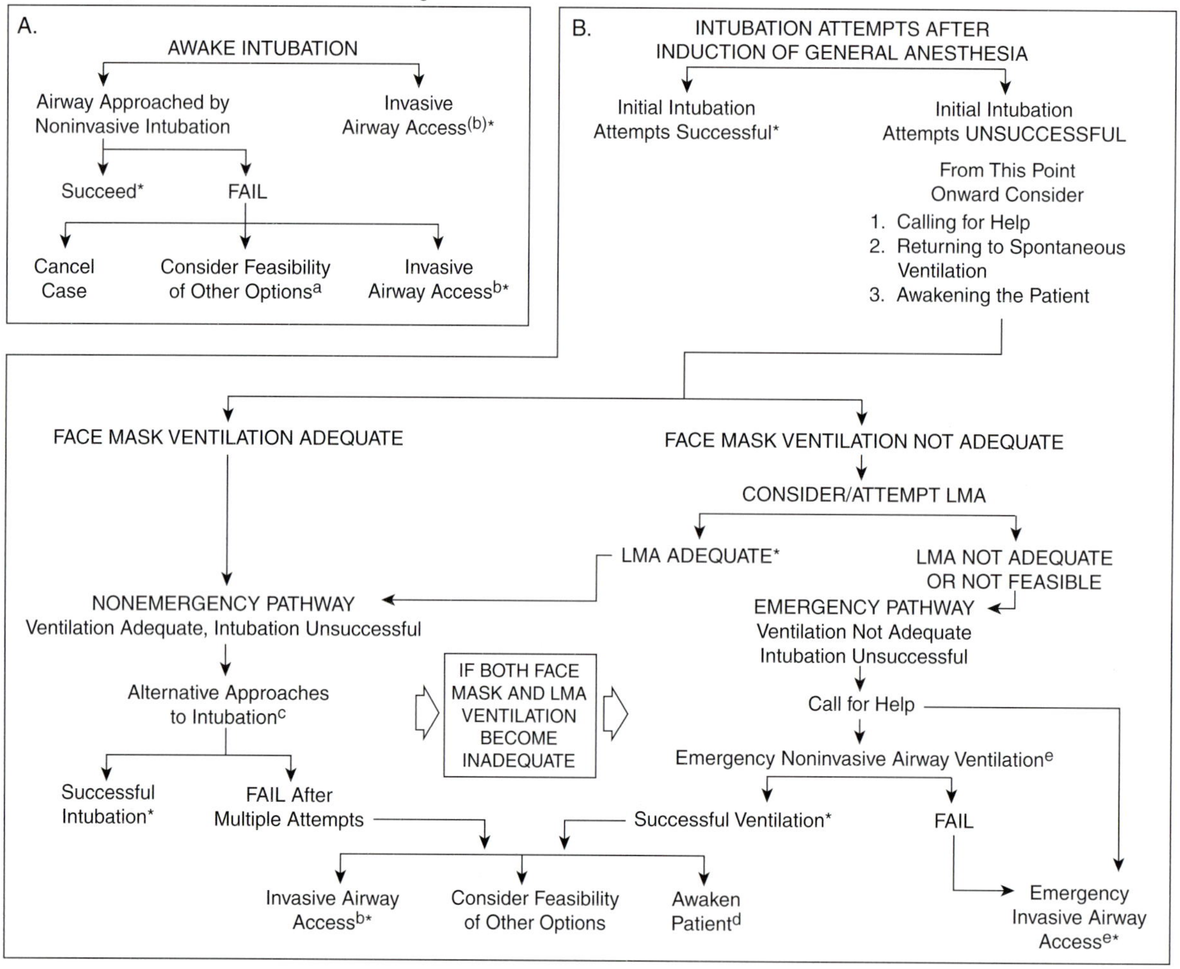

A.
AWAKE INTUBATION
Airway Approached by Noninvasive Intubation
Invasive Airway Access(b)*
Succeed*
FAIL
Cancel Case
Consider Feasibility of Other Options[a]
Invasive Airway Access[b]*

B.
INTUBATION ATTEMPTS AFTER INDUCTION OF GENERAL ANESTHESIA
Initial Intubation Attempts Successful*
Initial Intubation Attempts UNSUCCESSFUL
From This Point Onward Consider
1. Calling for Help
2. Returning to Spontaneous Ventilation
3. Awakening the Patient

FACE MASK VENTILATION ADEQUATE
FACE MASK VENTILATION NOT ADEQUATE
CONSIDER/ATTEMPT LMA
LMA ADEQUATE*
LMA NOT ADEQUATE OR NOT FEASIBLE
NONEMERGENCY PATHWAY
Ventilation Adequate, Intubation Unsuccessful
Alternative Approaches to Intubation[c]
Successful Intubation*
FAIL After Multiple Attempts
IF BOTH FACE MASK AND LMA VENTILATION BECOME INADEQUATE
EMERGENCY PATHWAY
Ventilation Not Adequate
Intubation Unsuccessful
Call for Help
Emergency Noninvasive Airway Ventilation[e]
Successful Ventilation*
FAIL
Invasive Airway Access[b]*
Consider Feasibility of Other Options
Awaken Patient[d]
Emergency Invasive Airway Access[e]*

*Confirm ventilation, tracheal intubation, or LMA placement with exhaled CO_2.

a. Other options include (but are not limited to): surgery utilizing face mask or LMA anesthesia, local anesthesia infiltration, or regional nerve blockade. Pursuit of these options usually implies that mask ventilation will not be problematic. Therefore, these options may be of limited value if this step in the algorithm has been reached via the Emergency Pathway.

b. Invasive airway access includes surgical or percutaneous tracheostomy or cricothyrotomy.

c. Alternative noninvasive approaches to diffcult intubation include (but are not limited to): use of different laryngoscopic blades, LMA as an intubation conduit (with or without fiberoptic guidance), fiberoptic intubation, intubating stylet or tube changer, light wand, retrograde intubation, and blind oral or nasal intubation.

d. Consider repreparation of the patient for awake intubation or canceling surgery.

e. Options for emergency noninvasive airway ventilation include (but are not limited to): rigid bronchoscope, esophageal-bracheal Combitube ventilation, or transtracheal jet ventilation.

FIGURE 36-37. The American Society of Anesthesiologist's difficult airway algorithm. LMA, laryngeal mask airway. [From Practice guidelines for management of the difficult airway: an updated report by the American Society of Anesthesiologists Task Force on Management of the Difficult Airway. *Anesthesiology*. 2003;98:1269-1277.]

skin adhesives may improve stability. An oropharyngeal airway or roll of gauze sponges placed between the teeth keeps the patient from biting the tube. Nasotracheal tubes should be taped securely without putting pressure on the nares. The position of the tube is verified each time the patient's position changes.

MANAGING THE DIFFICULT AIRWAY AND THE AMERICAN SOCIETY OF ANESTHESIOLOGISTS DIFFICULT AIRWAY ALGORITHM

The lungs of patients who are difficult to intubate often can be ventilated by face mask. When intubation has failed but ventilation is adequate, the anesthesiologist should weigh the available options to ensure that each new maneuver represents a logical, substantive change from steps that have failed. Repeated rigid laryngoscopy causes bleeding and rapidly evolving airway edema that frustrates subsequent attempts and may render mask ventilation impossible.[125] It is therefore essential to anticipate patients at risk for difficult intubation or mask ventilation so they can benefit from a controlled awake or sedated intubation. Proper preparation includes optimal positioning, thorough denitrogenation, glycopyrrolate pretreatment, and the presence of proper tools and personnel. Only 2 or 3 rigid laryngoscopy attempts generally are indicated before changing techniques.[2,3,125] A simple algorithm for tracheal intubation after 2 attempts at direct laryngoscopy with a Macintosh blade and fiberoptic intubation had a 99.96% success rate when both techniques were incorporated in daily use.[141] Allowing an anesthetized patient to awaken or maintaining or resuming spontaneous ventilation may be the wisest course. Experienced assistance is invaluable.

Morbidity and mortality surrounding airway management prompted the ASA to convene the Difficult Airway Task Force to develop a management algorithm (**Fig. 36-37**).[125] Subsequent to the publication of the ASA guidelines, other organizations have published guidelines for airway management.[142]

Key features of the ASA guidelines include 3 management choices made before the initiating the anesthetic: Should the airway be secured with the patient awake or after induction of general anesthesia? Should the initial technique be noninvasive, or should it include invasive elements? Should spontaneous ventilation be maintained or abolished? If problems are encountered after the induction of general anesthesia, the algorithm distinguishes between difficult ventilation (life threatening) and difficult intubation (rarely life threatening). In the 2003 revision of the guidelines, the LMA was mentioned as a means to establish or maintain ventilation and oxygenation and to facilitate intubation.

Because any patient may unexpectedly prove difficult to intubate or ventilate, proper denitrogenation before inducing general anesthesia should be routine. Maintaining skills at techniques of ventilation without tracheal intubation and mastering a variety of methods for tracheal intubation are a must for every anesthesiologist.[2,3] Each anesthetizing location should have rapid access to a difficult airway cart, including equipment to deal with a cannot intubate, cannot ventilate scenario.

EXTUBATING THE TRACHEA

THE ROUTINE AIRWAY

Extubation of an easily intubated patient who did not undergo airway surgery is performed as soon as extubation criteria are met (**Box 36-16**).[12,23,75] Breath holding and coughing elevate pulse, blood pressure, intracranial pressure, and intraocular pressure (**Box 36-17**).[143,144] IV lidocaine and esmolol are popular adjuncts to minimize coughing and the cardiovascular responses to laryngeal stimulation by the ETT during emergence from anesthesia.[45,145]

BOX 36-16

Tracheal Extubation in Patients With Uncomplicated Airways

Criteria for extubation

No ongoing indication to keep the patient intubated

Spontaneous ventilation is adequate

Muscle relaxant is fully reversed (demonstrated with strong 5-second head lift)

Airway reflexes are recovered

Patient follows commands

Technique of extubation

Suction oropharynx before patient is reactive.

Administer 100% oxygen until end-tidal level plateaus.

Remove tape.

Deflate the cuff.

Apply positive pressure to the breathing bag and gently remove the tracheal tube.

Suction again if secretions are present.

Apply mask with high-flow oxygen.

Check for airway patency and adequacy of ventilation.

BOX 36-17

Complications Related to Extubation

During extubation

Hypertension, tachycardia, arrhythmias, electrocardiographic ST-segment changes

Coughing, breath holding, cyanosis

Difficult extubation

Postextubation

- Laryngospasm
- Airway obstruction
  - Soft tissue obstruction
  - Laryngeal edema
  - Edema of stenotic trachea
  - Vocal cord malfunction
    - Bilateral palsy
    - Unilateral palsy
    - Dysfunctional vocal cords (paradoxical adduction during inspiration)
  - External compression
    - Hematoma
    - Bleeding
  - Laryngotracheomalacia
- Negative pressure pulmonary edema
- Aspiration of gastric contents
- Ventilatory depression
- Laryngeal incompetence
- Dysphonia, aphonia
- Dislocation of arytenoid
- Laryngotracheal stenosis
- Sore throat

Extubation of the trachea during deep anesthesia minimizes the cardiovascular response,[146,147] although ventilatory depression, upper airway obstruction, and difficulty with mask ventilation may be problematic. In patients who were difficult to intubate or in those at high risk of aspiration, extubation during deep anesthesia usually is contraindicated. Even properly treated patients with asthma tolerate conscious extubation.

Laryngospasm and airway obstruction are common after extubation, especially in children.[148] Although a patient with mild laryngeal spasm may have stridor, a severe episode results in complete airway obstruction and silence. To manage laryngeal spasm, positive pressure is applied with oxygen, oropharyngeal secretions are suctioned, and jaw thrust is applied. In patients with severe episodes, IV succinylcholine, 0.1 mg/kg, relieves the spasm for mask ventilation without causing apnea.[149] On rare occasions, reintubation may be necessary.

Laryngeal edema should be suspected when postextubation inspiratory stridor develops within 30 to 60 minutes after extubation.[150] Laryngeal edema caused by intubation is uncommon in adults. Overhydration, prolonged Trendelenburg position, and an allergic reaction to medications given before or during surgery should be considered. Management includes maintaining the head-up position, providing humidified oxygen, inhaled racemic epinephrine, IV dexamethasone, and possible reintubation.

Acute pulmonary edema may complicate tracheal extubation when severe airway obstruction coexists with vigorous spontaneous attempts at inspiration.[151,152] The negative intrathoracic pressure and possibly associated hypoxemia contribute to the development of pulmonary edema. Management consists of relieving the obstruction and administering supplemental oxygen while the congestion resolves. Tracheomalacia caused by thyroid disease may obstruct the airway after extubation.[153]

THE DIFFICULT AIRWAY

A 2005 closed claims analysis showed that since the introduction of the ASA practice guidelines for management of difficult airways in 1993, there has been a reduction in airway-related claims associated with the induction of anesthesia. There has been no change, however, in the rate of claims for airway misadventures during the maintenance, emergence, or recovery from an anesthetic. The authors call for the development of additional management strategies during these phases.[154]

Patients who are difficult to intubate, who have had major head and neck operations, or in whom airway access is restricted are at high risk after extubation. Proper timing of extubation, equipment availability, and the presence of a skilled anesthesiologist are vital for safe extubation of these patients. Should emergent reintubation be required, these patients are likely to be hypoxic, hypercarbic, and uncooperative, with gastric distension from failed ventilatory attempts or prior application of a continuous positive airway pressure device (**Box 36-18**).[127,155,156]

Extubation may proceed more easily if these patients are extubated when fully awake and after edema or hematoma has resolved. The presence of a leak around a deflated ETT cuff usually predicts that glottic edema will not complicate extubation in adult patients. Under most circumstances, the patient should be extubated after a negative cuff leak test result.[78] If the patient does not have a leak around a deflated cuff or if other risk factors are present, consideration should be given to extubating or over an introducer, fiberscope, or jet stylet.[157-162] A jet stylet, airway exchange catheter, or bougie may be left in the trachea to facilitate reintubation.[157-161] If reintubation fails, the hollow device can be used to oxygenate and ventilate the patient's lungs.[157-159] The jet stylet can be positioned in the lower trachea using the centimeter markings along its length. Side holes placed along its distal 5 cm prevent tissue trauma from catheter whip during jet ventilation.[158] If the anesthesiologist is confident that the subglottic larynx will not be obstructed, an LMA or similar device may be placed in the hypopharynx before extubation to reduce the risk of upper airway obstruction and serve as bridge to full extubation[163,164] (**Fig. 36-38**).

BOX 36-18

Challenges of Immediate Reintubation

Known difficult airway
Surgical distortion
Limited access
Edema
Uncooperative, combative patient
Emergent nature
Blood and secretions
Hematoma
Cervical immobilization or instability
Maxillomandibular fixation
Head and neck dressing
Halo vest
Inadequate experience
Difficult mask ventilation
Risk of aspiration
Poor oxygenation and ventilation
Poor topical anesthesia as a result of secretions
Residual nondepolarizing neuromuscular blocker or reversal agent
Occurrence during transportation
Unavailability of equipment

THE DIFFICULT EXTUBATION

Iatrogenic causes and mechanical failure on rare occasion can render extubation difficult or impossible.[161,165-168] Extubation may be difficult in patients with laryngeal abnormalities and those biting the ETT. Difficult extubation with a deflated cuff has been reported when the ETT tube

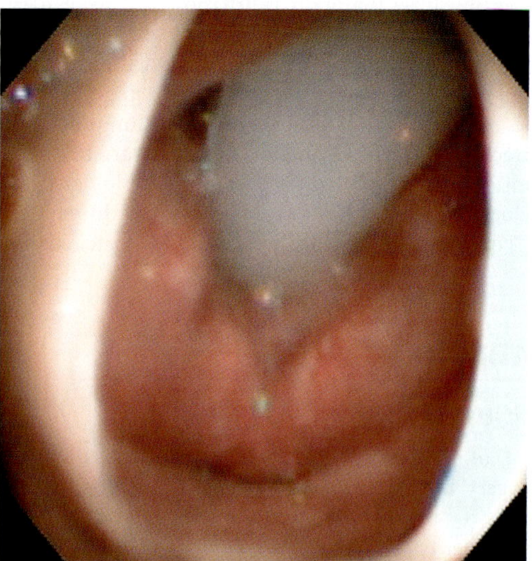

FIGURE 36-38. Endoscopic view of the LMA (laryngeal mask airway) Classic positioned behind the endotracheal tube.

BOX 36-19

Complications of Tracheal Intubation

Physiologic responses to laryngotracheal stimulation

Cardiovascular

Tachycardia, hypertension, myocardial ischemia

Reflex bradycardia

Bronchospasm and bronchorrhea

Intracranial hypertension

Intraocular hypertension or extrusion of vitreous humor

Trauma

Abrasion of the cornea

Lacerations of lips, gums, tongue, or pharynx

Epistaxis

Perforation of pharyngeal or esophageal mucosa

Chipping or avulsion of teeth or dental appliances

Persisting subluxation of the mandible

Laryngotracheal penetration with subcutaneous emphysema

Pneumothorax

Injury to the vocal cords and arytenoid cartilages

Tube malposition

Prolonged or failed intubation

Insufficient insertion

Bronchial intubation

Airway foreign bodies

Teeth

Laryngoscope bulb

Stylet

During tracheal tube maintenance

Unintended extubation

Obstruction

Unrecognized disconnection

Changes in position

With extubation

Physiologic responses (same as previous)

Difficult or impossible extubation

Laryngeal spasm

Negative pressure pulmonary edema

Common sequelae of a mild nature and lasting <48 hours

Hoarseness

Sore throat

Complications of prolonged intubation

Infections

Laryngotracheobronchitis

Sinusitis

Pneumonia

Laryngeal ulceration

Vocal cord granuloma

Tracheomalacia

Tracheal stenosis

Vocal cord paralysis

cuff folds below the vocal cords or from laryngeal edema after a difficult intubation. Persistent fixation of the tracheal tube with surgical wires, sutures, and screws also has been reported.[165]

FOLLOW-UP OF A DIFFICULT AIRWAY

For safe airway management in the future, patients with proven difficult airways should be identified and informed of the difficulty. Immediate application of a temporary wristband or flagging the medical record alerts health care providers to the special requirements of these patients.

A written statement with pertinent airway management information is given to the patient, with a copy filed in the patient's medical record. For future reference and availability of information for other health care organizations, the patient with a difficult airway can be enrolled in the Medic Alert Difficult Airway/Intubation Registry.[169]

COMPLICATIONS OF INTUBATION

The difficulties and complications of tracheal intubation arise from the act of intubation itself, maintenance of the ETT, or extubation (**Box 36-19**).[6,170-175] A closed claims analysis found that the larynx, pharynx, and esophagus are the most common sites of airway injuries. Pharyngoesophageal perforation injuries were the most severe. Early signs of perforation were found in only 51% of the claims. The authors of the analysis recommend extended observation of patients in whom tracheal intubation has been difficult. Patients should be instructed to watch for signs and symptoms of retropharyngeal abscess, mediastinitis, or both.[172]

KEY REFERENCES

- American Society of Anesthesiologists Task Force on Management of the Difficult Airway. Practice guidelines for management of the difficult airway: an updated report by the American Society of Anesthesiologists Task Force on Management of the Difficult Airway. *Anesthesiology.* 2003;98:1269.
- Asai T, Morris S. The laryngeal mask airway: its features, effects and role. *Can J Anaesth.* 1994;41:930.
- Benumof JL. Management of the difficult airway: with special emphasis on awake tracheal intubation. *Anesthesiology.* 1991;75:1087.
- Birmingham PK, Cheney FW, Ward RJ. Esophageal intubation: a review of detection techniques. *Anesth Analg.* 1986;65:886.
- Caplan RA, Posner KL, Ward RJ, et al. Adverse respiratory events in anesthesia: a closed claims analysis. *Anesthesiology.* 1990;72:828.
- Finucane BT, Tsui BCH, Santora AH. *Principles of Airway Management.* 4th ed. New York, NY: Springer; 2011.
- Hagberg CA. *Benumof's Airway Management: Principles and Practice.* 2nd ed. Philadelphia, PA: Mosby Elsevier; 2007.
- Hartley M, Vaughan RS. Problems associated with tracheal extubation. *Br J Anaesth.* 1993;71:561.
- Ovassapian A. *Fiberoptic Endoscopy and the Difficult Airway.* 2nd ed. New York, NY: Lippincott-Raven; 1996.

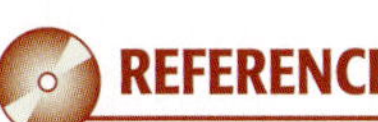

REFERENCES

Complete references available on DVD and online version at www.LongneckerAnesthesiology.com

SECTION C

Anesthesia Drugs and Drug Delivery Systems

CHAPTER 37 Mechanisms of General Anesthetic Action

Max B. Kelz
Slobodan M. Todorovic
Roderic G. Eckenhoff

KEY POINTS

1. The mechanisms by which the inhaled general anesthetics work are not fully understood. No single molecular target has been proven to transduce anesthesia.
2. Correlation of the physicochemical character of anesthetics with their potency suggests that target sites are dominantly hydrophobic, with a small degree of polarity and chirality. Internal or interfacial protein cavities best fit this description.
3. Inhaled anesthetic binding site character is not highly specific, predicting more than a few anesthetic binding targets. The interaction at some of these targets may not contribute significantly to anesthetic action but may contribute to side effects.
4. Use of the lipid membrane as a direct target for inhaled anesthetics has been dismissed prematurely. Some components of anesthetic action may occur via this interaction.
5. Many potential protein targets in the synapse have been identified, suggesting that inhaled anesthetic action results from disruption of the specific process of synaptic transmission rather than from a receptor-like interaction with a single molecular target.
6. Anesthetic effects on a process, such as synaptic transmission, may have a different system-level effect depending on placement in the neural circuitry. The circuits that regulate sleep and arousal are well positioned to mediate the hypnotic properties of anesthetics.

General anesthetics were formally introduced into medical practice more than 160 years ago and have been hailed as one of the most significant medical advances of all time. Yet there is still considerable mystery about how the drugs work and how to characterize the state that they produce. This should not be too surprising because a description of the transition from consciousness to unconsciousness necessarily requires an understanding of the former, and the neurobiology of consciousness is still in its infancy. Nevertheless, considerable progress has been made toward the characterization of anesthesia and the potential mechanisms of the drugs that produce it. In this chapter, we summarize the current body of evidence for the mechanism(s) of general anesthesia, with emphasis on the inhaled anesthetics because they are used most commonly. Excellent and comprehensive reviews summarize current knowledge of the molecular, cellular, and in vivo pharmacology,[1,2] so we have selected only a few of the putative molecular targets to illustrate the principles and to support the notion that alteration of a neurophysiologic process, rather than the activity of an individual protein, is responsible for the state of general anesthesia.

GENERAL ANESTHESIA

Mechanistic searches are greatly aided by clear physiologic or behavioral endpoints. Those associated with anesthesia, however, often are ambiguous and arbitrary. Most people associate anesthesia with unconsciousness or "sleep," but the transition to this state often is not apparent to the observer, so the lack of physical movement in response to a noxious stimulus is the most common endpoint associated with the term *anesthesia*. This is essentially the same endpoint used in Boston more than 160 years ago. But it is immediately apparent that many pathways can lead to such an endpoint, most notably paralysis, which itself is at the end of many pathways. Nevertheless, the mobility endpoint is well entrenched and has been useful as a practical comparison of the potency of different drugs. After all, surgery is greatly facilitated by a motionless patient. Thus was born the concept of minimum alveolar concentration (MAC; as described in this chapter), a useful tool for practitioners. Investigators, on the other hand, were hampered by such a concept and only now are starting to break the state of anesthesia into its many components in an attempt to relate them to the underlying targets and pathways. For example, most acknowledge the presence of hypnosis, amnesia, excitement, weakness, and analgesia in the state of anesthesia. These are distinct from the many arbitrarily assigned "side" effects of the drugs, including alterations in vascular, cardiac, respiratory, metabolic, and renal function. Also produced is a series of "toxic" effects, which might be unique or simply an enhancement of the primary or the side effects. This disassembly of effects is likely to facilitate the linkage with molecular targets and with their reassembly to the final in vivo state of anesthesia. At the very least, it facilitates the formation and testing of critical hypotheses. We return to these ideas toward the end of this chapter.

GENERAL ANESTHETICS

Mechanistic searches are also aided by clear structural motifs among the drugs that produce the endpoint. This permits a search for the complementary motif on the target macromolecules. Here too, general anesthetics fall short of the mark. A **structurally diverse** range of molecules is capable of producing a state of anesthesia (**Fig. 37-1**). Nonetheless, certain physicochemical features appear to be important. For example, **hydrophobicity** correlates exceedingly well with anesthetic potency, with only a few exceptions (**Fig. 37-2**). Although impressive, this only suggests that the domain(s) producing the effects is hydrophobic, limiting the choices to most proteins and all lipid membranes. Other more subtle features of the drugs seem to be important. Most inhaled anesthetics have an asymmetric distribution of hydrogen atoms, giving the molecule enough of a dipole moment to interact favorably with polarity within the hydrophobic environments. The few **nonimmobilizer** drugs (**Fig. 37-3**), introduced to allow for selection of relevant targets,[3,4] lack this feature and therefore are extremely insoluble in water.[4] Although the mechanism of their failure to cause anesthesia is not clear, it likely is related to their low dipole and poor solubility in water and therefore lower occupancy in targets. Also, there is a clear relationship between potency and the presence of halogens (and their size) on the anesthetic molecule. Given that the halogens are uncharged atoms, then polarizability must be important, another indication that the sites responsible for anesthesia have a degree of polarity. Despite a narrowing focus on protein as the molecular target (see below), lipids still cannot be excluded because the head group region has both polar and hydrophobic character.

Related to hydrophobicity is the **cutoff effect** (**Fig. 37-4**). In a homologous series of compounds, for instance, *n*-alcohols, anesthetic potency increases progressively as the hydrocarbon chain lengthens until a certain length is reached; then anesthetic potency is abruptly lost. This typically occurs at 10 to 14 carbons, depending on assay and endpoint, and has been used to implicate specific molecular targets.[5] Interpretation

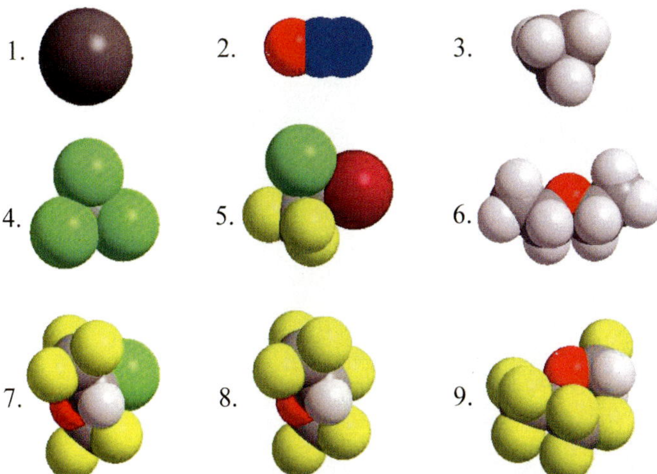

FIGURE 37-1. Space-filling representation of some inhaled general anesthetics. 1, xenon; 2, nitrous oxide; 3, cyclopropane; 4, chloroform; 5, halothane; 6, diethyl ether; 7, isoflurane; 8, desflurane; 9, sevoflurane. Atoms are color coded: *light gray*, carbon; *white*, hydrogen; *blue*, nitrogen; *red*, oxygen; *green*, chlorine; *yellow*, fluorine; *magenta*, bromine; *dark gray*, xenon.

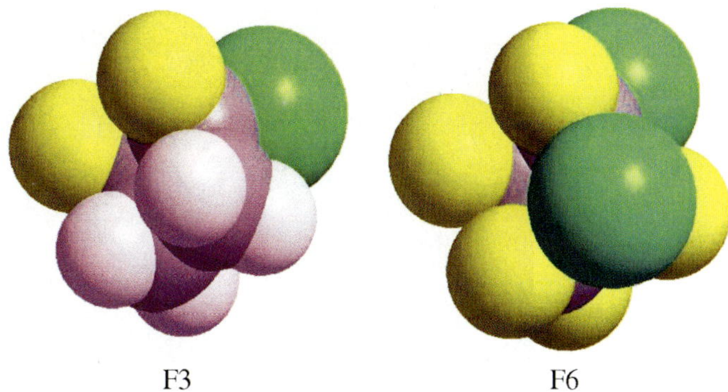

FIGURE 37-3. Two nonclinical molecules used for research purposes. Whereas the molecule on the left (chlorotrifluorocyclobutane [F3]) has anesthetic properties similar to isoflurane, the molecule on the right (dichlorohexafluorocyclobutane [F6]) is devoid of anesthetic activity despite being very soluble in oil. Because F6 is much less soluble in water that F3, this suggests the anesthetic site(s) on molecular targets transducing the minimum alveolar concentration endpoint has some polar character in addition to being hydrophobic.

of this phenomenon has varied, but is conventionally viewed as indicating the geometric capacity of a binding site—a molecular ruler. Of course, this interpretation requires that the alcohol actually bind to the target in question, a requirement that is almost never tested. In the 1 case in which it was, a cutoff effect was observed with no apparent loss in binding affinity,[6] suggesting that cutoff is attributable to mechanisms other than steric hindrance, perhaps (similar to the nonimmobilizers) to the extremely low solubility of the long compounds in water. The final blow to the cutoff effect being useful as a molecular ruler of important protein binding sites was the demonstration that polyhydric alcohols (essentially *n*-alcohol polymers) retained anesthetic activity at molecular sizes in large excess of the *n*-alkanol cutoff.[7]

The final drug feature that has been used to aid the search for targets is **enantioselectivity.** Many of the inhaled anesthetics have chiral carbons, indicating that mirror image molecules are possible (**Fig. 37-5**). Such pairs are identical from a physicochemical standpoint but have a different arrangement of atoms in space, which would be expected to interact with a unique spatial distribution of atoms in a protein binding site, for example, more specifically than in a more fluid-like assembly of lipid molecules. Small differences in the immobilizing potency of the isoflurane enantiomers were found[8] and in at least 1 species for the halothane enantiomers.[9] Although this has the potential for selecting relevant targets, the small degree of enantioselectivity (~20%), combined with the fact that many proteins display enantioselectivity for inhaled anesthetics, renders the potential small. It is even possible that the few chiral molecules in phospholipid bilayers (ie, cholesterol) or that very general and conserved chiral features of proteins (eg, L-α-amino acids and uniquely handed helices) contribute to this small degree of selectivity.

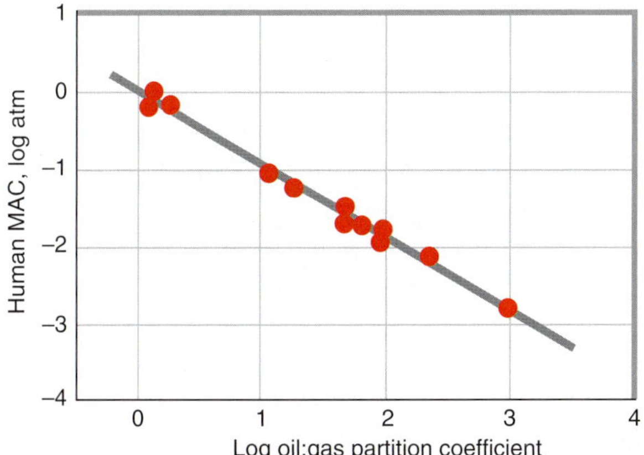

FIGURE 37-2. Log/log plot of the oil/water partition coefficient against human minimum alveolar concentration (MAC) in atmospheres for 12 inhaled anesthetics. Note the tight correlation over almost 5 orders of magnitude, strongly suggesting that the anesthetic site(s) are hydrophobic.

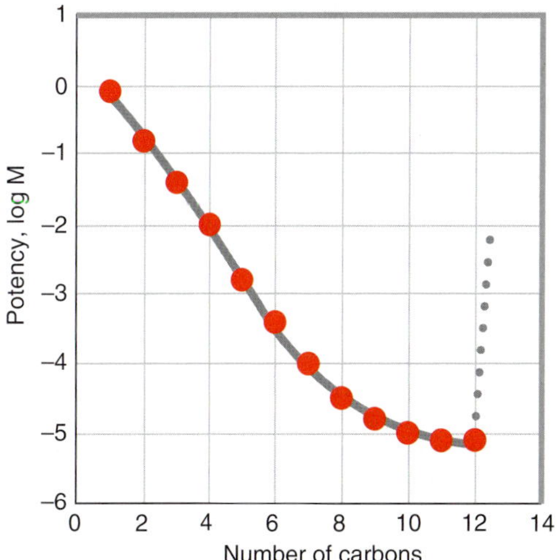

FIGURE 37-4. The cutoff effect. As one ascends a homologous series of compounds, such as the *n*-alkanols, anesthetic activity increases until about C_{12}, where activity is abruptly lost with the addition of just 1 more carbon. The cutoff point is different for different chemical series, in different in vitro systems, and in different organisms. Long interpreted as reflecting the dimensions of the anesthetic site on an important molecular target, a form of molecular ruler, the progressive decline in water solubility of the long-chain molecules suggests that occupancy of sites may decline for reasons unrelated to site dimensions. This suggests that the mechanism for failure of long hydrocarbons and nonimmobilizer molecules to produce immobility is similar.

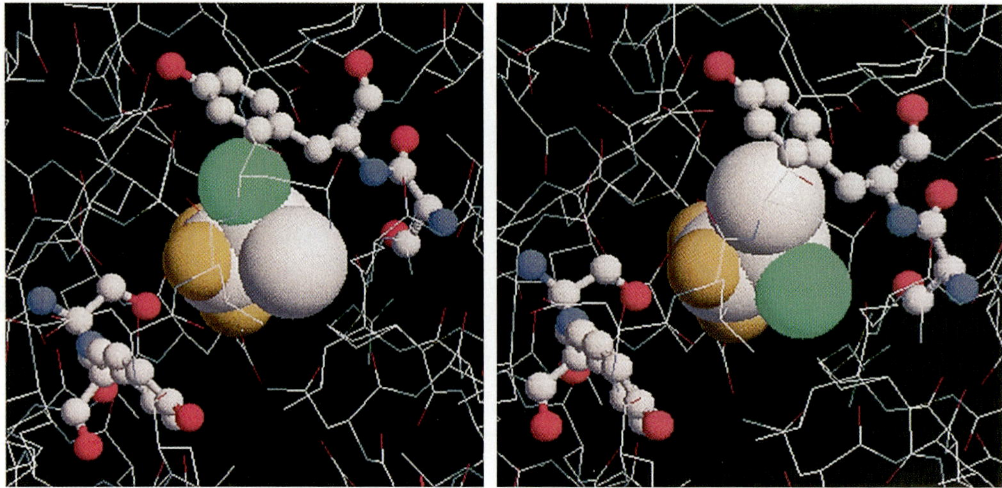

FIGURE 37-5. Stereoselective binding of halothane enantiomers. Binding of racemic halothane in hydrophobic cavity of apoferritin revealed a 2:1 preference for the *S*-enantiomer over the *R*-enantiomer. This provides credibility that the small degree of enantioselectivity observed in vivo is transduced through protein targets.

Thus, in general, drug features have given us only general clues to the identity of important anesthetic targets and the underlying mechanisms of their dysfunction.

ANESTHETIC TARGETS

LIPID BILAYERS

The dramatic correlation of hydrophobicity with anesthetic potency predated an understanding of protein interiors, so initial focus fell on the obvious oily candidate: the lipid bilayer (**Fig. 37-6**). The idea was that solubilization of the hydrophobic anesthetic into the thin lipid membrane altered a property sensed by the cell or by proteins wholly or partially embedded in the lipid. The crucial property was (and still is) unclear, so surrogate properties that could be easily measured, such as the gel–liquid phase transition, were studied extensively. Changes induced by the anesthetics in these properties could be demonstrated, but several features gradually emerged that dampened enthusiasm in the lipid membrane as an important transducer of anesthetic effects. First, measurable changes in phase transition at clinical concentrations of anesthetic were small, mimicked by only 1° to 2°C. Second, other compounds that dissolved well and produced similar effects in these bilayers (eg, nonimmobilizers) did not produce anesthesia. Finally, the emergence of protein-centered theories shifted attention away from the lipid bilayer.

A shift in attention, however, does not suffice to eliminate the potential for an important contribution. New theories, coupled with improved understanding of the lipid bilayer and its interaction with anesthetics and membrane protein, call for a return to the lipid bilayer at some point to test whether anesthetic modulation contributes to in vivo anesthetic effects. For example, it is clear that phase transitions are not a relevant feature of biologic membranes, so conclusions based on their measurement must be viewed cautiously. It now is clear that anesthetics distribute in the lipid bilayer heterogeneously, less in the center (acyl trough) and more toward the outer edges. This asymmetric distribution can influence lipid properties not easily measured, such as lateral pressure (**Fig. 37-7**) but posited to have a potent effect on membrane protein conformational transitions.[10] Interestingly, even though nonimmobilizers partition well into the lipid bilayer, the distribution within the bilayer is very different than that of an anesthetic,[11] yet again opening the door for lipid theories. Furthermore, lipid microdomains exist (eg, lipid rafts) that appear to organize specific proteins into functional groups may have a higher affinity for inhaled anesthetics (because of unique lipids or unique proteins), increasing the opportunity for anesthetic effects on signaling pathways.[12] Finally, in most assays of membrane protein activity (eg, ion channels), protein is functionally inseparable from the lipid. Cholesterol, for example, may contribute structurally essential roles in some membrane proteins by binding deep within the protein matrix.[13] Therefore, mutagenesis of membrane protein by itself cannot be directly used to implicate a protein target because the mutation also

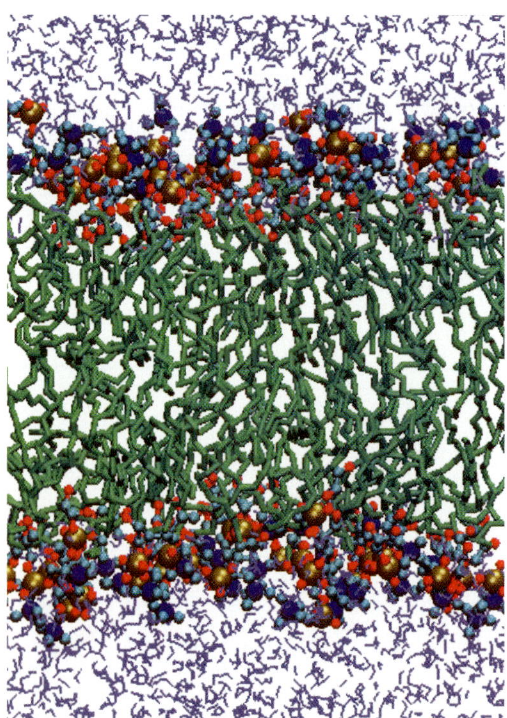

FIGURE 37-6. Snapshot of a lipid membrane in a molecular dynamics simulation. This gives an idea of the complexity and organization of this essential and widely distributed structure. Our poor understanding of its communication with proteins embedded in it and of effects of solutes distributed in it have conspired to make it difficult to eliminate the lipid bilayer as a viable potential target for transducing some anesthetic effects.

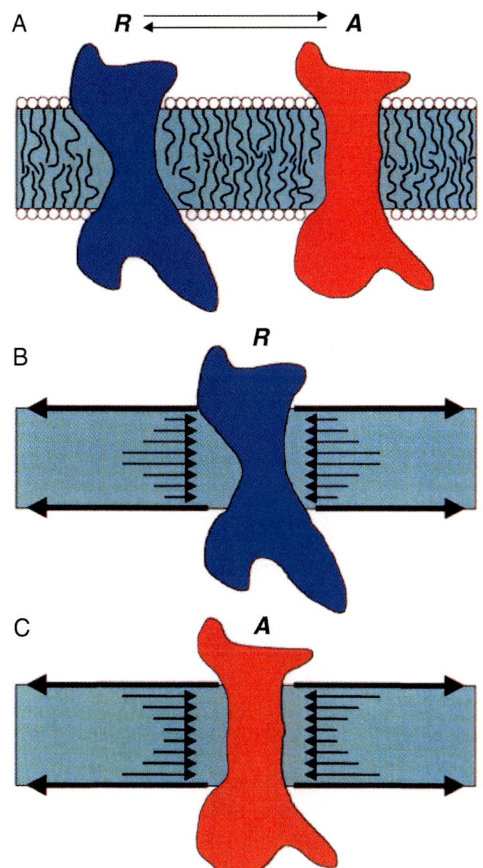

FIGURE 37-7. Lateral pressure hypothesis of membrane–protein communication. **A.** Membrane protein in 2 conformations: R for resting, and A for activated. The A conformer requires some expansion in the membrane center. **B.** Membrane lateral profile of vectors that favors the R state. **C.** Pressure profile that favors the A conformer. A solute that distributes unevenly across the membrane will, of necessity, alter this lateral pressure profile, resulting in a modulation of conformational state and therefore of activity. Molecular dynamics simulations predict that anesthetic molecules do distribute unevenly across the lipid bilayer. [Reprinted with permission from Gompf H, Chen J, Sun Y, et al. Halothane-induced hypnosis is not accompanied by inactivation of orexinergic output in rodents. *Anesthesiology.* 2009;111:1001-1009.]

might influence the interaction with lipid. Thus, it is premature to rule out the biologic lipid membrane as an important direct target for the inhaled anesthetics.

PROTEINS

Proteinaceous components of the cell as targets for anesthetics were first proposed by Claude Bernard in 1875 but did not gain favor until the demonstration that the activity of lipid-free preparations of protein were reversibly influenced by anesthetics and in a way that reproduced the correlation with hydrophobicity.[14] Because this paralleled the understanding that the interior of proteins is as hydrophobic as that of lipid membranes, this association should not have been surprising. When combined with enantioselectivity and an ability to measure and alter protein function, especially in ion channels, protein-centered theories rapidly became favored. Many protein targets have been proposed and studied, and we review some of them briefly. *However, at this time it is safe to conclude that not a single protein target or even class or family of protein targets has been proven to play the central role in inhaled anesthetic action.* This is not to say, however, that favored candidates have not emerged, especially for the injectable induction agents. We first review some essential basics of protein–ligand interactions as they relate to anesthetics and then present the evidence for specific targets.

Binding The submolecular mechanism by which the anesthetic causes a change in protein function or activity must first involve a binding event—formation of drug-target complex. This often is the initial criterion for establishing the relevance of any proposed drug target but has not been used for inhaled anesthetics because the affinity for protein targets is low, and they appear to be fairly promiscuous, binding to many targets. Both nuclear magnetic resonance spectroscopy and photolabeling have suggested a large number of protein binding targets (ie, 27) and no particular regional preference in the brain (**Fig. 37-8**).[15,16] This renders untenable the conventional radioligand binding approach for discovering targets. Whether anesthetics also significantly alter the function of a large number of proteins is not clear, but even if only a minority of the binding target pool, the number of contributing targets is still large.

Nature of the Binding Site Until recently, the nature of anesthetic binding sites has been inferred from correlations with anesthetic structural or physicochemical features. For example, the Overton-Meyer relationship suggested that sites are in the hydrophobic interior of proteins, and the relationship of halogen size and asymmetric hydrogens with potency suggested that polar amino acids must contribute to these sites. High-resolution structures of a clinically used inhaled anesthetic complexed to a protein target

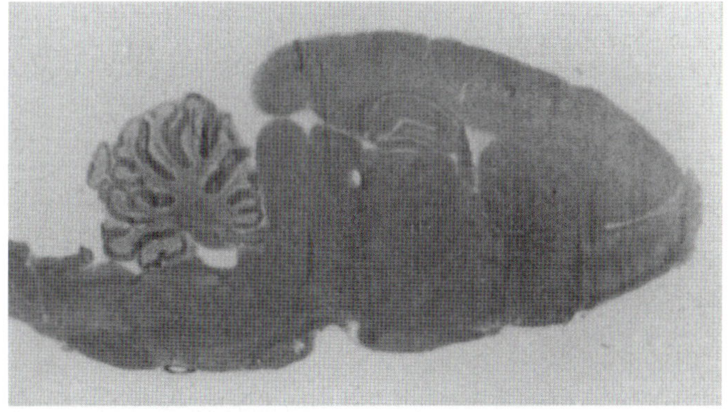

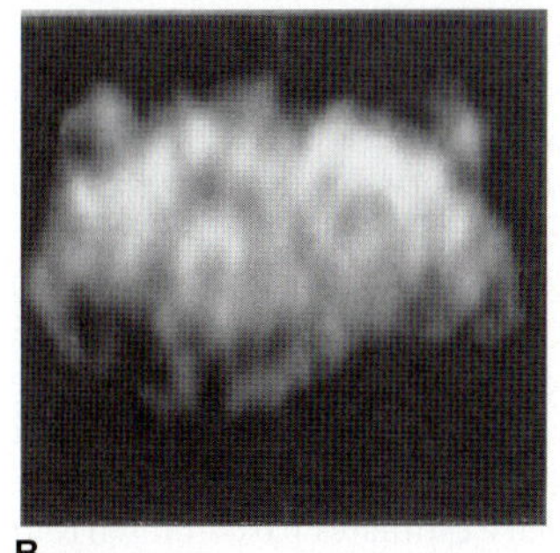

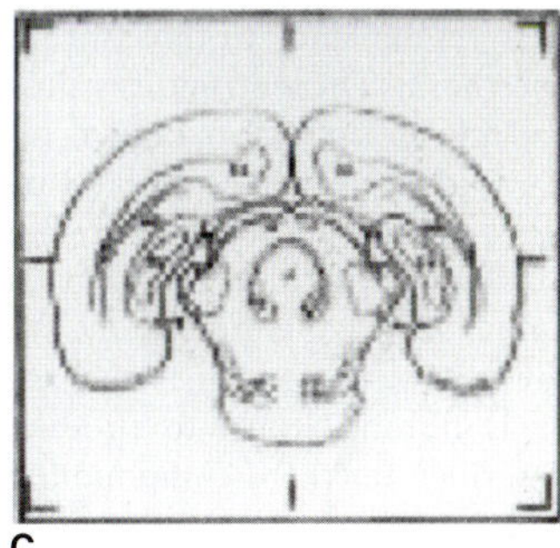

FIGURE 37-8. **A.** Autoradiogram of rat brain sagittal section photoaffinity labeled with ^{14}C-halothane. The degree of halothane binding is indicated by the level of darkness; no other stain has been applied to this section. There appears to be no regional preference, and excess unlabeled halothane reduces incorporation by approximately 70% (image not shown), indicating that this distribution represents specific binding. **B.** ^{19}F-Nuclear magnetic resonance coronal section of in vivo rat brain after equilibration with sevoflurane. **C.** Orientation of *B*. Both experiments demonstrate widespread anesthetic distribution in mammalian brain. [Part B from Eckenhoff MF, Eckenhoff RG. Quantitative autoradiography of halothane binding in rat brain. *J Pharmacol Exp Ther.* 1998;285; Fig. 2c.]

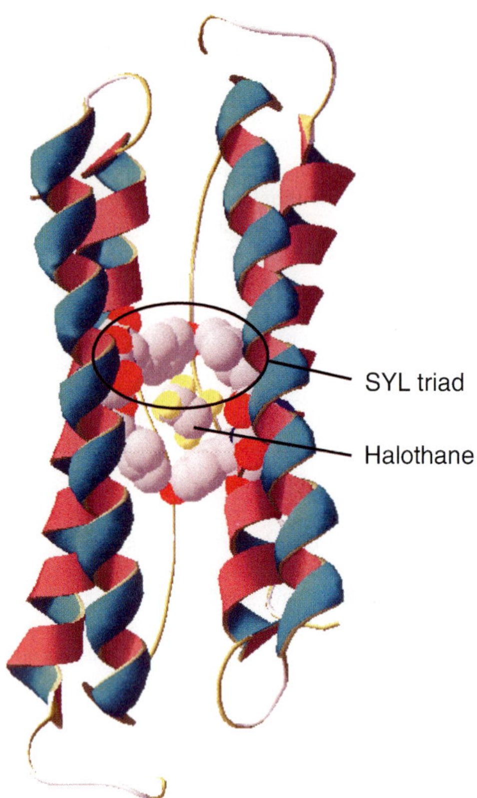

FIGURE 37-9. High-resolution structure of the high-affinity anesthetic binding site in an interface between 2 subunits of apoferritin. Halothane is shown in the middle, coordinated by 2 serine–tyrosine–leucine (SYL) triads (see text for details). Note that the parallel helical bundle motif of this binding domain is found in the transmembrane region of the ligand-gated ion channel subunits and in many receptors (see Figs. 37-14 and 37-15).

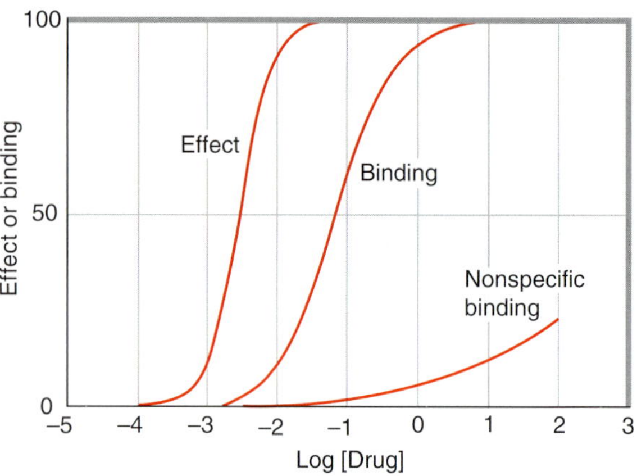

FIGURE 37-10. Sigmoid-shaped dose–response curve for a typical anesthetic-like drug. The effect curve often most left shifted is the steepest. The binding effects that underlie that the effect usually is shifted to the right and may or may not have the same slope, depending on the number targets, the number of sites per target, and whether the sites interact (cooperativity). This indicates that molecular sites underlying a specific effect do not necessarily need to be fully occupied to reach full (saturation) effect. Nonspecific binding (that generally not associated with the primary effect) is most right shifted and may appear to be linear in many experiments.

have been revealed for at least 3 protein models: serum albumin,[17] apoferritin (**Fig. 37-9**),[18] and integrin lymphocyte function-associated antigen 1 (LFA-1).[19] Although unlikely to transduce desirable effects of anesthesia, the affinity of these proteins (see later discussion) suggests substantial occupancy at clinical concentrations of anesthetic (~0.2 mmol/L), and thus the binding site architecture is likely to bear resemblance to those in targets underlying effects relevant to anesthesia. These structures show occupancy of preexisting internal packing defects, also known as *cavities*. The apoferritin example goes further to suggest that a packing density of just over half full represents an optimal balance between enthalpic and entropic forces. Finally, all of these examples suggest that polar (but uncharged) amino acids contribute to the strength of binding. In the apoferritin cavity, 2 serine–tyrosine–leucine triads interact with either halothane or isoflurane atoms to produce the highest affinity binding yet described for these compounds (Fig. 37-9). The stringency of these features is not yet clear, but preliminary estimates based on current entries in the Protein Data Bank (http://www.rcsb.org/pdb) suggest that less than 1% of the proteome (~3000 proteins) have comparable binding sites for volatile anesthetics.

Affinity and Stoichiometry Affinity of a drug for a site, indicated by the association constant (K_a) or, more commonly, the dissociation constant ($K_d = 1/K_a$), is experimentally defined as the drug concentration at which half the sites are occupied. It is more properly called "apparent" affinity because other aspects of the mixture can modify the true affinity of the ligand–site complex. Relevant to this is whether the binding event "causes" a conformational change (see later discussion) in the protein to which it binds. If so, the apparent affinity will be lowered by the amount of free energy used to change the protein conformation **(Fig. 37-10)**. Thus, a set of binding site features that produces a 10 μmol/L *absolute* K_d with an anesthetic perhaps will have an *apparent* K_d of 1 mmol/L if approximately 2 kcal/mol of free energy is required to change the protein conformation.

The slope of the relationship between drug concentration and occupancy, the Hill slope, is an indication of both the number of sites on a target and whether they interact. For example, a single site should always have a Hill slope of 1, reflecting a relationship in which the site goes from 0% to 100% occupancy over an approximately 100-fold change in drug concentration (Fig. 37-10). Multiple sites on a single target also can demonstrate a Hill slope of 1, or they can "cooperate," increasing the slope. In other words, if occupancy of the first site enhances occupancy of the second (as in oxygen binding by hemoglobin), the slope will rise, although rarely over 2 or 3. Although difficult to measure as indicated, anesthetic K_d values in model proteins typically are approximately 1 mmol/L, and Hill slopes are generally 1 or slightly greater even though more than 1 binding site has been found in most proteins studied. Serum albumin has at least 6 sites,[17] apoferritin 12,[18] and the intact nicotinic acetylcholine receptor (nAChR) 15 to 20.[20-23] As might be deduced from the preceding paragraph, occupancy of multiple sites is a potentially powerful method of donating free energy to the protein to alter its conformation. Occupancy of only 1 additional binding site in a protein contributes as much free energy as an approximately 10-fold increase in affinity at a single site.

An issue frequently causing confusion has been what affinity an important anesthetic target should display for anesthetics. Prevailing logic has suggested that for a target to be relevant to a particular endpoint (eg, immobility), the dissociation constant for the anesthetic–target complex should approximate that achieved at MAC. However, this logic holds only if one assumes that this target is alone capable of producing the endpoint, an assumption that rarely is valid. Furthermore, even if the target is wholly responsible for the endpoint, it is difficult to know the expected K_d because drug efficacy at this target is not known. It is rare for the relationship between receptor occupancy and median effective concentration (EC_{50}) to be linear; thus, predicting more than that some degree of occupancy should be anticipated at clinical concentrations is difficult. As our discussion on Hill slopes indicates, this limits the expected K_d to an approximately 100-fold range.

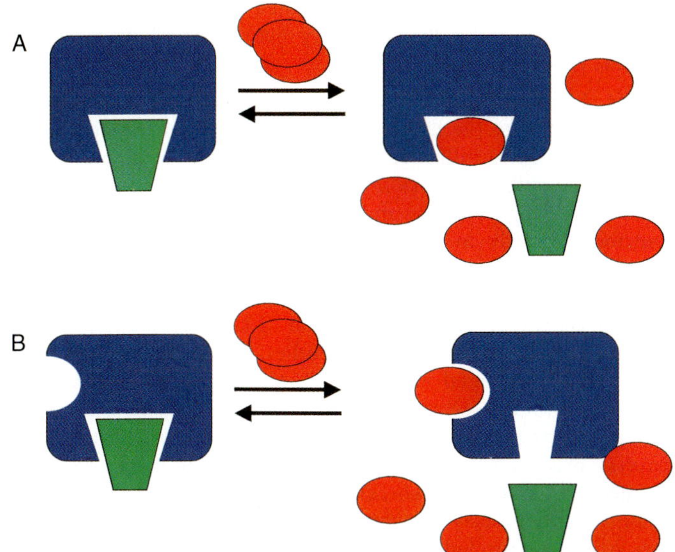

FIGURE 37-11. A. Example of isosteric competition in which the anesthetic (*red oval*) achieves a high enough concentration to actually replace the endogenous ligand (*green trapezoid*) in its site of action. **B.** Example of allosteric competition in which the anesthetic binds preferentially to a conformer that disfavors binding of the endogenous ligand, but at a distant site.

Coupling Mechanism As discussed earlier, the anesthetic can only alter the protein's activity through a contribution of binding energy—through either the affinity or the stoichiometry of the complex. This binding energy alters protein activity through at least 3 potential and partially overlapping mechanisms. The first mechanism, competition, occurs when the drug–protein complex is strong enough to compete with the binding of an endogenous ligand, therefore inhibiting the associated effect (**Fig. 37-11**). This was the mechanism initially proposed for anesthetic inhibition of firefly luciferase.[14] There are 2 forms of competition: isosteric and allosteric. In isosteric competition, the drug occupies the same binding site as the endogenous ligand, physically preventing binding. An anesthetic example is halothane occupancy of the retinal cavity in the G-protein coupled receptor (GPCR) rhodopsin.[24] In allosteric competition, the drug binds elsewhere in the protein, altering the structure sufficiently to disfavor ligand binding in its otherwise unoccupied site. A clear example is integrin LFA-1, in which isoflurane binds in a cavity that stabilizes a conformation with low affinity for the intercellular adhesion molecule (ICAM) receptor protein.[19] In a closely related form of allosterism, cooperativity, allosteric binding of anesthetic *favors* a conformation that binds the endogenous ligand more tightly. Thus, in firefly luciferase, the binding of adenosine triphosphate (ATP) and anesthetic is cooperative.[25] Cooperative effects of agonist and anesthetic in some receptors may also be attributable to binding cooperativity.[22,26]

The second general category of drug–effect coupling is **ensemble modulation** (**Fig. 37-12**). Functional proteins exist in an ensemble of conformations, each of which is associated with some aspect of activity. Resting, active, desensitized, and so on all describe states of activity with a specific underlying protein conformation. Some conformers may possess binding sites for anesthetics that are more attractive than others and therefore are populated to a greater extent when the anesthetic is present. The anesthetic changes protein activity by selecting the most favorable conformer for binding and increasing its stability and therefore prevalence. One can immediately see the overlap with allosterism. Similar to allosterism, ensemble modulation can explain either an enhancement or an inhibition in protein activity, depending on which conformer has the most attractive anesthetic binding sites.

The final general mechanism for coupling binding to a change in protein function is **oligomerization modulation** (**Fig. 37-13**). Much protein activity and signaling is controlled by interactions with other proteins. In general, these interactions are highly specific but relatively weak so that they can be readily reversed. The protein–protein interface may include features attractive to an anesthetic, such as cavities. If these features are optimal when the proteins are linked, then the anesthetic will enhance the interaction

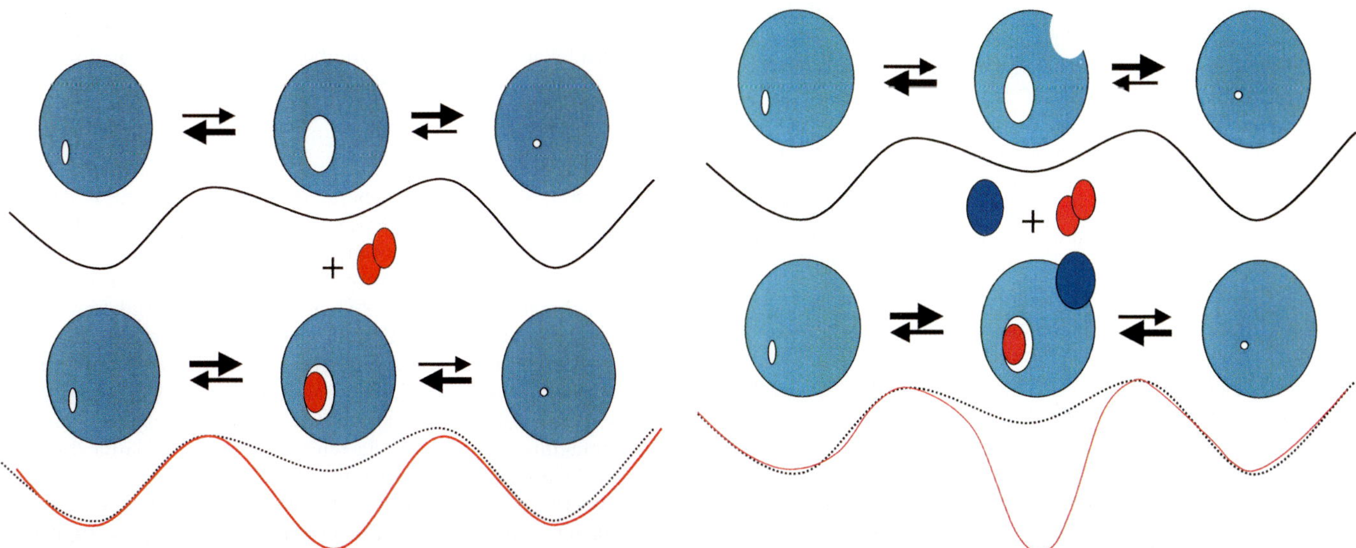

FIGURE 37-12. Simple ensemble of protein conformers, with the relative free energy shown beneath. **A.** Anesthetic favors the conformer with the most attractive cavities, lowering its free energy (*red line*) and increasing its concentration. **B.** Same schematic demonstrating cooperativity, but in this case, the anesthetic-preferred conformer also preferentially binds an endogenous ligand. Thus, free energy is lowered even further in the presence of both ligands, more dramatically enhancing the population and therefore activity associate with this conformer. [Part A reprinted with permission from Gompf H, Chen J, Sun Y, et al. Halothane-induced hypnosis is not accompanied by inactivation of orexinergic output in rodents. *Anesthesiology.* 2009;111:1001-1009.]

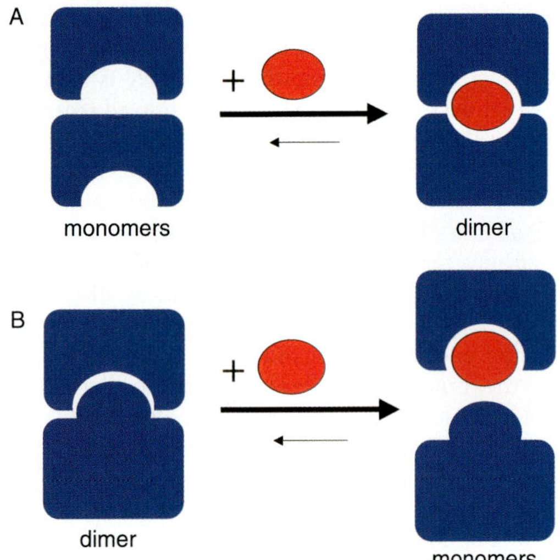

FIGURE 37-13. Example of oligomerization modulation. **A.** Anesthetic binding site is created by dimerization of a monomer that otherwise has no binding site. Thus, the anesthetic will be observed to increase the population of dimer. **B.** On the other hand, occupancy of an anesthetic site in the monomer disfavors binding of the second protein because of a steric clash. In this case, the anesthetic will be observed to decrease the population of dimer. Although both mechanisms may occur in vivo, the situation shown in A probably is more likely.

or oligomerization; if they are optimal when separated, anesthetics will disfavor oligomerization. Examples of the former appear to be the sarcoplasmic reticular calcium adenosine triphosphatase (ATPase)[27] and of the latter the PSD-95 PDZ domain proteins (see later discussion).[28] The synaptic vesicle machinery is highly dependent on these oligomerization events, and components that might be modulated by anesthetics in this way have been identified.[29] It should be apparent that this mechanism has important implications as to the number of potential effects these drugs might have. Whereas the set of all proteins expressed—the proteome—is very large (~300 000 proteins), the number of protein–protein interactions, the so-called *interactome*, is much larger. Thus, anesthetic effects at the interactome level produced by effects at the interface could dwarf those at the individual protein level.

An important caveat in this discussion is that all binding interactions do not necessarily result in an important change in protein activity.[30] It is possible that an anesthetic binding site is precisely preserved across the entire conformation or oligomerization ensemble, in which case anesthetic binding will not alter the distribution of conformers and therefore will have no effect on activity. How commonly this form of "unproductive" binding occurs is not clear.

Summary Any or all of these general coupling mechanisms may be involved in anesthetic-induced protein dysfunction. The distinction often is difficult but is important if we are to intelligently modify the drugs to favor or disfavor specific interactions.

POTENTIAL PROTEIN TARGETS

As suggested earlier, the anesthetic sensitivity of a number of protein systems has been studied over the past few decades, and, remarkably, many are altered within only a 10-fold range of clinical concentrations. We briefly review some of these systems and the evidence for inclusion. This discussion is not intended to be a comprehensive list of those proteins studied; many have come and gone. Rather, we focus on some of the more recent and compelling candidates, especially those with associated in vivo evidence for a contribution. Furthermore, we focus on targets associated with the desirable effects, such as hypnosis, rather than the many that might underlie less desirable side effects.

Soluble As pointed out earlier, proteins have domains as hydrophobic as those of the lipid bilayer, and it now is clear that anesthetics bind to and influence the activity of many soluble proteins. Much of the published work involved model systems, such as firefly luciferase, serum albumin, and apoferritin, which are unlikely to contribute directly to anesthesia. However, plausible candidates, centrally located in signal transduction cascades or cellular machinery, have emerged. For example, protein kinase C (PKC) transduces receptor activation to phosphorylation of key membrane proteins, such as certain ion channels and other receptors, and has been shown to bind general anesthetics.[31] Alteration of its activity by anesthetics would be expected to have generalized and widespread cellular effects that might contribute to anesthesia, although controversy exists as to both the expected and observed directions of effect (reviewed by Rebecchi and Pentyala[32] and Gomez and Guatimosim[33]). Initially thought to be inhibited by general anesthetics, later studies performed under physiologic conditions showed PKC to be activated. This one system demonstrates the complexity of sorting out anesthetic targets and effects. The observed effects in this relatively simple physiologic assay can result from anesthetic effects on membrane lipid, stimulus–kinase coupling, kinase–target coupling, or the phosphorylated target itself. Anesthetics might interact with any component. Studies in intact, genetically altered animals are in progress but to date have not provided unambiguous answers. Further studies on PKC isoform distribution and activity are required to sort out the influence of anesthetics and potential contribution to the anesthetic state.

Another attractive anesthetic target is any of the components of the cellular cytoskeleton, motility apparatus, and vesicle transport systems. These systems subserve a variety of basic cellular functions, the alteration of which would manifest as a decrease in cellular activity or communication. For example, tubulin forms microtubules, which are crucial elements of cellular scaffolding and motility. Anesthetics bind specifically to tubulin,[34] and the assembly of the monomer into the large tubular oligomer is altered by anesthetics, albeit at high concentration.[35] Entire mechanisms for general anesthesia based on microtubular dynamics and organization have been proposed,[36] and some experimental support has been reported.[37] Oligomerization of actin, a protein acting with myosin and other proteins to subserve cellular motion, is inhibited by anesthetics and is another relatively unexplored potential general mechanism of anesthesia.[38]

Anesthetics also affect the synaptic vesicle machinery. A decrease in synaptic transmission is generally agreed to accompany general anesthesia; therefore, inhibition of synaptic vesicle transport, fusion, and release is a plausible general mechanism of central nervous system (CNS) dysfunction. Evidence comes from several disparate sources. In a genetic screen of the nematode *Caenorhabditis elegans*, mutations in the vesicle fusion soluble *N*-ethylmaleimide sensitive attachment factor (SNARE) proteins were found to produce resistance to some anesthetic endpoints.[29] Furthermore, 1 component, syntaxin, and various SNARE assemblies have been shown to bind isoflurane using nuclear magnetic resonance approaches.[39] Transcript profiling[40] in mammals has shown an upregulation of synaptotagmin, another vesicle-release protein. The latter does not necessarily implicate synaptotagmin as a direct anesthetic target, but it lends credence to the idea that synaptic vesicle release is inhibited during general anesthesia. Other synaptic targets implicated are the PDZ domain proteins. These domains are responsible for fusion events (oligomerization) between proteins and are intimately involved in synaptic vesicle trafficking. Work has shown that anesthetics disrupt the oligomerization, and the probable anesthetic binding site responsible has been identified in a truncated version of PSD-95.[28]

Membrane

Ion Channels A variety of proteins embedded in, and dependent on, the lipid bilayer for their activity are altered by general anesthetics in in vitro assays. Most studied are the ion channels, largely because of the availability of electrophysiologic approaches for measurement of function. Of the ion channels, most emphasis has been placed on the ligand-gated cys-loop receptor–channel complex, the prototype of which is the nicotinic acetylcholine receptor (nAChR). These proteins are transmembrane heterooligomers of 5 subunits arranged around a central ion channel. A variety of anesthetics inhibit this excitatory channel, perhaps by promoting the desensitized state via cooperative binding with acetylcholine; the probable basis for the muscle relaxation associated with many general anesthetics. Volatile anesthetics bind this receptor specifically, and a site underlying cooperative binding behavior has been tentatively identified.[20,22] The nAChRs are also found in the brain, adding credibility to the possibility that alterations in their activity contribute to anesthesia. In vivo support of an important role for these receptors is still lacking.

γ-Aminobutyric acid (GABA)ergic neurotransmission was identified 20 years ago as a plausible substrate for anesthetic effects,[41] so recent emphasis has been placed on the inhibitory GABA type A ($GABA_A$) and glycine receptor–ion channel complex as potential contributors to at least the sedative or amnestic component of general anesthesia. Similar to the nAChR, many general anesthetics (most volatile ones and alcohols) probably bind cooperatively with agonist (either GABA or glycine). However, because these receptors undergo desensitization more slowly that the nAChR, the final effect is enhanced agonist-stimulated currents instead of inhibition (**Fig. 37-14**). These ion channels are inhibitory (produce hyperpolarization of neuronal membrane by opening of chloride channels), so enhancement of their activity is expected to inhibit synaptic transmission. The difficulty of isolating or expressing sufficient $GABA_A$ receptor of any subunit composition for biochemical studies so far has precluded the demonstration of specific volatile anesthetic binding, although an etomidate site has been identified at an intersubunit interface.[42]

Most studies to date have focused on the action of volatile anesthetics on $GABA_A$ receptors mediating rapid synaptic transmission. However, volatile anesthetics also act on $GABA_A$ channels mediating tonic inhibition. Tonic $GABA_A$ channels are found in many areas of the nervous system, including the hippocampus and the spinal cord interneurons. Although the precise receptor subunits composing the tonic $GABA_A$ channels remain unknown, the α_5- and δ-subunits likely are involved because tonic currents inhibited by bicuculline are not seen in null-mutant mice devoid of these subunits. These $GABA_A$ channels are more sensitive to agonists than the rapid type, requiring only low micromolar concentrations of GABA for opening, concentrations found in even extrasynaptic regions of a nerve cell. Similarly, tonic $GABA_A$ channels are more sensitive to volatile anesthetics than those mediating rapid synaptic transmission.[43] Because of this sensitivity and expression in the hippocampus, it is reasonable to hypothesize that these channels mediate the amnestic component of volatile anesthetic action. A thorough characterization of the volatile anesthetic effects on the various tonic $GABA_A$ null mutant mice has not been reported.

In an attempt to both find sites of action as well as to implicate anesthetic targets, site-directed mutagenesis has been coupled with electrophysiology. For example, an asparagine to methionine mutation at position 265 in the $GABA_A$ β_3 subunit largely eliminated enflurane enhancement of GABA action in vitro, but the knock-in mouse, in which the wild-type β_3-subunit was replaced by the point mutant, had minimally altered righting reflex sensitivity or MAC.[44,45] Greater success was obtained with the injectable general anesthetics (induction agents) in this same model. For example, similar to enflurane, etomidate and propofol failed to enhance GABA-evoked currents in vitro, but in this case, the whole-animal sensitivity to both injectable drugs was significantly diminished. The technology of mutant receptor knock-in is far superior to an overall elimination of the receptor produced by the knock-out technology because the normal cellular process that regulates expression of the wild-type receptor is preserved. Based on structure–activity studies demonstrating the role of both α- and β-$GABA_A$ subunits[46] as well as other ligand-gated channels in determining volatile anesthetic responsiveness in in vitro expressed receptors, a multiple knock-in mutant mouse in which many sites are simultaneously altered is more likely to exhibit relative resistance to the volatile anesthetics.

Interestingly, in contrast to prototypical volatile anesthetics such as isoflurane and injectable anesthetics such as propofol, etomidate and barbiturates, a group of agents called dissociative anesthetics, similar to ketamine and nitrous oxide (N_2O),[47] as well as xenon,[48] at clinically relevant concentrations, do not significantly affect $GABA_A$ currents, but they inhibit a major excitatory drive in the CNS via blockade of *N*-methyl-D-aspartate receptors (NMDAr). Thus, when ligand-gated ion channels are concerned, general anesthetics may inhibit CNS neurons either by potentiating inhibitory $GABA_A$ currents or inhibiting excitatory NMDAr-mediated currents. Because NMDA receptors play a key role in pain pathways in CNS, their blockade may contribute to the prominent analgesic properties of dissociative anesthetics.

Another hypothesis is that the 2-pore domain family of background K (KCNK) channels is involved in volatile anesthetic action. This gene family encodes for K^+-selective ion channels with a common structural feature of 2 protein domains putatively lining the ion channel and 4 transmembrane domains. Two 2-pore domain proteins are thought to assemble as a dimer, creating a complete protein complex with a functional K^+-permeable ion channel normally open at all physiologic membrane potentials, thus contributing to the background leak K channel critical in determining the resting membrane potential and regulating neuronal excitability.[49] Opening of channels encoded by 2 members of the KCNK family, TREK-1 and TREK-2, and more recently a third member, TRESK, are enhanced by volatile anesthetics, thereby hyperpolarizing the cell membrane. However, the enhancement is not seen in all the family TRESK because the channel activity of a closely related member, TRAAK, is not affected. As in the case for $GABA_A$ receptors, the hypothesis that the anesthetic-responsive KCNK

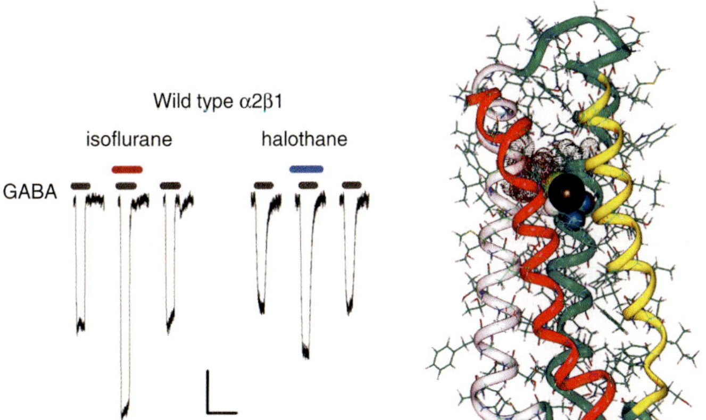

FIGURE 37-14. Enhancement of activity of γ-aminobutyric acid type A ($GABA_A$) chloride conductance by isoflurane and halothane. In both cases, the effect of an endogenous ligand, GABA, is significantly enhanced by the presence of the anesthetic. The probable basis for this is shown in Fig. 37-12B, and the region of the protein thought to transduce this effect is shown on the right by the hypothetical placement of an anesthetic in the interhelical space. Note the similarity of this hypothetical structural motif and binding site to the crystal structure shown in Fig. 37-9. [Reprinted with permission from Jenkins A, Greenblatt EP, Faulkner HJ, et al. Evidence for a common binding cavity for three general anesthetics within the GABAA receptor. *J Neurosci* 2001;21:RC136]

channels play a role in the general anesthetic action at the whole animal level was examined and confirmed in TREK-1 knock-out mice. For example, mice without the TREK-1 gene were approximately 20% less sensitive to halothane, sevoflurane, desflurane, and chloroform (but not pentobarbital) as defined by the loss of righting reflex (LORR) and withdraw to tail clamp. Interestingly, an invertebrate analog of this channel[41] was discovered a decade earlier in the pond snail,[49] pointing out the importance of information derived regardless of the model organism used. Voltage-gated potassium channels are generally insensitive to anesthetics, although a couple variants found in *Drosophila* and in mammalian orthologs are sensitive to clinical concentrations of both alcohols and anesthetics.[50]

Voltage-gated calcium channels (VGCCs) have been studied for years because of the central role of calcium in intracellular signaling. VGCCs, which are heteromeric complexes in the plasma membrane of virtually all cell types, show a high level of electrophysiologic and pharmacologic diversity. These channels consist of a pore-forming α_1-subunit and ancillary subunits β, γ, and α2–δ.[51] On the basis of the membrane potential at which they activate, these channels are subdivided into high voltage-activated (HVA) and low voltage-activated (LVA) or transient T-type Ca^{2+} channels (T channels). These channels in nerve tissue have a central function in sensory, cognitive, and motor pathways and controlling cell excitability and neurotransmitter release. These channels, which are products of different genes, give rise to α1 subunits that form the pore of the neuronal VGCCs. The HVA VGCCs are members of different families: Ca_V1 (α1C) encoding L-type, $Ca_V2.1$ (α1A) encoding P/Q-type, $Ca_V2.2$ (α1B) encoding N-type, and $Ca_V2.3$ (α1E) encoding R-type HVA current. Similarly, cloning of T-type channels has established that at least 3 isoforms exist based on the structure of α1 subunits: $Ca_V3.1$ (α1G), $Ca_V3.2$ (α1H), and $Ca_V3.3$ (α1I). Because of its importance, intracellular calcium is tightly controlled via many systems, including voltage- and ligand-gated channels, exchangers, ATPases, and soluble binding proteins. Many of these systems have been shown to be influenced by anesthetics, although early studies have shown that, in general, the magnitude of effect is modest at clinical concentrations.[33] However, in most instances, previous studies used only 1 general anesthetic; did not pharmacologically separate subtypes of VGCCs in native cells; and in many cases, did not obtain careful concentration-response curves. An important issue is that even small blockade of a particular VGCC by any general anesthetic may produce profound physiologic effects. When this has been examined, small changes in Ca^{2+} influx into presynaptic terminals can result in profound changes in transmitter release and synaptic efficacy.[51] Indeed, presynaptic transmitter release is proportional up to the fourth power of Ca^{2+} entry.[51] Thus, even if VGCCs are only partially inhibited by anesthetics in the clinically relevant range, this can profoundly alter neuronal signaling. The effects of volatile anesthetics on even 1 subset of VGCCs are variable, probably reflecting the molecular heterogeneity of these channels. Of the functionally characterized VGCCs, the N- and P/Q-type channels, which are major putative presynaptic channels regulating neurotransmitter release, were only partially inhibited by clinically relevant concentrations of inhaled anesthetics.[52,53] The recent evidence supporting a possible role of inhibition of N-type VGCCs in the pharmacology of inhaled anesthetics comes from the observation that N-type VGCCs knock-out mice exhibited increased sensitivity to halothane,[54] although as noted elsewhere in this chapter, this is an extremely common observation regardless of the target manipulated. Another recent study using in vitro recordings from intact thalamic slices and in vivo recordings using $Ca_V2.3$ R-type knock-out mice has established that presynaptic R-type VGCCs in the thalamus are potently inhibited by clinically relevant concentrations of isoflurane.[55] The T-type VGCCs channels, although not involved in synaptic neurotransmitter release, play an important role in controlling neuronal excitability and in generating spontaneous oscillatory bursting of groups of neurons in the thalamus thought to be involved in regulating the state of arousal and sleep. The thalamic T-type channels are significantly blocked by clinically relevant concentrations of the inhaled anesthetics.[56] The molecular mechanism of how these drugs inhibit the VGCCs channels is not known but appears to involve acceleration of channel inactivation and slowing of the recovery from this nonconducting state.[56] There is no evidence of anesthetic binding to these targets, so whether this electrophysiologic effect is mediated via anesthetic interactions with lipid or protein is uncertain.

Voltage-gated sodium channels (NaVs) play a key role in regulating neuronal excitability and therefore are a plausible target for the inhaled volatile anesthetics. However, NaVs were largely dismissed as a relevant target because initial studies indicated that high concentrations were required for inhibition in squid axons (reviewed by Elliott et al[57]). However, later studies of mammalian brain NaVs indicated that these channels are significantly inhibited by lower, more clinically relevant concentrations of volatile anesthetics.[58] In fact, these anesthetics influence specific ligand binding to $GABA_A$ receptors and the NaVs with approximately equal potency,[59] and rank-order effects appear to qualify the presynaptic NaV as a feasible target for contributing to general anesthesia (**Box 37-1**).

Receptors The dominant receptor type in the brain is the GPCR. This enormous family includes most of the neurotransmitter and sensory receptors, whether small molecule, peptide, or lipid. These receptors are monomeric and have 7 transmembrane domains arranged like an envelope around a central cleft, or cavity. On the cytoplasmic face, GPCRs couple to the heterotrimeric (3 different subunits) G-protein messenger systems. The native ligand binding site tends to be at various depths in the interhelical cavity, and although some features are conserved, the site can accommodate a wide variety of ligand structure and chemistry (**Fig. 37-15**). Ligands range from small molecules (volatile odorants, catecholamines) to small peptides (endogenous opioids). That anesthetics act on these receptors is suggested by the anesthetic-sparing effect of agonists for the dopamine and α_2-adrenergic receptors in addition to alterations of activity of the eicosanoid receptors.[61] Finally, volatile anesthetics have been shown to bind the conserved agonist site in many of these receptors (Fig. 37-15),[24] producing either inhibition or excitation.[62] Effects downstream of these receptors (eg, on the G-protein transduction pathway) are also possible. Evidence is ample for anesthetic effects on G-protein–mediated signaling[32,61] and the importance to function in vivo. For example, *C. elegans* with diminished Go activity (a negative modulator of synaptic activity) was 2-fold resistant to isoflurane.[63] These effects probably are related to effects on the receptor, or the receptor–G interface, because evidence for direct

BOX 37-1

Isoform and State Dependence of Anesthetic Action

It now is clear that voltage-gated sodium channels (NaVs) constitute a family of closely related proteins with distinct physiologic and pharmacologic properties, although which isoforms are present in the presynaptic terminal remains unknown. Systematic comparison of the sensitivity of different NaV isoforms with isoflurane confirmed the differential sensitivity of the different isoforms to this volatile anesthetic.[60] Of curiosity is the observation that volatile anesthetics had no effect on the NaV1.8 tetrodotoxin-resistant isoform predominantly expressed in the primary afferent neurons thought to play a critical role in pain signaling, which could explain why volatile anesthetics exhibit no analgesic property. An additional confounder that may explain some of the inconsistencies reported in the literature is the fact that halothane inhibition of NaV was dependent on coexpression of protein kinase C.[48] Therefore, both the state of the NaV itself (resting vs inactivated) and the presence or absence of other modulatory proteins most likely influence the effect of volatile anesthetics on NaVs. Similar arguments can be used when studies concerning voltage-gated calcium channels are interpreted.

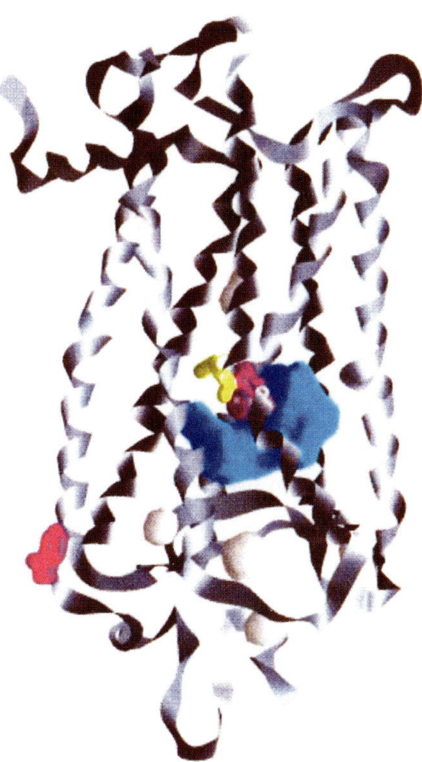

FIGURE 37-15. Structure of the prototypical G-protein coupled receptor (mammalian rhodopsin, PDB No. 1F88) showing the anesthetic binding site (*blue object*) located through photolabeling experiments. Occupancy of this interhelical hydrophobic site competes with native ligand (retinal), a mechanism shown in Fig. 37-11. The general motif of an interhelical site in a parallel bundle (see Figs. 37-9 and 37-14) is retained. [Reprinted with permission from Eckenhoff RG. An inhalational anesthetic binding domain in the nicotinic acetylcholine receptor. *Proc Natl Acad Sci U S A*. 1996;93:2807-2810.]

binding to any G-protein subunit or the heterotrimeric complex has not yet emerged.[32] This work is highly intricate because of the multiple complexes and states and at this time is unresolved.

Mitochondria Mitochondria have long been suspected as contributing to anesthetic action because of their obvious role in cellular energy production. However, the anesthetic concentrations required for inhibition of ATP production and the apparently slow kinetics for ATP depletion seemed to obviate their role. Recent evidence has renewed interest in the mitochondrion. First, signaling and feedback between mitochondria and cellular consumers of ATP is considerably more precise and rapid than originally thought, effectively eliminating the kinetic argument against their contribution to the anesthetic state. Second, mitochondrial genes have been implicated in unbiased genetic screens in simple organisms (see later discussion). For example, mutations in a mitochondrial complex I subunit gene dramatically increased sensitivity to halothane, enflurane, and isoflurane. As expected, mitochondria isolated from this mutant had a reduced rate of oxidative phosphorylation in the presence of halothane.[64] Furthermore, several subunits of the oxidative phosphorylation complexes, including complex I, were found to bind halothane specifically.[65] Perhaps most importantly, children with biopsy-proven complex I disease were found to be extraordinarily sensitive to the anesthetic sevoflurane,[66] rendering this anesthetic target the only to date that has supportive evidence from the gene, the binding interaction, to the human. The underlying mechanism for how the altered mitochondrial function affects anesthetic sensitivity is unclear, but given the recent evidence that mitochondria modulates synaptic transmission through the regulation of presynaptic Ca^{2+} dynamics,[67] it is possible that previously described mutations affect synaptic transmission. Another potential mitochondrial target is the voltage-dependent anion channel 1 (VDAC-1), an anion channel also related to mitochondrial steroid synthesis and synaptic activity and implicated through halothane and neurosteroid binding assays, although knock-out animals had unaltered anesthetic sensitivity.[65,68,69]

Summary A wide variety of molecular candidates have been examined, and although several are compelling, proof for dominant involvement in the in vivo anesthesia endpoint is still lacking. But how does one determine the relevance of a molecular interaction to the in vivo effect, especially when it is as complex as consciousness?

FROM MOLECULES TO BEHAVIOR

HOW TO DETERMINE THE RELEVANCE OF IN VITRO ASSAYS

The plethora of potential targets, the imprecise definitions of anesthesia, the variable endpoints, and the low-affinity drugs have conspired to make it difficult to judge the contribution of molecular targets to drug behavior, an already difficult task. As a start, 2 broad concepts of anesthetic action have been proposed: one favors a single molecular target site (the "unitary" hypothesis), and the other proposes that anesthesia results from the combination of actions at many molecular targets (distributed hypothesis). Lipid theories are an example of unitary theories, as are those that focus solely on the $GABA_A$ receptor. Distributed action hypotheses require careful dissection of more molecular targets. Historically, the hunt for the volatile anesthetic targets has taken 2 general approaches: the study of effects on a well-defined and functionally or physically isolated target (bottom-up approach) and those that start with the anesthetic effect on an organism with the goal of defining the target responsible for the observed effect using either genetic or pharmacologic probes (top-down approach). Although both approaches have merits and limitations, it is the complex, dynamic coupling between "top" and "bottom" that has so far made clear conclusions difficult. Next we discuss how information derived from one approach might contribute to testable hypotheses in the other and how when taken together, support for a neurophysiologic *process* (the "middle") rather than an individual protein or behavior emerges as a likely anesthetic target. It is important to realize that disruption of a process might have multiple contributing and interacting molecular events.

"Bottom-up" Approach This approach has dominated much of the literature on the mechanism of general anesthetic action. Examples are studies of the biochemistry of anesthetic action on a specific signaling cascade, such as activation of a G-protein coupled pathway, studies on the structural nature of anesthetic binding sites in synthetic proteins, and electrophysiology of heterologously expressed ion channels. An important weakness of this approach is that it requires the identification of a system for study based on the inherently biased criterion, plausibility.

Plausibility has driven studies on the effects of anesthetics on the electrophysiology of ion channels expressed in heterologous systems such as the *Xenopus* oocyte. Such electropharmacologic studies have demonstrated effects (enhancement or inhibition) of anesthetics on essentially all the ion channels examined, albeit some requiring higher concentrations of anesthetics than others. Herein lies the principal weakness of the bottom-up approach. How do we determine whether a given effect on a given target contributes to a particular behavioral endpoint? Discrepancy between the anesthetic concentration required for the effect on a given target protein and the clinical MAC (either positive or negative) has led to a call for dismissal of some putative targets as biologically irrelevant.[70] As we discussed for the relationship between K_d and EC_{50}, the relationship between EC_{50} and MAC is not likely to be linear. The nervous system is complex, and

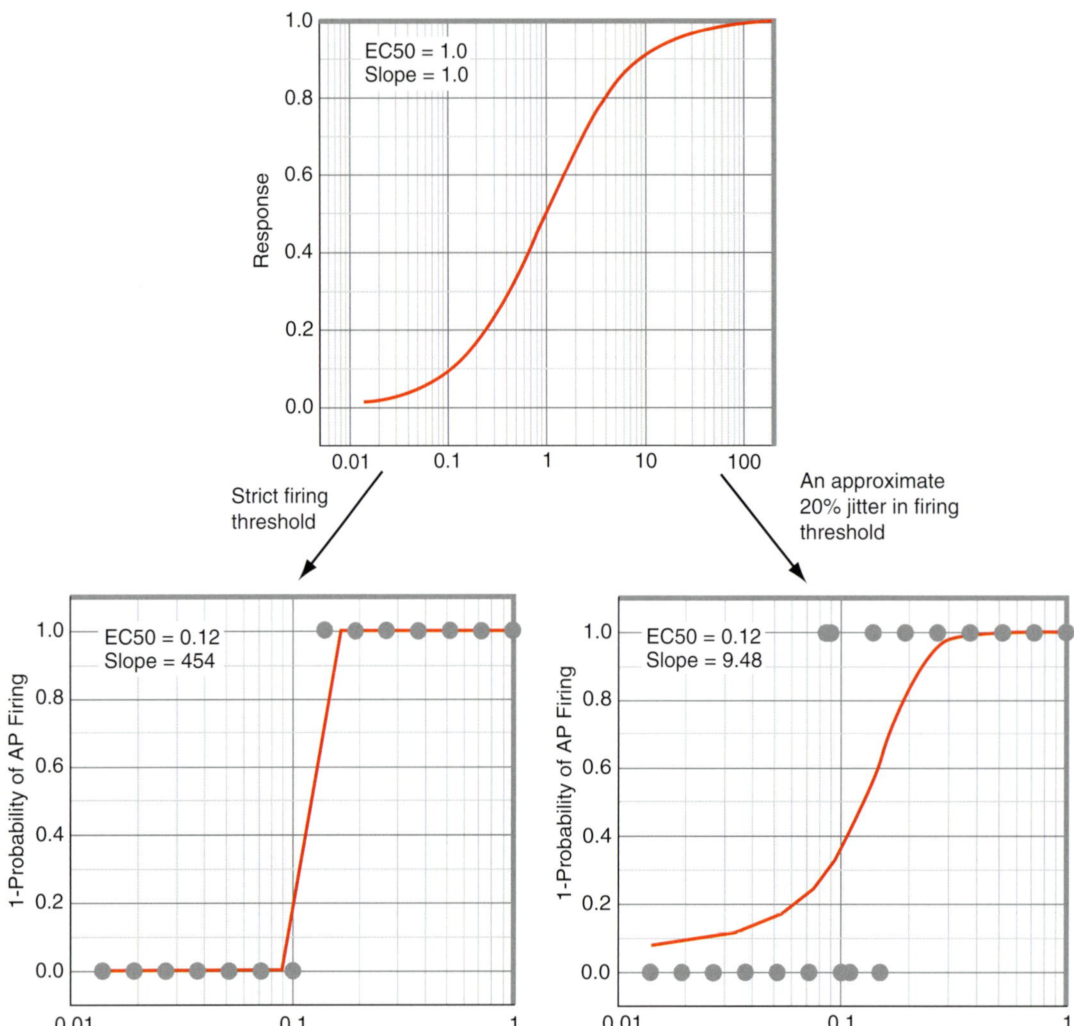

FIGURE 37-16. Effects of a single nonlinear threshold process on a continuous concentration–response relationship describing a volatile anesthetic (VA) action. **Top.** Simulated continuous concentration–response relationship of a VA action on a response described by Response = [VA]/([VA] + 1), yielding median effective concentration (EC_{50}) = 1.0 and slope = 1.0. Suppose the response represents enhancement of γ-aminobutyric acid (GABA)ergic inhibitory post-synaptic current (IPSC) decay rate and that initiation of an action potential (AP) is inhibited by a 10% increase in the IPSC duration. If the threshold for AP firing is set at exactly 10% with no variability, we obtain an effective concentration response described by a logistic equation with EC_{50} = 0.1 and slope = 454. **Bottom left.** If we incorporate an approximate 20% jitter in the AP firing so that on occasion IPSC prolongation slightly greater than 10% fails to inhibit and likewise a VA-induced event slightly less than 10% inhibits AP firing, we obtain the relationship on the right, described by EC_{50} = 0.1 and slope = 9.48. **Bottom right.** Further cascading of more threshold events in between the continuous concentration–response, such as those obtained in in vitro studies, and the final anesthetic endpoint, such as immobility to noxious stimulus surely to be present in even the simplest neural pathway, will result in a large transformation of the overall concentration–response relationship, giving little credence to using the sensitivity or the slope of a concentration–response relationship to include or exclude a putative VA target.

inclusion of even 1 simple nonlinear process, such as generation of an action potential in a synaptic transmission (a threshold effect), can easily shift an apparently irrelevant in vitro concentration–response relationship to one that is quantitatively consistent with clinical MAC (**Fig. 37-16**).[51] Even at the *single* synapse level, spatial and temporal integration of postsynaptic currents contributing to the generation of action potentials will interpose further nonlinear processes between a drug action at a receptor and an observable output. A simple cascading of multiple processes, each well described by a conventional continuous concentration–response curve (ie, Hill equation), will further shift the composite concentration–response curve to the left with an increase in the Hill slope.[71,72] Thus, a quantitative discrepancy in the experimentally and clinically observed concentration–response relationship cannot discredit the biologic relevance of a putative anesthetic target.

Given the apparent difficulty of linking molecular events and behavior, other "litmus test" criteria have emerged. For a target to be seriously considered as a candidate, most agree that the anesthetic must actually occupy a binding site in or on the target (see earlier). Thus, it is remarkable how many candidates are being favored in the complete absence of binding data. Other criteria used to establish relevance are Overton-Meyer behavior (correlation of potency with lipid solubility), enantioselectivity, sensitivity (correlation of in vitro EC_{50} with MAC), lack of response to nonimmobilizer compounds, hydrostatic pressure reversal, cutoff, and plausibility. For example, if differences in potency exist in the intact organism for the enantiomers of a given anesthetic, then the targets responsible for this anesthetic effect also should exhibit this difference in potency in vitro. If the organism fails to lose consciousness with a particular compound (eg, F6 or F8), then any underlying molecular target also should remain unaffected.[73]

However, this litmus test logic assumes that a single target can produce anesthesia, and now that several molecular targets have emerged that satisfy many of these criteria, such criteria should be viewed with considerable skepticism.

A final means of establishing linkage of the molecular event with the behavior involves use of specific pharmacologic probes. For example, concentration–effect experiments with anesthetics can be performed in the presence of other sedative drugs, and then the interaction can be characterized as synergistic, additive, or antagonistic through isobolographic analysis. If the second drug is known to be highly specific for a given molecular target, then some insight might be gained into the targets used by anesthetic. Although this approach has identified many potential targets for the inhaled anesthetics, its use has been somewhat reduced by the fact that the second drug rarely produces the same endpoint as that of the anesthetics. For example, the opioids and the benzodiazepines, unless given in very high doses, do not produce the MAC endpoint, but this is the standard endpoint for the volatile anesthetics. Yet in both cases, the second drug decreases the volatile anesthetic MAC by 10% to 50%. Agonism at the GPCR α_2-adrenergic receptors reduces anesthetic requirements by as much as 90%,[74] although whether synergistic or additive cannot be clear because these agents cannot independently reach this endpoint. Finally, this pharmacologic approach is further confounded by the fact that the effects are global, and it is now recognized that the same targets may have important influences only regionally (see later).

Summary Bottom-up studies allow for well-controlled experiments with well-defined endpoints (eg, examination of the extent of anesthetic potentiation of $GABA_A$ receptors) and for straightforward subsequent genetic manipulation of the target protein through conventional site-directed mutagenesis of the complementary DNA encoding the protein of interest expressed in vitro. However these approaches are primarily useful for generating *testable hypotheses,* in which the biologic relevance of the putative target can be proposed and then examined in a more intact system, such as with targeted pharmacologic or knock-out, knock-in, or knock-down genetic approaches.

"Top-down" Approach An alternative approach to determining the sites and mechanisms of drug action is a "top-down approach" in which the starting point is an individual or a population of intact organisms. Populations typically harbor mutations in their genome, and thus individuals with high or low sensitivity to volatile anesthetics can be identified through standard potency experiments and the potential molecular basis hypothesized based on the discovered genetic differences. For example, strain differences in mice have been demonstrated[75] but are small (<50%), and the underlying genetics appear to be complex. This approach is limited, however, because it requires that considerable variability exist within the population of organisms to clearly select for the differences. The Hill slopes of 20 in the human population suggest that sufficient variability in the response does not exist for this to be a productive approach unless enormous numbers of individuals can be tested.

Although difficult in human studies, such numbers can be easily studied in simple organisms, such as the fruit fly *Drosophila melanogaster* or the worm *C. elegans*. These systems give the added advantage of relatively easy identification of the genetic defect from the selected population, an approach called "forward genetic" screening. The primary advantage of such a system lies in the possibility of revealing a direct correlation between a genetic target and a complex behavior involving no a priori assumptions or biases. Furthermore, the natural prevalence of mutations often can be considerably enhanced by chemicals or ultraviolet light in these simple systems, greatly increasing the odds of finding interesting alterations. On the other hand, the fundamental limitation of simple model systems lies in the definition of the anesthetic state or the behavioral endpoint used and its relevance to the state of general anesthesia in higher organisms. For example, the yeast *Saccharomyces cerevisia* is an enormously useful eukaryote for genetic studies, but how can one possibly define anesthesia in the absence of behavior? Is anesthetic-induced immobility in a nematode analogous to anesthesia? Should similar endpoints be chosen across species (eg, immobility) independent of the anesthetic concentration dependence, or should arbitrary endpoints be chosen that happen to have similar concentration–response relationships across species? Will determining the genetic basis for anesthetic-induced growth inhibition in yeast or escape behavior in flies tell us anything about how anesthetics work in humans? Although such questions are legitimate and vexing, conservation of biologic processes throughout phylogeny has been proven time and again, and a fundamental biologic mechanism operating in simple organisms is likely to have a homologous mechanism in the more complex organisms. Research using the forward genetic approach to seek the volatile anesthetic site of action in simple organisms has yielded several exciting potential targets.

Similar to humans, nematodes have different behaviors that demonstrate different sensitivity to anesthetics. For example, whereas complex behaviors such as mating, chemotaxis, and coordinated movement are inhibited at halothane concentrations similar to human MAC values,[29] immobility occurs only at concentrations approximately 8 times higher (**Fig. 37-17**).[76] The top-down screening of a de novo mutagenized population using immobility as the endpoint has identified genes encoding the worm homologues of 2 mammalian proteins as the genetic basis for increased sensitivity to anesthetics (resistant organisms for the immobility endpoint have not been discovered): a subunit of mitochondrial complex I protein (see earlier) and stomatin, a transmembrane protein enriched in the lipid raft microdomains. Interestingly, these studies have clearly documented that these mutations do not affect sensitivity to all volatile anesthetics, the first solid evidence against a unitary hypothesis of volatile anesthetic action. A very powerful tool in these simple creatures is that suppressors (ie, strains with additional mutations that negate the phenotype of the original mutation) can be sought. Identification and function of the suppressor then can be reconciled with that of the original mutation to provide validation and further understanding of the underlying pathways and mechanisms. For example, a suppressor of the worm mitochondrial complex I mutation was found that increased the capacity for oxidative phosphorylation in isolated mitochondria and partially restored-wild type anesthetic sensitivity in the intact worm.[77] This, when combined with the observation that children with complex I disorders have unusual high anesthetic sensitivity,[66] strengthens the association between anesthetic sensitivity and mitochondrial function.

A similar screening of *C. elegans* mutants using the loss of more complex behaviors, such as coordinated movement, as the behavioral endpoint identified the syntaxin-1A gene, mentioned earlier,[29] as being associated with anesthetic resistance (≤ 6-fold). Further work, including binding studies and suppressors, has provided evidence for the involvement of syntaxin-1A in anesthetic action and has led to the attractive and intuitive hypothesis that anesthetics interfere with the release of neurotransmitters at the presynaptic terminal, producing a general reduction in synaptic transmission (see later).[78] Again, these simple creatures have provided compelling hypotheses for testing in higher organisms.

Moving up the complexity and evolutionary scale, studies in *D. melanogaster* have documented that specific ion channels can contribute to volatile anesthetic sensitivity (**Fig. 37-18**). For example, forward genetic screening has succeeded in isolating a putative ion channel resembling the voltage-gated sodium and calcium channels as important for anesthetic-induced immobility.[79] As in the worm, the different ion channels show variable sensitivity to different volatile anesthetics, suggesting that multiple neurophysiologic mechanisms mediate the action of different anesthetics even in simple organisms.

A final related approach that avoids investigator bias is assaying for the genes or proteins whose expression is altered during or after

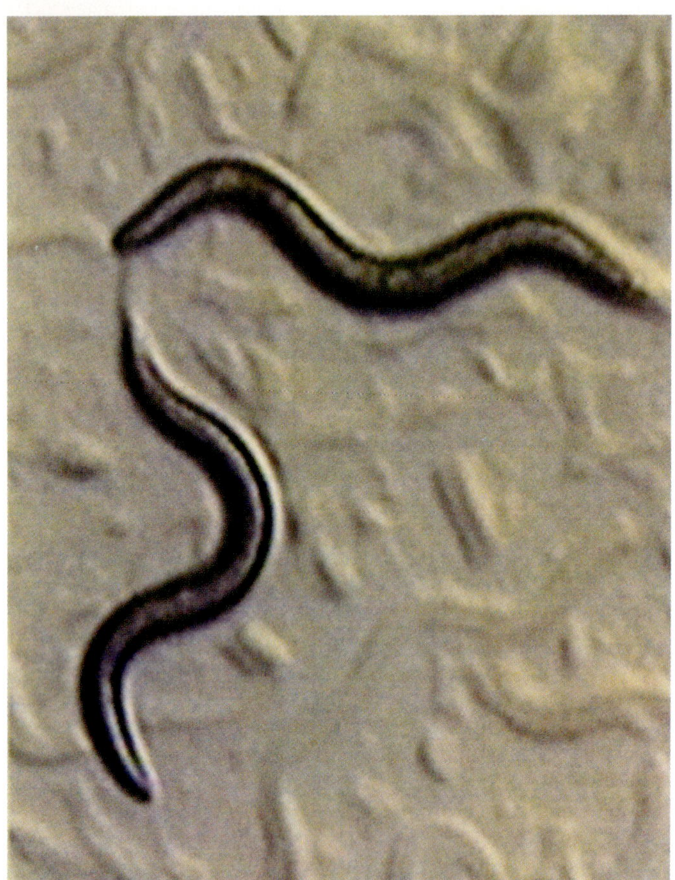

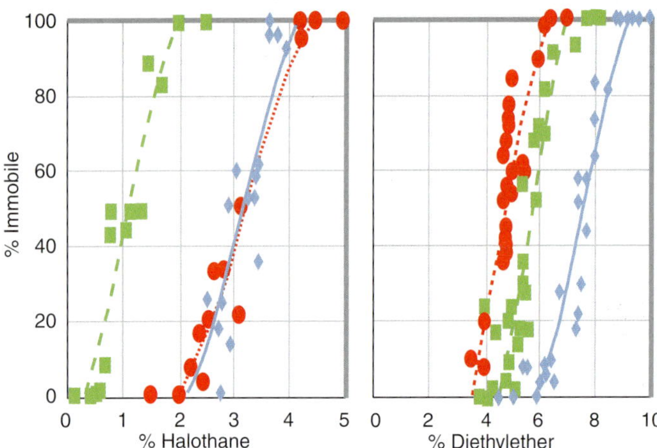

FIGURE 37-17. "Worm" model. *Caenorhabditis elegans* is only 1 mm long, but the short generation time, the ease of manipulation, the fully understood genome, and the presence of complex behaviors have made it a popular model for anesthetic studies. **Right.** Anesthetic dose–response curves for the wild-type and for more sensitive mutants (shifted to the left). [Reprinted with permission from Steriade M, McCormick DA, Sejnowski TJ. Thalamocortical oscillations in the sleeping and aroused brain. *Science*. 1993;262:679-685.]

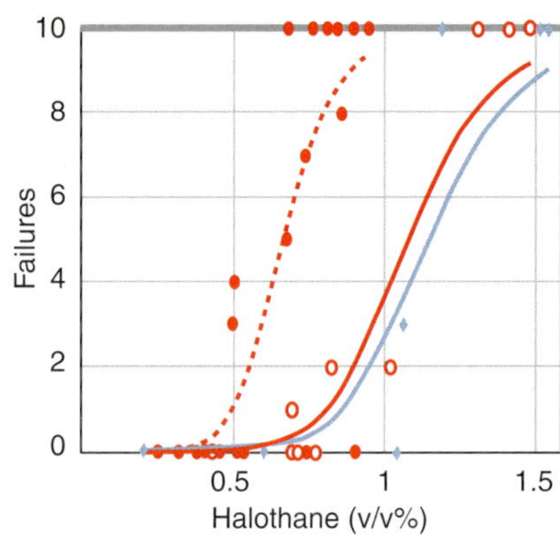

FIGURE 37-18. "Fly" model. *Drosophila melanogaster* is a similarly popular organism for anesthetic studies for the same reasons as is the worm but is a somewhat more complex organism. Median effective concentration (EC_{50}) concentrations in this assay are more analogous to those required for immobility in mammals and shown are hypersensitive mutants. [Reprinted with permission from Gottschalk A, Miotke SA. Volatile anesthetic action in a computational model of the thalamic reticular nucleus. *Anesthesiology*. 2009;110:996-1010.]

exposure to volatile anesthetics. This approach carries the tenuous assumption that the cells and organism will choose to alter the expression of those targets directly affected by the anesthetic in an attempt at homeostasis. In some published studies, the expression of many genes or proteins is altered.[80,81] However, using a more (perhaps overly) rigorous statistical approach, a study found only a modest transcriptional response after considerable exposure to either halothane or isoflurane in both animals and cells.[40] It is still too early to summarize this approach because the methodology, analysis, and interpretation are evolving.

Taken together with the evidence presented, observations from both bottom-up and top-down studies suggest that a search for a small number of targets for volatile anesthetic action in a complex organism is overly simplistic and unlikely to yield a satisfactory or interpretable answer. However, future studies using novel methods for confirming a critical role of a given genetic defect in determining the inhaled anesthetic sensitivity may yet prove that our arguments against the unitary hypothesis are incorrect.

INTEGRATION OF MOLECULAR RESPONSES

If anesthesia is an integrated response to a large number of molecular events, then validation at the molecular level or in translational attempts of single candidates will be difficult. For example, the most popular means of testing hypotheses from both bottom-up and top-down approaches is to produce genetically altered animals (usually mice). As mentioned for $GABA_A$ receptors, this form of validation suffers from at least 2 weaknesses. First, in a knock-out (null mutant) animal, developmental compensation may occur in multiple associated pathways, possibly providing new mechanisms for anesthetic-induced perturbations. However, this does argue against highly specific "unitary" targets because the likelihood that such adaptation in other components of the pathway will produce similarly unique and functionally active binding sites seems rather small. The second weakness, for both knock-out and knock-in strategies, is that the physiologic alteration may be of sufficient magnitude to render endpoint evaluation difficult (eg, seizures, lethality). Consistent with these concerns, this means of testing individual targets has generally yielded ambiguous results.

The existence of a large number of targets does not fully rule out a unitary mechanism of action, however. Such a mechanism might be found at a higher level of resolution, such as at the level of a neurophysiologic process. Candidates at this level are numerous but could include transcription or translation, mitochondrial activity, membrane resting potential, action potential conduction, and synaptic transmission, ultimately leading to changes in the output of neuronal circuits. Each process has multiple and overlapping molecular contributors.

Decades of study have implicated the *synapse* as a key neurophysiologic substrate affected by volatile anesthetics.[82] This idea initially was based on the simple observation that axonal conduction of action potentials was more resistant to volatile anesthetics than synaptic transmission. Insight gained from the large number of bottom-up and top-down studies of volatile anesthetics has supported and refined the notion that synaptic transmission is the most likely neurophysiologic *process* targeted by these drugs (Fig. 37-17).

Synaptic transmission, although the most fundamental unit of intercellular information transfer in the nervous system, is a highly complex process in itself (**Fig. 37-19**). When an action potential arrives at the presynaptic terminal, an increase in presynaptic Ca^{2+} concentration via voltage-gated calcium channels and release from intracellular stores activates the synaptic vesicle release machinery orchestrated by and consisting of a myriad of proteins. After release into the synaptic cleft, the concentration of transmitter available to the postsynaptic receptor is influenced by neurotransmitter uptake pumps and degradative enzymes for some synapses. On activation of the postsynaptic receptor (G-protein coupled or ligand-gated channel) and the consequent influx of ions and activation of cellular

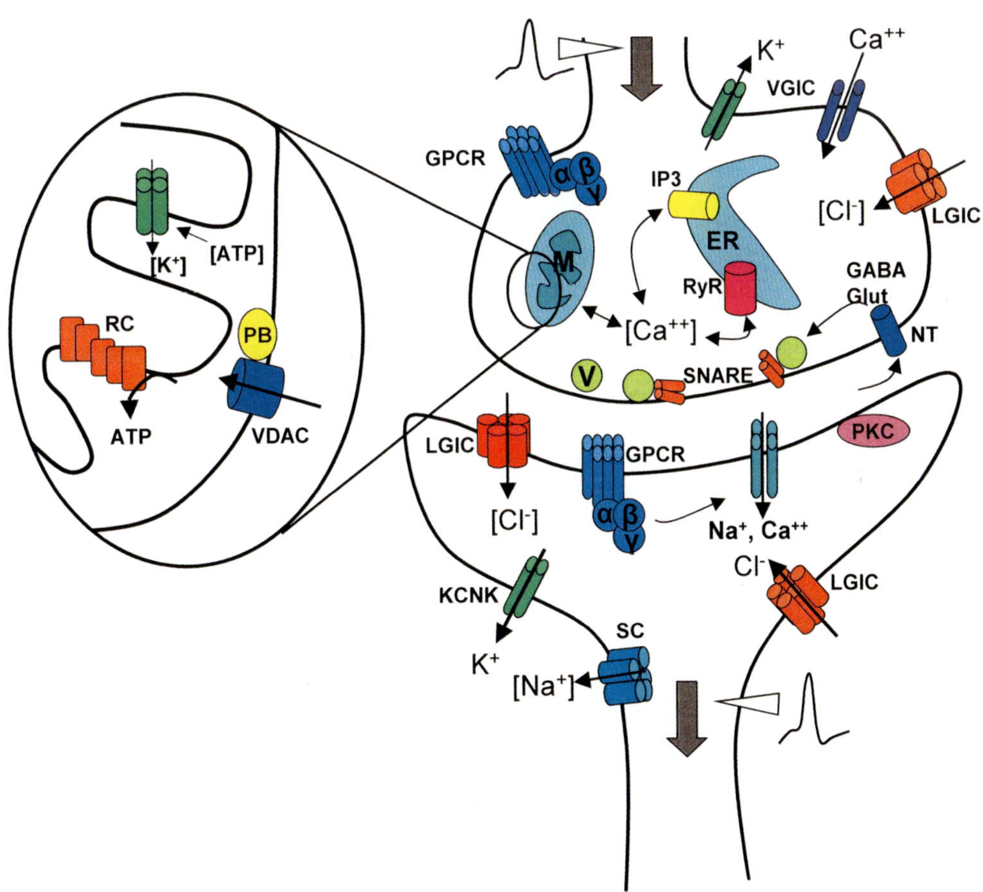

FIGURE 37-19. Some potential targets of inhaled anesthetics in the synapse. Synaptic transmission is a likely neurophysiologic process targeted by the inhaled anesthetics. On the presynaptic side, interference with calcium channels or mobilization of intracellular calcium[109] will reduce neurotransmitter release and perhaps cause synaptic failure. Interference with vesicle trafficking and fusion proteins[110] would clearly add to this effect. Heterotrimeric G-protein and G-protein coupled receptors (GPCRs) also are likely to affect anesthetic sensitivity, as already demonstrated in *Caenorhabditis elegans* and other systems. Thus, the seemingly unrelated putative protein targets of volatile anesthetics already revealed by both the bottom-up and top-down studies may play a key role in the presynaptic events of transmission. So too are the dynamics of transmitter concentrations in the synaptic cleft. The activity of all of the major neurotransmitter transporters is altered by volatile anesthetics, either raising or lowering synaptic cleft concentrations. This is important because of the apparent cooperativity with anesthetics in some postsynaptic receptors (ligand-gated channels [LGIC]) or the competition with others (some GPCRs). Finally, the effects on many postsynaptic receptors already alluded to are thought to contribute to anesthetic action. Likewise, increased "shunting" of the postsynaptic charge because of enhancement of the KCNK leakage channels or tonic γ-aminobutyric acid type A ($GABA_A$) channels will limit depolarization of the postsynaptic membrane and likely preclude the generation of postsynaptic action potentials. Anesthetic action on other lipophilic proteins, such as stomatin and others residing in lipid rafts enriched in signaling proteins, could disrupt the signaling initiated by neurotransmitter activation of the myriad of metabotropic receptors regulating synaptic transmission.

Presynaptic: ER, endoplasmic reticulum, containing ryanodine receptors (*magenta*) and inositol-trisphosphate channels (*yellow*); GPCR (*blue*), G-protein coupled receptor with associated heterotrimeric G-protein (αβγ); M, mitochondria, containing ATP-gated potassium channels (*green*), the respiratory complexes (RC, *orange*), and the voltage-dependent anion channel (VDAC, *dark blue*) with its associated peripheral benzodiazepine receptor (PB, *yellow*); VGIC (*green* and *purple*), voltage-gated ion channels, either calcium (Ca) or potassium (K); LGIC (*orange*), tonic ligand-gated ion channels; NT (*dark blue*), neurotransmitter transporters; SNARE (*orange*), synaptic vesicle transport and fusion proteins; V (*light green*), synaptic vesicles.

Postsynaptic: GPCR, neurotransmitter G-protein coupled receptor; KCNK, tandem pore potassium channels (TREK, TASK, and so on); LGIC (*red*), ligand-gated ion channels such as $GABA_A$, AMPA/KA, nicotinic cholinergic, and $5HT_3$; PKC, protein kinase C; SC, sodium channels.

signaling molecules, the change in charge distribution may produce depolarization of the postsynaptic membrane and formation of an action potential if the threshold is exceeded. Thus, it should be clear that anesthetics can and do have an effect at each of the many points in the process.

Given a focus on synaptic transmission as a key *process* targeted by volatile anesthetics, some predictions can be made on the anesthetic phenotype of some mice not yet examined. For example, the null-mutant mice for the various calcium channels or release mechanisms that regulate presynaptic calcium dynamics, all with impaired synaptic transmission, should demonstrate increased sensitivity to volatile anesthetics. In contrast, mouse mutants with enhanced synaptic transmission, which may result from mutations increasing neurotransmitter concentration in the synapse, should exhibit decreased sensitivity to anesthetics. If we assume that the state of clinical general anesthesia is a manifestation of all the downstream consequences of the failure of synaptic transmission, there will be many more yet unidentified target proteins and processes contributing to this complex drug action. However, interpretation of the anesthetic phenotype of any gene-targeted mice must take into consideration the likely redundancy built into any complex system and the possibility of compensatory changes in the conventional null-mutant mice.

A model in which a process is altered by widely distributed and perhaps small input effects also predicts difficulty in altering the output with isolated input manipulations. Analogy may be found on the Internet, where many coordinated small and essentially undetectable influences on router function (colluding routers) can have a considerably larger effect on Internet "function" than a few large and easily detected router "meltdowns."[86] A small-effects-at-multiple-targets model leads to predictions that so far have been largely verified. For example, altered plausible molecular targets with clear alteration of anesthetic effects in isolation, when introduced in a system or process context, produce little, if any, effect on anesthetic sensitivity. Although this is complicated in biologic systems by homeostasis and compensation, this observation appears to be consistent. In no case has a mutation of an individual target or highly specific drug altered anesthetic potency by more than 2-fold, usually much less. Furthermore, the facts that antagonists have not emerged, that there is little biologic variability, and that there is no adaptation even when the drugs are given continuously for weeks all argue for a highly distributed, redundant molecular effect. Redundancy is often used in systems design to produce reliability, a feature synonymous with low variation. The reliability of anesthetic action is a clinical feature we cannot afford to ignore, but its foundation in a distributed mechanism is a scientific feature that will be difficult to sort out.

NEUROANATOMIC SUBSTRATES

A process may be widely distributed within the nervous system (eg, synaptic transmission), but the influence of its dysfunction could be sensed and exhibited regionally. Although there is no evidence for regional binding of anesthetic (Fig. 37-8), binding targets may be positioned within networks and pathways that rely on their neurotransmitter types and regional interactions for higher functions, such as behavior. Thus, GABAergic enhancement in the spinal cord or the cerebellum may have very different functional effects than enhancement in the hippocampus. The different functional components of general anesthesia likely arise from such regionality (**Box 37-2**).

Thus, volatile anesthetics produce a composite state that can be subdivided into functional components, which include amnesia, unconsciousness, analgesia, muscle atonia, and autonomic nervous system modulation. Each may represent specific interactions of general anesthetics upon discrete neuronal loci. Just as the search for molecular targets of anesthetic action has revealed multiple sites of modulation, so too has the hunt for cellular sites of anesthetic action. In this section, we focus upon different features of the anesthetic state that arise from anesthetic actions in various parts of the CNS.

BOX 37-2

Further Definition of Targets Within the Process

Despite the logical appeal of a forward genetic approach to identifying volatile anesthetic sites of action, a well-defined population of mouse mutants amenable to this approach is not presently available, relegating the genetic approach to volatile anesthetic site-of-action research to a painstaking testing of many specific mouse mutants. However, a true forward genetic screening to allow identification of volatile anesthetic–sensitive gene products in mice may be possible in the near future. A concerted effort using state-of-art techniques, including gene targeting, gene trapping, and RNA interference to produce mouse mutants on a large scale with the ultimate goal of creating knock-outs covering a substantial portion of the entire genome, is under way.[83,84] Of course, we must be cognizant of the usual caveats of the inherent strain differences in anesthetic sensitivity[75] and genetic compensation in the traditional global knockout. A combination of gene trapping and site-specific DNA inversion methods[85] may allow large-scale production of conditional knock-out mice in animals from a uniform background that could overcome these limitations. The technical ingenuity of all these approaches is that the genetic basis for any observed phenotype can be traced back with relative ease because the site of gene disruption is traceable, similar to the fruit fly and the worm model systems. Such projects envision a systematic hierarchical phenotyping of every mutant, starting with a low-cost tier I screen (home-cage observation, physical examination, blood hematologic and chemistry profiles, and skeletal radiographs) followed by a more specialized tier II screening with all results publicly available. For the general anesthesia research community to take advantage of these upcoming international scientific resources, an inexpensive large-scale screening of volatile anesthetic sensitivity in mice must be developed. Integration of results garnered from the bottom-up and top-down approaches, particularly in mice, although cognizant of a "neurophysiologic process" as the true target for the complex action of volatile anesthetic, is likely to provide a clearer picture of how these clinically essential drugs produce clinical general anesthesia.

Anesthetics and Immobility The MAC endpoint is defined as the MAC of an agent that is required to suppress movement in response to a defined noxious stimulus. It should not be surprising then that anesthetics appear to exert their immobilizing effects most sensitively through interactions within the spinal cord. For example, transection of the brain at the level of the inferior colliculus does not alter the MAC of inhaled anesthetics in mammals.[87] Although such lesions ablate ascending and descending forebrain and midbrain communications with the spinal cord, they do not impair spontaneous ventilatory efforts because brainstem respiratory groups are left intact. This works suggests that MAC is primarily determined by a direct action of anesthetics upon the CNS at a level caudal to the brainstem—the spinal cord. Further work in multiple species supports this hypothesis. Surgical isolation of brain and spinal cord blood flow in goats (which lack significant cerebral perfusion from vertebral arteries) allowed independent determination of MAC. Delivery to the brain required a greater than 2-fold higher concentration than did whole-animal MAC, suggesting that immobility is produced via direct interactions within the spinal cord.[88,89] In vitro evidence of anesthetic effects on the spinal cord has also been obtained. All volatile anesthetics tested to date appear to suppress the excitability of spinal motor neurons; however, even within the spinal cord, different anesthetics exert their effects at multiple sites. For example, whereas halothane reduces noxious-evoked movement via depression of dorsal horn neurons, isoflurane appears to have smaller effects on these sensory neurons yet produces an identical inhibition of movement by exerting a relatively greater suppression of anterior horn motor neurons or interneurons.[90]

Anesthetics and Hypnosis Although the neural substrate responsible for generating consciousness remains unknown, much has been learned about the systems responsible for its nightly loss and subsequent return during the normal process of sleep. The physiologic changes associated with unconsciousness induced by both anesthesia and sleep are strikingly similar. They include decreased minute ventilation, blood pressure, heart rate, core body temperature, motor tone, and (most importantly) responsiveness to external stimuli. Studies of cortical function in both states reveal a similar breakdown of spatial and temporal information transfer.[91,92] The slow-wave oscillations in the electroencephalogram (EEG) that define the deepest stage of non–rapid eye movement (NREM) sleep bear striking resemblance to those seen under hypnotic doses of some anesthetics. In both instances, slow waves originate in the same "hotspots" and propagate in similar directions throughout the cortex.[93] Moreover, the spindle waves common to NREM sleep are also seen during general anesthesia.[94] Positron emission tomography, used to study cerebral blood flow during both sleep and anesthesia, has confirmed that similar alterations in regional cerebral blood flow, metabolism, and regional neuronal activity occur during both sleep and general anesthesia.[95] These similarities and others (documented in the following) have led to the speculation that sleep and general anesthesia share an underlying neural substrate. Consistent with this hypothesis is the observation that an individual's underlying state of arousal alters anesthetic sensitivity. In rodents, loss of consciousness typically is assessed by the LORR behavioral assay in which animals turned from supine to prone are unable to right themselves. Using this endpoint, Einon et al[96] noted that the hypnotic duration of pentobarbital was prolonged when the drug was administered to rats during their sleeping hours compared with their normally wakeful hours. Sleep deprivation acts synergistically with anesthetics, reducing the dose of anesthetic required for hypnosis and allowing recovery from sleep deprivation.[97]

Further linkage between sleep and anesthesia derives from pharmacologic studies. Endogenous somnogens such as adenosine, which can induce sleep, also potentiate the hypnotic effects of inhaled and intravenous anesthetics and delay emergence from anesthesia.[98] Moreover, anesthetic exposure appears to affect levels of endogenous somnogens, such as prostaglandin D_2.[99]

Despite these overlapping features, it is clear that sleep and general anesthesia have important differences. The most notable is that whereas sleep is readily reversed through external stimuli, anesthesia is reversed only upon discontinuation of the anesthetic drugs. Another primary difference is that anesthetics appear to inhibit systems required for rapid eye movement (REM) sleep as well as cortical arousal.[94] Hence, general anesthesia has been likened to a form of NREM sleep from which one cannot be easily aroused.[95]

The similarities between NREM sleep and general anesthesia extend to various measures of the EEG. For example, both power spectrum analysis and the bispectral index[100] show a high degree of similarity between NREM sleep and general anesthesia. EEG entropy, a measure of the disorder inherent in the EEG, declines during deep NREM sleep and during general anesthesia.[101,102] In both instances, as NREM sleep or anesthetic depth increases, the EEG becomes more ordered, further reducing EEG entropy.

Neural Circuitry of Arousal Similarities between general anesthesia and NREM sleep have led to the speculation that the 2 states share a common underlying neural network. As is the case with the molecular targets, there are many potential neuronal structures upon which anesthetics can act to produce unconsciousness. Because of bidirectional signaling (a neuron may send efferent fibers to and receive afferent fibers from its signaling partner), it has been difficult to unravel a primary site of anesthetic-induced hypnosis. Nonetheless, putative sites of action for the hypnotic effects of anesthetics are found along the entire neuroaxis from the brainstem through the thalamus, hypothalamus, basal forebrain, and cerebral cortex (**Fig. 37-20**). Distinct anesthetic drugs differentially alter activity of key arousal-promoting nuclei depending on the diverse set of molecular targets expressed in those nuclei.[95,103-105]

The extent of arousal is determined by the coordinated activity of many nuclei within the brain. Among the best studied are the thalamocortical, reticular, and corticothalamic circuit loops.[106,107] During wakefulness, descending excitatory input from the cortex together with ascending excitatory input from the reticular activating system (Fig. 37-20) drive thalamocortical neurons to fire tonically. Conversely, during deep slow-wave sleep or general anesthesia (with ketamine as a notable exception), thalamocortical neurons adopt a bursting pattern of activity. This switch is thought to underlie a dramatic synchronization of the cortex, which is heavily innervated by the thalamus, resulting in the slow 1- to 4-Hz delta waves that mark the deepest stage of NREM sleep and are also common to anesthetic hypnosis as well as the characteristic sleep spindles, 10- to 14-Hz oscillations that also accompany anesthesia.[94] This change in thalamic activity has been proposed to underlie the switch from conscious to unconscious states.[95] Moreover, in vivo electrophysiologic recordings in animals confirm that anesthetic-induced changes in neural activity are attributable to the hyperpolarization of thalamocortical resting membrane potential brought about partly by the reticular thalamic nucleus' inhibitory input.[1] Detailed understanding of natural thalamocortical oscillations and their physiologic significance in switching from tonic to burst firing has led to intense interest in the electrophysiologic properties of the thalamic nuclei and the recognition of the key role played by the GABAergic reticular nucleus as well as anesthetic-induced hyperpolarization of thalamocortical neurons arising from potentiation at 2 pore potassium and $GABA_A$ channels and inhibition at hyperpolarization-activated cyclic nucleotide-gated channels.[1] Knowledge of the function of these circuits also led to accurate predictions that voltage-gated calcium channels might also contribute to the clinical effects of anesthetics[55] and promising mathematical models.[108] One major feature of the midline thalamic nuclei is to integrate afferent reticular activating input from both sleep- and wake-active centers (Fig. 37-20) leading to modulation of both the arousal state and circuit output.

The prototypic sleep-promoting cluster of neurons is found in the ventral lateral preoptic (VLPO) nucleus located in the anterior hypothalamus and has been shown to contain a group of cells specifically active during non-REM sleep.[109] Subsequent studies in rodents using in vivo electrophysiologic recordings together with polysomnography have proved that VLPO neurons are sleep active, firing rapidly during sleep while being inhibited during wakefulness. VLPO neurons send projections to the orexinergic and all of the monoaminergic wake-active centers in the brain[110] (Fig. 37-20) and express the inhibitory neurotransmitters GABA and galanin. Hence, through GABA-mediated signaling, VLPO neurons together with sleep-promoting neurons in the median preoptic nucleus (MnPO) inhibit wake-active centers responsible for regulating vigilance and cortical arousal and thereby favor sleep.

The major arousal centers, located in the hypothalamus and brainstem, consist of the orexinergic neurons (Ox) concentrated around the perifornical and lateral hypothalamus as well as the histaminergic cells in the tuberomammillary nucleus (TMN), the noradrenergic cells in the pontine locus coeruleus (LC), the serotonergic cells in the raphe nuclei (RN), and the cholinergic mesopontine neurons in the lateral dorsal tegmentum (LDT) and pedunculopontine tegmentum (PPT). As a group, the TMN, LC, and DR (monoaminergic neurons) as well as the orexinergic neurons are maximally active during wakefulness, decrease their firing rate during NREM sleep, and are virtually silent during REM sleep. These neuronal groups send diffuse projections that innervate the entire neuraxis. The cholinergic brainstem arousal system also displays state-dependent activity. However, unlike the orexinergic and monoaminergic groups, the brainstem cholinergic neurons show highest activity during both wakefulness and REM sleep

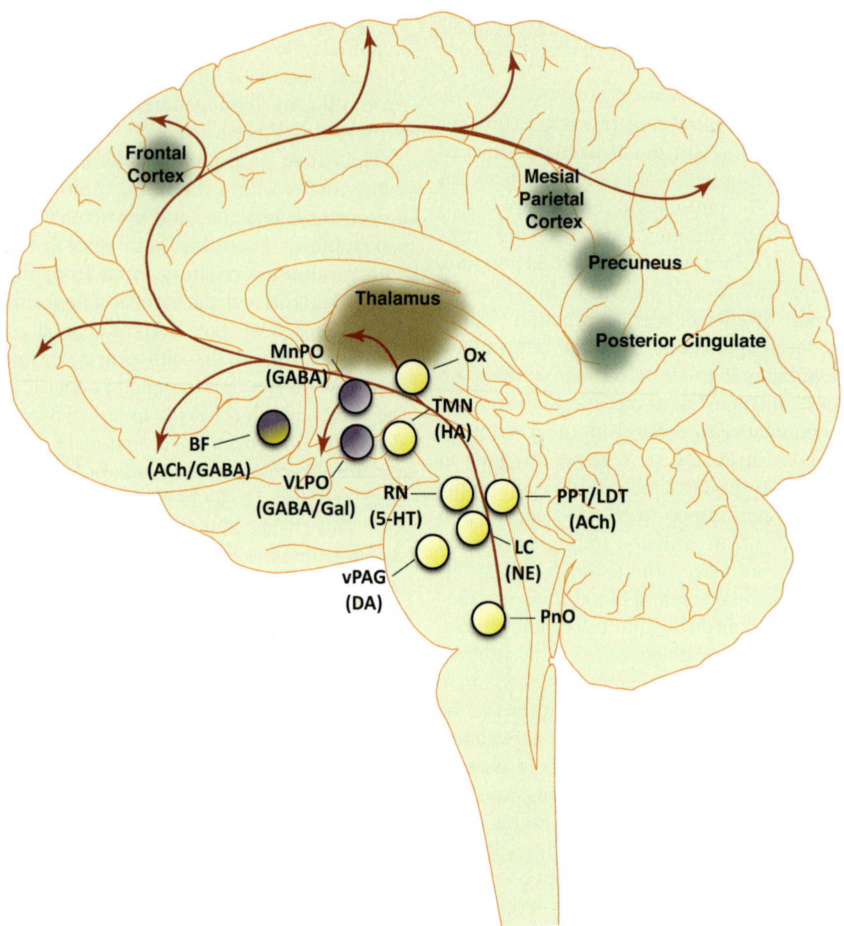

FIGURE 37-20. The extended reticular activating system modulates states of sleep and wakefulness and serves as a network upon which anesthetics act to produce unconsciousness. As at the synapse, there are multiple sites at which anesthetics could act to impair consciousness. Individual anesthetics initiate hypnosis through interactions at distinct sites; however, the drugs ultimately converge at the level of the net circuit output to transition an individual from wakefulness into anesthetic-induced unconsciousness. Under conditions of wakefulness, a ventral pathway of ascending input from the brainstem carries wake-promoting input from the yellow nuclei into the hypothalamus toward the basal forebrain and cortex, and a dorsal pathway carries input from the brainstem through the thalamus and up to cortex via corticothalamic afferent fibers (not shown). During non–rapid eye movement sleep and anesthetic-induced unconsciousness, the circuit output switches driven both by activity in the sleep-promoting ventrolateral preoptic nucleus (VLPO) and median preoptic nucleus (MnPO; purple nuclei) as well as by a change from tonic to burst firing in the thalamus (brown nucleus). Cortical sites shown in *green*, including the medial prefrontal, frontal, mesial parietal, precuneus, and posterior cingulated cortices, have all been implicated in conscious perception. During sleep or in the presence of hypnotic doses of anesthetics, processing at these sites is disrupted. The reticular activating system is wired as a series of bistable loops, such that mutual antagonism between nuclei with sleep-promoting function, such as the VLPO and wake-promoting function such as the hypothalamic orexinergic neurons, inhibits activity in the opposing groups to control the individual's state of arousal. ACh, acetylcholine; BF, basal forebrain contains both sleep- and wake-active neurons; 5-HT, serotonin; DA, dopamine; DpMe, deep mesencephalic nucleus; GABA, γ-aminobutyric acid; Gal, galanin; Glut, glutamane; HA, histamine; LC, locus caeruleus; LDTg, lateral dorsal tegmentum; MPTA, mesopontine tegmental anesthesia locus; NE, norepinephrine; Ox, orexin/hypocretin neurons; PnO, oral part of the pontine nucleus; PPTg, pedunculopontine tegmentum; RN, raphe nuclei; TMN, tuberomammillary nucleus.

and virtual quiescence during NREM sleep.[110] Another important neuronal target is the oral part of the pontine nucleus (PnO) located in the pontine reticular formation. The PnO receives critical cholinergic, GABAergic, and orexinergic innervation to modulate sleep and arousal.[111]

Anesthetic Effects on Arousal Centers As is the case for natural sleep, early pharmacologic, lesion, and more recent gene knock-out studies indicate that the hypnotic component of general anesthesia is modestly affected by modulation of any of the monoaminergic, orexinergic, or cholinergic wake-active systems. Thus, at the systems level, general anesthetics produce unconsciousness in part by inhibiting arousal. Disruption of cholinergic neurotransmission, in particular, appears to participate in the hypnosis associated with halothane, isoflurane, sevoflurane, propofol, opioids, and ketamine. Consistent with this is the observation that physostigmine, an acetylcholinesterase inhibitor that crosses the blood–brain barrier, partially antagonizes sevoflurane or propofol hypnosis.[112] In addition to interacting with other wake- and sleep-active groups, cholinergic brainstem nuclei such as the LDT and PPT project within the brainstem to PnO and ascend beyond it to the thalamus and cortex. When these brainstem centers are activated, desynchrony of the EEG typical of wakefulness or REM sleep occurs (reviewed by Jones[113]). Conversely, when cholinergic output of the LDT and PPT is inhibited, as occurs with general anesthesia (see discussion of anesthetic effects on nAChRs), EEG activity in the cortex assumes a striking similarity to that seen during NREM sleep.

Similar to the cholinergic centers, monoaminergic centers are most active during wakefulness. The noradrenergic LC has long been known as a region of the brain associated with vigilance. Whereas independent excitation of the LC enhances an individual's state of arousal, reduction in the LC firing rate decreases alertness.[114] Inhibition of the LC appears to be a primary mechanism of action through which the α_2-adrenergic agonist dexmedetomidine exerts its strong hypnotic effect.[115] Inhibition of the LC further destabilizes wakefulness by releasing inhibition of the sleep center VLPO. Classic pharmacologic studies over the past 5 decades have demonstrated that increasing central adrenergic output from the LC is associated with an increased anesthetic requirement, a fact known to any anesthesiologist caring for a patient who recently ingested cocaine, amphetamines, or similar psychostimulants. Conversely, decreasing catecholaminergic output reduces MAC, as evidenced by reserpine or α-methyldopa depletion experiments and by isolated destruction of the LC.

Modulation of serotonergic output from the DR also affects anesthetic sensitivity. As with the LC, lesion and pharmacologic inhibition of serotonergic signaling reduces MAC. Blockade of 5-hydroxytryptamine 2A (5-HT_{2A}) receptors with the 2 different antagonists has been shown to reduce the MAC of isoflurane and halothane. When combined with in vitro data demonstrating that inhaled anesthetics such as isoflurane inhibit signal transduction mediated through G-protein coupled 5-HT_{2A} receptors, these data suggest that 5-HT_{2A} receptors are in the neural circuitry influencing MAC.[116]

Similar to other aminergic nuclei, the histaminergic neurons of the TMN are part of a phylogenetically ancient arousal system conserved across vertebrates. The TMN is reciprocally connected to and tonically inhibited by other neurons of the VLPO. In brain slice studies, norepinephrine inhibits GABAergic activity in the TMN and thus releases inhibition. Serotonin and orexin depolarize the TMN through activation of an electrogenic sodium/calcium (Na/Ca) exchanger, suggesting that the TMN is excited by increased activity of the other wake-active arousal centers. Moreover, activity of TMN neurons has been linked to hibernation as well as to the hypnotic component of general anesthetic action.[117,118] As discussed earlier, one molecular mechanism shared by many (but not all) anesthetics is their ability to potentiate inhibitory GABAergic signaling. Nelson et al[118] established the TMN as an important neuronal site mediating the sedation of propofol, pentobarbital, and the classic $GABA_A$ agonist muscimol because the anesthetic facilitation of $GABA_A$ receptor signaling inhibits the tonic TMN inhibition of VLPO activity.

Orexinergic neurons release the neuropeptides orexin-A and orexin-B (also called hypocretin), thereby coordinating and stabilizing the activity of the entire reticular activating system during wakefulness. Orexinergic neurons are ideally positioned to be the master regulator of arousal. They send dense excitatory projections to all other monoaminergic and cholinergic arousal nuclei while also projecting to thalamus and PnO.[119-121] Thus, increased firing of orexinergic neurons stimulates activity of the other arousal nuclei and inhibits VLPO neurons, thereby driving the system toward wakefulness (Fig. 37-20). Mutual antagonism between VLPO and orexinergic neurons creates a bistable switch[110] that drives an organism either toward wakefulness (low VLPO activity in conjunction with increased orexinergic activity) or toward sleep (high VLPO activity in conjunction with decreased orexinergic activity).

Orexin receptors are GPCRs that, because of the binding and functional results discussed earlier, are reasonable direct anesthetic targets. Moreover, several reports suggest that modulation of orexinergic neurotransmission alters anesthetic responsiveness. Using the LORR behavioral assay as an endpoint, intrathecal administration of an orexin-A agonist and antagonist were shown to reduce and prolong, respectively, the duration of barbiturate induced hypnosis.[122] Direct evidence for orexin modulation of anesthetic hypnosis was also obtained when intracerebroventricular administration of orexin-A produced cortical arousal, opposing the depressive effects of 1.0 and 1.5 MAC of isoflurane.[123] Recently, direct effect of anesthetics on orexin-mediated signal transduction has been demonstrated.[124] Intriguingly, modulation of orexinergic signaling appears to asymmetrically alter emergence from some anesthetics without changing anesthetic induction.[103,104,125] This has led to the idea that the forward and reverse processes through which the state of general anesthesia arises and dissipates may not be identical.[126] Additional support for this notion comes from studies in midline central medial thalamus, where modulation of cholinergic signaling was shown to precipitate anesthetic emergence despite ongoing exposure to hypnotic doses of sevoflurane yet not altering induction.[127] It is becoming clear that reactivating endogenous arousal promoting systems may be a common means of facilitating anesthetic emergence.[128-130]

Anesthetics and Other Endpoints Although the majority of research on the mechanisms of anesthetic action has been focused at the molecular level, the interpretation of these findings in the context of the whole animal requires knowledge of the neuronal networks upon which anesthetics exert their site-specific effects to produce different behavioral endpoints. Toward that end, elegant and sophisticated studies are clarifying and standardizing endpoints for quantitative application and qualitative association with the networks. Using these approaches, future studies promise to unravel the neuroanatomic loci that mediate many anesthetic actions, both desired and undesired.

SUMMARY

Despite their importance and widespread application in medicine, the general inhalational anesthetics still defy a comprehensive description of their action. A rational explanation for this state of affairs is that inhalational anesthesia relies on a multitude of targets, a proposal well aligned with the results of binding, in vitro functional studies, and behavioral phenomenology. Nevertheless, substantial progress at the molecular level has allowed a pool of protein candidates to be proposed and a detailed understanding of the submolecular mechanisms of anesthetic action to be developed. Progress has been made in the linkage of specific endpoints to underlying targets and neuronal circuitry.

However, little progress has been made toward developing novel inhaled molecules with a more favorable therapeutic ratio. A reason for this lack of progress may be a fundamental dissociation between the pharmacology and the application. To date, the development of anesthetic molecules has been guided by more practical goals, including fast kinetics to facilitate rapid induction, emergence, and patient throughput; enhanced stability to reduce metabolic degradation and its associated toxicity and to prolong shelf-life; and operating room safety (eg, absence of flammability or toxicity from inhalation of trace amounts in the ambient air). These goals may have had the unintended consequence of actually reducing specificity for molecular targets and may not have achieved a lower toxic potential. It is clear that greater molecular complexity will be necessary to enhance specificity, but this may come at the price of slower kinetics, lower and less predictable efficacy, and a less "complete" anesthetic. Such an outcome predicts that combination drug therapy will assume a greater role in anesthetic care in the future.

KEY REFERENCES

- Eckenhoff RG. Promiscuous ligands and attractive cavities: how do the inhaled anesthetics work? *Mol Interv.* 2001;1:258-268.
- Franks NP. General anaesthesia: from molecular targets to neuronal pathways of sleep and arousal. *Nat Rev Neurosci.* 2008;9:370-386.
- Lydic R, Baghdoyan HA. Sleep, anesthesiology, and the neurobiology of arousal state control. *Anesthesiology.* 2005;103:1268-1295.

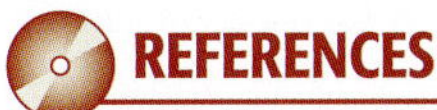

REFERENCES

Complete references available on DVD and online version at www.LongneckerAnesthesiology.com

CHAPTER 38

Pharmacology of Inhalational Anesthetics

Stuart A. Forman
Claudia Benkwitz

KEY POINTS

1. The most useful definition of "dose" for inhaled anesthetics is the partial pressure in alveolar gases, which is readily monitored in end-tidal gases.
2. All halogenated anesthetics break down, releasing carbon monoxide (CO) and heat when they contact *desiccated* alkaline chemicals, such as those in common CO_2 adsorbents. Potential harm to patients from this breakdown can be avoided by proper use and maintenance of anesthesia equipment and by using less alkaline CO_2 adsorbents.
3. The rate at which the alveolar anesthetic concentration (F_A or P_{alv}) approaches the inspired (circuit) concentration (F_I or Pcirc) depends on minute alveolar ventilation (increased ventilation accelerates equilibration), cardiac output (increased output slows equilibration), and the blood-gas partition coefficient of the anesthetic (high solubility slows equilibration).
4. Nitrous oxide (N_2O) diffuses into air-filled spaces in the body, causing expansion, increased pressure, or both.
5. The minimum alveolar concentration (MAC) is the alveolar concentration of inhaled anesthetic that blocks movement in half of subjects in response to a surgical incision. MAC is influenced by age, pharmacologic and physiologic factors (eg, temperature), and genetic factors.
6. MAC-awake is the alveolar concentration of anesthetic causing loss of response to verbal commands in half of subjects. Amnesia is produced by inhalational anesthetic concentrations lower than MAC-awake.
7. Awareness and explicit recall of intraoperative events is attributable to inadequate delivery of anesthetics for the patient's needs. Without preventive measures, awareness during anesthesia occurs in about 1 of 750 patients and may cause psychological disturbances leading to post-traumatic stress disorder.
8. All potent volatile anesthetics in current use decrease mean arterial pressure in a dose-dependent manner. Severe cardiovascular and respiratory depression can occur even at low volatile anesthetic concentrations in elderly, hypovolemic, or critically ill patients. Avoidance of these toxicities requires vigilant monitoring and anticipation of anesthetic requirements.
9. Volatile anesthetics may increase heart rate, both by a baroreceptor reflex in response to decreased arterial pressure and a direct vagolytic effect on the heart.
10. Volatile anesthetics tend to increase respiratory rate and decrease tidal volume and blunt ventilatory responses to hypercapnia and hypoxia.
11. Desflurane is very pungent, and its use can be associated with airway irritability, bronchoconstriction, and laryngospasm during induction. Among volatile anesthetics, sevoflurane causes the least amount of airway irritation.
12. Volatile anesthetics vasodilate cerebral vessels, increasing blood flow while reducing cerebral metabolic oxygen consumption. Cerebral vascular responses to altered pCO_2 are maintained in the presence of volatile anesthetics. N_2O increases cerebral metabolism.
13. Halothane undergoes the most hepatic metabolism of the inhaled agents. Whereas enflurane, isoflurane, and sevoflurane are also metabolized in the liver, desflurane and nitrous oxide are minimally metabolized. Oxidative metabolism of halothane and other volatile agents can induce a severe immune-mediated hepatitis.
14. All potent volatile agents may trigger malignant hyperthermia in susceptible individuals.

INTRODUCTION

Experimentation with inhalation of gases and vapors for the purpose of obtunding the distress associated with surgery began in the 19th century. The administration of inhaled anesthetics spread rapidly after the successful public demonstration of ether anesthesia by William T.G. Morton on October 16, 1846, at Massachusetts General Hospital.

Inhaled agents were the sole means of reliably inducing general anesthesia until the development of intravenous (IV) delivery techniques and drugs. Inhalants continue to be used in a large fraction of general anesthetics because of their ease of use and predictable effects. The inhalational route of administration is almost always available, and the same route is used for drug removal. Thus, inhaled anesthetics require no metabolic clearance (indeed, their metabolism is associated with toxicity). Modern equipment for administration of inhaled anesthetics is simple and robust, providing an elegant method for inducing, maintaining, and reversing general anesthesia. Furthermore, monitoring inhaled anesthetic concentrations in end-tidal gases provides an estimate of drug concentrations in the circulating blood and central nervous system (CNS). This ability to assess drug concentrations in the body reduces pharmacokinetic uncertainty when determining how much inhaled vapor to administer.

PURPOSE AND SCOPE OF THIS CHAPTER

This chapter describes the chemical and biophysical properties of commonly used inhaled anesthetics and relates these properties to the clinical pharmacology. Various properties of inhaled drugs influence their chemical stability, rate of pulmonary uptake, distribution to various body compartments, elimination, and metabolism (pharmacokinetics), as well as clinically important differences among their therapeutic actions and toxicities (pharmacodynamics). Understanding these pharmacologic relationships is crucial for the safe and effective delivery of inhaled anesthetics. An understanding of inhaled anesthetic pharmacology must begin with clear definitions of both the drug amount (dosage) and important effects (response).

ANESTHETIC DOSE-RESPONSE CONCEPTS

The "dosage" of an inhaled anesthetic can be a confusing concept. The dosage of inhaled anesthetic documented in an anesthetic record is most frequently the **delivered gaseous concentration** (in percent of total gas) in the vaporizer outflow (ie, fresh gas). Dosage may also be defined as the **inspired concentration** of inhaled anesthetic in the breathing circuit or, analogous to injected drugs, as the **amount absorbed** by the body via the lungs. However, these definitions are of limited use because several factors, including ambient atmospheric pressure, fresh gas flow (FGF) rate, minute ventilation, and the rate of uptake into the blood via the lungs, determine how these various "doses" affect patients. **The most useful and practical definition of dosage for inhaled anesthetic drugs is the partial pressure in alveolar gas, which is approximated in end-expiratory gas.** The partial pressure of an inhaled drug is directly proportional to its fractional concentration in a gas mixture (Dalton's law) and is measured on an absolute scale of pressure (see Biophysical Properties of Inhaled Anesthetics, later).

The common effects that all general anesthetics reversibly induce are hypnosis (loss of perceptive awareness), amnesia (anterograde loss of memory), and ablation of movement in response to pain (inhibition of nociceptive reflexes).[1] These therapeutic actions, which define the state of general anesthesia, are all mediated by the CNS (brain and spinal cord). Some anesthetics can provide additional therapeutic actions, such as analgesia, attenuation of autonomic reflexes, and protection of the heart and brain from ischemia and reperfusion. In addition, the nontherapeutic effects of anesthetics (side effects) must be considered because these often influence the choice of anesthetic drug and dosage, depending on the specific clinical setting.

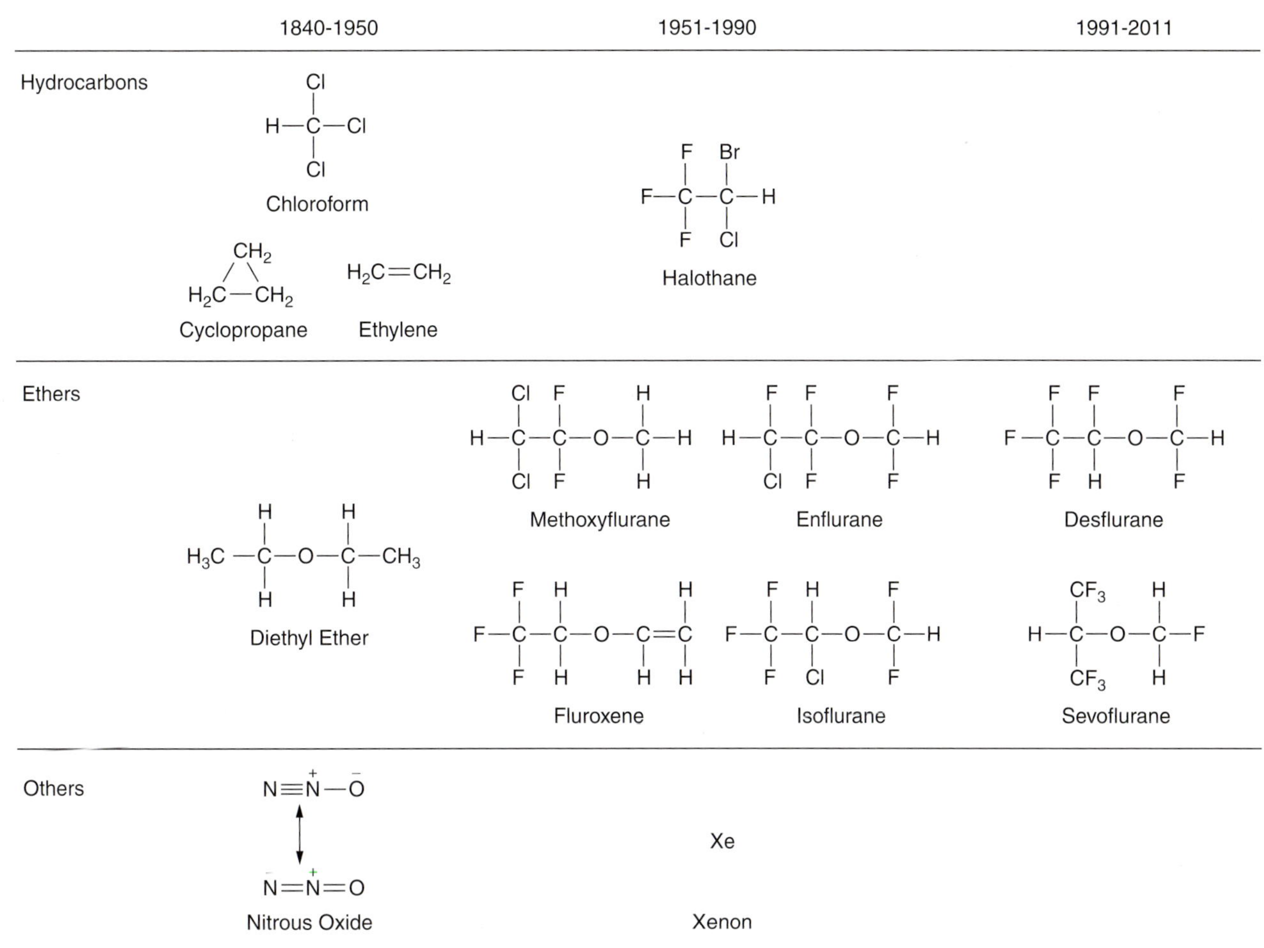

FIGURE 38-1. Structures of inhaled anesthetics. Of note, 3 different classes of inhaled anesthetics were identified in the 19th century.

CHEMICAL AND PHYSICAL PROPERTIES OF INHALED ANESTHETICS

The structures of various inhaled anesthetics, in 3 chemical categories, are depicted in **Fig. 38-1**. Three inhaled anesthetics (nitrous oxide [N_2O], diethyl ether, and chloroform) were used in the 19th century. In the early 20th century, more inhaled anesthetics were identified, including ethylene, ethyl chloride, and cyclopropane. Of these, only N_2O remains in use. The other early inhaled anesthetics in use up to 1950 were combustible, occasionally resulting in catastrophic outcomes for both patients and caregivers.[2] The chemical and physical properties of the gaseous and volatile anesthetics currently available for clinical use (N_2O, isoflurane, enflurane, halothane, desflurane, and sevoflurane) are summarized for comparison in **Table 38-1**.

NITROUS OXIDE

Nitrous oxide is a simple linear inorganic compound that is in the gas phase at normal ambient temperature and pressure and is chemically stable. N_2O has no odor or taste. The boiling point of N_2O is −88.5°C. At room temperature (25°C), N_2O condenses into a liquid at 745 psi (50 atm), making the storage and transport of large quantities in pressurized cylinders economical. A room temperature cylinder will display a pressure near 745 psi as long as liquid N_2O remains. The pressure will decrease if the temperature of the liquid drops or if the tank is completely depleted of liquid and nearly empty. Pressure within the cylinder may decrease during rapid delivery of N_2O as vaporization absorbs heat, cooling the tank and its contents. The amount of N_2O remaining in the cylinder can only be determined by its weight, not by a pressure reading. N_2O can support combustion, and the use of N_2O during surgery with

TABLE 38-1 Physicochemical Properties of Inhaled Anesthetics

Property	N_2O	Isoflurane	Enflurane	Halothane	Desflurane	Sevoflurane
Molecular weight	44	184.5	184.5	197.4	168	200.1
Boiling point (°C/°F)	−88.5/−127.3	48.5/119.3	56.5/133.7	50.2/122.4	22.8/74.3	58.6/137.5
Density (g/mL)	1.84×10^{-3} (gas)	1.5	1.52	1.86	1.45	1.50
Vapor pressure at 20°C (mm Hg)	43 879 (gas)	238	175	243	664	157
Oil-gas partition coefficient at 37°C	1.3	90.8	96.5	197	19	47–54

TABLE 38-2 Biophysical and Pharmacokinetic and Pharmacodynamic Properties of Inhaled Anesthetics

Property	N_2O	Isoflurane	Enflurane	Halothane	Desflurane	Sevoflurane
$\lambda_{blood/gas}$ at 37°C[a]	0.47	1.4	1.8	2.5	0.45	0.65
Blood V_{eff} (L)[b]	2.4	7.5	9.0	12.5	2.3	3.3
$\lambda_{brain/blood}$ at 37°C[a]	1.1	1.6	1.4	1.9	1.3	1.7
Brain V_{eff} (L)[b]	1.5	2.2	2.0	2.7	1.8	2.4
$\tau_{brain/blood}$ (min)[c]	2.1	3.0	2.6	3.5	2.4	3.2
$\lambda_{muscle/blood}$ at 37°C[a]	1.2	2.9	1.7	3.4	2	3.1
Muscle V_{eff} (L)[b]	36	87	51	102	60	93
$\tau_{muscle/blood}$ (min)[c]	62	147	87	174	103	159
$\lambda_{fat/blood}$ at 37°C[a]	2.3	45	36	51	27	48
Fat V_{eff} (L)[b]	29.7	580	464	658	348	619
$\tau_{fat/blood}$ (min)[c]	126	2470	1976	2800	1482	2635
MAC[d] (%/mm Hg) in O_2	105/800	1.28/9.7	1.58/12.0	0.75/5.7	6.0/45.6	2.05/15.6
MAC[d] (%/mm Hg) in 70%N_2O/30%O_2	--	0.56/4.26	0.57/4.33	0.29/2.20	2.5/19	0.66/5.02
MAC-awake[e] (%/mm Hg)	71/540	0.43/3.27	0.51/3.88	0.41/3.21	2.4/19	0.63/4.79
Metabolism (%)	0.0	0.2	2.4	20	0.02	2-5

[a]Partition coefficient at 37°C.

[b]Effective volumes and time constants were calculated based on a 70-kg adult with blood volume of 5.0 L; brain volume of 1.4 L, and brain blood flow of 0.75 L/min; muscle volume of 30 L and muscle blood flow of 0.59 L/min; fat volume of 12.9 L, and fat blood flow of 0.24 L/min. After Kennedy et al.[225]

[c]Time constants (τ) are for equilibration between the blood and the specified tissue, calculated using equation 2 and V_{eff}.

[d]Minimum alveolar concentration (MAC) is the anesthetic concentration inhibiting motor responses to skin incision in half of subjects.

[e]MAC-awake is the anesthetic concentration that inhibits appropriate motor responses to spoken commands in half of subjects.

electrocautery or lasers may accelerate the fire if flammable materials ignite.

Nitrous oxide produces analgesia, yet it has a low potency as an anesthetic. It must be delivered at nearly 0.7 atm (530 mm Hg) to ablate awareness in half of patients, and preventing movement during an incision would require more than 1 atm in most patients. Therefore, N_2O is frequently used in combination with other inhaled or IV anesthetic agents.

HALOTHANE

In the mid-20th century, efforts to develop safer inhaled anesthetics focused on reducing flammability by halogenation (adding bromine; chlorine, and fluorine) of alkanes and ethers.[3] Halothane is a halogenated alkane ($CF_3CHBrCl$) and became clinically available in 1956. It has a pleasant, nonpungent odor and is tolerated well during inhalation. Halothane is a liquid at room temperature and 1 atm pressure, and its high vapor pressure (243 mm Hg at 20°C) is many times that needed to induce anesthesia. Clinically used concentrations of halothane are not flammable, but higher concentrations (in anesthesia machines) can ignite. Halothane is slightly unstable, decomposing in the presence of light and oxygen. To prevent photo-oxidative breakdown, halothane is stored in dark glass bottles containing 0.01% thymol. Newer halogenated volatile anesthetics do not require such chemical stabilizers. Halothane undergoes significant metabolism in the liver (**Table 38-2**).

ENFLURANE AND ISOFLURANE

Enflurane and its isomer isoflurane were introduced to clinical practice in the 1970s. They are halogenated ethers that undergo much less metabolism and have faster onset and offset compared with halothane.

Enflurane is a halogenated ether ($CHFClCF_2OCHF_2$) and is more pungent than halothane but is reasonably well tolerated for inhalation induction. It is a clear liquid with a vapor pressure of 172 mm Hg at 20°C.

Isoflurane is a halogenated ether and an isomer of enflurane ($CF_3CHClOCHF_2$). It is a clear liquid with a vapor pressure of 238 mm Hg at 20°C. It is pungent and frequently stimulates coughing during inhalation induction.

DESFLURANE AND SEVOFLURANE

Desflurane and sevoflurane, introduced in the 1990s, are ethers that are halogenated exclusively with fluorine. Both are less potent and less blood soluble than other halogenated anesthetics. Low blood solubility provides rapid pulmonary uptake and elimination, which is highly desirable in clinical settings during which rapid emergence from anesthesia is valued.

Desflurane ($CF_3CHFOCHF_2$) is extremely resistant to biodegradation. Desflurane has a high vapor pressure at 20°C (664 mm Hg) and boils at 22.8°C (73°F). To prevent boiling, desflurane is stored in special bottles with valves that only open when fitted into the filling port of a vaporizer. The unique desflurane vaporizer heats the anesthetic to 39°C to control its vapor pressure and delivery rate.[4] Desflurane vapor is extremely pungent, and coughing and autonomic stimulation are frequently produced during inhalation induction.

Sevoflurane [$(CF_3)_2CHOCH_2F$] is a clear liquid with a vapor pressure of 157 mm Hg at 20°C. Sevoflurane has a pleasant odor and low pungency, making it well tolerated for inhalation induction of anesthesia.

BIOPHYSICAL PROPERTIES OF INHALED ANESTHETICS

The concepts of partial pressure and partition coefficients are central to understanding how gases distribute among various compartments in the body.

PARTIAL PRESSURE

Partial pressure is the pressure exerted by 1 component of a gas mixture, in which the sum of all the partial pressures equals the total pressure. For example, air contains about 79% nitrogen (fraction of

$N_2 = F_{N2} = 0.79$) and 21% oxygen ($F_{O2} = 0.21$), so at 1 standard atmosphere barometric pressure (P_{Bar} = 1 atm = 760 mm Hg), the partial pressure of N_2, P_{N2} = 0.79 atm = 600 mm Hg and P_{O2} = 0.21 atm = 160 mm Hg. Near sea level, where atmospheric pressure is about 760 mm Hg, the fractional concentration of a gas differs insignificantly from its partial pressure (in atm), and the 2 terms can be used interchangeably. At high altitudes, where ambient pressure is lower, air contains the same fractional concentrations of nitrogen and oxygen, and their partial pressures are reduced relative to those at sea level. For example, in Denver (P_{Bar} = 630 mm Hg), P_{N2} = 500 mm Hg and P_{O2} = 130 mm Hg. Similarly, gaseous anesthetics such as N_2O, when used at high altitudes, exert a lower partial pressure (and have a subsequently reduced anesthetic effect) relative to the same fractional concentration at sea level.

VAPOR PRESSURE

Volatile anesthetic vapor pressure is the gaseous partial pressure at the liquid–gas interface, such as that in a vaporizer. Vapor pressure remains independent of total ambient pressure and is solely a property of the anesthetic agent and its temperature. Thus, in relation to carrier gases, the fractional concentration of a saturated volatile anesthetic in a vaporizer is higher at high altitude (**Fig. 38-2**). When working at

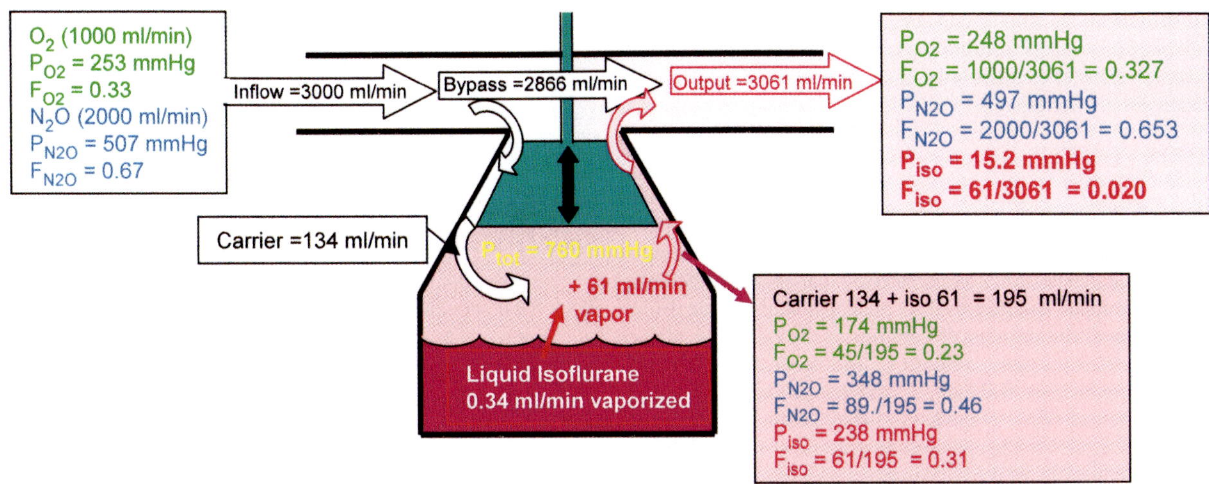

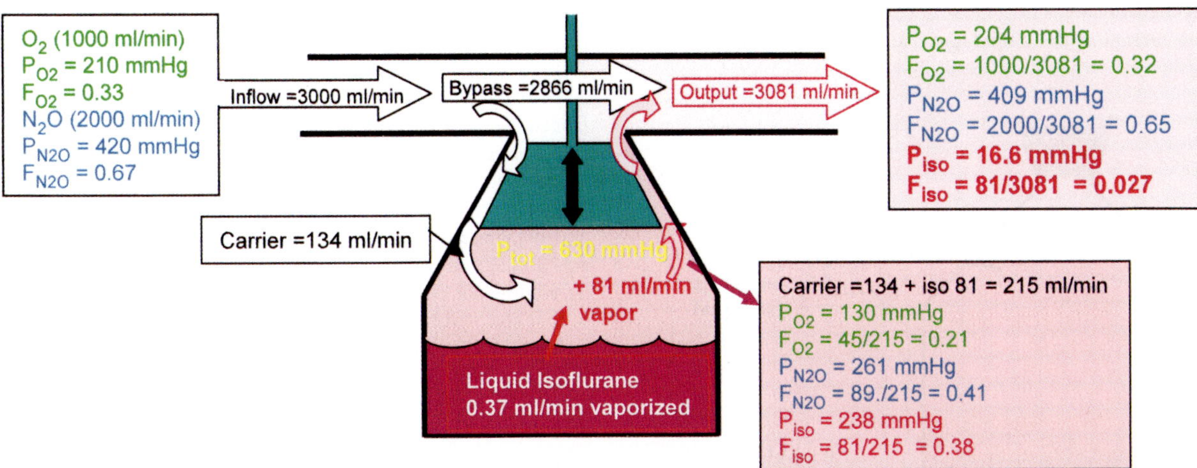

FIGURE 38-2. Vapor pressure, partial pressure, and concentration of inhaled anesthetics: The impact of atmospheric pressure on vaporizer output. **Top.** Variable bypass vaporizers are calibrated at 20°C and 1 atm (standard temperature and pressure). The partial pressure of isoflurane in the vaporization chamber is its vapor pressure, 238 mm Hg. Isoflurane vapor adds to the carrier gases (O_2 and nitrous oxide [N_2O]), and the sum of the partial pressures equals atmospheric pressure (~760 mm Hg at sea level) at all points in the flow path. With fresh gas flow of 3 L/min and the vaporizer set at 2.0%, the carrier flow through the vaporization chamber is 134 mL. About 61 mL/min of isoflurane vapor (0.34 mL/min liquid) is added to the carrier gases so that the output of the vaporizer after dilution is 3061 mL/min at 2.0% isoflurane (P_{iso} = 15.2 mm Hg). **Bottom.** With the same flow and vaporizer settings in Denver (5280 ft elevation; ambient pressure, 630 mm Hg), isoflurane comprises a larger portion of the carrier gas mixture, and after dilution, the output of the vaporizer is 3081 mL/min at about 2.6% isoflurane. Thus, in Denver, the *delivered concentration* of isoflurane is 30% higher than that at sea level. However, the delivered *partial pressure* of isoflurane in Denver is 16.7 mm Hg, only 10% higher than that at sea level. Similarly, liquid isoflurane is vaporized at 0.37 mL/min in Denver, about 10% more than that at sea level. Because its partial pressure directly determines the uptake and effect of isoflurane on patients, only minor changes in vaporizer settings are required at high altitudes. Partial pressures of N_2O and O_2 carrier gases in Denver are about 17% lower than those at sea level. Thus, at similar carrier gas flows, N_2O has a significantly reduced anesthetic action in Denver versus sea level. Moreover, the inspired O_2 concentration in Denver should be increased to reduce the risk of hypoxia, so increasing the N_2O concentration may not be possible.

ambient pressures that differ significantly from sea level, anesthetists must adjust the delivered oxygen concentrations and vaporizer settings appropriately.

Partial pressure is the driving force for the diffusion of gases across permeable barriers into other gases, liquids, or tissues. At equilibrium, the partial pressure of any gas is equal in all intercommunicating compartments within a closed system. In the operating room, intercommunicating compartments include the anesthesia machine, the breathing circuit, and the patient's body, which is further compartmentalized. The partial pressure of an inhaled anesthetic is directly proportional to its concentration in certain compartments that may be liquid phase (ie, blood) or tissue (eg, brain), where concentration is usually defined as the weight, volume, or moles of drug per volume of liquid or tissue. Importantly, various liquids (eg, blood or cerebrospinal fluid) and tissues may contain remarkably different anesthetic concentrations at the same partial pressure, depending on the solubility of the anesthetic gas in each liquid or tissue. The concentrations in 2 different compartments define a partition coefficient.

PARTITION COEFFICIENTS

A *partition coefficient* is defined as the ratio of concentrations of a drug in one compartment (gas, blood, or tissue) versus another intercommunicating compartment at equilibrium (ie, when the anesthetic partial pressure is equal in both compartments). Partition coefficients therefore have no units. Another useful concept is that the partition coefficient represents the number of volumes of the reference phase (eg, gas) that contains the same amount of anesthetic as the second phase (eg, blood), which we will call the *effective volume* (or relative volume) of the second phase (**Fig. 38-3**; Table 38-2). The effective volume concept is similar to the distribution volume of injected drugs when calculating metabolic or renal clearance and helps illustrate why drug equilibration in different tissues takes vastly different amounts of time. Both blood–gas partitioning and tissue–blood partitioning (see Table 38-2) determine the distribution of inhaled anesthetics within the body.

Blood–Gas Partitioning The *blood solubility* of inhaled anesthetics is another term for the blood–gas partition coefficient ($\lambda_{b/g}$). At equilibrium, the concentration (eg, volume of drug per volume of gas, liquid, or tissue = v/v) of most inhaled anesthetics is higher in blood than in surrounding gases. That is, $\lambda_{b/g}$ is greater than 1.0 (Table 38-2). Two notable exceptions are N_2O and desflurane, which have the lowest blood solubility of the commonly used inhaled anesthetics. Blood–gas partitioning varies depending on temperature, hematocrit, and the lipid content of blood. The solubility of most gases, including inhaled anesthetics, increases as the temperature of a liquid such as blood decreases.[5] Blood cells and plasma contain protein and lipids, which provide a higher capacity for anesthetics. Thus, hemodilution (decreased cell mass) reduces and hypertriglyceridemia increases the blood solubility of inhaled anesthetics. Elevated blood lipids after a fatty meal increase anesthetic solubility relative to that after fasting.[6]

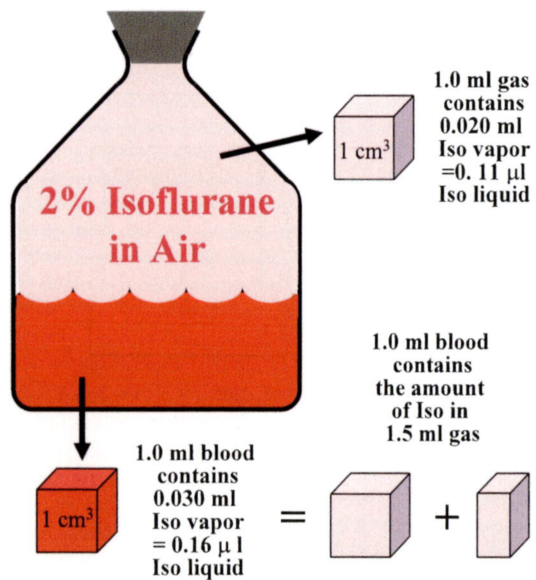

FIGURE 38-3. Blood–gas partitioning of isoflurane. After equilibrating a sealed container containing blood and isoflurane in air, a sample of blood will contain 1.5 times the amount of isoflurane as an equal volume of air.

Tissue–Blood Partitioning In general, the solubility of inhaled anesthetics in tissues depends on the fraction of tissue that is lipid[7] because most anesthetics are highly lipophilic. Thus, the more potent volatile anesthetics, which are also the most oil soluble (based on the Meyer-Overton correlation), tend to partition avidly into fatty tissues (Table 38-2).

PHARMACOKINETICS: INHALED ANESTHETIC UPTAKE AND DISTRIBUTION

A MULTICOMPARTMENTAL KINETIC MODEL

The inflows and outflows between the anesthesia machine circuit and the patient's lungs, blood, and tissues can be depicted as a cyclical multicompartmental system wherein the anesthetic partial pressure in 1 compartment is the upstream partial pressure driving anesthetic into downstream compartment(s) (**Fig. 38-4**). These compartments have different phases: gas in the anesthetic circuitry and airspace of the lung, liquid in blood, and mixed liquid and solid in organs and tissues.[8] The model depicted in Fig. 38-4 is complex and requires computer assistance to calculate how the anesthetic partial pressure in various compartments changes over time (for details, see the legend of Fig. 38-4). It is, however, relatively easy to understand how an anesthetic moves between 1 upstream compartment and 1 downstream compartment (a 2-compartment system).

Transfer of anesthetic gas from one compartment to another (eg, from a vaporizer to the breathing circuit) is proportional to both the bulk carrier flow (FGF in this example) and the partial pressure difference (eg, $P_{delivered} - P_{circuit}$). As more anesthetic gas is transferred, the partial pressure difference between the compartments becomes smaller, and the transfer rate slows. The time it takes a given compartment to equilibrate with upstream anesthetic partial pressure is determined by its volume (or effective volume) and the bulk flow carrying anesthetic to that compartment.

Equilibration between 2 compartments is quantitatively described by an exponential equation (Eq. 38-1), which is characterized by a time constant (τ). After each time constant, the difference between upstream and downstream concentrations is reduced by about 63%. A general equation describing this is

$$P_{downstream} = P_{upstream} \times (1 - e^{-t/\tau}) \qquad (38\text{-}1)$$

where t is the elapsed time measured from when the anesthetic is turned on during induction. The time constant (τ) is directly proportional to the downstream compartment volume (V): If the volume of the receiving compartment doubles, τ doubles and it takes twice as long for equilibration to occur. τ is inversely proportional to carrier flow (F): If the delivery flow doubles, τ halves and equilibration occurs twice as fast.

$$\tau(\text{min}) = \frac{V(L)}{F(L/\text{min})} \qquad (38\text{-}2)$$

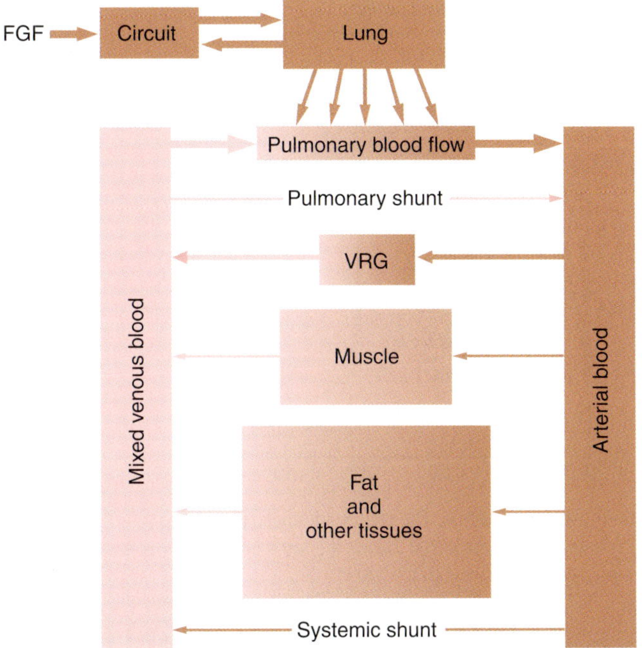

FIGURE 38-4. A model for uptake and distribution of inhaled anesthetics. The schematic depicts the flow of anesthetic gas from the vaporizer to the breathing circuit, its transfer into blood via the lungs, and distribution to various tissues. The sizes of tissue compartments are drawn in general proportion to their effective volumes ($V_{eff} = V_{anatomic} \times \lambda_{tissue/blood}$) and arrows of different width indicate relative blood flows. A variety of mathematical models have been devised to quantitatively illustrate anesthetic flow and distribution, and most are elaborations on the model introduced in 1963 by Mapleson.[226] The model shown here is not intended to replicate reality, although it approximates it and serves as a simple way of illustrating how the various input parameters (fresh gas flow [FGF], type of agent, vaporizer setting, minute ventilation, and cardiac output) affect the rate of gas uptake. The following differential equations were used to generate the uptake and clearance data displayed in figures throughout this chapter ($\dot{V}$ is minute ventilation, $\dot{Q}$ is cardiac output, and $\dot{q}$ is tissue perfusion).

The anesthetic partial pressure in the breathing circuit:

$$dP_{circ}/dt = FGF/V_{circ} \times (P_{del} - P_{circ}) - \dot{V}/V_{circ} \times (P_{circ} - P_{alv}) \quad (38\text{-}3)$$

The anesthetic partial pressure in alveolar gas:

$$dP_{alv}/dt = \dot{V}/V_{lung} \times (P_{circ} - P_{alv}) - (\dot{Q}\times\lambda_{b/g})/V_{lung} \times (P_{alv} - P_{mv}) \quad (38\text{-}4)$$

Uptake into a specific tissue (i):

$$dP_i/dt = \dot{q}_i/(V_i \times \lambda_{i/b}) \times (P_{alv} - P_i) \quad (38\text{-}5)$$

The anesthetic partial pressure in mixed venous blood:

$$P_{mv} = \frac{\sum_{i=1}^{n} P_i \times q_i}{\dot{Q}} \quad (38\text{-}6)$$

VRG, Vessel Rich Group, including brain, heart, liver, kidneys.

After 5 time constants have elapsed, anesthetic concentrations in upstream and downstream compartments differ by less than 1%. At this equilibrium state, the compartments have the same partial pressure of anesthetic, and no net anesthetic transfer between compartments occurs even though carrier flow continues.

Equilibration time is independent of the source partial pressure if this pressure is small (see the discussion of the concentration effect below). The time, however, to reach a target partial pressure in the downstream compartment (eg, to reach a specific depth of anesthesia) will be shorter if the upstream partial pressure is higher. A common practice is to deliver potent volatile anesthetics at 2 to 3 times the target partial pressure (*overpressure*) to reduce the induction time. When the desired depth of anesthesia has been achieved, the vaporizer is set to a lower concentration to prevent the toxic effects of overdosage.

THE INSPIRED PARTIAL PRESSURE OF ANESTHETIC GAS

The example cited above can be used to illustrate how long it takes to "prime" a breathing circuit with anesthetic, such as is done before a single breath induction. The upstream source is the output from a vaporizer ($P_{delivered}$), the drug carrier is FGF, and the breathing circuit volume is V_{circ}. The delivery of anesthetic is determined by the product of the FGF and $P_{delivered}$. The time needed to equilibrate the circuit with the delivered gas is determined by the ratio of V_{circ} to FGF. High FGFs and low circuit volume, such as that in open-circuit delivery systems, enable rapid control of the anesthetic concentration in the circuit that is inhaled by the patient (**Fig. 38-5**).

The most common breathing circuit configuration is a circle system that allows rebreathing of exhaled anesthetic gases while removing carbon dioxide. These circuits have total gas volumes of 6 to 8 L. If V_{circ} is 6 L and FGF is 6 L/min, then τ will be 1 minute, and it will take approximately 5 minutes for the anesthetic concentration in the circuit to closely approach the concentration delivered by the vaporizer. However, at FGF of 1 L/min, τ is 6 minutes, and it will take up to a half hour to fully equilibrate the circuit (Fig. 38-5A).

To illustrate the impact of additional compartments in our model, consider what happens if a patient is breathing circuit gases when the vaporizer is turned on. In this case, uptake of anesthetic into the patient's body reduces the rate of rise of the partial pressure of anesthetic in the circuit (Fig. 38-5B). These examples illustrate why a high FGF is most useful when rapid changes in inspired anesthetic concentration are needed, such as during induction and emergence. After the induction period, the rate of uptake of anesthetic into the patient slows, and if a rebreathing circuit is used, FGF can be reduced, usually in the range of 1 to 3 L/min. After FGF is reduced, modestly increasing the delivered anesthetic concentration will help maintain drug delivery to match the uptake of anesthetic into the body (**Fig. 38-6**). Reducing FGF has economic, environmental, and medical benefits. Lower FGF results in lower usage of inhaled gases, reducing costs as well as adverse environmental effects. The patient's airway humidity is also maintained, improving the clearance of bronchopulmonary secretions.

The extreme of low FGF is "closed circuit" anesthesia, wherein almost all inhaled gases are rebreathed and fresh gas is delivered with only sufficient oxygen to replace that metabolized by the patient (about 0.25 L/min for a typical normothermic 70-kg adult) and anesthetic vapor is added to match uptake and maintain the level of anesthesia. The practice of closed circuit anesthesia should be based on detailed knowledge of anesthetic gas uptake into patients (for a more thorough description, see Baum[9]).

THE ALVEOLAR PARTIAL PRESSURE OF ANESTHETIC GAS

The alveolar anesthetic partial pressure (P_{alv}) is important because it is the upstream source or driving pressure that rapidly equilibrates with the blood, brain, and other highly perfused tissues (see below) and because its level can be monitored in end-expired gases. Thus, P_{alv} represents the most useful definition of inhaled anesthetic "dose."

Transfer of Anesthetic From the Breathing Circuit to Alveoli The transfer of inhaled anesthetic from the breathing circuit into the lungs depends on the minute alveolar ventilation rate and the difference between the partial pressures in the circuit (P_{circ}) and the

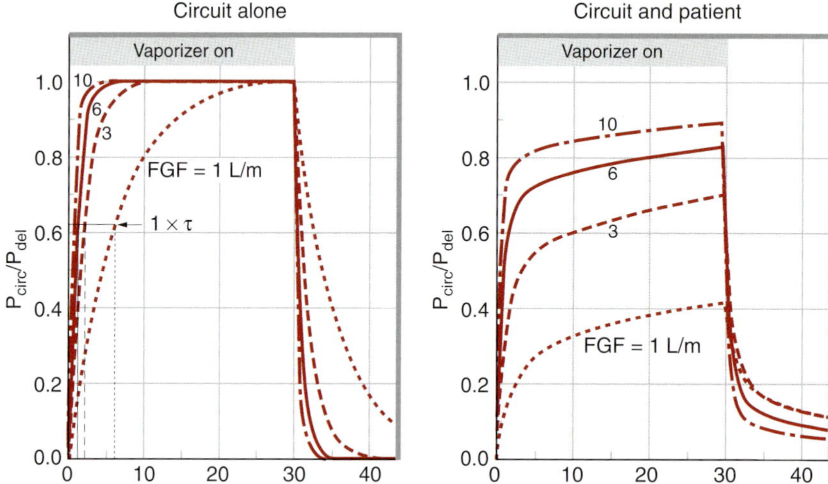

FIGURE 38-5. The impact of fresh gas flow (FGF) on the anesthetic concentration in the breathing circuit. **A.** The rise of anesthetic partial pressure follows a single exponential when there is only a single downstream compartment (the circuit). Anesthetic clearance from the circuit follows the same time course as its rise, depending on FGF. **B.** The rise of the inspired anesthetic (isoflurane in this example) partial pressure is slowed by uptake into the patient.

lung (P_{alv}). Thus, hyperventilation enables the rapid adjustment of P_{alv}. The impact of varying minute alveolar ventilation is illustrated in **Fig. 38-7**.

It is traditional to illustrate uptake with P_{alv} normalized to P_{circ} (inspired), which represents the case of high flow open-circuit anesthesia, wherein $P_{circ} \approx P_{delivered}$. However, with a rebreathing circuit, as we have described, $P_{circ}/P_{delivered}$ is not constant (Fig. 38-5). In this instance, a clearer illustration of how P_{alv} varies over time is obtained by normalizing to $P_{delivered}$, which is held constant in our uptake model calculations. The difference between open-circuit versus rebreathing models is illustrated in Fig. 38-7. Comparing the 2 panels, it is apparent that P_{alv} increases more slowly with moderate FGF using a rebreathing circuit, but the impact of changing minute ventilation is similar in both cases. For simplicity, we have adopted the traditional open-circuit model to illustrate the impact of other physiologic variables on anesthetic uptake (for washout in these figures, we have normalized to either $P_{delivered}$ or P_{circ} just before the agent is turned off).

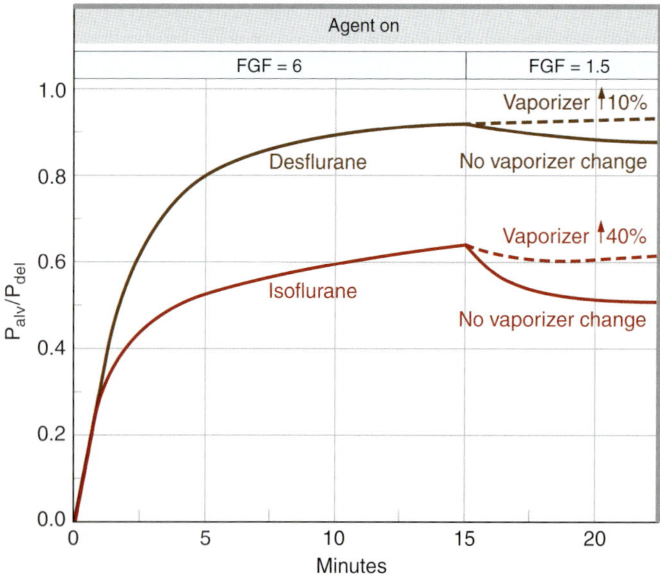

FIGURE 38-6. Lowering fresh gas flows (FGFs) after induction. After the initial rapid uptake of anesthetic, FGF may be dropped, reducing both drug delivery and waste. The decrease in anesthetic concentration that results is larger for highly soluble agents.

Anesthetic Uptake Into Pulmonary Blood Pulmonary blood rapidly takes up alveolar anesthetic gases. The uptake into blood depends on blood solubility (the blood–gas partition coefficient, $\lambda_{b/g}$), the rate of pulmonary blood flow (usually similar to cardiac output), and the difference between the anesthetic partial pressure in the lung and that of mixed venous blood entering the lung. The more blood-soluble anesthetics produce a slower rise of P_{alv} relative to the inspired concentration (P_{circ}) because more vapor needs to be transferred into blood before the blood compartment is "filled" (**Fig. 38-8**). Stated another way, the effective blood volume is larger for the more soluble anesthetics (see Table 38-2).

Whereas increased cardiac output (pulmonary blood flow) slows the rise in P_{alv} by more rapidly removing the anesthetic agent from alveolar gases, decreasing cardiac output will accelerate the rise in P_{alv}. This effect is most significant for the highly blood-soluble anesthetics, for which the rate of rise of P_{alv} is reduced more by vapor uptake into blood. Changes in cardiac output cause smaller changes in the rate of rise of P_{alv} for the less blood-soluble anesthetics such as N_2O and desflurane (**Fig. 38-9**).

The role of cardiac output in inhaled anesthetic uptake (and therefore inhalation induction) can seem counterintuitive. Increased cardiac output results in a more rapid delivery of anesthetic to the major sites of action in the nervous system, suggesting that anesthesia induction might be faster, not slower. The key to untangling this conundrum is to understand that during inhalation induction, P_{alv} is the driving force for anesthetic drug entry into the blood and nervous system. Because P_{alv} increases more slowly when cardiac output increases, partial pressure in the brain and spinal cord also increases more slowly. What happens to the "extra" anesthetic that is taken up via the lung at an elevated cardiac output? The brain and other highly perfused tissues (see below) equilibrate rapidly with P_{alv}. However, muscle and fat tissue, which typically take hours to equilibrate with P_{alv}, are absorbing most of the additional anesthetic agent.

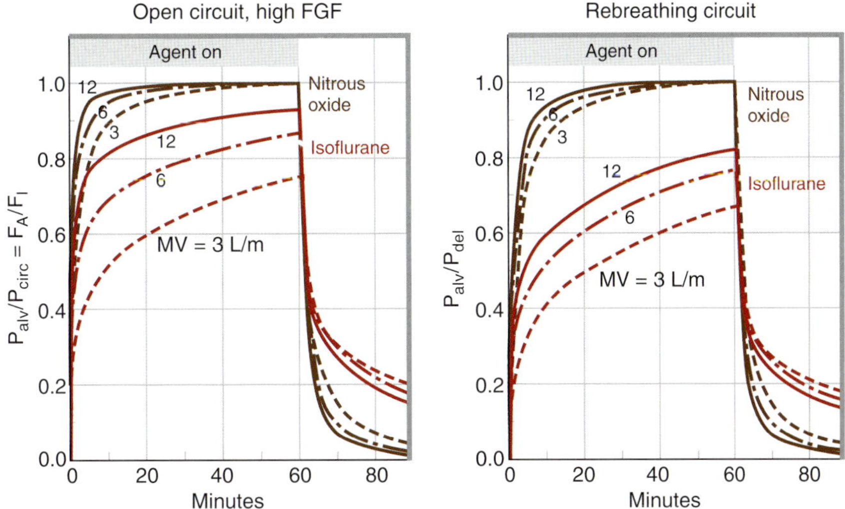

FIGURE 38-7. The impact of minute ventilation on the alveolar anesthetic concentration. **A.** The rise of P_{alv} is shown in the traditional manner, normalized to inspired concentration (P_{circ}), which is constant only with very high fresh gas flows (FGFs) and no rebreathing. Increased minute ventilation (MV) accelerates the rise of P_{alv} and increases clearance after delivery stops. **B.** P_{alv} is shown normalized to the constant delivered anesthetic concentration. This illustration better reflects the rise of P_{alv} during a typical induction when rebreathing occurs (FGF = 6 L/min).

In summary, the rate of equilibration between the alveolar partial pressure (P_{alv}) and the inspired anesthetic partial pressure (P_{circ}) depends on 3 factors: (1) Minute alveolar ventilation (as minute alveolar ventilation increases, the lung more rapidly equilibrates with the circuit), (2) cardiac output (as cardiac output increases, uptake from the pulmonary airspace into the blood and tissues slows the rate at which P_{alv} rises), and (3) blood–gas partitioning (high blood solubility, or $\lambda_{b/g}$, increases uptake into blood, removing a higher fraction of anesthetic from the pulmonary airspace and slowing the rate at which P_{alv} increases).

DISTRIBUTION OF INHALED ANESTHETICS IN BODY TISSUES

Mixed venous blood entering the pulmonary capillary bed rapidly equilibrates with the alveolar partial pressure of an inhaled anesthetic (P_{alv}) so that blood exiting from the pulmonary vein has a partial pressure close to P_{alv}. Anesthetic is then distributed to various tissues via systemic arterial blood. Delivery of anesthetic to each tissue is determined by its blood flow rate, its anatomic volume, and its tissue–blood partition coefficient (Table 38-2).

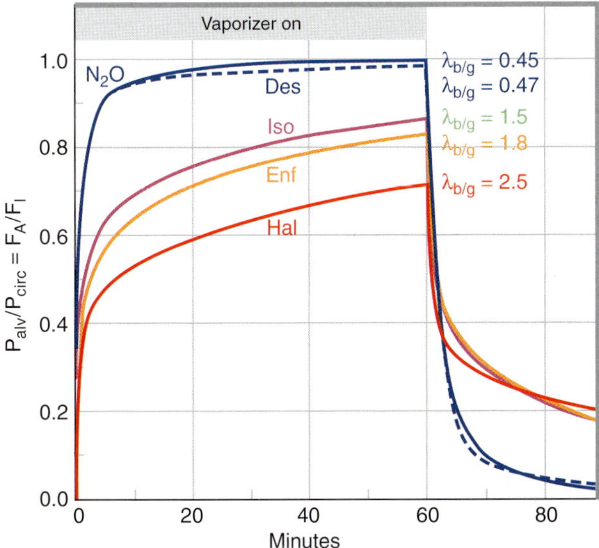

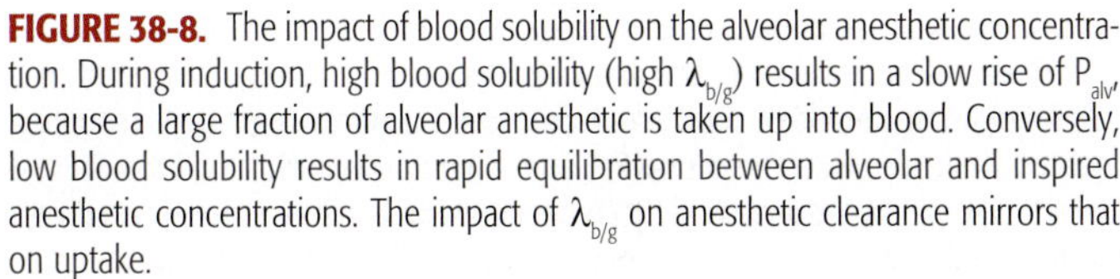
FIGURE 38-8. The impact of blood solubility on the alveolar anesthetic concentration. During induction, high blood solubility (high $\lambda_{b/g}$) results in a slow rise of P_{alv}, because a large fraction of alveolar anesthetic is taken up into blood. Conversely, low blood solubility results in rapid equilibration between alveolar and inspired anesthetic concentrations. The impact of $\lambda_{b/g}$ on anesthetic clearance mirrors that on uptake.

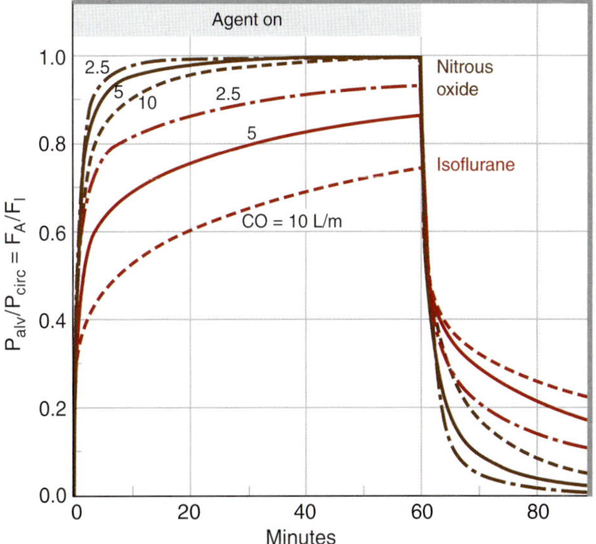

FIGURE 38-9. The impact of cardiac output (CO) on the alveolar anesthetic concentration. During induction, increased CO (pulmonary blood flow) results in a slower rise of P_{alv} because uptake from the alveoli into pulmonary blood is accelerated. The dependence of the P_{alv} rate of rise on CO is greatest for highly soluble anesthetics and minimal for insoluble drugs like nitrous oxide. The impact of CO on anesthetic clearance is similar to that on uptake.

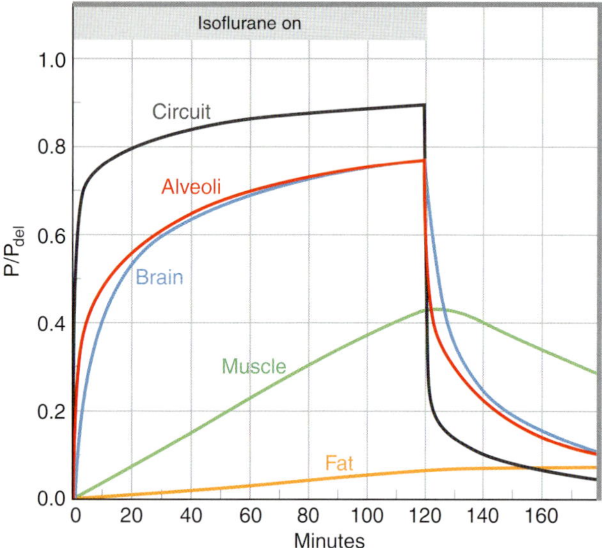

FIGURE 38-10. Uptake of anesthetics into different tissues. The partial pressure of isoflurane in different tissue beds is depicted during induction with fresh gas flow (FGF) = 6 L/min, $\dot{V}$ = 5 L/min, and $\dot{Q}$ = 5 L/min. Note that the isoflurane partial pressure in highly perfused tissues (brain) closely matches that in alveoli except when P_{alv} is changing very rapidly. Also note that the partial pressure of anesthetic in fat continues to rise after discontinuing isoflurane delivery, as long as P_{alv} is greater than P_{fat}. $\dot{V}$, minute alveolar ventilation; $\dot{Q}$, cardiac output.

The effective volume (V_{eff}) for uptake of anesthetic in a given tissue is the product of its anatomic volume and $\lambda_{tissue/blood}$. The time it takes for anesthetic partial pressure in a given tissue to equilibrate with P_{alv} is decreased when tissue perfusion is high and increased when V_{eff} is large (see Eq. 38-2).

Highly perfused tissues include the brain, spinal cord, kidney, liver, and heart, which comprise less than 10% of an adult body's mass while normally receiving about 70% of the cardiac output. Highly perfused tissues equilibrate within a few minutes with the arterial (alveolar) anesthetic partial pressure (**Fig. 38-10**, Table 38-2). As a result, the alveolar partial pressure of anesthetic, which can be measured in end-tidal gases, is usually close to the brain and spinal cord partial pressures (except when the anesthetic concentration in alveolar gas is changing rapidly).

Muscle represents a large anatomic volume (average, 35%-40% of body mass) and the muscle–blood partition coefficient for all inhaled agents ranges from 1.2 to 3.1. Because muscle normally receives only about 10% of cardiac output at rest, the anesthetic partial pressure in muscle rises slowly, and equilibration with P_{alv} takes hours for most clinically used anesthetics (Table 38-2).

Fat receives about 13% of cardiac output and represents about 25% of body mass in the average adult, with considerable variation. In addition, the potent volatile agents partition highly into fat ($\lambda_{fat/blood}$; range, 27-51), so that the effective volume for uptake of volatiles into fat is extremely large (Table 38-2). For the volatile anesthetics, uptake into fat is so slow that equilibration of the partial pressure with P_{alv} never occurs under normal clinical conditions. The only commonly used inhaled anesthetic with a low fat solubility is N_2O ($\lambda_{fat/blood}$ = 2.3), for which the equilibration time constant is about 2 hours.

The vessel-poor group of tissues include skin, ligaments, tendons, cartilage, and cortical bone. These represent about 14% of the average adult's body mass and receive less than 2% of cardiac output. As a result, their contribution to anesthetic uptake is negligible.

OTHER FACTORS AFFECTING THE UPTAKE AND DISTRIBUTION OF INHALED ANESTHETICS

Intrapulmonary right-to-left shunts (perfused but nonventilated lung regions) do not participate in anesthetic uptake. They slow the rate of uptake into blood and make P_{alv} increase more quickly, especially for the highly blood-soluble anesthetics. At the same time, pulmonary shunting results in an arterial admixture of mixed-venous blood with blood from gas-exchanging lung regions. As the fraction of pulmonary blood flow passing through right-to-left shunts increases, P_{art}, the direct upstream anesthetic pressure source for the nervous system, decreases relative to P_{alv}. For the highly soluble anesthetics, the increased P_{alv} somewhat compensates for admixing, and P_{art} increases only slightly slower than normal (**Fig. 38-11**). With less soluble agents, the impact of shunt on uptake from the lung (P_{alv}) is smaller and there is less compensation for admixing.

Systemic arteriovenous (left-to-right) shunting causes the anesthetic partial pressure in mixed venous blood to increase rapidly, slowing the uptake of anesthetic agent from alveolar gas. Alveolar anesthetic partial pressure therefore increases more rapidly, compensating for the reduced uptake rate. Overall, arteriovenous shunting modestly increases the rate of increase of anesthetic partial pressures in alveoli and in the highly perfused tissues.

Systemic right-to-left shunting, such as that in the lung, causes downstream arterial admixing. Right-to-left intracardiac shunts, such as patent foramen ovale or patent ductus arteriosus (PDA) with elevated right heart pressures, result in regional P_{art} lower than P_{alv}. PDA right-to-left shunting may result in different anesthetic partial pressures delivered to the brain and spinal cord. The overall effect of shunting can be difficult to predict because total cardiac output may also increase to compensate for the shunt.

Anatomic and physiologic deadspace (ventilated but nonperfused lung regions) effectively reduces alveolar ventilation relative to minute ventilation. This results in slower anesthetic uptake into blood from perfused lung areas, particularly for highly soluble drugs. At the same time, the lack of anesthetic uptake from nonperfused deadspace results in a faster increase in P_{alv}, which compensates for the slowed uptake.

Anesthetic-induced changes in cardiac and respiratory function affect the rate of anesthesia induction with volatile anesthetics. When spontaneous ventilation is maintained, the uptake of inhaled

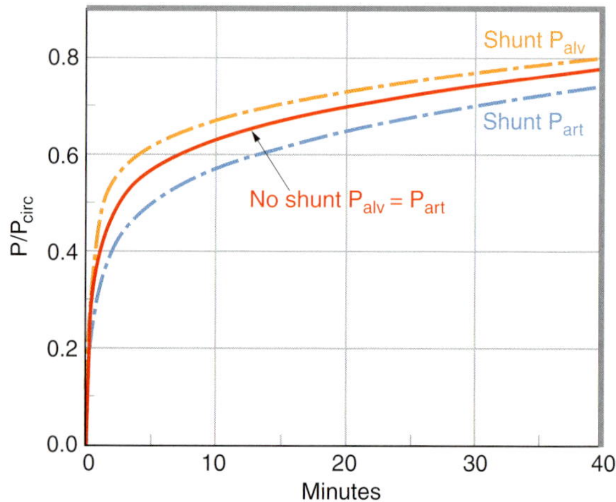

FIGURE 38-11. The impact of pulmonary right-to-left shunting on alveolar and arterial anesthetic concentrations. The impact of a 30% left-to-right shunt was calculated using a modified model from Fig. 38-4. Pulmonary right-to-left shunting reduces alveolar uptake, increasing P_{alv}, and mixing of shunted blood results in a lower P_{art}. However, the increased P_{alv} compensates for admixing, so compared with the zero shunt model, P_{art} is only about 10% reduced by the 30% shunt.

drug is reduced as anesthetic is absorbed, and minute ventilation decreases. Anesthetic depression of cardiac output is another dynamic factor altering both uptake and distribution of anesthetic, as discussed above.

CONCENTRATION EFFECT AND SECOND GAS EFFECT

Nitrous oxide represents a special case in clinical anesthesia because it is often the major constituent of the inhaled gas mixture. As a result, uptake of N_2O from the alveolar space into blood produces significant shifts of alveolar gas volume.[10] As alveolar gas volume diminishes, the alveolar concentration of N_2O is thus maintained (the concentration effect) as are the alveolar concentrations of other gases (the second gas effect). Consider a single breath of a gas mixture of 70% N_2O, 29% O_2, and 1% isoflurane near the start of an anesthetic when mixed venous blood does not contain N_2O (**Fig. 38-12**). When half of the alveolar N_2O is taken up into blood, the remaining alveolar gas volume will be 65% of the original volume with relative concentrations of 35 N_2O:29 O_2:1 Iso = 54% N_2O:45% O_2:1.5% Iso. Because of the reduction in alveolar gas volume, the alveolar N_2O concentration (and partial pressure) is more than half its original concentration (if 100% N_2O were inhaled, uptake would not reduce the alveolar concentration at all). The concentration effect therefore maintains the pressure gradient for uptake and increases the rate of rise of P_{alv} for N_2O toward the inspired concentration. The second gas effect is also illustrated in Fig. 38-12. With N_2O uptake, the alveolar concentrations of both oxygen and isoflurane can become higher than the inspired concentration, accelerating their uptake into blood.[11]

NITROUS UPTAKE INTO AIR SPACES IN THE BODY

Inhalation of N_2O at high concentrations leads to important effects on airspaces within the body. Airspaces usually contain mostly nitrogen (79% of air), which has a low solubility in blood ($\lambda_{b/g}$ = 0.015) such that bulk transfer of trapped nitrogen gas cannot occur on the timescale of most anesthetics. N_2O ($\lambda_{b/g}$ = 0.45) is delivered to airspaces 30 times faster than nitrogen leaves. As N_2O diffuses into the preexisting airspace, the volume or pressure in the airspace increases. In most cases, both airspace volume and pressure increase, but examples in which one or the other effect dominates are useful for illustration.

A compliant airspace, such as a small air embolus or pneumothorax, can increase its volume with minimal pressure change. It will continue to expand until the partial pressure of N_2O within the airspace equals that in surrounding blood. Theoretically, at 50% inspired N_2O, the preexisting volume of the gas bubble would double (half of its gas volume would then consist of N_2O). Similarly, 67% N_2O could lead to a tripling of volume, and 75% N_2O could quadruple the volume (**Fig. 38-13**). Small venous air emboli may thus become easier to detect with Doppler and echocardiographic monitors but may create more physiologic problems by obstructing blood vessels.[12,13] A small pneumothorax could also expand to compress mediastinal structures and impair oxygenation or create hemodynamic compromise. The rate of air-space expansion depends on the volume, geometry, and compliance of the airspace as well as the blood flow delivering N_2O to it. Small venous air emboli may expand within seconds, and a pneumothorax can expand toward equilibrium in less than an hour; airspaces in the bowel may take considerably longer to expand.

N_2O diffusion into noncompliant airspaces can also create clinical problems. In a noncompliant space, volume does not change, so pressure increases as N_2O enters. For example, after intravitreal injection of sulfur hexafluoride (SF_6) or perfluoropropane (C_3F_8) gases, N_2O administration can result in rapid increases of intraocular pressure, compromising retinal blood flow.[14,15] Intracranial air bubbles (after craniectomy or pneumoencephalography) and the inner ear also represent airspaces in noncompliant body compartments.

Other common inhaled anesthetics also diffuse into airspaces, but their low concentrations in clinical settings result in negligible impact on airspace volume and pressure. Xenon is an experimental anesthetic inhaled at high concentrations (60%-70%), and similar to N_2O, is associated with airspace expansion.[16]

ELIMINATION OF INHALED ANESTHETICS VIA VENTILATION

The removal of inhaled anesthetics via the lungs is essentially the reverse of uptake, and many of the factors affecting induction also affect elimination rates. High FGF promotes faster washout of anesthetic from the circuit, enhancing the gradient for removal from the lung (Fig. 38-5). High minute ventilation clears alveolar anesthetic, reducing P_{alv} and providing a gradient for movement of anesthetic from the blood to the alveoli (Fig. 38-7). Highly blood soluble anesthetics are retained longer than insoluble drugs because the effective volume of blood is higher as $\lambda_{b/g}$ increases (Fig. 38-8). Similarly, increasing the cardiac output retards recovery (Fig. 38-9).

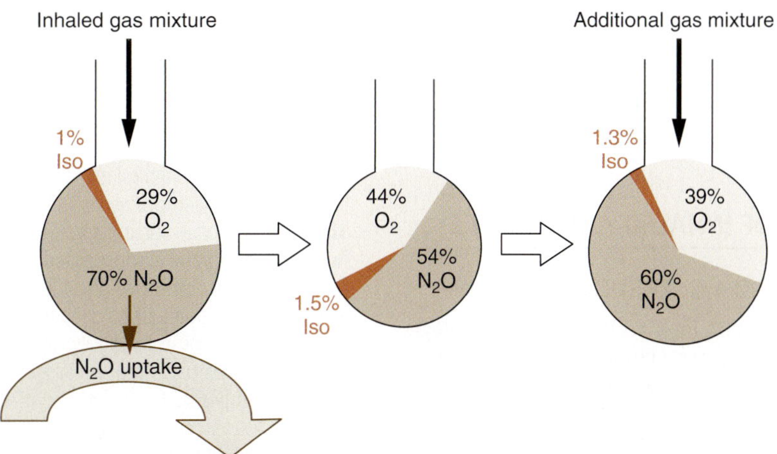

FIGURE 38-12. The concentration and second gas effects. When nitrous oxide (N_2O) is inspired at high concentrations, transfer from the lung into pulmonary blood causes the volume of alveolar gas to decrease, drawing in more of the gas mixture and concentrating the remaining gases. This *concentration effect* on N_2O itself results in a sustained alveolar driving pressure and more rapid uptake. The alveolar concentrations of other gases, such as isoflurane and oxygen, become higher than the inspired concentrations, which increases their uptake as well—the *second gas effect*.

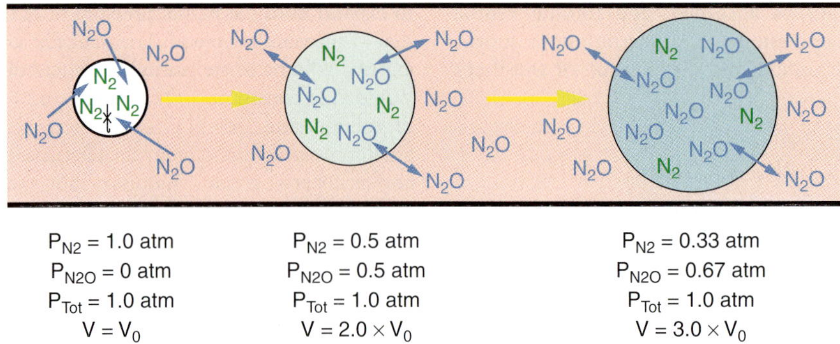

FIGURE 38-13. Expansion of venous air emboli by nitrous oxide. Nitrous oxide (N_2O) enters air pockets far faster than nitrogen leaves (because of low blood nitrogen-carrying capacity), causing airspace expansion. Expansion continues until the partial pressure of N_2O inside the air bubble matches that in surrounding blood. Thus, at 50% N_2O (P_{N2O} = 0.5 atm), air emboli can double in volume, and at 67% N_2O (P_{N2O} = 0.67 atm), they can triple in volume. Expansion of small venous air emboli can lead to occlusion of pulmonary capillaries, compromising both blood flow and gas exchange.

Some aspects of anesthetic elimination do not mirror the uptake during anesthetic induction. The use of overpressure to accelerate anesthetic induction has no parallel during recovery because the delivered concentration or partial pressure of anesthetic agent cannot fall below zero. Also, before induction, whereas the inhaled anesthetic partial pressure in all tissues is zero, different tissues will typically have reached different partial pressures when anesthetic delivery is discontinued. In particular, the partial pressures in muscle and fat may be far lower than P_{alv} after a brief anesthetic. Because an anesthetic will continue to be transferred into tissue as long as P_{alv} is greater than P_{tissue}, these compartments may continue to absorb the drug even after delivery is discontinued. This effect is illustrated in Fig. 38-10, where fat continues to take up isoflurane from blood long after delivery is discontinued, until P_{alv} is less than P_{fat}. This uptake helps reduce the anesthetic partial pressure within the highly perfused tissues and can shorten emergence time.

The longer anesthesia is maintained, the more drug is absorbed into muscle and fat, which are characterized by a slow uptake and release of agent. Thus, clearance of inhaled anesthetics is context sensitive: the longer the anesthetic, the slower the clearance. Theoretical modeling suggests that after 4 hours at 1 × minimum alveolar concentration (MAC) of various anesthetics, 99.9% brain elimination takes 33 hours for desflurane, 52 hours for sevoflurane, and 71 hours for isoflurane and that significant amounts of these drugs remain in the body for days after discontinuation of anesthetic delivery.[17] If fat and muscle reach high partial pressures (after many hours for most potent agents), recovery from anesthesia may be significantly delayed. Obese patients and those with a higher than normal muscle mass are therefore at risk for slowed emergence after long exposures to soluble anesthetics.

PHARMACODYNAMICS OF INHALED ANESTHETICS

THERAPEUTIC EFFECTS AND ANESTHETIC DEPTH

Although general anesthesia results in a multitude of physiologic alterations, there is no consensus among clinicians and researchers as to which actions are essential to the state of general anesthesia.[18] Our view is that the common desired outcomes of general anesthesia include hypnosis (loss of awareness), amnesia (loss of memory), and immobility (suppression of movement in response to pain). Some have argued that analgesia is also an essential component.[19] Pain is unquestionably a critical consideration in perioperative care, but the potent sedative–hypnotic effects of most general anesthetics confound the assessment of pain. Hypnosis and amnesia are produced via drug effects on neural networks within the brain, and immobility is primarily mediated by the spinal cord. In short, the major therapeutic actions of the volatile anesthetics take place in the CNS. Beneficial and toxic effects of inhaled anesthetics on other physiologic systems (eg, cardiovascular function, respiration) can thus be regarded as secondary. In this section, we discuss various measurements of anesthetic effects in the nervous system, as well as their limitations.

Because *general anesthesia* is defined as the loss of normal responses to environmental stimuli, *anesthetic depth* is most rigorously defined by stimulus–response testing using stimuli that range from benign (eg, spoken commands) to noxious (eg, laryngoscopy or surgical incision).[20] In addition, certain consistent pharmacologic effects of anesthetics that are stimulus independent are useful signs of anesthetic depth. Traditionally, both desired and undesired clinical effects have been associated with the various stages and planes of anesthesia introduced by Snow (1847)[21] and modified by Guedel (1937).[22] These descriptions (**Table 38-3**) were developed during the era of ether and chloroform anesthesia and are therefore not fully applicable to modern practice.

TABLE 38-3 Classic Stages and Planes of Inhalational Anesthesia

- **Stage 1** is defined as the time between the normal waking state and the loss of consciousness (**hypnosis**) caused by an anesthetic agent. There is also mild **analgesia** in stage 1 anesthesia.
- **Stage 2** is associated with loss of awareness and recall (**amnesia**). Stage 2 is associated with the undesired effects of cardiovascular instability, excitation, dysconjugate ocular movements, and emesis.
- **Stage 3** is defined as surgical anesthesia, a state during which **movement in response to pain is suppressed**. Various planes of anesthesia were described by Guedel[22] based on additional physiological signs:
  - **Plane 1** is associated with deep respiration, coordinated thoracic and diaphragmatic muscular activity, and pupillary constriction.
  - **Plane 2** is associated with diminished respiration, as well as fixed midline and dilated pupils.
  - **Plane 3** is associated with continued diaphragmatic movement, diminished thoracic movement, and further pupillary dilation.
  - **Plane 4** is associated with thoracic immobility and diminished diaphragmatic movement.
- **Stage 4** is associated with cessation of spontaneous respiration and medullary cardiac reflexes and may lead to death.

MINIMUM ALVEOLAR CONCENTRATION, MINIMUM ALVEOLAR CONCENTRATION AWAKE, AND MINIMUM ALVEOLAR CONCENTRATION BAR

Minimum Alveolar Concentration In 1965, Eger introduced the concept of MAC as a stimulus–response measure of anesthetic potency.[23,24] MAC is the alveolar concentration of inhaled anesthetic that prevents movement in half of subjects in response to a surgical incision. Thus, MAC is the equivalent of an ED50. (dose of a drug that produces an effect in 50% of subjects) inhibition of movement in response to a specific noxious stimulus. If different noxious stimuli (eg, varying point pressures or electric shocks) are used, the concentration of inhaled anesthetic required to suppress movement increases with stimulus intensity.[25] Thus, MAC is most useful for comparing potency among different inhaled agents under the same conditions, with potency being inversely related to MAC. During measurement of MAC, equilibrium between the alveolar gas compartment and the CNS must first be established. Other drugs that modulate awareness (eg, benzodiazepines), pain sensation (eg, opioids), or movement (eg, muscle relaxants) cannot be present. MAC as originally defined depends on atmospheric pressure, but when agent concentration is expressed as a partial pressure, MAC becomes independent of ambient pressure. The MAC values of common inhaled agents in oxygen (Table 38-2) show that N_2O is least potent followed by desflurane, sevoflurane, enflurane, isoflurane, and halothane. By definition, an exclusively inhalational anesthetic to a level of 1 × MAC will prevent movement in only 50% of patients. The ED95, which is roughly 1.3 × MAC, may be a more clinically useful value. The ED_{95} corresponds to 0.9% for halothane, 1.68% for isoflurane, and 1.88% for enflurane.

MAC is altered by age and physiologic, genetic, and pharmacologic factors. MAC decreases with age (**Fig. 38-14**). Standard MAC values are those for patients around age 40 years. MAC is highest within the first year of life (age 6-12 months) and decreases with advancing age.[26,27]

Physiologic factors such as temperature influence MAC. For each decrease in core temperature by 1°C, MAC decreases by 5%. Other physiologic extremes that affect CNS function (eg, hypoxia, hypercapnia, acidosis, hypotension) also decrease MAC.

Whether MAC is affected by gender is controversial. Elderly women require 26% less xenon than age-matched men. In young men and women, however, MAC for desflurane does not significantly differ.[28] MAC is reduced in parturient women.[29] Increases in either progesterone or endogenous opiates (endorphins) during pregnancy have been proposed to account for this decreased anesthetic requirement, but these theories have not been substantiated by experiment.

Genetic factors play a role in determining MAC. Mice of varying genomic backgrounds are differentially susceptible to volatile anesthetics such as halothane, isoflurane, and sevoflurane.[30] In humans, patients with naturally red hair have a significantly higher desflurane MAC than other patients (**Fig. 38-15**).[31] Ninety percent of the red heads tested had mutations reducing expression of the melanocortin-1 receptor gene. Genetically altered (knock-out) mice lacking the melanocortin-1 receptor gene also display a modest increase in MAC for desflurane, isoflurane, sevoflurane, and halothane.[32]

Pharmacologic factors alter MAC. The addition of 70% N_2O reduces the anesthetic requirements of other inhaled agents by 55% to 70% (Table 38-2). MAC is an additive phenomenon when 2 or more inhaled agents are combined.[33] Adjunct opiate or benzodiazepine administration reduces MAC. Whereas acute alcohol intoxication reduces MAC, chronic intake of alcohol or sedatives can increase MAC, a phenomenon known as cross-tolerance.[34]

MAC reflects the effects of inhaled anesthetics in the spinal cord. In animal models, MAC has been shown to be primarily dependent on anesthetic effects on the spinal cord and not the brain.[35,36] Anesthetic-induced immobility is likely attributable to suppression of spinal motor neuron function, observed as a diminished Hoffmann's reflex (H-reflex) and F-wave amplitudes.[37,38] Suppression of movement and H-reflex amplitude by sevoflurane follow similar dose-response relationships in humans.[39]

Minimum Alveolar Concentration–Awake MAC-awake is the concentration of inhaled anesthetic that inhibits appropriate responses to spoken commands in half of patients.[26] The ratio of MAC-awake to MAC is not consistent among inhaled agents. It is fairly constant for the halogenated volatiles (roughly 0.35 × MAC), and significantly higher for N_2O,[40] which likely reflects their different mechanisms of action (see Chapter 37).

Functional recovery from anesthesia is influenced by MAC-awake for the specific agent as well as its elimination kinetics. Therefore, the time required to awaken after an anesthetic, especially a long one, depends on what concentration of the anesthetic was used relative to its MAC-awake. If the inhaled concentration was 2 × MAC-awake,

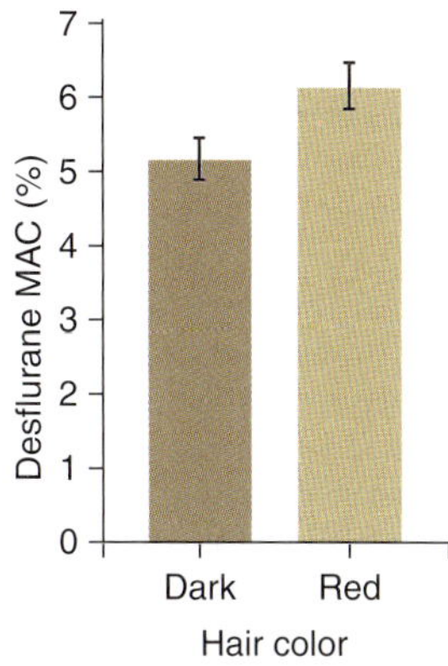

FIGURE 38-15. Minimum alveolar concentration (MAC) values are increased in natural redheads. The figure depicts data reported by Liem et al.[31] On average, red heads require about 20% higher alveolar concentrations of desflurane to prevent movement. Columns represent averages and error bars represent standard deviations.

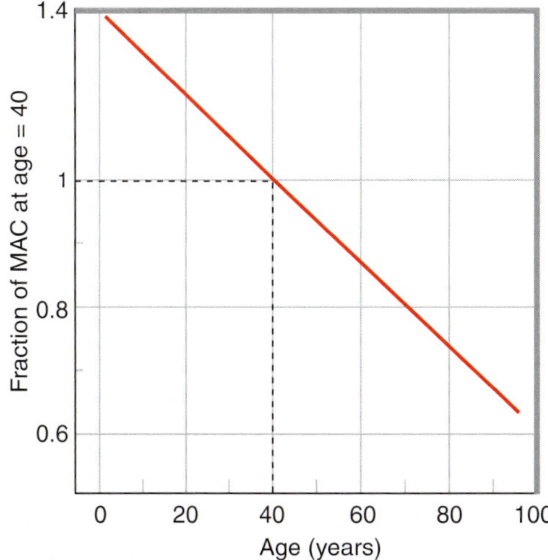

FIGURE 38-14. Minimum alveolar concentration (MAC) varies with age. MAC is maximal in the first year of life and decreases with age. The figure shows the relationship on a semi-logarithmic scale. The equation of the line is $MAC/MAC_{40} = 1.32 \times 10^{-0.00303Age}$, or a 6.7% decrease in MAC per decade.[26]

then only a 50% reduction in P_{alv} will be needed before the patient awakens, which is usually rapidly achieved for most agents. If higher concentrations were used, then emergence may be more than proportionately slowed because the slower phases of agent elimination will have a more dominant effect (see Elimination of Inhaled Anesthetics via Ventilation).

Similar to MAC, MAC-awake is reduced in elderly adults, by hypothermia and by the presence of other drugs with hypnotic activity (ethanol, benzodiazepines, anticonvulsants, antidepressants).[26] MAC-awake is also reduced by neuraxial blockade (spinal or epidural) despite intact cranial nerve function.[41-44] This effect is believed to be caused by diminished ascending signals from the spinal cord, which stimulate cortical arousal via the brainstem. MAC-awake is decreased by high doses of opiates, but this reduction is smaller than that of MAC.[45]

MAC-awake (hypnosis) is associated with volatile anesthetics effects on the cerebral cortex. Gamma range (25-100 Hz) signals from different cortical regions become desynchronized during the transition from conscious to unconscious states.[46,47] Synchrony in specific cortical circuits, particularly the thalamocortical network, is believed to be associated with higher cognitive function, and its interruption may account for loss of consciousness.[48] Loss of "functional connectivity" among various cortical networks during anesthesia has been demonstrated by functional brain imaging studies.[49,50]

Low concentrations of inhaled anesthetics block memory more than awareness.[40] When inhaled agents are given at MAC-awake, only a small fraction of "aware" experimental subjects (those responding to spoken commands) can recall events.[51] Amnesia is likely caused by effects on the limbic network, including the amygdala and hippocampus. Lesions in the basolateral amygdala produce resistance to the amnestic effects of sevoflurane in animals.[52] Volatile anesthetics both attenuate hippocampal activity and inhibit long-term potentiation of hippocampal synapses that is associated with memory formation.[53,54]

Minimum Alveolar Concentration for Blockade of Autonomic Responses

Minimum **alveolar concentration for blockade of autonomic responses** (MAC-BAR) is the alveolar anesthetic concentration that suppresses cardiovascular responses to surgical incision in half of patients.[55] MAC-BAR is typically greater than MAC. For example, MAC-BAR for desflurane is 1.66 × MAC.[55] Similar to MAC and MAC-awake, MAC-BAR is reduced by opiates.[20]

Limitations on Traditional Anesthetic Depth Measurements Stimulus–response testing is usually impractical in clinical settings. Neuromuscular blocking drugs ablate motor responses to both painful (MAC) and benign (MAC-awake) stimuli. Techniques for maintaining a motor response capability are laborious. As a result, autonomic signs such as blood pressure, heart rate, diaphoresis, tearing, and pupillary responses are often the only accessible data for assessing depth of anesthesia. These signs are valuable but unreliable guides to anesthetic depth and are confounded by drugs and diseases that impair cardiac or autonomic nervous system functions.

Numerous factors affect anesthetic sensitivity (including unknown genetic factors), resulting in widely varying individual anesthetic requirements. Too little anesthetic puts patients at risk for intraoperative awareness (see below). Conversely, deep anesthesia for all patients is neither feasible nor advisable. Deep inhalational anesthesia in patients with cardiac disease, hypovolemia, and other critical illnesses predictably causes profound hypotension and organ hypoperfusion. Healthy patients may tolerate deep anesthesia, but it may result in a slow emergence and a high incidence of side effects. Recent research suggests that excessively deep general anesthesia may accelerate the pathogenesis of neurodegenerative diseases such as Alzheimer dementia[56-58] and may be associated with increased late mortality.[59] The delivery of sufficient but not excessive anesthesia while providing optimal surgical conditions represents a central challenge for anesthetists.

ELECTROENCEPHALOGRAPHIC MEASUREMENT OF ANESTHETIC DEPTH

Given that the modern practice of general anesthesia frequently includes neuromuscular blockade to provide immobility, narcotics to provide analgesia, and other drugs to control autonomic activity, the essential therapeutic effects of general anesthetics are hypnosis and amnesia (ablation of awareness and memory). These effects, which are mediated in the brain, are also the most difficult to assess clinically. Monitors that analyze electrical signals from the brain can provide anesthetists with more data to individually titrate the depth of general anesthesia to achieve these endpoints. In addition, titration to individual needs has been shown to reduce anesthetic dosage, resulting in faster emergence in some settings.[60,61]

A number of techniques based on electroencephalography (EEG) have been developed and used. Fourier transformation of raw EEG data enables the derivation of median power and spectral edge frequencies.[62] Other EEG analyses assess bispectral phase relationships, burst suppression, and entropy. The bispectral index (BIS; Covidien, Boulder CO) is a proprietary algorithm based on burst suppression, near-burst suppression, beta-band power, and phase relationships between delta- and theta-waves.[63] The patient state index (PSI; Physiometrix, Inc., N. Billerica, MA) is based on EEG component relationships between the frontal and occipital regions.[64] Entropy monitors (eg, S/5, General Electric [Datex-Ohmeda], Helsinki, Finland) analyze entropy (randomness in frequency and phase relationships) using both EEG and frontal electromyography (EMG).[65] Some of these monitors are now available for clinical use to provide additional information and help prevent undesired side effects such as awareness during general anesthesia. For most patients, EEG indices such as BIS and spectral entropy correlate with the alveolar concentration of volatile anesthetics (**Fig. 38-16**).[66] Monitors based on stimulus–response are also being developed for clinical use. Auditory evoked potentials can be used to assess anesthetic-induced unconsciousness and may be used in conjunction with other EEG parameters.[67] A recent innovation is the use of transcranial magnetic stimulation in conjunction with EEG to detect loss of consciousness.[68] Nonetheless, all of these monitors have considerable limitations. Further research in identifying neural correlates of consciousness is needed to improve the utility of monitors that assess the depth of anesthesia.

INTRAOPERATIVE AWARENESS AND RECALL

The interindividual variability in sensitivity to general anesthetics and the difficulty in clinical assessment of anesthetic depth inevitably result in excessive or inadequate depth of anesthesia in some patients. Inadequate anesthesia can result in awareness and explicit recall of intraoperative events, a problem that is a subject of clinical, public, and scientific attention.[69]

INCIDENCE OF AWARENESS WITH RECALL DURING GENERAL ANESTHESIA

Large studies in both Sweden[70] and the United States[71] have used multiple postoperative interviews (eg, **Table 38-4**) to investigate intraoperative awareness. In a total of 31 360 combined patients, 40 cases of "definite" and "probable" awareness with recall were identified, an incidence of 0.13%. Given that 30 to 50 million general anesthetics are administered in the United States, the number of patients experiencing awareness with recall is estimated at around 50 000 per year.

PATIENT REPORTS AND POSTTRAUMATIC STRESS DISORDER AFTER INTRAOPERATIVE AWARENESS

Spontaneous reports by patients of intraoperative awareness are rare, highlighting the need to using a structured interview that probes for these events.[72] Patients report a variety of intraoperative experiences after general anesthesia. A high proportion of these experiences are

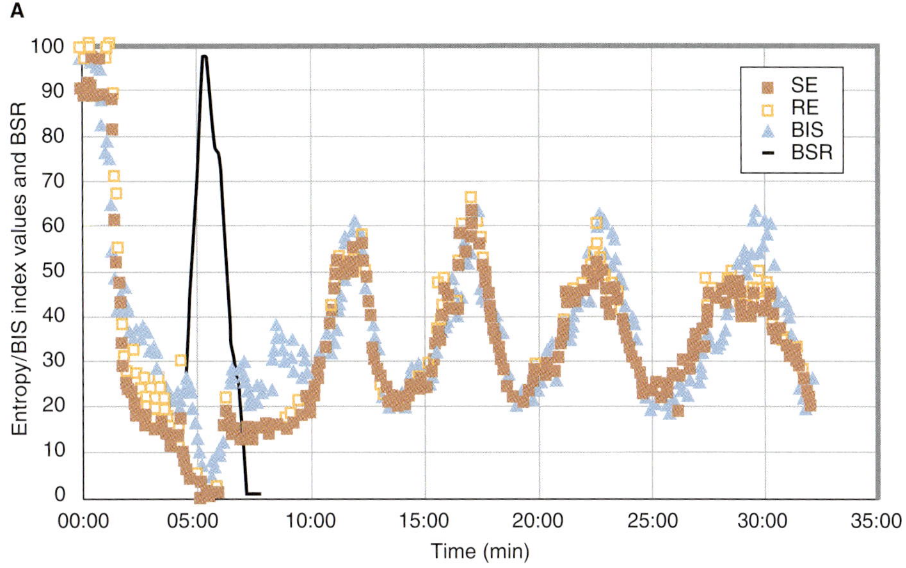

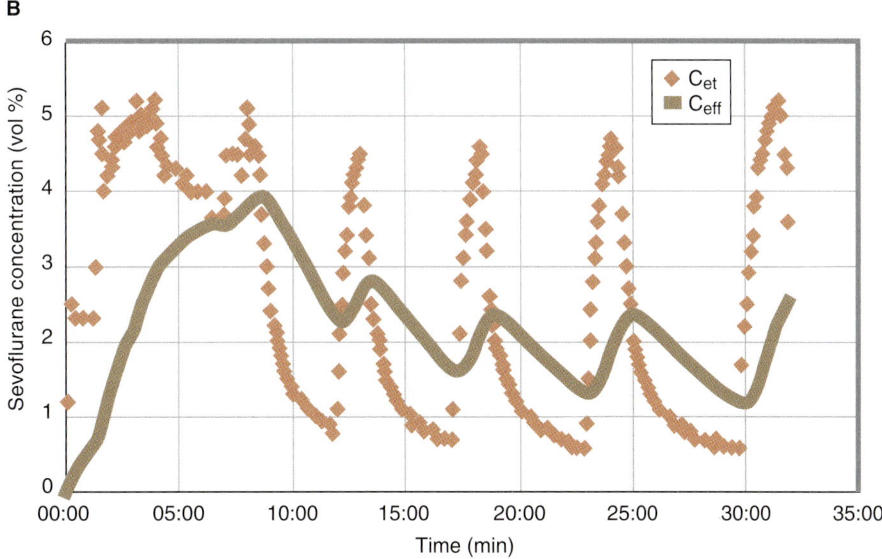

FIGURE 38-16. Correlation between processed electroencephalographic (EEG) parameters and volatile anesthetic concentration. **A.** Time course of state entropy (SE), response entropy (RE), bispectral index (BIS), and burst suppression ratio (BSR) of a single patient. Each symbol represents an EEG parameter of a 5-sec epoch. **B.** End-tidal sevoflurane concentration (Cet) and calculated effect site concentration (Ceff) during the same time course in the same patient. [Reprinted with permission from Ellerkmann RK, Liermann VM, Alves TM, et al. Spectral entropy and bispectral index as measures of the electroencephalographic effects of sevoflurane. *Anesthesiology.* 2004;101:1275-1282.]

vague and dreamlike, but others are explicit recollections of intraoperative events. Explicit recollections may include hearing conversations among operating room personnel; pain associated with intubation or surgery; and extreme anxiety, particularly in paralyzed patients. These experiences can lead to postoperative psychological problems. In the most severe cases, patients may develop posttraumatic stress disorder (PTSD). PTSD is characterized by recurrent episodes of anxiety, irritability, anger, and vigilance, often associated with flashbacks or nightmares, avoidance of cues related to the trauma, and sleep disturbances.[73] The incidence of PTSD after intraoperative awareness is not known, but it likely depends on the length of the awareness episode and the presence of pain, anxiety, and preexisting psychological problems. In a small study of 16 post-awareness patients, more than 50% developed symptoms of PTSD requiring psychotherapy.[74]

TABLE 38-4 The Modified Brice Interview

1. What is the last thing you remember before anesthesia?
2. What is the first thing you recall after waking up?
3. Do you recall anything in between?
4. Did you have any dreams during surgery?
5. What was the worst thing about your surgery and anesthesia?

From Brice DD, Hetherington RR, Utting JE. A simple study of awareness and dreaming during anaesthesia. *Br J Anaesth.* 1970;42:535-542.

RISK FACTORS FOR AWARENESS DURING GENERAL ANESTHESIA

Factors that contribute to intraoperative awareness include the use of muscle relaxants, high individual requirements for anesthetics,

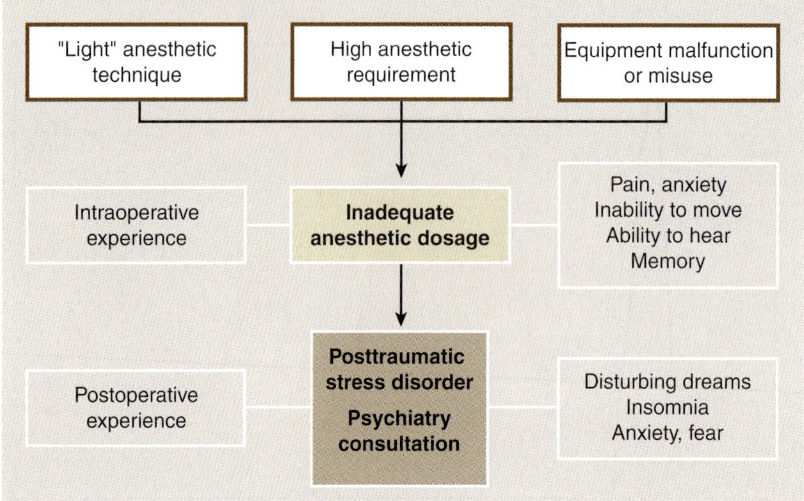

FIGURE 38-17. Causes and consequences of awareness during anesthesia.

surgical situations during which "light" anesthesia is typically used, and errors by the anesthesia care team (**Fig. 38-17**).[75] Awareness with recall has been reported in patients who were anesthetized without muscle relaxants, but the incidence is much higher when muscle relaxants were given.[76] Furthermore, severe psychological problems seem to develop primarily in patients who experience "awake paralysis" with anxiety and pain.[77] Patients receiving chronic therapy with sedatives, opiates, and some anticonvulsants can develop tolerance (resistance) to anesthetic drugs and require higher than normal anesthetic doses. Pharmacogenomic factors are likely to play a role, and patients with either a personal or a family history of awareness during general anesthesia may be at increased risk. Surgical procedures associated with high incidences of intraoperative awareness include major trauma, thoracoabdominal, and cardiac surgery. In these settings, hemodynamic instability often precludes the use of sufficient depth of anesthesia to prevent awareness, resulting in increased incidences of awareness ranging from 1% up to 40%.[78,79] Caesarean section under general anesthesia, during which a "light" anesthetic is often used to reduce depression of the newborn, is also associated with a high incidence of awareness (0.4%).[80] Inadequate dosing, misuse of equipment, and other human errors can also lead to patient awareness during general anesthesia. Many cases of awareness appear to occur during prolonged attempts at airway intubation when the hypnotic effect of IV induction agents wears off while patients remain paralyzed with a muscle relaxant. Other reports have described awareness when anesthetic vaporizers were empty or when drug pumps were not delivering proper doses of hypnotic agents. Reviews of awareness during general anesthesia incidents report that most cases were preventable.[81]

MONITORING AND PREVENTION OF INTRAOPERATIVE AWARENESS

There is evidence that 2 monitoring strategies may be effective at reducing the incidence of intraoperative awareness when inhaled anesthetics are used to produce hypnosis. These are based on 2 measurements, the EEG-derived BIS and end-tidal anesthetic partial pressures, both known to correlate with depth of hypnosis (perceptive awareness).

The BIS is the only EEG-based monitoring technique that has been extensively evaluated for its ability to reduce the incidence of awareness. Myles et al[82] conducted a prospective, randomized, double-blinded, multicenter trial of 2463 patients at high risk of awareness with recall who were assigned to either "standard care" or BIS-guided anesthesia groups. Postoperative interviews identified 2 patients (0.16%) who experienced awareness with recall in the BIS-guided group and 11 (0.9%) in the high-risk control group. Of note, use of the BIS monitor in this study did not reduce the total incidence of intraoperative experiences reported by patients (including reports judged as "possible awareness" or "no awareness") but only those with "confirmed" awareness with recall. A number of confounding factors can also affect the BIS, reducing its ability to accurately gauge depth of anesthesia. These factors include electrical artifact from electrocautery devices, physiologic alterations such as hypoglycemia, low-voltage EEG caused by genetic variation or drugs, and neurologic abnormalities such as Alzheimer disease.[83] A common confounding factor that can alter BIS and spectral entropy values is EMG (muscle) activity, which can be reduced with neuromuscular blockade.[84,85] Furthermore, appropriate interpretation and intervention are required for effective use of these monitors. In Sebel's et al's incidence study,[71] BIS monitors were used in about 40% of the patients, yet this group of patients did not have a reduced incidence of awareness reports. Finally, the value of BIS monitoring has been validated only for propofol and volatile anesthetics. When ketamine and N_2O are present, the relationship between BIS value and perceptive awareness can be significantly altered.[86]

End-tidal anesthetic gas (ETAG) monitoring, which is available in most modern anesthesia systems, appears to be also useful for reducing the incidence of intraoperative awareness. Avidan et al[87] conducted a prospective randomized trial that assessed explicit awareness in high-risk patients. The incidence of explicit awareness was similarly low (0.2%) in patients whose anesthetics were guided using BIS monitors and a comparison patient group who received ETAG concentration-guided anesthesia (0.7 – 1.3 × Age-adjusted MAC). However, there was no "standard care" control group included in this study, and thus, additional research is needed to verify that ETAG monitoring is effective at reducing the incidence of intraoperative awareness. A clear limitation of ETAG is that it is not applicable or reliable for patients receiving total IV anesthesia or a combination of IV infusions and inhaled anesthetic agents.

MANAGEMENT OF INTRAOPERATIVE AWARENESS

Prevention of intraoperative awareness with recall begins with recognizing and addressing known risk factors. Caregivers must be familiar with their equipment and its proper use. Amnestics, such as benzodiazepines, can reduce the incidence of awareness with recall and should be considered as premedication for most patients and when "light" anesthesia is unavoidable. Muscle relaxants should be used judiciously to provide adequate relaxation for surgery or avoided whenever possible. N_2O-relaxant anesthesia should be supplemented with volatile anesthetics or IV hypnotic agents to maintain adequate hypnosis (~2 × MAC-awake). When intubation is delayed or multiple attempts are required, consideration should be given to supplementing the induction bolus with additional inhaled or IV hypnotic agents. All patients should be routinely informed of the risk of awareness during general anesthesia. High-risk patients should be monitored using ETAG analysis or an EEG-based monitor when feasible and appropriate. If adjunct monitoring is used, it should be used according to manufacturer's guidelines, and indications of potentially inadequate anesthesia on the monitor should be treated with an increased dose of hypnotic agents unless other circumstances make this inadvisable.

Ideally, in the postoperative period, all patients should be interviewed and asked specific questions (Table 38-4) to assess for intraoperative awareness. When awareness is detected, the patient should be treated for this occurrence like any other complication that results in harm or potential harm to patients. A thorough debriefing of the patient is warranted, and the details of the patient's experiences should be documented in the medical record. All personnel involved in the surgery should be informed, and patient recollections should be corroborated as thoroughly as possible. The incident should also be reported to the departmental Quality Assurance Committee and possibly to the institutional legal counsel. Patients reporting awareness during anesthesia should be reassured that their experience is valid and provided with an explanation of why and how the intraoperative awareness occurred. Expressing sympathy for the patient's suffering and apology if indicated can help maintain a therapeutic relationship, and the patient should be offered professional psychological evaluation and therapy for his or her symptoms. Maintaining contact with the patient with daily visits or phone calls may facilitate their recovery and can reduce malpractice risk.

SYSTEMIC ACTIONS OF INHALED ANESTHETICS

In this section, we summarize both the therapeutic and toxic secondary effects of inhaled anesthetics on important physiologic systems.

CENTRAL NERVOUS SYSTEM

Cerebrovascular and Metabolic Effects The effects of anesthetics on cerebral metabolism and vascular tone are summarized in **Table 38-5**. Normal cerebral blood flow (CBF) is tightly autoregulated and coupled with cerebral metabolic demands. Volatile anesthetics interrupt this autoregulation by acting as direct vasodilators of the cerebral vasculature.[88] Volatile anesthetics dependently increase middle cerebral artery blood flow velocity, with sevoflurane causing less vasodilation than isoflurane or desflurane.[89,90] Both K^+ channels[91] and neuronal nitric oxide synthase[92] have been linked to these direct actions of anesthetics.

Volatile anesthetics also decrease the cerebral metabolic rate (CMR) of oxygen consumption.[18,88] Cerebral metabolism is decreased by halothane, isoflurane, sevoflurane, and desflurane.[93] The extent to which blood flow and metabolism are altered depends on the choice of agent. For example, halothane may increase CBF by almost 200% while reducing the CMR by only 10%.[94] Isoflurane, by contrast, increases CBF by about 20% while reducing CMR by 45%.[95,96] Volatile agents also partially uncouple flow–metabolism relationships and carbon dioxide reactivity.[97,98] These agents have not been shown to increase intracranial pressure (ICP) in normocapnic adults undergoing supratentorial brain tumor resection without a preoperative midline shift.[99] In children, isoflurane, sevoflurane, and desflurane have all been shown to increase ICP.[100] N_2O is distinguished from the potent volatile anesthetics in that it increases CBF and CMR and may increase ICP.[101,102] This is partly attributable to its sympathomimetic effects.[103]

Electroencephalographic Effects Volatile anesthetics alter the cortical EEG, decreasing high-frequency (gamma band) activity and increasing slower frequencies. Quantitative EEG analysis demonstrates that power shifts anteriorly.[46] In comparison, N_2O has little effect or increases the frequency of the cortical EEG.[104-106] Indeed, EEG-based monitors do not reliably detect the hypnotic effects of N_2O alone or in combination with other anesthetics.[107,108] Deep volatile anesthesia (1.5-2 × MAC) leads to burst-suppression or isoelectric EEG patterns. Although all volatile anesthetics have been used to suppress seizures, both enflurane and sevoflurane have been reported to augment epileptic brain activity and may induce EEG patterns associated with epilepsy in normal patients.[109-111] Enflurane and sevoflurane may be useful during cortical mapping for ablation of seizure foci but should otherwise be avoided in patients with seizure disorders.

The actions of anesthetics that are thought to produce the state of general anesthesia are discussed briefly above in this chapter and in more detail in Chapter 44. The long-term effects of anesthetics on cognitive function are reviewed in Chapter 84.

CARDIOVASCULAR SYSTEM

The effects of volatile anesthetics on the cardiovascular system are of paramount clinical importance intraoperatively, particularly in patients at risk for end-organ ischemia. The effects are summarized in **Table 38-6**.

Mean Arterial Pressure Volatile anesthetics decrease mean arterial pressure (MAP) in a dose-dependent manner[93] by direct vascular and autonomic nervous effects. Volatile anesthetics reduce MAP by decreasing systemic vascular resistance, increasing vascular compliance (the change in circulatory volume with changes in pressure), and inhibiting myocardial contractility. Halothane depresses myocardial contractility more than other volatile anesthetics. Whereas isoflurane and desflurane decrease systemic vascular resistance, halothane, isoflurane, and sevoflurane increase arterial compliance[112] (**Table 38-7**). Desflurane has been found to stimulate sympathetic nervous system activity (especially with rapid increases in vapor concentration), which may account for its minor effect on vascular compliance.[113] N_2O increases sympathetic activity and systolic blood pressure[114] and thus counters the vasodilatory and hypotensive effects of coadministered volatile agents.[115]

TABLE 38-5 Inhaled Anesthetic Effects on Central Nervous System Physiology

Effect	Nitrous Oxide	Desflurane	Sevoflurane	Isoflurane	Halothane
Cerebral blood flow	⇑	⇑	⇑	⇑	⇑
Cerebral perfusion pressure	⇓	⇓	⇓	⇓	⇓
Intracranial pressure	⇑	⇔/⇑	⇔/⇑	⇔/⇑	⇔/⇑
Metabolic demands	⇑	⇓	⇓	⇓	⇓
CO_2 reactivity	⇔	⇔	⇔	⇔	⇔

TABLE 38-6 Effects of Inhaled Anesthetics on Cardiovascular Physiology

Effect	Nitrous Oxide	Desflurane	Sevoflurane	Isoflurane	Halothane
MAP	⇔/⇑	⇓	⇓	⇓	⇓
SVR	⇔/⇑	⇓	⇔	⇓	⇔
Heart rate	⇔/⇑	⇑	⇑	⇑	⇔
Myocardial function	⇓	⇓	⇓	⇓	⇓
Epinephrine-induced arrhythmia	⇑	⇔	⇔	⇔	⇑

MAP, mean arterial pressure; SVR, systemic vascular resistance.

Heart Rate Volatile anesthetics increase heart rate, both by a baroreceptor reflex in response to decreased arterial pressure and by a direct vagolytic effect on the heart. In dogs, desflurane increases heart rate the most followed by sevoflurane, isoflurane, and halothane.[116] Rapid increases in the alveolar concentration of desflurane are associated with both an increased heart rate and blood pressure,[117,118] which is attributed to stimulation of sympathetic activity.[113] The minimal effect of halothane on heart rate is associated with its inhibition of the baroreceptor reflex.[119] N_2O is associated with only modest transient increases in heart rate,[120] which reflect its sympathetic effects and preservation of MAP.

Myocardial Contractility Volatile anesthetics cause myocardial depression, partly by inhibiting calcium ion influx in the myocardium.[121] Halothane causes a marked dose-dependent inhibition of myocardial contractility and reduces cardiac output.[122,123] Isoflurane, sevoflurane, and desflurane have lesser effects on myocardial contractility. In dogs, all of these anesthetics depress myocardial contractility, delay cardiac chamber relaxation, reduce chamber stiffness, and impair left atrial–left ventricular coupling.[124,125] N_2O administration also decreases intracellular calcium levels and depresses myocardial contractility.[126,127] Thus, although N_2O minimally affects blood pressure and heart rate, it has negative inotropic effects similar to those of potent volatile agents.

Cardiac Rhythm and Conduction Volatile anesthetics affect the function of cardiac ion channels, increasing the risk of arrhythmias.[128] Whereas halothane sensitizes the heart to the arrhythmogenic effects of epinephrine,[129] isoflurane, desflurane, and sevoflurane do not.[130,131] Halothane, isoflurane, desflurane, and sevoflurane all prolong the QT interval.[132,133] In dental outpatients, halothane produced more ventricular arrhythmias than isoflurane.[134,135] In pediatric dental outpatients receiving halothane anesthesia, 48% had ventricular dysrhythmias compared with 8% to 16% of those who received sevoflurane.[136] Furthermore, sevoflurane-induced arrhythmias were primarily single supraventricular ectopic beats, but ventricular tachycardia was observed in 12% of patients receiving halothane. N_2O may induce atrioventricular junctional rhythms[137] and can lower the threshold for epinephrine-induced arrhythmias in conjunction with halothane.[138]

Coronary Artery Perfusion Isoflurane is a coronary vasodilator and can thus potentially induce "coronary steal," a diversion of blood flow away from fixed stenotic lesions.[139] The clinical significance of this phenomenon appears to be mostly theoretical. Isoflurane has been observed to be safe in patients with coronary artery disease as long as adequate perfusion pressure is maintained. Isoflurane also provides beneficial effects via ischemic preconditioning.[140] Desflurane and sevoflurane do not cause coronary steal.[141,142]

RESPIRATORY SYSTEM

Ventilation Volatile anesthetics depress respiration through both central medullary and peripheral muscular effects. In general, inhaled anesthetics decrease tidal volume and increase respiratory rate. Halothane, isoflurane, desflurane, and sevoflurane dose dependently reduce tidal volume. The concomitant increase in respiratory rate is more pronounced with halothane, desflurane, and sevoflurane than with isoflurane.[141,143-145] Desflurane maintains minute ventilation with compensatory tachypnea up to alveolar concentrations of $1.6 \times$ MAC. Nonetheless, alveolar ventilation is reduced by all volatile anesthetics, resulting in an increased $Paco_2$. N_2O also causes tachypnea and decreased tidal volume but alone causes minimal changes in $Paco_2$. Ventilatory depression is additive when N_2O is administered in combination with other inhalational agents.[146]

Factors that contribute to hypoxia and hypercarbia during inhalational anesthesia include hypoventilation, atelectasis, airway closure, decreased functional residual capacity, and ventilation/perfusion (V/Q) mismatch.[147] Volatile anesthetics blunt hypoxic and hypercarbic respiratory drive, increasing the risk of severe hypoxia and hypercarbia in spontaneously breathing patients.[148-150] Depression of hypoxic and hypercarbic ventilatory drives occurs even at subanesthetic concentrations. N_2O blunts the respiratory drive to hypoxia and hypoventilation, but its clinical effects are minimal because of its low potency.[151] Rapid elimination of N_2O from blood after discontinuation dilutes alveolar gases, and if supplemental oxygen is not supplied, it can lead to *diffusion hypoxia.*[152,153]

Hypoxic Pulmonary Vasoconstriction Hypoxic pulmonary vasoconstriction (HPV) is a pulmonary vascular mechanism that diverts blood flow away from poorly ventilated areas of the lung, minimizing V/Q mismatch. The mechanisms underlying HPV are not yet fully understood, but cyclooxygenase, calcium channels, and potassium channels appear to be involved.[154] N_2O has been shown in vivo to

TABLE 38-7 Inhaled Anesthetic Effects on Vascular Resistance and Compliance: Comparison With Sodium Nitroprusside

Effect	Desflurane	Sevoflurane	Isoflurane	Halothane	Sodium Nitroprusside
Total arterial resistance	⇓	⇔	⇓	⇔	⇓
Total arterial compliance	⇔	⇑	⇑	⇑	⇑

Modified from Lowe D, Hettrick DA, Pagel PS, Warltier DC. Influence of volatile anesthetics on left ventricular afterload in vivo. Differences between desflurane and sevoflurane. *Anesthesiology.* 1996;85:112-120.

TABLE 38-8 Effects of Inhaled Anesthetics on Respiratory Physiology

Effect	Nitrous Oxide	Desflurane	Sevoflurane	Isoflurane	Halothane
Tidal volume	⇓	⇓	⇓	⇓	⇓
Respiratory rate	⇑	⇑	⇑	⇑	⇑
Hypoxic or hypercarbic responses	⇓	⇓	⇓	⇓	⇓
HPV (in vitro)	⇓	⇓	⇓	⇓	⇓
Airway resistance	⇔	⇑	⇓	⇓	⇓

HPV, hypoxic pulmonary vasoconstriction.

inhibit HPV.[155] In isolated lung models, halothane, isoflurane, sevoflurane, desflurane, and N_2O all inhibit HPV dose dependently.[156-158] In many animal studies, however, clinical concentrations of halothane, isoflurane, sevoflurane, and desflurane have not been shown to inhibit HPV.[159-162] In a few studies of chronically instrumented dogs, isoflurane was found to attenuate HPV.[163] The conflicting data regarding isoflurane effects on HPV may be attributable to different flow conditions in the pulmonary vasculature during different experiments.

Bronchial Tone Most volatile anesthetics, including halothane, enflurane, isoflurane and sevoflurane, are bronchodilators that decrease respiratory resistance and increase dynamic compliance (**Table 38-8**).[164] At equi-MAC concentrations, respiratory resistance is reduced by sevoflurane > halothane > isoflurane.[165] In contrast to the other volatile anesthetics, desflurane is associated with either no bronchodilatory effects or bronchoconstrictor effects at higher concentrations.[166] Inhalational induction with desflurane is associated with coughing and an increased risk of laryngospasm, which is likely caused by its pungency. Sevoflurane causes the least amount of subjective airway irritation and is well tolerated during inhalational induction.[167] N_2O has no effect on respiratory resistance.[165]

HEPATIC AND RENAL SYSTEMS

Liver Volatile anesthetics reduce overall hepatic perfusion by altering portal venous or hepatic arterial inflows. Most agents decrease portal venous flow. Isoflurane has the least overall effect on hepatic perfusion because of compensatory increases in hepatic artery flow.[168] In contrast, halothane causes hepatic artery vasoconstriction and decreases overall hepatic blood flow,[169] hepatic oxygen delivery, and hepatic vein blood oxygen saturation.[170] N_2O causes minimal circulatory effects on the liver.

Transient modest increases in liver enzymes are common after exposure to volatile anesthetics (halothane, desflurane, sevoflurane, and isoflurane). This effect is independent of surgical intervention and is almost always clinically insignificant.[171,172] The increase in liver enzymes after halothane may be caused by anaerobic reductive metabolism that generates free radicals.[173] More severe hepatic injury (halothane hepatitis) is described under Breakdown of Inhaled Anesthetics and Toxicity of By-products.

Kidney Volatile anesthetic agents cause dose-dependent decreases in renal blood flow, glomerular filtration rate, and urine output, which can be minimized with preoperative hydration.[174-176] Autoregulation of renal blood flow is preserved during halothane anesthesia.[175] Decreases in renal blood flow during inhalational anesthesia reflect a reduction in effective circulating volume secondary to increased vascular capacitance. Anesthetics do not directly stimulate antidiuretic hormone (ADH) release, but diminished urine production is associated with an increase in ADH because of surgical stress.[177] N_2O causes minimal effects on renal blood flow and function. Nephrotoxicity can be associated with breakdown of volatile anesthetics (see Breakdown of Inhaled Anesthetics and Toxicity of By-products).

OTHER SYSTEMIC AND ADVERSE EFFECTS

Muscular System Volatile anesthetics potentiate neuromuscular blockade via direct effects on the neuromuscular junction.[178] The muscle relaxant effect of volatile agents is stronger than that of IV anesthetics; N_2O has no relaxant action. In isolated diaphragmatic muscle, enflurane and sevoflurane enhance fatigability at high concentrations.[179,180] This may be mediated in part by cyclic adenosine monophosphate because administration of the phosphodiesterase inhibitor olprinone attenuates the effects of volatile anesthetics.

Malignant Hypothermia Malignant hypothermia (MH) is a life-threatening clinical myopathy triggered by all potent volatile anesthetics and succinylcholine. It is a genetic disorder associated with autosomal dominant transmission of genes encoding mutant forms of the skeletal muscle calcium release channel (the ryanodine receptor protein or RyR1).[181] Upon exposure to the triggering drugs, patients with MH develop an exaggerated increase in intracellular calcium, resulting in sustained skeletal muscular contracture, which is not inhibited by neuromuscular blocking agents. Sustained contracture produces a hypermetabolic state, leading to increased CO_2 production and eventually hyperthermia. This condition is fatal unless treated aggressively and rapidly with IV dantrolene.

Methionine Synthase Inhibition by Nitrous Oxide Nitrous oxide irreversibly oxidizes the cobalt atom of vitamin B_{12}, which inhibits the cobalamin-dependent enzyme methionine synthase. This pathway is essential for homocysteine breakdown, nerve myelination, methyl substitutions of neurotransmitters, and DNA synthesis. Most patients are unaffected by temporary inactivation of vitamin B_{12} after N_2O administration. Nonetheless, this reaction can be clinically significant in patients with poor nutrition, preexisting vitamin B_{12} deficiency, or other metabolic diseases that converge on the same metabolic pathways. N_2O exposure may lead to "anesthesia paresthetica," which is characterized by paresthesias, ataxias, and poor manual dexterity.[182] Widespread neuronal damage, status epilepticus, and death were reported in 1 infant with a preexisting deficiency of 5,10-methylenetetrahydrofolate reductase, an enzyme in the methionine synthetic pathway, after exposure to N_2O.[183]

Endocrine Function Halothane and enflurane impair glucose tolerance in animal models by reducing both insulin secretion and receptor sensitivity. Isoflurane has been shown to increase endogenous glucose production and decrease glucose utilization.[93,184] The selection of anesthetic may also play a role in modulating the stress responses to surgery. In a study of 20 women requiring laparoscopic surgery for ovarian cystectomy, sevoflurane was associated with less increase in cortisol and adrenocorticotropic hormone levels than isoflurane.[185]

Immune Function Potent inhalational anesthetics can alter immune cell functions in various ways, which in turn may affect recovery from surgery and tumor viability. Halothane depresses the neutrophil oxidative response to inflammatory mediators of infection; this effect is smaller with desflurane, sevoflurane, and isoflurane.[186] Sevoflurane impairs transcription factors in human lymphocytes, which may reduce the inflammatory response.[187] Volatile anesthetics can also induce apoptosis in human T cells in vitro[188] and may affect cytokine function.[189] However, clinical studies suggest that the impact of anesthesia on immune function is transient and of little clinical significance.[190]

Ischemic Preconditioning Volatile anesthetics induce cellular responses that protect against ischemia and biochemical stress mediators. For example, sevoflurane decreases markers of myocardial and renal damage after coronary artery bypass grafting.[191] Animal models of renal ischemic injury demonstrate differential preconditioning, with desflurane demonstrating less protective effects against tubular necrosis than sevoflurane, isoflurane, or halothane.[192] Volatile anesthetics can protect against neural ischemia in animal models through pathways involving both nitric oxide metabolism[193] and potassium channels.[194]

Genotoxicity and Teratogenicity Halogenated hydrocarbons and ethers can cause DNA damage. Halothane and isoflurane produce genotoxicity in proliferating blood lymphocytes in vitro; sevoflurane does not appear to be cytotoxic in an animal model.[195] The potential for anesthetic-induced teratogenicity has been studied. Prolonged N_2O exposure is teratogenic in a number of embryonic animal models.[196] N_2O inhibition of vitamin B_{12}–dependent DNA synthesis is the likely cause. Because of potential genetic damage after chronic exposure to inhaled anesthetics, it is currently recommended that operating room air contain less than 25 parts per million (ppm) of N_2O and less than 2 ppm of halogenated anesthetics. Under these conditions, there is little evidence of significant risk from workplace exposure to inhaled anesthetics.[197] Furthermore, approximately 75 000 pregnant women undergo nonobstetric surgery each year. Although there was once controversy over the effects of surgery and anesthesia in this population, volatile anesthesia appears to be safe for both the woman and the fetus.[198]

BREAKDOWN OF INHALED ANESTHETICS AND TOXICITY OF BY-PRODUCTS

Inhaled anesthetics represent a class of drugs that are eliminated largely via nonmetabolic pathways—for the most part, they leave the body as they entered, unaltered and via ventilatory gas exchange. Undesirable effects directly associated with anesthetics are summarized above, but others are caused indirectly by chemical decomposition of inhaled anesthetics into toxic by-products. The breakdown of volatile anesthetics into potentially harmful chemicals can occur in the presence of CO_2 adsorbents or via enzymatic biotransformation in the body. In general, greater breakdown of inhaled anesthetics leads to greater toxicity.

NONMETABOLIC DECOMPOSITION OF INHALED ANESTHETICS

Although inhaled anesthetics are chemically stable under normal storage conditions (including within vaporizers), decomposition can occur under certain environmental conditions.

Sevoflurane Breakdown and Compound A When sevoflurane contacts CO_2 adsorbents containing a strong base (Baralyme and Sodalime), chemical decomposition occurs, releasing volatile breakdown products.[199] The major degradation product, compound A (fluoromethyl-2-2-difluoro-1-[trifluoromethyl] vinyl ether), was shown to cause renal injury and death in rats when inhaled at high levels.[200] Renal injury is both dose and time dependent with a threshold for detectable injury in laboratory animals of 150 to 300 ppm hours. Nonetheless, in human volunteer and clinical studies, blood urea nitrogen (BUN) and creatinine levels remain unchanged after exposures that sometimes exceed 300 ppm hours. It is thought that humans sustain less renal injury than rats after compound A exposure because of lower levels of renal cysteine conjugated β-lyase enzyme activity.[201,202] Special laboratory markers for subtle renal tubular damage in humans are elevated after 300 ppm hours of compound A exposure, and these normalize within a few days.[203] In clinical settings, the inhaled concentration of compound A is proportional to the sevoflurane concentration and inversely related to fresh-gas flows. Whereas low gas flows allow compound A to accumulate in the breathing circuit, high gas flows wash out compound A with waste gases. At FGFs of 2 L/min or higher, concentrations of compound A are low enough that the conservative exposure threshold of 150 ppm hours is unlikely to be reached. Sevoflurane package labeling guidelines should be heeded. Clinical studies using standard renal function tests demonstrate that sevoflurane is no more harmful than isoflurane when administered with low FGFs to patients with preexisting renal disease.[204]

Volatile Anesthetic Breakdown and Desiccated Carbon Dioxide Adsorbents All of the halogenated volatile anesthetics degrade in the presence of dry alkaline CO_2 adsorbents in rebreathing circuits. (Only sevoflurane breaks down in the presence of moist adsorbent.) Decomposition in the presence of dry CO_2 adsorbents releases carbon monoxide (CO), formaldehyde, methanol, and heat. These exothermic reactions have resulted in the ignition of breathing circuit components[205] and acute respiratory distress syndrome in patients[206] and can lead to significant carboxyhemoglobin levels in patients.[207] These problems are avoidable and only arise when the CO_2 adsorbent is desiccated (eg if flushed overnight with high-flow oxygen) and depend on the type and quantity of strong base in the adsorbent (in descending order of reactivity these are KOH > NaOH >> $Ba[OH]_2$). Sevoflurane releases more heat than desflurane or isoflurane,[208] and carbon monoxide production is highest with desflurane > enflurane > isoflurane > sevoflurane > halothane.[209,210]

Photochemical Breakdown of Anesthetic Waste Gases Waste gases scavenged from anesthesia machines enter the atmosphere, where they are exposed to solar radiation and other gases.[211,212] Ultraviolet light catalyzes the reaction between N_2O and O_2, producing the free radical nitric oxide, which in turn destroys atmospheric ozone.[213] Waste N_2O from medical uses is about 3% of the total emissions (the majority results from agriculture and combustion of fossil fuels). Halogenated volatile anesthetics act as greenhouse gases.[214] Halogenated anesthetics also break down when exposed to ultraviolet light to form halogen free radicals, which deplete atmospheric ozone. Volatile anesthetic waste gases represent only a small portion of total atmospheric chlorofluorocarbons.

BIOTRANSFORMATION OF INHALED ANESTHETICS

Hepatic Drug Metabolism In the liver, enzymes can transform volatile anesthetics by oxidation, reduction, and conjugation. These reactions convert hydrophobic substrates into more hydrophilic metabolites that are excreted via the kidneys. Of these, the most important pathways for volatile anesthetics are oxidative, and the enzymes responsible are various members of the large cytochrome P450 (CYP) family. Neonates lack some enzymes that are present in older humans, and diverse other factors, such as genetic variation, can alter individual metabolic activities. Intrinsic liver disease or hepatic congestion caused by heart failure may result in diminished enzymatic capacity, and intrahepatic blood flow shunting may reduce the efficiency of drug metabolism. CYP enzyme activities may also be inhibited by drugs such as cimetidine and amiodarone or enhanced by prolonged exposure to "inducers" such as phenobarbital, phenytoin, and a wide range of other compounds, including inhaled anesthetics.

Hepatitis Associated With Volatile Anesthetics Among the currently available agents, halothane undergoes the most hepatic metabolism (20%-25%) and is associated most frequently with significant toxicity. Usually, less than 1% of halothane metabolism is reductive. Halothane's oxidative metabolism by CYP enzymes generates trifluoroacetic acid, bromide, and an intermediate metabolite, trifluoroacetic chloride, which can covalently modify proteins. Protein acetylation by these compounds primarily occurs within the liver, and modified proteins can act as neoantigens that stimulate the immune system to attack hepatocytes, resulting in fulminant hepatic necrosis. "Halothane hepatitis" occurs in 1 in 6000 to 1 in 35 000 adults after halothane anesthesia and is fatal in 50% to 75% of these cases.[215] Genetic factors are likely involved, and females are affected about twice as frequently as males. Hepatic necrosis has been reported in many cases after multiple exposures to halothane, consistent with an amplified secondary immune response. Halothane hepatitis has also been reported in pediatric patients, but its incidence in children is 10 to 20 times lower than in adults.

Other inhaled anesthetics are metabolized by CYP enzymes to reactive acetyl intermediates that can also modify hepatic proteins. Rare cases of fulminant hepatic injury after administration of enflurane, isoflurane, and desflurane have been reported and the incidence for each anesthetic is related to the degree of their metabolism (2.5%, 0.2%, and 0.02%, respectively).[216]

Fluoride Nephrotoxicity Metabolism of some inhaled anesthetics releases inorganic fluoride ions (F^-), which can cause polyuric renal failure and increased mortality. Clinical findings include hypernatremia, hyperosmolarity, and increased BUN and creatinine. This problem is primarily associated with methoxyflurane, a very blood- and tissue-soluble anesthetic that is no longer in use. Metabolic release of fluoride is linked to methoxyflurane nephrotoxicity in a dose-related manner, and its causal relationship is shown in animal experiments. Renal injury after methoxyflurane is rare at fluoride blood levels below 50 μM; moderate injury is seen at 50 to 80 μM and severe injury at higher levels. In rats, clinical and pathologic changes similar to those in human fluoride nephrotoxicity can be produced by IV administration of fluoride at similar levels.

Other fluorinated anesthetics, particularly enflurane and sevoflurane, release detectable amounts of fluoride when metabolized in the liver. Nephrotoxicity, however, is very rarely associated with these drugs. Serum fluoride levels during and after enflurane anesthesia are usually below 50 μM, but those during and after sevoflurane anesthesia often peak above 50 μM. However, sevoflurane is much less soluble in blood and tissue than methoxyflurane. Sevoflurane is eliminated rapidly at the end of anesthesia, which halts fluoride production. In contrast, methoxyflurane is retained in tissues, and fluoride concentrations continue to increase after delivery is halted, reaching peak levels 2 to 3 days after anesthesia (for a review, see Anders[217]). Moreover, methoxyflurane is decomposed to fluoride within the kidneys more than sevoflurane, so intrarenal fluoride levels are higher than those detected in blood samples.[218]

INERT GASES: FUTURE ANESTHETICS?

Although the safety of inhaled anesthetics has improved greatly since the 19th century, all of the currently used agents are far from ideal because of their toxic effects on various physiologic systems (**Table 38-9**). The inert gas xenon was shown to produce anesthesia in 1951, and further study has revealed a pharmacokinetic and pharmacodynamic profile that approaches the ideal for an inhalational anesthetic.[219,220] Xenon is an odorless, tasteless, nonflammable, and nonexplosive gas. Similar to other noble gases (helium, neon, argon, krypton, and radon), it

TABLE 38-9 Advantages and Disadvantages of Inhaled Anesthetics

Anesthetic	Advantages	Disadvantages
Nitrous oxide	• No odor, taste, or pungency • Rapid uptake and elimination • Analgesic effect • Minimal cardiovascular depression • Minimal biotransformation	• Airspace expansion • Increased nausea or vomiting • Inhibits methionine synthase • Environmental pollutant • Supports combustion
Halothane	• Inexpensive • Not pungent	• Myocardial depression • Arrhythmias • Halothane hepatitis risk • Very slow uptake and elimination
Enflurane	• Good muscle relaxation • Stable heart rate	• Pungent • Slow uptake and elimination • Epileptogenic
Isoflurane	• Good muscle relaxation • Maintains cardiac output • Low biotransformation • Inexpensive	• Pungent • Slow uptake and elimination
Desflurane	• Rapid uptake and elimination • Very low biotransformation	• Airway irritant • Sympathetic stimulant • Requires electric vaporizer • Breakdown to CO in circuit • Expensive
Sevoflurane	• Rapid uptake and elimination • Not pungent	• Breakdown to compound A in circuit • Potentially nephrotoxic • Expensive
Xenon	• No odor, taste, or pungency • Very rapid uptake and elimination • Analgesic effect • Minimal cardiovascular depression • No toxic metabolites • Environmentally safe • Inhibits combustion	• Limited worldwide supply • Expensive • Airspace expansion

is extremely chemically inert, undergoes no metabolic transformation, and has no direct negative environmental effects. Xenon does not cause airway irritation, and its blood–gas partition coefficient is 0.14, which makes inhalation induction significantly faster than with N_2O or desflurane. Xenon, similar to N_2O, produces minimal cardiovascular or respiratory depression. It produces no direct systemic organ toxicity, and there is evidence that xenon has neuroprotective effects,[221] including the attenuation of cognitive dysfunction after cardiopulmonary bypass in an animal model.[222] However, clinical studies have not demonstrated this benefit in patients.[223,224] Because MAC for xenon is about 0.7 atm for patients near age 40 years and $ED_{95} \approx 1.3 \times MAC \approx 0.9$ atm, its use as a sole anesthetic agent is likely limited to older patients who require lower concentrations. One of its few negative physiological effects is, similar to N_2O, airspace expansion. Xenon has analgesic effects, which are likely attributable to inhibition of *N*-methyl-D-aspartate (NMDA)–sensitive glutamate receptors. Unlike ketamine, an IV anesthetic that also acts on NMDA receptors, xenon is not associated with emergence delirium.

The main barrier to routine use of xenon is the high cost of its fractional distillation from air, where its concentration is about 1 part per 12 million. Xenon cannot be synthesized, so these factors are unlikely to change unless new sources are discovered. Energy expended in collecting xenon also creates secondary negative environmental impacts. Methods for conserving (closed circuit delivery) and recycling xenon may make its clinical use economically possible in the future.

KEY REFERENCES

- Anders MW. Formation and toxicity of anesthetic degradation products. *Annu Rev Pharmacol Toxicol.* 2005;45:147-176.
- Avidan MS, Zhang L, Burnside BA, et al. Anesthesia awareness and the bispectral index. *N Engl J Med.* 2008;358:1097-1108.
- Baum JA. *Low Flow Anaesthesia: The Theory and Practice of Low Flow, Minimal Flow and Closed System Anaesthesia.* 2nd ed. Boston, MA: Butterworth-Heinemann; 2001.
- Campagna JA, Miller KW, Forman SA. Mechanisms of actions of inhaled anesthetics. *N Engl J Med.* 2003;348:2110-2124.
- Eger EI. Uptake of inhaled anesthetics: the alveolar to inspired anesthetic difference. In: Eger EI, ed. *Anesthetic Uptake and Action.* Baltimore, MD: Williams & Wilkins; 1974:77-96.
- Eger EI 2nd. Age, minimum alveolar anesthetic concentration, and minimum alveolar anesthetic concentration-awake. *Anesth Analg.* 2001;93:947-953.
- Kenna JG, Jones RM. The organ toxicity of inhaled anesthetics. *Anesth Analg.* 1995;81(Suppl):S51-S66.
- Myles PS, Leslie K, McNeil J, et al. Bispectral index monitoring to prevent awareness during anaesthesia: the B-Aware randomised controlled trial. *Lancet.* 2004;363:1757-1763.
- Sebel PS, Bowdle TA, Ghoneim MM, et al. The incidence of awareness during anesthesia: a multicenter United States study. *Anesth Analg.* 2004;99:833-839; table of contents.
- Stoelting RK, Eger EI 2nd. An additional explanation for the second gas effect: a concentrating effect. *Anesthesiology.* 1969;30:273-277.

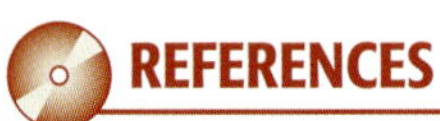

REFERENCES

Complete references available on DVD and online version at www.LongneckerAnesthesiology.com

CHAPTER 39

Anesthesia Delivery System

James B. Eisenkraft

KEY POINTS

1. A basic understanding of the anesthesia delivery system and its components is important to the provision of safe patient care.
2. The current voluntary consensus standard describing the features of a contemporary anesthesia workstation is the American Society for Testing and Materials (ASTM) F1850–00, published in 2000 and reapproved in 2005.
3. The ASTM F1850–00 standard calls for an integrated and prioritized alarm system, breathing pressure monitoring, and exhaled volume or ventilatory CO_2 monitoring.
4. Pin-index and DISS ensure that the correct medical gas enters the correct part of the anesthesia machine. The "fail-safe" valve (pressure sensor shut-off valve, O_2 failure protection device) prevents the flow of nitrous oxide (N_2O) or other gases if the O_2 supply pressure is not adequate, but it does not ensure O_2 flow. An O_2 analyzer in the patient circuit is essential to detect a hypoxic mixture. It should be automatically enabled and the low O_2 alarm set whenever the machine is capable of delivering an anesthetic gas mixture.
5. The O_2 and N_2O flow controls are interlinked so that a gas mixture containing 25% or greater of O_2 is created at the flowmeters when N_2O and O_2 are in use. Use of a third or fourth gas (eg, helium) may "defeat" this feature.
6. A variable bypass anesthesia vaporizer creates a saturated vapor concentration of the anesthetic and then dilutes it to clinically desirable concentrations. Contemporary vaporizers for halothane, isoflurane, enflurane, and sevoflurane are variable-bypass, concentration-calibrated, and temperature-compensated types.
7. Vaporizers are agent specific. Erroneous filling must be avoided; agent-specific filling devices should be used.
8. The anesthesia workstation should be checked each day before anesthetizing the first patient and whenever any change has been made to the system. A shortened checkout should precede each administration of anesthesia. The checkout procedure should follow the directions given in the machine's operation and maintenance manual. Because of the diversity of the newer workstations, in 2007, the American Society of Anesthesiologists published guidelines to act as a template for developing preanesthesia checkout procedures.
9. Use of free-standing vaporizers downstream from the common gas outlet can be hazardous and should be avoided. Such vaporizers are often used on pump oxygenators for cardiopulmonary bypass procedures.
10. Anesthesia ventilators are traditionally pneumatic and of "bag-in-a-bottle" or "double-circuit" design. In traditional ventilators, a standing bellows design, in which the bellows descend on inspiration and ascend on expiration, is preferred because it makes a leak in the breathing system more obvious (ie, the bellows do not refill). In Dräger workstations, an electronically driven piston in a cylinder replaces the traditional bellows.
11. In a traditional ventilators, the delivered tidal volume (VT) may differ from the VT setting because delivered VT is influenced also by the fresh gas flow, the inspiratory-to-expiratory ratio, the breathing circuit compliance, and the peak inspiratory pressure. Newer designs (eg, GE-Datex Anesthesia Delivery Unit [ADU], Aisys, Smart Vent, Dräger Apollo, Fabius GS, Narkomed 6400) use various approaches to ensure that VT is delivered as set on the ventilator controls.
12. Free-standing positive end-expiratory pressure (PEEP) valves may be hazardous if added to the circuit incorrectly. PEEP valves are safer when designed as an integral part of the circuit.

13. Waste anesthesia gases should be scavenged. The National Institute for Occupational Safety and Health recommends that exposure of operating room workers to halogenated agents should be kept below 2 ppm. N_2O levels should be controlled so that no worker is exposed at time-weighted average concentrations greater than 25 ppm. The latter guide should result in levels of approximately 0.5 ppm of the halogenated agents.
14. In the event of a severe machine or gas delivery system malfunction, an alternative means for ventilating the patient's lungs with O_2 (or room air) must be immediately available. Thus, a self-inflating bag whose function has been checked before use should be available in each anesthetizing location.
15. User error is the most common cause of adverse outcomes in relation to anesthesia gas delivery equipment. User education must be emphasized, and there must be thorough in-service training whenever there is a new user or new equipment is introduced.

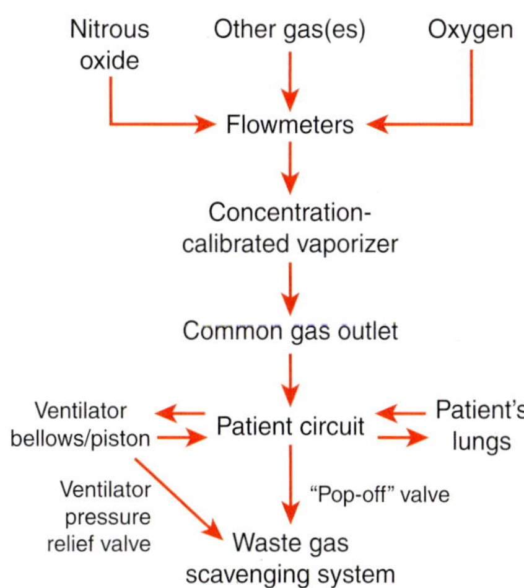

FIGURE 39-1. Schematic of a generic anesthesia gas delivery system.

The anesthesia delivery system comprises the anesthesia machine, anesthesia vaporizer(s), ventilator, breathing circuit, and waste gas scavenging system. It is the anesthesia caregiver's constant companion in the operating room or procedure room. Whether a patient is to receive general anesthesia, regional anesthesia, or monitored anesthesia care, the anesthesia delivery system must be properly checked and ready for immediate use. An understanding of the structure and function of the anesthesia delivery system is essential to the safe practice of anesthesia.

The anesthesia delivery system continues to evolve. The current voluntary consensus standard describing the features of a contemporary system is that published by the American Society for Testing and Materials (ASTM) and designated F1850–00. This document, published in March 2000 and reapproved in 2005, is titled *Standard Specification for Particular Requirements for Anesthesia Workstations and Their Components.*[1] The term *anesthesia workstation* is defined as a system for the administration of anesthesia to patients. It consists of the anesthesia gas supply device, anesthesia ventilator, monitoring devices, and protection device(s). This standard supersedes the F1161–88 anesthesia machine standard published in 1989 by ASTM.[2]

The above standards represent a consensus adopted voluntarily by the machine manufacturers. Certain accrediting and licensing bodies, however, may choose to adopt such standards in whole or in part and make them requirements for machines used in that locality. Readers are referred to the source documents for more details.

The recent evolution of the anesthesia workstation and advances in technology have led to many changes in design. Although all of the basic operations remain the same, the functions of many of the traditional "gas machine" components are now performed by more technologically advanced components. Thus, in many new models, the familiar rotameter tubes are replaced by virtual flowmeters displayed on a computer screen. The gas flow-control needle valves may be replaced by electronically controlled gas-mixing devices. Space does not permit a detailed description of each model of workstation; therefore, the basic components and functions of a traditional anesthesia workstation are described.

Figure 39-1 depicts the components of a contemporary basic anesthesia delivery system. These include the anesthesia machine itself, which receives the gases oxygen (O_2), nitrous oxide (N_2O), and perhaps a third and fourth gas (eg, air, heliox) delivered under pressure. A controlled gas mixture in terms of concentration of O_2 and other gas(es), as well as total gas flow rates, is created using the gas flow controls and delivered to a concentration-calibrated vaporizer, to which a measured amount of a potent inhaled anesthetic agent may be added. The resulting fresh gas mixture of known composition and metered production rate leaves the anesthesia machine at the common gas outlet and flows continuously to the patient breathing circuit. The breathing circuit represents a mini environment that allows respiratory exchange and control of anesthetic (eg, sevoflurane) and respiratory (ie, Po_2 and Pco_2) gas tensions in the patient's alveoli, blood, and tissues (eg, brain). An anesthesia ventilator bellows (or in recent Dräger models, a piston) may be connected to the breathing circuit by means of which the patient's lungs can be mechanically ventilated. Excess gases are vented from the breathing circuit via either the adjustable pressure-limiting (APL or "pop-off") valve or the ventilator pressure relief valve. The vented gases enter the waste gas scavenging system and are removed from the operating room, usually through the hospital suction.

Presently, in the United States, the 2 largest manufacturers of anesthesia delivery systems (machines, ventilators, vaporizers, scavenging systems) are Dräger Medical (Telford, PA) and GE-Datex (Madison, WI). Other manufacturers include Maquet (formerly Datascope), Blease, and Penlon. This chapter reviews the features of a basic anesthesia gas delivery system, referring to the model from a specific manufacturer when appropriate. The approach used is to trace the flow of gases from their pressurized storage sources and vapors through the various components of the delivery system and to understand the function of each component. In this way, readers can more readily appreciate the rationale for the various checkout procedures and have a framework from which to diagnose problems that may arise during use of the equipment. A review of problems with the delivery system is presented elsewhere.[3] The most comprehensive source of reference for any individual model of workstation is the workstation manufacturer's operator's and maintenance manuals, and readers are strongly encouraged to review the manual(s) relevant to the equipment. Additionally, an alternative means for delivering O_2 or room air to the patient should be kept immediately available in the event of a severe workstation malfunction. Thus, a self-inflating (eg, Ambu) resuscitation bag, previously tested for correct function and, ideally, a full tank of O_2 should be immediately available in each anesthetizing location.

BASIC ANESTHESIA MACHINE

Figure 39-2 depicts the flow arrangements of a basic 2-gas anesthesia machine. The machine receives each of the 2 basic gases, O_2 and N_2O, from 2 supply sources: a tank or cylinder source and a pipeline source.

OXYGEN

Oxygen has a molecular weight of 32 and a boiling point of −183°C at a pressure of 760 mm Hg (14.7 pounds per square inch absolute pressure [psia]). (Absolute pressure is designated in psia, and gauge pressure is designated in psig [pounds per square inch gauge pressure]. Gauges

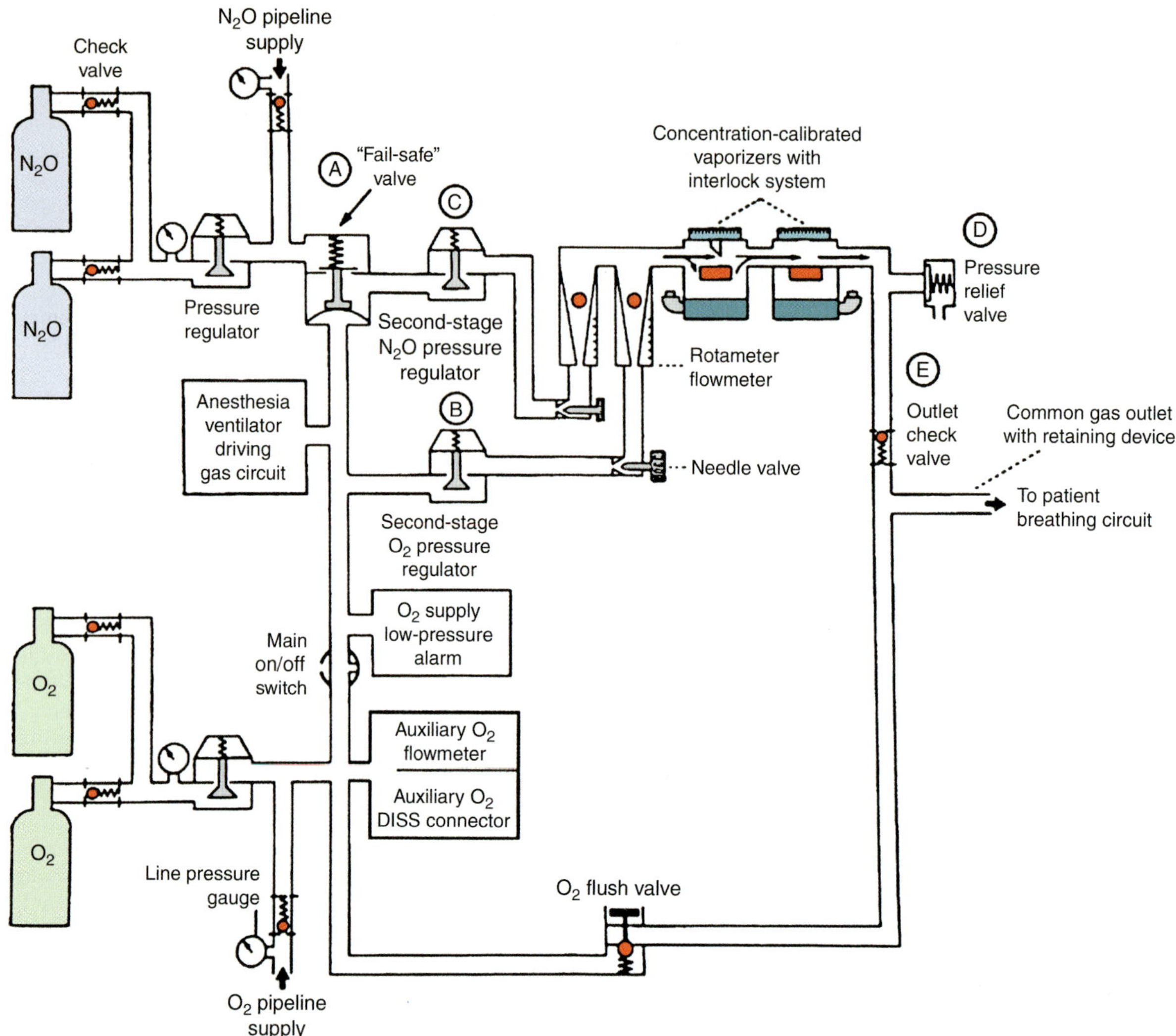

FIGURE 39-2. Schematic of flow arrangements of contemporary anesthesia machine. The "fail-safe" valve *A* in GE-Datex-Ohmeda machines is termed a *pressure sensor shutoff valve*. In Dräger machines, it is the *oxygen-failure protection device*. The second-stage O_2 pressure regulator *B* is used in GE-Datex-Ohmeda (but not Dräger Narkomed) machines. The second-stage nitrous oxide (N_2O) pressure regulator *C* is used in GE-Datex-Ohmeda Modulus and Excel machines with the Link-25 Proportion Limiting Control System; this is not used in Dräger Narkomed machines. The pressure relief valve *D* is used in GE-Datex-Ohmeda Modulus machines; it is not used in Dräger machines. The outlet check valve *E* is used in GE-Datex-Ohmeda machines except the Modulus II Plus and Modulus CD models; it is not used in Dräger machines. Datex-Ohmeda Excel machines have a pressure-relief valve located downstream from the outlet check valve, between this valve and the machine common gas outlet. DISS, diameter-index safety system.

record pressure above or below existing atmospheric pressure. Thus, 1 atmosphere [atm] pressure = 760 mm Hg = 14.7 psia = 0 psig.) Boiling point (the temperature at which O_2 changes from the liquid to the gas phase) is related to ambient pressure such that as pressure increases, so does the boiling point of O_2. However, a certain critical temperature is reached above which, no matter how much pressure is applied, the liquid O_2 boils to a gas. The critical temperature for O_2 is −118°C, and the critical pressure that must be applied at this temperature to keep O_2 liquid is 737 psia. Because room temperature is normally around 20°C and thus well above the critical temperature, O_2 can exist only as a gas at room temperature. This has certain implications for understanding the contents of an O_2 tank.

Oxygen tanks serve as the primary source of O_2 if there is no pipeline in the anesthetizing location and as a backup supply in case of pipeline failure. Machines are usually equipped with 1 or 2 E cylinders that hang on specific O_2 hanger yokes. The medical gas pin-index safety system ensures that the correct medical gas tank is hung in the correct yoke. The system consists of 2 pins that are fixed in the yoke and that fit into 2 corresponding holes in the tank valve (see Fig. 39-5E). The 2 pins are in a unique configuration for O_2 and should never be removed from the hanger yoke. Specific pin configurations exist for each of the medical gases supplied in small cylinders to prevent erroneous misconnections of gas supplies. A tank should never be force fitted to a hanger yoke.

Oxygen tanks are normally filled to a pressure of approximately 1900 psig (add 14.7 to convert to psia) at room temperature. After they are filled, they contain a fixed number of gas molecules (fixed mass of gas) that obey Boyle's law (ie, Pressure × Volume = Constant), provided that temperature does not change. A full E cylinder of O_2 at a pressure of 1900 psig will evolve 660 L of gaseous O_2 at 1 atm pressure (14.7 psia, or 760 mm Hg). The internal volume (V1) of an E cylinder is therefore approximately 5 L because, by Boyle's law, P1 × V1 = P2 × V2. Thus, 1900 × V1 = 14.7 × 660. If the O_2 tank pressure is 1000 psig, the tank is 1000/1900, or 52% full and will generate only 660 × 52%, or 340 L of gaseous O_2 at atmospheric pressure. If such a tank were being used at an O_2 flow rate of 6 L/min, it would empty in just under 1 hour (340/6 = 57 min).

If one assumes that the full E cylinder of oxygen has a pressure of 2000 psig, then the time to becoming empty can be approximated as follows:

Time to empty (in hours) = Tank pressure (psig)/(200 × Flow rate L/min)

The understanding and application of these principles are vital to safe practice whenever O_2 cylinders are in use to supply the machine or during patient transport. If the anesthesia machine is equipped with 2 E cylinders of O_2, only 1 should be open and in use at any one time so that both tanks are not emptied simultaneously.

There is a check valve in the hanger yoke for each O_2 (and other medical gas) cylinder to prevent leakage of gas out through the hanger yoke if no cylinder is hanging in place and the machine is being supplied by the pipeline or from a second O_2 tank (Fig. 39-2). If 2 O_2 tanks are hanging, the check valve in the yoke prevents transfilling of gas from one tank to the other. However, these check valves may leak, so if a hanger yoke does not have a tank hanging in it, a yoke plug should be inserted to prevent leakage of gas in the event of an incompetent check valve. These solid plastic block yoke plugs are usually attached to the back of the machine by a chain to prevent their loss. In the Dräger Apollo workstation, the tank pressures are measured using electronic pressure transducers, and the values are displayed on a screen.[4]

In many medical facilities, the O_2 pipeline is supplied from a bulk liquid O_2 source. This may be more economical for the institution, depending on rate and volume of O_2 used. Liquid O_2 is stored at temperatures of around −160°C under pressure in a storage vessel that resembles a large vacuum (Dewar) flask. When gaseous O_2 is drawn from the top of the storage vessel, liquid O_2 boils to replace it. The boiling (change of phase) helps to keep the remaining liquid O_2 cold. Because the O_2 gas evolved is very cold, it is first passed through a heating coil and then through a pressure regulator that maintains the hospital pipeline pressure at 50 to 55 psig. Alarms and safety devices, including relief valves and shut-off valves, ensure the safe functioning of the bulk O_2 storage and pipeline systems. Pipeline systems, although usually reliable, may fail. One report describes failure between the bulk liquid oxygen storage vessel and the pipeline, which resulted in the release of 8000 gal of liquid O_2 into the atmosphere.[5] Consequently, ensuring that a backup (tank) supply is available is an important part of the preuse checkout. Furthermore, an appropriate response to such a failure is an important component of an anesthesiologist's education.[6,7]

Pipeline O_2 is available in the operating rooms usually via gas-specific and manufacturer-specific "quick connectors" or via oxygen-specific diameter-indexed safety system outlets. The operating room wall pipeline "quick connectors" are both noninterchangeable among medical gases (so that an O_2 hose quick connector cannot be connected to a N_2O wall outlet) and are also manufacturer specific (eg, Schraeder, Ohmeda, Chemetron, Puritan-Bennett) (**Fig. 39-3**). At the machine end of the hose that conducts O_2 from the wall outlet to the machine is a connector that is gas specific by a national standard, the diameter-index safety system (DISS). The DISS specifies that at the machine end the medical gas connectors be of different diameters. The diameter- and pin-index safety systems are designed to ensure that the correct medical gas enters the correct part of the anesthesia machine.[8]

Although they are not as convenient as quick connect fittings, many institutions are now using DISS gas connection fittings at the wall outlets (**Fig. 39-4**).

As an alternative to the traditional backup E cylinders, lightweight E cylinders are available that are pressurized to 3000 psig and can therefore deliver about 1000 L of gaseous oxygen. These cylinders (**Fig. 39-5A**) have a permanently mounted Linde Integrated Valve (Life Gas, Atlanta, GA) that has a 50 psig DISS connector to which the machine's oxygen hose can be connected. The valve is also calibrated to deliver oxygen at low flows (0.25-25 L/min) for transporting a patient who requires supplemental oxygen.

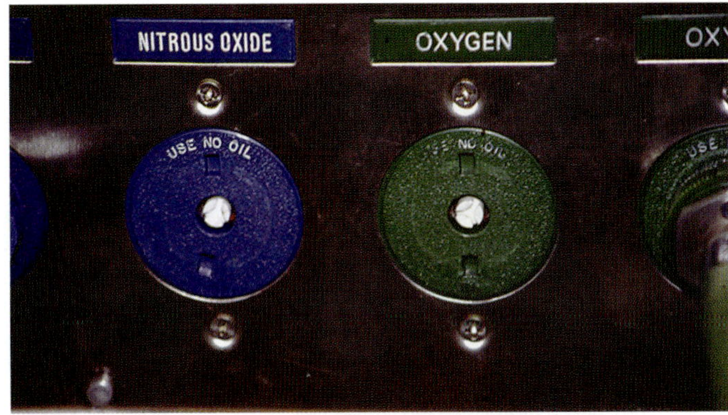

FIGURE 39-3. Gas-specific wall outlets for Ohmeda quick connect gas fittings. Quick connect systems are manufacturer and gas specific.

For simplicity, the anesthesia machine is described as consisting of 2 basic systems, a high-pressure system for each gas and a common low-pressure system for the gas mixture. Those parts upstream of the gas flow-control valves contain gas at relatively high pressures and are considered to be the high-pressure system. Those parts downstream of the flow-control valves (Fig. 39-2) contain gas at low pressure (measured in cm H_2O rather than psig) and constitute the low-pressure system. The low-pressure system extends from the flow-control valves to the machine common gas outlet. Although O_2 from the pipeline supply enters the machine O_2 high-pressure system at a pressure of approximately 50 psig, O_2 from a full tank enters the yoke at pressures of approximately 1900 psig. The O_2 tank source is therefore regulated (O_2 passes through a regulator valve) and enters the machine high-pressure system at a nominal pressure of 45 psig (Fig. 39-2).

A pressure regulator is a device that reduces a variable high input pressure (in this case, ~1900 psig from the O_2 tank) to a constant low-output pressure (in this case, 45 psig) for the gas whose pressure

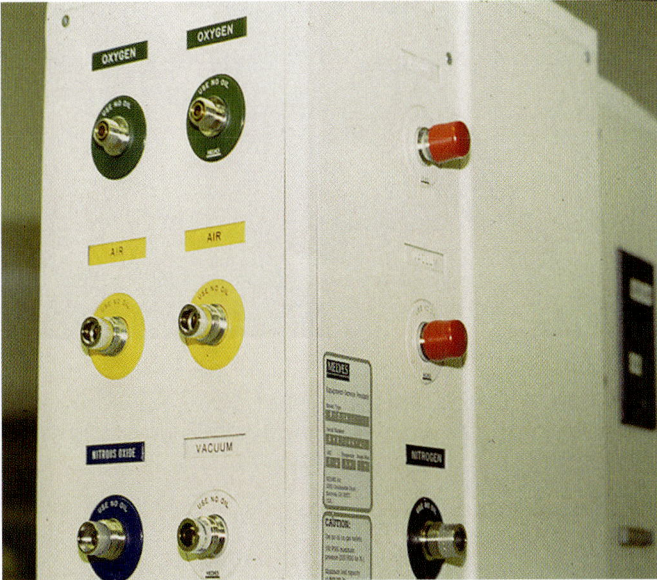

FIGURE 39-4. Diameter-index safety system wall outlets. These are not Quick-Connect fittings.

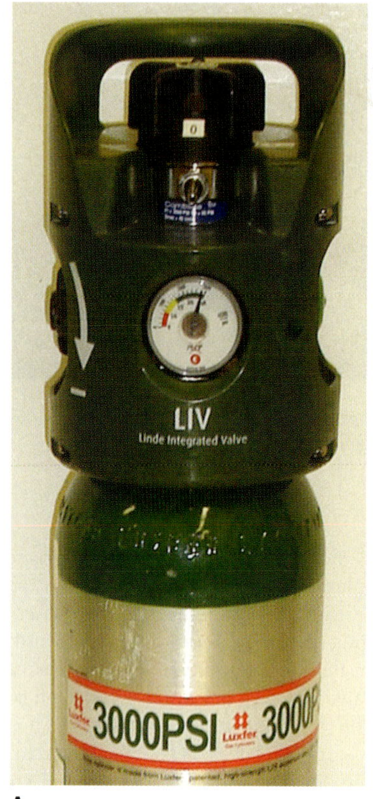

A

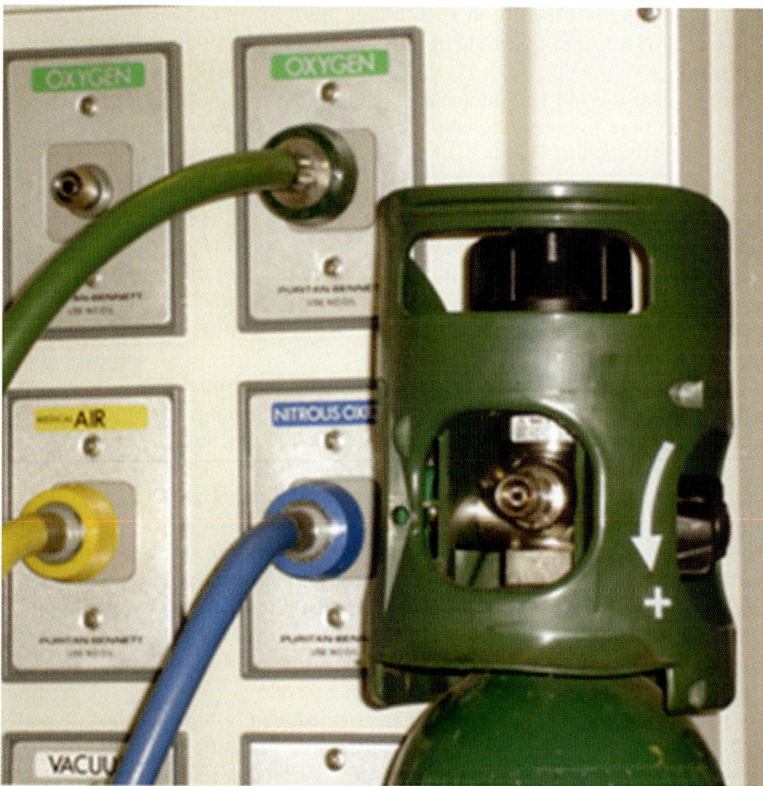

B

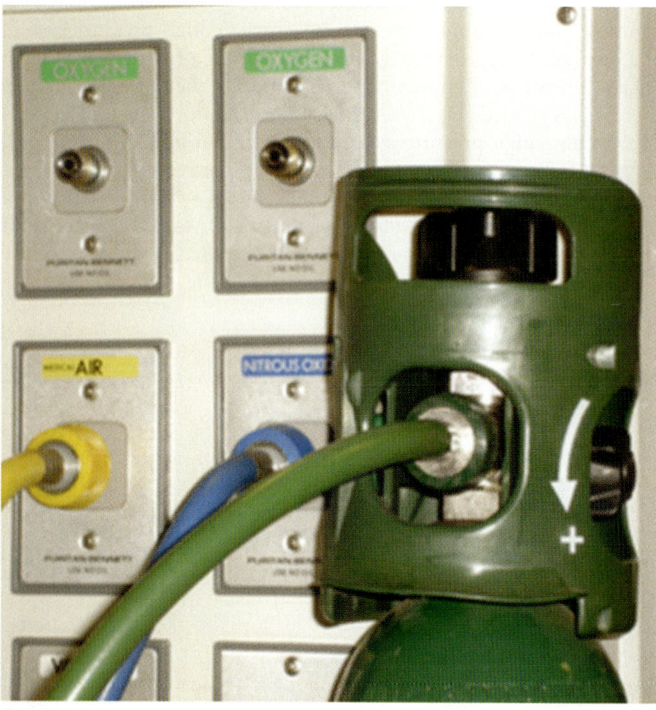

C

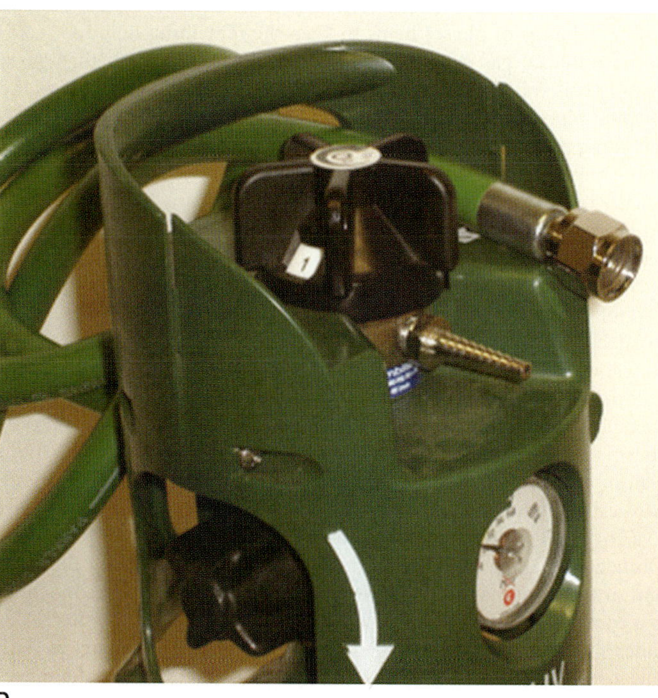

D

FIGURE 39-5. **A.** Lightweight oxygen tank filled to 3000 psig can deliver 1000 L of gas at 1 atm pressure. **B.** Oxygen can be delivered at 50 psig via a diameter-index safety system oxygen outlet. **C.** Can supply oxygen to the machine via the wall hose. **D.** Oxygen can also be delivered at flows of up to 25 L/min from the low-pressure nipple.

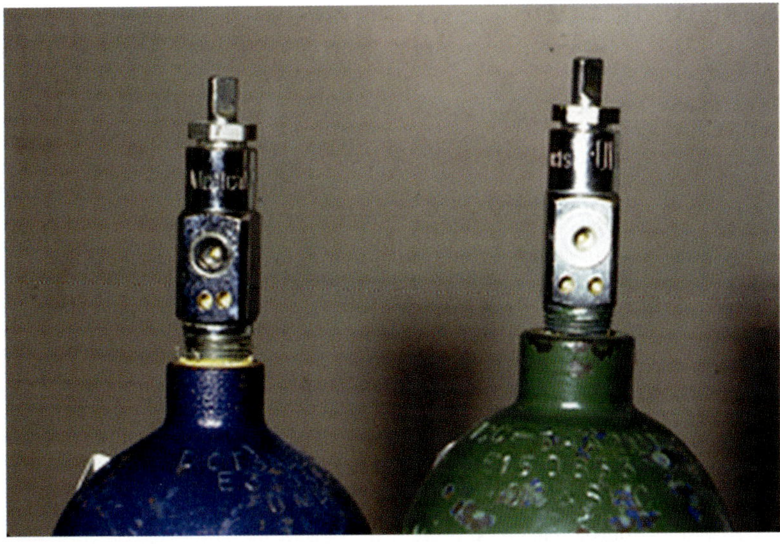

E

FIGURE 39-5. E. Pin-indexed safety system for a nitrous oxide tank (*left*) and an oxygen tank (*right*).

is being regulated. Because the tank supply serves as a backup in case the pipeline fails, after the tank pressures have been checked during the preuse checkout, the tank supply should be turned off if gas from the pipeline source is being used. If the O_2 tank(s) remains turned on while the machine is being supplied from the pipeline, O_2 is drawn preferentially from the pipeline supply (50–55 psig) because the regulator that controls flow from the O_2 tanks only permits flow into the machine high-pressure system for O_2 when the pressure in the machine high-pressure system falls below about 45 psig (Fig. 39-2). However, the pipeline pressure at times may fluctuate to below 45 psig, in which case O_2 would be drawn from an open tank. Thus, if the machine is being supplied from the O_2 pipeline, the O_2 tanks on the machine should be turned off to prevent the tank O_2 supply from being used and the backup tank supply from being unintentionally depleted.

When pipeline supply pressure (50–55 psig) exceeds the pressure downstream of the first-stage O_2 (tank supply) regulator, the O_2 tank source will not supply the machine. If one wants to use the tank O_2 to supply the machine, the O_2 pipeline connector must first be disconnected from the wall. Thus, if one should ever suspect that a hypoxic gas (ie, a gas other than O_2) is being delivered through the O_2 pipeline system at 50 to 55 psig (eg, because of pipeline crossover or misfilling of the bulk O_2 supply tank), the machine's O_2 pipeline connection must be disconnected from the wall outlet to permit the tank O_2 supply to flow into the high-pressure system.

Having entered the machine high-pressure system for O_2 at a pressure of 45 to 55 psig (from the tank or pipeline), O_2 may flow or pressurize in seven directions (Fig. 39-2):

1. It provides the power source for a pneumatically driven anesthesia ventilator. Most anesthesia ventilators (eg, those on GE-Datex-Ohmeda Modulus, Aestiva, Aespire, Excel, ADU, and Aisys machines; Dräger Narkomed 2, Narkomed 3, and Narkomed 4, Narkomed GS, Narkomed Mobile) use compressed oxygen as the driving gas. The driving gas is used to compress ("drive" or squeeze the ventilator bellows during the inspiratory phase of positive-pressure ventilation). It is important to realize this because if the machine and therefore the ventilator are being supplied from the tank rather than the pipeline, the tank will be depleted much more rapidly. Thus, if the pipeline oxygen supply fails during use of the ventilator and one switches to the tank supply, one should consider ways to limit the rate of use of the tank oxygen by ventilating the lungs using the reservoir bag, having the patient breathe spontaneously if possible, and using the lowest flow of oxygen necessary at the oxygen flowmeter.
2. It supplies the auxiliary oxygen flowmeter that is present on most contemporary workstations. This is the separate flowmeter that is commonly used to supply a nasal cannula.
3. It supplies oxygen to an auxiliary oxygen DISS fitting. This may be used to power a jet ventilator, or a Venturi design vacuum–suction system.
4. If the oxygen flush control (valve) is opened by pressing the oxygen flush button, oxygen flows directly (bypassing the flowmeters) to the common gas outlet of the machine at a rate of 35 to 75 L/min and potentially at a pressure of 50 psig. Consequently, the flush must not be activated if a patient is connected to the breathing system and there is no means for pressure relief. Activation of the flush during the inspiratory phase of ventilation, when gas can enter the breathing system but cannot leave, has the potential to cause positive-pressure barotrauma.
5. It pressurizes an oxygen supply pressure failure alarm system such that if oxygen pressure in the high-pressure system falls (usually to <30 psig), an audible alarm sounds. On modern machines, a pressure-operated electrical switch ensures a continuous audible (and visual) alarm when the oxygen supply pressure falls below 30 psig. This will alert to a possible problem with the machine's oxygen supply pressure, such as pipeline failure or if the tank in use is nearing empty.
6. It pressurizes and opens the "fail-safe" valve (Fig. 39-2 item A). This is a pressure-sensitive valve that can decrease or totally interrupt the supply of N_2O and other gases (eg, heliox and air in some machines) to their flow-control systems if the pressure of gas in the oxygen high-pressure system falls below a threshold level.

   In the GE-Datex-Ohmeda machines, this valve is called the pressure sensor shut-off valve (PSSV). These valves interrupt the gas supplies to the N_2O and other gas flowmeters when the oxygen pressure falls below a nominal 26 psig. In the GE-Datex-Ohmeda machines, these valves are either fully open or fully closed.

   In the Dräger Narkomed 2, Narkomed 3, and Narkomed 4 machines, the "fail-safe" valve is called the *oxygen-failure protection device* (OFPD), and there is 1 interfacing the high-pressure system for oxygen with the high-pressure systems for each of the other gases supplied to the machine (eg, N_2O). Unlike the GE-Datex-Ohmeda PSSV "fail-safe" valves, the OFPDs gradually reduce the supply pressure to the N_2O and other gas flowmeters as the oxygen supply pressure decreases. The supply of other gases to their respective flowmeters is completely interrupted when the oxygen supply pressure falls below 12 ± 4 psig. In this way, a hypoxic mixture arising from oxygen supply problems to the flowmeters should be prevented. In all contemporary workstations that are set to deliver N_2O and oxygen, when the oxygen supply pressure is low, only 100% oxygen is delivered.

7. It passes to the oxygen flow-control valve. In traditional machines, this is the needle valve that is connected to the oxygen flow-control knob used to set the oxygen flow at the oxygen flowmeter.

In GE-Datex-Ohmeda machines (eg, Modulus II, Modulus II Plus, Modulus CD, and Excel models), to reach the oxygen flow-control valve, oxygen in the high-pressure system must first pass through a second-stage regulator valve where the pressure is downregulated to about 16 psig. This second-stage regulator (Fig. 39-2 B) ensures that the oxygen flowmeter is supplied at a constant pressure of 16 psig. Thus, even if the oxygen supply pressure to the machine falls to below 45 to 50 psig, as long as it exceeds 16 psig, the oxygen flow set at the flowmeter will be maintained. Without this second-stage regulator, if the oxygen supply pressure to the machine were to fall, the oxygen flow would decrease at the flowmeter and, if N_2O were being used also, a hypoxic gas mixture might result at the level of the flowmeters. In summary, in GE-Datex-Ohmeda machines, if the oxygen supply pressure falls below 30 psig, the low-pressure supply alarm sounds (see #5 above); below 20 psig, the "fail-safe" valve will interrupt the flow of other gases to their flowmeters so that only oxygen can be delivered, and the oxygen flow set on the oxygen flowmeter will not decrease until the oxygen supply pressure falls below 16 psig.

Dräger Narkomed 2, Narkomed 3, and Narkomed 4 machines do not use a second-stage oxygen pressure regulator (Fig. 39-2, item B) to supply the oxygen flowmeter at constant pressure. Instead, they use OFPDs (see #6 above) to continually interface the pressure of oxygen in the high-pressure system with the pressure of N_2O just upstream of the N_2O flowmeter. A decrease in the oxygen supply pressure causes a proportionate decrease in the pressure of N_2O supplied to its flowmeter. Thus, as oxygen supply pressure decreases, the flow of oxygen and that of all other supplied gases will decrease in *proportion* so as to avoid creation of hypoxic gas mixture.

NITROUS OXIDE

Similar to O_2, N_2O may be supplied to the machine from the pipeline system at a pressure of approximately 50 psig or from a backup E cylinder supply on the machine. N_2O has a molecular weight of 44 and a boiling point of −88°C at 760 mm Hg (14.7 psia) pressure.[9] Because it has a critical temperature of 36.5°C (critical pressure, 1054 psig), N_2O can exist as a liquid at room temperature (20°C). E cylinders of N_2O are factory filled to 90% to 95% capacity with liquid N_2O. Above the liquid in the tank is N_2O vapor. Because the liquid agent is in equilibrium with its vapor or gas phase, the pressure exerted by the gaseous N_2O is its saturated vapor pressure (SVP) at the ambient temperature. At 20°C, the SVP of N_2O is 750 psig.[7]

A full E tank of N_2O generates approximately 1600 L of gas at 1 atm pressure at sea level (14.7 psia). As long as some liquid N_2O is present in the tank and the ambient temperature remains at 20°C, the pressure in the N_2O tank will remain at 750 psig, which is the SVP of N_2O at 20°C.

Unlike with O_2, the content of a N_2O tank cannot be determined by reference to the N_2O tank pressure gauge. Rather, it is determined by weighing the tank and subtracting the weight of the empty tank (tare weight) to determine the weight of the contained N_2O. By Avogadro's volume, 1 g molecular weight (ie, 44 g) of N_2O will occupy 22.4 L at standard temperature and pressure (STP, 760 mm Hg; 273.15 K or 0°C). After all of the liquid N_2O has been used and the tank contains only gas, Boyle's law may be applied. In this situation, where the tank pressure is approximately 750 psig (or 764.7 psia, from gas only) and the internal volume of the E cylinder is approximately 5 L (see Oxygen above), the volume of N_2O that will evolve at a pressure of 760 mm Hg (14.7 psia) can be calculated. Thus, $P1 \times V1 = P2 \times V2$; $750 \times 5 = 14.7 \times V2$, or $V2 = 255$ L. At this point, the N_2O tank is 255/1600, or 16%, full. At 20°C room temperature, an E tank of N_2O with a pressure of 400 psig would deliver ($400/750 \times 255$ L), or 136 L of N_2O gas.

Nitrous oxide from the tank supply enters the N_2O hanger yoke at pressures of up to 750 psig (at 20°C) and then passes through a regulator that reduces this pressure to 40 to 45 psig (Fig. 39-2). The pin-index safety system is designed to ensure that only a N_2O tank may hang in a N_2O hanger yoke. As with O_2, a check valve in each yoke prevents the back leakage of N_2O if no tank is hanging in the yoke.

The N_2O pipeline is supplied from a bulk storage container of liquid N_2O or from banks of large N_2O tanks, usually H cylinders. (Each H cylinder of N_2O evolves 16,000 L of gas at atmospheric pressure.) The pressure in the N_2O pipeline is regulated to approximately 50 psig to supply the outlets in the operating room. Having entered the anesthesia machine high-pressure system for N_2O, N_2O must flow past the fail-safe valve to reach the N_2O flow-control (traditionally a needle) valve and flowmeter (traditionally a rotameter) (Fig. 39-2).

In GE-Datex-Ohmeda anesthesia machines that have the Link-25 Proportion Limiting Control System (see next section), a second-stage N_2O regulator further reduces gas pressure so that N_2O is supplied to its flow-control (needle) valve at a nominal pressure of 26 psig (Fig. 39-2). The actual downstream pressure of this regulator is adjusted at the factory or by a field service representative to ensure correct functioning of the Link-25 Proportion Limiting Control System.

GAS FLOW-CONTROL SYSTEMS

The anesthesia machine is used to adjust the proportions of oxygen and N_2O, as well as total gas flows delivered to the patient. For each gas (eg, oxygen, N_2O, air, heliox), this is achieved in a traditional machine (**Fig. 39-6**) by means of a flow-control valve and a gas flow measuring system.

The flow-control knob is connected to a needle valve whereby gas flow is set and adjusted. Turning the knob counterclockwise opens the valve wider, permitting a greater flow of gas. The flow-control knob for oxygen is larger than those for the other gases, and it is fluted rather than knurled so that it is "touch coded." Thus, the oxygen knob feels different than the knobs for the other gases.

Traditionally, gas flows on the conventional anesthesia machine are measured using the rotameter flowmeter (Fig. 39-6). There may be 1 rotameter or 2 rotameters in tandem for each gas. If 2 are present for each gas, the first permits accurate measurement of low flows (usually up to 1 L/min) and the second of flows of 1 to 12 L/min. In North America, the oxygen rotameter(s) is (are) positioned on the right side of the rotameter bank to be downstream of the other gases. The rotameter is a constant pressure, variable orifice flowmeter based on the Thorpe tube principle. Each rotameter consists of a vertical tapered glass tube that is of small diameter at the bottom and wider at the top and contains a ball, float, or bobbin. The cross-sectional area between the outside of the float and the inside of the tapered glass tube represents the variable orifice. A certain pressure difference across the bobbin is required to "float" the bobbin in the upwardly flowing gas stream. As the orifice widens, increasing flows are required to create the same pressure difference across the bobbin, which floats at a higher level in the tapered glass tube. At low gas flow rates, flow is essentially laminar, and Poiseuille's law applies:

$$\text{Flow} = \frac{\pi \times P \times r^4}{8 \times \eta \times L}$$

where P is the pressure decrease across the bobbin, r is the radius of the tube, η is the viscosity of the gas, and L is the length of the bobbin or float.

When the orificial area (proportional to r^2) is larger and flows are greater, flow becomes turbulent, in which case flow is proportional to the $\sqrt{P}$, r^2, length^{-1}, and density$^{-0.5}$.

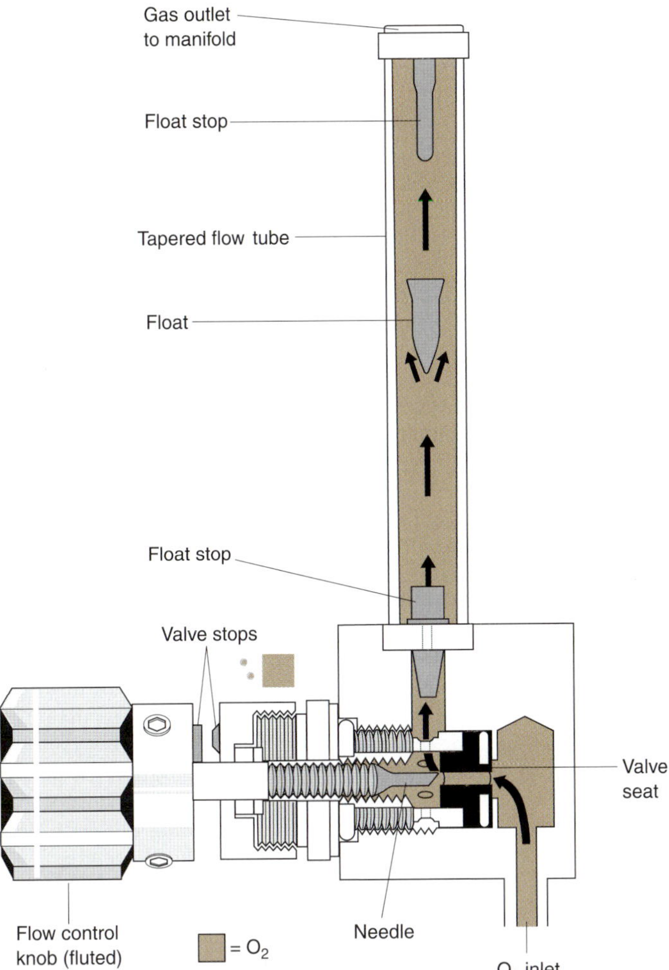

FIGURE 39-6. Conventional oxygen flow-control (needle) valve and flowmeter (rotameter).

Rotameter flowmeters are precision instruments. Flow tubes are manufactured for specific gases, calibrated with a unique float and for use within a certain range of temperatures and pressures. Flowmeters are *not* interchangeable among gases, and if a gas were passed through a rotameter for which it was not calibrated, the flows shown would likely be incorrect. Theoretical exceptions to this include that at *low (laminar) flows*, the flow rates of gases with *similar viscosities* would be read identically (eg, oxygen and helium have viscosities of 202 and 194 micropoise, respectively) and at *high flows* gases of *similar densities* (eg, N_2O and carbon dioxide, both of which have a molecular weight of 44 atomic mass units) would be read identically.

VIRTUAL FLOWMETERS

As the anesthesia workstation evolves, some of the traditional mechanical components are being replaced by more sophisticated electronic devices. For example, in some models of contemporary anesthesia workstation (GE-Datex-Ohmeda S5/ADU; Dräger Fabius GS), gas flows are still controlled by mechanical needle valves, but they are measured using electronic flow sensors. Flows are displayed on a screen in the form of a virtual graduated flowmeter together with a digital display. In the GE-Datex-Ohmeda S5/ADU (**Fig. 39-7**) and Aisys and the Dräger Apollo and some Fabius GS workstations, the virtual flow displays are color coded (eg, green column = O_2; blue = N_2O; yellow = air). Among the advantages of electronic flow sensors are that they are less expensive than rotameters, are very accurate, and the data can be used elsewhere

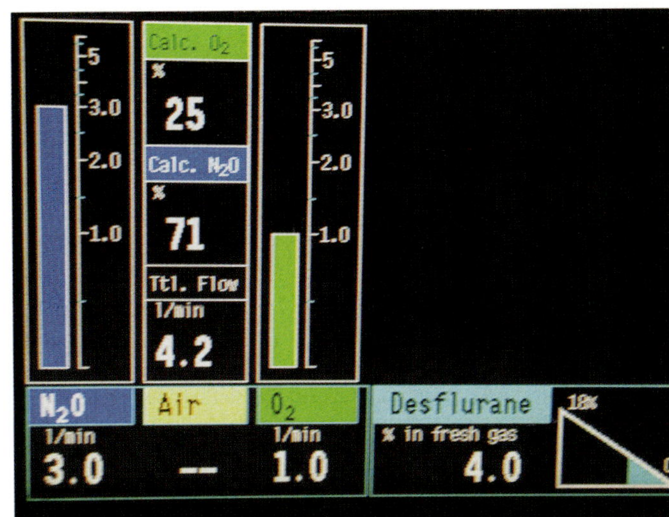

FIGURE 39-7. Virtual flowmeter display from a GE-Datex ADU workstation.

in the workstation to record gas and agent consumption or to adjust ventilator bellows tidal volume (as in the GE-Datex-Ohmeda ADU workstation).

One obvious concern with any electronically based system is what would happen if electrical power were totally lost. Also, many anesthesiologists are not completely comfortable unless they can see physical evidence of gas flowing. For these reasons, the workstation manufacturers provide as an option (GE-Datex Ohmeda ADU) or standard (Dräger Fabius GS and Apollo) a rotameter that displays the approximate total flow of gas leaving the machine to enter the breathing system (**Fig. 39-8**).

Some anesthesia workstations offer, as an option, an oxygen flow that cannot be discontinued completely because either a "stop" is provided on the oxygen flow-control valve to ensure a minimum oxygen flow of 200 to 300 mL/min past the needle valve (some GE-Datex-Ohmeda machines) or a gas flow resistor is provided (North American Dräger

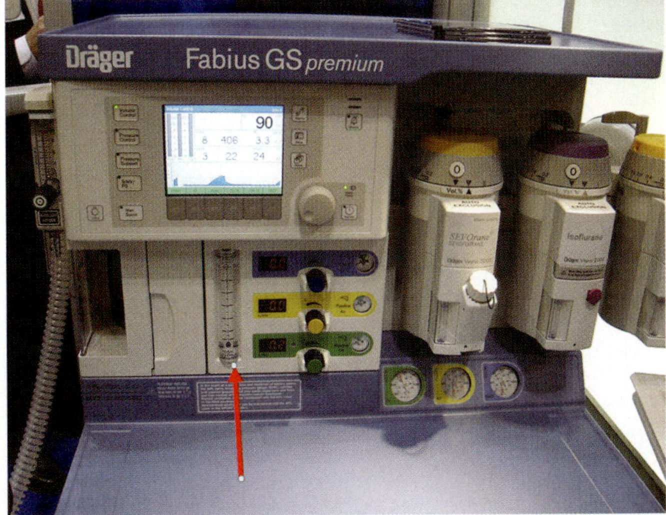

FIGURE 39-8. Virtual flowmeter display on a Dräger Fabius GS premium workstation. Note the vertical arrangement of the gas flow-control knobs, the lowest being the touch-coded oxygen knob. *Arrow* indicates rotameter showing approximate total gas flow.

Narkomed 2, Narkomed 3, and Narkomed 4 machines) that permits a similar flow of 200 to 300 mL/min to bypass a completely closed oxygen flow-control needle valve. In the North American Dräger Narkomed 2, 3, and 4 machines, the minimum oxygen flow feature functions only in the "O_2/N_2O" mode but not in the "ALL GASES" mode.

OXYGEN RATIO MONITORING AND PROPORTIONING SYSTEMS

A major consideration in the design of contemporary anesthesia machines is prevention of the delivery of a hypoxic gas mixture. The fail-safe system described previously only serves to interrupt (GE-Datex-Ohmeda pressure sensor shut-off valve) or proportionately reduce and ultimately interrupt (Dräger OFPD) the supplies of N_2O and (in some models) other gases (eg, air, He) to their flowmeters if the O_2 supply pressure to the machine is reduced. The fail-safe system is pressure sensitive, not flow sensitive. It does not prevent the delivery of a hypoxic mixture to the common gas outlet, making the term *fail-safe* somewhat of a misnomer.

In basic contemporary machines, N_2O and O_2 flow controls are physically interlinked either mechanically (GE-Datex-Ohmeda) or mechanically and pneumatically (Dräger), so that a fresh gas mixture containing 25% or more O_2 is delivered at the flowmeters when only N_2O and O_2 are being used.[10,11]

GE-Datex-Ohmeda anesthesia machines use the Link-25 Proportion Limiting Control System to ensure an adequate percentage of O_2 in the gas mixture created.[10] In this system, a gear with 14 teeth is integral with the N_2O flow-control spindle; a gear with 29 teeth is allowed to rotate ("float") on a threaded O_2 flow-control valve spindle (**Fig. 39-9**). The 2 gears are connected together by a precision stainless steel link chain. For every 2.07 revolutions of the N_2O flow-control spindle, an O_2 flow control, set to the lowest O_2 flow, rotates once because of the 14:29 ratio of gear teeth. Because the gear on the O_2 flow-control spindle is thread mounted so it can rotate on the control valve spindle similar to a nut on a bolt (rather than being integral with the spindle), O_2 flow can be increased independently of N_2O. However, regardless of the O_2 flow set, if the flow of N_2O is increased sufficiently, the gear on the O_2 spindle will engage with the O_2 flow-control knob, causing it to rotate and thereby causing O_2 flow to increase. If N_2O flow is now reduced, the O_2 flow remains at the increased setting unless it is deliberately decreased by the user. The 75% N_2O:25% O_2 proportioning is completed because the N_2O flow-control valve is supplied from a second-stage gas regulator that reduces N_2O pressure to a nominal 26 psig (adjusted as previously described) before it reaches the flow-control valve, whereas the O_2 flow-control valve is supplied at a pressure of 14 psig from a second-stage O_2 regulator (Figs. 39-2 and 39-9). The Link-25 Proportion Limiting Control System permits the N_2O and O_2 flow-control valves to be set independently of one another, but whenever a N_2O concentration of more than 75% would be accidentally set, the O_2 flow is automatically mechanically increased to maintain at least 25% O_2 in the resulting mixture. This system thus increases the minimum flow of O_2 according to the N_2O flow set. The Link-25 Proportion Limiting Control System interconnects only the N_2O and O_2 flow-control valves. If the anesthesia machine has flow controls for other gases (eg, He, air) (Fig. 39-9), a gas mixture containing less than 25% O_2 could potentially be set at the flowmeters.

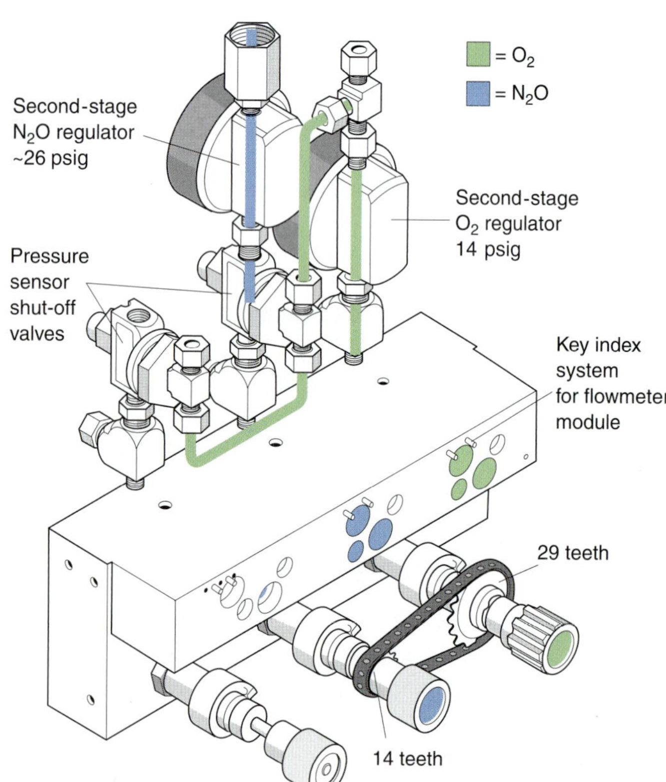

FIGURE 39-9. GE-Datex-Ohmeda Link-25 Proportion Limiting Control System, which ensures at least 25% O_2 concentration at the level of the flowmeters when O_2 and nitrous oxide (N_2O) are being used. When supply pressure to the second-stage O_2 regulator falls below a nominal 26 psig, the pressure sensor shut-off valves ("fail-safe" valves) cause the supply of N_2O and other gases to be shut off.

In the Dräger Narkomed 2A, Narkomed 2B, Narkomed 3, and Narkomed 4 machines, the oxygen ratio monitor controller (ORMC) (**Fig. 39-10**) serves to limit the N_2O flow according to the O_2 flow and create a mixture of at least 25% O_2 at the flowmeter level when these 2 gases are being used.[9] Contemporary Dräger workstations, the Fabius GS and the Apollo, use a similar system called the sensitive oxygen ratio controller (S-ORC). At O_2 flow rates of less than 1 L/min, even higher concentrations of O_2 are delivered. These ratio monitor controllers work as follows: As O_2 flows past its flow-control needle valve and up the rotameter tube, it encounters a resistor, which creates a back pressure that is applied to the O_2 diaphragm (Fig. 39-10). As N_2O flows past its flow-control valve and up the rotameter tube, italso encounters a resistor that creates a back pressure on the N_2O diaphragm. The 2 diaphragms are linked by a connecting shaft, the ultimate position of which depends on the relative back pressures and therefore *flows* of N_2O and O_2. The left-hand end of the connecting shaft controls the orifice of a slave valve, which, in turn, controls the supply pressure of N_2O to its flow-control valve. When the O_2 flow is high, the shaft moves to the left and opens the slave control valve (Fig. 39-10, lower). Conversely, if the N_2O flow is increased excessively, the shaft moves to the right, closing the slave valve orifice and decreasing the supply pressure of N_2O to, and thereby flow of N_2O from, its flow-control valve. When the ORMC is acting to prevent a hypoxic mixture, the leaf-spring contacts (Fig. 39-10) are closed, sounding an alarm. This alarm is disabled if the machine is in the "all gases" mode.[9]

The Dräger ratio controllers differ from the Link-25 Proportion Limiting Control System in several ways. First, the ORMC and S-ORC do not require second-stage O_2 and N_2O regulators. Second, whereas the ORMC and S-ORC limit the N_2O flow according to the O_2 flow, the Link-25 Proportion Limiting Control System increases the O_2 flow as the N_2O flow is increased. As with the Link-25 Proportion Limiting Control System, the ORMC and S-ORC function only with N_2O and O_2, and there is no interlinking of O_2 with other gases (eg, air, He) that might also be deliverable by the machine. Thus, when a third or fourth gas is in use, the gas flow proportioning systems afford no protection against a hypoxic mixture. Prevention of delivery of a hypoxic gas mixture when a third or fourth gas is supplied to the machine may be achieved by supplying

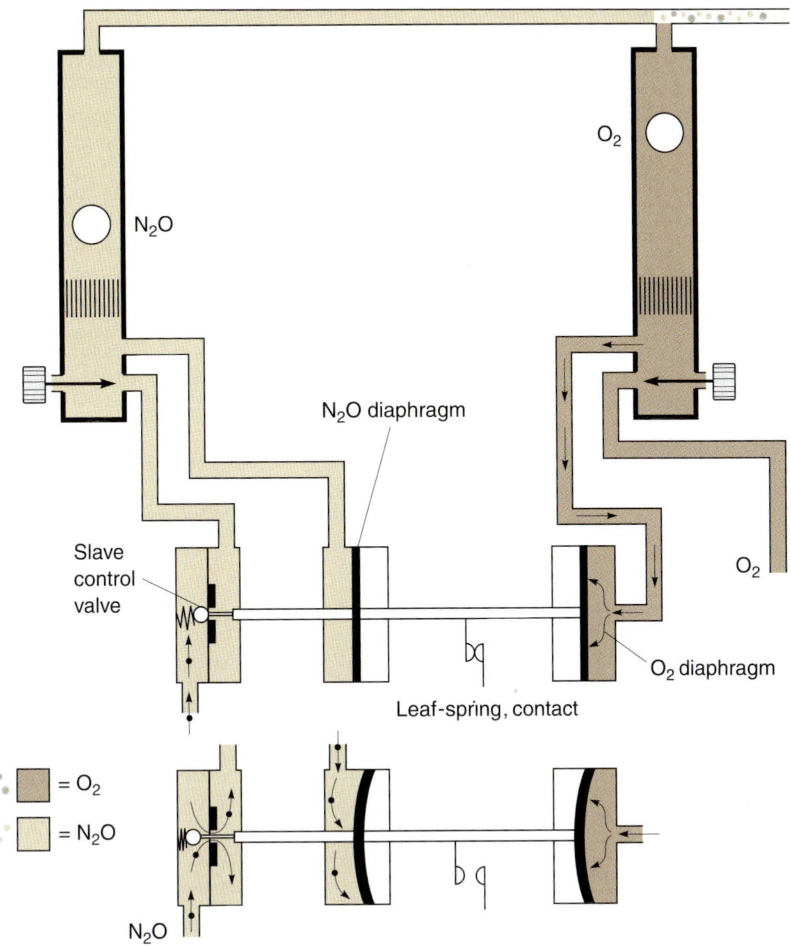

FIGURE 39-10. Dräger oxygen ratio monitor controller. See text for details of operation.

that gas in a tank premixed with O_2 (eg, heliox, a gas mixture of 75% He and 25% O_2).

Although elegant in design, the ORMC, S-ORC, and Link-25 Proportion Limiting Control Systems are subject to mechanical and pneumatic failure and should be tested according to the manufacturer's instructions during the preuse machine checkout. Furthermore, if the systems are functioning correctly, they only ensure adequacy of greater than 25% O_2 at the flowmeter level. An O_2 leak downstream from the flow-control valves (ie, from the low-pressure system of the machine) could result in a hypoxic mixture flowing into the breathing circuit. Consequently, an oxygen analyzer in the patient circuit is essential if a hypoxic mixture is to be detected. The controlled flows of O_2, N_2O, and other gas or gases are mixed in the manifold at the top of the flowmeter bank, and they flow to a concentration-calibrated anesthesia vaporizer (Fig. 39-2).

ANESTHESIA VAPORIZERS

A vapor is the gas phase of an agent that is normally a liquid at room temperature and atmospheric pressure. An anesthetic vaporizer facilitates the change of a liquid anesthetic into its vapor phase and adds a controlled amount of this vapor to the flow of gases passing to the patient circuit.

VAPOR, EVAPORATION, AND VAPOR PRESSURE

Consider isoflurane in a closed container at 1 atm pressure (760 mm Hg) and room temperature of 20°C. Although most is in liquid form, some isoflurane molecules escape from the surface of the liquid to enter the space above as a vapor. Under steady-state conditions of temperature, equilibrium is established between the molecules in the vapor phase and those in the liquid phase. The vapor phase molecules are in constant motion, striking the walls of the container to exert a vapor pressure. If the temperature is increased, more isoflurane molecules enter the vapor phase (evaporate), resulting in an increase in vapor pressure. When the gas phase above the liquid contains all of the isoflurane vapor that it can hold at that temperature, it is said to be saturated and the pressure exerted by the isoflurane is called its saturated vapor pressure (SVP) at that temperature.

The SVP exerted by the vapor phase of a potent volatile anesthetic agent depends only on the volatile agent and the ambient temperature (**Fig. 39-11**). The temperature at which SVP becomes equal to atmospheric pressure and at which all the liquid agent changes to the vapor phase is the liquid's boiling point. The most volatile agents are those with the highest SVPs for any given temperature, and they also have the lowest boiling points (eg, desflurane and diethyl ether boil at 22.8°C and 35°C, respectively, at an ambient pressure of 760 mm Hg). Boiling point decreases with decreasing ambient pressure, such as occurs at increasing altitude.

UNITS OF VAPOR CONCENTRATION

Anesthetic vapor presence may be quantified either as an absolute pressure (or tension), expressed in millimeters of mercury (mm Hg), or in volumes percent of 1 atm (ie, volumes of vapor per 100 volumes of total gas).

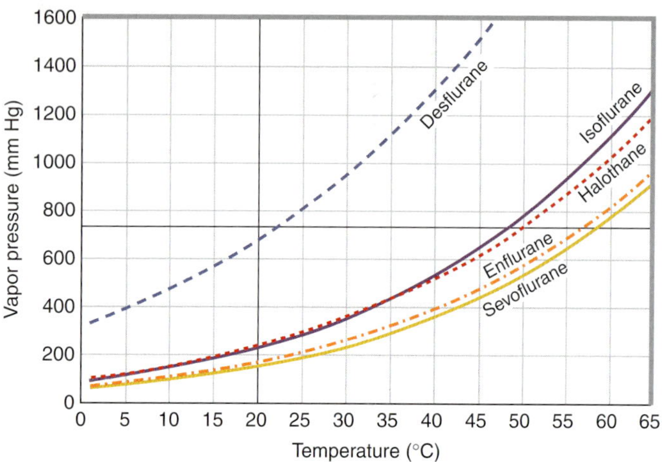

FIGURE 39-11. Vapor pressure curves for 5 potent inhaled anesthetics.

TABLE 39-1 Expression of Minimum Alveolar Concentration (MAC) of Anesthetic Agent As Partial Pressure at Concentration of a MAC (P_{MAC1}) Assuming Ambient Pressure of 760 mm Hg[a]

Anesthetic Agent	MAC (vol%)		P_{MAC1} (mm Hg)
Halothane	0.75 × 760	=	5.7
Enflurane	1.68 × 760	=	12.8
Isoflurane	1.15 × 760	=	8.7
Methoxyflurane	0.16 × 760	=	1.2
Desflurane[a]	6.0 × 760	=	45.6
	7.25 × 760	=	55.1
Sevoflurane	2.1 × 760	=	16.0

[a]MAC of desflurane is age dependent: 18-35 years, 7.25%; 31-65 years, 6.0%. See Rampil IJ, Lockhart SH, Eger EI II, et al. The electroencephalographic effects of desflurane in humans. *Anesthesiology.* 1991;74:429 and Eger EI II, Weiskopf RB, Eisenkraft JB. *The Pharmacology of Inhaled Anesthetics*. San Antonio, TX: Dannemiller Inc.; 2002:21-32.

Reprinted from Eisenkraft JB. Anesthesia vaporizers. In: Ehrenwerth J, Eisenkraft JB, eds. *Anesthesia Equipment: Principles and Applications*. St. Louis, MO: Mosby-Year Book; 1993:59, with permission from Elsevier.

By applying Dalton's law, volumes percent is similar to the agent's fractional partial pressure:

Vol % = (Partial pressure of agent/Total ambient pressure) × 100

Dalton's Law of Partial Pressures Dalton's law states that in a mixture of gases (or vapors) the pressure exerted by each gas is the same as that it would exert if it alone occupied the container.[7] Each gas (or vapor) exerts its pressure independently of the pressure of the other gases present. For example, in a container of dry air at atmospheric pressure (760 mm Hg), if O_2 represents 21% of all gases present, the pressure exerted by the O_2 (its partial pressure) is 21% of 760, or 159.6 mm Hg.

Now consider air that is fully saturated with water vapor at 37°C (normal body temperature). Vapor pressure depends on temperature. The SVP for water at 37°C is 47 mm Hg. O_2 now represents 21% of what remains (ie, 713, or 760 – 47), having a partial pressure of 21% of 713, or 149.3 mm Hg.

Whereas volumes percent expresses the ratio of gas molecules in a mixture, partial pressure is an absolute value. Anesthetic uptake and potency are directly related to partial pressure and only indirectly to volumes percent. This distinction will become more apparent when the use of vaporizers under hyperbaric and hypobaric conditions is considered in a later section (see Changes in Barometric Pressure).

MINIMUM ALVEOLAR CONCENTRATION

The minimum alveolar concentration (MAC) of a potent inhaled anesthetic agent that produces immobility in 50% of patients undergoing a surgical incision is used as a measure of anesthetic potency or depth. MAC is typically expressed as volumes percent of alveolar (end-tidal) gas at 1 atm pressure at sea level (760 mm Hg). **Table 39-1** shows how MAC in familiar volumes percent can be expressed as a partial pressure in millimeters of mercury. Readers are encouraged to think of MAC in terms of minimum alveolar pressure (MAP) or minimum alveolar partial pressure (MAPP) rather than volumes percent because it is the partial pressure (tension) of the anesthetic in the brain that determines the depth of anesthesia.[12,13] The term P_{MAC1} (Table 39-1) is used to express the partial pressure of a potent inhaled agent at a concentration of 1 MAC. Thus, 1 MAC of sevoflurane is equivalent to a P_{MAC1} of 16 mm Hg.

LATENT HEAT OF VAPORIZATION

Energy in the form of heat is needed to transfer molecules from the liquid to the vapor phase. This energy is called the *latent heat of vaporization* and is defined as the amount of heat (calories) required to convert unit mass (grams) of the liquid into vapor.[7] For example, the latent heat of vaporization at room temperature is 41 cal/g for isoflurane.

The heat of vaporization is inversely related to ambient temperature so that the lower the temperature, the more heat is required. Heat required to vaporize anesthetic agents is drawn from the remaining liquid and the surroundings. As vapor is generated, the temperatures of the vaporizer and remaining liquid decrease. This causes the vapor pressure to decrease and would result in decreased vaporizer output if no compensatory mechanism were provided.

SPECIFIC HEAT

Specific heat is the quantity of heat (calories) required to raise the temperature of unit mass (grams) of a substance by 1°C.[7] Heat must be supplied to the liquid anesthetic in the vaporizer to maintain its temperature while heat is being lost in the process of evaporation.

Specific heat is also important in choice of vaporizer construction material. Materials with high specific heat change temperature more gradually than those with low specific heats for the same amount of heat lost through vaporization. *Thermal capacity* is defined as the product of specific heat and mass and represents the total quantity of heat stored in the vaporizer body.[7]

The vaporizer construction material's ability to conduct heat from the environment through to the contained liquid anesthetic is also important. This is called *thermal conductivity*, defined in terms of how quickly heat is transmitted through a substance. The ideal material for vaporizer construction would have a high specific heat and high thermal capacity and conductivity. In this respect, copper comes close to the ideal (hence the Copper Kettle vaporizer). More recently, bronze and stainless steel have been used in vaporizer construction.

REGULATING VAPORIZER OUTPUT

The SVPs of the 4 potent inhaled agents—halothane, isoflurane, enflurane, and sevoflurane—at room temperature are 243, 238, 175, and 160 mm Hg, respectively, and far in excess of those required for clinical anesthesia (Fig. 39-11 and **Table 39-2**). Consequently, the vaporizer first creates a saturated vapor that must then be diluted by a larger bypass gas flow to result in clinically useful concentrations. If this were not done, a lethal concentration of agent could be delivered.

Contemporary anesthesia vaporizers for halothane, isoflurane, enflurane, and sevoflurane are concentration calibrated and of the variable-bypass design. The vaporizers for desflurane (GE-Datex-Ohmeda Tec 6; Dräger D-Vapor) are of a different design and are described

TABLE 39-2 Physical Properties of Potent Inhaled Volatile Anesthetic Agents

Parameter/Agent	Halothane	Enflurane	Isoflurane	Methoxyflurane	Sevoflurane	Desflurane
Structure	$CHBrClCF_3$	$CHFClCF_2OCHF_2$	$CF_2HOCHClCF_3$	$CHCl_2CF_2OCH_3$	$CH_2FOCH(CF_3)_2$	$CH_2HOCFHCF_3$
Molecular weight	197.4	184.5	184.5	165.0	200	168
Boiling point at 769 mm Hg (°C)	50.2	56.5	48.5	104.7	58.5	22.9
SVP at 20°C	243	175	238	20.3	160	669
Saturated vapor concentration at 20°C and 1 atmosphere absolute (vol %)	32	23	31	2.7	21	87
MAC at 1 atmosphere absolute (vol %)	0.75	1.68	1.15	0.16	2.1	6.0–7.25[a]
P_{MAC1} (mm Hg)	5.7	12.8	8.7	1.22	16	46–55[a]
Specific gravity of liquid at 20°C	1.86	1.52	1.50	1.42	1.52	1.46
Vapor (mL) per liquid at 20°C	226	196	195	204	182	207

[a]Age related; see Table 39-1.

MAC, minimum alveolar concentration; P_{MAC1}, partial pressure at concentration of 1 MAC; SVP, saturated vapor pressure.

Reprinted from Eisenkraft JB. Anesthesia vaporizers. In: Ehrenwerth J, Eisenkraft JB, eds. *Anesthesia Equipment: Principles and Applications*. St. Louis, MO: Mosby-Year Book, 1993:60, with permission from Elsevier.

separately in a later section (see Desflurane and the Tec 6 Vaporizer). In a variable-bypass vaporizer (eg, Datex-Ohmeda Tec series, Dräger Vapor 19.n series), the total fresh gas flow (FGF) from the anesthesia machine flowmeters passes to the vaporizer. The vaporizer splits the incoming gas flow into both a smaller flow, which enters the vaporizing chamber to emerge with the agent at its saturated vapor concentration, and a larger bypass flow, which when mixed with the vaporizing chamber output, results in the desired or "dialed-in" concentration (**Fig. 39-12**).

Measured-flow (ie, not concentration-calibrated) vaporizers, such as the Copper Kettle (Foregger/Puritan-Bennett) or Verni-Trol (Ohmeda) are considered obsolete, are not mentioned in the most recent machine and workstation standards,[1,2] and therefore are not discussed here.

An efficient system must exist to create a saturated vapor concentration in the vaporizing chamber. This is achieved by having a large surface area for evaporation of the liquid agent. In flow-over vaporizers (eg, Dräger Vapor series, GE-Datex-Ohmeda Tec series), the area is increased by the use of wicks and baffles.

Desflurane, because of its high SVP at room temperature (669 mm Hg at 20°C) and its low boiling point (22.8°C at 1 atm), cannot be safely delivered using a conventional variable bypass vaporizer. The physical properties of desflurane require that a special design of vaporizer (eg, Datex-Ohmeda Tec 6; Dräger D-Vapor) be used to deliver this agent in a controlled fashion (see Desflurane and the Tec 6 Vaporizer).

VARIABLE BYPASS

Assume that room temperature is kept constant at 20°C. The SVPs of each agent are as follows: halothane, 243 mm Hg; isoflurane, 238 mm Hg; enflurane, 172 mm Hg; and sevoflurane, 160 mm Hg (Table 39-2). If ambient pressure is 760 mm Hg, these vapor pressures represent 243/760, or 32% for halothane; 238/760, or 31% for isoflurane; 175/760, or 23% for enflurane; and 160/760, or 21% for sevoflurane in terms of volumes percent of each agent at 1 atm.

In a variable-bypass vaporizer, a given volume of carrier gas flowing into the vaporizing chamber over time will exit the chamber over the same period (Fig. 39-12). In the vaporizing chamber, however, anesthetic vapor at its SVP constitutes a mandatory fractional volume of the atmosphere (eg, 79% by volume in a sevoflurane vaporizer at 20°C and 760 mm Hg ambient pressure). Thus, the volume of carrier gas entering the vaporizing chamber constitutes the difference between 100% of the atmosphere in the vaporizing chamber

In the concentration-calibrated variable-bypass ("Tec-type") design, the vaporizer splits the incoming total flow of gas arriving from the machine flowmeters between a variable-bypass and the vaporizing chamber that contains the anesthetic agent (Fig. 39-12). The ratio of these flows—the splitting ratio—depends on the anesthetic agent, the temperature, and the dialed-in vapor concentration set to be delivered.

Consider a sevoflurane vaporizer set to deliver 1% sevoflurane at 20°C (**Fig. 39-13**). In the vaporizing chamber, sevoflurane vapor constitutes a mandatory 21% of the atmosphere and carrier gas the other 79%. Assume that carrier gas flows into the chamber at a rate of 79 mL/min. Emerging from the vaporizing chamber will be 100 mL/min (ie, 21 mL of sevoflurane vapor + 79 mL of carrier gas). To create 1% sevoflurane per minute, the 21 mL of sevoflurane vapor must be diluted in a total flow of 2100 mL because 21/2100 equals 1%. The bypass gas flow must therefore be 2000 mL, that is:

$$(21/[21+79+2000]) \times 100 = 1\%$$

If 2079 mL/min of gas enters the vaporizer and splits so that 2000 mL/min enters the bypass and 79 mL/min enters the vaporizing chamber

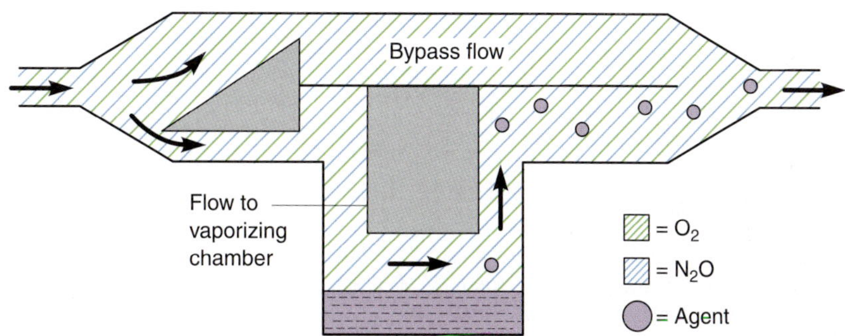

FIGURE 39-12. Variable-bypass vaporizer principle. These are concentration-calibrated and are of the flow-over design (see text).

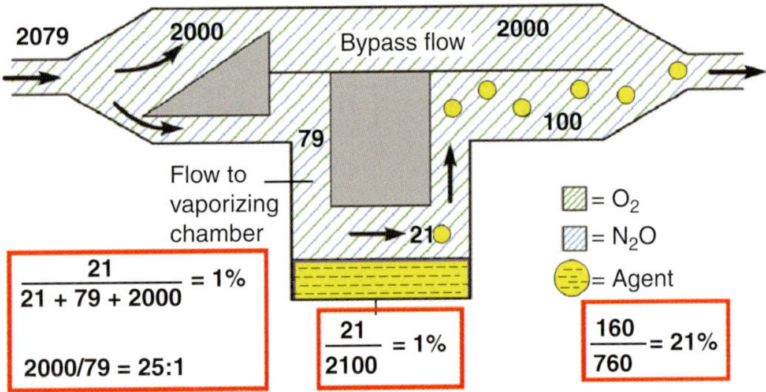

FIGURE 39-13. Variable-by pass vaporizer flow arrangement to deliver 1% sevoflurane by volume. See text for details. N_2O, nitrous oxide.

containing sevoflurane at 20°C, 1% sevoflurane would be produced. The incoming gas flow was split in the ratio 2000:79, or 25:1. A variable-bypass concentration-calibrated vaporizer is basically a gas flow splitting device, the flow split determining the concentration of agent produced (Fig. 39-13).

Figure 39-14 shows the schematic of a contemporary concentration-calibrated vaporizer, the Dräger Vapor 19.1. Anesthetic output concentration is increased by turning the concentration dial counterclockwise. This raises the control cone, decreases the split ratio, and allows more saturated anesthetic vapor to leave the vaporizing chamber.

Concentration-calibrated vaporizers are agent specific and designed to be used only with the agent for which the unit is designed and calibrated. To produce a 1% vapor concentration, whereas an isoflurane vaporizer makes a flow split of 44:1, a sevoflurane vaporizer makes a flow split of 25:1 (**Table 39-3**). If an empty sevoflurane vaporizer set to deliver 1% were filled with isoflurane, the concentration of the isoflurane vapor emerging would exceed 1% (44/25 = 1.7%). An understanding of splitting ratios enables fairly accurate prediction of the concentration output of an agent-specific variable-bypass vaporizer that has been erroneously filled with an agent for which it was not designed (see Incorrect Filling of Vaporizers below).

EFFICIENCY AND TEMPERATURE COMPENSATION

Agent-specific, variable-bypass, concentration-calibrated vaporizers are located in the fresh gas path between the flowmeters (eg, rotameters) on the anesthesia machine and the machine common gas outlet (Fig. 39-2). The vaporizers must be efficient and produce steady concentrations of the agent over a fairly wide range of incoming gas flows. However, as the agent is vaporized and the temperature decreases, SVP also decreases, and vaporizing chamber output tends to decrease.

Most contemporary variable-bypass vaporizers (eg, GE-Datex-Ohmeda Tec series, Dräger Vapor 19.n and 2000 series) have automatic temperature compensation achieved by a temperature-sensitive valve in the bypass gas flow. When temperature increases, the valve in the bypass opens wider to create a greater splitting ratio. More gas flows through the bypass, and less gas enters the vaporizing chamber. A smaller volume of a higher concentration of vapor emerges from the vaporizing chamber. When mixed with an increased bypass gas flow, this volume maintains a reasonably constant vaporizer output when temperature changes are gradual and not extreme.

The design of the temperature-sensitive valve varies among the different types of vaporizer. The GE-Datex-Ohmeda Tec series vaporizers use a bimetallic strip. This is a flap valve situated in the bypass flow composed of 2 different metals that have different coefficients of expansion (defined as change in length per unit length per unit change in temperature). As temperature increases, 1 surface of the flap expands more than the other, causing the flap to bend in such a way that the valve

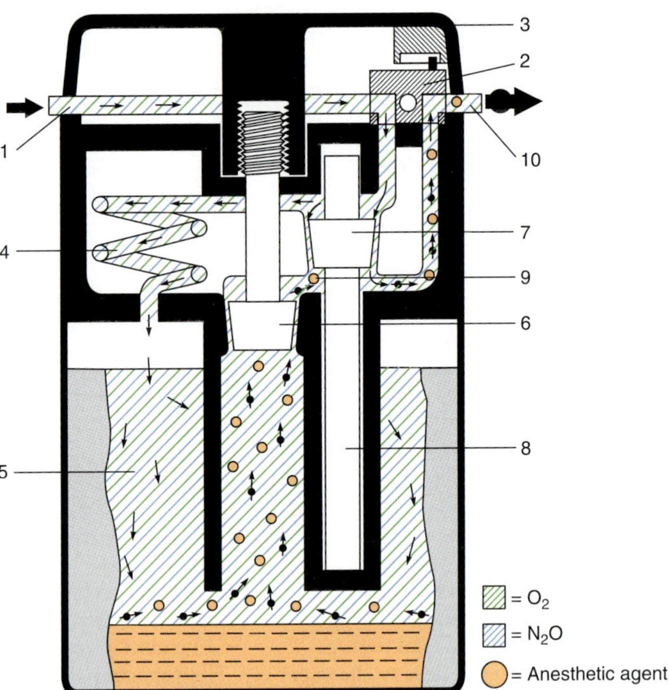

FIGURE 39-14. Schematic of Dräger Vapor 19.1 vaporizer. When concentration knob (*3*) is in 0 (zero) position, the on/off switch (*2*) is closed. Gas mixture enters the vaporizer at the fresh gas inlet (*1*) and leaves through the fresh gas outlet (*10*) without entering the vaporizer's interior. When concentration knob (*3*) is turned to any volume (%) concentration above 0.2 vol%, the on/off switch (*2*) automatically opens and allows fresh gas to enter the vaporizer's interior. Gas is immediately divided and follows 2 different routes. One part of the fresh gas moves through a thermostatically controlled bypass (*7*), which compensates for temperature changes and maintains correct volumes percent concentration vapor output as selected with concentration knob (*3*). The other part of the fresh gas moves through a pressure compensator (*4*), which prevents pressure changes that occur upstream or downstream from the vaporizer to be transmitted into the vaporizer and thus affect volumes percent vapor output. From the pressure compensator, gas continues into vaporizing chamber (*5*). This chamber contains liquid anesthetic agent, which is absorbed and evaporated by a special wick assembly. As fresh gas moves through the vaporizing chamber, it is fully saturated with anesthetic vapor. Saturated gas leaves the chamber through a control cone (*6*). The cone is adjustable with concentration knob (*3*). Saturated vapor and fresh gas that did not pass through the vaporizing chamber are combined and leave through the fresh gas outlet (*10*). Combination of the bypass opening (*7*) and control cone opening (*6*) determines volumes percent vapor output. The expansion element (*8*) reduces vaporizing chamber gas flow as temperature increases. N_2O, nitrous oxide.

TABLE 39-3 Gas Flow Splitting Ratios at 20°C[a]

	Halothane	Enflurane	Isoflurane	Methoxyflurane	Sevoflurane
1%	46:1	29:1	44;1	1.7:1	25:1
2%	22:1	14:1	21:1	0.36:1	12:1
3%	14:1	9:1	14:1	[b]	7:1

[a]Ratios are not given for desflurane because the vaporizer for this agent (Datex-Ohmeda Tec 6; Dräger D-Vapor) uses a different design from that used for the above agents.

[b]Maximum possible concentration is 2.7% at 20°C; see Table 39-2.

Reprinted from Eisenkraft JB: Anesthesia vaporizers. In: Ehrenwerth J, Eisenkraft JB, ed. *Anesthesia Equipment: Principles and Applications*. St. Louis, MO: Mosby-Year Book, 1993:63, with permission from Elsevier.

orifice opens wider.[14] The principle of differential expansion of metals is applied similarly in the Dräger Vapor 19.1 vaporizers, in which an expansion element increases bypass gas flow as temperature increases (Fig. 39-14, component 8).

The vapor pressures of the potent volatile anesthetics vary nonlinearly as a function of temperature (Fig. 39-11). The automatic temperature compensation mechanisms described are linear in terms of expansion coefficients of materials. When these affect the size of the orifice that they control, however, the compensation mechanisms become nonlinear. The situation is complex, depending on the geometry of the valves and the nature of the gas flow through them. The result is that the vapor output concentration at any given vaporizer setting remains constant only within a certain range of temperatures. For example, the Dräger Vapor 19.1 vaporizers are specified as accurate to ±15% of the concentration set when used within the temperature range of 15° to 35°C at normal atmospheric pressure.[9,11] At temperatures outside this range, the resulting concentration increases beyond the upper tolerance limit despite continuing compensation. The boiling point of the volatile agent must never be allowed to be reached in the current variable-bypass vaporizers designed for enflurane, halothane, isoflurane, and sevoflurane because the vapor output concentration would otherwise be totally uncontrolled and potentially lethal.

INCORRECT FILLING OF VAPORIZERS

Modern vaporizers are agent specific. If an empty vaporizer designed for 1 agent is filled with an agent for which it was not designed, the vaporizer output may be erroneous for both agents and delivered vapor concentration.

A dangerous situation would result if a vaporizer designed for methoxyflurane (very low SVP of 20.3 mm Hg at 20°C) were erroneously filled (Table 39-2). A methoxyflurane vaporizer filled with halothane and set to deliver 1% methoxyflurane (albeit 6 MAC; Table 39-2) would deliver 14.8% (20 MAC) halothane. Set to 1 MAC (0.16%) methoxyflurane, the vaporizer makes a flow split of 16:1, similar to that of a halothane or isoflurane variable-bypass vaporizer set to deliver 2.7%.

Table 39-4 lists the outputs of erroneously filled vaporizers. Erroneous filling affects the output concentration and consequently the MAC (MAP, MAPP) or potency output of the vaporizer. Thus, an enflurane vaporizer set to deliver 2% (1.19 MAC) but filled with halothane at 22°C will deliver 3.21% (4.01 MAC) halothane, that is, 3.3 times the anticipated anesthetic potency output.[15]

Erroneous filling of vaporizers can be prevented by careful attention to the specific agent and the vaporizer when filling is performed. In the United States, agent-specific filling devices are standard on modern vaporizers. Liquid anesthetic agents are commercially available packaged in bottles that have an agent-specific, color-coded collar. One end of the agent-specific filling device fits the collar on the agent bottle, and the other end fits only the vaporizer designed for that agent. An agent-specific filling system assumes even greater importance with desflurane (see Desflurane and the Tec 6 Vaporizer and Table 39-2). Keyed filling systems also decrease contamination of the operating room atmosphere during vaporizer filling.

TABLE 39-4 Output in Percent and Minimum Alveolar Concentration (MAC) in O_2 of Erroneously Filled Vaporizers at 22°C

Vaporizer	Liquid	Setting (%)	Output (%)	Output MAC
Halothane	Halothane	1.0	1.00	1.25
	Enflurane	1.0	0.62	0.37
	Isoflurane	1.0	0.96	0.84
Enflurane	Enflurane	2.0	2.0	1.19
	Isoflurane	2.0	3.09	2.69
	Halothane	2.0	3.21	4.01
Isoflurane	Isoflurane	1.5	1.50	1.30
	Halothane	1.5	1.56	1.95
	Enflurane	1.5	0.97	0.57

Reproduced with permission from Bruce DL, Linde HW. Vaporization of mixed liquids. *Anesthesiology.* 1984;60:342.

VAPORIZATION OF MIXED ANESTHETIC LIQUIDS

A more likely scenario is that an agent-specific variable-bypass vaporizer partially filled with correct agent is topped off with an incorrect agent.[16] The situation here is more complex, vaporizer output is less easily predicted, and large errors in vapor administration can occur. Halothane, enflurane, and isoflurane, when mixed, do not react chemically but do influence the extent of each other's ease of vaporization. Halothane facilitates the vaporization of both enflurane and isoflurane and in the process is itself more likely to vaporize.[17] The clinical consequences depend on the potencies of each of the mixed agents as well as the delivered vapor concentrations. If a halothane vaporizer 25% full is refilled to 100% with isoflurane and set to deliver 1%, the halothane output is 0.41% (0.51 MAC), and the isoflurane output is 0.9% (0.78 MAC) (**Table 39-5**).[18] In this case, the output potency of 1.29 MAC is not far from the 1.25 MAC (1% halothane) expected.

However, an enflurane vaporizer 25% full and set to deliver 2% (1.19 MAC) enflurane that is filled to 100% with halothane has an output of 2.43% (3.03 MAC) halothane and 0.96% (0.57 MAC) enflurane (Table 39-5).[19] This represents a total MAC of 3.6, or more than twice that intended. In any event, it is important that erroneous filling of vaporizers be avoided and that if suspected, the vaporizer be emptied, serviced, purged, and refilled with the correct agent.

FILLING OF VAPORIZERS

Vaporizers should only be filled as directed in their accompanying instructions. Overfilling or tilting of a vaporizer (free standing or by tilting the whole anesthesia machine) may result in liquid agent entering parts of the anesthesia delivery system (eg, vaporizer bypass flow) designed for gases or vapors only and might give rise to lethal concentrations of the agent.[16] If a vaporizer has been tilted and there is concern that liquid agent has leaked into the gas delivery system, then with no patient connected to the system, the vaporizer should be purged with a high flow rate of O_2 (10 L/min) from the machine flowmeter (not the O_2 flush, which bypasses the vaporizer) and with the vaporizer concentration dial set to the *maximum* concentration setting.[14] The most recent models of vaporizer (Datex-Ohmeda Tec 7; Dräger Vapor 2000 series) are designed with antispill mechanisms. Thus, to remove a Vapor 2000 vaporizer from the mounting manifold, the concentration dial must be turned past the OFF setting to the T setting, or transport mode.[18] In this setting, the sump that contains liquid agent is completely isolated from the other parts of the vaporizer, which can then be safely tilted.

Table 39-2 shows that 1 mL of liquid volatile anesthetic agent produces approximately 200 mL of vapor at 20°C. Thus, if small volumes of liquid agent enter parts of the delivery system intended for gas or vapor only, it is easy to see how potentially lethal concentrations of vapor could arise. For example, if 1 mL of liquid sevoflurane entered the patient breathing system, it would require 18.2 L of fresh gas to dilute the resulting vapor to a 1% concentration (0.5 MAC).

EFFECT OF CARRIER GAS ON VAPORIZER OUTPUT

The carrier gas used to vaporize the volatile agent in the vaporizing chamber may also affect vapor output concentration. Thus, when the carrier gas flow through a variable-bypass Ohio enflurane vaporizer (**Fig. 39-15**) was changed from N_2/O_2 to N_2O/O_2, the vapor concentration decreased for about 15 minutes and then returned to normal.[19] When the output concentration is stable with a carrier gas of N_2O/O_2, changing back to N_2/O_2 resulted in an increase in vapor concentration for about 15 minutes.

TABLE 39-5 Vaporizer Output after Incorrectly Refilling from 25% to 100% Full

			Vaporizer Outputs						
			Halothane		Enflurane		Isoflurane		
Vaporizer	Setting (%)	Refill liquid	%	MAC	%	MAC	%	MAC	Total MAC
Halothane	1.0	Enflurane	0.33	0.41	0.64	0.38	–	–	0.79
	1.0	Isoflurane	0.41	0.51	–	–	0.90	0.78	1.29
Enflurane	2.0	Halothane	2.43	3.03	0.96	0.57	–	–	3.60
Isoflurane	1.5	Halothane	1.28	1.60	–	–	0.57	0.50	2.10

MAC, minimum alveolar concentration.

Reproduced with permission from Bruce DL, Linde HW. Vaporization of mixed anesthetic liquids. *Anesthesiology.* 1984;60:342.

The explanation for this observed effect is the solubility of N_2O in the liquid volatile agents. When N_2O/O_2 first enters the vaporizing chamber, some N_2O gas physically dissolves in the liquid agent, and the vaporizing chamber output decreases until the liquid has become saturated with N_2O. Conversely, when N_2O is discontinued as the carrier gas, the N_2O gas that is dissolved in the liquid anesthetic comes out of solution and represents, in effect, additional gas flow to the vaporizing chamber. The solubility of N_2O is approximately 4.5 mL per mL of liquid anesthetic. Thus, 100 mL of halothane liquid, when fully saturated with N_2O, can dissolve approximately 450 mL of N_2O. Such a volume of N_2O, being added to the vaporizing chamber flow over a brief period when N_2O has been discontinued, causes the observed increase in vaporizer output concentration.

CHANGES IN BAROMETRIC PRESSURE

Although vaporizers are most often used at ambient pressures of approximately 760 mm Hg (1 atm at sea level), they may also be used under hypobaric (eg, at increased altitude) or hyperbaric (eg, in a hyperbaric chamber) conditions.[20]

Hypobaric Conditions Because few reports discuss the use of vaporizers under hypobaric conditions, the theoretic considerations applying to such use are discussed here. Consider a variable-bypass vaporizer set to deliver 1% sevoflurane (0.5 MAC at 760 mm Hg atmospheric pressure) that is being used at an ambient pressure of 500 mm Hg (equivalent to an altitude of approximately 10 000 feet above sea level) and at a temperature of 20°C (**Fig. 39-16**). In the vaporizing chamber, sevoflurane has an SVP of 160 mm Hg (at 20°C), but this now represents 160/500 = 32 vol%. The vaporizer, set to deliver 1% under normal conditions, creates a splitting ratio of 25:1 (Table 39-3) between bypass and vaporizing chamber flows. If the total gas flow to the vaporizer is 2600 mL/min (Fig. 39-16), 2500 mL/min enters the bypass and 100 mL/min of carrier gas enters the vaporizing chamber. This 100 mL represents 68% of the volume there because sevoflurane represents the other 32 vol% (100% – 68%). Emerging from the chamber is 100 mL/min of carrier gas plus ([100/68] × 32) = 47 mL/min of sevoflurane vapor. When the vaporizing chamber and bypass flows merge, the 47 mL/min of sevoflurane vapor are diluted in a total volume of 2647 mL/min (2500 + 100 + 47), giving a sevoflurane concentration of 1.8 vol%. This is almost double the dialed-in concentration in terms of volumes percent.

Now consider partial pressures. If sevoflurane represents 1.8% of the gas mixture by volume, its partial pressure in the emerging mixture is 1.8 × 500, or 9 mm Hg. In terms of anesthetic potency, this represents 9/16, or 0.6 MAC because the P_{MAC1} of sevoflurane is 16 mm Hg (Table 39-1). Thus, in theory, when used at an ambient pressure of 500 mm Hg, the variable-bypass sevoflurane vaporizer set to 1% (vol/vol) would deliver almost twice (1.8 vs.1.0) the dialed-in concentration in volumes percent but only 0.6/0.5 MAC, or 1.2 times the anesthetic potency expected.

Hyperbaric Conditions Consider a variable-bypass isoflurane vaporizer set to deliver 2% (1.74 MAC at 760 mm Hg atmospheric pressure) isoflurane vapor used at 20°C and 3 atm (3 × 760 = 2280 mm Hg), as may exist in a hyperbaric chamber (**Fig. 39-17**).

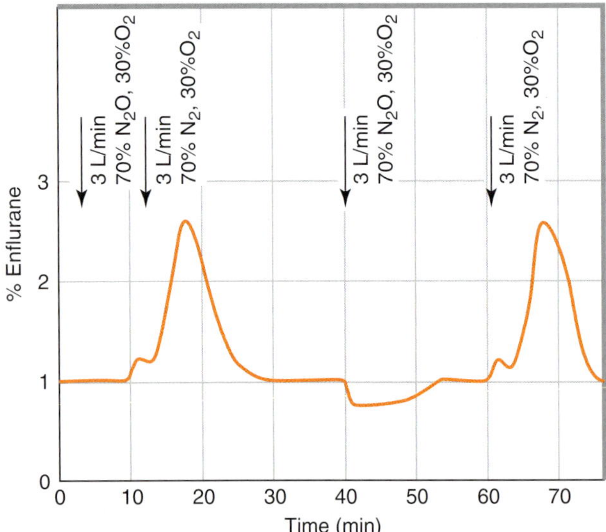

FIGURE 39-15. Effect of carrier gas composition on output of Ohio enflurane variable-bypass vaporizer. See text for details. N_2O, nitrous oxide.

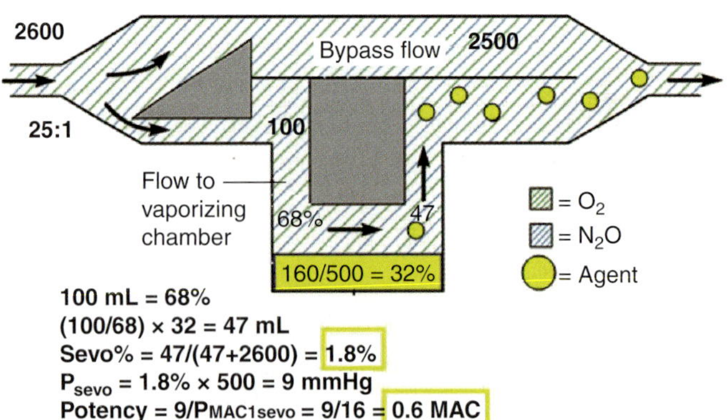

FIGURE 39-16. Use of variable-bypass sevoflurane vaporizer under hypobaric conditions. The vaporizer is set to deliver 1% (vol/vol) and is being used at ambient pressure of 500 mm Hg. See text for details.

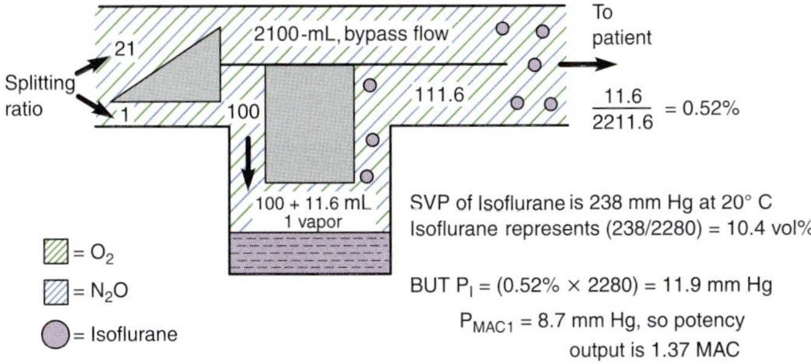

FIGURE 39-17. Use of a variable-bypass isoflurane vaporizer under hyperbaric conditions. The vaporizer is set to deliver 2% (vol/vol) and is being used at ambient P_I pressure of 2280 mm Hg (3 atm). See text for details.

In the vaporizing chamber, the SVP of isoflurane is 238 mm Hg (Table 39-2), and the isoflurane concentration is 10.4 vol% ([238/2280] × 100). A variable-bypass isoflurane vaporizer set to deliver 2% creates a splitting ratio of 21:1 for the FGF (Table 39-3). If the total gas flow to the vaporizer is 2200 mL/min, 2100 mL enters the bypass, and 100 mL of carrier gas enters the vaporizing chamber per minute (Fig. 39-17). This 100 mL represents 89.6% (100 – 10.4) of the total gas there; the remainder is isoflurane vapor. The amount of isoflurane vapor evolved is ([100/89.6] × 10.4) = 11.6 mL/min. This volume, diluted in 2100 + 100 + 11.64 gives 11.6/2211.6, or 0.52% isoflurane vapor by volume. This is 0.26 (0.52/2.0) of what was set on the concentration dial in terms of volumes percent.

How about potency? The partial pressure of isoflurane in the emerging gas mixture is 11.9 mm Hg (0.52% × 2280). Dividing by the P_{MAC1} for isoflurane of 8.7 mm Hg (Table 39-1) gives a potency output of 1.37 MAC (11.9/8.7). Thus, the isoflurane vaporizer, set to deliver 1.74 MAC under conditions of 1 atm pressure, delivers 1.37 MAC at 3 atm, or about 0.80 times the anesthetic potency expected.

These examples show that although changes in ambient pressure may have a great effect on vapor concentration output in terms of volumes percent, the anesthetic potency (MAC) output is changed less drastically. In the examples discussed, it was assumed that the set splitting ratios (Table 39-3) would be maintained constant as ambient pressure changed. In reality, changes in gas density occur with changes in ambient pressure and may affect the splitting ratios slightly. The anesthetic potency output expected for any given vaporizer setting is relatively unchanged, by ambient pressure, even though vapor concentration (vol/vol) may be altered considerably.[21] Again, vaporizer output concentration expressed in volumes percent is of limited value unless converted to MAC units using the concept of pressures as described in the foregoing examples.[12,13,21]

ARRANGEMENT OF VAPORIZERS

Some (now obsolete) anesthesia machines had up to 3 variable-bypass vaporizers arranged in series such that fresh gas from the flowmeters passed through each vaporizer to reach the common gas outlet of the anesthesia machine. Without an interlock system, which permits only 1 vaporizer to be in use at any time, it was possible to have all 3 vaporizers turned on simultaneously. Apart from potentially overdosing the patient, the agent from the upstream vaporizer could contaminate the liquid agent(s) in the downstream vaporizer(s). During subsequent use, the output of the downstream vaporizer would be contaminated. The resulting concentrations in the emerging gas and vapor mixture would be indeterminate and might even be lethal.[22]

With modern workstations, only 1 vaporizer can be on at any time. The recent standards require that a system must be provided that isolates the vaporizers from each other and prevents gas from passing through the vaporizing chamber of 1 vaporizer and then through that of another.[1,2] This specification is met by use of an interlock system. All contemporary workstations that permit the mounting of more than one vaporizer incorporate a manufacturer-specific interlock or exclusion system. In addition, one must never place a freestanding vaporizer in series between the machine common gas outlet and the patient circuit. Not only would this defeat the exclusion system, but operation of the oxygen flush might also cause delivery of undesirably large amounts of agent to the patient circuit.

CALIBRATION AND CHECKING OF VAPORIZER OUTPUTS

Vaporizers should be regularly serviced according to the manufacturer's recommendations and their outputs checked to ensure that a malfunction does not exist. Thus, the vaporizer dial is set to deliver a certain concentration in oxygen (GE-Datex) or air (Dräger). The actual output concentration is measured by an anesthetic agent analyzer that samples gas via a connector placed at the common gas outlet of the anesthesia machine.

DESFLURANE AND THE TEC 6 VAPORIZER

With an SVP of 669 mm Hg at 20°C and a boiling point of 22.8°C, desflurane is extremely volatile. Clearly, this agent cannot be administered using the conventional (mechanical flow splitting) variable-bypass design of vaporizer used for halothane, enflurane, isoflurane, and sevoflurane. If such a variable-bypass vaporizer were somehow filled with desflurane, an increase in temperature to above 22.8°C would result in the desflurane boiling in the vaporizing chamber and uncontrolled output from the vaporizer. The consequences of misfilling contemporary agent-specific variable-bypass vaporizers with desflurane at 22°C have been predicted.[21] Thus, an enflurane vaporizer set to deliver 3 MAC (~5% enflurane) would deliver 16 MAC (~96%) desflurane at 22°C.

Datex-Ohmeda (Steeton, UK) designed the Tec 6 concentration-calibrated vaporizer for the controlled administration of desflurane. It was designed to make the practical aspects of the clinical administration of desflurane no different from that of other potent inhaled agents using their Tec series of vaporizers (**Fig. 39-18A**).[23,24]

The principle of operation of the Tec 6 is that liquid desflurane is heated in a chamber (the sump) to 39°C to produce vapor under pressure (~1500 mm Hg or 2 atm absolute) analogous to having a reservoir of compressed gas in a tank (**Fig. 39-19**). The vapor leaves the sump (item 9) via a variable pressure-regulating valve (item 7), the opening of which is continuously adjusted according to the output from pressure transducers (items 3 and 4) to ensure that the pressure of the desflurane vapor entering the rotary valve in the user-controlled concentration dial is the same as the pressure generated by the fresh gas inflow (from the anesthesia machine flowmeters) into a fixed restrictor. The concentration dial and rotary valve control the quantity of desflurane vapor added to the FGF so that what emerges from the vaporizer outlet is the dialed-in concentration of desflurane. Unlike other concentration-calibrated vaporizers (eg, GE-Datex-Ohmeda Tec 5, Dräger Vapor 19.1), which are of variable-bypass design, no fresh gas enters the desflurane sump in the Tec 6.

The Tec 6 is calibrated by the manufacturer using 100% oxygen as the fresh gas. As the oxygen enters the vaporizer, it flows through a fixed restrictor (Fig. 39-19, item 2, and **Fig. 39-20**). This is a device that offers a fixed resistance, *resistance* being defined as change in pressure per unit of flow. The resistance is approximately 10 cm H_2O/L/min over a wide range of gas flows. The back pressure created by gas flowing through the fixed restrictor is therefore proportional to the main gas flow (as set on the machine flowmeters) and changes according to Poiseuille's law (see Gas Flow-Control Systems above). By sensing this back pressure (via a pressure transducer) and ensuring that the pressure of the desflurane vapor entering the variable restrictor is always made equal to this pressure (via the control electronics and variable pressure control valve), the variable restrictor provides a means to control the concentration of desflurane (Fig. 39-20).

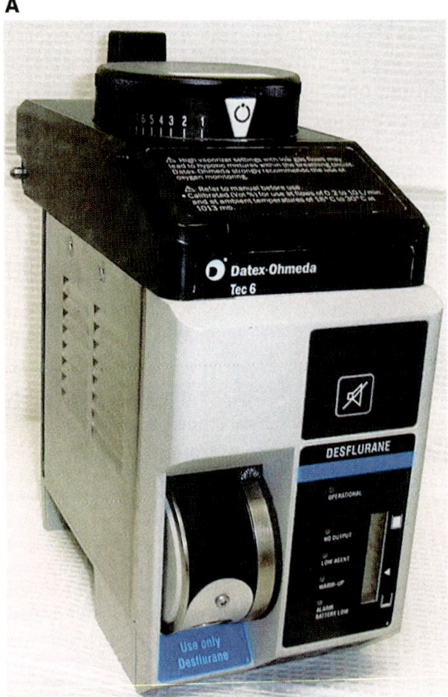

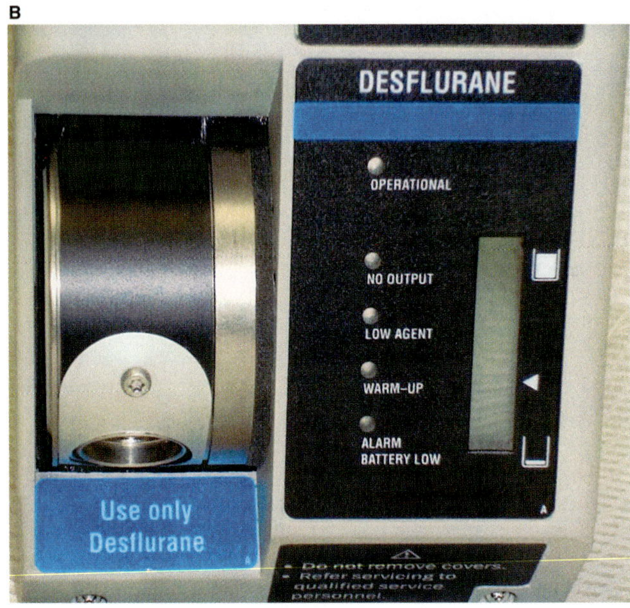

FIGURE 39-18. A. Tec 6 vaporizer for delivery of desflurane. **B**. Close-up of front panel showing status and warning lights and liquid crystal display of agent level.

Special Considerations

Design Features of the Tec 6 (Figs. 39-18 to 39-20) The sump, when full, contains 450 mL of liquid desflurane. Because the sump is pressurized to 1500 mm Hg, the agent level is sensed electronically and shown on a liquid crystal display (LCD) rather than the sight-glass used in variable-bypass vaporizers. When the vaporizer is energized by connecting the power cord to an electrical outlet, a heater in the sump heats the agent to 39°C and maintains that temperature via thermostatic controls. While the agent is being heated, the sump shut-off valve is held closed, keeping the agent in the sump. During the warm-up period, the vaporizer is not operational because the sump shut-off valve remains closed, and a solenoid-locking device prevents the concentration dial from being turned on. When it is operational (ie, at 39°C), the dial lock is released, and when the dial is turned on, the sump shut-off valve is opened, permitting desflurane vapor to flow to the pressure regulating valve.[23,24]

To prevent condensation ("rain out") of desflurane vapor, in addition to the heater in the sump, there are heaters in the rotary valve and in the vicinity of the pressure transducers that sense the back pressures created by the main gas flow and by the flow of desflurane vapor.

The Tec 6 thus differs considerably from variable-bypass vaporizers. None of the fresh gas flow enters the vaporizing chamber. The Tec 6 requires electrical power and incorporates sophisticated electronics to ensure normal operation and a display panel to inform the user about its operational status. It also has alarms to alert to any malfunction, in the event of which the sump shut-off valve closes (Fig. 39-20).

Filling System Because of its high SVP, desflurane is supplied in plastic-coated glass bottles to which a patented agent-specific filling device (Saf-T-Fill) is firmly attached. The vaporizer incorporates an agent-specific filling system that permits filling of the sump at any time, including when the vaporizer is in use. This may be important because of desflurane's low blood-to-gas partition coefficient.

During filling, the bottle is locked to the vaporizer-filling system and the high pressure of vapor in the sump at 39°C is transmitted to the interior of the bottle, which helps to drive liquid desflurane from the bottle into the sump. When filling is complete, the bottle is disconnected from the vaporizer fill system, and the valve on the bottle closes to avoid loss or spillage of agent. At this time, the bottle contains vapor at 39°C and a pressure of 1500 mm Hg. As the bottle and its contents cool to room temperature, the pressure in the bottle decreases toward atmospheric (760 mm Hg at 22.8°C).

Effect of Fresh Gas Composition on Performance The Tec 6 is calibrated at the factory using 100% O_2. Performance accuracy at 5 L/min oxygen is specified as ±0.5% of the delivered agent or ±15% of the dial setting, whichever is greater.[23]

The Tec 6 design uses back pressure from laminar gas flow through the fixed restrictor to infer flow (Fig. 39-20). If the viscosity of the gas flowing through the fixed resistor were to decrease, then the same flow would result in a lower back pressure. This back pressure is used to determine the pressure of desflurane into the variable restrictor in the concentration dial. A lower back pressure results in a lower flow of desflurane vapor through the variable restrictor.

Of the gases on the anesthesia machine, O_2 is the most viscous and N_2O the least viscous. Thus, changing the main gas flow composition from O_2 to O_2/N_2O decreases fresh gas viscosity and the output concentration of desflurane from that set on the dial. Differences between the actual concentration produced and the dial setting are greatest (≤20% of dial setting) with high concentrations of N_2O at low gas flow rates. The clinical implications of this are minimal, however, because the anesthetic effect lost by the decrease in desflurane is offset by the effect of the N_2O.[23]

Effects of Altitude on Output The Tec 6 accurately delivers the dialed-in concentration of desflurane in terms of volumes percent even at altitudes different than sea level. At sea level, 7% desflurane (1 MAC) creates a P_{des} of (7% × 760 mm Hg) = 53 mm Hg (the P_{MAC1}; Table 39-2). At high altitude, if the ambient pressure were 500 mm Hg, the same 7% desflurane would create a P_{des} of only 35 mm Hg (7% × 500), which is only 0.66 of the P_{MAC1}. To compensate for this decrease in potency output at increased altitude, a higher concentration (in this case, 10% because 10% × 500 = 50 mm Hg) must be set on the dial.

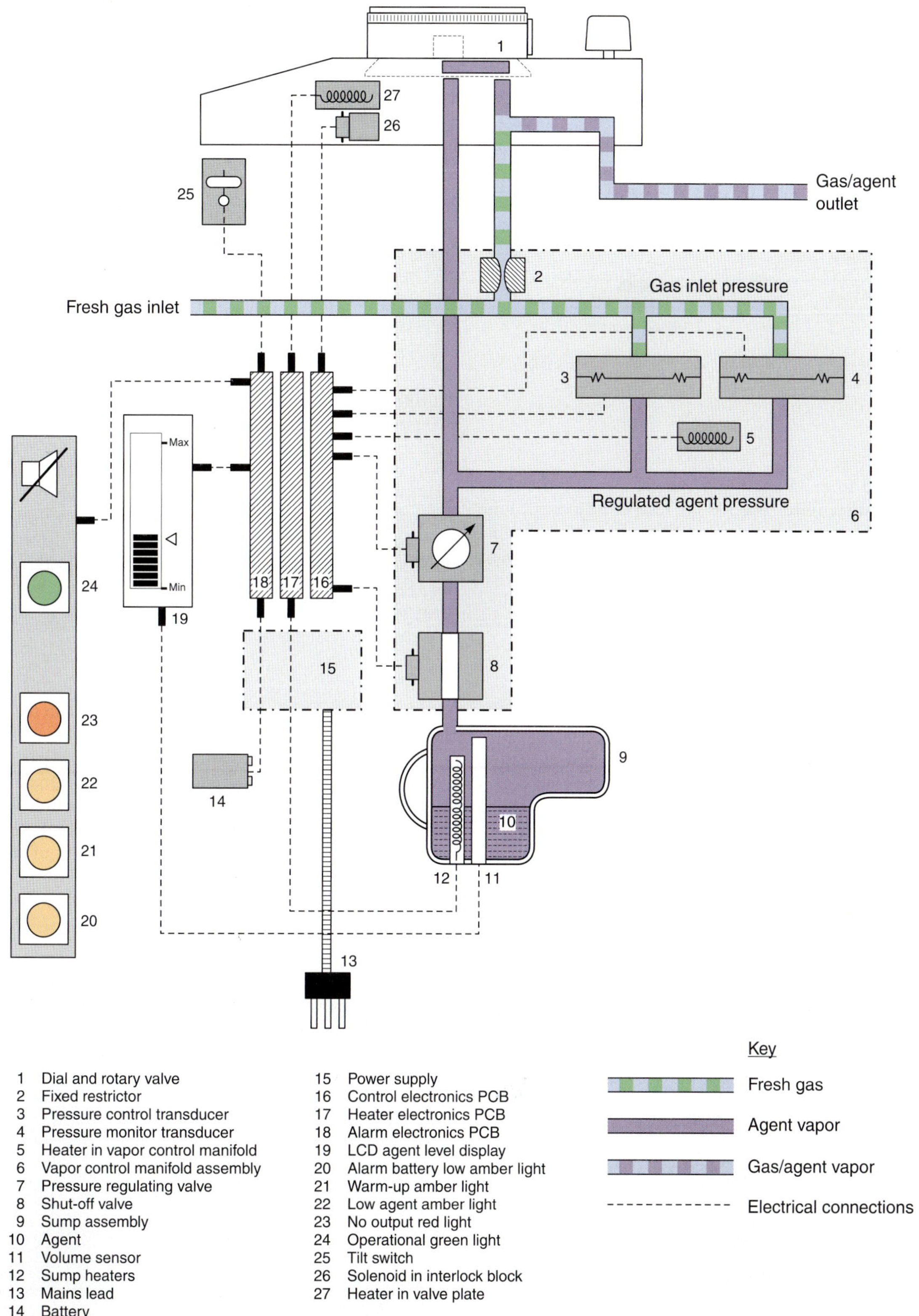

FIGURE 39-19. Schematic of the Tec 6 vaporizer for desflurane. LCD, liquid crystal display; PCB, printed circuit board.

Conversely, at higher ambient pressures, a lower concentration dial setting would be indicated. Recommendations as to how the dial setting should be changed at altitude are provided in the operator's manual.[23]

Interlock System and Dräger D-Vapor Although the Tec 6 is manufactured by GE-Datex-Ohmeda and is mountable on their patented Select-a-Tec manifold on a GE-Datex-Ohmeda anesthesia machine, a version is also available for mounting on Dräger anesthesia workstations. Recently, Dräger introduced the D-Vapor desflurane vaporizer to its Vapor 2000 series (**Fig. 39-21**). The operating principles are the same as in the Tec 6, but it weighs significantly less. Similar to other vaporizers in their Vapor 2000 series, the D-Vapor is hermetically

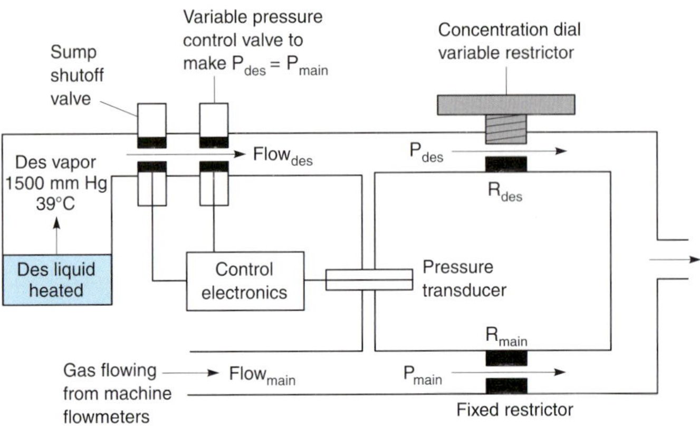

FIGURE 39-20. Tec 6 vaporizer simplified to illustrate principles of operation. See text for details.

sealed when removed from an anesthesia system, allowing transport in any position even when filled. The 300-mL reservoir capacity of the tank can hold the entire contents of a standard anesthetic agent bottle. Similar to the Tec 6, the D-Vapor is electrically powered, but it also features 5 minutes of emergency battery operation, which ensures that dose settings remain constant even during a brief power failure. Unlike the Tec 6, the D-Vapor has a sight glass through which the agent level can be seen directly.

ALADIN VAPORIZING SYSTEM

Advances in technology and computerization of the workstation have led to the development of a new design of variable-bypass, electrically powered Aladin vaporizing system that is used in the GE-Datex S5/ADU and Aisys workstations. The principles of operation differ from those of earlier variable-bypass vaporizers and from the Tec 6 design of vaporizers already discussed.

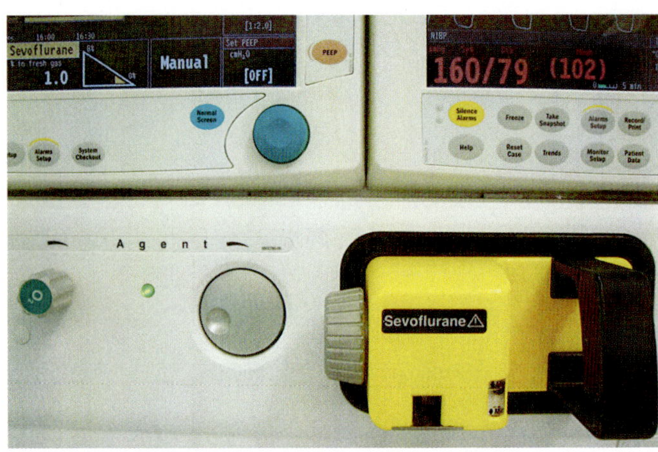

FIGURE 39-22. Aladin vaporizing system shown on a GE-Datex-Ohmeda Anesthesia Delivery Unit (ADU) workstation. The cassette is agent specific (in this case, sevoflurane). The dial to the left of the cassette is the concentration control. The (green) pilot light to the left of the dial indicates that the vaporizer is on. The dialed-in agent concentration (1%) is shown at the bottom of the left-hand screen. Although this is an electronically controlled vaporizing system, agent concentration in the ADU is *increased* by turning the dial in a *counterclockwise* direction, analogous to the dial on a traditional variable-bypass vaporizer (eg, Tec 7, Dräger Vapor 2000). (The Aladin system is also used in the GE Aisys workstations, but there, agent concentration is *increased* by turning the com wheel in a *clockwise* direction.)

The Aladin vaporizer consists of 2 separate parts that must be joined to produce a functioning vaporizer. One is a sump, the detachable agent-specific Aladin cassette, that can hold up to 250 mL of liquid agent (**Fig. 39-22**). Each anesthetic agent, including desflurane, has its own cassette made unique by means of an agent-specific fill system (eg, Saf-T-Fil for desflurane; key fill or Quick-Fill for other agents) (**Fig. 39-23**). Thus, 5 different cassettes are available,

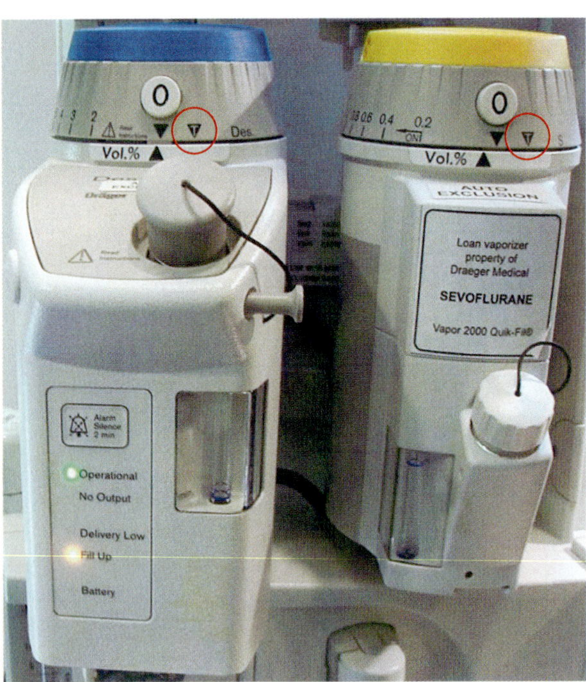

FIGURE 39-21. Left. Dräger D-Vapor desflurane vaporizer. **Right.** Dräger Vapor 2000 sevoflurane vaporizer. Note the T position (for Transport mode) on the concentration dial (*circled*).

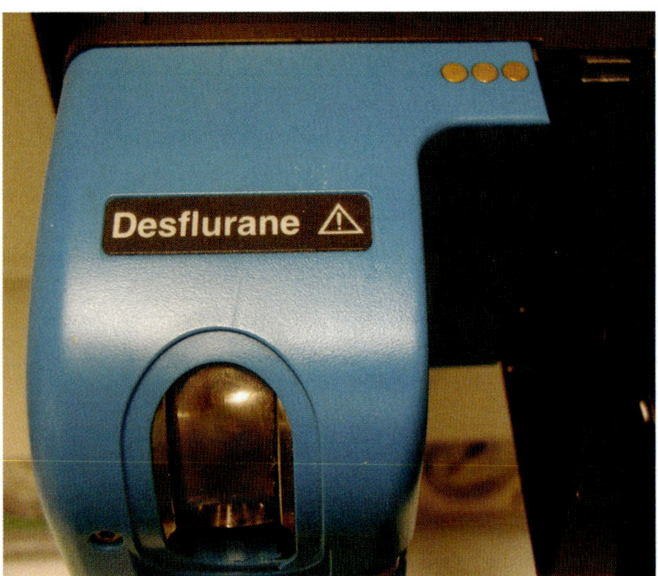

FIGURE 39-23. Aladin cassette for desflurane. Note the desflurane-specific Saf-t-fil port for filling the cassette. The 3 brass terminals allow the fill status to be monitored electronically and displayed on the screen of the workstation.

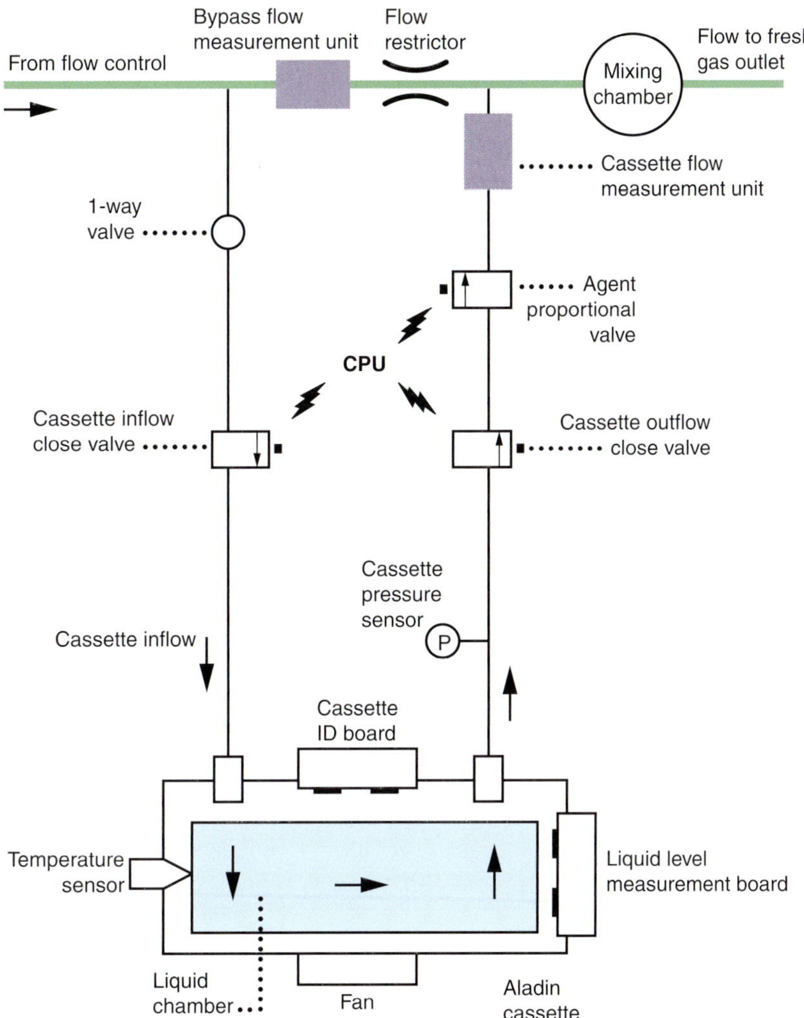

FIGURE 39-24. Schematic showing principles of operation of the Aladin vaporizing system used on some of the GE-Datex-Ohmeda workstations. CPU, central processing unit; P, pressure sensor.

1 for each of the presently available potent inhaled agents. The second part of the vaporizer is a component of the ADU or Aisys workstation and contains the concentration-control hardware and software. The agent-specific cassette identifies itself to the second part of the vaporizer by the arrangements of signature magnets at the top of the cassette. The ADU and Aisys workstations monitor and control gas and vapor at several points. They monitor and control flow through the N_2O, O_2, and air flowmeters and do not permit the delivered oxygen concentration to fall below 25% at the workstation's common gas outlet. Gas flow from these sources is delivered to or bypasses the anesthetic in the sump. The flow of agent at its saturated vapor concentration issuing from the sump, and the bypass flow are monitored and adjusted by hardware, as governed by software algorithms to produce the dialed-in concentration of anesthetic. The algorithms take into account the anesthetic agent, temperatures, and gas pressures in the sump and bypass (each separately measured) (**Fig. 39-24**). One-way valves at the inlet and outlet of the Aladin cassette ensure unidirectional flow of gas and vapor. Thus, vapor cannot leave the cassette through the gas inlet pathway. This is especially important in the desflurane cassette.

The agent wheel (an electronic control) on the front panel of the ADU or com wheel on the Aisys workstation is used to set the desired concentration of agent to be delivered to the breathing system. A green light-emitting diode (LED) indicates that the vaporizer is on (Fig. 39-22). The vaporizer is controlled via a central processing unit (CPU). See Figure 39-24 for principles of operation.[25] The flow restrictor in the bypass causes fresh gas from the gas flow controls to be split into a bypass flow and a flow that passes through a unidirectional valve (which prevents backflow) to the Aladin cassette. The latter is an agent-specific cartridge that contains liquid anesthetic at its saturated vapor concentration at the ambient temperature (eg, 21 vol% for sevoflurane at 20°C). Continuous monitoring of temperature and pressure in the cassette means that the agent vapor concentration there is always known. The concentration of anesthetic vapor delivered to the common gas outlet of the machine is determined by the concentration of agent vapor in the cassette and the ratio of cassette outflow to the bypass flow, both of which are measured continuously. The delivered concentration is controlled by the position of the agent proportional valve, which is set continuously according to information from the agent controller (ie, CPU).

Each Aladin cassette is essentially a flow-over vaporizer because it contains liquid agent that is vaporized as fresh gas flows between the agent-soaked wicks and baffles (**Figs. 39-25** and **39-26**). It is equivalent to the sump of a traditional variable-bypass vaporizer, but because it does not incorporate bypass flow channels, tilting the cassette during handling, changing, or filling is not hazardous.

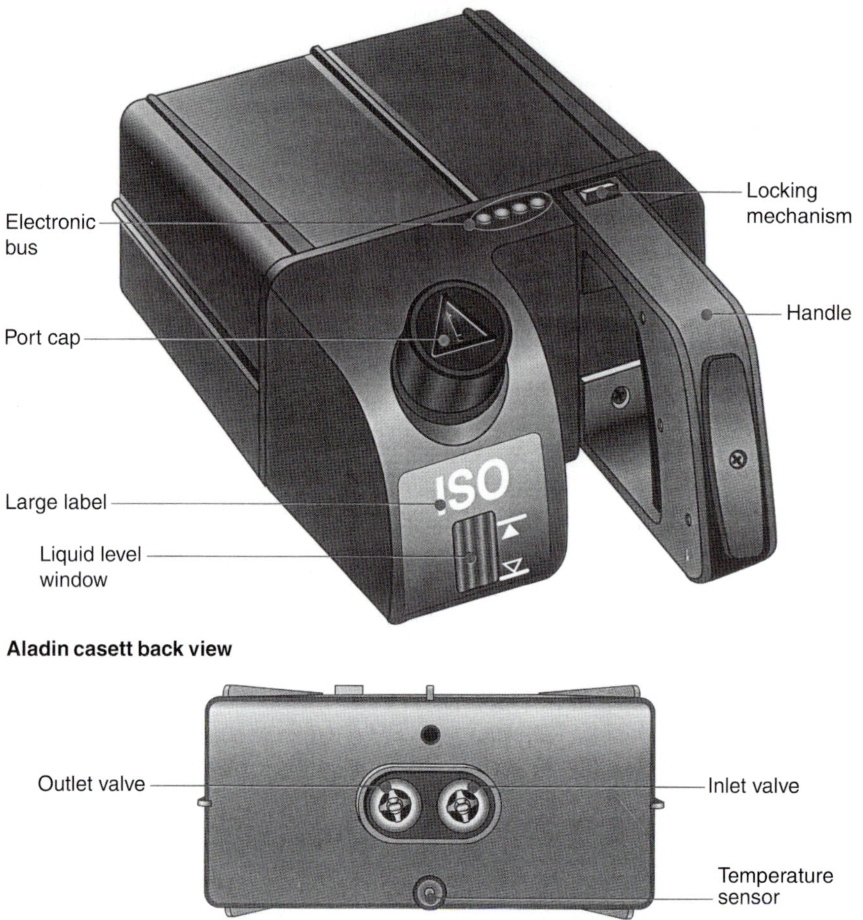

FIGURE 39-25. Aladin cartridge specific for isoflurane. The electronic bus (electrical contacts) allows the agent fill status to be monitored by the central processing unit (CPU); pressure sensor (p).

The Aladin cassette for desflurane incorporates an electronic liquid level measuring device so that if less than 10% liquid desflurane (<25 mL) remains, an alarm message is displayed (Fig. 39-23). If the temperature is below 22.8°C (boiling point of desflurane), fresh gas must enter the cassette for vapor to be delivered via the exit connection. If the temperature is above 22.8°C, no fresh gas inflow is needed, and the desflurane vapor is released by controlling the outflow valve. Desflurane vapor cannot exit the cassette via the gas inlet pathway because of the unidirectional valve. A fan is mounted inside the fresh gas control unit beneath the Aladin cassette housing and is required to heat the cassette when large amounts of agent are being vaporized. The fan operates when the cassette temperature is below 17°C and stops when it is above 20°C.

The Aladin vaporizing system offers certain advantages, the greatest of which is that the CPU can control the concentration of any of the available potent inhaled anesthetic agents. Separate vaporizers (or at least their flow-splitting mechanisms) are not required for each agent. An obvious disadvantage is that in the event of a prolonged power loss (ie, after the backup battery has been depleted), delivery of the volatile agent will cease. In contrast, conventional mechanical Tec-type vaporizers will function as long as there is a source of compressed gas to the machine.

COMMON GAS OUTLET AND OUTLET CHECK VALVES

The fresh gas mixture produced by the settings of the flow controls for O_2, N_2O, and other gases and vapor from one concentration-calibrated vaporizer exit the anesthesia machine via the common gas outlet. Situated between the vaporizer and the common gas outlet, some machines (Datex-Ohmeda Modulus I and Modulus II) have an outlet check valve and a pressure relief valve that opens at a pressure of 120 to 150 mm Hg (2.3-2.9 psig) (Fig. 39-2). The pressure-relief valve, as its name suggests, prevents the buildup of excessive pressures upstream of the outlet check valve. These components are located upstream from where the O_2 flush flow would join to pass to the common gas outlet. The Datex-Ohmeda Excel and Aestiva machines have an outlet check valve and a pressure relief valve (opening pressure threshold, 5 psig) that is located downstream of the outlet check valve.

The purpose of the outlet check valve, when present, is to prevent reverse gas flow, which would permit gas to go back into the variable-bypass (older Tec-type) vaporizer if the latter did not have its own outlet check valve or specialized design. This "pumping" effect, if not prevented, could cause increased vaporizer output concentrations.

Dräger Narkomed models 2A, 2B, 3, and 4 are designed so as not to require an outlet check valve. Any pumping effect is eliminated by special design of the Vapor vaporizer (Fig. 39-14, component 4). The Datex-Ohmeda Modulus II Plus and Modulus CD machines are equipped with Datex-Ohmeda Tec 5 or Tec 7 that incorporate a baffle system and a specially designed manifold to prevent the pumping effect, making an outlet check valve unnecessary on these machines. Nevertheless, the Datex-Ohmeda Modulus II Plus and Modulus CD machines do have pressure-relief valves (Fig. 39-2). Dräger Narkomed 2A, 2B, 3, and 4 machines do not require a separate pressure-relief valve.[11] In these machines, pressure-relief opening (threshold ~18 psig), if required, takes place through the specially designed Dräger Vapor

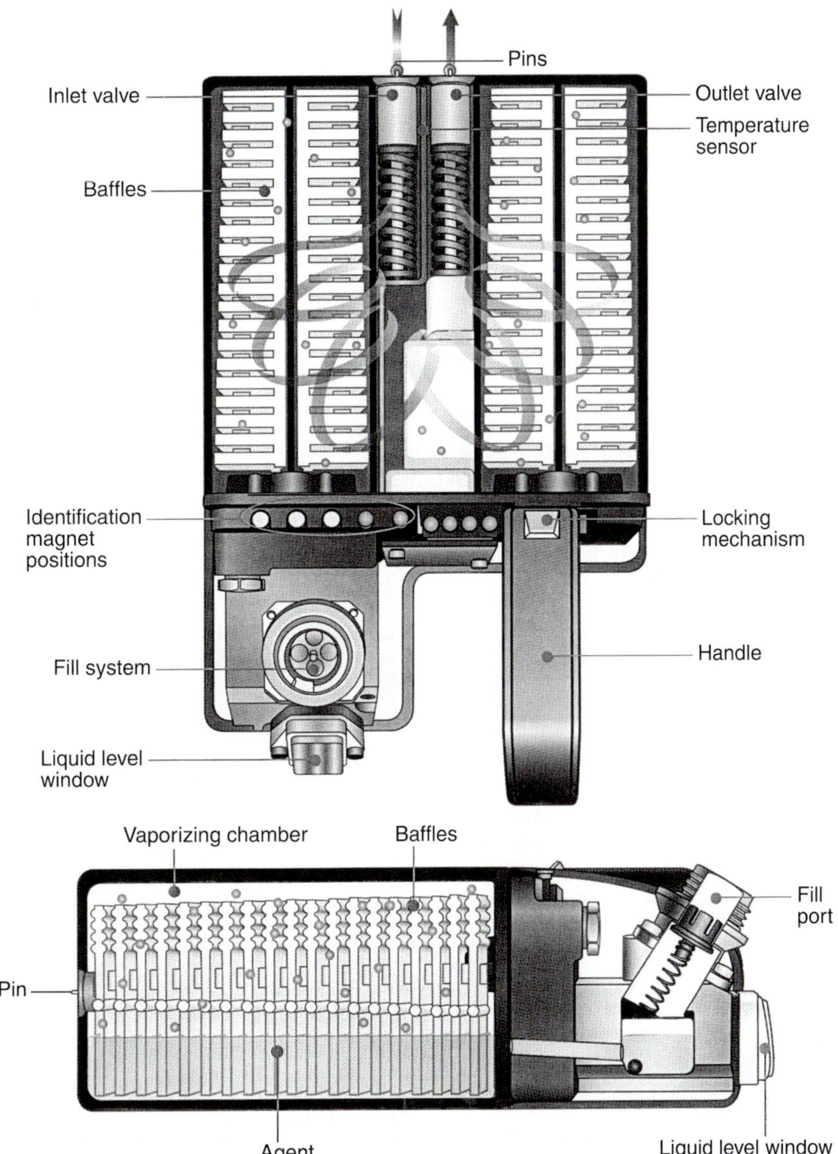

FIGURE 39-26. Schematic cross-section of Aladin cartridge showing that it is the same as the agent-specific sump of a standard variable-bypass vaporizer with wicks and baffles to increase the surface area for evaporation of the anesthetic agent. [Courtesy of GE-Datex-Ohmeda, a Division of GE Health Care, Madison, WI.]

vaporizers. The presence or absence of an outlet check valve and pressure-relief valve is important when considering how to test the low-pressure system of the anesthesia machine for leaks.

The workstation standard requires that when the common gas outlet is connected to the breathing system by a fresh gas supply hose (the usual arrangement in most workstations), the common gas outlet should be provided with a manufacturer-specific retaining device. It may have a 15-mm female fitting or a 15-mm or 22-mm coaxial fitting.[1,2] Machines should have only 1 common gas outlet. The retaining device's purpose is to help prevent disconnection or misconnections between the machine common gas outlet and the patient circuit, which could result in patient injury. Many contemporary workstations (eg, GE-Datex Aestiva, Aespire, Aisys; Dräger Apollo) do not have a visible CGO and hose connection between the machine and circle system. The GE-Datex Aestiva, however, has an auxiliary CGO that can be accessed if other than a circle system is used (eg, Bain) or to leak check the low-pressure system of the machine (see Anesthesia Machine Checkout; Testing for Leaks in the Anesthesia Machine and Breathing System). An auxiliary CGO is an option on the GE Aisys workstation.

ANESTHESIA BREATHING SYSTEMS

The anesthesia breathing system or circuit represents a mini environment for respiratory gas exchange. The FGF from the anesthesia machine delivers known volumes and concentrations of O_2, N_2O (and possibly air or helium), and potent inhaled anesthetic to the circuit, and gases are vented from the circuit to the waste gas scavenging system. In some arrangements, high FGFs are used, in which case the patient's inspired gas concentrations approximate those in the fresh gas supply. Other circuits, such as the adult circle system, use lower FGFs and rely on an absorption system for CO_2. In the circle breathing system, when low FGFs are used, the composition of the inspired gas may be quite different from that of the fresh gas inflow.

Adult anesthesia circuits are composed of corrugated 22-mm-diameter tubing, a reservoir bag, and connecting piece or elbow to the patient's airway. They may or may not also include a valve or valves. How these items are arranged gives the resulting circuit its functional characteristics. Breathing systems are generally classified as rebreathing, having no CO_2 absorption system (ie, Mapleson classification circuits A-F), or nonrebreathing, having a CO_2 absorber (eg, circle system).

REBREATHING SYSTEMS

Figure 39-27 shows the circuits assigned letters according to the Mapleson classification.[26] Whereas in circuits A, B, and C, the APL (pop-off) valve is located close to the patient, circuits D, E, and F are T-piece arrangements with gas leaving the circuit at a distance from the patient. Because there is no CO_2 absorber in any of these systems, the potential exists for the patient to inhale alveolar gas that has been previously exhaled and contains CO_2. The extent of rebreathing depends on the circuit anatomy, the patient's minute ventilation, the pattern of ventilation, the FGF rate, and whether ventilation is spontaneous or controlled.[27-29]

Mapleson A: Magill Attachment The Magill attachment (circuit A) is illustrated in Fig. 39-27. Fresh gas from the anesthesia machine enters at the end of the system farthest from the patient and closest to the reservoir bag and leaves via a spring-loaded adjustable pop-off valve located close to the patient. The system functions very differently during spontaneous than during controlled ventilation. During spontaneous ventilation, as the patient begins to exhale, deadspace gas enters the tubing and passes toward the reservoir bag. Meanwhile, fresh gas entering the system from the machine is stored in the reservoir bag. As exhalation continues, pressure increases in the system, and the pop-off valve opens to preferentially vent alveolar gas. If the FGF rate is high, deadspace gas stored in the tubing may also be vented via the pop-off valve. During the next spontaneous inspiration, the patient breathes in any deadspace gas stored in the tubing followed by fresh gas from the anesthesia machine and that stored in the reservoir bag. Mapleson[26] calculated and others[28] confirmed that during spontaneous ventilation, an FGF rate equivalent to alveolar ventilation (ie, ~70% of minute ventilation) will prevent rebreathing. However, as the FGF rate approaches alveolar ventilation, the system's vulnerability to producing rebreathing, as a result of an uneven ventilatory pattern, is increased.

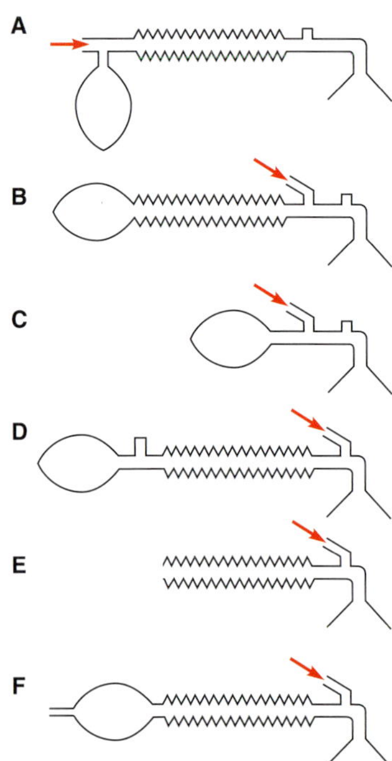

FIGURE 39-27. Mapleson classification of rebreathing systems (see text for details on A-F circuits). The Mapleson A circuit is also known as the Magill attachment. *Red arrows* indicate fresh gas inflow locations.

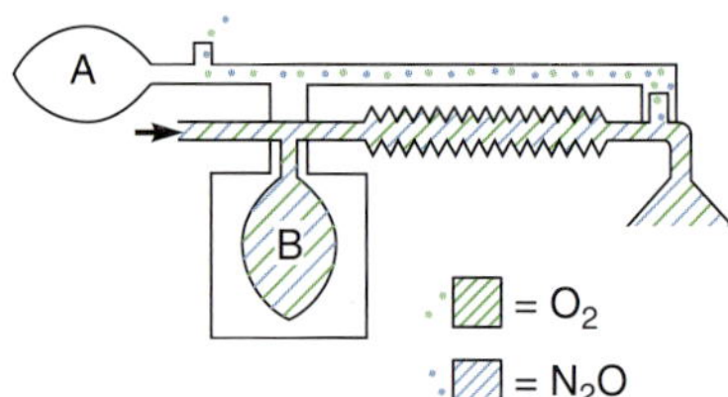

FIGURE 39-28. The enclosed Magill system. Squeezing the reservoir bag (*A*) causes the pop-off valve to be held closed and results in compression of enclosed reservoir bag (*B*). Note the similarity, in principle, to the "bag in a bottle ventilator" (see Fig. 39-35).

When used during controlled ventilation, the Magill attachment becomes very inefficient in terms of fresh gas requirements. During controlled inspiration, when the bag is squeezed, the pop-off valve opens, causing release of fresh gas.[29] Previously exhaled alveolar gas is not vented efficiently and is rebreathed. With controlled ventilation, the most efficient removal of CO_2 occurs with a short inspiratory-to-expiratory (I:E) ratio, a large tidal volume, and a high FGF.[28,30] Consequently, FGF rates of 3 times the estimated minute ventilation are recommended during controlled ventilation with the Magill attachment.[27] Such high flows are wasteful of anesthetic gases and pose additional problems for waste gas scavenging.

Enthusiasm for the Magill attachment resulted in potential modifications to address these problems. Thus, during controlled ventilation, the fresh gas requirement can be reduced by keeping the pop-off valve closed during inspiration. This is achieved by the Enclosed Magill System or the Miller modification (**Fig. 39-28**).[31] This is a system somewhat analogous to that used in contemporary double-circuit anesthesia ventilators (see Anesthesia Ventilators). This modified system is reported to be as efficient during controlled ventilation as the Magill attachment is during spontaneous ventilation.[32]

As noted, because the pop-off valve in the Magill attachment is close to the patient, waste gas scavenging is a potential problem. This is addressed in the coaxial Mapleson A or Lack Breathing System (**Fig. 39-29**), which is functionally similar to the Mapleson A.[33]

Mapleson B and C Systems In the Mapleson B and C systems (Fig. 39-27B and 39-27C), the site of fresh gas inflow and the pop-off valve are near the patient, and the circuit tubing and reservoir bag form a cul-de-sac in which a mixture of deadspace, alveolar, and fresh gas may collect. The Mapleson C system, with a shorter length of tubing between the patient and the bag, is also known as the Waters to-and-fro system without absorber. These systems function similarly during both spontaneous and controlled ventilation. Rebreathing is prevented with FGFs of at least twice the minute ventilation.[27,29] The Mapleson B and C systems are rarely used in contemporary anesthesia practice.

Mapleson D System The Mapleson D system (Fig. 39-27D) is basically a T piece with a long expiratory limb, the end of which has a reservoir bag and a pop-off valve. During spontaneous ventilation, it is less efficient than the A system but more efficient than the B or C systems.[27,29] On spontaneous exhalation, deadspace, alveolar, and fresh gas enter the

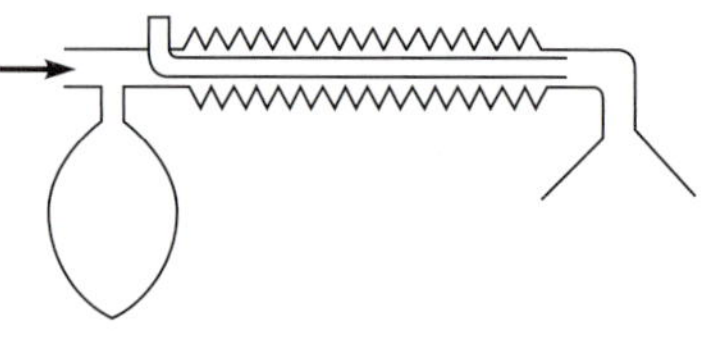

FIGURE 39-29. Coaxial Mapleson A or Lack Breathing System. FGF, fresh gas flow.

tubing, and as pressure increases, some of this gas mixture is vented. During the next spontaneous inspiration, the patient inhales fresh gas from the anesthesia machine mixed with gas from the tubing, the composition of which depends on FGF, tidal volume, and the duration of the patient's expiratory pause.

If the latter is long, the tubing is flushed with fresh gas, which is then available to be inhaled on the next inspiration. If the pause is short, less flushing occurs, and rebreathing of CO_2 becomes more likely. Large tidal volumes result in more alveolar gas entering the tubing, which also predisposes to rebreathing. Mapleson[26] calculated that an FGF of at least twice the minute ventilation was required to prevent rebreathing. This has been confirmed by others.[29,31]

When used during controlled ventilation, gas is distributed similarly in the circuit. Thus, manual compression of the reservoir bag ensures that alveolar and deadspace gas is released via the pop-off valve during inspiration and that fresh gas enters the patient's airway. During exhalation, deadspace gas and fresh gas tend to enter the reservoir bag first before the pop-off valve opens to vent the remaining (mainly alveolar) gas. As with spontaneous ventilation, an FGF of 2 to 3 times the minute ventilation prevents rebreathing.[29,31]

The Mapleson D circuit originally described is rarely used now in the United States. However, a coaxial modification, the Bain circuit, is sometimes used in pediatric anesthesia practice.

Bain Circuit: Coaxial Mapleson D This system, introduced by Bain and Spoerel in 1972,[34] is shown in **Figure 39-30**. Fresh gas from the anesthesia machine enters the inner (smaller bore) tubing and is delivered to the patient end. Exhaled gas is carried via the outer tubing to the reservoir bag and pop-off valve. Both reusable and disposable versions are available. The outer tubing is now made from transparent material so the inner tubing can be inspected for kinking or disconnection. Clearly, if disconnection occurred at the machine end, the whole system would become apparatus deadspace and result in excessive rebreathing.

The Bain system may be used for spontaneous or assisted ventilation, or the reservoir bag may be removed and an anesthesia ventilator hose attached to the bag mount for mechanical ventilation. Several studies have evaluated the FGF requirements of the Bain system. Although some have found that during spontaneous ventilation, an FGF of 100 mL/kg/min produces normocapnia at the cost of increased minute ventilation,[35] another study reported that an FGF of 2.5 to 3 times the minute ventilation prevents rebreathing during spontaneous ventilation.[36] The slightly higher FGF requirement of the Bain circuit compared with the basic Mapleson D system may be attributable to turbulence at the patient end of the coaxial system, in turn causing failure to store fresh gas in the outer corrugated tubing. During controlled ventilation, the Bain circuit behaves more as a Mapleson D system, and an FGF of 70 mL/kg/min results in normocapnia, provided minute ventilation is adequate (120 mL/kg/min). This applies in patients weighing more than 40 kg.[35]

A ventilation nomogram has been produced for the Bain circuit during controlled ventilation (**Fig. 39-31**).[37] This shows that the alveolar CO_2 tension (and therefore $Paco_2$) can be estimated from a combination of FGF and minute ventilation V_E. At high FGF, $Paco_2$ becomes independent of FGF and dependent on minute ventilation. At high minute ventilation, $Paco_2$ is independent of minute ventilation and becomes dependent on FGF.

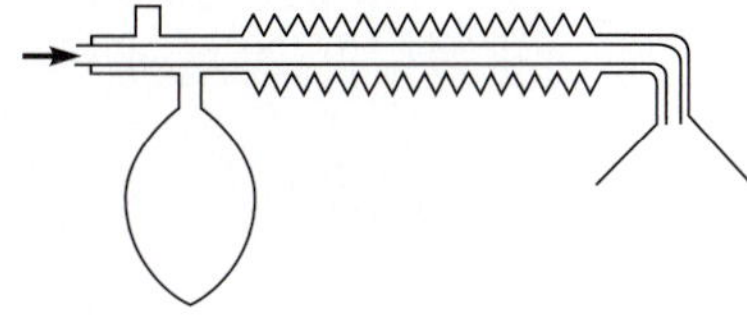

FIGURE 39-30. Bain circuit: coaxial version of Mapleson D.

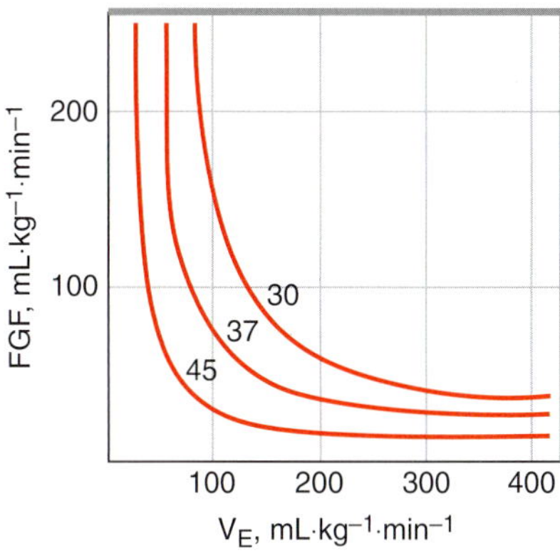

FIGURE 39-31. Nomogram for predicting $Paco_2$ from given combination of fresh gas flow and minute ventilation for Bain system. Three isopleths indicate $Paco_2$ of 30, 37, and 45 mm Hg. VE = minute ventilation.

The Bain circuit can thus be used to provide controlled rebreathing with hyperventilation, resulting in normal $Paco_2$. Such predictive nomograms, although useful guides, have become of less importance because monitoring of end-tidal CO_2 by capnometry has become the standard of care. Because the pop-off valve in the Bain circuit is located close to the machine, scavenging from the Bain circuit is not a problem.

A preuse check of the Bain circuit is essential to ensure that the inner gas delivery tube has not become disconnected. If this occurs, it would lead to rebreathing. Two checkout methods have been described. In one (Pethick's method), the patient end of the whole system is occluded, the pop-off valve is closed, and the system is filled with O_2 until the reservoir bag is distended. The patient end is then unoccluded, and O_2 is flushed into the circuit via the inner tube. The high O_2 flow produces a Venturi effect at the patient end of the circuit. The low pressure created at the end of the outer tubing causes O_2 to be drawn along the outer tubing from the bag, causing the reservoir bag to deflate. If a disconnection or a leak occurs in the inner tubing, flushing the circuit with O_2 would allow the high pressure to be transmitted from the inner to the outer tubing, and the reservoir bag would remain inflated or distend further.

A second method (Seed's method) for checking the Bain circuit is to set 50 mL/min of flow on the O_2 flowmeter and then occlude the distal (patient) end of the inner tube using the plunger of a small syringe. If the inner tube is intact, this should cause the gas flow to cease and the flowmeter bobbin to decrease. This (Seed's) method is preferred because if the inner tube has been omitted, Pethick's method may give no indication that anything is wrong.

Mapleson E and F Systems The Mapleson E and F systems are valveless, T-piece arrangements (Figs. 39-27E and 39-27F). The E system is modified from Ayre's original T-piece by the addition of corrugated tubing to the expiratory limb, which thereby becomes a reservoir of fresh gas during inspiration. During inspiration, the patient breathes fresh gas from the machine and gas stored in the expiratory limb. The latter should have a capacity greater than the patient's expected tidal volume to prevent entrainment of room air during inspiration. During exhalation, exhaled gas enters the expiratory limb; during the expiratory pause, this limb is flushed with fresh gas, which is then available for the next inspiration.

The E system may be used for either spontaneous or controlled ventilation, the latter being achieved by intermittent occlusion of the expiratory limb by a "mechanical thumb" ventilator. With the E system, rebreathing is avoided if an FGF of 3 times the minute ventilation is used.[29]

The Mapleson F circuit is a modification by Jackson-Rees[35] of the Ayre's T-piece (Mapleson E) system (Fig. 39-27E and 39-27F). In this system, a 2-tailed reservoir bag and a means for venting waste gases are added to the end of the expiratory limb tubing. The venting piece is usually a valve with an adjustable orifice that is connected to a waste gas scavenging system.

The Mapleson F system functions similarly to the Mapleson E except that during exhalation, a mixture of exhaled and fresh gas collects in the bag. On the next inspiration, the patient inhales fresh gas from the machine and that stored in the expiratory limb. Addition of the reservoir bag to the E system provides a means to qualitatively monitor ventilation during spontaneous breathing as well as a means to control ventilation by manually squeezing the reservoir bag. Prevention of rebreathing is achieved using FGFs of 2 to 3 times the minute ventilation.[29]

The Ayre's T-piece and Jackson-Rees' systems have been popular for pediatric anesthesia because they are simple to assemble; inexpensive; and because they are valveless, offer low resistance to breathing. However, because relatively high FGFs are needed, all T-piece systems are less desirable for use in adults. They also cause greater loss of moisture from the airway if dry gases are used.[29,31]

CIRCLE SYSTEM

In this system, the components form a circle into which fresh gas can enter and from which excess gas can leave. **Figure 39-32** shows the arrangement of the components of a contemporary circle system. Fresh gas enters just upstream from the inspiratory unidirectional valve and during inspiration passes down the circle's inspiratory limb to the Y-piece connector. During expiration, gas passes along the expiratory limb to the expiratory unidirectional valve. A spirometer is usually located between the expiratory limb of the circle and the expiratory unidirectional valve. In this location, it measures the expired tidal volume. Just beyond the expiratory valve are the adjustable pressure limit (APL or "pop-off") valve and a reservoir bag. Gas then passes through a canister containing a CO_2 absorbent (eg, soda lime) and emerges to rejoin fresh gas entering the circuit from the anesthesia machine just upstream from the inspiratory valve.

In the system described, rebreathing of CO_2 is prevented by its absorption from exhaled gas before it is reinspired. At high FGFs, however, CO_2 absorption becomes unnecessary, and some older circle systems even permitted bypass of the absorber canister. At lower FGFs, CO_2 absorption is necessary. Eger[37] proposed 3 basic rules for minimizing CO_2 rebreathing in a circle system: (1) a unidirectional valve must be present between the reservoir bag and the patient on both inspiratory and expiratory sides, (2) fresh gas must not enter the system between the expiratory unidirectional valve and the patient, and (3) the overflow (APL) valve must not be placed between the patient and the inspiratory unidirectional valve.

Unidirectional gas flow occurs only in that part of the circle between the unidirectional valves and the patient. In the part of the circuit between the fresh gas inlet and the APL valve, gas flow is bidirectional (Fig. 39-32). Incompetence of either unidirectional valve permits bidirectional gas flow in the corrugated patient circuit tubing, leading to rebreathing of previously exhaled CO_2.

The circle system is currently the most popular anesthesia system in use in the United States. It has the advantages of permitting low FGFs, reduction of operating room pollution, and conservation of heat and humidity. Disadvantages of the circle system include a somewhat complex design with multiple components that could malfunction or possibly be arranged incorrectly. It is also difficult to predict inspired gas composition within the circle, particularly if low FGFs are being used. The latter may cease to be a problem as monitoring of anesthetic gas and vapor concentrations becomes more common.

Absorption of Carbon Dioxide The CO_2 absorber is the central component in a circle system. Traditional absorber canisters are large, with a minimal gas space equal to the largest expected patient tidal volume. This design permits low gas flow rates and long dwell times and, as a result, more complete removal ("scrubbing") of CO_2. Traditional absorber canisters usually have 2 chambers so that half of the absorbent (that in the upstream chamber) can be completely exhausted before removal. The chambers are then reversed so that the previously downstream chamber now becomes upstream (**Fig. 39-33**).[38]

The CO_2 absorbent most commonly used is soda lime. The once popular absorbent Baralyme is no longer available. Soda lime consists of 4% NaOH, 1% KOH, 14% to 19% H_2O, and the remainder $Ca(OH)_2$.[38]

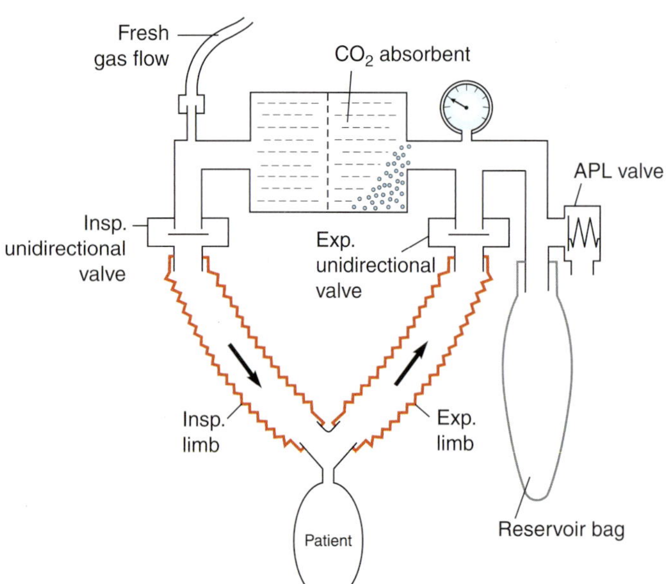

FIGURE 39-32. Contemporary standard anesthesia circle breathing system arrangement. APL, adjustable pressure-limiting; Exp, expiratory; Insp, inspiratory.

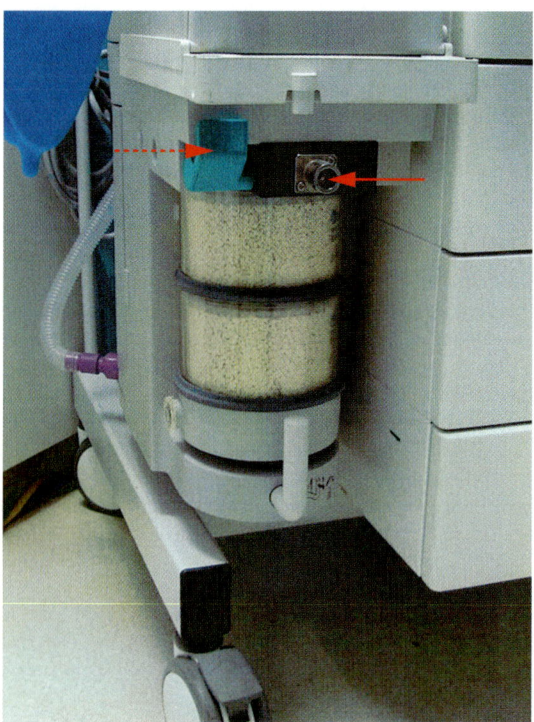

FIGURE 39-33. Traditional 2-compartment absorber canister as used on a GE-Datex Aestiva machine. *Solid arrow* indicates auxiliary common gas outlet. *Dotted arrow* indicates auxiliary common gas outlet selector lever.

In addition, small amounts of silica or kieselguhr are added for hardening to reduce the formation of dust. The absorptive efficacy of soda lime is inversely related to its hardness. The reaction of CO_2 with soda lime is as follows[38]:

$$(1) \quad CO_2 + H_2O \rightarrow H_2CO_3$$
$$(2) \quad H_2CO_3 + 2NaOH \rightarrow Na_2CO_3 + 2H_2O$$
$$(3) \quad H_2CO_3 + 2KOH \rightarrow K_2CO_3 + 2H_2O$$
$$(4) \quad Na_2CO_3 + Ca(OH)_2 \rightarrow 2NaOH + CaCO_3$$

or

$$K_2CO_3 + Ca(OH_2) \rightarrow 2KOH + CaCO_3$$

Considerable heat is liberated during the course of this reaction. The preservation of heat and moisture within the system is considered to be a desirable feature.

Absorptive surface area and gas flow through soda lime are functions of granule size. The smaller the size, the larger the area for absorption but the greater the resistance to gas flow. Conversely, large granules decrease absorptive surface area, offer less resistance to flow, and may encourage channeling of gases through the soda lime, thereby decreasing CO_2 absorption. The most frequently used size of soda lime granule is 4 to 8 mesh (ie, 0.25-in to 0.125-in diameter). In theory, 100 g of CO_2 absorbent (soda lime) can absorb 26 L of CO_2. In practice, the amount of CO_2 actually absorbed is less because of the channeling of gas through the absorber.

Indicators are added to the absorbent granules to show when they are becoming exhausted. These indicators are pH sensitive and are colorless when soda lime is fresh but become colored when pH decreases. The most frequently used indicator is ethyl violet, which changes to purple as absorption proceeds. It was chosen because the color change is conspicuous even under poor lighting conditions.[39]

Ethyl violet may be deactivated by fluorescent lighting and may possibly be temporally deactivated after a container is opened even with storage in the dark. Such deactivation increases the hazard of using CO_2 absorption, but such a hazard would be offset by continuous capnography.

When using CO_2 absorption, the absorbent must be compatible with the anesthetic gases in use. Sevoflurane is degraded by both soda lime and the now discontinued Baralyme.

Prolonged exposure of desflurane, enflurane, and isoflurane to desiccated CO_2 absorbents may result in anesthetic degradation, leading to the production of CO.[40] Use of dry absorbent produces more CO than standard absorbent with normal amounts of water. For any given water content, the now discontinued Baralyme produced more CO than does soda lime. Increased temperature increases CO production, as does use of higher anesthetic concentrations. Although there were no reports of patient harm resulting from CO found in the breathing system, CO is of concern because there is the potential for injury. To minimize exposure to CO from the degradation of anesthetics in the breathing system, only an absorbent with the full complement of water should be used. Drying of the absorbent can be minimized by using low FGF rates.

NEW ABSORBENTS AND THE PROBLEMS ASSOCIATED WITH STRONG BASES

Baralyme was a very popular absorbent and was used safely for many years. In late 2004, Allied Health Care, the manufacturer of Baralyme, halted its distribution. This was because desiccated Baralyme acting on sevoflurane can produce great amounts of heat that could result in temperatures in excess of 400°C, fires, and explosions.[39,41,42] Animal studies and a bench model have demonstrated fires and explosions with sevoflurane.[43] In August 2004, several reports documented fires and explosions in clinical practice with sevoflurane but none with desflurane or isoflurane.[44-47] In a bench study of the action of desiccated Baralyme on potent inhaled anesthetics at 1.5 MAC, sevoflurane degradation by Baralyme produced temperatures greater than 300°C and fires, but degradation of desflurane or isoflurane produced temperatures of approximately 100°C and no fires.[48]

Monovalent bases (potassium hydroxide and sodium hydroxide) in absorbents cause the exothermic degradation of potent inhaled anesthetics to compound A and carbon monoxide. In new absorbents, such as Amsorb, Drägersorb, and Drägersorb Free,[49,50] the elimination of such bases (but not calcium hydroxide) minimizes compound A or CO production with both moist and desiccated absorbents (**Table 39-6**).[51-53]

TABLE 39-6 Absorbent Comparisons[a]

Company	Product Name	H_2O%	NaOH%	KOH%	$Ca(OH)_2$%	Significant Other	US Availability
Allied Healthcare/Chemetron	Baralyme	11.0-16.0	0.0	<5	73	$Ba(OH)_2$	No longer available
Allied Healthcare	Carbolime[b]	12.0-19.0	3	0.0	>75	–	Yes
W.R. Grace and Company	Sodasorb	15.0-17.0	3.7	–	50-100	–	Yes
Intersurgical Ltd.	Intersorb Plus	13.5-17.5	2.6	0.0	81	–	Yes
Intersurgical Ltd.	Spherasorb	13.5-17.5	1.3	0.0	78	4% Zeolite	Yes
Intersurgical Ltd.	LoFloSorb	13.5-17.5	0.0	0.0	78	6.5% Silica	Yes
Armstrong Medical Ltd.	Amsorb	13.5-16.5	0.0	0.0	79-82	$CaCl_2$	No longer available
Armstrong Medical Ltd.	Amsorb Plus	13.0-18.0	0.0	0.0	>80	$CaCl_2$	Yes
Dräger Medical, Inc.	Drägersorb 800	–	~2	~3	–	–	No longer available
Dräger Medical, Inc.	Drägersorb 800 Plus	~16	1-3	NA	75-83	–	Yes
Dräger Medical, Inc.	Drägersorb Free	14-18	0.5-2	NA	74-82	$CaCl_2$	Yes
Airgas/Molecular Products	Sodalime	–	<3.5	2.6	>80	–	Yes
Molecular Products	Sofnolime	12-19	<3.5	0.0	–	–	No[d]
GE Medical[c]/Molecular Products	Medisorb	–	<3.5	0.0	–	–	Yes

[a]This table was formulated based on information supplied by the various manufacturers. The Anesthesia Patient Safety Foundation assumes no responsibility for variations in or deviations from the formulations that are represented in this table. The table is supplied for educational and conceptual purposes.

[b]Manufactured by Molecular Products.

[c]Distributor of product manufactured by Molecular Products.

[d]Not available in the US market as a medical product, although diving and military grades are available in the United States. Medical grade is available outside the United States.

More than one manufacturer reported variable absorption capacity based on canister design, shape, volume fresh gas flow, hydration, and carbon dioxide concentration. Nearly all reported price variability depends on marketing and type of fill.

Reprinted with permission from Absorbent Comparisons from *Anesthesia Patient Safety Foundation (APSF) Newsletter* 2005; 20(2); and Dr. Michael Olympio.

Although the new absorbents appear to be safer, compared with soda lime they are more expensive and absorb less CO_2. It is likely that the withdrawal of Baralyme (with its high content of KOH) from clinical use will minimize or eliminate the problem of fires and explosions. Amsorb has the additional advantage that it turns from white to purple when it becomes desiccated and when its capacity to absorb CO_2 is exhausted. Drägersorb Free, which contains no monovalent bases, may not only cause less anesthetic degradation but also may have a greater absorptive capacity for CO_2.[53-55]

In April 2005, the Anesthesia Patient Safety Foundation (APSF) convened a conference to discuss the safety of CO_2 absorbents. The stated goal of the conference was "to develop a consensus statement to share with anesthesia professionals on the use of carbon dioxide absorbents so as to reduce the risk of adverse interactions with volatile anesthetic drugs." The conclusions of the attendees were as follows.

The APSF recommends use of carbon dioxide absorbents whose composition is such that exposure to volatile anesthetics does not result in significant degradation of the volatile anesthetic.

The APSF further recommends that there should be institutional, hospital, or departmental policies regarding steps to prevent desiccation of the carbon dioxide absorbent if they choose conventional carbon dioxide absorbents that may degrade volatile anesthetics when absorbent desiccation occurs.

In such circumstances of using absorbents that may degrade volatile anesthetics, conference attendees generally agreed that users could take the following steps, consistent with Emergency Care Research Institute recommendations:

1. Turn off all gas flow when the machine is not in use.
2. Change the absorbent regularly, on Monday morning, for instance.
3. Change absorbent whenever the color change indicates exhaustion.
4. Change all absorbent, not just 1 canister in a 2-canister system.
5. Change absorbent when uncertain of the state of hydration, such as if the FGF has been left on for an extensive or indeterminate time period.
6. If compact canisters are used, consider changing them more frequently.

There was also support for the APSF to create an Expert Task Force to define further the characteristics of carbon dioxide absorbents that do not significantly degrade volatile anesthetics.

Mini-Absorbers Although traditional circle systems used large absorber canisters, some workstations (eg, GE-Datex-Ohmeda ADU, Aisys, and Dräger Apollo workstations) use smaller volume (600-mL) compact or "mini absorbers" that contain soda lime or one of the new absorbents shown in Table 39-6. These compact absorber canisters can be replaced without causing a leak in the breathing system because the absorber mount block is self-sealing (**Fig. 39-34**).

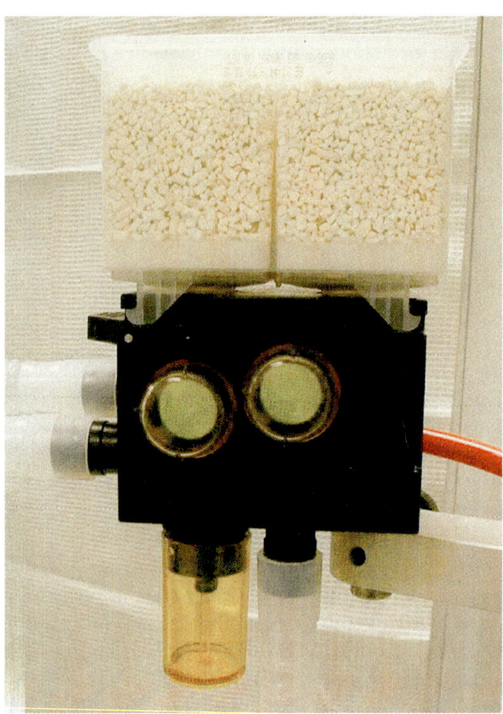

FIGURE 39-34. GE-Datex ADU Carestation Compact Block and mini-absorber. In this design of circle breathing system, the fresh gas flow from the CGO enters the circuit *downstream* (ie, on the patient side) of the inspiratory unidirectional valve (rather than upstream as shown in Fig. 39-32). The absorber block is self-sealing so there is no leak from the breathing circuit if the absorber canister is removed.

Variations on the Basic Circle System The 3 basic rules that must be followed to prevent rebreathing in a circle system[37] still allow some flexibility in design without compromising function. Several variations on the basic circle system are in clinical use; 2 examples follow.

A coaxial version of the circle system tubing is available (Universal F Circuit, King Systems, Noblesville, IN), analogous to the Bain circuit being a coaxial version of Mapleson D. In this system, the inspired gas flows from the inspiratory connector on the anesthesia machine through the inner tube to the patient's end, and exhaled gas flows back through the outer tube. The exhaled gas therefore warms the inspired gas. At the machine end, expired gas flows through a side tube that connects to the expiratory port on the anesthesia machine. The Universal F circuit can be easily reconfigured from a circle system to become a Bain circuit for patient transport or resuscitation. In the latter modes, a supply of oxygen is needed to fill the circuit and distend the bag to ventilate the patient's lungs.

The circle system design in the GE-Datex-Ohmeda ADU workstation is modified so that the FGF enters the circuit downstream (ie, on the patient side) of the inspiratory unidirectional valve rather than upstream of the valve (as shown in Fig. 39-32). This adaptation ensures a more efficient delivery of fresh gas to the patient so that any changes in fresh gas composition made on the machine flowmeters will be more rapidly reflected at the patient's airway. A further benefit is that if fresh gas is left flowing with no patient connected at the Y-piece, the dry fresh gas will not flow through the CO_2 absorbent and therefore will not cause it to become desiccated (Fig. 39-34). One problem with having fresh gas flowing continuously into the inspiratory limb of the circle system, rather than only during inspiration, is that readings from a spirometer placed between the expiratory limb of the circuit and the expiratory connector port on the machine would be inaccurate (**Fig. 39-35**), overestimating the tidal volume. This potential problem is resolved by placing a bidirectional gas flow sensing airway adapter (D-lite for adults; Pedi-lite for small patients) between the Y-piece of the circle and the patient's airway. This gas sampling bidirectional flow sensor is based on the Pitot tube principle and measures the patient's actual inspired and expired tidal volumes, as well as other spirometric parameters.

ANESTHESIA VENTILATORS

Anesthesia ventilators have evolved considerably over the past several years. The traditional anesthesia ventilator is a pneumatically powered, electronically controlled device. The visible bellows acts as a "counter-lung" that exchanges with the gas in the patient's lungs via the breathing circuit. Examples of traditional ventilators include the Dräger AV-E, the GE-Datex-Ohmeda 7900 series with Smart Vent used in the Aestiva and Aisys workstations, and GE-ADU models. These are sometimes described as "bag-in-a-bottle" respirators. The basic principle is that the reservoir bag of the anesthesia circle system is replaced by a bellows

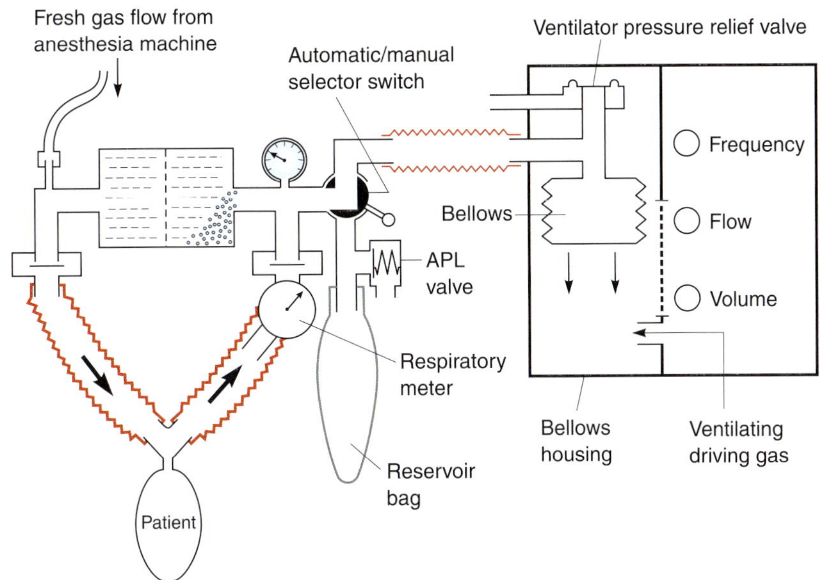

FIGURE 39-35. Schematic of typical "bag-in-a-bottle" double-circuit design of anesthesia ventilator. The reservoir bag and adjustable pressure-limiting (APL) valve are switched out of circuit and replaced by ventilator hanging bellows (bag) in bellows housing (bottle).

in a bellows housing, and the APL ("pop-off") valve is replaced by a ventilator pressure-relief valve (Fig. 39-35). Inspiration occurs when compressed (driving) gas enters the bellows housing. The bellows is compressed, and the pressure-relief valve is held closed (**Fig. 39-36**). Gas contained within the bellows, as well as fresh gas entering the patient circuit from the anesthesia machine, are forced into the patient's lungs. At end-inspiration, the bellows housing is no longer pressurized, the bellows refills (by gravity in the case of a hanging bellows, as in Figures 39-35 and 39-36), and the pressure-relief valve is able to open, permitting excess gas in the patient circuit to be vented to the waste gas scavenging system.

The traditional "bag-in-a-bottle" anesthesia ventilators are also described as double-circuit ventilators, one circuit being the driving gas circuit and the other the patient breathing system. The interface between these 2 circuits is the ventilator bellows itself. If the bellows rises as it refills during exhalation, it is called a *standing* or *ascending bellows*. If it falls during exhalation, it is called a *hanging* or *descending bellows*. Figure 39-35 shows a hanging bellows arrangement, where it is seen to replace the hanging reservoir bag in the circle system. An advantage of the standing bellows is that it will fail to rise if there is a significant leak in the breathing system. A hanging bellows ventilator will continue to descend fully in the presence of a leak.

In some recent models of Dräger anesthesia workstation (Narkomed 6400, Apollo, Fabius GS, Tiro), the ventilator bellows, bellows housing, and driving gas circuit are replaced by a piston in a cylinder. The movements of the piston are precisely controlled by a microprocessor and electric motor. This design is described in a later section (New Designs of Anesthesia Ventilator and Patient Breathing Systems).

TRADITIONAL ANESTHESIA VENTILATORS

Although the Dräger AV-E and the Datex-Ohmeda 7000 series, 7900 series, and ADU model ventilators are of the double-circuit design, their mechanisms of action differ in certain details.

Datex-Ohmeda 7000 The Datex-Ohmeda 7000 ventilator is shown in **Figure 39-37**. It consists of 2 basic units: a bellows housing and assembly and a control unit. The former may be separate from or be mounted on the control unit, as in Figure 39-37. The driving gas circuit is considered first (**Fig. 39-38**).[54]

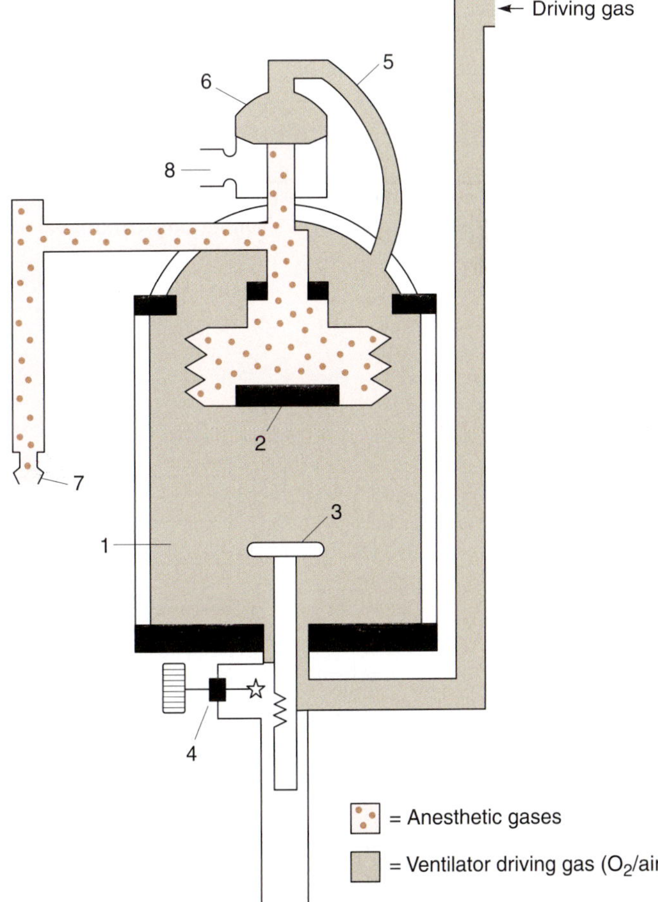

FIGURE 39-36. Schematic of North American Dräger AV-E hanging bellows ventilator during inspiration. *Hatched area* represents driving gas under pressure, which comes from ventilator control circuits, enters bellows housing to compress and empty the bellows, and pressurizes and thereby closes ventilator pressure-relief valve. *1*, Bellows housing; *2*, bellows; *3*, tidal volume adjustment plate; *4*, tidal volume control knob; *5*, relief valve pilot line; *6*, ventilator pressure-relief valve; *7*, connector to patient circuit; *8*, connector to waste gas scavenging system.

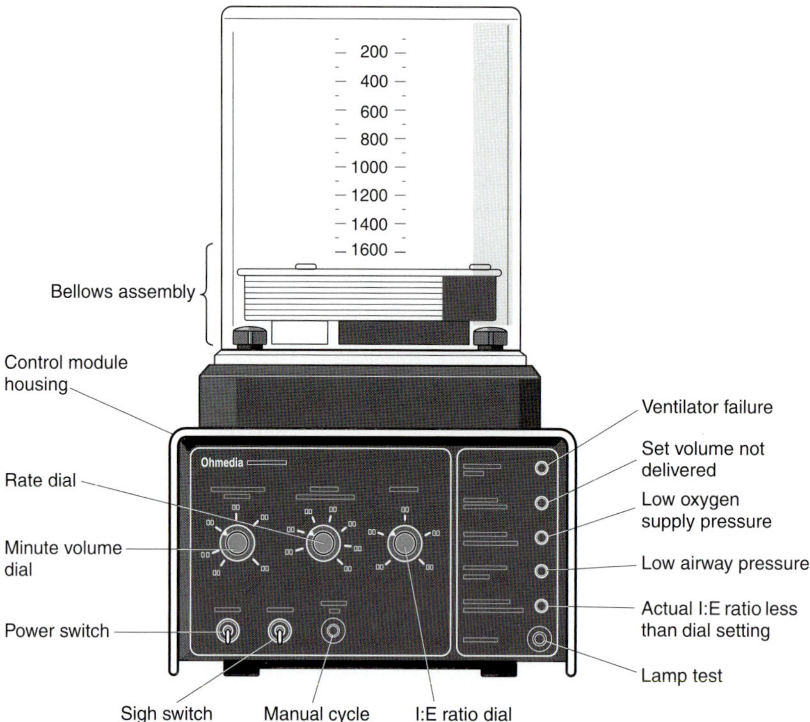

FIGURE 39-37. Ohmeda 7000 electronic anesthesia ventilator. I:E, inspiratory-to-expiratory. [Courtesy of Datex-Ohmeda, GE Health Care, Madison, WI.]

The driving gas supply of this ventilator, O_2 at a nominal pressure of 50 psig, passes to a pressure regulator whose output is set to 38 psig at 24 L/min of flow. From here the pressure-regulated O_2 flow passes to a block containing 5 solenoid flow-control valves connected in parallel. These flow-control valves are electronically opened during the inspiratory phase to direct O_2 flow through tuned orifices, which are calibrated for flows of 2, 4, 8, 16, and 32 L/min. The possible range for flow selection is 4 to 60 L/min in 2-L/min

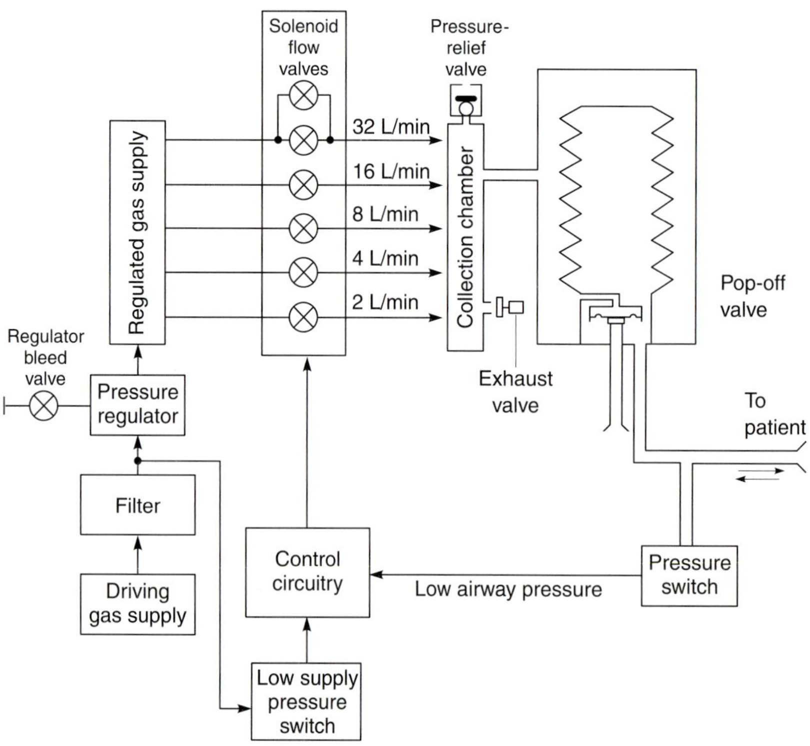

FIGURE 39-38. Ohmeda 7000 electronic anesthesia ventilator. Schematic of driving gas circuit. [Courtesy of Ohmeda, GE Health Care, Madison, WI.]

increments. By controlling the duration of opening of each of the 5 solenoid valves, the control module determines the O_2 volume that passes into the collection chamber. This metered O_2 volume then enters the bellows housing, where it exerts pressure on the bellows and displaces an equal volume of anesthesia gas mixture from the bellows into the patient circuit. This displaced volume is the ventilator tidal volume.

The Datex-Ohmeda 7000 ventilator uses a standing bellows. According to the settings on the ventilator panel, tidal volume (VT) equals set minute volume (MV) divided by set respiratory rate (RR), or VT = MV/RR; the bellows empties until the predetermined tidal volume has been delivered. The bellows therefore does not empty completely unless a tidal volume of 1600 mL or greater is selected (Fig. 39-37). During inspiration, the exhaust valve in the collection chamber is closed so that the driving gas does not escape. A ventilator pressure-relief valve (pop-off valve) located in the base of the bellows is held closed by the driving gas pressure during inspiration so gas passes from within the bellows to the patient circuit (**Fig. 39-39**).

Exhalation begins when the driving gas exhaust valve located in the control module opens, permitting driving gas to be vented from the bellows housing. This occurs because this gas is displaced by the bellows refilling with anesthesia gases from the patient's lungs during passive exhalation, and the FGF from the anesthesia machine. During exhalation, for the bellows to refill with anesthesia gases, a slight positive pressure must be maintained in the circuit. If the circuit were kept at atmospheric pressure during exhalation, circuit gas would preferentially flow out to the scavenging system, and the bellows would not reexpand. The ventilator pressure-relief valve therefore also incorporates a positive end-expiratory pressure (PEEP) valve that exerts a pressure of about 2.5 cm H_2O on the gas contained within the patient circuit. At end-expiration when the bellows has reached its limit of expansion and the circuit pressure has risen to greater than 2.5 cm H_2O, the ventilator pressure-relief valve opens, and excess gas from the patient circuit is vented to the waste gas scavenging system.

The pressure-relief valve in the driving gas collection chamber (Fig. 39-38) represents a safety feature such that if the pressure in the driving gas circuit becomes too high (>65 cm H_2O), the valve opens to relieve the excess pressure. This prevents such excessive pressure from being applied to the patient's airway.[54] The Ohmeda 7000 ventilator is electronically controlled and time cycled. Operator controls (Fig. 39-37) are for minute volume, respiratory rate (thus VT = MV/RR), and I:E ratio.

GE-Datex-Ohmeda 7800 Series The GE-Datex-Ohmeda 7810 ventilator (**Fig. 39-40**) is very similar to the model 7000 but differs in certain features.[55] Driving gas is O_2 at 50 psig nominal pressure (**Fig. 39-41**). The O_2 passes to a primary regulator whose output is controlled to 26 psig. From here the O_2 passes to a pneumatic manifold, where its flow into the bellows housing is controlled by a flow-control valve. This sophisticated mass flow valve varies the opening of a flow orifice according to the current supplied to the valve's coil, thereby controlling O_2 flow. A combination of the current supplied to the coil and the time for which it is applied (valve opening size and time) is determined by the microprocessor and based on the operator control settings.

The pneumatic manifold in the model 7810 replaces the 5 solenoid valves and tuned orifices of the model 7000 (Fig. 39-38). The operator controls also differ in that the model 7810 the limits of tidal volume, rate, inspiratory flow, and inspiratory pressure (maximum, 100 cm H_2O) may be set directly (Fig. 39-40). The I:E ratio, however, is not set directly but is calculated by the unit and displayed. The control unit contains an O_2 analyzer and displays the O_2 concentration sensed in the patient circuit. It also incorporates pressure and volume alarms. In other respects, the 7810 ventilator functions are similar to those of model 7000.

Datex-Ohmeda 7900 The Datex-Ohmeda 7900 ventilator is similar to the 7810 model in that it consists of a control unit (**Fig. 39-42**) and a separate bellows housing assembly. It uses compressed oxygen and a precision control valve to control the flow and pressure of gas delivered to the patient circuit. Inspiration may be volume or pressure preset and during exhalation, the ventilator controls the PEEP by regulating the exhalation pressure at the ventilator pressure-relief valve. Using signals from pressure, flow, and oxygen sensors, microprocessor circuits in the ventilator monitor the patient breathing circuit and display the

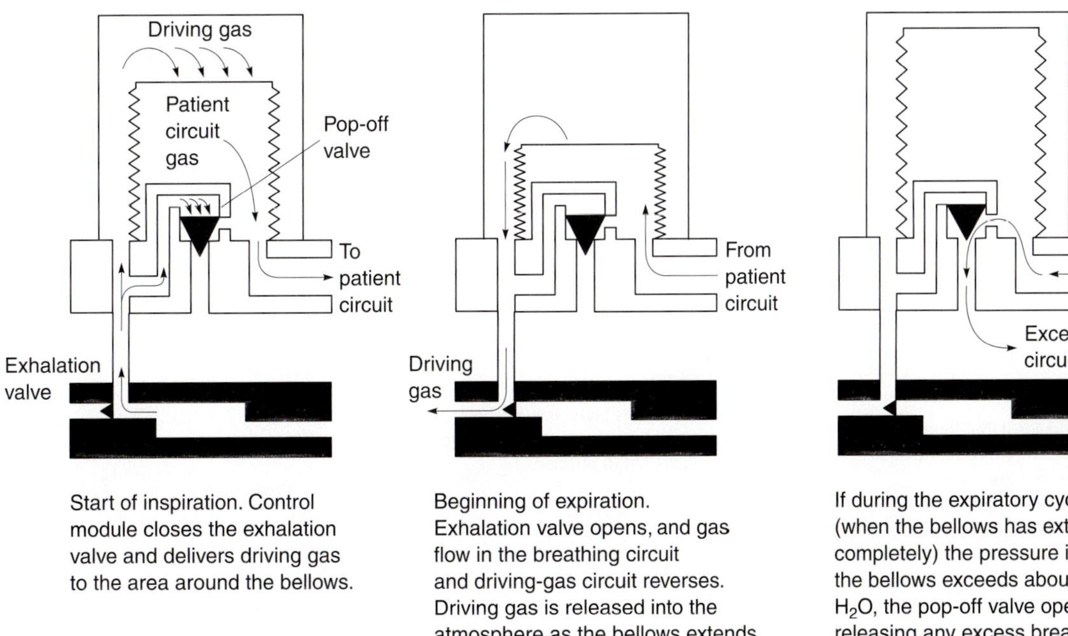

FIGURE 39-39. Ohmeda 7000 and 7810 ventilators. Schematic of function of pop-off (pressure-relief valve; ventilator pressure-relief) valve in bellows during inspiration and expiration. See text for details. [Courtesy of Ohmeda, GE Health Care, Madison, WI.]

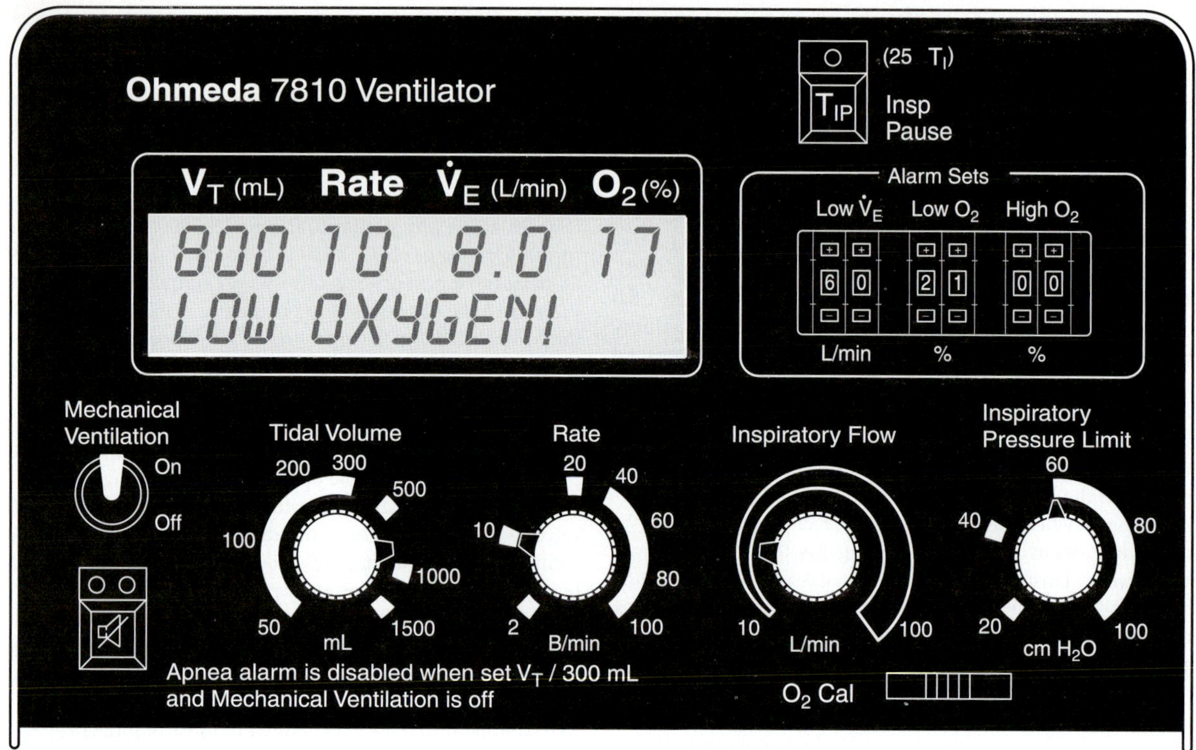

FIGURE 39-40. Datex-Ohmeda 7810 electronic anesthesia ventilator. Schematic of control panel. See text for details. [Courtesy of Datex-Ohmeda, GE Health Care, Madison, WI.]

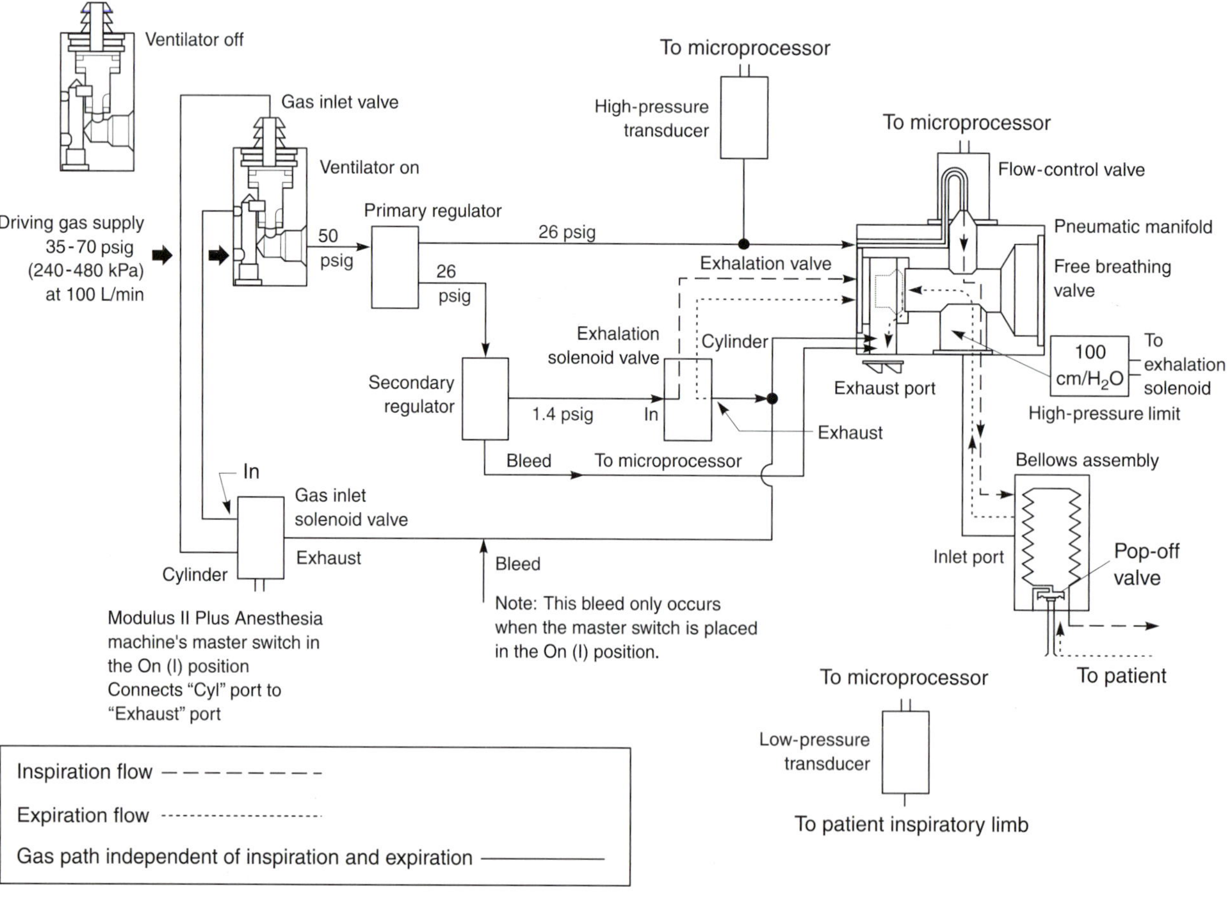

FIGURE 39-41. Datex-Ohmeda 7810 electronic anesthesia ventilator. Schematic of driving gas circuit. See text for details. [Courtesy of Ohmeda, BOC Health Care, Madison, WI.]

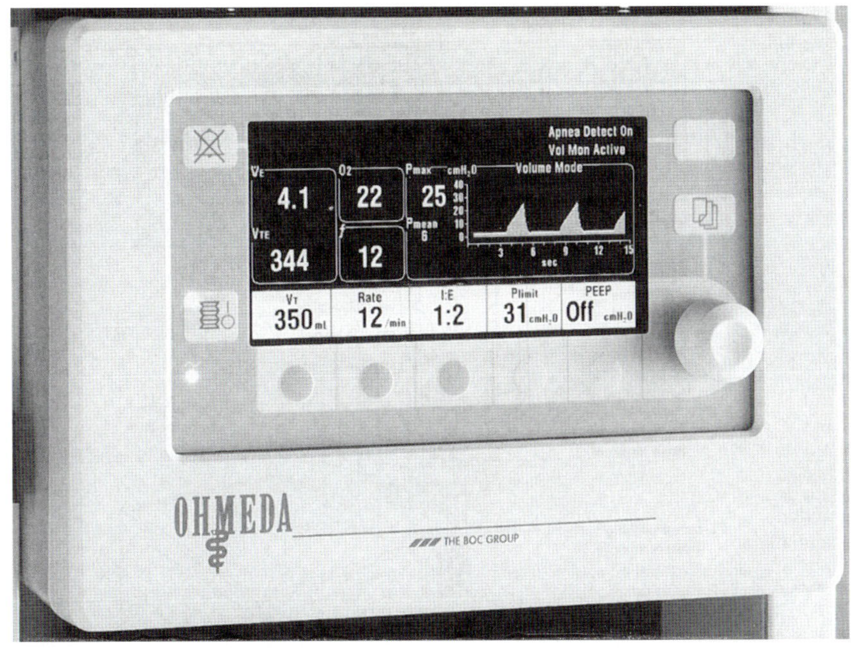

FIGURE 39-42. Datex-Ohmeda 7900 ventilator showing the control panel and display. See text for more details. [Courtesy of GE-Datex-Ohmeda, Inc., Madison, WI.]

measured variables. By comparing the operator set values for ventilatory parameters with those measured by the inspiratory and expiratory flow sensors, the ventilator automatically compensates for gas losses because of compression of gases in the ventilator, ventilator circuit, and absorber system but not for losses in the patient circuit. The system also compensates for gas gains as a result of anesthesia machine FGF (see Tidal Volume below). Thus, the user-set tidal volume is delivered to the patient circuit even when FGF, respiratory rate, or I:E ratios are altered. The most recent models of GE-Datex-Ohmeda workstations (Aestiva, Aespire, Aisys) use the 7900 series ventilator.

Dräger AV-E The Dräger AV-E ventilator (used on the Dräger Narkomed 2B, 2C, 3, 4, GS, and Mobile machines) is also a double-circuit, pneumatically powered design.[56] It consists of a control unit mounted above the flowmeters and vaporizers on a Dräger Narkomed machine and a bellows assembly (**Fig. 39-43**). A schematic illustration of this ventilator is shown in **Figure 39-44**. The following numbers in parentheses refer to Figures 39-44 and **39-45**. The driving gas circuit is described first.[57]

The ventilator is powered by O_2 at a driving pressure of 50 psig (2). When the ventilator on/off switch (3) is turned on, O_2 pressure is supplied to a 1 psig switch, which is activated and energizes the electronic circuit. The respiratory rate (7) and I:E ratio (6) controls (Fig. 39-43, *inset*) are set as desired. Inspiration (Fig. 39-44) occurs when the solenoid valve (9) receives an electrical signal from the control unit (5). This signal remains throughout inspiration and activates the solenoid valve (9) to allow O_2 at 50 psig to pass through it to activate the control valve (10). Opening the control valve allows O_2 that has passed through the adjustable flow regulator (11) to pass through the control valve (10) to the Venturi (13). The inspiratory flow rate is adjusted by the flow regulator (11) (flow-control knob, Fig. 39-43), and the flow rate is monitored on a flow indicator gauge (12). This indicator is really a pressure gauge, measuring pressure downstream from the flow regulator. The display on the gauge shows flow in 3 zones: high, medium, and low (Fig. 39-43). During inspiration, back pressure from the Venturi (13) is conducted to a pilot actuator (15), which is held closed. As the O_2 flows from the Venturi (13), room air is entrained through the muffler and entrainment port (14).

The mixture of O_2 and entrained air is directed into the bellows chamber (16). As pressure rises in the bellows chamber, the bellows is compressed. Anesthetic gases within the bellows are forced into the patient circuit via the breathing connector (22). At the same time, driving gas pressure from the bellows housing (16) is transmitted via the relief valve pilot line (20) to hold the ventilator pressure-relief valve (21) closed as long as the bellows housing is under pressure (ie, throughout inspiration). In this ventilator the bellows is emptied completely with each inspiratory cycle. Thus, tidal volume is determined by the extent to which the bellows is allowed to expand during exhalation, which in turn is adjusted by the tidal volume control knob (19) and bellows plate (18). During the inspiratory pause, the O_2 continues to flow from the Venturi (13). Because the bellows is now fully compressed, no further air is entrained, and pressure is maintained in the bellows housing by the pressure of the O_2 jet from the Venturi. Meanwhile, the chamber (16) contains a mixture of air and O_2 with an average O_2 concentration of 33%.

Expiration (Fig. 39-45) begins when the electrical signal from the control unit (5) to the solenoid valve (9) stops. The solenoid valve is deactivated and closes, interrupting the supply of 50 psig O_2 to the control valve (10), which therefore also closes. The preset O_2 flow from the flow regulator (11) is interrupted by the control valve (10), causing a pressure drop at the Venturi (13), and no back pressure is supplied to the pilot actuator (15). The latter opens to allow gas from the bellows chamber (16) to be vented through the pilot actuator (15) and the entrainment port (14) of the Venturi (13). This exhausted driving gas leaves the ventilator through a muffler. A clean, dry muffler is essential for normal function of this ventilator. As the pressure falls in the bellows chamber (16), the bellows (17) begins to refill. As long as any pressure remains in the bellows chamber (16), the ventilator relief valve (2) is also pressurized and held closed.

Figures 39-46 and **39-47** are schematic illustrations of the standing bellows version of the Dräger AV-E during inspiration and expiration, respectively. As with the standing bellows arrangement in the GE-Datex-Ohmeda ventilators, the Dräger AV-E ventilator relief valve applies about 2.5 cm H_2O PEEP to the gas in the patient circuit. When the standing bellows has reached its preset limit of expansion (the next tidal volume) and circuit pressure exceeds 2.5 cm H_2O, the PEEP valve opens, permitting excess circuit gas to enter the waste gas scavenging system (Fig. 39-47).

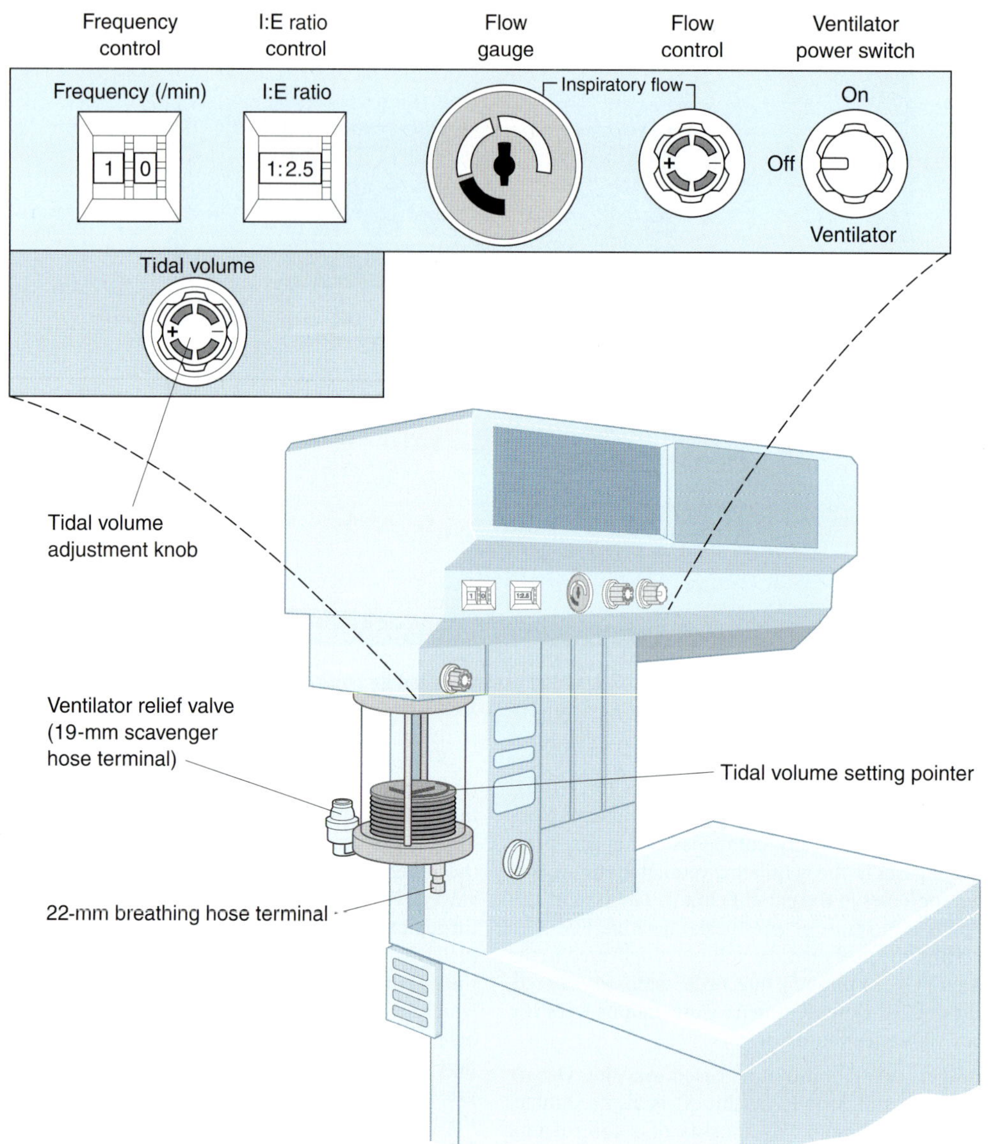

FIGURE 39-43. Dräger AV-E anesthesia ventilator. Note the standing bellows arrangement in this diagram. Figure 39-35 shows the hanging bellows version. [Copyright Dräger Medical AG & Co, KG, Lubeck-Germany.]

In the Dräger AV-E, the ventilator pressure-relief valve is controlled via an external relief valve pilot line (Figs. 39-44 and 39-45, item 20), which is essentially a short length of plastic tubing. Kinking this tubing can cause ventilator malfunction. Occlusion during inspiration when the valve is being held closed causes it to remain closed thereafter, and excess gas cannot leave the anesthesia circuit. Consequently, pressure in the circuit rises and, if not relieved, could result in barotrauma.[57,58] A circuit continuing pressure or high-pressure alarm should alert the clinician to such a situation. If the tubing is occluded during exhalation when the valve is not held closed, during the next inspiratory cycle, pressure cannot be transmitted through to the valve to hold it closed. Patient circuit gas can then leak out to the scavenging system rather than entering the patient circuit, which might result in hypoventilation. Incompetence of the pressure-relief valve itself may also result in hypoventilation.[57] Again, contemporary circuit pressure, volume, or ventilation (CO_2) alarms should alert one to these situations. More recent versions of Dräger ventilator (AV 2+) incorporate a high-pressure limit control capable of inverse I:E ratios with a built-in safety mechanism that allows application to a wider range of patient conditions.

DIFFERENCES AMONG TRADITIONAL DOUBLE-CIRCUIT VENTILATOR DESIGNS

Standing Versus Hanging Bellows Ventilators Contemporary traditional anesthesia ventilators are of the standing bellows design; that is, they rise (ascend as the bellows fills) during exhalation and descend (empty) during inspiration. With a disconnection in which circuit pressure becomes equal to atmospheric pressure, the bellows cannot refill during exhalation. Some consider this to be a desirable safety feature.

In the (older) hanging bellows design (Figs. 39-35 and 39-36), the bellows fills by gravity during exhalation so that the ventilator pressure-relief valve does not require a PEEP design. With a circuit disconnection, room air is entrained into the patient circuit via the leak, and the bellows refills, emptying through the leak on the next

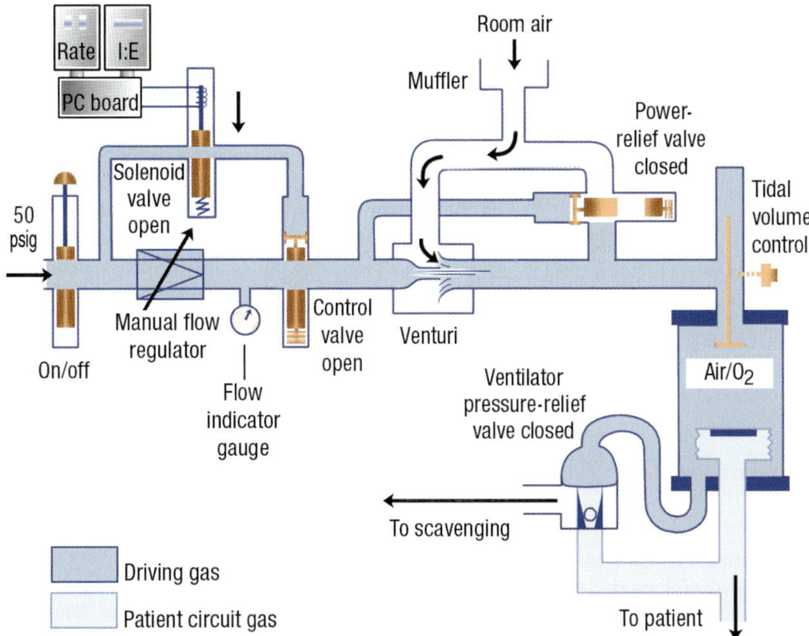

FIGURE 39-44. Dräger AV-E standing bellows design ventilator. Schematic of ventilator function during inspiration. See text for details of operation. [Copyright Dräger Medical AG & Co, KG, Lubeck-Germany.]

inspiration. For this reason, the standing bellows design is preferred, although it is not required by the standard describing specifications for anesthesia ventilators.

Dräger AV-E Versus GE- Datex-Ohmeda: Driving Gas The gas entering the bellows housing in a GE-Datex-Ohmeda ventilator is 100% O_2 (Figs. 39-37, 39-39, and 39-41), but in the Dräger AV-E, the gas is an air and O_2 mixture (Fig. 39-44). With a leak (hole) in the bellows, driving gas enters the patient circuit and dilutes the gases there. This can cause O_2 enrichment with a GE-Datex-Ohmeda ventilator but a decrease in the FIO_2 with a Dräger AV-E if an oxygen concentration of < 40% were set at the machine flowmeters.

In the Dräger ventilator, the tidal volume is determined by setting the expansion limit of the bellows during expiration because the bellows is emptied completely during inspiration. The bellows (Figs. 39-44 and 39-45) housing is graduated from 0 mL below to 2000 mL at the top of the housing. In the GE-Datex-Ohmeda design, the bellows is graduated from 0 mL at the top to 1600 mL at the bottom of the bellows housing

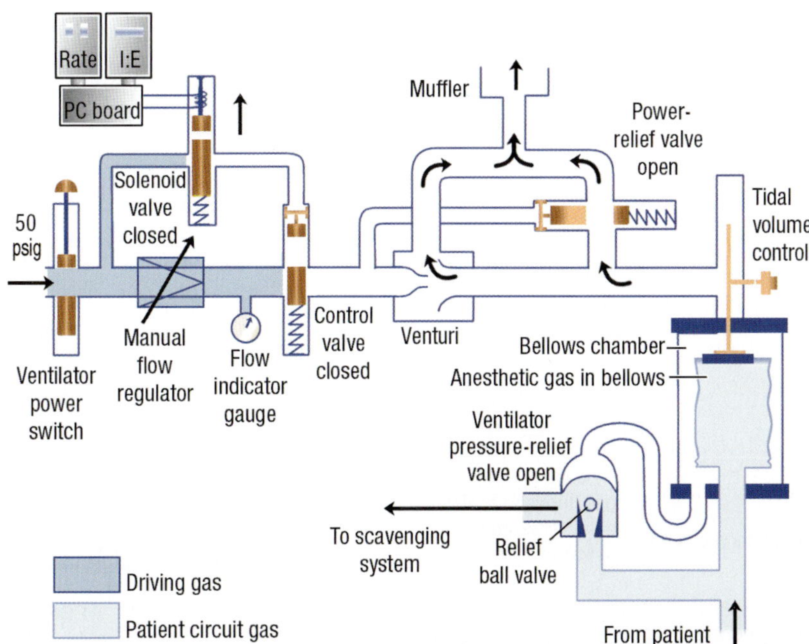

FIGURE 39-45. North American Dräger AV-E standing bellows design ventilator. Schematic of ventilator function during *exhalation*. I:E, inspiratory-to-expiratory. [Copyright Dräger Medical AG & Co, KG, Lubeck-Germany.]

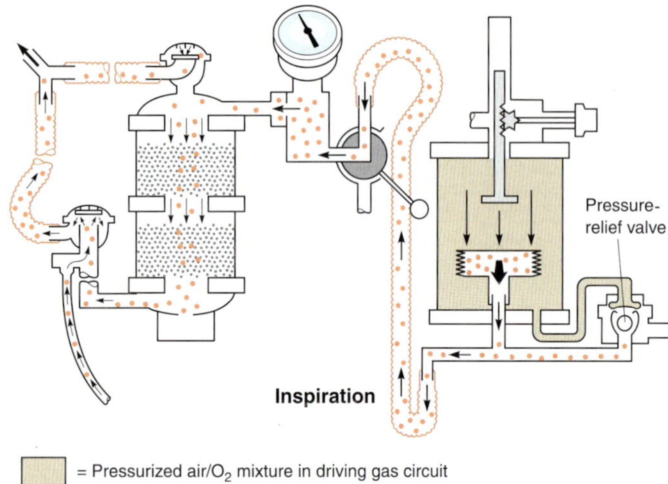

FIGURE 39-46. Dräger AV E standing bellows design showing events during inspiration. [Copyright Dräger Medical AG & Co, KG, Lubeck-Germany.]

because the tidal volume is displaced from the bellows by a metered volume of compressed O_2 during inspiration (Fig. 39-37).

The Dräger AV-E ventilator uses a Venturi and an air and O_2 mixture to compress the bellows. This economizes on the use of compressed O_2. In the GE-Datex-Ohmeda ventilator, O_2 consumption as the driving gas is a little greater than the set minute ventilation.[59]

In the GE-Datex-Ohmeda 7000, 7800, and 7900 series ventilators, the circuit pressure-relief ("pop-off") valve is flush mounted inside the bellows (Fig. 39-39). The design does not use a relief valve pilot line and is therefore not vulnerable to the effects of this line kinking (Fig. 39-44, item 20).[59] In the GE-Datex-Ohmeda ADU workstation, the ventilator pressure-relief valve is visible, but there is a direct rather than a pilot tube connection to the driving gas circuit.

GE-Datex-Ohmeda ventilators incorporate a pressure-relief valve in the driving gas circuit (Figs. 39-36 and 39-38). This may be preset to 65 cm H_2O (as in the Datex-Ohmeda 7000 model) or may be adjustable (Fig. 39-40, Ohmeda 7810 model, "Inspiratory Pressure Limit") as on the 7900 series. Most of the original Dräger AV-E ventilators do not have a pressure-relief valve in the driving gas circuit. Such a valve (Dräger Pressure Limit Control), with variable relief pressure settings, is available and may be retrofitted to standing bellows versions of these ventilators, thereby providing a pressure limit. It is now standard with the more recent model, the Dräger AV 2+.

Because the Dräger AV-E ventilator Venturi requires entrainment of air (Figs. 39-44 and 39-45), a clean (unoccluded) muffler is essential. If the muffler becomes blocked for any reason, room air is no longer entrained, and inspiration cannot be completed. If blockage occurs during exhalation, gas cannot leave the ventilator bellows housing, and the bellows remain collapsed.[60]

Tidal Volume During inspiration, the anesthesia ventilator pressure-relief valve is held closed so that gas contained in the bellows enters the patient circuit rather than the scavenging system (Fig. 39-44). Meanwhile, because the anesthesia machine is a continuous flow machine, fresh gas continues to enter the patient circuit from the anesthesia machine throughout the ventilatory cycle, according to the (O_2, N_2O, air) gas flow-control settings.

In the traditional design of anesthesia ventilator, when setting a certain VT to be delivered from the bellows to achieve a certain VT delivered to the patient's lungs, one must consider the FGF rate from the anesthesia machine to the patient circuit.[61,62]

Consider an anesthesia ventilator set to a frequency of 10 breaths/min, an I:E ratio of 1:2, and an FGF of 6 L/min (or 100 mL/s) to the anesthesia circle. Each breath lasts 6 seconds (60 s/10 breaths), with inspiration lasting 2 seconds and expiration 4 seconds (I:E = 1:2). During inspiration, the ventilator pressure-relief valve is closed so that both gas from the emptying bellows and FGF from the machine enter the patient circuit (Fig. 39-46). Because FGF is 100 mL/s and each inspiration lasts 2 seconds, the VT set on the ventilator bellows is potentially augmented by 200 mL. Consequently, changing the FGF, respiratory rate, or I:E ratio may have a profound effect on circuit VT, alveolar ventilation, and Pa_{CO_2}.[62,63] **Figure 39-48** illustrates the effect on Pa_{CO_2}.

The additional minute ventilation to the patient circuit when using an anesthesia ventilator is approximated by the formula:

$$\text{Additional ventilation} = (I/[I + E]) \times FGF$$

This is divided by the respiratory rate to determine the augmentation of each ventilator bellows VT.

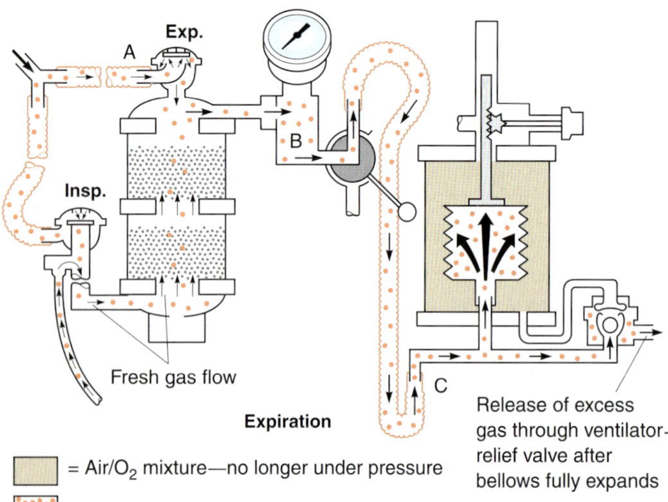

FIGURE 39-47. Dräger AV-E standing bellows design showing events during expiration. Insp., inspiratory unidirectional valve. Exp., expiratory unidirectional valve *A*, *B*, and *C* represent possible positions for positive end-expiratory pressure valve placement See text for details. I:E, inspiratory-to-expiratory. [Copyright Dräger Medical AG & Co, KG, Lubeck-Germany.]

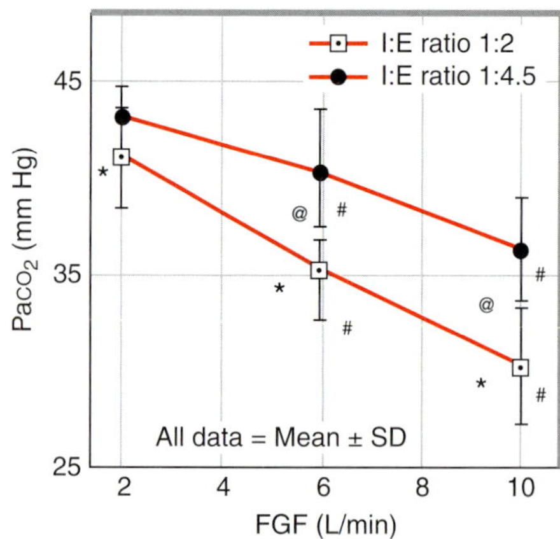

FIGURE 39-48. Effect of fresh gas flow (FGF) and inspiratory-to-expiratory (I:E) ratio on arterial CO_2 tension (Pa_{CO_2}) in patients ventilated with anesthesia ventilator set to constant tidal volume (VT). Increasing FGF or I:E ratio causes an increase in delivered VT, an increase in alveolar ventilation, and a decrease in Pa_{CO_2}.

In terms of VT actually delivered to the patient's airway, this formula provides an approximation only. The actual augmentation of VT also depends on the patient's total thoracic compliance compared with that of the anesthesia circuit components. If the patient's total thoracic compliance is low, additional fresh gas inflow from the machine may be accommodated mainly by compression in the circuit. Thus, patient MV is given by:

$$\text{Set MV} + (\text{FGF} \times [\text{I/I} + \text{E}]) - (\text{Gas volume compressed in circuit at peak inspiratory pressure} \times f)$$

where f is the respiratory rate in breaths per minute. The compressed gas volume term can be calculated as the product of circuit compliance and peak inspiratory pressure. Thus, volume compressed in the circuit equals compliance of circuit (mL/cm H_2O) times peak inspiratory pressure. These considerations do not apply to intensive care unit ventilators, which are designed to be minute volume dividers and whose VT is not affected by FGF, I:E ratio, or rate.

The GE-Datex-Ohmeda 7900 ventilator uses the SmartVent compensation system to compensate automatically for changes in FGF, I:E ratio, and RR as far as they affect the tidal volume delivered to the patient circuit. However, because the inspiratory flow transducer (which senses the inspired volume and provides feedback to the ventilator) is located at the inspiratory connection to the circuit, compression losses experienced in the patient circuit itself are not compensated. The uncompensated loss is the product of the peak inspiratory pressure and the compliance of the patient circuit. If during the preuse checkout, the compliance of the breathing circuit is measured, then compensation is made for these compression losses.

Positive End-Expiratory Pressure The deliberate application of PEEP to the patient's airway is common during anesthesia. PEEP may be applied by adding a free-standing PEEP valve between the circle system's expiratory limb and the expiratory valve. Although free-standing PEEP valves function well when used correctly, they are occasionally used erroneously and may totally occlude the circuit if incorrectly placed in the circle's inspiratory limb.[63] Because of this potential hazard, the use of free-standing PEEP valves is not recommended.

Contemporary workstations have PEEP valves that are an integral component of their ventilators. These valves are convenient to use and avoid the risk of erroneous PEEP valve placement. However, one must consider the possible effects of placement positions of a PEEP valve in the anesthesia circuit.

At end-exhalation, the pressure in an anesthesia circuit during positive-pressure ventilation using a standing bellows ventilator is +2.5 cm H_2O because of the PEEP effect of the ventilator pressure-relief valve (Fig. 39-47). If a 10-cm H_2O PEEP valve is now added by the expiratory unidirectional valve (Fig. 39-47, position A), that part of the circuit between the inspiratory and PEEP valves is at +10 cm H_2O compared with pressure beyond the valve. That part of the circuit between the PEEP valve and the ventilator is at +2.5 cm H_2O. On the next inspiration, gas from the compressed bellows enters the circuit and must compress that gas in the patient circuit that is at +2.5 cm H_2O by an additional +10 cm H_2O before any entering gas will flow past the inspiratory unidirectional valve to enter the circle's inspiratory limb. The volume of gas that leaves the ventilator bellows and is compressed in the part of the circuit that was at +2.5 cm H_2O represents wasted bellows VT because it is not available to ventilate the patient's lungs. If the PEEP valve is placed close to the ventilator bellows (Fig. 39-47, position C), at end-exhalation, most of the gas in the patient circuit is now at +10 cm PEEP. In this case, a much smaller volume of gas leaving the bellows during inspiration must be compressed in the circuit before the patient begins to receive a VT. Thus, when a VT has been set to be delivered from an anesthesia ventilator bellows, addition of PEEP to the basic circle system may decrease delivered VT, depending on the position of the PEEP valve in the circuit. In Figure 39-47, bellows VT loss would be greatest with position A and least with position C; position B is intermediate.[64] Decreases in VT may be reflected in spirometer readings or in other monitors of patient ventilation (eg, $Paco_2$; end-tidal CO_2).

Advantages of placing the PEEP valve near to the expiratory unidirectional valve (see Fig. 39-47, position A or B), however, are that in these positions, PEEP may be applied during spontaneous as well as during mechanical ventilation. The decrease in patient VT on application of PEEP at position A in Figure 39-47 (such as would be obtained with insertion of a free-standing PEEP valve) is greatest at low bellows VT settings.[64] It is also more significant with the GE-Datex-Ohmeda design of ventilator (models 7000, 7810) than with the Dräger AV-E. This is because the Dräger AV-E bellows empties completely during each inspiration, but the Datex-Ohmeda bellows empties only the set VT into the circuit. Because a Datex-Ohmeda bellows has a capacity of 1600 mL (Fig. 39-37), the compression volume in the circuit at end-inspiration is greater than in the Dräger AV-E ventilator system by a volume of 1600 mL – VT.

In the GE-Datex-Ohmeda 7900 ventilator, Aisys and the ADU, the PEEP is applied at the level of the ventilator pressure relief valve; therefore, the whole circuit is at PEEP and the tidal volume loss caused by application of PEEP at positions A, B, and C (shown in Fig. 39-47) does not apply. Furthermore, any deviation from the tidal volume set would be sensed by the inspiratory flow transducer, and a correction would be made via the SmartVent Compensation System.

NEW DESIGNS OF ANESTHESIA VENTILATOR AND PATIENT BREATHING SYSTEMS

As already discussed, several problems were inherent in the design of the traditional anesthesia ventilator. There was often a discrepancy between what was set as VT and what was delivered. Thus, with a Datex-Ohmeda 7000 ventilator and GMS absorber system, one might set a VT of 500 mL and observe a different value on the bellows housing graduations (which are inaccurate) and yet another value from the spirometer on the expiratory side of the circuit. The ventilators were not very accurate in small pediatric patients, in whom changes in FGF, I:E ratio, and RR could have profound effects that might lead to barotrauma.

Two basic approaches have been taken to compensate for unintentional changes in VT, computerized compensation and fresh gas decoupling. These require a more detailed discussion of some of the newer workstations.

Computerized Compensation: GE-Datex-Ohmeda Anesthesia Delivery Unit and 7900 with SmartVent The GE-Datex-Ohmeda ADU uses conventional needle valves to control gas flows (O_2, N_2O, air) but the flows are measured electronically and the information fed to the CPU. Information from the Aladin vaporizing system is also fed to the CPU. The total FGF and vapor leaving the CGO is therefore constantly measured. It may pass through an optional conventional rotameter located at the common gas outlet that reassures the user that O_2 is flowing in the event electrical power is lost.

The ADU uses a circle system with fresh gas inflow on the patient side of the inspiratory unidirectional valve. The ADU ventilator controls are integrated with the CPU so that when a VT is set to be delivered by the ventilator, the CPU can adjust the excursion of the bellows, adjusting it accordingly if FGF, RR, or I:E ratio is changed. If a high FGF is set at the gas flow controls and a small VT is set on the ventilator, the bellows may move only slightly because most of the VT is now being provided by the FGF. If the FGF is decreased, this is sensed by the CPU, which automatically increases the VT delivered from the ventilator bellows. In addition, during the automated preuse checkout, the user occludes the Y-piece, and the workstation measures the compliance of the breathing system so that this is also taken into account by the ventilator. The ADU Carestation achieves PEEP by controlling the ventilator pressure-relief valve.

The latest addition to the GE-Datex product line is the Aisys Carestation. Although it incorporates totally electronic gas flow control using a gas mixer (the user selects N_2O or air, F_{IO_2}, and total gas flow) and Aladin vaporizer controls, the ventilator used is the 7900. The SmartVent feature monitors the patient's breathing system by signals from pressure, flow, and O_2 transducers. Inspiratory and expiratory flow sensors measure the flow, and therefore volume, of gas to and from the patient circuit. By comparing the operator set value with the actual delivered inspired V_T, the ventilator compensates for gas compression losses and contributions from FGF. SmartVent compensation occurs over several breaths after a change in FGF, but in the ADU, compensation is immediate.

FRESH GAS DECOUPLING

Fresh gas decoupling is used in the Dräger Narkomed 6400, Fabius GS, and Apollo (**Fig. 39-49**) workstations, all of which use an electric motor-driven piston in place of the traditional gas-driven bellows. Fresh gas decoupling is used in the Datascope Anestar workstation, which has a hanging bellows design.

The principle of fresh gas decoupling is that during the inspiratory cycle of positive-pressure ventilation, a decoupling valve closes to divert FGF into the reservoir bag of the circle system so that only gas from the ventilator (piston or bellows) flows to the patient. **Figure 39-50** shows fresh gas decoupling in the Datascope Anestar circuit. During inspiration, the decoupling valve closes, bellows gas flows to the patient, and fresh gas is diverted into the reservoir bag. If the FGF is high such that the bag's capacity is exceeded, the excess flows through the absorber and is vented to the waste gas scavenging system. In other designs, the bellows can be replaced in function by an electric motor-driven piston (**Fig. 39-51**). During the expiratory phase (**Fig. 39-52**), the fresh gas decoupling valve opens, permitting the descending bellows (or retracting piston) to fill with fresh gas from the bag and FGF from the machine followed by exhaled gas that has passed through the absorber. After the bellows (piston) has descended (retracted) completely, additional exhaled gas (mainly alveolar) is vented to the scavenging system.

Unlike the traditional circle system (Figs. 39-32 and 39-35), in a fresh gas decoupling circuit, the reservoir bag is always in circuit whether ventilation is spontaneous or controlled.[65] It is important to understand the function of the reservoir bag. A case is reported of failure of a decoupling valve that resulted in inability to mechanically ventilate the lungs.[66] Manual bag ventilation was possible. In this case, during inspiration, when the piston ventilator delivered its tidal volume into the circuit, the gas took the path of least resistance into the reservoir bag rather than inflating the lungs.

In the fresh gas decoupling ventilator circuits that use a piston (Fig. 39-51) or a hanging bellows, negative pressure could potentially be applied during exhalation if FGF is inadequate. This is of particular concern with the piston ventilator when the piston withdraws as it attempts to refill the cylinder. To protect against possible negative pressure barotrauma, fresh gas decoupling circuits incorporate a negative pressure relief valve through which room air can be drawn when the negative pressure exceeds approximately −2 cm H_2O. When this occurs, an alarm sounds because unrecognized entrainment of room air could lead to an unintended low F_{IO_2} and dilution of the anesthetic. Consequently, monitoring of F_{IO_2} and anesthetic agent concentration at the airway is of particular importance.

During the preuse checkout of the workstation the integrity of the breathing system is pressure checked for leaks. A leak could result in anesthetic gases being released into the atmosphere, as well as room air being entrained as just described. In one report, the workstation was checked out correctly. The users then noted that the patient was allergic to latex, so the reservoir bag was replaced with one that was latex free. It was then noted that the F_{IO_2} and the anesthetic agent concentration were decreasing. The users concluded that air was being entrained, and a large hole was found in the latex-free bag. No alarm sounded, however, because the air entrainment was not occurring through the negative-pressure relief valve (**Fig. 39-53**).[65]

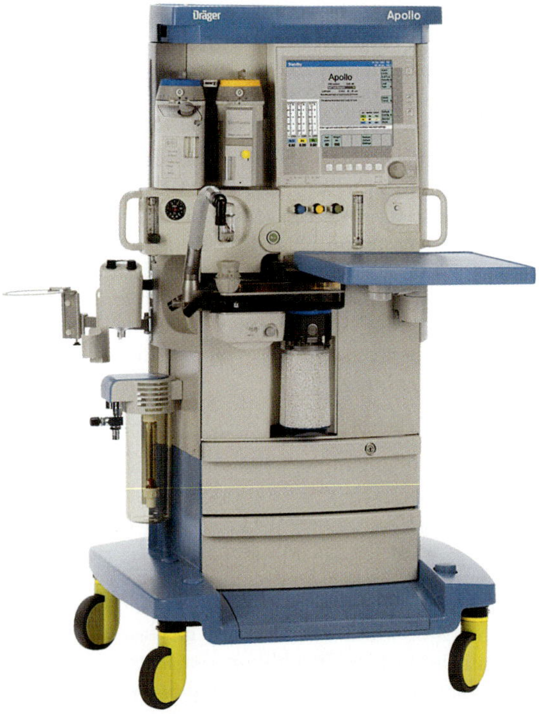

FIGURE 39-49. Dräger Apollo Anesthesia workstation. [Copyright Dräger Medical AG & Co, KG, Lubeck-Germany.]

WASTE GAS SCAVENGING

The anesthesia workstations in common use are all continuous flow devices, that is, fresh gas flows continuously from the common gas outlet to the breathing system. Because the FGF is usually more than that required either by the patient or to compensate for small leaks, the excess gas must be allowed to exit the breathing system and be scavenged by the waste gas scavenging system. Trace concentrations of anesthetic (waste) gases have neither been fully incriminated nor fully exonerated as health hazards to operating room personnel. However, all of the concerned agencies, such as the National Institute for Occupational Safety and Health (NIOSH), the American Hospital Association (AHA), The Joint Commission (formerly the Joint Commission on Accreditation of Healthcare Organizations, or JCAHO), and the American Society of Anesthesiologists (ASA), encourage reduction of exposure to waste gases, which includes waste gas scavenging and monitoring of measures to reduce exposure.

In a 1977 publication that to date has not been superseded, NIOSH recommended environmental limits for the upper boundary of exposure[67]:

> Occupational exposure to halogenated anesthetic agents shall be controlled so that no worker is exposed at concentrations greater than 2 parts per million (ppm) of any halogenated anesthetic agent.... When such agents are used in combination with nitrous oxide, levels of the halogenated agent well below 2 ppm are achievable. In most situations, control of nitrous oxide to a time-weighted average (TWA) concentration of 25 ppm during the anesthetic administration period will result in levels of approximately 0.5 ppm of the halogenated agent.... Occupational exposure to nitrous oxide, when used as the

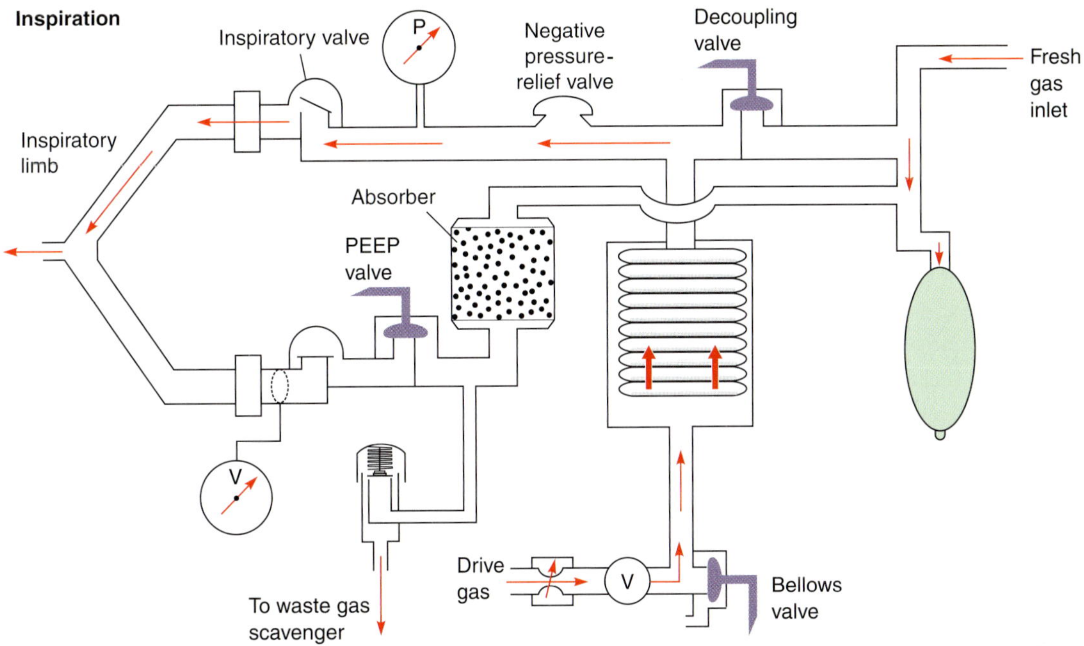

FIGURE 39-50. Fresh gas decoupling during the inspiratory phase of positive-pressure ventilation. During this phase, the decoupling valve, positive end-expiratory pressure (PEEP) valve and bellows valve are held closed. Fresh gas entering the breathing system is diverted into the reservoir bag, which therefore distends. [Reproduced with permission from Abramovich A. Fresh gas decoupling minimizes complexity. *APSF Newsletter.* 2005;20:35.]

> sole anesthetic agent, shall be controlled so that no worker is exposed at TWA concentrations greater than 25 ppm during anesthetic administration. Available data indicate that with current control technology, exposure levels of 50 ppm and less for nitrous oxide are attainable in dental offices.

These recommended exposure limits were based on 2 reports. Whitcher et al[68] showed that these levels were readily attainable in the operating room when certain precautionary measures were taken. Bruce and Bach[69] found no decrement in the psychomotor capacities of volunteers exposed for 4 hours at these levels. Because trace concentrations

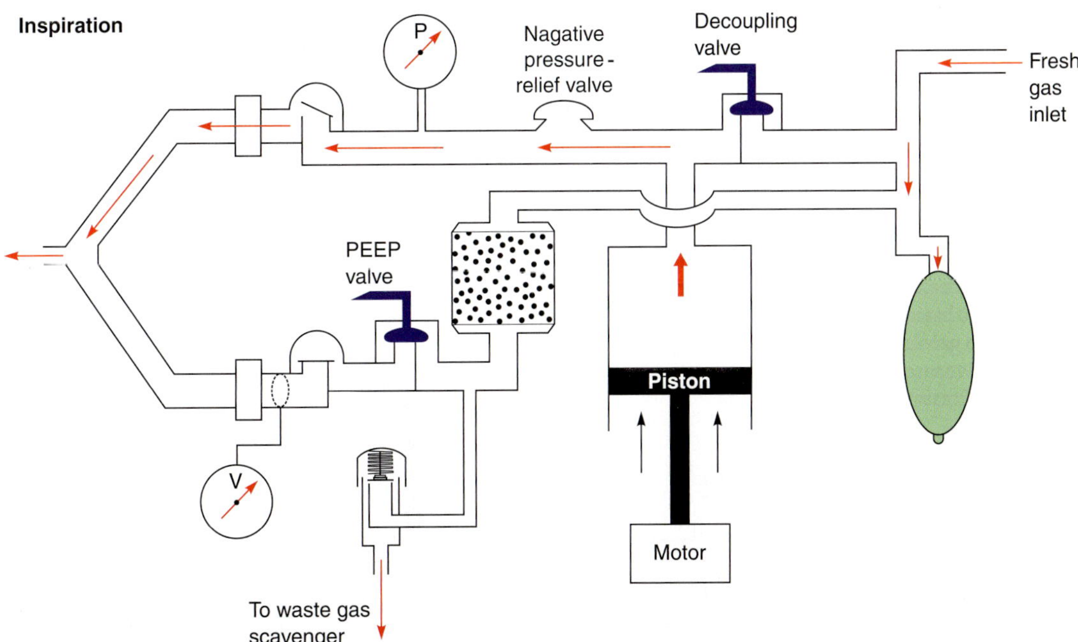

FIGURE 39-51. This figure shows that the function of the ventilator bellows can be performed by a piston in the same location. Piston ventilators are used in the Dräger Narkomed 6400 (Divan ventilator, horizontal piston), Fabius GS, and Apollo workstations (vertical pistons). Several potential advantages are afforded by a piston ventilator. Because they are driven by an electric motor, there is no need for a driving gas circuit, which economizes on the use of oxygen, particularly if a cylinder supply is in use. The electric motor can control the piston very accurately and provide versatility in ventilatory modes such as offered in intensive care unit ventilators. These ventilators are silent in operation, and many anesthetists are used to the familiar sounds of a pneumatic ventilator. Some models offer variable tones to simulate inspiration and expiration. PEEP, positive end-expiratory pressure. [Adapted with permission from Abramovich A. Fresh gas decoupling minimizes complexity. *APSF Newsletter.* 2005;20:35.]

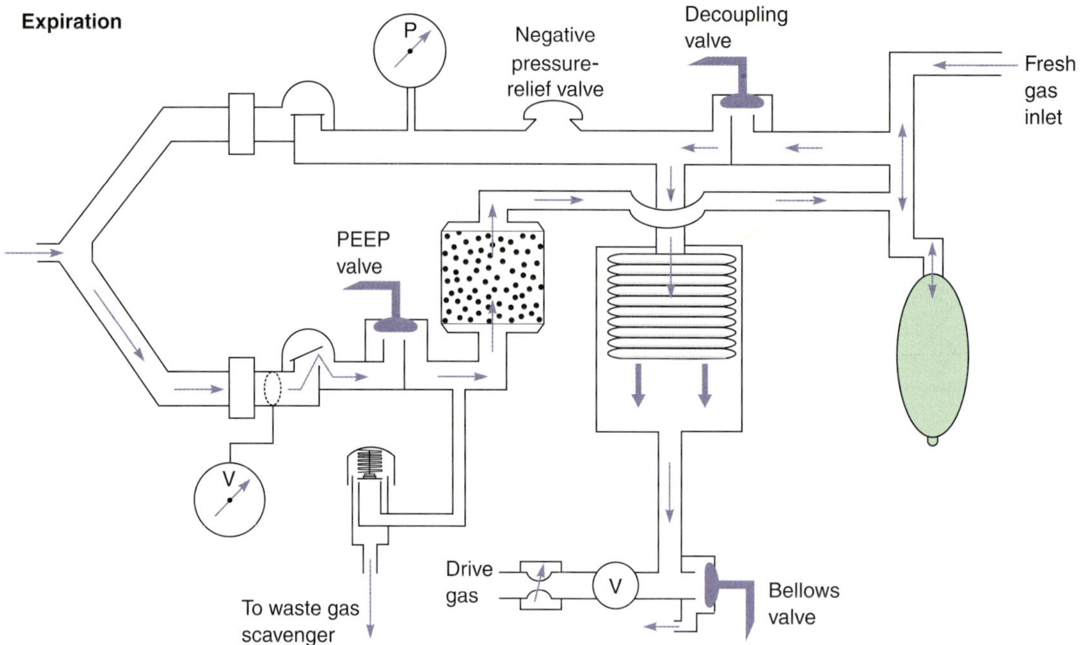

FIGURE 39-52. Fresh gas decoupling circuit during exhalation. The bellows refills (in this example by descending) and draws in fresh gas from the fresh gas inlet and fresh gas that was stored in the reservoir bag during the previous inspiration. PEEP, positive end-expiratory pressure. [Reproduced with permission from Abramovich A. Fresh gas decoupling minimizes complexity. *APSF Newsletter.* 2005;20:35.]

of anesthetic gases have never been proven to be a health hazard, the NIOSH-recommended limits were never promulgated into law and are therefore not enforceable by OSHA. In 1998, the ASA convened a Task Force on Trace Anesthetic Gases (of which this author was a member) to evaluate the status of this subject and make recommendations. The opinion and recommendations of the Task Force are summarized as follows:[70]

Studies have not shown an association between trace levels of waste anesthetic gases found in scavenged anesthetizing locations and adverse health effects to personnel.

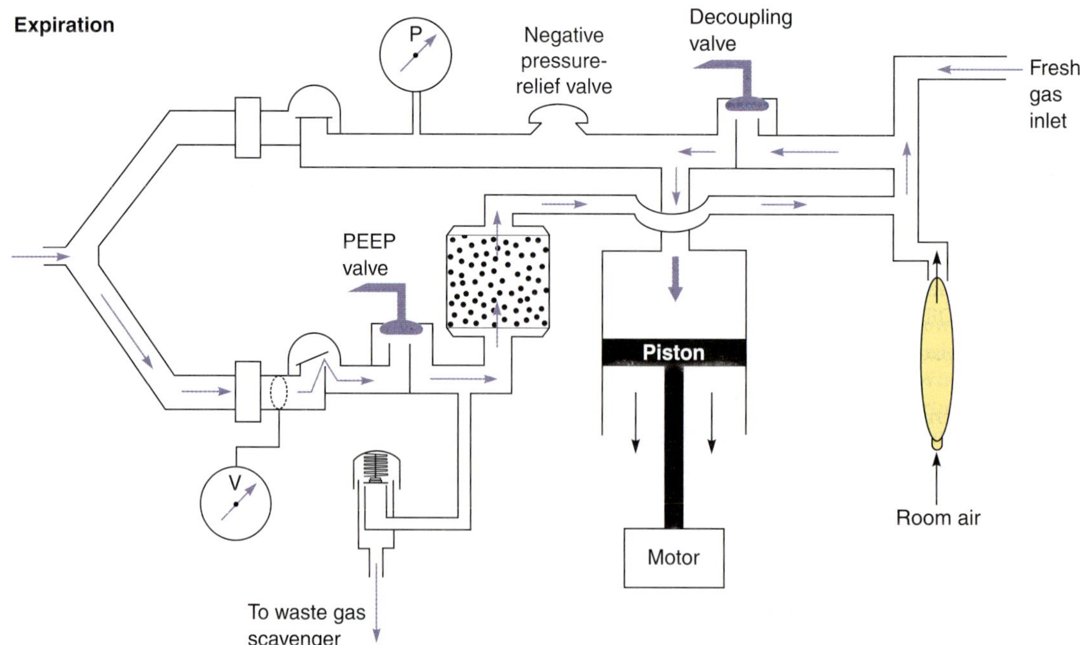

FIGURE 39-53. Figure shows in principle the situation described by Sandberg and Kaiser.[65] The reservoir bag that passed the machine checkout is replaced by one that is latex free but has a large hole in it. During exhalation, room air is entrained into the circuit via the hole in the bag as the piston descends to refill the cylinder with anesthetic gas mixture. Because the circuit is now at atmospheric pressure (because of the hole in the bag, no air is entrained through the negative-pressure relief valve, and therefore no alarm is annunciated. PEEP, positive end-expiratory pressure. [Adapted with permission from Abramovich A. Fresh gas decoupling minimizes complexity. APSF *Newsletter.* 2005;20:35.]

Recommendations of ASA Task Force on Waste Anesthetic Gases are:

1. Waste anesthetic gases should be scavenged.
2. Appropriate work practices should be used to minimize exposure to waste anesthetic gases.
3. Personnel working in areas where waste anesthetic gases may be present should be educated regarding current studies on health effects of exposure to waste anesthetic gases, appropriate work practices to minimize exposure, and machine checkout and maintenance procedures.
4. There is insufficient evidence to recommend routine monitoring of trace levels of waste anesthetic gases in the operating room and postanesthesia care unit.
5. There is insufficient evidence to recommend routine medical surveillance of personnel exposed to trace concentrations of waste anesthetic gases, although each institution should have a mechanism for employees to report suspected work-related health problems.

WASTE GAS SCAVENGING SYSTEMS

Waste gases may leave the anesthesia circuit via the APL valve or the ventilator pressure-relief valve. In either case, tubing of either a 19- or 30-mm internal diameter is used as distinct from the 22-mm internal diameter of the anesthesia circuit and ventilator tubing and the 15-mm internal diameter common gas outlet and tracheal tube connector sizes (**Fig. 39-54**). The scavenging system interfaces the gas flow out of the patient circuit with the hospital suction system. Scavenging systems may be open (to the atmosphere) or closed.

Closed systems use spring-loaded valves to ensure that excessively high or low pressures are not applied to the patient circuit (**Fig. 39-55**).[71,72] Thus, if not connected to negative pressure (suction), excess pressure in the closed interface caused by gas entering it from the circuit is vented via the positive-pressure (pop-off) relief valve, which opens at about +5 cm H_2O. If excessive suction might be applied to the circuit, 1 (GE-Datex-Ohmeda interface) or 2 (North American Dräger closed interface; Fig. 39-55) negative-pressure relief ("pop-in") valves (−0.25 to −1.80 cm H_2O, depending on the system) would open to preferentially draw in room air. This would minimize the potential for application of negative pressure to the patient circuit.

Open-reservoir scavenging interfaces are valveless (**Fig. 39-56**) and use continually open relief ports to provide pressure relief.[73] Waste gas that exits from the breathing circuit (via the APL or ventilator pressure-relief valve) is directed to the bottom of the canister (all anesthetic gases are more dense than air), and the hospital suction system aspirates gas from the bottom of the canister. In this type of interface, the reservoir canister contains the excess waste gas and thereby accommodates a range of waste gas flow rates from the patient circuit. Because this type of interface depends on open relief ports for pressure relief, care must be taken to ensure that these ports remain unoccluded at all times. Items 8a through 8e of the 1993 Food and Drug Administration (FDA) checklist describe, in principle, how the

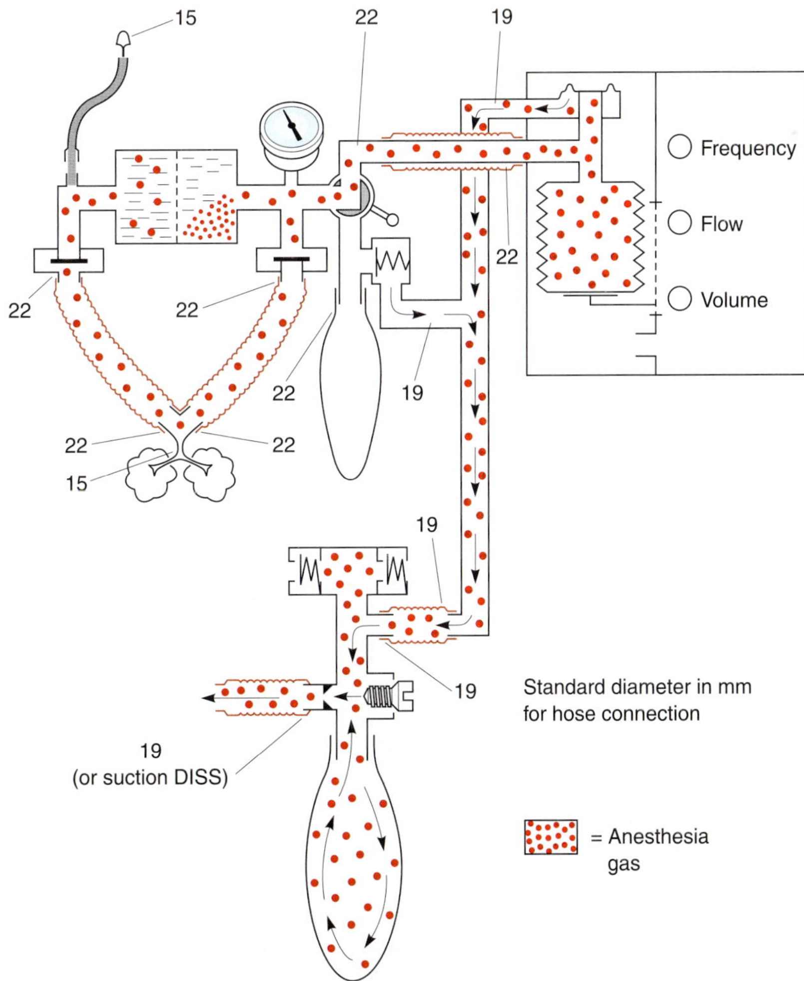

FIGURE 39-54. Schematic of anesthesia circuit and scavenging system tubing showing diameters for hose connections. [Copyright Dräger Medical AG & Co, KG, Lubeck-Germany.]

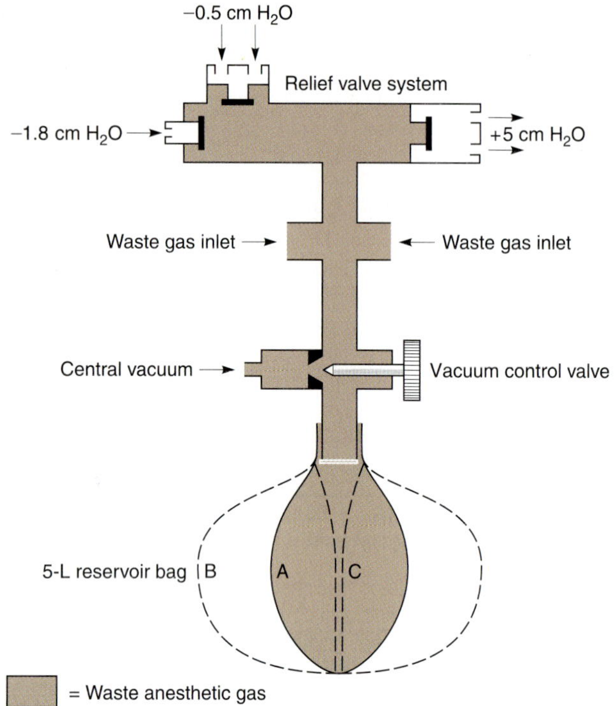

FIGURE 39-55. Dräger closed reservoir scavenger interface. *A*, Normal distension of bag–system working normally; *B*, inadequate suction–bag distends, and positive pressure-relief valve opens; *C*, excessive suction–bag collapses, and negative pressure relief valves opens. [Copyright Dräger Medical AG & Co, KG, Lubeck-Germany.]

scavenging system should be checked out (**Box 39-1** in Anesthesia Machine Checkout below).

In some recent workstation models (eg, GE-Datex ADU), the waste gas scavenging interface is internal to the machine and not visible to external inspection by the user. The principle of operation is that of an open reservoir system, and the checkout requires that the machine's scavenging connector is connected to the hospital vacuum and that the scavenging flowmeter indicates that flow is present. With the flowmeter indicator ball floating between the 2 line marks, the vacuum system is drawing about 25 L/min from the interface.

ANESTHESIA WORKSTATION CHECKOUT

The anesthesia delivery system should be checked each day before administering anesthesia to the first patient and whenever any change has been made to the system. Such changes include replacing the ventilator bellows, replacing the anesthesia circuit, changing the absorbent, and moving the anesthesia workstation even within the same operating room. Moving the machine may cause kinking or compression of tubing, which in turn may produce interference with gas delivery, ventilator function, or waste gas scavenging. Thus, in addition to a complete checkout at the start of each day, a shortened checkout of the delivery system should precede each administration of an anesthetic.

The FDA first published its anesthesia apparatus checkout recommendations, which had 24 steps, in August 1986.[74] A subsequent study reported that the mere introduction of the FDA 1986 checklist did not improve the ability of anesthesiologists to detect anesthesia machine faults.[75]

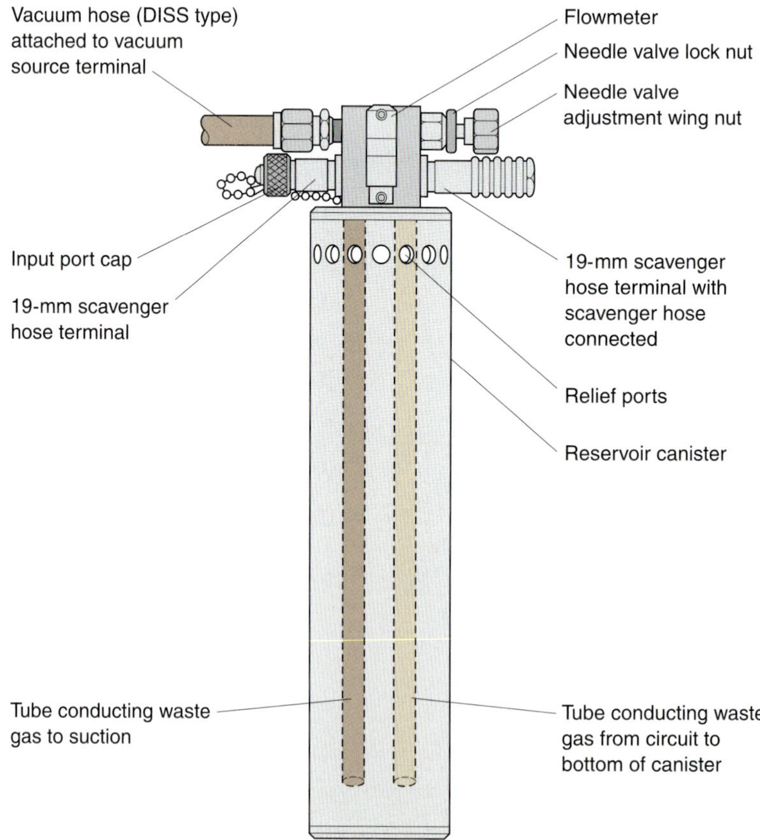

FIGURE 39-56. Dräger open-reservoir scavenging system. This interface uses continually open relief ports to provide positive and negative pressure relief (compare with the valves in Fig. 39-55). An adjustable needle valve regulates waste gas exhaust flow, which is indicated on uncalibrated flowmeter. The flowmeter reading halfway between 2 white lines corresponds to suction flow rate of about 25 L/min. [Copyright Dräger Medical AG & Co, KG, Lubeck-Germany.]

BOX 39-1

Food and Drug Administration Anesthesia Apparatus Checkout Recommendations of 1993

This checkout, or a reasonable equivalent, should be conducted before administration of anesthesia. These recommendations are only valid for an anesthesia system that conforms to current and relevant standards and includes an ascending bellows ventilator and at least the following monitors: capnograph, pulse oximeter, oxygen analyzer, respiratory volume monitor (spirometer), and breathing system pressure monitor with high- and low-pressure alarms. This is a guideline that users are encouraged to modify to accommodate differences in equipment design and variations in local clinical practice. Such local modifications should have appropriate peer review. Users should refer to the operator's manual for the manufacturer's specific procedures and precautions, especially the manufacturer's low-pressure leak test (step #5).

Emergency Ventilation Equipment

1. Verify that backup ventilation equipment is available and functioning.[a]

High-Pressure System

2. Check the oxygen cylinder supply.[a]
   a. Open the O_2 cylinder and verify that it is at least half full (~1000 psi).
   b. Close cylinder.
3. Check central pipeline supplies.[a]
   a. Check that hoses are connected and pipeline gauges read about 50 psi.

Low-Pressure Systems

4. Check the initial status of the low-pressure system.[a]
   a. Close the flow-control valves and turn off vaporizers.
   b. Check fill level and tighten the vaporizers' filler caps.
5. Perform a leak check of the machine's low-pressure system.[a]
   a. Verify that the machine master switch and flow-control valves are off.
   b. Attach a "suction bulb" to the common fresh gas outlet.
   c. Squeeze the bulb repeatedly until it is fully collapsed.
   d. Verify that the bulb stays fully collapsed for at least 10 seconds.
   e. Open 1 vaporizer at a time and repeat c and d as above.
   f. Remove the suction bulb and reconnect a fresh gas hose.
6. Turn on the machine master switch and all other necessary electrical equipment.[a]
7. Test the flowmeters.[a]
   a. Adjust flow of all gases through their full range, checking for smooth operation of floats and undamaged flow tubes.
   b. Attempt to create a hypoxic O_2/N_2O mixture and verify correct changes in flow or alarm (or both).

Scavenging System

8. Adjust and the check scavenging system.[a]
   a. Ensure proper connections between the scavenging system and both the APL (pop-off) valve and ventilator relief valve.
   b. Adjust the waste gas vacuum (if possible).
   c. Fully open the APL valve and occlude the Y-piece.
   d. With minimum O_2 flow, allow scavenger reservoir bag to collapse completely and verify that absorber pressure gauge reads about zero.
   e. With the O_2 flush activated, allow the scavenger reservoir bag to distend fully and then verify that absorber pressure gauge reads <10 cm H_2O.

Breathing System

9. Calibrate the O_2 monitor.[a]
   a. Ensure that the monitor reads 21% in room air.
   b. Verify that the low-O_2 alarm is enabled and functioning.
   c. Reinstall the sensor in the circuit and flush the breathing system with O_2.
   d. Verify that the monitor now reads >90%.
10. Check the initial status of the breathing system.
    a. Set the selector switch to "Bag" mode.
    b. Check that the breathing circuit is complete, undamaged, and unobstructed.
    c. Verify that the CO_2 absorbent is adequate.
    d. Install the breathing circuit accessory equipment (eg, humidifier, PEEP valve) to be used during the case.
11. Perform a leak check of the breathing system.
    a. Set all gas flows to zero (or minimum).
    b. Close the APL (pop-off) valve and occlude the Y-piece.
    c. Pressurize the breathing system to about 30 cm H_2O with an O_2 flush.
    d. Ensure that pressure remains fixed for at least 10 seconds.
    e. Open the APL (pop-off) valve and ensure that pressure decreases.

Manual and Automatic Ventilation Systems

12. Test ventilation systems and unidirectional valves.
    a. Place a second breathing bag on the Y-piece.
    b. Set appropriate ventilator parameters for the next patient.
    c. Switch to automatic ventilation (Ventilator) mode.
    d. Fill the bellows and breathing bag with O_2 flush and then turn on the ventilator.
    e. Set O_2 flow to minimum and other gas flows to zero.
    f. Verify that during inspiration the bellows deliver appropriate tidal volume and that during expiration the bellows fill completely.
    g. Set the fresh gas flow to about 5 L/min.
    h. Verify that the ventilator bellows and simulated lungs fill and empty appropriately without sustained pressure at end-expiration.
    i. Check for proper action of the unidirectional valves.
    j. Exercise the breathing circuit accessories to ensure proper function.
    k. Turn off the ventilator and switch it to manual ventilation (Bag/APL) mode.
    l. Ventilate manually and ensure inflation and deflation of artificial lungs and appropriate feel of system resistance and compliance.
    m. Remove the second breathing bag from the Y-piece.

Monitors

13. Check, calibrate, or set alarm limits of all monitors.
    a. Capnometer pulse oximeter
    b. Oxygen analyzer respiratory volume monitor (spirometer)
    c. Pressure monitor with high and low airway alarms

Final Position

14. Check the final status of the machine.
    a. Vaporizers off
    b. AFL valve open
    c. Selector switch to "Bag"
    d. All flowmeters to zero
    e. Patient suction level adequate
    f. Breathing system ready to use

[a]If an anesthesia provider uses the same machine in successive cases, these steps need not be repeated or may be abbreviated after the initial checkout.

APL, adjustable pressure-limiting; PEEP, positive end-expiratory pressure.

Anesthesia Apparatus Checkout Recommendations, 1993. Available at: http://www.osha.gov/dts/osta/anestheticgases/index.html#Appendix2. Accessed Sept. 18, 2011.

A revised version of the FDA preuse checkout with 18 steps was published in 1993 (Box 39-1).[76] Many potential problems with the machine can be detected if the FDA checkout is performed correctly, although the best checkout is always that recommended by the manufacturer for its particular model of machine.

TESTING FOR LEAKS IN THE ANESTHESIA MACHINE AND BREATHING SYSTEM

Item 5 in the 1993 FDA checkout recommendations (Box 39-1) describes how to check for leaks in the low-pressure system. This checkout evaluates the components of the delivery system that are downstream of the gas flow control and should detect gross leaks that may result from cracked rotameter tubes, leaking gaskets, and vaporizers. This leak check evolved from that in the 1986 checkout. In the 1986 test, the APL ("pop-off") valve is closed, and the patient circuit is occluded at the patient end. The system is then filled via the O_2 flush until the reservoir bag is just full but negligible pressure exists in the system. Oxygen flow is set to 5 L/min, and the oxygen flow is slowly decreased until pressure no longer rises above about 20 cm H_2O (**Fig. 39-57**). This set flow is said to approximate the total gas leak rate, which should be no greater than a few hundred mL/min. The reservoir bag should then be squeezed to a pressure of about 50 cm H_2O to verify that the system is gas tight. If a large enough leak is present, the circuit pressure may decrease to zero (**Fig. 39-58**).

The advantages of this test routine are that it can be performed quickly and that it checks the patient circuit as well as the low-pressure parts of the machine in those models without an outlet check valve. Disadvantages of this routine are that it is relatively insensitive to small leaks and that in machines with an outlet check valve (eg, Datex-Ohmeda Modulus I, Modulus II, Aestiva, and Excel models), only the patient circuit downstream of the outlet check valve is tested for leaks (**Fig. 39-59**).

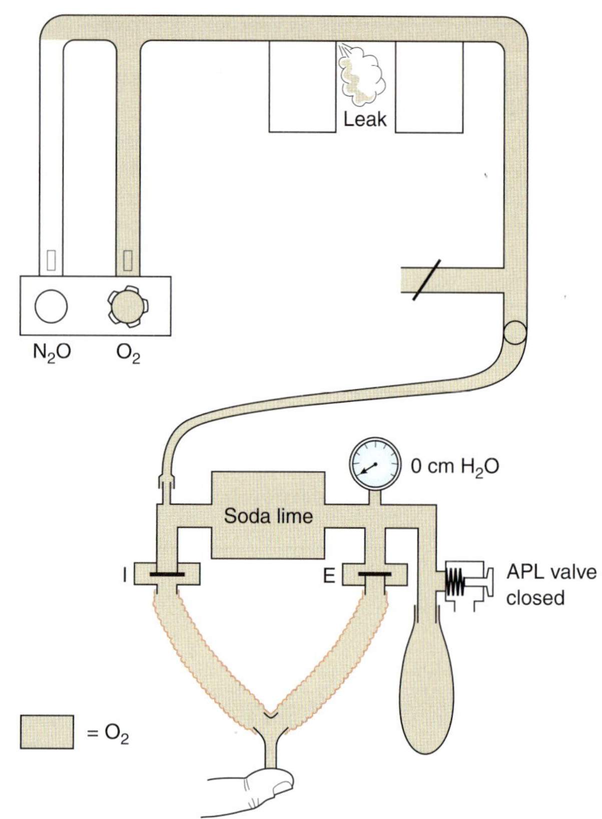

FIGURE 39-58. In the absence of outlet check valve, a leak at the vaporizer mount results in failure of the system to hold pressure, which in this case falls to zero. Such a leak would not be detectable by this test if an outlet check valve (see Fig. 39-59) were present. APL, adjustable pressure-limiting.

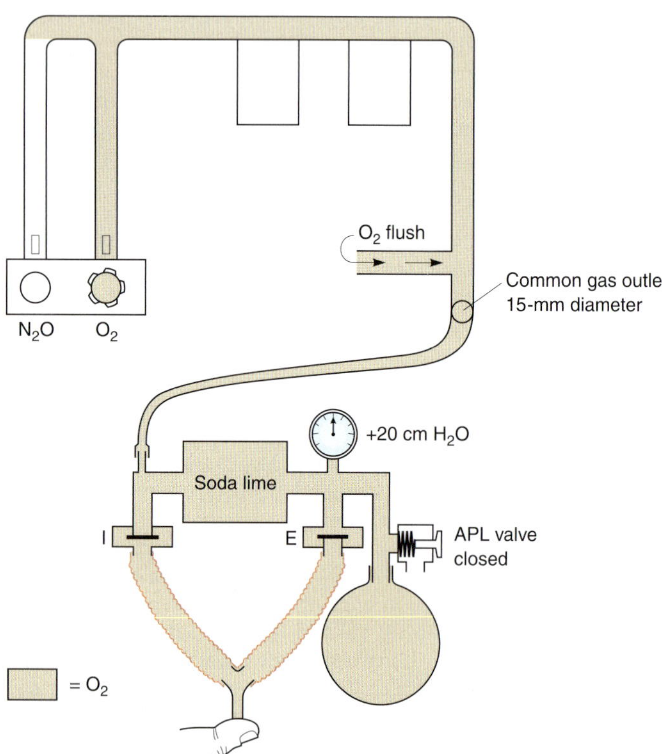

FIGURE 39-57. Food and Drug Administration 1986 generic leak test in a machine without an outlet check valve. In this case, a pressure of 20 cm H_2O is held with no gas flow, indicating that both the patient circuit and low-pressure parts of machine are gas tight. APL, adjustable pressure-limiting.

The FDA 1986 generic leak check also is insensitive because it is volume dependent. Thus, in this test, a large volume of gas (ie, that contained in the circuit tubing, absorber, and reservoir bag) is compressed, and a change in reading on the pressure gauge is sought. The term *compliance* expresses the relationship between volume and pressure and is defined as change in volume per unit change in pressure. Because of the large volume of gas compressed and the high compliance of the distensible reservoir bag, relatively large changes in volume (ie, leaks) may exist with minimal changes in pressure. The anesthetist performing the check is seeking a pressure decrease as an indicator of gas leakage, but large leaks may go undetected by this test. Such leaks may be unimportant while high FGFs are used but become more significant if gas flow rates are reduced subsequently during the maintenance of anesthesia.

The second limitation of the FDA 1986 generic checkout is related to the presence or absence of an outlet check valve, which, if present, separates the low-pressure part of the machine from the common gas outlet and circuit components downstream (Fig. 39-2). Application of the generic leak check in this situation may fail to detect leaks in components downstream of the outlet check valve (Fig. 39-59). The limitations of the FDA 1986 generic leak check demand that specialized leak checks of the low-pressure system must be used and that the machine operator's manual be consulted for details. The tests described for the traditional Dräger Narkomed and GE-Datex-Ohmeda machines are briefly reviewed to illustrate the differences in system design, function, and checkout.

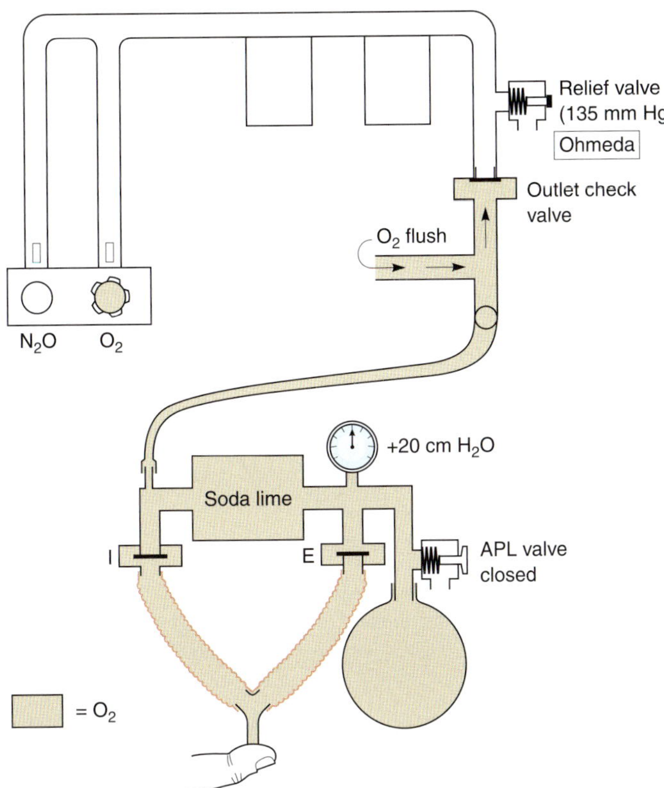

FIGURE 39-59. Application of Food and Drug Administration 1986 generic checkout to a system with an outlet check valve. In this case, application of positive back pressure of 20 cm H_2O causes the check valve to close so that only components downstream (ie, the circuit) are being tested for leaks. APL, adjustable pressure-limiting.

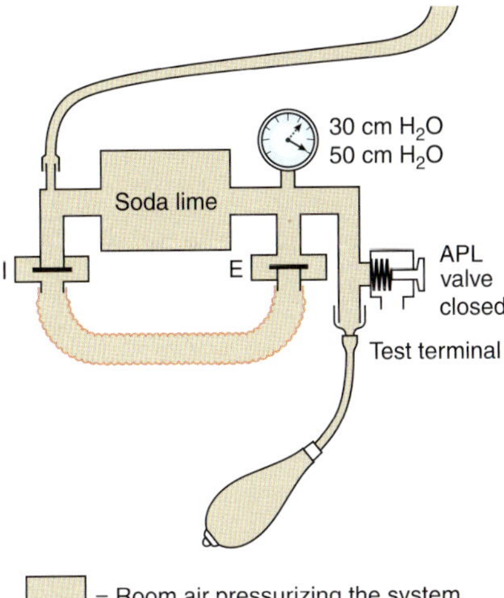

FIGURE 39-60. Dräger Narkomed positive-pressure leak check. It should take 30 seconds or longer for the pressure to decrease from 50 to 30 cm H_2O. APL, adjustable pressure-limiting.

Dräger Narkomed 2, Narkomed 3, Narkomed 4, and Narkomed GS Machines: No Outlet Check Valve Dräger recommends the following procedure for checking the anesthesia breathing system and fresh gas delivery system.[11] In this test, all gas flow-control (flowmeter) valves are closed, and the machine system's main power switch is turned to standby or off. This way, no gas should flow to the flowmeters or from the common gas outlet. All vaporizer concentration dials are set to zero. The inspiratory and expiratory valves are interconnected using a 22-mm-diameter circuit hose (**Fig. 39-60**). The shortest possible length of hose should be used to minimize contained gas volume. The "manual/automatic" selector valve is set to the manual (bag) position. The APL (pop-off) valve is closed (turned fully clockwise). The reservoir bag is removed, and the "test terminal" is attached to the bag mount. A sphygmomanometer squeeze bulb is connected to the hose barb on the test terminal.

The total volume of the circuit components has now been drastically reduced by removing the circle system tubing (a circle with each limb measuring 152 cm in length has a volume of about 1200 mL) and the reservoir bag (3 L). The sphygmomanometer bulb is then squeezed by hand until the pressure shown on the breathing system pressure gauge indicates a pressure higher than 50 cm H_2O. The gauge is then observed for a pressure decrease. The manufacturer specifies that 30 seconds or longer is required for a pressure decrease from 50 to 30 cm H_2O.[11] Because the volume of gas being compressed in this test is minimal, small gas leaks result in decreased pressure, which is observable on the circuit pressure gauge. The positive-pressure leak check should be repeated sequentially with each vaporizer turned on and set at any concentration above 0.4%. This will check for leaks in individual vaporizers (eg, filler caps, selector switches, vaporizer mounts).

The test specifications given in this section apply to an anesthesia breathing system without accessories (eg, spirometer, sidestream gas analyzer, other adapters).[11] Test limits are exceeded when accessory items are included in the test. (The supplier of the accessory items should be contacted for leak specifications.)

Leaks in the patient circuit components can be distinguished from leaks in the low-pressure part of the Dräger Narkomed machine (no outlet check valve) as follows: If a leak has been identified using the combined circuit/machine positive-pressure leak check just described, the sphygmomanometer bulb can be connected to the machine's common gas outlet using a 15-mm connector and to a pressure gauge using a 3-way stopcock. With this arrangement, only the machine (as opposed to machine and circuit in the previous test) is pressurized to 50 cm H_2O. A decrease in pressure then indicates a leak within the machine upstream of the common gas outlet. This test is possible because no outlet check valve is present in Dräger Narkomed machines.

Leaks in the patient circuit can be detected by systematically examining each component and connection in the circuit. If necessary, soap solution can be applied over joints suspected of leaking, with bubbles indicating the leakage site(s).

GE-Datex-Ohmeda Machines: Outlet Check Valve Present In certain Datex-Ohmeda anesthesia machines (Modulus I, Modulus II, Excel, and Aestiva), an outlet check valve (Fig. 39-2) complicates positive-pressure testing of the machine's low-pressure system (Fig. 39-59).

Application of positive pressure downstream from the valve causes it to close, and only components downstream of this valve (ie, beyond the common gas outlet) would then be checked for leaks. Positive-pressure ventilation and opening of the O_2 flush valve cause the check valve to close. For this reason, Datex-Ohmeda describes a negative-pressure leak test using a special suction bulb device that is supplied with each machine to which this test applies (**Fig. 39-61**).

First, the adequacy of the leak-testing device should be checked by sealing the bulb's inlet connector and squeezing the bulb until it is collapsed. The bulb is then released, and the time taken to reinflate is observed. If reinflation occurs in less than 60 seconds, the device should be replaced.[10] The device is checked periodically (at times of machine servicing) to ensure that the vacuum produced by the evacuated bulb is at least −65 mm Hg (Fig. 39-61).

The device is then used to check the machine. The anesthesia machine system's master switch and all vaporizers are turned off so that no gases flow into the machine's low-pressure system. Each gas

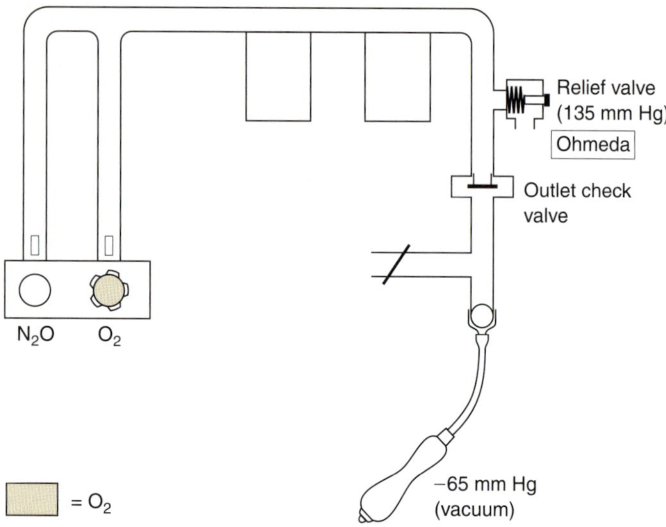

FIGURE 39-61. GE-Datex-Ohmeda negative-pressure leak check. See text for details.

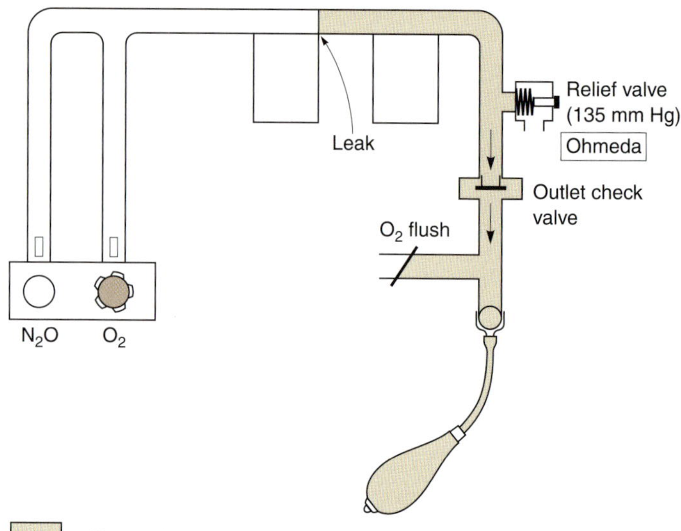

FIGURE 39-62. GE-Datex-Ohmeda negative-pressure leak check. With a leak in the low-pressure system of the machine, the evacuated bulb reinflates. See text for details.

supply is then opened by turning on the cylinder valves or by connecting the pipeline supply. The flow-control valves (rotameters) are turned fully open. The negative-pressure leak-testing bulb is attached to the machine's common gas outlet (or auxiliary common gas outlet, Fig. 39-33) via a 15-mm connector. The hand bulb is repeatedly squeezed and released until it remains collapsed. If the bulb reinflates within 30 seconds or less (Fig. 39-61), a leak of as little as 30 mL/min is present. The test procedure is repeated with each vaporizer on in turn to seek leaks in individual vaporizers. If the source is not obviously correctable, the machine should be withdrawn from service.

When the leak tests are completed, the negative-pressure bulb is removed from the common gas outlet, and residual vapors are purged from the machine by turning on O_2 flow at 1 L/min for 1 minute with all vaporizers off. Use of the O_2 flush control after this check does not purge vapors from the machine because the O_2 flush flow enters the system downstream from the vaporizers and from the outlet check valve. Because the leak check described is conducted with all the flow-control valves open, components up to and including the machine's main on/off control switch are also tested for leaks.

The negative-pressure leak check described for GE-Datex-Ohmeda machines results in the outlet check valve being held open by the −65 mm Hg vacuum (**Fig. 39-62**) and air or gas being sucked into the system through any leaks. If such leaks were present while the machine was in service, anesthesia gases would escape from the system through such leaks.

Considering the basic internal arrangement of the GE-Datex-Ohmeda machines that have an outlet check valve, one might suggest that an internal machine leak could be detected by occluding the common gas outlet (by thumb or by clamping the fresh gas delivery tubing, as shown in **Fig. 39-63**). The machine is then turned on and the O_2 flow rate observed, which is possible at the rotameter, assuming that the O_2 flow rate indicates the leakage rate (compare with FDA 1986 checkout procedure). The procedure described does not necessarily indicate the true leakage rate, because these Datex-Ohmeda machines also have a pressure-relief valve located between the vaporizers and the outlet check valve (see Figs. 39-61 to 39-63). This pressure-relief valve opens at a pressure of 135 ± 15 mm Hg (~2.3–2.9 psig) to release gas and prevent pressure buildup proximal to the outlet check valve. GE-Datex-Ohmeda Excel machines have a pressure-relief valve located downstream from the outlet check valve between this valve and the common gas outlet. This pressure-relief valve has an opening pressure of 5 psig. A pressure-relief valve limits the use of the procedure just described to testing for machine leaks only at pressures below the pressure-relief valve's opening pressure. Consequently, only the negative-pressure test described by GE-Datex-Ohmeda in its operator's manual for the particular model should be used.

If, after testing, the anesthesia machine is found to have a leak, it should be withdrawn from use until an authorized agent has repaired the leak, rechecked the system, and certified that it is ready to be put back into clinical service.

Datex-Ohmeda Modulus II Plus and Modulus CD Machines: No Outlet Check Valve Although the more recently introduced Datex-Ohmeda models (Modulus II Plus, Modulus CD) do not have an outlet check valve (Fig. 39-2), GE-Datex-Ohmeda recommends the negative-pressure leak-test procedure previously described to check for leaks in these models.[10] The negative-pressure leak check device can, in principle, be used to check for leaks in a Dräger Narkomed machine, but Dräger has not provided specifications for using such a device on their products. Indeed, Myers et al[77] reported that the negative-pressure leak test could be used to detect leaks in all traditional anesthesia machines, whether

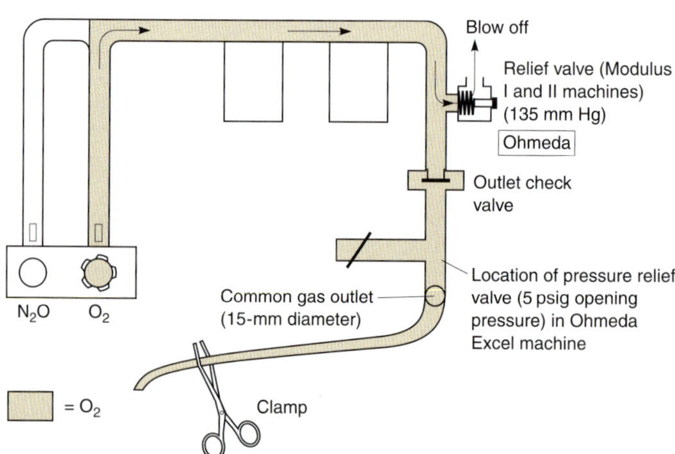

FIGURE 39-63. GE-Datex-Ohmeda system. The effect of occluding the common gas outlet and turning on the O_2 flowmeter is shown. Flow shown does not necessarily indicate leakage rate but may indicate rate of gas flow (blow-off) through the pressure-relief valve (pressure-relief valve). See text for details.

they have an outlet check valve or not. Item 5 of the FDA 1993 preuse checkout recommendations describes the use of the negative-pressure leak check bulb and states that it should stay fully collapsed for at least 10 seconds.

Automated Preuse Checkouts Although the preuse checkout of the workstation is very important, it is apparent that it is often performed inadequately. The most recently introduced anesthesia workstations (eg, GE ADU, Aisys; Dräger Fabius GS, Tiro, Apollo) use an automated checkout of many of the important functions. Advantages of an automated checkout are that it is performed correctly and alerts the user to faults and potential problems, the results are recorded in the memory of the workstation, and it enables certain parts of the checkout to be performed by an anesthesia technician so that an anesthetist who subsequently uses the workstation can see what has been checked and when.

Automated checkouts cannot, however, check all aspects of the workstation function. Certain procedures must still be performed by the user, and it is essential that the user understands what is checked automatically by the workstation and what is not (**Figs. 39-64** and **39-65**). The computerized checkout screen prompts and educates the user to perform certain checkout actions and to log that the actions have been done. For example, the user is expected to correctly assemble the breathing system and connect it to the workstation. The automated checkouts require that the Y-piece of the circuit be occluded so that the system can be pressurized to test for leaks and to measure compliance. This must be performed each time a change is made to the circuit. There may not be a leak in the circuit used in the first case, but there may be a leak in the next used disposable circuit. Breathing circuit function, as opposed to integrity, can be checked by attaching a second reservoir bag to the circuit Y-piece to act as a model lung and ventilating the bag in both manual and ventilator modes (see Box 39-1, FDA 1993 checkout, step 12, above). This is important because the circuit may pass an automated pressure check but not a functional flow check.

With the introduction of the new electronic workstations, the specific procedures recommended in the FDA 1993 checkout may not always be applicable, although the principles still apply. A subcommittee of the ASA Committee on Equipment and Facilities reviewed the previous recommendations in relation to the new workstations, and in 2008, the ASA published the Committee's report.[78] The report stated: ". . . Furthermore, anesthesia delivery systems have evolved to the point that 1 pre-anesthesia checkout (PAC) procedure is not

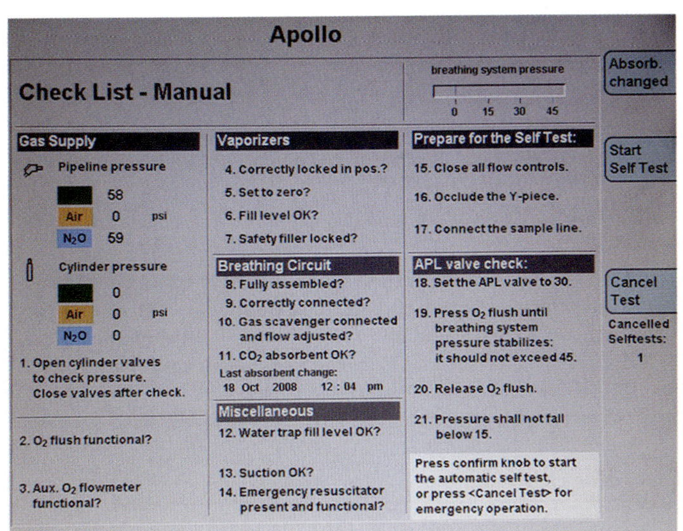

FIGURE 39-64. Dräger Apollo workstation preuse checkout screen showing the manual checklist.

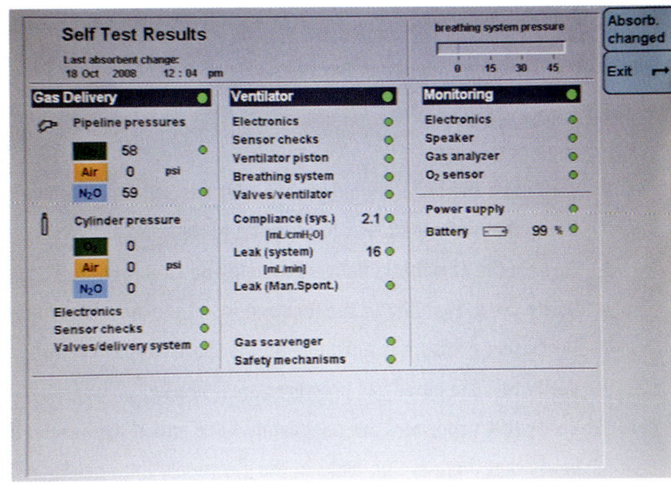

FIGURE 39-65. Dräger Apollo workstation screen showing self-test results from the automated checkout.

applicable to all anesthesia delivery systems currently on the market. For these reasons, a new approach to the PAC has been developed. The goal was to provide guidelines applicable to all anesthesia delivery systems so that individual departments can develop a PAC that can be performed consistently and expeditiously." The 2008 guidelines are intended to provide a template for developing checkout procedures that are appropriate for each individual anesthesia machine design and practice setting. They discuss which systems and components should be checked, the checkout interval (eg, before first case vs before every case), and who may be responsible for performing each checkout procedure (ie, anesthesiologist or technician). Regardless of who performs the checkout, the anesthesiologist bears the ultimate responsibility. A summary of the Committee's recommendations is shown in **Box 39-2**. Readers are encouraged to visit the ASA's website for the original and detailed (18-page) document, as well as examples of system-specific preuse checklists that were developed from the recommendations.[78]

SAFE USE OF THE ANESTHESIA WORKSTATION

Several studies have found that anesthesia caregivers' knowledge concerning the anesthesia delivery system is wanting.[7,79,80] Studies of critical incidents and adverse outcomes in relation to anesthesia gas delivery equipment have consistently shown that use error is the most common cause of such incidents and outcomes.[81-83] Because intensive training of anesthetists improves their ability to detect problems with anesthesia equipment, educational efforts must be emphasized.[84] User education is a major concern and priority of the manufacturers as new and increasingly sophisticated workstations are introduced. Human patient simulation has been reported to be an effective training device to ensure that practitioners are competent to use new equipment in both straightforward and crisis situations before using the equipment with human patients.[85]

SUMMARY

A basic understanding of the anesthesia delivery system and its components is important to the provision of safe patient care. Readers are encouraged to trace the flow of gases and vapors from their sources of storage, through their own particular delivery system, to waste gas scavenging. One should also consider the structure and function of each component in the gas pathway. In this way, malfunctions can be more readily identified and often more easily corrected by the user.

Readers are also strongly encouraged to review the operator's manual accompanying their anesthesia delivery systems and, in particular, to understand the rationale behind the specific checkout procedures described. Review of the manufacturer's product-specific educational materials is also encouraged.

BOX 39-2

Summary of American Society of Anesthesiologists 2008 Checkout Recommendations by Frequency and Responsible Party[79]

TO BE COMPLETED DAILY **ITEM TO BE COMPLETED**	Responsible Party
Item #1: **Verify that the auxiliary oxygen cylinder and self-inflating manual ventilation device are available and functioning.**	Provider and Tech
Item #2: **Verify that patient suction is adequate to clear the airway**	Provider and Tech
Item #3: **Turn on the anesthesia delivery system and confirm that AC power is available.**	Provider or Tech
Item #4: **Verify the availability of the required monitors, including alarms.**	Provider or Tech
Item #5: **Verify that pressure is adequate on the spare oxygen cylinder mounted on the anesthesia machine.**	Provider and Tech
Item #6: **Verify that the piped gas pressures are ≥50 psig.**	Provider and Tech
Item #7: **Verify that vaporizers are adequately filled and, if applicable, that the filler ports are tightly closed.**	Provider or Tech
Item #8: **Verify that there are no leaks in the gas supply lines between the flowmeters and the common gas outlet.**	Provider or Tech
Item #9: **Test the scavenging system function.**	Provider or Tech
Item #10: **Calibrate, or verify calibration of, the oxygen monitor and check the low-oxygen alarm.**	Provider or Tech
Item #11: **Verify that carbon dioxide absorbent is not exhausted.**	Provider or Tech
Item #12: **Perform breathing system pressure and leak testing.**	Provider and Tech
Item #13: **Verify that gas flows properly through the breathing circuit during both inspiration and exhalation.**	Provider and Tech
Item #14: **Document completion of the checkout procedures.**	Provider and Tech
Item #15: **Confirm ventilator settings and evaluate readiness to deliver anesthesia care. (ie, anesthesia time out).**	Provider
TO BE COMPLETED BEFORE EACH PROCEDURE **ITEM TO BE COMPLETED**	Responsible Party
Item #2: **Verify that patient suction is adequate to clear the airway.**	Provider and Tech
Item #4: **Verify the availability of the required monitors, including alarms.**	Provider or Tech
Item #7: **Verify that vaporizers are adequately filled and, if applicable, that the filler ports are tightly closed.**	Provider
Item #11: **Verify that carbon dioxide absorbent is not exhausted.**	Provider or Tech
Item #12: **Perform breathing system pressure and leak testing.**	Provider and Tech
Item #13: **Verify that gas flows properly through the breathing circuit during both inspiration and exhalation.**	Provider and Tech
Item #14: **Document completion of the checkout procedures.**	Provider and Tech
Item #15: **Confirm ventilator settings and evaluate readiness to deliver anesthesia care. (ie, anesthesia time out).**	Provider

KEY REFERENCES

- American Society for Testing and Materials. Standard specification for minimum performance and safety requirements for components and systems of anesthesia gas machines. F1850.00. West Conshohocken, PA: ASTM, 2005.
- Wabiszewski J. Explore the Anesthesia System: Aestiva/5. Datex-Ohmeda, GE Healthcare, Madison, WI, 2003.
- Cicman J, Himmelwright C, Skibo V, Yoder J. *Operating Principles of Narkomed Anesthesia Machines.* 2nd ed. Telford, PA: North American Dräger, 1993.
- Conway CM. Anaesthetic breathing systems. *Br J Anaesth* 1985; 57: 649.
- Dorsch JA, Dorsch SE. *Understanding Anesthesia Equipment.* 5th ed. Baltimore: Lippincott Williams & Wilkins, 2008.
- Ehrenwerth J, Eisenkraft JB, eds. *Anesthesia Equipment: Principles and Applications.* St. Louis, MO: Mosby-Year Book; 1993.
- Food and Drug Administration. *Anesthesia Apparatus Checkout Recommendations.* Rockville, MD: FDA, 1993.
- Schreiber P. Safety *Guidelines for Anesthesia Systems.* Telford, PA: North American Dräger, 1985.
- Sykes MK. Rebreathing circuits, a review. *Br J Anaesth* 1960;40: 666.
- ASA. Waste anesthetic gases. Information for management in anesthetizing areas and the postanesthesia care unit. Task Force on Trace Anesthetic Gases of the ASA Committee on Occupational Health of Operating Room Personnel. Park Ridge, IL: American Society of Anesthesiologists, 1999.

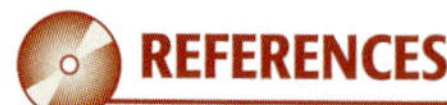

REFERENCES

Complete references available on DVD and online version at www.LongneckerAnesthesiology.com

CHAPTER 40

Principles of Pharmacokinetics and Pharmacodynamics: Applied Clinical Pharmacology for the Practitioner

Ken B. Johnson
Talmage D. Egan

KEY POINTS

1. The ultimate goal of pharmacokinetic–pharmacodynamic study is the accurate prediction of the time course and magnitude of drug effect so the clinician can answer a very simple and important question: "What is the appropriate dosing scheme for my patient?"
2. Pharmacokinetics, often thought of as "what the body does to the drug," is the study of the relationship between the drug dose and the drug concentrations that are produced over time.
3. Pharmacodynamics, often thought of as "what the drug does to the body," is the study of the relationship between the drug concentration and the drug effects that are produced.
4. Pharmacokinetic–pharmacodynamic models can be constructed that characterize drug behavior. These models are mathematical expressions of the relationship between drug dose and concentration (pharmacokinetics) and drug concentration and effect (pharmacodynamics). The models are composed of individual parameters (eg, clearance, distribution volume, effective concentration for 50% of maximal effect). Because of the complex interaction of the parameters, it is difficult to draw conclusions about drug behavior from a single parameter.
5. Because it is a mathematically based discipline, pharmacokinetics–pharmacodynamics is a distinctly unpopular subject among clinical anesthesiologists. This unpopularity is ironic considering that there is no medical specialty for whom the accurate prediction of the time course and magnitude of drug effect is more important (anesthesiologists produce profound, potentially dangerous drug effects that must be "turned on and off" in a rapid fashion).
6. Fortunately, the clinical implications of pharmacokinetic–pharmacodynamic models can be easily understood and conveyed through the use of computer simulation. Using computer simulation, a proposed dosing scheme can be "input" into a pharmacokinetic–pharmacodynamic model, producing a "picture" of the drug levels and drug effects that are expected to occur. These pictures (ie, computer simulations) are intuitively understandable and are easily applied to clinical situations.
7. The "biophase" is the theoretical site of drug action or "effect site" (eg, the brain, the neuromuscular junction, the spinal cord). It is important to consider drug concentrations in the biophase (and not just the plasma) because most drugs do not exert their effect in the blood. Pharmacokinetic–pharmacodynamic models account for this problem by linking the concentrations in the blood to theoretical concentrations in the biophase.
8. Because anesthetics are rarely administered alone (ie, anesthesia is usually at least a 2-process consisting of an analgesic and a sedative), characterizing the interaction between drugs is also an important goal of pharmacokinetic-pharmacodynamic study. Most anesthetics commonly used in combination, such as fentanyl and propofol, interact in a profoundly synergistic way (eg, where 2 + 2 = 7 or more …) so that much less of each drug is required (compared with the doses necessary when the drugs are used alone). Drug interaction models using "response surface" methods can be used to visualize these synergistic interactions and identify optimal dosing regimens.
9. Anesthesiologists have long recognized the need to adapt their anesthetic to account for differences in demographic factors and disease processes that influence drug disposition or effect. Comorbidities such as obesity, blood loss, presence of opioid tolerance, and differences in age are referred to as *covariates*. Covariates are descriptors of demographic factors or pathophysiologic states that impact anesthetic drug behavior.

CLINICAL PHARMACOLOGY: WHY BOTHER?

Clinical pharmacology is the science of predicting the magnitude and time course of drug effect. Given that anesthesiologists and other anesthesia providers spend their days administering low therapeutic index agents, clinical pharmacology is perhaps more important to anesthesiology than any other specialty. From a practical aspect, the ultimate goal of clinical pharmacology is to provide anesthesia practitioners with the information they need to make rational decisions about the selection and administration of anesthetics.

Anesthesia and reanimation necessitate a standard of precision and accuracy in drug administration not required in most areas of clinical medicine. Practitioners must profoundly depress the central nervous system to maintain the anesthetized state but then rapidly reanimate patients after an operation is complete. Although overdosing every patient within the constraints of acceptable hemodynamic variables is one approach to ensuring patients are adequately anesthetized, it comes at the cost of slow emergence from anesthesia, among others. Clinicians must therefore target drug levels that are within a relatively narrow therapeutic window to achieve the competing clinical imperatives of adequate anesthesia (without toxicity) and rapid emergence.

After an agent is selected (presumably because the agent's pharmacologic profile is well suited to the proposed application), the next challenge is the formulation of a scientifically grounded dosing strategy. What does the anesthetist need to know? **Table 40-1** catalogs some of the important considerations in determining the proper drug administration scheme in the context of anesthesia practice.

Anesthesiologists have long recognized that conventional, often simplified approaches to describing drug behavior such as "half-life" or "peak and trough" are not useful in answering these questions.[1] Perhaps no other specialty in medicine is more dependent on accurate predictions of a drug's pharmacokinetic and pharmacodynamic profile than is anesthesiology. Most settings in clinical medicine do not require immediate onset and rapid offset of pharmacologic effect. When an internist prescribes an oral medication for treatment of hypertension, for example, the fact that several days may be required for the development of a steady-state level of drug effect is of little consequence. The anesthetist, however, must rely on drugs with rapid onset and predictable offset of effect to ensure maintenance of an anesthetic state with return of responsiveness and other vital function at the appropriate time. In sum, an understanding of fundamental pharmacokinetic and pharmacodynamic concepts is of critical importance to the clinical practice of anesthesiology.

Modern clinical pharmacology techniques and concepts provide the scientific foundation to answer the questions listed in Table 40-1. Clinical pharmacologists have created tools using principles of pharmacokinetics and pharmacodynamics to construct models that predict drug behavior. Unfortunately, the often puzzling mathematical manipulations involved in estimating pharmacokinetic and pharmacodynamic parameters and the complex mathematics required to build models that predict drug behavior have made these techniques distinctly unpopular among most practitioners. Most practitioners have been slow to integrate the intricacies of kinetics and dynamics into their clinical practice and instead rely on training and experience to determine dosing. Thus, the determination of the proper dose in clinical anesthesia is often little more than a sophisticated guess based on the anesthesiologist's gestalt impressions.

TABLE 40-1 Questions to Consider When Formulating a Dose of Intravenous Anesthetic

1. What is an appropriate dose for my particular patient? Should I give the dose as a bolus or as a continuous infusion?
2. How soon will the intended effect start?
3. How long will it last?
4. How does the onset and duration of effect change in the presence of other anesthetics?
5. How do I minimize sedation yet optimize analgesia after surgical procedures associated with a painful postoperative course?
6. Do I know how to account for body weight, age, or other important factors (eg, blood loss, heart failure, kidney failure) that may alter the dosage requirements when I determine the dose?
7. How can I tailor my anesthetic to account for opioid tolerance in patients who chronically consume opioids or benzodiazepines?

Adapted from Sheiner LB. Learning versus confirming in clinical drug development. *Clin Pharmacol Ther*. 1997;61(3):275-291.

So why bother with clinical pharmacology? It is because this discipline provides the core scientific foundation for optimizing doses of intravenous (IV) anesthetics and should be a part of every practicing anesthetist's knowledge base. Fortunately, advances in pharmacologic computer simulation have revolutionized the way we apply complex pharmacokinetic and pharmacodynamic models. Simulations can be used to create meaningful pictures of drug behavior that are useful when considering the questions described in Table 40-1. Pharmacokinetic and pharmacodynamic model simulations get beyond the clinically unappealing mathematics associated with this area, providing an intuitively interpretable picture of drug behavior that clinicians can grasp and apply in day-to-day practice. Relying almost entirely on simulations (and not math), the purpose of this chapter is to empower practitioners with key concepts in pharmacokinetics and pharmacodynamics that influence the answer to: "What is an appropriate dose for my patient?"

PHARMACOLOGIC MODELING

PHARMACOKINETICS

To develop a *pharmacokinetic* model, clinical pharmacologists administer a drug and then repeatedly measure drug levels until the concentration is undetectable. The raw data are drug concentrations over time (**Fig. 40-1**). Using computerized pharmacokinetic tools, an equation is fit to the raw data. The equations used are simply a mathematical expression of the shape of the concentration versus time curve. The equations comprise parameters such as fractional coefficients and rate constants that are not much use to most providers.

To make parameters more meaningful, these equations are often "re-parameterized" (converted) in terms of *distribution volumes* and *clearances* or intercompartmental micro *rate constants.* Distribution volumes and clearances are used to create compartmental models that provide a schematic representation of drug behavior (**Fig. 40-2**A).

UNIMPORTANCE OF INDIVIDUAL PARAMETERS

It is difficult for clinicians to take advantage of compartment models and the mathematical equations that represent them in a clinical setting. Consideration of individual volumes of distribution or clearance parameters in formulating a dose of anesthetic that accounts for the complex interplay of the parameters is impossible for humans to do in real time.

As an example of this complexity, consider the illustration in Fig. 40-2B. As a metaphor of a compartment model, tracking loans and bank accounts over time provides insight into what is required to estimate drug concentrations in the body over time. Consider a person with an income of $2900 that is deposited into his or her bank account each month. From this bank account, there are 2 monthly withdrawals to pay for credit card debt and mortgage payments. The credit card debt has a high interest rate (18%) with a debt load of $10 000. The mortgage has a low interest rate (5.5%) and a balance of $100 000. The monthly payments to each are $200 and $900 to the credit card and mortgage companies, respectively. In addition, each month, there is a monthly expenditure of $1000 for savings and daily living operating costs. Assuming no other expenses, how much

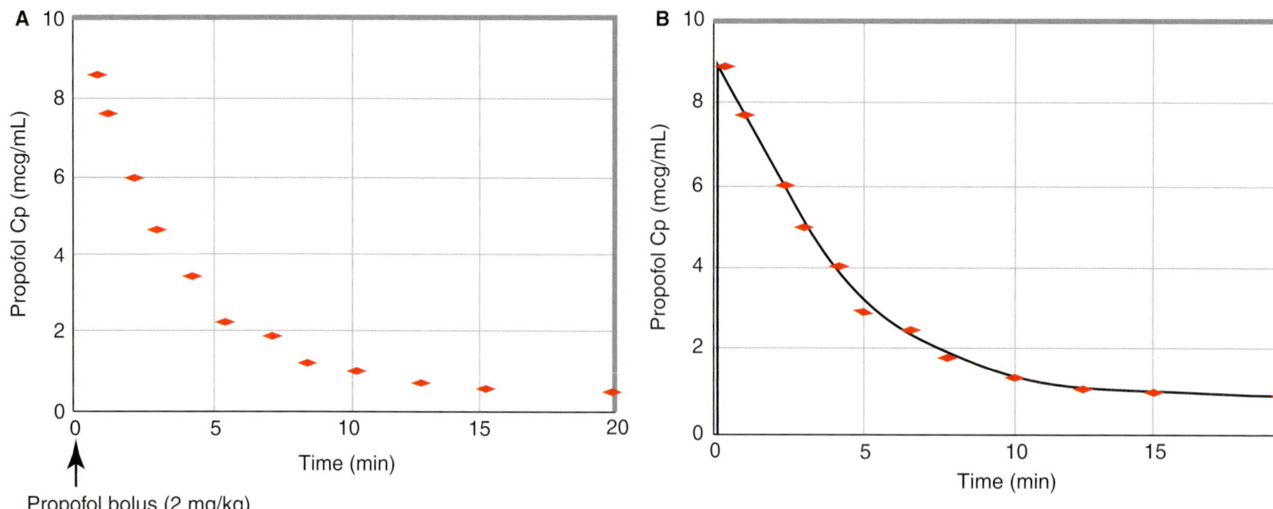

FIGURE 40-1. Development of a pharmacokinetic model (using propofol as an example). **A.** Raw data. Drug levels (*red dots*) are repeatedly measured over time. **B.** Analyzed data. A drug disposition curve (*black line*) is fit to the raw data using an exponential equation based on a computerized nonlinear regression analysis. **C.** The equation is simply a mathematical representation of curves of the general shape that "fit" the data. The nonlinear regression "curve fitting" exercise results in a set of parameters (in this example, A, B, α, and β) that when plugged into the equation reproduce the curve through the data. Cp(t) represents the plasma propofol concentration as a function of time (t). This is the mathematical basis of the pharmacokinetic model that clinicians need not worry about!

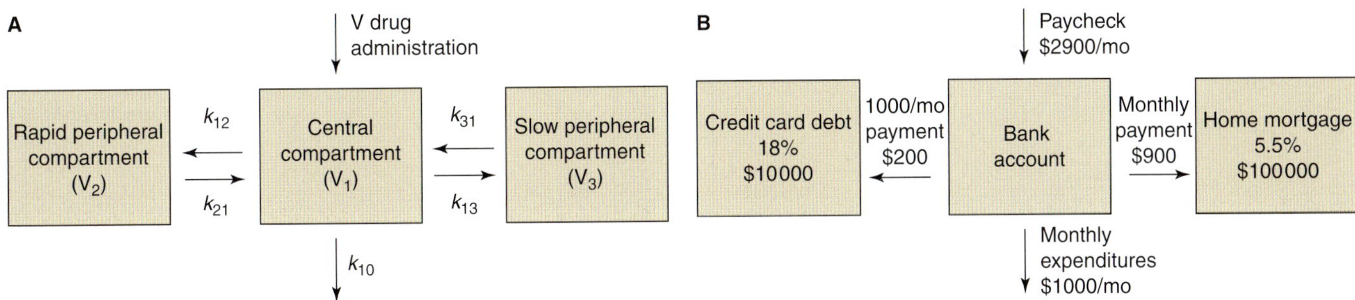

FIGURE 40-2. The mathematical complexity of the 3-compartment model. **A.** Schematic of a 3-compartment model. The k parameters represent rate constants. The V parameters represent the compartment volumes. **B.** Metaphor of a 3-compartment model: cash flow through multiple accounts. IV, intravenous.

money will be in the bank (central compartment) in 21 months? It is clear that without the use of a computer, calculating the answer to this question is impossible. Hence, using compartmental models without computer support makes them not very useful in a clinical environment.

IMPORTANCE OF SIMULATIONS

The real power from these pharmacokinetic parameters and compartment models comes through simulation. Because little insight into a drug's pharmacokinetic profile can be gleaned from simple inspection of its multicompartment pharmacokinetic parameters, computer simulation of the expected rise and fall of drug concentrations using a drug's pharmacokinetic parameters has assumed an important role in modern pharmacokinetic research and analysis. Making use of population pharmacokinetic parameters estimated in research studies, computers can be programmed to simulate the concentration versus time profile that results from any combination of boluses or continuous infusions. Although such simulations are subject to certain limitations, they are intuitive graphic representations of the time course of drug concentration.[2]

For example, **Fig. 40-3** illustrates a set of simulations of propofol using pharmacokinetic parameters from the literature.[3] In these simulations, the temporal profiles of plasma propofol levels that result from various bolus doses are plotted over time. From these plots, it is possible to visualize the peak plasma propofol concentration attained and the time propofol levels remain present in the plasma.

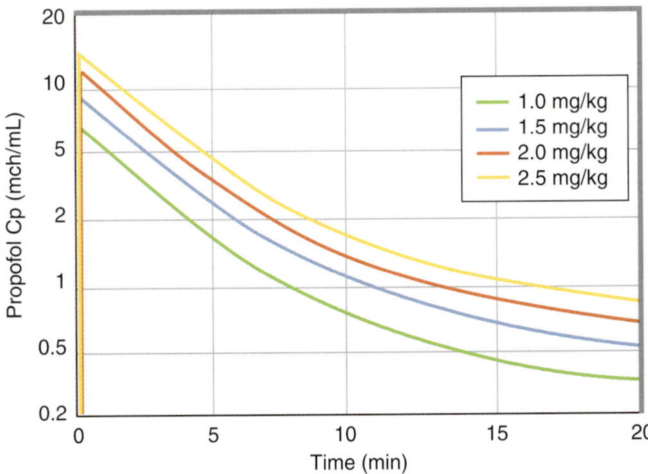

FIGURE 40-3. Simulations of 4 different bolus doses of propofol ranging from 1 to 2.5 mg/kg. The vertical axis is on a log scale. Cp, plasma concentration.

Without the aid of a computer, these simulations would be impossible. Although the simulations are limited by the quality of the original research from which the pharmacokinetic parameters were estimated and the inherent variability of pharmacokinetic parameters from patient to patient, the simulations are nonetheless graphic representations of a drug's expected clinical pharmacokinetic profile and provide an excellent framework within which to formulate a rational dosing strategy.

CONTEXT-SENSITIVE HALF-TIMES

Computer simulation has also been useful in demonstrating how estimating drug behavior based on individual kinetic parameters such as terminal half-lives can be misleading.[1] Clinicians have traditionally relied on terminal half-lives as a reflection of the duration of drug action when in fact terminal half-life alone is not a very useful pharmacokinetic parameter.[4] To that end, techniques have been used to predict the time necessary to achieve a 50% decrease in drug concentration after termination of a variable lengths continuous infusions. Simulation approaches have been developed to provide a *context-sensitive half-time* or *50% decrement time* in which *context* refers to the duration of a continuous infusion.[5] Such simulations are intended to provide more clinically relevant parameters than "half-life" or "volume of distribution."[6]

Figure 40-4 is a graphical representation of context-sensitive half-times for selected opioids and sedatives using parameters from the literature.[3,7-11] As can be appreciated in part A, clinically relevant information is easily gleaned from the plot that compares the context sensitive half-times for propofol, etomidate, and midazolam. Here propofol and etomidate have a more rapid decrement time than midazolam for any continuous infusion of duration longer than 30 minutes. This illustrates why a prolonged continuous infusion of midazolam is a poor choice if rapid emergence is an important anesthetic goal. By contrast, propofol and etomidate have much more forgiving profiles for prolonged continuous infusions. Even for infusions that last more than 8 hours, for example, the time required for propofol to decrease by 50% is less than 20 minutes. This feature of propofol makes it an attractive drug when delivering prolonged IV anesthetics. Etomidate, although it has a favorable pharmacokinetic profile for prolonged infusions compared with midazolam, has other features that make it unattractive for prolonged use such as nausea and vomiting, hemolysis, and adrenal suppression.[12]

With regard to opioids, sufentanil appears to have more favorable pharmacokinetics for infusions lasting less than 8 hours compared with fentanyl when the goal is to achieve a rapid 50% decrease in concentration. This difference can be explained by the fact that sufentanil's pharmacokinetic model has a large, slowly equilibrating peripheral compartment that continues to fill after termination of an infusion, thus contributing to the faster decrease in sufentanil central compartment concentration. In other words, central compartment sufentanil concentrations

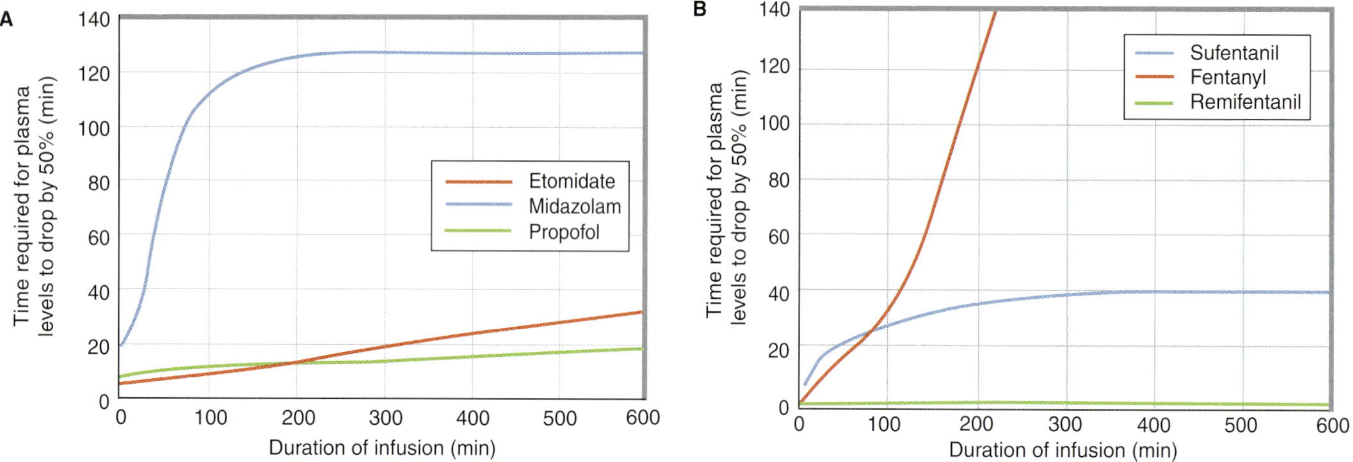

FIGURE 40-4. Simulations of the context-sensitive half-life (or 50% decrement time) for selected sedatives (**A**) and opioids (**B**). The vertical axis represents the time required for plasma concentrations to decrease by 50% after a continuous infusion is terminated. The *horizontal axis* represents the duration of a continuous infusion.

(which is the compartment that drives drug effect) decrease rapidly after an infusion of less than 8 hours is stopped because of continued elimination and distribution.[5,13]

Unlike sufentanil, fentanyl exhibits an early time-dependent increase in the context-sensitive half-time. Although fentanyl would be a poor choice for clinical situations in which a rapid decrease in concentration after infusion termination is desirable, in clinical scenarios in which prolonged opioid effect is the goal, fentanyl might well be the drug of choice. For example, fentanyl is well suited for cases after which the patient's trachea will remain intubated for a period of time after the procedure to promote a gradual emergence from anesthesia and a long-lasting level of significant analgesia.

Note that for cases of very brief duration, the context-sensitive half-times for sufentanil and fentanyl are nearly identical. Thus, for brief applications, when the opioid is administered by infusion (or by frequent small bolus doses), there would not be any substantial differences among these drugs in the time to a 50% decrease in concentration after stopping a continuous infusion.

Remifentanil, in contrast to both sufentanil and fentanyl, has a very short context-sensitive half-time for infusions of any duration. This feature may be attractive during procedures associated with varied surgical stimuli during which giving longer-acting opioids such as fentanyl or sufentanil to blunt the response to noxious stimulation may prolong emergence or increase the chance of unwanted respiratory depression. Remifentanil's short context-sensitive half-time may be useful in cases in which timely postoperative neurologic assessments are warranted to rule out developing neurologic deficits after neurosurgical procedures. Remifentanil, on the other hand, may be a poor choice as a prolonged infusion in cases associated with significant postoperative pain (ie, total hip arthroplasty). In this setting, when a continuous infusion of remifentanil is terminated, without the addition of a "transition" analgesic, patients can become remarkably uncomfortable when remifentanil plasma levels wane.

Although the 50% decrease in time is an improvement compared with the use of the terminal half-life for estimating how anesthetic drugs will behave, it is not always relevant. Depending on the dose and pharmacokinetic features of a particular drug, the 50% decrement time may not adequately describe drug behavior that is of clinical interest (eg, when will the analgesic effect of my IV opioid infusion dissipate after the infusion is terminated?). To get beyond this limitation, other decrement times can be used, such as the 20% or the 80% decrement time, to tailor the pharmacokinetic description of drug behavior to a clinical endpoint of interest.[6,13]

IMPORTANCE OF BIOPHASE

Biophase refers to the equilibration delay between peak drug levels in the blood or plasma and peak drug effect. The time lag (or hysteresis) between peak concentration in the plasma and peak drug effect is a function of drug movement into and action within the effect site.[14-16] The effect site represents a theoretical space without any definitive anatomic analog where drug exerts its effect. The lag time represents a summation of events that can impact the onset of pharmacologic effect such as drug diffusion to the effect site, receptor binding, and so on (**Fig. 40-5**A). Hysteresis is important to account for when forecasting drug effect. It is particularly important to consider when simulating bolus injections of drug; for long infusions, the time lag assumes less importance because the effect site and plasma are generally closer to equilibrium.

Consider again a 2-mg/kg bolus of propofol and the observed changes in a processed electroencephalogram (EEG) parameter such as the bispectral index scale (BIS). The maximal decrease in the BIS lags behind the peak plasma propofol level (Fig. 40-5B). The time delay, or *hysteresis*, represents the time required for propofol to go from the plasma to the site where it exerts an effect. In other words, most drugs do not work in the plasma.

For many drugs, including propofol, the equilibration delay between peak concentration in the plasma and peak effect has been characterized by estimating a parameter called the k_{eo}. The k_{eo} represents the rate constant for elimination of drug from a virtual compartment called the *effect site*.[14,17] (Fig. 40-5C). The effect site concept is schematically represented as an additional compartment in the 3-compartment model (**Fig. 40-6**). When the k_{eo} parameter is available for a drug, theoretical effect compartment concentrations can be simulated along with plasma concentrations, thus making the effect of the time lag easily appreciated. In essence, the time course of effect site concentrations should accurately predict the time course of drug effect.

One of the useful clinical features of simulating the effect site concentration is that the time required to reach peak effect can be easily visualized. **Figure 40-7** presents simulations of the effect concentration over time for selected sedatives and opioids after commonly used doses for each drug. It is readily apparent that some IV anesthetics reach their peak effect site concentrations for a given dose much later than others (**Table 40-2**).

Midazolam, for example, requires up to 9 minutes to reach peak effect in contrast to propofol and etomidate. This may explain why

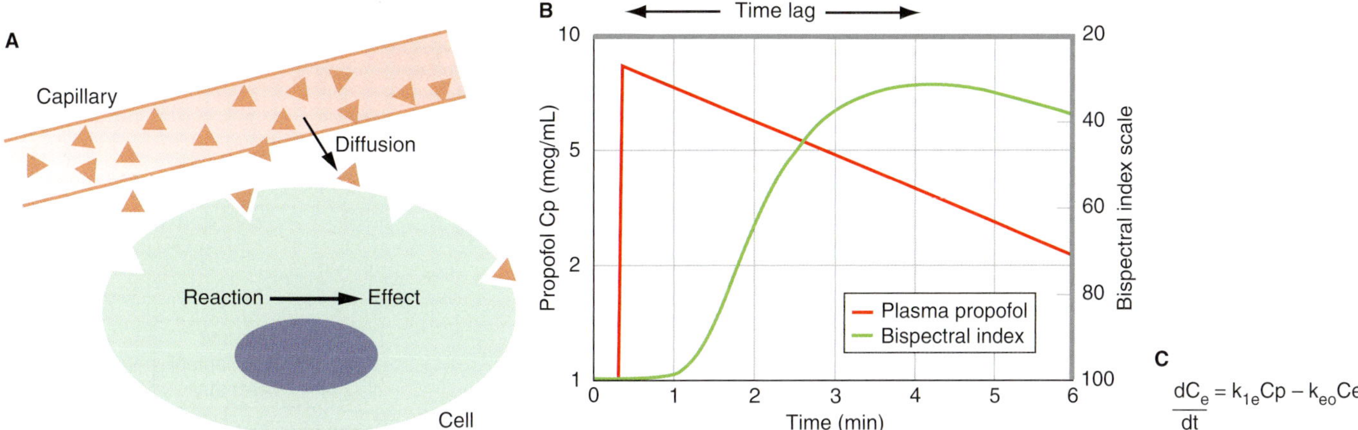

FIGURE 40-5. The biophase concept. **A.** Schematic of drug (*red triangles*) diffusion from a blood vessel to the site of action (effect site), in this case, a cell membrane. Drug interaction with a cell membrane receptor produces a biochemical reaction that leads to a drug effect. **B.** Simulation of plasma propofol levels and the bispectral index scale (BIS) after a 2-mg/kg propofol bolus to a 70-kg person. The *green* and *red lines* represent the plasma propofol concentration and BIS, respectively. The *right side* vertical axis for BIS has been reversed. Note the time (hysteresis) lag between the peak propofol plasma level and the peak BIS value. **C.** The mathematical expression used to compute the effect site concentration. k_{1e} and k_{eo} represent the elimination rate constants from the central (Cp) and effect site (Ce) compartments, respectively. Although important for modeling, this is another mathematical detail that clinicians need not worry about!

the early use of midazolam for endoscopic procedures was associated with adverse events related to excessive sedation.[18-20] One misleading characteristic of midazolam is that it has a rapid onset of effect (ie, some effect is apparent soon after injection), but the latency to peak effect is slower relative to some other sedatives. When a desired effect has not been reached within 90 seconds, practitioners may be tempted to administer additional midazolam. This may lead to a peak effect site concentration that is excessive and delayed in presentation compared with other sedative hypnotics. This underscores the importance of using caution when administering large doses of IV midazolam.

By contrast to midazolam, etomidate and propofol, given as a bolus dose under normal hemodynamic conditions, reach their peak effect within 2 minutes after administration and then quickly dissipate. With these agents, if a desired effect has not been achieved within 120 seconds, practitioners may be inclined to give additional drug knowing that the previous doses are already waning.

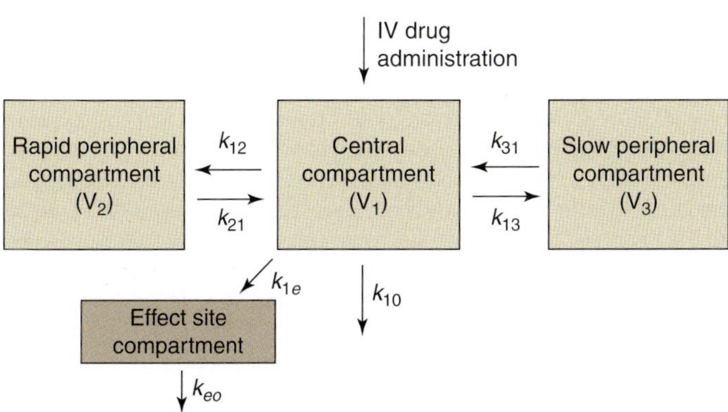

FIGURE 40-6. The effect site compartment concept. Addition of the effect site to a 3-compartment model. k_{1e} and k_{eo} (in *blue*) represent the elimination rate constants from the central and effect site compartments, respectively. Drug effect correlates with the concentration in the effect compartment. IV, intravenous.

With regard to opioids, after a bolus dose, the time required to reach peak effect site concentrations for remifentanil is considerably quicker than that of fentanyl and sufentanil. The clinical implications of this difference may be considerable when administered to patients breathing spontaneously. Remifentanil by bolus injection may lead to a more pronounced respiratory depression compared with equipotent doses of sufentanil or fentanyl. With the slower onset of effect for fentanyl and sufentanil, blood P_{CO_2} levels are given time to rise, providing some offset to the respiratory depression associated with opioids. With remifentanil, the onset of effect outpaces the accumulation of blood P_{CO_2}, leading to more pronounced respiratory depression.[21-23]

PHARMACODYNAMICS

Pharmacodynamic models have been constructed to describe the relationship between drug effect site levels and drug effect. Some important features of pharmacodynamic models are presented in **Fig. 40-8**. In this figure, a schematic illustrates how drug, when it reaches the effect site, interacts with a receptor to produce effect (Fig. 40-8A). This process is typically characterized graphically using a sigmoidal curve (Fig. 40-8B). Parameters used to describe the pharmacodynamic model (ie, the sigmoid curve) include the C_{50} and γ. The C_{50} represents the effect site concentration at which 50% of the maximal drug effect will be elicited, and γ represents the slope of the concentration–effect curve. The most important part of the sigmoid curve, the steep section of the curve, represents the dynamic range of drug effect. The dynamic range charts the concentration–effect relationship from E_0 (baseline effect) to E_{max} (maximal effect). In this region, small changes in drug concentration lead to large changes in drug effect. This is the region of particular interest to anesthesia providers. Increasing effect site concentrations beyond the dynamic range leads to minimal changes in drug effect. The mathematical expression that uses the C_{50} and γ to estimate drug effect is presented in Fig. 40-8C.

A surfing analogy is helpful in conceptualizing the application of pharmacodynamic models to rational drug administration.[24] Just as a surfer attempts to ride just in front of the crest of a wave to slide down the front edge of the wave, practitioners attempt to maintain their anesthetic drugs at effect site concentrations near the "crest" of the concentration–effect relationship (Fig. 40-8B). In so doing, clinicians

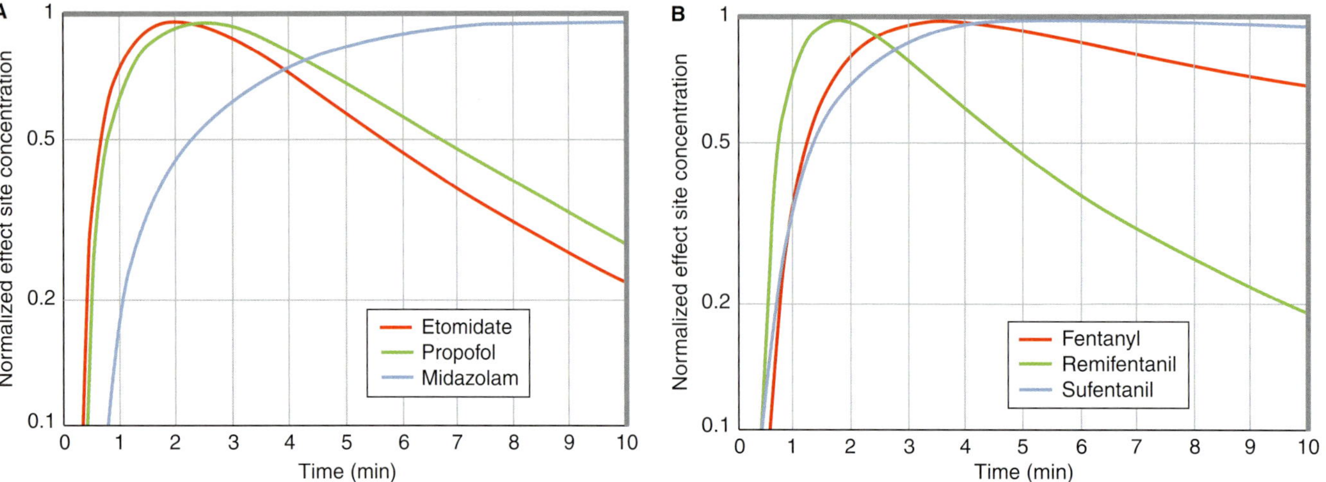

FIGURE 40-7. The latency to peak effect site concentration. Effect site concentrations over time for selected opioids (**A**) and sedatives (**B**) after conventional doses for each drug. The vertical axis has been normalized for all drugs such that a "1" indicates the maximal effect site concentration.

maintain significant drug effect but can "slide down" the concentration curve to promote recovery at the end of an anesthetic. From an efficacy and toxicity perspective, there is no advantage of being on the flat part of the concentration–effect relationship near E_{max}.

As an example, consider 3 bolus doses of propofol (0.5, 2, and 7 mg/kg). The resultant effect site concentrations for each bolus are presented in **Fig. 40-9**. Using a pharmacodynamic model for propofol, the effect of these boluses is plotted on a sigmoid curve. The C_{50} for this curve (1.8 μg/mL) represents the effect site concentration at which there is a 50% probability of loss of responsiveness.[25] Dosing regimens that maintain drug concentrations along the lower left portion of the sigmoid curve (ie, below the wave) are too low to be effective, as illustrated by the low-dose propofol bolus (0.5 mg/kg). Dosing regimens that maintain drug concentrations to the right side of the sigmoid curve (ie, before the wave breaks) are excessive and may produce unwanted hemodynamic depression or prolonged recovery. In this region, increasing drug concentration does not increase drug effect. This phenomenon is illustrated by the 7-mg/kg bolus dose of propofol. The ideal dosing strategy targets the upper portion of the steep part of the concentration–effect relationship: A concentration that produces

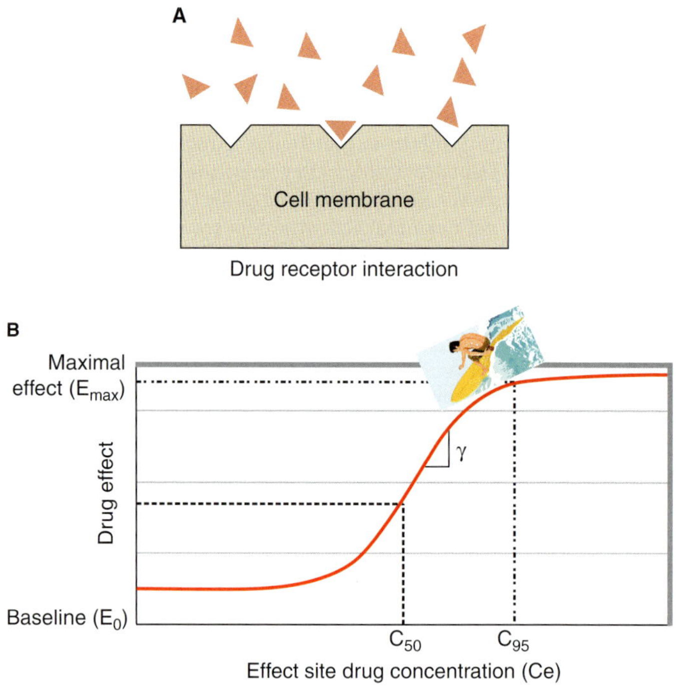

TABLE 40-2 Time to Peak Effect for Selected Opioids and Sedative–Hypnotics[a]

Drug	Dose	Peak Effect Site Concentration	Time Required to Reach Maximal Effect (min)
Opioids			
Fentanyl	150 μg	1.5 ng/mL	3.9
Sufentanil	15 μg	0.2 ng/mL	5.5
Remifentanil	150 μg	8.6 ng/mL	1.5
Sedatives			
Propofol	2 mg/kg	4.8 μg/mL	2.3
Etomidate	0.2 mg/kg	0.6 μg/mL	2.0
Midazolam	2 mg	22.0 ng/mL	9.5

[a]Simulations based on a body weight of 70 kg.

FIGURE 40-8. A typical pharmacodynamic model. **A.** Schematic of the pharmacodynamic process. Drug (*red triangles*) interacts with receptors in the effect site to elicit a drug effect. **B.** A graphical expression of pharmacodynamic drug behavior. E represents drug effect, C_{50} represents the effect site concentration necessary to produce 50% of the maximal drug effect, E_0 represents the baseline effect (with no drug present), and E_{max} represents the maximal effect. The *vertical axis* is on the log scale. The sigmoid shape of the concentration versus effect curve is characteristic of intravenous anesthetics. γ represents the maximal slope of the concentration versus effect curve. A surfing analogy is useful to understand the application of the pharmacodynamic model. As the surfer rides just below the crest of a wave, anesthesia providers attempt to dose their anesthetics to achieve near-maximal effect just at the point where the sigmoid curve starts to flatten out. The *dashed line* represents the concentration at which 50% of the maximal effect is achieved. The *dash-dot-dash* line represents the concentration at which 95% of the maximal effect is achieved. **C.** Mathematical expression of the pharmacodynamic model used to render the concentration versus effect curve in *B*. This is the mathematical basis of the pharmacodynamic model that clinicians need not worry about.

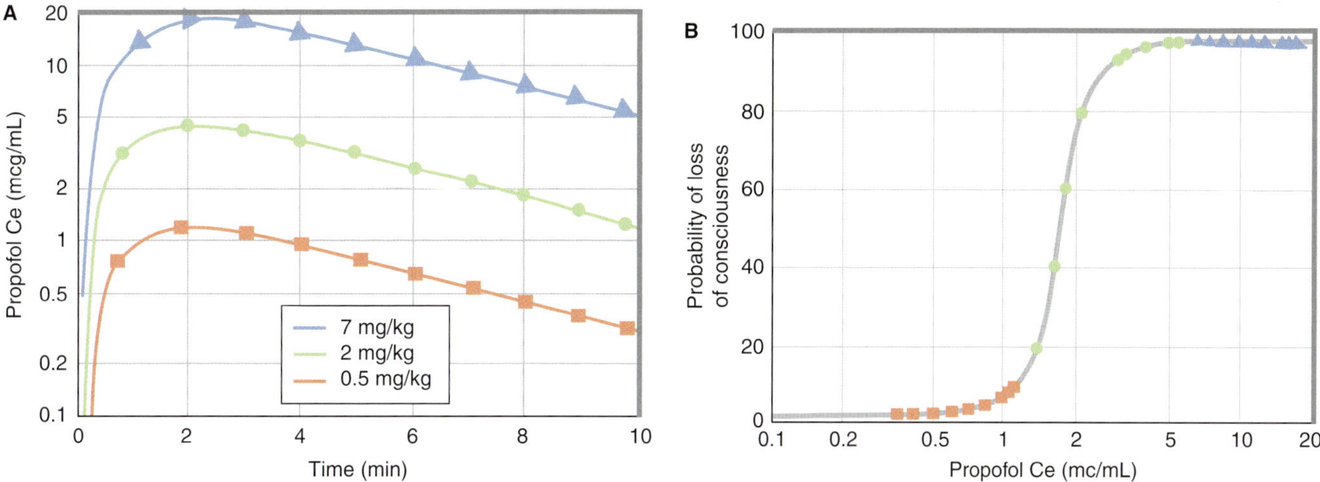

FIGURE 40-9. A simulation integrating pharmacokinetic and pharmacodynamic models illustrating the interplay between the dose–concentration (pharmacokinetic) relationship and the concentration–effect (pharmacodynamic) relationship. **A.** Simulation of the propofol effect site concentrations (Ces) over time for bolus doses of 0.5 mg/kg (*red squares*), 2 mg/kg (*green circles*), and 7 mg/kg (*blue triangles*). **B.** The corresponding concentration versus effect of the bolus doses in *A* superimposed over a pharmacodynamic model for propofol.

considerable drug effect but from which drug effect will recover quickly when drug administration is terminated as illustrated by an intermediate dose of propofol (2 mg/kg).

One practical aspect of anesthesia care that makes pharmacologic "surfing" difficult to do is that the concentration–effect relationship is not consistent across various stimuli. For some stimuli, much less drug is required to achieve a desired effect compared with other stimuli. For example, skin incision is typically less noxious than laryngoscopy.[26-28] In an effort to characterize how different stimuli vary, numerous pharmacodynamic models have been built for selected stimuli.

A schematic, presented in **Fig. 40-10**, plots out the relative difference between pharmacodynamic models for opioids across various stimuli. Effect measures used to characterize opioid behavior include mild to moderate analgesia (ie, blunting response to a noxious stimulus), respiratory depression, significant analgesia (ie, blunting response to laryngoscopy), and suppression of EEG activity. As expected, the pharmacodynamic relationship for each stimulus is very similar (a sigmoid curve), but the C_{50}s are shifted from left to right with increasing stimulus. Several important points flow from this schematic, especially for the meticulous clinician who seeks to "surf" near the ideal Ce and thus achieve the desired drug effect without

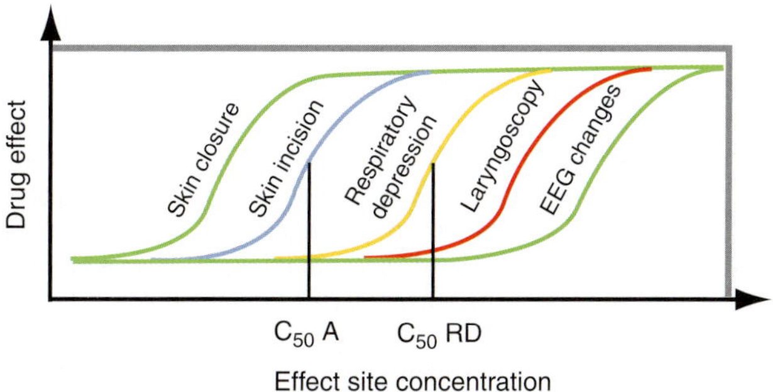

FIGURE 40-10. Schematic of the concentration–effect relationship for various stimuli.[26] Anesthesia is a dynamic process that requires frequent adjustments of drug levels. C_{50}A, C_{50} for analgesia; C_{50}RD, C_{50} for respiratory depression.

administering a relative overdose. These include (1) significant analgesia is required to blunt the response from laryngoscopy compared with other stimuli encountered in the operating room; (2) the C_{50} for the effect site concentration necessary to blunt a response to laryngoscopy is higher than the C_{50} for respiratory depression; (3) dosing anesthetics requires an appreciation of ongoing and anticipated stimuli; and (4) there is a window in opioid levels between which one can achieve analgesia yet avoid excessive respiratory depression. Investigators have demonstrated that the C_{50} for analgesia is approximately 30% of the C_{50} for respiratory depression.[26] This may be especially important during emergence from anesthesia.

IMPORTANCE OF COMBINING KINETIC AND DYNAMIC MODELS

To depict a patient's response to a dose of drug, it is necessary to combine pharmacokinetic–pharmacodynamic models and provide a quantitative description of each. Because most drugs do not act in the blood, pharmacokinetic and pharmacodynamic models must be linked so that concentrations in the plasma can be translated into effect site concentrations and thus drug effect. One approach to visualize the link between the pharmacokinetics and pharmacodynamic models is to plot a horizontal line on the pharmacokinetic plot of effect site concentrations over time that represents the C_{50} for a desired drug effect. Two key points of interest are now easily visualized through computer simulation: the time to onset of effect and the duration of drug effect.[4,29,30]

For example, using linked pharmacokinetic and pharmacodynamic models, the simulations of propofol bolus doses ranging from 1 to 2.5 mg/kg presented in Fig. 40-3 can be re-performed for effect site concentrations rather than plasma concentrations (**Fig. 40-11**). To visualize the onset and duration of effect, the C_{50} for loss of responsiveness is overlaid on the simulations of propofol effect site concentrations. Several investigators have estimated propofol effect site concentrations required for loss of responsiveness with C_{50}s ranging from 1.8 to 2.4 μg/mL.[25,31-33] For simulation and discussion purposes, the C_{50} for loss of responsiveness to be used in these simulations and throughout the remainder of this chapter will be 1.8 μg/mL. A summary of the time to onset and duration of effect for each propofol bolus dose is presented in **Table 40-3**. It is important to point out that this C_{50} for loss of responsiveness, similar to all pharmacokinetic and pharmacodynamic

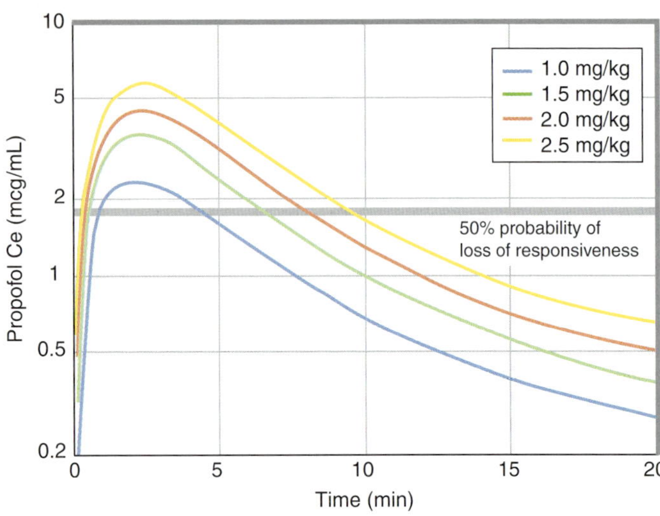

FIGURE 40-11. Simulations of the propofol effect site concentration (Ce) in response to bolus doses ranging from 1 to 2.5 mg/kg for a 70-kg person. The *vertical axis* is on the log scale. The *gray line* represents the propofol effect site concentration associated with a 50% probability of loss of responsiveness (LOR).[25,32,33,38] Note the time to LOR and the duration of the LOR for varying doses.

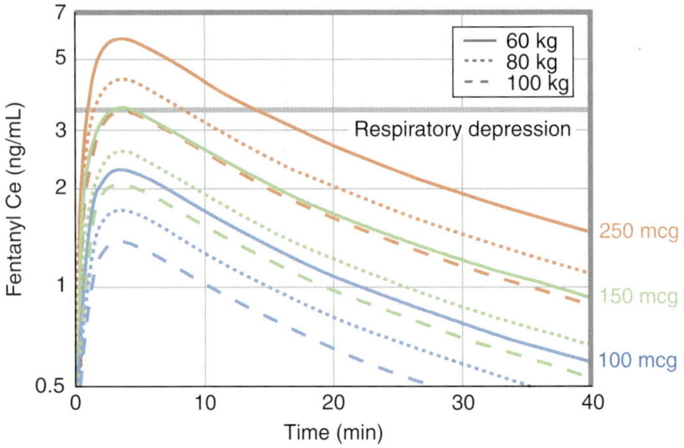

FIGURE 40-12. Simulations of the fentanyl effect site concentration (Ce) after a 100-, 150-, and 250-µg bolus in a 60-, 80-, and 100-kg person, respectively. The fentanyl effect site concentration associated with a 50% probability of substantial respiratory depression is plotted as a *gray line* (3.5 ng/mL).[34] The vertical axis is on a log scale. Note the implication of dose on the respiratory depression.

parameters, is a population estimate for the typical patient and as such is subject to intersubject variability and will not perfectly predict unresponsiveness in individuals.

Guided by simulations, the clinical implications of a given propofol dosing strategy become apparent. For example, using a higher dose of propofol as part of a rapid sequence induction, if hemodynamically tolerable, may prove useful in minimizing the time when the airway is unsecured because of faster onset of effect. By contrast, a lower dose may be useful when providing anesthesia for brief procedures associated with a noxious stimulus, such as a retrobulbar block, during which only brief unresponsiveness is required. When using the lower dose, however, practitioners need to recognize that it will take up to 50 seconds longer to achieve loss of responsiveness.

Simulations may also be useful in illustrating how drugs behave in relation to an unwanted toxic effect. Consider a plot of fentanyl effect site concentrations for various doses of fentanyl and the concentration at which probability of substantial respiratory depression exceeds 50% (ie, somewhere around 3.5 ng/mL) in 60-, 80-, and 100-kg people.[34] (**Fig. 40-12**). In this simulation, the bolus of 100 and 150 µg of fentanyl avoids respiratory depression for each weight. A 250-µg bolus, however, exceeds the effect site concentrations associated with a 50% probability of respiratory depression for people weighing 60 and 80 kg for 7 and 13 minutes, respectively. According to these simulations, persons weighing 100 kg or more briefly approach the fentanyl effect site concentration associated with a 50% probability of respiratory depression but do not exceed it.

Linked pharmacokinetic–pharmacodynamic models can also provide insight into how drugs behave after termination of continuous infusions.

TABLE 40-3 Onset and Duration of Effect After a Propofol Bolus

Dose (mg/kg)	Time to Onset (s)	Duration of Effect (min)
1.0	80	3.7
1.5	50	6.9
2.0	40	8.0
2.5	30	9.5

Factors that influence the duration of effect after termination of an infusion include the infusion rate and the duration of the infusion. For example, consider the time required to regain responsiveness after termination of a continuous infusion of propofol. **Figure 40-13** shows a series of simulations of the resultant propofol effect site concentration after continuous infusions at rates between 50 and 150 µg/kg/min for 1, 2, and 3 hours. As with the previous simulations of bolus dosing of propofol, the plot also charts the propofol effect site concentration associated with a 50% probability of loss of responsiveness (1.8 µg/mL).[25]

The area of interest is the segment of time from when the infusion is terminated until the propofol effect site concentration falls below the level associated with a loss of responsiveness. The results of these simulations are summarized in **Table 40-4**. When the infusion was terminated, longer propofol infusions at equivalent dosages required more time for propofol levels to drop below a level associated with unresponsiveness. As expected, once the infusion was terminated, higher propofol infusion rates required more time to drop below a level associated with unresponsiveness. With higher infusion rates, the time to regaining responsiveness can be quite long (ie, up to 13 minutes).

Conceptualizing this clinical issue in terms of compartmental models, these simulations illustrate how during prolonged infusions propofol gradually "fills" the slowly equilibrating peripheral compartments (extravascular tissues). When the infusion is terminated, the propofol in the peripheral compartments serves as a reservoir to maintain plasma propofol concentrations, thereby slowing the decline in drug effect. This may be clinically evident as a delay in emergence. These simulations also suggest that running a propofol infusion at a single continuous rate throughout an anesthetic will lead to propofol effect site levels that may be higher than desired. A prudent approach to dosing prolonged propofol infusion therefore is to reduce the infusion rate over time to minimize drug accumulation. This accumulation phenomenon emphasizes the advantage of target-controlled infusions (TCIs) that instead of delivering drug at a set rate (ie, µg/kg/min) deliver drug to achieve and maintain a set effect site concentration (ie, 2.5 µg/mL for propofol). In so doing, they avoid the accumulation of drug yet maintain an appropriate drug level for the desired duration. These types of infusion systems are widely used throughout the world,

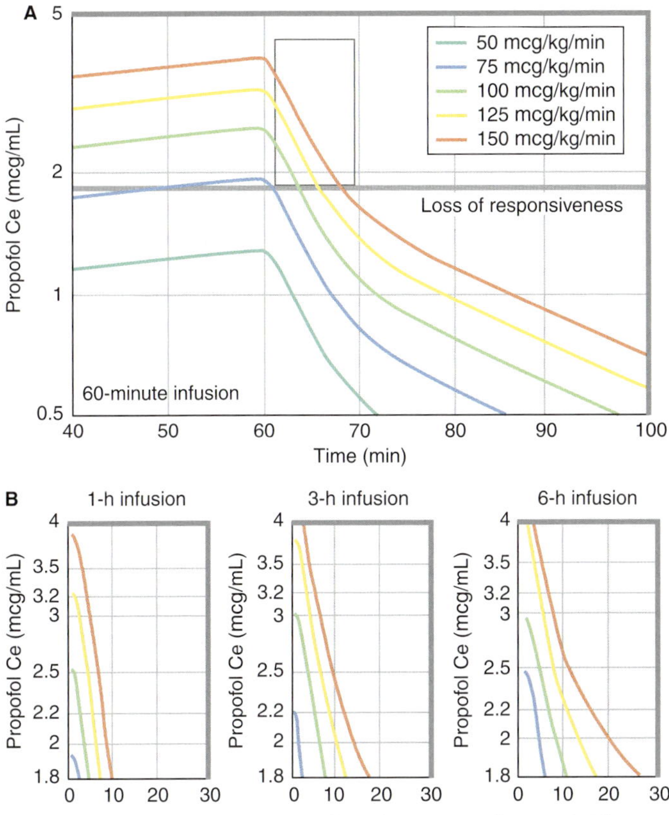

FIGURE 40-13. **A.** Simulation of a 60-minute infusion of propofol at rates ranging from 50 to 150 μg/kg/min. At 60 minutes, the infusion is terminated. Superimposed on this plot is the effect site concentration (Ce) associated with a 50% probability of loss of responsiveness (LOR; *gray line*).[25,32,33,38] Of interest is the time required after the infusion is terminated for the propofol effect site concentration to fall below the concentration associated with LOR (black box). **B.** The plot within the black box expanded for 3 different infusion durations (1-6 hours). After termination of the continuous infusion, the time on the *x*-axis has been reset to 0 for each plot. Each plot illustrates the time required for propofol effect site levels to drop below the propofol concentration associated with a LOR for infusion rates commonly used in clinical practice. Simulations used pharmacokinetic and pharmacodynamic parameters for propofol reported by Marsh et al [8] and Kern et al [25], respectively.

TABLE 40-4 Time Required for Propofol Effect Site Concentrations to Fall Below Levels Associated With Loss of Responsiveness for Various Infusion Rates Running for 1, 3, and 6 Hours

Infusion Rate (mcg/kg/min)	Time Required for Propofol Effect Site Concentrations to Fall below Effect Site Concentrations Associated With a 50% Probability of Loss of Responsiveness (min).		
	60-min infusion	180-min infusion	360-min infusion
50	–	–	–
75	1	3	4
100	4	7	9
125	6	11	17
150	9	17	23

yet unfortunately have not attained regulatory approval within the United States.[24]

This form of analysis may be also useful to use when exploring the duration of analgesic effect from fentanyl after surgical procedures of various durations. A common practice is to administer intermittent boluses of fentanyl starting at induction and then throughout a general anesthetic with the goal of providing perioperative analgesia during and after a stimulating procedure. Consider an anesthetic where fentanyl, in addition to a potent inhaled agent, is given as a bolus (3 μg/kg or ~200 μg for a 70-kg patient) on induction and then intermittently (ie, 1.5 μg/kg or ~100 μg for a 70-kg patient every 20 minutes) throughout a surgical procedure associated with significant painful stimuli.

Simulations of this fentanyl dosing regimen for anesthetics lasting 1, 2, and 3 hours reveal several clinical points of interest (**Fig. 40-14**). For a 1-hour anesthetic with an induction dose of 200 μg of fentanyl followed by 2 supplemental 100-μg doses during the anesthetic, the total fentanyl dose administered is 400 μg (8 mL). With this dosing regimen, the fentanyl effect site concentration intermittently rises above the fentanyl effect site concentration associated with analgesia (1.6 ng/mL)[35] but rapidly drops below the analgesic level after the anesthetic is terminated.

Simulations of the 2- and 3-hour anesthetics using a similar dosing scheme result in total fentanyl doses of 700 and 1000 μg (14 and 20 mL). With the longer duration, the fentanyl concentration rises above the effect site level associated with analgesia. In this simulation, what becomes apparent is that repetitive doses increase the fentanyl concentration at the end of a 3-hour anesthetic; the resulting effect site concentration of fentanyl is much higher than after the 1-hour anesthetic. After termination of the anesthetic, the time required for the fentanyl effect site concentrations to decrease below the level associated with analgesia was 9 and 57 minutes for a 2- and 3-hour anesthetic, respectively. Similar to what was learned in the simulations of the context-sensitive half-time for fentanyl, prolonged infusions or repetitive dosing of fentanyl over prolonged periods can lead to high fentanyl effect site concentrations. High fentanyl levels may be of clinical benefit (ie, adequate analgesia after a pain surgical procedure) or detriment (prolonged respiratory depression) in the early postoperative period. These simulations demonstrate the potential benefit of visualizing fentanyl effect site concentrations in real time when caring for patients in whom the anesthetic goals upon termination of a general anesthetic include adequate analgesia yet avoidance of unwanted respiratory depression. At present, many investigators are developing tools to allow clinicians to visualize both drug concentrations and effects over time.

One very important limitation of these simulations is that painful surgical procedures are rare if ever performed with fentanyl alone. Other anesthetics, such as potent inhaled agents or IV sedatives, are used as well. Inhaled agents and IV sedatives accentuate the analgesic effect of opioids in a synergistic fashion. This limitation is addressed in the following section. Thus, these simulations chart the effect of fentanyl alone and at best are representative of analgesic effect after other anesthetics that have been coadministered with the fentanyl have been allowed to dissipate. Hence, the segment of this simulation set reflective of the actual analgesic state are the fentanyl effect site concentrations well beyond (ie, 20-30 minutes) the termination of the anesthetic.

DRUG SYNERGISM

Anesthetics are typically administered as a combination of several different types of drugs to achieve a desired complete anesthetic. Anesthesiologists have long appreciated that the administration of 1 type of drug may enhance and prolong the effect of another type of drug. The concept of minimum alveolar concentration (MAC)

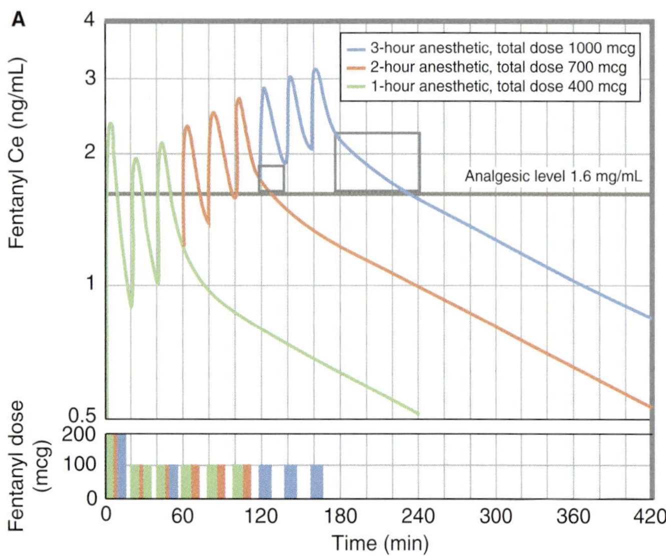

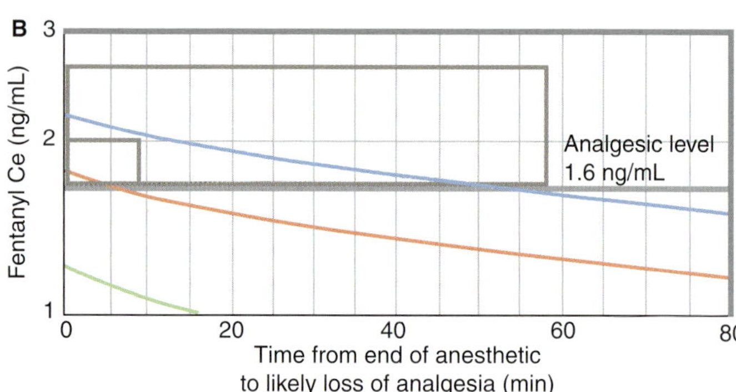

FIGURE 40-14. **A.** Simulation of intermittent doses of fentanyl for anesthetics lasting 1, 2, and 3 hours. The *red line* represents the fentanyl effect site concentration (Ce) that results from a 200-μg bolus on induction followed by intermittent 100-μg boluses throughout the remainder of the anesthetic. The *red bars* just above the *x*-axis represent the fentanyl dosing regimen. The *blue* and *green lines* represent the fentanyl Ce for similar dosing schemes that last for 2 and 3 hours, respectively. Superimposed on this plot is the Ce associated with analgesia (*gray line*). Of interest is the time required after the anesthetic is terminated for the fentanyl Ce to fall below the concentration associated with analgesia (*gray boxes*). **B.** The plots within the *gray boxes* have been expanded, and after termination of the anesthetic, the time on the horizontal axis has been reset to 0. This plot illustrates the time required for fentanyl Ce to drop below the fentanyl concentration associated with analgesia. These simulations used pharmacokinetic and pharmacodynamic parameters for fentanyl reported by Shafer et al.[99] and fentanyl Ce associated with analgesia (1.6 ng/mL) reported by Scott and Stanski.[73] Simulations were based on a patient weight of 70 kg.

reduction is well established and used to describe how the addition of an IV opioid reduces the amount of a potent inhaled agent required to achieve and maintain a desired MAC. This line of thinking is especially important when trying to avoid unwanted side effects associated with high doses of a single anesthetic such as hemodynamic depression, prolonged emergence from anesthesia, or persistent respiratory depression.

As clinical pharmacologists have become more sophisticated in their approach to characterizing the interaction between different anesthetic drug types, several tools have been developed to describe drug–drug interactions. One simple tool characterizes drug–drug interactions as additive (ie, 2 + 2 = 4), antagonistic (eg, 2 + 2 = 1), or synergistic (eg, 2 + 2 = 8). These can be graphically illustrated to allow visualization of the extent of antagonism or synergism present between 2 drugs (**Fig. 40-15**). These drug interaction plots present the effect site concentrations for 2 drugs that are necessary to achieve specified drug effects. In this schematic a desired effect is achieved at point A on the horizontal axis and point B on the vertical axis. The points labeled a and b represent the concentrations of *both* drugs required to achieve a similar effect to either drug A or B alone. As can be appreciated, there are an infinite number of drug–drug combinations that result in a similar drug effect. The line that runs through all the possible drug–drug concentration pairs and connects points A and B is known as an **isobologram**. The isobologram represents drug concentration pairs that would result in the same drug effect when the 2 drugs are used alone or in combination.

With drug–drug interactions that are additive, the isobologram is a straight line indicating that as drug A increases, proportionally less of drug B is required to achieve the same degree of effect (Fig. 40-15A). With drug–drug interactions that are synergistic, the isobologram is a curved line bowing toward the origin of the graph (Fig. 40-15B), indicating that when both drugs A and B are used, much less of both is required to achieve the same degree of desired effect. Conversely, with drug–drug interactions that are antagonistic, the isobologram is a curved line bowing away from the origin of the graph (Fig. 40-15C), indicating that when both drugs A and B are used, much more of each is required to achieve the same degree of desired effect. Most interactions between anesthetic drugs are synergistic.

Common anesthetic goals can be characterized in terms of isobolograms. For example, isobolograms can be used to plot effect site concentration pairs necessary to achieve a 50% or 95% probability of achieving a desired drug effect (ie, no response to laryngoscopy) or when a worrisome side effect may occur (ie, onset of respiratory depression). Using these isobolograms, it is possible to explore through computer simulations how well an anesthetic performs in terms of meeting desired anesthetic goals.

For example, consider a schematic of a combined anesthetic technique using drugs A (an opioid) and B (a sedative) that are known to have a synergistic interaction (**Fig. 40-16**). Drug delivery that yields concentration pairs to the left of 50% isobole for no response to painful stimuli do not meet analgesic goals. With drug pairs in this region, patients will most likely respond to painful stimuli. Drug delivery that yields concentration pairs between the 50% and 95% isoboles will likely meet analgesic goals, but some patients may respond to a painful stimulus. In this region, after the anesthetic is terminated, the analgesic effect will quickly dissipate. With drug delivery that yields concentration pairs to the right of the 95% isobole, a patient is very likely to be unresponsive to painful stimuli, and increasing the anesthetic target will not substantially increase the probability of adequate effect. A key point with regard to this region of the isobole plot is that administering additional anesthetic will not provide more analgesia but rather only prolong the time required for drug effect to dissipate, especially if the resultant concentrations have far exceeded the 95% isobole. A prolonged duration of effect may be a desired outcome (ie, adequate analgesia after a surgery associated with significant

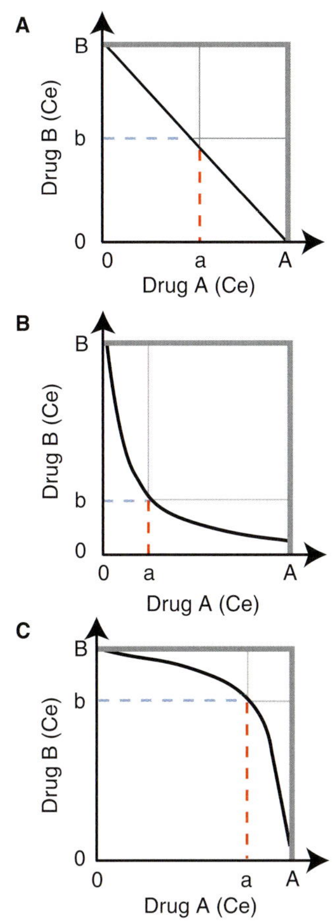

FIGURE 40-15. Schematic representation of drug–drug interactions. *A* represents an additive interaction, *B* represents a synergistic interaction, and *C* represents an antagonistic interaction. The horizontal and vertical axes represent the effect site concentration (Ce) of drugs A and B, respectively. *A* and *B* represent the concentrations of each drug required to achieve a similar effect when used alone. *a* and *b* represent the concentrations of drugs A and B, respectively, that result in a similar effect when combined. The *blue lines* represent an isobologram. An isobologram is a plot of all the drug–drug concentration pairs that result in the same level of drug effect. These schematics are patterned after schematics originally described by Minto et al.[36]

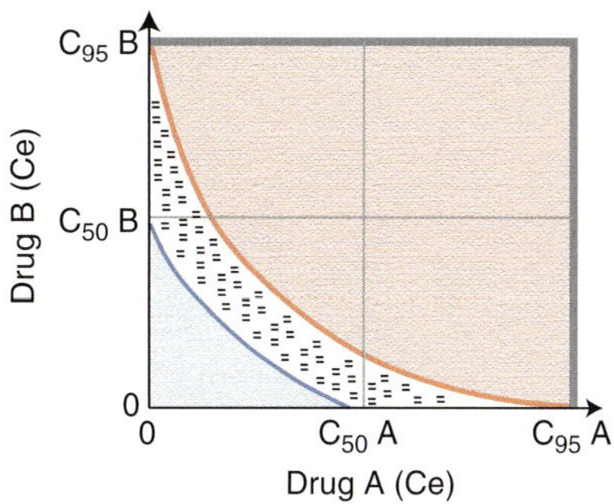

FIGURE 40-16. Schematic representation of a synergistic drug–drug interaction of drugs A and B for the probability of no response to a noxious stimulus. The *blue line* represents the 50% isobole, and the *red line* represents the 95% isobole. The area to the right of the 95% isobole (*shaded red*) represents drug–drug pairs that are higher than the 95% isobole. The area to the left of the 50% isobole (*shaded blue*) represents drug–drug pairs that are less than the 50% isobole. The area contained within the 50% and 95% isobole (*black hash marks*) represent drug–drug pairs that are in between the 2 isoboles. The C_{50} and C_{95} effect site concentrations for drugs A and B are marked on the horizontal and vertical axes, respectively. Any of the infinite number of combinations of drugs A and B along the isoboles yields the same probability of drug effect.

postoperative pain) or an undesired outcome (ie, delayed emergence after a prolonged surgery).

Because visualization of these complex interactions is currently not feasible in a clinical setting and clinicians are justifiably more frequently concerned with preventing awareness while patients are under anesthesia or exaggerated responses to painful stimuli than promoting rapid emergence from anesthesia, most anesthetic techniques target concentration pairs that are substantially above the 95% isobole. In sum, to avoid unwanted consequences of light anesthesia, most practitioners tend to administer relatively excessive doses of anesthetics. For the majority of anesthetics, this practice is well tolerated. However, in patients sensitive to adverse consequences of excessive anesthesia, administering an anesthetic beyond the 95% isobole may be associated with adverse consequences.

In order to visualize the concentration interaction 2 drugs have on a particular drug effect such as analgesia, recent work has focused on the development of 3-dimensional plots called *response surfaces*. Response surface portrays the concentration–effect relationship for each drug individually (similar to a simple pharmacodynamic model) as well as paired concentration–effect (drug–drug interaction). Plotted on these surfaces are the effect site concentrations for 2 drugs (ie, an opioid and a potent inhaled agent) over a range of concentrations of clinical interest and a measure of drug effect. The measure of drug effect is typically presented as a probability ranging from 0 to 1 (ie, the probability of loss of responsiveness with a selected drug pair is 0.8). Recently, many investigators have characterized response surfaces for a variety of drug–drug pairs and clinical relevant drug effects in human volunteers and patients. For example, surfaces have been developed for analgesia, loss of responsiveness to verbal and tactile stimulation, and laryngoscopy for propofol and remifentanil[25,33,36-41] and sevoflurane and remifentanil.[42]

To illustrate the visual power of response surfaces, consider a simulation of 90-minute total IV anesthetic using continuous infusions of propofol and remifentanil (**Fig. 40-17**). Simulated infusion rates are consistent with dosing recommendations for each drug. The resultant effect site concentrations for both drugs are plotted over time. With a bolus dose before starting a continuous infusion, therapeutic levels for each drug are quickly achieved and then maintained throughout the anesthetic. To visualize the combined analgesic effect of remifentanil and propofol, this anesthetic technique has been plotted out on a previously established response surface for analgesia.[25] (**Fig. 40-18**).

With the concentration pairs of remifentanil and propofol plotted for the entire anesthetic on this response surface, 2 important features of the anesthetic technique are easily observed. First, remifentanil and propofol have a pronounced synergistic interaction. When given together, much less of both drugs is required to achieve a desired analgesic effect than if given individually. This is best illustrated by the 50% and 95% isoboles in Fig. 40-18B. Here, the isoboles bow inward and reveal that propofol, when dosed to produce an effect site concentration of 1 μg/mL, decreases the remifentanil needed to meet an analgesic goal by more than half. Of note, a propofol effect site concentration of 1 μg/mL by itself is typically enough to sedate someone but not enough to render them unconscious.

Second, the dosing used in this total IV technique results in a combined drug–drug analgesic effect that for a majority of the anesthetic exceeds the 95% isobole for analgesia. The trajectory of the dosing

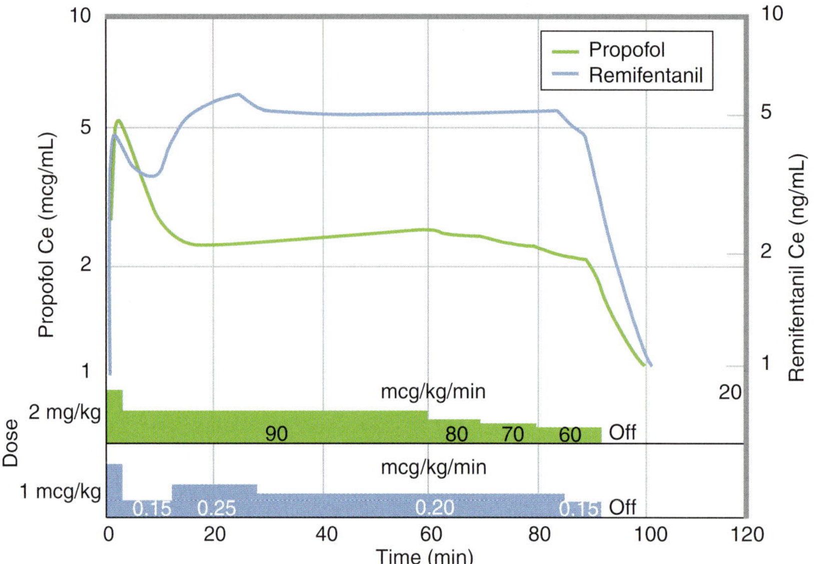

FIGURE 40-17. Simulation of a 90-minute total intravenous anesthetic with propofol and remifentanil. The propofol and remifentanil dosing regimens are presented along the horizontal axis. They include the induction bolus dose (in mg/kg for propofol and μg/kg for remifentanil) followed by the continuous infusion rates (in μg/kg/min) for each drug. The propofol and remifentanil effect site concentrations (Ces) that result from the dosing regimens are plotted over time.

regimen is color-coded into 3 segments: the induction (ie, bolus doses of both drugs), maintenance (continuous infusions of both drugs), and emergence (termination of both drug infusions). It is interesting to observe that the maintenance phase of the anesthetic exclusively occupies the relatively flat region on the surface. Maintaining an anesthetic that is so far removed from the 95% isobole is essentially unnecessary. With regard to analgesia, in this region, additional anesthetic would not be expected to increase the analgesic effect. In the case of remifentanil and propofol, this practice may not be overly worrisome because both drugs exhibit a rapid decline in drug effect when infusions are terminated. With other opioid–sedative drug pairs, however, overdosing an anesthetic onto the flat portion of the response surface will slow the decline of drug effect in most instances.

One of the challenges of drug synergism is to quantify the magnitude of drug–drug interactions in a clinically meaningful manner

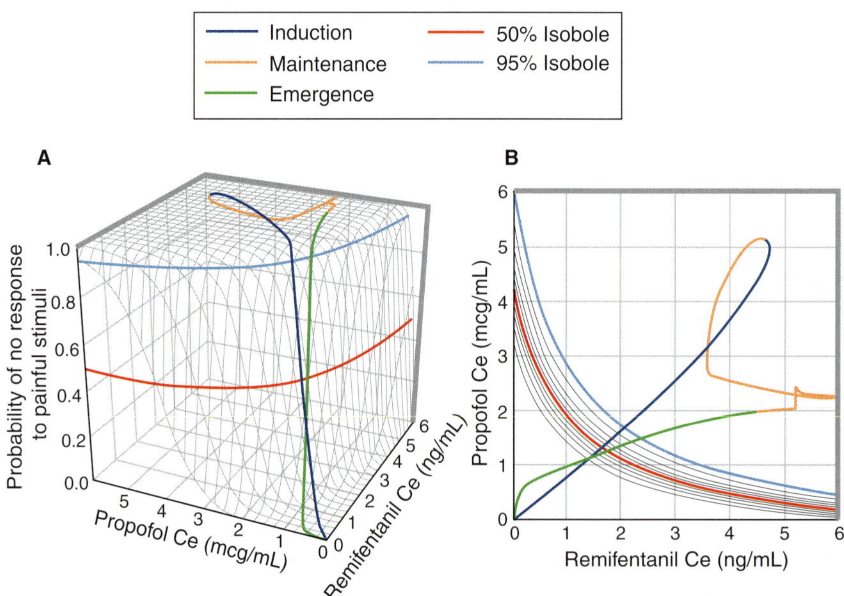

FIGURE 40-18. **A.** Response surface for remifentanil and propofol effect site concentration pairs and the probability of no response to a painful stimulus. **B.** Isobologram of the response surface presented in *A*. Superimposed on both plots are the remifentanil and propofol effect site concentrations that result from the simulated total intravenous anesthetic presented in Fig. 40-17. Segments of the anesthetic are color-coded to depict the induction, maintenance, and termination of anesthetic delivery.

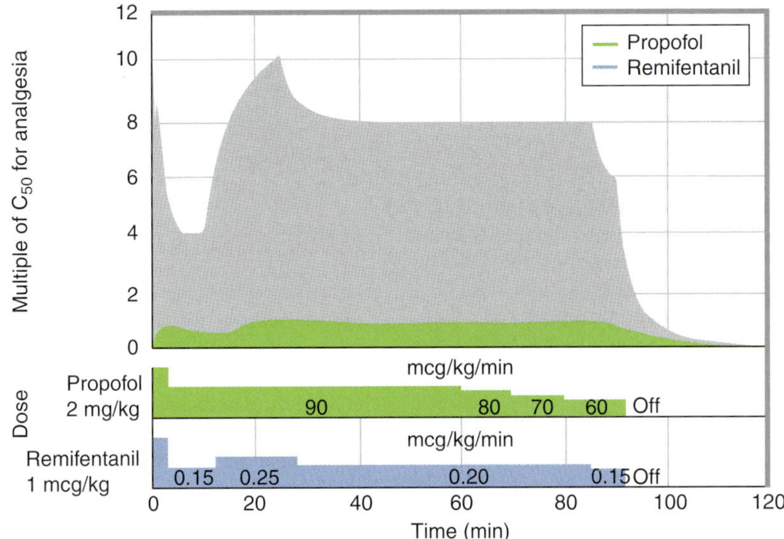

FIGURE 40-19. Simulation of the analgesic effect of remifentanil (*blue*) and synergistic effect of remifentanil and propofol on analgesia (*green*) over time. The analgesic effect is presented as multiples of the C_{50} for analgesia (8.8 ng/mL[25]). The dosing regimens for propofol and remifentanil are presented on the horizontal axis.

that will allow clinicians to reliably modify their dosing regimens to optimize a desired drug effect. Although response surfaces and isoboles provide useful tools for characterizing drug interactions, their clinical utility when delivering an anesthetic in real time has yet to be explored. Suspecting that anesthesia providers may have difficulty interpreting response surfaces and isoboles, investigators have explored other means of visually presenting synergistic effects in real time. Recent work has focused on plotting the contribution of simultaneously administered sedatives or potent inhaled agents and opioids to the overall analgesic and sedative effects over time.[43] With this approach, the overall analgesic effect, for example, is plotted over time as a function of the C_{50} for no response to a painful stimulus. Using this technique, the total IV anesthetic introduced in Fig. 40-17 has been replotted in terms of the contribution of remifentanil alone (*blue*) and remifentanil and propofol (*green*) to the overall analgesic effect (**Fig. 40-19**).

To gain a perspective of how synergistic these 2 drugs are with regard to analgesia, consider the contribution of remifentanil without the propofol to analgesia. The bolus and infusion of remifentanil rendered an effect site concentration that approached half of the effect site concentration (4-5 ng/mL) necessary to reach the C_{50} for analgesia (8.8 ng/mL).[25] By contrast, when added to the bolus and continuous infusion of propofol, the cumulative effect of both drugs exceeds the C_{50} for analgesia 8-fold during most of the anesthetic.

An important limitation of these simulations used to describe drug synergy is that they are inherently limited by pharmacokinetic and pharmacodynamic parameter variability within the population that was used to estimate them.[44,45] Population pharmacokinetic parameters should thus be viewed as an estimate of the population's typical parameters, recognizing that each individual will likely vary from the population parameters to some degree.[46] Some patients, of course, will vary greatly from the population mean. For these patients, the simulations are admittedly of little value. For most patients, however, the prediction based on the population pharmacokinetic and pharmacodynamic parameters are a good starting point for initial therapy. Adjustments in dosing scheme are then made on the basis of patient response.

VISUALIZING ANESTHETIC DRUG EFFECTS IN REAL TIME

Anesthesiologists often consult scientific journal articles and textbooks that describe drug behavior to develop general guidelines when formulating rational dosage schemes (ie, older patients require less propofol). However, the available kinetic-dynamic information is much more comprehensive and is likely to be of more value when applied in real time at the point of care. Most information regarding anesthetic drug behavior exists in the form of pharmacokinetic, pharmacodynamic, and response surface interaction models. These models are often complex and mathematically oriented and unfortunately appear in scientific journals that are not intended for practicing anesthesiologists. This means that perhaps only a small part of the information describing anesthetic drug behavior revealed in clinical pharmacology studies is ever translated into clinical practice. Until recently, the mathematical complexity of these models has precluded their practical introduction into the operating room.

Research is now being conducted to bring anesthetic pharmacologic models to the operating room through the use of drug interaction and conventional kinetic-dynamic models that visually display the time course of not only the effect site concentrations but also how anesthetic drugs interact and the resultant drug effects over time.[41,43,47-49] This technology automatically acquires from infusion pumps and anesthesia machines the drug doses administered by the anesthesiologist and shows the drug dosing history (bolus doses, infusion rates, and expired concentrations); the predicted drug concentrations at the site of action (past, present, and future); and the predicted drug effects, including sedation, analgesia, and neuromuscular blockade.[41,42,47,50]

Compared with TCI systems, visual display systems potentially represent a significant advance because they include not only pharmacokinetic predictions of drug concentrations but also pharmacodynamic predictions of the likelihood of certain anesthetic effects. Response surface models are at the core of these display systems; that is, the information these displays present is based on response surface drug interaction models.

A basic assumption of these displays is that anesthesia care providers cannot solve complex polyexponential equations in their head in real time to choose the best dose for each patient. A major goal of the drug display systems is to bring the sophisticated body of clinical pharmacology information to the point of care in a useable form in real time.[51-53] Existing prototypes of these display systems provide 3 forms of information: (1) drug concentrations (plasma, end tidal, or effect site) over time, (2) drug effects (as individual drugs and the resultant effect from drugs in combination) over time, and (3)

3-dimensional or topographic views of response surfaces for various drug effects.

A major advantage of these display views is that anesthesia care providers can visually appreciate the extent to which their anesthetic technique leads to synergistic effects between drug types. For example, sedatives or inhalation agents, when coadministered with an opioid, have a large synergistic effect on analgesia and, by comparison, a much smaller synergistic effect on sedation. Another advantage of the display is that it provides a more sophisticated way to assess the effectiveness of an anesthetic beyond what is offered on many physiologic displays through the use of the MAC concept. Anesthesiologists rarely dose their anesthetic so that 50% of their patients will move during incision. They always give more! The drug display provides not only a 50% probability of achieving an anesthetic goal but a 95% probability as well. The 95% probability is much more in keeping with how anesthesiologists dose their anesthetics.

In addition, the drug display separates the components of anesthesia into sedation, analgesia, and muscle relaxation and provides a probability of response for each component. This offers anesthesiologists a practical approach to designing and modifying anesthetics to meet the dynamic changes associated with various patients and surgical procedures. Additionally, these drug displays have the potential to simulate various therapeutic decisions immediately before they are implemented, thus allowing anesthesiologists to explore the consequences of a proposed change in therapy prospectively.

Figure 40-20 displays 2 prototype systems currently in development. Although somewhat different in terms of display format, the displays both use tabular and graphical presentation of predicted drug concentrations and drug effects, including a prediction of the synergistic interaction between hypnotics and opioids. Both systems include prediction modules that allow anesthesia care providers to explore various dosage regimens before administration to best meet the anesthetic needs of a surgical procedure. For example, it is possible to simulate the decay of drug concentrations and the projected time to recovery if the drug administration were stopped 5 minutes in the future.

Numerous challenges need to be overcome before these display systems can be adopted into widespread clinical practice. How these drug displays will improve clinical outcomes (eg, faster recovery, improved analgesia on emergence) and how they will gain clinician acceptance (eg, decreased physician workload) must be demonstrated in clinical testing before widespread adoption. Preliminary evidence suggests that they will perform reasonably well,[47-49] but much work remains to be done. One of the barriers to implementation involves the anesthesia care providers' level of understanding of the scientific basis of these complex models and what can be expected from their use during clinical care. Anesthesiologists will likely require education and training to fully use the information this technology offers.

Although it is too early to predict how drug display technology will be used in future anesthesia practice, the concept provides a promising potential to bring more sophisticated clinical pharmacology knowledge to the point of care. Similar to the pharmacokinetic component of these displays already widely implemented in the form of TCI systems, it is conceivable that in the future a real-time display of the predicted pharmacokinetics and pharmacodynamics of anesthetic drugs might be found alongside the traditional physiologic vital sign monitors.[54]

In summary, most practitioners tend to relatively overdose patients with their anesthetic technique because the current surrogate measures of anesthetic depth (ie, changes in heart rate, blood pressure, patient movement, processed EEGs) and display tools to visualize the time course of anesthetic drug concentrations over time are inadequate. Given that variations in surgical stimulus are often difficult to predict and that pharmacologic interpatient variability is substantial, clinical experience mandates that clinicians continue to administer generous doses of anesthetics. As pharmacokinetic and pharmacodynamic display systems become more effective at reliably communicating useful information in a timely manner regarding clinical endpoints of interest, perhaps anesthesiologists will be more inclined to tailor their technique to the precise needs of each patient and the demands of a given surgical procedure or, in other words, surf the 95% isobole.

SPECIAL POPULATIONS

Anesthesiologists have long recognized the need to adapt their anesthetic to account for differences in demographic factors and disease processes that influence drug disposition or effect. Increasingly, the scientific rationale to support these dosing changes is taking shape. Comorbidities in these special populations such as obesity, renal failure, heart failure, liver failure, blood loss, presence of opioid tolerance, and differences in age are referred to as *covariates*. Covariates are descriptors of demographic factors or pathophysiologic states used to estimate the impact these states have on anesthetic drug behavior. Although a significant amount of research has been dedicated to describing covariates and how they can be used to optimize dosing, there are still many gaps in our knowledge base, making the development of guidelines and dosing recommendations for commonly used anesthetics difficult. Nevertheless, as newer IV anesthetics have expanded the array of drugs available to practitioners, covariate analysis has become an increasingly useful tool to describe potential dosing pitfalls associated with these anesthetics.

The next segment of this chapter reviews comorbidities and demographic factors that have been described with covariate analysis for selected IV anesthetics (propofol, fentanyl, and remifentanil) as an example of how to account for disease states such as obesity and blood loss and commonly occurring patient conditions such as advanced age and opioid tolerance when formulating a dosing regimen. Unfortunately, our pharmacologic database is incomplete and does not allow us to generalize these examples to all IV anesthetics. Furthermore, some of the studies have been performed in animal models and are therefore difficult to translate to clinical practice. Nevertheless, this body of work does provide some insight into how IV anesthetics behave in the presence of commonly occurring covariates and is important to consider when formulating a dosing regimen.

BODY WEIGHT AND INTRAVENOUS ANESTHETIC PHARMACOLOGY: DEVELOPING RATIONAL DOSING STRATEGIES

The clinical relevance of accounting for differences in body mass is a result of the prevalence of obesity in the Western culture. Obesity is a major public health problem throughout the developed world. Since the early 1970s, the proportion of the American population that is overweight has steadily increased.[55] Among US adults ages 20 to 74 years, approximately 25% are overweight with a slightly higher prevalence among women.[56] Almost 5% of US adults are morbidly obese (ie, they weigh twice their ideal body weight [IBW]). Anesthesia providers thus frequently encounter obese patients in everyday practice.

Many investigators have explored the impact of weight on drug dosing for opioids[46,57-59] and sedatives[60] and have offered strategies on how doses should be formulated for patients who are overweight. Nonetheless, despite the high prevalence of obesity, practitioners often formulate dosage regimens for many drugs based on total body weight (TBW). Dosing according to TBW in obese patients, however, can lead to large doses and prolonged or toxic effect. Clinicians should recognize that most studies designed to determine appropriate doses of IV anesthetics have been conducted in healthy patients or volunteers at or near their IBW. A unique attribute of IBW is that it represents an estimate of appropriate body weight based on height only. For example, a popular formula to estimate

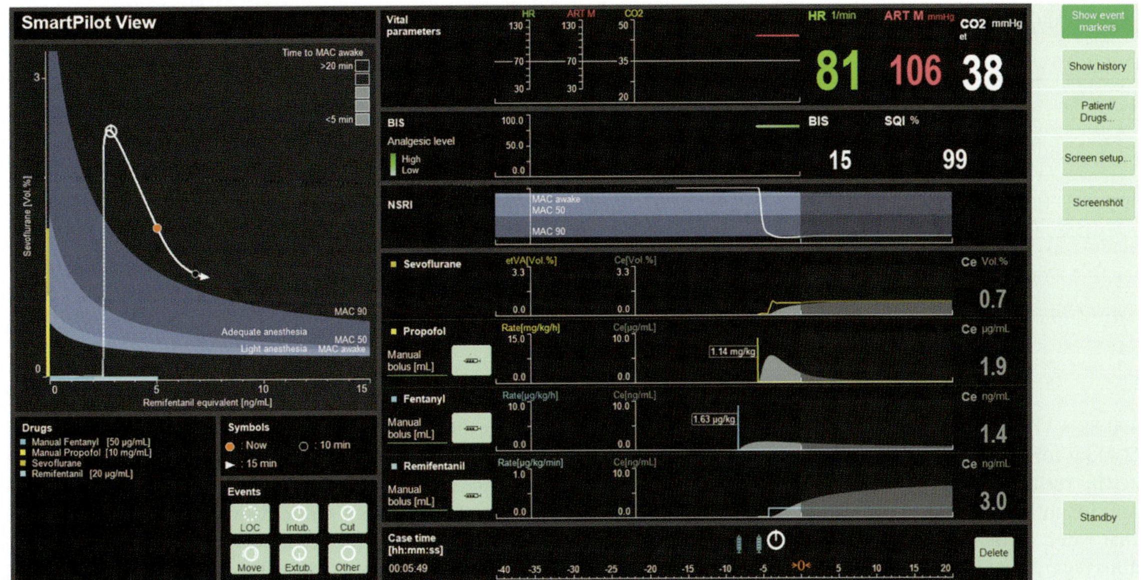

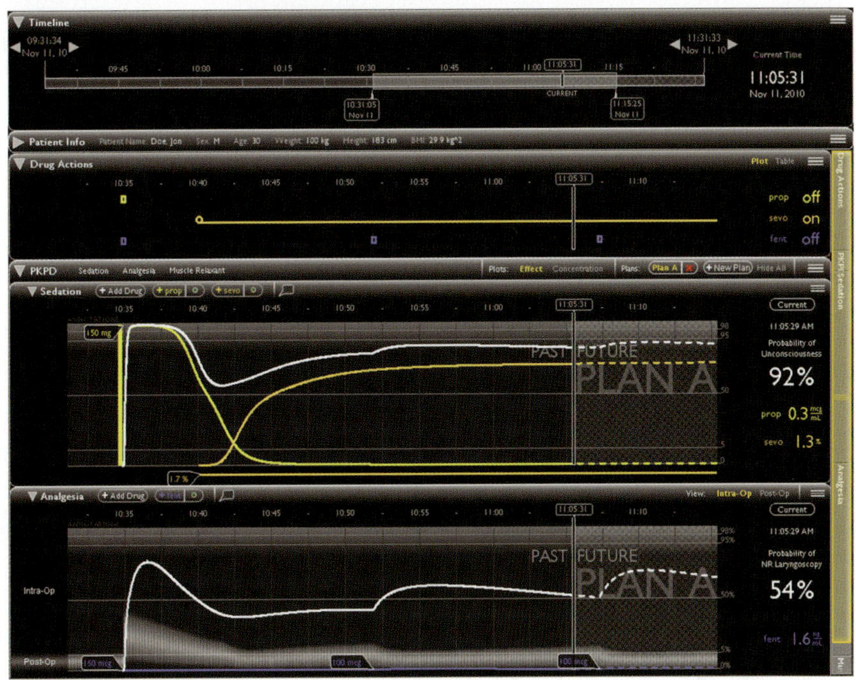

FIGURE 40-20. Examples of drug interaction displays. **A.** Smart Pilot Trainer. This display presents a total intravenous anesthetic using propofol, remifentanil, and fentanyl. It uses a topographical plot of the interaction between propofol and remifentanil (*left plot*) and the vital signs, bispectral index scale (BIS), probability of tolerating a painful stimulus (NSRI), and dose and effect over time (*right plots*). The *left plot* illustrates the synergistic interaction of propofol and remifentanil with gray-scaled isoboles. TOL 50 and 90 indicate the probability of loss of response to laryngoscopy. TOSS 90 indicates the probability of loss of response to a surgical stimulus. Fentanyl is converted into remifentanil equivalents so its contribution can be accounted for on the isobole plot. A series of symbols (light green buttons) are used as Event Markers during a surgical procedure (ie, loss of consciousness, intubation, incision) on both the topographic plot and the dose and effect over time plots. These markers are useful in calibrating the display to individual patients; they allow clinicians to mark the concentration pairs required to meet the anesthetic demands at that event. The series of plots on the *lower right* present the time course for each drug over the past 30 minutes and 30 minutes into the future. [Reproduced with permission from Smart Pilot Trainer, Dräger Medical, Telford, PA.]

B. PKPD Display. This display demonstrates drug effect over time (past, present, and future) as a result of a combined anesthetic technique, induction with propofol and fentanyl followed by maintenance with sevoflurane and fentanyl. Combined pharmacokinetic and pharmacodynamic models are used to predict drug effects. Anesthetic effects are divided into probability of unconsciousness (middle plot), analgesia framed in terms of loss of response to laryngoscopy (bottom plot), and muscle relaxation (not shown). Fentanyl effects are represented by the blue line. Sedative effects are represented by the bright yellow line for propofol and the dark yellow line for sevoflurane. White lines represent drug interactions. For example, the white line on the analgesia plot illustrates the large synergistic interaction between propofol, sevoflurane, and fentanyl on analgesia and to a lesser extent the synergistic interaction on loss of consciousness. The PLAN A refers to predictions of drug effect if the dosing scheme presented in the "future" window is carried out (ie, sevoflurane 1.8% with 100-µg fentanyl bolus). The 2 vertical lines represent a scrollable pointer to identify predicted drug effect at any point during the anesthetic (left line) and the current predictions (right line between the words "past" and "future"). [Reproduced with permission from Applied Medical Visualizations, Salt Lake City, UT.]

TABLE 40-5 Ideal Body Weights for Selected Heights in Men and Women

Height	Women	Men
4′9″ (145 cm)	85 lb (39 kg)	–
5′1″ (155 cm)	105 lb (48 kg)	115 lb (52 kg)
5′6″ (165 cm)	130 lb (59 kg)	140 lb (63 kg)
5′9″ (175 cm)	145 lb (66 kg)	155 lb (70 kg)
6′1″ (185 cm)	165 lb (75 kg)	174 lb (79 kg)
6′5″ (196 cm)	194 lb (88 kg)	–

TABLE 40-6 Pharmacokinetic Population Model Scaled to Lean Body Mass[a]

Parameter Name	Scale Pharmacokinetic Parameter
V1 (L)	(0.121 × LBM) – 0.0713
V2 (L)	(0.165 × LBM) – 0.0713
Cl1 (L/min)	(0.0185 × LBM) – 1.88
Cl2 (L/min)	1.04

[a]Equations used to describe lean body mass (LBM) include LBM = 1.1 × Weight – 128 × (Weight/Height)^2 for men and LBM = 1.07 × Weight – 148 × (Weight/Height)^2 for women.

IBW is 49.9 + 0.89 × (Height – 152.4) kg for men and 45.4 + 0.89 × (Height – 152.4) kg for women.[61]

To illustrate the resultant weights using these formulas, IBWs for several common heights are presented in **Table 40-5**. It is important to point out that when using these formulas for any given height, the IBW is the *same* regardless of weight. Formulating a dose according to the IBW for patients of equivalent height that are 70, 100, and 150 kg would be the same. By contrast to dosing patients according to their TBW, dosing according to the IBW has the potential for significant *underdosing*.

To get around the limitations of IBW for dosing anesthetics, investigators have used lean body mass (LBM) instead. Advantages of LBM are that it excludes weight associated with adipose tissue and accounts for patient height and TBW. For example, LBM has been used to scale pharmacokinetic parameters (ie, volumes and clearances) for remifentanil to predict drug levels in lean and obese patients (**Table 40-6**).[57]

Using these weight-adjusted pharmacokinetic parameters, simulations of remifentanil effect site concentrations in obese and lean patients can be compared when dosed according to TBW versus LBM (**Fig. 40-21**). This set of simulations was performed for a lean woman (125 lb) and an obese woman (220 lb) of the same height (5 ft, 5 in). The simulations used dosing regimens typical for remifentanil as part of a combined technique with a potent inhaled agent, nitrous oxide, or a continuous infusion of a sedative hypnotic. The dosing scheme included a bolus dose (1 μg/kg) followed by a continuous infusion at 0.25 μg/kg/min for 20 minutes and then 0.15 μg/kg/min for 60 minutes.

Key points illustrated by these simulations include (1) Dosing obese patients according to their TBW can yield remifentanil effect site concentrations that are substantially higher than equivalently dosed lean patients. The peak effect site concentrations after 20 minutes of the anesthetic were 9.5 and 5.4 ng/mL for the obese and lean patient, respectively. (2) With the dosing scaled to LBM, the resultant simulated

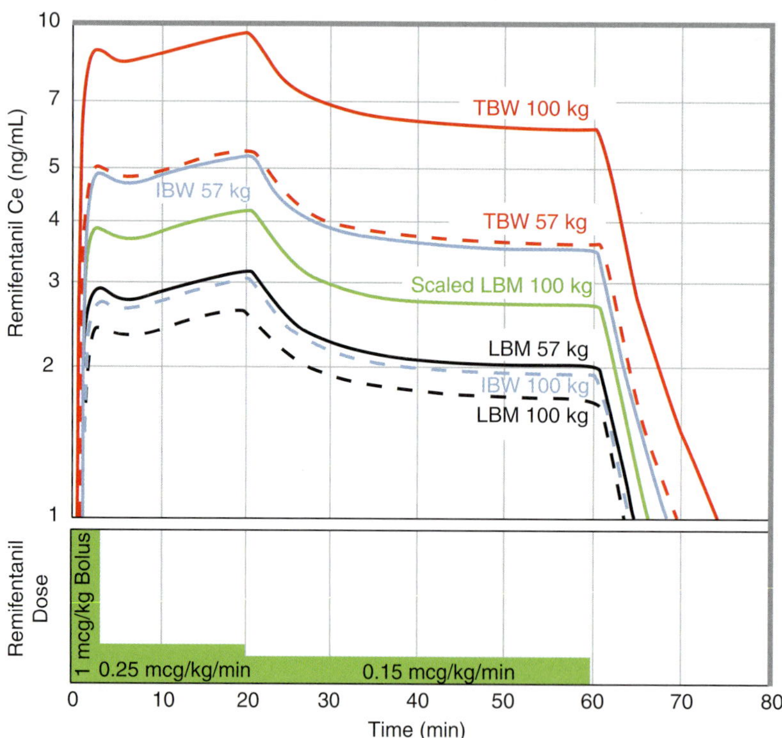

FIGURE 40-21. A computer simulation of a remifentanil infusion for 2 patients: a 5′5″ (165 cm) lean (57-kg) and a 5′5″ obese (100-kg) woman. *Solid lines* represent dosing to 100 kg, and *dashed lines* represent dosing to 57 kg. The dosing regimen is presented along the horizontal axis. The *red, blue,* and *black lines* represent the resultant remifentanil effect site concentration (Ce) when dosed according to the total body weight (TBW), ideal body weight (IBW), and lean body mass (LBM). The *green line* represents the resultant effect site concentration when remifentanil is dosed according to the scaled LBM for the 100-kg patient. The effect site concentration when remifentanil is dosed according to the scaled LBM for the lean patient is equivalent to the concentration for the lean patient dosed to TBW.

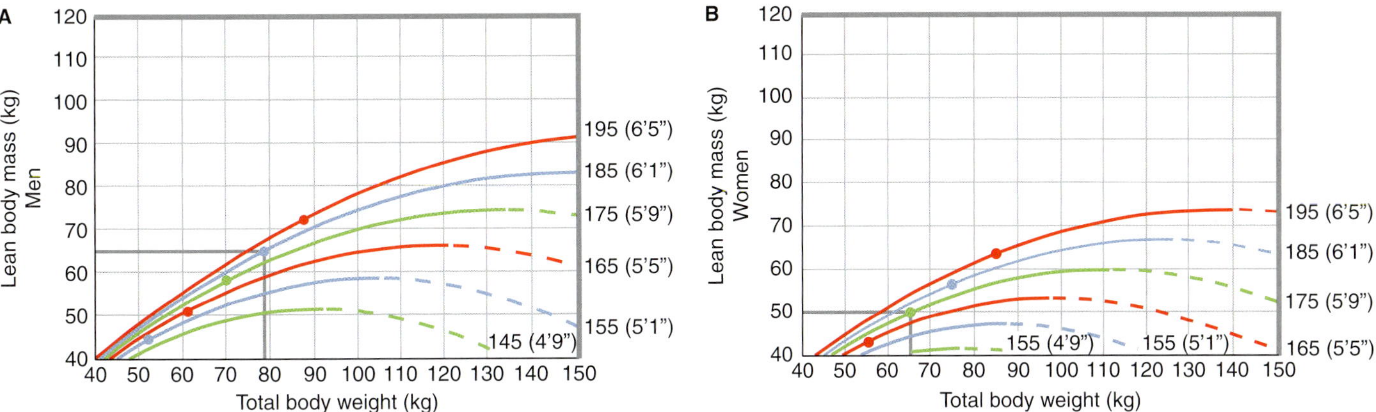

FIGURE 40-22. A normogram by height of the lean body mass (LBM) over a range of total body weights for men (**A**) and women (**B**). Height is presented in centimeters with feet and inches in parentheses. The *dots* represent the ideal body weight (IBW) at each height. The *solid lines* illustrate the LBM for an IBW for a 6'1" man and a 5'9" woman. The *dashed lines* represent the segment of each normogram in which the formula for LBM begins to generate LBMs that are smaller for increasing total body weight. Ideal body weights and LBM were calculated from standard formulas presented in the text.[61] These normograms are patterned after normograms originally described by Bouillon and Shafer[62] using different heights and weights.

effect site concentrations for both the lean and obese patients were *lower* than the effect site profile for a lean patient dosed to her TBW. These simulations suggest that dosing IV anesthetics to LBM, similar to IBW, may lead to significant underdosing.

LBM has an additional limitation. When a patient's weight approaches morbid obesity, dosing according to the LBM becomes increasingly inaccurate.[62] A unique and somewhat worrisome feature to the LBM equation is that for any given height, there is a maximum LBM. For TBWs that are above the maximum LBM, the LBM decreases. In **Fig. 40-22**, an LBM normogram, the LBM estimates that correspond to TBWs in which the LBM decreases with increasing TBW are plotted as a *gray dashed line*. This is most likely an artifact of the LBM equation. If not accounted for, very large patients would receive smaller doses than patients of equivalent height who are not as large. Another limitation of using the LBM normogram for dosing is that the LBM reports the patient mass in the absence of any fat tissue.

The LBM is always lower than the IBW. This is illustrated in the normogram with *solid gray lines*. These lines point out the resultant LBM for an IBW for a man who is 6 ft, 1 in tall and a woman who is 5 ft, 9 in tall. Because even lean people have some fat, this suggests that using the LBM for dosing anesthetics, as observed in Fig. 40-21, leads to some degree of underdosing. Hence, for clinical purposes, the LBM equation is perhaps only useful until reaching the maximum LBM for a given height with the expectation that many patients may require additional anesthetic.

With this limitation in mind, Bouillon and Shafer[62] recommended that estimates of the *ideal* dosing weight from which to formulate dosing regimen use a modified normogram of LBM. Their modified normogram uses the following guidelines: (1) Conventional LBM scales are adjusted to IBW (in other words, for a patient who is at his or her IBW, the LBM at a given height should be the IBW). In effect, this shifts the original normograms presented in Fig. 40-22 up and to the left. (2) The scaled or modified LBM normograms are truncated at the maximal estimates of LBM. This approach relies on the assumptions that recommended doses printed in package inserts are appropriate for patients who are at their IBW. The scaled normogram of LBM is presented in **Fig. 40-23**. Again, the **gray dashed lines** represent the point where the scaled LBM decreases with increasing weight. Scaled LBM estimates in this region should not be used to estimate the proper dosing weight.

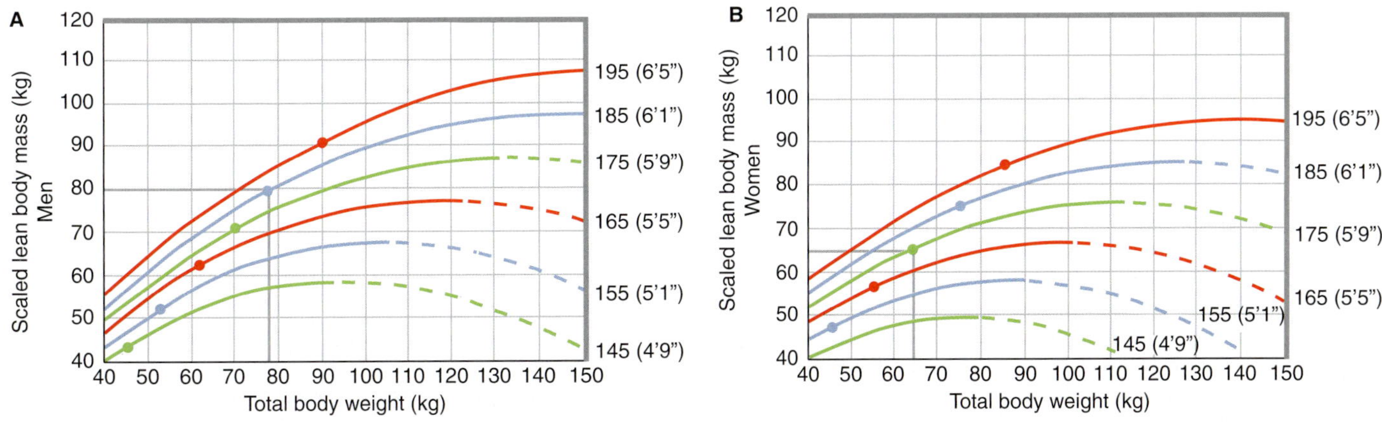

FIGURE 40-23. A modified normogram by height of the *scaled* lean body mass (LBM) over a range of total body weights (TBWs) for men (**A**) and women (**B**). This normogram represents weights that should be used when formulating a dosing regimen by weight. The normogram assumes that published dosing recommendations are correct for persons of ideal body weight (IBW). Height is presented in centimeters with feet and inches in parentheses. The dots represent the IBW at each height. Note that with the scaled normogram, the IBW plotted on the horizontal axis corresponds to the same scaled LBM on the vertical axis. The *solid lines* illustrate that the scaled LBM and the IBW for a 6'1" man and a 5'9" woman are the same. The *dashed lines* represent the segment of each normogram in which the formula for scaled LBM begins to generate scaled LBMs that are smaller for increasing TBW.

TABLE 40-7

Estimates of scaled Lean Body Mass From Ideal Body Weight and Total Body Weight

BMI (kg/m^2)	Increase in IBW as a percentage of TBW – IBW
Men	
≤27	IBW
28–35.1	IBW + 40% of (TBW – IBW)
36–42	IBW + 30% of (TBW – IBW)
≥43	IBW + 20% of (TBW – IBW)
Women	
BMI (kg/m^2)	**Increase in IBW as a percentage of TBW – IBW**
≤27	IBW
27–33	IBW + 30% of (TBW – IBW)
>33	IBW + 20% of (TBW – IBW)

BMI = body mass index; IBW = ideal body weight; TBW = total body weight.

Using this scaled normogram for dosing remifentanil when a person's weight is at or below his or her IBW is unnecessary. Using the person's actual weight will suffice. When a person's weight is above his or her IBW, using the normogram in Fig. 40-23 may be useful but probably not immediately practical if not readily available in a clinical setting. A more simplified approach based on the normograms presented in Fig. 40-23 is to use a patient's IBW or if approaching morbid obesity, consider using their IBW *plus* some fraction of the difference between TBW and IBW.[62] A simplified summary of scaled LBM normograms is presented by gender in **Table 40-7**. To account for height and weight, suggested scaled weights to use for dosing are presented as a function of the body mass index (BMI).

In Fig. 40-21, the *green line* represents the resultant remifentanil effect site concentration when dosing the 5-ft, 5-in (165-cm), 220-lb (100-kg) patient according to the suggested dosing weight in Table 40-6. Her IBW is 57 kg. Her BMI was calculated as 37. Twenty percent of the difference between the TBW and IBW is 8.6 kg. The suggested dosing weight is therefore 65.6 kg. The resultant effect site concentrations are in between the concentrations when dosing her according to her TBW and LBM, respectively. Using this approach, the inherent risks of underdosing using the LBM and overdosing using the TBW as well as avoiding the limitations of dosing according to the IBW are avoided.

AGE AND INTRAVENOUS ANESTHETIC PHARMACOLOGY: DEVELOPING RATIONAL DOSING STRATEGIES

Considering the aging of the world's population, the clinical significance of age in the practice of anesthesia is obvious. Practitioners are frequently faced with the clinical challenge of anesthetizing older adults, sometimes even patients in their ninth or tenth decades of life. Clinicians have long recognized that elderly patients usually require smaller dosages of most IV anesthetics to produce the desired therapeutic effect while minimizing adverse effects.

Of the frequently considered patient covariates (eg, gender, age, body weight, kidney function, hepatic function), age is perhaps one of the most valuable in terms of developing a therapeutic, nontoxic dosage strategy for many IV anesthetics. Age is easily measured (ie, just ask the patient), and its influence on the pharmacokinetics and pharmacodynamics of many IV anesthetics has been described in some detail.

With regard to age, both remifentanil and propofol can serve as prototypes to examine the impact of age on anesthetic pharmacology. Studies specifically designed to assess the influence of age on remifentanil and propofol pharmacokinetics and pharmacodynamics have been conducted, and complex models have been constructed that characterize the influence of age in quantitative terms.[11,32,60,62,63]

With regard to remifentanil, it is clear that the elderly do indeed require less drug to produce the desired spectrum of opioid effects. The reduced dosage requirement is a function of both pharmacokinetic and pharmacodynamic mechanisms, although pharmacodynamic factors dominate.[11] The concentration of remifentanil necessary for 50% of maximal effect as measured by the EEG is markedly decreased in elderly adults (C_{50} for EEG changes); in addition, remifentanil's clearance and volume of distribution are also decreased.[11] These age-related changes translate clinically into the need for a very substantial dosage reduction in elderly adults that is based largely on the increased potency of remifentanil in older patients (ie, a pharmacodynamic difference).

Using the pharmacokinetic–pharmacodynamic parameters from age-adjusted pharmacologic models of propofol and remifentanil, computer simulations can be performed to explore the suitability of various dosage schemes. **Figure 40-24** presents a set of simulations of propofol's pharmacologic behavior after an induction dose of propofol. Using age-adjusted pharmacokinetic and pharmacodynamic parameters,[32,60] 4 simulations of a 2-mg/kg propofol bolus for a 20-, 40-, 60-, and 80-year-old patient demonstrate that with the same dose, there is a subtle rise in the peak propofol effect site concentration and a small delay in reaching the peak with increasing age. By contrast, the concentration at which there is a 50% probability of losing unresponsiveness (C_{50} for unresponsiveness) drops by 50% from age 20 to 80 years (**Table 40-8**). Combining the pharmacokinetic and pharmacodynamic models, the duration of propofol effect (ie, the time above the effect site concentration associated with a loss of responsiveness) substantially increases with increasing age.

Similarly, **Fig. 40-25** is an illustration of simulations of remifentanil's pharmacologic behavior after a 1-hour infusion. Using age-adjusted pharmacokinetic and pharmacodynamic parameters,[11,63] 4 simulations

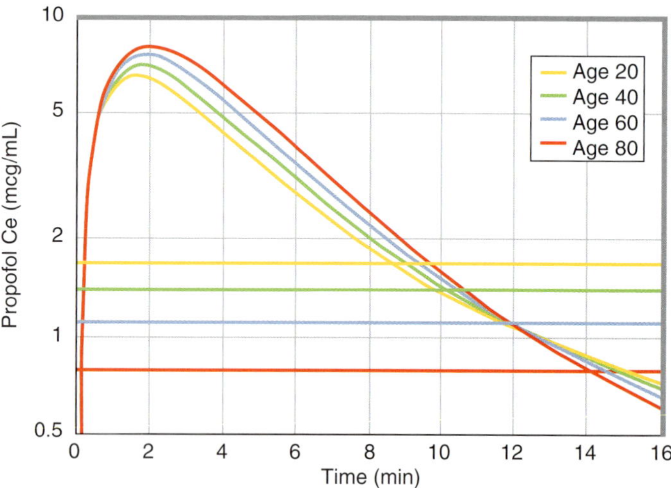

FIGURE 40-24. This plot illustrates a combined pharmacokinetic and pharmacodynamic simulation of the propofol effect site concentration that results from a 2-mg/kg bolus. The simulated patient is an 80-kg, 183-cm-tall man. Simulations were performed for patients of age 20, 40, 60, and 80 years old. The *horizontal lines* represent the effect site concentrations (Ces) associated with a 50% probability of loss of responsiveness. They are 1.7, 1.4, 1.1, and 0.8 μg/mL for ages 20, 40, 60, and 80 years, respectively. Pharmacokinetic and pharmacodynamic parameters for propofol by age were adapted for simulation from Schnider et al.[32,60]

TABLE 40-8 Influence of Age on the Pharmacologic Behavior of a 2-mg/kg Bolus of Propofol and a 1-Hour Remifentanil Infusion Set at 0.2 mcg/kg/min

Age (y)	20	40	60	80
Propofol[a]				
Peak propofol Ce (mcg/mL)	6.5	7.0	7.6	8.2
Time to peak Ce (min)	1.7	1.8	2.0	2.0
C_{50} for LOR (mcg/mL)	1.7	1.4	1.1	0.8
Time above the C_{50} for LOR (min)	9	10	12	14
Percent reduction in dose (%)	0	25	56	65
Remifentanil[a]				
Remifentanil Ce (ng/mL) upon termination of the infusion	5.6	6.6	8.0	10.2
C_{50} for analgesia (ng/mL)	2.0	1.6	1.3	0.9
Upon termination of the infusion, time above the C_{50} for analgesia (min)	8	13	19	29
Percent reduction in dose (%)	0	18	37	55

[a]Pharmacokinetic and pharmacodynamic parameters for propofol by age were adapted for simulation from Schnider et al.[32,60] Pharmacokinetic and pharmacodynamic parameters for remifentanil by age were adapted for simulation from Minto et al.[11,63]

Ce, effect site concentration; C_{50} for LOR, the effect site concentration associated with a 50% probability of loss of responsiveness; C_{50} for analgesia, the effect site concentration associated with a 50% probability of analgesia.

are presented of a 1-hour continuous infusion at a rate of 0.2 μg/kg/min for a 20-, 40-, 60-, and 80-year-old patient. With the same infusion rate, the remifentanil effect site concentration develops a substantial increase over time with increasing age (Table 40-8). Estimates of the C_{50} for analgesia allow for the prediction of duration of analgesic effect after termination of the 1-hour infusion. In Fig. 40-25, the C_{50} for each

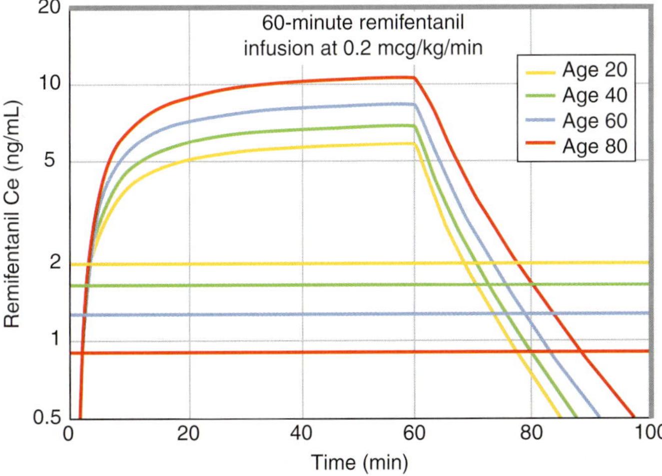

FIGURE 40-25. This plot illustrates a combined pharmacokinetic and pharmacodynamic simulation of the remifentanil effect site concentration (Ce) that results from a 1-hour infusion set at 0.2 μg/kg/min. The simulated patient is an 80-kg, 183-cm-tall man. Simulations were performed for patients of age 20, 40, 60, and 80 years old. The *horizontal lines* represent the effect site concentrations associated with a analgesia. The analgesic levels are 2, 1.6, 1.3, and 0.9 ng/mL for ages 20, 40, 60, and 80 years, respectively. Pharmacokinetic and pharmacodynamic parameters for propofol by age were adapted for simulation from Minto et al.[11,63]

simulated age is presented as a *horizontal line*. After termination of the infusion, the duration of analgesic effect markedly increases with age (>3-fold increase from age 20-80 years).

Additional simulations can be used to estimate the percent reduction in dose as a function of age for both propofol and remifentanil. As is illustrated in Table 40-8, achieving equipotent doses in 20- and 80-year-old adults requires that an 80-year-old patient receive a dose that has been reduced by 55% to 65% of that which would be given to a 20-year-old patient. These simulations emphasize the importance of considering age when formulating an appropriate dose in elderly patients.

Although physiologic mechanism of the pharmacodynamic changes in elderly people remains largely unexplored, the pharmacokinetic changes may be at least attributable to decreased cardiac output. The lower cardiac output associated with advanced age[64] presumably results in slower drug mixing and therefore higher peak concentrations after a bolus dose.[65-67] Lower cardiac output may also decrease drug delivery to metabolic organs, resulting in lower clearance for some drugs.

When generalizing to other drugs, whether reduced cardiac output is the primary underlying mechanism responsible for the pharmacokinetic changes observed in elderly adults, it is consistent with the observation that many IV anesthetics (thiopental, propofol, etomidate) appear to have a smaller distribution volume or slower clearance in elderly adults.[10,60,68,69]

It is, however, important to point out that reduced cardiac output is not a ubiquitous finding in elderly adults, particularly in the absence of heart disease in well-conditioned individuals.[70] Recognizing this has perhaps led to the common clinical notion of identifying a patient's "physiological" age instead of relying on chronological age alone.[71,72] Significant reductions in dosage may not therefore be necessary for physically robust elderly patients with normal body habitus and without substantial coexisting disease.

It is more difficult to generalize with regard to age-induced pharmacodynamic changes to other IV anesthetics. Although elderly adults clearly have a "left-shifted" concentration–effect relationship for opioids (ie, the opioids are more potent in elderly patients[11,73]), a good deal of data suggest that older patients are not more pharmacodynamically sensitive to the sedative–hypnotics. For example, there is no difference between old and young in terms of the EEG C_{50} for etomidate or thiopental.[10,68,69] On the other hand, recently published data suggest that both propofol and midazolam are more potent in elderly patients.[32,74] Thus, although there is certainly general consensus that elderly patients require less medication than younger patients, whether this reduced dosage requirement can be attributed to pharmacokinetic or pharmacodynamic mechanisms remains unclear for some individual agents.

BLOOD VOLUME AND INTRAVENOUS ANESTHETIC PHARMACOLOGY: DEVELOPING RATIONAL DOSING STRATEGIES

Dr Halford, a surgeon, wrote a letter to the editor of *Anesthesiology* after caring for several trauma victims after the attack on Pearl Harbor in 1941. He noticed that anesthetists had started using the IV anesthetic sodium pentothal. His comments included: "Then let it be said that intravenous anesthesia is also an ideal form of euthanasia. . . .With this heterogeneous mass of emergency anesthetists, it is necessary to choose an anesthetic involving the *WIDEST MARGIN OF SAFETY* for the patient. . . . Stick with *ETHER*."[75]

Anesthesiologists have long recognized the need to select certain IV anesthetics over others, to incrementally dose these anesthetics, and to moderate the overall dose for patients who have significant blood loss before or during surgery. Through experience, clinicians have learned that a full dose of selected IV anesthetics can lead to pronounced and often unwanted side effects with potentially disastrous consequences.

In the recent past, several researchers have attempted to quantify how the extent of blood loss impacts IV anesthetic pharmacokinetics

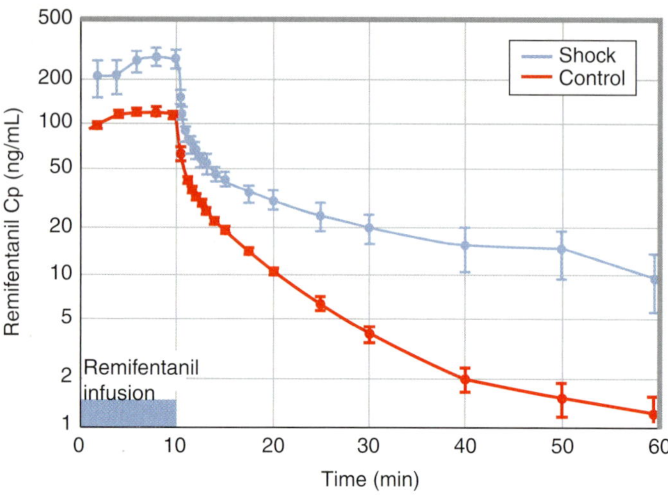

FIGURE 40-26. Resultant mean blood drug concentrations versus time from equivalent dosing of remifentanil in bled (42 mL/kg) and unbled swine. The *red* and *blue lines* represent the mean levels for bled and unbled animals, respectively. The *blue box* at the lower left corner represents the duration of the 10-μg/kg/min remifentanil infusion. The *error bars* indicate the standard error. The vertical axis is on the log scale. Cp, plasma concentration.

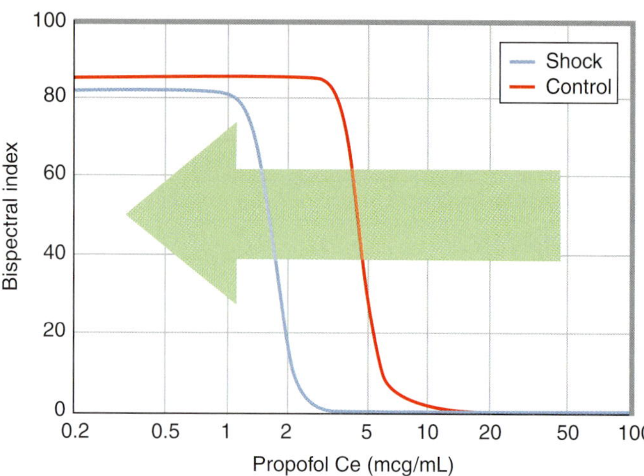

FIGURE 40-27. The concentration–effect relationship of propofol to the bispectral index scale (BIS) in bled (30 mL/kg) and unbled swine as characterized by a pharmacodynamic model. The *blue* and *red lines* represent the mean change in BIS over a range of propofol effect site concentrations (Ces) for unbled and bled swine, respectively. The *green arrow* illustrates the shift in the C_{50} between groups.

and pharmacodynamics to include work with opioids,[76-78] sedative-hypnotics,[79-83] benzodiazepines,[84,85] and local anesthetics.[86] The most important finding consistent throughout this body of work is that equivalent dosing leads to higher drug concentrations with severe blood loss compared with control participants without bleeding. In addition, although derived volumes and clearances from pharmacokinetic analyses do not reflect true organ drug distribution and clearance, they do indicate that in severe blood loss, blood flow to muscle, gut, liver, and connective tissue is markedly decreased such that anesthetics delivered IV are most likely pumped straight to the brain in higher concentrations. This phenomenon leads to higher brain concentrations of anesthetic drugs and a more pronounced or prolonged anesthetic effect.[87]

As an example, **Fig. 40-26** illustrates the differences in blood concentrations that result from identical doses of remifentanil in bled and unbled swine.[78] After severe blood loss (42 mL/kg), resultant remifentanil blood levels were 2-fold higher during and after a 10-minute remifentanil infusion. Of note in this study, the dose (10 μg/kg/min) is approximately 50- to 100-fold more than a typical dose of 0.1 to 0.2 μg/kg/min, yet all animals survived despite losing more than half of their blood. A decrease in blood volume and cardiac index (5-1.7 L/min/m^2) along with compensatory changes in regional blood flow are the likely physiologic mechanisms explaining these pharmacokinetic changes. Pharmacokinetic analyses revealed that the volumes of distribution and clearances were decreased in bled animals compared with unbled control subjects. Spectral edge changes in the EEG were used to measure drug effect. By contrast to the pharmacokinetic analysis, there was no difference observed in the pharmacodynamics between groups. As has been observed with fentanyl[77] and morphine,[76] these findings with remifentanil corroborate the relative forgiving posture of high-dose opioids on cardiovascular function even when used in hemorrhagic shock.

In contrast to opioids, blood loss has a more worrisome impact on propofol pharmacokinetics and pharmacodynamics. Similar to the experimental design used with remifentanil described above, investigators have bled animals and then administered propofol. Two major differences were observed when compared with remifentanil. First, the administration of propofol after severe hemorrhage (42 mL/kg) led to certain cardiovascular collapse. Second, the dose found to elicit a pharmacologic effect (ie, a change in the BIS of at least 50) in unbled animals was in no way tolerated in bled animals. To conduct experiments in bled animals, the propofol dose had to be reduced by more than 50%, and the extent of hemorrhage had be markedly reduced to 30 mL/kg. In this case, hemorrhage led to a decrease in the cardiac index from 5 to 2.6 L/min/m^2. Subsequently, animals received a 10-minute propofol infusion at 200 μg/kg/min. Of interest, with equivalent dosing, the hemorrhaged animals exhibited approximately 2-fold greater plasma concentrations of propofol throughout the study period. A pharmacokinetic analysis revealed that similar to remifentanil, propofol compartmental clearances and volumes were decreased in bled animals.

The BIS was used as a surrogate measure of propofol effect. As expected, changes in the BIS lagged behind the changes in plasma propofol concentrations. These data were used to estimate the k_{eo} for bled and unbled animals and construct previously described pharmacodynamic models to include estimates of the C_{50} and γ. Comparison of pharmacodynamic parameters between bled and unbled animals revealed a similar k_{eo} and γ but a 2.7-fold decrease in the C_{50} (4.6 μg/mL vs 1.7 μg/mL for the control and shock groups, respectively). This is emphasized by the leftward shift (*green arrow*) in the C_{50} for each study group in **Fig. 40-27**.

Perhaps one of the more dangerous uses of IV anesthetics is during the induction of anesthesia. Here bolus doses are used to rapidly render a patient analgesic or unconscious, but these doses can be associated with significant morbidity if dosing does not account for large changes in blood volume. For purposes of discussion, consider an induction dose of propofol. The pharmacokinetic and pharmacodynamic findings related to propofol during blood loss described previously will be used to illustrate how blood loss impacts conventional dosing of sedative hypnotics.

In Fig. 40-11, using pharmacokinetic parameters previously described in humans,[3] the onset and duration of loss of responsiveness after a propofol bolus of 2 mg/kg were 1 and 8 minutes, respectively, assuming that the necessary propofol effect site concentrations required for loss of responsiveness near 1.8 μg/mL.[25] Conducting a propofol bolus simulation after moderate blood loss (35% of the blood volume) yields a significantly different result (**Fig. 40-28**). Based on the impact of blood loss on propofol pharmacokinetics and pharmacodynamics, this simulation takes in account the 2.5-fold increase in effect site propofol

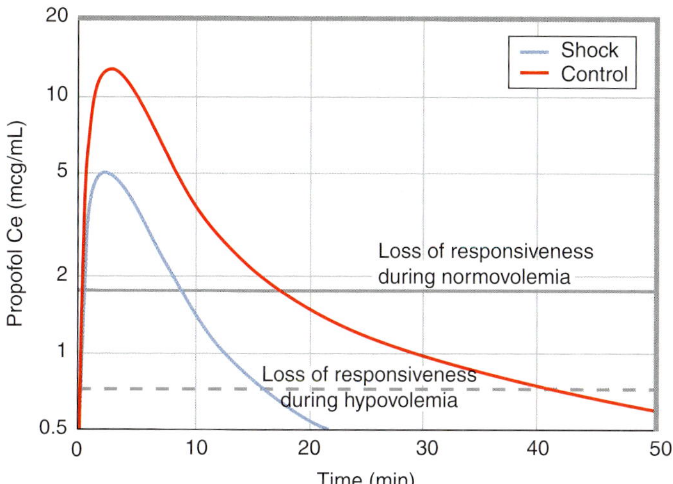

FIGURE 40-28. Combined pharmacokinetic and pharmacodynamic simulations of a propofol bolus dose 2 mg/kg under normal hemodynamic conditions and after moderate blood loss. The *blue* and *red lines* represent the effect site concentrations (Ces) under normal and hypovolemic conditions. The *gray solid* and *dashed lines* represent the propofol effect site concentration associated with a loss of responsiveness under normal and hypovolemic conditions.

concentration and the 2.7-fold decrease in concentration required for loss of responsiveness.

With this simulation, the impact of moderate blood loss on the duration of effect is easily appreciated. Of note, with blood loss, there is more than a 5-fold increase in the duration of effect (8-44 minutes). These simulations suggest that propofol should be used, if at all, with extreme caution! Estimating the dose that would provide an equivalent effect in a person with severe blood loss compared with a person with normal cardiovascular physiology yields a propofol dose reduction of 80% (eg, 0.4 mg/kg). Although the impact of blood loss on propofol is dramatic, it is important to recognize that this simulation is of a single propofol bolus and does not reflect the common practice of combining propofol with an opioid during the induction of anesthesia. In this scenario, it is likely that the pronounced increase in peak effect and duration of effect would only be larger and potentially more dangerous.

Perhaps the most important consequence of blood loss on propofol behavior is the exaggerated hemodynamic response after a bolus dose. Propofol is a peripheral vasodilator and suppresses contractility.[88] As observed in these simulations, a propofol bolus dose yields higher effect site concentrations that remain elevated for a prolonged period of time, thus amplifying propofol's cardiovascular depression. Sodium thiopental has a similar profile of cardiovascular depression, and this likely explains why Dr Halford was so adamant about the dangers associated with the induction of anesthesia with sodium pentothal.

What about resuscitation? Does volume resuscitation restore drug disposition and effect to baseline? In typical clinical practice, some fluid resuscitation is usually under way before the administration of an anesthetic. Based on the premise that resuscitation will restore cardiac output and systemic blood flow, the shock-induced pharmacokinetic and pharmacodynamic changes may be reversed. In a similar set of experiments, a comparison was made between unbled control subjects and bled and then partially resuscitated swine.[89] Hemorrhage was severe (42 mL/kg), and resuscitation constituted an infusion of crystalloid to maintain a mean arterial blood pressure of 70 mm Hg for 60 minutes. This resulted in a resuscitation volume of 59 mL/kg.

After a 10-minute high-dose (750 µg/kg/min) propofol infusion, the propofol plasma concentrations were nearly identical. Resuscitation restored the shock-induced changes in propofol pharmacokinetics to near baseline values. The pharmacodynamic parameters, however, remained altered. As with severe blood loss, the C_{50} was decreased 1.5-fold after hemorrhage and resuscitation. Although the mechanism for this phenomenon is not well understood, one explanation for the increase in end-organ sensitivity to propofol may be at least partly attributable to an unrecognized increase in unbound propofol. Thus, the leftward shift in the C_{50} of propofol may represent an undetected *pharmacokinetic* difference between groups. Although the plasma propofol levels were similar between the bled and then resuscitated animals and the unbled animals, the amount of unbound propofol available to exert a pharmacologic effect may have been increased.[90] After removing more than 50% of the estimated blood volume and replacing it with crystalloid, plasma protein content would most likely be decreased. Furthermore, alterations in organ blood flow, capillary wall integrity, and plasma pH may influence the levels of unbound propofol. Given that plasma protein content, propofol-plasma protein binding, or unbound propofol levels were not measured or estimated, the extent that changes in unbound propofol played in altering the observed differences in end-organ sensitivity remains unknown.

With this protocol, 60% of the estimated blood volume was removed. A total of 140% of the shed blood volume was replaced with lactated Ringer solution to maintain a near-normotensive blood pressure. *The near-normal blood pressure was deceiving!* Although hemodynamic function appeared near normal (ie, the central venous pressure and cardiac index were similar to those in unbled animals), the cardiovascular response to propofol remained exaggerated. During the propofol infusion, the cardiac index decreased by 1.7 L/min/m^2 in the shock-resuscitation group but only by 0.2 L/min/m^2 in the control group. The large hemodynamic changes in the shock-resuscitation group illustrate how severe blood loss followed by partial resuscitation can lead to potentially large cardiovascular changes with the administration of propofol. In fact, a significant clinical correlate from this analysis is that despite a near-normal hemodynamic profile after partial resuscitation for severe blood loss, resuscitation should continue to minimize the potentially severe hemodynamic depression that can be associated with the administration of propofol.

Figure 40-29 represents a simulation of the propofol effect site concentration after a propofol bolus dose in a patient with severe

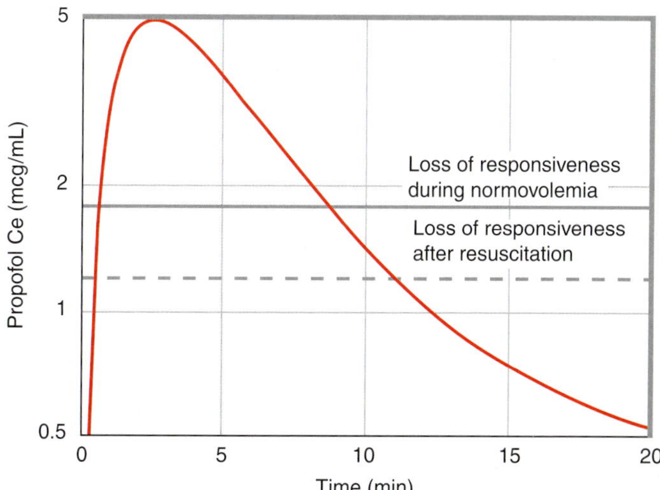

FIGURE 40-29. Combined pharmacokinetic and pharmacodynamic simulation of a 2-mg/kg propofol bolus dose after severe blood loss and resuscitation. The *solid* and *dashed gray lines* represent the effect site concentrations (Ces) at which there is a loss of responsiveness under normal and bled and then resuscitated conditions. E_{max}, maximal effect.

blood loss followed by partial resuscitation with crystalloid (1.5 mL of crystalloid per 1 mL of estimated blood loss). This simulation accounts for the pharmacodynamic changes as manifest by a 1.5-fold decrease in the effect site concentration required for loss of responsiveness. The duration of effect increases from 8 to 11 minutes.

Compared with propofol, both ketamine and etomidate have greater acceptance among clinicians who care for patients with significant blood loss. This is largely because the cardiovascular depression known to be exaggerated with propofol and sodium pentothal is not as apparent with etomidate and even to a lesser extent with ketamine. Although etomidate is known to produce mild cardiovascular depression, prior work surprisingly has revealed minimal cardiovascular change after a high-dose brief continuous etomidate infusion[81,83] during moderate hemorrhagic shock (30 mL/kg). In a similar fashion, the pharmacokinetic and pharmacodynamic profile of etomidate after blood loss was also minimally influenced by blood loss. This suggests that dosing requirements for etomidate do not require adjustment after moderate blood loss. This finding goes along with the widely held view that etomidate is a good choice in hemodynamically unstable patients.

What remains unknown is the impact of blood loss on ketamine. Preliminary work has revealed that, similar to etomidate, blood loss does not significantly impact the pharmacokinetics of ketamine. Ketamine is known to increase sympathetic tone, serve as a potent analgesic, and perform favorably in patients with poor cardiovascular function. These preliminary findings support the widely held view that ketamine is an important drug to maintain in our pharmacologic armamentarium when caring for patients with life-threatening blood loss.

The pharmacodynamic properties of ketamine, however, are difficult to assess. This is largely because ketamine is a racemic mixture that, when metabolized, has an active metabolite, norketamine. Hence, the contribution of both enantiomers and norketamine must be considered when assessing the overall drug effect of ketamine. An additional difficulty with measuring ketamine's drug effect is that it is difficult to identify surrogate measure for ketamine's effect. For example, the BIS is not a reliable measure of ketamine's sedative effects.

In summary, as clinicians manage patients with blood loss through often perilous anesthetics, hemorrhage and even hemorrhage followed by resuscitation that appears to restore hemodynamic function to near normal can lead to dramatic alterations in the pharmacologic behavior of commonly used sedative hypnotics and opioids. Duration of effect, peak effect site concentrations, and extent of cardiovascular depression should all be considered when selecting an IV anesthetic and formulating an appropriate dose. Hemodynamically compromised patients are especially susceptible to the cardiovascular suppression of selected sedative hypnotics, but other sedative hypnotics appear to be much safer. Propofol and sodium pentothal are especially poor choices even after some degree of resuscitation. By contrast, ketamine and etomidate tend to be immune to the deleterious effects of moderate to severe blood loss on their pharmacokinetic profiles. Severe blood loss alters opioid pharmacokinetics, leading to higher plasma concentrations, but opioids, in contrast to propofol and sodium pentothal, enjoy a wider therapeutic margin in the presence of blood loss. What remains unexplored, however, is the impact blood loss has on the resultant effect from the simultaneous administration of multiple drugs. As illustrated in the drug synergism section of this chapter, opioids and sedative-hypnotics can dramatically influence one another. How this interaction behaves in the presence of intravascular volume depletion remains unknown.

OPIOID-TOLERANT PATIENTS

One of the most vexing problems facing anesthetists is satisfactorily caring for patients who chronically consume opioids (see Chapter 24 for a general review of substance abuse and anesthesia practice). With chronic consumption of opioids, tolerance develops, and more drug is required to achieve a desired analgesic effect. This becomes especially problematic in the perioperative period when opioid dosing requirements for these patients often reach thresholds associated with significant morbidity in the nonopioid-tolerant population. Out of concern for patient safety, opioid doses are often administered in more conventional doses to avoid unwanted side effects associated with opioid toxicity, leading to often dramatically poor pain control in the postoperative period. In these types of patients, the population-based pharmacodynamic models used to describe opioid concentration–effect relationships become obsolete. Performing simulations to estimate opioid behavior either alone or in combination with other types of anesthetics using pharmacodynamic models built from studies evaluating an opioid-naïve population is bound to provide a faulty estimate of drug effect in patients who chronically consume opioids. The essential problem is that the magnitude of the right shift in the C_{50} and C_{95}, which are key parameters used to build the pharmacodynamic models, is unknown (**Fig. 40-30**).

With the widespread use of oral short-acting and time-contingent opioids, transdermal opioid delivery systems, and implantable opioid infusion pumps, opioid tolerance is recognized as a growing challenge in the perioperative environment. Nevertheless, there is a paucity of literature examining the phenomenon of opioid tolerance as a covariate in pharmacodynamic models. One potential reason for this is that opioid tolerance is a difficult feature of drug behavior to quantify and most likely varies substantially from person to person based on duration of opioid consumption and opioid dose.

With this problem in mind, investigators have explored methods of identifying the concentration-effect relationship for opioid on an individual basis.[91-93] Using principles of pharmacokinetics and pharmacodynamics, a technique has been developed called the *fentanyl challenge*. The fentanyl challenge was designed for use in patients with a known history of chronic opioid consumption who are scheduled to undergo surgical procedures associated with significant postoperative pain that will require a general anesthetic and are of moderate to long duration (ie, multilevel lumbar spine instrumentation). The fentanyl challenge protocol calls for a rapid continuous infusion of fentanyl (2 μg/kg/min) to be administered until the onset of respiratory depression in the absence of any other sedatives, anxiolytics, or opioids (**Fig. 40-31**). The optimal setting in which to perform the challenge is just before the induction of general anesthesia. The onset of respiratory depression as defined within the fentanyl challenge is a respiratory rate less than 6 breaths/min. A critical component of the challenge is to measure the time from the onset of the fentanyl infusion until the onset of respiratory depression.

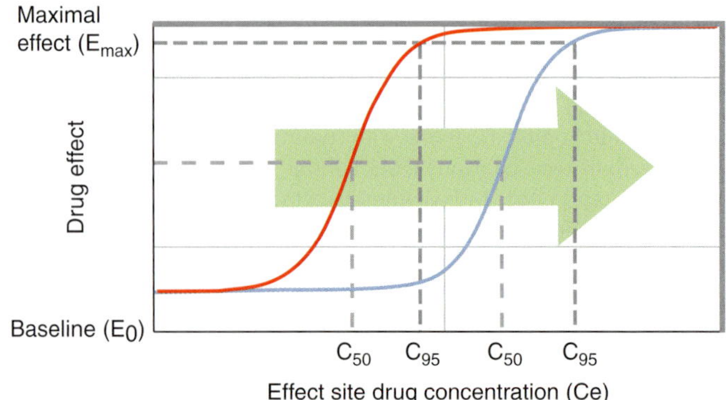

FIGURE 40-30. The effect of opioid tolerance on the concentration–effect relationship characterized by pharmacodynamic modeling. The C_{50} and C_{95} are shifted to the right indicating that the more drug is required to achieve the same level of drug effect.

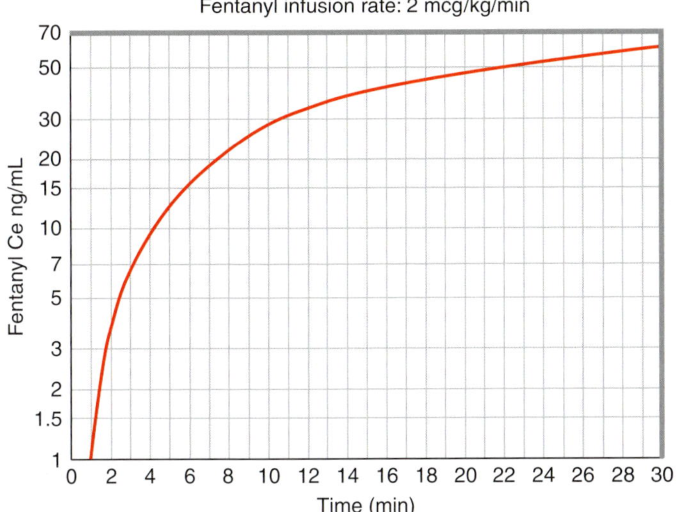

FIGURE 40-31. Computer simulation of the fentanyl challenge. The plot illustrates the fentanyl effect site concentration (Ce) that results from a continuous infusion of 2 μg/kg/min. This plot is used to estimate the fentanyl effect site concentration at the onset of respiratory depression. For example, if 8 minutes elapse before the onset of respiratory depression (ie, a respiratory rate <6 breaths/min), the associated fentanyl effect site concentration is approximately 20 ng/mL.

With the duration of the high-dose fentanyl infusion until respiratory depression identified, a pharmacokinetic simulation of the infusion is made to identify the fentanyl effect site concentration that is associated with respiratory depression. This process redefines the pharmacodynamic relationship between fentanyl effect site concentrations and drug effect that is unique to a particular patient. A major assumption of this protocol is that more drug will be required to achieve analgesia.

As previously described in the pharmacodynamic section, there are a series of pharmacodynamic relationships over an array of noxious stimuli encountered in the perioperative environment (Fig. 40-10). One interesting feature of this array of concentration relationships is that they can be quantified in terms of a percentage of the amount of drug required to elicit EEG changes.[26] For example, the fentanyl effect site concentration associated with C_{50} for changes in the spectral edge, a measure of EEG activity is approximately 9 ng/mL.[35,73,94,95] The fentanyl effect site concentration C_{50}s associated with analgesia and respiratory depression are 1.6 and 5.4 ng/mL, respectively. Hence, the fentanyl effect site concentrations for analgesia and respiratory depression are 17% and 60%, respectively, of the C_{50} for EEG changes. Taking advantage of this linearity, the analgesic fentanyl effect site concentrations are approximately 30% of those associated with respiratory depression.[96,97]

Although not well established, preliminary work has indicated that the linear relationship between analgesia, respiratory depression, and EEG changes remains intact despite a rightward shit in the concentration effect relationships associated with opioids in chronic opioid-consuming patients.[91-93] Using this linearity, the fentanyl challenge is able to predict analgesic effect site concentrations from estimated concentrations of fentanyl required to produce respiratory depression. For example, the fentanyl effect site concentration associated with analgesia is 30% of the effect site concentration associated with respiratory depression regardless of whether the fentanyl effect site concentration is required to achieve respiratory depression.

With the analgesic effect site concentration identified as a percentage of the concentration required for respiratory depression, the next step is to develop fentanyl dosing regimens to achieve and maintain analgesia. Dosing goals may be directed at providing intraoperative analgesia as part of a combined anesthetic technique or postoperative analgesia until the patient is able to take oral analgesics. Additional simulations are used to identify optimal infusion rates that will produce the target analgesic effect during the course of the anesthetic and into the postoperative period.

Unique features of fentanyl pharmacokinetics that are important to consider when initiating an infusion following a fentanyl challenge include

1. With prolonged continuous infusions (ie, >2 hours), effect site concentrations continue to rise. Simulations of continuous infusions reveal that effect site concentrations do not reach near steady state for at least 24 hours. Thus, it is important to anticipate the duration of a postoperative continuous fentanyl infusion and select an infusion rate that will not exceed the effect site concentrations associated with respiratory depression.
2. Upon completion of the fentanyl challenge before the induction of anesthesia, a significant amount of fentanyl can be delivered depending on the duration of the challenge. For example, an 8-minute infusion at 2 μg/kg/min in a 90-kg patient will result in the delivery of 1440 μg (29 mL) of fentanyl. This initial dose should be accounted for when formulating an intraoperative fentanyl infusion rate.

In **Fig. 40-32**, a set of simulations illustrate the fentanyl effect site concentrations that result from a fentanyl challenge. In this case, an 8-minute infusion was required to reach the onset of respiratory depression. After the challenge are 6 simulations of a fentanyl infusion ranging from 1 to 6 μg/kg/h for a 6-hour anesthetic. At 8 minutes, the fentanyl effect site concentration associated with respiratory depression is 20 ng/mL, giving a target effect site concentration of 6 ng/mL (ie, 30% of 20). Using this simulation, the fentanyl infusion that best approximates the target effect site concentration of 6 ng/mL is a continuous infusion at 3 μg/kg/h.

Information obtained from pharmacokinetic simulations after a fentanyl challenge can be used to improve intraoperative dosing of fentanyl to ensure adequate analgesia in the early postoperative period. In addition, this same information can be used to identify IV fentanyl dosing regimens for the first 24 to 48 hours after selected surgical procedures associated with significant postoperative pain and no or inadequate ability to use oral analgesics.

To improve intraoperative dosing of fentanyl, prior work has found that administering a continuous infusion of fentanyl that

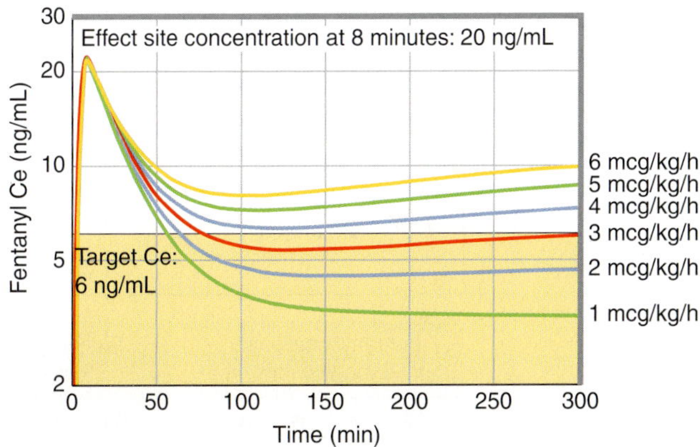

FIGURE 40-32. Computer simulation of the fentanyl challenge (2 μg/kg/min) for 8 minutes followed by continuous infusions at various rates for 6 hours. This plot is used to estimate the fentanyl infusion rate necessary to achieve analgesia. The target effect site concentration (Ce) is estimated as 30% of the fentanyl Ce associated with the onset of respiratory depression (20 ng/mL). For a 5-hour anesthetic, a continuous infusion of 3 μg/kg/h best achieves the target Ce.

maintains the analgesic effect site concentration throughout the duration of a surgical procedure leads to an adequate level of analgesia in the early postoperative period yet allows for timely emergence from anesthesia in patients who chronically consume opioids.[92] With regard to postoperative dosing of fentanyl, information gained from the fentanyl challenge can be used to identify dosing regimens for patient-controlled analgesia (PCA) combined with a basal continuous infusion to maintain analgesia while avoiding respiratory depression.[91-93] Infusion rates (in μg/kg/h) used intraoperatively to target the fentanyl concentrations associated with analgesia are divided in half. Half the infusion rate is administered as a continuous infusion, and the other half is administered as intermittent boluses using a PCA.

Preliminary exploration into the efficacy and safety of this technique has been encouraging. In a cohort of patients who reported chronic consumption of opioids, a fentanyl challenge was used to identify the intraoperative and postoperative dosing regimens for fentanyl. The number of interval doses delivered via the PCA was used as a metric of pain control. Interval dose requirements of 2 doses or fewer per hour were considered to provide adequate analgesia. No use of the PCA over a 4-hour period was considered to be an aggressive basal infusion and was decreased by 20%. PCA usage more than twice an hour was considered in inadequate basal infusion and was increased by 20%. After 24 hours of this dosing regimen, measures of respiratory function, arterial P_{CO_2} levels, and pain control were made. In all subjects, respiratory rates and blood oxygenation were normal. Arterial P_{CO_2} levels ranged from 40 to 47 mm Hg. PCA usage was within 1 to 2 doses per hour.

A computer simulation of a fentanyl challenge followed by the intraoperative and postoperative course is presented in **Fig. 40-33.** In this example, an 80-kg patient known to chronically consume opioids required 10 minutes to achieve the onset of respiratory depression. The corresponding fentanyl effect site concentration at this time was 27 ng/mL. The target effect site concentration for analgesia was therefore 30% of 27 or approximately 8 ng/mL. Subsequently, a basal infusion of fentanyl was administered during the 4-hour intraoperative period at 5 μg/kg/h as part of a combined technique with a potent inhaled agent. Upon completion of the intraoperative period, the patient was allowed to emerge from anesthesia. In the postoperative phase, a basal infusion was started at 2.5 μg/kg/h. In addition to the basal infusion, the PCA was set to deliver a demand dose of 50 μg every 15 minutes (2.5 μg/kg/h if using all 4 doses). The basal infusion and PCA were used for 36 hours after the anesthetic. The average PCA usage was 2 demand dose per hour. No adjustments were made in the PCA.

Several points of clinical interest are illustrated by this simulation. By starting a fentanyl infusion rate at 5 μg/kg/h immediately after the fentanyl challenge, the resultant effect site concentrations were well above the target concentration for nearly 90 minutes. This is an important feature to consider when delivering anesthetics of shorter duration. Also of interest, by the end of the 4-hour anesthetic, the effect site concentration was beginning to climb above 8 ng/mL. If an anesthetic requires more time, perhaps a more moderate infusion rate would be prudent (ie, 4 μg/kg/h). In the postoperative phase, the simulation reveals that the basal infusion rate in combination with the PCA maintained the target concentration well. On being turned off, the fentanyl effect site concentrations drop fairly slowly. The time required for the fentanyl effect site levels to drop by half is more than 5 hours. This dissipation time may be important to consider when initiating oral analgesic therapy after terminating a PCA and basal infusion.

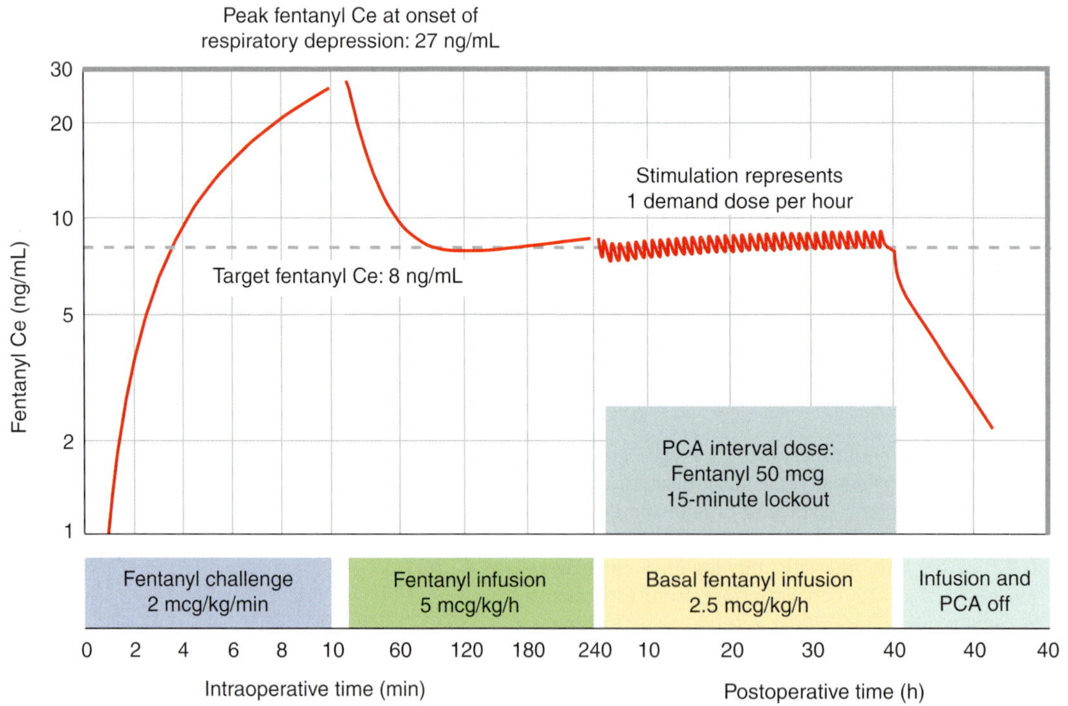

FIGURE 40-33. Computer simulation of the intraoperative and postoperative course after a fentanyl challenge for an 80–kg, 180-cm patient. The fentanyl challenge (2 μg/kg/min) required 10 minutes to achieve respiratory depression (respiratory rate <6 breaths/min). The fentanyl effect site concentration (Ce) at 10 minutes was 27 ng/mL. Subsequently, a fentanyl infusion was run at 5 μg/kg/h (8 mL/h) for 4 hours with a target analgesic concentration of 8 ng/mL. Upon completion of the anesthetic, a basal infusion at 2.5 μg/kg/h (4 mL/h) and a patient-controlled analgesia (PCA) pump with a 50-μg bolus dose on a 15-minute lockout were started. The average PCA dose was 1 bolus per hour.

KEY REFERENCES

- Bouillon T, Shafer SL. Does size matter? *Anesthesiology.* 1998;89(3):557-560.
- Davis JJ, Swenson JD, Hall RH, et al. Preoperative "fentanyl challenge" as a tool to estimate postoperative opioid dosing in chronic opioid-consuming patients. *Anesth Analg.* 2005;101(2):389-395; table of contents.
- Egan TD, Shafer SL. Target-controlled infusions for intravenous anesthetics: surfing USA not! *Anesthesiology.* 2003;99(5):1039-1041.
- Fisher DM. (Almost) everything you learned about pharmacokinetics was (somewhat) wrong! *Anesth Analg.* 1996;83(5):901-903.
- Krejcie TC, Avram MJ. What determines anesthetic induction dose? It's the front-end kinetics, doctor! *Anesth Analg.* 1999;89(3):541-544.
- Minto CF, Schnider TW, Egan TD, et al. Influence of age and gender on the pharmacokinetics and pharmacodynamics of remifentanil. I. Model development. *Anesthesiology.* 1997;86(1):10-23.
- Minto CF, Schnider TW, Short TG, et al. Response surface model for anesthetic drug interactions. *Anesthesiology.* 2000;92(6):1603-1616.
- Shafer SL. Shock values. *Anesthesiology.* 2004;101(3):567-568.
- Shafer SL, Stanski DR. Improving the clinical utility of anesthetic drug pharmacokinetics. *Anesthesiology.* 1992;76(3):327-330.
- Sheiner LB, Stanski DR, Vozeh S, et al. Simultaneous modeling of pharmacokinetics and pharmacodynamics: application to d-tubocurarine. *Clin Pharmacol Ther.* 1979;25(3):358-371.

REFERENCES

Complete references available on DVD and online version at www.LongneckerAnesthesiology.com

CHAPTER 41 Pharmacology of Intravenous Anesthetics

Mark Dershwitz
Carl E. Rosow

KEY POINTS

1. Propofol decreases cerebral metabolic rate for oxygen and cerebral blood flow. By causing vasoconstriction of central nervous system (CNS) blood vessels, propofol also significantly decreases intracranial pressure.
2. Propofol produces a dose-dependent decrease in ventilatory drive. It decreases tidal volume and minute ventilation and increases $Paco_2$. The ventilatory depressant effect is exaggerated in patients with underlying chronic obstructive pulmonary disease (COPD).
3. Propofol decreases myocardial contractility, leading to a reduction in cardiac output. It reduces smooth muscle tone, causing vasodilation in both systemic arteries and veins. Propofol also blunts the barostatic reflex, resulting in a slower heart rate for a given decrease in blood pressure.
4. Coexisting factors, such as other medications (eg, benzodiazepines and/or opioids), advanced age, or presence of concurrent disease (eg, cardiac dysfunction, COPD, hypovolemia), can increase the hemodynamic effects of propofol and decrease the amount needed to produce unconsciousness. Patients with acquired tolerance because of chronic use of other CNS depressants, anticonvulsants, or alcohol may require higher doses of propofol to produce unconsciousness.
5. Propofol causes the lowest incidence of postoperative nausea and vomiting of any general anesthetic agent, injected or inhaled. Propofol also has intrinsic antiemetic activity and has been used successfully as an antiemetic.
6. Propofol often causes pain on injection, which can sometimes be severe. Placing a tourniquet proximal to the injection site and administering lidocaine is the most effective way to prevent this pain.
7. Propofol is a very short-acting intravenous anesthetic. It undergoes relatively little accumulation, even after long-duration infusions. Because of its rapid recovery characteristics, it is an extremely useful drug for maintaining general anesthesia.
8. Fospropofol is a new, water-soluble prodrug of propofol. The onset of the sedative effect is slow.
9. The CNS effects of thiopental are qualitatively similar to those of propofol. When thiopental is given before a planned decrease in global cerebral perfusion, the likelihood of CNS damage appears to be reduced.
10. The cardiac and pulmonary effects of thiopental are qualitatively similar to those of propofol. Thiopental generally causes a smaller decrease in blood pressure.
11. The CNS effects of etomidate are similar to those of thiopental and propofol.
12. Etomidate is notable for its lack of cardiovascular effects. Given by itself, it has little effect on systemic arterial or venous vascular tone or on cardiac contractility, and usually little change in blood pressure or heart rate occurs. Cardiovascular stability is generally preserved in persons with hypovolemia or cardiac dysfunction.
13. Etomidate inhibits the enzyme responsible for performing the 11β-hydroxylation reaction in cortisol synthesis. A single induction dose of 0.3 mg/kg inhibits cortisol synthesis and the normal response to adrenocorticotropic hormone for up to 12 hours. Infusions of several days' duration in ventilated intensive care unit patients were associated with increased mortality.
14. Sedative doses of midazolam cause patients to become sleepy and calmer and to have anterograde amnesia. The amnestic effects of midazolam are variable but usually short-lived, and they should not be relied on to prevent recall of intraoperative events.
15. Intramuscular administration of midazolam results in reliable absorption and little injection pain. Its oral bioavailability is only approximately 15%.
16. Midazolam is synergistic with opioids or alcohol in depressing ventilatory drive. Patients with COPD are more sensitive to its ventilatory depressant effects.
17. Flumazenil is a benzodiazepine antagonist with a very short duration of action. When given by itself to healthy volunteers, mild anxiety and symptoms resembling those that occur during a panic attack may occur. When given to patients chronically taking benzodiazepines, acute withdrawal, including seizures, may occur.
18. Ketamine produces dissociative anesthesia. Under ketamine anesthesia, a patient may move, vocalize, open eyes, and make ocular tracking movements. Depth of anesthesia is difficult to assess. Also, in subhypnotic doses, ketamine produces profound analgesia. Ketamine is often preceded by an antisialagogue such as glycopyrrolate to reduce the large amount of salivation it produces.
19. Ketamine usually causes sympathetic activation leading to an increase in blood pressure, heart rate, cardiac contractility, cardiac output, and vascular resistance. It has little effect on ventilatory drive in normal patients or in patients with COPD, and it produces bronchodilation. Protective airway reflexes are less likely to be ablated than with other intravenous anesthetics.

20. Intramuscular administration of ketamine results in reliable absorption and little injection pain.
21. Droperidol produces a neuroleptic state in which behavior is diminished and responses to stimuli are fewer, slower, and smaller in magnitude. At high doses, it can produce catatonia, although consciousness and memory are preserved.
22. At very low doses, droperidol is an excellent antiemetic. At much higher doses, the drug can prolong cardiac repolarization (increase QTc interval), and this is the basis for a precaution from the US Food and Drug Administration regarding its use.
23. Dexmedetomidine is an α_2-adrenoceptor agonist that produces sedation without associated amnesia. Even at high doses, loss of consciousness may not occur.

HISTORY

For 90 years after the introduction of ether as a general anesthetic agent, almost all general anesthetics were administered via the inhalational route. That practice changed in 1935 following the description by Lundy[1] of the use of thiopental. During World War II, intravenous cannulation for the administration of blood products and crystalloid solutions was common, and it was increasingly utilized by physicians specializing in anesthesiology. Thiopental was widely used during surgery for battlefield wounds, and it was soon recognized that intravenous anesthesia with thiopental required greater skill and was not as "forgiving" as general anesthesia with ether.[2] Over the next 3 decades, induction by inhalation became less and less common (with the exception of pediatric anesthesia) while additional intravenous agents were introduced to compete with thiopental.

Thiopental is an excellent intravenous anesthetic, and its introduction revolutionized the practice of anesthesiology. Newer agents such as propofol have improved on thiopental and largely supplanted it in clinical practice. The characteristics of an "ideal" intravenous anesthetic agent are listed in **Box 41-1**. How each of the available intravenous anesthetics approaches this ideal is described in detail. The unique characteristics of the individual agents must be considered when choosing the best drug for a particular patient and a specific clinical setting.

BOX 41-1

The "Ideal" Intravenous Anesthetic Agent

Stable in aqueous solution

No pain on injection, venous irritation, or tissue damage from accidental perivenous administration

Very low potential to release histamine or precipitate hypersensitivity reactions

Rapidly metabolized to pharmacologically inactive substances, with minimal accumulation when administered by repeated bolus doses or continuous infusion

Rapid and smooth onset of action, without excitatory phenomena such as muscle movements, hypertonus, or hiccoughing

Produces a steep dose–response relationship so that changes in the rate of administration result in rapid changes in the depth of anesthesia when administered by continuous infusion

Rapid and smooth return of consciousness, even after prolonged administration for maintenance of anesthesia or sedation

Produces a decrease in cerebral metabolism proportional to the decrease in cerebral blood flow and does not increase intracranial pressure

Minimal cardiovascular and ventilatory depressant effects with no adverse effects on other organ systems

Allows rapid recovery without postoperative side effects, such as nausea and vomiting, psychomimetic symptoms, dizziness, headache, or prolonged sedation ("hangover")

PROPOFOL

CHEMISTRY

Propofol is 2,6-diisopropylphenol, a simple derivative of phenol (**Fig. 41-1** and **Table 41-1**). Propofol is an oil at room temperature and is essentially insoluble in water. Its initial formulation used a detergent called Cremophor, but this solubilizer was found to produce anaphylactoid reactions. Propofol subsequently was prepared as a 1% emulsion in Intralipid, a commonly used source of nutritional fat in patients receiving total parenteral nutrition. Intralipid contains 10% soybean oil, 2.25% glycerol, and 1.2% egg lecithin. The propofol emulsion readily supports bacterial growth, and the original formulation was associated with numerous cases of iatrogenic sepsis. Currently, all propofol formulations have a bacteriostatic agent added in low concentration to slow, but not prevent, bacterial growth. Depending on the manufacturer, the bacteriostatic agent is 0.005% ethylenediaminetetraacetic acid (EDTA), 0.025% metabisulfite, or 0.1% benzyl alcohol. Propofol undergoes dimerization and oxidation to a quinone when exposed to oxygen. These chemical reactions occur at a more rapid rate in the preparation containing metabisulfite.[3] When the metabisulfite-containing propofol preparation is exposed to room air, it becomes visibly yellow after approximately 6 hours because of the presence of quinone. Whether this oxidation product affects safety or efficacy is unknown, but all opened vials and syringes containing propofol (irrespective of preservative) should routinely be discarded after 6 hours in order to reduce the risk of bacterial contamination.

PHARMACODYNAMICS

Central Nervous System Propofol is a rapid-acting hypnotic whose effects after brief administration are terminated by rapid redistribution (Table 41-5). It exerts its central nervous system (CNS) effects primarily via the $GABA_A$ receptor, a ligand-gated ion channel. The $GABA_A$ receptor is coupled to a chloride channel; as the GABA effect increases, the postsynaptic membrane becomes hyperpolarized, and thus GABA acts as an inhibitory neurotransmitter. Propofol binds to a unique binding site and increases chloride conductance in a concentration-dependent manner. Thus propofol potentiates the inhibitory effects of GABA.[4] In vitro studies suggest that it also acts to inhibit glutamate action at *N*-methyl-D-aspartate (NMDA) receptors.[5]

In the CNS, neuronal activity is coupled to oxygen utilization and delivery as a result of autoregulation (**Table 41-2**). By decreasing neuronal activity, propofol decreases both CNS oxygen utilization, as measured by the cerebral metabolic rate of oxygen consumption ($CMRo_2$), and cerebral blood flow (CBF). By causing vasoconstriction of CNS blood vessels and therefore a reduction in cerebral blood volume, propofol also significantly decreases intracranial pressure (ICP). Although it has not been studied as well as thiopental for its neuroprotective activity, propofol appears to produce a similar effect.[6]

Cerebral perfusion pressure (CPP) is estimated to be the difference between the mean arterial pressure (MAP) in the carotid arteries and the ICP or, if low, the venous pressure in the jugular veins. It is significantly affected by the position of the patient with respect to gravity (see Chapter 51). Propofol must be used cautiously in this setting because it causes more hypotension than thiopental (see Cardiovascular System) and therefore is more likely to reduce CPP and thus CBF.

Propofol is an anticonvulsant, and it has been used to terminate status epilepticus. It probably does not produce this effect in sedative doses.[7]

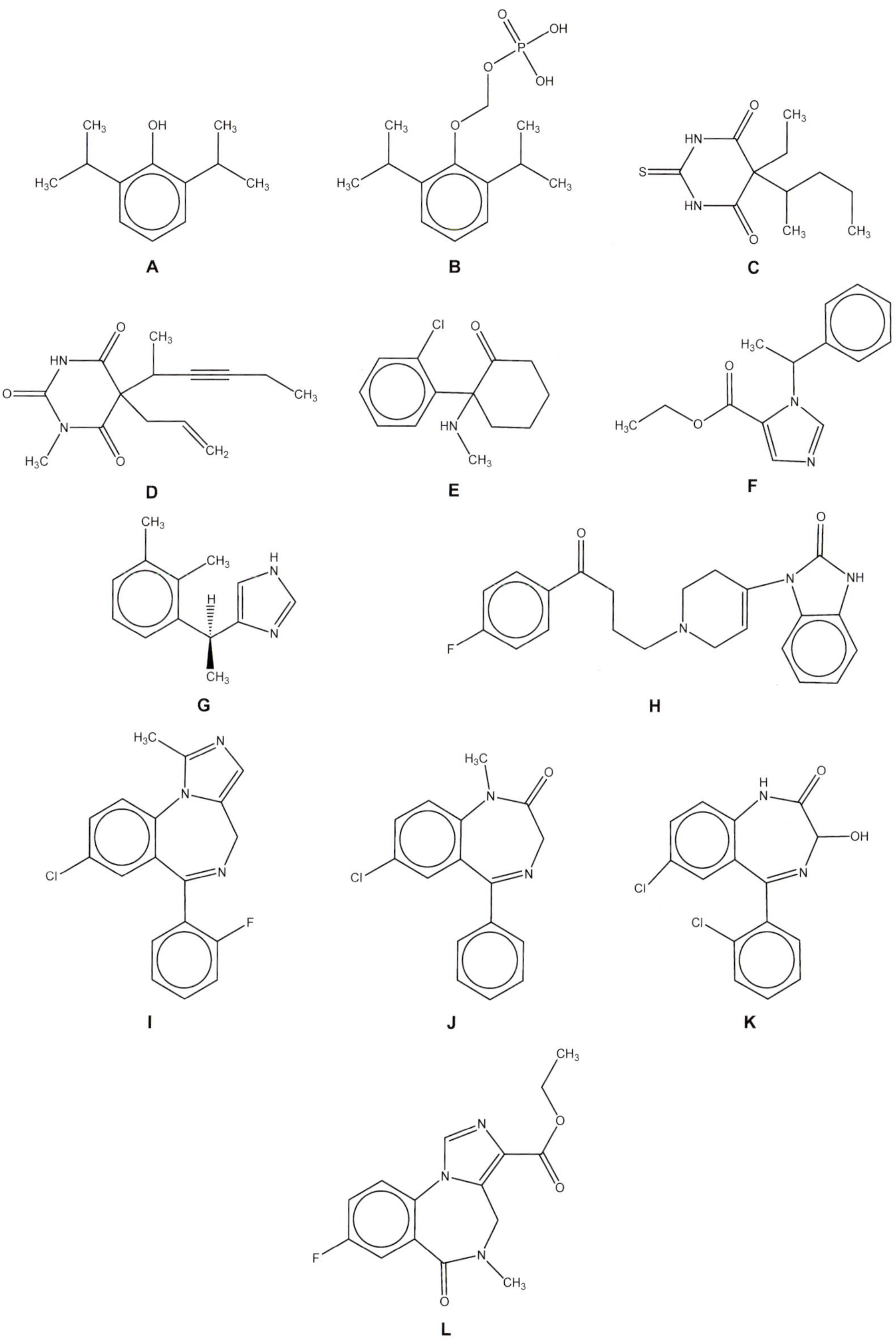

FIGURE 41-1. Chemical structures of the intravenous anesthetic agents: **A.** propofol, **B.** fospropofol, **C.** thiopental, **D.** methohexital, **E.** ketamine, **F.** etomidate, **G.** dexmedetomidine, **H.** droperidol, **I.** midazolam, **J.** diazepam, **K.** lorazepam, and **L.** flumazenil.

Although propofol shortens the duration of "therapeutic" seizure during electroconvulsive therapy (see Chapter 69), it still can be used in this setting.[8]

Propofol has pharmacodynamic effects that differ from those of thiopental in several ways. It does not produce hyperalgesia in sedative doses, and it is more likely to suppress movement responses to painful stimuli at concentrations achieved during routine administration. Unlike thiopental, sedative doses of propofol can produce significant amnesia.[9] At sedative and hypnotic concentrations, propofol is much more effective in reducing airway responsiveness, and the incidence of cough or laryngospasm is greatly reduced. On the other hand, induction of anesthesia with propofol often causes myoclonic

TABLE 41-1 Physicochemical Properties of Anesthetic Agents

Drug Group	Drug Name	Available Solutions (pH or pK_a)	Venous Irritation
Barbiturates			
Thiobarbiturate	Thiopental	pK_a = 7.5	+++
		Sodium salt, to be diluted in water or saline to create 2.5% solution, pH >10	
Oxybarbiturate	Methohexital	pK_a = 7.9	+++
		Sodium salt, to be diluted in water or saline to create 1% solution, pH >10	
Alkylphenols	Propofol	pK_a = 11	++
		1% solution in aqueous emulsion containing 10% soybean oil, 2.25% glycerol, 1.2% lecithin	
	Fospropofol	3.5% aqueous solution of disodium salt	–
Imidazole	Etomidate	pK_a = 4.3	+++
		0.2% solution in 30% propylene glycol	
Benzodiazepines	Diazepam	0.5% solution in 40% propylene glycol, 10% ethanol	+
	Lorazepam	0.4% solution in 80% propylene glycol, 18% polyethylene glycol, 2% benzyl alcohol	+
	Midazolam	0.1% or 0.5% aqueous solutions, pH 3-4	–
Arylcyclohexylamine	Ketamine	pK_a = 7.5	–
		1%, 5%, or 10% aqueous solutions, pH 3.3-5.5	

movements, an effect that is much less common with thiopental. Finally, even subhypnotic concentrations of propofol have a direct antiemetic effect (see Nausea and Vomiting). In this respect it is unlike any other intravenous anesthetic agent.

Respiratory System Propofol produces a dose-dependent decrease in ventilatory drive, with a decreased tidal volume and minute ventilation and an increased $Paco_2$ (**Table 41-3**). At the usual intravenous anesthetic induction dose of 1 to 3 mg/kg, most patients will become apneic for a few minutes. Accompanying this ventilatory depression is a decrease in protective airway reflexes. The ventilatory depressant effect of propofol is exaggerated in patients with underlying chronic obstructive pulmonary disease (COPD), and there is a synergistic effect between propofol and opioids in decreasing ventilatory drive.

Airway resistance after intubation is lower after induction with propofol than after thiopental.[10] Some persons with reactive airway disease become bronchospastic when exposed to sulfites in the environment, such as those found naturally in certain wines. Reports on the bronchospastic effects of the metabisulfite-containing propofol preparation are conflicting, but any such effects, if they exist, appear to be sporadic and minor.

Cardiovascular System Propofol causes a greater decrease in systemic blood pressure than does thiopental (**Table 41-4**).[11] Although the 2 drugs have similar depressant effects on cardiac contractility, propofol causes a larger reduction in venous and arteriolar systemic vascular resistance, resulting in decreases of both preload and afterload. Contributing to the hypotensive effect of propofol is its action in blunting the barostatic reflex, resulting in a slower heart rate for a given decrease in blood pressure compared with thiopental.[12] The decrease in blood pressure with propofol injection is exaggerated in older persons and those with preexisting cardiac dysfunction or hypovolemia, those given opioid or benzodiazepine premedication, or those receiving therapy with β-adrenergic blockers or vasodilators. Propofol does not alter the normal resting pulmonary vascular resistance in dogs; however, it potentiates the pulmonary vasoconstriction produced by phenylephrine.[13]

Nausea and Vomiting Propofol causes the least incidence of postoperative nausea and vomiting of any general anesthetic agent, injected or inhaled.[14] The use of propofol as a maintenance anesthetic is associated with a very low incidence of postoperative nausea and vomiting, perhaps because residual subhypnotic concentrations are antiemetic.[15] In addition, propofol has intrinsic antiemetic activity and has been used successfully as an antiemetic.[16] The mechanism of this effect is unknown, although it does not involve dopamine D_2 receptors such as with droperidol or metoclopramide.[17]

Other Effects Propofol decreases renal blood flow and causes increased secretion of antidiuretic hormone. Subhypnotic doses appear to be effective in reversing the itching produced by cholestasis or by epidural morphine.[18] Propofol is safe to give to patients with all types of porphyria and for those with malignant hyperthermia.

TABLE 41-2 Central Nervous System Effects of Intravenous Anesthetic Agents

Drug Name	$CMRO_2$	CBF	CPP	ICP
Thiopental	– –	– –	±	– –
Methohexital	– –	– –	±	– –
Propofol	– –	– –	–	–
Etomidate	– –	– –	+	– –
Benzodiazepines	–	±	0	–
Ketamine	+	+ +	±	+

CBF, cerebral blood flow; $CMRO_2$, cerebral metabolic rate for oxygen; CPP, cerebral perfusion pressure; ICP, intracranial pressure.

TABLE 41-3 Ventilatory Depressant Effects of Intravenous Anesthetic Agents

Drug Name	Healthy Patients	Patients with COPD
Barbiturates	++	+++
Propofol	++	+++
Etomidate	+	+
Benzodiazepines	+	+++
Ketamine	0	0

COPD, chronic obstructive pulmonary disease.

TABLE 41-4 Cardiovascular Effects of Intravenous Anesthetic Agents

Drug Name	MAP	HR	CO	Contractility (dP/dt)	SVR	Venous Dilatation
Thiopental	–	+	–	–	±	++
Methohexital	–	++	–	–	±	+
Propofol	– –	–	–	–	– –	++
Etomidate	0	0	0	0	0	0
Diazepam	0/–	±	0	0	–/0	+
Midazolam	0/–	±	0/–	0	–/0	+
Ketamine	++	++	+	±[a]	±[a]	0

CO, cardiac output; HR, heart rate; MAP, mean arterial pressure; SVR, systemic vascular resistance.

[a]Change depends on sympathetic reserve.

Adverse Effects

Pain on Injection Propofol often causes pain, sometimes severe, on injection. The importance of this problem to the anesthesia community is indicated by the fact that, in the 20 years since the introduction of propofol, hundreds of publications have addressed this adverse effect. No technique is universally reliable in preventing this adverse effect, and there is no general agreement on which technique is most recommended.

Mitigating the pain on injection of propofol has involved 3 general approaches: modifying the vehicle in which the propofol is contained, adding a drug to the propofol emulsion, or administering a drug before propofol injection.

There appears to be a correlation between the incidence and severity of pain and the free concentration of propofol in the aqueous phase of the emulsion. Modifications of the emulsion that increase the free propofol concentration (ie, decreasing the concentration of lecithin) are associated with increases in pain. Conversely, a modified emulsion product has been developed that uses a mixture of medium-chain and long-chain triglycerides instead of egg lecithin (Propofol Lipuro). It has a lower free concentration of propofol and causes less pain on injection.[19] Although not available in the United States (as of 2010), it is widely used in Europe and Japan.

Free propofol may exert its painful effect by stimulating the kallikrein-kinin system, resulting in the generation of bradykinin, which stimulates intravascular nociceptors. Administration of nafamostat, an inhibitor of kallikrein, before propofol injection has significantly decreased the incidence and severity of pain.[20]

Clinicians desiring a simple and practical method for alleviating pain on injection have studied numerous medications either given before propofol or mixed with the propofol emulsion. A meta-analysis of the published studies concluded that injection of lidocaine with a proximal tourniquet in place provided the highest efficacy.[21] The authors recommended that "IV lidocaine (0.5 mg/kg) should be given with a rubber tourniquet on the forearm, 30 to 120 seconds before the injection of propofol." This method was superior to mixing lidocaine with propofol, which itself was superior to giving lidocaine without a tourniquet before injecting the propofol.

Hypersensitivity Reactions Propofol does not cause histamine release and is only very rarely associated with hypersensitivity reactions. Although components of the emulsion are derived from eggs and soybeans, the product contains no egg albumin or soy protein (the proteins to which hypersensitive persons are most likely to react). Persons allergic to egg albumin or soy protein have been given propofol safely.

PHARMACOKINETICS

Lipid Solubility Propofol is one of the most lipid-soluble drugs used in medicine. Its oil/water partition coefficient of 4700 is almost 10-fold higher than that of thiopental. This high lipid solubility, coupled with the large fraction of cardiac output typically delivered to the brain, is responsible for the very rapid onset of effect, typically well under 1 minute, after intravenous administration (**Table 41-5**).

Protein Binding Protein-bound propofol is unable to diffuse across the blood–brain barrier and produce a pharmacologic effect. Propofol is approximately 98% bound to plasma protein. In clinical situations in which the plasma concentration of protein is decreased, as in hepatic disease or hemorrhage that has been treated only with crystalloid solutions and/or packed red blood cells, the free fraction of propofol will be elevated compared with normal, and lower doses of propofol may be needed. Despite being an extensively bound drug, propofol has a high hepatic extraction ratio (**Table 41-6**). The total clearance of propofol is greater than hepatic blood flow, indicating that there is significant extrahepatic metabolism (see Metabolism and Elimination).[22]

Redistribution The redistribution half-life of a drug, often abbreviated as $t_{1/2\alpha}$, is the time required for the central compartment concentration of the drug to decrease by 50% as the drug is distributed to peripheral compartment(s) (see Chapter 40). Propofol $t_{½\alpha}$ is approximately 1 to 2 minutes , indicating that the effect of a typical bolus injection will be terminated within 3 to 4 half-lives or approximately 3 to 8 minutes (Table 41-5).[23] This process of redistribution is the primary process by which the pharmacologic effect of propofol is terminated. Unless very large doses are given or a long infusion is given, the processes of metabolism and elimination are much less important in terminating the drug's effect.

Metabolism and Elimination The terminal half-life of a drug, often abbreviated as $t_{1/2\beta}$ for medications fitting a 2-compartment model (see Chapter 40), is a function of the processes of both metabolism and elimination. Propofol $t_{1/2\beta}$ is approximately 4 to 6 hours, substantially less than the corresponding value for thiopental.[23] The rapid plasma

TABLE 41-5 Pharmacokinetic Parameters for Intravenous Anesthetic Agents

Drug Name	Redistribution Half-Life (min)	Terminal Half-Life (h)	Clearance (mL/min)	Volume of Distribution (L)	Protein Binding (%)
Thiopental	2-4	6-12	120-180	100-200	85
Methohexital	5-6	2-5	700-900	60-80	85
Propofol	1-2	4-6	1400-2800	200-500	98
Etomidate	2-4	2-5	800-1400	200-400	75
Diazepam	10-15	20-40	15-35	60-100	98
Lorazepam	3-10	10-20	50-70	50-90	98
Midazolam	7-15	2-4	300-550	70-130	94
Ketamine	11-17	2-3	1250-1400	200-250	12

TABLE 41-6 Relative Hepatic Extraction Ratios for Intravenous Anesthetic Agents

Low	Intermediate	High
Diazepam: 0.01-0.025	Midazolam: 0.2	Etomidate: 0.7
Thiopental: 0.1-0.2	Methohexital: 0.5-0.6	Ketamine: 0.8
		Propofol: >1

clearance and relatively slow transfer of propofol from peripheral tissues into the plasma help explain why the propofol concentration drops so much more rapidly than thiopental after termination of a continuous infusion (see Maintenance of Anesthesia).

Approximately 60% of administered propofol is *para*-hydroxylated and then conjugated with glucuronide or sulfate at 1 of the 2 hydroxyl groups.[24] In persons with normal hepatic and renal function, approximately 60% of propofol metabolism occurs in the liver and approximately 40% occurs in the kidneys.[22] The overall clearance of propofol is not reduced in patients with end-stage renal disease[25] or with cirrhosis.[26] Significant propofol metabolism occurs in the lungs of some animals, but kidney rather than pulmonary metabolism of propofol may be more important in humans.[22]

Factors Affecting Pharmacodynamics and Pharmacokinetics Many factors may alter the pharmacodynamics and pharmacokinetics of propofol. Elderly patients require lower doses of propofol to produce unconsciousness. This altered response is due to both increased sensitivity of the brain to the drug's effect (pharmacodynamic alteration)[27] as well as decreased protein binding and decreased clearance (pharmacokinetic alterations).[28]

The pharmacokinetics of propofol in persons with significant impairment of hepatic function is complex. Despite a significant increase in volume of distribution, the total clearance rate is preserved.[26] Persons with cardiac dysfunction typically have an exaggerated hypotensive response to propofol, to a greater degree than with thiopental. In hypovolemic shock, a lower propofol dose is needed because a greater fraction of the cardiac output goes to the brain. The hypovolemic patient tolerates propofol-induced vasodilatation very poorly.

CLINICAL USE

Induction of Anesthesia Propofol is currently the most commonly used intravenous induction agent. The characteristics of propofol as an induction agent are listed in **Table 41-7**. An induction dose of 1 to 3 mg/kg is often given to the typical healthy patient undergoing elective surgery, but there is enormous variability between patients in the amount actually required. Coexisting factors, such as previous premedication (eg, with benzodiazepines and/or opioids), advanced age, or presence of concurrent disease (eg, cardiac dysfunction, COPD, hypovolemia), will decrease the required dose of propofol. Conversely, patients with acquired tolerance because of chronic use of medications that exhibit cross-tolerance with propofol (eg, benzodiazepines, barbiturates, anticonvulsants, alcohol) may require higher doses of propofol to produce unconsciousness.

If there is concern about a possibly exaggerated response to propofol and a rapid sequence induction is not planned, it may be prudent to administer the induction dose slowly or in divided doses, treating the initial bolus as a "test dose" and waiting 1 to 2 minutes to evaluate the effects.

After administration of the induction dose, consciousness is typically lost within 30 seconds, although this time may be longer in persons with a slow circulation time because of cardiac dysfunction. Recovery of consciousness usually occurs within 3 to 8 minutes; however, some degree of cognitive impairment may persist for hours. The time to awakening from propofol is slightly faster than that with thiopental, and patients are able to achieve recovery "milestones" (voiding, ambulation) more rapidly. A portion of the rapid recovery may be due to propofol's relative freedom from "hangover" and its tendency to cause an elevation in mood. Emergence from propofol is often accompanied by a sense of well-being,[29] and patients occasionally become euphoric. Occurrence of hallucinations and sexual fantasies during emergence also has been reported.

TABLE 41-7 Induction Characteristics for Intravenous Anesthetic Agents

Drug Name	Induction Dose (mg/kg)	Onset (s)	Duration (min)	Excitatory Activity	Injection Pain
Thiopental	4-7	<30	5-10	+	+
Methohexital	1-3	<30	5-10	++	++
Propofol	1-3	<30	3-8	+	+++
Etomidate	0.2-0.3	<30	5-10	+++	++
Diazepam	0.3-0.6	45-60	15-30	0	++
Lorazepam	0.03-0.06	60-120	60-120	0	++
Midazolam	0.2-0.4	30-60	15-30	0	0
Ketamine	1-2	45-60	10-20	++	0

Maintenance of Anesthesia General anesthesia can be maintained by either intermittent intravenous boluses or continuous intravenous infusion of propofol. After an induction bolus, infusion rates of 100 to 200 mcg/kg/min typically are used to maintain general anesthesia in healthy patients. If nitrous oxide and/or opioids are administered concurrently, a reduction in the required propofol infusion rate by one-third to one-half may be anticipated. To maintain a nearly constant blood (and brain) concentration of propofol during an infusion requires that the infusion rate be decreased as the infusion continues (see Target-Controlled Infusion). Autonomic signs are not reliable end points for determining the depth of hypnotic effect with propofol. Processed electroencephalograph (EEG) monitors, such as the bispectral index or patient state index, are correlated with the level of consciousness and facilitate titrating the infusion rate. Elderly patients and those with coexisting cardiopulmonary disease typically will require reduced infusion rates. Because of propofol's higher clearance compared with that of thiopental, it accumulates to a much lesser degree, and its recovery characteristics after an infusion, even of very long duration, permit it to be an extremely useful drug for maintaining general anesthesia.

The context-sensitive half-time (CSHT) describes the time required for the central compartment blood concentration to fall by half as a function of the duration of an infusion (of variable rate designed to maintain a constant blood concentration).[30] The CSHTs for propofol after 1-, 2-, and 6-hour infusions are approximately 11, 16, and 34 minutes, respectively (**Fig. 41-2**). Thus a "rule of thumb" for the CSHT for propofol would be to take the value of 11 minutes for a 1-hour infusion and add to that 4 minutes for each additional hour of infusion duration; this linear relationship remains valid for infusions up to approximately 10 hours in duration. Remember that CSHT is not the same as time to clinical recovery, which depends on the actual concentrations achieved.

Sedation Sedation during regional anesthesia or monitored anesthesia care can be achieved by the administration of intermittent boluses or a continuous infusion of 1 or more sedatives. Frequently an opioid is given to relieve the discomfort that may accompany a noxious procedure as well as decrease the required dose of the sedative. Intermittent bolus administration of rapid-acting hypnotics like propofol or thiopental is riskier than continuous infusion, because it is easier to overshoot and produce periods of unconsciousness that may be accompanied by diminished or absent airway reflexes.

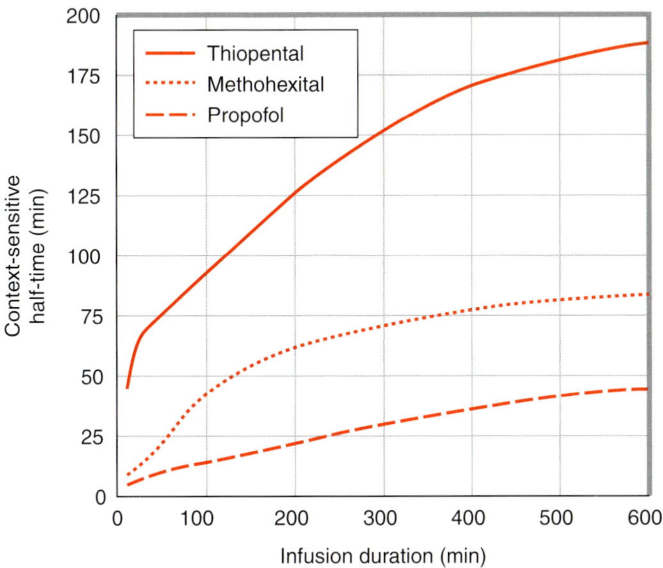

FIGURE 41-2. Context-sensitive half-times for thiopental, methohexital, and propofol as a function of the duration of infusion.

Propofol is commonly used for procedural sedation as well as for longer-term sedation in the intensive care unit (ICU). If loss of consciousness is to be avoided (as is the goal for most cases of procedural sedation), a loading dose of 0.5 to 1 mg/kg is used, followed by an infusion of 25 to 75 mcg/kg/min. Lower infusion rates will be required in persons given benzodiazepines and/or opioids, in elderly patients, and in those with coexisting cardiopulmonary disease.

Propofol is routinely used in the ICU for long-term (ie, weeks) sedation of patients requiring mechanical ventilation. Even in this setting, its recovery characteristics permit rapid recovery. For example, a patient who is sedated (but not rendered unconscious) for 2 weeks will recover in approximately 3 hours.[31] This property allows a patient to be awakened intermittently from relatively deep propofol sedation in order to perform neurologic examinations. Long-term infusion of propofol may result in a very large dose of lipid, and this has been associated with hypertriglyceridemia and pancreatitis.[32] Logically, propofol should be administered cautiously in patients with preexisting pancreatitis or hyperlipidemia. Long-term administration (particularly in critically ill children) has also been linked to a rare and often fatal disorder termed *propofol infusion syndrome.* The pathophysiology has not been well characterized, but typical features include rhabdomyolysis, metabolic acidosis, and cardiac and renal failure.[33]

Target-Controlled Infusion By using estimates of the pharmacokinetic parameters for propofol, it is possible to achieve and maintain a targeted blood (or "effect site") concentration using a computer-controlled infusion pump (see Chapter 43). Such a target-controlled infusion (TCI) pump, with the pharmacokinetic constants for propofol built in, is marketed as the Diprifusor in many countries (but not in the United States). The patient's age, body weight, and desired blood concentration are entered, and the pump delivers a propofol bolus followed by a variable-rate infusion. The rate is automatically adjusted to match predicted losses from distribution and elimination in order to maintain a constant propofol concentration. TCI pumps have been used successfully in closed-loop delivery systems with processed EEG signals as a control variable. For scientists interested in studying TCI, several public-domain computer programs are available that facilitate this process.[34] Most modern infusion pumps have the ability to be controlled by a computer, so by connecting the pump to a portable computer and using one of the available programs, a TCI can be delivered. Despite more than a decade of routine clinical use in other parts of the world, it must be emphasized that TCI is still considered an experimental treatment in the United States.

FOSPROPOFOL

CHEMISTRY

Fospropofol is a water-soluble prodrug of propofol. It is metabolized by alkaline phosphatases in the liver to yield propofol, phosphate, and formaldehyde. A substantial fraction of the liberated propofol undergoes further metabolism to inactive products before reaching the systemic circulation. After the usual clinical doses of fospropofol, formaldehyde concentrations do not approach the toxic range. Fospropofol is supplied as a 3.5% isotonic aqueous solution with a pH between 8.2 and 9.0.[35] The sedative/hypnotic effects of fospropofol are due it its active metabolite propofol.

PHARMACOKINETICS

Unlike propofol, fospropofol has a small volume of distribution (0.33 L/kg). Like propofol, it is highly bound to plasma albumin (98%). Unfortunately, at the time of this writing, the kinetic behavior of fospropofol cannot be accurately described; all of the publications describing its kinetic behavior have been retracted due to a problem with the collection and preservation of the blood samples obtained from the volunteers.[36]

Thus far, fospropofol has been studied after bolus administration and short (10 minutes) infusion. There is clearly a significant lag time after bolus injection until sedative or hypnotic effects occur. For example, after a sleep dose of fospropofol, given as a bolus, approximately 3 to 4 minutes will elapse until consciousness is lost.[35]

CLINICAL USE

Fospropofol is approved for procedural sedation. The recommended dose is 6.5 mg/kg administered as a bolus, followed by intermittent bolus doses of 1.5 mg/kg. The loading dose should be decreased in the elderly and in persons with significant comorbidities. Unlike propofol, fospropofol is not associated with pain at the injection site. Bolus administration does, however, commonly cause a burning or itching sensation in the groin and perineum.

Interestingly, in the United States fospropofol is a controlled substance (Schedule IV), whereas its active metabolite, propofol, is not.[35]

Although fospropofol has not yet been adequately studied during prolonged infusion, it may ultimately find utility as a sedative in the ICU. Because it does not contain the lipid emulsion of propofol preparations, adverse effects related to prolonged lipid infusion (eg, pancreatitis) are unlikely.

BARBITURATES

CHEMISTRY

A large number of barbiturates have been introduced into clinical medicine, but only 2 remain in use as intravenous anesthetics: thiopental (a thiobarbiturate) and methohexital (an oxybarbiturate; Fig. 41-1 and Table 41-1). Both of these medications are practically insoluble in water; however, they are weak acids, and their sodium salts are freely soluble in water. Thiopental is no longer available in the United States.

The usual concentrations of the sodium salts used clinically are 2.5% thiopental and 1% methohexital. Thiopental is soluble at higher concentrations, but pain on injection is likely to occur. The 2.5% thiopental solution usually is painless when given intravenously. This solution is irritating to tissues if it extravasates because it has a pH between 10 and 11. If accidentally injected intra-arterially, vasospasm and thrombosis may occur that can lead to limb loss if not treated rapidly. Recommended treatments include intra-arterial injection of a vasodilator (eg, papaverine or nitroglycerin) and an anticoagulant (eg, heparin). The 1% methohexital solution is more likely to cause pain after intravenous injection; however, it is well tolerated after intramuscular injection and can be given via this route in a patient who does not have intravenous access. Methohexital is also hazardous if inadvertently injected intra-arterially.

Both thiopental and methohexital are supplied in powdered form and usually are reconstituted with sterile, preservative-free water (although normal saline can be used). Neither reconstituted solution is stable in the long term, and the manufacturer's package inserts state that they are stable at room temperature for 24 hours. Despite this conservative recommendation, thiopental has been shown to be both chemically stable and bacteriologically sterile for at least 1 week after reconstitution when refrigerated.[37] Under refrigeration, methohexital remains chemically stable and microbiologically sterile for at least 6 weeks.[38]

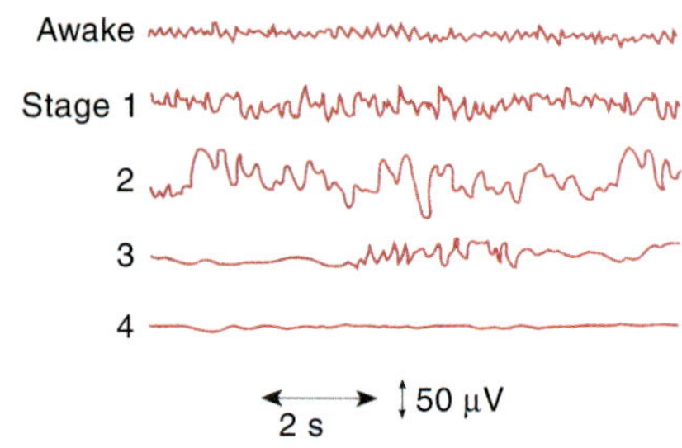

FIGURE 41-3. Changes in electroencephalographic pattern with increasing concentrations of thiopental. Loss of consciousness (hypnosis) occurs early during stage 1. [Redrawn from Hudson RJ, Stanski DR, Saidman LJ, et al. A model for studying depth of anesthesia and acute tolerance to thiopental. *Anesthesiology.* 1983;59:301-308.]

PHARMACODYNAMICS

Central Nervous System Like propofol, thiopental has its primary neuronal action at the γ-aminobutyric acid $(GABA)_A$ receptor. Although barbiturates allosterically affect GABA binding (and vice versa), GABA is not necessary for barbiturate action on the channel.[39]

The barbiturates are classified as sedative–hypnotics; they produce dose-related depression of the CNS, ranging from mild sedation to unconsciousness. Thiopental or methohexital rapidly produces unconsciousness, and awakening will occur in minutes unless additional drugs are given. When administered in subhypnotic doses, barbiturates can sometimes produce disinhibition and "paradoxical" excitation. These drugs are not analgesics, and suppression of movement or hemodynamic responses to painful stimuli requires plasma concentrations in excess of those needed to cause unconsciousness. Like propofol, thiopental decreases ICP, CBF, and $CMRo_2$. In some instances thiopental may exert a "neuroprotective" effect (see later) in which decreased oxygen delivery to the CNS (eg, during clamping of an intracranial artery) may be less likely to result in CNS damage because there has been a profound drug-induced decrease in oxygen utilization.

Because of its effects on $CMRo_2$, CBF, and ICP, intravenous thiopental injection may produce beneficial effects in patients with intracranial space-occupying lesions or cerebral edema associated with a brain tumor, intracranial hemorrhage, or head trauma (Table 41-2). The effect of thiopental on CPP in the supine patient is unpredictable. Thiopental decreases mean arterial pressure in a dose-dependent manner (see Cardiovascular System); however, if CPP is low in a patient because of an elevated ICP, the overall effect of thiopental may be beneficial.[40]

The ability of thiopental to produce "neuroprotection" is both variable and controversial. When thiopental is given *in advance* of a planned reduction or interruption of cerebral perfusion, the likelihood or severity of subsequent CNS damage appears to be less.[41] In contrast, when thiopental is given *after* the onset of cerebral ischemia, such as following a cardiac arrest, no apparent beneficial effect is seen.[42] Protective efficacy appears to be superior when the size of the ischemic area is smaller and when the total duration of ischemia is shorter (see Chapter 85 for detailed considerations on this topic).

Thiopental produces a dose-dependent effect on the EEG (**Fig. 41-3**).[43] At sedative doses or at doses associated with excitation or disinhibition ("stage 2" anesthesia), median EEG frequency increases because alpha waves (7-13 Hz) typical of the awake state change to beta waves (13-30 Hz). As the depth of hypnosis increases, there is a decrease in frequency and an increase in amplitude (power) of the EEG waves. Surgical anesthesia is associated with an EEG characterized by a predominance of delta waves (0.5-3.5 Hz). Increasing the dose of thiopental further leads to burst suppression (characterized by alternating periods of delta waves and electrical inactivity) and, finally, a completely isoelectric ("flat-line") EEG. An isoelectric or burst suppression EEG pattern is associated with a profound decrease in both $CMRo_2$ and CBF, and this end point has been used to titrate the dose of thiopental for brain protection studies. Some studies suggest that alternative mechanisms (eg, decrease in amino acid–induced excitotoxicity) are more important than reducing cerebral metabolic rate.[44]

Thiopental is an excellent anticonvulsant. The typical intravenous anesthetic induction dose of 4 to 7 mg/kg usually is effective in rapidly terminating seizures. Refractory status epilepticus is often treated with repeated boluses or with continuous infusion of thiopental; such patients usually also require mechanical ventilatory support and may require infusion of vasopressors (see Cardiovascular System).

In contrast to thiopental, methohexital may cause abnormal spiking activity of the EEG and may elicit seizures in patients with a seizure disorder, especially in those with psychomotor epilepsy. For this reason, methohexital has long been used as the hypnotic agent to render patients unconscious for electroconvulsive therapy. Methohexital is also associated with abnormal motor activity during induction of general anesthesia, such as myoclonic jerks, muscle tremors, and hiccoughs.

Respiratory System The respiratory effects of thiopental are very similar to those of propofol (Table 41-3). At the usual intravenous anesthetic induction dose of 4 to 7 mg/kg, most patients will become apneic for a few minutes. Accompanying this ventilatory depression is a decrease in protective airway reflexes, although overall responsiveness of the airway is increased. The incidence of coughing and laryngospasm during induction is higher with barbiturates than with most other sedative–hypnotics.

Thiopental produces an increase in the circulating concentration of histamine (see Hypersensitivity Reactions). The effect of histamine on the respiratory musculature is to cause constriction in the trachea and dilation in smaller airways. Typically no net alteration in bronchial resistance occurs.[45]

Cardiovascular System Thiopental typically causes a transient, although significant, decrease in systemic blood pressure when it is administered to induce general anesthesia (Table 41-4).[46] This decrease in blood pressure is exaggerated in persons with preexisting cardiac dysfunction or hypovolemia, those given opioid or benzodiazepine premedication, or those receiving therapy with β-adrenergic blockers or vasodilators. Thiopental-induced hypotension is more pronounced in older patients and when the drug is administered rapidly. Thiopental has a direct effect on the heart, decreasing contractility and leading to a decrease in cardiac output. It also has a direct effect on both systemic arteries and veins, causing vasodilatation. This vasodilatation results in decreased systemic arterial pressure as well as decreased venous return to the heart, the latter effect compounding the decrease in cardiac output and blood pressure. An equipotent dose of methohexital causes slightly less hypotensive effect than does thiopental. Thiopental increases the pulmonary vascular resistance in rat lung,[47] although this effect may not be significant in humans.[48]

Adverse Effects

Hypersensitivity Reactions In an *anaphylactic* reaction, there is IgE-mediated release of vasoactive and immune mediators from mast cells and basophils. An *anaphylactoid* reaction results when a drug directly causes the release of some of these mediators from mast cells or basophils. Anaphylaxis and other true immunologic reactions to barbiturates are extremely rare. They occasionally produce an *anaphylactoid* reaction by displacing vasoactive mediators from tissue mast cells or basophils. Thiopental injection increases the circulating concentration of histamine 3.5-fold, with the histamine concentration returning to baseline within 10 minutes.[49] This effect contributes to the overall decrease in systemic vascular resistance produced by the drug. Anaphylactic or anaphylactoid reactions to thiopental are much less common than are perioperative reactions to latex exposure or injection of muscle relaxants and antibiotics.[50]

Porphyria Barbiturates are the prototypical inducers of the hepatic microsomal enzyme system, including the cytochromes P450 (CYP) and the glucuronyl transferases. The rate of metabolism of some medications may be increased in the postoperative period if a patient is given thiopental for anesthesia induction, although this effect is rarely of clinical consequence. Thiopental is also an inducer of the enzyme δ-aminolevulinic acid (ALA) synthase, an enzyme that catalyzes the initial step in the biosynthesis of heme. Thiopental is absolutely contraindicated in persons with certain porphyrias (**Fig. 41-4**). In 3 of the clinically important porphyrias, there is a deficiency in a heme biosynthetic enzyme that follows ALA synthase in the pathway, and ALA, which is neurotoxic, then accumulates. These 3 porphyrias are acute intermittent porphyria, hereditary coproporphyria, and variegate porphyria,[51] and the enzyme deficiencies responsible for them are shown in Fig. 41-4. Each of these is transmitted as an autosomal-dominant trait, so affected individuals usually are heterozygotes with approximately half the normal amount of enzyme. Interestingly, a fourth variety, porphyria cutanea tarda, also due to a deficiency in a heme biosynthetic enzyme, is not a contraindication to use of a barbiturate.[51] Anesthetic medications generally considered safe or unsafe in persons with porphyria are listed in **Box 41-2**.

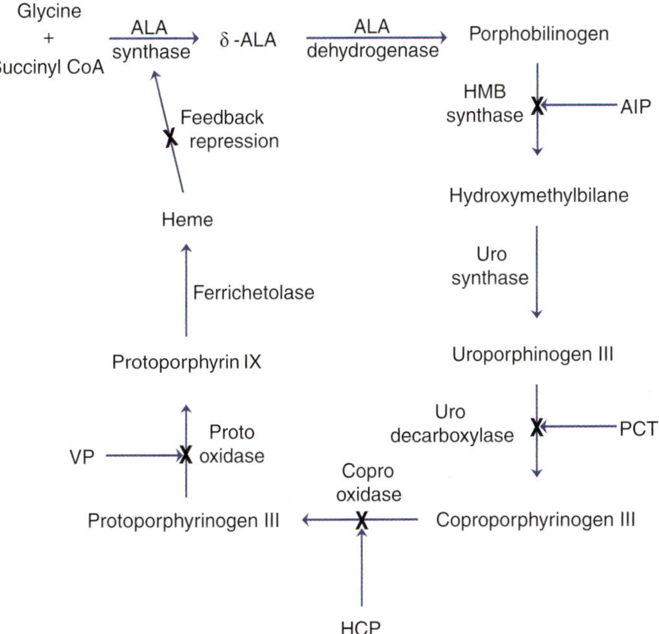

FIGURE 41-4. Heme biosynthesis pathway. The enzyme deficiencies that result in the various forms of porphyria are indicated with an "X." AIP, acute intermittent porphyria; ALA, aminolevulinic acid; HCP, hereditary coproporphyria; HMB, hydroxymethylbilane; PCT, porphyria cutanea tarda. [Redrawn from Desnick RJ. The porphyrias. In: Kasper DL ed. Harrison's Principles of Internal Medicine. 16th ed. New York: McGraw-Hill, 2004.]

BOX 41-2

Safety of Anesthetic Medications in Porphyria[a]

Unsafe	Safe	Inadequate Data[b]
Alcohol	Acetaminophen	Atracurium
Barbiturates	Aspirin	Diazepam
Carbamazepine	Atropine	Halothane
Etomidate	Bupivacaine	Isoflurane
Pentazocine	Droperidol	Ketamine
Valproic acid	Nitrous oxide	Lidocaine
	Opioids	Midazolam
	Phenothiazines	Vecuronium
	Procaine	
	Propofol	
	Scopolamine	
	Succinylcholine	

These recommendations are based on the authors' review of the available literature.

[a]Acute intermittent porphyria, hereditary coproporphyria, and variegate porphyria.

[b]These medications probably are safe in that there are no case reports that have linked them to exacerbations of porphyria; however, the number of reports suggesting that they are safe is inadequate to justify a generalized recommendation as safe.

Renal Effects Thiopental decreases renal blood flow and increases the secretion of antidiuretic hormone. The actions act together to decrease urine output.

Other Effects In comparison with propofol (see Propofol, Nausea and Vomiting), thiopental used for anesthesia induction results in a higher incidence of postoperative nausea and vomiting. In sedative (ie, subhypnotic) doses, thiopental causes hyperalgesia (ie, it decreases the threshold to pain).[52] This effect (and thiopental's tendency to accumulate) makes it a poor choice for intraoperative sedation during regional anesthesia or monitored anesthesia care. Thiopental is safe to use in patients susceptible to malignant hyperthermia.

PHARMACOKINETICS

Lipid Solubility Thiopental is administered as the alkaline (pH 10-11) solution of its sodium salt, but it is buffered to physiologic pH immediately upon contacting the circulation. Because its pK_a is 7.5, at physiologic pH slightly more than 50% of the thiopental molecules are uncharged and therefore lipid soluble. Its oil/water partition coefficient of approximately 500 is more than twice that of halothane, indicating that it is highly lipid soluble. This high lipid solubility, coupled with the large fraction of the cardiac output typically delivered to the brain, is responsible for the very rapid onset of effect, typically well under 1 minute, after intravenous administration.

Protein Binding Thiopental is approximately 85% bound to plasma protein. Protein-bound thiopental is unable to diffuse across the blood–brain barrier and produce a pharmacologic effect. In addition, the extensive binding of thiopental limits overall hepatic clearance, as only free drug is taken up by the liver to be metabolized. In clinical situations in which the plasma concentration of protein is decreased (eg, hepatic disease or hemodilution due to fluid resuscitation), the free fraction of thiopental is elevated, and lower doses of thiopental may be needed.

Redistribution Thiopental has a redistribution half-life ($t_{½\alpha}$) of approximately 2 to 4 min,[53] indicating that, after a typical bolus injection, the effect of the drug will be terminated within 3 to 4 half-lives or approximately 6 to 16 minutes (Table 41-5). Redistribution out of the CNS is the primary process by which the pharmacologic effects of thiopental are terminated. Unless the drug is given in very large doses (eg, barbiturate coma), in repeated doses, or by a long continuous infusion, metabolism and elimination are much less important in terminating its effect.

Metabolism and Elimination Thiopental has a terminal half-life ($t_{1/2\beta}$) of approximately 6 to 12 hours.[53] Thiopental undergoes an interesting metabolic reaction catalyzed by CYP. The initial step is oxidation of the sulfur atom, forming a sulfoxide derivative that spontaneously rearranges, leaving oxygen in place of the sulfur in the barbiturate ring. This metabolite is the active barbiturate, pentobarbital. Because of slower redistribution, pentobarbital is a longer-acting drug than thiopental. Thus, when large cumulative doses of thiopental are given, clinically significant concentrations of pentobarbital occur. Pentobarbital contributes to the overall effect and makes thiopental appear as a much longer-acting medication.[54] Other inactive hydroxylated metabolites of thiopental also are produced. Methohexital has a lower volume of distribution and a higher hepatic clearance than thiopental, and it is metabolized to inactive hydroxylated metabolites (Table 41-5).

Factors Affecting Pharmacodynamics and Pharmacokinetics Many factors affect the pharmacodynamics and pharmacokinetics of thiopental. For example, elderly patients require lower doses of thiopental to produce unconsciousness. This altered response is due to the decreased rate of distribution from the central compartment to the rapidly equilibrating compartment.[55]

The pharmacokinetics of thiopental in persons with significant impairment of hepatic function is complex. The fraction of unbound thiopental is increased because of decreased plasma albumin concentrations, but hepatic clearance of unbound drug is decreased. Total clearance remains normal.[53] Persons with cardiac dysfunction typically have an exaggerated hypotensive response to thiopental. In patients who are hypovolemic, a lower thiopental dose is needed because a greater fraction of the cardiac output goes to the brain. The hypovolemic patient may tolerate thiopental-induced vasodilatation very poorly.

CLINICAL USE

Induction of Anesthesia The characteristics of thiopental as an induction agent are listed in Table 41-7. An induction dose of 4 to 7 mg/kg is reasonable in the typical healthy patient undergoing elective surgery. Coexisting factors, such as previous premedication (eg, with benzodiazepines and/or opioids), advanced age, or presence of concurrent disease (eg, cardiac dysfunction, COPD, hypovolemia) will decrease the required dose of thiopental. Patients with acquired tolerance because of chronic use of barbiturates or cross-tolerance to benzodiazepines, anticonvulsants, or alcohol may require higher doses of thiopental to produce unconsciousness.

If there is concern about a possibly exaggerated response to thiopental, a prudent practice would be to administer the induction dose slowly or in divided doses, using a small initial bolus as a "test dose" and waiting 1 to 2 minutes to evaluate the central nervous and hemodynamic responses.

After administration of the induction dose, consciousness typically is lost within 30 seconds, although this time may be longer in persons with a slow circulation time because of cardiac dysfunction. Recovery of consciousness usually occurs within 6 to 16 minutes; however, some degree of cognitive impairment (a "hangover") may persist for hours.

The induction dose of methohexital is 1 to 3 mg/kg. Onset and awakening are similar to those with thiopental; however, the duration of cognitive impairment will be somewhat shorter. As mentioned previously, excitatory effects like twitching and hiccoughs are often seen during induction.

Maintenance of Anesthesia General anesthesia can be maintained by either intermittent intravenous boluses or a continuous intravenous infusion of thiopental; however, a rapid recovery should not be anticipated. Giving any rapidly redistributed medication by intermittent bolus results in a series of peaks and troughs in both blood concentration and effect, typically causing alternating periods of overmedication and undermedication. A continuous infusion, typically following a loading dose, permits a more constant blood (and brain) concentration and effect (see Chapter 43).

The CSHTs for thiopental after 1- and 2-hour infusions are approximately 80 and 100 minutes, respectively (Fig. 41-2). Thus thiopental is not a good choice for a maintenance infusion when rapid emergence and recovery are desired.

Methohexital has shorter CSHT values than does thiopental. The CSHTs for methohexital after 1- and 2-hour infusions are approximately 26 and 48 minutes, respectively (Fig. 41-2). Although shorter than for thiopental, emergence and recovery after an infusion of methohexital are still prolonged.

Sedation Barbiturates are infrequently used for procedural sedation (except perhaps the use of methohexital during office-based oral surgical procedures). In subhypnotic doses, thiopental is less likely than propofol to produce anterograde amnesia[9] (usually considered a desirable effect), and there may be hyperalgesia to pain.

ETOMIDATE

CHEMISTRY

Etomidate is an imidazole derivative whose structure is unlike that of any other anesthetic (Fig. 41-1 and Table 41-1). Its imidazole nucleus permits it to bind to, and inhibit, certain isozymes of CYP (see Endocrine Effects). It contains an ester linkage that is hydrolyzed to produce an inactive metabolite. With a pK_a of 4.2, it is ionized and water soluble at acidic pH and lipid soluble at physiologic pH. It is supplied as a 0.2% solution in 35% propylene glycol.

PHARMACODYNAMICS

Central Nervous System Etomidate works via $GABA_A$ receptors to produce rapid onset of unconsciousness. It has a brief duration of effect, similar to that of thiopental and propofol. The drug has virtually no analgesic effects, so usually it must be combined with other drugs to suppress autonomic or somatic responses to painful surgical stimulation. Induction of anesthesia is frequently accompanied by myoclonic movements (Table 41-7). Such myoclonic movements may be substantially mitigated by the prior administration of a small dose of midazolam.[56]

Cardiovascular System Etomidate is notable for its lack of cardiovascular effects, although the reasons for this remain obscure (Table 41-4).[57,58] At the typical induction dose of 0.3 mg/kg, it has little effect on arterial or venous vascular tone or on cardiac contractility. After induction of general anesthesia with etomidate, usually little change in blood pressure or heart rate occurs. It must be emphasized that etomidate is almost never administered alone, and the addition of other drugs may substantially alter the cardiovascular effects. Cardiovascular stability usually is preserved in persons with hypovolemia or cardiac dysfunction. Etomidate does not release histamine. At the higher dose of 0.7 mg/kg needed to produce EEG burst suppression, hypotension due to vasodilatation has been reported.[59]

Respiratory System Etomidate has less of a ventilatory depressant effect than does thiopental or propofol; however, an induction dose is still likely to result in transient apnea particularly when an opioid has also been administered (Table 41-3). The ventilatory depressant effect is not exaggerated in persons with COPD.

Endocrine Effects In 1984, Watt and Ledingham[60] reported a 2-fold increase in mortality among ventilated ICU patients who were given etomidate for 5 days or longer. This excess mortality subsequently was confirmed and attributed to the production of adrenal insufficiency. At clinically relevant concentrations, etomidate inhibits the mitochondrial CYP isozyme (CYP11B) responsible for catalyzing the 11β-hydroxylation reaction in cortisol synthesis. Etomidate is also able to inhibit the 17α-hydroxylase isozyme, although not at the plasma concentrations achieved during clinical infusions.[61] The duration of suppression of cortisol synthesis by etomidate is dependent on the cumulative dose. A single induction dose of 0.3 mg/kg inhibits cortisol synthesis and the normal response to adrenocorticotropic hormone for up to 12 hours. However, the effects are not large, and there is no convincing evidence that this effect is deleterious in normal persons undergoing elective surgery. The clinical relevance of this effect remains controversial over 25 years after its description. Nevertheless, fear of adrenal suppression has significantly limited the popularity of etomidate over the years (see Clinical Use). Analogues of etomidate that do not inhibit cortisol synthesis are being investigated (see Future Horizons: Experimental Drugs).

In 2005, Jackson warned against the use of etomidate in patients with septic shock.[62] Since then there have been several studies that have attempted to confirm or refute the safety of etomidate in critically ill patients, including those with sepsis. Unfortunately, these studies disagree: some confirm the danger of etomidate,[63-66] whereas others support its continued use.[67-71]

Other Effects Etomidate produces changes in $CMRo_2$, CBF, and ICP similar to those seen with thiopental and propofol. In contrast, etomidate will not likely lower, and may actually increase, CPP because it has minimal effect on blood pressure while decreasing ICP. Etomidate may be useful in the short-term management of the neurosurgical patient in whom cardiovascular stability is desired.

Etomidate is associated with the highest incidence of postoperative nausea and vomiting among the intravenous anesthetics (30%-40%, by some estimates). The propylene glycol solvent can cause pain on injection and superficial phlebitis. Excitatory phenomena, such as hiccoughs and myoclonic movements, are common during induction. The safety of etomidate in patients with porphyria is questionable. Although a few case reports have described its safe use in patients known to have porphyria, etomidate induces the synthesis of ALA synthase in rats. Etomidate is safe to give patients with malignant hyperthermia.

PHARMACOKINETICS

After an induction dose of 0.3 mg/kg, loss of consciousness and recovery will be similarly rapid, as with thiopental and propofol. Because of the long duration of adrenal suppression associated with etomidate infusions, continuous administration has not been as extensively studied. Its redistribution half-life is similar to that of thiopental, whereas its terminal half-life is shorter than that of thiopental and similar to that of propofol (Table 41-5).

Etomidate is approximately 75% bound to plasma proteins, a fraction that is significant but not as high as for thiopental or propofol. Most of an administered dose of etomidate is metabolized via ester hydrolysis, yielding an inactive carboxylic acid that is excreted in the urine. Despite the presence of high concentrations of esterases throughout the body, hydrolysis of etomidate occurs primarily in the liver. It has a high extraction ratio of 0.7, so alterations in hepatic blood flow should affect clearance. Because the effects of a bolus are terminated by redistribution and repeated doses or infusions are unlikely to be given, hepatic clearance of etomidate is unlikely to play an important role in recovery (Table 41-6).

CLINICAL USE

Etomidate is a popular choice for induction of anesthesia in patients compromised by cardiac dysfunction or hypovolemia (Table 41-4). Hemodynamic stability after induction with etomidate is superior to that of any alternative method of induction. In theory, etomidate's pharmacokinetics should make it an excellent drug for use during short surgical procedures, but the high incidence of nausea and vomiting is a major disadvantage for patients undergoing same-day surgery. The occurrence of myoclonus and hiccoughs is annoying but similar in frequency to that seen with methohexital.

After more than 25 years of using etomidate, what can we conclude about the importance of adrenal suppression? When etomidate is used for induction and short-term maintenance, reduction in cortisol historically has not been a problem, although there is substantial conflict in the literature on this issue. As mentioned, a single induction dose of etomidate may be hazardous in patients with established or evolving septic shock. In contrast, a review concluded that there was no harm from etomidate infusions during coronary surgery and that the stress of a major operation overcomes the inhibition of cortisol synthesis.[72] Some investigators have proposed the concurrent administration of etomidate plus a glucocorticoid, but in the absence of adequate studies, this routine practice cannot be recommended.

Ultimately, the decision to use etomidate must rest on the proven benefits of this drug, that is, cardiovascular and respiratory stability. These benefits are most likely to be seen when higher doses are used during induction. In our opinion, there is little compelling reason to use etomidate for maintenance of anesthesia or for procedural sedation.

BENZODIAZEPINES

CHEMISTRY

Three injectable benzodiazepines are used in the perioperative period: midazolam, diazepam, and lorazepam (Fig. 41-1 and Table 41-1). Diazepam and lorazepam are "classic" benzodiazepines that are lipid soluble and difficult to solubilize for injection. Diazepam injection is supplied as a 0.5% solution in 40% propylene glycol and 10% ethanol. Lorazepam is supplied as a 0.4% solution in 80% propylene glycol, 18% polyethylene glycol, and 2% benzyl alcohol. Midazolam has unique properties as a result of its substituted imidazole ring. The imidazole nitrogen has a pK_a of 6.2, so it becomes protonated and water soluble when buffered in a solution of pH 3 to 4 (as supplied in the vial).[73] At physiologic pH, more than 90% of the midazolam molecules exist in the unprotonated lipid-soluble form. Hydroxylation of the methyl group on this imidazole ring decreases the pharmacologic activity of midazolam and increases its clearance, permitting this drug to be shorter acting than the other injectable benzodiazepines.

The water solubility of midazolam at low pH has erroneously been attributed to opening of one of the rings in the benzodiazepine nucleus. In fact, all benzodiazepines undergo ring opening at low pH. At pH 2, 75% of the midazolam molecules are in the open-ring configuration, whereas at pH 4, that percentage decreases to 9%.[61] Because midazolam is supplied at a pH of 3 to 4 in the vial, ring opening can account for only a small percentage of its water solubility at that pH.

PHARMACODYNAMICS

Central Nervous System Benzodiazepines bind to a specific site located at the interface between the α- and γ-subunits of the pentameric $GABA_A$ receptor. GABA itself appears to bind at a different site between the α- and β-subunits.[39] Unlike the relatively nonselective barbiturates or propofol, the benzodiazepines bind preferentially to $GABA_A$ receptors containing $\alpha_{1,2,3,5}$ and γ-subunits. Binding by endogenous benzodiazepine ligands (endozepines) or by benzodiazepine agonists to this benzodiazepine receptor acts allosterically to increase the affinity of the GABA receptor for GABA. Thus benzodiazepines potentiate the inhibitory effects of GABA, thereby increasing chloride conductance and hyperpolarizing neuronal membranes. Unlike barbiturates, benzodiazepines have a much more limited effect on neuronal hyperpolarization. The limited effect and selective CNS binding probably account for the great safety of benzodiazepines; they lack significant toxicity, even when they are taken in very high doses. At higher doses, such as those necessary to produce hypnosis or anticonvulsant effects, benzodiazepines may be working by non-GABA mechanisms such as inhibition of adenosine reuptake[74] or inhibition of neuronal Ca^{2+} currents.[75] Benzodiazepines also have agonist activity at the glycine receptor, an important inhibitory neurotransmitter in the spinal cord. Some of the effects of benzodiazepines, such as muscle relaxation, likely are mediated by their actions in the spinal cord. Benzodiazepine receptors in the periphery appear to regulate the initial step in the synthesis of steroid hormones from cholesterol.[76] The physiologic significance of this action remains unclear.

Patients who are chronically taking benzodiazepines can become tolerant to some, but not all, of the effects. The initial drowsiness usually decreases, although some degree of psychomotor impairment seems to persist. Tolerance develops to the muscle relaxant and anticonvulsant effects, and the latter has limited the use of benzodiazepines in chronic seizure disorders. Alcohol, barbiturates, and benzodiazepines exhibit some cross-tolerance, so higher doses of these sedatives will be needed in patients with significant alcohol or barbiturate intake.

Benzodiazepines have effects on $CMRo_2$ and ICP qualitatively similar to the effects of propofol; however, the magnitude of these effects is far less (Table 41-2). The effect of benzodiazepines on CBF and CPP is variable and is more of a function of their effects on blood pressure. Benzodiazepines are excellent anticonvulsants, although their primary use is limited to initial control of seizures and not prophylaxis. All of them raise the threshold for seizures induced by local anesthetics. Unlike thiopental and propofol, benzodiazepines, even in very high doses, do not cause burst suppression on the EEG or an isoelectric tracing, and they are not used for neuroprotection. Benzodiazepines given in subhypnotic doses produce amnesia for events after drug administration (anterograde amnesia).

Benzodiazepines are classified as "anxiolytics" because they are active in various animal models thought to represent anxiety. In patients who have chronic anxiety states, benzodiazepines can reduce anxiety at doses that are not highly sedating. Of note, the same effects may not occur in surgical patients. Many patients scheduled for surgery do not have high levels of self-rated anxiety, and the effect of midazolam is more likely to produce dizziness or sleepiness.[77] An occasional patient may find the feeling of drunkenness or dizziness to be unpleasant.

Other Effects Benzodiazepines produce much smaller cardiovascular effects than do thiopental or propofol, even when used for general anesthesia induction (Table 41-4). Some dilation of capacitance vessels leads to a decrease in venous return; however, there is little or no effect on myocardial contractility. Thus the overall effect on blood pressure and heart rate will depend on the volume status of the patient. Elevated blood pressure in the anxious patient is often lowered by low doses of benzodiazepines by virtue of their sedative properties (see later, Clinical Use).

Although benzodiazepines cause a dose-dependent decrease in hypoxic ventilatory drive, subhypnotic doses given alone rarely cause apnea. Doses of midazolam sufficient to induce unconsciousness produce apnea with a frequency similar to that of thiopental.[78] There is profound synergy in depressing ventilatory drive between benzodiazepines and opioids or ethanol. Patients with COPD are more sensitive to the ventilatory depressant effects of benzodiazepines (Table 41-3).

Benzodiazepines, given alone, have a very low risk for causing nausea and vomiting. They are safe in patients with malignant hyperthermia, but they should be used with caution in persons with acute intermittent porphyria, hereditary coproporphyria, and variegate porphyria because some benzodiazepines induce ALA synthase in rats. Hypersensitivity reactions to benzodiazepines are rare.

PHARMACOKINETICS

After an induction dose of 0.3 mg/kg midazolam, loss of consciousness is rapid; however, awakening will be much slower and hangover more prolonged than after thiopental or propofol. Simultaneous pharmacokinetic–pharmacodynamic modeling using an EEG end point suggests that midazolam is slightly slower in onset than is diazepam. The half-time to achieve steady-state effect was over 4 minutes, compared with 90 seconds for diazepam.[79] The $t_{1/2\alpha}$ for midazolam is 7 to 15 minutes, much longer than the 2- to 4-minute values for thiopental or propofol. The $t_{1/2\beta}$ for midazolam is 2 to 4 hours. When given by infusion, recovery after termination of a midazolam infusion will be longer than after propofol but shorter than after thiopental (Table 41-5).

Midazolam is metabolized primarily via hydroxylation of the *N*-methyl group on the imidazole ring. Although this metabolite has some residual benzodiazepine activity, circulating concentrations are low because midazolam is rapidly conjugated with glucuronic acid, yielding an inactive and rapidly excreted metabolite. Midazolam has high first-pass metabolism after oral administration, with an oral bioavailability of approximately 15%.[80]

Diazepam and lorazepam are metabolized and eliminated much more slowly than midazolam because of a high degree of protein binding (98%) and a much lower hepatic clearance. Whereas lorazepam is metabolized to an inactive glucuronide, diazepam is metabolized to several active metabolites. The most important of these active metabolites is nordazepam, which has an extremely long terminal half-life (100 hours vs 20 hours for diazepam). The processes of metabolism and elimination of these medications become important only when repeated doses or long infusions are given.

CLINICAL USE

Midazolam is the most commonly used preoperative sedative in anesthesia. It replaced diazepam largely because it does not produce pain on injection. Given as a single intravenous bolus, the effects of diazepam and midazolam are quite similar and have about the same duration. Lorazepam is slower in onset and longer in duration, and its tendency to cause prolonged amnesia may be undesirable for patients undergoing short procedures. After administration of 1 to 2 mg of midazolam, most patients become sleepy and calmer and have anterograde amnesia, effects that persist for 30 to 60 minutes. At these doses and in the absence of other medications, there are few significant effects on cardiorespiratory parameters. Sedation can be maintained by repeating intermittent boluses of 0.5 to 1 mg or by giving a continuous infusion. As with barbiturates, administration of benzodiazepines can sometimes produce paradoxical excitation.

The amnestic effects of benzodiazepines are dose related and often occur in patients who remain conscious and capable of normal conversation. The amnestic effects of midazolam (when given in usual doses for premedication) are variable but usually short lived, and they should not be relied on to prevent recall of intraoperative events. Although lorazepam has a shorter plasma half-life than does diazepam, its amnestic effects are more prolonged. This may be a function of higher affinity for benzodiazepine receptors.

Midazolam is commonly given by mouth for preoperative sedation in pediatric patients. The usual dose is 0.5 to 0.75 mg/kg, and a significant effect is apparent within 15 to 30 minutes. However, the peak effect may occur up to 1 hour after oral administration, so there might be significant postoperative sedation after short procedures.[80] An official oral preparation of midazolam is unavailable in many countries. The intravenous solution can be mixed with fruit juice or flavored syrup; however, there is no completely effective way to mask the bitter taste.

Midazolam is 1 of only 2 induction agents (the other being ketamine) whose administration by the intramuscular route is well tolerated without pain and whose absorption is both reliable and predictable. Doses ranging from those that produce mild sedation up to those required to induce general anesthesia can be given intramuscularly. Doses in excess of a few milligrams should be given using the more concentrated 10 mg/mL preparation to minimize injected volume.

Diazepam is an excellent oral preoperative sedative and anxiolytic agent for patients undergoing inpatient surgery. A dose of 10 to 20 mg in an adult, or 0.2 to 0.4 mg/kg in a child, given by mouth an hour before transport to the operating room usually results in a drowsy and calm patient. Both diazepam and lorazepam are associated with significant pain when given intravenously, and the propylene glycol solvent can cause superficial phlebitis. Both medications are absorbed erratically when administered by intramuscular injection.

Midazolam can be used in higher intravenous doses (0.05-0.15 mg/kg) to induce anesthesia, or it can be given via continuous infusion during maintenance (see Chapter 42). The slower onset and offset of effect compared with propofol or thiopental are counterbalanced by midazolam's modest cardiovascular effects. The drug is not an analgesic, so it is usually administered with opioids. This significantly reduces the required dose of midazolam but usually causes a greater decrease in peripheral vascular resistance than seen with the individual drugs. This vasodilatation may be due to an increased effect on central sympathetic tone or possibly to a decrease in plasma catecholamines.[81,82]

The doses of midazolam and diazepam should be reduced in the elderly because of their increased sensitivity and reduced clearance. Hepatic disease or drugs that inhibit the oxidative metabolism of diazepam (eg, cimetidine) can significantly increase the intensity and duration of sedation.[83] Because the hepatic clearance of midazolam is moderately high, elimination is not greatly affected by enzyme induction or inhibition. Renal disease, on the other hand, can delay the excretion of hydroxymidazolam and cause an increase in effect. Lorazepam is glucuronidated and has no active metabolites, so its effects are not markedly altered by moderate hepatic or renal disease.

FLUMAZENIL

Flumazenil (Fig. 41-1) is a benzodiazepine antagonist.[84] It has high affinity for the benzodiazepine binding site on the $GABA_A$ receptor, which prevents or reverses the effects of benzodiazepines and endozepines. There is no evidence that flumazenil will reverse nonbenzodiazepine CNS depression. The usual initial dose in a patient who has been given a therapeutic dose of a benzodiazepine is 0.1 to 0.2 mg intravenously. The initial dose can be repeated every 1 or 2 minutes up to a total dose of 1 mg to antagonize benzodiazepine-induced sedation. The various actions of benzodiazepines require different concentrations of agonist, and effects that require high doses (eg, hypnosis) are most sensitive to flumazenil reversal. Some effects, such as depression of hypoxic ventilatory drive, appear to be incompletely antagonized (see bulleted list that follows, second bullet).[85]

Reports that flumazenil is a weak partial agonist or inverse agonist are inconsistent. Healthy volunteers given a relatively high dose (2 mg) of flumazenil alone experienced mild anxiety and symptoms resembling those that occur during a panic attack.[86] These symptoms are more likely to occur in patients with previously diagnosed panic attacks. These effects may indicate tonic activity in some critical $GABA_A$ pathways, and flumazenil may be acting weakly as an inverse agonist (ie, producing an effect opposite to that of the benzodiazepine). This action likely is not clinically important in the typical anesthesia setting in which flumazenil is used to reverse midazolam. Persons on chronic benzodiazepine therapy who are given flumazenil have been reported sporadically to have seizures,[87] sometimes progressing to status epilepticus.[88] This finding suggests that some patients develop physical dependence on the benzodiazepine, and flumazenil can precipitate withdrawal. A few cases of flumazenil-induced seizures in persons not on chronic drug therapy have been reported.[87]

Flumazenil is rapidly cleared by hepatic metabolism, with a half-life of approximately 1 hour. Therefore, it has a shorter duration than the benzodiazepines that are used to antagonize, so repeated doses usually are necessary.

The appropriate clinical roles for flumazenil are relatively limited:

- If a patient receiving midazolam for sedation becomes disoriented or uncooperative, reversal may be helpful. In contrast, planned use of flumazenil, that is, giving excessive amounts of benzodiazepines for a procedure and then relying on reversal at the end, will produce risk with little benefit. Such treatment risks ventilatory depression and loss of airway reflexes during the procedure and recurrence of depressant effects when reversal by the short-acting antagonist decays.
- Excessive sedation and ventilatory depression most often occur when benzodiazepines are combined with opioids. Flumazenil only partially reverses the depression of hypoxic ventilatory drive produced by midazolam, and it has no effect on ventilatory depression due to an opioid. In this setting, support of ventilation and administration of naloxone are more appropriate treatments.
- When flumazenil has been used empirically for treatment of suspected drug overdoses, deaths due to status epilepticus have occurred. Risk factors in such deaths include concurrent ingestion of tricyclic antidepressants and prior long-term therapy with benzodiazepines or anticonvulsants. Unless an overdose is known to be due to the acute ingestion of only a benzodiazepine, flumazenil treatment may be riskier than simply supporting blood pressure and ventilation until the drug effects wear off.

KETAMINE

CHEMISTRY

Ketamine is a derivative of aminocyclohexanone whose chemical structure is related to phencyclidine (Fig. 41-1 and Table 41-1). It is a weak base with a p*K* of 7.5 and is supplied in solution as the hydrochloride salt. The 3 concentrations available—10 mg/mL, 50 mg/mL, and 100 mg/mL—are typically used for monitored anesthesia care, intravenous anesthesia, and intramuscular injection, respectively. Ketamine is compatible in solution with atropine or glycopyrrolate, with which it is often mixed.

The commercial preparations of ketamine contain a racemic mixture of its 2 isomers. The *S*-isomer is a more potent anesthetic with fewer adverse effects,[89] which is available in Europe, but not the United States.

PHARMACODYNAMICS

Central Nervous System Whereas all the previously discussed intravenous anesthetics potentiate the inhibitory effects of GABA, ketamine produces its inhibitory effects by blocking the NMDA receptor.[90] The NMDA receptor is, like GABAA, a ligand-gated ion channel, but it is gated by the excitatory neurotransmitter glutamate. When open, it passes a current carried by calcium ions.

The anesthetic state induced by ketamine is called *dissociative anesthesia*. It does not resemble normal sleep; rather, patients appear to be dissociated from their environment. Under ketamine anesthesia,

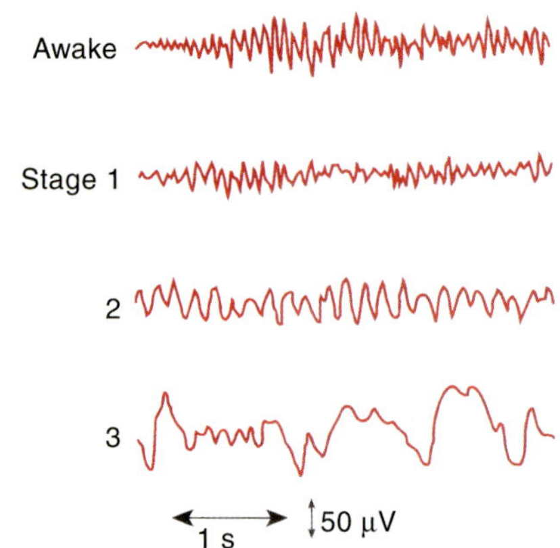

FIGURE 41-5. Progressive changes in the electroencephalogram produced by ketamine. Stages 1 to 3 are achieved with racemic ketamine and its *S*(+) isomer. With *R*(–) ketamine, stage 2 was the maximal electroencephalographic depression produced. [Redrawn from Kilpatrick GJ. New drugs for sedation and hypnosis. 2005 EuroSIVA Annual Scientific Meeting, Vienna, Austria, May 27-28, 2005.]

patients may move, vocalize, have their eyes open, and make ocular tracking movements. However, patients are anesthetized and do not respond to noxious stimuli or have any recall of events that occurred during the anesthetic. Ketamine causes profound analgesia that persists well into the postoperative period. Vivid dreams or hallucinations that may be perceived as unpleasant often accompany ketamine anesthesia, and hallucinations and/or dysphoria may occur in the postoperative period.

In contrast to the other intravenous anesthetics, ketamine produces increases in $CMRo_2$, CBF, and ICP. Thus ketamine is relatively contraindicated in patients with an intracranial mass or increased ICP or who have suffered recent head trauma (Table 41-2).

Ketamine produces dose-dependent changes in the EEG that are quite different from those resulting from thiopental or propofol (**Fig. 41-5**).[91] For this reason, EEG-based monitors of the depth of anesthesia (see Chapter 33) are not accurate when ketamine is the primary anesthetic. As seen with thiopental, light anesthesia with ketamine is associated with an increase in EEG frequency so that beta waves predominate. As the depth of anesthesia increases, high-amplitude theta waves, with intermittent delta waves, can occur. An isoelectric EEG does not occur with ketamine anesthesia.[92]

Cardiovascular System In contrast to the other intravenous anesthetics, ketamine usually causes an increase in blood pressure, heart rate, cardiac contractility, cardiac output, and systemic vascular resistance (Table 41-4). These are indirect effects by virtue of increased centrally mediated sympathetic tone and increased centrally mediated release of catecholamines from the adrenal medulla. In the critically ill or injured patient whose circulating catecholamine concentration has reached its maximum value, ketamine may cause a decrease in blood pressure and cardiac output because the drug and its major metabolite have a direct negative inotropic effect. Ketamine may increase myocardial oxygen demand more than it increases oxygen delivery, and in some patients with coronary artery disease, this effect may lead to ischemia.

Respiratory System Ketamine differs from the other intravenous anesthetics in its respiratory effects (Table 41-3). Ketamine has little effect on ventilatory drive in normal patients or in those with COPD. It produces bronchodilation and has proved useful in patients with, or prone to, bronchospasm. Protective airway reflexes are less likely to be ablated by ketamine, even in the presence of surgical anesthesia, although aspiration remains a risk. Ketamine causes copious salivation, and for this reason it is usually administered with an antisialagogue (eg, an anticholinergic drug such as glycopyrrolate).

Other Effects Like etomidate, ketamine is associated with a high risk for postoperative nausea and vomiting. Ketamine is safe in patients with malignant hyperthermia and, based on a number of case reports, probably is safe in patients with porphyria.

PHARMACOKINETICS

After an intravenous induction dose of 1 to 2 mg/kg of ketamine, loss of consciousness is rapid; however, awakening will be much slower and the hangover more prolonged than after any other intravenous anesthetic. Ketamine has a redistribution half-life $t_{1/2\alpha}$ of 11 to 17 minutes, much longer than the values for either thiopental or propofol (Table 41-5).

Ketamine is extensively metabolized, primarily by *N*-demethylation. The resulting active metabolite, norketamine, is approximately one-fourth as potent. Norketamine is further metabolized to an inactive glucuronide.

In contrast to the other intravenous anesthetics, only a small fraction of circulating ketamine is bound to plasma protein. Ketamine has a high hepatic extraction ratio, and other medications or coexisting diseases that decrease hepatic blood flow would be expected to prolong its duration of action (Table 41-6). Ketamine has high first-pass hepatic metabolism after oral administration, although it is sometimes administered by this route.

CLINICAL USE

Like etomidate, ketamine is most commonly used for induction of general anesthesia in patients compromised by concurrent cardiac dysfunction or hypovolemia (Table 41-4). It has been used extensively for acute and chronic treatment of burn victims. Infusions are used for analgesia and hypnosis as part of balanced anesthesia. Because increasing doses of ketamine do not produce consistent changes in hemodynamics, respiration, eye signs, or movement, the depth of anesthesia may be difficult to assess. Unless there is maximal sympathetic tone, ketamine usually causes an increase or no change in blood pressure. Ketamine is a good choice for patients with, or prone to, bronchospasm. A slow emergence, often accompanied by hallucinations and/or dysphoria, is a common adverse effect that must be balanced against the desire for a lack of cardiovascular depression. The unpleasant psychological effects may be mitigated, but not completely eliminated, by concurrent administration of propofol or a benzodiazepine.

In subhypnotic doses (0.15-0.3 mg/kg), ketamine is commonly used for monitored anesthesia care. It produces profound analgesia without the concurrent ventilatory depression produced by opioids. In combination with a low dose of propofol or a benzodiazepine, the unpleasant psychological effects are minimal, and the ventilatory depressant effects are much less than the combination with an opioid.

Ketamine is commonly used, either alone or in combination with midazolam, as an oral medication in children, especially as the sole agents for conscious sedation for a short but noxious procedure (eg, upper endoscopy). Typical doses of the combination are 3 to 6 mg/kg of ketamine plus 0.25 to 0.5 mg/kg of midazolam.

Ketamine is 1 of only 2 induction agents (the other being midazolam) that have reliable and predictable absorption with minimal pain after intramuscular injection. Doses ranging from those that produce mild sedation to those required to induce general anesthesia may be given intramuscularly. The preparation containing 100 mg/mL usually is given, especially in adults, to minimize the injected volume. A rapid onset after intramuscular injection makes ketamine a frequent choice for induction of anesthesia in children and adults with mental disabilities who will not tolerate a mask or the placement of an intravenous catheter. After intramuscular administration of 2 to 4 mg/kg of ketamine, the patient will lose consciousness, thus allowing placement of an intravenous catheter within approximately 5 minutes.

ADJUNCTS

BUTYROPHENONES

Droperidol and the closely related antipsychotic agent haloperidol exert their CNS effects via antagonism of the dopamine D_2 receptor. Unlike their predecessors, the phenothiazines, they have less affinity at other sites, such as α-adrenoceptors or muscarinic cholinergic receptors. They are classified as *neuroleptic* agents because of their distinct behavioral effects. When a neuroleptic agent is given to a "normal" individual, behavior is diminished and responses to stimuli are fewer, slower, and smaller in magnitude. In high doses, a catatonic state is induced, although consciousness and memory are preserved. These drugs should generally not be given by themselves. Patients treated this way usually appear sleepy and comfortable when drug concentrations are maximal, but they often describe an intensely dysphoric experience after the effects have worn off. This is in distinct contrast to the benzodiazepines, which often produce anterograde amnesia. When a neuroleptic agent is given to a psychotic patient, the thought disorder usually improves. In schizophrenia, the delusions and auditory or visual hallucinations become less pronounced or disappear, and thinking becomes more orderly. Even if some hallucinations remain, the patient is far more likely to recognize them as unreal.

Droperidol is a highly effective antiemetic at doses (0.625-1.25 mg) that do not cause sedation or dysphoria. In rare instances, it may be useful in higher doses for its neuroleptic effect. Droperidol is a very safe sedative, albeit one often associated with dysphoria. It causes no ventilatory depression and, in contrast to the benzodiazepines, does not potentiate the ventilatory depressant effects of opioids.[93] It has few cardiovascular side effects other than very mild vasodilatation due to its weak interaction with α-adrenoceptors. Butyrophenones can lower the seizure threshold and cause extrapyramidal symptoms (see next paragraph), so they are generally avoided in patients with seizure disorders or Parkinson disease. Many clinicians find droperidol useful for sedation during monitored anesthesia care or regional anesthesia in patients with dementia, psychosis, or mental retardation. In addition, droperidol may be useful to facilitate procedures such as line placement or awake intubation in uncooperative and/or intoxicated trauma patients. In such cases, its overall safety renders the possible later dysphoria a tolerable adverse effect.

Like all dopamine antagonists, droperidol has the potential to cause extrapyramidal reactions. These may include involuntary facial grimacing, neck stiffness, and limb movements such as akathisia ("restless legs"). These effects usually are not seen with antiemetic doses unless they are repeated, and they can be treated by administration of diphenhydramine or trihexyphenidyl, drugs with central anticholinergic effects.

An anesthetic technique rarely used today is neuroleptanesthesia, which involves the concurrent administration of droperidol, fentanyl (an opioid), and nitrous oxide. Anesthesia induction is accomplished via administration of 10 to 15 mg of droperidol and 250 to 500 mcg of fentanyl. Loss of consciousness and a lack of awareness are unlikely unless a high concentration of nitrous oxide is also given, and even then awareness still may occasionally occur. The neuroleptanesthetic state is accompanied by cardiovascular stability, and for this reason the technique gained some popularity before the use of invasive monitoring and intensive care units. The technique is associated with prolonged emergence and frequent dysphoria.

Although droperidol has been used as a neuroleptic for more than 4 decades, its ability to cause cardiac dysrhythmias has only recently been appreciated. Droperidol causes a dose-dependent prolongation of the QTc interval, and, in a subset of the population (of unknown incidence), this may lead to polymorphic ventricular tachycardia (torsade de pointes). Antiemetic doses of droperidol almost certainly are safe, but there is the possibility that larger, sedating doses may be associated with this dysrhythmia.[94] In the United States, droperidol is labeled with a boxed warning that mandates continuous electrocardiographic monitoring for 2 to 3 hours after droperidol administration in doses above 2.5 mg; such doses are above those needed for a reliable antiemetic effect.

α_2-ADRENOCEPTOR AGONISTS

Clonidine was the first centrally acting α_2-adrenergic agonist widely used in medicine. Introduced as an antihypertensive, a common adverse effect was sedation to which the patient became tolerant after 1 to 2 weeks of therapy. Because one person's adverse effect may be another person's therapeutic effect, clonidine was later investigated and used as a preoperative sedative (see Chapter 9). In some studies, such use was associated with diminished intraoperative requirements for hypnotic and analgesic medications and less intraoperative tachycardia and hypertension.

Dexmedetomidine is the first α_2-adrenoceptor agonist specifically marketed as a sedative. It is considerably more selective for α_2-adrenoceptors than clonidine. The primary site of its action as a sedative is in the locus ceruleus, where its effect is to mimic physiologic sleep.[95] Dexmedetomidine decreases inhibitory neuronal outflow from the locus ceruleus to the ventrolateral preoptic nucleus, resulting in increased GABA release from the latter. In rats, dexmedetomidine produces analgesia at the spinal cord level by activating descending inhibitory pathways originating in the midbrain, thereby reducing pain impulses that would otherwise ascend in the cord. Additionally it acts synergistically with nitrous oxide to potentiate the latter's analgesic activity in the spinal cord.[96]

Dexmedetomidine produces intense sedation, although it cannot reliably produce amnesia, hypnosis, or general anesthesia.[97] It does not have anticonvulsant properties. As would be expected, dexmedetomidine lowers blood pressure and heart rate, and dramatic decreases have occasionally occurred in patients without preexisting cardiovascular disease. Like clonidine, higher doses of dexmedetomidine can produce an initial increase in blood pressure that is believed to result from stimulation of α_{2B}-adrenoceptors. Sympathetic stimulation is also responsible for the common side effect of dry mouth. In animals and humans, dexmedetomidine can markedly reduce the requirement for volatile or intravenous anesthetics and opioids. Sedative doses have very little effect on ventilation and do not appear to increase the ventilatory depressant effects of opioids.[98]

Dexmedetomidine is approved for sedation of mechanically ventilated adult patients, but only for up to 24 hours. The infusion typically is started near the end of an operative procedure before the patient is transported to the ICU or shortly after arrival. A bolus dose of 1 mcg/kg is given over 10 minutes, followed by an infusion of 0.003 to 0.012 mcg/kg/min. No ventilatory depression is associated with this sedation, and patients should require less opioid for management of postoperative pain. The heart rate usually is slow, although symptomatic bradycardia occasionally occurs, and dexmedetomidine should not be given to patients with preexisting heart block. Postoperative hypertension usually is well controlled; however, some patients experience hypotension and require pressor infusion, especially if they have preexisting ventricular dysfunction. Dexmedetomidine has also been evaluated for procedural sedation, and it was recently approved for this indication.[99] Both clonidine and dexmedetomidine are able to suppress postoperative shivering, probably via stimulation of α_{2B} receptors in the hypothalamus.

An intriguing possibility is that perioperative administration of an α_2-adrenoceptor agonist decreases cardiovascular mortality. A meta-analysis concluded that such use decreases mortality and myocardial infarction after vascular surgery.[100]

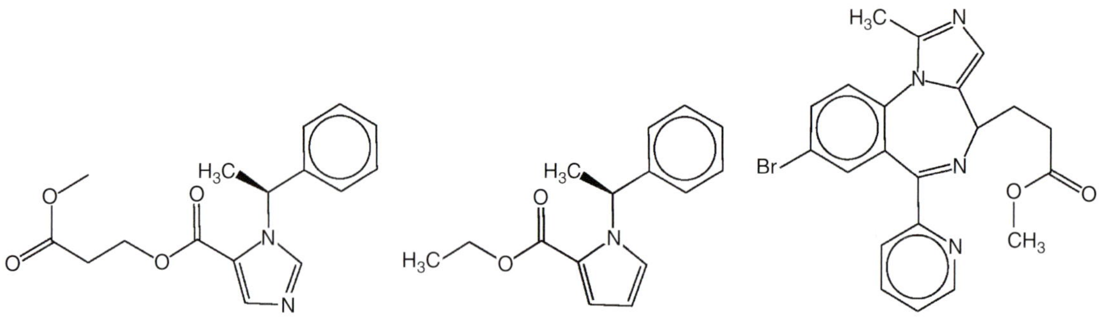

FIGURE 41-6. Structures of some investigational intravenous anesthetic agents: **A.** MOC-etomidate, **B.** carboetomidate, and **C.** CNS 7056X.

FUTURE HORIZONS: EXPERIMENTAL DRUGS

ETOMIDATE DERIVATIVES

In order to take advantage of the desirable properties of etomidate without producing adrenal suppression, Cotten and colleagues have synthesized and evaluated 2 derivatives of etomidate that avoid adrenal suppression via 2 different mechanisms. The structures of methoxycarbonyletomidate (MOC-etomidate) and carboetomidate are shown in **Fig. 41-6**. Note that both are optically active. Thus far these novel compounds have been primarily evaluated in rats.

MOC-etomidate is an esterase-metabolized analogue of etomidate that, like other esterase-metabolized drugs, has a very short duration of action. When compared with etomidate in rats at equipotent doses, the duration of the loss of righting reflex was about 1 minute with MOC-etomidate and about 24 minutes with etomidate. Furthermore, there was no detectable adrenocortical suppression 30 minutes after administration.[101]

Carboetomidate is a simple but elegant analogue of etomidate in which 1 nitrogen atom of the imidazole ring is replaced with a carbon. It is this nitrogen atom in etomidate that binds to the heme iron atom of CYP11B, thereby preventing the binding of 11-deoxycortisol, the precursor to cortisol. Carboetomidate is approximately 3 orders of magnitude loss potent an inhibitor of CYP11B than is etomidate.[102]

ESTERASE-METABOLIZED BENZODIAZEPINE (CNS 7056X)

CNS 7056X (Fig. 41-6) is an esterase-metabolized benzodiazepine. It is metabolized by nonspecific tissue esterases, as is remifentanil (see Chapter 42). The carboxylic acid metabolite that results from its hydrolysis is approximately 400 times less potent than the parent medication. The duration of the effect of CNS 7056X in sheep is less than that of midazolam after equisedating doses.[103]

KEY REFERENCES

- Avram MJ, Krejcie TC, Henthorn TK. The relationship of age to the pharmacokinetics of early drug distribution: the concurrent disposition of thiopental and indocyanine green. *Anesthesiology.* 1990;72:403-411.
- Brain Resuscitation Clinical Trial I Study Group. Randomized clinical study of thiopental loading in comatose survivors of cardiac arrest. *N Engl J Med.* 1986;314:397-403.
- Coursin DB, Coursin DB, Maccioli GA. Dexmedetomidine. *Curr Opin Crit Care.* 2001;7:221-226.
- Dershwitz M, Rosow CE, Di Biase PM, et al. Comparison of the sedative effects of butorphanol and midazolam. *Anesthesiology.* 1991;74:717-724.
- Gan TJ, Glass PS, Howell ST, et al. Determination of plasma concentrations of propofol associated with 50% reduction in postoperative nausea. *Anesthesiology.* 1997;87:779-784.
- Hoffman EJ, Warren EW. Flumazenil: a benzodiazepine antagonist. *Clin Pharm.* 1993;12:641-656.
- Hudson RJ, Stanski DR, Saidman LJ, et al. A model for studying depth of anesthesia and acute tolerance to thiopental. *Anesthesiology.* 1983;59:301-308.
- Hughes MA, Glass PS, Jacobs JR. Context-sensitive half-time in multicompartment pharmacokinetic models for intravenous anesthetic drugs. *Anesthesiology.* 1992;76:334-341.
- Jackson WJ. Should we use etomidate as an induction agent for endotracheal intubation in patients with septic shock? A critical appraisal. *Chest.* 2005;127:1031-1038.
- Picard P, Tramèr MR. Prevention of pain on injection with propofol: a quantitative systematic review. *Anesth Analg.* 2000;90:963-969.
- Russo H, Bressolle F. Pharmacodynamics and pharmacokinetics of thiopental. *Clin Pharmacokinet.* 1998;35:95-134.
- Veselis RA, Reinsel RA, Feshchenko VA, et al. The comparative amnestic effects of midazolam, propofol, thiopental, and fentanyl at equisedative concentrations. *Anesthesiology.* 1997;87:749-764.
- Watt I, Ledingham IM. Mortality amongst multiple trauma patients admitted to an intensive therapy unit. *Anaesthesia.* 1984;39:973-981.

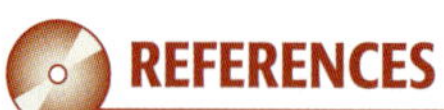

REFERENCES

Complete references available on DVD and online version at www.LongneckerAnesthesiology.com

CHAPTER 42

Pharmacology of Opioid Analgesics

Carl Rosow
Mark Dershwitz

KEY POINTS

1. An *opioid* is any natural or synthetic compound that has effects similar to those of morphine or that acts as an antagonist at the same receptors to which morphine binds.
2. Because opioid agonists relieve pain, they are classified as *analgesics*. In contrast to the local anesthetics (which interrupt the transmission of all nerve impulses, including pain) and the anti-inflammatory analgesics such as aspirin (which decrease some of the pathologic processes leading to pain), the opioid analgesics act primarily to alter the *perception* of pain as a noxious entity.
3. The "classic" pharmacologic effects of morphine, such as analgesia and ventilatory depression, are mediated by μ receptors. The κ receptor shares a number of effects with the μ receptor, including analgesia, sedation, and ventilatory depression. The δ receptor is responsible for mediating some of the analgesic effects of the endogenous opioid peptides, especially in the spinal cord.
4. All opioid receptors are G-protein coupled receptors. The actions of both μ and δ agonists result in overall neuronal depression, and they share several signal transduction mechanisms, including inhibition of adenylyl cyclase, activation of K^+ currents, and suppression of Ca^{2+} currents.
5. Five families of endogenous opioid peptides bind to the various opioid receptors. Although some of these peptides undoubtedly function in nociceptive pathways, they also appear to play fundamental roles in processes like thermoregulation and hormone release, as well as gastrointestinal and cardiovascular control.
6. The most widely used opioid analgesics are the pure agonists that are relatively selective for μ-opioid receptors. Unlike the volatile anesthetics, opioid agonists produce a group of highly specific depressant and stimulant effects by acting at discrete sites within the central nervous system.
7. Opioid analgesic effects result from actions at several different levels of the neuraxis. Patients given morphine will typically report that pain is still present, but the intensity is decreased and it no longer bothers them as much. Sufficient doses of opioids will relieve almost any pain, although some types of pain are typically more responsive than others. Prolonged, burning pain, for example, is more effectively blunted than the brief, sharp pain of an incision. Neuropathic pain (eg, pain of nerve root compression) can be very resistant to opioid treatment. Intraoperatively the opioids can produce sufficient analgesia to reduce or abolish autonomic and somatic responses to surgical stimuli.
8. In usual analgesic doses, morphine-like drugs may produce drowsiness, feelings of heaviness, and difficulty concentrating. Unlike benzodiazepines, opioids do not usually produce anterograde amnesia. Doses of opioids that are sufficient to produce apnea and profound analgesia do not reliably produce unconsciousness in healthy individuals.
9. True seizures have been reported after repeated doses of meperidine because its major metabolite, normeperidine, is a potent convulsant.
10. Opioids produce a dose-related depression of the ventilatory response to CO_2 by a direct effect on ventilatory centers in the medulla. Morphine also blunts the response to hypoxia. It is important to remember that a decrease in ventilatory rate is not a very sensitive indicator of opioid effect. A patient's drive to breathe may be abnormal despite an apparently normal ventilatory rate and state of consciousness. Sleep will further depress the response to CO_2 and potentiate the ventilatory depression caused by opioids.
11. Equianalgesic doses of all opioids produce equivalent amounts of ventilatory depression. There is no convincing evidence that any analgesic is more or less dangerous than morphine in this regard.
12. Tolerant individuals who require large amounts of opioid for relief of pain are not at a proportionately increased risk of ventilatory depression.
13. It is very difficult to reverse ventilatory depression without reversing some analgesia.
14. Opioids suppress cough by depressing putative cough centers in the medulla. This effect apparently involves different receptor mechanisms than those mediating analgesia.
15. The pinpoint pupil is a pathognomonic sign of opioid overdose (unless hypoxia is severe enough to produce mydriasis).
16. Opioids produce complex effects on vomiting centers in the medulla. There is direct stimulation of the chemoreceptor trigger zone (CTZ) in the area postrema on the floor of the fourth ventricle. This, in turn, activates the vomiting center proper, which is a deeper structure. The emetic effects are markedly potentiated by stimulation of the vestibular apparatus, so ambulatory patients are much more likely to vomit than those patients who are lying quietly.
17. Generalized hypertonus of skeletal muscle can be produced by large intravenous doses of most opioid agonists. Although morphine can produce rigidity, the problem is most commonly associated with fentanyl, alfentanil, sufentanil, and remifentanil. In its most severe form, "lead pipe" muscle rigidity can totally prevent mechanical ventilation. There is very little loss of compliance when opioids are given to patients with tracheotomies, suggesting that the primary etiology is supraglottic obstruction from constriction of laryngeal and pharyngeal muscles.
18. At normal analgesic doses opioids produce modest cardiovascular effects. Bradycardia and peripheral vasodilatation are seen at higher doses and when opioids are combined with other anesthetic drugs. The combination of slow heart rate, peripheral vasodilatation, minimal myocardial effects, and preservation of autonomic function makes opioid-based anesthesia particularly useful for critically ill patients with cardiac ischemia or failure.
19. In dogs, rabbits, rats, and mice, exposure to brief periods of ischemia reduces the size of a myocardial infarct from a subsequent ischemic insult–so-called ischemic "preconditioning." Stimulation of δ opioid receptors appears to mediate both the acute and delayed phases of this effect, although various studies have implicated κ receptors as well.
20. Some opioids, particularly morphine and meperidine, produce a nonimmunologic release of histamine from tissue mast cells. This is most often seen as local itching, redness, or hives near the site of intravenous injection, signs that patients will often mistake for true allergy. Sometimes a patient will experience generalized flushing. If sufficient histamine is liberated, it may cause a short period of decreased systemic vascular resistance, hypotension, and tachycardia. The potent opioids fentanyl, sufentanil, alfentanil, and remifentanil do not release histamine.
21. Opioids decrease the passage of fluids and solids at every level of the GI tract–so-called opioid bowel dysfunction (OBD). They delay gastric emptying and increase antral tone, and these effects may slow the absorption of oral medications that are administered concomitantly. Food might not pass into the proximal jejunum for many hours, so surgical patients given opioids preoperatively may remain at risk for aspiration despite nominal NPO status. Chronic administration of opioids usually necessitates the administration of laxatives and stool softeners to treat constipation.
22. Opioids cause contraction of smooth muscle in the gall bladder and spasm of the sphincter of Oddi. In some individuals this can precipitate biliary colic.
23. Opioids increase the contractions of the ureter although they relieve the pain caused by ureteral stones. They also decrease detrusor contraction in response to bladder distension (the voiding reflex) and increase the tone of the urinary sphincter by both central and peripheral mechanisms.

24. Opioids have no specific teratogenic effects, but chronic opioid use by the mother can lead to physical dependence by the fetus. Neonatal withdrawal may occur shortly after delivery and in some instances may be life-threatening.
25. When tolerance to an opioid occurs, there is simultaneous development of *cross-tolerance* to all other opioid agonists. In general, tolerance develops most rapidly to the effects we have described as depressant (analgesia, ventilatory depression, euphoria), but much less tolerance occurs to some of the stimulant effects, like constipation or pupillary constriction.
26. Physical dependence is not the same thing as *psychological dependence* or *addiction,* which includes the dimension of compulsive drug-seeking behavior. The data of Porter and Jick suggest that addiction resulting from appropriate medical treatment is a very unusual event.
27. Morphine is the least lipophilic of the opioids, which has 2 important implications for its pharmacokinetics: morphine penetrates biologic membranes more slowly than lipophilic opioids, and it is less likely to accumulate in lipid membranes or fatty tissues. The plasma pharmacokinetics of morphine does *not* parallel its clinical effects. In spite of morphine's rapid distribution and elimination from plasma, the changes in brain concentration are small and delayed. As a result, the onset and offset of analgesia are slow.
28. Morphine 6-glucuronide (M6G), which may constitute 15% of total morphine metabolites, possesses morphine-like analgesic and respiratory depressant activity, although higher doses are required.
29. Meperidine is significantly more lipid soluble than morphine, although its plasma pharmacokinetics is similar. The onset of analgesic effect is faster than morphine, and the duration is shorter (2 to 3 h). Meperidine is rapidly *N*-demethylated to form normeperidine. Seizures have occurred in patients with renal failure (who could not excrete normeperidine) and in cancer patients who received high doses of meperidine over long periods of time.
30. Austin et al titrated meperidine to analgesic effect in postsurgical patients. For each individual, the change from no pain relief to excellent pain relief occurred over a very narrow range of plasma concentrations, and this level was fairly consistent over a 2-day period. In contrast, there was a large variability (400%) in meperidine requirement between individuals.
31 Meperidine (or one of its metabolites) inhibits SERT, the transporter mediating presynaptic reuptake of serotonin. Patients chronically taking nonselective monoamine oxidase inhibitors who are given meperidine may suffer a serotoninergic crisis manifested as clonus, agitation, hyperreflexia, and hyperthermia.
32. Hydromorphone is a hydrophilic drug with an octanol–water partition coefficient only slightly higher than morphine's. Its water solubility means that it can be prepared in concentrated solutions (up to 100 mg/mL) that are useful for highly tolerant patients or delivery with implanted infusion pumps. The low lipid solubility gives hydromorphone some of morphine's characteristics as a selective spinal analgesic.
33. Methadone is a long-lasting synthetic μ opioid approximately equipotent with morphine. Unlike most other opioids, methadone has very high oral bioavailability (approximately 80%). Repeated oral or parenteral doses may result in substantial accumulation; subsequent doses appear to last much longer than the initial dose.
34. Fentanyl is extremely fat soluble, which accounts for its rapid onset and relatively short duration. The effects of low doses (eg, 100-200 μg) are brief because they are terminated by rapid redistribution. After much higher doses (eg, >20 μg/kg) redistribution may be insufficient to bring plasma concentrations to subtherapeutic levels. In this circumstance, termination of effect depends on the much slower elimination process, and the drug appears long-acting.
35. Alfentanil is a slightly less potent congener of fentanyl and has an extremely rapid onset and short duration of effect. Peak analgesic and ventilatory depressant effects occur in less than 2 minutes, and the duration of the effects of small doses (10 μg/kg) may last only 15 minutes.
36. Sufentanil is a thienyl derivative of fentanyl that is more potent and even more fat soluble. Despite a terminal half-life of approximately 10 hours (longer than that of fentanyl and much longer than that of alfentanil), sufentanil has the shortest context-sensitive half-time of the 3 when given by infusion for up to 10 hours.
37. Pharmacodynamically, remifentanil is similar to the other fentanyl derivatives, but it has an extremely short duration of action due to rapid metabolic inactivation. It is hydrolyzed by nonspecific esterases primarily in skeletal muscle. The context-sensitive half-life is less than 5 minutes, regardless of the duration of the infusion. There is essentially no accumulation of remifentanil after infusions or repeated boluses. The ultrashort duration of this analgesic can be a drawback: patients who are expected to have postoperative pain will need a longer-acting opioid for pain relief. This should be administered *prior* to stopping remifentanil.
38. Clinically available preparations of tramadol contain the racemic mixture of 2 isomers. (+)-Tramadol is a weak agonist at μ receptors and an inhibitor of serotonin reuptake. It is also demethylated to yield a metabolite with greater μ opioid efficacy. (−)-Tramadol more selectively inhibits norepinephrine reuptake. The effects on neurotransmitter reuptake enhance inhibitory effects on pain transmission in the spinal cord.
39. The administration of opioids potentiates the hypnotic effects of barbiturates, benzodiazepines, and propofol. By reducing the amount of hypnotic administered, an opioid can sometimes produce more rapid emergence. The opioids also produce a dramatic, dose-related decrease in the need for volatile anesthetics, and they are frequently used for this specific purpose.
40. The amount of opioid analgesic required varies tremendously from patient to patient, so anesthetic "recipes" with a predetermined opioid dose are not advisable.
41. How does one titrate an opioid intraoperatively? Decreasing ventilatory rate and depth are not very sensitive measures of opioid effect, and they have never been validated as guides to dosing during surgery. More commonly, the rise in blood pressure and other autonomic responses to a "painful" stimulus are gauged. This requires good clinical judgment because autonomic responses are nonspecific and may be produced by many conditions that do not involve pain. Unlike the volatile anesthetics, the opioids do not produce graded cardiovascular depression as depth increases. Normal blood pressure does not necessarily mean that the anesthetic level is appropriate, because large overdoses of most opioids are well tolerated as long as ventilation is supported.
42. Naloxone acts as a competitive antagonist at all opioid receptors, but it has greatest affinity for μ receptors. Small doses of naloxone reliably reverse or prevent the effects of pure opioid agonists and most mixed agonist–antagonists. The block is reversible and competitive, so it can be overcome by additional agonist. The onset of antagonist effect is extremely rapid, but the duration of action is quite brief. An intravenous dose of 0.4 mg will usually antagonize morphine for less than 1 hour; increasing the dose does not increase the duration appreciably. With the exception of remifentanil, the duration of naloxone is shorter than the opioids it is used to antagonize.
43. The agonist–antagonist opioids are synthetic and semisynthetic analgesics that are structurally related to morphine. They have been used primarily for moderate to severe acute pain, although buprenorphine has now been approved for maintenance therapy in opioid addiction. All these compounds produce some degree of competitive antagonism to morphine and the other pure agonists.

44. Most of the clinically available agonist–antagonists bind to both μ and κ receptors, but they have different intrinsic activities at each site. Nalorphine, pentazocine, butorphanol, and nalbuphine produce analgesia and sedation by a partial agonist effect at μ receptors. All of them are competitive antagonists at μ receptors and therefore reverse the effects of morphine. Buprenorphine binds to μ receptors with extremely high affinity but has limited efficacy. When given alone, its effects are similar to those of morphine. When given after morphine, it competes with the full agonist and causes a reduction in opioid effect.
45. The subjective effects of buprenorphine are similar to morphine throughout the dose range. The κ-type agonists have been described as producing "apathetic sedation." Patients given pentazocine, nalbuphine, or butorphanol may experience floating and dissociation, but usually do not experience mood elevation. After analgesic doses these patients often appear extremely sedated, yet remain capable of surprisingly lucid conversation. With pentazocine, patients are increasingly likely to experience "weird" feelings, dysphoria, or even hallucinations as the dose is raised. These unpleasant effects occur less frequently with butorphanol or nalbuphine. Lack of a morphine-like mood effect makes these analgesics much less desirable for opioid addicts, and it is thought to be a key factor in their low abuse liability.
46. Nalbuphine and buprenorphine are strong antagonists, and they have been used clinically for this purpose. Administration of an opioid antagonist to an opioid-dependent patient will precipitate withdrawal, and this has occurred after therapeutic doses of pentazocine, nalbuphine, and buprenorphine.
47. There has been renewed interest in chronic sublingual administration of buprenorphine since 2002 when the FDA approved it for maintenance therapy of opioid addicts. To reduce the possibility that the buprenorphine will be diverted or abused during chronic maintenance, one formulation, Suboxone, combines buprenorphine with naloxone. In the event that a patient taking buprenorphine/naloxone presents for surgery, treatment of acute pain may present a significant problem. These patients are highly tolerant to opioids, and residual levels of the partial agonist may antagonize other opioids for a long time.

HISTORY AND CHEMISTRY

With perhaps the exception of ethanol, the opioids have enjoyed the longest history of use of any of the groups of medicinal agents. In 300 BC, Theophrastus wrote of the medicinal effects of the juice extracted from the poppy. This elixir was known to the Arabs and Chinese of medieval times and was described in the writings of Paracelsus in the 16th century. Morphine was isolated and purified from poppy extract in 1806 by Sertürner, and Wood's introduction of the hypodermic needle a half-century later enabled the parenteral administration of morphine. Based on his battlefield experiences, Beecher described, in 1946, the dramatically smaller morphine requirements in seriously wounded soldiers as compared with persons having elective surgery. His observations are now understood in terms of how stress and the humoral responses to stress modify intrinsic analgesic pathways.

Opioid analgesics are used in nearly every facet of modern anesthesia practice. They are used as premedicants or sedatives (Chapter 69), intravenous anesthetics (Chapter 43), postoperative analgesics (Chapter 72), intraspinal analgesics (Chapter 47), and in the management of chronic pain (Chapters 91 and 93). Unfortunately, they are also abused by patients (Chapter 24) and physicians (Chapter 95).

The initial suggestion that more than a single mechanism may be operative in opioid-mediated analgesia came in 1954, when Beecher and Lasagna reported that nalorphine had the characteristics of both an agonist and an antagonist. In the succeeding 2 decades, a number of agonists and antagonists were synthesized, permitting the description of 3 opioid receptor types by Martin in 1967. Goldstein hypothesized the existence of endogenous opioid compounds in 1970, and 3 years later, independent research teams led by Terenius, Snyder, and Simon identified stereospecific binding sites for opioids. Hughes, Kosterlitz, Goldstein, and their respective colleagues then isolated peptide molecules having morphine-like effects from brain and pituitary gland.

The term *narcotic* has long been used to describe morphine and related analgesics, but it is best avoided for the purposes of pharmacologic discussions. *Narcosis* implies sleep (which may certainly occur when opioids relieve pain), but opioids are not reliable hypnotics. Furthermore, under US law, a narcotic is any substance deemed likely to be abused, and the class includes such obviously "nonnarcotic" agents as amphetamine, cocaine, and marijuana. Morphine and codeine are *opiate* analgesics—naturally occurring alkaloids obtained from the juice of the poppy, *Papaver somniferum*. An *opioid* is any natural or synthetic compound that has effects similar to those of morphine or that acts as an antagonist at the same receptors to which morphine binds.

An opioid *agonist*, such as morphine or fentanyl, binds to one or more of the opioid receptors and elicits the typical response mediated by that receptor. The opioid *antagonists*, such as naloxone, are competitive, meaning they produce a block of opioid effect that is surmountable when a sufficient amount of agonist is present. Some clinically used opioids, such as buprenorphine, are *partial agonists*. Such drugs have lower efficacy than full agonists, even when given at extremely high doses. Their dose–response curves plateau at a lower maximal effect than do those of full agonists (**Fig. 42-1**A). In some circumstances a partial agonist may act like an antagonist: In the presence of a full dose of an agonist, the partial agonist may displace the agonist from its receptor binding sites and reduce the overall effect (Fig. 42-1B).

Because opioid agonists relieve pain, they are classified as analgesics. In contrast to the local anesthetics (which interrupt the transmission of

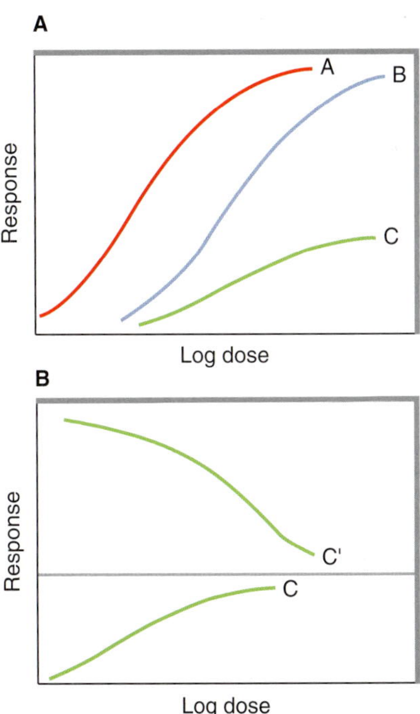

FIGURE 42-1. A. Idealized log dose–response curves for 2 agonists (*A* and *B*) and a partial agonist (*C*) with an intrinsic activity of approximately 0.4. **B.** Idealized log dose–response curve for the interaction of a partial agonist with a pure agonist. Curve (*C*), the partial agonist alone; curve (*C'*), increasing doses of the partial agonist in the presence of a high concentration of pure agonist. The final level of response is 0.4 × maximum. [Reproduced with permission from Rance MJ. Multiple opiate receptors–their occurrence and significance. *Clin Anaesthesiol.* 1983;1:183.]

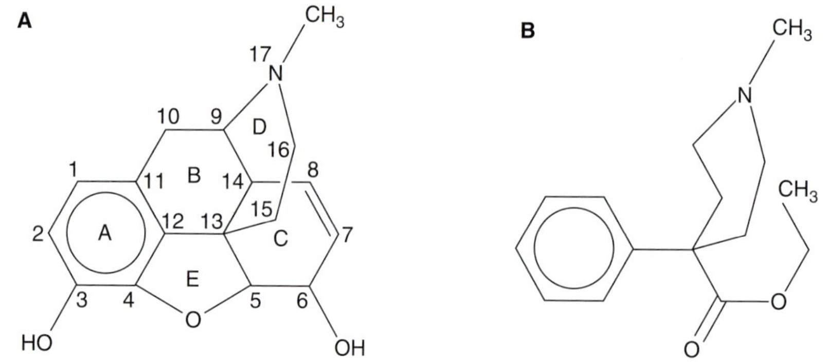

FIGURE 42-2. Structural formulas of (A) morphine and (B) meperidine.

all nerve impulses, including pain) and the anti-inflammatory analgesics such as aspirin (which decrease some of the pathologic processes leading to pain), the opioid analgesics act primarily to alter the perception of pain as a noxious entity. A patient's overall response to pain is a function of many simultaneous processes. These include the magnitude of the noxious stimulus, the patient's individual threshold for experiencing suffering in response to pain, what the patient anticipates will be the result of the noxious stimulus, and the presence or absence of agents (such as opioids) capable of modulating the integration of these processes. As we shall see, the opioid analgesics are also used to decrease "pain" responses in individuals who are unconscious.

Figure 42-2A shows the structure of morphine. It is a 5-ring molecule, 3 rings of which lie in 1 plane, whereas the other 2 (labeled *C* and *D*) lie nearly perpendicularly, forming a T shape. There are 2 hydroxyl groups (1 phenolic and 1 alcoholic), a quaternary carbon atom at position 13, and a piperidine ring with a methyl group on the nitrogen. Morphine is optically active, and only the levorotatory form is analgesically active. Codeine is morphine that has been *O*-methylated at position 3. The first semisynthetic opioids (heroin, hydromorphone) were made by simple substitution, but the morphine molecule may be much simplified while retaining opioid agonist activity. Meperidine (Fig. 42-2B) is a phenylpiperidine that contains only fragments of the original morphine structure. Fentanyl and its derivatives are anilidopiperidines, closely related to meperidine (**Fig. 42-3**). Note that when the piperidine ring is opened, the ensuing molecule is structurally analogous to tyrosine, the amino acid required to be in the terminal position for peptide opioid activity.

When the piperidine nitrogen has a bulkier chemical group (eg, allyl, cyclopropyl, cyclobutyl), the compound often takes on opioid antagonist properties. For example, the *N*-allyl derivatives of morphine and oxymorphone are the antagonists, nalorphine and naloxone, respectively.

OPIOID RECEPTORS

Four broad classes of opioid receptors are currently accepted, each encoded by a different gene. Most of the clinically important pharmacologic effects of opioid alkaloids are mediated by μ, κ, and δ receptors. The international names for these receptors are MOP, KOP, and DOP, but in this chapter we will use the Greek letter designations. The fourth receptor, called the nociceptin-orphanin FQ receptor (NOP), may also be involved in pain processing (see Endogenous Opioids). Older literature describes a σ receptor, but this is no longer considered to be a true opioid receptor.

Studies with knockout mice confirm that the "classic" pharmacologic effects of morphine, such as analgesia and ventilatory depression, are mediated by μ receptors. Other μ effects include sedation, euphoria, tolerance, and physical dependence; decreased gastrointestinal motility; biliary spasm; and miosis. Studies with selective agonists and antagonists support the concept that there are many subclasses of μ receptors,

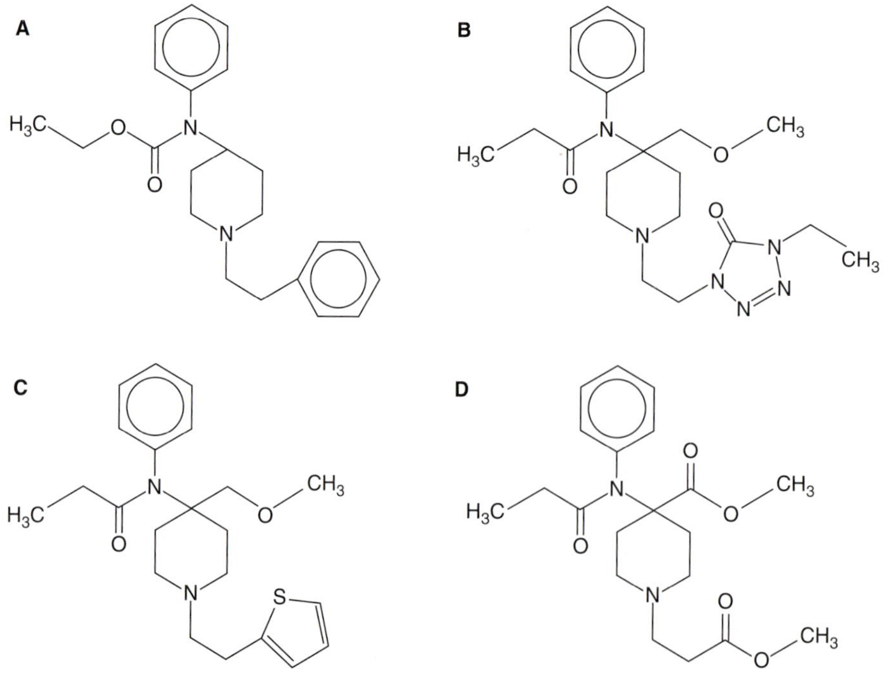

FIGURE 42-3. Structural formulas of (A) fentanyl, (B) alfentanil, (C) sufentanil, and (D) remifentanil.

and specific functions have been ascribed to a few of these subclasses. For example, ventilatory depression and spinal opioid analgesia are mediated by μ_2 receptors, whereas supraspinal analgesia is a μ_1-opioid effect.[1] A μ_3 receptor is found in vascular tissue and in leukocytes,[2] and it may have roles in vascular control and immunomodulation. For nearly 40 years since the original description of opioid receptors, researchers have been seeking a receptor-specific agonist that has greater analgesic efficacy or less toxicity than morphine. Despite the evaluation of hundreds of compounds, no such agent has been developed for clinical use.

All μ receptors are encoded by a single gene, denoted OPRM1, found on chromosome 6q24-q25 (**Fig 42-4**). Although genetic polymorphisms exist,[3] most receptor variants arise from posttranscriptional or posttranslational modifications.[1,4] The transcribed messenger ribonucleic acid (mRNA) may be modified by splicing or polyadenylation, whereas the receptor may be covalently modified by phosphorylation or conjugation to ubiquitin. More than 20 μ-receptor variants have been identified and cloned. This heterogeneity may explain why opioids have variable efficacy and toxicity in different patients, and it may also account for the fact that patients who are tolerant to the effects of one μ agonist can sometimes get relief with another.

There is a great deal of interest in the possibility that μ receptor single nucleotide polymorphisms (SNPs) will be found to explain much of the variability in opioid requirement. The most common SNP for the μ receptor is the substitution of guanine for adenine at position 118

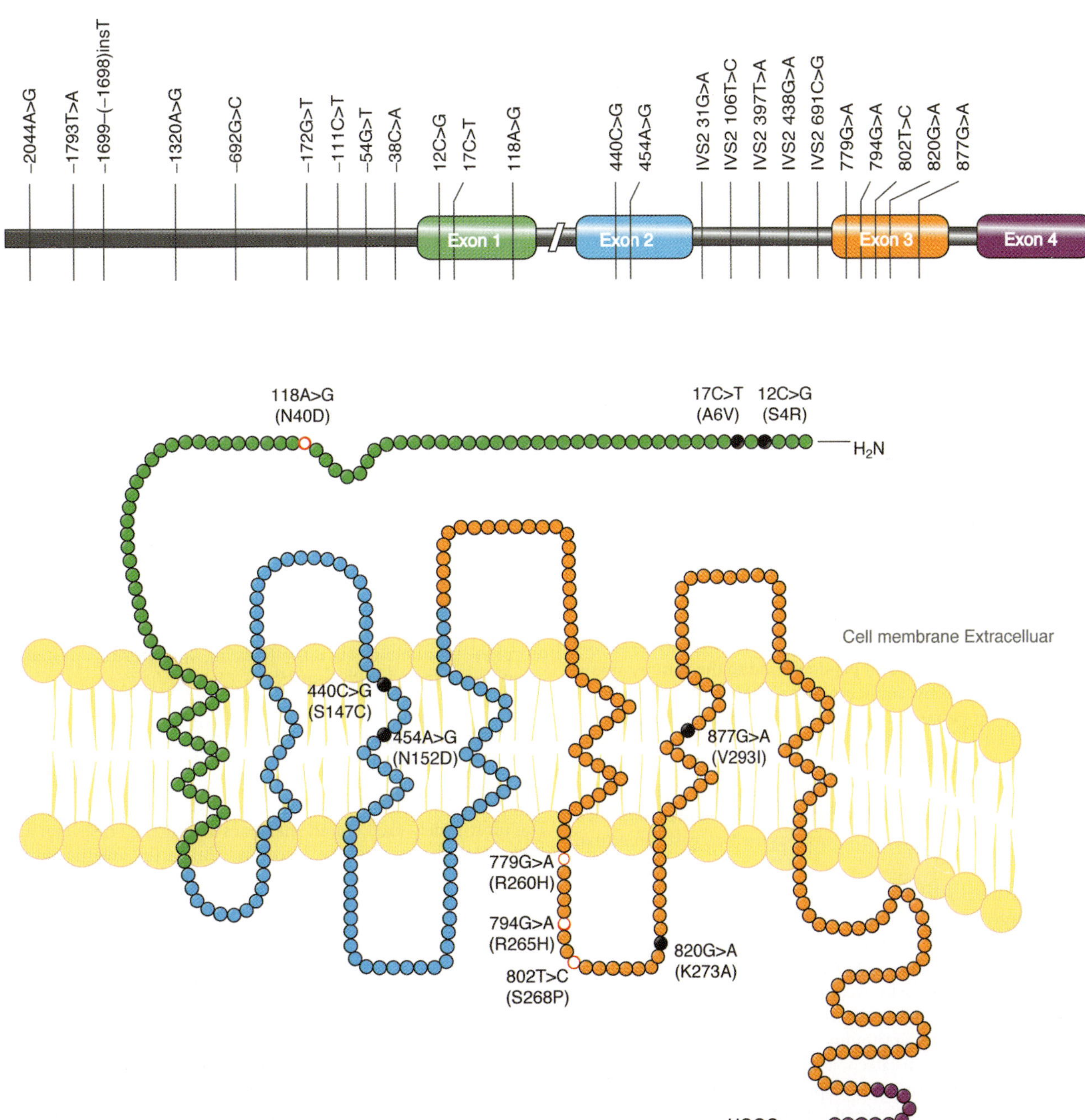

FIGURE 42-4. Structure of the *OPRM1* gene and the μ-opioid receptor. The amino acids are colored according to the 4 exons that encode them. Twenty-four mutations are each indicated by the nucleotide exchange and the resulting amino acid exchange. Black circles denote a naturally occurring mutation at that amino acid, and red circles indicate mutations where functional consequences have been demonstrated. The most frequent mutation is 118A>G, which causes an asparagine to aspartate substitution at position 40. [Modified with permission from Lötsch J, Geisslinger G. Are μ-opioid receptor polymorphisms important for clinical opioid therapy? *Trends Mol Med.* 2005;11:82-89.]

(A118G), causing a single amino acid change at position 40 in the peptide extracellular tail.[3] A rapidly growing body of animal and clinical studies suggest that homozygous substitution at this site may alter some effects of either morphine or morphine 6 glucuronide.[5-7] The clinical data, thus far, do not suggest any simple relationship between this SNP and any important opioid action.

The κ receptor shares a number of effects with the μ receptor, including analgesia, sedation, and ventilatory depression. It now appears that the ability of some opioids to cause dysphoria is caused by action at κ receptors. All κ receptors are encoded by a single gene that may theoretically produce at least 6 mRNA variants.[4] The κ receptors have been subdivided into several subclasses, 2 of which (κ_1 and κ_3) are relevant to opioid analgesics that are used clinically. The κ_1 receptor mediates spinal analgesia,[8] whereas activation of the κ_3 receptor results in supraspinal analgesia,[9] sedation, and ventilatory depression. The κ_3 receptor is the most prevalent opioid receptor in the brain.

The δ receptor is responsible for mediating some of the analgesic effects of the endogenous opioid peptides, especially in the spinal cord.[10,11] The majority of opioid receptors in myocardium appear to be δ, and this receptor may play a role in the phenomenon of ischemic preconditioning (discussed later). Only a few of the clinically used opioid alkaloids have significant affinity for δ receptors at usual analgesic doses. If a μ-selective opioid is administered in a sufficiently high dose (to treat a tolerant patient, for example), the drug may be less selective and produce significant δ effects.

All opioid receptors are G-protein coupled receptors. All have 7 transmembrane domains and significant structural homology. The actions of both μ and δ agonists result in overall neuronal depression, and they share several signal transduction mechanisms, including inhibition of adenylyl cyclase, activation of K^+ currents, and suppression of Ca^{2+} currents. The ability of opioids to inhibit inward calcium currents in presynaptic neurons limits the release of various neurotransmitters, including putative pain transmitters like substance P. Opening of the inwardly rectifying K^+ channel serves to hyperpolarize postsynaptic neuronal membranes and reduce their responsiveness. Other mechanisms have been demonstrated, including stimulation of phospholipase C[12] and mitogen-activated protein kinase,[13] as well as blockade of L-type calcium channels. The κ receptor elicits similar cellular responses,[12,14] and it may also block N-type calcium channels.[15]

ENDOGENOUS OPIOIDS

Five families of endogenous opioid peptides bind to the various opioid receptors. The peptides show some binding selectivity, but there is no consistent association between a peptide family and a particular receptor mechanism. In 4 of the families, large precursor polypeptide molecules are cleaved to yield several opioid (and some nonopioid) peptides. Although some of these peptides undoubtedly function in nociceptive pathways, they also appear to play fundamental roles in processes such as thermoregulation and hormone release, as well as gastrointestinal and cardiovascular control.

1. The *enkephalins* are pentapeptides derived from proenkephalin A. Each molecule of proenkephalin contains 4 sequences of met-enkephalin (Tyr-Gly-Gly-Phe-Met), 1 copy of leu-enkephalin (Tyr-Gly-Gly-Phe-Leu), and some slightly larger enkephalin-like peptides. The enkephalins are moderately selective for δ receptors and probably act as neurotransmitters released from short interneurons within the spinal cord and brainstem. They are found in the adrenal medulla and in nerve terminals that contain catecholamines. Enkephalins (and exogenous opioids) bind to presynaptic opioid receptors on nociceptive neurons and modulate the release of various pain neurotransmitters. The naturally occurring enkephalins are hydrolyzed extremely rapidly by peptidases in plasma. Stable analogues of the enkephalins have been synthesized, permitting in vivo experiments on their actions.
2. *Prodynorphin* (also called proenkephalin B) contains the sequences for dynorphin A and dynorphin B. The dynorphins show selectivity for the κ receptor. Their distribution is similar to that of the enkephalins. The 5 amino acids at the *N*-terminus of the dynorphins are identical in sequence to leu-enkephalin.
3. Proopiomelanocortin (POMC) contains a multitude of opioid and nonopioid peptides and is found in high concentrations in the anterior pituitary gland and the hypothalamus. The *N*-terminus of POMC is identical to met-enkephalin, although POMC is not cleaved to yield met-enkephalin. The final 31 amino acids form β-endorphin, the most important of the humoral endogenous opioids and an important endogenous ligand at the μ receptor. In addition, selective cleavage of POMC yields many nonopioid hormones, including adrenocorticotropic hormone (ACTH), several varieties of melanocyte-stimulating hormone (MSH), and the lipotropins.
4. *Proorphanin* is cleaved to orphanin FQ (also called nociceptin), a peptide containing 17 amino acids. Although proorphanin has significant sequence homology with the other 3 parent opioid peptides, orphanin FQ does not bind to μ, κ, or δ receptors. It binds to a G-protein coupled receptor (NOP) and causes cellular responses similar to other opioids, including inhibition of adenylyl cyclase, opening of the inwardly rectifying potassium channel, and blockade of N-type calcium channels.[16] Orphanin FQ is found in unusual places like hippocampus and sensory cortex. It has a supraspinal antianalgesic effect while producing spinal analgesia. The possible roles for this system in pain modulation, learning, and drug reward are topics for much current research.
5. The *endomorphins* appear to be endogenous agonists that have high affinity and high selectivity for the μ receptor. A precursor molecule for the endomorphins has not yet been identified. The tetrapeptide Tyr-Pro-Trp-Phe-NH_2 is called endomorphin-1, and a related peptide, Tyr-Pro-Phe-Phe-NH_2, is called endomorphin-2.[17] In vivo studies suggest that endomorphin-1 acts via stimulation of μ_2 receptors. Endomorphin-2 is less specific, acting at both μ and κ receptors. These peptides have both in vitro and in vivo cardiovascular effects. They decrease spontaneous neuronal discharge in the rostral ventrolateral medulla (RVLM), an area important in the central control of blood pressure. Peripherally, they decrease norepinephrine release from vascular sympathetic neurons.

There is some evidence that mammals have the ability to synthesize morphine from tyrosine precursors, using apparently the same reaction scheme as the opium poppy.[18] The significance of endogenous morphine is unknown, but it is interesting that arthritic rats make more morphine than do healthy ones.[19]

OPIOID AGONISTS

GENERAL PROPERTIES

The most widely used opioid analgesics are pure agonists that are relatively selective for μ-opioid receptors. Unlike the volatile anesthetics, opioid agonists produce a group of highly specific depressant and stimulant effects by acting at discrete sites within the central nervous system. For example, morphine stimulates the vagal nuclei in the medulla while depressing ventilatory centers only a few millimeters away. The opioids consistently depress cellular function, so it should be understood that a "stimulant" effect is produced by depression of inhibitory neurons. **Box 42-1** lists the acute and chronic effects of opioids.

Given their common mechanism of action, it is easy to see why morphine, meperidine, fentanyl, and the fentanyl congeners have very similar pharmacodynamic effects. The few qualitative differences between them (eg, histamine release) usually do not involve opioid receptor mechanisms. The various opioids differ greatly in their physicochemical properties, as well as in speed of onset and duration of action, so the clinical selection of an opioid is usually based on pharmacokinetic considerations and the desired route of administration. Opioid pharmacokinetics will be considered later in the discussion of specific agonist drugs.

BOX 42-1

Acute and Chronic Effects of Opioids

Acute

Analgesia
Ventilatory depression
Sedation
Euphoria
Vasodilatation
Bradycardia
Cough suppression
Miosis
Nausea and vomiting
Skeletal muscle rigidity
Smooth muscle spasm
- Constipation
- Urinary retention
- Biliary spasm

Chronic

Tolerance
Physical dependence

TABLE 42-1 Dose, Time to Peak Effect, and Duration of Analgesia for Intravenous Opioid Agonists and Agonist-Antagonists[a]

Opioid	Dose (mg)[b]	Peak (min)	Duration (h)[c]
Morphine	10	>30	3-4
Meperidine	80	5-7	2-3
Hydromorphone	1.5	10-20	2-3
Oxymorphone	1	10-20	2-3
Methadone	10	5-10	(see text)
Tramadol[d]	100	<30	4-6
Fentanyl	0.1	3-5	0.5-1
Sufentanil	0.01	3-5	0.5-1
Alfentanil	0.75	1.5-2	0.2-0.3
Remifentanil	0.1	1.5-2	0.1-0.2
Pentazocine	60	15-20	2-3
Butorphanol	2	15-20	2-3
Nalbuphine	10	15-20	3-4
Buprenorphine	0.3	<30	5-6

[a]Data for fentanyl derivatives are derived from intraoperative studies, the remainder from postoperative pain studies.

[b]Approximately equianalgesic doses (see text).

[c]Average duration of first, single dose. Value is highly dose-dependent.

[d]Intravenous tramadol is not available in the United States.

CNS Effects

Analgesia and Mood Effects The opioids produce selective relief of pain at doses that do not produce sleep or impair sensation. Opioid analgesic effects result from actions at several different levels of the neuraxis. The processing of pain information is inhibited by a direct spinal effect at the dorsal horn; the rostrad transmission of pain signals is decreased by activation of descending inhibitory pathways in the brainstem[20]; finally, the emotional response to pain is altered by opioid actions on the limbic cortex. Opioids also act at receptors located peripherally on sensory and smooth muscle motor neurons.[21]

Opioids affect both the perception of pain and the response to pain, but it is difficult to make the distinction in most clinical circumstances. Patients given morphine will typically report that pain is still present, but the intensity is decreased and it no longer bothers them as much. The relief of pain and anxiety will often result in sleep, but sometimes mood elevation or frank euphoria can occur. The euphoriant effect or sense of well-being produced by opioid agonists is thought to be one of the most important reasons for their abuse.

Sufficient doses of opioids will relieve almost any pain, although some types of pain are typically more responsive than others. Prolonged, burning pain, for example, is more effectively blunted than the brief, sharp pain of an incision. Neuropathic pain (eg, pain of nerve root compression) can be very resistant to opioid treatment.[22,23] Because many chronic pain states involve neuropathic pain, there has been a great deal of debate about the appropriate role for opioids in these conditions.[24] Opioids are highly effective for the acute pain states encountered perioperatively. Intraoperatively, the opioids can produce sufficient analgesia to reduce or abolish autonomic and somatic responses to surgical stimuli. In this circumstance, they are almost always combined with other central nervous system depressants (see discussion on Intraoperative Use of Opioids).

Table 42-1 lists some commonly used opioid agonists along with their recommended doses and durations of action. The relative potencies of most older opioids have been determined in postoperative pain, whereas those for the fentanyl series are from intraoperative studies. The doses in the table are for comparison only, and the actual doses given during administration of anesthesia will vary greatly depending on the application. Several of the opioids have active metabolites that accumulate over time, so their relative potencies and oral-to-parenteral dose ratios may change significantly when repeated doses are given. For this reason, the doses recommended for patients with chronic cancer pain can sometimes be different from the doses used during surgery. "Equianalgesic" doses can also be very difficult to determine when bolus doses of opioids with very different analgesic time-effect curves are being compared. For example, fentanyl is often stated to have 80 to 100 times the potency of morphine, a figure that takes into account both the intensity and duration of effect (ie, the area under the time-effect curve is measured). If one considered only the peak intensity of effect, fentanyl might appear to be 200 times more potent than morphine (**Fig. 42-5**). Because the anesthesiologist is typically concerned with the peak analgesic and toxic effects following an intravenous bolus, the latter estimate might be more useful.

Sedation–Hypnosis In usual analgesic doses, morphine-like drugs may produce drowsiness, feelings of heaviness, and difficulty concentrating. Unlike benzodiazepines, opioids do not usually produce anterograde amnesia. At higher doses sedation becomes more pronounced, and, eventually, hypnosis may occur. Doses of opioids that are sufficient to produce apnea and profound analgesia do not reliably produce unconsciousness in healthy individuals.[25] The use of opioids alone to produce

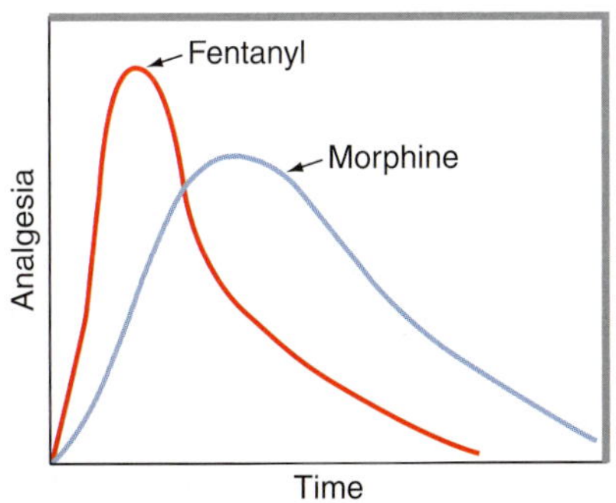

FIGURE 42-5. Idealized time-effect curves for fentanyl and morphine. Estimated potency of fentanyl is higher if only peak analgesia is considered and duration ignored (see text).

both hypnosis and analgesia has resulted in numerous cases of intraoperative awareness. Hypnosis is much more likely to occur in elderly or debilitated patients or in those given small doses of benzodiazepines.[26] High doses of morphine, fentanyl, or its congeners produce a cortical electroencephalogram (EEG) pattern that is superficially similar to deep sleep.[27] The average frequency decreases, and large-amplitude delta waves predominate. Unlike the intravenous or inhaled anesthetics, even very high doses of opioids will not produce EEG burst suppression.

CNS Toxicity Dysphoria and agitation occur infrequently after analgesic doses of most opioids, although their incidence is thought to be higher with meperidine and codeine. In laboratory animals, extremely high doses of morphine or fentanyl can produce seizure activity, but this does not occur at the concentrations achieved in clinical practice.[28] Opioid-induced hypertonus of skeletal muscle (see Muscle Rigidity) can sometimes lead to myoclonic limb movements that have been mistaken for seizures. True seizures have been reported after repeated doses of meperidine because its major metabolite, normeperidine, is a potent convulsant.[29] (see Specific Drugs).

Administration of opioids can raise cerebrospinal fluid pressure if ventilation is not controlled and $Paco_2$ is allowed to rise. Opioid premedication should generally be avoided when elevated intracranial pressure (ICP) is suspected; ICP may rise further, and the opioid effects may mask changing neurologic signs. These drugs are very useful, however, during induction of anesthesia in neurosurgical patients. When ventilation is controlled, fentanyl and sufentanil have little effect on cerebral metabolic rate and blood flow, and therefore do not increase ICP.[30,31]

Ventilatory Depression Opioids produce a dose-related depression of the ventilatory response to CO_2 (actually, hydrogen ion concentration).[32] This occurs, in part, by a direct effect on μ receptors expressed in and around the pre-Bötzinger complex, a small area in the ventrolateral medulla that mediates inspiratory rhythm.[33] Morphine also blunts the response to hypoxia.[34] In an awake subject given an analgesic dose of morphine, the intercept of the CO_2 response curve is shifted to the right, and (depending on the measurement technique) there may also be a decrease in slope (**Fig. 42-6**). Both the rate and the rhythm of breathing are affected: As the dose of opioid is increased, ventilatory rate will slow, but the effect of this may be partially offset by an increase in tidal volume. It is important to remember that a decrease in ventilatory rate is not a very sensitive indicator of opioid effect. A patient's drive to breathe may be abnormal despite an apparently normal ventilatory rate and state of consciousness. Sleep will further depress the response to CO_2 and potentiate the ventilatory depression caused by opioids.[35]

At usual analgesic doses, the opioids do not usually cause clinically significant ventilatory depression unless there is preexisting pathology (such as hypothyroidism or pulmonary or CNS disease) or concomitant administration of CNS depressant drugs (alcohol, general anesthetics, or benzodiazepines). Volunteers with obstructive sleep apnea (OSA) who were given infusions of remifentanil actually had fewer obstructive episodes, possibly because the opioid decreased the amount of time spent in REM sleep. However, remifentanil significantly increased the risk for central apneic episodes in these subjects.[36] In most cases, perioperative use of longer-acting opioid analgesics in patients with OSA will warrant increased respiratory monitoring.[37,38]

Very large doses of opioids eventually cause inadequate ventilation. Breathing may become irregular or even take on a Cheyne-Stokes pattern. There may be striking inattention to breathing: Otherwise responsive patients may hypoventilate to the point of cyanosis unless they are reminded to breathe. Ventilatory depression is, of course, the major toxicity of opioids and nearly always the cause of death from overdose.

Equianalgesic doses of all opioids produce equivalent amounts of ventilatory depression. There is no convincing evidence that any analgesic is more or less dangerous than morphine in this regard. Despite experimental evidence that analgesia and ventilatory depression may be mediated by different receptor subtypes (μ_1 and μ_2, respectively), no highly selective agonist or antagonist has been developed for clinical use.[1]

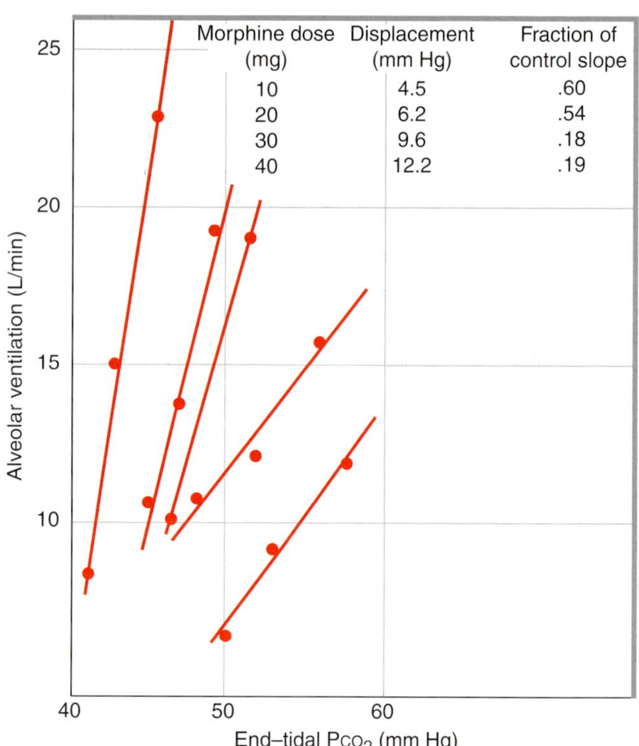

FIGURE 42-6. CO_2 response curves from 1 subject who received 4 doses of morphine 10 mg intravenously at 40-minute intervals. [Reprinted with permission from Keats AS. The effect of drugs on respiration in man. *Ann Rev Pharmacol Toxicol.* 1985;25:41.]

Both analgesia and ventilatory depression are reduced by administration of an opioid antagonist or by the development of opioid tolerance. This has 2 important clinical implications:

1. Tolerant individuals who require large amounts of opioid for relief of pain are not at proportionately increased risk of ventilatory depression.
2. It is very difficult to reverse ventilatory depression without reversing some analgesia (see Naloxone). A recent clinical study found that an experimental glutamate (AMPA) modulator could selectively reverse alfentanil-induced ventilatory depression without affecting analgesia.[33]

A number of case reports have described "recurrent" or "delayed" ventilatory depression after administration of anesthetics with fentanyl or alfentanil. Becker et al[39] showed that CO_2 sensitivity could recover after fentanyl-N_2O anesthesia, only to decline once again over the next hour (**Fig. 42-7**). It is likely that these events are actually caused by varying levels of stimulation. Opioid-induced ventilatory depression can be antagonized by pain and the many types of stimulation that occur during emergence and transfer to the recovery area; depression may reappear when the patient is allowed to go back to sleep.

Cough Suppression Opioids depress putative cough centers in the medulla. This effect involves different receptor mechanisms than those mediating analgesia, because weak analgesics such as codeine may be effective cough suppressants. The molecular modification that selectively increases antitussive potency is replacement of the 3-hydroxyl group on morphine with a bulkier group. Thus cough suppression is strong with heroin (3-acetoxy) and codeine (3-methoxy), but weak with meperidine (no functional group). For many years, cough has been treated with stereoisomers of opioids (eg, dextromethorphan) that have no analgesic activity. Recently, questions have been raised about the clinical effectiveness of these compounds.[40]

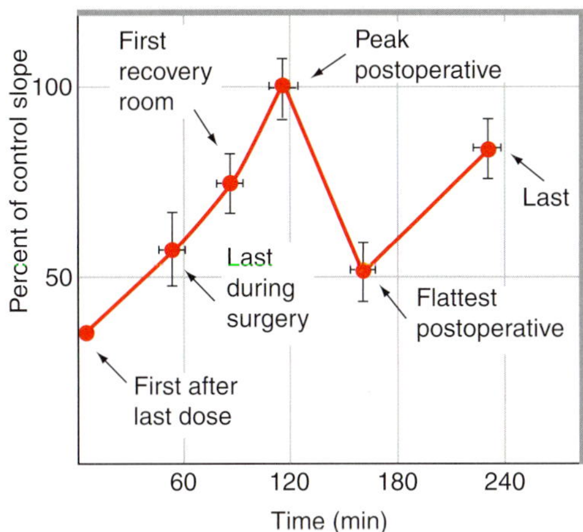

FIGURE 42-7. Recurrent ventilatory depression expressed as slope of CO_2 response curve (percentage of awake control) versus time. First data point obtained after last intraoperative dose of fentanyl. Response recovered, then subsequently declined when patients were no longer stimulated (see text). [Reproduced with permission from Becker LD, Paulson BA, Miller RD, et al. Biphasic respiratory depression after fentanyl-droperidol or fentanyl alone used to supplement nitrous oxide anesthesia. *Anesthesiology.* 1976;44:291.]

Pupillary Constriction Opioids stimulate the Edinger-Westphal nucleus of the oculomotor nerve to produce miosis.[41] The pinpoint pupil is a pathognomonic sign of opioid overdose (unless hypoxia is severe enough to produce mydriasis). Miosis is rapidly reversed with naloxone. Because it is easily measured, it has proven to be a sensitive method for experimental modeling of opioid effect.[42-44] Pupil constriction is maximal after relatively small opioid doses, so it is not a very useful way to grade the intensity of opioid effect. Absence of miosis, however, strongly suggests absence of opioid effect.

Nausea and Vomiting Opioids produce complex effects on vomiting centers in the medulla (**Fig. 42-8**). There is direct stimulation of the chemoreceptor trigger zone (CTZ) in the area postrema on the floor of the fourth ventricle. This, in turn, activates the vomiting center proper, which is a deeper structure.[45] The emetic effects are markedly potentiated by stimulation of the vestibular apparatus, so ambulatory patients are much more likely to vomit than those patients who are lying quietly. Postoperatively, patients frequently become nauseated when they have to move from stretcher to bed. The dose–response for emesis is not straightforward, because patients given very high doses of fentanyl (eg, during cardiac surgery) do not typically vomit. Costello and Borison[46] have shown in animals that high doses of opioids can actually block emesis by depressing the vomiting center proper. It is not clear at which dose a given opioid becomes antiemetic.

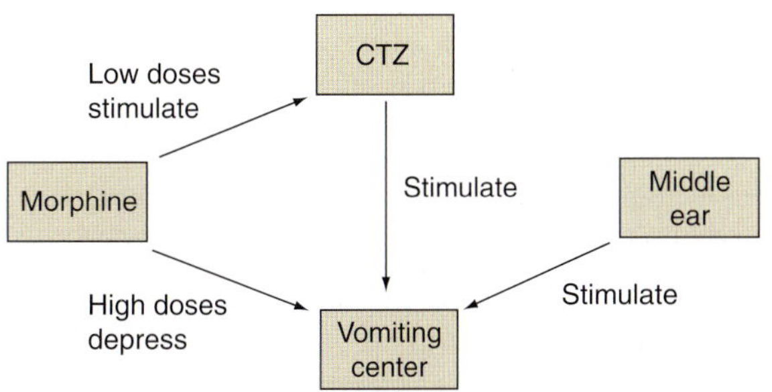

FIGURE 42-8. Mechanisms of opioid-induced nausea and vomiting (see text for details). [Reproduced with permission from Rosow CE. Newer synthetic opioid analgesics. In: Smith G, Covino BG, eds. *Acute Pain*. London, UK: Butterworths; 1985:74.]

Tolerance can occur to the emetic effects, but treatment with antagonists such as naloxone may often elicit more nausea and vomiting. These effects involve complex interactions of dopaminergic, cholinergic, and serotonergic mechanisms, and no single type of antiemetic has proven to be highly specific for opioid-induced nausea and vomiting.

Muscle Rigidity The opioids have no significant effects on nerve conduction, neuromuscular transmission, or the skeletal muscle membrane. In animals they produce some depression of monosynaptic and polysynaptic spinal reflexes, but the clinical relevance of this is probably minimal. A much more important effect is the generalized hypertonus of skeletal muscle, which can be produced by large intravenous doses of most opioid agonists. Although morphine can produce rigidity, the problem is most commonly associated with fentanyl, alfentanil, sufentanil, and remifentanil.

This effect was called "chest wall rigidity" because it was originally thought to be restricted to the abdominal and thoracic musculature. It is now known that all striated muscle—including muscles of the neck and extremities—can be involved.[47] The incidence and severity of the problem are greatest when high doses are infused rapidly, but rigidity can occur with doses of only 1 to 2 μg/kg of fentanyl. It usually occurs during induction of anesthesia, just at loss of consciousness. When very large amounts of opioid have been administered (eg, for cardiac surgery), rigidity may occur on emergence. It is thought more likely to happen in older patients and when nitrous oxide is administered (although evidence for this is largely anecdotal).[48]

In its most severe form, "lead pipe" muscle rigidity can totally prevent mechanical ventilation. Substantial amounts of positive pressure are sometimes needed for effective ventilation, which can lead to decreased venous return, gastric insufflation, and so forth. Such rigidity is substantially mitigated by pretreatment with midazolam or diazepam (and to a lesser degree with thiopental). There is very little loss of compliance when opioids are given to patients with tracheotomies, suggesting that the primary etiology is supraglottic obstruction from constriction of laryngeal and pharyngeal muscles.[49]

Opioids are believed to produce rigidity by actions at μ receptors in the striatum. Opioids increase the rate of striatal dopamine biosynthesis and inhibit the release of the inhibitory neurotransmitter γ-aminobutyric acid (GABA).[50] Antagonism of this effect on GABA may account for the beneficial effects of sedative–hypnotics. In the rat, microinjection of opioid antagonists at certain raphe nuclei will selectively block rigidity.[51]

Cardiovascular Effects At normal analgesic doses opioids produce modest cardiovascular effects. Bradycardia and peripheral vasodilatation are seen at higher doses and when opioids are combined with other anesthetic drugs.

Opioids selective for μ receptors (eg, fentanyl) produce bradycardia by a direct action on the central nuclei of the vagus nerves. In animals, microinjection of naloxone at these central sites antagonizes the bradycardia, but not the analgesia, produced by intravenous fentanyl.[52] The opioid-induced increase in vagal tone leads to a prolongation of atrioventricular (AV) conduction. There is also evidence of a direct depressant effect on the sinoatrial (SA) node.[53] In the dog there are abundant enkephalins in myocardium, and these appear to modulate vagal transmission by binding to large numbers of presynaptic δ receptors in AV and SA nodal tissue.[54] Morphine and fentanyl decrease central sympathetic tone, which raises the threshold for ventricular fibrillation in the dog.[55]

Bradycardia is most likely to occur when large doses of opioids are administered rapidly. It may be prevented or reversed by atropine, pancuronium, and other vagolytic drugs. Opioid-induced bradycardia may be more frequent when a relaxant such as vecuronium is used because it lacks vagal blocking effects. Meperidine, which is weakly atropinic, does not usually cause bradycardia.

Opioids produce peripheral vasodilatation by depressing vasomotor centers in the medulla. Analgesic doses frequently cause orthostatic hypotension, and higher doses may significantly reduce venous return.

The peripheral vascular effects involve both resistance and capacitance vessels.[56] Zelis showed that an analgesic dose of morphine increases blood flow through forearm skeletal muscle without altering systemic pressure.[57] This effect is thought to represent a centrally mediated lysis of sympathetic tone. In dogs, decreases in skeletal muscle vascular resistance produced by either morphine[58] or sufentanil[59] are neurally mediated and markedly increased under conditions of high sympathetic activity. These experimental findings are consistent with clinical observations that opioids are more apt to cause hypotension in patients with conditions that elevate the baseline level of sympathetic tone (eg, hypovolemia, coronary artery disease, congestive failure).

A number of studies suggest that opioids may have a direct action on vascular smooth muscle, but the clinical significance of this effect is unclear. Morphine, but not enkephalin analogues, can bind to a μ_3 receptor on arterial endothelial cells and cause vasodilatation by releasing nitric oxide.[2] When large doses of morphine are administered, some vasodilatation may be caused by the release of histamine.

Venodilation may lead to significant pooling of blood, especially in the splanchnic vasculature.[60] There is evidence in the dog that morphine causes blood to be sequestered in hepatic sinusoids.[61] In both humans and animals, opioid-induced venodilation seems to occur later and last longer than the effect on arterioles.[56,62]

At clinically relevant concentrations, the opioids do not produce significant myocardial depression, and they do not block α or β adrenergic receptors. Unlike the volatile anesthetics, morphine does not block arteriolar constriction in response to sympathetic nerve stimulation or circulating catecholamines.[63] Fentanyl, even when combined with a benzodiazepine, does not block high- or low-pressure baroreceptor responses.[64] The combination of slow heart rate, peripheral vasodilatation, minimal myocardial effects, and preservation of autonomic reflexes makes opioid-based anesthesia particularly useful for critically ill patients with cardiac ischemia or failure. When hypotension does occur, it frequently responds to simple measures such as administration of intravenous fluids.

A growing literature indicates that opioids may either mimic or play a complex physiologic role in various mechanisms that protect the heart from ischemic insults:

- In dogs, rabbits, rats, and mice, exposure to brief periods of ischemia reduces the size of a myocardial infarct from a subsequent ischemic insult—so-called ischemic preconditioning. Stimulation of δ opioid receptors appears to mediate both the acute and delayed phases of this effect, although various studies have implicated κ receptors as well.[65,66] The opioid effect occurs by activation of protein kinase C and by activation of mitochondrial ATP-regulated potassium channels (K_{ATP}), a signaling pathway that attenuates oxidant stress and cell death in cardiomyocytes.[67] The possibility that opioids may produce a cardioprotective effect in patients was investigated by Murphy et al, who administered morphine or fentanyl before bypass in patients undergoing coronary artery bypass grafting (CABG).[68] These investigators found a postoperative improvement in global ventricular function after morphine, but not fentanyl. Compared with morphine, fentanyl has less affinity for δ opioid receptors and less ability to activate the K_{ATP} channel.
- Opioids can also confer protection by a "postconditioning" effect that occurs when opioids are given during reperfusion. The mechanism may also involve δ and κ receptors.[69-71] It is much less clear that opioids are protective when they are administered after the ischemic insult has occurred. A dog model indicates that κ agonists can actually cause ventricular dysfunction if they are administered after myocardial stunning.[72]
- Finally, it appears that κ opioid receptors may be involved in the phenomenon of "remote preconditioning."[73] Repeated occlusion of the femoral artery can confer myocardial protection in rats undergoing subsequent coronary artery ligation. This effect is mimicked by a κ opioid agonist and blocked by a κ antagonist. δ Receptors do not appear to be involved.

Histamine Release True allergic responses to opioids are very rare, and only 1 or 2 cases of anaphylaxis to fentanyl and meperidine have been reported. Some opioids, particularly morphine and meperidine, produce a nonimmunologic release of histamine from circulating basophils and tissue mast cells. This is most often seen as local itching, redness, or urticaria near the site of intravenous injection, signs that patients often mistake for true allergy. Sometimes a patient will experience generalized flushing. If sufficient histamine is liberated, it may cause a short period of decreased systemic vascular resistance, hypotension, and tachycardia.[74] The cardiovascular effects (but not the histamine release) may be prevented by pretreatment with H_1 and H_2 antagonists such as chlorpheniramine and cimetidine.[75]

The histamine release is a nonspecific effect that depends on competitive displacement of the amine by opioid molecules. Mast cell degranulation is more likely to occur in some sites (eg, skin) than others (lung, gastrointestinal [GI] tract).[76] Because highly potent opioids expose tissue mast cells to lower opioid concentrations, they are less likely to cause release. The potent opioids fentanyl, sufentanil, alfentanil, and remifentanil do not release histamine.[77,78] Chemical structure also influences this process, because even equimolar concentrations of fentanyl and morphine do not cause equivalent histamine release.[79]

Histamine release does not usually cause bronchospasm, but opioids should still be used with great care in patients with asthma. Opioids may exacerbate preexisting bronchospasm by depressing cough and ventilatory drive and by drying airway secretions.

Pruritus Patients given opioids frequently complain of itching and warmth over the neck and face, especially over the malar area. Neuraxial administration of opioids (especially intrathecal) can often produce very troublesome generalized itching.[80] This effect is an opioid receptor–mediated dysesthesia, and it can be produced by opioids such as fentanyl that do not release histamine. The itching is not antagonized by antihistamines, but it may be reversed with opioid antagonists.

Smooth Muscle Effects

Intestine and Stomach Opioids decrease the passage of fluids and solids at every level of the GI tract—so-called opioid bowel dysfunction (OBD). They delay gastric emptying and increase antral tone, and these effects may slow the absorption of oral medications that are administered concomitantly. Food may not pass into the proximal jejunum for many hours, so surgical patients given opioids preoperatively may remain at risk for aspiration despite nominal NPO status. Chronic administration of opioids usually necessitates the administration of laxatives and stool softeners to treat constipation. Some of the agonist–antagonist opioids are less likely to cause this effect. OBD can be reversed or prevented by the use of opioid antagonists that act peripherally (see Methylnaltrexone).

The constipating effect is caused by a combination of decreased intestinal fluid production and increased fluid absorption as the passage of intestinal contents is delayed. Opioids decrease GI secretory activity by direct effects on intestinal secretory cells and by modulation of sympathetic transmission in the enteric nervous system. The decrease in GI motility involves both CNS effects and peripheral actions on opioid receptors in the bowel.[81] In the small bowel, there is initial stimulation of activity followed by atony. The stimulation produces segmenting, nonpropulsive contractions that prolong intestinal transit time. Opioids increase GI sphincter tone and cause an increase in colonic tone. The increase in resting colonic tone is especially pronounced in patients with ulcerative colitis, and opioids may predispose these patients to the development of toxic megacolon.

Opioids may also be used therapeutically in the treatment of diarrheal syndromes. Treatment of diarrhea is usually accomplished with orally administered drugs such as diphenoxylate or loperamide. Therapeutic doses of these drugs do not usually produce central effects because they are poorly absorbed, and loperamide is actively pumped from the CNS by P-glycoprotein (P-gp), an energy-dependent transporter molecule responsible for the efflux of many cationic compounds out of cells.[82]

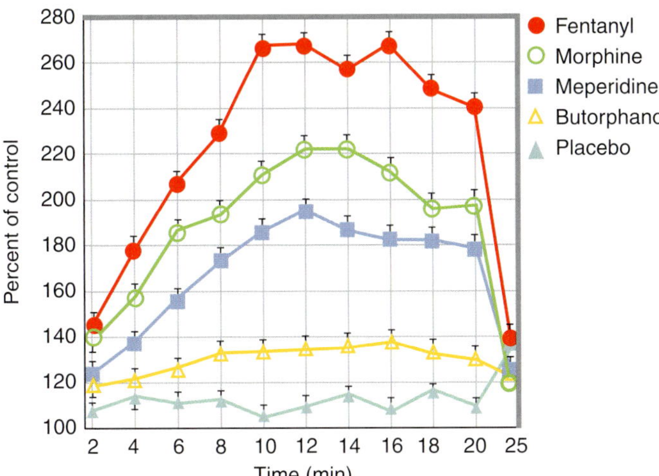

FIGURE 42-9. Percentage change in common bile duct pressure versus time following equianalgesic doses of several opioids. Patients were undergoing cholecystectomy with basal enflurane anesthesia. After 20 minutes, the effect was reversed by naloxone. [Reproduced with permission from Radnay PA, Duncalf D, Novakovic M, et al. Common bile duct pressure changes after fentanyl, morphine, meperidine, butorphanol and naloxone. *Anesth Analg.* 1984;63:441.]

Biliary System Opioids cause contraction of smooth muscle in the gall bladder and spasm of the sphincter of Oddi. In some individuals this can precipitate biliary colic. Intraoperatively, the same effect has been reported to cause false-positive cholangiograms and even to prevent instrumentation of the common duct. The biliary effects may be completely antagonized by naloxone and partially reversed by glucagon, nitroglycerin, or atropine.[83] The biliary effects of full agonists (including meperidine) appear to be similar when the medications are given at equianalgesic doses, whereas the agonist–antagonist opioids have much smaller smooth muscle effects (**Fig. 42-9**).

Urinary Tract Opioids increase the contractions of the ureter, although they relieve the pain caused by ureteral stones. They also decrease detrusor contraction in response to bladder distension (the voiding reflex) and increase the tone of the urinary sphincter by both central and peripheral mechanisms.[84,85] Postoperatively, patients may complain of a sense of urinary urgency but an inability to void. Urinary retention occurs much more commonly in men, and it is an especially frequent side effect when opioids are administered into the subarachnoid or lumbar epidural spaces. Sufficient opioid may also eliminate urgency; that is, the patient may become inattentive to the stimulus of bladder distension.

Hormonal Effects Morphine inhibits the release of gonadotropin-releasing hormone and corticotropin-releasing factor by actions on the hypothalamus. The concentrations of testosterone and cortisol in plasma are decreased because the secretion of pituitary trophic hormones is inhibited. In the rat, morphine increases the expression of aromatase mRNA in brain and testis, and this causes a prolonged decrease in testosterone concentrations.[86] Opioids also increase plasma levels of certain hormones such as growth hormone and prolactin. In the perioperative period, most of these hormonal changes are probably not clinically significant. Perhaps more importantly, surgery and pain can produce large increases in many hormones (the so-called stress response), and opioids are able to blunt or abolish these responses (see Intraoperative Use of Opioids later).

Immune Effects For many years there have been reports about the immunosuppressive effects of opioids. In animal models, there is evidence that opioids suppress resistance to infection and may promote metastatic spread of tumors. Heroin addicts have increased incidences of many different infections, although multiple factors are undoubtedly involved in this setting. Neuraxial opioids can reactivate herpes zoster, and pregnant women receiving neuraxial morphine are at increased risk for reactivation of oral herpes simplex.[87] Opioid-induced immunosuppression is probably mediated by effects on both peripheral immune cells and the central nervous system. Opioids decrease natural killer cell activity, lymphocyte proliferation, antibody production, and nuclear factor kappa B (NF-κB) activation in neutrophils.[88] Many of these effects are blocked in μ-receptor knockout mice, and some are blocked by opioid antagonists.[89]

The clinical impact of all this is still unknown, and it is likely to be complex. Opioid agonists do not all produce the same effects on immune cells, and untreated pain can also be immunosuppressive. This research may ultimately have important implications, particularly for patients with chronic pain, those in methadone programs, and hospitalized patients given very large doses of opioids.

Effects on Pregnancy and the Neonate Opioids have no specific teratogenic effects, but chronic opioid use by the mother may lead to physical dependence in the fetus. Neonatal withdrawal may occur shortly after delivery, and in some instances it may be life-threatening. Parenteral opioids are commonly used to treat labor pain. Because opioids cross the placenta readily, they can cause ventilatory depression in the neonate. Morphine produces more depression in the neonate than meperidine.[90] The newborn infant has an incompletely developed blood–brain barrier, so a dose of morphine that has somewhat restricted distribution into the CNS of the mother may produce excessive effects in the baby. Meperidine is much more lipophilic than morphine, so its effects in mother and infant are more comparable. Opioids take time to accumulate in the fetus, so the neonate may actually be less affected if the opioid is given very close to the time of delivery. Naloxone may be required to reverse the effects of opioids given repeatedly during a long labor. One alternative is the use of remifentanil, because it is cleared very rapidly by both mother and fetus. Despite its extremely short duration of action, experimental data suggest that remifentanil is effective when administered via patient-controlled analgesia during labor.[91]

Opioid agonist–antagonist agents such as nalbuphine and butorphanol are popular for use in laboring women because they produce less ventilatory depression at higher doses than full agonists (See Opioid Agonist-Antagonists). They are thought to be safer for mother and child; however, convincing controlled trials are lacking.

Tolerance There appear to be 2 types of tolerance to opioid action. When a large dose is administered by bolus or rapid infusion, *acute tolerance* or *tachyphylaxis* may occur. Acute tolerance to a brief infusion of remifentanil has been reported by several investigators,[92] but the data are inconsistent,[93,94] and the clinical relevance has been difficult to confirm.

The more important problem of *chronic tolerance* occurs when opioids are administered frequently over longer periods of time. The first indication of tolerance is often a decrease in the duration of analgesia after each dose, but eventually the intensity of effect also declines. Tolerance may be overcome, in most cases, by an increase in the dose of the opioid. Cancer patients receiving very high doses or continuous neuraxial opioid administration can acquire profound tolerance, and huge doses may be needed to produce an adequate analgesic effect. Regional blocks and nonopioid analgesics may be necessary to produce adequate pain relief in these circumstances. In recent years, opioid tolerance has also become a common problem for mechanically ventilated patients in the intensive care unit who receive fentanyl or morphine infusions for sedation.

When tolerance to an opioid occurs, there is simultaneous development of cross-tolerance to all other opioid agonists. In general, tolerance develops most rapidly to the effects we have described as depressant (analgesia, ventilatory depression, euphoria), but much less tolerance occurs to some of the stimulant effects like constipation or pupillary constriction. For example, a heroin addict who is placed on chronic methadone treatment becomes tolerant to the euphoriant effect but frequently continues to have miosis and constipation. Similarly, constipation is a common problem for the terminal cancer patient who requires large doses of morphine for relief of pain. As previously discussed, cross-tolerance among full agonists is often incomplete, perhaps because of the heterogeneity of μ-receptor subtypes. A patient who is tolerant to one opioid can often get additional relief by switching to another—a process known as *opioid rotation*.[95]

The precise mechanisms of both acute and chronic tolerance are still unclear. Some of the mechanisms are similar to desensitization of other G-protein coupled receptors (GPCRs): receptor phosphorylation and internalization can occur, as well as activation of mitogen-activated protein kinases, adenylyl cyclase, and phosphokinase C. Confusingly, the mechanisms are not consistent for the various opioid receptors, not even for different ligands of the same receptor. Desensitization of GPCRs involves binding by the intracellular protein β-arrestin, and there is evidence that the analgesic effect of morphine in mice is increased and prolonged in knockout mice deficient in the β-arrestin-2 subtype.[96] Numerous compounds appear to decrease the development opioid tolerance in animals,[97] but the effects in man have been disappointing. Activation of glutamate (*N*-methyl-D-aspartate [NMDA]) receptors appears to play a role, and inhibitors of NMDA reduce tolerance development in animal models.[98] A growing literature now indicates that chronic administration of opioids activates pain pathways via NMDA activation and consequent nitric oxide production. This means that a part of what we have historically termed opioid "tolerance" is actually the result of a hyperalgesic effect.[99]

Physical Dependence After sufficient doses have been administered for an adequate period of time, all opioids induce a state of physical dependence. Abruptly stopping the drug or administering an antagonist then causes a stereotypic withdrawal syndrome. The symptoms of withdrawal can be rapidly terminated with small doses of intravenous morphine.

Some authorities believe that medically induced physical dependence is common, and clinically imperceptible dependence may actually be present after only a few injections of a potent opioid. In most cases, "withdrawal" may occur without the patient or physician being aware of it. Physical dependence is not the same thing as *psychological dependence* or *addiction*, which includes the dimension of compulsive drug-seeking behavior. The data of Porter and Jick[100] suggested that in 1980, addiction resulting from appropriate medical treatment was a very unusual event. The recent dramatic increase in abuse of prescription analgesics has now caused some rethinking about the risks of opioid treatment.[101] It is important to remember that undertreatment of pain is still a major problem, and inappropriate fear of causing addiction is often the cause.

When a patient with known physical dependence is to be detoxified (withdrawn), the patient is commonly switched to a long-acting agonist (usually methadone), and the dose is reduced slowly. This produces a mild, although protracted, withdrawal syndrome. However, a person addicted to heroin or methadone who presents emergently for medical treatment is generally not an appropriate candidate for detoxification (see Chapter 24).

TABLE 42-2 Physicochemical Properties of Some Opioid Agonists

Drug	pK_a	% Ionized at pH 7.4	Partition Coefficient[a]
Morphine	7.9/9.4	76	0.7,[104] 1.42[103]
Meperidine	8.5	93	38.8[103]
Hydromorphone	8.1[b]	83	1.28[104]
Oxymorphone	8.17	84	0.98[104]
Methadone	9.26	94	116.3[104]
Fentanyl	8.4	91	717,[104] 860[103]
Sufentanil	8.0	80	1778,[103] 2842[104]
Alfentanil	6.5	11	130[103]
Remifentanil	7.1	33	17.9[c]

[a]The *n*-octanol/water partition coefficient (at 98.6°F [37°C], corrected for the percentage of drug un-ionized at pH 7.4) is a measure of lipid solubility.

[b]Data on file, Purdue Pharma.

[c]Data on file, GlaxoSmithKline Beecham Pharmaceuticals.

SPECIFIC DRUGS

As discussed previously, the onset or duration of effect is most often the basis for selection of a particular opioid. Chapter 40 discusses many of the pharmacokinetic properties of opioids. The clinically available opioid agonists vary greatly in their physicochemical properties and therefore in their absorption and distribution. **Table 42-2** lists important physicochemical properties of several opioids, and **Table 42-3** lists pharmacokinetic parameters. It should be noted that there is tremendous variability in the published values for most of these pharmacokinetic parameters. Some of the variability reflects true differences between patient populations, whereas some is the result of sampling times and other technical aspects of measurement. The weak opioid, codeine (not covered here), has significant pharmacokinetic variability due to genetic polymorphisms in metabolism by the microsomal enzyme CYP2D6. Codeine is an inactive prodrug and must be demethylated to form morphine for its effect. As a result, poor metabolizers may have no pain relief from codeine, whereas extensive metabolizers (with multiple gene copies) can have an exaggerated effect or toxicity.[102]

TABLE 42-3 Pharmacokinetic Properties of Some Opioid Agonists

	Morphine	Meperidine	Hydromorphone	Fentanyl	Sufentanil	Alfentanil	Remifentanil
A[a]	94	34	87	90	84	83	90.3
B[a]	5	39	9	8	15	12	9.5
C[a]	1	27	4	2	1	5	0.2
$t_{1/2\alpha}$ (min)[a]	0.9	3.1	1.1	1.0	1.4	0.67	0.9
$t_{1/2\beta}$ (min)[a]	8.1	30	11	19	23	13	9.1
$t_{1/2\gamma}$ (min)[a]	96	330	151	475	562	111	48
VDss (L/kg)	3.2-4.7	2.8-4.2	4.1-4.4	3.2-4.2	2.5-3.0	0.4-1.0	0.2-0.3
Cl (mL/min/kg)	12.4-15.2	10.1-16.4	23-28	11.2-13.3	10-15	4-9	30-40
Protein binding (%)	30	64	8-19	84	92	92	80

Cl, clearance; $t_{1/2}$, half-life; VDSS, steady-state volume of distribution.

[a]The pharmacokinetic parameters A, B, C, $t_{1/2\alpha}$, $t_{1/2\beta}$, and $t_{1/2\gamma}$ describe the blood concentration of the drug after a bolus injection according to the equation:

$$\text{Conc} = Ae^{-\alpha t} + Be^{-\beta t} + Ce^{-\gamma t}$$

where the sum of A, B, and C equals 100%. The half-lives $t_{1/2\alpha}$, $t_{1/2\beta}$, and $t_{1/2\gamma}$ are related to the rate constants α, β, and γ, respectively, according to the following equations:

$$t_{1/2\alpha} = \frac{\ln 2}{\alpha} \qquad t_{1/2\beta} = \frac{\ln 2}{\beta} \qquad t_{1/2\gamma} = \frac{\ln 2}{\gamma}$$

Morphine Morphine is the least lipophilic of the opioids listed,[103,104] and this has 2 important implications for its pharmacokinetics: Morphine penetrates biologic membranes more slowly than lipophilic opioids, and it is less likely to accumulate in lipid membranes or fatty tissues. It is rapidly absorbed after intramuscular, subcutaneous, or oral administration. After an intravenous bolus, plasma concentrations decline rapidly as the drug is distributed into well-perfused tissues. Only approximately 25% to 35% is bound to plasma proteins, primarily albumin. The steady-state volume of distribution is very large, and it is probably made up of nonfatty tissues.

Morphine is a substrate for the P-gp transporter (see Opioid Agonists, Smooth Muscle Effects). What used to be called the blood–brain barrier for morphine is actually a combination of slow CNS penetration and rapid efflux. Together, these effects account for the relatively slow onset and low concentrations of morphine found in the brain after analgesic doses.[105]

Morphine is eliminated primarily by hepatic biotransformation, with approximately 5% to 15% excreted unchanged in the urine. The rate of hepatic clearance is very high and accounts for the relatively short 3-hour terminal half-life. The hepatic extraction of morphine is approximately 0.7; that is, 70% is cleared in one pass through the liver. Morphine therefore undergoes flow-dependent elimination, so factors that decrease hepatic blood flow will prolong its elimination. High hepatic clearance also means that morphine is subject to a large first-pass effect, and larger doses are required when the drug is given orally.

More than 90% of a dose of morphine is metabolized and excreted within 24 hours. The primary route of metabolism is conjugation in the liver to produce morphine 3-glucuronide (M3G) and morphine 6-glucuronide (M6G). A small amount of morphine is *N*-demethylated to form normorphine. These polar metabolites are then excreted in the urine and bile. M6G, which may constitute 15% of total morphine metabolites, possesses morphine-like analgesic and respiratory depressant activity, although higher doses are required.[106,107] M6G is a substrate for a transporter protein distinct from P-gp,[108] and it does not appear to contribute to the overall analgesia produced by morphine after a single or a few doses.[109] M6G accumulates slowly in the CNS and contributes progressively more to the overall analgesic effect when it is administered in repeated doses.[44] It may accumulate sufficiently to produce toxic effects in patients with renal failure.[110]

The plasma pharmacokinetics of morphine does not parallel its clinical effects. In spite of morphine's rapid distribution and elimination from plasma, the changes in brain concentration are small and delayed. As a result, the onset and offset of analgesia are slow. In a study in human volunteers, the peak pupillary effect occurred 86 minutes after intravenous injection, although 90% of that effect was achieved within 22 minutes.[42] Hug et al[111] demonstrated in dogs that peak ventilatory depression did not occur for 30 to 60 minutes after an intravenous bolus of morphine (**Fig. 42-10**). During the recovery period, Hug et al[111] showed that concentrations of morphine in cerebrospinal fluid declined more slowly than those in plasma, and the decline in ventilatory depression was slower still.

Meperidine This substituted phenylpiperidine is significantly more lipid soluble than morphine, although its plasma pharmacokinetics is similar. The onset of the analgesic effect is faster than morphine, and the duration is shorter (2-3 hours). Meperidine is rapidly distributed into a large apparent volume of distribution, and it has a very high rate of clearance by hepatic biotransformation.[112,113] The high hepatic extraction means that meperidine undergoes significant (48%-56%) first-pass metabolism. The terminal half-life has been estimated as 3 to 7 hours—which is similar to or longer than that of morphine. Meperidine is more highly protein bound than morphine (65%-80%), and it is bound mainly to α_1-acid glycoprotein.

Meperidine is rapidly *N*-demethylated to form normeperidine; the other major metabolites are meperidinic acid and normeperidinic acid. Less than 7% of a dose is excreted unchanged in the urine. The metabolism of meperidine plays a significant role in its pharmacodynamics.

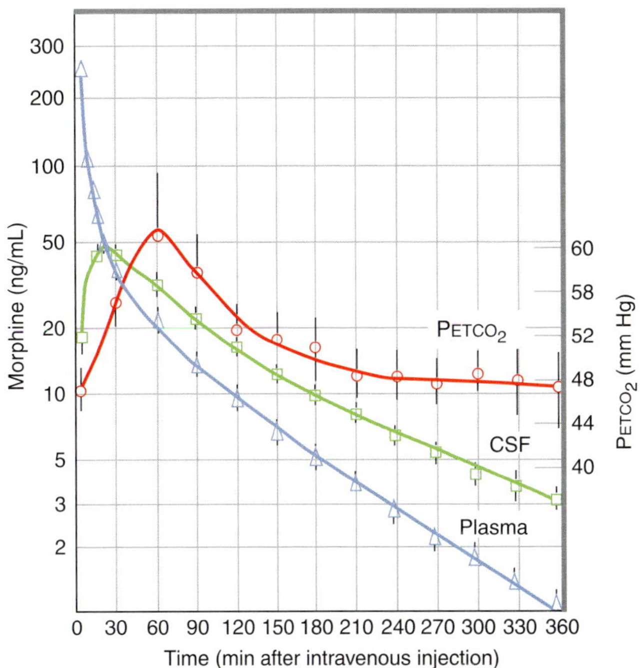

FIGURE 42-10. Concentration of morphine in plasma and cerebrospinal fluid (CSF), and end-tidal CO_2 (P_{ETCO_2}) versus time in 6 dogs given 0.3 mg/kg and allowed to breathe spontaneously (see text for details). [Reproduced with permission from Hug CC Jr, Murphy MR, Rigel EP, et al. Pharmacokinetics of morphine injected intravenously into the anesthetized dog. *Anesthesiology.* 1981;54:38.]

In the mouse, normeperidine is an analgesic with approximately half the potency of meperidine; unfortunately, in both mouse and man it is a potent convulsant. Normeperidine has a terminal half-life of 8 to 12 hours, so significant amounts of this toxic metabolite can accumulate. Seizures have occurred in patients with renal failure (who could not excrete normeperidine) and in cancer patients who received high doses of meperidine over long periods of time.[29]

In addition to its actions at opioid receptors, meperidine has significant effects at other receptor sites. It has agonist activity at the α_{2b} adrenergic receptor, and this probably accounts for the ability of meperidine (and clonidine) to lower thermoregulatory set point and stop shivering.[114] The dose needed to treat postoperative shivering is usually 12 to 25 mg, substantially less than the amount needed for analgesia. Meperidine (or one of its metabolites) also inhibits SERT, the transporter mediating presynaptic reuptake of serotonin.[115] Inhibition of SERT is the basis for a well-described and potentially fatal interaction between meperidine and monoamine oxidase inhibitors (MAOI). Administration of meperidine to a patient chronically taking one of the nonselective MAOI (tranylcypromine, phenelzine, or isocarboxazid) may result in a serotoninergic crisis manifested as clonus, agitation, hyperreflexia, and hyperthermia. This interaction has also been reported in patients taking higher doses of the selective MAOI, selegiline.

The use of meperidine has been declining in recent years due to the toxicity of its metabolite and the potential for adverse interactions. It is still of value for the treatment of postoperative shivering. Early studies of meperidine are still of great value for demonstrating the relationship between opioid plasma concentration and analgesic effect. Austin et al[116] titrated meperidine in patients with postoperative pain and described 2 important characteristics of opioid analgesia:

1. For each patient, opioid titration demonstrated a very sharp analgesic end point; that is, the change from no pain relief to excellent pain relief occurred over a very narrow range of meperidine concentrations
2. In contrast, there was a large variability (400%) in meperidine requirement between individuals.

These data demonstrate why traditional fixed-dosage regimens for relief of acute pain often result in inadequate or excessive plasma concentrations. The findings for meperidine are remarkably similar to those that describe the relationship of alfentanil concentration to intraoperative analgesic response[117] (see Intraoperative Use of Opioids).

Hydromorphone Hydromorphone is an older, semisynthetic μ agonist that has gained increasing popularity for a number of acute and chronic indications as an alternative to morphine. It is approximately 5 to 7 times more potent than morphine (although some data suggest as much as 10 times more potent), and it has a slightly shorter duration of action. It is cleared by hepatic glucuronidation with an approximate 62% first-pass metabolism. There is no active 6-glucuronide, but the 3-glucuronide can accumulate to produce neuroexcitation.

Hydromorphone is a hydrophilic drug with an octanol–water partition coefficient only slightly higher than that of morphine.[104] This probably explains the 10- to 20-minute delay in peak analgesic effect after an intravenous (IV) bolus dose, as well as the relatively poor correlation between plasma concentration and effect.[118] Its water solubility means that it can be prepared in concentrated solutions (up to 100 mg/mL), which are useful for highly tolerant patients or delivery with implanted infusion pumps. The low lipid solubility gives hydromorphone some of morphine's characteristics as a selective spinal analgesic. The epidural-to-parenteral equianalgesic ratio is 1:2, and the duration of a single epidural dose is estimated as being between 7.7 and 19.3 hours.[119] A few papers suggest that hydromorphone may produce fewer side effects (nausea, pruritus) than morphine, but the evidence for this is weak.

Oxymorphone This semisynthetic derivative of morphine is 7 to 10 times more potent, and it has been available for many years in intravenous and suppository formulations. It is quite hydrophilic and behaves much like hydromorphone when administered intravenously. There are very few studies comparing intravenous oxymorphone with other opioids for perioperative use. Recently, oxymorphone was approved in an immediate- and controlled-release oral tablet formulation. The immediate release form can produce measurable analgesic effects in 5 to 10 minutes. Oxymorphone is biotransformed to 6 hydroxy and 3-glucuronide metabolites, with a terminal half-life of 7 to 10 hours[120]

Fentanyl This potent synthetic opioid is extremely fat soluble, which accounts for its rapid onset and relatively short duration. After intravenous administration, fentanyl is rapidly distributed to the brain, heart, and other highly perfused tissues, and its half-time for effect site equilibration ($T_{1/2}k_{e0}$)is ~5 minutes.[121] Within a short time, the drug is distributed extensively throughout the body (steady-state volume of distribution is more than 4 L/kg), so plasma levels drop precipitously. Termination of effect occurs when fentanyl redistributes away from the central nervous system. Recent data from animal studies suggest that fentanyl transport between plasma and lung or brain is affected by both the organic anion transport protein (OATP) and P-gp. OATP and P-gp mediate transport of the drug into and out of the CNS, respectively.[82]

Plasma concentrations fall much more slowly during the terminal phase. Fentanyl is biotransformed in the liver to inactive metabolites, primarily norfentanyl and several hydroxylation products. Only 6% to 8% is excreted unchanged in the urine. The hepatic clearance of fentanyl is very high, and more than 60% is cleared in one pass. The large distribution volume, however, means that most of the drug remains extravascular and unavailable for biotransformation. The long terminal half-life of fentanyl (approximately 8 hours) is a function of the slow rate at which it reenters the central compartment.[122]

Fentanyl concentration in the plasma correlates well with cerebrospinal fluid (CSF) concentration and pharmacodynamic effect. Fentanyl plasma pharmacokinetics therefore predicts some of its more important pharmacodynamic properties:

- The effects of low doses (eg, 100-200 μg) are brief because they are terminated by rapid redistribution. After much higher doses (eg, >20 μg/kg) redistribution may be insufficient to bring plasma concentrations to subtherapeutic levels. In this circumstance, termination of effect depends increasingly on the much slower elimination process, and the drug appears long-acting[123] (**Fig. 42-11**). Although the duration increases, the distribution and terminal half-lives do not change with dosage (fentanyl obeys first-order kinetics throughout the clinical dose range).
- A long terminal half-life means that repeated intravenous boluses of fentanyl are very likely to produce cumulative effects.
- A high hepatic extraction ratio (0.6) means that the clearance of fentanyl is limited by hepatic blood flow. Factors that lower hepatic blood flow (eg, intra-abdominal surgery, cardiopulmonary bypass) can increase the terminal half-life of fentanyl.
- Fentanyl undergoes substantial first-pass metabolism, so the oral route is inefficient. The drug is well absorbed when given transdermally, intranasally, or via the oral mucosa. These routes bypass the portal circulation and result in high blood levels of fentanyl.

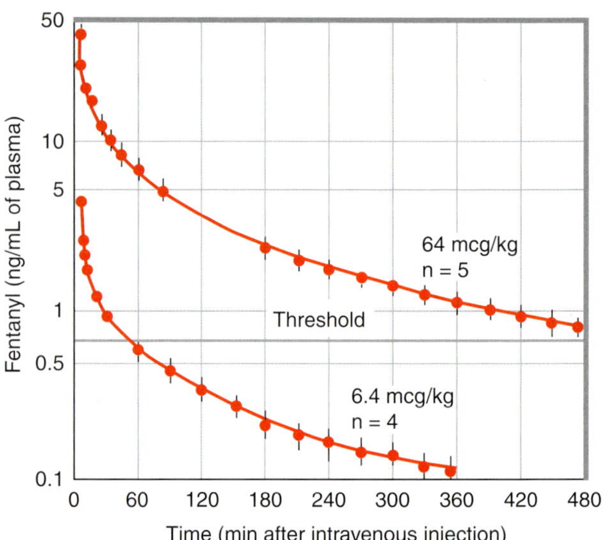

FIGURE 42-11. Plasma concentration of fentanyl versus time in dogs given either 6.4 or 64 μg/kg intravenously. Threshold represents the concentration above which depression of ventilation occurs (see text for details). Effects of the lower dose are terminated by redistribution; those of the higher dose are terminated by elimination. [Reproduced with permission from Murphy MR, Olson WA, Hug CC Jr. Pharmacokinetics of ^{3}H-fentanyl in the dog anesthetized with enflurane. *Anesthesiology.* 1979;50:13.]

Alfentanil Alfentanil is a slightly less potent congener of fentanyl and has an extremely rapid onset and short duration of effect. It was developed as an opioid suitable for infusion delivery during anesthesia, but remifentanil has largely replaced it for this indication. Peak analgesic and ventilatory depressant effects of alfentanil occur in less than 2 minutes ($T_{1/2}k_{e0}$ ~ 1 minutes), and the effects of small bolus doses (eg, 10 μg/kg) may last only 15 minutes. The pharmacokinetics of alfentanil is unusually well studied; Table 41-3 lists some of its more important pharmacokinetic parameters.

Like fentanyl, termination of alfentanil's effects after a small bolus dose mainly depends on redistribution, and the effects of larger doses (100-200 μg/kg) may be prolonged. Alfentanil has much less tendency than fentanyl to bind nonspecifically in most tissues. This is reflected in smaller initial and steady-state volumes of distribution.[124] It is rapidly metabolized by *N*-dealkylation and *O*-demethylation, and very little of the drug is excreted unchanged in the urine.[124]

The terminal half-life of alfentanil is only 1.5 to 2 hours in most healthy patients, so alfentanil is less likely than fentanyl to produce cumulative effects after repeated doses or continuous infusion.[125] For infusions of 2 hours or less, its context-sensitive half-time

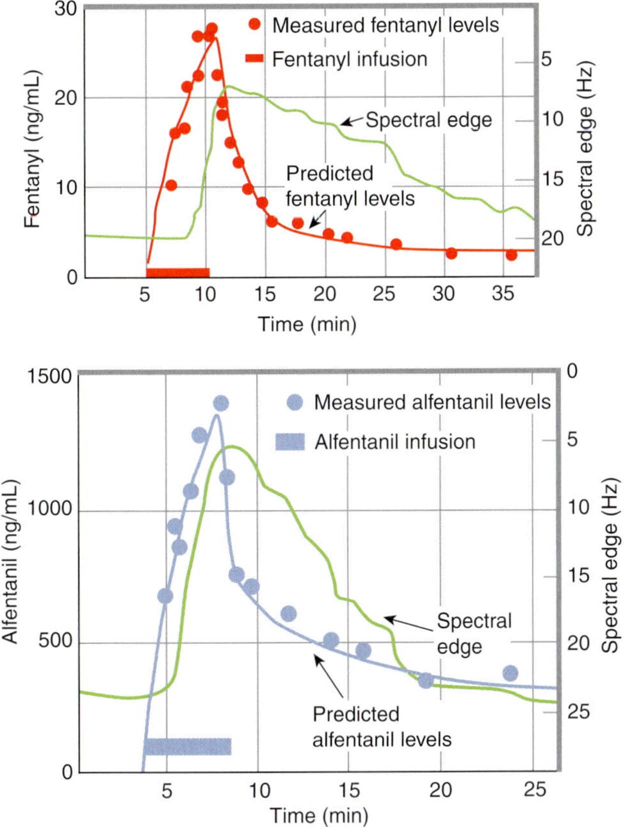

FIGURE 42-12. Plasma concentration of fentanyl or alfentanil versus time with simultaneous measurement of EEG spectral edge. Volunteers were given fentanyl 150 μg/min or alfentanil 1500 μg/min. Increasing opioid effect is depicted as a decrease in average EEG frequency and spectral edge. Changes in spectral edge follow plasma concentrations more closely for alfentanil (see text for details). [Reproduced with permission from Scott JC, Ponganis KV, Stanski DR. EEG quantitation of narcotic effect: the comparative pharmacodynamics of fentanyl and alfentanil. *Anesthesiology.* 1985;62:234.]

(see Chapter 40) is about half the infusion duration. For infusions longer than 2 hours, its context-sensitive half-time remains at approximately 1 hour.

Alfentanil was one of the very first drugs characterized by simultaneous pharmacokinetic–pharmacodynamic modeling. Scott et al gave volunteers a brief infusion of either fentanyl or alfentanil at a sufficient rate to produce slowing of the EEG[121] (**Fig. 42-12**). Both opioids produced a decrease in the median EEG frequency as the plasma level increased. When the infusions were terminated, the EEG reverted to normal fast frequencies. In the fentanyl group, there was a delay of 2 to 3 minutes before measurable slowing occurred, and the effects persisted for 20 to 30 minutes after the infusion was discontinued. In the alfentanil group, the onset and offset of effect were much more closely correlated with the rise and fall in plasma levels. There are a few possible reasons for this difference: diffusion of alfentanil into the CNS may be faster because most of the drug is not ionized (and therefore diffusible) at body pH (see Table 42-2), and it is also 22 times less soluble than fentanyl in rat brain.[126] Rapid effect-site equilibrium (see Chapter 40) may be due to the fact that alfentanil undergoes less nonspecific binding in brain tissue.

Sufentanil This thienyl derivative of fentanyl is more potent and even more fat soluble. Its high affinity and selectivity for μ opioid receptors have made it a common probe for μ effects in pharmacologic studies. Despite a terminal half-life of approximately 10 hours (longer than that of fentanyl and much longer than that of alfentanil), sufentanil has the shortest context-sensitive half-time of the 3 when given by infusion for up to 10 hours. For example, after a 2-hour infusion, the context-sensitive half-time of sufentanil is approximately 20 minutes, approximately a third the value for alfentanil. Hepatic clearance is very rapid (extraction ratio = 0.7). Sufentanil is metabolized by *N*-dealkylation and *O*-demethylation.

Other than a difference in potency and pharmacokinetics, the clinical properties of sufentanil are much like those of fentanyl. Sufentanil has had extensive use in cardiac surgery, where it was initially given in extremely large doses (up to 30 μg/kg). The distribution of the opioid is dramatically affected by cardiopulmonary bypass: Plasma concentrations of sufentanil drop with hemodilution, but the huge amounts sequestered in lung and muscle cause a secondary increase when the bypass is discontinued.[127] Large amounts of sufentanil are bound to oxygenators and tubing in the bypass circuit.

The fat solubility of sufentanil allows it to be absorbed rapidly through intact skin and mucous membranes. Although it has been used epidurally, its rapid absorption by spinal cord and vertebral plexus result in a very short duration.

Remifentanil Remifentanil is the newest opioid to be introduced into clinical use. Pharmacodynamically, it is similar to the other fentanyl derivatives, but it has an extremely short duration of action because of rapid metabolic inactivation. It is hydrolyzed by nonspecific esterases, primarily in skeletal muscle, and the resulting acid metabolite has only minor activity as a μ-opioid agonist. Remifentanil is not a substrate for pseudocholinesterase, and the dose does not need to be changed for patients with pseudocholinesterase deficiency. Its redistribution half-life is similar to that of other fentanyl derivatives, but metabolism is always the predominant mechanism for clearance. The capacity of the esterases to hydrolyze remifentanil is enormous, resulting in a total clearance of 2 to 3 L/min. The context-sensitive half-life is less than 5 minutes, regardless of the duration of the infusion.[128] There is essentially no accumulation of remifentanil after infusions or repeated boluses.

Remifentanil is more potent than alfentanil and less potent than sufentanil. In the presence of 70% nitrous oxide, infusion rates between 0.05 and 0.3 μg/kg/min will provide adequate analgesia for most surgical procedures. Higher doses have been approved, but they are usually not needed and may produce bradycardia and hypotension. Recovery from the opioid effects is essentially independent of the infusion rate or cumulative dose given (**Fig. 42-13**) and will occur within a few minutes of discontinuing the drug.[129] The ultrashort duration of this analgesic can be a drawback: Patients who are expected to have postoperative pain will need a longer-acting opioid for pain relief. If the postoperative analgesic has a slow onset (eg, morphine), it will need to be administered *prior* to stopping remifentanil.

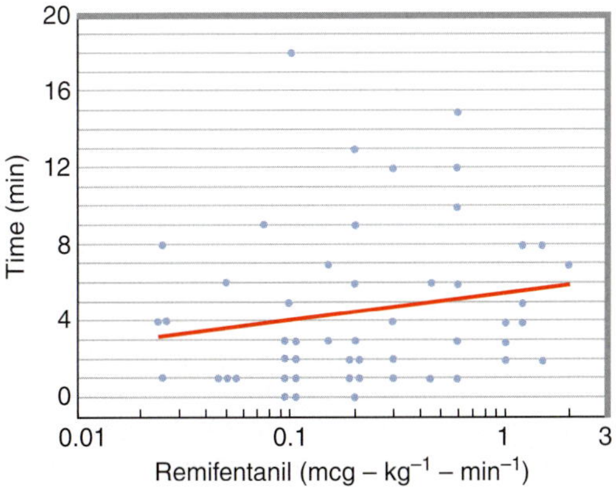

FIGURE 42-13. The time to spontaneous ventilation after discontinuing an infusion of remifentanil expressed as a function of the infusion rate. [Reprinted from Dershwitz M, Rosow CE. Remifentanil: a truly-short-acting opioid. *Semin Anesth.* 1996;15:88, with permission from Elsevier.]

Patients with hepatic or renal failure do not experience a prolongation in effect, and the dose of remifentanil does not need to be adjusted in such patients.[130,131] In fact, the dose of remifentanil does not need to be adjusted for age or weight except at the extremes of these parameters.

Methadone Methadone is a long-lasting synthetic μ opioid approximately equipotent with morphine. Unlike most other opioids, methadone has very high oral bioavailability (approximately 80%). Compared with morphine, methadone is much more lipid soluble and has higher tissue and plasma protein binding (to α_1-acid glycoprotein). The pharmacokinetics of methadone have been widely misunderstood, and many clinicians assume that a single dose has both a slow onset and a long duration. Methadone's half-time for effect-site equilibration ($T_{1/2}k_{e0}$) is only 4 minutes (similar to that of fentanyl), so the onset is considerably faster than that of morphine.[132] Like fentanyl, the redistribution half-life of methadone is quite fast (~ 6 minutes), and single small doses (<10 mg) may have a duration of less than an hour. These properties have led to renewed interest in methadone as a perioperative analgesic.[133] After larger doses, the duration increases dramatically due to the drug's extremely slow clearance via CYP2B6 (terminal half-life ~35 hours). Single bolus doses of 20 to 30 mg can produce detectable analgesic effects for 24 to 36 hours. Repeated oral or parenteral doses can result in substantial accumulation, with subsequent doses lasting much longer than the initial dose.

There is also renewed interest in methadone for the therapy of chronic pain. The drug is available as a racemic mixture, and the *d*-isomer was long thought to have no activity. Recently, *d*-methadone was demonstrated to be a noncompetitive glutamate (NMDA) antagonist in concentrations similar to those achieved when the drug is administered as the racemate. In animal models, *d*-methadone attenuates the development of opioid tolerance and blocks NMDA-induced hyperalgesia.[132] It is not known whether any of these benefits can be achieved in humans, but methadone does produce substantial tolerance when it is given in maintenance programs for heroin addicts.

Tramadol Tramadol is considered here with other opioid agonists, but it has multiple and unique mechanisms of action as an analgesic. Clinically available preparations of tramadol contain the racemic mixture of 2 isomers.

- (+)-Tramadol is a weak agonist at μ receptors and an inhibitor of serotonin reuptake through SERT. (+)-Tramadol is also demethylated to yield a metabolite with greater μ opioid efficacy.
- (−)-Tramadol selectively inhibits norepinephrine reuptake. The effects on neurotransmitter reuptake enhance inhibitory effects on pain transmission in the spinal cord.[134]

Tramadol is partially reversed by naloxone and exhibits incomplete cross-tolerance to opioid agonists. It does not have opioid antagonist properties and does not precipitate withdrawal when given to opioid-dependent addicts.

In the United States, tramadol is only available for oral administration, whereas a parenteral preparation is available in many other countries. Given orally, tramadol is effective in both acute postoperative pain and neuropathic pain. Given parenterally, it has been used epidurally, as part of a balanced anesthetic, and for patient-controlled analgesia.[134] The drug undergoes oxidative hepatic metabolism, then renal excretion of a glucuronidated metabolite. The active *O*-demethylated metabolite is formed by CYP2D6, so there are rapid and slow metabolizers. There is some evidence that these genetic polymorphisms will influence the drug effect.[135] Common side effects are sedation and nausea. It sometimes causes burning pain on injection, thought to be due to agonist activity at capsaicin (TRV1) receptors.[136] Because it inhibits serotonin reuptake, tramadol (like meperidine) can cause a serotonergic crisis in a patient taking an MAOI or another reuptake inhibitor such as fluoxetine or paroxetine.[115] Its effects on ventilatory drive and its potential to be abused appear to be less than those of the typical μ-opioid agonists.

INTRAOPERATIVE USE OF OPIOIDS

Although opium extracts were used hundreds of years ago in "soporific sponges," the modern concept of an opioid-based general anesthetic did not evolve until quite recently. Gray and Rees[137] defined general anesthesia as a "triad" consisting of narcosis (ie, hypnosis), analgesia, and muscle relaxation. The opioids by themselves do not produce muscle relaxation, and even high doses sometimes fail to produce unconsciousness. In the days before muscle relaxants, endotracheal tubes, and controlled ventilation, high doses of morphine were tried alone as total anesthetics and found to be both dangerous and only marginally effective.

BALANCED ANESTHESIA

In 1942, Griffiths introduced curare, which made it possible for muscle relaxation to be achieved during relatively light levels of anesthesia. The first attempts at "balanced" anesthesia used curare together with thiopental and nitrous oxide, but these techniques usually failed to block autonomic responses to surgical stimuli. In 1947, Neff et al[138] introduced a more satisfactory anesthetic that included small doses of meperidine in combination with thiopental, curare, and nitrous oxide. Although the individual components have changed over the years, this technique is the basis for modern balanced anesthesia.

In the 1950s the "major tranquilizers" (phenothiazines and butyrophenones) were introduced into clinical practice. De Castro and Mundeleer[139] described a technique called *neuroleptanalgesia* in which a butyrophenone (droperidol) was combined with fentanyl. This combination did not necessarily cause unconsciousness or amnesia, but it produced analgesia, apparent indifference to stimuli, immobility, and autonomic stability. When nitrous oxide was added to produce hypnosis, the resulting state was called *neuroleptanesthesia*. This anesthetic technique is infrequently used today.

In modern practice, nearly all anesthesia is "balanced." The term is no longer restricted to nitrous oxide–opioid anesthesia, but includes mixtures of opioids with volatile agents or infusions of intravenous hypnotics.

INTRAOPERATIVE ANALGESIA

Analgesia is sometimes difficult to assess—or even define—in a patient who is not awake. In general, we consider intraoperative analgesia to be a reduction in autonomic and somatic responses to noxious surgical stimuli. The cardiovascular responses to incision, laryngoscopy, and other painful events are blunted much more effectively by opioids than by most other intravenous agents[140] (**Fig. 42-14**).

Analgesia can also be measured by the decreasing requirement for other anesthetic agents. The administration of opioids potentiates the hypnotic effects of barbiturates, benzodiazepines, and propofol[141,142] (**Fig. 42-15**). By reducing the amount of hypnotic administered, an opioid can sometimes produce more rapid emergence. The opioids also produce a dramatic, dose-related decrease in the need for volatile anesthetics, and they are frequently used for this specific purpose. The minimum alveolar concentration (MAC) of isoflurane, for example, is decreased as the blood concentration of remifentanil is increased[143] (**Fig. 42-16**). The maximal effect of full opioid agonists seems to be approximately a 70% reduction in MAC, whereas the mixed agonist–antagonists have lower efficacy.[144]

The amount of opioid analgesic required varies tremendously from patient to patient, so anesthetic "recipes" with a predetermined opioid dose are inadvisable. Shafer et al[125] found that administration of alfentanil at a fixed infusion rate resulted in inadequate anesthesia in some patients and postoperative ventilatory depression in others. This variability is a result of both pharmacokinetic and pharmacodynamic factors. The requirement for opioid also depends on the nature of the surgical stimulus.

Ausems et al[117] demonstrated the nature of this variability in patients receiving nitrous oxide and a continuous infusion of alfentanil. The infusion was titrated to suppress various clinical responses, and plasma

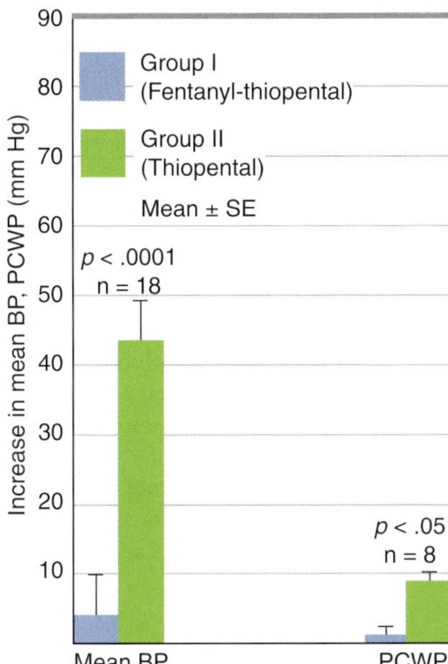

FIGURE 42-14. Fentanyl 8 μg/kg, administered intravenously, prevents the increase in mean systemic and wedge pressure after laryngoscopy and intubation. All patients were given thiopental and pancuronium. [Reproduced with permission from Martin DE, Rosenberg H, Aukburg SJ, et al. Low-dose fentanyl blunts circulatory responses to tracheal intubation. *Anesth Analg.* 1982;61:680.]

concentrations were measured simultaneously. The Cp50 (plasma concentration necessary to prevent a response in 50% of patients) was calculated for each stimulus. The study showed, for example, that the Cp50 for tracheal intubation was 475 ng/mL of alfentanil, but skin closure required only 150 ng/mL (**Fig. 42-17**A). When results were analyzed for individual subjects, the data for intraoperative analgesia bore a remarkable resemblance to those published by Austin et al[116] for postoperative analgesia (see Specific Drugs, Meperidine). For each patient, the change from inadequate to adequate analgesia occurred over a very small range of alfentanil concentrations, but there was more than a 4-fold difference in opioid sensitivity between individuals (Fig. 42-17B). The challenge for the anesthesiologist is to titrate the opioid and find this narrow range for the individual patient.

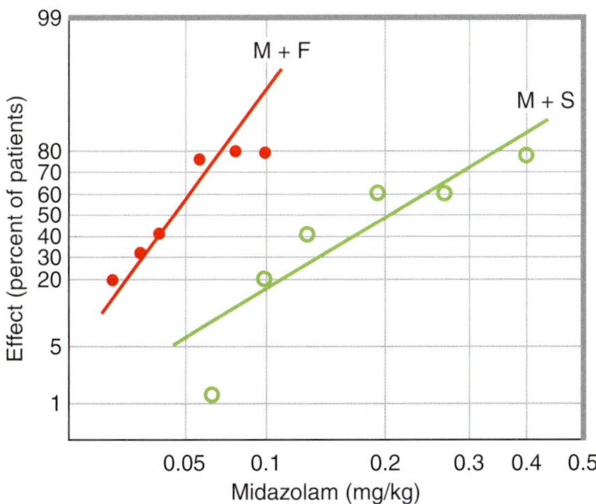

FIGURE 42-15. Percentage of patients asleep versus dose of midazolam on a log-probit plot. Curve is shifted to the left in the presence of fentanyl 1.9 μg/kg (*M* + *F*) compared with midazolam plus saline (*M* + *S*). [Ben-Schlomo I, abd-el-Khalim H, Ezry J, et al. Midazolam acts synergistically with fentanyl for induction of anesthesia. *Br J Anaesth.* 1990;64:45. By permission of Oxford University Press.]

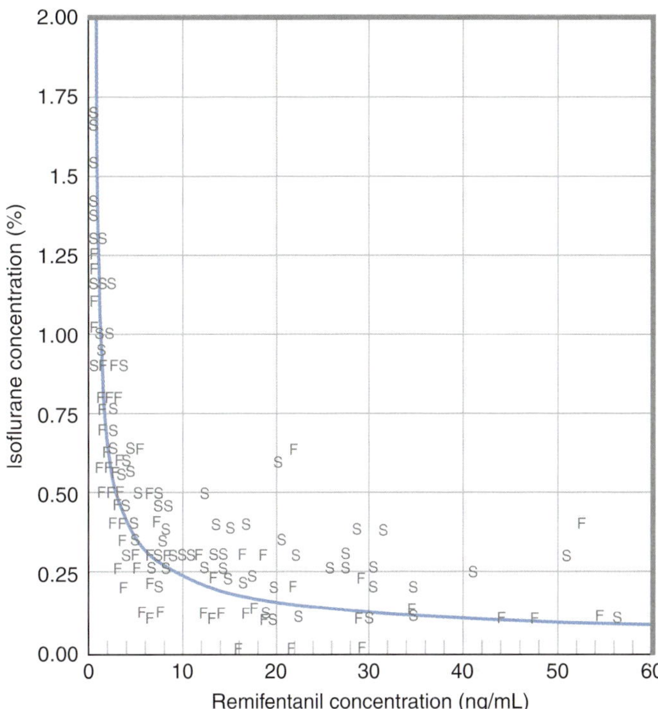

FIGURE 42-16. Decrease in minimum alveolar concentration (MAC) for isoflurane versus blood concentration of remifentanil in humans. *F* represents a patient who moved, and *S* a patient who did not move. [Reproduced with permission from Lang E, Kapila A, Shlugman D, et al. Reduction of isoflurane minimal alveolar concentration by remifentanil. *Anesthesiology.* 1996;85:721-728.]

How is an opioid titrated intraoperatively? Decreasing ventilatory rate and depth are not sensitive measures of opioid effect. They parallel analgesia but have not been validated as guides to opioid dosing during surgery. More commonly, blood pressure and other autonomic responses to "painful" stimuli are gauged. This requires good clinical judgment because autonomic responses are nonspecific and may be produced by many conditions that do not involve pain. Unlike the volatile anesthetics, the opioids do not produce graded cardiovascular depression as depth increases. Normal blood pressure does not necessarily mean that the anesthetic level is appropriate, because large overdoses of most opioids are well tolerated as long as ventilation is supported. In spite of substantial efforts to develop an "analgesia meter," neurophysiologic measurements such as cortical EEG, electromyography, cortical-evoked potentials, and evoked spinal reflexes have not been demonstrated to be reliable indices of opioid analgesia.

The dose of opioid may need to be modified according to the patient's age and physical condition. On average, opioid sensitivity is increased in patients who are elderly,[145] hypovolemic, or debilitated. Reduced doses are usually given to patients with significant CNS disease and those who have received other CNS depressants. The clearance of morphine, meperidine, fentanyl, and alfentanil is decreased in the elderly and the neonate; however, pharmacokinetic differences due to age can be much less than the unexplained variability between individual patients. This means that some elderly patients may require higher doses than some young patients. A frail older patient probably requires cautious opioid titration, but arbitrarily reducing the dose for all elderly patients can cause unnecessary suffering.[146]

A number of animal studies and a few clinical studies have examined the influence of sex on the response to opioids. Morphine appears to produce a greater analgesic and respiratory depressant effect in males, although once again, the variation between patients is larger than that attributable to sex.[147] Thus far, the data do not indicate any consistent sex-related differences among the opioid agonists.

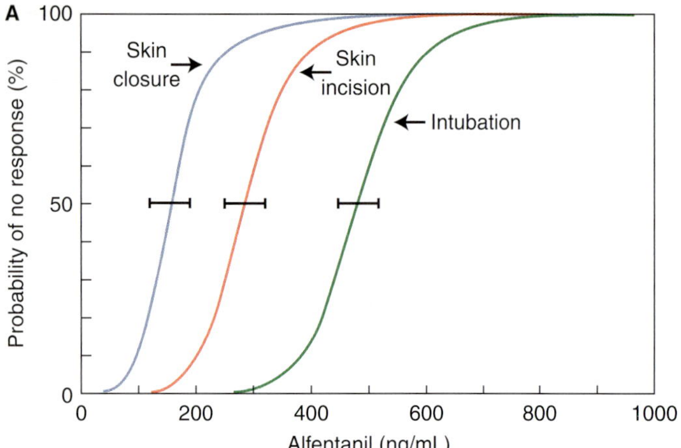

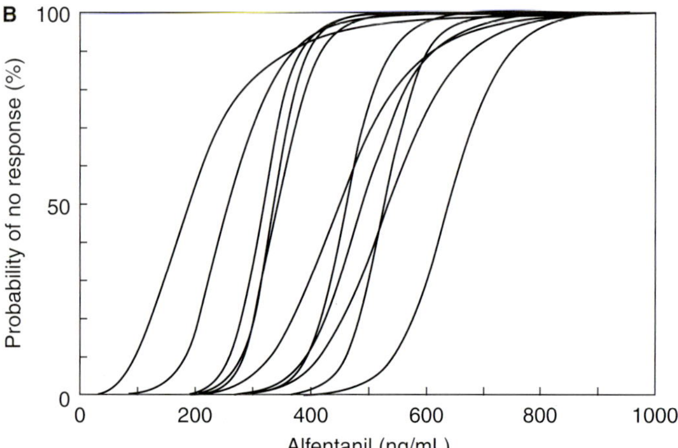

FIGURE 42-17. **A.** Alfentanil plasma concentration versus effect curves for the probability of responding to each of 3 intraoperative stimuli. Patients received 66% nitrous oxide, muscle relaxants, and a variable rate infusion of alfentanil. Curves were defined by quantal responses using logistic regression. During balanced anesthesia, much lower concentrations of alfentanil are required for skin incision and closure than for intubation. **B.** Alfentanil plasma concentration versus effect curves for each individual patient. The curves show the probability of responding during manipulation of the viscera in the upper abdomen. For each patient, the change from very high to very low probability of response occurred over a narrow range of alfentanil concentrations, but sensitivity to the opioid was highly variable between patients. [Modified with permission from Ausems ME, Hug CC Jr, Stanski DR, et al. Plasma concentrations of alfentanil required to supplement nitrous oxide anesthesia for general surgery. *Anesthesiology.* 1986;65:362.]

Hepatic dysfunction must usually be severe before it produces a substantial change in opioid pharmacokinetics. The clearances of morphine and alfentanil are reduced in cirrhosis, but fentanyl and sufentanil are not greatly affected.[148] As mentioned previously, renal failure can cause an increase in the effect of morphine, and there have been several cases of ventilatory depression reported in such patients. The mechanism may be delayed renal excretion of morphine's active metabolite.[110,149] As stated previously, remifentanil clearance is unaffected by hepatic or renal dysfunction.

HIGH-DOSE OPIOID ANESTHESIA

Some aspects of high-dose opioid anesthesia are discussed in greater depth in Chapter 52. Although this technique is no longer widely used, it taught us some valuable lessons about our intraoperative use of opioids. In 1969, Lowenstein et al[150] showed that high doses of morphine (>1 mg/kg) with only oxygen and a muscle relaxant could be used during cardiac surgery to produce profound analgesia and unconsciousness. In patients with left ventricular dysfunction as a consequence of valvular disease, large doses of morphine frequently improved hemodynamics because both preload and afterload were reduced. This anesthetic technique rapidly became popular for cardiac procedures, including the newly introduced CABG surgery. It soon became clear that morphine/oxygen "anesthesia" had a number of drawbacks, including hypotension, histamine release, occasional intraoperative awareness, and prolonged ventilatory depression. Even 1 to 2 mg/kg of morphine sometimes failed to block hypertensive responses to some intraoperative stimuli (eg, sternotomy).

In 1978, Stanley and Webster[151] proposed that 50 to 100 μg/kg of fentanyl with oxygen produced better intraoperative conditions than morphine for cardiac surgery. They found only modest decreases in systemic pressure and total peripheral resistance, and unlike morphine, high doses of fentanyl did not release histamine.[74] For a few years, fentanyl/oxygen was an extremely popular anesthetic technique for most open-heart surgery. In 1983, sufentanil was introduced with cardiac surgery as its specific indication. In doses as high as 30 μg/kg, it was used like fentanyl, as an opioid anesthetic.[78]

What was the logic behind administering such huge doses of these opioids?

- If no other sedative-hypnotic agents are administered, very large opioid doses are *required* to produce unconsciousness.[25,26]
- Unlike volatile anesthetics, opioids do not depress contractility or impair cardiovascular reflexes. Induction is usually smooth and well tolerated, even by patients with limited myocardial reserve.
- Most hemodynamic responses to surgery are suppressed, and the release of many "stress" hormones (catecholamines, insulin, growth hormone, antidiuretic hormone, cortisol, renin, etc) is blocked.[152]
- Opioids do not produce dangerous interactions with most vasoactive medications, and the myocardium is not sensitized to endogenous or exogenous catecholamines.
- The long duration of opioid effect allows for a smooth transition to mechanical ventilation in the immediate postoperative period.

Fentanyl and sufentanil provided excellent basal analgesia for cardiac procedures, but it became clear that they cannot be considered complete anesthetics. Intraoperative awareness occurred, even after fentanyl doses as high as 90 μg/kg.[153] Even extraordinarily high plasma concentrations of fentanyl or sufentanil failed to block some of the hemodynamic and hormonal responses to surgery[154] (**Fig. 42-18**). We now understand that it was a mistake to assume that all hypertensive or tachycardic events signified pain or an inadequate dose of analgesic. Many intraoperative stimuli, such as manipulation of the heart and great vessels, can elicit reflex cardiovascular responses that we now know to be opioid resistant. Similarly, the stress hormonal responses that occur during nonphysiologic conditions such as cardiopulmonary bypass cannot be eliminated by opioids.[152]

In clinical practice, "pure" opioid-oxygen anesthesia (without adjuvant anesthetic drugs) is rarely performed. The desire of most clinicians to be flexible and "fast-track" some of their patients makes such a long-lasting anesthetic less desirable. Most patients receive premedication and moderate doses of opioids, then inhalation or intravenous agents are added to control hemodynamics and to ensure unconsciousness. The addition of hypnotic agents creates a complete anesthetic, although cardiovascular depression is more likely. High-dose fentanyl, for example, produces a much larger fall in peripheral resistance when the patient has received intravenous diazepam.[155]

In summary, high-dose opioid anesthesia taught us several important lessons about the way we use these drugs intraoperatively:

1. Anesthesiologists rely on opioids during surgery for *both* suppression and preservation of autonomic function. Opioids suppress autonomic responses to painful stimuli, but we use them for critically ill patients because they preserve myocardial contractility and do not block essential hemodynamic reflexes.

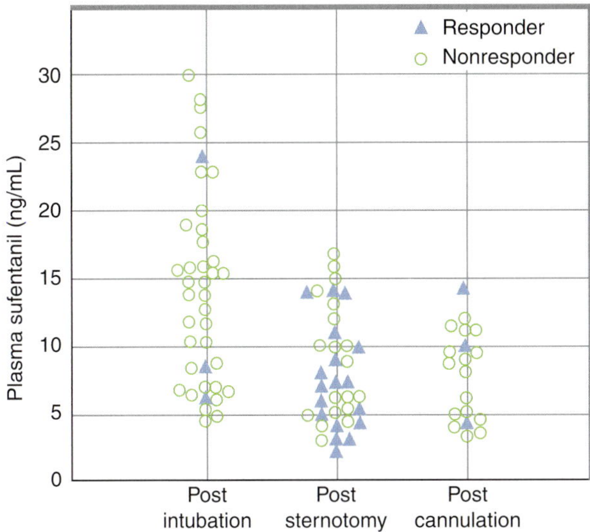

FIGURE 42-18. Presence or absence of hemodynamic response versus plasma concentration of sufentanil at 3 points during cardiac surgery. Patients undergoing coronary revascularization received only sufentanil, 100% oxygen, and muscle relaxant. Response was defined as a blood pressure increase of 15% or more over control value while awake. Given alone, even extremely high concentrations of sufentanil did not block all responses. [Reproduced with permission from Philbin DM, Rosow CE, Schneider RC, et al. Fentanyl and sufentanil anesthesia revisited: how much is enough? *Anesthesiology.* 1990;73:5.]

2. Opioids are not substitutes for β-blockers, intravenous vasodilators, or the controlled vasodilatation produced by inhalation anesthesia. In an otherwise fit patient who has hypertension, the *lack* of cardiovascular depression can sometimes make it difficult to control intraoperative hemodynamics with only opioid/nitrous oxide anesthesia.
3. Finally, we have learned that responses to surgical stimulation do not always signal the need for more opioid. This was elegantly demonstrated by Wynands et al,[156] who compared high-dose fentanyl anesthesia in patients with good or poor left ventricular function undergoing CABG. Plasma concentrations of fentanyl were high in all patients, but hypertensive episodes occurred almost exclusively in patients who had good left ventricular function. In this study, hypertension was not a sign of insufficient analgesia, it was an indicator of adequate myocardial function! These patients tolerated—and required—supplemental intravenous or inhaled anesthetic agents.

OPIOID ANTAGONISTS

NALOXONE

Naloxone, the *N*-allyl derivative of oxymorphone, was the first pure opioid antagonist to become available for parenteral use (**Fig. 42-19**A). Naloxone acts as a competitive antagonist at all opioid receptors, but it has greatest affinity for μ receptors. Small doses of naloxone reliably reverse or prevent the effects of pure opioid agonists and most mixed agonist–antagonists. The block is reversible and competitive, so it can be overcome by additional agonist.

Given alone, naloxone is nearly devoid of clinically demonstrable effects. In animal models, chronic treatment with low doses of naloxone can upregulate opioid receptors and increase the effect of agonists. The relevance of this for clinical care is uncertain. In humans, extremely large doses of naloxone (4 mg/kg) cause a mild increase in heart rate and systolic blood pressure, as well as slowing of EEG alpha-wave activity. Animal studies also show that naloxone can reduce

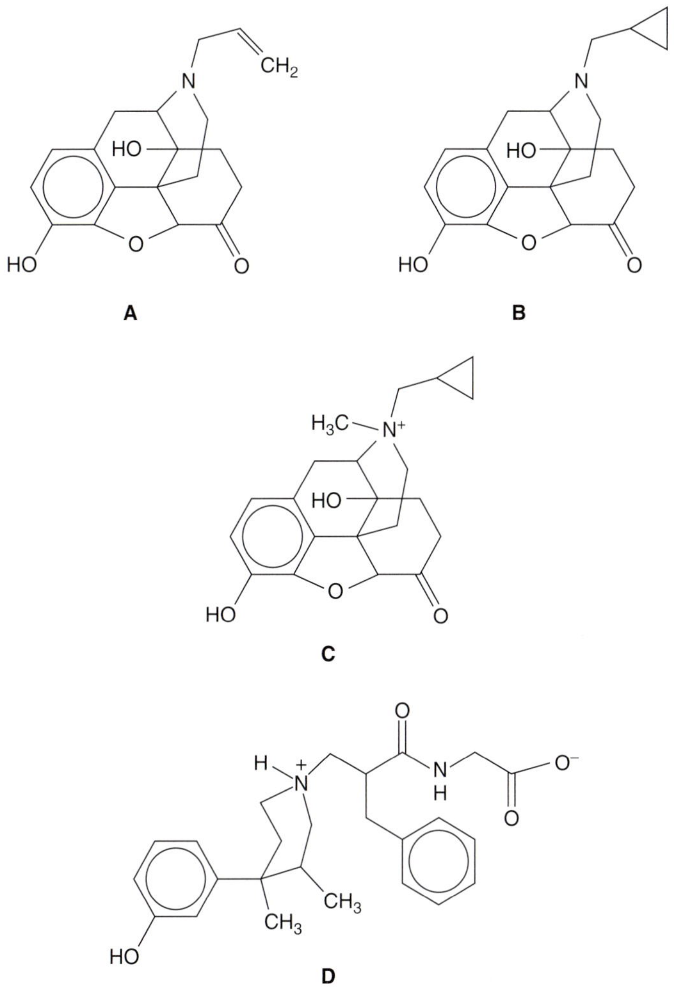

FIGURE 42-19. Structural formulas of (**A**) naloxone, (**B**) naltrexone, (**C**) methylnaltrexone, and (**D**) alvimopan.

food intake, alter sleep patterns, and improve spatial learning. In some disease states, such as septic shock, large doses can have a pressor effect. This may be the result of antagonism of elevated endogenous opioid peptides.

Naloxone is widely distributed and rapidly achieves effective concentrations in the CNS. Plasma and brain levels fall precipitously because of rapid redistribution. The drug is rapidly cleared by hepatic biotransformation, mainly to the 3-glucuronide. The clearance is very high (approximately 30 mL/kg/min), which suggests that extrahepatic elimination may be occurring. The terminal half-life is 1 to 2 hours. The onset of antagonist effect is extremely rapid, but the duration of action is quite brief. An IV dose of 0.4 mg will usually antagonize morphine for less than 1 hour; increasing the dose does not increase the duration appreciably. With the exception of remifentanil, the duration of naloxone is shorter than that of the opioids that are used to antagonize.

The presence of excessive opioid effects is a common problem in the postoperative setting. Small doses of naloxone (40 μg in an adult, repeated every 3 minutes) can be given intravenously, usually with dramatic improvement. In many cases there will also be partial reversal of analgesia, but this can be minimized by careful dosing. Patients who receive naloxone need continued observation and possibly repeated doses. Postoperative ventilatory compromise is frequently caused by a combination of factors, and therapy with naloxone does not eliminate the need to search for and treat conditions like residual paralysis, bronchospasm, and airway edema.

Naloxone is used to reverse opioids in several other clinical settings:

- In the delivery suite, naloxone can be used in depressed neonates whose mothers received opioids during labor. Clark et al[157] showed that 0.01 mg/kg via an umbilical vein catheter was usually sufficient. Acidotic infants were slower to reverse and sometimes required a second dose.
- In the emergency department, 0.4 to 0.8 mg of naloxone is usually administered in cases of suspected opioid overdose. Naloxone is also useful as an aid in the differential diagnosis of coma; if a patient fails to respond to naloxone, nonopioid causes should be considered.
- Patients who receive epidural or intrathecal opioids are frequently troubled by side effects such as pruritus and urinary retention (see Chapter 47). An IV infusion of naloxone prevents or reverses these side effects, but may also produce an unacceptable reduction in analgesia.[158]

Opioid reversal can sometimes have important hemodynamic consequences. Increases in systemic pressure, heart rate, and plasma levels of catecholamines can occur. This may be because of the sudden onset of pain, but these effects have been reproduced experimentally in the absence of painful stimuli.[159] There are several case reports of fulminant pulmonary edema, dysrhythmias, and even death in young, previously healthy individuals given naloxone. In one case, the dose of naloxone was only 0.1 mg.[160] The etiology of this rare, catastrophic response is unknown.

NALTREXONE

Naltrexone is the *N*-cyclopropylmethyl derivative of oxymorphone (Fig. 42-19B). Like naloxone, it is a relatively pure antagonist. The main clinical use of naltrexone is in the treatment of previously detoxified heroin addicts. When high doses are taken chronically, naltrexone will block the euphoriant effects of injected heroin and thus help to prevent relapse. It also decreases drug craving in former addicts. Naltrexone has been approved by the US Food and Drug Administration (FDA) for the maintenance of sobriety in alcoholics by blocking an opioid link in alcohol craving.[161] It is available orally and in a depot formulation for intramuscular injection.

Naltrexone is rapidly absorbed and undergoes 95% first-pass metabolism to 6-β-naltrexol. This is an active metabolite that probably accounts for most of naltrexone's activity. The metabolite accumulates during chronic treatment; it has a terminal half-life of 12.9 hours, so significant antagonist effects may persist for 2 to 3 days after naltrexone is stopped.

In the event that a patient on naltrexone requires emergency surgery or treatment for acute pain, the patient should be managed (if possible) with regional anesthesia, nonopioid analgesics, and other nonopioid methods. If opioids are necessary, naltrexone antagonism is competitive and may be overcome with high doses of morphine or fentanyl.

N-METHYLNALTREXONE

N-methylnaltrexone (MNTX) is a quaternary analogue of naltrexone that does not achieve significant concentrations in the CNS (Fig. 42-19C). It has been approved as a subcutaneous injection for the treatment of OBD in patients on chronic opioid therapy.[162,163] In healthy volunteers who were given morphine, intravenous MNTX reversed depression of gastric emptying and intestinal motility, but it did not interfere with analgesia against experimental pain.[164] It rapidly relieves constipation in subjects on methadone maintenance and in hospice patients who are taking opioids chronically. Efficacy of an experimental oral formulation suggests that this action is likely achieved via an intraluminal effect.[165] In healthy volunteers who had detrusor dysfunction induced by a remifentanil infusion, MNTX restored the ability to void in some of the subjects.[85] MNTX, like naloxone, has minimal effects on opioid-naïve persons.

ALVIMOPAN

Alvimopan is another permanently charged, peripheral opioid receptor antagonist (Fig. 42-19D).[163,166] It is poorly absorbed after oral administration, does not cross the blood–brain barrier, and does not reverse opioid analgesia. Alvimopan has been studied exclusively in an oral formulation for the treatment of OBD and also for the more general problem of postoperative ileus. Its efficacy in postoperative ileus may be because surgical insult releases endogenous opioid peptides in the bowel wall, which accounts for some of the decrease in intestinal motility. In both OBD and postoperative ileus, alvimopan significantly improves various indices of motility. The improvement in postoperative ileus decreases the time to hospital discharge.[167] One of the phase 3 studies suggested that alvimopan might be associated with cardiovascular morbidity, although this has not been confirmed, and no logical mechanism has been proposed. Until this is resolved, the FDA approval limits patient exposure to 15 doses of alvimopan.

OPIOID AGONIST–ANTAGONISTS

GENERAL PROPERTIES

The agonist–antagonist opioids are synthetic and semisynthetic analgesics that are structurally related to morphine (**Fig. 42-20**). They have been used primarily for moderate to severe acute pain, although buprenorphine has now been approved for maintenance therapy in opioid addiction. All these compounds produce some degree of competitive antagonism to morphine and the other pure agonists.

Nalorphine, the original agonist–antagonist, is no longer used clinically, but it has pharmacologic properties that illustrate the most important features of the class:

- A strong analgesic effect, sufficient for moderate to severe postoperative pain.
- A morphine antagonist effect that depends on the ratio of morphine to nalorphine. At very high doses of nalorphine, the agonist effects predominate.
- A very low potential for diversion or abuse. Administration to subjects who are physically dependent on opioids produces a violent "precipitated withdrawal" syndrome. Former heroin addicts given nalorphine do not experience euphoria or perceive the drug as being similar to morphine.
- A combination of typical and atypical opioid side effects. Nalorphine produces limited ventilatory depression and GI effects, but analgesic doses can cause severe psychotomimetic reactions.

The unusual mental effects—distressing hallucinations and dysphoria—made nalorphine clinically unacceptable as an analgesic, although it was used for many years as an opioid antagonist. Nalorphine was an important milestone in opioid pharmacology because it demonstrated, for the first time, that addiction liability and potent analgesia might be separated. All the more modern agonist–antagonist opioids are products of an intense search for strong analgesics that are less likely to be abused.

All of the agonist–antagonists behave as partial agonists; these drugs tend to have shallower dose–response curves and produce lower maximal effects than fentanyl or morphine[168] (Fig. 42-1A). This means there is a "ceiling" to the analgesic effects, but the toxic effects also are limited. Most of the clinically available agonist–antagonists bind to both μ and κ receptors, but they have different intrinsic activities at each site:

- κ Partial agonists: Pentazocine, butorphanol, and nalbuphine (and nalorphine) produce analgesia and sedation by a partial agonist effect at κ receptors. All of them are competitive antagonists at μ receptors and therefore reverse the effects of morphine.
- μ Partial agonists: Buprenorphine binds to μ receptors with extremely high affinity but has limited efficacy. When given alone, its effects are similar to those of morphine. When given after morphine, it competes with the full agonist and causes a reduction in opioid effect[168] (Fig. 42-1B). Buprenorphine is also an antagonist at κ-opioid receptors.

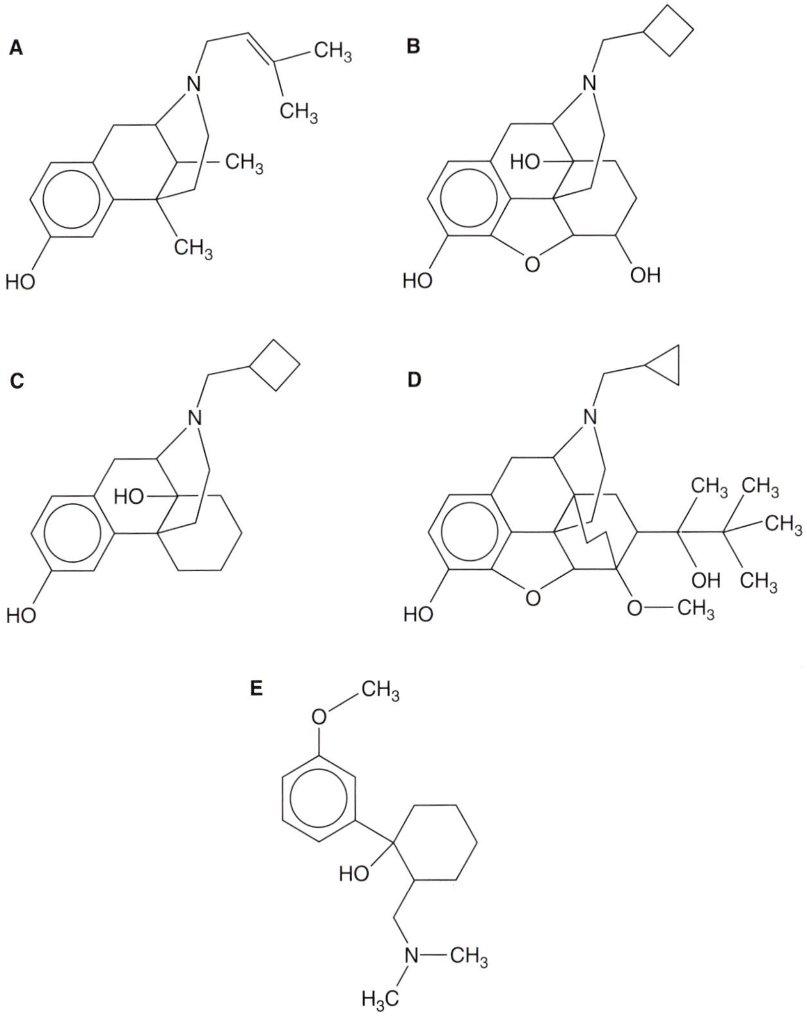

FIGURE 42-20. Structural formulas of (**A**) pentazocine, (**B**) nalbuphine, (**C**) butorphanol, (**D**) buprenorphine, and (**E**) tramadol.

These drugs vary widely in their potencies, both as analgesics and antagonists (**Table 42-4**). Neither agonist versus antagonist potency nor μ versus κ interaction has proved to be a predictor of clinical usefulness or patient acceptance.

ACUTE EFFECTS

Analgesia The agonist–antagonists are effective in a variety of acute and chronic pain states. They can be given intramuscularly, orally, sublingually, intranasally, intravenously by bolus or continuous infusion, and in patient-controlled analgesia systems. Table 42-1 lists the agents and their recommended intravenous doses. None of these drugs are currently approved for epidural or intrathecal use, although they have all been reported to be effective by this route.

The agonist–antagonist opioids have been used during balanced anesthesia, but their partial agonist properties are not a particular advantage in this setting. Even extremely large doses of nalbuphine or butorphanol will not produce the intensity of analgesia one expects from fentanyl or its derivatives. Compared with morphine or fentanyl, the agonist–antagonists produce more limited decreases in the requirements for potent volatile anesthetics.[144]

Sedation and Mood Effects The subjective effects of buprenorphine are similar to morphine throughout the dose range. The κ-type agonists have been described as producing "apathetic sedation"; this may reflect the localization of κ receptors in deeper layers of the cerebral cortex.[169] Patients given pentazocine, nalbuphine, or butorphanol may experience floating and dissociation, but usually do not experience mood elevation like that seen with morphine. After analgesic doses, patients often appear extremely sedated, yet remain capable of surprisingly lucid conversation. With pentazocine, patients are increasingly likely to experience "weird" feelings, dysphoria, or even hallucinations as the dose is raised. As stated previously, these unpleasant effects may also be mediated by κ receptors. They occur less frequently with butorphanol or nalbuphine.

Most physicians are familiar with the pleasant mental detachment produced by morphine and use it as a sign that the drug is working. Because mood elevation and euphoria do not usually occur with the κ-type agonist–antagonists, patient and physician acceptance of these

TABLE 42-4 Agonist Versus Antagonist Potential of Opioid Mixed Agonist–Antagonists

Drug	Analgesic Potency (Morphine = 1)	Morphine Antagonist Potency (Nalorphine = 1)
Pentazocine	0.2	0.02
Nalbuphine	1	0.25
Butorphanol	5	–[a]
Buprenorphine	25	10

[a]Weak antagonist; see text.

drugs has been somewhat limited. Ironically, lack of a morphine-like mood effect makes these analgesics much less desirable for opioid addicts, and it is thought to be a key factor in their low abuse liability.

The sedative effects of some agonist–antagonists may be used to advantage. Butorphanol was evaluated as a premedicant in elective surgical patients, and it produced useful sedation in doses lower than those routinely used for analgesia.[170] Its effects on body perception, anxiety, and psychomotor testing were similar to those of midazolam. Unlike the benzodiazepine, it produced very little anterograde amnesia. In this patient population, there was no evidence of dysphoria or hallucinations.

Ventilatory Depression As stated previously, these opioids are all partial agonists, and their toxic effects are limited in intensity. Ventilatory depression reaches a maximum after approximately 30 mg of nalbuphine[171] or 2 to 4 mg of butorphanol,[172] and even larger doses are well tolerated by most patients. Severe depression is still possible in sensitive individuals, those with concomitant CNS or pulmonary disease, and those receiving other depressant drugs. Ventilatory depression may be reversed with naloxone but *not* with another agonist–antagonist.

A ceiling effect on ventilation has also been demonstrated with the use of buprenorphine. This is important because buprenorphine has very high affinity for μ receptors and is not easily antagonized by naloxone.[173]

Smooth Muscle Effects Nalbuphine, butorphanol, and pentazocine do not cause significant elevation of intrabiliary pressure.[83,174] These agents may be particularly useful for patients who experience biliary colic after morphine. Buprenorphine is believed to cause biliary effects that are slightly more pronounced.[175] The agonist–antagonists appear to have small effects on smooth muscle in the intestine and bladder, and they cause less constipation than full opioid agonists.

Cardiovascular Effects The cardiovascular effects of buprenorphine and nalbuphine are similar to those of morphine. Pentazocine may increase heart rate, systemic and pulmonary artery pressure, and left ventricle end-diastolic pressure. Butorphanol (2 mg) can also increase pulmonary artery pressure, but heart rate and systemic pressure usually decrease slightly.[176] The rise in pulmonary artery pressure does not increase as the dose is raised.

Antagonist Effects Table 42-4 lists the approximate agonist versus antagonist potencies of these drugs. Nalbuphine and buprenorphine are strong antagonists and have been used clinically for this purpose. The available evidence does not suggest that reversal with an agonist–antagonist is safer or more reliable than reversal with naloxone.[177]

Administration of an opioid antagonist to an opioid-dependent patient will precipitate withdrawal; this has occurred after therapeutic doses of pentazocine, nalbuphine, and buprenorphine. Butorphanol is a weak antagonist, and it produces only mild withdrawal in addicts who are maintained on 30 mg/d of methadone.[178] A low level of physical dependence may occur in patients who receive opioid agonists over long periods, and this subclinical state may be unmasked by administration of an antagonist. During routine perioperative care, it seems prudent to avoid agonist–antagonists in patients who have had significant prior treatment with morphine, meperidine, oxycodone, and other such drugs.

CHRONIC ADMINISTRATION

In the United States, pentazocine is the only agonist–antagonist available in a typical oral tablet; butorphanol is available as a nasal spray, and buprenorphine is available only as a high-dose sublingual tablet for treatment of opioid abuse. It is possible to give agonist-antagonists parenterally for long periods of time, but there are few clinical data on such use.

Long-term studies on ex-heroin addicts showed that tolerance and physical dependence do occur after repeated administration of agonist–antagonist opioids. Withdrawal is usually qualitatively different from that of morphine and not usually accompanied by intense drug-seeking behavior. There has been renewed interest in chronic sublingual administration of buprenorphine since 2002 when the FDA approved it for maintenance therapy of opioid addicts (see Chapter 24). Chronic administration of buprenorphine in very high doses prevents withdrawal and reduces drug seeking.[179] Unlike methadone maintenance, buprenorphine treatment of addicts does not have to occur in a specially licensed clinic, although physicians who use it this way must have additional qualifications. The heroin addict is usually switched to sublingual buprenorphine under supervision because the partial agonist properties may sometimes elicit withdrawal symptoms. Chronic dosing is then done by the addict without direct supervision. To reduce the possibility that the buprenorphine will be diverted or abused during chronic maintenance, one formulation, Suboxone, combines buprenorphine and naloxone. Sublingual administration of this combination produces similar effects to buprenorphine alone, because sublingual naloxone undergoes high first-pass clearance and does not achieve effective concentrations in blood. If the addict attempts to dissolve the tablet and inject it intravenously, the naloxone will antagonize the euphoriant effect and possibly cause precipitated withdrawal.

In the event that a patient taking buprenorphine/naloxone presents for surgery, treatment of acute pain may present a significant problem.[180] These patients are highly tolerant to opioids, and residual levels of the partial agonist may antagonize other opioids for a long time. Regional anesthesia and nonopioid techniques should be used whenever possible. If opioid treatment is required, large doses of potent opioid agonists may be needed, and advice should be sought from a specialist in addiction medicine.

KEY REFERENCES

- Ausems ME, Hug CC Jr, Stanski DR, et al. Plasma concentrations of alfentanil required to supplement nitrous oxide anesthesia for general surgery. *Anesthesiology*. 1986;65:362.
- Austin KL, Stapleton JV, Mather LE. Relationship between blood meperidine concentrations and analgesic response: a preliminary report. *Anesthesiology*. 1980;53:460.
- Eisenberg E, McNicol ED, Carr DB. Efficacy and safety of opioid agonists in the treatment of neuropathic pain of nonmalignant origin: systematic review and meta-analysis of randomized controlled trials. *JAMA*. 2005;293:3043-3052.
- Forrest WH, Bellville JW. The effect of sleep plus morphine on the respiratory response to carbon dioxide. *Anesthesiology*. 1964;25:137.
- Kharasch ED. Intraoperative methadone: rediscovery, reappraisal, and reinvigoration? *Anesth Analg*. 2011;112:13-16.
- Kurz A, Sessler DI. Opioid-induced bowel dysfunction: pathophysiology and potential new therapies. *Drugs*. 2003;63:649-671.
- McClain DA, Hug CC Jr. Intravenous fentanyl kinetics. *Clin Pharmacol Ther*. 1980;28:106.
- Philbin DM, Rosow CE, Schneider RC, et al. Fentanyl and sufentanil anesthesia revisited: how much is enough? *Anesthesiology*. 1990;73:5.
- Romberg R, Olofsen E, Sarton E, et al. Pharmacodynamic effect of morphine-6-glucuronide versus morphine on hypoxic and hypercapnic breathing in healthy volunteers. *Anesthesiology*. 2003;99:788-798.
- Scott JC, Ponganis KV, Stanski DR. EEG quantitation of narcotic effect: the comparative pharmacodynamics of fentanyl and alfentanil. *Anesthesiology*. 1985;62:234.

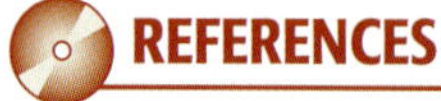

REFERENCES

Complete references available on DVD and online version at www.LongneckerAnesthesiology.com

CHAPTER 43

Total Intravenous Anesthesia

John Sear

KEY POINTS

1. The availability of drugs with short blood–brain equilibration times (especially those with an ester linkage) enables the clinician to use intravenous anesthetics and analgesics where controllability is easy and recovery rapid.
2. Total intravenous anesthesia (TIVA) offers some important advantages over inhalation anesthetics, including rapid recovery with minimal hangover and a low incidence of nausea and vomiting. TIVA may be the technique of choice for some operations.
3. Effective delivery of TIVA requires the clinician to have a good knowledge and understanding of pharmacokinetics, pharmacodynamics, and pharmacokinetic–pharmacodynamic (PK-PD) modeling.
4. Important drug characteristics include induction dose, rate of administration, and k_{e0} (rate constant for the elimination of drug from the effect compartment; drugs with small k_{e0} values take longer to equilibrate between the blood and the effect compartment or biophase). Thus for a rapid sequence induction, drugs with a large k_{e0} are preferable (viz., propofol, thiopental, remifentanil, and alfentanil compared with midazolam, ketamine, and fentanyl).
5. Drug interactions are important in TIVA. Excepting ketamine, opiates and hypnotics potentiate each other and can result in synergistic cardiovascular and respiratory depression. This means the doses of each can be reduced. There is a ceiling to the potentiating effect of the opiates, beyond which there is an increased incidence of adverse side effects and often delayed onset of spontaneous ventilation at the end of surgery.
6. Ketamine is the only hypnotic drug with established analgesic properties; there are few data suggesting that the S (+) isomer has major advantages over the racemic mixture.
7. If the patient shows signs of response during TIVA, additional IV supplementation can be achieved by bolus doses or by increasing the infusion rate, or the targeted concentration if using target-controlled infusion (TCI).
8. The elimination half-life and systemic clearance are not useful in TIVA for determining the offset of IV drugs. The context-sensitive half-time (CSHT) is more relevant, and modeled data and dynamic measurements correlate well.
9. Context-sensitive decrement times are useful indices of recovery from anesthesia. Recovery is influenced by other factors apart from the CSHT, including patient characteristics such as age, sex, body habitus, coadministered therapies, and disease states.
10. Knowledge of the context-sensitive decrement times for opiates and hypnotics allows appropriate choice of drugs for the maintenance of anesthesia. CSHT also helps determine which infusions should be terminated at the end of anesthesia, and which should be terminated some time beforehand.

In 2011 we are still without any one drug that can provide all the requirements of anesthesia (ie, unconsciousness, analgesia, amnesia, and muscle relaxation). Consequently, administration of several different agents is needed to produce the desired end result. The use of intravenous agents to achieve these goals began with the introduction of the rapidly acting barbiturates in 1934. Despite the disastrous consequences after the use of thiopental at Pearl Harbor in 1941, intravenous anesthesia is now well established as an appropriate alternative to the traditional approach of volatile anesthetics alone; indeed, sometimes it is the preferred alternative. Further, intravenous anesthesia is a fundamental component of "balanced anesthesia," in which volatile and intravenous anesthetics are combined to produce the anesthetic state.

The kinetics of the early barbiturates did not render the drugs ideal for the *maintenance* of anesthesia; the provision of analgesia could not be achieved by the barbiturates alone, and the addition of either meperidine or morphine (both drugs having slow blood–brain equilibration) led to overdosing and hence to poor clinical conditions, especially in the spontaneously breathing patient. The introduction of modern *volatile* agents, starting with halothane in 1956, with their easy titratability, encouraged the anesthetist to turn away from the intravenous agents for the maintenance of anesthesia.

The development of and present interest in total intravenous anesthesia (TIVA) owes much to a number of important studies. When considering the role of hypnotic agents, the contribution of Savege et al,[1] who, in 1975, used the steroid agent Althesin (alphaxalone and alphadolone acetate) (Glaxo, London, UK) with meperidine to supplement oxygen-enriched air in the spontaneously breathing patient, is of great importance. Subsequent drug developments included the use of infusions of thiopental, methohexital, the carboxylated imidazole etomidate, propofol, midazolam, and ketamine. With the exception of ketamine, none of these agents probably provided analgesia (although analgesic effects of alphadolone have been described by Goodchild et al[2] when administered by the enteral route).

Another approach to the provision of intravenous anesthesia was studied by Lowenstein et al[3] in 1969 using morphine *as a sole agent* to achieve anesthesia in patients undergoing cardiac surgery. This method of anesthesia (more popular in the United States and Europe than in the United Kingdom) was not reliably effective. It was associated with a high incidence of episodes of awareness during anesthesia, as well as intraoperative episodes of hypotension caused by histamine release, resulting in increased intraoperative and postoperative fluid and blood requirements. A reduction in the incidence of some of these side effects was seen when morphine was replaced with fentanyl or one of its congeners, but at the cost of increased truncal rigidity.

The selective and highly potent μ-receptor opiates (fentanyl, alfentanil, sufentanil, and more recently, remifentanil) have the advantage of less cardiovascular depression, as well as the ability to obtund the hemodynamic responses to laryngoscopy and intubation. However this apparent stability is less evident during major cardiovascular surgery, particularly during the period of sternotomy and aortic root dissection in patients undergoing cardiopulmonary bypass, where there are frequent episodes of significant hypertension and tachycardia that are not always remediable by increased doses of the opiates. Thus it became clear that use of high doses of opiates *alone* was inappropriate to provide anesthesia. Hence attempts to control the hemodynamic effects of surgical stimulation and to reduce the incidence of awareness have used either low inspired concentrations of volatile agents or infusions of a sedative-hypnotic agent as supplements to opiates.

Use of TIVA techniques are not without difficulties in these patients, as some combinations of opiates, such as fentanyl and diazepam, can result in significant reductions in both cardiac output and systemic vascular resistance. However, the effectiveness of the benzodiazepines in reducing the circulating levels of catecholamines may be important, and greater hemodynamic stability has been found in cardiac surgical patients in whom the combination of sufentanil with ketamine or midazolam has been employed. In noncardiac surgery, opiates remain popular as the basis of most neurosurgical anesthetic techniques, as they do not alter the carbon dioxide reactivity of the cerebral blood vessels. The kinetics and dynamics of remifentanil (and to less extent alfentanil) allow the anesthesiologist to titrate dose requirements more closely for a given surgical procedure during abdominal and other major body surface surgical procedures.

Over the past 3 decades, increased interest in intravenous anesthesia has been prompted by the availability of newer and more appropriate

TABLE 43-1 Adverse Properties of Volatile Agents

1. Organ toxicity is associated with the use of most of our present volatile agents, such as dose-related cardiovascular and respiratory depression, dose-related increases in cerebral blood flow and intracranial pressure, hepatic and renal toxicity, coronary blood-flow steal phenomena, and immune-modulation and depression.
2. Environmental issues related to trace concentrations of volatile agents and nitrous oxide as well as the effects of these trace concentrations on the health and work performance of anesthesiologists, surgeons, operating room, and recovery area personnel.

rapid-onset and short-acting IV sedative-hypnotics (eg, midazolam, propofol, etomidate), analgesics (alfentanil, sufentanil, remifentanil), and muscle relaxants (atracurium, vecuronium, mivacurium, and rocuronium). All these factors have refocused the anesthetist's attention on the *total* provision of anesthesia by the intravenous route. Furthermore, there are also a number of clinical situations in which intravenous anesthesia techniques are advantageous. These include

- Provision of sedation to supplement local or regional anesthetic techniques
- Provision of general anesthesia with accompanying minimal cardiovascular depression
- Use in anesthesia for office or ambulatory surgery, where the speed and completeness of recovery are important
- Use in situations in which volatile-based anesthetics may be difficult to administer because of the unavailability of resources, such as nitrous oxide; at sites of military or nonmilitary trauma; and for anesthesia at increased ambient pressure
- Use in circumstances in which nitrous oxide may either be undesirable (eg, because of the need for high inspired oxygen concentrations) or contraindicated (eg, for 1-lung anesthesia; for middle ear surgery, some neurosurgical operations, and prolonged abdominal surgery where nitrous oxide can cause closed-space effects as a result of increased volume and pressure; for relief of cardiac tamponade; for airway endoscopies [bronchoscopy and laryngoscopy]; and for bronchotracheal surgery), or where volatile agents may best be avoided (**Table 43-1**)
- Prevention of awareness during cardiopulmonary bypass and cerebral protection in patients at risk of episodes of brain ischemia
- Use in malignant hyperthermia-susceptible patients

However, the general application of TIVA techniques is not without important considerations and questions. These include the possibility and detection of awareness, the possibility of postoperative respiratory depression because of the persistent effects of concurrently administered analgesic agents, the requirement of a separate dedicated IV access site, appropriate infusion pumps, and the observation that some researchers consider depth of anesthesia as uncontrollable as that with the volatile agents.

WHAT ARE THE IDEAL DRUG PROPERTIES FOR AND ADVANTAGES OF TIVA?

Table 43-2 lists the ideal properties of a hypnotic drug for continuous infusion anesthesia. Although *none* of the present hypnotic or analgesic agents fulfills all of these criteria, some are more suitable than others under differing circumstances. **Table 43-3** lists some of the pharmacologic advantages of TIVA over inhalational agents.

DOSING STRATEGIES FOR TIVA

The administration of hypnotic, analgesic, and neuromuscular blocking components of TIVA can be provided in a number of different ways:

TABLE 43-2 Ideal Properties of a Hypnotic Drug for Use During Total Intravenous Anesthesia

1. Soluble in aqueous such that use of a solvent is avoided.
2. Stable in solution and on exposure to light for prolonged periods of time.
3. No absorption onto plastic tubing or giving sets.
4. No venous damage (pain on injection, venous phlebitis, or thrombosis) or tissue damage when administered either extravascularly or intra-arterially.
5. Sleep in 1 arm–brain circulation time.
6. Short duration of action and inactivation by metabolism in either the liver, blood, or other organs of the vessel-rich group of tissues.
7. Inactive, nontoxic, water-soluble metabolites.
8. Minimal cardiovascular and respiratory side effects.
9. If solvented in nonaqueous solution, the solvent should have no cardiorespiratory, allergenic, or other toxic side effects.

- Intermittent bolus doses of the drugs
- Continuous infusions using syringe infusion pumps or similar delivery systems
- Through the introduction (in most parts of the world, although not presently in the United States) of target-controlled infusion systems (TCI)

When given by intermittent bolus doses, there will be fluctuating drug concentrations that are associated with accompanying changes in the depth of anesthesia. Continuous infusions of IV hypnotics, opiates, and muscle relaxants can reduce these swings in drug concentrations, as well as minimize any relative under- or overdosing during drug administration. This offers a number of advantageous features to the anesthetized patient, including greater hemodynamic stability, fewer episodes of hemodynamic breakthrough and other signs of patient responsiveness, reduced need for supplemental anesthetics or vasoactive drugs, more rapid awakening and decreased incidence of requirements for naloxone or need for postoperative ventilatory support, decreased incidence of side effects, and a 25% to 30% lower total drug dose compared with bolus dosing.[5-9] Use of continuous drug infusions may also lead to decreased drug costs.

However, because modern IV agents exert profound pharmacologic effects and have short durations of action, frequent adjustments to drug dosage are necessary in order to match anesthetic effect to the varying noxious stimuli being perceived at different times during surgery, as well as the different noxious intensities of different surgical operations. This requires either frequent additional bolus dosing or the calculation of new infusion rates to achieve different drug targets.

TABLE 43-3 Advantages of TIVA

1. Smooth induction of anesthesia without coughing or hiccupping.
2. Easy control of depth of anesthesia when using drugs with short blood–brain equilibration times.
3. With most of the agents there is rapid and predictable emergence with minimal hangover and improved patient well-being.
4. Low incidence of postoperative nausea and vomiting.
5. Ideal operating conditions for neurologic surgery with reduced cerebral brain flow, decreased intracranial pressure, and decreased cerebral metabolic rate for oxygen, and in the case of propofol, preservation of cerebral autoregulation and vascular reactivity.
6. Minimal organ toxicity, although infusions of etomidate cause depression of adrenosteroidogenesis and red cell hemolysis. Infusions of propofol can lead to a metabolic syndrome.
7. However, a recent meta-analysis failed to show any advantage of TCI over manually controlled infusion regimens.[4]

Early studies using IV infusion anesthesia focused on providing fixed rate infusions that were adequate for 50% or more of a given population.[6,10] With the passage of time, these have been viewed as being less appropriate and flexible in output because they failed to allow easy titration of the achieved drug concentration to clinical effect in accordance with an individual patient's requirements. Indeed there is the probability that many patients received an overdosage because of the desire to design regimens that were "all-embracing" to all people! Nevertheless, the work of Prys-Roberts[11] and Sear[12,13] confirmed the usefulness of this approach to the provision of anesthesia with minimal cardiorespiratory depression and no reported cases of awareness.

With the hypnotic drugs currently available for continuous infusion, several manual protocols for anesthesia delivery have been developed. For example, there is the regimen for propofol described by Roberts et al[14] based on an infusion protocol to maintain a plasma propofol concentration of approximately 3 μg/mL. This was achieved by an initial 1 mg/kg induction dose, then 10 mg/kg/h for 10 minutes, 8 mg/kg/h for 10 minutes, and maintained at 6 mg/kg/h. Because this scheme is designed to achieve a fixed plasma propofol concentration, there is often a need for supplementation with additional propofol boluses and/or opiates during abdominal or other major operations. Similar manual regimens have been described for midazolam infusion. Persson et al[15,16] used an induction dose of 0.25 mg/kg, followed by a fast infusion of 0.65 mg/kg/h for 15 minutes and maintained with 0.13 mg/kg/h. This provided a hypnotic plasma concentration of 300 to 400 ng/mL. In a separate study, Thiel et al[17] described an infusion of midazolam (0.1-0.15 mg/kg then 0.02 mg/kg/h) supplemented with an opiate infusion of sufentanil for cardiac surgery.

PHARMACOKINETIC PRINCIPLES OF TIVA

Simplistically, the design of infusion protocols for TIVA is based on 2 important equations that define the loading dose and the maintenance infusion rate.

$$\text{Loading dose} = V_d \times Cp$$
$$\text{Maintenance infusion rate} = Cp \times Cl$$

where V_d = initial apparent volume of distribution, Cp = the desired plasma drug concentration, and Cl = the systemic clearance of the drug.

However, these calculations of drug requirements to reach a given target concentration are flawed for several reasons. First, the plasma is not the site of action of IV drugs; the site where the drugs produce their effects is in the brain and is termed the *biophase*. To reach the biophase, drug redistributes from the blood to the brain. At the same time, drug is also being redistributed to other tissues of the body. Hence the loading dose necessary to produce a desired pharmacologic effect cannot usually be calculated based on the initial volume of drug distribution (which is primarily the blood volume), but should use the apparent volume of distribution into which the drug has distributed once it has equilibrated with the biophase (ie, this will, of necessity, be a larger volume). (See Chapter 40 for a detailed discussion of pharmacokinetic [PK] and pharmacodynamic [PD] principles.)

When a drug is given by rapid infusion, there may be a simultaneous pharmacologic effect; however, the measure of drug effect (be it the electroencephalogram [EEG] spectral edge frequency, minute ventilation volume, or change in blood pressure or heart rate) does not always parallel the rapid increase and decrease in the plasma drug concentration. This implies "hysteresis" in the relationship between drug concentration and effect. From studies that provide continuous measurement of plasma drug concentration and effect, it is possible to relate the plasma drug concentration to the effect produced in the biophase[18] and, in turn, to calculate the volume of distribution of this effect compartment.

Further, by complex mathematical manipulation, the hysteresis loop can be "collapsed" to derive a linear relationship between concentration

TABLE 43-4 Typical Values for the k_{e0}, $t_{½}k_{e0}$, Time-to-Peak Effect After a Bolus Dose, and the Apparent Volume of Distribution Incorporating the Effect Compartment

	k_{e0} (min^{-1})	$t_{½}k_{e0}$ (min)	Time-to-Peak Effect (min)	V_{de}
PROP	0.291	2.4	2.2	37
THIOP	0.46	1.5	1.4	
ETOM	0.48	1.5	2.0	
MIDAZ	0.124	5.6	3.0	
REMI	0.46	1.5	1.5	
ALF	0.77	0.9	1.4	5.9
FENT	0.147	4.7	3.6	75
SUF	0.227	3.0	5.6	89

ALF, alfentanil; ETOM, etomidate; FENT, fentanyl; KET, racemic ketamine; MIDAZ, midazolam; PROP, propofol; REMI, remifentanil; SUF, sufentanil; $t_{½}k_{e0}$, half-time for blood–brain equilibration; THIOP, thiopental; V_{de}, volume of distribution incorporating the effect compartment.

and effect. The value that causes the hysteresis loop to collapse represents the rate of equilibration of the drug concentration between the plasma and the biophase. This is termed k_{e0} or the blood–brain equilibration rate constant. **Table 43-4** shows the values of k_{e0}, $t_{½}k_{e0}$, time to peak effect, and the apparent volume of the effect compartment.

TIME TO PEAK EFFECT

Plasma drug concentration targeting is associated with a temporal delay between the equilibration of concentrations in the plasma and at the effect site. The rate of equilibration depends on 2 factors: the rate of drug delivery to the effect site (which is influenced by cardiac output and cerebral blood flow) and the pharmacologic properties of the drug with respect to passage across the blood–brain barrier.

Although the $t_{½}k_{e0}$ is the time for blood–brain equilibration, this can only be defined if both the kinetic and dynamic properties of the drug are measured simultaneously. Because of the interindividual variability of both of these properties, it is recommended that if PK and PD data are not available from the same subjects that the *time to peak effect* (TTPE), a model-independent parameter, be used to estimate the average k_{e0} for a given kinetic model and given patient group.[19] In general, the TTPE for a drug is independent of drug dosage.

For simple infusion models (eg, the Marsh kinetic model used in the Diprifusor[20] [Zeneca Pharmaceuticals, Macclesfield, United Kingdom]), the same bolus dose will have the same predicted drug concentration profile, the same peak concentration, the same TTPF, and therefore the same k_{e0}. For more complex models (as those described by Schnider et al [21] and Minto et al,[22] in which there are included a number of covariates such as age, height, weight, and lean body mass), there will be different peak concentrations, different drug time courses, and different TTPF for patients with different characteristics (ie, each patient will have a unique k_{e0}).

For optimal dosing strategies, clinicians need to know the TTPF when giving IV drugs during both the induction and maintenance phases of anesthesia (**Fig. 43-1**). For example, during a rapid sequence induction, the anesthesiologist should use drugs with short times to peak effect. The combination of thiopental or etomidate and alfentanil or remifentanil is probably more appropriate than a combination of propofol and fentanyl. With the latter combination, the effect of the fentanyl (if given immediately before the hypnotic agent) would not be maximal by the time of intubation, leading to an initial hypertensive response to the noxious stimulus of laryngoscopy. This might then be followed by a hypotensive response when the peak effect of the fentanyl is achieved and airway stimulation is minimal. In addition, when giving drugs by bolus dosing, the interval between doses needs to be of a

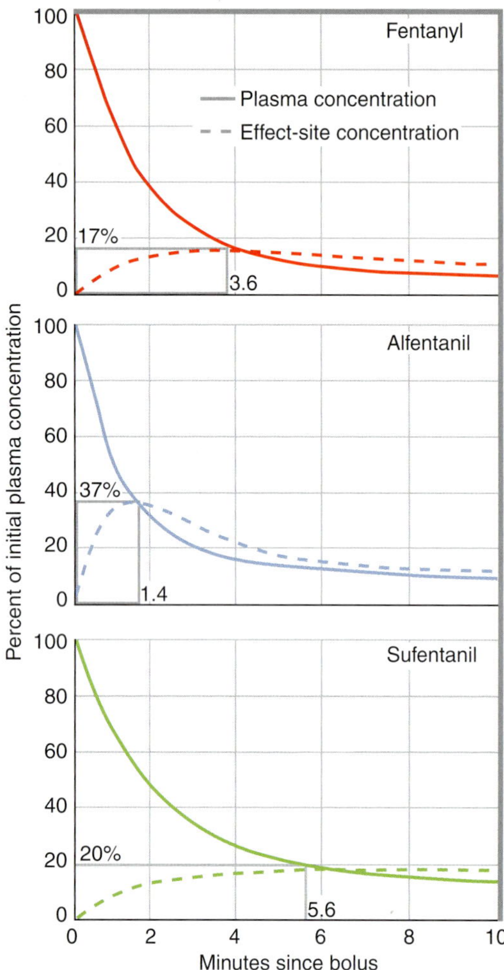

FIGURE 43-1. Computer-simulated plasma and effect-site concentrations for fentanyl, alfentanil, and sufentanil for the first 10 minutes after a bolus injection, as a percent of initial plasma concentration. [Adapted with permission from Shafer SL, Varvel JR. Pharmacokinetics, pharmacodynamics and rational opioid selection. *Anesthesiology.* 1990;74:53-63.]

TABLE 43-5 Plasma Drug Concentrations of Hypnotics and Analgesics Needed for Provision of Adequate Anesthesia for Different Noxious Stimuli During Surgery in Patients Receiving TIVA

	Incision	Major Surgery[a]	Minor Surgery[b]
Hypnotics (μg/mL)			
Propofol	5-6	2.5-7.5	2-6
Methohexital	5-10	5-15	5-10
Thiopental	35-45	10-20	10-20
Etomidate	0.4-0.6	0.5-1.0	0.3-0.6
Midazolam	–	0.05-0.20	0.02-0.25
Ketamine (racemic)	–	–	1-2
Opiates (ng/mL)[c]			
Alfentanil	200-300	250-450	100-300
Fentanyl	3-6	4-8	2-5
Sufentanil	1-3	2-5	1-3
Remifentanil	2-6	4-8	2-4

[a]Major surgery includes abdominal and vascular surgery, thoracic surgery, major orthopedic surgery, and neurosurgery.

[b]Minor surgery is body surface surgery.

[c]In the case of the opiates, adequate spontaneous ventilation will occur at concentrations ≤200 to 250, ≤1 to 2, ≤0.2, and ≤1 to 3 ng/mL, respectively.

sufficient duration to allow the peak effect of 1 bolus to be observed before the next dose of the drug is administered.

For most of the drugs used as the hypnotic and analgesic components of TIVA, plasma (blood) concentration–effect relationships have now been determined. From these, and using appropriate kinetic data sets, the clinician can derive manually controlled dosing schedules (**Tables 43-5** and **43-6**). However, these protocols do not really take account of time delays in the concentration–effect relationship. Hence many anesthesiologists view TIVA using manually controlled infusion systems and devices as a more complex strategy for maintaining anesthesia than using a vaporizer in the case of volatile agents!

COMPUTERIZED DRUG ADMINISTRATION: TARGET-CONTROLLED INFUSIONS

One of the most significant and recent advances in the delivery of infusion anesthesia over the last decade is the introduction of TCI systems that allow the anesthesiologist to set the target concentration of anesthetic. This target can be defined as either the blood or the effect-site (ie, brain) concentration. In many respects, these systems function in a similar manner to the setting of the inspired concentration of the volatile agents using a vaporizer. To achieve a given target concentration requires a greater initial infusion rate followed by a declining maintenance rate over time.

A number of publications describe a theoretical approach to attaining and maintaining steady-state drug concentrations,[23-26] with different algorithms used for targeting blood concentrations[5,27-29] and incorporating effect-site concentrations into model-driven automated delivery systems.[30,31] Several different systems for computerized drug delivery have been described. For example, Schwilden et al[32] formulated a system to maintain anesthesia using the hypnotic agent etomidate. Other systems include the computer-assisted continuous infusion (CACI) system for fentanyl[5]; the target-controlled infusion-based anesthesia (TIAC) system, also for fentanyl[6]; and the various systems for propofol.[33]

A TCI system consists of an infusion pump linked to a microprocessor containing the disposition pharmacokinetic parameters for the drug in question. The equations describing disposition are based on the bolus-elimination-transfer (BET) scheme of Schuttler et al.[34] TCI combines sequential BET schemes for maintaining or increasing the target concentration and periods of discontinuation of the infusion

TABLE 43-6 Dosing Strategies (μg/kg or μg/kg/min) of Hypnotics and Analgesics When Given by Manual Infusion Regimens to Achieve the Concentrations Needed for Major Surgery as Identified in Table 43-5

	Induction or Loading Dose	Maintenance Infusion Rates
Hypnotics		
Propofol	1000-2000	50-150
Methohexital	1500-2500	50-150
Midazolam	50-150	0.25-1.5
Ketamine (racemic)	1500-2500	25-75
Opiates[a]		
Alfentanil	50-150	0.5-3.0
Fentanyl	5-15	0.03-0.10
Sufentanil	1-5	0.01-0.05
Remifentanil	0.5-1.0	0.1-0.4

[a]For the opiates, the induction of loading dose is best given over 2 minutes to avoid marked cardiorespiratory depression.

when the target concentration has to decrease. Infusion halts are mandatory if a new lower drug concentration is to be achieved as fast as possible. The first commercially available TCI system is the Diprifusor (Zeneca Pharmaceuticals),[35] which was introduced in 1996 and uses prefilled glass syringes of propofol tagged with a unique metallic strip. More recently, open TCI systems that allow use of the various available generic formulations of propofol have been developed. Such systems include the Asena PK system (Alaris Medical Systems, San Diego, CA), the Base Primea system (Fresenius Kabi, Bad Homburg, Germany), and the FM System (B Braun, Melsungen, Germany).

At present, no drugs apart from propofol are licensed for use for TCI; in addition, approval for TCI is still awaited in the United States. However, research or developmental computer-driven delivery systems have been described for both sufentanil and remifentanil.[36–41] Sufentanil has been administered by TCI in combination with isoflurane, propofol, and midazolam, with targeted concentrations, in most studies, of sufentanil between 0.2 and 1.5 ng/mL for noncardiac surgery and 3 and 10 ng/mL for cardiac surgery. Most studies report good-quality anesthesia with hemodynamic stability and satisfactory times to return of spontaneous ventilation and extubation. Remifentanil by TCI has been assessed in combination with both IV hypnotics and volatile agents,[19,42–44] the most appropriate kinetic model for drug delivery being that of Minto et al.[22] For analgesia, concentrations between 1 and 1.5 ng/mL are needed. In combination with propofol for noncardiac surgery, remifentanil concentrations in the range of 4 to 8 ng/mL are appropriate. However, these data need confirmation in larger clinical trials.

A TCI drug delivery system has 4 key components:

1. A calculator (computer or microprocessor) and a software program, either separate with cables linking to a syringe pump, or an "all-in-one" system (as is the case with the Diprifusor)
2. Data sets of pharmacokinetic parameters for each drug to be infused
3. An infusion device
4. A user interface

For TCI delivery, the anesthesiologist needs to enter the patient's age and weight into the device and then select the desired target drug concentration. On pressing "start," the TCI system delivers precisely the amount of drug to achieve the target drug concentration and then continues to infuse drug at an appropriate rate to maintain that concentration.

Unlike using a manual fixed-infusion system, the anesthesiologist can easily either increase or decrease the target drug concentration at any time, thereby facilitating the titration of the drug concentration according to the patient's response to differing noxious stimuli.

One fundamental principle underlies the TCI pump—namely, the relationship between the infusion rate and achieved drug concentration:

$$\text{Drug concentration} \quad \frac{\text{Infusion rate}}{\text{Drug clearance}}$$

If a higher target concentration is selected, the system automatically delivers a further small bolus of drug and then infuses at a faster rate to achieve and maintain the higher drug concentration. When a lower target is chosen, the device discontinues the infusion of drug until the system predicts that the patient's drug concentration has decreased to the new value (by a combination of drug redistribution and clearance). The system then restarts the infusion at the appropriate rate for the new target concentration. With a TCI system, the anesthesiologist does not control the device's infusion rates and the size of bolus doses; rather, the anesthesiologist titrates the depth of anesthesia by selecting target drug concentrations appropriate to the patient's needs. A number of different algorithms are used in the different systems to calculate the required infusion rate.[28,31,33,45]

KINETIC MODEL SELECTION

TCI systems tend to incorporate population-averaged pharmacokinetic parameters to drive the infusion pump. This can lead to considerable variability in the observed drug concentration compared with the targeted concentration. The mean variation between these 2 concentrations (targeted and observed) is usually of the order of 20% to 30%, with a maximum of 50% to 60% considered clinically acceptable. It seems likely that greater accuracy is not going to be achievable. The sources of this variability include the differences in the parameter estimates of the polyexponential equation that is used to describe the concentration–time relationship. At the present time, there are several different commercial systems on the market for the delivery of propofol and the opiates sufentanil and remifentanil. Two types of systems exist presently—those incorporating the Diprifusor module, using tagged Diprivan (propofol; AstraZeneca, London, United Kingdom) prefilled syringes with the fingergrip tag and the original Diprifusor kinetics and "open" systems that do not require the tagged syringes and use different pharmacokinetic data sets for the delivery of propofol, remifentanil, and sufentanil (**Table 43-7**). For further discussion of TCI open systems, the reader is referred to the Open TCI Initiative (www.opentci.org).

EFFECT-SITE TARGETING

Initial drug-targeting technology was based on the plasma concentration, but as this is not the site of anesthetic action, it is more logical to target the effect site or biophase. This has been described by several authors and reviewed by Jacobs and Williams.[30] Effect-site control should allow for a faster induction time and during maintenance a more rapid increase in the depth of anesthesia. However, there are some limitations to effect-site compartment targeting, including that of overshoot of the arterial drug concentration with associated adverse consequences. Effect-site TCI has been described by a number of different research groups.[8,30,46]

Wakeling et al[47] have compared the efficacy of plasma and effect-site targeting. Twenty American Society of Anesthesiologists (ASA) classification PS-I or PS-II patients were randomized to receive TCI propofol targeted at one or the other site. In this study, the delivery system was modeled according to the kinetic data set of Gepts et al[48] and a

TABLE 43-7 TCI Systems Currently Available for the Delivery of Propofol, Remifentanil, and Sufentanil in the United Kingdom and Other Parts of the World[a]

Diprifusor TCI systems incorporate use of tagged prefilled syringes:

1. Graseby 3500 system (Graseby Medical, Watford, UK) – k_{e0} 0.26 min^{-1}
2. Vial Medical Master TCI (Fresenius Vial, Brezins, France)
3. Alaris IVAC TIVA TCI (Alaris Medical Systems, Basingstoke, UK)
4. Terumo TERUFUSION TE-372 TCI TIVA (Terumo Corporation, Tokyo, Japan)

Open TCI systems have the advantages of being able to use "generic" formulations of propofol:

1. **Alaris Asena PK Syringe Pump.** This has the same pharmacokinetic model as in the Diprifusor, with a k_{e0} of 0.26 min^{-1}. It also incorporates modeling for effect-site control.
2. **Base Primea (Fresenius Vial, France).** This includes 2 kinetic sets for propofol delivery. These are the kinetic model included in the diprifusor but with a modified value for k_{e0} of 1.21 min^{-1} and a second model system based on the kinetics of Schnider et al[90] where the kinetics are corrected for patient age and weight. The k_{e0} is also different (0.456 min^{-1}), which leads to a faster rise in brain propofol concentration.
3. **B Braun (FM System–"Space Station," Meslungen, Germany).** Incorporating the "ProTiva" pump system.

[a]At the time of writing (August 2011), none of these delivery systems are licensed for use in the United States.

k_{e0} value of 0.63 min^{-1}. At a target concentration of 5.4 μg/mL (the predicted effect-site concentration associated with loss of consciousness in 95% of subjects),[49,50] Wakeling found a median time to loss of consciousness of 3.02 minutes in the plasma-targeted group, but only 1.23 minutes in the effect-site targeted group. However, loss of consciousness occurred at the same predicted effect-site concentration in both groups.[47] Other studies of effect-site drug control have found similar results.[46,51,52]

Although an advantage of these systems is that drug delivery is optimized to a given effect-site concentration, the speed of achieving this concentration varies with the k_{e0} value incorporated into the different delivery systems. At present, several different models with different k_{e0} values are in use for the delivery of propofol. If the Diprifusor is used with the Marsh model kinetics, the blood–brain equilibration half-life ($t_{½}$ k_{e0}) is 2.6 minutes (k_{e0} 0.26 min^{-1}).[53] However, modifications of the Diprifusor algorithm in the 2 new open-TCI systems (the Base Primea and Asena PK systems) with a longer k_{e0} of 1.2 min^{-1} gives a $t_{½}$ k_{e0} of 34 seconds. When the slower k_{e0} is used, any increase in the target effect-site concentration requires higher blood drug concentrations to generate a bigger gradient to drive drug to the effect site.

A second effect-site model, based on the kinetics of Schnider et al,[21] incorporates additional details into the algorithms (including patient age, height, weight, and calculated lean body mass). In this system, the k_{e0} varies with the age of the patient. Although most studies suggest that effect-site targeting provides faster control, it is only true if there is an accurate value for k_{e0}! The recent studies of Kazama et al[54] show that k_{e0} values have a wide interindividual variability with regard to age and end point assessed. This may be a result of a number of factors, including poor delineation of early distribution kinetics and failure to accurately define the EEG hysteresis effect; this will clearly limit the accuracy of any effect-site TCI delivery system in a given individual. Use of effect-site TCI will, of necessity, lead to an overshoot of the plasma drug concentration, which can result in hemodynamic depression. Although this overshoot has little effect in patients younger than age 60,[46] further study is needed in the elderly.

As a further development in effect-site targeting, Van Poucke et al[55] have described modified delivery algorithms that target the effect-site but limit the peak plasma concentration. This should have the advantage of reducing the acute hemodynamic effect of intravenous anesthetic drugs on the heart and circulation. Simulations suggest that this approach will reduce the plasma overshoot by approximately 60%, with an accompanying 20% delay in the time to peak effect and hence the onset of drug effect. In vivo studies are clearly needed to confirm the efficacy of this method of TCI delivery.

INDUCTION OF ANESTHESIA WITH TIVA

Several factors affect the speed of induction by TIVA, including the size of the induction dose and important drug interactions.

FACTORS DETERMINING THE INDUCTION DOSE OF HYPNOTIC AGENTS

The onset of anesthesia requires the brain drug concentration to reach a given level; this can be achieved either slowly or rapidly. Rapid achievement is usually accompanied by significant adverse effects such as hypotension, bradycardia, and respiratory depression. The greater the gradient, the greater the time needed to induce anesthesia. Conversely, any marked overshoot in the effect-site concentration leads to a greater incidence and severity of the adverse effects. The transfer of drug from the blood to the effect site is governed by simple diffusion. The time needed to achieve this transfer varies with the concentration gradient and the k_{e0}.

The rate of infusion of the induction dose is another determinant governing the size of the induction dose; an infusion rate designed to only just achieve a desired effect-site concentration causes a loss of consciousness but at the cost of a slow onset. The loss of consciousness is only transient, and is maintained only for the duration that the targeted effect-site concentration is maintained. A faster rate of infusion provides a more rapid onset of anesthesia and a longer duration of loss of consciousness, but again involves administration of a larger induction dose and hence a greater likelihood of adverse effects.

Variations in induction dose requirements also occur because of interindividual pharmacokinetic differences and because of pharmacodynamic differences that are the result of age, sex, cardiac output, smoking, concomitant medications, and the presence of coexisting disease states.[56]

DRUG INTERACTIONS

Because no single IV drug (with the possible exception of ketamine) can provide hypnosis, amnesia, and analgesia, total intravenous anesthesia will be, by definition, provided by a combination of drugs.[57] However, in contrast to the simply additive effects of the different gaseous and volatile anesthetics (see Chapter 38), IV anesthetics may interact in either additive or synergistic manners (see Chapters 41 and 42). In the case of most IV agents, this interaction is synergistic. One example used to good effect is the combination of a hypnotic and benzodiazepine or other sedative drug (eg, an α_2-agonist) for induction of anesthesia (the technique of *coinduction*).[57] One major advantage of this technique is the provision of an adequate depth of anesthesia for a noxious stimuli such as laryngoscopy and intubation *without* any associated significant cardiovascular depression.

Also clinically useful is pretreatment with a rapid-acting opiate (eg, fentanyl, sufentanil, alfentanil, or remifentanil), which will reduce the amount of hypnotic agent needed for loss of consciousness and provide analgesia to reduce the adrenergic stimulus caused by the instrumentation of the airway (whether by laryngoscopy and intubation or insertion of the laryngeal mask airway). However, the combination of an opiate with an IV hypnotic agent can cause both positive and negative side effects (namely, cardiovascular stability *or* profound cardiovascular and respiratory depression). Respiratory depression is of little importance in the mechanically ventilated patient, but is a significant and unwanted effect in the spontaneously breathing individual.

Although the combination of benzodiazepines with nitrous oxide produces minimal cardiovascular effects for induction of anesthesia, the combination of benzodiazepines with opiates results in a synergistic depression of most hemodynamic parameters. Because opiates *alone* are not complete anesthetics, they cannot be used reliably to induce anesthesia and amnesia in the absence of supplements. In clinical practice, a second anesthetic drug (eg, an IV hypnotic) should always be given to ensure loss of consciousness. Thus the main functions of opiates are to provide analgesia *and potentiate* the effects of IV anesthetic agents, both at induction and during the maintenance phase.

TERMINATION OF IV ANESTHETIC ACTION

The duration of drug effect of a bolus dose of IV drugs is terminated predominantly by redistribution of drug from the blood and brain to the lean tissues. This redistribution occurs by a series of different compartmental clearances, and to a lesser extent, metabolic clearance, the sum of these depending on cardiac output in the case of lipid-soluble hypnotic agents. However, if the dose of the induction agent causes a significant reduction in cardiac output, the offset of the drug effect is delayed.

DRUGS FOR INDUCTION OF ANESTHESIA

(Note: Detailed discussions of the following drugs appear in Chapters 41 and 42.)

THIOPENTAL

This thiobarbiturate was the most popular of all IV anesthetic induction agents, although propofol may now be more appropriate in circumstances where rapid recovery from anesthesia is a prerequisite (eg, in ambulatory surgical practice). Thiopental has a number of drawbacks as it is highly alkaline in solution and therefore extremely irritating if injected extravascularly or intra-arterially, and it has a low therapeutic index of about 4. When given IV, the barbiturates achieve onset of hypnosis within 1 arm–brain circulation time. Because of their high lipid solubility and low percentage of ionization at physiologic pH, there is rapid uptake into the brain. The maximum effect of thiopental is seen within approximately 1 minute of a single induction dose of 3 to 6 mg/kg. There then follows a similarly rapid decline in the brain concentration as a consequence of redistribution into the "lean" body tissues, making the duration of effect of an induction dose about 5 to 10 minutes. However, at the time of awakening, only 18% of the injected thiopental dose will have undergone metabolism (compared with approximately 38% of a dose of methohexital and nearly 70% of propofol).

Population kinetic data for thiopental have been described by Stanski and Maitre, with a mean clearance value of 0.0031 L/min/kg and apparent volume of distribution at steady state of 2.73 L/kg.[58] A number of different factors influence thiopental elimination. Although age influenced the kinetics of thiopental, it had no effect on brain responsiveness or dynamics when the spectral edge frequency was used as the measure of drug effect. The induction dose requirements for thiopental anesthesia vary with patient age and weight, and, most importantly, cardiac output. Lower doses are indicated in the premedicated patient, in patients with severe anemia or burns, in malnourished patients, in patients with uremia or liver failure, and in the hypovolemic individual regardless of cause. Both circulatory failure and hypothermia slow the circulation time, prolonging the induction period for thiopental. Moreover, the total dose needed in such patients is also reduced.

The blood–brain equilibration rate constant for thiopental is rapid (0.46-0.58 min^{-1}). The effect-compartment concentration associated with dropping a loaded syringe is approximately 17 μg/mL, and the duration of effect of an induction dose of 320 mg is approximately 4 minutes. Induction with thiopental causes a decrease in cardiac output, and a compensatory 10% to 15% increase in heart rate. Thiopental also causes venodilation, but has no effect on systemic vascular resistance.[59] Another feature of thiopental induction is the decrease in respiratory responsiveness to hypoxia and hypercapnia. Opiates potentiate these effects. When anesthesia is induced with the combination of thiopental and midazolam, the 2 hypnotics act synergistically; when thiopental is given with an opiate such as alfentanil, there is greater potentiation of the antinociceptive response than hypnosis.[60]

THIAMYLAL

Thiamylal (another thiobarbiturate used mainly in the United States and Japan) has pharmacologic characteristics similar to thiopental with regard to potency, incidence of laryngospasm and respiratory depression, cardiac toxicity, and recovery time. Like thiopental, it is formulated as a racemic mixture, with the potency of the S enantiomer about twice that of the R+ form. There are also enantiomeric kinetic differences. The plasma protein binding of the R+ isomer is 82.5%, and of the S– isomer 88.3%. The elimination half-life of the R+ enantiomer is 20.2 hours, the apparent volume of distribution is 3.66 L/kg, and clearance is 0.27 L/kg/h. The corresponding values for the S– compound are 24.1 hours, 2.60 L/kg, and 0.15 L/kg/h, respectively.

METHOHEXITAL

This is an oxybarbiturate with a faster recovery profile than thiopental because of a greater systemic clearance and a shorter elimination half-life. Compared with thiopental, methohexital has a more appropriate kinetic profile for both induction and maintenance of IV anesthesia (elimination half-life of 420-460 minutes, clearance of 700-800 mL/min). Because its main metabolite, 4-OH methohexital, has no pharmacologic activity (unlike thiopental's major metabolite, pentobarbital), methohexital may be usefully given by continuous infusion for maintaining anesthesia or sedation (see Drugs for Maintenance of TIVA).

Induction of anesthesia with methohexital requires doses of 1 to 2 mg/kg, giving it a potency of 2.7 times that of thiopental. The side-effect profile of methohexital is more significant than that of thiopental and includes increased incidences of pain on injection, a tendency to venous thrombophlebitis, and exaggerated involuntary movements, especially in the unpremedicated patient. Inadequate induction doses can also cause excitatory phenomena because the inhibitory areas of the brain are thought to be depressed at lower drug concentrations.

ETOMIDATE

Etomidate is a carboxylated imidazole compound formulated as the R+ enantiomer. The approximate potency ratio of the enantiomers is R+:S– = 1:10.[61] As an induction agent, etomidate has important advantages over the barbiturates, showing many ideal properties for an IV agent (cardiostability; reduction in cerebral blood flow, cerebral metabolic rate, and intracranial pressure; no release of histamine and low rate of allergic reactions; only transient and minimal respiratory depression and no inhibition of the hypoxic pulmonary vasoconstrictor reflex) and offers hemodynamic advantages during induction of anesthesia in patients with poor cardiac reserv, and hypovolemia. The drug has one of the widest margins of safety in animals of all the present hypnotic agents, with a high therapeutic index of 26.4.

Because it is unstable in water, etomidate is presently solubilized either in 33% propylene glycol or as an emulsion. The drug has a pH of 8.1 and pK_a of 4.2. It is a base, and approximately 99% of the drug is un-ionized. Plasma protein binding is approximately 75% (mainly to albumen). Metabolism occurs predominantly in the liver and plasma by esterase hydrolysis, and hence etomidate shows the expected high systemic clearance.

Induction doses of 0.2 to 0.4 mg/kg provide hypnosis for 5 to 15 minutes, with only minor alterations in cardiovascular parameters in healthy patients and in those with valvular or ischemic heart disease. Little is known about the interaction of etomidate and opiates or other hypnotics for loss of consciousness. Etomidate alone does not obtund the sympathetic responses to laryngoscopy and intubation,[62] and for a smooth hemodynamic profile, etomidate is best combined with an opiate or benzodiazepine.

However, its use as an induction agent is also associated with a number of minor disadvantages, with significant incidences of pain on injection, thrombophlebitis, myoclonia, and a high incidence of postoperative nausea and vomiting. When given either as a single induction dose or by infusion, etomidate suppresses adrenal steroidogenesis,[63-65] and low plasma cortisol levels are found after use of the agent. Does this matter? In patients receiving etomidate by infusion for intensive therapy unit sedation, Ledingham and Watt[66] found that its use was associated with increased mortality. However these findings were *not* based on a double-blind, randomized, controlled trial. There are no data to support this association when etomidate was administered by continuous infusion to anesthetized surgical patients.

The role of etomidate was further confused by an unreasoned and unsupported editorial in *Anaesthesia* expressing the view that the drug had no place in current anesthetic practice.[67] This view is *not* shared by the present author in the absence of properly conducted clinical outcome trials in nonseptic patients. But what evidence is there? In 2010, Ray et al[68] retrospectively reported on 176 patients admitted to an intensive care unit (ICU) after an emergency laparotomy. Fifty-two of the patients had anesthesia induced with etomidate. There was no association between use of etomidate and in-hospital mortality, and the risk of developing hypotension after the induction of anesthesia or the need for vasopressors to treat hypotension was least following etomidate. However, a second study (in the form of a randomized controlled trial of single doses of etomidate or ketamine in critically ill patients requiring emergency intubation) reported a greater percentage of patients with evidence of adrenal insufficiency in the etomidate group (odds ratio 6.7, 95% CI, 3.5-12.7).[69]

Use of etomidate for induction of anesthesia in the critically ill *septic* patient is probably contraindicated (despite the drug's minimal cardiovascular effects) because of data taken from a subpopulation within the CORTICUS trial that suggest an increased mortality.[70,71]

Alternate Formulations of Etomidate Attempts at improving the side-effect profile of etomidate have focused primarily on the solvent. Development of an emulsion formulation does not change the drug's dynamic properties, but is associated with lower incidences of pain on injection, myoclonus, and local thrombophlebitis.[72,73] Another advantage of the emulsion formulation is its lower osmolality and higher pH (400 mOsm/kg and pH 7.6 compared with 4965 mOsm/kg and pH 5.1 for the propylene glycol formation), which means less red cell hemolysis.[74,75] A second reformulation of etomidate has used 2-hydroxypropyl-β-cyclodextrin as the solvent.[76] Again, there was a lower incidence of myoclonia (17% vs 92%) and pain (8% vs 58%), and thrombophlebitis (0% vs 42%) and no hemolysis. None of these formulations appears to show alterations in the kinetics or dynamics of etomidate.

Although it is widely believed that use of etomidate is associated with an increased incidence of postoperative nausea and vomiting, this was not supported by a comparison in which etomidate-lipuro and propofol were used for induction of anesthesia to supplement isoflurane/fentanyl in air in patients undergoing orthopedic procedures.[77] There were no differences in rates of nausea, vomiting, or the intensity of any nausea during the early postoperative period to 24 hours. However, the rates of vomiting after etomidate were higher (27% vs 10%).

Because it causes cortisol suppression, etomidate by infusion is contraindicated in many countries including the United States, and its use in that manner must be considered as off-label.

MIDAZOLAM

Midazolam is the only currently available benzodiazepine suitable for induction of anesthesia. It has a faster onset and lower incidence of venous complications than either diazepam or lorazepam, but a slower onset than the other IV hypnotic agents (30-60 seconds for loss of consciousness). Induction of anesthesia (as is the case with the barbiturates) coincides with loss of the eyelash reflex. Induction occurs with doses of 0.1 to 0.2 mg/kg midazolam given over 20 to 30 seconds; smaller doses are sufficient in premedicated patients, in the elderly, and in patients of ASA groups PS-III to PS-IV. However, emergence from midazolam-induced anesthesia may be prolonged.[78]

Midazolam has some advantages over thiopental, including improved perioperative amnesia and hemodynamic stability. However, the combination of midazolam and an opiate can result in significant cardiovascular depression. Although a single induction dose of midazolam does not suppress the adrenal steroidogenesis,[79] data from Crozier et al[80] and Desborough et al[81] suggest that high doses of midazolam given by infusion prevent the increase in plasma cortisol concentrations in response to surgical stress. As with etomidate, the significance of this finding during TIVA is uncertain in the absence of appropriate outcome data.

Another advantage of midazolam over other hypnotic agents is the availability of a specific antagonist, flumazenil, which is devoid of any intrinsic effects on the respiratory or cardiovascular systems. However, it has a short duration of action, with peak effect occurring 1 to 3 minutes after IV injection. Because of its shorter elimination half-life (40-70 minutes) and faster clearance rate than midazolam, flumazenil may produce an initial arousal from sedation or anesthesia, followed by resedation.[82] Thus, if larger doses of midazolam are used for induction and/or maintenance of anesthesia, flumazenil preferably should be given as the combination of a loading dose and continuous infusion to maintain a plasma drug concentration in excess of 20 to 40 ng/mL.

PROPOFOL

This sterically hindered alkyl phenol was originally formulated as an emulsion containing soybean oil and egg phosphatide (Diprivan).

Propofol (as Diprivan) has a neutral pH of 7.4 and pK_a of 11.0; this means that the drug is 99.7% nonionized and highly lipid soluble at pH 7.0. It is rapidly broken down to inactive metabolites (the glucuronide and the corresponding quinol glucuronide and sulphate) in the liver and possibly in other organs, such as the lungs.[83,84] Other minor metabolites detected in the urine include 2-(ω-propanol)-6-isopropylphenol and 2-(ω-propanol)-6-isopropyl-1,4-quinol. It is not known whether any of these have anesthetic potencies. The hydroxylation of propofol by hepatic cytochrome P450 (CYP) involves the isoform 2B6, which shows wide individual variability.[85] Another isoform that shows high binding for propofol is CYP 2C9.[86]

Despite its rapid and complete offset of effect, propofol has a long elimination half-life (of up to ≥45 hours), an apparent volume of distribution of 1000 to 3940 L, and a systemic clearance between 1.0 and 1.8 L/min. Because of its high extraction ratio, propofol shows flow-dependent clearance, and its own clearance is reduced secondary to its action on myocardial contractility and cardiac output. Population kinetic analyses by Schuttler and Ihmsen[87] indicate weight to be a significant covariate for the elimination clearance, the 2 intercompartmental clearances of a 3-compartment model, and the apparent volumes of the central and 2 peripheral compartments, whereas in older patients (age >60 years), both elimination clearance and the central volume compartment decrease linearly with age.

Induction of anesthesia with propofol is smooth and associated with a low incidence of excitatory side effects. Doses of 1 to 2.5 mg/kg (depending on patient age, physical status, and use of premedicant drugs) induce anesthesia in approximately 30 seconds; however, lower induction doses should be used in patients with cardiovascular disease. Loss of consciousness occurs at propofol concentrations between 2.5 and 5.5 μg/mL, with the concentration for loss of response to verbal command being between 2.5 and 3.5 μg/mL. The speed of onset and the dose of propofol needed for induction are dependent on the administration rate. Stokes and Hutton[88] compared induction times when propofol was infused at 50, 100, and 200 mg/min and as a 2-mg/kg bolus. Times to loss of consciousness were 124, 92, 62, and 32 seconds, respectively, with the corresponding total induction doses being 1.4, 1.96, 2.61, and 2.15 mg/kg.

The size of the induction dose depends on many physiologic factors. Kazama et al[89] determined 4 factors to be independent variables influencing the size of the induction dose (namely age, lean body mass, central blood volume, and liver blood flow). When the dynamics of propofol are related to age, 3 functions correlate in a linear manner: the blood–brain equilibration rate constant and time to peak effect, the steepness of the concentration–response relationships for EEG activation and depression, and the effect-site concentration associated with 50% of peak EEG activation.[90]

The hemodynamic effects after induction doses of propofol are similar to those of the thiobarbiturates, although propofol additionally decreases systemic vascular resistance. In contrast to the barbiturates, propofol has little effect on heart rate. In contrast to the barbiturates, propofol has little effect on heart rate, the combination of the drug's vagotonic effect and the fall in vascular resistance predisposing to significant falls in blood pressure when used in the hypovolemic patient or in patients receiving other vagotonic drugs (eg, opiates).[91] The ventilatory effects of propofol are comparable to those of other hypnotic agents. Induction doses cause significant decreases in tidal and minute volumes, coupled with episodes of apnea often greater than 30 seconds, in 25% to 30% of patients. Comparative studies indicate the duration of apnea after propofol is longer than with thiopental.[92] All induction agents decrease the rib cage and abdominal components of ventilation to a similar amount. The ventilatory depressive effects of propofol are synergistic with those of midazolam and fentanyl and with the combination alfentanil-midazolam.

One advantage of propofol as an induction agent is the greater depression of pharyngeal and laryngeal reactivity than is seen with thiopental, methohexital, or etomidate. This can be of benefit during upper airway instrumentation and insertion of the laryngeal mask airway.

Pain on injection is commonly observed during induction of anesthesia with propofol, with incidences of up to 50% when administered into the small veins on the dorsum of the hand. The incidence may be reduced by use of large veins, by mixing with lignocaine (10-20 mg) and by pretreatment with drugs such as fentanyl and alfentanil. Other side effects of induction include excitatory myoclonic phenomena and occasional epileptiform fits reported during recovery. Like etomidate, propofol appears to have in vitro potential for inhibition of adrenal steroidogenesis, but this is not relevant in clinical anesthetic practice.

KETAMINE (2-*O*-CHLOROPHENYL-2-METHYLAMINOCYCLOHEXANONE HCL)

This phencyclidine derivative is formulated as a racemic mixture. It is unique among the induction agents in that it produces both dose-related unconsciousness and analgesia. After induction with ketamine, patients have little recall of surgery or anesthesia.

The 2 stereoisomers, R(−) and S(+), show differing anesthetic potencies (1:3 to 4), but have similar kinetics. The pH of ketamine is 3.5 to 5.5, and the pK_a is 7.5. At physiologic pH, ketamine is highly lipid soluble, with 12% to 35% being plasma protein bound and 44% nonionized. Recovery from ketamine anesthesia occurs as a result of both distribution and degradation by demethylation and hydroxylation by hepatic cytochrome P450 2B6 and 2C9. The metabolic breakdown of ketamine is complex, but 1 metabolite (norketamine; metabolite I) is pharmacologically active with a potency of approximately 30% that of the parent drug and a longer elimination half-life. The main excretory metabolites are ketamine and metabolite I and II glucuronides. The efficacy of ketamine is enhanced in patients with renal impairment with an accompanying delayed recovery. Most of the ketamine is excreted in the urine as the glucuronides; only 2.5% is unchanged.

Ketamine causes rapid induction of anesthesia by the IV route. However, its cardiovascular effects differ from other hypnotic agents; ketamine causes increases in heart rate, blood pressure, and cardiac output. These inotropic and chronotropic effects are seen in both healthy patients and in those with heart disease and are mediated via central mechanisms. Ketamine blocks the reuptake of noradrenaline by both the uptake 1 (extraneuronal) and uptake 2 (intraneuronal) mechanisms, as well as causes the release of noradrenaline from the sympathetic ganglia. The in vivo effects are obtunded in patients receiving adrenergic antagonists (both α and β) and vasodilators, as well as by pretreatment with benzodiazepines.

Ketamine has advantages over propofol and etomidate because it is water soluble. However, although it lacks the cardiorespiratory depressive properties of other IV agents, its usefulness is limited by high incidences of disturbing emergence reactions (up to 30% of patients). Ketamine also causes increases in intracranial pressure and salivation. The psychomimetic effects of ketamine may be attenuated by benzodiazepine premedication, although these drugs appear to prolong the elimination half-life of ketamine and increase its recovery time.

Stereoisomers of Ketamine The potency ratio for anesthesia is approximately 4:2:1 for S(+) ketamine, ketamine racemate (ie, mixture), and R(−) ketamine enantiomers. Some data suggest that administration of S(+) ketamine is accompanied by a lower median EEG power spectrum, a greater rise in blood pressure and heart rate, decreased locomotor activity, shortened recovery times, and equipotent analgesia compared with the racemate at similar doses.[93-96]

OPIATES

As already mentioned in the section on induction of anesthesia with TIVA, these are not complete IV hypnotics and do not produce anesthesia in the absence of other supplements. However, all opiates potentiate the effects of hypnotics when used for induction of anesthesia (this is seen less with thiopental, but is most important with midazolam).

DRUGS FOR MAINTENANCE OF TIVA

In modern anesthesia, the dosing of both hypnotics and analgesics is by titration to clinical effect, measured either by effects on the cardiovascular system or the EEG (or one of its surrogates). The changes in heart rate and blood pressure tend to be "agent specific" (for *most* IV agents, increasing depth of anesthesia causes a reduction in heart rate and blood pressure, although with ketamine, the heart rate may increase with increasing plasma drug concentrations). However, of all the markers of inadequate anesthesia, patient movement remains the most reliable.

Despite the availability of pharmacokinetic-based infusion regimens, it is the dynamic responses of the individual patient to any given surgery that governs the rate of drug infusion. No single plasma drug concentration results in satisfactory anesthetic and surgical conditions for all patients and all operations.

Titration of the infusion rate should reflect the anticipated intensity of the applied stimulus and likely observed patient responses. In general, drug requirements are greatest during endotracheal intubation and decrease during surgical preparation and draping. The infusion rates will need to be increased before skin incision, whereas during anesthesia, drug dosing should be titrated according to signs of patient movement, hemodynamics, and autonomic responses. In the absence of any response over a given period of time, the anesthesiologist may consider reducing the infusion rate by 15% to 20%.

Table 43-8 shows typical infusion regimens used to achieve the steady drug concentrations required to provide analgesia using IV analgesic drugs given by infusion. If the dose of drug administered is clearly too high in the presence of continuing signs of inadequate anesthesia, then the anesthesiologist should examine for a disconnection of the delivery system or delivery to a subcutaneous rather than vascular site. Other causes could include incorrect programming of pumps or mechanical errors of the delivery systems.

During TIVA, use of combinations of drugs poses questions over which one to increase or decrease and for what reasons. In general,

TABLE 43-8 Typical Drug Concentrations and Manual Infusion Regimens to Provide Adequate Analgesia for Major Noncardiac Surgery Under TIVA and Other Target Analgesic Concentrations

	Cp50 (ng/mL) for Surgery	Cp50 (ng/mL) for Adequate Spontaneous Respiration
Alfentanil	200-300	10-30
Fentanyl	4-6	0.5-1.0
Remifentanil	4-6	0.5-1.0
Sufentanil	0.3-0.4	0.025-0.05

Dosing strategies

	Target Concentration (ng/mL)	Loading Dose (mg/kg)	Maintenance Infusion (mg/kg/min)
Alfentanil	40	20	0.25
	160	80	1.0
	320	160	2.0
Fentanyl	1	3	0.02
	4	10	0.07
Remifentanil	6	1	0.02
	12-20	1-2	0.04-1.0
Sufentanil	0.15	0.15	0.003
	0.5	0.5	0.01

the dosing of opiates should be aimed at achieving analgesic drug concentrations at the effect site, whereas the hypnotic infusion should be titrated to individual patient requirements and to the intensity of the surgical stimulation. At the end of surgery, the anesthesiologist should reduce the infusion rates of the hypnotic and analgesic during skin closure to allow restoration of spontaneous respiration by the end of surgery.

THIOPENTAL AND THIAMYLAL

Early recovery from thiopental occurs because of a decline in the blood (and brain) concentrations as a result of drug redistribution. After bolus doses and after short or low-dose infusion regimens, thiopental is eliminated by first-order kinetics, and the patient promptly awakens. However, at rates in excess of 300 μg/kg/min, thiopental concentrations increase nonlinearly because of the peripheral tissue stores becoming saturated. Maintaining anesthesia with infusions of thiopental requires rates of 150 to 300 μg/kg/min in combination with an opiate. This will achieve thiopental concentrations of 15 to 25 μg/mL.[27] In the absence of an analgesic supplement, thiopental concentrations of the order of 40 to 50 μg/mL are needed to abolish the response to squeezing the trapezius muscle (which has been equated with the initial surgical incision). Besides the changes in pharmacokinetics, high doses of thiopental also lead to the formation of significant blood concentrations of its active metabolite, pentobarbital. Other inactive metabolites occur after C_5 side-chain oxidation. Renal excretion of thiopental is very low (approximately 0.3%).

Possible advantages to the use of thiopental infusions include minimal cardiovascular depression and cerebral protection during ischemic episodes, with blood thiopental concentrations on the order of 70 μg/mL resulting in EEG burst suppression.[97]

When given by continuous infusion for TIVA, thiopental has a low systemic clearance (2.2-5.5 mL/kg/min) and an apparent volume of distribution at steady state of 1.3 to 2.4 L/kg.[26, 98-100] Larger volumes of distribution, coupled with altered kinetics, have been observed after prolonged or high-dose infusions.[97]

METHOHEXITAL

Plasma methohexital concentrations of 3 to 4 μg/mL result in hypnosis, and concentrations between 10 and 12 μg/mL cause EEG burst suppression. Based on dose–response data from Sear and Prys-Roberts,[101-103] infusion rates of 50 to 65 μg/kg/min supplemented by opiates or of 100 μg/kg/min methohexital alone are required for anesthesia. Methohexital infusions depress both blood pressure and cardiac output; they also decrease baroreceptor reflex sensitivity with a resetting of the response to allow a more rapid heart rate at lower arterial pressures than when awake.[104] Side effects include excitatory movements, pain on injection, and predisposition to convulsions. Epileptiform activity has been recorded by EEG, but clinical fitting is rare. Methohexital also causes pain if accidentally injected into arteries, but unlike thiopental, this does not normally lead to thrombosis.

The combination of methohexital and opiates can cause significant respiratory depression. No untoward effects of methohexital infusions on liver, renal, or adrenal function have been described.

MIDAZOLAM

Continuous infusions of midazolam have been used to provide both sedation and maintenance of anesthesia. When used as the hypnotic component to supplement alfentanil in a TIVA technique and compared with propofol, Vuyk et al observed similar hemodynamic effects but slower recovery.[105] For the maintenance of anesthesia, infusions on the order of 10 mg/h (resulting in plasma drug concentrations of 200-350 ng/mL) are needed to supplement opiate infusions.[7,16,78,80,106] There are few data describing the disposition of midazolam during TIVA for noncardiac surgery; typical clearance estimates range from 5.0 to 11.0 mL/kg/min and distribution 1.3 to 1.7 L/kg.[107-110]

Several of these studies showed that infusions of midazolam and opiates together may cause myocardial depression; this does not appear to be dose dependent, and there is an apparent ceiling effect at midazolam concentrations greater than 100 ng/mL. Clinically relevant rates of infusion of midazolam in combination with alfentanil have no significant effect on the plasma cortisol response during lower abdominal surgery.[111] A major disadvantage of midazolam for TIVA is the slow recovery. Awakening occurs at drug concentrations of approximately 50 to 80 ng/mL. Nilsson et al[82] showed that recovery can be improved by reversal with bolus doses of flumazenil, but re-sedation may subsequently occur as a consequence of the faster elimination of the antagonist and rebinding of the agonist.

KETAMINE

Although widely used throughout the world for the maintenance of anesthesia, there are few concentration-effect data for continuous infusions of ketamine. Most studies suggest that hypnotic and analgesic thresholds are approximately 1.5 to 2.5 μg/mL and 150 to 200 ng/mL, respectively. Awakening from anesthesia occurs in the concentration range 600 to 1100 ng/mL. As sole agent, infusion rates of 60 to 80 μg/kg/min will provide clinical anesthesia.

The use of TCI ketamine for sedation and maintenance of anesthesia was described by Bowdle et al[112] and Gray et al.[113] For examination of the psychomimetic effects of ketamine, Bowdle et al designed a BET delivery scheme based on the kinetic parameters of Domino et al[114] to achieve a stepwise series of plasma target concentrations between 0 and 200 ng/mL. Bowdle et al showed a good correlation and relationship between the targeted and observed drug concentrations. Increasing ketamine concentrations were associated with greater psychedelic effects for a variety of symptoms. Interestingly, there was no apparent threshold concentration and no concentration at which these effects plateaued.[112]

In the second study, Gray et al[113] developed a TCI scheme for ketamine to provide the analgesic component of a TIVA technique with propofol in spontaneously breathing patients undergoing body-surface surgery, using the kinetic parameters of Wieber et al.[115] The target concentration of ketamine was 300 ng/mL, with propofol delivered according to the manual BET scheme of Roberts et al.[14] Clinically this combination provided good cardiovascular control throughout the surgery, with an average end-tidal carbon dioxide of 5.8 kPa. There were episodes of involuntary movements (although these did not interfere with the surgery being undertaken) and no episodes of recall. However, recovery to giving date of birth was prolonged in some patients. There were no reports of unpleasant dreams or other psychomimetic side effects.

Schuttler et al[116] described a similar technique in patients undergoing lower abdominal surgery under propofol-ketamine anesthesia. They describe satisfactory anesthesia without any significant psychic disturbances or cardiovascular stimulation. Recovery was not significantly delayed.

A major development in the use of ketamine as part of TIVA has been the separation of the hypnotically active S(+) ketamine enantiomer from the racemic mixture.[94] In a crossover volunteer study, White et al[96] examined the pharmacologic effects of infusions of racemic, S(+), and R(−) ketamine, with measurement of cardiovascular parameters, the raw EEG, and a battery of psychometric tests. S(+) ketamine was approximately 2 times more potent in terms of anesthesia and was associated with faster recovery compared with both the racemic mixture and the R(−) isomer. This is in agreement with subsequent kinetic studies showing inhibition of metabolism of S(+) ketamine by its R(−) isomer.[117] Ketamine enantiomer concentrations at time of regaining consciousness and orientation are consistent with an S-to-R potency ratio of 4:1, whereas for impairment of psychomotor function, the ratio was between 3:1 and 5:1. When administered at equipotent doses, S(+) ketamine produces longer hypnosis than the R(−) isomer, with the racemate being intermediate. Improved recovery was seen after S(+) ketamine by infusion compared with the racemate.

However, cardiovascular stimulation and psychotomimetic effects are seen with both stereoisomers.

When the racemate is given by infusion, the terminal or elimination half-life of ketamine is 2.2 to 3.5 hours and clearance 14.0 to 20.0 mL/kg/min.[118-120] Similar values have been described for the S+ enantiomer.[121,122]

When given alone as part of an anesthetic technique to surgical patients, ketamine can cause considerable side effects. Emergence reactions are commoner after infusions of the R(−) enantiomer than after the racemate and S(+) isomer. However the incidences of dreaming with all 3 treatment groups were comparable.[123] There are no apparent differences between the enantiomers and racemate in their hemodynamic effects, but recovery is faster after the S(+) isomer. The EEG effects of both racemic ketamine and the S(+) isomer are similar; both cause increased fast activity (21-30 Hz) with an accompanying reduction in Δ power. The IC_{50} (concentration that inhibits 50%; in this instance, the plasma ketamine concentration necessary to achieve a 50% depression of the maximal EEG median frequency reduction) was 0.8 μg/mL for S(+) ketamine, compared with 1.8 and 2.0 μg/mL, respectively, for the R(−) and the racemic preparations.[95] The concentration–effect relationships show the curve for S(+) ketamine to lie to the left of the racemate and to be steeper.

PROPOFOL

Propofol is the most widely used hypnotic for the maintenance of TIVA. Infusion rates of 2 to 10 mg/kg/h are needed when administered with bolus doses or an opiate infusion, whereas drug concentrations > 8 μg/mL will be necessary if propofol is used as a sole anesthetic agent. Recovery occurs rapidly after cessation of an infusion at blood concentrations of approximately 1.0 μg/mL.[91] Because of the wide variability in the therapeutic drug concentration window (related to both age and type of surgery) and intersubject drug kinetics, propofol dosing must be titrated to effect. This is easily achievable as it has a short blood–brain equilibration time ($t_{½}\,k_{e0}$).

The disposition of propofol has been studied extensively during TIVA or for sedation during regional anesthesia.[48,87,124-126]

A number of other formulations (apart from Diprivan) are either available or undergoing clinical evaluation (**Table 43-9**). The efficacy of these newer formulations has not been evaluated in large outcome studies, but there appears to be little difference in their kinetic and dynamic properties.

TABLE 43-9 Different Formulations of Propofol (di-Isopropyphenol) Presently in Preclinical Trials, Current Clinical Practice, or Under Development[a]

1. Original preclinical formulation: 2% propofol in 16% Cremophor EL and 8% ethanol (withdrawn after initial preclinical evaluation)
2. 1% propofol in 16% Cremophor EL (preclinical and early phase I use only; withdrawn after administration to 1151 patients because of adverse reactions)
3. 1% propofol in lipid emulsion (containing 10% soybean) [= Diprivan]; emulsion preservatives include ethylenediaminetetracetic acid (EDTA), metabisulfite.
4. 0.5% formulation for use in pediatrics.[127]
5. Modified lipid emulsions containing medium-chain triglycerides (MCTs) and 1% propofol; IDD-D propofol (Skye Pharma Inc., New York, NY)[128] and Propofol-lipuro (B Braun, Meslungen, Germany).[129] The latter formulation is not presently available in the United States due to the lack of EDTA or metabisulfite in the solvent.
6. 6% propofol in MCTs-LCTs (long-chain triglycerides) (Lipofundin, B Braun).
7. AM 149 (Amrad Operations Pty Lyd, Richmond, Victoria, Australia): 1% propofol in MCT alone.
8. 1% "Aquafol" micro-emulsion.[130,131]
9. Albumin-containing emulsions (under development).[132]
10. Non-emulsion formulations (under development): β cyclodextrin,[133,134] micelle formulations.[135]
11. Propofol prodrugs formulated as the hemisuccinate, hemiglurate, hemiadipate, mono- or di-phosphate.[136,137]

[a]Data so far suggest little difference between formulations with regard to pharmacokinetics and pharmacodynamics.

When used to maintain anesthesia, infusions of propofol cause dose-related decreases in blood pressure, cardiac output, and systemic vascular resistance.[91] One important difference when compared with methohexital is that infusions of propofol do not show the normal baroreflex increase in heart rate to a decreased blood pressure. Propofol causes a resetting of the baroreceptor reflex such that slower heart rates are seen for a given arterial blood when compared with awake values.[91,138] As well as these central hemodynamic effects of propofol by infusion, other cardiac effects, including severe bradycardia, sinus arrest, heart block, and asystole, have been reported, which usually occur when propofol is coadministered with vagotonic drugs.[91,132] During TIVA, propofol affects ventilatory control, causing a reduction in the ventilatory response to carbon dioxide and in the acute ventilatory response to isocapnic hypoxia.[139,140]

Although bolus doses of propofol have no effect on renal or portal venous blood flows, dose-related changes in liver blood flow have been reported in dogs during graded infusions to concentrations greater than those needed clinically in people.[141] However, in patients, clinically relevant infusion rates of propofol appear to cause no significant changes of liver blood flow or liver function tests.[142]

Propofol–Drug Interactions During TIVA Because TIVA normally depends on the coadministration of more than 1 IV drug, there is always the potential for drug–drug interactions, which may result in changes to drug distribution, metabolism and elimination, or drug dynamics. In vitro, propofol inhibits drug metabolism at clinical concentrations.[143-145] The magnitude of this inhibition varies from 30% to 71%, with the greatest effect on biotransformations mediated by hepatic isocytochrome P450 2B1. Other cytochromes (P450 1A1 and 2A1) are also inhibited, and Chen et al[146] showed that clinical concentrations of propofol inhibit renal monooxygenase and defluorinase activities. There are 4 types of drug interaction in vivo between propofol and opioids. Besides the interaction of propofol and cytochrome P450 to inhibit drug metabolism, there is also competition between propofol and fentanyl for pulmonary binding sites.

As infusions of propofol decrease liver blood flow,[141] they also decrease clearance of flow-dependent drugs. Capacity-limited drug clearance is also decreased by action of propofol on the hepatic extraction ratio.[33] These findings are relevant during TIVA, because propofol may decrease the systemic clearance of other coadministered drugs through changes in effective liver blood flow or in the hepatic extraction ratio. However, simulation studies by Schnider et al[21] suggest that significant changes will not be associated with propofol infusion rates used in clinical practice, as the kinetics of propofol appear linear with regard to infusion rate at those concentrations. Schnider's simulations are in general agreement with the data of Sear and colleagues[141] in an open-chested dog model.

In vivo there are significant interactions between propofol and alfentanil that lead to alterations in drug clearance.[147] Pavlin et al[148] found that an infusion of alfentanil caused an increase in the predicted propofol concentration and led to greater than predicted alfentanil concentrations when compared with those when alfentanil was infused alone. In male volunteers, Mertens et al[147] showed that addition of a propofol infusion (at a steady-state concentration ranging between 0.85 and 1.75 μg/mL) to alfentanil infused at 25 μg/kg/h resulted in a decrease in mean arterial pressure. In turn, this influenced the disposition of the alfentanil, resulting in a 15% decreased systemic clearance, a 68% reduction in the rapid distribution clearance, and a 51% reduction in slow distribution clearance.

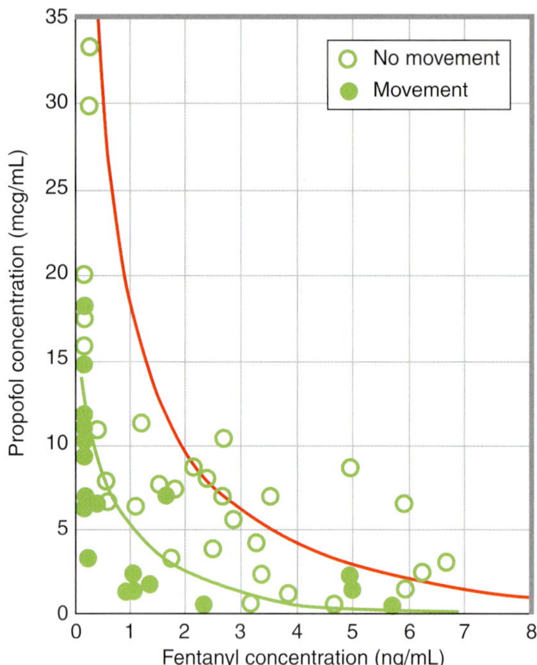

FIGURE 43-2. Increasing concentrations of fentanyl reduces the propofol concentration at which 505 patients (95%) did not move at skin incision (Cp50i and Cp95i, respectively). *Solid lines*, logistic regression solution. [Adapted with permission from Smith C, McEwan AL, Jhaveri R, et al. The interaction of fentanyl on the Cp50 of propofol for loss of consciousness and skin incision. *Anesthesiology.* 1994;81:820-828.]

A similar interaction is seen with the combination propofol-remifentanil, where there is a significant reduction in the initial volume of distribution of the opiate and reductions in both systemic clearance and the intercompartmental distributional clearance. Because this effect is not concentration dependent, it does affect the dosing strategy when using this opiate.[19,149]

Of greater importance, however, are the dynamic interactions between the hypnotics and opiates during the maintenance phase of anesthesia. One of the earliest studies examining the hypnotic–opiate interaction was by Smith et a[49] (**Fig. 43-2**). Other clinical studies and computer simulations by Vuyk et al[50,150-152] from Leiden, the Netherlands, confirm a synergism between these groups of drugs. They also indicate that regardless of an opiate's relative potency, the optimal effect-site concentration should be one that (1) prevents responses to noxious stimulation and (2) allows the rapid recovery of spontaneous ventilation at the end of anesthesia and surgery. Although the original interaction studies focused mainly on the combination propofol-alfentanil,[147,148,150-152] more recent studies confirm similar interactions for propofol with remifentanil and sufentanil.[39,149] A further dynamic interaction is seen between the 2 groups of drugs, with the frequent need for vasoconstrictor drugs to correct hypotension after the induction of anesthesia.

Adverse Effects of Propofol During TIVA Although widely used as the main hypnotic component of TIVA, propofol exhibits a number of significant adverse effects, including pain on injection (especially when given into small veins and to children), hypotension and bradycardia (which are exaggerated in the presence of other vagotonic drugs, such as opioids and hypovolemia), apnea in up to 40% of patients after induction, and reports of epileptiform movements and true convulsions.

Nonhypnotic Effects of Propofol In addition to its anesthetic effects, propofol has other properties that may be advantageous. These include:

1. *Mood-altering effects:* Subhypnotic doses of propofol administered by a patient-controlled analgesia (PCA) system (10 mg with a 1- to 5-minute lockout) exert sedative and anxiolytic effects in anxious patients presenting for ambulatory surgery and thus can be useful as premedication in ambulatory patients.[153]
2. *Antiemetic effects:* Although several authors have suggested an antiemetic effect of propofol (in both hypnotic and subhypnotic doses), the site of this action of the drug remains uncertain.[154] It is probable that propofol does not act at dopaminergic receptors. Subhypnotic infusions of the hypnotic are also effective in the prevention of nausea and emesis after cisplatin chemotherapy.[154]
3. *Antipruritic effects:* Again, subhypnotic doses (10-20 mg IV) of propofol are equally as effective as naloxone in relieving pruritus caused by both epidural and spinally administered opiates.[155,156]
4. *Effects on the cerebral circulation and metabolism*: Although in vitro studies demonstrate a vasodilating effect of propofol, in vivo measurement shows that infusions of propofol act to decrease cerebral blood flow and intracranial pressure (ICP) and decrease the cerebral metabolic rate. Infusions of propofol have no effect on cerebrovascular autoregulation to carbon dioxide, although the slope of the curve is decreased. There is some evidence for a cerebral protective effect of propofol, and high doses of propofol have been used to afford protection during cerebral aneurysm surgery in patients requiring cardiopulmonary bypass and deep hypothermic arrest, as well as in patients undergoing nonpulsatile bypass for cardiac surgery.[157,158]

α_2-AGONISTS AND OTHER SEDATIVE DRUGS

α_2-Agonist drugs are widely used as part of TIVA techniques in veterinary practice; however, few of these agents are presently licensed for clinical use for sedation or hypnosis in people. Dexmedetomidine (DMD) is presently undergoing evaluation for both its sedative and hypnotic properties. It also has analgesic properties in animals.

In humans, DMD interacts with both opiates and hypnotics to reduce drug requirements needed to maintain sedation or anesthesia. Peden et al[159] examined the combination DMD and propofol. They found that an infusion of 3 ng/kg/min of DMD reduced the median effective (ED_{50}) infusion rate of propofol for loss of consciousness from 5.79 to 3.45 mg/kg/h and the resulting plasma median effective concentration (EC_{50}) from 2.3 to 1.69 µg/mL. However, at these infusion rates, DMD caused significant side effects (with 2 cases of sinus arrest and 1 case of severe postural hypotension persisting for 24 hours postanesthesia). Sinus arrest has also been observed in other studies. Consequently, it is appropriate to pretreat patients (especially those younger than 40 years) with an anticholinergic agent. At an infusion rate of 3 ng/kg/min, DMD blunted the hemodynamic responses to intubation and surgical incision, with the blood pressure and heart rate remaining stable throughout surgery and into the recovery period.

In a separate study, Dutta et al[160] determined the EC_{50} of propofol for loss of motor response to an electrical stimulus to be 6.63 µg/mL; when DMD was infused to a steady plasma concentration of 0.66 ng/mL, the EC_{50} of propofol was reduced by 41% to 3.89 µg/mL.

A number of other clinical studies describe the use of DMD as part of TIVA techniques. Ramsey and Luterman[161] used variable-rate DMD infusions to provide hypnosis for surgery in patients with upper airway pathology. When infused at rates up to 10 µg/kg/h, DMD caused no respiratory depression, none of the patients experienced severe hypotension or bradycardia, and recovery was not excessively prolonged (although the patients, who were ages 50 to 66 years, required 2 to 3 hours for complete recovery).

Clomethiazole (a derivative of the thiazole part of vitamin B_1) can be used by continuous IV infusion to supplement both regional and spinal anesthesia. It permits ease of titration of the depth of sedation and anesthesia, with minimal cardiovascular effects. However, widespread use is limited because of the large fluid loads that occur when administered as a 0.8% infusion in 4% glucose; increased red cell fragility when given as infusions of greater than 5%; a high incidence of peripheral thrombophlebitis, necessitating central venous administration; and minor side effects of nasal irritation and stuffiness. After prolonged infusions, recovery may be delayed.[162]

OPIATES

When used in TIVA, the opiates act synergistically with most hypnotic agents. Studies by Vuyk et al,[6,19,50,147,150-152] Smith et al,[49] and Lentschener et al[163] show that even very small doses of opiates can markedly reduce the requirements of the hypnotic component. These studies also demonstrate a significant "ceiling effect"—such that above a given opiate dose or plasma concentration, little further reduction in hypnotic requirement can be achieved. During TIVA, the ability to prevent autonomic responses appears to be largely dependent on increasing the amount of the opiate drug.[164] Examples of "useful" interactions between the hypnotic and analgesic components of TIVA can be found in the cited work of Vuyk et al and Mertens et al (see earlier). Table 43-8 shows the typical plasma opiate concentrations needed to obtund responses to noxious stimuli during TIVA (and the associated opiate concentrations needed for adequate spontaneous ventilation in the recovery room), together with the regimens needed to achieve other drug concentrations.

RECOVERY FROM TIVA

The rapidity of recovery after TIVA depends on how well the clinician is able to keep the effect-site drug concentrations near to those concentrations found in the awake or spontaneously breathing subject. If intraoperative concentrations are kept at approximately 20% above those associated with wakefulness, rapid recovery will occur.

CONTEXT-SENSITIVE HALF-TIME

In 1992, Hughes et al[165] offered a different approach to the anesthesiologist's understanding of the recovery profile after infusions of intravenous anesthetic agents. Rather than relating recovery to elimination half-life or systemic clearance, they defined a new term: *context-sensitive half-time* (CSHT). Compared with the various half-lives of a kinetic model, the CSHT describes what is happening to the plasma drug concentration.

Termination of drug effect is dependent on 2 separate kinetic processes: drug distribution and drug elimination. An IV drug with a short elimination half-life is not necessarily a short-acting drug, as drug redistribution can affect the dynamic profile of the agent. The CSHT is dependent on the 3 rate constants—k_{el}, k_{12}, and k_{21}—of a 2-compartment mamillary model in which drug elimination occurs only from the central kinetic compartment. The CSHT is a "half-time" rather than "half-life," as the time needed for plasma or effect-site drug concentration to decrease by 40% will not be twice that required to decrease by 20%! The term *context* refers to the duration of the drug administration, with the half-time measured from the moment of cessation of the infusion (**Fig. 43-3**). One limitation of the CSHT is that it describes the time to a 50% decrease in the plasma or central compartment drug concentration. This may not be the required decrement in the drug concentration needed to achieve recovery, although the studies of Prys-Roberts and Sear[10] suggest that it may certainly be appropriate when predicting the behavior of hypnotic agents given by infusion.

The study of Kapila et al[166] comparing the modeled CSHT for both alfentanil and remifentanil with values determined from volunteers where the effect measured was that of depression of minute ventilation validated the predictive accuracy of the CSHT. The modeled values of the CSHT after a 3-hour infusion were 2.0 and 51.9 minutes, respectively, for remifentanil and alfentanil, compared with measured values of 3.2 and 47.3 minutes, respectively.

Youngs and Shafer[167] further elaborated on the concept of CSHT. They produced simulations of the time courses not just for a 50% decline in the plasma drug concentration, but also for the 20% and 80% declines after varying-length infusions of 3 opiates (alfentanil, fentanyl, and sufentanil), giving rise to the 20%, 50%, and 80% decrement times. Examination of the relationship between 6 derived components

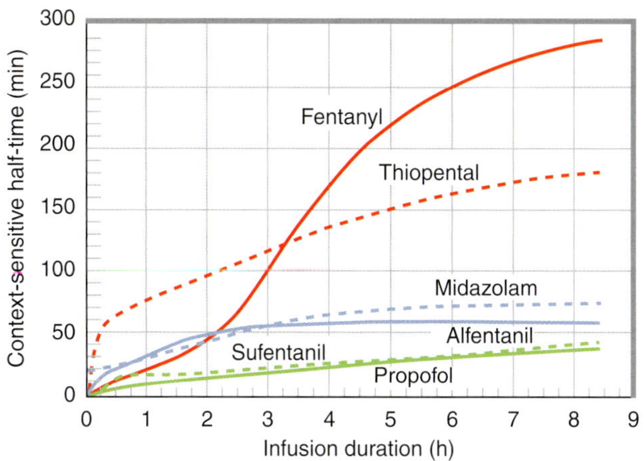

FIGURE 43-3. Context-sensitive half-times as a function of infusion duration from computer simulations of pharmacokinetic models. *Solid* and *dashed* lines are used only to permit overlapping lines to be distinguished. [Adapted with permission from Hughes MA, Glass PSA, Jacobs JR. Context-sensitive half-time in multicompartment pharmacokinetic models for intravenous drugs. *Anesthesiology.* 1992;76:334-341.]

of a 3-compartment mammillary model (namely V_1, V_2, V_3, Cl_{10}, Cl_{12}, and Cl_{13}) on these decrement times show that increases in the initial volume of drug distribution (V_1) lead to longer decrement times. The reverse is true after increases in the clearance constant Cl_{10}. Similarly, increases in the peripheral volumes of distribution (V_2 and V_3) and the intercompartmental clearances Cl_{12} and Cl_{13} lead to shorter decrement times when the infusion is of limited duration, but longer times after prolonged infusions.

For rapid recovery from TIVA, drugs with a small initial volume of distribution (V_1) and high clearance (Cl_{10}) are the most suitable. After prolonged anesthesia, the fastest recovery times are seen after infusion of drugs with small apparent peripheral volumes of distribution and small intercompartmental clearances. Because the "biophase" concentration is always related to the plasma drug concentration, the "decrement times" are also a good descriptor of drug effect *except* after bolus doses or very short infusions.

Bailey described another descriptor of recovery after intravenous infusions: the "mean effect time."[168] The mean effect time is based on whether a patient responds to a given parameter or end point. For a given plasma drug concentration, the "probability (*p*) of a given drug effect" is described by a logistic regression equation of the type:

$$p = C^{\gamma}/C^{\gamma}_{50} + C^{\gamma}$$

where C = drug concentration, C_{50} = drug concentration at which there is a 50% probability of a given effect, and g = a parameter estimate describing the steepness of the concentration–probability relationship. From this equation, Bailey calculates the mean effect time as the integral of p against time.

Whereas the 50% decrement time of Youngs and Shafer will be, by definition, the median recovery value for a given population of patients after a given dosing regimen, it will also be the *mean* recovery index based on the probability of that event occurring. A large steepness coefficient g indicates a steep drug concentration–response relationship. Under such circumstances, the difference between the mean effect time and the 50% decrement times will be insignificant. However, if the concentration–response relationship is flatter, recovery times will tend to be right-skewed, and the mean effect time will be significantly greater than the 50% decrement time.

Although determination of decrement times is straightforward, the calculation of the 50% value for the intraoperative maintenance drug concentration or determination of the mean effect time requires the anesthetist to have a clear understanding of the nature of the

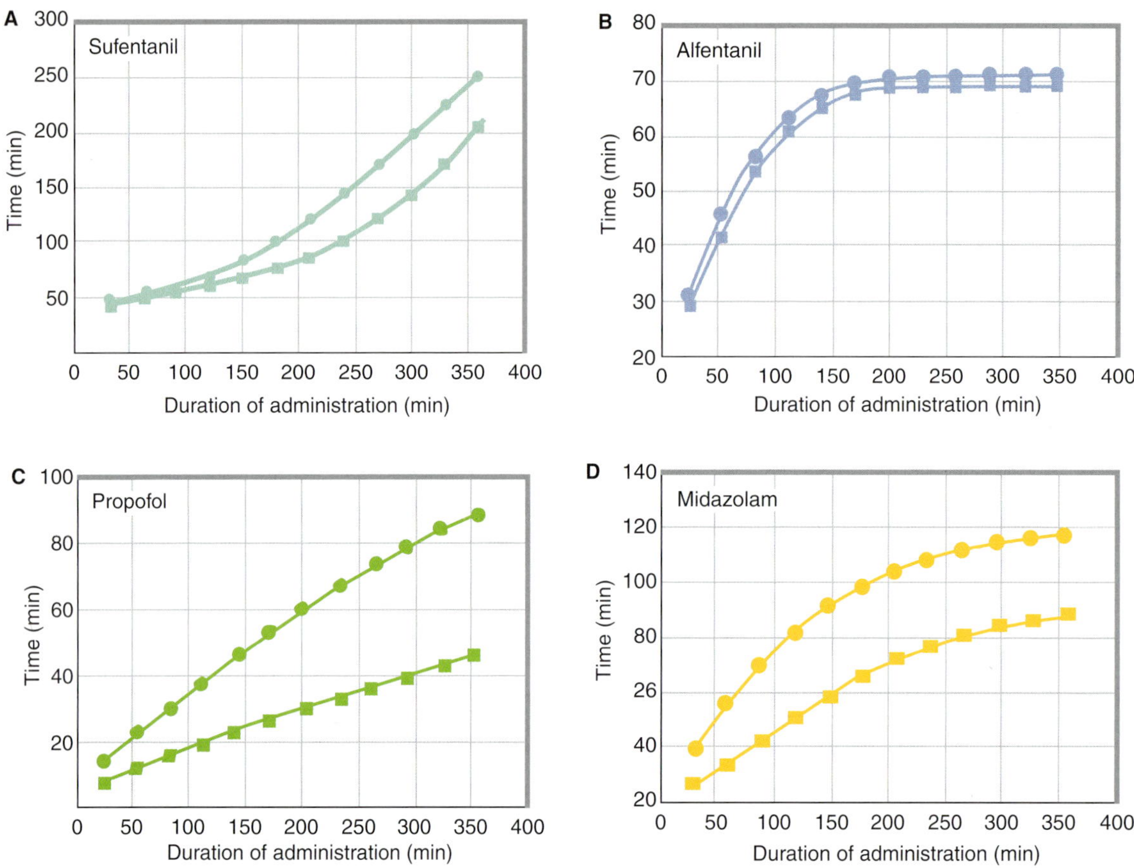

FIGURE 43-4. Comparison of mean effect time (MET) (•) and 50% decrement times (▪) as a function of length of administration of (**A**) sufentanil, (**B**) alfentanil, (**C**) propofol, and (**D**) midazolam when maintained as an infusion maintaining a constant plasma concentration equal to the Cp90 for surgery. [Adapted with permission from Bailey JM. Technique for quantifying the duration of intravenous anesthetic effect. *Anesthesiology.* 1995;83:1095-1103.]

concentration–response relationship (and hence be able to determine *g*). For low values of γ, the anesthetist needs to "overdose" the patient to make sure that *all* patients are adequately asleep or pain free. This necessitates a greater decline in the maintenance drug concentration in order to achieve concentrations where there is a 50% probability of recovery occurring. Alfentanil is an example of a drug with a high *g* value (9.2), whereas sufentanil, propofol, and midazolam have flatter dose–response curves (with γ values of 5.99, 3.27, and 3.05, respectively). Thus the mean effect time and the 50% decrement times for alfentanil are similar, whereas those for propofol, midazolam, and sufentanil differ, depending on the duration of drug administration, with the mean effect time being increasingly greater as the dosing time increases[168] (**Fig. 43-4**).

HOW DO ALL THESE SIMULATION DATA COMPARE WITH IN VIVO OBSERVATIONS FOR DIFFERENT IV AGENTS?

Hypnotics Propofol has a CSHT of less than 25 minutes for infusions lasting up to 3 hours duration (Fig. 43-3), and hence recovery will be prompt; in contrast, thiopental has a longer CSHT, and after infusions to achieve plasma concentrations of 10 to 20 μg/mL, recovery takes 40 to 300 minutes.[100]

Methohexital has a CSHT similar to that for propofol, and its recovery profile is similar to that of propofol after short-duration procedures. On the other hand, as the studies of Vuyk et al[105] demonstrate, midazolam has a CSHT approximately twice that of propofol. The computed CSHT for ketamine appears to be similar to that for propofol, although its rate of elimination is slower.[169] This is because ketamine equilibrates faster with the peripheral compartments. The modeled CSHT of ketamine after a BET infusion for 8 hours is approximately 50 minutes. However, its recovery profile is influenced by the high incidence of psychological reactions (seen in between 5% and 30% of patients).

Etomidate has a CSHT of approximately 50% that seen with propofol. This should lead to fast recovery after TIVA, but, again, there are associated high incidences of adverse recovery sequelae, including nausea and vomiting (15%-20% of patients), twitching and restlessness, and venous sequelae such as thrombophlebitis. The occurrence of these postoperative side effects will slow the completeness of recovery after etomidate.

Opiates The rational use of opiates in TIVA has been well discussed by Shafer and Varvel.[170] If a dosing strategy of providing analgesic concentrations is adopted, then a 20% to 30% decrease in the opiate concentration will allow adequate postoperative ventilation. Fentanyl concentrations show a rapid initial decline followed by a slower decrease, permitting spontaneous ventilation at the end of the procedure while maintaining analgesia for a considerable time thereafter. When a rapid and maximal decline in opiate concentration is desirable (as in ambulatory and day surgery), remifentanil, alfentanil, and sufentanil are more suitable (**Fig. 43-5**).

With infusions of less than 8 hours' duration, the decline in the sufentanil concentration is more rapid than that of alfentanil, although alfentanil has the shorter CSHT for infusions lasting 6 to 8 hours or longer. For infusions of less than 1-hour duration, fentanyl and sufentanil have CSHTs that are both shorter than alfentanil. However, for infusions of variable duration, the CSHT of remifentanil is virtually independent of its duration, with no adjustment apparently required for weight, age, or sex. Its high systemic clearance is because of its rapid metabolism by

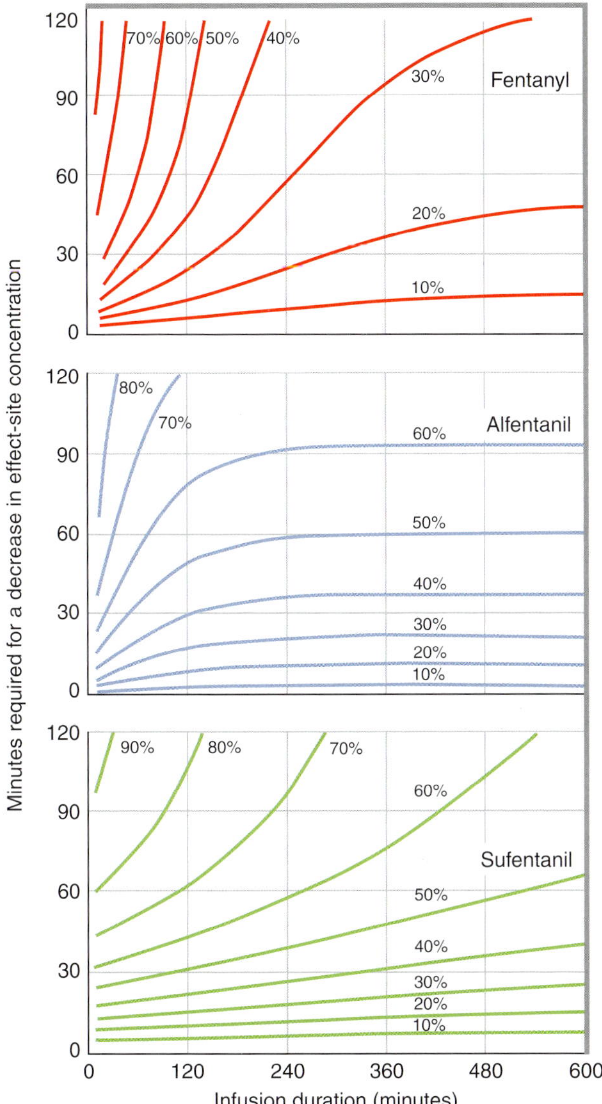

FIGURE 43-5. Recovery curves for fentanyl, alfentanil, and sufentanil showing the time required for decreases of a given percentage (labeled for each curve) from the maintained effect-site concentration after termination of the infusion. [Adapted with permission from Shafer SL, Varvel JR. Pharmacokinetics, pharmacodynamics and rational opioid selection. *Anesthesiology.* 1990;74:53-63.]

plasma esterases. The short CSHT means that most patients will achieve spontaneous ventilation within 3 to 5 minutes of stopping the infusion. However, there remains the *major* postoperative problem of how to provide adequate analgesia after the offset of action of the remifentanil. Although a number of strategies to overcome this have been suggested, several cases of abreaction-type responses to remifentanil have been described in the literature.[164,171]

FUTURE TRENDS IN TOTAL INTRAVENOUS ANESTHESIA

These will be focused in several distinct areas. First, there is need to develop kinetic models for patient populations other than the healthy adult (ie, the young, the elderly, and those patients with comorbidities). One example is the Paedfusor for propofol administered to children.[172] An alternative will be further development of existing models to allow these covariates to be taken into account (as is presently the case when they are incorporated into TCI systems that use the Schnider kinetic model for propofol delivery).[21] Another major problem is obese patients, as weight alone is a poor covariate against which to determine infusion rates or target drug concentrations.

TCI technology was originally focused on propofol using the Diprifusor system. The different kinetic models for propofol questions the appropriateness of the kinetic parameters included in that system. The recent development of generic or open TCI systems allows not only use of different kinetic data sets, but also infusion of other drugs (eg, remifentanil). Whereas different equipment manufacturers produce different delivery systems, the choice of the mathematical model driving the syringe is the responsibility of the anesthesiologist. The Open TCI Initiative is an attempt to allow academics and clinicians to share data sets and develop the most appropriate parameters for given patients.

New IV drug developments will focus on those compounds with short context-sensitive half-times and that are not significantly affected by any of the major comorbidities of renal or hepatic impairment, heart failure, or diabetes mellitus. Ideally, future new IV hypnotic drugs will possess minimal cardiovascular and respiratory depression, no pain on injection, and be water soluble. However, recent studies modeling the pharmacophores for different end points of intravenous anesthesia suggest that it may not be possible to separate immobilizing activity and cardiovascular depression.[173] New analgesics should not cause nausea and vomiting or prolonged or delayed respiratory depression.

Drugs fulfilling these desired kinetic and dynamic properties will either be reformulations of present compounds or new esterase-metabolized compounds similar to remifentanil.

NEW PROPOFOL FORMULATIONS

Any new formulation should aim to improve the drug's profile by reducing the incidence of pain on injection; using a less toxic solvent than intralipid (which has been incriminated with the development of the so-called propofol infusion syndrome after prolonged infusion in the ICU); showing a faster onset of effect; or reducing the risk of bacterial contamination when the drug is given by continuous infusion.[126] The support of bacterial growth can be blunted by the addition of benzyl alcohol, meta-bisulphite, or EDTA. The pain on injection may relate to the compound itself, as the lipid solvent is not associated with pain when used to solubilize other agents or when given alone.[174]

Most new formulations of propofol have focused on lipid solubilization. The Lipuro formulation (B Braun) is made up of medium-chain rather than long-chain triglycerides, has a similar PK-PD profile to Diprivan, and is associated with less pain on injection. This formulation is not presently available in the United States because of a lack of EDTA in the solvent. IDD-D propofol is another medium-chain triglyceride formulation but is prepared as a 2% solution. Studies have shown a slower onset of effect compared with Diprivan and increased pain on injection.[128]

Current propofol formulations are manufactured with an oil droplet size of 0.15 to 0.5 μm (fine macroemulsions)[132]; smaller microemulsions (<0.1 μm) are highly stable but require added surfactants. Aquafol (Daewon Pharmaceutical Co. Ltd, Seoul, South Korea) is such a formulation, containing polyethylene glycol 600 hydrostearate as a non-ionic surfactant, with 5% glycofural (Roche, Basel, Switzerland) as a co-surfactant.[130,131] Its pharmacologic profile is similar to that of Diprivan; however, there are issues over the safe maximum-tolerated daily dose of both the surfactant and co-surfactant, which might limit its use in the ICU.

Three aqueous formulations of propofol solubilized in cyclodextrans have been described, with the hydroxypropyl-β cyclodextrin having the most favorable physicochemical and biologic properties.[133] Studies in the pig show a similar PK/PD profile to Diprivan[134]; studies in man are awaited.

Other propofol formulations use co-solvent mixtures (propofol solubilized in propylene glycol: water; or the prolinate ester of propofol and

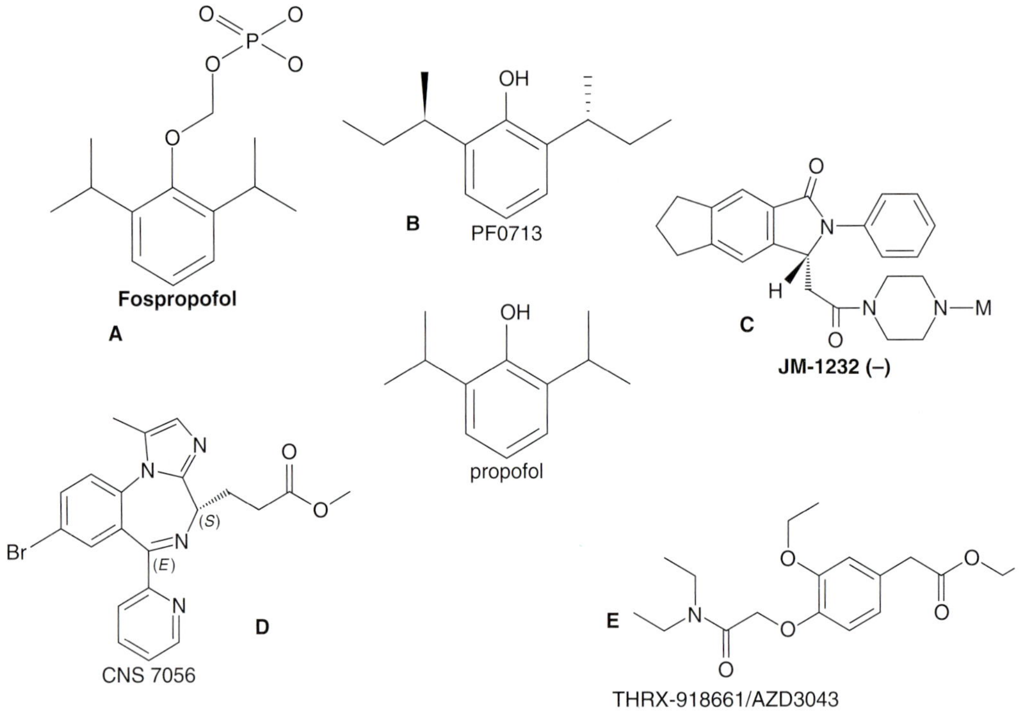

FIGURE 43-6. Chemical structures of (**A**) fospropofol, (**B**) PF 0713, (**C**) JM-1232 (–), (**D**) CNS 7056, and (**E**) THRX 918661 (AZD3043).

its water-soluble derivative dissolved in water in equimolar concentrations). A polymeric micelle formulation has also been described,[135] but again, there are no data to date in man.

The development of propofol prodrugs has been studied in laboratory animal, based on para-substituted propofol analogues. A phosphate ester formulation looks the most promising.[136,137]

Fospropofol This is the only clinically approved propofol analog. It is the water-soluble phosphono-ester of propofol (phosphono-*O*-methyl-2,6-diisopropylphenol) (**Fig. 43-6**). It is broken down to propofol, inorganic phosphate, and formaldehyde by alkaline phosphatases that are widely distributed in the body. There are no reports of pain on injection, but some subjects have described transient and painful sensations in the perineal region.

In phase III studies, doses of 6.5 mg/kg of fospropofol followed by subsequent titrated doses have been used to provide procedural sedation, with fentanyl 50 μg given prior to dosing.[53] Recovery was rapid and without any noticeable hangover effect. The drug has also been associated with a low incidence of postoperative nausea and vomiting. Comparison with propofol shows the new drug to have a lower incidence of adverse effects, with only minor respiratory depression. It has a slower onset of action than propofol, and the metabolic products cause no clinically significant drug-related sedative effects.

Fospropofol has some apparent advantages over propofol and is associated with a lower risk of bacterial contamination, as well as the absence of the infused lipid load that has been associated with organ toxicity during long-term infusions of Diprivan. Fospropofol was approved in the United States by the US Food and Drug Administration (FDA) in December 2008 for use in monitored anesthesia care sedation in adult patients undergoing diagnostic or therapeutic procedures. There are few comparative data relating to fospropofol and no reliable PK-PD studies. (See useful reviews by Campion and Gan[175] and Garnock-Jones and Scott[176] for additional information.)

OTHER NEW INTRAVENOUS ANESTHETICS

At the time of writing (August 2011), there are several other agents being investigated for their total intravenous anesthesia.

PF0713 PF0713 is a potent $GABA_A$ receptor agonist which, in animal species so far tested, shows a hypnotic potency comparable to that of propofol, but with a slower onset of action and duration of effect. It is a sterically hindered phenol (R,R 2′6′ di-*sec*butyl phenol) and is therefore similar in structure to propofol (Fig. 43-6). Indeed in its racemic form, it was one of the original compounds evaluated during the development of propofol. It is water insoluble and formulated as a 1% lipid emulsion. It is presently in phase I human volunteer clinical testing. When given to male subjects in doses of 1 to 2 mg/kg, it produces rapid loss of consciousness without injection pain or agitation. The depth and duration of anesthetic effect, as assessed by the bispectral index and the Richmond Agitation Sedation Score, was dose-related, and blood pressure and heart rate were adequately maintained.[177] Although bolus dose recovery is predictable, there are no available data when given by infusion.

JM-1232 (–) JM-1232 (–) is an isoindolin-1-one derivative and one of a series of water-soluble sedative–hypnotics presently being evaluated by the Maruishi Pharmaceutical Company (Osaka, Japan)[178] (Fig. 43-6). It has a wide margin of safety, with a hypnotic ED_{50} of 3.1 mg/kg and LD_{50} of greater than 120 mg/kg (therapeutic index >35). In vitro binding data suggest that the compound has a high affinity for the benzodiazepine receptor, but not at the same binding site as midazolam. Its effect is fully reversed by flumazenil.

JM-1232 has recently undergone early clinical evaluation. When given as a 10-minute infusion to 6 male volunteers, it had a rapid onset and short duration of action.[179] Doses between 0.05 and 0.8 mg/kg caused sedation, with the higher doses producing a deeper and longer reduction in the bispectral index.

Preliminary kinetic data indicate a clearance of approximately 0.78 L/min and an apparent steady-state volume of distribution of 77.3 L. Simulated context-sensitive half-times to 120-minute infusion suggest a drug with a similar profile to propofol. Further studies in a larger population of volunteers have confirmed the drug's kinetic profile and estimated an EC_{50} effect-site concentration for anaesthesia of 162 ng/mL (95% CI, 121-203) and a $t_{1/2}k_{e0}$ of 4.2 minutes (95% CI, 3.1-6.7).[180] The latter compare with 0.9 to 5.6 minutes for midazolam and 1.2 to 3.3 minutes for propofol.

CNS 7056 CNS 7056 is an ultra–short-acting benzodiazepine hypnotic agent hydrolyzed by esterases in the blood to the metabolite 7054 (Fig. 43-6). The parent compound has a very predictable offset of effect in animals with a low risk of oversedation and is reversible by the benzodiazepine antagonist flumazenil. Metabolism of 7056 occurs rapidly by human, rat, mouse and the mini-pig liver tissue. Rapid metabolism also occurs in organs other than the liver (kidney, lung, brain), but there is no metabolism by plasma in human, mini-pig or dog. This metabolite profile is in keeping with CNS 7056 being a substrate for carboxylesterases rather than butyrylcholinesterase.[181] In a kinetic and dynamic comparison with midazolam in the pig,[182] both drugs rapidly induced sedation, but recovery was faster after 7056. Midazolam was eliminated more slowly (33 vs 18 min half-life) and was more widely distributed (1038 vs 440 mL/kg volume of distribution at steady state).

The first human study with CNS 7056 has been reported.[183] CNS 7056 was well tolerated in doses between 0.01 and 0.35 mg/kg, although episodes of hypoxia were seen with higher doses. There was no hypo- or hypertension. Plasma drug clearance was approximately 3 times that of midazolam, and there was a linear dose-kinetic relationship. There was rapid onset of sedation (after approximately 1 minutes, with a peak at 4 minutes) and also rapid recovery (10 min vs approximately 40 minutes for equipotent doses of midazolam). A double-blind randomized controlled trial of 100 patients undergoing upper gastrointestinal endoscopy has compared midazolam and CNS 7056. Full outcome data are awaited.

THRX-918661 (also known as TD4756 and AZD3043) This is another designer-built water soluble drug that is a congener of the hypnotic agent propanidid, with about twice the potency (Fig. 43-6). The structure of THRX-918661 is that of an acetic acid propyl ester broken down by tissue and plasma esterases to inactive metabolites. When given to the rat by infusions ranging from 20 minutes to 5 hours, the time to recovery of the righting reflex was approximately 3 minutes. In contrast, the recovery from propofol anesthesia ranged between 30 and 60 minutes. Faster recovery when compared with propofol has also been demonstrated in the pig.[184] Kinetic studies in the pig after a 3-hour continuous infusion indicated a clearance estimate of approximately 3.4 L/kg/h and an elimination half-life of 0.4 hour, with recovery faster than after propofol at equipotent doses.[185] However, the anesthetic appears to have a low potency, with doses for the maintenance of anesthesia in the pig being of the order of 1.5 mg/kg/min. Clinical studies in man are presently being conducted.

Other New Hypnotic Agents Three further drugs (Alphaxalone formulated in cyclodextrin; MOC-etomidate; Carbo-etomidate) have all been studied in animals, but clinical trials in man are awaited.

Although Althesin in Cremophor EL continues to be used by veterinarians in some animal species, a formulation of one of the steroids (alphaxalone) in cyclodextrin is available and licensed for use in cats and dogs.

There are also a number of etomidate congeners being studied.[186-189] Two potentially useful compounds are methoxy-carbonyl etomidate (MOC-etomidate) and carbo-etomidate. In a rat model, the latter appears not to cause adrenocortical suppression.[186] Should this be the case in humans, the agent may be suitable for maintenance of anesthesia and/or sedation.

Other developments may include use of closed-loop control systems for the delivery of anesthesia using physiologic biomarkers such as auditory evoked potentials and the bispectral index to provide better control of the depth of sedation and anesthesia.[190-194]

Comparable indicators of the depth of analgesia may also be developed. It is obvious that the TIVA has become a major technique in anesthetic practice only because of the availability of drugs with potent hypnotic or analgesic effects, minimal side effects, and kinetic profiles that allow easy and rapid titration to different noxious stimuli. There are still advances to be made, including identification of the best and most accurate method of monitoring depth of anesthesia.

One of the stated advantages of TCI is the facilitation of the transition from induction to maintenance of anesthesia. However, the Cochrane Database Systematic Review by Leslie and colleagues[4] does not provide any evidence showing advantages of TCI when compared with manually controlled drug delivery. Hence the striving for technological advances in drug administration in order to enable relatively accurate drug dosing should be tempered by the need to reduce the increased cost of health care delivery.

KEY REFERENCES

- Absalom A, Sutcliffe N, Kenny GN. Closed-loop control of anaesthesia using Bispectral Index performance assessment in patients undergoing major orthopaedic surgery under combined general and regional anaesthesia. *Anesthesiology.* 2002;96:67-73.
- Bailey JM. Technique for quantifying the duration of intravenous anesthetic effect. *Anesthesiology.* 1995;83:1095-1103.
- Garnock-Jones KP, Scott LJ. Fospropofol. *Drugs.* 2010;70:469-477.
- Kazama T, Ikeda K, Morita K, et al. Comparison of the effect-site k(e0)s of propofol for blood pressure and EEG bispectral index in elderly and younger patients. *Anesthesiology.* 1999;90:1517-1527.
- Leslie K, Clavisi O, Hargrove J. Target-controlled infusion versus manually-controlled infusion of propofol for general anaesthesia or sedation in adults. *Cochrane Database Syst Rev.* 2008;3:CD006059.
- Mertens MJ, Olofson E, Engbers FHM, et al. Propofol reduces perioperative remifentanil requirements in a synergistic manner. Response surface modeling of perioperative remifentanil-propofol interactions. *Anesthesiology.* 2003;99:347-359.
- Mertens MJ, Vuyk J, Olofsen E, Bovill JG, Burm AG. Propofol alters the pharmacokinetics of alfentanil in healthy male volunteers. *Anesthesiology.* 2001;94:949-957.
- Schuttler J, Ihmsen H. Population pharmacokinetics of propofol: a multicenter study. *Anesthesiology.* 2000;92:727-738.
- Sear JW. Development of pharmacophoric maps for cardiovascular depression by intravenous anaesthetic agents: comparison with maps for immobilizing activity. *Br J Anaesth.* 2010;104:684-690.
- Struys MM, De Smet T, Depoorter B, et al. Comparison of plasma compartment versus two methods for effect compartment-controlled target-controlled infusion for propofol. *Anesthesiology.* 2000;92:399-406.
- Struys MM, De Smet T, Versichelen L, et al. Comparison of closed-loop controlled administration of propofol using Bispectral Index as the controlled variable versus "standard practice" controlled administration. *Anesthesiology.* 2001;95:6-17.
- Youngs EJ, Shafer SL. Pharmacokinetic parameters relevant to recovery from opioids. *Anesthesiology.* 1994;81:833-841.

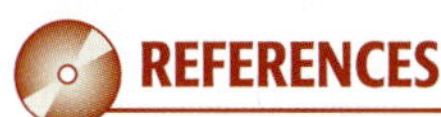

REFERENCES

Complete references available on DVD and online version at www.LongneckerAnesthesiology.com

CHAPTER 44 Cardiovascular Drugs

David Bronheim
Alina Nicoara
Mark Abel

KEY POINTS

1. Patients with preoperative blood pressure elevation have exaggerated perioperative blood pressure fluctuations, which may be associated with electrocardiogram (ECG) evidence of myocardial ischemia. The American College of Cardiology/American Heart Association (ACC/AHA) Guidelines for Perioperative Cardiovascular Evaluation for Noncardiac Surgery recommend that antihypertensive medication be continued during the perioperative period. Particular care should be taken to avoid withdrawal of β-blockers and clonidine because of the potential for withdrawal syndromes.
2. Recommendations for patients taking diuretics call for withholding diuretics on the day of surgery unless evidence suggests volume overload or signs and symptoms of overt congestive heart failure (CHF). In stable patients with chronic mild-to-moderate hypokalemia without signs or symptoms of hypokalemia (eg, muscle weakness, ileus, and nephropathy) and in the absence of dysrhythmias or digitalis use, anesthesia and surgery can proceed.
3. α_2-Agonists have many desirable effects, such as minimum alveolar concentration (MAC) reduction, analgesia, anxiolysis, sedation, and sympatholysis. Recent studies evaluating the perioperative effect of α_2-agonists during noncardiac surgery show less perioperative myocardial ischemia. The ACC/AHA guidelines introduced the use of α_2-agonists as a class IIb recommendation for perioperative control of hypertension or risk reduction in patients with known coronary artery disease (CAD) or major risk factors for CAD.
4. During the perioperative period, patients maintained on angiotensin-converting enzyme (ACE) inhibitors and angiotensin II receptor blockers through the morning of the surgery have an increased number of hypotensive episodes requiring treatment with vasopressors.
5. Perioperatively, intravenous (IV) nitroglycerin may be used for treatment of myocardial ischemia, CHF, acute volume overload, systemic and pulmonary hypertension, and coronary artery spasm. It enhances blood flow to the subendocardium and areas of ischemia by both decreasing preload and left ventricular end-diastolic pressure and volume.
6. The recent focus on perioperative β-blockade has led to mounting evidence that their *prophylactic* use will reduce cardiac mortality and morbidity. β-Blockers reduce ischemia by decreasing myocardial oxygen demand caused by increased stress and catecholamine release in the perioperative period. However, their aggressive prophylactic use without proper titration may result in an increased incidence of hypotension, stroke, and mortality. The ACC/AHA guidelines state that β-blockers should be titrated to effect preferably days to weeks before elective surgery in patients at risk for or with evidence of ischemia.
7. The calcium channel blockers represent a diverse group of compounds with dissimilar structures and pharmacologic effects. Unlike β-blockers, which all depend on blockade of receptors for their activity, the sites and mechanisms of action of the individual calcium channel blockers vary, as do their individual actions on different tissues.
8. Over the past decade, the use of most antidysrhythmic drugs has been reassessed and dramatically limited as a result of increased awareness of their proarrhythmic potential and advances in ablation techniques. Moreover, recent clinical trials have demonstrated negative effects on survival in many situations when these drugs may have been administered in the past. Finally, implantable cardiodefibrillators have largely replaced antidysrhythmic medications in the management of ventricular dysrhythmias.
9. Amiodarone is considered by some the most efficacious antidysrhythmic agent available; unfortunately, however, it is associated with a high incidence of side effects. In the intraoperative and postoperative settings, IV amiodarone may be used to treat a variety of ventricular and supraventricular arrhythmias. It may be used to convert new-onset atrial fibrillation into sinus rhythm. In addition, its use is now advanced cardiac life support (ACLS) recommended for the treatment of pulseless ventricular tachycardia and ventricular fibrillation refractory to defibrillation, stable ventricular tachycardia, wide-complex supraventricular tachycardia, and atrial fibrillation.
10. Multiple studies have evaluated the effect of statin agents on perioperative mortality during the perioperative period. Results of these studies largely show a reduction in perioperative mortality with minimal adverse effects. As such, they should be continued through the perioperative period.

Cardiovascular disease in some form affects the majority of adults past the age of 60 years, the fastest growing segment of the US population. Today, because advanced age and concurrent cardiovascular diseases are almost never viewed as absolute contraindications to even the most complex surgical procedures, optimal anesthetic management depends on an anesthesiologist's intimate knowledge of a large variety of cardiovascular medications and the implication of their use during the perioperative period.

This chapter reviews the many classes of cardiovascular medications and the anesthetic considerations associated with their concurrent use during the perioperative period.

ANTIHYPERTENSIVES

Hypertension is a powerful predictor of cardiovascular mortality and death from all causes and a major risk factor for nonfatal events, such as stroke, kidney failure, myocardial infarction, and congestive heart disease. National Health and Nutrition Examination Survey (NHANES) IV data from 1999 to 2004 showed that 67% of US adults aged 60 and older were classified as having hypertension. This represents a 10% increase over the earlier NHANES III survey conducted from 1988 to 1994.[1] Fortunately, the most recent analysis of the 2007 to 2008 NHANES data provides evidence that treatment and control of hypertension has improved since the earlier survey.[2]

Many agents are currently available for treatment of essential hypertension. The optimal choice of one agent over another depends on the effectiveness of certain drugs within a given population, the incidence of side effects, and the presence of concurrent diseases. Most patients will require 2 or more antihypertensive medications to achieve proper blood pressure control.[3]

The Seventh Report of the Joint National Committee on Prevention, Detection, Evaluation, and Treatment of High Blood Pressure (JNC7) has provided guidance in the treatment of patients with hypertension and specific comorbidities. For certain high-risk conditions there are compelling data that show that the use of a particular class of antihypertensive treatment has benefit in terms of reduction in mortality and morbidity.[4] Some of these compelling indications are listed in **Table 44-1**.

Numerous studies have shown that stage 1 and stage 2 hypertension (systolic blood pressure <180 mm Hg and diastolic blood pressure <110 mm Hg) are not an independent risk factors for perioperative cardiovascular complications.[5] However, patients with preoperative blood pressure elevation have exaggerated perioperative blood pressure fluctuations, which may be associated with electrocardiogram (ECG) evidence of myocardial ischemia.[5] As perioperative myocardial ischemia has been linked to subsequent increased cardiac morbidity and mortality, anesthesiologists have viewed preoperative control of blood pressure

TABLE 44-1 Compelling Indications and the Corresponding Recommended Antihypertensive Drug Class

Compelling Indication	Drug Treatment
Post–myocardial infarction	ACE inhibitor, β-blocker
Angina pectoris	β-Blocker, calcium channel blocker
Heart failure	ACE inhibitor, ARB, β-blocker, diuretic, aldosterone inhibitor
Chronic renal disease	ACE inhibitor, ARB
Diabetes	ACE inhibitor, ARB and others
High coronary artery disease risk	ACE inhibitor, ARB, β-blocker, calcium channel blocker, diuretic

ACE, angiotensin-converting enzyme; ARB, angiotensin receptor blocker.

Modified from Mensah GA, Bakris G. Treatment and control of high blood pressure in adults. *Cardiol Clin.* 2010;28:609-622.

as optimal practice for over a generation. The American College of Cardiology/American Heart Association (ACC/AHA) Guidelines for Perioperative Cardiovascular Evaluation for Noncardiac Surgery guidelines for medical therapy recommend that antihypertensive medication be continued during the perioperative period. In addition, particular care should be taken to avoid withdrawal of β-blockers and clonidine because of the potential for catastrophic withdrawal syndromes.

DIURETICS

Patients with evidence of cardiovascular disease frequently are treated with a regimen that includes a diuretic for control of hypertension, for treatment of congestive heart failure (CHF) and fluid overload states, and for related diseases. Diuretics are among the most commonly used drugs. **Table 44-2** lists dosage schedules and side effects for the more commonly prescribed diuretics.

Thiazides Although thiazide-type diuretics were recommended in the JNC 7 as the preferred initial therapy for most patients with hypertension, recent studies such as Losartan Intervention for Endpoint Reduction in Hypertension (LIFE),[6] Anglo-Scandinavian Cardiac Outcomes Trial (ASCOT),[7] and Avoiding Cardiovascular Events through Combination Therapy in Patients Living with Systolic Hypertension (ACCOMPLISH)[8] showed that several drug classes with reasonable side-effect profiles can reduce cardiovascular complications to a degree similar to that associated with diuretics.[9]

The thiazide diuretics primarily inhibit sodium transport in the distal tubule, the connecting segment at the end of the distal tubule, and possibly the cortical collecting tubule. This, however, is not the direct mechanism by which thiazides treat hypertension; chronically administered thiazides inhibit a maximal reabsorption of 3% to 5% of the filtered sodium. The initial hypotensive response is mediated by a modest reduction in plasma volume and cardiac output. However, the fall in blood pressure is blunted by hypovolemia-induced activation of the renin-angiotensin system, resulting in a partial reversal of the initial hemodynamic changes. Long-term maintenance of the decrease in

TABLE 44-2 Diuretics

Agent	Usual Daily Dose (mg)	Precautions and Special Considerations	Side Effects
Thiazides and related sulfonamide diuretics			
Bendroflumethiazide	2.5-5	May be ineffective in renal failure except for metolazone; hypokalemia increases digitalis toxicity; may cause an increase in blood levels of lithium; decrease urinary excretion of calcium; may precipitate acute gout	Hypokalemia, hypomagnesemia, hyperuricemia, glucose intolerance, hypercholesterolemia, increased low-density lipoprotein cholesterol, hypertriglyceridemia, hypercalcemia, sexual dysfunction, weakness, photosensitivity (except for ethacrynic acid), leucopenia, allergic skin rash
Benzthiazide (Exna)	12.5-50		
Chlorothiazide (Diuril)	125-500		
Chlorthalidone (Hygroton)	12.5-50		
Hydrochlorothiazide (HydroDIURIL, Esidrix)	12.5-100		
Hydroflumethiazide (Saluron, Dixardin)	12.5-50		
Indapamide (Lozol)	2.5-5		
Methyclothiazide	2.5-5		
Metolazone (Zaroxolyn)	2.5-5		
Polythiazide (Renese)	1-4		
Quinethazone (Hydromox)	25-100		
Trichlormethiazide	1-4		
Loop diuretics			
Bumetanide (Bumex)	0.5-5	Effective in chronic renal failure; increase urinary calcium excretion	As noted above, except for hypercalcemia
Ethacrynic acid (Edecrin)	25-100		
Furosemide (Lasix)	20-320		
Torsemide (Demadex)	2.5-50		
Potassium-sparing agents			
Amiloride (Midamor)	5-10	Danger of hyperkalemia in patients receiving a potassium supplement, a potassium-containing salt substitute, or an angiotensin-converting enzyme inhibitor, and in patients with renal failure; can cause renal failure in patients treated with a nonsteroidal anti-inflammatory drug (indomethacin and triamterene); may increase blood levels of lithium; spironolactone interferes with digoxin immunoassay	Hyperkalemia for all 3 agents; for spironolactone only: gynecomastia, mastodynia, gastrointestinal irritation, drowsiness, lethargy, irregular menses or postmenopausal bleeding, hirsutism
Spironolactone (Aldactone)	25-100		
Triamterene (Dyrenium)	50-200		
Eplerenone (Inspra)	50-100		

Modified with permission from Gifford RW. Treatment of patients with systemic arterial hypertension. In: Schlant RG, Alexander RW, eds. *Hurst's The Heart.* New York, NY: McGraw-Hill; 1994:1430.

blood pressure with thiazide diuretics is mostly due to arteriolar dilation and decrease in systemic vascular resistance.

Thiazide diuretics, and particularly chlorthalidone, have a greater antihypertensive effect than loop diuretics; this is probably related to their longer duration of action.[10] Thiazide diuretics must reach the lumen or the urinary side of the nephron in order to exert their effects. This process is hindered by the buildup of organic acids in renal insufficiency.[11] Therefore, a loop diuretic is more effective as an antihypertensive agent in patients with a glomerular filtration rate below 30 mL/min.

Thiazide diuretics act on the distal nephron to increase calcium reabsorption and reduce calcium excretion. They may be useful in preventing the formation of calcium-containing renal stones, and this may also explain their protective effects on rates of bone mineral loss and prevention of hip fracture.[12] Side effects may include hypokalemia, hypomagnesemia, hyperuricemia, hyperglycemia, metabolic alkalosis, hyponatremia, orthostatic hypotension, dysrhythmias, and gout. In the current treatment of patients with essential hypertension and normal renal function, thiazide diuretics are used at low doses to minimize the metabolic complications.[4]

Loop Diuretics Furosemide, bumetanide, ethacrynic acid, and torsemide are unrelated chemically but act on the kidney at the level of the medullary and cortical aspects of the thick ascending limb of the Henle loop to prevent reabsorption of sodium, chloride, and water. Loop diuretics are substantially more potent diuretics than thiazides, resulting in superior fluid clearance for the same degree of natriuresis. Therefore, loop diuretics are preferentially indicated in treatment of acute and chronic heart failure, as well as in treatment of edema of hepatic or renal origin. Loop diuretics are less effective than thiazides in treatment of hypertension, except when the hypertension is associated with chronic renal insufficiency. In this setting, fluid retention frequently plays a major role in the elevation in blood pressure and thiazides become less effective when the glomerular filtration rate (GFR) falls below 30 mL/min.

Side effects include ototoxicity, hypokalemia, hypomagnesemia, hyperuricemia, metabolic alkalosis, dehydration, and hyponatremia. Treatment with loop diuretics may lower serum calcium levels by increasing calcium excretion. In combination with hydration, they are used in the acute therapy of hypercalcemia.

Finally, loop diuretics have been used to decrease intracranial pressure and to convert acute oliguric renal failure to nonoliguric renal failure.[13]

Potassium-Sparing Agents Triamterene and amiloride inhibit the sodium-proton exchanger in the distal and collecting tubules, resulting in decreased sodium absorption and a concurrent decrease in potassium and hydrogen ion excretion. Spironolactone and eplerenone are both aldosterone antagonists and have the same effect by competitively inhibiting the mineralocorticoid receptor. When compared with spironolactone, eplerenone has a higher specificity for the aldosterone receptor and a low affinity for the progesterone and androgen receptor, resulting in less endocrine side effects (eg, gynecomastia, sexual dysfunction) than spironolactone.[14] All these drugs may cause hyperkalemia.

The potassium-sparing agents have relatively weak natriuretic activity, leading to the maximum excretion of only 1% to 2% of the filtered sodium. Consequently, they are commonly used in combination with a loop or thiazide diuretic, either to diminish the degree of potassium loss and metabolic alkalosis or to increase the net diuresis in patients with refractory edema. Aldosterone antagonist therapy also reduces mortality in selected patients with heart failure by blocking the damaging effects of aldosterone on heart, kidney, and vasculature.[15] The 2005 American College of Cardiology/American Heart Association heart failure guidelines with 2009 update recommended addition of an aldosterone antagonist in selected patients with moderately severe to severe symptoms of heart failure and a reduced left ventricular ejection fraction who can be monitored for preserved renal function and a normal plasma potassium concentration.[16]

Anesthetic Considerations The major anesthetic considerations with diuretics pertain to their effects on fluid balance and electrolytes. Recommendations for patients taking diuretics call for withholding diuretics on the day of surgery unless evidence suggests volume overload or signs and symptoms of overt congestive heart failure. Because intravascular volume may be decreased after diuretic administration, physical examination should include careful evaluation of vital signs, with particular attention to orthostatic blood pressures and other signs or symptoms of dehydration. If hypovolemia is unrecognized, anesthetic induction may result in significant hypotension and tachycardia.

Diuretics can cause profound electrolyte disturbances, and serum electrolyte levels must be verified preoperatively. Patients receiving chronic therapy with loop diuretics or thiazides may have decreased total-body potassium and evidence of low serum potassium levels. Rapid correction of mild-to-moderate hypokalemia before surgery in asymptomatic patients is not indicated for the following reasons:

1. Acute replacement may itself be dangerous and cause life-threatening hyperkalemia.
2. Little can be done to rapidly correct total-body potassium. (The difference between a serum potassium level of 2.5 mEq/L and 3.5 mEq/L may be 200 to 400 mEq in a 70-kg individual.)
3. Some studies suggest that chronic hypokalemia does not increase the incidence of intraoperative dysrhythmias.[17] However, antiarrhythmics that prolong the QT interval, such as class IA or III agents, may precipitate torsade de pointes in the presence of diuretic-induced hypokalemia.
4. In stable patients with chronic mild to moderate hypokalemia without signs or symptoms of hypokalemia (eg, muscle weakness, ileus, and nephropathy) and in the absence of dysrhythmias or digitalis use, anesthesia and surgery can proceed.

CENTRALLY ACTING α_2-AGONISTS

Table 44-3 lists some of the centrally acting α_2-agonists.

Clonidine Clonidine is an antihypertensive agent with a complex mode of action. Its major effect is to activate presynaptic central α_2 receptors with a α_2-to-α_1 selectivity ratio and reduce norepinephrine (NE) release by peripheral sympathetic nerve terminals. This leads to a 60% to 80% reduction in sympathetic outflow and catecholamine levels. Part of the antihypertensive effect of clonidine is a result of its action as an agonist of the imidazoline-1 receptors located in the rostral ventrolateral medulla, a vasopressor area of the descending reticular formation.[18] Clonidine decreases heart rate, systemic vascular resistance, plasma renin activity, and epinephrine and norepinephrine levels. Side effects include orthostatic hypotension, sedation, dry mouth, and dizziness.

TABLE 44-3 Centrally Acting α_2-Adrenoreceptor Agonists

Agent	Dosage (mg)	Duration of Action	Elimination
Clonidine	0.1-1.0 BID	6-12 h	Hepatic/renal
Clonidine TTS (patch)	3.5, 7.0, 10.5 cm² weekly	7 d	Hepatic/renal
Dexmedetomidine	IV: 1 μg/kg loading dose over 10 min; maintenance 0.2-0.7 μg/kg/h		Hepatic
Guanabenz	4-64 BID	6-12 h	Hepatic
Guanfacine	1-3 daily	12-24 h	Renal
α-Methyldopa	250-1000 BID	6-12 h	Renal/hepatic

BID, twice a day.

Clonidine is notable in that sudden discontinuation may result in a severe withdrawal syndrome, which includes rebound hypertension or hypertensive crisis. Restlessness, insomnia, agitation, nausea, and sweating may also occur. These disturbances usually occur 18 to 36 hours after the last dose. The transdermal clonidine patch allows continued administration in those unable to take oral medication, thereby avoiding withdrawal. Administered orally, clonidine reaches peak plasma concentrations in approximately 90 minutes, whereas when administered topically, it takes approximately 2 to 3 days to reach therapeutic levels. The clonidine patch is available in 3.5-, 7.0-, and 10.5-cm sizes, equivalent to oral doses of 0.1, 0.2, and 0.3 mg/d, respectively. Clonidine may also be administered via the intrathecal or epidural route to enhance the efficacy of regional anesthesia.

α_2-Agonists have many desirable effects, such as minimum alveolar concentration (MAC) reduction, analgesia, anxiolysis, sedation, and sympatholysis.[19] Substantial reductions in the need for various anesthetics (volatile agents, propofol, narcotics) while providing hemodynamic instability have been demonstrated after administration of clonidine in patients undergoing cardiac or noncardiac surgery.[20,21] In addition, clonidine attenuates sympathetic outpouring during drug addiction withdrawal.[22] A recent Cochrane review of randomized controlled trials that compared α_2-adrenergic agonists (clonidine, dexmedetomidine, or mivazerol) with placebo or non–α_2-adrenergic agonists found that α_2-agonists were associated with statistically significant reductions in all-cause mortality, cardiac mortality, and myocardial ischemia after surgery. Subgroup analysis, however, suggested that these effects applied mostly to patients undergoing vascular surgery. In addition, there was a significantly increased risk for perioperative hypotension and bradycardia.[23]

Although evidence supporting the routine use of α_2-agonists is not as compelling as that for perioperative β-blockade, the ACC/AHA guidelines introduced the use of α_2-agonists as a class IIb recommendation for perioperative control of hypertension or risk reduction in patients with known coronary artery disease (CAD) or major risk factors for CAD.[5] Unfortunately, the effects of clonidine are long acting and are not quickly reversed if severe hypotension or bradycardia develops. Recently, there has been resurgence in interest in clonidine because of its analgesic properties, both alone and in combination with other agents.

Dexmedetomidine Dexmedetomidine is a highly selective α_2-adrenergic receptor agonist (an α_2-to-α_1 selectivity ratio of 1600:1) with pharmacologic properties similar to those of clonidine. It decreases sympathetic tone, with associated decreases in heart rate and blood pressure. Like clonidine, it produces anxiolysis and sedation with minimal respiratory depression.[24] Dexmedetomidine and other α_2-agonists are known to interrupt nociceptive processing in the periphery, in the spinal cord, and in supraspinal sites, thereby explaining its analgesic properties.

Dexmedetomidine has an elimination half-life of approximately 2 hours with a distribution half-life of approximately 6 minutes. Its short half-life makes it particularly suitable for intravenous (IV) infusion. In adult patients, treatment is generally initiated with a loading infusion of 1 µg/kg over 10 minutes, followed by a maintenance infusion of 0.2 to 0.7 µg/kg/h. The rate of the maintenance infusion is adjusted to achieve the desired level of sedation. It is not indicated for infusions lasting longer than 24 hours. When administered to patients who are volume depleted or vasoconstricted or who have severe heart block, dexmedetomidine may result in hypotension and bradycardia.[25]

Transient hypertension may occur during administration of the loading dose. This is due to activation of the α_{2b}-adrenoceptor located in the smooth muscle cells of the resistance vessels and resulting in vasoconstriction. Treatment of this hypertension is not usually necessary, although reduction in the loading infusion rate may be beneficial.

Dexmedetomidine may be a useful adjuvant during general anesthesia due to its sedative, hypnotic, analgesia, and sympatholytic properties by promoting hemodynamic stability and decreasing the doses of volatile agents and narcotics.[26] It can be used in some of the following clinical situations: during intracranial surgical procedures that require neurophysiologic testing, awake intubation in patients with potentially difficult airway, procedural sedation in the pediatric population, bariatric surgery, sedation, and ventilator weaning in the intensive care unit (ICU).[27]

A number of studies have shown that dexmedetomidine may be a useful adjunct in cardiac surgery. A 2003 meta-analysis comprising 23 trials and more than 3000 patients investigated the effects of α_2-adrenergic receptor agonists, including dexmedetomidine, clonidine, and mivazerol, on patients undergoing vascular and cardiac surgery.[27] During cardiac surgery, α_2-adrenergic receptor agonists reduced the number of ischemic episodes and were associated with a reduced risk of myocardial infarction and a trend toward reduced mortality.

Mivazerol Mivazerol is another intravenous α_2-agonist, which is administered by continuous infusion (α_2-to-α_1 receptor selectivity of 119:1). It has been studied along with other α_2-adrenergic receptor agonists for perioperative myocardial protection.[28]

α-Methyldopa α-Methyldopa is an antihypertensive agent that was widely used in the past. Its major pharmacologically active metabolite, α-methylnorepinephrine, is a potent α_2-agonist that stimulates brainstem postsynaptic α_2 receptors. This decreases sympathetic tone and systemic vascular resistance. As with clonidine, α-methyldopa should be used with diuretics to prevent tolerance secondary to volume expansion. Common side effects include orthostatic hypotension, dizziness, sedation, dry mouth, nasal congestion, headache, and impotence. Less common but more serious side effects include leukopenia, hepatitis, thrombocytopenia, and a lupus-like syndrome. Rebound syndromes may occur after discontinuation of α-methyldopa, but much less frequently than with clonidine.[29]

Guanabenz and Guanfacine Guanabenz and guanfacine are centrally acting agonists with modes of action and anesthetic considerations similar to those of clonidine, including similar withdrawal syndromes.[30]

PERIPHERALLY ACTING SYMPATHOLYTIC AGENTS

α-Adrenergic Blockers **Table 44-4** lists α-adrenergic blocking agents. Prazosin, terazosin, and doxazosin competitively block postsynaptic α_1-adrenergic receptors in vascular smooth muscle, their main cardiovascular action being arterial and venous dilation. They reduce blood pressure with little effect on cerebral and renal vascular blood flow or heart rate. Prazosin, terazosin, and doxazosin have been used for treatment of hypertension and for afterload reduction in patients with congestive heart failure. Fluid retention may occur during chronic therapy requiring the addition of a diuretic. Today, these drugs are most commonly and successfully used for the treatment of benign prostatic hypertrophy.[30] Side effects include occasional tachycardia, orthostatic hypotension, dizziness, and even frank syncope after the initial dose, especially in patients already receiving other antihypertensive medications. Side effects may be significantly reduced by the administration of small initial doses.

Phenoxybenzamine and phentolamine are combined α_1- and α_2-receptor antagonists. Whereas phenoxybenzamine has a half-life of 24 hours, phentolamine has duration of action of 10 to 15 minutes, making

TABLE 44-4 α-Adrenergic Blocking Agents

Agent	Dosage (mg)	Duration of Action
Prazosin	1-10 BID	4-8 h
Terazosin	1-20 daily	12-24 h
Doxazosin	1-16 daily	24 h
Phenoxybenzamine	10-40 BID or TID	3-4 d
Phentolamine	IV: bolus 30-70 µg/kg, maintenance 1-20 µg/kg/min	10-15 min

BID, twice a day; TID, 3 times a day.

it suitable for continuous intravenous infusion. Phenoxybenzamine is predominantly used for long-term control of hypertension associated with pheochromocytomas. Phentolamine is used intravenously for perioperative management of hypertension associated with pheochromocytomas[31] and for reversal of deleterious effects secondary to drug extravasation (ie, norepinephrine, dopamine).[32] Common side effects of these drugs include hypotension and tachycardia. Tachycardia occurs secondary to baroreceptor reflex activation and blockade of the presynaptic α_2 receptors interfering with the normal feedback inhibition of norepinephrine release. This tachycardia responds well to β-blockers.

Adrenergic Neuronal Blocking Agents Guanethidine, guanadrel, and reserpine are antihypertensive agents more often used in the past. They have limited current use because of availability of drugs with fewer side effects. They exert their antihypertensive effect at the level of the postganglionic adrenergic neurons; however, their exact mechanism of action is incompletely understood. Guanethidine must be actively transported into the neuron, where it accumulates in neuronal storage vesicles and causes norepinephrine (NE) storage depletion. Reserpine acts by inhibition of NE and dopamine (DA) uptake into terminal vesicles; therefore, it results in NE depletion due to increased NE degradation and decreased conversion of DA to NE. Reserpine also crosses the blood–brain barrier and decreases central nervous system (CNS) serotonin and DA. Although this effect is thought to be unrelated to its antihypertensive effect, it may be the mechanism by which reserpine causes depression, nightmares, and sedation.

Other side effects include expansion of intravascular volume, necessitating the addition of a diuretic, as well as orthostatic and exercise-induced hypotension, diarrhea, and sexual dysfunction.[30]

The anesthetic implications of guanethidine and reserpine involve the decrease in NE concentration, which may cause the pharmacologic equivalent of denervation hypersensitivity. Therefore, direct-acting sympathomimetics may cause exaggerated hemodynamic responses. Decreased NE neuronal tissue stores render indirect-acting agents (eg, ephedrine) less effective.

VASODILATORS

Table 44-5 lists direct-acting vasodilators.

Hydralazine Hydralazine is one of the oldest antihypertensives still in use. It is a direct arteriolar vasodilator with little or no effect on the venous circulation. Although angiotensin-converting enzyme (ACE) inhibitors and angiotensin receptor (ATR) blockers have largely usurped its use, hydralazine is still used in patients who cannot tolerate these other agents or in hypertension during pregnancy. Several mechanisms of action have been proposed for its direct action on arteriolar smooth muscle, including preventing the accumulation of intracellular free Ca^{2+}, promoting influx of potassium, and reduction in nitric oxide (NO) consumption.[33]

In response to arteriolar vasodilatation, a baroreceptor-mediated increase in plasma volume, heart rate, cardiac output, and stroke volume often occurs, accompanied sometimes by vasodilatory edema. As a result, β-blockers and/or diuretics are given concurrently to minimize reflex sympathetic stimulation and fluid retention. Additional side effects include palpitations, headaches, flushing, and nasal congestion, and, in patients with coronary artery disease, worsening angina. In higher dosages, it may cause a lupus-like syndrome, which is completely reversible on discontinuation.

TABLE 44-5 Direct-Acting Vasodilators

Agent	Dosage	Duration of Action (h)
Minoxidil	PO: 10-40 mg daily	8-12
Hydralazine (PO)	PO: 40-300 mg daily	6-12
Hydralazine (parenteral)	IV: 2.5-10 mg q20-30min, max 30-40 mg IM: 10-20 mg q4-6h	4-8

IM, intramuscularly; IV, intravenously; PO, orally; q, every.

Several clinical trials have shown that hydralazine plus nitrate therapy when added to β-blockers and neurohormonal blockers (ACE inhibitors, angiotensin receptor blockers [ARBs]) may provide symptomatic and mortality benefit in selected patients with heart failure due to systolic dysfunction.[34,35]

Perioperatively, hydralazine is titrated intravenously for control of hypertension. It may take up to 30 minutes for an intravenous dose of hydralazine to exert its full effect, and the decrease in blood pressure may persist for up to 12 hours; therefore, it should be administered in doses divided by appropriate time intervals.

Minoxidil Minoxidil, like hydralazine, is a direct arterial vasodilator that has no effect on the venous circulation. It is used to control hypertension resistant to multidrug regimens. Like hydralazine, minoxidil may increase heart rate and cause fluid retention. To minimize these effects, it is generally administered with a diuretic and a β-blocker. Other side effects include facial hirsutism, hypertrichosis, and, infrequently, pericardial effusion.[36,37]

Sodium Nitroprusside Sodium nitroprusside (SNP) is one of the most effective parenteral drugs for treatment of hypertensive emergencies and acute congestive heart failure. SNP dilates both arterioles and veins, reducing both preload and afterload. SNP is a nitric oxide donor. In vascular smooth muscle, NO activates the enzyme guanylate cyclase, resulting in increased intracellular cyclic guanosine monophosphate (cGMP), which inhibits calcium entry into the smooth muscle cell and may increase calcium uptake by the endoplasmic reticulum producing vasodilatation.[38]

While dissociating to produce NO, SNP produces also cyanide ions and interacts with oxyhemoglobin to produce cyanmethemoglobin. The cyanide ions are converted to thiocyanate via transsulfuration within the liver by the enzyme rhodanese using thiosulfate as sulfur donors. In the face of SNP infusion rates exceeding 2 μg/kg/min, sulfur donors and methemoglobin are exhausted and cyanide radicals may accumulate, producing clinical cyanide toxicity by binding and inactivating tissue cytochrome oxidase. Cyanide toxicity prevents oxidative phosphorylation; thus tissue hypoxia, anaerobic metabolism, and lactic acidosis may result despite adequate available oxygen. Patients receiving SNP who show subsequent central nervous system dysfunction, cardiovascular instability, and increasing metabolic acidosis should be assessed for cyanide toxicity, and sodium nitroprusside should be discontinued.[39]

Because availability of thiosulfate is the rate-limiting step in cyanide metabolism, a concomitant infusion of sodium thiosulfate is advocated to prevent toxicity.[39] Thiocyanate itself can cause toxicity in patients with impaired renal function, but only at concentrations that are seldom reached. Other agents used in the treatment of cyanide toxicity are sodium nitrite, which converts hemoglobin in methemoglobin and hydroxocobalamin. Both methemoglobin and hydroxocobalamin bind cyanide radicals, forming cyanmethemoglobin and cyanocobalamin, respectively.

SNP produces direct venous and arterial vasodilatation with a dose-dependent decrease in blood pressure and a marked decrease in systemic vascular resistance (SVR). It produces pulmonary vasodilatation, decreases pulmonary vascular resistance (PVR), and directly inhibits hypoxic pulmonary vasoconstriction (HPV). The effect on cardiac output is dependent on end-diastolic volume. With increased end-diastolic volumes, as in patients with CHF, cardiac output may increase, whereas with normal volumes, cardiac output may be unchanged. SNP can produce "coronary steal" with shunting of blood away from areas of ischemia; it was associated with increased mortality when administered in patients with acute myocardial infarction and elevated left ventricular filling pressures.[39] Because of dilation of the large capacitance vessels in the cerebral circulation, SNP may increase the cerebral blood volume, leading to an increase in the intracranial pressure and decrease in the cerebral perfusion pressure in patients with brain injury and altered intracranial compliance.[39] In addition, although SNP appears to impair platelet aggregation via NO[40] in a dose-related manner, the duration of the effect is apparently limited to 5 to 25 minutes. The clinical importance of this effect has been questioned, as studies have not shown an increase in blood loss or blood transfusions with the use of SNP.[41]

SNP has an immediate onset and a very short duration of action (1-2 minutes). The initial dose of sodium nitroprusside is 0.3 to 0.5 μg/kg/min, with increases in increments of 0.5 μg/kg/min to reach the desired hemodynamic effect. The duration of treatment should be as short as possible, and it is best to avoid doses exceeding 2 μg/kg/min.[39]

SNP is a popular agent for induced intraoperative hypotension. Concern regarding its toxicity has prompted many anesthesiologists to supplement SNP with β-adrenergic blockers, calcium channel blockers, nitroglycerin, or volatile agents so as to maintain a rate of SNP infusion of less than 2 μg/kg/min. Because of concerns of cyanide toxicity, SNP should be avoided in patients with liver and kidney insufficiency. SNP has also found use in hypertensive emergencies, management of acute and congestive heart failure, pheochromocytomas, and blood pressure control during cardiac and aortic surgery.

Other Vasodilators

Fenoldopam Fenoldopam is a selective DA type 1 (DA1) receptor agonist 10 times more potent than DA. It does not act as an agonist at DA type 2 (DA2) receptors or at α and β receptors. Onset of action is within 5 minutes, with a maximal response achieved within 15 minutes. Duration of action is 30 to 60 minutes and does not cause rebound hypertension when the infusion is discontinued.

Fenoldopam decreases blood pressure without increasing heart rate and cardiac contractility. It dilates a variety of arteries, including coronary arteries, afferent and efferent arterioles of the kidney, and mesenteric arteries.[42] Consequently, it increases renal blood flow, creatinine clearance, urinary flow, and sodium excretion.[43] Fenoldopam can be safely used in hypertensive emergencies and may be particularly beneficial in patients with renal insufficiency. The infusion is initiated at 0.1 to 0.3 μg/kg/min and the dose titrated in increments of 0.05 to 0.1 μg/kg/min every 15 minutes until the target blood presure is reached.

Fenoldopam should be given cautiously to patients with glaucoma or high intraocular pressure because it may increase intraocular pressure. Other side effects are related to the vasodilator effect and can include headache, dizziness, tachycardia, or bradycardia.[43]

Fenoldopam has demonstrated nephroprotective properties in critically ill patients and in patients undergoing major surgery. A recent meta-analysis including more than 1200 patients undergoing cardiac surgery, vascular surgery, liver transplant, or renal transplant showed that fenoldopam reduced the risk of renal replacement therapy and all-cause mortality as compared with best medical therapy.[44] A second meta-analysis included more than 1000 patients undergoing cardiac or vascular surgery and showed that fenoldopam reduced the risk of renal replacement therapy and overall mortality.[45]

Nesiritide Nesiritide is a recombinant B-type natriuretic peptide structurally identical to the brain natriuretic peptide (BNP) produced by the cardiac ventricles in response to increased wall stress, hypertrophy, and volume overload. It reduces preload and afterload, increases cardiac output without having inotropic effects, and decreases dyspnea in patients with decompensated congestive heart failure and pulmonary edema.[39]

Several clinical trials have proved the efficacy of nesiritide when compared with standard vasoactive agents in improving hemodynamic parameters (eg, pulmonary capillary wedge pressure) and symptoms (eg, dyspnea) in patients with decompensated congestive heart failure.[46,47] However, a post hoc analysis of the pooled results of several large trials raised concern about the effect of acute nesiritide therapy on 30-day mortality when compared with treatment with other noninotropic vasodilators (nitroglycerin or nitroprusside).[48] A recent large study of serial infusions of nesiritide for chronic severe heart failure (The Second Follow-up Serial Infusions of Nesiritide [FUSION II]) showed no difference in all-cause mortality or hospitalization from cardiac or renal causes in patients treated with nesiritide compared with placebo.[49] These findings are the subject of further investigation.

For treatment of patients with acute decompensated heart failure, nesiritide is given as an initial intravenous bolus of 2 μg/kg, followed by a continuous infusion of 0.01 μg/kg/min. If the desired therapeutic response is not achieved, at 3-hour interval, the dosage may be increased by 0.005 μg/kg/min after a bolus of 1 μg/kg up to a maximum of 0.03 μg/kg/min.[50]

ANGIOTENSIN-CONVERTING ENZYME INHIBITORS

ACE inhibitors (**Table 44-6**) have become the cornerstone of heart failure and hypertension treatment. They competitively inhibit the ACE (**Fig. 44-1**), which mediates the conversion of angiotension I to angiotensin II. Angiotensin II is responsible for arterial vasoconstriction and increased aldosterone secretion. The decrease in plasma angiotensin II causes vasodilation of both venous capacitance and arteriolar resistance vessels without reflex increases in heart rate. ACE inhibitors also decrease aldosterone levels and increase the level of local bradykinin by decreasing its breakdown. Bradykinin has vasodilatory properties by increased formation of nitric oxide and increased formation of vasodilatory prostaglandins.[50]

Side effects include hypotension, acute renal failure, and hyperkalemia.[51] Other complications, including cough, bronchospasm, angioneurotic edema, and anaphylactoid reactions, are believed to be related to increased bradykinin levels. Precipitous reductions in blood pressure may occur after initiation of therapy, particularly in hypovolemic patients.

In patients with normal renal function, ACE inhibitors generally raise plasma potassium concentrations by less than 0.5 mEq/L. More prominent hyperkalemia may be seen in patients with renal insufficiency, concurrent use of a potassium-sparing diuretic or a nonsteroidal anti-inflammatory drug, and in the elderly.[53] Declines in renal function occur in patients with bilateral renal artery stenosis, hypertensive nephrosclerosis, congestive heart failure, polycystic kidney disease, or chronic renal insufficiency. Nevertheless, as a result of the favorable effects on the progression of diabetic and nondiabetic renal disease, an increase in serum creatinine of as much as 35% above baseline is acceptable, unless hyperkalemia develops.[53]

Several clinical trials support the use of ACE inhibitors in patients with diabetes and hypertension based on their favorable impact on cardiovascular and renal outcomes.[53] In addition to lowering blood pressure, the ACE inhibitors have the following effects: decrease the progression of chronic renal disease,[54] decrease morbidity and mortality in patients with heart failure caused by systolic dysfunction,[55]

TABLE 44-6 Angiotensin-Converting Enzyme Inhibitors

Agent	Dosage	Duration of Action (h)	Elimination
Captopril	12.5-50 mg BID-TID	4-8	Renal
Enalapril	5-20 mg BID	12-24	Renal
Enalaprilat	1.25 mg IV QID	6	Renal
Lisinopril	10-40 mg daily	24	Renal
Benazepril	10-40 mg daily BID	24	Renal/hepatic
Fosinopril	10-40 mg daily BID	24	Renal/hepatic
Quinapril	5-80 mg daily BID	24	Renal/hepatic
Ramipril	1.25-20 mg daily BID	24	Renal/hepatic
Moexipril	7.5-30 mg daily BID	>24	GI tract/hepatic
Perindopril	4-8 mg daily BID		Renal/hepatic
Trandolapril	2-4 mg daily	72	Renal

BID, twice a day; GI, gastrointestinal; IV, intravenously; QID, 4 times a day.

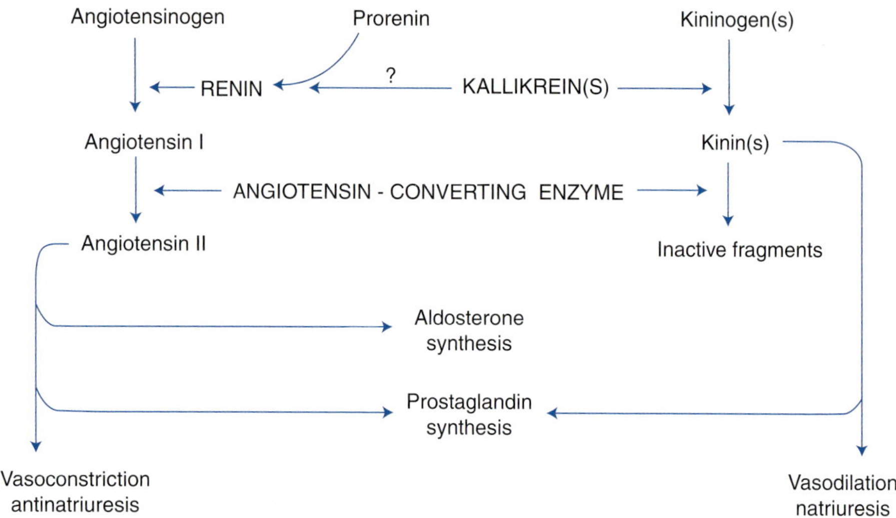

FIGURE 44-1. Schematization of the renin–angiotensin–aldosterone system and the kallikrein–kinin system and their interaction with the angiotensin-converting enzyme. [Mensah GA, Bakris G. Treatment and control of high blood pressure in adults. *Cardiol Clin*. 2010;28(4):609-622.]

improve survival after myocardial infarction with reduced systolic function, and induce regression of left ventricular hypertrophy.[56] Also, ACE inhibitors seem to reduce the rate of recurrence of atrial fibrillation after cardioversion and to protect against development of atrial fibrillation in patients with left ventricular dysfunction.[57] It has also been shown that increased bradykinin levels improve insulin sensitivity, which may result in better glycemic control in diabetic patients.[58]

ANGIOTENSIN II RECEPTOR BLOCKERS

Table 44-7 lists the angiotensin II receptor blockers (ARBs). There are 2 well-described subtypes of angiotensin II receptors, designated AT1 and AT2, both of which have a high affinity for angiotensin II. The AT1 subtype mediates the vasoconstrictor effect of angiotensin II and may mediate angiotensin II-induced growth in the left ventricle and the arterial wall. The AT2 receptor has a less well-understood role. ARBs are selective blockers of AT1 receptors on the cell membrane.[59] Because the formation of angiotensin II may result from a non–ACE-dependent pathway, ARBs result in a more complete blockade of the action of angiotensin II than the ACE inhibitors.

The ARBs have been primarily evaluated for the treatment of hypertension, where they appear to have an effect similar to other antihypertensive drugs. In fact, ARBs are more effective than β-blockers in reducing the long-term risk of cardiovascular morbidity and mortality in patients with hypertension, diabetes, and left ventricular hypertrophy.[60] The role of ARBs in heart failure has been extensively studied. As in heart failure there is a strong activation of the renin–angiotensin–aldosterone system (RAAS), and a complete blockade of angiotensin II at the level of the AT1 receptors should be of special benefit. However, large randomized clinical trials failed to show superior outcomes with ARBs when compared with ACE inhibitors.[61,62] ARBs have a special role in patients with diabetic nephropathy. Several large-scale randomized clinical trials demonstrated the benefit of ARBs in patients who had early- or late-stage diabetic nephropathy and type 2 diabetes. Based on these results, it has been recommended that ARBs, as a class, should be the therapy of choice for most diabetic patients who have microalbuminuria or advanced nephropathy.[63]

The angiotensin II receptor blockers are generally well tolerated. They exhibit side effects similar to ACE inhibitors, with the exception of those mediated by kinins, particularly cough, which is the most common reason that patients discontinue ACE inhibitors. It should be recognized, however, that multiple cases of angioedema have been described in patients taking losartan, typically characterized by swelling of the mouth, tongue, pharynx, and eyelids, and occasional laryngeal obstruction. Consequently, physicians should proceed with caution when choosing an antihypertensive for patients who have discontinued ACE inhibitors because of angioedema.[64]

In the perioperative setting, induction of general anesthesia in patients with angiotensin blockade may result in significant hypotension requiring the administration of vasopressors.[65,66] A recent prospective, observational study that included more than 9000 patients on ACE inhibitor/ARB therapy demonstrated that patients receiving ACE inhibitor/ARB therapy and concomitant diuretic therapy had more episodes of hypotension intraoperatively.[67] These data suggest that hypovolemia may play a role in the hypotension observed during surgery. Withholding ACE inhibitors for 10 hours or more before surgery may result in less intraoperative hypotension.[68]

TABLE 44-7 Angiotensin II Receptor Blockers

Agent	Dosage	Half-Life (h)
Losartan	50-100 mg daily BID	6-9
Valsartan	80-320 mg daily BID	9
Irbesartan	150-300 mg daily BID	11-15
Telmisartan	40-80 mg daily BID	24
Candesartan	16-32 mg daily BID	3-11
Eprosartan	400-800 mg daily	5-7
Telmisartan	20-80 mg daily	24

BID, twice a day.

RENIN INHIBITORS

Chronic activation of the RAAS is a major factor in the pathogenesis of many cardiovascular and renal diseases. Also, RAAS blockade by ACE inhibitors and ARBs may result in increased plasma renin activity and concentration and incomplete angiotensin II activity suppression.[69] Therefore, blockade of the RAAS at the rate-limiting step by direct renin inhibitors (DRI) is an attractive and logical therapeutic approach. DRIs directly inhibit the catalytic activity of renin, resulting in decreased plasma renin activity, which in turn reduces the production of angiotensin I, angiotensin II, and aldosterone.

Aliskiren is the only orally active direct renin inhibitor that is currently approved for the treatment of hypertension. Aliskiren (either as monotherapy or in combination therapy) has been compared with representatives of several different classes of antihypertensive medications and has been shown to produce comparable or greater reductions in blood pressure.[70,71] Beyond its effect on blood pressure, evidence from preclinical and clinical studies has shown that aliskiren may have renal and cardioprotective effect, as demonstrated by a decrease in proteinuria and albuminuria and a reduction in left ventricular mass.[72]

Aliskiren is generally well tolerated. The most common adverse effects are headache, fatigue, and diarrhea. As with other drugs that interfere with the RASS, aliskiren may result in hyperkalemia.[71]

DIGOXIN

Digoxin is part of the mainstay therapy for chronic heart failure. It inhibits the neurohumoral response present in patients with heart failure and has a positive inotropic effect.

The mechanism of action of digoxin is unique. It directly inhibits the membrane-bound sodium-potassium adenosine triphosphatase (Na-K ATPase) pump of the myocardial cell, causing transient increase in intracellular sodium and decrease in intracellular potassium. The increase in intracellular sodium changes the sodium concentration gradient and produces decreased exchange of extracellular sodium for intracellular calcium. This leads to net increased inward calcium current and intracellular calcium concentration, resulting in enhanced isolated myocyte contractile performance (increased shortening velocity) and left ventricular (LV) systolic function. Digitalis remains the only inotrope available for chronic oral use and has been shown clinically to decrease symptoms of CHF as well as the number of hospitalizations.[73] Unlike other inotropes, digoxin has an overall neutral effect on mortality.

Digoxin also has substantial electrophysiologic effects. It substantially enhances parasympathetic tone while causing some decrease in cardiac sympathetic activity. These effects result in sinoatrial (SA) slowing and atrioventricular (AV) nodal inhibition. By affecting the Na-K ATPase pump, digitalis may also have effects on conduction independent of vagal tone. In normal subjects, digoxin has only a small effect on the SA node. It may be safely used in patients with sinus bradycardias without decreasing heart rates. However, patients with evidence of sick sinus syndrome given digoxin may have lengthened SA node conduction and recovery time. In patients with Wolff-Parkinson-White (WPW) syndrome and atrial fibrillation, digitalis may accelerate antegrade conduction over the bypass tract, resulting in ventricular tachycardia or fibrillation.

The most common indication for digoxin is the combination of chronic heart failure and atrial fibrillation.[74] In patients with chronic heart failure and sinus rhythm, digoxin has been shown to have limited benefit on mortality. The Digitalis Investigation Group Study is the largest randomized trial designed to evaluate the effects of digoxin in patients with heart failure in sinus rhythm with reduced or preserved systolic function. The study has shown that digoxin had a bidirectional effect on mortality; it reduced mortality from heart failure but possibly increased mortality from sudden death.[73] In the treatment of acute supraventricular tachycardias, digoxin has been replaced by more modern approaches, and in the treatment of chronic atrial fibrillation, digoxin is no longer the drug of first choice.[74]

The usual dose of digoxin is about 0.25 mg/d, with half that dose prescribed for the elderly (age >65 years) and patients with renal insufficiency. When acute therapy is necessary, a loading dose of 1 to 1.5 mg is given over 24 hours. Digoxin-induced arrhythmias and other toxic manifestations occur at progressively increasing frequency as the plasma digoxin concentration rises above 2.0 ng/mL, the upper limit of normal.

Digitalis possesses a very low therapeutic index. At toxic levels, in addition to causing anorexia, nausea, fatigue, visual disturbances, and confusion, digitalis may cause severe conduction disturbances. The electrocardiogram manifestations may include sinus bradycardia or SA node exit block, AV block, premature atrial contractions, junctional tachycardias, premature ventricular contractions, ventricular tachycardia, and fibrillation.

The risk of digitalis intoxication can be increased by certain factors, such as renal insufficiency, electrolyte abnormalities (hypokalemia, hypomagnesemia, and hypercalcemia), hypothyroidism, pulmonary disease, and pharmacokinetic interactions with other drugs that can affect digoxin metabolism (quinidine, cyclosporine, verapamil, rifampin).

Treatment of digitalis toxicity can include several measures, ranging from simply stopping further dosages to aggressively treating hypokalemia and hypomagnesemia, oral therapy with activated charcoal, or placement of a transvenous pacemaker in patients with symptomatic bradycardia or AV dissociation. It has been suggested, however, that transvenous cardiac pacing might precipitate cardiac dysrhythmias and deterioration, and should, if possible, be avoided.[75] Atrial, junctional, and ventricular ectopy are amenable to therapy with phenytoin or procainamide. Ventricular ectopy is usually treated successfully with lidocaine. Amiodarone can displace digoxin from binding sites and increase the blood levels of digoxin. Other drugs that increase serum digitalis levels (eg, quinidine, propafenone, verapamil) and administration of calcium salts should be avoided.

The availability of digoxin-specific Fab fragments has dramatically changed therapy for severe toxicity. The Fab fragments bind to digoxin intravascularly and in the tissues. The digoxin-Fab fragments complexes are small, so they can be rapidly excreted by glomerular filtration in patients with normal renal function.[76]

In the perioperative period, in patients receiving digoxin therapy, the possibility of digoxin toxicity as the dysrhythmia source must always be considered. Under this suspicion, one should avoid the use of drugs that increase digoxin levels (eg, verapamil) or cardioversion, which may precipitate ventricular fibrillation in the presence of digoxin toxicity.

Some data suggest that halothane, enflurane, ether, methoxyflurane, ketamine, droperidol, and curare may reduce the likelihood of digitalis-induced ventricular dysrhythmias. Thiopental and fentanyl have no effect, whereas succinylcholine, neostigmine, and diazepam may induce dysrhythmias in patients taking digitalis. No reports are available regarding the interaction of digoxin with sevoflurane or desflurane to our knowledge. More important in the perioperative period is the prevention of hypokalemia, acid–base imbalance, hypoxia, hypercalcemia, catecholamine excess states, and avoidance of medications that acutely increase digitalis serum levels.[77]

ANTIANGINALS

Three groups of drugs—nitrates, β-adrenergic blocking agents, and calcium channel blockers—alone or in combination, are effective and are commonly used to manage angina. Choosing a class of drugs, or a particular drug within each class, depends primarily on patient tolerance of side effects, ventricular function, presence or absence of conduction disease, and relative indications or contraindications caused by additional comorbidities.

NITRATES

Nitrates have been used under many forms for the treatment and prevention of angina for more than 100 years. Nitrates are potent dilators of the vascular smooth muscle that affect venous capacitance more than arterial resistance. By causing pooling in the peripheral veins, nitrates cause decreases in preload and ventricular volumes. At higher doses, nitrates may cause decreases in systemic and pulmonary vascular resistance.[78] Low doses of nitrates have little effect on cardiac output and heart rate in patients with normal or increased intravascular volume. Rapid administration or high doses of nitrates, especially in patients with volume-contracted states, may decrease left ventricular end-diastolic pressure, stroke volume, cardiac output, and mean arterial pressure and cause reflexive increases in heart rate and sympathetic tone. Nitroglycerin inhibits hypoxic pulmonary vasoconstriction, but to a lesser extent than nitroprusside.

The antianginal use of nitroglycerin stems from its effect on the relationship between myocardial oxygen supply and demand. By increasing venous capacitance, and thus decreasing left ventricular end-diastolic pressure and volume, nitroglycerin decreases systolic ventricular wall tension, which is the major determinant of myocardial oxygen demand. Nitrates improve oxygen supply by increasing blood flow to areas of ischemia through several mechanisms. By lowering the left ventricular end-diastolic pressure and decreasing the resistance in collateral vessels, nitrates result in redistribution of coronary blood flow to the subendocardial tissue and increased ratio of endocardial-to-epicardial blood flow. Nitroglycerin is also a direct coronary arterial vasodilator, especially of large epicardial vessels.[79] Dilation of large coronary arteries explains the beneficial effects of nitrates in patients with angina caused by coronary vasospasm. However, in patients with angina caused by coronary insufficiency, the administration of nitroglycerin does not result in net coronary blood flow increase. It has been postulated that dilation of large epicardial vessels in patients with coronary insufficiency causes an autoregulated increase in coronary vascular resistance in well-perfused arteriolar resistance vessels distal to large coronary arteries. This increased resistance shunts coronary flow to areas of ischemia, where the arterioles are already maximally dilated. Effects of nitrates on coronary blood flow distribution are different (indeed opposite) from those of sodium nitroprusside and dipyridamole. The latter drugs dilate arteriolar resistance vessels and can lead to myocardial steal phenomenon.

The mechanism of action of nitrates is by providing an exogenous source of the vasodilator nitric oxide. Nitrates enter the vessel wall and are ultimately converted in nitric oxide. Nitric oxide together with tissue thiols forms *s*-nitroso-thiol; nitrosothiols in turn activate guanylate cyclase, the enzyme that catalyzes the formation of cGMP (**Fig. 44-2**).[80] Increased cGMP causes smooth muscle relaxation. Higher intracellular levels of cGMP also mediate bronchial, biliary, gastrointestinal, ureteral, and uterine smooth muscle relaxation. Nitrates also have beneficial antiplatelet and antithrombotic properties. The antiplatelet effect of nitrates seems to be due to an increased cGMP level in platelets resulting in a reduction in fibrinogen binding to the platelet glycoprotein IIb/IIIa receptor, which is essential for platelet aggregation.[81]

Nitrate therapy has an important role in the management of patients with an acute coronary syndrome, despite the absence of a mortality benefit.[82,83] It can be used for reducing or potentially eliminating pain (either initial or recurrent) due to myocardial ischemia, improving symptoms of pulmonary congestion, lowering blood pressure in hypertensive patients, and aiding in the diagnosis and management of the rare patient who presents with variant angina (coronary artery spasm). Nitrates can be used transdermally or orally for chronic therapy, on an intermittent basis via the sublingual route, or intravenously for acute therapy (**Table 44-8**).

TABLE 44-8 Nitrate Preparations

Nitroglycerin	
Sublingual tablets–Nitrostat	0.3-0.6 mg PRN (up to 3 tablets)
Translingual spray–Nitrolingual	0.4 mg/spray (up to 3 sprays)
Transmucosal tablets–Nitrogard (Forest)	1-3 mg q5h TID
Oral extended-release	2.5-6.5 BID to QID
Ointment–2%	1" to 2" q4h for 12-14 h/d
Transdermal patches	1 patch 12-14 h/d
Isosorbide dinitrate	
Sublingual tablets–immediate release	2.5-10 mg q2-3h
Oral tablets	30 mg BID or 20 mg TID in morning and afternoon
Extended-release tablets and capsules	40-80 mg once daily to TID
Isosorbide-5-mononitrate	
Immediate release	20 mg in morning and afternoon, 7 h apart
Extended-release	60-120 mg once daily
Pentaerythritol tetranitrate	
Sublingual	10 mg PRN
Erythritol tetranitrate	
Sublingual	5-10 mg PRN
Oral	10-30 mg TID

BID, twice a day; PRN, as needed; q, every; QID, 4 times a day; TID, 3 times a day.

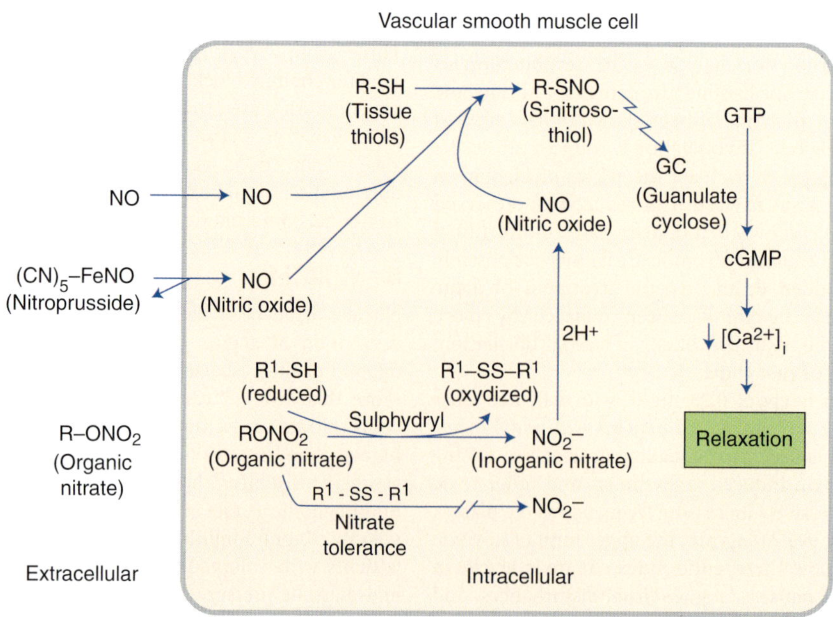

FIGURE 44-2. Cellular mechanism of action of nitroglycerin and nitroprusside. [Reproduced with permission from Ignarro LJ, Lippton H, Edwards JC, et al. Mechanism of vascular smooth muscle relaxation by nitrates, nitroprusside and nitric oxide. *J Pharmacol Exp Ther.* 1981;218:739.]

Continuous administration of nitrates is associated with tolerance, which is characterized by blunting of the hemodynamic response seen with nitrate therapy. The exact mechanism of tolerance is not known but may involve impaired bioconversion of nitrates to the active form, vascular sulfhydryl depletion or activation of RAAS, and the more recently described formation of free radicals through oxidative stress, resulting in endothelial dysfunction.[84] Common adverse effects in patients taking nitrate therapy are headache, flushing, and hypotension. Nitrates must be used cautiously in patients with severe aortic stenosis and volume depletion.

In the perioperative period, patients taking nitrates should continue to receive therapy until and possibly throughout surgery. If a substantial perioperative or postoperative lapse is expected, nitrate ointments or IV nitroglycerin may be used.

Perioperatively, IV nitroglycerin may be used for treatment of myocardial ischemia, CHF, acute volume overload, systemic and pulmonary hypertension, and coronary artery spasm. Patients receiving acute nitroglycerin therapy may exhibit exaggerated hemodynamic responses to anesthetics, possibly related to its effects on preload. Prolonged use or excessive doses of nitroglycerin rarely may cause methemoglobinemia,[85] but to a much lesser extent than sodium nitroprusside. More recently, the Evaluation of Clevidipine in the Perioperative Treatment of Hypertension Assessing Safety Events (ECLIPSE) trial was performed to compare the safety and efficacy of the ultra–short-acting calcium channel blocker clevidipine with nitroglycerin, sodium nitroprusside, and nicardipine in the treatment of perioperative acute hypertension in patients undergoing cardiac surgery. There was no difference in the incidence of myocardial infarction, stroke, or renal dysfunction for clevidipine-treated patients compared with the other treatment groups. There was no difference in mortality rates between the clevidipine, nitroglycerin, and nicardipine groups. Mortality was significantly higher, though, for nitroprusside-treated patients. Clevidipine was more effective compared with nitroglycerin or nitroprusside in maintaining blood pressure within a prespecified range.[86]

β-ADRENERGIC BLOCKING AGENTS

β-Adrenergic blocking agents are among the most widely prescribed cardiac medications and have a wide spectrum of therapeutic uses beyond treatment of hypertension, angina, and dysrhythmias.

There are at least 3 distinct types of β receptors:

- Activation of β_1 receptors, found primarily in the heart muscle, increases heart rate, contractility, and AV conduction and decreases AV node refractoriness.
- Activation of β_2 receptors, present in cardiac muscle but more prominently found in bronchial and peripheral vascular smooth muscle, results in bronchodilatation and vasodilatation.
- Activation of β_3 receptors, found in adipose tissue and the heart, may induce thermogenesis[87] and may have cardiodepressant effects.[88]

The major therapeutic effects of β-adrenergic blockers are on the cardiovascular system.

Variations among β-adrenergic blocking agents result from their differing pharmacologic properties in regard to β_1 selectivity, α-adrenergic blocking activity, presence of intrinsic sympathomimetic activity (ISA) or membrane-stabilizing activity (MSA), potency, lipid solubility, first-pass effect, half-life, and mode of metabolism and excretion. All β-adrenergic blocking agents competitively block effects of catecholamines on receptors in the heart, lung, vasculature, kidney, brain, and eye, and their therapeutic value stems from these effects.

β-Adrenergic blockers lower blood pressure in patients with hypertension, although the mechanism is still debated. β-Blockers decrease myocardial contractility and heart rate, and thus cardiac output, but even at dosages lower than necessary to cause substantial decreases in cardiac output, they can be effective antihypertensives. β-Blockers with ISA such as pindolol decrease cardiac output less, yet are similarly effective antihypertensives. β-Blockers decrease the release of renin from the juxtaglomerular apparatus. This action contributes to the antihypertensive effect. However, even though hypertensive patients with high plasma renin activity (PRA) respond well to propranolol, which decreases PRA, β-blockers that do not decrease PRA (eg, pindolol) are also effective.

Evidence suggests that β-blockers cross the blood–brain barrier, and a CNS mechanism involving reduction in receptor-mediated sympathetic outflow has been proposed. On the other hand, lipophilic drugs such as propranolol and metoprolol are no more effective than hydrophilic compounds such as atenolol. Other proposed mechanisms of action include resetting of baroreceptors, attenuation of pressor responses to stress and exercise, and blockade of prejunctional receptors that normally facilitate norepinephrine release.[89,90] Despite unclear mechanisms, β-blockers are among the most useful and commonly prescribed cardiovascular medications.

With the recent introduction of the so-called third-generation β-blockers, other additional antihypertensive mechanisms have been proposed, such as release of nitric oxide, antioxidant action, Ca entry blockade, and opening of K channels.[91]

In angina pectoris, β-adrenergic blocking agents decrease heart rate, blood pressure, and contractility and therefore reduce myocardial O_2 consumption. They may improve perfusion by increasing diastolic coronary filling time. Although β-blockers have little effect on the factors influencing plaque vulnerability, they may decrease the incidence of plaque rupture by reducing mechanical stress.[92] Other mechanisms have been suggested (**Box 44-1**). Not all the actions of β-blockers are beneficial in all patients. In patients with very poor ventricular function, worsening failure may negate other gains. Similarly, in Prinzmetal angina, β-blockade is ineffective and may even be harmful because of unopposed α-tone in the large coronary arteries.[93] Treatment of angina pectoris with β-blockers, in combination with nitrates, aspirin, and/or calcium channel blockers, represents the current standard of care, if no contraindications exist. Competitive β-receptor inhibition has useful antidysrhythmic effects. β-Blockers decrease the phase IV depolarization slope of the action potential and thus decrease automaticity. They slow the rate of discharge of the sinus and ectopic pacemakers and increase the effective refractory period of the AV node. The membrane-stabilizing effect of β-blockers does not appear to be relevant in the management of arrhythmias because it is manifested at concentrations well above therapeutic levels. β-Blockers are particularly effective in dysrhythmias caused by increased circulating catecholamines such as pheochromocytomas, anxiety, exercise, myocardial ischemia, and heart failure caused by cardiomyopathy; in those caused by increased

BOX 44-1

Possible Mechanisms by Which β-Blockers Protect the Ischemic Myocardium

Reduction in myocardial oxygen consumption, heart rate, blood pressure, and myocardial contractility

Augmentation of coronary blood flow

Increase in diastolic perfusion time by reducing heart rate

Augmentation of collateral blood flow

Redistribution of blood flow to ischemic areas

Alterations in myocardial substrate utilization

Decrease in microvascular damage

Stabilization of cell and lysosomal membranes

Shift to oxyhemoglobin dissociation curve to the right

Inhibition of platelet aggregation

Reproduced with permission from Frishman WH. *Clinical Pharmacology of the β-Adrenoceptor Blocking Drug*. 2nd ed. Norwalk, CT: Appleton-Century-Crofts; 1984:306.

cardiac sensitivity to catecholamines such as thyrotoxicosis; and in the dysrhythmias of mitral valve prolapse. They control heart rate in atrial fibrillation, flutter, and paroxysmal atrial tachycardia.[94,95] β-Blockers reduce sudden death, especially in patients with prior myocardial infarction or heart failure.[96] Survivors of myocardial infarctions have decreased morbidity, less sudden death, and fewer recurrent infarctions when treated with β-blockers. Although the reasons for this are not completely clear, a combination of the anti-ischemic and antidysrhythmic effects seems to play a key role.[97]

Other cardiovascular syndromes in which β-blocker therapy has proved useful include mitral valve prolapse, preexcitation syndromes, hypertrophic cardiomyopathy,[98] tetralogy of Fallot, aortic aneurysm, prolonged QT interval syndromes, and advanced cardiomyopathies. Noncardiac uses have included prevention of bleeding in patients with portal hypertension and treatment of glaucoma, thyrotoxicosis, migraines, essential tremors, delirium tremens, and anxiety.

These important drugs are not without significant side effects. β-Blockers may precipitate CHF in patients with preexisting ventricular dysfunction. Patients with sinus node dysfunction or AV block may develop symptomatic bradycardias; consequently, β-blockers are relatively contraindicated in patients with sick sinus syndrome. Stimulation of $β_2$ receptors in lungs causes bronchodilation; conversely, treatment with β-blockers may induce bronchospasm. Even β-blockers with relative $β_1$ selectivity (eg, metoprolol, atenolol, betaxolol, esmolol, acebutolol, bisoprolol) occasionally induce bronchoconstriction in therapeutic doses. Nevertheless, they are preferred in patients with chronic lung disease.[99] β-Blockade may decrease cardiac output and block $β_2$-mediated coronary or peripheral arterial dilation, allowing unopposed constriction (eg, spasm). Symptoms of peripheral vascular disease may worsen after β-blocker therapy, although this concern might be overstated in patients with mild to moderate peripheral vascular disease.[100] Additional concerns include impotence and decreased sympathetic manifestations of hypoglycemia in patients taking insulin or hypoglycemic agents. CNS effects such as depression, psychosis, and obtundation may occur. Depression, fatigue, and sexual dysfunction are common causes of β-blocker discontinuation.

Multiple interactions between β-adrenergic blocking agents and other drugs have been described, particularly ones that depress myocardial function and automaticity, such as calcium channel blockers and antiarrhythmic drugs.

Propranolol Propranolol is the prototype against which all other β-adrenergic blocking agents are measured. It is noncardioselective and has no ISA. Although propranolol possesses MSA, this occurs only at doses far beyond therapeutic and is not clinically relevant except after massive overdoses. Propranolol is almost completely absorbed after oral administration, but undergoes extensive first-pass hepatic metabolism. Thus the usual oral dosage of propranolol is 40 to 320 mg/d, whereas the IV dosage is only 0.025 to 0.15 mg/kg. Cimetidine decreases hepatic metabolism and blood flow and may decrease propranolol's therapeutic dose. Propranolol is highly lipophilic and crosses the blood–brain barrier, which may explain its many CNS effects. Its usual oral half-life is approximately 4 hours. Propranolol is available as a long-acting preparation, a marked advantage for treatment of patients with angina pectoris.[101] Propranolol may be slowly administered intravenously to patients under anesthesia in incremental doses of 1 mg with frequent monitoring of blood pressure.

Metoprolol Metoprolol is a moderately $β_1$ selective blocker with no ISA or MSA. It is primarily metabolized by the hepatic cytochrome P450 system with a half-life of 3 to 7 hours. When used in low doses, metoprolol may be preferable to propranolol for smokers and other patients who may have bronchospastic diseases but who require therapy with β-blockers. Although relatively cardioselective, metoprolol still may precipitate bronchospasm. It is less likely than propranolol to mask symptoms of hypoglycemia. Its usual oral dosage is 50 to 200 mg twice daily, although an extended-release formulation is also available and widely prescribed. Like propranolol, metoprolol is available in IV form, with usual dosage of 0.025 to 0.15 mg/kg. Metoprolol is used in the treatment of hypertension, stable angina, acute myocardial infarction, and chronic heart failure. The efficacy of metoprolol in heart failure management was studied in several randomized clinical trials, which showed an improved survival, reduced need for hospitalizations as a consequence of worsening heart failure, improved New York Heart Association (NYHA) functional class, and beneficial effects on patient well-being.[102,103]

Atenolol Atenolol is a long-acting, cardioselective β-blocker with no ISA or MSA. It is eliminated by renal excretion and has a half-life of 6 to 7 hours. Its usual dosage is 50 to 200 mg daily. It is available in an IV form, with a recommended dosage of 5 to 10 mg given slowly. Besides being cardioselective and requiring only a single daily intake, other possible advantages include relative hydrophilia and minimal blood–brain barrier crossing. Unfortunately, in clinical trials with atenolol, this has not been reflected by a lower incidence of CNS side effects.[104]

Bisoprolol Bisoprolol is a very highly selective, long-acting, cardioselective β-blocker, without any ISA or MSA. It is well-absorbed after oral administration and is eliminated by renal excretion, with 50% unchanged in the urine and the remaining 50% eliminated as inactive metabolites.[105] Its half-life of 9 to 13 hours makes it suitable for once-daily administration. Recent randomized clinical trials show that bisoprolol prevents major cardiovascular events in patients with CHF.[106]

Betaxolol Betaxolol is an oral, long-acting, cardioselective β-blocker with no ISA or MSA. Undergoing mainly hepatic metabolism, its half-life of 16 to 22 hours makes it suitable for once-daily administration. As with timolol, betaxolol is available for topical ophthalmic use and may be better tolerated by patients with bronchospastic disease because of its $β_1$ selectivity.

Nadolol Nadolol is a long-acting, noncardioselective β-blocker with no ISA or MSA. Unlike propranolol, it is renally excreted, with a half-life of 20 to 24 hours, allowing for once-daily administration. The usual dosage is 40 to 240 mg/d; dosage should be reduced in patients with renal failure.

Timolol Timolol is a noncardioselective β-blocker with no MSA or ISA. Its usual dosage is 10 to 30 mg twice a day, with a half-life of 4 to 5 hours. It undergoes both hepatic and renal excretion. Otherwise, it is similar to propranolol. Timolol is frequently used as an eye-drop therapy for open-angle glaucoma. In this form, it is often systemically absorbed and produces effects similar to those after oral ingestion.

Acebutolol, Carteolol, Penbutolol, and Pindolol Acebutolol, carteolol, penbutolol, and pindolol are nonselective β-blockers with ISA and partial agonist effects. With the patient at rest, these drugs may decrease heart rate to a lesser extent than other β-blockers. They are efficacious in blunting exercise-induced hemodynamic response. These drugs are thought to produce fewer lipid abnormalities and peripheral vascular complications, with less myocardial depression and bronchospasm. Specifically, pindolol produces less depression of heart rate and fewer nocturnal pauses in patients with sick sinus syndrome as compared with agents lacking agonist effects.[107,108] Another possible advantage may be the absence of rebound after discontinuation; however, no large-scale trials are available to support these claims. No data are available to support the use of these drugs after myocardial infarction (MI). **Table 44-9** lists the dosages for these drugs.

Labetalol Labetalol is a nonselective β-blocker unique among β-blockers for its β-adrenergic blocking properties in a ratio of approximately 7:1(β:α). In addition, labetalol has partial agonist activity at $β_2$ receptors.[109] This blocking can be used to decrease arterial pressure with somewhat better maintenance of cardiac output. Labetalol is available in both IV and oral forms, and its use is well established in acute therapy of severe hypertension in the emergency room, operating room, and recovery suite, but it is seldom used as a long-term medication.

Esmolol Esmolol is a highly cardioselective adrenergic blocker with little ISA and no MSA. It has a distribution half-life of 2 minutes and

TABLE 44-9 Pharmacologic Properties of β-Blockers

Agent	Relative β_1 Selectivity	ISA	MSA	α Activity	Elimination Half-Life Charts	Predominant Mode of Elimination	Oral Dosage (mg)	IV Dosage
Acebutolol	+	+	+	–	3-4 h	Renal/hepatic	200-600 BID	
Atenolol	++	–	–	–	6-7 h	Renal	50-200 daily	5-10 titrated at 1 mg/min
Betaxolol	++	–	+	–l	16-22 h	Hepatic/renal	10-40 daily	
Bisoprolol	++	–	–	–	9-13 h	Renal/hepatic	10-20 daily	
Carteolol	–	+	–	–	5-6 h	Renal	2.5-10 daily	
Carvedilol	–	–	+	+	7-10 h	Hepatic	3.125-25 BID	
Esmolol	++	–			9 min	Red blood cell esterases	–	0.5-1 mg/kg bolus, then 100-300 μg/kg/min
Labetalol	–	–	–	+	6-8 h	Hepatic	200-1200 BID	5-20 mg initially, then 40 mg q10min up to 300 mg as boluses or 2 mg/min as infusion
Metoprolol	+	–	–	–	3-7 h	Hepatic	50-200 BID	0.1-0.15 mg/kg titrated slowly to effect
Metoprolol extended release	++	–	–	–	?	Hepatic	50-400 daily	
Nadolol	–	–	–	–	20-24 h	Renal	40-240 daily	
Oxprenolol	–	+	+		4-6l	Hepatic	40-80 TID	
Penbutolol	–	+	–	–	5 h	Renal	20 daily	
Pindolol	–	++	+	–	3-4 h	Renal/hepatic	5-30 BID	
Propranolol	–	–	++	–	4 h	Hepatic	40-320 daily, 0.1-0.15 mg/kg BID or QID titrated slowly to effect	
Propanolol extended release	–	–	++	–	10 h	Hepatic	80-320 daily, BID	
Timolol	–	–	–	–	4-5 h	Renal	10-30 BID	

BID, twice a day; ISA, intrinsic sympathomimetic activity; IV, intravenous; MSA, membrane-stabilizing activity; q, every; TID, 3 times a day.

an elimination half-life of 9 minutes as a result of rapid hydrolysis by red blood cell (RBC) esterases. Its short duration of action makes it particularly valuable in management of perioperative patients. Esmolol is typically used as a bolus, with or without an infusion. Steady-state plasma levels are obtained within 5 minutes. Usual bolus dosages are 0.5 to 1 mg/kg. Infusion rates of 50 to 300 μg/kg/min are titrated to clinical effect. On discontinuation of an esmolol infusion, significant recovery occurs within 10 to 20 minutes, and blood concentrations are undetectable within 30 minutes. Because esmolol is metabolized by red blood cell esterase, *plasma* cholinesterase inhibitors do not affect metabolism and elimination. Esmolol has been used intraoperatively to attenuate response to intubation, prevent and/or treat tachycardia and ischemia, and produce deliberate hypotension. The time course for attainment of decreases in heart rate is faster than that for changes in blood pressure.[110] It has been used to attenuate the increased heart rate and mean arterial pressure associated with rapidly increased desflurane concentrations.[111] Postoperatively, it has been used in treatment of hypertension, myocardial ischemia, and supraventricular dysrhythmias.

Celiprolol Celiprolol is a third-generation cardioselective β-blocker without MSA but with evidence of ISA at the β_2 receptor. It is an effective drug in the treatment of hypertension and angina.[112] It is a weak bronchodilator and vasodilator as a result of its β_2-receptor effect. It may prove superior to other β-blockers for asthmatic patients.[113]

Carvedilol Carvedilol is a nonselective β-blocker that also blocks α_1 receptors in a manner similar to that of labetalol. It has MSA but no ISA. Carvedilol is also a potent antioxidant and antiproliferative, which inhibits vascular smooth muscle proliferation.[114] This property makes it useful in the treatment of chronic CHF. In numerous clinical trials, carvedilol significantly reduced morbidity and mortality in patients with heart failure.[115] Favorable effects on the remodeling process in heart failure were seen, with a decrease in left ventricular size and improvement in ejection fraction.[116] A recent clinical trial comparing metoprolol and carvedilol in patients with chronic heart failure showed that carvedilol extends survival.[117]

Bucindolol Bucindolol is a third-generation nonselective β-blocker with α_1 blocking and β_2-agonist capabilities. In contrast to other β-blockers studied, bucindolol failed to show any significant overall survival benefit in patients with advanced cardiac failure.[118]

Nebivolol Nebivolol is a third-generation, highly selective β_1-receptor blocker, which can be distinguished from other β-blockers by its hemodynamic profile. It combines β-blocking activity with a vasodilating effect, which is mediated at least in part by endothelial NO. The blood-pressure-lowering effect of nebivolol is linked to a reduction in peripheral resistance and an increase in stroke volume with preservation of cardiac output.[119] Recent clinical trials show that it is an effective and well-tolerated treatment for heart failure in the elderly (age >65 years).[120] It may reduce mortality in patients with heart failure.[121]

Anesthetic Considerations Anesthetic considerations regarding β-blocker therapy are numerous. Initially, β-blockers and antihypertensives were discontinued before anesthesia and surgery because of concerns that their effects would be additive with those of general anesthetic agents. Unfortunately, this sudden withdrawal tended to result in rebound effects with worsening of both angina and hypertension. There is little doubt that preoperative initiation of β-blocker therapy decreases the risk of perioperative ischemia and MI. Nevertheless, there is a raging controversy over whether *acute* perioperative β-blockade should be initiated in patients who have high or intermediate risk for a perioperative MI. Earlier research supported such of administration of β-blockers in these patients, demonstrating a decreased incidence of postoperative ischemia and lower mortality at 2-year follow-up in the group of patients who received β-blockers.[122,123] More recently, the POISE study and others raise the question of whether the reduced incidence of perioperative ischemia and nonfatal MI occurs at the expense of increased stroke risk and death rates in patients randomized to receive β-blockers compared to with controls.[124,125] Other investigators disagree, saying that the purported increased stroke and death rates are due to study design. They say that moderate rather than high-dose β-blockers administered starting 30 days before rather than the day of surgery improves cardiac outcomes without any increased risk in both high- and intermediate-risk patients undergoing noncardiac surgery.[126-128] Badgett et al[129] conducted a meta-analysis of existing trials and suggested that disparate results between trials may be due to differences between individual β-blockers. Trials using β-blockers with reduced β_1 selectivity and increased metabolic dependence on cytochrome P450, with its high degree of genetic polymorphism, seem to result in poorer outcomes than those which are more selective and less cytochrome P450 dependent. Hence bisoprolol, which is not cytochrome dependent and highly β_1 selective, may be a better choice than metoprolol, which is less β_1 selective and very cytochrome dependent as compared with bisoprolol. Atenolol is intermediate with respect to these properties. Badgett et al[129] recommend comparison of metoprolol with other β-blockers in survival and morbidity trials. Whether these differences are due to study design, including dosage and timing of various β-blockers, remains to be determined. As of this writing, the American Heart Association 2009 guidelines aver that several class IIa recommendations exist to initiate β-blockade in patients with inducible ischemia, known coronary disease, or multiple risk factors who are undergoing intermediate-risk surgery. In light of the conflicting results outlined previously, they suggest *considering* early preoperative initiation of β-blockers in such patients in doses titrated to avoid bradycardia and hypotension. They specifically do not advocate high-dose regimens initiated on the day of surgery, such as that of the POISE study.[130]

There is, however, a strong consensus that β-blockers should be continued in patients who are chronically β-blocked.[130,131] Abrupt discontinuation of β-blockers can result in a withdrawal syndrome caused by upregulation of β-receptors. This increased sensitivity to endogenous catecholamines can result in hypertension, tachycardia, or exacerbation of anginal syndromes, and even MI or death.

The β-adrenergic blocking agents most frequently used in the United States today are described in the following sections (Table 44-9).

Because of their pharmacologic effects, β-blockers interact with many anesthetic agents. β-Blockers have additive negative inotropic effects with potent inhalation agents. In dogs at 1.0 MAC of enflurane, propranolol causes mild decreases in myocardial contractility, heart rate, and cardiac output. These changes are more pronounced at deeper anesthetic concentrations. Circulatory depression, although present, is less when halothane or isoflurane is combined with propranolol compared with enflurane. In dogs anesthetized with halothane, isoflurane, or enflurane, propranolol produces additive slowing of heart rate and AV node conduction.[132]

Patients maintained on β-blockers, particularly when combined with calcium channel blockers, are at risk for severe bradyarrhythmias when anesthesia is induced with high-dose fentanyl or sufentanil. These bradyarrhythmias especially occur when muscle relaxants lacking vagolytic effects are used. When high-dose narcotics are given to patients who take β-blockers, with or without calcium channel blockers, it is recommended that vagolytic muscle relaxants (eg, pancuronium) be used.[133] β-Blockers are also associated with bradycardia during neuraxial anesthesia.[134]

The currently available IV β-blockers—propranolol, metoprolol, atenolol, labetalol, and esmolol—may be administered perioperatively to attenuate hemodynamic responses to intubation or surgical stress, treat hypertension and ischemia, slow heart rates, or treat dysrhythmias, in addition to the prophylactic uses described earlier.

CALCIUM CHANNEL BLOCKERS

The calcium channel blockers represent a diverse group of compounds with dissimilar structures and pharmacologic effects (**Table 44-10**). They inhibit voltage-sensitive calcium channel function (L-type or slow channels), which mediates the entry of extracellular calcium into smooth muscle (**Fig. 44-3**), cardiac myocytes, and SA and AV nodal cells in response to electrical depolarization. They therefore have vasodilatory properties, especially in arterial beds, and have negative chronotropic and inotropic effects to varying degrees.[135,136] Unlike β-blockers, which all depend on blockade of receptors for their activity, the sites and mechanisms of action of the individual calcium channel blockers vary, as do their individual actions on different tissues. They are not nearly as interchangeable as β-blockers.

Used predominantly in antianginal and antihypertensive therapy (**Fig. 44-4**), calcium channel blockers are also used in the treatment of syndromes as diverse as paroxysmal supraventricular tachycardia,

TABLE 44-10 Pharmacologic Effects of the Calcium Channel Blockers

	HR Acute	SA Node	AV Node	Myocardial Contractility	PVR	CO	CBF	MVO_2	Oral Dosage	Intravenous Dosage	$T_{1/2}$ (h)
Diltiazem	↓	↓	↓	↓	↓	V		↓	30-90 mg q6-8h	0.25 mg/kg (bolus) then 0.15 ng/kg/h	2-6
Bepridil	↓	↓	↓	V	–	V		↓	200-400 mg QD	–	24-48
Verapamil	↓	↓	↓	↓↓	↓	↓		↓	80-120 mg q6-2h	0.75-0.15 mg/kg (bolus) then 0.075-0.15 ng/kg/h	3-7
Amlodipine		–	–	↓–	↓↓			V	2.5-10 mg QD	–	36-45
Felodipine		–	–	–	↓↓			V	2.5-10 mg QD	–	tri-exponential: 4.8 min; 1.5 h; 9.1 h
Isradipine		–	–	–	↓↓			V	2.5-10 mg QD	–	6-11
Nicardipine		–	–	–	↓↓			V	10-20 mg q8h	5-15 mg/h	2
Nifedipine		–	–	↓–	↓↓			V	10-40 mg q8h	–	1.5-5
Nimodipine		–	–	–	↓↓			V			
Nisoldipine		–	–	–	↓↓			V	20-40 mg QD	–	10

↓, decrease; –, no change; AV, atrioventricular; CBF, coronary blood flow; CO, cardiac output; HR, heart rate; MVO_2, myocardial oxygen consumption; PVR, peripheral vascular resistance; q, every; QD, every day; SA, sinoatrial; $T_{1/2}$, terminal half-life; V, variable.

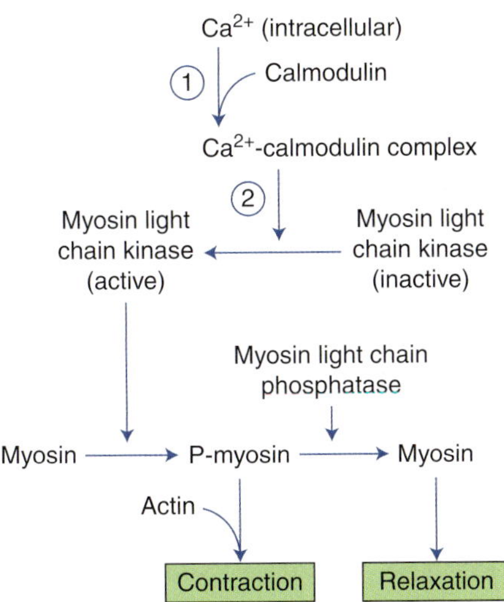

FIGURE 44-3. Activation sequence of mechanical contraction in vascular smooth muscle. The calcium ($Ca^{2|m+}$) calmodulin complex (*1*) activates myosin light-chain kinase (*2*), which catalyzes the phosphorylation of myosin (*P-myosin*). Cross-bridge formation between P-myosin and actin produces mechanical contraction.

hypertrophic obstructive cardiomyopathy, Raynaud phenomenon, preterm labor, and migraine headache prophylaxis.[137,138] The currently available calcium channel blockers can be categorized into 4 groups based on different chemical structures: dihydropyridines (which include nifedipine, nisoldipine, nicardipine, nimodipine, amlodipine, isradipine, felodipine, nitrendipine), verapamil (a phenylalkylamine), diltiazem (a benzothiazepine), and bepridil (a diarylaminopropylamine).

Verapamil Verapamil, which is structurally similar to papaverine, has a complex mode of action. It is a racemic mixture, with L-verapamil being a more potent calcium channel blocker than D-verapamil.[139] The net effect is depression of both slow channel activation and recovery from inactivation. Via its effects on the calcium channels, verapamil decreases myocardial contractility and dilates coronary and peripheral vascular beds, increasing coronary blood flow and decreasing systemic vascular resistance. Reflex tachycardia, secondary to decreased systemic vascular resistance, does not occur as a result of its negative chronotropic effect. Like other calcium channel blockers, verapamil has little effect on venous capacitance vessels in clinical doses. By decreasing heart rate, contractility, and peripheral resistance, verapamil decreases myocardial O_2 consumption. By increasing diastolic filling time and coronary blood flow while decreasing coronary vascular resistance, it increases myocardial O_2 delivery. In patients with CHF, intravenous verapamil can cause a *marked decrease* in contractility and left ventricular function. By directly antagonizing coronary vascular spasm, verapamil is useful in treatment of classic and Prinzmetal angina. Verapamil is useful in managing patients after myocardial infarction without CHF, and its use may decrease long-term mortality.[140]

The electrophysiologic effects of verapamil are substantial. It slows spontaneous rates of firing and increases SA node recovery time, thereby decreasing heart rate. The velocity of AV node conduction decreases as a consequence of both decreased conduction and increased refractoriness. Because of this effect on the AV node conduction, verapamil can terminate paroxysmal supraventricular tachycardia and slow the ventricular response in atrial flutter, fibrillation, and multifocal atrial tachycardia. It can successfully convert paroxysmal supraventricular tachycardias (PSVTs) to sinus rhythm with an effectiveness of greater than 90%. It is also of prophylactic value in preventing recurrences of PSVT and controlling the ventricular response in atrial flutter and fibrillation during long-term oral therapy.[141] It should be noted that in patients with Wolff-Parkinson-White syndrome, verapamil might increase heart rate by preferential AV slowing, which may increase conduction through accessory pathways in patients who develop atrial fibrillation.

The net effect of verapamil in lowering both systolic and diastolic blood pressure with few side effects makes it efficacious for treatment of hypertension, although calcium channel blockers are currently not recommended as first-line therapy for hypertension. Possibly as a result of its improvement in diastolic function, verapamil improves exercise tolerance and decreases the severity of symptoms in patients with hypertrophic obstructive cardiomyopathy (HOCM). It is mainly used in HOCM patients who cannot tolerate β-blockers.[114]

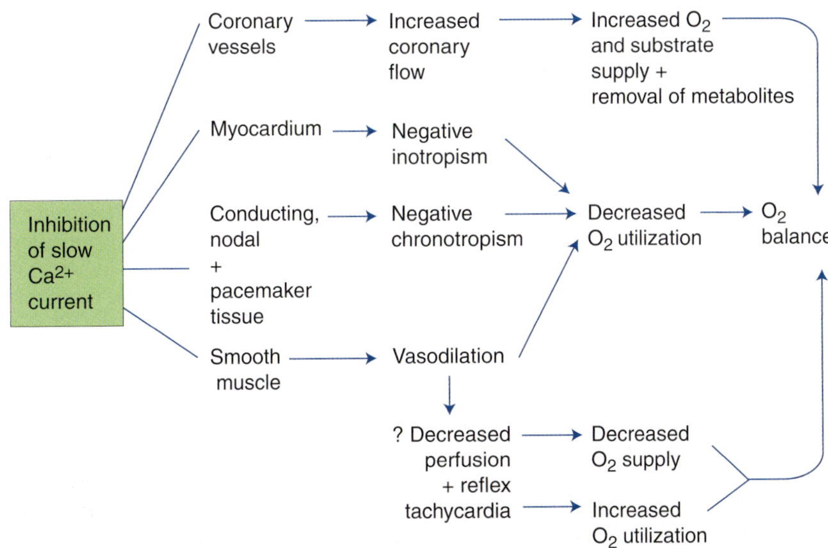

FIGURE 44-4. Consequences of calcium channel blockers on myocardial O_2 balance. Because of reflex responses, negative chronotropism and inotropism may not be important. [Reproduced with permission from Nayler WG, Dillon JS, Daly MF. Cellular sites of action of calcium antagonists and β-adrenoceptor blockers. In: Opie LH, ed. *Perspectives in Cardiovascular Research. Vol 9. Calcium Antagonists and Cardiovascular Disease*. New York, NY: Raven Press; 1984:188.]

In acute IV therapy, the recommended dose of verapamil is 0.075 to 0.15 mg/kg titrated to effect. Peak vasodilatory effect occurs at approximately 5 minutes and may persist for 30 minutes, although the antidysrhythmic effect may persist substantially longer. IV distribution half-life is 3.5 minutes and elimination half-life 110 minutes. Anesthetics or other drugs that decrease liver blood flow will increase the half-life of verapamil.

The side effects of verapamil are related to its pharmacologic and therapeutic actions. Verapamil may exacerbate SA and AV node dysfunction, especially in patients with underlying disease or those treated with digitalis or β-blockers. Verapamil may worsen symptoms of CHF, especially if used in combination with β-blockers.[147] Digitalis levels increase by an average of 70% after initiation of therapy with verapamil.

Diltiazem Diltiazem, a benzothiazepine, is a calcium channel blocker with a spectrum of pharmacologic effects between verapamil and the dihydropyridines. Diltiazem, like all calcium channel blockers, is an effective coronary artery dilator, but has less effect on peripheral vessels than the dihydropyridines. It is a mild negative inotrope, but less so than verapamil.[142] Reflex tachycardia is also blunted because diltiazem decreases sinus node automaticity and AV nodal conduction, albeit to a lesser extant than verapamil. Although diltiazem can be used in combination with β-blockers, the effects may be additive, causing SA and AV node dysfunction in patients with underlying conduction disease.

Diltiazem is approved for rapid conversion of paroxysmal supraventricular tachycardia to sinus rhythm and for temporary control of rapid ventricular rate in atrial flutter or fibrillation. The usual dose of IV diltiazem is 0.25 mg/kg as a slow loading dose, followed by an infusion of 0.15 mg/kg. An additional bolus of 0.35 mg/kg may be given if needed. Oral diltiazem can be used for the chronic management of these problems.

THE DIHYDROPYRIDINES

Nifedipine In vitro, nifedipine has significant effects on both smooth muscle and myocardium. In vivo, however, it is an effective coronary and systemic arterial dilator at doses that have little effect on myocardial contractility or conduction tissue. The vasodilatation and increase in coronary artery blood flow result from the blockade of calcium influx, as well as an increase in the levels of nitric oxide and bradykinin.[143] Because of its afterload reduction, nifedipine may cause reflex sympathetic increases in heart rate and cardiac output.[144] This sympathetic stimulation is more evident with short-acting preparations than it is with sustained-release nifedipine.[145]

Clinically, with the exception of short-acting formulations, which may occasionally worsen angina, nifedipine effectively improves exercise tolerance, prolongs the time to the onset of angina in exercise, and decreases the frequency of episodes of angina.[147] Concurrent therapy with nifedipine and a β-blocker is more effective than either agent given alone. Indeed, β-blockers eliminate nifedipine's potentially detrimental reflex increases in heart rate.[146] Although it is an effective antihypertensive, nifedipine—and generally all calcium channel blockers—is not currently recommended as first-line therapy, unless there are contraindications to other antihypertensives.[6] Even though nifedipine has fewer negative chronotropic or inotropic effects than verapamil or diltiazem, in long-term studies, hemodynamic deterioration occurred in some patients with CHF who were treated with dihydropyridines.[147]

Because it is light sensitive, IV nifedipine is not commercially available in the United States. Nifedipine's side effects include headaches, pedal edema, hypotension, and exacerbation of angina. Like verapamil, nifedipine increases serum digitalis levels. Because a higher rate of cardiac events was reported among patients who were treated with short-acting nifedipine after myocardial infarction, this preparation is no longer recommended in patients with angina.[148]

Nicardipine Nicardipine has structural and pharmacologic properties similar to those of nifedipine. Like nifedipine, nicardipine is a potent coronary and systemic vasodilator with little effect on contractility. It is available as an IV agent for treatment of hypertension in acute care settings, including the perioperative period and neurologic emergencies.[149-151] An initial intravenous bolus of 2 mg is followed by an initial infusion rate of 5 mg/h, which may be increased in 2.5-mg increments every 15 minutes, up to a maximum infusion rate of 15 mg/h. Nicardipine administered intra-arterially reverses vasospasm in subarachnoid hemorrhage and interventional coronary procedures.[152,153]

Nimodipine Nimodipine, a nifedipine analogue, is a calcium channel blocker with high lipid solubility and apparent preference for cerebrovascular smooth muscle. It is useful in inhibiting cerebral vasospasm and improving outcome in patients with neurologic defects associated with cerebral vasospasm after subarachnoid hemorrhage.[154] Its usefulness in patients with acute ischemic stroke has not been proven.[155]

Amlodipine, Isradipine, Felodipine, Nisoldipine, and Nitrendipine Amlodipine, isradipine, felodipine, nisoldipine, and nitrendipine are structurally and pharmacologically similar to nifedipine, the dihydropyridine prototype. They dilate coronary and peripheral arteries with minimal effect on cardiac conduction and contractility. Like nifedipine, these drugs are used to treat hypertension and angina and may be safely used in patients with CHF.[156]

The individual agents are distinct from each other in many ways. Because isradipine has an inhibitory effect on the SA node but not on the cardiac myocytes, it produces little or no reflex tachycardia. Felodipine and nisoldipine have a higher degree of vascular specificity than the rest of the dihydropyridines. Several trials have shown that amlodipine increases exercise duration, decreases the number of anginal attacks, and reduces the consumption of nitroglycerin.[157] The Systolic Hypertension in Europe (Syst-Eur) Trial reported that antihypertensive therapy initiated with the nitrendipine reduced the risk of fatal and nonfatal stroke, as well as all cardiovascular events combined, in older patients (age >65 years) with isolated systolic hypertension.[158]

Clevidipine Clevidipine is a new, lipophilic, short-acting, third-generation dihydropyridine calcium channel blocker. It is an intravenous agent designed for immediate control of blood pressure in a monitored setting. Clevidipine should be initiated with a dose of 1 to 2 mg/h and then titrated to the desired effect. It is a selective arterial dilator without effects on the venous circulation and minimal effects on cardiac contractility or conduction. It has a half-life of approximately 2 minutes, resulting in a rapid onset and offset of its effects. It is metabolized by blood and tissue esterases and is therefore not end-organ dependent for its elimination. Headache, nausea, and vomiting are the most frequent side effects. Patients should be monitored for rebound hypertension once the drug is discontinued.[159-161]

Mibefradil Mibefradil is an antagonist of T-type calcium channels. This arterial dilator has negative chronotropic effects but minimal inotropic effects. Mibefradil is an effective antianginal whose vasodilatory effects are associated with a reduction in heart rate.[162,163] There are case reports of QT interval prolongation and ventricular dysrhythmias during treatment with mibefradil.[164]

Monatepil Monatepil is a calcium channel blocker similar to nifedipine, which also has α_1-adrenoreceptor–blocking properties. It decreases systolic and diastolic pressure without changes in heart rate. Furthermore, it significantly decreases levels of low-density lipoprotein (LDL) cholesterol, apolipoprotein B, and glycosylated hemoglobin ($HgbA_{1c}$).[165]

Bepridil Bepridil is structurally unrelated to other calcium channel blockers. It blocks slow calcium channels in both cardiac and vascular smooth muscles as well as fast sodium channels in cardiac muscle. It has negative chronotropic and dromotropic and mild negative inotropic effects.[166] Bepridil reduces blood pressure and heart rate, improves left ventricular performance in patients with angina, and decreases the frequency of exercise-induced angina attacks. Bepridil can prolong QT interval, especially in the setting of hypokalemia or bradycardia, and can precipitate polymorphic ventricular tachycardia. Bepridil is also associated with agranulocytosis and pancytopenia. Because of these serious side effects, it should be used only in cases of angina refractory to other therapies.

Anesthetic Considerations There are limited data regarding the risks and benefits of calcium channel blockers in the perioperative setting. Although a classic withdrawal syndrome has not been described, there are case reports of severe coronary vasospasm after abrupt discontinuation of the calcium channel blockers.[167] Overall, the continuation of calcium channel blockers in patients already taking them preoperatively is recommended, despite the paucity of information in relation to their interaction with the process of anesthesia and surgery.

There is considerable potential for drug interaction between anesthetic drugs and calcium channel blockers. When used in combination with high-dose narcotics in patients with normal conduction systems and ventricular function, IV verapamil decreases systemic vascular resistance and mean arterial pressure with no change in cardiac output or pulmonary capillary wedge pressure. Although lengthening of the PR interval has been observed, neither first-degree nor more advanced AV block has occurred.

In combination with inhalation agents, verapamil may produce varying degrees of AV block and must be given carefully in patients anesthetized with enflurane, halothane, and, to a lesser degree, isoflurane in patients with AV nodal block or in patients chronically taking β-blockers.[168]

Verapamil has many perioperative uses. It has been used for intraoperative control of paroxysmal supraventricular tachycardia. During cardiopulmonary bypass, verapamil terminates refractory ventricular fibrillation after aortic cross-clamp removal. Verapamil successfully treats intraoperative myocardial ischemia refractory to IV nitroglycerin.[169]

In vitro, diltiazem may depress left ventricular function in the presence of enflurane or desflurane, whereas the incidence of bradyarrhythmias is higher with enflurane than with equivalent levels of desflurane.[170] Combined with enflurane, diltiazem is particularly depressant to conduction. Together, they may cause first-degree AV block, Mobitz I AV block, or sinus node dysfunction.[171]

Nifedipine administered in dogs during fentanyl/nitrous oxide anesthesia decreased systemic vascular resistance accompanied by an increase in cardiac index and heart rate. In vitro, the combined treatment of nifedipine and volatile anesthetics, especially enflurane, additively depresses atrial rate and contractility. However, these effects appear less pronounced than the combination of volatile agents with diltiazem and especially verapamil.[172]

Nicardipine has a longer duration of action in the presence of isoflurane and produces greater initial hypotension with sevoflurane.[173]

Calcium channel blockers may potentiate effects of depolarizing and nondepolarizing neuromuscular blocking agents, although this is controversial. In contrast with β-adrenergic blocking agents, calcium channel blockers have not been shown to be effective in prevention of intraoperative ischemia.[174]

OTHER ANTIANGINALS

Novel therapeutic strategies have been developed for patients with ischemic heart disease and angina pectoris that were unsuccessfully managed with conventional medical or interventional approaches.

Ivabradine Ivabradine is the first of a new class of drugs called I_f inhibitors. It selectively and specifically inhibits I_f, a sinus node–specific sodium-potassium inward current. It reduces heart rate at rest or exercise without decreasing myocardial contractility, atrioventricular conduction, and ventricular repolarization duration.[175] A double-blind trial comparing the anti-ischemic and antianginal effects of ivabradine to atenolol showed that ivabradine is as effective as atenolol in preventing exercise-induced angina in patients with chronic stable angina.[176] Ivabradine preserves ejection fraction better than metoprolol when given to patients who were revascularised after STEMIs.[177] Ivabradine has been approved in Europe for the symptomatic treatment of chronic stable angina pectoris in patients with normal sinus rhythm who have a contraindication or intolerance to β-blockers. Ivabradine interacts with retinal currents, causing visual side effect. These include reversible, transient symptoms described mainly as increases in brightness in limited areas of the visual field. Extreme sinus bradycardia is very uncommon.[178] No other adverse effects are attributed to ivabradine therapy.

Nicorandil Nicorandil is a nicotinamide ester, which activates the adenosine triphosphate (ATP)–sensitive potassium channel. It dilates peripheral and coronary resistance arterioles, and because of a nitrate-like effect, it dilates systemic veins and epicardial coronary vessels. Consequently, nicorandil increases coronary blood flow, reduces preload and afterload, and has antianginal efficacy similar to that of oral nitrates, β-blockers, and calcium antagonists.[179] By opening ATP-dependent potassium channels, nicorandil may also mimic a natural process of ischemic preconditioning, protecting the heart from subsequent ischemic attacks. The IONA (Impact of Nicorandil in Angina) trial showed a significant improvement in outcome as a result of reduction in major coronary events by adding nicorandil to standard antianginal therapy in patients with stable angina.[179] Nicorandil is not available in the United States.

Inhibitors of Fatty Acid Oxidation Two agents, ranolazine and trimetazidine, are presently available and represent this new class of drug. During episodes of acute myocardial ischemia, fatty acid levels rise, promoting their uptake and use as energy source by the myocardium. Because fatty acid oxidation is more oxygen inefficient than carbohydrate oxidation, this abrupt increase in circulating free fatty acids imposes a further deleterious effect on an already imbalanced oxygen supply–demand situation. Inhibition of fatty acid oxidation may increase glucose oxidation, which generates more ATP for each molecule of oxygen than fatty acid oxidation, thereby minimizing lactate accumulation.[180] Both drugs are virtually devoid of hemodynamic effects.

The efficacy of ranolazine has been studied in several clinical studies, such as the MARISA (Monotherapy Assessment of Ranolazine in Stable Angina) and CARISA (Combination Assessment of Ranolazine in Stable Angina) trials. Both MARISA and CARISA showed that ranolazine increases exercise capacity and provides antianginal effects on symptomatic patients with chronic angina.[181]

Similar benefits were shown in the TRIMPOL (Trimetazidine in Poland) II trial, which studied trimetazidine in patients already receiving metoprolol. The addition of trimetazidine produced significant improvement in exercise stress tests and anginal symptoms relative to metoprolol monotherapy.[182]

Ranolazine but not trimetazidine is available in the United States.

ANTIDYSRHYTHMIC AGENTS

Antidysrhythmic agents are indicated for prevention and treatment of symptomatic dysrhythmias and for therapy of asymptomatic dysrhythmias with malignant potential. Reasons for selecting one drug over another are frequently complex; the choice may depend on type of dysrhythmia, a particular drug's therapeutic index, a medication's effectiveness during electrophysiologic studies, or a patient's tolerance to side effects.

Antidysrhythmic drugs are classified on the basis of their major pharmacologic effects on myocardial electrophysiology, as originally proposed by Vaughan Williams[183] and now modified to include newer agents (**Box 44-2**). Although now loosely used to group drugs, this classification was originally proposed to rigorously classify patterns of pharmacologic action. This is a subtle but important difference. Many antidysrhythmics, although classified into one group or another, have (1) multiple actions in a given tissue, (2) different actions in different heart tissues, and (3) active metabolites with different actions than the parent compound.

BOX 44-2

Vaughan-Williams Classification of Antiarrhythmic Agents

IA	IB	IC
Quinidine	Lidocaine	Flecainide
Procainamide	Mexiletine	Encainide
Disopyramide	Tocainide	Propafenone
Moricizine	Phenytoin	

Class II

All β-blockers except Sotalol

Class III

- Bretylium
- Amiodarone
- Acecainide (*N*-acetylprocainamide)
- Dofetilide
- Ibutilide
- Azimilide
- Sotalol

Class IV calcium channel blockers

- Verapamil
- Diltiazem
- Bepridil

Other agents not formally classified

- Digoxin
- Adenosine

Since the early 1990s, the use of most antidysrhythmic drugs has been reassessed and dramatically limited because of increased awareness of their proarrhythmic potential and advances in ablation techniques. Moreover, clinical trials have frequently demonstrated adverse effects on survival in many situations in which these drugs might have been given in the past. Finally, implantable cardiodefibrillators have largely replaced antidysrhythmic medications in the management of ventricular dysrhythmias.[184]

Agents with class I actions include drugs that affect the fast inward sodium current of phase O, the period of rapid depolarization of the action potential (**Fig. 44-5**). They have been further divided into 3 groups: IA, IB, and IC.

Class II actions refer to antidysrhythmic effects associated with β-adrenergic antagonism. Therefore, class II agents include all β-adrenergic blocking agents except sotalol.

Class III agents block potassium repolarization currents and increase action potential duration (APD) and effective refractory period (ERP) in atrial and ventricular muscle, as well as in Purkinje fibers. The ERP-to-APD ratio is increased.

Class IV agents are represented by blockers of the L-type calcium channel, that is, calcium channel blockers. Among them only verapamil and diltiazem are effective for antidysrhythmic use.

Some newer drugs, such as adenosine and ibutilide, do not fit neatly into any of these categories (although ibutilide is categorized by most as a class III drug).

CLASS IA AGENTS

Antidysrhythmics with class IA action include quinidine, procainamide, and disopyramide (**Table 44-11**). They all decrease the maximal velocity (V_{max}) and amplitude of phase 0 depolarization of the action potential. The ERP, APD, and ERP-to-APD ratio are increased. Automaticity, represented by the decreased slope of phase 4 of the action potential, is decreased with these drugs. These agents produce measurable increases in refractoriness of cardiac tissue and lengthening of the QTc interval on the ECG.

Quinidine Quinidine decreases automaticity in atrial and ventricular tissue and in the His-Purkinje and pacemaker fibers. Quinidine's direct effects on SA node automaticity are balanced by its anticholinergic effects, which speed conduction through the SA and AV nodes, causing little change in heart rate. ECG changes occur with quinidine; most noticeably, it prolongs the QT interval by up to 25% at therapeutic levels.

Quinidine also blocks the rapid component of the K channel, prolonging action potentials in most cardiac cells, especially at slow heart rates.[185] It has been used effectively for conversion of atrial fibrillation, atrial flutter,[186] and PSVT and for maintenance of sinus rhythm after conversion.[187] In addition, it suppresses ventricular ectopy, tachycardia, and fibrillation.

Quinidine is available orally as a sulfate, gluconate, or polygalacturonate salt with 83%, 62%, and 60% quinidine content, respectively. Quinidine sulfate is typically initiated at 200 mg every 6 hours and increased to 800 to 2400 mg/d, titrated to drug levels and therapeutic

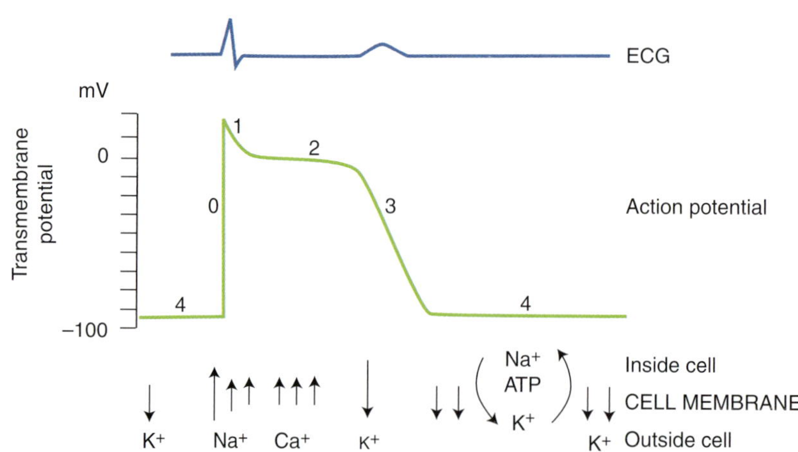

FIGURE 44-5. Schematic of the action potential in a ventricular myocardial cell as it correlates with the electrocardiogram (ECG). Arrows indicate times of major ionic movement across the cell membrane.

TABLE 44-11 Class Ia Antidysrhythmic Agents

Drug	Usual Dosage and Interval	Effect on Electrocardiogram	Adverse Effects	Concentrations	Metabolism	Indications	Half-Life (h)
Quinidine	PO: 200-400 mg q4-6h	Prolongs QRS, QT, and PR (+)	Diarrhea and other GI symptoms; cinchonism; hepatic granulomas and necrosis; thrombocytopenia; rashes; hypotension; heart blocks; tachyarrhythmias; torsade de pointes; fever; lupus-like syndrome	2-7 μg/mL	Hepatic (60%-80%); renal (20%-40%)	Ventricular and supraventricular arrhythmias, including PAT, AF atrial flutter, WPW, junctional tachycardias	4-10; increased in elderly
Procainamide	PO: 50 mg/kg/d in divided doses q3-4h or q6h (long-acting); IV loading no more than 100 mg q5min to 1 g (12 mg kg); IV maintenance 2-4 mg/min	Prolongs QRS, QT, and PR (+)	Lupus-like syndrome; confusion; disorientation; GI symptoms; rash; blood dyscrasias; fever hypotension; arrhythmias; torsade de pointes	4-10 mg/mL NAPA 10-20 μg/mL	Hepatic, excreted in urine by filtration and active secretion	As above	2-5; increased in renal failure
Disopyramide	PO: 100-200 mg q6h	Prolongs QRS, QT, and PR (+)	Anticholinergic effects; hypotension; heart failure; tachyarrhythmias; torsade de pointes; heart block; nausea; vomiting; diarrhea; hepatic toxicity; acute psychosis; agranulocytosis; constipation; hypoglycemia	2-8 μg/mL	Hepatic; 50 excreted unchanged in urine	As above	4-10; 8-18 with renal dysfunction
Moricizine	200-300 mg TID	Prolongs QRS interval	May be prodysrhythmic; Congestive heart failure; intraventricular conduction delays	0.2-1.5 μg/mL	Hepatic; biliary and urinary excretion	Ventricular dysrhythmias	9.2

AF, atrial fibrillation; GI, gastrointestinal; IV, intravenously; NAPA, *N*-acetylprocainamide; PAT, paroxysmal atrial tachycardia; PO, orally; q, every; TID, 3 times a day; WPW, Wolff-Parkinson-White syndrome.

Data from Abramowicz M. Drugs for cardiac arrhythmias. *Med Lett Drugs Ther.* 1991;33:60.

effect. It undergoes hepatic metabolism (60%-80%) and renal excretion (20%-40%), with a variable half-life of 4 to 10 hours. The metabolites of quinidine also possess antidysrhythmic activity. Although it is available in an IV form, this route is usually avoided because of profound hypotensive and negative inotropic effects.

As with all antidysrhythmics, quinidine may be prodysrhythmic. Patients with CHF are at greater risk. With congenital prolongation of the QT interval or bradycardia associated with hypokalemia, quinidine, by further lengthening the QT interval, may initiate torsade de pointes, a serious, potentially lethal dysrhythmia.[188] If torsade de pointes occurs, therapy should include increasing heart rate with isoproterenol or pacing, correction of hypokalemia and hypomagnesemia, and discontinuation of quinidine.

Because of its anticholinergic effects on the AV node, quinidine may increase ventricular response in atrial fibrillation and flutter. Consequently, if it is used for conversion of atrial dysrhythmias, digoxin, diltiazem, verapamil, or a β-blocker should be administered concurrently. If quinidine therapy is initiated in a patient receiving digitalis, one must be aware that quinidine may double the digitalis plasma concentration, possibly leading to digitalis toxicity. Digitalis dosages should therefore be decreased by half. Evidence of quinidine-induced cardiac toxicity may be manifested by greater than 50% increase in QT interval, widening of QRS complexes, and SA or AV node disturbances. Noncardiac adverse effects typically occur with quinidine. In 30% to 40% of patients, therapy must be withdrawn because of gastrointestinal (GI) intolerance. Quinidine may cause CNS toxicity, as manifested by tinnitus and delirium. Other adverse effects include fever, rash, anaphylaxis, thrombocytopenia, hemolytic anemia, and agranulocytosis.

In surgical patients, quinidine should be continued preoperatively and resumed as soon as possible after surgery. If oral intake is impossible, IV procainamide or lidocaine may be substituted, depending on the original reason for initiating quinidine therapy. Quinidine increases the neuromuscular blockade of succinylcholine and may worsen neuromuscular blockade in myasthenia gravis. Quinidine has fallen into disfavor because it worsens survival in patients with ventricular dysrhythmias.[189] Even in the presence of atrial dysrhythmias, where quinidine may be highly successful in maintaining sinus rhythm, it still has a negative effect on survival.[190]

Procainamide Procainamide, an analogue of the local anesthetic procaine, has a pharmacologic effect and a set of clinical indications similar, but not identical, to those of quinidine. Although both are class IA agents, each may be effective in suppression of dysrhythmias that are unresponsive to the other drug. This is not surprising, because procainamide's major metabolite, *N*-acetylprocainamide (NAPA), actually has class III actions.[191] In addition, because procainamide is readily available in stable IV form, it was used extensively in the past for acute management of atrial fibrillation and flutter, PSVT, and dysrhythmias associated with Wolff-Parkinson-White syndrome, as well as for acute suppression of ventricular dysrhythmias after acute MI and in treatment of ventricular tachycardia. When given intravenously, it may produce vasodilatation by a mild ganglionic blocking action; consequently, loading doses should be given slowly over approximately 20 to 30 minutes while monitoring the QRS duration. A loading dose up to 1 g may be given, followed by an infusion at 1 to 4 mg/min. Procainamide undergoes acetylation to NAPA, with half the population being fast acetylators. Subsequently, both substances are renally excreted. Therefore, dosage should be adjusted in patients with renal dysfunction. Procainamide and NAPA levels may prove useful to facilitate dosage adjustment.

Procainamide has fewer anticholinergic properties than quinidine and disopyramide. As with quinidine, procainamide may be prodysrhythmic and may cause torsade de pointes.[195] Consequently, it should not be used in patients with prolonged QT interval, hypokalemia, or history of torsade de pointes. Chronic administration is associated with positive antinuclear antibody titers; however, only 15% to 20% of patients develop a lupus-like syndrome. It usually resolves with discontinuation of the drug. Preoperatively, procainamide should be continued until surgery. In the perioperative period, procainamide may be given as an IV infusion and used as a substitute for quinidine or disopyramide in treatment of atrial and ventricular dysrhythmias. Like quinidine, procainamide increases long-term mortality and is now seldom used on a chronic basis.[196]

Disopyramide Disopyramide is used to maintain sinus rhythm in patients with atrial flutter or atrial fibrillation and to prevent recurrence of ventricular tachycardia or ventricular fibrillation. Unlike quinidine and procainamide, it has significant negative inotropic effects. Even more than quinidine, it has substantial anticholinergic effects. If it is tolerated, little additional chronic toxicity occurs.

The usual dosage of disopyramide is 100 to 400 mg, 3 to 4 times daily, up to 800 mg total. Its half-life elimination is 4 to 10 hours and is usually increased in patients with cardiac or renal disease. Fifty percent is excreted unchanged by the kidney and the remainder as an active metabolite.

As with all class IA agents, disopyramide should not be used in patients with congenital prolongation of the QT interval, hypokalemia, or history of torsade de pointes. It may cause severe bradycardia in patients with sinus node dysfunction or conduction system disease. Because of negative inotropic effects, disopyramide is contraindicated in patients with CHF. Disopyramide is still sometimes used in management of dysrhythmias in patients with HOCM, for which its negative inotropic effect is an advantage. In HOCM, it can decrease the subaortic gradient and ameliorate symptoms without increasing mortality.[191] Like other class IA agents, disopyramide has largely been abandoned as a treatment of chronic dysrhythmias. Because of its anticholinergic effects, it is contraindicated in patients with glaucoma and obstructive uropathy. In addition, disopyramide may cause dry mouth, constipation, urinary retention, and esophageal reflux.

Moricizine Moricizine, a phenothiazine derivative, has characteristics of class IA, class IB, and class IC agents. Moricizine decreases V_{max} to an extent similar to class IA agents. As with IB agents, it shortens APD and increases the ERP-to-APD ratio. On the ECG, moricizine prolongs the QRS complex with little effect on the QT interval, a characteristic of class IC agents.

In clinical studies, moricizine has been effectively used for treatment of chronic complex ventricular dysrhythmias and prevention of ventricular tachycardia and fibrillation. However, in the Cardiac Arrhythmia Suppression Trial (CAST) II trial, moricizine was shown to increase mortality in patients shortly after a myocardial infarction and did not improve survival during long-term therapy.[193] Moricizine use has therefore been largely abandoned.

Moricizine is well absorbed orally and undergoes hepatic metabolism and biliary and urinary excretion. In healthy volunteers, the half-life was 1.5 to 3.5 hours; however, cardiac disease may increase this to as long as 13 hours.

Recommended dosages are 600 to 900 mg 3 times daily. Adverse reactions include dizziness, nausea, and headaches. Intraventricular conduction delays may occur in up to 9% of patients. Moricizine may be prodysrhythmic or worsen CHF in 2% to 5% of patients.[186] Few data are available regarding interactions with anesthetic agents.

CLASS IB AGENTS

Drugs with class IB actions, such as lidocaine, mexiletine, tocainide, and phenytoin, have more moderate effects on phase O of the action potential (**Table 44-12**). Unlike class IA agents, they shorten APD and ERP and increase the ERP-to-APD ratio in the Purkinje fibers, but have little effect on the refractory periods in sinus node, atrium, and AV node, thus being ineffective against supraventricular tachycardias. They show little ECG effect. They exhibit rapid association and dissociation from the sodium channels.[186]

Lidocaine Although lidocaine, the prototypical class IB agent, was first introduced as a local anesthetic, it was widely used in acute treatment and suppression of all ventricular dysrhythmias, except those associated with prolonged QT intervals and torsade de pointes. As with all class I agents, lidocaine decreases V_{max} to some extent.

In addition to its typical type IB effects, lidocaine decreases the slope of phase 4 of the action potential, reducing automaticity. Like other IB agents, lidocaine has little effect on atrial tissue and thus is ineffective against supraventricular tachycardias.

Because lidocaine undergoes rapid first-pass elimination, it is unavailable as an oral agent. IV lidocaine is usually given as a 1-mg/kg bolus, followed by repeat small boluses of an additional 2 mg/kg over 15 minutes and an infusion of 1 to 4 mg/min. An infusion is necessary because of lidocaine's rapid distribution out of the central compartment with termination of the antidysrhythmic activity. Because elimination is significantly longer than central compartment redistribution, a steady-state lidocaine infusion can be discontinued without "tapering." The blood levels will gradually decrease over 8 to 10 hours.

Modifications of infusion rates are required in the elderly and in patients with liver disease or CHF with decreased liver blood flow. Normal individuals show great variability in plasma levels. Thus the patient's ECG, blood pressure, and mental status should be carefully monitored so that infusions or boluses may be discontinued if toxicity develops. If dysrhythmias persist at usual doses and no toxic symptoms are present, lidocaine administration may be increased after a drug level has been obtained. If dysrhythmias persist with plasma lidocaine concentrations greater than 9 μg/mL, another agent should be used, even without symptoms of toxicity. Lidocaine provides little antidysrhythmic effect at levels less than 1.5 μg/mL, and toxicity often occurs at levels greater than 5 μg/mL.

Lidocaine has been used for the treatment of life-threatening ventricular arrhythmias, especially when associated with myocardial ischemia.

Although shown to be effective in prevention of ventricular fibrillation after acute myocardial infarction, meta-analyses of the effects of lidocaine on in-hospital mortality among patients with acute myocardial infarction suggest that despite a reduction in primary ventricular fibrillation, there is a small *increase* in the risk of death in the hospital among patients treated with lidocaine.[194] In light of this, its prophylactic use after myocardial infarction has fallen into disfavor. Lidocaine is inferior to amiodarone (see Amiodarone, later) in the management of pulseless ventricular tachycardia/fibrillation.[195] Potential adverse reactions to lidocaine include drowsiness, dizziness, confusion, delirium, dysarthria, dysesthesias (especially periorally), and even coma and seizures. Seizures may occur with nontoxic doses if they are given too quickly. Lidocaine may occasionally cause sinus and AV nodal dysfunction in patients with underlying conduction disease. In patients with atrial fibrillation, lidocaine may increase ventricular response rates. Multiple animal model studies have evaluated cardiac toxicity

TABLE 44-12 Class IB Antidysrhythmic Agents

Drug	Usual Dosage and Interval	Effect on Electrocardiogram	Adverse Effects	Usually Effective Plasma Concentrations	Indications	Half-Life (h)	Metabolism
Lidocaine (Xylocaine and others)	IV loading: 1 mg/kg given over 2 min, then 2 mg/kg over 20 min or 50 mg given over 1 min and repeated every 5 min × 3 or 20 mg/min infused over 10 min IV; maintenance for 24-30 h 30 μg/kg each min	No significant change	Drowsiness or agitation; slurred speech; tinnitus; disorientation; coma; seizures; paresthesia; cardiac depression, especially with excessive accumulation in heart failure or liver failure or infusions for >24 h	1.5-6 μg/mg	Ventricular dysrhythmias	1.5-2.0	Hepatic; <10% excreted in urine
Phenytoin (Dilantin and others)	PO loading: 14 mg/kg; PO maintenance: 200-400 mg/d; IV loading: 50 mg q5min to total dose of 1000 mg (up to 12 mg/kg); IV maintenance: 200-400 mg/d	No significant change	Ataxia, nystagmus; drowsiness; coma blood dyscrasias; cardiac toxicity with rapid IV injection; fever; rash; hepatic granulomas and necrosis	5-20 μg/mL	Dysrhythmias associated with Digitalis toxicity	22	Hydroxylated in liver, excreted in urine
Mexiletine (Mexitil)	PO initial dose: 100-200 mg q8h taken with food; PO maintenance: 100-300 mg q6-12h, maximum 1200 mg/d	No significant change	GI upset; fatigue; nervousness; dizziness; tremor; sleep upset; convulsions; infrequent aggravation of arrhythmias; visual disturbances psychosis; fever; hepatic toxicity; blood dyscrasias	0.5-2 μg/mL	Ventricular dysrhythmias	10-12	Hepatic
Tocainide (Tonocard)	PO initial dose: 200-400 mg q8h; PO maintenance: 200-600 mg q8h, maximum 2400 mg/d	No significant change	GI upset; paresthesia; dizziness; tremor; confusion; nightmares; psychotic reactions; coma; seizures; rash; fever; arthralgia; infrequent cytosis; aplastic anemia; thrombocytopenia; hepatic granulomas; interstitial pneumonitis	3-10 μg/mL	Ventricular dysrhythmias	15	Hepatic biotransformation 55%; excreted unchanged in urine 45%

GI, gastrointestinal; IV, intravenously; PO, orally; q, every.

Data from Abramowicz M. Drugs for cardiac arrhythmias. *Med Lett Drugs Ther.* 1991;33:60.

associated with lidocaine. Lidocaine clearly has cardiac toxicity, but this occurs at levels approximately 4 times higher than those associated with CNS toxicity. Characteristic ECG findings in these studies were sinus arrest, increased PR intervals and AV block, widening QRS complexes, ectopy, and tachydysrhythmias. In dogs, lidocaine, in combination with isoflurane and calcium channel blockers, caused hypotension and AV block, which was reversed with calcium chloride.[196]

Mexiletine and Tocainide Mexiletine is an orally active congener of lidocaine with similar indications and modes of action. Mexiletine is indicated in the treatment of life-threatening ventricular arrhythmias in combination with class IA and even class II and class III agents.[197] It may be safer for patients with prolonged QT syndrome than class IA or IC agents. It undergoes predominantly hepatic elimination, with a half-life of 10 to 12 hours and may be safely administered to patients with renal failure.[198]

Mexiletine has little hemodynamic effect and is well tolerated in patients with CHF. Adverse reactions, such as dizziness, tremor, visual blurring, and nausea, are usually dose related. Rash occurs less often with mexiletine than with tocainide, but thrombocytopenia and positive antinuclear antibody testing occur occasionally. Mexiletine may be prodysrhythmic in 10% of patients. It should be continued perioperatively and restarted as soon as possible postoperatively. If oral intake is not possible, a lidocaine infusion may be substituted. Like other class IA agents, mexiletine increases long-term mortality and is infrequently used.[199]

Tocainide is an orally active analogue of lidocaine indicated in the chronic treatment of complex ventricular dysrhythmias. Response to lidocaine is often, but not always, predictive of response to tocainide and mexiletine. Like lidocaine, tocainide is ineffective against supraventricular dysrhythmias. Tocainide and mexiletine are not necessarily interchangeable.

After oral administration, peak blood concentrations occur at 1 to 2 hours. Tocainide undergoes both hepatic metabolism and renal elimination, with a 15-hour half-life. Adverse reactions after oral administration occur in approximately 40% of patients. These include nausea, vomiting, tremor, paresthesia, and rash. Tocainide worsens symptoms of CHF in approximately 5% of patients and may be prodysrhythmic in 1% to 8% of patients. *Because tocainide can cause potentially fatal bone marrow aplasia and pulmonary fibrosis, it is no longer available in the United States.*

Phenytoin Although mainly used as an anticonvulsant, phenytoin has been used in patients with prolonged QT syndromes, atrial and ventricular dysrhythmias, and chronic ventricular dysrhythmias. Since the advent of Fab fragments, phenytoin is now rarely used to treat digoxin toxicity. In addition to its class IB effects, much of phenytoin's antidysrhythmic activity is a result of centrally mediated sympatholysis. It is well tolerated orally in doses of 300 mg/d, titrated to serum blood levels and side effects. A usual loading dose is 1000 mg given at a rate that does not exceed 50 mg/min, while the ECG and blood pressure are monitored to prevent hypotension and cardiovascular collapse.

Phenytoin undergoes hepatic metabolism with excretion in the bile, enterohepatic reabsorption, and subsequent urinary excretion. It has a 22-hour half-life. Common adverse effects include nystagmus, ataxia, slurred speech, confusion, and dizziness. Rarely, reactions that are more serious include severe dermatitis, Stevens-Johnson syndrome, and possibly hematologic malignancies. In patients with liver disease or any altered metabolic state, or when given with a wide range of other medications, phenytoin levels should be reassessed.

CLASS IC AGENTS

Available class IC agents, such as flecainide and propafenone, have the greatest effect on phase 0 of the action potential with minimal effect on repolarization (**Table 44-13**). As previously mentioned, moricizine shares many of these properties as well. These drugs suppress automaticity of the SA node, slow AV node, His-Purkinje, and ventricular conduction. On the ECG, PR and QRS intervals are lengthened, but QTc intervals are largely unchanged. Data from the CASTs that suggest increased mortality with class IC agents after MI have limited their use.[200] Type IC agents all profoundly suppress cardiac conduction, which may explain their proarrhythmic effects.

Flecainide Flecainide is indicated in suppression of both ventricular and supraventricular tachycardias, including Wolff-Parkinson-White syndrome. Usual doses are 200 to 400 mg daily given in divided doses. Although it undergoes hepatic metabolism, approximately 30% of flecainide is renally excreted, with a usual half-life of 12 to 27 hours.[201]

As with all antidysrhythmics, flecainide has prodysrhythmic effects. Data from the CASTs have limited its use to pharmacologic cardioversion and maintenance of sinus rhythm in symptomatic atrial fibrillation in patients without heart disease and in patients with hypertension but no left ventricular hypertrophy.[200] Flecainide has a negative inotropic effect, can aggravate CHF in approximately 15% of patients, and can cause sinus arrest, AV block, and intraventricular conduction disturbances.[202] Because flecainide can increase pacemaker thresholds up to 200%, it should be used with caution in patients with conduction disease. Other adverse effects include dizziness, blurred vision, GI upset, and neutropenia. Flecainide dosages may need to be reduced when given with cimetidine or amiodarone. Conversely, digoxin and propranolol doses must be reduced when flecainide is introduced. Finally, β-adrenergic blocking agents and flecainide may have additive negative effects on myocardial contractility. Few data are available about interaction with anesthetics.

Encainide Encainide is no longer readily available in the United States because the CASTs showed increased incidence of fatal arrhythmias with encainide.[200] It remains available for compassionate use for those who were taking encainide before its discontinuation. Encainide's mode of action and indications are similar to those of flecainide. Its pharmacokinetics are complex. Ninety-three percent of the population (normal metabolizers) metabolizes encainide to active metabolites, yielding a 25% bioavailability and half-life between 1 and 12 hours for the various metabolites. In the remaining 7% of the population (slow metabolizers), encainide has a 90% bioavailability and a half-life as long as 20 hours.[203]

Propafenone Propafenone, an antidysrhythmic agent approved for management of ventricular dysrhythmias, is a sodium channel blocker with mode of action similar to the other approved class IC agents, flecainide and encainide.[204] Because data from the CAST Investigators[200] suggested increased mortality in patients taking encainide and flecainide, these drugs were relabeled. Currently, they are only approved in patients with life-threatening dysrhythmias. Because propafenone has a mode of action similar to these 2 agents, it is also generally used for the same indications.

TABLE 44-13 Class IC Antidysrhythmic Agents

Drug	Usual Dosage and Interval	Effect on Electrocardiogram	Adverse Effects	Usually Effective Plasma Concentration	Indications	Half-Life (h)	Metabolism
Flecainide (Tambocor)	PO initial dose: 100 mg q12h, increase q4-6d if required, by 50 mg q12h; PO maintenance: up to 400 mg/d	Prolongs PR and QRS	Bradycardia; heart block; new ventricular fibrillation; sustained ventricular tachycardia; heart failure; dizziness; blurred vision; nervousness; headache; GI upset; neutropenia	0.2-1 μg/mL	Ventricular dysrhythmias	12-27; unchanged renally	Hepatic; 10%-50% excreted
Encainide (Enkaid)	PO initial dose: 25 mg q8h, increase q4-6d if required to 35 mg q8h, and then to 50 mg q8h; maintenance: up to 200 mg/d	Prolongs PR and QRS	Bradycardia; heart block; new ventricular fibrillation; sustained ventricular tachycardia; heart failure; dizziness; headache visual disturbances; diarrhea; GI upset; glucose intolerance	Active metabolites preclude establishment	Ventricular dysrhythmias	12	Hepatic metabolism; renal excretion
Propafenone (Rythmol)	PO initial dose: 150 mg q8h, increase q3-4d if required; PO maintenance: 150-300 mg q8h	Prolongs PR and QRS	Bradycardia; heart block; new ventricular fibrillation; sustained ventricular tachycardia; heart failure; dizziness; light-headedness; metallic taste; dysgeusia; GI upset; bronchospasm	Active metabolites preclude establishment	Ventricular dysrhythmias	6-7	Hepatic metabolism; renal excretion

GI, gastrointestinal; PO, orally; q, every.

Data from Abramowicz M. Drugs for cardiac arrhythmias. *Med Lett Drugs Ther.* 1991;33:60.

Propafenone has shown evidence in vitro and in vivo of β-adrenergic blocking properties. Oral propafenone increases human lymphocyte B-cell adrenoreceptor density, a phenomenon observed with other β-blockers. In healthy patients and asthmatic persons, propafenone decreases heart rate during exercise, increases airway reactivity to methacholine, and decreases hemodynamic response to isoproterenol. As with other class IC agents, propafenone increases the QRS interval, even at normal heart rates. QT intervals are increased only to the extent that QRS intervals increase. The PR, AH, and HV intervals may also increase. Propafenone depresses sinus node automaticity and increases refractoriness in atrium, AV node, ventricle, and accessory pathways. It has a negative inotropic effect, which may reduce ejection fraction in normal subjects and produce symptoms of CHF in approximately 0.8% to 2.5% of patients. As with other class IC agents, propafenone may worsen conduction system disease.

After oral administration and absorption, propafenone undergoes a cytochrome P450 metabolism that varies genetically. In 93% of the population, the half-life is 6 to 7 hours; in the remaining 7% of the population, the elimination half-life is 12 to 32 hours. Usual starting doses are 150 mg every 8 hours, which may be increased up to 1200 mg/d. Propafenone increases plasma concentrations of digoxin, warfarin, and metoprolol; consequently, dosages of these drugs may need adjustment.

In clinical studies, propafenone has been effective in suppression of frequent ventricular ectopy, nonsustained ventricular tachycardia, and exercise-induced ventricular ectopy. Propafenone has proven useful in prevention of atrial fibrillation and suppression of AV node and accessory pathway supraventricular dysrhythmias. Even when propafenone is not able to suppress these dysrhythmias, it is effective at slowing the heart rate.

Other adverse effects include worsening of asthma and bronchoconstriction, dizziness, and CNS and GI disturbances. Rare cases of cholestatic jaundice have been reported.[204]

CLASS III AGENTS

Class III agents include amiodarone, bretylium, sotalol, ibutilide, dofetilide, and azimilide (**Table 44-14**). Their predominant effect is

TABLE 44-14 Class III Antidysrhythmic Agents

Drug	Usual Dosage and Interval	Effect on Electrocardiogram	Adverse Effects	Usually Effective Plasma Concentration	Indication	Half-Life	Metabolism
Amiodarone (Cordarone)	PO loading:800-1600 mg/d 1-3 wk then 600-800 mg/d for 4 wk; PO maintenance: 100-400 mg/d cardia IV 150 mg over 10 min then 1 mg/min × 6 then 0.5 mg/min; may be rebolused for breakthrough arrhythmias	Prolongs PR, QRS, and QT	Bradycardia; heart block; new ventricular fibrillation; sustained ventricular tachycardia; torsade de pointes; GI upset; alcoholic-like hepatitis; phospholipidosis; ataxia; tremor; dizziness; acute pulmonary toxicity; pulmonary fibrosis; photosensitivity; blue-gray skin; corneal microdeposits; hyper- or hypothyroidism; increased serum cholesterol	Not established	Ventricular and supraventricular dysrhythmias	26-107 d	Hepatic
Bretylium (Bretylol and others, Bretylate in Canada)	IV loading: 5 mg/kg with additional doses of 10 mg/kg to maximum of 30 mg/kg (effect must be delayed); IV maintenance: 5-10 mg/kg q6h or continuous infusion 1-2 mg/min	No change; sinus bradycardia	Orthostatic hypotension; nausea and vomiting; increased sensitivity to catecholamines; initial increase in dysrhythmias	Not established	Ventricular dysrhythmias	8 h; increased in renal failure	Renal
Sotalol	PO: 40-80 mg q12h increased to 320 q12h as necessary; IV: 0.2 mg/kg initially, increasing to 1.5 mg/kg over 5 min	Prolongs PR and QT interval	Bradycardia; heart block; torsade de pointes; congestive heart failure; bronchospasm; worsening arrhythmics	0.8-2.6 mg/mL	Ventricular dysrhythmias (used for supraventricular arrhythmias in Europe)	12 h	Renal
Ibutilide	IV: 1-2 mg	Prolongs QT interval	Torsade de pointes		Atrial fibrillation and atrial flutter	2-12 h	Hepatic/renal
Dofetilide	PO: 0.125-0.5 mg q12h IV: 4-8 μg/mL	Prolongs QT interval	Torsade de pointes		Conversion of atrial fibrillation and atrial flutter to sinus rhythm and prevention of recurrence	7-13 h	Hepatic/renal

GI, gastrointestinal; IV, intravenously; PO, orally; q, every.

Data from Abramowicz M. Drugs for cardiac arrhythmias. *Med Lett Drugs Ther.* 1991;33:60.

to prolong APD and increase ERP via action on potassium channels; ERP to APD ratio is also increased. However, each of these agents has additional effects on other channels and receptors, rendering this class of agents a very heterogenic one.

Amiodarone Some physicians consider amiodarone to be the most efficacious antidysrhythmic agent available; unfortunately, however, it is associated with a high incidence of side effects. It is a structural analogue of thyroid hormone and is highly lipophilic. Many of its side effects are caused by either its thyroxin-like structure or its large volume of distribution and affinity for many tissues.

The electrophysiologic effects of amiodarone are complex. Like all class III agents, amiodarone delays repolarization and increases duration of the action potential. Its primary mechanism involves blocking K channels, thereby prolonging repolarization. In doing so, the ERP is increased and the incidence of reentry rhythms decreased in all cardiac tissues.[205] In addition to blocking K channels, amiodarone is a vasodilator, acting on cardiac and vascular smooth muscle. Consequently, it dilates coronary arteries and causes decreased afterload and oxygen consumption. It also noncompetitively antagonizes α and β receptors, blocks conversion of thyroxin to triiodothyronine, and blocks inactivated Na and Ca channels. As such, amiodarone's effects on the ECG are complex; it slows the sinus rate, prolongs PR interval and AV node conduction, widens QRS complex, and prolongs QT interval.[206]

Amiodarone is effective in prevention of ventricular tachycardia and fibrillation, in treatment of supraventricular tachycardias with and without preexcitation syndromes, and in conversion and control of paroxysmal atrial fibrillation and flutter or other dysrhythmias associated with hypertrophic cardiomyopathies. It does decrease the incidence of postoperative atrial fibrillation after open-heart surgery.[207] Intravenous amiodarone may improve short-term survival in patients with ventricular fibrillation or hemodynamically unstable ventricular tachycardia that persists despite defibrillation or recurs promptly after successful defibrillation.[195,208] The Antiarrhythmics Versus Implantable Defibrillator (AVID) trial, which included patients with an ejection fraction less than 40% and who had suffered spontaneous hypotensive ventricular tachycardia or cardiac arrest, showed an improved survival in patients in the implantable cardioverter-defibrillator (ICD) group. Nevertheless, despite its toxicity, the use of amiodarone is appropriate for the management of recurrent ventricular fibrillation or unstable ventricular tachycardia in patients with ICDs. In the intraoperative and postoperative settings, IV amiodarone can be used to treat a variety of ventricular and supraventricular arrhythmias. It can be used to convert new-onset atrial fibrillation into sinus rhythm. In addition, its use is now advanced cardiac life support (ACLS) recommended for the treatment of pulseless ventricular tachycardia and ventricular fibrillation refractory to defibrillation, stable ventricular tachycardia, wide complex supraventricular tachycardia, and atrial fibrillation.[209]

Amiodarone is highly lipophilic, with a very large volume of distribution; consequently, it needs a long time to reach stable plasma concentrations and has a very long and variable elimination half-life—26 to 100 days. The North American Society of Pacing and Electrophysiology (NASPE) has published guidelines for the use of amiodarone. With oral therapy, the recommended loading dose for ventricular arrhythmias is 800 to 1600 mg/d (usually in divided doses) for up to 3 weeks, followed by a maintenance level of 400 to 600 mg/d during the first year. The maintenance level can be further decreased to 200 to 300 mg/d. With intravenous therapy, an initial loading dose of 150 mg is given over 10 minutes. The loading dose should be followed by a continuous infusion of 1 mg/min for 6 hours followed by 0.5 mg/min thereafter. Amiodarone should be mixed in a 5% dextrose solution and the amiodarone concentration kept below 2 mg/mL if given through a peripheral vein so as to minimize the development of local phlebitis.[210] In pulseless ventricular tachycardia and fibrillation, 300 mg is given as a bolus.

Amiodarone has little negative inotropic effect and is frequently used with caution in patients with CHF. It may cause symptomatic heart block, requiring permanent pacemaker insertion in approximately 4% of patients. Its incidence of prodysrhythmic effects is 1% to 2%; this is less than that associated with other antidysrhythmics.

Noncardiac effects of amiodarone are dose related and occur often. These include photosensitivity dermatitis (which sometimes results in an iridescent blue-gray discoloration), corneal micro deposition, hyper- and hypothyroidism, pulmonary infiltration and fibrosis, tremor, ataxia, neuropathies, myopathies, hepatitis, and gastrointestinal symptoms.[206] The very long half-life makes preoperative discontinuation impossible. In the past, serious adverse effects have been reported for patients anesthetized while receiving amiodarone. This likely represents the degree of underlying disease in this patient population rather than the drug itself. A poorly understood postoperative acute respiratory distress syndrome (ARDS) has been described in patients taking oral amiodarone who undergo cardiac or noncardiac surgery.[211] Whereas the hemodynamic consequences of chronic oral amiodarone therapy during noncardiac surgery are usually limited to hypotension, in the cardiac surgery AV nodal blockade, left ventricular dysfunction and extreme systemic vasodilatation have been reported. As a result, AV pacing, inotropes, and vasoconstrictors should be available and administered as necessary. In an isolated animal heart model, amiodarone in conjunction with potent inhalation agents caused an additive decrease in heart rate and inotropy, along with prolongation of AV conduction time.[211] Despite its hemodynamic and pulmonary side effects, amiodarone remains a valuable therapy for perioperative life-threatening ventricular arrhythmias refractory to conventional therapy.

Bretylium Bretylium has been approved for parenteral use in patients with life-threatening ventricular arrhythmias unresponsive to other therapies. Its use has been, by and large, usurped by amiodarone in newer ACLS protocols.

Bretylium has a direct class III action, with increased APD and ERP. In addition, after initially causing norepinephrine release from postganglionic adrenergic nerve terminals, it blocks further release of norepinephrine, producing a state resembling chemical sympathectomy.[206] When given intravenously to patients without cardiac arrest, bretylium is administered as a 5-mg/kg loading dose over 10 to 20 minutes, which may be repeated up to a total dose of 20 mg/kg if no response occurs. Subsequently, a maintenance infusion of 1 to 4 mg/min may be used. Because bretylium is eliminated unchanged in the urine, maintenance infusions must be decreased if creatinine clearance is reduced. In cardiac emergencies, bretylium is given as a rapid bolus in doses of 5 to 10 mg/kg.

After an initial increase in blood pressure, bretylium can cause significant hypotension, especially in volume-depleted patients. Orthostatic hypotension occurs in almost all patients and may persist for days after drug discontinuation. It has minimal effects on myocardial contractility. Rapid infusion can cause nausea and vomiting in awake patients.

The anesthetic implications for patients receiving bretylium are worth noting. By blocking catecholamine release, bretylium causes the equivalent of a denervated state. Direct-acting catecholamines may cause exaggerated responses, and indirect agents may be less effective. Bretylium may also be used to treat bupivacaine-induced ventricular arrhythmias.[213]

Sotalol Sotalol is another class III antiarrhythmic agent with mixed properties. It is a racemic mixture of *d*- and *l*-sotalol isomers. The *d*-isomer has class III antiarrhythmic properties, blocking K channels and prolonging repolarization, whereas the *l*-isomer prolongs repolarization and has noncardioselective β-blocking capabilities without any intrinsic sympathomimetic activity or membrane-stabilizing effects.[214] The β-blocking effects of sotalol occur at considerably lower doses than the class III effects.[215]

The electrophysiologic effects of sotalol include an increase in APD and prolongation of ERP. The prolongation of the APD is greater at slower heart rates (reverse use dependence). Automaticity is decreased and, in a manner similar to other β-blockers, sotalol decreases heart rate and slows conduction through the AV node. On ECG, the PR and QT intervals may increase.

The hemodynamic effects of sotalol are secondary to a combination of β-adrenergic antagonist–mediated negative inotropic effects and a propensity to increase contractility secondary to prolonged repolarization, which occurs maximally at slower heart rates.

Sotalol is approved by the US Food and Drug Administration (FDA) for treatment of life-threatening ventricular arrhythmias. It is also effective for treating supraventricular arrhythmias, as it slows sinus tachycardia, slows the ventricular response rate to atrial fibrillation, and converts atrial flutter and fibrillation to normal sinus rhythm. Sotalol appears to be as effective as β-blockers and amiodarone for the prevention of atrial fibrillation after cardiac surgery.[216]

Table 44-14 summarizes the usual dosage, effective plasma concentration, half-life metabolism, and side effects of sotalol. Notably, many of the adverse effects of sotalol are secondary to its β-blocking activity. These include fatigue, dizziness and dyspnea, aggravation of bronchospasm, hypotension, and bradycardias, much like other β-blockers. However, exacerbations of CHF occur less frequently with sotalol.[214]

Like all other class III antiarrhythmic drugs, sotalol has an arrhythmogenic potential; ventricular tachyarrhythmias occur in approximately 4% of patients, and torsade de pointes occur in approximately 2.5% of patients.[206] Predisposing factors include electrolyte disorders (hypokalemia, hypomagnesemia), diuretic therapy, female sex, bradycardia, and concurrent therapy with other drugs that prolong repolarization (eg, amiodarone, disopyramide, and flecainide).

Studies using an animal heart model show that halothane may sensitize the heart to pharmacologic K channel blockade.[217] Caution should probably be taken when using halothane in patients taking sotalol, although there are no studies to support this. No data exist on the interactions between sotalol and anesthetics.

Ibutilide Ibutilide has been approved for acute termination of atrial fibrillation or flutter of recent onset. Like other class III agents, it blocks outward potassium currents; however, unlike other class III drugs, ibutilide also blocks inward sodium currents through slow inward sodium channels. It thereby prolongs repolarization, the action potential duration, and the refractory period. It does not affect AV conduction or QRS duration on the ECG, but it does prolong the QT interval.[218]

The drug undergoes extensive first-pass metabolism and is renally excreted. It is not used orally. Intravenous dosage is usually 1 mg over 10 minutes and may be repeated a second time. Half-life varies between 2 and 12 hours.

In addition to the use for pharmacologic conversion or facilitation of electrical cardioversion of conventional atrial fibrillation, ibutilide may be used to convert atrial fibrillation that occurs after cardiac surgery.[219]

Ibutilide has no significant hemodynamic effects. Its major side effect is QT prolongation and torsade de pointes, which happens in approximately 2% of patients, especially those with left ventricular dysfunction. In light of this, its use is limited to patients with preserved left ventricular function and normal QT intervals.

Dofetilide Dofetilide is approved for acute conversion of atrial fibrillation and atrial flutter to sinus rhythm and for prevention of recurrence of atrial fibrillation.[220] It is a very potent K channel blocker that prolongs repolarization more prominently in the atria than in the ventricle.[206] Because it is a pure blocker of outward potassium currents, it does not have significant hemodynamic effects, does not depress cardiac function, and lacks extra cardiac effects.

It is partially metabolized in the liver and excreted predominantly in the urine, with an elimination half-life of 7 to 13 hours. The recommended dose is 0.125 to 0.5 mg twice daily, initiated under continuous ECG monitoring.[206] Higher than usual doses may be required in patients taking drugs that accelerate hepatic metabolism, such as phenytoin.

The most significant adverse effect is QT prolongation and torsade de pointes. Because of its proarrhythmic capabilities, the American College of Chest Physicians guidelines do not recommend it for prevention and management of atrial fibrillation after cardiac surgery.[221]

OTHER NONCLASSIFIED AGENTS

Adenosine Adenosine is an endogenous nucleotide natural to all cells of the body (**Table 44-15**). In pharmacologic doses, it slows conduction through the AV node and is proven highly efficacious as acute IV therapy for patients with paroxysmal supraventricular tachycardia in both reentry and accessory pathway (Wolff-Parkinson-White) dysrhythmias. Although adenosine does not convert atrial fibrillation or atrial flutter to sinus rhythm, it may be useful in their diagnosis. It may also terminate adrenergic-sensitive ventricular tachycardias originating from the right ventricular outflow tract.[186]

After IV administration, adenosine undergoes rapid redistribution to erythrocytes and cells of the vascular endothelium, with a half-life estimated at less than 10 seconds. Subsequently, it is metabolized to inosine or adenosine monophosphate. After a bolus of 6 mg, approximately 60% of patients with paroxysmal supraventricular tachycardia will convert to sinus rhythm within 1 minute. If the initial bolus is unsuccessful, 12 mg given intravenously will convert most of the remaining patients, for a cumulative effectiveness of 92%. Transient high-grade blocks, and even asystole, may be seen after adenosine administration. These usually resolve rapidly and without therapy. Dipyridamole blocks reuptake of adenosine, delaying its clearance and potentiating its effects, whereas caffeine and methylxanthines are competitive

TABLE 44-15 Unclassified Antiarrhythmic Agents

Drug	Usual Dosages	Effects on Electrocardiogram	Adverse Reactions	Usually Effective Plasma Concentration	Indications	Half-Life	Metabolism
Adenosine	6-12 mg IV (may repeat 12 mg × 2)	Increased PR interval; AV block	High-grade block; asystole; hypotension; dizziness; nausea; headaches	0.5-2 μg/mL	Paroxysmal supraventricular tachycardias including Wolff-Parkinson-White syndrome	10 s	Metabolized to inosine and adenosine monophosphate

Data from Abramowicz M. Drugs for cardiac arrhythmias. *Med Lett Drugs Ther.* 1991;33:60.

antagonists, necessitating larger doses of adenosine to achieve clinical effect.[206]

Adenosine is contraindicated in patients with sick sinus syndrome and second- or third-degree AV block. Hypotension may develop, especially when higher dosages are used. Other adverse side effects include facial flushing, headache, chest pain, dyspnea, dizziness, and nausea. Adenosine may precipitate ventricular fibrillation in patients with Wolff-Parkinson-White syndrome when administered during preexcited atrial fibrillation.[222]

Adenosine is also used to induce ischemia in both laboratory models of coronary steal with flow-limiting stenosis and clinically to elicit ischemia in adenosine-thallium scan. Adenosine is not FDA approved for use as a vasodilator or for deliberate intraoperative hypotension. Preclinical studies showed that intrathecal adenosine might be effective in the treatment of acute and chronic pain.[223]

STATINS

Because patients with dyslipidemias are at an increased risk of developing atherosclerosis and subsequent coronary artery disease, lipid lowering is beneficial for both primary and secondary prevention of coronary heart disease, as shown in several studies involving large populations.[224-226] The statins are the most effective and best-tolerated agents for treating dyslipidemias and have revolutionized the treatment in lipid abnormalities (**Table 44-16**).

The mechanism of action is competitive inhibition of 3-hydroxy-3-methylglutaryl coenzyme A reductase, which catalyzes an early, rate-limiting step in cholesterol biosynthesis, resulting in reduction in low-density lipoprotein cholesterol (LDL-C) levels, the major effect exerted by the statins.

The protective effect related to the use of statins cannot be completely explained by the lowering of LDL-C at baseline. Among the nonlipid-related mechanisms that may be involved are regression of atherosclerotic lesions, plaque stabilization, reduced inflammation, reversal of endothelial dysfunction, and decreased thrombogenicity.[227] Nonlipid properties may be observed earlier than lipid effects.

Several mechanisms may be responsible for the development of coronary ischemia and myocardial infarction in the perioperative setting, but there is evidence that coronary plaque rupture, which leads to thrombus formation and coronary artery occlusion, is the most important mechanism.

Recently, several studies analyzed the effect of statin agents on perioperative cardiovascular mortality and morbidity in patients undergoing noncardiac surgery.[228-232] Results of these studies, most of them retrospective, showed a reduction in the perioperative cardiovascular events or mortality.

Statins are effective and generally safe. However, certain side effects are associated with their use, particularly hepatotoxicity and myopathy. Although the incidence of myopathy is low (0.01%), the risk of myopathy, and even of rhabdomyolysis, increases in proportion to plasma statin concentration. Although there are case reports of perioperative myopathy and rhabdomyolysis in patients treated with statins,[233] the benefits of continuing these agents through the perioperative period have been demonstrated in both randomized clinical trials and large observational studies. In light of the high benefit to risk ratio, the data strongly suggest that statins should be continued through the perioperative period.

TABLE 44-16 Statins

Drug	Dose	Side Effects
Atorvastatin (Lipitor)	10-80 mg/d	Hepatotoxicity (elevation of aminotransferases); myopathy (factors associated with increased risk include advanced age, hepatic or renal dysfunction, perioperative periods, multisystem disease especially diabetes mellitus, hypothyroidism); proteinuria; headache; nausea
Fluvastatin (Lescol)	20-80 mg/d 80 mg SR/d	
Lovastatin (Mevacor)	20-80 mg/d	
Pravastatin (Pravachol)	10-180 mg/d	
Rosuvastatin (Crestor)	5-40 mg/d	
Simvastatin (Zocor)	5-80 mg/d	

KEY REFERENCES

- Chobanian AV, Bakris GL, Black HR, et al. The Seventh Report of the Joint National Committee on Prevention, Detection, Evaluation, and Treatment of High Blood Pressure: the JNC 7 report. *JAMA.* 2003;289:2560-2572.
- Chobanian AV. Shattuck Lecture. The hypertension paradox—more uncontrolled disease despite improved therapy. *N Engl J Med.* 2009;361:878-887.
- Dahlof B, Devereux RB, Kjeldsen SE, et al. Cardiovascular morbidity and mortality in the Losartan Intevention for Endpoint reduction in hypertension study (LIFE): a randomised trial against atenolol. *Lancet.* 2002;359:995-1003.
- Dahlof B, Sever PS, Poulter NR, et al. Prevention of cardiovascular events with an antihypertensive regimen of amlodipine adding perindopril as required versus atenolol adding bendroflumethiazide as required, in the Anglo-Scandinavian Cardiac Outcomes Trial-Blood Pressure Lowering Arm (ASCOT-BPLA): a multicentre reandomised controlled trial. *Lancet.* 2005;366:895-906.
- Egan BM, Zhao Y, Axon RN. US trends in prevalence, awareness, treatment, and control of hypertension, 1988-2008. *JAMA.* 2010;303:2043-2050.
- Fleisher LA, Beckman JA, Brown KA, et al. ACC/AHA 2007 Guidelines on Perioperative Cardiovascular Evaluation and Care for Noncardiac Surgery: Executive Summary: a report of the American College of Cardiology/American Heart Association Task Force on Practice Guidelines (Writing Committee to Revise the 2002 Guidelines on Perioperative Cardiovascular Evaluation for Noncardiac Surgery) Developed in Collaboration with the American Society of Echocardiography, American Society of Nuclear Cardiology, Heart Rhythm Society, Society of Cardiovascular Anesthesiologists, Society for Cardiovascular Angiography and Interventions, Society for Vascular Medicine and Biology, and Society for Vascular Surgery. *J Am Coll Cardiol.* 2007;50:1707-1732.
- Jamerson K, Weber MA, Bakris GL, et al. Benazepril plus amlodipine or hydrochlorothiazide for hypertension in high-risk patients. *N Engl J Med.* 2008;359:2417-2428.
- Mensah GA, Bakris G. Treatment and control of high blood pressure in adults. *Cardiol Clin.* 2010;28:609-622.
- Ostchega Y, Dillon CF, Hughes JP, Carroll M, Yoon S. Trends in hypertension prevalence, awareness, treatment, and control in older U.S. adults: data from the National Health and Nutrition Examination Survey 1988 to 2004. *J Am Geriatr Soc.* 2007;55:1056-1065.
- Reyes AJ, Taylor SH. Diuretics in cardiovascular therapy: new clinicopharmacological bases that matter. *Cardiovasc Drugs Ther.* 1999;13:371-398.

REFERENCES

Complete references available on DVD and online version at www.LongneckerAnesthesiology.com

CHAPTER 45

Pharmacology of Local Anesthetics*

James E. Heavner

KEY POINTS

1. Pharmacodynamics–Local anesthetics stop the propagation of action potentials in nerve axons by preventing the influx of sodium through voltage-gated sodium channels in the axon membrane. Other actions of local anesthetics (eg, effects on other voltage-gated ion channels and ligand-gated ion channels) may be important for their analgesic action and/or for undesired side effects.
2. Chemistry–Local anesthetics are weak bases with 3 structural parts: a hydrophilic end and a lipophilic end linked by an amino ester or an amino amide bond. The bond is the basis for classifying local anesthetics into 2 groups: the amino esters and the amino amides. Optical isomers of local anesthetics with an asymmetric carbon atom usually differ in potency, duration of action, and toxicity.
3. Expression of local anesthetic action–In vitro, there generally is a positive correlation between molecular weight of local anesthetic molecules and lipophilicity, protein binding, duration of action, potency, and toxicity; there is an inverse relation with speed of onset. In vivo expression of local anesthetic action is dependent on other factors as well, such as injection site, dose, intrinsic vasoactivity, and formulation. The manifestation of sensory versus motor block varies and is dependent on many factors, including the agent and type of block performed.
4. Pharmacokinetics–Local anesthetics usually are injected near the target site instead of relying on systemic circulation to carry them there (except, eg, intravenous regional anesthesia and treatment of certain neuropathic pain states). Barriers to the diffusion of local anesthetics to their target vary and are dependent on injection site (eg, epidural vs intrathecal), influence dose, speed of onset, and duration of action. Local anesthetics that reach systemic circulation are widely distributed in the body. Hydrolysis of the amino ester bond by esterases in blood is the primary biotransformation process for amino ester-linked local anesthetics. Hepatic extraction and biotransformation are important elimination and biotransformation pathways for amino amide-linked local anesthetics.
5. Toxicity–Local anesthetic toxicity can be categorized as allergic, tissue, cardiovascular, central nervous system, and methemoglobinemia. Clinically, manifestations of local anesthetic systemic toxicity do not occur in a predictable order, and which occur and how soon after local administration are variable. Concerns about cardiovascular toxicity related to bupivacaine have driven a search for long-acting local anesthetics with less cardiotoxic action.
6. Formulation–Substances are sometimes added to local anesthetic formulations to preserve the molecules, to prevent microbial growth, to prevent systemic absorption, to enhance and/or prolong local anesthetic action, and to enhance spread of the local anesthetic.

Local anesthetics are widely used to prevent or treat acute pain; to treat inflammatory, cancer, and chronic pain; and for diagnostic and prognostic purposes. Drugs classified as local anesthetics reversibly block action potential propagation in axons by preventing the sodium entry that produces the potentials.[1] However, other actions of these drugs, such as anti-inflammation by interaction with G-protein receptors[2] and analgesic effect in the spinal cord by blocking postsynaptic ionotropic receptor function mediated by extracellular receptor-activated kinase,[3] also are thought to be relevant to their use to prevent or treat pain. Nociceptive pain, as well as neuropathic pain, is targeted with this group of drugs. Any part of the nervous system, from the periphery to the brain, may be where local anesthetics act to produce a desired anesthetic or analgesic effect. A variety of formulations of local anesthetics, routes of administration, and methods of administration are used. The drugs are formulated commercially or by medical personnel according to the intended route of administration and/or to address specific concerns or needs. This chapter provides a concise review of the pharmacology of local anesthetics.

DISCOVERY AND EVOLUTION OF LOCAL ANESTHETICS

COCAINE, PROCAINE, AND LIDOCAINE

Koller is credited with introducing local anesthetics into medical practice when he used cocaine to numb the cornea before operating on the eye.[4] Fundamental to the development of synthetic local anesthetics was isolation of cocaine by Neimann, in 1860, from coca beans, and elucidation of its chemical structure. Procaine was first synthesized in 1904, and lidocaine was first synthesized in 1943. Synthesis of molecules with local anesthetic activity paved the way for "tinkering" with the molecules by systematically modifying chemical structure and testing for a desired result, for example reducing toxicity, in developing new local anesthetics.

ROOTS OF MODERN USE

Figure 45-1 presents a chronology of the introduction of local anesthetics into clinical practice. Four amino ester–linked local anesthetics (see Three Parts of Local Anesthetic Molecules) appear in the figure: cocaine, procaine, tetracaine, and chloroprocaine. The other local anesthetics are amino amide linked. What is evident from the figure is the focus since 1955 on the development of amino amide– and not amino ester–linked local anesthetics. Reasons for this include the allergenic potential of amino ester–linked local anesthetics and the instability of amino ester bonds.

IMPORTANT CHEMICAL FEATURES

THREE PARTS OF LOCAL ANESTHETIC MOLECULES

All local anesthetic molecules in clinical use have 3 parts: lipophilic (aromatic) end, hydrophilic (amine) end, and a link between the ends (**Fig. 45-2**). The link contains either an amino ester or an amino amide bond, and local anesthetics are designated as belonging to 1 of 2 groups: the amino ester–linked local anesthetics or amino amide–linked local anesthetics. Procaine is the prototypic amino ester–linked local anesthetic, and lidocaine is the prototypic amino amide–linked local anesthetic (**Fig. 45-3**).

Amino amides are extremely stable agents, whereas amino esters are relatively unstable in solution. Consequently, aqueous solutions of amino ester agents have relatively short shelf lives as compared with solutions of amino amides and are sensitive to exposure to high temperatures. The amino esters are hydrolyzed in plasma by cholinesterase enzymes, whereas the amino amide compounds undergo enzymatic biotransformation in the liver.

There are 2 varieties of amino amide local anesthetics based on the structure of the amino amide link. One variety is the aminoacyl amides, such as lidocaine and bupivacaine, and the other is the amino alkyl amides, such as dibucaine. The different structures influence the duration of action and biotransformation. Further distinction within the aminoacyl amide class is made based on whether the hydrophilic amino end is a straight carbon chain (eg, lidocaine) or the amino nitrogen is within a ring structure (pipecoloxylidide, eg, mepivacaine)

*This chapter includes substantial material from Covino BG. Pharmacology of local anesthetic agents. In: Rogers MC, Tinker JH, Covino BG, et al, eds. *Principles and Practice of Anesthesiology, Vol 2*. St. Louis, MO: Mosby Year Book; 1993:1235-1257.

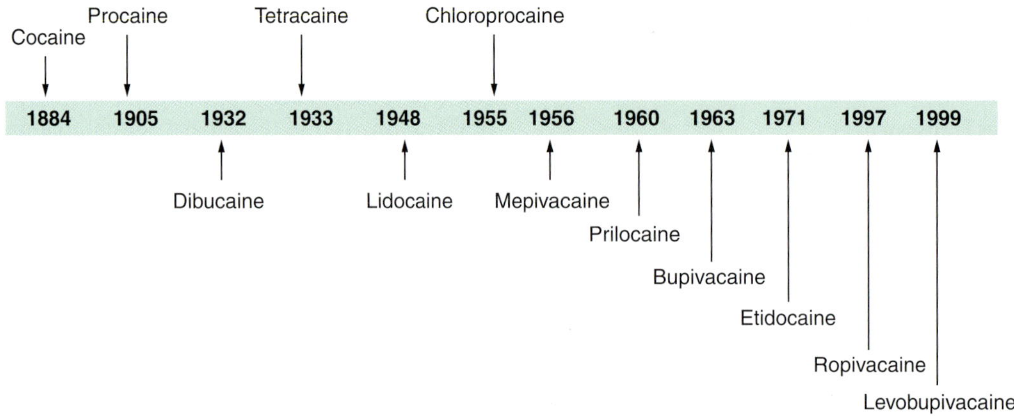

FIGURE 45-1. Chronology of the introduction of different anesthetics into clinical practice. Chloroprocaine (1955) is the last amino ester–linked local anesthetic introduced that is still in clinical use. [Courtesy of David A. Scott, Melbourne, Australia, 2000.]

CHIRAL FORMS

The newest additions to clinically available local anesthetics, ropivacaine (**Fig. 45-4**) and levobupivacaine, represent (1) the exploitation of technology that permits cost-favorable separation of racemic mixtures of local anesthetics into pure enantiomers and (2) the search for local anesthetics with greater safety margins. Simplistically stated, molecules with an asymmetric carbon atom exist in forms that are mirror images (ie, exhibit "handness, chirality"), with images (enantiomer, stereoisomers) distinguished by how they rotate light according to the orientation of the structures in 3 dimensions. Various terms are used to refer to the different enantiomers; this chapter uses S and R to designate 2 different enantiomers. A racemic mixture contains equal amounts of the R and S isomers. Commercial formulations of ropivacaine and levobupivacaine contain the S enantiomer. Note that levobupivacaine is the S form of bupivacaine. The motive for marketing pure enantiomers is evidence that the S form is less toxic, more potent, and longer acting than the R form or the racemic mixture (**Table 45-1**).

LIPID SOLUBILITY AND PROTEIN BINDING

Testing modifications to the basic procaine and lidocaine structure revealed that increasing the molecular weight of the molecules by adding carbon atoms to either end of the structure or to the link generally increases lipid solubility, protein binding, and duration of action and toxicity and influences biotransformation of the molecule (**Figs. 45-5** and **45-6**). There is a positive correlation between intrinsic local anesthetic potency and lipid solubility of local anesthetics.

CATION AND BASE FORMS

Most local anesthetics have a tertiary amine on the hydrophilic end. Exceptions include prilocaine, which has a secondary amine, and benzocaine, which has a primary amine. Tertiary amines have a positive charge (*cation*) or are uncharged (*base*). The ratio of cation to base is determined by the pK_a of the local anesthetic and the pH of the solution (**Table 45-2**). The unchanged forms of local anesthetics

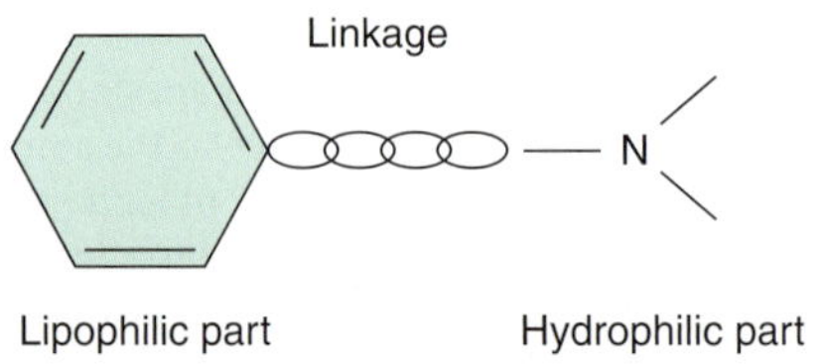

Linkage
Lipophilic part
Hydrophilic part

FIGURE 45-2. General structure of all local anesthetic molecules showing 3 parts.

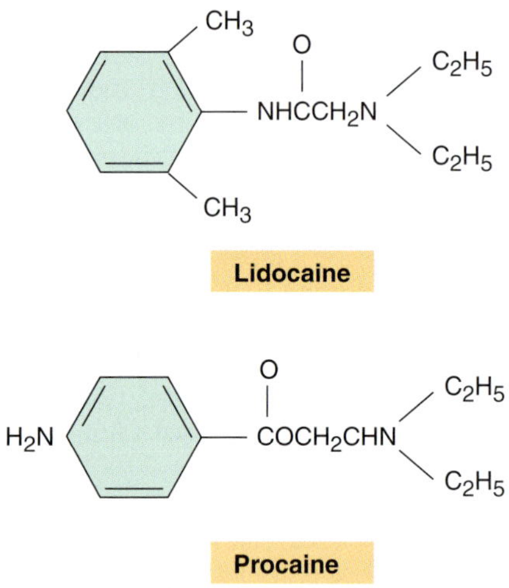

Lidocaine

Procaine

FIGURE 45-3. Structure of lidocaine and procaine

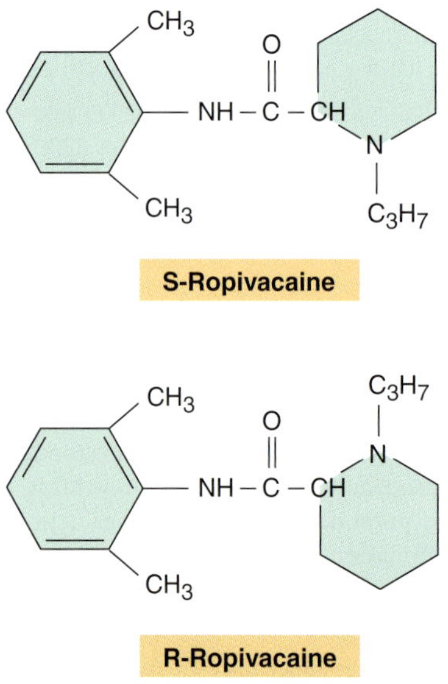

S-Ropivacaine

R-Ropivacaine

FIGURE 45-4. Clinical forms of ropivacaine. The only difference between the S- and R-isomers is their spatial orientation.

TABLE 45-1 Anesthetic Duration and Toxicity of Local Anesthetic Isomers

Drug	Duration	Toxicity
Etidocaine	S = R	S = R
Mepivacaine	S > R	S = R
Bupivacaine	S > R	S < R
Ropivacaine	S > R	S < R

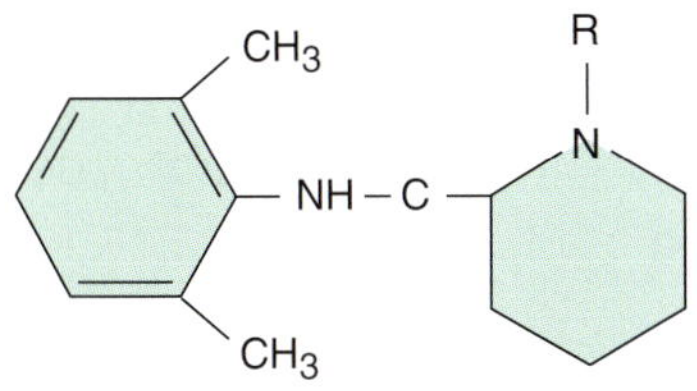

	Mepivacaine	Ropivacaine	Bupivacaine
R =	CH_3	C_3H_6	C_4H_9
Equieffective	1	0.37	0.25
Lipid/H_2O	0.8	2.8	27.5
Protein bound (%)	77.5	94	95.6

FIGURE 45-5. Results of structure alterations–amide linked. The amino amide–linked local anesthetics mepivacaine, ropivacaine, and bupivacaine vary only by substitution at R on the basic molecule shown. As the number of carbon atoms increases at R, potency, lipid solubility, and protein binding increase. [Reprinted from Heavner JE. Pain mechanisms and local anesthetics: scientific foundations for clinical practice. In: Raj PP, ed. *Textbook of Regional Anesthesia*. New York, NY: Churchill Livingstone; 2002:105-124, with permission from Elsevier.]

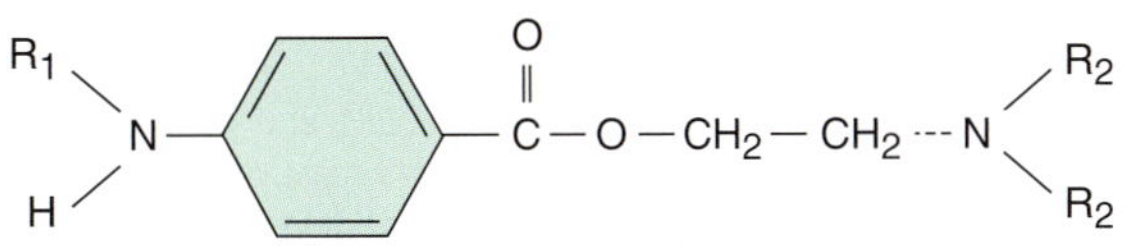

	Procaine	Tetracaine
R_1	H	C_4H_9
R_2	C_2H_5	CH_3
Hydrolysis rate (μmol/mL/h)	1.1	0.25
= potent	2	0.25
Duration (min)	50	175
LD50 (mice)	615	48

FIGURE 45-6. Results of structure alterations–ester linked.

TABLE 45-2 Cation-to-Base Ratio

	pK_a	pH 7.4
Procaine	8.9	32:1
Lidocaine	7.9	3:1
Mepivacaine	7.6	2:1
Tetracaine	8.5	13:1
Benzocaine	3.5	All base
Bupivacaine	8.1	5:1
Ropivacaine	8.1	5:1

pass readily through cell membranes and hence speed of onset of local anesthetic block, at least theoretically, is increased by increasing the concentration of uncharged local anesthetic molecules injected.

Because local anesthetics are weak bases, increasing the pH ("alkalinization") of solution increases the ratio of base to cation. The Henderson-Hasselbalch equation can be used to quantitate the ratio:

$$pK_a\text{(local anesthetic)} - \text{pH(solution)} = \text{Log ([cation]/[base])}$$

Sodium bicarbonate is used clinically to increase the pH of local anesthetic solutions.

Important to note is that commercial aqueous solutions of local anesthetics are acidified, so the hydrophilic (cationic) state, which is water soluble, is favored. Overzealous alkalinization can cause local anesthetic molecules to precipitate from solution.

PHARMACODYNAMICS OF LOCAL ANESTHETICS

NEUROPHYSIOLOGIC AND NEUROANATOMICAL CONSIDERATIONS

Reversible block of fast voltage-gated sodium channels in axons is generally thought to be how local anesthetics block sensory and motor function (**Fig. 45-7**). Some of the evidence supporting this is the following: (1) action potentials do not develop in axons exposed to local anesthetic; (2) sodium currents responsible for generation of action potentiations are blocked by these drugs; and (3) local anesthetics do not affect the transmembrane potential of axons. The "state" of the sodium channel (resting, open, inactivated) changes during the cycle of polarized, depolarized, repolarized. The order of affinity of local anesthetics for different channel states is open > inactivated > resting. Many investigators have shown that the block of propagation of action potentials is a function of frequency of depolarization, which supports the conclusion that the open state of the sodium channel is the primary target of local anesthetic molecules. This is referred to as "state-dependent block."

VOLTAGE-GATED SODIUM CHANNELS

Voltage-gated ion channels are ion channels (Na^+, K^+, Ca^{2+}, etc) whose permeability is a function of transmembrane potential. There are a number of sodium channel subtypes that generally are divided into those that are tetrodotoxin sensitive (TTXs) and tetrodotoxin resistant (TTXr). A standard nomenclature was adopted for voltage-gated Na^+ channels that uses a numerical system to define subfamilies and subtypes based on similarities between the amino acid sequences of the channels. Nine mammalian sodium channel isoforms have been identified (Na_V1.1 through Na_V1.9). Na_V1.1, Na_V1.2, Na_V1.3, and Na_V1.7 are broadly expressed in neurons and are highly TTXs; Na_V1.5, Na_V1.8, and Na_V1.9 are highly expressed in heart and dorsal root ganglia neurons.[5] Most sensory neurons generate TTXs currents. However, TTXr currents are present in a high proportion of smaller dorsal root ganglion neurons associated with nociceptive Aδ and C fibers. Available evidence indicates that channels from both groups are involved in pain states as a result of changes in channel function and expression caused by disease or injury.

Existing local anesthetics lack specificity for Na^+ channel subtypes However, there are ongoing efforts to develop Na^+ channel blockers specific for Na_V1.7, Na_V1.8, and Na_V1.9, which are expressed extensively on peripheral nociceptors. Na_V1.7 is of particular interest, as this channel determines the ability of a nerve to transmit nociceptive information.[6]

Arguments have been put forth that local anesthetics might exert their pharmacologic action not only on Na^+ conductance, but also on other ionic conductances (eg, K^+ and Ca^{2+}).[7]

DIFFERENTIAL BLOCK

Differential block, the block of pain perception without motor block for example, is observed clinically, but the mechanism responsible for this is poorly understood. The clinical manifestations of differential block vary depending on the local anesthetic used.[9] Etidocaine has a propensity

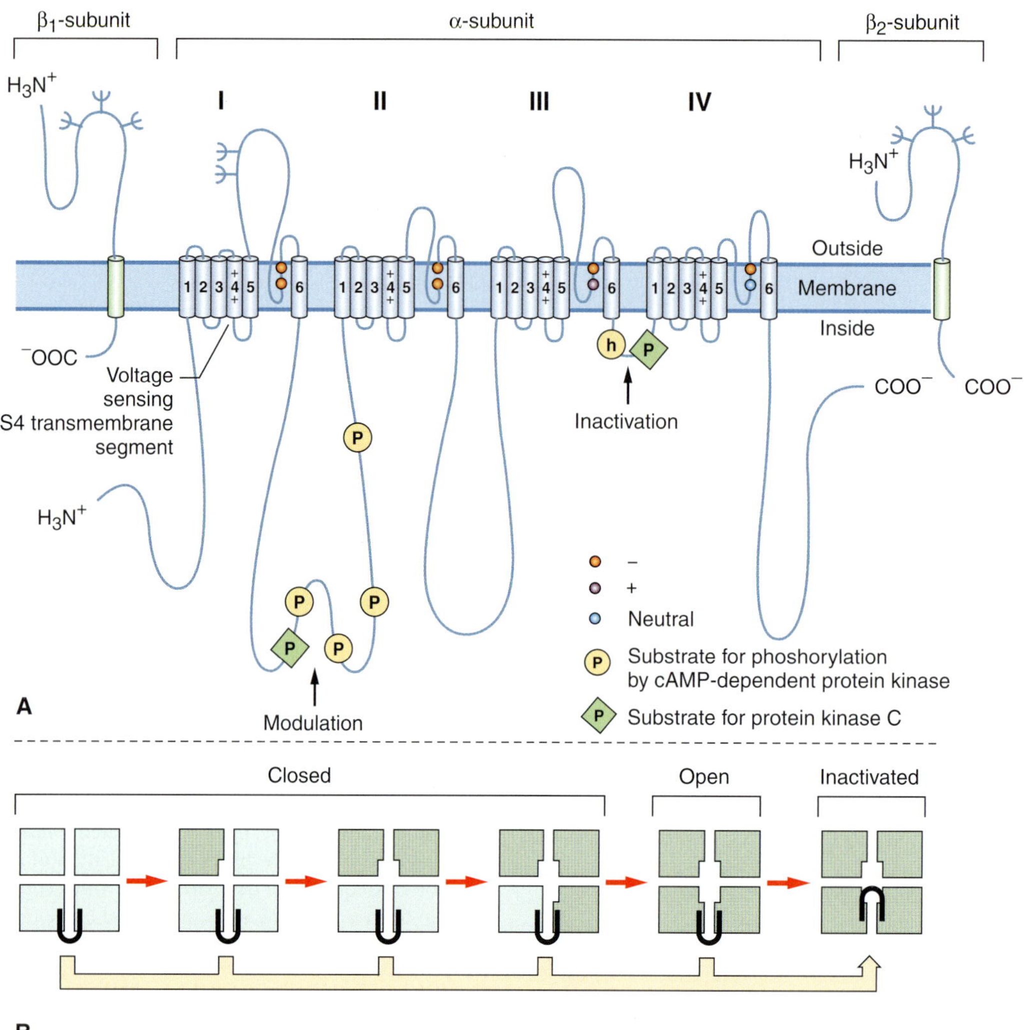

FIGURE 45-7. Structure and function of voltage-gated Na+ channels. **A.** A 2-dimensional representation of the α (center), β_1 (left), and β_2 (right) subunits of the voltage-gated Na+ channel from mammalian brain. The polypeptide chains are represented by continuous lines with length approximately proportional to the actual length of each segment of the channel protein. Cylinders represent regions of transmembrane α helices. Ψ indicates sites of demonstrated *N*-linked glycosylation. Note the repeated structure of the 4 homologous domains (I through IV) of the α-subunit. Voltage sensing: The S4 transmembrane segments in each homologous domain of the α-subunit serve as voltage sensors. (+) Represents the positively charged amino acid residues at every third position within these segments. An electrical field (negative inside) exerts a force on these charged amino acid residues, pulling them toward the intracellular side of the membrane. Pore: The S5 and S6 transmembrane segments and the short membrane-associated loops between them (segments SS1 and SS2) form the walls of the pore in the center of an approximately symmetrical square array of the 4 homologous domains (see *B*). The amino acid residues indicated by circles in segment SS2 are critical for determining the conductance and ion selectivity of the Na+ channel and its ability to bind the extracellular pore blocking toxins tetrodotoxin and saxitoxin. Inactivation: The short intracellular loop connecting homologous domains III and IV serves as the inactivation gate of the Na+ channel. It is thought to fold into the intracellular mouth of the pore and occlude it within a few milliseconds after the channel opens. Three hydrophobic residues (isoleucine–phenylalanine–methionine [IFM]) at the position marked *H* appear to serve as an inactivation particle, entering the intracellular mouth of the pore and binding to an inactivation gate receptor there. Modulation: The gating of the Na+ channel can be modulated by protein phosphorylation. Phosphorylation of the inactivation gate between homologous domains III and IV by protein kinase C slows inactivation. Phosphorylation of sites in the intracellular loop between homologous domains I and II by either protein kinase C ◈ or cyclic adenosine monophosphate (AMP)–dependent protein kinase Ⓟ reduces Na+ channel activation. **B.** The 4 homologous domains of the Na+ channel α-subunit are illustrated as a square array as viewed looking down on the membrane. The sequence of conformational changes that the Na+ channel undergoes during activation and inactivation is diagrammed. Upon depolarization, each of the 4 homologous domains undergoes a conformational change in sequence to an activated state. After all 4 domains have activated, the Na+ channel can open. Within a few milliseconds after opening, the inactivation gate between domains III and IV closes over the intracellular mouth of the channel and occludes it, preventing further ion conductance. [Reproduced with permission from Catterall W, Mackie K. Local Anesthetics. In: Hardman JG, Limbird LE, Gilman AF, eds. *The Pharmacological Basis of Therapeutics*. 10th ed. New York, NY: McGraw-Hill; 2001:370.]

to produce more profound motor block than sensory block. For many years, differential block was ascribed to smaller axons being more sensitive than large ones to local anesthetics,[10] but this "size principle" was challenged.[11] Strichartz and Berde[9] cite a number of different factors that might contribute to differential block, including anatomical and relative sensitivity to sodium and potassium channels of different local anesthetics. Oda et al[12] suggested that preferential block of TTXr sodium channels by ropivacaine in small dorsal root ganglia neurons (associated with nociceptive sensation) underlies differential block observed during epidural anesthesia with this drug.

Using a combination of local anesthetic and another drug to produce nociceptive selective block is under investigation. For example, activating transient receptor potential vanilloid subtype 1 channels on C-fibers with capsaicin to deliver the local anesthetic, QX-314, into the fibers is effective in animal models.[13] Another approach combining local anesthetic and α_2-adrenergic agonist such as dexmedetomidine has yielded favorable results. The mechanism for the α_2-adrenergic agonist action is not known but may include direct inhibition of TTXr Na^+ channel or through hyperpolarization activated cation current.[14]

PAIN RELIEF BY SYSTEMIC ADMINISTRATION

Another pharmacodynamic puzzle is the mechanism whereby systemically administered local anesthetic relieves pain. Analgesic effect has been reported after intravenous lidocaine administration in many acute and chronic conditions.[15-23] Subcutaneously injected bupivacaine reportedly produces analgesia via a systemic effect.[24] Normal or altered sodium channels located in various areas of the brain, spinal cord, or dorsal root ganglia, or in peripheral axons, are mentioned most frequently as the action sites. Zhang et al[25] reported that in rats systemic lidocaine delivered via implanted osmotic pump reduces sympathetic nerve sprouting in dorsal root ganglion that is associated with some neuropathic pain behaviors. Takatori et al[26] presented evidence that inhibition of nerve growth factor (NGF)–stimulated tyrosine kinase activity of TrkA, a high-affinity receptor of NGF, might be involved in the suppression of neurite outgrowth by local anesthetics.

Frolich et al[27] suggested that intravenous lidocaine may be effective against deep tissue pain but has limited value for treating superficial pains except neuropathic conditions.

LIGAND-GATED ION CHANNELS

Ligand-gated ion channels are channels whose permeability status depends on the interaction between a ligand and a receptor that influences channel function. Many of these receptors interact with G proteins. Local anesthetics affect a number of biologic processes, including inhibition of G-protein coupled receptor signaling, that are potentially important pharmacodynamic actions of value in treating pain.

PHARMACOKINETICS OF INJECTED LOCAL ANESTHETICS

DISTRIBUTION TO THE TARGET SITE

The usual pharmacokinetics parameters (**Table 45-3**) presented for local anesthetics incompletely describe important details regarding distribution of these drugs from application sites to target and nontarget structures. It is well established that systemic absorption of local anesthetics correlates positively with the vascularity of the injection site (intravenous > tracheal > intercostal > paracervical > epidural > brachial plexus > sciatic > subcutaneous). The spinal cord meninges influence distribution of local anesthetics from the epidural and subarachnoid spaces. Intact skin is nearly a complete barrier to local anesthetic penetration. In the latter case, special local anesthetic formulations (eg, eutectic mixture of local anesthetics [EMLA] cream, an eutectic mixture of lidocaine and prilocaine) or delivery methods (eg, electrophoresis) are employed to facilitate transcutaneous transfer. The large number of different injection sites used (eg, epidural, intrathecal, intrapleural, intra-articular, intramuscular, perineural, topical) and the variety of dosing methods (eg, single shot, continuous infusion, intermittent infusion) make comprehensive discussion of all pharmacokinetic considerations beyond the scope of this chapter.

ABSORPTION

In addition to the injection site, the vascular absorption of local anesthetic agents is related to dosage, addition of a vasoconstrictor agent, and specific agent employed. The high blood concentrations after intercostal administration are probably related to the multiple injections required for intercostal nerve blocks. As a consequence of this, local anesthetic solution is exposed to a greater vascular area, which results in a greater rate and degree of absorption. After thoracic paravertebral block, ropivacaine demonstrates a biphasic fast and slow absorption pattern.[28] The fast phase approximates the speed of intravenous injection and accounts for nearly half of ropivacaine absorption. When epinephrine (5 µg/mL) is added, systemic absorption and peak plasma concentration of ropivacaine are significantly reduced.

For most local anesthetic agents, a linear relationship exists between the amount of drug administered and the resultant peak venous plasma concentration. The mean venous plasma concentration of lidocaine increases from approximately 1.5 to 4 µg/mL as the total dose administered into the lumbar epidural space is increased from 200 to 600 mg. Depending on the site of administration, a peak blood concentration of 0.5 to 2.0 µg/mL is achieved for each 100 mg of lidocaine or mepivacaine injected. Simon et al[29] reported that systemic absorption of ropivacaine after epidural administration was biphasic, with higher absorption kinetics in younger than in older patients. The absorption kinetics were in the same range as for other long-acting local anesthetics. Buffington and Blix[30] recently suggested that the early peak seen after epidural injection of local anesthetic might be due in part to bulk transfer from the epidural space to the bloodstream.

In general, the addition of epinephrine to local anesthetic solutions decreases the rate of vascular absorption of these agents.[31] Epinephrine 5 µg/mL (1:200 000) significantly reduces the peak blood concentrations of lidocaine and mepivacaine, regardless of the site of administration. However, peak blood concentrations of bupivacaine and etidocaine are minimally influenced by the addition of epinephrine after injection into the lumbar epidural space. On the other hand, the rate of vascular absorption of these agents is significantly decreased when epinephrine-containing solutions are employed for brachial plexus blockade.[32,33]

The rate of vascular absorption also varies and is dependent on the specific local anesthetic agent. Lidocaine is absorbed more rapidly after brachial plexus and epidural blockade than is prilocaine, whereas bupivacaine is absorbed more rapidly than etidocaine.[31,33] Prilocaine is a less potent vasodilator than lidocaine, which partly accounts for lower blood concentrations of prilocaine. The lower peak blood concentrations of etidocaine compared with bupivacaine may be related to the greater lipid solubility of etidocaine, which results in its sequestration by adipose tissue and a decreased rate of absorption. The differences

TABLE 45-3 Disposition Kinetics in Adult Human

Local Anesthetic	V_{dss} (L)	Cl (L/min)	$T_{½}\gamma$ (h)	Hepatic Extraction	Lipid Solubility	Protein Binding (%)	Blood/Plasma Partitioning
Mepivacaine	84	0.78	1.9	0.40	0.8	78	0.92
Ropivacaine	59	0.73	1.8	0.40	2.8	94	0.69
Bupivacaine	73	0.58	2.7	0.51	27.5	96	0.73
Lidocaine	91	0.95	1.6	0.72	2.9	60	0.84
Prilocaine	261	2.84	1.5	–	–	55	–
Etidocaine	133	1.22	2.6	0.74	–	94	0.58

in absorption rates are of practical clinical significance, as they permit the use of larger doses of prilocaine compared with lidocaine and of etidocaine compared with bupivacaine.

SYSTEMIC DISTRIBUTION

The distribution of local anesthetic agents from systemic circulation can be described by a 2- or 3-compartment model.[34] The rapid disappearance (α) phase is believed to be related to uptake by rapidly equilibrating tissues, that is, tissues with a high vascular perfusion. The slower phase of disappearance from blood (β phase) is mainly a function of distribution to slowly equilibrating tissues and the biotransformation and excretion of the compound (**Fig. 45-8**). The α half-life ($T_{½}α$) of prilocaine is shorter than that of lidocaine and mepivacaine, which indicates that prilocaine is redistributed at a significantly more rapid rate from blood to tissues than either of the other 2 drugs (Table 45-3). The $T_{½}α$ of lidocaine and mepivacaine are similar. The half-life of the β disappearance phase ($T_{½}β$) of prilocaine is more rapid than that of lidocaine and mepivacaine, suggesting a more rapid rate of biotransformation. A comparison study reveals that etidocaine has a more rapid rate of tissue redistribution and biotransformation than bupivacaine.[35] The clearance of ropivacaine is closer to that of mepivacaine and faster than that of bupivacaine, and the terminal $t^{1/2}$ of mepivacaine and ropivacaine are less than that of bupivacaine.[36]

Local anesthetic agents are distributed throughout all body tissues, but the relative concentration in different tissues varies as a function of time, vascular perfusion, and tissue mass. Initially, local anesthetic agents are rapidly extracted by lung tissue so that the whole blood concentration of local anesthetics decreases greatly as they pass through the pulmonary vasculature.[37,38] Ultimately, the highest percentage of an injected dose of a local anesthetic agent is found in skeletal muscle, simply because the mass of skeletal muscle makes it the largest reservoir for local anesthetic agents.

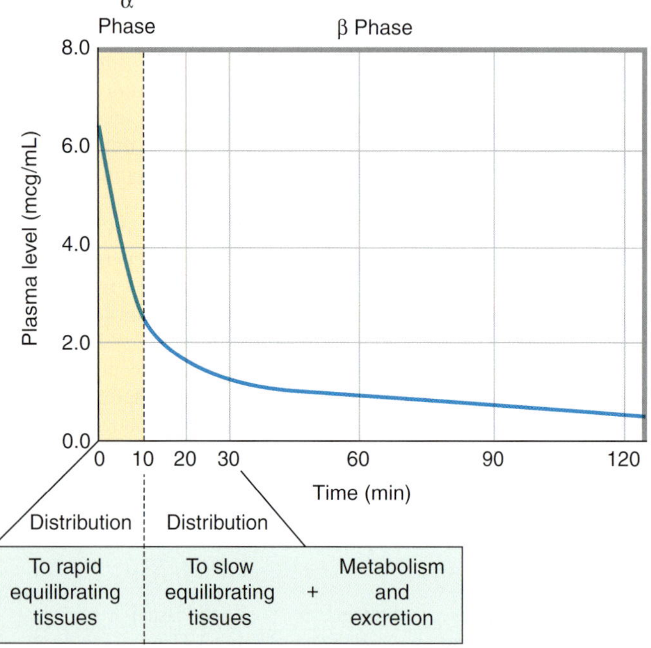

FIGURE 45-8. Plasma concentration curve of lidocaine after IV administration showing initial rapid rate of disappearance related to distribution to rapidly equilibrating tissues and slower rate of disappearance caused by distribution to slowly equilibrating tissues and biotransformation and excretion. [Reprinted from Covino BG. Pharmacology of local anesthetic agents. In: Rogers MC, Tinker JH, Covino BG, et al, eds. *Principles and Practice of Anesthesiology, Vol. 2*. St. Louis, MO: Mosby Year Book; 1993:1245, with permission from Elsevier.]

BIOTRANSFORMATION AND ELIMINATION

The degradation of local anesthetic agents varies according to their chemical classification. Amino ester local anesthetic drugs are hydrolyzed in plasma by cholinesterase enzymes. Chloroprocaine shows the most rapid rate of hydrolysis (4.7 μmol/mL/h), compared with a rate of 1.1 μmol/mL/h for procaine and 0.3 μmol/mL/h for tetracaine.[39] Less than 2% of unchanged procaine is found in urine, whereas approximately 90% of *p*-aminobenzoic acid, which is a primary product of procaine hydrolysis, appears in urine. Only 33% of dimethylaminoethanol, the other hydrolysis product of procaine, is excreted unchanged.

The amino amide agents are biotransformed primarily in the liver.[40] Elimination depends both on hepatic blood flow and enzyme activity.[36] Prilocaine undergoes the most rapid rate of hepatic metabolism, and lidocaine is biotransformed somewhat more rapidly than mepivacaine. In humans, the hepatic clearance of etidocaine is greater than that of bupivacaine, which suggests a more rapid rate of hepatic biotransformation for etidocaine. Evidence also exists that prilocaine may be biotransformed in the kidney, which would explain the rapid clearance of this agent compared with all other amino amides.[41]

The biotransformation of the amino amide–type agents results in the formation of a variety of metabolites. The biotransformation of lidocaine has been studied most extensively. The main pathway of lidocaine biotransformation in humans involves oxidative de-ethylation of lidocaine to monoethylglycinexylidide by cytochrome P450 IIIA4, followed by a subsequent hydrolysis of monoethylglycinexylidide to xylidine.

The excretion of the amino amide–type local anesthetic drugs occurs by way of the kidney. Less than 5% of the unchanged drug is excreted via the kidney into the urine. The major portion of the injected agent appears in the urine in the form of various metabolites. The renal clearance of the amino amide local anesthetic agents appears to be inversely related to their protein-binding capacity. Prilocaine, which has a lower protein-binding capacity than lidocaine, has a substantially higher clearance value than lidocaine.[42] Renal clearance also is inversely proportional to the pH of urine, suggesting that urinary excretion of these agents occurs by nonionic diffusion.

Patient age may influence the physiologic disposition of local anesthetics. The half-life of lidocaine after IV administration increased from an average of 80 minutes in human volunteers 22 to 26 years of age to 138 minutes in subjects ages 61 to 71 years.[43] Age-dependent disposition kinetics have been reported for ropivacaine after epidural administration, with elimination half-life significantly longer and clearance significantly decreased in older (>61 years) than in younger patients (18-40 years).[29]

The elimination of local anesthetic agents also is influenced by the individual patient's hepatic and cardiac function. For example, an average lidocaine half-life of 1.5 hours was reported in volunteers with normal hepatic function, whereas patients with liver disease demonstrated an average half-life of 5 hours.[44] In patients with congestive heart failure (CHF), the IV infusion of lidocaine results in significantly higher plasma concentrations of lidocaine than occurs in patients with normal cardiovascular function, indicating a decreased plasma clearance in patients with CHF.[45]

CLINICAL CONSIDERATIONS

ROUTES OF ADMINISTRATION

The clinical profile of local anesthetic drugs varies and is dependent on the type of regional anesthetic technique performed (**Fig. 45-9**). The shortest duration of action occurs after the intrathecal or subcutaneous administration of local anesthetics. The longest latencies and durations are observed after major peripheral nerve blocks, such as brachial plexus blockade. Intrathecal bupivacaine usually produces anesthesia within 5 minutes and persists for 3 to 4 hours.[46] For brachial plexus blockade, the onset time of bupivacaine is approximately 20 to 30 minutes, whereas the duration of anesthesia averages approximately 10 hours.[47]

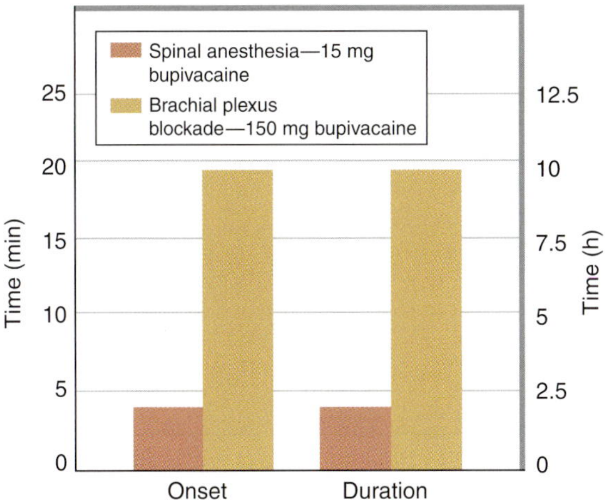

FIGURE 45-9. Comparison of onset and duration of spinal anesthesia and brachial plexus blockade with bupivacaine. [Reprinted from Covino BG. Pharmacology of local anesthetic agents. In: Rogers MC, Tinker JH, Covino BG, et al, eds. *Principles and Practice of Anesthesiology, Vol. 2*. St. Louis, MO: Mosby Year Book; 1993:1242, with permission from Elsevier.]

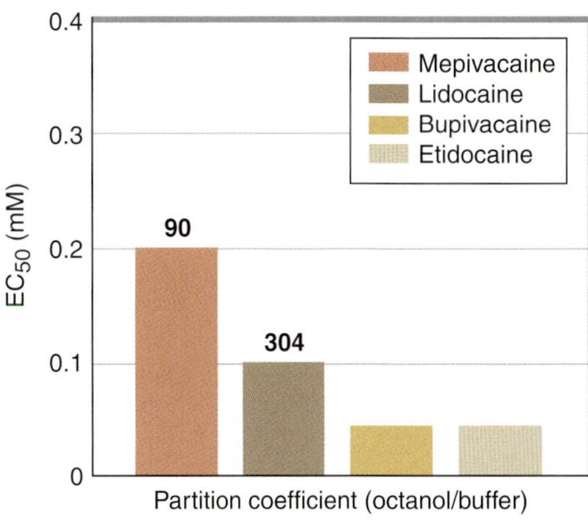

FIGURE 45-10. Relationship between concentrations of various local anesthetics required to cause 50% depression in amplitude of isolated nerve action potential (median effective concentration [EC_{50}]) and partition coefficient values. [Reprinted from Covino BG. Pharmacology of local anesthetic agents. In: Rogers MC, Tinker JH, Covino BG, et al, eds. *Principles and Practice of Anesthesiology, Vol. 2*. St. Louis, MO: Mosby Year Book; 1993:1236, with permission from Elsevier.]

These variations in the onset and duration of anesthesia result from differences in the anatomy of the injection sites and the amount of drug employed for various types of regional anesthesia. In the subarachnoid space, the lack of a nerve sheath around the spinal cord and the placement of the local anesthetic solution in the immediate vicinity of the spinal cord is responsible for the rapid onset of action. The relatively small amount of drug employed for spinal anesthesia probably accounts for the short duration of conduction block. For example, 50 to 75 mg of lidocaine and 10 to 15 mg of bupivacaine are usually employed for most spinal anesthetic procedures.

The onset of brachial plexus blockade is slow, as the anesthetic agent is usually injected some distance from the nerve roots and must diffuse through various tissue barriers before reaching the nerve membrane. The prolonged blockade is probably related to the decreased rate of vascular absorption from that site and the larger dose of drug employed for this regional anesthetic technique. For example, 400 to 600 mg of lidocaine and 100 to 150 mg of bupivacaine are usually employed for brachial plexus blockade. Techniques (eg, ultrasound guided) that allow more precise placement of local anesthetic near nerves theoretically will produce more rapid onset of block and clearly reduce volume required to produce a block. Using ultrasound for needle placement, Latzle et al[48] found that when the ED_{99} volumes of 1.5% mepivacaine were used for sciatic nerve blocks, local anesthetic volume had no impact on sensory onset times, but sensory block duration was shortened.

CLINICAL MANIFESTATIONS OF POTENCY

In vitro studies show a general positive correlation between lipid solubility of local anesthetics and potency (**Fig. 45-10**).[49,50] This presumably is because the nerve membrane that represents the site of action of local anesthetics consists primarily of lipids. However, the hydrophobicity and anesthetic potency are not as well correlated in intact animals and humans. The EC_{50} (median effective dose) of lidocaine, for example, is significantly less than that of mepivacaine in an isolated nerve, but in humans, little difference in anesthetic potency is apparent between these agents.[31]

The difference between potency in an isolated nerve and in a clinical situation is probably a function of the vasodilator or tissue redistribution properties of the various local anesthetics. Lidocaine is a more profound vasodilator than mepivacaine in humans. More rapid vascular absorption of lidocaine as a result of vasodilatation causing increased blood flow results in fewer lidocaine molecules being available for neural blockade. Hence lidocaine and mepivacaine appear to possess similar anesthetic potencies clinically. The profound conduction-blocking activity of etidocaine in vitro is a result of its high lipid solubility. However, sequestration of etidocaine in adipose tissue in vitro, such as in the epidural space, results in fewer etidocaine molecules being available for neural blockade compared with bupivacaine.

SPEED OF ONSET

In isolated nerves,[50,51] onset time of conduction block is correlated with the pK_a of the various agents (**Fig. 45-11**), and lipid solubility influences onset of action, too. The pK_a of local anesthetics and the pH of the anesthetic solution determine the degree of ionization of specific agents. This is because the degree of ionization influences the rate of diffusion of local anesthetics across the nerve sheath and membrane. The uncharged base form diffuses more easily than the charged cationic form.[52,53]

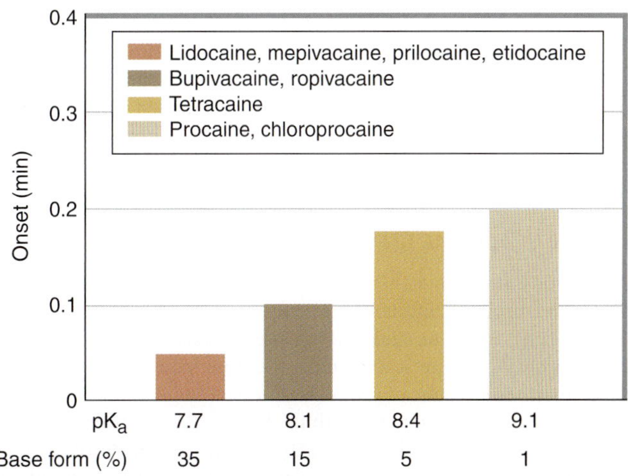

FIGURE 45-11. Relationship between onset of conduction block in isolated nerve and pK_a and percentage of local anesthetic present in base form. [Reprinted from Covino BG. Pharmacology of local anesthetic agents. In: Rogers MC, Tinker JH, Covino BG, et al, eds. *Principles and Practice of Anesthesiology, Vol. 2*. St. Louis, MO: Mosby Year Book; 1993:1236, with permission from Elsevier.]

TABLE 45-4 Dissociation Constants (Rounded)

Local Anesthetic	pK_a
Benzocaine	3.5
Mepivacaine	7.7
Lidocaine	7.8
Etidocaine	7.9
Prilocaine	7.9
Ropivacaine	8.1
Bupivacaine	8.1
Tetracaine	8.4
Cocaine	8.6
Dibucaine	8.8
Procaine	8.9
Chloroprocaine	9.1
Hexylcaine	9.3
Procainamide	9.3
Piperocaine	9.8

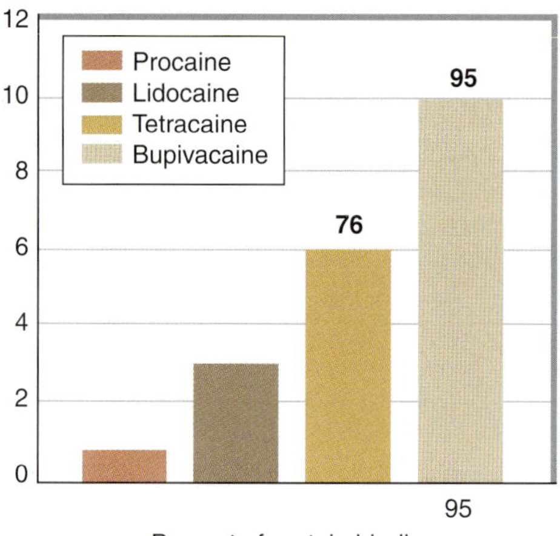

FIGURE 45-12. Relationship between duration of brachial plexus blockade of various local anesthetics and their degree of protein binding. [Reprinted from Covino BG. Pharmacology of local anesthetic agents. In: Rogers MC, Tinker JH, Covino BG, et al, eds. *Principles and Practice of Anesthesiology, Vol. 2*. St. Louis, MO: Mosby Year Book; 1993:1238, with permission from Elsevier.]

The pK_a of all local anesthetics, except benzocaine, varies from 7.6 to 9.1 and is greater than the physiologic pH (7.4) of tissue (**Table 45-4**). At a pH of 7.4, approximately 2% of procaine (pK_a of 9.1) exists in the base form. In contrast, 35% of mepivacaine, lidocaine, etidocaine, and prilocaine, which possess a pK_a of approximately 7.6, are present in the un-ionized forms. The pH of most local anesthetic solutions is approximately 5 to 6 because of the relatively low solubility of local anesthetics in solutions of higher pH. The inclusion of epinephrine in local anesthetic solutions results in a further decrease in pH to approximately 3 to 4.

Studies in vitro clearly demonstrate the relationship among the pK_a of specific agents, the pH of anesthetic solution, and the onset of conduction block.[51-53] Agents with a relatively low pK_a, such as lidocaine and mepivacaine, show the most rapid onset of conduction block. Procaine, chloroprocaine, and tetracaine, which possess high pK_a values, demonstrate a longer latency. The onset of conduction blockade is also reduced by increasing the pH of the bathing solution.[52] Clinically, onset time may be influenced by the dose or concentration of local anesthetic employed.[54] For example, increasing the concentration of bupivacaine from 0.25% to 0.75% results in a significant acceleration in anesthetic effect. Despite its pK_a being approximately 9 and its onset of action in isolated nerves being relatively slow, chloroprocaine demonstrates a rapid onset of action in humans. This is because chloroprocaine's low systemic toxicity allows the use of high concentrations such as 3%. Lidocaine has been shown in some studies to produce a more rapid onset of epidural anesthesia than chloroprocaine when employed at the same concentrations. However, use of a 3% chloroprocaine solution results in a more rapid onset of conduction block compared with 2.0% lidocaine.[55]

DURATION OF ACTION

The various local anesthetics have greatly different durations of action, and protein binding apparently is a determinant of duration (**Fig. 45-12**).[51] Procaine and chloroprocaine have a short duration of action; lidocaine, mepivacaine, and prilocaine have a moderate duration of anesthesia. Tetracaine, bupivacaine, levobupivacaine, etidocaine, and ropivacaine are associated with the longest durations of anesthesia. Procaine produces duration of brachial plexus blockade of 30 to 60 minutes—approximately 10 hours of anesthesia has been reported after the use of bupivacaine, etidocaine, and ropivacaine for brachial plexus blockade.

Local anesthetics are believed to act by binding to a protein receptor in the sodium channel,[4] and thus the greater protein binding of a specific agent presumably results in a longer period of sodium channel blockade and a longer duration of anesthesia. Plasma proteins have been used to measure protein binding of local anesthetics, assuming that binding to membrane proteins is similar to plasma protein binding.

Duration of action of the various agents is influenced by their peripheral vascular effects. Local anesthetics except cocaine generally tend to have a biphasic effect on vascular smooth muscle.[56-58] These agents cause vasoconstriction at low concentrations and vasodilatation at clinically employed concentrations. The protein kinase C Rho and p44/42 mitogen-activated protein kinase signaling pathways in calcium sensitization mechanisms may be involved in the biphasic action.[59] Choi et al[60] reported that levobupivacaine-induced contraction of rat aorta smooth muscle is mediated mainly by activation of the lipoxygenase pathway and in part by the activation of the cyclooxygenase pathway. Lipoxygenase pathway activation by levobupivacaine apparently facilitates calcium influx via L-type channels and endothelial nitric oxide attenuates levobupivacaine-induced contractions.

Differences exist in the vasodilator activity of the various drugs. Lidocaine is a more potent vasodilator than mepivacaine or prilocaine. In vivo, the duration of anesthesia produced by lidocaine is shorter than that of mepivacaine or prilocaine. If epinephrine is added to solutions of these agents, the duration of action for all 3 drugs is similar. The duration of action of ropivacaine is similar to that of bupivacaine when the agents are administered for peripheral or central neural blocks.[61,62] However, ropivacaine produces a significantly longer duration of infiltration anesthesia than bupivacaine in animals, which appears related to ropivacaine's cutaneous vasoconstrictor effects (**Fig. 45-13**).[58,61]

DIFFERENTIAL SENSORY/MOTOR BLOCK

Differential block is observed clinically but is poorly understood. Local anesthetic agents differ with respect to producing motor versus sensory block. The most significant separation between sensory anesthesia and motor blockades is produced by bupivacaine.[63] Depending on the concentration of bupivacaine employed, significant sensory anesthesia may be obtained with little inhibition of motor activity. Ropivacaine appears to provide a similar degree of sensory/motor separation.[64]

Bupivacaine and etidocaine are notably different in terms of their differential sensor/motor fiber–blocking activity (**Fig. 45-14**). Bupivacaine is widely used epidurally for obstetric procedures and relief of pain postoperatively because of its ability to provide adequate analgesia with minimal muscle weakness or paralysis, particularly as a 0.125% or 0.25% solution. In contrast, etidocaine shows little separation between blockade of sensory and motor fibers and thus achieved limited popularity.[65]

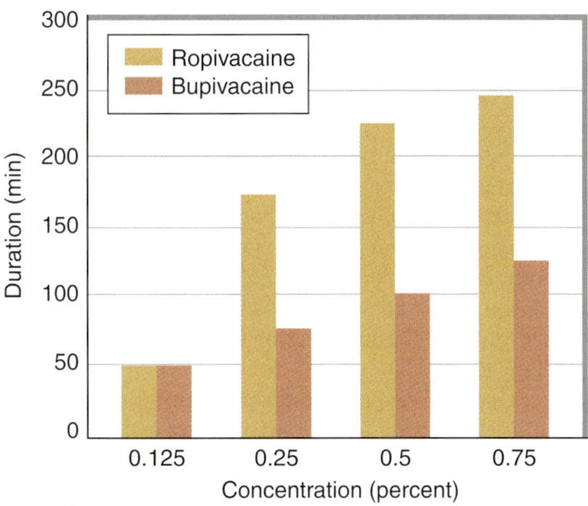

FIGURE 45-13. Relationship between duration of infiltration anesthesia and concentration of bupivacaine and ropivacaine. [Reprinted from Covino BG. Pharmacology of local anesthetic agents. In: Rogers MC, Tinker JH, Covino BG, et al, eds. *Principles and Practice of Anesthesiology, Vol. 2*. St. Louis, MO: Mosby Year Book; 1993:1239, with permission from Elsevier.]

INFLUENCE OF DOSE

An increase in the dose of local anesthetic usually results in a more profound depth of block, a prolongation of satisfactory anesthesia, and a decrease in the onset of block.[63,64] No clinically significant differences in onset, depth, and duration of anesthesia appear to exist when the same dose of local anesthetic is administered as a large volume of dilute solution or as a small volume of concentrated solution. A comparison of 15 mL of 2% prilocaine with 10 mL of 3% prilocaine (300 mg) and 30 mL of 2% prilocaine with 20 mL of 3% prilocaine (600 mg) for epidural blockade showed no difference in onset, adequacy, or duration of anesthesia and onset, depth, and duration of motor blockade if the dose was maintained constant (**Fig. 45-15**).[66] However, the increase in total dose from 300 to 600 mg of prilocaine did result in a more rapid onset, a greater degree of satisfactory anesthesia, and a prolonged duration of anesthesia.

Similar studies of spinal anesthesia indicate little difference between the use of varying volumes of 0.5% and 0.75% bupivacaine if the total dose was constant (**Fig. 45-16**).[46] The volume of anesthetic solution

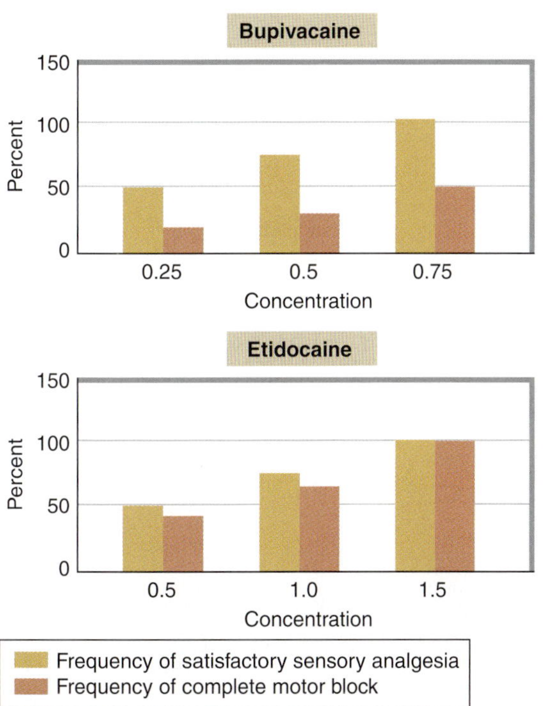

FIGURE 45-14. Frequency of satisfactory sensory analgesia and frequency of motor block produced by bupivacaine and etidocaine at various concentrations. [Reprinted from Covino BG. Pharmacology of local anesthetic agents. In: Rogers MC, Tinker JH, Covino BG, et al, eds. *Principles and Practice of Anesthesiology, Vol. 2*. St. Louis, MO: Mosby Year Book; 1993:1239, with permission from Elsevier.]

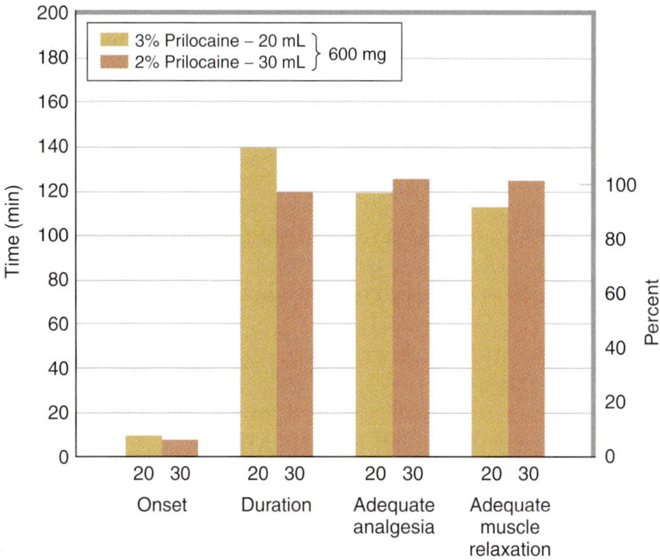

FIGURE 45-15. Relationship between onset, duration, and frequency of adequate analgesia and frequency of adequate muscle relaxation produced by prilocaine when used as either a 3% solution or a 2% solution for epidural blockade. [Reprinted from Covino BG. Pharmacology of local anesthetic agents. In: Rogers MC, Tinker JH, Covino BG, et al, eds. *Principles and Practice of Anesthesiology, Vol. 2*. St. Louis, MO: Mosby Year Book; 1993:1240, with permission from Elsevier.]

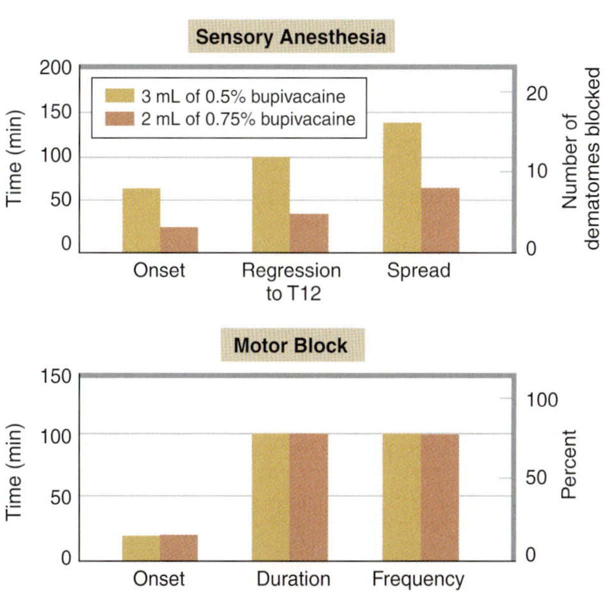

FIGURE 45-16. Relationship between onset, duration, and spread of sensory anesthesia and onset, duration, and frequency of motor block produced by bupivacaine when employed as either a 0.5% or a 0.75% solution for intrathecal use. [Reprinted from Covino BG. Pharmacology of local anesthetic agents. In: Rogers MC, Tinker JH, Covino BG, et al, eds. *Principles and Practice of Anesthesiology, Vol. 2*. St. Louis, MO: Mosby Year Book; 1993:1240, with permission from Elsevier.]

may influence the spread of anesthetic in the epidural or subarachnoid space. For example, the level of anesthesia was 4.3 dermatomes higher when 30 mL of 1% lidocaine was injected epidurally compared with 10 mL of 3% lidocaine.[67] In general, increased dosage is usually achieved by the use of more concentrated anesthetic solutions, as the volume of solution that can be administered is usually restricted by the anatomy of the specific injection site.

More recently, Latzke et al[48] used ultrasound-guided sciatic nerve block with 1.5% mepivacaine to examine the effect of volume on sensory block onset and duration of sensory block. As compared with larger volumes, the ED_{99} volume had no effect on onset but shortened block duration.

FORMULATIONS

PURPOSE OF DIFFERENT FORMULATIONS

Local anesthetics are mixed with other substances during the manufacturing process or just prior to administration. Some objectives of this practice are to shorten onset time, limit absorption, increase intensity of action, stabilize local anesthetic molecule, and inhibit microbial growth. A 2004 issue of *Techniques in Regional Anesthesia and Pain Medicine* discussed in detail additives to local anesthetics.[68]

MIXTURES OF LOCAL ANESTHETICS

Mixtures of local anesthetics have been employed by adding an agent, such as chloroprocaine or lidocaine, which have a relatively rapid onset, to a solution of bupivacaine, which has a slow but long duration of action. A mixture of 3% chloroprocaine and 0.5% bupivacaine was reported to produce a rapid onset and prolonged duration of brachial plexus blockade.[69] Subsequent epidural studies indicated that a mixture of chloroprocaine and bupivacaine resulted in a slower onset than chloroprocaine alone and a shorter duration than bupivacaine alone.[70] Isolated nerve studies demonstrate that the addition of a metabolite of chloroprocaine to bupivacaine significantly decreased the duration of conduction block compared with bupivacaine alone (**Fig. 45-17**).[71] To date, no similar antagonism has been demonstrated when lidocaine or mepivacaine is mixed with bupivacaine. One should remember that in terms of the potential systemic toxicity of mixtures of local anesthetics, the toxicity of local anesthetics is additive if an unintentional IV injection occurs.

USE OF VASOCONSTRICTORS

Epinephrine (1:200 000; 5 μg/mL) is frequently added to local anesthetic solutions to decrease the rate of vascular absorption.[31] This allows more anesthetic molecules to diffuse to the nerve membrane and thus improves the depth and duration of anesthesia. Epinephrine 1:200 000 has been reported to be the optimal concentration for prolonging the duration of anesthesia of lidocaine for epidural or intercostals use. Other vasoconstrictor agents, such as norepinephrine and phenylephrine, have been used but do not appear to be superior to epinephrine. For example, equipotent concentrations of epinephrine and phenylephrine similarly prolong the duration of spinal anesthesia produced by tetracaine (**Fig. 45-18**).[72]

Epinephrine's ability to prolong the duration of anesthesia depends on the local anesthetic employed and the injection site. Epinephrine significantly extends the duration of both infiltration anesthesia and peripheral nerve blocks with most agents.[73,74] The duration of surgical epidural anesthesia, however, is not greatly prolonged when epinephrine is combined with prilocaine, bupivacaine, or etidocaine, but does result in a significant increase in the duration of epidural blockade produced by agents such as lidocaine.[75,76] Diluted solutions of bupivacaine employed for epidural analgesia in obstetric patients may be improved with the addition of epinephrine. The depth and duration of epidural analgesia in obstetric patients were improved when epinephrine 1:300 000 was added to 0.25% bupivacaine.[77] Although the addition of epinephrine may not significantly prolong the duration of surgical epidural anesthesia produced by 0.5% to 0.75% bupivacaine, a more profound degree of motor blockade has been observed after the use of bupivacaine with epinephrine.[75]

Epinephrine's ability to prolong spinal anesthesia may be partly related to a direct antinociceptive effect in the spinal cord. Adrenergic receptor agents exert a direct antinociceptive action in the spinal cord. For example, clonidine, an α_2-adrenergic agonist, produces analgesia after epidural administration.[78]

Epinephrine's effect on the onset of regional anesthesia is controversial. Some studies demonstrate a more rapid onset of conduction blockade, presumably because of the decreased vascular absorption of local anesthetics.[73] Others fail to demonstrate any difference in onset time.[79] This is attributed to the low pH of epinephrine-containing local anesthetic solutions, which favor the formation of the local anesthetics cationic form, which does not easily diffuse through nerve sheaths.

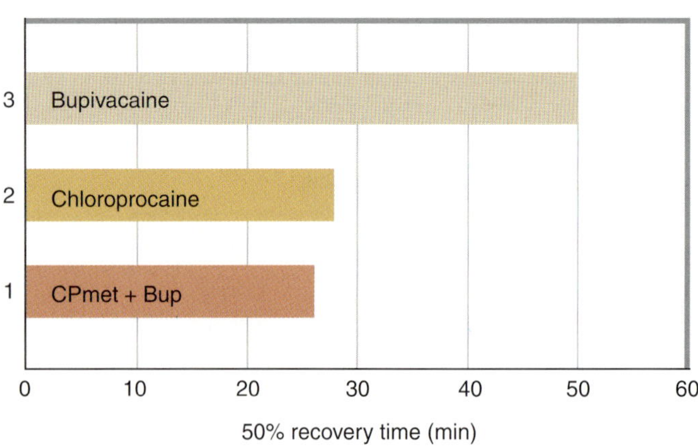

FIGURE 45-17. Recovery of conduction blockade in isolated nerve after exposure to bupivacaine alone, chloroprocaine alone, and mixture of a chloroprocaine metabolite and bupivacaine. [Reprinted from Covino BG. Pharmacology of local anesthetic agents. In: Rogers MC, Tinker JH, Covino BG, et al, eds. *Principles and Practice of Anesthesiology, Vol. 2*. St. Louis, MO: Mosby Year Book, 1993:1243, with permission from Elsevier.]

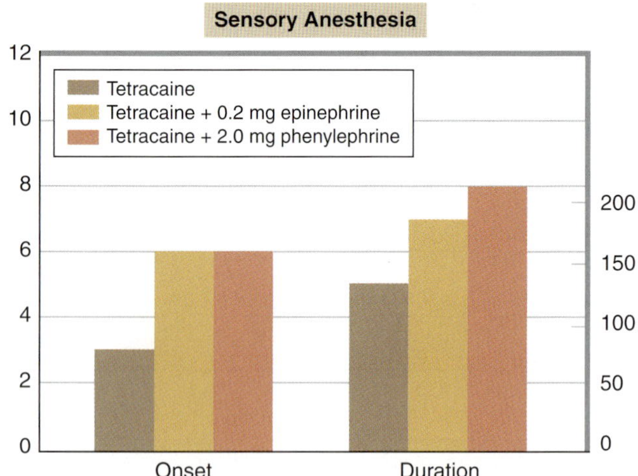

FIGURE 45-18. Relationship between onset and duration of spinal anesthesia after use of plain tetracaine, tetracaine with epinephrine, and tetracaine with phenylephrine. [Reprinted from Covino BG. Pharmacology of local anesthetic agents. In: Rogers MC, Tinker JH, Covino BG, et al, eds. *Principles and Practice of Anesthesiology, Vol. 2*. St. Louis, MO: Mosby Year Book; 1993:1241, with permission from Elsevier.]

CARBONATION AND PH ADJUSTMENT OF LOCAL ANESTHETICS

Carbonation of local anesthetics results in a more rapid onset and a more profound degree of conduction blockade in an isolated nerve preparation.[52,80,81] The enhanced onset is believed to be related to a more rapid dissociation of the local anesthetic to the base form, a direct depressant effect of carbon dioxide (CO_2) on the nerve membrane, and a decrease in the axoplasmic pH from the diffusion of CO_2 intraneurally. The lower axoplasmic pH increases the rate of formation of the local anesthetic's active cationic form within the nerve. Although CO_2 clearly enhances the onset of local anesthetic-induced conduction block in an isolated nerve, discrepancies exist among clinical studies in which hydrochloride and carbonated local anesthetic solutions have been compared. Several investigations have demonstrated a significant decrease in the onset of epidural blockade with lidocaine carbonate compared with lidocaine hydrochloride.[82,83] However, other researchers have failed to observe a significant reduction in onset of epidural anesthesia with lidocaine carbonate.[84] Similarly, differing results concerning onset time have been reported when bupivacaine hydrochloride and bupivacaine carbonate were employed for brachial plexus blocks.[85,86] Although controversy may exist regarding the effect of carbonation on onset of anesthesia, most studies show that carbonated solutions do improve the depth of sensory and motor blockade when administered into the epidural cavity. Also, these solutions produce a more complete blockade of the various nerve roots when employed for brachial plexus blockade.

Alkalinization of local anesthetic solutions by the addition of solution bicarbonate has also been reported to decrease the onset of conduction blockade (**Fig. 45-19**).[87,88] An increase in the pH of the local anesthetic solution increases the amount of drug in the uncharged base form, which should enhance the rate of diffusion across the nerve sheath and nerve membrane. The use of pH-adjusted solutions of bupivacaine or lidocaine has been reported to significantly decrease the latency of brachial plexus and epidural blockade.[87,88] Again, controversy surrounds the improved onset of pH-adjusted local anesthetic solutions. Some investigators have failed to demonstrate an improved onset of brachial plexus or epidural blockade with the use of pH-adjusted solutions of bupivacaine or lidocaine.[89,90] The differences between these studies might be related to the magnitude of the pH change produced by the addition of bicarbonate. In the original study in which onset time for brachial plexus blockade was significantly reduced, the pH of bupivacaine with epinephrine was increased from 3.9 to 6.4.[88] In the subsequent study in which no effect on latency was observed, the pH of plain bupivacaine was increased from 5.5 to 7.0.[89] The amount of bicarbonate added to local anesthetic solutions depends on the particular local anesthetic. One milliliter of sodium bicarbonate is added to 10 mL of lidocaine, whereas 0.1 mL of bicarbonate is added to every 10 mL of bupivacaine. The latter agent is insoluble at a high pH, and the addition of excess bicarbonate will result in a precipitation of bupivacaine.

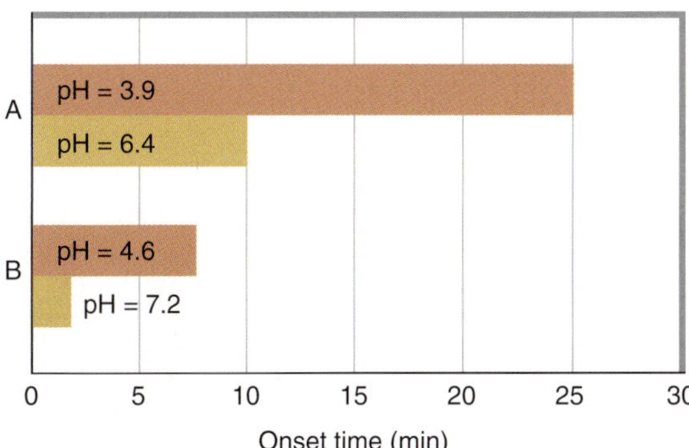

FIGURE 45-19. Comparison of onset of brachial plexus blockade with bupivacaine (**A**) and onset of epidural blockade with lidocaine (**B**) using solutions of varying pH. [Reprinted from Covino BG. Pharmacology of local anesthetic agents. In: Rogers MC, Tinker JH, Covino BG, et al, eds. *Principles and Practice of Anesthesiology, Vol. 2.* St. Louis, MO: Mosby Year Book; 1993:1243, with permission from Elsevier.]

HYALURONIDASE, LIPOSOMES, MICROENCAPSULATION

Hyaluronidase (tissue spreading factor) is sometimes added to local anesthetic solutions to facilitate spread of solution at the injection site, thereby affecting speed of onset and extent of a block. This seems only to be useful when local anesthetic is injected in the orbit preparatory to ophthalmologic surgery. Hyaluronidase may be injected with local anesthetic during epidural neurolysis to treat pain with positive benefit. Various attempts have been made to prolong the duration of action of local anesthetics by loading them into liposomes or microcapsules, but no such formulations have been approved by the US Food and Drug Administration (FDA) for marketing.

TOXICITY

Table 45-5 shows categories of the toxic effects of local anesthetics.

ALLERGIC REACTIONS

True allergic reactions are associated with amino ester–linked local anesthetics, not amino amide–linked ones. In a study of anaphylactic and anaphylactoid reactions (n = 789) occurring during anesthesia, Mertes et al[91] found no such reactions to local anesthetics. However, Mackley et al[92] reported that of 183 patients who were patch tested, 4 had positive reactions to lidocaine, 2 of whom had histories of sensitivity to local injections of lidocaine manifested by dermatitis. They concluded that contact-type IV sensitivity to lidocaine might occur more frequently than previously thought. It is common, but inappropriate, to refer to all adverse events as "allergic reactions."

TISSUE TOXICITY

Tissue toxicity, primarily myotoxicity and neurotoxicity, can be produced by all local anesthetics if "high" concentrations are used. Signs and symptoms of varying degrees of neuropathy (eg, transient neurologic symptoms, cauda equina syndrome) have been reported after spinal anesthesia with, for example, 2% and 5% lidocaine. In a systematic review, Zaric et al[93] compared the frequency of transient neurologic symptoms and neurologic complications after spinal anesthesia with lidocaine with that after other local anesthetics. The results showed that the risk for developing transient neurologic symptoms after spinal anesthesia with lidocaine was higher with lidocaine than with bupivacaine, prilocaine, procaine, or mepivacaine.

SYSTEMIC TOXICITY

Methemoglobinemia A variety of local anesthetics reportedly may produce methemoglobinemia. Prilocaine is the local anesthetic for which there appears to be greatest risk for this to occur. A dose–response relationship exists between the amount of prilocaine administered epidurally and the degree of methemoglobinemia. In general, doses of prilocaine of 600 mg are required for the development of clinically significant levels of methemoglobinemia.[94] The formation of methemoglobinemia is believed to be related to prilocaine's chemical structure. This agent lacks a methyl group in the benzene ring. The metabolism of

TABLE 45-5 Categories of Local Anesthetic Toxic Reactions

Localized or Systemic	Systemic	Localized
Allergic reactions	Cardiac/vascular Central nervous system Methemoglobin	Tissue toxicity

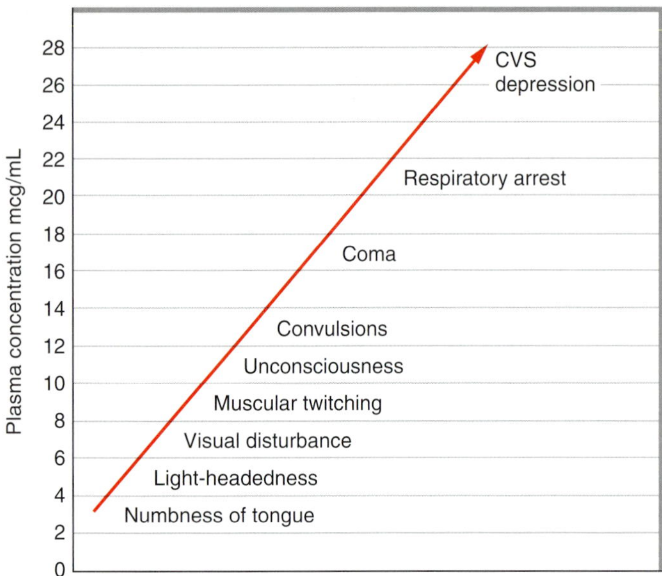

FIGURE 45-20. Plasma concentration of lidocaine versus systemic toxicity. CVS, cardiovascular system.

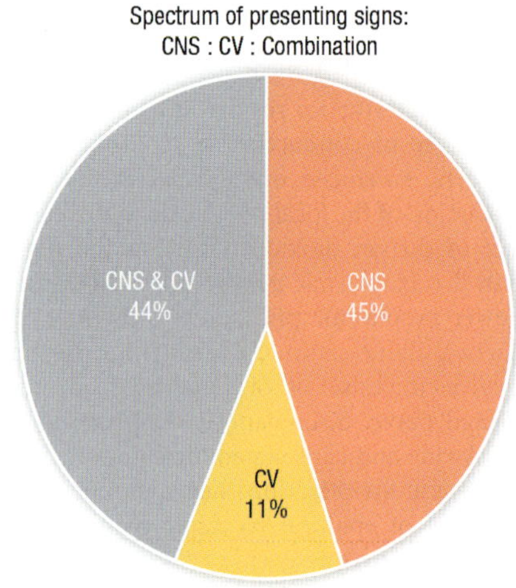

FIGURE 45-21. The frequency of symptoms and signs referable to cardiovascular system (CV), central nervous system (CNS), or both. [Reprinted from Neal JM, Weinberg GL, Bernards CM, et al. ASRA practice advisory on local anesthetic systemic toxicity. *Reg Anesth Pain Med.* 2010;35:152-161, with permission from American Society of Regional Anesthesia and Pain Medicine.]

prilocaine in the liver results in the formation of O-toluidine, which is responsible for the oxidation of hemoglobin to methemoglobin.[95] The methemoglobinemia associated with prilocaine is spontaneously reversible or may be treated by IV methylene blue.

Cardiovascular and Central Nervous System As concentration of local anesthetic in systemic circulation increases, various cardiovascular system and central nervous system (CNS) signs and symptoms appear (**Fig. 45-20**). The relative CNS and cardiovascular toxicity of local anesthetics has been of interest, especially after Albright[96] reported unexpected cardiovascular toxicity of bupivacaine. Most animal studies show that the ratio of doses of bupivacaine that produced convulsive activity and cardiovascular collapse are lower than for other local anesthetics.[97] Human volunteer studies of doses required to produce early features of CNS and cardiovascular system toxicity by ropivacaine and levobupivacaine demonstrated the doses were about equal and higher than for bupivacaine.[98-100]

Brown et al[101] reviewed records of patients who had seizures while undergoing brachial plexus, epidural, and caudal regional anesthetics. No adverse cardiovascular, pulmonary or nervous system events were associated with any of the seizures, including in 16 patients who received bupivacaine blocks. Clinically, which of the usual features of systemic local anesthetic toxicity occurs, the order in which they occur and how soon after local anesthetic administration are quite variable (**Fig. 45-21**).[102] This is not surprising given what is known about how various health conditions, other drugs, and rate of increase of local anesthetic concentration in systemic circulation influence the manifestation and progression of signs and symptoms of local anesthetic toxicity.

In dogs, the relative CNS toxicity of bupivacaine, etidocaine, and lidocaine is 4:2:1,[103] which is similar to the relative potency of these agents for the production of regional anesthesia in humans. The convulsant doses of bupivacaine and ropivacaine are similar.[104] IV infusion studies in human volunteers have also demonstrated an inverse relationship between the intrinsic anesthetic potency of various agents and the dosage required to induce CNS toxicity.[105,106]

The rate of IV administration alters the toxicity of local anesthetic agents.[106] In human volunteers, an average dose of 236 mg of etidocaine and a venous blood concentration of 3.0 μg/mL resulted in CNS symptoms when 10 mg/min was infused. When the infusion rate was increased to 20 mg/min, an average of 161 mg of etidocaine, which produced a venous plasma concentration of approximately 2 μg/mL, caused symptoms of CNS toxicity.

Acid–base status can alter the CNS activity of local anesthetic agents. In cats, the convulsive threshold of various local anesthetics is inversely related to the arterial CO_2 tension ($Paco_2$)[107] (**Fig. 45-22**). An increase in $Paco_2$ from 25 to 40 mm Hg to a range of 65 to 81 mm Hg decreases the convulsive threshold of procaine, mepivacaine, prilocaine, lidocaine, and bupivacaine by approximately 50%. A decrease in arterial pH also decreases the convulsant threshold of these agents. Respiratory acidosis, with a resultant increase in $Paco_2$ and a decrease in arterial pH, consistently decreases the convulsant threshold of local anesthetic agents. However, an elevation in both $Paco_2$ and arterial pH, as may occur during metabolic alkalosis, does not increase CNS toxicity to the same degree.

Hypercarbia increases cerebral blood flow, which probably results in a greater uptake of local anesthetic by the brain. In addition, diffusion

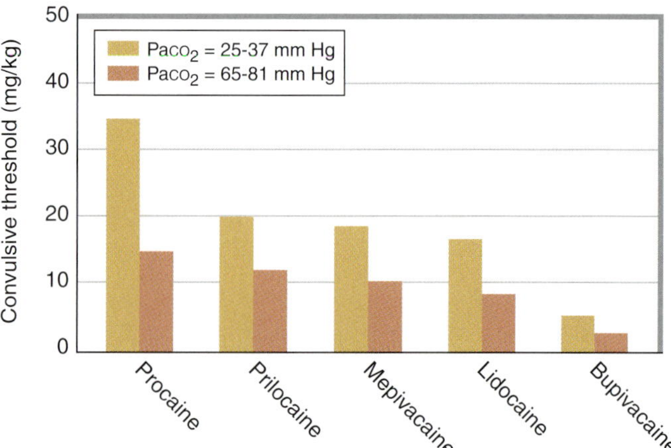

FIGURE 45-22. Relationship between convulsive threshold doses of various local anesthetics and arterial CO_2 tension ($Paco_2$). [Reprinted from Covino BG. Pharmacology of local anesthetic agents. In: Rogers MC, Tinker JH, Covino BG, et al, eds. *Principles and Practice of Anesthesiology, Vol. 2.* St. Louis, MO: Mosby Year Book, 1993:1247, with permission from Elsevier.]

of CO_2 into neuronal cells decreases intracellular pH and thus increases the intracellular cationic form of the local anesthetic agents. This form does not diffuse well across the nerve membrane, so ion trapping occurs. Hypercarbia and/or acidosis also decrease the plasma protein binding of local anesthetic agents, which will increase the proportion of free drug available for diffusion into the brain.[108,109] On the other hand, acidosis also decreases the percentage of the local anesthetic existing in the base form, which should decrease the rate of diffusion into neuronal cells.

Local anesthetics have a direct effect on both cardiac muscle and vascular smooth muscle.[97] These agents alter the heart's electrical and mechanical activity. Studies using the intact, isolated mammalian heart in vitro show that highly lipid-soluble, extensively protein-bound, highly potent local anesthetics (eg, tetracaine, bupivacaine, etidocaine) are much more cardiotoxic than are the less lipid-soluble, protein-bound, potent local anesthetics (eg, lidocaine, mepivacaine, prilocaine).[110] Bupivacaine has a potent depressant effect on electrical conduction in the heart primarily via an action on voltage-gated sodium channels that generally govern the initial rapid depolarization (phase 0) of cardiomyocytes. The S forms of bupivacaine are less cardiotoxic than the R form. Bupivacaine actions other than on voltage-gated sodium channels probably also contribute to dose-dependent cardiotoxic effect of this local anesthetic.

Local anesthetics decrease the maximal rate of depolarization in Purkinje fibers and ventricular muscle because of an inhibition of sodium channels in cardiac membranes.[111-113] Action potential duration and the effective refractory period are also decreased by local anesthetics. However, the ratio of effective refractory period to action potential duration is increased both in Purkinje fibers and in ventricular muscle.

Qualitative differences exist between the various local anesthetic agents. Bupivacaine depresses the rapid phase of depolarization (V_{max}) in Purkinje fibers and ventricular muscle to a greater extent than does lidocaine.[111-113] In addition, the rate of recovery from a use-dependent block is slower in bupivacaine-treated than in lidocaine-treated papillary muscles.[114] This slow rate of recovery results in an incomplete restoration of V_{max} between action potentials, particularly at high heart rates. In contrast, recovery from lidocaine is complete, even at rapid heart rates. These differential effects of lidocaine and bupivacaine may explain the antidysrhythmic properties of lidocaine and the dysrhythmogenic potential of bupivacaine.

Bupivacaine, and to a lesser degree etidocaine and ropivacaine, can produce severe cardiac dysrhythmias, including ventricular fibrillation, in various animal species.[97,115-119] Ventricular dysrhythmias are rarely seen with lidocaine, mepivacaine, or tetracaine. Although the dysrhythmogenic action of bupivacaine is probably related primarily to an inhibition of the fast sodium channels in the cardiac membrane, evidence also exists that this agent may block the slow calcium channels.[120] These electrophysiologic effects of bupivacaine may result in conduction abnormalities, leading to a reentrant type of dysrhythmia similar to a torsade de pointes dysrhythmia.[116]

The dysrhythmogenic activity of bupivacaine is believed to result primarily from a direct cardiac effect. Isolated guinea pig hearts perfused with bupivacaine revealed evidence of conduction block, bigeminy, and trigeminy.[121] In addition, ventricular fibrillation occurred in intact pigs in which bupivacaine was injected directly into the left anterior descending coronary artery.[118] On the other hand, the injection of bupivacaine directly into certain regions of the brain may result in cardiac dysrhythmias, which may indicate a relationship between the CNS and cardiotoxic effects of bupivacaine.[122,123]

Electrophysiologic studies in intact dogs and in people have shown that high blood levels of local anesthetics prolong conduction time through various parts of the heart as indicated by an increase in the PR interval and QRS duration. Extremely high concentrations of local anesthetics depress spontaneous pacemaker activity in the sinus node, resulting in sinus bradycardia and sinus arrest.

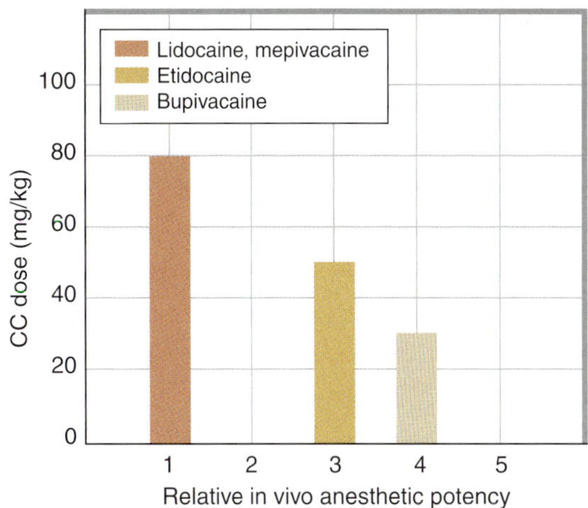

FIGURE 45-23. Relationship between dose of various local anesthetics that causes cardiovascular collapse (CC) and in vivo anesthetic potency of these agents. [Reprinted from Covino BG. Pharmacology of local anesthetic agents. In: Rogers MC, Tinker JH, Covino BG, et al, eds. *Principles and Practice of Anesthesiology, Vol. 2.* St. Louis, MO: Mosby Year Book; 1993:1249, with permission from Elsevier.]

Local anesthetic agents also depress myocardial contractility. All local anesthetics exert a dose-dependent negative inotropic action on isolated cardiac tissue that is proportional to the conduction blocking potency of the various agents in isolated nerves (**Fig. 45-23**).[124] For example, bupivacaine, tetracaine, and etidocaine produce the greatest degree of myocardial depression. The agents of moderate anesthetic potency (ie, lidocaine, mepivacaine, prilocaine) are intermediate in terms of their negative inotropic action. Procaine and chloroprocaine, which are the least-potent local anesthetics, require the highest concentration to decrease cardiac contractility.

In dogs, tetracaine is approximately 8 to 10 times more potent than procaine as a local anesthetic and as a myocardial depressant.[125] Hemodynamic studies in closed-chest anesthetized dogs have shown that tetracaine, etidocaine, and bupivacaine caused a 50% decrease in cardiac output at doses of 10 to 20 mg/kg, whereas doses of 30 to 40 mg/kg of lidocaine, mepivacaine, prilocaine, and chloroprocaine were required for a similar decrease in cardiac output. A dose of 100 mg/kg of procaine was needed to reduce cardiac output to 50%.

Most local anesthetic agents exert a biphasic effect on peripheral vascular smooth muscle.[56,57] Low concentrations of lidocaine and bupivacaine produced vasoconstriction in the cremaster muscle of rats, whereas high concentrations increased arteriolar diameter, indicative of vasodilatation. In vivo studies also demonstrate that low doses of local anesthetics decrease peripheral arterial flow without any change in blood pressure, whereas higher doses increase blood flow. Cocaine causes vasoconstriction because of its ability to inhibit the uptake of norepinephrine by storage granules.[126] Studies indicate that ropivacaine causes cutaneous vasoconstriction, whereas bupivacaine produces vasodilatation.[59]

In a review of the cardiotoxicity of modern local anesthetics, Mather and Chang[127] concluded that as compared with bupivacaine, although ropivacaine and levobupivacaine may be seen as "safer," they must not be regarded as totally "safe."

FACTORS INFLUENCING CARDIOVASCULAR TOXICITY

Specific Agents Although the CNS is more susceptible to the toxic effects of local anesthetics than the cardiovascular system, differences exist in the margin between the dose of various agents that causes convulsions and the dose that results in cardiovascular collapse (**Fig. 45-24**). A cardiovascular collapse (CC)-to-convulsive (CNS) dose ratio of 7.1 + 1.1 was reported for lidocaine in adult sheep, indicating

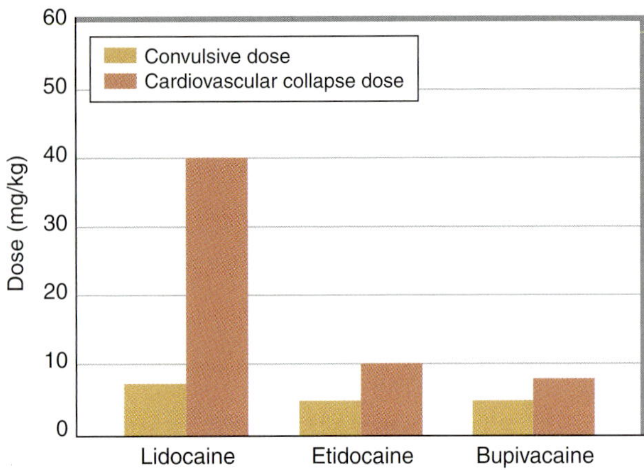

FIGURE 45-24. Relationship between dose of lidocaine, bupivacaine, and etidocaine that causes CNS toxicity and dose that produces cardiovascular collapse. [Reprinted from Covino BG. Pharmacology of local anesthetic agents. In: Rogers MC, Tinker JH, Covino BG, et al, eds. *Principles and Practice of Anesthesiology, Vol. 2.* St. Louis, MO: Mosby Year Book; 1993:1249, with permission from Elsevier.]

that 7 times as much drug was required to induce irreversible cardiovascular collapse as to cause convulsions.[128] The CC:CNS ratio for bupivacaine was 3.7 + 0.5 and for etidocaine, 4.4 + 0.9. The CC:CNS blood level ratio of lidocaine was 3.6 + 0.3, compared with values of 1.6 to 1.7 for bupivacaine and etidocaine. At the time of cardiovascular collapse, high concentrations of bupivacaine and etidocaine were present in the myocardium compared with lidocaine, which suggests that the enhanced cardiac toxicity of these more potent agents may result from a greater myocardial uptake.

Pregnancy Data regarding the effects of pregnancy on the cardiovascular toxicity of local anesthetic are not conclusive.

Acidosis and Hypoxia Hypercarbia, acidosis, and hypoxia potentiate the negative chronotropic and inotropic action of lidocaine and bupivacaine in isolated cardiac tissue.[129] The combination of hypoxia and acidosis greatly potentiates the cardiodepressant effects of bupivacaine. Hypoxia and acidosis also increase the frequency of cardiac dysrhythmias and the mortality rate in sheep after the IV administration of bupivacaine.[130] Hypercarbia, acidosis, and hypoxia occur very rapidly in some patients after seizure activity because of the rapid unintentional intravascular injection of local anesthetic agents.[131] Thus the cardiovascular depression observed in some patients after the accidental IV injection of bupivacaine may be related in part to the severe acid–base changes that occur during toxic reactions to this agent.

Measures to prevent systemic toxic reactions to local anesthetics include following dose recommendations, injecting aliquots over time, avoiding unintentional intravascular injections, and monitoring vital signs during injection. Blanket recommended doses versus block-specific recommended doses were discussed recently.[132,133] Drug administration must be stopped should signs or symptoms of toxicity develop. Seizures induced by local anesthetics are usually self-limiting and require maintenance of respiratory gas exchange and control of muscle contractions (eg, intubation, oxygenation, short-acting muscle paralysis). Drugs such as propofol, thiopental, and benzodiazepines are effective against these seizures.

Cardiovascular toxicity is treated according to American Heart Association guidelines, depending on the nature of the toxicity. Recent evidence suggests that in some instances, lipid emulsion infusion may be beneficial.[134] Recently published recommendations by the American Society of Regional Anesthesia and Pain Medicine for treatment of local anesthetic systemic toxicity are summarized in **Table 45-6.**[135]

TABLE 45-6 Practice Advisory on Treatment of Local Anesthetic Systemic Toxicity for Patients Experiencing Signs or Symptoms of Local Anesthetic Systemic Toxicity (LAST)

Get Help
Initial Focus
- ***Airway management:*** ventilate with 100% oxygen
- ***Seizure suppression:*** benzodiazepines are preferred
- ***Basic and advanced cardiac life support (BLS/ACLS)*** may require prolonged effort

Infuse 20% lipid emulsion (values in parenthesis are for a 70-kg patient)
- ***Bolus 1.5 mL/kg*** (lean body mass) intravenously over 1 min (~100 mL)
- ***Continuous infusion at 0.25 mL/kg/min*** (~18 mL/min; adjust by roller clamp)
- Repeat bolus once or twice for persistent cardiovascular collapse
- Double the infusion rate to 0.5 mL/kg/min if blood pressure remains low
- ***Continue infusion*** for at least 10 min after attaining circulatory stability
- Recommended upper limit: approximately 10 mL/kg lipid emulsion over the first 30 min

Avoid vasopressin, calcium channel blockers, β-blockers, or local anesthetic
Alert the nearest facility having cardiopulmonary bypass capability
Avoid propofol in patients having signs of cardiovascular instability

Modified from Neal JM, Weinberg GL, Bernards CM, et al. ASRA practice advisory on local anesthetic systemic toxicity. *Reg Anesth Pain Med.* 2010;35:152-161, with permission from American Society of Regional Anesthesia and Pain Medicine.

SPECIFIC LOCAL ANESTHETICS

LOCAL ANESTHETICS IN CLINICAL USE

Table 45-7 lists generic and trade names of local anesthetics. Undoubtedly, lidocaine is most commonly used to prevent procedure-related pain and for diagnostic tests. Intermediate- to long-acting local anesthetics, such as ropivacaine, levobupivacaine, and bupivacaine, are used for therapy.

TABLE 45-7 Generic and Trade Names of Local Anesthetics

Generic Name	Trade Name(s)
Benoxinate	Dorsacaine; Novesine
Bupivacaine	Marcaine; Sensorcaine
Butacaine	Butyn
Chloroprocaine (2-chloroprocaine)	Nesacaine
Cyclomethycaine	Surfacaine
Dibucaine	Nupercaine; Percaine
Etidocaine	Duranest
Hexylcaine	Cyclaine
Levobupivacaine	Chirocaine
Lidocaine	Xylocaine; Xylotox
Mepivacaine	Carbocaine; Polocaine
Piperocaine	Metycaine
Prilocaine	Citanest
Procaine	Novocain; Planocaine
Proparacaine	Ophthaine; Ocu-Caine
Ropivacaine	Naropin
Tetracaine	Pontocaine; Pantocaine

Because these local anesthetics are administered chiefly as the chloride or sulfate slats, it is more accurate to specify procaine hydrochloride than just procaine. Because the latter is the active species, it is the usually used term.

Modified with permission from deJong RH. *Local Anesthetics*. St. Louis, MO: Mosby-Year Book; 1994.

TABLE 45-8 Topical: Local Anesthetics and Available Dosage Forms

Benzocaine	Lidocaine/prilocaine
Cream	Cream
Ointment	Lidocaine/tetracaine
Topical aerosol	Patch
Benzocaine and menthol	Pramoxine
Lotion	Cream
Topical aerosol solution	Lotion
Butamben	Pramoxine and menthol
Ointment	Gel
Dibucaine	Lotion
Cream	Tetracaine
Ointment	Cream
Lidocaine	Tetracaine and menthol
Film-forming gel	Ointment
Ointment	
Patch	
Cream	

Table 45-8 lists topical anesthetics and dosage forms. Most of the forms are available without prescription. A 5% lidocaine patch (Lidoderm) is approved by the FDA for controlling postherpetic neuralgia.

AMINO ESTER AGENTS

Local anesthetics in this class have an ester linkage to benzoic acid or its derivatives. The amino ester–linked local anesthetics most commonly used clinically are procaine, chloroprocaine, and tetracaine. All of these agents were introduced into clinical practice by 1955.

Procaine Procaine was the first synthetic local anesthetic agent introduced into clinical practice. It is a relatively weak local anesthetic with a slow onset and a short duration of action. Its systemic toxicity is relatively low because of rapid plasma hydrolysis. Procaine is hydrolyzed to *p*-aminobenzoic acid, which is responsible for the allergic reactions associated with repeated use of procaine. Procaine is used primarily for infiltration anesthesia, diagnostic differential spinal blocks in certain pain states, and obstetric spinal anesthesia.

Chloroprocaine Chloroprocaine has rapid onset of action, short duration, and low systemic toxicity. It undergoes hydrolysis by human plasma esterases approximately 4 times faster than procaine. Chloroprocaine is primarily employed for epidural analgesia and anesthesia in obstetrics because of its rapid onset and low systemic toxicity in the mother and fetus. However, frequent injections are required to provide adequate pain relief during labor. Sometimes, epidural analgesia is established in the pregnant patient with chloroprocaine, followed by a longer-acting agent such as bupivacaine. Chloroprocaine has also proved of value for various regional anesthetic procedures in ambulatory surgical patients for whom surgery is not expected to exceed 30 to 60 minutes.

Concern about potential myotoxicity and neurotoxicity has haunted chloroprocaine.

Tetracaine Tetracaine is used primarily for spinal anesthesia. It may be employed as an isobaric, hypobaric, or hyperbaric solution for spinal blockade, although hyperbaric solutions of tetracaine are probably employed most often. Tetracaine provides a relatively rapid onset of spinal anesthesia, excellent qualities of sensory anesthesia, and a profound block of motor function. Plain solutions of tetracaine produce an average duration of spinal anesthesia of 2 to 3 hours, whereas the addition of epinephrine can extend anesthesia to 4 to 6 hours.

Tetracaine is rarely used for other forms of regional anesthesia because of its extremely slow onset of action and the potential for systemic toxic reactions when larger doses are employed.

Cocaine Cocaine was the first agent successfully employed clinically for the production of local anesthesia. It has limited use in modern anesthesia practice because of its relatively high potential for systemic toxicity and addiction liabilities. It is listed as a schedule II drug in the United States. Cocaine is an excellent topical anesthetic agent, and it produces vasoconstriction at clinically useful concentrations. As a result, it is still sometimes employed to anesthetize and constrict the nasal mucosa before nasotracheal intubation, and otolaryngologists use cocaine during nasal surgery because of its topical anesthetic and vasoconstrictor properties. It is the only local anesthetic that inhibits the reuptake of catecholamines in the central and peripheral nervous systems.

AMINO AMIDE AGENTS

Amino amide–linked local anesthetics most commonly used clinically are lidocaine, mepivacaine, ropivacaine, bupivacaine, and levobupivacaine. The first step in the biotransformation of the tertiary amine forms typically is dealkylation of the amino nitrogen by cytochrome P450 in the liver.

Lidocaine Lidocaine, the first of the amino amide–type local anesthetics to be introduced into clinical practice, remains the most versatile and most frequently used drug in this class. It is popular because of its inherent potency, rapid onset, moderate duration of action, and topical anesthetic activity. Solutions of lidocaine are available for infiltration, peripheral nerve blocks, and epidural anesthesia. In addition, hyperbaric lidocaine is useful for spinal anesthesia of 30 to 60 minutes' duration. Lidocaine is also used in ointment, jelly, viscous, and aerosol preparations for a variety of topical anesthetic procedures. Lidocaine currently is still the only agent officially approved in the United States for IV regional anesthesia.

Lidocaine is sometimes given intravenously as an antiepileptic agent, as an analgesic for certain chronic pain states, and as a supplement to general anesthesia. It is administered intravenously for the treatment of ventricular dysrhythmias.

Mepivacaine Mepivacaine has a local anesthetic profile similar to that of lidocaine. It can produce a profound depth of anesthesia with a relatively rapid onset and a moderate duration of action. Mepivacaine may be used for infiltration, peripheral nerve blocks, and epidural anesthesia, and in some countries, 4% hyperbaric solutions of mepivacaine are also available for spinal anesthesia.

It is ineffective as a topical anesthetic agent. The metabolism of mepivacaine is greatly prolonged in the fetus and newborn; thus this agent is not usually employed for obstetric anesthesia. Mepivacaine appears to be somewhat less toxic in adults than lidocaine and has less vasodilator activity than lidocaine. Because of the difference in vasoactivity, mepivacaine provides a somewhat longer duration of anesthesia than lidocaine when used without epinephrine. Mepivacaine seems to be particularly useful for brachial plexus blockade when large volumes of anesthetic solutions without epinephrine are given.

Ropivacaine Ropivacaine is prepared as the pure S isomer rather than a racemic mixture. Onset of action, potency, and duration of sensory nerve blockade appear similar for ropivacaine and bupivacaine, but ropivacaine is a less potent and short-acting agent in terms of motor fiber blockade. Toxicity studies suggest that ropivacaine is less cardiotoxic than bupivacaine, although ropivacaine still possesses some dysrhythmogenic potentia.

Bupivacaine Bupivacaine was the first local anesthetic that combined the properties of an acceptable onset, long duration of action, profound conduction blockade, and significant separation of sensory anesthesia and motor blockade. This agent is used for various regional anesthetic procedures, including infiltration, peripheral nerve blocks, and epidural and spinal anesthesia. The average duration of surgical anesthesia with bupivacaine varies from approximately 3 to 10 hours. Its longest duration of action occurs with major peripheral nerve blocks such as brachial plexus blockade.

The major advantage of bupivacaine appears to involve epidural obstetric analgesia for labor when satisfactory pain relief for 2 to 3 hours is achieved, which significantly decreases the need for repeated injections in the pregnant patient. Moreover, adequate analgesia is usually achieved without significant motor blockade such that the patient in labor is able to move her legs. This differential blockade of sensory and motor fibers is also the basis for the widespread use of bupivacaine for postoperative epidural analgesia and for certain chronic pain states.

Levobupivacaine The clinical profile of levobupivacaine, the S isomer of bupivacaine, is essentially the same as the profile of racemic bupivacaine except with somewhat wider therapeutic index for cardiac toxicity and systemic toxicity.

Prilocaine The clinical profile of prilocaine is also similar to that of lidocaine. Prilocaine has a relatively rapid onset of action while providing a moderate duration of anesthesia and a profound depth of conduction blockade. Because this agent causes significantly less vasodilatation than lidocaine, it can be used without epinephrine.

Prilocaine biotransformation produces aminophenols that oxidize hemoglobin to methemoglobin thus limiting its clinical use. The primary use of prilocaine is in EMLA cream, a eutectic mixture of prilocaine and lidocaine for topical application.

Etidocaine Etidocaine is characterized by very rapid onset, prolonged duration of action, and profound sensory and motor blockade. It has a significantly more rapid onset of action than bupivacaine. Concentrations of etidocaine required for adequate sensory anesthesia produce profound motor blockade. As a result, etidocaine is primarily useful as an anesthetic for surgical procedures in which muscle relaxation is required. Consequently, this agent is of limited use for obstetric epidural analgesia and postoperative pain relief, as it does not provide a differential blockade of sensory and motor fibers. The drug is used infrequently in North America.

Dibucaine Dibucaine is only available for topical anesthesia in the United States. It is more potent than tetracaine, although the onset of action of the 2 agents is similar. The duration of spinal anesthesia is slightly longer with dibucaine. The degree of hypotension and depth of motor blockade appear to be less in patients receiving intrathecal dibucaine than in those receiving tetracaine into the subarachnoid space, although the spread of sensory anesthesia is similar in the 2 groups.

Benzocaine This local anesthetic is used exclusively for topical anesthesia. Benzocaine is available in a variety of proprietary and nonproprietary preparations. The most common forms used in an operating room setting are aerosol solutions for endotracheal administration and ointments for lubrication of endotracheal tubes. One should remember that benzocaine also can cause methemoglobinemia.

KEY REFERENCES

- Albright GA. Cardiac arrest following regional anesthesia with etidocaine or bupivacaine. *Anesthesiology.* 1979;51:285-287.
- Butterworth JF. Models and mechanisms of local anesthetic cardiac toxicity. *Reg Anesth Pain Med.* 2010;35:167-176.
- Drasner K. Local anesthetic systemic toxicity. A historical prospective. *Reg Anesth Pain Med.* 2010;35:162-166.
- Gerner P, Above all, do no harm. *Anesthesiology.* 2008;109:939-939.
- Heavner JE, guest ed. Additives to Local Anesthetics. *Techniques Reg Anesth Pain Manage.* 2004;8:105-140.
- IUPHAR database: Voltage-gated sodium channels: Introduction. http://iuphar-db.org/DATABASE. Accessed June 18, 2010.
- Mackley CL, Marks JG, Anderson BE. Delayed-type hypersensitivity to lidocaine. *Arch Dermatol.* 2003;139:343-346.
- Moller RA, Covino BG. Cardiac electrophysiologic effects of lidocaine and bupivacaine. *Anesth Analg.* 1988;67:107-114.
- Stewart J, Kellett N, Castro D. The central nervous system and cardiovascular effects of levobupivacaine and ropivacaine in healthy volunteers. *Anesth Analg.* 2003;97:412-416.
- Zaric D, Christiansen C, Pace NL, et al. Transient neurologic symptoms after spinal anesthesia with lidocaine versus other local anesthetics: a systematic review of randomized, controlled trails. *Anesth Analg.* 2005;100:1811-1816.

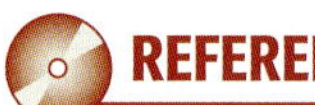

REFERENCES

Complete references available on DVD and online version at www.LongneckerAnesthesiology.com

SECTION D
Regional Anesthesia

Incorporating Regional Anesthesia Into Anesthetic Practice

Richard W. Rosenquist
David L. Brown

KEY POINTS

1. The one overriding benefit of regional anesthesia techniques is that they do not need to end as the patient leaves the operating room at the end of the intraoperative period.
2. The patient education and expectation-setting process is most effective if started in the surgeon's office at the time of the visit at which the decision for operation is completed. Both the surgeon and the nurses need to understand the general concepts and goals of anesthesia and are often strong coadvocates of better perioperative analgesia for their patients.
3. The perioperative period should be designed so that regional anesthesia does not delay or slow down a surgical day. Perceived surgical delay is one of the most important items to avoid if you desire to successfully add regional anesthetic techniques to your practice.
4. Regional anesthesia techniques should be selected and performed on the basis of clear indications to maximize benefit and minimize complications.
5. The preoperative anesthetic note should clearly outline that the patient has been informed of the risks and benefits of the entire anesthetic experience, including the regional anesthetic portion, if that is applicable to the patient. In addition, any preexisting neurologic deficits should be documented on the preanesthetic assessment.
6. Patients should have regional anesthetics performed in settings where full monitoring, resuscitation equipment, and supplies are available.
7. When a practice adds continuous regional anesthetic techniques (either epidural or continuous peripheral nerve block techniques), it is important that round-the-clock coverage and follow-up is available to the patient and hospital if the patient remains as an inpatient or the patient is discharged to an out-of-hospital setting.
8. One of the most important technical items in the intraoperative period with regional anesthesia is to recognize that if a block is not 100%, the anesthesiologist should be the only individual aware of that fact. This means that if the block is not working as well as desired, general anesthesia or deep sedation should be added efficiently.
9. If a patient is to be discharged with a continuous catheter technique, a clear understanding of catheter and pump management, limb protection, catheter removal, breakthrough pain control, and contact numbers must be assured.
10. Anesthesiologists need to continue their own regional anesthesia education by attending continuing education conferences and workshops that help them to have a more complete understanding of the topic and learn new techniques for introduction into their practice. This enables anesthesiologists to continue the education of physicians, nurses, and others regarding regional anesthesia advances.

Incorporating regional anesthesia into an established anesthesia practice demands that the physicians involved understand and make preparations to address the following:

- Management of regional anesthesia through the entire perioperative period
- Clinical indications for the regional anesthetic chosen
- Resources necessary to perform the blocks efficiently, effectively, and safely
- Establishing of an institutional strategy to optimize the introduction of new techniques

Physicians often desire to immediately transfer "techniques" they have learned in workshops into their own practices. That strategy is often destined to fail, as the 4 areas of understanding clearly need to be managed to predictably and reliably introduce regional anesthesia into established practices. This chapter explores each of these necessary steps for successful introduction of regional anesthesia into a practice and expands on them so that you are able to individualize a plan for your own institution and practice.

CONCEPT OF THE CONTINUUM OF ANESTHESIA CARE: THE PERIOPERATIVE PERIOD

Physicians who desire to add regional anesthesia techniques to their own practice are most successful if they fundamentally are truly outstanding physicians and, as a result, excellent anesthesiologists. These physicians must be true perioperative physicians. They *must* be able to understand patient medical problems, surgeons' operative requirements, and regional anesthesia techniques, as well as recovery pattern, nursing requirements, rehabilitation, and potential complications from the surgical procedure performed. Only if all of these are incorporated into decisions about regional anesthesia will the patient, surgeon, anesthesiologist, and nursing staff be coadvocates of the proposed new technique.

In today's surgical and anesthetic environment, our intraoperative general anesthetic care has advanced to a level where it is unusual to validate clear advantages for regional anesthesia when considering the isolated intraoperative period. There are exceptions, of course. Nevertheless, regional anesthesia may be better termed "regional analgesia," as one seeks to incorporate that concept into an anesthetic and surgical practice. The one overriding benefit of regional anesthesia techniques is that they do not need to end as the patient leaves the operating room at the end of the intraoperative period. Rather, when effectively chosen, these regional techniques can be extended either through appropriate drug selection or via catheter insertion and continuous infusion of medication. Either of these choices may help transition the patient from the intraoperative to the postoperative period and to nearly full recovery with manageable pain. The most obvious example is by inserting *home going* peripheral nerve plexus catheters to provide local anesthetic-induced analgesia into the immediate and more distant postoperative period.[1-4]

A key step in successfully introducing regional anesthesia to an established practice is ensuring that preoperative evaluation and education of the patient includes an explanation of regional anesthesia and that realistic patient expectations are established. Far too often patients are under the misunderstanding that because they choose a regional anesthesia technique, they will be "awake" during their surgical procedure. Experts in regional anesthesia are nearly always capable of providing outstanding sedation and anxiolysis for the entire perioperative period for patients undergoing a regional technique. This observation fits with these anesthesiologists being excellent physicians and understanding that it is a rare patient who wants to be, or should be allowed to be, completely unsedated for a surgical procedure. The patient education process is most effective if started in the surgeon's office at the time of the visit at which the decision for operation is completed. Both the nurses and the surgeon need to understand the general concepts and goals of anesthesia, including regional anesthesia techniques. Once they understand these concepts, they are often strong coadvocates of better perioperative analgesia for their patients and help to set appropriate patient expectations for the perioperative period.

When considering patient education, the most important concept is that realistic expectations for both patient and the patient's family are outlined. The patient's expectations should be focused around anesthesia, sedation, postoperative analgesia, and what side effects the patient might experience so that, for example, a "numb" arm does not bother the patient on arrival in the recovery room or discharge to the floor or home. In setting these expectations, it is important that the anesthesiologist and institution design an analgesia transition program that addresses resolution of the regional anesthetic and follow-up analgesia. As an example, outstanding brachial plexus anesthesia and analgesia for an upper-extremity operation can frustrate a patient and the patient's family if the block abruptly wears off while the patient is expecting to sleep through the night and no oral medication regimen has been planned to ease that transition. When setting expectations for surgeons, a key element is that the perioperative period is designed so that regional anesthesia does not delay or slow down a surgical day. This demands that anesthesiologists and institutional leaders be creative about incorporating regional blocks and techniques into their practices. Our experience is that surgical delay is one of the most important items to avoid if you desire to successfully add regional anesthesia techniques to your practice. Avoidance of delay will demand that an effective team approach be designed that allows induction of regional anesthetic techniques to be carried out prior to moving patients into the operating room.

CLINICAL INDICATION FOR REGIONAL ANESTHESIA

After considering the continuum of anesthesia care in the entire perioperative period, the next step for successful introduction of regional techniques into a practice is to develop clear indications for the use of these techniques. It must be remembered that the dominant focus for regional anesthesia is regional analgesia and the ability to minimize opioids and other intravenous agents in the immediate perioperative period. Additional advantages of regional anesthesia techniques include the ability to avoid airway manipulation in patients who evidence difficult airway characteristics or those with full stomach considerations. This does not mean that regional anesthetics should be applied in every full-stomach situation, but a mature clinical risk-to-benefit approach for many emergency patients suggests that the use of effective regional anesthesia does modify risk. As example, in a patient with obstructive cardiomyopathy, the intravascular volume shifts from both general anesthetic vasodilatation and/or neuraxial anesthetic vasodilatation may be avoided, to the patient's advantage, by the use of a brachial plexus nerve block. Another example might be a patient with end-stage pulmonary disease, who requires open reduction with internal fixation of a hip fracture. This clinical setting might be effectively handled with a continuous spinal anesthetic and minimal sedation, rather than a general anesthetic with tracheal intubation. Finally, there is developing evidence that typical general anesthetics may in selected patients have lasting adverse cognitive effects that make regional anesthetics more appropriate.[5]

In a patient who is undergoing regional anesthesia, there must be clear documentation of both the technical procedure and the indications for the regional technique in the patient's chart. This is another opportunity for the anesthesiologist to educate both surgeons and nurses about the primary reason why the regional anesthesia technique was chosen. In our opinion, anesthesiologists frequently do not take advantage of the educational opportunities present in writing clear and effective progress notes in a patient's record. The preoperative anesthesia note should clearly outline that the patient has been informed of the risks and benefits of the entire anesthesia experience, including the regional anesthesia portion, if applicable to the patient. In addition, any preexisting neurologic deficits should be clearly documented.

The increasing number of drugs being developed that impact coagulation demands that anesthesiologists interested in adding regional techniques to their practice fully understand the implications of these anticoagulants and platelet-active drugs. For example, consensus statements for the use of neuraxial anesthesia techniques in relation to the use of anticoagulant and antiplatelet agents were recently updated and published by the American Society of Regional Anesthesia and Pain Medicine (ASRA) in 2010.[6] Recent data outlining a 10-year Swedish experience with anticoagulants and neuraxial anesthesia underscore the need to understand the potential risks and benefits of this drug and technique combination.[7] The Swedish results reiterated the danger of using more than 1 agent with anticoagulant or antiplatelet activity in combination. They also identified subgroups of patients at markedly increased risk; for example, elderly females with osteoporosis undergoing total knee arthroplasty under epidural analgesia and receiving once-per-day low-molecular-weight heparin have a 1 in 3600 incidence of epidural hematoma. The data to develop clear consensus statement guidelines regarding the use of anticoagulants and antiplatelet agents in conjunction with peripheral regional anesthetics is extremely limited. It has been suggested that the ASRA consensus guidelines for neuraxial anesthesia be applied to all regional anesthesia techniques. This may be too restrictive. In most cases, techniques performed in areas that are easily compressed in the event of bleeding may be appropriate. Others, such as paravertebral or subclavian blocks, should be avoided unless coagulation parameters are normal.

RESOURCES REQUIRED FOR EFFICIENT PRACTICE

A common stumbling block for practices desiring to add regional anesthesia expertise to their practice is being limited by having too few anesthesiologists skilled in the techniques. There must be a critical mass of personnel, resources for the techniques, and interest in the techniques for these to be added successfully to an anesthesia practice. Many practices often seek to have a single individual provide the regional anesthesia expertise. This is nearly always doomed to failure as that individual cannot be present 24 hours a day, year-round. Rather, it seems important to have enough physicians with the technical skills and interest in these anesthesia approaches to be able to provide consistent delivery of regional anesthesia throughout the day, week, and year. In general, this means that at least 3 to 4 physicians with significant regional expertise are available within a practice to ensure continuous provision of sophisticated regional anesthetic care is possible. In addition to the physician resources, it is often helpful to have allied health personnel help to prepare patients and supplies for the regional techniques to optimize timing of the technical performance of the regional anesthetic. This may be with a technician who is well trained in assisting the physicians, a nurse anesthetist who is skilled in this area of practice, or a registered nurse who works for the practice or hospital and has an interest in and a desire to grow this part of the practice.

For the physicians, there must be a complete understanding of anatomy and regional anesthesia technical skills to safely and reliably perform the nerve blocks. Patients should have regional anesthesia performed in settings where full monitoring, resuscitation equipment, and supplies are available. These are major anesthesia techniques and need to be treated as such. Monitoring should meet American Society of Anesthesiologists (ASA) standards for performance of an anesthetic.[8] Delays in the surgical day can often be minimized if many of the regional anesthesias are performed outside the operating room itself. This serves 2 functions. First, it allows the regional anesthesia to be performed while the surgical team is still preparing the operating room. Second, it gives the injected local anesthetic additional time to effectively anesthetize the desired region. This, of course, demands that regional anesthesia block rooms, or at least regional anesthesia block areas, are established outside the operating room. In many practices, this could be accomplished in areas of the preoperative holding or of postoperative anesthesia recovery. The ideal is to have induction rooms near the operating rooms. Within these areas of the hospitals, regional anesthesia carts with supplies easily at hand and with appropriate monitoring and resuscitation gear are critical for effectively caring for these patients.

As the regional anesthetic practice is established, allied health staff assisting physicians with the technical features of these nerve blocks need to be trained and to have regional block protocols developed so that they are most effective. This demands significant planning and communication to effectively implement this practice.

When a practice has added continuous regional anesthesia techniques (either epidural or continuous peripheral nerve block techniques), it is important that round-the-clock coverage and follow-up are available to the patient and hospital if the patient remains as an inpatient. Even the most successful technical regional anesthetic can be viewed as unsuccessful if this part of the practice is not accounted for in the development phase of adding regional anesthesia to a practice. Other ideas to ease the transition of regional anesthetic techniques into a practice are to use regional anesthesia continuous infusion pumps that differ from general intravenous infusion pumps used throughout the hospital with tubing that has no injection ports. This difference helps to minimize the inappropriate administration of other intravenous drugs through regional block catheters. Drug swaps remain one of the dilemmas of modern medicine, and the use of different pumps and tubing helps to minimize this type of error and potential neurotoxicity. New devices with the capability to read barcodes and recognize appropriate or inappropriate drugs for the device may provide additional safety in the future. Successful introduction and continued use of regional anesthetic techniques require that physicians stay abreast of the latest technologies, such as ultrasound guidance or the use of stimulating catheters for catheter placement.[9-11] The increasing use of ultrasound-guided regional anesthetics demands that physicians incorporate a means to stay abreast of developments in ultrasound as well as providing their assistants with a means of gaining ultrasound fundamentals so the ultrasound equipment can be most effectively used.[12,13]

OPTIMIZING INSTITUTIONAL INTRODUCTION OF REGIONAL ANESTHESIA

Once the preceding 3 major elements are understood and a group decides to move ahead with introduction of regional anesthesia or expansion of regional anesthesia into its practice, strategies need to be developed to optimize this introduction. First, a core group of regional anesthesia physicians who agree, in principle, on the plan must be established. It is most effective if, as a system is rolled out, a small number of surgeons and surgical procedures are used as the initial clinical settings so that "success" can be validated more quickly. One of the easiest ways to cause an introduction of regional anesthesia to a practice to fail is to try to be all things to all patients and all surgeons at the outset. It is important to emphasize that successful introduction of regional anesthesia to a practice demands that all involved perceive that regional anesthesia is truly an advantage to the patient, to the surgeon, to the anesthesiologist, and to the institution. Collins et al[14] provided clear evidence for this as they examined the impact of a regional anesthesia–analgesia program for outpatient foot surgery. They documented a marked increase in regional anesthesia use, no decrease in operating room efficiency, reduced postanesthesia care unit and discharge time, decreased analgesic use, and decreased nursing interventions for analgesia.

An important technical item in the intraoperative period with regional anesthesia is to recognize that if a block is not 100%, the anesthesiologist should be the only individual aware of that fact. This means that if the block is not working as well as desired, general anesthesia or deep sedation should be added efficiently. This demands that anesthesiologists interested in this practice understand enough about regional anesthesia and sedation to blend the 2 techniques so that patients are effectively sedated and do not have any painful memories of either block insertion or eventual surgical manipulations. The potential for this transition from conscious sedation to deep sedation or general anesthesia should be explained in advance so that patients have realistic expectations regarding the plan of management.

Successful use of regional anesthesia also requires education and training of the nursing staff and development of care protocols. This often begins in the postanesthesia care unit where the limb must be protected. If the patient is to be discharged, the patient and family must be educated about how to protect the limb until recovery from the block has occurred. If the patient is to be discharged with a continuous catheter technique, a clear understanding of catheter and pump management, limb protection, catheter removal, breakthrough pain control, and contact numbers must be assured. In some settings, this may require training home health nurses to facilitate the process. On the inpatient side, education regarding limb protection, neurologic evaluations, breakthrough pain, fall prevention, and issues with anticoagulation and ambulation must be completed.

Once the techniques are well established within an institution and the anesthesiologists are interested, the anesthesiologists need to continue their own regional anesthesia education by attending continuing education conferences and workshops that help them to an even more complete understanding of the topic and to learn new techniques for introduction into their practice. This enables these anesthesiologists to continue the education of nurses and others interested in regional anesthesia advances. This is a critical component of successful introduction of the practice of regional anesthesia.

Once it is effectively introduced, the registered nurses within an institution often are its most vocal advocates, as they see firsthand the difference between patients having effective regional anesthesia and those having either ineffective regional anesthesia, excessive opioid analgesia, or uncontrolled pain in the perioperative period.

CONCLUSION

The introduction of regional anesthesia to an established anesthesia practice is no different from the introduction of any new technique to a practice. There must be expertise, planning, and a group of physicians and support staff interested in the entire perioperative period that can coordinate the necessary personnel and resources to provide state-of-the-art medical care.

KEY REFERENCES

- Collins L, Halwani A, Vaghadia H. Impact of a regional anesthesia program for outpatient foot surgery. *Can J Anaesth.* 1999;46:840-845.
- Gray AT. Ultrasound-guided regional anesthesia: current state of the art. *Anesthesiology.* 2006;104:368-373.
- Horlocker TT, Wedel DJ, Rowlingson JC, et al. Regional anesthesia in the patient receiving antithrombotic or thrombolytic therapy: American Society of Regional Anesthesia and Pain Medicine Evidence-Based Guidelines (Third Edition). *Reg Anesth Pain Med.* 2010;35:64-101.
- Ilfeld BM, Enneking FK. Continuous peripheral nerve blocks at home: a review. *Anesth Analg.* 2005;100:1822-1833.
- Liu SS, Ngeow JE, Yadeau JT. Ultrasound-guided regional anesthesia and analgesia: a qualitative systematic review. *Reg Anesth Pain Med.* 2009;34:47-59.
- Moen V, Dahlgren N, Irestedt L. Severe neurological complications after central neuraxial blockades in Sweden 1990–1999. *Anesthesiology.* 2004;101:950-959.

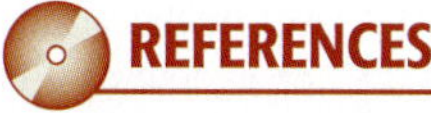

REFERENCES

Complete references available on DVD and online version at www.LongneckerAnesthesiology.com

CHAPTER 47

Neuraxial Anesthesia

Daniel T. Warren
Joseph M. Neal
Christopher M. Bernards

KEY POINTS

1. A systematic and rational approach based on a thorough 3-dimensional understanding of anatomy should be used when accessing the subarachnoid or epidural space.
2. Anesthetic doses, agents, and combinations of agents should be individualized to optimize neuraxial blockade for a given clinical setting.
3. Hypotension and bradycardia associated with neuraxial anesthesia should be identified early and treated aggressively to minimize development of cardiovascular collapse and poor outcome.
4. Our understanding of potential neurotoxicity and the nature of transient neurologic symptoms (TNS) are continuing to evolve. However, there is growing consensus that TNS may not represent direct neural toxicity.
5. Evaluating the appropriateness of neuraxial procedures in patients receiving anticoagulant and antiplatelet medications is a challenge. Clinicians should be familiar with the recommendations presented by the American Society of Regional Anesthesia and Pain Medicine in the consensus statement addressing these issues.
6. When suspicion of spinal hematoma or abscess is credible, definitive diagnosis with appropriate imaging and prompt surgical decompression within 4 to 8 hours of onset of neurologic symptoms is crucial to improve chances of recovery of function.
7. Developing an understanding of the nature of combined spinal–epidural anesthesia and facility with its techniques can expand a clinician's armamentarium to provide neuraxial anesthesia and optimize patient care.

With more than 100 years of use, neuraxial anesthesia has enjoyed much success and endured controversy. With the stage set by the developments of the hollow needle and syringe, the discovery of neuraxial anesthesia began in 1885 when Corning was experimenting with effects of cocaine on the spinal nerves of dogs. Bier brought spinal anesthesia into clinical use for surgery in 1898, but only after self-experimentation and a personal experience with a well-described postmenigeal puncture headache. Epidural anesthesia gained widespread attention in the setting of labor analgesia, maintaining the medical community's interest in neuraxial blockade despite rapid advancements in techniques for general anesthesia in the 1940s and 1950s. More recently, the introduction of continuous catheter techniques, combined spinal–epidural anesthesia, and various neuraxial anesthetic adjuvants has presented further opportunities to provide our patients the many benefits of neuraxial blockade.

ANATOMY

NEURAL STRUCTURES

A thorough appreciation for the anatomy of spinal structures is necessary for appropriate technique, patient selection, and management of neuraxial anesthesia. The spinal structures are identified by cervical, thoracic, lumbar, sacral, and caudal regions (**Fig. 47-1**). The spinal cord begins at the base of the brainstem and continues caudad terminating as the conus medullaris, typically at the L1-L2 level in the adult, although the terminus rarely may be as high as T12 or as low as L4. The spinal cord has cervical and lumbar enlargements to accommodate the increased neuronal supply to the limbs. Rootlets emerge from the dorsal and ventral surface of the spinal cord and converge to form the respective ventral and dorsal roots of the spinal nerves at each spinal level (**Fig. 47-2**).

CEREBROSPINAL FLUID

As with the brain, the spinal cord and portions of the spinal nerves are bathed in cerebrospinal fluid (CSF), which provides protection for these structures and participates in maintaining homeostasis. The CSF is secreted by the choroid plexuses located on the roofs of the lateral, third, and fourth ventricles, accounting for 40% to 60% of production. Water derived from glucose metabolism is also a major CSF source. CSF is reabsorbed mainly through arachnoid villi, which project into the parasagittal venous sinuses, and to a much lesser extent into the epidural veins accompanying spinal nerves. CSF typically has a density range of 1.00028 to 1.00100 g/mL.[1] CSF volume and its clinical significance are discussed in the Clinical Pharmacology section.

MENINGES

As with the brain, the spinal cord, nerve roots, and CSF are enveloped by 3 membranes: the pia mater, arachnoid mater, and the dura mater (Figs. 47-2 and **47-3**). The innermost pia mater is intimately applied to the surface of the cord and nerve roots. It is a vascular and permeable membrane. The arachnoid mater approximates the outermost membrane, the dura mater. Between the pia and the arachnoid is the subarachnoid space, home to the CSF, arachnoid trabecular network, and dentate ligaments. The subarachnoid space extends laterally with the dura as nerve root "sleeves," with the accompanying CSF as far as the dorsal root ganglion. The spinal dura mater extends from the level of the foramen magnum, where it is contiguous with cranial dura, to the level of S2 in most adults. Here the subarachnoid space terminates as the dura fuses with the filum terminale (pial extension) and then with the coccygeal periosteum. Between the dura mater and arachnoid mater resides the subdural space, which contains little more than a small amount of serous fluid. This space is often implicated, though not proved, as a link in complications such as a total spinal after an intended epidural administration of local anesthetic and failed spinal anesthetics.

VERTEBRAE

The neural structures of the spinal cord are protected by the bony vertebral column, which is composed of 7 cervical, 12 thoracic, 5 lumbar, 5 sacral, and 4 coccygeal vertebrae (Fig. 47-1). The vertebrae of the sacral and coccygeal regions are fused to form the sacrum and coccyx, respectively. Cervical and lumbar lordotic curves and thoracic kyphotic curves of the normal spine allow for distribution of mechanical forces and spinal movements. A typical vertebra consists of a pillar-like vertebral body joined by the pedicles to the posterior elements, namely the laminae, superior and inferior articular processes, transverse processes, and the spinous process. The vertebrae have regional characteristics that are relevant to the techniques used to access the neuraxis in clinical situations. The figures depict relevant features of representative thoracic and lumbar vertebrae (**Fig. 47-4**).

INTERVERTEBRAL DISKS AND LIGAMENTS

The endplates of the vertebral bodies are joined to one another by the intervertebral disks (Fig. 47-2), consisting of the outer annulus fibrosus and the inner nucleus pulposus. Further structural support comes from the anterior and posterior longitudinal ligaments running along the ventral and dorsal aspects of the vertebral bodies respectively. Along with the supraspinous ligament traversing superficially, the deeper interspinous ligament joins the spinous processes to one another (Fig. 47-3). Adjacent laminae are interconnected by the ligamentum flavum, together forming the posterior wall of the spinal canal. The ligamentum flavum forms embryologically from 2 (right and left) separate neural crest structures. These ligamenta meet in the midline at an acute angle,

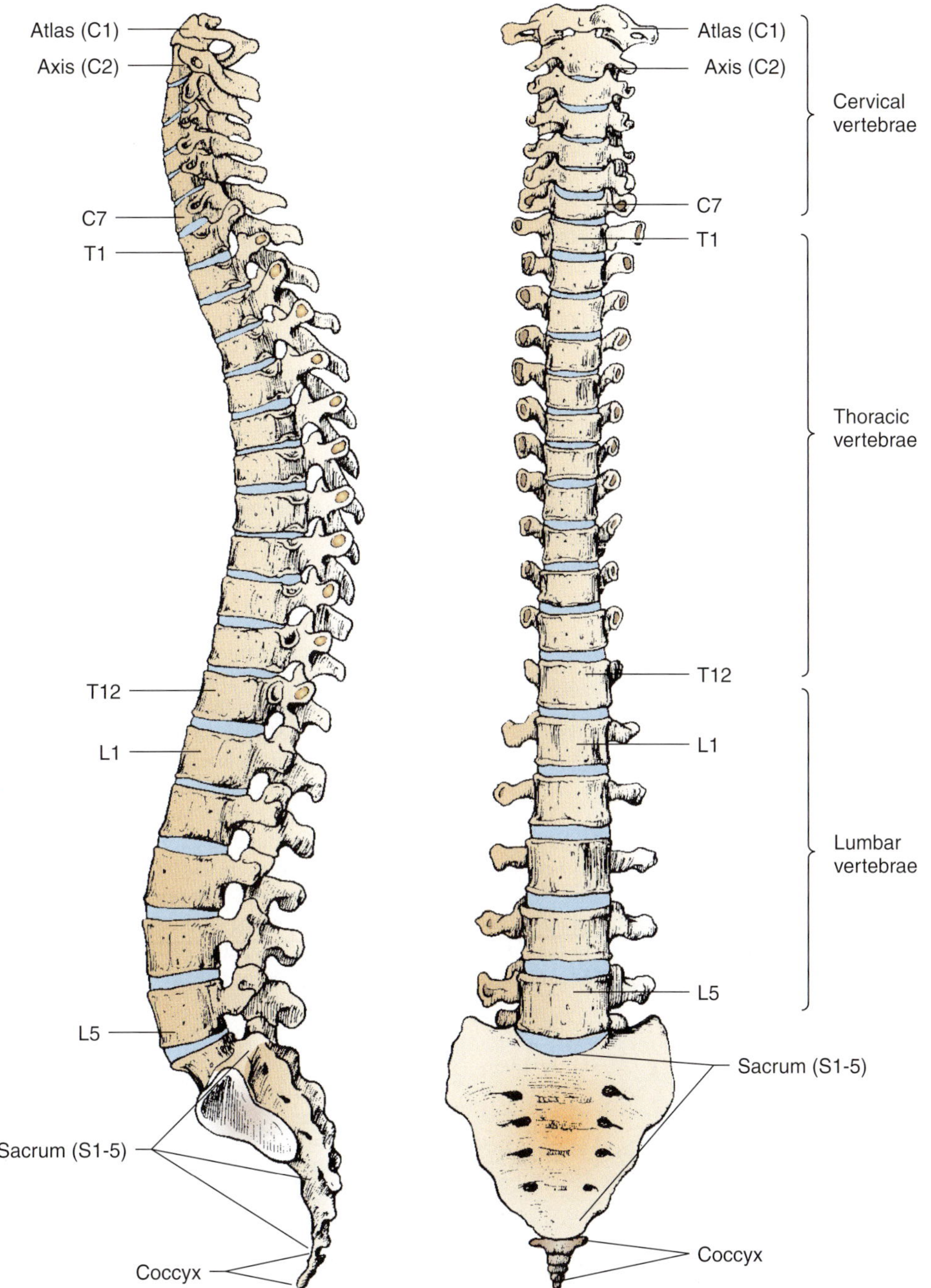

FIGURE 47-1. Regions of the spinal column.

but have an inconsistent degree of fusion. Incomplete fusion results in sagittal gaps, which are variable not only between individuals, but also among spinal levels within a given patient. Cervical and upper thoracic levels have a higher rate of failed fusion compared with levels below T3-T4 (as high as 50%-70%) and are thus perhaps more difficult for epidural access using the loss or resistance technique.[2]

EPIDURAL SPACE

The epidural space (also referred to as extradural and peridural space) lies between the dura and the borders of the spinal canal (Fig. 47-3). Anteriorly, this border is formed by the posterior longitudinal ligament; posteriorly, by the vertebral lamina and adjoining ligamentum flavum (Fig. 47-3). The spinal epidural space runs from the level of the foramen magnum to the sacral hiatus, which is bound by the sacrococcygeal ligament. The lateral borders of the epidural space are partially delineated by the vertebral pedicles, but this space extends laterally through the intervertebral foramina to communicate with the paravertebral spaces on each side. The epidural space is somewhat compartmentalized by the sections of the dura abutting the ligamentum flavum, vertebral lamina, and other borders of the vertebral canal (Fig. 47-3B). However, these compartments are joined by a "potential space" that is opened by injection of fluid or air, thus connecting the compartments and revealing a more continuous communication.

The contents of the epidural space include epidural fat, venous plexus, and segmental arteries. The epidural fat is largely located in

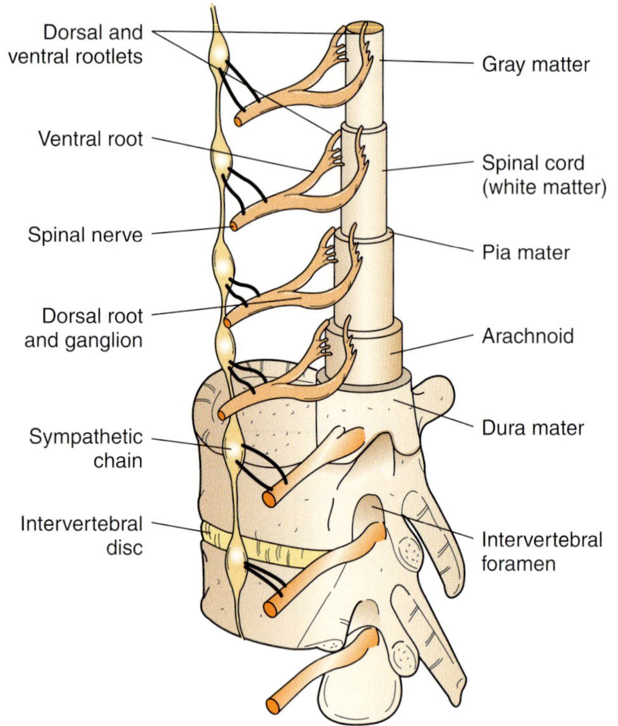

FIGURE 47-2. The spinal cord, along with the emerging root structures, is enveloped by the meninges, as depicted in this figure.

the posterior and lateral aspects of the epidural space. This fat can be a site for sequestration of epidurally administered local anesthetics and opioids as a function of the lipid solubility of the drug.[3] The plexus of epidural veins (Batson's plexus) is principally within the anterior and lateral portions of the epidural space, with rare presence in the posterior aspect. These veins communicate with the azygous system, which can become engorged in the setting of increased intra-abdominal or intrapelvic pressure.

EQUIPMENT

SPINAL NEEDLES

Although many designs have been introduced throughout the history of spinal anesthesia, the needles commonly used today can be generally classified as either *cutting needles* or *pencil-point needles* (**Fig. 47-5**). The Quincke-style needle, one of the most frequently used cutting needles, has a medium-length bevel, coming to a sharp point. In contrast, pencil-point needles, such as the Whitacre, Sprotte, and Gertie-Marx, have a rounded, noncutting tip. The latter 3 needles have openings on the side rather than at the tip. Efforts to minimize the incidence of postmeningeal puncture headache have driven the advancement of needle design. More recent designs include tapered needles and return of stylet-point needles, such as the Ballpen needle (Rusch, France). Needle gauge usually ranges from 27 to 18, with the thinner needles requiring an introducer needle to prevent spinal needle deflection.

EPIDURAL NEEDLES AND CATHETERS

Needles for accessing the epidural space need to have a large enough diameter (eg, 16-20 gauge) to permit catheter insertion and facilitate loss of resistance techniques to identify the epidural space.

Currently, the most commonly used needle is the Tuohy needle (Fig. 47-5D). The design of this needle has undergone many modifications, but is characterized by a curved, or Huber, tip. This curved tip decreases coring of tissue during insertion, but has been used chiefly in an effort to provide directional control of catheter insertion. Epidural needles have a tight-fitting stylet, which prevents coring of the skin with subsequent transfer to the epidural space where it can grow and cause mass effects. Larger-gauge needles are less likely to be deflected by firm ligaments and osseous structures and may provide a more reliable "loss-of-resistance" for identification of the epidural space.[4]

Commercially available catheters for cannulation of the epidural space are composed of polyurethane, nylon, or silicone-based material.

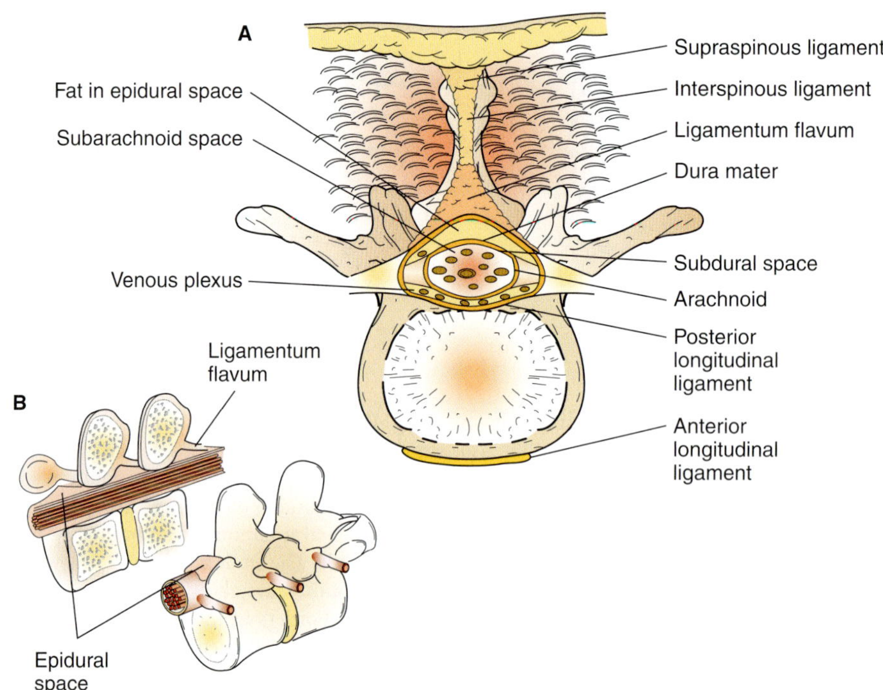

FIGURE 47-3. **A.** Cross-sectional view of the lumbar region depicting the location of the epidural space and other anatomical structures associated with neuraxial procedures. As demonstrated in **B**, the epidural space is somewhat compartmentalized, but continuous via "potential space" pathways, which expand with injection of liquid.

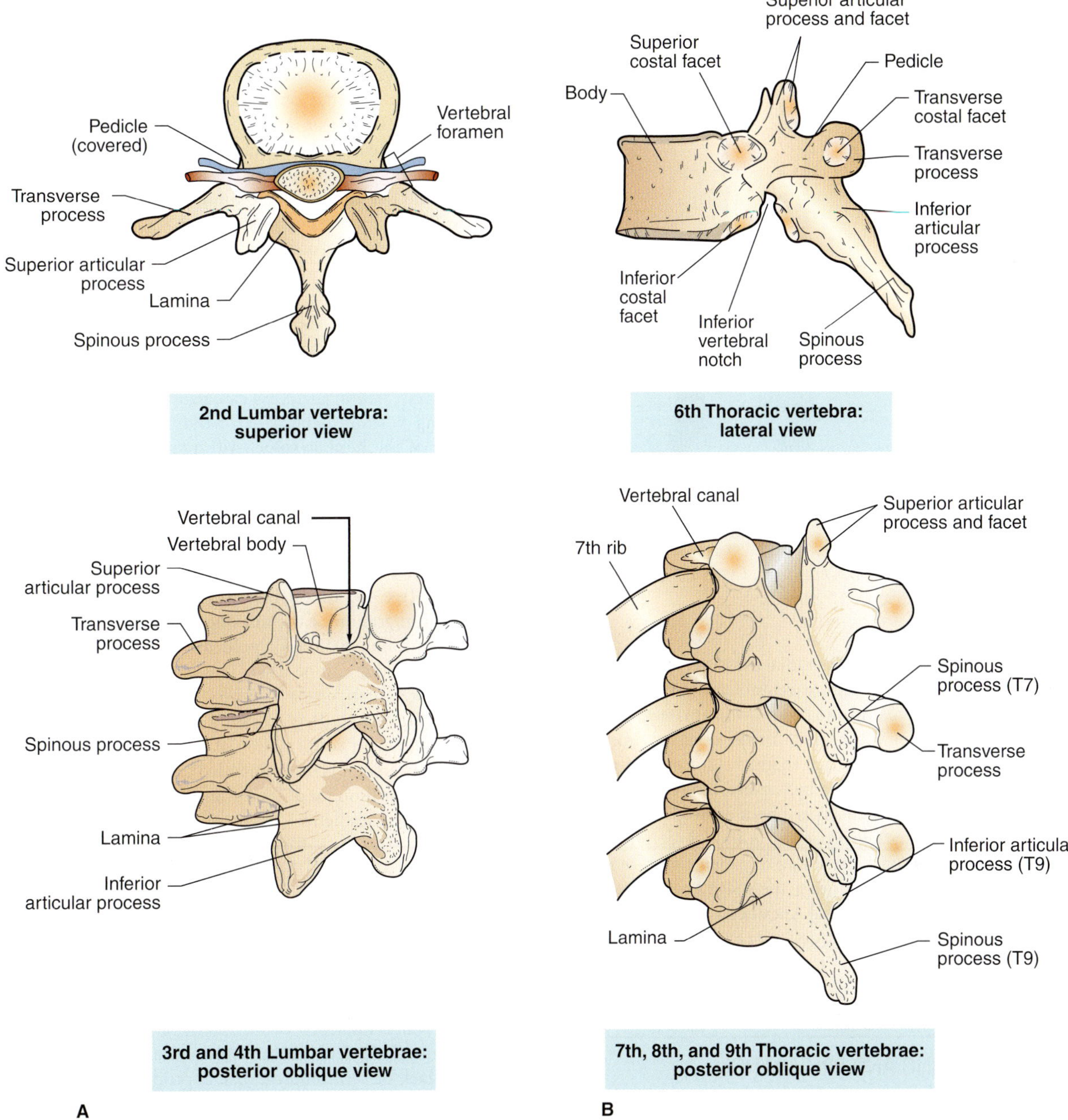

FIGURE 47-4. Anatomical structures associated with (**A**) lumbar and (**B**) thoracic vertebrae.

Catheters with wire-wound reinforcement are designed to prevent kinking of the lumen and to increase durability, thus making them useful for postoperative analgesic infusions. Several variations of catheters have been brought to the market, with options for multi-orifice tips, metal stylets, and varying stiffness. Although the many available needles and catheters have various purported advantages, definitive, consistent data for superiority for any particular product are limited. Therefore, selection among these is primarily driven by subjective preference or availability.

PATIENT SELECTION

The clinical success of neuraxial anesthesia begins with proper patient selection and creation of an environment that is conducive to regional anesthetic techniques. Principally, the surgical procedure should be able to be performed with a sensory and motor block level that is tolerable and safe for the patient under the appropriate positioning, monitoring, and supplemental medication. Lower-extremity, pelvic, and lower-abdominal procedures are often appropriate for spinal or epidural anesthesia. Procedures in the perineum, or involving the foot, usually are more suited to spinal anesthesia because of the potential for sacral nerve sparing with epidural anesthesia. Upper abdominal procedures usually require sensory levels that are not comfortably attainable with regional techniques alone and would require "supplementation" with light general anesthesia.

It is imperative that the patient be able to cooperate and tolerate the experience, from placement of the block, to block resolution. This can be accomplished through proper preoperative evaluation of the patient's maturity and affect and appropriate informed consent discussions regarding risks, benefits, alternatives, and patient expectations in light of the requirements of the procedure.

Absolute contraindications to neuraxial anesthesia are few in number, but include patient refusal, significant hypovolemia, infection at the

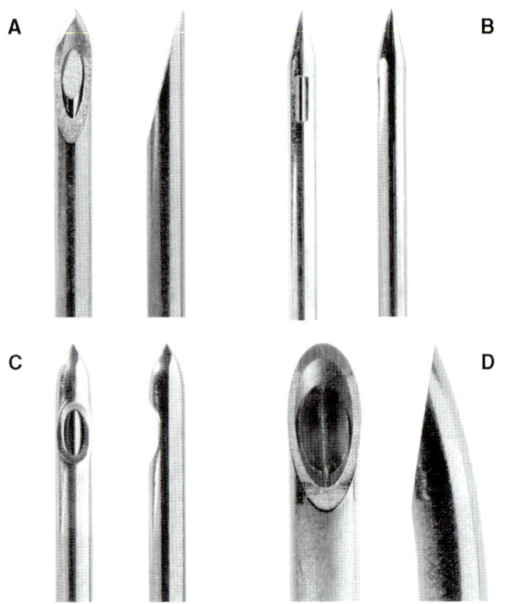

FIGURE 47-5. Close-up views of the tips of a "cutting-tip" spinal needle: **A.** Quincke, and 2 "pencil-point" needles: **B.** Whitacre, **C.** Gertie-Marx. Also shown is the tip of a common epidural needle: **D.** 17-gauge Tuohy.

site of needle entrance, increased intracranial pressure, and significant coagulopathy. Relative contraindications require analysis of the risks and benefits for a given patient and situation. Unfortunately, this often needs to be done in light of the current medicolegal environment. Commonly encountered conditions that might be considered relative contraindications are minor coagulopathy, sepsis/bacteremia, and preexisting neurologic conditions, such as peripheral neuropathy, multiple sclerosis, and other demyelinating processes. Although definitive data for the relative safety of neuraxial anesthesia in patients with central or peripheral neurologic disorders are lacking, the ASRA Practice Advisory in Neurologic Complications in Regional Anesthesia and Pain Medicine suggests that the risk of new neurologic deficit or exacerbation of a present condition appears to be extremely rare in these conditions.[5]

TECHNIQUE FOR NEURAXIAL ANESTHESIA

PATIENT POSITIONING AND PREPARATION

In addition to confirming patient consent and understanding, one should also verify the immediate availability of equipment and medications to manage airway compromise and hemodynamic perturbations. The patient should have proper monitoring and supplemental oxygen during neuraxial anesthesia. Most patients prefer to have sedation administered before beginning neuraxial anesthesia, and this is typically achieved with judicious use of agents such as midazolam and fentanyl, maintaining the patient's ability to report paresthesia. Performance of neuraxial anesthesia on anesthetized or heavily sedated patients is considered routine in pediatric anesthesia, but remains controversial in adult care. Although wakefulness is suggested for adults as a means of decreasing the risk of neurologic injury,[5] some clinical situations may present with extenuating circumstances that justify deep sedation while performing neuraxial procedures after a careful consideration of the risks and benefits of the practice.

The lateral decubitus position (**Fig. 47-6**) is most often used for spinal anesthesia. The patient should have hips and knees flexed with head approximating the knees in an effort to relax the lumbar lordotic curve and accentuate the interlaminar aperture.

Alternatively, neuraxial access can also be obtained with the patient in the sitting position (**Fig. 47-7**), bending forward to relax the lordotic curve of the lumbar spine. Advantages of this position are that it facilitates the identification of the midline in obese or anatomically distorted patients and augments CSF pressure at the needle entrance site, enhancing CSF flow through the needle when performing lumbar puncture. It is also used to accomplish "saddle block" anesthesia for procedures limited to the perineum by administering hyperbaric spinal preparations (see section on Baricity) to the intrathecal space to promote caudal migration of the anesthetic agent. If the patient is going to be in the prone position for procedures such as perianal surgery, a hypobaric technique can be used. This is accomplished by positioning the patient for surgery prone with hips flexed and lumbar spine relaxed (jackknife) (**Fig. 47-8**), then accessing the subarachnoid space, using a syringe to aspirate for confirmation of CSF flow. Once a hypobaric solution is administered, it is recommended that the patient remain in a flat or head-down position for at least 1 hour to prevent unintended rostral migration of the anesthetic.

ACCESSING THE SUBARACHNOID SPACE

It is recommended that all procedures for neuraxial anesthesia begin with foundational elements of safety, including protective masks for all participants (US Centers for Disease Control and Prevention [CDC] guideline), marking of the target site (if lateralized), setup of procedural tray and equipment (including labeling of all medications and solutions), and a final procedural pause immediately before starting the procedure to review critical information (correct patient, correct procedure, lack of contraindications, appropriate equipment available, etc) Several techniques have been described for inserting a needle percutaneously into the subarachnoid space, each having specific advantages in different clinical situations. By developing skill with multiple

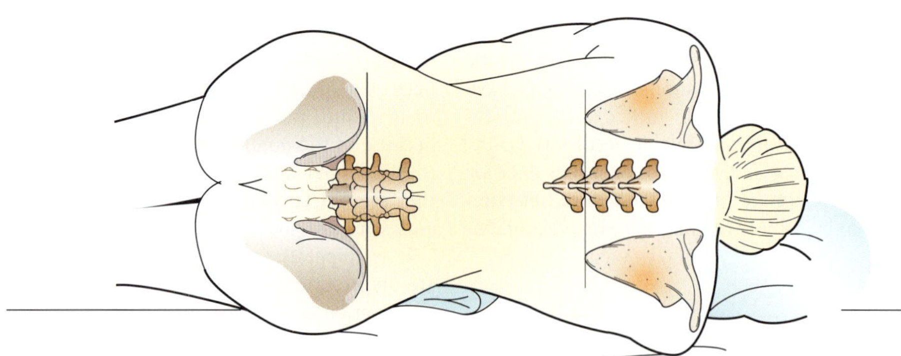

FIGURE 47-6. Lateral decubitus position for neuraxial procedures. The patient is positioned with the head tucked down, hips flexed, and back rounded in efforts to maximize the aperture of the interlaminar space. Lines depicting the levels of the iliac crests and scapulae are commonly used anatomical landmarks to identify the levels of L4 and T7, respectively. However, these landmarks are often unreliable.

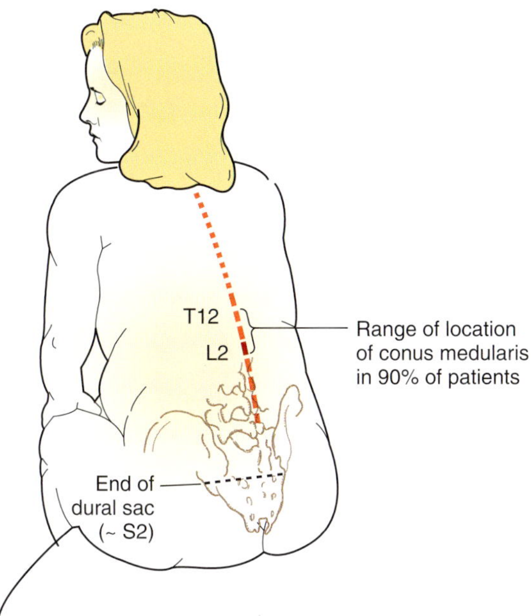

FIGURE 47-7. A patient in the sitting position, with the spine curved to relax the lordotic curve on the lumbar region. The approximate range of cord termination in 90% of patients is from T12 to L2.

techniques, the practitioner can be prepared to adapt to the clinical challenges presented. Regardless of the position and technique to be used, the procedure should begin with identifying the midline and palpating the iliac crests. The intercrestal line (Fig. 47-6) is classically described as crossing the level of the fourth lumbar vertebra, or the L3-L4 or L4-L5 interspace, which are the preferred levels of entry, due to increased risk of spinal cord injury when entering at higher vertebral levels. The most commonly used and easily mastered technique for needle insertion is the midline approach. After identification of the desired interspace, a skin wheal is raised over the interspace, and appropriate infiltration of local anesthetic is fanned along the midline. It is useful to firmly place 2 fingers of the nondominant hand parallel to the axis, straddling the lateral borders of the interspace (**Fig. 47-9**). When using small-diameter spinal needles, an introducer needle is first inserted in the sagittal plane between the spinous processes, initially parallel to the plane of the surface of the back. The introducer is then stabilized by grasping the hub with the digits of the nondominant hand as the spinal needle is passed through the bore of the introducer and advanced in the sagittal plane. The path of travel for the needle in the midline approach is through

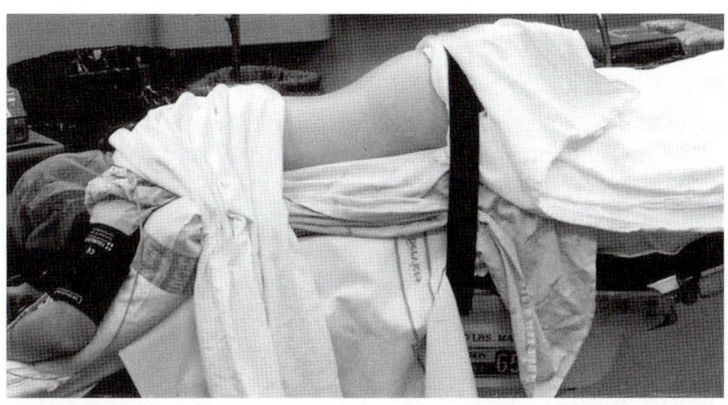

FIGURE 47-8. Patient positioned in the prone-jackknife position for surgery to be performed under hypobaric spinal anesthesia. Note that the head is below the level of the hips to ensure that the anesthetic "floats" to the caudad portion of the intrathecal space.

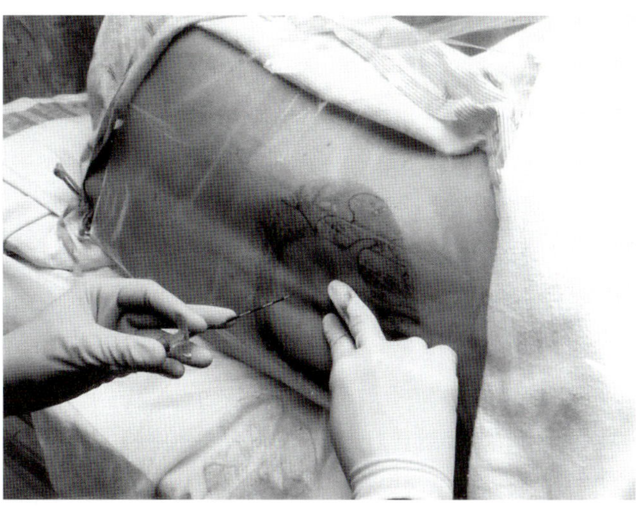

FIGURE 47-9. Fingers of the nondominant hand are used to identify the lateral borders of the interspace of interest. This will aid in developing a 3-dimensional mental image of the anatomical structures to facilitate neuraxial access.

skin, subcutaneous tissue, supraspinous ligament, interspinous ligament, ligamentum flavum, and, finally, through the dura and arachnoid mater into the subarachnoid space. As the needle tip passes beyond the ligamentum flavum and through the dura, a change in resistance, and possibly a "pop," can be appreciated. At this point, the stylet is withdrawn from the spinal needle, and the hub is inspected for free flow of CSF. If bone is contacted before entering the thecal sac, the practitioner should reassess the angle of projection and ensure that it is within the sagittal plane. If no correction toward the midline is needed, the most fruitful adjustment is usually an attempt to gradually "walk" the needle tip in a cephalad direction until the subarachnoid space is encountered. If progress in the cephalad direction leads to contacting bone at a more shallow depth, then a caudad direction should be attempted because it is likely that you have contacted the more superior lamina. If free flow of CSF is in question, rotating the bevel or side hole of the needle through the 4 quadrants can help ensure proper placement of the needle opening. In addition, because the holes of the pencil-point needles are located proximal to the tip, it is possible for the tip to be in the subarachnoid space but not the needle hole. Consequently, advancing a pencil-point needle a 1 or 2 mm may result in free flow of CSF.

Once satisfied with needle placement, the dosing syringe (typically a Luer slip style), which was previously prepared with the intended agent(s), is firmly attached to the hub of the spinal needle. Aspiration of CSF into the syringe is final confirmation of subarachnoid placement; the agent is slowly injected while keeping the needle tip immobile. Once the injection is complete, the patient should be placed in the intended position to impact the spread of the agent or into the appropriate position for surgery. The advantages of the midline approach include simplicity and the stability provided by the relatively avascular sagittal plane through the interspinous ligament.

The paramedian technique (**Fig. 47-10**), which is routinely used by some, should be mastered to the same level as the midline technique because of its advantages in common clinical situations. When the midline approach is difficult, the paramedian approach may still allow access to the subarachnoid space in patients who are unable to maintain ideal positioning, are obese or pregnant, or who have heavily calcified interspinous ligaments (common in elderly patients), compression fracture, or scoliosis. This advantage is a consequence of the larger interlaminar aperture presented via the path of the paramedian approach, especially when lumbar lordosis is retained. Although variations have been described, in the lumbar region this approach begins with identification of the superior aspect of the caudad spinous process of the interspace to be accessed. The percutaneous entry point is

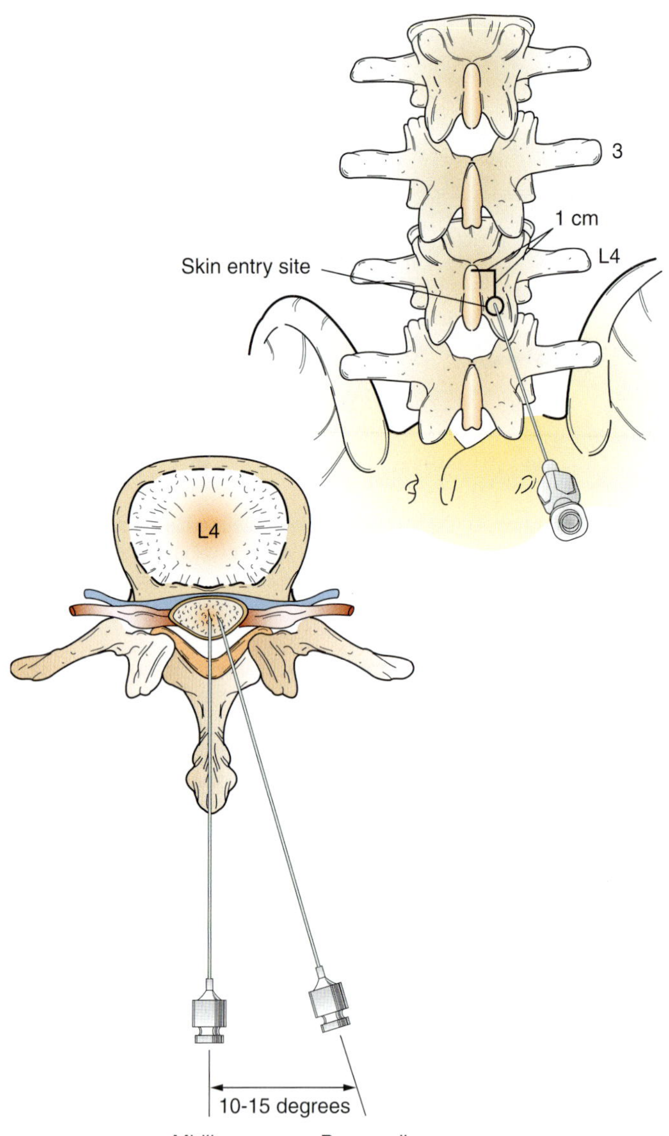

FIGURE 47-10. In the paramedian approach for neuraxial access, an entrance site is identified 1 cm lateral and caudad to the inferior aspect of the superior spinous process. After appropriate local anesthetic is infiltrated, the needle is typically inserted to touch-down on the lamina, then walked first medially, then cranially to step off of the lamina.

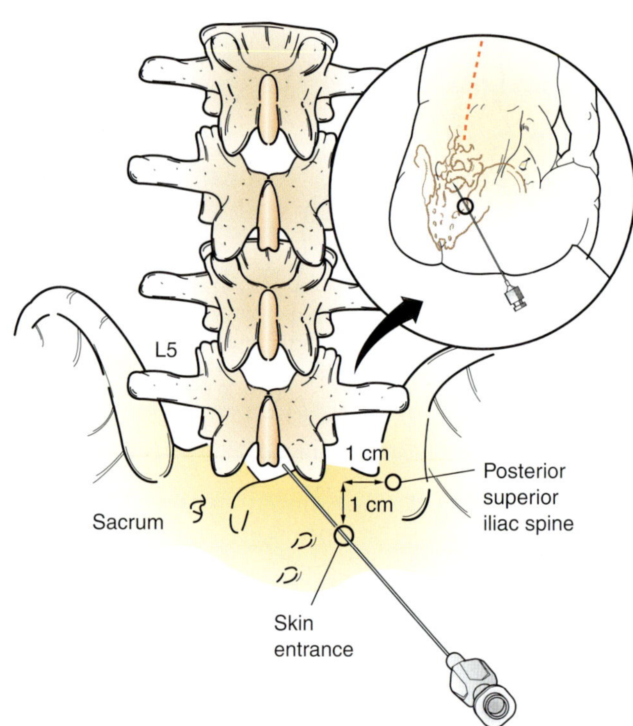

FIGURE 47-11. The Taylor approach begins with identification of the posterior superior iliac spine (PSIS). The skin entrance site is 1 cm medial and 1 cm caudad to the PSIS. The needle is then directed approximately 45 degrees medial and cephalad to enter the L5-S1 interspace.

identified 1 cm lateral to this superior tip of the spinous process. After raising a skin wheal and appropriate infiltration with local anesthetic, the introducer and/or spinal needle are advanced through the anesthetized region, directed approximately 10 to 15 degrees toward midline and at a slightly cephalad angle. This path will traverse skin, subcutaneous tissue, paraspinous muscle, ligamentum flavum, dura, and arachnoid mater to reach the subarachnoid space. If bone is encountered prior to dural puncture, it is most likely the caudad lamina, in which case the needle should be "walked" cephalad, then medial, until the thecal sac is breached.

The Taylor approach (**Fig. 47-11**) is a variation of the paramedian technique; it capitalizes on the breadth of the L5-S1 interspace (typically the largest interspace) and the palpable and relatively constant location of the posterior superior iliac spines (PSISs). Once a PSIS is identified, a skin wheal is raised 1 cm medial and caudad to its inferior border. After appropriate infiltration of local anesthetic, the spinal needle (typically at least 22 gauge) is directed approximately 45 degrees medial and cephalad toward the L5-S1 interspace. Again, if bone is contacted, the correction needed is a greater cephalad angle to "walk off" of the superior aspect of the sacrum.

ACCESSING THE EPIDURAL SPACE

Although the pathway and approach to the epidural space are the same for the subarachnoid space, the technical skills to correctly and reliably access and identify the epidural space require more experience to develop than those for dural puncture.[6] Again, both midline and paramedian approaches are used for needle placement, and the patient can be placed in either the sitting or lateral position. In contrast to spinal anesthesia with increasing risk of cord injury above the L2 level, the epidural space theoretically can be accessed at any vertebral level (though there remains the risk of spinal cord injury above L2 if the clinician fails to correctly identify the epidural space or control the advancing needle). Because of the differences in the projecting angles of the spinous processes in the lumbar and midthoracic regions, an angle of approach closer to the plane of the surface of the back is used when performing thoracic epidural placement.

With the midline approach, the desired interspace is identified by palpation as described previously, and a skin wheal is raised with local anesthetic at the site of intended needle entrance, which should be in the sagittal plane at the midpoint between the spinous processes. The needle is inserted through the skin, subcutaneous tissue, and supraspinous ligament and into the interspinous ligament. With the blunter tip of the larger-diameter needles used for epidural anesthesia, passage into the interspinous ligament is typically met with a "crunchy" sensation. Patients who are not sedated might either hear or feel this "crunching" and should be reassured if report of this is elicited. If in the sagittal plane, further advancement of the needle should place the tip in the ligamentum flavum, which provides increased resistance to needle advance.

Alternatively, if the paramedian approach is used, as may be required in the thoracic region due to the acutely angled spinous processes, the interspinous ligament is not typically encountered. If attempting access in the thoracic region, the appropriate needle entrance site is 1 cm lateral to the inferior aspect of the superior spinous process of the interspace desired. The needle is advanced through an anesthetized skin wheal, subcutaneous tissues, paraspinous muscle, and to the lamina of the inferior vertebra, providing a reference depth. The needle tip is walked medially until the base of the spinous process is encountered, which will be noted to have a shallower depth. The needle tip is then marched superiorly until it "walks off" of the lamina, and it should encounter resistance as it meets the ligamentum flavum.

With either approach, correct passage of the needle tip through the ligamentum flavum and into the epidural space without breaching the dura can be accomplished by using several different methods for identifying the epidural space. The most commonly used method is the loss of resistance (LOR) technique using saline or air, although saline may be preferred, given the risk of headache if air is unintentionally injected into the subarachnoid space. A low-resistance syringe made of glass or plastic is filled with 1 to 2 mL of sterile saline, as well as a small (0.2 mL) air bubble (**Fig. 47-12**). This syringe is attached to the epidural needle once the tip has been placed in the ligamentum flavum. The degree of resistance to injection of the saline is assessed by determining whether the bubble can be compressed without allowing injection of fluid. If little resistance is encountered, the needle tip is either not yet within the ligamentum flavum, or perhaps has passed through to the epidural space. If uncertain, careful advancement of the needle by a few millimeters could be considered in an attempt to reach the ligament, but one might wish to withdraw and reattempt placement. Once this ligament is identified, the needle is advanced slowly, with constant pressure on the syringe plunger, until the resistance to injection is reduced. A dramatic loss of resistance is reassuring for passage of the needle tip just beyond the ligamentum flavum and into the epidural space.

An alternative technique is the "hanging drop" of Gutierrez. This relies on negative pressure in the epidural space to aspirate a visible drop of fluid "hanging" from the hub of the needle and into the lumen of the epidural space itself (**Fig. 47-13**). This negative pressure is encountered just as the tip of the needle enters the epidural space and is much more reliable in the thoracic and cervical regions. One theory for the origin of this negative pressure is that it is created by the tip of the needle tenting the dura, thus increasing risk of dural puncture. This technique is best used in the thoracic region with a sitting patient. It may be helpful in the setting of combined spinal–epidural anesthesia because of minimal saline entering the epidural space and less chance of a "false return" being interpreted as CSF.[7]

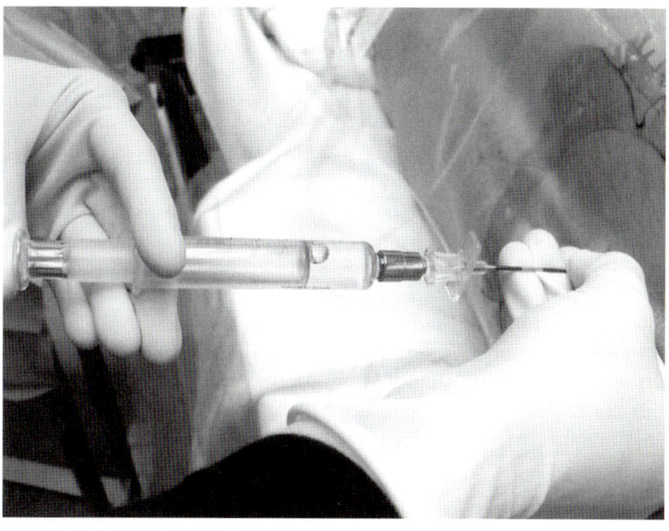

FIGURE 47-12. Photo depicting a glass loss-of-resistance syringe attached to an epidural needle. The syringe is filled with saline and a small (0.2 mL) bubble of air. The bubble will provide visual indication of "compression" resultant of resistance to injection that is characteristic of the ligamentum flavum.

Newer techniques for identifying the epidural space are being described. The use of electrical nerve stimulation via a conducting catheter allows for confirmation of placement of the catheter within the epidural space by confirming appropriate stimulation threshold.[8] Additionally, the myotomal distribution of the stimulation can provide information regarding the spinal level of the catheter tip. Lechner et al[9] describe an apparatus for use in epidural access that produces both audible and visual indication of the pressure encountered at the tip of

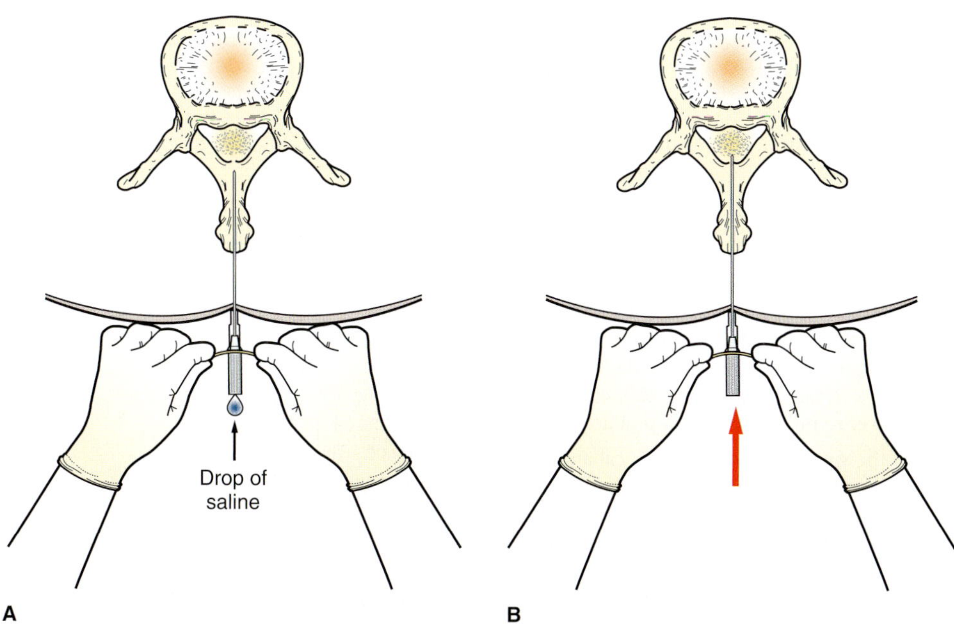

FIGURE 47-13. The "hanging drop" technique is performed by first placing a drop of saline at the "mouth" of the needle hub (**A**). The needle is then advanced while monitoring the drop of fluid. The drop will be drawn into the needle when the epidural space is entered (**B**).

an attached epidural needle. Using this device allows a 2-handed (which facilitates control) advancement of the epidural needle while awaiting the drop in pressure that is characteristic of entering the epidural space. Further testing and study are needed to determine the appropriate role for these new methods.

As ultrasound-guided regional anesthesia continues to gain popularity, some have attempted to apply these tools to the performance of neuraxial anesthesia. At the time of this writing, the use of ultrasound for neuraxial anesthesia is primarily described in pediatric and obstetric anesthesia for initial evaluation of anatomic landmarks and estimation of depth of the epidural space. In these populations, it has been demonstrated that the use of ultrasound can result in fewer passes at fewer interspaces, but there is no support for the blocks being more successful or safer.[10] Further studies are under way that will help determine the clinical utility of and impact of ultrasound imaging on neuraxial anesthesia.

CLINICAL PHARMACOLOGY

DISTRIBUTION, UPTAKE, AND ELIMINATION

Before reaching the site of action, anesthetic agents injected into the subarachnoid space undergo dilution within the CSF via mass effect. It has long been postulated that CSF circulation played a role in distribution of anesthetic agents; however, this has not been reliably demonstrated. In fact, is now known that CSF motion is primarily a rostral-caudad oscillation with no net movement,[11] rather than a circuitous flow, as has been traditionally described. The uptake of anesthetic agents by nerve roots depends on the concentration of agent at a given point, lipid content of the tissue, and hydrophobicity of the local anesthetic. Drug elimination from the subarachnoid space and spinal cord is determined by regional blood flow (primarily spinal cord and dura mater) and vascular reabsorption, not metabolism of the anesthetic within the intrathecal space. Drugs administered into the epidural space must diffuse across the spinal meninges (primarily the arachnoid mater which is the primary permeability barrier) to reach the CSF and neural tissues, where it produces conduction blockade. The rate and extent to which any drug distributes from the epidural space to the subarachnoid space depends on how much drug is taken up via competing pathways; in particular, clearance via the capillary network in the dura mater (particularly for hydrophilic drugs) or uptake into the epidural fat (particularly for hydrophobic drugs).

FACTORS AFFECTING BLOCK HEIGHT

Spinal Anesthesia

Patient Characteristics The ability to affect and predict sensory block height is important for producing reliable and manageable spinal anesthesia. Many parameters have been studied as potential determinants of block height (**Table 47-1**). Current data suggest that the most significant physiologic parameter determining block height is CSF volume. Unfortunately, easily measurable physical features, such as height, weight, sex, and age, do not correlate well with CSF volume.[12] However, it has been observed that obese individuals have lower CSF volumes than those who are not obese. Although some studies show a slight influence of age and height on peak block levels,[13,14] these are weak correlations with inadequate predictive power to influence clinical practice.

Baricity Baricity (the ratio of the specific gravity of the local anesthetic solution to the specific gravity of CSF), drug dose (mass), and patient position relative to baricity of the agent are the most important factors influencing block height. Hyperbaric solutions will migrate within the CSF in the direction of gravity. Conversely, hypobaric solutions will rise opposite gravitational force in the CSF column.

Solutions with a density greater than 1.0015 g/mL (3 standard deviations above mean human CSF density) can be expected to reliably behave as a hyperbaric solution (**Table 47-2**). Hyperbaric solutions are typically prepared by adding dextrose to the solution. However, it should be noted that room temperature 2% 2-chloroprocaine may behave in a hyperbaric fashion. Once injected into the subarachnoid space, hyperbaric solutions distribute to the dependent portions of the spinal column. Thus, for a patient in the sitting position, the agent sinks to the sacral regions to produce a "saddle block." In the supine patient, hyperbaric agents injected at or above the apex of the lumbar lordotic curvature will migrate to the thoracic kyphosis, hence the tendency for a peak block of T4-6 in most supine patients. Manipulation of patient position after hyperbaric subarachnoid injection can enhance either

TABLE 47-1 Various Factors Proposed as Determinants of Spinal Block Height

Factors
Patient characteristics
Height
Weight
Age
Sex
Intra-abdominal pressure
Pregnancy
Technical variations
Patient positioning
Site of injection
Speed of injection
Direction of bevel
Barbotage
CSF characteristics
Volume
Density
Velocity/circulation
Characteristics of the local anesthetic solution
Baricity
Volume of injection
Concentration of solution
Drug dose (mass)
Temperature

TABLE 47-2 Baricity of Solutions for Spinal Anesthesia

Agent	Baricity
Hypobaric	
Bupivacaine 0.3% in water	0.9946
Tetracaine 0.2% in water	0.9922
Lidocaine 0.5% in water	0.9985
Isobaric	
Bupivacaine 0.5% in saline	0.9983
Bupivacaine 0.75% in saline	0.9988
Tetracaine 0.5% in saline	0.9997
Lidocaine 2% in saline	0.9986
Hyperbaric	
Bupivacaine 0.75 % in 8.25% dextrose	1.0227
Tetracaine 0.5% in 5% dextrose	1.0133
Lidocaine 5% in 7.5% dextrose	1.0265
Procaine 10% in water	1.0104
2-Chloroprocaine 2% in saline	1.0012

Data from Horlocker TT, Wedel DJ. Density, specific gravity, and baricity of spinal anesthetic solutions at body temperature. *Anesth Analg.* 1993;76:1015-1018; Bodily MN, Carpenter RL, Owens BD. Lidocaine 0.5% spinal anaesthesia: a hypobaric solution for short-stay perirectal surgery. *Can J Anaesth.* 1992;39:770-773; Greene NM. Distribution of local anesthetic solutions within the subarachnoid space. *Anesth Analg.* 1985;64:715-730; and Na KB, Kopacz DJ. Spinal chloroprocaine solutions: density at 37 degrees C and pH titration. *Anesth Analg.* 2004;98:70-74.

migration of the agent to the thoracic region (head down position) or to the sacral region (head up or sitting position).

Isobaric solutions have a density that is clinically equivalent to that of CSF. Thus, once injected into the subarachnoid space, the agent neither sinks nor floats. This can be advantageous because patient position does not affect block height. In such a scenario, peak block height is more determined by dose of anesthetic agent (mass effect), but individual CSF density and volume contribute.[19] It should be noted that it may be difficult to achieve block heights above the midthoracic region because of the tendency of isobaric solutions to remain in the lumbar region after injection due to the lack of sufficient forces promoting mixing and migration.

Hypobaric solutions have a distinct advantage in perianal surgery or other procedures that require a head down or jackknife position or for lateralized procedures when the patient cannot lie on the operative side (eg, hip fracture). Hypobaric solutions are produced by diluting anesthetic agents in distilled water to produce a density less than 0.9990 g/mL. For perirectal and perineal surgery that will be performed in the prone jackknife position, the patient is positioned prone with the head down, and an intrathecal injection is performed with a hypobaric local anesthetic solution, which will rise within the CSF to the sacral region. As mentioned previously (see Patient Positioning and Preparation), the patient must be recovered in the head-down or flat position for at least 60 minutes from time of injection to prevent unintentional rise of the block.[16]

Other Factors The volume and concentration of isobaric spinal local anesthetics have been shown not to affect block height when using a constant dose.[20] In contrast, when using hyperbaric preparations, baricity seems to overcome alterations in dose and volume, showing similar block heights with a range of doses if concentration is held constant. This highlights the propensity for hyperbaric preparations to settle to the dependent portions of the spinal canal.

Injection site can influence the nature of spinal blockade. If using hyperbaric solutions, injection low in the lumbar region can cause failure to achieve expected block height and cephalad block density as a result of sacral pooling and absence of agent above the lordotic curve. However, if injection is made at or above L2-3, then block height and success are more reliable, though it must be noted that risk of spinal cord injury theoretically increases above L3-4. For isobaric solutions, block height can be reduced by as much as 2 dermatomes per interspace when comparing administrations at L2-3, L3-4, and L4-5.[14] The manner of injection is thought to have little influence on block characteristics. Investigations into the effect of barbotage show no impact on peak block height, although it does seem to reduce the time from injection to achievement of peak block height.[21]

Epidural Anesthesia Most procedures that are amenable to spinal anesthesia can also be served by an epidural anesthetic that produces a similar block height (**Table 47-3**). However, unlike spinal anesthesia, lumbar epidural anesthesia is likely to spare or delay onset in sacral dermatomes, which can make its use in perineal procedures and surgeries involving the foot or lower leg problematic. Thus, when planning an epidural anesthetic, the choice of local anesthetic, dose, and injection site must be appropriate for the given procedure and the clinical context.

TABLE 47-3 Required Block Height for Common Surgical Procedures

Surgical Procedure	Block Height
Upper abdominal surgery	T4-5
Cesarean section	
Lower abdominal (appendectomy, inguinal herniorrhaphy)	T6-8
Pelvic procedures	
Transurethral resection of prostate	T10
Obstetric vaginal delivery	
Hip and lower extremity (with thigh tourniquet)	
Lower extremity	L2-3
Perineal procedures (limited to exterior)	S1-2

In contrast to spinal anesthesia, epidural anesthesia produces a segmental block that is closely related to physical spread of local anesthetic within the epidural space, which in turn is related to the site of local anesthetic injection. For example, Visser et al[22] administered 3 mL of 2% lidocaine into the low, middle, and high thoracic epidural space and found that spread was primarily caudad from the high thoracic injection, primarily cephalad from the low thoracic injection, and equally distributed cephalad and caudad after the midthoracic injection. Similar results were reported by Masataka et al, who additionally measured spread after lumbar injection and found that spread was primarily cephalad from the injection site. This finding helps to explain the sacral sparing noted previously. These injection site–related differences in spread within the epidural space are presumably related to differences in epidural compliance.

Clinically, the best injection site is that which falls in the middle of the range of dermatomes targeted. Thus, for an incision extending from T9 to L1, a T11-T12 injection site would be ideal, although low to midthoracic dermatomes can be reached from lumbar injection sites if a sufficient local anesthetic dose is used.

In general, one can think of administering 2 mL of local anesthetic solution for each additional dermatome to be blocked. When administering anesthetic to the thoracic region, the dose is typically reduced by 30% to 50% as compared with the lumbar region to accommodate the greater spread of solution in the thoracic epidural space and thereby avoid unwanted cephalad spread. Greater spread is thought to be caused by the decreased volume and compliance of the thoracic epidural space.

When considering the ranges that are typically used for surgical anesthesia, concentration of the anesthetic solution has little effect on extent of the epidural block, but increased block density is observed with higher concentrations. Increasing the volume of solution injected for a given total dose will have a minor, and nonlinear, effect on cephalad spread (approximately 4 dermatomes when increasing from 10 to 30 mL), but will compromise density and quality of the block. Patient position also has no demonstrable effect on lateralization of the block or cephalad spread, but is often incorrectly used clinically.

The effect of patient age on epidural block height and dose requirement seems to be only clinically relevant in extremes of age, but some studies suggest as much as a 40% reduction in dose requirement when comparing 60- to 79-year-old patients with 20- to 39-year-old patients.[24] This is attributed to the increased likelihood of spinal canal stenosis and decreased epidural volume, resulting in greater spread in the older population. Similarly, the influence of height and weight on the spread of epidural block is small[25] and usually not clinically relevant unless considering the extremes of the spectrum.

The effect of pregnancy on the spread of epidural blockade is unclear. Several studies suggest greater spread and density of epidural block per milligram of local anesthetic during pregnancy. The mechanism responsible for this observation is unclear. Some early reports suggest that the gravid uterus compresses pelvic and abdominal veins, forcing blood into the epidural venous plexus and decreasing the volume of the epidural space. However, the fact that the increase is seen in early pregnancy before the uterus is significantly enlarged suggests this may not be the case.[26] Interestingly, local anesthetic block of peripheral nerves is also enhanced beginning in early pregnancy,[27] suggesting that sex steroid potentiation of local anesthetic action may be responsible for exaggerated epidural and spinal block in pregnancy.

In summary, patient physical characteristics seem to have little if any predictable clinical effect on epidural block spreads over the relatively narrow range of human sizes and ages typically encountered clinically. However, clinical judgment may allow for reducing the initial epidural dose for a patient who is very short, very old, and morbidly obese. Conversely, more aggressive dosing can be used for the patient who is

TABLE 47-4 Typical Dose–Response Effects of Spinal Local Anesthetics

Local Anesthetic	Dose (mg)	Peak Block	Duration of Sensory Block (min)[a]	Duration of Motor Block (min)	Time Until Discharge (min)	Anesthetic Success Rate (%)[a]
Lidocaine	30					0[b]
	40	T4 (T2-10)	130(26)	93(24)	178(34)	90
	60	T3 (T2-10)	162(32)	128(31)	216(33)	90
	80	T3 (T1-7)	170(24)	142(32)	236(46)	97
Bupivacaine[c]	5	T5 (T4-7)	123(27)	50(20)	181(30)	75
	7.5	T8 (T4-11)	144(25)	75(24)	202(28)	100
	10	T8 (T6-10)	194(26)	100(24)	260(30)	100
	15	T5 (T4-7)	343(28)	150(24)	471(35)	100
Mepivacaine	30	T9(T2-L5)	158(32)	116(38)	180(34)	72
	45	T6(T2-12)	182(38)	142(37)	191(29)	100
	60	T5(T2-L1)	203(36)	168(36)	203(35)	100
Ropivacaine	8	T9(T4-L1)	130(27)	107(25)	165(45)	63
	10	T8(T4-L2)	152(44)	135(31)	174(38)	83
	12	T8(T4-L1)	176(42)	162(37)	199(52)	93
	14	T9(T3-L1)	192(48)	189(44)	233(52)	100
Procaine	100	T5(T1-10)	120(23)	100(30)	244(43)	83
Prilocaine	50	T6(T1-10)	128(38)	165(37)	253(55)	100
2-Chloroprocaine	30	T8(T6-L1)	103(12)	54(23)	103(12)	65
	40	T7(T3-T10)	114(14)	69(16)	113(14)	87
	60	T4(C6-T6)	132(23)	100(13)	141(21)	100

Increasing doses of spinal local anesthetics increase duration of both anesthesia and recovery. Dose–response data allow selection of appropriate dose for planned anesthetic duration. Isobaric solutions are glucose free. Hyperbaric solutions contain glucose or dextrose.

[a]Anesthetic success rate is defined as ability to perform the surgical procedure as planned, without resorting to general anesthesia. Definition duration of sensory block is variable among the studies, ranging from 2-dermatome regression to complete resolution of block.

[b]Without adjuvants.

[c]Levobupivacaine is equipotent.

Data from Liu SS, McDonald SB. Current issues in spinal anesthesia. *Anesthesiology*. 2001;94:888-906; except for data from 2- chloroprocaine, which is from Wang BC, Hillman DE, Spielholz NI. Chronic neurological deficits and Nesacaine-CE: an effect of the anesthetic 2-chloroprocaine, or the antioxidant, sodium bisulfite? *Anesth Analg*. 1984;63:445-447; and Casati A, Danelli G, Berti M, et al. Intrathecal 2-chloroprocaine for lower limb outpatient surgery: a prospective, randomized, double-blind, clinical evaluation. *Anesth Analg*. 2006;103(1):234-238.

very young, tall, and thin. Comorbidities and other clinical challenges may help guide the appropriate dosing regimen (ie, will it be easier/safer to deal with a failed block [inadequate spread and/or duration] or to treat the complications and side effects resulting from a block that is higher or longer than intended).

CLINICAL ASPECTS OF NEURAXIAL AGENTS

LOCAL ANESTHETICS

Local anesthetic agents are discussed in Chapter 45 in detail, but some clinical points relating to neuraxial anesthesia are addressed here. The choice of neuraxial agents is determined by the nature and estimated duration of the surgical procedure, as well as postoperative issues such as planned discharge. **Tables 47-4** and **47-5** list representative durations for doses of spinal and epidural agents. For spinal anesthesia, increasing the dose of agent administered prolongs the block, and unless counteracted by positioning and baricity, it may also increase peak block height. Longer-acting local anesthetics, such as bupivacaine, levobupivacaine, tetracaine, and ropivacaine, are typically chosen for longer procedures (>120 minutes). Lidocaine, mepivacaine, and prilocaine are considered to be of intermediate duration (60-120 minutes). Short-acting local anesthetics include procaine and 2-chloroprocaine, which are used for appropriately brief procedures (<60 minutes), particularly in outpatients.

Long-Duration Agents Bupivacaine and levobupivacaine have the benefit of a very low incidence of transient neurologic symptoms[29] (TNS; see section on Neurologic Complications); however, the variability in time to complete block resolution and achievement of discharge criteria provides a challenge in the ambulatory setting. Bupivacaine and levobupivacaine are used in epidural anesthesia when a longer block is desired. The use of 0.5% solutions is typical, but 0.75% solutions or adding epinephrine may provide increased motor block. Levobupivacaine is approximately equipotent to bupivacaine, with the exception of less systemic toxicity in animal models.

Ropivacaine was released for clinical use in 1996. When used as a spinal agent, ropivacaine has a clinical profile similar to bupivacaine at equipotent doses (ropivacaine is 60% as potent as bupivacaine) with little risk of TNS.[30] Ropivacaine is used in concentrations of 0.5% to 1% for epidural anesthesia, providing blockade of somewhat shorter duration

TABLE 47-5 Duration of Sensory Block for Commonly Used Local Anesthetics for Epidural Anesthesia

Local Anesthetic	Concentration (%)	Time Until 2 Dermatome Regression (min)	Time Until Complete Regression
2-Chlorprocaine	2-3	45-60	100-160
Lidocaine	1.5-2	60-100	160-200
Mepivacaine	1.5-2	60-100	160-200
Bupivacaine	0.5-0.75	120-240	300-460
Levo-bupivacaine	0.5-0.75	105-290	390-780
Ropivacaine	0.5-1	90-180	240-420

than bupivacaine. There is some evidence that ropivacaine may have less motor block when compared with bupivacaine when used for labor analgesia[31]; however, this effect is not reliably demonstrated when comparing equipotent doses.

Although tetracaine is used less commonly at this time, it remains the agent that provides the most reliable isobaric spinal anesthetic when the crystalline powder is reconstituted with the patient's cerebrospinal fluid. It should be noted that the use of vasoconstrictors might increase the risk of TNS with tetracaine.[32]

Investigators have modified use of long-acting agents as spinal anesthetics for short duration procedures by reducing the administered dose and thus reducing the duration of spinal blockade. When these agents are used for low-dose spinal anesthesia, this typically requires adjuvants (usually fentanyl) to have reliable block success.

Intermediate-Duration Agents Lidocaine has enjoyed widespread popularity and perceived safety as a neuraxial agent, but it has undergone increasing scrutiny given the high incidence of TNS seen when used for ambulatory spinal anesthesia (see Neurologic Complications, later). In an attempt to avoid this problem, lower doses of lidocaine have been investigated, usually requiring adjuvant agents to provide suitable reliability of spinal blockade. Lidocaine is used in concentrations of 1.5% and 2% for epidural anesthesia to provide reliable blockade for procedures lasting less than 120 minutes. However, continuous catheter techniques commonly use lidocaine, with reinjection typically required every 60 to 90 minutes.

Mepivacaine has a clinical profile similar to that of lidocaine when used as a neuraxial agent, although it has higher potency (1.3:1 compared with spinal lidocaine).[33] It also may have similar concerns regarding the high incidence of TNS when used for outpatient spinal anesthesia, depending on concentration of agent.[34] It is used in concentrations of 1% to 2% for epidural anesthesia, again with a clinical profile similar to lidocaine.

Prilocaine is an amide local anesthetic with pharmacologic properties similar to those of lidocaine when used as a spinal anesthetic.[35] However, it shows a much lower incidence of TNS compared with spinal lidocaine and thus may be a favorable agent for ambulatory spinal anesthesia. Because of the risk of methemoglobinemia at required doses, prilocaine is generally considered unsuitable for epidural anesthesia. Currently, prilocaine is not available in the United States, but it is used commonly in Europe.

Short-Duration Agents As the first synthesized local anesthetic, procaine has been used for spinal anesthesia since the early 1900s. Procaine provides brief spinal anesthesia, but has limited clinical usefulness given the high incidence of block failure (see Table 46-4) and side effects. For reasons that are poorly understood, spinal procaine carries a higher risk of nausea than do other local anesthetics (odds ratio [OR] 3:1).[36] Although it has a lower incidence of TNS than spinal lidocaine (**Table 46-6**), spinal procaine is clearly not enticing as an agent for outpatient spinal anesthesia.

2-Chloroprocaine has received increased attention as a spinal anesthetic because of the challenges of ambulatory spinal anesthesia and concerns of relative neurotoxicities of other local anesthetics (eg, lidocaine). One year after its introduction into clinical use (1952), Foldes and McNall described successful use of a preservative-free preparation of 2-chloroprocaine for spinal anesthesia in 214 patients. Subsequently, 2-chloroprocaine enjoyed increasing popularity as an agent for epidural anesthesia, particularly in the obstetric population. Unfortunately, reports of accidental intrathecal injection of large volumes of Nesacaine-CE (chloroprocaine hydrochloride; AstraZeneca, Mississauga, Ontario, Canada) intended for the epidural space, resulting in several cases of neurotoxicity with lower-extremity paralysis and sacral nerve dysfunction, came to attention in the 1980s. Studies in dogs suggest that the combination of the antioxidant sodium bisulfite in the presence of low pH was responsible for the neurotoxicity,[37,38] and the formulation of 2-chloroprocaine was changed. Interestingly, a more recent laboratory study observed direct neurotoxicity from high doses of preservative-free 2-chloroprocaine in a rat model that was equivalent to 2% lidocaine and suggested that bisulfite was neuroprotective when added to 2-chloroprocaine.[39] Currently, 2 of the commercially available formulations of 2-chloroprocaine (Nesacaine-MPF, Astra Pharmaceuticals, Wilmington, DE, and generic chloroprocaine, Bedford Pharmaceuticals, Bedford, OH) are preservative-free and antioxidant-free. Given the availability of these new preparations and growing concerns about the TNS associated with lidocaine, 2-chloroprocaine has been reinvestigated for off-label use as a short-acting spinal anesthetic. Work by Kopacz et al shows 2-chloroprocaine to be a reliable spinal anesthetic, with consistent time to block resolution and achievement of discharge criteria without identifiable occurrence of TNS.[40-45] It should be noted that 2% 2-chloroprocaine may behave in a hyperbaric fashion,[43] and that the addition of epinephrine to spinal 2-chloroprocaine is not recommended because of reports of flu-like symptoms in volunteers receiving this combination.[40] As with fentanyl and plain bupivacaine, 2-chloroprocaine as a spinal anesthetic is currently an off-label use. However, the very low incidence of TNS and the rapid, dependable spinal block resolution is a very attractive profile for spinal anesthesia in ambulatory surgery. Given that the complete risk-to-benefit ratio of spinal 2-chloroprocaine is not known, clinicians should be mindful of restricting doses to not more than 40 mg, which is the most widely studied dose and ensure that only preservative-free, antioxidant-free preparations are utilized.

The use of 2% and 3% 2-chloroprocaine is an appropriate and US Food and Drug Administration (FDA)–approved choice for epidural anesthesia of short duration. After the release of Nesacaine-MPF, which contains ethylenediaminetetraacetic acid (EDTA), back pain following block resolution was reported with the use of high volumes of injected agent (>40 mL).[47] One proposed mechanism for this observation is tetanic spasm of the paraspinous muscles resulting from chelation of calcium by the EDTA. However, this was never proved and reports of back pain persist, despite the use of EDTA-free solutions. Given the potential for any solution intended for the epidural space to be accidentally injected into the subarachnoid space, it may be prudent to use only 2-chloroprocaine preparations that are preservative- and antioxidant-free for neuraxial blockade.

TABLE 47-6 Typical Incidences of TNS With Outpatient Spinal Anesthesia

Local Anesthetic	Patient Position	TNS(%)
Lidocaine 2-5%	Supine	6
Lidocaine 3%	Prone	0.4
Lidocaine 0.5%	Knee arthroscopy	17
Lidocaine 5%	Knee arthroscopy	16
Lidocaine 5%	Lithotomy	24
Bupivacaine (0.25%-0.75%)	Supine	0-1
	Knee arthroscopy	0-1
	Lithotomy	0-1
Mepivacaine 1.5%	Knee arthroscopy/Mixed	6-8
Mepivacaine 4%	Mixed	30
Ropivacaine 0.25%	Supine	1
Ropivacaine 0.2%-0.35%	Knee arthroscopy	0
Procaine 5%	Knee arthroscopy	6
2-Chloroprocaine 1%	Lower limb/mixed	0
Prilocaine (2%-5%)	Mixed	3-4

Bupivacaine, ropivacaine, and 2-chloroprocaine consistently result in low incidences of TNS, whereas lidocaine typically results in the highest incidences. Other local anesthetics are intemediate in incidence of TNS.

Data from Liu SS, McDonald SB. Current issues in spinal anesthesia. *Anesthesiology.* 2001;94:888-906; YaDeau JT, Liguori GA, Zayas VM. The incidence of transient neurologic symptoms after spinal anesthesia with mepivacaine. *Anesth Analg.* 2005;101:661-665; and Casati A, Danelli G, Berti M, et al. Intrathecal 2-chloroprocaine for lower limb outpatient surgery: a prospective, randomized, double-blind, clinical evaluation. *Anesth Analg.* 2006;103(1):234-238.

TABLE 47-7 Analgesic Adjuvants for Neuraxial Anesthesia

Agent	Dose	Typical Anesthetic Effect	Comments
Clinically Useful			
Fentanyl	Spinal 10-25 μg	25% increase in duration of surgical anesthesia 33% increase in anesthetic success with small doses of local anesthetic 60% incidence of easily treated pruritus	No delay of anesthetic recovery
	Epidural 1-2 μg/kg	2-fold reduction in volatile anesthetic requirements Decreased visceral pain with Cesarean section	Bolus administration may act at spinal level, infusions act via systemic uptake and redistribution to brainstem
Clonidine	Spinal 15-45 μg	29% increase in duration of motor block 37% increase in anesthetic success with small doses of local anesthetic Mild perioperative sedation and decrease in heart rate and blood pressure	No delay of anesthetic recovery
	Epidural 150 μg	2-3 fold increase in duration of sensory anesthesia Increased time to first analgesic request	Less oxygen desaturation, pruitis, and urinary retention compared to opioids
Epinephrine	Spinal 0.1-0.6 mg	Dose-related increase in surgical anesthesia and motor block	Dose-related increase in time until recovery of the same or greater magnitude
	Epidural 5 μg/mL	Increased duration, intensity of block with lidocaine and 2-chloroprocaine Will intensify block, but less effect on duration with bupivacaine Minimal effect with ropivacaine	Decreased plasma levels with lidocaine and bupivacaine, but not ropivacaine
Investigated			
Neostigmine	Spinal 6.25-50 μg	Dose related increase in surgical anesthesia and motor block 60% incidence of nausea and vomiting	Dose-related increase in time until recovery of the same or greater magnitude
	Epidural 1-4 μg/kg	Dose-dependent analgesic effect Increased time to first analgesic request	Reports of sedation with higher doses, less nausea than with intrathecal administration

Utility and safety of other agents (ketamine, ketorolac.) not fully determined.

Data from references 48, 50-53, 55, 63-64, 67, 69, 72-81, 83, 96, and 101.

ANALGESIC ADJUVANTS

Initially, interest in adjuvant medications for neuraxial anesthesia centered around increasing the duration and intensity of blockade (eg, epinephrine, phenylephrine). As the percentage of operations performed in the ambulatory setting increases, interest is shifting to identifying adjuncts that will augment block depth and reliability without prolonging recovery, especially motor block recovery (eg, fentanyl) (**Table 47-7**).

Opioids The potent analgesic effects of neuraxial opioids have been exploited to improve perioperative analgesia and reduce the supraspinally mediated side effects of sedation and respiratory depression seen with systemic opioids. Neuraxial opioids that diffuse into the spinal cord exert spinal analgesia by modulating C-fibers to decrease afferent nociceptive input,[48] inhibiting Ca^{2+} influx presynaptically, and increasing K^+ conductance and hyperpolarizing ascending neurons postsynaptically.[49]

Owing to its relative hydrophilic nature, neuraxial morphine provides highly selective, prolonged spinal analgesia, but is not typically used to augment intraoperative anesthesia because of slow onset. The lipophilic opioids, such as fentanyl (note that intrathecal use is not FDA-approved), are more suited for intraoperative use in the intrathecal space because of rapid onset, modest duration, and lower risk of delayed respiratory depression (though greater risk of early respiratory depression). The rapid onset of fentanyl is due to multiple factors, including the relatively large dose typically used, noting that 25 μg of fentanyl is roughly equivalent to 2.5 mg of morphine. The addition of 10 to 25 μg fentanyl to low-dose lidocaine and bupivacaine spinal anesthetics dramatically improves anesthetic success without delaying achievement of discharge criteria for ambulatory patients.[50,51] However, when used with the ultra–short-acting spinal anesthetic 2-chloroprocaine, fentanyl can slightly delay discharge (95 vs 104 minutes) and increase pruritus.[42]

The administration of epidural fentanyl can reduce volatile requirements more than intravenous fentanyl (>2-fold at 2 μg/kg).[52] The method of delivery of epidural fentanyl may be important for optimal effect. Ginosar et al[53] showed that when epidural fentanyl is given as a bolus, it imparts segmental analgesia consistent with spinal level of action, but if given as an epidural infusion, the analgesia is mediated through systemic uptake and supraspinal effect, as is seen with sufentanil and alfentanil.[54]

α_2-Agonists Interest in α_2-agonists, such as clonidine, has been rising in the field of regional anesthesia given their ability to enhance neuraxial analgesia without the respiratory depression and pruritus common to opioids. As with analgesia, the sedation, hypotension, and bradycardia seen with neuraxial clonidine are dose dependent.[55] Additionally, less urinary retention is seen with intrathecal clonidine than with intrathecal morphine.[56] Clonidine exerts its analgesic effects by binding to α_2-adrenoreceptors (on primary afferents, substantia gelatinosa, and several brainstem nuclei attributed to analgesic mechanisms), attenuating A-δ and C-fiber nociception, producing conduction blockade via increased potassium conductance,[57,58] as well as by increasing acetylcholine and norepinephrine in the CSF, inhibiting the release of substance P.[58] Although clonidine rapidly redistributes systemically to the periphery after epidural or spinal administration, the analgesic effect is spinally mediated, as evidenced by the lack of correlation between time of analgesia and peripheral blood levels. Through extensive testing for neurotoxicity and safety in several animal models, neuraxial clonidine shows no histopathologic or behavioral evidence of injury or toxicity and is FDA approved for epidural infusion for inadequately controlled cancer pain.

Although previously investigated as a sole anesthetic,[59] the majority of the clinical use of intrathecal clonidine is in combination with local anesthetics to produce dose-dependent prolongation of both sensory and motor block.[60-63] Showing a promising role in ambulatory anesthesia, De Kock et al[64] demonstrated that the addition of as little as 15 μg of clonidine to 8 mg of ropivacaine for spinal anesthesia in outpatients undergoing knee arthroscopy produced a considerable increase in anesthetic success (from 70% to 90%) without significant effect on recovery time. However, increasing the dose to 45 μg increased time to resolution of motor and sensory block and time to void from

170 to 215 minutes. Adding clonidine to local anesthetics intensifies and prolongs epidural blockade and can reduce local anesthetic dose requirement.[65,66] The typical dose of clonidine for addition to local anesthetics for epidural bolus administration is 150 μg, or 2 μg/kg.[67-69] Klimscha et al[68] demonstrated that the addition of 150 μg of clonidine to 10 mL of 0.5% bupivacaine for epidural anesthesia increased the mean duration of anesthesia from 1.8 to 5.3 hours, reduced pain scores, and increased time to first postoperative analgesic request. These benefits of clinical doses of neuraxial clonidine typically persist for approximately 3 hours and can be achieved without increasing hemodynamic instability more than local anesthetic alone or significantly altering responsiveness to resuscitation drugs.[69-72]

Vasoconstrictors Vasoconstricting agents, namely epinephrine and phenylephrine, are commonly added to local anesthetic solutions and have a long history of clinical use to prolong the anesthetic effect, provide more reliable block, and intensify anesthesia and analgesia.[73-76] Drugs with α-adrenergic activity appear to accentuate local anesthetic block by both pharmacokinetic and pharmacodynamic mechanisms. Pharmacokinetically, vasoconstriction of the arterioles in the dura mater,[77] and thus decreased blood flow, can reduce uptake of local anesthetics into the circulation, thus maintaining concentrations at the site of injection and reducing peak plasma concentrations. Additionally, intrinsic analgesic effects of epinephrine are exerted via stimulation of presynaptic α_2 adrenoreceptors found at the terminals of primary afferents. These receptors are also found centrally on neurons in the superficial laminae of the spinal cord and several brainstem nuclei that participate in analgesic mechanisms. α_2-Agonists can also produce motor block via actions on primary motor afferents.[78]

Epinephrine For spinal anesthesia, epinephrine is commonly used in a dose of 0.2 mg (although doses of 0.1-0.6 mg have been described), which, when added to a bupivacaine spinal anesthetic, increases time of regression to L2 by 25%.[79,80] The addition of epinephrine to spinal anesthetics prolongs motor block and delays the return of bladder function, which is problematic for ambulatory surgery patients trying to meet discharge criteria. Chiu et al,[81] using volunteers, showed that adding 0.2 mg of epinephrine to 50 mg of hyperbaric lidocaine prolonged surgical anesthesia (as demonstrated by tolerance of transcutaneous electrical stimulation) by 30 minutes, whereas time to void and discharge time were increased by 80 minutes.

As for safety, intrathecal epinephrine by itself, in clinically relevant doses, shows no neurotoxicity in humans. Spinal cord blood flow is well maintained in the dog and cat model in doses up to 0.5 mg.[77] However, animal studies suggest that epinephrine may worsen the degree of injury associated with local anesthetic neurotoxicity.[82] Smith et al[40] reported consistent flu-like symptoms (myalgias, malaise, arthralgias, back stiffness, loss of appetite) when epinephrine was added to spinal 2-chloroprocaine in a volunteer study. Phenylephrine may increase the risk of TNS, as suggested by Sakura et al[32] in a study of tetracaine spinal anesthesia.

With epidural anesthesia, the typical use of epinephrine is in concentrations of 1:200 000, or 5 μg/mL. The clinical effect of epinephrine on duration of anesthesia depends on the local anesthetic used. Epinephrine is more effective at prolonging the anesthetic duration of shorter-acting agents, such as lidocaine and 2-chloroprocaine. Adding 1:200 000 epinephrine to 2% lidocaine will nearly double the time to resolution of blockade.[83] Agents with longer duration of action show much less prolongation of anesthesia with the addition of epinephrine. Adding epinephrine to ropivacaine will intensify the block, but will not prolong the duration of epidural anesthesia or affect plasma concentrations.[74] This is likely a result of the inherent vasoconstricting effects of ropivacaine, as well as the clearance of ropivacaine not being dependent on blood flow. Other agents do show reduction of plasma concentrations when epinephrine is added.[73,75] Epinephrine 1:200 000 will decrease plasma lidocaine and chloroprocaine concentrations by 20% to 30%, but will decrease plasma bupivacaine concentrations only by 10% to 20%. The effect of epinephrine on plasma concentrations of local anesthetics has long been thought to be caused by constriction of the epidural venous plexus, reducing blood flow and slower uptake of local anesthetics. More recent evidence implies that reduced dural blood flow and increased hepatic clearance may be more important in this phenomenon.[84] Furthermore, work by Bernards et al[85] suggests that systemic effects on vasculature of epidurally administered epinephrine may alter volume of distribution and thus contribute to the altered plasma concentrations of local anesthetics. Its potential to prolong discharge times and delay bladder function limits the usefulness of adding epinephrine to epidural agents for ambulatory surgery. The premixed solutions of local anesthetics with epinephrine that are commercially available are prepared more acidic to prevent spontaneous epinephrine oxidation. Because this lower pH slows the onset of block and inhibits the vasoconstricting actions of epinephrine, adding "fresh" epinephrine to local anesthetic solutions at the time of use is preferred. When phenylephrine is added to epidural solutions, the systemic absorption results in increased vascular resistance (as opposed to the decrease in systemic vascular resistance [SVR] seen with epidural epinephrine at 1:200 000 concentration), without the benefit of increased contractility or chronotropy seen with epinephrine. Consequently, phenylephrine is typically only used in the subarachnoid space.

Neostigmine The acetylcholinesterase inhibitor neostigmine has been investigated as a neuraxial analgesic adjunct because of its ability to provide analgesia without hemodynamic depression. Unfortunately, its tendency to induce nausea and delay recovery from neuraxial blockade limits clinical use. Intrathecal neostigmine inhibits the breakdown of acetylcholine in the meninges and spinal cord via reversible inhibition of acetylcholinesterase. Animal models suggest that acetylcholine plays a role in spinal analgesia through stimulation of cholinergic receptors in the substantia gelatinosa and superficial laminae of the spinal cord dorsal horn[86-88] and perhaps through stimulating nitric oxide production in the spinal cord.[89] Whereas intrathecal injection of cholinergic agonists stimulates all receptors of a particular class, neostigmine increases endogenous acetylcholine in a manner dependent on the tonic release of this neurotransmitter within each particular region of the spinal cord. Hood et al[90] evaluated safety, analgesic efficacy, and side effects of intrathecal neostigmine in volunteers. All doses produced analgesia without sedation, pruritus, respiratory depression, hypotension, or bradycardia; however, there was dose-related motor weakness, decreases in deep tendon reflexes, urinary incontinence, and nausea and vomiting. Further studies in patients revealed similar incidence of nausea and vomiting that proved to be both prolonged and difficult to treat.[91-93] Liu et al[93] showed that when added to low-dose (7.5 mg) bupivacaine spinal anesthetics, 50 μg of neostigmine enhanced motor and sensory block, but delayed achievement of discharge criteria. Doses of 6.25 and 12.5 μg did not prolong anesthesia but still elicited nausea and delayed discharge. Intrathecal neostigmine does counteract hypotension resulting from bupivacaine spinal anesthesia in rats,[94] but these effects are not reproducible in human subjects.[95] Low and moderate doses of neostigmine are considered to have little or no cardiovascular effects.

Lauretti et al[96] studied the analgesic effect of epidural neostigmine, in doses from 1 to 4 μg/kg added to epidural lidocaine, and showed a dose-independent analgesic effect, increasing time to first analgesic request from 3.5 to 8 hours, with less nausea and vomiting than seen with intrathecal administration. Other studies report similar results with doses in the range of 1 to 10 μg/kg, without reporting increased nausea,[97-102] but reporting some suggestion of sedation.[101]

Alkalinization and Carbonation Alkalinizing local anesthetic solutions to raise the pH closer to the pK_a of the local anesthetic, thereby increasing the proportion of the nonionized form available to cross cell membranes, is thought to speed the onset of epidural anesthesia. Although this is well demonstrated with peripheral nerves in vitro,[103] studies attempting to demonstrate this clinically in epidural anesthesia are conflicting.

Most studies show that alkalinization speeds onset of epidural blockade with lidocaine,[104-109] bupivacaine,[104,110,111] mepivacaine,[104,112,113] and chloroprocaine[114,115] by up to 10 minutes. Ropivacaine seems not to show faster onset with alkalinization,[116] but as with the other drugs, there is evidence that alkalinization can intensify epidural anesthesia and improve spread to sacral dermatomes.[105,108,109,117] One trend that is noted is that the effects of alkalinization are greatest on solutions containing epinephrine, whether freshly added or prepackaged. This is perhaps a result of pH-dependent vasoconstrictive actions of epinephrine. Alternatively, this may be attributed to the fact that commercially available epinephrine-containing solutions are prepared at lower pH (usually with bisulfite), ranging from 3.2 to 4.2, in efforts to preserve the epinephrine.

Typically recommended volumes of 8.4% sodium bicarbonate to be added to local anesthetic solutions are 1 mL per each 10 mL of lidocaine or mepivacaine, 0.1 mL per 10 mL of bupivacaine, and 0.3 mL per 10 mL of 2-chloroprocaine. Because of the tendency to precipitate, adding sodium bicarbonate to ropivacaine solutions is not recommended. It should be noted that the degree of alkalinization is limited by precipitation, and all preparations should be inspected for precipitation before administration. Alternatively, the carbonate salts of local anesthetics have a more rapid onset of epidural blockade than standard hydrochloride preparations.[118] However, carbonated drugs are of limited availability and may be more prone to induce hypotension with epidural administration.[119]

PHYSIOLOGY OF NEURAXIAL ANESTHESIA

NEUROPHYSIOLOGY

Neural blockade by local anesthetics is discussed in Chapter 45, and thus this section highlights some of the clinical aspects specific to neuraxial blockade. After intrathecal injection of local anesthetics, drug is found in the spinal cord as well as in the spinal nerve rootlets within the CSF. After epidural injection, local anesthetic is found in spinal nerves in the epidural space, spinal nerve rootlets within the CSF, and within the spinal cord. Consequently, conduction blockade may take place at multiple sites along the neural pathway for both spinal and epidural anesthesia, and the exact site(s) of action are not precisely known.[120] However, previous studies do provide some insight into primary sites of action. After spinal anesthesia, somatosensory evoked potentials from the tibial nerve (peripheral nervous system) are abolished, whereas direct spinal cord stimulation remains unchanged.[121,122] These findings lend support to the theory that the spinal nerve rootlets are the primary site of action of spinal anesthesia and not the spinal cord. Animal studies suggest that the mechanism of action of epidural anesthesia is similar to that of spinal anesthesia. Measurement of evoked potentials in monkeys again indicates that the primary site of action of epidural anesthesia is the spinal nerve rootlets.[123] Interestingly, epidural anesthesia does not produce complete conduction block, as somatosensory evoked potentials from the tibial nerve are only modestly changed after induction of surgical epidural anesthesia. Furthermore, the magnitude of change in somatosensory evoked potentials does not correlate with intensity of epidural block.[124] This finding is similar to peripheral nerve block, and investigators suggest that anesthesia occurs from loss of information coding inherent in the oscillations of the action potential instead of from complete loss of conduction. Finally, the ability of spinal but not epidural anesthesia to completely suppress somatosensory evoked potentials from the tibial nerve offers objective support for the clinical impression that spinal anesthesia produces a more intense and complete block than epidural anesthesia.

In addition to direct conduction blockade within the CNS, spinal and epidural anesthesia produce sedation that is unrelated to systemic concentrations of local anesthetic, but which correlates with block height.[125] Animal studies using electroencephalogram (EEG) monitoring and direct brain stimulation during spinal anesthesia suggest that this is the result of a decrease in reticular activating system activity from decreased tonic afferent input from the anesthetized region.[126] One may note decreased requirements for supplemental sedation during high spinal blockade from this direct sedative effect. Previous clinical studies examining use of propofol and midazolam suggest that spinal anesthesia per se decreases sedative requirements by approximately 30% to 50% with clinically relevant spinal block heights.[127,128] This direct sedative effect of epidural anesthesia also becomes clinically relevant when a combined epidural-general anesthetic technique is performed. The use of epidural anesthesia reduces volatile anesthetic requirements by 20% to 30% during surgery when general anesthesia is titrated to either hemodynamics or bispectral index monitoring.[129,130]

RESPIRATORY PHYSIOLOGY

With spinal or epidural blockade to midthoracic levels, pulmonary function, gas exchange, and control of breathing are generally preserved in patients without preexisting respiratory disease.[131] Many patients will report a subjective sensation of dyspnea as a consequence of reduced sensation of expansion of the chest wall with inspiration. However, resting tidal volumes, respiratory rate, minute ventilation, and lung volumes are maintained in healthy patients.[132,133] Preservation of gross pulmonary function—even with relatively high thoracic level blocks—is explained by the fact that the diaphragm is the primary muscle of ventilation and is innervated by the cervical plexus (C3-5). In contrast, accessory respiratory muscles (abdominal, intercostal) do play a role in active expiratory function, and small block height–dependent decreases in peak expiratory flow can be observed (11% reduction at T8 vs 17% reduction at T4).[134] Active expiratory function plays a role in ability to cough; thus spinal anesthesia may impair ability to clear secretions.[131] Overall, healthy patients easily tolerate these mild changes, but patients with severe pulmonary disease may not. However, previous studies indicate that patients with chronic lung disease do not suffer from significant reductions in vital capacity or forced expiratory volume at 1 second (FEV_1) during spinal anesthesia.[131]

Control of breathing during spinal anesthesia is not altered significantly, although earlier studies demonstrated a small decrease in resting end-tidal PCO_2.[135] Although hyperventilation as a consequence of anxiety may cause lowering of the PCO_2, the hypocapnia is speculated to result from a lack of proprioceptive input from the abdomen and chest wall during spinal anesthesia, resulting in an increased drive to breathe.[135] It has been reported that spinal anesthesia with bupivacaine in unpremedicated patients increases ventilatory responsiveness to CO_2.[136] The rare respiratory arrest after spinal anesthesia is thought to result from brainstem hypoperfusion secondary to decreased cardiac output rather than the direct effects of local anesthetics on the brainstem, as the concentration of local anesthetic in the ventricular fluid is not high enough to result in medullary depression.

Preoperative discussions usually encourage tolerance of the subjective dyspnea, but at times judicious sedation can be used to quell anxieties. It should be noted that sedative medications used to facilitate neuraxial blockade are more likely to impact the patient's respiratory status than the blockade itself.[140] This is likely a result of both reduction in respiratory drive and initiation of paradoxical respiration from upper airway obstruction.

CARDIOVASCULAR PHYSIOLOGY

The perturbations of cardiovascular function during neuraxial anesthesia are perhaps the most critical factors to consider in evaluating the risk to patients and in preventing adverse outcomes. In the nonobstetrical population, the incidences of hypotension and bradycardia after spinal anesthesia are approximately 33% and 13%, respectively.[28,119] Large epidemiology studies from France, Scandinavia, and the United States

TABLE 47-8 Risk Factors for Moderate Bradycardia (Pulse <50 beats/min) and Hypotension During Spinal Anesthesia

Risk Factor	Odds Ratio
Bradycardia	
Baseline heart rate <60 beats/min	4.9
ASA physical status I (vs ASA physical status III or IV)	3.5
Prolonged PR interval	3.2
Use of β-blocking drugs	2.9
Sensory level above T5	1.7
Hypotension	
Sensory level above T5	3.8
Age > 40 y	2.5
Baseline SBP < 120 mm Hg	2.4
Spinal puncture above L2-3	1.8

Data from Carpenter RL, Caplan RA, Brown DL, et al. Incidence and risk factors for side effects of spinal anesthesia. *Anesthesiology.* 1992;76:906-916 and Salinas FV, Sueda LA, Liu SS. Physiology of spinal anaesthesia and practical suggestions for successful spinal anaesthesia. *Best Pract Res Clin Anaesthesiol.* 2003;17:289-303.

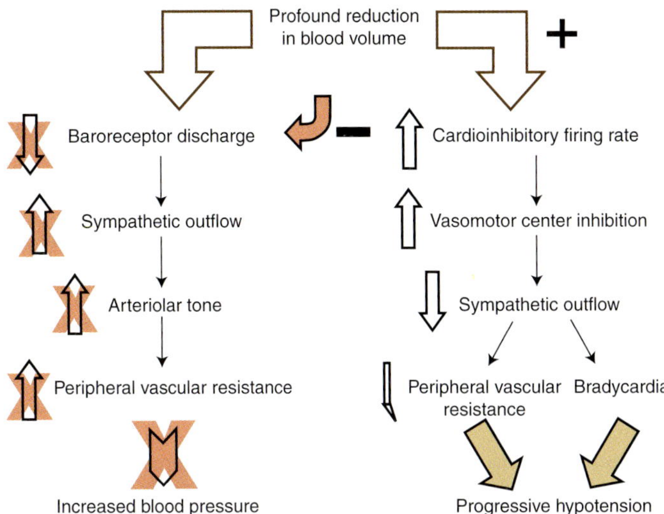

FIGURE 47-14. A proposed mechanism for the participation of the Bezold-Jarisch Reflex (BJR) type Cardioinhibitory pathways (right) in the cardiovascular collapse after neuraxial anesthesia. It is suggested that the redistributive hypovolemia produced by neuraxial blockade results in paradoxical bradycardia and inhibition of the baroreceptor reflex pathway (left), resulting in progressive hypotension.

indicate that the risk of cardiac arrest after spinal anesthesia is approximately 0.1-1:1000 and 1:10 000 after epidural anesthesia.[137] Although cardiac arrest after spinal anesthesia appears to be distressingly common, a recent study suggests that survival is better for cardiac arrest during neuraxial block than during general anesthesia (65% vs 31%).[138] This may be a result of enhanced vigilance, as several risk factors for bradycardia and hypotension have been identified for spinal anesthesia (**Table 47-8**). Risk factors for epidural anesthesia are probably similar but have not been fully identified because of the decreased frequency of occurrences. An appreciation for the mechanisms involved in these physiologic derangements allows early recognition and prompt treatment of potentially detrimental situations.

Cardiovascular changes seen with spinal anesthesia are caused by blockade of the sympathetic efferent fibers and thus generally are related to block height.[139] Both arterial and venous relaxations contribute to hypotension, resulting from decreases in SVR and cardiac output. SVR decreases to a greater degree in patients aged 69 to 80 years (26% from baseline) than in young, healthy subjects (13%-18% from baseline).[140] Venodilation causes increased pooling of blood in the capacitance vessels, thus reducing central blood volume.

Although heart rate is typically maintained, bradycardia can occur with spinal anesthesia in 10% to 15% of cases, and unexpected circulatory collapse remains a dreaded complication with a potentially grave outcome. In addition to the risk factors of age younger than 50 years, American Society of Anesthesiologists (ASA) physical status P1, and concomitant use of β-blockers, the incidence of bradycardia increases with increased block height with 75% of occurrences associated with sensory block above T5[36] (Table 47-8). Cardioaccelerator fibers originate from T1 to T5, and thus sympathetic blockade above T5 is thought to allow parasympathetic predominance over heart rate, mediated via the vagus nerve. However, some studies of heart rate variability demonstrate that even with high thoracic blockade, the activity of sympathetic and parasympathetic systems can remain in balance.[141,142] Reports of bradycardia/asystole and circulatory collapse in patients with blocks too low to be attributed solely to sympathectomy are further evidence that other factors may play important roles. Bradycardia may be induced by an increase in baroreceptor reflex activity.[143] With redistribution of blood to capacitance vessels and decreased venous return to the heart, resulting in decreased filling pressures, intracardiac stretch receptors within the right atrium and left ventricle have been suggested to participate in a bradycardic response (Bezold-Jarisch reflex; **Fig. 47-14**).[144,145] Maintaining preload and aggressive treatment of bradycardia may help improve the safety of spinal anesthesia.[146]

Efforts have been made to investigate the usefulness of heart rate variability analysis for predicting hypotension after spinal anesthesia for cesarean section to assess the underlying balance of patients' autonomic systems.[147,148] Although small and limited, these studies demonstrate that measurements of heart rate variability are predictive of hypotension in this patient population. Heart rate variability is extracted from the patient's electrocardiogram (ECG) and analyzed based on the preponderance of low versus high frequencies to determine subsets of patients who are at risk and who would benefit from additional prophylactic interventions (see next paragraph). Computer-aided analysis is being developed, as currently this is not a common ECG analysis. More research is needed, but this appears to be a promising clinical tool to direct selective therapy aimed at preventing hypotension with spinal anesthesia.

The prevention and prompt treatment of hypotension and bradycardia during spinal anesthesia is essential in protecting the patient from untoward outcomes. The practice of administering a crystalloid bolus before spinal anesthesia has been a standard method for preventing hypotension induced by neuraxial blockade. Behind this is an effort to maintain central blood volume, and, therefore, venous return to the heart, so as to preserve cardiac output. However, studies reveal a more complicated interaction between fluid loading, hemodynamic effects, and efficacy for preventing hypotension in the nonobstetric population. For example, prophylactic bolusing of 500 to 1500 mL of crystalloid may be ineffective for prevention of hypotension in normovolemic patients if performed before induction of spinal anesthesia,[149-151] but may be effective if performed later during the actual performance of spinal anesthesia.[152] This may be a result of the rapid redistribution of crystalloids out of the intravascular compartment, thus providing only a fleeting contribution to venous return.[153] Furthermore, a crystalloid bolus does not adequately address other factors contributing to hypotension, namely heart rate and SVR, and may actually decrease SVR.[154] In contrast, the administration of colloid solutions is more effective in maintaining intravascular volume caused by favorable pharmacokinetics[154,155] and may actually increase SVR.[154] Prophylactic administration of 500 to 1000 mL of colloid solution before induction of spinal blockade more effectively prevents hypotension but can grossly affect fluid balance in the patient. In regards to treatment of hypotension in the setting of established hypovolemia, crystalloid remains a suitable choice because of altered volume kinetics in such a setting.[156]

The technique of spinal anesthesia may also be altered to attenuate resultant vasodilatation and hypotension. Sympathetic block is somewhat dose dependent; thus selection of an appropriate dose is helpful. The use of unilateral spinal anesthesia for unilateral lower-extremity procedures allows limited spread of sympathetic block and has been investigated. Typically, a small dose of hyperbaric local anesthetic is injected and the patient is kept in the lateral position (operative side down) for 15 minutes. Casati et al[157] showed a decreased rate of hypotension in patients with intentionally asymmetric spinal blocks as compared with conventional bilateral blockade (5% vs 22%). Incidence of hypotension is reduced with epidural compared with spinal anesthesia, and placement of a catheter with gradual titration of epidural local anesthetic dose allows time for treatment of the gradual sympathectomy.

Effective treatment of hypotension should be tailored to the clinical situation at hand, with consideration of alterations in SVR and cardiac output. Vasopressors with α-adrenergic agonist activity, such as phenylephrine and metaraminol, are quite effective for increasing SVR. However, this may be at the expense of a further decrease in cardiac output as a response to the increase in afterload.[158] In light of this, it is thought that the use of mixed α- and β-adrenergic agonist drugs, like ephedrine, may be more appropriate for the treatment of hypotension induced by neuraxial blockade as a result of the ability to augment heart rate and cardiac output as well as SVR. Ephedrine is most often administered as an intermittent intravenous bolus of 5 to 10 mg, but may also be given via continuous infusion or intramuscularly as a depot of 25 to 50 mg. Atropine in doses of 0.4 to 1 mg intravenously can be used to treat moderate bradycardia if ephedrine is ineffective. In the case of precipitous bradycardia, or in situations unresponsive to the previously mentioned interventions, one should not hesitate to consider administration of epinephrine. Although clinical data are lacking, closed claims data analysis suggests that the lack of early administration of epinephrine is a management pattern in spinal anesthesia that leads to cardiac arrest with poor outcome.[159]

Although similar hemodynamic changes are seen with epidural anesthesia, these tend to be better tolerated than changes seen with spinal anesthesia, perhaps because of a more gradual and titratable onset. Nonetheless, sudden bradycardiac cardiac arrest has been described with epidural anesthesia.[160] Risk of sudden cardiovascular collapse from epidural anesthesia may be influenced by the addition of epinephrine to the epidural solution. With the typical dose range used for epidural anesthesia, systemic levels of epinephrine remain low, producing a β_2-adrenergic effect of vasodilatation, increased heart rate, and myocardial contractility. Ward et al[161] evaluated the cardiovascular effects of epidural blockade to T5 using lidocaine with and without epinephrine. Mean arterial pressure decreased 20% in the epinephrine group, compared with 10% in the plain lidocaine group. However, the group with epinephrine also showed a 20% to 30% increase in cardiac output. Bonica et al [162] suggested that this systemic β-adrenergic effect of epinephrine might prevent the potential cardiovascular collapse from epidural blockade, though this has not been demonstrated in studies of sufficient power.

GASTROINTESTINAL, HEPATIC, AND GENITOURINARY PHYSIOLOGY

The sympathectomy of spinal anesthesia results in a relaxation of sphincters, constriction of the bowel, and an increase in secretions caused by "parasympathetic dominance." This imbalance of the autonomic nervous system is also thought by some to explain the occurrence of nausea seen with spinal anesthesia. Hepatic blood flow is related to mean arterial pressure and is thus maintained if the patient is hemodynamically stable.[163] Likewise, renal blood flow and renal function are preserved during spinal anesthesia when perfusion pressure is adequate.[164] Urinary retention after spinal anesthesia is the most noteworthy and clinically significant concern in regard to the genitourinary system. Postoperative urinary retention occurs in approximately 16% of patients in the recovery unit.[165]

After the induction of spinal anesthesia, the urge to void (normal detrusor function) is abolished within 60 seconds.[166,167] Recovery of the ability to void normally does not return until sensory anesthesia has regressed to the S3 sacral segment.[166] Prolonged inhibition of normal detrusor function with the use of long-acting local anesthetics such as bupivacaine may allow bladder overdistension and urinary retention. In a study of healthy male patients undergoing nonurologic surgery after spinal anesthesia comparing 100 mg lidocaine with 10 mg bupivacaine, the time to return of normal detrusor function was significantly longer in the bupivacaine group (233 ± 31 vs 462 ± 61 minutes).[166] The cystometric capacity (the bladder volume at which patients feel an urge to void before spinal anesthesia) in this study was between 500 and 600 mL, and the patients in the bupivacaine group generated an average of 875 ± 385 mL of urine, far exceeding the cystometric capacity and suggesting that the use of long-acting local anesthetics may lead to bladder overdistension and urinary retention. Furthermore, the use of epinephrine as an adjuvant for spinal anesthesia has been identified as a factor in delayed voiding ability.[81] Other factors such as age (>50 years), volume of intraoperative fluid administration, and type of surgical procedure also influence rate of urinary retention.[165]

Concern for postoperative urinary retention is especially important in the ambulatory setting, where the traditional requirement to void after spinal anesthesia often leads to prolonged delays in discharge.[168] However, optimal use of short-acting local anesthetics for ambulatory spinal and epidural anesthesia has not been associated with urinary retention.[169] A study of ambulatory surgery patients discharged before voiding after short-acting spinal anesthesia demonstrated significantly shorter discharge times, with no reports of urinary retention.[170] Thus the risk of urinary retention appears to be low after short-acting spinal anesthesia, and further prospective study is needed to confirm this practice (discharging patients before voiding after short-acting spinal anesthesia) in a large population.

COMPLICATIONS OF NEURAXIAL ANESTHESIA

POSTMENIGEAL PUNCTURE HEADACHE

Appreciated since perhaps the first spinal anesthetic, postmeningeal puncture headache (PMPH) remains a complication of spinal anesthesia and is seen in as much as 50% of cases of unintentional meningeal puncture during attempted epidural anesthesia. Reported incidence of PMPH after spinal anesthesia varies greatly, depending on the types of needles used and patient population. Although rates as high as 40% are seen with 22-gauge beveled-tip needles,[171] the use of smaller-diameter pencil-point needles has decreased the risk of PMPH after spinal anesthesia to approximately 1%.[172] The traditional mechanism of PMPH is believed to involve the loss of CSF from the thecal sac and a "sagging" of the brain while standing or sitting upright. This is thought to result in traction on the cranial meninges, meningeal vessels, and, at times, traction on the cranial nerves, leading to cranial nerve palsy. Magnetic resonance imaging (MRI) studies demonstrating reduced CSF volume[173] and meningeal enhancement postgadolinium during PMPH[174] lend support to this theory of CSF loss and meningeal irritation. There are also data suggesting that vasodilatation of cerebral vessels may be important in etiology of PMPH.[175] A persistent hole in the dura mater has traditionally been blamed for PMPH, but there is no evidence that the dural hole is more important than the arachnoid hole in this regard. Consequently, we use the more general term *postmeningeal puncture headache*.

The headache is typically positional, being most severe while standing or sitting and nearly eliminated when supine. Patients usually describe a band-like aching pain in the frontal and occipital regions, posterior neck pain, and at times nausea, tinnitus, photophobia, and diplopia. Differentiation from infectious meningitis or intracranial mass lesions is important and usually based on positional nature of symptoms, absence of lateralizing neurologic findings, lack of fever, and, if necessary, normal peripheral white blood cell count and CSF profile.

Although traditionally held to the contrary, patient sex and postoperative recumbency are not related to incidence of PMPH.[176] Although the incidence of PMPH decreases with increasing patient age,[176] factors that are in the control of the clinician to reduce the occurrence of PMPH include the use of smaller-gauge needles, pencil-point needles, and longitudinal orientation of the bevel if a cutting needle is used.[176,177] The mechanisms in play for the latter 2 factors are not entirely clear. The classically described scenario is that of more dural fibers being cut by a transversely oriented cutting bevel and thus a more substantial hole in the dura. However, given that the dural fibers are not actually longitudinally arranged, rather, randomly, the number of these fibers cut will not depend on bevel orientation. It has been suggested that the longitudinal tension placed on the meninges tends to pull open a transversely oriented defect and thus allow for more CSF leakage. As for pencil-point needles, the supposition that they cause less trauma to the meninges is questionable. Reina et al[173] suggest that Whitacre needles produce more trauma, as evidenced by electron microscopy images, and that the reduced loss of CSF may be a result of an "edematous plug" resulting from greater inflammatory reaction.

Conservative management of PMPH includes bed rest, oral analgesics, adequate hydration, and caffeine (because of its ability to constrict cerebral arterioles). Although these measures are often ineffective, patients should be reassured that the symptoms are likely to resolve within 1 week without further invasive treatments. If the patient is not responding adequately to conservative treatments or is having prolonged symptoms, then an epidural blood patch can be considered. This is usually performed by accessing the epidural space within 1 interspace of the suspected meningeal hole and injecting 10 to 20 mL of autologous blood in an aseptic fashion. This is intended to form a clot, or "patch," over the dural defect, preventing further leakage of CSF. Additionally, this volume will tamponade the dural sac and restore buoyant support to the brain, explaining the near-immediate relief that many patients report. The success of epidural blood patch is reported to be in the range of 70% to 95%, with those who fail to improve with an initial patch showing the same range of response to a repeat procedure. Large needle causing the meningeal puncture and early administration of the treatment (delay of <4 days from puncture) are factors suggested to be associated with failure of epidural blood patch.[178] The effectiveness of prophylactic blood patch administration is controversial, with some studies showing no benefit and others reporting greater than 50% success in preventing PMPH.[179,180] More recent evaluations demonstrate that prophylactic blood patch will not prevent PMPH, but might at best shorten the duration of symptoms in obstetric patients with inadvertent meningeal puncture with a large-diameter needle.[181]

In the search for alternatives to epidural blood patch, administration of saline[182] and dextran[183] has been performed, but without prolonged relief of symptoms. Other substances, such as fibrin glue, have been used in the epidural space with some success,[184,185] but further investigation is needed to determine the potential benefits and safety of such procedures.

INFECTIOUS

Infectious complications after neuraxial anesthesia are rare, but can arise in the form of meningitis and epidural abscess.[186,187] In a large and relatively complete retrospective review, Moen et al[188] estimated the incidence of meningitis to be less than 1 in 50 000 after spinal anesthesia and approximately 1 in 90 000 after epidural procedures and the incidence of epidural abscess to be 1 in 37 000 after epidural blocks. The source of microorganisms can be from contaminated equipment or injected solutions, or from patient source, namely bacteremia. The concern for potential inoculation from the performer's oral or nasopharyngeal flora has led to a CDC recommendation and the American Society of Anesthesiology Practice Advisory regarding the use of masks covering nose and mouth when performing neuraxial techniques.[187] It is speculated that lumbar puncture may disrupt the blood–brain barrier and allow transfer of blood-borne bacteria into the spinal space. Animal studies support this theory, but also show pretreatment with antibiotics to drastically reduce this risk.[189]

Epidural anesthesia for surgical procedures may have a similar risk profile, but the use of indwelling epidural catheters for continuous analgesic infusions provides an additional risk of serving as a wick for surface infections to migrate along the tract to become a deep infection or epidural abscess. Although some surveillance studies and studies examining rates of bacterial contamination of epidural catheter tips indicate that risk is low,[188,190] a survey by Wang et al[191] reported an incidence of 1 in 1930 catheters, with prolonged duration of catheterization identified as a risk factor. Patients with postoperative catheters should be under surveillance for signs of infection, having the catheter site inspected daily. If signs of skin infection are present, the catheter should be removed and the site monitored for improvement, with or without the initiation of antibiotics as deemed suitable. If the patient presents with severe back pain, and/or new neurologic deficits that are not explained by the analgesic infusion, then the diagnosis of epidural abscess must be considered, and MRI or computed tomography (CT) performed if appropriate. Du Pen et al[192] showed successful nonsurgical management of infections associated with chronic tunneled epidural catheters. However, in the setting of neurologic compromise, prompt diagnosis and surgical evacuation is imperative to permit recovery if an epidural abscess is identified.

HEMORRHAGIC COMPLICATIONS

With any invasive procedure, the possibility of inducing bleeding, especially in a noncompressible region, enters the risk-to-benefit analysis. With neuraxial procedures, hematoma can develop in the epidural, subdural, or intrathecal space, with the potential for devastating neurologic outcome. The estimated incidence of spinal hematoma in the absence of anticoagulant and antiplatelet medications is less than 1 in 150 000 neuraxial blocks,[193] although Moen and colleagues[194] identified significantly higher rates in elderly females and patients with concurrent coagulation-modifying factors. The majority of cases of spinal hematoma are in patients receiving anticoagulants or with hemostatic abnormalities from hepatic dysfunction or thrombocytopenia.

The usual presenting signs/symptoms are motor or sensory deficits or bowel/bladder dysfunction that are not explained by the administered anesthetic/analgesic agents. In patients with such symptoms, especially in the setting of anticoagulants, definitive diagnosis should be sought without delay. A review by Vandermeulen et al[195] indicated that early identification by MRI or CT and surgical decompression performed within 4 to 8 hours of presentation is associated with good neurologic recovery. This review also highlighted the importance of coagulation status at the time of epidural catheter removal, with nearly 50% of the epidural hematomas in patients with indwelling catheters manifesting clinical symptoms after removal of the catheter.

The American Society of Regional Anesthesia and Pain Medicine has released an updated consensus statement to address the concerning issues surrounding neuraxial procedures in patients receiving anticoagulant and antiplatelet medications.[193] Some of the recommendations from this statement are presented here, but this in no way substitutes for a full review of the information provided by the Consensus Conference, which can be downloaded for free at www.asra.com. One should also consider that any patient who is receiving combinations of the following medications is likely at further increased risk and appropriate caution taken.

Warfarin therapy should be stopped 5 days before planned intervention and international normalized ratio (INR) measured before neuraxial procedures. In patients with indwelling epidural catheters who have had warfarin therapy initiated, a lower-extremity neurologic examination protocol should be followed, and the INR should be confirmed to be less than 1.5 before epidural catheter removal.

The use of aspirin and nonsteroidal anti-inflammatory drugs is not considered to increase the risk of hemorrhagic complications with neuraxial procedures. However, clopidogrel should be discontinued for at least 7 days before neuraxial techniques. Given shorter half-lives, the glycoprotein (GP) IIb/IIIa antagonists only need to be held for 24 to 48 hours to allow return of platelet function.

Patients receiving twice-daily 5000 units of subcutaneous heparin for thromboprophylaxis are not considered to be at increased risk for spinal hematoma, but considerations should be made with regard to timing of procedures in light of the peak onset of 2 hours after administration of heparin dose. The safety of subcutaneous heparin administration in a 3-times daily regimen or in larger doses has not been determined. Intraoperative anticoagulation with IV heparin is acceptable if given 1 hour after and discontinued 2 to 4 hours (and normal partial thromboplastin time [PTT] confirmed) before block placement or catheter removal.

Low-molecular-weight heparins (LMWHs) present added management concerns given the prolonged action (especially in patients with decreased renal clearance) and difficulty in measuring the induced alterations in coagulation status. Current recommendations state that patients receiving thromboprophylactic doses should have neuraxial procedures delayed 10 to 12 hours after last dose. If receiving "treatment" dosing (1 mg/kg twice a day), a delay of 24 hours is recommended. After neuraxial procedures, initiation of LMWH therapy should be delayed 6 to 8 hours for daily dosing or 24 hours for twice-daily dosing.

NEUROLOGIC COMPLICATIONS

Neurologic injury from neuraxial procedures is rare, but it remains a fervently held fear among many patients. The overall incidence of persistent neurologic injury associated with neuraxial blocks is reported to be approximately 0.08% to 0.16%; however, the vast majority of these reported cases fail to show evidence that the block was directly causative.[196] Potential mechanisms of neurologic injury after neuraxial anesthesia include direct needle or catheter trauma, neurotoxicity of injected substances (intended agents or unintended chemicals), infectious complications, hemorrhagic complications, or spinal cord ischemia. The majority of perceived injuries are related to persistent paresthesia or motor weakness, but cauda equina syndrome is also rarely reported.

Although paresthesia is reported in as many as 13.6% of patients during needle placement for spinal anesthesia,[197] this rarely results in persistent neurologic deficit.[198] Similarly, most paresthesias associated with indwelling epidural catheters are likely to dissipate after removal of the catheter.[199] Despite its rare occurrence, paresthesia during block placement is considered a risk factor for persistent paresthesia. Patients experiencing this should be reassured and queried postoperatively regarding their neurologic status.

Attention has been focused on the issues surrounding neurotoxicity of local anesthetics and common additives because of identification of several cases of cauda equina syndrome associated with continuous spinal anesthesia via microcatheters. Although the injuries in these cases have been attributed to supranormal doses of local anesthetic, pooling and maldistribution of the local anesthetic within the thecal sac caused by the nature of administration through the small diameter catheter,[200] there are reports of similar injuries from single-shot lidocaine spinal anesthetics using relatively high doses (>75 mg) with epinephrine.[201] Despite the long history of relative safety, animal data exist to suggest that all local anesthetics have some potential to cause neural injury; however, lidocaine and tetracaine appear to have a greater potential for neurotoxicity than bupivacaine at clinically relevant concentrations.[202] Drasner[203] has presented recommendations for lidocaine spinal anesthesia, including limiting the dose to 60 mg, avoiding epinephrine, and restricting concentrations to 2.5% or less, although little human evidence exists to support these proposals. The concerns of dose, concentration, and adjuvants might be applicable to all local anesthetics.

A much more commonly reported complication after neuraxial anesthesia is transient neurologic symptoms (TNS). These symptoms, initially termed *transient radicular irritation* in 1993,[204] are described as back pain radiating to the buttocks and/or the lower extremities. Although TNS has been reported after spinal anesthesia with all local anesthetics, it is far more common with lidocaine, showing an incidence in prospective studies to be between 4% and 36%.[29] Drastic variation in the observed rates of TNS (Table 47-6) lends support to the theory that multiple factors are involved in its development. Factors demonstrated to contribute to the incidence of TNS include the use of lidocaine (relative risk of 4.35 compared with other local anesthetics),[205] lithotomy position, knee arthroscopy, and early ambulation (as in outpatient surgery) (Table 47-6).[204]

The etiology of TNS remains elusive, but proposed culprits include direct neurotoxicity of local anesthetics, stretching of neural structures via positioning and muscle relaxation, and muscular spasm. The evidence against neurotoxicity being the principal cause of TNS includes lack of motor deficit or electrophysiologic changes during acute symptoms,[206] as well as its response to nonsteroidal anti-inflammatory drugs and other modalities targeting muscular discomfort.

LOCAL ANESTHETIC SYSTEMIC TOXICITY AND EPIDURAL TEST DOSE

It is important to verify correct placement of needles and catheters in the epidural space before initiating epidural anesthesia. Unintentional subdural or subarachnoid dosing can result in high blocks or "total spinals," whereas intravascular injection can result in local anesthetic systemic toxicity (LAST), which can progress to seizures or cardiovascular collapse.[207] Subdural injection is rare and may be difficult to recognize, as CSF will not be aspirated from the needle or catheter. The clinical pattern is one of an unusually high block after administration of local anesthetic.[208] Unintentional subarachnoid injection is a more common occurrence with incidences of "total spinals" ranging from 0.3% to 0.6%. It is important to realize that an epidural catheter may migrate into the subarachnoid space at any time during use. Unintentional intravascular injection is probably more common, with incidences of systemic toxic reactions (ranging from mild CNS symptoms to seizures) ranging from 0.01% to 2%.[208] Again, it is important to realize that an epidural catheter may migrate into the intravascular space at any time during use.

Although efficacy for improving safety is uncertain, it is standard practice to administer a test dose before initiating full epidural anesthesia.[209] This test dose is intended to detect unintentional placement of the needle or catheter into either the subarachnoid or intravascular space. A 3-mL volume of local anesthetic is the primary component of a test dose. Theoretically, subarachnoid injection of this local anesthetic will produce a much more rapid and profound sensory and motor block than epidural injection. However, changes can be subtle and will require time to develop. Previous reports indicate that 2 to 4 minutes are required before development of sensory or motor block after subarachnoid injection of 3 mL of 1.5% lidocaine.[208,210] Subarachnoid injection of a bupivacaine test dose (3 mL 0.25%-0.5%) produces spinal blocks with highly variable onset time and spread and is probably not a reliable indicator.[208] Use of a test dose to detect subarachnoid placement is not without risk, as previous publications have reported high spinal anesthesia requiring tracheal intubation after 3 mL of 1.5% lidocaine or 0.5% bupivacaine.[208] The local anesthetic component of the test dose has been suggested to aid in detection of intravascular injection by producing classic symptoms of systemic toxicity, such as tinnitus, perioral tingling, metallic taste, and dizziness; however, the presenting symptoms of LAST are variable and possibly delayed.[211] Detection ability is limited, as the standard 3-mL test dose (45 mg of lidocaine or 15 mg of bupivacaine) contains insufficient local anesthetic to reliably produce such symptoms. Previous studies suggest that larger doses, such as 100 mg or 1 mg/kg of lidocaine or more than

TABLE 47-9 Use of Epinephrine Test Doses to Detect Intravascular Injection

Patient Type	Hemodynamic Criteria for Intravascular Injection of 15 μg of Epinephrine
Healthy surgical patient	HR increase > 20 beats/min SBP increase > 15 mm Hg T wave amplitude decrease by ≥ 25% on ECG
Beta adrenergic blockade	HR unreliable SBP increase > 15 mm Hg
Age >60 y	HR increase > 9 beats/min SBP increase > 15 mm Hg
General anesthesia	HR increase > 8 beats/min SBP increase > 13 mm Hg
Spinal anesthesia	HR increase > 20 beats/min SBP unreliable

All responses occur within 2 minutes of injection.

HR, heart rate; SBP, systolic blood pressure.

25 mg of bupivacaine, levobupivacaine, or ropivacaine, are required in the unsedated patient.[208,212] Administration of even modest doses of sedation further reduces the ability of patients to report these symptoms (40% reduction in sensitivity).[213]

Epinephrine is commonly added to the local anesthetic dose to increase sensitivity for detection of intravascular injection. Addition of 15 μg is the standard dose of epinephrine; it will consistently produce increases in heart rate and systolic blood pressure and reduction in T-wave amplitude within 60 to 120 seconds in healthy patients (**Table 46-9**).[208,214] Use of β-blockers, advanced age, and concurrent general or spinal anesthesia all decrease the hemodynamic response to this dose of epinephrine, and reduced criteria, or larger epinephrine doses, should be applied in these circumstances.[208,215,216] Intravascular injection of epinephrine may be of concern in patients with hypertension, patients at risk for myocardial ischemia, and in obstetrical patients, and potential risks should be considered in these patients.

The best method for avoiding systemic toxicity from local anesthetics is through prevention.[207,209] Toxic systemic concentrations can occur by unintentional intravenous or intra-arterial injection or by systemic absorption of excessive doses placed in the correct area. Unintentional intravascular injections can be minimized by frequent syringe aspiration for blood, use of a local anesthetic test dose (see earlier discussion), and either slow injection or fractionation of the rest of the dose of local anesthetic.[209] Detailed knowledge of local anesthetic pharmacokinetics will also aid in reducing the administration of excessive doses of local anesthetics. Ideally, heart rate, blood pressure, and ECG should be monitored during administration of local anesthetics. Pretreatment with a benzodiazepine might also lower the probability of seizure by raising the seizure threshold. The administration of intravenous lipid emulsion in the treatment of cardiovascular toxicity has gained much attention after demonstrated benefit in experimental animals and case reports in human patients.[217] Although acceptance of this treatment is rapidly taking hold in clinical practice, further evaluation is needed to identify optimal administration and potential adverse effects. A treatment algorithm for LAST can be accessed for free at www.asra.com through the Practice Advisory section.

CONTINUOUS SPINAL ANESTHESIA

Because of the density and reliability of spinal anesthetic blockade, attempts to extend the duration and graduate the dosing of agents led to techniques for continuous spinal anesthesia (CSA). A century ago, malleable spinal needles were left within the subarachnoid space to allow redosing during prolonged procedures, and later, Tuohy placed catheters in the intrathecal space. The development of microcatheters (29-32 gauge) in the 1980s led to a revisiting of this technique, with hopes of titrating and prolonging spinal blockade with reduced incidence of PMPH as compared with Tuohy's 15-gauge catheters. Unfortunately, beyond the problems of breakage and knotting, these catheters are associated with several reports of cauda equina syndrome, usually with 5% hyperbaric lidocaine used as the agent. The hypothesis is that the small-bore catheters reduced local anesthetic mixing in the CSF, which in turn led to a "sacral pooling" of the hyperbaric agents, limiting spread and dilution of the drug in the CSF, unmasking the neurotoxic potential of lidocaine at such a concentration. The FDA subsequently removed these microcatheters from the market, as did the Canadian authorities. However, a recent evaluation of bupivacaine and sufentanil via 28-gauge intrathecal catheters by Arkoosh et al[218] encourages renewed interest in microcatheters, demonstrating superior analgesia without evidence of neurologic complications, but with increased technical difficulty with placement and removal. Although some practitioners still use continuous spinal anesthesia using larger-gauge catheters, the risks and benefits must be weighed carefully for the given situation. If CSA is to be undertaken, precautions should be taken to not advance the catheter beyond 3 cm within the intrathecal space, avoid dextrose-containing preparations, give adequate time for spread and distribution of the agent befre additional dosing, and be prepared to abandon the technique if sacral pooling is suspected.

COMBINED SPINAL–EPIDURAL ANESTHESIA

Combined spinal–epidural anesthesia (CSEA) is an increasingly popular technique owing to its advantages of rapid onset, dense neuraxial block, ability to titrate spread and duration of block, and lower total drug dosage when compared with epidural anesthesia. Potential disadvantages include increased time to perform the dual technique, intrathecal migration of epidural drug and/or catheter, effects of increased epidural pressure from injection of solutions on spinal block, and decreased ability and reliability of epidural test dosing. Although a seemingly simple combination of 2 routine techniques for neuraxial anesthesia, the interactions between the 2 can be subtle, can impact clinical management, and have not been fully determined.

PATIENT SELECTION AND CLINICAL APPLICATIONS

Obstetrics CSEA has been most widely accepted in the obstetric population. The concept of the "walking epidural" has become popular among patients, where intrathecal opioid allows rapid onset of analgesia without motor blockade. Lipid-soluble opioids, such as fentanyl (up to 25 μg) and sufentanil (up to 10 μg), are commonly used to provide dose-dependent analgesia for 60 to 90 minutes. Opioids are also commonly combined with small doses of local anesthetics, such as bupivacaine, to either prolong this initial spinal analgesia or to reduce side effects by decreasing the required dose of opioids. Previous dose–response studies indicate that 2.5 mg of bupivacaine combined with either 15 μg of fentanyl or 2.5 μg of sufentanil provides satisfactory analgesia while reducing incidences of nausea and pruritus, when compared with larger doses of opioid.[219,220] Preservation of motor function is an important goal after CSEA for labor analgesia, and sophisticated testing of positional sense and motor function after CSEA indicates little effect from the initial spinal dose (2.5 mg of bupivacaine + 5 μg of fentanyl).[221] However, subsequent injection of a standard test dose (45 mg of lidocaine + 15 μg of epinephrine) to confirm epidural catheter placement or the initiation of continuous epidural analgesia appears to degrade motor function and positional sense.[221,222] Addition of other less commonly used adjuncts to standard doses of opioids can also increase duration of analgesia. For example, addition of 200 μg of epinephrine or 50 μg of clonidine to opioid is equivalent to adding 2.5 mg of bupivacaine and can provide an additional 30 minutes of analgesia.[223] Despite the apparent preservation of motor function, large clinical trials have not observed a decrease in incidence of cesarean section when CSEA is compared with conventional epidural analgesia, although the incidence is similar to systemic analgesia.[224-226]

As an anesthetic for cesarean section, CSEA offers a rapid, titratable block, good muscle relaxation if an appropriate local anesthetic concentration is used, and the ability to use reduced doses of local anesthetic. Several clinical trials have compared CSEA with epidural anesthesia with lidocaine or bupivacaine combined with fentanyl. These studies report more rapid onset, better motor block, decreased anxiety levels, decreased shivering, and greater patient satisfaction with CSEA.[227,228] Incidences of side effects were similar in that the severity of hypotension did not differ, nor did the incidence of postmenigeal puncture headaches, backaches, nausea, or vomiting.[227,228] When compared with conventional single-shot spinal anesthesia, use of CSEA offers the potential advantage of using a smaller initial dose of spinal anesthetic with the epidural catheter available, should the block be insufficient. Such an approach theoretically offers the advantage of greater individual titration with reduced side effects and faster recovery from conduction block. However, results from studies are inconsistent, with some trials observing faster motor recovery with this approach[229] and others not discerning a reduced dosing need for spinal anesthesia with epidural supplement.[230,231] A potential disadvantage of the CSEA technique versus the single-shot technique is an increased incidence of transient paresthesia during placement of the spinal needle. A previous study randomizing patients undergoing cesarean section to CSEA versus conventional spinal anesthesia observed incidences of paresthesia of 37% versus 9%. There were no long-term complications, and the authors speculated that the CSEA technique might lead to deeper tissue penetration as a mechanism for increased incidence of transient paresthesia.[232]

Ambulatory Anesthesia The dose of local anesthetic determines both anesthetic success and duration of recovery. Availability of the epidural catheter for a rescue anesthetic allows use of minimal doses of spinal local anesthetic with resultant rapid recovery and discharge (Table 47-4) and represents an alternative or complementary strategy to use of analgesic additives. Several clinical trials have determined minimally effective doses for ambulatory knee arthroscopy using this approach. For example, initial doses of spinal lidocaine 40 mg or mepivacaine 45 mg[233,234] have been determined to be optimal doses for CSEA by previous dose–response studies. However, induction of a CSEA technique probably takes more time than conventional spinal anesthesia, and no current data are available to assess relative cost benefit of increased induction time versus decreased recovery time with CSEA. Thus final conclusions on the role of CSEA in a busy ambulatory surgery center remain to be determined.

TECHNIQUES AND EQUIPMENT

The most widespread approach used in the literature is the needle-through-needle technique, in which an epidural needle is placed and then a spinal needle is inserted through it into the subarachnoid space. The spinal injection is made, and subsequently the spinal needle is removed from the epidural needle and an epidural catheter placed. A number of commercial kits are available. The simplest version is a Tuohy needle (or equivalent) through which a long, small-diameter spinal needle (24-30 gauge) is passed. Epidural needles with a "back hole" are also available, configured to allow placement of the spinal needle through a separate conduit to avoid bending of the spinal needle tip as it exits the curved epidural needle tip (**Fig. 47-15**). Recent studies suggest that use of a back-hole needle may offer advantages over a conventional needle-through-needle technique. A randomized trial in parturients observed decreased incidence of paresthesia (14% vs 42%) and failure to obtain CSF on the first attempt (8% vs 28%) with the back-hole needle.[235] The separate conduit for the spinal needle may also reduce risk of toxicity from metal fragments caused by needle friction.[236] Metal fragments have been proposed as a cause of aseptic meningitis,

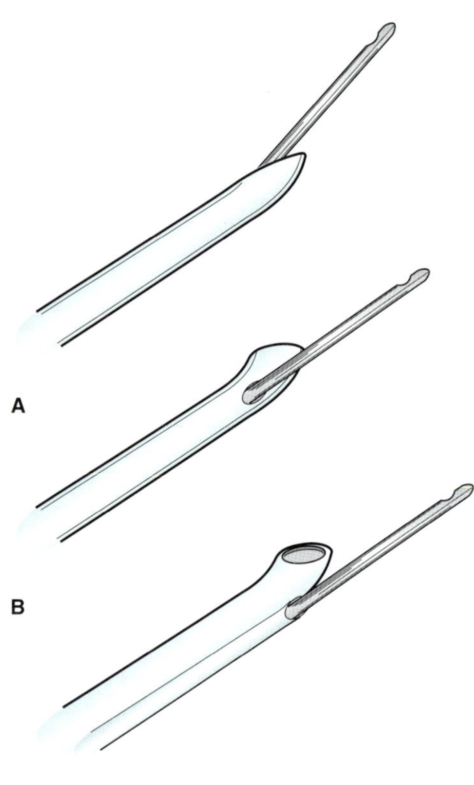

FIGURE 47-15. Styles of needles for combined spinal-epidural anesthesia. Depicted are: **A.** "conventional" Touhy with a long spinal needle exiting the curved tip, **B.** "back-eyed" needle with spinal needle exiting through the eye, and **C.** "double barrel" design, with a separate bore for passage of a spinal needle. Notice the difference in the angle of projection of the spinal needle passing out of the "conventional Tuohy" tip, as compared with B and C.

following the observation of notches in epidural needle tips.[237] However, subsequent evaluations using atomic absorption spectrography and photomicrography did not demonstrate metal fragments, even after up to 5 spinal needle passes, and suggest that the notches were caused by malleability of the metal.[238]

As an alternative to the needle-through-needle technique, the double-segment method also offers the ability to place the epidural catheter and administer a test dose before placing the spinal block. Typically, the epidural and spinal blocks are performed separately at different interspaces. By first introducing the catheter, there exists the potential risk of damaging the catheter with the spinal needle. Furthermore, creating 2 separate cutaneous punctures could lead to increased incidence of adverse events, including backache, headache, infection, and hematoma.[239] However, the double-segment technique has been shown to elicit fewer paresthesias as compared with a needle-through-needle approach.[240] However, one study demonstrated greater acceptance by surgical patients of the needle-through-needle over the double-segment technique (85% vs 67%).[241] That same study also showed a significantly longer time to perform the double-segment technique without decreasing the failure rate of spinal anesthesia, although other studies suggest a higher failure rate with the needle-through-needle technique.[241]

POTENTIAL COMPLICATIONS

Failure of Spinal Anesthesia The combined technique is associated with a higher failure rate of spinal anesthesia than conventional spinal anesthesia. There are a number of reasons for failure: (1) Smaller-diameter spinal needles with long lengths are typically used. These needles lead to slower return of CSF and a greater resistance

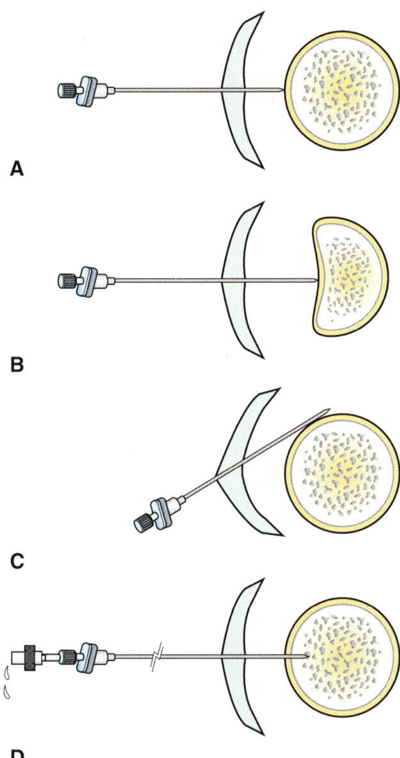

FIGURE 47-16. Various reasons for not achieving successful spinal anesthesia when attempting combined spinal-epidural anesthesia. **A.** Inadequate length of spinal needle, or epidural needle not advanced far enough. **B.** Spinal needle tents the dura, but does not achieve puncture. **C.** Angle of advancement is too far deviated from midline. **D.** Successful dural puncture with return of CSF.

to injection. (2) Because the epidural needle has penetrated the tissue planes, there is little to anchor the spinal needle in place. Although a Luer lock apparatus is available, it locks at a fixed needle length, which can prevent the spinal needle from reaching or traversing the meninges.[33] (3) Any deviation from midline can lead to missing the dura altogether (**Fig. 47-16**). (4) If loss-of-resistance technique uses saline, a false return of saline in the spinal needle rather than CSF can occur. Kopacz and Bainton[7] recommend the hanging drop method within the epidural needle to aid identification of dural puncture in this situation. Negative pressure from tenting the dura with the spinal needle will cause an inward movement of the drop of fluid followed by return of CSF. (5) Finally, patient positioning and duration between spinal injection and completion of epidural catheter placement can change the characteristics of the spinal block.

Failure of Epidural Anesthesia There are no controlled randomized prospective studies addressing the failure of epidural anesthesia or analgesia with the combined technique.[28] The incidence of failure is unlikely to be higher with the combined technique, given the identical approach for standard epidural catheter placement. However, the difficulty in early testing with a needle-through-needle technique may lead to late recognition of a misplaced catheter. Prior injection of spinal anesthetic precludes testing the epidural catheter for intrathecal placement, and epidural injection of a test dose can lead to increased height of spinal block (see Intrathecal Effects of Epidural Agent).[244] Reliability of detecting an intravascular test dose using 15 μg of epinephrine remains intact in healthy individuals using heart rate and systolic blood pressure criteria, although the developing spinal block will reduce the magnitude of hemodynamic response to epinephrine.[216]

Intrathecal Effects of Epidural Agent The intrathecal effects of epidurally administered drugs can occur through migration of the epidural catheter through the meningeal puncture, leakage of epidural anesthetic through the meningeal hole, and pressure from the epidural injection displacing CSF and the local anesthetic suspended within it. The likelihood of passing an epidural catheter through a meningeal hole is very small, provided a 24-gauge or smaller spinal needle is used. This has been demonstrated using in vitro models and in vivo epiduroscopy.[245] However, intrathecal catheter placement is possible if the epidural needle (17-18 gauge) initially rented the meninges. Migration later in the anesthetic course appears no more likely than with conventional epidural techniques.

Although Kamiya et al[246] demonstrated that lidocaine concentrations in CSF are not different between epidural administration with or without prior meningeal puncture, significant leakage of epidural agents can occur through large meningeal rents, such as with a "wet tap."[247,248]

Pressure effect is the observation that increasing epidural volume can "squeeze" the CSF compartment and thus raise the cephalad spread of spinal drugs. A recent myelographic evaluation demonstrated that the subarachnoid space's diameter decreased to 25% after 10 mL of normal saline was injected through an epidural catheter.[249] The ability to increase dermatomal spread by epidural volume appears to be time dependent. Sensory block extension can be significant (3-4 dermatomes) if epidural saline or air is injected soon after or before bupivacaine spinal anesthesia.[243,250] This block enhancement may be clinically significant, as a clinical trial reported that CSEA required 20% less local anesthetic than single-shot spinal anesthesia.[251] However, if delayed until 2-segment regression has begun, there is no increase in sensory blockade level[252]; in fact, it can even result in shorter duration of anesthesia.[253]

KEY REFERENCES

- Auroy Y, Benhamou D, Bargues L, et al. Major complications of regional anesthesia in France: the SOS Regional Anesthesia Hotline Service. *Anesthesiology*. 2002;97:1274-1280.
- Carpenter RL, Caplan RA, Brown DL, et al. Incidence and risk factors for side effects of spinal anesthesia. *Anesthesiology*. 1992;76:906-916.
- Curatolo M, Scaramozzino P, Venuti FS, et al. Factors associated with hypotension and bradycardia after epidural blockade. *Anesth Analg*. 1996;83(5):1033-1040.
- Hebl JR. The importance and implications of aseptic techniques during regional anesthesia. *Reg Anesth Pain Med*. 2006;31(4):311-323.
- Horlocker TT, Wedel DJ, Rowlingson JC, et al. Regional anesthesia in the patient receiving antithrombotic or thrombolytic therapy: American Society of Regional Anesthesia and Pain Medicine Evidence-Based Guidelines (Third Edition). *Reg Anesth Pain Med*. 2010;35(1):64-101.
- Liu SS, McDonald SB. Current issues in spinal anesthesia. *Anesthesiology*. 2001;94:888-906.
- Neal JM, Bernards CM, Butterworth JF, et al. ASRA practice advisory on local anesthetic systemic toxicity. *Reg Anesth Pain Med*. 2010;35(2):152-161.
- Neal JM, Bernards CM, Hadzic A, et al. ASRA Practice Advisory on Neurologic Complications in Regional Anesthesia and Pain Medicine. *Reg Anesth Pain Med*. 2008;33(5):404-415.

REFERENCES

Complete references available on DVD and online version at www.LongneckerAnesthesiology.com

CHAPTER 48

Paravertebral Anesthesia

Holly Evans
Steve Melton
Stephen M. Klein

KEY POINTS

1. A paravertebral nerve block involves conduction block of the spinal nerve within the paravertebral space.
2. Dense sensory, motor, and sympathetic block results.
3. Unilateral or bilateral, thoracic, or lumbar segmental block can be obtained.
4. Common indications include thoracic surgery, breast surgery, and hernia repair
5. Benefits include diminished stress response to surgery, decreased opioid consumption, reduced opioid-related side effects (nausea, vomiting, sedation), and hemodynamic stability as well as preservation of pulmonary mechanics, lower extremity strength, and bladder function.
6. Potential adverse effects are rare and include pleural puncture, pneumothorax, epidural or intrathecal injection, and local anesthetic toxicity.

Paravertebral nerve blockade (PVB) involves injection of local anesthetic close to the spinal nerve roots within the paravertebral space (PVS). The resultant unilateral or bilateral segmental anesthesia and analgesia of thoracic or lumbar dermatomes have multiple applications. In this chapter, paravertebral anatomy and PVB techniques are described. The physiologic effects are discussed in relation to the advantages, disadvantages, and contraindications for PVB. The existing literature outlining the use of PVB for a variety of surgical procedures is summarized.

PARAVERTEBRAL ANATOMY

THORACIC PARAVERTEBRAL ANATOMY

The thoracic PVS is a wedge-shaped space that lies on each side of the vertebral column. Detailed descriptions of the anatomic features of the PVS are available.[1-7]

Figure 48-1 illustrates the wedge-shaped boundaries of the thoracic PVS. Posteriorly, the space is limited by the superior costotransverse ligament. At each thoracic level, the superior costotransverse ligament extends from the lower border of the transverse process above to the upper border of the rib below (**Fig. 48-2**). Anterolaterally, the thoracic PVS is limited by the parietal pleura. The medial base of the thoracic PVS is defined by the posterolateral segment of the vertebral body, the intervertebral disk, the intervertebral foramen, and its contents.

The PVS is continuous medially with the epidural space via the intervertebral foramen; in addition, dural sleeves may extend into the PVS.[1,5,8] Laterally, the thoracic PVS is continuous with the intercostal space, lateral to the transverse processes. Communication with the contralateral PVS may occur by contact through the prevertebral[9,10] or epidural spaces.[2] The PVS is continuous superiorly and inferiorly across the heads and necks of adjacent ribs. The precise cranial limit of the PVS has not been fully elucidated; however, cervical spread of injectate has been observed after thoracic PVB.[2] It was previously thought that, caudally, the thoracic PVS was limited by the origin of the psoas major muscle[11]; however, continuity with the PVS below the diaphragm has been supported by studies documenting the lumbar spread of dye after thoracic injection.[2,12,13]

The contents of the thoracic PVS include the endothoracic fascia, the spinal nerves, the sympathetic chain, the intercostal vessels, lymphatics, and loose fatty tissue (**Fig. 48-3**). The endothoracic fascia is the deep, fibroelastic fascia of the thoracic cavity.[14,15] It is continuous medially with the prevertebral fascia that covers the vertebral bodies and intervertebral disks,[15] superiorly with the scalene fascia, and inferiorly with the fascia transversalis of the abdomen.[2,14] Karmakar[2] described the endothoracic fascia dividing the thoracic PVS into 2 potential fascial compartments—the anterior *extrapleural paravertebral compartment* and the posterior *subendothoracic paravertebral compartment*. The anterior compartment is thought to contain loose areolar connective tissue (subserous fascia)[7] and the sympathetic trunk.[2,16] The posterior compartment is thought to contain the intercostal nerves.[2,16]

The spinal nerves emerge from the intervertebral foramina and course through the thoracic PVS as a collection of small nerve rootlets devoid of fascial covering.[2,4,17,18] Early in the course of the spinal nerve, the posterior primary ramus branches to supply the posterior vertebral muscles, ligaments, facet joints, and the overlying skin (Fig. 48-3). The sympathetic chain traverses anteriorly within the thoracic PVS[2] and communicates with the spinal nerves through the preganglionic white rami communicantes and the postganglionic grey rami communicantes (Fig. 48-3). The intercostal arteries (originating from the descending aorta) as well as the hemiazygos and accessory hemiazygos veins[19] also pass through the thoracic PVS. Lymphatic drainage is to local nodes and subsequently to tributaries of the thoracic duct, which form a plexiform network around the vertebral bodies.[20]

Several features of the thoracic spine, serving as landmarks for PVB, are important to note. The spinous processes in the thoracic spine are steeply angulated. As a result they lie in the same transverse plane as the transverse processes of the vertebra below (ie, spinous process of T5 is at the same horizontal level as the transverse process of T6) (Fig. 48-2). A spinal nerve exits through its intervertebral foramen to enter the PVS caudal to the transverse process of the same level (ie, T5 nerve root passes inferior to the T5 transverse process). In adults, the thoracic transverse processes project laterally a mean distance of 3.18 cm from midline (range 2.1-4.2 cm),[8] and the mean depth from skin to thoracic PVS is 55 mm.[21] Depth is greater in the upper thoracic spine (mean 77 mm at T1) compared with the mid and lower thoracic spine (mean 50 mm at T6)[21]; in addition, considerable variation exists as a result of body habitus (mean depth to T1 PVS 67.5 mm if body mass index [BMI] <25, 78 mm if BMI 25-30, and 84 mm if BMI >30).[21]

LUMBAR PARAVERTEBRAL ANATOMY

A number of pertinent differences exist between thoracic and lumbar paravertebral anatomy. In the lumbar region, there are no ribs or superior costotransverse ligament to mark the posterior boundary of the PVS. The anterior margin of the lumbar PVS is the fascial lining of the abdomen. The endothoracic fascia above the diaphragm is continuous with the fascia transversalis, which lines the abdominal wall[14] (**Fig. 48-4**). In the abdomen, the fascia transversalis blends medially with the anterior layer of the quadratus lumborum fascia and the psoas fascia[22] (**Fig. 48-5**). The cephalad part of the psoas and quadratus lumborum fascias are thickened to form the medial and lateral arcuate ligaments, respectively. The medial arcuate ligament is attached medially to the body of L2 and laterally to the transverse process of L1. The lateral arcuate ligament passes from the lateral aspect of the L1 transverse process to the inferior border of the twelfth rib. The transversalis fascia is in direct communication with the endothoracic fascia at the medial and lateral arcuate ligaments as well as at the aortic hiatus. It is via these communications that there exists continuity between the thoracic and abdominal PVS.[2,14,23]

The lumbar nerve roots course through the lumbar PVS and subsequently combine to form the nerves of the lumbar plexus. The subcostal, iliohypogastric, ilioinguinal, and lateral femoral cutaneous nerves course anterolaterally over the quadratus lumborum muscle. The genitofemoral and, more distally, the femoral and obturator nerves pass over the anterolateral surface of the psoas muscle. Accordingly, local anesthetic injected into the PVS has the potential to block a segment of the lumbar plexus.

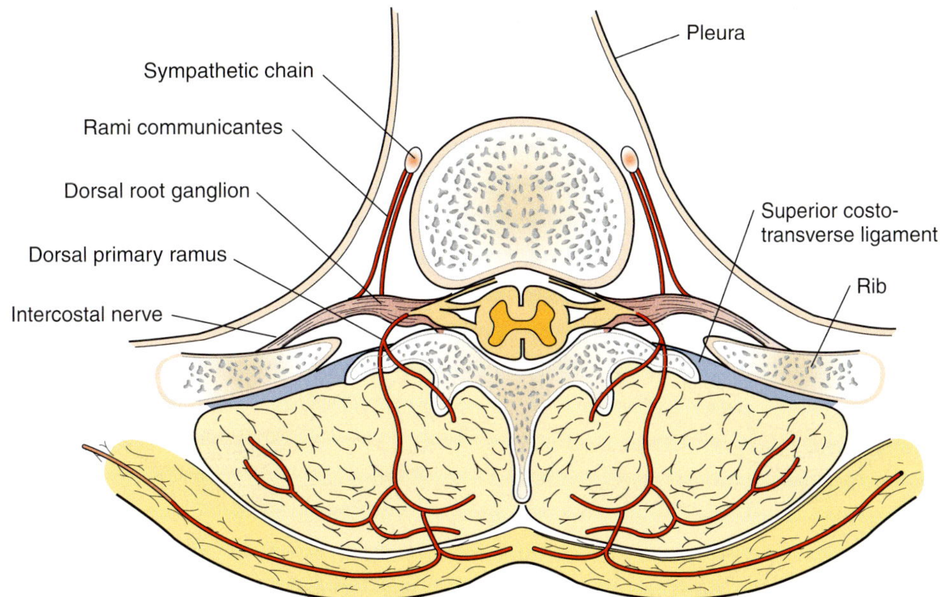

FIGURE 48-1. Transverse section of the thoracic spine depicting the boundaries, contents, and structures surrounding the paravertebral space. [Reproduced from Eason MJ, Wyatt R. Paravertebral thoracic block-a reappraisal. *Anaesthesia.* 1979;34:638-642.]

Several features of lumbar spinal anatomy deserve mention. The spinous process of a lumbar vertebra projects posteriorly with less angulation as compared with the thoracic spine (**Fig. 48-6**). As a result, a given transverse process lies at the same horizontal level as its corresponding spinous process. In addition, the transverse processes in the lumbar region do not articulate with the ribs and are much smaller and thinner in the anteroposterior plane in contrast to the thoracic spine.

Lung

Superior costotransverse ligament

Superior costotransverse ligament (medial portion removed)

Paravertebral space

FIGURE 48-2. Posterior view of the thoracic spine depicting the relationship between the superior costotransverse ligament and the paravertebral space. [Reprinted from Greengrass R, Steele S. Paravertebral blocks for breast surgery. *Tech Reg Anesth Pain Manage* 1998;2:8–12, with permission from Elsevier.]

HISTORY

Hugo Selheim, an obstetrician, is credited with the development of paravertebral anesthesia in 1905.[2] Arthur Lawen, a surgical resident, subsequently refined Sellheim's technique[2] and performed PVB on patients presenting with abdominal pain. This provided acute pain relief that facilitated abdominal muscle relaxation and palpation. Subsequent laparotomy or autopsy allowed identification of the underlying pathology. As a result, detailed information was collected on the segmental innervation of various thoracic and abdominal organs. These pioneers are credited with early development of the familiar segmental dermatome map (**Fig. 48-7**). Selheim, Lawen, and subsequently Kappis further expanded the use of PVB for surgical anesthesia in an attempt to reduce complications and improve survival in the early years of general and spinal anesthesia.[2] The technique fell into disfavor for several decades until a publication by Eason and Wyatt renewed interest.[3]

NERVE BLOCK TECHNIQUE

The patient can be positioned sitting, prone, or lateral decubitus (side to be blocked uppermost). The neck is flexed, the back is rounded, and the shoulders are rounded forward, similar to positioning for a thoracic epidural. Conscious sedation is useful for anxiolysis and analgesia.

The levels (spinal nerve roots) to be blocked are selected based on the surgical procedure as summarized in **Table 48-1** (ie, T1 to T6 for mastectomy and axillary dissection) (Fig 48-7). The spinal nerve root is located after identification of its corresponding transverse process. In the thoracic spine, a given transverse process is located in the same transverse plane as the spinous process of the vertebra above (ie, the T4 transverse process is beside the T3 spinous process) (Fig. 48-2). Spinous processes are generally palpable in the midline with the most prominent spinous process in the neck representing C7, the lower border of the scapula corresponding to T7, and the intercristal line marking L4. The superior aspect of the desired spinous process is identified in the midline, and from this point (in adults) a mark is

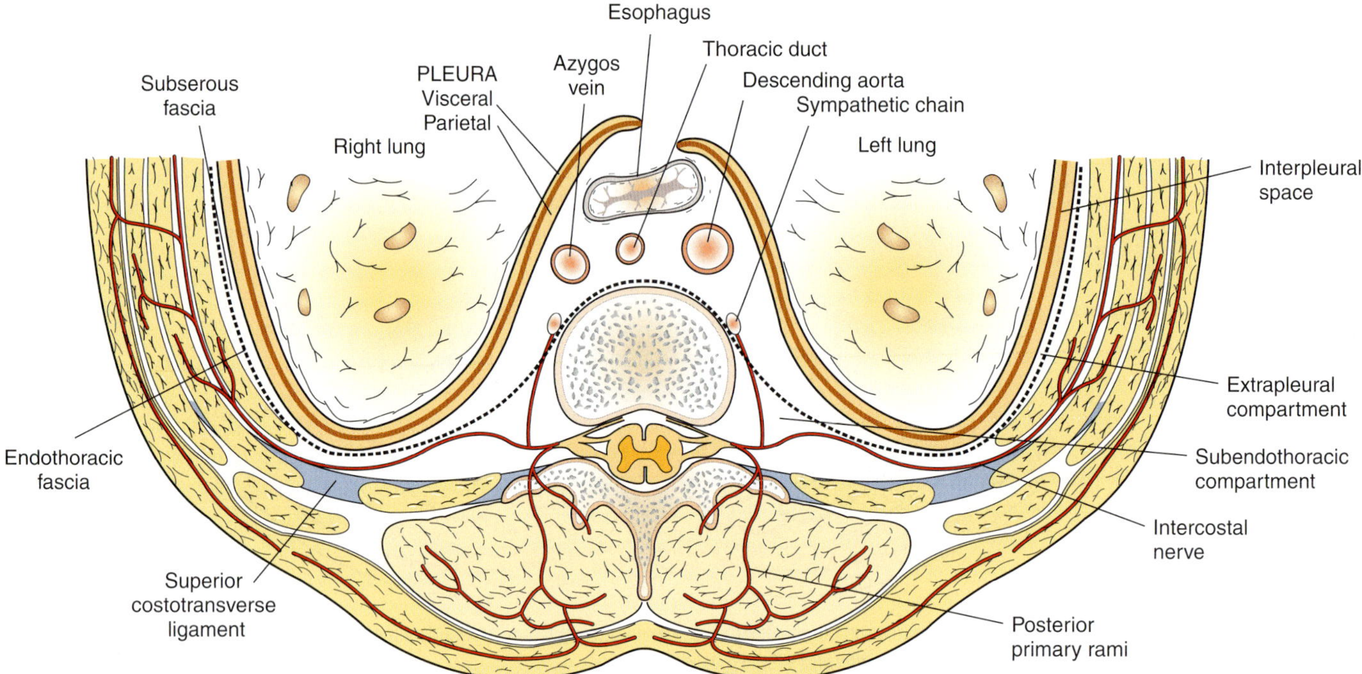

FIGURE 48-3. Mid-thoracic transverse section depicting the contents of the paravertebral space (including the endothoracic fascia) and surrounding structures. [Reproduced with permission from Karmakar MK. Thoracic paravertebral block. *Anesthesiology*. 2001;95:771-780.]

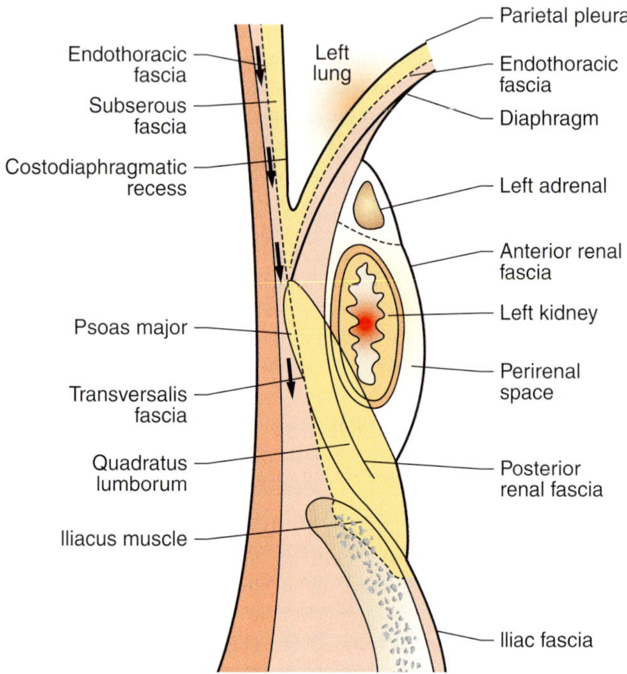

FIGURE 48-4. Thoracoabdominal sagittal section showing the relationship between the endothoracic fascia in the chest and the transversalis fascia in the abdomen. [Karmakar MK, Gin T, Ho AM. Ipsilateral thoraco-lumbar anaesthesia and paravertebral spread after low thoracic paravertebral injection. *Br J Anaesth* 2001;87:312–316. © The Board of Management and Trustees of the British Journal of Anaesthesia. Reproduced by permission of Oxford University Press/British Journal of Anaesthesia.]

drawn 2.5 cm lateral (**Fig. 48-8**). The skin is cleaned with disinfectant, and subcutaneous infiltration of local anesthetic is given at all needle entry sites.

A number of techniques have been described to identify the PVS, as described next.

ANATOMIC OR LOSS OF RESISTANCE

For thoracic PVB, the superior border of the appropriate spinous process is palpated and its midpoint identified. In adults, 2.5 cm lateral from this midpoint, a 10-cm, 22-gauge Tuohy needle is inserted and advanced in the parasagittal plane to contact the transverse process. Upon contact with the transverse process, the block needle is withdrawn to the subcutaneous tissue and redirected caudad to "walk-off" the transverse process (**Fig. 48-9**). After this caudad redirection, the needle is slowly advanced until the PVS is identified. This occurs approximately 1 cm past the depth at which the transverse process is contacted. Identification of the PVS can be made as the needle traverses the superior costotransverse ligament either by perception of a tactile change in resistance or utilization of a loss of resistance to injected air or saline. The end point with the latter is more subtle and subjective than with epidural anesthesia.[3,23,24] As an alternative approach, the block needle may be safely advanced by a fixed distance (1 cm) after caudal redirection from the transverse process,[25] followed by tactile identification of the appropriate resistance with initial local anesthetic injection. The depth from skin to thoracic PVS varies by vertebral level and patient size.[21]

A cautious approach is warranted if bone is contacted deep to the transverse process, as this may represent the rib. Further advancement of the block needle past the rib can result in pleural puncture and pneumothorax. This risk can be minimized by caudad redirection (as opposed to cephalad redirection) of the needle after initial bony contact. If the rib is unintentionally contacted first, caudal redirection will bring the block needle in contact with the transverse process at a shallower depth (**Fig. 48-10**). Subsequently, a more accurate estimation of the depth of the PVS is provided, and the risk of pleural puncture is

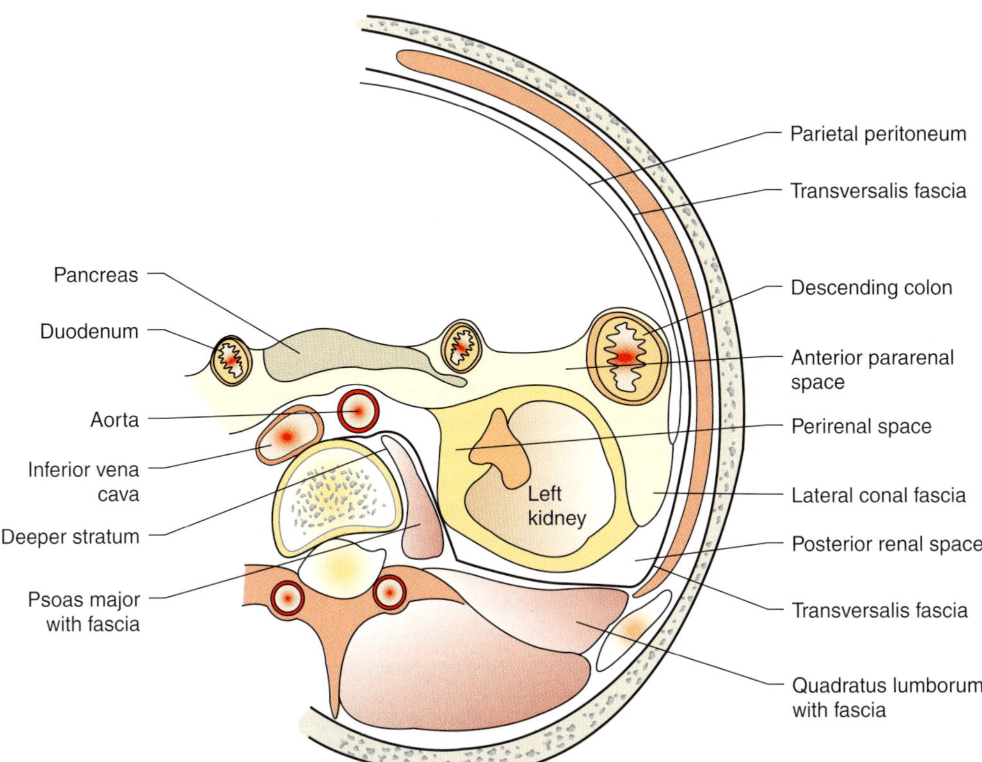

FIGURE 48-5. Upper abdominal transverse section depicting the relationship between the fascia transversalis and the fascia of the psoas major and quadratus lumborum muscles. [Karmakar MK, Gin T, Ho AM. Ipsilateral thoraco-lumbar anaesthesia and paravertebral spread after low thoracic paravertebral injection. *Br J Anaesth* 2001;87:312–316. © The Board of Management and Trustees of the British Journal of Anaesthesia. Reproduced by permission of Oxford University Press/British Journal of Anaesthesia.]

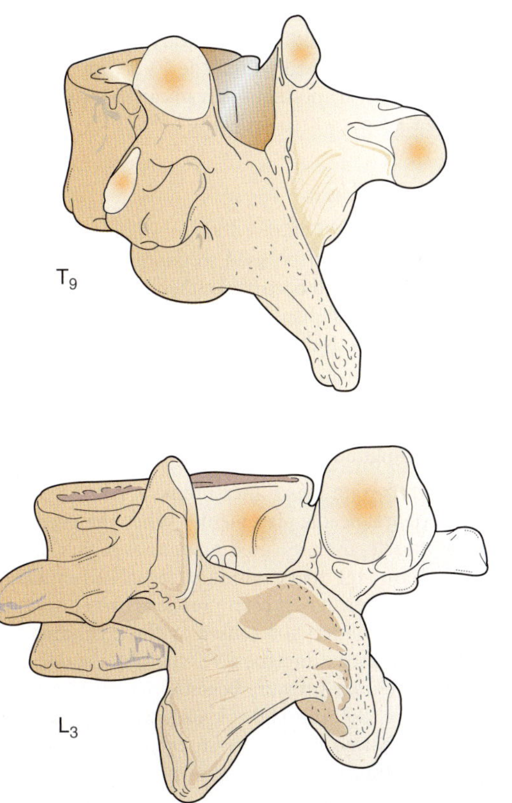

FIGURE 48-6. Oblique views of a thoracic and a lumbar vertebra. [Reprinted from Covino BG, Scott DB, Lambert DH. In: *Handbook of Spinal Anaesthesia and Analgesia*. Philadelphia, PA: WB Saunders, 1994, with permission from Elsevier.]

decreased. In contrast, an alternative approach has been described in which the needle is redirected cephalad to the transverse process. If initial contact is made with the rib, cephalad redirection will not bring the needle into contact with the transverse process. Further advancement of the needle deep to the rib increases the possibility of pleural puncture and possible pneumothorax.

When the thoracic PVS has been located, 3 to 5 mL of local anesthetic is typically injected at each level. Injection should occur without resistance. Deliberate aspiration to detect pleural puncture or intravascular or subarachnoid needle placement is important. Local anesthetic doses may need to be adjusted when multiple-level or bilateral PVB is performed.

Nerve block adequacy is confirmed by appropriate thoracic dermatomal sensory block, intercostal muscle motor block, and sympathectomy-related changes such as vasodilation and increased skin temperature.

Lumbar PVB involves a modification of the thoracic technique. In contrast to the thoracic level, needle entry site for each spinal nerve at the lumbar level corresponds to the spinous process of the same level. Correction for spinous process angulation is unnecessary in the lumbar region. In addition, after contact with the lumbar transverse process, the block needle is advanced no more than 0.5 cm anteriorly. This is because the lumbar transverse processes are thinner in the anteroposterior plane as compared with the thoracic spine. Finally, the loss of resistance upon entrance into the lumbar PVS is even less defined as compared with that felt in the thoracic spine. This may be related to absence of the costotransverse ligament in the lumbar region.

NERVE STIMULATION

The spinal nerve can be located in the PVS using a nerve stimulator and a 21- or 22-gauge short bevel insulated stimulating needle. The needle is inserted as previously described. Direct paraspinal muscle stimulation

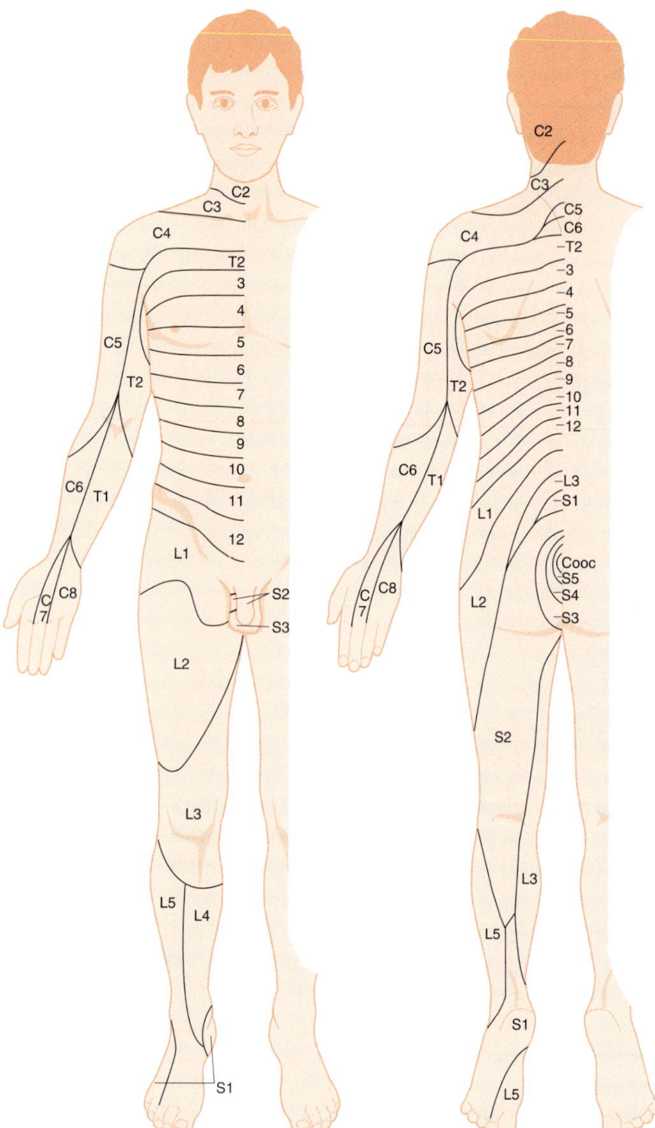

FIGURE 48-7. Dermatomal distribution of spinal nerves. [Reprinted from Covino BG, Scott DB, Lambert DH. In: *Handbook of Spinal Anaesthesia and Analgesia*. Philadelphia, PA: WB Saunders, 1994, with permission from Elsevier.]

is observed initially as the needle passes through these muscles. Further advancement caudad to the transverse process brings the stimulating needle in close proximity to the spinal nerve and leads to intercostal or abdominal muscle contractions depending on the level of the block. Similar to other peripheral nerve block technique, appropriate needle placement is confirmed when muscle contractions persist with a current 0.5 mA or less. Isolated posterior spinal muscle contraction should not be accepted, as this may represent direct muscle activation or stimulation of the posterior ramus of the spinal nerve root after it diverges from the spinal nerve.

Proponents of this technique describe its usefulness in challenging cases (ie, morbid obesity, ankylosing spondylitis) and as a way to minimize the occurrence of pneumothorax, though this has yet to be proven.[26]

ULTRASOUND GUIDED

Ultrasound-guided single-injection and continuous paravertebral blockade may prove beneficial to one skilled in its application. Ultrasound guidance allows for real-time identification of pertinent anatomy, visualization of needle-tip advancement, and local anesthetic spread. Ultrasound imaging can be used to provide an estimate of transverse process location and depth.[27,28] Pusch et al[28] found a close correlation between the ultrasound estimated and the actual demonstrated needle depth from skin to transverse process, thoracic PVS, and parietal pleura. Ultrasound guidance, however, is not without limitations: Hara et al[27] visualized both transverse process and parietal pleura at T4 in all patients, but only the transverse process alone at T1.[27]

Ultrasound guidance can be performed using a transverse or saggital paramedian ultrasound-guided technique.

Transverse Ultrasound-Guided PVB With the patient in the sitting, prone, or lateral decubitus position, place a low-frequency linear or curvilinear ultrasound probe in the transverse plane at a position lateral to the spinous process on the rib/transverse process of the desired level. While maintaining the transverse orientation, slide the ultrasound probe slightly caudad to a position between adjacent transverse processes to visualize the PVS. Using an in-plane technique, a needle is directed toward the PVS from the lateral aspect of the probe (**Fig. 48-11**A and 48-11B). Local anesthetic spread is visualized within the PVS with anterior displacement of the pleura and lateral spread to the intercostal space. Alternatively an out-of-plane technique may be used with this approach. Upon subsequent saggital scan, local anesthetic spread can be visualized at contiguous paravertebral spaces with a widening of the PVS.

Paramedian Saggital In-Plane Ultrasound-Guided PVB With the patient in the sitting, prone, or lateral decubitus position, place a low-frequency linear or curvilinear ultrasound probe in the saggital plane at a position 2 to 3 cm lateral to the spinous process. Rotate the probe to a slight oblique axis orientation from the saggital plane to achieve visualization of the PVS.[29] The needle is directed toward the PVS using an in-plane technique (Fig. 48-11C and 48-11D). Alternatively, the needle may be advanced to make contact with the lower border of the transverse process and then redirected toward the PVS, advancing the needle a predetermined distance of 1 cm beyond the transverse process as with the anatomic or loss of resistance approach.[25,29] Upon injection, local anesthetic spread is visualized within the PVS with anterior displacement of the pleura. Local anesthetic spread can be visualized at contiguous paravertebral spaces with a widening of the PVS.

OTHER TECHNIQUES

Injection of Radiographic Contrast Dye Injection of contrast dye and radiologic examination can be used to confirm proper paravertebral needle location. Dye spread occurs in either a longitudinal distribution or a segmental, cloud-like dispersal[7] (**Fig. 48-12**). Naja et al[30] hypothesized that dye dispersion is dependent on the location of the needle with respect to the endothoracic fascia. They conjectured that needle position posterior to the endothoracic fascia would be associated with segmental, cloud-like dye spread and needle position anterior to the endothoracic fascia with more longitudinal dye distribution.[30]

Pressure Transduction Pressure measurement has been described to confirm paravertebral needle placement.[24] When the needle tip is in the erector spinae muscle, the measured pressure is higher during inspiration (mean 29.6 mm Hg) than expiration (mean 19.4 mm Hg).[24] This is thought to occur as a result of greater muscle activity during inspiration or due to muscular compression caused by the expanding chest cage.[23] As the needle is advanced into the PVS, there is a sudden lowering of pressures, and expiratory pressure becomes higher (7.6 mm Hg) than inspiratory pressure (3.3 mm Hg).[24] Unintentional pleural puncture is identified when subatmospheric pressures are recorded, both during inspiration and expiration.

Continuous PVB Placing a continuous catheter into the PVS can be used to extend the duration of postoperative analgesia provided by PVB. This is typically reserved for more invasive surgery associated with intense postoperative pain, such as thoracotomy and subcostal incisions.

TABLE 48-1 Clinical Applications for PVBs[2,23,49]

Surgical Procedure	Levels Blocked
Thoracotomy	T4-T9
Thoracoscopy	T4-T9
Rib fractures	Level of fracture with 1 level above and below
Cardiac surgery	T2-T6 bilaterally
Mastectomy, breast surgery	T2-T6
Mastectomy with axillary dissection	T1-T6 with superficial cervical plexus block
Breast biopsy	Level of lesion with 1 level above and below
Inguinal hernia repair	T10-L2
Umbilical hernia repair	T9-T11 bilaterally
Incisional hernia repair	According to level of repair
Ileostomy closure	T8-T12
Nephrectomy	T8-T12
Cholecystectomy	T6-T10
Appendectomy	T10-T12
Adjunct for shoulder surgery (subdeltoid incision)	T1-T2
Adjunct for hip surgery	T11-T12 with lumbar plexus block
Bone marrow aspiration	T11-L2 bilaterally
Iliac crest bone harvesting	T11-L1
Labor analgesia	T10 bilaterally for first stage of labor
Chronic pain	According to condition

PVBs, paravertebral nerve blocks.

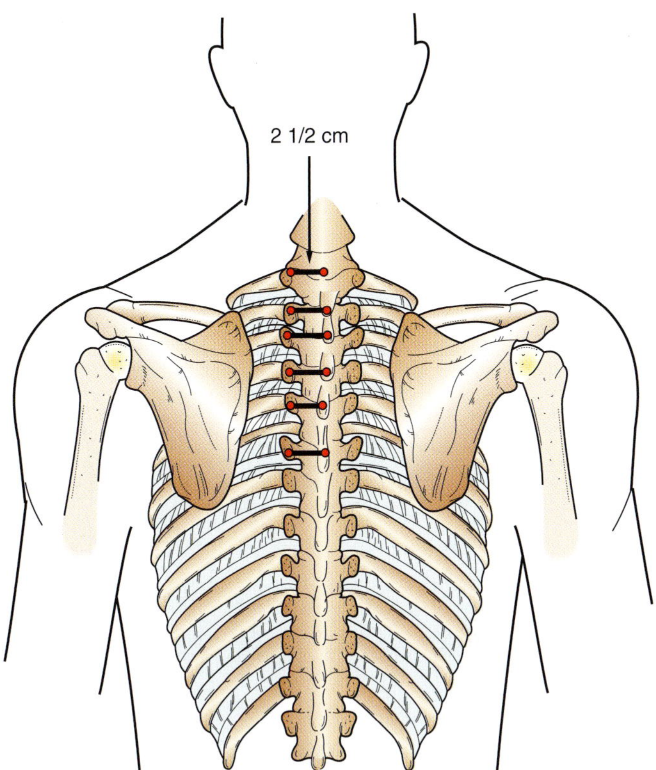

FIGURE 48-8. Skin markings for paravertebral blocks performed for left mastectomy. [Reprinted from Greengrass R, Steele S. Paravertebral blocks for breast surgery. *Tech Reg Anesth Pain Manage* 1998;2:8-12, with permission from Elsevier.]

Insertion methods are usually modifications of single-injection techniques. A single-injection 22-gauge, 10-cm Tuohy needle is initially used to estimate the depth of the transverse process and paravertebral space. A larger-bore Tuohy (ie, 18 gauge) capable of accommodating a 20-gauge epidural catheter is then substituted. Extension tubing or a hemostatic valve is used to create a closed circuit with the needle to mitigate entrainment of air if the pleura is punctured. The catheter is threaded 1 to 2 cm into the paravertebral space to minimize the risk of migration. Consequently, a catheter with a single distal orifice is used in order to reduce leakage of local anesthetic solution outside of the paravertebral space.

Final catheter position is variable. A cadaveric study by Luyet et al[31] revealed correct paravertebral spread of contrast in only 11 of 20 cases, with 1 catheter found in the pleural space, 6 in the epidural space, and 2 with prevertebral spread of contrast dye. A cadaveric study by Riain et al[32] demonstrated 8 of 10 catheters correctly placed within the PVS. Ultrasound-guided continuous paravertebral catheters placed in fresh cadavers were found outside of the paravertebral space in 40% of cases.[33] In contrast, Renes et al[34] determined 100% PVB correct catheter position within the thoracic PVS in 36 patients using a transverse in-plane ultrasound-guided technique with radiologic confirmation.[34]

An alternative to the classic approach is an intercostal approach to paravertebral catheterization as described by Burns et al.[35] At the midpoint of the anticipated surgical incision, the appropriate rib is identified and marked 8 cm lateral to the midline. An 18-gauge Tuohy needle is advanced to come in contact with the rib. With the bevel directed medially (the tip angled 45 degrees cephalad and 60 degrees medial to

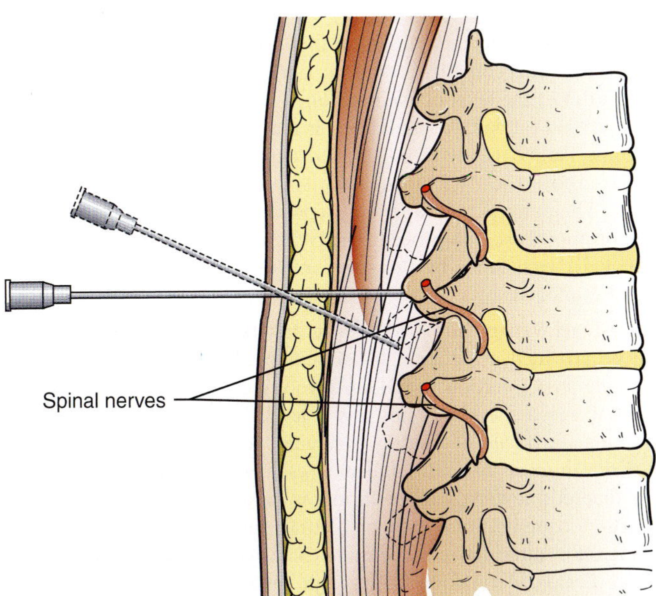

FIGURE 48-9. Paravertebral nerve block technique. After identification of the transverse process, the block needle is redirected inferiorly and advanced into the paravertebral space. [From Greengrass R, Steele S. Paravertebral blocks for breast surgery. *Tech Reg Anesth Pain Manage.* 1998;2:8-12. Used with permission from Elsevier.]

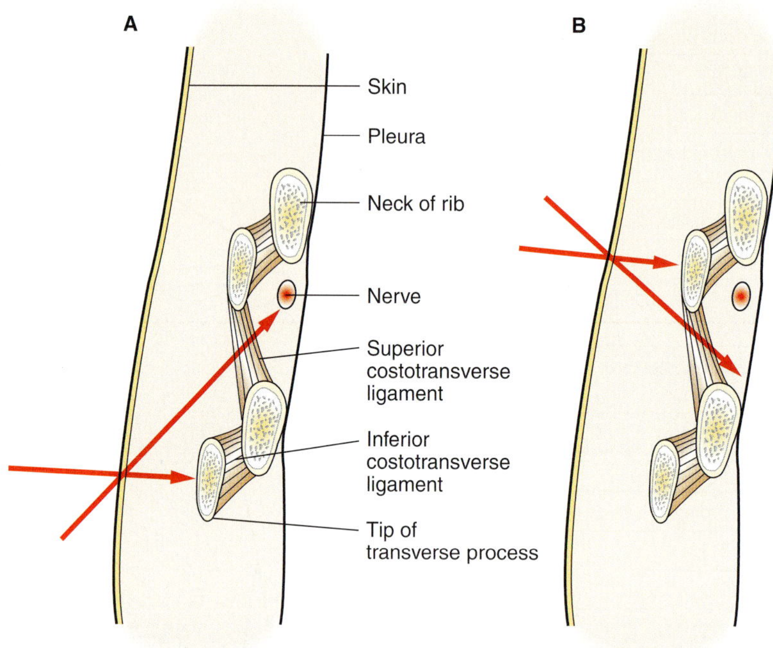

FIGURE 48-10. Paravertebral nerve block technique. Longitudinal section depicting insertion of the block needle (**A**) above and (**B**) below the transverse process or rib. [From Eason MJ, Wyatt R. Paravertebral thoracic block-a reappraisal. *Anaesthesia.* 1979;34:638-642. Used with permission from Blackwell Publishing.]

the saggital plane) in effort to place the bevel and tip away from the pleura, the needle is "walked-off" the inferior border of the rib. Once under the rib, the needle is advanced, maintaining the aforementioned position, 5 to 6 mm to enter the intercostal neurovascular space. After injection of local anesthetic, a 20-gauge epidural catheter is advanced through the needle and inserted 8 cm past the needle tip, brining it to the PVS.[35]

A novel insertion method described for thoracic surgery is to place the catheter under direct vision in the surgical field[4,23,36-40] (**Fig. 48-13**). At the completion of the thoracotomy just before chest closure, the surgeon strips away the parietal pleura in the paravertebral gutter at the level of the incision, 2 dermatomes cephalad and 2 dermatomes caudad. A small defect is made in the extrapleural fascia. Then, a Tuohy needle is introduced percutaneously and a catheter is placed into the PVS through the small defect in the extrapleural fascia. The parietal pleura is then repositioned and sutured in place. During thoracoscopic procedures, catheter placement may be done with video assistance by the surgeon[41] or in combination with the anesthesiologist.[42]

Single-Level Versus Multiple-Level Technique Paravertebral anesthesia can be provided using a single- or multiple-level injection technique. A single-level injection technique involves depositing a large volume of local anesthetic (10-20 mL) at 1 level. A multiple-level injection technique involves depositing a smaller volume of local anesthetic (3-5 mL thoracic; 5-7 mL lumbar) at each involved dermatomal level. The theoretic advantage of the former is a reduction in potential needle insertion complications such as pleural puncture or pneumothorax, whereas the latter may provide more extensive and complete anesthesia of the desired dermatomes. Although single-level injection PVB has been shown to reduce postoperative pain and hospital stay,[3-45] several authors have recommended using a multiple-level injection technique for surgical anesthesia.[23,25,46-50] In a study by Naja et al,[50] 97% of patients had complete loss of sensation with 4-level injection as compared with 11% with single-level injections. In an ultrasound-guided study of fresh cadavers, contrast dye spread more extensively across intercostal segments with a dual-injection technique as compared with a single-injection technique (6 vs 4.5; $p < .03$).[33] There was 40% frequency of epidural spread of contrast associated with paravertebral injection in both techniques.[33]

EFFECT OF TECHNIQUE ON DISTRIBUTION OF INJECTATE

A single-level paravertebral injection of 10 to 15 mL of local anesthetic in adults[12,48,51] and 0.5 mL/kg in children[7] achieves a mean sensory block of 4 to 5 dermatomes independent of age, height, weight, or sex. Naja et al,[50] in a prospective randomized trial investigating radiographic and clinical differences in local anesthetic spread as a function of injection number, concluded that increasing the number of paravertebral injections results in more reliable radiographic and sensory-block distribution compared with a single-injection technique. In this study they demonstrated vertical contrast spread with 4 injections to be a mean (SD) of 6.5 (2.01) dermatomes as compared with 3.0 (1.19) dermatomes achieved with 1 injection. The vertical distribution pattern for both single-injection and multiple-injection techniques is slightly asymmetric, with a more extensive caudad spread of the block,[50] as previously identified.[12]

Few studies have been designed to rigorously investigate the potential effect of dose or volume of injectate on spread within the PVS. One study in adults has shown no association between these variables,[48] whereas another study of pediatric patients has found a moderate to strong correlation between injected volume and segmental spread of dye.[7] It has been proposed that there may be an age-related loss of connective tissue leading to greater spread of injectate in adults.[48]

Additional factors do affect the spread of injectate within the PVS. Purcell-Jones et al[8] studied single-injection PVB using the loss of resistance technique. They radiographically showed greater craniocaudal distribution of solution (5.5 mL) when the PVB was associated with epidural spread. They found sensory anesthesia in a mean 1.43 dermatomes when injectate was confined to the PVS, 2.27 dermatomes when injectate

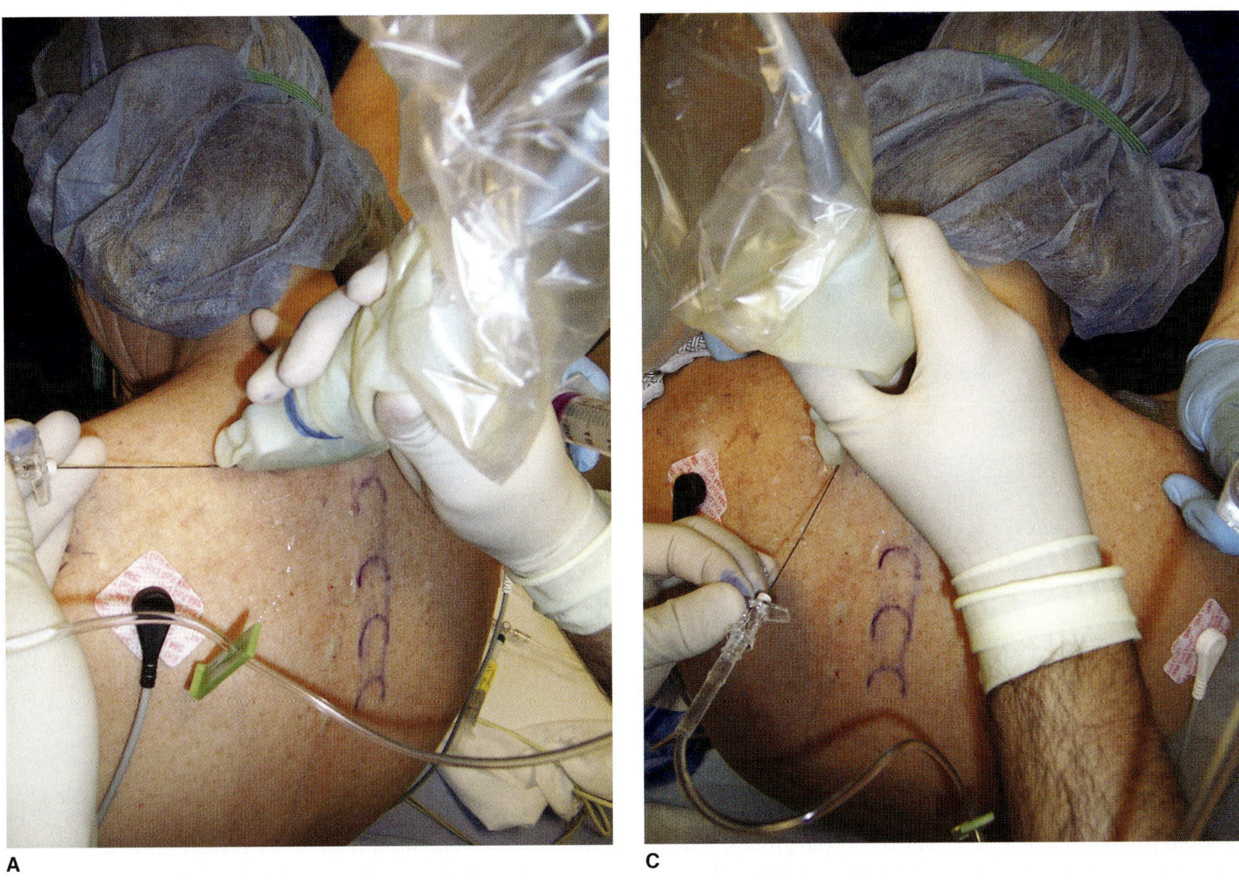

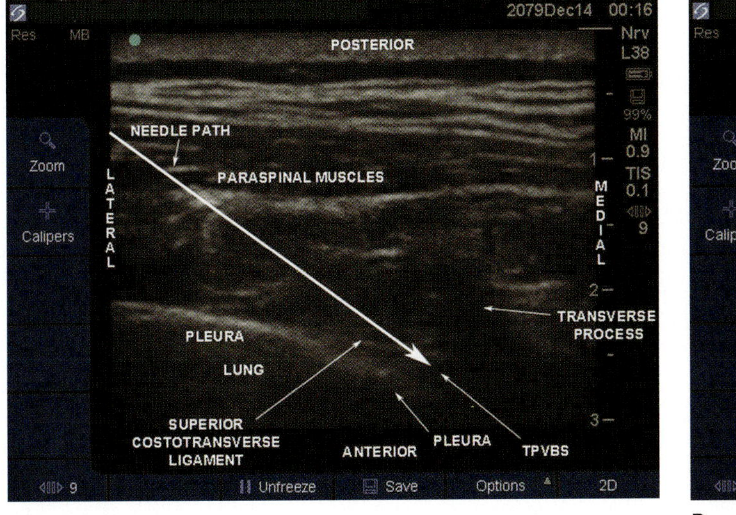

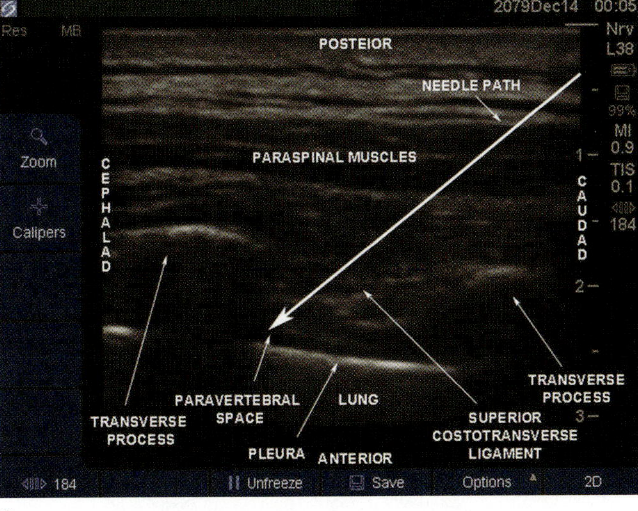

FIGURE 48-11. A. Transverse in-plane ultrasound-guided PVB technique. **B.** Sonographic landmarks for transverse in-plane ultrasound-guided PVB technique. **C.** Paramedian sagittal in-plane ultrasound-guided PVB technique. **D.** Sonographic landmarks for paramedian sagittal in-plane ultrasound-guided PVB technique.

was primarily in the PVS but also spread to the epidural space, 4.66 dermatomes when injectate was confined to the epidural space, and 6.6 dermatomes when the injectate was primarily in the epidural space but also spread to the PVS. In all instances, the spread of contrast dye was greater than the observed sensory block. Cheema et al[12] studied patients who received a single-injection PVB using loss of resistance with 15 mL of local anesthetic and dye. They found that the mean extent of vasodilation (sympathetic block) was 8 dermatomes and exceeded the mean sensory block of 5 dermatomes.

LOCAL ANESTHETIC REGIMEN

Bupivacaine and ropivacaine are the most frequently used local anesthetics for PVB, and the duration of analgesia is similar to that obtained with brachial plexus anesthesia, a length of 12 to 24 hours. In a study by Hura et al,[52] ropivacaine was associated with a more rapid onset of sensory blockade, with 53% of patients demonstrating dermatome coverage to undergo modified radical mastectomy 5 minutes after block completion as compared with 20% in the bupivacaine group ($p < .01$).

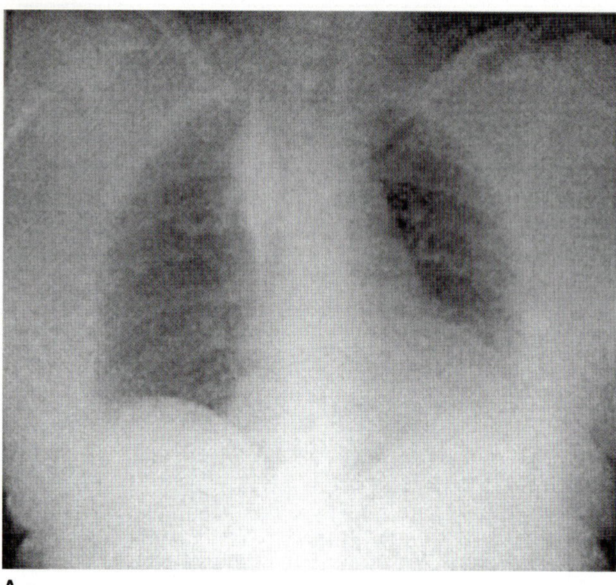

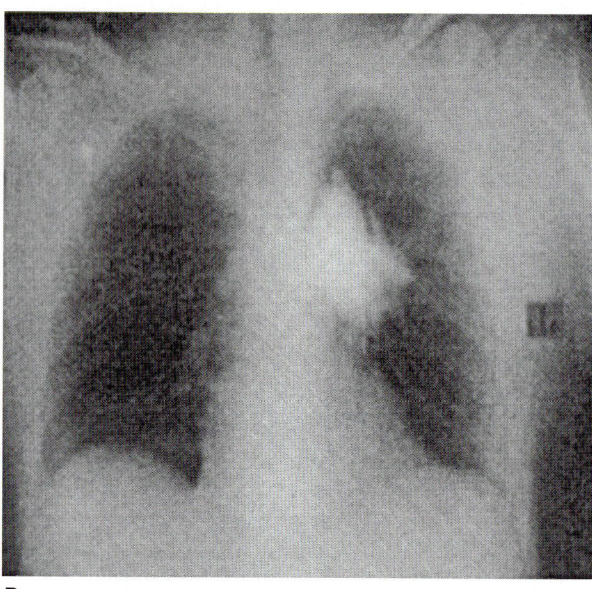

FIGURE 48-12. Chest radiographs taken after injection of radiocontrast dye into the paravertebral space depicting (**A**) longitudinal and (**B**) cloud-like spread. [From Naja MZ, Ziade MF, El Rajab M, El Tayara K, Lonnqvist PA. Varying anatomical injection points within the thoracic paravertebral space: effect on spread of solution and nerve blockade. *Anaesthesia.* 2004;59:459-463. Used with permission from Blackwell Publishing.]

Although ropivacaine demonstrated a longer duration of analgesia and a wider extent of segmental anesthesia ($p < .05$), degree of postoperative pain and analgesic consumption were similar between groups.[52] Navlet et al[53] concluded that both bupivacaine 0.25% and ropivacaine 0.3% are equally effective to control post-thoracotomy pain at rest with a continuous paravertebral block, but suggested that higher concentrations of both drugs during the first 24 hours might improve visual analog scale (VAS) scores on coughing and spirometry values, including forced vital capacity and forced expiratory volume in 1 second (FEV_1). Indeed, a systemic review and meta-regression by Kotze et al[54] demonstrated that the use of higher doses of bupivacaine (890-990 mg/24 h compared with 325-472.5 mg/24 h) was found to predict lower pain scores (50%) at all time points up to 48 hours after the operation ($p < .006$ at 8 h, $p < .001$ at 24 h, $p < .001$ at 48 h) and faster recovery of pulmonary function by 72 h (20% improvement in FEV_1 ($p < .029$). Continuous infusions of local anesthetic predicted lower pain scores compared with intermittent boluses ($p < .04$ at 8 h, $p < .003$ at 24 h, $p < .001$ at 48 h). Epinephrine is frequently added to the local anesthetic solution to indicate intravascular injection, to reduce the peak local anesthetic blood level,[55] and to improve analgesia. Epinephrine produces a 25% reduction in the mean peak arterial concentration of ropivacaine and delays the time to peak arterial and venous concentrations.[55] Some add opioids or clonidine to local anesthetic solutions[46,57]; however, this has not been extensively studied with PVB. Standard dosing regimens are outlined in **Table 48-2**. A single-level injection is typically performed with 0.5 mL/kg of dilute local anesthetic solution in children and 10 to 20 mL in adults. Multiple-level injections are accomplished in adults with 3 to 4 mL of local anesthetic per segment in the thoracic region and 5 to 7 mL per segment in the lumbar area. Continuous PVB is dosed with 0.1 to 0.2 mL/kg/h of dilute local anesthetic.

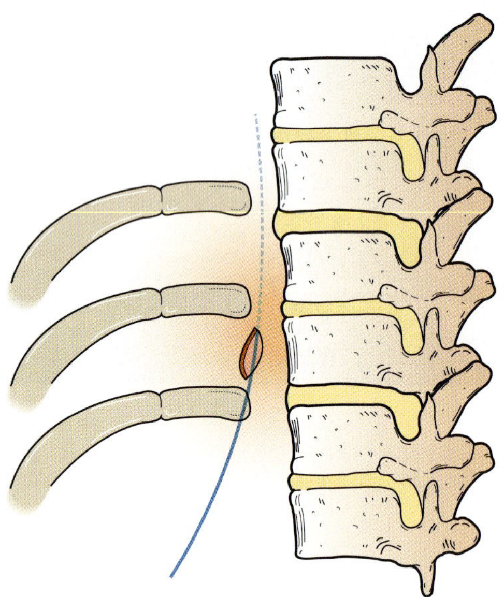

FIGURE 48-13. Placement of a paravertebral catheter under direct vision. The extrapleural fascia (stippled) is exposed by raising the parietal pleural from the posterior chest wall. The epidural catheter is lying within the paravertebral space (broken line), introduced through the small defect. [From Berrisford RG, Sabanathan SS. Direct access to the paravertebral space at thoracotomy [comment]. *Ann Thorac Surg.* 1990;49:854. Used with permission from Elsevier.]

TABLE 48-2 Local Anesthetic Regimen for PVBs

Single-level injection	Children: 0.5 mL/kg up to 20 mL of local anesthetic Adults: 10-20 mL of local anesthetic (ie, ropivacaine 0.5% with epinephrine 1:400 000)
Multiple-level injections	Thoracic spine: 3-4 mL of local anesthetic per segment Lumbar spine: 5-7 mL of local anesthetic per segment (ie, ropivacaine 0.5% with epinephrine 1:400 000)
Continuous infusion	0.1-0.2 mL/kg/h of local anesthetic (ie, ropivacaine 0.2%)

PVBs, paravertebral nerve blocks.

TABLE 48-3 Beneficial Effects of PVBs

Dense sensory, motor, and sympathetic nerve block
Unilateral or bilateral segmental block
Wide application for various surgical procedures
Decreased stress response to surgery[62]
Low postoperative opioid requirements[68,101,133]
Infrequent opioid-related side effects (nausea, vomiting, sedation)[68,101,133]
Postoperative analgesia similar to or better than epidural[101,140]
Hemodynamic stability[69,101]
Preservation of pulmonary function[99,101]
Preservation of lower extremity motor strength
Preservation of bladder function[69,101]
Enhanced perioperative efficiency[43,46]

PVBs, paravertebral nerve blocks.

ADVANTAGES

The advantages of PVB are summarized in **Table 48-3**. PVB provides blockade of afferent nerves, leading to dense anesthesia and postoperative analgesia. Richardson et al[57] performed somatosensory evoked potential testing on patients before and after they received a single injection block. They discovered complete abolition of the evoked potentials at the level of the paravertebral injection in 100% of patients (**Fig. 48-14**). As a result, PVB may be associated with a reduced development of chronic postsurgical pain after breast surgery. In a study by Iohom et al[59] at 10 weeks, 80% of patients (12 of 15) not receiving PVB analgesia developed chronic postsurgical pain as compared with 0% (0 of 14) in those receiving PVB analgesia ($p < .009$). Preoperative PVB may reduce the incidence of chronic pain 1 year after breast cancer surgery[60] and reduce the incidence of post-thoracotomy neuralgia.[61]

PVB also modifies the stress response to surgical stimulation. Giesecke et al[62] studied patients having open cholecystectomy under general anesthesia and discovered that those who received single-injection PVB for postoperative pain control had lower plasma adrenaline and cortisol concentrations ($p < .05$), as well as a smaller rise in plasma glucose concentration ($p < .025$) compared with patients who did not receive PVB.

PVB is associated with reduced postoperative opioid consumption and incidence of opioid-related side effects when compared with intravenous opioid analgesia[43,46,63-68] and preservation of lower-extremity motor strength, greater hemodynamic stability, and less urinary retention when compared with epidural analgesia.[69] This technique has the potential to provide improved analgesia with a reduced risk of pleural puncture and local anesthetic toxicity compared with intercostal and intrapleural analgesia.

A retrospective analysis suggested that paravertebral anesthesia and analgesia for breast cancer surgery reduced the risk of recurrence or metastasis during the initial years of follow-up. The proposed mechanism was maintenance of perioperative immune function by attenuation of the stress response and reduction in volatile anesthetic and postoperative opioid requirements.[70] Prospective trials are necessary to investigate the conclusions of this retrospective analysis.

CONTRAINDICATIONS

ABSOLUTE CONTRAINDICATIONS

Similar to other percutaneous techniques, PVB should be avoided in patients with skin infections at the proposed needle entry site and in those with an empyema or a deep infection within the chest.[2,71] A paravertebral tumor also contraindicates PVB due to the risk of tumor seeding. In addition, this technique is avoided in the setting of local anesthetic allergy, patient refusal, and severe hemodynamic instability.

RELATIVE CONTRAINDICATIONS

A severe chest deformity, such as kyphoscoliosis, increases the risk of pneumothorax or unintentional subarachnoid injection and should be considered a relative contraindication to PVB.[2,71] Similarly, patients who have had a prior thoracotomy are at higher risk of pleural puncture and pneumothorax due to paravertebral scarring and obliteration of the thoracic PVS. Nevertheless, operator experience and/or imaging adjuncts can result in successful blocks in these circumstances with few complications. Coagulopathy represents a relative contraindication to PVB. Based on the increased compliance of the PVS compared with the epidural space, the neurologic impairment from a paravertebral hematoma will be less than that from an epidural hematoma.[71]

ADVERSE EFFECTS

Two large series provide incidence rates for adverse events after PVB in both adults and children.[72,73] (**Table 48-4**). Naja and Lonnqvist[72] provide data on multilevel PVB performed on 662 adult and pediatric patients using nerve stimulation. Lonnqvist et al[73] reported their results from single-level PVB performed with a loss-of-resistance technique in 367 adult and pediatric patients. Additional adverse event data can be gleaned from other studies.[25,47,68]

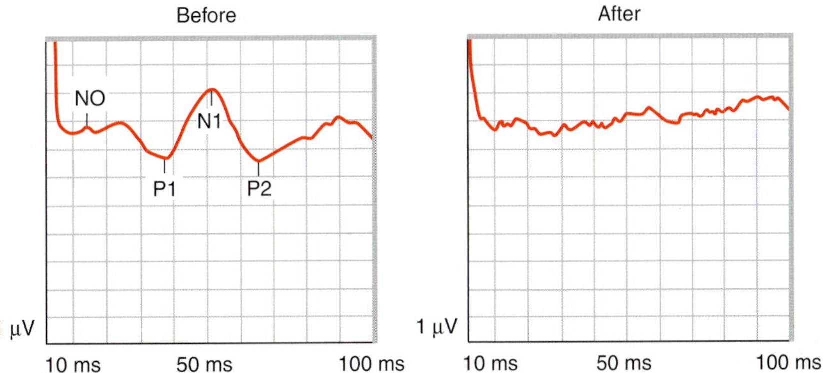

FIGURE 48-14. A somatosensory evoked potential recording from T3 before and after deposition of paravertebral bupivacaine at T2. Latencies and amplitudes were measured, and the evoked potential was abolished after the block. [Richardson J, Jones J, Atkinson R. The effect of thoracic paravertebral blockade on intercostal somatosensory evoked potentials. *Anesth Analg*. 1998;87:373-376.]

TABLE 48-4 Incidence of Complications After PVBs

Complication	Mean Incidence (Unilateral PVBs) (%)	Mean Incidence (Bilateral PVBs) (%)	Overall Mean Incidence (%)
Block failure[25,47,68,72,73]			6.1-10.7
Inadvertent vascular puncture[72,73]	5.4	8.7	3.8-6.8
Hypotension[72,73]	3.9	3.6	4.0-5.0
Localized hematoma[72]	1.9	3.1	2.4
Localized pain[72]	1.1	1.5	1.3
Pleural puncture[72,73]	0.2	2.0	0.8-2.1
Pneumothorax[47,72,73]	0.2	1.0	0.3-2.1
Pulmonary hemorrhage[74]	Case report		
Intrathecal or epidural spread[8,72,73]	1.1	0.5	1.0-70 (epidural spread)
Dural puncture headache[76]	Case report		
Brachial plexus block[9]	Case report		
Horner syndrome[8,9,68,80]	Case report		
Local anesthetic toxicity[44]	Case report		
Nerve injury[87]	Case report		
Infection			

PVBs, paravertebral nerve blocks.

The most common reported adverse event is technique failure. A failure occurs when a PVB does not succeed in providing adequate surgical anesthesia or when general anesthesia is required to complete the procedure. The published incidence of block failure is 6.1% to 10.7%[25,47,68,72,73] and is relatively similar among different operators and different institutions. Interestingly, the incidence of failure was slightly higher in the series in which a single level PVB was performed with the loss-of-resistance technique (10.7%)[73] compared with the study in which multiple PVB was performed using nerve stimulation (6.1%).[72]

Unintentional vascular puncture occurs in up to 6.8%[72] and when recognized before injection of local anesthetic is of little consequence. Blood pressure and heart rate are generally maintained within normal limits after both unilateral and bilateral PVBs.[2] Hypotension has been reported in up to 5.0% of patients[73]; however, it is usually mild and easily managed. Other common side effects of PVB includes localized hematoma or pain at the site of injection. These are usually self-limiting and do not require treatment.

Unintentional pleural puncture can result from deep insertion of the nerve block needle. A pneumothorax may result and is considered a serious adverse event. An early warning sign includes cough during needle insertion. Aspiration of air occurs if the lung has been punctured or if air has been introduced into the pleural cavity by the needle.[2] Shortness of breath or pleuritic chest pain may follow the PVB. To establish the diagnosis and estimate the size of a pneumothorax, a chest x-ray is often required. Many pneumothoraces that result from PVB are small and can be managed conservatively.[2] Although there are no studies directly comparing the incidence of pleural puncture or pneumothorax using various PVB techniques, the incidences in 2 large series can be contrasted. The incidence of pleural puncture and pneumothorax were 2.1% and 0.3% to 2.1%, respectively, in the series who received single-level PVB with loss of resistance[73]; in contrast, these adverse effects occurred in 0.8% and 0.5% in the series of patients who received multilevel PVB using nerve stimulation.[72] Pulmonary hemorrhage is a rare respiratory complication that has been reported after PVB.[74] The risk of both pneumothorax and pulmonary hemorrhage is thought to be increased in patients who have an obliterated PVS from scar tissue as a result of previous thoracotomy.[74]

Studies on the spread of injectate within the PVS have shown spread of contrast dye into the epidural space in a variable proportion of patients[8]; however, the magnitude with which epidural block contributes to paravertebral anesthesia is unpredictable.[2,72,73] Subarachnoid injection,[75] total spinal anesthesia, and postdural puncture headache[76] are also rare adverse events. They can result either from needle entry into the subarachnoid space or into dural extensions around the spinal nerve roots. The hemodynamic effects of an unintentional thoracic subarachnoid injection may require efficient resuscitation.

Cephalad spread of local anesthetic to the brachial plexus or the stellate ganglion frequently occurs and may result in a brachial plexus block[2] or Horner syndrome,[77] respectively. These effects are temporary, and patients should be reassured.

Systemic absorption of local anesthetic with resulting toxicity is rare.[44] Local anesthetic plasma levels after paravertebral injections have been extensively studied. After a bolus dose of 0.75 to 1.5 mg/kg of bupivacaine, mean peak serum levels varied from 0.705 μg/mL[78] to 1.45 μg/mL[79] in adults and from 1.03 μg/mL[80] to 1.60 μg/mL[81] in children. Karmakar et al[82] administered a single-level PVB with 2 mg/kg of ropivacaine and randomized patients to receive a solution with or without epinephrine. They found that epinephrine decreased mean peak serum concentration of ropivacaine from 2.47 μg/mL to 1.85 μg/mL and increased mean time to peak serum concentration from 7.5 minutes to 11.25 minutes.[82] In other studies, the median time to peak plasma bupivacaine levels ranged from 5 minutes[78] to 25 minutes.[79] Continuous infusion of 0.2 to 0.5 mg/kg/h of bupivacaine for up to 4 days results in variable mean peak plasma bupivacaine levels. Several studies of adult and pediatric patients report levels between 1.6 μg/mL and 2.5 μg/mL.[80,81,83] However, other investigators have found mean peak plasma bupivacaine concentrations as high as 4.92 μg/mL[79] to 5.43 μg/mL,[84] with some individuals as high as 7.48 μg/mL.[79] Despite these high plasma concentrations, no patients in these studies manifested clinical signs of local anesthetic toxicity. Although total bupivacaine increases steadily during paravertebral infusion, free bupivacaine remains unchanged[83] due to a perioperative increase in α_1-acid glycoprotein, a serum protein that binds local anesthetic molecules. This may explain the low incidence of clinical local anesthetic toxicity seen even among patients with plasma bupivacaine concentrations that are considered above the toxic threshold.

There are published case reports of serious neurologic complications related to PVB: incomplete transverse myelitis occurred in association with the use of efocaine,[85] and a Brown-Séquard syndrome resulted from paravertebral injection of alcohol.[86] In more recent publications, neurologic injury is rarely reported.[72,73] There is only 1 case report of chronic segmental pain after PVB[87]; however, some authors[23] believe that this complication occurs more frequently, but is often attributed to nerve injury from surgical dissection.

CLINICAL APPLICATIONS

The various indications for PVB are summarized in Table 48-1 and described in detail next. The most common indications include breast surgery, hernia repair, and thoracic surgery. A systematic review of the literature, which included 8 randomized clinical trials evaluating PVB for breast surgery or herniorrhaphy, concluded that PVB for surgical anesthesia is associated with less pain during the immediate postoperative period, as well as less postoperative nausea and vomiting and greater satisfaction as compared with general anesthesia.[88] A systematic review of randomized trials evaluating regional anesthetic techniques for post-thoracotomy analgesia concluded that continuous paravertebral block was comparable to thoracic epidural analgesia with local anesthetic, but was associated with a reduced incidence of hypotension and a reduced incidence of pulmonary complications compared with systemic analgesia, whereas thoracic epidural analgesia was not.[89]

THORACIC SURGERY

The use of PVB for postoperative analgesia after thoracoscopy or thoracotomy has been investigated in both adults[36,37,41,63-67,90-95] and children.[80,96] A commonly used approach involves preoperative PVB to provide intraoperative analgesia in addition to a continuous local anesthetic infusion via a paravertebral catheter for postoperative analgesia. Preoperative PVB is performed using either a single- or multiple-level injection technique with the goal to provide sensory block from T4 to T9. A paravertebral catheter can be placed preoperatively by the anesthesiologist percutaneously, intraoperatively by the thoracic surgeon under video assistance during thoracoscopy[41] or in combination with the anesthesiologist,[42] or under direct visualization at the time of chest closure.[36-40]

Hill et al[92] investigated multilevel PVB after thorascopic procedures in a prospective, double-blinded, randomized, placebo-controlled study. The benefits of PVB included less intraoperative fentanyl ($p < .003$), reduced cumulative opioid consumption ($p < .03$), and lower maximum pain scores at 6 hours ($p < .02$). No significant difference in cumulative morphine consumption was reported at 12 or 18 hours after block placement, and there was no difference in spirometry, cortisol levels, or cytokine production between groups. A prospective, randomized, blinded, placebo-controlled study by Vogt et al[94] demonstrated a significant difference in VAS scores at rest and coughing over a 48-hour time course with single-level injection PVB ($p < .05$). There was no difference with regard to peak expiratory flow rate at 24 and 48 hours between groups. Kaya et al[95] demonstrated that preoperative multiple-level injection PVB for postoperative analgesia after video-assisted thorascopic surgery procedures was associated with lower intraoperative fentanyl use ($p < .01$), longer time to first analgesic requirement ($p < .05$), lower VAS at first analgesic requirement ($p < .01$), lower maximum VAS pain scores during the 48-hour study period ($p < .01$), improved patient satisfaction ($p < .05$), decreased time to first mobilization ($p < .01$), and decreased time to hospital discharge ($p < .05$).

In a prospective, randomized, placebo-controlled trial, Berrisford et al[63] documented the beneficial effects of continuous PVB for thoracotomy patients. They found lower pain scores ($p < .01$), reduced opioid consumption (8.6 mg vs 119 mg over 5 days), fewer postoperative pulmonary complications (8% vs 52.4%; $p < .05$) and better preservation of pulmonary function ($p < .01$) in the group who received bupivacaine compared with saline. Comparable results were obtained in a number of studies with similar design[64-67] and a non–placebo-controlled study.[91] The moment of insertion of PVB catheter, before or after rib-spreading, did not affect analgesic quality after thoracotmy.[97] An additional advantage of PVB involves a potential reduction in the incidence of post-thoracotomy neuralgia.[61]

Continuous PVB has a number of theoretical advantages over both continuous interpleural and intercostal blocks. PVB more reliably achieves block of the dorsal ramus of the spinal nerve. This is important because much of the pain that results from thoracotomy stems from the paraspinal muscles and other areas innervated by the dorsal ramus. In addition, greater cephalocaudal spread of local anesthetic occurs and results in more extensive block with continuous PVB compared with the other 2 modalities.[98] Despite these theoretical advantages, prospective studies comparing continuous PVB versus interpleural[99] and intercostal[100] infusions of local anesthetic failed to show a difference between groups in pain scores and opioid consumption. Nevertheless, PVB was associated with better preservation of lung function as measured by forced vital capacity and FEV_1.[99]

PVB continuous catheters have been compared with incisional (subcutaneous) catheters and a combination of the 2 for postoperative analgesia after thoracotomy.[37] VAS reports were lower at rest, on coughing, and on movement at 12 ($p <.01$, $p < .05$, and $p < .05$, respectively) and 24 hours ($p < .05$, $p < .05$, and $p < .05$, respectively) after surgery when incisional catheters were used to supplement paravertebral analgesia. However, excluding the first 4 hours, there was no significant difference in daily morphine use to improve analgesia between the 3 groups. There was no significant difference in spirometry testing observed between groups.

Continuous PVB has also been compared with intermittent boluses of epidural morphine for post-thoracotomy analgesia. Dauphin et al[38] found that these 2 modalities resulted in similar pain scores and supplemental intravenous morphine consumption.

A number of prospective, randomized trials exist comparing continuous PVB (local anesthetic alone) versus epidurals (local anesthetic with or without opioid).[36,40,69,90,101,102] In a study by Richardson et al,[101] the group who received PVB had lower postoperative pain scores at rest ($p = .02$) and with coughing ($p = .0001$) as well as lower cumulative morphine consumption over 48 hours ($p \leq .008$). However, other studies[36,40,90] failed to replicate these findings. Messina et al[90] demonstrated increased morphine consumption with PVB as compared with epidural with local anesthetic and opioid infusion; however, VAS scores were not significantly different between the 2 groups. Opioid-related side effects were not reported. Gulbahar et al[36] found no significant difference between the 2 groups with regard to VAS, serum cortisol and glucose levels, necessity for additional analgesia, and hospital stay duration. There was a significant difference in side effects, with no side effects in the PVB group ($p < .01$).[36] A number of investigators have shown a lower incidence of side effects such as nausea,[36,101] vomiting,[36,101] hypotension,[36,69,101] and urinary retention[36,40,69,101] with PVB as compared with epidurals.

Studies of the effects of PVB on postoperative lung function have been conflicting. Richardson et al[101] documented that the postoperative peak expiratory flow rate as a fraction of preoperative value was 0.73 in the PVB group compared with 0.54 in the epidural group ($p < .004$), suggesting better preservation of lung function with PVB. In contrast, Messina et al[90] reported improved spirometry values at 72 hours with return of forced vital capacity to 83% of the preoperative value in the epidural group, as compared with 31% in the paravertebral group. Other studies[36,102] found no significant difference between the 2 analgesic modalities.

In addition to their utility for thoracoscopies and thoracotomies, PVB has also been used successfully for other indications. In a prospective, randomized, placebo-controlled trial of patients having pleurectomy, Mozell et al[103] established that continuous PVB with bupivacaine provided lower pain scores, reduced opioid consumption, and better preservation of pulmonary function than placebo. In a retrospective study by Patel et al,[104] the addition of PVB to general anesthesia after first rib resection demonstrated decreased postanesthesia care unit (PACU) pain scores. PVB has also been used to provide analgesia for rib fractures. Mohta et al[105] demonstrated that continuous PVB provided comparable analgesia and respiratory function to continuous thoracic epidural analgesia (TEA) in patients with unilateral multiple rib fractures with a decreased incidence of hypotension. There was no significant difference in VAS scores at rest and on coughing, respiratory rate, morphine requirement, peak expiratory flow rate, incidence of pulmonary complications, infusion duration, length of intensive care unit stay, and length of hospital stay.[105] Additionally, PVB has been used to provide analgesia for rib fractures in patients with head[106] and spinal cord[107] injuries. In patients with head injury, paravertebral analgesia reduced the need for potentially sedating analgesics and enhanced neurologic assessment.[106] Unilateral PVBs were administered instead of an epidural block in patients with lumbar spinal cord injury because the PVB enhanced assessment of lumbosacral spinal cord function.[107] Moreover, paravertebral analgesia provides quality analgesia and has beneficial effects on pulmonary function among patients with traumatic chest injury.[108] Additional applications have been in the management of chest pain caused by pleural effusion.[109]

BREAST SURGERY

PVBs can be used as the sole intraoperative anesthetic or as an analgesic supplement to general anesthesia for breast surgery. The block may be performed as a single-level injection or as injections at multiple levels. The dermatomal levels blocked depend on the surgical procedure (Table 48-1). Block of T2-T6 is required for mastectomy. When mastectomy and axillary dissection is scheduled, extending the block to include the T1 dermatome is essential. Supplementing with a superficial cervical plexus block can also enhance analgesia at the superior aspect of the incision. Breast biopsy requires block of the dermatome involved in addition to 1 level cephalad and 1 level caudad. Long-acting local anesthetics such as bupivacaine can provide postoperative analgesia for up to 23 hours.[110]

A number of prospective, randomized trials exist comparing general anesthesia versus PVB for breast surgery.[43,45,46,59,68,111,112] Pusch et al[68] performed a single-injection block with bupivacaine using the loss-of-resistance technique at T4 in patients having breast cancer surgery. They found rapid onset of block, with skin incision occurring within 15 minutes of the block. They also documented a shorter emergence time in the group who had PVB ($p < .01$). The PVB group had lower pain scores during the 13 hours of the study ($p < .05$) and received fewer analgesics ($p < .01$). There was less painful restricted motion ($p < .001$) and a reduced incidence of postoperative nausea and vomiting ($p < .05$) in the PVB group. Paravertebral anesthesia with propofol sedation was inadequate in 6% of patients; however, supplemental analgesia with intravenous fentanyl was sufficient to avoid conversion to general anesthesia. Naja et al[46] used a nerve stimulator and performed injections at multiple levels with a mixture of lidocaine, bupivacaine, epinephrine, fentanyl, and clonidine. They showed an analgesic benefit for the first 5 days postoperatively and also documented a shorter length of hospital stay among patients who received PV ($p < .01$). Klein et al[43] studied patients having unilateral or bilateral cosmetic and reconstructive breast surgery and also showed similar benefits, including lower verbal pain scores up to 72 hours after surgery. In addition, they were able to reduce intraoperative induction time from 24 minutes with general anesthesia to 4 minutes with PVBs by using a preoperative block area. Terheggen et al[45] studied patients having minor breast surgery and performed PVB with bupivacaine via a catheter placed at T3-T4. The PVB reduced intraoperative fentanyl requirements and lowered postoperative pain scores only in the first 90 minutes postoperatively for this group of patients having surgery that may be considered less stimulating. Boughey et al[111] compared general anesthesia with general anesthesia with multilevel PVB at T1 to T6 for patients undergoing breast cancer surgery. This was a prospective study in follow-up to a retrospective analysis that demonstrated improved postoperative analgesia up until the morning after surgery and a decreased proportion of patients requiring overnight stay after major breast operations.[111] The prospective study demonstrated decreased pain scores and a greater percentage of pain-free patients at 1 hour (1 vs 3, $p < .014$; 44% vs 17%, $p < .006$) and 3 hours (0 vs 2, $p < .001$; 54% vs 17%, $p < .005$) after surgery; however, at 6 hours the difference was no longer evident. The overall worst pain score was lower with PVB (3 vs 5, $p < .02$), and there was a greater number of subjects in the PVB group reporting to be pain-free during hospital stay (33% vs 12%, $p < .032$). At 24 hours, there were more subjects reporting to be pain-free in the general anesthesia–alone group (23% vs 54%, $p < .011$), which might be representative of inadequate analgesia with block resolution. There was no difference in opioid consumption, nausea/vomiting, and hospital length of stay between groups. This study was limited in that it did not include a standardized surgical procedure. An underpowered subgroup analysis of the more extensive surgeries failed to demonstrate a difference between groups at any time. Moller et al[112] in a prospective, randomized, double-blind, placebo-controlled study also demonstrated duration of postoperative analgesia provided with PVB to be less than that described in previous studies. Intraoperatively, PVB was associated with a significant decrease in intraoperative fentanyl ($p < .0001$) and propofol ($p < .001$). In the PACU, PVB was associated with decreased opioid consumption $p < .001$) and improved pain control (patients reporting VAS <3; $p < .0001$). There was no difference in postoperative nausea and vomiting between groups. No benefits were demonstrated beyond the PACU. Another, randomized, placebo-controlled trial[44] studied patients scheduled for breast cancer surgery receiving single-injection PVB at T3 with bupivacaine 0.5% (1.5 mg/mL) or saline before general anesthesia. Pain scores were low in both groups; however, patients receiving PVB with bupivacaine had less postoperative pain in the PACU and up to 12 hours after surgery, as measured by longer time to first analgesic (20 min vs 10 min; $p < .019$) and lower VAS (PACU, 3.0-1.7 vs 4.8-1.4, $p < .025$; 12 h, $p < .096$). Postoperative pain was minimal in both groups of this study, as evident by low PACU pain scores and zero opioid consumption after discharge from PACU in either group. There was no significant difference in the number of patients with postoperative nausea and vomiting (PONV) between groups. Iohom et al[59] demonstrated improvement of postoperative VAS pain scores with PVB continuous catheters at rest up to 12 hours ($p < .035$) and movement at 12 hours and on postoperative days 1, 2, 3, 4, and 5 ($p < .04$.)

A prospective comparison of continuous wound infiltration with ropivacaine versus single-level injection PVB after modified radical mastectomy[113] demonstrated low pain scores in both groups. PVB was associated with reduced pain scores at 4 hours ($p < .02$) and less PONV. Continuous wound infiltration was associated with reduced pain scores at 16, 20, and 24 hours. There was no difference in opioid consumption between groups at any time point.

PVB may be associated with a reduced development of chronic postsurgical pain after breast surgery. In a study by Iohom et al[59] at 10 weeks, 80% of patients (12 of 15) not receiving PVB continuous catheters developed chronic postsurgical pain as compared with 0% (0 of 14) in those receiving PVB catheters ($p < .009$). Preoperative PVB may reduce the incidence of chronic pain 1 year after breast cancer surgery.[60]

HERNIA REPAIR

PVB can be used for surgical anesthesia or for analgesia as a supplement to general anesthesia for inguinal, umbilical, or incisional hernia repair. When performed for inguinal hernia repair, block of the T10 through L2 dermatomes is typically required. This can be achieved by a single-level injection in the low thoracic PVS or by injections at multiple levels.

PVB may be used as the sole anesthetic for inguinal hernia repair.[114,115] Klein et al[114] demonstrated that bupivacaine PVB provided surgical anesthesia within 15 to 30 minutes and prolonged postoperative analgesia with a mean time to first opioid of 22 hours. In a study by Weltz et al,[115] the failure rate requiring conversion to general anesthesia was 6.7%; however, these investigators documented low pain scores for 48 hours postoperatively.

Studies have evaluated the efficacy of PVB compared with other anesthetic techniques, including general anesthesia, spinal anesthesia, ilio-inguinal block, and local field block for inguinal hernia repair. As compared with general anesthesia, multilevel PVB from T9 to L1 was associated with shorter time to home readiness, greater phase 1 PACU bypass, less postoperative pain, faster ambulation, and quicker discharge home.[116] Single-level injection PVB at L1 demonstrated shorter time to ambulation, increased recovery room bypass, and decreased postoperative urinary retention as compared with spinal anesthesia with 12.5 mg of 0.5% bupivacaine.[117] Multilevel PVB from T9 to L1 versus unilateral spinal anesthesia with 8.0 mg of 0.5% bupivacaine provided statistically significant shorter hospital stays with shorter time to home readiness (with and without voiding), shorter discharge time, and prolonged postoperative analgesia with a mean time to first analgesic of 16 hours as compared with 7 hours in the spinal group.[118] Naja et al[119] compared multilevel PVB from T12 to L2 versus general anesthesia versus spinal anesthesia. Again, patients in the PVB group had a shorter duration of hospital stay (1.2 d vs 2.9 d for general anesthesia vs 2.5 d for subarachnoid block; $p < .0001$), better postoperative analgesia, and a lower incidence of postoperative nausea and vomiting (0 vs 21% for general anesthesia vs 19% for subarachnoid block; $p < .001$). In a randomized trial, Wassef et al[120] compared lidocaine PVB versus lidocaine/bupivacaine field block. The PVB was associated with less frequent intraoperative supplementation (20% vs 41%; $p < .01$), a lower rate of conversion to general anesthesia (0 vs 6.7%), and greater patient satisfaction ($p < .05$).

Alternatively, PVB can supplement another primary anesthetic technique (ie, general or spinal anesthesia) to provide postoperative analgesia. In a prospective, randomized study of subjects undergoing inguinal hernia repair under general anesthesia, Klein et al[121] compared postoperative analgesia from ropivacaine PVB with ilio-inguinal-iliohypogastric nerve blocks with wound infiltration. They found reduced opioid consumption intraoperatively ($p = .02$) and in the PACU ($p = .002$), as well as a lower antiemetic use ($p < .001$) in the PVB group; however, there was no subsequent difference in pain scores and opioid use. In children undergoing inguinal herniorrhaphy under general anesthesia, multilevel PVB from T12 to L1 as compared with general anesthesia with systemic analgesia (GA/SA) demonstrated improved postoperative analgesia during the first 48 hours, increased same day discharge (80% PVB group vs 52% GA/SA), and greater parental and surgeon satisfaction.[122] As compared with ilio-inguinal block, multilevel PVB from T12 to L2 in children undergoing inguinal herniorrhaphy under general anesthesia demonstrated a significant improvement in intraoperative hemodynamic stability, postoperative analgesia with decreased consumption of analgesic drugs during the first 36 hours after surgery, and again greater parental and surgeon satisfaction.[123]

Ozkan et al[124] comparing 2-level (T10, L1) PVB versus 4-level (T10-L1) PVB demonstrated shorter block performance time (5 min [SD 1] vs 16 min [SD 4]; $p < .001$) with 2-level injection but no difference in the other parameters investigated, including intraoperative propofol and remifentanil use, VAS scores, postoperative analgesics consumed, sensory block duration adverse effects, PONV, and patient satisfaction.

When PVB is used for umbilical hernia repair of moderate size, a bilateral block from T9 to T11 is required. In a nonrandomized study, Naja et al[56] compared PVB versus general anesthesia. PVB was performed using a nerve stimulator and a mixture of lidocaine, bupivacaine, epinephrine, fentanyl, and clonidine. Interestingly, 10% of patients in the PVB group required supplemental analgesia due to unanticipated extension of the surgical field. Nevertheless, PVB had a number of benefits, including lower pain scores and reduced opioid requirements up to 48 hours ($p < .001$). PVB was also associated with a decreased incidence of PONV (3.3% vs 26.7%; $p < .05$) and shorter length of hospital admission (2.3 d vs 4.1 d; $p < .05$).

Finally, PVB can be used for incisional hernia repair and are performed according to the dermatomal levels involved. Block from T8 to T12 has also been used for ileostomy closure.[125]

RENAL SURGERY

Unilateral PVB is well suited to provide postoperative analgesia after renal surgery. A PVB continuous catheter can be placed preoperatively, or alternatively, a catheter can be placed under direct vision by the surgeon at the time of wound closure.[126] In a randomized, prospective, placebo-controlled trial, Awwad and Atiyat[126] found reduced pain scores for 3 days ($p < .026$) and decreased opioid consumption (13.3 mg vs 40.13 mg over 3 d; $p < .001$) in the continuous PVB catheter with bupivacaine versus saline. Lonnqvist[127] and Lonnqvist and Olsson[128] have used continuous PVB in children having renal surgery. In a nonrandomized study, they compared the postoperative analgesia obtained from paravertebral versus epidural bupivacaine[128] and found decreased opioid consumption in the PVB group. In a case report of 30 patients, PVB as a part of a multimodal analgesia regimen provided significant opioid sparing as compared with previous studies[129,130] after hand-assisted laparoscopic nephrectomy.[131]

Jamieson and Mariano[132] reported pain scores of zero for 24 hours and no opioid rescue analgesia in 2 patients undergoing lithotripsy under PVB.

CHOLECYSTECTOMY

Few studies exist evaluating the efficacy of PVB for postoperative analgesia after open cholecystectomy by subcostal incision. Giesecke et al[62] suggest that PVB reduces the stress response to surgery; however, Bigler et al[87] found no benefit from continuous PVB when compared with thoracic epidural. More recently, PVB has been used to provide postoperative analgesia for laparoscopic cholecystectomy. In a prospective, randomized study, Naja et al[133] randomized patients receiving general anesthesia to have PVB or opioid analgesia. Although there was no difference between groups in time to first oral intake or length of hospital stay, patients who received PVB had lower pain scores ($p < .05$), reduced opioid consumption over 36 hours ($p < .05$), and a decreased incidence of PONV ($p < .05$). Paleczny et al[134] in a randomized, prospective study compared general anesthesia alone with PVB performed before the induction of general anesthesia. PVB demonstrated a significantly lower mean pain score during the first 72 hours after surgery ($p < .005$) and improved patient satisfaction.

APPENDECTOMY

Splinter and Thompson[135] demonstrated in children (3-16 y) undergoing appendectomy that PVB T11 to L1 using ropivacaine 0.2% 0.25 mL/kg with 1:200000 epinephrine was associated with decreased opioid consumption ($p < .001$) with an increased time to first opioid dose ($p < .001$). There was no significant difference in vomiting and no other adverse effects observed in the 2 groups.

ORTHOPEDIC SURGERY

PVB can be used as an adjunct to other peripheral nerve blocks or as the sole regional technique for the treatment of postoperative pain in orthopedic patients. In patients receiving an interscalene brachial plexus block for shoulder surgery, the addition of T1 to T2 PVB provides more complete shoulder analgesia. And, in combination with a lumbar plexus block, T11 to T12 PVB provides more comprehensive analgesia for patients having hip surgery. Alternatively, PVB from T12 to L4 and from L2 to S1 has been used to provide postoperative analgesia after total hip and knee arthroplasty, respectively.[136] For hip arthroscopy, Lee et al presented 2 cases in which they performed 2-level (L1 and L2) PVB with 5 mL of ropivacaine 0.5% preoperatively in combination with general anesthesia and injection of 20 mL of 0.25% bupivacaine with epinephrine into the hip joint by surgery at the end of the procedure. This regimen provided postoperative analgesia of approximately 36 hours and greater with no opioid requirement.

BONE MARROW ASPIRATION

Bilateral PVB from T11 to L2 can be used to provide intraoperative anesthesia and postoperative analgesia for patients having bone marrow aspiration. This technique provides an alternative option when general and/or spinal anesthesias are contraindicated (ie, mediastinal tumor and chemotherapy-related thrombocytopenia).

CARDIAC AND VASCULAR SURGERY

PVB has been used both for analgesia after cardiac surgery as well as peripheral vascular procedures. In a prospective, observational study, Canto et al[137] performed continuous bilateral ropivacaine PVB at T3 to T4 for patients having open-heart surgery with cardiopulmonary bypass. They reported excellent analgesia, a low complication rate, and facilitation of early tracheal extubation. Moderate hypotension and bradycardia were repeatedly observed and presumed due to sympathectomy; however, dopamine support was required in only 6.4%.

Bilateral T4 to T5 continuous PVB has also been successfully used for postoperative analgesia after minimally invasive coronary artery bypass[138] and may facilitate early extubation.[139] In a prospective, randomized trial, Dhole et al[140] compared continuous PVB versus epidural and found no significant differences between the techniques with respect to analgesia.

A prospective randomized study in patients undergoing elective robotic-assisted coronary artery bypass grafting comparing thoracic epidural analgesia with PVB revealed no significant difference with regard to hemodynamics, arterial blood gases, pulmonary functions, and analgesia.[141]

Thoracic PVB with mild sedation was successfully used for implantable cardioverter-defibrillator and laser lead extraction in a patient who had a high opioid tolerance and desired prolonged analgesia.[142]

Richardson et al[143] described paravertebral analgesia after major abdominal vascular surgery in an observational study. They placed bilateral PVB catheters at T10 in 8 patients and administered an infusion of bupivacaine. The continuous PVB provided excellent postoperative analgesia with preserved hemodynamic stability.

A retrospective review comparing paravertebral blockade with propofol sedation with general anesthesia for elective endovascular abdominal aortic aneurysm repair demonstrated decreased intraoperative hypotension ($p < .05$) and blood pressure lability ($p < .01$), as well as postoperative nausea ($p < .01$).[144]

HEPATIC SURGERY

A prospective, randomized, placebo-controlled study compared bilateral PVB injection of 25 mL of 0.25% bupivacaine with epinephrine to saline before induction of general anesthesia in 24 patients undergoing right lobe donor hepatectomy. PVB was associated with a 50% decrease in opioid consumption, a significant increase in time to rescue analgesia, and decreased PONV.

In a case report, Ho et al[146] described the use of a right thoracic paravertebral catheter for hepatectomy and cite their preference for this technique over epidural analgesia in patients who have or may develop a coagulopathy.

In an additional case report, Hall and Leach[147] illustrated the use of continuous paravertebral analgesia for the pain associated with a traumatic liver fracture managed conservatively.

In a feasibility study performed by Culp et al,[148] PVB at T8 to T9 and T9 to T10 under fluoroscopic guidance in combination with intravenous sedation was successfully performed for 10 consecutive patients undergoing biliary drainage procedures. This group also performed multilevel PVB injection with 15 mL of 0.25% bupivacaine at T7 and T9 for analgesia after liver mass radiofrequency ablation, with no additional analgesic requirements. Sensory blockade of the T4 to T12 dermatomes was reported.[149]

PROSTATE SURGERY

A retrospective study of 100 patients undergoing radical retropubic prostatectomy under general anesthesia compared 50 patients (group 1) receiving local anesthetic wound infiltration with 30 mL of 0.25% bupivacaine, intravenous ketorolac, and opioids for postoperative pain management with 50 patients (group 2) who had received an amended analgesia protocol to include, in addition to the preexisting protocol, the use of preoperative, multiple-injection PVB at T10 to T12 bilaterally and a single preoperative oral dose of a COX-2 inhibitor. The study suggested that the analgesic protocol of group 2 might significantly reduce intraoperative and postoperative opioid requirements and reduce hospital length of stay.

LABOR ANALGESIA FOR OBSTETRICS

Bilateral PVB has been used to provide analgesia for laboring obstetrical patients in whom epidural anesthesia is impossible or contraindicated. In a case series, Nair and Henry[150] described using bilateral T11 and T12 PVB to obtain labor analgesia for patients with coagulation abnormalities (prolonged bleeding time, syndrome of hemolysis, elevated liver enzymes, and low platelets) and lumbar spinal anomalies (neuroblastoma, spina bifida occulta). Suelto[151] underlines the limitation of this technique in providing analgesia for the second stage of labor as well as for cesarean section.

CHRONIC PAIN

Several authors have published descriptions of the use of PVB in the management of chronic pain. Kirvela and Antila[152] provided retrospective information on 32 patients having 281 PVBs for chronic chest wall pain. Results were similar for those patients with post-thoracotomy chest pain and those with postmastectomy pain. Among the thoracic surgical patients, immediate pain relief occurred in 99% of cases; however, prolonged pain relief was rare. Fifty-eight percent were pain-free at 1 month, 30% at 2 months, 8% at 4 months, and only 3% at 5 months. Among the breast cancer patients, 88% were pain-free for less than 1 month and only 6% were pain-free for more than 5 months. Antila and Kirvela [153] observed similar results in a population of patients who had chronic thoracic pain related to malignant disease with poor prognosis. PVB may offer a useful treatment for thoracic myofascial pain syndrome refractory to traditional therapeutic approaches.[154] Limited data exist on the use of PVB for pain relief from acute herpes zoster[155] and post-herpetic neuralgia.[156]

CONCLUSION

PVB is a technique that offers dense, long-lasting, segmental anesthesia and analgesia. This block takes advantage of the anatomical structure and contents of the PVS. Local anesthetic is delivered at discrete locations to achieve site-specific block of both the dorsal and ventral rami as well as the sympathetic chain. In contrast to neuraxial techniques, PVB offers the flexibility of either unilateral or bilateral blockade and avoids many of the side effects associated with centrally administered local anesthetics.[40,69,101] The density of the achieved block is highlighted in the profound analgesia that results and in the mitigation of the surgical stress response.[62] Additionally, preoperative PVB may reduce the incidence of chronic pain after breast cancer surgery[60] and reduce the incidence of post-thoracotomy neuralgia.[61] Further prospective investigation is necessary to determine whether PVB for breast cancer surgery may reduce the risk of cancer recurrence or metastasis.[70] By peripherally targeting individual nerve roots or segmental innervation, the technique has wide-scale applicability for nearly all procedures of the thorax and abdomen as well as the lower extremities. Despite these advantages, the greatest impediments to wider scale adoption of this technique are the low but consistent failure rate of up to 10%[73] and the concern of pneumothorax.

It has been most extensively studied after thoracotomy, demonstrating profound block, excellent analgesia, opioid sparing, and reduction in opioid- and epidural-related side effects.[63-67] In addition, PVB offers better preservation of pulmonary function and a reduced incidence of postoperative pulmonary complications.[63-67] The magnitude of these outcome differences suggests that PVB is underutilized, particularly in procedures such as thoracic surgery where iatrogenic pneumothorax is of limited concern.

PVB has also been validated as an effective sole intraoperative anesthetic or as an analgesic adjunct for breast surgery[43,45,46,68] and inguinal hernia repair,[114,115,119,120] 2 of the most commonly performed outpatient surgical procedures. When used for ambulatory surgery, PVB facilitates recovery and has the potential to hasten discharge and reduce costs. Efficacious results have also been produced for procedures as diverse as cardiac surgery,[137,138] cholecystectomy,[62,87,133] and labor.[150] In short, the ability to provide site-specific segmental anesthesia makes PVB one of the most useful and broadly applicable peripheral nerve block techniques.

KEY REFERENCES

- Cheema S, Richardson J, McGurgan P. Factors affecting the spread of bupivacaine in the adult thoracic paravertebral space. *Anaesthesia.* 2003;58:684-687.
- Eason MJ, Wyatt R. Paravertebral thoracic block-a reappraisal. *Anaesthesia.* 1979;34:638-642.
- Karmakar MK. Thoracic paravertebral block. *Anesthesiology.* 2001;95:771-780.
- Karmakar MK, Ho AM, Law BK, Wong ASY, Shafer SL, Gin T. Arterial and venous pharmacokinetics of ropivacaine with and without epinephrine after thoracic paravertebral block. *Anesthesiology.* 2005;103:704-711.
- Naja Z, Lonnqvist PA. Somatic paravertebral nerve blockade. Incidence of failed block and complications. *Anaesthesia.* 2001;56:1184-1188.
- Naja MZ, Ziade MF, Lonnqvist PA. Nerve-stimulator guided paravertebral blockade vs. general anaesthesia for breast surgery: a prospective randomized trial. *Eur J Anaesthesiol.* 2003;20: 897-903.
- Richardson J, Sabanathan S, Jones J, Shah RD, Cheema S, Mearns AJ. A prospective, randomized comparison of preoperative and continuous balanced epidural or paravertebral bupivacaine on post-thoracotomy pain, pulmonary function and stress responses. *Br J Anaesth.* 1999;83:387-392.

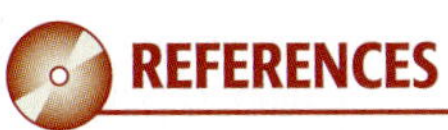

REFERENCES

Complete references available on DVD and online version at www.LongneckerAnesthesiology.com

CHAPTER 49 Peripheral Nerve Blocks

Brian C. Spence
Michelle C. Parra

KEY POINTS

1. The duration of the surgical procedure, patient comorbidities, and postoperative factors, such as the early need for the use of the operative extremity and potential for significant postoperative discomfort, should all be used to determine the selection of local anesthetic and technique.
2. The lowest clinically effective dose of a local anesthetic should be used whenever possible to minimize toxicity.
3. Studies to date have shown that ultrasound decreases the time for placement of peripheral nerve blocks, increases the speed of block set-up, and improves the "quality" of the block by modest amounts when compared with the traditional landmark techniques or nerve stimulation.
4. Because the frequency of neurologic injury is low with peripheral nerve blocks, no single technique has been shown to be "safer" than another.
5. The use of ultrasound does not replace the need for a fundamental understanding of anatomy when placing peripheral nerve blocks.
6. The interscalene approach to the brachial plexus, unlike the supraclavicular approach, will most likely miss the ulnar distribution of the hand; thus it is not suitable as a complete anesthetic distal to the elbow.
7. Femoral nerve block is a relatively easy block to perform and its success rate is high. A femoral nerve block is usually performed in conjunction with other lower-extremity blocks.
8. The popliteal approach to the sciatic nerve can be done with the patient supine or prone and is ideal for surgeries involving the lower leg and/or foot. If the medial aspect of the lower leg or foot is required for surgical anesthesia, then the saphenous portion of the femoral nerve must be included.

INTRODUCTION

Peripheral nerve blocks are a powerful component of the practice of anesthesia. No other anesthetic technique allows a precise targeting of anesthetic to the surgical site while sparing non–procedure-involved locations. This not only allows one to create tailored area of surgical anesthesia, but also to avoid, or reduce, the risk of systemic complications from general anesthesia such as nausea and vomiting.[1,2] To perform a peripheral nerve block, one must have a local anesthetic, a means to administer the anesthetic, and a target nerve structure.

The modern knowledge of anatomy can be traced to the Renaissance, when scholars once again began using cadavers to teach their students anatomy after the Church banned cadaveric dissection during the Middle Ages. It was the "reawakening" of such scholars as Andreas Vesalius and the publication of his *De Humani Corporis Fabrica* (*On the Structure of the Human Body*) that shaped the modern day study of anatomy.[3] However, the mapping of dermatomes and the understanding of peripheral nerve anatomy would not begin until the late 1800s. The combination of the observations of French neurologist Jean Martin Charcot and the American scholar Silas Weir Mitchell would begin to suggest the need for "cutaneous nerve mapping."[4] Mitchell especially seemed to be a keen observer and was interested in peripheral nerve anatomy as he cared for injured veterans from the American Civil War.[4] However, it was the English surgical registrar William Thorburn who published some of the first dermatomal maps in the 1880s based on observation of patients with spinal cord lesions.[4]

The discovery and development of local anesthesia can be traced back to the jungles of South America with the coca leaf, first described to the West by Amerigo Vespucci in the log of his 1499-1500 expedition.[5] It was not until 1855 that the German chemist Friedrich Gaedke isolated the cocaine alkaloid, and it would take another 29 years before Karl Köller, a Viennese ophthalmologist, would use it first in a clinical setting in 1884.[5] The early 1900s witnessed further local anesthetic discoveries, the most significant being procaine in 1904 by Alfred Einhorn. It was the Swedish chemist Nils Löfgren who synthesized lidocaine, the first of many amide local anesthetics.[5]

The invention of the hypodermic needle and syringe is credited to 2 individuals who developed their respective devices independently in 1853, the Scottish physician Alexander Wood and the French surgeon Charles Gabriel Pravaz. However, it was Wood who first published the medical use of the device when he used it to inject morphine to treat neuralgia.[5,6]

Modern day regional anesthesia techniques did not take foot in the United States until Gaston Labat published *Regional Anesthesia: Its Technic and Application* in 1922.[7] Labat's book was written while he was teaching regional anesthesia techniques at the Mayo Clinic under the invitation of Charles Mayo. The text was the first of its kind published in the United States and would be the standard reference for the performance of peripheral nerve blocks through the first half of the 20th century.[7,8] In deference to his contributions, it was proposed that the American Society of Regional Anesthesia be named the Labat Society when it was founded in 1923.[9]

Modern regional anesthesia techniques have grown from the solid and broad foundation established in the early 20th century with the further development and introduction of the amide local anesthetics and modern nerve localization techniques, such as nerve stimulation and ultrasound guidance. What has not changed is the dedication of anesthesiologists to their patients' safety and comfort.

SELECTION OF LOCAL ANESTHETICS

The primary variable used in selection of local anesthetics is arguably the duration of the surgical procedure. It should be obvious that a peripheral nerve block that resolves before the conclusion of the surgical procedure has a negative clinical impact on the patient. A long-acting peripheral nerve block may not be ideal either, especially if a patient will need to ambulate or use the affected limb in the early postoperative period. Studies have also shown that total dosage or mass of local anesthetic is the primary contributor to block density.[10-12] Thus a block with a higher concentration and lower volume of local anesthetic may provide a more profound block than a lower concentration, higher volume block.[10]

Another variable to be cognizant of when selecting a local anesthetic is toxicity. The overall volume and concentration of injected local anesthetic both contribute to the potential risk of toxicity (**Table 49-1**). Commonly cited maximum dosage limits (such as 3 mg/kg for bupivacaine and 4.5 mg/kg for lidocaine without epinephrine) have not been rigorously studied or confirmed except in the pediatric population.[13] In addition, absorption of local anesthetics differs throughout the human body and from individual to individual. Therefore, the "toxic dose" in one location that has higher systemic absorption (eg, the intercostal space) may be much lower than an area with more limited systemic absorption (eg, around the sciatic nerve). Regardless, when injecting any local anesthetic for a peripheral nerve block, one should attempt to use the lowest dose possible for a successful block and perform the injection in a slow, deliberate manner with repeated aspiration during the course of injection to confirm that the needle has not migrated into a vascular structure. Traditionally, a vascular injection "indicator" such as epinephrine has been added to the local anesthetic solution to hint at an intravascular injection. The new technology of ultrasound guidance allows one to visualize the spread of local anesthetic to confirm correct placement and therefore may replace the need for an indicator in the future. Patients should also be monitored closely both during and after the injection for signs of toxicity. An unintended intravascular injection can show almost immediate signs of toxicity, whereas toxicity from systemic absorption (eg, a large volume placed correctly for a peripheral nerve block) may take 30 minutes to an hour to manifest.

TABLE 49-1 Local Anesthetic Maximum Dosages

Local Anesthetic	Maximum Dosage (mg/kg)
Lidocaine	4.5 (without epinephrine) 7 (with epinephrine)
Mepivacaine	4.5 (without epinephrine) 7 (with epinephrine)
Bupivacaine	3
Ropivacaine	3
Chloroprocaine	12

Adapted From Morgan GE, Mikhail MS, Murray MJ. *Clinical Anesthesiology*. 3rd ed. New York, NY: McGraw-Hill; 2002:236-237.

Lidocaine has a fairly short onset and duration of action, making it ideal for stimulating surgical procedures of less than a couple hours duration. However, these properties are its weakness as well. It is not the best option for prolonged procedures or for postoperative pain control. Typically 2% lidocaine is the concentration selected for short-duration profound surgical anesthesia.

Bupivacaine has a slower onset of action compared with lidocaine. However, its duration of action can be up to 24 hours with an appropriate volume and placement. It is a good choice for peripheral nerve blocks placed for postoperative pain control or surgical anesthetics for procedures that are expected to be more than a couple of hours. Higher volumes and concentrations of bupivacaine may cause a profound block to be formed that can be used as a surgical anesthetic. Many early studies of peripheral nerve blocks typically used volumes of 30 to 40 mL of 0.5% bupivacaine; however, dosages of 0.25 mL/kg with the maximum of 30 mL are now being used. Bupivacaine does have serious toxic potential when contrasted with shorter-acting local anesthetics. Its affinity for blocking sodium channels in the cardiac conduction fibers resulting in sudden cardiac death should be approached with vigilance by practitioners. (Recent case reports and a small study in dogs have suggested that infusion with 20% lipid emulsion may rescue patients suffering from bupivacaine toxicity.[14,15]) Higher concentrations may also prolong a peripheral nerve block longer than intended, thus interfering with the patient's ability to ambulate or perform postoperative physical therapy. Typically 0.5% bupivacaine is used for a surgical anesthetic, with 0.2% to 0.3% used through a catheter or single shot for postoperative pain control in order to provide some muscle sparing.

Ropivacaine is an enantiomer of bupivacaine with similar properties as bupivacaine in terms of onset and duration of action. It has been suggested that ropivacaine provides more profound sensory than motor block as compared with bupivacaine, and ropivacaine has also been shown to have a slightly shorter duration of action as compared with bupivacaine.[16] One potential advantage of ropivacaine compared with bupivacaine is that it is not as cardiotoxic as bupivacaine.[17] Thus it is good selection for blocks that are placed with high volumes or for blocks where there is going to be significant systemic uptake. As with bupivacaine, 0.5% ropivacaine is a suitable choice for a surgical anesthetic, and 0.2% to 0.3% ropivacaine is a good choice for a continuous catheter or a single-shot block for postoperative pain control.

Chloroprocaine is a very short-onset and short-duration local anesthetic. It is a suitable choice for surgical procedures of 30 to 45 minutes in duration and for procedures with minimal expected postoperative pain. Chloroprocaine can also be bolused through a continuous nerve catheter to ensure proper function or as a "rescue" injection.

Mepivacaine 2% is also used for peripheral nerve blocks, as its onset is similar to lidocaine; however, its duration of action is longer. It is a good choice for surgical procedures in which a block of 2 to 3 hours duration is needed with postoperative return of limb function being necessary and postoperative pain not expected to be severe.

ADDITIVES

Additives can prolong the duration of the sensory component or both motor and sensory components of a peripheral nerve block. However, additives are not without their own side effects and contraindications; thus their selection must also be carefully considered before their inclusion in a local anesthetic "cocktail" for a peripheral nerve block.

Epinephrine is probably one of the most commonly used additives with peripheral nerve blocks. It is typically added in a concentration that is 1:200 000 to 1:400 000 parts per solution (5-10 µg/mL). It decreases the local anesthetic uptake by causing vasoconstriction at the site of injection, thus prolonging the duration of peripheral nerve blocks when added to the local anesthetic solutions of short- and mid-duration local anesthetics. Epinephrine is a potent vasoconstrictor, so it should be avoided in distal extremity blocks such as an ankle block or a forearm block. It also can cause systemic hypertension and tachycardia if injected intravascularly; thus it should be used with caution in patients with cardiac disease. However, it has been traditionally added to local anesthetic solutions as an indicator for intravascular injection because of these very properties.

Clonidine is an α_2-agonist that has been shown to provide prolongation of peripheral nerve blocks when used in doses between 10 and 150 µg.[18,19] This prolongation is more sensory than motor in nature and provides a relatively small increase in duration of bupivacaine when compared with the shorter-acting local anesthetics such as lidocaine and mepivacaine.[18,19] The "ideal" dose has not been conclusively demonstrated; however, with increasing dosages, there are increasing side effects.[19] Most notable are hypotension, bradycardia, sedation, and low body temperature.

Dexamethasone has been shown in a small study to prolong the duration of an axillary nerve block when used with lidocaine. However, this study did have a very small sample size.[20] This has not been replicated in studies with bupivacaine except when the dexamethasone was combined with bupivacaine in microspheres.[21] Although the exact mechanism of action is unknown, the prolongation of the nerve block with dexamethasone in microspheres can be several days. Thus this area of active research portends to have a potential significant impact on peripheral nerve blocks in the future.

Opioids have been routinely added to peripheral nerve blocks for their presumed synergistic effects; however, they have not been shown to increase the duration, onset, or quality of the block.[22-24]

Nonsteroidal anti-inflammatory drugs (NSAIDs) have been proposed to be added to peripheral nerve blocks to prolong the analgesic duration of the block. To date there have been very few studies to support the use of NSAIDS as additions to local anesthetic solutions for peripheral nerve blocks.[23,25]

TECHNIQUES

The choice of technique has evolved over the last 30 years. Originally landmark techniques were the only methods for placing peripheral nerve blocks. In fact, the nomenclature that is used for the majority of peripheral nerve blocks owes its existence to the landmark technique. Descriptions of *supraclavicular*, *infraclavicular*, *interscalene*, and *axillary* do not correlate to a particular nerve structure, but to the area of the body where the brachial plexus will be encountered. The true landmark techniques are techniques where the needle is placed and directed into the body based on certain surface anatomical landmarks. The clinician, through tactile stimulation of "clicks and pops," ascertains whether he or she is in the correct position to inject local anesthetic. Daniel C. Moore, MD, astutely coined the phrase "No paresthesia, no analgesia" to describe the performance of these techniques.[26]

Nerve stimulation was the next "evolution" for facilitating the placement of peripheral nerve blocks. Nerve stimulation is founded on the landmark technique; however, an insulated needle is used, connected to a pulse generator with an additional lead attached to the patient to complete a circuit (**Fig. 49-1**). When the needle is advanced within the proximity of a nerve, a muscle twitch is witnessed in the distribution of the stimulated nerve. This helped increase the accuracy of peripheral nerve blocks; however, it still remains a blind technique. It also should be noted that there is a false-negative rate of between 10% and 15% when a nerve simulator is used.[27]

Ultrasound-guided regional anesthesia is the most recent technique used to place peripheral nerve blocks (**Fig. 49-2**). The technique uses

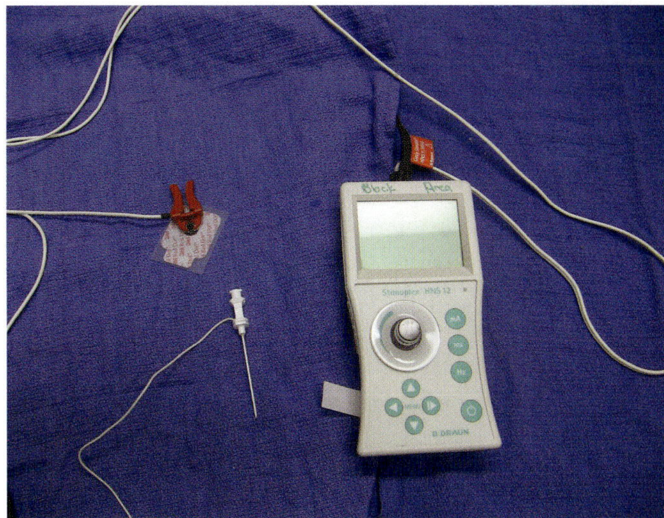

FIGURE 49-1. Example of a nerve stimulator with needle and electrocardiogram pad connected.

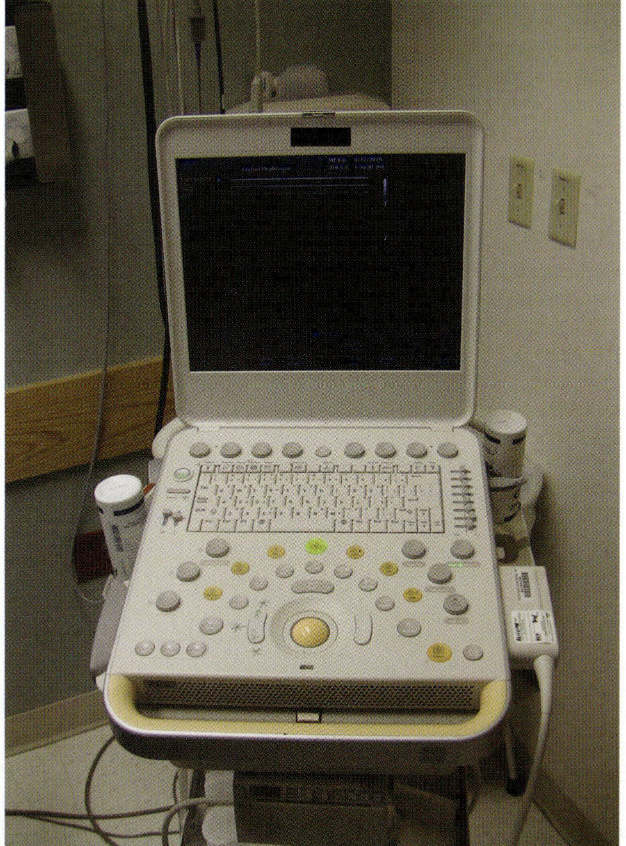

FIGURE 49-2. Example of an ultrasound machine used for peripheral nerve blocks.

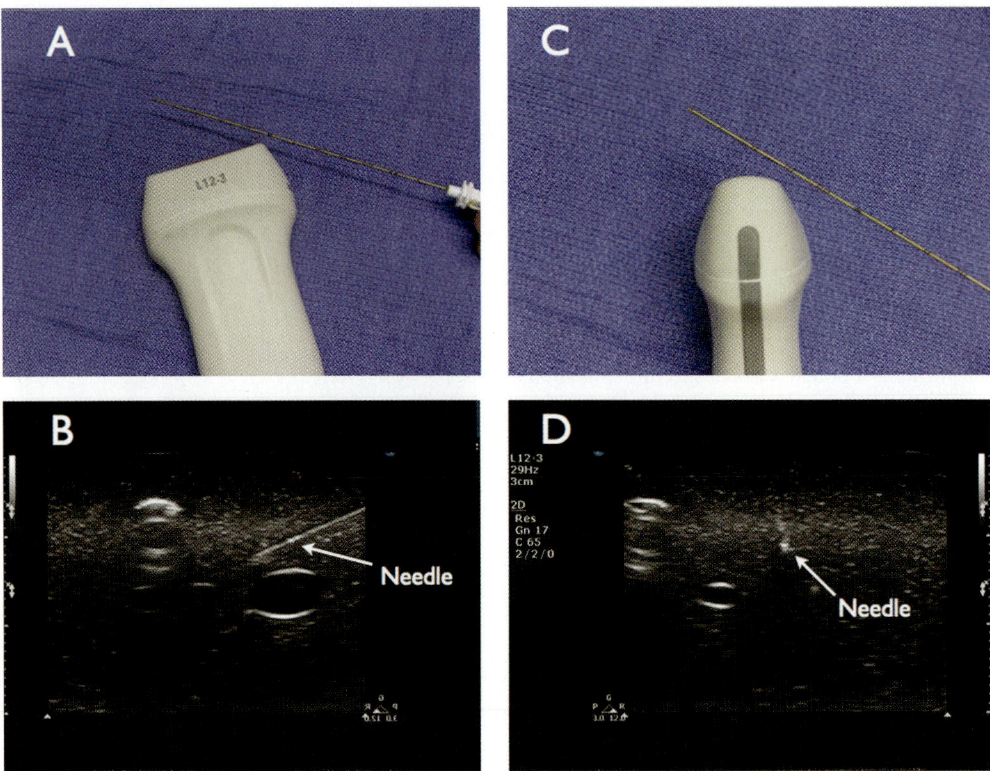

FIGURE 49-3. Example of needle and probe orientation for ultrasound-guided regional anesthesia. **A.** In-plane orientation with (**B**) the corresponding in-plane ultrasound image. **C.** Out-of-plane image with the (**D**) corresponding out-of-plane image of the needle.

ultrasound to identify the target nerve structure and the needle such that the needle can be guided near the nerve structure accurately. More importantly, ultrasound allows one to see the spread of local anesthetic around the target nerve structure. Ultrasound was first used to facilitate the placement of peripheral nerve blocks in 1978 by La Grange when he used a Doppler to map the subclavian artery when placing a supraclavicular nerve block.[28] It would be another decade before the 2-dimensional ultrasound was used in the placement of peripheral nerve blocks.[29] Currently the popularity of ultrasound-guided techniques is rapidly expanding. Studies to date have shown that ultrasound decreases the time for placement of peripheral nerve blocks, increases the speed of block set-up, and improves the "quality" of the block as compared with the traditional landmark techniques or nerve stimulation by modest amounts.[30–32] It should be pointed out, however, that the available randomized, controlled studies have low patient numbers and that their overall number is rather limited. It also should be stressed that to date there has been no conclusive evidence that one technique is "safer" as compared with another because the number of patients that would need to be enrolled to ensure adequate power would be in the hundreds of thousands. Perhaps the greatest contribution of ultrasound is that it enables moderately experienced regional anesthesiologists to have success rates similar to those of expert regional experts.

With ultrasound there are 2 ways to orientate the needle with the beam of the ultrasound probe (**Fig. 49-3**). The in-plane technique has the needle imaged along its entire course from the hub to the point. It is believed that this adds safety because the needle is imaged its entire length, and thus objects such as veins and arteries can be avoided. The other technique is the out-of-plane technique, in which the needle is imaged in cross section. This technique demands vigilance by the operator to make sure that the needle tip is known because the needle could be bisected anywhere along the needle shaft. Thus it is possible that with this technique the needle may appear to be outside a vascular structure; however, in reality it may be lodged within it. To avoid this complication when using the out-of-plane technique, it can also be useful to slide the probe down the trajectory of the needle to help identify the needle tip. Another technique is to give a "puff" of saline while advancing the needle and look for the spread on the ultrasound image. If the needle is in view, but the saline puff is not visualized, then it is the needle shaft and not the tip that is being imaged. Echogenic needles with etched patterns at the tip that display a characteristic pattern on ultrasound have recently been developed to help the practitioner identify the needle tip as well (**Fig. 49-4**).

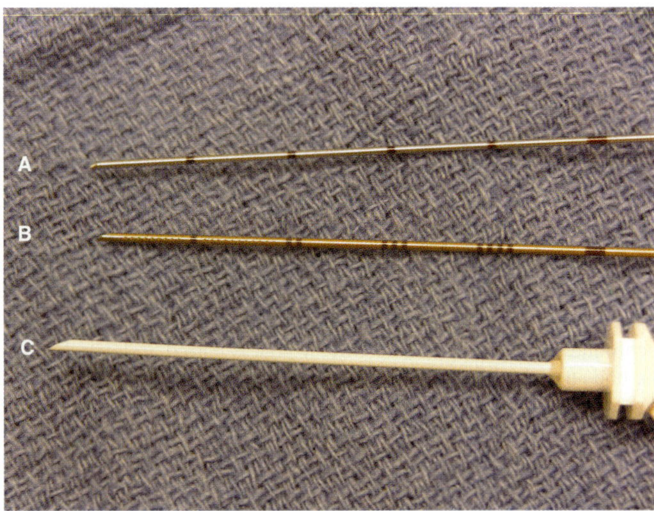

FIGURE 49-4. Example of 3 different needles for the performance of regional anesthesia: (**A**) B-bevel needle, (**B**) B-bevel "ultrasound-lucent" needle (notice etchings on the 2 cm proximal to the tip), (**C**) insulated B-bevel needle.

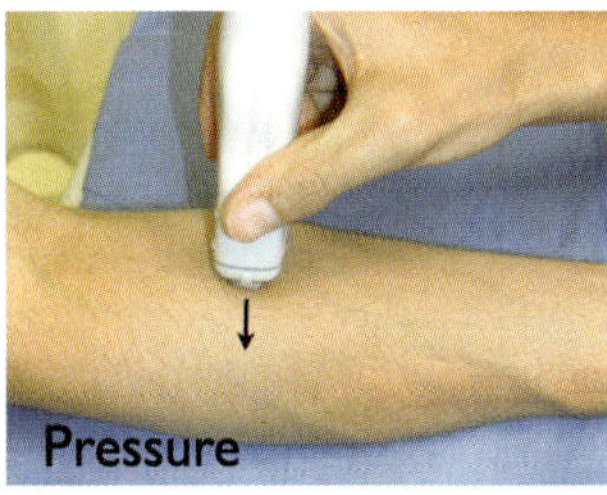

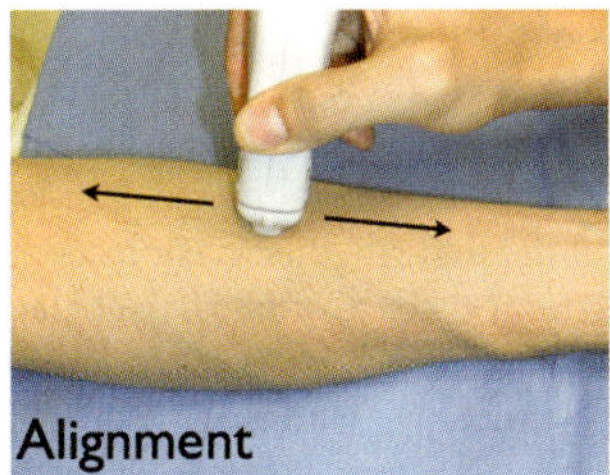

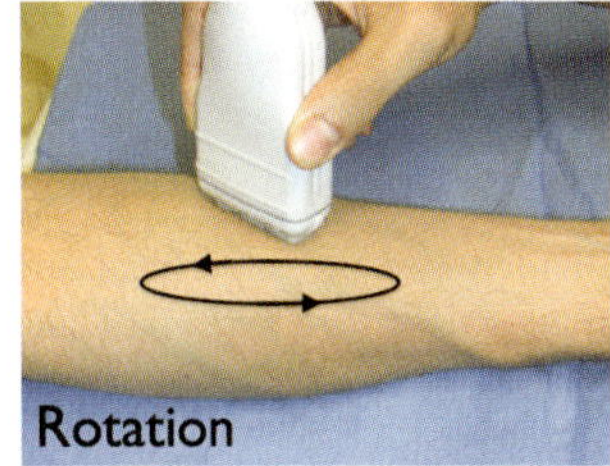

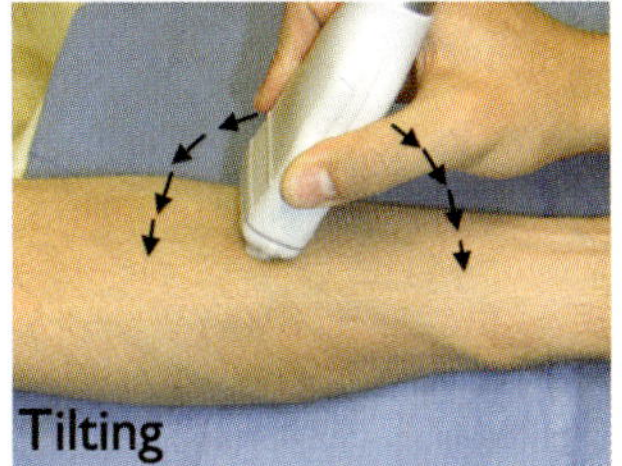

FIGURE 49-5. PART maneuvers: pressure, alignment, rotation, and tilting.

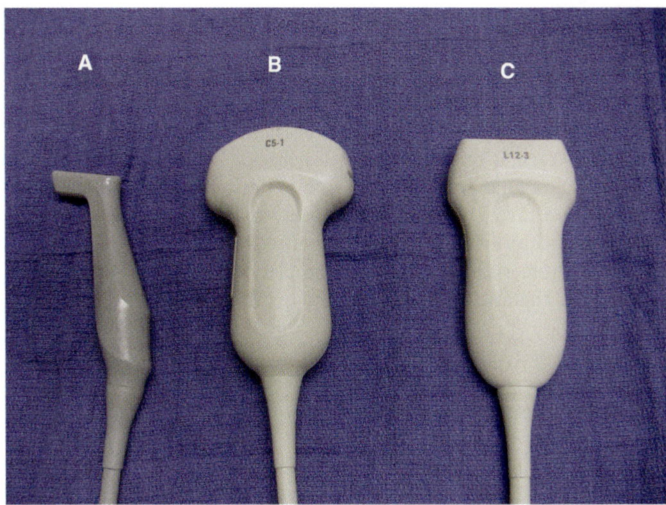

FIGURE 49-6. Example of 3 different types of ultrasound probes: (**A**) linear transducer, small footprint, "hockey stick" probe for superficial blocks and small working areas; (**B**) curvilinear probe for improved penetration but lower frequency and resolution; (**C**) linear transducer for superficial to moderately deep blocks.

Regardless of which needle approach is selected, it is useless without an optimized ultrasound image with the target nerve structure and structures to avoid identified. The transducer manipulation technique by which an ultrasound image is formed and optimized has also been recently standardized as the PART maneuvers (Pressure, Alignment, Rotation, and Tilting)[33] (**Fig. 49-5**). Pressure is applied to the patient to improve contact between the probe and the patient. Alignment relates to characterizing the course of the target nerve structure in a longitudinal axis. Rotation is achieved by rotating the transducer either clockwise or counter-clockwise to optimize the image of the target structure. Tilting describes the tilting of the transducer probe to improve the angle of incidence upon the target nerve structure.[33] It is only after the ultrasound image has been optimized that the needle should be placed in the patient.

Only time will show whether the traditional landmark and nerve stimulation techniques will be completely replaced by ultrasound guidance or a new hybrid technique of ultrasound with nerve stimulation will become the new gold standard. It should be mentioned, however, that no matter what nerve location technique is used (ultrasound vs nerve stimulation vs landmark), none are a substitute for the fundamental knowledge of anatomy.

EQUIPMENT

Needle selection for peripheral nerve blocks is not standardized. Certainly insulated needles are optimal for nerve stimulation techniques and there are ultrasound-lucent needles for ultrasound-guided techniques, although the clinical benefit over a standard needle has yet to be demonstrated. Touhy needles are great choices for placement of nerve catheters regardless of nerve localization technique used to place the block. We use B-bevel needles for single-shot nerve blocks because we believe the blunted bevel adds an extra degree of safety, although this has never been demonstrated. Lengths of 50 to 100 mm are usually more than adequate to place the standard blocks in all but the largest patients.

Nerve stimulators are modestly priced pulse generators that should be able to generate a current from 0.1 to 10 mA. A nerve stimulator should also have the ability to adjust this current in small 0.1-mA increments, thus allowing the practitioner to be able to adjust the needle for nerve localization with accuracy.

The purchase of an ultrasound machine is a major expenditure. There are stand-alone machines that must be wheeled to the patient and portable machines that can be carried. The images on the stand-alone tend to be of higher fidelity; however, this probably does not have a clinical impact except in the most difficult morphologic patients. Portable machines allow one to perform peripheral nerve blocks in other nontraditional locations in the hospital and can be moved easily and expeditiously between operating rooms as needed. The selection of transducer probe is also vitally important (**Fig. 49-6**). We prefer a linear probe that is 25 to 38 mm in length with the capability of 8 to 12 MHz at a minimum. The lower frequency allows deeper penetration for blocks of the lower extremity, and the higher frequency is better for more peripheral structures, such as the brachial plexus. Curvilinear probes are good for performing neuraxial blocks or very deep blocks in the extremities such as the infragluteal or transgluteal sciatic block. Generally the frequency of such probes is lower than 8 MHz, which is necessary to penetrate several centimeters of tissue.

CLINICAL DECISION MAKING

There are many branch points that must be traversed in the decision-making process before placing a peripheral nerve block. The first question that must be answered is whether a regional anesthetic is appropriate to place in the selected patient. The patient may not wish to have a regional anesthetic, the surgical site may not be easily anesthetized with a regional technique, or the patient may have a high potential for a nerve injury either intraoperatively or postoperatively that could be masked by a peripheral nerve block. The next question is whether to sedate the patient for the peripheral nerve block. Our personal preference is to sedate the patient with a low-dose opioid and benzodiazepine (fentanyl and midazolam). This relieves the discomfort of placing the block as well as patient anxiety. However, be careful not to oversedate, as the patient then will not be able to help with positioning and more importantly will be unable to communicate discomfort with the block placement. It is because of this latter point that some practitioners refuse to sedate their patients before placing a regional anesthetic, as they would like the added safety measure of a responsive patient. Traditionally peripheral nerve blocks have not been placed in anesthetized patients due to the lack of input being perceived as a possible safety hazard. However, with the advent of ultrasound, placing peripheral nerve blocks in anesthetized patients has begun to emerge once again as a possibility. This has been demonstrated by several recent regional anesthesia studies in anesthetized pediatric patients.[34-36]

The next decision that has to be made is whether a single-shot or catheter is more appropriate for the patient. Single-shot blocks have variable durations depending on volume and selected local anesthetic agent. The continuous catheter, when functioning properly, gives the practitioner the ability to provide consistent regional anesthesia to a patient for several days. Potential drawbacks, however, remain infectious risks and follow-up.[37-39] There is also the question of the safety of a continuous catheter in an anticoagulated patient.[40-42]

Selection of a local anesthetic also needs to address postoperative factors as well, such as need for ambulation, need for participation in physical therapy, and the need to perform tasks of daily living. Concentration appears to influence the duration as well as the quality of the block. Lower concentrations provide analgesia but have been shown to have some motor sparing, thus allowing the patient to ambulate or perform basic tasks sooner postoperatively, which may have benefits to the patient's overall outcome.[43-47] Lower concentrations are predominately used in blocks primarily placed for postoperative pain control and for nerve catheter infusions. Likewise, higher concentrations may provide a more profound block and thus be more appropriate for blocks placed for a primary surgical anesthetic.

An additional factor for the selection of a local anesthetic is speed of onset of the block. This can have major clinical implications if not selected properly. If the operating room will be ready for the patient within 10 minutes and you are placing a block for a surgical anesthetic, then selection of a slower-onset local anesthetic may not be efficient enough, and thus a rapid onset local anesthetic should be chosen. The difficulty then is what to do with a patient who will be in the operating room shortly, but needs a prolonged block for postoperative pain control. Clearly bupivacaine would be ideal for its duration of action; however, its slower onset may not be efficient enough. Likewise, lidocaine's rapid onset may be necessary; however, its short duration of action would not be in the patient's interest. The mixing of local anesthetics has shown that their properties are affected by the presence of an additional local anesthetic.[40] In the preceding combination of 1:1 bupivacaine and lidocaine, the resulting mixture would have an onset longer than lidocaine, but its duration of action would be reduced from that of bupivacaine. Other techniques that can be used to prolong block duration are the use of continuous catheters, the use of adjuvants within the local anesthetic solutions (eg, epinephrine), and the placement of the local anesthetic itself in relation to the target nerve structures.

Toxicity is another factor that needs to be addressed with the selection of a local anesthetic. The placement of large volumes in highly vascular areas increases the risk of toxicity from local anesthetics. Thus it may be wise to reduce volumes or use a less catastrophically toxic local anesthetic when performing a block that requires a large dose of local anesthetic. Typically volumes of 5 to 30 mL are used for placement of peripheral nerve blocks.

There is not a large volume of randomized controlled studies to support or refute the placement of peripheral nerve blocks in anticoagulated patients. For years some practitioners extrapolated the 2002 American Society of Regional Anesthesiologists (ASRA) consensus statement for placement of neuraxial anesthetics to peripheral nerve blocks.[41] In 2010 ASRA submitted a practice advisory for the placement of a peripheral nerve block in an anticoagulated patient.[42] Although these 2 documents only provide recommendations, it is in the regional anesthesia provider's and patient's interest to adhere to them when possible.

UPPER-EXTREMITY BLOCKS

The brachial plexus is derived primarily from the cervical nerve roots of C5, C6, C7, C8, and T1, although there are variable contributions from C4 and T2 as well. As the roots emerge from between the anterior and middle scalene muscle, they form 3 trunks that are cephalad and posterior to the subclavian artery. At the level just above the clavicle, each trunk begins to transition to an anterior and posterior division; however, there is a high degree of variability between individuals at this level, and some continue to have trunks to just below the clavicle. Once the brachial plexus passes under the clavicle, at the lateral border of the first rib, the divisions combine to form the medial, posterior, and lateral cords around the subclavian artery. They then emerge from the lateral border of the pectoralis minor and become the peripheral nerves of the upper extremity. The ulnar, radial, and median nerves lie adjacent to the axillary artery in most individuals with the musculocutaneous between the muscle bellies of the biceps and the coracobrachialis (**Fig. 49-7**).

CERVICAL PLEXUS

Anatomy The cervical plexus can be divided into the superficial and deep branches, both of which have their origins from the anterior rami of C2, C3, and C4 that lie directly under the sternocleidomastoid muscle. It is the superficial plexus that innervates the skin of the neck, posterior head, and superior shoulder. The deep cervical plexus innervates the muscles and other structures of the neck. It should be noted that C4 can participate in the formation of the brachial plexus in certain individuals. It also should be mentioned that with the deep cervical plexus block, it is possible to partially block the phrenic nerve because its origins are from C3, C4, and C5.

Technique First position the patient supine with the neck turned away from the surgical site with the practitioner on the ipsilateral side. To block the deep cervical plexus, identify the mastoid process and the prominent transverse process of C6 (Chassaignac tubercle) (**Fig. 49-8**). The first of 2 lines is drawn from the mastoid to the Chassaignac tubercle. The C2 transverse process should then be palpated along this line approximately 1 cm caudal to the mastoid and then marked. This should be repeated with the C3 and C4 transverse processes as well by palpating down the line between the mastoid and the C6 transverse process. Once all of the processes are marked, a needle should be inserted over the C4 process until it contacts the C4 process at roughly 2 to 3 cm of depth (**Fig. 49-9**). A paresthesia may be obtained upon which 10 mL of local anesthetic should be injected with intermittent aspiration. If no paresthesia is obtained, then the needle can be walked along the line in a superior or anterior direction until a paresthesia is elicited. To block the superficial cervical plexus, asking the patient to lift their head should identify the lateral border of the sternocleidomastoid muscle. The midpoint of this border should be marked. The needle should then be advanced approximately 1 cm deep to the sternocleidomastoid muscle. It then can be withdrawn slightly and then redirected superior and inferior along the lateral border of the sternocleidomastoid muscle (**Fig. 49-10**).

The ultrasound technique requires one to identify the anterior scalene muscle and trace it cranially up the neck until it tapers off at C3 or C4. The longus capitus muscle should be anterior to the remnant of the anterior scalene at this level (**Fig. 49-11**). The needle should be directed into the longus capitus muscle and an injection of 5 to 10 mL should be performed.[49] For the superficial plexus, the sternocleidomastoid muscle should be identified at the level of the interscalene groove. The needle should be directed immediately under the lateral border of the sternocleidomastoid muscle, and 10 mL of local anesthetic should be injected (**Fig. 49-12**).

Pearls and Pitfalls Because the phrenic nerve will most likely be blocked with the deep cervical plexus block, it should go without saying that bilateral plexus blocks should be avoided. This block also is near several structures that must be avoided, such as the vertebral artery, the intrathecal space, and the spinal cord itself. Standard safety techniques should be used with vigilance, such as intermittent aspiration upon injection of local anesthetic and the use of epinephrine in the local anesthetic solution. This block provides excellent coverage for carotid endarterectomies and for supplementation for the superior shoulder if necessary after an interscalene block.

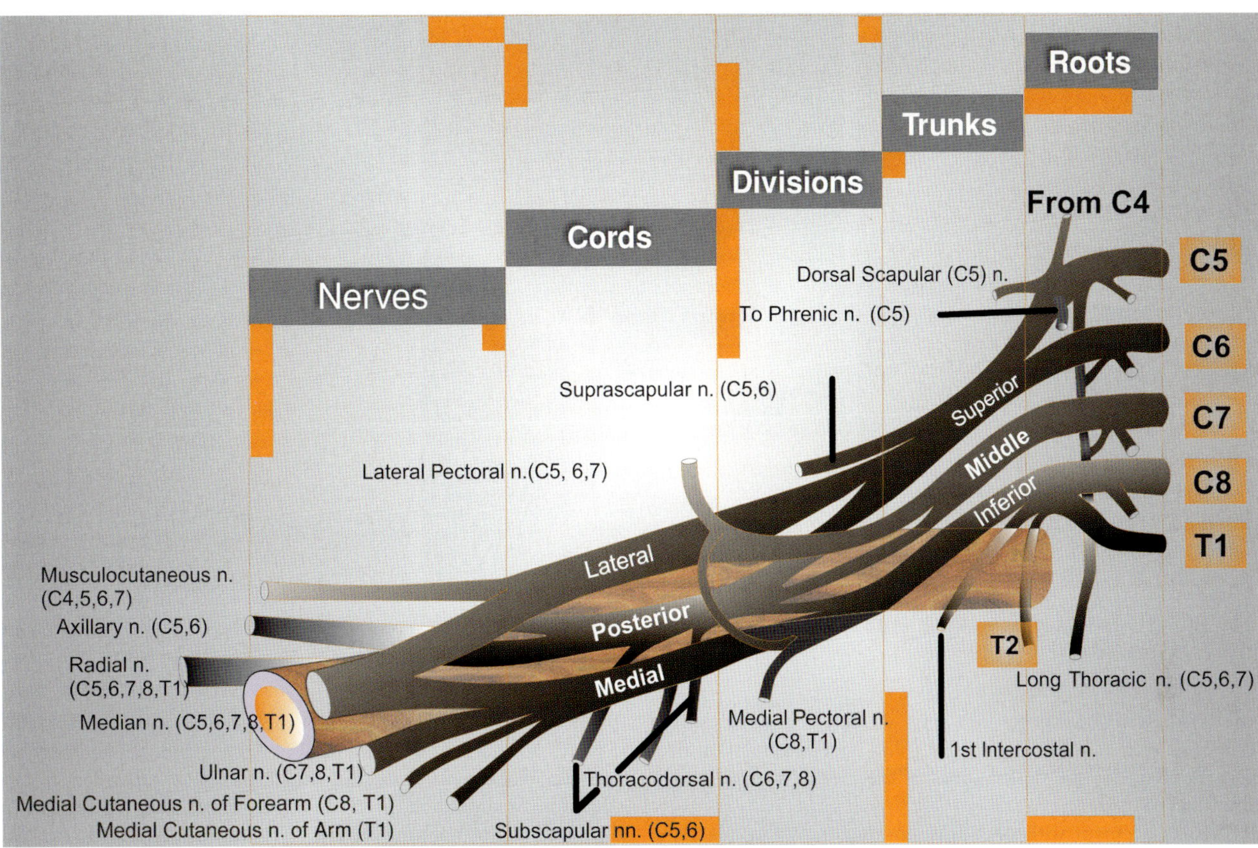

FIGURE 49-7. Organization of the brachial plexus. [Reprinted with permission from Hadzic A. *Textbook of Regional Anesthesia and Acute Pain Management*. New York, NY: McGraw-Hill; 2007.]

INTERSCALENE

Anatomy The C5, C6, and C7 nerve roots represent the brachial plexus at the level of the interscalene groove as they emerge from between the anterior and middle scalene muscles in the lateral neck. There are several documented variations to the brachial plexus at this level, one of the most common being perforation of the anterior scalene muscle by the C5 nerve root itself.[50] The interscalene groove may be palpated by moving one's fingers posterior and laterally from the lateral edge of the sternocleidomastoid muscle at the level of the cricoid cartilage. To facilitate identification of these landmarks, the patient should be asked to turn their head away from the side to be blocked and should be asked to raise their head off of the bed momentarily in order to identify the lateral edge of the sternocleidomastoid muscle (**Fig. 49-13**).

Technique With traditional landmark techniques initially described by Winnie, a needle is advanced in the interscalene groove at a 45-degree

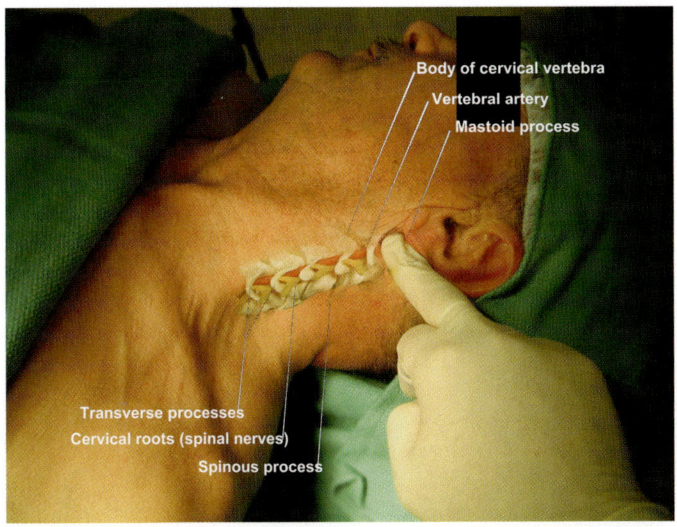

FIGURE 49-8. Anatomic landmarks for the cervical plexus block. [Reprinted with permission from Hadzic A. *Textbook of Regional Anesthesia and Acute Pain Management*. New York, NY: McGraw-Hill; 2007.]

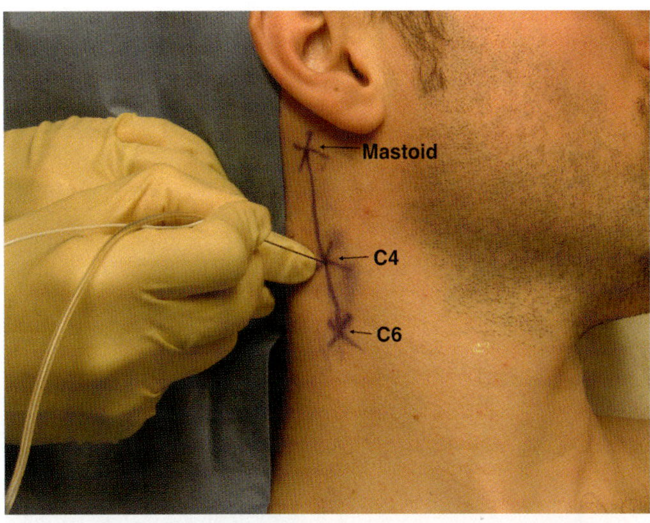

FIGURE 49-9. Line drawn between mastoid process and the transverse process of C6 (Chassaignac tubercle); the C4 process has been palpated and marked.

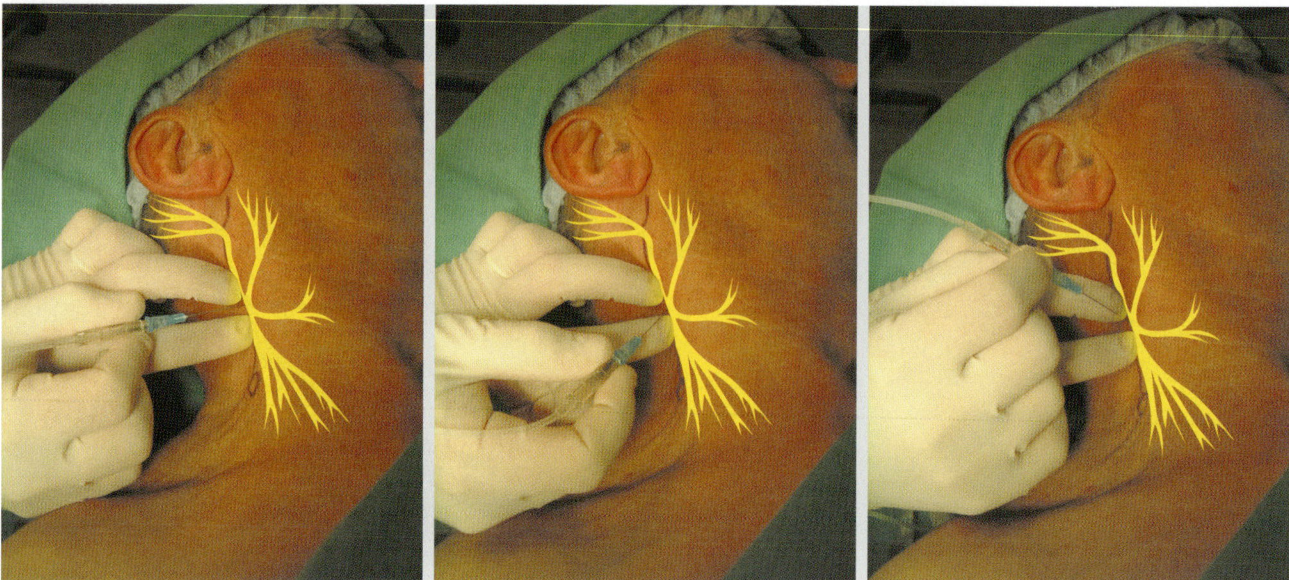

FIGURE 49-10. Technique of superficial cervical plexus block. [Reprinted with permission from Hadzic A. *Textbook of Regional Anesthesia and Acute Pain Management*. New York, NY: McGraw-Hill; 2007.]

angle caudad and slightly posterior[51] (**Fig. 49-14**). A contraction of the shoulder or arm should be elicited if using nerve stimulation or a paresthesia over one of the dermatomes of the plexus if using only a blunted needle.

To facilitate placement with the ultrasound technique, we place the patient in the full lateral position with the nonoperative side dependent or slightly rotated, with a bump under the operative side depending on patient body habitus. The ultrasound probe is then placed over the interscalene groove in a medial/lateral plane at the level of the cricoid cartilage (**Fig. 49-15**). The nerve roots of the brachial plexus should appear as 3 distinct hypoechoic or dark circles between the anterior and middle scalene muscles (**Fig. 49-16**). The needle should be advanced in-plane in a posterior to anterior direction with the needle tip aiming between the C5 and C6 nerve root. When a distinct "pop" is felt or observed into the fascia around the nerve roots and injection should commence after negative aspiration, local anesthetic should be observed surrounding the nerve roots.

For a continuous-catheter technique, the procedure is the same as a single shot; however, a 19-gauge Touhy needle should be used. Once the needle has penetrated the fascia between C5 and C6, a small bolus of 5 mL of normal saline should be placed to expand the sheath to facilitate catheter placement. Once the sheath has been expanded, a stimulating catheter should be inserted and visualized near the brachial plexus and potentially "hooking around" one of the nerve roots. This catheter will only be inserted 1 to 2 cm. Once in place, the needle is removed. Confirmation of correct placement comes with bolusing the catheter and watching the circumferential spread of local anesthetic during ultrasound imaging.[52]

Pearls and Pitfalls With traditional techniques, if bone is contacted within 2 cm of the skin, it is likely that one has contacted the transverse process of a cervical vertebrae and the needle should be angled either more caudad or cephalad to find the plexus. If using nerve stimulation, beware of mistaking contraction of the diaphragm as the intended twitch, as this is an indication that the needle is located too anterior.

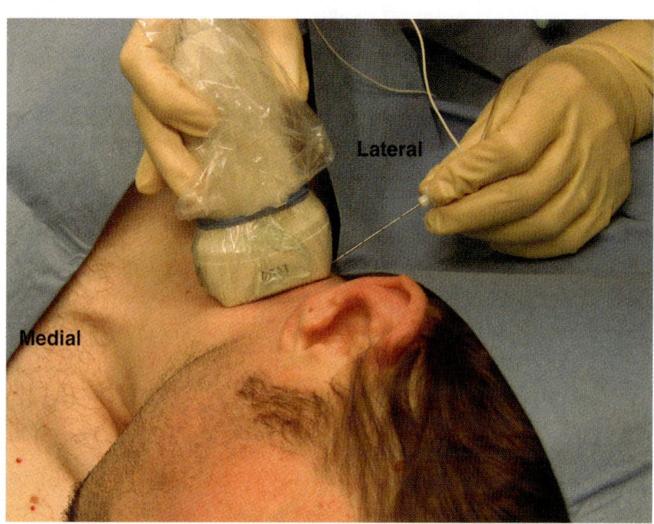

FIGURE 49-11. Ultrasound-guided cervical plexus block.

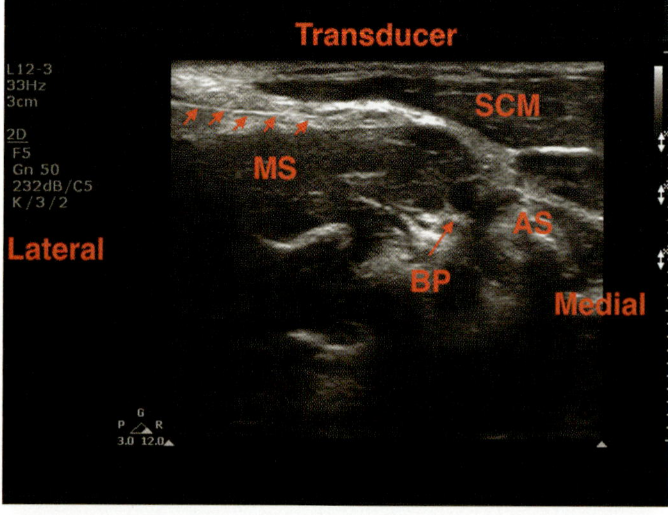

FIGURE 49-12. Ultrasound image for superficial cervical plexus block. Arrows, needle; AS, anterior scalene muscle; BP, brachial plexus; MS, middle scalene muscle; SCM, sternocleidomastoid muscle.

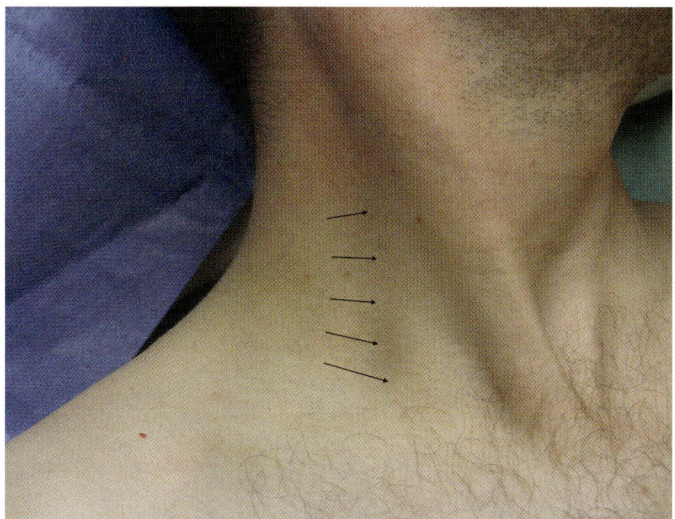

FIGURE 49-13. Patient with their head rotated away from side to be blocked and head raised off of bed to help identify lateral border of the sternocleidomastoid muscle (arrows).

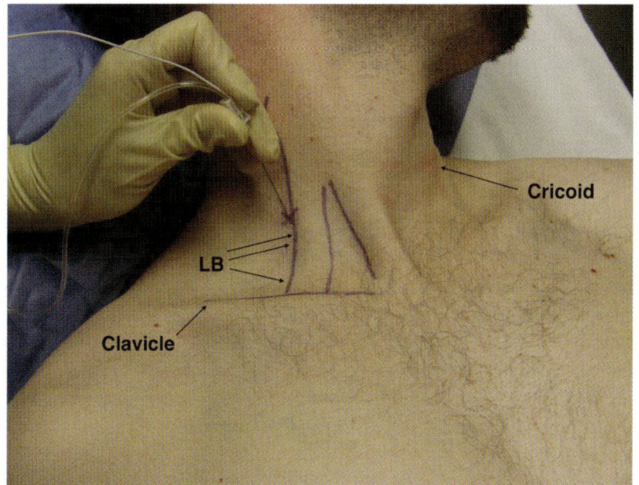

FIGURE 49-14. Interscalene nerve block using landmark techniques. LB, lateral border of the sternocleidomastoid muscle.

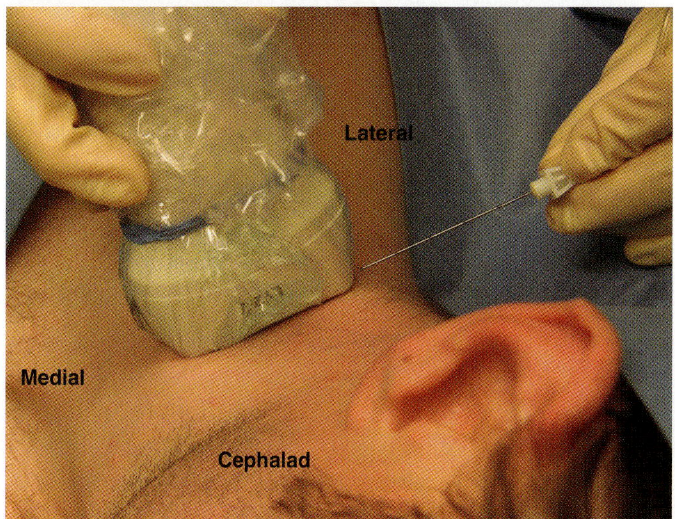

FIGURE 49-15. Ultrasound-guided interscalene nerve block probe position and needle approach.

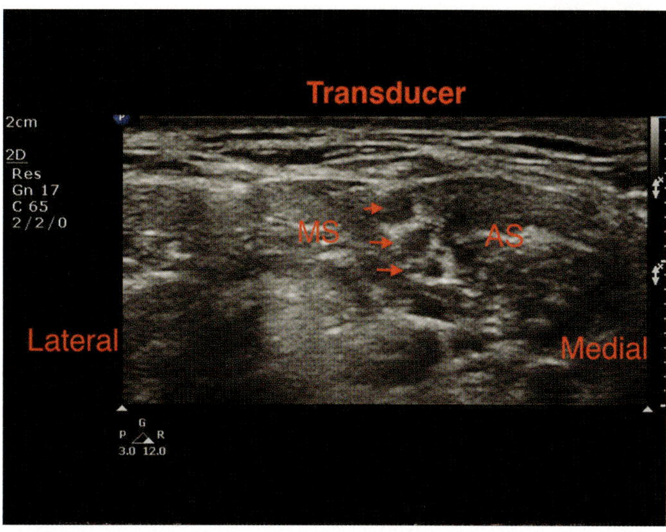

FIGURE 49-16. Ultrasound image of the interscalene approach to the brachial plexus. Arrows, nerve roots of the brachial plexus; AS, anterior scalene muscle; MS, middle scalene muscle.

With ultrasound techniques, it is possible to approach with the needle from the medial to lateral direction. However, the medial approach should be avoided because the carotid artery and internal jugular vein are immediately under your insertion site and thus are at risk of puncture. Also the phrenic nerve lies on the anterior border of the anterior scalene muscle and may be injured with this trajectory.

Interscalene nerve block, if performed correctly, should spare the ulnar distribution; thus it is not an appropriate block for surgeries distal to the elbow. The interscalene block also carries an almost certain risk of transient ipsilateral diaphragm paralysis and thus should be avoided in patients whose respiratory mechanics are depleted to such an extent that the loss of diaphragm mechanics would cause them respiratory distress. There is also a risk of ipsilateral Horner syndrome (ptosis, miosis, anhidrosis). There is also a small risk of injection into the vertebral artery or the intrathecal space; thus equipment for emergent airway management should be readily available when performing this block.

SUPRACLAVICULAR

Anatomy Several authorities have referred to the supraclavicular block as "the spinal of the arm," as it is a very powerful technique for performing complete anesthesia distal to the elbow, as well as covering an upper-arm tourniquet site. In the supraclavicular fossa, the brachial plexus is transitioning between the trunks and the divisions; however, it is in a small, tight bundle, as it lies over the first rib cephalad and slightly posterior to the subclavian artery. The clavicle remains anterior to the neurovascular bundle. It should be stated that the first rib lies between the plexus and pleural space, and thus caution should be used when placing this block using traditional landmark techniques. However, with ultrasound the rib can be easily imaged and the needle can be directed away from the rib, thus potentially decreasing the risk of pneumothorax.

Technique Patient positioning is once again a key component to success for placing this block. A 22-gauge 4-cm B-bevel needle is our choice for this block. The traditional landmark approach has the patient supine, with the arms at the sides and head rotated away from the side that the block is being placed. The needle should be inserted at the mid clavicle approximately 1 cm cephalad to the clavicle itself with a trajectory parallel with the patient's neck (**Fig. 49-17**). The end point will be either a paresthesia or nerve twitch of the muscles of the fingers if using a nerve stimulator. The insertion depth will be approximately 2 to 3 cm and should not be exceeded unless the patient is very large. Because there are several objects that should be avoided with this block (ie, the pleura and subclavian artery), if you fail to elicit either end point with your

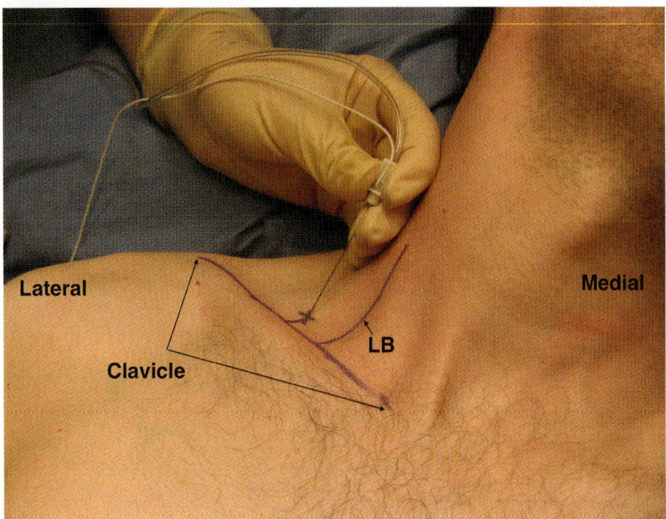

FIGURE 49-17. Traditional approach for supraclavicular nerve block. The ends of the clavicle are identified by arrows. LB, lateral border of the sternocleidomastoid muscle; needle insertion is 1 cm cephalad from the mid clavicle with trajectory parallel with the patient's neck.

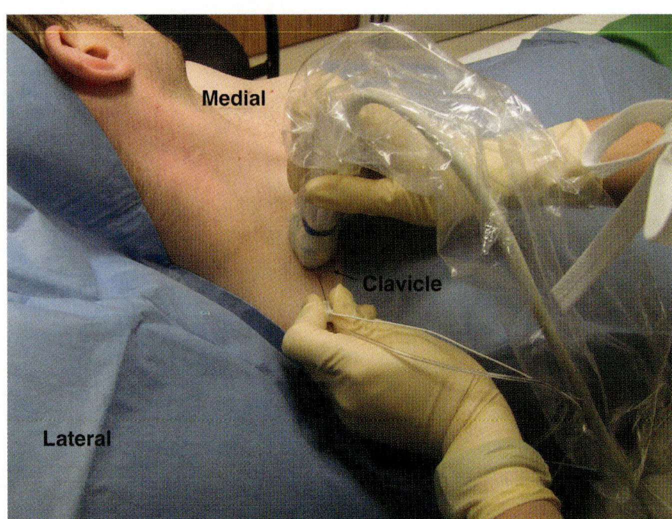

FIGURE 49-19. Ultrasound-guided supraclavicular nerve block probe orientation and needle approach.

first pass and contact the first rib, withdraw the needle and recheck your landmarks. The needle can then be walked anterior or posterior along the rib in an effort to locate the brachial plexus. Do not direct the needle medially toward the apex of the lung.

The "plumb bob" or vertical technique is another landmark technique that was developed as a way to simplify the anatomical landmarks needed for the block. Once again the patient should turn his or her head away from the side being blocked and be in the supine position. The patient should be asked to raise his or her head off of the pillow in order to identify the insertion point of the lateral sternocleidomastoid muscle with the clavicle. The needle should be inserted directly superior to the clavicle at this point; however, unlike the classic approach, the needle will now be directed perpendicularly to plain of the floor (thus 90 degrees to the trajectory of the classic approach) (**Fig. 49-18**). Once again, a paresthesia or nerve twitch of the fingers should be elicited. If neither of these end points is achieved on the first pass, but the first rib is contacted, you may walk along the rib in an anterior-posterior direction. The needle should never be directed medially in order to avoid puncturing of the pleura.

The ultrasound technique is distinctly different from either landmark technique and was first described by Chan et al.[53] The ultrasound probe should be placed on the patient immediately cephalad to the clavicle (**Fig. 49-19**). The subclavian artery should be imaged with the application of the PARTs maneuvers to form the subclavian artery into a circle.[33] The brachial plexus should be located immediately lateral and slightly superior to the artery as 3 hypoechoic or dark circles (trunks) arranged in an inferior to superior direction or as a collection of 5 or 6 smaller hypoechoic circles or "cluster of grapes" that represent the divisions. The first rib will be immediately distal to the neurovascular bundle. In petite patients, the pleura may be imaged beyond the rib (**Fig. 49-20**). The rib is considered the "hard deck," and the needle should never be advanced beyond it in order to minimize the risk of pneumothorax. The needle will then be directed from the lateral to medial direction, in-plane with the ultrasound beam such that the

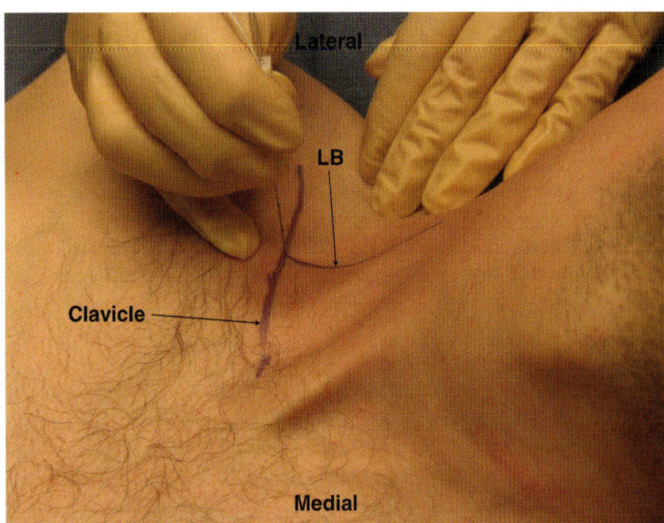

FIGURE 49-18. "Plumb Bob" approach to the brachial plexus in the supraclavicular fossa. LB, lateral border of the sternocleidomastoid muscle; notice trajectory is now perpendicular to the floor, unlike the classic approach of parallel to the neck.

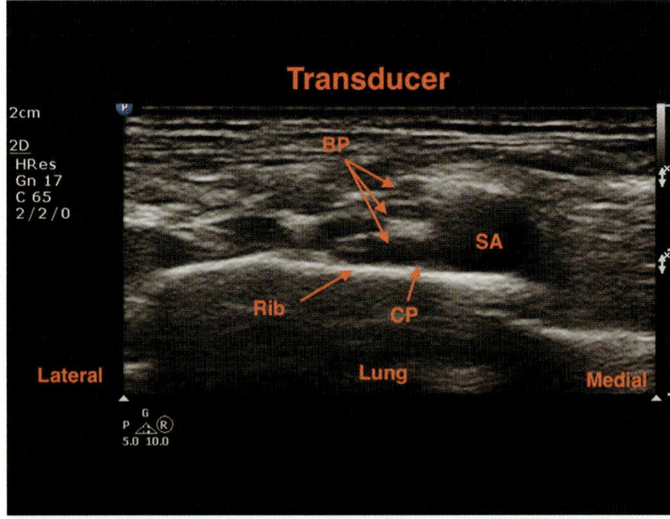

FIGURE 49-20. Ultrasound image of the supraclavicular approach to the brachial plexus. BP, brachial plexus identified by arrows; CP, corner pocket; Rib, first rib; SA, subclavian artery.

needle can be seen in its entire course as it approaches the plexus. The first target should be the "corner pocket" or the extreme inferolateral border of the plexus adjacent to the rib. It has been observed in several institutions, including ours, that if this location is not addressed, then there is a high probability of missing the ulnar distribution.[54] If spread of the local anesthetic appears to be spreading circumferentially within the nerve sheath, then one injection is necessary. Otherwise repositioning the needle cephalad to extend the local anesthetic placement in the sheath is recommended. Typical volumes for this block are 10 to 30 mL depending on duration needed for the surgical procedure.

Pearls and Pitfalls Traditionally this block was avoided in favor of the axillary block for procedures distal to the elbow due to the risk of pneumothorax (reportedly between 0.5% and 5%) and the risk of phrenic nerve paralysis (between 30% and 50%). To avoid the risk of pneumothorax, the needle should never be walked medially along the first rib, only anterior or posterior. If a pneumothorax should occur, it will usually take several hours to establish; thus patients should be informed of possible signs and symptoms if they are to be discharged within 24 hours of block placement. The risk of pneumothorax with the ultrasound-guided technique appears to be lower and thus the supraclavicular block has become more common with practitioners using ultrasound-guided regional techniques. Lower volumes of local anesthetic can be used in an effort to avoid phrenic nerve paralysis. It also should be mentioned that patient selection is important, and this block should be carefully considered in those patients who have decreased pulmonary function. Vascular puncture of the subclavian artery is always a possibility as well; however, pressure can be applied to the site to minimize hematoma size, as the subclavian artery is superficial at this location.

With ultrasound-guided techniques, if you are having difficulty imaging the plexus in the supraclavicular fossa, find the plexus in the interscalene groove and trace it down to the supraclavicular fossa with the ultrasound probe. The first injection should always be as distal to the probe as possible, such as in the corner pocket. This allows one's remaining image not to be obscured and distorted by cavitations or air introduction from the first injection so that the remaining injections may be performed. We also do not recommend placing catheters at this level, as the plexus is fairly superficial and there is a fair amount of movement in this area from the neck and shoulder, thus making it very easy for a catheter to become dislodged.

INFRACLAVICULAR

Anatomy As the brachial plexus descends below the clavicle, it becomes 3 distinct cords that are named in their relation to the axillary artery. The posterior divisions become the posterior cord, the anterior division of the inferior trunk becomes the medial cord, and the anterior divisions of the superior and medial trunks become the anterior cords. Several less prominent, but important neural structures branch from the brachial plexus at this level, they are nerves to the pectoralis major and minor, the subscapularis nerve, the medial brachial cutaneous nerve, medial antebrachial cutaneous nerve, and the axillary nerve. These "lesser" nerves are important to block in order to cover an upper-arm tourniquet site. It should be noted that the brachial plexus is now 5 to 6 cm deep to the patient's surface.

Technique With a classic landmark technique, the patient should be placed supine, and the patient's arm can be abducted up to 90 degrees at the shoulder, but this is not necessary, although palpation of the coracoid process will be facilitated by arm abducted. The coracoid technique requires the coracoid process being palpated and marked. The insertion site will be 2 cm caudad and 2 cm medial to that mark at the coracoid process (**Fig. 49-21**). The needle should be directed posterior until a nerve twitch or the muscles of the hand or a paresthesia is elicited, which should occur at a depth of 4 to 5 cm.[55] The modified Raj technique requires the jugular notch and the acromioclavicular joint be marked and a line drawn between the two. A second line should then be drawn

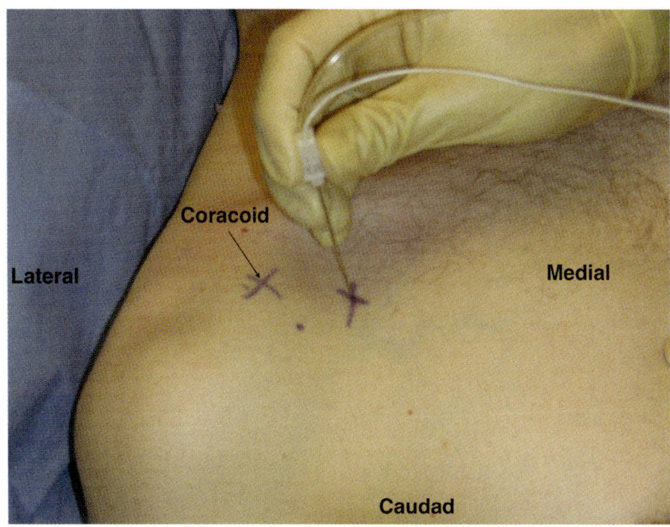

FIGURE 49-21. Traditional "coracoid" approach for an infraclavicular block. Needle insertion is 2 cm caudad and 2 cm medial to palpated coracoid process.

perpendicular to this line, from the midpoint, approximately 2.5 cm in length, and a mark placed at the end. This will be the needle insertion site. The needle is then directed laterally toward the axilla with a nerve twitch or paresthesia being elicited at 5 to 6 cm of depth (**Fig. 49-22**). If the first pass fails to elicit the desired end point, the needle should be redirected cephalad or caudad.[56]

With the ultrasound-guided technique, the probe is placed below the clavicle and the PART maneuvers are used to form the subclavian artery and vein into circular cross sections. Color flow Doppler should be engaged to confirm the artery from the vein; however, the artery is usually the more cephalad structure. The needle should be inserted from the superior border of the ultrasound probe almost adjacent to the clavicle (**Fig. 49-23**). (If the probe is in direct contact with the clavicle, it should be moved slightly caudad to allow needle insertion.) The needle is then advanced in-plane with the ultrasound beam, with the target location being at the inferior border of the subclavian artery at the 7 o'clock position (**Fig. 49-24**). The cords remain perivascular at this location, so

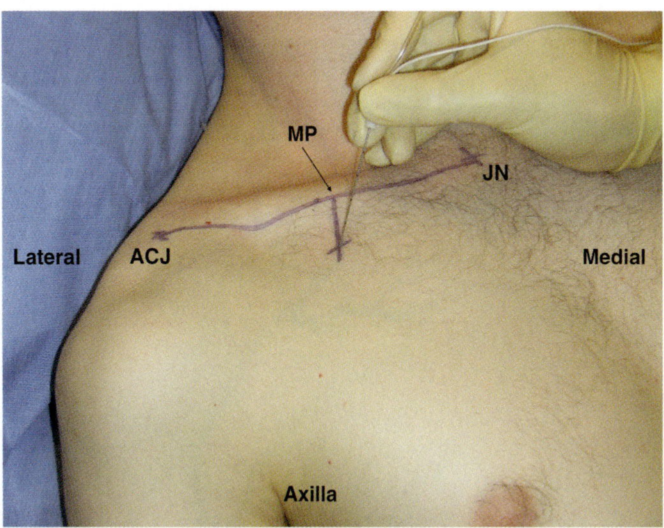

FIGURE 49-22. Modified "Raj" technique for infraclavicular block. ACJ, acromioclavicular joint; JN, jugular notch; MP, midpoint of line between ACJ and JN demarcated by arrow; 2.5-cm line is drawn perpendicular from MP, with needle insertion site at the end of this line directed toward the axilla.

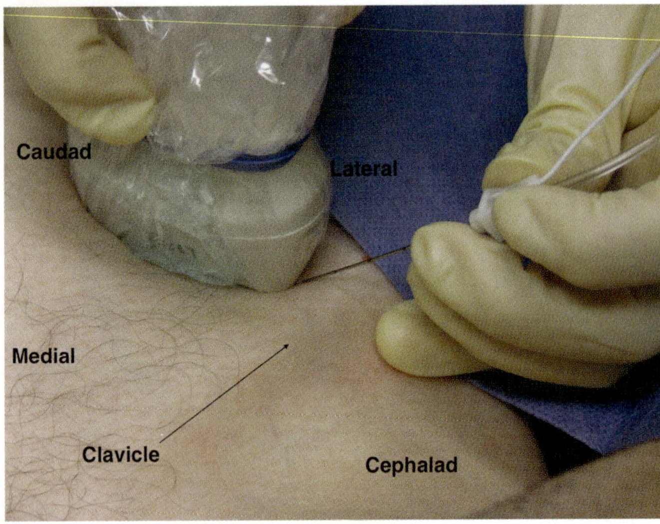

FIGURE 49-23. Ultrasound-guided infraclavicular block probe orientation and needle trajectory.

circumferential spread of local anesthetic around the artery should be sufficient, even if you are unable to visualize the individual cords.[57] This approach also allows one to easily thread a catheter 2 to 3 cm such that the tip "hooks" around the artery and the tip lodges between the artery and vein. After the needle has been removed, catheter placement can be confirmed by visualizing circumferential spread around the artery with a small bolus of local anesthetic through the catheter.

Pearls and Pitfalls The infraclavicular approach to the brachial plexus is usually the deepest block of the upper extremity and thus can be uncomfortable for patients if inadequate local anesthesia is given along the needle path. With the ultrasound-guided technique, the depth of the block will entail a lower frequency setting for adequate tissue penetration, thus decreasing the resolution. The reason for a superior opposed to an inferior approach for the ultrasound-guided technique is to facilitate catheter placement around the subclavian artery. With the inferior approach, one would have to aim between the subclavian artery and vein, which increases the risk of vascular puncture; however, this is still a viable option for a single shot as long as perivascular spread of local anesthetic is observed around the subclavian artery. The further lateral the block is placed, the higher the likelihood of missing the distribution of the musculocutaneous nerve, thus negating one of the advantages of the infraclavicular block over the axillary block.

The infraclavicular approach is excellent for catheter placement for surgical procedures distal to the elbow, regardless of what placement technique is selected. The added tissue between the patient's exterior and the plexus provides enough friction to maintain a catheter in place. The catheter exit is also in an area that can be cleaned and maintained with minimal annoyance to the patient.

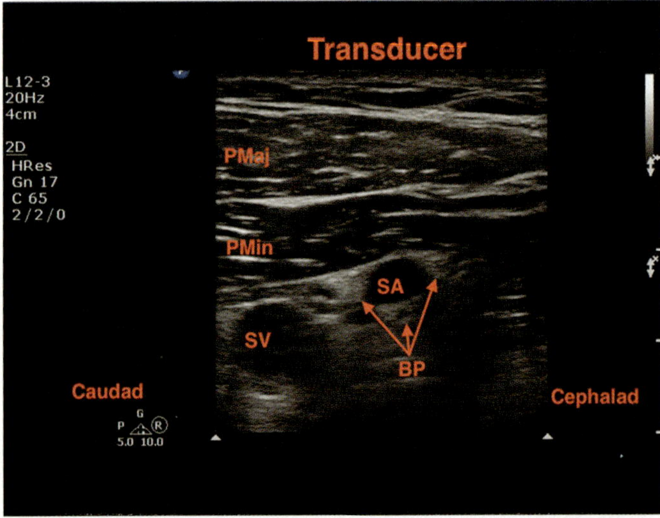

FIGURE 49-24. Ultrasound image of the infraclavicular approach to the brachial plexus. BP, brachial plexus cords identified with arrows; PMaj, pectoralis major; PMin, pectoralis minor; SA, subclavian artery; SV, subclavian vein.

AXILLARY

Anatomy The brachial plexus finally evolves into the peripheral nerves of the upper extremity once it exits from under the lateral border of the pectoralis minor muscle. The radial, median, and ulnar nerves surround the axillary artery, with the musculocutaneous nerve now located between the bellies of the biceps and coracobrachialis muscles. Despite the classical teaching of the radial nerve being the nerve on the opposite side of the axillary artery from the axilla, the median nerve anterior and cephalad to the artery and the ulnar nerve anterior and caudad to the artery, recent ultrasound investigations have shown that there is a large degree of variability regarding where the nerves lie in relation to the artery[58] (**Fig. 49-25**). It should also be mentioned that there is variability among the vascular structures at this level in the axilla as well in that we have seen patients with bifurcation of both axillary artery and vein at this level when using ultrasound. It also should be stressed that the neurovascular bundle at this level is not 1 contiguous compartment, but several different compartments. Thus multiple injections are usually required.

Technique The axillary block is a good choice for those patients having surgery distal to the elbow. However, you must remember that the upper-arm tourniquet site will not be covered with this block, so an additional "ring block" may have to be placed subcutaneously in the axilla to cover the tourniquet site. All the different techniques require the patient to be placed supine with the ipsilateral arm abducted 90 degrees at the shoulder and the forearm flexed at the elbow such that the hand is almost behind the patient's head. The transarterial technique is a blind landmark technique that allows the perivascular placement of local anesthetic using a deliberate puncture of the axillary artery.[59] If the transarterial technique is used, we would stress using epinephrine in the local anesthetic solution to indicate intravascular injection. With the transarterial technique, a small 25-gauge butterfly (or similar sized) needle is advanced toward the pulsation of the axillary artery. Once pulsatile blood is seen in the needle, the needle is advanced further until the blood stops being pulsatile. At this point the needle should be aspirated. If no blood comes back through the needle, then a 3-mL "test dose" should be injected and the patient monitored for increased heart rate or signs of an intravascular injection. If there are no indications of an intravascular injection, then half of the local anesthetic solution can be placed with intermittent aspiration. Once the injection is completed, the needle is slowly extracted with the return of pulsatile blood flow. Once the pulsatile blood flow stops, the needle should be aspirated and once again a 3-mL test dose should be administered. If the test dose is negative, the remainder of the local anesthetic solution can be deposited with intermittent aspiration.

Other methods using either nerve stimulation or blind techniques require the palpation of the axillary artery and marking its course on the skin (**Fig. 49-26**). A needle should be advanced on either side of the artery to either elicit a muscle twitch if using a nerve stimulator, in the appropriate peripheral nerve distribution, or a paresthesia if using the traditional technique.[60] Five to 10 mL of local anesthesia can be deposited at each site. The musculocutaneous nerve will be blocked by a separate injection either in the body of the coracobrachialis muscle or in the antecubital fossa.

The ultrasound-guided approach requires similar patient positioning as the traditional approaches with the transducer placed over the

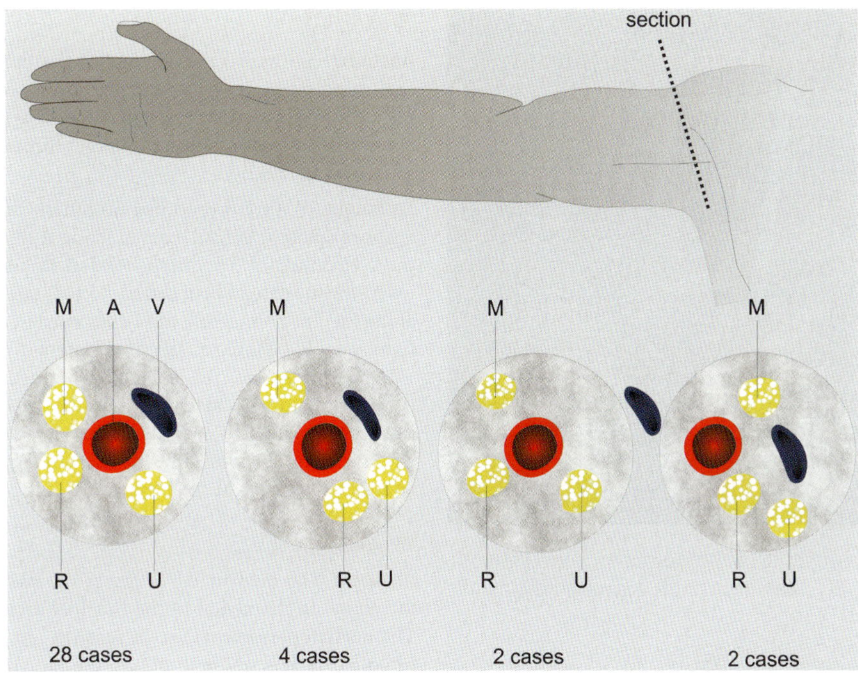

FIGURE 49-25. Spatial arrangement of the terminal nerves of the brachial plexus in the axilla. A, artery; M, median nerve; R, radial nerve; U, ulnar nerve; V, vein. [Reprinted with permission from Hadzic A. *Textbook of Regional Anesthesia and Acute Pain Management*. New York, NY: McGraw-Hill; 2007.]

patient's axilla and the PARTs maneuvers used until the axillary artery rests in the center and is in a circular cross section (**Fig. 49-27**). Because there is such a high degree of variability in the location of the different nerves in relation to the artery, a nerve stimulator may be helpful to confirm which nerve is being visualized and approached with the needle.[61] Once again, this is an in-plane technique, with the needle advanced to each peripheral nerve, which should appear as a white, hyperechoic structure with black fascicles located in the interior, or a "popcorn" appearance. Once the radial, ulnar, and median nerves have been located and blocked, the probe should be moved cephalad and lateral to identify the musculocutaneous nerve, which has a similar popcorn appearance but is located in the body of the coracobrachialis muscle[62] (**Fig. 49-28**).

Pearls and Pitfalls The axillary approach to the brachial plexus was developed primarily as a means to provide anesthesia to the forearm and hand, but avoid the risk of pneumothorax and phrenic nerve paralysis. The drawback, however, is that the musculocutaneous nerve can be missed and that placement of the block requires several needle passes, which has shown to reduce patient satisfaction. Toxicity is also a factor, especially with the transarterial technique, because large dosages have traditionally been used in order to cover the musculocutaneous nerve as well as ensure circumferential spread around the axillary artery. The success rate of the axillary approach has also been called into question. Claims of 100% success are probably exaggerated, with more typical success rates of 60% to 80% being more typical. Whether the block is placed for surgical anesthetic or postoperative pain control and the very definition of "success" can all affect this number. Certainly the success rate is not as high as that of the supraclavicular block.

It is because of this last point that the axillary block has fallen out of favor with the ultrasound-guided regional anesthesiologist. When

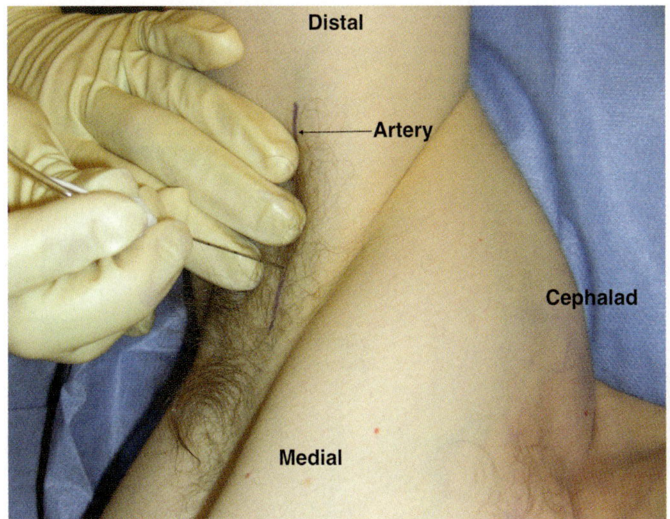

FIGURE 49-26. Axillary block using traditional techniques. Artery, line illustrating the course of the axillary artery as identified by palpation.

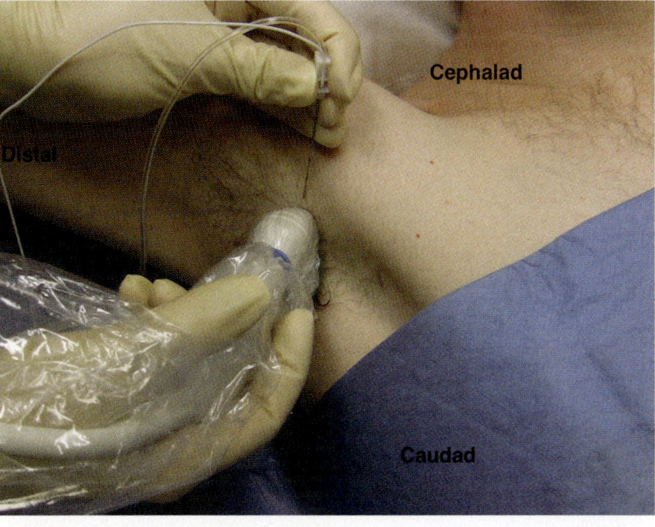

FIGURE 49-27. Ultrasound-guided axillary approach to the brachial plexus, probe orientation and needle trajectory

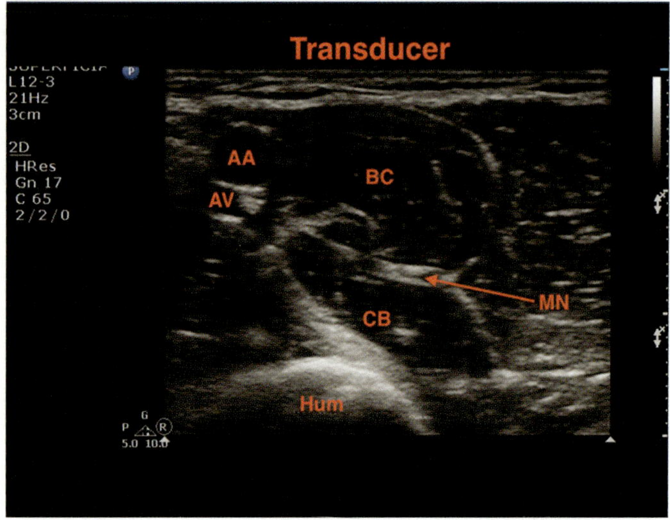

FIGURE 49-28. Ultrasound image for the musculocutaneous nerve (MN). AA, axillary artery; AV, axillary vein; BC, biceps muscle; CB, coracobrachialis muscle; Hum, humerus.

compared with the supraclavicular approach, the axillary block requires more time and more needle passes and has decreased fidelity with the higher likelihood of needing a "rescue block" distal to the elbow. All of these components contribute to a decrease in patient satisfaction. However, the axillary block still has some uses for patients when a supraclavicular or infraclavicular block is not a possibility.

RADIAL

Anatomy The radial nerve supplies the dorsum of the thumb, index, and middle fingers, as well as the lateral half of the ring finger. The radial nerve leaves the axilla and courses between the brachialis and brachioradialis muscles before it emerges through the lateral intramuscular septum (**Fig. 49-29**).

Technique With conventional landmark techniques, the radial nerve is approached in the antecubital fossa. A line should be drawn between the 2 epicondyles. The biceps tendon should be identified. The needle insertion site should be inserted 1.5 to 2 cm lateral to the biceps tendon along the line connecting the 2 epicondyles, and 3 to 5 mL of local anesthetic should be injected in a "fan" lateral to medial (**Fig. 49-30**).

With ultrasound, the nerve can be identified as the white, hyperechoic structure located between the brachialis and brachioradialis muscles proximal to the elbow. Its appearance is more oblong than circular at this location (**Fig. 49-31**). Once again, only 3 to 5 mL of local anesthetic needs to be injected.

MEDIAN

Anatomy The median nerve leaves the axilla and it courses down to the elbow to lie medial to the brachial artery in the antecubital fossa. The median nerve provides the sensory component of the palm and the proximal fingers of the thumb to the radial half of the ring finger. The median nerve provides the motor component to the forearm flexors, the thenar eminence, and the lumbrical muscles of the first and second digits.

Technique Once again, a line should be drawn between the 2 epicondyles. The traditional landmark technique requires the identification of the brachial artery by palpation or Doppler ultrasound. Once the

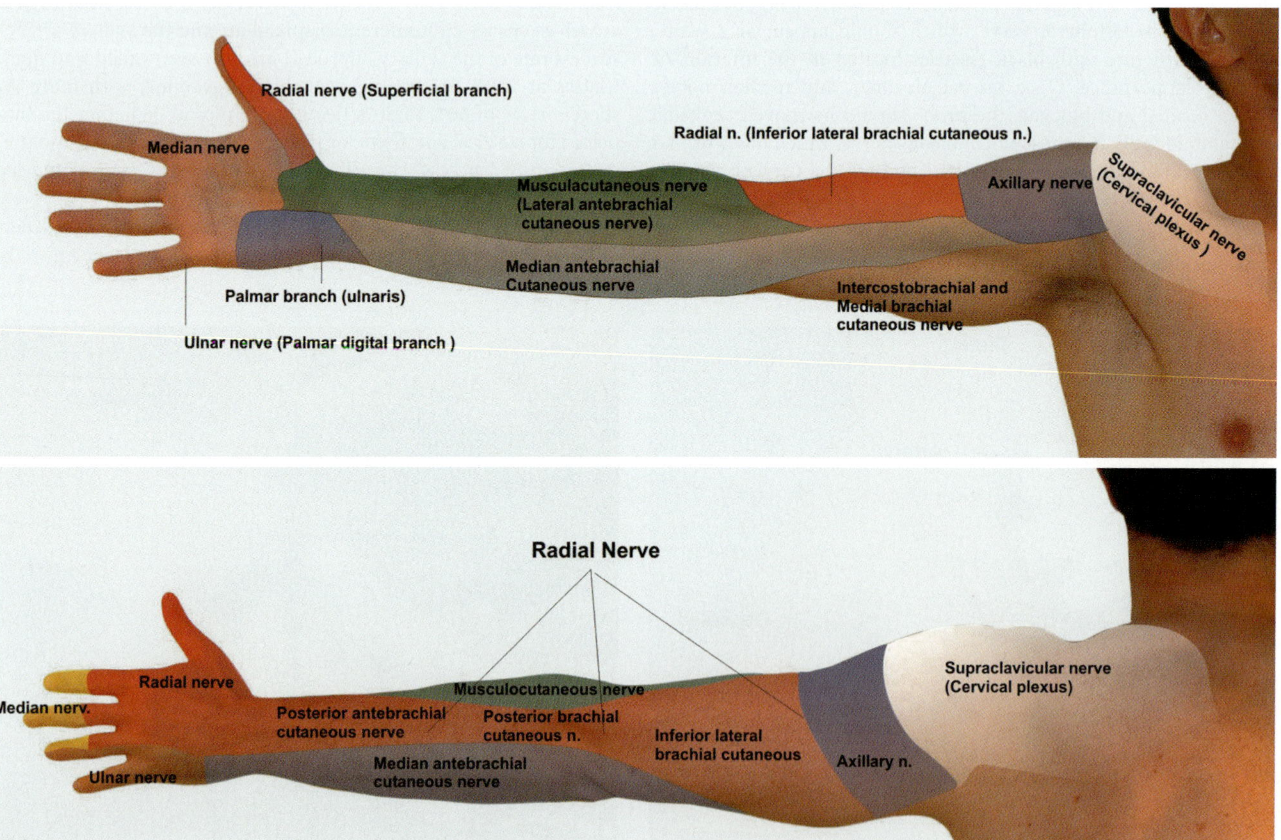

FIGURE 49-29. Sensory innervation of the upper extremity. [Reprinted with permission from Hadzic A. *Textbook of Regional Anesthesia and Acute Pain Management*. New York, NY: McGraw-Hill; 2007.]

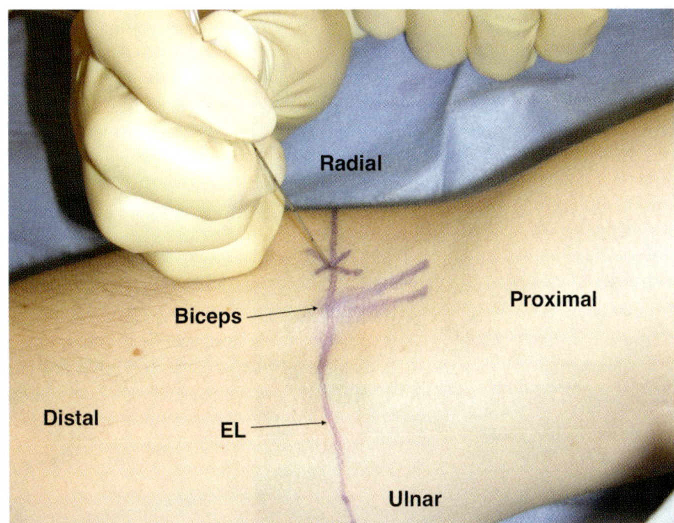

FIGURE 49-30. Traditional landmark approach to the radial nerve. Biceps, biceps tendon; EL, epicondylar line.

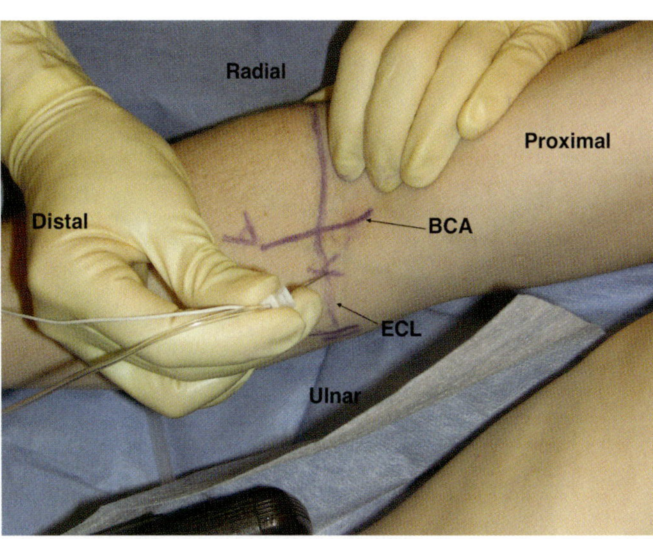

FIGURE 49-32. Traditional landmark approach to the median nerve. BCA, brachial artery as identified by palpation; ECL, epicondylar line.

brachial artery has been identified on the intercondylar line, 3 to 5 mL of local anesthetic should be injected medial to the brachial artery pulse (**Fig. 49-32**). A paresthesia or nerve stimulation of wrist flexors should be the end point before injection, although an injection in a fan pattern may be effective.

The ultrasound technique entails placement of the ultrasound probe over the antecubital fossa in a medial to lateral direction and identification of the brachial artery by color flow Doppler. The median nerve should appear as a white, hyperechoic structure immediately adjacent to the medial side of the artery (**Fig. 49-33**). Either an in-plane or out-of-plane technique can be used at this location. An injection of 3 to 5 mL of local anesthetic should be placed around the nerve. The median nerve can also be blocked at the wrist using ultrasound. Place the ultrasound probe approximately 1 to 2 cm proximal to the crease of the wrist. The surrounding tendons can be mistaken for the nerve; however, the nerve should be about 0.5 cm deep to the tendons and should not change its shape when the patient makes a fist. Either an in-plane or out-of-plane approach is acceptable to place 3 mL of local anesthetic solution.

ULNAR

Anatomy The ulnar nerve leaves the axilla and courses to the posterior aspect of the medial epicondyle, where it lies in the ulnar groove. It then continues proximally, where it joins the ulnar artery approximately 5 cm distal to the elbow and continues down to the hand. The ulnar nerve supplies the sensory component of the ulnar side of the hand, the ulnar side of the ring finger, and the little finger. The ulnar provides the motor component of the all the remaining intrinsic muscles of the hand.

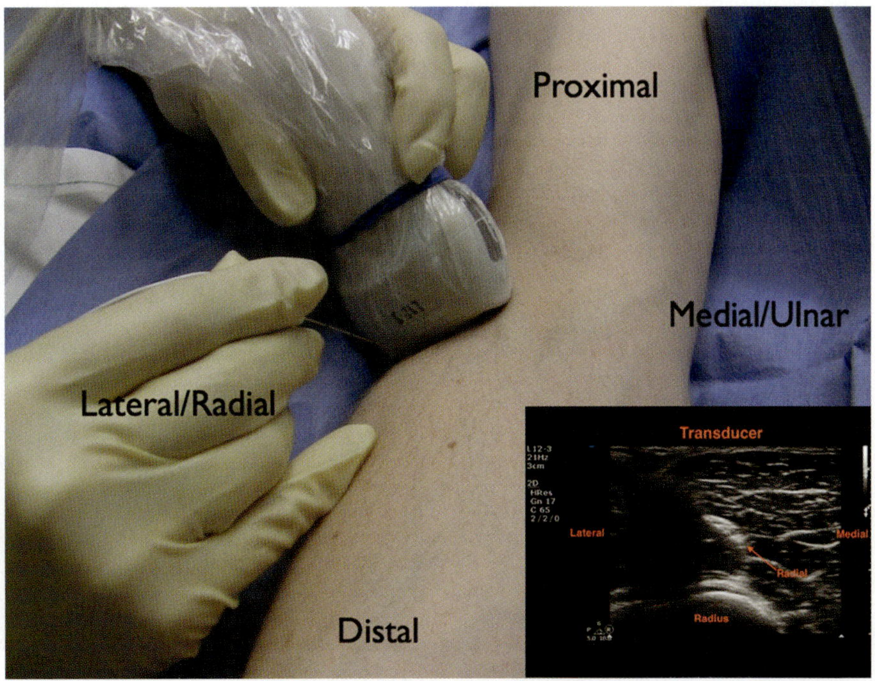

FIGURE 49-31. Ultrasound-guided approach to the radial nerve, probe orientation, and needle trajectory with corresponding image of the radial nerve (radial).

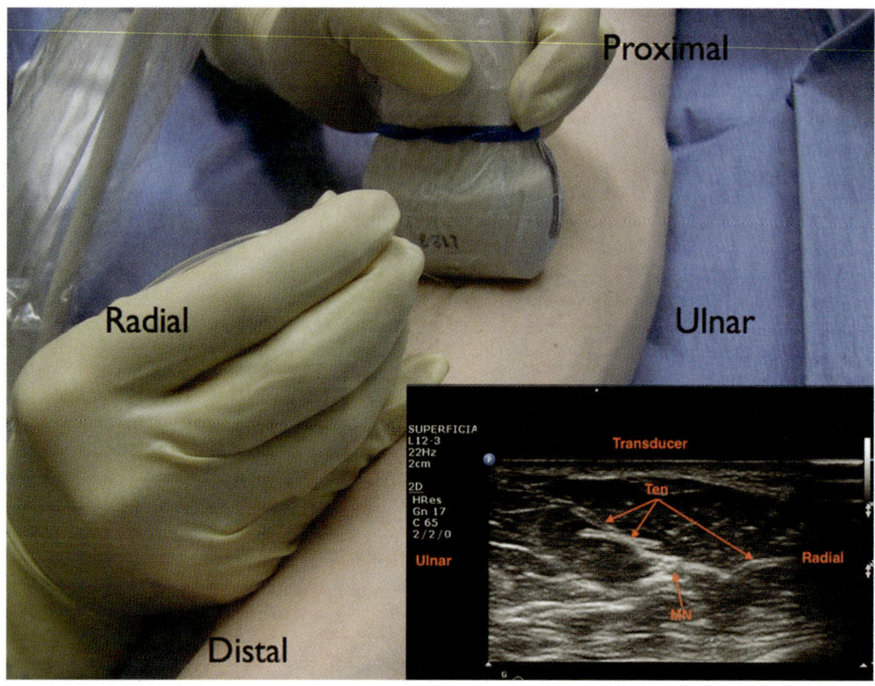

FIGURE 49-33. Ultrasound-guided median nerve block, probe orientation, needle trajectory, and corresponding ultrasound image. MN, median nerve; Ten, tendons identified by arrows.

Techniques Classic landmark techniques entail palpating the ulnar groove and then injecting 1 cm proximal to minimize the chance of nerve injury, as the ulnar groove is a tightly confined space. A paresthesia should be elicited without difficulty in this location (**Fig. 49-34**). There are descriptions of using very fine needles in this location to perform this block because of the almost certainty of entering the ulnar nerve when performing this block. The ulnar nerve can also be blocked at the wrist. The ulnar nerve lies between the ulnar artery and the pisiform bone. Both of these structures can be palpated, and 3 to 5 mL of local anesthesia can be placed in this location. With ultrasound, the ulnar nerve can be imaged 1 to 2 cm proximal to the wrist crease adherent to the ulnar artery on the ulnar side of the artery. The nerve should then be traced proximal, up the arm, to where it separates from the artery (**Fig. 49-35**). At this location using either an in-plane or out-of-plane technique, 3 to 5 mL of local anesthesia can be injected.

Pearls and Pitfalls With any of the blocks of the distal upper extremity, it is important to be cognizant of the fact that the nerves in this location are in tighter anatomical compartments, and thus large local anesthetic doses should be avoided due to the risk of causing ischemia or nerve injury from increased compartmental pressure. Usually only 3 to 5 mL of local anesthetic is required for a successful block. It should also be noted that these tighter compartments make it more difficult for the nerve to "get out of the way" of a needle as it attempts to penetrate the nerve sheath, thus making it theoretically more likely to cause injury due to mechanical trauma. Even though relatively small volumes of local anesthetics are being used to perform these peripheral nerve blocks,

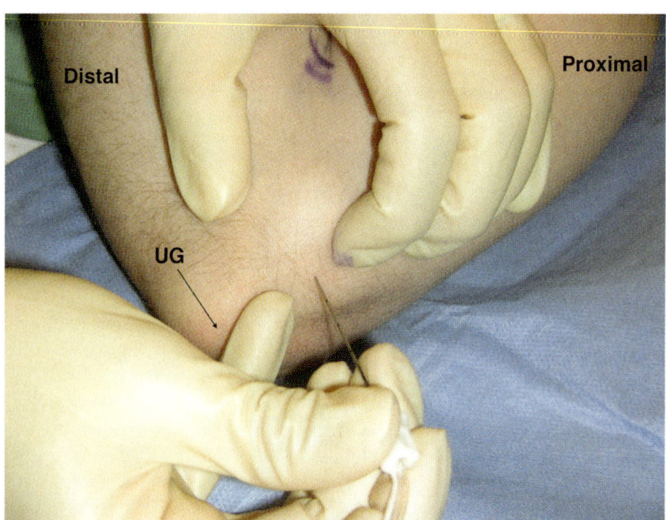

FIGURE 49-34. Traditional approach for the ulnar nerve at the elbow. UG, ulnar groove.

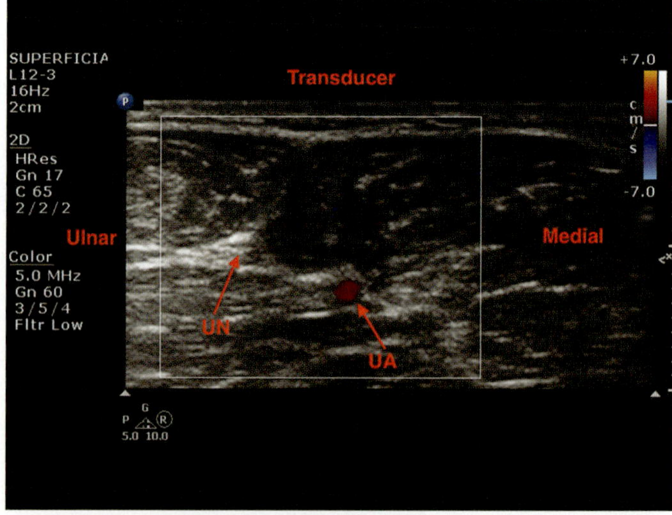

FIGURE 49-35. Ultrasound image of the ulnar nerve (UN) and ulnar artery (UA) at the forearm.

many of these blocks are performed around vascular structures. Thus the practitioner should continue to remain vigilant for the possibility of an intravascular injection or vascular injury while performing these blocks.

Because many of these blocks distal to the elbow do not cover an upper-arm tourniquet site, we find these blocks for surgical anesthesia, by themselves, to be of limited value. Where these blocks add value are as supplemental blocks for missed distributions of more proximal blocks. A good example is blocking the ulnar nerve for a procedure on the hand after a supraclavicular block has failed to set up in the ulnar distribution. The other advantage of these blocks is for postoperative pain control when the motor block of the entire upper extremity from a more proximal block is to be avoided, yet preemptive pain control is necessary in a proximal nerve distribution in the hand.

LOWER-EXTREMITY BLOCKS

There are several important considerations for regional anesthesia involving the lower extremity. First, it is important to clarify the goals of the block: a surgical block versus supplementation to a general anesthetic primarily for postoperative pain control. It is also important to consider the surgical use of tourniquets. This is especially important if the regional anesthetic goal is to provide a surgical block, as a tourniquet placed outside the field of the regional anesthetic will limit the time that a patient can tolerate the surgical procedure. Similar to upper-extremity nerve blocks, aseptic practice should be used during regional anesthesia involving the lower extremity. This includes use of sterile gloves, thorough cleansing of the skin, and barrier precautions when appropriate. In addition, one should always deposit local anesthetic at the site of needle entry. For the remainder of the discussion, we will assume that these considerations have been addressed.

LUMBAR PLEXUS

A lumbar plexus block may be used as an analgesic option for surgeries of the hip, anterior thigh, and/or knee. It can provide anesthesia to the entire lower extremity when combined with a sciatic nerve block.

Anatomy The lumbar plexus is primarily derived from the anterior or ventral rami of the L1 to L4 nerve roots, but there are also contributions from T12 in 50% of patients. This neural plexus is formed within the psoas major muscle[63] and includes the iliohypogastric, ilioinguinal, genitofemoral, lateral femoral cutaneous, femoral, and obturator nerves. Local anesthetic blockade of the femoral, lateral femoral cutaneous, and the obturator nerves is most important for lower-extremity regional anesthesia. The sciatic nerve, discussed later in the chapter, receives contributions from the lower lumbar and sacral plexuses **(Fig. 49-36)**.

Two basic approaches have been described for blockade of the lumbar plexus: (1) a posterior approach and (2) a perivascular approach. Although the posterior approach is most often used for procedures involving hip or femoral neck repair, the perivascular approach is most commonly utilized for surgical procedures involving the knee.

Technique

Psoas Compartment Block (posterior) With the patient in a lateral decubitus position (operative site up), the hips are flexed. A line connecting the iliac crests (Tuffier line) is drawn. The spinous process at midline is most often the L4. On the operative side, a line is drawn 5 cm parasagittal to the midline **(Fig. 49-37)**. A point 3 cm caudal to the Tuffier line on this parasagittal demarcation is then made. This will be the entry point of a 10-cm, 21-gauge insulated needle for the purpose of nerve stimulation. The needle is inserted perpendicular to the skin until the L5 transverse process is encountered. The needle is then directed cephalad in a manner that allows the regionalist to walk off the transverse process. A quadriceps motor response confirms correct needle position, and approximately 30 mL of local anesthetic is then injected after careful, sequential aspiration attempts confirming that the needle is not intravascular.

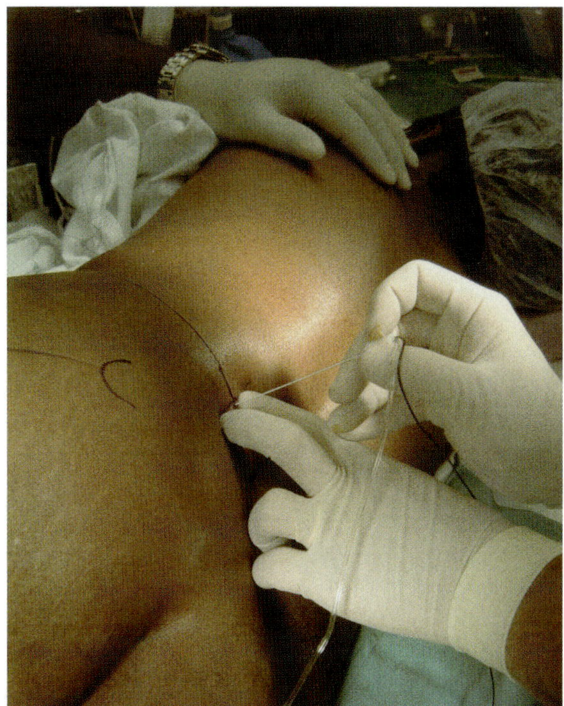

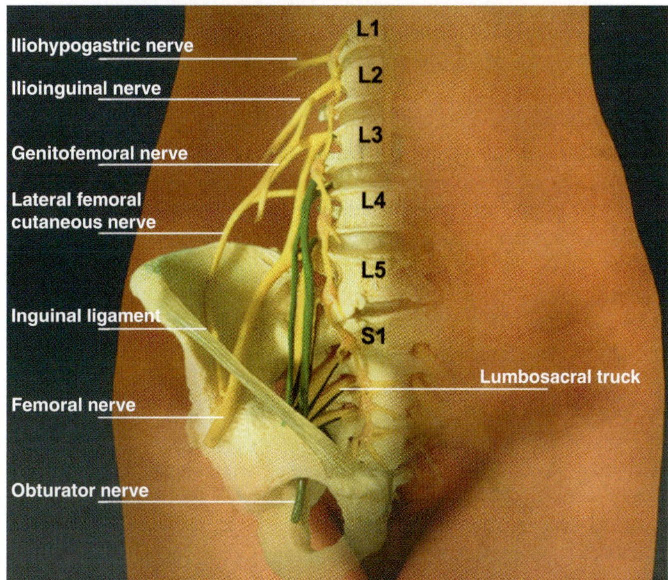

FIGURE 49-36. Anatomy of the lumbar plexus and the cutaneous innervation of the lumbar plexus. [Reprinted with permission from Hadzic A, Vloka J. *Peripheral Nerve Blocks: Principles and Practice*. New York, NY: MCGraw-Hill; 2004.]

A modification of the above technique involves use of a Touhy needle to identify the psoas compartment via stimulation and loss of resistance techniques. As above, this modified technique uses quadriceps contraction to signify proper location of the needle.[64]

INGUINAL PERIVASCULAR APPROACH (THREE-IN-ONE BLOCK)

This block is based on the premise that injection of local anesthetic in sufficiently large amounts will track up fascial planes between the iliacus muscle and the psoas muscle, ultimately anesthetizing the nerves of the lumbar plexus that exit at the level of the inguinal ligament (the femoral, lateral femoral cutaneous, and the obturator). The approach is identical to the femoral nerve block described later, with the caveat that

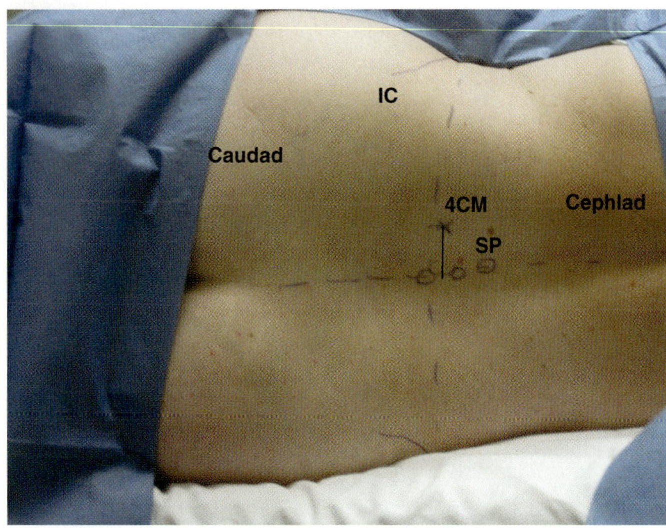

FIGURE 49-37. Posterior approach to the lumbar plexus (psoas compartment block). IC, iliac crest; SP, spinous process.

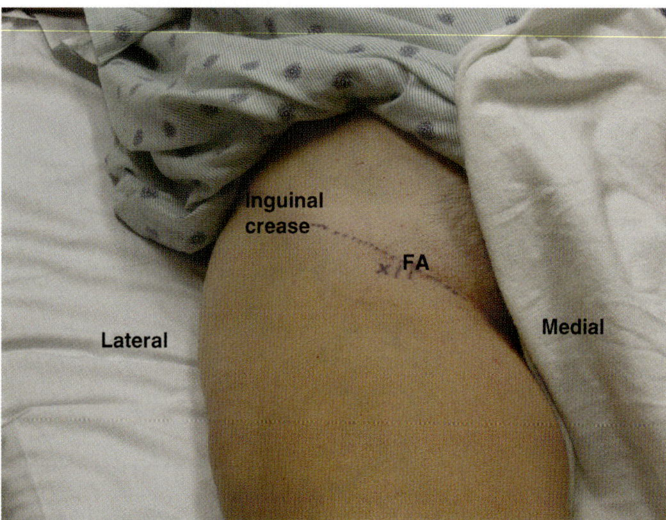

FIGURE 49-38. Femoral nerve block: landmark technique. FA, femoral artery.

firm pressure is applied distal to the needle insertion to allow fascial tracking of the local anesthetic. Some authors have advocated high volumes of local anesthetic as a means of greater spread. Imaging studies have demonstrated that medial and lateral spread of the local anesthetic provide blockade of the obturator and lateral femoral cutaneous nerves, respectively.[65]

Pearls and Pitfalls As with any regional anesthetic technique, local toxicity can occur secondary to vascular absorption and/or direct intravascular injection. The lumbar plexus block is associated with increased risk of local anesthetic toxicity due to proximity of vascular structures and use of large volumes of local anesthetics to obtain the desired spread.

It is important to note that the depth of the lumbar plexus for men and women can differ. Median depth for men is 8.5 cm and for women is 7.0 cm.[66]

FEMORAL

The femoral nerve block is used to provide analgesia to the lower extremity, often in combination with other nerve blocks. Occasionally, it may be used as the sole anesthetic for isolated procedures involving the thigh. More often, it is used for postoperative analgesia in cases of midshaft femoral fracture repair and/or after surgical procedures involving the knee.

Anatomy The femoral nerve arises from the posterior branches of L2, L3, and L4 of the lumbar plexus. From the plexus, it travels between the psoas and iliacus muscles until it passes under the inguinal ligament. At this point, it assumes a position lateral and somewhat posterior to the femoral artery, where the division to anterior and posterior branches occurs. The anterior branches are largely cutaneous, whereas the posterior branches supply motor input to the quadriceps muscle and provide articular branches to the knee.

The terminal branch of the posterior division of femoral nerve is the saphenous nerve, which supplies sensory input to the medial aspect of the leg from the knee to the medial malleolus.

Technique With the patient supine, the anterior superior iliac spine (ASIS) is identified on the ipsilateral side to be blocked. A line is then identified from the ASIS to the public tubercle. This is commonly known as the approach of Labat.[67] After the skin is anesthetized, a 3- to 4-cm 22-gauge needle is inserted perpendicular to the skin at a point below the inguinal ligament and lateral to the pulse of the femoral artery. A path through the fascia iliaca will be denoted by a pop (**Fig. 49-38**). A contraction of the sartorius muscle in the medial aspect of the thigh will be appreciated if a nerve stimulator is being used. The path should continue deeper with redirection laterally. A patellar "snap" from contraction of the quadriceps muscle is confirmation that the posterior branch of the femoral nerve has been encountered.

An alternative approach to blockade of the femoral nerve is to elicit a paresthesia, which might be encountered using the nerve stimulation technique as well. Once a paresthesia is obtained, 20 mL of local anesthetic can be injected in a fan-like distribution.

Yet another approach to femoral nerve blockade is an ultrasound-guided approach.[68,69]

A linear transducer is placed at the level of the inguinal ligament in order to identify the femoral vessels and to achieve medial and lateral orientation. Using an in-plane technique, a 22-gauge bevel needle (2-4 cm) is used to approach the femoral nerve from the lateral aspect. The ultrasound is then used to guide the needle under the fascia lata, a linear, hyperechoic structure, toward the fascia iliaca (**Fig. 49-39**). Once the fascia iliaca is identified, the needle is advanced until a "pop" is felt and confirmed visually, indicating penetration of the fascia iliaca. The local anesthetic is then injected. Another finding consistent with correct needle placement is circumferential spread of the local anesthetic around the nerve after injection.

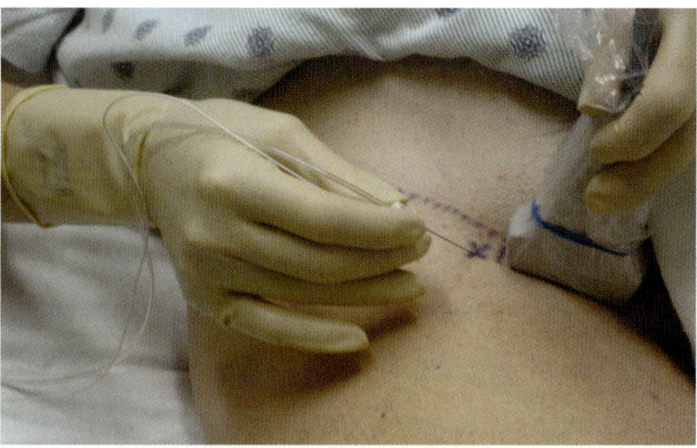

FIGURE 49-39. Femoral nerve block: ultrasound surface anatomy and ultrasound pictures. **A.** Surface anatomy. **B.** Ultrasound anatomy.

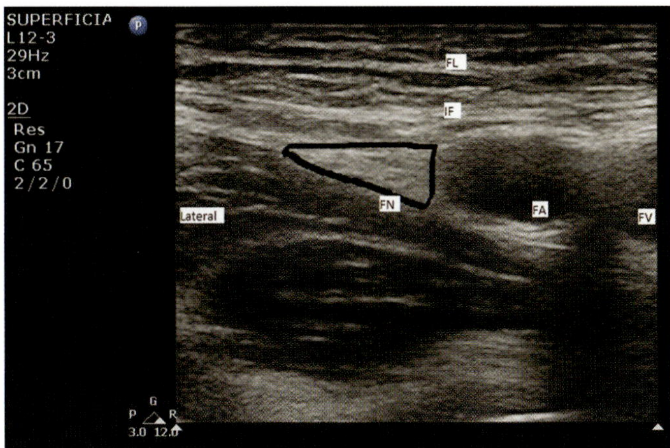

FIGURE 49-39. *(Countinued)*

SAPHENOUS NERVE

The saphenous nerve can act as a supplement to a sciatic nerve block for a lower-extremity surgery involving the medial portion of the leg or foot.

Anatomy The saphenous nerve is the largest sensory component of the femoral nerve, and it is the only component to innervate below the level of the knee. The saphenous nerve courses through the femoral triangle and becomes more superficial as it travels between the sartorius and gracilis muscles in the thigh. The saphenous nerve also has a close relationship with the saphenous vein as it progresses caudally. Thus the trans-sartorial and perivenous are 2 common approaches to saphenous nerve blockade (**Fig. 49-40**).

Trans-Sartorial Approach to Saphenous In the supine position with leg extension, the sartorius muscle is identified on the medial aspect of the upper leg. An 18-gauge loss-of-resistance needle is inserted 1 to 2 cm above the level of the patella, and with a posterior and caudad direction, it is passed through the body of the sartorius muscle. A sub-sartorial loss of resistance, usually achieved at 1.5 to 3.0 cm, indicates the usual plane where the nerve is located. Ten milliliters of local anesthesia is then deposited. This approach has been demonstrated to have an 80% success rate.[70]

Perivenous Approach to Saphenous The patient is placed in the supine position and the tibial tuberosity identified. At this level, there is a close relationship between the saphenus nerve and tibial vein; the saphenous nerve lies medial and posterior to the vein. A tourniquet may aid in identification of the perivenous anatomy. Once identified, a small amount of local anesthetic is deposited on either side of the vein. Five to 10 mL of local anesthesia should be sufficient. This can also be done with ultrasound visualization (**Fig. 49-41**).

An alternative approach is a field block. With the tibial tuberosity identified, a subcutaneous wheal of local anesthetic is injected from the medial aspect of the tibial tuberosity to the medial portion of the gastronomies muscle.

Pearls and Pitfalls The proximity of the femoral nerve to the vascular bundle generates some risk for vascular puncture and subsequent hematoma development. Thus special care should be taken to ensure proper understanding of the new anatomy in patients who have had femoral revascularization procedures. In fact, the presence of a new graft can be considered a relative contraindication if the anatomy cannot be identified using ultrasonography.

Femoral and lower-extremity nerve blocks have also been implicated as coexisting risk factors for falls.[71] As such, patients, family, and health care providers should be informed of this potential risk in order to minimize the chance of a fall in the postoperative period.

In addition, because blockade of the femoral nerve is commonly used in conjunction with a sciatic nerve block to achieve complete lower-extremity analgesia, the total amount of local anesthetic used should be carefully considered in order to avoid local anesthetic toxicity.

It is important to also note that prolonged tourniquet time may increase the risk for nerve palsy,[72] a complication that may be confounded by the addition of a local anesthetic.

Finally, continuous femoral nerve techniques, as compared with intravenous narcotics, have been shown to reduce hospital duration in patients undergoing total knee arthroplasty.[73]

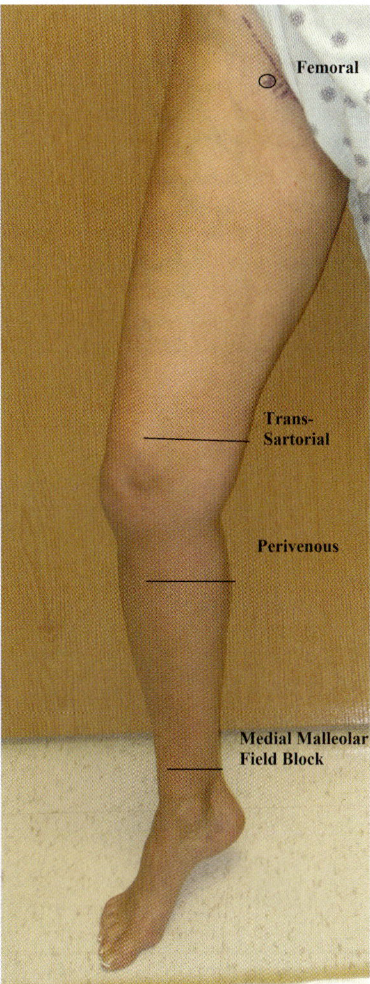

FIGURE 49-40. Levels of saphenous nerve blockade.

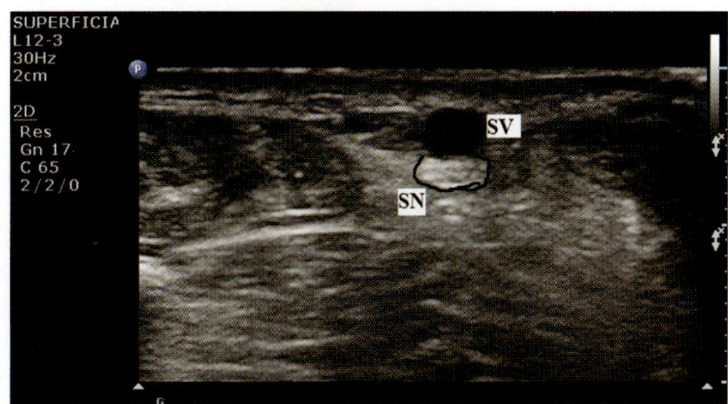

FIGURE 49-41. Ultrasound paravenous examination and corresponding surface anatomy. SN, saphenous nerve; SV, saphenous vein.

LATERAL FEMORAL CUTANEOUS

This block is used primarily in conjunction with other blocks of the lower extremity to offer complete lower-extremity analgesia. It may act as a supplement to skin graft harvesting, although it has been reported as the sole anesthesia for these procedures.[74]

Anatomy The lateral femoral cutaneous nerve (LFCN) arises as a direct branch from the lumbar plexus (L2 to L3) and courses via the lateral edge of psoas muscle to enter the thigh deep to the inguinal ligament. It emerges from the fascia inferior and medial to the anterior superior iliac spine (ASIS). As it travels beneath the fascia lata, it divides into an anterior and posterior branch. The anterior branch provides sensory innervation to the anterolateral thigh, whereas the posterior branch provides sensory innervation to the true lateral portion and a small posterior portion of the thigh from the hip to the knee (**Fig. 49-42**).

Technique

Landmark With the patient supine, the ASIS is identified on the ipsilateral side to be blocked. A mark approximately 2 cm medial and 2 cm caudad to the ASIS is made. A 22-gauge, 4-cm needle is advanced perpendicular to the surface of the skin until the fascia lata is encountered, as noted by a pop. Local anesthetic is then injected in a fan-like maneuver in a lateral to medial direction. Ten to 15 mL of local anesthetic should be sufficient.

Nerve Stimulator There have been descriptions of using nerve stimulator techniques with improved success with localization.[75]

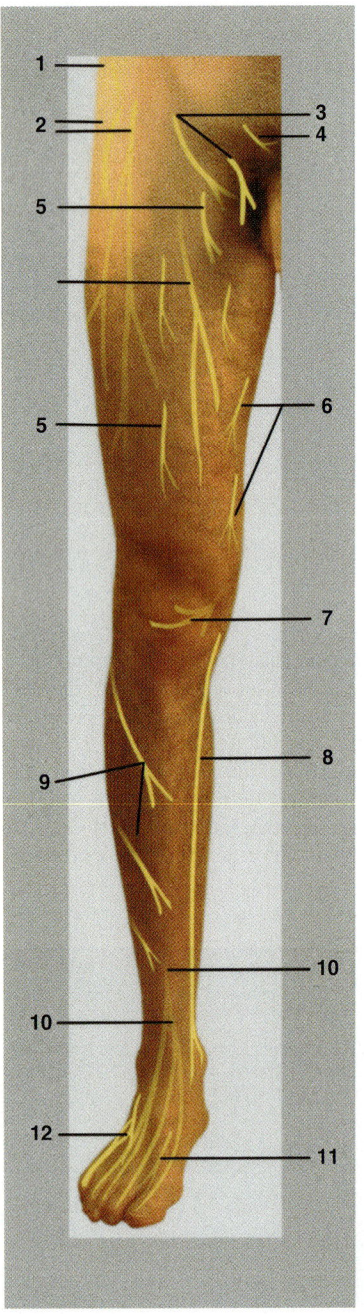

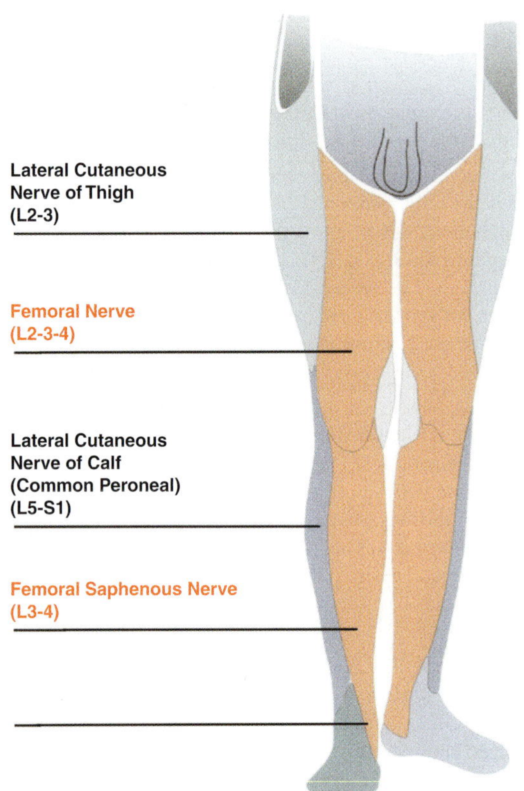

LEGEND

1. Subcostal nerve (lateral cutaneous branch)
2. Lateral femoral cutaneous nerve
3. Femoral branch of the genitofemoral nerve
4. Genital branch of the genitofemoral nerve
5. Anterior femoral cutaneous nerve (from femoral nerve)
6. Cutaneous branches of the obturator nerve
7. Infrapatelar branch of the saphenous nerve
8. Saphenous nerve (terminal cutaneous branch of the femoral nerve)
9. Lateral sural cutaneous nerves (from common peroneal nerve)
10. Superficial peroneal nerve
11. Deep peroneal nerve
12. Lateral dorsal cutaneous nerve (branch of sural nerve)

FIGURE 49-42. Distribution of anesthesia for the anterior lower extremity. Lateral cutaneous nerve of the thigh. [Reprinted with permission from Hadzic A, Vloka J. *Peripheral Nerve Blocks: Principles and Practice*. New York, NY: McGraw-Hill; 2004.]

Ultrasound Guided Ultrasound localization of the LFCN is possible with knowledge of its intrafascial location.

Pearls and Pitfalls If the block is to be used as a sole anesthetic for a skin graft collection procedure, it is clearly important to determine the field of sensory blockade before starting the collection.

OBTURATOR NERVE BLOCK

The obturator nerve provides sensory innervation to the articular surfaces of the knee. Therefore, blockade of this nerve is an important consideration for total knee arthroplasties and anterior cruciate ligament repairs. However, obturator nerve blockade should not be thought of as a complete anesthetic for these procedures due to contributions from the femoral nerve.

Anatomy The obturator nerve is formed from the anterior divisions of L2, L3, and L4 of the lumbar plexus. These anterior divisions organize within the body of the psoas muscle and emerge on the medial border as the obturator nerve. As such, the obturator nerve can be found situated within the obturator canal, where it divides into anterior and posterior divisions. The anterior division provides sensory innervation to the hip via an articular branch and motor supply to the adductor muscles of the thigh. The anterior branch also provides a highly variable sensory component to the medial thigh.[76] The posterior division supplies the motor component to deep adductors and sensory innervation via an articular branch to the posterior knee joint.

Technique The classic description involves nerve stimulator techniques, but paresthesias are not an uncommon associated finding. With a supine patient, the pubic tubercle is identified. A mark is placed 2 cm lateral and 2 cm caudad to the pubic tubercle.

A 22-gauge needle (8-10 cm) is then inserted perpendicular to the skin with a medial slant. When the inferior pubic ramus is encountered, the needle is withdrawn slightly and walked off caudad and lateral. The needle will walk off the rami into the obturator canal (after approximately 3 cm), identified by adductor contraction. Approximately 10 mL of local anesthetic should be injected.

Wassef[77] described an interadductor approach. A skin mark delineating the obturator canal is made below the inguinal ligament and 1 to 2 cm lateral to the palpated femoral artery. The adductor longus tendon is identified near the pubic insertion and an 8-cm, 22-gauge needle is inserted behind the tendon, directed laterally and superiorly using the skin mark as a guide. Adductor contraction is the end point.

Ultrasound-guided obturator block has recently been used as an adjunct to femoral blocks for knee surgery (**Fig. 49-43**).

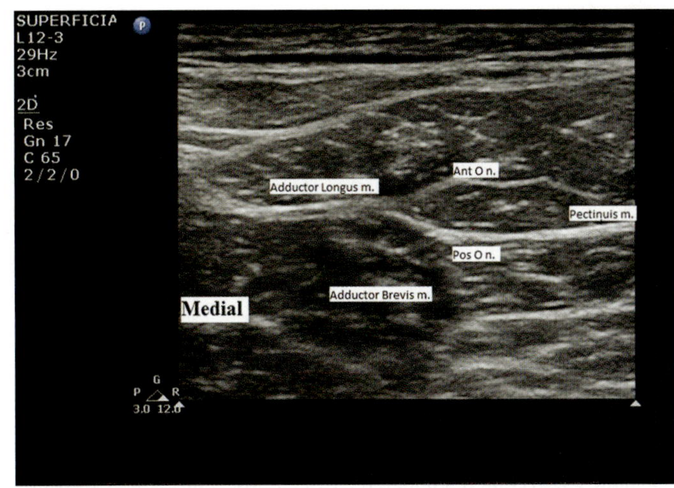

FIGURE 49-43. Ultrasound view of obturator block. In-plane, obturator nerve at the confluence of the adductor longus muscle, adductor brevis muscle, and pectineus muscle. Ant O n., anterior branch of obturator; Pos O n., posterior branch of obturator.

Pearls and Pitfalls Neurovascular bundles place patients at risk for intravascular injections and/or hematoma formation. In the case of spasticity, obturator nerve blockade and/or neurolytics may be used. It may also prove useful as an aide in ascertaining patients who may benefit from additional modalities for relief of spasticity, such as Botox injections.

SCIATIC

The sciatic nerve is the largest of the lower-extremity nerves and has several well-described levels that can be approached for blockade. Sciatic nerve blockade can be used as a complete anesthetic for surgeries of the foot or ankle where a lower-leg tourniquet will be needed and an ankle block would not be sufficient. However, a sciatic nerve block should be used in conjunction with a saphenous nerve block if the medial portion of the leg or ankle is in the surgical field.

Anatomy The sciatic nerve is composed of the ventral rami from L4 to S3, which join on the anterior surface of the piriformis muscle. The sciatic nerve is the largest nerve in the body, with a width of 2.0 cm. As it passes through the greater sciatic foramen, it passes lateral to all of the other structures that emerge inferior to the piriformis (inferior pudendal vessels, pudendal nerve, inferior gluteal nerve and vessels) (**Fig. 49-44**).

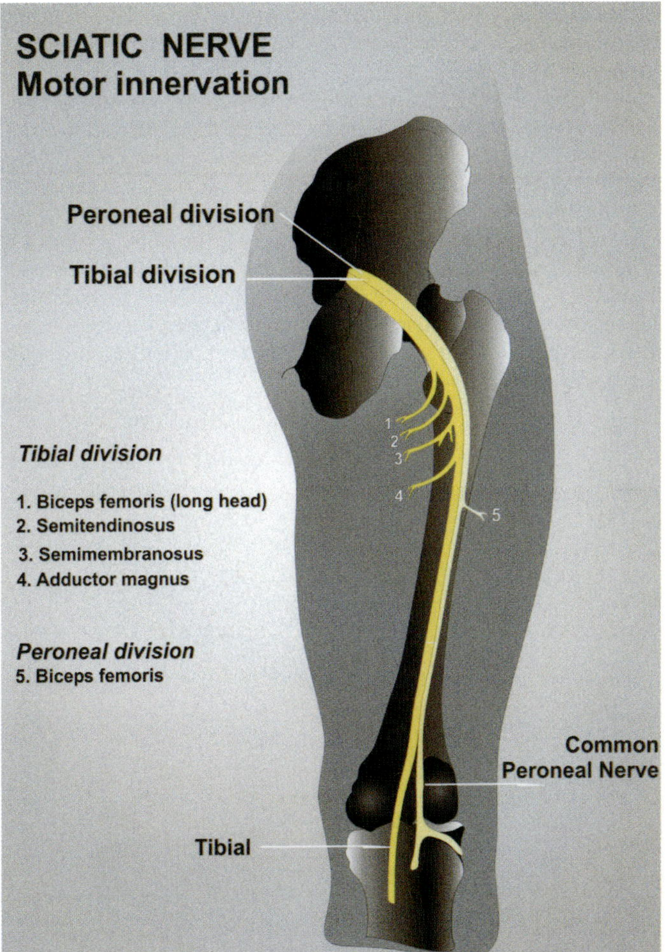

FIGURE 49-44. Sciatic nerve motor innervation. [Reprinted with permission from Hadzic A, Vloka J. *Peripheral Nerve Blocks: Principles and Practice*. New York, NY: McGraw-Hill; 2004.]

The posterior femoral cutaneous nerve courses with the sciatic and the inferior gluteal nerves and vessels and is important because this nerve supplies the posterior portion of the thigh. It is important to note that the posterior cutaneous nerve will only be anesthetized via a high sciatic block.

The sciatic nerve courses inferolaterally deep to the gluteus maximus at a midpoint between the ischial tuberosity and the greater trochanter of the femur. The sciatic nerve itself is a combination of the common peroneal (lateral) and the tibial (medial) nerves joined by an epineurial sheath. These 2 nerves separate approximately 8 cm superior to the popliteal fossa.

Technique There are many different approaches to the sciatic nerve. Several considerations are given to which technique is chosen: patient ability to roll over or aid in positioning, level of the surgery, and body habitus are important factors

Anterior Approach With the patient supine and neutral position of the leg, a line connecting the pubic tubercle and the anterior superior iliac spine is drawn at the level of the inguinal ligament. A second parallel line is drawn inferomedially from the greater trichinae toward the lesser trochanter. A perpendicular line one-third the initial distance is then drawn perpendicular. This is the point of insertion for a 22-gauge, 10- to 15-cm needle. The lesser trochanter is contacted and the needle directed slightly medial. Five centimeters past the point of the lesser trochanter, a paresthesia or a contraction consistent with a sciatic nerve stimulation is encountered. Injection of 20 to 25 mL of local anesthetic is done incrementally (**Fig. 49-45**).

Posterior Approach (Classic Approach of Labat) The positioning for the classic approach to the sciatic may make it impractical in patients who are suffering with a lower-extremity trauma. With the patient positioned in the lateral decubitus position (operative side up), the hip is flexed with the heel of the operative side resting on the non-operative knee. Marking is done to identify the posterior superior iliac spine (PSIS) and the greater trochanter. A line connecting these 2 is bisected perpendicularly, and a point 5 cm caudad is identified (**Fig. 49-46**). This is the point of insertion with a 22-gauge, 10-cm needle. Paresthesia, sciatic motor response, and/or bone is contacted as the needle is advanced. If a paresthesia or motor response is elicited, then slow injection of 20 to 30 mL of local anesthetic is performed. If bone is contacted, methodical redirection of the needle is performed, with a medial and then lateral redirection until paresthesia or motor response is encountered.

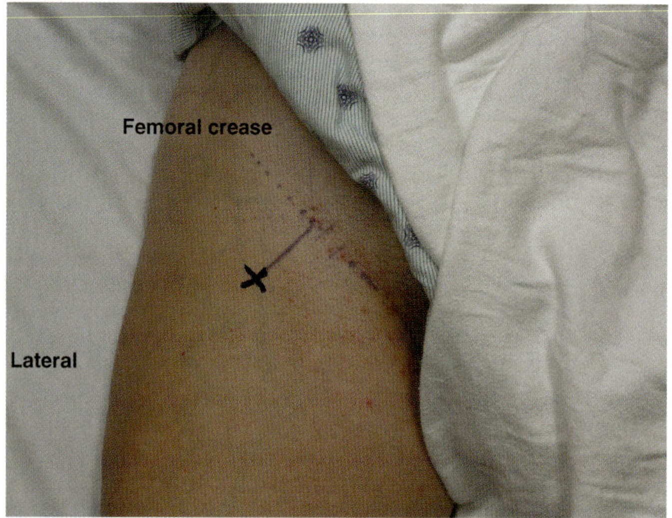

FIGURE 49-45. Surface anatomy for anterior approach to the sciatic. X, needle insertion site.

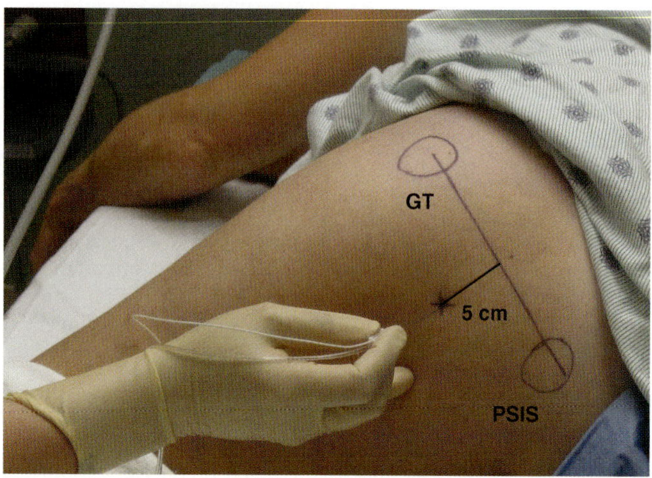

FIGURE 49-46. Posterior approach to the sciatic nerve. GT, greater trochanter; PSIS, posterior superior iliac spine; X, point of needle insertion.

Subgluteal Approach A description of a subgluteal approach to the sciatic was given by Di Benedetto et al[78] and has been used with success. With the patient in the lateral decubitus position, operative side up and hips flexed, and the operative knee at 90 degrees, a line is drawn connecting greater trochanter and the ischial tuberosity. At the bisection of this line, a perpendicular line is then drawn 4 cm caudal. This is the entry point of the 22-gauge, 10-cm needle. Surface anatomy indicates that this is below the bulk of the gluteal muscles in a depression that represents the biceps femoris and the lateral border of the vastus lateralis. In the original description, a nerve stimulator technique was used. However, several descriptions have recently been published discussing ultrasound-guided techniques.[79-81] A curvilinear probe (2-5 MHz) with the patient in the above semilateral position has been used with an in-plane and out-of-plane approach to the nerve (**Fig. 49-47**). Single-injection and catheter-based techniques have been described.

Popliteal Fossa Approach to the Sciatic

Posterior Approach For the posterior approach, the patient is positioned prone. With the knee in a flexed position, the base of a triangle is delineated by the skin crease of the posterior knee. The medial border of the triangle is the semimembranosus muscle and the lateral border is the biceps femoris muscle. In order to block the sciatic nerve before it separates into its 2 smaller components, it is recommended that the point of needle insertion be 7 to 10 cm above the skin crease.[82]

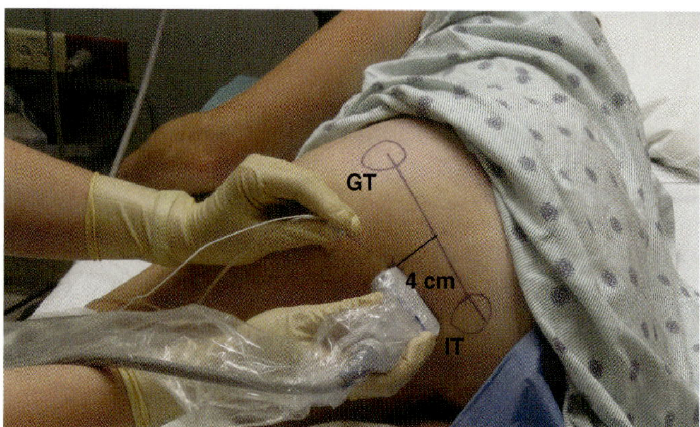

FIGURE 49-47. Subgluteal approach. Surface anatomy and ultrasound imaging. GT, greater trochanter; IT, ischial tuberosity.

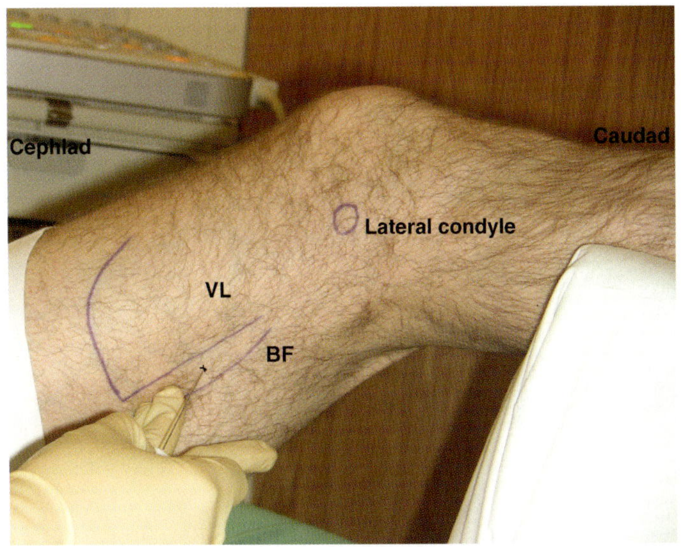

FIGURE 49-48. Lateral approach to the sciatic nerve. BF, biceps femoris; VL, vastus lateralis.

A paresthesia or muscle twitch confirming either sciatic component is accepted.

Lateral Approach Ichiyanagi[83] originally described a lateral approach to the popliteal fossa. The patient is supine with the leg in a neutral position. The leg may be supported so it is flexed at the knee to ease identification of structures (**Fig. 49-48**). The groove between the vastus lateralis and biceps femoris muscles is identified. A 22-gauge, 10-cm needle is inserted until contact with the femur is made. Once the femur is contacted, the needle is redirected posterior and the sciatic nerve should be encountered 1 to 2 cm beyond the femur contact distance. Acceptable nerve stimulation is either tibial nerve (plantar flexion at ankle, inversion of foot) or common peroneal nerve (ankle dorsiflexion or eversion of the foot).

Some authors[84] have advocated for separate stimulation of each component of the sciatic, citing a greater success rate (88% for double stimulation vs 54% for only tibial). The volume of local anesthetic for the lateral and posterior approaches has widely varied in the literature from 20 to 40 mL.

Ultrasound in-plane techniques have also been used with great success for both the posterior and lateral approaches. The positioning for the lateral approach necessitates having the patient in 90-degree flexion in order to place the ultrasound probe on the posterior portion of the popliteal fossa. The entry point of the needle is exactly the same as in the lateral approach, but direct visualization of the local anesthetic ensures circumferential spread (**Fig. 49-49**).

Pearls and Pitfalls Unlike other lower extremity blocks, the time required for the sciatic nerve analgesia to become apparent may be considerable. It is not unusual to have analgesia after 30 to 40 minutes. In contrast, femoral nerve sensory deficits can be appreciated relatively quickly.

As stated above, patient ability to position certainly guides the level at which the sciatic nerve is blocked. Patients with a body mass index greater than 35 may prove difficult for subgluteal approaches using ultrasound technology.

ANKLE

The femoral and sciatic nerves terminate in the lower extremity into 5 terminal branches. The saphenous is the only contribution from the femoral nerve; the other 4 terminal branches—the deep peroneal, superficial peroneal, posterior tibial, and the sural—originate from the sciatic nerve.

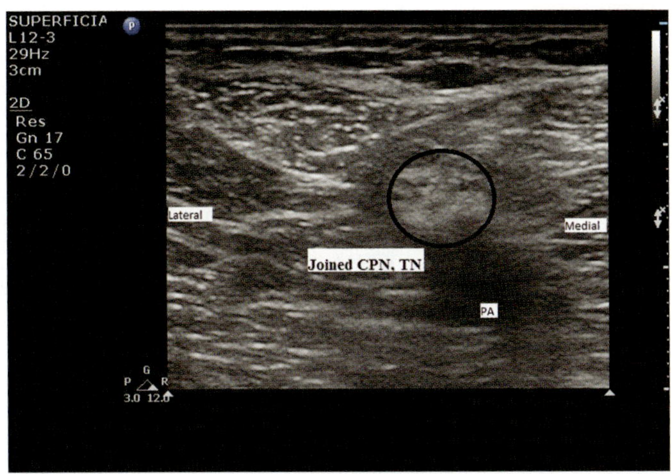

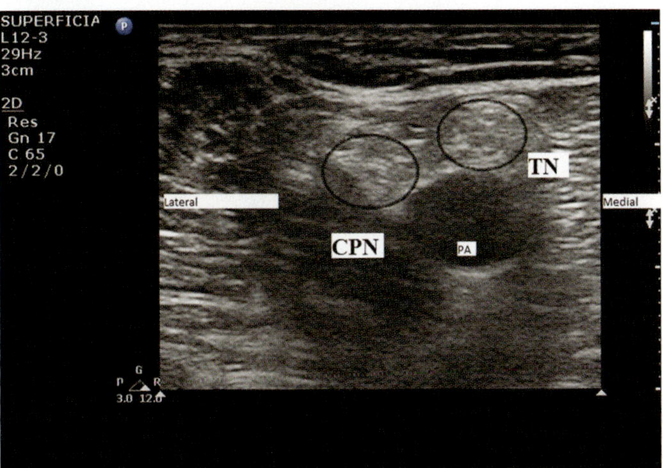

FIGURE 49-49. Ultrasound images of sciatic nerve. **A.** Common peroneal and tibial prior to divide in popliteal fossa. **B.** After divide into common peroneal and tibial nerves. CPN, common peroneal nerve; PA, popliteal artery; TN, tibial nerve.

The sensory innervation of the foot is provided by these 5 nerves (**Fig. 49-50**). Local anesthetic blockade of any one of these nerves or a combination will provide anesthesia and/or analgesia for surgery of the foot. Consideration must be paid to the possible use of a tourniquet. An ankle block is ideal for surgery on the toes or metatarsals.

Anatomy The sciatic nerve branches into the common peroneal and the tibial nerves at the level of the popliteal fossa. The common peroneal further divides into the superficial and deep peroneal nerves. The tibial nerve is the larger of the 2 branches of the sciatic, and it terminates as the posterior tibial nerve and the sural nerve. It courses through the lower extremity in a neurovascular bundle accompanied by the posterior tibial artery and vein. At the ankle level, the posterior tibial nerve can be found posterior to the medial malleolus.

Technique

Posterior Tibial Nerve Classic description is with a patient in the prone position, although this procedure can be accomplished in the supine position with the lower leg resting on a table or elevated. The posterior tibial artery is palpated, and a 22-gauge, 4-cm needle is inserted medial to the Achilles tendon, directed anteriorly toward the medial malleolus. If a paresthesia is elicited, a small volume of local anesthetic is injected (5 mL). In no paresthesia, then the needle is advanced until it contacts the medial malleolus and then the local anesthetic is deposited. This is essentially a field block.

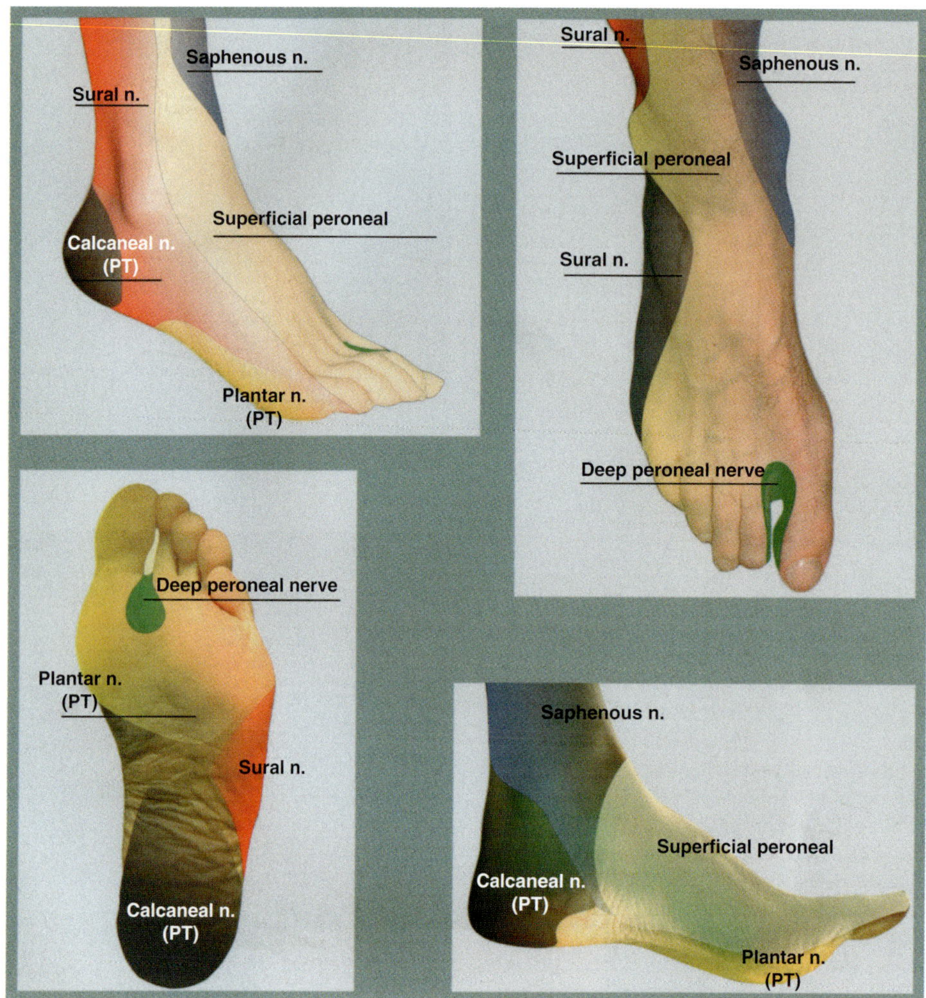

FIGURE 49-50. Ankle block distribution of anesthesia. [Reprinted with permission from Hadzic A, Vloka J. *Peripheral Nerve Blocks: Principles and Practice*. New York, NY: McGraw-Hill; 2004.]

Deep Peroneal and Superficial Peroneal Nerves The patient is positioned as discussed earlier with the foot elevated, resting on a bump. Extension of the great toe identifies the extensor hallicis longus (EHL) tendon. A 22-gauge, 4-cm needle is inserted perpendicular to the skin lateral to the EHL tendon in the groove between the EHL and the extensor digitorum longus tendon (**Fig. 49-51**). The needle is advanced until bone is contacted, and then 5 mL of local anesthetic is injected as the needle is slowly pulled back. This raised skin wheal serves as an initiation point for the superficial peroneal nerve. A superficial wheal is made to the lateral malleolus, and then the needle is redirected toward the medial malleolus. Approximately 5 mL of local anesthetic should be appropriate.

Sural Nerve An approach similar to the posterior tibial nerve is used for the sural nerve. A 22-gauge, 4-cm needle is inserted lateral to the Achilles tendon, directed anteriorly toward the malleolus, and approximately 5 mL of local anesthetic is injected.

Descriptions of the use of ultrasound guidance have been noted. A proposed use of ultrasound is in limiting the amount of local anesthesia necessary with deposition near nerves as opposed to the "field" block, where large volumes may be used to provide complete foot anesthesia. Specifically, ultrasound has been used to identify the sural nerve in association with the lesser saphenous vein. Injection of small amounts of local anesthetic (5 mL) according to these anatomical landmarks using ultrasound guidance has been shown to generate a denser and longer-lasting block as compared with traditional landmark techniques alone.[85]

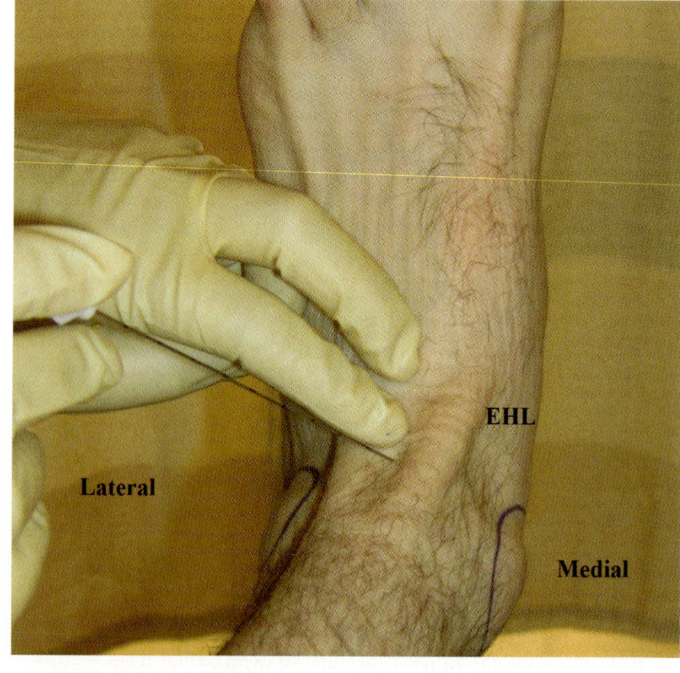

FIGURE 49-51. Surface anatomy with deep peroneal nerve block. The initial needle puncture is also the site for the superficial peroneal nerves.

Pearls and Pitfalls As with all other blocks, knowing the anatomy is essential. Ankle blocks can be quite uncomfortable for patients, and they require multiple injection sites. Local anesthetic volumes need to be monitored.

The saphenous nerve is the only contribution from the femoral that has a terminal branch at the level of the ankle. For procedures on the medial aspect of the foot or ankle, this nerve is important to block.

OTHER USES FOR PERIPHERAL NERVE BLOCKS

Peripheral nerve blocks are being used more frequently in the pain literature for diagnostic[86] and therapeutic[87] purposes. As mentioned previously, interruption of obturator nerve conduction can aide in diagnosis or treatment of adductor spasm.

KEY REFERENCES

- Enneking FK, Chan V, Greger J. Lower-extremity nerve blockade: essentials of our current understanding. *Reg Anesth Pain Med.* 2005;30(1):4-35.
- Horlocker TT, Wedel DJ, Rowlingson JC, et al. Regional anesthesia in the patient receiving antithrombotic or thrombolytic therapy: American Society of Regional Anesthesia and Pain Medicine Evidence-Based Guidelines (Third Edition). *Reg Anesth Pain Med.* 2010;35(1):64-101.
- Neal JM, Brull R, Chan V, et al. The ASRA evidence-based medicine assessment of ultrasound-guided regional anesthesia and pain medicine. *Reg Anesth Pain Med.* 2010;35(2):S1-S9.
- Neal JM, Hebl JR, Gerancher JC, et al. Brachial plexus anesthesia: essentials of our current understanding. *Reg Anesth Pain Med.* 2002;27(4):402-428.

REFERENCES

Complete references available on DVD and online version at www.LongneckerAnesthesiology.com

CHAPTER 50 Managing Adverse Outcomes During Regional Anesthesia

Ban C.H. Tsui
Adam M. Dryden
Brendan T. Finucane

KEY POINTS

1. Safe regional anesthesia begins with a thorough knowledge of anatomy. In Labat's words, "anatomy is the foundation upon which the entire concept of regional anesthesia is built." Studying the anatomy of the major plexuses and peripheral nerves is critical for learning regional anesthesia and avoiding its complications.
2. Prior to performing regional anesthesia, it is imperative to thoroughly discuss the techniques, and their limitations, with the patient. Assessing which patients are most appropriate for performing these techniques on is important, as some are not suitable candidates (eg, those with major anatomic distortion or serious mental illness).
3. One of the most important principles for safe regional anesthesia is provision of a comfortable patient environment. If a patient suffers as a result of one's intervention, a basic principle of the practice of anesthesia has been violated.
4. Resuscitation equipment must be immediately available when performing regional anesthesia, and one must be prepared, at all times, to anesthetize and resuscitate the patient when necessary.
5. A skilled clinician must be willing to abort their technique in the face of excessive challenge. Dogged persistence is inadvisable. One must seek assistance when faced with difficulties and be prepared to change to an alternative route of anesthesia if persistent failure (more than 3 attempts or 20 minutes) occurs.
6. Do not perform regional anesthesia procedures in anesthetized adult patients unless the benefits outweigh the risks. If this principle is violated, the reasoning must be documented in the patient's file.
7. Always be accompanied by a skilled assistant when performing regional anesthesia.
8. The patient must be adequately monitored at all stages during regional anesthesia. Close monitoring can only be discontinued when the block has adequately resolved.
9. If neurologic injury is suspected after regional anesthesia, the cause should be determined quickly to minimize injury. Timely advice should be sought from appropriate consultants (neurologists, radiologists).
10. One must not assume that all patient injury is from regional anesthesia, as other possibilities exist. Do not hesitate to involve other disciplines in the quest to determine the cause of injury.

INTRODUCTION

No matter how skillful an anesthesiologist may be, adverse perioperative events are inevitable in anesthesia practice. Adverse events have been associated with regional anesthesia since local anesthetics were first introduced by Koller in 1884[1] and will persist despite advances in technique, skill, and safety mechanisms. It is nearly impossible to address all of the described and potential complications of regional anesthesia; instead, we focus here on those most relevant to current practice.

GENERAL PRINCIPLES

IMPORTANCE OF PREVENTION

The time-honored statement that "an ounce of prevention is worth a pound of cure" is essential to remember[2] when considering the management of adverse outcomes in regional anesthesia practice. It is most effective to prevent and minimize the risk of regional anesthesia complications. Neurologic injury is one of the most dreaded complications associated with all anesthesia techniques, including regional anesthesia, and it is important to realize that once a serious neurologic injury occurs, the chances of full recovery are unlikely.

Safe regional anesthesia begins with the first encounter with the patient. The first task at hand is to perform a thorough preoperative assessment of the patient. Good outcomes are obtained when a *skilled* anesthesiologist uses appropriate equipment and technique and sound judgment. Skilled intraoperative sedation and monitoring are vital to the practice of regional anesthesia. To this end, we advocate for specialized regional anesthesia areas in the operating room space where the appropriate equipment, monitoring, and assistance are readily available. Resuscitation drugs and equipment must always be immediately available in the event of a problem, and one must always be ready to convert to general anesthesia if required. Patients must be carefully observed during the postoperative period by appropriately trained postanesthetic care team when most of the serious complications become evident.

Early identification and intervention are of the utmost importance in preventing neurologic injury.

Poor outcomes and serious complications are *not* prima facie evidence of negligence. However, the risk of litigation in contemporary anesthesia practice is closely associated with the severity of patient injury rather than the occurrence of negligence; this is particularly true of regional anesthesia injuries. The American Society of Anesthesiologists (ASA) Closed Claims study in the United States reported a high incidence of successful suits against anesthesiologists involved in regional anesthesia cases, even though the standard of care was met.[3] The importance of effective communication and truthful disclosure with the patient and the patient's family cannot be overemphasized. Litigation is more frequent with the combination of an adverse event and a poor physician–patient relationship. A patient who feels that the physician has the patient's best interests at heart is less likely to pursue litigation than is a patient who does not respect or trust the physician; thus the anesthesiologist should pay particular attention to developing a good rapport with the patient in the limited time allotted. **Table 50-1** summarizes basic recommendations for maintaining a standard of care in regional anesthesia practice. Maintaining a standard of care at all times does not guarantee against legal action, but it certainly will minimize the risk and is to be encouraged at all times.[4]

TABLE 50-1 Maintaining a Standard of Care During Regional Anesthetic Practice

Preoperative patient selection
Informed consent
Appropriate use of equipment and technique
Monitoring regional anesthesia practice
Accurate and meticulous anesthesia documentation
Physician–patient communication
Appropriate and timely postoperative follow-up

Patient Selection Proper patient selection is a critical consideration for the safe and successful performance of regional anesthesia, as not all patients are suitable candidates for regional anesthesia (**Fig. 50-1**).[5] Some patients are not psychologically suitable for regional anesthesia.

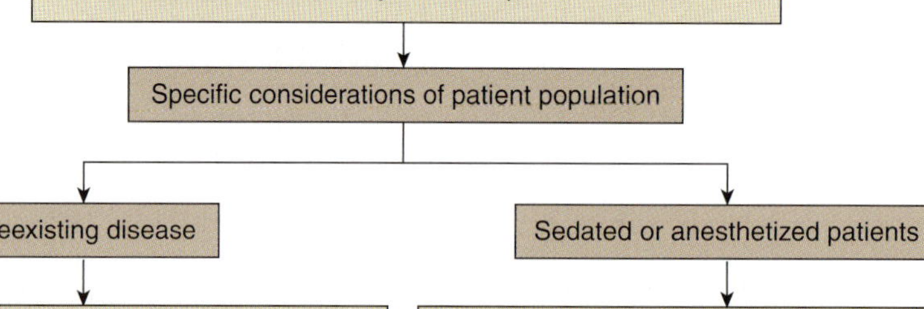

FIGURE 50-1. Patient selection factors for the prevention of complications of regional anesthesia techniques.

A number of patients suffer from needle phobias and faint at the least provocation. In general, patients with severe mental illness are not suitable candidates for regional anesthesia unless it is combined with general anesthesia. Gross anatomic distortion may hinder the performance of regional anesthesia in some patients. Neuraxial techniques may be associated with hemodynamic disturbances such as bradycardia and hypotension; therefore, they are contraindicated in hemodynamically unstable patients and in those with fixed cardiac outputs. Regional anesthesia should be used cautiously in patients with preexisting neurologic disease, and if regional techniques are used in these patients, neurologic deficits must be clearly documented before the performance of regional anesthesia. Some patients are rigidly opposed to regional anesthesia, and it is important not to sell them on it. If it is clearly evident that a patient will benefit from regional anesthesia, it is reasonable to explain in detail the rationale behind the procedure; however, the decision to undergo regional anesthesia must be finally left to the discretion of the patient. It is very important to discuss the options of anesthesia with patients even if they are undergoing minor operative procedures. It is imperative to follow national and international guidelines pertaining to regional anesthesia practice (eg, ASA monitoring, American Society of Regional Anesthesia and Pain Medicine [ASRA] guidelines for anticoagulated patients, etc.), and if there is any deviation, it is important to specify the reasons and to document them. **Table 50-2** summarizes the important factors involved in selecting suitable patients for regional anesthesia.

Consent Informed consent and an explanation of the risks and alternatives to regional anesthesia must be provided to the patient (the anesthesiologist should never coerce a patient to accept or reject any anesthetic plan). Potentially serious complications associated with regional anesthesia should be disclosed to patients, including convulsions and the risk of cardiac toxicity from systemic injections of local anesthetics, spinal cord/nerve injury leading to paralysis or neurologic deficit, pneumothorax, hematoma, infection, cardiac arrest, and death. Interestingly, a recent study revealed that fewer than half of anesthetists disclose the risks of seizures, respiratory failure, and cardiac arrest before the administration of either neuraxial blocks or peripheral nerve blocks.[6] Any common side effects specific to certain procedures such as the failure to achieve surgical anesthesia, patient awareness during conscious sedation, nausea, pruritus, headache, shivering, backache, dizziness, and urinary retention should also be discussed. However, anesthesiologists should bear in mind that even with informed consent, proper disclosure, effective communication, and an appropriate ethical approach, there is no guarantee that they will be legally protected.[7]

Use of Appropriate Equipment and Technique As advances in regional anesthesia continue, techniques used must be continuously revised in light of any new, clinically relevant information and developments. For years, we have been percutaneously inserting needles toward neural targets and have relied solely on our knowledge of anatomy and techniques of paresthesia and the loss of resistance (LOR). The introduction of nerve stimulation was an important advance in regional anesthesia because it provided some objective evidence that the needle tip was close to the neural target. One of the most exciting recent advances has been the introduction of ultrasonography as a method to accurately place needles in close proximity to neural targets. Ultrasonography allows real-time visualization of anatomical structures and offers the potential to guide needle and catheter placement in regional anesthesia. This section highlights recent advances in nerve stimulation and ultrasonography that may play an important role in preventing complications during regional anesthesia practice.

Nerve Stimulation in Regional Anesthesia: Peripheral Nerve Blockade Despite years of clinical use, the electrophysiologic effect of injectates on nerve stimulation has never been fully explained. The classic unanswered question concerning electrical stimulation is why is it that one may not be able to consistently stimulate a nerve with a current of less than 0.5 mA, even after eliciting a paresthesia in that nerve? Another phenomenon that is poorly understood is the "Raj test." The Raj test is when nerve stimulation is used to locate a nerve and a twitch is observed when the needle tip is close to the neural target. Ideally, the twitch is required to persist at a current of 0.5 mA. The clinician then injects a small volume of local anesthetic or normal saline through the needle. If the needle tip is in the correct location, the muscle twitch disappears immediately.[8] Until very recently, the disappearance of the twitch was thought to be caused by physical displacement of the nerve by the injectate.[9] We recently learned that this mechanism is best explained in electrical terms and is not entirely a result of the physical displacement of the nerve.[10] In a porcine model, the injection of 0.9% sodium chloride solution (NaCl) abolished the motor response, and a subsequent injection of 5% dextrose reestablished a motor response during peripheral nerve stimulation.[10] Simulation and in vitro experiments show that injections of 0.9% NaCl and 5% dextrose alter the electrical field in different ways.[11] It was concluded that the injection of electrically conducting solutions (saline or local anesthetic) increases the conductive area surrounding the stimulating needle tip, leading to a decrease in the current density surrounding the target nerve (**Fig. 50-2**). The current density surrounding the needle tip is then no longer sufficient to stimulate the desired nerve.[10] This observation suggests that effective nerve stimulation is sensitive to changes that occur at the needle–tissue interface,

TABLE 50-2 Patient Selection Factors

Factors Involved in Patient Selection	Relative Contraindications	Absolute Contraindications
Patient cooperation	Anxiety states; needle phobias; poorly controlled psychiatric disease; language barriers; pediatric patients	Patient refusal
Anatomic and physiologic considerations	Anatomical anomalies; technical challenges: obesity, severe arthritis, degenerative joint disease	
Anesthetic considerations		Lack of experience and skills; lack of appropriate equipment for performing the block (eg, nerve stimulator, ultrasonogram); lack of appropriate equipment for resuscitation and monitoring (eg, oxygen, mask, drugs)
Coexisting diseases	Preexisting progressive neurologic disease; comatose states; sepsis; coagulopathy	Infection at the site of injection; allergy to local anesthetics; coagulopathy (although an international normalized ratio [INR] of <2 is acceptable for ophthalmic procedures)
Surgical procedures	Lengthy procedures that outlast the duration of action of the local anesthetic (single-injection techniques; uncomfortable positioning for an extended period of time)	

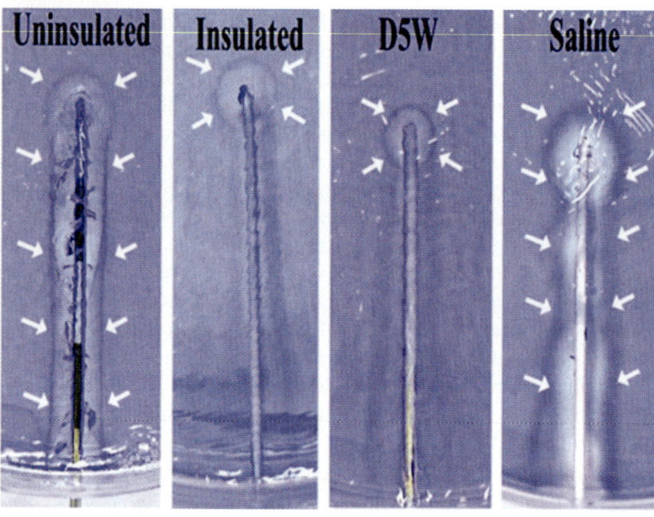

FIGURE 50-2. Gel electrophoresis: changes in the electrical field with uninsulated and insulated needles after 5% dextrose in water (D_5W) and saline injection. Arrows show the margin of the clear zone/electric field. *Far left*: Diffuse electric field with an uninsulated needle; *center left*: narrow electric field with an uninsulated needle; *center right*: electric field with an insulated needle after D_5W injection remains narrow; *far right*: diffuse electric field with an insulated needle after normal saline injection. [Adapted from Tsui BC, Wagner A, Finucane B. Electrophysiologic effect of injectates on peripheral nerve stimulation. *Reg Anesth Pain Med.* 2004;29(3):189-193. Copyright May 2004, with permission from American Society of Regional Anesthesia and Pain Medicine.]

TABLE 50-3 Comparison of the Standard Test Dose With the Epidural Stimulation (Tsui) Test for Confirming Epidural Catheter Location

Catheter Location	Test Dose	Epidural Stimulation Test
Subarachnoid	Hypotension/total spinal	Positive unilateral/bilateral motor response (<1 mA)
Subdural		Diffuse motor response in many segments (<1 mA)
Epidural space close to the nerve root		Unilateral motor response (<1 mA)
		Positive motor response (1-10 mA); threshold current increased after local anesthetic injection
Not intravascular	↑ Heart rate	Remain or return to baseline positive motor response (1-10 mA) even after local anesthetic injection
Intravascular	↑ Blood pressure	Electrocardiogram changes
Subcutaneous		Negative response

Black box indicates insensitive or undefined response.

Reprinted and modified from Tsui BC, Finucane B. Epidural stimulator catheter. *Tech Reg Anesth Pain Manage.* 2002;6(4):150-154. Copyright 2002, with permission from Elsevier.

such as the angle of the needle or the injection of the local anesthetic. The net effect of these changes is to alter the current density at the tip of the needle or the path of the electric current, ultimately resulting in a change in the quality of the motor response.[12] This phenomenon has also been reported in a clinical setting.[13,14] In a clinical study, the mean current required to stimulate the supraclavicular, axillary, femoral, and sciatic nerves when using an insulated needle was significantly higher (up to 6 times) after the injection of normal saline.[15] This effect has also been verified by others in the femoral and sciatic nerves.[16] The clinical implications are as follows:

- One may use a nonconducting solution, such as 5% dextrose in water (D_5W), rather than saline to open up the perineural space.[10]
- Reports of the use of nonconducting injectates (eg, D_5W) in peripheral nerve block are promising and appear to provide stability when using electrical stimulation techniques.[13,14,16]
- The motor response resulting from electrical stimulation is augmented after an injection of D_5W in a very high percentage of cases (96%). This allows one to increase the accuracy of placement of continuous catheters.[14,16]

Nerve Stimulation in Regional Anesthesia: Neuraxial Blockade Epidural stimulation has been used to confirm and guide catheter placement in the epidural space. The epidural stimulation test confirms catheter placement through stimulation of the spinal nerve roots (not the spinal cord) with a low-amplitude electrical current conducted through normal saline via an electrically conducting catheter.[17] Correct placement of the epidural catheter tip (1-2 cm from the nerve roots) is indicated by a motor response elicited with a current between 1 and 10 mA.[17,18] There has been 1 case report of a current response indicating epidural placement with radiologic evidence of subdural placement.[19] Any motor response observed with a significantly lower threshold current (<1 mA) suggests that the catheter is in the subarachnoid or subdural space or is in close proximity to a nerve root[20-22]; in these rare cases, a motor response is elicited with a significantly lower threshold current because the stimulating catheter may be very close (<1 cm) to the nerve roots or because it may be in direct contact with highly conductive cerebrospinal fluid (CSF) (**Table 50-3**).

Electrical stimulation has been applied to neural structures for neurophysiologic evaluation and pain control for many years[23-26] and has proven to be safe. Although no known complication or patient discomfort has resulted from the epidural stimulation test, it has been recommended to keep the current below 15 mA and the stimulation time as brief (less than a few minutes) as possible.[17,18,27,28] In particular, the current output must be carefully increased from zero and stopped once motor activity is visible to ensure that all motor responses, even those elicited with a low current (<1 mA), are detected. The nerve stimulator must allow a gradual increase in current output to at least 10 mA.

Table 50-3 compares features of the epidural "test dose" (lidocaine with 1:200 000 epinephrine) and the epidural stimulation test. Epidural stimulation is a tool for clinician use that may have a significant impact on 3 of the most significant complications associated with epidural anesthesia: systemic toxicity, accidental subarachnoid or subdural injections of local anesthetics, and neural damage.

Ultrasound Imaging in Regional Anesthesia The application of ultrasound in regional anesthesia was first published in 1989 by Ting and Sivagnanratnam.[29] Since then there has been an increasing number of reports in the world literature on this exciting application in regional anesthesia. With the widespread availability of highly portable ultrasound machines, ultrasound techniques have taken hold as a mainstay in the practice of regional anesthesia.

Ultrasound-Guided Peripheral Nerve Blockade With the use of ultrasonography, one can observe neural targets, vascular structures, the advancing needle, and the actual spread of the local anesthetic solution after the injection of the local anesthetic in real time. Brachial plexus anesthesia is one of the most challenging techniques in regional anesthesia; therefore, ultrasound has potential to improve success rates with this technique. The application of ultrasound in regional anesthesia has renewed interest in the classic supraclavicular brachial plexus block (**Fig. 50-3**).[30,31] Advances in this technology and, more importantly, familiarity with it (via appropriate training programs)[32] continue to facilitate better

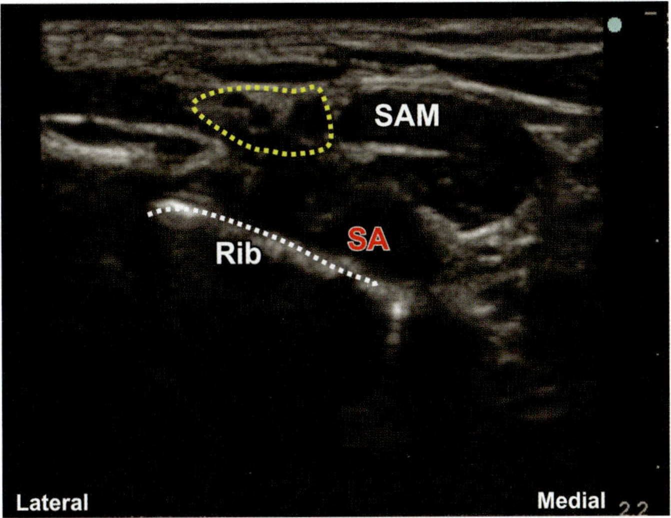

FIGURE 50-3. Ultrasonogram of supraclavicular region. The trunks of the brachial plexus can be identified as a cluster of circles (ie, a honeycomb shape) positioned lateral and superior to the subclavian artery. If the identity of the hollow structure was in doubt, the color flow Doppler provided further verification (*left bottom*).

imaging of nerve trunks, blood vessels, pleura, and the approaching needle.[33,34] The safety advantages to ultrasound have been studied with great fervor.[35] It seems that ultrasound convincingly can decrease the amount of local anesthetic used, it can decrease the incidence of unintentional vascular punctures, and it can significantly decrease the number of needle passes to perform a block.[36-40] One can draw all sorts of conclusions regarding the positive effects that ultrasound-guided blocks will have on patient outcomes, but this has not yet been proven.[41] Ultrasonographic technology is an undeniable advance in regional anesthesia; however, it does not completely eliminate difficulty in accurately identifying structures and observing the advancing needle in detail in all cases.

To minimize risks of regional anesthesia, potential exists to combine ultrasound and nerve stimulation techniques when performing regional anesthesia. Ultrasonography allows the clinician to see the advancing needle approaching what appears to be the target nerve or trunk. Nerve stimulation allows one to identify which nerve is being approached and, if indeed, what is being approached is a neural structure. Needle/catheter-tip visibility is enhanced using D_5W as a preinjectate. Moreover, by using ultrasonography, one can observe the pattern of spread of D_5W before committing to the injection of local anesthetic. Individually, ultrasonography (anatomic locating tool) and nerve stimulation techniques (physiologic response aid) have their limitations, but, when used in combination, these techniques may serve to compensate for each other's weaknesses and may facilitate optimal needle placement for peripheral nerve blocks, although this remains to be proven.[35]

Ultrasound Imaging for Neuraxial Blockade Ultrasonography is useful for guiding peripheral nerve block placement in adult patients[42,43]; however, its application for guiding neuraxial blockade in adults and children remains limited, despite increasing interest.[44]

- Real-time ultrasound imaging of the lumbar spine is a simple procedure. Ultrasound aids the placement of lumbar epidural catheters and enhances the performance of combined spinal–epidural anesthesia.[45,46]
- Ultrasonography use improves the learning curve of obstetric lumbar epidural catheter placement for anesthesia trainees.[47]
- In patients with anticipated difficult epidural localization, this technology is helpful for estimating lumbar epidural depth; it also facilitates ease of placement.[48,49]
- Although ultrasound imaging has been used to guide lumbar epidural needle placement, it may be of limited value in the thoracic region, particularly in older children and adults, when visualization of the spinal cord and relevant structures is sought.[50,51] Calcification of the posterior vertebral bodies in children older than 6 months of age prevents reliable imaging of the spinal cord.[50]

At the present time, ultrasonography guidance is helpful for viewing the lumbar region of selected patients, although its use for thoracic epidural placement is of value only in infants and small children, as their vertebrae are not fully ossified.

Monitoring Regional Anesthesia We believe it is important to have an assistant observe and aid the patient at all times during the performance of regional anesthesia. As many as 15% of patients have a fear of needles and vasovagal episodes occur when performing regional anesthesia.[52]

- Standard electrocardiogram and pulse oximetry are essential monitors while performing regional anesthesia.
- Before performing the neural block, a baseline blood pressure reading should be obtained. Once the regional anesthesia procedure is complete, the monitors should remain attached. In conscious patients, end-tidal carbon dioxide monitoring is not used; however, there are special nasal prongs available for monitoring spontaneously ventilating patients.
- Evidence of regressing sensory and motor blockade and stable vital signs must be present to fulfill the criteria for discharge from the recovery area.
- Local anesthetic infusions are now routinely used in many medical centers. Patients receiving local anesthetic infusions should be visited regularly by a qualified physician postoperatively (ie, Acute Pain Service).

Record Keeping/Documentation Accurate and meticulous recording of anesthesia information is essential for maintaining the quality of care in regional anesthesia. When determining the true nature and extent of complications, an accurately documented preoperative examination is important.

- Detailed documentation of patient consent and the clinical procedure is very important.
- Open and honest communication with the patient is essential for providing good quality patient care.

Physician–Patient Communication Effective communication with each patient is essential for the prevention and early diagnosis of any potential complications. Patients undergoing regional anesthesia may report anxiety, and appropriate preoperative education for the patient can help mitigate this.[53] Discussing the procedures, including their benefits and any significant risks involved, is the legal and professional responsibility of all anesthesiologists. It is equally important to maintain good rapport with the patient during the postoperative period.

- A telephone call to the patient on the first postoperative day is a reasonable and practical alternative to a visit.
- Specific common risks for certain blocks should be discussed with the patient before discharge. For example, patients undergoing supraclavicular blocks should be warned about the risk of pneumothorax and be informed about potential symptoms and what to do if they develop.
- Caution patients about the risk of burns (ie, from radiators) or the consequences of applying pressure to desensitized areas when sensory anesthesia continues after discharge.
- Warn patients about lying on paralyzed extremities for any length of time or letting them become dependent.
- Patients should receive written instructions and information about when to seek medical attention before discharge from the hospital.

- As per hospital policy in local practice areas, ambulatory patients should be discharged to the care of a family member or guardian. The consequences of being left unmonitored must be made clear to patients.

SYSTEMIC COMPLICATIONS INVOLVED WITH LOCAL ANESTHETIC ADMINISTRATION IN REGIONAL ANESTHESIA

ALLERGIC REACTIONS

Although allergies to local anesthetics are rare, a full array of allergic symptoms and signs ranging from mild skin irritation to full-blown anaphylaxis have been described. These signs and symptoms are almost always associated with amino ester preparations or preservatives (eg, methylparaben). Allergic reactions are more common after exposure to ester compounds than amides.[54]

It is quite difficult to obtain good statistical information on the problem of allergic reactions to local anesthetics, and most anesthesiologists are convinced that the risk of allergic reactions to lidocaine is infinitesimal. Lidocaine is frequently administered intravenously by cardiologists, emergency medicine specialists, and anesthesiologists, and reports of allergic reactions using it in this fashion are indeed rare.

The United Kingdom uses a tracking system for adverse reactions to all medications referred to as the ADROIT system (Adverse Drug Reporting on Line Tracking System). Nazir and Holdcroft[55] accessed that database and studied adverse reactions to local anesthetics between the years 1967 and 2005 and recently published their findings. What was really surprising was that of 797 reports of adverse events to lidocaine, 331 of the reports involved lidocaine with no additives, and 96 of 331 of these were considered to be *allergic* reactions. Lidocaine in combination with methylprednisolone or prilocaine generated the most allergic reactions. There were 16 deaths linked with lidocaine alone, and at least 4 of them were deemed to be anaphylactic reactions. Allergic reactions were reported in 16% of the adverse events associated with bupivacaine. One can argue of course that most of these allergic reactions were not true allergies, but merely systemic effects mislabeled as "allergic" reactions.

SYSTEMIC TOXIC REACTIONS

Nazir and Holdcroft's report provided further evidence of the minimal risk of local anesthetics.[55] They report approximately 1 fatality per year in the United Kingdom by all users of local anesthetic drugs since 1967. Unfortunately, we do not have a denominator for the number of local anesthetics administered in the United Kingdom each year, but we can assume that it would be a large number. This study again proved that lidocaine caused fewer deaths than bupivacaine. There were 17 bupivacaine fatalities of 160 adverse events as compared with 20 of 797 for lidocaine. Fifteen of these fatalities had a cardiovascular origin. Ropivacaine was released for clinical use worldwide in 1996. Since that time there were 16 adverse events reported to the ADROIT tracking system, including 1 allergic reaction and no fatalities, though the editor is aware of ropivacaine-related deaths.

Systemic toxic reactions to local anesthetic drugs occur almost always as a result of unintentional intravascular injection and rarely follow the injection of an excessive quantity of local anesthetic into an appropriate site. The incidence of systemic toxicity has substantially decreased within the past 30 years. In 1969, Dawkins[56] reported the incidence of seizures after local anesthetic injections to be 0.2% after epidural anesthesia. A recent study from France reported an incidence of seizures of 0.01%, which represents a 20-fold decline in a 40-year period.[56,57] A higher occurrence of systemic reactions is after peripheral nerve blocks, especially brachial plexus and caudal blocks in adults.[58] The maximum plasma concentration of local anesthetic (C_{max}) resulting from an unintentional intravascular injection depends on a number of factors,[59] including the total dose of local anesthetic injected, the speed and site of injection, and whether the injection is administered intravenously or intra-arterially. The lungs are an important repository for local anesthetic drugs; plasma concentrations of these drugs will be substantially higher if the lungs are bypassed (eg, an accidental intra-arterial injection in the head, face, or neck region).[60] Plasma concentrations of local anesthetics are also influenced by the tension of carbon dioxide (CO_2) and the pH. An elevated arterial CO_2 tension increases cerebral blood flow, and an acidotic state increases intracellular ion trapping and the amount of free drug available. This combination of factors has a synergistic effect on the seizure threshold.[61]

Systemic toxic reactions occur much less frequently when local anesthetics are administered in peripheral sites. A number of factors influence the degree of absorption taking place from the periphery to the central circulation. The most important factor influencing absorption is the site of injection—absorption is more rapid in highly vascular tissues and less so in poorly perfused tissue. Rapid absorption also occurs from intrapleural injections, and very slow absorption occurs from the bladder and skin. Consequently, local anesthetic absorption increases from the highest to the lowest rates in the following anatomic sites: intercostal, epidural, brachial plexus, lower extremity, and subcutaneous tissue (**Fig. 50-4**).

The rate of absorption is reduced by the addition of epinephrine to local anesthetic drugs, but this also depends on the local anesthetic used. Furthermore, the addition of epinephrine itself may lead to other complications (see Complications of Peripheral Nerve Blocks later). As the plasma concentration of lidocaine increases, there is a typical progression of effects on the CNS and the cardiovascular system. This pattern of symptomatology is not typically seen with the more potent local anesthetics (**Fig. 50-5**).[62] CNS excitation after epidural

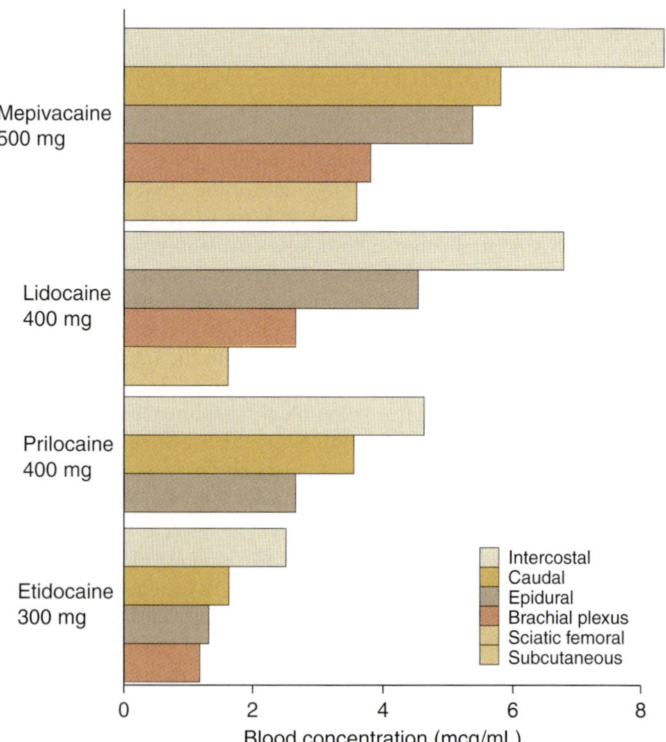

FIGURE 50-4. Comparative peak blood concentrations of several local anesthetic agents after administration into various anatomical sites. Subcut, subcutaneous. [Modified from Covino BG, Vassalo HG. Pharmacokinetic aspects of local anesthetic agents. In: *Local Anesthetics. Mechanisms of Action and Clinical Use*. New York, NY: Grune and Stratton; 1976:95-123. Copyright 1976 Grune and Stratton, with permission from Elsevier.]

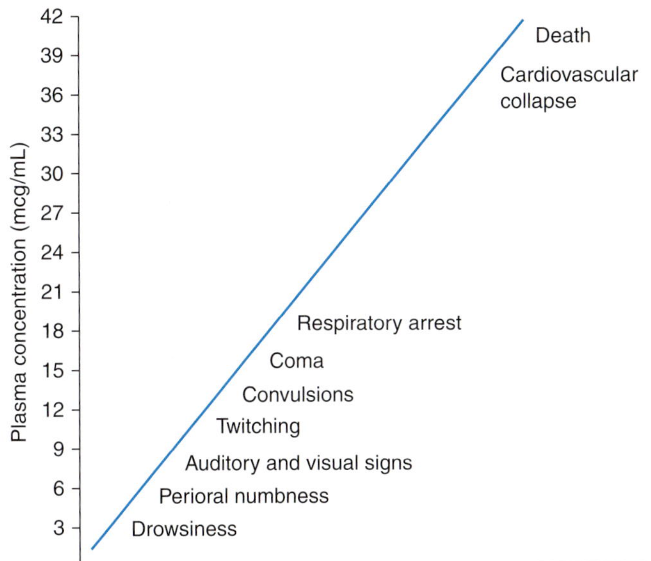

FIGURE 50-5. Concentration–toxicity profile of lidocaine. [Reprinted with permission from Covino BG. Clinical pharmacology of local anesthetic agents. In: Cousins MJ, Bridenbaugh PO, eds. *Neural Blockade in Clinical Anesthesia and Management of Pain*. 3rd ed. Baltimore, MD: Lippincott Williams & Wilkins; 1998:107.]

anesthesia almost always arises as a result of unintentional intravascular injections. Local anesthetics are amphiphilic molecules, having both lipophilic and hydrophilic properties; these drugs enter a variety of cellular compartments and have the potential to interact with a wide variety of molecules, including inotropic signaling pathways (sodium, potassium, and calcium ion channels), and also influence adrenergic and lysophosphatide signaling systems, cardiac bioenergetics, and mitochondrial dynamics.[63] As plasma concentrations of local anesthetic increase, signs of local anesthetic toxicity increase in severity. Concurrent treatment with CNS depressant medications may modify the typical clinical signs of a toxic reaction and can mask some of the early warning signs (**Table 50-4**).

The cardiovascular system is more resistant to the toxic effects of local anesthetics than the CNS, especially after toxic doses of lidocaine. Local anesthetics affect both electrical and mechanical cardiac activity. Tachycardia and hypertension are early signs of cardiac toxicity, and with increasing doses patients develop bradycardia and hypotension; however, this pattern of symptomatology may not be seen when the patient receives a rapid intravascular injection and this pattern of symptoms and signs is not evident with potent local anesthetics.

PREVENTION

Early recognition of an intravascular injection is the key to prevention. Aspiration should be performed before any injection of local anesthetic. The aspiration should be repeated with any change in needle position.

The administration of epinephrine and isoproterenol with the local anesthetic can aid in ruling out an intravascular injection.[64] Increased heart rate and systolic blood pressure in addition to T-wave changes are considered sensitive and specific end points in response to an intravascular injection of a test dose containing epinephrine. A single injection of 15 μg of epinephrine produces a heart rate increase of greater than 10 beats/min, a blood pressure increase greater than 15 mm Hg, and a decrease in T-wave amplitude of 25%.[65] In the sedated patient, changes in heart rate may not be as reliable as T-wave and blood pressure changes.[66] Older patients (>60 years of age) and those on β-blockers and anesthetized patients are less sensitive to β-adrenergic stimulation.

TABLE 50-4 Signs of Early Accidental Intravascular Injection

Early Signs	Late Signs
Light-headedness	Muscle twitching
Tinnitus	Drowsiness
Blurred vision	Generalized tonic-clonic convulsions
Perioral numbness	

The accurate deposition of local anesthetic, in potentially smaller doses than traditionally used, holds promise to reduce the incidence of systemic toxicity. Ultrasound guidance may help to prevent intravascular needle placement and, more importantly, injection of local anesthetic.[67] This has yet to be proven, although there is 1 report of a reduction in the number of seizures associated with ultrasound versus nerve stimulation guidance.[68]

Recently, an additional measure to warn of intravascular needle placement has been investigated, making use of simple observation of electrical impedance (as displayed on currently available nerve stimulators) during block placement.[69] The failure to observe a rise in impedance upon injection of a test dose of D_5W seems highly predictive of intravascular needle placement. The basis for this observation is that the injected fluid is quickly dispersed within the systemic circulation and does not increase the current density in the local vicinity as does a nonconducting solution (D_5W). Although this "test" would not replace other precautionary measures, it may provide an additional warning sign of intravascular injection before *any* local anesthetic is injected.

Following the precautions outlined next can minimize the chances and impact of unintentional intravascular injection.

- Incremental administration of the local anesthetic
- Frequent aspiration
- Observation of heart rate, systolic blood pressure, and T-wave changes
- Observation of the patient

MANAGEMENT OF LOCAL ANESTHETIC TOXICITY

The initial treatment recommended for the management of patients with systemic toxicity is very similar to that used for any resuscitation. The SAVED mnemonic outlined in **Fig. 50-6** can be used to guide the management of allergic reactions and systemic toxicity to local anesthetics.[70]

Because hypoxia, hypercapnia, and acidosis exacerbate all local anesthetic toxic reactions,[71,72] control of the airway and ventilation is of paramount importance in the treatment of local anesthetic toxicity. Recent studies demonstrate improved hemodynamics and survival in animal models of bupivacaine toxicity with the administration of intravenous lipid emulsion.[73,74] It is suggested that lipid emulsions function to remove local anesthetic molecules from binding sites that are responsible for cardiovascular depression.[75] This has been verified clinically in one instance in which the serial serum concentrations of bupivacaine decreased faster than its half-life would predict after the administration of a lipid emulsion.[76] It is likely by this same mechanism that lipid emulsions have been used to treat other toxidromes. Lipid emulsions may also act by reversing the local anesthetic inhibition on myocardial fatty acid oxidation.[77] In this manner, they would restore myocardial adenosine triphosphate supply. Propofol, which is formulated in lipid, may reduce susceptibility to local anesthetic toxicity; however, its negative inotropic effects may mitigate against its use as an antidote in the face of cardiovascular collapse, and its use is not recommended for the treatment of local anesthetic systemic toxicity.[78] Vasopressin is no longer recommended for treatment during resuscitation from local anesthetic toxicity.

Of course, studies to fully evaluate the use of lipid emulsions are difficult given the nature of its use. Regardless, there is a large and growing body of evidence to support its efficacy. It has been used in cases to treat local anesthetic-induced cardiac arrest due to bupivacaine, levobupivacaine, ropivacaine, and mepivacaine.[79-81] It has even been reported

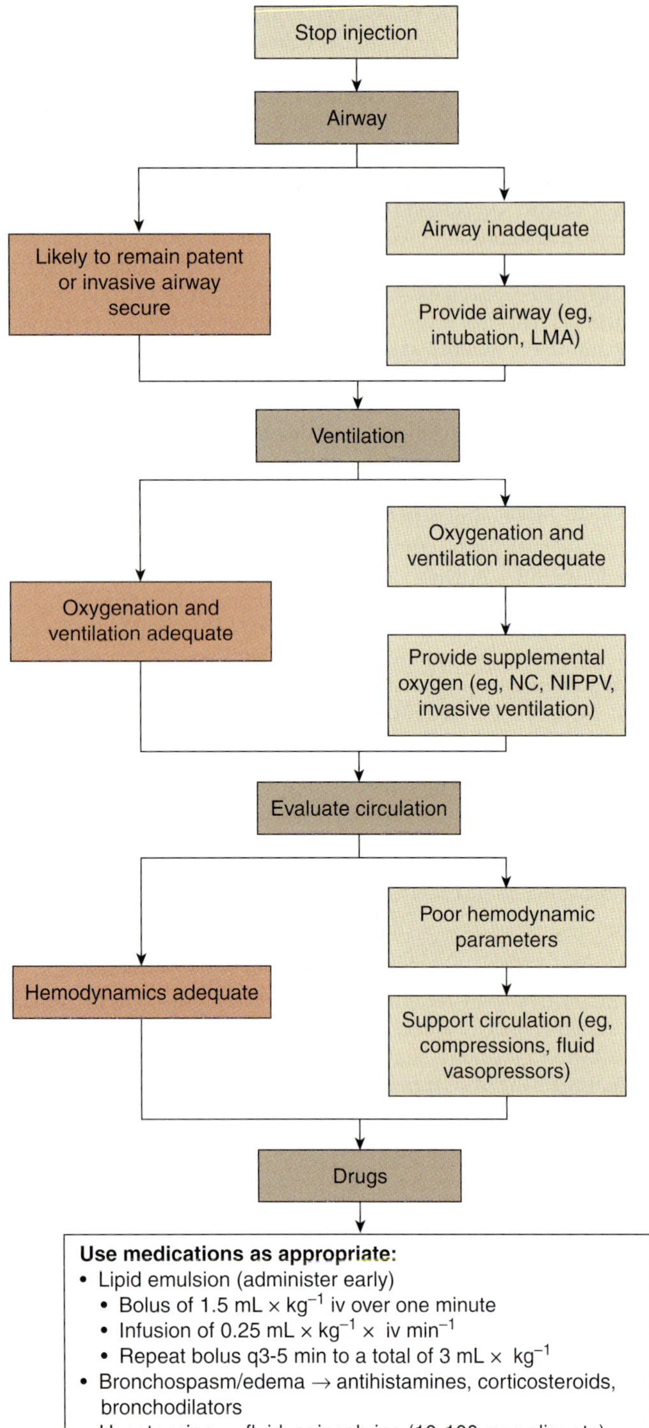

FIGURE 50-6. SAVED mnemonic for management of systemic toxicity to local anesthetics.[82] LMA, laryngeal mask airway; NC, nasal cannula; NIPPV, noninvasive positive pressure ventilation.

to reverse the neurologic effects of local anesthetics.[82] The use of lipid emulsions in pediatrics has not been extensively reported, but there are case reports of successful outcomes.[83] Thus far, the safety profile of lipid emulsions seems to be quite good. There has been a case of an elevated amylase without clinical sequelae after its administration.[84]

The limits of safe dosing and systemic adverse effects of high-volume lipid emulsion administration are unknown at this time, and there is caution for administering high volumes in patients with abnormal pulmonary, renal, hepatic, and pancreatic function. The recommended dosing for Intralipid ® 20% (Fresenius Kabi, Uppsala Sweden) is to first administer a bolus of 1.5 mL $\times$ kg^{-1} IV over 1 minute and then start an infusion of 0.25 mL $\times$ kg^{-1} $\times$ min^{-1}. Compressions should be maintained to circulate the lipid. Bolus doses can be administered every 3 to 5 minutes to a total of 3 mL $\times$ kg^{-1}. Lipid emulsions should be administered (during resuscitation) to patients in cardiac arrest due to local anesthetic toxicity, and, preemptively, to those displaying overt neurologic toxicity.

The following are some recommendations for the management of significant local anesthetic systemic toxicity:

- Bronchospasm and generalized edema, sometimes associated with allergic reactions, may require use of bronchodilators, antihistamines, and corticosteroids.
- Ventilation and oxygen are required to correct acidosis and prevent hypoxia and hypercarbia; tracheal intubation should be individualized.
- Chest compressions and defibrillation may be required to restore organ perfusion and should be instituted based on patient hemodynamics.
- Lipid emulsion therapy can be lifesaving and should be administered early. Lipid emulsions should be available in locations where local anesthetics are used in potentially toxic doses.[85]
- Seizures may be managed with benzodiazepines (eg, midazolam 0.05-0.1 mg/kg), but alternatively with propofol (0.5-1.5 mg/kg) or barbiturates (thiopentone 1-2 mg/kg). Evidence exists that lipid emulsions can halt local anesthetic induced seizures, though this needs further evaluation.
- Profound hypotension can occur in both allergic reactions and systemic toxicity and usually responds well to vasopressors (eg, epinephrine) and plasma "expansion."
- Because reduced cardiac contractility is a core element in this condition, it is thought that the maintenance of coronary perfusion with the administration of epinephrine and norepinephrine improves outcome.[86] There is now laboratory evidence to suggest that epinephrine may impair resuscitation and reduce the efficacy of lipid therapy.[87]
- Animal model evidence exists that epinephrine can interfere with lipid emulsion rescue.[87] Current recommendations are to use epinephrine bolused in 10- to 100-mcg aliquots in the treatments of local anesthetic-induced hypotension.[85]
- However, malignant dysrhythmias, which particularly occur with bupivacaine systemic toxicity, should be controlled in a timely fashion because epinephrine can exacerbate these dysrhythmias.
- Therapeutic agents that are less arrhythmogenic have been investigated, including the use of vasopressin[88,89] and phosphodiesterase inhibitors such as milrinone and amrinone, though their use still needs to be validated clinically.[89,90]
- In addition to lipid treatment, ventricular arrhythmias should be suppressed primarily with amiodarone 300 mg IV, with repeat administration of up to 150 mg 3 to 5 minutes later.
- Effective resuscitation in this setting is difficult, and atrioventricular pacing and cardiopulmonary bypass are additional options in refractory cases.[91]

COMPLICATIONS OF PERIPHERAL NERVE BLOCKS

DIRECT NEEDLE TRAUMA TO THE NERVE

Auroy et al[57] reported an incidence of serious nerve injury (permanent sensory and/or motor loss) after peripheral nerve blocks (PNBs) as 1.9 per 10 000 nerve block cases; in this study, all patients with serious injury experienced either pain on injection, paresthesia, or both during the performance of the block. A more recent analysis of nearly 7000 blocks reported a similar incidence of 0.04% for late neurologic deficits after PNBs.[92] The incidence of minor neural injury after PNBs is in the range of 1% to 2%; most of these injuries are transient neurapraxias, which represent axonal disruption. Typically neurapraxia injuries are observed postoperatively when patients complain of persistent numbness in the distribution of a peripheral nerve. One cannot simply assume that all neurapraxia injuries are anesthesia related, as patient positioning, surgical trauma, and tourniquet application can all give rise to these symptoms. Numbness gradually regresses over a period of weeks and is rarely observed beyond 3 months, which is the amount of time required for axonal regeneration to occur.[93] Regional anesthesia-related injuries may be the result of needle trauma, injection pressure, or the toxic effects of local anesthetics or additives. It is generally agreed that the location within the nerve which is most sensitive to injury is the intrafascicular compartment.

Prevention Some suggest that most neural injuries are associated with either paresthesia or pain on injection. Needle damage or pressure generated during injection of local anesthetics account for most of these injuries.[57,94] Needle insertion without injection is a routine technique used during microneurography and surgical repair procedures, which results in insignificant nerve damage. It is more likely that significant nerve damage is caused or worsened by both mechanical and chemical injury during intraneural injections of neurotoxic substances (ie, local anesthetics). High-pressure injections cause mechanical destruction of the neural fascicular architecture, pathophysiologic damage, and neural scarring.[95] Chemically induced damage is also possible from high concentrations of local anesthetics, vasoconstrictors, preservatives, and other additives.

There is an ongoing debate among anesthesiologists about the safety of deliberately seeking paresthesia in regional anesthesia.[96] There is also concern about performing regional anesthesia in comatose/anesthetized patients because of the inability to detect paresthesia. Currently, there is no substantial evidence that performing nerve blocks in awake patients is any safer than performing them in anesthetized patients, and attitudes are shifting toward the acceptance of performing blocks in anesthetized individuals as the safety of PNBs in general continues to increase.[97]

Ultrasound imaging has been used to examine the location of needle placement as positioned using paraesthesia[98] and nerve stimulation as localization techniques.[99,100] The resounding finding has been that intraneural injection of local anesthetic may occur with a greater frequency than previously thought, without inevitably leading to neurologic complications. Moreover, the generally held assumption that nerve stimulation thresholds of less than 0.3mA may not reliably prevent intraneural injection. Comparing intraneural and extraneural stimulation thresholds in ultrasound-guided supraclavicular block, Bigeleisen et al[101] found that a stimulation current of 0.2 mA or less reliably predicts intraneural needle placement, but that a threshold current greater than 0.2 mA does not preclude intraneural placement. These results are based on the assumption that ultrasound can reliably visualize intraneural injection. Studies using pigs have shown that ultrasonographic nerve expansion during injection is consistent with intraneural injection as confirmed by histologic analysis.[102,103] It is important to note that at this time it is wise to avoid intraneural needle placement, particularly because ultrasound imaging at this time cannot ensure avoidance of the intrafascicular compartment, which has been shown to be the principal location for nerve trauma via mechanical or chemical means.

Common sense dictates that small-gauge needles are less likely to damage nerves than larger-gauge ones. More than 30 years ago, Selander et al[104] recommended using blunt needles when performing regional anesthesia, as it was thought that blunt needles were less likely to penetrate neural structures, and resultant intraneural injections would be less likely to occur; this recommendation was based on information derived from animal experiments. Selander's influence on this topic persists to this very day, even though subsequent studies showed that blunt needles, although far less likely to penetrate neural structures, are far more disruptive to neural tissue than sharp needles.[105] Nevertheless, there are no clinical trials supporting any recommendations regarding what type of needle is best for regional anesthesia procedures. Most clinicians prefer small-gauge, short, blunt needles.

Injection pressures may influence the amount of damage inflicted on a nerve. One study suggested that persistent motor deficits were observed in animals injected with pressures of 1293 mm Hg or greater.[106] Monitoring injection pressures is possible, although it is neither specific or sensitive enough to reliably predict neural injury.[106] Clinicians should avoid rapid and high-pressure injections. The difficulty with monitoring injection pressures is that subjective "resistance" is often relied on, which has shown to be unreliable.[107] One standardized technique that one of the authors (B.T.) routinely uses is the compressed air injection technique.[108] Using Boyle's law, the pressure can be kept significantly below 1293 mm Hg (mean was 745 mm Hg) by compressing air, previously aspirated above the fluid, to 50% of its initial volume before and during injections.

Sterilizing agents, skin-cleansing substances, detergents, and certain preservatives (eg, metabisulfite) all cause neurotoxicity and should be carefully avoided when introduced into perineural spaces.

The neurotoxicity of a local anesthetic is related to its potency and its concentration.[109] High-concentration local anesthetics such as 2% lidocaine and 0.75% bupivacaine should be avoided in peripheral nerve blocks. The addition of vasoconstrictors (eg, epinephrine) to local anesthetics may enhance the damage caused by an intraneural injection.[110-112]

Generally, neural damage resulting from peripheral nerve blocks is rare; consequently, it may be difficult to clearly demonstrate the safest equipment and techniques to be used. However, **Table 50-5** summarizes several measures to prevent nerve injuries.

Management When a neurologic injury is suspected postoperatively, a thorough history must be taken, and a complete physical examination must be performed and documented. Because most regional anesthesia procedures involve the percutaneous insertion of needles toward nerves, the burden often lies with the anesthesiologist to prove that damage was not caused as a result of improper technique and unsafe practice. Clinicians are obliged to maintain a very open mind when dealing with such challenging cases, as there can be a variety of causative factors (**Table 50-6**). The anesthesiologist should play a major role in determining the cause of the injury, as anesthesiologists have far more information concerning preoperative and intraoperative events than do most neurologists. Symptoms and signs of compression of the spinal cord must be dealt with urgently (within 6-8 h); otherwise, permanent paraplegia or quadriplegia may result. The anesthesiologist, neurologist, neurosurgeon, and radiologist must work as a team and strive to arrive at a diagnosis before serious permanent injury occurs. Diagnostic tools should be used judiciously to support the team of clinicians in arriving at a correct diagnosis; this is when we must rely on our neurology and radiology colleagues to guide us. Electrodiagnostic and imaging techniques can often take the guesswork out of many diagnostic dilemmas

TABLE 50-5 Suggested Methods/Equipment for Preventing Peripheral Nerve Injuries When Performing Regional Anesthesia

Needle type: small gauge, short beveled
Patient: awake with appropriate level of sedation
Nerve stimulation: use accurate nerve stimulators and insulated nerve needles (current at least >0.2 mA)
Ultrasonography: direct visualization of nerves and surrounding structures by using high-resolution ultrasound equipment if available
Paresthesia: injection should be stopped and needle repositioned if persistent
High injection pressure: avoid rapid and high-pressure injections (pressure <20 psi)
Local anesthetic: avoid high concentrations (ie, lidocaine 2% or bupivacaine 0.75%)

TABLE 50-6 Potential Causes of Neurologic Injury

Surgical causes to consider:

- Surgical trauma to neural structures from retractors, a scalpel blade, or tension within the surgical site may not have been mentioned to the anesthesiologist.
- Long-acting local anesthetics may have been injected by the surgeon.
- Compartment syndrome resulting from edema, or bleeding around the wound caused by dressings or casts, can compromise neural function.
- Vascular injury during the surgery could result in nerve injury (eg, spinal cord injury after thoracic aneurysm repair). Because of this, it is probably desirable to let the local anesthetic blockade abate after aortic surgery.
- Patient positioning must be reviewed to rule out direct pressure (eg, peroneal nerve at the fibular head) or tension on nerves (eg, traction on the brachial plexus from hyperextension of the shoulder during thoracotomy); improper patient positioning may produce nerve injury that might otherwise be attributed to a regional anesthetic mishap.

Anesthetic causes to consider:

- The details of anesthesia management should be thoroughly reviewed, especially if portions of the anesthetic care were delivered by other anesthesiologists.
- Drug choice, dose, and last time of administration should be recorded.
- Duration of nerve blockade should be noted; a long duration of blockade can result in neural injury.
- High concentrations of agents probably increase the risk of neural complications.
- Multiple nerve-blocking attempts can increase the risk of injury.
- The presence of paresthesia during needle insertion and the subsequent injection of local anesthetic can be a warning sign indicating neural injury.
- The level of sedation must be appropriated without compromising the ability to observe a paresthesia.

and allow for quick and precise diagnoses. **Figure 50-7** summarizes the key steps involved in determining neurologic injury.

Diagnostic Tools for the Determination of Nerve Injury The initial step in the diagnostic workup is to perform a thorough and well-documented history and physical examination, paying careful attention to the muscles innervated by the nerve(s) in question. Direct injury to the spinal cord, nerve roots, or peripheral nerves is best evaluated using imaging techniques, especially in the early stages of an injury. Electrophysiologic techniques are more useful in the later phases of an injury. The most common imaging modalities used are computerized tomography (CT)

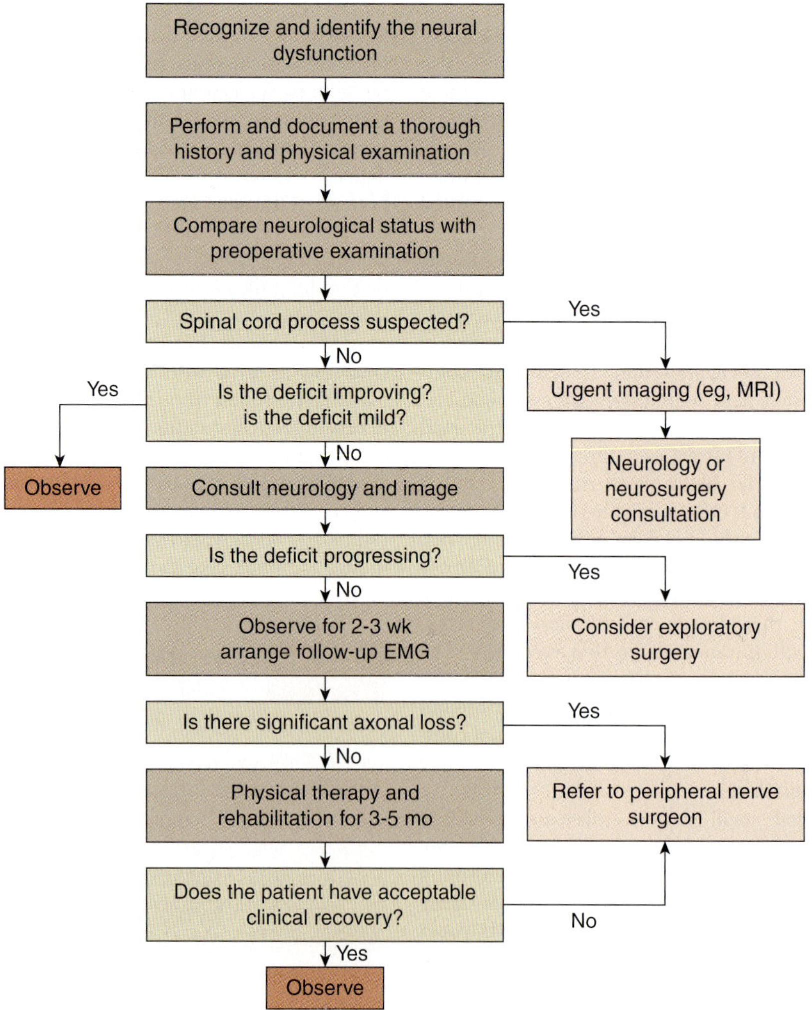

FIGURE 50-7. Algorithm outlining the steps to investigating and managing neurologic injury. EMG, electromyography; MRI, magnetic resonance imaging.

and magnetic resonance imaging (MRI). Electrodiagnostic techniques include evoked potentials, nerve conduction studies, and needle electrode examination of muscles (electromyography [EMG]). The use of these tools should complement the clinical examination, rather than replace an examination. Choosing the best tools/technologies for diagnosis should be a joint decision made with the neurologist, surgeon, and radiologist.

- CT is best suited for evaluating bony abnormalities.
- MRI is ideally suited for the examination of soft-tissue abnormalities, especially the spinal cord.
- For peripheral nerve, nerve plexus, and peripheral nerve complications, imaging is less likely to be useful for the demonstration of nerve injury.
- MRI may demonstrate the accumulation of blood and edema fluid, which can lead to compartment syndrome; MRI may also indicate neural compression caused by injury from the needle and local anesthetic injection.
- Nerve conduction studies test the function of large sensory and motor nerve fibers. Evaluating nerve conduction can reveal axonal loss or demyelination of the nerve; however, nerve conduction is less useful in timing lesions when the injury occurs.
- EMG is preferentially used for evaluating smaller motor units. EMG can be useful for the diagnosis of axonal injury and is also useful for quantitating the severity of the neurologic injury and for identifying the actual site of injury. EMG studies are typically recommended 2 to 3 weeks after an injury, although an early EMG studies are recommended 2 to 3 weeks after an injury.

The only effective way to manage neurologic complications is to prevent any mishaps from occurring in the first place, as there is limited chance of recovery once the damage has occurred. Neurologic consultation and testing should be considered if there are any persistent symptoms or signs after a procedure. If symptoms are mild and do not interfere with the patient's daily activities, reassurance can be offered after evaluating the extent and severity of the patient's symptoms. It is of prime importance to continue to follow patients suffering from nerve injury after discharge from the hospital; it is also necessary to instruct patients to seek medical attention if their symptoms worsen or do not improve. Most residual dysthesias or hypesthesias resolve in 4 to 6 weeks, and the majority are resolved (>99%) within 1 year.[113,114]

NEEDLE TRAUMA TO SURROUNDING STRUCTURES

Tissues within the vicinity of the PNB may be unintentionally injured. Vascular injury can also occur during PNB because many peripheral nerves travel in parallel with vascular structures. Other injuries may be caused by direct needle trauma, including pneumothorax and direct spinal cord injury.

SPINAL CORD INJURY

Permanent spinal cord injury after brachial plexus block is the most severe complication resulting from PNB. There are a number of reported spinal injuries associated with peripheral nerve blocks: an interscalene block performed with an 8-cm needle resulted in a permanent neural deficit at the C8-T1 level.[115] In another instance, an anesthetized patient suffered permanent spinal cord injury after an interscalene block.[116] A patient has suffered from Brown-Séquard syndrome after an attempted interscalene block using a spinal needle.[117] Other peripheral blocks may also increase the risk of spinal cord injury. Permanent spinal cord injuries may occur after paravertebral blocks because the needles used for paravertebral blocks are inserted in close proximity to the spinal cord.

Prevention It is important to note that most of the serious nerve injury cases reported involve deviations from the recommended anesthetic practice standards. Currently, it is recommended to perform these blocks in awake patients to detect paresthesia or pain on injection. Ultrasonography may help to reduce the risk of spinal injury as needle advancement can be observed in real time. It is important to note here that the use of ultrasound visualization should not preclude other precautionary means during performance of PNB. When performing ultrasound-guided techniques in close proximity to the spine, using a technique that directs the needle toward to spine should still be avoided. For instance, when aligning the needle to a sagittally positioned probe during lumbar plexus blockade, it is important to avoid out-of-plane technique from lateral to medial, which would direct the needle toward the spinal column.

The best option for avoiding the risk of nerve injury is to select a block insertion site remote from the spinal cord. Axillary blocks appear to be safer than supraclavicular blocks; however, supraclavicular approaches to the brachial plexus are required in shoulder surgery.

Small-gauge needles and short needles are strongly recommended when performing brachial blocks in the supraclavicular region. Longer-than-usual needles were associated with many of the spinal cord injuries associated with brachial plexus blocks.

Management There is no specific treatment for primary needle damage to the spinal cord. Nevertheless, the initial step in the management of spinal cord injury is the recognition and identification of neural dysfunction. Acute, potentially reversible causes of spinal cord injury, such as nerve compression from hematomas, must be identified and dealt with early (within 6-8 h); otherwise permanent paraplegia or quadriplegia may result. The anesthesiologist, neurologist, and radiologist must work as a team to arrive at a correct diagnosis. Appropriate electrodiagnostic and imaging techniques must be used to make a quick and precise diagnosis.

PNEUMOTHORAX

Any regional technique requiring needle insertion toward the lung involves the risk of pneumothorax. Pneumothorax has been an unwelcome complication of supraclavicular techniques since Kulenkampff[118] first described the classic supraclavicular approach in 1911. The incidence of pneumothorax is difficult to determine and varies depending on the approach. Brand and Papper[119] reported an incidence of 6.1% in a large teaching hospital using the classic Kulenkampff technique. The risk of pneumothorax has deterred many anesthesiologists from using the supraclavicular approach and is the most likely reason that axillary and infraclavicular approaches are popular. The risk of pneumothorax is much lower following the interscalene approach to the brachial plexus compared with the classic supraclavicular approach.[120] Ward[121] reported a 3% incidence of symptomatic pneumothorax following the interscalene technique. The risk of pneumothorax is reduced following the vertical technique mainly because the needle is not directed toward the lung.[122] More recently, however, case series of supraclavicular blocks performed with ultrasound guidance have reported the absence of any single clinically significant pneumothorax.[20,123] Although these studies are not large enough to detect the true incidence, the practice of supraclavicular blocks is being revisited.

Prevention Anesthetic techniques requiring the insertion of a needle directed toward the lung in the supraclavicular region all carry the risk of pneumothorax. Extra care should be exercised in tall, thin patients, as they appear to be at greater risk of pneumothorax. For all patients, a right-sided pneumothorax occurs more frequently because the cupola of the lung is higher on the right side. Patients should be warned in advance of this risk, and ambulatory patients should be given careful instructions on how to proceed should symptoms develop.

Supraclavicular approaches should be avoided in patients with severe impairment of pulmonary function. Blocks should never be performed bilaterally. Intuitively, complications can be avoided or reduced if clinicians are able to visualize the advancing needle approaching the target nerve or trunk. Ultrasonographic technology facilitates this goal in real time. However, this technique requires significant training and practical experience.

Management Because upper-extremity operations are carried out on ambulatory patients who are discharged within a few hours of surgery, it is important that patients be warned about the risk of pneumothorax before leaving the hospital. Patients who develop chest pain, dyspnea, or cyanosis after discharge should be instructed to go to the nearest emergency center. Symptoms and signs may not develop for hours, and patients may not become symptomatic until a 20% pneumothorax is present. Evacuation of the pneumothorax is usually required when the degree of lung collapse is 25% or greater.

Ultrasound Detection of Pneumothorax Ultrasound imaging can rule out or confirm pneumothorax both effectively and efficiently and is better than bedside chest radiographs.[124] This said, acquiring the prerequisite imaging technique to master interpretation of both normal and pathologic lung signs requires time and effort. Ultrasonography to detect pneumothorax should be performed at the anteroinferior aspect of the thorax in a supine patient; a large majority of cases involve the anterior zone, and this area is involved in most if not all life-threatening cases.

TOXIC EFFECTS OF LOCAL ANESTHETICS ON NERVES AND SURROUNDING STRUCTURES

NEURAL TOXICITY

Local anesthetics are considered harmless substances when injected perineurally in appropriate concentrations and quantities. High concentrations of local anesthetics can permanently damage neural tissue in some instances.[125] Preservatives in local anesthetic drugs may also damage nerves and other surrounding tissues. In the United States during the 1970s, it was noted that a change in the constitution of a sodium metabisulfite, a preservative found in chloroprocaine, resulted in several cases of cauda equina syndrome.[126] The addition of ethylenediaminetetraacetic acid (EDTA) to chloroprocaine is associated with severe back pain in some patients after epidural anesthesia.[127,128] Studies show that 5% hyperbaric lidocaine for spinal anesthesia is linked to the syndrome transient neurologic symptoms (TNS).[129]

MYOTOXICITY

Myotoxicity is a recognized complication of intramuscular injections of local anesthetics.[130] Local anesthetics are proposed to cause a pathologic efflux of Ca^{2+} from the sarcoplasmic reticulum, resulting in contracture, cell destruction, and necrosis. After this occurrence, the regeneration of fibrils occurs within a few weeks. Among the local anesthetics tested, bupivacaine caused the most damage, and procaine caused the least.[131] Injury was noted to be worse with repeated injections and when epinephrine was used.[132-134] In clinical practice, myotoxicity is largely unnoticed except in ophthalmic regional anesthesia. Diplopia has been reported after retrobulbar blocks; however, this symptom is short-lived in most cases, and permanent damage is rare. Ropivacaine was found to be less myotoxic than bupivacaine in an animal model.[135] The full implications of the effects of local anesthetics on muscle have not yet been evaluated.

PHRENIC NERVE PARALYSIS

The incidence of hemidiaphragmatic paresis and decreased respiratory function after supraclavicular blocks in 8 healthy volunteers was noted; the overall incidence of paresis was 50% after the administration of 30 mL of lidocaine 1.5% with epinephrine, and none of the volunteers reported respiratory symptoms.[152] However, anecdotal reports exist concerning patients who are devoid of respiratory disease and who later became symptomatic after an interscalene block.[121,137-139]

Temporary phrenic nerve paralysis after interscalene brachial plexus block is expected in up to 100% of cases. Permanent phrenic nerve palsy has been observed after interscalene block,[140] but is extremely rare.[141]

Phrenic nerve paresis is common after supraclavicular blocks, regardless of the technique used, yet patients do not usually become symptomatic.[142,143] In another study, the effects of ipsilateral hemidiaphragmatic paralysis on respiratory function after continuous interscalene blocking showed that all patients had a 27% reduction in forced vital capacity, a reduced forced expiratory volume of 26%, and a decreased peak expiratory flow rate.[144]

Thus the use of supraclavicular techniques in certain groups of patients must be considered carefully. Supraclavicular techniques may need to be avoided in patients with advanced pulmonary disease. Bilateral supraclavicular techniques are *absolutely* contraindicated.

Detection of Hemidiaphragmatic Paresis Using Ultrasonography By observations of diaphragmatic excursion, ultrasound is a practical, sensitive, and low-risk method for detecting ipsilateral hemidiaphragmatic paresis after PNB.[142,145] The primary diagnosis is paradoxical cephalad motion as compared with normal active caudad motion on inspiration.

HORNER SYNDROME

Horner syndrome (ipsilateral, miosis, ptosis, enophthalmos, loss of sweating) is frequently observed after supraclavicular approaches to the brachial plexus, although its incidence may be lower when ultrasound is used to guide the supraclavicular approach,[30,146] and patients and other caregivers should be informed of this temporary distortion to avoid diagnostic confusion.

HOARSENESS

Hoarseness may occur if the local anesthetic spreads to the recurrent laryngeal nerve. Specific management is not required, as the symptoms will abate as the anesthetic wears off. Persistent hoarseness should urge the clinician to consider an alternative cause.

PREVENTION/MANAGEMENT OF LOCALIZED TRAUMA/TOXICITY

The key to preventing complications associated with PNB is to increase the accuracy of needle placement and to use the minimum volume and concentration of local anesthetic required to produce a successful and high-quality block. Ultrasonography has revolutionized regional anesthesia, as sonography makes it possible to directly visualize the needle tip and local anesthetic spread in real time while ensuring the avoidance of critical structures. Perhaps the greatest advantage of ultrasound guidance is the ability to reposition the needle after injecting a test dose of local anesthetic or alternative (D_5W) and failing to observe adequate or appropriate spread.[146] Although the evidence base at this time is limited for improved safety with ultrasound-guided brachial plexus blocks,[147] and although there have been reports of nerve injury after and vascular punctures during ultrasound-guided PNB,[41,42] our increasing experience as well as others' has shown promise in this area. Like any other technological advance, receiving proper training and gaining experience is critical with real-time ultrasonography. This is particularly critical for obtaining and maintaining needle control and visibility. As with other adverse effects, careful diagnosis of brachial plexus complications and the provision of supportive measures are essential for proper clinical management.

COMPLICATIONS OF NEURAXIAL BLOCKS (EPIDURAL/SPINAL)

DIRECT NEEDLE TRAUMA

As a needle or catheter is advanced into the epidural space, direct trauma to the spinal cord, conus medullaris, and spinal nerve roots can occur. Sensory loss and, less commonly, motor deficits occur as a result of spinal cord trauma. Some patients recover completely; however, the injury persists in the many of patients. The incidence of spinal cord trauma is very low, and much of the data available comes from retrospective sources. In a prospective multicenter study, Auroy et al[57] found 5 cases of radiculopathy after 30 413 epidurals. In each of these patients, pain or paresthesia was noted during needle insertion and drug administration, and the radiculopathy was observed in the distribution of the associated paresthesia. One of the most disturbing complications of neuraxial blockade is neurologic injury. Three well-known syndromes are associated with damage to the spinal cord, roots, and coverings: cauda equina syndrome, adhesive arachnoiditis, and anterior spinal artery syndrome. These syndromes are addressed in other chapters.

Prevention To avoid nerve trauma, a studied technique and accurate anatomic knowledge is a prerequisite.[149] Although epidural placement in the anesthetized child is considered safe, similar placement in the adult population remains controversial. Recent case reports highlight the potential for neurologic trauma when performing epidural anesthesia in the anesthetized patient.[150-152] The use of the stimulating epidural catheters allows pediatric anesthesiologists to place lumbar or thoracic epidurals from the caudal space, minimizing the risk of needle-mediated nerve injury.[28] When performing an epidural in an awake, cooperative adult, needle advancement should be halted if the patient complains of pain. In most adults, the spinal cord terminates at the lower portion of the body of L1; however, there are considerable variations among individuals. The ability of the clinician to correctly identify lumbar spinous interspaces has been questioned by Broadbent et al[153] using magnetic resonance imaging. In this study, only 29% of the interspaces were correctly identified, whereas 51% of the time clinicians were at a higher vertebral level than anticipated; furthermore, the spinal cord terminated below L1 in 19% of subjects. One explanation for inaccuracy in determining the level of needle placement in the lumbar region is that the Tuffier line is not a fixed landmark, nor is the conus medullaris.[154-156] Fortunately the variation in these landmarks is such that there is almost always a safety margin of 2 to 4 vertebrae between the Tuffier line and the conus medullaris. With advancing age, however, this safety margin narrows. Furthermore, with the increasing incidence of obesity in our population, there is a tendency to estimate the Tuffier line to be at a higher level. Therefore, one should be particularly attuned to anatomic variation when performing spinal anesthesia in elderly obese patients. There are very few reports of spinal cord damage caused by errant needle placement in the literature, the reason being that many of these cases enter the court system and are subsequently not published, at least in the medical literature. Reynolds[157] published some information about this problem about 10 years ago. She accumulated 7 case reports (6 of which were obstetric) of spinal cord trauma after spinal anesthesia and indicated that there were several more cases pending in the United Kingdom. It is very important to take the time to identify the landmarks in every patient and if in doubt seek verification of the landmarks using ultrasonography, performed by an experienced spinal sonographer, or just a plain x-ray.

Although the use of ultrasound has been used to assess determination of the intervertebral level through palpation,[153] the learning curve for having accuracy with determining interspaces is shallow, with only 27% of anesthesiologists achieving competency within 20 trials (2 min each).[158] Paresthesia associated with spinal cord injury can occur at the time of needle placement, yet it may also occur during the injection of the solution or as a secondary consequence of irritation, edema, or hematoma.[159,160] Pain is more commonly associated with extra-axial lesions affecting the nerve roots or blood vessels that are innervated by pain-mediating sensory neurons.[161] In contrast, because there are no pain receptors within the spinal cord (or the brain), intra-axial trauma may be painless[161]; this allows percutaneous cervical cordotomy to be performed in awake patients.[162,163] During this procedure, the cervical cord is typically punctured multiple times with a 22-gauge needle electrode, yet the patient generally describes neither pain nor paresthesia.[164] In addition, pain after dural puncture is rare in clinical practice. Thus anesthesiologists should be reminded that they should not simply assume that paresthesia will always be reported as the needle encroaches on the spinal cord.[165,166] However, one might expect a motor response if a needle encroaches on a motor tract during attempts at epidural anesthesia. Electrical stimulation during epidural needle advancement may provide an additional warning sign.[147,148]

Ischemic injuries are among the rarest complications reported after regional anesthesia procedures; however, when such injuries occur, several factors play a role, including hypotension, abnormal positioning, vascular disease, diabetes mellitus, and the clamping of major vessels.[94,169] In short, the addition of epinephrine to local anesthetic solutions has both advantages and disadvantages.[170] In an animal study in which epinephrine and phenylephrine were administered, a significant reduction in dural blood flow but no reduction in spinal cord blood flow occured.[171]

Management The management of postoperative neurologic sequelae requires the cooperation of the anesthesiologist, surgeon, and neurologist. Advice may also be required from the radiologist and neurosurgeon. Although it is easy to blame an adverse neurologic outcome on the presence of an epidural, it should be borne in mind that other factors can lead to demonstrable nerve injury, including undiagnosed preexisting neurologic disorders, ligation of nutrient spinal cord vessels during abdominal or thoracic surgery, injury to the femoral nerve during pelvic surgery, injury to the lateral cutaneous nerve of the thigh during retraction close to the inguinal ligament, and pressure on the fibular head leading to neurapraxia of the lateral popliteal nerve. If an adverse outcome occurs, the lesion should be localized by taking the patient's history and by performing a thorough neurologic examination. Some factors enabling differential diagnosis are as follows:

- Bilateral symptoms associated with pain should alert one to the possibility of neuraxial pathology.
- Injury at the nerve roots affects both posterior and anterior rami.
- Preservation of sensation over the paraspinous muscles suggests a more distal injury.
- Investigations should include blood cultures and coagulation studies.
- Immediate MRI is the standard for evaluating neuraxial lesions.
- EMG can be used to determine the site of injury and the degree of axonal loss, although it may take up to 3 weeks for changes to appear on the electromyogram. It may be useful to perform this immediately upon recognition of neural dysfunction to establish the possibility of a preexisting lesion.

HEMATOMA

Epidural hematoma after neuraxial anesthesia is a rare event. Bleeding from an epidural vein may occur on needle or catheter insertion, but is usually self-limiting. Neurologic symptoms and signs caused by an epidural hematoma are atypical in the presence of normal coagulation. The true incidence is unknown, but is estimated to occur in fewer than 1 in 150 000 cases of neuraxial anesthesia.[172] Vandermeulen et al[173] reviewed 61 case reports between 1906 and 1994 and found that two-thirds of the cases had a hemostatic abnormality. Early diagnosis and intervention are essential to preventing any long-term adverse outcomes.

Prevention In recent years, new anticoagulant and antiplatelet drugs have been introduced and have given rise to new challenges in the management of the anticoagulated patient undergoing neuraxial blockade. The American Society of Regional Anesthesia has released guidelines in response to this evolving shift in medical practice[172]; it is important to follow these guidelines to minimize the risk of hematoma.

Management Similar to the peripheral nerve injury, the evaluation of neurologic injury after regional anesthesia is a vital part of adverse outcome management. Several issues should be considered:

- Back pain with lower-limb weakness and sensory deficit should alert the clinician to the presence of a central compressing lesion.
- Bowel and bladder incontinence can be an associated finding.

- Painless evolution of this complication has been reported, and early warning signs may be masked by the administration of local anesthetic via an epidural catheter and the presence of a urinary catheter.
- If MRI confirms the diagnosis, then rapid surgical intervention within 6 to 8 hours is recommended.
- Epidural catheters containing metal elements should be avoided while undergoing MRI, as it will generate artificial interference and inaccurate diagnoses and poses other additional risks.[174] Such catheters should be removed if it is safe to do so; if catheter removal is unsafe, a CT scan should be considered instead of an MRI.

INFECTION

Epidural abscess formation, although rare, is a serious, potentially devastating complication. Kane's[175] retrospective review of 50 000 epidurals found no case of abscess formation, whereas Moen et al[176] reported 12 cases of abscess formation from an estimated 250 000 patients after epidural insertion. Nine of these patients had risk factors predisposing them to infection. Six of the patients received their epidural for analgesia after trauma, and of these, 5 were thoracic epidurals for chest trauma. The authors speculated that the overrepresentation of thoracic trauma patients might in part be a result of a lesser hygienic standard being observed, where placement likely occurred outside the "cleaner" environment of the operating suite.

Although the immunocompromised patient may carry a greater risk of developing infective complications with epidural use, extensive experience using epidural analgesia and anesthesia with patients who have HIV has countered early fears surrounding regional anesthesia in this population. Regional anesthesia is particularly beneficial for the HIV carrier population, as it eliminates delayed metabolism of systemic opioids caused by protease inhibitors.[177] Patients with AIDS often have neurologic manifestations of their disease, and the prevalence of peripheral neuropathy increases as the disease progresses.[178] Attention should be given to assessing preoperative neurologic status, as this allows the clinician to correctly attribute post-block neurologic sequelae to the true underlying cause.

Epidural abscess presentation can be variable, but the cardinal symptoms and signs involve back pain with localized tenderness and fever that often develop days after the puncture. Leukocytosis would be expected in the presence of an epidural-induced abscess and may occur several days or months after needle and catheter insertion. After the formation of an epidural abscess, the patient can develop progressive weakness and may develop paraplegia if untreated. Meningitis may develop if the patient has endured a lumbar puncture in this setting. The most common pathogen involved in abscess formation is *Staphylococcus aureus*; it should act as a standard for guiding antibiotic treatment until definitive culture results are available. As with an epidural hematoma, prompt surgical consultation is warranted for potential abscess drainage.

In pediatric patients, there is some concern regarding catheter infection with prolonged use of caudally placed catheters because of the proximity of the sacral hiatus to the anal region. Although studies have not found clinical evidence of greater infection rates with the caudal approach to catheter placement, increased bacterial colonization has been reported with this technique. *Staphylococcus epidermidis* was the predominant microorganism colonized on the skin and catheters of lumbar and caudal epidurals, and gram-negative bacteria were also found on tips of caudal catheters.[179] Although the overall infection rate associated with caudal epidural catheters appears to be quite low, tunneling caudal catheters or simply fixing the catheter with occlusive dressing in an immediate cephalad direction has been recommended to reduce the risk of contamination by stool and urine.[28,180]

Prevention Epidural abscesses can occur spontaneously (a reported incidence of 0.2 to 2 per 10 000 hospital admissions per year),[181] and lumbar puncture has been safely performed in potentially bacteremic patients.[182] Following is a list of guidelines for the prevention of epidural abscess formation:

- Sound aseptic technique, monitoring of the infection site, antibiotic prophylaxis, and bacterial filter use all contribute to a lower incidence of epidural space infections.
- Although both lidocaine and bupivacaine are bactericidal in high concentration, this property is likely not clinically significant at the concentrations used in practice.[183]
- The performance of neuraxial block should be avoided where local infection exists at the needle entry site.

Management Following is a list of guidelines for the management of epidural abscess formation:

- Daily catheter site inspection is essential for the early identification of epidural abscess formation.
- Prompt removal of the catheter is essential when erythema and local discharge are present.
- Carefully assess any symptoms or signs of back pain.
- If any neural dysfunction occurs, a diagnosis must be immediately made in order to evaluate infective causes.
- Once a diagnosis of epidural abscess is made, a combination of medical (antibiotic) and surgical (incision and drainage) treatment may be needed.

TOTAL SPINAL ANESTHESIA

Total spinal anesthesia occurs when an excessive dose of local anesthetic is injected into the subarachnoid space; this is usually the result of an unintentional injection of a dose of local anesthetic intended for the epidural space. A high spinal may be seen when a small epidural dose or a large spinal dose of local anesthetic enters the subarachnoid space. Obstetric patients are particularly vulnerable because the engorged epidural venous plexus reduces spinal CSF volume and predisposes this population to cephalad local anesthetic spread. Total spinal anesthesia is rarely seen in nonobstetric cases, as observed by Dawkins, who reported an incidence of 0.2% of total spinal anesthesia in 48 000 patients undergoing epidural anesthesia.[56]

Prevention To prevent total spinal anesthesia from occurring, it is essential to use standard technique when aspirating, and an epidural test dose should be used. The subsequent use of small, incremental doses of local anesthetics may reduce the risk of this complication. The use of electrical stimulation is a useful and reliable real-time technique that can be used as an adjuvant tool for ruling out intrathecal placement before the administration of a potentially large test dose (Table 50-3).

Management Total spinal anesthesia is a true medical emergency, as patients become profoundly hypotensive, apneic, and unconscious with remarkable pupillary dilation. Resuscitation with endotracheal intubation, mechanical ventilation, and vasopressor therapy is frequently required, and recovery may take between 30 minutes and 6 hours, depending on the agent used and the type of dose administered. Cerebrospinal fluid lavage via an epidural catheter has been used to successfully treat a total spinal in a 14-year-old child; in this case, the patient recovered within 30 minutes.[184]

With a high spinal, the patient may complain of numbness in the hands or may have difficulty breathing; if this occurs, the situation can usually be managed with reassurance, careful use of sedation, and treatment of hypotension. Respiratory function should be closely monitored with pulse oximetry, and measurements of adequate airflow should be made.[185] The potency of sedative agents is increased in the presence of a high spinal,[186-188] and one should be prepared to intervene in the event of significant respiratory compromise.

SUBDURAL INJECTIONS OF LOCAL ANESTHETIC DRUGS

The subdural space is a potential space between the dura and the arachnoid that extends from the level of the second sacral vertebra up to the

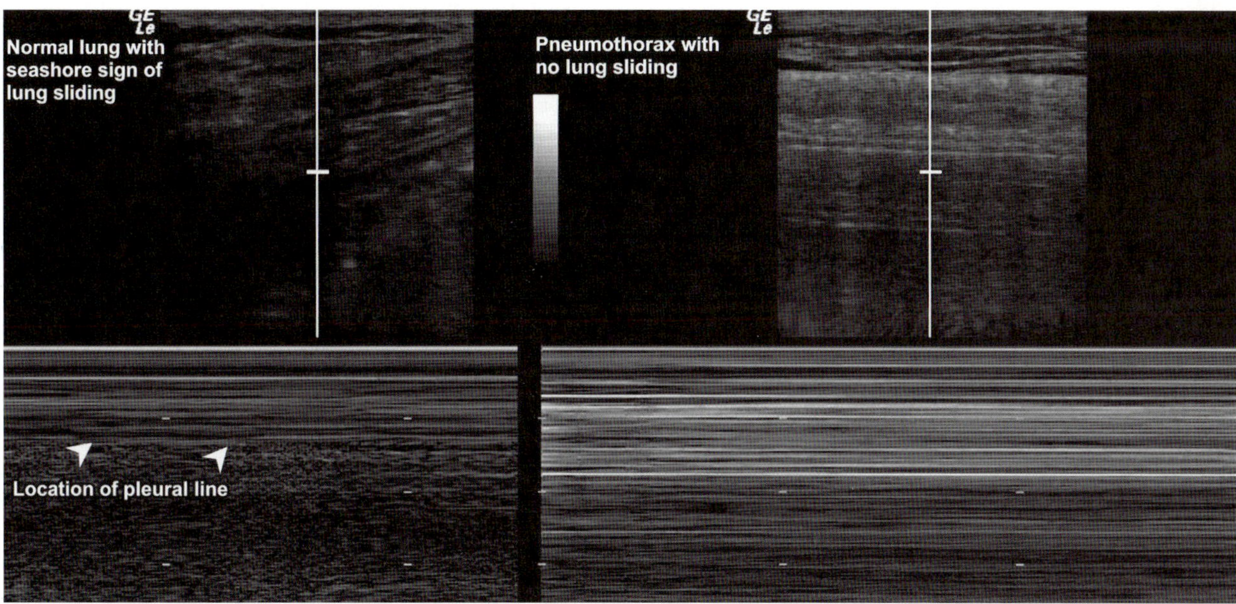

FIGURE 50-8. Ultrasound images of normal lung with the "seashore" appearance of lung sliding (*left*) and of left pneumothorax with abolished lung sliding (*right*).

floor of the third ventricle; the subdural space differs from the epidural space in that it is both extra- and intracranial. This space envelops the cranial and spinal nerves for a short distance and is widest in the cervical area. The incidence of subdural injections of local anesthetic drugs is reported to range from 0.1% to 0.8%,[189] and this occurs more frequently after epidural injections.[190] However, subdural injection may be an explanation for the occasional failed spinal anesthesia when pencil-point needles with side apertures are used. The design of a pencil-point needle with side apertures makes it possible for the opening to exist partially in both the subarachnoid and the subdural spaces.[191] The diagnosis of a subdural catheter placement is best achieved using an injection of radiopaque dye. A typical radiologic pattern is pathognomic of subdural catheter placement (**Fig. 50-9**).

Prevention Extra care should be exercised in patients who have had previous back surgery or a dural puncture at the same or adjoining interspace, as subdural injections are more likely to occur in these patients. Clinically, the subdural injection of local anesthetic drugs should be suspected when motor or sensory changes do not follow the expected pattern. Subdural injections result in a very slow onset of motor and sensory anesthesia and extensive and/or patchy sensory blocking.[22] Patients may also complain of respiratory difficulties and may appear obtunded. The degree of cardiovascular depression may vary but hypotension is usually not severe; however, rapid onset of cardiovascular depression with concurrent loss of consciousness can result within 2 minutes, and cardiorespiratory arrest has been reported in the obstetric setting.[192] Based on cases reported, the epidural stimulation test appears to be a potential diagnostic test providing information about the location of the needle or catheter in the subdural space.[21,22]

Management The treatment of subdural injections of local anesthetics is predominantly supportive. Patients sometimes require intubation, ventilation, and sedation and usually recover within 6 hours of the injection.

SYSTEMIC AND LOCAL TOXICITY

Unintentional intravascular catheter placement can go unrecognized and may lead to local anesthetic toxicity. There has been a dramatic decline in the incidence of systemic toxic reactions to local anesthetics after epidural anesthesia within the past 30 years. Dawkins[56] reported a 0.2% incidence of toxicity in a retrospective analysis of 48 292 cases of epidural anesthesia in 1969; this series included thoracic, lumbar, and sacral epidurals. More recently, Brown et al[193] reported a 0.01% incidence of toxicity after lumbar epidural anesthesia in a retrospective study of 16 870 cases and a 0.69% incidence of toxicity after caudal epidural anesthesia in a series of 1295 cases. This 20-fold reduction in toxic reactions after epidural anesthesia during the past 30 years is explained, in part, by significant changes in regional anesthesia practice and by the influence of regional anesthesia societies in North America, Europe, Asia, Australia,

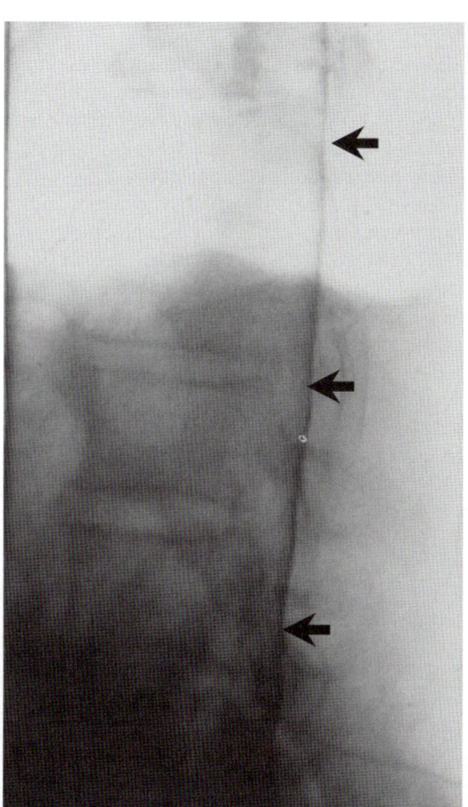

FIGURE 50-9. Radiograph showing pathognomic patten of subdural catheter placement.

and New Zealand. In the early 1980s, several deaths were reported in the United States after accidental intravascular injections of bupivacaine while performing epidural anesthesia. These deaths occurred as a result of cardiac toxicity that had not been previously reported with bupivacaine.[194] Several deaths were also reported in the United Kingdom when bupivacaine was used for intravenous regional anesthesia.[195] These tragedies led to a practice change in regional anesthesia. Single-injection epidural techniques commonly practiced 30 years ago have been replaced by continuous techniques involving injections of small incremental doses of local anesthetics; subsequently, "test dosing" has become a standard when using local anesthetics in regional anesthesia. Bupivacaine was implicated in 50% of toxic reactions reported by Auroy et al[57] and in a large percentage of cases in Brown et al's study.[193]

Prevention/Management To avoid potential local toxicity, local anesthetic free of preservatives in an appropriate concentration should be considered for use in the neuraxial space.

For epidural catheter anesthesia, using soft-tipped catheters (eg, metal-reinforced catheter) may reduce the introduction of the catheter into the vessel.[196] The most important aspects of prevention were discussed in the local anesthetic section earlier. In summary, aspiration, test doses, and incremental dosing are vital to preventing local and systemic toxicity.

The epidural stimulation test has the potential to detect intravascular catheter placement and should not be overlooked.[20]

POSTDURAL PUNCTURE HEADACHE

Postdural puncture headache (PDPH) is a widely discussed and published topic in regional anesthesia; it is also one of the most common complications of epidural and spinal anesthesia. Advances in needle design and gauge, as well as a better understanding of the physiologic mechanism of PDPH, have dramatically reduced the incidence of PDPH associated with spinal anesthesia, even in the obstetric population.[197] However, the incidence of PDPH after epidural anesthesia in obstetric patients remains unchanged, with headaches ranging from 0 to 2.6% of cases.[197]

Prevention Prevention of PDPH relies on the education of clinicians regarding the factors influencing the incidence of PDPH; such information is based on previous clinical case reports and studies. There is a strong link between onset of headache and needle gauge, age, sex, pregnancy, bevel design, and bevel orientation.

The dura consists of a mixture of elastic collagen and elastin fibers contained in a viscous intercellular ground substance[196]; it is primarily a longitudinally oriented structure, and its greatest tensile strength and stiffness exists in the longitudinal orientation. When a needle penetrates the dura, the size of the defect will be dependent on the number of elastin fibers cut, as well as by the tendency of those cut fibers to recoil in opposing directions, creating a crescent-shaped defect. As the gauge of the needle increases, more elastic fibers are cut. Fink[197] examined the dura of elderly cadavers and found less viscoelastic material and more fibrous connective tissue. Young patients are at greatest risk of PDPH, as their greater dural elasticity maintains a patent defect compared with the less elastic dura of the elderly.

Norris et al[200] demonstrated the importance of bevel orientation in relation to the incidence of PDPH after penetration of the dura with an epidural needle. Lybecker et al[201] suggested that bevel orientation may be even more important than needle gauge and was unable to show any difference in PDPH when using 22- and 25-gauge needles, provided that the bevel was vertically oriented. Ready et al[202] suggested that the incidence of PDPH is reduced when the needle is placed in an oblique direction. The arachnoid is closely adherent to the dura, and when a needle is advanced perpendicularly, the holes made by the bevel in the dura and arachnoid regions are directly in line with one another. When a needle is directed obliquely, the dural puncture does not line up with that in the arachnoid layer, thus obstructing CSF leakage.

Needle design has been implicated as a factor in the development of PDPH. Blunt-pointed needles (eg, Sprotte, Whitacre) are linked to a reduced incidence of PDPH as opposed to sharp cutting-point needles (eg, Quincke). Blunt needles rather than sharp needles are the tool of choice, particularly in patients with a high risk of developing PDPH (eg, adolescent and young adult patients). The most effective way to treat PDPH is to prevent this problem in the first place. The principal factor responsible for the development of PDPH is the size of the dural perforation. Thus smaller, blunt needles should be used for spinal anesthesia. On the other hand, the most commonly used epidural needle used is the 16- or 17-gauge Tuohy needle for continuous epidural anesthesia.

Treatment After unintentional dural puncture with a Tuohy needle during epidural catheter placement, some authors suggest that the epidural catheter should be advanced through the puncture hole in an effort to reduce the incidence of PDPH. Intrathecal placement of the epidural catheters after accidental dural puncture in the obstetric setting is common practice in some centers.[203] It is thought that the presence of the epidural catheter generates an inflammatory response, leading to early closure of the dural defect.[204] Because the epidural catheter is in the intrathecal space in this circumstance, extreme caution should be exercised to treat this catheter as a spinal catheter to avoid possible neurologic complications and infection.[197] Conservative measures, including bedrest and oral hydration, remain popular therapies for PDPH, despite no evidence to support them. Bedrest may postpone the occurrence of the headache, yet it does not prevent the onset.[205] Obstetric patients should be encouraged to mobilize soon after delivery, so that PDPH, if present, can be diagnosed and treated while yet in the hospital.

Mild headaches can be treated with intravenous fluids, caffeine, and theophylline; methylxanthines may block cerebral adenosine receptors, leading to cerebral vasoconstriction, although this proposed mechanism is controversial.[206] Camann et al[207] have demonstrated the efficacy of caffeine in 40 postpartum patients. A single oral dose of caffeine is safe, less expensive than intravenous caffeine, and may offer temporary relief. The evidence for both the therapeutic and prophylactic use of caffeine has been called into question after a systematic review of the literature.[206] Caffeine is a potent CNS stimulant and should be avoided in women who have pregnancy-induced hypertension, as it may lower the seizure threshold.[208] When considering the usage of caffeine as treatment for mild headache, it is worth noting that the cerebral vasoconstrictive properties of caffeine are transient, and the headache may return after 48 hours.

Sumatriptan is a serotonin type 1-*d* receptor agonist and has been used for cluster headaches and migraine and has been suggested as a treatment of PDPH.[209] Currently, it is not routinely recommended for use for the treatment of PDPH.[210] Further analysis of frovatriptan is required before it can be considered a useful prophylactic agent.[211]

Cosyntropin, the synthetic form of adrenocorticotropic hormone, has been used to treat PDPH; this pharmaceutical is thought to work by stimulating CSF production and β-endorphin output.[212]

EPIDURAL BLOOD PATCH

The epidural blood patch (EBP) was introduced by Gormley in 1960 and is known to be the most effective treatment for PDPH. Gormley[213] observed that patients who bled during myelography had a lower incidence of PDPH, and when he himself subsequently developed PDPH, he requested an injection of autologous blood into his epidural space with the positive result of the alleviation of his headache. In 1970, the report of DiGiovanni and Dunbar[214] of the successful use of epidural blood patching in 41 of 45 patients led to its popularization. This form of treatment is indicated when conservative measures have failed and the headache is severe or is likely to extend the hospital stay. The success rate for a first epidural blood patch is 85%, rising to 98% after a second patch.

DiGiovanni et al[215] suggested that an epidural blood patch acts as a gelatinous tamponade, and when injected, the blood generates sufficient pressure to lift the brain; this author has suggested that blood acts as a sealant, plugging the hole created by the needle, thus preventing further CSF leakage. Magnetic resonance images displaying the lumbar region after blood patching show a mass effect that compresses the thecal sac and conus. The blood spreads 3 to 5 spinal segments from the injection site and spreads mostly in the cephalad direction. This finding was confirmed by Szeinfeld et al[216] using tagged red cells demonstrating extension of the blood 6 segments in the cephalad direction and 3 in the caudad direction after the injection of an average of 14.8 mL of autologous blood. The mass effect persists beyond 3 hours, and clot resolution occurs in 7 hours.[217] Symptoms are frequently relieved within minutes of the procedure, and this response supports the counterpressure theory.

When performing an EBP, care should be taken to maintain a sterile field, and the epidural space should be identified in the usual manner. An assistant draws 15 to 20 mL of autologous blood aseptically. The administration of blood should be done at a rate of 1 mL/3 s. The end point of injection occurs when the patient complains of back, neck, or buttock pain as classically described by Szeinfeld et al.[216] Much less blood is required for blood patches in the midthoracic region than in the lumbar region, usually in the order of 5 to 10 mL.

To ensure adequate healing, the patient should remain recumbent for 1 to 2 hours after a blood patch and may resume ambulation thereafter; the patient should refrain from any strenuous activity for several days.

Complications from EBPs are rare, but can be serious. Transient bradycardia, lumbovertebral syndrome, and facial palsy have all been reported.[218-221] One case of cauda equina syndrome has been reported in a patient who was subjected to 6 blood patches; the patient made a full recovery after evacuation.[222]

EBP has been successfully performed in children. A caudal blood patch has been reported by Kowbel in a 4-year-old child who developed a subarachnoid cutaneous fistula after repeated lumbar punctures for chemotherapy.[223] In this situation, the epidural blood patch was performed by passing an epidural catheter via the caudal canal and by injecting 8 mL of blood. A lumbar EBP has been performed in a 7-year-old child.[224]

Blood patches have been safely performed in HIV-positive patients. HIV crosses the blood–brain barrier and infects the CNS early in the clinical course. EBP is unlikely to introduce HIV into the CNS.[203]

Prophylactic Epidural Blood Patching Prophylactic blood patches are controversial and have supporters and detractors.[225,226] The effectiveness of using EBP as a prophylactic depends on the proximity of the catheter tip to the dural tear. Although blood patching is a relatively safe procedure, there are some risks associated with its use, and patients do not always get a headache after dural puncture, even with a large-gauge needle. Aldrete and Brown[227] describe a case of intrathecal hematoma and arachnoiditis after prophylactic blood patching through a catheter. Meta-analysis of studies considering the prophylactic use of EBPs concluded that there are not enough trial participants to reliably draw conclusions.[228]

Alternatives to the Epidural Blood Patch

- Epidural saline treatment has been used for PDPH, but it is significantly less effective than EBP.[228] Successful use of prolonged saline infusion has been reported in patients with failed EBP.[229,230]
- Fibrin glue, a pooled plasma product, has been used to treat CSF leak in cancer patients[229] and in PDPH cases after spinal anesthesia where 2 EBPs had failed.[230]
- Dextran-40 has also been used to treat PDPH as it undergoes delayed absorption from the epidural space because of its high viscosity and molecular weight.[231]

FAILURE OF SPINAL/EPIDURAL ANESTHESIA

Failure of neuraxial blockade is more common with epidural rather than spinal anesthesia. Thus this section focuses on discussing failed epidural anesthesia. Anesthesiologists recognize entry into the *subarachnoid space* by the tactile sensation produced and the visual element of CSF. On the other hand, anesthesiologists generally recognize entry into the *epidural space* by the tactile sensation produced when using the LOR technique and the ease of epidural catheter insertion. Thus entry into the epidural space is purely tactile in many cases, and the end point of entry is subject to more misinterpretation than that of spinal anesthesia. In epidural anesthesia, false LOR may occur, and quite often the only proof that the needle is correctly positioned is that a successful block occurs. False losses of resistance are more frequently encountered in obese patients in whom anatomy may be ill-defined. The less fibrous tissue planes in neonates limit tactile feedback.[234] Moreover, Sharrock[235] suggested that false loss of resistance may also occur in the elderly who have a high incidence of cyst formation within the interspinous ligaments.

Prevention An important distinction that should be made during epidural anesthesia is that of complete failure versus a partial blockade/failure. The inability to pass a catheter into the epidural space frequently indicates that the needle is not in the epidural space. Catheters may become occluded with blood, or the catheter may kink, take a unilateral course, break, or become knotted, all of which can contribute to the complete failure of epidural anesthesia. The presence of a midline epidural band has been suggested[236] and may explain why difficulty may be encountered when threading the catheter through the Tuohy needle. When epidural local anesthetic dosing for anesthesia approaches the maximum safe limit without noticeable analgesia, a failed epidural must be considered and should prompt the clinician to pursue an alternative course of anesthesia.

Careful matching of the dermatomal level of the catheter tip to that of the surgical site will yield greater success of epidural blockade. The epidural stimulation test has been used to verify accurate epidural tip placement,[28] ensuring that the dermatomes involved in the surgical procedure are selectively blocked.

Management Effectively managing partially working and/or failed epidurals is very important in patient satisfaction and safety, particular in obstetric patients. The partially working epidural is commonly encountered when undergoing anesthesia for cesarean sections; reported failure rates are in the order of 2% to 13.1%.[237] A poorly functioning epidural or partially working spinal should be identified early before the decision to proceed to cesarean section is made. In an emergency situation, the anesthesiologist has a number of options available to rescue the situation; such options include converting to general anesthesia, supplemental epidural or caudal injections, and local infiltration anesthesia. Intraoperative discomfort and visceral pain may occur in up to 50% of cesarean patients.[238] A block to the T4 level is considered optimal in most cesarean patients; however, debate exists concerning the best modality with which to test the upper level of the block. Loss of pinprick and cold sensation are popular testing options, but may have poor predictive value.[239,240] The loss of touch is considered by some to best equate with surgical anesthesia.[241]

Surgical factors increasing the likelihood of intraoperative discomfort include exteriorization of the uterus and round ligament stretching, both of which exceed the analgesia provided during an apparently adequately dense nerve block. Subdiaphragmatic blood or amniotic fluid may cause back, chest, or shoulder discomfort.

Intervention by the clinician should involve direct communication with the patient. Pharmacologic management may be necessary depending on the level of distress. Intravenous ketamine in 10- to 20-mg increments and small doses of fentanyl or benzodiazepines are considered safe, although some advise waiting to administer these medications until the umbilical cord is clamped.[237] Nitrous oxide has been used in the treatment of patients with breakthrough pain, but this treatment is controversial in obstetric anesthetics.[242] If rescue efforts fail, general anesthesia should be considered, paying special attention to preoxygenation and potential airway difficulties.

For postoperative epidural analgesia, it is also important to confirm the working condition of epidural analgesia (sensory test, epidural stimulation test, low pain scores).

HYPOTENSION

Hypotension is a common physiologic change associated with neuraxial blockade. Its presence predicts block success, but as a side effect, if left untreated or poorly managed, hypotension can lead to serious morbidity or death. Hypotension results from preganglionic sympathetic blockade that leads to a reduction in systemic vascular resistance (SVR) and cardiac output if the venous return is not maintained. SVR decreases as a result of a reduction in sympathetic tone, the extent of which is related to the number of spinal segments blocked. Cardiac output is altered by changes in heart rate and stroke volume. The reduction in stroke volume is a result of a fall in preload and contractility, which is load dependant. If the block involves the cardiac sympathetic nerve supply, bradycardia and reduced contractility can be expected.

High thoracic epidural anesthesia has the potential to block cardiac afferent and efferent fibers originating at the first to fifth thoracic levels. Interest has evolved concerning the potential positive effects of cardiac sympathetic blockade in patients with coronary artery disease: dilation of coronary vessels, reduced heart rate, and decreased myocardial oxygen demand.[243] Clinically, improvement in cardiac function when using high thoracic epidural anesthesia is likely due to improved diastolic function of the left ventricle.[242] Although measures of cardiac function can be improved with a high thoracic epidural, there does not appear to be a decrease in mortality or myocardial infarction incidence after coronary artery bypass grafting.[244]

Prevention The effect of prophylactic administration of intravenous fluid, ephedrine, and methoxamine on cardiovascular responses to both epidural and combined epidural and general isoflurane anesthesia in 45 adult patients undergoing knee arthroplasty has been examined.[245] In Wright and Fee's study,[246] systolic blood pressure was significantly greater after ephedrine administration than after fluid preloading or methoxamine administration. An increase in plasma volume triggered by epidural-induced hypotension has been observed as a result of fluid movement from the interstitial to the intravascular space.[244] A larger percentage of fluid administered is retained by hypotensive than normotensive patients,[248] resulting in hemodilution. Holte et al's study[249] showed that it was not the epidural that leads to changes in blood volume, but rather the infusion of fluid that effects blood volume. Hydroxyethyl starch and ephedrine have similar hemodynamic effects; ephedrine may be the preferred option for patients when excess fluid administration is undesirable. Fluid administration before induction of spinal and epidural analgesia usually can reduce the risk of hypotension. Patient position is crucial in preventing low cardiac output states in patients undergoing epidural anesthesia. If severe hypotension occurs during the course of epidural anesthesia, the most likely cause is inadequate venous return as a result of blood loss, an unfavorable patient position, or surgical obstruction.

Management The first step in the management of hypotension is making sure that there is no interference with venous return. Place the patient in 5 degrees of Trendelenburg (and in the case of a pregnant patient, a leftward roll) to improve return. Subsequent treatment with fluid or pressor administration should be used to restore the systemic blood pressure to acceptable levels.

Significant changes in blood pressure are uncommon in pediatric patients after the proper administration of epidural analgesia. A high sympathetic single-shot caudal block to T6 caused no significant changes in heart rate, cardiac index, or blood pressure in children.[250,251] Even when thoracic epidural blockade is combined with general anesthesia, cardiovascular stability is usually maintained in otherwise healthy pediatric patients.

RESPIRATORY COMPLICATIONS

Several studies have examined high thoracic epidurals in both healthy people and in those with chronic obstructive airway disease. Peak expiratory flows, forced vital capacity, forced expiratory volume in 1 second, and maximum expiratory pressures are reduced[252,253] in those suffering from this disorder. Kochi et al[254] investigated the effect of high thoracic epidural anesthesia on the hypercapnic ventilatory response and ventilation pattern; duration of inspiration, rib cage excursion, and its contribution to tidal volume decreased significantly, whereas mean inspiratory flow rate and minute ventilation increased. Furthermore, end-tidal P_{CO_2} and the tidal excursion of the abdomen remained unchanged, whereas hypercapnic ventilatory response decreased significantly. Lumbar and high thoracic region–induced epidurals do not interfere with the ventilatory response to hypoxemia.[255] Gruber et al[256] demonstrated the safety of thoracic epidural anesthesia with bupivacaine 0.25% in patients with severe chronic obstructive pulmonary disease. The potential for phrenic (C3 to C5) palsy is low with an epidural block, except during unintentional blockade after an interscalene brachial plexus block.[257] Cervical epidural anesthesia has been used for upper limb, parathyroid, and carotid operations.[258-260]

Bonnet et al[258] reported respiratory difficulties in 3 of 394 patient undergoing carotid endarterectomy using 15 mL of 0.5% bupivacaine or 0.37% to 0.40% bupivacaine plus fentanyl (50-100 µg). Many case series, although smaller in number than this study published by Bonnet, have not reported respiratory difficulties to be a significant problem.[259,260]

Capdevila et al[261] reported that both 0.25% and 0.375% cervical epidural bupivacaine impaired diaphragmatic excursion, tidal volume, forced vital capacity, and hand grip strength in patients having postoperative hand rehabilitation and did not recommend the technique for this purpose.

The incidence of respiratory depression is closely associated with the use of neuraxial opioids. The rate of incidence of respiratory depression requiring intervention after conventional opioid dosing is approximately 1%.[262]

Prevention To prevent respiratory complications, do the following:

- Avoid the use of high doses of opioids.
- Limit opioid dosages, especially in the intrathecal space.
- Avoid the concomitant use of parenteral opioids or sedatives.
- Avoid or limit doses in the patient with advanced age (>60 years of age), sleep apnea, and other coexisting diseases.
- Use hydrophilic drugs (eg, morphine) with caution.

Management To manage respiratory complications, do the following:

- Treat mild respiratory depression with oxygen.
- If an infusion is used, then reduce the rate.
- Depending on the severity of respiratory complications, consider ventilatory support, the administration of narcotic antagonists, and the discontinuation of the opioid infusion.

NAUSEA AND PRURITUS

Nausea and pruritus are common side effects seen with the administration of neuraxial opioids. The reported incidence of postoperative nausea and vomiting (PONV) with opioid administration is 30% to 65%[263-265] and for pruritus is 80%.[266] Pruritus is thought to be multifactorial in nature and is speculated to operate via an "itch center" in the CNS via medullary dorsal horn activation and antagonism of inhibitory transmitters.[267] Pruritus is a dose-dependant phenomenon; its onset involves possible mediators including C fibers in the skin, serotonin (5-HT_3) receptors, prostaglandins, and micro-opioid receptors.[268] The obstetric population seems to be at greater risk for developing pruritus.

PONV is a complex, multifactorial problem:

- Epidural administration of local anesthetics alone carries a low risk of causing the occurrence of PONV.[269]
- Factors such as surgery, age, and sex influence the reported incidence of PONV associated with epidural anesthesia.[270]

- Within 5 to 15 minutes of epidural administration, peak plasma opioid concentrations can reach levels similar to those seen after an intramuscular injection.[271]
- In patients receiving epidural morphine, there have been no differences in PONV onset or duration when different doses up to 5 mg were administered,[272] whereas higher doses have been shown to lead to both an increase and a decrease in reported PONV.[270]
- Epidural fentanyl and meperidine do not appear to influence PONV in the same way that morphine does; as reported, fewer PONV cases have been documented with the use of fentanyl and meperidine after orthopedic surgery when compared with morphine.[273]

Prevention/Management To prevent and/or manage PONV and pruritus, do the following:

- Reduce the dose administration and avoid neuraxial opioid administration. Doing so is effective in reducing the incidence of nausea and pruritus.
- Use antihistamines, opioid antagonists (naloxone and nalbuphine), propofol, nonsteroidal anti-inflammatory drugs (NSAIDs), and 5-HT_3 receptor antagonists as both preventative and therapeutic measures.
- Dexamethasone has been shown to be a superior antiemetic for PONV-associated epidural morphine as compared with metoclopramide[274] and 5-HT_3 receptor antagonists.[275]
- Investigation into acupressure point P6 for the prevention of PONV has revealed inconsistent findings. There may be a reduction in nausea, but there is currently no evidence that it decreases postoperative vomiting.[276]

POSTOPERATIVE URINARY RETENTION

Postoperative urinary retention (POUR) is common after major surgery and occurs in

- 20% to 68% of patients after abdominoperineal resection.
- 16% to 80% of patients after radical hysterectomy.
- 20% to 25% of patients after anterior resection.
- 10% to 20% of patients after proctocolectomy.[277]

POUR is a multifactorial condition and involves factors such as age, pain, bladder outlet obstruction, detrusor-inhibiting medication, pelvic autonomic nerve damage, and the inhibition of sympathetic reflexes.[278] A single episode of bladder overdistension can result in significant POUR morbidity. Overfilling of the bladder can stretch and damage the detrusor muscle, leading to atony of the bladder wall, so that recovery of micturition may not occur when the bladder is emptied. On the other hand, the excessive use of an indwelling catheter can lead to urinary tract infection, urethral stricture, prolonged hospital stay, or death.[279,280] Epidural use for postoperative pain management is usually reserved for patients undergoing major surgery, where urinary catheter placement may be performed for reasons other than anticipated postoperative urinary retention. Stenseth et al[281] found an incidence of 42% for POUR in 1085 uncatheterized patients having epidural morphine for a variety of major operations. Epidural morphine relaxes the detrusor muscle with a corresponding increase in the maximal bladder capacity, whereas intramuscular and intravenous morphine have no effect on detrusor contraction. This is further supported by the fact that detrusor changes occur 15 to 30 minutes after epidural morphine administration and are reversed by intravenous naloxone, suggesting that spinal opioid receptors have an important role.[278]

Prevention/Management Other epidural opioids such as fentanyl, meperidine, and methadone may also contribute to POUR, but contribute to a lesser degree than that observed with morphine.[273,283] Diagnosis of POUR is best made with a portable ultrasound bladder scanner.[278] There is a suggestion that use of the bladder scanner ought to be routine in the postanesthetic care unit for patients at high risk of retention.[284,285] A threshold of 600 mL has been suggested as a diagnostic threshold.[286] In addition to bladder catheterization, treatment options for opioid-mediated POUR may include intravenous naloxone administration.[287] Nalbuphine is an opioid-mixed agonist–antagonist and has been used to restore detrusor function without reversing the analgesic effects of epidural morphine.[288] Short-term (24 hours) urinary catheterization for major surgery involving morphine epidural analgesia may help prevent the morbidities associated with both POUR and longer-term epidural catheterization.[289]

BACKACHE

Backache is a common complaint after epidural anesthesia, and its incidence ranges between 2% and 30% of patients.[139,290] The causal relationship between epidural anesthesia and backache has been suggested by some studies[291,292] and refuted by others.[293,294] The etiology of backache is multifactorial in nature. Drug use, abnormal posture, muscle relaxation, and, in obstetric cases, exaggerated lumbar lordosis and the process of undergoing labor have been implicated as causes.[205]

In a retrospective study, MacArthur et al[291] looked at 11 701 patients. Of the 1634 women who reported backache, 1132 (69%) had experienced it for more than 1 year. In this study, a significant association was found between backache and epidural anesthesia (relative risk: 1.8); 903 of 4766 women (18.9%) who had had epidural anesthesia reported this symptom, compared with 731 of the 6935 women (10.5%) who had not undergone epidural anesthesia. However, prospective data refute the findings of Macarthur, as noted by Breen,[293] who interviewed 1185 women and found that of the 1042 (88%) for whom follow-up data were available, the incidence of postpartum back pain in those who received epidural anesthesia was equivalent to that of those who did not (44% vs 45%). Multiple logistic regressions revealed that postpartum back pain was associated with a history of back pain, younger age, and greater weight. Russell[240] demonstrated that new-onset postpartum back pain was not associated with regional anesthesia. Among the women in Russell's study who received either 0.125% bupivacaine or 0.0625% bupivacaine, the incidence of new long-term back pain was 7.6% when compared with controls, and there was no difference found between the groups. Women who are seeking analgesia for labor should be reassured that back pain after epidural analgesia is minimal and is usually limited to the early postpartum period.

In 1987, 2-chloroprocaine was marketed by AstraZeneca in a new formulation (Nesacaine-MPF) involving disodium EDTA as a chelating agent for epidural and caudal use. Reports linking this new formulation with backache emerged[128,294] and gave way to a possible explanation that the EDTA could cause hypocalcemic tetany of the paraspinous muscles. The drug now comes preservative-free and is prepared in dark-glass bottles to prevent light-induced disintegration. Despite the elimination of EDTA from this medication, backache continues to be reported with its use.[296]

Prevention/Management Backache after epidural placement should not be ignored, as it can be a cardinal symptom of a space-occupying lesion within the spinal canal. Complications such as an epidural hematoma and abscess, although rare, can have catastrophic outcomes if unrecognized and untreated.

COMPLICATIONS OF INTRAVENOUS REGIONAL ANESTHESIA

Intravenous regional anesthesia (IVRA) is one of the oldest techniques used in anesthesia practice today; Bier[297] first described IVRA in 1908. The technique was not widely practiced for the first 50 years of its inception because it was not practical to perform a venous cut down on patients undergoing relatively minor extremity procedures. Holmes[298] made a very simple adjustment to the technique in 1963 and demonstrated that Bier's technique could be performed using a percutaneous intravenous approach. IVRA is now widely used for minor upper- and lower-extremity procedures all over the world,[298] as it is relatively easy to perform and has a very high success rate. There are a number of recognizable risks associated with this procedure, the most serious being compartment syndrome and local anesthetic toxicity. A primary limitation of the technique is the duration of tolerability of the tourniquet, which, without opioid supplementation, is about 45 minutes. The addition of ketamine in very low doses (0.1 mg/kg) greatly extends the time that patients can tolerate the tourniquet. Clonidine and Ketoralac have also been recommended for this purpose. Fortunately systemic toxicity and compartment syndrome are rare complications when IVRA is properly administered.

COMPARTMENT SYNDROME

Compartment syndrome has been reported after IVRA of the upper and lower extremities.[299,300] In 1 reported case, hypertonic saline was mistakenly used as a diluent for the local anesthetic. Long-bone fractures of the forearm or leg increase the risk of compartment syndrome, and IVRA should not be used in this circumstance. Severe ischemia of the upper extremity has been reported in at least 1 case after IVRA in an otherwise healthy young female, where the etiology was unclear.[301] **Table 50-7** lists some of the possible causes of compartment syndrome.

Venous thrombosis is a recognized complication of tourniquet application. There are anecdotal reports of subclavian steal syndrome after sudden LOR in the upper extremity, leading to transient cortical blindness.[302]

LOCAL ANESTHETIC TOXICITY

The risk of local anesthetic toxicity is quite low after IVRA. Auroy et al[57] reported an incidence of 2.7 seizures per 10 000 cases after IVRA in their study. Deaths have been reported when increased amounts of toxic cardiac drugs (eg, bupivacaine) have been used for IVRA.[195] The main cause of this complication is faulty tourniquet technique.

Inadequate exsanguination before the inflation of the tourniquet allows the operator to exceed the tourniquet inflation pressure during the injection, thereby allowing local anesthetic solution to escape into the circulation. Interosseous escape of the local anesthetic can occur during injection. Accidental or premature deflation of the tourniquet (within 20 minutes) allows the local anesthetic to enter the circulation in toxic concentrations. When an excessive dose of local anesthetic is injected, toxicity may occur on release of the tourniquet, even when following appropriate recommendations.

Prevention Intravenous regional anesthesia is easy to perform, yet one must pay particular attention to the details surrounding the procedure. Preventing complications begins with appropriate patient selection and surgical indication. Good intravenous access is important, as is proper exsanguination of the limb. **Table 50-8** lists points to consider for proper patient and surgical selection.

Proper techniques for effective and safe IVRA that are essential to prevent complications are as follows:

- Place the tourniquet above the elbow (tourniquet application is less reliable in the distal portion of the extremity).

TABLE 50-7 Causes of Compartment Syndrome

Excessive tourniquet pressures
Allergic reactions
Undiagnosed Raynaud disease
Sickle cell disease
Intra-arterial injection
Drug administration error

TABLE 50-8 Factors for Proper Patient/Surgical Selection

The upper-limb surgical procedure should not last longer than 1 h. Surgical procedures lasting longer than 1 h are not recommended because patients become very intolerant of the tourniquet.
Failed IVRA occurs more frequently in lower-extremity procedures.
The risk of toxicity is much greater in lower-limb surgery where larger quantities of drug are required.
In addition to the usual contraindications of regional anesthesia, physicians should avoid the use of IVRA in patients who have the following: sickle cell disease, Raynaud disease, sickle cell anemia, or allergies to local anesthetics.
Patients with gaping venous wounds, those with infected lesions, and those with long bone fractures of the extremities are not suitable for IVRA.
IVRA is generally not recommended in lengthy procedure.

IVRA, intravenous regional anesthesia.

- Thorough exsanguinations should take place before injection of the local anesthetic. Appropriate doses of preservative-free local anesthetic should be administered.
- Lidocaine free of preservatives is one of the most frequently used local anesthetics for IVRA; the recommended dose is 3 mg/kg.
- Other drugs, such as prilocaine, have been used because of their favorable pharmacokinetic profile; however, some of these drugs, such as prilocaine, are no longer available in many countries.
- A preservative-free form of chloroprocaine was recently introduced in Europe and has many potential benefits, especially with regard to toxicity.[303]
- Ropivacaine has also been studied as a potential local anesthetic for IVRA and may offer better tourniquet tolerance and better postoperative analgesia compared with lidocaine.[304]
- Bupivacaine is contraindicated in IVRA.

Management The management of local anesthetic toxicity is the same as that discussed in the previous section. The clinician must have dedicated intravenous access to inject other medications if required. Proper equipment and personnel must be available for emergency cardiopulmonary support (airway, breathing, circulation).

COMPLICATIONS OF OPTHALMIC REGIONAL ANESTHESIA

Like other types of nerve blocks, there are some serious risks associated with the use of ophthalmic regional anesthesia. Common complications include hemorrhage, brainstem anesthesia, and myotoxicity. These complications vary with the mode of regional opthalmic anesthesia. The clinician should be aware of other less frequently occurring complications of ophthalmic regional anesthesia that include globe ischemia, perforation of the globe, optic nerve and facial nerve damage, and elicitation of the oculocardiac reflex.

GENERAL PREVENTION

To prevent complication as a result of ophthalmic regional anesthesia, do the following:

- Inform the patient of the procedures and its likely outcomes during anesthesia. For instance, many patients experience visual alterations with sub-Tenon's anesthesia, which can be terrifying.
- Provide sedation to those patients who require it. Routine use of sedation is discouraged.[305]
- Consider only selected patients who are taking anticoagulant medication with a current international normalized ratio of less than 2 as a potential candidate for ophthalmic regional blocks.[306]

- Carefully weigh the benefits and risks of performing ophthalmic regional anesthesia in patients who have discontinued their anticoagulant medication.
- Consider alternative methods of applying ophthalmic anesthesia if there is risk of thrombotic complications after discontinuation of anticoagulant medication.[307,308]
- Let patients on antiplatelet therapy continue their medications if medically indicated.[309]
- Postpone surgery in severely hypertensive patients.
- Consider using small-gauge disposable needles (25 gauge), less than 31 mm in length.[310,311]
- Consider the site of anesthetic injection. Vascular structures are larger in the apex of the orbit, and also the upper nasal area is particularly vascular. Areas with increased vascular architecture should be avoided to prevent complications during the induction of ophthalmic regional anesthesia.

GENERAL MANAGEMENT

As with other nerve blocks, once damage has occurred as a result of ophthalmic regional anesthesia, it is difficult to reverse. If complications do occur, supportive measures are recommended for patient care.

RETROBULBAR HEMORRHAGE

The reported risk of retrobulbar hemorrhage varies substantially in anesthetic literature.[312] In one of the largest reported series, Hamilton reported an incidence of 0.44% hemorrhages in 12000 ophthalmic regional anesthesia cases.[313] The severity of retrobulbar hemorrhage varies depending on the origin of the bleeding. Arterial bleeding is the most dangerous complication of retrobulbar injections because tamponade can occur, which leads to ischemia of the globe. In this situation, lateral canthotomy may be required to relieve the pressure. The site of injection is also important to consider in avoiding hemorrhage.

SUBCONJUNCTIVAL HEMORRHAGE

The risk of subconjunctival hemorrhage in sub-Tenon's anesthesia has been reported as high as 100%, and as low as 19%.[316,317] Its incidence is influenced by the type of cannula used (anterior cannulae causing more hemorrhage than others) and patient factors such as age as well as steroid, antiplatelet agent, and NSAID use. This complication can be prevented with careful dissection as well as the use of epinephrine locally.[318] Some advocate for the use of bipolar cautery, but this remains controversial.[305] Fortunately, this complication tends to be self-limiting, and ocular compression is often enough for treatment.

BRAINSTEM ANESTHESIA

When local anesthetic spreads directly into the brain from the orbit, brainstem anesthesia occurs. The incidence of brainstem anesthesia is 1 case for every 350 to 1500 ophthalmic cases,[310] and symptoms may appear within 2 minutes of the injection. Maximum effects usually occur within 20 minutes, and recovery occurs in 2 to 3 hours. Symptoms and signs can vary greatly and include those listed in **Table 50-9**.

TABLE 50-9 Signs and Symptoms of Brainstem Anesthesia, Prevention, and Management

Brainstem anesthesia	• Confusion • Shivering • Convulsions • Paralysis • Loss of consciousness • Apnea • Hypotension • Bradycardia • Nausea/vomiting
Prevention and management	• Use short needles (<31 mm) and small doses of local anesthetics. • Surgery should be postponed and the patient should be observed and treated appropriately if symptoms of brainstem anesthesia develop. The treatment varies depending on the symptoms and is mostly supportive in nature.

GLOBE PERFORATION

Blindly inserting a needle into the orbit is associated with the risk of globe perforation. The site of injection and the axial length of the globe must be carefully considered before needle insertion to prevent damaging the globe. In 1 reported series, there were no globe perforations in 2000 cases of ophthalmic regional anesthesia,[319] whereas another study reported an incidence of 1 case of globe perforation per 12000 ophthalmic cases.[313]

Prevention The risk of globe perforation can be reduced by presurgically assessing the axial length of the patient's eye. Patients susceptible to perforation of the globe include those with elongated globes (>26 mm), which occur in myopic patients; in those with retinal detachment; and in those who require refractive surgery. Myopic patients with staphyloma are particularly vulnerable to globe perforation.[320]

The clinician should attempt to visualize in the "mind's eye" the equator of the globe and to avoid repositioning the needle until it is located past the equator. All needles should be directed tangentially with the bevel facing the globe. Pain or resistance to needle advancement is a warning sign of perforation of the sclera. Some experts suggest aiming the needle midway between the inferior and lateral rectus muscles to allow a clear point of entry to the intraconal space. The inferior rectus muscle should be carefully avoided to prevent diplopia.

Management The key to successful management of globe perforation is early diagnosis and treatment. The patient may report paresthesia at the time of needle insertion. Funduscopic examination by an ophthalmologist may confirm the diagnosis of globe perforation. Depending on the severity of damage, globe perforation can be managed by laser photocoagulation therapy, cryotherapy, and other prompt surgical procedures. Because the appropriate management of globe perforation is complex, careful consultation should take place with the ophthalmologist.

MYOTOXICITY

Myotoxic effects of local anesthetic drugs were discussed in this chapter's section on Toxic Effects of Local Anesthetics on the Nerves and Surrounding. Typically, diplopia and ptosis can occur for up to 48 hours when using long-acting local anesthetics. However, direct injection of these drugs into the highly sensitive eye muscles can permanently damage them. The inferior rectus muscle appears to be particularly vulnerable to injury.[139,321]

MISCELLANEOUS COMPLICATIONS RESULTING FROM OPHTHALMIC REGIONAL ANESTHESIA

Globe ischemia, optic nerve, and facial nerve damage and oculocardiac reflex are less frequent complications of ophthalmic regional anesthesia.

SUMMARY

This chapter provides a comprehensive review of the management of complications after regional anesthesia.

- Although the overall incidence of complications after brachial plexus anesthesia is low, the proportion of complications after supraclavicular methods is higher than that reported after axillary blocks (ie, the incidence of seizure activity after interscalene or subclavian perivascular methods is at least 6 times that of the axillary approach).

- Many of the complications of supraclavicular methods have an impact on pulmonary function; consequently, supraclavicular methods should be avoided in patients with significant pulmonary dysfunction. In a sense, there should always be a clear-cut indication for selecting supraclavicular methods because of the risk of pulmonary complications.
- Local anesthetic drugs must be injected slowly and incrementally, and patients must be observed carefully for signs of local anesthetic toxicity. The addition of epinephrine to local anesthetics is a useful marker for detecting accidental intravascular injections.
- Persistent pain on injection of local anesthetics is a potential sign of intraneural injection.
- Large-gauge and long needles should be avoided, and brachial blocks should be avoided in comatose adult patients.

Finally, brachial plexus anesthesia is not yet an exact science. Ultrasound-guided needle insertion is renewing interest in regional anesthesia as a result of this advance. We can expect success rates close to 100% in the near future. However, complications will still occur.

Primary factors for consideration with respect to adverse outcomes during regional anesthesia are as follows:

- Patients must be selected carefully.
- Patients must provide informed consent.
- The safest approach must be selected.
- The appropriate dose of local anesthetic should be given.
- Patient discomfort must be minimized.

Drug delivery via neuraxial block is an effective method for providing analgesia for lower-extremity, abdominal, and thoracic procedures, as well as for managing labor pain. In the perioperative setting, epidural analgesia has numerous benefits in addition to providing effective pain relief. These benefits include earlier ambulation, rapid weaning from mechanical ventilation, reduced time spent in a catabolic state, and lowered circulating stress hormone levels.[316] Although serious complications are uncommon, patients should be informed about common side effects, such as urinary retention and pruritus, and should be counseled concerning the risks of major neurologic complication such as paralysis. Newer technologies such as sonography and the stimulating epidural catheter may increase the safety and ease of catheter placement. For the individual patient, the risks and benefits of epidural analgesia should be carefully considered, and prevention of patient injury is the highest priority.

KEY REFERENCES

- Atlee JL. *Complications in Anesthesia.* 2nd ed. Philadelphia, PA: Elsevier/Saunders; 2007.
- Horlocker TT, Wedel DJ, Benzon H, et al. Regional anesthesia in the anticoagulated patient: defining the risks (the second ASRA Consensus Conference on Neuraxial Anesthesia and Anticoagulation). *Reg Anesth Pain Med.* 2003;28:172-197.
- Neal JM, Bernards CM, Butterworth JFt, et al. ASRA practice advisory on local anesthetic systemic toxicity. *Reg Anesth Pain Med.* 2010;35:152-161.
- Neal JM, Bernards CM, Hadzic A, et al. ASRA Practice advisory on neurologic complications in regional anesthesia and pain medicine. *Reg Anesth Pain Med.* 2008;33:404-415.
- Neal JM, Brull R, Chan VW, et al. The ASRA evidence-based medicine assessment of ultrasound-guided regional anesthesia and pain medicine: executive summary. *Reg Anesth Pain Med.* 2010;35:S1-S9.
- Tsui BC, Finucane B. Epidural stimulator catheter. *Tech Reg Anesth Pain Manage.* 2002;9:150-154.

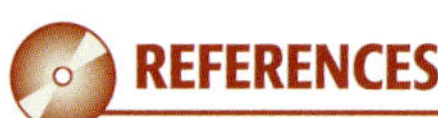

REFERENCES

Complete references available on DVD and online version at www.LongneckerAnesthesiology.com

SECTION E

Specialty Areas of Anesthetic Practice

CHAPTER 51 Neuroanesthesia

Rafi Avitsian
Ehab Farag

KEY POINTS

1. The most important anatomic and physiologic characteristic of the cranium is its closed system. In order to provide adequate blood flow, the volume of the brain, the brain's interstitium, and cerebrospinal fluid should not increase.
2. Cerebral blood flow (CBF) and cerebral blood volume are separate but related entities. Maintaining adequate CBF is important for neurons, but high CBF can increase the intracranial pressure.
3. Anesthesiologists can manipulate CBF by changing the factors controlling it, namely $Paco_2$, Pao_2, autoregulation, cerebral metabolic rate, and the autonomic nervous system.
4. The management of most neurosurgical procedures requires invasive and specialized monitoring methods that can give information about blood supply, oxygen utilization, and electrical activity of the brain and spinal cord.
5. Maintaining the proper cerebral perfusion pressure and proper surgical conditions are the most important key point for anesthetic management during supratentorial and infratentorial craniotomies.
6. Both secreting and nonsecreting pituitary tumors can cause significant changes in the function of all organ systems, which affects the perioperative care of patients undergoing surgical procedures.
7. Intracranial aneurysms and arteriovenous malformations are the 2 main intracranial vascular abnormalities, each of which has special characteristics requiring specific perioperative care.
8. Interventional neuroradiology is a new specialty for the nonsurgical management of cerebral aneurysms and arteriovenous malformations. Understanding interventional neuroradiological techniques and ensuring hemodynamic stability are the most important points during anesthetic management.
9. The shunt and neuroendoscopy for obstructive hydrocephalus might cause hemodynamic problems such as severe bradycardia and surgical problems like hemorrhage and massive increase in intracranial pressure.
10. The prone position during spine surgery is accompanied by a decrease in cardiac index. The upper airway management for cervical spine surgery needs meticulous attention to maintain the neutral position during intubation and positioning. The main causes for postoperative visual loss after spine surgery are hypotension, anemia, and massive face edema.

INTRODUCTION

Neuroanesthesia involves patients undergoing surgical procedures on the central and peripheral nervous system. It includes craniotomies, spine surgeries, and surgical procedures on the cranial and peripheral nervous system, as well as interventional neuroradiology procedures. The neuroanesthesiologist should be insightful about the anatomy and physiology of the central nervous system, pathophysiologic mechanisms of diseases, monitoring, and the effect of anesthetics on the nervous system.[1] The past decade showed a swift acceleration of progress in this field. Improvements in the speed of transporting patients with acute intracranial and spinal traumatic or vascular problems to tertiary hospitals have increased the patient population undergoing neurosurgical procedures. The development of new interventional methods has increased anesthetic challenges specific to this therapeutic modality.[2] As much as we would like to introduce and describe these advances in detail, that is not the aim of this chapter. In this chapter our goal is to describe the essentials of neuroanesthesia, focusing on the important features that make this area unique when compared to anesthesia for other organs. It can offer a review of neuroanesthesiology for general anesthesiologists who practice neurosurgical cases occasionally, as well as residents rotating through the neurosurgical anesthesia course.

ANATOMY

Knowing the anatomical structure of the operating site in neuroanesthesiology is important. Although it is not required to know the anatomy of the central nervous system in as much detail as the neurosurgeon, the anesthesiologist should have adequate knowledge of the anatomy because it might affect the anesthetic and monitoring plan, and the plan for postoperative care. A tumor involving the left parietal lobe has a higher chance of being scheduled as an awake craniotomy, or a suboccipital craniotomy may have a higher chance of intraoperative hemodynamic changes or a more challenging positioning.

CRANIUM AND BRAIN

The frontal, parietal, temporal, and occipital sphenoid and ethmoid bones join to make the framework of the cranium. The inner surface of this bony structure overlies the *meninges*, which has 3 layers. The innermost layer, the pia mater, is closely adherent to the brain. The midsection or the arachnoid is a lacelike structure below which is the subarachnoid space. The outer layer or the nonelastic dura has an endosteal layer connected to the periosteum and the meningeal layer. Between these two is the epidural space. The potential space under the dura or the subdural space has a lot of vascularity with little supporting structure and may bleed with injury (**Fig. 51-1**). The dura is sensitive in the vicinity of its blood vessels.

The tentorium is a horizontal folding of the dura separating the upper supratentorial cavity and lower infratentorial space. The supratentorial space is also divided into the right and left side for each cerebral hemisphere by an interhemispheric fissure occupied by an invagination of dura, the falx cerebri. The cerebral hemispheres have an uneven surface caused by infoldings called the sulci and bulges in between them called gyri. The cerebrum is divided into anatomical lobes by sulci, namely the frontal, temporal, parietal, and occipital lobes. Identification of the large central sulcus is important, especially in brain mapping because the somatomotor and motor cortexes are in the gyri posterior and anterior to it, respectively. The lateral sulcus (or sylvian fissure) is another important invagination dividing the temporal lobe from the frontal and parietal lobes. The speech comprehension (Wernicke) area is below this fissure at the parietal lobe level and the speech motor (Broca) area is above and more anteriorly at the frontal lobe level. Almost all right-handed and 80% of left-handed people have left hemispheric dominance for speech. The visual cortex is in the occipital lobe in the region of the calcarine sulcus, mostly on the medial side of the cerebral hemisphere. The thalamus is a small nuclear mass mainly of gray matter within the cerebral white matter at the base of the hemispheres. It acts as

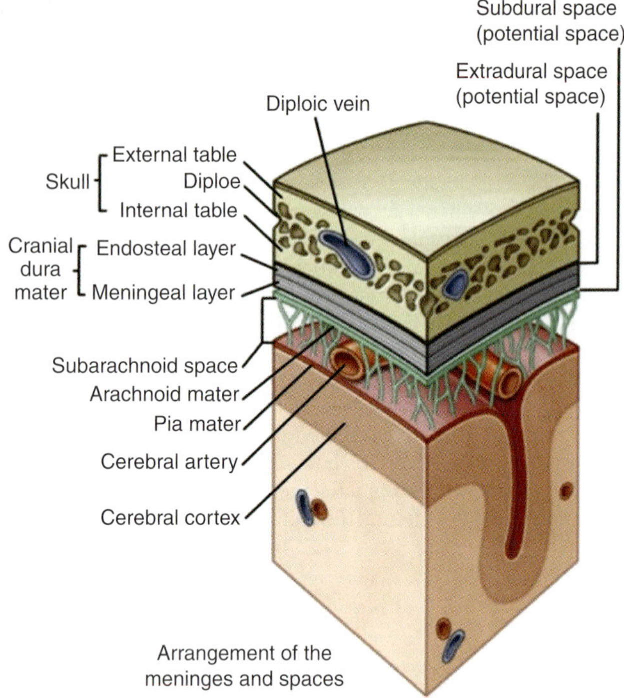

FIGURE 51-1. Brain covering and vessels. [Reprinted with permission from Drake RL, Vogl AW, Mitchell AWM. *Gray's Anatomy for Students*. 2nd ed. Churchill Livingstone; 2009.]

a relay station for all (except olfactory) sensory tracts. Below the thalamus is the hypothalamus, which has important endocrine, autonomic, and visceral control function. Another important part, the hypophysis, is located beneath and connected to the hypothalamus. The significance of the hypothalamus is its proximity to the optic chiasm, which causes visual disturbances when affected by tumors, as well as unique surgical approaches, which frequently are transsphenoidal or translabial.

The brainstem consists of the medulla, pons, and midbrain and is home for all but the first 2 cranial nerve nuclei (**Fig. 51-2**). It also has the essential role of maintaining alertness, and generating and controlling the vital respiratory activity. Thus in surgical procedures close to this area, one should not rush extubation because edema or injury to this part can cause respiratory depression or even arrest. Some of the important reflexes in determining the eligibility of a patient for extubation, such as pupillary, gag, and corneal reflexes, have their control center in the brainstem.

The cerebellum is in the infratentorial space divided into right and left cerebellar hemispheres by falx cerebelli. It is connected to the midbrain via 3 cerebellar peduncles and has a major role in regulating movement. Ataxia or tremors can result from cerebellar lesions.

The basal ganglia, namely the caudate nucleus, amygdala, putamen, and globus pallidus are embedded in the cerebral hemispheres. Their main function is the modulation of the information received from the cortex and spinal cord, processing it and then relaying it to the thalamus, cortex, and midbrain. Lesions in these parts can cause motor and muscular tone abnormalities as well as emotional and cognitive changes. Parkinson disease is an example of abnormal functioning of the basal ganglia. Recently, placement of deep brain stimulators for treatment of these motor abnormalities has become popular. Anesthesia for these procedures has unique challenges because most are performed with the patient under monitored anesthesia care and at times with the patient awake for examination.

Cerebral ventricles comprise 4 cavities that communicate with each other and contain the cerebrospinal fluid. The 2 lateral ventricles are within the cerebral hemispheres and communicate with the third ventricle through the foramen of Monro. The third ventricle is inside the substance of the thalamus, dividing it to 2 lateral parts. The floor of this ventricle is the optic chiasm. The fourth ventricle, which communicates with the third ventricle via the aqueduct of Sylvius, lies anterior to the cerebellum and has a connection to the subarachnoid space through the median foramen of Magendie and 2 lateral foramen of Luschka.

The brain receives its arterial supply from the 2 internal carotid arteries anteriorly and 1 basilar artery formed by the joining of the 2 vertebral arteries posteriorly. In order to provide an adequate blood supply to the brain, even in situations where one of the major feeding arteries of the brain is getting insufficient flow, although not always complete, there is a connective system between all arteries at the base of the cranium called the circle of Willis (**Fig. 51-3**). The anterior cerebral arteries, which are branches of the internal carotid artery, communicate through the anterior communicating artery to form the anterior part of the circle. Laterally, the internal carotid artery gives off the posterior communicating arteries, which travel posteriorly on each side and anastomose to the posterior cerebral arteries, which are branches of the basilar artery. After giving off its branches, the internal carotid artery continues as the middle cerebral artery. The middle cerebral artery has an important role in supplying the sensory motor area of the brain; because it does not have many anastomoses, a blockage above the circle of Willis can cause major focal neurologic signs.

Most of the blood in the cranium is in the venous system. The superficial cerebral veins receive their blood supply from the brain substance and run in the pia until they puncture the arachnoid and dura to enter the venous sinuses. The diploic veins are channels within the cranial bone, and the emissary veins connect them to the veins of the surface of the skull and venous sinuses. The venous sinuses are at dilated parts of the dura and contain venous blood. Knowledge of the proximity of the operating site to these sinuses can help in the estimation of blood loss as well as the estimation of the possibility of venous air embolism. The cavernous sinus is one that is in close proximity to the operating site of transsphenoidal excision of the pituitary.

SPINE

The spinal column is made up of an assembly of 7 cervical, 12 thoracic, and 5 lumbar vertebrae and each group has specific anatomic characteristics. The first and second cervical vertebrae are different in shape to allow neck mobility and attachment to the skull base. The anterior portion of C2 (axis) has an upright protrusion (dens), which is attached to the anterior portion of C1 by ligaments. Any traumatic injury, degenerative disease, or congenital malformation that disrupts the integrity of this anatomical arrangement can cause an unstable cervical spine (**Fig. 51-4**). When there is concern about the stability of the cervical vertebrae and there is time, radiologic evaluation to confirm the stability can help in guiding the tracheal intubation plan. Although fiberoptic intubation while the patient is awake and breathing spontaneously is a safe method in this situation, the decision will depend on the experience of the anesthesiologist. Currently there are multiple intubating devices available to decrease the range of motion of the cervical spine during intubation.

The transverse processes in cervical vertebrae are relatively larger and include the transverse foramen through which the vertebral arteries pass. An injury to the cervical spine can injure these arteries and disrupt the blood supply of the cervical spine causing ischemia. The thoracic vertebrae are distinct because they have the costal facets on the sides. The vertebral foramina are smaller and rounder, and the spinous processes are long with more caudad inclination. In the lumbar region the vertebrae are larger with short and strong pedicles.

There are multiple ligaments connecting the vertebrae from the cervical to the lumbar region. In some disease states, as well as in the elderly, calcification of these ligaments can make the neuraxial blocks more challenging.

The blood supply of the spinal cord stems from the single anterior and 2 posterior spinal arteries, which originate from radicular arteries. Six to ten anterior radicular arteries supply blood to the anterior spinal artery. The radicular arteries pass through the vertebral foramina

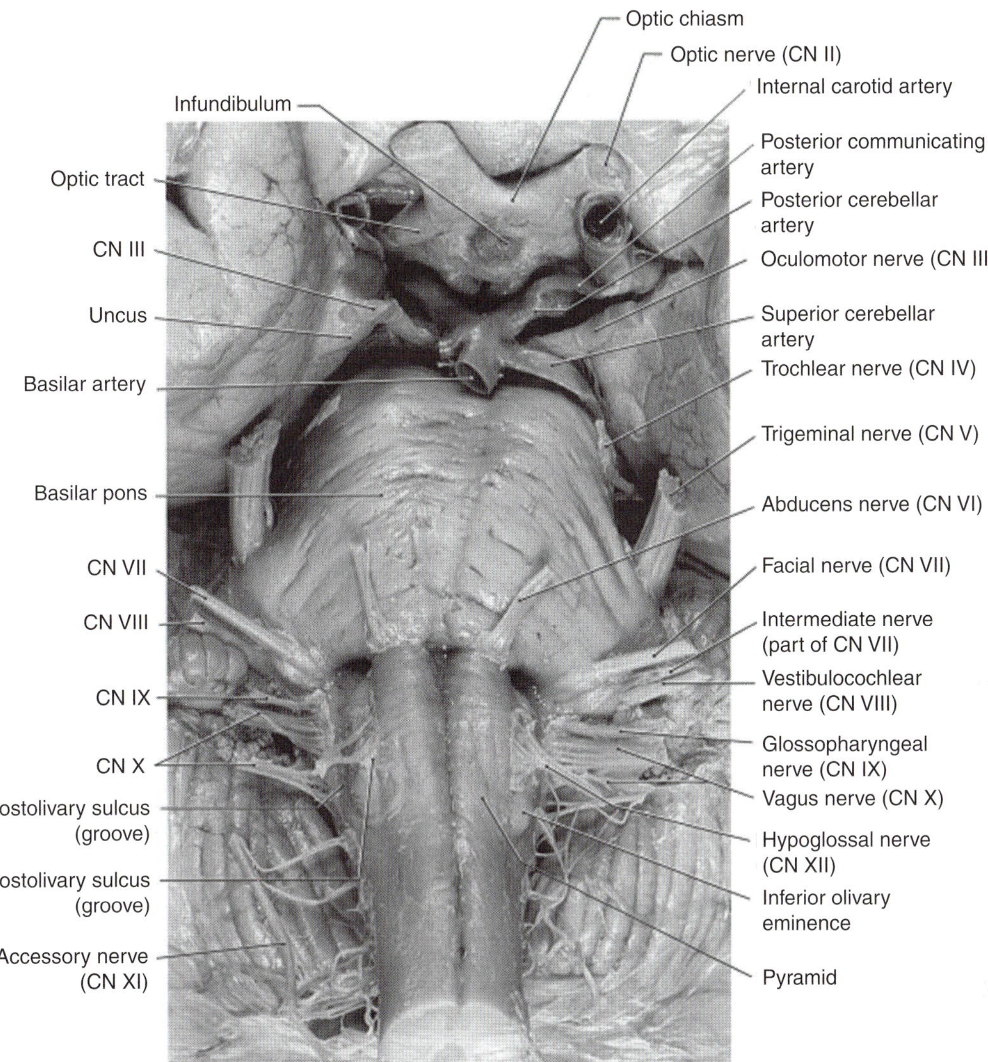

FIGURE 51-2. Brain stem and cranial nerves.

along with the nerve roots. The anterior spinal artery gives blood to the anterior two-thirds of the substance of the spinal cord. In contrast, the posterior spinal arteries are paired and get their blood from 10 to 23 posterior radicular arteries. Thus ischemia of the anterior part of the spinal cord is more concerning, especially during intravascular procedures on the aorta such as stenting, which can obstruct the supply of anterior radicular arteries.

BASIC NEUROPHYSIOLOGY

The neurons are one of the most demanding cells in the body when it comes to oxygen use. The adult brain, with a weight of about 1350 g, uses 3.5 mL of oxygen for every 100 g of its weight, thus generating a need for a continuous high blood supply. The blood supply to the brain is about 50 mL a minute for every 100 g. This can be calculated as 15% of the cardiac output. Not to be mistaken with the blood flow is the blood volume or content of the brain, which is about 50 mL but can vary according to the position of the head.

The overall goal is to meet the high demand of neurons for oxygen and avoid ischemia, meaning there should be enough oxygen (Fio_2), enough hemoglobin (Hgb) to carry the oxygen, and enough perfusion to the brain to direct the oxygen-rich Hgb to the brain. The Fio_2 and Hgb concentration are easier to measure and control. Perfusion to the brain will depend on the blood pressure driving blood toward brain and the resistance inside the cranium that will work against this driving pressure, namely the intracranial pressure (ICP). Thus the basic equation determining the blood perfusion to the brain is

$$CPP = MAP - ICP$$

where CPP is the cerebral perfusion pressure, MAP is the mean arterial pressure, and ICP is the intracranial pressure. Each is discussed in detail as follows.

INTRACRANIAL CONTENTS AND PRESSURE

In simplified terms, the contents of the cranium are the brain and its covering membranes, cerebrospinal fluid (CSF), and blood. The cranium is a closed space and an increase in any of its components will cause an increase in the intracranial pressure (**Fig. 51-5**). Thus the intracranial compliance curve is steep, showing a rapid increase in pressure with minimal increase in volume (**Fig. 51-6**). Although this is commonly known as a low compliance of the cranium, in fact it is a reference to a rapid increase in pressure (ΔP) with a slight change of pressure (ΔV), causing a high $\Delta P/\Delta V$ or elastance.

The *brain* mass with the interstitial fluid is about 1100 g and occupies nearly 78% of the intracranial volume. An increase in this part can be either an increase in the cerebral mass via tumor, a foreign body, or abscesses, or by an increase in the interstitial fluid.

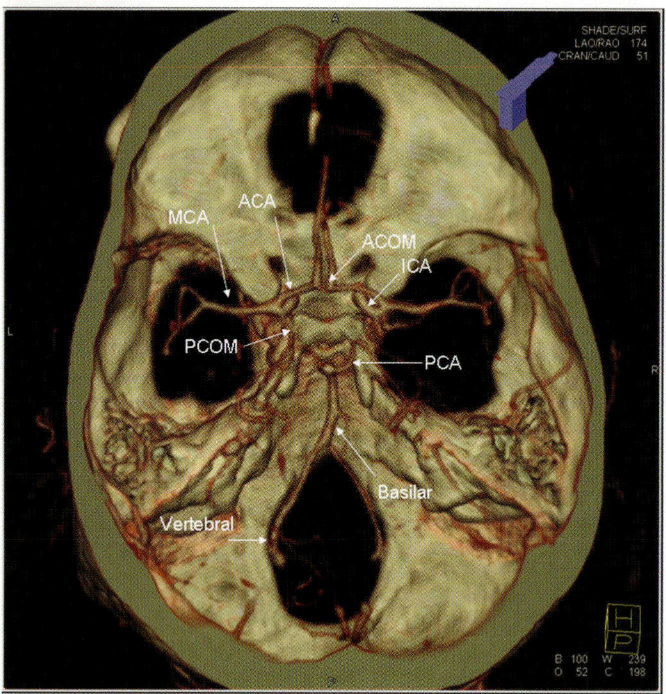

FIGURE 51-3. Circle of Willis. ACA, anterior cerebral artery; ACOM, anterior communicating artery; ICA, internal carotid artery; MCA, middle cerebral artery; PCA, posterior cerebral artery; PCOM, posterior communicating artery.

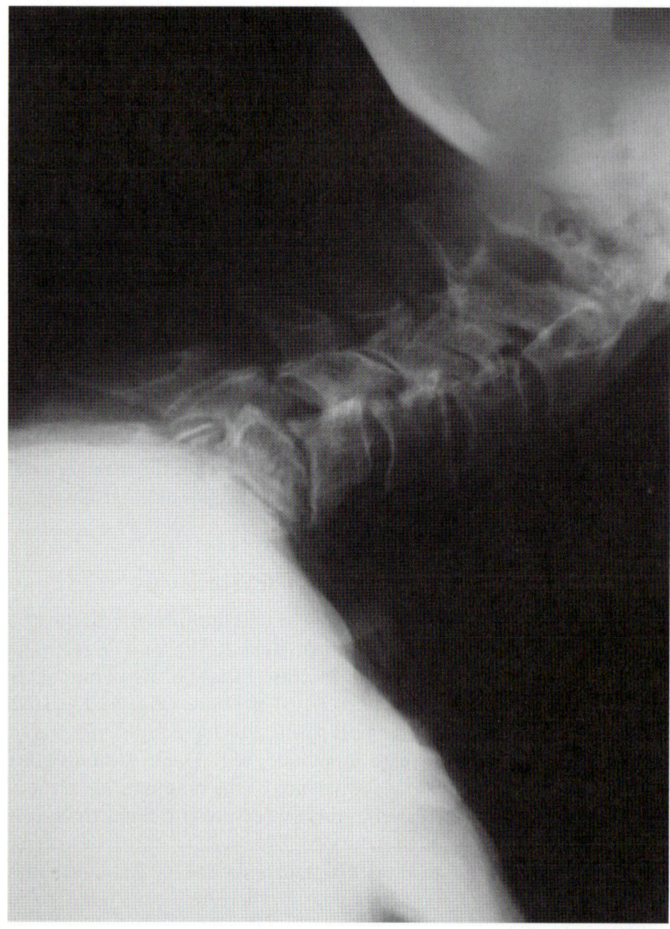

FIGURE 51-4. Traumatic subluxation of cervical spine.

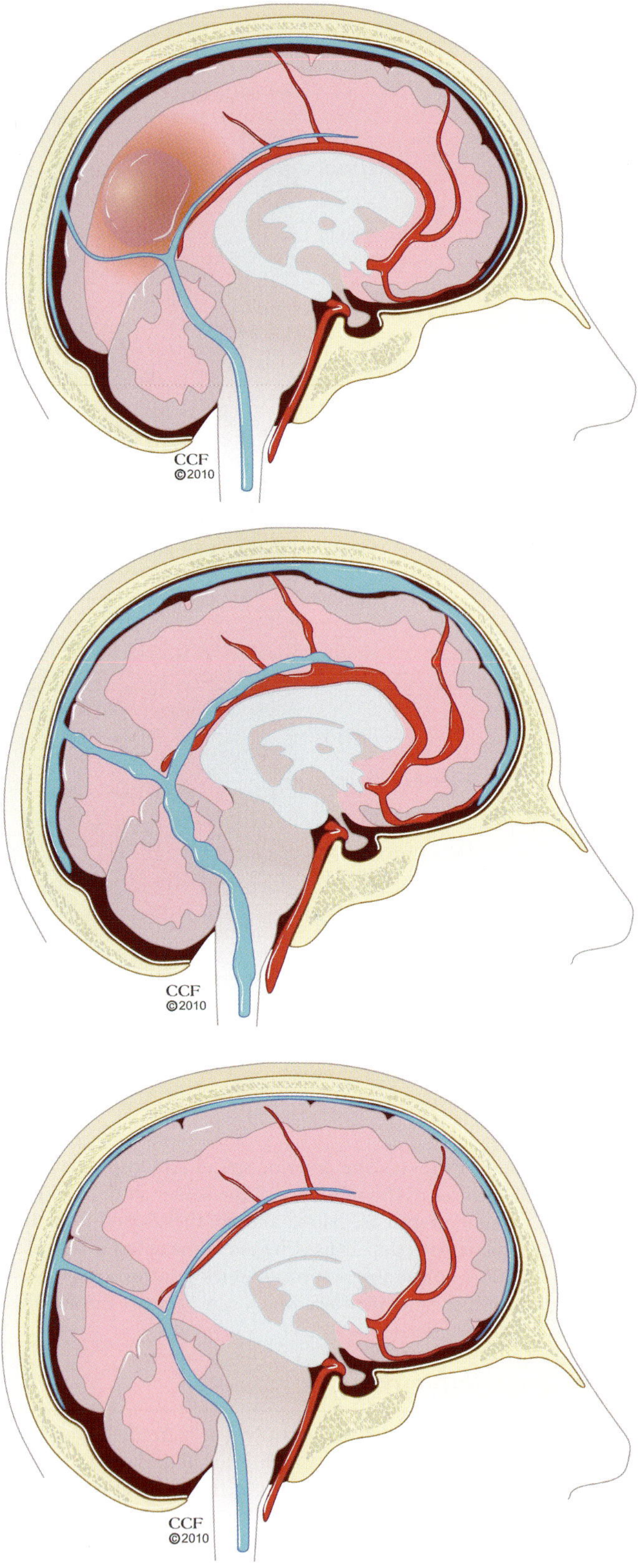

FIGURE 51-5. Intracranial space has 3 major components: brain and interstitial fluid, blood, and cerebrospinal fluid. An increase in intracranial pressure can be seen with an increase in volume of each. (**A**) represents a tumor or cerebral edema (eg, following a stroke); in (**B**) there is an increase in blood volume increasing pressure on the brain tissue and contracting the ventricle; and (**C**) represents an increase in cerebrospinal fluid dilating the ventricles and pressurizing the brain and blood vessels. [Reprinted with permission, Cleveland Clinic Center for Medical Art & Photography © 2010. All rights reserved.]

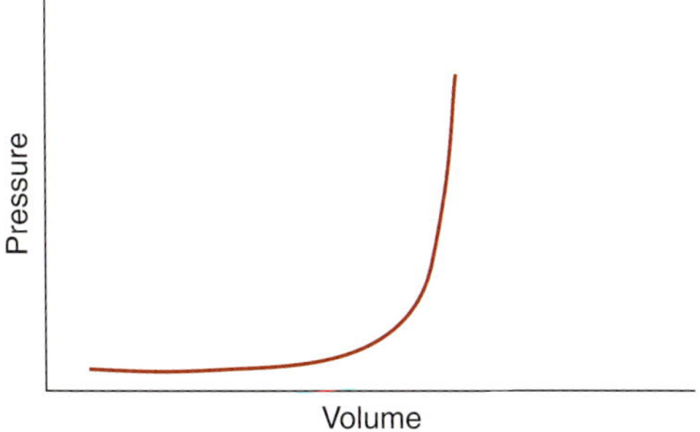

FIGURE 51-6. Intracranial compliance (or better, noncompliance) curve. An increase in intracranial volume content can increase the intracranial pressure very rapidly.

The *CSF* is produced by the choroid plexus in the ventricles, as well as minimally in the interstitium from transependymal perfusion. The intracranial part of the CSF is about 75 mL and helps protect the brain by its cushioning effect. It also provides an excretory pathway within the brain. After circulating, it is reabsorbed by the arachnoid villi in the subarachnoid space. The CSF is made at a rate of about 20 to 30 mL/h and it is renewed 3 to 4 times in 24 hours. Although an increase in CSF production per se is rare, there are many pathologic situations where the drainage of CSF is hindered. During noncommunicating hydrocephalus, there is an obstruction to the flow of CSF from the ventricles, which could be secondary to tumor, infection, or bleeding. In communicating hydrocephalus there is open flow of CSF from the ventricles; however, CSF absorption in the arachnoid villi is hindered. This commonly occurs after a subarachnoid hemorrhage (SAH). Some anesthetics can influence the production and absorption of CSF (**Table 51-1**); animal studies show that halothane can decrease the secretion and absorption of CSF, isoflurane does not affect secretion but increases absorption, and etomidate decreases secretion and increases absorption. The volatile agent least appropriate in the scenario of increased ICP is enflurane, which increases the production and decreases the absorption of CSF.

The third component within the intracranial vault is *blood*. The volume of blood in the cranial space averages about 50 mL depending on the body position with only 7 to 8 mL being arterial. This shows that the brain is dependent on *blood flow* to renew the supply of oxygenated blood in the brain. Blood volume (CBV) and blood flow (CBF) are 2 separate entities even though their numeric values are similar, 50 mL for CBV and about 50 mL/100 g/min for CBF; it is important to see the time variable in the CBF. The CBV is related directly to the flow of blood inside the cranium and indirectly to the amount of blood leaving it. Any change that increases brain blood flow or decreases the outflow of blood from the brain can increase CBV. Obstructions to the internal jugular vein (IJ) such as thrombosis, extreme neck rotation, and external pressure can decrease blood flow from the brain. Head positioning is also important and maintaining a head-up position may be the fastest way to decrease the intracranial pressure. Some anesthesiologists avoid the steep Trendelenburg position in patients with high ICP when accessing

TABLE 51-1 Effect of Anesthetics on Production and Absorption of CSF per Animal Studies

	CSF Production	CSF Absorption
Halothane	↓	↓
Enflurane	↑	↓
Isoflurane	–	↑
Desflurane	↑ (only with hypocapnia)	–
Fentanyl	–	↑
Etomidate	↓ (higher doses)	↑

CSF, cerebrospinal fluid.

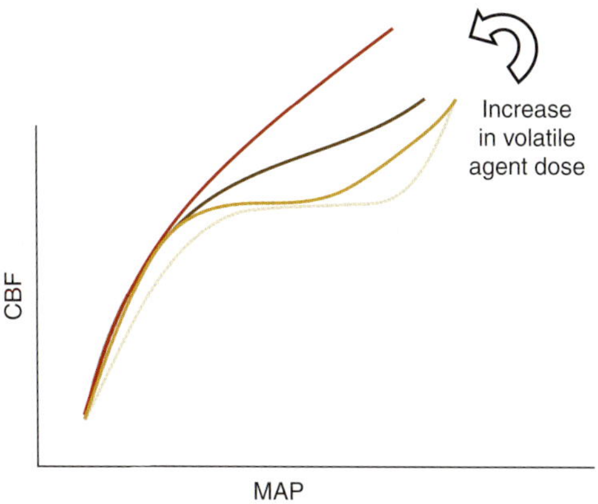

FIGURE 51-7. Change of autoregulation with volatile anesthetics. CBF, cerebral blood flow; MAP, mean arterial blood pressure.

the jugular vein for central catheterization. Right heart failure, pulmonary venous thrombosis or emboli, and high positive end-expiratory pressure (PEEP) can also decrease the amount of blood return from the brain.

An increase in CBF can also increase the CBV and thus ICP. According to Ohm law, the pressure (P) difference depends on flow (I) as well as resistance (R):

$$P = I \cdot R$$

For a given blood pressure the flow depends on the resistance of a vessel. An intact brain changes its resistance to maintain adequate flow across a wide range of pressure. This is called *autoregulation* and produces constant blood flow with MAP ranging between 50 and 150 mm Hg. There is a time lag between a pressure change and leveling of flow; abrupt changes in pressure can cause a significant drop in CBF and CPP. Also, one should keep in mind that the MAP measured by conventional monitoring systems may not accurately reflect the blood pressure in the brain, especially in the elderly population where the stenosis of arterial supply decreases the perfusion pressure. Volatile anesthetics can alter autoregulation in a dose-dependent manner (**Fig. 51-7**). Pathologic situations can disrupt the autoregulation, including tumors, trauma, stroke, vascular malformations such as arteriovenous malformations (AVMs), and ruptured intracranial aneurysms (IAs). When treating these patients the blood pressure should be controlled more closely to optimize the CPP. With hypotension, the intracranial vessels might not be able to dilate enough to allow more flow, and with hypertension the ability to vasoconstrict may not be adequate to decrease excessively high blood flow. For emphasis, CBV is not the same but is highly dependent on CBF, and variables affecting the CBF can influence CBV and as a result change ICP.

FACTORS AFFECTING CBF

Low CBF may disrupt adequate brain perfusion causing ischemia. On the other hand, a high CBF can result in increased CBV and ICP, which can be deleterious in patients with already elevated ICP, increasing the chance of brain herniation. Therefore a neuroanesthesiologist or a neurointensivist should have a solid understanding of all variables affecting the CBF (**Table 51-2**).

One of the main determinants of cerebral blood flow is the cerebral metabolic rate. The cerebral metabolic rate for oxygen ($CMRO_2$) demonstrates the amount of oxygen utilization in neurons to produce adenosine triphosphate (ATP). In adults the normal rate of oxygen utilization is 3.0 to 3.8 mL/100 g/min and is higher in the gray matter. Normally this is coupled with the blood flow of 50 mL/100 g/min with a ratio of 15:1. This *coupling* causes an increase in CBF during neuronal activity. The increase in blood flow exceeds the increase in oxygen

TABLE 51-2 Factors Influencing Cerebral Blood Flow[a]

Factor	Comment
Chemical/Metabolic/Humoral	
CMR	CMR influence assumes intact flow-metabolism coupling, the mechanism of which is not fully understood
Anesthetics	
Temperature	
Arousal/seizures	
$Paco_2$	
Pao_2	
Vasoactive drugs	
Anesthetics	
Vasodilators	
Vasopresors	
Mygenic	
Autoregulation/MAP	The autoregulation mechanism is fragile, and in many pathologic states CBF is regionally pressure passive
Rheologic	
Blood viscosity	
Neurogenic	
Extracranial sympathetic and parasympathetic pathways	

CBF, cerebral blood flow; CMR, cerebral metabolic rate; MAP, mean arterial pressure.

[a]See text for discussion.

From Miller RD. Miller's Anesthesia, Vol. 1. 7th ed. Elsevier; 2009:307.

metabolism causing some hyperoxygenation and decreased deoxygenated Hgb, thus creating the basis of functional neuroimaging.[3] Many theories have been suggested for the coupling mechanism, including accumulation of adenosine, nitric oxide (NO), cyclooxygenases, astrocytic cytochrome P450, and potassium concentration. Factors affecting the CMR include the state of arousal, seizure, temperature, and anesthetics. There is a higher degree of CMR in an awake state compared to sleep; seizures can cause a very high metabolic rate demanding a high oxygen supply.[4] Hypothermia decreases $CMRO_2$[5]; for every degree of centigrade drop in temperature there is a 6% to 7% decrease in the CMR; however, the neurometabolic and neurovascular coupling are preserved during hypothermia[6]; in contrast an increase in temperature up to 42°C increases the metabolic rate. In neurons 60% of ATP production is utilized for electrophysiologic activity and the remaining 40% is used for cellular homeostasis.

Anesthetics also can change the $CMRO_2$.[7] All volatile anesthetics decrease the $CMRO_2$, thus decreasing the need for oxygen, and if autoregulation remains intact they will decrease the CBF, CBV, and ICP. However, it is also known that all volatile anesthetics can decrease the vascular tone, thus increasing intracranial volume. It appears that these 2 effects (a decrease in CBF following a decrease in $CMRO_2$ and an increase in CBF following the vasodilatory effect) act in opposition. This is true, and in a less than 1.5 minimum alveolar concentration (MAC) of volatile anesthetics the vasoconstrictive effect following decreased $CMRO_2$ is the dominant arm. At higher levels of MAC the vasodilatory effect predominates and the CBF change becomes *uncoupled* with $CMRO_2$. This is why during craniotomies a balanced anesthetic method, including the use of opioids (often in a continuous infusion), is desirable to decrease the amount of volatile agent necessary for general anesthesia. Nitrous oxide use increases the global CBF, but mainly in the frontal region, and reduces the CO_2 responsiveness. In addition, there may be an increase in $CMRO_2$ with N_2O.[8] Regional blood flow changes are different with volatile anesthetics.[9]

Almost all intravenous anesthetics decrease the $CMRO_2$ and concomitantly the CBF, the exception being ketamine.[10] Ketamine can increase $CMRO_2$ in parts of the brain, and, because the autoregulation remains intact with ketamine, the CBF can increase. Some other anesthetics can attenuate this effect of ketamine. Thiopental can decrease the electrical activity during electroencephalogram (EEG), and at complete electrical silence the $CMRO_2$ will decrease to about 60%. Thiopental acts on reducing the ATP requirement by acting on the electrical activity of the brain and only minimally on the cellular homeostasis part. Thus after producing a flat EEG, additional doses of thiopental will not further decrease the $CMRO_2$.

One of the most widely used and perhaps misused methods of changing the CBF is changing the $Paco_2$. Hypoventilation can increase $Paco_2$, causing intracranial vasodilation and increasing the CBF; in contrast, hyperventilation decreases the $Paco_2$, causing vasoconstriction. Cerebral blood flow changes 1 to 2 mL/100 g/min with each millimeter of mercury change in $Paco_2$. Cerebral blood volume also changes with $Paco_2$ in the same direction of CBF but by a different percentage.[11] The degree of change in CBF depends on resting CBF. Volatile anesthetics can alter the vascular responsiveness to hyperventilation; there is also regional variability in blood flow reduction.[12] Below $Paco_2$ of 25 mm Hg, CBF change is attenuated because severe vasoconstriction can cause local ischemia. In patients with increased ICP, one should take into consideration that administration of opioids in the perioperative period in nonintubated patients further increases ICP by causing hypoventilation. An important and often missed fact is the temporary nature of this phenomenon. Hyperventilation can cause alkalosis of CSF and extracellular space because CO_2 can easily cross the blood–brain barrier (BBB). In the course of time, after more than 6 hours, the bicarbonate decreases following changes in the activity of the enzyme carbonic anhydrase and the pH returns to normal, and the effect of hyperventilation is diminished. At this point if the ventilation is returned to normal, accumulation of CO_2 will cause acidosis and intracranial vasodilation. Thus, after prolonged hyperventilation, the return to normal ventilation should be made gradual.

The effect of Pao_2 on vascular tone and CBF is not apparent until its levels decrease to 60 mm Hg, below which vasodilation can increase the CBF. Vasoactive drugs can also change the vascular tone and thus the CBF. Systemic vasodilators can cause vasodilation, hypotension, and a decrease in CBF. There are mixed reports regarding the effect of nitroprusside on intracranial CBF.[13,14] Angiotensin-converting enzyme inhibitors typically do not affect the CBF. The intracranial vasculature does not have α_1 receptors, and α_1 stimulation does not cause intracranial vasoconstriction. This along with an increase in systolic blood pressure (SBP) following injection of α_1-agonists can increase CBF. Alternatively, β-receptor agonists in large doses can increase $CMRO_2$ and CBF, but β-blockers can either reduce or have no effect on CBF and $CMRO_2$. Dobutamine can increase the CBF, but high-dose dopamine does not cause vasoconstriction in cerebral vessels. Dexmedetomidine, a selective α_2-agonist, has been shown to cause cerebral vasoconstriction without affecting $CMRO_2$.

Blood viscosity can also affect CBF. Low hematocrit (Hct) can decrease the viscosity, providing an improved flow; however, it can also decrease blood oxygen content. An Hct of 30% to 34% produces the optimal O_2 delivery.

MONITORING

One of the most common questions asked by anesthesia trainees concerns the optimal blood pressure in patients with increased ICP. The question comes up often in patients with increased ICP following an intracranial hemorrhage (ICH). If the CPP equation suggests a need for increased MAP when ICP is elevated to maintain the CPP, wouldn't this increase the CBF, expand the ICH, and cause a higher ICP? Conversely, if we decrease the MAP to decrease the intracranial bleed in a patient with ICH which has disrupted autoregulation, wouldn't this cause a low CPP, especially because ICP is elevated?

Both are logical questions as far as they go; the answer is to find the optimal blood pressure to provide the best possible perfusion and not increase the ICP. In addition to measuring blood pressure this would require knowledge of cerebral oxygenation and intracranial pressure, neither of which are easy to measure.

An invasive method of measuring the arterial pressure is preferable in intracranial and multilevel spine procedures when the potential for large amounts of blood loss or blood pressure variation is present. When deciding on placement of an invasive blood pressure monitor the same principles apply in neurosurgery as in other subspecialties. Indications for arterial line placement include patients with a history of poorly controlled hypertension, expectation for sudden and major changes in blood pressure and intravascular fluid, a need for frequent arterial blood gas measurements, problems with using a noninvasive method, or to plan for induced hypertension or hypotension. Placement of a central venous catheter also follows the general rules of monitoring central venous pressure in other surgical procedures; however, there are some special considerations in neurosurgical patients. In most spine procedures patients are placed in the prone position. The measured central venous pressure in this position might not provide an accurate central venous pressure. In patients undergoing thoracic spine surgery where there is a chance of entering the pleural space during the surgical procedure, a chest x-ray (CXR) after central line placement may be helpful. In anterior or lateral approaches to the thoracic spine where 1-lung ventilation is part of the surgical plan, it is better to place the central line on the side of surgery. The possibility of air embolism is another indication for a central venous catheter. Air embolism is possible in spine procedures where air can enter the epidural venous system or cancellous tissue in the vertebral body; adequate hemostasis and the use of "bone wax" can decrease the chance of air embolism. Air embolism, however, is also common in craniotomies where the position of the head with open veins and cranial diploë may be significantly higher than the cardiac level, especially in sitting craniotomies. A central venous catheter can be helpful in withdrawing the air and relieving the air lock caused by embolized air. This central catheter should be placed so the distal tip is at the entrance of the right atrium. Appropriate positioning of the catheter is confirmed by using a modified central venous catheter, conducting the electrocardiogram (ECG) electrical waveform produced at the catheter tip. Positioning of the catheter tip adjacent to the SA node will record a large biphasic P wave. These central catheters are also multiperforated at the distal end to allow better aspiration of air. Detection of air embolism is also facilitated by the use of precordial Doppler. Compared to the transesophageal echocardiogram, the sensitivity of the precordial Doppler in detecting air within the central venous system entering the heart is lower; however, it is less cumbersome and allows continouous auditory monitoring throughout the procedure. The Doppler should be placed in the second to fourth intercoastal space at the left or right parasternal position. Use of a pulmonary artery catheter should be limited to cases where proper information about preload and cardiac function is essential in clinical management. Intracranial vasospasm after subarachnoid hemorrhage, especially in patients with cardiac dysfunction, is an example of a situation where a high preload is desirable as part of the *triple H* (hypertension, hypervolemia, hemodylution) therapy despite the risk of fluid overload.

There are also some specific monitoring methods used in neurosurgery. In patients who need ICP measurement and access to CSF, a ventriculostomy drain or spinal drain can be used. A spinal drain can measure the pressure transferred from the intracranial part of CSF to the subarachnoid space in the spine. It may not accurately reflect the ICP. It is important to note that placement of a spinal drain in patients who have increased ICP can risk brain herniation. In comparison with other ICP monitors such as an intraparenchymal probe, epidural probe, or subarachnoid probe, ventriculostomy is counted as the "gold standard" and can be used to measure pressure and drain the CSF, although not simultaneously. It is important to remember to close the CSF drain during transportation of patients to avoid overdrainage. Intraparenchymal probes have also been introduced to monitor the ICP, oxygenation, and metabolism. Most of these probes are invasive, are susceptible to artifacts, increase the chance of infection, and only monitor the focal brain area. These probes are placed through a burr hole and can also be used to measure the brain tissue oxygen pressure ($pBtO_2$); however, the measured pressure is very local and may not be a good determinant of the global oxygenation of the brain. Microdialysis catheters are also used to measure the local oxygen concentration as well as any other substance that is dialyzable within the brain tissue. Metabolic end products, concentrations of drugs, neurotransmitters, and markers of tissue damage and inflammation can be measured using this method (**Table 51-3**).

Measurement of the difference in oxygen content between the arterial and venous side of the brain is an indicator of the brain's oxygen need. A jugular bulb catheter can be used for this purpose. This catheter is placed in a retrograde manner into the internal jugular vein and the tip is positioned within the jugular bulb beyond the entry of venous drainage of extracranial origin. Analysis of this blood for oxygen content and lactate will reflect the global brain oxygen supply-and-demand relationship. A low oxygen content and high lactate demonstrates a higher demand-to-supply ratio. One of the drawbacks of this monitoring method is that small changes representing focal ischemia may not be evident. An EEG is another way of monitoring the brain during craniotomies. Sometimes this method is used for intraoperative mapping and defining of a seizure focus. It is also used to detect intraoperative ischemia during cranial vascular procedures including carotid endarterectomy. Ischemic changes can help in decision making to put a temporary shunt during this procedure. Other neuromonitoring methods including evoked potentials are also used in monitoring the functional integrity of neurons in intracranial as well as spinal procedures. The sensory evoked potentials are divided into somatosensory (SSEP), auditory (AEP), and visual evoked potentials (VEP). Stimulation of a sensory nerve, peripheral in the case of SSEP, auditory by headphones in the case of AEP, and visual by flashing light in the case of VEP, can stimulate an evoked potential. Measurement of the amplitude of waveform and the latency or time required for the potential to reach the proximal end of the neuron group being monitored can denote functional integrity in that nerve. In some situations the cortical motor areas in the brain are stimulated to monitor the descending motor pathways. The recording electrodes in this method are placed in the muscles of the patient's arms or legs. Most anesthetic agents can affect the evoked potentials (EP) and this should be kept in mind during anesthetic planning in procedures when this type of monitoring will be used as part of the surgical procedure.

NEUROPHARMACOLOGY

All medications given during anesthesia may have a direct or indirect effect on the central nervous system. Not all pharmacologic agents pass the blood–brain barrier (BBB); however, this barrier may be disrupted in central nervous system (CNS) diseases or injury. The anesthesiologist should be aware of the effects of medications on the CNS used within the perioperative period. After neurosurgery the best indicator of adequacy of the surgical outcome is a mental and neuromuscular examination. In cranial surgery this includes gross mental status and motor and sensory evaluation, as well as speech testing commonly known as a "neuro check." In spine procedures the surgeon is usually keen to evaluate sensory and motor nerves as soon as possible. Information about pharmacodynamic and pharmacokinetic properties of drugs can help in choosing the best anesthetic plan. In this section medications commonly used in the perioperative period with specific emphasis on physiologic changes in CBF, CBV and $CMRO_2$ are discussed.

PROPOFOL

Propofol is a sedative hypnotic, a γ-aminobutyric acid (GABA) receptor agonist, which is used for induction as well as maintenance of anesthesia. Induction is rapid, and intravenous injection of 1.5 to 2.5 mg/kg can cause unconsciousness in 30 seconds. Although the elimination half-life is up to 1.5 hours, emergence is very rapid and complete following redistribution. Propofol can decrease the $CMRO_2$, CBF[15], and ICP[16] in large doses and if there is inadequate preload, it can decrease the MAP and CPP. It significantly decreases the intraocular pressure, and the CO_2 responsiveness and autoregulation remains intact. It slows the cortical EEG waves and can even cause burst suppression in large doses;

TABLE 51-3 Brain Monitoring Methods

Method	Spatial Resolution	Temporal Resolution	Purpose	Advantages	Disadvantages
Intracranial pressure	Global	Continuous	Measuring intracranial compliance	Reliable Quantitative Allows monitoring of CPP	Invasive Risk of infection Risk of hemorrhage
Jugular oximetry ($Sjvo_2$)	Global	Continuous	Measuring adequacy of hemispheric oxygenation	Quantitative Allows monitoring of A-VDo_2 and O_2ER	Susceptible to artifacts Local complications (eg, infection, thrombosis)
EEG	Global	Continuous	Monitoring electrical brain activity Detection of seizures	Technique well standardized Only method to diagnose nonconvulsive seizures	Qualitative Relatively insensitive to secondary insults
SSEPs	Global	Continuous	Monitoring integrity of sensory pathways	Technique well standardized Simple	Qualitative Fairly insensitive to secondary insults
Bedside Xe-133 cerebral blood flow	Regional	Discontinuous	Measuring hemispheric CBF	Quantitative	Accurate only if radiotracer injected into carotid artery Radioactivity
TCD	Regional	Continuous	Measuring CBF velocities	Simple Noninvasive Allows measuring PI, VMR	Qualitative and indirect assessment of CBF Difficult to keep probes in place
Laser Doppler flowmetry	Local	Continuous	Measuring cortical CBF	Accurate Dynamic information	Qualitative Invasive Susceptible to artifacts
Thermal diffusion flowmetry	Local	Continuous	Measuring cortical CBF	Simple Dynamic information	Qualitative Invasive Monitors small volume of tissue
Brain tissue Po_2	Local	Continuous	Measuring cerebral oxygenation	Quantitative Sensitive Probes also measure brain temperature	Invasive Susceptible to artifacts Monitors small volume of tissue
NIRS	Local	Continuous	Measuring cerebral oxygenation	Noninvasive	Measures only relative changes Susceptible to artifacts
Microdialysis	Local	Discontinuous	Measuring cerebral metabolism	Sensitive Quantitative	Invasive Complicated technique Labor intensive Unclear which is the best parameter to monitor

A-VDo_2, arteriovenous oxygen difference; CBF, cerebral blood flow; CPP, cerebral perfusion pressure; NIRS, near-infrared spectroscopy; O_2ER, oxygen extraction rate; PI, pulsatility index; Po_2, partial pressure of oxygen; $Sjvo_2$, jugular vein oxygen saturation; SSEPs, somatosensory evoked potentials; TCD, tanscranial Doppler; VMR, vasomotor reactivity.

From Bradly WG. Neurology in Clinical Practice, Vol. 1. 5th ed. Elsevier; 2008:922.

however, it is useful in awake craniotomy because EEG recording will be back to baseline 15 minutes after stopping the infusion. In the case of intraoperative seizure it can act as an antiepileptic, stopping the seizure activity even in small doses. It affects the SSEP and motor evoked potentials (MEPs) more than the AEP. Propofol can also cause some subcortical excitatory movements, which are not seizures[17]; it can cause dyskinesia or temporarily improve tremors in Parkinson disease.[18]

THIOPENTAL

Thiopental is a barbiturate used as a sedative hypnotic. It is an agonist on the GABA receptor. Following a very rapid redistribution, it can cause a fast awakening after a bolus dose. After a bolus injection the concentration in the brain reaches a maximum in 40 seconds and redistribution decreases it to 50% in 5 minutes and 10% in 30 minutes. $CMRO_2$, and coupled with it CBF and CBV, will decrease with the use of thiopental; thus the ICP will also decrease. The EEG will show a slow waveform and will progress to burst suppression and flatline EEG. At this point there will be a 60% decrease in brain oxygen consumption. Additional doses of thiopental will not further decrease the oxygen consumption.[19] This means that as long as the EEG shows brain activity, administration of thiopental can have a brain protectant effect by decreasing the $CMRO_2$, but no further protection is seen with a flat EEG. That is why thiopental has not been helpful in global ischemia such as that seen in cardiac arrest,[20] although this effect may be influenced by underlying cardiac disease.[21] Thiopental does have a protectant effect in focal ischemia, and it has been widely used intraoperatively when focal temporary ischemia is induced specifically in intracranial vascular procedures. There is no standard dose for brain protection; however, monitoring methods such as EEG can help in directing the treatment.[19]

Thus in an intact autoregulation scenario, because there is a decrease in $CMRO_2$, less CBF is needed and there is an increase in the perfusion-to-metabolism ratio; however, a severe drop in blood pressure can decrease the CPP. The CO_2 response and autoregulation remain intact with thiopental. Although thiopental can change evoked potentials in a dose-dependent manner, it is an acceptable medication to use during EP monitoring.

ETOMIDATE

Etomidate is associated with cardiovascular stability[22] and is usually used when strict blood pressure control is needed during induction. Etomidate does not have analgesic properties and it can cause adrenal suppression. It has a rapid awakening after metabolism and redistribution. It decreases the $CMRO_2$ and is a potent cerebral vasoconstrictor decreasing the CBF and ICP.[23] Etomidate can cause spike waveforms in the EEG and because it can also cause myoclonus, it may be mistaken for a seizure. In high doses it can cause an isoelectric EEG, although it can activate seizure foci and it can also be used to terminate status epilepticus. Etomidate has recently been used to help in the localization of seizure foci.[24] It can augment amplitude during SSEP monitoring.

KETAMINE

Ketamine can cause dissociation between thalamic and limbic systems; ketamine-induced anesthesia can resemble a cataleptic stage. Ketamine has an effective analgesic and amnestic effect, and acts rapidly after intravenous and intramuscular administration. It increases $CMRO_2$ in regional parts of the brain including the frontal lobe. Global CMR is also increased. In patients with intact autoregulation this can cause an increase in CBF that may be disproportionate to the increase in CMR.[10] Although this can in turn increase the ICP, it is dependent on the use of other anesthetics and $Paco_2$.[25] This effect can be attenuated by the use of benzodiazepines and propofol. However, specifically in patients with an increased ICP, it is not often the ideal induction agent. It does not affect the CBF response to CO_2. It can slow the EEG waveforms and in high doses can cause burst suppression. It does not change the seizure threshold, and although it is considered an antiepileptic, it can cause myoclonic movements. The amplitude on SSEP increases, but it can depress the AEP and VEP.

OPIOIDS

Opioids are an important part of the anesthetic plan in neurosurgical procedures. A common effect of all opioids is hypoventilation. In patients with an increased ICP, an elevated $Paco_2$ can further increase the ICP. This should be kept in mind when premedicating patients before a craniotomy. However, untreated pain can increase the sympathetic response, which may increase ICP by elevating blood pressure (BP) in patients in whom autoregulation is disrupted. In neurosurgical cases it is desirable to maintain a steady infusion of opioid as an adjunct to anesthesia to avoid significant changes in concentration, with boluses resulting in sudden alterations in hemodynamic parameters. Opioid infusions are used during anesthetic maintenance as an adjunct to volatile or other intravenous anesthetics. By decreasing volatile anesthetic use, opioids can decrease vasodilatory effect. Opioids can decrease the mean arterial pressure; however, reports on the effect of opioids on ICP are varied. Although they are known to have minimal, if any, effect on ICP, in some reports an elevated ICP has been noted after use in patients with head trauma.[26] Another important effect of opioids is an increase in rigidity, which can make ventilation difficult, although priming with muscle relaxants may prevent this effect.[27] An infusion of remifentanil as an adjunct for general anesthesia has been widely favored due to its ultra-short half-life,[28] which enables an early neurologic examination postoperatively. This can also produce an earlier start of postoperative pain.[29]

BENZODIAZEPINES

Benzodiazepines can cause anxiolysis, sedation, and amnesia. They also have spinal cord–mediated muscle relaxation as well as antiseizure activity. The main concern in using benzodiazepines in neurosurgical patients is the potential for changing the mental status, which may confuse the neurologic examination. The most common short-acting benzodiazepine used is midazolam, although diazepam and lorazepam have also commonly been used. Benzodiazepines enhance the action of GABA, which acts as an inhibitory neurotransmitter. Midazolam decreases the $CMRO_2$ and in parallel CBF,[30] but does not affect the ICP. Interestingly, positron emission tomography (PET) scans show the decrease in the CBF to be in regions of arousal, memory, and attention. The benzodiazepine antagonist flumazenil can reverse the sedative effects, but it can also reverse the decreased CBF and $CMRO_2$ effect and should be used cautiously in patients with concerned intracranial compliance issues. Although midazolam has not been shown to depress ventilation in healthy volunteers in regular doses, it can suppress ventilation in higher doses and has a synergistic effect on ventilatory depression when administered with opioids. This suppression can be more pronounced in patients with chronic obstructive pulmonary disease. Because midazolam can cause sedation, in patients with obstructive sleep apnea it can cause hypoventilation. Benzodiazepines can decrease the α activity and increase the low-voltage rapid β activity in EEG, but a flat EEG is not seen with midazolam.

DEXMEDETOMIDINE

Studies show this selective α_2-agonist to be a cerebral vasoconstrictor.[31] Because studies in animals showed no effect on $CMRO_2$, there is a concern about brain hypoperfusion. However, in humans a decrease in CBF/CMR ratio has not been shown. A transient increase in blood pressure during the loading dose of dexmedetomidine followed by hypotension may be a concern in patients who should have strict blood pressure control following intracranial hemorrhage or increased ICP. The most valuable characteristic of this agent is the ability to induce sedation without respiratory depression, making it useful in awake craniotomies.[32] Although the effect of dexmedetomidine on respiration is similar to normal sleep, it should be kept in mind that patients with obstructive sleep apnea as well as obese patients might have hypoventilation and hypercapnea with the use of this agent. Currently, several studies are under way in determining the neuroprotective effect of dexmedetomidine. This agent is also useful in sedation for deep brain stimulator placement.

ANTIEPILEPTICS

The use of antiepileptics (AED) is a common practice in the perioperative period in neurosurgical patients. In some instances the presenting symptom of an intracranial mass is seizure. Some patients may have recently been placed on these medications and plasma drug levels may not be in the therapeutic range. Following craniotomy the concentration of AED may also change.[33] Patients with sudden onset of seizures may have received a loading dose of AED, and because these medications have side effects that can influence the anesthetic plan, it is important to direct the physical examination and laboratory studies toward evaluation of these side effects. Some AEDs including barbiturates, primidone, clonazepam, and gabapentin can cause sedation. Nausea, vomiting, and gastrointestinal disturbances are seen in phenytoin, carbamazepine, gabapentin, lamotrigine, ethosuximide, and valproic acid. Many of these medications also can cause idiosyncratic reactions such as Stevens-Johnson syndrome (phenobarbital, phenytoin, carbamazepine, lamotrigine), agranulocytosis (phenobarbital, phenytoin), aplastic anemia (carbamazepine, ethosuximide, valproic acid), or thrombocytopenia (primidone, clonazepam). Hepatotoxicity is also seen with some of these medications and a hepatic function panel may be indicated because many anesthetic medications depend on hepatic metabolism or excretion. Many AEDs bind to albumin and a change in the concentration of this protein can change the free drug concentration. Because valproic acid can induce hemostatic disorders such as thrombocytopenia, platelet disfunction, and hypofibrinogenemia, patients who are chronically treated and are scheduled for an elective procedure with a higher risk of surgical hemorrhage (such as deep brain stimulator placement or major spine surgery) may need to change their AED under the supervision of a neurologist; however, sudden discontinuation of these medications is not advised because it can cause severe relapse of seizures.

Patients on chronic AED will need more frequent administration of nondepolarizing muscle relaxants.[34,35] This could be as a result of hepatic enzyme induction, change in plasma protein binding, decreased sensitivity of acetylcholine binding, or direct competition for binding sites. Most studies show that recovery from neuromuscular blockade of atracurium is not affected by AED; however, there is a need for higher rate of infusion of cisatracurium in these patients.

Another important consideration in the intraoperative administration of AED is the potential for hypotension, especially in the presence of anesthetic agents.

MUSCLE RELAXANTS

Succinylcholine increases the ICP as well as CBF. The use of nondepolarizing muscle relaxants as a pretreatment can decrease this increase in ICP.[36] Nondepolarizing muscle relaxants especially in high doses can cause histamine release. Histamine can increase the ICP by intracranial vasodilation; it can also decrease the blood pressure, which can lead to low CPP.[37] Atracurium can metabolize to laudanosine, which has been shown to be a seizure-inducing agent in animals but not in humans in clinical doses. Vecuronium may be a better muscle relaxant in the neurosurgical setting because it lacks the deleterious hemodynamic effects of histamine release. Antiepileptics can cause rapid metabolization of muscle relaxants by enzyme induction.

INHALED ANESTHETICS

All inhaled anesthetics are vasodilators and can increase CBF. However, if autoregulation is not intact the intracranial blood flow response will follow the $CMRO_2$. Apart from nitrous oxide (N_2O), all other commonly used halogenated anesthetics and xenon decrease the $CMRO_2$, thus decreasing CBF. The net result of the difference between the vasodilatory effect of volatile agents and the vasoconstrictive effect secondary to decreased $CMRO_2$ determines the net CBF change.[38] The vasodilatory effect of volatile agents, although not fully understood, may be the result of nitric oxide (NO) release. However, the change in regional blood flow shown by PET scan in different parts of the brain is varied. Nitrous oxide causes an increase in $CMRO_2$, CBF,[39] and ICP. This effect can be attenuated with concurrent use of other volatile anesthetics. The increase in CBF and ICP can be counteracted by hyperventilation. Some intravenous anesthetics also decrease the effect of N_2O on $CMRO_2$ and CBF.[40] However, some look at this situation differently and conclude that adding N_2O to these anesthetics counteracts their protective effect on the brain, thus the use of this agent as an adjunct for intracranial procedures is still under debate. As an *N*-methyl-D-aspartate (NMDA) blocker, N_2O has a neuroprotective potential because neuronal death after ischemia depends on NMDA receptor activation. Up to a certain concentration N_2O and xenon (another NMDA inhibitor) can decrease ischemia-associated brain damage and NMDA-associated Ca^{++} influx in cortical cells.[35] On the other hand, NMDA blockers have been shown to have neurotoxic properties that can be attenuated by short-term use as well as concurrent use of GABA-ergic agents such as diazepam or isoflurane.[41] However, the use of N_2O does increase the rate of postoperative nausea and vomiting, which is an undesired side effect because it can elevate ICP. In patients who have an intracranial air trap, the use of N_2O can increase the size of the air pocket. Isoflurane, like other volatile anesthetics, can decrease the $CMRO_2$ in a dose-dependent manner until a flat EEG is achieved (~2.0 MAC). A decrease in $CMRO_2$ can also decrease the CBF, but with higher doses its vasodilatory effect overpowers causing an increase in CBF. This is why anesthetic adjuncts, such as opioids (fentanyl, remifentanil, or sufentanil) are being used with volatile anesthetics to decrease the MAC level. Isoflurane has been studied for its preconditioning effect,[42] as a GABAergic agent and depressor of cerebral metabolism it can have a neuroprotective effect, the clinical value of which still has to be proven. Sevoflurane has similar effects to isoflurane in increasing the CBF and decreasing the $CMRO_2$, but the increase in CBF is less than isoflurane. With sevoflurane, the increase in ICP is also less than isoflurane; however, in patients with elevated ICP, propofol may be a better agent to use. Similar to isoflurane, the neuroprotective[43] and preconditioning[44,45] effects of sevoflurane are under study and the clinical value still has to be demonstrated. Desflurane is another volatile anesthetic with similar effects to isoflurane and sevoflurane. It can decrease the $CMRO_2$ and CBF at 1 MAC, but with increased concentration, when the $CMRO_2$ is maximally suppressed, it can increase the CBF. Compared to isoflurane and sevoflurane it increases the ICP more. The neuroprotective effect of desflurane is comparable to isoflurane.

NEUROPROTECTION

Neurological injury has a negative impact on the patient's quality of life and health resources. There is a considerable risk of cerebral ischemia in patients who undergo neurosurgical, cardiac, and vascular surgery. In cardiac surgery, perioperative neurocognitive dysfunction is a relatively common event with an incidence ranging from 30% to 79% at 2 weeks and 24% to 57% at 6 months, and can result in significant morbidity.[46] The annual cost of neurological injury following cardiac surgery is estimated to be in the range of \$2 to \$4 billion. To date there has been little clinical success with pharmacological neuroprotection; benefits were demonstrated in preclinical studies; however, they failed to materialize in human trials.[47]

PATHOGENISIS OF NEURONAL INJURY

Following an ischemic insult, there appears to be 2 distinct injuries. The central area or core has rapid cell death and is generally believed not amenable to neuroprotection. The area of tissue surrounding the central core is known as the penumbra. Cell death in the penumbra is considered an active process that can potentially be altered by neuroprotective therapies. The penumbra has sufficient blood supply to maintain ion channel integrity but not enough to maintain electrical activity. During hypoxic-ischemic injury, cellular function is largely unregulated and does not match demand, resulting in dysfunction of ATP-dependent ion channels leading to cellular depolarization and the release of excitatory neurotransmitters such as glutamate, in addition to the failure of energy-dependent glutamate uptake by astrocytes. Excess glutamatergic excitatory neurotransmission induces excitotoxic cell death as extracellular concentrations of glutamate rise by 3- to 10-fold. Activation of the NMDA receptor subtype of the glutamatergic receptor produces an influx of sodium and calcium ions, contributing to depolarization and neural overactivation. During ischemia the high concentrations of junctional glutamate spill out of the synaptic cleft, stimulating extra synaptic NMDA receptors to induce excitotoxic cell death.[48] Necrosis is thought to occur in the acute phase in the core of cerebral infarct. In the penumbra region the neurons die slowly by apoptosis. This process involves the increase in permeability of the mitochondrial membrane with increased influx of sodium and calcium into the mitochondria, resulting in depolarization. The increased permeability of the mitochondrial membrane leads to the release of cytochrome *c* into the cytoplasm, which activates the caspases enzyme system. The activation of caspases leads to programmed cell death or apoptosis. Consequently, one important action of neuroprotective agents during the ischemia and reperfusion period is to maintain the integrity of the mitochondrial membrane during those periods, which will prevent the release of cytochrome *c* into the cytoplasm and subsequent programmed cell death. In addition, there is an immunological response to the insult with released cytokines, such as interleukin (IL)-1, contributing to ongoing neurodegeneration.[49] Within minutes following initial vessel occlusion, there is an increase in the expression of transcription factors such as c-fos and c-jun, followed by a second wave of heat shock proteins (HSP-70) that increase their expression in the 1- to 2-hour to 1- to 2-day period. An increase in chemokine expression (IL-1, IL-6, IL-8, tumor necrosis factor [TNF]-α, etc.) is observed in the first 24 hours after occlusion.[50] The involvement of gray versus white matter in the ischemic zone has an important impact on outcome, as ischemia in deep white matter is generally severe due to the lack of collateral blood supply in this area.

Inflammation may promote repair through the ability of T cells to produce neurotrophic factors such as brain-derived nerve growth

(BDNF), nerve growth factor (NGF), and neurotrophins 3, 4, and 5, which facilitate neural cell proliferation and differentiation.[51] Macrophages also play a role in this process through secretion of cytokines (IL-1β and IL-6), chemokines, and TNF-α. Increased activity of contralateral or undamaged adjacent brain areas may attenuate the long-term effects of ischemic injury on outcome.

ANESTHETIC-INDUCED NEUROPROTECTION

Barbiturates can produce isoelectricity of the electrocorticogram (ECoG) and they have been studied extensively. In the early 1970s, Yatsu et al first demonstrated that methohexital was neuroprotective.[52] In the setting of global ischemia, barbiturates induced ECoG burst-suppression doses do not reduce ischemic injury.[53] This is not particularly surprising because the ECoG is rendered isoelectric rapidly after the occurrence of global ischemia. The mechanism of neuroprotection of barbiturates can be attributed to glutamate receptor blockage, potentiation of GABA-ergic activity, and inhibition of calcium influx, similar to other anesthetic agents.[54] It should be noted that the magnitude of the protective efficacy is modest. In addition, doses that produce burst suppression of the ECoG may not be necessary to achieve protection. It was shown that one-third of the dose required to achieve ECoG suppression yielded injury reduction similar to that achieved with much larger doses.[55] The administration of barbiturates for the purpose of neuroprotection has many disadvantages, including the potential need for inotropes to maintain the blood pressure and the possible need for postoperative mechanical ventilation secondary to delayed emergence from anesthesia.[56]

Propofol has been shown to be neuroprotective in vivo in both focal and global[57,58] models of cerebral ischemia. This neuroprotective effect may be due to antioxidant effects (enabled by its phenolic hydroxyl group) or by effects on glutamate uptake, dopamine release, or GABA receptors. No clinical data exist that establish neuroprotection by propofol in humans. A small study comparing propofol with isoflurane anesthesia during coronary artery bypass grafting (CABG) in 20 patients found no difference in early neurocognitive performance (3-6 days postoperative) and even saw a transient increase in serum S100β levels (a surrogate marker for neuronal damage) in the propofol group.[59]

The α_2-agonist dexmedetomidine was shown to have a neuroprotective effect in animal models of ischemia. Dexmedetomidine exerts its neuroprotective effects via a myriad of mechanisms. It lowers plasma catecholamine levels and improves neurological outcome in rat models of ischemia assessed functionally and histopathologically. It also enhances the astrocyte uptake and metabolism of glutamate. Dexmedetomidine maintains the integrity of the mitochondria membrane during ischemia by upregulating the expression of antiapoptotic factors Bcl-2 and mdm-2 and downregulating the expression of apoptotic factors like Bax.[31,60,61]

The potential neuroprotective effect of ketamine is due to its antagonistic effect on the NMDA receptor. However, its psychomimetic side effects are associated with vacuolation of neurons in the posterior cingulate and retrosplenila cortex (PC/RS). These side effects may worsen during ischemia, adding concern for the use of ketamine as neuroprotective agent.

Comparison of ketamine sedation with fentanyl or sufentanil after traumatic brain injury failed to find effects on functional outcome after 6 months.[62] Similarly, the addition of S+ ketamine to propofol/remifentanil anesthesia in 106 patients during open-heart surgery showed no effects on neurological outcome 10 weeks after surgery.[63]

Etomidate was used in the past as a neuroprotective agent during cerebral aneurysm clipping; however, experimental studies showed that etomidate actually increased the volume of brain infarction.[64] Etomidate enhances the neuronal injury by reducing nitric oxide levels in ischemic brain tissue, thereby reducing the blood supply to the vulnerable ischemic brain tissues and resulting in greater reduction in tissue Po_2.[65] Based on these investigations, the use of etomidate as a neuroprotective agent is no longer recommended.

Neuroprotection by *lidocaine* has been attributed to Na^+-channel blockade. In a model of focal ischemia, clinically used concentrations of lidocaine reduced the extent of cerebral infarction and improved neurological outcome. The neuroprotective effects are accompanied by the preservation of mitochondrial membrane integrity, thereby lidocaine reduced early release of cytochrome *c* and caspase-3 activation.[66,67] In spite of these supportive data, the use of lidocaine as a neuroprotective agent in the operating room setting has not gained wide acceptance.

Volatile anesthetics reduce ischemia, induce glutamate release,[68] antagonize postsynaptic glutamate receptors, and enhance GABA-A mediated hyperpolarization. They increase the levels of antiapoptotic factors like Bcl-2 that reduce mitochondrial membrane permeability and consequently the release of cytochrome *c* into the cytoplasm. Volatile anesthetics also have a preconditioning effect. Administration of volatile anesthetics prior to ischemia either immediately or up to 1 to 4 days before induction of ischemia attenuates injury. Such preconditioning has been demonstrated for isoflurane and sevoflurane. The mechanisms for preconditioning are mainly due to volatile anesthetic activatation of sarcolemmal and mitochondrial potassium–ATP channels, adenosine receptors, and signaling cascades, such as ERK1/2, AKt, PKC, and p38 signaling pathways, that have prosurvival effects.[69] Isoflurane-mediated preconditioning may be more effective in men than in women.[70] Recently, part of the neuroprotective and even the anesthetic effects of volatile anesthetics have been attributed to their agonistic action on TREK1 (a subtype of potassium 2-pore[71] channels). This leads to presynaptic terminal hyperpolarization by TREK1 activation, thus reducing the neurotransmitter release. Similarly, hyperpolarization of the postsynaptic cell might reduce calcium influx via voltage-dependent calcium channels and NMDA receptors.[71,72] Increasing the activity of the TREK channels with neuroprotection induced by halogenated agents and agents like polyunsaturated fatty acids and riluzole, an antiglutamate and anesthetic agent, may improve the outcome of amyotrophic lateral sclerosis.[50]

Although volatile anesthetics have neuroprotective effects, there is clear evidence of their harmful effects on the growing brain. NMDA-receptor blockade during synaptogenesis in the immature brain can induce widespread neuronal degeneration. It is suggested that NMDA antagonistic effects of volatile anesthetics cause cerebral damage in neonates.[73]

The noble gas *xenon* exerts its anesthetic effects by noncompetitive anatogonism of the NMDA receptors. In the studies of neonatal hypoxic-ischemic encephalopathy models, xenon not only improved neurologic outcome but also led to histologic protection.[74] Like volatile anesthetics, xenon can also precondition the brain against ischemic injury.[75] Xenon is considered to have potential as a new neuroprotective agent during cerebral ischemia.

RECENT ADVANCES IN EXPERIMENTAL PHARMACOLOGICAL NEUROPROTECTION

Lithium improves neurological outcome and even inhibits the neurotoxic effects of volatile anesthetics on the growing brain. Lithium downregulates tau (a phosphoprotein involved in the path physiology of Alzheimer disease) in cultured cortical neurons. This effect may explain the efficacy of lithium in the treatment of neurological disorders, such as amyotrophic lateral sclerosis.[76]

Erythropoietin (EPO) has a prominent role in neuroprotection, neurogenesis, and acting as a neurotrophic factor in the brain. It also exhibits anti-inflammatory and angiogenetic properties. Encouraging clinical results have been obtained for EPO as a neuroprotectant in acute stroke and brain trauma.[77] Derivatives of EPO without hematopoietic properties have shown promising results.[78] *Minocycline* is in early clinical trials for neuroprotection as it is found to offer benefit in animal models of brain injury and chronic disease. Minocycline inhibits cytochrome *c*.[79] *Dexamethasone* has also been found to inhibit caspase-3 activity in rats with brain injury secondary to meningitis.[80]

ROLE OF HYPOTHERMIA AND NORMOBARIC HYPEROXIA

Mild hypothermia has been shown to protect the brain in a large number of experimental models of both global and focal ischemia. The use of mild hypothermia is recommended in comatose survivors of out-of-hospital cardiac arrest.[81] The use of mild hypothermia failed to significantly improve neurologic outcome in patients undergoing intracranial aneurysm surgery. The failure of mild hypothermia to show its effect may be due to rapid rewarming.[82] The important issue to remember in order for mild hypothermia to be effective is that it should be maintained for a reasonable time and the rewarming rate should be conducted at a slow rate.

Normobaric hyperoxia may increase the therapeutic window for thrombolysis and neuroprotectant drugs. Pilot clinical magnetic resonance imaging (MRI)–based data suggested that 8 hours of normobaric hyperoxia is effective in reducing infarct volume and National Institutes of Health Stroke Scale score (NIHSSS) within 12 hours of the onset of symptoms, even in the absence of recanalization of the occluded vessel.[83] However, the beneficial effects of normobaric hyperoxia seem to be only transient.

ANESTHESIA FOR SUPRATENTORIAL AND INFRATENTORIAL CRANIOTOMIES

The most important aims during intracranial surgery are first to provide adequate cerebral perfusion pressure (CPP) and cerebral blood flow (CBF) to meet the tissue demands of oxygen and glucose, and second, for the occasion of a decreased supply, to protect the brain. Avoiding brain swelling during surgery is very important as brain swelling can impair the working conditions of the neurosurgeon. Fast emergence after craniotomy has considerable importance because immediate neurological examination is desirable to reveal such new deficiencies that may need an added intervention.

CPP, CBF, AND AUTOREGULATION

In the healthy brain, the CBF is well autoregulated to meet the demands for brain metabolism. With intact autoregulation, the CBF remains constant within a wide range of CPP, and with sudden changes in the arterial pressure and consequently in the CPP, dynamic autoregulation restores the CBF to normal.

Traditionally, CPP has been calculated as mean arterial pressure (MAP) minus intracranial pressure (ICP); however, this is only valid in conditions with high ICP. In conditions with normal ICP the major determinant of the effective downstream pressure is the vascular tone. In normal conditions the CPP can be calculated according to the following formula: CPP = MAP – ZEP, where ZEP (zero flow pressure) represents the MAP at which the blood flow through the cerebral circulation ceases. Transcranial Doppler is a noninvasive method that can be used to measure CPP and ZEP utilizing the middle cerebral artery flow velocity (FV). CPP can be calculated according to the following formula: CPP = [(BP mean – BP diastolic)/(FV mean – FV diastolic)] × FV mean, and thus ZEP = BP mean – CPP.[84,85]

ICP AND BRAIN SWELLING

Controlling the high ICP, or preventing any further increases in the ICP, is essential during anesthesia induction to avoid even short periods of insufficient perfusion and to improve the working conditions for the neurosurgeon. In craniotomy for supratentorial brain tumors, subdural ICP is measured at the start of surgery. The degree of midline shift and histopathological diagnosis of either glioblastoma or a metastasis are independent risk factors for intraoperative brain swelling. At an ICP of greater than 13 mm Hg, brain swelling is highly probable.[86] Reverse Trendelenburg and head elevation positions usually help to decrease ICP and reduce brain swelling. Avoiding hypercarbia, hypoxia, obstruction of brain venous drainage induced by extreme neck positions, and endotracheal tube kinking or obstruction are very crucial to avoid brain swelling during the craniotomy. In patients with supratentorial tumors, the cerebral autoregulation (measured by transient hyperemic response ratio [THRR]) and CO_2 reactivity are usually preserved as long as the tumor is medium sized (<40 cm^3) and midline shift is 5 mm or less on preoperative computed tomography (CT) or MRI.[87]

THE DRUGS USED TO DECREASE HIGH ICP AND BRAIN SWELLING

Indomethacin, a cyclooxygenase inhibitor, is a cerebral vasoconstrictor and reduces CBF without affecting cerebral oxygen metabolism ($CMRO_2$). The injection of indomethacin reduces ICP and improves CPP in patients with intracranial tumors during isoflurane anesthesia[88] and in patients with severe head injury. In a recent study indomethacin given as a bolus of 0.2 mg/kg followed by infusion of 0.2 mg/kg/h during propofol anesthesia in patients subjected to craniotomy for supratentorial brain tumors did not show any evidence of brain ischemia as assessed by diffusion-weighted imaging (DWI) MRI.[89]

DIURETICS

Mannitol is an osmotic diuretic widely used during neurosurgery to reduce increased ICP. Mannitol is effective only when some degree of blood–brain barrier (BBB) integrity is preserved in a significant portion of the brain. The dose of mannitol varies from 0.25 to 1 g/kg. During mannitol administration, especially in multiple doses, no further doses should be given if serum osmolarity reaches to 320 mOsm/L to avoid hyperosmolar acute kidney injury (AKI). Mannitol should be administered by infusion over 10 to 15 minutes. Sudden exposure of the cerebral circulation to extreme hyperosmolarity can have a vasodilatory effect, which can produce brain engorgement and further increased ICP that does not occur with slower infusions. Enhancing the effect of mannitol and reducing the rebound brain swelling after mannitol administration can be achieved by adding a loop diuretic, like furosemide. These effects can be explained by 2 mechanisms. First, loop diuretics enhance the water excretion, thus helping to maintain the gradient between the intravascular compartment and the brain parenchyma across the BBB. Second, *furosemide* inhibits the chloride channels in neurons and glia cells, thus reducing their ability to reaccumulate idiogenic osmoles like chloride ions; this effect will inhibit their ability to draw water into them in order to restore their original size.[90]

THE EFFECTS OF ANESTHETICS DURING CRANIOTOMIES FOR BRAIN TUMORS

Volatile anesthetics have a dual effect on cerebral vasculature. In low concentrations *halothane*, *isoflurane*, and *sevoflurane* constrict the cerebral vessels secondary to suppression of metabolism. With high concentration the direct vasodilatory effect will increase the CBF and ICP. In pigs, 1 minimal alveolar concentration (MAC) of desflurane has the most profound vasodilating effect, resulting in increased CBF and ICP.[91] However, in humans undergoing craniotomies for supratentorial mass lesions who received 1.2 MAC of either desflurane or isoflurane for maintenance of anesthesia, desflurane and isoflurane had similar effects on CPP and MAP. Additionally, desflurane in the setting of hyperventilaton ($Paco_2$ 30 ± 2 mm Hg) did not cause significant changes in lumbar cerebrospinal fluid pressure (LCSFP).[92] In patients undergoing craniotomy for supratentorial tumors randomized to receive either 1.2 MAC of sevoflurane or desflurane, those receiving desflurane had a shorter extubation and recovery time but similar intraoperative and postoperative incidences of complications compared with those who received sevoflurane.[93] Sevoflurane has fewer cerebral vasodilatory effects than isoflurane at the same depth of anesthesia.[94] It is now generally accepted that the order of cerebral vasodilating potency among the volatile anesthetics is approximately halothane > enflurane > desflurane ≈ isoflurane > sevoflurane.[95] Therefore, among all volatile anesthetics, sevoflurane seems to be most suitable for neuroanesthesia.[96]

CBF AND METABOLISM

At equipotent concentrations of sevoflurane (1.5 vol%) compared with propofol (3.7 mcg/mL), the reduction in CBF with propofol is associated with decreases in jugular bulb venous oxygen saturation close to the lower threshold of 50%. With further vasoconstriction during hypocapnia ($Paco_2$ = 33 mm Hg), propofol reduces jugular bulb venous oxygen saturation below 50%, indicating critical cerebral perfusion. With sevoflurane, decreases in jugular bulb venous oxygen saturation do not occur with normo- or hypocapnia. At equipotent concentrations, cerebral metabolism is reduced to the same extent with the same anesthetics. Coupling between regional CBF and $CMRO_2$ is maintained with both sevoflurane and propofol.[97-101]

CBF AND AUTOREGULATION

Autoregulation is impaired with higher concentrations of isoflurane, desflurane, and sevoflurane. This is likely related to reduced baseline tone due to increased availability of brain tissue nitric oxide by inhalation anesthetics.[102] Propofol does not alter cerebrovascular autoregulation independent of the concentration used. This makes propofol most suitable for patients with reduced intracranial.[97]

RECOVERY FROM ANESTHESIA

In a multicenter randomized trial, patients undergoing craniotomy for supratentorial tumor were enrolled to either sevoflurane-remifentanil or propofol-remifentanil for the maintenance of anesthesia. There was no clinically relevant difference between the groups in the time to emergence. Moreover, shivering, postoperative nausea and vomiting, pain, and seizure during the first 3 postoperative hours were not significantly different between the study groups, nor was intraoperative brain relaxation.[103]

The use of propofol for total intravenous anesthesia (TIVA) is not without complications. The use of propofol infusion can cause the development of propofol-related infusion syndrome.[104] Characterized by the development of lactic acidosis, rhabdomyolysis, renal failure, and cardiac failure, propofol infusion syndrome occurs in patients who receive a high dose of propofol (>5 mg/kg/h) in the intensive care unit for more than 58 hours.[105] Another potential complication of TIVA is the potential for a significant decrease in cerebral blood volume (CBV).[106,107] This becomes significant during stereotactic-guided craniotomies, where brain shift may ensue. Additionally, a large decrease in CBV may worsen epidural bleeds; however, the average decrease in CBV during propofol-remifentanil anesthetic is only 25%.[97]

VENTILATION STRATEGY DURING CRANIOTOMY

Hyperventilation should not be an automatic component of every craniotomy for brain tumors. Hyperventilation is not without adverse effects. It induces cerebral alkalosis and CBF decreases abruptly. The time course for cerebral alkalosis is short, only 6 to 18 hours, due to the reduction in carbonic anhydrase enzyme activity to restore the pH of the cerebrospinal fluid (CSF) back to normal level.[108] If hypocapnia is required as an adjunct to brain relaxation during craniotomy, $Paco_2$ should be allowed to increase when the retractors are removed to avoid the residual intracranial pneumatocele.

Steroids are used to decrease ICP by reducing the edema and BBB permeability associated with brain tumors.[109] The administration of steroids is not for acute intervention for controlling elevated ICP. Steroids usually should be given 48 hours before an elective surgery, to reduce edema formation and improve the clinical condition by the time of craniotomy.[110] Perioperative steroids can induce hyperglycemia so perioperative blood glucose concentration monitoring should continue for a least 12 hours postoperatively if intraoperative dexamethasone is used.[111]

IMPORTANT POSITIONS DURING CRANIOTOMY

The *sitting position* is used mainly for infratentorial craniotomy; the sitting position has many advantages but at the same time has potential life-threatening complications. *Advantages*: (1) It provides excellent surgical exposure, particularly of midline structures and those in the brainstem. (2) It provides less pooling of blood and CSF in the surgical field. (3) It has better ventilation-perfusion matching and lower peak airway pressure than the prone position.

Complications of Sitting Position

Venous Air Embolization (VAE) VAE can occur whenever the pressure within an open blood vessel is subatmospheric. Significant VAE is rare unless the surgical site is elevated by more than 20 to 40 cm. In addition, the risk of VAE increases when open veins cannot collapse, as is encountered with injury to the venous sinuses, cerebellar bridging veins, epidural veins, emissary veins, and marrow spaces in the skull or cervical vertebra. During posterior fossa procedures done in the sitting position, VAE is detected by precordial Doppler in approximately 40% of patients and by transesophageal echocardiography (TEE) in 76% (**Fig. 51-8**).[112]

Monitoring and the Physiology of VAE If the air embolus is large and cannot be cleared it will result in occlusion of the pulmonary vascular bed. This results in an increase in pulmonary vascular resistance and pulmonary artery pressure, and consequently right ventricle (RV) afterload. If obstruction is severe, cardiac output will fall, caused by airlock in the RV, RV failure, or impaired left ventricle (LV) filling caused by displacement of the intraventricular septum by a distended RV. Detection of VAE can be monitored by TEE and precordial Doppler. TEE is the most sensitive tool for VAE detection, even more so than precordial Doppler. In our practice we routinely use a right atrial catheter in the sitting position. The use of multiorifice catheters will allow more air aspiration in the event of VAE. The tip of the right atrial catheter should be at the junction between the superior vena cava (SVC) and the right atrium. The proper catheter position can be detected by the use of TEE, electrocardiography (ECG), or by chest x-ray. In TEE, the bicaval view will determine the proper position of the catheter tip by visualizing the SVC and the right atrium. While in the chest x-ray, the proper position of the catheter tip should be at the same level of the carina. We prefer the chest x-ray method; it is accurate and universally available. In the ECG technique the right arm lead of a standard ECG monitor is attached to the catheter via a fluid column (sodium bicarbonate). The catheter is advanced until a biphasic P wave is seen, then withdrawn until the P wave is slightly shorter than the R wave.

Positioning and the Response to VAE When a major VAE is encountered, the initial response is to ask the surgeon to flood the wound or pack it with wet gauze, discontinue N_2O (if used), and aspirate from the right atrial catheter. The addition of PEEP and/or bilateral jugular compression is helpful to decrease the air entry by increasing the head venous pressure. If hemodynamic deterioration occurs, the patient must be moved into a horizontal position. A horizontal posture can be achieved by moving the table into a head-down position (**Fig. 51-9**).

Paradoxical Air Embolism There is a potential for the passage of air from the right to the left of the heart, with subsequent entry into the coronary or cerebral circulation. This can occur in either the pulmonary vascular bed or more commonly via a patent foramen ovale (PFO). It was observed that paradoxical air embolism (PAE) occurred only in the context of major air embolic events, suggesting that significant increases in right heart pressures are an important predisposing factor of the occurrence of PAE.[113] PFO can be detected preoperatively by contrast bubble studies using either preoperative transthoracic echocardiography (TTE) or intraoperative TEE. Detection of PFO is crucial before the

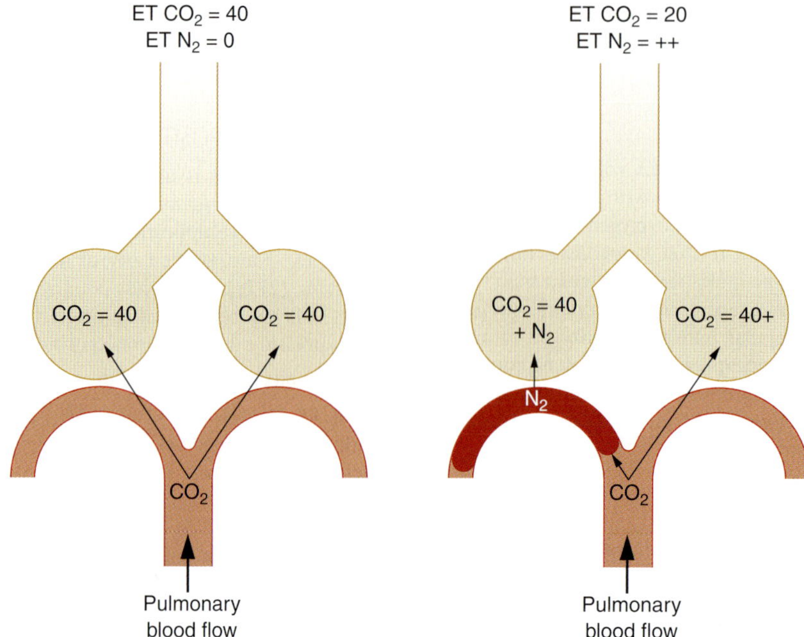

FIGURE 51-8. Changes in expired CO_2 and N_2 in alveoli (*left* diagram). A VAE does 2 things (*right* diagram). First, it occludes a portion of the pulmonary circulation, preventing the delivery of CO_2 to the alveoli. As a result, end-tidal CO_2 (which should represent an alveolar gas sample) will decrease (even though $Paco_2$ may rise). In addition, N_2 present in the gas bubble will diffuse into the alveoli and appear in exhaled gas.

institution of PEEP during the sitting position to prevent paradoxical emboli. The use of PEEP increases the right atrial pressure (RAP) in relation to the left atrial pressure (LAP) and consequently increases the incidence of PAE in the presence of PFO. Even when the mean LAP exceeds mean RAP, PAE can still occur because transient reversal of the interatrial pressure gradient can occur during each cardiac cycle.[114]

Transpulmonary Passage of Air Air can occasionally traverse the pulmonary vascular bed to reach the systemic circulation in the absence of PFO. Transpulmonary passage is more likely to occur when large volumes of air are presented to the vascular filter. The threshold for transpulmonary passage may decrease in the presence of pulmonary vasodilators including volatile anesthetics.

Hemodynamic Deterioration The sitting position is accompanied by a decrease in cardiac output with an increase in systemic vascular resistance. Black et al[115] found a 20% incidence of hypotension requiring vasopressors in 330 sitting patients. Measures to avoid hypotension include prepositioning hydration, wrapping of the legs with elastic bandages to counteract venous pooling in the legs, and the use of vasopressors to maintain the required MAP.

Some degree of *pneumocephalus* occurs in all craniotomies performed in the sitting position and in other postoperative craniotomy/craniectomy patients regardless of operative position.[116] In our practice we prefer to not use N_2O during craniotomies to avoid the development of tension pneumocephalus. Tension pneumocephalus is difficult to diagnose, but should be suspected when a patient fails to awaken after an uneventful procedure, deteriorates after awakening, or suffers unexplained cardiovascular catastrophe. In suspected conditions a CT scan should be done to confirm the diagnosis. The treatment can be achieved either by simple observation, administration of high O_2 concentrations, and/or surgical evacuation in severe conditions.

Cases of *quadriplegia/paresis* have been reported after sitting position. This might be due to the combination of cervical cord compression from extreme neck flexion and reduced arterial perfusion pressure. Allowing at least a 2-finger breadth between the patient's chin and chest and maintaining adequate perfusion pressure at the level of the surgical site can minimize extreme head flexion.

Other Problems *Peripheral nerve injuries* and severe *swelling of the base of the tongue*, soft palate, and pharynx have been described after posterior fossa craniotomies. Nerve injuries can be minimized by careful positioning and padding. The main cause of tongue and upper airway edema is impairment of head venous return due to extreme head flexion. Avoidance of extreme flexion by allowing adequate distance between the patient's chin and sternum is important to minimize this complication.

PRACTICAL POINTS FOR ANESTHETIC MANAGEMENT DURING CRANIOTOMIES

1. Monitoring during craniotomies is via American Society of Anesthesiologists (ASA) standard monitors; in our practice we use direct arterial monitoring by inserting an intra-arterial catheter to measure the arterial blood gases and continuous monitoring of the blood pressure. We do not routinely use a central venous pressure catheter except for patients in the sitting position, lack of proper peripheral venous access, or in craniotomies for large tumors with expected major blood loss.
2. The maintenance of anesthesia is usually accomplished by using sevoflurane with remifentanil infusion. In cases of severe intracranial hypertension, we prefer to use TIVA and remifentanil infusion.
3. In our practice, sevoflurane is considered the preferred inhalation anesthetic during neuroanesthesia. During sevoflurane anesthesia, CO_2 reactivity is preserved up to 1.3 MAC (2.5%) with minimal effect on ICP.[117]
4. Head elevation or reverse Trendelenburg position (RTP) is usually adopted during the procedure as an effective means to reduce ICP.[118]
5. We usually maintain $Paco_2$ between 30 and 35 mm Hg, and we use hyperventilation ($Paco_2$ 30-25 mm Hg) only during cases with severe elevation of ICP.
6. Blood pressure should be tightly controlled during craniotomies to maintain adequate CPP, especially in cases with increased ICP.

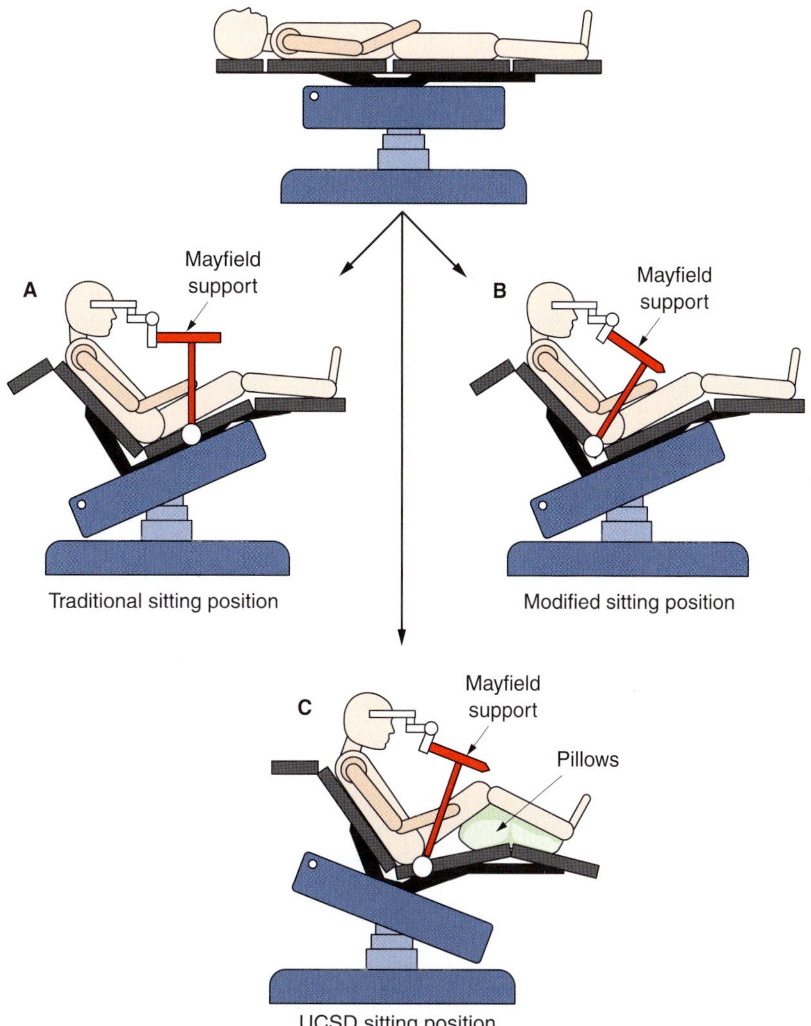

FIGURE 51-9. Three variations of the sitting position. **A.** In the "traditional sitting position," the table is placed in a steep Trendelenburg, the back is elevated, and the Mayfield support is attached to the midsection of the table. It is possible to return the patient to a horizontal position after a severe VAE without removing the head from pin fixation. To facilitate a return to a horizontal position, 2 alternatives are suggested. **B.** In the first (modified sitting position), the same table position is used, but the Mayfield support is attached to the back section of the table. The horizontal position can now be achieved simply by lowering the back. **C.** In the "UCSD (University of California at San Diego) position" the table base is placed in reverse Trendelenburg, the back is elevated, and the legs are supported on pillows. In the event of a serious VAE, the horizontal position can be achieved simply by placing the table in the Trendelenburg position.

The arterial pressure transducer is usually zeroed at the level of the external auditory meatus.

7. Fluid management during craniotomy should be aimed toward providing proper tissue perfusion and at the same time avoiding increased ICP and cerebral edema.
8. We prefer to use a mixture of colloid and crystalloids. Albumin 5% is our preferred colloid, as hydroxyethylstarch solutions, even the new low-molecular-weight solutions, have harmful effects on the coagulation process. Maintaining normal coagulation is very crucial after brain or spine surgeries.[119-121]
9. Supratentorial craniotomy requiring incision of the temporalis muscle is associated with the risk of limitation of mandibular opening (pseuodoankylosis) and may result in difficult intubation if subsequent surgery is required after a short interval.[122]
10. Cerebellar hemorrhage following supratentorial craniotomy is a very seldomly described but very serious complication. There is no single presurgical factor, such as a history of hypertension, or a surgical factor like CSF leak (which results in cerebral hypotension) that can reliably predict the occurrence of cerebellar hemorrhage after supratentorial craniotomy. The etiology of this entity still remains unclear. The most important keys to minimizing the hazardous sequelae are to be aware of this potential complication and to diagnose it early.[123]
11. Postoperative pain control after craniotomies can be accomplished by using acetaminophen in addition to tramadol or nalbuphine.[124]
12. Meningiomas have been described to be most frequently complicated by hemorrhagic postoperative manifestations, probably because of abnormal hyperfibrinolysis.[123,125]

TRANSSPHENOIDAL SURGERY

Although excision of some pituitary tumors may require open craniotomy, most of these procedures are being performed through a transsphenoidal approach. Pituitary tumors encompass about 10% of intracranial neoplasms. Most of these tumors are hypersecreting adenomas, about 20% to 25% are null cells with no secreting hormones, and about 20% are other tumors including mixed cell adenomas. The adenomas are also classified as macroadenomas and microadenomas depending on their size—larger or smaller than 1 cm. Pressure on adjacent structures of the brain can also be the presenting symptom, such that headache or visual field disturbance (as a result of pressure on optic chiasma) is common in these patients.

The most common functioning adenoma is the *prolactin*-secreting prolactinoma. Recent data show an even higher than expected prevalence in the general population.[126] In addition to prolactinomas, all other tumor space-occupying lesions can increase the prolactin level by impeding the inhibitory pathway of the hypothalamus on prolactin-secreting cells.

The symptoms caused by nonsecreting adenomas such as null cells and other more infrequent space-occupying lesions of the pituitary (eg, Rathke cleft cyst, craniopharyngioma) are secondary to pressure on adjacent structures and decrease of secretion in bordering cell types.[127] In rare instances pressure to the posterior pituitary can cause diabetes insipidus.

An increase in the production of *growth hormone* after the fusion of epiphysial growth plates can cause acromegaly. These tumors account for 10% to 15% of all pituitary adenomas and diagnosis may be delayed due to slow progression of the disease. Early diagnosis can improve survival and quality of life.[128] An increase in the secretion of *adrenocorticotropic hormone* (ACTH) can cause Cushing disease. These adenomas represent only up to 15% of all pituitary adenomas, but their diagnosis requires special laboratory evaluation[129] and is important for deciding on perioperative steroid therapy. Thyrotropic *TSH*-secreting adenomas are both the most rare of all pituitary-secreting adenomas and a rare cause of hyperthyroidism. Thus treatment of associated hyperthyroidism may be directed toward other more common causes of hyperthyroidism[130] and its symptoms, allowing time for this adenoma to grow with some invasion of adjacent structures and increasing the chance of intraoperative bleeding. Faulty excision of the thyroid gland may in fact increase the size of this tumor.

PREOPERATIVE CONSIDERATIONS

In addition to the routine preoperative evaluations of patients scheduled for craniotomy, history and physical examination, as well as radiologic and laboratory evaluation should be directed toward end-organ involvement. Evaluation of pituitary function is essential before surgery.[131] The anesthesiologist should direct the preoperative assessment toward organs affected by the excess or shortage of secreted hormones. Pressure on the optic chiasm can manifest as visual field disturbance. Macroadenomas, especially if complicated by an ischemic or hemorrhagic accident within the adenoma, can compress other cranial nerves including the third, fourth, and sixth cranial nerves. Pressure on the third cranial nerve can cause mydriasis, limitation of gaze, and ptosis.[132] Symptoms will depend on the increase in prolactin or decrease in follicle-stimulating hormone (FSH) and luteinizing hormone (LH) and include amenorrhea, decreased libido, and galactorrhea in women, and impotence, decreased libido, and oligospermia in men. The medical therapy for prolactinoma is bromocriptine, a dopamine agonist with an inhibitory effect on the secretion of prolactin.[133]

Patients with acromegaly can present with widening of bones and the excessive growth and hypertrophy of soft tissue. Enlarged mandible, lips, tongue, and upper airway soft tissue can make airway management including ventilation and intubation difficult. A higher incidence of obstructive sleep apnea can also be seen in these patients. Enlargement of bones and the soft tissue of hands and feet raises the concern of pressure on the peripheral nerves and necessitates caution during positioning. An important part of evaluation of acromegalic patients is the degree of involvement of the cardiovascular system. Left ventricular hypertrophy can be isolated or be associated with hypertension, which is seen in 40% of patients.[134] A thick myocardium can lead to diastolic dysfunction[135] as well as conduction abnormalities, resulting in arrhythmias. Osteoporosis and skeletal muscle weakness can also be seen. Acromegalic patients may be hyperglycemic and have electrolyte abnormalities. Medical treatment is directed toward a decrease in production of this hormone or blocking its action at the end-organ level. Analogs of somatostatin, octreotide, and lanreotide can be used to decrease the secretion of growth hormone. The dopamine agonist bromocriptine can also be used; however, it is less effective than the somatostatins. The growth hormone receptor antagonist pegvisomant has also been used for the medical therapy of acromegaly.

Patients with excess ACTH may show signs and symptoms of Cushing disease including central obesity with accumulation of fat in the face, fragile skin, skeletal muscle weakness, osteoporosis, hypertension, hyperglycemia, and electrolyte changes. Part of the perioperative assessment of patients suspected of having Cushing disease is measurement of daily urine cortisol. In a dexamethasone suppression test, exogenous dexamethasone is administered to see the suppression effect on ACTH.[136] The low-dose dexamethasone suppression test is a screening test to diagnose Cushing syndrome. The high-dose suppression test can differentiate between Cushing disease and Cushing syndrome from nonpituitary ACTH-secreting tumors. Although dexamethasone does not interfere with postoperative serum cortisol assay, it is better to communicate with the surgeon before administering any steroids in the perioperative period. Currently the practice is to avoid any steroids to observe remission postoperatively.[137] Ketokonazole had been used for medical treatment of Cushing syndrome, which can block cortisol synthesis, but drugs that inhibit ACTH secretion (cyproheptadine, valproic acid, somatostatin analogs, vasopressin antagonist) are used much less. Glucocorticoid receptor antagonists are used in patients with ectopic ACTH-secreting tumors or those not amenable to surgery.[138]

Patients with thyrotropic adenoma present with signs and symptoms of hyperthyroidism, including goiter, tachycardia, weight loss, heat intolerance, tremor, and anxiety. Patients are usually on medications to control the hyperthyroidism symptoms. The somatostatin analog octreotide has been used in the medical management of this tumor and to decrease its size.[130]

INTRAOPERATIVE CONCERNS

The different methods for surgical access in the transsphenoidal excision of pituitary tumors include through the nasal cavity or sublabial, the transseptal approach using a microscope, and endoscopic resection.[139,140] In many cases the surgical approach to the tumor is performed by a head and neck surgeon. A preoperative sign-in with both scheduled surgical teams, anesthesiologists, and intraoperative nursing teams can help in outlining the plan and ascertain preparedness to ensure patient safety. In most instances a stereotactic method is used by the surgeon for navigation and confirmation of the tumor position intraoperatively, thus immobility of the head is an important component of the surgical plan. The head is usually placed in a Mayfield holder for this. The patient is usually placed in a sniffing position and care must be taken to elevate the legs above the operative site to increase lower extremity venous return and minimize air embolus. The anesthetic plan usually is a balanced general anesthesia with opioids in combination with volatile anesthetics or other intravenous anesthetics. Muscle relaxation is provided with intermittent boluses or continuous infusion of a nondepolarizing muscle relaxant. Although pituitary tumors are space-occupying lesions, their small size and relatively gradual growth rate cause a much lower incidence of increased ICP compared to other intracranial tumors; however, precautions to avoid an increase in ICP during induction are still suggested. Close monitoring of arterial blood pressure is possible with placement of an invasive arterial line. Large-bore intravenous accesses are recommended, especially in cases that have a potential for blood loss. Subglottic stenosis is also seen in patients with acromegaly, and using a correct size endotracheal tube and measuring the cuff pressure is advisable.

After induction and intubation the surgical team should inform the anesthesia provider before placement of the head frame to ascertain the adequate depth of anesthesia to avoid movement[141] or sudden sympathetic discharge, which could increase the ICP. The sympathetic discharge could also be intensified by placement of local anesthetics with epinephrine, phenylephrine, or cocaine swabs in the nasal cavity in order to achieve local anesthesia and vasoconstriction to avoid excessive bleeding during dissection. In some instances, for example, large tumors, where there is a higher incidence of postoperative CSF leak, the surgeon may place a spinal drain to decrease the CSF pressure. Positioning the patient in a lateral position for this purpose can cause intravenous or arterial line dislodgment or unwarranted endotracheal tube displacement and should be performed with care. Placement of a gauze pad in the oropharyngeal area can decrease the extension of hemorrhage into the stomach and potentially decrease postoperative nausea; however, the surgeon should remember to remove it before emergence to avoid suffocation. A Foley catheter is usually placed to monitor urine output, especially when involvement of the posterior pituitary can cause diabetes insipidus. In some instances fat, usually from the abdominal area, is taken to fill the excised pituitary space and further decrease the chance of postoperative CSF leak. At the end of a surgical procedure the nares are packed with dressing, the oropharyngeal pack is removed, and in some instances gastric contents are aspirated with an oropharyngeal tube. Although conventionally the anesthetic level is decreased toward the end of the procedure, patient movement or cough while still in the head holder can be disastrous. We advocate the use of intravenous lidocaine to decrease the chance of cough during extubation; also, a smooth extubation can decrease the chance of a nasal or intracranial bleed or CSF leak. A neurologic examination focusing especially on cranial nerves postoperatively can help in the early detection of surgical complications and the need for emergent cranial imaging such as CT scan.

Postoperative care of patients is usually in the postanesthesia care unit, where special attention should be paid to blood pressure control.

INTRACRANIAL VASCULAR SURGERY

Intracranial vascular surgical procedures are usually performed to correct or excise a vascular malformation or create an alternative route for blood flow bypassing the affected arterial supply. The main intracranial vascular malformations are intracranial aneurysms (IA), or arteriovenous malformations (AVM)s. An alternative method of treatment for intracranial vascular pathologies is by endovascular treatment.

INTRACRANIAL ANEURYSM

Although surgical methods have improved, anesthetic techniques have advanced, and the transportation and management of critical patients has progressed, mortality and morbidity following SAH from an IA still remains high. Different reports claim the incidence of IA between 0.2% and 9.9%, but the incidence of SAH is 5 to 10 in 100,000.[142] The most common cause of SAH is IA. Intracranial aneurysms mostly appear at the branching of cerebral vessels, mainly in the anterior communicating artery or middle cerebral artery. About 10% of these aneurysms are at the internal carotid artery bifurcation or at the tip of the basilar artery. In 30% of patients presenting with SAH there is more than one aneurysm. There may be familial or genetic[143] patterns in IA and screening is advisable in relatives of patients, especially if more than 1 family member has an IA. In some genetic disorders, such as polycystic kidney disease and collagen abnormalities, a higher incidence of IA is seen. Heavy smoking, moderate to heavy alcohol consumption, hypertension, female gender (most men with SAH present before the fifth decade of life), and pregnancy can increase the chance of SAH. Certain characteristics of aneurysms also increase the chance of rupture including size, position, transmural pressure, and history of previous bleed. Aneurysms larger than 10 mm and those in the basilar tip or vertebrobasilar system have a higher chance of bleeding. Transmural pressure is the pressure on the aneurysm wall: the difference between the pressure inside (the arterial pressure trying to expand the aneurysm) and pressure outside (ICP trying to contain the aneurysm). You may notice a similarity between this equation and what was described for CPP; however, in transmural pressure the systolic pressure, which adds to the shear force, is also important. For example, a balloon expanding with air will rupture earlier outside the swimming pool compared to one underneath the water. Thus similarly decreasing the pressure outside the aneurysm (ICP) can increase the chance of aneurysm rupture. The dilemma arises when the ICP is elevated acutely after SAH; although this elevation can contain the aneurysm, decreasing further bleeding (for which it is desirable to lower the blood pressure), it can also decrease the CPP (promoting an increase in blood pressure). That is, management of ICP and blood pressure can be difficult. Determining the best level to ensure an adequate perfusion while decreasing the chance of rebleeding requires information from invasive monitors. Autoregulation is also impaired in SAH, and this should be kept in mind in deciding the best blood pressure for an adequate CPP.

TABLE 51-4 Hunt and Hess Grading for Patients Presenting With SAH[a]

Grade	Criteria
I	Asymptomatic or minimal headache and slight nuchal rigidity
II	Moderate to severe headache, nuchal rigidity, no neurologic deficit other than cranial nerve palsy
III	Drowsiness, confusion, or mild focal deficit
IV	Stupor, moderate to severe hemiparesis, possibly early decerebrate rigidity and vegetative disturbances
V	Deep coma, decerebrate rigidity, moribund appearance

SAH, subarachnoid hemorrhage.

[a]Note that if the patient has a serious systemic disease, such as hypertension, diabetes, severe arteriosclerosis, chronic pulmonary disease, or severe vasospasm on angiography, the next lower grade is selected.

The most important primary information regarding IA that affects all aspects of perioperative care, as well as selecting an anesthetic plan, is the presenting picture of the patient. Management of patients presenting comatose from a SAH is obviously different compared to a patient with an asymptomatic, incidentally found IA. Many systems have been developed for the grading of SAH.[144] Hunt and Hess developed a grading system based on presenting signs and symptoms (**Table 51-4**). This grading can be used to evaluate the prognosis as well as the improvement or regression of severity of involvement. Another grading system commonly used is the World Federation of Neurological Surgeons (WFNS) grading for SAH, which is based on the Glasgow Coma Scale score and motor deficit (**Table 51-5**). Obviously, in both grading systems the higher the grade, the poorer the outcome. The Fisher Scale (**Table 51-6**) relies on CT findings of location and amount of intracranial hemorrhage and can help in determining the likelihood of vasospasm. This association is more pronounced when the initial CT scan is performed within the first 24 hours of SAH.[145] It should be noted that Fisher grade 3 has the highest chance of vasospasm.[146]

There has been a long debate regarding the best timing of treatment for SAH.[147] Although according to some earlier belief that waiting for the acute stage of SAH to subside can help in decreasing the intracranial pressure and, theoretically, early operation may increase the risk of vasospasm, delaying the surgical procedure can increase the chance of rebleeding. According to the International Cooperative Study on

TABLE 51-5 World Federation of Neurologic Surgeons Classification of SAH

WFNS Grade	GCS Score	Motor Deficit
I	15	Absent
II	13-14	Absent
III	13-14	Present
IV	7-12	Present or Absent
V	3-6	Present or Absent

GCS, Glasgow coma scale; SAH, subarachnoid hemorrhage; WFNS, World Federation of Neurological Surgeons.

TABLE 51-6 Fisher Grading Scale Regarding Amount of Blood Seen in Head CT Scan

Grade	Description
1	No subarachnoid blood visualized
2	Diffuse deposition or thin layer, no clots >3-mm-thick or vertical layers >1 mm
3	Dense collection of clot >1 mm thick in vertical or >5 × 3 mm in longitudinal and transverse dimension in horizontal plane
4	Intraparanchymal or intraventricular clots, but only diffuse and no blood in basal cistern

CT, computed tomography.

Timing of Aneurysm Surgery[148] the worst outcome is seen when surgery is performed on postbleed days 7 to 10; currently, in order to get the best results in patients with good grades, the belief is to operate on the first 3 to 4 days postbleed.[149]

Preoperative Evaluation Preoperative evaluation of patients scheduled for craniotomy is similar to other craniotomies but again dependent on presenting symptoms. In patients who present with an unruptured aneurysm scheduled for an elective procedure, time for a more liberal evaluation including history, physical examination, laboratory, and imaging can help in the optimization of the patient. Even in this group of patients, the urgency of the surgical procedure varies and there may not be enough time for adequate optimization. Neurogenic pulmonary edema may accompany SAH[150]; although the pathophysiologic mechanism is not yet totally understood,[151] it could be related to the sympathetic discharge. Cardiac involvement may contribute to the development of pulmonary edema.[152] A sudden increase in sympathetic discharge can cause significant changes in cardiac function. *Cardiac* involvement can manifest as stunned myocardium.[153] ECG changes are frequent and vary from rate and rhythm alterations to signs of myocardial strain such as ST depression and T inversion. QTc prolongation and ventricular arrhythmias can also be present.[154] ECG abnormalities could be of neurogenic origin and not necessarily as a result of myocardial dysfunction. A subset of patients show apical akinesia and concomitant sparing of basal segments, which is also known as "takotsubo" cardiomyopathy.[153] There may be release of cardiac troponin as well as echocardiographic signs of ischemia including wall motion abnormalities. Although the CK-MB levels are elevated in stunned myocardium as well as myocardial infarction, the inconsistencies of echocardiographic abnormalities with ECG findings and lower values of troponin in patients with ejection fraction lower than 40% may point to stunned myocardium.[154] Differentiation between stunned myocardium and myocardial infarction is important in surgical decision making. The ECG abnormalities can also be a result of *electrolyte* disturbances and should be corrected. Cerebral salt wasting syndrome[155] can cause hyponatremia; other electrolyte disturbances include hypokalemia or hypocalcemia. A true myocardial infarction as a result of the SAH or coincidentally secondary to a preexisting coronary artery disease may occur. Anesthetic consideration is similar to patients with a recent cardiac ischemic event undergoing emergent surgery.

Patients presenting with SAH may have coexisting chronic medical conditions such as hypertension, diabetes mellitus (DM), and chronic renal insufficiency. Information regarding these conditions can be critical in establishing the anesthetic plan and are useful prognostic indicators (see Table 51-4). The 2 important complications after a SAH are rebleeding and vasospasm. Rebleeding has the highest rate in the first 24 hours (up to 8%).[156] Risk of rebleed is higher in females with higher grade, poor medical condition, and elevated blood pressure. More than half of patients who rebleed may die.[157] Close blood pressure control and early surgery can decrease the rate of rebleeding. The mechanism of vasospasm is still under debate. It is thought, however, that the accumulation in the basal cisterns of vasoactive substances released in the blood can induce vasospasm in the arteries, leading to a decrease blood flow and ischemic changes. Clinical vasospasm is usually apparent 72 hours after bleeding.

Patients with SAH are often already under treatment for vasospasm. It is important to continue the treatment during transport to the operating room. Realization that patients with vasospasm are entirely dependent on optimal blood pressure control for adequate CPP is important in determining the intraoperative hemodynamic goals. Medical treatment for vasospasm is by pharmacologic means or *triple-H* therapy. Multiple pharmacologic agents have been suggested to decrease the mortality and morbidity after vasospasm, but only a few have shown any promising results. The calcium channel blocker nimodipine is shown to improve the outcome[158]; some have also suggested using magnesium because it has a vasodilatory effect. There are mixed reports regarding the effectiveness of statins in decreasing the incidence of vasospasm after SAH.[159,160] Still, *triple-H* therapy with hemodilution, hypertension, and hypervolemia is a commonly used treatment in intensive care units. Because the flow of blood through the vasospastic vessels is dependent on blood pressure, a drop in blood pressure may worsen the clinical picture. Hypervolemia has the potential to cause pulmonary edema, especially in patients whose cardiac function reserve is reduced. In such situations the use of a pulmonary artery catheter can help in guiding the fluid therapy. Hemodilution usually follows with the expansion of intravascular volume; a decrease in hematocrit can improve the blood rheology and lower the viscosity to enhance perfusion through vasospastic vessels. It is important to keep in mind that a hematocrit of less that 30 may by itself cause an ischemic effect by decreasing the oxygen content of the blood. Interventional radiology has also been helpful in the treatment of vasospasm. Angioplasty as well as selective intra-arterial injection of vasodilators such as papaverine, verapamil, milrinone, and nicardipine have shown improvement in the vasospasm.[158,161]

Intraoperative Considerations Regardless of presentation, the goal for induction of general anesthesia is to avoid an increase in transmural pressure as a result of hypertension or decrease in ICP, thus preventing aneurysm rupture. Hyperventilation at the time of induction may decrease the ICP and theoretically increase the chance of bleeding; however, in patients with a ruptured aneurysm a decrease in ICP to reach an effective CPP may be necessary. An intravenous induction is usually the method of choice. Intravenous lidocaine (0.5-1 mg) can help in preventing sympathetic discharge in response to intubation. The anesthesiologist should confirm that the patient has reached an anesthetic depth enough to avoid a sudden increase in blood pressure and heart rate in response to positioning the head in the frame. Maintenance of anesthesia is achieved by a balanced method. An opioid infusion such as remifentanil or sufentanil accompanied by a volatile anesthetic is a common practice in many institutions, although the use of total intravenous anesthesia is also advocated. Remifentanil has the advantage of a very short half-life, allowing early postoperative neurological examination; however, postoperative hyperalgesia should be taken into account. Postoperative pain can increase the blood pressure and cause a risk of intracranial hemorrhage. Muscle relaxation can be achieved by nondepolarizing muscle relaxant boluses or infusion. After the dura is opened, slight hyperventilation can help in decreasing the tightness of the brain, especially in patients with SAH, although there may be a need for mannitol or diuretics to achieve a relaxed brain. Ample effort on the surgeon's side to remove blood and clots especially from cisternae can decrease postoperative vasospasm.[162] Placement of temporary clips can facilitate dissection and decrease the chance of bleeding. Close communication between the surgeon and the anesthesiologist is important for maintaining the hemodynamic parameters in accordance with the procedure stage. Because temporary clips can impede blood flow to a large portion of the brain, a brain protective method is usually used. Although many protective methods have been suggested, currently the common practice is infusion of thiopental to decrease the $CMRO_2$; a dosing method still has to be agreed upon, but if EEG monitoring is available, the goal is to trigger burst suppressions.[163] However, in a recent study on patients who had undergone the Intraoperative Hypothermia for Aneurysm Surgery Trial (IHAST), neither hypothermia nor other protective medications showed any change in short- or long-term neurologic outcomes,[164] although in this study the supplemental pharmacologic protective measure was neither randomized nor standardized. The time of temporary clips should be recorded and the surgeon informed periodically. Temporary clips are also used if intraoperative bleeding of the aneurysm in noticed. In such situations an initial decrease in blood pressure can decrease the pool of blood in the surgical field to allow visualization and placement of the temporary clip. After placement of temporary clips, a slight elevation in blood pressure can help in collateral perfusion to the ischemic parts of the brain. After placement of the permanent clip, the hemodynamic goal is to return the blood pressure to the baseline and optimal level that can provide adequate CPP. A temporary increase in blood pressure can help the surgeon identify any bleeding in the field. Recently, intravenous dyes such as indocyanine green have become available and allow the surgeon to visualize the anatomy of the aneurysm and adjacent vessels with a specialized camera.[165]

Postoperative Period The decision on emergence and extubation depends on the preoperative condition, the presence of SAH and vasospasm, the operative course, blood loss, and if the patient meets the routine extubation criteria. In some cases intraoperative barbiturates given for brain protection as well as antiepileptics may cause delayed emergence. Patients with asymptomatic IA undergoing elective surgery are usually extubated in the operating room. A slow, controlled emergence to decrease sympathetic discharge and cough reflex is again the optimal goal. Even in cases that may not be ready for extubation, it is desirable to decrease the anesthetic level so that a neurologic examination becomes possible. Although a slow wake-up may be attributed to the intraoperative medications used, a delay in accepting a surgical complication can be harmful. The surgical team may decide on transportation to the CT scan suite to rule out surgical causes of delayed emergence such as intracranial bleeding or pneumocephalus.

Most postaneurysmal clipping patients are admitted to a close-monitoring unit where skilled nursing for frequent neurological examination is available. Transport should be in a controlled manner with the ability for continuous monitoring and resuscitative measures if necessary.

ARTERIOVENOUS MALFORMATIONS (AVM)

An AVM by definition is a tangled cluster of thin-walled vessels that connect the high-pressure arterial to the low-pressure venous system. The pathophysiologic result follows the principle of flow to the path of least resistance, that is, because blood has a low-pressure path to flow, it bypasses the normal arteriolar and capillary system in the adjacent tissue, causing a "steal syndrome" and ischemia.[166] Because the etiology is congenital there is compensation in the brain tissue and no relevant ischemic symptoms are apparent in an intact AVM; however, an ischemic site can give rise to a seizure focus with some patients presenting with seizures. Many AVMs are discovered incidentally after brain imaging. Complications arising from AVM include seizures and intracranial hemorrhage. Seizures could be a result of focal ischemia or hemorrhage. Intracranial hemorrhage in AVM, unlike IA, causes a SAH, is usually intraparenchymal or intraventricular. Intracranial hemorrhage could be as a result of venous blockade or an increase in the arterial blood pressure. Signs and symptoms are secondary to increased intracranial pressure including headache, mental status change, and focal neurological deficit. Some AVMs are associated with 1 or more aneurysms.

In neurosurgical practice a specific grading system, Spetzler Martin grading,[167] is used to identify a therapeutic plan. The grading is based on the size, eloquence, and pattern of venous drainage. Twelve combinations for grading are possible in this system (**Table 51-7**). Treatment strategies include radiosurgery, interventional, and open surgical, or a combination of these.[166] Selection of treatment modality depends on patient age, medical condition, pattern of venous drainage, and size and location of the AVM.

TABLE 51-7 Spetzler Martin Grading[a]

Graded Feature	Points
Size of AVM	
Small (<3 cm)	1
Medium (3-6 cm)	2
Large (>6 cm)	3
Eloquence of Adjacent Brain	
Noneloquent	0
Eloquent	1
Pattern of Venous Drainage	
Superficial only	0
Deep	1

AVM, arteriovenous malformation.

[a]The total grade is the addition of points in each graded feature of size, eloquence, and venous drainage.

Preoperative Evaluation The goals for the management of AVM are to eliminate the chance of bleeding and maximize neurological function in the patient.[168] In patients who present with an intracranial hemorrhage, the main focus is to stabilize their clinical picture and improve their CPP. Although it seems reasonable to aim for the excision of abnormal tissue that not only can cause seizure but also has the potential for a devastating intracranial hemorrhage, this may not be a simple procedure. In these patients, the normal blood flow (arterial → capillary → venous) is replaced by a high-pressure arterial side to sudden low-pressure venous circulation. This can cause a steal phenomenon in the surrounding area. Sudden blockage of a large amount of the feeding arterial supply can cause bleeding and/or edema. Two mechanisms have been suggested for this complication. The *normal perfusion pressure breakthrough* explanation suggests diversion of blood flow to vasculature not accustomed to high-pressure blood flow, causing brain edema.[169] Another explanation, *occlusive hyperemia*, attributes the swelling to the occlusion of draining veins during surgery, which can result in brain edema.[170] Thus the reason to perform the intravascular treatment in stages. Through angiographic access the feeding arteries are identified[171] and cyanoacrylate glue is injected. The glue can occlude the feeding arteries permanently; however, to decrease the chance of intracranial edema by the mechanism explained, this procedure is usually performed in stages. At each stage some arterial supply is occluded and the final excision is performed after it is determined that there will be a lower chance of brain edema or hemorrhage after excision.

Perioperative consideration in patient selection, evaluation, and optimization is similar for patients with IA; however, the hemodynamic goals may be different. In patients presenting with intracranial bleeding, the principle of improving the CPP and decreasing the $CMRO_2$ is still in effect. Determination of the best hemodynamic parameter for improvement of perfusion to the brain without increasing the chance of enlarging the intracranial bleed requires monitoring methods of cerebral oxygenation. Intubation and sedation, barbiturate coma, and hypothermia have been suggested in the management of these patients. In patients who have asymptomatic AVM, preoperative evaluation and optimization should accompany medical treatment directed toward decreasing the chance of AVM hemorrhage, including, blood pressure control.

Intraoperative Considerations Patients may arrive to the operating room from home in an elective situation or be transported from an intensive care setting. Patients admitted in the ICU may have an intracranial hemorrhage or be admitted after a neuroangiographic interventional staging procedure with the goal of close hemodynamic control. In either case the intraoperative goals are summarized as (1) close hemodynamic monitoring and intervention to optimize perfusion and decrease cerebral oxygen need, (2) decrease the chance of intraoperative bleeding and be prepared to treat excessive blood loss, and (3) lower the possibility of brain edema by normal perfusion pressure breakthrough or hyperemia after excision of the AVM.

Postoperative Period Emergence should avoid an increase in blood pressure. In some instances where there is a high possibility of normal perfusion pressure breakthrough, it may be beneficial to keep the patient intubated and sedated. Decision on extubation depends on preoperative condition, AVM grade, intraoperative course, and hemodynamic goals; this decision should be mutually made after communication with the surgeon and neurointensivist. Dexmedetomidine, a selective α_2-agonist used as a sedative agent, can help control the blood pressure while allowing serial neurologic examinations in the intensive care unit. Patients sedated with dexmedetomidine in some reports were awakened easily to perform neurologic examination during awake craniotomies[172]; however, some reports mention that it may impair neurocognitive testing during endovascular embolization of AVM.[173]

EXTRACRANIAL-INTRACRANIAL BYPASS

Intravascular or open surgical treatment may not be feasible in all intracranial vascular lesions such as moyamoya disease, giant or complex aneurysm, or those inaccessible for surgical extraction. Sacrificing an arterial supply or diverting the intracranial blood flow may also be needed with large or inaccessible intracranial tumors.[174] In such cases an arterial bypass connecting an extracranial artery to an intracranial one is the treatment of choice. Usually the superficial temporal artery is connected to the ipsilateral middle cerebral artery. In pediatric patients with small arteries or in patients with inadequate extracranial arterial supply the procedure of choice is encephaloduroarteriomyosynostosis or EDAMS. The aim of this procedure is to allow the arterial growth and migration from the muscle flap through the dura to the cerebral surface. The same principles of all intracranial vascular surgeries regarding adequate collateral perfusion and maintenance of acceptable cerebral perfusion, as well as decrease in intracranial oxygen demand are also in effect. During the surgical procedure a drop in blood pressure, especially during the stages where surgical arterial anastomosis is facilitated by temporary clips, can decrease the collateral blood flow and cause ischemia. Use of brain protection modalities such as thiopental may be indicated in the ischemic period.

AWAKE CRANIOTOMY

Awake craniotomy is one of the most challenging procedures for the neuroanesthesiologist. Awake craniotomy is not a new technique; it was performed in the early 20th century by neurosurgeons Cushing and De Martell. The enthusiasm for awake craniotomy has surged in the last 2 decades with the advancs in functional neurosurgery. Awake craniotomy is the preferred setting for functional neurosurgery including deep-brain stimulation for the treatment of Parkinson disease and, more recently, for the treatment of other conditions including obesity, depression, and obsessive compulsive disorders.[175] It is also indicated for the surgical management of epileptic foci in the dominant hemisphere, minimizing the risk of postoperative language disturbance. Similarly, during surgery for tumor resection nearby or involving Broca and Wernicke speech areas, awake craniotomy while maintaining verbal contact with the patient is considered the most accurate monitor for optimizing neurological outcome.[172] The aim of anesthetic management during awake craniotomy is to ensure optimal patient comfort, adequate sedation, analgesia, and hemodynamic control without interfering with electrophysiologic monitoring and patient cooperation. Guaranteeing adequate ventilation and a patent upper airway are important challenges during the procedure. In the past, alternating asleep-awake-asleep (AAA) techniques were used. Patients were fully anesthetized during a major part of the craniotomy, usually during the opening of the cranium, and then were awakened during stimulation; after the resection of the tumor the patients were returned to sleep during closure. The maintenance of the upper airway during AAA technique is usually by using either endotracheal tube or laryngeal mask airway (LMA). We believe the AAA technique has problems that minimize its benefit during awake craniotomy. Current techniques include continuous sedation with infiltrative anesthesia of the scalp. The commonly used drugs during awake craniotomy are propofol, fentanyl, remifentanil, midazolam, and dexmedetomidine. A combination of propofol with remifentanil is usually administered during the AAA technique.

REGIONAL ANESTHESIA AND SCALP NERVE BLOCKS DURING AWAKE CRANIOTOMY

During sedation, block of the auriculotemporal, zygomaticotemporal, supraorbital, supratrocheal, occipital, and greater occipital nerves can allow for minimal discomfort during skin incision. Doses of up to 4.5 mg/kg of ropivacaine appear safe.[176,177]

Propofol has a rapid onset of action and fast clearance from the plasma by redistribution and metabolism, so the level of sedation can be easily titrated. However, its prolonged use can adversely affect the mitochondrial function.[178] Dexmedetomidine is a highly selective α-agonist that offers cooperative sedation, anxiolysis, and analgesia without respiratory depression. Patients can be awakened easily by verbal stimulation after administration of dexmedetomidine. It is particularly valuable when the eloquent areas of the brain are stimulated; the patient is able to perform neurocognitive tasks.[179] Dexmedetomidine produces cerebral vasoconstriction by stimulating α-2b receptors in the cerebral blood vessels. Dexmedetomidine inhibits the cerebral vasodilatation induced by hypercapnia, thus avoiding increased intracranial pressure and brain bulging during the procedure. Dexmedetomidine also has anticonvulsant effects that might be helpful during epilepsy surgery or tumor resection.[180]

Our preferred technique is the combination of dexmedetomidine and propofol infusions during the period of patient positioning, application of head pin, and opening of the cranium. During the tumor resection period where the awake, cooperative patient is capable of performing neurocognitive tests, we stop the propofol infusion while reducing the dexmedetomidine infusion dose. During the procedure we usually give minimal doses of benzodiazepines and opioids to avoid respiratory depression and allow the patient to be able to perform the required neurocognitive tests.

Complications The average incidence of intraoperative seizure during awake craniotomy is 9.5% with a range of 0% to 24%.[181] Most of the seizures can be resolved by irrigation of the surgical field with cold saline or administration of propofol. Prophylaxis with antiepileptic drugs is helpful to prevent intraoperative seizures.[182] Intraoperative hypertension and tachycardia are usually encountered during painful phases and emergence from anesthesia; they can be managed by short-acting β-blockers like esmolol or with labetalol.

Deep Brain Stimulation (DBS) In the late 1980s it was discovered that DBS with high- frequency electrical stimulation was able to have the same effect as surgical lesioning of the basal ganglia for treatment of Parkinsons disease (PD).[183,184] The targets for DBS are the subthalamic nucleus (STN) or globus pallidus interior (GPi). DBS has been shown to improve intractable epilepsy, cephalgias, restless legs syndrome, multiple sclerosis, major depressive disorders, obsessive-compulsive disorders, and essential disorders.[185]

Anesthetic Management During DBS The neuronal circuitry between the striatum and the GPi and STN contains the γ-aminobutyric acid (GABA)-ergic pathways which are involved in PD. The avoidance of drugs with GABA-ergic activity, like benzodiazepines or opioids, is crucial for proper electrode insertion. Drugs for PD should be stopped in the preoperative period for proper target identification; this period is called the off period. The off period causes PD patients to suffer from depression, delirium, rigidity, tremors, and laryngospasm, which causes airway obstruction.[186] PD patients might have dysarthria and impaired vocal cord function, which makes them prone to aspiration during the procedure. The patient's head is usually fixed in a head frame and sedation is administered until the burr hole is made. At this time the

TABLE 51-8 Complication Rate

Complication	No. of Events	Complication Rate Percentage per Patient
Respiratory	4	1.60
Cardiac	1	0.40
Neurologic	9	3.60
Intracranial hemorrhage	7	2.80
Seizure	2	0.80
Psychologic/psychiatric	8	3.20
Confusion/lack of cooperation	7	2.80
Severe anxiety	1	0.40
Patient-requested procedure termination	4	1.60
Coughing/moaning/sneezing	3	1.20
Total	29	11.6

From Khatib R, Ebrahim Z, Rezai A, et al. Perioperative events during deep brain stimulation: the experience at Cleveland Clinic. *J Neurosurg Anesthesiol*. 2008;20(1):36-40.

sedation is usually stopped or decreased to allow for proper target identification. The systolic blood pressure should be kept less than or equal to 140 mm Hg to minimize intracrebral hemorrhage. Dexmedetomidine provides sedation and anxiolysis with minimal effect on respiration. Also, the sympatholytic effect of dexmedetomidine provides control of the blood pressure during DBS. In a recent analysis of 258 DBS cases, the complication rate was found to be 11.6%, including airway, respiratory, neurologic, and psychological problems. Age (≥64) was determined to be an independent risk factor for anesthetic complications during DBS. Intracrebral hemorrhage and seizures occurred in 3.6%. Aspiration has been reported in 1.6%; propofol induced sneezing in 1.2% (**Table 51-8**).[187]

ANESTHETIC CONSIDERATIONS FOR INTERVENTIONAL NEURORADIOLOGY

Interventional neuroradiology (INR) or endovascular neurosurgery, a hybrid of traditional neurosurgery and neuroradiology, has emerged as a distinct specialty. INR can be broadly defined as treatment by endovascular access for the purpose of delivering therapeutic drugs and devices.

Procedures amenable to INR can be broadly classified as the basis of the aim of treatment. Closing or occluding procedures include embolization of aneurysms, arteriovenous malformations (AVMs), and fistulae of the brain, as well as preoperative embolization of vascular tumors such as meningiomas. Opening procedures include treatment of vasospasm or stenosis by angioplasty and stenting, and chemical and mechanical thrombolysis in stroke.

IMAGING TECHNOLOGY

INR requires high-resolution fluoroscopy and high-speed digital subtraction angiography (DSA). Road mapping is used to facilitate placement of superselective catheters in the distal circulation. To make a road map, a bolus of contrast is injected into the circulation from the guide catheter to obtain an image of the vascular anatomy. The computer then superimposes this image onto live, bone subtracted fluoroscopy so that the radiologists can see the progress of the radio-opaque microcatheter (especially the tip) against the roadmap (**Fig. 51-10**). Good-quality road maps are dependent on the patient being motionless.

RADIATION SAFETY

It is important to know that DSA delivers considerably more radiation than fluoroscopy. Ionizing radiation follows the inverse square law that the radiation exposure drops off proportionally to the square of the distance from the source.[188] Therefore, activity near the head of the patient should be kept to a minimum during fluoroscopy and the use of extension tubing is required for infusion and monitoring lines.

MATERIALS USED FOR EMBOLIZATION OR INFUSION

Coils The coils most commonly used for occlusion of aneurysms are detachable or retrievable coils. The basic principle is that the coil can be advanced into position through a microcatheter using a pusher wire to which the coil is attached. If the coil position is suboptimal, it can be retrieved and redeployed or replaced by a more appropriate one. The coils are usually made of platinum. After satisfactory placement of the coil in the aneurysm, the coil is detached from the pusher wire. The common deployment method is electrical as in the Guglielmi Detachable Coil (GDC). Recent advances include the development of bioactive coils, which are coated with materials that promote thrombus formation and endothelial growth.

MATERIALS USED FOR MANAGEMENT OF AVMs

Cyanoacrylates (Hisoacryl, Braun) These are rapidly polymerizing adhesives. The polymerization process is exothermic, which results in heat

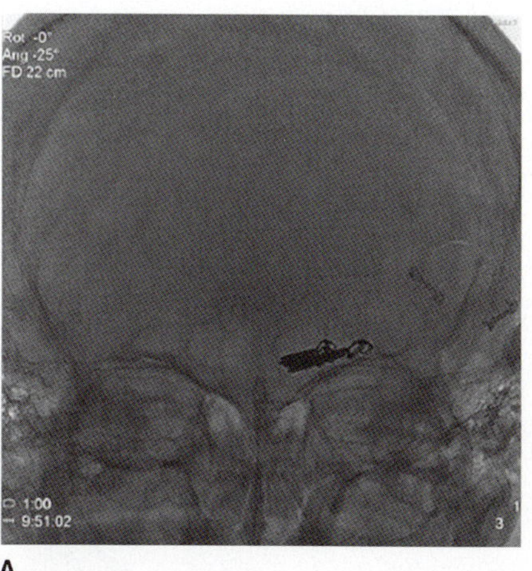

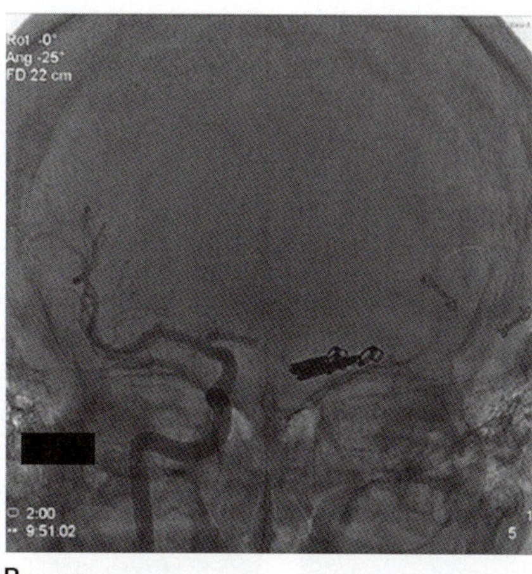

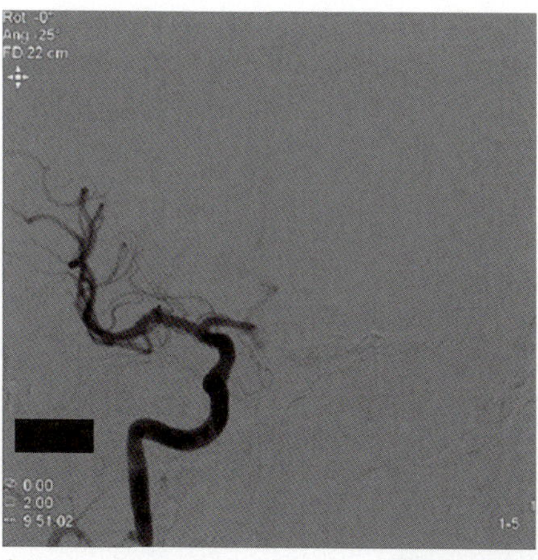

FIGURE 51-10. **A.** Anterioposterior scout film showing bone. This image is used as the "mask." **B.** The same view showing contrast injected through the coaxial carotid catheter. **C.** Subtraction of mask image (**A**) from (**B**) results in the "road map." The digital image is superimposed on live fluoroscopy, which will reflect the course the microcatheter takes as it is advanced distally. [From Varma MK, Price K, Jayakrishnan V, Manickam B, Kessell G. Anaesthetic considerations for interventional neuroradiology. *Br J Anaesth*. 2007;99:75-85, by permission of Oxford University Press.]

liberation into surrounding tissues during embolization. Because of its adhesive properties, the catheter has to be withdrawn immediately after cyanoacrylate injection to avoid it sticking.

Onyx Liquid Embolic System Onyx is a biocompatible liquid embolic agent consisting of ethylene vinyl alcohol copolymer (EVOH) dissolved in dimethyl sulfoxide. It solidifies through the process of precipitation. Precipitation of onyx begins immediately after injection, creating a skin that solidifies from outside in. Precipitation of onyx does not produce heat. Because onyx is nonadhesive, the controlled injection and filling of the vascular abnormality can take place over several minutes, and concurrent angiography can be performed with the catheter left in place. The advantages of onyx are its ability to reach difficult anatomical locations, the ability to penetrate a larger number of feeding vessels in one injection, and more precise control when delivering the material (access, handling, delivery, and visibility).[189]

Polyvinyl Alcohol Particles (PVA) PVA produce the temporary occlusion of blood vessels and are the preferred agents for preoperative embolization of tumors such as meningiomas.

ENDOVASCULAR TREATMENT OF CEREBRAL ANEURYSMS

Aneurysmal disease can be classified into 3 categories: (1) small (<12 mm in diameter), (2) large (12-24 mm), and (3) giant (>24 mm). Complete thrombosis can be achieved in 57% to 85% of aneurysms with neck diameter less than 4 mm after endovascular occlusion of the aneurysms.[190,191] The total occlusion rate of aneurysms with neck diameter greater than 4 mm is only 15% to 35%. The incidence of subsequent hemorrhage following coiling is 0% for small aneurysms, 4% for large aneurysms, and 33% for giant aneurysms (**Fig. 51-11**).[190-192]

International Subarachnoid Aneurysm Trial (ISAT) and Its Implications ISAT compared the safety and efficacy of endovascular coiling versus clipping for cerebral aneurysms. The study showed in the final 1-year results that in patients presenting with ruptured intracranial aneurysms and who were suitable for coiling and clipping, endovascular coil treatment reduces the relative risk of dependence or death by 23.9% with an absolute risk reduction of 7.4% at 1 year following SAH as compared to surgical clipping.[193] Overall, case mortality rates were similar between the 2 groups, with 10.1% and 8.1% in the clipping and coiling groups. In spite of these favorable data, IAST has problems in its methodology. Only 22.4% of the initially screened 9559 patients underwent randomization. Fewer than 10% of the patients were at high risk and 95% of them had an aneurysm in the anterior communicating artery with a size less than 10 mm. Complete occlusion was achieved more often in the surgically treated group compared with the endovascular treated group (82% vs 66%). Rebleeding occurred more often in the endovascular treated group compared with the clipping one (52% vs 41%).

COMPARISON OF CLIPPING AND COILING

Risks of Clipping Clipping of an unruptured aneurysm has been associated with morbidity and mortality rates of 4.0% to 10.9% and 1.0% to 3.0%, respectively. Intraoperative leak and frank rupture aneurysms occurred in approximately 6% and 13% of cases, respectively.[194]

Risks for Inserting Detachable Coils Minor risks are similar to those of diagnostic catheter angiography, like reactions to contrast material, groin hematomas, infections, or pseudoaneurysms of the femoral artery. Major risks include arterial dissection (0.7%), parent artery occlusion (20%), thromboembolic phenomena (2.4%), and intraprocedural rupture with associated mortality rates varying between 1% to 2.7% and 0% to 40%, respectively. Overall, procedural morbidity and mortality rates for coiling have been reported as 3.7% to 5.3% and 1.1% to 1.5%, respectively.[194]

Coiling is not indicated or possible in approximately 3% to 15% of cases. Large aneurysms or aneurysms with wider necks or with unusual tortuosity are not suitable for coiling.

Recent Technological Advances in Coiling Coils are now better able to conform in aneurysms with atypical morphology, the use of balloons, and intracranial stents (**Fig. 51-12**).

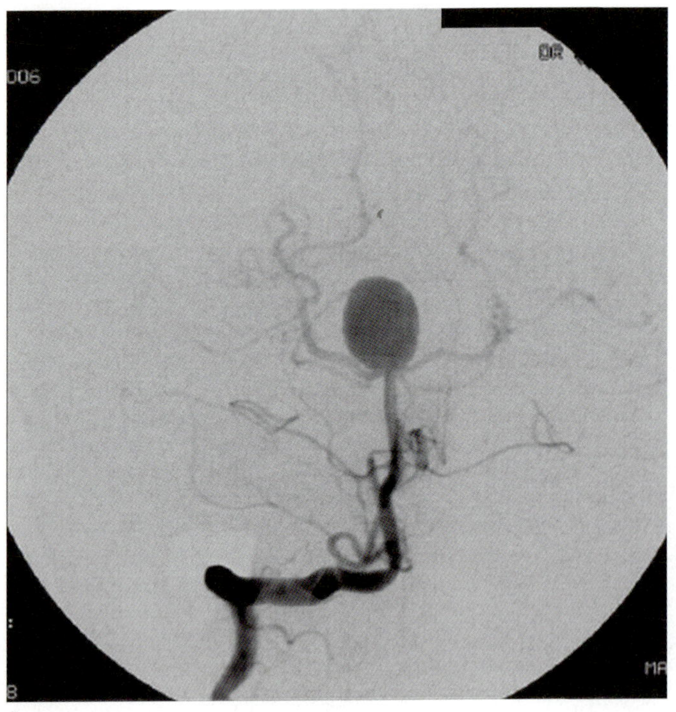

A

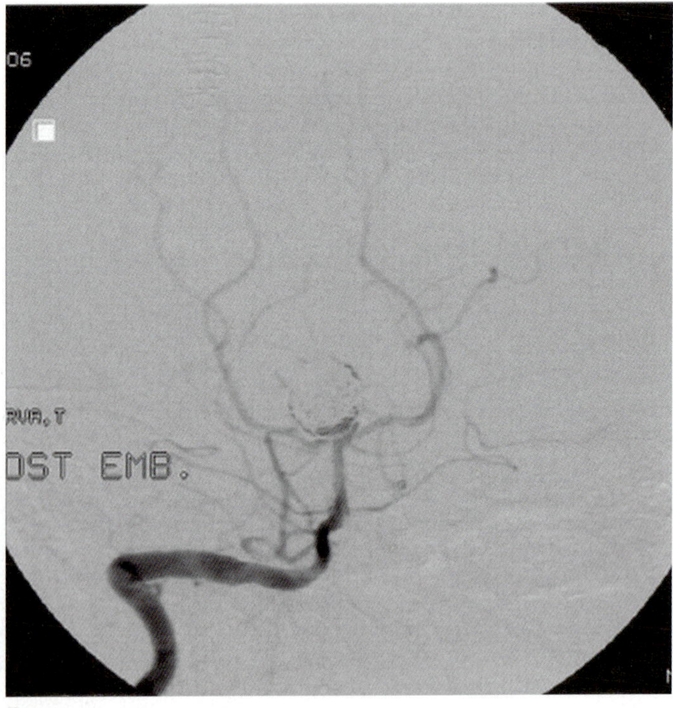

B

FIGURE 51-11. **A.** Saccular aneurysm at basilar artery bifurcation. **B.** Postembolization of saccular aneurysm at basilar artery bifurcation. [From Varma MK, Price K, Jayakrishnan V, Manickam B, Kessell G. Anaesthetic considerations for interventional neuroradiology. *Br J Anaesth.* 2007;99:75-85, by permission of Oxford University Press.]

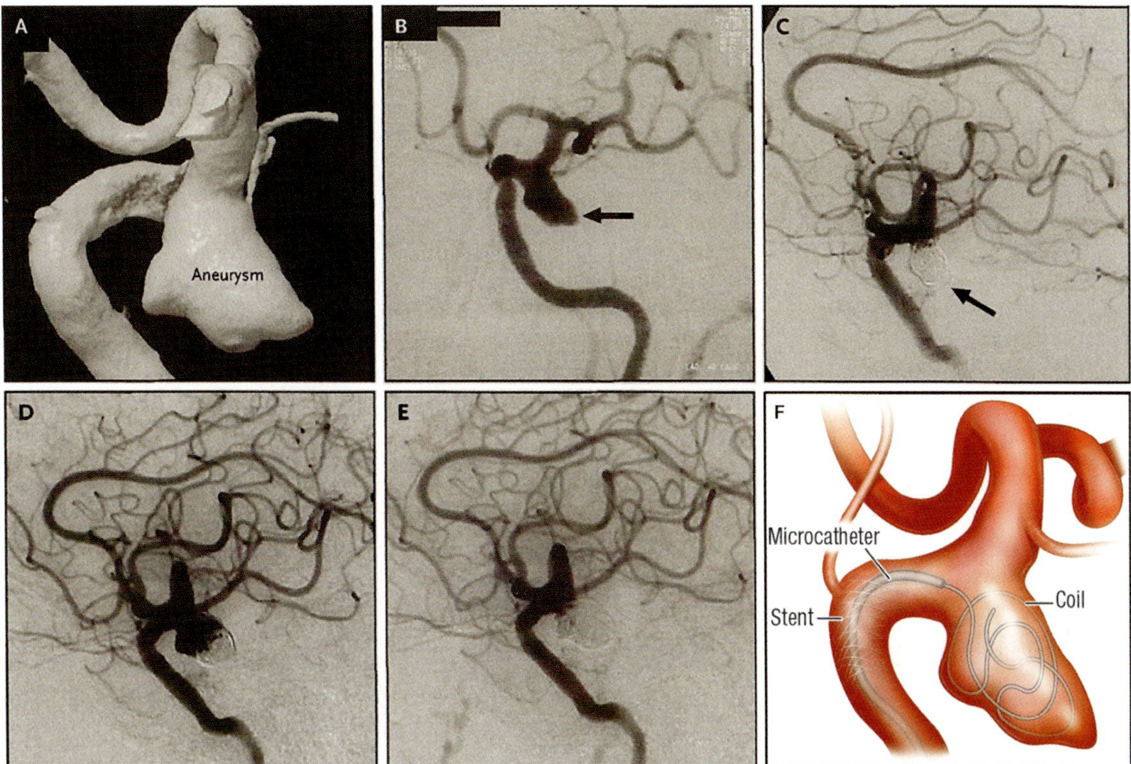

FIGURE 51-12. Stent-assisted recoiling after recurrence of an aneurysm initially treated with coiling. (**A**) (3-dimensional rotational catheter angiogram) and (**B**) (left carotid injection, 2-dimensional catheter angiogram, oblique view) show an aneurysm of the posterior communicating artery (**B,** *arrow*). (**C**) (2-dimensional catheter angiogram, lateral view) shows the successful coiling of the aneurysm (*arrow*); this was followed 8 months later with marked coil compaction and recanalization of the aneurysm (**D**, 2-dimensional catheter angiogram, lateral view). (**E**) (2-dimensional catheter angiogram, lateral view) shows successful recoiling of the aneurysm with the assistance of a stent (too small to visualize). (**F**) shows the configuration used for the stent and the coil. [Reprinted with permission from Brisman JL, Song JK, Newell DW. Cerebral aneurysms. *N Engl J Med.* 2006;355:928-939. Copyright© 2006 Massachusetts Medical Society. All rights reserved.]

Recanalization Over time, blood flow can compress the coil within the aneurysm, and as a result the aneurysm refills with blood. Recanalization rates appear to be in the range of 20.9% to 33.6%. The risk of hemorrhage from a coiled aneurysm due to recanalization is higher than after confirmed clipped aneurysm (**Figs. 51-13** and **51-14**). Surface active and bioactive coils have been developed to address the problem of recanalization. They are impregnated with substances intended to interfere with the vessel endothelium and form a collagenous matrix at the entrance of the aneurysm. Another solution is a new flexible, self-expandable, microcatheter-delivered, nitinol stent that is placed in the artery in which the aneurysm arises, thereby blocking it.[194]

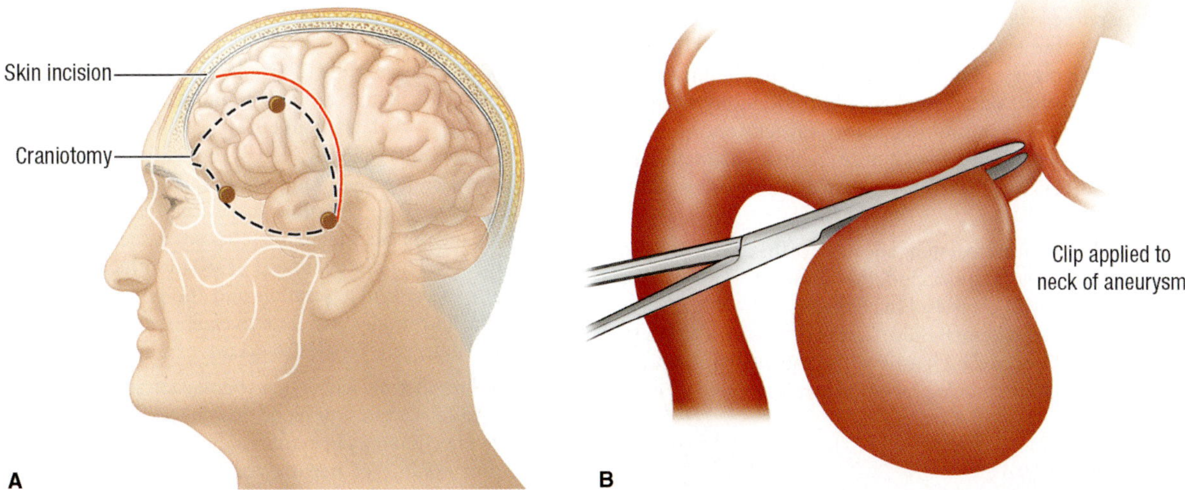

FIGURE 51-13. Microsurgical clipping of an aneurysm of the posterior communicating artery. (**A**) shows the typical skin incision (*unbroken curved line*) and craniotomy (*dashed lines*) needed to access the aneurysm. (**B**) shows the application of the clip blade to the neck of the aneurysm. [Reprinted with permission from Brisman JL, Song JK, Newell DW. Cerebral aneurysms. *N Engl J Med.* 2006;355:928-939. Copyright© 2006 Massachusetts Medical Society. All rights reserved.]

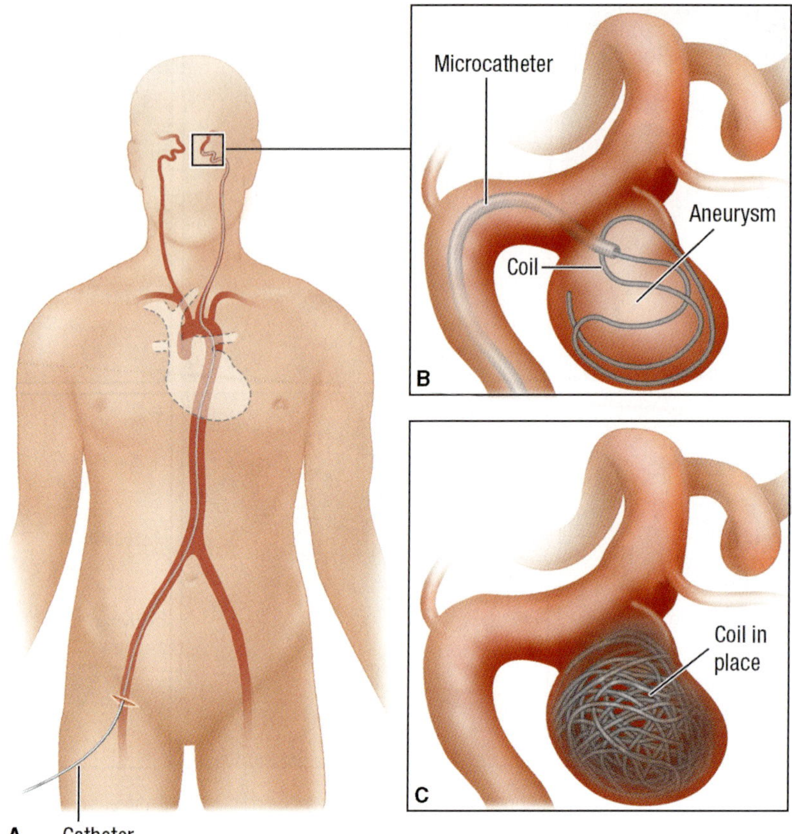

FIGURE 51-14. Endovascular occlusion of an aneurysm of the posterior communicating artery with Guglielmi Detachable Coils. (**A**) and inset show the route of the microcatheter into the aneurysm through the right femoral artery, aorta, and left carotid artery and the beginning of the coil deployment. (**B**) & (**C**) shows the final occlusion of the aneurysm with coils. [Reprinted with permission from Brisman JL, Song JK, Newell DW. Cerebral aneurysms. *N Engl J Med.* 2006;355:928-939. Copyright© 2006 Massachusetts Medical Society. All rights reserved.]

MANAGEMENT OF AVMS

A small AVM can be cured by embolization alone; large ones need embolization to shrink their size followed by surgery. Mortality and morbidity after embolization of an AVM are 1% to 1.6% and 5% to 7%, respectively. Embolization of glue into the draining vein may result in venous obstruction and pulmonary glue embolization. General anesthesia is preferred during the procedure to facilitate visualization of the structures and prevent the patient's movement. Controlled hypotension may be required to reduce the flow across the AVM. After AVM, treatment can be followed by normal perfusion pressure breakthrough as feeding arteries supply a variable amount of normal brain; abrupt restoration of normal systemic pressure to a chronically hypotensive vascular bed may overwhelm the autoregulatory capacity and result in hemorrhage or brain edema. Therefore, it is desirable to maintain arterial pressure at about 15% to 20% below the patient's normal level after the procedure.[195,196]

Carotid Occlusion Test It is used to test the adequacy of the cerebrovascular collateral circulation before electing to occlude the carotid artery. Combining the carotid occlusion test with controlled hypotension (10%-20% of baseline) increases the predictive value of the test. Complications include bradycardia, hypertension, and loss of consciousness. The patient must be awake for the procedure; continuous neurological evaluation is required to assess the effects of occlusion.

ANESTHETIC TECHNIQUE

The Options for Anesthetic Management of Interventional Neuroradiology

General Anesthesia *Advantages* of general anesthesia are that it provides an immobile patient with improved image quality and patient comfort, and better control of the respiratory and hemodynamic profile. *Disadvantages* of this method are the inability to perform neurological assessment intraoperatively. Other disadvantages are the consequences of endotracheal intubation and extubation, producing hypertension, coughing, or straining, which can lead to raised ICP. A recent study comparing the speed of recovery after maintenance of anesthesia for neuroradiology with sevoflurane or propofol found that sevoflurane was associated with a more rapid recovery.[205] Nitrous oxide is preferably avoided as there is a risk of enlargement of micro air bubbles during injection of contrast or irrigation fluid.

Sedation Dexmedetomidine is an ideal agent for sedation during the procedure as patients are arousable and cooperative when stimulated. A lack of respiratory depressant effect is another advantage. It has been used in endovascular embolization of AVMs.

Using the sedation technique will enable one to perform neurological testing repeatedly. The other advantage of the sedation technique is the avoidance of hemodynamic changes associated with intubation and emergence. The *disadvantages* of sedation include an unprotected airway with the risk of aspiration and the potential for hypoxia and hypercapnia, and sudden patient movements, and delays in managing a neurological emergency may also occur.

Conduct of Anesthesia Deliberate hypertension for occlusion and vasospasm, or hypotension to slow blood flow in feeding the artery of an AVM before glue injection may be required during interventional procedures. A significant volume of heparinized flush solution and radiographic contrast is often used, and administration of diuretics such as mannitol and furosemide may be required intraoperatively. Hypothermia can occur in the neuroradiology suite, and measures should be taken to keep the body temperature near normal and core temperature measured.

COMPLICATIONS OF INR PROCEDURES

Hemorrhagic Complications Hemorrhage is often accompanied by an abrupt rise in MAP. Immediate reversal of heparin may be required and lowering of systemic arterial pressure. Aneurysm perforation is usually treated by packing the defect with coils. Emergency craniotomy and clipping may be required if coiling fails.

Occlusive Complications In the event of occlusion, the arterial pressure should be raised to increase collateral blood flow and maintain normocarbia.

Treatment of vasospasm can be either medical (triple therapy: hypertension, hypervolemia, and hemodilution), pharmacological, or by angioplasty.

Intra-arterial papaverine is associated with side effects including mono-ocular blindness, mydriasis, seizures, transient increase in ICP, hypertension, tachycardia, and paradoxical worsening of vasospasm.

Angioplasty is the most effective procedure, especially if it is performed within 2 hours of symptomatic ischemia. Complications include vessel rupture (2%-5%) and rebleed from an unprotected aneurysm (5%).

Contrast Reactions The most commonly used contrast for INR is iohexol (nonionic) with an osmolality of 672 mOsm/kg. Fatal reactions occur at a frequency of 1 in 10,000 exposures. Reactions can be due to hypertonicity, direct cardiac depression, or idiosyncratic anaphylactoid reactions.

Contrast Nephropathy This is the third most common cause of hospital-acquired renal failure and occurs in 12% of patients. The risk factors include DM, high-dose contrast volume depletion, coadministration of nephrotoxic medications, and preexisting renal disease. To prevent renal complications, perioperative fluid management should be aimed at maintaining normovolemia to offset the diuretic effect of the injected contrast. Isotonic bicarbonate infusion may also reduce the incidence of contrast-induced nephropathy by alkalizing renal tubular fluid and thereby minimizing tubular damage.

Postoperative Care Maintenance of modest hypotension is required post-AVM embolization to prevent cerebral edema and hemorrhage. The MAP should be kept 15% to 20% below the baseline for 24 hours. A MAP 20% to 30% above normal may be required in patients with occlusive conditions or with vasospasm to maintain cerebral perfusion pressure. This can be achieved with the use of phenylephrine or norepinephrine. Postoperative nausea and vomiting can be a problem due to the effect of contrast and anesthetic agents used during the procedure.

INTRACRANIAL ENDOSCOPIC PROCEDURES

NEUROENDOSCOPY

The first endoscopic neurosurgical procedure was performed by Lespinasse, a urologist, in 1910. He used a cystoscope to fulgurate the choroid plexus in 2 children, 1 of whom died during the operation, and the other survived for 5 years.[206] In the 1970s advances in fiberoptics led to the construction of steerable neuroendoscopes, allowing the neurosurgeon to perform complex surgery within the confines of the ventricular space in adults, children, and even in neonates.[207]

HYDROCEPHALUS

Patients with uncomplicated noncommunicating hydrocephalus due to aqueductal stenosis or to space-occupying lesions of the midbrain or posterior fossa can have their cerebrospinal fluid (CSF) flow internally corrected through the creation of an opening of the third ventricle. A common complication of the traditionally placed shunt system is the obstruction of the ventricular catheter tip from adjacent tissue. The rigid fiberoptic endoscope was found to be a safe and efficient method of inserting the ventricular catheter, with improved accuracy over conventional methods.[208] Relative contraindications include patients with abnormal ventricular anatomy and those with an intraventricular hemorrhage or a history of meningitis. Damage to the walls of the third ventricle may occur in patients with smaller ventricular size.

SURGICAL APPROACH

Patient position for endoscopic entry into the third ventricle is usually supine with slight flexion of the neck, or with the head tilted from 45 to 90 degrees, depending on the planned procedure. The cranium may be fixed in a head frame. Through a coronal burr hole, the endoscope is introduced into the ventricle system via the frontal horn and advanced into the third ventricle where the mammillary bodies, an important landmark, can be visualized. The tuber cinereum is located immediately beyond these structures. Beneath this membrane are the basilar artery and the basal cisterns. In patients with aqueduct stenosis, fenestration of this membrane creates an opening through which CSF can be drained, bypassing the aqueduct of Sylvius. Operating in fluid-filled cavities requires intermittent or continuous warmed (37°C) irrigant fluid (either Ringer lactate or normal saline) to maintain adequate ventricular pressure and good visibility. The fluid is usually infused under pressure or gravity feed and allowed to egress passively through an open port of the endoscope. Inadequate venting of the irrigant fluid leads to marked increases in ICP. Increased ICP can be detected by increased blood pressure and bradycardia (Cushing reflex). Toxic reactions such as high fever and headaches have been described due to meningeal irritation, which can occur with large volumes of saline irrigation. Artificial CSF has been used to reduce the incidence of these toxic reactions. Surgical complications, such as acute increases in transcranial pressure and injury to brain structures, including the basilar artery and hemorrhage, have been described. Intracranial bleeding secondary to instrumentation can be catastrophic. Intracranial hypotension may follow sudden ventricular decompression and removal of CSF, causing pressure changes at the midbrain and hypothalamus level. This in turn can lead to sudden alterations in heart rate and blood pressure. Hypothermia can occur, especially with the use of large volumes of irrigation.

Cardiac arrhythmias in the form of bradycardia, and even asystole can occur during stimulation of the floor of the third ventricle due to its proximity to the vasomotor center or inadequate venting of the irrigant fluid. Injury to brain structures may result in short-term memory loss due to injury to the fornix,[209] syndrome of inappropriate secretion of antidiuretic hormone (SIADH) due to injury of hypothalamus,[210] and bleeding or pseudoaneurysm formation after injury to the basilar artery. Postoperative complications including transient confusion, headaches, and unresponsiveness have also been described.[206]

ANESTHETIC CONSIDERATIONS IN BRAIN NEUROENDOSCOPY

Patients with hydrocephalus may have hypovolemia due to vomiting, fluid restriction, contrast agents, or osmotic diuretics. Adequate volume replacement is a necessary consideration prior to induction. General anesthesia with endotracheal intubation and controlled ventilation is essential to ensure immobility and because sudden intracranial pressure changes may lead to vomiting. Nitrous oxide is avoided to prevent its effusion into air trapped in the ventricles and the subdural space following decompression of the ventricles, resulting in tension pneumocephalus. Anesthesia can be maintained with sevoflurane with remifentanil infusion or propofol with remifentanil infusion. Intra-arterial monitoring is recommended in view of the hemodynamic variability frequently seen and the need for arterial blood sampling.

OTHER USES FOR NEUROENDOSCOPY

Neuroendoscopy, which can be utilized for the management of arachnoid cyst, is an effective treatment. The introduction of the endoscope to assist strip craniotomies for the treatment of cranial synostosis has led to a significant reduction in blood loss and operative time, and has reduced the incidence of venous air embolism during the procedure. Endoscope-assisted microsurgery of cerebral aneurysms has been described.[211]

SPINE SURGERY

PHYSIOLOGICAL CHANGES IN THE PRONE POSITION

Prone positioning is the most common position in spine surgery; it is associated with major physiological changes. Understanding these changes allows one to reduce the incidence of complications associated with the prone position.

Cardiovascular There is decreased cardiac index (CI) and venous return[212] in the prone position. The measured cardiac index was decreased using a noninvasive cardiac output monitor in unanesthetized healthy volunteers in the prone position. CI decreased compared to the supine position as follows: knee-chest position (20%); onto pelvic props from a modified Relton-Hall frame under the anterior superior iliac spine and padded support under the chest (17%); onto the evacutable mattress (11%); and on pillows (1 pillow under the thorax and 1 under the abdomen leaving the abdomen free to move) (3%). Toyota and Amaki[213] studied transesophageal echocardiograms in 15 healthy patients undergoing prone-position lumbar laminectomy. The prone position caused left ventricular volume and compliance to decrease. These changes were attributed to a decrease in the venous return due to inferior vena caval compression, and decreased left ventricular compliance due to increased intrathoracic pressure in the prone position. These results had been confirmed by other studies using thermodilution pulmonary artery catheters to measure cardiac index when transferring from the spine to the prone position. The cardiac output in these studies decreased 17% to 24%.[214,215,216] Pearce[217] observed renal caval pressures to be 0 to 40 mm H_2O in patients who are in the prone position with the abdomen hanging free. In contrast, patients with abdominal compression had vena caval pressures greater than 300 mm H_2O. The increase in venous pressure not only will increase bleeding during spine surgery due to congestion of vertebral veins but also can also impair spinal cord perfusion.

The use of the prone position with abdominal compression was identified as a plausible cause of spinal cord ischemia leading to neurologic deficits after cervical laminectomy. The authors of this case series recommended the avoidance of abdominal compression and hypotension, especially in myelopathic patients for whom maintenance of spinal cord perfusion pressure is paramount.[218]

Changes in Respiratory Physiology In an elegant study, Nyren et al[219] studied the regional distribution of pulmonary blood flow in 10 healthy volunteers. The subjects were studied in both prone and supine positions with and without lung distension caused by 10 cm H_2O of continuous positive airway pressure (CPAP). The results of this study demonstrated that ventilation-perfusion matching during both normal breathing and positive pressure is more favorable in the prone than in the supine position. As perfusion is more evenly distributed in the prone position, the recruitment of dorsal airways results in an increase in lung units and consequently increased functional residual capacity (FRC) with near-normal ventilation-perfusion matching and a reduction in shunt.[220] By turning the patient prone and recruiting airways in the dorsal lung, prone positioning achieves similar beneficial effects as PEEP but without the risks of barotrauma or interference with cardiac function; the prone position is sometimes used in patients with autorespiratory distress syndrome (ARDS) to improve oxygenation and decreased shunt.[220] The same findings had been confirmed by Pelosi et al[221] during general anesthesia. Prone positioning during general anesthesia did not negatively affect respiratory mechanisms and improved lung volumes and oxygenation.

ANESTHESIA FOR CERVICAL SPINE SURGERY

Movement of C Spine With Intubation The primary force applied by the laryngoscopist is upward lift with a little bit of angular force. This force can be as high as 50 to 70 N (40 N is enough to lift 10 lb). The more difficult the exposure, the greater the force usually applied. Intubation needs extension of the occiput-on-C1, combined with flexion at lower vertebrae (the fulcrum is probably at C7-T1).[222] Direct laryngoscopy with a MAC 3 blade results in near maximal extension at occiput and C1 (with the posterior arch of C1 touching the skull).[222,223]

As an ideal method for intubation, Sahin et al[224] studied upper cervical vertebral motion with 3 intubation devices. Comparisons were made between direct laryngoscopy, the intubating laryngeal mask (ILMA), and fiberoptic intubation. In their study, the mean motion at the C1/C2 level was 10.2 ± 7.3, 5.0 ± 6.3, and 1.6 ± 3.2 degrees, respectively. The fiberoptic method was found to produce the least motion in the upper cervical spine. The authors conclude that fiberoptic laryngoscopy is the most suitable intubation technique when C-spine movement is not desired.

There are a few degrees less extension at C1/C2 with use of a straight blade.[225] It is unlikely that this difference is clinically meaningful. During intubation under general anesthesia with neuromuscular blockade and manual in-line stabilization, the use of a GlideScope produced better glottic visualization, but did not significantly decrease movement of the nonpathologic C spine when compared with direct laryngoscopy.[226]

Cervical Spine Movement and LMAs Keller et al[227] implanted microchip sensors into the pharyngeal surfaces of C2 and C3 in 20 cadavers to determine the pressures exerted against the C spine by the LMA and ILMA. The authors concluded that these devices exert high pressures against the upper cervical vertebrae during insertion, during inflation, and while in situ. These pressures could produce posterior displacement of the upper C spine.

Manual In-line Stabilization (MILS) and Cricoid Pressure The goal of MILS is to apply force to the head and neck equal in magnitude and opposite in direction to those generated by the laryngoscopist so as to limit the movement that might result during airway management; traction forces should be avoided. MILS failed to reduce movement at the site of instability in cadaver models.[228] Cricoid pressure (as long as not excessive) did not result in movement in a cadaver model of an injured upper cervical spine.[229]

Maintaining the head in neutral or near neutral position can be very important in maintaining proper cervical cord blood supply. Flexion of the spine causes elongation of the cord with narrowing of the diameter of the longitudinal vessels.[230] Extension causes an increase in diameter of the cervical cord and folding of the ligamentum flavum, which may exert pressure on the cord and posterior longitudinal vessels.[231] Rau et al[232] described a case of quadriplegia in a patient who underwent posterior fossa surgery in the prone position. The authors state that during a prolonged period in which the neck was in hyperflexion, overstretching of the cervical spinal cord and compromise to its blood supply likely caused this devastating complication.

Practical Points to Remember

- Awake fiberoptic intubation is ideal for most patients with *unstable* neck injuries.
- Surveys indicate that most American anesthesiologists would prefer to use a fiberoptic bronchoscope to intubate at-risk patients and to do so with the patient awake.[233]
- Induction of anesthesia diminishes the protective stabilization of the neck musculature. Neck motion during this phase can be substantial, sometimes producing dynamic cord compression that could result in cervical cord injury.
- If the cervical spine is grossly unstable, consideration should be given to both intubating the trachea and positioning the patient while he or she is still awake. If new neurological symptoms develop during positioning, repositioning should be attempted. During that period tight control of the patient's blood pressure and even inducing hypertension can help resolve these new symptoms.
- Airway complications are common after anterior cervical spine surgery and may range from acute airway obstruction to chronic vocal cord dysfunction. Recurrent laryngeal nerve injury after anterior cervical spine surgery can be due to direct nerve injury at the time of neck dissection, surgical retractor placement, and endotracheal balloon insufflation pressure.[214,234]

- C-spine surgery in the prone position could result in laryngeal edema and macroglossia.[235,236]
- The use of fiberoptic intubation results in fewer airway complications after C-spine surgery, thought to be due to a reduction in soft-tissue trauma.[237]
- For patients with subaxial spondylotic myelopathy, neck extension can narrow the diameter of the spinal canal, whereas in patients with atlantoaxial subluxation, such as those with rheumatoid arthritis and Down syndrome, neck flexion will widen the atlantodental interval, narrowing the spinal canal.
- Maintaining adequate spinal cord perfusion is crucial during cervical spine surgery in spondylitic myelopathy patients. Chronic mechanical compression inhibiting spinal cord blood supply leads to gradual, intermittent microinfarction of the cord. In this setting, invasive blood pressure monitoring using an arterial line and maintaining close attention to maintaining adequate perfusion pressure are very important.[214]

POSTOPERATIVE VISUAL LOSS (POVL) AFTER SPINE SURGERY

Vision loss or impairment after spine surgery is a devastating problem with an incidence between 0.1% and 1%.[238] The causes remain poorly understood but appear to be multifactorial and may include impaired perfusion of the eye or occlusion of retinal vessels from improper positioning.

Retinal Perfusion Pressure The main source of blood supply to the optic nerve head is the posterior ciliary circulation via the pericapillary choroids and the short posterior ciliary arteries. The blood supply in the optic nerve head has a sectoral distribution, which helps to explain why visual loss is usually segmental in anterior ischemic optic neuropathy. The blood supply to the optic nerve head shows marked interindividual variation, and even varies within an individual from eye to eye. This anatomical variability may explain why some people develop vision loss or impairment after spine surgery while others do not, despite exposure to similar conditions. Posterior ciliary arteries in vivo behave as end arteries. They also have watershed zones between their distributions (no anastomoses between the arteries in these areas). These areas are most vulnerable to ischemia when perfusion pressure is inadequate.[239]

Perfusion pressure of the eye is defined as the difference between mean systemic arterial pressure and intraocular pressure.[239] Decreased mean arterial pressure or elevated intraocular pressure will thus decrease ocular perfusion pressure. Most commonly, perfusion pressure is impaired by a combination of decreased mean arterial pressure and increased intraocular pressure.[239]

Arterial Blood Pressure Arterial hypertension, as well as arterial hypotension, may influence the blood flow in the optic nerve head. In hypertensive individuals, autoregulation of ocular blood vessels usually shifts to higher levels to maintain constant blood flow. Although this improves the patients' tolerance to high blood pressure, this upward shift in the autoregulation range makes hypertensive patients less tolerant to low blood pressures. In the optic nerve head, reduction in blood pressure below the critical autoregulatory level decreases blood flow.[239] As might thus be expected, hypotension is associated with perioperative vision loss.[240-242]

Intraocular Pressure (IOP) Intraocular pressure is the other factor that determines ocular perfusion pressure. Intraocular pressure usually increases over time in the prone position. Cheng et al[243] showed that intraocular pressure can reach up to 40 mm Hg (normal 8-20 mm Hg) after 6 hours in the prone position. Hunt et al[244] confirmed that intraocular pressure increases in the prone position. However, they could not find a relationship between an increase in intraocular pressure and duration of the procedure as did Cheng et al.[243] The causes for increased intraocular pressure during prone positioning might be due to increased episcleral venous pressure,[245] but also might be related to positive intraoperative fluid balance. In healthy volunteers, acute water loading (14 mL/kg) increased intraocular pressure,[246] whereas exercise-induced dehydration reduced intraocular pressure.[247]

Types of Visual Loss and Impairment Associated With Spinal Surgery The principal visual defects associated with spine surgery are ischemic optic neuropathy, cortical blindness, central retinal artery occlusion, and central retinal vein occlusion.

Ischemic Optic Neuropathy Ischemic optic neuropathy occurs either in the anterior part of the optic nerve where the nerve enters the globe, or the posterior part where the optic nerve lies within the orbit. Blood flow to the optic nerve is autoregulated[239] to maintain a nearly constant blood flow despite changes in perfusion pressure. However, autoregulation operates effectively only over a particular range of perfusion pressures. Above and below this range, blood flow depends directly on perfusion pressure, so ischemic damage can result. Anterior ischemic optic neuropathy can also result from a low hematocrit because choroidal blood flow decreases with hemodilution, whereas the blood flow to the retina increases.[248] Anterior ischemic optic neuropathy is frequently first noticed immediately upon awaking from normal sleep, which corresponds to a diurnal peak of intraocular pressure.[249] The true incidence of postoperative anterior ischemic optic neuropathy may be underestimated because small areas of anterior optic nerve infarction may produce only small visual defects that pass unnoticed during the postoperative period. These patients present later with low-pressure glaucoma with multiple areas of optic atrophy.[250]

Posterior ischemic optic neuropathy is relatively rare and presents clinically as a retrobulbar optic neuropathy. It is believed to result from infarction of the intraorbital portion of the optic nerve. Visual impairment is most often severe because the optic nerve swells as a consequence of ischemia. Posterior extension of swelling along the nerve involves the portion of the optic nerve within the sphenoidal optic canals where the nerve is encased in bony, nonelastic structures. Diagnostic criteria for posterior ischemic optic neuropathy include

- An acute deficit in visual acuity, visual field, or both
- An ipsilateral relative afferent papillary defect with unilateral disease and sluggish or nonreactive pupils with bilateral symmetric involvement
- Visual deficit in the presence of a normal optic disc and funduscopic examination
- Normal electroretinogram
- Abnormal visual evoked response
- Development of optic atrophy within 4 to 8 weeks of the onset of visual loss

The main causes of posterior ischemic optic neuropathy are hypotension, anemia, and facial edema. Posterior ischemic optic neuropathy has been described after bilateral neck dissection due to ligation of bilateral internal jugular veins, which led to facial edema, venous congestion, and increased intraorbital venous pressure.[242,251,252]

Cortical Blindness Cortical blindness results from damage to the occipital cortex or optic radiation; the main causes of cortical blindness are ischemic or traumatic. Clinically, loss of visual sensation is accompanied by retention of pupillary reaction to light and a normal funduscopic examination.[253] Cortical blindness is usually best diagnosed by CT or MRI, which helps identify infarcted areas in the occipital lobe. Cortical blindness has been described after cardiopulmonary bypass due to generalized hypoperfusion or emboli. It also has been described after craniotomy and laryngectomy surgery due to hypoperfusion caused by hemorrhagic hypotension.[253,254] Cortical blindness has been recorded during spine surgery due to hypotension, anemia, and abnormal head position jeopardizing vertebrobasilar circulation.[255,256]

Central Retinal Artery Occlusion Central retinal artery occlusion is often caused by an embolic ulcerated plaque from the ipsilateral carotid artery.[254] The main cause of central retinal artery occlusion after spine surgery is external ocular pressure from a headrest combined with arterial hypotension, resulting in obstruction to flow in the retinal artery.[257] Central retinal artery occlusion typically presents as a complete loss of vision in one eye that usually improves with time. Funduscopic examination reveals pallor and edema of the retina, with a cherry-red spot at the fovea.

Central Retinal Vein Occlusion Central retinal vein occlusion has been reported in the postoperative period after spine surgery due to external pressure on the globe from a headrest in the prone position.[258] Funduscopic findings usually include retinal hemorrhages in all quadrants, cotton-wool spots, and dilated tortuous retinal veins.[259]

Factors Contributing to Vision Loss and Impairment After Spine Surgery Case reports and studies of postoperative vision loss after spine surgery suggest that hypotension and anemia are major culprits in developing ischemic vision loss. This can be explained by the nature of posterior ciliary arteries as end arteries with no collaterals to compensate for low perfusion pressure.[240,241,260]

This is consistent with findings by Lee et al who used a porcine optic nerve model to show that the optic nerve has a limited compensatory mechanism to maintain the blood flow and oxygen delivery in the presence of anemia and hypotension. Also, in the presence of severe anemia and hypotension, there is a steal from the ophthalmic artery to the brain to maintain perfusion of the brain in preference to the eye.[261]

Increased resistance to blood flow can also decrease ocular perfusion pressure. As mentioned above, increased intraocular pressure during spine surgery in the prone position can lead to decreased ocular perfusion pressure.[238,262] Another finding is that blindness has been observed following bilateral ligation of the internal jugular veins. Blindness in these patients was attributed to increased intraocular pressure due to impaired drainage of the orbital venous plexus into the ophthalmic veins.[252,263] During extensive spine surgery, the excessive use of crystalloids to maintain the intravascular compartment and to replace blood loss has been suggested as contributory to vision loss after surgery.[241]

Roughly two-thirds of administered crystalloid volume distributes to the extravascular compartment shortly after administration; the eye socket is part of this compartment. Accumulation of fluid in the eye socket can thus lead to increased intraocular pressure, along with facial edema, and therefore the development of eye compartment syndrome, which compromises the retinal blood supply.[264] It has been shown that a decrease in plasma oncotic pressure results from using crystalloid as the primary solution for cardiopulmonary bypass rather than colloid.[265] The American Society of Anesthesiologists' practice advisory for perioperative vision loss associated with spine surgery recommends increased use of colloids to maintain intravascular volume in patients who have substantial blood loss.[266]

The Effect of the Type of Fluid on Facial Edema, Chemosis, and IOP Fluid management during spine surgery in the prone position plays a crucial role in determining the degree of facial edema, accumulation of fluid in the eye socket, chemosis, and IOP. It has been shown that large amounts of intravenous fluids and prolonged duration of the prone position can result in fluid collection in the face, especially the globe, because of venous stasis in the dependent soft tissues.[251] Furthermore, a recent report of vision loss after spine surgery attributed the defect to excessive use of crystalloids, and massive facial edema with severe chemosis, which could increase IOP to a degree that would jeopardize the eye perfusion in spite of the patient's BP and Hct levels being kept within normal levels.[267] Jeon et al have demonstrated that patient position, intraoperative fluid balance, and duration of surgery all influence the severity of postoperative chemosis.[268]

The type of fluid used in spine surgery in the prone position is likely to determine the extent to which facial edema and chemosis develop. After crystalloid infusion, only a third remains in the intravascular compartment, while two-thirds distributes to the extravascular compartment and to soft tissues. This leads to tissue edema and aggravates facial swelling, accumulation of fluid in the globe, and chemosis, and increases IOP. The potential for edema is aggravated by the fact that blood loss is usually replaced 3 to 1 with crystalloid. In contrast, a major advantage of using colloids is that they stay mainly in the intravascular compartment, thus potentially decreasing facial edema, chemosis, and accumulation of fluid in the eye socket that would lead to increased IOP. Consistent with this theory, the use of crystalloids for priming bypass machines increases IOP by decreasing the colloid oncotic pressure (COP), whereas priming with colloid solutions does not increase COP.[265]

Head Position and Compartment Syndrome Ocular chemosis (ie, conjunctival edema) can be a cause of short-term decreased visual acuity, patient discomfort, and increased risk for bacterial keratitis.[269] The risk factors for chemosis after prone spine surgery are (1) head-down position (OR = 8.8 [CI = 2.3-33.5]; $p = 0.001$ vs neutral position), (2) positive fluid balance greater than 700 mL (OR = 6.3 [CI = 1.6-24.1]; $p = 0.007$ for <700 mL vs 700-1399 mL) and OR = 32.8 ([CI = 2.7-403]; $p = 0.006$ for <700 mL vs >1400 mL), (3) surgical duration ± 180 minutes.[268]

In a recent case report, a patient underwent a 4-hour L3-L3 decompression with fusion in the prone position. His head was positioned on a C-shaped headrest soft bed with the left side of the face up. Postoperatively, the patient developed ischemic orbital compartment syndrome, manifested in his right eye with proptosis, ptosis, loss of light perception, visual acuity, and complete ophthalmoplegia. The right eye IOP was 33 mm Hg, which reached 40 mm Hg after 24 hours postoperatively, despite emergency use of mannitol and acetazolamide. The apparent reason for the development of the compartment syndrome in this case was that the patient's face was turned to one side, which occluded the right internal jugular vein and resulted in impaired venous drainage and increased IOP in the right eye.[270]

This case highlights the importance of keeping the head in the neutral position with elevation of the head to avoid the development of an ocular compartment syndrome. In a French survey of ophthalmic complications following spinal surgery, the authors proposed 2 preventive measures to avoid vision loss after spine surgery in the prone position. The first was to avoid eye compression when using a horseshoe-shaped headrest and the second was to avoid lateral rotation of the head in patients with suspected carotid atheroma.[271]

iMRI

In part because of challenges posed by surgical navigation systems, iMRI (intraoperative MRI) systems have developed.[272] iMRI allows imaging of changes during surgery, accurate navigation, immediate assessment of complications such as hemorrhage, and verification of the planned resection. iMRI systems can be classified according to the magnet's field strength; magnets can be described as low-field (0.12-0.5 T), midfield (0.5 T), and high-field (1.5-3.0 T) systems. The field strength of a magnet is quantified in the middle of the magnet when imaging is undertaken. However, this field extends beyond the margins of the magnet, decreasing in strength with distance from the magnetic bore. This is called the fringe field. The magnetic field strength drops more than the square of the distance to approximately the third or fourth power.

THERAPEUTIC/DIAGNOSTIC USES

Intracranial Lesions IMRI is mainly used for 2 types of lesions: *transsphenoidal (TPH) pituitary lesions* and *gliomas*.[273] Classic TPH surgery has several limitations. First, visually judging the extent of suprasellar and parasellar resection is difficult, if impossible. Second, in cases where there is cavernous sinus involvement where tiny tumor remnants are below the detection level of current imaging technology. The use of iMRI in patients with large intrasellar or suprasellar macroadenomas increased the rate of complete tumor removal.[274]

Gliomas present a different challenge due to the difficulty to assess their margin visually. Low-grade gliomas can look identical to normal brain parenchyma, whereas high-grade gliomas infiltrate beyond the visual margins. Gross total tumor resection (GTR) is associated with improved survival times and better quality of life.[275] iMRI is very useful for low- and high-grade glioma resection.

Cerebral Aneurysm Surgery iMRI allows the complete clipping of the aneurysm, and the use of diffusion-weighted imaging also helps to evaluate intraoperative blood supply, thus preventing reduced perfusion and ischemia.[276]

Functional Neuronavigation and Functional Imaging Functional neuronavigation (integrating functional data into the navigation data sets) is an important add-on to iMRI because it prevents resections that are too extensive, which would otherwise result in new neurologic deficits. iMRI was described in implanting a deep brain stimulator (DBS) in the subthalamic nucleus. This technique offers several advantages over the traditional technique. iMRI allows verification of lead placement intraoperatively rather than postoperatively and the ability to confirm a lack of an intracranial hemorrhage. This method also allows the patient to be anesthetized and obviates the need for a painful stereotactic frame placement.[277]

Monitoring Complications At the end of the procedure, iMRI can be used to exclude immediate operative complications such as cerebral edema, brain hemorrhage, acute hydrocephalus, and ischemia.

FEATURES OF AN iMRI SYSTEM

Newer iMRI systems allow surgery in the vicinity of the MR imaging machine but outside of the crucial 5-Gauss line (outside the 5-Gauss line, one is relatively safe from drawing ferromagnetic equipment into the magnet). When scanning is required, a rotating operating table mechanism brings the patient into the magnetic core for scanning. Other features to be taken into consideration include flexibility in patient positioning yet ensuring good positioning of the head. The surgeons' mobility and the ability to use surgical microscopes are important considerations.[278] A MRI-compatible operating table with MRI-compatible 4-point head holder made of fiberglass-reinforced plastic for head fixation during craniotomy and burr hole procedures, and radiofrequency coil are vital parts of the iMRI system. The patient's head is fixed in an MRI-compatible head clamp with a head coil. During surgery, the head of the patient is positioned outside the 5-Gauss line, thus allowing for the use of standard surgical instruments. During MRI scanning, the table is rotated 160 degrees and the patient's head is positioned in the center of the scanner. At the end of scanning, the operating table swings back in place, with the patient's head outside the 5-Gauss line. The monitoring cables and ventilation circuits have to be of sufficient length to allow for this rotational movement, and care must be taken during this movement to avoid disconnections.[279]

iMRI Anesthetic Induction Room The presence of an induction room with its own set of anesthetic equipment and monitors in the iMRI suite for the induction of anesthesia prior to MRI scanning has many advantages. It eliminates the stress of conducting an anesthetic and inserting invasive lines in the vicinity of the MRI scanner. It is a safe room because when patient complications occur, the patient can be moved to the induction room for resuscitation, as it is fully equipped. In addition, equipment such as defibrillators are not safe in the vicinity of the MRI scanner. Finally, reversal after anesthesia and transfer to the recovery unit with its oxygen source is safer and easier in this anesthetic induction room.

Screening of Patients and Staff Screening of people entering the iMRI helps to prevent injuries from projectile effects of ferromagnetic items brought into the iMRI accidently, because there have been reports of injury and lethal outcomes.[280,281] Certain groups of people must be excluded from working or being treated in the presence of strong magnetic fields. Implanted ferromagnetic devices or objects including pacemakers, intracranial aneurysm clips, tissue expanders with metallic ports, implantable defibrillators, cochlear implants are generally contraindicated.[282]

Anesthetic Equipment in the iMRI There are considerations regarding the use of anesthetic equipment in the iMRI. First, the hazardous effects of the strong magnetic field on the equipment can cause malfunction. Second, there is risk of thermal injury to the patient. All monitoring modes using long cables can potentially cause currents to be induced by the magnetic fields of the iMRI scanner. Recent monitors use wireless ECG and pulse oximetry to avoid the hazard of potential thermal burns and avoid lengthy electrode cables getting in the way during the rotation of the MR table into the MR core during scanning. All monitors should provide visual alarms because auditory alarms are not useful during scanning. The anesthesia machine should be MR compatible. TEC 5 and 7 vaporizers are MR compatible while a TEC 6 is not. E gas cylinders, nonferrimagnetic regulator yokes, and self-inflating bags with an oxygen source should be available. Long breathing circuits, extension tubings for invasive line transducer systems, and infusion lines should be available as well.

Other Considerations During scanning, noise levels may average 95 dB in 1.5 T. Protective earplugs are required for staff and patients. This noise also limits auditory sense as a monitoring tool and interferes with communication. As warming devices may not be suitable in the iMRI, good padding and blankets are essential for keeping the patient warm. As mentioned earlier, thermal injury is a hazard during iMRI and preventive measures should include padding to prevent direct skin contact, placing sensors and cables away from the magnetic coil, and keeping cables off the patient and running them on blankets.

IN CONCLUSION

iMRI is considered the third most significant technological advance in brain surgery after the bipolar coagulation for hemostasis and the operating microscope for vision improvment. Anesthesiologists are commonly involved in the setting up of this clinical service. Because an iMRI service has many considerations that involve anesthesia, the anesthesiologist is an integral member of the team during the planning and setting up of this specialized service.

POSTOPERATIVE CARE OF NEUROSURGICAL PATIENTS

After each neurological procedure, besides general postoperative considerations that are common in all patients undergoing anesthesia, there are specific postoperative challenges for the neuroanesthesiologist. Because the most important indicator of operative success as well as a marker of absence of a surgical complication is through an examination of the nervous system, the goal of a neuroanesthesiologist is to be able to emerge the patient in a timely manner so a neurologic examination is possible. The anesthetic plan usually includes using short-acting anesthetics and anesthetic adjuncts including volatile anesthetics, which are cleared by ventilation and intravenous agents with short context-sensitive half-lives (eg, remifentanil).

The goal in the neurosurgical postoperative period is to maintain adequate oxygenation, ventilation, and provide optimal hemodynamic parameters for tissue perfusion according to preoperative diagnosis, operative procedure, and comorbidities, while controlling the pain and preserving the mental status for adequate neurologic examination.

EMERGENCE

A plan for a successful emergence is a requirement in preparation for the postoperative care of neurosurgical patients. The best indicator of the surgical outcome is a neurological examination. In cranial surgeries this includes a gross mental status, motor, and sensory evaluation, as well as speech testing, which collectively are commonly known as a "neuro check." In spinal surgeries the surgeon evaluates the sensory as well as motor strength in extremities innervated by the segments operated on. As discussed previously, emergence especially from craniotomies should be in a controlled manner to avoid sudden hemodynamic changes and cough reflex due to the endotracheal tube (ETT), the commonly called "smooth wake-up." Both of these situations can increase the ICP as well as cause intracranial hemorrhage in a newly operated brain. In patients who will be intubated postoperatively there is still a desire to perform a postoperative neurologic examination; the patient is emerged to follow commands and then resedated to tolerate the ETT and control the hemodynamics.

DESTINATION AND TRANSPORT

The final postoperative destination depends on a mutual decision by the surgeon and the anesthesiologist, and should take into consideration the nature of the disease, surgical procedure, length of surgery, fluid shifts, comorbidities, and postoperative outcome.

A very important part of postoperative patient transport is early communication between the anesthesia provider and the ICU team. A complete report of patient diagnosis, surgical procedure, and important occurrences during the operative period, as well as the postoperative plan should be given by the anesthesiologist to the ICU physician.

KEY REFERENCES

- Avitsian R, Schubert A. Anesthetic considerations for intraoperative management of cerebrovascular disease in neurovascular surgical procedures. *Anesthesiol Clin.* 2007;25(3):441-463.
- Bilotta F, Rosa G. 'Anesthesia' for awake neurosurgery. *Curr Opin Anaesthesiol.* 2009;22(5):560-565.
- Engelhard K, Werner C. Inhalational or intravenous anesthetics for craniotomies? Pro inhalational. *Curr Opin Anaesthesiol.* 2006;19(5):504-508.
- Johnson JO. Anesthesia for minimally invasive neurosurgery. *Anesthesiol Clin North America.* 2002;20(2):361-375.
- Lakhani S, Guha A, Nahser HC. Anaesthesia for endovascular management of cerebral aneurysms. *Eur J Anaesthesiol.* 2006;23(11):902-913.
- Mantz J, Degos V, Laigle C. Recent advances in pharmacologic neuroprotection. *Eur J Anaesthesiol.* 2010;27(1):6-10.
- Nemergut EC, Dumont AS, Barry UT, Laws ER. Perioperative management of patients undergoing transsphenoidal pituitary surgery. *Anesth Analg.* 2005;101(4):1170-1181.
- Randell T, Niskanen M. Management of physiological variables in neuroanaesthesia: maintaining homeostasis during intracranial surgery. *Curr Opin Anaesthesiol.* 2006;19(5):492-497.
- Rasmussen M, Bundgaard H, Cold GE. Craniotomy for supratentorial brain tumors: risk factors for brain swelling after opening the dura mater. *J Neurosurg.* 2004;101(4):621-626.
- Sloan TB. Anesthetics and the brain. *Anesthesiol Clin North America.* 2002;20:265-292.

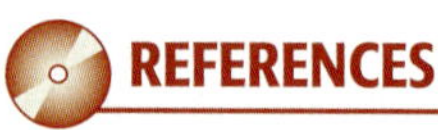

REFERENCES

Complete references available on DVD and online version at www.LongneckerAnesthesiology.com

CHAPTER 52

Cardiac Anesthesia

Mark A. Chaney
Albert T. Cheung
Christopher A. Troianos
Jessica L. Willert
David A. Zvara
Stanton K. Shernan

KEY POINTS

1. Initiation of cardiopulmonary bypass triggers an extremely complex and multifactorial response involving activation of complement, platelets, neutrophils, monocytes, and macrophages, thus initiating the coagulation, fibrinolytic, and kallikrein cascades. The systemic inflammatory response to cardiopulmonary bypass is further amplified by subsequent stimulated release of various endotoxins and cytokines, including interleukins and tumor necrosis factor, which further promote endothelial cell permeability.
2. Preparation for separation from cardiopulmonary bypass must be based on a clear understanding of the patient's preoperative condition and events of the operative course. Weaning from cardiopulmonary bypass is initiated after review and adjustment of numerous physiologic and technical variables, including temperature, laboratory data, heart rate and rhythm, myocardial contractility, and mechanical ventilation.
3. The anesthetic management of patients undergoing coronary artery bypass graft surgery requires an understanding of myocardial oxygen supply and demand, patient monitoring, and the anesthetic techniques that provide myocardial protection and favor oxygen supply over demand.
4. Patients with coronary artery disease presenting for coronary artery bypass graft surgery require special considerations in their anesthetic management. First and foremost are techniques that minimize myocardial oxygen demand while maximizing myocardial oxygen delivery. These considerations include preoperative preparation, intraoperative monitoring, and the use of anesthetic agents with hemodynamic effects that favor oxygen supply over demand and allow for myocardial protection. Postoperative management that provides particular attention to pain management, temperature control, and hemodynamic monitoring to avoid tachycardia, hypotension, and hypertension also must be considered.
5. Modern practices that focus on early extubation and "fast-tracking" cardiac surgical patients through the postoperative period use smaller narcotic doses, with supplementation by short-acting hypnotic agents.
6. Patients at risk for increased mortality after coronary artery bypass graft surgery are identified by preoperative factors. The most significant risk factors that increase mortality are older than 80 years of age, emergent surgery, prior cardiac surgery, and renal failure.
7. The unifying concept in all valve surgery includes the principles of preserving myocardial function and the influence of preload, afterload, inotropy, rate, rhythm, and diastolic function on myocardial performance and mechanics.
8. Intraoperative transesophageal echocardiography is an essential diagnostic tool and monitor of cardiac performance for patients undergoing heart valve procedures.
9. Cardiac anesthesia for heart valve surgery is associated with a number of special considerations not found in other aspects of cardiothoracic anesthesiology. Among these considerations is familiarity with the type of repair technique or prosthetic valve used.
10. The process of repairing or replacing a portion of the thoracic aorta typically requires the temporary or permanent interruption of blood flow through the aorta or its major branch vessels, creating the potential for ischemia or infarction of almost any major organ system. Techniques to protect organs

during temporary interruption of blood flow in the thoracic aorta include deep hypothermic circulatory arrest, selective antegrade cerebral perfusion, retrograde cerebral perfusion, and partial left heart bypass for distal aortic perfusion. Intraoperative neurophysiologic monitoring and lumbar cerebrospinal fluid drainage are recognized techniques commonly used for repairs involving the descending thoracic or thoracoabdominal aorta to decrease the risk of spinal cord ischemia and infarction.

11. Preoperatively, the anesthesiologist must identify any neurologic deficits and ascertain the extent of major organ dysfunction, including renal or hepatic insufficiency, which are common in patients undergoing placement of a ventricular assist device. Any further deterioration in the perioperative period may prevent a full recovery and eliminate the possibility of a patient qualifying for subsequent heart transplantation at a later date.
12. Right heart failure is one of the most important causes of perioperative death in patients undergoing placement of a left ventricular assist device. Right ventricular dysfunction and failure may develop in up to 20% to 30% of patients implanted with an isolated left ventricular assist device. β-Adrenergic agonists, phosphodiesterase inhibitors, as well as nitric oxide should be initiated to improve right ventricular contractility and decrease right ventricular afterload in an attempt to improve transpulmonary blood flow. A supplemental temporary right ventricular assist device may be necessary if right ventricular dysfunction persists.

CARDIOPULMONARY BYPASS: PATHOPHYSIOLOGY AND PATIENT MANAGEMENT CONSIDERATIONS

Despite the introduction and perseverance of off-pump coronary artery bypass graft surgery (OPCABG), cardiopulmonary bypass (CPB) remains an essential technique for most cardiac surgical patients.[1] Although the past 50 years have brought improvements in extracorporeal technology, including improved gas exchange devices, venous reservoir construction, and heparin-coated circuits, the modern extracorporeal circuit is still remarkably similar to that developed a half-century ago.[2] Despite such advances, fundamental questions remain regarding the management of CPB (pump flow, arterial blood pressure, temperature, acid-base strategy, hematocrit, or glucose level). A comprehensive understanding of the CPB circuit, pathophysiology, and important patient management issues is essential for anesthesiologists responsible for the perioperative care of these patients.

FUNDAMENTAL COMPONENTS OF A CPB CIRCUIT

Traditionally, the CPB circuit removes blood from the body via the venous circulation and returns blood to the body via the arterial circulation.[3] Thus CPB must function "physiologically" as the patient's heart and lungs. Most commonly, blood is drained by gravity via cannulae in the superior and/or inferior vena cavae and then is similarly returned by a cannula in the ascending aorta. Although the CPB circuit consists of many important components, the 2 most important components are the pump, which functions as the patient's heart, and the oxygenator, which functions as the patient's lungs.

The 2 most common types of pumps used are roller pumps and centrifugal pumps. Roller pumps induce blood flow by compressing the tubing via rollers, thereby pushing the blood ahead through the tubing. Flow rate depends on the size of the tubing, length of the roller track, and rotation rate of the rollers (ie, revolutions per minute). Alternatively, centrifugal pumps induce blood flow by either a vaned impeller or a group of cones that reside inside a plastic housing. The impellers or cones are magnetically coupled with an electric motor and, when rotated rapidly, generate a pressure differential that may cause movement of blood through the tubing. Thus, unlike roller pumps, centrifugal pumps are afterload dependent, such that increases in resistance decreases forward flow delivered to the patient.

The 2 most common types of oxygenators used are membrane oxygenators and bubble oxygenators. Membrane oxygenators attempt to achieve separation between blood and gas in a manner analogous to the natural lung. Bubble oxygenators physically mix blood and gas, allowing sufficient time for adequate gas exchange to occur prior to defoaming and delivery to the patient. A heat exchanger usually is an integral part of the oxygenator. The type of oxygenator used influences the configuration of the CPB circuit. Membrane oxygenators typically are positioned after the pump because the resistance in most membrane oxygenators requires blood to be pumped through them. Thus a venous reservoir collects venous return from the patient before delivery to the pump, followed by the membrane oxygenator, then back to the patient. Alternatively, bubble oxygenators typically are positioned before the pump because they do not require blood to be pumped through them, and they contain a reservoir of oxygenated blood that supplies the pump before it directly delivers blood back to the patient.

Over the past 4 decades, CPB technology has undergone a dramatic metamorphosis and can no longer be simply viewed as "the pump."[4,5] Additional vital components of the CPB circuitry include the arterial line filter, bubble detector, cardioplegia lines, suction lines, temperature monitor, arterial line pressure monitor, anesthetic vaporizer, and oxygen monitor, among others. Needless to say, the perfusionist plays an important role in intraoperative patient management during cardiac surgery.

PATHOPHYSIOLOGY OF CPB

Substantial controversy surrounds questions regarding "optimal" flow and pressure during CPB.[6] Each patient must be individualized, with specific goals determined by numerous factors, including age, comorbidity, temperature, and body mass. However, most clinicians aim for flows in the range of 2.4 to 2.8 L/min/m^2 and pressures in the range of 50 to 80 mm Hg. It has been known for many years that CPB induces a systemic inflammatory response syndrome (SIRS) in patients following cardiac surgery that can lead to major organ injury and postoperative morbidity.[7,8] Initiation of CPB triggers an extremely complex and multifactorial response involving activation of complement, platelets, neutrophils, monocytes, and macrophages, thus initiating the coagulation, fibrinolytic, and kallikrein cascades. The SIRS response to CPB is further amplified by subsequent stimulated release of various endotoxins and cytokines, including interleukins (ILs) and tumor necrosis factor (TNF), which further promote endothelial cell permeability. Transvascular migration of activated leukocytes into tissues associated with SIRS results in the release of various proteases and neutrophil elastases, which cause additional vascular and parenchymal damage that can exacerbate ischemia-reperfusion injury associated with CPB and cardiac surgery.[9] These physiologic changes associated with exposure to CPB are thought to initiate the detrimental changes seen in major organ systems (brain, heart, lung, kidneys) during the postoperative period.

The basic physiologic insults caused by CPB have been associated with major postoperative morbidity, including neurologic dysfunction, pulmonary dysfunction, renal dysfunction, and/or hematologic abnormalities. Additional clinical manifestations associated with SIRS include increased metabolism and fever, fluid retention, myocardial edema, and detrimental hemodynamic alterations. Recent controversies surrounding clinical management of patients exposed to CPB have focused on the potential detrimental physiologic effects of hemodilution,[10,11] hyperglycemia,[12,13] and use/non-use of colloids[14,15] on postoperative morbidity. Over the years, a wide variety of anti-inflammatory treatment options have been used in patients subjected to CPB in hopes of attenuating SIRS, including leukocyte depletion techniques, neutrophil adhesion molecule blockade, heparin coating of CPB circuitry, and use of monoclonal antibodies directed specifically against various inflammatory mediators. Although results from animal work appear promising, the demonstration of a definite clinical benefit in humans has not been consistent.[16-19]

MANAGEMENT OF ANTICOAGULATION

Heparin Dosing Anticoagulation is used during cardiac surgery to prevent thrombosis of the CPB circuit and to minimize excessive CPB-related activation of the hemostatic system. Heparin is used routinely because it is effective, immediately reversible, generally well tolerated, and inexpensive.[20,21] Heparin induces anticoagulation primarily by potentiating the activity of antithrombin III. Most heparin preparations are "unfractionated," meaning that the heparin compound isolated from animal tissues, including porcine intestine and bovine lung, contains heparin molecules of various lengths. Because the relationship between mass (milligrams) and potency (units) varies among heparin preparations, most clinicians record heparin doses in units rather than milligrams. The anticoagulant effect of an intravenous dose of heparin occurs within minutes, and the intravenous heparin bolus dose administered prior to initiation of CPB may decrease arterial pressure and/or systemic vascular resistance.

Much controversy surrounds appropriate heparin dosing and monitoring of anticoagulation in patients exposed to CPB.[22,23] Somewhat surprisingly, the literature does not consistently support the importance of anticoagulation monitoring techniques during CPB.[24] However, bleeding and transfusion outcomes likely can be improved by refining heparin monitoring techniques, either by sustaining better anticoagulation during CPB or by optimizing reversal of anticoagulation with protamine. Most clinicians administer an initial dose of 200 to 400 U/kg heparin and maintenance doses are determined by the particular laboratory test used for assessment of anticoagulation. The activated clotting time (ACT) is perhaps the most widely used method, and most clinicians administer additional heparin periodically in order to maintain the ACT greater than 400 to 480 seconds. However, numerous other clinical conditions can affect the ACT, including hypothermia, hemodilution, and thrombocytopenia. Heparin concentration measurement techniques also are commonly used. Whatever laboratory test is used, most clinicians assess anticoagulation every 30 minutes during CPB.

Protamine Protamine neutralizes heparin-induced anticoagulation. Salmon milt provides the pharmaceutical source of protamine, which neutralizes the antithrombin III effect of heparin by forming large complexes with heparin's sulfate groups. Protamine may exhibit antihemostatic properties by affecting platelets and by releasing tissue plasminogen activator from endothelial cells.

Much controversy surrounds the recommended dose of protamine to adequately neutralize heparin. Questions regarding the optimal ratio of milligrams of protamine to units of heparin, and how much heparin remains in the patient, are central to this controversy. Most clinicians use protocols that call for administration of protamine in slight excess doses of the usual ratio of 1 mg of protamine to 1 mg of heparin in order to ensure return of normal coagulation. Subsequent postoperative administration of protamine may be required to prevent "heparin rebound."[25]

A spectrum of adverse reactions may be associated with protamine use; the most important is hypotension and/or anaphylactoid/anaphylactic reaction.[26] Hypotension following administration of protamine is fairly common and may be related to rate of injection, subsequent decreased systemic vascular resistance, and perhaps myocardial depression. True anaphylactoid/anaphylactic reactions to protamine are rare. Patients receiving protamine-containing insulins and/or previously exposed to protamine may be at slightly increased risk of developing anaphylactic reactions. Pulmonary vasoconstriction causing pulmonary hypertension may be associated with protamine use. Heparin–protamine complexes and complement activation may be the primary mediators of these adverse reactions. Slow administration of protamine may limit adverse reactions. If sudden hypotension and/or pulmonary hypertension occur, protamine administration should immediately cease. Heparin may be considered in order to reduce heparin–protamine complex load. Hemodynamic support with vasopressors and inotropes may be required in addition to reinitiation of CPB. Milder cases may resolve without intervention.

Heparin-Induced Thrombocytopenia Unfractionated heparin given during CPB is remarkably immunogenic. In fact, 25% to 50% of cardiac surgical patients may develop heparin-dependent antibodies postoperatively over the first 5 to 10 days after exposure. This immunogenic response can strongly activate platelets and coagulation, causing the prothrombotic disorder known as heparin-induced thrombocytopenia (HIT).

HIT is defined as thrombocytopenia with a potential for associated thrombosis (HITT). A definitive diagnosis usually requires 1 or more positive tests for HIT antibodies.[27] An otherwise unexplained perioperative platelet count fall of 50% or more from baseline or any thrombosis that occurs 5 to 14 days after cardiac surgery is suggestive of HIT, even when heparin is not still being given (ie, delayed-onset HIT). Regarding laboratory testing, commercially available enzyme immunoassays and washed platelet activation assays (ie, platelet serotonin release or heparin-induced platelet activation) are highly sensitive for detecting HIT antibodies such that a negative test result essentially rules out HIT. Antibody seroconversion of no clinical consequence is common following cardiac surgery. Thus the presence of HIT antibodies in the absence of thrombocytopenia or thrombosis does not indicate HIT. However, patients with acute HIT usually have strong positive HIT antibody results. In general, the greater the magnitude of a positive HIT antibody test result, the greater the likelihood the patient has HIT. Following cardiac surgery, the frequency of HIT in patients is approximately 2%. Although HIT antibodies are transient, at least half of patients with HIT develop thrombotic complications. Porcine intestine heparin has been associated with a lower risk of HIT than bovine lung heparin.

If high suspicion of HIT exists, all heparin should be discontinued. In general, patients with HIT or HITT who require urgent anticoagulation should be treated with 1 of the following alternative anticoagulants: lepirudin, argatroban, danaparoid, or bivalirudin.[27] Warfarin and other oral anticoagulants are generally contraindicated during acute HIT and should be delayed pending substantial recovery of the platelet count. The alternative anticoagulant should be stopped only when platelet count recovery is complete and therapeutic oral anticoagulation is achieved. For patients strongly suspected of having HIT but without clinical evidence of thrombosis, an alternative anticoagulant in therapeutic doses is recommended because of the high risk of developing thrombosis.

Standard anticoagulation with heparin is recommended for cardiac surgical patients with previous HIT in whom HIT antibodies are no longer detectable (or only weakly detectable) by enzyme immunoassay. In patients with acute or subacute HIT who require cardiac surgery, and in whom the platelet count has recovered yet HIT antibodies remain detectable, 2 general approaches are available. One approach is administration of an alternative anticoagulant (ie, lepirudin, argatroban, danaparoid, bivalirudin) and avoidance of heparin exposure. The other is administration of standard heparin anticoagulation along with a platelet antagonist, including epoprostenol or tirofiban. Given the absence of prospective comparative studies, no single option can be generally recommended in these patients.

Antifibrinolytics Antifibrinolytic agents, including the lysine analogues ε-aminocaproic acid and tranexamic acid, and the serine protease inhibitor aprotinin have become mainstay prophylactic therapies for reducing bleeding and blood product transfusions for cardiac surgical patients.[28,29] Although many studies have demonstrated beneficial effects of these agents in reducing perioperative bleeding and morbidity,[30] others have reported adverse side effects associated with multiorgan dysfunction and prothrombotic outcomes,[31] especially among patients with a genetic predisposition to a hypercoagulable state.[32] Aprotinin, in fact, was taken off the market because of these detrimental effects.[33] Thus, similar to all pharmacologic agents, the decision to administer

TABLE 52-1 Common Cardiac Drugs Used During Weaning From Cardiopulmonary Bypass

Inotropic Agents
Dopamine
Dobutamine
Epinephrine
Isoproterenol
Milrinone
Norepinephrine
Vasopressor Agents
Norepinephrine
Phenylephrine
Vasopressin
Vasodilator Agents
Nitroglycerin
Nicardipine
Nitroprusside

any antifibrinolytic should include a thorough risk-to-benefit consideration that is individualized to each patient.[34]

MANAGEMENT OF PATIENTS DURING WEANING AND SEPARATION FROM CPB

Weaning from CPB should represent a smooth transition from the mechanical pump back to the patient's heart and lungs as the source of blood flow and gas exchange. The process should always be conducted in a coordinated fashion with all members of the team, including the surgeon, anesthesiologist, and perfusionist. Preparation for separation from CPB must be based on a clear understanding of the patient's preoperative condition and events of the operative course. Weaning is initiated after review and adjustment of numerous physiologic and technical variables, including temperature, laboratory data, heart rate and rhythm, myocardial contractility, and mechanical ventilation, among others. The patient should be normothermic and demonstrate normal laboratory values for hemoglobin, potassium, calcium, and acid–base balance. Myocardial function, including heart rate, cardiac rhythm, myocardial contractility, and preload, should be optimized, which may require administration of intravenous medications, depending on the desired goal (**Table 52-1**). Many patients usually require medications that increase myocardial contractility during separation from CPB. In extreme cases, mechanical devices may be required (eg, intra-aortic balloon pump [IABP], ventricular assist device [VAD]). It now is clear that information obtained from transesophageal echocardiography (TEE) is far superior in quality and quantity to that obtained from a pulmonary artery catheter (PAC) and may be very helpful in guiding therapy toward optimizing hemodynamics and guiding de-airing procedures during weaning from CPB. Furthermore, TEE has proved invaluable in assessing the quality of the surgical procedure following separation from CPB, especially among patients with significant ventricular dysfunction and those undergoing valve procedures, congenital heart surgery, and aortic surgery.[35-39]

ANESTHETIC MANAGEMENT DURING CORONARY ARTERY BYPASS GRAFTING

The anesthetic management of patients undergoing coronary artery bypass graft surgery (CABG) requires an understanding of myocardial oxygen supply and demand, patient monitoring, and the anesthetic techniques that provide myocardial protection and favor oxygen delivery over consumption. Myocardial ischemia results when there is an imbalance between the oxygen supply of the coronary circulation and the metabolic demand of myocardial tissue. Ischemia initially leads to contractile dysfunction. However, if ischemia is severe or prolonged, it can lead to cell death, tissue necrosis, and permanent loss of contractile function of the affected myocardial region. This section reviews the basic pathophysiology of myocardial ischemia, the anesthetic management of patients at risk for developing myocardial ischemia, and anesthetic considerations during CABG surgery.

CORONARY ARTERY ANATOMY

Coronary artery anatomy is particularly relevant to the anesthesiologist caring for patients with coronary artery disease. The severity of the coronary obstruction correlates with the margin of reserve for tolerating tachycardia and hypotension. Patients with coronary lesions obstructing 99% of the lumen (subtotal occlusion) may not tolerate even mild degrees of tachycardia and hypotension, whereas patients with lesions in the 70% to 75% range may tolerate some degree of hemodynamic compromise before developing ischemia. Knowledge of specific coronary lesions also allows for focused monitoring of targeted myocardial regions at increased risk for myocardial ischemia.

The 2 major coronary arteries are the first arterial branches of the aorta, which arise from 2 of the 3 sinuses of Valsalva in the aortic root (**Fig. 52-1**). The right coronary sinus is anteriorly located, and the left coronary sinus is located laterally and slightly posterior. The left coronary artery (LCA) divides into the left anterior descending coronary artery (LAD) and left circumflex artery (LCx). The LAD gives rise to the diagonal branches and supplies the anterior wall of the right ventricle (RV), the anterior two-thirds of the interventricular septum, the anterior wall of the left ventricle (LV), and the ventricular apex. The LCx gives rise to the obtuse marginal branches and supplies the left atrium (LA), and the posterior and lateral walls of the LV. Patients are described as having "a left main" if they have a significant lesion in the LCA. These patients are at particular risk for developing myocardial ischemia that affects a large portion of the LV, which would cause rapid hemodynamic compromise and cardiac arrest. Patients described as having a "left main equivalent" have high-grade obstructions in both the LAD and LCx arteries. These patients potentially have the same risk of coronary ischemia and rapid hemodynamic compromise as patients with left main disease.

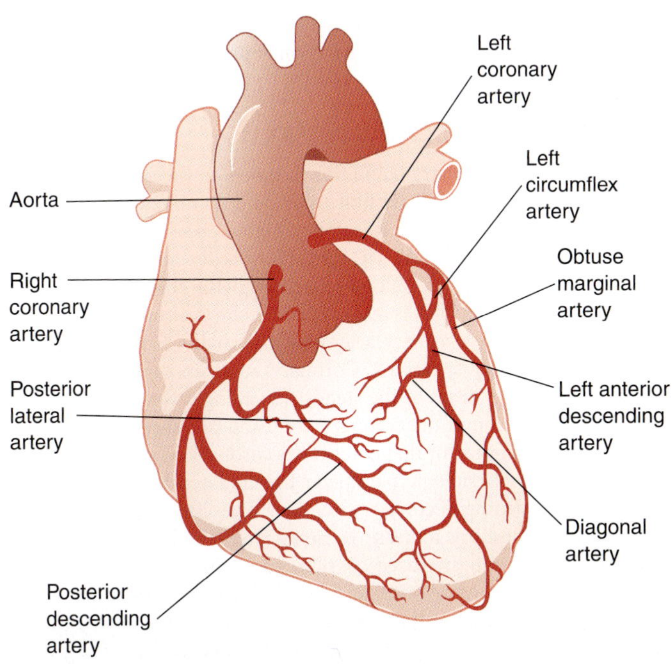

FIGURE 52-1. Coronary anatomy.

The right coronary artery (RCA) supplies blood to the lateral and posterior walls of the RV, the inferior wall of the LV, and the posterior third of the interventricular septum. The RCA terminates as the posterior descending artery (PDA) in 85% to 90% of the population. The blood supply of the PDA determines the pattern of coronary dominance: RCA for right dominant and LCx for left dominant. Most patients have an RCA-dominant or balanced pattern of blood supply to the PDA. A balanced pattern is used to describe coronary anatomy with no particular dominance in terms of the blood supply to the PDA. The presence of a right-dominant or balanced system during OPCABG frequently leads to bradycardia and hypotension during RCA occlusion because it supplies blood to the sinoatrial node in 55% of patients, whereas the PDA supplies the atrioventricular node in right-dominant patients.

Myocardial blood collects in the coronary veins, which drain into the coronary sinus, and subsequently the right atrium (RA). The coronary sinus is often used as a conduit for the delivery of cardioplegia to the myocardium in a retrograde fashion. This is possible because the coronary veins lack valves, allowing blood to flow in either direction. Retrograde cardioplegia is used in patients with aortic insufficiency (AI), during aortic valve (AV) surgery, in the presence of high-grade coronary obstructions, and in patients with previous CABG who have a patent internal mammary artery graft. All of these situations limit the antegrade delivery of cardioplegia to the myocardium from the aortic root. Retrograde delivery of cardioplegia via the coronary sinus also has limitations. A coronary sinus catheter inserted beyond the small cardiac vein will prevent delivery of cardioplegia to the RV. Subsequently, the right heart may be poorly protected from myocardial ischemia during aortic cross-clamping.[40] Coronary sinus catheters that are directed into the small or middle cardiac vein may cause coronary sinus rupture.

The LAD is positioned on the anterior aspect of the heart. The obtuse marginal branches of the LCx and diagonal branches of the LAD are located on the lateral or posterior aspect of the heart (see Fig. 52-1). The surgeon must rotate or lift the heart to gain access to these vessels, causing hemodynamic compromise if the cardiac chambers are compressed. The pulmonary outflow tract also may be compressed with cardiac rotation, again resulting in severe hypotension by dramatically reducing preload. Additionally, the electrocardiographic (ECG) axis changes during cardiac manipulation and may change the ECG–coronary artery anatomic relationship, limiting the ability to use ECG for ischemia monitoring. Use of TEE for ischemia and ventricular function monitoring may be compromised when the heart is lifted or manipulated within the surgical field. The PAC may be malpositioned during these maneuvers, providing erroneous data regarding cardiac output and filling pressures.

CORONARY BLOOD FLOW PHYSIOLOGY

The physiology of coronary blood flow is based on the assumption that coronary arteries are nondistensible tubes, and that blood is a homogeneous fluid. Blood flows from a region of higher pressure (aorta) to one of lower pressure (capillaries). The rate of flow is dependent on the pressure gradient that moves red blood cells through the coronary arteries in a laminar flow pattern. Flow is most dependent on the radius of the blood vessel, which is why coronary arterioles maximally dilate in response to coronary arterial stenosis.[41] Coronary stenosis causes the vessel to maximally dilate distal to the stenosis, creating a vessel with a fixed radius. Manipulation of the coronary perfusion pressure then becomes the most important factor that determines coronary blood flow and the most important physiologic parameter manipulated by the anesthesia provider in the setting of coronary ischemia. Exercise-induced ischemia causes a compensatory increase in heart rate, α_1-adrenergic–induced vasoconstriction, and increased LV filling pressure, all of which reduce coronary blood flow.[42] Adequate coronary perfusion pressure is the most important factor in the prevention and treatment of myocardial ischemia, both in the operating room and during exercise.

A second important factor is blood viscosity, determined rheologically as the concentration or suspension of erythrocytes within the blood. Patients with coronary artery disease (CAD) have disturbed blood flow patterns that create an increased tendency for coronary arterial thrombosis.[43] These abnormal flow patterns underscore the importance of aspirin therapy in the medical management of patients with CAD by reducing platelet adhesion and aggregation at the site of coronary stenoses.

Coronary blood flow has a characteristic phasic perfusion pattern, 70% to 80% of which occurs during the diastolic phase of the cardiac cycle. Cardiac contraction during systole impedes myocardial perfusion by increasing intraventricular cavitary pressure and coronary artery resistance, thus producing a nonlinear relationship between heart rate and diastolic time.[44] β-Blockade is a very effective medical therapy for patients with CAD by preventing even small increases in heart rate during the perioperative period, reducing mortality with heart rate reduction, and improving outcome.[45]

Heart rate reduction improves subendocardial coronary artery blood flow,[46,47] allowing for better matching of myocardial oxygen supply and demand (myocardial perfusion–contraction coupling), thus preserving regional myocardial contractility.[48] Recovery of stunned or hibernating myocardium in patients with ischemic heart disease occurs with restoration of myocardial perfusion–contraction coupling.

MYOCARDIAL OXYGEN DELIVERY

Myocardial oxygen delivery depends on the oxygen content in the blood and is composed of hemoglobin-bound oxygen and dissolved oxygen. Hemoglobin-bound oxygen composes most of the blood's carrying capacity. However, delivery of oxygen to myocardial cells is dependent on release of oxygen from hemoglobin and is represented by the oxygen–hemoglobin dissociation curve. A leftward shift of this curve from normal indicates a greater affinity of oxygen by hemoglobin, which has the effect of drawing more oxygen into the blood as it passes through the lungs but reducing oxygen release at the cellular level. A leftward shift is caused by alkalosis (both metabolic and respiratory), hypothermia, carboxyhemoglobinemia, methemoglobinemia, and decreased red blood cell 2,3-diphosphoglycerate (DPG), which may be observed after transfusion of a large volume of old blood stored in acid-citrate-dextrose. A rightward shift indicates less affinity of the red cells for oxygen, which has the effect of greater oxygen release to the tissues but at the expense of drawing less oxygen into the blood as it passes through the lungs. A rightward shift is caused by acidosis (both metabolic and respiratory), hyperthermia, and increased 2,3-DPG in the red blood cells.

Although anemia clearly reduces the oxygen-carrying capacity of blood, clinical studies have not determined the lowest acceptable level of anemia that does not produce myocardial ischemia. The degree of anemia that produces myocardial ischemia is dependent on factors that are specific for each patient and the loading conditions of the ventricle. Factors include the severity of CAD, myocardial wall thickness and tension, heart rate, and perfusion pressure. Isovolemic reduction in hemoglobin to 4.6 to 5.3 mg/dL in healthy volunteers produced ST-segment changes on Holter monitoring in 2 of 11 subjects, whereas hemoglobin levels of 5.0 mg/dL led to myocardial ischemia infrequently.[49] In another investigation, ECG ST-segment changes suggestive of ischemia occurred in only 3 of 55 subjects during acute reduction in hemoglobin concentrations to 5 g/dL. These authors attributed the imbalance of myocardial oxygen supply and demand to tachycardia.[50] Although excessive hemodilution (median lowest hematocrit below 25%) during CPB is a risk factor for major morbidity even in the absence of blood transfusion, preoperative anemia may not be associated with an increased risk of morbidity, provided that the lowest hematocrit during cardiopulmonary bypass is maintained above 28%.[12]

Patients with ischemic heart disease require a higher hemoglobin concentration to minimize perioperative complications. A higher incidence of postoperative mortality was found in cardiac surgical patients older than 75 years whose preoperative systemic oxygen delivery was less than 320 mL/min/m^2 and who had anemia on the second postoperative day.[51] Bracey et al found no increase in morbidity, mortality, or patient self-assessment of fatigue when the hemoglobin threshold for red cell transfusion was lowered to 8.0 g/dL after CABG.[52] Therefore, the lower limit of hemoglobin concentration depends on multiple factors, such as the patient's age, heart rate, perfusion pressure, clinical evidence of myocardial ischemia, and success of coronary revascularization. Moderate exposure to allogenic blood products is not associated with reduced long-term survival after coronary artery bypass surgery.[53]

MYOCARDIAL OXYGEN DEMAND

Myocardial oxygen demand is primarily determined by heart rate, ventricular wall tension, and myocardial contractility. Acting on the myocardial β receptors, β-blockers decrease heart rate and reduce contractility and thus are the primary treatment for patients with CAD at risk for myocardial ischemia. Although treatment with atenolol in the perioperative period does not significantly alter the neuroendocrine stress response,[54] perioperative β-blockade reduces mortality and myocardial infarction (MI) among patients undergoing noncardiac surgery.[55-57] Patients treated with metoprolol for whom ventricular filling pressures were unchanged had an up to 40% reduction in myocardial oxygen consumption.[45] Metoprolol also improves survival, patient well-being, and New York Heart Association (NYHA) functional class in patients with congestive heart failure (CHF).[58,59] β-Blockade and subsequent heart rate reduction clearly decrease myocardial oxygen consumption and increase oxygen supply in patients with CHF. Although most anesthesiologists recognize the benefits of perioperative β-blockade, few institutions have formalized protocols for administering β-blockers to surgical patients.[60]

Preload Preload is the ventricular volume at end-diastole that determines myocardial fiber length, which in part determines the force of ventricular contraction. Manipulation of preload is an important therapeutic option in the care of patients with myocardial ischemia. Nitroglycerin is commonly used for treatment of myocardial ischemia, primarily exhibiting its antianginal effect by preload reduction through venodilation and coronary vasodilation. Morphine is useful for treating myocardial ischemia by causing vasodilation (preload reduction) and providing pain relief, thereby leading to reduced heart rate. Furosemide reduces preload through both its diuretic action and venodilation.[61]

Determination of end-diastolic volume is problematic in the clinical arena. Pulmonary artery occlusion pressure (PAOP) is commonly used for approximating LV end-diastolic volume (LVEDV), but multiple assumptions must be made in order to use PAOP to estimate preload. Use of a pressure measurement to estimate volume must take into account LV compliance, which is the change in unit pressure for each change of unit volume. Both LVEDV and the compliance of the myocardium determine the LV end-diastolic pressure (LVEDP). Myocardial ischemia decreases ventricular compliance, thereby increasing LVEDP for the same LVEDV. This change may be reflected in PAOP measurements, allowing the use of PAOP as an ischemia monitor.

Other factors that affect the relationship between PAOP and LVEDP are mitral stenosis (MS), LA compliance, and intrathoracic pressure. Although the severity of MS does not change over the course of an anesthetic or surgical procedure, the pressure gradient between the LA and LV is dynamic, dependent on the cardiac output, heart rate, and flow though the mitral valve (MV) during the diastolic phase of the cardiac cycle. Tachycardia decreases diastolic time, thereby increasing flow through the MV during diastole and thus increasing the pressure gradient between the LA and LV. An increase in PAOP in this circumstance is due to an increase in the pressure gradient across the MV rather than an increase in preload. Actual LV preload may be reduced because tachycardia impedes LV filling in patients with MS. When PAOP is used for ischemia monitoring, trends in pressure changes must be taken in the context of these other hemodynamic variables in patients with MS.

Figure 52-2 shows a normal central venous pressure waveform and the relationship of the waveform with the ECG. PAOP appears similar but reflects LA pressure rather than RA pressure. The presence of large,

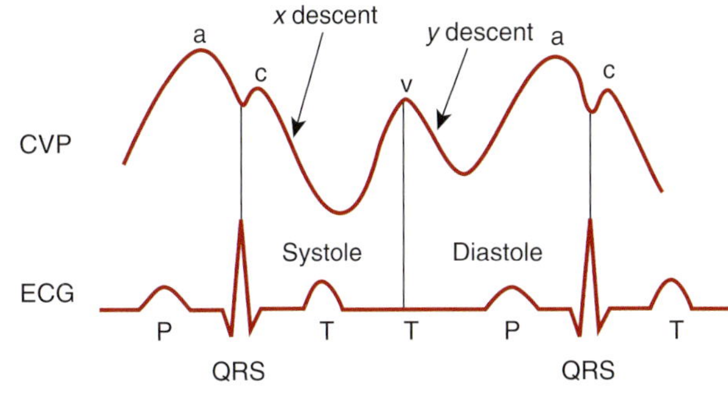

FIGURE 52-2. A normal central venous pressure (CVP) waveform consists of 3 systolic components (c wave, *x* descent, and v wave) and 2 diastolic components (*y* descent, a wave). ECG, electrocardiogram. [Reprinted and modified from Mark JB. Central venous pressure monitoring: clinical insights beyond the numbers. *J Cardiothorac Vasc Anesth.* 1991;5:163-173. Copyright 1991 Elsevier.]

prominent V waves is indicative of mitral regurgitation (MR), which can occur with ischemic papillary muscle dysfunction. This acute increase in LA volume decreases the compliance of the LA and pulmonary veins.

Large changes in intrathoracic pressure also affect PAOP.[62] During spontaneous inspiration, mean PAOP declines because of the decrease in intrathoracic pressure. Positive-pressure ventilation causes increased intrathoracic pressure, which is reflected in the pulmonary venous pressure. Measurement of PAOP is made at the end of expiration to minimize the effects of inspiration on intrathoracic pressure and the pulmonary vasculature.

Afterload Afterload is impedance to ventricular ejection and is best described with pressure–volume loops. The ratio of end-systolic pressure to stroke volume defines the elastance of the arterial tree. In the absence of aortic stenosis (AS), this is primarily determined by arterial vasculature tone. Afterload conditions that allow more fiber shortening allow greater metabolic efficiency and reduced oxygen consumption.[63] The clinician can manipulate afterload by changing the size or radius of the LV through preload manipulation or more commonly by affecting systemic vascular resistance or blood viscosity. Although systemic vascular resistance is only 1 component of afterload, it is the only factor that is easily measured and readily changed clinically.

Contractility Inotropy describes the contractile state of the ventricle and is measured using either the ejection or isovolumic phase of ventricular contraction. Pressure–volume loops consisting of ejection, relaxation, and isovolemic pressure are drawn under different loading conditions. The slope of the serial end-systolic pressure–volume relationship describes the myofibril contractile state independently from preload or afterload (**Fig. 52-3**). Simple clinical tools for measuring contractility independent of preload and afterload do not exist; however, some investigators have used simultaneous pressure and echocardiography area relationships to provide measurements of contractility.[64]

ANESTHETIC CONSIDERATIONS FOR PATIENTS UNDERGOING CABG

Patients with CAD presenting for CABG require special considerations in their anesthetic management. First and foremost are techniques that minimize myocardial oxygen demand while maximizing myocardial oxygen delivery, as described in previous sections. These considerations include preoperative preparation, intraoperative monitoring, and the use of anesthetic agents with hemodynamic effects that favor oxygen supply over demand and allow for myocardial protection. Postoperative management that provides particular attention to pain management, temperature control, and attentive hemodynamic monitoring to prevent tachycardia, hypotension, and hypertension, must also be considered. Many of these considerations apply to patients undergoing CABG, with or without CPB. However, certain considerations apply to patients who

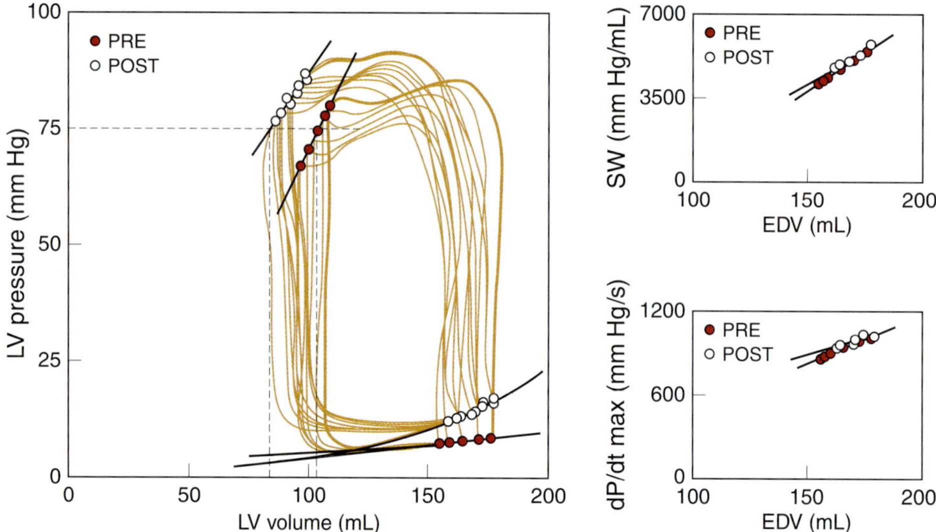

FIGURE 52-3. Example of end-systolic pressure–volume relations (ESPVRs) derived by caval vein occlusion before and after cardiopulmonary bypass (CPB). The ESPVRs (left) show the increased contractile performance after CPB in this patient. Although the slope of the ESPVR (Ees) is slightly decreased, the position of all end-systolic pressure–volume points to the left and above the pre-CPB ESPVR suggests higher contractility. Dotted lines indicate the position of the ESPVR at 75 mm Hg. The same holds for the preload recruited stroke work (PRSW) relation (upper right) and the dP/dt_{max}–end-diastolic volume (EDV) relation (lower right), although the differences are much less pronounced. The EDPVRs (left panel) provide clear evidence for a substantial increase in chamber stiffness after CPB, as observed in all patients. [From Tulner SA, Klautz RJ, van Rijk-Zwikker GL, et al. Perioperative assessment of left ventricular function by pressure–volume loops using the conductance catheter method. *Anesth Analg.* 2003;97:950-957, with permission.]

undergo CABG with CPB, although others apply if coronary revascularization is performed without CPB (ie, OPCABG).

Preoperative Evaluation Most patients presenting for CABG undergo extensive preoperative testing of their cardiac disease and other medical problems. Medical conditions that predispose patients to the development of CAD also affect other organ systems. They include smoking, hypertension, hypercholesterolemia, diabetes, obesity, and advanced age. It is particularly important to identify comorbidities that may prolong or complicate the patient's postoperative course. One comorbidity that deserves particular attention is respiratory insufficiency. Patients with CAD often complain of dyspnea due to ventricular dysfunction caused by myocardial ischemia. Dyspnea related to myocardial ischemia should resolve with adequate revascularization. However, patients with a long-standing smoking history who develop underlying pulmonary disease may not derive the same benefit after CABG, but instead experience exacerbation of their pulmonary disease and require prolonged postoperative mechanical ventilation and suffer pulmonary complications after surgery.

Diabetes is a progressive metabolic disorder that leads to the development of CAD, cerebral vascular disease, neuropathy, nephropathy, and retinopathy. An important aspect of diabetes in the patient with CAD is that myocardial ischemia may occur in the absence of classic symptoms. Patients may suffer from ischemic episodes without therapy, leading to potentially irreversible cardiac damage. They may have prolonged recovery from CABG surgery because of the increased need for inotropic support. Tight control of glycemic blood levels during the perioperative period is important for reducing the incidence of wound infection following cardiac surgery.

Hypertension is another medical condition common in patients with CAD. It also is a risk factor for cerebral vascular disease, renal failure, and CHF. This condition may be asymptomatic, yet it carries the risk of end-organ damage if untreated for prolonged periods. Patients with uncontrolled hypertension often are more difficult to manage because of wide swings in blood pressure associated with events such as sternotomy and pericardotomy. Their vasculature is more responsive to catecholamines causing an exaggerated response, and the relatively volume contracted state leads to exaggerated hypotension in response to vasodilator therapy. Intraoperative blood pressure variability is associated with 30-day postoperative mortality in patients undergoing coronary bypass surgery,[65] and an increased perioperative pulse pressure is associated with poor long-term survival after CABG.[66]

Renal disease is associated with cardiac surgical patients, especially in those with hypertension and diabetes. Development of renal failure after cardiac surgery is a concern, which occurs in 0.9% of CABG patients and 2.0% of patients undergoing valve procedures. More importantly, operative mortality has been reported to be 63.7% in patients who develop acute renal failure versus 4.3% for patients who do not develop renal failure.[67] The risk of postoperative MI, reoperation for bleeding, and mediastinitis is higher in patients who develop postoperative renal failure.[68]

Monitoring Continuous ECG monitoring, along with blood pressure measurement, pulse oximetry, and end-tidal carbon dioxide (CO_2) analysis are standard monitors for all anesthetized patients. It is preferred that cardiac surgical patients have a display monitor that allows viewing of 2 ECG leads simultaneously with automated ST-segment analysis. ECG limb leads II and V_5 allow for monitoring of myocardial regions supplied by the RCA and LAD coronary arteries, respectively. Automated ST-segment trending has only moderate sensitivity and specificity (75% for both) in detecting changes found by off-line Holter monitoring[69] but is a marked improvement over mere observation by the clinician, whose attention must also be directed at providing anesthetic care. Monitoring 2 ECG leads simultaneously increases the sensitivity of detecting ischemia to 80% if leads II and V_5 are monitored, 82% if leads II and V_4 are monitored, and 90% if leads V_4 and V_5 are monitored (**Fig. 52-4**).[70] Factors such as LV hypertrophy, cardiac conduction changes, electrolytes, and drugs such as digitalis all can affect the interpretation of ST segments,[71] but the primary concern is acute ST-segment changes that occur during the perioperative period (**Fig. 52-5**).

All cardiac surgical patients require invasive arterial blood pressure monitoring. Although the radial artery is used at many institutions, consideration must be given to the possibility of harvesting the radial artery as a conduit for CABG. When used for this purpose, the radial artery is harvested from the patient's nondominant hand, so radial artery cannulation should be performed in the dominant hand. Femoral artery cannulation

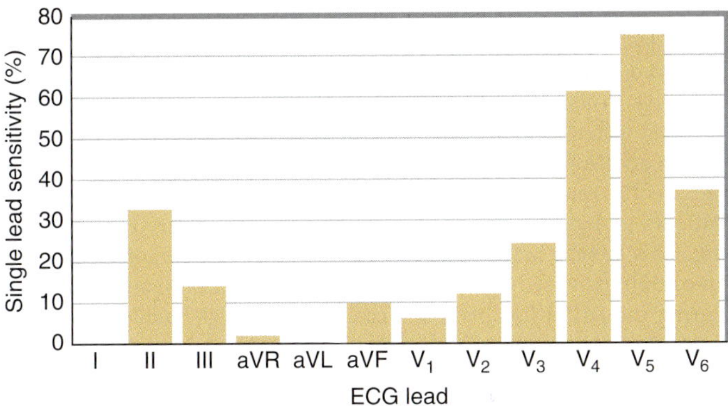

FIGURE 52-4. Distribution of ischemic ST-segment changes in each of the 12 ECG leads of 105 patients with known or suspected coronary artery disease undergoing noncardiac surgery with general anesthesia. Sensitivity was calculated from the number of changes in a single lead as a percentage of the total number of episodes obtained with continuous intraoperative recording. [From London MJ, Hollenberg M, Wong MG, et al. Intraoperative myocardial ischemia: localization by continuous 12-lead electrocardiography. *Anesthesiology.* 1988;69:232-241, with permission.]

TABLE 52-2 American Society of Anesthesiologists Task Force on Pulmonary Artery Catheterization Practice Guidelines

Indications Related to the Patient
- Clinical evidence of significant cardiovascular disease
- Pulmonary dysfunction
- Hypoxia
- Renal insufficiency
- Other conditions associated with hemodynamic instability (eg, advanced age, endocrine disorders, sepsis, trauma, burns)

Indications Related to Surgery
- Surgical procedures associated with an increased risk of hemodynamic changes, including damage to the heart, kidneys, lungs, or brain

Indications Related to Practice Setting
- Physician skills
- Duration of procedure
- Technical support
- Training and experience of nursing staff
- Ability to manage potential complications

Data from American Society of Anesthesiologists Task Force on Pulmonary Artery Catheterization. Practice guidelines for pulmonary artery catheterization: an updated report by the American Society of Anesthesiologists Task Force on Pulmonary Artery Catheterization. *Anesthesiology.* 2003;99:988-1014.

can be used and is preferred by some clinicians and institutions. The benefits of using femoral artery cannulation include a better correlation with mean arterial pressure in the immediate post-CPB period and access to the femoral artery if an IABP must be inserted. The intra-arterial catheter can be placed prior to or immediately after induction, but preinduction placement allows the clinician to respond more rapidly to the changing hemodynamic conditions that often occur during induction of anesthesia. Preinduction placement of the arterial catheter is preferred in the setting of a potentially difficult airway and for patients with a greater risk of rapidly changing hemodynamics (left main disease or severe ventricular dysfunction).

All cardiac surgical patients should have central venous access for the purpose of administering important vasoactive medications into the central circulation and for assessing volume status. The issue of whether to place a central venous pressure (CVP) catheter versus a PAC is controversial. A PAC measures pulmonary artery (PA) pressure and provides a means for sampling mixed venous oxygen saturation (Svo_2). PA pressure is not easily determined with TEE, and Svo_2 cannot be obtained with a CVP catheter or by TEE. Some studies have not demonstrated improved cardiac surgical outcomes with the use of a PAC.[72] However, prolonged pre-CPB pulmonary hypertension and post-CPB elevation of PA diastolic pressure are predictors for the development of perioperative MI.[73] Early treatment of pulmonary hypertension is presumed to improve outcome.

The American Society of Anesthesiologists (ASA) Task Force on Pulmonary Artery Catheterization has provided practice guidelines for PAC insertion (**Table 52-2**).[74] PA pressure monitoring is indicated based on the medical condition of the patient or the nature of the surgery (**Table 52-3**) but is not recommended when the patient, procedure, and practice setting each poses a low risk for hemodynamic complications.[74] Cardiac surgical patients with unstable angina, recent MI, active CHF, severe CAD or valvular heart disease, and severe pulmonary or renal disease should have PA pressure monitoring. However, routine PA catheterization is not necessary in all patients undergoing CABG. Outcome after CABG is not influenced by routine use of a PAC, suggesting its use can be delayed until a clinical need develops.[72]

Right bundle-branch block occurs in approximately 3% of patients undergoing PA catheterization.[75] For this reason, placement of a PAC in patients with a previous left bundle-branch block is not recommended unless precautions are taken for managing the patient should complete heart block occur. A decision-making algorithm for inserting a PAC in patients with a preexisting left bundle-branch block is shown in **Fig. 52-6**.

TEE can be used to assess global and regional myocardial contractility, volume status, and valvular function during cardiac surgery. Although TEE has revolutionized the intraoperative assessment and management of patients undergoing cardiac surgery, few data suggest that routine use of TEE for all patients with normal ventricular

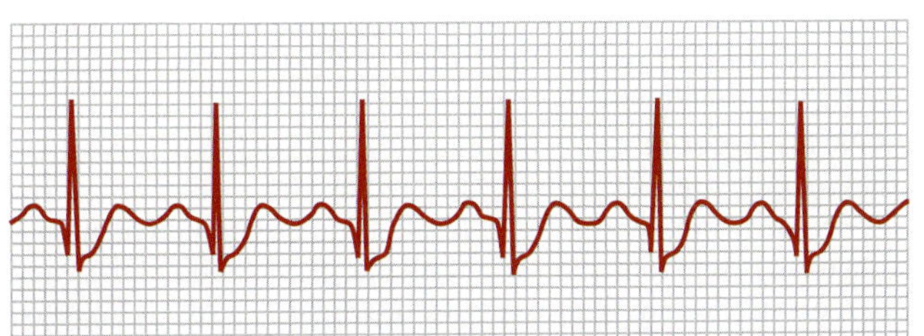

FIGURE 52-5. Electrocardiogram with ST-segment depression indicating myocardial ischemia.

TABLE 52-3 Indications for Pulmonary Arterial Pressure Monitoring

Indications Related to the Patient
- Right heart failure
- Pulmonary hypertension
- Pulmonary embolism
- Unstable angina
- Recent myocardial infarction
- Acute congestive heart failure
- Severe coronary artery disease
- Shock (cardiogenic, septic, or hemorrhagic)
- Massive trauma
- Severe lung disease
- Severe renal disease

Indications Related to Surgery
- Major organ transplantation
- Aortic cross-clamping procedures
- Large fluid shifts
- Massive blood loss
- Implantation/explantation of ventricular assist devices

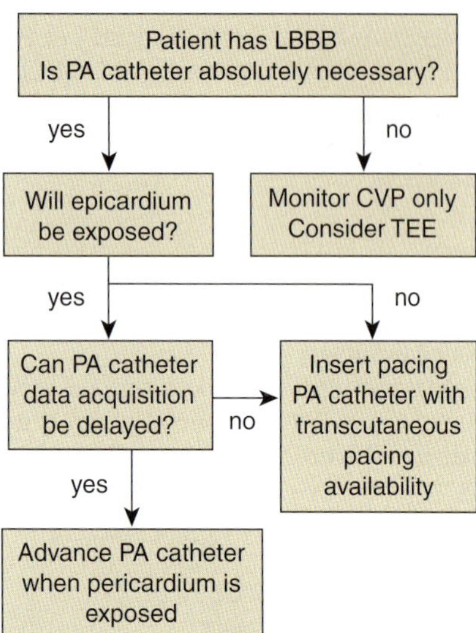

FIGURE 52-6. Algorithm for pulmonary artery (PA) catheter insertion in patients with left bundle-branch block (LBBB). CVP, central venous pressure; TEE, transesophageal echocardiography. [Reprinted from Troianos CA. Intraoperative monitoring. In: *Anesthesia for the Cardiac Patient*. St. Louis, MO: Mosby; 2002:106, with permission from Elsevier.]

function undergoing elective CABG improves outcome. Regional wall-motion assessment by qualitative inspection of radial shortening and wall thickening is subjective. Accurate diagnosis is dependent on observer experience and having the ischemic myocardial segment in the imaging plane during the ischemic episode. More sophisticated techniques such as computerized digitations, color kinesis, and tissue Doppler imaging may allow for better assessment, but these techniques are not readily available or familiar to all users. Nonetheless, information obtained from TEE is far superior in quality and quantity to that obtained from a PAC and may be very helpful in guiding therapy toward optimizing hemodynamics in the perioperative period. Furthermore, TEE has proven invaluable for assessing the quality of the surgical procedure following separation from CPB, especially among patients undergoing CABG surgery who have significant ventricular dysfunction and those undergoing concurrent valve procedures, congenital heart surgery, and/or aortic surgery.[35-39]

Near-infrared reflectance spectroscopy has been used to demonstrate a correlation between low bifrontal regional cortical oxygen saturation and cognitive dysfunction, prolonged hospital stay, and perioperative stroke. Intraoperative cerebral oxygen desaturation is associated with an increased risk of cognitive decline and prolonged hospital stay after coronary artery bypass surgery.[76] Thus some clinicians have advocated monitoring of cerebral oximetry in CABG patients as a technique for preventing profound cerebral desaturation and associated morbidity.[77]

Anesthetic Induction Induction of general anesthesia for CABG patients can be accomplished using a variety of medications, provided the goals of preventing tachycardia, hypotension, and hypertension are achieved. The worst combination of hemodynamic perturbations is tachycardia with hypotension. Although hypertension increases ventricular wall tension and therefore myocardial oxygen demand, it also increases coronary perfusion pressure. Myocardial depression and the vasodilating effects of the anesthetic agents are the most important considerations in patients with severely impaired ventricular function or valvular heart disease. Laryngoscopy and intubation are the first intraoperative events after induction of anesthesia that test the effects of the anesthetic technique used. Coincident with these events is the institution of positive-pressure ventilation, which may result in hypotension among hypovolemic patients or in patients with air trapping due to pulmonary disease.

Patients with CAD benefit from a narcotic-based technique because of the lack of myocardial depression, a tendency for decreased heart rate, and an attenuated response to laryngoscopy and intubation. Fentanyl probably is the most frequently used opioid in cardiac surgery, although sufentanil is also a reasonable choice. The prebypass addition of remifentanil to a fentanil and propofol anesthetic reduces the release of biochemical markers of myocardial damage to patients undergoing elective on-pump coronary artery bypass grafting. This benefit may be attributed to either remifentanil itself or to an overall increased opioid dose.[78] Use of remifentanil and sufentanil during induction has been associated with a high incidence of bradycardic/asystolic complications in patients who have been treated with β-blockers and calcium channel blockers.[79,80] Many patients with CAD are likely to be taking 1 or both types of drugs. A nondepolarizing muscle relaxant devoid of cardiovascular side effects is used to facilitate intubation. Pancuronium can be used with a large dose of narcotic because the tachycardic side effects of pancuronium are balanced by the bradycardic side effects of the large-dose narcotic. Use of vecuronium or rocuronium is prudent when the initial narcotic dose is smaller because the bradycardic effects of the narcotic are not as pronounced. Pancuronium use with only a small narcotic bolus may result in undesirable tachycardia.

Modern practices that focus on early extubation and "fast-tracking" the patients through the postoperative period use smaller narcotic doses, with supplementation by short-acting hypnotic agents such as midazolam. Dexmedetomidine can also be used as an adjunct to anesthetic induction to attenuate the hemodynamic response to tracheal intubation, which is particularly important when low-dose fentanyl is used for induction.[81] An intraoperative awareness protocol should be used to minimize the incidence of intraoperative recall, which is more of a concern with a low-dose narcotic-based anesthetic technique. A low concentration of a potent inhalational agent or intravenous propofol is used for hypnosis and amnesia. Reduced doses of opioids often are administered with small doses of hypnotic drugs such as benzodiazepines, thiopental, propofol, or etomidate to promote early postoperative extubation. Care must be taken when hypnotics are administered concomitantly with opioids. Mean arterial pressure can drop precipitously in hypovolemic patients. Midazolam significantly decreases blood pressure and increases heart rate when used as an induction agent.[82] Propofol causes venodilation and can profoundly decrease blood pressure.[83] A vasoactive drug such as ephedrine or phenylephrine should be readily available to treat hypotensive episodes during the induction of anesthesia. Although regional anesthesia for cardiac surgery may provide superior postoperative analgesia, shorter postoperative ventilation, reduced incidence of supraventricular dysrhythmias, and lower rates of perioperative MI, most clinicians use general anesthesia during CABG procedures.[84]

The same hemodynamic goals must be achieved for the patient with a difficult airway who requires an awake/sedated fiberoptic intubation prior to general anesthesia. The patient's airway should be well anesthetized with local anesthetics and the patient sedated with short-acting intravenous agents that blunt the response to laryngoscopy and intubation. An inhalational induction also might be considered in some patients. Alternatively, an intubating laryngeal mask airway can be used to secure the difficult airway under general anesthesia. The particular technique or approach is individualized to the patient's anatomy and medical condition, and the experience of the clinician in using 1 or more of these techniques.

Pre-CPB Management Once the airway is secured and general anesthesia induced, anesthesia care is directed toward maintaining a stable blood pressure and heart rate. If access to the central circulation was not obtained before induction of anesthesia, cannulation of the internal jugular or subclavian vein is performed, and a PAC is inserted if indicated. The right internal jugular vein is often used because of its predictable location, accessibility, and direct route into the RA. The patient is placed in the Trendelenburg position during central venous cannulation, which increases preload and helps maintain blood pressure at an acceptable range following the induction of anesthesia, in the absence of surgical stimulation. Use of surface ultrasound for guiding the insertion and placement of a central venous cannula has become more popular.[85] Blood pressure frequently declines as the operating room table is leveled following central venous cannulation. A fluid bolus or small doses of vasoactive drugs may be required.

Additional tasks for the anesthesia provider before surgical incision include placement of a TEE probe, antibiotic administration, determination of a baseline ACT, and infusion of antifibrinolytic drugs. Although many studies have demonstrated the beneficial effects of antifibrinolytic agents in reducing perioperative bleeding and morbidity,[30] others have reported adverse side effects associated with multiorgan dysfunction and prothrombotic outcomes,[31,32] especially among patients with a genetic predisposition to a hypercoagulable state.[33] Thus, similar to all pharmacologic agents, the decision to administer any antifibrinolytic should include a thorough risk-to-benefit consideration that is individualized to each patient.

Patients must be anesthetized to a depth that avoids a tachycardic and hypertensive response to surgical incision. Small doses of short-acting agents such as esmolol (50-100 mg) or nitroglycerin (50-100 mcg) can be administered, or the anesthetic depth can be deepened with additional narcotic or potent inhalational agent. The patient's response to skin incision is a gauge to his or her subsequent response to the more stimulating event of median sternotomy. If the anesthetic depth was not adequate for skin incision, then additional narcotic or a bolus of esmolol should be administered before sternotomy. The lungs typically are deflated during sternotomy to prevent the sternal saw from cutting the lung parenchyma. Another complication that can occur during sternotomy is accidental tearing of the innominate vein or the RV. Sternotomy is especially hazardous during repeat CABG, where adhesions from previous surgery placed the heart immediately posterior to the sternum. Banked packed red blood cells must be immediately available at the time of sternotomy, particularly for patients at increased risk for this complication.

Maintenance of anesthesia during the pre-CPB period can be accomplished with a variety of techniques. Isoflurane–fentanyl anesthesia and propofol–fentanyl anesthesia both are acceptable techniques for maintaining anesthesia during CABG.[86] Postoperative troponin release, cardiac morbidity, and mortality were similar between anesthetic regimens consisting of propofol-opioid versus isoflurane-opioid in patients undergoing CABG surgery.[87] Use of sevoflurane and desflurane has been shown to result in shorter intensive care unit (ICU) and hospital length of stay.[88] This finding seemed to be related to better preservation of early postoperative myocardial function. Considerable research has recently focused on the myocardial protective effects of potent inhalational anesthetics. Isoflurane protected the myocardium during ischemic episodes in an experimental model.[89,90] Isoflurane and other volatile anesthetics may mimic the protective effects of a process called *ischemic preconditioning.*[91] Brief periods of ischemia activate the protein kinase C–mediated pathway that confers cardioprotection during subsequently longer periods of ischemia.[92] Sevoflurane decreases the inflammatory response after CPB, as measured by the release of IL-6, neutrophil β-integrins (CD11b/CD18), and TNF-α. Myocardial function after CPB, as assessed by regional wall motion and LV stroke work index, also is improved with sevoflurane.[93] Both halothane and isoflurane have been shown to provide significant preservation of adenosine triphosphate (ATP) levels during ischemia, but this preservation did not improve hemodynamic recovery.[94] In a comparative study in which patients received either propofol or inhalational anesthesia during CABG surgery, patients who received inhalational anesthesia (sevoflurane or desflurane) but not propofol had preserved LV function after CPB, with less evidence of postoperative myocardial injury.[95] The cardioprotective effects are clinically most apparent when the inhalational agent is administered throughout the operation.[96] Although recent evidence suggests that remifentanil may play a similar role in protective preconditioning, the effect may be attributable to an overall increased opioid dose rather than to remifentanil itself.[79]

Important activities that occur during the pre-CPB period include surgical dissection of the left internal mammary artery, opening of the pericardium, and placement of the aortic and venous cannulas in preparation for CPB. Sternal retraction that exposes the internal mammary artery may affect the function of intravenous and arterial catheters placed in the ipsilateral arm. This most commonly affects the left arm with harvesting of the left internal mammary artery. Papaverine is commonly injected into the ligated internal mammary artery to prevent vasospasm but may cause hypotension. This decrease in blood pressure usually is brief but may require treatment with a small dose of phenylephrine. Hypertension may develop during surgical manipulation of the pericardium and aorta as a result of sympathetic activation. A small bolus of narcotic or esmolol can blunt this hypertensive response.

Heparin is administered prior to ligation of the internal mammary artery (if used) and cannulation of the aorta to prevent thrombus formation. Heparin is a polyanionic mucopolysaccharide that increases the rate of anticoagulant effect of antithrombin III on factors II, X, XI, XII, and XIII. It usually is given in a dose range of 300 to 400 U/kg to achieve ACT greater than 400 seconds. The adequacy of anticoagulation must be determined prior to initiating CPB. For patients undergoing OPCABG, some surgeons administer a smaller dose of heparin, with the goals of achieving ACT greater than 300 seconds.

CABG WITHOUT CPB

CABG without CPB (OPCABG) was first reported during the 1960s and 1970s.[97,98] Advancements in the safety of CPB with better equipment and techniques allowed surgical access to more distal coronary target sites and a quiet surgical field, thereby eliminating the need for CABG without CPB.[1,2] Developments in mechanical stabilization devices during the 1990s renewed the interest among surgeons to return to this technique in order to avoid the deleterious effects of CPB, particularly as the age of the surgical population increased to include more elderly patients with calcified aortas. OPCABG also allows faster recovery and fewer ICU days, providing an economic incentive to using this technique.

The anesthetic management of patients undergoing OPCABG encompasses the same hemodynamic goals as the pre-CPB management of patients undergoing CABG with CPB, but the goals are more difficult to achieve, particularly when distal coronary anastomoses are being performed. Myocardial protection with the use of inhalational agents remains an important consideration. Compared to patients who receive propofol, patients receiving sevoflurane have less myocardial injury in the first 24 postoperative hours.[99] Similarly, patients who received isoflurane during OPCABG had lower troponin-T leakage than patients who received a propofol infusion.[100] OPCABG requires more attention, vigilance, and intervention on the part of the anesthesia provider while the surgeon is performing the distal coronary anastomoses. Maintenance of perfusion pressure, cardiac output, and normothermia, while avoiding profound myocardial ischemia, is challenging during surgical manipulation that produces ventricular compression and temporary coronary occlusion. Ischemia monitoring is compromised by cardiac displacement that alters ECG polarization and affects the anatomic relation with a TEE probe. Vasoactive medications and the Trendelenburg position are used to maintain blood pressure and cardiac output. Despite the best efforts, however, decreases in cardiac output with elevations in central venous pressure and PAOP are commonly observed during surgical manipulation. Cardiac dysrhythmias are not uncommon and are treated by increasing the perfusion pressure and using medications such as lidocaine, amiodarone, and magnesium. Sevoflurane anesthesia is associated with less atrial fibrillation or supraventricular arrhythmias after OPCABG surgery than an equivalent dose of desflurane.[101] Malignant dysrhythmias that are not corrected by medications or electrical cardioversion may prompt the need for CPB. Temporary cardiac pacing may be required in patients with right coronary dominant anatomy because of bradycardia or cardiac arrest during right coronary occlusion. Upon successful completion of all distal coronary anastomoses, the blood pressure is lowered before application of the partial aortic clamp for the proximal anastomoses. Release of this clamp after all of the proximal grafts are completed may produce reperfusion dysrhythmias or send air through the coronary grafts, if they were not adequately de-aired by the surgeon.

Anticoagulation is reversed with protamine after the surgeon is satisfied with the grafts and the absence of surgical bleeding. The surgical wound is closed, and the patient is transported to the ICU. Some patients may be candidates for extubation immediately after surgery, but this should be individualized according to the patient's temperature, need for inotropic and mechanical support of the circulation, coexisting medical problems, and degree of mediastinal bleeding.[102] Although extubation within 2 to 4 hours after surgery is a reasonable goal for most patients, immediate extubation is possible after OPCABG using either opioid-based or thoracic epidural-based anesthesia.[103] Thoracic epidural analgesia may be of particular benefit in obese patients (>30 kg/m^2 body mass index) by providing early tracheal extubation and shorter ICU stays.[104] The benefits of thoracic epidural analgesia must obviously be weighed heavily against the risks associated with anticoagulation and appropriate management of the epidural catheter.

CABG WITH CPB

For patients undergoing CABG with CPB, a 2-stage cannula is placed in the RA to direct blood away from the patient to the CPB circuit, and a cannula is placed in the aorta to return oxygenated blood to the patient's circulatory system. The patient must be fully heparinized before cannulation to avoid thrombus formation. The arterial blood pressure is lowered to 85 to 90 mm Hg systolic pressure prior to aortic cannulation to reduce aortic wall tension and minimize the risk of aortic dissection as the aortic wall is punctured. The surgeon may request hand-bag ventilation to provide better visualization of the RA for insertion of the venous cannula. Atrial fibrillation may develop during placement of the venous or coronary sinus catheters. Cardioversion with internal paddles may be required if the patient becomes hypotensive prior to CPB.

Some institutions "retrograde prime" the CPB circuit by allowing the patient's blood to displace the clear fluid priming volume from the aortic and venous lines to the CPB machine. This process nearly always causes hypotension due to volume depletion and requires vigilance and treatment by the anesthesia provider to avoid profound hypotension. Small boluses of phenylephrine are effective for raising blood pressure during this process. Once the retrograde priming is complete, pump volume is infused through the aortic cannula and the venous cannula is unclamped, thereby initiating CPB.

Cardiopulmonary Bypass Mechanical ventilation of the lungs is no longer necessary for oxygenation and ventilation during CPB because the bypass machine provides these physiologic functions. Mechanical ventilation of the lungs is usually discontinued when a calculated circulation flow through the bypass machine is achieved. Although some have suggested that continued pulmonary ventilation during CPB might mitigate reperfusion injury to the lungs, recent evidence in humans did not demonstrate a significant difference in pulmonary vascular resistance between patients mechanically ventilated during CPB versus those who were not.[105] Dexamethasone may have a beneficial effect on A-a oxygen gradient, respiratory index, and Pao_2/Fio_2 ratio at 12 and 24 hours, but no effect on extubation time or lung compliance following CPB.[106]

The surgical field is observed for complications related to cannulation such as venous obstruction, aortic dissection, bleeding, and cardiac distension. Anesthesia is maintained by volatile anesthetics administered through a vaporizer on the CPB machine or by continuous infusion of hypnotic drugs such as propofol, titrated according to mean arterial blood pressure and readings on the awareness monitor. Some clinicians routinely administer hypnotics with initiation of CPB and during rewarming to reduce the incidence of intraoperative awareness. Additional muscle relaxation helps reduce oxygen consumption by minimizing shivering as the patient is cooled. ECG, systemic and pulmonary pressures, urine output, and temperature are monitored. PA pressure may increase with cardiac distension or because the PAC has migrated to more peripheral regions in the lung during cardiac manipulation. In the absence of cardiac distension, the PAC should be withdrawn until the pressure measured in the distal port decreases.

The clinician should use the CPB time to prepare for post-CPB events. Most patients with good ventricular function do not require inotropic support following successful coronary revascularization. However, patients with poor preoperative ventricular function and those who undergo complicated surgical procedures and prolonged prebypass ischemia often require inotropic or IABP support in the postbypass period. Prior to termination of CPB, the surgeon places epicardial atrial and ventricular pacing leads, to be used as needed to establish an adequate cardiac rhythm and rate.

POST-CPB MANAGEMENT

The patient is rewarmed to normothermia with CPB as the surgeon completes the coronary anastomoses. The rewarming process may take longer in patients with a higher body mass index and more profound hypothermia. Mechanical ventilation is resumed upon the surgeon's request, after inspection of the anastomotic sites reveals the absence of a surgical cause for bleeding. If inhaled anesthetics are being used in the CPB circuit, their delivery should be continued via the anesthesia machine. The dose of the potent inhalational agent used should be minimal to avoid myocardial depression. Vasoactive infusions should be started or maintained. Communication between the surgeon and the anesthesiologist is paramount to confirm that both are ready to begin the process to separate the patient from CPB. Venous drainage to the pump is reduced, and the patient's heart begins to receive more blood from the circulation. Preload is adjusted by observing mean arterial pressure, cardiac distension, and PA or central venous pressure. The physician performing TEE provides information to the surgeon regarding volume status and contractility, which also aids the separation from CPB. A cardiac index is determined if a PAC is used. The venous cannula is removed from the RA with satisfactory separation from CPB. The surgeon, perfusionist, and anesthesiologist all must be aware when protamine is administered to reverse the anticoagulant effects of heparin. CPB must not be reinitiated once protamine administration has started without administering another dose of heparin. Once it is determined that the patient will not return to cardiopulmonary bypass, the administration of protamine is completed. With adequate neutralization of the heparin, the surgeon inspects the surgical field for bleeding and closes the surgical wound with adequate hemostasis. The patient is transported to the ICU for postoperative care.

POSTOPERATIVE OUTCOME AFTER CABG

Postoperative myocardial ischemia occurs in up to 48% of cardiac surgical patients and is associated with adverse cardiac outcomes.[107] Thirty-eight percent of ischemic episodes occur during the first 2 postoperative days and peak within the first 2 hours of revascularization. These findings have important implications for monitoring, diagnosis, and treatment. Treatment of myocardial ischemia is directed toward adjusting the factors that determine myocardial oxygen supply and demand. Ischemia that develops immediately upon termination of CPB usually is related to air or particulate emboli in the bypass grafts. Elevation of mean arterial pressure and incremental increases in boluses of nitroglycerin are effective for treating ischemia caused by air in the venous grafts. The surgeon should confirm graft patency with Doppler flow probes or palpation. Persistent myocardial ischemia is treated with placement of an IABP. "Stunned myocardium" may be the result of reperfusion injury or intraoperative MI. These patients will require support of cardiac function until myocardial function improves.

Patients at risk for increased mortality after CABG are identified by several factors that evolve and are more prevalent or less over time. For example, patients undergoing myocardial revascularization between 1999 and 2004 were older and more likely to have metabolic syndrome or diabetes and peripheral vascular disease but fewer were smokers, compared with patients undergoing myocardial revascularization between 1993 and 1998. In terms of complications, the latter cohort had a higher rate of postoperative infarction and renal insufficiency, but a lower incidence of stroke and shorter duration of mechanical ventilation and hospital stays.[108] Preoperative risk factors that increase mortality include age older than 80 years, emergent surgery, prior cardiac surgery, and renal failure.[68,108] Mediastinitis is more common among patients with chronic obstructive lung disease, severe obesity, diabetes, renal failure, emergent surgery, and preoperative ejection fraction less than 40%.[68,109] Renal failure is associated with advanced age, history of CHF, and preexisting renal disease.[68,109]

Growing areas of development are genomic predictors and other proteins that can be used to identify patients at risk for complications. For example, noncoding single-nucleotide polymorphisms within the chromosome 4q25 region are independently associated with atrial fibrillation after CABG.[110] Preoperative C-reactive protein levels as low as 3 mg/L are associated with increased long-term mortality and extended hospital length of stay in patients undergoing primary CABG.[111] Similarly, heart-type fatty acid–binding protein peaks earlier and is a superior independent predictor of postoperative mortality and ventricular dysfunction after CABG.[112]

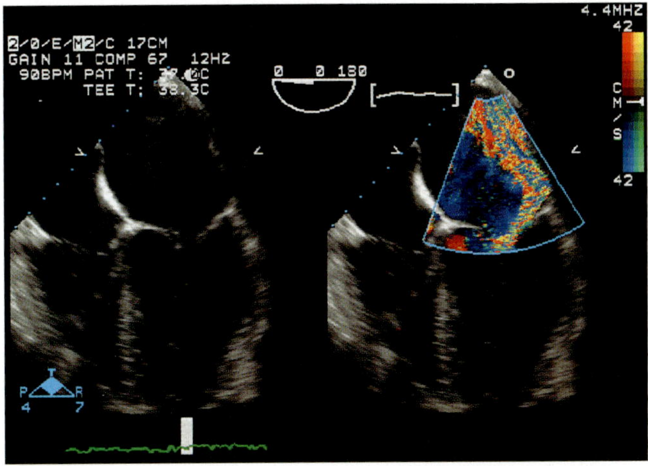

FIGURE 52-7. Mid-esophageal transesophageal echocardiographic 2-dimensional (*left*) and color-flow Doppler (*right*) view demonstrating mitral regurgitation associated with posterior leaflet tethering secondary to left ventricular dilation after a myocardial infarction. A coronary artery bypass grafting procedure was performed and the valve was repaired with a ring annuloplasty.

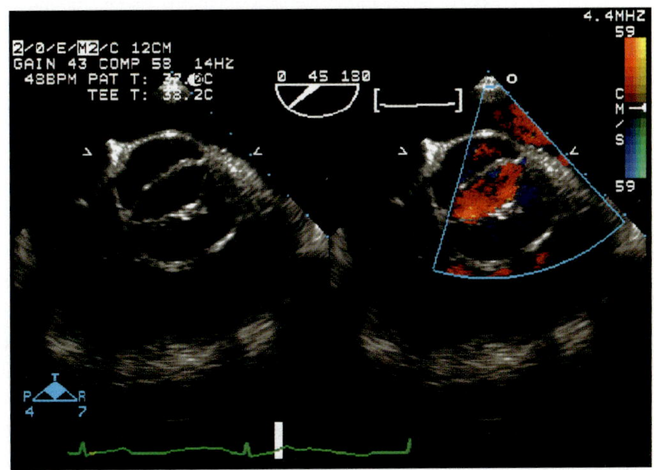

FIGURE 52-8. Transesophageal midesophageal aortic valve short-axis 2-dimensional (*left*) and color-flow Doppler (*right*) views demonstrating a bicuspid aortic valve.

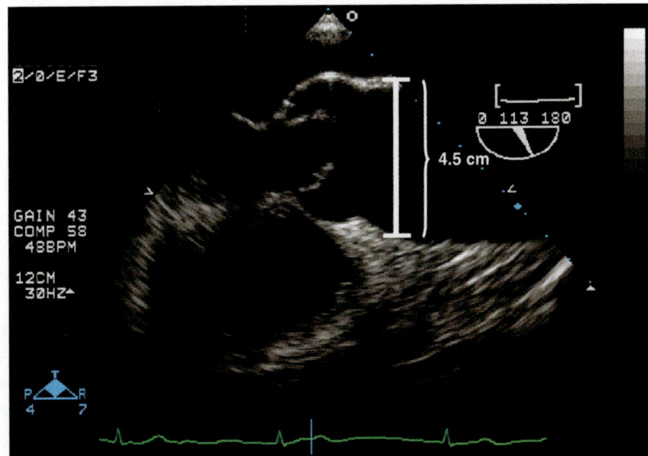

FIGURE 52-9. Transesophageal midesophageal ascending aortic long-axis view demonstrating a bicuspid aortic valve and a dilated aorta measuring 4.5 cm just beyond the sinotubular junction. Aortic dilation is commonly associated with a bicuspid aortic valve defect.

CARDIAC ANESTHESIA FOR VALVE SURGERY

OVERVIEW

Isolated valve surgery and valve surgery in combination with CABG are increasingly more common than CABG alone. The overall incidence of all valvular disease is unknown, but the progression and manifestation of symptoms is more common as the population ages.[113] This combination of an aging population, expanding indications for surgery, improvements in prosthetic valve construction, and reduced patient morbidity and mortality after surgical intervention all suggest that valve surgery will continue to increase in coming years.

The 2 most common valves requiring surgical intervention are the MV and AV. Over 5 million persons have moderate to severe valvular regurgitation in the United States.[114] Myxomatous MV disease is the most common cause of pure MR.[115] The defect is usually associated with advancing age and degenerative changes. The pathophysiology includes elongated and/or ruptured chordae with generous leaflet tissue, a dilated annulus, and severe regurgitation. The defect is associated with increased mortality, even in asymptomatic patients.[116] Most of these patients are amenable to valve repair rather than valve replacement (**Fig. 52-7**). Aortic valve disease is a common indication for surgery. Calcific aortic stenosis (AS) is seen in elderly patients, and in younger patients as well, especially with a bicuspid AV. Bicuspid AVs are found in approximately 0.5% of the population.[117] The bicuspid AV is a heritable condition, often associated with a defect in fibrillin and matrix metalloproteinase-2, which leads to weakening and aneurysm formation (**Figs. 52-8** and **52-9**).[118,119] These patients often present for replacement of both the AV and ascending aorta, requiring deep hypothermic circulatory arrest.

The spectrum of valve surgery extends well beyond this limited review. There are both regurgitant and stenotic lesions of all heart valves. The etiology varies widely from congenital birth defects, senile calcific stenosis, infective endocarditis, rheumatic disease, trauma, and other causes. However, the unifying concepts in all valve surgery include the principles of myocardial function and the influence of preload, afterload, inotropy, heart rate/rhythm, and diastolic function on myocardial performance and mechanics (**Table 52-4**). In valve defects that present acutely (ie, endocarditis, traumatic rupture), the compensatory ability

TABLE 52-4 Valve Abnormalities and Hemodynamic Goals

	Preload	Afterload	Contractility	Heart Rate	Diastolic Function[a]
Aortic stenosis	↑	↑	↔	↓	Impaired relaxation
Aortic regurgitation	↑	↓	↔	↑	Restrictive
Mitral stenosis	↑	↔	↔	↓	Normal
Mitral regurgitation	↓, ↔[b]	↓	↔	↑	Restrictive
HOCM	↑	↑	↓	↓	Impaired relaxation
Tricuspid stenosis	↑	↑, ↔	↔	↓, ↔	Normal
Tricuspid regurgitation	↑	↔	↔	↑, ↔	Normal
Pulmonic stenosis	↑	↔	↔	↑, ↔	Normal
Pulmonic regurgitation	↑	↔	↔	↑, ↔	Normal

↑, increase; ↓, decrease; ↔, maintain; HOCM; hypertrophic obstructive cardiomyopathy with systolic anterior motion of the mitral valve.

[a]Typical transmitral Doppler flow velocity profile pattern.

[b]Augmentation of preload usually is required to maintain forward stroke volume. However, excessive preload can induce further left ventricular dilation and exacerbate mitral regurgitation and left atrial hypertension.

of the heart and vascular system is limited. In chronic conditions (myxomatous MR, senile calcific AS), the ability to compensate can be remarkable. In caring for these patients, the clinician must understand these principles of myocardial performance, the acuity of the defect, the extent and mechanism of compensation, and the interplay of anesthetic drugs and surgery on the patient's condition.

Valve surgery will remain a mainstay of the contemporary cardiothoracic anesthesiology. This section reviews the preoperative evaluation of patients presenting for heart valve surgery, perioperative management techniques, and special considerations relating to the perioperative care of these complex patients.

PREOPERATIVE EVALUATION

In heart valve disease, there are a number of questions that must be answered that will directly influence anesthetic management. Typically, procedures are posted on the operating room schedule as "Aortic Valve Replacement" or "Mitral Valve Replacement." There is no information on whether this is for AS, aortic insufficiency (AI), or both; MS, MR, or both. Understanding the specific pathology of the valve preoperatively is essential in preparing hemodynamic goals for the induction, maintenance, and postoperative care of these patients. Obtaining a focused history and performing a physical examination are critical in preparing for the care of these patients. Patient outcome is dependent on a number of variables; however, understanding baseline status is the first step in ensuring the best possible outcome.

In addition to the usual anesthetic concerns (ie, airway, "NPO" status, comorbidities, etc), much additional information is required that may be unrelated to the valve pathology. For example, will there be other procedures during this repair including a carotid endarterectomy, CABG, septal myomectomy, a MAZE procedure, or other intervention? What is the clinical condition of the patient? Is the patient in a compensated or uncompensated state? For example, with AS, the timing of surgery will have a great impact on outcome depending on the patient's condition. A patient in the early to mid-stages of AS may have a hyperdynamic, hypertrophied heart that will likely perform well after CPB. In contrast, a patient in the late stages of AS may be in CHF, have a reduced ejection fraction (EF), and will likely require extensive inotropic support after CPB.

There are a number of essential imaging and laboratory studies that must be reviewed preoperatively. Imaging of the heart will provide the diagnosis and degree of the structural abnormality. Preoperative echocardiography will establish the type of lesion (stenosis versus regurgitant), valve gradients, and global heart function. Knowledge of the valve area is of critical importance in assessing any stenotic valve. In patients with normal LV function, AV gradients in severely stenotic lesions may be very high (**Figs. 52-10** and **52-11**). Alternatively, in

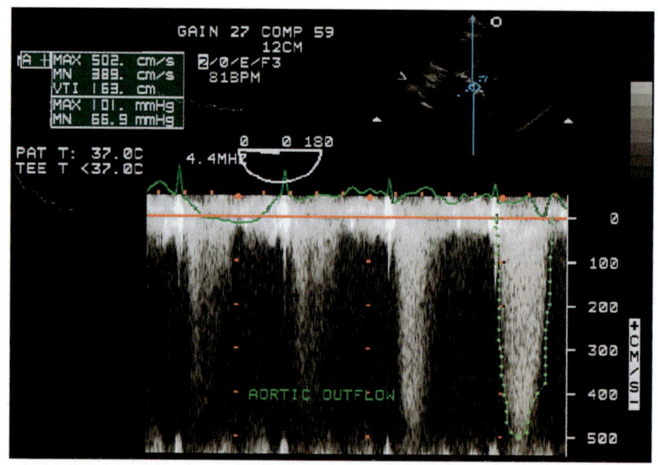

FIGURE 52-10. Intraoperative transesophageal deep transgastric long-axis view using continuous-wave Doppler obtained prior to cardiopulmonary bypass in a patient with aortic stenosis scheduled for an aortic valve replacement. Peak (101 mm Hg) and mean (66.9 mm Hg) transaortic valve (AV) pressure gradients (ΔP) are demonstrated. ΔP is obtained from the peak velocity (V = 502 cm/s) using the simplified Bernoulli equation: $\Delta P = 4\ V^2$.

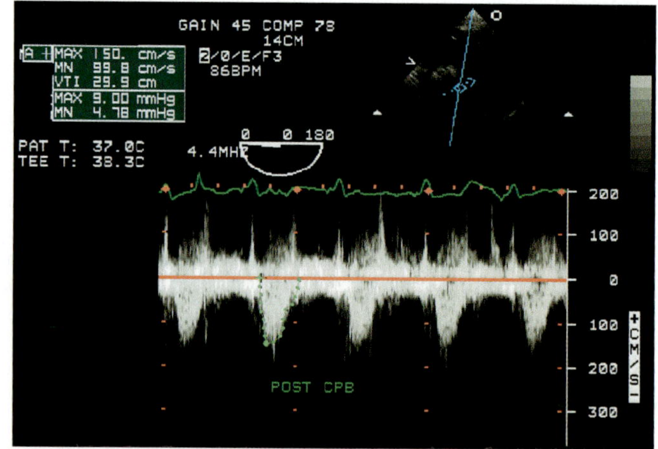

FIGURE 52-11. Intraoperative transesophageal deep transgastric long-axis view using continuous-wave Doppler obtained prior to cardiopulmonary bypass in the same patient shown in Fig. 52-4 now following aortic valve replacement for aortic stenosis. Peak (9 mm Hg) and mean (4.78 mm Hg) transaortic valve (AV) pressure gradients are significantly reduced and consistent with a normal prosthetic valve area.

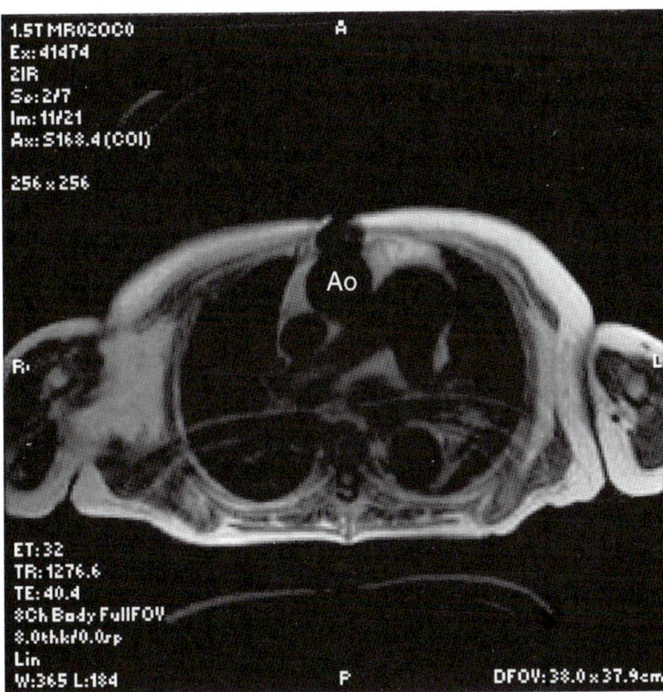

FIGURE 52-12. Preoperative MRI demonstrating the close proximity of the aorta (Ao) to the sternum in a patient scheduled for a fourth reoperation for mitral regurgitation. Sternotomy in this patient poses an extreme risk of aortic trauma and hemorrhage. Consequently, the surgical approach was via a right thoracotomy to avoid this complication.

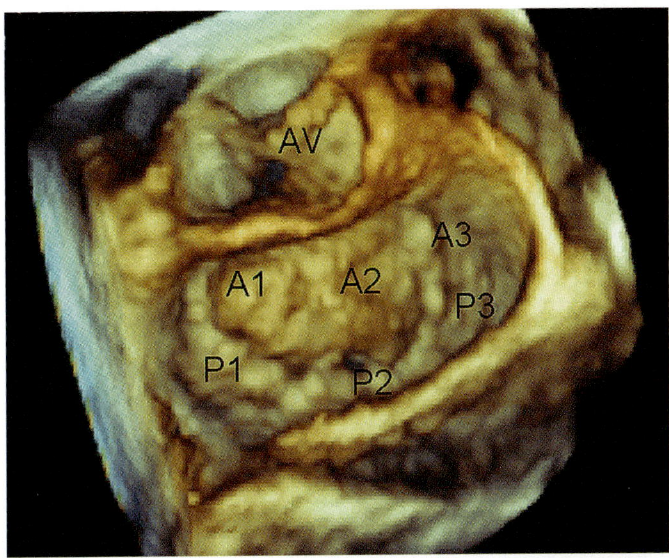

A

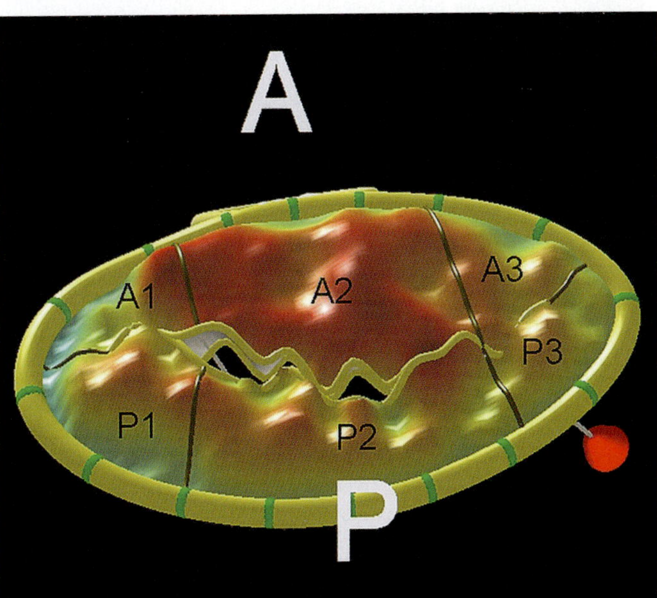

B

FIGURE 52-13. A. Transesophageal 3-dimensional echocardiographic full-volume *en face* view of a mitral valve obtained with a matrix array that demonstrates diffuse prolapse of both leaflets in a patient with myxomatous degeneration. **B.** Computer-generated model of the MV (Q-Labs; MVQ; Philips Healthcare, Inc) demonstrating diffuse prolapse of both anterior (A) and posterior (P) leaflets. A1, anterior-lateral; A2, anterior-middle; A3, anterior-medial; AV, aortic valve; P1, posterior-lateral; P2, posterior-middle. P3, posterior-medial.

patients with poor ventricular performance, there may be anatomically critical lesions (AV area <0.7 cm^2) and a low gradient. These patients are especially prone to intraoperative instability with the induction of general anesthesia and may require significant inotropic support post CPB. Other important imaging modalities include coronary angiography to rule out concurrent coronary artery disease, a chest radiograph, and perhaps thoracic computed tomography (CT) or magnetic resonance imaging (MRI) to evaluate thoracic anatomy. A chest x-ray is essential in "redo" operations involving the heart and mediastinum. The heart may be adherent to the posterior margin of the sternum, rendering sternotomy quite hazardous (**Fig. 52-12**). All precautions including adequate venous access, immediate availability of blood products, and intraoperative awareness and vigilance are required in these situations.

MONITORING

Monitoring during heart valve surgery varies little from monitoring required during other types of heart surgery including CABG. Outside of the American Society of Anesthesiologists standard monitors, an arterial line and a central venous line are essential. Many institutions routinely use PACs to monitor cardiac output, mixed venous oxygenation, pulmonary artery pressures, and PAOPs. Although this is standard practice by many clinicians, outcome data supporting pulmonary artery catheterization are lacking.

Intraoperative TEE is an essential component of anesthesia for all heart valve procedures. Extensive preoperative evaluation by TEE often reveals previously unknown structural or functional defects (**Fig. 52-13**). In addition, TEE can provide instant assessment of the status of a valve repair procedure. TEE may also diagnose perivalvular leaks requiring prompt intervention (**Fig. 52-14**). The assessment of air in the left side of the heart is important after an open-heart procedure. TEE may assist in locating the air, thereby facilitating direct venting procedures. TEE is helpful in guiding post-CPB hemodynamic intervention and treatment. In recognition of this tool's utility in cardiac surgical procedures, the American Society of Echocardiography and the American Heart Association provide a Class 1 recommendation for TEE use in all heart valve surgical procedures.[120]

The assessment of diastolic dysfunction by TEE is important in all patients presenting for cardiac surgical procedures. Dourvas et al reported 40 consecutive cases of right ventricular (RV) diastolic dysfunction in patients with significant AI, LVEF greater than 55%, LV end-diastolic pressure less than 15 mm Hg, RV systolic pressure less than 30 mm Hg, and normal coronary arteries.[121] The pathophysiology of this defect may be related to rapid dilation of the LV in early diastole, a bulging septum, and interference with RV filling. On examination, these patients show a small RV and a large right atrium.[122] An awareness of diastolic dysfunction may guide intraoperative and postoperative hemodynamic therapy.

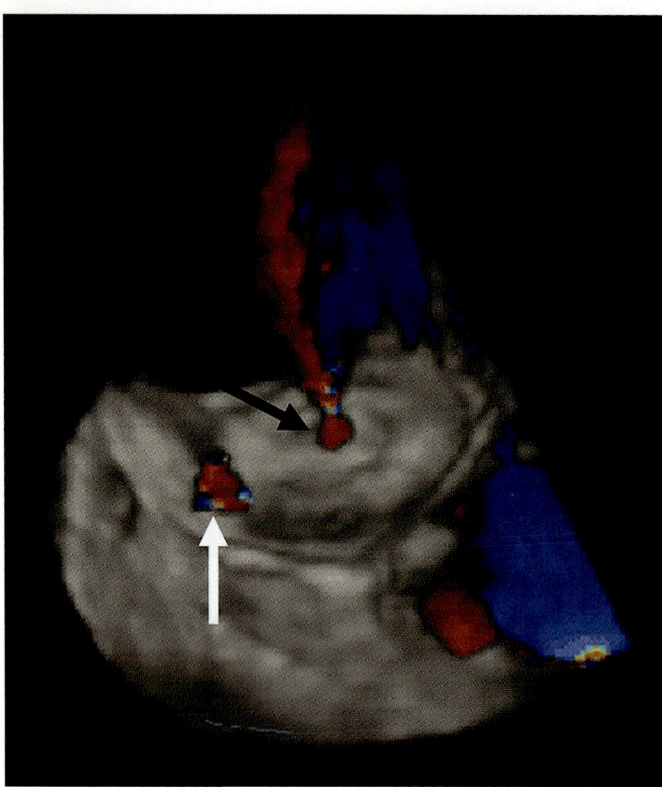

FIGURE 52-14. Transesophageal 3-dimensional echocardiographic *en face* view with color-flow Doppler obtained with a matrix array, demonstrating a single-tilting-disc mechanical mitral valve with a normal central washing jet (*black arrow*) and large perivalvular leak (*white arrow*).

In addition to newer TEE imaging modalities including 3-dimensional echocardiography,[123,124] other special monitoring devices in heart valve surgery may include processed EEG monitoring for either patient awareness or for EEG activity during procedures in which it is desirable to induce an isoelectric state (ie, hypothermic circulatory arrest). In addition, many clinicians find the data provided by cerebral oxymetry to be useful in preventing perioperative neurological injury.

INDUCTION OF ANESTHESIA

Heart valve disease poses an additional burden on the anesthesiologist when planning for the induction of general anesthesia. The clinician should have a clear understanding of how preload, afterload, inotropy, heart rate and rhythm, and diastolic function all interacted in the patient during the time of induction and maintenance of anesthesia. Table 52-4 outlines several basic considerations regarding these parameters. On occasion, a patient will present with a constellation of disease processes. For example, the patient may have severe AS with moderate to severe AI. This same patient may also have obstructive CAD requiring a CABG procedure, as well as moderate MR. How should the information in Table 52-4 be applied to such a patient? There are 2 approaches. One approach identifies the lesion that poses the greatest proximate risk. For example, in a patient with AS and tricuspid regurgitation (TR), it is most likely that the patient will be symptomatic from the effects of the AS rather than the low pressure, high volume lesion of TR. When caring far a patient like this, it is sometimes best to apply the hemodynamic recommendations supplied by the AS algorithm. Another approach is to identify those hemodynamic parameters at which the patient appears compensated. For example, in a patient who presents with compensated AI, it is wise to try to keep the patient in an unaltered hemodynamic condition, that is, keep preload, afterload, inotropy, and rate and rhythm unchanged from the conscious, compensated condition.

Much has been written on specific induction agents, contrasting dose schemes, and medication management for induction of anesthesia. Despite these data, no specific induction agents are indicated in any of the heart valve conditions. Careful titration, attention to the hemodynamic alterations, and prompt intervention when necessary are the key elements in induction of anesthesia for valvular surgery. More important than a specific agent is the adherence to identifying and maintaining clear hemodynamic goals. In certain disease states, abrupt alteration of hemodynamics can lead to catastrophic results. For example, in patients with severe LV hypertrophy, AS, and CAD, a decrease in arterial blood pressure may lead to significant myocardial ischemia and cardiovascular collapse. These patients are unable to alter ejection due to the outflow obstruction, and therefore any drop in preload and afterload may reduce both stroke volume and coronary perfusion. In a hypertrophied heart subject to increased myocardial oxygen demands, the resulting ischemia will be magnified in severity and hastened in onset.

MAINTENANCE OF ANESTHESIA

No agents or techniques (ie, "high-dose" narcotic technique vs inhalation-based anesthesia) are specifically indicated for maintenance of anesthesia in any specific valve disease condition. Again, adherence to the hemodynamic goals outlined in Table 52-4 will provide appropriate guidance when maintaining anesthetic depth. The sound principles of anesthesia apply, that is, loss of consciousness, muscle relaxation, and hemodynamic stability (blunting of the autonomic nervous system).

Patient awareness during cardiac surgical procedures requires special attention. Awareness, especially auditory recollection, may occur in up to 6% of patients requiring cardiopulmonary bypass.[125] Sebel et al reported an incidence of operative awareness of 0.13% in a broad population of 19 575 surgical patients.[126] Multivariate logistic regression identified increasing ASA status and type of procedure as risk factors for recall. For cardiac surgical procedures the odds ratio for recall was 3.58 with a 95% confidence interval of 0.72 to 17.9. As with any procedure, attention to hemodynamic signs, depth of anesthesia, the use of benzodiazepines, and at least one-half MAC of an inhalational agent will likely reduce the risk of operative recall.

There is good evidence to support the concept of "fast-track" or early extubation protocols in the care of patients presenting for CABG.[127] These benefits include reduced hospital length of stay, intensive care unit length of stay, and cost of care. Data on early extubation protocols in valve surgery are less common, although one might expect similar benefits to those observed in CABG.[128] One should be aware, however, that many valvular procedures are complex in nature, in elderly populations, requiring extended CPB time, potential deep hypothermic circulatory arrest, and increased requirements for blood and blood product transfusion. All of these factors may limit the opportunity for early extubation.

WEANING FROM CPB AND THE POST-CPB PERIOD

Once the valve is repaired or replaced, the hemodynamic goals of the patient may be fundamentally different from the pre-CPB period. A more normal hemodynamic profile is usually immediately observed while in the operating room (**Fig. 52-15**). The anticipation is that the heart will now perform normally; however, this is frequently not the case. The heart may suffer from an acute insult associated with the surgical intervention, aortic cross-clamping, and the myocardial depressant effects of the various anesthetic agents. As with any cardiac surgical procedure, there may be evidence of new regional wall motion abnormalities, global cardiac dysfunction, and peripheral vascular dysfunction. In valvular heart surgery, the heart often requires time to remodel before significant improvement is observed.

In some patients, hemodynamics may be greatly improved post CPB. In simple, compensated AS, the patient may be hyperdynamic and hypertensive after weaning from CPB. It may also be possible, however, that due to the LV hypertrophy, cardioplegia may have been incomplete for total myocardial protection, and the patient may emerge from CPB with transient myocardial dysfunction. In complex repairs, or surgery on more than 1 valve, an extended CPB run may be required, thereby

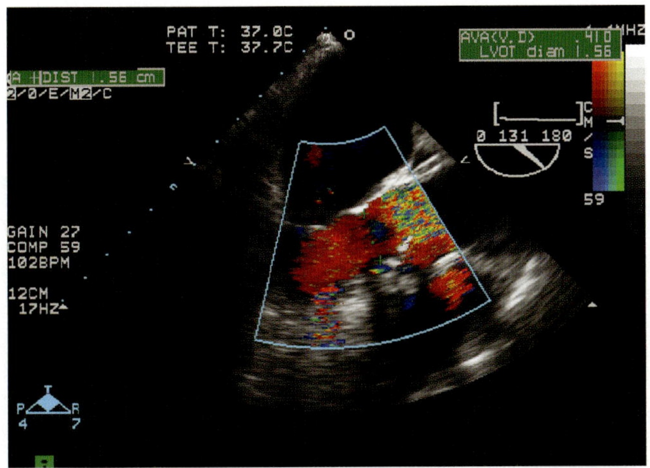

A

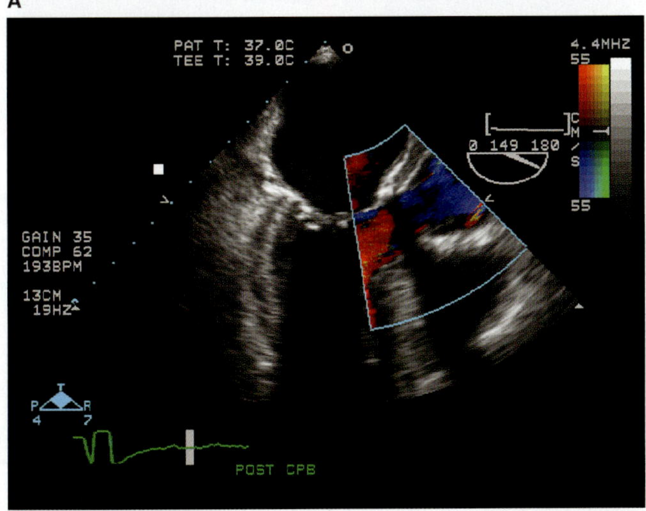

B

FIGURE 52-15. Transesophageal midesophageal aortic valve (AV) long-axis view before and after AV replacement with an allograft. **A.** Preoperatively, the color-flow Doppler pattern reveals laminar flow in the left ventricular outflow tract and highly turbulant flow distal to the AV. The continuity equation was used to calculate the AV area (AVA) as 0.41 cm^2. **B.** Following an AV replacement with an allograft, the color-flow Doppler pattern is now laminar in both the left ventricular outflow tract and the proximal aorta. LVOT diam, left ventricular outflow tract diameter.

increasing the risk of immediate postoperative cardiac dysfunction and the requirement of inotropic support. Ejection fraction and LV function may decline after surgery for MR. Once thought to be due to the new loading conditions imposed on the heart after removal of the "pop-off" associated with MR outflow, emerging data from MV repair procedures, in which there is sparing of the MV apparatus, show little alteration in EF.[129] This preservation of mitral annular integrity stabilizes LV shape and contractility, thereby preserving function. The diminished performance is likely secondary to other factors including extended cross-clamp time, inadequate myocardial protection, and myocardial stunning. Combined CABG and valvular heart surgery is associated with inotrope use during separation from CPB. In a retrospective study of 1009 consecutive patients undergoing either isolated CABG or CABG and valve surgery requiring CPB, a multivariate risk analysis revealed extended cross-clamp time, worsening wall motion score index, reoperation, combined procedures, severe MR, and low EF as predictors of inotrope use during separation from CPB.[130]

TEE is especially useful in the immediate postbypass period. TEE will facilitate the assessment of myocardial function and filling parameters, rendering important information affecting decisions about inotropes and volume management. TEE can also assess the condition of the valve repair or replacement. On every case in which TEE is used, a complete evaluation of the heart and valve is required. This examination includes an assessment of structure and function. In a valve repair, the degree of regurgitation must be documented. A gradient across the valve is required, and images of the valve movement are necessary. In a valve replacement, all of the above are essential and a further evaluation for a perivalvular leak is required. After mitral valve repair, an assessment for systolic anterior motion (SAM) of the mitral valve is required. These examinations should be recorded and a report generated for the patient's record.

The post-CPB period may be a time of unstable hemodynamics. The heart is adjusting to new conditions of preload, afterload, and inotropy. There is usually ongoing bleeding that, in many patients, and especially repeat procedures, may be severe. Constant vigilance regarding hemodynamics, blood volume, blood gas chemistry, and metabolic state (ie, ionized calcium, glucose concentrations, and urine output) are required. There may be new rhythm disturbances. Patients with preoperative atrial fibrillation may now be converted to sinus rhythm after mitral valve repair and a Maze procedure. These patients may be dramatically improved. Other patients, however, may suffer from third-degree heart block, bradycardia, tachycardia, or other rate and rhythm abnormalities, making management difficult.

In the ICU, the usual considerations of temperature management, metabolic and hemodynamic management, vigilance for excessive chest tube bleeding, and evidence of cardiac tamponade must be performed. Elderly patients and those with additional risk factors may require additional support.

SPECIAL CONSIDERATIONS AND LONG-TERM PROGNOSIS

Cardiac anesthesia for heart valve surgery carries numerous special considerations not found in other aspects of cardiothoracic anesthesiology. Among these considerations is familiarity with the type of valve used in the operative repair. There are a number of prosthetic valve types including mechanical and bioprosthetic valves. The choice of valve is up to the surgeon; however, the anesthesiologist may be asked to provide TEE measurements that may guide the surgeon in valve selection. For example, the measurement of the AV annulus size is important when determining the size of a prosthetic valve. In the assessment for a possible Ross procedure, the pulmonary annulus size and the degree of pulmonary insufficiency are important factors before committing to the procedure. After the repair, it is important to assess the new valve function. Bioprosthetic valves are accompanied with a complete hemodynamic profile in their packaging, which should be consulted when rendering a decision on the function of a new valve. The expected gradients are sometimes higher, and the calculated valve area may be less than one might expect. The impact of valve prosthesis-patient mismatch (PPM) on mortality is as high as 25%.[131] In a follow-up study of 1563 patients undergoing aortic valve replacement (AVR), the adjusted hazard ratio (95% confidence interval) at 5 years for heart failure with a PPM mismatch was 1.64 (1.01-2.56), $p = 0.047$, and for heart failure deaths was 2.09 (1.03-4.27), $p = 0.043$.[132] Reference to the packaging insert will guide the clinician as to whether intraoperative gradients and calculated valve areas are acceptable. In valve repair procedures, one must not only look for the cessation of regurgitation, but also ensure that there is no new stenosis. Measurement of valve gradients and orifice areas will help in this regard.

Valve repair for patients with endocarditis presents all of the aforementioned hemodynamic considerations in addition to the frequently septic condition of the patient (**Fig. 52-16**). Patients with endocarditis usually have acute regurgitant lesions and present in heart failure. The in-hospital mortality for acute endocarditis is 20%, and 82% of patients have endocarditis of a native heart valve.[133] The early predictors of in-hospital mortality include embolic events, diabetes mellitus, *Staphylococcus aureus*, and APACHE II score. The use of intraoperative TEE is especially helpful in the diagnosis of endocarditis and quantification of the valve defect. Valve surgery reduces 6-month mortality. In a study by Iung et al, 513 patients

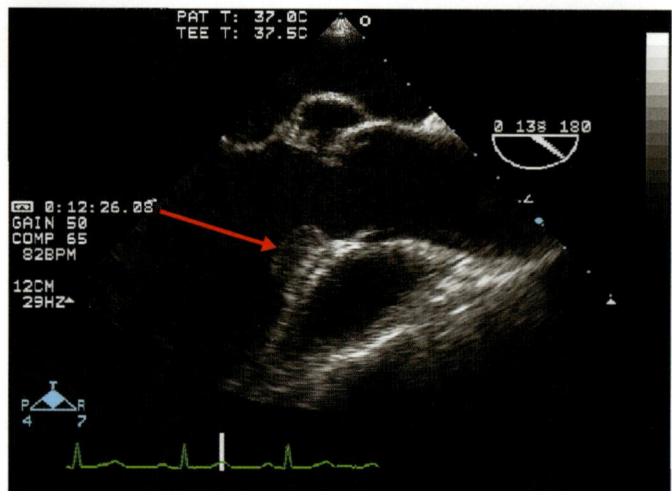

FIGURE 52-16. Intraoperative transesophageal midesophageal aortic valve (AV) long-axis view demonstrating an AV vegetation and abscess formation (*arrow*) in a patient who presented with sepsis.

with complicated left-sided infective endocarditis were treated with antibiotics; 45% underwent valve surgery and 55% received medical therapy alone.[134] The 6-month mortality was 16% in the surgery group compared to 33% in the medical group, $p < 0.01$. Patients with the most severe heart failure demonstrated the greatest reduction in mortality with surgery (14% vs 51%, $p = 0.001$).[134]

There are significant data to support valve repair and replacement in patients with heart valve disease over medical management.[115,135] After surgery for AS, initial remodeling of the heart is associated with subsequent LV mass reduction.[136-138] Between 1986 and 2001, 1410 patients had surgery for severe AI, of whom 160 (11%) had valve repair.[139] There was 1 operative death (0.6%), and 2 patients required early re-repair. At 7 years after repair, the survival was 89% and the reoperation rate on the AV was 15%.[139]

Patients with a history of MR often experience symptomatic relief and improvement in LVEF postoperatively.[140] Although there is known early mortality with heart valve surgery, the long-term benefit remains superior to medical management. As the population ages, more patients will present for valve procedures. Although advancing age is associated with poor outcome, there is no upper limit of age at which time valve surgery is contraindicated. In summary, these data and others indicate that surgery offers an opportunity for improved mortality, symptomatic relief, and hemodynamic improvement in nearly all patients with valve dysfunction.

Percutaneous approaches to valve repair and replacement are becoming more popular, especially in higher-risk populations.[141-144] It is unknown what impact percutaneous valves and other nonconventional valve repair procedures will have on the volume of heart valve surgeries. Anesthetic management is complicated by the duration of the procedures, the interruption of flow during deployments, and rhythm disturbances.[145] In such cases, all of the hemodynamic principles described above apply. In addition, advanced competency in perioperative TEE is required for both percutaneous AV replacement procedures (**Fig. 52-17**) and percutaneous mitral annular reduction for mitral regurgitation, as well as endovascular mitral valve repair.[146]

ANESTHETIC CONSIDERATIONS FOR AORTIC SURGERY

Thoracic aortic diseases are generally surgical problems (**Table 52-5**).[147] The most common operations performed on the thoracic aorta are repair of aortic dissection, aortic aneurysm, traumatic aortic injury, and aortic coarctation. Operative repairs involving the aortic root, ascending aorta, or transverse aortic arch typically are approached through a median sternotomy. Operative repairs involving the distal aortic arch or descending thoracic and thoracoabdominal aorta typically are approached through a left thoracotomy or thoracoabdominal incision.

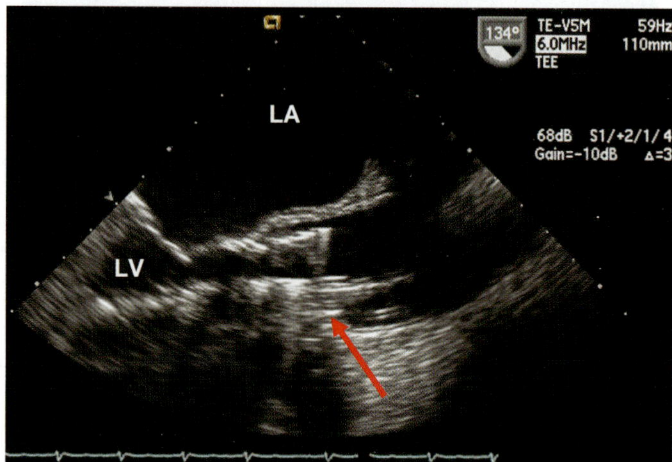

A

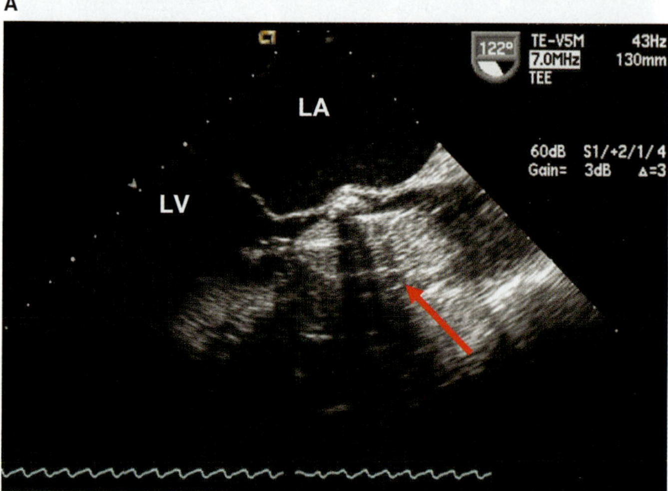

B

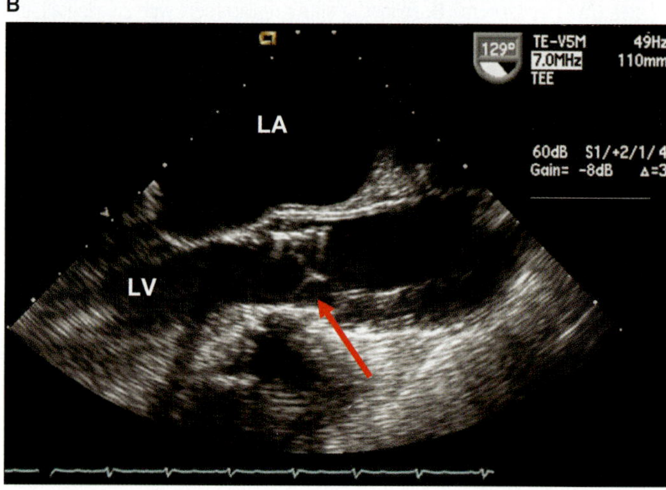

C

FIGURE 52-17. Sequential transesophageal midesophageal aortic valve (AV) long-axis views during a percutaneous aortic valve replacement procedure. **A.** Catheter (*arrow*) positioned across the AV prior to prosthetic valve deployment. **B.** Deployment of prosthetic valve (arrow). **C.** Prosthetic aortic valve (*arrow*) in position. LA, left atrium; LV, left ventricle.

TABLE 52-5 Diseases of the Thoracic Aorta That Are Amenable to Surgical Treatment

Aneurysm
Congenital or developmental Marfan, Ehlers-Danlos, Loeys-Dietz, Turner syndrome Familial thoracic aortic aneurysm or dissection Bicuspid aortic valve
Degenerative Cystic medial degeneration Annuloaortic ectasia Atherosclerotic
Traumatic Blunt and penetrating trauma
Inflammatory Takayasu arteritis, Behçet syndrome, Kawasaki disease Microvascular diseases (polyarteritis) Giant cell arteritis Ankylosing spondylitis (spondyloarthropathies)
Infectious (mycotic) Bacterial, fungal, spirochetal, viral
Mechanical Poststenotic, associated with arteriovenous fistula
Anastomotic (postarteriotomy)
Pseudoaneurysm
Aortic dissection Stanford type A Stanford type B
Intramural hematoma
Penetrating atherosclerotic ulcer
Atherosclerotic disease
Traumatic aortic injury
Aortic coarctation

Adapted from Kouchoukos NT, Dougenis D. Surgery of the thoracic aorta. *N Engl J Med.* 1997;336:1876-1888. Copyright 1997 Massachusetts Medical Society. Adapted with permission.

Endovascular stent graft techniques for repair of descending thoracic aortic aneurysm (TAA) and dissection have been developed that are accomplished by access through the femoral or iliac arteries.[148,149] Hybrid repairs that combine both endovascular and open techniques with extra-anatomic bypass of aortic branch vessels have also been developed for the treatment of aortic arch aneurysms.[150]

Specialized anesthetic management of patients undergoing thoracic aortic operations has contributed to the overall success of these operations and requires knowledge of several unique techniques that are practiced routinely in few other areas of medicine. Clinical application of TEE and ultrasound imaging performed by the anesthesiologist provides a means to emergently diagnose acute aortic syndromes, identify associated life-threatening complications, and detect cerebral malperfusion, permitting early surgical intervention and treatment.[147,151] The process of repairing or replacing a portion of the thoracic aorta typically requires the temporary or permanent interruption of blood flow through the aorta or its major branch vessels, creating the potential for ischemia or infarction of almost any major organ system. Techniques to protect organs during temporary interruption of blood flow in the thoracic aorta include deep hypothermic circulatory arrest (DHCA), selective antegrade cerebral perfusion, retrograde cerebral perfusion, and partial left heart bypass for distal aortic perfusion. Intraoperative neurophysiologic monitoring and lumbar cerebrospinal fluid (CSF) drainage are recognized techniques commonly used for repairs involving the descending thoracic or thoracoabdominal aorta to decrease the risk of spinal cord ischemia and infarction.

TABLE 52-6 Indications for Surgical Repair of Thoracic Aortic Aneurysm

	Condition
Ascending Aortic Diameter (cm)	
≥4.5	Marfan syndrome, collagen vascular disease, familial aortic dissection, bicuspid aortic valve
≥4.5	Requiring CABG or valve procedure
≥5.5	Any patient
Descending Aortic Diameter (cm)	
≥5.5	Chronic dissection, Marfan syndrome, or connective tissue disorder
≥5.5	Endovascular stent graft repair, saccular aneurysm
≥6.0	Any patient

THORACIC AORTIC ANEURYSM

Aortic aneurysm is a dilation of the aorta containing all 3 layers of the vessel wall that has a diameter at least 1.5 times that of the normal diameter of the corresponding aortic segment. TAAs are common. They are detected in 10% of autopsies, have an incidence of 5.9 per 100 000 person-years, and are the most common reason for thoracic aortic operation.[152] TAAs can be characterized by etiology, location, diameter, and extent of aortic involvement. Aortic pseudoaneurysms are caused by a contained rupture of the aorta or arise from intimal disruptions, penetrating atherosclerotic ulcers, or partial dehiscence of the suture line at the site of a previous aortic vascular graft. Aortic aneurysms can be associated with dissection of the vessel wall.

Surgical repair of TAAs is performed for acute rupture, AI, refractory pain, or to prevent eventual rupture. Rupture of the aortic root or proximal ascending aorta will cause cardiac tamponade because the first several centimeters of the ascending aorta lies within the pericardial sac. Dilation of the proximal ascending aorta may cause AI by distortion of the aortic root and outward tethering of the AV cusps.[152,153] Because the risk of aortic rupture or dissection is associated with aneurysm size, aortic diameter is commonly used as a clinical indication for elective repair (**Table 52-6**). In general, indications for operative repair are ascending aortic aneurysm diameter 4.5 cm or greater in patients with Marfan syndrome, collagen vascular disease, bicuspid AV, or a family history of aneurysm; ascending aortic aneurysm diameter 4.5 cm or greater in patients requiring CABG or valve procedures; ascending aortic aneurysm diameter 5.5 cm or greater in any patient; symptomatic aneurysms; or aneurysm growth rate greater than 0.5 cm per year.[147,154-156] Because the operative risks associated with open repair of the descending thoracic aorta is greater, endovascular repairs should be considered, and repair is usually not performed until an aneurysm size of 5.5 to 6.0 cm is reached.[147,155,156] Very large aneurysms of the ascending aorta, aortic arch, or descending thoracic aorta may produce a mediastinal mass effect, causing extrinsic compression of the trachea, left mainstem bronchus, right PA, RV outflow tract, or esophagus (**Fig. 52-18**). In contrast to patients with collagen vascular or familial aortic aneurysms, patients with atherosclerotic aneurysms generally are elderly and have more comorbid conditions and peripheral vascular disease.

ASCENDING AORTA AND AORTIC ARCH ANEURYSM

Aortic aneurysms limited to the aortic root and proximal ascending aorta can be repaired using standard CPB with cannulation of the aneurysm, ascending aorta, or femoral artery and cross-clamping of the distal ascending aorta. Based on assessment of the AV, the AV may

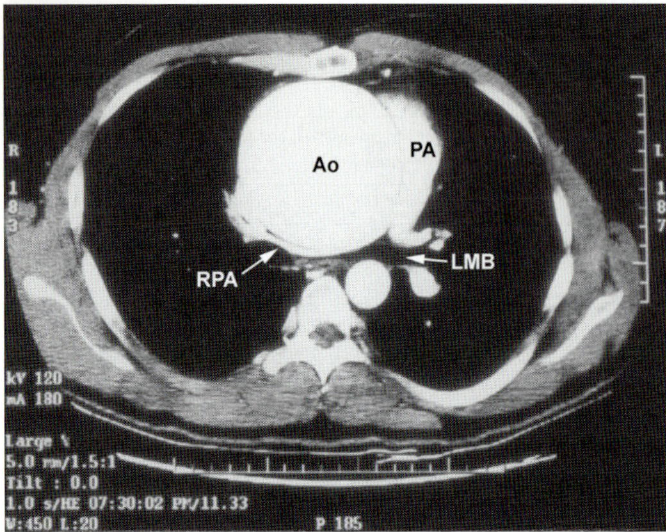

FIGURE 52-18. CT angiogram of the chest showing a large ascending aortic aneurysm (Ao) causing compression of the right pulmonary artery (RPA), distal trachea, and left mainstem bronchus (LMB). PA, main pulmonary artery.

be replaced, resuspended, or reimplanted within the prosthetic vascular graft. Replacement of the aortic root requires reimplantation of the right and left coronary arteries. Intraoperative TEE is useful for evaluating the native AV prior to repair and for determining the presence of residual AI after valve-sparing operations.

Operative repair of aortic aneurysms that extend into or involve the aortic arch require temporary interruption of cerebral perfusion. The primary technique used to protect the brain from ischemic injury in the absence of cerebral blood flow is DHCA. In the conduct of DHCA, achieving a satisfactory level of hypothermia is considered the most important intervention for brain protection, but the optimal temperature for DHCA, best site for temperature measurement, and safe duration of DHCA have not been established. EEG during the conduct of DHCA has demonstrated that the average nasopharyngeal temperature required to produce electrocortical silence was approximately 18°C, but a nasopharyngeal temperature of 12.1°C or cooling on CPB for at least 50 minutes was necessary to achieve electrocortical silence in 95% of patients (**Fig. 52-19**).[157] Clinical studies indicate that the cerebral metabolic rate decreases by a factor of approximately 2.6 for each 10°C decrease in temperature (Q_{10} ratio for adults).[158] Assuming the brain can tolerate an ischemic period of approximately 3 to 5 minutes at 37°C, the reduction in cerebral metabolism at a temperature of 17°C would predict that the brain should tolerate approximately 20 to 34 minutes of ischemia. Clinical studies support this prediction and have detected the onset of neuronal ischemia at approximately 18 minutes after DHCA (**Fig. 52-20**).[159] Other studies have indicated that postoperative neurocognitive dysfunction was more frequent when DHCA duration exceeded 25 minutes.[160]

Strategies for improving the safety of DHCA to facilitate operations requiring temporary interruption of blood flow in the aortic arch include techniques to provide retrograde cerebral perfusion (RCP) or selective antegrade cerebral perfusion. Retrograde cerebral perfusion can be provided immediately after initiation of DHCA by infusing cold oxygenated blood into the superior vena cava at flow rates averaging 150 to 250 mL/min.[161] During RCP, the pressure within the superior vena cava is generally maintained at or below 25 mm Hg to decrease the risk of cerebral edema, the aortic arch is opened to atmospheric pressure to prevent pressurization of the arterial system, and the patient is positioned in an 8- to 10-degree Trendelenburg to prevent air entry into the aortic arch branch vessels. Experimental and clinical studies have demonstrated that RCP via the superior vena cava provides perfusion to the brain, but existing evidence indicated that the flow achieved with RCP was insufficient to prevent cerebral ischemia.[161] Nevertheless, advocates of RCP argue that even some substrate delivery increases the margin of safety of DHCA, that cerebral hypothermia is maintained with RCP, and that RCP decreases the risk of cerebral embolization by flushing out particulate matter in the cerebral arteries prior to resumption of antegrade cerebral perfusion.

Selective antegrade cerebral perfusion can be accomplished by arterial cannulation and perfusion of the axillary artery, innominate artery, subclavian artery, or even the internal carotid arteries.[162,163] Antegrade perfusion into a single arch branch vessel provides flow to the contralateral cerebral hemisphere through a functional circle of Willis, but contralateral perfusion pressures may vary among patients.[163] Selective antegrade cerebral perfusion is generally performed in combination with deep hypothermia for operations where the duration of DHCA is anticipated to exceed 30 minutes. Flow rates for antegrade cerebral perfusion typically range from 400 to 1000 mL/min at radial artery pressures of 50 to 80 mm Hg.

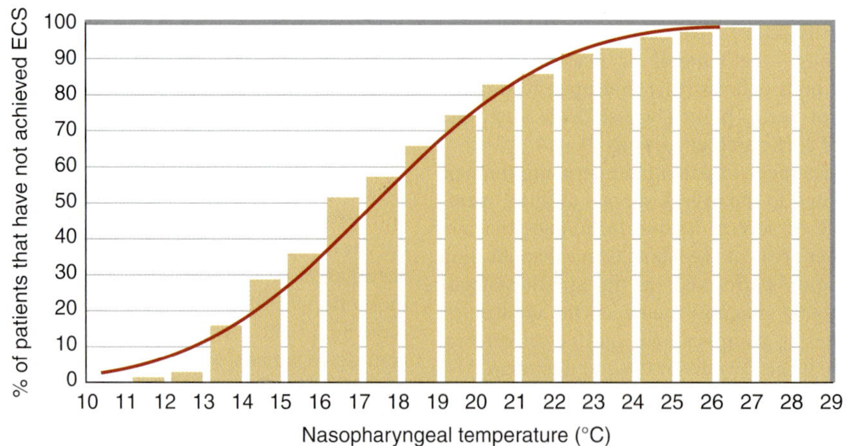

FIGURE 52-19. Relationship between electroencephalographic (EEG) activity and nasopharyngeal temperature prior to deep hypothermic circulatory arrest in 109 patients undergoing thoracic aortic operations requiring circulatory arrest. Electrocortical silence (ECS) was achieved by EEG in all patients after 50 minutes of cooling or at a nasopharyngeal temperature of 12.5°C. At a nasopharyngeal temperature of 18°C, only 50% of patients had electrocortical silence by EEG. [Adapted from Stecker MM, Cheung AT, Pochettino A, et al. Deep hypothermic circulatory arrest: I. Effects of cooling on electroencephalogram and evoked potentials. *Ann Thorac Surg.* 2001;71:14-21. Copyright Elsevier 2001.]

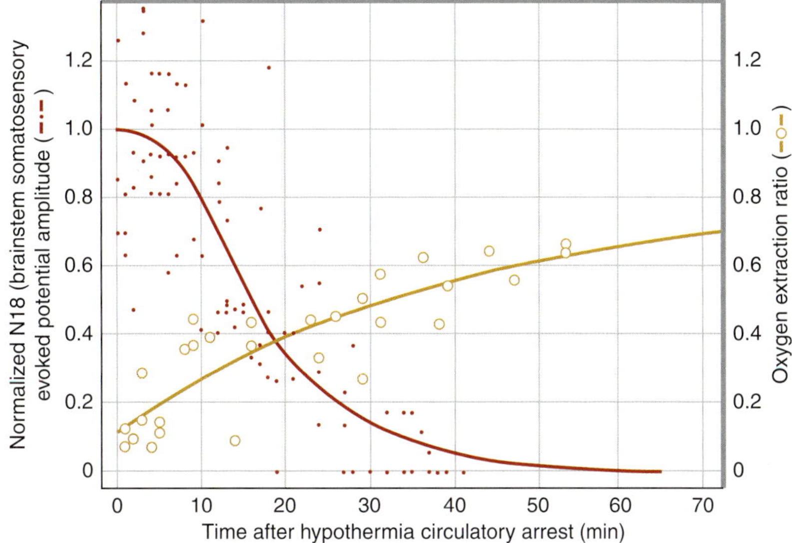

FIGURE 52-20. Changes in brainstem (N18) somatosensory evoked potential amplitudes after initiation of deep hypothermic circulatory arrest with retrograde cerebral perfusion superimposed on the change in brain oxygen extraction ratio (OER) in patients during retrograde cerebral perfusion (O; n = 19). The N18 somatosensory evoked potential decayed to half its original amplitude at 16 minutes after interruption of antegrade cerebral perfusion. OER decreased to half its maximal value of 0.66, also at 16 minutes after interruption of antegrade cerebral perfusion. [Adapted from Cheung AT, Bavaria JE, Pochettino A, et al. Oxygen delivery during retrograde cerebral perfusion in humans. *Anesth Analg.* 1999;88:8-15, with permission.]

Clinical studies supporting the efficacy of antegrade cerebral perfusion demonstrated acceptable outcomes despite antegrade cerebral perfusion duration times greater than 45 minutes at a temperature of 25°C.[163]

Attempts to further improve the safety of DHCA by manipulating pH, blood viscosity, or hemoglobin concentration or by administration of pharmacologic agents often are practiced, but no clinical evidence has supported the efficacy of these other interventions. Barbiturates or other central nervous system depressants are sometimes administered in an effort to decrease cerebral oxygen demands. Glucocorticoids, magnesium sulfate, lidocaine, and mannitol are sometimes administered in an effort to protect against cerebral and end-organ injury. In general, the existing evidence suggests that pharmacologic neuroprotection is unproven and should not be considered a substitute for hypothermia or selective antegrade cerebral perfusion to protect against cerebral ischemia during operative repairs of the aortic arch.

DESCENDING THORACIC AND THORACOABDOMINAL AORTIC ANEURYSM

Classification of TAAs and thoracoabdominal aortic aneurysms (TAAAs) according to anatomic extent provides a useful guide to surgical approaches, anesthetic management, and estimate of perioperative mortality and postoperative paraplegia associated with operative repair (**Table 52-7**).[147,164,165] In the Crawford classification, extent I TAAA involves the entire descending thoracic aorta from the origin of the left subclavian artery to the level of the diaphragm; extent II TAAA involves the entire descending thoracic aorta with extension across the diaphragm through the abdominal aorta to the aortic bifurcation; extent III TAAA involves the distal half of the descending thoracic aorta and most of the abdominal aorta; and extent IV TAAAs are confined to the upper abdominal aorta (**Fig. 52-21**). Isolated TAAs are those confined to the descending thoracic aorta between the origin of the left subclavian artery and the diaphragm. TAAAs can be further distinguished into those with dissection and those without dissection.

Operative repair of TAAA with an interposition tube graft is approached through a left thoracoabdominal incision and requires single-lung ventilation. Repairs originally were accomplished by cross-clamping the thoracic aorta proximal to the aneurysm. Modifications of this technique included passive arterial shunting (Gott shunt) or partial left heart bypass using extracorporeal circulation to provide distal aortic perfusion while the proximal descending thoracic aorta was cross-clamped.[166] CPB with DHCA may be necessary for aneurysms that extend into the distal aortic arch,[167,168] Endovascular stent graft repair has become an option for repair of isolated TAA and TAAA.[148,149,165] One of the major complications of operative repair is spinal cord ischemia or infarction resulting in postoperative paraplegia. The risk of spinal cord ischemia is a consequence of

TABLE 52-7 Mortality and Paraplegia After Thoracic and Thoracoabdominal Aortic Aneurysm Repair

Aneurysm Extent[a]	n	30-Day Mortality	1-Year Mortality	Spinal Cord Ischemia
Open Surgical Repair				
Isolated TAA	136	8 (4%)	15 (11%)	1 (1%)
Crawford extent I	51	1 (2%)	2 (4%)	7 (14%)
Crawford extent II	59	10 (17%)	13 (22%)	13 (22%)
Crawford extent III	62	8 (12%)	13 (21%)	6 (10%)
Crawford extent IV	64	4 (6%)	16 (22%)	1 (2%)
Total Open Surgical Repair	372	31 (7%)	59 (15%)	28 (8%)
Endovascular Repair				
Isolated TAA	163	8 (5%)	20 (12%)	1 (1%)
Crawford extent I	82	6 (7%)	15 (19%)	8 (10%)
Crawford extent II	16	1 (6%)	5 (36%)	3 (19%)
Crawford extent III	22	2 (9%)	7 (34%)	1 (5%)
Crawford extent IV	69	3 (4%)	8 (12%)	2 (3%)
Total Endovascular Repair	352	20 (6%)	55 (16%)	15 (4%)

[a]See text for description of classification of aneurysm extent.

Data from Greenberg RK, Lu Q, Roselli EE, et al. Contemporary analysis of descending thoracic and thoracoabdominal aneurysm repair: a comparison of endovascular and open techniques. *Circulation.* 2008;118:808-817.

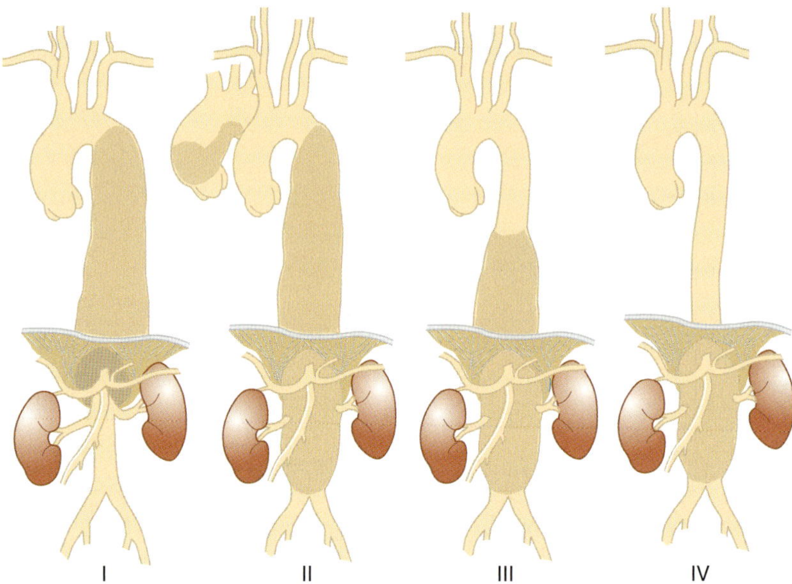

FIGURE 52-21. Crawford classification of thoracoabdominal aortic aneurysm extent. [From Coselli JS. Descending thoracoabdominal aortic aneurysms. In Edmunds LH, ed. *Cardiac Surgery in the Adult*. New York, NY: McGraw-Hill; 1997:1232, with permission.]

the interruption of distal aortic perfusion or the sacrifice of intercostal, lumbar, and sacral artery branches that provide collateral flow supplying the spinal cord. Strategies to prevent, detect, and treat spinal cord ischemia are important aspects in the anesthetic management of patients undergoing TAA and TAAA repair. Spinal cord protection strategies include deliberate hypothermia, surgical techniques to minimize ischemia time, arterial pressure augmentation, avoiding hypotension, lumbar CSF drainage, and perioperative neurophysiologic monitoring of spinal cord function.[147] Deliberate hypothermia is an established technique to protect against neuronal ischemia and can be accomplished by passive cooling to 32°C, active cooling using extracorporeal circulation, or selective cooling by infusion of cold saline into the epidural space (**Table 52-8**).[147,168,169] Passive arterial shunting using an ascending aorta to distal aortic shunt or partial left heart bypass using extracorporeal circulation to direct blood from the LA to the femoral artery can be used to provide distal aortic perfusion during construction of the proximal aortic anastomosis and decreases the duration of lower body ischemia. While the descending aorta is cross-clamped, spinal cord perfusion via the vertebral arteries can be augmented by maintaining the proximal aortic pressure at or above 90 mm Hg. Intraoperative neurophysiologic monitoring of somatosensory evoked or motor evoked potentials from the posterior tibial nerves has been advocated for detection of spinal cord ischemia during operation in the anesthetized patient, to permit early intervention or to prompt the reattachment of intercostal artery branches.[170,171] Pharmacologic agents such as glucocorticoids or even naloxone have been administered for spinal cord protection, but their efficacy remains unproven. Patients with delayed-onset paraplegia or paraparesis after TAA, TAAA, or endovascular stent graft repair often respond to strategies to improve spinal cord perfusion by increasing the arterial pressure and drainage of CSF.[168,169] One rationale for the routine use of lumbar CSF drainage is that the lumbar CSF pressure may increase during repair as a consequence of aortic cross-clamping or spinal cord edema during reperfusion. Hypotension associated with spinal cord ischemia may be a consequence of general anesthesia, regional anesthesia, blood loss, vasodilation, or even neurogenic shock from spinal cord ischemia and requires prompt treatment. The effectiveness of lumbar CSF drainage for treatment of spinal cord ischemia may be improved when combined with arterial pressure augmentation. Interventions to increase spinal cord perfusion pressure appear to be most effective when applied immediately upon detection of spinal cord ischemia. The effectiveness of lumbar CSF drainage as a therapeutic adjunct to decrease the risk of spinal cord ischemia is supported by several randomized controlled trials, case series, and meta-analyses.[172-174] Complications of lumbar CSF drainage are uncommon and include intracranial hypotension, subdural hematoma, catheter fracture, meningitis, and hemorrhagic complications.[175-177] Precise

TABLE 52-8 Strategies to Decrease the Risk of Paraplegia From Spinal Cord Ischemia After Thoracic or Thoracoabdominal Aortic Procedures
Distal Aortic Perfusion
Passive shunt (Gott)
Partial left heart bypass
Partial cardiopulmonary bypass
Minimize aortic cross clamp time
Deliberate Hypothermia
Mild to moderate systemic hypothermia (32°C-35°C)
Deep hypothermic circulatory arrest (14°C-18°C)
Selective spinal cord hypothermia (epidural cooling, 25°C)
Increase Spinal Cord Perfusion Pressure
Reimplantation of critical intercostal and segmental arterial branches
Lumbar cerebrospinal fluid (CSF) drainage (CSF pressure ≤10 mm Hg)
Arterial pressure augmentation (mean arterial pressure ≥85 mm Hg)
Avoid hypotension
Intraoperative Monitoring of Lower Extremity Neurophysiologic Function
Somatosensory evoked potentials
Motor evoked potentials
Postoperative Neurologic Assessment for Early Detection of Delayed-Onset Paraplegia
Serial neurologic examination
Pharmacologic Neuroprotection
Glucocorticoid
Barbiturate or central nervous system depressants
Magnesium sulfate
Mannitol
Naloxone
Lidocaine
Intrathecal papaverine

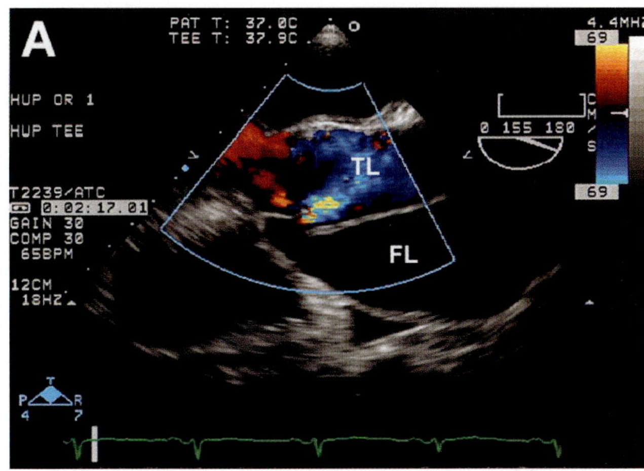

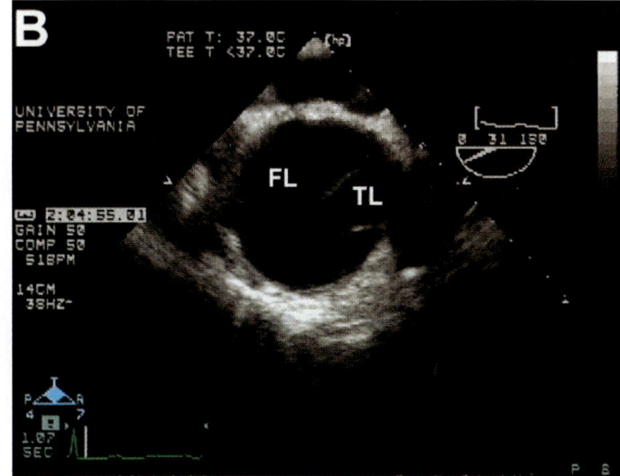

FIGURE 52-22. Transesophageal midesophageal long-axis view of the aortic valve (**A**) and short-axis views of the ascending aorta (**B**) in a patient with a type A aortic dissection. An intimal flap separating the true lumen (TL) of the aorta from the false lumen (FL) was shown in the aortic root and ascending aorta. Extension of the dissection into the aortic root may cause aortic regurgitation or coronary insufficiency.

monitoring of CSF pressure, controlled drainage of CSF to maintain a lumbar CSF pressure of at least 10 mm Hg, and supervised insertion and removal of catheters may decrease the risk of complications. Considering the morbidity associated with paraplegia, the application of lumbar CSF drainage, arterial pressure augmentation, and neurophysiologic monitoring can be justified in patients at risk for postoperative spinal cord ischemia.[147] Patients at risk for spinal cord ischemia include those undergoing Crawford extent I, II, and III open TAAA repair and endovascular stent graft repairs with prior distal aortic operations.[165,169,172]

AORTIC DISSECTION

Aortic dissection evolves from a tear in the intima that allows blood to enter the medial layer of the vessel, causing the intima to separate or dissect circumferentially and longitudinally within the aorta. Aortic dissection is diagnosed by imaging studies demonstrating a true and a false lumen separated by an intimal flap within the aorta (**Fig. 52-22**).[178,179] Aortic intramural hematoma is a variant of aortic dissection characterized by hemorrhage into the medial layer producing circumferential thickening of the aortic wall.[180] Aortic dissection affects a wide demographic population and age range. The most common associated diseases are hypertension, atherosclerosis, and cystic medial degeneration. Other associated conditions include collagen vascular disease, familial aortic dissection, bicuspid AV, aortic coarctation, pregnancy, cocaine abuse, arteritis, and aortic trauma. Early complications of aortic dissection include dissection into aortic branch vessels causing malperfusion, resulting in myocardial, cerebral, mesenteric, or limb ischemia (**Table 52-9**). Dissection into the aortic root may cause acute aortic regurgitation. Rupture of the proximal ascending aorta causes cardiac tamponade. Dilation and expansion in the diameter of the aorta over time as a consequence of a weakened vessel wall is a long-term complication of aortic dissection.

Aortic dissection is classified according to location. Dissections involving the ascending aorta and aortic arch are classified as Stanford type A or DeBakey type I or II. Dissections confined to the descending aorta are classified as Stanford type B or DeBakey type III (**Fig. 52-23**). Aortic dissections involving the ascending aorta (Stanford type A or DeBakey type I or II) are considered surgical emergencies. According to an international registry for acute aortic dissection, mortality rates for patients with Stanford type A aortic dissection managed without surgery was approximately 1% to 2% per hour following the initial symptom onset for the first 48 hours, 60% by day 6, 74% by 2 weeks, and 91% by 6 months.[181] When managed with surgery, the mortality rate for type A aortic dissection was 26% (**Fig. 52-24**).[181] Aortic dissections confined to the descending thoracic aorta (Stanford type B) are considered surgical emergencies only if there is evidence of a life-threatening complication such as malperfusion or aortic rupture. Mortality in patients with acute type B aortic dissection managed surgically was 31.4% at 30 days compared to a mortality rate of 10.7% at 30 days in medically managed patients (see Fig. 52-24).[181]

Acute management of patients with suspected aortic dissections requires establishing the diagnosis, distinguishing Stanford type A from Stanford type B aortic dissection, and detecting malperfusion or rupture. In an international registry of aortic dissection, the initial diagnosis was established by computed tomography in 61% of patients.[179] Echocardiography was used as the initial diagnostic technique in 33% of cases but was used as a secondary diagnostic technique in 56% of cases.[179] TEE is useful for intraoperative diagnosis and classification of dissection in unstable patients. Intraoperative TEE also is useful for detecting AI, cardiac tamponade, and myocardial ischemia. Surgery for type A aortic dissection involves replacement of the ascending aorta or aortic arch together with AV repair or replacement. Patients with type B aortic dissection are preferentially

TABLE 52-9 Complications of Acute Stanford Type A Aortic Dissection (n = 513)

Complications	Percent
All neurologic defects	18.0
Coma/altered consciousness	14.0
Myocardial ischemia/infarction	10.0
Limb ischemia	10.0
Mesenteric ischemia/infarction	4.0
Acute renal failure	6.2
Hypotension	26.0
Cardiac tamponade	17.0
Mortality	30.0

Adapted from Bossone E, Rampoldi V, Nienaber CA, et al. Usefulness of pulse deficit to predict in-hospital complications and mortality in patients with acute type A aortic dissection. *Am J Cardiol.* 2002;89:851-855. Copyright Elsevier 2002.

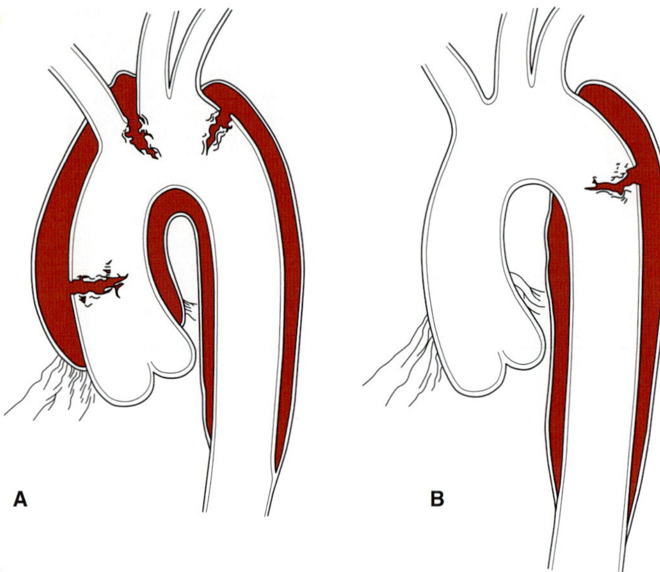

FIGURE 52-23. Stanford classification of aortic dissection. In type A aortic dissection, the ascending aorta is dissected regardless of the location or number of intimal tears (**A**). In type B aortic dissection, the dissection is limited to the descending aorta (**B**) distal to the origin of the left subclavian artery. [Reprinted with permission from Daily PO, Trueblood HW, Stinson EB, et al. Management of acute aortic dissections. *Ann Thorac Surg.* 1970;10:237-247.]

managed medically unless they have evidence of aortic rupture or malperfusion. Endovascular stent graft repair has become an alternative to open repair in patients with type B aortic dissection complicated by malperfusion or rupture.[149] The anesthetic management of operations for the repair of type A aortic dissection is similar to the management of patients undergoing repair of ascending aortic and arch aneurysms, and typically requires temporary interruption of cerebral perfusion and DHCA. A rare but lethal complication of CPB in patients with aortic dissection is acute cerebral malperfusion caused by inadvertent cannulation of the false lumen of the aorta or compression of the true lumen by expansion of the false lumen.[182] This complication can be detected by intraoperative TEE evaluation of blood flow in the aorta and ultrasound confirmation of carotid artery flow during initiation of CPB. Treatment consists of immediate discontinuation of CPB, cannulation of the contralateral femoral artery for CPB, or open fenestration of the intimal flap within the aorta. The anesthetic management of operations for type B aortic dissections requires the same strategies and techniques used for patients undergoing TAA and TAAA repair.

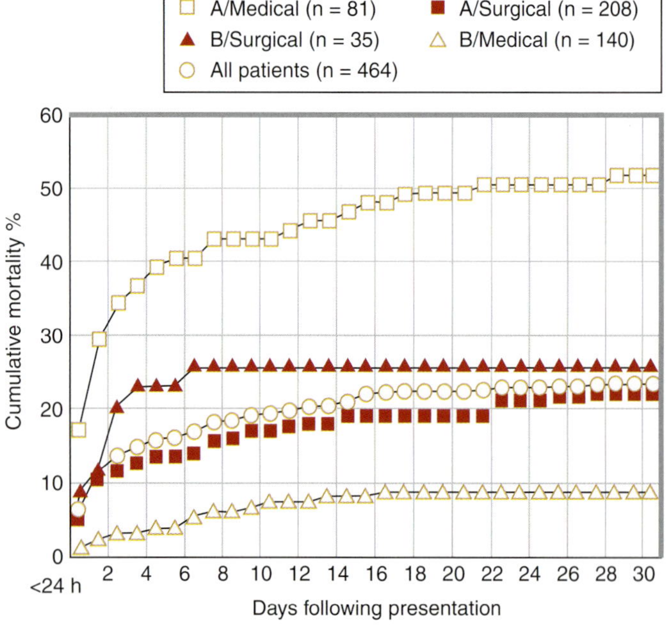

FIGURE 52-24. Thirty-day mortality in 464 patients from the International Registry of Aortic Dissection (IRAD) stratified by medical and surgical treatment in both type A and type B aortic dissection. [From Nienaber CA, Eagle KA. Aortic dissection: new frontiers in diagnosis and management: part I. From etiology to diagnostic strategies. *Circulation.* 2003;108:628-635, with permission.]

CARDIAC ANESTHESIA FOR HEART FAILURE AND VENTRICULAR ASSIST DEVICES

BRIEF HISTORY OF VENTRICULAR ASSIST DEVICES

The first left ventricular assist device (LVAD) was implanted by DeBakey in 1966 as a "bridge to recovery" in a patient suffering from postcardiotomy cardiogenic shock.[183] The decompressed and rested native ventricle recovered after 6 days of support and the device was explanted. Barnard performed the first orthotopic cardiac transplantation a year later. During the 1970s the development of heart transplantation as a viable therapy for end-stage heart failure was hindered by the use of nonspecific immunosuppressive agents, which resulted in patient deaths from opportunistic infections. By the early 1980s, with the introduction of cyclosporine, a specific T-cell inhibitor, heart transplantation became a viable therapy for end-stage heart failure with risk-adjusted survival rates equaling 50% at 10 years.[184] Ventricular assist devices subsequently assumed a new role as a "bridge to transplant." End-stage heart failure patients on transplant waiting lists, if supported by an assist device prior to transplantation, could wait longer, recover secondary organ function, be discharged home, and enjoy improved survival after transplantation.[185] Over 500 000 Americans are diagnosed each year with heart failure, but only 2200 donor hearts become available each year worldwide for transplantation.[186] In the late 1990s the REMATCH (Randomized Evaluation of Mechanical Assistance for the Treatment of Congestive Heart Failure) trial demonstrated that the HeartMate pulsatile pneumatic (Thoratec Corporation, Pleasantville, California) LVADs could be used as an alternative to transplantation (ie, "destination therapy") in end-stage heart failure patients who were not candidates for transplantation. Use of the device conferred a survival and quality-of-life benefit when compared to optimal medical therapy. Over the next decade LVAD technology continued to evolve and the next-generation continuous-flow LVADs were smaller and more durable than their pulsatile predecessors. An original randomized study (Clinical Trials.gov NCT00121485) by Slaughter et al demonstrated superiority of continuous-flow over pneumatic LVADs at 2 years in patients receiving an LVAD for destination therapy.[187] Fifty-eight percent of end-stage heart failure patients receiving the continuous-flow HeartMate II LVAD were alive after 2 years versus 23% for pulsatile pneumatic (HeartMate XVE) versus 8% for medical therapy. Actuarial–survival analysis performed by means of the Kaplan-Meier method demonstrated a 2-fold increase in survival with continuous-flow devices over pulsatile pneumonic, and a 4-fold increase in survival over optimal medical therapy.

In 2009 the PROTECT I trial demonstrated yet another application of LVAD technology. The Impella RECOVER LP 2.5 System (Abiomed Inc, Danvers, Massachusetts) could be delivered via a catheter-based technique and provide temporary support (averaging 2 h) during high-risk percutaneous coronary intervention (PCI) in patients with unprotected left main coronary artery disease or last patent coronary conduit.[188] The VAD is used to maintain a mean arterial blood pressure above 60 mm Hg during occlusion of the target vessel. The PROTECT II trial is designed to compare the use of the Impella 2.5 LVAD versus IABP for high-risk PCI. However, the true benefit of left main PCI has yet to be validated using adequately powered studies.

Most VADs placed in community hospitals are implanted for rapid stabilization of patients in acute cardiogenic shock who, despite multiple inotrope therapy and insertion of intra-aortic balloon pump, continue to deteriorate. These VADs are generally implanted as a "bridge to a bridge" or a "bridge to decision," or simply a "bridge to explantation" in that they are meant to serve as a short-term solution to cardiogenic shock and resultant multisystem organ failure until decisions can be made regarding possible cardiac recovery, neurologic status, feasibility of transfer to a tertiary facility for long-term assist device implantation, and possible heart transplant.[189] A disadvantage of temporary support is that multiple surgeries and the need for anticoagulation are required. An advantage, at least in patients with multisystem organ failure or neurologic status that does not recover, is that permanent LVAD implantation is avoided. The cost of LVAD implantation and follow-up is estimated to be between $500,000 and $1.4 million per patient.[190] The Bio-Medicus systems (Medtronic Inc, Minneapolis, Minnesota), CentriMag (Levitronix LLC, Waltham, Massachusetts), and ABIOMED devices have all demonstrated relative successes with 30-day survival rates ranging from 31% to 75%.[189,191,192] Extracorproal membrane oxygenation (ECMO) may also be used to support patients in acute cardiogenic shock. Hoefer et al reported a 50% mortality rate in patients with ECMO support who were bridged to permanent VAD implantation.[193] Which device is best for short-term support and which patients will benefit from the technology continue to be matters for debate.

GENERAL PRINCIPLES

In general VADs are pumps that collect blood returning to the heart and then eject it downstream of the failing ventricle. They differ from CPB and ECMO in that they do not provide any direct respiratory function. The goal of VAD implantation is to decompress the acutely ischemic failing or the chronically failing ventricle, thereby diminishing radius, wall tension, and oxygen consumption. The ventricle may recover while perfusion to the body is maintained by the assist device. For left ventricular support the inflow cannula is generally placed in either the left atrium (LA) or LV and drains into the device. Better drainage and decompression occur when the cannula is placed in the ventricular apex; however, postinfarction ventricular tissue may not be durable enough to hold sutures. Furthermore, LA inflow cannulation may result in a higher incidence of LV clot.[186,194] The outflow cannula is generally placed in the ascending aorta. Notable exceptions include the Jarvik 2000 in which the outflow cannula can be sutured to the descending aorta,[195] and the TandemHeart (CardiacAssist, Inc, Pittsburgh, Pennsylvania) in which the inflow cannula is in the LA and the outflow cannula is in the iliac artery (**Table 52-10**).[196] The Impella 2.5 catheter crosses the AV and aspirates blood from the LV and ejects it into the ascending aorta with the inflow and outflow orifices being contained in a single catheter. For RV support, blood is drained from the right atrium (RA) or ventricle to the pump and returned to the main pulmonary artery. The pumps come in 2 basic varieties: pulsatile and axial (continuous) flow.

HOW VADs ARE SELECTED

The duration of support, patient body habitus, ventricle(s) to be supported, surgical preference, and reliability are the main determinants for choosing a particular VAD (Table 52-10). Some devices, such as the pVAD and the Impella 2.5 device, are meant for short-term LV support and can be implanted percutaneously in the cardiac catheterization laboratory or operating room. These devices provide time to transfer the patient to a tertiary center, or may be used for support during high-risk interventions in the cardiac cath laboratory. The ABIOMED BVS 5000, CentriMag, and BioMedicus VADs provide an intermediate duration of support, from 7 to 14 days. They can support the right, left, or both ventricles. Because only a slit is made in the ventricle or atrium and a purse string suture is used to secure the inflow cannula, insertion of these VAD cannulas is less traumatic to the tissue, and explantation is much easier compared to the Thoratec or HeartMate devices in which the LV apex must be cored out in order to place the inflow cannula and upon explantation a patch repair of the apex made. The Thoratec (Thoratec Laboratories, Pleasantville, California) is the only Food and Drug Administration (FDA)–approved device that can provide long-term (months to years) *biventricular* support to serve as a bridge to transplant. It can be used to support the right, left, or both ventricles. The pneumatic HeartMate XVE provides only left ventricular support and provides long-term support as either a bridge to transplant or as destination therapy. Because the HeartMate XVE is implanted intracorporeally, in the left upper quadrant of the abdomen in the preperitoneal or intra-abdominal compartment, it is only suitable for patients with a body surface area greater than 1.8 m^2. The HeartMate II continuous-flow device may be used for long-term support in patients awaiting heart transplant[185] or as an alternative to the HeartMate XVE for destination therapy.[187] The advantages of the HeartMate II are that it can be implanted in patients whose body surface area is less than 1.8 m^2. It requires less dissection to implant than the HeartMate XVE. This may translate into lower infection rates. It has no bearings, and this design has translated into less mechanical failure, less need for reoperation, and higher 2-year survival rates when compared to the HeartMate XVE. In a study by Slaughter et al, 21 out of 59 HeartMate XVE pneumatic LVADs implanted required replacements because of bearing wear, valve malfunction, or infection.[187] In the same study, 13 out of 133 HeartMate II continuous-flow LVADs required replacement owing to breakage of the percutaneous lead (n = 11), pump thrombosis (n = 2), and outflow elbow disconnection (n = 1).[187] Pump thrombosis and thromboembolism are issues for both devices, but the HeartMate II requires higher levels of anticoagulation and is associated with an increased risk of bleeding secondary to anticoagulation. Continuous-flow pumps with diminished pulsatile flow have not been shown to have unfavorable effects on major organ function.[197]

MODES OF OPERATION

Most pneumatic VADs operate in a "volume mode" in which the VAD ejects as soon as the chamber is filled. VADs function best with slightly increased intravascular volume and slightly decreased intravascular resistance. Hypovolemia slows the rate of filling, thereby decreasing the number of pump cycles per minute and overall VAD output. Increased vascular resistance may impede VAD ejection, resulting in prolonged ejection or decreased chamber emptying and decreased pump output. Incomplete chamber emptying may result in blood stasis in the pump chamber with resultant thromboembolic risk. In the case of the LVAD, systemic vascular resistance is the main component of afterload, and for RVAD, pulmonary vascular resistance is the major determinant of afterload.

The ABIOMED pump fills by continuous gravity drainage. The pump will automatically eject when full. It is preprogrammed to deliver approximately 5 L/min of flow. There are no dials to adjust. Anticoagulation with heparin is mandatory to prevent thrombus formation on the mechanical valves in the pump. The goal activated clotting time (ACT) is between 180 and 200 seconds. ABIOMED filling is independent of the underlying cardiac rhythm. Patients with malignant arrhythmias with biventricular support will remain hemodynamically stable.

The Thoratec pump is filled by vacuum-assisted drainage. The pump can operate in 1 of 3 operating modes. In "volume mode" the pump will eject as soon as it is full-similar to the ABIOMED. In "asynchronous mode" the device operates in a fixed manner according to defined variables. The "external synchronization mode" is used to provide counterpulsation during device weaning. Anticoagulation is initially achieved with heparin with a goal ACT of between 180 and 200 seconds, but once the patient is tolerating oral medications, anticoagulation can be maintained with coumadin with a goal INR of 2.5 to 3.5.[198]

The HeartMate XVE pneumatic LVAD has an extremely sophisticated control algorithm that adjusts device output to the patient's needs. As long as intravascular volume and the RV are functioning properly, there is no need to adjust the control settings. The CentriMag continuous-flow VAD is based on the "bearingless motor" technology that combines the drive, magnetic bearing, and rotor function in a single unit. The motor generates the magnetic bearing force that levitates the

TABLE 52-10 Ventricular Assist Device Characteristics

Device	Pump Location	Ventricle Support and Duration	Pulsatile	Uses	Cannula Position	Device Output	Special Features
Impella *(ABIOMED)*	Intracorporeal	Left 7 d	No	Cardiogenic shock after surgery BTR, BTT	LV: either directly (recover LD 5.0) or percutaneously (2.5) via groin and positioned across the AV in LV	Max: 2.5 L/min for perc. (2.5) to the 5 L/min for (5.0)	Microaxial pump at distal tip of 9-Fr catheter Can be inserted percutaneously Potential for MS caused by catheter malposition preventing anterior MV leaflet opening
TandemHeart pVAD *(Cardiac Assist Inc.)*	Extracorporeal	Left 14 d	No	BTB, BTR	Inserted percutaneously via FV, advanced across the interatrial septum into LA Drains oxygenated blood from LA and propels it by impeller pump to iliac arteries	3.5 L/min	Possible right-to-left shunting if LA inflow cannula falls back into the RA
ABIOMED BVS 5000 *(ABIOMED)*	Extracorporeal	Right Left Bi Days to weeks	Yes	BTR, BTT	Variable	5 L/min	
CentriMag *(Levitronix LLC)*	Extracorporeal Magnetically Levitated radial pump	Right Left Bi 7 d	No	BTR BTB BTE	Wide variety of cannula size options for matching to body surface area	10 L/min	Fewer shear forces
Thoratec PVAD and TLC II *(Thoratec)*	Paracorporeal Intracorporeal	Right Left Bi Weeks to months	Yes	BTR, BTT	Variable	7 L/min	Mechanical valves requiring higher levels of anticoagulation
HeartMate IP, VE, XVE *(Thoratec)*	Intracorporeal	Left Months to years	Yes	BTT, BTR, Destination Therapy	Inflow cannula: LV apex Outflow cannula: Ascending aorta	10 L/min	BSA >1.8 m squared. XVE has a titanium inner coating and bioprosthetic valves making it less thrombogenic Patients can be discharged home on aspirin alone
Jarvik 2000 *(Jarvik Heart Inc)*	Intracorporeal	Left Months to years	No	BTT	Inflow cannula: LV apex Outflow cannula: Ascending aorta	5 L/min	
HeartMate II *(Thoratec)*	Intracorporeal	Left Months to years	No	BTT, Destination Therapy	Inflow cannula: LV apex Outflow cannula: Ascending aorta	10 L/min	High durability compared to HeartMate XVE Twice the 2-y survival when compared to HeartMate XVE Aspirin and coumadin (goal INR 2-3)

impeller in the pump housing while also generating the torque necessary for unidirectional flow. The maximal flow rate is 10 L/min. The Impella 2.5 is a continuous-flow device that can deliver 2.5 L/min of flow.

The HeartMate II and Jarvik 2000 are axial-flow devices using an impeller rotating at 6000 to 15 000 rpm (revolution per minute) with maximum outputs of 10 L/min. The impeller of the device continues at its set speed regardless of inflow to the ventricular cannula. Delivery of blood to the inflow cannula is dependent on adequate intravascular volume, RV function, and a properly positioned cannula.

PREANESTHETIC CONSIDERATIONS

Most patients presenting for VAD implantation are critically ill whether they are arriving from intensive care units, emergency rooms, or the cardiac catheterization laboratory, or have developed postcardiotomy cardiogenic shock (PCCS) in the operating room. When indicated, VAD insertion should be performed early in the setting of PCCS. If a patient is weaned from CPB on 2 high-dose inotropes, hospital mortality is 42% and increases to 80% if 3 high-dose inotropes are used to separate from CPB.[191,192] If these patients undergo VAD insertion within 3 hours of the first attempt to wean from CPB, a VAD wean rate of 60% and a hospital discharge rate of 43% can be achieved.[191,192] If VAD insertion is delayed, a VAD wean rate of 27% and hospital discharge rate of 7% are to be expected. The delay in VAD insertion results in end-organ damage and decreased survival.[191,192]

The anesthesiologist must identify any neurologic deficits and ascertain the extent of major organ dysfunction (renal or hepatic insufficiency), which is very common in this patient population. Any further deterioration in the perioperative period may prevent a full recovery and eliminate the possibility of a patient qualifying for heart transplantation at a later date.[198]

Strict sterile technique for all invasive procedures and appropriate antibiotic prophylaxis is mandatory in this high-risk population. Antibiotic therapy is ineffective in treating assist device infection once it occurs.

Central venous pressure monitoring may be of questionable accuracy in patients with an RVAD. However, central access may still be useful for drug and volume infusions. Pulmonary artery catheters provide little useful information in the patient with an LVAD (that displays cardiac output). However, they may be of some use in patients with pulmonary hypertension at risk for developing RV failure post LVAD implantation. PA catheters should not be placed in patients with a functioning RVAD. Transesophageal echocardiography is the intraoperative monitor of choice.

THE PRE-CPB INTRAOPERATIVE TEE EXAMINATION

The pre-CPB transesophageal echocardiographic assessment occurs in the operating room prior to assist device implantation. The goal of this assessment is to identify anatomic and physiologic abnormalities that could lead to postoperative complications or VAD malfunction.[199,200]

Aortic Insufficiency (AI) Over 20% of patients scheduled for LVAD insertion have some degree of AI.[199,200] Aortic insufficiency status post LVAD implantation results in high pump-flow rates secondary to increased LVAD preload from the regurgitant volume but decreased systemic blood flow. Hypotension, organ hypoperfusion, and metabolic acidosis may occur despite high VAD output. Some centers report oversewing the valve shut, or repairing or replacing the aortic valve if AI is at least mild to moderate. Oversewing the AV is considered if the LVAD is being implanted as a bridge to transplant. However, the outcome of LVAD failure in the setting of an oversewn AV is ominous. If the valve cannot be repaired and is to be replaced, bioprosthetic valves are preferred to mechanical valves because of their lower thrombotic potential. Perioperative TEE is used to identify and quantify the severity of AI. General anesthesia, blood loss, and low cardiac output can result in an underestimation of load-dependent echocardiographic measurements. Therefore, if AI is suspected or mild, an LV vent may be used instead of echocardiography to evaluate the severity of AI. Vent flow rates exceeding 1.5 L/min indicate the need for surgical correction.[201]

There are a number of reasons why AI can worsen after LVAD implantation. After LVAD implantation the aorta to left ventricular pressure gradient is increased because the device ejects blood into the aorta at arterial pressures, but during device diastole, subphysiologic pressures are recorded in the LV. Additionally a properly functioning LVAD unloads the LV. Aortic valve opening is minimized and commissural fusion is accompanied by valve distortion, and AI may result.

Patent Foramen Ovale and Interatrial Septal Aneurysm A patent foramen ovale (PFO) is found in up to 9% of all prepump TEEs for VAD placement.[199,200] Under normal physiologic conditions, LA pressure is greater than RA pressure, and flow is left to right through the defect. Arterial saturation remains normal. However, with initiation of LVAD inflow, LA and LV pressures fall dramatically and frequently become lower than right-sided pressures. Right-to-left shunting through the PFO occurs. Undiagnosed or unrepaired PFOs may result in significant arterial hypoxemia presenting during separation from CPB and LVAD device activation (**Fig. 52-25**).[202] The presence of a PFO presents an additional risk of paradoxical embolism, particularly in LVAD patients.

Interatrial septal aneurysm (IASA) is defined echocardiographically as protrusion of the aneurysm 10 mm beyond the plane of the atrial septum. According to 1 study, as many as 85% of patients with IASA have a coexisting PFO.[203] IASA is associated with PFO and may be a cardiogenic source of thromboembolus.[204] A bubble test in which 10 cc of agitated saline is injected into the RA immediately after release of a Valsalva maneuver is considered the gold standard for PFO identification. However, this test occasionally fails to identify a PFO, and it is possible that a PFO may only be identified after VAD insertion and the associated changes in hemodynamics.[199,200] Repair of a PFO or interatrial septal aneurysm requires dual cannulation and necessitates prompt identification and communication with the surgical team. A PFO identified post CPB necessitates a return to CPB for repair.

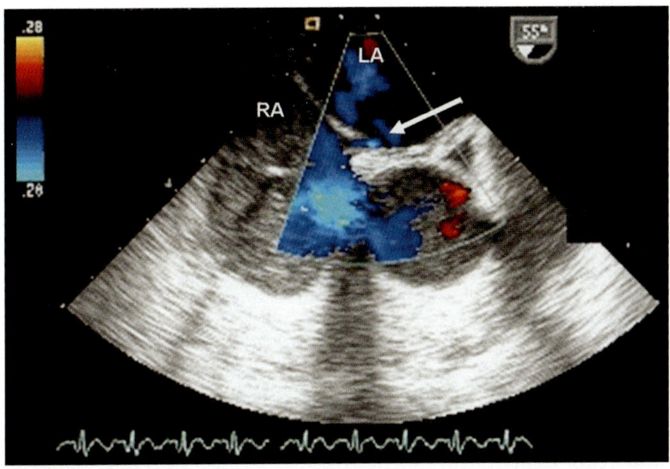

FIGURE 52-25. Transesophageal echocardiographic view showing an undiagnosed patent foramen ovale (*arrow*), which can result in arterial hypoxemia and paradoxical embolus following left ventricular assist device activation. LA, left atrium; RA, right atrium.

Right Heart Failure There is a 20% to 30% incidence of RV failure in patients implanted with an isolated LVAD.[206] Decompression of the left side of the heart after LVAD activation can lead to altered RV geometry. A leftward shift of the interventricular septum after LV decompression results in increased RV compliance and decreased RV contractility.[205] Additionally, although an LVAD should decrease RV afterload and thereby improve RV function in patients with normal PVR, patients with fixed PVR may actually experience an increase in RV afterload as increased left-sided output from the VAD increases venous return and flow through the pulmonary vasculature.

Right heart failure is one of the most important causes of perioperative death in LVAD patients.[206,207] Blood flow into the LVAD is dependent on adequate pressure gradients to drive blood flow between the LV and device reservoir/pump. Right heart failure leads to diminished transpulmonary flow and decreased left-sided heart pressures, thus reducing the driving force for LVAD filling. A preoperative RV fractional area change less than 20% is associated with RV failure upon LVAD device activation.[199,200] Low preoperative mean PA pressures and RV stroke work index may also be used to identify patients at risk for developing RV failure post LVADimplantation.[208]

Previous studies have demonstrated that female gender, nonischemic etiology of LV dysfunction, elevated central venous pressure, low mean pulmonary pressure, and low RV stroke work index are independent predictors of RV failure or need for RV assist device (RVAD) support after LVAD implantation. Preoperative evaluation of TR and RV geometry may help select patients who would benefit from biventricular support even if it is temporary. In a case series by Loforte et al, the authors reported using the CentriMag VAD for RVAD support in patients receiving a HeartMate II for LV support.[209] In cases of preoperative alteration of RV function as assessed by echocardiography, RVADs should be placed even prophylactically to avoid RV dilation and irreversible cardiomyocyte stretching that occur with a delayed RVAD insertion. RVADs were successfully explanted in these study patients on an average of 17 days postoperatively following weaning from nitric oxide in a stepwise fashion on postoperative days 1 to 2, administration of sildenafil, and weaning from CentriMag starting on postoperative day 13 by reducing RVAD flow by about 10% every 12 hours.

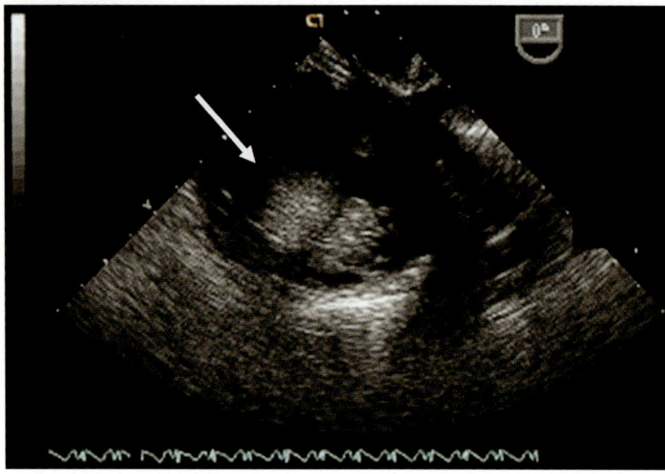

FIGURE 52-26. Large left ventricular thrombus (*arrow*) identified during precardiopulmonary bypass intraoperative transesophageal echocardiographic examination in a patient about to receive a left ventricular assist device.

Thrombus In addition to sepsis and device malfunction, neurologic dysfunction including stroke and transient ischemic attacks is one of the most common adverse events following assist device implantation.[210] Intracavitary thrombus has been identified as a thromboembolic risk factor in patients with assist devices (**Fig. 52-26**).[211] Ventricular or LA thrombus was found in 9.4% and 3%, respectively, of patients prior to LVAD insertion.[199,200]

Left ventricular thrombus may develop under conditions of blood stasis or low-velocity flow. Apical akinesis, ventricular aneurysm, and diffuse ventricular dysfunction (EF <20%) are conditions associated with blood flow stasis and thrombus formation. The sensitivity of echocardiography for detecting LV thrombi is operator dependent. Even when an LV thrombus is not identified on echocardiographic examination, the likelihood of thrombus formation remains high in the aforementioned patient population. Evidence of apical flow stasis or of continuous swirling of flow around the apex identifies patients at risk for apical thrombus. Certain clues should help the operator identify apical thrombus and distinguish it from apical trabeculations. A thrombus is somewhat more echogenic than myocardium, has a distinct contour from the endocardial border, and is located in a region of wall motion abnormality. Intracavitary thrombus can also lead to VAD inflow cannula obstruction and mechanical pump failure.[212] Thus it is important to communicate with the surgical team regarding the intended site of cannula insertion and to inspect that area carefully.

Miscellaneous Valvular Pathology Tricuspid regurgitation is commonly found in patients prior to VAD insertion. However, unless ascites is present, no benefit has been found in repairing this lesion.[207] As LV failure improves with device support, restoration of RV function and resolution of TR often follow. Mitral stenosis can compromise device inflow and should be corrected at the time of implant. Of note, for patients temporarily supported by an Impella 2.5 device, a catheter-induced incidence of MS has been reported. Impella catheter migration can lead to the prevention of normal anterior mitral leaflet excursion and result in MS. Mitral regurgitation often improves with LVAD activation and with prolonged support.[213]

Coronary Artery Disease Coronary artery disease is common in LVAD candidates. Adequate evaluation of CAD is important to ensure the best outcome after VAD implantation. Right-sided bypass grafts may be particulary necessary to support RV function after LVAD implantation. If a CABG is to be performed, placement of the proximal anastamosis site should take into account the LVAD outflow cannula anastomosis site. The lesser curvature of the aorta has been suggested as a good location for the proximal anastomosis site if the VAD outflow cannula is to be sutured to the anterolateral aspect of the ascending aorta.[207]

Ascending Aorta The ascending aorta should be evaluated for atheromatous plaque as well as aneurysm. Grade 3 plaque or higher has been identified as increasing the incidence of postoperative stroke from embolization associated with manipulation of the ascending aorta. Sites with the lowest plaque burden should be identified for LVAD outflow cannula anastomosis.

WEANING FROM CPB AND INITIATING VAD OPERATION

De-airing Before activation of the LVAD, the outflow graft is slowly unclamped and the pump is hand cranked. A modified TEE AV long-axis view at 130 degrees is used to monitor air efflux from the outflow graft into the ascending aorta (**Fig. 52-27**). If large quantities of air are observed, the hand cranking is stopped, the outflow graft is reclamped, and the aorta is vented. This process is repeated until minimal air is observed. The pump is then activated at a low rate, approximately 4 L/min.

Assessing RV Function In the early minutes after LVAD pump activation, the critical issue is RV function. RV failure is often associated with significant dilation and is often accompanied by acute TR. If transpulmonary blood flow does not improve and the device continues to empty the left-sided chambers, these 2 chambers will collapse, which may lead to obstruction of the inflow cannula. If the device pump continues to operate, air may be entrained from the sewing ring or the inlet cannula connections and ejected in large quantities into the aorta.[199,200] If these conditions exist, the device should be turned off and the patient returned to CPB. β-Adrenergic agonists, phosphodiesterase inhibitors, and nitric oxide should be initiated to improve RV contractility and decrease RV afterload in an attempt to improve transpulmonary blood flow. After several minutes, the LVAD can be restarted. If the same hemodynamic conditions persist, a supplemental temporary RVAD should be considered.

Inflow Cannula Position Inflow cannula patency is essential to adequate stroke volume and device output. The LVAD inflow cannula orifice should be directed at the mitral opening and be located in the center

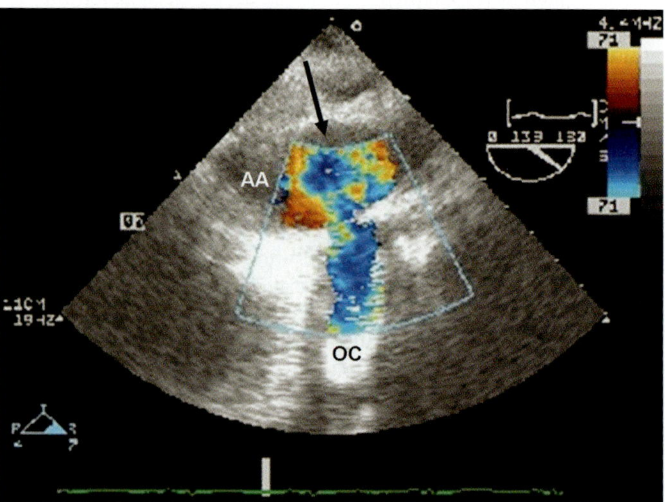

FIGURE 52-27. Transesophageal midesophageal ascending aortic long-axis view showing a normal color-flow Doppler jet (*arrow*) at the anastomotic site between a left ventricular assist device (LVAD) outflow cannula (OC) and the ascending aorta (AA). This same view can be used to monitor air efflux from the outflow graft into the ascending aorta prior to full activation of the LVAD.

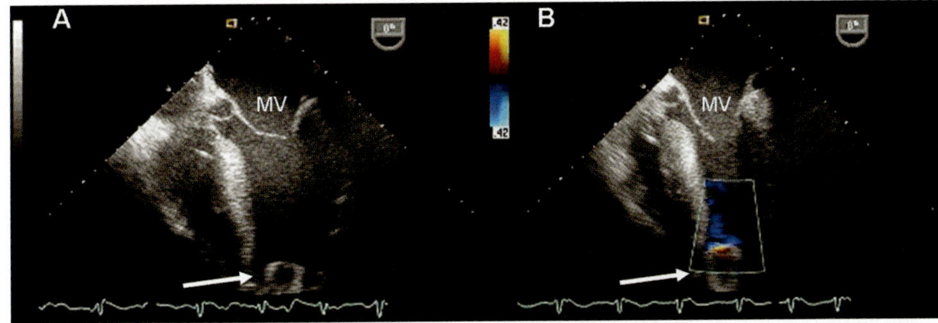

FIGURE 52-28. Transesophageal midesophageal 4-chamber, 2-dimensional (**A**) and color-flow Doppler (**B**) images showing correct positioning of the inflow cannula (arrows), oriented in the direction of mitral valve inflow.

of the apex (**Fig. 52-28**).[195] In practice, the inflow cannula is often misdirected anteroseptally (**Fig. 52-29**). Apical trabeculations, thrombi, papillary muscles, and surgical misplacement can lead to cannula obstruction and LVAD stroke volume reduction.

Inflow cannula obstruction can be assessed using color-flow Doppler and looking for turbulent flow. Continuous-wave Doppler in the midesophageal TEE 4-chamber view may be used to identify cannula obstruction. Using continuous-wave Doppler and orienting the ultrasound beam down the center of the cannula, peak velocities greater than 2.5 m/s are consistent with obstruction and require repositioning of the cannula.[199,200]

Patent Foramen Ovale PFOs may go undetected in the preoperative examination, as discussed previously. Arterial oxygen desaturation following LVAD initiation should raise suspicion of an undiagnosed PFO. Under these conditions, color-flow Doppler and contrast studies should be performed again, and if a PFO is identified, CPB should be reinstituted and the defect should be repaired.

Troubleshooting

Hypotension and Low Pump Flow Rates Hypovolemia, RV failure, inflow cannula obstruction, pulmonary embolus, and cardiac tamponade are the most frequent causes of hypotension associated with low pump flow rates. TEE clues to pericardial tamponade include pericardial effusion, systolic collapse of the RA, and diastolic collapse of the RV. These echocardiographic findings should be correlated with low QRS voltage on the ECG and equalization of chamber pressures by catheterization.[214]

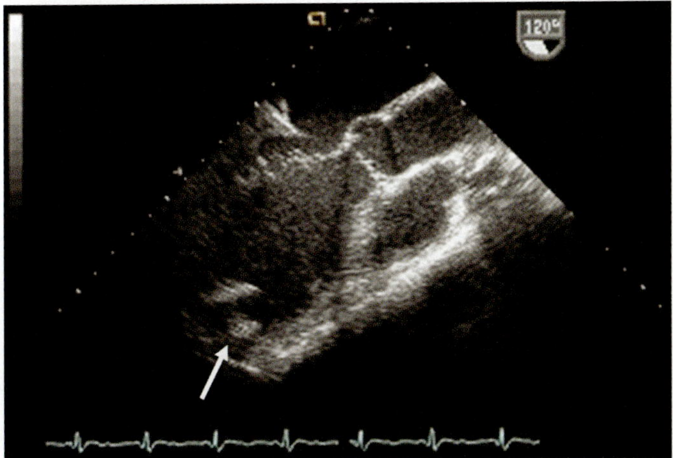

FIGURE 52-29. Transesophageal midesophageal long-axis view showing anteroseptal malalignment of a left ventricular assist device (LVAD) inflow cannula (*arrow*), which can cause obstruction and hypotension associated with low LVAD output.

Pulmonary embolus may be difficult to distinguish from acute RV failure because both result in RV dilation and severe TR. However, in pulmonary embolus it may be possible to identify an echogenic density in the main or proximal branch right pulmonary artery. Hypovolemia is best assessed by TEE. The end-diastolic area is a more accurate measure of LV preload than the PA catheter occlusion pressure. The range of normal values for the end-diastolic area is wide. Therefore, a fluid challenge may be needed.

Device malfunction is the third most common cause of death in long-term HeartMate pulsatile pneumatic VAD-assisted patients. Two fairly uncommon device malfunctions may also lead to hypotension with decreased pump flow rates: inflow graft obstruction and outflow graft kinking. Clues to inflow conduit obstruction can be gained by assessing color-flow Doppler of the normal laminar diastolic filling pattern into the apical cannula. In cases of cannula obstruction this flow pattern is intermittently interrupted. Pulsed Doppler of the inflow cannula may also indicate periods of obstruction to flow. The most common cause of inflow cannula obstruction is deviation of the inflow cannula toward the interventricular septum (see Fig. 52-29). Outflow graft obstruction may occur and is best diagnosed using contrast angiography to demonstrate an acute angle bend or "kinking."

Hypotension and High Pump Flow Rates Hypotension and high pump flow rates may present in either immediately post-CPB or after patients have been discharged from the hospital when the natural course of assist device decline and malfunction occurs. In LVAD patients who are both hypotensive and demonstrate high VAD flow rates, it is important to determine whether or not the right- and left-sided cardiac outputs are equal. This may mean placement of a PA catheter to determine the right-sided cardiac output, or performance of a TEE or transthoracic echocardiographic (TTE) examination with calculation of right-sided cardiac output. High biventricular flow rates suggest sepsis. If left-sided is greater than right-sided cardiac output, 1 of 3 etiologies must be ruled out: AI (**Fig. 52-30**), inflow valve regurgitation (IVR), or outflow valve regurgitation (OVR). In 1 prospective study, 26% of HeartMate pulsatile pneumatic LVAD patients discharged from the hospital developed inflow valve regurgitation, 32% developed new aortic insufficiency, and 0% were identified as having outflow valve incompetence.[215]

As mentioned earlier, AI may develop in LVAD patients secondary to native valve distortion, after LV decompression and diminished ejection through the native valve. Inflow valve incompetence may be caused by endocarditis, a torn cusp, or commissural dehiscence of the prosthetic. Although the inflow valve cannot be directly viewed by TEE, clues to incompetency may be gained by placing the color Doppler window over the orifice of the inflow cannula during device systole. Backflow into the ventricle during device systole suggests inflow valve incompetence (**Fig. 52-31**).[216] Aortic valve opening may be a clue that inflow valve regurgitation exists. Sixty-five percent of LVAD patients with IVR had frequent AV opening compared with only 19% in patients without

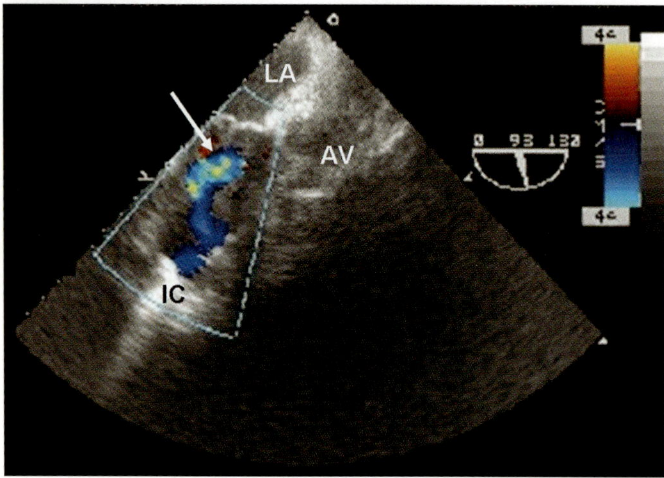

FIGURE 52-30. Transesophageal midesophageal aortic valve (AV) long-axis view showing a color-flow Doppler jet of aortic regurgitation (AR; *arrow*) directed apically toward the inflow cannula (IC) of a left ventricular assist device (LVAD). AR in LVAD patients may lead to hypotension and increased output. LA, left atrium.

IVR.[215] The outflow graft velocity, velocity time integral, and stroke volume are all significantly diminished in patients with IVR.

Of special note is a phenomenon with the continuous-flow Jarvik 2000 (Jarvik Heart, New York, New York) coined the "suckdown effect."[217] This effect may occur in any continuous-flow devices, including the CentriMag and the HeartMate II. If the revolutions per minute of the device are increased too quickly, without adequate preload a "suckdown" effect occurs in which the ventricular walls collapse and contact the LVAD inflow, leading to obstruction. The ventricular septum bows to the left and RV assumes an unfavorable geometry, leading to RV dysfunction further worsening LV preload. Although the natural tendency may be to increase the revolutions per minute on a continuous-flow device with a patient who is hemodynamically unstable, it will actually worsen the clinical picture if the cause is inadequate volume. The correct maneuver is to decrease the revolutions per minute and restore intravascular volume.[217]

Another unusual complication of a continuous-flow device was reported by Badiwala et al.[218] Three days post implantation of a HeartMate II device, the patient became profoundly hypotensive despite the LVAD at 9800 rpm. Echocardiography showed a poorly decompressed LV with paradoxical motion of the interventricular septum. The LVAD was adjusted to increase flow with decompression of the LV and septum returning to midline. Despite these maneuvers, the patient continued to deteriorate over the next several days and was started on pressors. Echocardiographic examination again showed a dilated LV with a dyskinetic septum and mild to moderate RV hypokenisis with a CVP of 19 mm Hg. Shortly thereafter the patient became profoundly hypotensive and expired. On autopsy the cause of death was determined to be an acute ventricular septal defect caused by erosion of the LVAD's inflow cannula into the interventricular septum.

ANESTHETIC MANAGEMENT OF VAD PATIENTS FOR NONCARDIAC SURGERY

As the population of assist-device patients grows, more of them will be requiring anesthesia for percutaneous insertion[219] and for noncardiac surgery. These patients can be managed using basic anesthetic principles with a few minor adjustments. Because infection and thromboembolic events are the 2 most common causes of morbidity in long-term VAD-assisted patients, every effort should be made to correctly manage antibiotic prophylaxis, ensure the strictest sterile technique for invasive procedures, and manage anticoagulation therapy appropriately.

Patients with long-term intracorporeal devices, such as the HeartMate XVE, suffer from delayed gastric emptying and early satiety because of the proximity of the device to the stomach. Cricoid pressure and a rapid sequence induction should be performed for these individuals if general anesthesia is desired. Except for the HeartMate XVE, which has a titanium-covered pump chamber and requires only aspirin for anticoagulation, most other VADs will require the maintenance of some level of anticoagulation to avoid thromboembolic complications. Increased intraoperative bleeding should be anticipated. A discussion should occur between the surgeon and the anesthesiologist regarding coagulation management prior to surgery. Giving small amounts of fresh frozen plasma to achieve the lower limits of anticoagulation recommended by the device manufacturer may be helpful in controlling excessive blood loss. Regional techniques are usually contraindicated secondary to the need to maintain anticoagulation.

Basic anesthetic principles regarding decisions to intubate and extubate patients apply in VAD-assisted patients. Although positive pressure ventilation may affect venous return to the left heart and diminish LVAD filling, in most circumstances this is only a minor consideration and mechanical ventilation should be implemented if needed. In general, invasive monitoring is not necessary because the VAD control console continuously displays the device output. An arterial line may be inserted under strict sterile precautions if frequent blood gases will be needed or if large alterations in blood pressure are anticipated. Otherwise, a noninvasive blood pressure cuff is usually adequate. Finally, because the VAD-assisted patient likely was transported to the operating room on battery-assisted power, it is important to remember to reconnect the VAD to the power supply in the operating room to avoid battery failure.

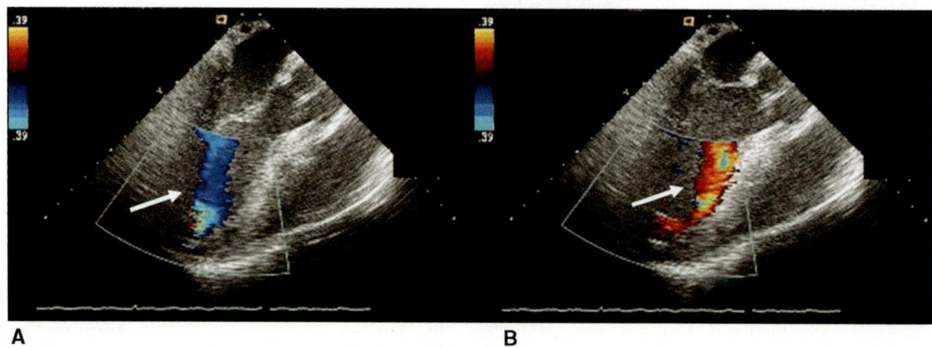

FIGURE 52-31. Transesophageal midesophageal long-axis views demonstrating normal laminar diastolic left ventricular assist device inflow (**A**; *arrow*) and a high-velocity jet of inflow valve regurgitation seen during device systole (**B**; *arrow*). Inflow valve regurgitation is the most common form of malfunction in HeartMate VE and XVE devices.

KEY REFERENCES

- Borer JS, Bonow RO. Contemporary approach to aortic and mitral regurgitation. *Circulation*. 2003;108:2432-2438.
- De Hert SG, Van der Linden PJ, Cromheecke S, et al. Choice of primary anesthetic regimen can influence intensive care unit length of stay after coronary surgery with cardiopulmonary bypass. *Anesthesiology*. 2004;101:9-20.
- Duncan AE, Abd-Elsayed A, Maheshwari A, et al. Role of intraoperative and postoperative blood glucose concentrations in predicting outcomes after cardiac surgery. *Anesthesiology*. 2010;112:860-871.
- Eltzschig H, Rosenberger P, Löffler M, et al. Impact of intraoperative transesophageal echocardiography on surgical decision making in 12,566 cardiac surgical patients. *Ann Thorac Surg*. 2008;85:845-852.
- Estrera AL, Sheinbaum R, Miller CC, et al. Cerebrospinal fluid drainage during thoracic aortic repair: safety and current management. *Ann Thorac Surg*. 2009;88:9-15.
- Fukamachi K, McCarthy PM Smedira NG, et al. Preoperative risk factors for right ventricular failure after implantable left ventricular assist device insertion. *Ann Thorac Surg*. 1999;68:2181-2184.
- Hiratzka LF, Bakris GL, Beckman JA, et al. 2010 ACCF/AHA/AATS/ACR/ASA/SCA/SCAI/SIR/STS/SVM guidelines for the diagnosis and management of patients with thoracic aortic disease: a report of the American College of Cardiology Foundation/American Heart Association Task Force on Practice Guidelines, American Association for Thoracic Surgery, American College of Radiology, American Stroke Association, Society of Cardiovascular Anesthesiologists, Society for Cardiovascular Angiography and Interventions, Society of Interventional Radiology, Society of Thoracic Surgeons, and Society for Vascular Medicine. *Circulation*. 2010;121:e266-e369.
- Levy J, Dutton R, Hemphill J, et al. Multidisciplinary approach to the challenge of hemostasis. *Anesth Analg*. 2010;110:354-364.
- Mckinlay KH, Schinderle DB, Swaminathan M, et al. Predictors of inotrope use during separation from cardiopulmonary bypass. *J Cardiothorac Vasc Anesth*. 2004;18:404-408.
- Practice guidelines for perioperative transesophageal echocardiography. An updated report by the American Society of Anesthesiologists and the Society of Cardiovascular Anesthesiologists Task Force on Transesophageal Echocardiography. American Society of Anesthesiologists and Society of Cardiovascular Anesthesiologists Task Force on Transesophageal Echocardiography. *Anesthesiology*. 2010;112:1084-1096.
- Rady MY, Ryan T, Starr NJ. Perioperative determinants of morbidity and mortality in elderly patients undergoing cardiac surgery. *Crit Care Med*. 1998;26:225-235.
- Smith RC, Leung JM, Mangano DT. Postoperative myocardial ischemia in patients undergoing coronary artery bypass graft surgery. S.P.I. Research Group. *Anesthesiology*. 1991;74:464-473.
- Stone ME, Soong W, Krol M, Reich DL. The anesthetic considerations in patients with ventricular assist devices presenting for noncardiac surgery: a review of eight cases. *Anesth Analg*. 2002;95:42-49.

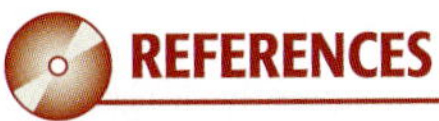

REFERENCES

Complete references available on DVD and online version at www.LongneckerAnesthesiology.com

CHAPTER 53 Anesthesia for Surgical Treatment of Congenital Heart Disease: A Problem-Oriented Approach

James S. Harrington
Avinash C. Shukla
Paul R. Hickey

KEY POINTS

1. Congenital heart diseases that decrease cardiopulmonary reserve include intracardiac shunting, hypoxemia from inadequate pulmonary blood flow or intracardiac shunting, congestive failure from volume or pressure overload, vascular obstructive disease from excessive pulmonary blood flow, various kinds of stenoses, and occasional coronary ischemia.
2. Many of the determinants of shunting (its magnitude and direction) may change considerably during anesthesia and operative manipulations.
3. There are simple shunts, bidirectional shunts, and occasionally complex shunts. The key for anesthesia providers is to understand the effects of vasodilators, cardiac depressants, and surgical manipulation on these various shunts.
4. "Bubble discipline" is an important concept for patients with congenital heart disease.
5. Chronic hypoxia leads to polycythemia, which in turn leads to dramatic increases in blood viscosity.
6. The anesthesia provider should understand the hemodynamic consequences of pulmonary vascular hypertrophy, the end stage of which is the Eisenmenger syndrome.
7. Even though a child with congenital heart disease may not have frank failure, cardiac reserves may be dramatically decreased, especially if episodes of prolonged congestive failure have been a part of the patient's history and have resulted in cardiomegaly or ventricular hypertrophy.
8. "Transitional circulation" keeps neonates with severe life-threatening congenital heart disease alive. In this context, therapy with prostaglandin E_1 infusion should be understood, especially the possibility of side effects such as apnea and major vasodilatation.
9. The functional capacities of the immature heart should be of particular interest to anesthesia providers. The immature noncompliant ventricle is extraordinarily sensitive to increases in volume and is considerably restricted in its ability to respond to the same by increasing stroke volume. The Starling curve plateau in neonates is reached at left ventricular end-diastolic pressures of 4 mm Hg. Therefore, cardiac compliance values in neonates do not correspond to values for adult patients.
10. Adult arterial pressures, especially during bypass, do not apply to neonates and infants.
11. The procedures for weaning from bypass and using deep hypothermic circulatory arrest or low-flow hypothermic bypass are important and should be reviewed in detail.
12. The anesthesia provider should fully understand the hemodynamic consequences and purpose of various pulmonary artery banding procedures and various kinds of transcatheter management of congenital lesions. Transcatheter procedures require anesthetic care in the interventional cardiac catheterization laboratory.
13. Halothane has been a successful induction anesthetic in children with various kinds of transcatheter treatment of congenital lesions.
14. Intravenous anesthetics, including high-dose opioids and ketamine, may provide increased margins of safety in some infants with congenital heart disease.

15. Intramuscular ketamine 3 to 5 mg/kg is reasonably well tolerated, even in sick children with cyanotic congenital heart disease.
16. Inhaled nitric oxide is a clinically useful and efficacious selective pulmonary vasodilator for many, but not all, patients with congenital heart disease.

The goal of anesthetic management in the treatment of patients with congenital heart disease (CHD) is maintenance of circulatory homeostasis despite the destabilizing events accompanying therapeutic procedures. Anesthesia for management of CHD is complicated by the diversity of lesions and the variety of therapeutic approaches. Congenital cardiac defects vary widely in severity, anatomic combinations, and pathophysiologic conditions. Complex cardiovascular pathophysiologic conditions change dynamically with time and with organ development and therapeutic interventions. In these circumstances, simple formulas for anesthetic management are not valid. The pathophysiology of each lesion and its alteration by previous medical and surgical treatment and by the proposed procedure should be individually considered in planning anesthetic management. Major interventional procedures in the catheterization laboratory are increasingly replacing or supplementing surgical procedures. Their anesthetic management also should be considered. Such transcatheter procedures can cause profound changes in homeostasis and often require anesthesia, particularly in children. Thus anesthetic considerations for these transcatheter interventional procedures are included. Anesthetic management of CHD is first approached by focusing on common pathophysiologic problems related to specific cardiac defects and previous therapeutic interventions. Understanding these problems is critical for determining anesthetic management priorities. Knowledge of the effects of anesthetics, manipulations, and adjunctive agents on the pathophysiologic and therapeutic procedure is essential for anticipating the responses of any patient.

SPECIFIC PROBLEMS RESULTING FROM CHD

Although many different lesions in varying combinations occur in patients with CHD, problems that decrease cardiopulmonary reserve include intracardiac shunting with increases and decreases in pulmonary blood flow, hypoxemia from inadequate pulmonary blood flow or intracardiac shunting, congestive heart failure from volume or cardiac pressure overload, pulmonary vascular obstructive disease (PVOD) from excessive pulmonary blood flow and pressure, obstruction to left or right heart outflow from stenosis at various sites, and coronary ischemia from congenital defects and iatrogenic intrusions. Of the 8 of 1000 live births with CHD, one-third have critical diseases requiring catheterization or surgery in the first year, so anesthetic management for CHD frequently involves immature neonatal circulatory and pulmonary physiology.[1] Physiologic limitations of the immature heart, circulation, and lungs are superimposed on CHD problems. **Table 53-1** shows problems encountered with CHD patients usually seen in the operating room or catheterization laboratory and frequencies of occurrence. In long-standing or particularly severe lesions, problems may occur more frequently than indicated in Table 53-1.

INTRACARDIAC SHUNTING

Shunting within the heart and between the great vessels gives rise to many of the problems seen in patients with CHD. These include hypoxemia, excessive pulmonary blood flow, high volume loads, and CHD. Thus control of intracardiac shunting is a central issue in CHD and its anesthetic management. The hemodynamics of intracardiac shunts are complex and depend on numerous factors determining shunt magnitude and direction (**Fig. 53-1**). Complete description of the dynamics of a particular shunt requires more data than are ordinarily clinically available. The determinants of shunting, such as ventricular compliance, may change considerably during anesthesia and operative manipulations, but the changes may not be readily measurable. A simplified view of shunt hemodynamics is useful in clinically assessing the hemodynamic importance of shunts and their probable alterations during therapeutic procedures.

Shunt orifice and outflow resistance are important determinants of shunting. By considering outflow resistance and the size of the shunt orifice, intraoperative changes in shunt magnitude and direction can be predicted for simple and complex shunts. Manipulation of pulmonary or systemic outflow resistances can alter shunt directions and magnitudes, depending on the type of shunt. Influences of cytokines, activated complement, and other endogenously released humoral agents such as nitric oxide also are important in determining pulmonary vascular resistance (PVR) and systemic vascular resistance (SVR). Local and circulating levels of such agents can be profoundly altered by surgical procedures and cardiopulmonary bypass (CPB).[2] Effects of such agents on vascular resistances may overwhelm clinical efforts to manipulate vascular resistances.

Simple Shunts In simple shunts (without associated obstructive lesions), outflow resistance is equivalent to PVR on the right and SVR on the left. The effects of shunt orifice and vascular resistances on simple shunts are schematically shown in **Fig. 53-2**. Shunts with small orifices are relatively fixed in magnitude and are restrictive by definition. As the communication becomes larger and nonrestrictive (equal to or exceeding the aortic valve area), shunt direction and magnitude depend more on the ratio of outflow resistances, that is, the relative resistances of the pulmonary versus systemic vascular beds (PVR/SVR).[3]

In many forms of CHD, hypoxemia requires additional pulmonary blood flow from surgically constructed aortopulmonary anastomoses. Aorta-to-pulmonary artery flow through a small diameter (restrictive). Blalock-Taussig shunt increases moderately with elevations in systemic arterial pressure when PVR remains constant or alternatively by decreasing PVR with a constant systemic arterial pressure. These changes increase pulmonary blood flow and arterial oxygen saturation (Sao_2) and probably are beneficial in increasing tissue oxygen delivery when oxygen saturations are very low (>70%). In contrast, when Sao_2 values are greater (eg, 85%-90%, approaching the plateau of the oxyhemoglobin dissociation curve), further increases in Sao_2 require high levels of pulmonary blood flow and may not improve tissue oxygen delivery because of concomitant decreases in systemic flow (**Fig. 53-3**). High pulmonary flow through large, unrestrictive shunts is required for greater levels of Sao_2, and it increases cardiac volume loading. This volume loading often may exacerbate congestive heart failure, producing a net decrease in systemic cardiac output and net oxygen delivery despite the small increases in Sao_2 produced by increased pulmonary flow. Thus the same relative changes in SVR and PVR could be detrimental with a large, nonrestrictive aortopulmonary shunt. Also, with large, nonrestrictive ventricular septal defects (VSDs), the same relative changes in PVR/SVR can increase left-to-right shunting, subjecting the heart to further increased volume loads, worsening congestive heart failure.

In contrast, with tetralogy of Fallot, because pathophysiology consists of right-to-left complex shunt flow through a VSD, the same changes, namely, increasing SVR and decreasing or holding PVR constant, decrease right-to-left shunting and improve the clinical picture. Sao_2 increases by decreasing systemic venous blood shunted into the left atrium and mixing with pulmonary venous blood, improving the patient's clinical condition. Relative levels of PVR and SVR needed to optimize the patient's clinical status with an intracardiac shunt become clearer when the pathophysiologic condition of the defect is detailed. Characteristics and examples of simple shunts of various sizes are listed in **Table 53-2**.

Mixing If the intracardiac communication is sufficiently large, the 2 cardiac chambers or great vessels effectively become a common chamber. More or less complete mixing (bidirectional shunting) occurs. This

TABLE 53-1 Frequency of Hemodynamic Problems in Various Forms of Congenital Heart Disease

Lesion	Hypoxemia	Intracardiac Shunting	Excessive Pulmonary Blood Flow	Congestive Heart Failure	Left-Sided Obstruction	Coronary Ischemia	Immature Circulation	Obstruction to Pulmonary Flow
Atrial septal defect	Rarely	Always (L → R)	Usually	Rarely	Not seen	Not seen	Not seen	Rarely
Patent ductus arteriosus	Rarely	Always (L → R)	Usually	Sometimes	Not seen	Not seen	Sometimes	Rarely
Ventricular septal defect	Rarely	Always (L → R)	Usually	Often	Not seen	Not seen	Often	Late (PVOD)
Tetralogy of Fallot	Often	Always (L → R)	Rarely	Sometimes	Not seen	Rare	Occasionally	Usually
Atrioventricular canal (partial or complete)	Rarely	Always (L → R)	Usually	Often	Not seen	Rare	Often	Late (PVOD)
Transposition of the great arteries	Always	Always (mixing)	Sometimes	Sometimes	Rare	Sometimes	Often	Rarely
Coarctation of aorta	Not seen	Occasionally (through PDA)	Not seen	Rarely	Always	Occasionally	Sometimes	Not seen
Interrupted aortic arch	Always (in lower half of body)	Always (through PDA)	Not seen	Rarely	Always	Rarely	Usually	Not seen
Pulmonary atresia	Always	Always (L → R)	Sometimes	Sometimes	Rare	Occasionally	Usually	Always
Truncus arteriosus	Usually	Always (mixing)	Usually	Often	Rare	Sometimes	Usually	Late (PVOD)
Anomalous of original coronary artery	Not seen	Not seen	Not seen	Often	Not seen	Always	Occasionally	Not seen
Single ventricle	Usually	Always (mixing)	Often	Often	Occasionally	Sometimes	Usually	Occasionally
Aortic stenosis	Not seen	Not seen	Not seen	Occasionally	Always	Not seen	Occasionally	Sometimes
Critical aortic stenosis	–	Usually (PDA)	Not seen	Usually	Always	Not seen	Frequently	Always
Pulmonic stenosis	Occasionally	Not seen	Not seen	Occasionally	Not seen	Always	Not seen	Sometimes
Critical pulmonary stenosis	Always	Usually (PDA)	Not seen	Usually	Not seen	Always	Not seen	Always
Tricuspid atresia	Always	Always	Frequently	Occasionally	Not seen	Always	Rarely	Frequently
Total anomalous pulmonary venous return	Occasionally	Always	Sometimes	Frequently	Not seen	Frequently	Rarely	Always

L, left; PDA, patent ductus arteriosus; PVOD, pulmonary vascular obstructive disease; R, right.

usually causes some degree of hypoxemia, despite normal or increased pulmonary blood flow. Mixing implies equal shunting in both directions for any period greater than a few cardiac cycles. If shunting is bidirectional but quantitatively unequal for any long period, there is a net transfer of blood into the pulmonary or systemic circulation. Continued for more than a few minutes (several hundred cardiac cycles in the infant), this theoretically puts the patient's entire blood volume on one side of the circulation. However, this does not occur because changes in compliance resulting from large shifts of blood tend to counteract shunt inequality. Thus for periods longer than a few cardiac cycles, shunting is equal in both directions.

With complete mixing in a common chamber and with no outflow obstruction, the amount of pulmonary and systemic blood flow depends on PVR/SVR. Because normal PVR often is much less than SVR (as little as 1/20 of SVR in older children and adults), pulmonary blood flow can become large with a nonrestrictive simple shunt, even in neonates. In these situations, it can become important to limit pulmonary blood flow because pulmonary volume overload can lead to congestive heart failure, inadequate systemic flow, and progressive acidosis. With mixing, Sao_2 is determined by the relative amount of pulmonary blood flow and systemic blood flow (Qp/Qs). Because of the shape of the oxyhemoglobin dissociation curve, increasingly large amounts of pulmonary blood flow are required to further increase Sao_2 as it increases. This is shown in Fig. 53-3 and explains why high Sao_2, 90% or higher, when CHD is present with mixing physiology can occur only with very high pulmonary blood flows. This high flow frequently leads to congestive heart failure from volume overload, which in turn results in net decreased systemic cardiac output.

Complex Shunt Lesions In complex shunts (**Fig. 53-4**), fixed central outflow obstruction is present at some level on one or the other side of the circulation. Fixed resistance additively increases downstream vascular outflow resistance, which increases shunting to the opposite side. When the fixed resistance is high, it largely dictates total shunting; only part of shunt flow in complex shunts is related to relative resistances in the distal pulmonary and systemic beds. As outflow obstruction increases and becomes a greater component of total resistance to flow, changes in ipsilateral vascular resistance (PVR or SVR) become progressively less important in determining flow because they become smaller components of total resistance. This is particularly true on the right side, where normal PVR is only a fraction of the resistance offered

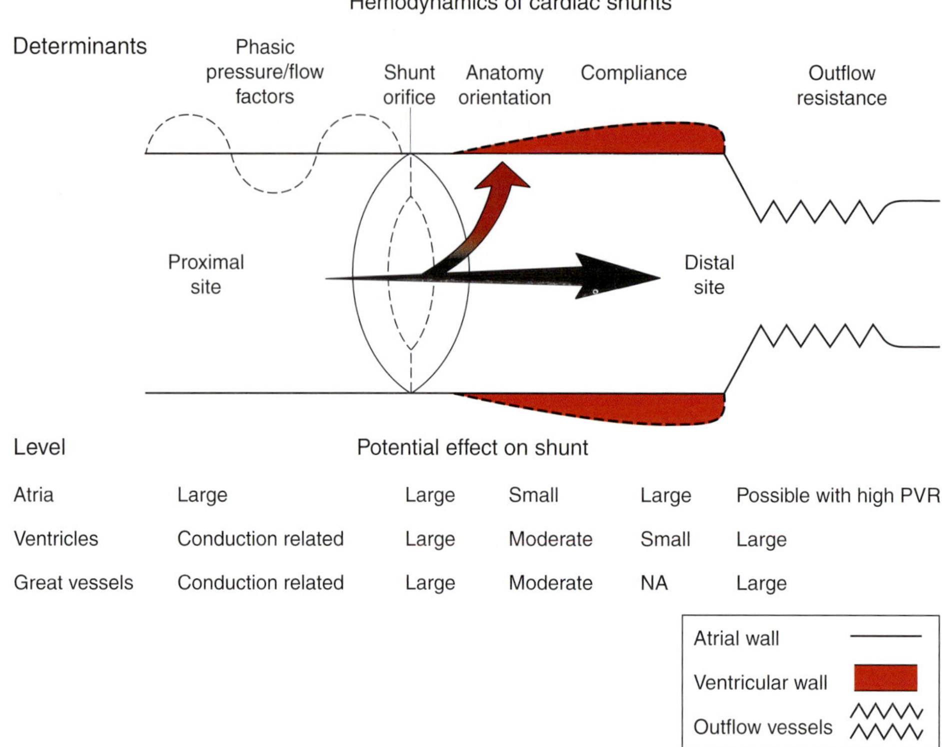

FIGURE 53-1. Effects of the many determinants on central cardiac shunting at various levels. PVR, pulmonary vascular resistance. [From Berman WJ. The hemodynamics of shunts in congenital heart disease. In: Johansen K, Burggren WW, eds. *Cardiovascular Shunts: Phylogenetic, Ontogenetic, and Clinical Aspects.* New York, NY: Raven Press; 1985:399-410, with permission.]

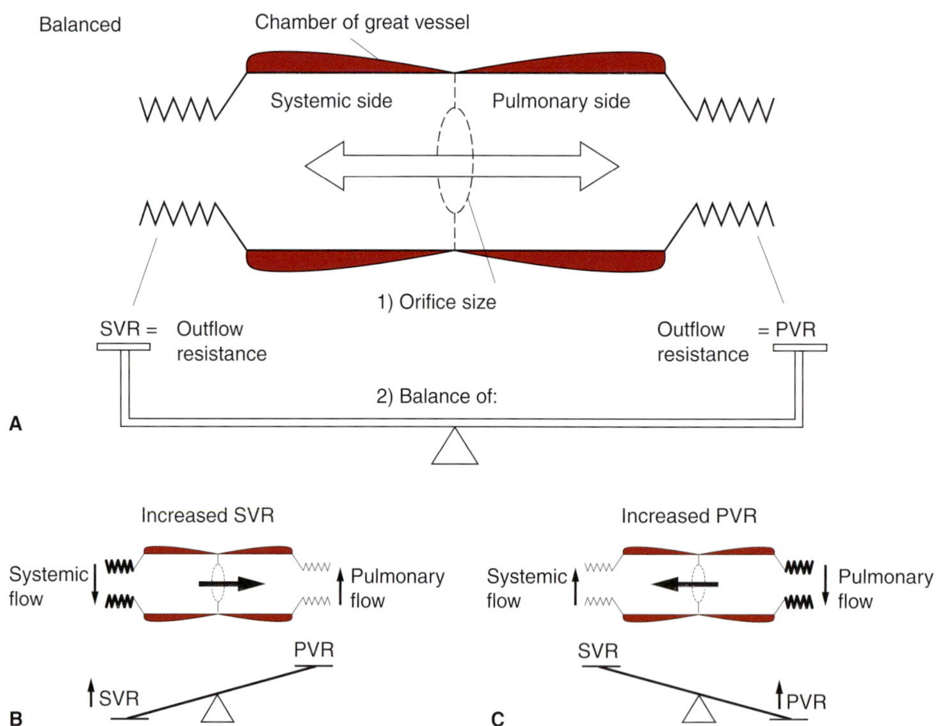

FIGURE 53-2. Determinants of magnitude and direction of simple central shunts. (1) Orifice size is important in determining magnitude of shunting and pressure gradient across the shunt and is generally fixed. (2) Balance of pulmonary vascular resistance (PVR) and systemic vascular resistance (SVR) is dynamic and determines the direction of shunt and variations in magnitude around limits fixed by orifice size. **A.** Balanced PVR/SVR. **B.** Increased pulmonary flow with increased SVR. **C.** Increased systemic flow with increased PVR. [Reprinted from Hickey PR, Wessel DL. Anesthesia for treatment of congenital heart disease. In: Kaplan JA, ed. *Cardiac Anesthesia*. 2nd ed. New York, NY: Grune & Stratton; 1987, with permission from Elsevier.]

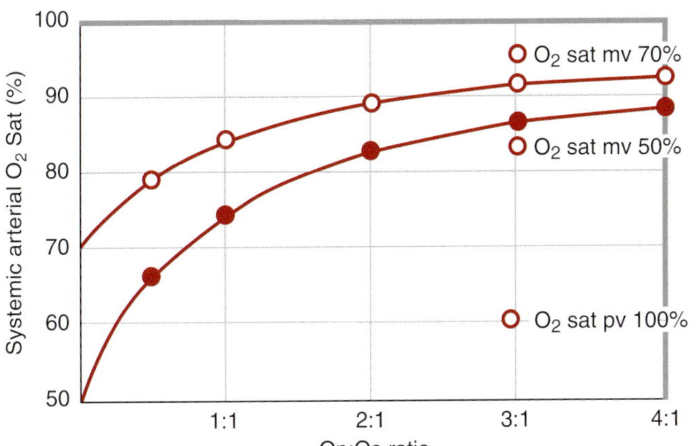

FIGURE 53-3. Changes in systemic arterial O_2 saturation with mixing lesions as the ratio of pulmonary flow to systemic flow (Qp:Qs) changes, assuming different levels of mixed venous (mv) O_2 saturation. This assumes a pulmonary venous (pv) O_2 saturation of 100%.[3]

TABLE 53-2 Simple Shunts (No Obstructive Lesions)

Restrictive Shunts (Small Communication)	Nonrestrictive Shunts (Large Communication)	Common Chambers (Complete Mixing)
Characteristics		
Large pressure gradient	Small pressure gradient	No pressure gradient
Direction and magnitude more independent	Direction and magnitude more dependent on PVR/SVR	Bidirectional shunting
Less subject to control	More subject to control	Net Qp/Qs totally dependent on PVR/SVR
Examples		
Small VSD, small PDA, Blalock shunts, small ASD	Large VSD, large PDA, large Waterston shunts	Single ventricle, truncus arteriosus, single atrium

ASD, atrial septal defect; PDA, patent ductus arteriosis; PVR, pulmonary vascular resistance; Qp, pulmonary blood flow; Qs, systemic blood flow; SVR, systemic vascular resistance; VSD, ventricular septal defect.

by most right-sided obstructive lesions seen in CHD. In contrast, changes in vascular resistance (PVR or SVR) contralateral to the fixed obstruction become relatively more important in determining shunting in complex shunts. For example, in tetralogy of Fallot with severe pulmonic stenosis, a large component of the right-to-left VSD shunting is caused by fixed pulmonary valve stenosis. An additional variable aspect of shunting may be caused by variations in PVR or dynamic right outflow infundibular obstruction. Dynamic changes in variable portions of the total right ventricular outflow obstruction may increase or decrease total right-to-left shunting, thereby increasing or decreasing hypoxemia. At baseline, when dynamic obstructive components are minimal, right-to-left shunting is determined largely by this large, fixed pulmonic obstruction. This presumes constant SVR and cardiac output; large changes in SVR markedly change shunting by altering the balance contralateral to the final obstruction (see Fig. 53-4). Characteristics and examples of complex shunts are listed in **Table 53-3**.

Complete Obstruction When obstruction to central outflow becomes complete, as in patients with tricuspid atresia, pulmonary atresia, or aortic atresia, shunting across communications proximal to the obstruction becomes total and obligatory, and can be considered an extreme type of simple shunt, as listed in Table 53-3. This should be associated

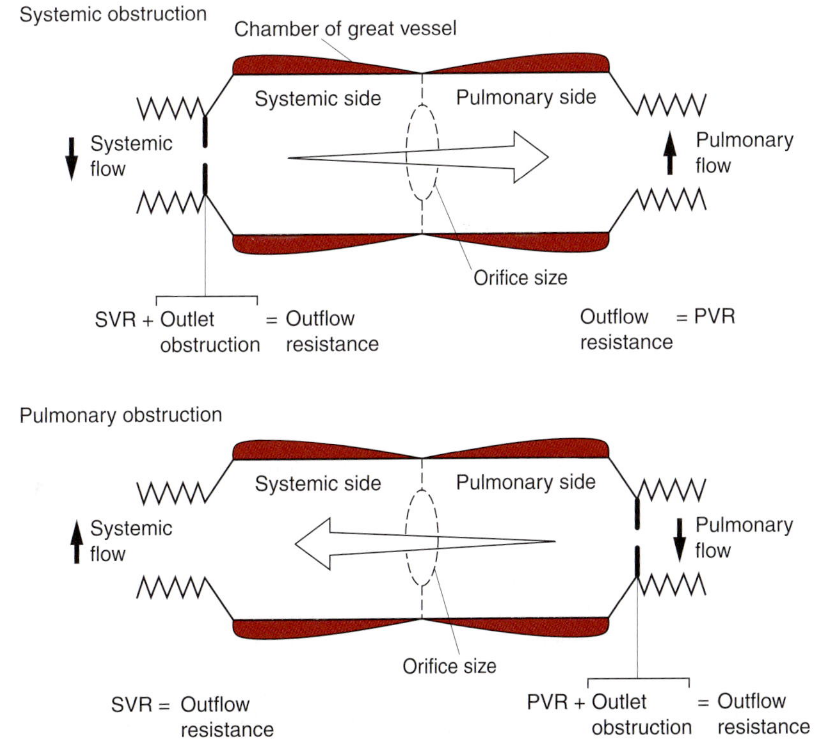

FIGURE 53-4. Determinants of complex shunting with systemic or pulmonary outflow obstruction. Orifice size again limits magnitude, but balance of outflow resistances include outlet obstruction on either side of the circulation in addition to systemic vascular resistance (SVR) or pulmonary vascular resistance (PVR). Addition of outlet obstruction increases flow on the opposite side and decreases flow on the same side. [Reprinted from Hickey PR, Wessel DL. Anesthesia for treatment of congenital heart disease. In Kaplan JA, ed. *Cardiac Anesthesia*. 2nd ed. New York, NY: Grune & Stratton; 1987, with permission from Elsevier.]

TABLE 53-3 Complex Shunts (Shunt and Obstructive Lesions)

Partial Outflow Obstruction	Total Outflow Obstruction
Characteristics	
Shunt magnitude and direction largely fixed by obstruction	Shunt magnitude and direction totally fixed
Shunt depends less on PVR/SVR	All flow goes through shunt
Orifice and obstruction determine pressure gradient	Pressure gradient depends on orifice
Examples	
Tetralogy of Fallot, VSD and pulmonic stenosis, VSD with coarctation	Tricuspid atresia, mitral atresia, pulmonary atresia, aortic atresia

PVR, pulmonary vascular resistance; SVR, systemic vascular resistance; VSD, ventricular septal defect.

with another downstream shunt that provides flow to the obstructed side of the circulation. The associated shunt can be a patent ductus arteriosus (PDA), which provides pulmonary blood flow in pulmonary valvular atresia or provides systemic blood flow in aortic valvular atresia. Downstream shunting variably depends on PVR/SVR, depending on the restrictive nature of the "compensatory" shunt, that is, a small patent ductus constitutes most of the resistance when the ductus is the site of the compensatory shunt in pulmonic atresia. In this situation, the small ductus limits pulmonary blood flow.

Intracardiac Shunting and Air Emboli Systemic air embolus is a constant danger in patients with CHD regardless of nominal left-to-right shunting patterns because anesthetic and surgical manipulations can dynamically alter shunts. Air traps are advisable for all intravenous (IV) lines but are not substitutes for meticulous attention and constant vigilance in the purging of air bubbles. Systemic air emboli are a relative contraindication to the use of nitrous oxide in patients with CHD. Right-to-left shunts may occur during some portions of the cardiac cycle or during straining or coughing in patients with open communications and nominal left-to-right shunts, because normal transatrial pressure gradients are transiently reversed. Right-to-left shunting may occur even across functionally "closed" communications. A "probe patent" foramen ovale is common in children (and adults) with and without CHD. Transient right-to-left shunting across such a foramen ovale has even been documented in a healthy child during emergence from anesthesia.[4] In many patients with CHD, direct shunting of microbubbles and macrobubbles of air into the systemic intracerebral arterial circulation from multiple IV lines and injections can be readily documented with transcranial Doppler (TCD). "Bubble-free" room temperature solutions may "rain out" bubbles at 37°C. The cerebral effects of such arterial air emboli have not been ascertained except in patients with massive cerebral arterial air emboli.

SEVERE HYPOXEMIA

Severe hypoxemia in patients with CHD results from inadequate pulmonary blood flow or defects that allow mixing, as defined previously. Chronic hypoxemia requires adaptations to provide adequate tissue oxygen transport. Although moderate hypoxemia is well tolerated in neonates, hypoxemia after infancy produces special problems, including polycythemia; increased blood volume; and vasodilatation, neovascularization, and alveolar hyperventilation with chronic respiratory alkalosis. Chronic hypoxemia and its accompanying adaptive mechanisms may limit cardiac reserve and oxygen delivery during the stress of anesthetic induction and surgery. Additionally, in such patients, the margin for error and tolerance for loss of airway is decreased.

Polycythemia increases blood hematocrit and blood viscosity to dangerously high levels that cause vascular stasis and worsen tissue hypoxia.[5] Although an increased hematocrit improves blood oxygen-carrying capacity, resultant increased blood viscosity decreases cardiac output when the hematocrit is above 60%. Patients with polycythemia and cyanosis have increased risk for renal or cerebral thrombosis because of increased viscosity, particularly if they become dehydrated. Hematocrits above 70% generally are associated with increased risk of cerebrovascular accidents and coagulopathies. These patients may have a history of cerebrovascular accidents and sometimes already have residual neurologic deficits. They require IV hydration starting on the evening before anesthesia and also postoperatively until oral intake is adequate. Some patients may benefit from erythropheresis before surgery if hematocrits are above 60% to 70%. Polycythemic CHD patients also have coagulopathies in part because of decreased levels of platelets and fibrinogen.[6] These coagulopathies increase the risk of excess intraoperative bleeding, and appropriate arrangements should be made for intraoperative transfusion of clotting factors when necessary.

Patients with severe hypoxemia caused by intracardiac shunting generally undergo anesthesia for procedures designed to improve their pulmonary blood flow and Sao_2. Induction of anesthesia itself using a variety of techniques markedly increases arterial saturation. This induction-related increase in arterial saturation probably results from greater systemic venous oxygen saturation caused by greater inspired oxygen concentrations plus decreased oxygen consumption with induction of anesthesia and muscle paralysis. Systemic venous blood with a greater oxygen saturation is shunted into the systemic circulation, decreasing the degree of hypoxemia seen. Thus induction of anesthesia itself may be therapeutic for patients with CHD with severe hypoxemia and sometimes can be used to temporize until correction or palliation can be accomplished surgically.

EXCESSIVE PULMONARY BLOOD FLOW

Excessive pulmonary blood flow is common in patients with CHD and produces cardiac and pulmonary complications. Volume overload always compromises cardiac reserve regardless of the presence of frank congestive heart failure. Increased pulmonary artery (PA) pressure and blood flow can limit gas exchange by several mechanisms. Compression of large bronchi by distended pulmonary vessels may obstruct large and small airways and increase the work of breathing. The increased pulmonary venous return distends the left atrium and may obstruct the left main stem bronchus. Most important, increased pulmonary blood flow and pressure combine with elevated left atrial pressure to produce pulmonary venous congestion and increased interstitial and alveolar lung water. Resultant lung compliance deterioration and increased airway resistance can produce tachypnea and sometimes wheezing. Regions of the lung with atelectasis and intrapulmonary shunt then contribute to systemic arterial desaturation, even in a child with "acyanotic" heart disease and left-to-right shunting.

PVOD is produced by prolonged high pulmonary flows and pressures. The anatomic lesion is hypertrophy of the medial layer of pulmonary arteries and intimal thickening, with resultant increased PVR and reactivity.[7] **Figure 53-5** shows normal progression of pulmonary flows, pressures, and vascular resistance during early childhood and alterations in the normal progression with a large VSD. **Figure 53-6** indicates normal evolution of pulmonary arteries during infancy and alteration caused by high pulmonary flows and pressures resulting from left-to-right shunting through a VSD. Smaller pulmonary arteries are anatomic substrates of increased pulmonary vascular reactivity and high PVR seen in patients with PVOD. When PVR eventually equals or exceeds SVR, a left-to-right shunt then becomes a right-to-left shunt (Eisenmenger syndrome). PVOD can occur during the first year of life in patients with some lesions, such as an atrioventricular canal, but may require decades to develop in patients with atrial septal defects (ASDs). Depending on the severity and duration of these changes, correction of the underlying lesion may result in varying degrees of reversal of pulmonary vascular changes and decreases in pulmonary hypertension.

In neonates with a wide PDA and a single source of blood supply to the systemic and pulmonary circulations, pulmonary blood flow may become particularly excessive intraoperatively. This is signaled

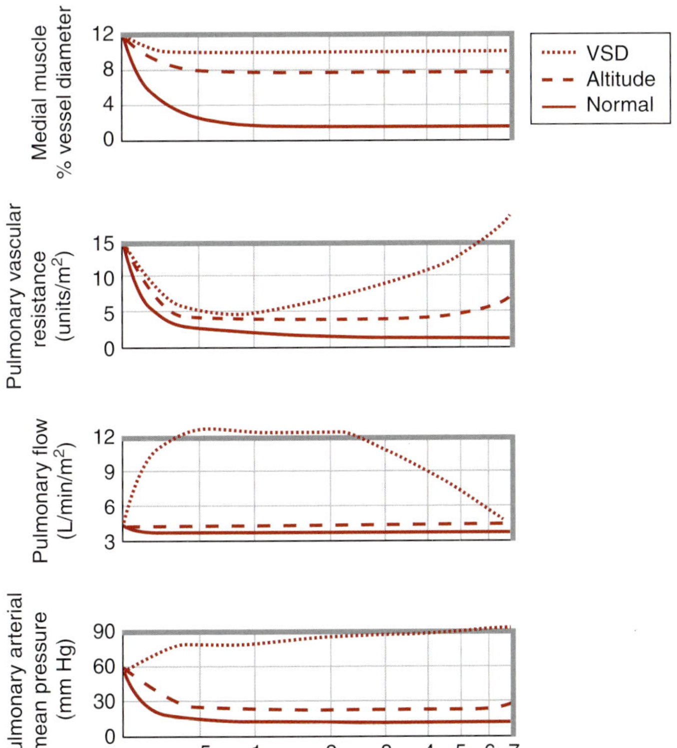

FIGURE 53-5. Normal and abnormal developmental changes in pulmonary arterial tree during the first years of life. Pulmonary vascular resistance, percentage of arterial smooth muscle, and pressure normally decrease in the first year of life. A large, nonrestrictive ventricular septal defect with a large left-to-right shunt results in an immediate increase in flow and a later increase in vascular resistance.[3]

by high systemic arterial saturations (>90%) in these mixing types of pathophysiologic conditions. It occurs in patients with lesions, such as truncus arteriosus or hypoplastic left heart syndrome (HLHS) and results in acute congestive heart failure with ventricular enlargement, low systemic output, high Sao_2, and hypotension. This can produce myocardial ischemia in neonates. The myocardial ischemia seen in this situation can be remedied only by acutely increasing PVR by placing a tourniquet on one of the branch pulmonary arteries or by applying a partially occluding PA clamp. These maneuvers mechanically increase PVR, decrease the excessive pulmonary blood flow and arterial saturation, increase systemic (coronary) perfusion pressure, and decrease cardiac volume load and reduce ventricular diameter. In patients with CHD with tendencies toward excessive pulmonary blood flow and only mild hypoxemia, anesthetic management is planned to avoid major decreases in PVR because such decreases exacerbate the increased pulmonary flow and lead to cardiovascular decompensation.

CONGESTIVE HEART FAILURE

The child with CHD develops congestive heart failure because of increased pressure, volume, or combined pressure and volume loads. Increased volume loads can result from intracardiac shunting or valvular insufficiency. Increased pressure loads can result from valvular obstruction, stenosis of major systemic or pulmonary arteries, or diffuse PVOD. Patients compensate by well-known mechanisms. Increased catecholamine production redistributes cardiac output to favored organs, increases heart rate, decreases skin temperature, and frequently induces a catabolic nutritional state.[8] Pulmonary congestion increases the work of breathing and caloric demand, whereas tachypnea limits intake of calories. Derangements vary with severity of congestive heart failure. In severe cases, growth is retarded and body weight is well below the third percentile for age. These patients often are tachypneic, tachycardic, and dusky in room air and may have chest wall retractions, expiratory wheezes, and diffuse rhonchi. Capillary refill may be prolonged and extremities cool to the touch, with palpable hepatomegaly. Preoperative chest radiographs demonstrate cardiac enlargement and increased pulmonary vascular markings with areas of atelectasis despite hyperexpansion of the lungs. In severe cases, medical management consisting of administration of digoxin and diuretics is indicated before surgery, which may induce a profound metabolic hypochloremic alkalosis with potassium depletion.

Other children with lesser degrees of congestive heart failure caused by CHD may be only mildly symptomatic but still have substantially decreased cardiovascular reserves. The additional stress of anesthesia and surgery may result in cardiac decompensation, particularly when compensation depends on maximal sympathetic tone. Reversibility of ventricular dysfunction accompanying congestive heart failure in those with CHD varies depending on the severity of the defect, degree of correction, and duration of ventricular dysfunction.

Prolonged congestive heart failure and attendant ventricular dysfunction result in cardiomegaly and ventricular hypertrophy. The amount and location of cardiomegaly or hypertrophy occurring depends on the combination of cardiac pressure and volume loads and intracardiac anatomy. Long-standing cardiomegaly and hypertrophy jeopardize the myocardium in children, particularly in those with chronic hypoxemia. In the young, growing heart, pressure-overload hypertrophy appears to occur in association with myocardial angiogenesis rather than with diminished myocardial capillary density, as occurs in adults.[9] Despite the former compensatory mechanism, microscopic areas of myocardial infarction eventually appear in young hearts subjected to chronic overload, particularly in those with chronic hypoxemia. This results in progressive ventricular dysfunction in the affected ventricle, as working muscle mass is depleted and is replaced by fibrous tissue. Some ventricular dysfunction may be reversible, depending on timing of correction of the underlying defect. For example, VSDs and tetralogy of Fallot defects repaired during early infancy before myocardial damage occurs subsequently have better ventricular function than those repaired later in childhood.

In patients with any degree of congestive heart failure, anesthetic treatment is planned to avoid large doses of myocardial depressants and alterations of PVR or SVR that exacerbate cardiac failure. The detrimental alterations depend on individual pathophysiology findings. In patients with severe congestive heart failure or in those with detrimental alterations in pathophysiologic conditions that cannot be avoided, appropriate pressor and inotropic support is included in the anesthetic plan.

OBSTRUCTIONS TO SYSTEMIC BLOOD FLOW

Congenital lesions producing obstruction to left heart outflow include interruption of the aortic arch, coarctation of the aorta, aortic stenosis (subvalvar, valvar, or supravalvar), mitral stenosis and atresia, and HLHS. These patients may have left ventricular hypertrophy, coronary ischemia, and limited systemic ventricular reserve. Systemic perfusion in neonates with these problems often depends on a PDA that may be rapidly narrowing. Such infants usually present with shock and metabolic acidosis, requiring resuscitation with prostaglandin E_1 (PGE_1) preoperatively. Ventricular fibrillation is a distinct risk. Older children with less severe forms of stenosis often are asymptomatic, with only mild hypertension in coarctation of the aorta or mild aortic stenosis. They may have dysrhythmias, syncope, fatigue, or chest pain in various forms of aortic stenosis.

OBSTRUCTIONS TO PULMONARY BLOOD FLOW

Pulmonary flow obstructions occur at many levels in the right side of the circulation. Right ventricular hypertension, pulmonary hypertension, and hypoxemia may result, depending on the location of obstructions and the presence of intracardiac shunting. Combinations of these

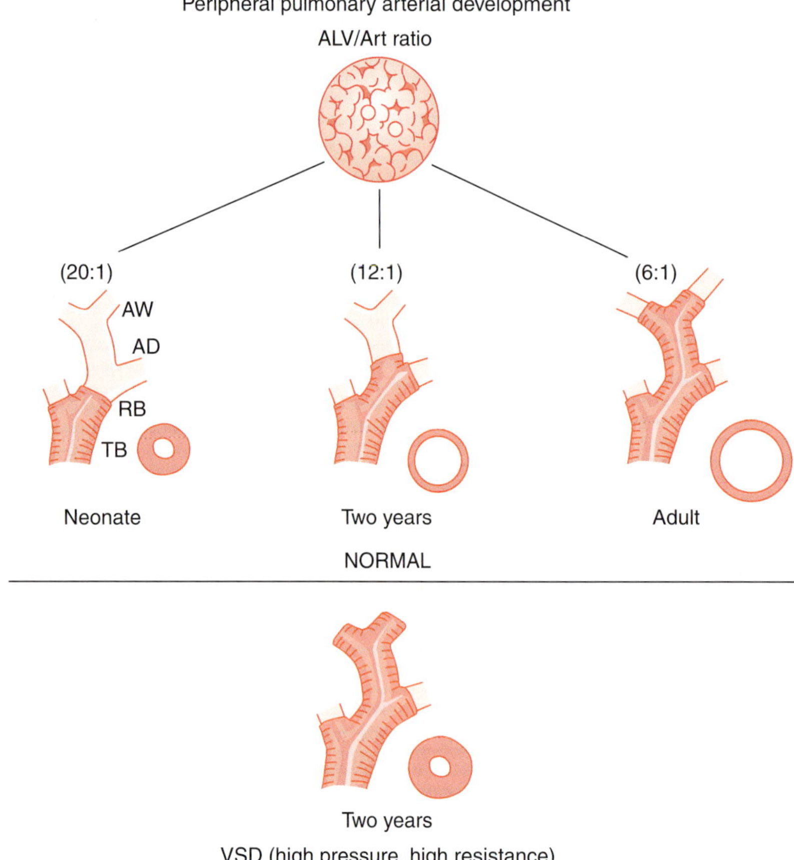

FIGURE 53-6. Developmental changes in peripheral pulmonary arterial tree in normal patients and in the presence of a ventricular septal defect (VSD) with a large left-to-right shunt. Alveolar-to-arteriolar (ALV/Art) ratio decreases with age because of extensive arborization of arterial tree as arteriolar lumen increases and muscle layer thins and spreads distally. Pulmonary hypertension with high flow from left-to-right shunt in a VSD causes pulmonary vascular obstructive disease marked by decreased numbers of pulmonary arterioles (ALV/Art = 25:1), decrease in vessel lumen, increase in muscle thickness, and more distal spread of muscle. Letters indicate arteriole from level of the terminal bronchiolus (TB) to the alveolar wall (AW).[3,148]

problems are seen in pulmonary valve and subvalvular stenosis, PA stenosis, PVOD, tetralogy of Fallot, and pulmonary atresia. High levels of right ventricular afterload result in a hypertensive, hypertrophied right ventricle that is prone to myocardial ischemia. As right ventricular intracavitary pressures approach and then exceed systemic arterial pressures, coronary perfusion pressures become inadequate, and right ventricular failure results from myocardial ischemia. Acute therapy is aimed at increasing systemic arterial pressure with α-adrenergic agents, such as phenylephrine, to improve coronary perfusion of the right ventricle. Lowering of PVR also is beneficial if it can be accomplished without decreasing systemic (coronary) perfusion pressure.

Patients with right ventricular hypertension resulting from outflow obstruction or obstruction of the larger pulmonary vessels can be effectively treated with balloon dilation in the cardiac catheterization laboratory or with a surgical procedure. Unilateral or segmental pulmonary edema requiring management may be seen after such procedures. When PVR at the small vessel level is markedly elevated and irreversible, as in patients with end-stage PVOD, therapy frequently is ineffective. Patients with a markedly hypertensive pulmonary circulation of any duration have cor pulmonale or dysrhythmias and are prone to sudden, poorly understood increases in PVR. Such pulmonary hypertensive crises may occur without warning, resulting in refractory acute right ventricular failure and sometimes in death. When systemic levels of pulmonary arterial pressure are encountered in the operating room, despite corrective procedures, every effort should be made to correct this problem because of the associated high risks of sudden decompensation and death.

CORONARY ISCHEMIA

Although acquired coronary artery disease is rare in children with CHD, except in those with transplanted hearts, coronary ischemia may occur with left heart outflow obstruction, surgical retraction, "pulmonary steal" in neonates with a single source of pulmonary and systemic flows, or anomalous coronary arteries arising from the PA. In neonates with truncus arteriosus, intraoperative decreases in PVR can lead to decreased systemic flow and diastolic pressure, which produces ST-segment changes indicative of acute myocardial ischemia.

Maneuvers to decrease pulmonary flow, such as temporarily ligating the left or right PA, can increase diastolic pressure and reverse the ischemia and ST-segment changes seen on electrocardiography (ECG).[10] In anomalous coronary arteries, retrograde flow into the PA occurs via anastomotic connection with normal coronary arteries (ie, those with aortic origin) when flow is "stolen" from the high-pressure origin and diverted to the low-pressure pulmonary circulation. Myocardial infarcts and ventricular dysfunction can result. These problems may be preventable or reversible if the anomalous coronary arteries are detected and corrected early in life.

Rarely, patients have aberrant sinusoidal coronary arteries originating directly from the right ventricular cavity. These arteries provide nutrient, antegrade (albeit hypoxemic) flow into the coronary bed as long as high (systemic) pressures are maintained in the right ventricle. Any intervention that substantially decreases right ventricular intracavitary pressure results in intractable and even fatal coronary ischemia. When perfusion pressure decreases, flow from these vessels becomes retrograde into the right ventricular cavity as flow is "stolen" from adjacent, communicating systemic coronary arterial beds.

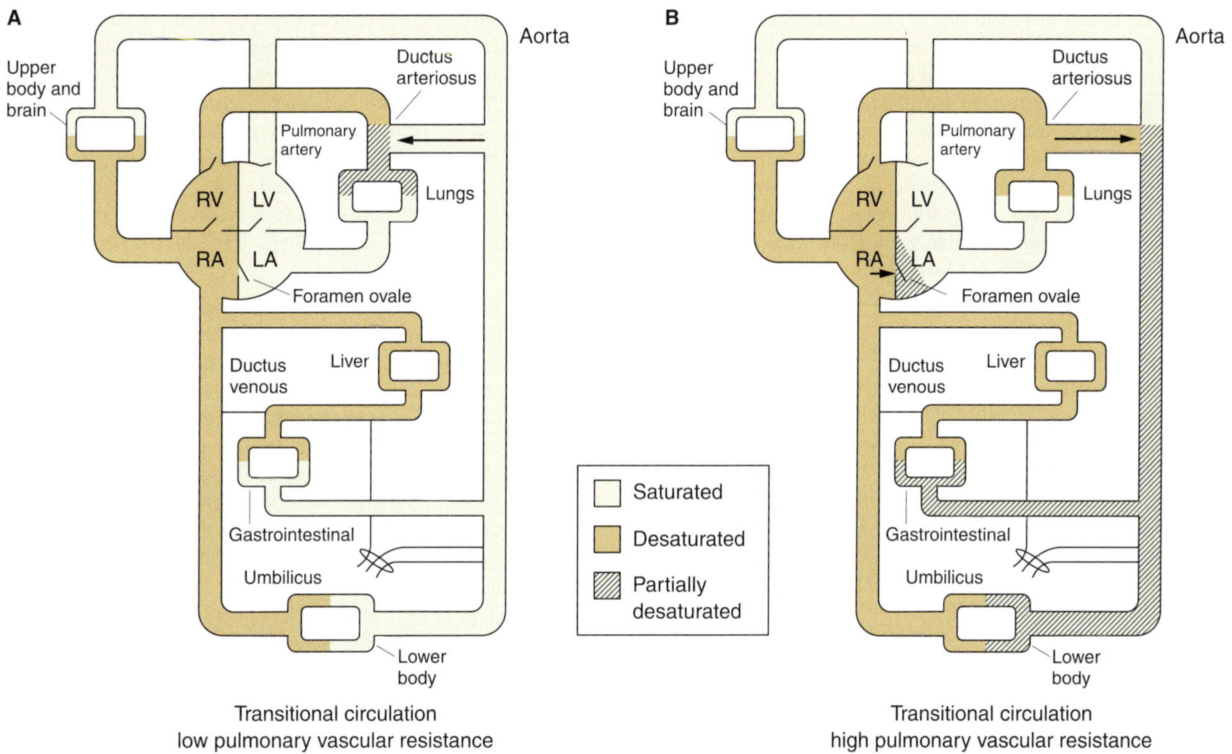

FIGURE 53-7. Schematic diagram of central shunting and blood saturations that occur normally in the transitional circulation in the first few hours and days after birth. **A.** In the first few hours, the foramen ovale is widely patent and pulmonary vascular resistance is high, leading to right-to-left shunting. **B.** Later stage of transitional circulation when pulmonary vascular resistance decreases and the ductus remains patent, resulting in left-to-right shunting. Foramen ovale is functionally closed. [Reprinted from Hickey PR, Crone RK. Cardiovascular physiology and pharmacology in children. In: Ryan JR, Todres PS, Coté C, et al., eds. *A Practice of Anesthesia for Infants and Children*. New York, NY: Grune & Stratton; 1986, with permission from Elsevier.]

IMMATURITY OF CIRCULATION

Transitional Circulation Transitional circulation consists of a PDA, patent foramen ovale, and high PVR, as shown schematically in **Fig. 53-7**. In neonates with severe, life-threatening CHD, the transitional circulation plays a major role in maintaining viability because its persistence is required to sustain functional circulation until therapeutic interventions can be undertaken. Particularly important in maintaining an intact circulation is patency of the ductus arteriosus. Before anatomic (as opposed to physiologic) closure occurs at several weeks of age in the normal sequence, the ductus may remain open in response to hypoxemia or PGE_1 infusion.[11] Reopening of the ductus has been documented in infants older than 7 days in whom the ductus has been kept open with PGE_1 infusions for many weeks when necessary.

The PDA plays a critical role in maintaining life by providing either systemic or pulmonary blood flow in neonates with severe congenital heart lesions (**Box 53-1**). Acute decompensation occurs in these infants when the ductus closes. When systemic and coronary perfusion depend on a PDA, closure results in reduction of systemic flow, coronary insufficiency, rapidly progressive metabolic acidosis, and death. When pulmonary flow depends on a patent ductus, closure results in acute reduction of pulmonary flow, progressive hypoxemia, and death. In neonates with ductus-dependent lesions who decompensate after closure, therapy with PGE_1 infusion for 24 to 48 hours provides effective resuscitation and correction of metabolic deficits. Side effects of PGE_1 infusion include apnea and vasodilatation; many neonates receiving PGE_1 infusions need intubation and ventilatory support, and supplementation of intravascular volume.

High PVR in the transitional circulation is particularly important when the congenital defect has only a single, nonrestrictive source of pulmonary and systemic blood flow, as in truncus arteriosus, HLHS, or pulmonary atresia. When the ductus arteriosus is kept widely patent with PGE_1 or when no ductus is involved (truncus arteriosus), decreases in high PVR from the immediate postnatal levels produce "pulmonary steal" of systemic blood flow and low diastolic blood pressure. This leads to systemic hypoperfusion, coronary ischemia, and progressive metabolic acidosis despite good Sao_2.[12]

The Immature Heart At birth, the immature heart is markedly different from the mature heart. Right and left ventricles have approximately equal size and wall thickness; the right ventricle is slightly heavier. The increased afterload on the left and decreased afterload on the right, occurring with birth, lead to progressive thickening of the left ventricular wall. By 4 weeks of age, the left ventricle weighs more than the right

BOX 53-1

Ductus-Dependent Neonatal Congenital Heart Defects

PDA Provides Systemic Flow
- Critical coarctation of the aorta
- Interrupted aortic arch
- Hypoplastic left heart syndrome
- Critical aortic stenosis

PDA Provides Pulmonary Flow
- Pulmonary atresia
- Critical pulmonic stenosis
- Severe subpulmonic stenosis with ventricular septal defect
- Tricuspid atresia with pulmonic stenosis

PDA, patent ductus arteriosus.

ventricle.[13] By 3 or 4 years of age, the left ventricle is approximately twice as heavy as the right, the normal adult relationship. These changes are accompanied by myocyte ultrastructural development. Small immature myocytes with chaotically arranged myofibrils accounting for 30% of gross muscle mass evolve into larger mature myocytes with organized, longitudinally oriented myofibrils that make up 60% of muscle mass. The larger mass of noncontractile elements in immature myocytes results in noncompliant cells with diminished contractile capacity. Myocardial contractility and compliance increase with development; immature myocardium develops less force during contraction than does adult myocardium, and velocity and magnitude of shortening also are less in immature myocytes.

Other changes include development of the transverse tubular system, essentially absent in the neonatal heart, and development of sarcoplasmic reticulum, increasing its capacity to store and release calcium. Contractile proteins, namely, myosin, tropomyosin, and troponin T, required for myocardial contraction also change their isoforms during this period.[14] Ultrastructural changes occurring in maturing myocytes result in improved myocardial function, but until myocytes fully mature, cardiac reserve is limited. This should be appreciated in the anesthetic treatment of infants with CHD, who have additional sources of decreased cardiac reserve in addition to immaturity. Despite these factors, immaturity confers some "advantage" for cardiac function during hemodynamic stress because during acidosis, contractile function is less affected and intracellular myocardial pH is better maintained.[15]

Functional capacities of the immature heart are well defined. The immature, noncompliant ventricle is highly sensitive to increases in filling volume and is relatively restricted in its ability to respond with increased stroke volume. Although stroke volume improves with increased filling pressure, the range over which this occurs is narrow. The Starling curve is reached at filling pressures of 4 mm Hg, and stroke volume actually decreases at filling pressures near 7 mm Hg. This Starling plateau may be a result of increased afterload effects as mean arterial pressure increases with increased preload.[16] The immature ventricle is highly sensitive to increased afterload. With constant afterload, stroke volume improves with progressive increases in left atrial pressure from 5 to 10 mm Hg. Because the immature heart is noncompliant, small increases in intravascular volume rapidly increase filling pressures to the plateau of the Starling curve where stroke volume is fixed. At the level of filling pressure where stroke volume is fixed, cardiac output becomes rate dependent. Additional increases in volume push filling pressures to the descending portion of the curve, and the ventricle begins to fail. Although the Starling curve of the neonate is clearly shifted to the left compared with the curve of older children and adults, it still does apply.[17] Because of this, cardiac output is not entirely rate dependent at lesser filling pressures and rates within neonatal physiologic range. Increases or decreases in heart rate within physiologic ranges result in changes in stroke volume without major changes in cardiac output in the term human fetus and in the lamb.[18] It is only when the plateau of the Starling curve is reached that the immature heart becomes truly rate dependent.

Reduced compliance and similarity in size and wall thickness of the ventricles during the first month lead to an intimate interrelationship between right and left ventricular function.[19] Failure of 1 immature ventricle quickly causes septal shift, and, in contrast to adults, congestive heart failure quickly becomes biventricular. This has important implications for ventilatory management, namely, the fact that inadequate ventilation in infants rapidly leads to increased right ventricular afterload and biventricular failure because of the muscular, hyperreactive pulmonary circulation. This also applies to small infants with CHD. As a result of the poor tolerance of the immature heart for increased afterload, right ventricular failure of some degree may result, which in turn rapidly compromises function of the left ventricle. Thus adequacy of ventilation in the infant frequently determines cardiac function even if severe hypoxemia has not yet occurred.

In summary, the functional capacity of the immature infant heart and cardiac reserve improve with age. Increasing preload or afterload results in ventricular failure sooner in neonates and infants than in adults, and failure quickly becomes biventricular. By 3 or 4 years of age, adult levels of systemic arterial pressure and PVR are achieved, and the previously mentioned functional limitations probably no longer apply. Additional stresses and loads placed on the immature heart by various forms of CHD further reduce cardiac reserves in infants, thus reducing their already compromised ability to deal with the stresses of anesthesia and surgery.

Combined Problems Combinations of the previously mentioned problems are found in many patients with CHD. Excessive flows caused by intracardiac shunting and flow obstruction often lead to congestive heart failure. In older children with long-standing complex lesions that cannot be readily corrected, ventricular function may gradually deteriorate because of long-standing ventricular pressure or volume overload. Chronic volume loading is seen in those with aortic or mitral valve regurgitation or in patients with long-standing pulmonary-to-systemic arterial shunts. The latter patients may have only mild to moderate hypoxemia despite complete mixing when there is a large shunt and excessive pulmonary blood flow.

The price paid for near-normal levels of Sao_2 is chronic ventricular dilation and potential development of PVOD. These patients may have combined problems of hypoxemia and mild cyanosis, some degree of PVOD, and left ventricular dilation with progressively decreasing ejection fractions.

In infants and especially neonates, problems of transitional circulation and limited functional capacity of the immature heart are invariably added to physiologic problems created by the CHD itself. Because the most severe forms of CHD generally are present in neonates, such congenital heart problems are complicated by physiologic limitations of the immature heart and lungs.

In patients with complex congenital disease in whom a number of previously discussed problems are present, assessment should be directed at myocardial performance and reserve, quantification of pulmonary blood flow, degree of cyanosis, and evaluation of PVR. For example, a patient with a long-standing Waterston shunt who is only mildly cyanotic but easily fatigued and who has a heaving precordium with bounding pulses may be expected to have a high-normal hematocrit with oxygen saturation in the upper 80s. Pulmonary blood flow is torrential, and PVR is elevated. This patient may not be a candidate for reparative cardiac procedures because of high (and irreversible) PVR resulting from progressive PVOD.

MANAGEMENT OF PROBLEMS ASSOCIATED WITH CPB

Management of CPB in children with CHD differs considerably from treatment of adults with acquired heart disease. Aortopulmonary communications, abnormal intracardiac anatomy, small body size, and immature cardiovascular systems alter CPB management. Historically, the morbidity of CPB in neonates and small infants has been a major limiting factor to surgical treatment.[20] Substantial evidence indicates that nonepithelial surface–induced damage to formed blood elements and blood proteins is proportionally greater in small children and infants, who have large surface area–to-body mass ratios. In recent years, technologic refinements have lowered the contribution of CPB-related problems to pediatric mortality, but CPB remains a substantial issue, particularly in small infants. Growing knowledge about the roles of cytokines, activated leukocytes, platelets, and endothelial cells in the inflammatory response to CPB holds promise for reducing the morbidity rate.[21]

Potential Perfusion Problems Because of the factors of scale related to surface area and blood volume, substantial hemodilution and multiple exchanges of the entire circulating blood volume are required when conventional pediatric CPB circuits are used in small infants. The minimum pump prime required even by current infant-sized pump oxygenator circuits (250-500 mL) is very large compared with the neonate native circulating blood volume (~300 mL). CPB results in an exchange of 1 or more blood volumes in neonates and small infants, plus hemodilution to hematocrits of 20%. This extensive dilutional exchange may make postbypass hemostasis difficult without fresh blood products and also imposes large crystalloid and metabolic loads. CPB priming solution has substantial metabolic consequences because of its large volume. Depending on the constituents of the pump prime solution, large glucose, lactate, and osmotic loads are imposed. These loads can be substantially reduced with modern washing and ultrafiltration techniques.[22] Ultrafiltration techniques likely reduce bypass morbidity in infants by decreasing the levels of cytokines and other inflammatory mediators.[2]

Pump perfusion in children is regulated primarily by flow rate in most institutions. Because of the greater relative cardiac output of infants and their greater surface area–to–body mass ratio, pump flow rates as high as 150 to 200 mL/kg/min are used in neonates weighing 2 to 3 kg to provide normal cardiac output. Despite these high flows, mean arterial pressures during bypass often are approximately 30 mm Hg in infants, particularly during deep hypothermia when hemodilution markedly decreases blood viscosity. In older children, lesser flows are used, and perfusion pressures increase until the standard adult flows (50-70 mL/kg/min) and pressures are achieved in patients weighing more than 50 kg. Because of the low mean arterial pressures frequently used during bypass surgery in infants, unobstructed venous return to the pump oxygenator reservoir is critically important during bypass surgery, particularly in the superior vena cava. The presence of high venous pressures in the cerebral circulation can markedly hamper cerebral perfusion in children when mean arterial pressures are low during bypass surgery. This is particularly true during deep hypothermia in children when pressure-flow autoregulation of cerebral perfusion may not be present.[23] When caval occlusion tapes are tightened around venous cannulae, it is especially important to check for signs of superior or inferior vena caval obstruction or alternatively to monitor pressures in central venous lines positioned superior to the caval tape.

In the absence of inferior or superior vena caval obstructions, with normal venous pressures, low arterial perfusion pressures cause no problem in hemodiluted children receiving adequate flow. However, the margin of error is small for proper positioning of inferior and superior vena cava cannulae in the small infant heart. Obstruction of hepatic or jugular veins can easily occur, so signs of caval obstruction should not be ignored, particularly when venous pump return is inadequate.

The frequent presence of aortopulmonary collaterals in patients with CHD makes the definition of adequate bypass flow rates uncertain. In assessing perfusion during CPB in patients with CHD, the potential effect of aortopulmonary shunts or collaterals on systemic perfusion should be considered. A high perfusion rate may be indicated by pump head revolutions, but unless all sources of aortopulmonary shunting are controlled, much of the aortic perfusion from the pump passes into the lungs through shunts and collaterals, and returns to the pump from the pulmonary veins through the intracardiac defect to the right atrial venous cannula. Blood traveling this route does not perfuse the systemic circulation and especially does not perfuse the brain. This may constitute a large proportion of apparent pump flow. Although well-defined shunts, such as PDA, Blalock-Taussig shunt, or Waterston shunt, may be ligated before bypass, many children with cyanotic disease have extensive aortopulmonary collaterals that are not easily controlled. During these conditions, pump flow rates may bear little relation to actual systemic perfusion.

Abnormally low perfusion pressure during bypass surgery despite high pump flows should suggest open systemic-to-pulmonary shunts. Sources of such shunts should be sought and controlled. Other indices of flow adequacy should be followed to ensure adequate perfusion of vital organs. Evidence indicates, for example, that systemic arterial collaterals to the lungs originating from the vertebral arteries may "steal" flow from the basilar artery and the brain during CPB, causing cerebral ischemia and choreoathetosis.[24]

During bypass cooling and warming, the rate of change recorded from temperature probes placed in various parts of the body provides an index of regional perfusion. Core temperature, measured by distal esophageal temperature, generally changes most quickly, followed by a lag of several degrees for nasopharyngeal or tympanic temperatures, the latter 2 better indicating brain perfusion. Rectal or extremity skin temperatures lag further because these areas reflect more peripheral perfusion. Temperature gradients between these regional beds decrease as steady state is approached and generally are seen in reverse order during warming. Deviations from normal temperature gradients seen on cooling and warming may indicate perfusion problems. However, such variations from normal temperature gradients do not predict the adequacy of cooling when jugular venous bulb oxygen saturations are measured during bypass cooling in small children.[25] In the absence of bypass warming or cooling, urine output and systemic acid–base balance are reasonable indicators of perfusion. Oxygen saturation of the venous outflow to the pump also is an important indicator of tissue perfusion. This value should be approximately 70% or greater, particularly during hypothermic bypass surgery.

Management of ventilation of the lungs during bypass surgery has been controversial. During partial bypass surgery, some ventilation probably is indicated if the pulmonic ventricle is demonstrably ejecting blood. This serves to oxygenate the small amount of blood being ejected so that the coronary arteries, which receive the bulk of this blood, are perfused with saturated blood. Low flow of 100% oxygen into the lungs should continue, even if no mechanical ventilation takes place, so that apneic oxygenation occurs as long as pulmonary blood flow continues. Frequent visual checks of arterial and venous lines at the pump provide estimates of the arteriovenous oxygen saturation difference and oxygen consumption. These estimates are periodically confirmed by measurement of venous and arterial blood gases, along with electrolytes, glucose, hematocrit, ionized calcium, and activated thromboplastin time (activated clotting time) during bypass surgery. Addition of blood, sodium bicarbonate, calcium, heparin, potassium, and crystalloid solutions to the pump reservoir, along with gas flow through the oxygenator, are guided by these measurements. Instruments that provide continuous Pao_2, PVo_2, pH, and Pco_2 are available for use during bypass but may not be as accurate as in vitro blood gas analysis.

Brain Damage The mortality after pediatric cardiac surgery has decreased significantly over the past few decades. As a result, attention has turned to the issue of morbidity, particularly neurologic morbidity. A survey of 6 major North American hospitals was conducted from 1988 to 1989. The conclusion drawn from this study was that the incidence of brain injury in children who had undergone pediatric cardiac surgery ranged from 2% to 25%.[26] Although significant improvements have been made in the perioperative management of children, the incidence remains significant. The most common problem seen is choreoathetosis, which has been reported with deep and moderate hypothermia, with long and short circulatory arrest, and with low and normal bypass flows.[27] Thus the exact cause of this problem is unclear, but it is almost certainly the result of disturbances of brain perfusion in the basal ganglia. Although it is known that brain blood flow is altered by temperature, $Paco_2$ levels, and the use of prolonged circulatory arrest periods,[28] among other factors, how these factors may interact to produce brain damage, such as choreoathetosis, in the isolated cases in which it occurs is not known. Studies have identified cerebral steal from systemic arterial collaterals to the pulmonary arteries originating from the vertebral–basilar artery system and short cooling times as a possible cause, but this remains to be confirmed.[10] In brain damage other than choreoathetosis, a relationship between high cooling rates and short cooling times before circulatory arrest and subsequent decreases in neurodevelopmental test scores in infants has been shown.[29] Even in the absence of overt neurologic injury, studies have shown that periods of hypothermic circulatory arrest longer than 30 to 40 minutes during bypass repairs of CHD in infants are associated with a greater incidence of postoperative seizures and lesser neurodevelopmental scores at 1 year of age.[30] In addition, the etiology of cerebral injury in adults usually is secondary to embolic phenomenon but in children is less clear. Preoperative, intraoperative, and postoperative factors all contribute to the final neurologic insult in children.

PREOPERATIVE FACTORS

Children with CHD may have some preexisting neurologic impairment or neurodevelopmental delay. Such abnormality has been known for some time with regard to the well-known syndromes, such as Down syndrome, Williams syndrome, and trisomy 13, but is being found with increasing frequency in patients with CHD as the ability to detect it improves. Limperopoulos et al[31] studied 131 newborns and infants before surgery for CHD. This group reported neurobehavioral abnormalities in more than half of the newborns, with more than 38% of the infants also showing neurodevelopmental abnormalities.

In addition to congenital abnormalities, acquired causes seem to make a significant contribution. The immature brain is extremely susceptible to the cardiorespiratory imbalance that often occurs in the preoperative patient before surgery.[29] Poor cardiac output, elevated central venous pressure (CVP), chronic hypoxia, and possible embolic phenomena all put the immature brain at risk. Limperopoulos et al[31] also noted that infants who had a saturation less than 85% preoperatively had a significantly greater incidence of neurologic abnormalities than those whose saturation was more than 85%. In a more recent study of babies with HLHS, 22 full-term neonates were examined by magnetic resonance imaging before surgery. Ischemic lesions were demonstrated in 23% of the patients.[32] Finally, the diagnosis itself has a significant prognostic effect. Patients with single ventricle physiology and arch obstruction have the highest risk of perioperative cerebral injury compared with all other forms of CHD.[33]

INTRAOPERATIVE FACTORS

Intraoperative cerebral injury usually is the result of ischemia and associated reperfusion injury. Some degree of inflammatory effect also may play a part. Current evidence suggests that management of the CPB aspect of the operation can substantially influence the outcome.

Deep Hypothermic Circulatory Arrest and Low-Flow Bypass In an effort to lower the high morbidity rate historically associated with CPB in young children undergoing intracardiac repairs for CHD, deep hypothermia with circulatory arrest or low-flow continuous bypass has been used. Deep hypothermic circulatory arrest (DHCA) with core and cerebral temperatures lower than 20°C in children weighing less than 10 kg and in selected older patients provides ideal operating conditions for the surgeon, reduces bypass time and blood trauma, and maximizes myocardial protection. These advantages are offset by the risk of central nervous system (CNS) damage from prolonged ischemic times. Studies, both animal and human, suggest that arrest times longer than 40 minutes increase the likelihood of severe injury.[34] Some centers have abandoned DHCA in favor of hypothermic low-flow CPB techniques because of concerns about subclinical neurologic damage and impairment of intellectual development, whereas others advocate using shorter periods of arrest interrupted by periods of perfusion to replace cerebral energy stores; however, this technique has not been conclusively proven in human studies.[35]

The potential disadvantages of DHCA are prolonged periods of ischemia to vital organs. As a practical matter in the large clinical experience with DHCA during the past 20 years, the only organ at appreciable risk is the brain. Most studies of neurologic outcome with DHCA in children and adults show no overt cerebral damage resulting from DHCA.[36] A minority of these studies have shown some evidence of effects on subsequent intellectual development, but usually only at circulatory arrest periods longer than 45 minutes. Neurologic outcome studies of DHCA patients have been criticized as being poorly controlled and nonrigorous in their assessment of neurologic injuries and of combining heterogeneous groups of patients. The most recent study that avoids these problems shows evidence of intellectual impairment at 1-year follow-up evaluations in infants subjected to DHCA periods of 30 minutes or lonoger.[30] Because mechanisms of ischemic protection of the hypothermic brain are incompletely understood, there are no accepted optimal techniques for cerebral protection and there is no well-defined "safe" period of circulatory arrest; however, circulatory arrest is being used less frequently in favor of low-flow bypass techniques. DHCA periods longer than 30 minutes are avoided whenever possible.

The alternative to DHCA, low-flow hypothermic CPB, in theory should allow for a reasonable surgical field while still providing adequate tissue perfusion to prevent cerebral injury. This has been demonstrated to be true metabolically, but recent studies in children have shown some significant deleterious effects of low-flow CPB.[37] In addition, there is no "standard" for "low-flow" bypass. Experimental studies have established that with decreasing total bypass flow during moderately hypothermic CPB surgery, the brain takes an increasingly larger fraction for itself to preserve normal cerebral oxygen consumption levels. When flow becomes sufficiently low, oxygen consumption decreases because of ischemia. Several studies have demonstrated that low-flow bypass resulted in loss of somatosensory-evoked potentials and intracellular adenosine triphosphate (ATP), and was associated with decreased intracellular pH when flow levels were sufficiently lessened.[38] In experimental studies measuring brain levels of high-energy phosphates in vivo, very low flows (down to 10 mL/kg/h) maintained normal brain creatinine phosphate and ATP levels in sheep during hypothermic low-flow bypass surgery.[39] In contrast, no middle cerebral artery (MCA) flow has been detected using TCD in clinical studies of infants and using greater levels of flow during hypothermic low-flow bypass surgery in 1 institution. A clinical study showed inconsistent perfusion of the MCA during hypothermic low-flow bypass surgery in infants in whom flows less than 30 mL/kg/min were used.[40]

Rossi et al[41] showed that creatine kinase levels were equally elevated after DHCA and after low-flow hypothermic bypass in infants, suggesting no difference between the 2 techniques using this measure of brain injury. Thus without any established "safe" level of low-flow bypass surgery, some degree of cerebral ischemia and damage may occur even when low-flow bypass surgery is used in preference to DHCA. Thus continuous low-flow bypass surgery may well provide a false sense of security about brain protection. Together with less favorable operating conditions obtained with low-flow bypass surgery, this false security can markedly prolong low-flow bypass time, bypass damage, and potentially cerebral ischemic time that may occur during low-flow bypass surgery. Because the mechanisms of cerebral injury and the physiology of low-flow bypass surgery during hypothermia in infants and children are not well understood, the cerebral protective effects of low-flow bypass surgery may not always be better than DHCA.

Cerebral blood flow studies in children undergoing DHCA and low-flow bypass surgery by Greeley et al[28] have shown that cerebral pressure-flow autoregulation is lost in children during deep hypothermia but that metabolism-flow regulation is retained. After prolonged circulatory arrest, cerebral blood flow and metabolism subsequently remain depressed during and after bypass compared with more normal recovery of metabolic rate and cerebral blood flow with continuous low-flow bypass.[23] These findings are consistent with delayed recovery of electroencephalographic (EEG) and somatosensory-evoked potentials after prolonged DHCA.[42] Despite delayed recovery of these functional measures and low cerebral blood flow and metabolism immediately after DHCA, gross neurologic deficits are seen infrequently.

DHCA provides optimal conditions for precise surgical repairs of complex intracardiac problems in tiny hearts, minimizes the formidable morbidity of CPB in small infants, improves myocardial protection, and lessens the incidence of cannulation-related problems and obstruction in the inferior and superior vena cavae. Low-flow bypass should provide less cerebral risk, with most of the surgical benefit associated with visualization of anatomy. In the Boston Circulatory Arrest Study, which compared these 2 support strategies in patients diagnosed with D-transposition of the great arteries, results were less conclusive. The patients in the DHCA group had worse outcome with respect to seizure activity postoperatively, motor skills at 1 year of age, and behavior, speech, and language at 4 years of age. However, at 8-year follow-up, the low-flow CPB group demonstrated more impulsive behavior, and although the DHCA group still fared worse with regard to manual dexterity and speech, IQ was similar across both groups but below the average for the normal population.[30]

GLUCOSE MANAGEMENT

Evidence suggests that management of glucose levels is important in cerebral protection. Recovery from cerebral ischemia occurring during hyperglycemia is impaired, suggesting that hyperglycemia in the mature brain should be avoided in DHCA.[43] In addition, children often have hyperglycemic responses to the stress of hypothermic CPB surgery, and deep levels of anesthesia can markedly attenuate both the hyperglycemic stress responses and other hormonal and metabolic stress responses seen with CPB in children.[44] In a study[45] that attempted to evaluate the effect of glucose levels on children undergoing the arterial switch procedure, patients were randomized to low-flow versus DHCA and a retrospective analysis of glucose versus outcome was performed. This study suggested that lower blood glucose in the early postbypass period tended to predict EEG seizures but was not associated with an increase in clinical seizures. The report concluded that because glucose levels in the perioperative period were not associated with neurodevelopmental outcome at 1, 4, and 8 years of age, perhaps avoidance of hypoglycemia should be more of a priority in the perioperative period than should avoidance of hyperglycemia. Anesthetic management should emphasize the use of muscle relaxants and barbiturates, and the reduction of stress responses to minimize oxygen consumption and hyperglycemia during the ischemic period, but avoidance of hypoglycemia should remain a priority.[45] Pharmacologic protective agents, such as high-dose steroids and barbiturates, have not been shown to be protective against DHCA-related brain damage despite theoretical support for their use.

ACID–BASE MANAGEMENT

Although cogent theoretical reasons exist for why acid–base management, through its influences on cerebral blood flow and cerebral intracellular pH in the brain, may affect such damage, clinical studies of its effects during DHCA have not yet been performed. Acid–base management thus far has not been shown to have an important effect on the incidence of cerebral complications in hypothermic open heart surgery, at least in adults in whom circulatory arrest has not been used.[46] A large prospective trial comparing pH-stat and α-stat strategies for patients undergoing surgery requiring DHCA demonstrated a lower incidence of seizures, shorter time to first EEG activity, lower postoperative morbidity and mortality, and better cardiac output perioperatively in the pH-stat group. Thus pH-stat is the recommended technique at present.[47]

TEMPERATURE MANAGEMENT

Temperature management has the most significant effect on cerebral homeostasis. Decreasing temperature provides for luxury perfusion of the brain. An increase in temperature above normal provides for an equally deleterious medium. Any excess in temperature increases the release of excitatory amino acids resulting in increased reperfusion injury and apoptosis.

POSTOPERATIVE FACTORS

Temperature management, inhibition of inflammatory mediators, and maintaining adequacy of cerebral oxygen delivery remain the mainstay by which cerebral injury is prevented in the postoperative period. As a result of this, the concept of multimodality neurophysiologic monitoring in the perioperative period has emerged. Although none of these modalities has been shown to predict cerebral injury individually, use of a combination may serve as a surrogate marker predictive of injury. The combination required is not yet decided.

NEAR-INFRARED SPECTROSCOPY

Near-infrared spectroscopy (NIRS) is a technique that enables continuous monitoring of regional cerebral oxygenation. Similar to pulse oximetry, cerebral oximetry uses the fact that oxygenated and deoxygenated hemoglobin absorb near-infrared light to differing degrees. With more than 1 wavelength, the oxyhemoglobin fraction can be determined. Currently 2 types of monitors are available for NIRS: a concentration monitor that measures the concentration of oxyhemoglobin and reduced hemoglobin and the relative redox state of cytochrome aa_3, and the saturation monitor that measures the ratio of oxyhemoglobin and deoxyhemoglobin.

The skull is translucent to infrared light, so intracranial measurement is possible. The device uses a light-emitting diode (near-infrared light 700-1000 nm) and 2 light sensors placed 3 and 4 cm away from the light source. The diode emits near-infrared light, which passes through a tissue volume to the detectors. The proximal detector detects light absorbed by extracranial tissues and is subtracted from the total signal, thus allowing determination of intracranial absorption.

Although 2 instruments, the INVOS 4100 (and 5100 for pediatrics; Somanetics, Troy, MI) and the NIRO 300 (Hamamatsu, Hamamatsu City, Japan) are commercially available, only the INVOS has Food and Drug Administration (FDA) approval. The INVOS is a continuous-wave, spatially resolved spectrometer that measures change in regional oxygen saturation (rSo_2). Although the device appears to provide continuous monitoring of cerebral oxygenation, the technology has some drawbacks. Because the range of values has not been established, only a trend can be followed, and absolute values are not available. Thus rSo_2 is reported as a percentage on a scale from 15% to 95%. This in itself may expose the patient to the risk of hyperperfusion at high cerebral rSo_2 values.[48] In addition, the proprietary algorithm used to calculate the rSo_2 value is based on the assumption that 25% of the intracranial blood is arterial and 75% is venous. In attempting to validate this assumption in children, Watzman et al[49] found a ratio closer to 15:85, with much interindividual variation. Finally, obtaining an estimate of cerebral blood volume is possible but not yet completely validated, so its accuracy and usefulness remain uncertain. Despite this, the INVOS instrument is increasingly used in the pediatric operating room, with a deviation of 20% from baseline suggestive of an abnormal event.

TCD ULTRASOUND

TCD ultrasound allows noninvasive continuous monitoring of cerebral blood flow velocity and emboli in the proximal segment of the MCA. This artery provides 70% of the blood flow to the ipsilateral cerebral hemisphere.[50] When using this device, the assumption is made that the diameter of the MCA remains constant, and that there is an association between blood velocity and actual blood flow that is independent of variables such as cerebral vascular resistance and temperature.

Comparing TCD with the xenon technique for measuring cerebral blood flow, Bishop et al[51] found a poor correlation between absolute values of cerebral blood flow velocity and cerebral blood flow. However, a good correlation was found during hypocapnia, leading the authors to conclude that changes in cerebral blood flow velocity expressed as a reactivity index, not an absolute number, should be used as an indicator of cerebral blood flow.[51] A study using TCD to examine the effect of temperature on cerebral blood flow during CPB found that autoregulation was maintained at normothermia, was partially lost with moderate hypothermia, and was totally lost with profound hypothermia under α-stat conditions.[52] TCD has also been used to detect emboli reaching the cerebral circulation. True emboli are designated high-intensity transient signals and have characteristic audio and visual signals that differentiate them from false positives. However, distinguishing between true emboli and false positives is difficult in practice, and the problem remains that detection occurs after the insult and thus does not in itself prevent the incident. Cannula malposition, however, causes a sudden reduction in blood flow velocity and thus is detected very quickly by TCD. Overall, although TCD can provide a gauge by which changes in cerebral blood flow can be monitored, its use as a preventative tool is yet to be determined.

Weaning From Bypass During rewarming, air is vented from the heart before ejection of blood into the systemic circulation is allowed. Arterial blood gases, electrolytes, glucose, and coagulation parameters are checked periodically during bypass surgery, but especially during rewarming. Electrolytes, especially ionized calcium, are adjusted to normal ranges before separation from bypass. Adequacy of rewarming is judged by temperature recording from multiple sites and is particularly important when deep hypothermia has been used.

The need for vasopressor and inotropic support to accomplish weaning from bypass is first estimated by close observation of the heart's behavior during rewarming. Dysrhythmias, coronary perfusion problems, and the state of myocardial contractility can be estimated from the appearance of the heart. Separation from bypass should be accomplished in close concert with the surgical team using all available sources of information about hemodynamic status. Monitoring appropriate intracardiac and intra-arterial pressures and waveforms and transesophageal echocardiogram may provide good information about the adequacy of the operative repair, myocardial preservation, ventricular function, and the state of the pulmonary circulation.[53] Slavish adherence to numbers produced by intracardiac catheters and pressure-monitoring systems without visual confirmation of cardiac performance can lead to numerous errors. Small size and presence of unsuspected congenital defects make interpretation of pressures from monitors difficult.[54,55] When rewarming is complete and cardiac function is judged adequate, weaning from extracorporeal circulation is accomplished by slowly allowing the heart to fill and eject while reestablishing ventilation. Optimal ventricular filling pressures are estimated using filling pressures from preoperative catheterization data, appearance of the heart, and infusion of small volume increments while watching filling and systemic arterial pressures. Using this latter technique, a mental Frank-Starling curve can be constructed.

If systemic arterial pressure or gas exchange is inadequate, CPB is reinstituted while problems are analyzed. Problems with oxygenation after bypass surgery are caused as frequently by deficiencies in pulmonary blood flow as by deficiencies in ventilation. With low Pao_2, adequacy of pulmonary blood flow and ventilation should be critically assessed. Analysis of problems with weaning should start with reassessment of surgical repair, adequacy of ventilation, and verification that inotropic support is reaching the heart. Measurement of PA and atrial and intraventricular pressures often is helpful, along with pullback pressure gradient measurement across aortic and pulmonic valves if indicated.

In patients who are doing poorly after the bypass period, missed or residual lesions are likely. This possibility should be carefully considered before committing the child to prolonged inotropic support postoperatively. Residual defects are by far the most frequent cause of immediate hemodynamic problems and instability after repair, even in institutions with superb diagnostic and surgical expertise in CHD.

Questions of inadequate repair should be resolved using intraoperative echocardiography, including Doppler assessment of intracardiac shunts, with either epicardial or transesophageal approaches.[56-58] In complex CHD, a physician specially trained and expert in the echocardiographic assessment of CHD should interpret such studies. When the problem is identified, appropriate corrective measures are taken and weaning is again attempted. If no anatomic problems are readily apparent and if the difficultly with weaning appears to be a result of reversible myocardial dysfunction or reversible pulmonary hypertension that cannot be adequately managed, use of a left or right VAD or ECMO should be considered.

ANESTHETIC PROBLEMS DURING CLOSED CARDIAC PROCEDURES

Anesthesia for closed cardiac procedures may be more demanding than for those involving CPB because bypass support can temporarily solve many hemodynamic problems that otherwise cause intraoperative deterioration. Monitoring requirements are just as stringent, and venous and arterial access is even more important. Pulse oximetry is invaluable to help evaluate the infant's condition. PDA and coarctation of the aorta are the only lesions corrected with closed surgical procedures; ductus ligation and other closed procedures now can be performed using video-assisted thoracoscopic surgery. Closed palliative procedures are used in patients with hypoxemia to increase pulmonary blood flow by constructing surgical shunts, to decrease excessive pulmonary blood flow using a PA band, and to improve atrial mixing of pulmonary and systemic venous return (Blalock-Hanlon atrial septectomy) in transposition of the great arteries. Palliative surgical procedures now are performed less frequently because early correction of many severe cases of CHD has become possible with accompanying low mortality rates and because of the efficacy and safety of interventional cardiac catheterization. Such palliative procedures, when used in preference to reparative procedures, have appreciable mortality and morbidity rates of their own.[59] Reparative operations that correct the intracardiac pathophysiologic conditions are increasingly feasible and preferable even in newborns.[60]

Acid–base and electrolyte balance are meticulously maintained throughout closed procedures. When these procedures are performed via thoracotomy, the operative field is rarely visible to the anesthesia care team. Marked deterioration in cardiopulmonary status may result from surgical manipulation and retraction. Any deterioration of the infant's condition should be immediately communicated to the surgical team, which has a better view of the surgical field. Serious deterioration should prompt solicitation of surgical help. Release of retraction usually results in return to hemodynamic stability. Some compromise of ventilation and pulmonary blood flow inevitably occurs in these procedures, sometimes with severe decreases in Sao_2. Inadvertent compression of coronary arteries during these procedures may cause severe cardiac ischemia and dysfunction, which is readily correctable by adjustment of retraction. Anesthetic management using deep levels of anesthesia that minimize oxygen consumption and support cardiovascular stability usually minimizes intraoperative problems but may prolong postoperative ventilation. In extreme cases, periods of inotropic and pressor support may be required intraoperatively.

Ductus Arteriosus and Vascular Ring Interruption PDA ligation and other procedures, such as interruption of vascular rings, now can be performed thoracoscopically, with either 1-lung anesthesia or 2-lung anesthesia with lung retraction.[61] In either case, transient decreases in Sao_2 that may occur can be managed with brief reexpansion of the collapsed lung. Visualization of the operative field is superior when thoracoscopy is used. Conversion to open thoracotomy occasionally is required if exposure is not adequate or if bleeding occurs. Transesophageal echocardiographic confirmation of interruption of flow is useful to ensure complete closure of the vessel.[62]

Surgical Shunts Severe hypoxemia occurring in the operating room during or after creation of the shunt implies inadequate pulmonary blood flow. Intrapulmonary shunting should be considered in lungs that are retracted, but mechanical obstruction of flow into the PA because of retraction or actual shunt obstruction (kinking or thrombosis) is the usual cause. Reinflation of the retracted lung segment eliminates intrapulmonary shunting. If hypoxemia persists, hyperventilation can minimize PVR and optimize gas exchange until pulmonary blood flow can be improved. Systemic-to-PA shunts are inherently inefficient, recirculating oxygenated blood into the lungs and placing a volume load on the heart.

Pulmonary blood flow should be several times greater than systemic flow to substantially reduce hypoxemia (see Fig. 53-3). When the surgically created shunt is too large, pulmonary flows are excessive. This is manifested by pulmonary edema (sometimes unilateral) on chest radiography obtained postoperatively. Intraoperatively, large pulse pressures, excessively low diastolic arterial pressures, and sometimes inadequate systemic output result in children whose Sao_2 is relatively high despite complete mixing of systemic and pulmonary venous return. Maneuvers to increase PVR can compensate for excessive pulmonary flow to a limited degree, but early or late shunt revision often is necessary. Other reported acute complications of systemic-to-PA shunts include Horner syndrome, chylothorax, and acute ischemia of the ipsilateral arm when the subclavian artery is sacrificed.

The Glenn shunt (superior vena cava to right PA with no pump in between) is limited to patients with low PVR because venous pressure is used to provide pulmonary blood flow. Consequently, its use in newborns and infants is excluded. Other problems with Glenn shunts include thrombosis, occlusion, and elevation of PVR leading to superior vena cava syndrome. The Glenn shunt is more efficient than an arterial shunt and is useful in patients who have congestive heart failure stemming from volume overload. In general, for other patients, the Blalock-Taussig shunt has proven the most reliable of the surgical shunts, with good long-term patency rates regardless of age. Early mortality and the incidence of late postoperative complications are less than those for alternative shunt procedures.[63]

PA Banding When pulmonary blood flow is excessive and high pressure is communicated to the pulmonary vasculature, surgical intervention may be necessary to prevent progressive PVOD or to lessen symptoms of high-output congestive heart failure and inadequate systemic output. When early complete repair is not possible, pulmonary blood flow is restricted by banding the PA. This adds pulmonary outflow resistance, which converts simple, nonrestrictive shunting situations into complex shunts with limited pulmonary flow. During induction of anesthesia before the band is applied, PVR occasionally may decrease enough to result in massive pulmonary flow and systemic hypotension ("pulmonary steal"). In this case, a partial occlusion of the PA with a clamp aids in maintaining hemodynamic stability until the band can be applied.

However, the banding procedure is unsatisfyingly crude, and results are hemodynamically unpredictable.[59] Adequacy of the band in the operating room is assessed by observing an increased systemic blood pressure and an acceptable decrease in systemic oxygen saturation. Direct measurement of PA pressure beyond the band is made, and the pressure is adjusted to approximately half the systemic arterial pressure. Continuous monitoring of Sao_2 is helpful in rapidly assessing critically low levels of pulmonary blood flow that may occur during band tightening.

TRANSCATHETER MANAGEMENT IN THE CARDIAC CATHETERIZATION LABORATORY

Congenital heart problems are frequently managed today by transcatheter interventions in the catheterization laboratory. Physiologic derangement and complications during such interventions may approach that seen in the cardiac operating room.[64] Anesthesia is often advisable for patient comfort and safety and for the monitoring and management of complications.[65] **Table 53-4** lists the lesions currently managed using interventional cardiac catheterization, the procedures used, and their effects and complications.

Evolving techniques of nonsurgical management of CHDs have markedly altered pediatric cardiac anesthesia. ASDs, VSDs, PDA, and coarctation of the aorta commonly form the bulk of pediatric cardiac surgery performed in many programs. These lesions now can be managed in the interventional catheterization laboratory using nonsurgical transcatheter techniques. A number of these procedures, including closure of ASDs and PDA, can even be performed on an outpatient basis.[64] In centers

TABLE 53-4 Interventional Procedures Performed in the Cardiac Catheterization Laboratory Affecting Pathophysiology of Congenital Heart Disease

Procedure	Structure/Lesion	Effects	Complications
Coil embolizations	Aortopulmonary collateral	Reduce pulmonary flow	Hypoxemia, systemic embolization
	Blalock-Taussig shunts	Reduce pulmonary flow	
	Anomalous coronary arteries	Increase coronary flow, reduce pulmonary flow	
Transcatheter device closures	Patent ductus arteriosis	Eliminate shunt, reduce pulmonary flow	Air embolization, device embolization, interference with mitral and tricuspid valve function
	Atrial septic defect	Eliminate shunt, reduce pulmonary flow, prevent paradoxic embolization	
	Ventricular septal defect	Eliminate shunt, reduce pulmonary flow	
Balloon and stent dilations	Pulmonary stenosis	Increase pulmonary flow	Embolization of stent, pulmonary artery disruption, unilateral pulmonary edema, pulmonary insufficiency, aortic insufficiency, mitral insufficiency, tricuspid insufficiency, aortic dissection
	Blalock-Taussig shunt	Increase pulmonary flow	
	Pulmonary valve stenosis	Increase pulmonary flow	
	Tricuspid valve stenosis	Increase pulmonary flow	
	Aortic valve stenosis	Increase pulmonary flow	
	Mitral valve stenosis	Increase systemic flow	
	Aorta (coarctations and others)	Increase systemic flow	
Atrial septostomies (balloon and blade)	Interatrial septum	Increase pulmonary blood flow	Perforation of heart, tamponade
Radiofrequency transcatheter mapping and ablation	Anomalous conduction pathways	Eliminate dysrhythmias, especially supraventricular tachycardia	Complete heart block; supraventricular tachycardia

that perform large numbers of interventional catheterization procedures, these common congenital heart lesions are seen less frequently in the operating room. Transcatheter closures of ASDs have been successfully done in hundreds of patients. Smaller number of VSDs, including multiple VSDs, are frequently closed with these techniques.[65]

Newer techniques continue to move this field forward. Patients with tetralogy of Fallot (and its subtypes) require relief of right ventricular outflow tract obstruction or restoration of continuity between the right ventricle and the pulmonary arteries. Whether the repair is conducted as a primary neonatal procedure or after a palliative arteriopulmonary connection is largely related to institutional bias. However, the end result appears very similar. In particular, this subgroup progresses very well toward adulthood, but the life span of prosthetic conduits is finite. Conduit stenosis and valve regurgitation appear to be the most problematic, requiring intervention before end-stage right ventricular dysfunction.

Balloon dilation of conduit stenosis may provide many months, if not years, of delay in the need for surgical conduit replacement, and transcatheter pulmonary valve replacement using bovine jugular valves (Melody valve) has become common. The procedure is new enough that it is currently unclear how many years' delay in pulmonary valve replacement may be gained by this technique. Percutaneous stenting is already used as a technique to delay surgical replacement. Further development in this area has included the development of percutaneous pulmonary valve insertion. A biologic valve is harvested from a bovine jugular vein. A section of this vein containing the trileaflet valve is then mounted in a stent for percutaneous insertion. Current studies have successfully demonstrated this technique, with low morbidity and mortality. The long-term durability of this stent and the ability to perform sequential percutaneous pulmonary valve implantation will determine its eventual place in the armamentarium, but at present it certainly should help to delay surgery to such a time that a 16-mm valve can be inserted rather than performing earlier and repetitive surgery with the obvious associated risks.[66] Interventional catheterization techniques listed in Table 53-4 also are used increasingly in conjunction with surgical procedures to improve the results of surgical management of CHD and to extend therapy to previously unmanageable lesions.

Anesthetic Care Catheterization procedures have become more invasive, use larger and multiple catheters, involve greater blood loss, and produce more pain in smaller and sicker patients. The cardiac catheterization laboratory has effectively turned into an operating room in which major problems and complications can result from increasingly invasive procedures. Although many patients seen in the pediatric catheterization laboratory can be adequately sedated by cardiologists, complex procedures in sick children require anesthetic care. Anesthesia, monitoring, and hemodynamic management are needed for many of these invasive procedures performed in children and contribute substantially to a successful procedure.[67] Many patients can be treated with monitored IV sedation techniques, but others require general endotracheal anesthesia. Indications for using either technique are not yet well defined but depend on patient condition, procedure, and anticipated complications.

Anesthetic management is handicapped by the catheterization laboratory environment. Problems include poor patient access, poor lighting, radiation hazards, and lack of communication with cardiologists. Independent monitoring, independent IV and sometimes intra-arterial access, independent light sources, and adequate access to the patient's airway should be sought. Prevention or prompt management of complications is a major anesthetic task in this setting. Without a thorough understanding of transcatheter procedures, their complications, and their management, the anesthesia provider is handicapped in coping with the accelerating development of these new techniques.

Problems and Hemodynamic Complications Complications of various interventional procedures are related partly to the type of interventional procedure, but all share risks associated with percutaneous access to major veins and arteries. Specific problems that may occur during various interventional transcatheter procedures are listed in Table 53-4. Many problems are sudden, occur without warning, and are potentially life threatening. As in the operating room, successful management of complications depends heavily on prompt action by anesthesiologists cooperating closely with interventional cardiologists and radiologists.

Loss of control of embolic and closure devices can result in systemic and pulmonary arterial embolization. Embolized devices usually can be retrieved using a variety of retrieval catheters, but in a minority of patients, surgical removal is required. If the device is lodged in the heart or a great vessel, CPB may be required for removal. Such device embolizations usually do not cause extreme hemodynamic instability or cardiovascular decompensation requiring emergency surgical removal, but urgent surgical procedures may be necessary. Even after successful transcatheter retrieval, femoral artery and vein reconstructions occasionally are necessary when embolized devices or large dilation balloons are removed through these vessels.[68] When deliberate embolization of aortopulmonary collaterals excessively decreases pulmonary flow and produces severe hypoxemia, general anesthesia and muscle paralysis can increase Sao_2 to acceptable levels by decreasing oxygen consumption, at least until surgical intervention.

Disruption and avulsion of major blood vessels occurs, particularly PA disruption during balloon dilation procedures.[69] PA disruption is signaled by hemoptysis or appearance of contrast media in the pleural space or major lung fissures. Substantial hemoptysis calls for immediate endotracheal intubation for airway control and ventilation. Positive end-expiratory pressure (PEEP) may be useful. Intrapulmonary hemorrhage often is self-limited, but hemothorax can be severe and can result in death.[69] Transient unilateral pulmonary edema can occur during PA dilation because of sudden increases in flow after dilation to a previously underperfused lung.[69] Unilateral pulmonary edema and disruption of PA integrity can occur abruptly. Both can cause the appearance of frank blood or blood-tinged edema or fluid in substantial quantities in the airway. Management starts with endotracheal intubation and positive-pressure ventilation unless symptoms are only minimal.

Intracardiac air embolization may be a particular problem when clamshell devices are used for PDA, ASD, and VSD closures because the large delivery sheath in the heart is transiently open to atmosphere. Transcatheter closure of an ASD using a clamshell device is shown schematically in **Fig. 53-8**. In patients with intracardiac shunts, air embolization may be life threatening. The large delivery sheath is a potential space for air accumulation and subsequent delivery into the heart. In addition, when the entry port of the large delivery sheath is open during removal and reinsertion of various catheters and devices, extreme inspiratory efforts may entrain intracardiac air. Air delivered into the right atrium may be shunted across the ASD even in the presence of nominal left-to-right shunting. Left atrial air embolization during these procedures can be seen with fluoroscopy. Resultant ST-segment changes, hypotension, arterial desaturation, and bradycardia generally respond to air aspiration followed by sealing the entry port, along with administration of atropine and inotropic support to maintain coronary perfusion. Meticulous purging of air from the catheter system, with sealing of open ports, should minimize air embolism. Controlled positive-pressure endotracheal ventilation in anesthetized, paralyzed patients may decrease the potential for air entrainment.

Tricuspid or mitral regurgitation with hemodynamic compromise may occur acutely when large catheters impinge on atrioventricular valves. These large catheters can cause dynamic stenosis as they pass across small valves. These problems usually respond to inotropic support and repositioning of the delivery catheter and device. Acute myocardial perforation with tamponade occurs occasionally during the course of interventional cardiac catheterization procedures. Prompt support of the circulation with volume infusions and pressor support, along with immediate catheter drainage of the pericardial space, are essential.

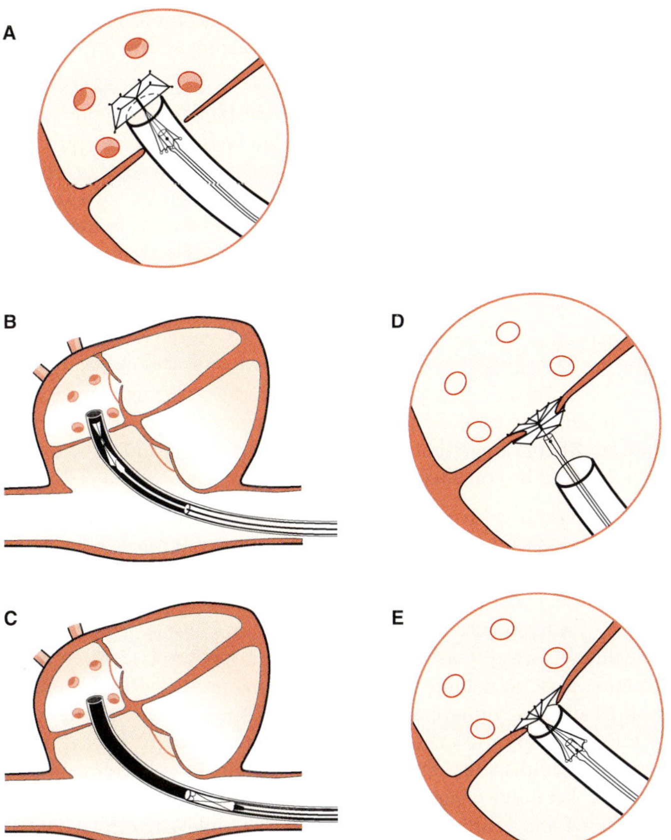

FIGURE 53-8. Technique of transcatheter atrial septal defect closure. **A.** Collapsed clamshell device is through the sheath. **B.** Device and sheath as a unit are positioned on the left atrial side of the defect using previously determined fluoroscopic landmarks. **C.** Sheath is pulled partially back, allowing 1 set of flexible, spring-loaded arms (covered with Dacron mesh) to spring open in the left atrium. **D.** Sheath, delivery system, and half-opened clamshell device are pulled back as a unit until the open arms engage the left atrial septal surface. **E.** Sheath is pulled farther back to expose the proximal half of the device, allowing it to spring open and engage the right atrial septal surface. Subsequently, the clamshell device is released and the delivery system withdrawn.

EFFECTS OF ANESTHESIA AND RELATED MANIPULATIONS ON PATHOPHYSIOLOGY

ANESTHETICS

Individual pathophysiology and the proposed therapeutic procedure largely dictate anesthetic management. Often the skill with which the technique is used determines the success of the anesthesia team in maintaining cardiovascular stability. Several anesthetic techniques provide good cardiovascular stability in children with severe CHD, but cardiovascular stability may not be the only criterion for a successful anesthetic.[70] Stress responses to pain and other noxious stimulation are profound even in the youngest neonates.[71] Extreme hormonal and metabolic stress responses during cardiac surgery and CPB can be pathologic in magnitude and are associated with poorer outcome in neonates undergoing cardiac surgery, despite hemodynamic stability.[72] Anesthetic techniques clearly have an effect on stress responses—metabolic and hormonal. It is important that children of all ages be given adequate anesthesia for suppression of hormonal and metabolic responses to noxious stimulation and for humane considerations.

Inhalational Anesthetics Inhalational anesthetics should be used cautiously in children with CHD because of their myocardial and circulatory depression. This is particularly true for induction of anesthesia before adequate access to the circulation and complete hemodynamic monitoring are established. Safe use of conventional inhalation induction with potent anesthetics depends on evaluation of the child's cardiac lesion and understanding the effects in young children with CHD. In children of any age with marginal cardiovascular reserve, myocardial depression caused by potent inhalational agents may produce systemic hypotension, but these agents are still unquestionably useful in small, titrated concentrations to control hypertensive responses after induction when the airway is secure after monitoring and hemodynamic stability is established.

Even in cyanotic children, if they have reasonable functional cardiac reserve, anesthesia can be induced with halothane and oxygen, even with 70% nitrous oxide (the latter relatively contraindicated because of air bubble expansion), without clinically significant decreases in Sao_2.[73] Dramatic decreases in arterial pressures occur with these techniques, sometimes to severe degrees. In infants, such induction techniques are of special concern because of the immature circulatory system. Use of these agents may considerably narrow the margin of safety in infants and younger children with severe CHD. At least in those given halothane, the levels tolerated by sick infants provide little suppression of the stress responses to cardiac surgery and CPB.[74]

Numerous studies have shown that even the normal immature cardiovascular system of infants without CHD does not tolerate isoflurane well; approximately 50% of infants with normal cardiovascular systems develop substantial hypotension and bradycardia during induction with these agents unless cardiovascular function is supported.[75] Ventricular function declines during isoflurane induction in normal infants; stroke volume and ejection fraction decrease by as much as 38%.[76]

Sevoflurane is a fluoridated derivative of methyl isopropyl ether and has rapidly become the inhalational agent of choice for children. This is largely because it is the only ethereal anesthetic that does not trigger a reflex response or cause airway irritation during inhaled induction. This, combined with its rapid recovery and minimal metabolism, makes sevoflurane an ideal agent in general pediatrics. It does cause myocardial depression in children, although stroke volume and ejection fraction are somewhat less depressed with sevoflurane than with other potent inhalational agents.[77] In adults, isoflurane appears to decrease SVR more than sevoflurane does. Although this decrease occurs, cardiac index appears to be preserved with both agents, and patients undergoing cardiac or thoracic procedures appear to tolerate either anesthetic safely.[78] In 1 of the few studies comparing isoflurane and sevoflurane in children with CHD, similar results were found. Fifty-four children undergoing cardiac surgery received sevoflurane, isoflurane, halothane, or fentanyl-midazolam. Only sevoflurane and isoflurane maintained cardiac index, with sevoflurane producing less reduction in SVR than any other agent in the study.[79]

Few published studies of desflurane in children with CHD are available, but studies in healthy children suggest that the effects of desflurane on ejection fraction and stroke volume are little different from those of halothane.[80] Isoflurane may be an unwise choice for inhalation induction in cyanotic children because increased airway problems and laryngospasm during induction, due to its pungency, may lead to increases in PVR. Somewhat less myocardial depression occurs in older children.

Nitrous Oxide Use of nitrous oxide may cause expansion of intravascular air emboli, exaggerating their circulatory effects, even without additional systemic embolization.[81] In patients with systemic embolization of air to the coronary circulation, nitrous oxide has been shown experimentally to be deleterious.[82] In children with intracardiac shunts, the potential exists for systemic shunting of microbubbles and macrobubbles of air from IV lines and from exposure of the left heart to the atmosphere during open cardiac surgical procedures. Although clinical problems from enlargement of air emboli by nitrous oxide have not been reported in this setting, avoidance of its use is prudent in patients in whom systemic air embolization is a strong possibility.

Nitrous oxide in adults decreases cardiac output, systemic arterial pressure, and heart rate, and increases PVR, especially in patients with elevated PVR.[83] In children with right-to-left shunts who have decreased pulmonary flow or pulmonary hypertension, increases in PVR with nitrous oxide are detrimental. However, at least in 1 study, no increase in PA pressure or PVR was observed in infants given 50% nitrous oxide, regardless of preexisting PVR.[84] Mild but notable decreases in cardiac output, systemic arterial pressure, and heart rate were seen in these infants. Inhalation induction with 70% nitrous oxide and halothane in cyanotic children does not decrease Sa_{O_2}, suggesting that pulmonary blood flow is not decreased and that PVR is not substantially increased by nitrous oxide.[85] Although use of nitrous oxide prevents the use of 100% O_2, this may not actually decrease arterial saturation in cyanotic children without lung disease because increases in the fraction of inspired oxygen (F_{IO_2}) have little effect on arterial desaturation caused by large central intracardiac cardiac shunts.[86] The effects of F_{IO_2} on arterial saturation for different levels of right-to-left shunting are shown in **Fig. 53-9**.

Use of inhalational agents in children with intracardiac shunting is theoretically complicated by differences in uptake and distribution. A complex computer model suggests that inhalation induction is slowed in the presence of central right-to-left shunts, is slowed less in mixed shunts, and is little changed in pure left-to-right shunts, all in proportion to the size of the shunt.[87] These models assume constant cardiac output and are most marked for insoluble gases such as nitrous oxide. In children with left-to-right shunts, speed of inhalation induction actually is altered little clinically. Experimental data in animals with right-to-left shunts confirm slowing of induction, but data in children with right-to-left shunts are not available.[88] Inhalation induction often seems somewhat slow in children with pure right-to-left shunts, but this effect is not marked, probably because of the effects of multiple other variables affecting uptake. Relatively slow induction of anesthesia in children with pure right-to-left shunts is a consideration in

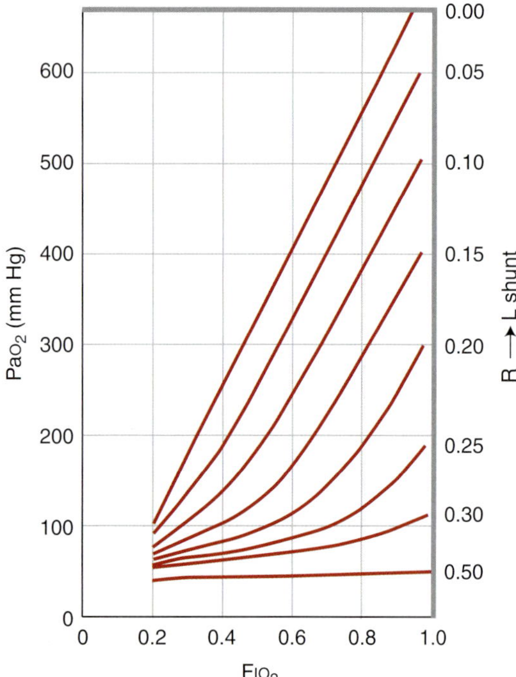

FIGURE 53-9. Iso-shunt graph depicting relationship between fraction of inspired oxygen (F_{IO_2}) and arterial Pa_{O_2} with different amounts of right-to-left shunting. Assumes normal values of pH, Pa_{CO_2}, pulmonary venous saturation, and mixed venous saturation. [Modified from Lawler PG, Nunn JF. A reassessment of the validity of the iso-shunt graph. *Br J Anaesth.* 1984;56:1325-1335. © The Board of Management and Trustees of the *British Journal of Anaesthesia*. Reproduced by permission of Oxford University Press/*British Journal of Anaesthesia*.]

deciding how rapidly to increase the inhaled concentrations of potent anesthetics during induction without producing severe myocardial depression.

Intramuscular and IV Anesthetics Some IV anesthetics, such as ketamine and high-dose opiates, can provide improved safety margins for induction of anesthesia in the immature and compromised cardiovascular system of neonates and infants with severe cardiac disease and in older children with minimal cardiovascular reserve. Very high transient arterial, cardiac, and brain concentrations of IV agents can result from normal IV doses given as a bolus in children with known right-to-left shunts because mixing, uptake, and pulmonary metabolism are bypassed. For example, IV lidocaine in a 1-mg/kg antiarrhythmic bolus dose administered in dogs with right-to-left shunts resulted in arterial concentrations higher than those reported to cause irreversible myocardial toxicity.[89] The potential for transiently high arterial levels of IV anesthetics in patients with intracardiac mixing and right-to-left shunts should be considered in planning.

Ketamine When IV access is a problem, intramuscular ketamine 3 to 5 mg/kg is well tolerated in sick children with cyanosis or congestive heart failure.[90] In contrast to older literature, experimental studies of isolated ventricular muscle show that ketamine has a positive inotropic effect.[89] Concomitant intramuscular succinylcholine can be used to facilitate airway control. Atropine or glycopyrrolate given with ketamine may be helpful to offset secretions produced by ketamine. A small dose of midazolam (0.1 mg/kg) can be used to attenuate ketamine's dysphoric effects. Although increases in PVR have been reported in adults after ketamine administration, in well-premedicated children, ketamine causes no change in PVR when the airway is maintained and ventilation is supported.[91] In children with CHD, the ejection fraction has been shown to be well preserved during ketamine anesthesia. Our clinical experience with intramuscular ketamine has been excellent with most forms of heart disease, including patients with limited pulmonary blood flow and cyanosis in whom arterial saturation usually improves with ketamine. Ketamine has long been used for cardiac catheterization procedures. Ketamine combined with midazolam has been used for interventional cardiac catheterization procedures such as PDA and ASD closures.

When IV access is available in patients with marginal cardiac reserve, ketamine (1 or 2 mg/kg IV) is an excellent induction agent in patients with most forms of CHD. Relative contraindications are coronary insufficiency caused by an anomalous coronary artery, severe critical aortic stenosis, and HLHS with aortic atresia and hypoplasia of the ascending aorta. These patients are at risk for ventricular fibrillation because of relative coronary insufficiency; tachycardia and catecholamine release with ketamine may predispose these patients to ventricular fibrillation.

Etomidate This imidazole derivative is being used frequently in patients with CHD. Studies in children are rare, but 1 study has examined the use of etomidate as an induction agent in children with limited hemodynamic reserve. The study concluded that etomidate was safe for use in children with limited hemodynamic reserve but suggested the need for studies in neonates and children with substantial ventricular dysfunction.[92] In another study comparing etomidate with ketamine and γ-hydroxybutyrate as the sole anesthetic for cardiac catheterization in children, no difference could be demonstrated among the 3 groups with regard to hemodynamic or respiratory effects. However, etomidate produced recovery that was more rapid and of better quality than in either of the other groups.[93] Induction with etomidate is generally as rapid as with thiopental, and with a distribution half-life of 2 to 3 minutes, recovery is very rapid for procedures such as cardioversions, which are common in this subgroup.

One presumed disadvantage of etomidate is the temporary suppression of adrenocortical function associated with its use, particularly when patients receive a continuous infusion. This is subject to interpretation. One study compared etomidate and ketamine induction with regard to cortisol production in the postoperative period. These investigators demonstrated reduced cortisol levels in the etomidate group but believed that this finding may be beneficial and certainly not detrimental in the context of pediatric cardiac surgery.[94]

Opiates As in adults with severe cardiac disease, high-dose IV opiates, given together with pancuronium and 100% oxygen, or air and oxygen, are excellent as induction agents in very sick children with all forms of CHD. High-dose opiates in infants and neonates provide excellent hemodynamic stability with suppression of hormonal and metabolic stress responses.[71] Anesthetic techniques based primarily on high doses of opiates have become standard care for infants and small children with severe forms of CHD, especially if they are critically ill. Hyperglycemic responses to cardiac surgery in children are suppressed by greater doses of fentanyl, so blood glucose measurements are necessary.[95] High-dose fentanyl technique has been reported to be effective in premature neonates undergoing patent ductus ligation and has been shown to effectively attenuate stress responses for this procedure.[71] Fentanyl doses as low as 10 mcg/kg may be sufficient for effective baseline anesthesia in neonates, but larger doses are necessary for prolonged anesthesia.[96] In high-risk, full-term neonates and older infants with severe CHD, use of high-dose fentanyl in doses up to 75 mcg/kg, given with pancuronium, results in minimal hemodynamic changes on induction and intubation; only mild hemodynamic responses to surgical incision generally occur.[97] Additional doses or infusions of potent opiates may be necessary for procedures involving CPB because narcotic levels decrease markedly in children on CPB.

Evidence indicates that suppression of stress responses and amnesia is better if another anesthetic, such as a benzodiazepine (midazolam), is used during high-dose opiate anesthesia. With the use of high-dose opiate anesthetic techniques, oxygen saturation levels are well maintained and may actually improve during induction, intubation, and surgical stimulation even in cyanotic children. Changes in cardiac index, SVR, and PVR in infants given 25 mcg/kg of fentanyl have been shown to be minimal.[98]

Use of pancuronium with the high-dose fentanyl technique is recommended; the vagolytic effects of pancuronium offset the vagotonic effects of fentanyl. When other muscle relaxants are used with high-dose opiates, hemodynamic stability may not be obtained.[99] When fentanyl or other opiates are used with nitrous oxide, the negative inotropic effects of nitrous oxide may appear, especially in sicker patients.[100] Sufentanil (5-20 mcg/kg) is an alternative to fentanyl and provides roughly equivalent hemodynamic stability, suppression of stress responses, and postoperative analgesia.[101] The use of a high-dose fentanyl or sufentanil technique usually necessitates continuous postoperative ventilatory support. Alfentanil, a shorter-acting potent opiate used as a continuous infusion, can be useful for providing hemodynamic stability and stress suppression in children in whom postoperative ventilatory support is not needed. A loading dose of 20 mcg/kg and an infusion of 1 mcg/kg/min as a supplement to nitrous oxide–halothane has been reported in children undergoing surgery for CHD.[102]

Remifentanil, an ultrashort-acting opiate, has been shown to be a useful agent in patients with CHD undergoing surgical correction, with no clinical differences in hemodynamic and respiratory parameters both intraoperatively and 24 hours postoperatively compared with fentanyl.[103] This opiate has clearly been shown to have no negative inotropic effect on the failing myocardium and has allowed for full response to β-adrenergic stimulation at all concentrations.[104] Remifentanil has been shown to be very predictable in the post-CPB period, with little change in the coefficient of variation despite 20% increased postbypass clearance values.[105]

Propofol Its short duration of action makes propofol attractive for brief procedures in patients with CHD. In the isolated heart, propofol has myocardial depressant properties somewhat greater than those of thiopental and substantially more than those of ketamine.[106] Its use in patients with CHD should be restricted to those with adequate cardiovascular reserve. For patients with marginal cardiovascular reserve, use of propofol can precipitate cardiovascular decompensation and even collapse.

Successful use of propofol for pediatric patients with CHD undergoing cardiac catheterization and transesophageal echocardiography has been reported,[107] but in 1 study, a substantial percentage of patients given propofol had decreases in blood pressure more than 20% from baseline.[108] These mild deleterious effects on blood pressure are confirmed in other studies.[109] Increased incidences of bradycardia and junctional rhythm have been reported in children receiving propofol compared with those receiving barbiturates.[110] In one specific study of propofol's effects on cardiac conduction in pediatric patients, no substantial effects were seen.[19] These data, taken together with clinical experience, suggest that the use of propofol in patients with CHD should be restricted to those with good levels of cardiovascular reserve because of the drug's cardiac depressant properties.

Dexmedetomidine Dexmedetomidine is an α_2-agonist approved by the FDA in 1999 for short-term (<24 hours) sedation and analgesia in critically ill patients. It has been shown to be highly effective for sedating children after cardiac and thoracic surgery who were either ventilated or spontaneously breathing.[111] The infusion rate of 0.3 mcg/kg/h (range 0.1–0.5 mcg/kg/h) provided mild to moderate sedation in 93% of the children for a range of 3 to 26 hours. Higher mean dosing was required in children younger than 1 year, and these children required more rescue medications compared with older children.[111] For painful interventions, adjunct pain medication frequently is required because the sedative properties of this medication are clearly higher than the analgesic effect. However, it is useful for very sick pediatric patients undergoing nonpainful procedures (eg, MRI or transthoracic echocardiography) and allows completion of the procedure without subjecting these children to intubation and mechanical ventilation. Finally, increasing evidence indicates that dexmedetomidine may be useful in facilitating the acute discontinuation of opioids and/or benzodiazepines in children in the ICU setting.[112]

Thiopental and Other IV Agents IV induction with thiopental generally is not used in patients with severe cardiac defects. However, a reduced dose of thiopental 1 or 2 mg/kg may be safe for induction in patients with moderate defects and may actually result in improved Sao_2 in cyanosis. In pediatric patients with minimal or mild cardiac defects, IV induction with larger doses of thiopental (3-5 mg/kg) usually are well tolerated, provided the patient is not hypovolemic.

Muscle Relaxants Pancuronium dosage requirements are unchanged in children with CHD and intracardiac shunts; it produces no heart rate or blood pressure changes when given slowly in these patients.[113] Through its vagolytic effect, a bolus dose of pancuronium can produce tachycardia and hypertension in children, which may be desirable to support cardiac output in infants with relatively fixed stroke volumes.[114] For patients in whom a short-acting nondepolarizing muscle relaxant is desirable, atracurium, vecuronium, and cisatracurium at the lower end of their dose ranges have few cardiovascular side effects in children.[115] Use of the latter 2 muscle relaxants rather than pancuronium during induction combined with a high-dose opiate anesthetic may produce clinically significant bradycardia, as reported in adults. Bradycardia and even sinus arrest can be problems with the use of succinylcholine in children with CHD, particularly those given large doses of opiates. To avoid these problems in vagotonic young children, atropine should be used with succinylcholine.

Novel Inotropic Drugs The increased sympathetic drive in these patients inevitably leads to an elevation in catecholamine levels. The continued stimulation of α- and β-receptors by both endogenous and exogenous catecholamines leads to a decreased effect via downregulation and ultimately causes irreversible destruction of receptors. Once this level of desensitization has occurred, recovery requires RNA-directed new receptor synthesis. The options available to support the circulation become limited. Either mechanical support must be initiated or nonadrenergic receptor–mediated inotropic support is instituted. Current therapy is discussed.

Phosphodiesterase Inhibitors Phosphodiesterase inhibitors are the most commonly used noncatecholamine-mediated inotropic agent. The mechanism of action of these agents is also the most straightforward. Phosphodiesterases degrade cyclic adenosine monophosphate (cAMP) to 5-adenosine monophosphate (5-AMP). Phosphodiesterase inhibitors prevent this degradation, thus allowing the concentration of cAMP to increase. The increased levels of this secondary messenger lead to increased calcium availability and thus increased contractility. Because the response is related to an increase in cAMP and not purely to inhibition of phosphodiesterase, the greatest effect is seen if initial levels of cAMP are higher than normal. Thus synergy is seen with β-agonists. In addition, phosphodiesterase inhibitors reduce afterload and improve coronary perfusion without any change in myocardial oxygen consumption.

Triiodothyronine The hormone triiodothyronine (T_3) is essential for maturation of sarcolemmal calcium channels, myosin, actin, and troponin. Hypothyroid rats demonstrate reduced numbers of β-receptors, as well as a reduction in stimulatory secondary messenger protein density with an increase in inhibitory secondary messenger protein density. T_3 is mostly produced by monodeiodination of thyroxine. This process is inhibited by surgery, hypothermia, catecholamines, propranolol, and amiodarone. Thus postoperative T_3 levels are reduced.

T_3 replacement acts via 2 pathways, intranuclear and extranuclear. Intranuclear effects include increased mitochondrial density and respiration, increased contractile protein synthesis, and upregulation in β-adrenoceptors. Extranuclear effects include improved glucose transport, increased stimulation of L-type calcium channels with subsequent calcium mobility, and increased efficiency in calcium reuptake with subsequent improvement in diastolic relaxation.

A randomized, double-blind, placebo-controlled study by Bettendorf et al[116] examined 40 children undergoing both simple and complex cardiac surgery. Results demonstrated that the group allocated to receive T_3 had better myocardial function with a decreased duration of ICU stay. T_3 provides improved contractility without any associated increase in oxygen consumption. In addition, the Bettendorf group demonstrated no delay in recovery of thyroid function secondary to exogenous administration.

Levosimendan Levosimendan is a novel drug with a unique mechanism of action. The levosimendan molecule binds to the N-terminal domain of troponin C in cardiac muscle. This process allows for stabilization of the troponin C molecule and maintains tropomyosin in an elevated position. This allows for prolongation of the contractile effect of a set dose of calcium. In addition, levosimendan acts via ATP-sensitive potassium channels, thus causing peripheral vasodilatation, coronary vasodilatation, and myocyte myocardial activation.

Follath et al[117] reported a multicenter, randomized, double-blind trial comparing levosimendan with dobutamine. Two hundred three patients with severe low-output heart failure were randomly allocated to receive levosimendan or dobutamine. The levosimendan patients reported a significant improvement in cardiac output and subsequent reduction in pulmonary capillary occlusion pressure with an associated reduction in mortality at 180 days. Two other large-scale studies found similar benefits in acute and chronic heart failure patients.[118] Levosimendan in adults improves systolic and diastolic function and reduces preload and afterload without any demonstrated increase in myocardial oxygen consumption. Studies in children are required.

Brain Natriuretic Factor and Nesiritide Brain natriuretic peptide (BNP) is a member of the natriuretic peptide family, which includes atrial natriuretic peptide, BNP, and C-type NP. These peptides together play a large role in maintaining hemodynamic and neurohumoral equilibrium. BNP is secreted from cardiac ventricles in response to increased stimulation of cardiac stretch receptors and increased intraventricular tension and acts mostly via natriuretic peptide receptors (NPRs) present in large vessels and kidneys. Once stimulated, NPRs promote diuresis, natriuresis, and vasodilatation and inhibit the renin-angiotensin-aldosterone system. BNP is used as a marker for heart failure in adults and as a method for monitoring therapeutic progress. Its usefulness in children is less obvious as there is no consensus regarding the normal range. Two studies attempting to determine the predictive value of BNP in acute heart failure in children came to directly opposing conclusions.[119]

Nesiritide is the recombinant form of BNP, thus it acts via the same receptors and has the same end results. Studies suggest that patients with decompensated heart failure may benefit from nesiritide administration, with demonstrated improvement in cardiac output, reduction in pulmonary capillary occlusion pressure, arterial and venous dilation, and minimal associated increase in heart rate or myocardial oxygen consumption. Pediatric studies are awaited.

NONPHARMACOLOGIC SUPPORT

The failing pediatric heart may require more support than is possible with medical management alone. The need for alternative assist devices is increasing dramatically for 2 reasons. The chief reason is that increasing numbers of pediatric patients with severe, complicated congenital cardiac anomalies are no longer considered inoperable. As a result, patients now frequently survive long enough to present for surgery and are smaller and much sicker than previously seen. Significant morbidity and mortality in these patients result from postcardiotomy cardiogenic shock, which may necessitate mechanical support of the sick ventricle(s) even if it did not require support preoperatively. Second, heart transplantation in the pediatric population has become much more successful in the past few years as the result of improved pretransplant diagnosis, better rejection prevention, and more sophisticated monitoring of rejection, leading to a vast increase in the potential recipient pool.[120] The donor pool has not increased with the demand, however, and is even more disparate in the pediatric population than in the adult population; therefore, patients are waiting longer for transplants and tend to be much sicker before they receive a new heart.[121] The number of pediatric patients that potentially could benefit from VADS as a bridge to transplant has been estimated to be 7000 to 30 000 patients per year in the United States alone.[122]

EXTRACORPOREAL MEMBRANE OXYGENATION

ECMO is the most widely used ventricular support modality in the United States. It has been shown to be quite successful and technically easier to initiate and discontinue, and it has the ability to provide oxygenation support in associated pulmonary failure/inadequacy. One study reported that approximately 40% of pediatric patients requiring ECMO for myocardial failure recovered sufficient function to allow them to be discharged from the hospital intact.[123] This includes patients with palliative anatomy, such as bidirectional Glenn, and those post Fontan. ECMO use within 24 hours of cardiac arrest suffered in the ICU has been shown to be associated with reduced mortality (odds ratio, 0.8%; confidence interval, 0.04-0.76).[124] ECMO is highly successful and technically feasible for use as a rescue device in patients undergoing interventional cardiac procedures, and successful outcomes have been demonstrated even with extended pre-ECMO cardiopulmonary resuscitation times.[125] ECMO has been used and shown to be safe in neonates as small as 1.6 kg.[126] Favorable outcomes as high as 48% for ECMO have been reported when used as a bridge to transplant.[127] Preprimed ECMO circuits may remain clear primed and stagnant for up to 30 days and still be able to far exceed the required minimum of 6 mL O_2/kg/min required by neonates for the first 6 hours of support.[128]

ECMO is associated with multiple, serious potential liabilities that can lead to increased frequency and acuity of complications. The nonpulsatile flow delivered by ECMO is nonphysiologic and associated with slower, more hemodynamically unstable, and longer recovery times. The list of liabilities includes requirement for anticoagulation and associated increased bleeding, embolization (air and/or thromboembolism), need for deep sedation and immobilization, and need for constant sophisticated physiologic and laboratory monitoring. Finally, ECMO cannulation of the carotid vessels is controversial and may lead to increased incidence of neurologic deficits via cerebral infarcts and/or hemorrhage. Venovenous ECMO cannulation is useful when cardiac output support is not required, as pulsatile blood flow is preserved and there is no arterial compromise and no direct route for embolization to the arterial system (barring intracardiac atrial or ventricular right-to-left shunting), all of which may contribute to a lower incidence of neurologic complications.[129] There is also increased oxygen delivery to the myocardium and pulmonary vascular bed with venovenous ECMO, and it may be delivered through a single cannula in tiny neonates. Venovenous ECMO does present the disadvantage of requiring ongoing, possibly intense respiratory/mechanical ventilation support.

The invasive nature of ECMO cannulation increases the risk of potentially fatal infections. The risk of these complications is magnified as the patient's time on ECMO increases, making ECMO generally unsuitable for long-term support (more than a few weeks at most).[130] These complex associated difficulties have helped fuel the search for alternative support modalities.

VADs

VADs for pediatric patients have become much more sophisticated and more available in the past few years as their size has decreased, but they still are trailing adult devices in the development process. This is primarily secondary to the smaller number of patients requiring the devices and the historically superior results in pediatric patients, compared with adult patients, treated with ECMO in the United States. Smaller devices operated at low flow rates historically have shown increased propensity for thrombosis and embolus formation[131]; this is improving with better anticoagulation protocols, more postoperative care experience, and improved device materials that are less thrombogenic.[132]

Use of VADs is more common in Europe than in the United States, and the results have been very encouraging. Multiple new devices are now in common use as the result of these recent successes. The Thoratec VAD (Thoratec Corporation, Pleasanton, CA) is still the most common, having been used in more than 1000 patients worldwide since its launch. Thoratec VADs are paracorporeal devices attached to a large driving console and are less suited to long-term support. They have been used in patients with a body surface area as small as 0.7 m^2. In a large series, survival rates in small patients were higher (~72%) for patients with cardiomyopathy or myocarditis than for patients with congenital cardiac anomalies (~14%).[133] A previous multicenter study showed that 60% of patients survived to transplant, but only 10% survived after recovery of their native heart.[134] The most common complication associated with the Thoratec VAD is infection, and the most common cause of death is multiorgan failure; embolization is always possible. The Berlin Heart VAD and the Medos VAD (MEDOS Medizintechnik AG, Stolberg, Germany) have been used with good results in Europe as a bridge to ventricular recovery and transplantation, and are now arriving for use in the United States. They are favorable for use in the pediatric population because they are available in multiple ventricle and cannula sizes.

The Medos DeltaStream DP1 VAD (MEDOS Medizintechnik AG) is an extracorporeal rotary pump with a diagonal flow impeller capable of both continuous and pulsatile blood flow. It has a very small priming volume (~30 mL) and a high pumping capability (≤8 L/min).[135] Clinical trials now under way have initially shown faster lactate recovery, reduced need for inotropic support, reduced assistance duration needed in bridge-to-recovery cases, and smoother, more physiologic hemodynamics in patients receiving pulsatile flow delivery.[135]

The Berlin Heart VAD is pneumatically driven, delivers pulsatile flow, and has been implemented in patients as small as 4 kg.[136] Complications associated with VAD use include minor infection at cannula exit sites, generalized sepsis, hemorrhagic events, and thromboembolic events. These complications have been shown to be less common with VADs than with ECMO.[137] Patients with the Berlin Heart VAD consume fewer red blood cell units, platelets, and fresh-frozen plasma compared with ECMO, which decreases exposure to potential blood-borne pathogens.[138] Potential advantages of VADs compared with ECMO are increased patient mobility (possibly even return to home and/or school), increased level of physical activity, and longer complication-free use time. Recent data suggest lower wait list mortality, longer duration of complication-free support, and higher survival to transplant and hospital discharge with VADs versus ECMO. However, use of these devices is just as expensive as ECMO and dramatically increases the cost of hospitalization and the overall costs of cardiac transplantation.

INTRA-AORTIC BALLOON PUMPS

Use of intra-aortic balloon pumps (IABPs) in the pediatric patient population has been reported, but in general their effectiveness is limited in this setting. Infants and small children have small vessels for access and exhibit increased aortic elasticity, rapid heart rates (which makes synchronization difficult), and small stroke volumes. They also frequently suffer from right heart dysfunction, which is not supported by IABP.

CONDUCT OF THE ANESTHETIC

Anesthetic Plan and Goals Virtually all children with CHD tolerate well-managed anesthetics, but their tolerance for events, such as loss of airway patency, hypoventilation, inappropriate amounts and choices of anesthetics, and major intraoperative surgical insults, often is limited. The anesthetic plan should be aimed at maintaining or improving existing circulatory homeostasis throughout the procedure, but particularly during induction of anesthesia. Because resuscitation may be very difficult in patients with CHD once cardiovascular collapse occurs, prevention of circulatory decompensation is the priority. This makes anticipation of potential problems a particularly important part of the anesthetic plan.

Preoperative Assessment An important aim of preoperative assessment is identifying those patients with CHD who are likely to develop problems. Cardiac catheterization and echocardiographic data are most useful. **Box 53-2** lists the critical indices of severe circulatory impairment in CHD. Patients who have any 1 of these indices are at risk for perioperative hemodynamic problems. If a patient has 2 or more of the listed criteria of critical impairment, particular care should be taken with planning the anesthetic. In such patients, depending on the experience of the anesthesia team, consultation with the patient's cardiologist to clarify critical aspects of the patient's pathophysiology may be

BOX 53-2

Indices of Critical Impairment in Congenital Heart Disease

Arterial saturation <75%

Qp/Qs >2:1

Left ventricular outflow tract gradient >50 mm Hg

Right ventricular outflow tract gradient >50 mm Hg

Pulmonary vascular resistance >6 Woods units

Polycythemia with hematocrit >60%

Qp, pulmonary flow; Qs, systemic flow.

BOX 53-3

General Associated Risk Factors in Congenital Heart Disease

Severe form of isolated lesion

Complex lesions

Concurrent infectious disease

Metabolic derangements

Congestive heart failure

Previous palliative or corrective procedures

Acute hemodynamic deterioration

advisable. In patients who have CHD that does not include any of the criteria listed in Box 53-2, the chances of hemodynamic problems with anesthesia are relatively low. Additional risk factors for patients with CHD undergoing anesthesia are listed in **Box 53-3**.

Preoperative Preparation and Medication Before surgery, patients should be in the optimum condition allowed by their underlying disease. Emergency operations in critically ill, severely hypoxemic, and acidotic neonates are rarely necessary because of the advent of PGE_1 treatment of ductus-dependent circulation in those with CHD. A period of 24 to 48 hours of medical therapy markedly improves the condition of most critically ill children with CHD and lessens perioperative morbidity. Such therapy should be considered part of the preoperative preparation of sick children with CHD.

Patients with more chronic problems, such as congestive heart failure and chronic pulmonary infections resulting from excessive pulmonary blood flow and congestion, should be at their pulmonary baselines if possible. Children taking cardiac medications should continue doing so up to and including the morning of surgery, except for diuretics. Preoperative medication can take many forms. A good preoperative visit may establish sufficient rapport with parents and child to eliminate the need for preoperative medication, whereas relatively large doses of IV sedation may be needed for the extremely anxious child. The goal should be a lightly sedated patient without respiratory depression. In patients with severe hypoxemia and cyanosis or with pulmonary hypertension, premedication should be relatively light to prevent depression of ventilation that may exacerbate their decreased hypoxic ventilatory drive or further increase their PVR. When the anxiety level is high and severe hypoxemia, severe congestive heart failure, or pulmonary hypertension precludes heavy premedication before the patient arrives in the preoperative holding area, intramuscular ketamine and midazolam are given just before the child is taken to the operating room. Such premedication is well tolerated by all but critically ill children and can ease the difficulties experienced by children and parents. Properly monitored transport should be available, with an anesthesia caregiver in constant attendance. This combination of drugs is quickly effective so that a deeply sedated child can be separated from anxious parents. Use of portable pulse oximetry and a precordial stethoscope often are advisable for the trip to the operating room. If there is any question of cardiac stability during this period, an IV line is started immediately after sedation is given or, in extreme cases, even before sedation. With the availability of eutectic mixture of local anesthetics (EMLA) cream, preoperative IV insertion for premedication has become much easier.

Alternatively, oral midazolam at a dose of 0.75 to 1.0 mg/kg can be given to small children in the presence of the anesthesia provider. This often results in excellent premedication and may be supplemented by intramuscular ketamine, if needed, mixed with atropine or glycopyrrolate.

Induction of Anesthesia Because of the potential for rapid and dramatic hemodynamic changes in young patients with CHD, especially infants, complete preparation of anesthetic and monitoring equipment and required drugs is essential. Adequate assistance should be immediately available during induction, particularly if the patient meets a number of the criteria of severe disease listed in Table 53-1. Flexibility is needed in the choice of induction techniques because response to premedication and emotional needs of parents and children facing a cardiac procedure can place constraints on choices.

Choice of induction technique is influenced by response to premedication and the parent–child–anesthesia provider relationship and to the anesthetic management plan. In older patients who are not hypoxemic and have minimal compromise of cardiac reserve, choice of induction techniques is large. Rectal, intramuscular, IV, or inhalation induction techniques using various agents can be used with reasonable safety if individual pathophysiologic limitations are respected. Choices decrease for younger, sicker, and less cooperative patients. In older children with only mildly compromised cardiac function, rectal administration of anesthetics, such as barbiturates, can be a useful technique, but lack of control and potential for circulatory depression make this technique unacceptable for sick infants.

In children with good IV access, quick insertion of a small-bore IV needle for induction can be virtually painless if sufficiently long applications of EMLA cream are used. Cooperative small children who have adequate cardiac reserve but difficult IV access or a morbid fear of needles can be induced cautiously with inhalational anesthetics, even if they are cyanotic. An IV catheter is then inserted expeditiously to facilitate intubation with adjunctive IV agents, avoiding the risk of deep levels of inhalational anesthesia in circulatory systems with little reserve, particularly in the immature circulation of the infant. Such use of an inhalational anesthetic for induction of patients with severe CHD without the presence of a working IV heavily depends on the judgment of the anesthesia provider for safety.

Maintenance of Anesthesia Maintenance of anesthesia in the pediatric heart patient depends on preoperative status and response to induction and on the surgical procedure and intraoperative events. Whether inhalational agents, additional narcotics, or other IV agents are used for maintenance depends on patient tolerance and postoperative plans for ventilatory management. In children with CHD, intraoperative changes in cardiac shunting are unique problems during maintenance of anesthesia. Whether clinical deterioration is caused by changes in shunting or by primary myocardial depression or dysfunction is not always clear, the intraoperative events and progress of the anesthetic usually suggest a cause. Hypotension and hypoxemia, particularly during induction of anesthesia, should be managed aggressively and immediately. Decreases in arterial oxygenation or systemic blood flow may be caused by alterations in intracardiac shunting in these children and usually can be managed by manipulations of PVR/SVR; however, inotropes are needed in some patients, assuming their circulating blood volume is adequate.

Manipulation of PVR and SVR Manipulation of PVR/SVR allows some control over shunting, depending on specific pathophysiology. PVR is particularly important because of the frequency of disturbances of pulmonary blood flow and right-sided defects in patients with CHD. Usually the goal is to decrease PVR in order to improve pulmonary flow, right heart function, and oxygenation, but in some lesions, pulmonary flow is excessively high at the expense of systemic output, requiring increases in PVR.[139] Many intraoperative manipulations tend to alter PVR. Manipulations that increase PVR are frequent problems because of the increased reactivity of the abnormal pulmonary vasculature often found in patients with CHD. These manipulations include sympathetic stimulation, encroachments on lung volumes that produce atelectasis (surgical retraction, pleural and peritoneal collections, and abdominal packing), CPB, alveolar hypoxia, and hypoventilation. Manipulations that increase and decrease PVR are listed in **Box 53-4**. Ventilation is important because it is subject to control by the anesthesia provider and is crucial in attempts to control PVR via airway

BOX 53-4

Manipulations Altering Pulmonary Vascular Resistance

Increased PVR
- Hypoxia
- Hypercapnia
- Acidosis
- Hyperinflation
- Atelectasis
- Sympathetic stimulation
- High hematocrit
- Mechanical pulmonary artery constriction

Decreased PVR
- Oxygen
- Hypocapnia
- Alkalosis
- Normal functional residual capacity
- Blockage of sympathetic stimulation
- Low hematocrit
- Inhaled nitric oxide

pressure, lung volumes, alveolar $Paco_2$ and Pao_2, and other, less well-understood variables.

The effects of various anesthetics on PVR are poorly understood. Ketamine and nitrous oxide increase PVR in adults, but studies of ketamine and nitrous oxide in infants with normal or elevated PVR have shown no increase in PVR when ventilation and Fio_2 are constant.[84] Stress responses in the pulmonary circulation of patients with CHD are a primary concern in some patients. Large doses of potent narcotics, such as fentanyl, attenuate pulmonary vascular responses to noxious stimuli, such as endotracheal suctioning in infants, but they do not change baseline PVR. Reactive pulmonary hypertensive responses are partially mediated by the sympathoadrenal axis and thus are attenuated by an adequate depth of anesthesia. CPB increases PVR through activation of the inflammatory response, cytokine release, and ischemia of the endothelium in the pulmonary circulation. After bypass surgery, elevated PVR can be a substantial problem.

PVR can be controlled independently of SVR by manipulating various aspects of ventilation (see Box 53-4). Nitric oxide delivered through alveoli has been shown to be a pulmonary vasodilator and to be effective in patients with CHD. In contrast to inhaled nitric oxide, even selective infusions of rapidly metabolized vasodilators (eg, nitroprusside) into the pulmonary circulation can result in systemic drug concentrations and systemic hemodynamic effects without desired effects on PVR.[140] Nitric oxide has been shown to be effective in selectively reducing PVR in a variety of different CHD lesions accompanied by high PVR; this can be accomplished without altering SVR.[141] Not all patients with CHD and high PVR respond to inhaled nitric oxide, particularly after the neonatal period, but nitric oxide therapy should be tried whenever high PVR is a substantial problem in patients of any age with CHD.[142] High levels of inspired oxygen, especially 100% O_2, also decrease elevated PVR in infants without changing SVR, whereas inspired oxygen levels 21% or lower increase PVR.[142] Hypoventilation, with associated acidosis and hypercapnia, increases PVR. Hyperventilation to alkalotic pH greater than 7.50 and low $Paco_2$ reliably decreases PVR in infants and improves right ventricular function.[143] This maneuver increases pulmonary blood flow and decreases right-to-left shunting in neonates, increasing Pao_2. Although prolonged hyperventilation to decrease PVR theoretically may cause problems from decreased cerebral blood flow, clinical and experimental studies in hyperventilated infants show no evidence of cerebral damage.[144] The pattern of ventilation and PEEP can alter PVR. PVR is lowest at normal functional residual capacity. At low lung volumes with atelectasis and at high lung volumes with hyperinflation of alveoli, PVR increases.[145] High levels of PEEP increase PVR primarily by hyperinflation of alveoli, but if atelectasis and pulmonary edema are corrected by PEEP, PVR may decrease. Different patterns of ventilation may further reduce PVR by releasing prostacyclin in the pulmonary vasculature.

Manipulation of SVR with vasopressors is useful when there is a need for increased coronary perfusion pressure or a need to decrease right-to-left shunting that causes severe systemic hypoxemia. Phenylephrine has been shown effective in reducing right-to-left shunting in patients with tetralogy of Fallot and increasing Sao_2.[146] A mechanical method for increasing SVR to decrease right-to-left shunting in tetralogy of Fallot is compression of the abdominal aorta. This can be done immediately and can be used to gain time while other pharmacologic therapy is started or while the child is prepared for CPB.

KEY REFERENCES

- Anand KJ, Hickey PR. Halothane-morphine compared with high-dose sufentanil for anesthesia and postoperative analgesia in neonatal cardiac surgery. *N Engl J Med.* 1992;326(1):1-9.
- Berman WJ. The hemodynamics of shunts in congenital heart disease. In: Johansen K, Burggren WW, eds. *Cardiovascular Shunts: Phylogenetic, Ontogenetic, and Clinical Aspects.* New York, NY: Raven Press; 1985:399-410.
- Chang AC, Zucker HA, Hickey PR, Wessel DL. Pulmonary vascular resistance in infants after cardiac surgery: role of carbon dioxide and hydrogen ion. *Crit Care Med.* 1995;23(3):568-574.
- Greeley WJ, Ungerleider RM, Smith LR, Reves JG. The effects of deep hypothermic cardiopulmonary bypass and total circulatory arrest on cerebral blood flow in infants and children. *J Thorac Cardiovasc Surg.* 1989;97(5):737-745.
- Hickey PR, Hansen DD. Fentanyl- and sufentanil-oxygen-pancuronium anesthesia for cardiac surgery in infants. *Anesth Analg.* 1984;63(2):117-124.
- Newburger JW, Jonas RA, Wernovsky G, et al. A comparison of the perioperative neurologic effects of hypothermic circulatory arrest versus low-flow cardiopulmonary bypass in infant heart surgery. *N Engl J Med.* 1993;329(15):1057-1064.
- Rivenes SM, Lewin MB, Stayer SA, et al. Cardiovascular effects of sevoflurane, isoflurane, halothane, and fentanyl-midazolam in children with congenital heart disease: an echocardiographic study of myocardial contractility and hemodynamics. *Anesthesiology.* 2001;94(2):223-229.
- Sarkar M, Laussen PC, Zurakowski D, Shukla A, Kussman B, Odegard KC. Hemodynamic responses to etomidate on induction of anesthesia in pediatric patients. *Anesth Analg.* 2005;101(3):645-650, table of contents.

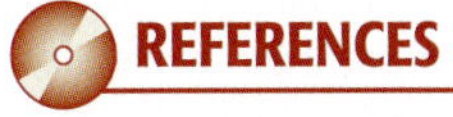

REFERENCES

Complete references available on DVD and online version at www.LongneckerAnesthesiology.com

CHAPTER 54 Thoracic Anesthesia

Stuart J. Weiss
E. Andrew Ochroch

KEY POINTS

1. Thoracic surgery is being performed on patients with more severe pulmonary disease than in earlier years. Previous exclusion criteria for undergoing general anesthesia now are considered overly conservative.
2. Because the mortality rate of untreated lung cancer approaches 100%, it is difficult to assign definitive exclusion criteria for lung resection. Parameters used to predict patients at increased risk for postoperative complications include forced vital capacity (FVC), forced expiratory volume in 1 second (FEV_1), split lung functions, and exercise tolerance.
3. Patients undergoing thoracic surgical procedures often have preexisting pulmonary and cardiac disease.
4. The preoperative symptoms of dyspnea, shortness of breath, and hoarseness of voice may be related to thoracic tumor pathology. Possible etiologies include superior vena cava obstruction, mediastinal mass, tracheal compression, tracheomalacia, and malignancy. Anesthetic management should include an adequate preoperative evaluation to assess extent of disease, severity of symptoms, and effects of supine positioning on respiratory and cardiac function.
5. One goal of preoperative preparation is to improve pulmonary function by use of bronchodilators for reactive airway disease, antibiotics for infection, and education to promote the cessation of smoking. Smoking should stop at least 4 to 8 weeks preoperatively.
6. Routine diagnostic procedures that are performed to confirm and evaluate the extent of pulmonary and thoracic disease include bronchoscopy, mediastinoscopy, and video-assisted thoracoscopic surgery (VATS).
7. The anesthetic plan should be coordinated with the surgeon and support staff to limit perioperative risk. In high-risk patients, anesthesia may proceed with a slow, controlled, and staged induction to cease if respiratory difficulties ensue.
8. Lateral decubitus position has a negative impact on the physiology of ventilation and circulation and is associated with position-related injuries.
9. Fiberoptic bronchoscopy is the most reliable method for ascertaining correct positioning of the double-lumen endotracheal tube and assuring pulmonary toilet.
10. When using single-lung ventilation, the anesthesiologist should be especially alert to problems with ventilation or oxygenation. Most problems are related to malposition of the double-lumen tube. Once proper position of the tube is confirmed, management strategies include (1) increased oxygenation to dependent lung (positive end-expiratory pressure [PEEP], increased tidal volume [VT], increased FIO_2), (2) increased oxygenation of blood flowing to the nondependent lung (continuous positive airway pressure [CPAP], intermittent ventilation), (3) decreased blood perfusion to nondependent lung (discontinue drugs that inhibit hypoxic pulmonary vasoconstriction [HPV], ligature to pulmonary artery [PA]), increased oxygen content of blood (transfusion, improve SvO_2), and (4) increased perfusion of the dependent lung (increased cardiac output and administer a pulmonary vasodilator).
11. Hypoxic pulmonary vasoconstriction (HPV) is a homeostatic mechanism that limits perfusion of unventilated nonoxygenated atelectatic alveoli, thereby decreasing the shunt admixture. HPV is activated by decreased alveolar oxygen tension, but is inhibited by certain anesthetic agents and vasodilators.
12. Volume reduction surgery and other sophisticated intrathoracic operations require extraordinarily careful and complex planning and constant vigilance to maintain adequate ventilation, oxygenation, and hemodynamic stability.
13. Postoperative management after thoracotomy or thoracoscopy is directed to the delicate balance between pain relief and respiratory depression associated with opioids. Epidural analgesia represents best practice in these patients.

INTRODUCTION

Advances in management of thoracic disease parallel the advances in thoracic anesthesia and surgery. In the early 20th century, thoracic surgery was limited to rib resection, decortication, and drainage of empyema as management for tuberculosis. During the first part of this century, pulmonary resections were accomplished by tightening a snare or tourniquet around the lesion and subsequently removing the necrotic tissue several days later. These procedures depended on the iatrogenic development of a passive pneumothorax in spontaneously ventilating patients. As expected, the unilateral pneumothorax was poorly tolerated and associated with mediastinal shift, dyspnea, and rapid ineffective spontaneous respiratory movements. A high incidence of perioperative morbidity resulted from infection, hemorrhage, and air leak.

The period of 1930 to 1950 saw major advancements in surgery and anesthesia. In the 1930s, Drs Gale and Waters in the United States and Magill in the United Kingdom developed the techniques of endobronchial intubation and placement of bronchial blockers, respectively, to selectively ventilate 1 lung. In addition, the introduction of muscle relaxants and controlled ventilation improved patient safety and surgical operating conditions. The development of single-lung isolation techniques accelerated from 1950 to 1960 with the development of double-lumen endotracheal tubes. In addition, patient safety and anesthetic management were markedly improved by the introduction of halogenated inhalational anesthetics and the dramatically increased use of perioperative physiologic monitoring. More recently, use of the fiberoptic bronchoscope greatly increased the success of single-lung ventilation by facilitating the placement and confirmation of position of double-lumen endotracheal tubes and bronchial blockers.

Thoracic surgery and anesthesia continue to evolve. The development of endoscopic surgery has revolutionized thoracic surgery by providing for the relatively noninvasive access to the contents of the thoracic cavity. Although endoscopic surgery has not replaced open thoracotomy for major pulmonary surgical resections, its use has further expanded to nonpulmonary surgery, such as thymectomy, pericardectomy, and sympathectomy. Surgical management of end-stage disease by lung reduction and transplantation are additional current challenges for thoracic anesthesiologists.

This chapter focuses on important perioperative considerations for the patient undergoing thoracic surgery. The initial portion of the chapter presents the relevant anatomy and pathophysiology. The next sections focus on specific anesthetic concerns and perioperative management issues of operative procedures. The approach to the anesthetic management of these patients should be flexible to allow for either the short diagnostic procedure or the prolonged anatomic tumor resection. Current strategies for staging and management of lung tumors call for sequential bronchoscopy, mediastinoscopy, and pulmonary resection. In addition, nonpulmonary thoracic operations, such as thymectomy, pericardectomy, and sympathectomy, use many of the same techniques and management strategies.

ANATOMY/PHYSIOLOGY

THORACIC CAVITY

The thoracic cavity is formed by the ribs laterally, sternum anteriorly, vertebral column posteriorly, and by the diaphragm and thoracic inlet inferiorly and superiorly, respectively. The thoracic cavity encompasses the lungs, which provide oxygenation of venous blood, excretion of carbon dioxide, and metabolism of endogenous compounds.

AIRWAY

The trachea is the initial conduit for airflow. Its cross section is outlined by the horseshoe shape of the cartilage anteriorly and the membranous portion posteriorly. The membranous portion consists of a fibrous envelope containing smooth muscle and epithelium. The location of the membranous trachea and the vertical orientation of the exposed muscle fibers guide fiberoptic-assisted placement of double-lumen endotracheal tubes into the appropriate side. The innominate artery lies just anterior to the trachea. Tracheal-innominate fistulae are rare but lethal complications of tracheal resection, tracheostomy, or prolonged intubation.

The trachea initially bifurcates into the right and left mainstem bronchi and then into the lobar and segmental bronchi. The right bronchus is shorter, wider, and more inline with the trachea as compared with the left bronchus. Because of the more oblique orientation of the left bronchus, inhaled foreign bodies and aspirated fluid are more likely to go into the right bronchus. The right bronchus provides access to 3 lobes (the upper, middle, and lower lobes) that are separated by major fissures. On the left, a major fissure separates the lower and upper lobes. The lobes of the lung are subdivided into bronchial pulmonary segments, each of which has its own bronchus, artery, and vein. The movement of air progresses through a series of branching tubes, which become narrower and more numerous as they penetrate deeper into the lung. The conducting airways contain no alveoli and therefore contribute a portion, about 50 mL, of the anatomic dead space.

MEDIASTINUM

The mediastinum is the region between the 2 pleural sacs and contains the heart, the great vessels, and the thymus gland. For purposes of description, the mediastinum is divided into 4 subdivisions (middle, posterior, anterior, and superior compartments). The middle mediastinum contains the pericardium with the adjacent phrenic nerves, the heart, and the great vessels emanating to and from it. The superior mediastinum lies between the thoracic inlet and the horizontal plane connecting the sternal angle with the lower border of the fourth thoracic vertebrae. The main contents of the superior mediastinum are the thymus, great vessels, and several nerves. The posterior mediastinum, which is bounded anteriorly by the pericardium and posteriorly by the vertebral column, contains the thoracic aorta, thoracic duct, azygos and hemiazygos veins, esophagus, and bifurcation of the trachea with the 2 bronchi. The anterior mediastinum, which lies between the sternum and the pericardium, contains lymphatic vessels, lymph nodes, and branches of the internal thoracic artery.

PULMONARY VASCULATURE

The lungs are blood vessel–rich structures with extensive capillary networks that allow gas exchange. The main pulmonary artery branches and follows the bronchial tree, decreasing in size with each bronchial generation. The arteries branch to supply the respiratory bronchioles and alveolar sacks, which provide for gas exchange. The vascular endothelial surfaces form boundaries of the capillaries and occupy about 50% of the surface of the alveolar wall.

The pulmonary capillary network not only provides an enormous surface area for gas exchange but also for active metabolism, synthesis, and release of stored vasoactive substances. The lung also maintains an active role as a biochemical filter, inactivating exogenous and endogenous substances by metabolic elimination or cellular uptake. The release of vasoactive substances can be stimulated either by manipulation during surgery or by hypo- or hyperinflation. One such example is that of hypoxic pulmonary vasoconstriction, which functions in a homeostatic capacity to normalize the perfusion to ventilation inhomogeneity caused by alveolar hypoxia.

The metabolic functions of the pulmonary circulation also can trigger pathologic consequences. Anaphylactoid response to protamine is of particular importance to the cardiac anesthesiologist. The biologically active substances (histamine, slow-reacting substance of anaphylaxis, prostaglandin E [PGE]1, PGE2, prostaglandin F [PGF]2, and bradykinin) are released in response to specific biochemical and mechanical triggers.

BRONCHIAL VESSELS

The bronchial vasculature normally accounts for about 1% of the cardiac output, but it may increase its flow in response to acute lung disease or injury. The origin of the bronchial arteries is variable, coming from the aorta or intercostal, subclavian, or innominate arteries. The bronchial arteries enter the hilus of the lung and form a communicating arc around the main bronchus. The vessels follow the bronchi distally, supplying the vasovasorum of the pulmonary arteries and bronchi. The dominant deep bronchial venous system drains into the pulmonary veins, and the lesser superficial system of bronchial veins drains into the azygos, hemiazygos, and mediastinal veins. The clinical importance of the bronchial vasculature system is appreciated under conditions of acute lung stress or injury. Neovascularization and increased blood flow occurs in response to acute and chronic lung disease. This response may help preserve normal pulmonary ventilation-to-perfusion ratio and protect the lung from ischemia. The absence of an intact bronchial arterial circulation in patients receiving a lung transplant places the new lung at increased risk of ischemic injury immediately after surgery.

LYMPHATIC SYSTEM

The lymphatic circulation has a major role in maintaining the balance of fluids across the endothelial membrane. Transcapillary flow (F) is proportional to the difference between pulmonary capillary hydrostatic pressure (inside pressure – outside pressure) and the difference between the capillary oncotic pressure and the interstitial oncotic pressure (Fa [P (inside – outside) – P (capillary – interstitial)]). Transcapillary flow also depends on the capillary filtration coefficient (K), which is a function of the effective capillary surface area and membrane permeability. Any clinical situation that impedes lymphatic flow increases the risk of pulmonary edema and pleural effusion. Abnormal clinical states that increase capillary permeability increase the flow of fluid into the interstitial space and increase the chance of developing pulmonary edema. In addition, pulmonary interstitial edema also may result from marked increases in negative pleural pressure. Markedly increased negative pressures can result from upper airway obstruction (tumors, laryngospasm, epiglottis), rapid reexpansion of the lung, or aggressive suctioning.

The lymphatic drainage pattern is from the periphery toward more proximal lymph nodes, which are located at the carina and points of bifurcation of the bronchi and alongside the trachea and great cardiac vessels. The location of the lymph nodes is classified for prognostic assessment of primary pulmonary cancers. The lowest number is assigned to the most central nodes and progresses to greater numbers at the periphery. The pattern of lymphatic drainage has an impact on the sensitivity and specificity of mediastinoscopy to diagnose and detect the spread of disease. Malignant disease of the right lung spreads ipsilaterally up the chain from the pulmonary nodes in the periphery to the paratracheal, scalene, or tracheal nodes more proximally. In contrast, disease from the left lung can either spread ipsilaterally or contralaterally up the chain or proceed subdiaphragmatically to the para-aortic lymph nodes. Biopsying of a lymph node unilateral to the lesion may provide false-negative results if spread occurs contralaterally or subdiaphragmatically.

WORK OF BREATHING

During normal spontaneous inspiration, the major contribution to respiratory mechanics is by the contraction and downward excursion of the diaphragm, which increases the vertical dimension of the thorax. The dimensions of the thorax also are increased by the outward and upward swinging movement of the ribs during inspiration. The importance of diaphragmatic excursion and chest wall movement is most easily appreciated in patients with compromised respiratory function related to positioning. The patient in a flexed lateral decubitus or Trendelenburg position experiences increased abdominal pressure, which limits diaphragmatic excursion and chest wall movement. In addition, patients undergoing thoracic operations are at increased risk of phrenic nerve injury or diaphragmatic dysfunction, which may result in postoperative ventilatory compromise.

The mechanics of respiration are divided into the inspiratory and expiratory phases. The work of normal breathing is associated with the inspiratory phase, whereas expiration normally is a passive process related to elastic recoil of the lung and chest cage structures. The work of inspiration depends on overcoming airway resistance and the elastic forces created by the lung and chest wall mechanics. During normal quiet breathing, the work of respiration constitutes only 2% to 3% of total energy expenditure. During heavy exercise, pulmonary ventilation and total body energy expenditure may increase some 15- to 20-fold, but the energy expended for ventilation increases only slightly to 3% to 4%. Pulmonary disease or dysfunction that alters compliance, airway resistance, or lung or chest wall mechanics can dramatically increase the work of breathing to one-third or more of the total body energy expenditure. For example, the patient with preexisting respiratory disease having minimal reserve is at increased risk of postoperative ventilatory failure and may require reintubation because of diaphragmatic dysfunction and atelectasis.

COUGH REFLEX

A normal cough reflex is critical for maintenance of pulmonary toilet. Afferent impulses from the respiratory passages are conducted centrally by the vagus nerve. Efferent impulses trigger closure of the epiglottis, apposition of the vocal cords, and contraction of abdominal, chest, and diaphragmatic muscles to produce an explosive exhalation of air. Patients having postoperative dysfunction related to recurrent laryngeal or phrenic nerve injury, trauma to the diaphragm, or pain and who cannot cough effectively are at risk for respiratory failure related to aspiration or poor pulmonary toilet resulting in pneumonia. Such patients may benefit from conservative measures, such as breathing humidified gases to prevent inspissated secretions, chest physiotherapy, and nasal tracheal suctioning to clear secretions.

PREOPERATIVE EVALUATION OF THE PATIENT UNDERGOING THORACIC SURGERY

The preoperative evaluation of patients undergoing noncardiac thoracic surgery is similar to any patient undergoing general anesthesia. The anesthesiologist should perform a history and physical examination and be familiar with current laboratory studies, electrocardiogram (ECG), and radiologic studies of the chest. The anesthesiologist also should understand the evaluation of pulmonary function and the prediction of postoperative pulmonary function. This knowledge will help formulate a rational anesthetic and perioperative plan.

HISTORY

Most patients with lung cancer have a smoking history and therefore have some degree of chronic bronchitis and emphysema. This history is important because the management of infections and reactive airway disease preoperatively will have a positive impact by decreasing the incidence of postoperative complications. Exercise tolerance also should be assessed because this will estimate a patient's cardiovascular and pulmonary reserve.[1-5]

PHYSICAL EXAMINATION

Along with a routine assessment of the airway and cardiovascular systems, the anesthesiologist should pay particular attention to the respiratory system during the physical examination. Observation of the respiratory rate and pattern may give insight into the pulmonary reserve of the patient. The auscultation of wheezes, rales, or rhonchi indicates abnormalities that can be managed preoperatively. Clubbing of the fingernails may indicate chronic hypoxia or lung cancer. Deviation of the trachea may indicate a mediastinal mass, hemothorax, pneumothorax, or fibrothorax. The anesthesiologist also should assess the patient's ability to tolerate the supine position, because an intolerance to this position may indicate congestive heart failure or major airway obstruction from a mediastinal mass.

DIAGNOSTIC STUDIES

Laboratory tests should be ordered based on positive findings elicited from history and physical examination. The complete blood count may reveal polycythemia, reflecting prolonged smoking and hypoxia, or leukocytosis, indicating an active infection. Liver function studies may be altered, indicating hepatic metastases or drug or alcohol effects.

The ECG should be assessed for the presence of cardiac or pulmonary disease. Signs and symptoms of ischemia may indicate the need for further cardiac workup. Manifestations of cor pulmonale may indicate the presence of pulmonary hypertension, which may alter intraoperative management or portend intolerance to major pulmonary resection.[6] However, the futility of subsequent therapeutic intervention is controversial. Recent research concerning patients undergoing aortic or peripheral arterial bypass graft surgery indicates that in some instances coronary revascularization does not decrease the rate of perioperative myocardial infarction or long-term mortality.[7]

Abnormal chest radiographs frequently antedate the first sign or symptom of lung cancer by many months. The radiograph may reveal tumor, secondary changes in lung parenchyma distal to an obstructed airway, or other abnormalities caused by intrathoracic and extrapulmonary tumor spread. Radiographic findings that may have implications to perioperative anesthetic management are listed in **Table 54-1**. The tumor may impinge on the trachea or the mainstem bronchi and thus influence the induction of anesthesia, or choice and placement of an endotracheal tube (**Fig. 54-1**). For example, tumor involvement of the trachea would suggest the use of awake, sedated fiberoptic intubation, whereas isolated impingement of the left bronchus would suggest the use of a right-sided double-lumen endotracheal tube.

In addition, patients will have a computed tomographic (CT) scan of the chest, which is helpful in delineating the presence or absence of high-level nodes and extrapulmonary spread of the disease. Further diagnostic workup is guided by these studies. If mediastinal nodes are suspected, mediastinoscopy or parasternal mediastinotomy may be performed to confirm the diagnosis and to determine the extent of tumor spread. If clinical manifestations of distant organ involvement are present, appropriate investigations, such as bone scan and scan of the brain, liver, and upper abdomen, also should be performed.

ASSESSMENT OF RESPIRATORY FUNCTION

Preoperative evaluation of pulmonary functional reserve is used to estimate the patient's ability to tolerate thoracotomy and lung resection. Patients undergoing thoracotomy for lung resection usually have a long-standing history of smoking and varying degrees of underlying lung disease. Therefore, they have decreased pulmonary reserve and are at increased risk for operative and postoperative morbidity and mortality. Smokers have a significantly increased risk of postoperative pulmonary complications, 8% for nonsmokers and 23% for smokers.[8] Carcinoma of the lung is associated with an average survival period of 18 months and a mortality rate of 100% after 5 years if not surgically treated. Therefore, every effort should be made to give the patient the benefit of surgical resection. It is difficult to answer the question,

TABLE 54-1 Radiographic Findings With Important Anesthetic Complications

Abnormality	Anesthetic Implication
Tracheal deviation	Difficulty with intubation Identify cause: mediastinal mass, nodal metastasis, thyroid gland, aortic aneurysm, other
Mediastinal mass	Difficulty with intubation Difficulty with ventilation even after successful intubation (see section entitled Anesthesia for Patients With Mediastinal Masses) Possibility of superior vena cava syndrome and obstruction Cardiac and vascular compressions
Pleural effusion	Cor pulmonale congestive heart failure Need for additional monitoring Careful assessment of response to myocardial depression from anesthetic drugs
Bullae	Risk of rupture with positive pressure and creation of pneumothorax Wasted ventilation, increased dead space Compression of healthy adjacent lung
Abscess	Need for separation of 2 lungs to prevent spillage and contamination of healthy lung
Consolidation and atelectasis	Need to manage infections aggressively with antibiotics Ventilation/perfusion mismatch admixture and hypoxia
Normal chest radiograph	Patient still may have chronic, diffuse infiltrative lung disease with normal chest radiograph Computed tomography is superior to chest radiography in diagnosing diffuse infiltrative lung disease and should be done before lung biopsy

"What is an appropriate risk for rendering the patient a respiratory cripple postoperatively when managing a disease with a mortality rate of almost 100%?" Although most patients do not undergo a complete pneumonectomy, they should be evaluated as potential candidates. It is not uncommon that a more extensive resection is needed than initially anticipated. The next section discusses the tests available to assess respiratory function and the criteria for eligibility to undergo thoracotomy and pulmonary resection (**Fig. 54-2**).

Arterial Blood Gas Analysis Arterial carbon dioxide tension of more than 40 mm Hg suggests increased risk for postoperative complications. Because hypercapnia may be reversible, attempts should be made to correct all potential reversible conditions, such as bronchospasm or infection. In contrast, hypoxemia is not a consistent criterion for increased risk. The change in Pao_2 after thoracotomy and lung resection varies. Lung resection beyond the tumor may not be associated with any further decrement in oxygenation, but it may increase oxygenation by improving ventilation perfusion matching. Tumors that have already occluded the bronchus and the blood supply have already caused a functional resection.

Spirometry Spirometry has proved to be an effective, inexpensive, and noninvasive way of measuring pulmonary reserve and predicting postoperative pulmonary function. Abnormal spirometry results that suggest an increased risk for postoperative pulmonary complications include forced vital capacity (FVC) less than 50% of predicted, forced expiratory volume in 1 second (FEV_1) less than 2 L and FEV_1/FVC ratio less than 50%. Other tests having predictive value are the maximum voluntary ventilation (MVV) and diffusing lung capacity for carbon monoxide (DLCO). The MVV is effort dependent, requiring the patient to breathe as fast and as deeply as possible for 6 to 12 seconds. This test is similar to an exercise test because it reflects the entire cardiorespiratory system and the patient's cooperation and motivation. The DLCO is reemerging as an important predictor of risk in patients undergoing pulmonary resection. A recent study has confirmed that the DLCO may be the best predictor of postoperative complications, including death and respiratory failure (**Fig. 54-3**).[9] DLCO less than 50% to 60% of the predicted value is an indication for further testing with split lung function studies before undertaking major pulmonary resection (see Fig. 54-3).

Split Lung Function and Ventilation: Perfusion Studies Patients who are deemed to be at increased risk after the initial phase of the pulmonary function evaluation should receive additional testing to assess the effect of lung resection. The goal is to predict the impact of resection on postoperative lung function. The involved lung tissue may contribute little to existing lung function, and therefore its removal may not cause further deterioration of pulmonary function. Thus some patients who would be denied operations based on the initial results maybe considered surgical candidates after more specific evaluation.

The effect of anticipated lung resection can be predicted using radioisotope ventilation scans, perfusion scans, or a combination of both. More recently, dynamic perfusion magnetic resonance imaging (MRI)[10] and quantitative CT have been shown to be as accurate as perfusion scintigraphy at predicting postoperative FEV_1.[11] Most authorities consider that the minimal predicted postoperative FEV_1 that will be tolerated by a patient is 800 mL (**Box 54-1**). This is based on the observation that patients with chronic obstructive pulmonary disease (COPD) having an FEV_1 value less than 800 mL had a dramatic reduction in their level of daily function.[12] Additionally, patients with COPD start retaining CO_2 and developing hypercapnia when their FEV_1 value is less than 800 mL.[12,13] These previous studies may have been overly conservative.[13,14] Because an absolute value for FEV_1 does not account for persons of different gender, height, and age, some physicians base their decision on an FEV_1 greater than 30% to 40% of the predicted value.[15]

The radioactive technetium-99 scan yields data about regional perfusion, and the xenon-133 ventilation scan provides data about regional ventilation and lung volumes. The results allow estimation of the fraction of lung function that is contributed by the lung segments to be removed. The equation for calculating the predicted postpneumonectomy lung function is postoperative FEV_1 = preoperative $FEV_1 \times$ perfusion (%) to the remaining lung. A modification of this equation has been proposed to predict the decrement in lung function after lobectomy: loss of function = preoperative $FEV_1 \times$ functional segments in the lobe to be resected/total number of segments in both lungs.

Exercise Studies In contrast with some previous studies, preoperative maximal and submaximal exercise testing has been shown to be a good predictor of postoperative pulmonary complications in patients undergoing pulmonary resection.[16-19] Exercise testing may better predict adverse outcomes by uncovering deficits in O_2 transport or cardiac function. A maximal oxygen consumption of less than 1 L/min is associated with a 75% mortality rate, whereas death is rare if oxygen consumption is more than 1 L/min. Additional exercise-related criteria indicating increased risk for pulmonary resection include (1) pulmonary vascular resistance more than 190 dynes/s/cm^5 (with exercise), (2) arterial oxygen desaturation more than 2% with exercise, and (3) maximal oxygen consumption less than 15 mL/kg/min. Disadvantages of exercise testing are that it depends on patient effort and cooperation, and it requires special equipment and trained personnel to administer the tests.

RIGHT HEART FUNCTION

Patients who are to undergo thoracotomy and lung resection frequently have a long-standing history of smoking and underlying COPD, which can lead to pulmonary arterial hypertension and its sequelae. Pulmonary arterial hypertension results from an increase in pulmonary vascular resistance (PVR) caused by a reduction of cross-sectional area of the pulmonary vascular bed associated with the destruction of the alveolar septa and hypoxemia-induced pulmonary vasoconstriction.

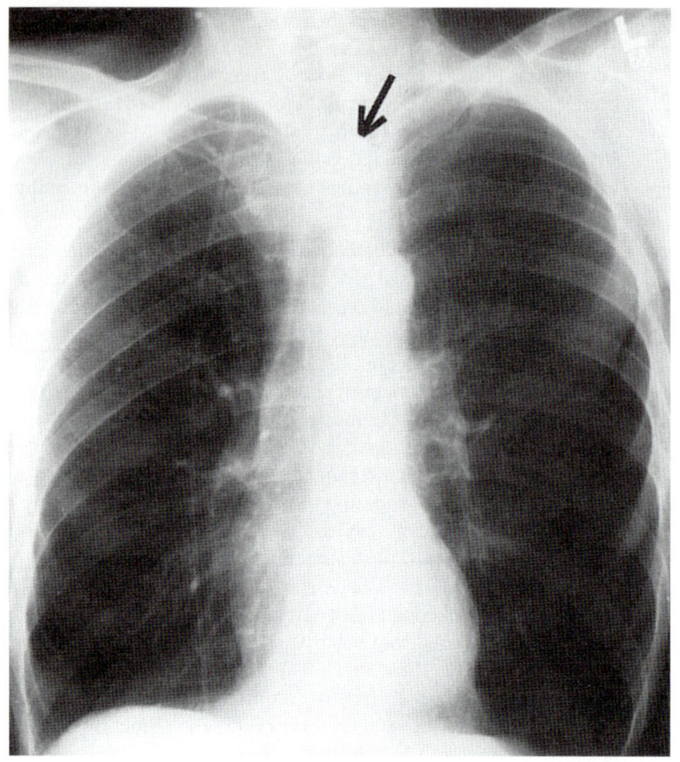

A

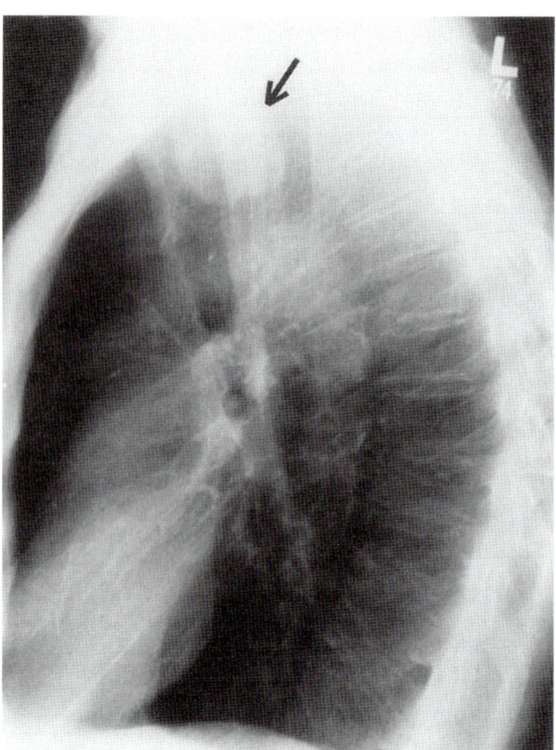

B

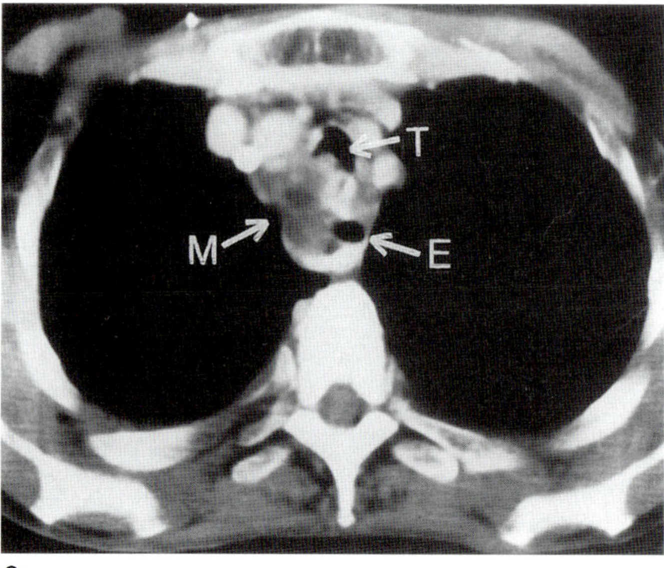

C

FIGURE 54-1. Patient is a 62-year-old man with esophageal cancer who presented with dysphagia and progressive shortness of breath. Panels **A** and **B** show enlarged lung fields with flattened hemidiaphragms consistent with COPD. A mass, designated by an arrow, arises from a structure posterior to the trachea at the level of the manubrium, causing partial opacification and deviation of the trachea, which is better visualized with the lateral chest radiography, panel **B**. The CT scan of the chest, panel **C**, shows a large tumor mass (M) in the mediastinum arising from the esophagus (E) and invading the right side and membranous portion of the trachea (T).

Over time, pulmonary hypertension can lead to right ventricular hypertrophy, cor pulmonale, and eventually right ventricular failure. The normal pulmonary vascular bed can tolerate an increase in cardiac output of 250% without an increase in pulmonary artery pressure. In contrast, even a small increase of cardiac output causes a large increase in pulmonary artery pressure in patients with a restricted pulmonary vascular bed. Preexisting impairment of pulmonary vascular compliance associated with congestive heart failure and cor pulmonale may be exacerbated after extensive lung resection, leading to serious pulmonary hypertension and right-sided heart failure. The preoperative evaluation of these patients should assess for signs and symptoms of pulmonary hypertension, right ventricular and right atrial hypertrophy, cor pulmonale, and congestive heart failure (**Boxes 54-2 and 54-3**). A fixed elevated PVR has been associated with an increased risk of complications.[6] In an attempt to simulate the cardiovascular effects of pneumonectomy, patients can undergo a right heart catheterization with occlusion of the affected pulmonary artery. The criteria for inoperability include (1) an increase in mean pulmonary artery pressure to more than 35 to 40 mm Hg, (2) an increase in $Paco_2$ to greater than 60 mm Hg, and (3) a decrease in Pao_2 to less than 45 mm Hg (see Box 54-1).[6,20,21]

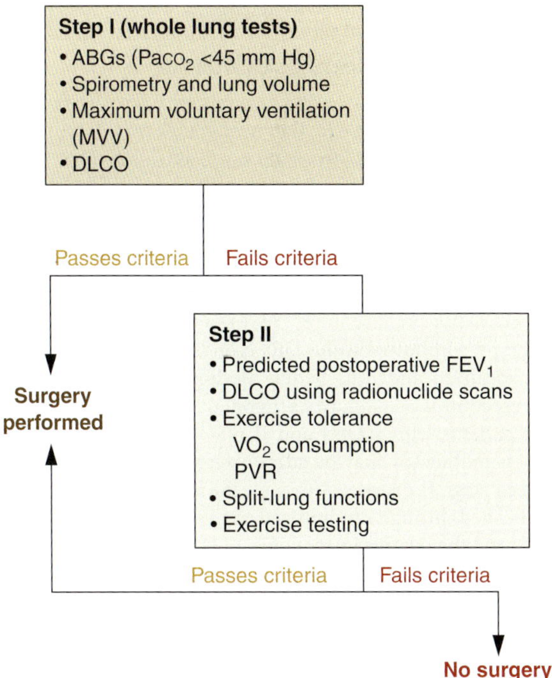

FIGURE 54-2. Sequence of tests for lung resection.[1,6,12,15-17,19,58,59,240,350-361]

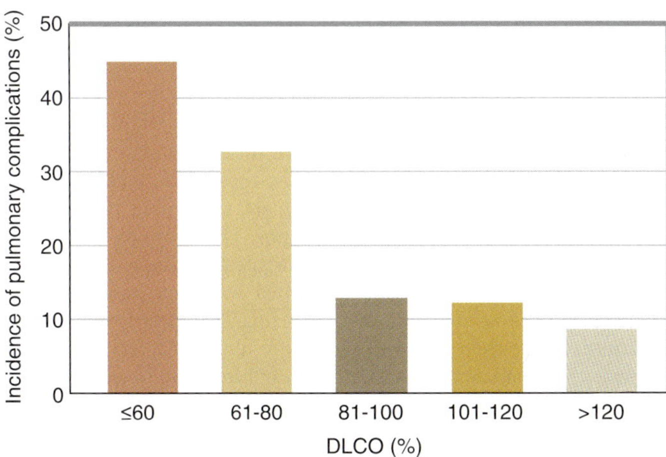

FIGURE 54-3. Prevalence of pulmonary complications after major pulmonary resection vs DLCO% for 165 patients.[356]

BOX 54-1

Factors That Predict Increased Perioperative Morbidity and Mortality

$Paco_2$ >45 mm Hg

Pao_2 <50 mm Hg on room air

Inability to walk 2000 ft in 6 minutes

Inability to ascend 2 flights of stairs

Inability to attain 7.5 mL/kg/min O_2 consumption

Predicted postoperative FEV_1 <30% of expected normal value for patient

Combined predicted postoperative FEV_1 <35% and predicted postoperative DLCO <35% of expected normal value for patient

Measures of right heart catheterization after balloon occlusion of PA of a mean PA pressure >35 mm Hg, Pao_2 <45 mm Hg, $Paco_2$ >60 mm Hg)

DLCO, diffusing lung capacity for carbon monoxide; FEV_1, forced expiratory volume in 1 second; PA, pulmonary artery; Pao_2/$Paco_2$, arterial oxygen/carbon dioxide tension.

BOX 54-2

Clinical Signs and Symptoms of Pulmonary Hypertension, Right Ventricular Hypertrophy, and Cor Pulmonale

Patient has prominent neck veins and prominent A waves, and perhaps prominent V waves are seen on electrocardiogram.

Prominent left parasternal heave and rocking motion synchronous with heart beat may be present.

Dullness to percussion over left second intercostal space near sternum may be present, indicating dilation of main pulmonary artery. However, if too much emphysema is present, entire precordium may be resonant because of hyperinflation of lungs.

On auscultation, pulmonary component of second heart sound increases, with narrowing or loss of normal splitting in second heart sound.

High-pitched, early systolic ejection click is heard.

Systolic ejection murmur is present.

Right-sided atrial S_4 gallop usually indicates increased right ventricular end-diastolic pressure and may coincide with prominent A waves in jugular venous pulse. S_4 gallop usually is not ominous.

Mid-diastolic right-sided S_3 gallop usually is evidence of impaired right ventricular function and is usually ominous. Right-sided gallops can be differentiated from left-sided gallops because they increase in intensity with inspiration.

Early diastolic, pulmonary regurgitant murmur may indicate functional pulmonary insufficiency caused by dilation of root of pulmonary artery and pulmonic valve.

Right-sided heart failure with chronic, dependent edema; large, tender liver; ascites; positive, hepatojugular reflex; and dilated, distended, pulsating neck veins are signs.

PREOPERATIVE PREPARATION OF THE PATIENT UNDERGOING THORACIC SURGERY

The preoperative preparation of the patient for thoracic surgery should focus on treatable conditions.[2-5,22] Stein et al[23] found that postoperative complications developed in 4 of 17 well-prepared patients compared with 13 of 17 unprepared patients. Prophylactic measures, such as bronchodilator therapy, hydration, and chest physical therapy, decrease the incidence of postoperative complications and should be started preoperatively and continued postoperatively. In addition, preoperative patient education about the importance of cessation of smoking, incentive spirometry, and bronchodilator therapy also are beneficial.

Cessation of smoking for at least 4 to 8 weeks before surgery is associated with decreased incidence of postoperative respiratory complications.[8,24] Although cessation of smoking for 12 to 24 hours preoperatively does not decrease the incidence of postoperative respiratory complications, it still may have a salutary effect by decreasing the concentration of carboxyhemoglobin. Other beneficial effects of

BOX 54-3

Radiographic Signs of Pulmonary Hypertension

Dilation of main pulmonary vessels

Attenuation of peripheral pulmonary vasculature, leading to oligemic peripheral lung zones

Radiographic findings characteristic of chronic obstructive pulmonary disease, such as hyperinflated lungs and low, flat diaphragms

Manifestations of right ventricular hypertrophy, clockwise cardiac rotation, and loss of air space behind sternum on lateral chest radiograph stopping smoking several weeks before surgery include decreasing sputum production and improving ciliary activity.[24,25]

Elective operations should be postponed in patients with acute exacerbation until proper management has been instituted. Sympathomimetic drugs can be administered to activate β_2-adrenergic receptors, increasing intracellular cyclic adenosine monophosphate (AMP) and leading to bronchodilation. Bronchodilation also can be produced by parasympatholytics, like ipratropium bromide, which inhibit parasympathetic vagal tone of the tracheobronchial tree. Other management for wheezing includes the administration of steroids to suppress inflammation and decrease mucosal edema. Because they are slow to act, their benefit in a patient with acute bronchospasm is debatable.

Mobilization of secretions and improved pulmonary toilet improve perioperative pulmonary function. Mobilization of secretions is achieved by a combination of deep breathing, vigorous coughing, postural drainage, hydration, and chest percussion.[26,27] However, chest physical therapy is relatively contraindicated in patients with lung abscesses, pulmonary metastases, or a history of hemoptysis.

Acute and chronic infection should be managed vigorously with antibiotics before operation. A change in the color and quantity of sputum produced by a patient with COPD may indicate infection. One prospective study reported decreased incidence of postoperative pulmonary complications and mortality rate in patients treated with prophylactic antibiotics before pulmonary operations.[28]

Preoperative pulmonary rehabilitation should be considered for all patients. It typically includes all of the steps reviewed previously along with structured exercise. Compared with education alone, comprehensive pulmonary rehabilitation has produced a significant increase in 6-minute walk test,[29] maximal exercise tolerance,[30] maximal oxygen uptake,[30] and quality of life measures.[29,30] Although these interventions have been shown to decrease postoperative pulmonary complications,[31] the programs need to be initiated 24 weeks prior to surgery to achieve maximal effectiveness.[29] Even then the effect on perioperative morbidity and postoperative outcome remain controversial.[32-35]

LUNG CANCER

CLASSIFICATION

Lung cancer is currently the most common cause of cancer mortality in the United States and throughout the world. The World Health Organization (WHO) classification of lung tumors, revised most recently in 2004, remains the foundation for lung carcinoma nomenclature.[36] The characterization of lung carcinomas by histopathologic subtype is the basis of formal classification and has implications for management and prognosis. Lung cancer is divided into several broad categories based on histology: adenocarcinoma (25%), squamous cell carcinoma (SCC, about 35%), large cell carcinoma, adenosquamous carcinoma, carcinoid tumors, and carcinomas with pleomorphic elements.

Classically, the therapeutic approach to lung cancer depends on the histologic type of tumor and its extent (stage). The most common staging classification, the TNM system, is based on cell type (T), extent of lymph node involvement (N), and metastatic spread (M) (**Box 54-4**). The TNM system is used to group patients into subsets or stages that have implications on treatment options, surgical resectability, and prognosis. Clearly, the revolution in genetics and move toward individualized targeted therapy will necessitate the inclusion of advanced diagnostics alongside classic TMN staging in determining potential therapies and outcome.[37,38]

The approaches to therapy for small cell lung carcinoma (SCLC) and for non–small cell lung carcinoma (NSCLC) differ. Small cell carcinomas account for about 25% of all bronchogenic carcinomas and have a strong correlation with cigarette smoking. In general, SCLC has metastized by the time of diagnosis and is managed primarily by chemotherapy without radiotherapy. Non–small cell carcinomas often are more localized and thus better candidates for curative resection. Surgical resection is a standard component in an attempt to cure lung cancer in patients with stage I and II NSCLC. In addition to surgery, adjuvant chemotherapy may be administered for selected patients with stage IB and stage II disease. Although the value of resection has never been established through randomized trials, the favorable results in surgical series and the relative infrequency of long-term survival in patients treated without surgery establish surgery as the treatment of choice.[39]

Lobectomy, the surgical removal of an anatomic lung segment, is generally accepted as the optimal procedure for early-stage NSCLC, because of its ability to preserve pulmonary function.[40] Limited (sublobar) resection is increasingly used to treat patients who cannot tolerate a full lobectomy because of severely compromised pulmonary function, advanced age, or other extensive comorbidity. In addition, advances in video-assisted thoracoscopic surgery (VATS) have facilitated the utilization of limited resections in selected patients.

BOX 54-4

Definitions for Staging Bronchogenic Carcinoma

Recent proposed changes in the classification system will potentially add subgroups based on tumor size (T) with cutoffs of 0-2 cm, 2-3 cm, 3-5 cm, and >5 cm in greatest dimension due to increasingly poor prognostic outcome.

Data adapted from Spiro SG. The diagnosis and staging of lung cancer. In: Smyth JR, ed. *The Management of Lung Cancer*. London, UK: Edward Arnold; 1984.

INTRATHORACIC METASTATIC MANIFESTATIONS

Clinical manifestations of lung cancer are varied. Common symptoms include shortness of breath, hemoptysis, chest pain, and increasing dyspnea (**Table 54-2**). Pleural effusions are a common but nonspecific finding observed on chest radiographs. The effusions result from obstruction of lymphatic drainage or malignant extension of the tumor to the lung surface. Chest pain associated with lung cancer usually is a dull or mild nonspecific pain occurring ipsilateral to the tumor. Metastasis to the chest wall and ribs can result in local tenderness and pleuritic chest pain. Shoulder pain may result from tumor growth at the lung apex and invasion or encroachment of the brachial plexus (such as in Pancoast tumor). Tumor extension into the pericardium can result in pericarditis, cardiac dysrhythmias, and pericardial effusions that cause tamponade. In addition, superior vena cava obstruction by local growth or lymphatic metastases will impede venous return from the head and upper extremities. Its implications to clinical management will be discussed later in this chapter.

Other manifestations of lung cancer include neurologic symptoms caused by mechanical encroachment or invasion of the nerve plexus. Involvement of the brachial plexus may result not only in shoulder pain but also in upper arm weakness. Involvement of the phrenic nerve can lead to unilateral diaphragmatic dysfunction, and involvement of the recurrent laryngeal nerve can result in hoarseness of voice.

EXTRATHORACIC METASTATIC MANIFESTATIONS

Common extrathoracic sites of metastases include lymph nodes, brain, bone, liver, skin, and suprarenal glands. The neurologic manifestations of metastatic brain tumors include hemiplegia, personality changes, cerebellar disturbances, seizures, headache, and confusion. Metastases to bone occur primarily in ribs, vertebra, humerus, and femur. Although metastases to the spinal cord and vertebral column are less common, they have implications for positioning and postoperative management of pain.

TABLE 54-2 Incidence of Various Clinical Manifestations on Initial Examination of Patients With Bronchogenic Carcinoma

Clinical Manifestation	Incidence (%)
Asymptomatic	5
Bronchopulmonary	75
Cough	
Hemoptysis	57
Chest pain	40
Dyspnea	30
Wheezing	10
Extrapulmonary intrathoracic	
Hoarseness	5
Superior vena cava syndrome	4
Chest wall pain	5
Pain radiating into upper extremity	<5
Horner syndrome	<5
Dysphagia	1
Pleural effusion	10
Extrathoracic metastatic	3-6
Liver skeleton	
Adrenals	
Gastrointestinal tract	
Kidneys	
Pancreas	
Extrathoracic nonmetastatic (paraneoplastic)	2
Endocrine/metabolic	
Neuromuscular	
Skeletal	
Dermatologic	
Hematologic	
Nonspecific	10-22
Weight loss	
Weakness	
Anorexia	
Lethargy	
Malaise	
Fever	

Based on data from Landais A, Morin JP, Roche A, et al. Measurement of cardiac output by the thermodilution method during left horacotomy in the lateral position in the dog. *Acta Anaesthesiol Scand*. 1990;34:158-161; Hoppin FG Jr, Green ID, Mead J. Distribution of pleural surface pressure in dogs. *J Appl Physiol*. 1969;27:863-873; and Rehder K, Wenthe FM, Sessler AD. Function of each lung during mechanical ventilation with ZEEP and with PEEP in man anesthetized with thiopental-meperidine. *Anesthesiology*. 1973;39:597-606.

BOX 54-5

Classification of Extrapulmonary Manifestations of Lung Carcinoma

Metabolic
Cushing syndrome
Excessive antidiuretic hormone
Carcinoid syndrome
Hypercalcemia
Ectopic gonadotropin
Insulinlike activity
Neuromuscular
Carcinomatous myopathy
Peripheral neuropathies
Subacute cerebellar degeneration
Encephalomyelopathy
Skeletal
Clubbing
Pulmonary hypertrophic osteoarthropathy
Dermatologic
Acanthosis nigricans
Scleroderma
Other dermatoses
Vascular
Migratory thrombophlebitis
Nonbacterial verrucal endocarditis
Arterial thrombosis
Hematologic
Anemia
Fibrinolytic purpura
Nonspecific leukocytosis
Polycythemia

Data adapted from Shields TW. Carcinoma of the lung. In: Shields TW, ed. *General Thoracic Surgery*. 2nd ed. Philadelphia, PA: Lea & Febiger; 1983.

EXTRATHORACIC NONMETASTATIC MANIFESTATIONS

The extrapulmonary manifestations of lung cancer affect the metabolic, neuromuscular, skeletal, dermatologic, vascular, and hematologic systems. Although uncommon, the systemic manifestations of such paraneoplastic syndromes can have an impact on the perioperative treatment. The metabolic and neuromuscular manifestations are more likely to affect perioperative management (**Box 54-5**). In general, the symptoms resolve and laboratory studies return to normal after a successful tumor resection.

Metabolic manifestations usually result from endocrine secretions by the tumor.

- Cushing syndrome most often is associated with small cell carcinoma of the lungs; it is characterized by increased elevations in adrenal corticotrophic hormone (ACTH).
- The syndrome of excessive antidiuretic hormone (ADH), which is associated with small cell carcinoma, may manifest as nausea, vomiting, anorexia, hyponatremia, seizures, or other neurologic disturbances.
- Carcinoid syndrome is associated with the production of serotonin; it is diagnosed by elevated 5-hydroxyindoleacetic acid (5-HIAA).
- Hypercalcemia, which is associated with hypophosphatemia, results from a parathyroid hormone–like polypeptide secreted most often by bronchogenic carcinoma.
- Hypoglycemia and ectopic gonadotropin production are rare manifestations.
- The neuromuscular manifestations are the most frequent extrathoracic nonmetastatic effects of lung cancer, most often small cell carcinoma of the lung.[41] The paraneoplastic myopathy, Eaton-Lambert syndrome, may appear as a myasthenic-like syndrome characterized by proximal muscle weakness, particularly of the pelvic and thigh muscles. The defect in neuromuscular transmission is a result of an antibody-mediated impairment of presynaptic neurocalcium channel activity, which reduces the release of acetylcholine.[42,43] Patients with this syndrome do not respond as well to anticholinesterase drugs as do patients with myasthenia gravis. In contrast, these patients exhibit an increased sensitivity to succinylcholine and nondepolarizing muscle relaxants.

- Other neuromuscular manifestations include subacute cerebral degeneration, encephalomyelopathy, and polymyositis. The cause and the pathogenesis of these neuropathies are not completely understood. Immunologic factors are believed to be important because antibody and T-cell responses are directed against shared antigens that are ectopically expressed by the tumor, but otherwise are exclusively expressed by the nervous system.[44,45]

MONITORING DURING THORACIC ANESTHESIA

The treatment of patients undergoing thoracic surgery is one of the most challenging aspects of anesthesiology. The patients usually have underlying respiratory and cardiac disease, which is altered further by surgical manipulations, operative position, and periods of lung collapse and 1-lung ventilation, which worsen V/Q mismatches. Thus it is extremely important to constantly monitor oxygenation and ventilation. There is disagreement about the need for invasive monitoring for patients undergoing thoracotomy. Monitoring should be individualized, depending on the extent of operation and the patient's underlying cardiovascular and respiratory disease (**Table 54-3**). (Please refer to Chapters 30-32.)

Monitoring for patients undergoing thoracic surgery includes ECG, pulse oximetry, blood pressure, and capnography. Other noninvasive monitors provide crucial information. Auscultation for wheezing, rales, or rhonchi assist in the diagnosis of endotracheal tube malposition, congestive heart failure, airway disconnect, or bronchospasm. Airway pressures give valuable information about changes in lung compliance, the occurrence of bronchospasm, or malposition of the double-lumen endotracheal tube. Perioperatively, pulse oximetry is the most valuable monitor for early diagnosis of problems with oxygenation. Capnography gives a continuous display of the CO_2 waveform and alerts the anesthesiologist to apnea, airway disconnects, and hypoventilation. End-tidal CO_2 is usually 5 mm Hg less than the arterial Pco_2; the difference between them will increase as ventilation perfusion matching worsens as in the case of 1-lung ventilation or pulmonary disease.

The anesthesiologist may require additional monitoring, such as systemic arterial or pulmonary arterial catheters, when caring for patients with a history of pneumonia, cardiac disease, or major anatomic pulmonary resection. Intra-arterial catheters are routinely used to monitor arterial blood gases and hemodynamics during major anatomic resections.

The pulmonary artery (PA) catheter is used to monitor cardiac output, left ventricular function, pulmonary artery pressures, and mixed venous oxygenation. It can be used to assess the effect of pulmonary resection on right ventricular function because patients with preoperative cardiac dysfunction are at risk of acute right ventricular failure after a pulmonary resection. A dramatic increase in pulmonary artery pressures during temporary clamping of vessels might contraindicate such resection. More than 90% of PA catheters float into the right lung.[46] During a right thoracotomy with the patient in the left lateral decubitus position, the PA catheter is in the nondependent lung. Although 1 study found that the pulmonary artery catheter in the nondependent lung underestimated measured cardiac output values, other clinical and animal studies found no difference whether the thermistor was located in the main trunk or branches of the pulmonary artery or in the dependent or nondependent lung.[47-49] Thus accuracy and clinical interpretation of PA pressures and PA occlusion pressures must account for the location of the PA catheter in relation to the patient positioning, mode of ventilation, blood flow, and hypoxic pulmonary vasoconstriction (HPV). It is exceedingly rare for the authors to use a PA catheter during thoracic surgery due to its variable reliability and risk of inclusion in the arterial staple line.

LATERAL DECUBITUS POSITION

The lateral decubitus position (or some variation of it) is common during thoracic surgery (**Table 54-4**). It allows for complete access to the hemithorax and permits extending the incision anteriorly and

TABLE 54-3 Use of Monitoring to Detect and Diagnose Intraoperative Events

Respiration	
Pattern, respiratory rate	Apnea, respiratory difficulty, rales
Auscultation	Wheezing, rhonchi, apnea, compliance
Airway pressure	Obstruction, pneumothorax, bronchospasm, secretions
Oxygenation	
Fio_2 analyzer	Inadvertent hypoxia
Pulse oximetry	Hypoxia, integrity of pulse
Arterial blood gas	Acidosis (metabolic, respiratory)
Ventilation	
Capnography	Bronchospasm Hypoventilation and apnea Confirm endotracheal intubation Return of spontaneous ventilation during controlled ventilation
Cardiovascular Function	
Electrocardiography	Arrhythmia, ischemia
Intra-arterial catheter	Hypotension or hypertension Arterial compression
Pulmonary artery catheter	Pulmonary hypertension, filling pressures, assess cardiac performance
Svo_2	Adequacy of cardiac output
Transesophageal echocardiography	Ischemia, volume status, right ventricular dysfunction

TABLE 54-4 Various Patient Positions Used During Thoracic Surgery

Position	Possible Surgical Incisions	Clinical Application
Supine	Median sternotomy	Cardiac surgery, mediastinal, major liver, vascular trauma
	Bilateral intercostal transverse sternotomy	Repair pectus excavatum, bilateral lung transplant
	Anterior or anterolateral incisions: side to be incised can be slightly elevated	Pericardial tamponade, lung biopsy
Upright	For minor thoracic procedures during local anesthesia	Used in high-risk patients (eg, open drainage of empyema) and for biopsy of lung or pleura
Lateral decubitus (90 degree angle to table)	Anterolateral and posterolateral thoracotomy incisions	Standard thoracotomy position
To provide optimal access for cardiac, thoracic, vascular, or gastrointestinal pathology, the obliqueness of the patient's back to the table can vary between 45 degree and 135 degree.	Anterolateral and posterolateral thoracotomy	To improve exposure in certain cardiothoracic, vascular, or gastroesophageal procedures
	Anterior thoracotomy	Tracheal or esophageal surgery, thyroid or vascular trauma, penetrating neck injuries
	Thoracoabdominal incisions	Thoracoabdominal aortic surgery

posteriorly. It offers access to the pleural cavity, the hilar vessels, the lateral pericardium, and the descending thoracic aorta. The lateral decubitus position is used for patients undergoing pulmonary surgery and operations on the esophagus, thoracic aorta, thoracic spine, and certain cardiac procedures. This position may affect pulmonary, cardiovascular, and neurologic physiology. Orientation of 1 lung in a more dependent position alters pulmonary mechanics and increases the risk of contaminating the dependent lung with blood and purulent materials. The dependent lung has decreased functional residual capacity (FRC) and increased airway closure and atelectasis. Increased pulmonary blood flow and reduced ventilation to the dependent lung results in ventilation and perfusion abnormalities when both lungs are ventilated, although the increased blood flow to the dependent lung is advantageous during single-lung ventilation.

The lateral decubitus position is associated with serious hazards (see Chapter 27). To avoid complications, special attention should be given to the orientation of the cervical spine, positioning of the extremities, and placement of straps to anchor the body. A chest roll should be placed under the axilla to prevent compression of neurovascular structures by the head of the humerus. Such compression decreases the fidelity and accuracy of the systemic blood pressure monitoring in the dependent arm. The use of a soft contour bag ("bean bag") is advocated because it not only functions as a chest roll but also supports the patient and decreases the risk of pressure necrosis by molding to the patient's body. Patients often are flexed to open the intercostal spaces and to facilitate the introduction of cameras or surgical instruments. Additionally, slight flexion of the dependent hip and knee help stabilize the patient and decrease stretch of the sciatic nerve. The nondependent leg is positioned on a pillow to avoid pressure on the dependent leg. Positioning of the upper extremities and the head require special attention to avoid compression or stretch injury to the brachial plexus and peripheral nerves. The cervical spine is placed in a neutral position, and the dependent arm is outstretched (**Fig. 54-4**). The nondependent arm is elevated superiorly on an arm board to bring the vertebral border of the scapula forward. The decubitus position is further stabilized by placing straps or tape across the table at the level of the hip and across the leg, paying attention to avoid compression of tissue.

The standard lateral decubitus position may be modified to facilitate surgical exposure. Slight rotation of the upper chest from 90 degree permits better access for more anterior or posterior incisions. Positioning of the nondependent arm in a more cephalad and abducted orientation permits a surgical approach that preserves the integrity of the latissimus and pectoralis muscles, "muscle-sparing approach."

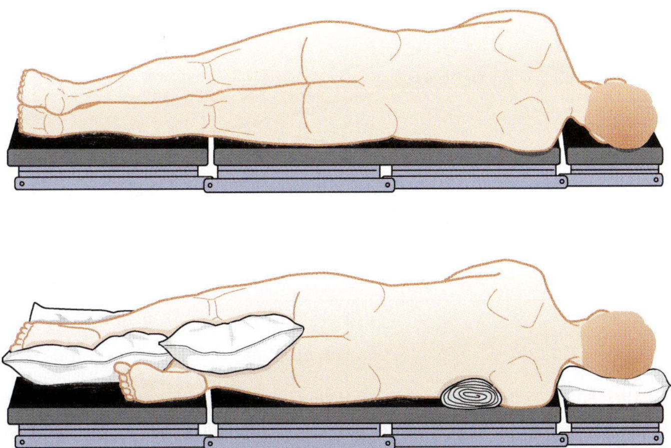

FIGURE 54-4. Standard right lateral decubitus position. **A.** Improper head position and inadequate padding. **B.** Proper padding over bony prominences, chest roll to protect axilla, proper alignment of cervical spine. Flexed lower leg stabilizes torso.

Proper positioning of the endobronchial tube should be reconfirmed after patient repositioning, because slight flexion or extension of the neck can displace the endotracheal tube. Flexion of the neck moves the endotracheal tube distally, whereas extension of the neck moves the tube proximally. Confirmation of tube position with fiberoptic endoscopy decreases the incidence of inadequate lung isolation.

PHYSIOLOGY: PRINCIPLES OF VENTILATION AND PERFUSION

Disparity between the greater gravitational pressures at the base and the greater negative intrapleural pressure at the apex are major factors in understanding normal ventilation and perfusion. Gravitational hydrostatic pressure causes distention of vessels and increased perfusion in the more dependent portions of the lung (**Fig. 54-5**). The apices of the lung may have little or no perfusion. In addition, the effects of gravity tend to collapse the apex of the lung inward and create a negative intrapleural pressure, whereas the lower dependent regions tend to push outward toward the chest wall and create a relatively positive pressure. Because the density of the lungs is 25% that of water and because the height of the upright lung is about 30 cm, the difference between the intrapleural pressure at the base of the lung versus the apex is approximately 7.5 cm water.[50] Because the intra-alveolar pressure is the same throughout the lung, the transpulmonary distending pressure is greatest at the top of the lung and decreases toward the bottom. Therefore, the alveoli in the apices are largest, and those in the base are the smallest. Approximately a 4-fold alveolar volume difference exists between the base and the apex of the lung (**Fig. 54-6**). The small alveoli in the base of the lung are on the steep portion of their compliance curve, whereas the nondependent alveoli are on the relatively flat, noncompliant portion of the curve. Therefore, in the upright position, the tidal volume is preferentially distributed to the basilar alveoli, because they expand more per unit pressure change than the apical alveoli. These physiologic effects result in greater increases in blood flow (Q) than the increase in ventilation (V), and the ventilation-to-perfusion ratio decreases from the lung apex to the base (**Figs. 54-7 and 54-8**).

PHYSIOLOGY: LATERAL DECUBITUS POSITION

Patient Awake, Spontaneously Breathing Gravity causes a vertical gradient in the distribution of pulmonary blood flow in the lateral decubitus position for the same reason it does in the upright position (**Fig. 54-9**). The vertical hydrostatic gradient is less than it is in the upright position because the distance from the most dependent to the most nondependent part of the lung is less. Nevertheless, blood flow to the dependent lung still is much greater than blood flow to the nondependent lung. Normally, in the upright position, the right lung, because of its larger size, receives 55% of the total blood flow, whereas the left lung receives 45% of total blood flow.[51,52] When the right lung is nondependent, it receives approximately 45% of total blood flow, whereas the dependent left lung receives 55% of the total blood flow. When the left lung is nondependent, it receives approximately 35% of the total blood flow, whereas 65% goes to the dependent right lung. As in the upright position, ventilation also is relatively increased in the dependent lung zones (**Fig. 54-10**).

In addition, in the lateral decubitus position, the dome of the lower diaphragm is pushed higher into the chest than the dome of the upper diaphragm and is therefore more stretched and sharply curved than the upper diaphragm. This gives the dependent diaphragm more efficiency during spontaneous ventilation. Thus in the lateral decubitus position with an awake, spontaneously breathing patient, the dependent lung is better ventilated than the nondependent lung, and V/Q still is well matched.[53]

Patient Anesthetized, Chest Closed In the anesthetized, spontaneously breathing patient in the lateral decubitus position, the dependent lung continues to receive relatively more perfusion than the nondependent

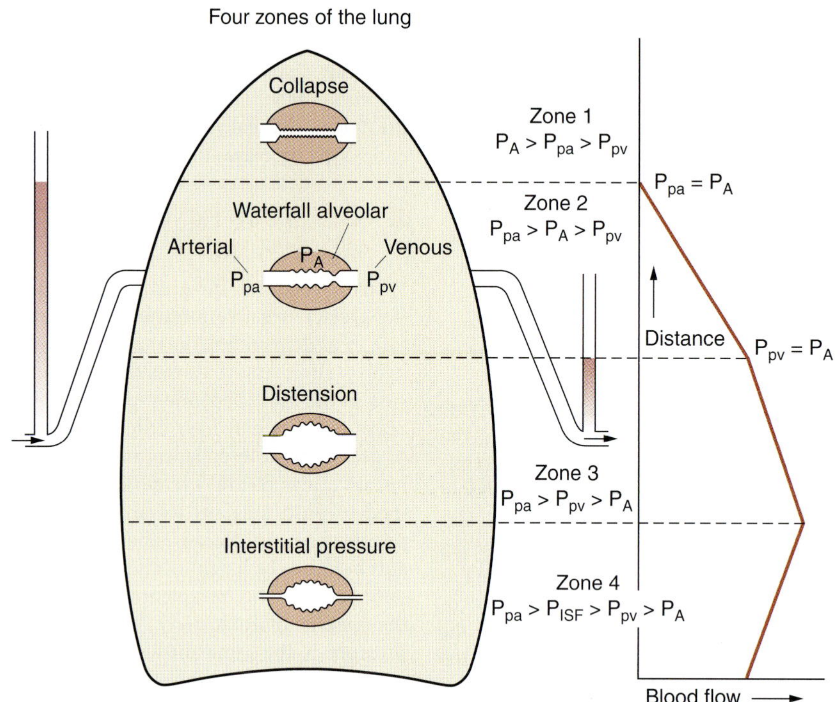

FIGURE 54-5. Schematic diagram shows the distribution of blood flow in the upright lung. In zone 1, alveolar pressure (P_A) exceeds pulmonary artery pressure (P_{pa}), and no flow occurs because the intra-alveolar vessels are collapsed by the compressing alveolar pressure. In zone 2, arterial pressure exceeds alveolar pressure, but alveolar pressure exceeds pulmonary venous pressure (P_{pv}). Flow in zone 2 is determined by the arterial-alveolar pressure difference ($P_{pa} - P_A$) and has been likened to an upstream river waterfall over a dam. Because P_{pa} increases down zone 2 and P_A remains constant, the perfusion pressure increases, and flow steadily increases down the zone. In zone 3, pulmonary venous pressure exceeds alveolar pressure, and flow is determined by the arterial-venous pressure difference ($P_{pa} - P_{pv}$), which is constant down this portion of the lung. The transmural pressure across the wall of the vessel increases down this zone so that the caliber of the vessels increases (resistance decreases), and therefore flow increases. Finally, in zone 4, pulmonary interstitial pressure becomes positive and exceeds pulmonary venous pressure and alveolar pressure. Consequently, flow in zone 4 is determined by the arterial-interstitial pressure difference ($P_{pa} - P_{ISF}$). [Redrawn from West JB. *Ventilation Blood Flow and Gas Exchange*. 4th ed. Oxford: Blackwell Scientific and Journal of Applied Physiology; 1985.]

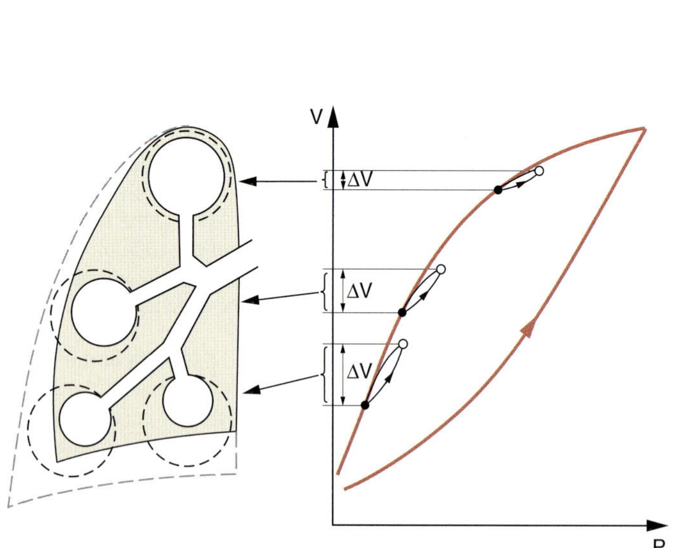

FIGURE 54-6. During quiet breathing, the lower parts of the lung show greater volume changes (ventilation) than the upper parts. [From Weibel ER, ed. *The Pathway for Oxygen: Structure and Function in the Mammalian Respiratory System*. Cambridge, MA: Harvard University Press; 1984.]

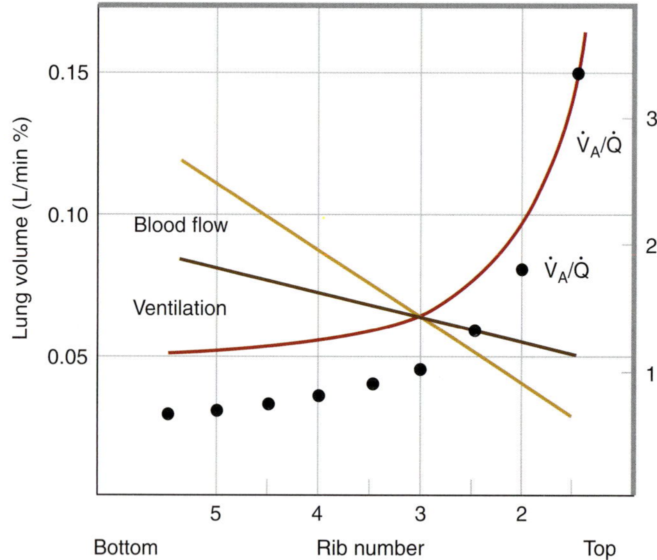

FIGURE 54-7. Distribution of ventilation and blood flow (left vertical axis) and the ventilation-to-perfusion ratio (right vertical axis) in normal upright lung. Blood flow and ventilation are expressed in liters per minute percentage alveolar volume and have been drawn as smoothed out linear functions of vertical height. The closed circles mark the ventilation-to-perfusion ratios of horizontal lung slices (3 of which are shown in Fig. 54-8). A cardiac output of 6 L/min and a total minute ventilation of 5.1 L/min were assumed. [From West JB. *Ventilation/Blood Flow and Gas Exchange*. 4th ed. Oxford: Blackwell Scientific; 1985.]

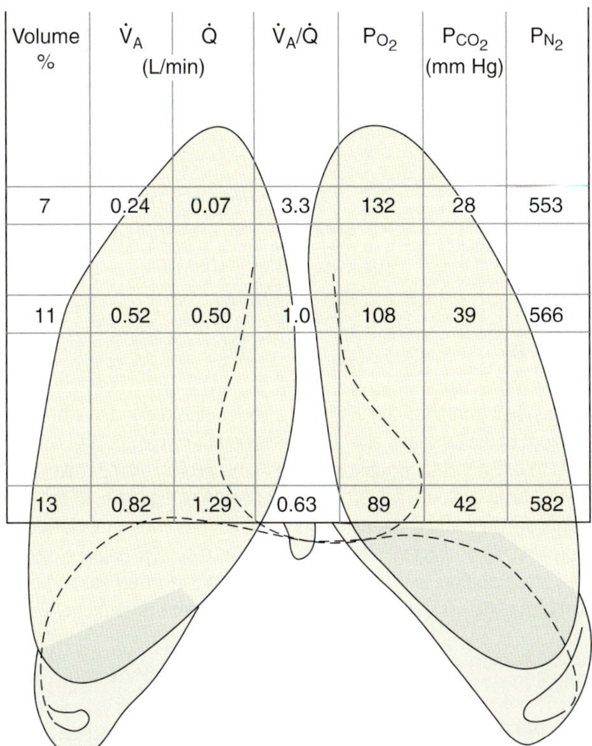

FIGURE 54-8. Ventilation-to-perfusion ratio ($\dot{V}/Q$) and the regional composition of alveolar gas. Values for the regional flow ($\dot{V}/Q$), ventilation (V_A), Po_2, and Pco_2 are derived from Fig. 54-7. PN_2 has been obtained by what remains from the total gas pressure (which, including water vapor, equals 760 mm Hg). The volumes (vol [%]) of the 3 lung slices also are shown. Compared with the top of the lung, the bottom of the lung has a low V/Q ratio and is relatively hypoxic and hypercapnic. [From West JB. Regional differences in gas exchange in the lung of erect man. *J Appl Physiol.* 1962;17:893.]

lung. The distribution of ventilation changes after the induction of anesthesia (**Fig. 54-11**).[51,54] With the induction of general anesthesia, FRC decreases. Both lungs share in the loss of lung volume and move to a lower location on the pressure–volume curve. The dependent lung now occupies the low, flat portion of the curve (ie, is less compliant). The nondependent lung, initially in the noncompliant part, now moves to the steep compliant part of the curve. Compression by the weight of the mediastinum and the abdominal contents contribute to the decrease in FRC of the dependent lung. Therefore, with the induction of anesthesia, little change occurs in perfusion distribution, whereas dramatic change occurs in ventilation distribution. Now the nondependent lung receives most of the ventilation but still is less perfused, whereas the dependent lung receives less ventilation but continues to be more perfused, which leads to an increase in shunt (dependent lung has a low V/Q ratio) and dead space ventilation (nondependent lung has a V/Q ratio >1).

Patient Anesthetized, Paralyzed, Mechanically Ventilated Mechanical ventilation causes further deterioration in the V/Q relationship. Perfusion continues to be more to the dependent lung because of gravitational effects, but now there is even more distribution of ventilation to the nondependent lung. With the institution of mechanical ventilation, the highly curved diaphragm in the dependent hemithorax no longer confers any advantage in ventilation because it is no longer actively contracting.[55] In addition, the weight of the abdominal viscera physically restricts expansion of the dependent lung, leading to further preferential distribution of ventilation to the nondependent, less-perfused lung. The anesthetized patient in the lateral decubitus position has an unfavorable V/Q ratio that is made worse by muscle relaxation and controlled ventilation. The application of PEEP to both lungs restores their FRC and most ventilation to the dependent lung.[51] The lower lung returns to a steeper, more favorable part on the pressure–volume curve, and the upper lung resumes its original position on the flat, unfavorable portion of the curve.

Patient Anesthetized, Chest Open In the spontaneously ventilating patient with an open chest, the inspiratory tidal volume in the dependent lung is decreased by the downward displacement of the mediastinum, which leads to impairment in ventilation to the dependent lung and paradoxic respiration. Paradoxic respiration refers to the movement of air between the dependent lung and the nondependent lung during respiration and the ambient atmosphere in and out of the open chest cavity. These physiologic changes also can affect circulatory performance by decreasing venous return and triggering associated sympathetic reflexes, resulting in a clinical picture similar to shock. The reflex symptoms of hypotension, pallor, cold and clammy extremities, and pupillary dilatation can be lessened by local anesthetic infiltration of the pulmonary plexus at the hilum. Most commonly, the ventilatory

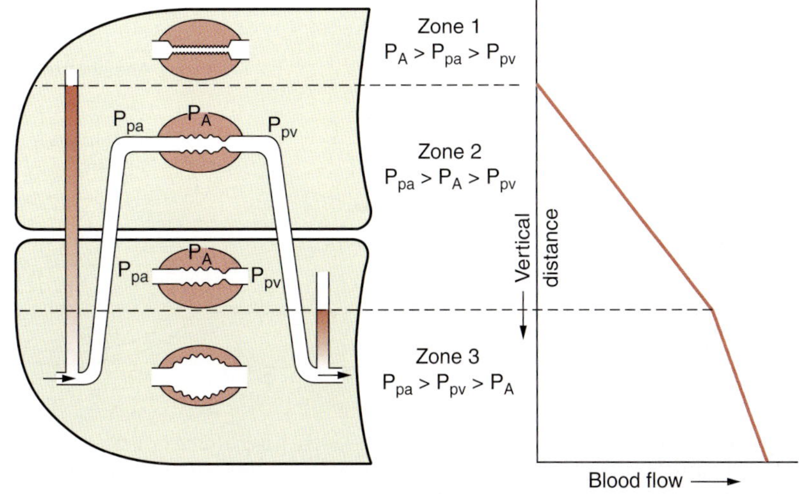

FIGURE 54-9. Schematic representation of the effects of gravity on the distribution of pulmonary blood flow in the lateral decubitus position. Vertical gradients in the lateral decubitus position are similar to those in the upright position and cause the creation of zones 1, 2, and 3. Consequently, pulmonary blood flow increases with lung dependency and is largest in the dependent lung and least in the nondependent lung. [Modified from Benumof J. *Anesthesia for Thoracic Surgery*. Philadelphia, PA: Saunders; 1987.]

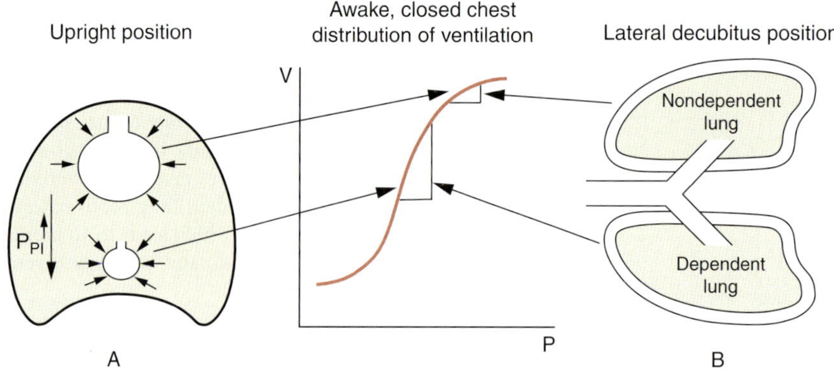

FIGURE 54-10. Pleural pressure in the awake patient (closed chest) is most positive in the dependent portion of the lung, and alveoli in this region therefore are most compressed and have the least volume. Pleural pressure is least positive (most negative) at the apex of the lung, and alveoli in this region therefore are least compressed and have the largest volume. When these regional differences in alveolar volume are translated to a regional transpulmonary pressure-alveolar volume curve, the small dependent alveoli are on a steep (large-slope) portion of the curve, and the large nondependent alveoli are on a flat (small-slope) portion of the curve. In this diagram, regional slope equals regional compliance. Thus for a given and equal change in transpulmonary pressure, the dependent part of the lung receives a much larger share of the tidal volume than the nondependent part of the lung. In the lateral decubitus position (right side of diagram), gravity also causes pleural pressure gradients and therefore similarly affects the distribution of ventilation. The dependent lung lies on a relatively steep portion, and the upper lung lies on a relatively flat portion of the pressure–volume curve. Thus in the lateral decubitus position, the dependent lung receives most of the tidal ventilation. [Modified from Benumof J. *Anesthesia for Thoracic Surgery.* Philadelphia, PA: Saunders; 1987.]

and circulatory changes associated with mediastinal shift are abolished by positive-pressure ventilation.

Patient Anesthetized, Mechanically Ventilated, Chest Open Opening the chest results in a marked increase in the compliance of the upper lung, with a slight but still important increase in the compliance of the dependent lung. Airway pressure decreases in the dependent and the nondependent lung. As a result, ventilation of the nondependent lung increases further compared with the closed-chest state.[56] The cardiac index increases with opening of the chest and pleura, but mean arterial pressure does not change drastically.[57]

The upper lung eliminates more CO_2 shortly after the pleura has been opened.[57] The increased elimination of CO_2 from the upper lung is proportionately greater than the increase in ventilation. Also, the end-tidal P_{CO_2} measured from the upper lung increases more than that of the lower lung, which reflects a marked increase in the blood flow to the upper lung. The decrease in airway pressure on opening the pleura, along with the increase in cardiac index, results in increased blood flow to the nondependent lung.

Effect of PEEP Selective PEEP application to the dependent lung can improve oxygenation by decreasing the shunt fraction. The explanation is that PEEP to the dependent lung increases the FRC of that lung, moving it to a steeper, more favorable portion on its pressure–volume curve and leading to improved ventilation of the dependent lung. Even if the increase in pulmonary vascular resistance caused by the application of PEEP shifts blood flow from the dependent to the nondependent lung, that portion of the cardiac output diverted to the nondependent lung still participates in gas exchange as long as it is ventilated or exposed to CPAP.

Effects of Surgical Manipulation With the onset of surgical manipulations, compliance and distribution of ventilation to the upper lung decrease dramatically. End-tidal P_{CO_2} and CO_2 elimination from the upper lung decrease greatly, but changes in Pa_{CO_2} are minimal.[57]

Summary The anesthetized, paralyzed patient in the lateral decubitus position with an open chest may have considerable V/Q mismatch. The nondependent lung receives greater ventilation and less perfusion and has a V/Q ratio of more than 1. The dependent lung has more perfusion

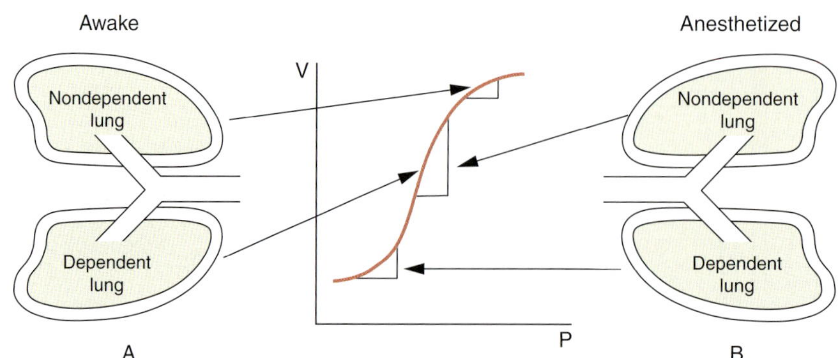

FIGURE 54-11. The left side of the schematic shows the distribution of ventilation in the awake patient (closed chest) in the lateral decubitus position, and the right side shows the distribution of ventilation in the anesthetized patient (closed chest) in the lateral decubitus position. The induction of anesthesia has caused a loss in lung volume in both lungs, with the nondependent (up) lung moving from a flat, noncompliant portion to a steep, compliant portion of the pressure–volume curve and the dependent (down) lung moving from a steep, compliant part to a flat, noncompliant part of the pressure–volume curve. Thus the anesthetized patient in a lateral decubitus position has most of the tidal ventilation in the nondependent lung (where there is the least perfusion) and the minority of the tidal ventilation in the dependent lung (where there is the most perfusion). [Modified from Benumof J. *Anesthesia for Thoracic Surgery*. Philadelphia, PA: Saunders; 1987.]

and less ventilation (ie, a low V/Q ratio) and therefore acts as a physiologic shunt. The blood flow distribution is mainly determined by effects of gravity. Causes of poor ventilation of the dependent lung are (1) loss of FRC because of induction of general anesthesia, (2) compression of the dependent lung by the mediastinum, (3) upward shift of the abdominal contents and paralysis of the diaphragm, (4) suboptimal positioning effects, (5) impaired ciliary clearance of mucus, and (6) absorption atelectasis from the use of high FIO_2. Consequently, 2-lung ventilation in these patients may result in an increased alveolar-to-arterial PO_2 difference and less than optimal oxygenation.

ONE-LUNG ISOLATION

INDICATIONS

The techniques of lung isolation are used to selectively ventilate the lung within 1 hemithorax while the nearly motionless lung is operated on in the contralateral hemithorax. Collapse of the nondependent lung produces less trauma than surgical retraction and offers better exposure of structures within the hemithorax.[58,59] The airways of the operated lung can be incised while positive pressure ventilation continues in the other lung. During thoracoscopic surgery, collapse of the operated lung is essential to provide adequate visualization of structures within the pleural cavity. Although many surgical procedures are greatly facilitated by the use of isolation techniques, most procedures are feasible without isolation.

Single lung isolation is absolutely indicated under certain clinical conditions. When one lung contains either blood or infectious secretions, isolation of the lungs becomes imperative to prevent spillage of contents into the unaffected lung. Isolated lung ventilation is essential when a bronchopleural or bronchocutaneous fistula would render positive pressure ventilation difficult or impossible. Further, directing ventilation toward the healthier lung may result in better oxygenation and ventilation.[60] Some procedures require isolated ventilation, including open procedures on the trachea and mainstem bronchi, such as sleeve and carinal resections, and bronchopulmonary lavage for pulmonary alveolar proteinosis.

DESIGN OF DOUBLE-LUMEN TUBES

Isolated lung ventilation usually is accomplished through a double-lumen endotracheal tube. The central shaft of a double-lumen endotracheal tube is cylindrical and contains a septum that divides it into 2 symmetric "D"-shaped lumens. At the proximal end of each lumen is a short length of tubing that creates a "Y" shape that permits independent attachment for ventilatory apparatus, clamping, or opening to atmospheric pressure. At the distal end, the shaft is surrounded by an inflatable tracheal cuff. The tracheal lumen terminates just below the tracheal cuff. The other lumen has a cylindrical extension, curved to fit into 1 of the mainstem bronchi, and carries an inflatable circumferential bronchial cuff. After the double-lumen endotracheal tube has been properly placed within the patient's airway, the bronchial cuff permits the bronchial lumen to be used for positive pressure ventilation or exclusion of the hemithorax in which it resides. The tracheal cuff provides a seal that directs pressurized gas from the tracheal lumen into the other bronchus. Thus a properly placed double-lumen endotracheal tube permits selective ventilation or collapse of either lung.

Double-lumen endotracheal tubes are manufactured with selective bronchial extensions intended for placement into either the left or right mainstem bronchus. The left main stem bronchus arises at a more acute angle with reference to the tracheal axis, but it is long enough to easily accommodate the endobronchial extension with its inflatable cuff. In contrast, the right mainstem bronchus is nearly a direct extension of the trachea, but it contains a branch to the right upper lobe bronchus that arises very close to the tracheal bifurcation (**Fig. 54-12**). A right-sided double-lumen endotracheal tube has a fenestration within the bronchial extension and an elaborately shaped cuff to permit a seal without airflow obstruction. Because of these considerations, right-sided tubes are more difficult to insert and require more maintenance to ensure continuous ventilation of all lobes of the right lung. In the absence of a specific indication for a right-sided double-lumen endotracheal tube, a left-sided tube is strongly preferred.

PLACEMENT OF DOUBLE-LUMEN TUBES

Before placement of a double-lumen endotracheal tube, all necessary equipment including a laryngoscope, several double-lumen endotracheal tubes, and a fiberoptic scope should be assembled and tested. The type of tube is chosen based on the surgical procedure, and its size is based on the patient's body habitus (**Table 54-5**). Direct laryngoscopy with a curved (Macintosh) laryngoscope blade is preferred because the glottic opening is better exposed by it as compared to a straight blade. The double-lumen endotracheal tube is held with its bronchial curve oriented anteriorly and its tracheal-pharyngeal curve oriented to the right. The tube is advanced through the glottic opening until the bronchial cuff just passes the vocal cords. If a stylet was used, it is removed.

There are 2 methods for the cannulation of the desired bronchus, empiric or "blind placement" and direct vision using fiberoptic assistance. In the first method, the tracheopharyngeal curve is then rotated anteriorly until the proximal end of the double-lumen endotracheal tube just passes the midsagittal axis. The bronchial curve should now be oriented to the side dictated by the type of tube, after which it is then advanced until moderate resistance to further insertion is encountered. A bifurcated connector is attached to the 2 lumens, and the tracheal cuff is inflated. Intubation of the trachea is then confirmed by capnography, auscultation, and observation of chest excursion. Once it has been determined that both lungs can be adequately ventilated, it is safe to proceed with confirmation that the tube is positioned to allow isolation of the 2 lungs. Correct placement can be determined by a series auscultation maneuvers whereby the tracheal and bronchial lumens are ventilated independently. However, this technique is time-consuming and may often prove inaccurate. The alternative method uses a bronchoscope to confirm placement. Each lumen of the bifurcated double-lumen endotracheal tube connector is fitted with a fenestrated membrane covered by a removable cap. While the lungs are ventilated with positive pressure, the fenestrated membrane on the tracheal lumen is uncovered, and the bronchoscope is passed through it into the double-lumen endotracheal tube to confirm placement. The alternative method of tube placement, which uses direct observation via a fiberoptic bronchoscope, is the most efficient method for confirming appropriate anatomic placement. The bronchoscope is steadily advanced through the tracheal lumen until its tip just exits from the distal opening. If the tube is properly positioned, the carina should be seen just beyond the opening, and the medial wall of the endobronchial extension should be seen entering the contralateral bronchus. The bronchial cuff should be entirely contained within the contralateral bronchus, while an unobstructed view of the opening into the ipsilateral bronchus is enjoyed. Disposable double-lumen tubes usually feature a prominent band around the endobronchial extension several millimeters above the endobronchial cuff to facilitate positioning. When ideally positioned, the band should lie at the level of the carina. It may be necessary to slightly advance or withdraw the tube to achieve the ideal position. Once anatomically correct tube position has been confirmed, it is secured in place and the endobronchial cuff is gently inflated under direct bronchoscopic visualization to ensure that the cuff does not herniate into the trachea. Each time the patient is repositioned, it is advisable to verify the position of the double-lumen endotracheal tube.

An alternative method of tube placement eliminates the possibility of placing the endobronchial extension in the wrong bronchus. The tube is passed through the cords and rotated as for the first method. It is advanced only until the tip of the bronchial extension is 20 to 22 cm beyond the central incisors as determined by markings on the shaft. The bronchial cuff is then inflated to seal against the wall of the trachea. An anesthetic circuit is attached to the connector for the bronchial lumen,

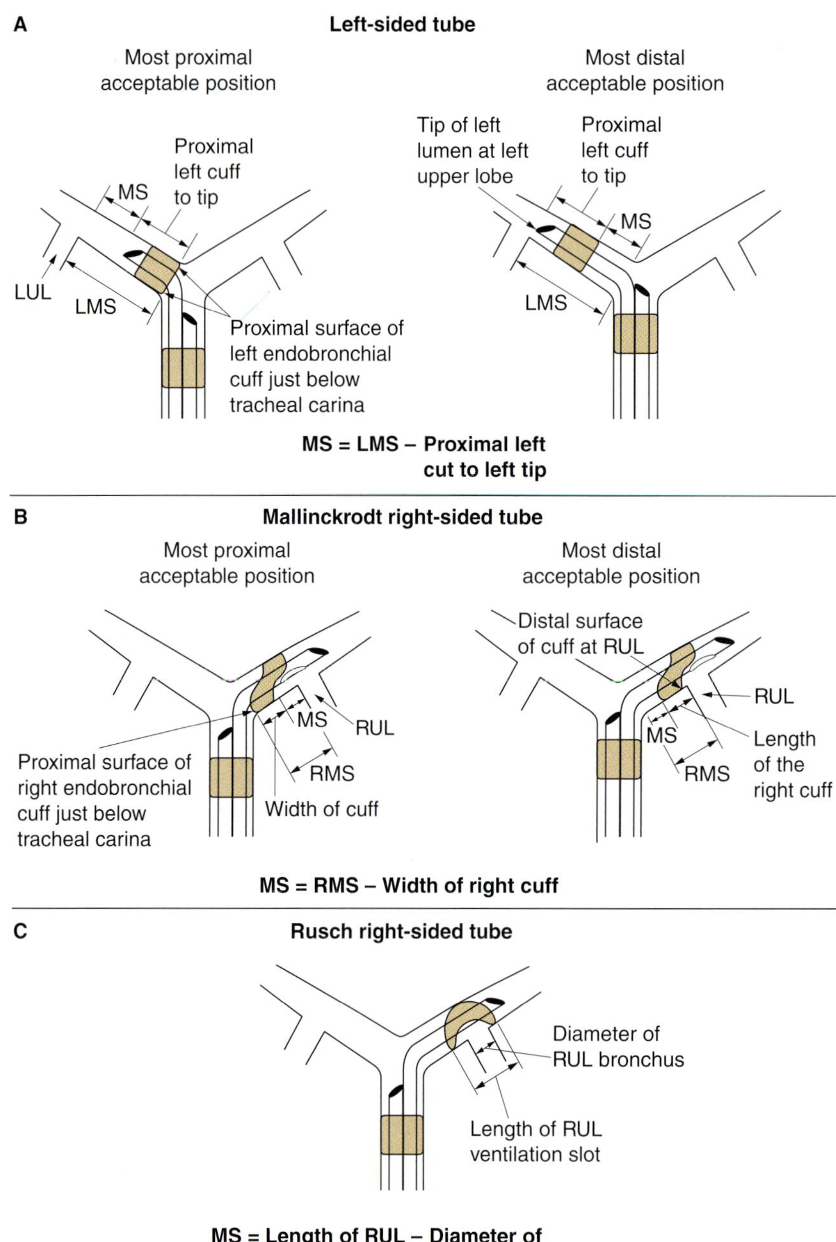

FIGURE 54-12. Schematic representation of the most proximal and most distal acceptable positions of left- and right-sided double-lumen tubes and the relative margins of safety in positioning the various tubes. **A.** All left-sided double-lumen tubes. **B.** Mallinckrodt right-sided double-lumen tube has an "s"-shaped balloon for the occlusion of the right mainstem bronchus. **C.** Rusch right-sided double-lumen tubes use a "c"-shaped cuff on the endobronchial tube that seals off the right mainstem and isolates the right upper lobe. LMS, length of mainstem bronchus; LUL, left upper lobe; MS, margin of safety; RMS, length of right mainstem bronchus; RUL, right upper lobe.

TABLE 54-5 Choice of Double-Lumen Endotracheal Tube

Patient Height	Tube Size (Fr) M	Tube Size (Fr) F	Depth of Insertion (cm)
136-164 cm 4′5.5″-5′4.5″	37	35	27
165-179 cm 5′5″-5′10.5″	39	37	29
180-194 cm 5′11″-6′4.5″	41	39	31

F, female; Fr, French; M, male.

Modified from Brodsky JB, Benumof JF, Ehenworth J, et al. Depth of placements of left double-lumen endobronchial tubes. *Anesth Analg.* 1991;73:570-572, with permission.

and intubation of the trachea is confirmed. The bronchoscope is then passed into the bronchial lumen. After the tip of the bronchoscope has entered the trachea, it is advanced under direct visualization past the carina into the desired mainstem bronchus (**Figs. 54-13 and 54-14**). After the bronchoscope is advanced as far as possible, the bronchial cuff is deflated. Using the bronchoscope as a directing stylet, the double-lumen endotracheal tube is advanced until gentle resistance is met. The bronchoscope is withdrawn and placed in the tracheal lumen to confirm unimpeded access to the ipsilateral bronchus as in the first method. Once placement is confirmed, the tube is secured.

Occasionally, double-lumen endotracheal tubes may be malpositioned. Three possible reasons are (1) the tube is so deeply inserted that the tracheal opening is beyond the carina; (2) the tube is not inserted far enough so that the bronchial cuff is above the carina; or

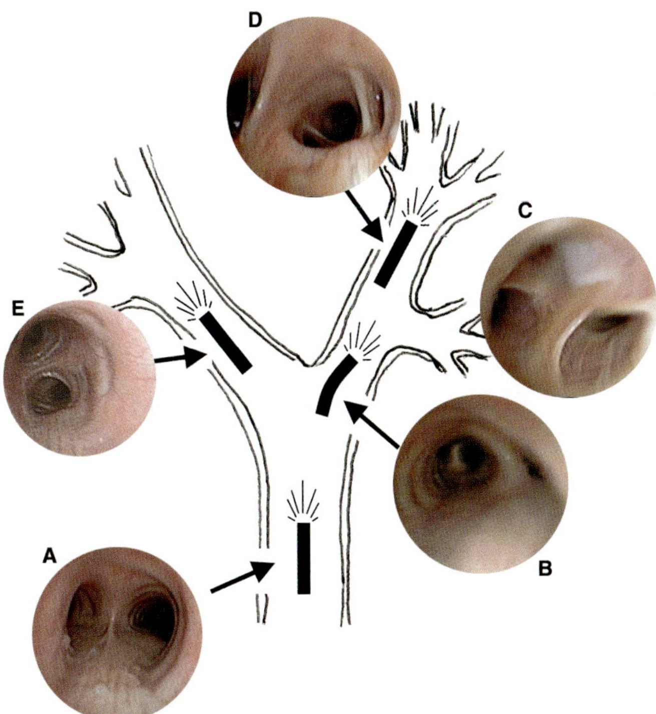

FIGURE 54-13. Bronchoscopic guide for placement of single-lung ventilation devices. **A.** The bronchoscope is situated in the distal trachea. In this view, the carina is clearly visualized along with the anterior cartilaginous rings and the posterior striated membranous portion of the trachea. The takeoff of the right mainstem bronchus is more aligned with the trachea, predisposing for endobronchal intubation of the right mainstem bronchus when an endotracheal tube is advanced too far. **The easiest way of absolutely identifying the main carina is to locate the right upper lobe** (or the scar of the previously resected right upper lobe). Confirmation of the "true" left and right mainstem bronchi is the best way to ensure proper placement of the selective lung ventilation device. **B.** The bronchoscope is in the right mainstem bronchus, just proximal to the bronchus intermedius, which begins below the origin of the right upper lobe. Origin of the right upper lobe is variable but usually arises 1 to 1.5 cm past the carina between 2 and 4 o'clock. **C.** The bronchoscope is in right upper lobe bronchus. The right upper lobe branches into 3 segments: apical, posterior, and anterior. These 3 orifices are typically arranged in a "V" pattern, but they can also be oriented in a line. **D.** The bronchoscope is in the distal bronchus intermedius. The right middle lobe, which is to the right, immediately splits into the lateral and medial segments. It is possible to advance a double-lumen endotracheal tube distal enough down the right side that the endobronchial lumen will be in the right inferior lobe and that the tracheal lumen will expose the right middle lobe. The right middle lobe's lateral segment orifice could be confused for the right upper lobe orifice, but the right middle lobe's lateral segment does not subdivide like the right upper lobe. **E.** The bronchoscope is in the distal left mainstem bronchus. This view reveals the left upper and lower lobe bronchi. It is important to ensure that left-sided double-lumen tubes have not been too far advanced, leading to selective intubation of the left upper or lower lobes.

(3) the endobronchial extension has entered the incorrect bronchus so that the tracheal lumen opening is trapped against the lateral wall of the trachea on the ipsilateral side (**Fig. 54-15**). Gently withdrawing or advancing the tube under direct bronchoscopic visualization should reveal and correct either of the first 2 causes. If the endobronchial extension is not in the correct bronchus, the tube is repositioned by inserting the fiberoptic bronchoscope in the endobronchial lumen and withdrawing the tube and scope until the carina is encountered, after which the tube and scope are advanced down the appropriate mainstem bronchus.

Right-sided tubes require more vigilance and confirmation that the fenestration supplying the right upper lobe bronchus is positioned correctly. This is accomplished by passing the bronchoscope into the endobronchial lumen and observing the upper lobe bronchial orifice through the fenestration in the lateral wall of the endobronchial extension (**Fig. 54-16**).

Although confirmation of position through direct visualization with a fiberoptic bronchoscope usually is rapid and definitive, it is not always feasible. Further, although it assures anatomically correct position, it does not ensure functional isolation of the left and right lungs. Functional isolation is tested by selectively ventilating 1 lung while the other is vented to the atmosphere, and unilateral ventilation of the intended lung is confirmed by auscultation and visual or tactile observation. The opposite lung then is ventilated, and the test is repeated. A test for functional isolation should always be used when the double-lumen endotracheal tube is placed to prevent spillage of liquid from one lung to the other.

Complications Complications associated with double-lumen endotracheal tubes can be divided into 2 types, those resulting from malposition of the tube and those caused by trauma to the tracheobronchial tree.

Malposition Malposition may lead to failure either to ventilate segments of the dependent lung or to collapse the operative lung. Failure to ventilate segments of the ventilated lung can occur if the bronchial lumen obstructs the origin of the upper lobe bronchus, which frequently manifests by hypoxemia and increased peak airway pressures. A common cause of upper lobe obstruction is distal migration of the endobronchial lumen associated with flexion of the neck. Upper lobe obstruction is more common when a right-sided double-lumen endotracheal tube is inserted. Failure to collapse the nonventilated lung may interfere with the operation.

Cephalad migration of the double-lumen endotracheal tube can be caused by surgical manipulation, neck extension (occurs with placement of patient into lateral decubitus position), or by traction on an inadequately secured tube. As the tube withdraws, the bronchial cuff herniates over the carina into the trachea. When partially herniated, increased cuff pressure may force the cuff further into the trachea. The herniated cuff may partially or fully obstruct the contralateral mainstem bronchus, making that lung difficult or impossible to collapse (or ventilate).

Malposition of the tube should be suspected when there is a sudden increase in peak airway pressure, when hypoxemia occurs, or when inflation of the nonventilated lung is detected. Vigilance should be heightened immediately after repositioning the patient and during surgical manipulation near the hilum of the lung. At the first suspicion of a malpositioned double-lumen endotracheal tube, tube position should be confirmed immediately by fiberoptic bronchoscopy. If it is difficult to discern anatomy during an open thoracotomy, the surgeon may be able to manually guide the endobronchial lumen of the double-lumen endotracheal tube into the desired mainstem bronchus.

Traumatic Damage Trauma to the tracheobronchial tree by double-lumen endotracheal tubes may include minor insults, such as ecchymosis of the mucous membranes, and more severe ones, like arytenoid dislocation or vocal cord rupture. Catastrophic tracheobronchial rupture has been reported.[61-66] The multiple lumen design and relatively large size of double-lumen endotracheal tubes make them stiffer than conventional endotracheal tubes, thus increasing the risk of damage from forceful advancement against resistance. The stiffness is further increased by use of a rigid stylet during tube placement. Therefore, when use of a stylet is required for intubation of the trachea, it should be withdrawn before the bronchial lumen of the double-lumen endotracheal tube is advanced into the mainstem bronchus.

Injuries also may result from excessive pressure in either the tracheal or bronchial cuffs, leading to tissue necrosis or rupture. The small size and high-pressure bronchial cuff increases the risk of tissue injury from overinflation. Cuff pressure should be regularly monitored by palpation of the pilot balloon or by use of a calibrated device.

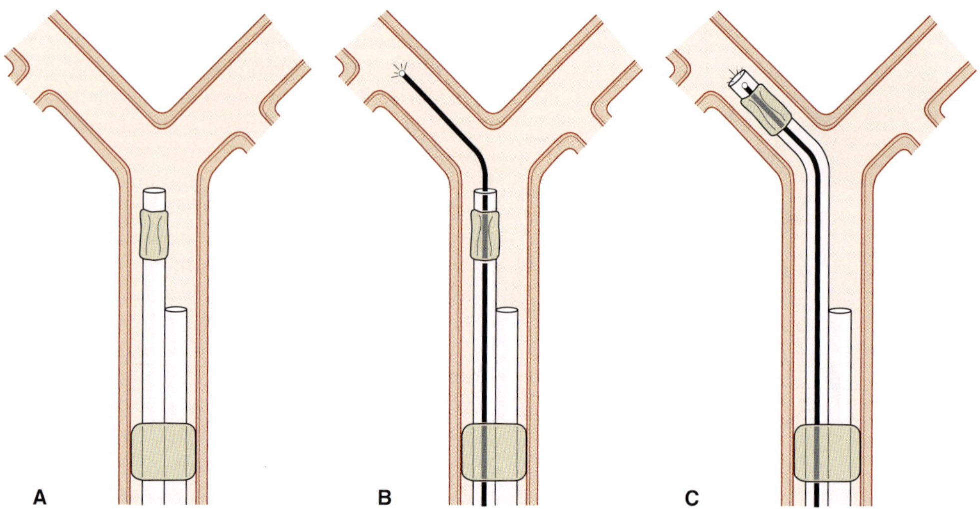

FIGURE 54-14. Schematic diagram portraying the use of the fiberoptic bronchoscope to insert a left-sided double-lumen tube. **A.** The double-lumen tube can be put into the trachea in a conventional manner, and both lungs can be ventilated by both lumens. The fiberoptic bronchoscope may be inserted into the left lumen of the double-lumen tube through a self-sealing diaphragm in the elbow connector to the left lumen; this allows continued positive pressure ventilation of both lungs through the right lumen without creating a leak. After the fiberoptic bronchoscope has been passed into the left mainstem bronchus (**B**), it is used as a stylet for the after-coming left lumen (**C**). The fiberoptic bronchoscope is then withdrawn. Final precise positioning of the double-lumen tube is performed with the fiberoptic bronchoscope in the right lumen. [From Benumof JL. Separation of the two lungs (double-lumen tube and bronchial blocker intubation). In: Benumof JL, ed. *Anesthesia for Thoracic Surgery*. Philadelphia, PA: WB Saunders; 1995.]

Failure to obtain a complete seal is especially hazardous when the double-lumen endotracheal tube is used to protect 1 lung from liquid contents within the other. The leak may allow spillage of liquid into the unaffected lung. Liquids include saline during bronchopulmonary lavage, pus from unilateral empyema, and blood from airway hemorrhage. In patients in whom a spillage occurs, a failed seal can lead to severe morbidity or death.

Contraindications The principal contraindication to the use of a double-lumen endotracheal tube is the presence of a lumenal airway mass that may be dislodged or may prevent passage of the tube. Relative contraindications

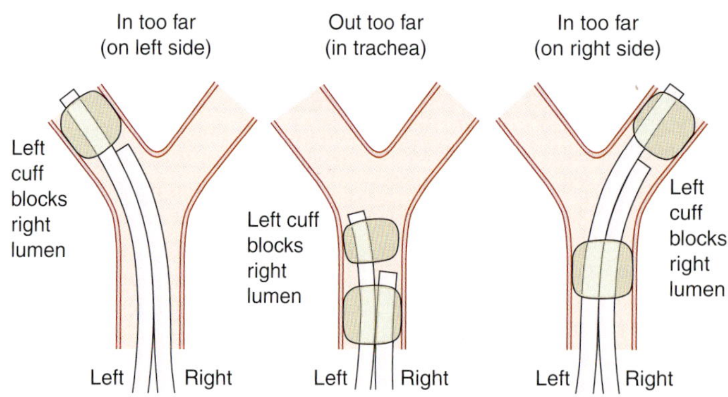

Procedure	Breath sounds heard		
Clamp right lumen (both cuffs inflated)	Left	Left and right	Right
Clamp left lumen (both cuffs inflated)	None or very ↓↓	None or very ↓↓	None or very ↓↓
Clamp left lumen (deflate left cuff)	Left	Left and right	Right

FIGURE 54-15. There are 3 major (involving a whole lung) malpositions of a left-sided double-lumen endotracheal tube. The tube can be in too far on the left (both lumens are in the left mainstem bronchus), out too far (both lumens are in the trachea), or down the right mainstem bronchus (at least the left lumen is in the right mainstem bronchus). In each of these 3 malpositions, the left cuff, when fully inflated, can completely block the right lumen. Inflation and deflation of the left cuff while the left lumen is clamped creates a breath sound–differential diagnosis of tube malposition. (See text for full explanation). L, left; R, right; -, decreased. [From Benumof JL. Separation of the two lungs (double-lumen tube and bronchial blocker intubation). In: Benumof JL, ed. *Anesthesia for Thoracic Surgery*. Philadelphia: WB Saunders; 1987.]

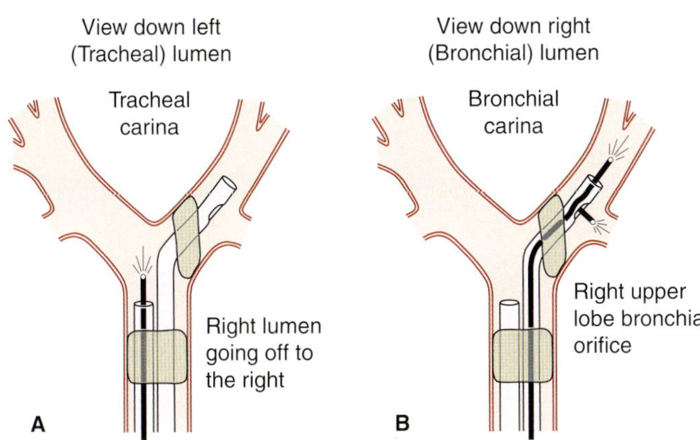

FIGURE 54-16. Schematic diagram portraying the use of a fiberoptic bronchoscope to determine precise right-sided double-lumen tube position. **A.** When the fiberoptic bronchoscope is passed down the left (tracheal) lumen, the endoscopist should see a clear straight-ahead view of the tracheal carina and the right lumen going off into the right mainstem bronchus. **B.** When the fiberoptic bronchoscope is passed down the right (bronchial) lumen, the endoscopist should see the bronchial carina off in the distance; when the fiberoptic bronchoscope is flexed cephalad and passed through the right upper lobe ventilation slot, the right upper lobe bronchial orifice should be visualized. [From Benumof JL. Separation of the two lungs (double-lumen tube and bronchial blocker intubation). In: Benumof JL, ed. *Anesthesia for Thoracic Surgery*. Philadelphia, PA: WB Saunders; 1995.]

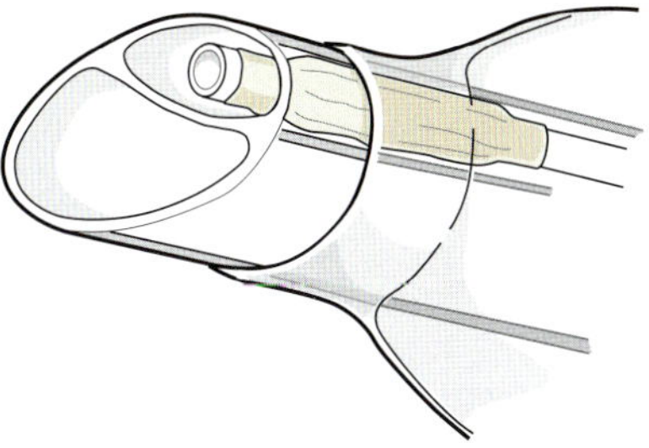

FIGURE 54-17. Close-up of the Univent tube shows 2 lumens. The small tube is retracted into the small lumen before intubation. [Modified from Kamaya H, Krishna PR. New endotracheal tube (Univent tube) for selective blockade of one lung. *Anesthesiology.* 1985;63:342.]

include critical dependence on bilateral mechanical ventilation in patients unable to tolerate its interruption, patients requiring rapid placement of an endotracheal tube to avoid aspiration of gastric contents, and patients in whom conventional tracheal intubation is judged to be difficult.

ALTERNATIVE METHODS OF LUNG ISOLATION

When collapse of the left lung and ventilation of the right is required or use of a double-lumen endotracheal tube is not feasible, a bronchial blocker can be placed in the left mainstem bronchus. In addition, this strategy eliminates the risk of losing the airway while changing the endotracheal tube at the end of the case for patients requiring postoperative ventilation. Specific bronchial blockers having a patent central lumen to permit deflation of the distal airway have been developed. The Ardnt® catheter has a nylon loop that is used to ensnare the distal portion of the fiberoptic scope as it is advanced in the selected mainstem bronchus.[67,68] The loop is loosened and advanced distal to the fiberoptic scope. Another variation, the Cohen endobronchial blocker®, incorporates a small wheel that is used to deflect the tip of the catheter into the selected bronchus.[69,70] Under direct vision, the catheter is slowly withdrawn until the inflated balloon is just distal to the level of the carina. In an emergency, an angled Fogarty catheter is inserted through the endotracheal tube under radiographic or fiberoptic guidance into the desired bronchus.[71] Absence of a patent lumen extending below the balloon of Fogarty catheters prevents suctioning or oxygen delivery to the occluded lung segment. Bronchial blockers produce less risk of hoarseness and vocal cord injury,[72] but they are more difficult to use when the surgeon requests intermittent insufflation or for application of continuous positive airway pressure (CPAP) to the operative lung.

Endobronchial intubation with a single-lumen tube offers an alternative to the double-lumen endotracheal tube that can be especially useful in emergencies. Disadvantages of using a single-lumen tube include loss of ability to selectively ventilate or suction the contralateral lung and increased difficulty in placing or ascertaining correct placement of the tube. Endobronchial intubation is especially useful for patients who require emergent tracheal intubation for massive hemoptysis. For adults, endobronchial intubation requires a tube of adequate length, often more than 31 cm, to ensure that the entire cuff is placed below the carina. Occasionally, it may be necessary to extend the tube using a length of tubing and a connector. Although endobronchial intubation of the right side is easier, there is inherent difficulty in preserving ventilation to the right upper lobe. Mainstem intubation is facilitated using a fiberoptic bronchoscope as a directing stylet. Blind left mainstem placement can be achieved with a 92% success rate by turning the head to the right after the tube has passed through the vocal cords and by then rotating the tube 180 degree so that the convex curve faces posteriorly before advancing it.[73]

The Univent tube is a single-lumen endotracheal tube that contains a bronchial blocker that passes through a small channel within the wall of an endotracheal tube. The bronchial blocker carries a low-pressure, high-volume cuff and has an internal lumen that can be used for suctioning the collapsed lung or for providing CPAP or high-frequency jet ventilation (**Fig. 54-17**).[74] Initial tube placement in the trachea is accomplished as for any single-lumen tube, then it is rotated 90 degree toward the lung into which the blocker will be passed and advanced (**Fig. 54-18**). The blocker is then advanced into the targeted mainstem bronchus, after which the tracheal cuff is inflated and the tube is secured. The depth of the blocker is adjusted and confirmed using a flexible bronchoscope passed through the main lumen of the tube. Additional techniques to assist in placing the blocker include rotation of the head and placing the fiberoptic scope in the opposite lung to divert the blocker into the contralateral side. The tube offers the advantage of allowing easy conversion from single- to 2-lung ventilation (and vice versa), and it is suitable for long-term use in an intensive care unit (ICU) setting. The mobility of the blocker and large volume of its cuff increase the likelihood of proximal migration, with herniation of the cuff into the trachea.

HYPOXIC PULMONARY VASOCONSTRICTION

Humans encounter hypoxia throughout their lives. This occurs by destiny in utero, through disease, and by desire, in our quest for altitude. Hypoxic pulmonary vasoconstriction (HPV) is a widely conserved, homeostatic, vasomotor response of resistance of pulmonary arteries to alveolar hypoxia. HPV mediates ventilation-perfusion matching and, by reducing shunt fraction, optimizes systemic Po_2.

Although total pulmonary blood flow is directly proportional to right ventricular cardiac output, its distribution within the pulmonary vasculature can be altered dynamically. Hypoxia, caused by either atelectasis or ventilation with a hypoxic gas mixture, diverts blood flow to better-ventilated, nonhypoxic lung segments. This phenomenon of HPV, first noted by Von Euler and Liljestrand in 1946, is of great importance to the anesthesiologist, particularly during thoracic anesthesia. In the absence of inhibiting factors, HPV can divert blood flow away from nonventilated regions.[75] When a patient is in the lateral decubitus position, the dependent lung receives 60% of the cardiac output, whereas the nondependent lung receives 40%. If the nondependent lung is not ventilated and atelectatic, a maximal HPV response can reduce its blood supply by 50%. As a result, the dependent lung receives 80% of the cardiac output, and the atelectatic nondependent lung receives only 20% of the cardiac output (**Fig. 54-19**). Therefore, the arterial oxygen tension (Pao_2)

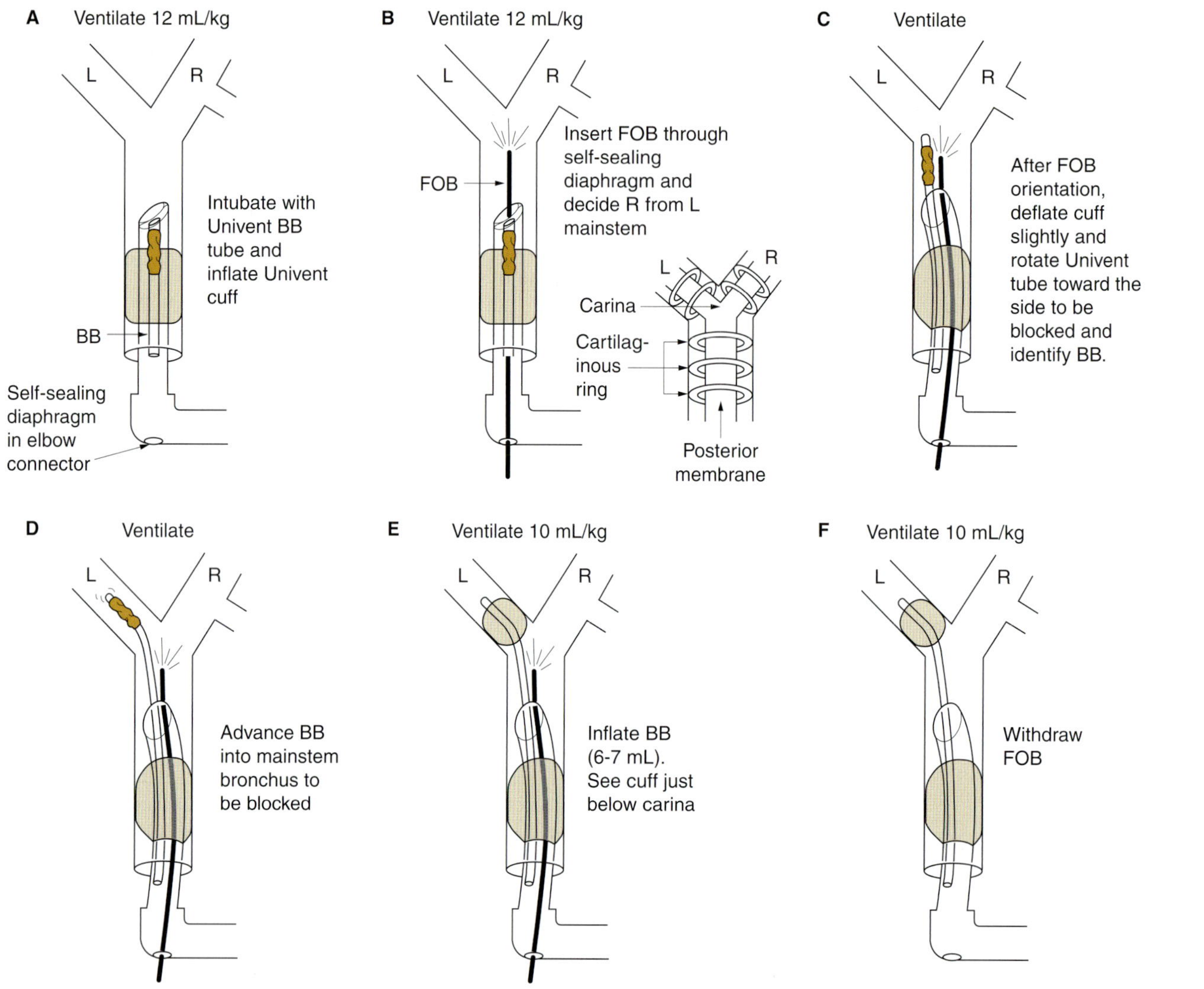

FIGURE 54-18. The sequential steps of the fiberoptic-aided method of inserting and positioning the Univent bronchial blocker in the left mainstem bronchus are illustrated. One- and two-lung ventilation is achieved by simply inflating and deflating, respectively, the bronchial blocker balloon. FOB, fiberoptic bronchoscope. [From Benumof JL. Separation of two lungs (double-lumen and bronchial blocker intubation). In: Benumof JL, ed. *Anesthesia for Thoracic Surgery*. Philadelphia, PA: WB Saunders; 1995.]

observed during regional lung hypoxia is much greater than would be expected if the HPV response were not present (**Fig. 54-20**).

MECHANISMS

HPV is mediated by the smooth muscle cells throughout the lung. Although modulated by the endothelium, the core mechanism is in the smooth muscle cell. The Redox Theory for the mechanism of HPV proposes the coordinated action of a redox sensor (the proximal mitochondrial electron transport chain) that generates a diffusible mediator (a reactive O_2 species) that regulates an effector protein (voltage-gated potassium [K(v)] and calcium channels). The subsequent inhibition of O_2-sensitive K(v) channels, particularly K(v)1.5 and K(v)2.1, depolarizes

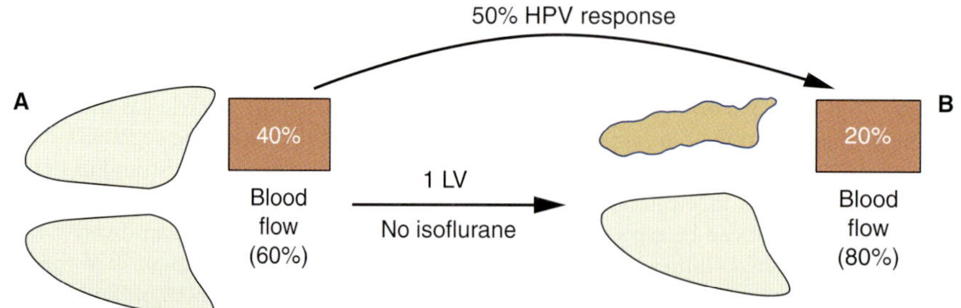

FIGURE 54-19. A. Schematic diagram showing that the 2-lung ventilation nondependent-to-dependent lung blood flow ratio is 40% to 60%. **B.** When 2-lung ventilation is converted to 1-lung ventilation (as indicated by atelectasis of the nondependent lung), the HPV response decreases the blood flow to the nondependent lung by 50%, so that the nondependent-to-dependent lung blood flow ratio is now 20% to 80%. [From Wernly JA, et al. Clinical value of quantitative ventilation-perfusion lung scans in the surgical management of bronchogenic carcinoma. *J Thorac Cardiovasc Surg.* 1980;80:535.]

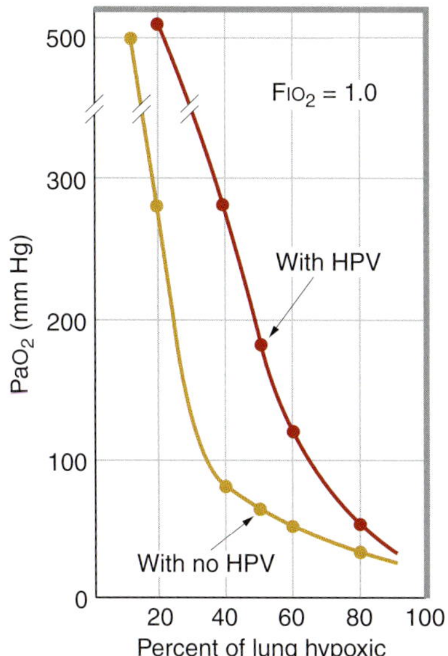

FIGURE 54-20. Effect of HPV on Pao_2. As the percentage of lung that is hypoxic increases (x-axis), the arterial Po_2 (Pao_2) decreases (y-axis). When the amount of lung that is hypoxic 30% to 70%, which is in the 1-lung ventilation/anesthesia range, the decrease in Pao_2 is much greater if there is no HPV compared with the normal expected amount of HPV. HPV, hypoxic pulmonary vasoconstriction. [From Benumof JL. One-lung ventilation and hypoxic pulmonary vasoconstriction: Implications for anesthetic management. *Anesth Analg.* 1985;64:821.]

pulmonary artery smooth muscle, activating voltage-gated Ca^{2+} channels and causing Ca^{2+} influx and vasoconstriction.[76] A similar mechanism for regulating O_2 uptake/distribution is partially recapitulated in simpler organisms and in the other specialized mammalian O_2-sensitive tissues, including the carotid body and ductus arteriosus.[77]

Hemodynamic variables can influence the magnitude of HPV. The pulmonary vasoconstrictor response to hypoxia is decreased with increases in PA pressure, cardiac output, left atrial pressure, or central blood volume.[78] Increases in pulmonary vascular pressures can mechanically open and recruit closed vessels in hypoxic lung regions, overcoming part of the active pulmonary vasoconstriction.[79] An increase in cardiac output can mask the HPV response by recruiting pulmonary vessels or by increasing Pvo_2. Alternatively, HPV may increase pulmonary vascular resistance and PA pressures as flow is diverted from a proportionately large section of hypoxic lung to a smaller section of normoxic lung.[79] When flow is diverted from small hypoxic segments, the high compliance of the pulmonary circulation prevents clinically significant changes in pulmonary vascular resistance or PA pressure.

Drugs and anesthetics may modulate HPV and interfere with ventilation-perfusion matching. Calcium channel blockers and vasodilators, such as sodium nitroprusside, attenuate the HPV response (**Table 54-6**).

TABLE 54-6 Effect of Vasodilators on Hypoxic Pulmonary Vasoconstriction

Drug	Effect	References
Hydralazine	No change	86
Nifedipine	Inhibited	86-89
Verapamil	Inhibited	90, 91
Nitroglycerin	Inhibited	93
Sodium nitroprusside	Inhibited	94
Nicardipine	No change	95
Labetalol	No change	96

These drugs increase the A-a gradient, often leading to hypoxemia perioperatively. Other perioperative conditions, such as hypocapnia and hypothermia, also decrease the normal HPV response.[78,80]

EFFECTS OF ANESTHETICS

Extensive studies have been performed to examine the effect of inhalation and intravenous anesthetics on HPV. The results and implications of these studies differ according to the type of experimental preparation used. In human studies and in more physiologic in vivo investigations with an intact systemic circulation, inhalation anesthetics produced either no effect or only a mild decrease in HPV.[81,82] In part, the discrepancy between the more complex in vivo studies and simpler in vitro models occurs because the additional factors that can modulate the HPV response, such as pulmonary vascular pressure, cardiac output, Pco_2, and temperature, are absent. In the more biologically complex in vivo models, these factors seem to diminish the inhibitory effect of inhaled anesthetics on HPV.[83,84]

Intravenous agents such as ketamine and propofol do not dramatically affect HPV.[83,85] HPV is also not directly affected by thoracic epidural analgesia. Any changes that have been observed during epidural may be attributable to alterations in cardiac function and loading conditions.[86]

Nitric Oxide Nitric oxide (NO) is a unique endogenous compound that is found in endothelium and smooth muscle cells. NO induces vasodilation by activation of protein kinases and guanylate cyclase and reduction or resequestration of intracellular Ca+. There is a class of intravenous vasodilators, including nitroglycerine and nitroprusside, that produces muscle relaxation in a similar manner.

The most common clinical uses of NO are for the management of pulmonary hypertension and ventilation-perfusion mismatching. Intravenous therapy nonselectively produces pulmonary and systemic vasodilation. In contrast, NO administered as an inspired gas or NO donor Flolan (see Prostacyclin section) selectively dilates the vascular supply to those areas, thereby improving ventilation-to-perfusion matching. Nitric oxide has been used clinically in cases of primary pulmonary hypertension, lung transplantation, cardiac transplantation, cardiac disease, adult respiratory distress syndrome (ARDS), acute pulmonary hypertension, congenital heart disease, and idiopathic pulmonary hypertension. Its clinical potential has been hampered by the complexity and cost of the gas and its delivery system.

Delivery systems require an adequate scavenging system to reduce the risk of occupational exposure and continuous gas concentration monitoring. The potential toxicity of NO focuses on its conversion from the free radical form to NO_2, which is associated with lung toxicity, and the formation of nitrosylhemoglobin, which is rapidly converted to methemoglobin.[87-90] Clinical reports of NO-associated toxicity include methemoglobin toxicity, paradoxical deterioration in oxygenation related to edema or worsening of right-to-left shunting,[74,91-95] and rebound pulmonary hypertension.[87,96,97] Because of these latter responses, the dose of NO should be gradually decreased to avoid deterioration in oxygenation or rebound pulmonary hypertension.

Prostacyclin Prostacyclin (PGI_2, Epoprostanol, Flolan) is a member of the prostaglandin family of lipid mediators derived from arachadonic acid and is synthesized predominantly by endothelial cells, including the pulmonary vascular endothelium.[98] PGI_2 produces vasodilation in low-resistance vascular beds such as the pulmonary circulation.[99] Not only has PGI_2 been shown to stimulate endothelial release of NO,[100] but NO has been shown in turn to enhance the production of PGI_2 in human pulmonary artery smooth muscle cells. It has a good safety profile; PGI_2 is spontaneously hydrolyzed in plasma to its inactive metabolite, 6-keto-prostaglandin-F. The in vitro half-life of prostacyclin in human blood at 37°C and pH of 7.4 is approximately 6 minutes.[101] Animal studies demonstrate that intravenous PGI_2 has a high clearance (93 mL · min^{-1} · kg^{-1}), small volume of distribution (357 mL/kg), and a short half-life (2.7 min).[101]

Prostacyclin, which can be delivered as an aerosol, has replaced NO as the preferred inhaled selective pulmonary vasodilator due to lower cost and absence of toxic metabolites.[98,102,103] It has minimal effects on systemic arterial pressure and dramatic improvements in arterial oxygenation and lowering pulmonary arterial pressures.[102,103] Its use during 1-lung anesthesia can improve V/Q matching, but it is not nearly as effective as CPAP to the nonventilated (nondependant, operative) lung (see the following section) deterioration in oxygenation or worsening of pulmonary hypertension.

STRATEGIES TO IMPROVE OXYGENATION DURING 1-LUNG VENTILATION

The occurrence of arterial hypoxemia during 1-lung ventilation (OLV) is difficult to predict clinically. Previous studies have attempted to identify predictive preoperative and intraoperative factors of Pao_2 during single-lung ventilation. Some variables (relative perfusion to the operative lung, intraoperative Pao_2 during 2-lung ventilation) were strongly identified as predictors of low Pao_2 during 1-lung ventilation, whereas others (side of operation, preoperative pulmonary function tests) have been controversial.[104,105] Interestingly, patients with a hematocrit value of greater than 45% are reported to have lower Pao_2 values during 1-lung ventilation.[106] The occurrence of hypoxia mainly depends on factors such as residual shunt to the nonventilated lung, cardiac output, and degree of pulmonary vasoconstriction. There are, however, strategies to decrease the occurrence of hypoxemia during 1-lung ventilation and manage it when present.

The basic principles for management of 1-lung ventilation include (1) delay initiation until after turning the patient to the lateral decubitus position, while still allowing sufficient time for the nondependent lung collapse, (2) confirm correct positioning of the double-lumen tube by fiberoptic bronchoscopy, (3) use high-inspired O_2 concentrations to decrease the risk of systemic hypoxemia, (4) using a large tidal volume while controlling peak inspiratory pressure to less than 30 mm Hg and adjusting respiratory rate to keep $Paco_2$ at approximately 35 mm Hg, (5) continuously monitor oxygenation using pulse oximetry, and (6) continuously monitor ventilation by noting changes in end-tidal CO_2 concentrations and peak inspiratory pressures.

Measures to improve oxygenation during 1-lung ventilation include 1 or more of the following strategies: (1) improve the V/Q distribution in the dependent lung (ie, lung recruitment maneuver, PEEP to the dependent lung), (2) increase Pao_2 in the nondependent lung (ie, CPAP), (3) decrease blood flow to the nondependent lung (ie, placement of a ligature on the pulmonary artery), and (4) increase blood flow and perfusion to the dependent lung (ie, prostacyclin or nitric oxide).

PREVENTION OF ABSORPTION ATELECTASIS

Absorption atelectasis, caused by increased Fio_2, can be decreased or prevented by ventilation using large tidal volumes, application of PEEP to the dependent lung, and ventilation with an Fio_2 less than 100%.[84] The use of 10% to 20% nitrogen with 80% to 90% O_2 has been suggested to decrease the possibility of absorption atelectasis, because nitrogen splits open the alveoli in areas of low V/Q ratio. The small reduction in the Fio_2 causes only a small decrease in Pao_2. Nitrogen is more efficacious than N_2O in splitting the alveoli because it is less soluble.

VERIFICATION OF LUNG ISOLATION

The most important factor in assuring adequate oxygenation and ventilation is the proper positioning of the double-lumen endotracheal tube or bronchial blocker. Tube position should be reconfirmed after turning the patient. In addition, secretions that could interfere with ventilation and increase inflation pressure also should be suctioned from the airway.

RECRUITMENT MANEUVER

Progressive atelectasis associated with decreasing Pao_2 is a common problem of the patient undergoing single-lung ventilation during thoracic surgery. These patients are at increased risk of atelectasis due to single-lung ventilation, lateral decubitus positioning, inhibition of HPV, and periodic disconnection from the ventilator. Recruitment maneuvers are used to reinflate collapsed alveoli, which results in improved oxygenation and ventilation. A sustained pressure of about 35 to 40 cm H_2O, which would be above the tidal ventilation range, is applied for a period of 30 to 60 seconds in order to inflate lung units. After this maneuver, it should not be necessary to increase the tidal volume or PEEP, as the subsequent lung volumes should be greater. A successful procedure will result in improved oxygenation, reduced end-tidal CO_2, and improved compliance. Profound hypotension can occur due to inhibition of right heart filling.

VENTILATION USING LARGE TIDAL VOLUMES

Small tidal volume ventilation to the dependent lung can decrease FRC and promote airway closure and atelectasis. The development of a hypoxic area in the dependent lung interferes with the overall effectiveness of HPV in the nondependent lung, to optimize oxygenation of the dependent lung. The tidal volume at initiation of 1-lung ventilation should be about 6 to 8 mL/kg. The tidal volume is then adjusted upward or downward according to the airway pressures and arterial blood gas values. Delivering an excessively large tidal volume to the dependent lung can paradoxically worsen oxygenation and ventilation of the dependent lung. Increased airway pressures with the associated the risks of pneumothorax or barotrauma and increased PVR can divert blood, that is, perfusion, to the nonventilated nondependent lung.[107-110] Increased airway pressures have been associated with postoperative inflammatory lung disease such as postlobectomy and postpneumonectomy pulmonary edema.[111,112]

MAINTENANCE OF NORMOCAPNIA

Respiratory rates should be adjusted to maintain normocapnia. Because the tidal volume is decreased with initiation of 1-lung ventilation, the respiratory rate should be increased to maintain the same minute ventilation and $Paco_2$. The change from 2-lung ventilation to 1-lung ventilation usually causes no problem with CO_2 elimination because of the high diffusibility of CO_2 across the alveolar membrane.[110,113,114] Theoretically, hypocapnia should be avoided because it can directly dilate the pulmonary vessels, interfering with HPV in the nondependent lung. Alternatively, hypercapnia will increase PVR and can increase right heart strain.

DEPENDENT-LUNG PEEP

Because the dependent lung often has a decreased volume during 1-lung ventilation, several attempts have been made to improve oxygenation by managing the ventilated lung with PEEP. The application of PEEP to the dependent lung maintains recently recruited atelectatic alveoli to increase FRC and lung compliance. The disadvantage of applying PEEP to the dependent lung is that the associated increased mean airway pressure and PVR could divert some blood flow to the nondependent, atelectatic, nonventilated lung. Therefore, the effect of using PEEP is a balance between its potential beneficial effects and the possible deleterious effects of decreasing HPV, causing the redistribution of blood flow to the nondependent nonventilated lung. In a patient with a very diseased dependent lung, the positive effect of selective dependent-lung PEEP may outweigh its negative effects. In contrast, patients who have a relatively normal dependent lung may have decreased oxygenation if PEEP is selectively applied to that lung (**Fig. 54-21**).

SELECTIVE NONDEPENDENT-LUNG CPAP

The application of CPAP to the nonventilated nondependent lung improves oxygenation during 1-lung ventilation (**Fig. 54-22**). Even with a maximal HPV response, 20% of the cardiac output still flows through the nondependent lung. The use of an inhalation agent, such

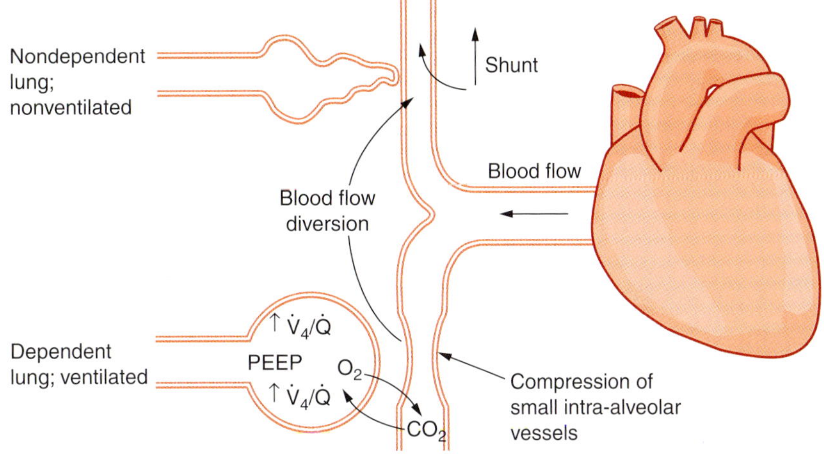

FIGURE 54-21. Selective positive end-expiratory pressure (PEEP) to the ventilated-dependent lung can increase dependent-lung ventilation-to-perfusion ratios (–A/). Dependent-lung PEEP also can cause compression of the small intra-alveolar vessels in the dependent lung, causing blood flow diversion to the nonventilated, nondependent lung, thereby increasing the shunt through the nonventilated, nondependent lung. Therefore, the overall arterial oxygenation effect of dependent-lung PEEP will be a trade-off between the good effect of an increase in dependent-lung A/ and the bad effect of increased nonventilated-lung blood flow. [From Benumof JL, ed. *Anesthesia for Thoracic Surgery*. Philadelphia: WB Saunders; 1987.]

as isoflurane, may increase the nondependent lung blood flow to 24% of the cardiac output. Application of CPAP during 1-lung ventilation leads to the oxygenation of blood that perfuses the nondependent lung and thereby dramatically increases Pao_2. CPAP is initiated during the deflation phase of a large tidal volume breath to maintain uniform expansion and avoid the need to overcome critical opening pressures of collapsed alveoli. The application of 5 to 10 cm H_2O CPAP may not interfere with surgical exposure during open thoracotomies, but will significantly impede visualization during thoracoscopy. In addition, CPAP at less than 10 cm H_2O does not compress small intra-alveolar vessels nor produce significant hemodynamic effects, but 15 cm H_2O of CPAP decreases blood flow through the nondependent lung, diverting flow to the dependent lung.[115]

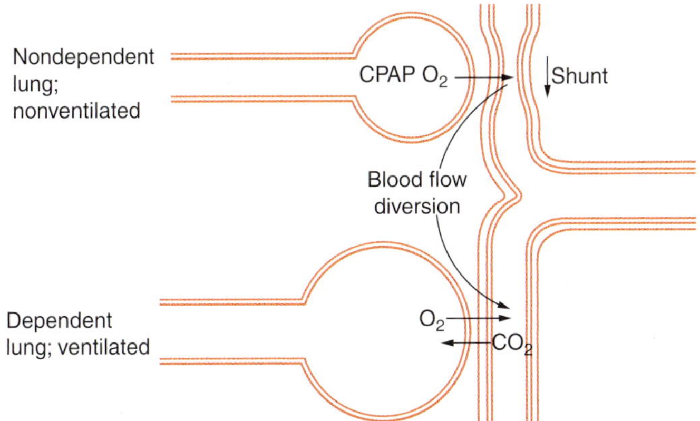

FIGURE 54-22. Selective continuous positive airway pressure (CPAP) to the nonventilated, nondependent lung (static distension without tidal movement) allows this lung to participate in oxygen uptake and markedly decreases the shunt through the nonventilated, nondependent lung. Even if the nonventilated, nondependent lung CPAP causes blood flow diversion to the ventilated, dependent lung, the diverted flow can still participate in oxygen uptake and CO_2 elimination in the ventilated, dependent lung. Usually 5 to 10 cm H_2O of nondependent lung CPAP is all that is clinically needed, and this amount of CPAP does not cause any serious surgical interference. [From Benumof JL, ed. *Anesthesia for Thoracic Surgery*. Philadelphia, PA: WB Saunders; 1995.]

During 1-lung ventilation, the nondependent lung does not remain totally unventilated. Each time the dependent lung is inflated, the mediastinum is displaced upward into the nondependent thorax. During the exhalation phase, the mediastinum falls away from the nondependent side. The effect of the mediastinal movement created by ventilation produces asynchronous, "pendelluft" ventilation of the nondependent lung. This phenomenon may be observed as a small puff of air emanating from the lumen of the nondependent endotracheal tube, which may be misinterpreted as a failed seal of the bronchial cuff. Because the nondependent lung is ordinarily open to the atmosphere, the pendelluft ventilation introduces room air into the tracheobronchial tree. Thus, even in the absence of CPAP, delivering 100% oxygen via T-piece may improve oxygenation of blood flowing through the nondependent lung.

The conventional method for instituting CPAP during 1-lung ventilation uses an O_2 source and a manometer or PEEP valve (**Fig. 54-23**).[116] Alternatively, delivery of oxygen at high flows via a catheter placed in the mainstem bronchus of the nondependent lung produces CPAP without need for a PEEP valve. In most situations, an O_2 flow rate of 5 to 10 L/min, which creates CPAP of 5 to 10 cm H_2O, is sufficient for improving oxygenation. One advantage of this system is that the elimination of CO_2 is proportional to the flow rate of the gas in the CPAP system. A very high O_2 flow rate delivered at or below the carina may improve gas exchange without any tidal exchange, which is known as "continuous high-flow apneic ventilation."

STRATEGIES TO IMPROVE OXYGENATION DURING SINGLE-LUNG VENTILATION

The strategies to maintain oxygenation are individualized to account for patient factors and surgical considerations. Although the application of CPAP during video thoracoscopy is contraindicated, its use for an open thoracotomy is better tolerated. The first step to improve arterial oxygenation is to confirm proper double-lumen tube placement. If oxygenation is still inadequate, the strategies of applying CPAP to the dependent lung and PEEP to the dependent lung can be sequentially and additively applied. If arterial oxygenation remains poor, the patient's hemodynamic status should be assessed. A decrease in cardiac output, leading to a decrease in mixed venous oxygen saturation (Svo_2), can magnify the effect of shunt on arterial oxygenation.

If hypoxemia still persists after differential CPAP/PEEP, the nondependent lung may be intermittently ventilated with positive pressure and 100% O_2. Intermittent reinflation of the collapsed lung with O_2 is

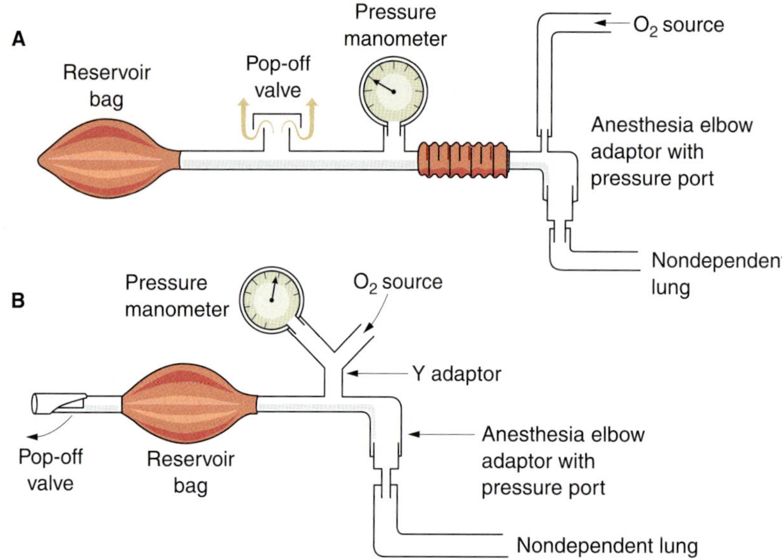

FIGURE 54-23. **A.** and **B.** Schematic diagram showing 2 nondependent lung continuous positive airway pressure (CPAP) systems without reservoir bags. Both contain an oxygen source and a pressure relief valve, but **A** has a pressure manometer to measure the CPAP, whereas **B** does not. [From Benumof JL. Conventional and differential lung management of one-lung ventilation. In: Benumof JL, ed. *Anesthesia for Thoracic Surgery*. Philadelphia, PA: WB Saunders; 1995.]

beneficial but its beneficial value was found to decline with repeated inflations.[117] Finally, most of the V/Q mismatch and arterial hypoxemia can be eliminated by decreasing blood flow to the nondependent lung by temporarily ligating its pulmonary artery (**Fig. 54-24**). Caution should be taken as this further increases right ventricular afterload and may cause acute cardiac decompensation.

SELECTIVE NONDEPENDENT-LUNG HIGH-FREQUENCY VENTILATION

Any method that results in splitting the alveoli and air spaces of the nondependent lung will lead to an improvement in arterial oxygenation and a decrease in the transpulmonary shunt. High-frequency

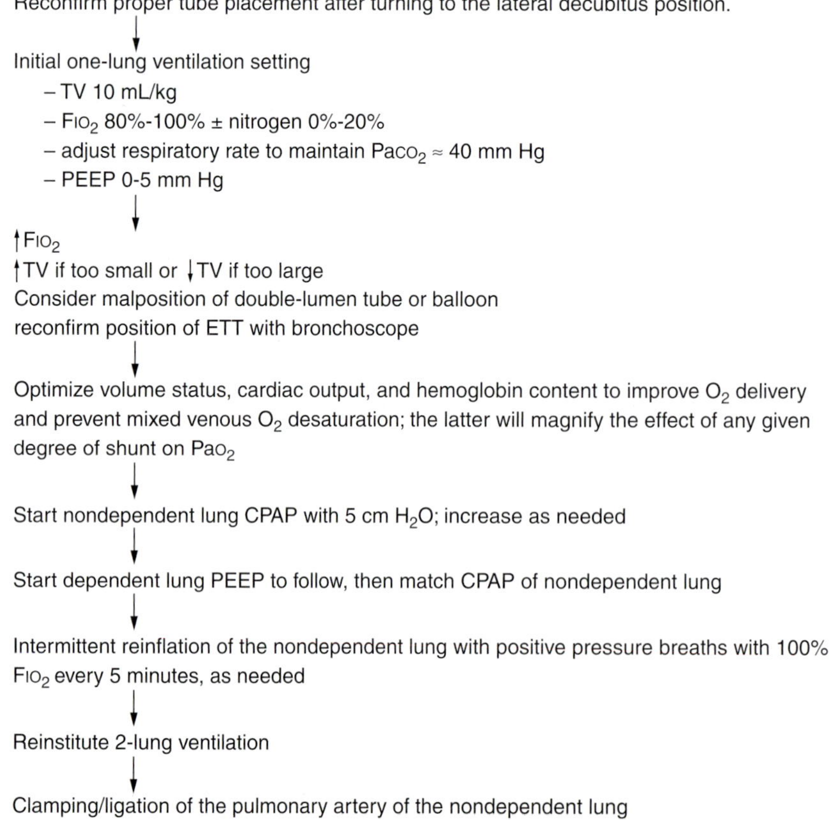

FIGURE 54-24. Algorithm for managing 1-lung ventilation and improving oxygenation.

ventilation of the nondependent lung has been studied in combination with conventional positive-pressure ventilation of the dependent lung. Using this combination, Pao_2 was much better than with intermittent positive-pressure ventilation of the dependent lung with total collapse of the nondependent lung.[118] In most patients, the same increase in arterial oxygenation can be achieved using selective nondependent lung CPAP, which requires much simpler equipment compared with high-frequency ventilation apparatus. In some situations, high-frequency ventilation may be more advantageous:

If the nondependent lung has a major bronchopleural fistula, high-frequency ventilation to the nondependent lung using low airway pressures helps to decrease the air leak and improve oxygenation and ventilation.[119]

During operation on the major conducting airways, high-frequency ventilation permits the use of small ventilation catheters that pass through the operating field.[119-122]

Unilateral high-frequency jet ventilation with contralateral intermittent positive-pressure ventilation has been used in the anesthetic treatment of patients with severely compromised respiratory reserve. The technique provided satisfactory anesthesia, good operating conditions, and adequate gas exchange.[123]

ANESTHETIC TECHNIQUES

Although thoracic surgery can be performed solely using a regional block, most thoracotomies are performed during general anesthesia with controlled ventilation. Epidural or other regional anesthetic techniques often are used to decrease the intraoperative anesthetic requirement to facilitate emergence and extubation and for postoperative pain control.[124] Recent evidence suggests that the use of epidural or paravertebral anesthesia for perioperative analgesia improves short-term outcomes up to several months.[125]

GENERAL ANESTHESIA

The choice of induction agent and dosage is influenced by the patient's medical condition. In patients in whom extensive airway instrumentation or manipulation precedes thoracotomy, an antisialogogue, glycopyrrolate, can reduce secretions. Opioids supplement the inhalational anesthetic, although the dosage of any narcotic should be reduced in patients who will receive epidural opioids. The incidence of postoperative respiratory depression is related to the total dosage of narcotics administered systematically and epidurally. After the induction of general anesthesia, controlled manual ventilation with mask is started using an inhalation anesthetic. N_2O is only occasionally used during the induction phase and during prepping, draping, and positioning of the patient. Because large intrapulmonary shunts are anticipated with initiation of 1-lung ventilation, it is prudent to increase the inspired concentration of oxygen. N_2O should be avoided in patients who have marginal preoperative oxygenation or in those with large bullae and emphysematous lungs to avoid expansion of bullae by N_2O.

After the induction of anesthesia, the trachea is intubated with a single-lumen or double-lumen tube as indicated by the surgical procedure. Position of the endotracheal tube is confirmed by careful auscultation, capnography, and, if indicated, by fiberoptic bronchoscopy.

Volatile, halogenated anesthetic drugs have several desirable properties for use during thoracic procedures. They decrease airway irritability and obtund airway reflexes in patients who usually have reactive airways, and they maintain adequate anesthesia while allowing increased inspired oxygen concentrations. They can be eliminated rapidly, allowing tracheal extubation in the operating room with less concern for postoperative respiratory depression. Although volatile anesthetics allow high inspired O_2 concentrations, at minimum alveolar concentration (MAC) values greater than 1 they may reduce Pao_2 by increasing the shunt related to partial inhibition of HPV.[81,82,126] The inhibition of HPV by inhaled anesthetics may exhibit substantial variability.

Patients with mediastinal and airway tumors may be at risk for airway obstruction during induction of anesthesia. In such patients, the anesthetic plan and emergency treatment strategies should be discussed with the surgeon preoperatively. If emergent tracheostomy, rigid bronchoscopy, or extracorpeal oxygenation are anticipated, the entire operating team should be prepared to act smoothly and efficiently. Patients at increased risk of airway obstruction may require awake fiberoptic intubation or spontaneous ventilation to avoid airway obstruction. Special management concerns for mediastinal tumors are discussed later.

REGIONAL ANESTHESIA

Epidural anesthesia, paravertebral block, intercostal nerve blocks, or field blocks have been occasionally used as the sole anesthetic for various thoracic procedures, including thoracotomy. Thoracic epidural blockade in awake, sedated patients has been used successfully for open thoracotomies or thoracoscopies.[127,128] Crawford et al described 677 patients with tuberculosis in whom epidural anesthesia was used for thoracotomy.[129] Others successfully used this technique. The most surprising results were the absence of paradoxical respiration and dyspnea. The breathing pattern and speech appeared normal even when an upper lobe bronchus was transsected and held open. Several factors may have contributed to the success of this unorthodox technique: (1) the patients were extremely cooperative and had a good rapport with the anesthesiologist; (2) analgesia was complete, and patients were comfortable; (3) the use of premedication and sedation avoided the pitfalls of oversedation and excitability; (4) supplemental O_2 was administered by positive pressure mask if the patient reported any shortness of breath; and (5) operation was remarkably gentle and swift. It is doubtful that all of the above conditions could be fulfilled during an anatomic resection in the routine patient by the average surgeon.

COMBINED EPIDURAL BLOCKADE AND GENERAL ANESTHESIA

It is unlikely that the routine patient would tolerate the sole use of regional anesthesia, especially during an open thoracotomy. The techniques of general and epidural anesthesia often are combined to achieve the benefits of each. The relative contribution of each technique to a combined anesthetic can vary. The epidural blockade may either be used for postoperative analgesia or as the major anesthetic, with light general anesthesia used for amnesia and sedation. Epidural anesthesia has the advantages of reduction in afterload,[130] improved pulmonary function, decreased incidence of venous thromboembolism,[131,132] and suppression of the stress response.[81,133] Potential disadvantages include the time required to establish the block, increased fluid requirements and relative decrease in blood pressure associated with sympathectomy, and the potential for technical complications such as epidural hematoma. A prospective, randomized, controlled clinical study examined the effect of epidural anesthesia and postoperative analgesia on postoperative morbidity rate in high-risk surgical patients.[134] When compared with control patients, those who received epidural anesthesia and analgesia had fewer overall complications and fewer cardiovascular or major infectious complications, lower urinary cortisol secretion (a marker of the stress response), and lower hospital costs.[134]

Vital capacity and lung compliance decrease after general anesthesia and neuromuscular blockade in patients undergoing thoracotomy. Epidural analgesia with light general anesthesia results in less decrease in static compliance and fewer alterations in postoperative pulmonary function.[135] The perioperative use of epidural anesthesia is also associated with fewer major postoperative infections. This may result from (1) decreased duration of endotracheal intubation and mechanical ventilation, which diminishes many of the defense mechanisms against infection[136,137]; (2) decreased duration of ICU stay postoperatively and reduced risks of nosocomial infection; and (3) suppression of the endocrine stress response to operation, which has an inhibitory effect on the immune system.[138] Immune competence is less disturbed postoperatively when epidural anesthesia is used compared with other anesthetic and analgesic techniques.[139,140]

Patients who received epidural anesthesia had fewer cardiovascular complications, including congestive heart failure.[134] A comparison of epidural analgesia with general anesthesia noted a decrease in the size of myocardial infarctions, probably related to improved regional subendocardial perfusion.[130] Possible mechanisms include afferent sensory blockade, decreased adrenergic tone, and coronary and systemic vasodilation with a reduction in cardiac preload and afterload.[141-143]

An epidural catheter can be inserted in the midthoracic (T4-T9) or low thoracic-lumbar (T9-L2) regions. To date, no studies have demonstrated overwhelming superiority of 1 approach. In the experience of the authors, the midthoracic level, about T7, provides excellent conditions for thoracic and thoracoabdominal procedures. The low thoracic region is suitable for thoracoabdominal procedures, such as gastrectomy. Use of a lumbar epidural blockade in patients undergoing thoracic surgery requires a greater dosage of local anesthetics or narcotics to provide analgesia in the thoracic regions and is not routinely recommended. Because of the multiple advantages conferred by thoracic epidural analgesia, the anesthetic plan for open thoracotomy should always include placement of a thoracic epidural catheter unless an absolute contraindication is present.

Paravertebral block with the placement of a catheter for continuous analgesia has been found to provide pain control as good as epidural analgesia with less hypotension and nausea.[144-147] These catheters can be placed with the aid of ultrasound. They are usually dosed with local anesthetic only as opioid does not improve analgesia. They may be safer to place in patients continued on platelet inhibiting drugs (Plavex) as hematoma formation will not directly impinge on the spinal cord. An alternative is to have the surgeon place these catheters from within the chest and externalize the catheter.

THORACOSCOPY VERSUS THORACOTOMY

Evolution of surgical technique and technical advances in electronics and instrumentation have led to renewed interest in thoracoscopy. In a health care environment that values cost and patient outcome, video-assisted thoracoscopy (VAT) has advantages beyond open thoracotomy, including decreased postoperative pain, pulmonary impairment, and hospital stay. Thoracoscopy permits the visualization of the pulmonary cavity through several small portals. These portals provide access for the video camera and allow manipulation of thoracic structures and use of surgical instruments such as staplers, dissectors, coagulators, and lasers. Although initially used for only minor surgical procedures, the application of VATs has expanded considerably for both diagnostic and therapeutic procedures (**Box 54-6**). If access is inadequate or if bleeding complications occur, VATs are easily converted to a limited open thoracotomy.

BOX 54-6

Applications of Video-Assisted Thoracoscopy

- Pulmonary
  - Lung biopsy
  - Resection mass
  - Bleb resection
  - Volume reduction pneumoplasty
- Pleura
  - Diagnostic evaluation
  - Pleurodesis
  - Decortication
- Pericardium
  - Pericardial drainage
  - Pericardectomy
- Cardiac
  - Automatic implantable cardiovertor/defibrillator placement
  - Cryoablation, radiofrequency ablation for treatment of atrial fibrillation
  - Cardiac pacemaker placement
- Mediastinum
  - Lymph node biopsy
  - Biopsy and resection of mediastinal mass
  - Vagotomy
- Esophageal surgery
  - Thoracic duct ligation
- Miscellaneous
  - Sympathectomy
  - Microdiscectomy

Anesthetic treatment for patients undergoing thoracoscopy is similar to that for open thoracotomy (**Table 54-7**). Although limited thoracoscopy has been performed in spontaneously breathing, sedated patients, this procedure usually is performed during general anesthesia with placement of a double-lumen endotracheal tube for lung separation. Good lung isolation is even more critical than in an open procedure because the surgeon cannot "pack the lung away." Many patients have obstructive lung disease that impedes passive deflation of the nonventilated lung. To foster deflation, the nondependent lung should be carefully suctioned of secretions that may cause air trapping, then denitrogenated by ventilating with 100% oxygen, with single-lung ventilation initiated before skin incision. The tidal volume delivered to the ventilated dependent lung should be decreased to prevent upward shift of the mediastinum during single-lung ventilation. If deflation is inadequate, CO_2 can be insufflated into the nondependent thoracic cavity. Hypercarbia and hypotension may develop if excessive gas inflation causes mediastinal shift and reduction in venous return to the heart. The use of VAT over open thoracotomy has several advantages. Analgesic requirements and length of hospital stay are less than those for open thoracotomy.[148-152] Adequate postoperative analgesia can be obtained with a combination of parenteral opiates, nonsteroidal anti-inflammatory drugs (NSAIDs), or paravertebral, epidural, or intercostal nerve blocks. We will typically place an epidural or paravertebral catheter for patients with respiratory compromise to facilitate postoperative pulmonary toilet.

ANESTHESIA FOR PATIENTS UNDERGOING BRONCHOSCOPY

BACKGROUND

Although introduced in the 1890s, it remained for Chevalier Jackson to perfect the therapeutic application of rigid bronchoscopy for retrieval of foreign bodies and diagnostic use in patients with neoplastic and inflammatory disease. The rigid bronchoscope is a hollow, metal tube with a blunted and beveled distal tip that allows insertion into the airway with minimal trauma. The proximal end is adapted for observation of the airway, maintenance of gas exchange, and introduction of surgical instruments. The proximal side arm is adapted for administration of oxygen or other gases, and also enables mechanical ventilation during bronchoscopy. Within the wall of the bronchoscope, there is a series of channels for the illumination of the distal field and for suctioning secretions and blood. The large size of the rigid bronchoscope permits insertion of sponges, snares, knives, scissors, electrodes, and other special devices. The most common uses of a rigid bronchoscope are for retrieval of large foreign bodies, evaluation and debulking of bronchial tumors, access to bleeding sites, and overall evaluation of the airways.

TABLE 54-7 Anesthetic Guidelines for Video-Assisted Thoracoscopic Surgery and Thoracotomy

	Video-Assisted Thoracoscopic Surgery	Thoracotomy
Indication	Diagnostic, therapeutic (see Box 54-6)	Same[a]
Monitors	Standard monitors Optional (arterial, pulmonary artery catheter, Foley catheter)	Same[a]
Anesthesia	General anesthesia Optional (combined regional/general anesthesia)	Same[a]
Additional equipment	Fiberoptic bronchoscope Arm board Pillows Bean bag or chest roll	Same[a]
Ventilation	Double-lumen endotracheal tube Bronchial blockers	
Position	Later decubitus position (check and pad pressure points)	Same[a]
Incision	Several portals for the introduction of equipment	Lateral thoracotomy Anterior thoracotomy Posterior thoracotomy Muscle-sparing incision
Unique considerations	Single-lung ventilation	Same[a]
Intraoperative complications	Hypoxia Hypercapnia Bleeding	Same[a]
Estimated blood loss	<300 mL	Variable
Postoperative analgesia	Parenteral opiates Nonsteroidal anti-inflammatory drugs Intrapleural catheter, intercostal nerve block	Epidural > parenteral opiates NSAIDs
Postoperative morbidity	Hypoxia (atelectasis, pneumothorax, pleural effusion) Bleeding	Same[a]
Postoperative case	Adequate analgesia Supplemental O_2 Chest radiography May require close follow-up evaluation overnight	Same[a]

[a]Same as video-assisted thoracoscopic surgery.

The introduction of the fiberoptic bronchoscope has had a dramatic impact by supplanting the use of the rigid instrument in many patients. The flexible fiberoptic bronchoscope initially contained clusters of glass fibers that illuminate the airway and transmit the visual image. Now they have an LED for light source and a photosensitive chip for image capture. Several hollow ports or channels are incorporated for suctioning, the instillation of medications or lavage fluid, and the introduction of accessory instruments. Flexion of the distal tip by cables allows the instrument to be directed to all segments of the tracheobronchial tree. Indications for fiberoptic bronchoscopy are listed in **Box 54-7**. Bronchoscopy often is only the first of several diagnostic or therapeutic procedures. After bronchoscopy, mediastinoscopy or thoracoscopy may be performed to further evaluate the presence of disease or for its management.

FLEXIBLE FIBEROPTIC BRONCHOSCOPY

Anesthetic Management Flexible fiberoptic bronchoscopy can be performed during local anesthesia in sedated, spontaneously breathing patients or during general anesthesia with or without placement of an endotracheal tube (**Table 54-8**).

Awake fiberoptic bronchoscopy is performed after administration of sedation, an antisialagogue, and adequate topical local anesthesia. If the correct balance of these components is not achieved, serious trauma can result from coughing and movement of the uncomfortable patient. Techniques of anesthetizing the airway include

- Topical application of local anesthetic to the nose, mouth, or oral pharynx
- Internal or percutaneous block of the superior laryngeal nerve
- Glossopharyngeal nerve block

BOX 54-7

Indications for Fiberoptic Bronchoscopy

Diagnostic indications
- Staging and characterization of pulmonary disease
- Evaluation of the site and etiology of pulmonary symptoms

Therapeutic indications
- Tracheal intubation
- Positioning of the double-lumen endotracheal tube
- Removal of secretions and bronchial toilet
- Laser of tumors

TABLE 54-8 Anesthetic Guidelines for Fiberoptic Bronchoscopy and Rigid Bronchoscopy

	Fiberoptic Bronchoscopy		Rigid Bronchoscopy
Indications	Diagnostic, biopsy, lavage, confirm placement of endotracheal tube		Therapeutic, laser, retrieval or foreign body, pulmonary toilet
Monitors	Standard monitors		Same[a]
Anesthesia	General anesthesia, sedation with block		General anesthesia
Additional equipment			Shoulder roll
Airway	Awake spontaneous ventilation, single-lumen endotracheal tube (≥8 mm)		Apneic ventilation Intermittent positive pressure ventilation Jet ventilation
Position	Semirecumbent (awake patients)		Cervical extension
Unique considerations	Local and nerve block, antisialagogue		Lidocaine intravenously or intratracheal, muscle relaxation, antisialagogue
Intraoperative complications	Bronchospasm Bleeding Pneumomediastinum Pneumothorax Subcutaneous emphysema Barotrauma Hypoxia Hypercapnia	Vasovagal (bradycardia) Arrhythmias Fever (bacteremia)	Same[a] Dental trauma
Analgesia	Minimal pain (parental opiates)		
Postoperative morbidity	Atelectasis Bleeding and hemoptysis Bronchospasm Fever		Same[a]
Postoperative care	Chest radiography Humidified O_2 No eating or drinking until protective airway reflexes have returned		Same[a]

[a]Same as fiberoptic bronchoscopy.

- Recurrent laryngeal nerve block either by spraying of the tracheal bronchial mucosa from inside with local anesthetic or percutaneous transcricothyroid membrane injection
- Inhalation of nebulized local anesthetic to the mucous membrane of the mouth, pharynx, larynx, trachea, and bronchi

The use of sedation and an antisialagogue improves bronchoscopic conditions. An anticholinergic, such as glycopyrrolate, is preferred because of the lack of central nervous system (CNS) side effects. A benzodiazepine is useful for anxiolysis and increasing the threshold for CNS toxicity to local anesthetics. Intravenous infusions of dexmedetomidine, remifentanyl, or propofol have also been successfully used to provide an adequate level of sedation. Sedation should be used with caution, especially in elderly debilitated patients or in those with serious underlying respiratory compromise. Cardiac and respiratory function should be monitored during the procedure by a person who is not responsible for the endoscopy. Because capnography often is unreliable during bronchoscopy, pulse oximetry is the most important monitor to assess the adequacy of oxygenation. After the procedure, the patient should be placed in a monitored environment initially to evaluate for complications from the procedure or the sedation.

Ventilation Management When performed during general anesthesia, fiberoptic bronchoscopy usually is accomplished through an endotracheal tube. The resulting marked reduction in the effective functional internal diameter of the endotracheal tube available for ventilation is associated with increased airway resistance and can result in distal air trapping. To reduce complications, the anesthesiologist should avoid spontaneous ventilation, eliminate PEEP from the circuit, ventilate with a prolonged expiratory phase (inspiratory/expiratory [I/E] ratio of 1:3), and use the largest endotracheal tube possible. Suppression of airway reflexes to prevent laryngospasm and bronchospasm can be accomplished by the use of inhaled anesthetic agents and by the administration of lidocaine. A helium-O_2 mixture will decrease airway resistance, but is usually not necessary.

RIGID BRONCHOSCOPY

Anesthetic Management Maintenance of anesthesia can be achieved with mixtures of intravenous sedatives and narcotics or in combination with potent inhalational anesthetics. Use of inhaled anesthetics has the obvious disadvantage of exposing personnel to the escaping anesthetic vapors. In the authors' experience, an infusion of remifentanyl and propofol provides very acceptable anesthetic conditions characterized by a quick emergence and negligible residual sedation. Topical anesthesia with lidocaine can be used to suppress cough reflexes and prevent bronchospasm. Patients undergoing rigid bronchoscopy should be paralyzed to prevent sudden movement or cough, which can result in major morbidity.

Ventilation Management Intermittent positive pressure ventilation can be delivered during rigid bronchoscopy by connecting the standard anesthesia circuit to the ventilating side-port of the rigid bronchoscope (**Fig. 54-25**). This ventilating technique requires no special equipment,

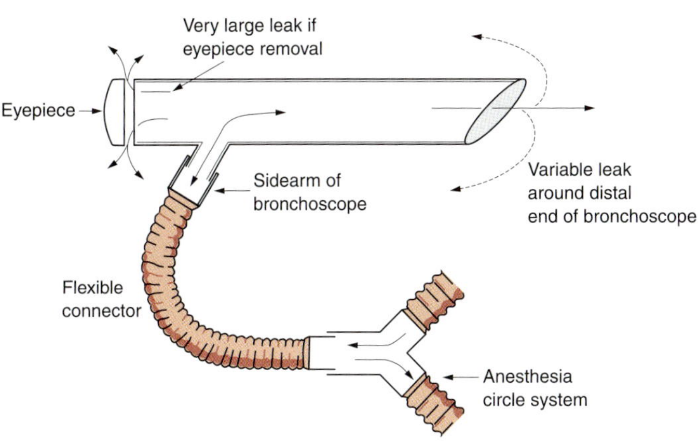

FIGURE 54-25. Schematic diagram showing a rigid ventilating bronchoscope system, which consists of the anesthesia circle system attached to a flexible connector that is attached to the sidearm of the bronchoscope. With the proximal eyepiece in place, most of the inspired gas goes into the patient. Because the bronchoscope cannot fully fill the area of the trachea, there is a variable leak around the distal end of the bronchoscope. Exhaled gases are through the anesthesia circle system. When the eyepiece is removed, there is a very large leak out the proximal end of the bronchoscope. [Modified from Benumof JL. Anesthesia for special elective diagnostic procedures. In: Benumof JL, ed. *Anesthesia for Thoracic Surgery*. Philadelphia, PA: WB Saunders; 1995.]

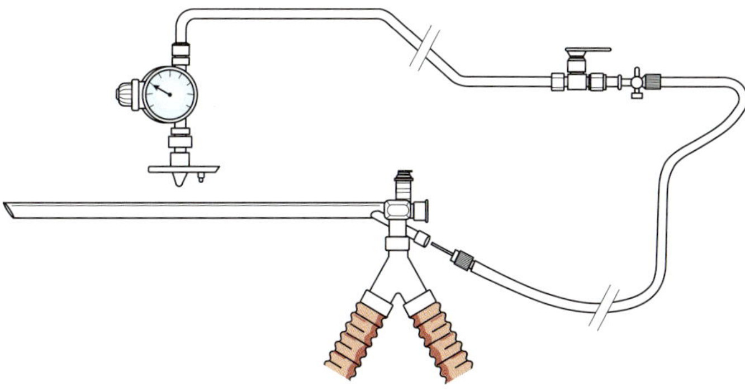

FIGURE 54-26. Components needed for jet ventilation through the bronchoscope (Sanders injector). Wall connector for oxygen supply, reducing valve and pressure gauge, high-pressure tubing, toggle switch, needle injector jet.

allows for accurate measurement of the FIO_2 and inhaled anesthetic concentration, and provides adequate oxygenation in most patients. The ventilating gases may leak through the space between the bronchoscope and the tracheal wall. To compensate for the leak, gas flows should be increased, and the posterior pharynx and larynx can be packed with gauze. Because ventilation is only possible when the eyepiece is in place, the cumulative effect of multiple periods of apnea may result in hypercapnia and cardiac dysrhythmias.

Jet Ventilation The use of jet ventilation has been advocated for prolonged rigid bronchoscopy. The Venturi (jet) ventilation technique allows the surgeon an unhurried, undisturbed period of viewing without need for an eyepiece. A potential disadvantage is that jet ventilation can result in spillage of blood and other debris into the tracheobronchial tree.

An intermittent high-velocity jet of oxygen entrains air into the bronchoscope, resulting in expansion of the lungs. If the lungs are noncompliant or if the bronchoscope is small in relation to the trachea, large amounts of the tidal volume will escape between the bronchoscope and tracheal wall, resulting in poor alveolar ventilation. Careful observation of the patient's chest movement is necessary to ensure adequate tidal volumes. The adequacy of ventilation, a function of total thoracic compliance, can be monitored by obtaining an arterial blood sample, by transcutaneous CO_2 monitoring, or by intermittent capnography. It is difficult to know the inspired concentration of oxygen because of the variable entrainment of room air, but the adequacy of oxygenation can be monitored by pulse oximetry or arterial blood gas sampling.

The intraluminal pressure is a function of the driving pressure from the in-line reducing valve, size and length of the needle jet, and design of the bronchoscope. In addition, a decrease in the effective intraluminal diameter by the introduction of suction catheters or biopsy forceps can prevent the escape of gas introduced by the jet and results in a dramatic increase in intratracheal pressure. If the instruments are tight fitting, the driving pressure should be decreased to prevent barotrauma.

The apparatus described by Sanders used a high-pressure oxygen source of 50 psi, which was delivered through a 16- or 18-gauge needle located within the rigid bronchoscope (**Fig. 54-26**). The original jet ventilation system has been improved by connecting the side arm to the anesthesia circuit, thereby entraining an oxygen anesthetic gas mixture. Increasing the size of the jet port (the Carden side arm) results in increased inflation pressure and increased FIO_2 at the distal tip of the bronchoscope.[153] Jet ventilation at low frequencies can provide for adequate oxygenation and ventilation. Commercial high-frequency jet ventilators (HFJV) have been used with the rigid bronchoscope. Rates of 150 to 300 breaths/min result in ventilation and oxygenation comparable with intermittent low-frequency jet ventilation,[154] but rates greater than 300 breaths/min result in a decrease in oxygenation and an increase in $PaCO_2$. The major advantage of HFJV over low-frequency jet ventilation is that there is less movement of the tracheobronchial tree, providing better surgical conditions for such procedures as laser therapy.

Apneic Oxygenation In the absence of ventilation, adequate oxygenation can be maintained for a prolonged period at the expense of increasing $PaCO_2$. Initially, the patient is hyperventilated with 100% inspired oxygen until relative hypocapnia and complete denitrogenation is achieved. A period of hyperventilation, to a $PaCO_2$ of approximately 30 mm Hg, will increase the period of apnea that can be tolerated before respiratory acidosis ensues. A small catheter is placed above the carina and insufflated with O_2 at 10 to 15 L/min. The adequacy of oxygen reserve and generation of CO_2 are functions of pulmonary mechanics and body size.

COMPLICATIONS

Aside from the inherent risks of local and general anesthetics, bronchoscopy of the airway may be associated with perioperative morbidity. Patients may exhibit decreases in FEV_1, FVC, peak expiratory flow rate, and peak inspiratory flow rate. Additional factors that may contribute to decreased lung function or bronchospasm include airway mucosal edema and mechanical activation of irritated airway reflexes.[155] These responses may in part be mediated by the vagus nerve because preoperative administration of an anticholinergic agent, such as glycopyrrolate or atropine, has been shown to prevent or attenuate them.

Rigid bronchoscopy is associated with more trauma than flexible fiberoptic bronchoscopy. Positioning of the patient and placement of the rigid bronchoscope can result in dental trauma or laceration of the mucosa of the larynx, trachea, or bronchi. The trauma has been associated with pneumomediastinum, pneumothorax, and perforation of the esophagus. The cervical hyperextension that is required for placement of the rigid bronchoscope can cause injury to the cervical spine, vasovagal reaction, and cerebral ischemia by occlusion of vertebral arteries.

Hypoxia and hypercarbia are common complications during rigid bronchoscopy.[108,156,157] Inadequate ventilation during rigid bronchoscopy can result from large air leaks along the space between the bronchoscope and the tracheal wall or from periods of apnea. There can be a serious loss of lung volume associated with plugging and atelectasis, which may be minimized by pulmonary toilet and ventilation with large tidal volumes. At the end of a procedure during general anesthesia, a single-lumen endotracheal tube should be placed, and the lung should be suctioned and ventilated with large tidal volumes to relieve atelectatic alveoli.

Transient cardiac dysrhythmias are common in patients undergoing bronchoscopy.[158,159] Their causes include hypoxia, intense stimulation, hypoventilation with hypercapnia, inadequate depth of anesthesia, vasovagal reaction, β_2-adrenergic agonists, and bronchodilators.

POSTOPERATIVE CONCERNS

Barotrauma with resultant interstitial emphysema, pneumomediastinum, and pneumothorax can occur after fiberoptic and rigid bronchoscopy. Postoperatively, patients may manifest dyspnea or evidence of airway obstruction. Subglottic and mucosal airway edema can result from mechanical irritation.[160,161] In addition, bleeding into the airway can result in reactive bronchospasm. Physical examination should confirm the absence of wheezing or stridor and the presence of bilateral breath sounds. A chest radiograph should be obtained to look for signs of pulmonary emphysema, mediastinal emphysema, or pneumothorax. Initial strategies for management include inhalation of cool moisturized oxygen and use of a bronchodilator. Further specific therapies may entail placement of chest tubes, administration of diuretics, pulmonary toilet, or repeat bronchoscopy.

ANESTHESIA FOR PATIENTS UNDERGOING BRONCHOALVEOLAR LAVAGE

Bronchopulmonary lavage is indicated for management of alveolar proteinosis.[162-168] The long-term improvements in arterial oxygenation, exercise tolerance, and level of activity vary from patient to patient. Some patients require annual or semiannual lavage, whereas others remain in remission for years.[169] The pathophysiology of the disease is characterized by the abnormal bilateral accumulation of alveolar surfactant.[169,170] Its accumulation is attributed to a failure of clearance mechanisms rather than increased formation. Most patients are diagnosed between the ages of 20 and 50 years and have symptoms of cough, fever, and chest pain. Pulmonary function tests and chest radiographs are abnormal, but definitive diagnosis requires lung biopsy.

INTRAOPERATIVE MANAGEMENT

Unilateral lung lavage is performed by irrigation of the tracheobronchial tree with chest physiotherapy during general anesthesia (**Table 54-9**). The preoperative assessment should include ventilation-perfusion scans to characterize the distribution of impairment. Unilateral lung lavage requires placement of a double-lumen endotracheal tube to prevent spillage to the contralateral lung. After induction of general anesthesia, the trachea is intubated with the largest left-sided double-lumen endotracheal tube that can be positioned properly. Correct tube position is essential; it should be confirmed with a fiberoptic bronchoscope. To prevent leakage of lavage fluid into the contralateral lung, it has been suggested that the bronchial cuff be inflated to functionally separate the lungs at 50 cm/water. The patient should be ventilated with 100% oxygen to minimize the risk of hypoxemia and eliminate nitrogen from the lung. Failure to adequately denitrogenate before lavage may leave residual pockets of intra-alveolar nitrogen and thus limit the effectiveness of the procedure.

The positioning of the patient is somewhat controversial. Lavage of the nondependent lung in the lateral decubitus position has the advantage of improving oxygenation by decreasing blood flow to the nonventilated lung. However, this arrangement also increases the risk of displacement of the bronchial cuff and spillage from the nondependent to the dependent lung. Lavage of the dependent lung decreases the possibility of spillage, but it may be associated with hypoxia resulting from shunt flow. The supine position balances the risk of aspiration against the risk of hypoxia.

TABLE 54-9 Anesthetic Guidelines for Bronchial Alveolar Lavage

Indication	Diagnostic Therapeutic (alveolar proteinosis, cystic fibrosis)
Monitors	Standard monitoring, optional (arterial catheter)
Anesthesia	General anesthesia (allows for sequential lavages on both sides) Awake, sedated (lavage by bronchoscopy limited to lobe)
Ventilation	Left double-lumen endotracheal tube
Position	Lateral decubitus Supine
Unique considerations	Single-lung ventilation To prevent spillage to the opposite lung, endobronchial balloon should be inflated to functionally separate lungs (~50 cm H_2O) (1) Drain 700-1000 mL warm saline into lung (2) Manual chest percussion (3) Drainage of fluid in Trendelenburg position (4) Repeat until turbidity clears (5) Repeat for contralateral lung (6) Maintain accurate account of infusion and drainage volumes (7) After lavage is completed, suction both lungs thoroughly, ventilate, and positive end-expiratory pressure
Intraoperative complications	Spillage of lavage fluid to contralateral lung Hypoxia Decrease pulmonary compliance Pneumothorax, hydropneumothorax Pulmonary edema
Analgesia	None required
Postoperative care	Supplemental O_2 Chest radiography

The choice of which lung to lavage first is based on the ventilation and perfusion studies; the lung with the least perfusion is chosen to be lavaged first. The procedure is performed by instilling warm, isotonic saline by gravity from a height of 30 cm. The adult lung will accept 700 to 1000 mL of lavage fluid. Vigorous manual chest percussion is applied to the hemithorax throughout the lavage. Then the lavage fluid is drained passively into a collecting system. The lavage procedure is repeated until the drainage decreases in turbidity to near clarity so that it is possible to read fine print through a 0.25-in-diameter column of fluid. Typically, 12 to 30 L of saline are required. We warm the fluid to prevent cooling the patient. Accurate records of fluid administration and drainage are kept. After the effluent lavage fluid clears, the procedure is terminated, the lavaged lung is thoroughly suctioned, and ventilation is reestablished. Because the lavaged lung has decreased compliance, it is ventilated with a large tidal volume (15-20 mL/kg) to reexpand the alveoli. To improve compliance during the immediate postprocedure period, the patient should be positioned to enhance drainage, and secretions should be suctioned from the airway.

During the lavage procedure, most patients remain hemodynamically stable, although this procedure may increase right heart strain and decrease left ventricular filling and systemic blood pressure.[171] Arterial oxygen saturation increases during lung filling and decreases with drainage. The increase in intra-alveolar pressure, resulting from fluid administration, causes an increase in pulmonary vascular resistance, thereby diverting blood flow to the ventilated side and decreasing the venous admixture. When the lavage fluid is drained, the pulmonary vascular resistance decreases, and the venous admixture increases.

Spillage of lavage fluid into the untreated lung is a serious complication. Leakage is detected by the appearance of bubbles in the lavage fluid, rales or rhonchi in the ventilated lung, discrepancy between the drained lavage fluid volumes, and arterial desaturation. If spillage is suspected, lavage should be stopped, the lung drained, and position of the double-lumen endotracheal tube confirmed. Massive spillage produces acute decreases in lung compliance and severe arterial desaturation. An unusual but serious complication of lung lavage is hydropneumothorax that is characterized by increased peak airway pressures, decreased oxygen saturation 20 minutes after an uneventful lung lavage, and a chest radiograph revealing mediastinal shift and a left pneumothorax. It was hypothesized that lung lavage decreased lung compliance by washing out surfactants, making it more susceptible to barotrauma. A chest radiograph should be obtained routinely within the first hour after lavage and compared with prelavage examination.[172]

ANESTHESIA FOR PATIENTS WITH BRONCHOPLEURAL FISTULA

ETIOLOGY

The possibility of a bronchopleural fistula should be considered after pneumonectomy, lobectomy, bullectomy, volume reduction surgery, or high-speed deceleration injury. The symptoms and findings of a clinically significant bronchopleural fistula include dyspnea, subcutaneous emphysema, contralateral deviation of the trachea, expectoration of purulent material, a persistent air leak, and purulent drainage from the chest tube. Diagnosis is confirmed by bronchoscopy. Predisposing factors in patients developing air leaks after lung resection include cancer, malnourishment, debilitation, poor general condition, trauma, barotrauma, lung abscesses, immunosuppression, steroid therapy, diabetes, preoperative or postoperative radiation therapy, and pulmonary resection for tuberculosis. A continued air leak can lead to infection in the pleural space and dehiscence of the bronchial stump.[173]

THERAPEUTIC MANAGEMENT

When bronchopleural fistula occurs early after resection, prompt resuturing of the bronchial stump may correct it. If the fistula develops later after operation it may be secondary to infection, and adequate drainage and reduction of the pleural space constitute initial therapy. Many small fistulas will close spontaneously using conservative therapy consisting of nutritional support, pulmonary toilet, antibiotics for infection, and spontaneous ventilation. If the lung expands to fill the thoracic cavity, the leak usually can be controlled with passive chest tube drainage. A persistent space indicates a leak from a larger bronchus, usually requiring surgical treatment.[173] Sepsis should be controlled with antibiotics and adequate chest drainage.

Surgical options include (1) decortication if the lung is entrapped by a thick purulent layer; (2) revision of a long bronchial stump; (3) closure of the bronchopleural fistula with a pedicled muscle flap, usually in the form of an intercostal or serratus flap[174,175]; (4) thoracoplasty to obliterate the pleural space, usually combined with a pedicled muscle flap to cover the bronchial stump; (5) bronchoscopic application of fibrin glue to seal the communication; and (6) temporary deployment of a silastic stent.

VENTILATION

Anesthesiologists care for patients with bronchopleural fistula either in the ICU when respiratory failure and sepsis require ventilator management or in the operating room. Goals include maintenance of adequate ventilation and oxygenation and protection of the contralateral lung from spillage of purulent material.

Application of positive pressure by a mask or a mechanical ventilator may lead to an apparent inadequate ventilation because the tidal volume is lost through the fistula. Several methods have been developed to improve the ventilation of patients with bronchopleural fistula and decrease the risk of pneumothorax. Chest tubes with unidirectional valves have been used to prevent air leak during spontaneous inspiration. During positive pressure ventilation, low inflation pressures should be used, and spontaneous ventilation with pressure support should be encouraged to decrease the air leak and to promote closure of the bronchopleural fistula. High-frequency ventilation has also been used to manage bronchopleural fistula but with varying results.[176-178]

The proposed advantage of high-frequency ventilation is that lower inspiratory pressures and smaller tidal volumes may result in less gas leak through the fistula. It appears to be less effective when patients have bilaterally diseased, noncompliant lungs. The improvement in the air leak depends on a decrease in peak and mean airway pressures; it is recommended that tracheal pressures and airflow through the leak be measured during HFJV and compared with values obtained during conventional mechanical ventilation.

ANESTHETIC MANAGEMENT

Intraoperative treatment of patients with bronchopleural fistula presents unique challenges. Management strategies for induction and intubation depend on the severity of the bronchopleural fistula and presence of infection. If a chest tube is not in place or is malfunctioning, accumulation of escaping air into the enclosed pleural space will result in a tension pneumothorax. Because positive pressure ventilation increases the air leak and risks contaminating the noninfected lung, patients often are induced using rapid sequence induction to minimize the time before tracheal intubation and lung isolation. An alternative approach is to intubate a spontaneously ventilating patient with a double-lumen tube. Awake, sedated intubation may be considered for patients at increased risk for aspiration of gastric contents caused by full stomach or a bronchopleuroenteric fistula.[179] Once the tube has been positioned, the healthy lung should be isolated immediately, and the head placed slightly raised to decrease the likelihood of contamination of the healthy lung.

In patients with a small chronic bronchopleural fistula with a minimal air leak and no associated infection or empyema, a standard endotracheal tube can probably be used safely. If intermittent positive pressure ventilation is then found to be inadequate, the tube can be advanced into the bronchus of the healthy side or replaced with a double-lumen tube. If an empyema is present, it should be drained before induction of anesthesia. Decreasing the amount of pus in the pleural cavity reduces the chance of contaminating the contralateral lung and developing a tension pneumothorax. If intermittent positive pressure ventilation using a double-lumen tube provides inadequate oxygenation or ventilation, HFJV to the affected lung through the double-lumen tube is another option.[119] When a double-lumen tube cannot be used, as in small pediatric patients or in those with difficult airway anatomy, lung separation can be achieved by endobronchial placement of a single-lumen endotracheal tube.

Our choice is to thoroughly denitrogenate/preoxygenate, and if no difficulty in managing the airway is expected we place and position the double-lumen tube immediately after induction so we can exclude the fistulae from positive pressure ventilation.

ANESTHETIC IMPLICATIONS OF SPONTANEOUS PNEUMOTHORAX

Patients who develop spontaneous pneumothorax usually are young, healthy, and sometimes athletic, with no preexisting lung disease and no previous lung resections. Surgical treatment for spontaneous pneumothorax includes pleurectomy and chemical pleurodesis.[180]

Surgical treatment is indicated in the following situations: (1) failure of the pneumothorax to resolve with chest tube drainage and suction, which indicates that bronchopleural fistula has formed; (2) if a second ipsilateral or a first contralateral spontaneous pneumothorax occurs; and (3) if the patient's lifestyle is such that a recurrence may be life threatening or highly inconvenient (recurrence rate for spontaneous pneumothorax is 10%-25%).

When patients with pneumothorax come to the operating room, they typically have a chest tube in place, and therefore tension pneumothorax usually is not a major concern. Patients usually are treated with a double-lumen endotracheal tube to facilitate surgical exposure for either thoracoscopy or thoracotomy. If a single-lumen tube is placed and if the air leak is too large, a then that tube can be advanced into the bronchus of the unaffected side with the guidance of a fiberoptic bronchoscope or replaced with a double-lumen tube.

ANESTHESIA FOR PATIENTS UNDERGOING BULLECTOMY AND VOLUME REDUCTION PNEUMOPLASTY

There was a resurgence in the surgical management of bullous disease and emphysema from 1995 to 2005. Multiple studies have documented the efficacy of this procedure for patients with isolated large bullae, although the benefits of resection of diseased peripheral lung tissue in the presence of bullous emphysema are less certain. Large multicenter trials are under way to assess the efficacy of this therapeutic modality.

Bullae are air-filled spaces within the lung parenchyma. As bullae expand, the volume of the remaining lung is reduced (**Fig. 54-27**). The rationale for the surgical resection of the diseased lung is to remove areas of nonfunctional lung to permit reexpansion of compressed functional alveoli and to improve diaphragmatic function.[18,181] Preoperative evaluation includes pulmonary function testing, chest radiograph, CT, and ventilation-perfusion scanning to predict which patients will benefit from bullectomy. Patients most likely to benefit from the plication of large bullae are those in whom the bullae occupies greater than 30% of the hemithorax,[182-184] those with progressively enlarging nonfunctional pulmonary units and recurrent pneumothoraces, and those with moderate to severe dyspnea that is refractory to conventional medical therapy.[183] A prospective trial with 20 patients reported an increase in FEV_1 (0.77-1.4 L), FVC (2.2-2.8 L), and arterial oxygenation on inspired room air (64-70 mm Hg). The patients experienced less dyspnea and improved quality of life during the next 6 months. The beneficial effects were attributed to expansion of the remaining lung and improved diaphragmatic function, resulting in improved respiratory mechanics and decreased ventilation-to-perfusion mismatching. Another study reported more modest improvements in symptoms and pulmonary function analysis (FEV_1, 1.74-1.85 L; FVC, 1.82-2.21 L) and was associated with a mortality rate of 5.5%.[184] It is not known whether the difference between these 2 studies reflected patient selection or a difference in surgical technique. In the first study, resection was performed by open thoracotomy using a stapler, and in the latter study, resection was accomplished by thoracoscopy using laser technology. The goals of future studies will be to improve surgical techniques, ascertain the efficacy of volume reduction surgery, and define the patient population who would benefit most from the procedure.

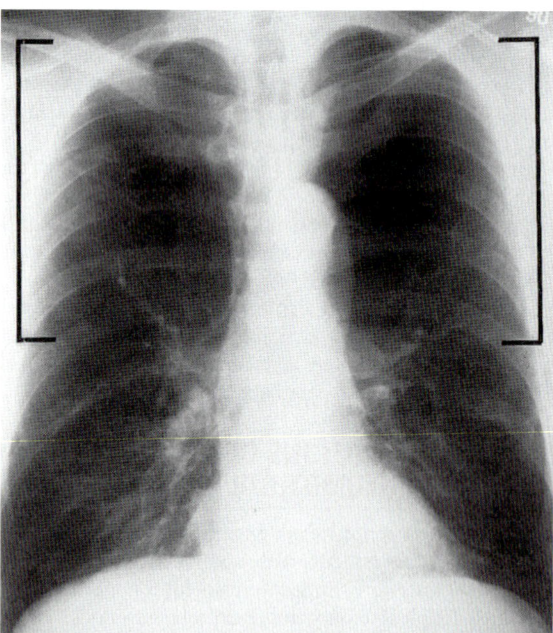

FIGURE 54-27. Characteristic radiographic findings of patients with bullous disease. Typical findings in patients with chronic obstructive pulmonary disease (COPD) include an increased size of lung fields and flattened hemidiaphragms. The appearance of hyperaeration of both apical lung fields (bracketed area), decreased vascular marking in upper lung fields, and compressive atelectasis of the lower lung fields also are consistent with severe bullous lung disease.

LUNG VOLUME REDUCTION SURGERY

In 1995 Cooper initiated a renewed interest in lung volume reduction surgery (LVRS), the technique of removing hyperinflated emphysematous lung to allow normal lung more space to function properly.[185] From this case series, many institutions started offering this invasive procedure to this high-risk patient population. Although many centers reported good results, increased rates of morbidity and mortality raised a need for a comprehensive multicenter trial.

The National Emphysema Treatment Trial (NETT)[186] was designed to determine if LVRS in combination with pulmonary rehabilitation led to greater improvements in functional capacity compared to pulmonary rehabilitation with medical therapy alone. The trial was a 4-year, multicenter study. Inclusion criteria were crafted to enroll patients with severe obstructive lung disease of varying anatomic distributions. Exclusion criteria eliminated patients at very high risk for perioperative morbidity, mortality, or other medical conditions that would decrease the likelihood of completing the trial. Once enrolled, all subjects went through 6 to 10 weeks of pulmonary rehabilitation prior to randomization.

Surgical management consisted of bilateral stapling of diseased lung, but the surgical approach was not consistent between centers. Eight centers performed LVRS by median sternotomy only, 3 centers performed LVRS by video-assisted thoracoscopy (VATS) only, and 6 centers randomized patients to either median sternotomy or VATS. The goal of surgery was the removal of 25% to 30% of lung tissue from each side. Anesthetic management was standardized to general anesthesia and a thoracic epidural. Although epidural analgesia was originally planned only for patients undergoing median sternotomy, the use of epidural analgesia in VATS patients was center dependent.

An interim analysis of the first 1033 subjects showed that there was excessive surgical mortality in the group of very high-risk patients[187] as defined by FEV_1 less than 20% predicted and either a homogeneous distribution of emphysema or a DLCO less than 20% predicted.[32] LVRS in this group resulted in a 30-day mortality rate of 16% compared to a 30-day mortality rate of 0% in the medically treated group. Although the survivors of surgery did exhibit modest improvements in FEV_1 and distance walked in 6 minutes, their quality of life did not improve.

Analysis of the completed study of 1218 randomized subjects showed that the risk of death was equal in the surgical and the medical treatment groups.[188] The surgically treated subjects had a greater improvement in exercise capacity compared to the medically treated patients. A greater than 10-W increase in exercise capacity was observed in 15% of patients treated with LVRS compared to only 3% of patients treated medically. When the high-risk patients who were identified in the aforementioned interim analysis were excluded (140 patients), there was no difference in mortality between surgical and medical groups. Exercise capacity had improved by more than 10 W in 16% of surgical patients as compared to 3% in medical patients.[186]

Further subgroup analysis examining the effect of distribution of emphysema produced exciting results. Patients with poor exercise capacity and predominantly upper-lobe emphysema based on CT scan had a significant decrease in mortality as compared to their medically treated matches. The risk ratio for death was 0.47; $P = 0.005$. Patients with non–upper-lobe predominant emphysema and high exercise had increased surgical mortality with a risk ratio for death of 2.06; $P = 0.02$.

Based on the subgroup analysis, the current trend is to offer patients with upper-lobe emphysema and poor exercise tolerance the option of LVRS. However, it is not clear from the publications how exercise capacity less than 15 W was determined to be poor exercise capacity. Similarly, the exact criteria used to define upper-lobe predominance of emphysema based on the CT scan of the chest needs to be described in detail. Once these additional data become available, the risks and benefits of LVRS in individual patients can be predicted with greater accuracy. This is critically important as this technique is being used more commonly as a bridge to transplant.

Surgery These procedures may be performed as single unilateral, sequential unilateral, or bilateral operations. Single unilateral bullectomy and volume reduction procedures are performed using the lateral decubitus position and video thoracoscopy or open thoracotomy. Sequential unilateral procedures can be performed by repositioning the patient to the contralateral decubitus position after the first side is completed. Bilateral procedures can be performed through a median sternotomy. Median sternotomy does not require repositioning and provides access to the contralateral pleural space in patients with pneumothorax. Plication of bullae and resection of peripheral lung tissue are accomplished with the use of a stapler. A major complicating factor in postoperative recovery is persistent air leaks at the suture line. This problem is decreased by using a stapler with a pericardial buttress.[182]

Anesthetic Considerations Patients presenting for bullectomy or LVRS have poor respiratory reserve and challenge the anesthesiologist during induction, single-lung ventilation, and extubation.[189,190] Before operation, the patients often are dyspneic and require supplemental oxygen. Many may have been considered for lung transplantation, but they were excluded because of their age or presence of coexisting diseases. Their tenuous cardiopulmonary status requires judicious use of any benzodiazepines or narcotics. In addition to the standard monitors, an arterial catheter should be placed to assess adequacy of oxygen and ventilation perioperatively.

Either thoracotomy or thoracoscopy requires general anesthesia and single-lung ventilation (**Table 54-10**). The combination of general anesthesia and epidural analgesia decreases the anesthetic requirement intraoperatively, thereby minimizing postoperative residual sedation. Patients with end-stage emphysema tend to have increased endogenous catecholamines caused by hypoxia and hypercapnia, often are hypovolemic, and are at risk for marked hypotension after induction of general anesthesia. General anesthesia can be maintained with either inhalation of intravenous agents or with a combination of techniques. Nitrous oxide should be avoided because of the risk of increasing the size of bullae, further compressing the adjacent lung or causing rupture. Communications between bullae and the airway may function as one-way valves, resulting in air trapping with rapid enlargement and compression of the surrounding lung. Initiation of controlled ventilation may be associated with hypoxia and hypercapnia. Acute rupture of bullae with resulting pneumothorax is a constant threat. An acute decrease in blood pressure associated with increased inspiratory pressures and loss of breath sounds should be considered a pneumothorax unless proven otherwise. The prompt placement of a chest tube can avert catastrophe. Low inflation pressures, that is, inspiratory pressures less than 25 cm H_2O, will decrease the risk of pneumothorax.

One-lung ventilation with a double-lumen tube facilitates bilateral volume reduction by providing selective ventilation, yet retaining the capacity for intermittent ventilation of the operative lung to manage hypoxia or hypercapnia or to assist the surgeon in identifying the location of bullae. Initiation of single-lung ventilation is associated with an increase in airway pressure and the concomitant risk of pneumothorax. Jet ventilation has been used to decrease airway pressures. The nonoperated, ventilated lung should be prepped and draped to allow access in case of a pneumothorax. Increased concentrations of halogenated anesthetics may worsen the venous admixture by inhibition of HPV. Anesthetic agents are chosen to permit quick emergence and minimal postoperative sedation, an important factor in causing respiratory embarrassment.

Postoperative Ventilation Extubation of the trachea at the end of operation can be accomplished in most patients and should be attempted to reduce the risk of air leak from continued positive pressure ventilation. The need for continued mechanical ventilation is greater after volume reduction pneumoplasty as compared with plication of bullae. The beneficial effects of operation are not realized immediately after operation. Volume reduction patients may decompensate in response to the usual decrement in postoperative pulmonary function associated with thoracic surgery and pain. They also seem to be more sensitive to residual sedation, respiratory depression from analgesics, residual muscle relaxants, or hypercapnia. The presence of a major air leak can interfere with respiratory function. Criteria for extubation include the presence of a regular respiratory pattern, adequate patient strength, alertness, ability to respond to command, and measurement of an arterial blood gas. If mechanical ventilation is required postoperatively, positive airway pressure should be minimized to decrease the chance of producing pneumothorax from rupture of residual bullae or suture lines. If air leak remains an important factor, airway peak pressure may be minimized by changing the mode of ventilation to pressure control. In addition, the chest tube suction should be put to water seal or at least the suction pressure should be minimal.

ANESTHESIA FOR PATIENTS UNDERGOING DECORTICATION AND PLEURODESIS PROCEDURES

CLINICAL FEATURES

The pleural space is a virtual cavity between the visceral and parietal pleura. Pleural inflammation, either infectious or noninfectious, increases permeability and results in the collection of high protein pleural fluid. Lymphatic obstruction, altered central venous pressures, and low oncotic pressure contribute to pleural fluid accumulation. Large effusions may dramatically decrease pulmonary function. Additionally, the collection of blood or empyema precipitates deposition of a fibrin layer on the pleura. As the fibrin layer (peel) matures, the underlying lung is entrapped and lung expansion is decreased, necessitating surgical intervention to release and expand collapsed lung and to manage infection.

The signs and symptoms of pleural disease include fever, chills, pleuritic chest pain, dyspnea, hemoptysis, and expectorate foul-smelling purulent sputum. Such patients may be cyanotic, hypovolemic, and hypotensive because of bacteremia and release of endotoxins. Preoperative studies include chest radiography and CT scans to locate the site of effusion or empyema.

Patients with a simple nonloculated empyema may be treated conservatively with antibiotic therapy and chest tube drainage. Once the empyema becomes loculated or develops into a fibrous peel, surgical intervention by thoracotomy or thoracoscopy is performed during general anesthesia. The access provided by VAT may be limited, and open thoracotomy may be required for a more definitive procedure. Perioperative complications include sepsis, chest tube bleeding, wound infection, bronchopleural fistula, and air leaks. Failure to adequately manage a chronic draining empyema may require the placement of an open window thoracostomy for long-term care. This procedure consists of suturing a flap of skin to the pleura, creating an epithelial-lined sinus into the empyema cavity.

Occasionally, additional intervention, pleurodesis, is required either because reaccumulation of the effusion causes respiratory compromise or is refractory to medical therapy as in the case of malignancies. A number of agents have been used intrapleurally to produce a chemical pleurodesis that leads to formation of adhesions and obliteration of the pleural space. Common sclerosing agents include tetracycline, talc, and bleomycin. Fever and chest pain are the most common complications of pleurodesis.

TABLE 54-10 Anesthetic Guidelines for Bullectomy and Volume Reduction Pneumoplasty

	Bullectomy/Volume Reduction Pneumoplasty	Volume Reduction Pneumoplasty
Indication	Bullectomy–large bullae >30% of hemithorax Volume reduction–severe bullous emphysema	Severe bullous emphysema
Preoperative concerns	Review preoperative pulmonary function tests and check arterial blood gases Pulmonary symptoms may mask presence of coronary artery disease	Same[a]
Monitors	Standard monitors and A-line	Same[a]
Anesthesia	General anesthesia Combined regional/general anesthesia	Same[a]
Additional equipment	Optional (jet ventilator)	Same[a]
Ventilation	Double-lumen endotracheal tube	Same[a]
Position	Bullectomy (lateral decubitus) Volume reduction pneumoplasty (lateral, supine)	Lateral decubitus Supine (median sternotomy)
Incision	Bullectomy (thoracotomy, VATS) Volume reduction pneumoplasty (thoracotomy, VATS, median sternotomy)	Thoracotomy VATS Median sternotomy
Unique considerations	Single-lung ventilation Avoid positive end-expiratory pressure Minimize use of long-lasting respiratory depressants Restrict administration of intravenous fluids	Same[a] Same[a]
Intraoperative complications	Tension pneumothorax Pneumothorax Hypoxia Hypercarbia	Same[a]
Blood loss	Minimal <500 mL	Same[a]
Postoperative analgesia	Epidural Parenteral opiates/NSAIDs	Same[a]
Postoperative morbidity	Persistant air leak Respiratory dysfunction Hypoxia Hypercarbia Pneumothorax Difficulty weaning from ventilator	
Postoperative care	Monitor respiratory status overnight for signs of decompensation Supplemental O_2 Chest radiography Adequate analgesia Minimize air leak by placing chest tubes to water seal or minimizing suction	

VATS, video-assisted thoracoscopic surgery.

[a]Same as bullectomy/volume reduction pneumoplasty.

ANESTHESIA MANAGEMENT

Surgical decortication requires the differential ventilation of the healthy and diseased lung to facilitate surgical exposure and to permit complete reexpansion after surgical intervention.[191] After induction and tracheal intubation, patients usually are placed in a lateral decubitus position with the affected lung in the nondependent position. In patients with a lung abscess, placement of an infected lung in the nondependent position increases the risk of contamination to the dependent lung. Most common management issues involve hypovolemia related to bleeding or sepsis and pain associated with decortication and pleurodesis. Inability to remove the fibrous peel may result in failure to reexpand the entrapped lung. After the decortication procedure is completed, positive pressure can be applied to the diseased lung to help break residual fibrous deposition, thus enabling lung reexpansion. We commonly place an epidural or paravertebral catheter for analgesia.

ANESTHESIA FOR PATIENTS UNDERGOING ESOPHAGEAL SURGERY

Dysphagia is the most common symptom of esophageal disease. When present for any major length of time, dysphagia can result in weight loss, dehydration, hypoalbuminemia, anemia, and depressed immune status. Postprandial heartburn, another common symptom of esophageal disease, is related to reflux of gastric contents into the esophagus.

BOX 54-8

Common Lesions of the Esophagus

- Tumors
  - Squamous cell
  - Adenocarcinoma
  - Hiatal hernia
- Benign strictures
  - Reflux esophagitis in the lower one-third of the esophagus
  - Caustic fluid ingestion in the upper one-third of the esophagus
- Motility disorders
  - Achalasia
  - Schatzki ring
- Collagen diseases (eg, scleroderma)
- Diverticuli
- Trachea esophageal fistula (congenital or malignant)
- Traumatic perforation or rupture
- Foreign bodies

Symptoms may manifest with change in position, exercise, or belching. Patients who experience such symptoms usually are evaluated by barium swallow under fluoroscopy, followed by esophagoscopy and tissue biopsy. Common esophageal lesions are summarized in **Box 54-8**.

ESOPHAGOSCOPY

Esophagoscopy is used for tissue biopsy or clarification of esophageal lesions detected after barium contrast studies. In addition, esophagoscopy is used for removal of foreign bodies, dilation of esophageal strictures, sclerotherapy of esophageal varices, diagnosis and management of bleeding lesions, and placement of prosthetic stents across malignant strictures.

Esophagoscopy can be performed using either a rigid or a flexible fiberoptic esophagoscope. Flexible esophagoscopy allows for greater comfort while examining the upper gastrointestinal tract and usually is performed on awake, slightly sedated patients. Although rigid esophagoscopy can be performed on awake, sedated patients, it is more readily accomplished during general endotracheal anesthesia. Rigid esophagoscopy is particularly valuable for removal of foreign bodies and for the examination and management of massive esophageal bleeding.

Anesthetic Management Fiberoptic esophagoscopy can easily be performed during topical anesthesia of the mouth and pharynx combined with mild sedation and an antisialagogue (**Table 54-11**). Patients should not be allowed to eat or drink until several hours after the procedure when the effect of topical anesthesia has dissipated and when protective airway reflexes have returned.

Rigid esophagoscopy usually is performed on patients during general anesthesia with endotracheal intubation and muscle relaxation. An anticholinergic agent is administered to decrease airway secretions and vagal responses to airway manipulation and gastric distention. Cricoid pressure should be used during induction because many patients are at risk for regurgitation from esophageal diverticuli, stenosis, or obstruction. Awake, sedated endotracheal intubation is an option. To avoid injury to the esophagus during passage of the esophagoscope, a small endotracheal tube is used, and the patient is paralyzed before introduction of the esophagoscope. It also may be necessary to temporarily deflate the endotracheal tube cuff to facilitate passage of the esophagoscope. Complications during esophagoscopy include hemorrhage, cardiac dysrhythmias, aspiration pneumonia, and perforation of the esophagus. Perforation can result in pneumothorax, pneumomediastinum, pneumoperitoneum, or subcutaneous emphysema. At the conclusion of the procedure, the trachea should remain intubated until protective reflexes have returned.

TABLE 54-11 Anesthetic Guidelines for Esophagoscopy

Indication	Diagnostic (biopsy mass, evaluate esophagus) Therapeutic (removal of foreign body, arrest bleeding, sclerosis)
Monitors	Standard monitors
Anesthesia	Awake, sedated (flexible fiberoptic) General anesthesia (flexible fiberoptic and rigid)
Additional equipment	None
Ventilation	Awake spontaneous respiration Single-lumen endotracheal tube (may require small size or cuff deflation to pass scope)
Position	Supine
Incision	None
Unique considerations	Antisialagogue Aspiration precautions
Intraoperative complications	Dysrhythmia Aspiration Hematemesis Pneumomediastinum Pneumoperitoneum Pneumothorax Dental trauma Respiratory compromise Perforation esophagus
Postoperative analgesia	Minimal pain (parenteral opiates, nonsteroidal anti-inflammatory drugs)
Postoperative morbidity	Hematemesis Respiratory distress (vocal cord paralysis)
Postoperative care	Chest radiography No eating or drinking until protective airway reflexes have returned

Esophageal Cancer Patients with esophageal malignancy often are malnourished with nutritional status predictive of poor outcome. Preoperative improvement in nutritional status has been shown to decrease the incidence of wound sepsis and perioperative morbidity and mortality.[161,192] Indications for total parenteral nutrition include inability to swallow food, 10% or greater decrease in body weight, serum albumin less than 3 g, cachexia and anergy, leukopenia, and low transferrin value.

Patients with esophageal cancer often are treated with chemotherapeutic agents before surgery. The perioperative implications of the previous use of antineoplastic agents for management of esophageal cancer include anemia, leukopenia, and thrombocytopenia. Drugs such as doxorubicin (Adriamycin), bleomycin, and mitomycin C have additional side effects that are important to the anesthesiologist.

Adriamycin administration can result in acute and chronic toxic cardiac effects. Acute cardiac toxicity from Adriamycin is characterized by supraventricular and ventricular dysrhythmias, abnormal conduction patterns, and ST-T wave changes. These acute changes usually resolve 1 or 2 months after cessation of therapy,[193] although Adriamycin administration also may result in irreversible cardiomyopathy and congestive heart failure. To avoid this complication, the total cumulative dose of Adriamycin usually is limited to a maximum of 300 mg/m^2. Adriamycin-induced cardiomyopathy is diagnosed by obtaining an endomyocardial biopsy and by determining the ejection fraction using a multigated nuclear scan (MUGA scan). If the usual maximal dose is exceeded or if patients demonstrate evidence of cardiomyopathy, then dexazoxane (Zinicard) is given before future Adriamycin therapy.

Bleomycin and mitomycin C395 administration can result in pulmonary toxicity. Early symptoms include cough, dyspnea, and rales. The toxic signs may progress to severe hypoxemia at rest and a radiologic picture similar to those with ARDS, followed by pulmonary fibrosis. Predisposing factors include age more than 20 years, dosage greater than 400 units, underlying pulmonary disease, and previous radiation therapy. O_2 in high concentrations can predispose the patient to pulmonary toxicity from bleomycin. Because the duration of O_2 sensitivity after the conclusion of bleomycin therapy is unknown, the lowest FIO_2 necessary to maintain adequate arterial saturation should be used perioperatively.

ESOPHAGEAL SURGERY: ESOPHAGEAL CANCER

Management Strategies Tumors of the lower third of the esophagus are managed by esophagogastrectomy through a left-sided thoracotomy or transhiatal esophagogastrectomy and gastric pull-through technique (**Fig. 54-28**).[194] Lesions of the middle third of the esophagus are managed by a combined laparotomy and right-sided thoracotomy.[195] Lesions of the upper third of the esophagus may be managed by combined laparotomy and cervical incision (**Fig. 54-29**).[194] Esophagogastrectomy with colon interposition is a 2-stage procedure used for lesions in the upper third of the esophagus when insufficient stomach length or gastric disease prevents performing an esophagogastrostomy. During the first stage, the esophagogastrectomy is performed through a midline laparotomy and right thoracotomy. The patient is then turned supine, and a cervical esophagostomy is performed. During the second stage, an antiperistaltic segment of the colon is passed into the retrosternal space and anastomosed to the cervical esophagus above and to the stomach remnant below (see Fig. 54-29).

The approach to surgical management of esophageal cancer is controversial. Major issues involve whether the goal is cure or merely palliation. The transthoracic approach, which involves complete resection of lymph nodes, is potentially curative, whereas the transhiatal approach is considered palliative. Other controversies include whether the patient should undergo immediate reconstruction with colon or stomach to restore continuity or delayed repair. Long-term survival appears to be a function of the stage and aggressiveness of the tumor at the time of operation rather than the type of operation. Surgical resection is associated with a local recurrence rate of 30% to 60% and 5-year survival of 20% to 25%. The addition of induction therapy of any kind does not significantly alter these survival rates.[196]

Anesthetic Management Preoperative evaluation should concentrate on the hematologic, nutritional, and cardiopulmonary systems. Preoperative improvement of nutritional status improves outcome. Hypoalbuminemia, an indicator of poor nutritional status, is associated with increased tissue edema, and anemia may increase the risk of ischemia. Because the operation may be associated with episodes of hemodynamic instability and cardiac arrhythmias, the patient should receive a thorough cardiac evaluation preoperatively. Accompanying respiratory disease should be managed if possible, and strong consideration should be given to placement of an epidural catheter for postoperative analgesia.

Preoperative medication is given according to the patient's general condition to allay anxiety. The use of an anticholinergic drug may be helpful if awake intubation is planned. Guidelines for anesthetic management are presented in **Table 54-12**. Use of central venous catheterization is encouraged for monitoring of central venous pressure, administration of antiarrhythmics or vasopressors, and fluid resuscitation. A pulmonary artery catheter should be placed if indicated, based on the patient's cardiopulmonary status; it may prove beneficial postoperatively for optimizing fluid therapy. Arterial lines are strongly recommended, particularly for transhiatal esophagogastrectomy where surgeons bluntly dissect behind the heart and often induce profound hypotension.

Before induction of anesthesia, a large-bore nasogastric tube should be placed and the proximal esophageal pouch should be emptied. The patient should still be considered to have a full stomach because it is impossible to completely empty the esophagus through a nasogastric tube. Awake intubation during topical anesthesia or induction with cricoid pressure is indicated. If airway compression by large mediastinal lymph nodes is noted, the patient should be treated as described in the section on mediastinal tumors (see Fig. 54-1). Anesthesia is maintained using inhalation anesthetics in O_2, supplemented with intermittent or continuous infusion of narcotics and nondepolarizing muscle relaxants. The combination of epidural and general anesthesia can dramatically decrease inhalation anesthetic and muscle relaxant requirements.

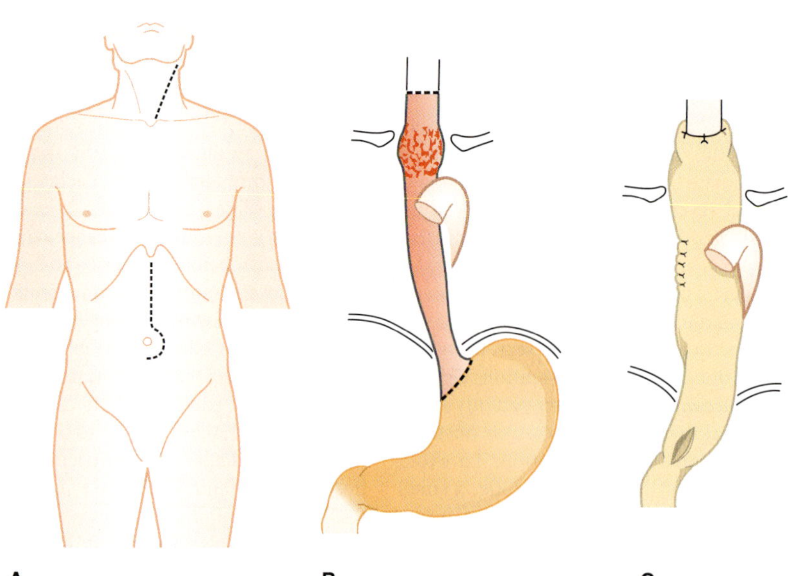

FIGURE 54-28. For esophagectomy without thoracotomy, the patient is in the supine position. **A.** Upper midline and left cervical incision (broken lines) are made. **B.** The extent of resection (shaded area) is shown. **C.** Completed anastomosis. [From Ellis FH Jr. Esophagogastrectomy for carcinoma: technical considerations based on anatomic location of lesion. *Surg Clin North Am.* 1980;60:275.]

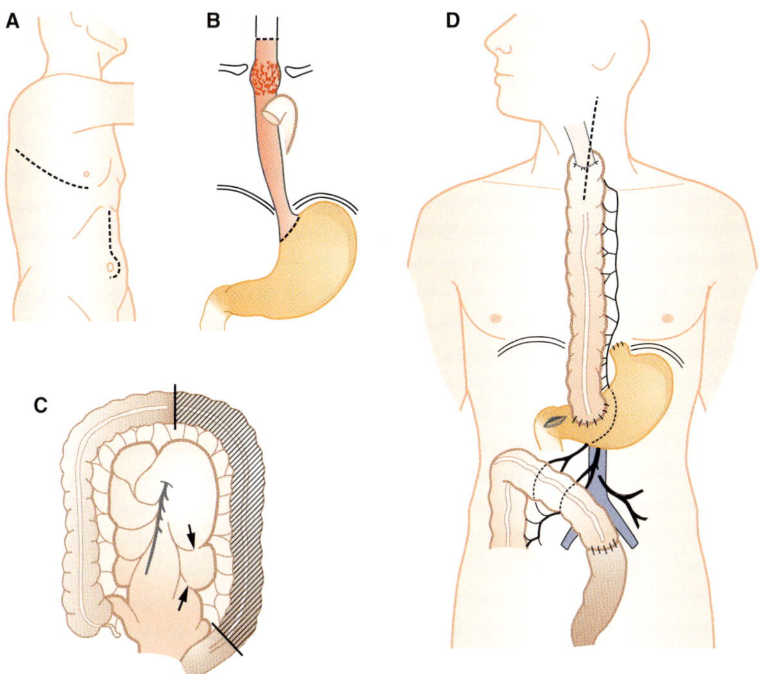

FIGURE 54-29. Esophagectomy with interposition of antiperistaltic segment of left colon. **A.** Incisions used in performance of esophagectomy, cervical esophagostomy, pyloromyotomy, and gastrostomy. **B.** Extent of esophageal resection (shaded area). **C.** Preparation of segment of left colon (shaded area) for interposition based on middle colic artery (note sites of vascular interruption, which maintain the integrity of the vascular arcade). **D.** Completed operation. [From Ellis FH Jr. Esophagogastrectomy for carcinoma: technical considerations based on anatomic location of lesion. *Surg Clin North Am.* 1980;60:277.]

If thoracotomy is planned for esophageal surgery, a double-lumen endobronchial tube or bronchial blocker to permit single-lung ventilation facilitates surgical exposure. Whether a right-sided or left-sided thoracotomy is performed, a left-sided double-lumen endobronchial tube is recommended because it is easier to position and offers less risk of obstruction of the upper lobe bronchial orifice. In patients having nonpulmonary surgery, the nondependent lung usually is not severely diseased and thus contributes greatly to normal respiratory function. Paradoxically, this increases the incidence of hypoxemia during single-lung ventilation as compared with that during pulmonary surgery, and the hypoxemia may persist as long as the lung is collapsed.[114]

Marked fluctuating cardiovascular responses are observed frequently during transhiatal esophagectomy. Bradycardia and hypotension may result from stimulation of carotid sinus reflexes during neck dissection and mobilization of the esophagus. They are easily managed with an anticholinergic drug such as atropine. Blunt manual dissection of the esophagus through the diaphragmatic hiatus is associated with hemodynamic lability. Arterial hypertension often occurs during manual dissection of the esophagus and when the stomach is brought up through the posterior mediastinum, whereas hypotension may result from impaired venous return and cardiac function during manual dissection. These relatively long-lasting alterations in hemodynamics could be deleterious to patients with cardiac disease, and they mandate careful intraoperative hemodynamic monitoring. Patients with advanced cardiac dysfunction may not tolerate these manipulations and therefore are not good candidates for a transhiatal esophagectomy. Sudden severe intraoperative hemorrhage also can occur, and therefore large-bore venous access is essential. Other complications include tracheal damage and recurrent laryngeal nerve palsy. Tracheal damage has been reported during transhiatal esophagectomy without thoracotomy and during dissection of the middle third of the esophagus during thoracotomy.

Postoperative Concerns Because esophagogastrectomy is associated with extensive visceral manipulations, difficulty in clearing secretions, advanced patient age with concomitant debilitation, and cardiorespiratory impairment, these patients may remain intubated overnight in the ICU. They often have increased fluid requirements during the initial postoperative period, and central venous monitoring is useful in guiding fluid management. Postoperative complications include pleural effusions, wound infection, pneumonia, and leak from the anastomotic site, resulting in mediastinitis, sepsis, hydrothorax, or pyrothorax.[197] Impaired pulmonary function, airway closure, atelectasis, and hypoxemia typically occur postoperatively because of lung manipulation, residual anesthesia, and postoperative incisional pain. Effective postoperative pain control is essential to facilitate deep breathing, cough, mobilization of secretions, participation in chest physiotherapy, and early ambulation. Postoperative analgesia is most effectively achieved using a thoracic epidural. For transhiatal esophagectomy we will often use a T10 epidural with dilute bupivacaine and a separate opioid intravenous patient-controlled analgesia (IVPCA) to cover the neck incision.

ANESTHESIA FOR PATIENTS UNDERGOING LASER SURGERY OF THE AIRWAY

Laser technology has been applied extensively for procedures on the upper and lower airways. It has been used successfully in the management of laryngeal tumors, subglottic stenosis, recurrent laryngeal papillomatosis in children, and for the removal and debulking of obstructing airway tumors.[198-205]

PHYSICS OF LASERS

LASER is an acronym for light amplification by stimulated emission of radiation. Laser light is a monochromatic coherent form of electromagnetic radiation that does not occur naturally. To produce a laser beam, atoms are stimulated by electrical, optical, or thermal energy. The stimulated lasing medium radiates energy in the form of light, which is then repeatedly reflected, amplified, and emitted as a laser beam.

TABLE 54-12 Anesthetic Guidelines for Esophagogastrectomy and Esophagectomy

Indication	Therapeutic (palliative and curative procedures for esophageal cancer)
Preoperative considerations	Assessment of nutritional status Presence of coexisting cardiopulmonary disease Implications of preoperative chemotherapy
Monitors	Standard monitors, optional (arterial catheter, central venous, or pulmonary artery catheters)
Anesthesia	General anesthesia, optional (combined regional and general anesthesia)
Additional equipment	Shoulder roll
Ventilation	Double-lumen ETT or bronchial blocker Single-lumen ETT
Position	Supine Lateral decubitus
Incision	Left thoracotomy–mobilize distal esophagus and stomach without changing positions Right thoracotomy–good exposure of upper and mid-esophagus, easy access to the azygous vein Abdominal transhiatal, abdominal and neck incisions, esophagus mobilized by blunt dissection
Unique considerations	Single-lung ventilation Anticholinergic drug to block carotid sinus reflex (vagal-mediated response) Avoid N_2O with abdominal surgery Increased risk for aspiration
Intraoperative complications	Aspiration Hypotension Bradycardia Dysrhythmia Hemorrhage Tracheal tears Recurrent laryngeal nerve injury Hypoxia and hypercapnia during 1-lung ventilation
Blood loss	1000 mL, but potential for large acute blood loss
Postoperative analgesia	Epidural > parenteral opiates
Postoperative morbidity	Aspiration Pneumothorax Respiratory compromise Hemoptysis Infection Anastomotic leaks
Postoperative care	Chest radiography Elevate head of bed to decrease edema and improve respiratory function Increased fluid requirements during early postoperative procedures

ETT, endotracheal tube.

The lasing medium can be a gas (eg, helium, argon, CO_2) or a solid medium (eg, ruby, neodymium ytrium-aluminum-garnet [Nd-YAG]).

The effect of the laser beam on tissues depends on its wavelength and its power density. Laser beams with long wavelengths are strongly absorbed by tissues and therefore are converted into heat energy with a very shallow depth of penetration. In contrast, laser light of short wavelength penetrates more deeply into the tissues. Therefore, a CO_2 laser that has a long wavelength (10 600 nm) is absorbed at the very superficial tissue layer, which allows for precise cutting and relatively little edema formation. The Nd-YAG laser has a short wavelength (1064 nm) and penetrates more deeply into the tissues, allowing its use for tumor-debulking procedures. The potassium titanyl-phosphate (KTP) laser emits green light with a wavelength of 552 nm. This lasing medium is produced by adding KTP to Nd-YAG crystals. The KTP laser beam is absorbed by blood and is therefore more effective than an argon laser beam for operation on vascular tumors (eg, subglottic hemangiomas).

LASER SURGERY OF THE AIRWAY

Malignant tumors of the tracheobronchial tree lead to progressive obstruction of major airways that manifest as progressive stridor. Laser resection has been used in the treatment of partially or totally occluding airway lesions with partial or complete relief of symptoms.[206-208] In patients with a totally obstructing airway lesion, lasers can be used to bore through the tumor to reestablish an airway. A serious risk of bronchial perforation and hemorrhage exists. On the other hand, a partially obstructing tumor can be approached tangentially and gradually resected, resulting in widening of the available airway lumen. For partially obstructing lesions, laser resection often provides immediate and dramatic relief of symptoms with a low incidence of bleeding complications. The Nd-YAG laser is the most frequently used laser to resect obstructing tracheobronchial tree tumors.[206-208] If a CO_2 laser is to be used for a subglottic lesion, a rigid bronchoscope or laryngoscope is required because the CO_2 laser beam cannot be transmitted along fiberoptic bundles. For supraglottic lesions being managed with a CO_2 laser, a small endotracheal tube can be used for patient ventilation, but the tube should be protected from the laser beam to prevent ignition.

INTRAOPERATIVE CONSIDERATIONS

Safety Issues The use of a laser in the operating room poses safety hazards for patients and operating room personnel. Warning signs on the operating room door should be clearly visible. The most common major complication of CO_2 laser surgery is the risk of explosion or fire.[209,210] The anesthesiologist should therefore limit the O_2 concentration to the minimum needed to maintain adequate oxygenation, even if the endotracheal tube is a specific "laser" stainless steel model. For a more complete discussion the reader is encouraged to review Chapter 67.

Use of Helium The use of helium and O_2 mixtures (60%/40% to 75%/25%) during CO_2 laser application has been reported to prevent ignition and fires with unwrapped PVC tubes.[201,211] Helium has greater thermal conductivity, thermal capacity, and thermal diffusivity than nitrogen. These properties of helium inhibit the increase in temperature around the site of laser exposure and thus prevent spontaneous ignition. Besides protecting against airway fire, helium may improve ventilation across an obstructing airway lesion because of its lower density compared with nitrogen, thereby decreasing turbulent gas flow across the stenotic area. The problem of delivering a hypoxic gas mixture of helium in certain anesthesia machines can be circumvented by using Heliox, a commercially available O_2-helium mixture.

Anesthetic Management Laser surgery often is performed on patients who have underlying respiratory compromise, a long-term history of smoking, and a malignant process encroaching on the airway. Because many of these patients have associated COPD, it is important to evaluate their respiratory function preoperatively and treat with bronchodilators and antibiotics if indicated. Because of the risk of life-threatening airway obstruction during induction of anesthesia or manipulation of the airway, the anesthesiologist should carefully examine the radiologic and other studies to define precisely the site and extent of airway compromise. Good communication with the surgeon or pulmonologist is necessary to plan anesthetic (eg, choice of endotracheal tube will depend on the size of bronchoscope and type of laser) and management strategies in case of emergencies.

Patients at risk of developing airway obstruction or those with severe pulmonary disease should be premedicated with an antisialagogue and minimal sedation only. If the patient is not at risk for airway obstruction, sedative premedications can be administered more liberally. Some ventilation techniques described in the next section do not allow the use of capnography. In these patients, monitoring of ventilation is done by careful auscultation of breath sounds, observation of chest movements, or monitoring of arterial blood gases.

Patients with minimal or no airway obstruction can receive a routine induction of anesthesia, followed by muscle relaxation and endotracheal intubation or placement of a laryngeal mask airway. The choice of anesthetic induction technique depends on the extent of airway compromise. Patients who have major airway obstruction should maintain spontaneous ventilation during induction. Induction therefore can be achieved by inhalation agents or by administering incremental doses of intravenous hypnotics and narcotics followed by the gradual introduction of inhalational anesthetics by mask. Alternatively, fiberoptic bronchoscopy can be performed in an awake, sedated patient whose airway has been topically anesthetized (**Table 54-13**).

Local anesthesia can be used for laser resection of an airway tumor via flexible fiberoptic bronchoscopy. Adequate anesthesia can be achieved by topicalization of the mouth and oropharynx, spraying of the larynx and vocal cords with local anesthetics, superior laryngeal nerve block, or transtracheal injection of a local anesthetic. To avoid serious potential complications, adequate sedation is imperative when awake, sedated anesthesia is used. This technique is not recommended for patients undergoing laser airway surgery performed with a rigid bronchoscope. The degree of discomfort is greater than that with fiberoptic bronchoscopy, and patient movement resulting in trauma and misdirection of the laser beam is more likely to occur.

TABLE 54-13 Anesthetic Guidelines for Laser Ablation

Indication	Therapeutic (palliative of airway obstruction related to tumor)
Monitors	Standard monitors Optional (arterial)
Anesthesia	General anesthesia
Additional equipment	Anesthetic ventilator capable of blending an O_2 and air mixture
Ventilation	Rigid bronchoscope Single-lumen ETT (special laser tube, but may be less important when using laser way distal to the ETT)
Position	Supine
Unique considerations	Maintain FIO_2 <40% Avoid nitrous oxide (N_2O; also supports combustion)
Intraoperative complications	Hemoptysis Hemorrhage Airway fire Airway obstruction Bronchospasm Hypoxia Perforation of the tracheobronchial tree
Analgesia	Opiates
Postoperative morbidity	Hemoptysis Bronchospasm Airway edema
Postoperative care	Humidified O_2

ETT, endotracheal tube.

Use of Fiberoptic Bronchoscopy During Laser Therapy Fiberoptic bronchoscopy for laser resection of airway tumors can be done during local anesthesia and sedation or during general anesthesia with the fiberoptic bronchoscope introduced through the lumen of the endotracheal tube or laryngeal mask airway. The device with largest lumenal diameter should be used to allow for sufficient ventilation after the fiberoptic bronchoscope is introduced. Because resistance to airflow occurs with the introduction of the bronchoscope into an endotracheal tube, patients should either receive total mechanical or pressure support ventilation to overcome the resistance created by the bronchoscope. The administration of muscle relaxants may be relatively contraindicated in patients with partial airway obstruction.

Hypercapnia is a common complication of transfiberoptic laser tumor resection, with $Paco_2$ ranging from 45 to 60 mm Hg.[204] Long-acting opioids and benzodiazepines should be avoided because of prolonged postoperative somnolence and respiratory depression. Short-action inhalation anesthetics and sedatives allow for rapid emergence without postoperative respiratory depression or sedation.

Use of Rigid Bronchoscopy During Resection of Airway Tumors Many laser resections are performed using a rigid, open-tube bronchoscope.[208] It allows easy manipulation of the laser beam and provides a greater field of vision, greater access for suction catheters, removal of tumor fragments, and promotion of homeostasis. The rigid bronchoscope can be used to establish an airway. If airway obstruction occurs, the bronchoscope is advanced distally to the site of obstruction, thereby reestablishing airway patency. The absence of a combustible endotracheal tube decreases the chance of an airway fire. Although the steel bronchoscope will not burn, carbonized tissue may flare.[212] It is important to use the lowest O_2 concentration needed to maintain adequate arterial saturation. The rigid bronchoscope facilitates homeostasis because the bronchoscope can be gradually withdrawn while the endoscopist coagulates bleeding sites as they appear.

Maintenance of ventilation can be achieved using 1 of several techniques. Conventional intermittent positive pressure ventilation can be maintained by connecting the anesthesia circuit to the ventilating side arm of the rigid bronchoscope, which allows the administration of O_2. If a major leak occurs around the rigid bronchoscope, interfering with the adequacy of ventilation, packing the distal pharynx with gauze is helpful. Typically, anesthesia is provided by the use of intravenous agents to avoid exposing the surgical staff to any inhalational agents. Often, the patients are paralyzed to eliminate the risk of sudden, unexpected movement. Ventilation and oxygenation may be further compromised if the rigid bronchoscope is advanced into the mainstem or distal bronchi. Inadequate ventilation to the contralateral lung will result unless the bronchoscope has side holes that allow ventilation of the opposite lung.

Ventilation during periods of rigid bronchoscopy may be provided by jet ventilation. Low-frequency manual jet ventilation using the Sanders' jet injector at a frequency of 20 breaths/min has been shown to provide adequate oxygenation and ventilation.[154] Total intravenous anesthesia can be achieved with intermittent or continuous infusions of propofol, etomidate, alfentanil, or remifentanil. Disadvantages of low-frequency jet ventilation include the lack of precise control of the FIO_2 because of entrainment of ambient air and Venturi effect, which can lead to distal migration or aspiration of blood and tissue debris. Alternatively, HFJV at rates of 150 to 300 breaths/min can achieve satisfactory surgical conditions and provide adequate gas exchange in patients with tracheobronchial stenosis.[154] At a faster rate, some hypoxemia and hypercapnia are noted, especially when the bronchoscope is advanced into a mainstem bronchus. The use of a small tidal volume at a high rate results in an immobile surgical field and decreases the chance of misdirection of the laser beam with trauma to healthy tissues. Additionally, unlike low-frequency ventilation using the Sanders' injector, which creates a Venturi effect, HFJV is associated with a continuous egress of gas to the outside, thus decreasing the chance of aspirating blood and tissue debris or forcing it into the distal airway. When arterial desaturation occurs during laser resection, the surgeon should stop the resection, thoroughly suction blood and tissue debris out of the airway, and hyperventilate with 100% O_2. When adequate arterial oxygenation is reachieved, the O_2 concentration can again be decreased, and the surgeon can resume laser resection.

ANESTHESIA FOR PATIENTS UNDERGOING MEDIASTINOSCOPY

Mediastinoscopy and mediastinotomy are performed to diagnose and stage lung cancer to determine resectability. These procedures provide access to paratracheal, subaortic, and bronchial lymph nodes to detect metastatic spread of lung carcinomas. Lymphatics of the lung initially drain into the subaortic and paratracheal areas and then to the sides of the trachea, supraclavicular areas, and thoracic ducts. The surgical site is chosen based on likely path for regional spread of metastatic disease. Cervical mediastinal exploration (mediastinoscopy) yields a greater percentage of positive results for tumors affecting the right upper and middle lobes, and to a lesser extent left lower lobes. Anterior mediastinotomy is recommended for those patients suspected of tumor in the left upper lobe.

Mediastinoscopy is performed in patients in the supine position with the neck extended. Access is gained through an incision in the suprasternal notch, and a tunnel is created by blunt dissection anterior and slightly lateral to the trachea into the mediastinum. The rigid mediastinoscope passes posterior to the innominate and aortic pulmonary arteries down to the subcarinal area. The mediastinoscope can injure adjacent structures (**Fig. 54-30**). Increased risk of complications during mediastinoscopy has been noted in patients with major collateral vascular flow and in patients with abnormal or altered anatomy (**Table 54-14**).[213]

ANESTHETIC MANAGEMENT

Preoperative assessment should include inspection for the presence of occult airway obstruction or distortion, superior vena cava outlet obstruction, evidence of paraneoplastic syndromes, and cerebral vascular disease. The standard anesthetic plan is designed to permit rapid emergence and extubation after surgical pathology confirms adequacy of the specimen. General anesthesia with mechanical ventilation is the most commonly applied technique (**Table 54-15**). However, mediastinoscopy can be performed using local anesthesia with sedation in rare cases (ie, mediastinal masses with airway compromise). Muscle relaxants are advantageous for facilitating intubation, controlling ventilation, and preventing sudden movement or coughing that would increase the risk of surgical complications.[214] The negative intrathoracic pressure associated with spontaneous ventilation may increase the risk of air embolism through open venous structures. Manipulation of the mediastinoscope can compress the innominate artery, thereby decreasing arterial blood flow to the right upper extremity and the right common carotid arteries, and obliterating the pulse and pressure in the right arm.[215] It is recommended that a noninvasive blood pressure cuff be placed on the patient's left arm and either a pulse oximetry probe or an arterial catheter (if indicated) be placed in the right upper extremity. Waveform analysis of the arterial pressure or pulse oximeter plethysmograph trace can detect compression of the innominate artery.[216]

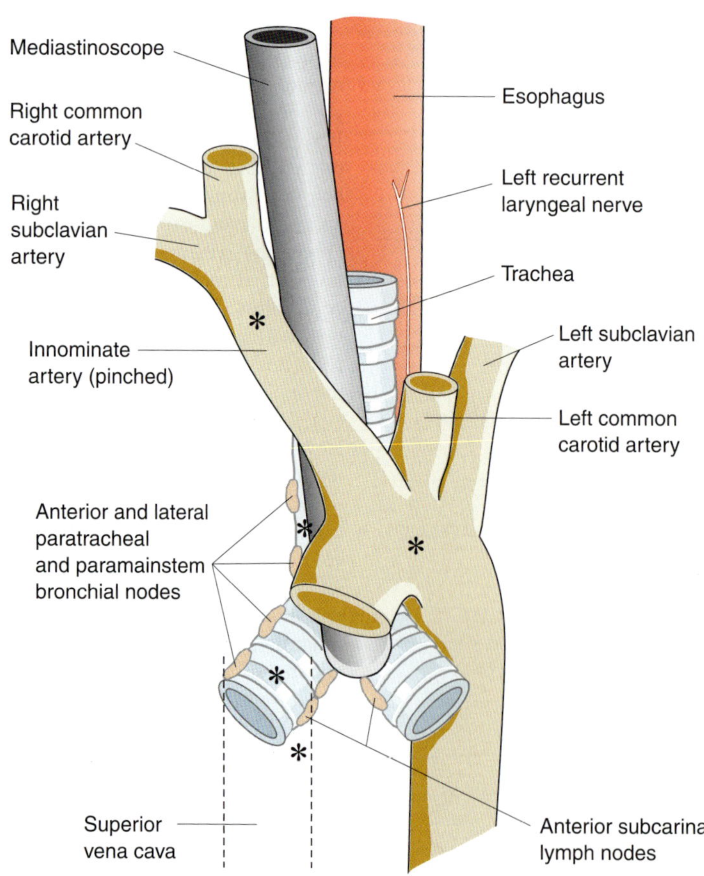

FIGURE 54-30. Mediastinoscope within the mediastinum. Note the pinched innominate artery. [Modified from Petty C. Right radial artery pressure during mediastinoscopy. *Anesth Analg.* 1979;58:428.]

TABLE 54-14 Complications of Mediastinoscopy From Review of 14 Mediastinoscopy Series (1968-1970)

Complications	No. of Patients
Bleeding	
Moderate	15
Necessitating thoracotomy	4
From superior vena cava	1
From brachiocephalic artery	1
Wound hematoma	1
Vocal cord paralysis	
Left vocal cord	7
Side not given	4
Bilateral	4
Hoarseness, possible vocal cord paralysis	1
Pneumothorax	11
Pleural tear	3
Tumor seeding in incision line	1
Perforation of esophagus	1
Myocardial infarction (postoperative)	1
Bradycardia	4
Cardiac arrest (anesthetic error)	1
Wound infection	2
Left hemiparesis (transient)	1
Total	60

From Foster ED, Munro DD, Dobell AR. Mediastinoscopy. A review of anatomical relationships and complications. *Ann Thorac Surg*. 1972;13:273-286.

TABLE 54-15 Anesthetic Guidelines for Mediastinoscopy and Mediastinotomy

Indication	Diagnostic (biopsy mass, lymph nodes)
Monitors	Standard monitors, optional (arterial catheter)
Anesthesia	General anesthesia
Additional equipment	Shoulder roll
Ventilation	Single-lumen endotracheal tube
Position	Supine with cervical extension
Incision	Mediastinoscopy (suprasternal) Mediastinotomy
Unique considerations	To avoid artifact induced by innominate artery compression, place noninvasive blood pressure cuff on left To detect innominate artery compression, place pulse oximeter on right hand
Intraoperative complications	Dysrhythmia Asthma Hemorrhage Pneumothorax Recurrent laryngeal nerve injury Respiratory compromise Air embolism Perforation of esophagus or bronchus Neurologic event (compression of innominate artery or hyperextension of the neck)
Blood loss	Usually minimal
Postoperative analgesia	Parenteral opiates
Postoperative morbidity	Pneumothorax Hemoptysis Respiratory distress (vocal cord paralysis)
Postoperative care	Chest radiography Elevate head of bed to decrease edema and improve respiratory function

COMPLICATIONS

The overall complication rate for mediastinoscopies ranges from 1.5% to 3%.[213,217-219] Appreciation for the surgical risks associated with mediastinoscopy comes from an understanding of the anatomy relevant to the procedure. The most common and potentially serious complications are bleeding, cardiac tamponade, and air embolism. Compromise of other structures such as the trachea, bronchi, esophagus, laryngeal nerve, or innominate artery can lead to temporary or permanent complications. Massive hemorrhage can result from laceration of a pulmonary artery or a thoracic aortic artery.[219] Therefore, a large-bore IV access catheter should be secured before induction of anesthesia. Clinical situations that increase collateral vascular flow, such as superior vena cava syndrome or aortic coarctation, predispose to bleeding and are relative contraindications to the procedure. Hemorrhage may be temporarily controlled by packing the surgical wound. Immediate mediansternotomy may be required to control bleeding. In patients with superior vena cava obstruction, intravenous access should be secured in the lower extremity to avoid distending the thoracic venous vasculature and increasing the risk of bleeding.

Laceration of venous structures in the mediastinum increases the risk of air embolism.[220]

Compression of the vertebral arteries from hyperextension of the cervical spine or compression of the innominate artery that feeds the right common carotid artery can cause CNS complications.[216,221,222] One study documented transient decreases in blood flow for periods ranging from 15 to 35 seconds in 4 of 7 patients.[221] However, the clinical significance of such transient effects is unknown.

Tracheal laceration can lead to mediastinal emphysema and loss of effective ventilation. If it is suspected, fiberoptic bronchoscopy should be used to define the site and to guide advancement of the endotracheal tube beyond the laceration. Tracheomalacia resulting from long-standing compression of the trachea by mediastinal tumor can predispose to acute tracheal injury or collapse.

Pneumothorax is the second most common complication of mediastinoscopy. It may be unilateral or bilateral, and the use of positive pressure ventilation can rapidly increase its size, causing hemodynamic compromise. It should be suspected if the patient exhibits an increase in peak airway pressures, hypotension, dysrhythmias, deviation of the trachea, or unilateral absence of breath sounds. A chest radiograph can be obtained to confirm the diagnosis if time permits. If the patient exhibits hemodynamic instability, rapid placement of a chest tube is indicated.

POSTOPERATIVE CONCERNS

Dyspnea and respiratory difficulty may occur in the initial postoperative period. Intraoperative bleeding or edema can cause compression of the airway, especially in patients with tracheomalacia.[218] Raising the head of the bed improves ventilatory mechanics, facilitates venous return, and decreases edema. Damage to the recurrent laryngeal nerve during mediastinoscopy does not become evident until after extubation. If injury to the recurrent laryngeal is suspected, the vocal cords should be visualized during extubation with the patient breathing spontaneously. Unilateral nerve damage without airway obstruction is managed conservatively.[220,223] Bilateral nerve injury requires reintubation to prevent airway obstruction. Laryngeal nerve injury during these conditions is permanent in 50% of patients.[224]

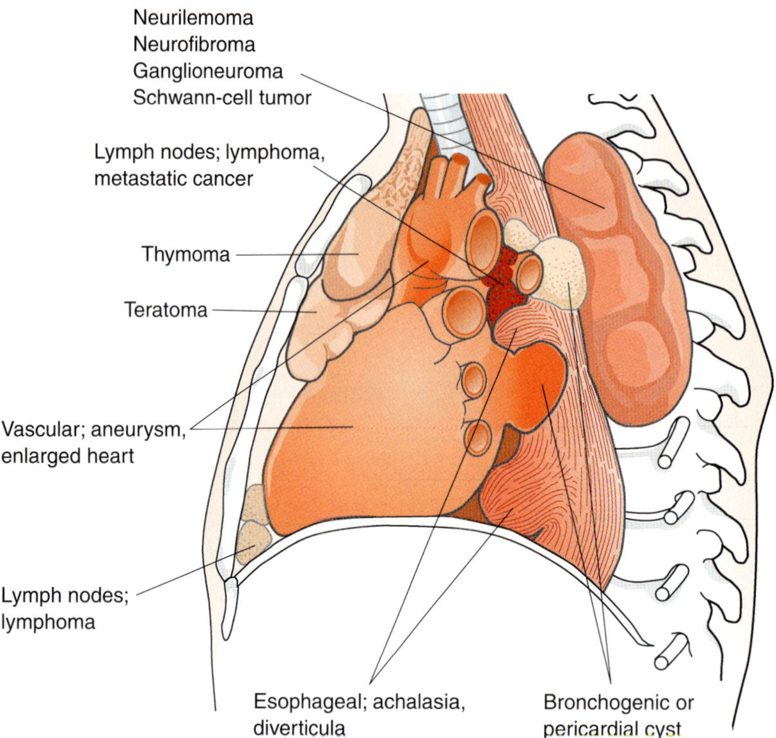

FIGURE 54-31. Anatomic location of commonly encountered mediastinal masses.

ANESTHESIA FOR PATIENTS WITH MEDIASTINAL MASSES

Patients with mediastinal masses may experience catastrophic complications during general anesthesia. Some of the most terrifying moments in the practice of anesthesiology occur while caring for patients who have mediastinal masses and undergo diagnostic procedures, especially those in the pediatric age group.

The mediastinum is divided into the superior, anterior, middle, and posterior mediastina. The most common tumors in the anterior mediastinum are thymomas, mesenchymal tumors, dermoid cysts, thyroid and parathyroid tumors, and lymphomas (**Fig. 54-31** and **Table 54-16**). In the middle and posterior mediastinum, tumor pathologies include pericardial cysts, bronchogenic cysts, lymphomas, neurogenic tumors, and aortic aneurysms.

SIGNS AND SYMPTOMS

The mechanisms postulated for the clinical symptoms of respiratory and cardiovascular compromise in awake patients include (**Table 54-17**) (1) progressive airway obstruction caused by compression of the distal trachea or bronchi, (2) loss of lung volume, (3) compression of the pulmonary artery or the heart, (4) superior vena cava obstruction,

TABLE 54-16 Mediastinal Mass Location

Superior	Anterior	Middle	Posterior
Children			
Lymphoma	Lymphoma	Lymphoma	Neurogenic tumors
Thymoma	Teratoma	Tuberculous nodes	Esophageal duplication cysts
Retrosternal thyroid	Cystic hygroma		Diaphragmatic hernia (Bochdalek)
Parathyroid tumor	Thymoma		
	Pericardial cysts		
	Diaphragmatic hernia (Morgagni)		
Adults			
Lymphoma	Lymphoma	Lymphoma	Neurogenic tumors
Thymoma	Metastatic carcinoma	Metastatic carcinoma	Lymphoma
Retrosternal thyroid	Teratoma	Teratoma	Hernia (Bochdalek)
Metastatic carcinoma	Bronchogenic cyst	Bronchogenic cyst	Aortic aneurysm
Parathyroid tumors	Aortic aneurysm	Aortic aneurysm	
Zenker diverticulum	Pericardial cyst	Pericardial cyst	
Aortic aneurysm			

TABLE 54-17 Clinical Findings in Patients With Mediastinal Masses

History	Physical Examination	Laboratory
Airway		
Cough	Decreased breath sounds	Chest radiograph (posteroanterior and lateral to look for tracheal deviation or compression)
Cyanosis	Wheezing	Flow-volume loops, supine and sitting
Dyspnea	Stridor	
Orthopnea	Cyanosis	
Cardiovascular		
Fatigue	Neck or facial edema	Chest radiographic changes in cardiac silhouette
Faintness	Jugular distension	Echocardiogram, supine and sitting
Headache	Papilledema	
Shortness of breath, orthopnea	Blood pressure changes or pallor with postural changes	
Cough	Pulsus paradoxus	

(5) involvement of the important nervous system elements in the mediastinum (eg, recurrent laryngeal nerves, sympathetic chain), and (6) spinal cord compression from intraspinal extension of neurogenic tumors of the posterior mediastinum.

The incidence of perioperative complications generally is related to the size of the mediastinal mass and to the extent of disease within the thoracic cavity. In 1 large series, clinical manifestations included (1) cough and pain, 40% each; (2) weight loss and fever, 24% each; (3) dyspnea and dysphagia, 20% each; (4) superior vena caval obstructions, 16%; (5) tracheal deviation, 12%; (6) Horner syndrome, 7%; (7) spinal cord compression, 5%; and (8) cyanosis, mediastinal widening, and hoarseness, 3% each. Twenty percent of patients were asymptomatic. Not all patients with mediastinal masses who have acute life-threatening airway complications during anesthesia are symptomatic preoperatively. Some are asymptomatic and show no airway compression on chest radiographs. Therefore, the severity of the patient's preoperative respiratory symptoms may be unrelated to the extent of respiratory or cardiovascular compromise encountered during anesthesia.[225-227]

DIAGNOSTIC EVALUATION

A careful preoperative diagnostic evaluation should be performed, even in the asymptomatic patient, to determine the extent of mediastinal pathology. A flow chart describing the preoperative evaluation of patients with mediastinal masses is shown in **Fig. 54-32**. Most patients

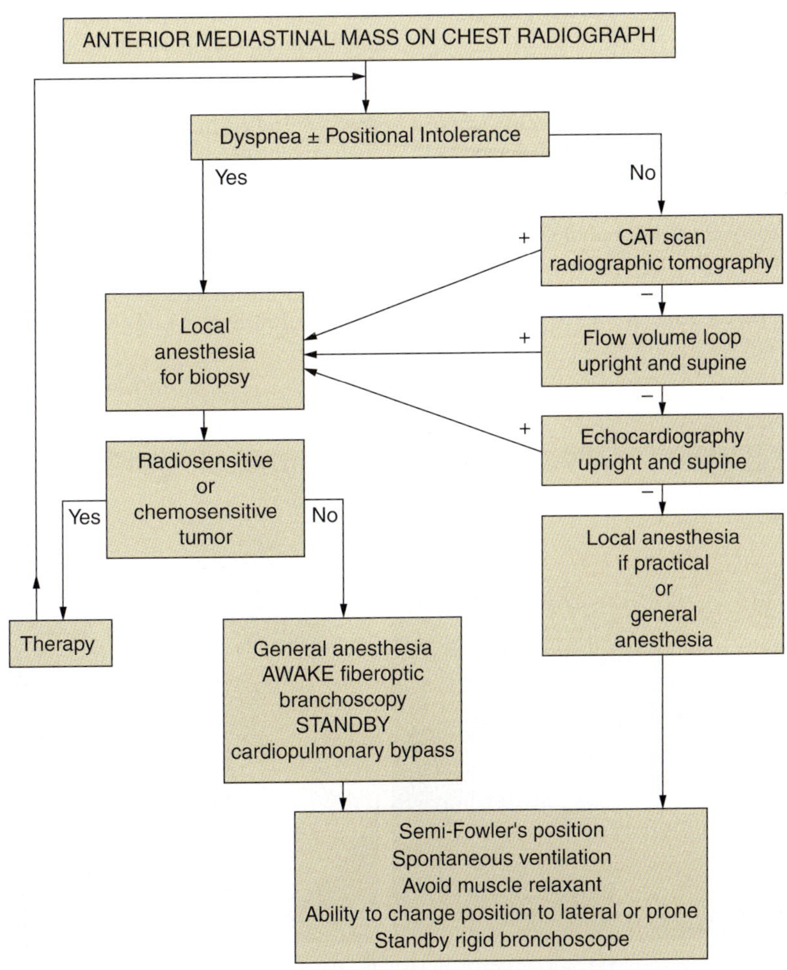

FIGURE 54-32. Flow chart describing the preoperative evaluation of the patient with an anterior mediastinal mass. +, positive finding; –, negative workup. [From Neuman GG, Weingarten AE, Abramowitz RM, et al. The anesthetic management of the patient with an anterior mediastinal mass. *Anesthesiology.* 1984;60:144.]

with mediastinal masses require scans to delineate the tumor size and location. The anesthesiologist should evaluate the extent of compression of the airway, heart, and vascular structures preoperatively.[228,229] The extent of tracheal compression is a reliable predictor of whether difficulty with the airway may be expected. In 1 series, all of the patients who developed total or near-total airway obstruction during induction or emergence from anesthesia had greater than a 50% decrease in tracheal cross-sectional area as measured on CT scan.[230]

In addition to the chest radiograph and CT scan, a series of noninvasive studies may be performed to evaluate the risk of occult airway or cardiac involvement. Upright and supine flow-volume loops are simple, noninvasive, and sensitive studies for the diagnosis of occult airway obstruction. The dynamic nature of this study makes it an extremely sensitive tool for evaluating obstructive lesions of major airways. The inspiratory limb of the flow-volume loop is useful in diagnosing extrathoracic airway obstruction, whereas the expiratory limb is sensitive to intrathoracic airway obstruction. Maximal inspiratory and expiratory flow-volume loops obtained with the patient in the upright and supine positions enable the extent of functional impairment to be quantitated and help distinguish fixed from variable intrathoracic airway obstruction.[231] A disproportionate reduction in maximal expiratory flow should alert the physician to the presence of tracheomalacia and the inherent risk of airway collapse after extubation of the trachea. In addition, echocardiography in the upright and supine positions can reveal encroachment of tumor on the heart and intrathoracic vessels. Flexible fiberoptic bronchoscopy is another method of evaluating dynamic airway obstruction (**Fig. 54-33**). It allows assessment of the functional anatomy of the entire airway and the response of the airway to variations in intrathoracic pressure and position.

Pretreatment with radiotherapy or chemotherapy to reduce the size of the tumor decreases the risk of perioperative complications. Several investigators have suggested that patients receive empiric treatment of mediastinal pathology for the presumed diagnosis.[232] Dramatic decrease in postoperative respiratory complications and improvement in risk category were achieved by preoperative radiation therapy for patients with severe clinical or radiologic findings.[233] Such views are controversial, and most clinicians advocate obtaining a biopsy before initiating therapy, even if this requires administration of general anesthesia with its inherent risks. An accurate pathologic diagnosis may be compromised if patients are empirically pretreated. In addition, the option of administering radiotherapy or chemotherapy to reduce the size of the mediastinal mass is not applicable to all patients. Some patients have large, benign mediastinal masses, such as a large dermoid cyst that cannot be managed except by surgical excision. Transcarinal aspiration of a large cystic subcarinal mass can be performed through a fiberoptic bronchoscope. This technique can be used preoperatively in patients who have cystic subcarinal masses to decrease the size of the mass before anesthetic induction. It has been reported to facilitate anesthetic management intraoperatively when a patient developed airway obstruction after induction of anesthesia.[234]

ANESTHETIC IMPLICATIONS AND MANAGEMENT

Symptomatic and asymptomatic patients are at risk of developing severe, life-threatening complications after induction of general anesthesia (**Table 54-18**). Infants and small children may have obstructive symptoms earlier than adults because their small airway size increases the magnitude of airway resistance produced by decreases in airway dimensions. To avoid the risk of complications inherent with general anesthesia, alternate diagnostic techniques can be used. Alternative methods that can be performed in awake, sedated patients include percutaneous needle aspiration of the hilum and mediastinum, mediastinotomy, and thoracoscopy.[235]

When the surgical procedure requires general anesthesia, the anesthesiologist and surgeon should discuss the plan and confirm the availability of equipment for emergency airway management (eg, fiberoptic and rigid bronchoscopes). Difficulties may occur during induction when the patient position is changed, when positive pressure is applied, after the administration of muscle relaxants, after intubation, during emergence, or after extubation. The patient should undergo a slow, controlled inhalational induction, with a staged approach that confirms an adequate airway before progressing. Induction may begin in a semirecumbent or seated position and progress to the supine position. After a deep anesthetic plane has been achieved, the anesthesiologist should attempt to gradually control ventilation. If wheezing or stridor ensues, the patient should be returned to spontaneous ventilation. If muscle relaxation is required to facilitate tracheal intubation, an ultrashort-acting relaxant such as succinylcholine should be

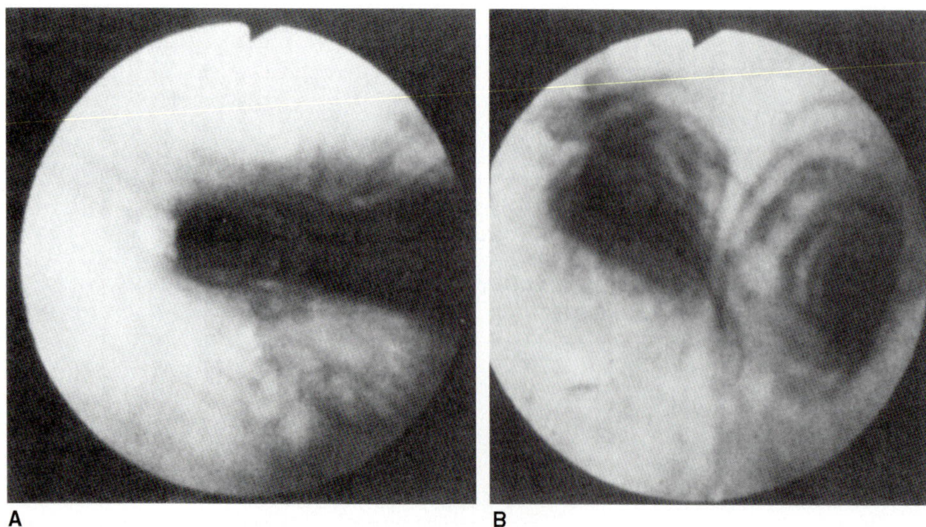

FIGURE 54-33. Fiberoptic bronchoscopic appearance of lower trachea with patient in supine position (**A**) exhibiting almost total obstruction of trachea in the anteroposterior plane. With patient in sitting position (**B**), lumen appears normal. [From Prakash UBS, Abel MD, Hubmayr RD. Mediastinal mass and tracheal obstruction during general anesthesia. *Mayo Clin Proc*. 1988;63:1004.]

TABLE 54-18 Anesthetic Guidelines for Mediastinal Mass

Indication	Biopsy or resection of mediastinal mass
Monitors	Standard monitors, arterial catheter
Anesthesia	Preferably awake, sedated using local anesthesia If general anesthesia is necessary, spontaneous ventilations should be maintained[a]
Additional equipment	Fiberoptic and rigid bronchoscope Multiple-sized endotracheal tube Standby of cardiopulmonary bypass or extracorporeal membrane oxygenation[239]
Ventilation	Spontaneous ventilation preferred Intubation does not guarantee a secure patent airway Use of flexible bronchoscope to evaluate and intubate airway
Position	As tolerated by patient (sitting, semirecumbent, or supine)
Incision	Depends on location and size of tumor Surgical options include biopsy during local anesthesia, mediastinoscopy, mediastinotomy, median sternotomy
Unique considerations	Inability to ventilate Risk of cardiovascular collapse Superior vena cava syndrome (increased risk of airway edema, bleeding, placement of IV access in lower extremity) Avoid use of muscle relaxants Maintenance of spontaneous ventilation
Intraoperative complications	Hypoxia Bleeding Hypotension Obstruction of airway
Postoperative morbidity	Airway edema, inability to extubate
Postoperative care	Monitor in intensive care environment

[a]Until one can demonstrate that controlled ventilation does not cause airway obstruction or cardiovascular instability.

used. The anesthetic technique should include the use of short-acting agents and avoidance of bolus administration of large doses of drugs. Intubation does not eliminate the risk of complications. Obstruction may even occur distal to a properly placed endotracheal tube that interferes with the normal protective glottic mechanism of physiologic PEEP that increases the tracheal distending pressure and reduces the possibility of dynamic collapse. Dynamic collapse of a tracheal segment also may occur with rapid respirations or cough during awakening from anesthesia.

Compression of the Tracheobronchial Tree Neither the presence nor the severity of the patient's preoperative respiratory symptoms reliably predicts the extent of respiratory compromise that could be encountered during anesthesia, although most patients with severe respiratory symptoms have dramatic decreases in tracheal cross-sectional area.[230] The supine position, anesthesia, and muscle paralysis are associated with decreased dimensions of the rib cage, cephalad displacement of the dome of the diaphragm, and a reduction in thoracic volume limiting the space available for the trachea.[236-238] At low lung volumes, the decreased tracheal distending pressure can lead to tracheal collapse, particularly with tracheomalacia. Spontaneous ventilation is preferred to positive-pressure ventilation because the negative intrapleural pressure of spontaneous ventilation exerts a distending force that opposes bronchial and tracheal collapse. The supine position increases the central blood volume, which can further increase tumor volume and size. Edema, bleeding, and hematoma formation in the tumor as a result of surgical biopsy also can contribute to airway compromise.

Compression of Pulmonary Artery and Heart Compression of the main pulmonary artery is relatively rare, partly because of the protective effect of the aorta. Compression of the pulmonary trunk or one of the main pulmonary arteries can result in sudden hypoxemia, hypotension, and cardiac arrest. Syncope during forced Valsalva maneuvers, such as occurs with a bowel movement, should alert the physician to the possibility of cardiovascular compression. Important factors contributing to a reduction in right ventricular output, hypotension, and severe hypoxemia include patient position, induction of anesthesia, and gravitational effects of the tumor on the heart and pulmonary artery.

SUPERIOR VENA CAVA SYNDROME

Pathophysiology Superior vena cava syndrome occurs in approximately 6% to 7% of patients with lung carcinoma. Other causes include bronchial carcinoma, malignant lymphoma, and benign conditions that include multinodular goiter, mediastinal granulomas, idiopathic mediastinal fibrosis, and catheter-induced thrombosis of the superior vena cava.[240] Obstruction of the superior vena cava impedes venous flow from the head and upper extremities. Clinical features are reviewed in **Box 54-9**. The symptoms of dyspnea, dysphasia, and stridor may be associated with ruddy complexion and dilated veins across the upper chest and neck (**Fig. 54-34**). The severity of clinical manifestations depends on the rate at which the SVC is occluded. Slow gradual obstruction is associated with mild signs and symptoms, whereas more

BOX 54-9

Clinical Features of Superior Vena Caval Syndrome

Neurologic

Headache, dizziness, decreased mentation, visual changes, restlessness, agitation, Horner syndrome, stupor, convulsions

Pathophysiology

Low cardiac output, decreased cerebral perfusion, increased cerebral venous pressure, cerebral edema

Respiratory

Shortness of breath, cough, hoarseness, hypoxemia, tachypnea, stridor

Pathophysiology

Upper airway edema, tracheal obstruction, vocal cord paralysis

Cardiac

Tachycardia; thoracic and cervical venous distention; plethoric face; edema of the face, neck, upper extremities, and trunk; cyanosis; distended veins over chest wall

Pathophysiology

Decreased venous return, development of collateral venous circulation, increased peripheral venous circulation, increased peripheral venous pressure, as high as 40 mm Hg

Gastrointestinal

Nausea, vomiting, dysphagia

Pathophysiology

Fluid imbalance, upper airway edema

Renal

Decreased urine output

Pathophysiology

Low cardiac output

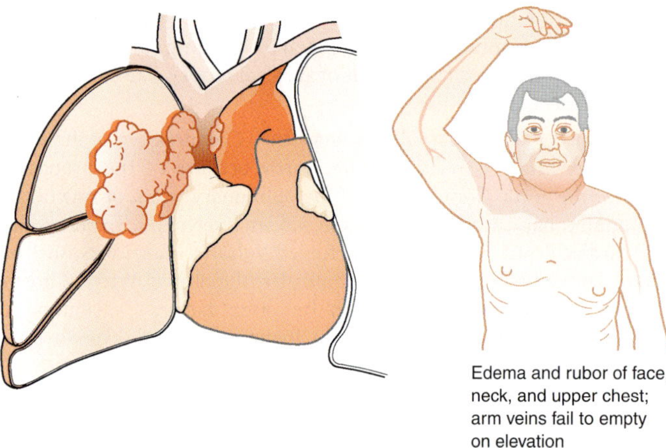

FIGURE 54-34. Bronchogenic carcinoma producing superior vena caval obstruction. Superior vena cava syndrome is characterized by edema and rubor of face, neck, and upper chest. Arm veins fail to empty on elevation.

severe symptoms occur with rapid onset of obstruction. The severity also depends on the extent of obstruction, site of obstruction (above or below the azygous vein), and integrity of the azygous venous system. Occlusion of the azygous venous system often is symptomatic and may require surgery to bypass the spinal vein and to resect the obstructing lesion.

Choice of therapy depends on etiology. Therapeutic options include radiation, chemotherapy, and thrombectomy. Once obstruction has produced complete thrombosis, thrombectomy is of little benefit. Patients having total or near total obstruction are at risk for cerebral vascular and airway compromise, both predictors of poor outcome. A tissue diagnosis should be obtained before the institution of therapy if possible. This can be done in most patients, noninvasively by bronchoscopy or lymph node biopsy. Occasionally, an open procedure requiring general anesthesia is necessary. Magnetic resonance imaging (MRI) and contrast venography are used to define the type and location of obstruction. If biopsy of the mediastinal mass is required, an open mediastinotomy should be performed instead of mediastinoscopy because the increased venous pressure increases the risk of bleeding during cervical exploration.

Anesthetic Management Patients with superior vena cava syndrome are at increased risk of airway compromise resulting from acute laryngospasm, bronchospasm, and airway edema caused by tumor edema or surgical manipulation.[241] Venous distention and symptoms are exacerbated by changes in positioning (supine or Trendelenburg) and by administration of intravenous fluids, especially through a catheter placed in the upper extremity. All venous access should be placed in the lower extremity, and an arterial catheter should be placed to monitor blood gases and blood pressure. Venous congestion increases the risk of airway compromise, bleeding, and hypotensive episodes. The preoperative evaluation should include a careful assessment of the airway. Edema of the oral pharynx, larynx, and trachea may be more severe than the external edema and swelling of the face and neck. Venous engorgement and tumor may involve the recurrent laryngeal nerve and cause external compression of the airway. These patients should be regarded in a manner similar to those with mediastinal masses. Premedication should be limited to the administration of an antisialagogue, and the patients should be transported in a semiseated position to decrease airway edema and facilitate venous drainage. If major airway edema is present, general anesthesia should be induced in a sitting position, and fiberoptic bronchoscopy may be required for airway access. Intraoperative management may be complicated by an abnormal response to the use of muscle relaxants related to a paraneoplastic myasthenic syndrome.[242] Many of these patients remain intubated postoperatively until edema of the airways and laryngeal structures is decreased.

ANESTHESIA FOR PATIENTS WITH THORACIC OUTLET SYNDROME

Thoracic outlet syndrome refers to neurologic and vascular symptoms affecting the upper extremity resulting from compression of the neurovascular bundle at the thoracic outlet between the first rib and the clavicle or between the anterior scalene muscle and the medial scalene muscle.[73,243,244] The etiology is classified either as noncancerous or cancerous.

Most noncancerous causes are related to either trauma or the presence of a cervical rib. A less frequent etiology is hypertrophy of the scalene and subclavian muscles. Clinical manifestations usually are vague and obscure, and may be misinterpreted as angina. Pain may be localized to the shoulder or extend along the medial aspect of the arm and forearm, along the proximal shoulder girdle, or to the neck and face. Symptoms may include weakness, numbness, and paresthesias. Conservative management includes rehabilitation exercises, anti-inflammatory drugs, and analgesics. In those with vascular insufficiency or if symptoms are refractory to medical therapy, operation may be indicated. Surgical approaches include resection of the first rib, partial resection of the scalene muscles, or removal of anomalous fibromuscular bands.

The presentation of lung cancer with symptoms of thoracic outlet syndrome is known as Pancoast syndrome. The most common etiology is a bronchogenic carcinoma originating in or near the superior pulmonary sulcus. These tumors invade the lymphatic system and spread by direct extension to entwine the brachial plexus intercostal arteries, stellate ganglia, and sympathetic chain, thereby producing Horner syndrome. If the tumor is considered resectable, the pulmonary tumor and extension into the chest wall and brachial plexus should be excised.

Anesthetic management includes the use of routine monitoring and may require 1-lung isolation (**Table 54-19**). The patient is placed in the lateral decubitus position, and an incision is made in the lower margin of the anterior axilla. Intraoperative complications include hemorrhage,

TABLE 54-19 Anesthetic Guidelines for Thoracic Outlet Syndrome

Indication	Therapeutic (syndrome characterized by lateral upper extremity weakness, numbness, paresthesias, pain)
Monitors	Standard monitors Noninvasive cuff on opposite side Ipsilateral pulse oximetry
Anesthesia	General anesthesia
Ventilation	Single-lumen or double-lumen endotracheal tube
Position	Supine or lateral decubitus position, determined by surgical approach
Incision	Cervical region (partial resection of first rib) Scalene muscles
Unique considerations	Intravenous access on opposite side
Intraoperative complications	Pneumothorax Pleural effusion Vascular injury Neural injury Cervical sympathectomy
Blood loss	Minimal <500 mL
Postoperative analgesia	Parenteral opiates
Postoperative morbidity	Temporary phrenic nerve palsy Pneumothorax Brachial plexus neuralgia or palsy Injury to long thoracic nerve and T1 roots
Postoperative care	Chest radiography

pneumothorax, brachial nerve injury with resulting nerve dysfunction, temporary phrenic nerve palsy, injury to the subclavian artery, and cervical sympathectomy on the ipsilateral side. Because of the position of the nondependent arm and the site of surgery, stretch and surgical trauma to the brachial plexus is a major risk.

ANESTHESIA FOR PATIENTS UNDERGOING THYMECTOMY: MYASTHENIA GRAVIS

CLINICAL FEATURES

The thymus is a central lymphoid gland that functions in the development and maintenance of immunologic competence. Surgical resection of the thymus most often is performed for myasthenia gravis and less often for primary neoplasm, carcinoid tumor, or multiple endocrine neoplasm syndrome. Seventy-five percent of the patients with myasthenia gravis have associated thymic hyperplasia or thymomas.

One-third of myasthenic patients have bulbar symptoms including difficulty swallowing and clearing secretions, which predispose to pulmonary aspiration (**Table 54-20**).

Therapy for myasthenia gravis includes anticholinesterase drugs, corticosteroids, other immunosuppressants, plasmapheresis, and thymectomy. These therapies may be used individually or in combination. Anticholinesterase drugs, such as neostigmine or pyridostigmine, most often are selected because they provide immediate symptomatic relief. These drugs inhibit the enzyme responsible for hydrolysis of acetylcholine and thereby increase the concentration of neurotransmitter at the neuromuscular junction.[245,246] Surgical resection of the thymus gland may result in complete remission or dramatic improvement in symptoms.[247]

ANESTHETIC CONSIDERATIONS

Management of anesthesia for patients with myasthenia gravis should consider the severity of symptoms, presence of other associated disorders (**Box 54-10**), and preoperative drug therapy. Considerations for the perioperative period are presented in **Table 54-21**. An assessment of preoperative pulmonary function should be obtained as a baseline for comparison. The patient's preoperative medications should be reviewed for those drugs that could interfere with neuromuscular function (**Box 54-11**). Drugs that have the potential to exacerbate muscle weakness in these patients include calcium channel blockers, aminoglycosides, and antiarrhythmic agents.[248-250] Most authors recommend that patients continue their usual dose of anticholinesterase therapy the night before surgery. On the day of operation, patients who are severely symptomatic should receive a full morning dose. Those patients who are only mildly affected should receive half a dose or none at all. The rationale for withholding the morning dose is to prevent antagonism of muscle relaxants that may be used to facilitate tracheal intubation. Patients receiving systemic steroids should continue their steroid supplementation on the day of surgery.

TABLE 54-20 Clinical Classification of Myasthenia Gravis

Stage	Term	Description
I	Ocular myasthenia	Involvement of ocular muscles only; mild symptoms of ptosis and diplopia
II	Mild to moderate generalized myasthenia	Slow onset; usually ocular, spreading to skeletal and bulbar muscles; no respiratory involvement; good response to drug
III	Acute fulminating myasthenia	Rapid onset of severe bulbar and skeletal weakness with involvement of respiratory muscles; poor response to therapy
IV	Late severe myasthenia	Severe disease developing 2 years after onset of stage I or II symptoms; poor response to therapy and poor prognosis

BOX 54-10

Disorders Associated With Myasthenia Gravis

- Thyroid disease
    - Hyperthyroidism
    - Hypothyroidism
    - Thyroiditis
- Thymoma
- Anemias pernicious
- Multiple sclerosis
- Ulcerative colitis
- Leukemia
- Lymphoma
- Autoimmune disorders
- Systemic lupus erythematosus
    - Idiopathic thrombocytopenic purpura
    - Rheumatoid arthritis
    - Scleroderma
    - Polymyositis
    - Sjögren syndrome

TABLE 54-21 Anesthetic Guidelines for Thymectomy: Myasthenia Gravis

Indication	Therapeutic (myasthenia gravis, thymoma, multiple endocrine neoplasm syndrome)
Monitors	Standard monitors
Anesthesia	General anesthesia
Preoperative considerations	Review use of anticholinesterase medications Evaluate strength Assess respiratory function
Ventilation	Usually single-lumen ETT Double-lumen ETT if by video-assisted thoracoscopic surgery
Position	Supine with shoulder roll Occasionally by left lateral decubitus (thoracoscopy)
Incision	Sternotomy, transcervical Portals for video-assisted thoracoscopic surgery
Unique considerations	Myasthenia gravis (increased sensitivity to muscle relaxants, risk of remaining intubated postoperatively, avoid neuromuscular blocking effects of antiarrhythmics, diuretics, and aminoglycosides)
Intraoperative complications	Myasthenia gravis (residual weakness or sedation leading to inability to extubate)
Blood loss	Minimal
Postoperative analgesia	Parenteral opiates, epidural
Postoperative morbidity	Respiratory insufficiency (inadequate reversal of muscle relaxants, excessive sedation, not received daily dose of anticholinesterase)
Postoperative care	Chest radiography Optimize respiratory function (analgesics, raise head of bed) Observe in monitored environment

ETT, endotracheal tube.

BOX 54-11

Drugs That Can Exacerbate Myasthenia Gravis

Acetylcholinesterase in high doses

Aminoglycosides

Other antibiotics (eg, clindamycin, colistin, polymyxin B, tetracycline, trimethaphan)

Antidysrhythmics (eg, procainamide, quinidine, propranolol, lidocaine)

Thyroid hormones

Quinine (tonic water)

Lithium

Phenytoin (Dilantin)

Oxytocin

Chlorpromazine

Chloroquine

Special attention should be given to the psychological preparation of these patients. They should be told about the increased risk of prolonged muscle weakness and respiratory depression that may uncommonly require temporary postoperative ventilation.

All patients undergoing thymectomy require general anesthesia regardless of the surgical approach. In patients undergoing a transmediastinal approach, the use of an epidural block as an adjunct to general anesthesia has been found to decrease the intraoperative MAC, lessen postoperative analgesic requirements, improve respiratory mechanics, and dramatically decrease the frequency of prolonged intubation.[251] Use of a muscle relaxant is not required but may facilitate tracheal intubation. Patients with myasthenia gravis have a marked sensitivity to nondepolarizing muscle relaxants, increasing their sensitivity and duration of action. If muscle relaxation is required, a small dose of a short-acting nondepolarizing drug such as cisatracurium should be used. Although muscle relaxation is usually less sensitive to succinylcholine in patients receiving anticholinergic therapy, its duration of action may be extended. If succinylcholine is to be used, the dose should be reduced to avoid prolongation of the response and associated phase-2 block.[251-254] Halogenated inhaled anesthetics have muscle relaxing properties. One study found that patients with myasthenia gravis were more sensitive to the neuromuscular depressant effects of isoflurane.[255] Recovery of the electromyographic response was still incomplete 1 hour after terminating isoflurane, despite satisfactory clinical recovery.

The most common surgical approaches are the transcervical and transsternal approaches; a minority of cases is performed by thoracotomy or VAT. The transcervical approach has the advantage of avoiding the immediate postoperative alterations in pulmonary mechanics.[252,256,257] Mediastinotomy may be necessary when resecting a hypertrophied thymus that extends substernally. If mediastinotomy or the cervical approach is to be used, a single-lumen tube is appropriate. Alternatively, a double-lumen endotracheal tube or bronchial blocker is indicated if lateral thoracotomy is planned.

POSTOPERATIVE CONCERNS

Improvement in myasthenic symptoms after thymectomy may take weeks to months. Therefore, the patient should receive any missed dose of anticholinesterase from the morning of operation. At the end of the operation, neuromuscular transmission is assessed using a nerve stimulator; nondepolarizing muscle relaxants are reversed. Residual weakness from an inhaled anesthetic can cause fade in the response to tetanic stimulation. Suitability for extubation is judged by measuring the patient's pulmonary function and comparing the results with preoperative values. Negative inspiratory force, tidal volume, and vital capacity should be measured immediately before induction and used as the basis for comparison. To improve respiratory mechanics, the patient is placed in a semirecumbent position with the head of the bed raised about 30 degree, is suctioned for secretions, and receives adequate analgesia without inducing respiratory depression. The patient should be monitored closely for 18 to 24 hours after operation. A chest radiograph is obtained immediately postoperatively to rule out the presence of a pneumothorax.

ANESTHESIA FOR PATIENTS UNDERGOING TRACHEAL RESECTION AND TRACHEOBRONCHIAL RECONSTRUCTION

Indications for tracheal resection include

- Tracheal tumors, most of which are malignant
- Carinal tumors or carinal involvement with a bronchogenic carcinoma
- Tracheal involvement with a thyroid carcinoma
- Traumatic disruption of the trachea and bronchi, which may occur as a result of blunt trauma, penetrating injuries, iatrogenic manipulations, and aspirated sharp foreign bodies
- Tracheal stenosis after prolonged intubation, trauma, etc

Patients undergoing surgical resection of the trachea, main bronchi, or both impose special anesthetic management problems. The surgical procedure often is prolonged, and episodes of ventilatory insufficiency may be unavoidable. Communication between the anesthesia and surgical teams, with emphasis on the ventilatory treatment of the patient during each phase of the procedure, is imperative. The most challenging aspect of these procedures is to design an effective method of ventilating the lungs during the resection and reconstruction of the airway that does not interfere with surgical exposure and that provides adequate ventilation and oxygenation. Patients with large intratracheal or carinal masses may develop total airway obstruction on the induction of anesthesia. Fortunately, many of these patients undergo laser debulking procedures before undergoing surgical resection. Because an inflated cuff and positive-pressure ventilation adjacent to the suture line may interfere with healing or cause disruption of the anastomosis, after the procedure the patient should breathe spontaneously and be extubated in the operating room or shortly thereafter.

Surgical techniques may include resection and primary anastomosis, resection, and reconstruction with prosthetic material or with the insertion of a T-tube stent.

Therapeutic adjuncts may include radiotherapy (preoperatively or postoperatively), radioactive seed implantation, and preoperative laser debulking.

SURGICAL CONSIDERATIONS

Surgery on the trachea and bronchi usually is done through a right thoracotomy to avoid the aortic arch, although if the left bronchus is involved or a left pulmonary resection may be done, a left thoracotomy may be performed. The surgical procedure requires extensive hilar dissection, mobilization of the lungs, and possibly opening of the pericardium. The omentum, serratus muscle, or intercostal muscle may have to be used to wrap the anastomosis or to cover defects in the tracheobronchial tree. Mobilization of the omentum requires an additional abdominal incision. Thoracoabdominal exposure substantially increases fluid requirements. On occasion, pericardium may be used to patch sections of the pulmonary artery involved with tumor. Every effort should be made to maintain normothermia and minimize heat loss. After the procedure, to decrease tension on the anastomosis, it may be necessary to maintain the patient's neck in a flexed position by suturing the skin and soft tissues of the chin to the anterior chest wall. Even in this situation, it is advantageous to extubate the trachea as soon as possible after surgery to minimize airway pressures. Therefore, the anesthetic should be planned with the goal of rapid emergence and recovery from muscle relaxants. Thorough suctioning of the tracheobronchial tree, via a fiberoptic bronchoscope if indicated, should be performed immediately before emergence from anesthesia.

Postoperative complications, particularly pulmonary infections and air leaks through the airway anastomosis, can lead to the development of a bronchopleural fistula and respiratory failure. Factors that predispose to poor healing of the tracheobronchial anastomosis include cancer, previous steroid and antineoplastic chemotherapy, preoperative radiotherapy, extensive dissection and devascularization of the tracheobronchial stump, and poor nutritional status and debilitation. In selecting the technique for airway management, the anesthesiologist should consider the need to provide appropriate surgical conditions. Constant cooperation and communication between the surgical and anesthesia team are extremely important during these procedures.

PERIOPERATIVE MANAGEMENT ISSUES

Preoperative Assessment and Preparation Patients should be evaluated for airway patency and cardiopulmonary reserve. Unless airway obstruction is imminent, requiring emergency surgery, pulmonary function studies should be obtained (**Figs. 54-35 and 54-36**). Flow-volume loops are very helpful in detecting fixed or variable intrathoracic or extrathoracic obstructions. Most of these patients have serious underlying pulmonary disease that may further compromise gas exchange intraoperatively and postoperatively. Reversible conditions that alter pulmonary function should be managed with antibiotics and bronchodilators preoperatively. All considerations that apply to patients with airway obstruction resulting from extrinsic compression by mediastinal masses also apply to patients with intrinsic obstruction of the airways. Preoperative ABG values should be obtained. Mucosal edema frequently contributes to airway obstruction in these patients, and preoperative steroids and diuretics may be beneficial.

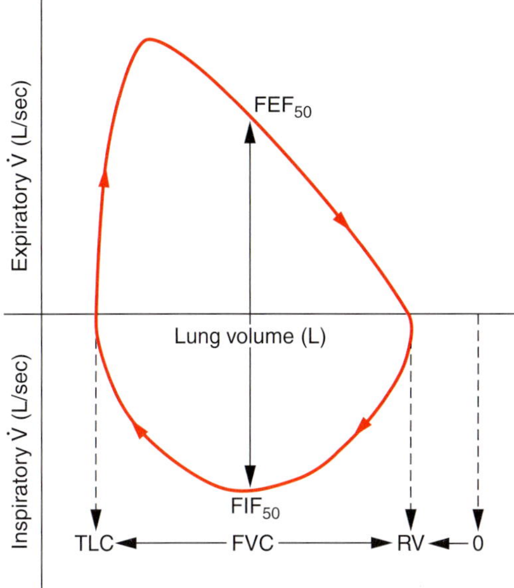

FIGURE 54-35. Idealized flow-volume loop. During forced expiration, the rate of airflow increases rapidly at volume close to TLC. As lung volume decreases, flow progressively falls in a near-linear fashion caused by increasing airway resistance. With maximum inspiratory effort, flow normally peaks at a lung volume near the midportion of FVC. At midpoint lung volume, the forced inspiratory flow (FIF_{50}) and forced expiratory flow (FEF_{50}) should normally be equal. When the ratio (FIF_{50}/FEF_{50}) is less than unity, it suggests an extrathoracic obstruction, compromising inspiratory flow. If greater than 1, it supports a diagnosis of intrathoracic airway obstruction.

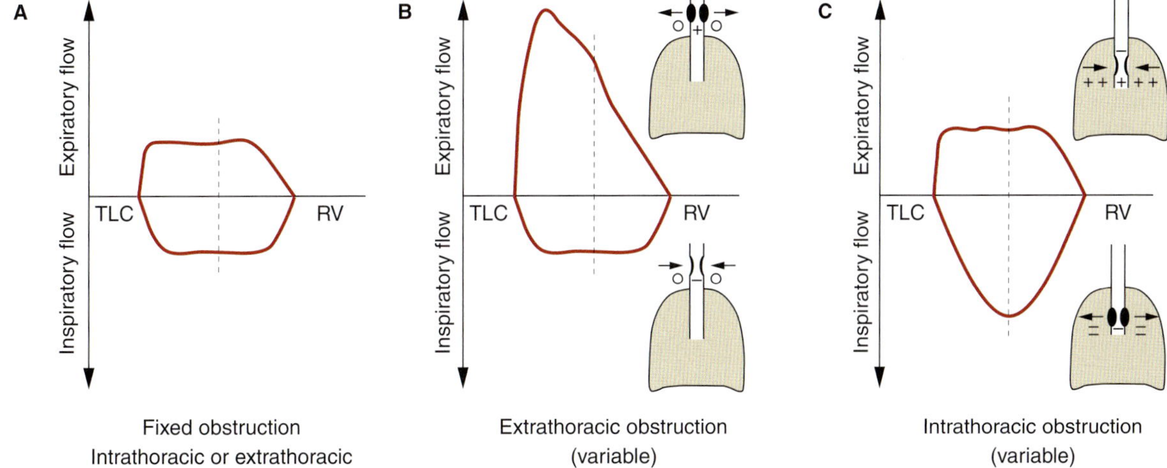

FIGURE 54-36. Maximal inspiratory and expiratory flow-volume curves in fixed obstruction (intrathoracic or extrathoracic), in which airway diameter does not change with inspiration or expiration, extrathoracic variable obstruction, or intrathoracic variable obstruction. The dotted line indicates 50% of the vital capacity; the ratio of expired-to-inspired flow at this point is the mid-VC ratio and is normally 0.9 to 1.0. **A.** With a fixed obstruction, expiratory and inspiratory flows are equally altered, and the mid-VC ratio remains normal. **B.** With a variable extrathoracic obstruction, forced expiration results in a slightly positive (+) intratracheal pressure that is greater than the pressure around the airway (atmospheric or 0), resulting in a decrease of the obstruction (airway dilates). During forced inspiration, when pressure around the airway (0) exceeds the intratracheal pressure (–), the obstruction is increased (airway narrows). Because the expiratory curve is normal and the inspiratory curve is altered, the mid-VC ratio is much greater than normal. **C.** With a variable intrathoracic obstruction, forced expiration results in a very positive (++) pleural pressure that is greater than the slightly positive (+) intratracheal pressure, resulting in an increase of the obstruction (airway narrows). During forced inspiration, the intratracheal pressure (–) is greater than the pleural pressure (– –), thus decreasing the obstruction (airway dilates). Because the inspiratory curve is normal and the expiratory curve is attenuated, the mid-VC ratio is much less than normal. Normal flow-volume curve (**A**) is a composite of the inspiratory curve in **B** and the expiratory curve in **C**. TLC, total lung capacity; RV, residual volume. [Benumof JL. Anesthesia for special elective therapeutic procedures. In: Benumof JL, ed. *Anesthesia for Thoracic Surgery*. Philadelphia, PA: WB Saunders; 1995.]

Induction of Anesthesia Induction of anesthesia follows the same guidelines as discussed in the section on anesthesia for patients with mediastinal masses. The anesthesiologist should know precisely the site and the size of the lesion and the extent of airway lumen compromise before induction of anesthesia. The anesthesiologist should review the chest radiographs, tomograms, CT scans, flow-volume loops, and results of bronchoscopy or bronchography preoperatively. A skilled endoscopist usually can pass a small-diameter ventilating bronchoscope past the lesion, allowing ventilation of at least 1 lung. Once ventilation and oxygenation have been satisfactorily established, intubation of the trachea may be attempted, perhaps over a stylet introduced via the rigid bronchoscope.

Modes of Ventilation The major challenge during operation for tracheobronchial resection and reconstruction is the maintenance of ventilation. The options include (1) a single-lumen endotracheal tube; (2) a single endobronchial tube or 2 endobronchial tubes, 1 into each mainstem bronchus distal to the area of resection; (3) low-frequency jet ventilation; (4) high-frequency ventilation to 1 or both lungs, above the site of the lesion; or (5) cardiopulmonary bypass through the femoral approach during resection of the carina.[258,259] Because of the risk of intrapulmonary hemorrhage with heparinization, cardiopulmonary bypass should be used only in selected patients when absolutely necessary.

Use of Conventional Ventilation for Tracheobronchial Reconstruction When planning to use conventional ventilation during tracheobronchial reconstructive surgery, the anesthesiologist should have several different sizes of armored endotracheal tubes available, some of them still sterile. A long, sterile anesthesia circuit is required because it often is necessary for the surgeon to intubate the trachea or bronchus within the sterile field. Airway management depends on the location of the lesion and its distance from the carina.

Resection of a High Tracheal Lesion A single-lumen, uncut endotracheal tube is placed above the tracheal lesion after induction of general anesthesia. If the obstruction is mild or if the area of obstruction can be bypassed, mechanical positive-pressure ventilation is safe. The surgeon may help guide the endotracheal tube past the area of stenosis when the trachea is open. Alternatively, a sterile tube can be passed through the field into the distal trachea after the trachea has been transsected below the lesion. That tube is then connected, via sterile anesthesia hoses and Y piece, to the anesthesia machine. Armored endotracheal tubes should be used to decrease the possibility of kinking and obstruction. If the distal segment of the trachea is short, the tip of the endotracheal tube can be cut distal to the cuff to allow the tube to remain above the carina (**Fig. 54-37**).

Repair of a high tracheal lesion usually is done through a cervical incision, possibly combined with a median sternotomy. After excision of the tracheal lesion and placement of the posterior tracheal suture line, the distal endotracheal or endobronchial tube is removed from the trachea. The proximal endotracheal tube then is advanced past the anastomotic lines and reconnected to the anesthesia circuit, and the anastomosis is completed.

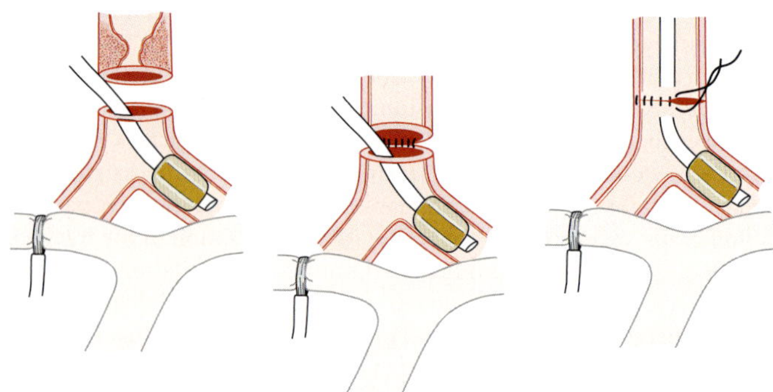

FIGURE 54-38. Procedure for resection of lower tracheal lesions. [Modified from Geffin B, Bland J, Grillo HC, et al. Anesthetic management of tracheal resection and reconstruction. *Anesth Analg.* 1969;48:884.]

Resection of a Low Tracheal Lesion This usually is performed through a right thoracotomy incision. A single-lumen endotracheal tube is placed with its tip above the lesion. If sufficient length of trachea distal to the area of resection is available, a Foley catheter with its tip removed just distal to the balloon may be used as a single-lumen endotracheal tube. It is inserted by the surgeon and maintained in place above the carina, thereby avoiding endobronchial intubation and the need for 1-lung ventilation. If the distal tracheal stump is very short, the tube should be advanced into the bronchus of the dependent (usually the left) lung. If oxygenation is inadequate, the shunt can be decreased by temporarily clamping the pulmonary artery of the nondependent side (**Fig. 54-38**).[260,261] When the posterior tracheal suture line has been completed, the distal endobronchial tube or Foley catheter is removed, and the original orotracheal tube is advanced across the suture line into the bronchus of the dependent lung. The anterior suture line then is completed. The endotracheal tube is then pulled proximally so that its tip lies above the suture line.

For carinal resection, a single-lumen endotracheal tube is inserted through the larynx (**Fig. 54-39**). After the carina is resected, the surgeon places a second endotracheal tube into the bronchus of the dependent lung, usually the left. The tube is connected by a set of sterile anesthesia

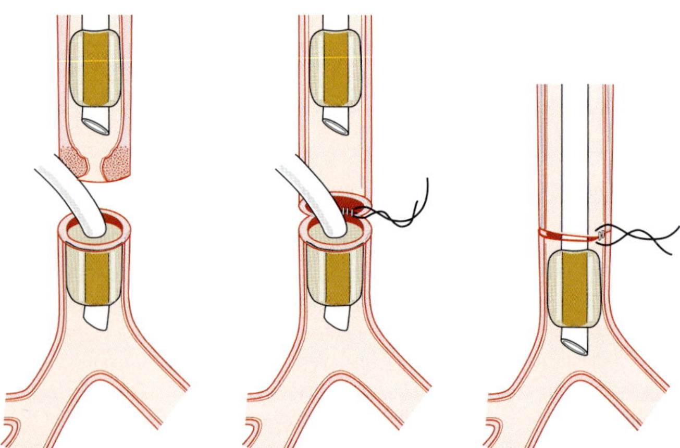

FIGURE 54-37. Procedure for resection of high tracheal lesion. [Modified from Geffin B, Bland J, Grillo HC, et al. Anesthetic management of tracheal resection and reconstruction. *Anesth Analg.* 1969;48:884.]

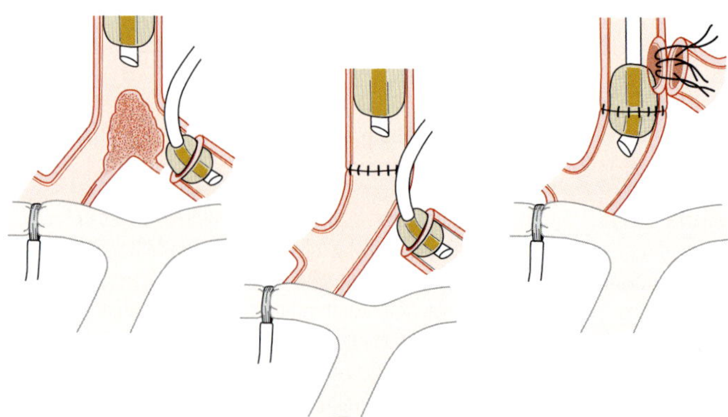

FIGURE 54-39. Procedure for resection of carinal lesions. [Modified from Geffin B, Bland J, Grillo HC, et al. Anesthetic management of tracheal resection and reconstruction. *Anesth Analg.* 1969;48:884.]

hoses and Y piece to the anesthesia machine. The left lung is ventilated through the endobronchial tube, whereas the right lung is collapsed as the right bronchus is attached to the trachea. After the right mainstem bronchus has been reattached to the trachea, the original translaryngeal endotracheal tube is advanced past the suture line into the right mainstem bronchus. Cutting the tip of this endotracheal tube helps to prevent obstruction of the right upper-lobe bronchus. The left endobronchial tube then is removed, and the left mainstem bronchus is attached to the trachea by an end-to-side anastomosis. The endotracheal tube then is pulled proximally so that its tip is above both anastomotic lines.

Alternatively, after the carina is resected, the anesthesiologist can independently ventilate each lung through the distal bronchial stumps. The surgeon places a single-lumen endotracheal tube into each bronchial stump. A plastic Y connector is used to deliver the tidal volume to both endotracheal tubes. A good air seal can be achieved by using stay sutures to pull the bronchial stump against the distal end of the inflated cuff. As the posterior layer of the anastomosis is performed, ventilation is maintained through the accessible distal bronchi. To attach the lateral wall of a bronchus to the trachea, the corresponding endobronchial tube is removed and 1-lung ventilation is used for a limited period. As the anastomosis of the anterior wall nears completion, ventilation from above is restored. The remaining air leak will progressively diminish as the incision is closed. If the air leak is too large, the proximal translaryngeal endotracheal tube may be passed across the anastomotic line into the distal bronchus for short periods. When the anastomosis of 1 side is complete, that side then is ventilated and the other endobronchial tube is removed to allow surgical access. Once the second anastomosis is complete, ventilation through the trachea is reestablished. Airway stents may be left in the trachea postoperatively to maintain airway patency.

Low-Frequency Jet Ventilation/Low-Frequency Interrupted High-Flow Ventilation Low-frequency jet ventilation has been used to maintain ventilation during tracheal resection.[262,263] Intermittent O_2 jets at a rate of 10 to 20 breaths/min with a pressure of 40 to 60 psi are delivered into the lungs via a small-bore catheter inserted through the endotracheal tube.[262] The pressure is regulated to produce adequate chest expansion and oxygenation. After the tracheal anastomosis is complete, the catheter is removed and the endotracheal tube above the suture line is used conventionally.

High-Frequency Ventilation High-frequency positive-pressure ventilation (HFPPV) usually uses a respiratory rate of 60 to 100 breaths/min administered with a volume-cycled ventilator. It does not depend on gas entrainment. Inspiration is active and expiration is passive. HFJV uses jet pulsations at a rate of 100 to 400 breaths/min. It depends on gas entrainment. Again, inspiration is active, and expiration is passive. Several reports have described the successful use of HFPPV or HFJV in the treatment of patients having tracheobronchial reconstructions.[264-267]

HFJV depends on gas entrainment for adequate ventilation and can result in distal aspiration of blood and tumor debris. With HFPPV, a continuous flow of gas occurs to the outside, which protects against distal aspiration of blood and debris. HFPPV provides adequate oxygenation and ventilation by the generation of eddy flows in the airway. It may lead to improved distribution of gas flow compared with conventional mechanical ventilation. Airway pressure during HFPPV is continuously positive. Intrapleural pressure is continuously subatmospheric, with minimal effect on pulmonary and systemic hemodynamics. The principal advantage of HFPPV in tracheobronchial resection is the ability to deliver ventilation through small catheters located either free in the airway or passed through standard endotracheal tubes. These catheters provide less interference with the surgical technique than standard single-lumen or double-lumen endotracheal tubes do. In addition, as soon as the lesion is resected, jet ventilation catheters can be passed into 1 or both bronchi, providing independent ventilation to both lungs.

HFPPV is likely to be beneficial in patients undergoing (1) carinal resections, (2) sleeve pneumonectomies or sleeve upper-lobe resections, (3) tracheal reconstruction supported by Montgomery T-tubes, and (4) tracheal resections (**Fig. 54-40**). For left-sided sleeve pneumonectomy, endobronchial intubation, with a small catheter passed through an endotracheal tube, provides the surgeon with an unobstructed field of vision. The catheter is passed through the operative field and guided by the surgeon into the left mainstem bronchus. The continuous outflow of gas through the open bronchus during HFPPV minimizes soiling with blood. Ventilation of the right lung with HFPPV via a thin catheter inside the right main bronchus eliminates the problem of right upper lobe collapse associated with the use of right-sided endobronchial tubes.

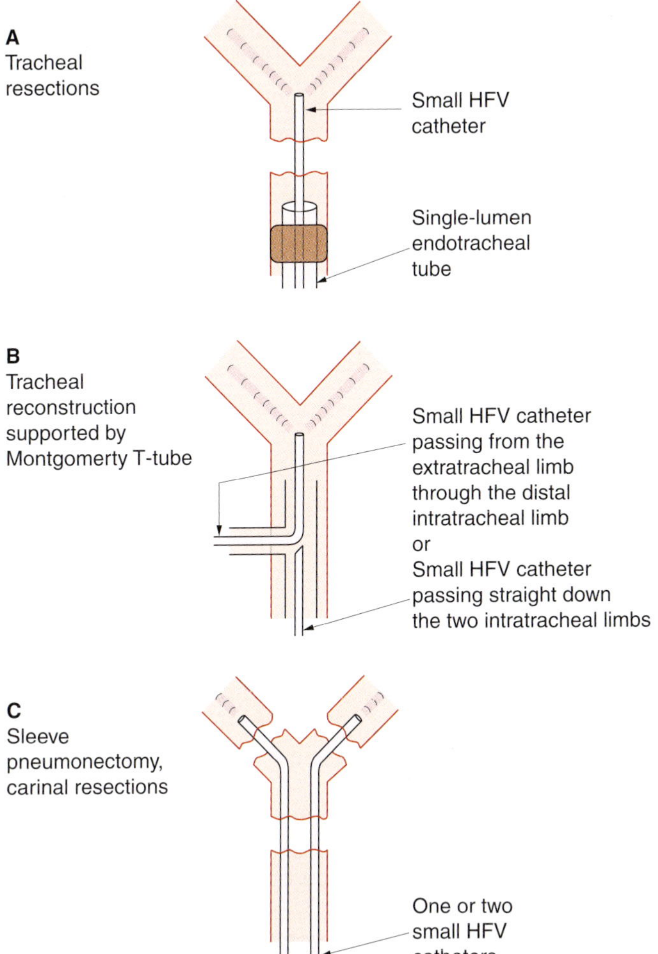

FIGURE 54-40. The 3 types of airway surgery aided by small high-frequency ventilation (HFV) are tracheal resections, tracheal reconstructions that require support by a Montgomery T-tube, and carinal procedures (sleeve pneumonectomy, carinal resections). With tracheal resections (**A**), a simple HFV catheter can be passed beyond the point of airway interruption, but above the tracheal carina, and used to ventilate both lungs with HFV. With tracheal reconstructions supported by a Montgomery T-tube (**B**), the small HFV catheter can be passed from either the extraluminal limb or from the proximal intraluminal tracheal limb to the distal intraluminal tracheal limb and can be used to ventilate both lungs with HFV. With carinal procedures (**C**), 1 or 2 HFV catheters can be passed into 1 or both of the mainstem bronchi and can be used to ventilate 1 or both of the lungs with HFV. [From Benumof JL. High-frequency and high-flow apneic ventilation during thoracic surgery. In: Benumof JL, ed. *Anesthesia for Thoracic Surgery*. Philadelphia, PA: WB Saunders; 1995.]

Carinal resection has been performed using 2 high-frequency jet ventilators and 2 catheters, 1 into each bronchus, to provide independent ventilation to both lungs (**Fig. 54-41**).[264] This is particularly advantageous when a large carinal tumor dramatically obstructs 1 or both bronchi, preventing delivery of adequate tidal volume to either lung. In this situation, a catheter is passed into 1 or both bronchi under fiberoptic bronchoscope

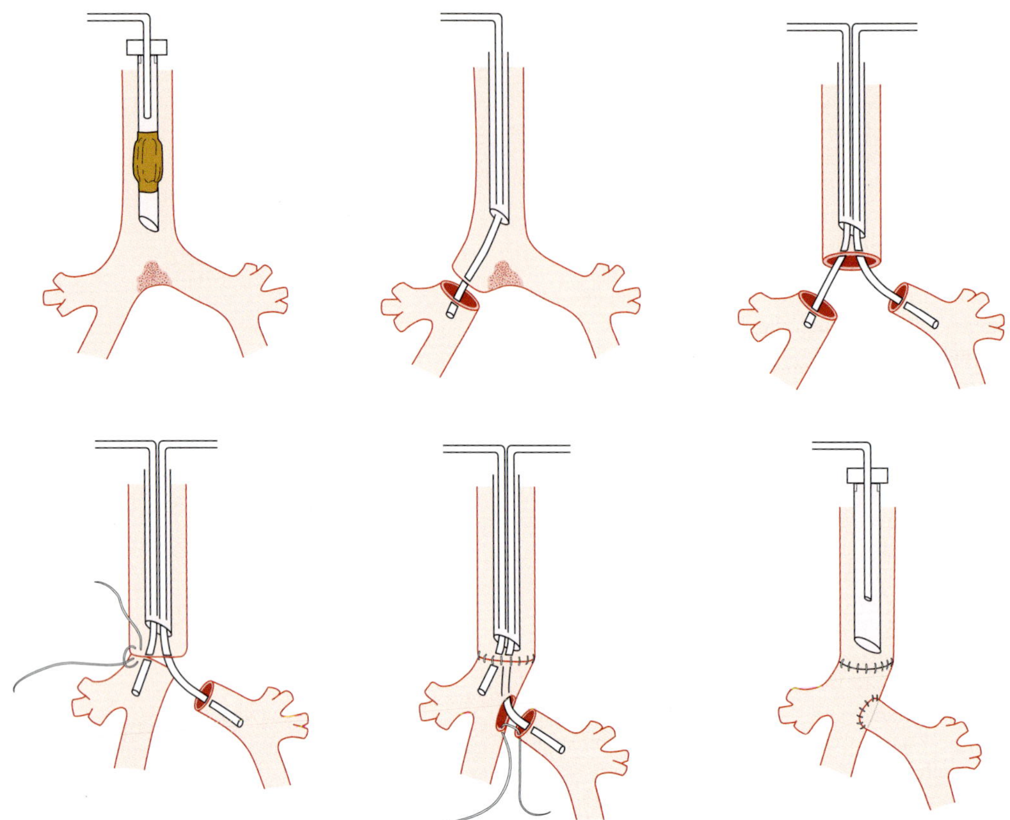

FIGURE 54-41. Arrangement of the HFJV catheters during the different phases of the operation. At the end of the right tracheobronchial anastomosis, the left catheter passes between 2 membranous sutures. It is then withdrawn and introduced into the left main bronchus via the bronchotomy of the right middle bronchus. [Modified from Crinquette V, Wurtz A, Leroy S, et al. Resection et reconstruction de la bifurcation tracheale sous jet ventilation a haute frequence, separee sur les deux poumons. *Ann Chir.* 1989;43:673.]

guidance. The presence of even two HFJV catheters through the surgical field does not interfere with surgical exposure.

Patients with major tracheal stenosis may not accommodate a large enough endotracheal tube to permit adequate ventilation. Several solutions exist for this problem. First, a special long endotracheal tube that has a small internal diameter can be used; for example, a long 5-mm oral endotracheal tube may pass through the tracheal lesion. Ventilation of an adult through such a small endotracheal tube requires high proximal airway pressures and may not be effective. Second, HFPPV with a small catheter passed through the stenotic area can be used. The anesthesiologist should ensure that enough space exists between the stenotic lesion and the catheter to allow for the adequate outflow of gas; otherwise, barotrauma will occur. Third, the surgeon first can perform laser resection of the stenotic lesion to increase airway diameter.

HFPPV also facilitates tracheal reconstruction supported by a Montgomery tracheal T-tube.[268] The Montgomery tracheal T-tube is used as a stent to maintain the patency of the upper airway in patients with subglottic and upper tracheal stenosis. The intraluminal limb also maintains the circumference of the airway and supports the tissue graft applied during the reconstruction of the larynx and cervical trachea. Because of the design and shape of the Montgomery endotracheal tube, it is difficult to establish an adequate airway for the administration of conventional mechanical ventilation. The use of the extraluminal limb as an airway for delivery of large tidal volumes is associated with a large gas leak through the open upper intraluminal limb and around the uncuffed tracheal limb. This can be circumvented by 2 methods. Occlusion of the superior part of the intraluminal limb can decrease the air leak. The occlusion can be accomplished with a Fogarty embolectomy catheter or with a tight pharyngeal pack. Alternatively, the anesthesiologist can perform translaryngeal intubation of the upper intraluminal limb with a small, cuffed endotracheal tube. Occlusion of the extraluminal limb then allows the use of positive-pressure ventilation.[269]

HFPPV through a catheter with a 2-mm internal diameter can provide adequate alveolar ventilation and oxygenation during tracheal reconstruction with a tracheal T-tube. The T-tube and open trachea around it function as expiratory ports for the continuous outflow of gas. If the patient already has a tracheal T-tube in place before operation, translaryngeal intubation of the intraluminal limb and trachea can be easily accomplished with the small HFPPV catheter. Alternatively, the catheter can be introduced through the extraluminal limb and gently flexed to direct the catheter to lie above the carina.[266]

Differential lung ventilation with HFJV has been used in patients undergoing tracheobronchial reconstructive surgery, such as pneumonectomy, sleeve lobectomies, and tracheal reconstruction, and who have compromised pulmonary reserve. For example, a patient undergoing a right upper sleeve lobectomy is ventilated through an endotracheal tube until resection of the right bronchus and the right upper lobe begins. The endotracheal tube then is advanced into the left mainstem bronchus, and unilateral intermittent positive-pressure ventilation (IPPV) is continued to the left lung. At the same time, HFJV is delivered to the right intermediate bronchus to ventilate the residual right, middle, and lower lobes and thereby maintain better oxygenation.

ANESTHESIA FOR PATIENTS UNDERGOING URGENT SURGERY

ANESTHESIA FOR PATIENTS WITH MASSIVE HEMOPTYSIS

Therapeutic Approaches Massive hemoptysis is an uncommon but life-threatening event that requires rapid management. Massive hemoptysis

BOX 54-12

Causes of Massive Hemoptysis

Infection
Tuberculosis
Bronchiectasis
Bronchitis
Lung abscess
Necrotizing pneumonia
Neoplasm
Bronchogenic carcinoma
Metastatic carcinoma
Mediastinal tumor
Endobronchial polyp
Cardiovascular disease
Mitral stenosis
Pulmonary arteriovenous malformation
Pulmonary embolus
Pulmonary vasculitis
Miscellaneous causes
Pulmonary artery catheterization
Exploratory needling
Cystic fibrosis
Pulmonary contusion, laceration
Reperfusion of pulmonary vasculature after pulmonary embolectomy and after cardiopulmonary bypass

From Benumof L. *Anesthesia for Thoracic Surgery*. Philadelphia, PA: WB Saunders; 1987.

TABLE 54-22 Anesthetic Guidelines for Patients With Massive Hemoptysis

Indication	Hemoptysis
Monitors	Standard monitors, arterial catheter
Anesthesia	General anesthesia
Additional equipment	Shoulder roll or bean bag
Ventilation	Double-lumen endotracheal tube (if possible)
Position	Lateral decubitus, supine
Incision	Thoracotomy, median sternotomy
Unique considerations	Frequently hypoxic; "full stomach" precautions, hypotensive, tachycardic Infectious precautions Type and cross for blood products Check coagulation status
Intraoperative complications	Hypoxia Hypotension Hemorrhage Dysrhythmia Syndrome of inappropriate antidiuretic hormone secretion Possibility of extensive lung resection
Blood loss	Variable >500 mL
Analgesia	Epidural thoractomy
Postoperative morbidity	Respiratory insufficiency Aspiration pneumonia Hemoptysis Acute respiratory distress syndrome Hypoxia
Postoperative care	Chest radiography Monitor in intensive care environment

refers to bleeding that ranges from greater than 200 mL during 1 episode to 1000 mL within 24 hours.[270-272] The most common associated diseases are tuberculosis, bronchiectasis, lung abscesses, and lung cancer (**Box 54-12**). The cause of hemoptysis is either direct invasion by infection or tumor into blood vessels or trauma (eg, bleeding after use of a pulmonary artery catheter). Patients at increased risk for perforation of the pulmonary artery by a pulmonary artery catheter include those with pulmonary hypertension, hypothermia, or coagulopathy.[273]

Death from hemoptysis usually results from asphyxia but rarely from exsanguination. The most effective way to stop bleeding from pulmonary sources is definitive pulmonary resection. The site of bleeding can be identified with either a rigid or flexible bronchoscope. Rigid bronchoscopy is preferred because it provides more access for suctioning of blood and removal of clots. The endoscopist may perform therapeutic interventions by the administration of topical saline, vasoconstrictors, laser therapy, or placement of a balloon-tipped Fogarty catheter. Alternative management includes transcatheter embolization of the bronchial and intercostal arteries, but this risks embolization of the spinal cord via collateral circulation. The placement of a pulmonary artery catheter under fluoroscopic guidance may be used in conjunction with other therapies to decrease bleeding by occluding the branch of the pulmonary artery feeding the bleeding site.

Anesthetic Management Management strategies are presented in **Table 54-22**. Patients with massive hemoptysis often are hemodynamically unstable as a result of hypovolemia and hypoxia. They require resuscitation with a large-bore intravenous catheter for rapid infusion of fluids to restore cardiac preload, blood products to correct any coagulopathies, and vasoactive drugs. If time permits, an arterial catheter should be placed for monitoring of blood pressure and arterial blood gases. One of the major goals is to isolate the source of bleeding to prevent contamination of the healthy lung and prevent further hypoxia.

Patients with massive hemoptysis are at grave risk for aspiration. These patients should undergo either awake intubation or rapid sequence induction followed by tracheal intubation during cricoid pressure. The use of ketamine or etomidate for induction of anesthesia may be indicated because the patients are hypovolemic and at risk for cardiovascular collapse. Intubation may be complicated by blood in the airway, obscuring laryngeal structures. Suctioning may be unable to provide adequate visualization. Air bubbles exiting the trachea may serve as the only guide to the site of the glottic orifice. Choice of endotracheal tube depends on the proposed management. Lung separation is best accomplished by placement of a left double-lumen endotracheal tube, but it may be technically difficult in emergency situations. If the bleeding is from the left side, a single-lumen tube can be blindly advanced into the right mainstem bronchus. If bleeding originates from the right side, intubation of the left mainstem bronchus may be guided with the assistance of a fiberoptic bronchoscope.

If definitive surgical intervention is required, the patient is placed in a lateral decubitus position for resection of the bleeding lung segment. Placement of the bleeding lung in a nondependent position mandates complete separation of the lungs to prevent soilage of the dependent nonbleeding lung. Aggressive suctioning of the tracheobronchial tree improves ventilation and oxygenation of the dependent nonbleeding lung. At the end of operation, the double-lumen endotracheal tube should be left in place, and the patient should be mechanically ventilated. Patients should be observed for recurrent bleeding and impaired oxygen exchange during the early postoperative period.

ANESTHESIA FOR PATIENTS UNDERGOING REMOVAL OF A FOREIGN BODY FROM THE AIRWAYS

Aspiration of foreign bodies is a common problem, particularly in children, and is associated with considerable morbidity and mortality rates.[29] In adults, acute alcoholism, dementia, bulbar muscle dysfunction, and previous history of aspiration are common predisposing factors.[158,274,275] The location of the aspirated object depends on the patient's posture at the time of aspiration. The right lung most often is involved because the axis of the right mainstem bronchus is more in line with the trachea. If the patient is upright at the time of aspiration, the right lower lobe most frequently is affected. The right upper lobe most often is involved in patients in the supine position.

More than 80% of the aspirated foreign bodies are organic material. Organic material, particularly peanuts and other nuts, produce severe mucosal irritation and swelling around the foreign body. The clinical sequelae of foreign body aspiration include acute airway obstruction, atelectasis, inflammation, pneumonia, and abscess formation (**Fig. 54-42**). The foreign body may act as a one-way valve, resulting in air trapping and regional hyperinflation.

Clinical Features and Diagnosis Acute signs and symptoms of aspiration include cough, wheezing, dyspnea, stridor, fever, cyanosis, and hemoptysis. Alternatively, there may be a history of recurrent or intractable pneumonia, unexplained atelectasis, or emphysema.[158,275] Physical examination may reveal unilateral decreased air entry, unilateral localized wheezing, or aphonia.[158,275,276] Most foreign bodies are radiolucent but are associated with an abnormal chest radiograph. Findings may include atelectasis, localized hyperinflation, pneumonia, or mediastinal shift.[274]

Therapeutic Approach The urgency of proceeding to bronchoscopy is dictated by the severity of the patient's respiratory distress. If the object is in the larynx or the proximal trachea, it causes considerably more distress and is associated with greater mortality than objects lodged more peripherally.[277] Foreign bodies are removed within the first 24 hours to avoid dislodging them into a more critical position and to decrease the incidence of secondary pneumonia. If possible, removal should be delayed long enough to allow for gastric emptying and patient preparation.[267] Use of bronchodilators, postural drainage, and chest physiotherapy to dislodge and expel the foreign body is contraindicated. These procedures occasionally resulted in total airway obstruction and cardiac arrest and are no longer recommended.[278,279]

Bronchoscopy for removal of the foreign body is successful about 95% of the time, but may need to be repeated either because the foreign body was not found initially or because it was incompletely removed.[278,279] Fluoroscopic guidance during bronchoscopy can aid in the removal of small radiopaque objects.[280] Rarely, thoracotomy is necessary for retrieval of the foreign body.

Anesthetic Management The anesthetic management depends on the patient's age, presence of a full stomach, the severity of respiratory distress, and the location of the foreign body. All patients should be premedicated with an anticholinergic to decrease airway secretions, H_2-antagonists to decrease gastric acid secretion, and metoclopramide to promote gastric emptying (**Table 54-23**). The endoscopist should be prepared for immediate rigid bronchoscopy in case of total airway obstruction.

Adults receive preoxygenation, intravenous induction, and direct laryngoscopy. A technique of intravenous anesthesia would address the concerns of providing adequate doses of inhaled agents. If the foreign body is in the larynx, it often can be removed during direct laryngoscopy, and the patient is allowed to emerge from anesthesia. A foreign body in the trachea or the bronchus requires rigid or fiberoptic bronchoscopy for removal. When a rigid bronchoscope is introduced into the airway, its ventilating side arm is attached to the anesthesia circuit to provide O_2 and inhaled anesthesia. The use of a helium-O_2 mixture can be helpful in patients with partial airway obstruction because the decreased density of the inhaled mixture decreases turbulence and improves flow across the stenotic airway. The maximal effect is obtained with a helium-O_2 mixture of 80% to 20%, but helium also is therapeutic when used in lesser concentrations. After the trachea is intubated, a large-bore nasal or oral gastric tube is inserted into the stomach, and the gastric contents are thoroughly suctioned.

Children are more difficult to manage because of their small airway, which makes them more susceptible to major airway obstruction. In children with severe respiratory distress, the risks of total airway obstruction that can occur during rapid-sequence induction should be weighed against the risk of aspiration during a slow inhalation induction with spontaneous ventilation. Attempting to place an intravenous catheter before induction can trigger violent struggling, straining, and crying and can precipitate total airway obstruction. A gentle inhalation

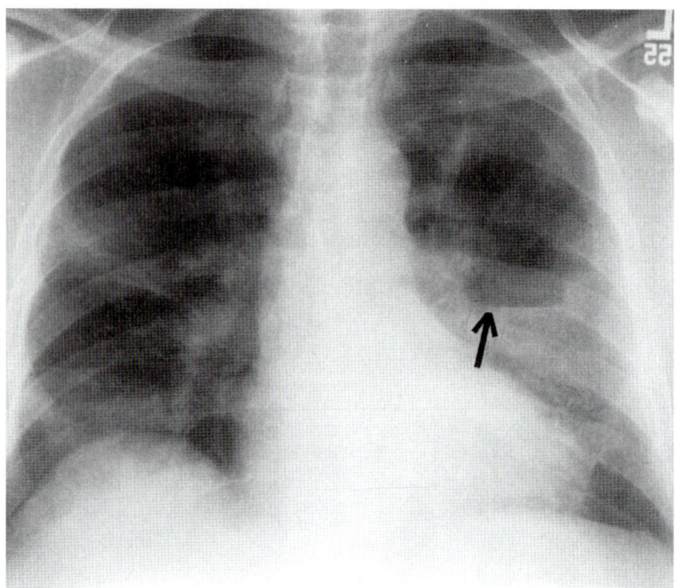

A

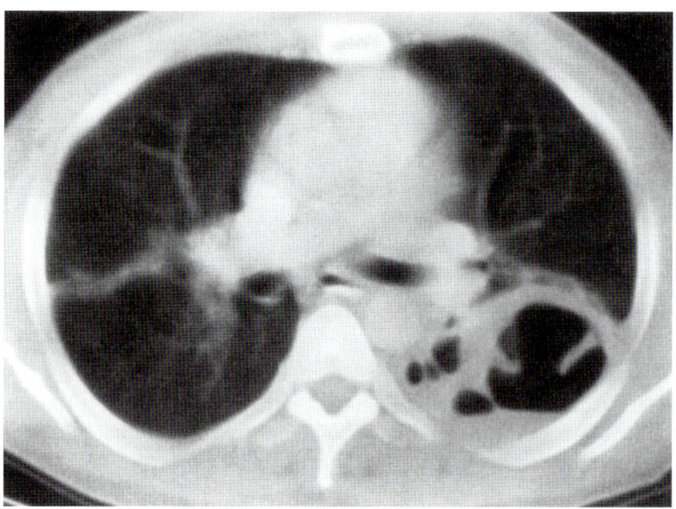

B

FIGURE 54-42. An aspiration pneumonia in a 58-year-old man with a history of alcohol abuse progressed to a suppurative cavitary lesion. The patient presented with progressive shortness of breath, fevers, and foul-smelling sputum. The chest radiograph (**A**) shows cavitary lesion with an air fluid level in the left lung and several pneumonic infiltrates in the right lung. The chest CT (**B**) shows the large cavitation in the left lower lobe that is consistent with a diagnosis of abscess or tumor. The patient subsequently underwent pulmonary resection that required placement of a double-lumen endotracheal tube to prevent soilage of the contralateral lung.

TABLE 54-23 Anesthetic Guidelines for Retrieval of Foreign Body

Indication	Aspiration of foreign body
Monitors	Standard monitors
Anesthesia	Pediatric (general anesthesia) Adult (awake, sedated, general anesthesia)
Additional equipment	Fiberoptic bronchoscope Rigid bronchoscope
Ventilation	Usually try to maintain spontaneous ventilation Controlled ventilation may be appropriate if mass is distal in tracheobronchial tree
Position	Seated or semirecumbent (positioned to optimize respiratory status)
Unique considerations	Respiratory status Sedation as tolerated Antisialagogue Precautions for "full stomach" H_2-blocker, metoclopramide, cricoid pressure Anesthetize airway for awake, sedated approach Availability of additional support personnel Place gastric tube to empty stomach after airway is secured
Complications	Loss of airway Hypoxia Cardiac arrest Aspiration Hemoptysis Soilage from contents distal to obstruction
Postoperative morbidity	Hemoptysis Postoperative edema (steroids, raise head of bed) Bronchospasm (racemic epinephrine, bronchodilators) Pneumonia Atelectasis
Postoperative care	Observe in monitored environment Aggressive pulmonary toilet, physical therapy Supplemental O_2 Chest radiography

induction, using cricoid pressure, can be used even in children with a full stomach. In the absence of intravenous access, intramuscular ketamine may be used for induction. As soon as the child becomes sleepy, cricoid pressure is applied, and inhalation of anesthetic agents is started while continuing spontaneous ventilation.

If the patient is minimally symptomatic with no serious respiratory distress and if the foreign body is thought to be peripherally located, the anesthesiologist can wait 6 to 8 hours before bronchoscopy, although some surgeons or endoscopists do not agree with this approach and prefer to proceed immediately to prevent a local inflammatory reaction to the foreign body. In the absence of a full stomach and if symptoms are minimal, the child may be heavily premedicated to facilitate a smooth inhalation induction. Spontaneous ventilation can facilitate detection of airway obstruction and prevents distal migration of the foreign body caused by positive-pressure ventilation. When using a rigid bronchoscope, many anesthesiologists administer muscle relaxants to prevent airway trauma induced by patent movement.

Some objects, such as beads, are hard to grip and may slip during removal, resulting in occlusion more proximally. The object should then be pushed back to its original location to allow adequate ventilation. Multiple instrumentations of the airway may produce mucosal edema and respiratory distress postoperatively. Therapy includes the administration of steroids (dexamethasone, 0.5-1.5 mg/kg), humidification of inspired gases, nebulized racemic epinephrine, and initiation of broad-spectrum antibiotic therapy.

ANESTHESIA FOR PATIENTS UNDERGOING ENDOSCOPY FOR INGESTED FOREIGN BODIES

The incidence of occurrence of ingested foreign bodies in the hypopharynx or esophagus in young children is as common as aspirations in the airway. Coins and fish bones are the most frequent foreign bodies in the esophagus. Most foreign bodies initially cause laryngeal irritation, coughing, or choking. Subsequent signs and symptoms include refusal to eat, increased salivation, pain or discomfort during swallowing, and vomiting.

The anesthesiologist should determine the nature and the location of the foreign body. Lateral neck radiographs should be obtained to determine the extent of impingement on the airway. In the absence of respiratory distress or airway compression, the anesthesiologist should consider waiting 4 to 8 hours for gastric emptying.[281] The child then is sedated, and anesthesia is induced with either inhalation or intravenous anesthetic agents. Emergency endoscopy should be performed in patients with respiratory distress and airway compression. In spontaneously ventilated patients, preoperative sedation is omitted and general anesthesia is induced. For patients with foreign bodies located in the hypopharynx or in the upper esophagus, cricoid pressure is contraindicated. The endotracheal tube size chosen should be slightly smaller than usual to facilitate endoscopy and decrease subsequent subglottic swelling.[281] In addition, a prophylactic dose of dexamethasone (0.5-1.0 mg/kg) may be given to decrease laryngeal edema.

A foreign body that is located high in the esophagus may dislodge into the larynx and produce an airway obstruction. Therefore, children with high esophageal foreign bodies should be heavily sedated, intravenous access obtained, and anesthesia induced. In the absence of major airway compression, an intravenous induction with muscle relaxants may be used.

ANESTHESIA FOR PATIENTS WITH ZENKER DIVERTICULUM

CLINICAL FEATURES

Zenker diverticulum is an outpouching of the pharyngeal mucosa between the inferior constrictor muscles of the pharynx, the thyropharyngeus, and the cricopharyngeus muscles. The etiology is believed to result from dysfunction or spasm of the cricopharyngeus muscle. Patients complain of food sticking in the throat, difficulty swallowing, noisy swallowing, regurgitation of food, and bouts of coughing when lying supine. Neck radiographs may reveal a collection of air anterior to C5 and C6, but diagnosis is confirmed with a barium swallow. Physical examination may reveal a compressible swelling as the sac enlarges. Patients usually are elderly, malnourished,[282] debilitated with coexisting cardiac and respiratory diseases, and susceptible to recurrent pneumonias and lung abscesses from aspiration. Symptomatic lesions are managed by surgical resection.

INTRAOPERATIVE MANAGEMENT

Oral premedications are not suitable because tablets may lodge in the pouch or be aspirated into the lungs.[283] The risk of regurgitation and aspiration of diverticular contents into the lungs during the immediate preoperative and intraoperative periods is a major concern for the anesthesiologist. The contents of the pouch usually have an alkaline pH and therefore are unlikely to benefit from H_2-receptor antagonists, antacids, or metaclopramide. Regurgitation and aspiration may occur even after successful tracheal intubation because of seepage of fluid around the endotracheal tube cuff during surgical manipulation. Measures to decrease the risk of aspiration during anesthesia include fasting overnight, preoperative emptying of the pouch by manual external pressure, and tilting the head of the bed upward 10 to 30 degree.

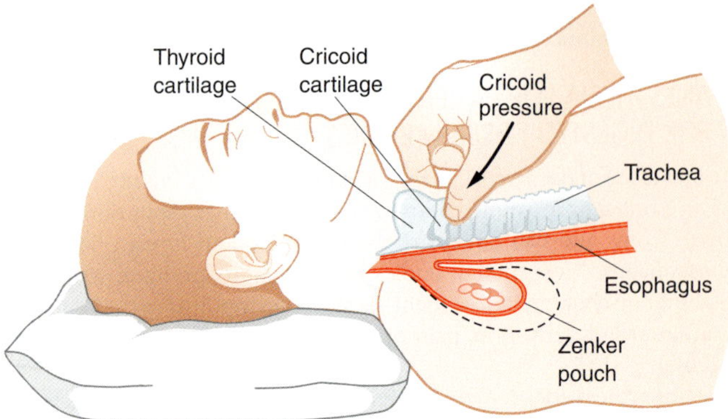

FIGURE 54-43. Zenker pouch in the hypopharynx, with the opening at the level of cricoid cartilage. [From Thiagarajah S, Lear E, Keh M. Anesthetic implications of Zenker's diverticulum. *Anesth Analg.* 1990;70:709.]

Awake intubation is an option, but coughing and straining may result in regurgitation and aspiration. The risk of aspiration may be increased by topical anesthesia and sedation, which blunt airway reflexes. Therefore, some authors advise against awake intubation.[284] Use of topical anesthesia should be limited to either the supraglottic or infraglottic part of the airway, leaving part of the airway responsive as a protection against aspiration. Transtracheal administration of local anesthetics is relatively contraindicated.

Use of cricoid pressure may precipitate aspiration in some patients. Careful preoperative examination of the barium swallow image may help determine whether cricoid pressure will be beneficial or harmful by defining the size and location of the pouch. If the sac is large, extending down into the mediastinum with its orifice at the level of the cricoid cartilage, cricoid pressure should obliterate the opening and protect against regurgitation. If the sac is small and the opening is cephalad to the cricoid cartilage, the application of cricoid pressure may actually squeeze the sac, resulting in regurgitation of its contents into the hypopharynx (**Fig. 54-43**).

The preferred approach is a smooth induction with a 30 degree upward head tilt and avoidance of coughing, bucking, and straining. The combination of intravenous hypnotics (ie, thiopental or etomidate) supplemented with narcotics and lidocaine and slow, gentle manual mask ventilation should result in a smooth, uneventful induction. A nondepolarizing muscle relaxant is administered, and endotracheal intubation is performed after complete relaxation has been achieved. The pharynx around the endotracheal tube can be packed with gauze to prevent seepage of the contents of the diverticulum into the hypopharynx with collection above the endotracheal tube cuff. Surgical access usually is through a cervical incision. A large diverticulum may extend into the mediastinum. Great care and gentleness should be exercised when inserting a nasogastric tube because of the potential for perforation of the diverticulum. Likewise in patients with a difficult airway, blind attempts at intubation of the trachea risk perforating the pouch. Perforation of the diverticulum results in mediastinitis and sepsis. Other complications include air embolism if major vessels are opened during the dissection or bradycardia and hypotension resulting from stimulation of baroreceptors during retraction near the carotid bifurcation.

An alternative is to perform the procedure during regional anesthesia using deep and superficial cervical plexus blocks.[285] A recent report describes the use of this approach in 58 patients undergoing repair of a Zenker diverticulum. The risk of aspiration is minimized by preserving protective airway reflexes. Provided the block is limited to one side, the awake, sedated patient is able to cooperate with the surgeon and to swallow on command, allowing the surgeon to view the pathology and assess the adequacy of repair.

COMPLICATIONS OF THORACIC SURGERY AND STRATEGIES FOR THEIR MANAGEMENT

The postoperative complications of thoracic surgery can be characterized as pulmonary, cardiovascular, neurologic, or miscellaneous (**Box 54-13**). Some of these are medical and surgical emergencies that require prompt diagnosis and management. Conditions requiring emergent intervention include pneumothorax, pulmonary edema, torsion of a residual lobe, herniation of the heart, malignant arrhythmias, or major hemorrhage. Early diagnosis and efficient management depend on the cooperative efforts of the anesthesia, surgical, and nursing staff. In the following section, the order of presentation is based on the system involved and the severity of symptoms.

CARDIOVASCULAR

Herniation of the Heart Cardiac herniation is a rare and rapidly fatal injury if not immediately diagnosed and managed. This complication occurs more often after right pneumonectomy in which the pericardium was opened to gain better access to the pulmonary vessels. It may occur after the creation of a pericardial window for management of a pericardial effusion. This complication has been associated with changing of patient position (lateral decubitus to supine position or placement of the operative lung in the dependent position) or a differential change in intrapleural pressures caused by suctioning of the chest tube after pneumonectomy or vigorous coughing.[286,287]

BOX 54-13

Complications of Thoracic Surgery

- Hemodynamic
  - Arrhythmias
  - Cardiac herniation
  - Right-sided failure
  - Tension pneumothorax
  - Bleeding
- Pulmonary
  - Pneumothorax
  - Atelectasis
  - Shunting
  - Pulmonary edema
  - Torsion of lobe
  - Damage to phrenic nerve
  - Damage to recurrent laryngeal nerve
  - Pain
- Neurologic
  - Positioning injuries
  - Brachial plexus, ulnar nerve, peroneal nerve
  - Phrenic nerve
  - Recurrent laryngeal nerve
  - Paradoxical embolization
  - Spinal cord
- Miscellaneous
  - Alopecia
  - Necrosis ear, nose
  - Infection

The clinical features of cardiac herniation include acute cardiovascular collapse, evidence of superior vena cava obstruction (distention of neck veins, facial flushing, and edema), altered axis of ECG, bulging of cardiac silhouette, and unusual positioning of pulmonary artery catheter on chest radiograph. A differential diagnosis includes tension pneumothorax, cardiac tamponade, dysrhythmia, pulmonary emboli, and massive hemorrhage. These patients require immediate operation, but they may be stabilized by placing the patient in a lateral position with the operated lung in the nondependent position.[288,289] Even if the heart does not fall back into its normal position, repositioning may relieve aortocaval kinking and increase cardiac output. The tidal volume should be decreased and use of PEEP should be discontinued to decrease any mediastinal shift. Additionally, suctioning of the chest tubes should be discontinued, and injection of air to counter cardiac herniation should be considered.

Definitive management requires that the thorax should be reexplored and pericardial defect repaired by primary closure, autograft, or prosthetic material.[290] Anesthesia should be carefully induced with either ketamine or etomidate and a muscle relaxant. To decrease mediastinal shift, the lungs should be ventilated with small tidal volumes.

Cardiac Dysrhythmias Supraventricular dysrhythmias, primarily sinus tachycardia and atrial fibrillation or flutter, which occur after thoracic surgery, are associated with an increase in postopertaive morbidity. Significant risk factors include male sex, advanced age, history of congestive heart failure or arrhythmias, and type of surgery (pneumonectomy > bilobectomy > lobectomy > esophagectomy > resection of mediastinal tumor or thymectomy).[291,292] Manipulation of the pulmonary veins, a major nidus for atrial fibrillation, is thought to be a significant factor.[293] Other potential causes include retraction and trauma of the heart (intrapericardial dissection), increased sympathetic tone related to inadequate postoperative analgesia, and postoperative respiratory or metabolic imbalance (hypoxia, hypercapnia, respiratory acidosis, and electrolyte imbalances). Although the use of digitalis for thoracic surgery is not supported by clinical trials, calcium channel and β-blockers are effective in reducing postoperative atrial tachyarrhythmias.[294] However, the use of such medications should be individualized to account for the possible adverse consequences of using β-blockers in this patient population. Interestingly, the preoperative use of statins has also been associated with a protective effect against postoperative atrial fibrillation, but its mechanism has yet to be elucidated.[295]

The appropriate management strategies for a new dysrhythmia are directed to stabilizing hemodynamics and managing the underlying problem. Hemodynamic instability resulting from new dysrhythmias may require emergent cardioversion. Normotensive patients having atrial fibrillation may be chemically converted to sinus rhythm with β-blockers, procainamide, or amiodarone.

Right Ventricular Failure The postoperative course after anatomic pulmonary resection may be complicated by right ventricular failure and acute cor pulmonale. Decreases in the vascular cross-sectional area caused by pulmonary resection increase the pulmonary vascular resistance and right ventricular afterload. Preoperative right heart catheterization or echocardiography may predict patients at risk for this postoperative complication. Operative risk is increased if the pulmonary vascular resistance is greater than 190 dynes/s/cm^{-5} or if the pulmonary artery pressure increases by more than 40 mm Hg in response to balloon occlusion. In addition, hypercapnia, acidosis, and increases in airway pressure may increase the risk of developing right heart failure. Patients with right heart failure have distended neck veins, peripheral edema, and new onset of atrial dysrhythmias. Echocardiography can be used to differentiate right heart failure from cardiac tamponade. Increased right heart volume and ventricular dysfunction can lead to a shift of the intraventricular septum and impede left ventricular filling and function. A decrease in left ventricular preload caused by the increased pulmonary vascular resistance and abnormal septal wall motion will result in a decreased cardiac output and peripheral perfusion pressure. Patients who have chronic right-sided heart failure with right ventricular hypertrophy may be at increased risk for developing myocardial ischemia and dysfunction related to decreased coronary perfusion. Increased oxygen demand related to wall stress and the decreased coronary perfusion resulting from decreased cardiac output and hypotension may exacerbate preexisting right ventricular dysfunction.

The treatment strategies for patients with right ventricular failure differ from those for patients with primary left ventricular dysfunction. Volume expansion in patients with increased pulmonary vascular resistance will increase wall stress and further exacerbate right ventricular dysfunction. The management goals are to improve right ventricular function by decreasing pulmonary vascular resistance, increasing myocardial contractility, and maintaining coronary perfusion. Vasodilating agents, such as milrinone, prostacyclin I2, nitric oxide, and nitroglycerin, have been used to decrease pulmonary vascular resistance. Often agents such as dobutamine or milrinone are chosen for their combined inotropic and vasodilator properties. In patients with decreased systemic blood pressure and inadequate coronary perfusion, vasopressors such as epinephrine, dopamine, phenylephrine, or norepinephrine can be added to enhance coronary perfusion.

Intracardiac Shunting The incidence of a probe-patent foramen ovale is about 25% in adults. During normal conditions, there is negligible right-to-left shunt across the atrial septal defect because the left atrial pressure exceeds that of the right. If the gradient between the right atrium and left atrium is reversed, oxygenated blood can flow from right to left, resulting in paradoxical embolization and hypoxia. The reversal of atrial pressures can occur during conditions of increased peripheral vascular resistance related to the use of PEEP or during the occurrence of pulmonary emboli, pulmonary hypertension, valvular stenosis, ARDS, or even coughing. Reversal of pressures may occur after pneumonectomy or lobectomy.[296-298] The occurrence of intracardiac shunt should be suspected in those with unexplained postoperative dyspnea and systemic oxygen desaturation. Transesophageal echocardiography can confirm the diagnosis and visualize the atrial septal defect.

Management goals are to decrease shunt flow by decreasing right-sided pressures and pulmonary vascular resistance. Initial management should involve correction of hypoxia, hypercapnia, acidosis, and increased sympathetic tone related to inadequate postoperative analgesia. In addition, the administration of pulmonary vasodilators and preload reduction can be used to decrease right heart pressures. In patients who are mechanically ventilated, the use of PEEP should be avoided if possible. When conservative measures fail, open surgical or percutaneous closure of the atrial septal defect may be necessary. Because the presence of an intracardiac shunt predisposes to paradoxical embolization, all intravenous solutions should be rigorously free of air bubbles, and blood products should be administered through filters to exclude particulate matter.

Major Hemorrhage Postoperative bleeding that requires surgical intervention is uncommon. The postoperative findings are those of hypovolemia (tachycardia, hypotension, respiratory variation, and absence of jugular venous distension). Most major hemorrhage results from slippage of ligatures around major pulmonary vessels. Bleeding from raw pleural surfaces is likely when vascular adhesions between the visceral and parietal pleura have been divided. Other sites of potential bleeding include the bronchial and intercostal arteries. Although chest tube drainage is an indicator of the extent of bleeding, the absence of chest tube drainage does not rule out major hemorrhage. Chest tubes may be malpositioned or occluded by clot, thus hiding the resulting hemothorax. If suspected, repositioning the patient and obtaining a chest radiograph will confirm the presence of serious pleural effusion with blood.

PULMONARY

Pneumothorax Pneumothoraces are common complications occurring intraoperatively and postoperatively. The presence of a large pneumothorax is a medical emergency. Clinical signs and symptoms include respiratory distress, decreased breath sounds unilaterally, increased airway pressure with decreased chest compliance, and decreased arterial oxygen saturation. Pneumothorax can expand to the point of tension pneumothorax, which is characterized by hypotension, tracheal shift, and cardiovascular collapse. If sufficient time is available, a chest radiograph is obtained to confirm diagnosis.

Management entails placement of a chest tube for evacuation of intrapleural air. In a spontaneously ventilating patient, the indications for placement of a chest tube are for pneumothorax occupying 15% or more of the hemithorax or for the presence of symptoms. Because mechanically ventilated patients are at risk of the pneumothorax increasing in size, they usually require placement of a chest tube. In emergency situations, decompression of the hemothorax can be accomplished by placement of a 14-gauge intravenous catheter into the intercostal space in the anterior axillary line.

Torsion of Residual Lobe Pulmonary torsion refers to lung rotation on its bronchovascular pedicle. If uncorrected, it will result in pulmonary infarction. Patients undergoing lung resection are at increased risk for torsion of the remaining lobe. The right middle lobe and lingula are at greatest risk for torsion after right upper or left upper lobectomy.[299] Chest radiograph reveals an area of atelectasis or an expanding intrathoracic mass. If suspected, bronchoscopy should be performed followed by immediate surgical reexploration. A double-lumen endotracheal tube should be placed to allow for complete pneumonectomy or untwisting of the rotated bronchial vascular pedicle.

Postoperative Respiratory Failure The risks of postoperative respiratory dysfunction increase as the incidence of coexisting disease increases and the economic pressure to extubate and streamline the postoperative period continues to grow. The increase in risk is related to the decrement in preoperative pulmonary function. The postoperative respiratory complications associated with smoking may be reduced with cessation of smoking at least 8 weeks before operation.[300,301]

The importance of such factors as age, obesity, and malnutrition are less clear. Advanced age alone does not appear to be a risk factor, but it may be a confounding variable. Respiratory mechanics and pulmonary functions are altered in obese patients.[302,303] The accumulation of fat in respiratory structures reduces compliance and increases the work of breathing. Although obesity may influence the risk of postoperative pulmonary complications, its importance is minor except with morbidly obese patients. Malnutrition is not a major risk factor for postoperative pulmonary complications, although it impairs immunity, decreases diaphragmatic muscle function, and diminishes the ventilation response to hypoxia.[304] Even though aggressive nutritional support improves biochemical parameters, it has not been shown to improve pulmonary function.[305,306]

Pulmonary Edema Pulmonary edema occurs because of altered balance of the Starling forces, resulting in a net movement of fluid into the interstitial space. Risk factors for pulmonary edema include cardiac, pulmonary, and anatomic reasons.

Pneumonectomy or reexpansion of atelectatic lung is associated with postoperative pulmonary edema. The etiology of these complications most likely is multifactorial and involves changes in hydrostatic pressure, oncotic pressure, cardiac output, and vascular permeability. Reexpansion pulmonary edema is unilateral and follows the reinflation of atelectatic lungs caused by removal of effusions, evacuation of a pneumothorax, or reinflation after use of a double-lumen endotracheal tube.[307,308] This type of edema has been related to increased vascular permeability caused by an inflammatory reaction to the endothelium and mechanical changes to the blood vessels.[309,310] To avoid mechanical damage caused by excess stretching and increased pressure gradients, the lung should be expanded slowly and gradually.[282] The factors associated with postoperative pulmonary edema are more complicated. Postpneumonectomy pulmonary edema has been commonly attributed to increased cardiac output and fluid overload. Pneumonectomy dramatically decreases the cross-sectional area of the vascular bed, increasing hydrostatic pressure. During normal conditions, the vascular bed can accommodate, although the presence of preexisting cardiac disease combined with aggressive fluid replacement and reduction of lymphatic drainage may predispose to the transudation of edema fluid. More recently, it has been recognized that a change in permeability is a major contributing factor to edema after pneumonectomy.[311] Occurrence of acute reexpansion pulmonary edema can be quite severe, resulting in mortality.[308] Patients become tachypneic, tachycardic, and hypoxic. These patients often remain intubated and require postoperative ventilatory support. The therapy is generally supportive. Mechanical ventilation with PEEP, diuresis, and hemodynamic support may be appropriate.[312] Patient positioning also may be therapeutic when pulmonary edema is unilateral. Lateral decubitus positioning with the affected side up will reduce intrapulmonary shunting and improve oxygenation.[313]

NERVE INJURIES

Phrenic Nerve Injury The phrenic nerve originates from C3, C4, and C5, passing into the chest anteriorly to the hilium of the lung within the pericardium. It is susceptible to damage during median sternotomy or thoracotomy. Phrenic nerve injury manifests as respiratory failure or failure to wean from mechanical ventilation. Diagnostic tests include chest radiography and fluoroscopic examination of diaphragmatic movement. Chest radiography shows a clear lung with an elevated hemidiaphragm, whereas fluoroscopy documents paradoxical movement of the diaphragm during inspiration. Most patients with normal lung function can tolerate unilateral phrenic nerve injury, although those patients with preexisting lung disease or those who have undergone extensive pulmonary resection may be debilitated. If lung function does not return within 2 to 9 months, alternative therapies, including diaphragmatic pacing and diaphragmatic plication, may be considered.

Recurrent Laryngeal Nerve Injury The left recurrent laryngeal nerve is susceptible to injury during hilar dissection and mediastinoscopy. Unilateral laryngeal nerve injury usually is asymptomatic or manifests by hoarseness of voice, although bilateral nerve injury could result in apposition of the vocal cords and inspiratory obstruction, requiring emergent reintubation of the trachea. If vocal cord function does not return after several months, the involved vocal cord may be injected to improve its function.

Spinal Cord Injury Spinal cord injury is a rare complication after thoracic surgery.[314] The mechanisms of injury include nerve compression and vascular ischemia. Epidural hematomas and nerve compression can result from placement of epidural catheters or from surgical bleeding into the epidural space. Disruption of the major intercostal artery supplying the anterior spinal artery can result in anterior spinal artery syndrome, leading to paralysis.

Brachial Plexus Injury The brachial plexus is susceptible to injury caused by surgical trauma and indirectly caused by positioning.[315] Stretch injury of the plexus can occur with extreme abduction, external rotation, and dorsal extension of the arm. For further discussion, the reader is referred to Chapter 27 (on positioning).

POSTOPERATIVE PAIN MANAGEMENT

The pain that accompanies thoracic surgery is notable for its intensity and duration. Acutely, moderate to severe levels of pain may not decrease substantially over the course of hospitalization and the first postoperative month.[316] Noxious input associated with thoracic surgery is conveyed to the central nervous system (CNS) along the intercostal, vagus, and phrenic nerves. Afferent phrenic activity is believed to be the source of the shoulder pain that frequently accompanies thoracic procedures because this is curtailed by phrenic[317] but not suprascapular or epidural blockade.[318] Intercostal nerve dysfunction resulting from incision, retraction, trocar placement, or suture is common[319] and likely plays a significant role in the pain accompanying thoracic surgery. In addition, the need for constant respiratory effort and enhanced pulmonary toilet produces an intense and relentless barrage of noxious input to the CNS. Although utilized with increasing frequency, thoracoscopic approaches have not had the favorable impact on pain that many had anticipated.[320,321]

Postoperative pain control is one of the most important management goals for preventing postoperative respiratory complications. Inadequate pain control leads to shallow respirations, tachypnea, inability to cough effectively, retention of secretions, and atelectasis. These symptoms contribute to postoperative hypoxia, hypercapnia, and respiratory failure in postthoracotomy patients. Effective postoperative pain management decreases these deleterious effects and abates the increase in norepinephrine levels associated with sympathetic outflow. The associated tachycardia, hypertension, and postoperative hypercoagulability increase the risk for adverse cardiac events in patients with ischemic heart disease. We are strong advocates of epidural analgesia utilizing local anesthetic and opioid that are intiated intraoperatively and continued postoperatively. This can be supplemented with NSAIDs, acetaminophen, α_2-adrenergic agonists and ketamine. Other options are patient-controlled analgesia (PCA), intercostal nerve blocks, cryoanalgesia, intrapleural catheters, and paravertebral block.

INTERCOSTAL NERVE BLOCKS

Intercostal nerve block is an effective technique to provide postoperative analgesia without central respiratory depression and to attenuate the decrease in pulmonary function after thoracic surgery.[322] Postthoracotomy pain is not completely managed with intercostal analgesia; it requires supplemental use of parenteral narcotics or NSAIDs. Complications of this technique are few, but they include pneumothorax, local anesthetic toxicity, and neuroaxonal spread of local anesthetics that can result in unintentional hypotension.[78,323]

The intercostal nerve block can be performed intraoperatively by intrathoracic injection or percutaneously by the anesthesiologist after the operation. Nerve blocks are performed at the levels above and below the site of chest tube insertion and incision (**Fig. 54-44**). Nerve blocks are performed at the midaxillary line by injection of 2 or 3 mL of bupivacaine, 0.5%, with epinephrine (1:200 000 concentration). Because the average duration of these nerve blocks is 4 to 8 hours, placement of indwelling catheters in the intercostal space is used to provide analgesia for up to 6 days.

A variation in providing postoperative intercostal analgesia is that of cryogenic analgesia. The efficacy of this technique is debatable compared with epidural or intravenous anesthesia.[127,324] Problems associated with cryoanalgesia of the intercostal nerves include long-term neuralgias, prolonged paresthesia, dysesthesias, and loss of intercostal muscle tone. Other possible options are paravertebral and intrapleural analgesia, which are variations of intercostal nerve block.[325-329]

THORACIC PARAVERTEBRAL BLOCK

An alternate method of achieving multiple intercostal nerve blockade is placement of a thoracic paravertebral block, either by single injection or continuous catheter.[330,331] Unilateral analgesia is achieved by depositing local anesthetic in the paravertebral space, which is the locus of the primary ramus of the intercostal nerve. Paravertebral catheters provide at least equianalgesic therapy as compared to epidural catheters and have some distinct advantages. Paravertebral catheters are dosed solely with local anesthetic so there is less nausea, vomiting, and constipation from

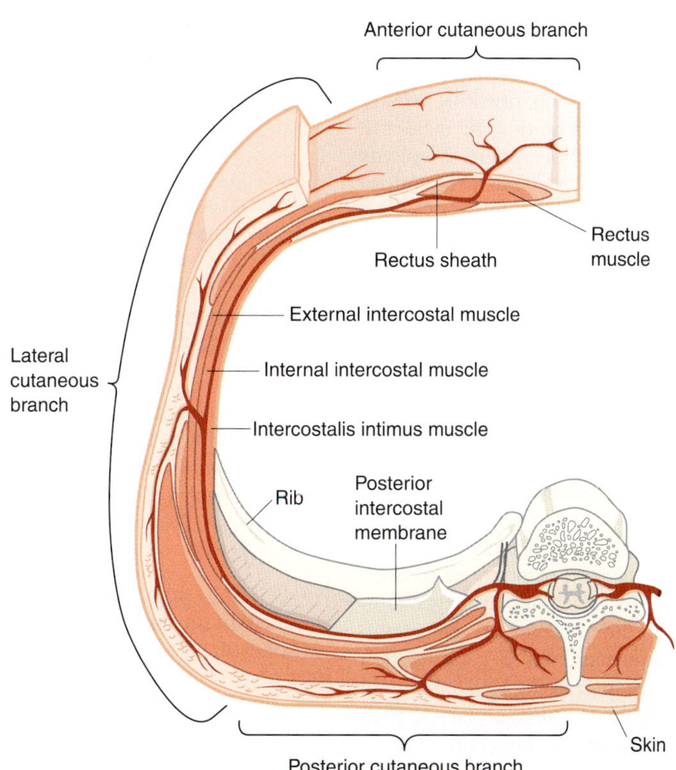

FIGURE 54-44. An intercostal nerve and its branches. Approximate area of skin supplied by branches also is shown. There is evidence that local anesthetic injected near the lateral cutaneous branch diffuses posteriorly to reach the posterior cutaneous branch. Note also the spinal nerves and dorsal root ganglia in the region of intervertebral foramen, with risk of perineural spread into spinal fluid after intraneural injection in this region. Direct injection into an intervertebral foramen may reach spinal fluid by means of a dural cuff. Local anesthetic may gain access to epidural space by diffusing into an intervertebral foramen; close to the midline, the intercostal nerve lies directly on the posterior intercostal membrane and pleura. [From Cousins MJ, Bridenbaugh PO, eds. *Neural Blockade*. 2nd ed. Philadelphia, PA: JB Lippincott; 1988.]

opioids. The typically unilateral nature of the local anesthetic block reduces the risk of hypotension. Furthermore, its position lateral to the spinal cord allows for use of this technique in patients who are maintained on antiplatelet drugs (ie, Plavix®) due to coronary drug eluding stents or other reasons.[144,145,332,333]

Paraveretebral catheters can be placed with traditional landmark plus loss-of-resistance techniques or with ultrasound guidance. No best ultrasound approach has been developed, and the technology is still improving. An alternative is for the surgeon to place the catheter at the conclusion of the resection.

EPIDURAL ANESTHESIA

Epidural anesthesia is a commonly used technique for the management of postthoracotomy pain; it has potential benefits for pulmonary and cardiovascular systems.[334-338] Surprisingly, video-assisted thoracic surgery (VATS) is associated with postoperative pain and a prevalence of chronic pain comparable to that of open procedures, with rates of pain ranging from 22% to 63%,[320,321] which is probably due to intercostal nerve and muscle damage from trocar insertion. Consequently, epidural analgesia is strongly recommended for patients undergoing VATS who are deemed high risk due during preoperative evaluation.

It is the clinical practice in many institutions to combine the use of epidural opioids with local anesthetics. Theoretically, the combination of the 2 agents would act synergistically to provide better analgesia while minimizing the side effects of either agent. The combination of epidural bupivacaine plus morphine or fentanyl provides better analgesia than local anesthetic alone.[339-344] Addition of bupivacaine to an opioid epidural infusion did not improve postthoracotomy analgesia when compared with an epidural infusion of narcotic alone.[345] Epidural narcotics appear to provide the predominant analgesic effect.

Side effects associated with neuraxial administration of local anesthetics include hypotension and bradycardia, caused by sympathectomy and peripheral vasodilation, and blockade of the cardiac accelerator nerve fibers at T1 to T4. Administration of opioids is associated with the side effects of nausea, vomiting, pruritus, urinary retention, central narcosis, and respiratory depression. The incidence of respiratory depression from neuraxial administration of opioids varies from 0.1% to 3%.[295] Depending on the agent used, respiratory depression from opioids may peak from 4 to 10 hours, but may persist up to 24 hours. Patients at increased risk for developing respiratory depression include older, sicker patients having lengthy surgical procedures and those receiving major parenteral narcotics perioperatively, or more than 6 mg of epidural morphine or 0.5 mg of intrathecal morphine (**Box 54-14**).[334] To decrease complications associated with respiratory depression, the patient should be monitored and cared for by knowledgeable staff with clear instructions for the management of respiratory depression.

The acute and chronic pain that accompanies thoracic surgery is significant but often underappreciated, with a well-established level of significant physiologic and functional impact, and unknown social and economic costs. It is likely that an aggressive perioperative analgesic regimen, apart from its more immediate benefits with respect to comfort and pulmonary function, will lead to reductions in longer-term pain. Therefore, we strongly recommend thoracic epidural analgesia in all patients scheduled for open thoracotomy, and serious consideration for the use of epidural analgesia in patients undergoing VATS. Epidural analgesia needs to be combined with NSAIDs and/or acetaminophen to reduce pain as much as possible to reduce risk and promote wellbeing. Patients whose pain is not well controlled (<3 out of 10) need to be assessed for epidural function and the need to add alternate analgesics including intravenous opioids, ketamine, and α_2 agonists. These aggressive regimens should be directed by physicians trained in pain management who will be immediately available to best care for these high-risk patients.

BOX 54-14

Factors Predisposing to the Development of Respiratory Depression After Epidural Opioids

Drug factor
- Hydrophilic drug (ie, morphine)
- Large doses
- Repeated doses
- Concomitant administration of parenteral opioids or other CNS depressants

Patient factors
- Elderly or debilitated
- Coexisting respiratory disease
- Thoracic epidural
- High sensitivity to opioids (ie, no previous exposure to opioids)
- Intrathecal administration
- Increased intrathoracic pressure (eg, controlled ventilation, coughing, vomiting)

From Etches RC, Sandler AN, Daley MD. Respiratory depression and spinal opioids. *Can J Anaesth*. 1989;36:165.

MULTIMODAL PAIN THERAPY

Due to the potential negative impact on health and recovery from the profound pain of thoracic surgery and the inability of effective regional anesthesia to block pain of vagal, phrenic, and pleural origin, most patients undergoing thoracic surgery receive multimodal analgesic therapy.[346,347] In addition to regional analgesia, typical regimens include NSAIDs and/or acetomenophen. The use of ketamine, clonidine, or dexmedetomidine is variable. Although there is no clear best regimen, there are clear advantages to incorporating nonopioid medications in addition to epidural or paravertebral blockade.[145,346,348,349] Although the regimen needs to be created for the individual patient, the goals of a comfortable patient who will be able to actively participate in pulmonary toilet and ambulate and the decrease of perioperative morbidity remain clear.

KEY REFERENCES

- Benumof JL, Augustine SD, Gibbons JA. Halothane and isoflurane only slightly impair arterial oxygenation during one-lung ventilation in patients undergoing thoracotomy. *Anesthesiology.* 1987;67:910-915.
- Gottschalk A, Cohen SP, Yang S, Ochroch EA. Preventing and treating pain after thoracic surgery. *Anesthesiology.* 2006;104:594-600.
- Pate P, Tenholder MF, Griffin JP, et al. Preoperative assessment of the high-risk patient for lung resection. *Am J Thor Surg.* 1996;61:1491-1500.

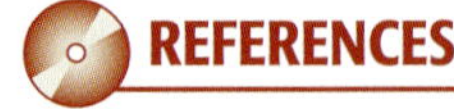

REFERENCES

Complete references available on DVD and online version at www.LongneckerAnesthesiology.com

CHAPTER 55

Anesthesia for Major Vascular Surgery

Alina Nicoara
Madhav Swaminathan

KEY POINTS

1. Atherosclerosis is the primary process leading to myocardial infarction, stroke, chronic mesenteric ischemia, renovascular hypertension, extremity ischemia, and aneurysmal disease. These pathologic states occur years after the slow onset of plaque formation in the vascular wall. The precise mechanism of final injury is 1 or more of the following: (a) plaque enlargement reducing blood flow; (b) complete occlusion of arteries at sites of advanced plaques; and (c) arterial embolism of plaque-associated thrombi or atheromatous debris.
2. The assessment of the surgical patient undergoing vascular surgery is a complex process that requires integration of multiple areas of expertise. The classic concept of clearing a patient for surgery has been replaced with an integrated approach of interdisciplinary cooperation that focuses on assessment of existing disorders, optimization of resilience and reserve in anticipation of increased preoperative demand, avoidance of therapeutic conflicts, and identification of potential procedure-specific risks.
3. Patients presenting for major vascular surgery usually have either overt or occult involvement of several organ systems. The vascular patient population has a high incidence of significant coronary artery disease (CAD), for example, left ventricular systolic dysfunction (left ventricular ejection fraction less than 40%) is 5 times more common in patients with cerebrovascular disease or peripheral arterial disease compared with matched controls.
4. The current standards for preoperative cardiac evaluation of these patients are the guidelines published by the American College of Cardiology and the American Heart Association initially in 1996 and revised in 2002 and in 2007. As stated in these guidelines, "patients who require vascular surgery appear to have an increased risk for cardiac complications because (a) many of the risk factors that contribute to peripheral vascular disease (eg, diabetes mellitus, tobacco use, and hyperlipidemia) are also risk factors for CAD; (b) the usual symptomatic presentation for CAD in these patients may be obscured by exercise limitations imposed by advanced age, intermittent claudication, or both; and (c) major open vascular surgery may be associated with substantial fluctuations in intravascular/extravascular fluid volumes, cardiac filling pressures, systemic blood pressure, heart rate, and thrombogenicity."
5. Vascular surgery patients require intensive perioperative monitoring for 2 primary reasons: (a) these patients often have systemic manifestations of atherosclerotic vascular disease and are at risk for cardiac, cerebral, renal, and spinal cord ischemia, all of which can be diagnosed and treated using appropriate monitors; and (2) vascular procedures involve major physiologic changes, including significant third-space losses, blood loss, and the complications of transfusion (coagulopathies, hypocalcemia, hypothermia, and acidosis). There can also be significant changes in the hemodynamic profile associated with the application and release of vascular clamps.
6. Monitoring of the awake patient is the gold standard for neurologic assessment during carotid endarterectomy (CEA) and may allow for the prompt identification of patients who would benefit from shunt placement. Change in contralateral strength or consciousness in the setting of adequate mean arterial pressure is an indication for shunt placement.
7. One of the goals of anesthesia for CEA is to avoid hemodynamic extremes during induction, incision, surgical manipulation, emergence, and extubation. The blood pressure during carotid occlusion should be maintained at or up to 20% higher than the patient's highest recorded resting blood pressure when awake in order to maintain adequate collateral blood flow. The patient should be sufficiently responsive immediately after surgery to follow commands and thereby facilitate neurologic evaluation.
8. Individuals undergoing lower extremity vascular surgery present a dilemma to the anesthesia provider. The procedure itself is associated with far less (intraoperative and postoperative) nociceptive stimulation than aortic surgery and less hemodynamic fluctuation than carotid or aortic surgery, and can be performed with a pure regional anesthetic. On the other hand, patients may have severe CAD and other systemic disorders and are at high risk for perioperative complications.
9. The physiology of aortic cross-clamping includes changes in blood pressure, cardiac output, myocardial perfusion, acid-base status, and tissue perfusion of the spinal cord, kidneys, and viscera. Conflicting findings have been obtained and likely reflect species variation, patient characteristics, degree of collateralization, location of the cross-clamp, baseline cardiac function, type of anesthesia, the use and type of vasodilators, and the presence or absence of CAD.
10. Preservation of renal function is a primary concern during aortic aneurysm surgery. Preoperative optimization of renal function, attention to intraoperative fluid balance, and the use of "renoprotective" agents are some of the methods that have been used in an effort to prevent this serious complication of vascular surgery.
11. Modalities of spinal cord protection during aortic surgery include identification of ischemia by monitoring evoked potentials, reimplantation of segmental vessels, sequential aortic clamping, maintaining aortic distal aortic perfusion through shunt or bypass, cerebrospinal fluid drainage, epidural cooling or hypothermic cardiopulmonary bypass, and circulatory arrest.
12. Endovascular repair of the aorta (EVAR) avoids the hemodynamic lability associated with major abdominal incision and aortic cross clamping and unclamping, and also presents other subtle benefits such as significantly smaller changes in plasma catecholamine levels, improved acid-base homeostasis, and a decreased metabolic stress response.
13. Various types of anesthesia can be used for stent repair, specifically general anesthesia, regional anesthesia, and monitored anesthesia care with local anesthetic infiltration at the incision site. Goals of an anesthetic plan should be providing hemodynamic stability, adequate oxygenation, and ventilation; preserving organ function; and maintaining normothermia.

The management of anesthesia for surgery of the aorta and its major branches is multifaceted, challenging, and dynamic. The pathologic processes that give rise to aneurysmal and occlusive disease are largely systemic; therefore, patients presenting for major vascular surgery usually have either overt or occult involvement of several organ systems. Coexisting coronary artery disease (CAD) is of particular concern because myocardial ischemia, myocardial infarction (MI), and myocardial failure constitute most of the perioperative morbidity. The stress response of surgery must also be aggressively controlled in both the intraoperative and the postoperative periods to minimize complications.

Vascular surgery necessitates the temporary interruption of arterial blood flow by isolation of the diseased vessel segment with occluding clamps; therefore, it results in dramatic physiologic changes superimposed on complex disease states.

The success and continuous development of the minimally invasive and hybrid (both intra- and extraluminal) surgical techniques led to the expansion of complex procedures that require the collaboration of various specialties (thoracic surgery, vascular surgery, interventional radiology). Knowledge of the indications, challenges, and consequences of these procedures is mandatory for the anesthesiologist involved in the management of these patients.

This chapter details the fundamental considerations surrounding the perioperative evaluation, preparation, and management of major vascular surgery.

PATHOPHYSIOLOGY OF VASCULAR DISEASE

PATHOGENESIS OF ATHEROSCLEROSIS

Atherosclerosis represents progressive thickening and hardening of the arterial walls in different vascular beds, leading to loss of elasticity, gradual stenosis of the luminal diameter, and clinical cardiovascular disease. It begins in childhood with the development of fatty streaks and continues through the adult life. Fatty streaks are commonly observed in young adults and have been identified in the coronary artery intima of children. Isolated lipid-laden monocytes and macrophages, called *foam cells*, have been identified in the intima of infants as young as 1 month of age.[1] Fatty streaks develop due to focal proliferation of smooth muscle cells in the intima and accumulation of lipids. Maturation of the fatty streak into fibroatheroma is due to macrophage migration from blood to intima, intimal macrophage lipid accumulations, smooth muscle cell migration from media to intima, intimal smooth muscle cell proliferation, lipid-laden macrophage necrosis, and organic calcium precipitation.

Multiple factors contribute to the pathogenesis of atherosclerosis including endothelial dysfunction, dyslipidemia, inflammatory and immunologic factors, diabetes, hypertension, and cigarette smoking.

Endothelial dysfunction is a systemic, reversible disorder characterized by an impairment of the endothelium-dependent vasodilation due to an imbalance in the bioavailability of vasodilators compared to the endothelium-derived contracting factors. A dysfunctional endothelium results in a proinflammatory, proliferative, and prothrombotic environment, which favors atherogenesis.[2] Dyslipidemia, especially high levels of low-density lipoprotein (LDL) and low levels of high-density lipoprotein (HDL), plays a crucial role in the development of atherosclerosis. Accumulation of oxidized LDL in cholesterol-enriched macrophages leads to mitochondrial dysfunction, apoptosis, and necrosis, with the resultant release of cellular proteases, inflammatory cytokines, and prothrombotic molecules.[3] The presence of inflammation also plays an important role in the development of atherosclerosis. The interleukins and the C-reactive protein are some of the more investigated inflammatory markers. Interleukin-6, a circulating cytokine, has been identified as a marker of inflammation in coronary atherosclerotic plaques. Interleukin-6 stimulates platelet aggregation and the expression of tissue factor, macrophage LDL receptors, C-reactive protein, and fibrinogen. Interleukin-6 also regulates the expression of other inflammatory cytokines, such as interleukin-1 and tumor necrosis factor-α. C-reactive protein, one of many human acute-phase reactants, is produced in the liver in response to interleukin-6, interleukin-1 β, and tumor necrosis factor-α. It activates the classic complement cascade, mediates phagocytosis, regulates inflammation, and is a nonspecific but sensitive marker of infection and tissue inflammation.[4]

PATHOPHYSIOLOGY OF ATHEROSCLEROSIS

Atherosclerosis is the primary process leading to myocardial infarction, stroke, chronic mesenteric ischemia, renovascular hypertension, extremity ischemia, and aneurysmal disease. These pathologic states occur years after the slow onset of plaque formation in the vascular wall. The precise mechanism of final injury is 1 or more of the following: (a) plaque enlargement reducing blood flow; (b) complete occlusion of arteries at sites of advanced plaques; and (c) arterial embolism of plaque-associated thrombi or atheromatous debris.

Atherosclerosis is a multifactorial disease. The impact of traditional risk factors such as age, sex, elevated blood pressure, smoking, and dyslipidemia has been demonstrated beyond any doubt. Newer risk factors, such as impaired fasting glucose, triglycerides and triglyceride-rich lipoprotein remnants, lipoprotein (a), homocysteine, and the C-reactive protein also contribute to an increased risk of coronary and cardiovascular diseases (**Table 55-1**).[5] Correction or modification of some of these may arrest or lessen the progression of the disease.

TABLE 55-1 Risk Factors for Atherosclerosis

Old	Old/New	New
Sex (men > women)	High-normal blood pressure	Apolipoprotein B; apolipoprotein A-1
Age	Metabolic syndrome	Triglycerides; triglyceride-rich lipoprotein remnants
Family history of premature cardiovascular disease	Diabetes mellitus; impaired glucose tolerance; impaired fasting glucose	Small, dense LDL; oxidized LDL; antibodies against oxidized LDL
Total cholesterol; LDL cholesterol; HDL cholesterol (negative risk factor)		Lipoprotein(a)
Hypertension		Homocysteine
Smoking		High-sensitivity C-reactive protein
Overweight/obesity		

HDL indicates high-density lipoprotein; LDL, low-density lipoprotein.

From Fruchart JC, Nierman MC, Stroes ES, Kastelein JJ, Duriez P. New risk factors for atherosclerosis and patient risk assessment. *Circulation.* 2004;109:III15-III19.

The Committee on Vascular Lesions of the American Heart Association identifies 6 histologic types of atherosclerotic lesions. The initial lesion (type I) contains enough atherogenic lipoprotein to elicit an increase in macrophages and the formation of scattered macrophage foam cells. Type II (fatty streak) lesions consist primarily of layers of macrophage foam cells and lipid-laden smooth muscle cells. In addition to the lipid-laden cells present in the type II lesions, type III (intermediate) lesions contain scattered collections of extracellular lipid droplets and particles that disrupt the coherence of some intimal smooth muscle cells. This extracellular lipid is the immediate precursor of the larger, confluent, and more disruptive core of extracellular lipid that characterizes type IV (atheroma) lesions. Beginning around the fourth decade of life, lesions that usually have a lipid core may also contain thick layers of fibrous connective tissue (type V lesion—fibroatheroma) and/or fissure, hematoma, and thrombus (type VI—complicated lesion; **Fig. 55-1**).[6]

Atherosclerotic plaques tend to occur in several specific anatomic locations, and plaque development at other sites is uncommon. The coronary arteries, the carotid bifurcation, the infrarenal abdominal aorta, the iliac arteries, and the superficial femoral artery are the most usual sites of development (**Fig. 55-2**).[7] The predilection for lesion formation at arterial branching points indicates the importance of rheologic factors in atherosclerosis formation.[2]

Atherosclerotic lesions can progress without compromise of the vascular lumen due to compensatory vascular enlargement (positive remodeling). Atherosclerosis is generally asymptomatic until the plaque stenosis exceeds 70% or 80%, which can produce a critical reduction in flow as with coronary blood flow to the myocardium. These large lesions can produce typical symptoms of angina pectoris. However, acute coronary and cerebrovascular syndromes (unstable angina, MI, sudden death, and stroke) are typically caused by plaque disruption and subsequent thrombus formation. The magnitude of thrombus formation depends on certain factors such as velocity, shear stress, pulsatility, elasticity, and microbiochemical environment at the endothelial surface.

Atherosclerosis is a very heterogeneous disease and the "high-risk" plaque of each vascular bed has certain characteristics. In the coronary circulation, the rupture-prone plaques have a large core of extracellular

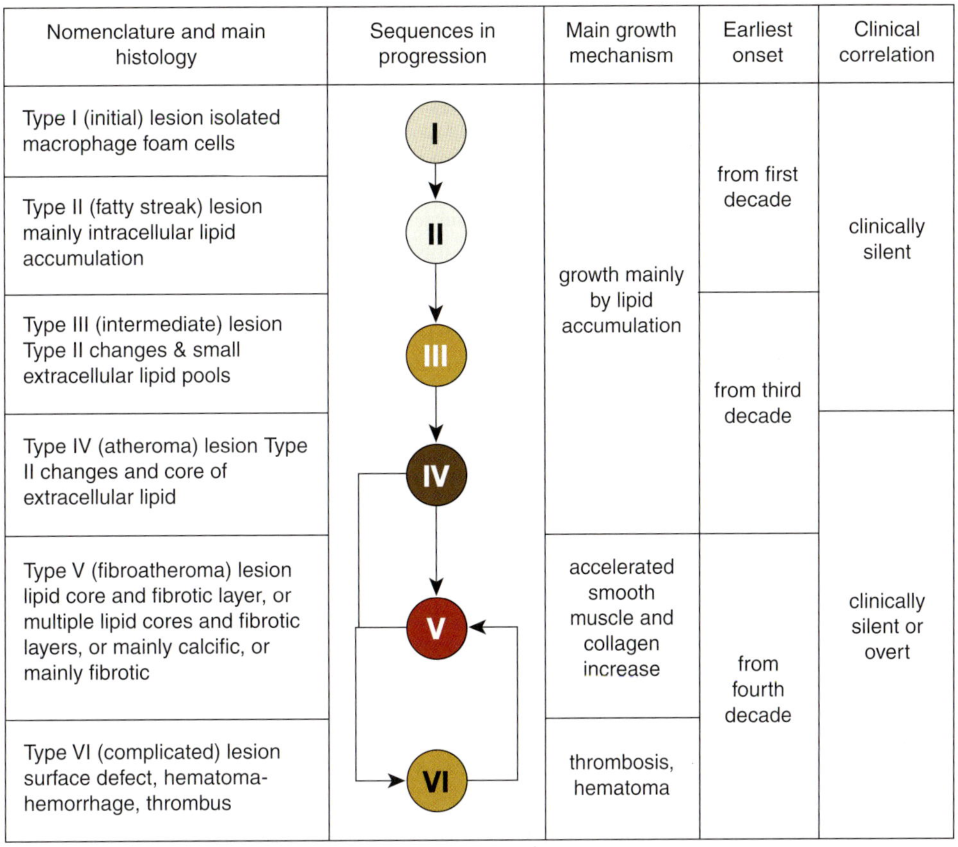

Nomenclature and main histology	Sequences in progression	Main growth mechanism	Earliest onset	Clinical correlation
Type I (initial) lesion isolated macrophage foam cells	I	growth mainly by lipid accumulation	from first decade	clinically silent
Type II (fatty streak) lesion mainly intracellular lipid accumulation	II			
Type III (intermediate) lesion Type II changes & small extracellular lipid pools	III		from third decade	
Type IV (atheroma) lesion Type II changes and core of extracellular lipid	IV			clinically silent or overt
Type V (fibroatheroma) lesion lipid core and fibrotic layer, or multiple lipid cores and fibrotic layers, or mainly calcific, or mainly fibrotic	V	accelerated smooth muscle and collagen increase	from fourth decade	
Type VI (complicated) lesion surface defect, hematoma-hemorrhage, thrombus	VI	thrombosis, hematoma		

FIGURE 55-1. Flow diagram in center column indicates pathways in evolution and progression of human atherosclerotic lesions. Roman numerals indicate histologically characteristic types of lesions enumerated in the text and defined at left of flow diagram. The direction of arrows indicates sequence in which characteristic morphologies may change. From type I to type IV, changes in lesion morphology occur primarily because of increasing accumulation of lipid. The loop between types V and VI illustrates how lesions increase in thickness when thrombotic deposits form on their surfaces. Thrombotic deposits may form repeatedly over varied time spans in the same location and may be the principal mechanism for gradual occlusion of medium-sized arteries. [From Stary HC, Chandler AB, Dinsmore RE, et al. A definition of advanced types of atherosclerotic lesions and a histological classification of atherosclerosis. A report from the Committee on Vascular Lesions of the Council on Arteriosclerosis, American Heart Association. *Circulation.* 1995;92(5):1355-1374.]

lipids, a high density of lipid-laden macrophages, a reduced number of vascular smooth muscle cells, and a thin, fibrous cap. The high-risk carotid plaques are significantly stenotic and very fibrous. Plaque disruption in this vascular bed is often due to intramural hematoma or dissection related to the systolic stroke of the blood in the presence of high resistance due to the stenotic lesion. The plaques at high risk in the lower extremities appear to be highly stenotic and fibrotic. Acute ischemic syndromes in the lower extremities are mostly due to plaque stenosis associated with hyperthrombogenicity of the blood.[2]

Additional comments on pathophysiology are presented at the beginning of the separate sections on carotid, lower-extremity, and aortic surgery.

PREOPERATIVE EVALUATION OF THE VASCULAR SURGERY PATIENT

The assessment of the surgical patient undergoing vascular surgery is a complex process that requires integration of multiple areas of expertise. The classic concept of clearing a patient for surgery has been replaced with an integrated approach of interdisciplinary cooperation that focuses on assessment of existing disorders, optimization of resilience and reserve in anticipation of increased preoperative demand, avoidance of therapeutic conflicts, and identification of potential procedure-specific risks. Silverman and Rosenbaum identify 4 separate phases of the preoperative assessment: *documentation* of existing conditions, *optimization* of the conditions identified, *risk assessment*, and *planning*.[8]

Risk assessment combines information obtained by documentation and changes due to optimization with the anticipated physiologic disturbance of the planned surgery (and accompanying anesthetic),[8] and will have value only if it leads to risk modification or otherwise influences the decisions regarding surgical or anesthetic procedures.

Although occasionally the atherosclerotic process manifests itself in a discrete vascular segment, the more common presentation is diffuse involvement of several organ systems. The vascular patient population has a high incidence of significant CAD, for example, left ventricular systolic dysfunction (left ventricular ejection fraction less than 40%) is 5 times more common in patients with cerebrovascular disease or peripheral arterial disease compared with matched controls.[9]

In addition, vascular patients often report a heavy smoking history, and some degree of pulmonary compromise is expected. Diabetes mellitus is frequently associated with vascular disease, necessitating appropriate evaluation and treatment in the preoperative period. Hypertension is both a predisposing factor for vascular disease and a consequence of its development.

These risk-assessment models are based on findings from the history, physical, and additional information from diagnostic studies. As cardiac complications pose one of the most significant risks to patients undergoing major vascular surgery, the continuing debate concerns the appropriate management sequence to be followed once the risk is

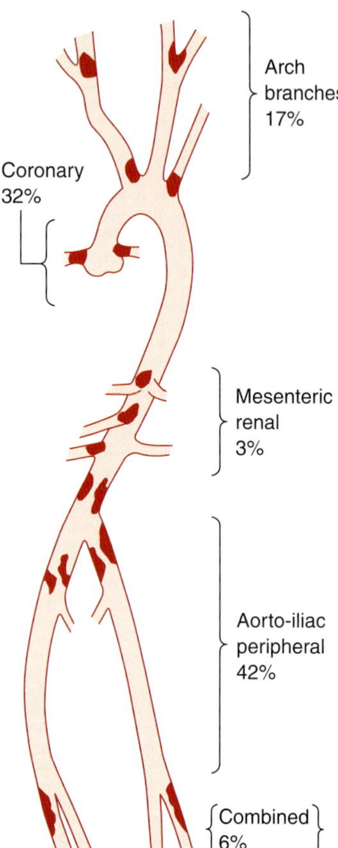

FIGURE 55-2. Distribution of atherosclerotic lesions. [Zwolak RM, Cronenwett JL: Pathophysiology of vascular disease. In Yeager MP, Glass DD [eds]: *Anesthesiology and Vascular Surgery*. East Norwalk, CT, Appleton & Lange, 1990.]

predicted. That is, should other tests, such as dipyridamole-thallium imaging (DTI) or dobutamine stress echocardiography (DSE) be performed toward selection of a subset of patients to be revascularized with percutaneous transluminal angioplasty or coronary artery bypass graft (CABG) prior to vascular surgery, or rather, should the patient proceed directly to vascular surgery with aggressive perioperative medical management in an attempt to reduce risk.

CLINICAL PREDICTORS OF PERIOPERATIVE RISK

Coronary Artery Disease Patients undergoing major vascular surgery constitute a particular challenge, because these are high-risk operations in a patient population with a high prevalence of significant CAD. Hertzer et al showed that only 8% of 1000 vascular surgery patients in whom coronary angiography was performed had normal coronary arteries, 30% had severe coronary artery disease, and more than 90% had significant (>70% stenosis) disease in at least 1 major coronary artery.[10]

Peripheral vascular surgery is associated with greater cardiac morbidity and overall mortality than other forms of noncardiac surgery. Physiologic factors associated with surgery predispose to myocardial ischemia, which is more pronounced in patients with underlying coronary disease. Myocardial ischemia can result from increases in myocardial oxygen demand secondary to increases in blood pressure and heart rate, elevated preload, and increased contractility, or from decreases in oxygen supply due to hypotension, tachycardia, increased filling pressure, anemia, hypoxemia, and obstructed coronary blood flow due to acute thrombosis or spasm. It is important to keep in mind that the leading causes for acute coronary and cerebrovascular syndromes (unstable angina, MI, sudden death, and stroke) are plaque disruption and thrombus formation in mildly stenotic lesions that may not be detectable by angiography or cardiovascular testing.[2]

Perioperative myocardial infarction (MI) is reported to occur in 4% to 15% of patients undergoing peripheral vascular surgery and accounts for more than 50% of perioperative mortality.[11,12] Cardiac risk also remains high in the subsequent months for patients who have suffered a perioperative cardiac event. Mangano et al have found that patients surviving a postoperative in-hospital MI had a 28-fold increase in the rate of cardiac complications within 6 months following surgery.[13] L'Italien et al investigated 547 patients undergoing vascular surgery from 2 medical centers who underwent aortic, infrainguinal, or carotid vascular surgery. Perioperative MI occurred in 6% of patients undergoing aortic and carotid artery surgery and in 13% of patients undergoing infrainguinal procedures. Although patients undergoing infrainguinal procedures exhibited more than twice the risk for perioperative MI compared with patients undergoing aortic surgery, this value was reduced to insignificant levels after adjustment for comorbid factors.[14] Using the Medicare National Inpatient Sample from 1994 through 1999, Birkmeyer et al noted that in high-volume hospitals, the perioperative mortality rates for carotid endarterectomy, lower-extremity bypass, and aneurysm surgery were 1.5%, 4.1%, and 3.9%, respectively.[15]

As stated in the guidelines on perioperative cardiovascular evaluation and care for noncardiac surgery published by the American College of Cardiology (ACC) and the American Heart Association (AHA), "patients who require vascular surgery appear to have an increased risk for cardiac complications because (1) many of the risk factors that contribute to peripheral vascular disease (eg, diabetes mellitus, tobacco use, and hyperlipidemia) are also risk factors for CAD; (2) the usual symptomatic presentation for CAD in these patients may be obscured by exercise limitations imposed by advanced age, intermittent claudication, or both; and (3) major open vascular surgery may be associated with substantial fluctuations in intravascular/extravascular fluid volumes, cardiac filling pressures, systemic blood pressure, heart rate, and thrombogenicity."[16]

Multivariate analysis, initially developed by Goldman and based on routine clinical information and laboratory tests, identified combinations of factors that could estimate the risk of cardiac complications. More recently, Lee et al derived and validated a Revised Cardiac Risk Index (RCRI) for the prediction of cardiac risk in stable patients undergoing nonurgent major cardiac surgery. It is currently the most used model of risk assessment in noncardiac surgery. The authors identified 6 independent predictors of complications: high-risk type of surgery (intrathoracic, intra-abdominal, suprapubic vascular), history of CAD, history of congestive heart failure, history of cerebrovascular disease, preoperative treatment with insulin, preoperative serum creatinine greater than 2 mg/dL. These predictors were validated later in a cohort of 1422 patients. The predictive value was significant in all types of elective major noncardiac surgery except for abdominal aortic aneurysm surgery. Cardiac event rates for 0, 1, 2, and 3 or more than 3 of the 6 factors were 0.4%, 0.9%, 7%, and 11%, respectively.[17]

The current standards for preoperative cardiac evaluation of these patients are the guidelines published by the ACC and the AHA initially in 1996 and revised in 2002 and in 2007.[16] The 2007 ACC/AHA guidelines identify a group of active cardiac conditions that when present indicate major clinical risk (**Box 55-1**) and for which patients should undergo evaluation and treatment before noncardiac surgery. Based on the widespread use of RCRI, the ACC/AHA 2007 perioperative guidelines have replaced the intermediate-risk category from the 2002 version of the guidelines with the following clinical risk factors: history of ischemic heart disease, history of compensated or prior heart failure, history of cerebrovascular disease, diabetes mellitus, and renal insufficiency. Also, the 2007 guidelines do not segregate clinical risk factors into major, intermediate, and minor. The guidelines provide a 5-step algorithm for determining which patients should undergo further cardiac testing based on functional capacity (**Box 55-2**), the surgery-specific risk (**Box 55-3**), and the presence of clinical risk

BOX 55-1

Active Cardiac Conditions for Which the Patient Should Undergo Evaluation and Treatment Before Noncardiac Surgery

Condition	Examples
Unstable coronary syndromes	Unstable or severe angina (CCS class III or IV)[a]
	Recent MI[b]
Decompensated HF (NYHA functional class IV; worsening or new-onset HF)	High-grade atrioventricular block
	Mobitz II atrioventricular block
	Third-degree atrioventricular heart block
Significant arrhythmias	Symptomatic ventricular arrhythmias
	Supraventricular arrhythmias (including atrial fibrillation) with uncontrolled ventricular rate (HR greater than 100 bpm at rest)
	Symptomatic bradycardia
	Newly recognized ventricular tachycardia
Severe valvular disease	Severe aortic stenosis (mean pressure gradient greater than 40 mm Hg, aortic valve area less than 1.0 cm^2, or symptomatic)
	Symptomatic mitral stenosis (progressive dyspnea on exertion, exertional presyncope, or HF)

[a]May include stable angina in patients who are unusually sedentary.

[b]The American College of Cardiology National Database Library defines recent MI as more than 7 days but less than or equal to 1 month (within 30 days).

CCS, Canadian Cardiovascular Society; HF, heart failure; HR, heart rate; MI, myocardial infarction; NYHA, New York Heart Association

From Fleisher LA, Beckman JA, Brown KA, et al. ACC/AHA 2007 guidelines on perioperative cardiovascular evaluation and care for noncardiac surgery: executive summary: a report of the American College of Cardiology/American Heart Association Task Force on Practice Guidelines (Writing Committee to Revise the 2002 Guidelines on Perioperative Cardiovascular Evaluation for Noncardiac Surgery) developed in collaboration with the American Society of Echocardiography, American Society of Nuclear Cardiology, Heart Rhythm Society, Society of Cardiovascular Anesthesiologists, Society for Cardiovascular Angiography and Interventions, Society for Vascular Medicine and Biology, and Society for Vascular Surgery. *J Am Coll Cardiol.* 2007;50:1707-1732.

BOX 55-3

Cardiac Risk[a] Stratification for Noncardiac Surgical Procedures

Risk Stratification	Procedure Examples
Vascular (reported cardiac risk often more than 5%)	Aortic and other major vascular surgery
	Peripheral vascular surgery
Intermediate (reported cardiac risk generally 1% to 5%)	Intraperitoneal and intrathoracic surgery
	Carotid endarterectomy
	Head and neck surgery
	Orthopedic surgery
	Prostate surgery
Low[b] (reported cardiac risk generally less than 1%)	Endoscopic procedures
	Superficial procedure
	Cataract surgery
	Breast surgery
	Ambulatory surgery

[a]Combined incidence of cardiac death and nonfatal myocardial infarction.

[b]These procedures do not generally require further preoperative cardiac testing.

From Fleisher LA, Beckman JA, Brown KA, et al. ACC/AHA 2007 guidelines on perioperative cardiovascular evaluation and care for noncardiac surgery: executive summary: a report of the American College of Cardiology/American Heart Association Task Force on Practice Guidelines (Writing Committee to Revise the 2002 Guidelines on Perioperative Cardiovascular Evaluation for Noncardiac Surgery) developed in collaboration with the American Society of Echocardiography, American Society of Nuclear Cardiology, Heart Rhythm Society, Society of Cardiovascular Anesthesiologists, Society for Cardiovascular Angiography and Interventions, Society for Vascular Medicine and Biology, and Society for Vascular Surgery. *J Am Coll Cardiol.* 2007;50:1707-1732.

BOX 55-2

Estimated Energy Requirements for Various Activities

	Can you…
1 MET	Take care of yourself?
	Eat, dress, or use the toilet?
	Walk indoors around the house?
	Walk a block or 2 on level ground at 2 to 3 mi/h (3.2 to 4.8 km/h)?
4 METs	Do light work around the house like dusting or washing dishes?

	Can you…
4 METs	Climb a flight of stairs or walk up a hill?
	Walk on level ground al 4 mi/h (6.4 km/h)?
	Run a short distance?
	Do heavy work around the house like scrubbing floors or lifting or moving heavy furniture?
	Participate in moderate recreational activities like golf, bowling, dancing, doubles tennis, or throwing a baseball or football?
Greater than 10 METs	Participate in strenuous sports like swimming, singles tennis, football, basketball, or skiing?

From Fleisher LA, Beckman JA, Brown KA, et al. ACC/AHA 2007 Guidelines on perioperative cardiovascular evaluation and care for noncardiac surgery: executive summary: a report of the American College of Cardiology/American Heart Association Task Force on Practice Guidelines (Writing Committee to Revise the 2002 Guidelines on Perioperative Cardiovascular Evaluation for Noncardiac Surgery) developed in collaboration with the American Society of Echocardiography, American Society of Nuclear Cardiology, Heart Rhythm Society, Society of Cardiovascular Anesthesiologists, Society for Cardiovascular Angiography and Interventions, Society for Vascular Medicine and Biology, and Society for Vascular Surgery. *J Am Coll Cardiol.* 2007;50:1707-1732.

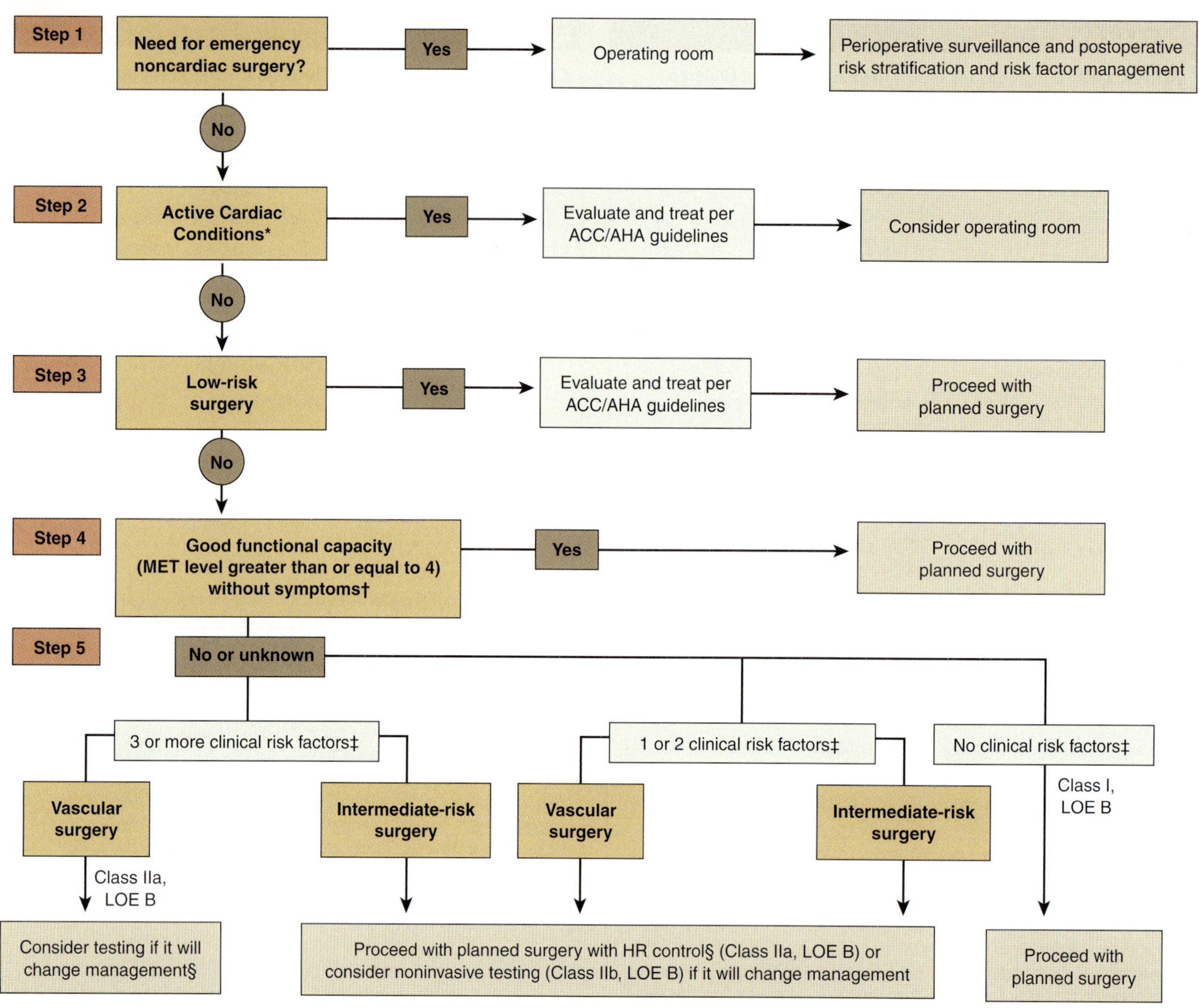

FIGURE 55-3. Cardiac evaluation and care algorithm for noncardiac surgery based on active clinical conditions, known cardiovascular disease, or cardiac risk factors for patients 50 years of age or older.
*See Box 55-1 for active clinical conditions.
†See Box 55-2 for estimated MET level equivalent.
‡Clinical risk factors include ischemic heart disease, compensated or prior heart failure, diabetes mellitus, renal insufficiency, and cerebrovascular disease.
§Consider perioperative beta blockade for populations in which this has been shown to reduce cardiac morbidity/mortality.
ACC/AHA, American College of Cardiology/American Heart Association;HR, heart rate; LOE, level of evidence; and MET, metabolic equivalent.
[From Fleisher LA, Beckman JA, Brown KA, et al. ACC/AHA 2007 guidelines on perioperative cardiovascular evaluation and care for noncardiac surgery: executive summary: a report of the American College of Cardiology/American Heart Association Task Force on Practice Guidelines (Writing Committee to Revise the 2002 Guidelines on Perioperative Cardiovascular Evaluation for Noncardiac Surgery) developed in collaboration with the American Society of Echocardiography, American Society of Nuclear Cardiology, Heart Rhythm Society, Society of Cardiovascular Anesthesiologists, Society for Cardiovascular Angiography and Interventions, Society for Vascular Medicine and Biology, and Society for Vascular Surgery. *J Am Coll Cardiol.* 2007;50:1707-1732.]

factors (**Fig. 55-3**). Several studies have assessed the utility of the ACC/AHA guidelines for risk stratification. Licker et al compared data from 2 consecutive 4-year periods (1993-1996 control period vs 1997-2000 intervention period). The introduction of ACC/AHA protocols was associated with increased preoperative myocardial scanning (44.3% vs 20.6%) and coronary revascularization (7.7% vs 0.8%) as well as a significant decrease in the incidence of cardiac complications (11.3%-4.5%) and an increase in event-free survival at 1 year after surgery (91.3%-98.2%).[18,19]

Recent Myocardial Infarction and Angina Acute MI is defined as a documented MI 7 days or less before the examination, and a recent MI is defined as a documented MI more than 7 days but less than or equal to 1 month before the examination.[16] Recent myocardial infarction and unstable and severe angina represent active cardiac conditions for which patients should undergo evaluation and treatment before noncardiac surgery.[16]

Traditionally, risk assessment for noncardiac surgery was based on the time interval between the MI and the surgery. Older studies found as much as a 36% risk of reinfarction or cardiac death when patients underwent surgery within 3 months of a previous MI. The risk fell to 15% to 25% at 3 to 6 months, and 5% when surgery was performed after more than 6 months.[20] However, due to preoperative optimization and intensive perioperative monitoring, the risk was lower in later studies.[21]

The ACC/AHA guidelines for perioperative evaluation of the cardiac patient undergoing noncardiac surgery advocate a wait period of 4 to 6 weeks after MI and before proceeding with an elective surgery; after that period, risk stratification is based on the presentation of the disease.

Risk stratification of patients with acute coronary syndromes such as unstable or severe angina begins upon presentation and continues throughout to predict those who are at high risk for further ischemic events or adverse outcomes. Such patients should not undergo noncardiac surgery except in the most emergent of circumstances.

Valvular Diseases Severe valvular disease is considered by the 2007 ACC/AHA guidelines as an active cardiac condition that when present may indicate major clinical risk. However, when the clinician is aware of the pathophysiologic implications of the disease and uses individual clinical judgment, patients can undergo surgery with a risk that is not so high, and may not be different from controls.

Severe aortic stenosis deserves special attention as it represents a risk factor for preoperative cardiac complications.[22,23] The 2007 ACC/AHA guidelines recommend that in patients with symptomatic severe aortic stenosis elective noncardiac surgery "should generally be postponed or canceled" and such patients should undergo aortic valve replacement. If the aortic stenosis is severe but asymptomatic, elective surgery should be postponed if the valve has not been evaluated within the year.[16]

Diabetes Diabetes has been strongly suggested as a predictor for perioperative cardiac morbidity after vascular surgery, and insulin therapy for diabetes mellitus has been identified as a significant risk factor for cardiac morbidity in the RCRI.[17] Altered autonomic function in diabetes may predispose to greater intraoperative risk of blood pressure lability, variation of heart rate, gastroparesis, and decreased esophageal sphincter tone. Diabetic autonomic neuropathies can obscure symptoms of myocardial ischemia, thus adding to the already high incidence of "silent" ischemia seen in the perioperative period. The presence of diabetes in vascular surgery patients may identify a population in whom DTI is useful.

Pulmonary Disease Preoperative evaluation of patients with pulmonary disease allows for optimization, risk stratification, and designing of strategies for reduction of postoperative pulmonary complications. The most important components of preoperative assessment of patients with known pulmonary disease are a thorough history and a comprehensive physical examination.[24] Pulmonary function tests (PFT) may be useful to assess severity of disease and adequacy of bronchodilator therapy in patients in whom it is difficult to elicit this from history or physical examination.[24] Arterial blood gases may be used to evaluate the degree of pulmonary disease and provide a baseline for subsequent clinical decisions.

Many vascular patients are chronic smokers; cigarette smoking increases the risk for postoperative pulmonary and nonpulmonary complications even in the absence of chronic lung disease.[24] The risk of pneumonia is twice as high in smokers as in nonsmokers, and the development of hypoxemia in the postoperative period occurs more frequently and more severely in smokers as compared with nonsmokers.

Renal Disease The presence of preexisting renal disease (preoperative serum creatinine levels ≥2 mg/dL) increases the rates of morbidity and mortality for patients undergoing major vascular surgery[16,25]; therefore, a comprehensive preoperative evaluation of a vascular surgical patient should include an assessment of renal function.

Causes of baseline renal insufficiency include atherosclerosis of the renal arteries, hypertension, diabetic nephropathy, and depressed myocardial function. Contrast-enhanced imaging studies performed before surgeries also alter renal function by both a direct toxic effect and by a hyperosmolar-induced diuresis that reduces the intravascular volume. Intravascular volume expansion before, during, and after the angiographic study minimizes renal effects.

In the vascular patient undergoing abdominal aortic surgery there are several causes of renal impairment superimposing on an already precarious renal function. These additional causes of renal impairment include wide fluctuations in the intravascular volume and cardiac output; altered neuroendocrine milieu with increased epinephrine, norepinephrine, and renin secretion; and emboli shower dislodged by the aortic clamp and dysfunctional effects on renal hemodynamics from aortic cross-clamping.

Evolving technology and progress in surgical and anesthetic management has decreased the incidence of renal failure.

DIAGNOSTIC TESTING

Electrocardiogram Preoperative electrocardiogram (ECG) abnormalities are observed in 40% to 70% of patients with CAD undergoing noncardiac surgery such as ST-segment and T-wave abnormalities (65%-90%) and Q waves (0.5%-8%). Abnormal ECG can be due to several other causes such as metabolic and electrolyte disturbances, pulmonary disease, conduction disturbances, and medications. Although some studies have demonstrated that the presence of ECG abnormalities such as Q waves, significant ST-segment elevation or depression, and left ventricular hypertrophy pattern have been associated with an increased incidence of cardiac complications in patients undergoing major noncardiac surgery,[17] other studies have failed to demonstrate the predictive value of the preoperative 12-lead ECG.[26]

Exercise Electrocardiography Noninvasive diagnostic tests have been proposed to evaluate the extent of CAD before noncardiac surgery and permit further stratification in patients deemed to be at intermediate risk after clinical evaluation. Detailed cardiac assessment and treatment are not feasible in the emergent setting. However, according to the 2007 ACC/AHA guidelines for preoperative evaluation of patients undergoing elective vascular surgery, noninvasive stress testing is reasonable in patients with 3 or more clinical risk factors (class IIa) or at least 1 to 2 clinical risk factors (class IIb) and poor functional capacity (<4 metabolic equivalents [METs]) who require vascular surgery if it will change management.[16] One caveat of interpreting stress testing in the overall preoperative evaluation of the patient is that for the purpose of predicting perioperative cardiac events, stress testing has a high negative predictive value (90%-100%) but low positive predictive value (6%-67%), thus being more useful in reducing estimated risk if negative (or normal) than for identifying patients at very high risk if positive.[27]

Exercise ECG without myocardial imaging has been the traditional method for evaluating CAD, and is the standard method for determining functional capacity and detecting myocardial ischemia with a sensitivity of 68% to 81% and a specificity of 66% to 77%. Exercise tolerance appears to be more important than the ECG response to exercise. McPhail et al showed that the ability to perform moderate exercise or to achieve greater than 85% of predicted maximal heart rate during treadmill exercise testing is associated with a low risk of a postoperative cardiac event even in the presence of ST-segment depression more than 1 mm.[28]

Two groups of patients are excluded from performing exercise ECG testing: patients who cannot exercise (due to leg claudication, arthritis, deconditioning, or associated pulmonary disease) and patients who have abnormalities on the resting ECG such as preexcitation (Wolff-Parkinson-White) syndrome, a paced ventricular rhythm, more than 1 mm of ST-segment depression at rest, complete left bundle branch block, or ECG criteria for left ventricular hypertrophy. These patients may undergo pharmacological stress testing. The 2 most commonly used tests are dipyridamole-thallium myocardial perfusion imaging (DTI) and dobutamine stress echocardiography (DSE).

RADIONUCLIDE MYOCARDIAL PERFUSION IMAGING METHODS

Radionuclide myocardial perfusion imaging (MPI) involves the visualization of a radiopharmaceutical that is distributed throughout the myocardium in proportion to coronary blood flow, thereby permitting the determination of relative blood flow in various regions of the heart. The vasodilators used for pharmacologic myocardial perfusion imaging are adenosine, regadenoson, and dipyridamole. Adenosine and dipyridamole are equally effective, but adenosine has the advantages of a very short half-life, rapid reversal of side effects after the test is completed, and possibly more predictable vasodilation. The vasodilator agents should be avoided in patients with resting hypotension (because these drugs lower the blood pressure), sick sinus syndrome, or a high degree atrioventricular (AV) block in the absence of backup pacing. In addition, adenosine and dipyridamole should not be used in patients with bronchospastic airway disease. The most frequently used myocardial perfusion agents are thallium-201 and technetium 99–labeled agents. Thallium-201 is taken up by cells similarly to potassium and is readily assimilated by healthy myocardial cells, and thus infarcted, ischemic, or hypoperfused areas appear as defects. After injection of thallium or 99-technetium, normal myocardium will show up on initial imaging while areas of infarction or hypoperfusion distal to a stenosis will appear as a defect. After dissipation of the dilatory effect and after a second injection of technetium, defects caused by ischemia will resolve while those caused by scarred infarcted tissue will persist.

MPI has a high sensitivity for detecting patients at risk for perioperative cardiac events. The negative predictive value for MI or cardiac death of a normal scan is very high at approximately 99%, and the positive predictive value of an abnormal scan with reversible defects is very low, varying between 2% and 20%.[16] Given the low positive predictive value, this test is best used on patients at high clinical risk for perioperative cardiac events. The ability to identify patients at risk may be improved when taking into account the extent of ischemia rather than only its presence. A recent meta-analysis showed that the probability of MI or cardiac death ranged from 3% to 4% in patients with no or only fixed defects, to 9% in patients with reversible defects involving less than 20% of the left ventricle, to 18% and 45% in patients with reversible defects involving 30% to 49% and more than 50% of the left ventricle, respectively.[29] In a meta-analysis of dypiridamole MPI for risk stratification before elective vascular surgery, Shaw et al showed that the pretest coronary disease probability was correlated with the positive predictive value of a reversible DTI, increasing 6-fold from low- to high-risk patient subsets. Cardiac event rates were low in patients without a history of coronary artery disease (1% in 176 patients) compared with patients with coronary disease and a normal or fixed-defect pattern (4.8% in 83 patients) and 1 or more thallium-201 redistribution abnormality (18.6% in 97 patients).[30]

Conversely, Baron et al studied a large consecutive population of patients undergoing abdominal aortic surgery and were unable to demonstrate an association between thallium redistribution and perioperative cardiac morbidity. In this study the presence of definite CAD and age greater than 65 years were better predictors of cardiac complications than perfusion imaging, raising the need for caution regarding the indiscriminate evaluation with DTI of patients undergoing vascular surgery.[98]

DOBUTAMINE STRESS ECHOCARDIOGRAPHY

Dobutamine stress echocardiography (DSE) is preferred in patients with bronchospastic lung disease and in those with severe carotid stenosis because adenosine and dipyridamole may induce bronchospasm and hypotension. It also provides information about left ventricular function or valvular heart disease. As opposed to DTI, which is limited in its methodology by not increasing myocardial oxygen consumption, the administration of dobutamine mimics intraoperative conditions by increasing the heart rate. Similarly to other noninvasive testing, DSE had a high negative predictive value ranging from 93% to 100% and a relatively low positive predictive value up to 33%.[16] Kertai et al performed a meta-analysis of studies looking at perioperative cardiac risk stratification in patients undergoing major vascular surgery (8119 patients). They concluded that DSE showed a positive trend toward better diagnostic performance than the other tests, but this was only significant in the comparison with MPI.[31] The predictive value appears to vary with patient risk. This was illustrated in a recent analysis of 1097 patients who were assigned 1 point for each of the following clinical risk factors: age older than 70 years, current or prior angina and prior MI, congestive heart failure, or cerebrovascular event. The study showed that the additional predictive value of DSE is limited in clinically low-risk patients (<3 clinical risk factors) receiving β-blockers such that DSE may be avoided in a large number of patients who can proceed safely for surgery without delay. In patients with 3 or more risk factors, DSE provided additional prognostic information; patients without stress-induced ischemia had a much lower risk of events than those with stress-induced ischemia (among those receiving β-blockers, 2.0% vs 10.6%). Moreover, patients with limited stress-induced ischemia (1-4 segments) experienced fewer cardiac events than those with more extensive ischemia (≥5 segments).[32] Other studies have suggested that the extent of the wall-motion abnormality and/or wall-motion change at low ischemic thresholds, particularly at a heart rate of less than 60% of age-predicted maximum, are important predictors of long-term or short-term outcomes.[16]

TRANSTHORACIC ECHOCARDIOGRAPHY

Transthoracic echocardiography (TTE) may add predictive information about the risk of postoperative cardiac complications in selected patients.[33]

A recent study evaluated the prevalence of left ventricular (LV) dysfunction in 1005 consecutive patients undergoing vascular surgery. Left ventricular dysfunction was diagnosed in 506 (50%) patients. Of the patients with LV dysfunction, 403 (80%) patients had asymptomatic LV dysfunction and 103 (20%) had symptomatic heart failure. Of the patients with asymptomatic LV dysfunction, 209 (52%) had asymptomatic isolated diastolic LV dysfunction and 194 (48%) had asymptomatic systolic LV dysfunction. This study also looked at the association of asymptomatic heart failure with perioperative cardiac events in patients undergoing vascular surgery and found that in open vascular surgery both asymptomatic systolic and isolated left ventricle diastolic dysfunctions were associated with 30-day cardiovascular events and long-term cardiovascular mortality. In endovascular surgery, only symptomatic heart failure was associated with 30-day cardiovascular events and long-term cardiovascular mortality.[34]

The 2007 ACC/AHA guidelines for preoperative evaluation of patients undergoing elective vascular surgery recommend preoperative evaluation of LV function in patients with dyspnea of unknown origin or in patients with current or prior heart failure with worsening dyspnea or change in clinical status (class IIa recommendation). However, based on recent findings some investigators suggest a move toward more routine cardiac echocardiography evaluation, especially in patients undergoing open vascular surgery.[34]

CORONARY ANGIOGRAPHY

In the perioperative setting, many infarctions are the result of acute thrombosis of a noncritical stenosis, therefore limiting the value of routine angiography prior to major noncardiac surgery. The 2007 ACC/AHA guidelines for preoperative evaluation of patients undergoing elective vascular surgery state that indications for preoperative coronary angiography are similar to those identified for the nonoperative setting.[16]

PREOPERATIVE THERAPY

Prophylactic preoperative coronary revascularization, through either coronary artery bypass grafting (CABG) or percutaneous coronary intervention (PCI), to decrease perioperative complications is controversial. Some earlier studies have indicated that CABG before major elective surgery may improve long-term survival and reduce the incidence of perioperative cardiac complications in patients with multiple cardiac risk factors and/or multiple vessel disease.[35,36] However, in some patients the risk of coronary artery bypass surgery and the added risk of delaying the needed vascular surgery might outweigh the benefits of such an approach. Furthermore, these studies did not take into account the effectiveness of cardioprotective medication such as β-blockers and statins for the reduction of perioperative and long-term cardiac complications.

PREOPERATIVE CORONARY ARTERY BYPASS GRAFTING

The Coronary Artery Revascularization Prophylaxis (CARP) trial was the first large, randomized trial to assess the long-term benefit of preoperative coronary artery revascularization in patients with stable CAD undergoing elective vascular surgery. This study prospectively randomized 510 patients with stable coronary disease to either coronary revascularization by CABG surgery, PCI, or medical therapy before undergoing major vascular surgery. Two-thirds of the enrolled patients had either 1- or 2-vessel disease. Excluded from the study were patients who had unstable coronary disease, left main coronary artery stenosis, severe left ventricular dysfunction, or severe aortic stenosis. Potentially beneficial medications, including β-blockers, antiplatelet agents, angiotensin-converting enzyme inhibitors, and statins, were widely used in both groups. Eighty-four percent of the patients in the revascularization group and 86% of the patients in the medical therapy group received β-blockers. The study found no significant difference in long-term outcome. After 2.7 years, mortality was 22% in the revascularization group and 23% in the nonrevascularized group. However, the study was also not large enough to provide a conclusive analysis of the potential benefit of revascularization in high-risk subgroups, such as those with a large stress-induced defect on MPI or those with 3-vessel disease plus left ventricular dysfunction.[37]

The Dutch Echocardiographic Cardiac Risk Evaluation Applying Stress Echo-V (DECREASE-V) pilot study reported similar results in a high-risk cohort of patients undergoing vascular surgery. In this study, 430 patients were identified as being high-risk due to 3 or more cardiac risk factors (similar to risk factors from the RCRI) and underwent DSE or MPI. Of these patients, 101 (23%) had extensive stress-induced ischemia (≥5 segments on dobutamine echo or ≥3 walls on stress nuclear imaging) and were randomized to the best medical therapy and revascularization or the best medical therapy alone. Optimized medical therapy consisted of aspirin, β-blocker, angiotensin-converting enzyme inhibitor, and statin. There was no difference in mortality and nonfatal MI at 30-days and 1-year between the 2 groups.[38]

In contrast to these findings, other reports suggest that surgical revascularization may provide a net reduction in perioperative and, in particular, long-term morbidity and mortality in selected patients with coronary disease who undergo major noncardiac surgery. Landesberg et al, in a retrospective observational study of 502 consecutive patients undergoing major vascular surgery, found that patients with moderate to severe ischemia on MPI who underwent subsequent coronary revascularization (by either CABG or PCI) had better long-term survival than patients with similar preoperative thallium scanning results who did not undergo revascularization.[39] The difference in results compared with the CARP trial may be due to the fact that, while only 33% of the patients enrolled in the CARP trial had triple-vessel disease and the patients with left main disease were excluded, 73% of the patients enrolled in this study had triple-vessel or left main disease.

The 2007 ACC/AHA guidelines for preoperative evaluation of patients undergoing elective vascular surgery recommend coronary revascularization in patients with stable angina who have significant left main coronary artery stenosis, 3-vessel disease, 2-vessel disease with significant proximal left anterior descending (LAD) stenosis plus either an ejection fraction less than 50% or demonstrable ischemia on noninvasive testing, high-risk unstable angina, non–ST-segment-elevation MI (NSTEMI), or acute ST-elevation MI (STEMI) (class I indication).[16]

PREOPERATIVE PERCUTANEOUS CORONARY INTERVENTION

Percutaneous coronary intervention (PCI) can be performed either through stenting or angioplasty (percutaneous transluminal coronary angioplasty [PTCA]). Drug-eluting stents are now implanted in most PCI procedures because of a much lower expected rate of restenosis and target vessel revascularization than that seen with angioplasty alone or bare-metal stents. However, recent studies have questioned whether long-term outcomes, including stent restenosis, MI, and cardiac death, are lower with drug-eluting stents compared with bare-metal stents.[40-42]

The role of PCI in preventing perioperative cardiac events in patients undergoing noncardiac surgery is less well established and appears to be limited to patients with unstable active CAD (unstable angina, STEMI, NSTEMI) in whom PCI would be independently indicated, irrespective of the scheduled surgery.[16]

Coronary stenting poses unique challenges related either to perioperative bleeding due to postprocedural antiplatelet therapy or to stent thrombosis that may be associated with withholding or reducing antiplatelet therapy in order to minimize bleeding. The reason for the increased risk of stent thrombosis in patients undergoing noncardiac surgery may be multifactorial and includes incomplete endothelialization of the stent, premature interruption of dual antiplatelet therapy, and the prothrombotic state associated with surgery. When it occurs, stent thrombosis is a feared complication associated with significant morbidity and mortality. The incidence of death or MI was 64.4% in patients with bare-metal stent thrombosis, and mortality as a result of drug-eluting stent thrombosis ranged from 20% to 45%.[43] For patients who require revascularization before noncardiac surgery, the timing and bleeding risk of surgery needs to be carefully considered before catheterization. For PTCA, delaying noncardiac surgery for at least 2 weeks allows for healing of the vessel injury at the balloon treatment site. However, postponing noncardiac surgery for more than 8 weeks after balloon angioplasty may raise the likelihood of restenosis at the angioplasty site, theoretically raising the chances of perioperative ischemia or MI.[16] After bare-metal stent placement, elective surgery should be postponed for 4 to 6 weeks for proper dual antiplatelet therapy (aspirin and clopidogrel) during stent endothelialization in order to reduce the risk for coronary stent thrombosis. For drug-eluting stent placement, it is recommended that elective noncardiac surgery be delayed for at least 12 months due to delayed endothelialization and risk for early and late stent thrombosis with premature discontinuation of dual antiplatelet therapy; premature discontinuation of dual antiplatelet therapy markedly increases the risk for catastrophic stent thrombosis, resulting in death or MI.[44]

PERIOPERATIVE MEDICAL THERAPY

Nitrates, β-blockers, and calcium channel blockers are common chronic medications in vascular surgery patients. Perioperative discontinuation of these therapies may lead to perioperative ischemia, dysrhythmias, MI, and cardiac death. Therefore, it is recommended to continue all significant cardiovascular medications up to and including the morning of surgery.

β-Blockers β-blockers have been the most studied and advocated perioperative medical therapy. Clinical studies have shown that perioperative beta-blockade can reduce mortality and cardiovascular complications in high-risk patients who must undergo noncardiac surgery.[45,46] β-blockers reduce myocardial oxygen demand by decreasing heart rate, contractility, and afterload; decrease the incidence of plaque rupture by reducing mechanical stress via hemodynamic effects; exert antiarrhythmic and anti-inflammatory effects; alter gene expression; and protect against apoptosis.[47]

The PeriOperative Ischemic Evaluation (POISE) trial was the first large trial of perioperative beta-blockade, which randomized 8351 patients with, or at risk of, atherosclerotic disease to receive either extended-release metoprolol succinate or placebo. Treatment was started 2 to 4 hours before surgery and continued for 30 days. The primary composite end point (cardiovascular death, nonfatal MI, and nonfatal cardiac arrest) was lower at 30 days in the metoprolol group than in the placebo group due mostly to a reduction in nonfatal MI. However, there were more deaths in the metoprolol group and more strokes. The increased mortality seems to have been secondary to sepsis or infection, but the mechanism by which β-blockers increase death in the setting of sepsis is not entirely clear. Additionally, clinically significant hypotension and bradycardia were increased in the metoprolol group. The investigators in this trial recommended reconsideration of the perioperative guidelines in light of the findings of this trial.[48]

The 2007 ACC/AHA perioperative guidelines recommend that β-blockers should be continued in patients undergoing surgery who are receiving β-blockers to treat angina, symptomatic arrhythmias, hypertension, or other ACC/AHA class I guideline indications (class I indication). Also, β-blockers should be given to patients undergoing vascular surgery who are at high cardiac risk owing to the finding of ischemia on preoperative testing (class I indication). Beta-blockers are recommended for vascular surgery patients in whom preoperative assessment identifies coronary heart disease or high cardiac risk as defined by the presence of multiple clinical risk factors (class IIa indication). Beta-blockers should be started days to weeks before elective surgery, and accumulating evidence suggests that heart rate control less than 65 beats per minute should be targeted.[49,50]

α_2-Agonists Although evidence supporting the routine use of α_2-agonists such as clonidine is not as compelling as that for perioperative beta-blockade, the ACC/AHA perioperative guidelines have introduced the use of α_2-agonists as a class IIb recommendation for perioperative control of hypertension in patients with known CAD or at least 1 clinical risk factor.

Statins Statins inhibit hydroxy-methylglutarate coenzyme A activity and decrease serum lipid levels. Recently, attention has focused on the role of statins in reducing adverse perioperative cardiac events. Beyond their lipid-lowering effects, statins have pleiotrophic effects, which include improvement of endothelial function, atherosclerotic plaque stabilization, decreased oxidative stress, and decreased vascular inflammation. These effects may prevent plaque rupture and MI in the perioperative period. Several studies have evaluated the perioperative use of statins in vascular surgery patients. Kertai et al retrospectively evaluated 570 patients undergoing open repair for infrarenal abdominal aortic aneurysm and found that statins reduced the incidence of the composite end point (perioperative mortality and MI).[51] The Dutch Echocardiographic Cardiac Risk Evaluation Applying Stress Echocardiography-III (DECREASE-III) trial looked at the beneficial role of long-term statin therapy on perioperative cardiac outcome. This study randomized 497 statin-naïve patients to fluvastatin XL 80 mg daily or placebo for a median of 37 days before noncardiac vascular surgery (abdominal aortic aneurysm repair, distal aortoiliac reconstruction, lower-limb arterial reconstruction, or carotid-artery endarterectomy) and continued for at least 1 month following surgery. The combined end point of cardiovascular mortality or nonfatal MI was significantly lower in the group receiving fluvastatin XL.[52]

The 2007 ACC/AHA guidelines recommend continuation of statin therapy perioperatively in patients already receiving it (class I indication) and suggest that prescribing a statin is reasonable in patients undergoing vascular surgery whether or not they have other risk factors (class IIa indication).[16]

GENERAL CONSIDERATIONS

Modern developments in risk assessment, surgical risk modification, physiologic monitoring, anti-ischemic therapies, techniques of anesthesia and analgesia, and postoperative intensive care and rehabilitation can all produce clinical pathways that truly optimize patient care. Full realization of this potential requires an integrated approach and collaboration between vascular surgery, cardiac surgery, cardiology, anesthesiology, and critical care medicine to a degree not easily achievable in most institutions.

Vascular surgery patients require intensive perioperative monitoring for 2 primary reasons: (1) these patients often have systemic manifestations of atherosclerotic vascular disease and are at risk for cardiac, cerebral, renal, and spinal cord ischemia, all of which can be diagnosed and treated using appropriate monitors; and (2) vascular procedures involve major physiologic changes, including significant third-space losses, blood loss, and the complications of transfusion (coagulopathies, hypocalcemia, hypothermia, and acidosis). There can also be significant changes in the hemodynamic profile associated with the application and release of vascular clamps.

In order to reduce cardiac morbidity, appropriate ECG monitoring is mandatory. A more recent study showed that monitoring the standard leads II and V5 detects 80% of ST-segment changes caused by ischemia, although V4 is preferable to V5 and the concomitant monitoring of 3 leads increases the sensitivity to 95% or higher. The following discussions presume that the American Society of Anesthesiology (ASA) standards of basic monitoring are met by using pulse oximetry, capnography, ECG, and body temperature measurement.[53]

CAROTID ENDARTERECTOMY

PATHOPHYSIOLOGY OF CAROTID DISEASE

Occlusive disease of the carotid system is commonly caused by atherosclerosis and involves the origins of both the internal and external carotid arteries as well as the bifurcation of the common carotid artery. Carotid atherosclerosis is usually most severe within 2 cm of the bifurcation of the common carotid artery, and predominantly involves the posterior wall of the vessel. The plaque encroaches on the lumen of the internal carotid artery and often extends caudally into the common carotid artery. Various theories have been proposed to explain atheromatous plaque formation at the carotid bifurcation. Impedance mismatch, with altered hemodynamic conditions that accompany the division of a vessel into conduits of substantially different sizes, may be implicated in the vessel injury. Plaque formation may produce symptoms either through low flow due to the stenosis with inadequate collateral compensation or by exhibiting degenerative changes that lead to atheromatous emboli and thromboemboli.

INDICATIONS

Although successful carotid endarterectomy (CEA) may reduce the risk of stroke in selected patients, it is always important to balance the risk of operation with the risk of stroke from the unoperated lesion.

Three major trials have investigated the efficacy of CEA in selected patients with symptomatic carotid atherosclerosis: the North American Symptomatic Carotid Endarterectomy Trial (NASCET), the European Carotid Surgery Trial (ECST), and the Veterans Affairs Cooperative Trial 309. These major clinical trials defined symptomatic carotid disease as focal ischemic symptoms that are referable to the appropriate carotid artery distribution, including 1 or more transient ischemic attacks characterized by focal neurologic dysfunction or transient monocular blindness, or 1 or more minor (nondisabling) ischemic strokes.[54,55] A recent pooled analysis of these 3 trials using the same measurements and definitions yielded highly consistent results. CEA is of some benefit for patients with 50% to 69% symptomatic stenosis and is highly beneficial for those with 70% symptomatic stenosis or greater but without near-occlusion. Benefit in patients with carotid near-occlusion is marginal in the short term and uncertain in the long term. CEA was not beneficial for symptomatic carotid stenosis of 30% to 49% stenosis, and was harmful for symptomatic patients with less than 30% stenosis.[56]

Three high-quality major trials—the Veterans Affairs Cooperative Study Group, the Asymptomatic Carotid Atherosclerosis Study (ACAS), and the Asymptomatic Carotid Surgery Trial (ACST)—have evaluated the efficacy of CEA in patients with asymptomatic high-grade carotid stenosis (≥60%). A meta-analysis of these 3 trials showed that despite a 3% perioperative stroke or death rate, CEA for asymptomatic carotid stenosis reduces the risk of any stroke by approximately 30% over 3 years. However, the absolute risk reduction is small for the first few years of follow-up.[57] The ACST showed that significant benefit for the population is not evident until 2 years after surgery. Early after CEA, perioperative morbidity outweighs the modest, though significant, reduction in stroke risk that accompanies this procedure. One of the major concerns among clinicians regarding the ACAS and ACST trials was that the low operative risk in the 2 trials (<3%) is not routinely matched in clinical practice. A meta-analysis of 46 surgical case series that published operative risks during the ACAS trial and 5 years after its publication found that operative mortality was 8 times higher than in the ACAS trial.[58] Therefore, institution-specific assessment of the risk of CEA should be a prime consideration when implementing results of clinical trials.[59]

Carotid artery stenosis can be managed either by established surgical treatment such as CEA or by nonsurgical approaches such as angioplasty or stenting. The Carotid Revascularization Endarterectomy versus Stenting Trial (CREST) was a randomized controlled trial that compared the outcomes of carotid artery stenting (CAS) with those of CEA among patients with symptomatic or asymptomatic extracranial carotid stenosis. The results indicated that CAS and CEA were associated with similar rates of the primary composite outcome—periprocedural stroke, myocardial infarction, or death and subsequent ipsilateral stroke within 4 years from randomization. However, periprocedural stroke was more likely in the carotid stenting group, whereas periprocedural myocardial infarction was more likely in the endarterectomy group, the latter having a lesser impact on the quality of life than stroke.[60]

Data from several studies identified clinical predictors for adverse outcome. Although not validated in other studies, 1 or more of the following characteristics have been associated with an increased risk of poor outcome of stroke, MI, or death at 30 days after CEA: age older than 80 years, congestive heart failure, chronic obstructive pulmonary disease, renal failure (serum creatinine concentration >2.0 mg/dL), contralateral carotid artery occlusion, recurrent ipsilateral carotid artery stenosis.[61]

INTRAOPERATIVE MONITORING

Monitoring for Cerebral Ischemia The beneficial effects of CEA over medical therapy are partially dependent on low perioperative morbidity. It is recommended that the perioperative stroke and death rate should be less than 6% for symptomatic patients and less than 3% for asymptomatic patients in order to maintain this benefit.[62]

The carotid artery must be temporarily completely occluded by a cross-clamp in order to perform the CEA. Although 80% to 85% of patients tolerate clamping of the carotid artery without symptoms, assessment of collateral circulation occurring contralaterally via the circle of Willis is needed in all patients. The most common technique to restore flow across the carotid artery is a temporary Javid shunt, which is inserted through the arteriotomy distally in the internal carotid artery and proximally in the common carotid artery. Although beneficial in restoring blood flow, shunt insertion may incur an embolism-associated stroke, can be associated with intimal dissection leading to acute occlusion, and by limiting exposure of the plaque may affect the adequacy of the endarterectomy. Several authorities argue that any monitoring modality that could reliably indicate inadequate cerebral blood flow would allow a more conservative use of the shunting procedure.

Electroencephalography Electroencephalography (EEG) is the gold standard for monitoring patients under general anesthesia (GA). Cerebral ischemia produces neuronal dysfunction, leading to slowing of frequencies or reduced amplitude in the EEG tracing. These changes may be generalized (global ischemia) or regional (focal ischemia). The depth of ischemia is associated with the severity of EEG changes. EEG cannot assess the whole cerebral cortex, however, and is less reliable at assessing subcortical structures. In the setting of CEA, the focal EEG changes after cross-clamping the carotid artery may be defined as none, mild (increase in theta waves <25% or decrease in amplitude >50%), moderate (increase of theta waves >25% or increase of delta waves <25%), or severe (increase of delta waves >25%, severe flattening of amplitude or isoelectric curve).[63] Pinkerton evaluated the efficacy of continuous intraoperative EEG monitoring in a group of 1661 CEA operations in which the EEG was the sole criterion for shunt insertion. Intraoperative stroke rate in the study group was 0.3% (5 strokes). Intraoperative EEG monitoring has accurately identified (99.92%) patients who may safely undergo CEA without the need of a shunt. A statistically significant increase in intraoperative stroke rate was associated with the development of an abnormal EEG, contralateral internal carotid artery occlusion, and the combination of both abnormal EEG and contralateral internal carotid occlusion.[64] One explanation for the high sensitivity of the EEG monitoring in this study may be the technique used (16-channel EEG interpreted by experts). A more recent study attempted to correlate neurologic changes in awake patients undergoing CEA under cervical block anesthesia with EEG and measurement of carotid artery stump pressure (SP). EEG identified cerebral ischemia in only 59.4% of patients needing shunt placement, with a false-positive rate of 1.0% and a false-negative rate of 40.6%. The study concluded that EEG as a guide to shunt placement has a poor sensitivity.[65]

Anesthetic agents and changes in temperature and blood pressure affect EEG. Additionally, the value of EEG monitoring is limited by the fact that most neurologic deficits after CEA is caused by thromboembolism rather than occlusion of blood flow during carotid clamping.

Processed EEG, such as compressed spectral array, density spectral array, and spectral edge frequency, is easier to monitor and interpret. Although there is still insufficient data, studies so far have shown that these techniques have a lower sensitivity than raw EEG.

Somatosensory-Evoked Potentials The most commonly used electrophysiologic technique to monitor functional continuity of nerve, spinal cord, and brain is somatosensory-evoked potentials (SSEPs). The use of SSEP monitoring during CEA is still inconclusive. Although some studies found similar sensitivity in their ability to detect postoperative neurologic defects when compared with EEG,[66] others have shown SSEP to be less sensitive than EEG in predicting the need for shunting.[67] Inhalational agents depress the cortical SSEP under general anesthesia, with increase in amplitude and latency in a dose-dependent manner. Accurate SSEP monitoring can be obtained, however, in most patients with 0.5 minimum alveolar concentration (MAC) of a volatile anesthetic supplemented by intravenous medications, usually narcotics or intravenous hypnotics. Furthermore, the technique is dependent on the availability of specialized equipment and trained staff.

Transcranial Doppler Transcranial Doppler (TCD) provides noninvasive assessment of the middle cerebral artery (MCA) by insonating the MCA through the temporal bone using a specially designed Doppler probe. As long as fluctuations in arterial blood pressure and arterial CO_2 content are small, changes in flow velocity reflect changes in cerebral blood flow. Hemodynamic compromise is indicated by a reduction in mean flow velocities or when there is slow flow acceleration. In addition, TCD has the unique ability to detect cerebral microembolic signals, reflecting the presence of gaseous or particulate matter in the insonated cerebral artery, which occur most commonly during the dissection phase, during shunting and unclamping, during wound closure, and in the first few hours postoperatively.[68]

Data regarding the reliability of TCD in monitoring for cerebral ischemia is controversial. Ackerstaff et al showed that stroke was independently associated with emboli during dissection and wound closure, greater than 90% decrease in MCA peak systolic velocity at cross-clamping, or greater than 100% increase of the pulsatility index of the Doppler signal at clamp release.[69] TCD may be used as a complementary monitoring technique to EEG. Although there is high overlap between low flow velocities and ipsilateral EEG slowing, neither technique alone may identify all candidates for shunting or prevent all strokes.[63] Technical difficulties or an inappropriate visualization window make TCD difficult to interpret in 15% to 20% of cases.

Near-Infrared Spectroscopy Near-infrared spectroscopy (NIRS) is a noninvasive technique that allows continuous monitoring of regional cerebral oxygenation (rSo_2) through the scalp and skull.

Although easy to use and interpret, noninvasive NIRS has several limitations related to the fact that NIRS primarily measures venous oxygen saturation at the level of the frontal lobes, and there is a wide range of values that are not associated with a clinically detectable neurologic dysfunction. Samra et al noted that although there was a significant change in ipsilateral rSo_2 during carotid cross-clamping as compared with preclamp and postclamp values, there was a highly variable patient-to-patient change in rSo_2 after carotid cross-clamping, with no relation to neurologic dysfunction.[70] A recent systematic literature review looking at the value of NIRS during CEA in perioperative stroke prevention found that a threshold for obtained NIRS values below which shunting should be indicated could not be determined in a valid manner, because criteria used for shunting varied considerably across studies. Similarly, a NIRS value, based upon which cerebral ischemia was likely to occur postoperatively, could not be determined from the literature due to large variability in patients and approaches taken.[71] Moritz et al compared the accuracy of different cerebral monitoring systems in detecting cerebral ischemia during CEA. The authors compared TCD, NIRS, SP measurement, and SSEP in 48 patients undergoing carotid surgery during regional anesthesia by performing receiver-operating characteristic (ROC) analysis and measuring the area under the ROC curve (AUC). The study found that no single monitoring method provided 100% sensitivity and 100% specificity compared with awake patient monitoring. TCD (AUC = 0.973), NIRS (AUC = 0.905), and SP (AUC = 0.925) measurement provided similar accuracy for the detection of cerebral ischemia during carotid surgery, but lesser accuracy was found for SSEP monitoring (AUC = 0.749). However, because of the high rate of technical difficulties encountered with TCD, it appears that NIRS and SP may be more practical in the clinical setting.[72]

NIRS is a simple and noninvasive method to indirectly assess cerebral perfusion in patients undergoing CEA. It correlates with the development of clinical and EEG signs of cerebral ischemia; however, because of low sensitivity and specificity, it should not be used alone to predict the need for shunt placement.[73]

The Awake Patient Monitoring of the awake patient is the gold standard for neurologic assessment and may allow for prompt identification of patients who would benefit from shunt placement. Change in contralateral strength or consciousness in the setting of adequate mean arterial pressure is an indication for shunt placement. Intraoperative neurologic changes in the awake patient may predict a 6-fold increase in the incidence of postoperative stroke.[74] A more recent study attempted to correlate neurologic changes in awake patients undergoing CEA under cervical block anesthesia with EEG and measurement of carotid SP and found that, compared with intraoperative neurologic monitoring of the awake patient, both EEG and carotid SP had poor sensitivity.[65] However, this method of monitoring requires the absolute cooperation of surgeon, anesthesiologist, and patient.

GENERAL CONSIDERATIONS

Standard cardiovascular monitoring should include continuous ECG with 2 leads displayed (usually II and V5) and invasive continuous measurement of arterial blood pressure.

The American Society of Anesthesiology (ASA) revised practice guidelines for the use of pulmonary artery catheters (PACs) do not support the use of PACs in peripheral vascular surgery unless indicated by comorbidities.[75] As changes in pulmonary capillary occlusion pressure are relatively insensitive to myocardial ischemia, some advocate the continuous use of transesophageal echocardiography (TEE) in patients with severe CAD.

Intravenous access may be limited to large-bore peripheral intravenous catheters. The use of central venous catheters should be parsimonious, weighing in risks and benefits. It may be more appropriately reserved for patients with documented or suspected severe CAD or valvular heart disease in which the need for administration of vasopressors or inotropes may arise. The contralateral internal jugular vein should be preferably and cautiously cannulated under ultrasound guidance to avoid carotid puncture.

ANESTHETIC TECHNIQUES

The goals of anesthesia should balance concerns related to both the brain and the heart and may be summarized as follows:

1. Hemodynamic extremes should be avoided during induction, incision, surgical manipulation, emergence, and extubation.
2. The patient should be sufficiently responsive immediately after surgery to facilitate neurologic evaluation.

Clearly, these 2 objectives narrow the range of acceptable anesthetic options and require clinical expertise. The impact of the anesthetic technique on outcome remains controversial with proponents of both regional and general anesthesia.

Some investigators have found that regional anesthesia by cervical plexus block obviates the use of a shunt in more than 80% of patients and facilitates safe, simple, and effective intraoperative cerebral function monitoring.[76-78] Regional anesthesia may be associated with shorter hospital stays, decreased intensive care costs, and less cardiovascular morbidity.[79,80]

A meta-analysis of the available randomized clinical trials comparing CEA under local anesthesia (LA) versus general anesthesia (GA) showed that, although LA was associated with a significant reduction in local postoperative hemorrhage, there were no significant differences in morbidity and mortality outcomes. These results should be interpreted with caution because of small sample sizes and insufficient power.[81]

Probably the strongest evidence comes from the General Anesthesia versus Local Anesthesia (GALA) trial. This is a multicenter, randomized controlled trial in which 3526 patients with symptomatic or asymptomatic carotid stenosis were randomly assigned to surgery under regional or general anesthesia. The primary outcome measure was a composite of stroke (including retinal infarction), MI, or death between randomization and 30 days after surgery. There was no statistically significant difference in the primary outcome between the regional and general anesthesia groups (4.4% vs 4.8%). However, local anesthesia seems to be more effective than general anesthesia for patients with contralateral carotid occlusion. The primary outcome of a stroke, including retinal infarction, MI, or death, at 30 days was 10% for GA versus 5% for LA in patients with contralateral carotid occlusion.[82]

Regional anesthesia is performed by blocking the superficial and deep cervical plexus formed from C2 to C4 anterior rami of the ipsilateral spinal roots. Proponents of this technique believe that an awake patient is the best monitor of neurologic function during carotid surgery. To achieve this goal the patient must be minimally sedated, and the procedure requires a high degree of patient cooperation, a profound blockade, and an expeditious surgeon. Intraoperatively, the internal, external, and common carotid arteries are clamped sequentially followed by neurologic assessment. If neurologic deficit is noted by monitoring speech and upper extremity motor function, surgery may proceed either with elevation of systemic blood pressure, reocclusion, and reassessment of the patient or with placement of a Javid shunt that bypasses the operative area. Practitioners may prefer one block to another (superficial cervical plexus block, deep cervical plexus block, or a combined superficial and deep block), but no consensus exists on the efficacy of one block when compared with another. A recent systematic review of the literature assessed the complication rate associated with superficial and deep (or combined deep plus superficial) cervical blocks. Deep/combined block was associated with a higher rate of complications related to the injecting needle when compared with the superficial block. The conversion rate to general anesthesia was also higher with deep/combined block probably due to the higher rate of direct complications. Of the specific complications that occurred with placement of the deep block, the most common was intravascular injection, followed by respiratory failure or distress (due to presumed or confirmed diaphragmatic or vocal cord paralysis). There were several criticisms brought to this meta-analysis, including the fact that it included only 2 randomized clinical trials, the rest being nonrandomized trials, case series, and case reports.[83]

Complications associated with regional anesthesia include infection, hematoma, local anesthetic toxicity, nerve injury, inadvertent spinal anesthesia, and phrenic nerve blockade, which can result in loss of function of the ipsilateral hemidiaphragm and consequent respiratory insufficiency, especially in patients with chronic respiratory disease.

Disadvantages of regional anesthesia include patient discomfort and loss of cooperation, confusion, panic, or seizures. Management of intraoperative problems may be more difficult and theoretically may be associated with increased morbidity.

General anesthesia allows reliable airway control and better control of ventilation, and thus nearly eliminates the possibility of hypoxemia and hypo- or hypercapnia, and provides optimal operating conditions for the surgical team. A potential benefit of using GA is the ability to use intraoperative monitoring of myocardial ischemia with TEE and guide therapy in patients with severe CAD.

Induction of GA should proceed slowly with medications titrated to the desired effect. Propofol, and etomidate are the induction agents used more frequently. Addition of a short- or intermediate-acting narcotic, depending on the proposed duration of surgery, is recommended. Moderate doses of narcotic allow for better hemodynamic control during intubation and incision, and permit a lower dose of inhalational agent to be used for anesthetic maintenance. The choice of neuromuscular blocking agents is not important as long as the duration of action of the agent does not delay emergence and it is not associated with hemodynamic disturbances related to the vagolytic or histamine release effects. Vecuronium seems to be the ideal muscle relaxant for procedures lasting 90 minutes or less.

The use of a laryngeal mask airway (LMA) may lessen perioperative hemodynamic responses associated with airway management during intubation and extubation, but this decision must be based individually on the pros and cons related to the use of either an endotracheal tube (ETT) or LMA.

Maintenance of general anesthesia can be achieved with various agents depending on hemodynamic stability provided, rapidity of emergence, and interference with the methods of monitoring used. The rapid elimination of desflurane and sevoflurane may allow earlier postoperative neurologic assessment compared with isoflurane. However, desflurane may be associated with tachycardia and hypertension, and may therefore increase cardiovascular risk. A study investigating hemodynamic and recovery characteristics in patients scheduled for CEA anesthetized with isoflurane, sevoflurane, or desflurane found no significant perioperative differences on ST-segment analysis. The times to extubation, movement on command, and consciousness were shorter after desflurane and sevoflurane than after isoflurane.[84] As mentioned above, moderate amounts of opioids can be used to enhance hemodynamic stability during maintenance of anesthesia, with care not to compromise rapid emergence at the end of the procedure. Researchers have found that although fentanyl, sufentanil, and remifentanil offered similar intra- and postoperative hemodynamic stability, remifentanil allowed faster recovery and earlier neurologic examination and was superior in blunting the sympathetic response to intubation.[85,86]

Blood pressure and heart rate changes during and after CEA surgery are quite variable and can even be extreme. Surgical manipulation of the carotid sinus can cause an increase in afferent impulses to the brainstem and trigger an abrupt bradycardic response and hypotension. This may be prevented by infiltration of the sinus with local anesthetic by the surgeon. If infiltration has not been performed, then clamp application may cause hypertension and tachycardia because the sinus now senses a low pressure. The reverse may or may not be observed with unclamping. The variability between individuals in this reflex behavior may be due to differences in sinus insensitivity secondary to the atherosclerotic process.

Control of the arterial partial pressure of carbon dioxide in the arterial blood is controversial. Hypocapnia produces nondiscriminatory bilateral cerebral vasoconstriction and hypercapnia may induce a "steal" phenomenon. Most authors therefore recommend the maintenance of normocarbia during CEA.[87]

A number of animal studies of traumatic brain injury, focal cerebral ischemia, and global cerebral ischemia demonstrate that glycemic control is a critical factor in terms of outcome.[88] Glycemic control with insulin has been shown to improve neurologic outcome in patients who are critically ill and in those undergoing cardiac surgery. Although there is relative lack of evidence to support the tight control of glucose in diabetic patients undergoing CEA, the adverse impact of hyperglycemia on cerebral ischemic injury suggests that the perioperative management of glucose is vital in these patients.

It is universally accepted that blood pressure during carotid occlusion should be maintained at or up to 20% higher than the patient's highest recorded resting blood pressure when awake in order to maintain adequate collateral blood flow. This may be achieved by titration of vasoconstrictors or inotropes, or infusion of intravenous fluids. No evidence is available to help choose one intervention over another.[87]

Nowhere are emergence issues more important and complex than in CEA. It is desirable to have the patient alert and responsive immediately after the procedure in order to permit neurologic assessment; however, hypertension, which can stress and rupture the surgical anastomosis, is an ever-present threat. The patients undergoing CEA are frequently smokers with hyperreactive airways and copious airway secretions. Unless thorough precautions are taken, stimulation from the ETT at the time of emergence from GA will cause coughing and straining, and can result in severe hypertension. Residual effects from previously administered narcotics are particularly helpful at this time. Early extubation could be considered in selected patients. Careful evacuation of oropharyngeal secretions, instillation of 60 to 80 mg of 2% lidocaine in the ETT during the surgical closure, and careful adjustment to minimal pressure in the ETT cuff are partially effective techniques to blunt hypertension with emergence. Aggressive pharmacologic intervention may be necessary with short-acting agents.

POSTOPERATIVE CONSIDERATIONS

There are several potential complications that may occur postoperatively, notably stroke, MI, and respiratory dysfunction. Hypertension is common, can have a multifactorial etiology, and is associated with increased incidence of cardiac and neurologic complications. An avoidable consequence of poorly controlled hypertension is wound hematoma necessitating prompt evaluation and possible wound exploration.

Patients with severe hypertension are also at risk of developing hyperperfusion syndrome, which is an abrupt increase in blood flow with loss of autoregulation in the surgically reperfused brain. Reports describe a spectrum of findings, including severe headache, transient ischemia, seizures, and intracerebral hemorrhage, which presents as headache, seizures, and cerebral edema, and often occurs several days after surgery.[89] TCD can detect changes in the cerebral blood flow (CBF). An increase greater than 100% of the postoperative CBF, as compared to preoperative CBF values, has been associated with a 10 times higher risk for cerebral hypertension syndrome. TCD, however, cannot be performed in all patients, because a temporal bone window is missing in 10% to 15% of CEA patients. Studies have also looked at the value of NIRS in the detection of cerebral hypertension syndrome.[90,91] In all patients with cerebral hypertension the NIRS values exceeded 105% of the postclamping value and exceeded 110% of the preclamping values by the end of the procedure.

Hypotension and bradycardia may occur secondary to carotid sinus hypersensitivity after plaque removal. Respiratory distress may be caused by an expanding neck hematoma, laryngeal dysfunction from superior laryngeal or recurrent laryngeal paralysis, pneumothorax, or the loss of carotid body chemoreceptor-mediated hyperventilatory response to hypoxia. The latter complication is particularly likely after bilateral CEA, and such patients are especially prone to opioid-induced central respiratory depression.[92]

A number of nerve injuries can complicate CEA: recurrent laryngeal, hypoglossal, and marginal mandibular nerve injury may result in hoarseness, tongue deviation on protrusion, and drooping of the corner of the mouth; superior laryngeal nerve injury may present as impaired phonation; spinal accessory nerve injury may result in ipsilateral shoulder weakness.

LOWER EXTREMITY VASCULAR SURGERY

PERIPHERAL ARTERIAL DISEASE—OVERVIEW

Peripheral arterial disease (PAD) is a constantly growing clinical problem in the United States and its prevalence is only likely to increase as the population ages. PAD prevalence increases dramatically with age from 0.9% between the ages of 40 and 49 to 14.5% in those 70 and older. African American ethnicity, current smoking, diabetes, hypertension, hypercholesterolemia, and low kidney function were significantly associated with prevalence of PAD.[93]

Atherosclerosis is the most common etiology of peripheral arterial disease. Other less common causes are acute arterial disease (embolism, thrombosis, dissection, trauma), adventitial cystic disease, arterial fibrodysplasia, occluded limb aneurysms, and tumors. Ninety percent of the cases of embolism to the lower extremities are due to emboli that originated in the heart in patients with cardiac dysrhythmias, recent MIs, ventricular aneurysms with intracardiac thrombus, or diseased or prosthetic cardiac valves.

Patients are candidates for elective surgery to correct peripheral occlusive disease if they exhibit (1) intermittent, activity-limiting claudication; (2) ischemic rest pain; (3) ischemic ulceration; or (4) gangrene. According to the 2005 ACC/AHA and the 2007 revised TransAtlantic Inter-Society Consensus (TASC II) guidelines for management of patients with PAD, certain issues have to be considered before revascularization: morphology of the lesions, projected natural history and prognosis of the patient, projected improvement in quality of life from alleviation of claudication, and inadequate response to exercise rehabilitation and medical therapy.[94,95]

Patients with intermittent claudication have normal flow to skeletal muscle at rest but markedly impaired flow to meet metabolic demands during exercise. The location of pain varies with the anatomic site of obstruction: buttock and hip pain is usually due to aortoiliac disease; thigh pain is due to common femoral artery disease; calf pain is due to either superficial femoral artery or popliteal artery disease; and foot pain is due to tibial or peroneal artery disease. Over time PAD affects the neurologic and metabolic function of the skeletal muscle, leading to further impairments in muscle performance and patient functional status.

Modifiable atherosclerotic risk factors for PAD include smoking, diabetes, obesity, hyperlipidemia, hypertension, and homocysteine elevation.[95]

Although over 70% of the patients with PAD have no progression of symptoms with conservative management such as smoking cessation, exercise rehabilitation, or antiplatelet therapy,[94] the remainder have progression of their symptoms that mandates revascularization. Given the availability of less invasive percutaneous procedures, the 2005 ACC/AHA guidelines and the 2007 TASC II consensus document on the management of PAD recommended initial revascularization with surgery only when the arterial anatomy is not favorable for a percutaneous approach.

Percutaneous transluminal angioplasty (PTA) results in a "controlled" dissection of the arterial media. PTA has been traditionally limited to the treatment of focal, short segmental stenoses or occlusions. With advancements in technology, PTA is now routinely applied to more extensively diseased segments to attempt limb salvage before a distal surgical bypass. PTA can also be used in patients who are poor surgical candidates.

Individuals undergoing lower extremity vascular surgery present a dilemma to the anesthesia provider. The procedure itself is associated with far less (intraoperative and postoperative) nociceptive stimulation than aortic surgery and less hemodynamic fluctuation than carotid or aortic surgery, and can be performed with a pure regional anesthetic. On the other hand, patients may have severe CAD and other systemic disorders, and are at high risk for perioperative complications. The CAD in these patients may be undiagnosed due to limited mobility and low activity level. In a large study, patients undergoing infrainguinal bypass had a 30-day mortality rate of 5.8% and a 1-year mortality of 16.3%.[96] Thus the perioperative management of this group, including the anesthetic technique, must proceed with considerable caution.

ANESTHETIC CONSIDERATIONS

Monitoring Standard monitoring should include continuous ECG with 2 leads displayed (usually II and V5), pulse oximetry, noninvasive blood pressure capnography, and temperature. In patients with cardiac risk factors who are undergoing noncardiac surgery, the perioperative maintenance of normothermia is associated with a reduced incidence of morbid cardiac events and ventricular tachycardia.[97]

Arterial cannulation and continuous pressure monitoring are considered standard. Central venous pressure (CVP) monitoring is frequently helpful. Volume status can be difficult to judge, especially in long, complicated cases, which can evolve unpredictably. Improved response time to the administration of vasoactive agents is often sufficiently important to justify central venous cannulation.

Pulmonary artery catheterization is not routinely used. Although monitoring with pulmonary artery catheters (PACs) provides more hemodynamic data, its benefit has not been demonstrated in several outcome studies, so it is not routinely used.[98] The 2003 ASA revised practice guidelines for the use of PACs do not support their use in peripheral vascular surgery unless indicated by comorbidities or in major surgical procedures associated with significant hemodynamic fluctuations.[75] As changes in pulmonary capillary occlusion pressure are relatively insensitive to myocardial ischemia, some advocate the continuous use of transesophageal echocardiography (TEE) in patients with severe CAD.

Anesthetic Techniques Lower extremity vascular surgery patients have been the subjects of several studies comparing regional and general anesthesia due to their high-risk status and the nature of the surgery, which allows a pure regional technique. However, both prospective, randomized clinical trials and retrospective studies have been plagued with several limitations; therefore, most investigations have produced findings that vary widely and must be carefully interpreted.

Spinal and epidural anesthesia using local anesthetic agents have long been believed to provide overall better operative conditions for a variety of reasons, including avoidance of airway and pulmonary morbidity, lower blood loss, and ablation of the surgical stress response. The latter effect presumably produces more stable hemodynamics, reduced hypercoagulability, better wound healing, and less immune suppression. Further, vasodilation, secondary to sympathetic blockade, should be particularly helpful in sustaining graft patency.

A meta-analysis of 141 randomized trials comparing neuraxial anesthesia with GA for all types of patients has shown that neuraxial blockade reduced the odds of deep vein thrombosis by 44%, pulmonary embolism by 55%, transfusion requirements by 50%, pneumonia by 39%, and respiratory depression by 59% (all $P < 0.001$). There were also reductions in MI and renal failure.[99]

The landmark study by Yeager et al showed much less morbidity and mortality in a group of patients undergoing diverse major surgical procedures who received regional anesthesia and analgesia postoperatively compared with those who received general anesthesia followed by on-demand parenteral narcotics. Only a few vascular surgery subjects were included in this study, and the morbidity and mortality in the general anesthesia group was much higher than reported in other studies.

No management techniques were specified, and the general anesthesia group actually received a wide variety of techniques.[100] Tuman et al randomized patients undergoing lower extremity vascular surgery or aortic abdominal aneurysm surgery to receive epidural-supplemented GA followed by postoperative epidural analgesia or GA followed by on-demand parenteral narcotics.[101] The investigators found somewhat higher cardiac morbidity in the GA group, but the difference was much less dramatic than in the study by Yeager et al. The most remarkable outcome was a larger number of reoperations for inadequate lower extremity flow in the GA group (20%). Tuman et al have speculated that the mechanism for this morbidity was attributable to perioperative hypercoagulability in the GA group that was not seen in the regional anesthesia group. It has been long believed that regional blockade with local agents blunts certain components of the surgical stress response, including procoagulant activity. Establishing the ability of regional anesthesia to attenuate this phenomenon would be significant; however, caution is warranted in the attribution of the prevention of hypercoagulability to the reduced revascularization rates because other possibilities include sympathetic blockade, or other aspects of management may participate. Two other studies comparing regional and GA[102,103] in which neuraxial analgesia was not continued in the postoperative period found no benefit in terms of vascular graft patency.

Christopherson et al conducted the Perioperative Ischemia Randomized Anesthesia Trial (PIRAT) in which 100 patients were randomized to undergoing lower extremity grafts either under epidural or general anesthesia. Postoperative analgesia included epidural fentanyl in the regional group and intravenous (IV) patient-controlled analgesia (PCA) in the general group. Cardiac morbidity and mortality in each group was low; however, the revascularization rate was high in the GA group.[104] Rosenfeld et al, using patients from the PIRAT study, reported an increase in plasminogen activator inhibitor (PAI-1) in the general anesthesia patients but not the regional anesthesia patients on the morning after surgery (**Fig. 55-4**).[105] This finding confirms the hypercoagulable state found by Tuman et al postoperatively in the GA group, as well as the ability of regional anesthesia and analgesia to prevent the phenomenon. Also reporting from the PIRAT study, Breslow et al showed that norepinephrine levels rose at the end of surgery in the general anesthesia but not the regional anesthesia group, and remained elevated through the postoperative period. Clearly, in this study regional anesthesia/analgesia was effective in blocking the stress response after surgery.[106]

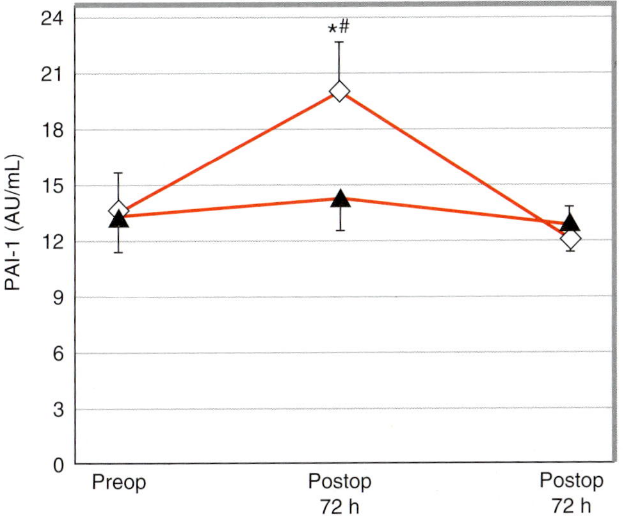

FIGURE 55-4. Plasminogen activator inhibitor-1 levels in activity units per milliliter for general and regional anesthesia groups over time. Values are mean ± SEM. #*P*, 0.001 compared to preoperative and 72 hours. **P* = 0.05 general anesthesia (GA) compared to regional anesthesia (RA). [From Rosenfeld BA, Beattie C, Christopherson R, et al. The effects of different anesthetic regimens on fibrinolysis and the development of postoperative arterial thrombosis. Perioperative Ischemia Randomized Anesthesia Trial Study Group. *Anesthesiology.* 1993;79(3):435-443.]

Bode et al conducted a trial larger than the previous studies in which he randomized 423 patients undergoing lower extremity grafts to either regional (spinal or epidural) or general anesthesia. They found low cardiac morbidity and mortality, and low revascularization rates in both groups. In this study, however, all patients were monitored with pulmonary artery catheters intraoperatively and for the first 48 hours postoperatively. This permitted aggressive optimization of hemodynamic status and probably contributed to the excellent results in both groups.[107]

Anticoagulant therapy is an important adjunct in the perioperative period in the maintenance of vascular graft patency. As the anticoagulant therapy has implications in the choice of anesthetic technique, the 2010 American Society of Regional Anesthesia and Pain Medicine guidelines regarding neuraxial anesthesia and anticoagulants make a few recommendations regarding neuraxial anesthesia in the anticoagulated patient.[108]

1. Combining neuraxial techniques with intraoperative anticoagulation with heparin during vascular surgery is acceptable with the following recommendations: (a) unfractionated heparin should not be given at least 1 hour after needle placement; (b) epidural catheters should be removed at least 1 hour before a heparin dose and at least 2 to 4 hours after a heparin dose after evaluation of patient's coagulation status; (c) there should be careful monitoring of the patient's neurologic status in the postoperative period, and minimal concentration of local anesthetic should be used.
2. Although the occurrence of a bloody or difficult neuraxial needle placement may increase risk, there are no data to support mandatory cancellation of a case. Direct communication with the surgeon and a specific risk-benefit decision about proceeding in each case is warranted.
3. There are no current contraindications to using neuraxial techniques in patients on subcutaneous heparin prophylaxis.
4. Because heparin-induced thrombocytopenia may occur during heparin administration, we recommend that patients receiving heparin for more than 4 days have a platelet count assessed before neuraxial block and catheter removal.
5. For patients on low-molecular-weight heparin (LMWH), needle placement should occur at least 12 hours after the last thromboprophylactic dose of LMWH and at least 24 hours after the last therapeutic dose (enoxaparin 1 mg/kg every 12 hours, enoxaparin 1.5 mg/kg daily, dalteparin 120 U/kg every 12 hours, dalteparin 200 U/kg daily, or tinzaparin 175 U/kg daily).
6. The presence of blood during needle and catheter placement does not necessitate postponement of surgery. We suggest that initiation of LMWH therapy in this setting should be delayed for 24 hours postoperatively and that this consideration be discussed with the surgeon.
7. In patients administered a dose of LMWH 2 hours preoperatively (general surgery patients), we recommend against neuraxial techniques because needle placement would occur during peak anticoagulant activity.
8. Warfarin therapy should be discontinued 4 to 5 days before block placement and coagulation status should be checked.
9. Nonsteroidal anti-inflammatory drugs (NSAIDs, including aspirin) do not create a level of risk that will interfere with the performance of neuraxial blocks. In patients receiving these medications, we do not identify specific concerns as to the timing of single-shot or catheter techniques in relationship to the dosing of NSAIDs, postoperative monitoring, or the timing of neuraxial catheter removal.

10. Clopidogrel should be discontinued for 7 days and ticlopidine for 14 days prior to neuraxial anesthesia. If a neuraxial block is indicated between 5 and 7 days of discontinuation of clopidogrel, normalization of platelet function should be documented.

Although regional anesthesia has desirable effects, there is not sufficient data to recommend one technique over another. With the advent of new anesthetic agents, general anesthesia can be safely used with attention to detail throughout the perioperative period and aggressive management of hemodynamic changes.

ANEURYSMS

PATHOPHYSIOLOGY AND MANAGEMENT

Aneurysms are arterial expansions that occur as the vascular wall becomes weakened from atherosclerosis or other degenerative processes. The abdominal aorta is the most common site of arterial aneurysm. Abdominal aortic aneurysms (AAA) most often occur in the segment of aorta between the renal and inferior mesenteric arteries. Approximately 5% involve the renal or visceral arteries. Thoracoabdominal aneurysms involve the thoracic and abdominal aorta together.

Recently, the role of atherosclerosis in the pathogenesis of aneurysms has become less defined and the underlying cause of aneurysmal aortic dilation is uncertain in most patients. A genome scan of 36 families with abdominal aortic aneurysm identified a possible gene locus for this disease on chromosomes 19q13 and 4q31.[109] Other investigators suggested that destruction of elastin in the aortic wall is a key event that shifts the load produced by blood pressure on collagen. This is exacerbated in the presence of hypertension. Smoking and age are other important factors. The location of the aneurysm is also important, as elastic lamellae are relatively less common in the abdominal aorta. Once the shielding effect of elastin is lost, further dilation and rupture of the aorta depend on the physical properties of the collagen present.[110] Although the infrarenal portion may exhibit atherosclerosis, the suprarenal aorta often shows degenerative changes of the media called mucoid degeneration, myxomatous degeneration, or cystic medial necrosis.

The natural progression of untreated aneurysm is expansion and eventual rupture. This is because with equal distending pressure within a vessel, the wall tension is higher when the vessel radius is larger, as described by Laplace law. This physical principle states that the tension (T) sustained by a vessel wall due to blood pressure (P) is directly proportional to the vessel radius (R) as given by the relationship $T \sim P \times R$.

Perioperative mortality after elective aneurysm repair is low (5.8% and 2.7% in the UK Small Aneurysm trial and the Aneurysm Detection and Management [ADAM] trial, respectively).[111,112] In contrast, perioperative mortality is much higher with emergency surgery, occurring in 37% of 81 patients in a large screening trial.[113] It is therefore important to identify individuals at greatest risk for rupture and appropriately time the surgical repair.

The likelihood that an aneurysm will rupture is influenced by a number of factors including aneurysm diameter, rate of expansion, and gender. According to a statement from the Joint Council of the American Association for Vascular Surgery and Society for Vascular Surgery, the estimated annual risk of rupture, according to AAA diameter, is 0.5% to 5% for AAAs that are 4.0 to 4.9 cm, 10% to 20% for those 6.0 to 6.9 cm, 20% to 40% for those 7.0 to 7.9, and 30% to 50% for those greater than 8.0 cm.[114] Other factors include continued smoking, uncontrolled hypertension, increased wall stress, and rate of expansion (a rate of growth of more than 0.5 cm in 6 months).[94]

Two randomized trials, the UK Small Aneurysm trial and the ADAM trial, investigated the management of medium-sized aneurysms (4.0-5.5 cm), comparing early surgery with ultrasound surveillance. Both trials showed no long-term difference in mean survival between the early surgery and surveillance groups, although in the UK Small Aneurysm trial, after 8 years there was a lower total mortality in the early surgery group, probably attributable to changes in lifestyle adopted by patients in this group.

In 2005 the ACC/AHA published guidelines on the diagnosis and management of peripheral arterial disease in collaboration with major vascular medicine, vascular surgery, and interventional radiology societies. Some of these recommendations are as follows:

1. Aneurysms 4.0 to 5.4 cm in diameter should be monitored by ultrasound or tomographic scanning every 6 to 12 months.
2. Aneurysms 3.0 to 4.0 cm in diameter should be monitored by ultrasound every 2 to 3 years.
3. Aneurysms with diameter more than 5.5 cm should be repaired.
4. Patients with asymptomatic aneurysms that are more than twice the size of the normal segment should be considered for repair.
5. Earlier repair may be beneficial in patients with increases in diameter more than 0.5 cm in 6 months.
6. Patients with symptomatic aneurysms should undergo repair, regardless of aneurysm diameter.
7. AAA repair may be reasonable in patients with medium-sized aneurysms who also have iliac or femoral artery aneurysms requiring treatment, and in patients with severe coexistent occlusive disease or thrombotic or embolic complications.
8. Repair of suprarenal and/or thoracoabdominal aneurysms involves more extensive surgery and greater operative risk. Repair of such aneurysms may be beneficial at diameters greater than 5.5 to 6.0 cm in diameter.

ANESTHETIC CONSIDERATIONS

Monitoring All patients undergoing aortic surgery should have continuous intravascular monitoring of arterial pressure. As with other types of surgery, the first site considered is the radial artery of the arm with the highest pressure, determined by sphygmomanometry. Reasons for choosing other sites include inadequate collateral flow to the hand (Allen test), poor radial pulsations due to previous trauma or proximal vascular disease, and site of cross-clamping above the left subclavian artery. The axillary artery offers an excellent alternative. Cannulation of the axillary artery is usually performed with the Seldinger technique. Caution is warranted in flushing an axillary artery catheter because the tip is rather more proximate to the carotid and vertebral system, and air or particulate matter could enter these vessels.

In addition to radial or axillary pressure monitoring, a femoral arterial cannula should be strongly considered in thoracic or thoracoabdominal aneurysm surgery where shunt or bypass procedures are used. Knowledge of arterial pressure distal to the cross-clamp permits a considerably more rational approach to hemodynamic manipulations during surgery. Although embolization and arterial occlusion can occur, studies have shown that complication rates are similar for ulnar, brachial, axillary, femoral, and dorsalis pedis cannulation, and are very low.[115]

The use of PACs in the perioperative setting and their impact on morbidity and mortality is still under intense scrutiny and debate. Although some clinicians advocate the use of PACs in all patients undergoing an aortic cross-clamp procedure, others moderate their use based on the cross-clamp level and extent of comorbid disease. Several clinical trials have compared outcomes in vascular surgical patients monitored with central venous pressure (CVP) only versus PACs. Multiple small studies have evaluated prospectively the efficacy of the intraoperative use of PACs in patients undergoing vascular surgery and have shown conflicting results. A meta-analysis of these small studies concluded that in moderate-risk vascular surgery patients, routine preoperative PA catheterization is not associated with improved outcomes.[98] One other prospective trial randomized abdominal aortic reconstructive surgery patients to monitoring with a central venous catheter or with a PAC and showed that the choice of central venous catheter or pulmonary artery catheter monitoring made little difference in outcome.[116] Sandham et al and the Canadian Critical Care Trials Group published a landmark study that looked at the routine use of PACs and found no benefit to therapy directed by PAC over standard care in elderly, high-risk surgical patients requiring intensive care. They also found a higher rate of pulmonary emboli among the catheter group.[117] A rational approach is to use a PAC in those cases requiring a suprarenal (or above) cross-clamp and reserve its use in infrarenal aneurysms and occlusive disease in those individuals with significant cardiac, renal, or pulmonary pathology. This endorsement presumes that the venous cannulation and balloon flotation are initiated safely; the pressure transducers are properly leveled, zeroed, and calibrated; thermodilution cardiac outputs are technically sound; calculated and measured parameters are interpreted correctly; and therapeutic interventions reflect appropriate understanding of physiology and pharmacology. If any 1 of these requisites is missing, PACs are best omitted.[118]

TEE is a valuable tool, increasingly available in the noncardiac operating rooms. According to the 2010 revised Practice Guidelines for Perioperative TEE by the American Society of Anesthesiologists and Society of Cardiovascular Anesthesiologists Task Force, TEE should be used for noncardiac surgical patients when the patient has known or suspected cardiovascular pathology that might result in hemodynamic, pulmonary, or neurologic compromise; during unexplained persistent hypotension; when persistent, unexplained hypoxemia occurs; and when life-threatening hypotension occurs.[119] TEE is a sensitive monitor for detecting myocardial ischemia, considered by many to be more sensitive than ECG, PACs, or other means of hemodynamic monitoring.[120] Smith et al determined that intraoperative TEE could successfully demonstrate myocardial ischemia by revealing acute segmental wall-motion abnormalities; in many instances the wall motion abnormalities occurred before or were not accompanied by the appearance of ST changes on the ECG, demonstrating the superiority of TEE for the intraoperative detection of myocardial ischemia.[121] There are certain risks involved with a TEE exam, such as anatomic damage from insertion and manipulation of the probe, incomplete examination, or incorrect interpretation of the images, which can lead to decisions detrimental to the patient.

Despite tremendous development in surgical and anesthetic techniques, resection of the thoracic and thoracoabdominal segments of the aorta remains associated with the risk of paralysis. Procedures that require aortic cross-clamping above the celiac axis or more cephalad incur a progressively higher risk of major neurologic sequelae. Although the number of reported incidents of paraplegia following aortic surgery varies from approximately 1 in 1000 for elective repair of uncomplicated abdominal aortic aneurysm,[122] the risk of spinal cord ischemia or infarction as a consequence of open repair of thoracoabdominal aneurysms is in the range of 8% to 28%.[123,124] Early detection of spinal cord ischemia is paramount. Monitoring of functional continuity of the spinal cord would allow for implementation of hemodynamic or cytoprotective interventions to minimize spinal cord injury. Detection of intraoperative spinal cord ischemia requires intraoperative monitoring of somatosensory-evoked potentials (SSEPs) or motor evoked potentials (MEPs). SSEP monitoring is performed by placing stimulating electrodes on the skin adjacent to the peripheral nerves in the arms and legs. Electrical stimulation of the peripheral nerves generates action potentials that can be measured from recording electrodes over the spine, brainstem, thalamus, and cerebral cortex.[125] SSEPs monitor only the posterior column of the spinal cord; therefore, spinal cord ischemia confined to the anterior spinal cord may not be detected. Intraoperatively, SSEPs can be influenced by temperature, hypoxia, vascular malperfusion of the lower extremities, peripheral nerve ischemia, and acute intraoperative stroke. Cortical SSEPs can be attenuated by high concentration of inhaled anesthetics, thiopental, or propofol. The fidelity of SSEPs is improved with neuromuscular blockade and a balanced general anesthesia with inhaled anesthetics maintained at 0.5 MAC.[125]

To complement SSEPs in monitoring spinal cord functional integrity, MEPs were introduced. MEPs are produced by delivering electrical stimulation to the scalp overlying the motor cortex. The evoked potentials travel through the cortical spinal tracts and peripheral nerves, and the response typically is recorded near the muscle as a compound muscle action potential. Some investigators state that although SSEPs show delayed ischemia detection and may have a high rate of false-positive results, MEPs have been proven to indicate reliably instantaneous changes of spinal cord perfusion.[126] Similar to SSEPs, MEPs are influenced by hypothermia, malperfusion of the limbs, and peripheral nerve ischemia. Transcranial MEPs are also exquisitely sensitive to anesthesia. Total intravenous technique with propofol/ketamine and opioid continuous infusions without neuromuscular blockade or controlled incomplete neuromuscular blockade is required when MEP monitoring is used. Certain risks are associated with MEP monitoring such as skin burns at electrode sites, development of cardiac arrhythmias and hypertension, and rarely excitotoxic injury to the brain and seizure activity.[127]

Blood loss during aneurysm surgery is highly variable. Central venous access and large-bore peripheral venous access for the administration of large blood volumes is necessary. A rapid infusion system, which can administer up to 1500 mL/min of warmed fluids, should be available. Blood-salvaging techniques for autotransfusion have proven useful in aortic aneurysm repair. Systems that use cell separation and return only red blood cells result in fewer coagulation abnormalities than systems that return whole blood. Given the high cost of current technology, it becomes cost-effective (when compared to the cost of providing allogeneic blood) when at least 2 or more units of blood can be salvaged and reinfused. Major vascular surgery offers the best opportunity for appropriate use of blood-scavenging units. Although no randomized, prospective studies of efficacy have been reported, it is obvious that the use of these devices would decrease the exposure of the patient to multiple donors.

Some degree of hypothermia is commonly observed in patients undergoing aneurysm surgery. This is caused by the exposure of abdominal contents, the administration of large amounts of fluid, and disturbances in thermoregulatory mechanisms caused by both inhaled and intravenous anesthetics. Although hyperthermia is associated with increased metabolic rates and with deleterious cerebral and spinal cord effects, hypothermia is associated with adverse myocardial events, coagulopathy, wound infection, and delayed wound healing. In a review of patients undergoing elective AAA repair, Bush et al[128] noted significantly more organ dysfunction (53% vs 29%) and a higher mortality rate (12% vs 1.5%) in hypothermic patients (temperature <34.5°C) than in normothermic patients. Active measures should be taken to maintain normothermia. However, during aortic cross-clamping, the lower body should not be actively warmed.

PHYSIOLOGY OF CROSS-CLAMPING

The hemodynamic and metabolic alterations caused by acute interruption of aortic blood flow have been the subject of both animal and human investigations for many years. Features of particular relevance to anesthetic management include changes in arterial blood pressure, cardiac function, myocardial perfusion, and acid-base status, as well as tissue integrity of the kidneys, viscera, and spinal cord. Conflicting findings have been obtained and likely reflect species variation, patient characteristics, degree of collateralization, location of the cross-clamp, baseline cardiac function, type of anesthesia, the use and type of vasodilators, and the presence or absence of CAD. In this section, we review the classic and conflicting findings from the literature and present arguments for making rational clinical decisions.

Blood Pressure The degree of hypertension caused by application of an aortic cross-clamp depends on the location of the clamp, the degree of collateralization, and the preocclusion aortic flow. Thus an infrarenal clamp in a patient with aortic occlusive disease may cause virtually no elevation in the blood pressure because distal preclamp flow was minimal. Also, aortic clamping above a thoracic coarctation may result in no pressure change proximal (or distal) to the clamp because of adequate collateral flow. In the case of AAA repair, runoff is usually good and collateralization minimal. Therefore, an increase in blood pressure should be expected, the magnitude of which is proportional to how proximal the location of the cross-clamp is in relation to the heart. Clamping below the renal arteries is common and usually produces only a small increase in blood pressure, but supraceliac occlusion can result in significant hypertension. Other factors may contribute to the observed hypertension. During proximal aortic occlusion, increased concentrations of catecholamines, angiotensin, and renin have been observed. These agents, as well as other mediators released from ischemic tissues below the clamp, may influence the vascular tone above the clamp.[129,130]

Venous Return and Cardiac Output It may seem intuitive that cardiac output should decrease with acute occlusion of a major arterial conduit caused by an increase in afterload. However, reflex mechanisms, venous return, and left heart function may modify this response. For example, location of the cross-clamp is important. If the clamp is placed in the supraceliac region, evidence suggests that venous return and cardiac output actually increase. This is probably due to splanchnic venous collapse distal to the cross-clamp and blood volume redistribution above the level of the clamp with increased filling pressures (central venous pressure, pulmonary capillary wedge pressure, or left ventricular end-diastolic pressure). However, an infrarenal cross-clamp may redistribute blood volume back to the compliant splanchnic bed, decrease preload, and cause a decrease in cardiac output.[129]

Other mechanisms have been suggested to explain an increase in cardiac output with thoracic aortic clamping, including an aortic-cardiac reflex,[131] which increases contractility, and elimination of slow time-constant vascular beds (splanchnic) from the circulation.[132] Conversely, an increase in aortic pressure should stimulate baroreceptors to depress heart rate, contractility, and vascular tone. Previous studies have shown a decrease in cardiac output with aortic occlusion, and this finding has come to represent the common understanding. **Figure 55-5** summarizes the issues surrounding blood volume distribution during application of supra- and infraceliac cross-clamps.

Myocardial Effects The effects of aortic cross-clamping on cardiac function and myocardial perfusion have been the subject of several investigations. In the absence of any underlying disorder of contractility or coronary flow, the heart can generate and withstand very high arterial pressures.

However, serious deterioration of pump function could be produced if a high afterload is superimposed on a myocardium depressed by cardiomyopathic processes. Moreover, myocardial ischemia itself could be precipitated during clamping, leading to regional wall-motion abnormalities or infarction if afterload elevation occurs in the presence of coronary artery stenosis. The presumed mechanism for this ischemia is subendocardial hypoperfusion caused by the high intercavitary pressures during diastole and systole, in conjunction with impaired inflow due to stenotic coronary lesions.

One investigation using monitoring with TEE determined that occlusion of the aorta at the supraceliac level caused major increases in left ventricular end-systolic and end-diastolic dimensions, decreases in ejection fraction, and frequent wall motion abnormalities. These changes were not detected by conventional monitoring devices. Occlusion at the suprarenal-infraceliac level caused similar but smaller changes, and occlusion at the infrarenal level caused only minimal cardiovascular effects. The hemodynamic effects of clamping the aorta were managed by administration of vasodilating drugs, anesthetics, and fluids to keep systemic and pulmonary arterial pressures normal.[133]

It is quite possible that aortic occlusion could have effects on ventricular function even if mean arterial pressure and systemic vascular resistance (SVR) were normalized to baseline. The blood pressure

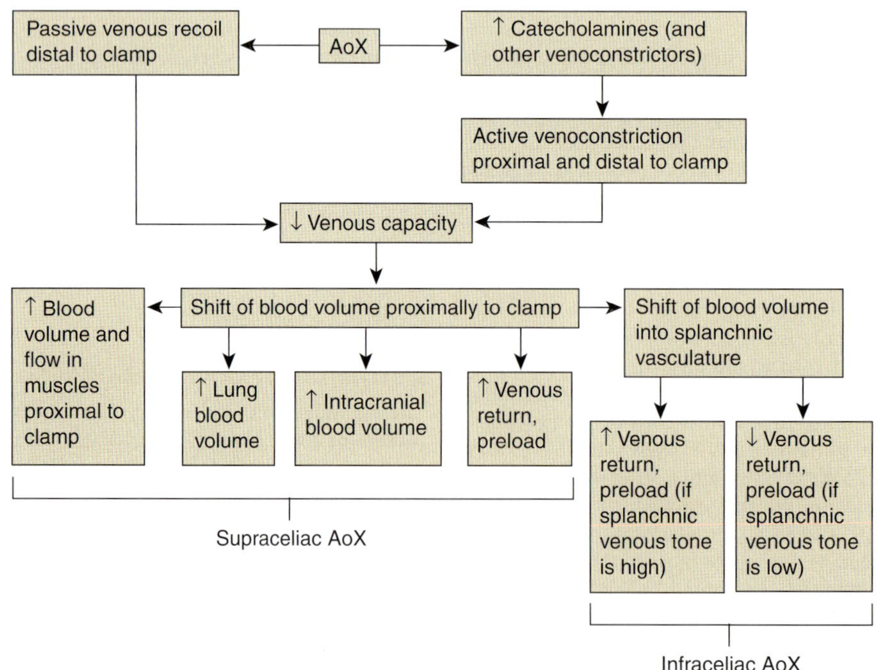

FIGURE 55-5. Blood volume redistribution during aortic cross-clamping. This scheme depicts the reason for the decrease in venous capacity, which results in blood volume redistribution from the vasculature distal to aortic occlusion to the vasculature proximal to aortic occlusion. If the aorta is occluded above the splanchnic system, the blood volume travels to the heart, increasing preload and blood volume in all organs and tissues proximal to the clamp. However, if the aorta is occluded below the splanchnic system, blood volume may shift into the splanchnic system or into the vasculature of other tissues proximal to the clamp. The distribution of this blood volume between the splanchnic and nonsplanchnic vasculature determines changes in preload. AoX, aortic cross-clamping; ↑, increase; ↓, decrease. [From Gelman S. The pathophysiology of aortic cross-clamping and unclamping. *Anesthesiology.* 1995;82(4):1026-1060.]

wave form, as observed in the ascending aorta, is created by characteristics of ventricular ejection and vascular resistance and compliance, as well as by pressure waves returning retrograde from major reflecting sites in the periphery. If sufficiently delayed, reflected waves may appear in diastole, thus augmenting myocardial perfusion. Return during systole, however, would add to wall stress during ejection and increase myocardial oxygen demand. By moving the major reflecting site closer to the heart, aortic cross-clamping could thus cause myocardial dysfunction in the face of a mean aortic pressure normalized by therapy.

Aortic cross-clamping is associated with increases in preload and afterload, leading to an increase in myocardial oxygen demand. The intact coronary vasculature responds to this increase in demand by an increase in flow. In 1 set of experiments, cross-clamping of the aorta was associated with a greater than 65% increase in the coronary blood flow, which probably represents coronary blood flow autoregulation, and increases in myocardial oxygen demand and consumption.[134]

The responses to cross-clamping differ in patients with and without CAD. In conditions of increased systolic left ventricular pressure and left ventricular dilation, the normal ventricle responds with a positive inotropic effect (the "Anrep effect").[129] In contrast, with the presence of CAD, left ventricular decompensation ensues due to the inability to increase subendocardial blood flow in response to an increase in intraventricular pressure.

Metabolic Changes Two fundamental interconnected metabolic effects characterize aortic cross-clamping: (1) lowered total-body oxidative metabolism (Vo_2) and (2) conversion to anaerobic metabolism of the hypoperfused body mass distal to the clamp. Gelman[129] showed that application of an infrarenal cross-clamp caused a 16% decrease in Vo_2, whereas other studies have shown that supraceliac cross-clamping causes a 55% reduction.[135] Presumably, a suprarenal occlusion would cause a reduction similar to the infrarenal occlusion because the kidneys do not consume oxygen in proportion to their flow.

The effects of aortic cross-clamping on mixed venous oxygen saturation depend on the therapeutic modalities used to control blood pressure. If arteriolar dilation is the dominant therapy, then aerobically functioning tissue will be overperfused, its extraction will decrease, and the saturation and partial pressure of oxygen of mixed venous blood will increase substantially. Conversely, preload reduction techniques maintain both oxygen extraction ratio and mixed venous saturation at approximately their preclamp values.

Anaerobic metabolism by tissue below the aortic cross-clamp produces lactic acid that reaches the proximal circulation by collaterals, leading to a progressive rise in blood lactate presumably reaching the proximal circulation by collaterals. For infrarenal cross-clamps, the buildup in systemic lactate during occlusion, as well as its release with unclamping, is noticeable but rarely clinically significant. Exceptions to this occur with grossly prolonged ischemic times. Cross-clamps above the celiac axis not only produce a larger anaerobically functioning tissue mass, but also, by excluding the liver and kidneys, greatly attenuate the elimination of lactate.[136]

THERAPEUTIC STRATEGIES

Most clinicians view the physiologic problem of aortic cross-clamping as a consequence of increased left ventricular afterload and propose interventions that reverse this effect. Vasodilators, notably sodium nitroprusside, are routinely used to control hypertension.[137]

Arteriolar dilation in vessels supplying organs proximal to the clamp can, in most circumstances, cause them to accommodate a sufficient increase in blood flow to maintain blood pressure within an acceptable range. Obviously, this produces a relative overperfusion of the affected organs. Problems with this method include (1) partial failure (eg, inability to adequately control pressure); (2) requirement for high doses of sodium nitroprusside; and (3) exceedingly low pressures in the circulation distal to the lowest clamp.

Alternate strategies involve manipulating the venous return. During the period of cross-clamp, that portion of the body supplied by the occluded arterial flow is unavailable for oxidative metabolism. Thus the heart does not need to maintain its preclamp output, and interventions that would reduce output seem appropriate.[129] Simultaneous interventions to decrease the venous return and minimize blood redistribution may solve the problem.

Venodilation with nitroglycerine sufficient to lower filling pressure and reduce cardiac output appears to be the most attractive alternative. In experimental aortic cross-clamping in animals, despite the severe myocardial depression observed, nitroglycerin maintained transmural distribution of flow favoring the endocardium. The benefit probably reflected decreased ventricular wall tension resulting from an increase in venous capacitance and subsequent preload reduction.[138]

Although nitroglycerin is an attractive alternative given its coronary vasodilatory and preload reduction effects, it is a weak arteriodilator and may not be sufficient in controlling blood pressure in situations of high aortic occlusion. The use of a combination of low-dose nitroprusside along with nitroglycerine as a titratable technique to control pressure will benefit both afterload and preload reduction with rapid termination of the pharmacologic effects before aortic unclamping.

Isoflurane, which mildly depresses contractility and causes vasodilation of both resistance and capacitance vessels, has been safely used for anesthesia and blood pressure control in patients with good myocardial function undergoing thoracic aneurysm repair.[139]

Bypass and shunting techniques that divert flow from the left atrium, left ventricle, or proximal aorta to the aorta distal to the lowest clamp have been used to blunt the effects of cross-clamping. Because these methods are not devoid of complications, they are usually reserved for surgery that necessitates thoracic aortic clamping.

Femoral vein–femoral artery bypass uses femoral venous inflow by gravity to a reservoir/oxygenator and roller-pump-generated outflow to the femoral artery, thus retrogradely perfusing vasculature below the most distal clamp (femoral–femoral bypass). Hypertension caused by clamp application is quickly resolved by increasing volume in the venous reservoir, which reduces venous return to the heart and lowers cardiac output.[140] The requirement for full systemic anticoagulation can be a disadvantage in terms of postoperative bleeding. Technical problems with cannula size and placement that limit the venous return will decrease the bypass pump flows and will limit the distal perfusion and the effectiveness of the circuit in controlling proximal blood pressure.

A Gott shunt is a heparin-coated conduit that passively shunts blood from the proximal to the distal aorta without the need of systemic coagulation. One end of the conduit is placed in the ascending aorta or in the aortic arch, and the distal end is placed in the distal descending aorta.[141] Although it is a simple and inexpensive technique, distal flow is limited by the size of the shunt and dislodgement of atheromatous plaque, vessel injury, bleeding, kinking, and malpositioning of the conduit can occur.

Partial left heart bypass uses extracorporeal circulation to shunt flow from the left atrium to the distal circulation. The left atrium is cannulated most commonly via a left pulmonary vein and oxygenated blood is diverted either through a centrifugal pump or through an oxygenator/reservoir and a roller pump to the femoral artery. Although using a reservoir requires full systemic anticoagulation, using a centrifugal pump requires minimal or no heparin. Bypass flow rates ranging from 25 to 40 mL/kg/min seem to be sufficient to normalize proximal aortic pressures and maintain adequate distal perfusion.[130]

Renal Protection Renal dysfunction after vascular surgery remains a serious complication. Godet et al reported a 20% to 25% incidence of acute postoperative renal failure after aortic surgery in 475 patients.[142] Huynh et al found a 13% incidence of renal failure requiring dialysis in 540 thoracoabdominal aneurysm repairs over a 10-year period.[143] Therefore, preservation of renal function is a primary concern during aortic aneurysm surgery. Preoperative optimization of renal function, attention to intraoperative fluid balance, and the use of "renoprotective" agents are some of the methods that have been used in an effort to prevent this serious complication of vascular surgery.

Several intraoperative events may precipitate renal dysfunction either alone or in concert, such as hypovolemia, the use of contrast agents, hypotension and hypoperfusion due to hemodynamic instability, aortic occlusion for aneurysm repair, atheroembolic occlusion of the renal vessels, and the inflammatory response activated during periods of visceral ischemia.[144]

Most strategies of renal protection have focused on the preoperative optimization and manipulation of intraoperative anesthetic and surgical techniques to minimize postoperative renal dysfunction. The most significant progress toward reducing renal injury has come from the widespread adoption of the endovascular technique of aortic aneurysm repair. Wahlberg et al have reported that aortic clamp time was the strongest predictor of postoperative renal dysfunction, especially if the clamp time exceeded 50 minutes.[145]

In animal experiments, preischemia administration of mannitol exerts a protective effect on renal function.[146] Because the mechanisms that produce acute tubular necrosis (ATN) are complex, it is not surprising that controversy exists regarding the exact manner in which mannitol or other agents might prevent ATN. It is possible that mannitol, a potent osmotic diuretic, exerts its protective effect by the scavenging of free radicals produced upon reperfusion of the kidney with cross-clamp release and by shifting blood flow to the renal cortex by its vasodilatory properties. As there is some evidence to support a beneficial effect of intravenous mannitol given before aortic clamping,[147] it is common clinical practice to administer 12.5 g/70 kg 10 to 15 minutes before aortic cross-clamping.

The use of furosemide is more controversial. Although a protective effect of furosemide has not been established per se, it is generally believed that this agent may result in a conversion of low output–to–high output renal failure, the latter being much easier to manage in the postoperative period. When diuretics are used, increased fluid requirements and hypokalemia should be anticipated throughout the perioperative period.

For the more common infrarenal aneurysms, where cross-clamp application would not seem to impede renal perfusion, renal vascular resistance increases and renal blood flow decreases.[129,148] The distribution of renal blood flow is altered during infrarenal aortic cross-clamping, and this phenomenon can result in impairment of function.[148] Renal blood flow is reduced not only during cross-clamp, but also post–cross-clamp.[129] All of these factors combine to increase the risk of postoperative renal dysfunction. Patients with preoperative renal insufficiency are at greatest risk of developing renal failure.

Maintenance of adequate intravascular volume and a short cross-clamp time have been shown to be the most important factors in avoiding renal dysfunction postoperatively. Many clinicians advocate the use of low-dose dopamine (3 mcg/kg/min) to increase renal blood flow during aneurysm surgery, although there is no evidence to support this approach.[144] Fenoldopam mesylate, a highly selective dopamine type-1 agonist that preferentially dilates the renal and splanchnic vasculature, has been found to have renoprotective effects and has been associated with relatively rapid return of renal function to baseline values in this setting.[144]

Other methods of renal protection include hypothermic renal perfusion, partial left heart bypass and intermittent arterial blood renal perfusion.

Spinal Cord Ischemia and Protection The spinal cord receives blood via radicular arteries that supply the anterior spinal artery and the posterolateral spinal arteries. The upper part of the spinal cord receives most of its blood supply via the vertebral arteries and in a small proportion via the ascending and deep cervical arteries and through the costovertebral arteries. The lower half of the spinal cord is supplied entirely by branches of the intercostal, lumbar, iliolumbar, and lateral sacral arteries. The paired posterior arteries supply the posterior one-third of the spinal cord, and the anterior spinal artery supplies the anterior two-thirds of the spinal cord.

The single anterior artery commences from the spinal branches of the vertebral arteries and receives variable blood supply through radicular arteries derived from ascending cervical, intercostal, lumbar, and iliolumbar arteries. The largest and most developed radicular artery is the arteria radicularis magna or the artery of Adamkiewicz, which can originate from T9 to L3 levels, but most commonly arises from T9 to T12.[122] Based upon anatomic distribution of segmental vessels supplying the spinal cord, the tenuous collateral flow to the anterior spinal artery in the midthoracic region makes the spinal cord vulnerable to ischemia during aortic occlusion or hypotension.

In a recent elegant review, Sinha and Cheung recommend the following strategies in order to prevent or treat spinal cord ischemia after thoracic aortic surgery[125]:

1. Minimize spinal cord ischemia time by (a) segmental reconstruction of the descending aorta, (b) distal aortic perfusion with a passive shunt (Gott shunt), and (c) partial left heart bypass.
3. Increase tolerance to ischemia by (a) deliberate mild systemic hypothermia, (b) deep hypothermic circulatory arrest, (c) selective spinal cord hypothermia by epidural cooling, and (d) pharmacologic neuroprotection.
3. Augment spinal cord perfusion by (a) deliberate hypertension, (b) lumbar cerebrospinal fluid drainage, (c) reimplantation of intercostals and lumbar segmental arteries, and (d) preservation of subclavian artery flow.
4. Detect spinal cord ischemia early by (a) intraoperative MEP and SSEP monitoring and (b) serial postoperative neurologic examination.

UNCLAMPING

Release of the aortic cross-clamp results in metabolic and hemodynamic changes that vary in magnitude according to (1) the extent and nature of the tissue reperfused, (2) the total occlusion time, (3) administration of fluids and therapeutic agents during the cross-clamp period and at the moment of unclamping, and (4) the use of shunts or bypass. The most consistent cardiovascular response to clamp release in the absence of shunts or bypass is an acute fall in systemic blood pressure. The dominant influence is a decrease in systemic vascular resistance due to opening of the previously minimally perfused vascular beds, which may be maximally dilated due to reactive hyperemia.

Release of an infrarenal clamp usually causes a small drop in blood pressure that is transient and well tolerated, although treatment with fluid infusion or small increments of a vasopressor may be occasionally necessary. Removal of a supraceliac cross-clamp can result in profound hypotension, which should be anticipated by vigorous prerelease intravascular volume administration, and frequently requires transient vasopressor support. However, the indiscriminate use of vasopressors may result in excessive vasoconstriction above the aortic clamp compared with below the clamp because the former, which is nonischemic, would respond better to vasopressors than the latter, which is acidotic. This would promote redistribution of blood volume from the upper to the lower part of the body, further reducing the flow above the aortic clamp.[129] **Figure 55-6** summarizes the hemodynamic responses to aortic unclamping.

Several different mediators have been suggested as being responsible for the hemodynamic effects seen after the release of the aortic cross-clamp including acidosis, lactate production, renin-angiotensin system, oxygen-free radicals, prostaglandins, complement activation, and myocardial depressant factors.[129] Unless the myocardium becomes ischemic or failure ensues, stability usually returns within several minutes with conservative therapy. Disseminated intravascular coagulation is an unusual but devastating complication. The etiology of the condition is largely unknown but is likely related to cross-clamp duration and intestinal ischemia.

Total-body oxygen consumption increases with unclamping as below-clamp tissues return to aerobic metabolism. Mixed venous blood

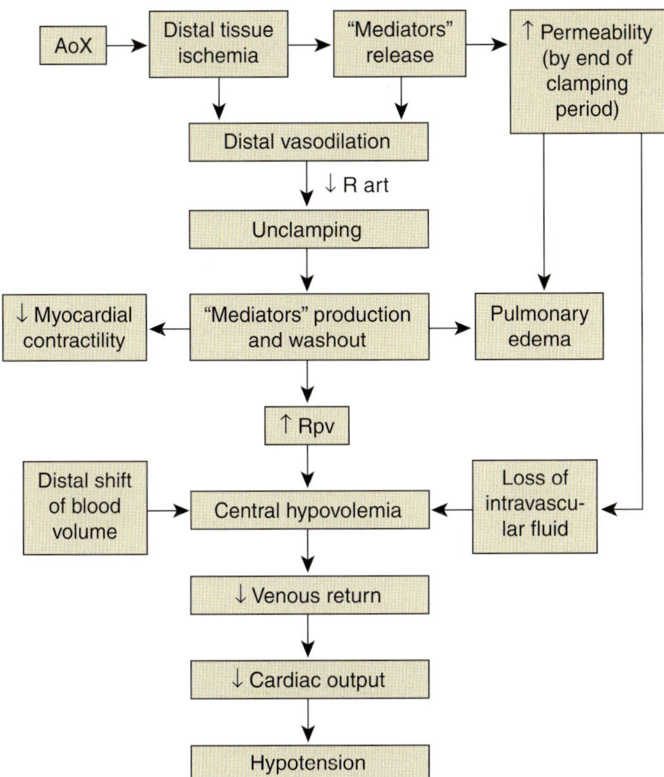

FIGURE 55-6. Systemic hemodynamic response to aortic unclamping. AoX, aortic cross-clamping; Cven, venous capacitance; R art, arterial resistance; Rpv, pulmonary vascular resistance; ↑, increase; ↓, decrease. [From Gelman S. The pathophysiology of aortic cross-clamping and unclamping. *Anesthesiology.* 1995;82(4):1026-1060.]

shows an abrupt desaturation within minutes after release of a supraceliac clamp and rapidly returns to preclamp values. The transient rise in oxygen extraction implied by this finding may only reflect "reloading" of oxygen-depleted hemoglobin, myoglobin, and cytochromes rather than actual energy production. Investigators have addressed the issue of "oxygen debt," wherein reperfusion of a previously ischemic tissue mass may result in an overshoot of oxygen consumption to "repay" a deficit incurred during the anaerobic period.[149]

Carbon dioxide is elevated in arterial and venous blood within moments of unclamping, and this is reflected in the end-tidal partial pressure. Two principal sources contribute to the appearance of CO_2: (1) as the end product of aerobic metabolism and (2) from the buffering (through carbonic acid) of organic acids that are washed out during reperfusion. It was formerly common clinical practice to administer a bolus of sodium bicarbonate just before unclamping in an attempt to buffer the expected fall in pH. Unfortunately, additional CO_2 produced by the exogenous sodium bicarbonate buffering adds to the CO_2 produced by aerobic metabolism and dramatically increases $Paco_2$ levels. Carbon dioxide readily diffuses across cell membranes and could worsen intracellular acidosis, resulting in organ dysfunction (eg, cardiac conduction and contractility disturbances). Bicarbonate should be administered, if desired, when volume resuscitation, perfusion, and ventilation are adequate.

Blood lactate levels often increase after release of the aortic clamp. Higher concentrations occur with prolonged ischemia and higher levels of clamping. Lactate levels rapidly return to normal after complete restoration of hepatic and liver flow, and elimination of continued excess production. It is uncommon for significant lactate elevation to persist into the postoperative period.

Gradual release of the aortic clamp and its reapplication has been recommended to allow time for volume replacement and washout of the vasoactive and cardiodepressant mediators from the ischemic tissues.[129]

ANESTHETIC TECHNIQUES

The anesthetic plan should take into consideration the comorbidities of the patient and knowledge of intraoperative physiologic changes, as well as specific plans for postoperative care.

General Anesthesia After institution of appropriate monitoring, induction of general anesthesia can be induced with etomidate, or propofol while avoiding hemodynamic extremes. Intravenous opioids such as fentanyl and sufentanil can be titrated to blunt the hemodynamic effects of endotracheal intubation. Neuromuscular blockade may be introduced at any time during this process after the loss of consciousness. Tachycardia and/or hypertension that may be triggered by laryngoscopy and intubation can be controlled with short-acting β-blockers such as esmolol. Brisk fluid administration may be necessary during induction to prevent hypotension. Preoperative antihypertensive medications, recent use of intravenous contrast agents, and fasting can result in intravascular volume depletion. The generalized withdrawal of sympathetic tone that accompanies anesthetic induction can then lead to hypotension. Anesthesia may be maintained with volatile agents in combination with opioids and neuromuscular blocking agents. The choice of volatile agent may be based on its secondary effects. Isoflurane causes mild vasodilation and minimal myocardial depression, and seems to be the agent of choice. More importantly, both isoflurane and sevoflurane have been shown to protect the myocardium from ischemia by means of preconditioning.

Total intravenous anesthesia (TIVA) can be used with titrated, continuous infusion of propofol and short-acting opioids such as remifentanil and alfentanil. TIVA should be considered when intraoperative neurologic monitoring with SSEP and MEP is used. This technique is also appealing in patients who have renal insufficiency or in cases involving suprarenal aortic clamping due to the lack of dependency of these agents on renal clearance for recovery. Additionally, it allows rapid emergence and extubation. Although there may be concerns with TIVA because of its tendency to cause hypotension, this can be prevented by ensuring euvolemic status before induction.

Combined Techniques The introduction of intrathecal and epidural narcotics and local anesthetic agents for both intraoperative and postoperative analgesia has proved to be a major advance in perioperative anesthetic management. The use of epidural anesthesia provides certain physiologic effects and may attenuate some of the detrimental pathophysiologic effects associated with surgery. The benefits of epidural analgesia include efficient pain management, decrease in adrenocortical stress response, and a reduction in protein catabolism, immunosuppression, and pulmonary and cardiac morbidity. Due to blocking the cardiac sympathetic fibers (T1-T4), thoracic epidural analgesia leads to dilation of both normal and stenotic coronary vessels, and results in a reduction of the myocardial work and oxygen demand.[150] Thoracic epidural extending above T12 blocks the activity of sympathetic fibers innervating the mesenterial blood vessels and improves the intestinal mucosal blood flow, even under conditions of reduced perfusion pressure.[151] Thoracic epidural anesthesia and postoperative analgesia also increase wound tissue oxygen tension compared with general anesthesia and intravenous morphine analgesia.[152] Studies have disagreed on the influence of anesthetic technique on perioperative morbidity in this patient population. Although some studies involving high-risk surgical patients undergoing elective abdominal aortic surgery have reported significant reductions in cardiac morbidity associated with the use of intraoperative and postoperative epidural analgesia using local anesthetics and opioids,[101,153] others did not show a decrease in cardiac morbidity.[154,155]

Intraoperative use of this modality may influence anesthetic management. Any significant dose of parenteral opiates given to blunt the stimuli of intubation and incision may act synergistically with the neuraxial narcotic to produce prolonged or delayed respiratory depression at the end of the procedure, therefore delaying emergence. Epidural anesthesia using local anesthetic agents is an attractive adjunct to general anesthesia and has been advocated for vascular surgery. Experience has shown, however, that extreme hypotension can result with combined regional and general anesthesia in patients undergoing aortic surgery. The drop in blood pressure that accompanies removal of an aortic cross-clamp is exacerbated by any degree of sympathetic blockade. Adequate fluid resuscitation before cross-clamp or the use of vasopressors with declamping may be required. Although excessive fluid administration may predispose to hypervolemia in the postoperative period, the use of vasopressors may cloud clinical judgment when organ or limb perfusion is in doubt. Hypotension can be minimized by optimizing intravascular volume and by administering much smaller volumes of local anesthetics in the epidural space than normally required for a "pure" regional anesthetic.

It is becoming increasingly evident that the postoperative period is associated with a high risk of morbidity in patients with cardiac disease undergoing noncardiac surgery.[156] Several possible sequelae of major vascular surgery may make emergence and extubation problematic. These include "third-space" fluid accumulation, postoperative pulmonary dysfunction, coagulopathy, hypothermia, and renal failure. The ideal goal is to have an extubated, comfortable, well-oxygenated, ventilating patient who is normothermic and normovolemic, has good renal function, and has stable vital signs.

POSTOPERATIVE CARE

Although there is wide variation in clinical practice, emergence technique, need for mechanical ventilation, and postoperative analgesia are critical determinants of postoperative morbidity. Relevant issues to consider are the anesthetic technique, extent of aneurysm repair, and patient stability with regard to certain physiologic parameters including body temperature, pulmonary function, urine output, blood loss, and intravascular volume.

Many patients will be ready for extubation at the termination of surgery. However, several factors may complicate what would otherwise appear to be a simple decision. Several patients have a significant smoking history with resulting respiratory compromise. Postoperative deterioration of pulmonary function superimposed on preexisting dysfunction can result in poor oxygenation immediately after surgery. Further, varying degrees of fluid shift occur commonly during aortic aneurysm repair and continue postoperatively. Even if intravascular volume has been carefully maintained, extravascular fluid must be mobilized and eliminated over time. It is not always possible to monitor and control this process with a sufficient degree of precision. Thus patients who seem to be doing well may develop problems several hours after the procedure and require reintubation after an apparently "normal" recovery. The use of postoperative epidural analgesia may have a beneficial effect in reducing pulmonary morbidity. Ballantyne et al found that postoperative epidural analgesia was associated with a decrease in the incidence of atelectasis, pneumonia, and overall pulmonary complications, and an increase in the arterial partial pressure of oxygen when compared with systemic opioid administration.[157]

Myocardial ischemia is common in the postoperative period, although much of it may be "silent" and require careful surveillance to detect. There is also a strong association between postoperative ischemia and adverse outcome.[156]

Postoperative care of vascular surgery patients can be challenging. Coagulopathy in the perioperative period can become a major problem requiring reexploration. Hypothermia may persist and require treatment with heating blankets. Electrolytes and blood gases should be followed closely and hemodynamic profiles optimized. Patients who have experienced a ruptured aneurysm and/or prolonged suprarenal cross-clamping are at high risk of acute renal failure. Adequate attention to these details is essential for ensuring a successful outcome.

ANESTHETIC CONSIDERATIONS FOR ENDOVASCULAR AORTIC ANEURYSM REPAIR

Endovascular aortic repair (EVAR) has steadily gained popularity as a reliable alternative to conventional surgical repair of aortic aneurysms. Endovascular repair of abdominal aneurysms was developed to reduce morbidity and mortality, and to provide an alternative to patients who cannot undergo standard surgical therapy.

EVAR was initially developed to provide an alternative for patients who could not undergo the standard open surgical repair. However, the use of EVAR has increased dramatically and by 2006 EVAR was used more frequently than open repair in patients of all ages. Two randomized trials of patients who were considered suitable candidates for either elective open surgery or endovascular repair investigated both short- and long-term outcome. The EndoVascular Aortic Repair (EVAR 1) trial included 1082 patients who were at least 60 years of age with aneurysms at least 5.5 cm in diameter. The results showed that the 30-day mortality was significantly lower with endovascular than with open repair (1.8% vs 4.3%). However, no differences were seen in total mortality or aneurysm-related mortality at 4 years. Endovascular repair was associated with increased rates of graft-related complications and reinterventions and was more costly.[158]

Similar findings were reported by the Dutch Randomized Endovascular Aneurysm Management (DREAM) trial. The DREAM trial evaluated 345 patients with aneurysms of at least 5 cm in diameter and found a significant trend toward lower operative mortality with EVAR than with conventional surgery (1.2% vs 4.6%). There was no difference in cumulative survival at 2 years of follow-up (89.7 vs 89.6 with surgical repair), an effect that was present at 1 year.[159] However, at 6 years survival rates were similar in the endovascular-repair group and the open-repair group, but there was a significantly higher rate of secondary interventions in the endovascular-repair group.[160] Therefore, based on the patient's life expectancy and comorbidities, the decision to choose one technique over the other may need to be individualized.

EVAR avoids the hemodynamic lability associated with major abdominal incision and aortic cross-clamping and unclamping, and also presents other subtle benefits such as significantly smaller changes in plasma catecholamine levels, improved acid-base homeostasis, and a decreased metabolic stress response.

In 2005 the ACC/AHA published practice guidelines for the management of patients with peripheral arterial disease (lower extremity, renal, mesenteric, and abdominal aortic).[94] The following recommendations were made with regard to the type of intervention:

1. Open surgical repair was recommended for patients at low or average risk of operative complications.
2. EVAR was suggested in patients at high risk of complications from open operations.
3. EVAR was suggested for patients who are not at high surgical risk, but evidence of benefit is less well established in this setting.

For the deployment of the graft, a femoral or iliac arteriotomy is performed, and a sheath is passed into the aorta over a guidewire. The endovascular stent is threaded over the guidewire and is positioned under fluoroscopic guidance. An inflatable balloon catheter is positioned inside the proximal attachment system. The balloon is inflated for a period of 30 to 60 seconds during which time aortic blood flow is occluded. This expands the stent and imbeds the hooks into the normal arterial wall. Newer, approved devices are self-expanding once released from the sheath and use a tri-lobed balloon for stent fixation. This combination results in less hemodynamic stress because the aorta is never totally occluded during balloon expansion.

Endovascular repair is suitable for patients who meet certain anatomic criteria: at least 1.5 cm of aneurysmal neck below the renal arteries; at least 1 cm of aneurysmal neck above the aortic bifurcation; femoral artery free from limiting occlusion and at least 8 mm in diameter; and, if the distal attachment is the iliac artery, a minimal length and maximum diameter of healthy artery as specified by the manufacturer.

Surgical complications can include damage to iliofemoral vessels (dissection, ischemia), distal embolization of atheromatous debris, adverse reactions to radiographic contrast, rupture of aneurysm, or displacement of the proximal stent to occlude the renal or mesenteric arteries or other arteries in repair of the thoracic aorta.

Endoleak is defined as the persistence of blood flow outside the lumen of the endograft but within an aneurysm sac. Endoleak may occur due to misplacement or poor sizing of an endograft (technical error), fatigue, displacement or distortion of the endograft material (device failure), or by reactions to the endograft within the aneurysmal sac environment. Endoleaks are classified based on location/mechanism and timing of occurrence. Type I endoleak is a persistent flow around the attachment sites (proximal or distal) of the endograft due to inadequate or ineffective seal at the graft ends. Type II endoleak is due to retrograde flow into the aneurysmal sac from a patent collateral branch vessel. Type III is defined as flow into the aneurysmal sac due to tear or defect in the endograft fabric or due to leakage between modular segments of an endograft, and type IV is flow detected in the aneurysmal sac due to the highly porous graft material.[161]

Anesthetic Techniques General anesthesia, regional anesthesia, and monitored anesthesia care with local anesthetic infiltration at the incision site have all been used successfully for EVAR. Goals of an anesthetic plan should be to maintain hemodynamic stability, provide adequate oxygenation and ventilation, preserve organ function, and maintain normothermia.[161]

Certain concerns related to the procedure should be addressed. Careful positioning of the device over guidewires for accurate deployment and the utilization of fluoroscopy require the patient to be perfectly still, sometimes for longer periods of time than anticipated. Care must be taken to ensure that tachycardia and hypertension are avoided. During the transient balloon occlusion of the aorta, the surgeon may request that the mean blood pressure is maintained at about 60 mm Hg so that the force pushing the stent distally is minimized. Also at this time the patient may experience significant hemodynamic stress, especially if baseline cardiac function was poor. Vasopressors and inotropes must be available at hand to manage hemodynamic emergencies. Preparation must be made for sudden massive blood loss, following major disruption of the aorta, and immediate laparotomy with aortic cross-clamping.

Blood loss can be difficult to quantify, as it is often lost around the sheaths and catheters, and can be retroperitoneal in the case of injury to femoral or iliac vessels. Hemoglobin should be checked during the procedure, especially if the patient becomes unstable. Endovascular procedures involve the liberal use of radiographic contrast to assist in appropriate deployment of the graft, to ensure exclusion of the aneurysmal sac, and to determine branch vessel patency. It is important to ensure that patients are adequately hydrated during the procedure and in the postoperative period to minimize contrast-induced nephropathy.

At the time of instrumentation of the aorta the patient must be anticoagulated with intravenous heparin. This, however, should not restrict the use of regional anesthesia as long as the recommendations made by the American Society of Regional Anesthesia and Pain Medicine regarding neuraxial anesthesia and anticoagulation are followed.

Anesthetic techniques were compared in various studies. A recent retrospective analysis based on the European registry of patients undergoing EVAR (the EUROSTAR registry) showed that a benefit in systemic complications, hospital stay, and admission to the intensive care unit could be documented both for local and regional anesthesia compared with general anesthesia.[162] De Virgilio et al compared cardiopulmonary mortality and mortality rates in a retrospective study of 200 patients undergoing infrarenal EVAR and found no overall difference.[163] This study as well as other studies noted lower fluid requirements and less need for vasopressor support associated with local anesthesia.[164] Also, by avoiding mechanical ventilation, patients with pulmonary comorbidities may benefit from a regional or local anesthesia technique.

From the preceding discussion, it is apparent that a variety of anesthetic techniques may be used, as long as specific goals of EVAR are met. Future randomized trials are needed, however, to further address the issue of impact of anesthetic technique on outcomes.

CONCLUSION

The patient undergoing major vascular surgery can be both challenging and rewarding for the anesthesiologist. The pathophysiology of vascular disease is complex and involves several organ systems. Predictive factors for vascular disease like smoking, hypertension, and diabetes must also be considered when planning perioperative anesthesia management. Temporary flow interruption of major diseased vessels may induce dramatic physiologic changes that can be a challenge during the intraoperative phase. Adequate knowledge of the pathology of vascular disease, operative technique, and monitoring modalities available is essential in ensuring favorable outcomes in this high-risk patient population.

KEY REFERENCES

- Devereaux PJ, Yang H, Yusuf S, et al. Effects of extended-release metoprolol succinate in patients undergoing non-cardiac surgery (POISE trial): a randomised controlled trial. *Lancet.* 2008;371:1839-1847.
- Fleisher LA, Beckman JA, Brown KA, et al. ACC/AHA 2007 Guidelines on perioperative cardiovascular evaluation and care for noncardiac surgery: executive summary: a report of the American College of Cardiology/American Heart Association Task Force on Practice Guidelines (Writing Committee to Revise the 2002 Guidelines on Perioperative Cardiovascular Evaluation for Noncardiac Surgery) developed in collaboration with the American Society of Echocardiography, American Society of Nuclear Cardiology, Heart Rhythm Society, Society of Cardiovascular Anesthesiologists, Society for Cardiovascular Angiography and Interventions, Society for Vascular Medicine and Biology, and Society for Vascular Surgery. *J Am Coll Cardiol.* 2007;50:1707-1732.
- Gelman S. The pathophysiology of aortic cross-clamping and unclamping. *Anesthesiology.* 1995;82:1026-1060.
- Greenhalgh RM, Brown LC, Powell JT, Thompson SG, Epstein D, Sculpher MJ. Endovascular versus open repair of abdominal aortic aneurysm. *N Engl J Med.* 2010;362:1863-1871.
- Horlocker TT, Wedel DJ, Rowlingson JC, et al. Regional anesthesia in the patient receiving antithrombotic or thrombolytic therapy: American Society of Regional Anesthesia and Pain Medicine Evidence-Based Guidelines (Third Edition). *Reg Anesth Pain Med.* 2010;35:64-101.
- Lewis SC, Warlow CP, Bodenham AR, et al. General anaesthesia versus local anaesthesia for carotid surgery (GALA): a multicentre, randomised controlled trial. *Lancet.* 2008;372:2132-2142.
- Kertai MD. Preoperative coronary revascularization in high-risk patients undergoing vascular surgery: a core review. *Anesth Analg.* 2008;106:751-758.
- Practice guidelines for perioperative transesophageal echocardiography. An updated report by the American Society of Anesthesiologists and the Society of Cardiovascular Anesthesiologists Task Force on Transesophageal Echocardiography. *Anesthesiology.* 2010;112:1084-1096.
- Sinha AC, Cheung AT. Spinal cord protection and thoracic aortic surgery. *Curr Opin Anaesthesiol.* 2010;23:95-102.
- Sweitzer BJ, Smetana GW. Identification and evaluation of the patient with lung disease. *Anesthesiol Clin.* 2009;27:673-686.

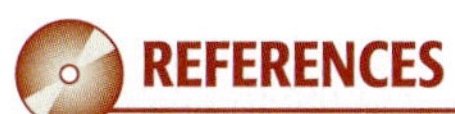

REFERENCES

Complete references available on DVD and online version at www.LongneckerAnesthesiology.com

CHAPTER 56

Anesthesia for Gastrointestinal Surgery

Martin Slodzinski
William T. Merritt

KEY POINTS

1. Diseases of the gastrointestinal system frequently result in abnormal gastric function, with potentially increased anesthetic risk caused by increased intragastric pressure, delayed gastric emptying, gastric dilation, and increased gastric secretion.
2. Although volume, pH, and amount of particulate matter in the aspirate appear to be the 3 most important factors determining the severity of the pulmonary insult, overall the medical fragility of the patient is often the most important determinant influencing the clinical course and outcome of pulmonary aspiration.
3. Extensive bowel, pancreatic, or esophageal resections entail considerable morbidity, with potential serious postoperative complications such as hemorrhage, coagulopathy, and hepatic, renal, pulmonary, or cardiovascular failure.
4. Laparoscopy entails the installation of gas (usually CO_2) into the peritoneal cavity with physiologic changes resulting from this gas under pressure and subsequent surgical positioning. Hemodynamic compromise can occur, which, although rare, can be catastrophic.
5. The systemic inflammatory response syndrome/multiorgan dysfunction syndrome continuum is often accompanied by gastrointestinal mucosal ischemia and the release of mediators that further compromise both splanchnic and systemic perfusion. Anesthetic care of these patients is especially challenging.
6. If the lower esophageal sphincter is not functioning properly, or if a hiatal hernia exists, stomach contents may reflux into the esophagus and pharynx during anesthesia and surgery, increasing the potential for serious aspiration pneumonia.
7. Narcotics have intestinal side effects that are well recognized. Lower esophageal sphincter tone is decreased. Gastric emptying is impaired because of decreased propulsive motility and increased tone in the antrum of the stomach.
8. During laparoscopy, the development of pneumothorax and/or pneumomediastinum is a serious and/or potentially life-threatening complication. When either is suspected, from hemodynamic deterioration or from the presence of subcutaneous emphysema, especially of the neck and face, aggressive investigation (auscultation, chest radiograph) and management (eg, chest tube for tension pneumothorax) should be undertaken. Procedures on the lower esophagus may be more likely to result in these complications. Conversion to an open procedure is usually required.
9. Approximately 40% of patients with gastroesophageal reflux have delayed gastric emptying, and in approximately one-third of these, the delay is clinically significant.
10. Maneuvers necessary for blunt esophagectomy are capable of causing serious hemodynamic and ventilatory compromise and require appropriate monitoring of blood pressure and respiration.
11. Bariatric surgery patients may have significant medical problems and their perioperative care can be quite challenging. Newer procedures continue to lessen morbidity and mortality.

Gastrointestinal (GI) surgical practice has evolved dramatically with experience and technology. Newer techniques result in less physiologic trespass and more rapid return to full activities, and the trend continues. Current robotics-assisted laparoscopic surgery will be augmented by remotely controlled natural orifice transluminal endoscopic surgery (NOTES).[1]

The GI system includes an amazingly complex neurochemical system with far-reaching implications on homeostasis and well-being.[2] Furthermore, from routine appendectomies to advanced robotic-assisted natural orifice hepatic resections,[3] GI surgery occupies a major percentage of the operative time in most hospitals. Therefore, providing anesthesia care for patients requiring these procedures represents a great portion of the anesthesiologist's time and attention. From routine to sophisticated procedures, this chapter illustrates and discusses preoperative, intraoperative, and postoperative considerations. A discussion of the effects of anesthesia administration on GI function is followed by important surgical and anesthetic considerations of specific GI surgical procedures.

OROPHARYNX

Mastication begins the process of digestion. Inadequately swallowed and regurgitant material may be in the pharynx. Pulmonary aspiration of oropharyngeal, esophageal, or gastric contents is an extremely important issue for all patients receiving anesthesia care, and especially those with gastrointestinal disorders/symptoms.

Local and general anesthesia depress sensation of the upper digestive system, starting with trigeminal innervations of the nasopharynx. The posterior third of the tongue and oral pharynx are innervated by the glossopharyngeal nerve, which accompanies the carotid sheath emerging from the jugular foramen. The superior laryngeal nerve innervates the tongue base and inferior epiglottis to the vocal cords. The recurrent laryngeal nerve innervates from the vocal cords distally. The remaining larynx and trachea are innervated by penetrating branches of the vagus. Any local (eg, pharyngeal tumor) or general (eg, cerebral vascular accident or metabolic toxin) pathology affecting the innervation of these areas increases risks of perioperative mishandling of oropharyngeal secretions and fluids, and an increased potential aspiration pneumonitis.

ESOPHAGUS AND STOMACH

Proper functioning of the esophagus and the lower esophageal sphincter (LES) is a concern during anesthesia care. If the esophagus is dilated because of obstruction by tumor, destruction of neural mechanisms (eg, achalasia), or existence of a diverticulum (**Fig. 56-1**), particulate matter will remain for hours (if not days) after ingestion, and secretions will not pass normally to the stomach. **If the LES is not functioning properly and/or if a hiatal hernia exists, stomach contents may reflux into the esophagus and even the pharynx during anesthesia and surgery, increasing the potential for serious aspiration pneumonia.** During an operative procedure, placement of a cuffed endotracheal tube during surgical procedures protects the airway from such materials. When an obstruction(s) is present, endotracheal intubation should occur with the patient awake (eg, direct oral, blind nasal, or fiberoptic bronchoscopy) or via a rapid sequence method with the patient anesthetized. With the awake method, sedation should be limited or avoided altogether, especially in patients with a "full" stomach, proximal obstruction, esophageal diverticulum, or altered consciousness. Emptying the gastric or esophageal contents (eg, nasogastric tube, Sengstaken-Blakemore tube) when feasible should decrease the volume and nature of any fluid available for reflux.[4] In any patient with known hiatal hernia or LES dysfunction, or when the stomach or esophagus is suspected to contain fluid or particulate matter, an attempt should also be made to aspirate the material before *emergence* from anesthesia. In addition, extubation should occur only after swallowing, adequate strength, and the ability to follow commands are apparent.

Many surgical approaches to the esophagus require a thoracotomy and a laparotomy, the lateral position, and a method of collapsing 1 lung. In addition, a temporary esophageal dilator may be requested intraoperatively by the surgeon; a nasogastric or naso-"intestinal" tube will need to be positioned at some point during the procedure to

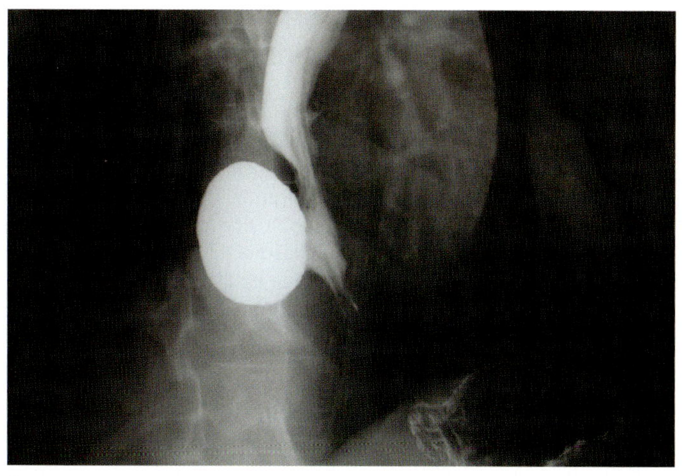

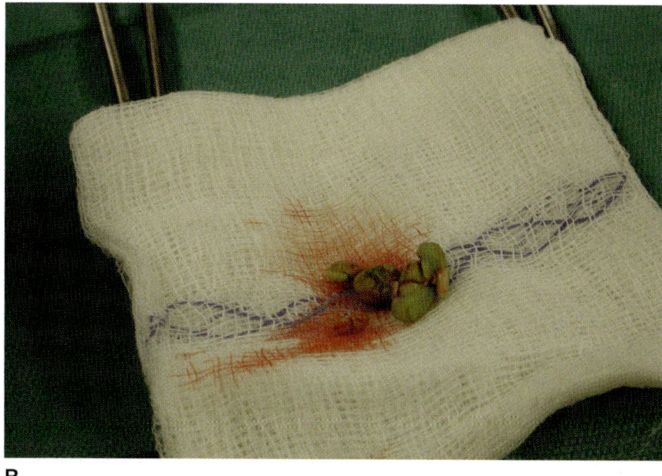

A B

FIGURE 56-1. **A.** Contrast material in clinical diverticulum surgery. **B.** Particulate material noted at time of removal.

maintain continuity above and below the anastomosis. Such procedures can be demanding and require considerable preoperative planning. Discussion with the primary surgeon both before arriving in the operating room and during the "Team Time Out" can be very helpful for all involved.

ISSUES OF CONCERN IN ANESTHESIA FOR GASTROINTESTINAL PROCEDURES

MANAGEMENT OF ACID REFLUX

Abdominal surgery has been associated with as much as 75% of the perioperative mortality related to aspiration pneumonitis.[5] In addition, fasting gastric volume can be large in patients with GI disorders, especially duodenal ulcer disease.[6] Many other conditions, some directly related to the GI tract, are associated with some risk of regurgitation of esophageal or stomach contents and ultimate pulmonary aspiration (**Box 56-1**). In these conditions, an inadequate initial clearance or the return of a substance to the pharynx may be followed by ineffective removal with subsequent passage through the glottic opening into the lungs.[7] Mortality associated with aspiration ranges from 3% to 70%[8] and the true incidence and morbidity are not well quantified. A large European study suggests that the actual incidence is considerably lower, approximately 0.05%.[9] Unrecognized or "silent" regurgitation typically occurs, as does subsequent aspiration.[10,11]

BOX 56-1

Conditions Associated With Aspiration Pneumonia

Abdominal distension
Abdominal infection
Abdominal trauma
Abnormal esophageal function
Abnormal LES
Altered state of consciousness
Anesthesia induction, intubation
"Full" stomach
Inadequate muscle relaxant reversal
Inadequate pharyngeal reflexes
Intestinal obstruction, dysmotility
Obesity
Pain
Poor cough
Pregnancy
Recent extubation (dysfunctional vocal cords/hypopharynx/sedation, dyspnea)

The volume, pH, and amount of particulate matter in the aspirate appear to be the 3 most important factors determining the severity of the pulmonary insult. Particulate matter obstructs airways and quickly leads to ventilation and perfusion mismatching, hypoxia, hemorrhagic edema, and sometimes acute pulmonary hypertension.[12] Traditionally, gastric volumes greater than 25 mL and pH less than 2.5 have been associated with the most severe pneumonitis,[13] although more recent data suggest that greater volumes of nonparticulate aspirated fluid would be tolerated when the pH is greater than 2.5.[12,14]

In addressing the problem of aspiration during the delivery of anesthesia, anesthesiologists have focused on 4 areas: (1) reduction of the acid content and volume of the stomach contents, (2) improvement of intestinal motility, (3) prevention of reflux into the pharynx, and (4) a better understanding of gastric emptying.

Although antacids increase gastric pH, particulate (ie, opaque) antacids produce severe aspiration damage similar to that of gastric acid.[21] The use of clear antacids is just as effective in increasing pH but is associated with only mild pulmonary changes if aspirated.[15]

Histamine-2 (H_2)-blocking agents are effective in reducing the acidity and, to a lesser extent, the volume of gastric fluid. Typical agents used include cimetidine and ranitidine.[16,17] None of these agents has much effect on the acidity of material already present in the stomach (eg, that found in the trauma patient or patients requiring other emergency surgery) but may decrease intraoperative acid production if given before surgery. Oral therapy seems to be as effective (and considerably less expensive) as intravenous (IV) or intramuscular forms when premedication by the oral route is suitable. Administration the night before and the morning of surgery consistently increases gastric pH to above 2.5. Rapid administration of cimetidine is associated with hypotension,[18] bradycardia, and cardiac arrest. Ranitidine appears to have a lesser incidence of similar side effects. Mechanisms may include blockage of the inotropic and chronotropic responses of stimulation of myocardial H_2 receptors.[19] These agents alter the metabolism or kinetics of various drugs, including the cytochrome P450 system,[20] lidocaine,[21] nifedipine,[22] theophylline, warfarin, and phenytoin. Although atropine and glycopyrrolate decrease gastric acid production somewhat, they generally are not used for this specific purpose because they also decrease LES tone.

Rapid-acting intravenous *proton pump inhibitors* are effective in reducing gastric volume and increasing gastric pH. In a prospective, randomized, controlled trial, proton pump inhibitors were compared with H_2 antagonists. After intravenous administration 1 hour prior to surgery, pantoprazole 40 mg (Protonix) and ranitidine 50 mg (Zantac) were compared. Gastric aspirate pHs were 5.3 and 4.8 and residual volumes 8 mL and 15 mL, respectively, measured just after induction of anesthesia. This was compared with an IV saline control. Patients receiving pantoprazole and ranitidine had statistically greater gastric pH and less gastric volume than control patients (5 mL IV saline with gastric aspirate pH 3.7 and 29 mL volume), but there was no statistical difference between the pantoprazole and ranitidine groups.[23] Although both proton pump and H_2 inhibition may be used to reduce perioperative gastric acid, neither seems to be superior.

Gastric and intestinal motility are stimulated by metoclopramide, which acts centrally by inhibiting dopamine and in the gut by releasing acetylcholine. LES tone also increases, but the pylorus and duodenum relax. Metoclopramide usually is administered concurrently with an H_2 blocker.

Preventing refluxed material from reaching the pharynx is the goal of cricoid pressure (the Sellick maneuver) and rapid sequence intubation. When properly performed, cricoid pressure should provide a barrier for at least 100 cm H_2O of esophageal pressure.[24] Pressure should not be released until the cuff is inflated and until correct placement has been verified by appropriate observations, including auscultation and capnometry. However, a meta-analysis of 241 peer-reviewed articles found little evidence that rapid-sequence intubation provided protection against aspiration. Furthermore, in a controlled, blinded, randomized crossover study comparing the Sellick and BURP (backward, upward, and right-sided pressure on the thyroid cartilage) maneuvers, the BURP maneuver and cricoid pressure worsened the laryngoscopic view in 30% of cases, cricoid pressure alone worsened the view in 12.5% of cases, and there was no difference in 65% of cases.[25,26] Although the protocol of rapid-sequence intubation is generally valued as an important tool to prevent aspiration, anesthesiologists continue to evaluate the relative values of drug dosage, manual ventilation, cricoid pressure, and patient position in an attempt to maximize patient safety A recent volunteer study suggests that compression of the alimentary tract does occur during both midline and lateral displacement of the cricoid cartilage.[6] The application of cricoid pressure appears to have a net positive value, but experience in its application is important.

As more is learned about the physiology of gastric emptying, the tradition of overnight fasting for elective surgery has come into question.[27-31] Residual gastric volumes may be acceptable after 2 to 4 hours of fasting, and the addition of H_2 blockers lowers pH as well. One should not extrapolate from such information directly to the emergency patient or the patient with a full stomach. **The aspiration of particulate matter produces such a devastating insult in the lung that, except for the most urgent situations, 6 to 8 hours of fasting after solid foods is recommended.** Even after this waiting period, the stomach often still contains food and large amounts of fluid.

BOWEL DISTENSION

Nitrous oxide (N_2O) administration is associated with an increase in intraluminal gas volume. Experimentally, in dogs, *bowel gas* volume increases approximately 75% to 100% after 2 hours of 70% to 80% N_2O, and by 100% to 200% after 4 hours.[32] Normally, luminal contents include approximately 100 mL of gas, mostly swallowed air; aerophagia or bowel obstruction greatly increases this volume. Clinically, N_2O use results in a slow increase in bowel distension and intraluminal pressure. The principal surgical consequence is difficulty with abdominal closure at the completion of a procedure. During extreme conditions (eg, obstruction with distended bowel), increased intraluminal pressure may lead to bowel ischemia. N_2O use during abdominal surgery, if needed, should be limited to the initial 10 to 15 minutes at induction and intubation, and during the period of abdominal wall closure at the completion of the surgical procedure. (See Endoscopy section for issues regarding N_2O during laparoscopy.)

BOWEL MOTILITY

Anticholinesterase drugs (eg, neostigmine) are necessary for the reversal of residual nondepolarizing muscular blockade. Although relatively safe, the parasympathetic stimulation of anticholinesterase drugs can have undesirable side effects. Bradycardia occurs so often that it is anticipated and managed before its occurrence by the administration of a parasympatholytic drug (eg, atropine or glycopyrrolate) prophylactically before administration of a neuromuscular blockade reversal agent. This parasympathetic stimulation also affects intestinal motility, increasing the frequency and pressure of peristaltic waves, especially in the colon. For unknown reasons, diseased colon (eg, from ulcerative colitis, diverticulitis) appears to be more susceptible to this effect. This has led to considerable debate over the potential for cholinesterase inhibitors to cause breakdown of colonic anastomoses.[33] Fortunately, residual anesthetic agents and pretreatment with parasympatholytic agents (atropine, glycopyrrolate) attenuate this response. Inadequate perfusion of the anastomotic site, infection, and underlying tissue abnormality are now thought to be more significant issues.

Thiopental increases the electrical and mechanical activity of the duodenum and jejunum in experimental studies, and atropine premedication decreases the response. Ketamine has little effect on GI motility, and oral diazepam reduces gastric emptying and increases small bowel transit time.[34]

Narcotics have significant intestinal side effects. LES tone is decreased.[35] Gastric emptying is impaired[36] because of decreased propulsive motility and increased tone in the antrum of the stomach. The duodenum and the small intestine undergo a decrease in propulsive contractions, whereas the amplitude of rhythmic segmental nonpropulsive contractions often is enhanced, which results in an increase in resting tone and can cause peristaltic spasms. The proximal small bowel is more affected than the distal part, and the tone of the ileocecal valve is increased. Parasympatholytic agents can partially abolish these effects. In the large intestine, the narcotic effects can be more pronounced; peristaltic waves are decreased or absent. The amplitude of rhythmic nonpropulsive contractions is increased, often to the point of spasm. Anal tone also is increased. Again, diseased bowel appears more susceptible to such effects.[37]

High spinal or epidural anesthesia promotes hyperperistaltic activity because of blockade of sympathetic innervation. The unopposed parasympathetic activity may cause nausea and vomiting in approximately 20% of patients, for whom atropine may be effective. Because of the increased peristaltic activity, controversy has arisen over the effects of spinal or epidural anesthesia on anastomotic breakdown, especially in colon surgery. Some data suggest that this problem is not significantly increased with regional anesthesia and that colonic blood flow is improved by spinal or epidural anesthesia.[38] Others disagree with these findings. Many believe that axial anesthesia is the emerging standard for early postoperative pain control.

Postoperative ileus is probably associated with manual trauma during laparotomy or from increased splanchnic nerve discharge in other procedures. Gastric peristalsis returns within 24 to 48 hours, and colonic activity returns after 48 hours, beginning at the cecum and progressing caudally. Small bowel motility returns more rapidly, and sometimes enteral tube feedings can be initiated within 24 hours. This ileus can lead to mild abdominal distension and absent bowel sounds for as long as 48 to 72 hours. Passage of flatus, cramping, and return of appetite suggest the return of normal peristaltic activity.[39]

Although neuraxial narcotics generally are recommended for pain relief in most patients, the side effects of pruritus, urinary retention, and especially respiratory depression are problematic in some. Effects are presumably through local spinal cord receptors and via more central mechanisms after rostral spread in the cerebrospinal fluid or systemic absorption. Although used extensively and successfully in patients undergoing all forms of surgery, including many varieties of abdominal surgery,[19,40] there are animal data that document alterations in intestinal motility associated with neuraxial narcotics,[41] and at least 1 note of caution in humans.[41] Most studies conclude that postoperative epidural anesthesia and analgesia directed by an anesthesiologist, compared with intravenous anesthesia administered by a surgeon, provides superior analgesia and decreases postoperative ileus, but does not reduce mortality or major morbidity, especially after major abdominal and cardiac surgical procedures[43,44] Postoperative epidural analgesia, in conjunction with a comprehensive program of preoperative counseling, no bowel preparation, carbohydrate clear liquids (until 2 hours before surgery), perioperative oxygen supplementation, nonopioid analgesia, minimal surgical drains and nasogastric tubes, early removal of urinary catheters, standard laxatives and prokinetic agents, and early ambulation, can reduce length of stay.[44]

BILIARY EFFECTS

Therapeutic doses of the opioids can cause a marked increase in biliary tract pressure in susceptible patients. For example, 10 mg of subcutaneous morphine can produce a 10-fold increase in common bile duct pressure within 15 minutes that can last 2 or more hours.[45] This effect results from opiate receptor-mediated mechanisms that cause spasm of the sphincter of Oddi. Fentanyl and alfentanil also increase common bile duct pressure.[46,47] The general importance of this effect on intraoperative cholangiograms is uncertain, but fentanyl-supplemented anesthesia is associated with a 3% surgical failure rate.[48] Considering the possibility of opioid-induced sphincter of Oddi spasm after a cholycystectomy or endoscopic retrograde cholangiography may avoid additional unnecessary and/or potentially dangerous procedures.[49]

Meperidine increases biliary tract pressure via mechanisms that are not receptor mediated. Opiate antagonists (eg, naloxone) can reverse this opiate-related increase in biliary tract pressure (except for that caused by meperidine)[50] but also may reverse general analgesic effects. Sublingual nitroglycerin (0.6 mg) decreases the elevated intrabiliary pressure, but atropine only partially attenuates the response. Glucagon (1-3 mg), titrated to effect, also reverses opiate-related biliary spasm.

RESPIRATORY FUNCTION

Frequently, abdominal procedures are conducted with the patient supine, which decreases functional residual capacity (FRC) by 0.5 to 1.0 L. The relationship of FRC to closing volume contributes to the alveolar–arterial oxygen difference and shunt.[51,52] This augments the 15% to 20% decrease in FRC associated with general anesthesia,[53] which continues postoperatively.[54,55] The Trendelenburg position, along with intra-abdominal retractors or packings, aggravates this problem even further[56] because more of the lung assumes zone III conditions. Patients with elevated pulmonary arterial pressure (eg, mitral stenosis) generally do not tolerate the Trendelenburg position. Diaphragmatic impairment and abdominal pain contribute to the potential for major respiratory embarrassment after abdominal surgery and, at least initially, are intensified by any negative effects from residual inhalation agents, IV anesthetics, and neuromuscular blockade. After upper abdominal surgery, vital capacity remains abnormal for more than 1 week.[57,58] Experimental data demonstrate that excessive fluid administration contributes to hypoxemia if fluid accumulates in the lungs and leads to increasing arteriovenous shunting.[59] However, no rigorous evidence exists favoring either the amount or type (colloid vs crystalloid) of intravenous fluid, in spite of decades of controversy.[60,61]

GASTROINTESTINAL ENDOCRINOLOGY

The understanding of GI endocrine tumors has expanded dramatically since original descriptions of the *carcinoid syndrome* several decades ago. That clinical syndrome (including flushing, diarrhea, telangiectasias, bronchoconstriction, and fibrous endocardial plaques) has traditionally been said to originate from metastatic carcinoid tumors in the GI system, pancreas, biliary vessels, bronchi, ovaries, and testes via release of vasoactive hormones into systemic circulation. Cardiac involvement (primarily right-sided valvular) is actually noted in more than 50% of patients by echocardiography and may require valvular surgery.

In the gastrointestinal tract, at least 14 endocrine cell types produce numerous peptide hormones such as gastrin, glucagon, somatostatin, secretin, and vasoactive intestinal peptide (VIP). The hormonal and/or neurotransmitter functions are complex and tumor presentation is uncommon; excellent references detail their complexity, management, and uncommon clinical syndromes.[62-65] Most produce small amounts of neuroendocrine substances and do not result in clinical symptoms until late stages of disease. Fortunately, aggressive malignancy is relatively infrequent; these tumors tend to have an indolent course. An increasing number of such lesions are being discovered before biochemical clinical symptoms. In addition to these endocrine/neuroendocrine tumors (terms considered synonymous), there are also pancreatic islet cell tumors. Duodenal gastrinomas can be associated with multiple endocrine neoplasia type-1 and may or may not result in the Zollinger-Ellison syndrome. Somatostatinomas may be associated with neurofibromatosis.

These gastroenteropancreatic neuroendocrine tumors have a yearly incidence of 1.0 to 2.6 per 100 000 people from gastrointestinal origin, with an additional 0.2 to 0.4 per 100 000 people from the pancreas. Because only approximately 10% of the 100 000 people produce bioactive hormones, diagnosis often occurs late after metastasis has occurred. There is emerging evidence of distinct molecular genetic differences between GI and pancreatic neuroendocrine tumors.[66]

Therapy of functional tumors involves controlling symptoms, which includes somatostatin analogues for carcinoid syndrome, watery diarrhea syndrome ("VIPomas"), and hyperglucagonemia.[67] For those with gastrinoma (Zollinger-Ellison syndrome), proton pump inhibitors have improved therapy of high acid production. In addition to true insulinomas, some other neuroendocrine tumors may secrete a chemical that behaves like insulin.

Surgical treatment includes attempts to discover/remove the primary tumor, regional lymph nodes, and appropriate distant metastases, for example, liver tumors. This includes liver resection and both cryoablation and radiofrequency ablation. Impressive improvements in symptomatology can occur, and depending on cell type, meaningful 5-year survival may result.[68]

Anesthesia management of this broad group of patients requires an understanding of the biochemical abnormalities noted, the clinical/potential clinical manifestations, the medical therapy being used, the surgical/diagnostic procedure(s) contemplated, and the ability to monitor hemodynamics and lab values (eg, glucose) closely in the operating room/perioperative environment.

For the carcinoid syndrome, a nonhistamine-releasing anxiolytic can be used to reduce the catecholamine levels. The somatostatin analogue octreotide,[69] odansetron (5-HT_3 antagonist),[70] and remifentanil[71] have been found useful in perioperative suppression of carcinoid signs and symptoms.

MEDICAL AND SURGICAL CONCERNS IN GI ILLNESS

THE ESOPHAGUS

The esophagus extends from the pharynx at the level of C6 to the gastroesophageal junction. The hypopharynx courses from the level of the epiglottis to the upper border of the esophagus and funnels food into the esophagus. Swallowing begins as a voluntary process as food and liquid pass through the mouth, which initiates a complex and normally coordinated sequence of involuntary discharges through cranial nerves V, VII, X, and XII to the oropharynx and the esophagus. The upper third of the esophagus contains striated musculature, the lower third has smooth muscle, and the middle third has a mixed muscular supply.

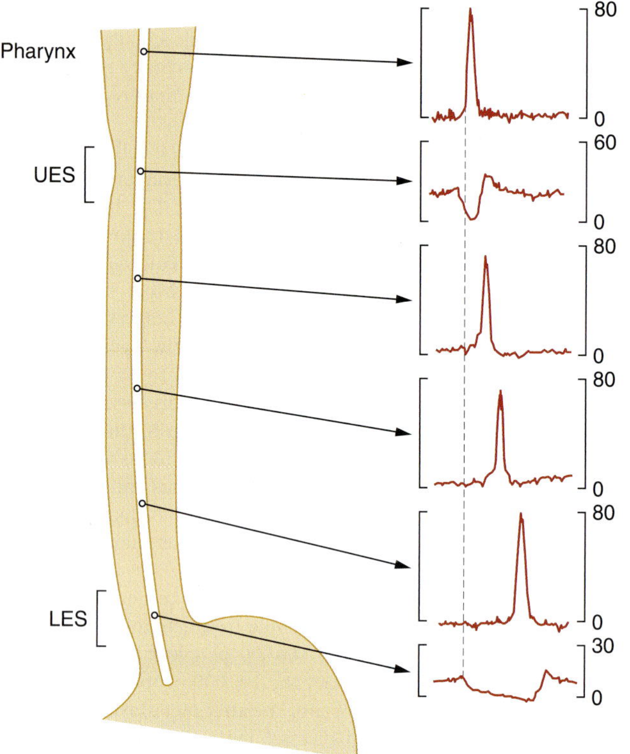

FIGURE 56-2. Esophageal manometry. Simplified representation of normal physiologic pressures in pharynx, upper esophageal sphincter (*UES*), esophagus, and lower esophageal sphincter (*LES*). On right, high-pressure zones are noted as the pressure catheter is withdrawn from stomach. On left, normal peristalsis occurs after a swallow, with relaxation followed by contraction and return to resting tone for UES and LES.

Motor innervation is supplied by the vagus nerves. Striated muscle is innervated by preganglionic fibers and smooth muscle by postganglionic fibers from the Auerbach plexus.

In adults, the upper esophageal sphincter (UES) is approximately 3 cm in length and consists of the cricopharyngeal muscle (striated), a portion of the inferior constrictor muscle superiorly, and circular esophageal muscles inferiorly.[72,73] The primary function of the UES is controlled by the swallowing mechanism in general, but its resting tone is increased in response to esophageal distension or acid from gastroesophageal reflux[74] and decreases during sleep.[75]

The lower end of the esophagus (3-5 cm in length) acts as a functional LES. Thickness of the smooth muscle layers increases in this area, and circular fibers develop considerable tension. Control of the LES tone is complex and chiefly results from vagal cholinergic and myogenic mechanisms, although prostaglandins,[76] neuropeptides (eg, vasoactive intestinal peptide),[77] GI hormones (eg, gastrin, motilin),[78] the progesterones and estrogens of pregnancy, and thyroid-stimulating hormone[79] are among substances known or suspected of affecting LES tone. Material enters the esophagus after voluntary propulsion by the tongue into the hypopharynx. With relaxation of the UES (resting tone, approximately 20-60 mm Hg), food enters the esophagus and is moved along by primary peristaltic waves (25-80 mm Hg). LES relaxation (resting tone, 10-20 mm Hg) occurs, and the bolus enters the stomach. This whole process takes only 4 to 8 seconds. Secondary peristaltic waves serve to move residual matter through and into the stomach. **Figure 56-2** depicts normal esophageal motility.

ACID REFLUX AND HIATAL HERNIATION

Reflux of material from the stomach into the esophagus is a complex topic and is covered in depth in other texts.[80] Criteria for diagnosis include those of reflux symptoms (**Box 56-2**) and the results of various tests, including radiographic studies, endoscopy, biopsy, manometry, and prolonged esophageal pH monitoring. **The pH test demonstrates that virtually all healthy subjects have episodes during daily activity when their esophagus is exposed to pH less than 4.** This exposure is increased during awake upright activity, especially after eating, and occurs during supine sleep activity,[115] when swallowing frequency is diminished and less effective (**Table 56-1**). Reflux is associated with pressure gradients between the abdomen (positive pressure) and the thorax (intermittently negative pressure), and with poorly understood episodes of "transient lower esophageal relaxation."[82-86] pH testing also detects those patients with reflux of alkaline duodenal material into the stomach and esophagus.[87]

The etiology for increased exposure of the esophagus to acid material and ultimately to the risks of acid and particulate matter aspiration can involve 1 of several mechanisms (**Box 56-3**). The mechanical competence of the LES depends on intrinsic tone (normally >5 mm Hg[88]), the overall length of the LES muscular segment (normally ≥3 cm), the portion of that segment that is intra-abdominal (at least 1 cm), and interaction with the cardia of the stomach, which should transmit intra-abdominal pressure to the distal LES.[87,89-91] The most common abnormality is decreased LES tone, but even normal LES tone can be affected by the other mechanisms.[100]

Esophageal clearance of reflux material depends on swallowing, gravity, intrinsic motor activity, salivation, and whether a hiatal hernia is present. Although the frequency of acid reflux may be greater during the day, the duration of episodes is longer when the patient is in the supine position because of loss of gravitational effects. Additionally, any disease that affects the motor activity of the esophagus may lead to

BOX 56-2

Symptoms of Acid Reflux

Anginal type of chest pain
Coughing or wheezing from aspiration
Dysphagia
Heartburn
Regurgitation with bending or in supine position
Vagally induced bronchoconstriction
Water brash

TABLE 56-1 Exposure of Esophagus to pH <4 (n = 50)[a]

Segment of 24-Hour pH Test	Mean	SD	95%
Total time (%)	1.51	1.36	4.45
Upright time (%)	2.34	2.34	8.42
Supine time (%)	0.63	1.0	3.45
Number of episodes/24 hours	19.00	12.76	46.90
Number of episodes >5	0.84	1.18	3.45
Longest episode (usually in supine position)	6.74	7.85	19.80

95%, asymptomatic volunteers; SD, standard deviation.

[a]This represents a "normal" level of reflux in healthy subjects. Those with gastroesophageal reflux disease have more "frequent" and longer episodes (>5 min) representing a greater percentage of time.

Modified from DeMeester TR, Stein HJ. Gastroesophageal reflux disease. In: Moody FG, ed. *Surgical Treatment of Digestive Disease*. Chicago, IL: Year Book Medical Publishers; 1990:68.

BOX 56-3

Etiology of Acid Reflux

Abnormal gastric function

Ineffective esophageal clearance of refluxed material

Mechanically incompetent lower esophageal sphincter

Transient lower esophageal relaxation

impaired clearance of acid material (**Box 56-4**), with resultant effects on the esophageal mucosa and potential for aspiration. Saliva is important in neutralizing the small amounts of acid refluxed with peristalsis even in healthy persons, and clearance of this acid is prolonged when saliva is removed by suctioning.[93] The salivation stimulated by heartburn (termed *water brash*) can lead to repetitive swallowing, aerophagia, and gastric distension with further reflux.[94] Perioperatively, the presence of a nasogastric/orogastric tube may contribute to reflux of gastric contents and the risk of aspiration, and has been challenged as a routine practice.[95,96]

The presence of a hiatal hernia is associated with additional abnormalities (**Fig. 56-3**). The hernia produces a defect in esophageal propulsion that results in inadequate acid clearance and longer transit time.[97] The retreat of all or part of the distal LES into the chest impairs the ability of the lower third of the LES, in concert with the cardia of the stomach, to impart extrinsic abdominal pressure and enhance sphincter function. If intrinsic LES tone also is decreased, a setup exists for major reflux of acid material and, ultimately, for the development of aspiration pneumonia. Despite this, most patients with hiatal hernias are asymptomatic.[98]

Certain abnormalities of gastric function also can result in acid reflux through a normal gastroesophageal junction or by exacerbating preexisting LES abnormalities (**Box 56-5**). Normally, the body and fundus of the stomach are able to adapt to a large volume of material with minimal increases in pressure, although a previous vagotomy interferes with the active relaxation necessary for this to occur, and greater intragastric pressures occur with lesser volumes.[99] Outlet obstruction of the stomach more obviously leads to increases in pressure, which occurs normally with vomiting, but also with pyloric stenosis in newborns and obstructing ulcers or tumors in patients of any age.

Delayed gastric emptying leads to persistence of gastric acid and foodstuffs. The causes are varied[80] (**Box 56-6**) but yield a similar effect. As larger volumes accumulate and persist for a longer period, the potential for reflux through either a normal or abnormal LES increases. Approximately 40% of patients with gastroesophageal reflux have delayed gastric emptying,[100,101] and in approximately one-third of these,

BOX 56-4

Diseases Affecting Esophageal Motility

Achalasia

Alcoholic neuropathy

Brainstem lesions

Chagas disease

Diabetes mellitus

Familial dysautonomia

Myotonia dystrophica

Polymyositis and dermatomyositis

Scleroderma

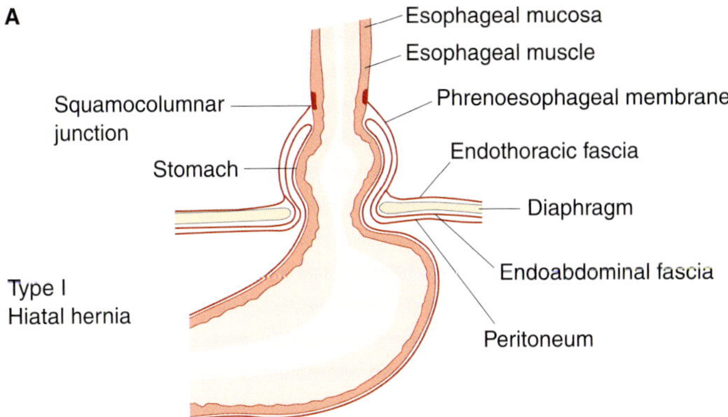

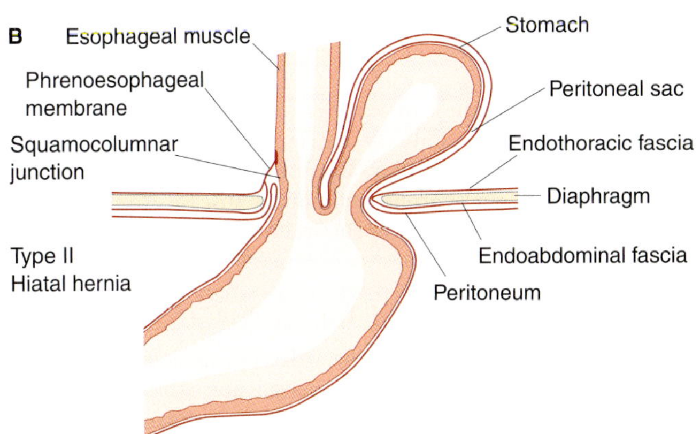

FIGURE 56-3. Types of hiatal hernia. **A.** Type I sliding, or axial, hiatal hernia. **B.** Rarer type II rolling, or paraesophageal, hernia.

the delay is clinically significant. Those rare patients with postviral gastroparesis also may have serious autonomic neuropathy.[102] Patients with various neurologic illnesses may manifest a variety of GI motility abnormalities.[103]

As the stomach dilates from any cause, the relationship between the cardia and abdominal portion of the LES changes, which results in decreased maintenance of proper LES tone and increased risk of reflux. In addition to the conditions already mentioned, aerophagia from several causes also may lead to gastric distension. Normally, each pharyngeal swallow results in several cubic centimeters of swallowed air. Patients with reflux may habitually swallow (water brash; some even chew gum to stimulate saliva) to clear acid and can develop air-induced gastric distension, which can exacerbate their reflux. Other patients with decreased saliva formation (eg, with Sjögren syndrome) or after head and neck irradiation may swallow excessively with resultant aerophagia. Loss of secondary peristalsis, which can occur with diabetes mellitus and collagen vascular diseases, also leads to inordinate swallowing in an effort to propel food along, again with resultant aerophagia.

BOX 56-5

Abnormal Gastric Function and Acid Reflux

Delayed gastric emptying

Gastric dilation

Increased acid secretion

Increased intragastric pressure

BOX 56-6

Etiology of Delayed Gastric Emptying

Altered duodenal motility
Diabetic gastric atony
Diffuse neuromuscular disorders
Myogenic abnormalities
Postvagotomy
Postviral gastroparesis
Pyloric dysfunction

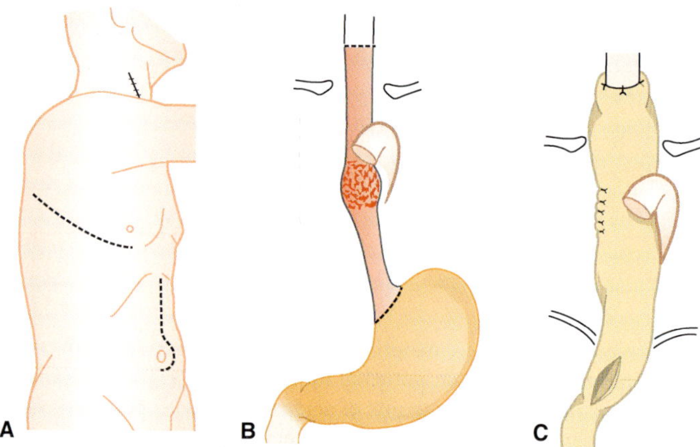

FIGURE 56-4. Ivor-Lewis/McKeown-type esophagectomy. After abdominal mobilization of stomach, the chest and neck are explored concurrently to allow total esophagectomy and cervical esophagogastrostomy.

Gastric acid hypersecretion plays a role in some patients with gastroesophageal reflux who have a mechanically normal LES, and is a complicating factor in other patients with abnormal LES function.[104,105]

The most serious acute consequence of acid reflux is the risk of aspiration of stomach contents. Chronic complications include esophagitis, stricture formation, Barrett esophagus (with risk of esophageal cancer), and chronic pulmonary disease from repeated episodes of aspiration. Aspects of surgical management are discussed next.

SURGICAL PROCEDURES OF THE ESOPHAGUS

Several surgical procedures for patients with esophageal disease are worthy of specific mention, but an extensive discussion of all approaches is beyond the scope of this text.[106] Patient positioning, site of incision, and whether the esophagus will be transected are important to the anesthesiologist in all esophageal procedures.

Several approaches exist for the management of reflux disease. The Nissen-type (360-degree gastric fundoplication) procedure may be approached abdominally (open or more commonly via laparoscopy) or through a left posterolateral thoracotomy. During the abdominal approach, severe liver retraction typically occurs, and the reverse Trendelenburg position is useful to the surgeon. The transthoracic approach may be used for repeat procedures, in obese patients, and when esophageal shortening is suspected. The Belsey-type (240-degree fundoplication) procedure also is approached from a left lateral chest incision. For any of these procedures, the anesthesiologist may be asked to pass a bougie through the pharynx into the distal esophagus to the area of surgical manipulation so that the repair can be sized. Should the restoration tend to slide back into the chest because the esophagus is too short, a lengthening procedure (eg, colon interposition) may be required. Except for this latter maneuver, the esophagus is not transected for these procedures. Laparoscopic and robotically assisted laparoscopic operations have increased in quantity and complexity.[107] Because of restrictions in patient positioning and the shear mass of the robotic devices, access to the patient during these procedures may be suboptimal. Attempts to use endoscopically placed devices have generally failed to produce long-term symptom relief.[108] Although 2-year data in a small study with the "Esophyx" device for treating small hiatal hernias with mild to moderate reflux disease demonstrated results comparable with the Nissen-type fundoplication, additional trials are needed.[109] As NOTES (natural orifice transluminal endoscopic surgery) technologies expand, antireflux surgery may be of historical interest, like vagotomy and antrectomy is for benign ulcers. Heightened awareness of the operative field is required by the anesthesiologist because the surgeon may be viewing only the video projection at a platform physically removed from the patient.

Several techniques are used for patients with esophageal cancer. For lesions of the distal esophagus, the Ivor-Lewis/McKeown-type repair (**Fig. 56-4**) includes an anterior abdominal incision followed by a right thoracotomy. The McKeown-type is similar but adds a right neck incision to facilitate the anastomosis of the stomach to the cervical esophageal remnant. Either procedure may include extensive node dissection in the chest, entry into the pericardium or the opposite chest, and thoracic duct ligation. Single-lung ventilation may facilitate operative exposure. Blunt esophagectomy (**Fig. 56-5**) is used for cervical esophageal disease, for lower-third esophageal carcinoma, and in early noninvasive disease. Abdominal and left cervical incisions are made, and extensive "blind" bimanual dissection through the chest is performed. Bleeding or tracheal injury may necessitate an emergent thoracotomy. Postoperative recurrent nerve injury is described in 10% of patients.[110] In 600 patients undergoing surgical resection for esophageal cancer with and without preoperative chemotherapy, aspiration pneumonia, adult respiratory distress syndrome, cardiovascular events, and neurological accidents were the most common complications: patients less than 60 years old had the fewest complications and patients older than 70 years had the most.[111]

PEPTIC ULCER DISEASE AND DUODENAL AND GASTRIC CARCINOMA

Millions of Americans have symptoms of acid and peptic ulcer disease,[112] and annual direct and indirect costs exceed $3.4 billion.[113] Duodenal ulcer disease (DUD) occurs 2 to 3 times more often in men than in women, and mortality rates may be somewhat greater in nonwhites aged up to about 65 years. Genetic (eg, family history, blood

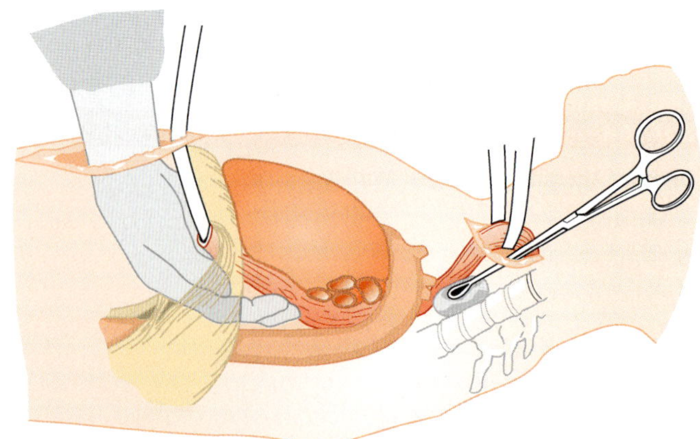

FIGURE 56-5. Blunt esophagectomy. Maneuvers necessary for this procedure are capable of causing serious hemodynamic and ventilatory compromise and require appropriate monitoring of blood pressure and respiration.

group O, human leukocyte antigen [HLA] types B_5 and B_{12}) and environmental (eg, smoking, aspirin, nonsteroidal anti-inflammatory drugs [NSAIDs]) factors are involved in DUD. Chronic pulmonary disease, cirrhosis, renal transplantation, and possibly high psychological stress also may increase the incidence of ulcer disease. Resting and stimulated secretion of acid are increased[114,115] in common DUD and in patients with gastrinoma (Zollinger-Ellison syndrome—see Gastrointestinal Endocrinology section). The number of parietal cells secreting acid may be increased. The rapid emptying of stomach contents in some patients with DUD may overwhelm duodenal buffering and clearance mechanisms. Because these patients appear to have reduced duodenal bicarbonate secretion,[116] they are predisposed to ulceration.[117]

Gastric ulcers occur only one-third to one-fifth as often as duodenal ulcers, and causal factors in gastric ulcer disease (GUD) are largely unrelated to those for DUD. Genetic, psychological, and hypersecretion of acid are not factors for most patients. The largest group of patients with GUD has normal to low secretion of acid and evidence of decreased gastric mucosal defenses against acid and pepsin-related endothelial injury. GUD tends to occur in older patients, and possibly as a result, the mortality rate is higher. GUD is associated with gastritis and with gastric carcinoma. Aspirin is clearly a risk factor,[118] as may be NSAIDs; both are thought to work via inhibition of prostaglandin synthesis. Pyloric function may be defective in patients with GUD, permitting reflux of duodenal, biliary, and pancreatic secretions into the stomach, initiating gastritis, and, ultimately, ulcerations.[119] Smoking reduces pyloric sphincter tone and increases the risk of bleeding from ulcers.[120] DUD and GUD are associated with *Helicobacter pylori* infection[121] and elimination of *H pylori* is a focus of treatment.

Medical Treatment The medical treatment of patients with ulcer disease involves dietary and environmental restrictions (eg, avoiding aspirin, NSAIDs, smoking, alcohol; limiting caffeine, anxiety) and medication. Antacids, H_2-receptor antagonists, and coating agents (eg, sucralfate) are useful in patients with DUD or GUD. Protein pump (H, K-ATPase) inhibition (eg, omeprazole) has become important as an extremely potent inhibitor of gastric acid secretion in the patient with DUD. Exogenous prostaglandins ultimately may have a role. Bleeding patients undergo endoscopic procedures with the potential for cauterization. At arteriography, selective administration of vasopressor (eg, vasopressin into the left gastric artery) or embolization may be warranted. Multiple trials support the suppression of acid production in the critically ill patient, especially those receiving anticoagulation or on mechanical ventilation. However, there is insufficient data to support proton pump inhibitors over H_2 antagonists, but in the acutely bleeding patient, proton pump inhibitors are quite effective as prophylaxis and superior to H_2 antagonists.[122] Although proton pump inhibitor treatment has been associated with rare reports of interstitial nephritis, hepatitis, and fundic gland polyps, long-term treatment with these drugs is safe when an indication exists for lengthy inhibition of acid secretion.[11]

Surgical Treatment Several procedures and variations are performed for the management of DUD (**Box 56-7**). Duration of symptoms, gastric outlet obstruction, perforation,[123] and hemorrhage impose specific considerations, as do various known complications of these procedures (**Box 56-8**). For example, after a truncal or selective vagotomy, approximately 20% of patients will have clinically impaired gastric emptying if a drainage procedure also is not performed.

BOX 56-7

Surgical Management of Duodenal Ulcer Disease

Vagotomy with drainage via pyloroplasty or gastrojejunostomy

Vagotomy with antrectomy (hemigastrectomy) and gastroduodenostomy (Billroth I) or gastrojejunostomy (Billroth II)

Subtotal gastrectomy and Billroth I or II

BOX 56-8

Complications of Procedures for Duodenal Ulcer Disease

Abdominal fullness and pain

Nausea

Heartburn

Reflux and regurgitation

Bile and food emesis

Dumping syndrome

Diarrhea

Erosive gastritis is a common problem. Therapy involves appropriate blood and volume resuscitation, gastric irrigation with saline, and instillation of antacids. When bleeding does not stop or recurs, endoscopic evaluation and cauterization may suffice. If not, angiography may allow visualization of the damaged vessel for embolization or continuous infusion of intraarterial vasopressin. Surgical procedures for hemorrhagic gastritis are required in 10% to 20% of patients. No single technique is considered the procedure of choice, and decisions regarding the nature of the procedure selected may require open visualization of the focal versus diffuse nature of the bleeding. Total gastrectomy, partial gastrectomy with vagotomy, vagotomy and pyloroplasty, devascularization, and simple oversew procedures all have advocates.

Surgical therapy for patients with gastric ulcer generally involves ulcer removal and antrectomy (ie, distal gastrectomy) with direct anastomosis to the duodenum (Billroth I procedure). Unless features of hypersection of acid exist, a vagotomy generally is not performed. Perforation can be managed with excision and simple closure in debilitated elderly patients or more definitively in younger stable patients. If malignancy is encountered, an appropriate procedure should be performed.

Gastric carcinoma generally is divided into 2 broad categories. Early carcinoma is confined to the gastric mucosa or submucosa, regardless of size or of lymph node seeding. Many of these patients are curable surgically. A subtotal gastrectomy is warranted for localized disease, and a total gastrectomy is needed for more extensive involvement. Surgical therapy for advanced gastric carcinoma is generally less successful because less than 10% of patients survive 5 years. Procedures vary as to the extent of gastric resection and to the aggressiveness of lymph node and adjacent organ resection.[124-125] Some studies suggest improved survival for patients undergoing palliative resections even when a cure is not possible.

CHOLECYSTITIS, GALLSTONE DISEASE, CHOLECYSTECTOMY, AND BILIARY DISEASE

Approximately 20 million Americans have cholelithiasis, and another 800 000 are diagnosed with it each year. Many predisposing factors exist (**Box 56-9**). The 3 basic types of gallstones are cholesterol, pigment, and mixed. The last category represents approximately 75% of all affected patients. Catalysts for stone formation include decreased gallbladder motility with stasis, increased gallbladder mucous secretion, altered epithelial ion transport, and possibly increased gallbladder synthesis of prostaglandins[126] and increased biliary calcium.[127]

Diagnosis Clinical cholecystitis is classically associated with obstruction of the cystic duct (eg, from stone, edema, sludge, fibrosis) and subsequent epithelial injury, enzyme release, and inflammatory response.[128] In approximately 75% of patients, cholecystitis is self-limiting and resolves over approximately 1 week, but 5% to 10% of patients develop serious complications, including empyema, cholangitis, gangrene, or

BOX 56-9

Factors Associated With Increased Incidence of Gallbladder Disease

- Increased age
- Female sex
- Pregnancy
- Obesity
- Hemolysis
- After truncal vagotomy
- Long-term parenteral nutrition
- Pima Indian

perforation. Positive cultures are found in approximately 20% to 30% of patients younger than 50 years of age, in greater than 50% of patients older than 70 years of age,[181] in 20% to 40% of those with chronic disease, and in 60% to 70% of those with acute cholecystitis.[129,130] Gram-negative organisms predominate. An overriding focus in evaluating patients is detecting cystic duct obstruction. Abdominal ultrasonography is extremely useful in detecting cholelithiasis, and technetium scans in detecting cystic duct obstruction (even in patients with elevated bilirubin levels). Plain abdominal films, oral cholecystography, and IV cholangiography are more limited as diagnostic tools.

Treatment Oral therapy using deoxycholic acid analogues results in cholelitholysis because of their ability to decrease the rate-limiting enzyme in cholesterol synthesis, coenzyme A reductase. This is effective in some patients. Although it is recognized that asymptomatic gallstones frequently exist, management options are debated. Some studies document that about one-third of these patients will develop complications requiring urgent surgery. Others note that morbidity and mortality are lower after elective procedures in younger patients,[103,131] although most suggest that routine prophylactic cholecystectomy for asymptomatic disease is not required.[132]

Cholecystectomy generally is performed within several days of onset of symptoms. Approximately 25% of patients develop recurrent cholecystitis if surgery is delayed, and 1 in 8 will require emergency cholecystectomy.[133-134] Despite the risks associated with older patients, conservative management (eg, delayed surgery) in the elderly population may be inadvisable; gallbladder empyema, perforation, sepsis, and cardiovascular complications occur more often in this group.[135-137]

Lithotripsy with high-frequency shock waves disintegrates some gallstones. General anesthesia usually is not needed, but sedation and analgesia with appropriate monitoring are required.[138] Although laparoscopic cholecystectomy[17] has become the staple of gallbladder removal, management considerations are similar to those of any laparoscopic procedure (**Box 56-10**).

BOX 56-10

Effects and Complications Associated With Laparoscopy

- Abnormal gastroesophageal junction competence from high intra-abdominal pressure
- Altered ventilatory dynamics caused by large volume of intra-abdominal carbon dioxide (CO_2)
- Bleeding (eg, at trocar insertion)
- Decreased venous return from increased intra-abdominal pressure/patient position
- Effects of patient positioning
- Hypercapnia from CO_2 absorption
- Venous CO_2 embolism, intraoperatively and in early postoperative period

Open laparotomy is generally reserved for more complicated considerations (eg, abscess, perforation, need for intraoperative cholangiogram or bile duct exploration, suspected anatomic abnormalities, obesity). In addition, laparotomy remains the backup procedure for other procedures that fail or for patients with complications. Surgical manipulation of the abdominal viscera has been associated with various circulatory changes, including bradycardia and hypotension.

Transvaginal NOTES (natural orifice translumenal endoscopic surgical) cholecystectomy minimizes visible scars and expands the surgeon's arsenal in the healthy patient.[12] In the high-risk patient, ultrasound-guided percutaneous cholecystostomy may be a valuable bridging alternative.[13] The surgical and anesthesia team must discuss appropriate patient selection for NOTES, standard laparoscopic, open, or percutaneous surgical care of cholecystitis.

Biliary Tract Cancer As many as 2000 new cases of gallbladder carcinoma may be seen in the United States annually. Patients are likely to be elderly women who have associated gallstones. Because of early metastasis, most patients are unresectable at presentation, and their 5-year survival rate is extremely low. Patients with microscopic disease have a much better prognosis. Palliative procedures are difficult for those with advanced disease; biliary decompression stents are placed for bile drainage.

Extrahepatic bile duct cancer survival rate depends on the location of the tumor. Survival improves from proximal to distal common duct sites and is best with a papillary morphology. Patients may undergo 1 or more laparotomies before arrival at a tertiary/definitive treatment center. Surgical management generally involves some form of biliary-enteric anastomosis (eg, Roux-en-Y hepaticojejunostomy, Roux-en-Y choledochojejunostomy, Whipple procedure, palliative silastic tube drainage) depending on the tumor's location.

Strictures of the Biliary Tract and Sclerosing Cholangitis Benign strictures of the biliary tract result from various causes, including surgical trauma, inflammation from calculi, biliary tract infection (eg, bacterial cholangitis), blunt or penetrating abdominal trauma, toxic injury during hepatic arterial infusion therapy, and sclerosing cholangitis. Eighty percent of patients have symptoms within 1 year of the associated surgery or trauma.[139] Symptoms and signs include abnormal biliary drainage or bile leakage immediately postoperatively and variable evidence of biliary obstruction and abnormal liver function in all patients. Painless jaundice and cholangitis are seen less often. Cholangiography should define biliary tree anatomy, and the placement of a ring catheter permits drainage and management of infection preoperatively.

When patients have an acute structure after surgery, operative treatment may consist of the resection of a short segment of bile duct or a segmental duct ligation. More involved injuries usually demand creation of a Roux-en-Y jejunal limb and T-tube of transhepatic drainage catheters. Later in the postinjury period, extensive adhesions often are present, necessitating tedious dissection. Again, surgical management requires the creation of a Roux-en-Y loop and decompression via T-tube, ring catheter, or a transhepatic silastic stent.

PROVIDING ANESTHESIA

ENDOSCOPIC PROCEDURES

Endoscopic abdominal procedures leave inconspicuous scars and result in less postoperative pain with shorter hospitalizations, decreased hospital costs,[140,141] and even immunologic advantages.[142] As "minimally invasive" surgical techniques, reduced risk is implied, but endoscopic surgery involves the instillation of gas under pressure into a "closed" cavity, a process that may initiate unique physiologic responses and potential complications.

Diagnostic examination, cholecystectomy, vagotomy, appendectomy, adrenalectomy, nephrectomy, bariatric procedures, liver resection, pancreatic surgery, colectomy and hiatal, diaphragmatic, and inguinal hernia repair are among the abdominal procedures being performed with laparoscopic equipment. Each procedure has its own indications and conversion rates to an open method (eg, 1.0%-6.9% conversion to laparotomy with laparoscopic cholecystectomy).[143]

The physiologic changes associated with laparoscopy include those associated with tilting the patient to facilitate instrumentation and surgical exposure, the pressure effects of instilled gas, and the systemic effects of the gas—almost universally CO_2—that is instilled (and absorbed or embolized). In addition, careful positioning of the extremities and torso is a shared responsibility of the surgical team and the anesthesia team.

The head-down position (ie, Trendelenburg) reduces vital capacity because of the increased weight of the abdominal contents on the diaphragm.[144] This effect is more pronounced in elderly, obese, and debilitated patients. In those undergoing *open* procedures, it is made worse by the placement of retractors and surgical packing under the diaphragm. In addition to this encroachment on lung expansion, right mainstem bronchial intubation can occur. Either of these can be associated with hypoxemia.[145] In contrast, the head-up position redistributes central blood volume peripherally and further aggravates any impairment of venous return created by the pneumoperitoneum.

The instillation of CO_2 to create an intentional pneumoperitoneum carries with it a number of physiologic side effects and complications (**Box 56-11**). Mechanical injury at the time of trocar insertion can lead to bleeding or bowel perforation. Bleeding also can occur from injury to vessels encountered during surgical instrumentation and dissection. With current laparoscopic equipment, intra-abdominal pressure is maintained between 12 and 15 mm Hg (17-22 cm H_2O). Because of leaks around the various cannulae, enormous gas volumes (≥50 L)[146] may be required during the course of the procedure to generate this relatively low pressure. Such pressures and the resulting abdominal distension may disturb the protective function of the gastroesophageal junction. The hemodynamic changes associated with this pneumoperitoneum depend on a number of factors, including the resulting intra-abdominal pressure, the amount of CO_2 absorbed, the patient's level of hydration, the type of ventilation, and the nature of the surgery. Cardiac function during insufflation of peritoneal CO_2 has been studied primarily in healthy (eg, no known cardiac disease) patients using a variety of cardiac function measurements (dye dilution, impedance cardiography, transesophageal echocardiography, and pulmonary artery catheters). Unfortunately, none of the studies have controlled well for the level of anesthesia at the various stages of the procedures and have managed hypercapnia differently. Most studies,[147-150] but not all,[151,152] report a decrease in left ventricular function and cardiac output (cardiac output decreased 7%-24%). Similarly, most studies found an increase in central venous pressure (redistribution of abdominal blood volume), with an increase in systemic vascular resistance and mean arterial pressure. In addition, with assumption of the reverse Trendelenburg position, cardiac index may decrease by 50% of preanesthesia and preinsufflation values.[149] Left ventricular end-diastolic, right atrial, and pulmonary capillary wedge pressures dramatically decrease after assumption of the reverse Trendelenburg position.[153] Venous stasis of the lower extremities also occurs, with attendant concerns for embolic phenomenon.[154] Patients with cardiovascular disease will have responses to laparoscopy that are affected by the extent of cardiac reserve, baseline medications, level of hydration, and their response to the anesthesia medications used.[155] The potential deleterious effects of hypercapnia on cardiac function (eg, increased sympathetic activity, myocardial depression) may further complicate laparoscopy in those with cardiovascular disease.

BOX 56-11

Reported Complications Associated With Laparoscopy

- Acidosis
- Airway obstruction
- Bradycardia (eg, increased vagal tone)
- Cardiac arrest
- CO_2 dissecting through tissue planes
- Hemorrhage
- Hypotension, decreased cardiac output
- Increased sympathetic activity secondary to increased CO_2
- Mainstem endobronchial intubation
- Pneumothorax
- Pneumomediastinum
- Regurgitation and aspiration
- Retroperitoneal CO_2
- Subcutaneous emphysema
- Venous stasis
- Venous CO_2 embolism (can be fatal)

During retroperitoneoscopic adrenalectomy (prone–jackknife position or lateral), a small (<10 cm) cavity in the lumbodorsal fascia is created with a distension balloon trocar. CO_2 is insufflated to a pressure of 15 to 20 mm Hg. Unlike laparoscopy, stroke volume and cardiac output appear to increase with insufflation, as do mean arterial pressure, central venous pressure, and pulmonary artery pressure. No change was noted in pulmonary capillary wedge pressure, heart rate, and systemic vascular resistance.[156]

Relatively small CO_2 emboli have been detected by transesophageal echocardiography in 69% of patients, classified by the American Society of Anesthesiologists as physical status P1 to P3, who undergo laparoscopic cholecystectomy.[157] Fatal massive CO_2 embolism has been reported,[158] including a report of death from delayed CO_2 embolism associated with gas trapping in the portal circulation.[159] With time, subcutaneous or mediastinal emphysema and pneumothorax may develop, with associated hypoxemia, hypotension, and cardiovascular collapse. The incidence of extraperitoneal insufflation of CO_2 has been reported to range from as little as 0.4% to 2%[160] to 20% to 64%,[161] and is more likely during lengthy procedures such as fundoplication.[162] **The development of pneumothorax and/or pneumomediastinum during endoscopic surgery is a serious and potentially life-threatening complication. When either is suspected, from hemodynamic deterioration or from the presence of subcutaneous emphysema, especially of the neck and face, aggressive investigation (auscultation, chest radiograph) and management (eg, chest tube for tension pneumothorax; conversion to an open procedure) should be undertaken. Procedures on the lower esophagus are more likely to result in these complications.**[163]

Ventilation and pulmonary function are important concerns during laparoscopy. With conventional open laparotomy, it is well accepted that upper abdominal surgery is associated with postoperative pulmonary dysfunction in approximately 50% of patients.[163] This dysfunction is related to impaired diaphragmatic function, pain, type of incision, and decreased FRC.[164-166] **Pulmonary function is also impaired after laparoscopic cholecystectomy, with sustained decreases in forced vital capacity, peak expiratory flow, and forced expiratory volume in 1 second (FEV_1) noted 24 hours after surgery; fortunately, these changes are only approximately 50% of those seen in conventional open cholecystectomy.**[167]

The exogenous CO_2 insufflated during laparoscopy is soluble in blood and after transperitoneal absorption is presented to the lungs for excretion. End-tidal CO_2 ($ETCO_2$) increases from 0% to 30%[168,169] when minute ventilation is held constant. Increasing ventilation by as much as 30% may be necessary to keep the $ETCO_2$ in the mid-30s (mm Hg) range.[170]

During laparoscopy, an overriding anesthetic concern is the preservation of ventilation, which tends to be impaired by surgical positioning and abdominal distension. This almost always means general anesthesia with endotracheal intubation.[17] Not only does this provide protection for the airway, but it permits adequate measurement of $ETCO_2$ and manipulation of ventilation as needed. Routine intraoperative monitoring ($ETCO_2$, pulse oximetry, blood pressure, airway pressure) should be adequate for the expected physiologic changes encountered in most patients. **The anesthesiologist should be aware of the insufflating pressure being used and should be alerted if an unusual amount of CO_2 is required.**

It is theoretically sound to avoid N_2O for at least 2 reasons. First, it diffuses into the abdominal cavity in concentrations sufficient to support combustion of intestinal gas[172,173]; second, it will diffuse into CO_2 bubbles and emboli, increasing their size and the potential for an obstructive event.

Adequate muscle relaxation is required during laparoscopy so that spontaneous respiratory effort does not impair the surgical procedure or risk increasing the gradient for embolic gas to enter the central circulation.

Despite the limited surgical incision(s), postoperative muscle pain remains a problem, even in children.[174] This has not been eliminated by avoiding succinylcholine or by manipulation of other anesthetic regimens.[175] Nausea and vomiting is common after laparoscopy, especially in women, and it appears that women are at increased risk for this during their menses.[176]

Droperidol, a dopamine receptor antagonist, has been found to decrease nausea and vomiting in nonmenstruating women, but not during menses. However, the low risk of QT interval prolongation and torsades des pointes has led to a recent Food and Drug Administration (FDA) black box warning, yet at lower dosages maintains clinical utility. Because serotonin has been implicated in several premenstrual syndromes, serotonin antagonist therapy (eg, ondansetron) can be beneficial.

In the rare event of catastrophic hemodynamic collapse during laparoscopy, several possible causes should be considered. **During laparoscopy, hemorrhage can be obvious or occult (eg, retroperitoneal). Pneumothorax, massive CO_2 embolus, and pneumomediastinum may occur. Initial therapy includes releasing the pressurized pneumoperitoneum (ie, conversion to open procedure). For pneumothorax, a thoracentesis should be performed. If massive embolization occurs, N_2O, if used, should be discontinued immediately and cardiopulmonary resuscitation should be performed.** The patient should be placed in the left lateral position. Attempts at embolus retrieval should be made through central venous access, if available. If these measures do not provide sustained benefit, even cardiopulmonary bypass, if available, may be necessary.

Laparoendoscopic single-site surgery (LESS) uses one port side to minimize pain. Natural orifice translumenal endoscopic surgery (NOTES) uses a natural orifice to access the abdominal cavity.[177] Endoscopists have experience in endoscopic ultrasound-guided pancreatic biopsy, endoscopic retrograde cholangiograms, and stenting. Gynecologists have experience with transvaginal hysterectomies. Gastrointestinal surgeons are using transvaginal and transgastric NOTES for cholecystectomies, sigmoidectomies, appendectomies, liver biopsies, and tubal ligation.[178] As instrumentation and techniques evolve, LESS and NOTES will be used more frequently. The GI anesthesiologist must remain cognizant of limitations and a steep learning curve for natural orifice surgery in order to minimize the risk of infection (eg, the perioperative administration of appropriate antibiotics), and must be prepared to recognize and manage intraperitoneal hemorrhage, compression syndromes, and more prolonged procedures.[179]

BARIATRIC PROCEDURES

Ten percent of all health costs in the United States are related to treating obesity and obesity-related complications.[180] Perioperative care of the extremely obese (body mass index [BMI] >40 kg/m^2) presents multiple challenges. A myriad of comorbidities including obstructive sleep apnea, diabetes, dyslipidemia, hypertension, atherosclerosis, cardiomyopathy, cholecystitis, nonalcoholic steatohepatitis, and certain cancers[181] make this a formidable group of patients.

Bariatric surgery refers to procedures of the stomach or intestines designed to result in weight loss. Initial attempts at such surgery (eg, jejunoileal bypass) induced malabsorption and rapid weight loss, but the resulting blind loop syndrome limited its long-term acceptability. Some advocate adjustable gastric banding, whereas others advocate a procedure involving the so-called duodenal switch. Variations on the theme of a Roux-en-Y gastric bypass may be the most frequently used method in the United States. With the advent and increasing use of laparoscopic approaches, the early postoperative course and recovery have been greatly improved. Ultimately, the goal has been to balance restriction of food intake and malabsorption for enhanced patient acceptance and success of therapy.[182] NOTES endoluminal and transgastric procedures are now being performed that include banding, botulism toxin injection, and electrode implantation.[183,184]

Peripheral venous access is often difficult or impossible and central venous access is required. Central access can be very challenging because of an inability to properly appreciate anatomical landmarks; however, such access has been greatly facilitated by the use of ultrasound guidance.[185,186] Measurement of an accurate blood pressure may require invasive access. Unsurprisingly, the physical mass of the extremely obese patient requires appropriate bed selection and positioning because of the risk of compression neurologic injuries.[187]

One misconception associated with anesthesia for the extremely obese involves airway management; with increasing bariatric surgical experience, extreme obesity no longer is an independent risk factor for difficult intubations. In more than 750 patients without airway pathology, no correlation between BMI and difficult intubation was noted.[188] In fact, of 100 direct laryngoscopies of patients with BMI greater than 40 kg/m^2, only 1 intubation failed and only 12 intubations were deemed challenging (not significantly different from the general population).[189] Morbidities associated with obstructive sleep apnea include hypoxemia, pulmonary hypertension, and cor pulmonale.

Extreme obesity is associated with significant cardiovascular perioperative risks. More than 50% of these patients are hypertensive.[190] (See Chapter 23 for a detailed discussion of the preoperative assessment of the obese patient.) The Framingham study indicated that for every increased increment in body mass index (weight in kg/height in m^2), a 5% to 7% increased risk of congestive heart failure exists.[191] An "X" syndrome of massive obesity that includes glucose intolerance, hypertension, hyperlipidemia, and microalbuminemia has been described; it is strongly associated with coronary artery disease.[16] Such findings suggest the potential positive benefits of bariatric surgery: for example, for every kilogram of weight loss, systolic pressure decreases 0.5%, serum glucose decreases 0.2 mM, low-density lipoprotein cholesterol decreases 0.7%, and high-density lipoprotein cholesterol *increases* 0.25.[192] In spite of these potential long-term benefits, bariatric surgery still has significant perioperative risk: mortality 1.5%, pulmonary embolism 1.14%, and small bowel obstruction and anastomotic leaks 3% each.[193] In addition, there are both short- and long-term metabolic and nutritional issues that vary with the procedure type and can be of concern.[194,195]

Mean weight loss for patients undergoing all forms of bariatric surgery has been reported to be approximately 61% of excess body weight, and maintenance of weight loss far exceeds that from medical treatments alone. Significant improvements in diabetes, hyperlipidemia, hypertension, and obstructive sleep apnea are usually expected. Improvements in other comorbidities, such as fatty infiltration of the liver, respiratory and asthmatic symptoms, and cardiomyopathy are more modest. Emerging studies suggest a reduction in mortality associated with bariatric surgery and a clear improvement in quality of life.[183,196] and many consider such surgery the only cure for morbid obesity (**Fig. 56-6**).

Advances in bariatric surgery using endoscopy and NOTES have the potential to improve cosmesis and postoperative recovery. The natural orifice incision used in NOTES procedures may be very beneficial in obese patients if it reduces the high rate of incision-related hernia

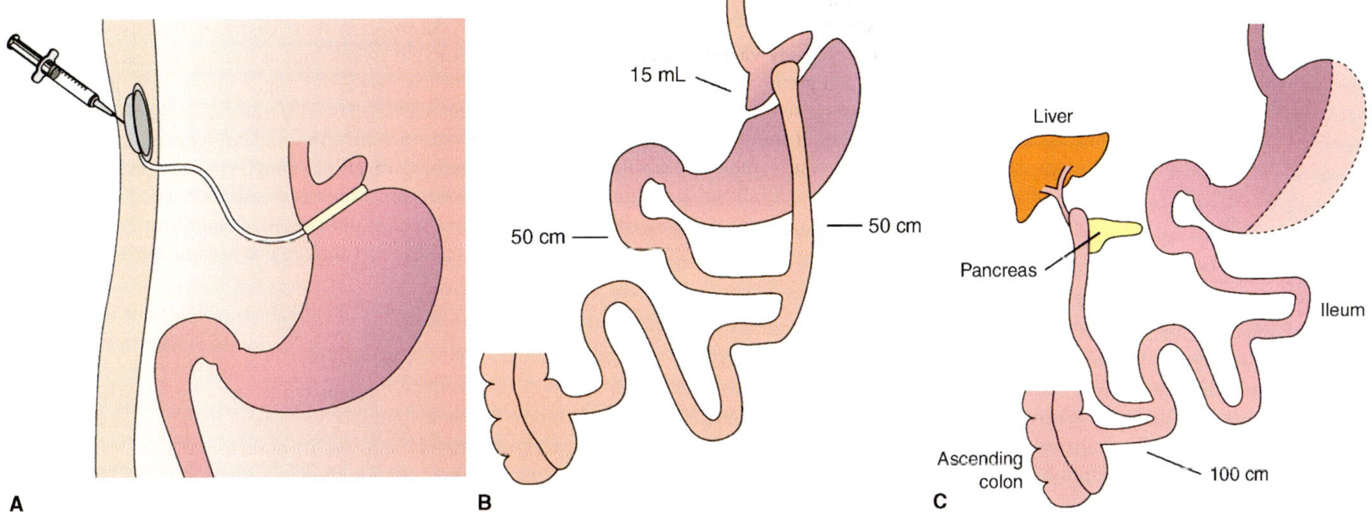

FIGURE 56-6. Among the procedures for bariatric surgery are the following: (**A**) adjustable gastric banding (least invasive); (**B**) Roux-en-Y gastric bypass (can be done laparoscopically); and (**C**) biliopancreatic diversion with sleeve resection of greater curvature and postpyloric, duodenoileal anastomosis ("duodenal switch").

formation.[197] The first human transvaginal endoscopic sleeve gastrectomies were reported in 4 patients, taking 90 to 100 minutes to perform and a 2-day hospital stay.[198] Note that intrinsic challenges include entry visualization, complication management, infection prevention, and patient positioning; these are magnified in the bariatric population, but provide a promising future.

THE PANCREAS AND PANCREATIC SURGERY

Pancreatitis Although the treatment of acute pancreatitis is primarily medical, surgery may be required for such conditions as draining an abscess. Emerging evidence suggests that early surgery may not be as high a risk as previously thought.[199] Patients with pancreatitis are extremely ill with severe abdominal pain and may have fever, nausea and vomiting, jaundice, hypotension, ileus, and external distortion of the stomach on radiographs. Management includes nasogastric suction, maintenance of intravascular volume, anticipation of respiratory insufficiency,[200-202] analgesia, and nutritional support.

The patient with chronic pancreatitis may have incapacitating upper abdominal pain radiating to the back, which can be continuous or intermittent, especially after eating. Forty percent of patients have diabetes from loss of pancreatic tissue.[203] Exocrine function may be sufficiently abnormal to require pancreatic enzyme replacement. Obstructions, strictures, and dilations of the pancreatic ductal system are thought to produce the pain through sympathetic pathways. Several surgical procedures have evolved to decompress the ducts and remove damaged pancreas. A caudal pancreatojejunostomy[204] uses a Roux-en-Y loop to decompress the tail of the pancreas. With the Puestow-type[205] procedure (**Fig. 56-7**), the Roux-en-Y limb envelops the pancreas distally, allowing pancreatic ducts to be opened longitudinally for drainage into the loop. For both of these procedures, a splenectomy and excision of the tail of the pancreas are necessary for technical reasons. A modification of the Puestow procedure[206] (Partington procedure) allows the tail of the pancreas and the spleen to be spared. Postoperatively, some patients require insulin and pancreatic enzyme replacement. Other patients with severe chronic pancreatitis require a near-total pancreatectomy or a pancreatoduodenectomy to remove sufficient tissue to relieve pain. Patients with pseudocyst of the pancreas require drainage of the cyst through a Roux-en-Y loop or directly into the stomach. Alternatively, a distal cyst may be removed by a partial pancreatectomy.

Other Conditions Cancer of the pancreas and periampullary area is a frequently diagnosed problem with, unfortunately, an increasing incidence. Approximately 25 000 patients are diagnosed each year in the United States. Diagnosis usually is suggested by ultrasonography or computed tomography. Magnetic resonance imaging, endoscopic retrograde cholangiopancreatography, or percutaneous transhepatic cholangiography may yield information concerning the site and etiology of bile duct obstruction. Percutaneous fine-needle aspiration biopsy may be performed with the aid of ultrasound examination or computed tomography. Despite this array of tests, determination of the

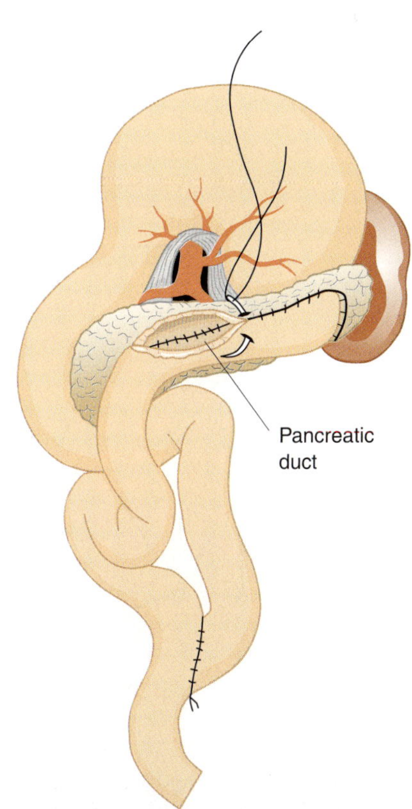

FIGURE 56-7. Puestow procedure: lateral or longitudinal pancreatojejunostomy. Roux-en-Y limb of jejunum is sutured to open pancreatic duct along its length.

extent of disease and often the tissue diagnosis should await a thorough intraoperative examination. Only then can the necessary procedure be decided. The cure rate is 5% or less, largely because of relatively vague and general symptoms before the onset of jaundice, which greatly narrows the diagnostic possibilities. By the time the diagnosis is suspected, the lesion may be unresectable. Because only small lesions of the head of the pancreas or ampullary area are resectable, and because many of the remaining patients still require a palliative procedure to relieve obstructive jaundice, a considerable number of these patients undergo laparotomy.

Most procedures aimed at a cure are termed a *pancreatoduodenectomy* (**Fig. 56-8**; ie, Whipple procedure). Variations include total pancreatectomy, regional pancreatectomy, and similar procedures that preserve the pylorus of the stomach. **These are long, extensive bowel resections that cause considerable morbidity. Serious postoperative complications include hemorrhage, coagulopathy, and hepatic, renal, pulmonary, and cardiovascular failure.** Invasive monitoring and postoperative intensive care are generally required. Thoracic epidural analgesia can be an important component of postoperative management.

With the advent of improved laparoscopic instrumentation and techniques, a comparison of laparoscopic to open distal pancreatectomies demonstrated no differences in the positive margin (eg, remaining local malignancy) rate, operative time, or fistula formation rate. Laparoscopic distal pancreatectomies were associated with less blood loss, shorter hospital stay, and overall fewer complications.[207,208]

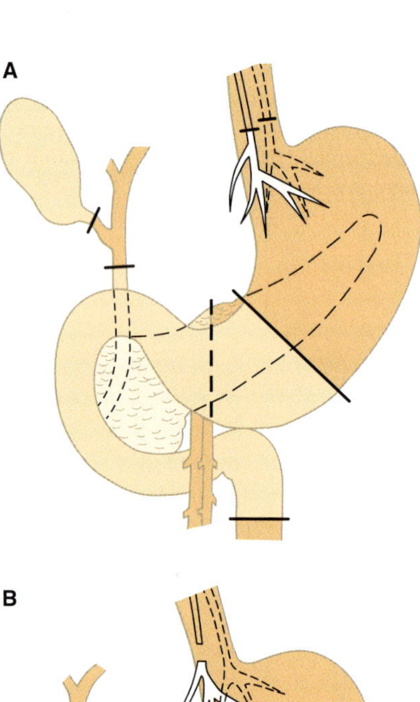

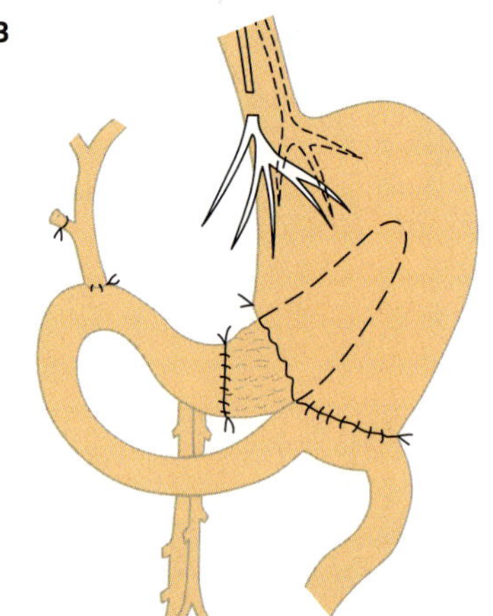

FIGURE 56-8. Pancreatoduodenectomy (Whipple procedure). **A.** Presurgical anatomic relationships. **B.** Reconstruction demonstrating biliary, pancreatic, and gastric anastomoses. If distal stomach and pylorus are preserved, truncal vagotomy is unnecessary. Gallbladder is removed if diseased.

Endocrine disease of the pancreas also is managed surgically. An insulinoma is the most common of these diseases. Because this tumor secretes insulin autonomously, spontaneous hypoglycemia is seen, with symptoms caused by decreased blood sugar levels and the resultant burst of catecholamine release. The differential diagnosis for hypoglycemia is extensive, but once insulinoma is diagnosed, management is surgical. Benign tumors are either enucleated or resected with a margin of pancreas. When no tumor is found at laparotomy, a distal or near-total pancreatectomy is performed, depending on the histology. Malignant disease may be surgically debulked with subsequent chemotherapy.

The Zollinger-Ellison syndrome results from a pancreatic or duodenal tumor (gastrinoma) that secretes excessive gastrin. Symptoms usually are abdominal pain and possibly diarrhea. Associated endocrinopathies include multiple endocrine neoplasia syndrome type 1 (MEN 1: parathyroid, pituitary, adrenal) and MEN 2 (medullary carcinoma of the thyroid, parathyroid adenoma, pheochromocytoma). Medical management involves H_2-receptor antagonists or proton pump blocker therapy. Surgical management involves vagotomy and pyloroplasty when no tumor is discovered at laparotomy or major resection procedures when a localized tumor is found. The presence of metastatic disease and MEN syndromes dictates medical therapy.

Other endocrine tumors of the pancreas include VIP (VIPoma), glucagonoma, and somatostatinoma. Surgical considerations are similar to those for insulinoma and gastrinoma (see Gastrointestinal Endocrinology section).

Pancreas Transplantation Pancreas transplantation (PTX)[209] has become a surgical treatment for type 1 diabetes mellitus.[210] Most patients receive their PTX with or shortly after a renal transplantation, although some have received a pancreas before becoming uremic (such treatment is controversial).[211]

Evaluation of patients before PTX includes extensive assessment of the cardiovascular system because the incidence of coronary artery disease in young diabetic patients with end-stage renal disease is high.[212] Active infection (eg, dental abscess, peritonitis, osteomyelitis, decubitus ulcers) should be sought and managed before transplantation. Secondary diabetic complications (eg, retinopathy) should be documented and quantified in an effort to gauge the effects of the transplant process on their progression. Recipient contraindications include malignancy and active infection, with concern for those with blindness, advanced cardiovascular disease, and major amputation.

Donor organs typically come from patients younger than 55 years of age without major atherosclerosis of the celiac axis, abdominal contamination, pancreatic injury or pancreatitis, or diabetes. Neither donor serum glucose nor amylase appears to have predictive value for ultimate function in the recipient.[213] Earlier competition between harvesting teams for the liver or pancreas has been largely resolved by techniques permitting simultaneous retrieval of the liver and the pancreas.[214]

There are several approaches to implanting the pancreas. Some drain the pancreas enterically via a Roux-en-Y loop. Reexploration is frequent with this procedure because of a high incidence of complications. Assessment of organ function and rejection is difficult. Other centers perform PTX via a bladder drainage procedure (**Fig. 56-9**). Some use direct draining of the pancreatic duct into the ureter or bladder, whereas others use a small "button" of duodenum or a closed duodenal segment for union with the bladder. Vascular anastomoses are with the iliac vessels, similar to a renal transplantation. Hypertension, abnormal renal function, and all the sequelae of diabetes mellitus and its management make this a challenging group of patients.

Perioperatively, patients undergoing PTX need to have appropriate cardiovascular monitoring and a regimented approach to managing serum glucose levels. This may entail insulin infusion protocols and frequent intraoperative glucose determinations in an attempt to prevent hypoglycemia and hyperglycemia. Glucose-containing solutions

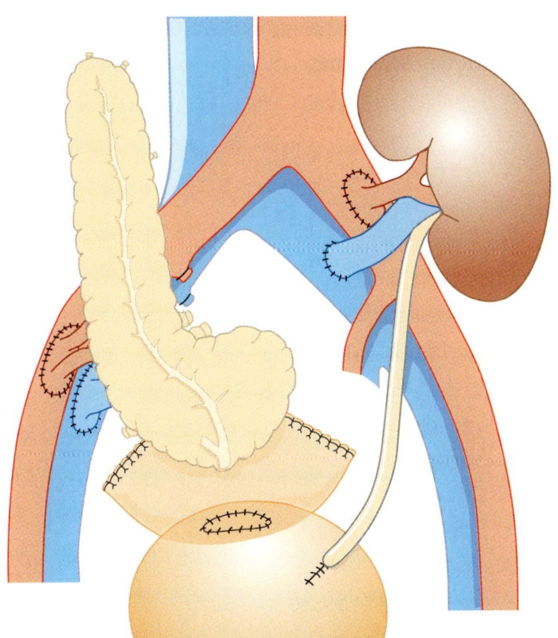

FIGURE 56-9. Pancreas transplantation. Pancreas transplanted with bladder drainage via a pancreatic duodenocystostomy. Concurrent renal transplantation also is depicted.

are avoided unless the glucose level is lowered to less than 60 mg/dL. With reperfusion of the new pancreas, a dramatic increase occurs in blood sugar levels for reasons not entirely understood, so it is also prudent to monitor glucose levels frequently for the first hour or so after reperfusion. Postoperatively, the patient is treated in an intensive care setting.[215-217] (See Chapter 59 for an in-depth discussion of pancreas transplantation.)

SMALL BOWEL TRANSPLANTATION

Because of extremely poor outcomes in patients with extensive bowel resection for acute and chronic disease, and because of success in other solid-organ transplantation, small bowel transplantation has been pursued by a few selective academic centers. Candidate patients have intestinal failure and have significant complications from total parenteral nutrition. Furthermore, these patients have one of the highest mortality rates of any patients waiting for solid organs.[218] Candidate organs are difficult to acquire because the intestine is sensitive to pressor-induced ischemia that may occur during aggressive intensive care, both before and after brain-death declaration. (See Chapter 59 for a detailed discussion of small bowel transplantation.)

Small bowel transplantation may be coupled with liver or en bloc visceral organ transplantation. Anesthesia for small bowel transplantation with liver or en bloc visceral transplantation is similar to orthotopic liver transplantation. (See Chapter 57 for a detailed discussion of liver transplantation.) For isolated small bowel transplantation, significant lysis of adhesions and vascular anastomoses require adequate perfusion pressure and fluid resuscitation.[219]

Children with intestinal failure and total parenteral nutrition–induced liver disease who are without venous access have the highest mortality of solid organ candidates. A recent small report of living related hepatic/intestinal transplantation in 13 donors and 10 recipients noted no donor complications, 100% 1- and 2-year recipient survival, and 80% intestinal graft survival (1 intestinal graft was successfully reimplanted). The same institution reported a 60% and 50% 1- and 3-year survival, respectively, for living related intestinal transplantation.[220]

Surgical technique of en bloc visceral transplantation and the exclusion of the colon aided the improvement of small bowel transplantation.[219] But the greatest advances, as with other solid-organ transplantation, have occurred because of improvements in immunosuppression, which have led to longer organ and patient survival. Tacrolimus, mycophenolate, rapamycin, daclizumab, alemtuzumab, interleukin-2 antagonists, and steroids represent novel increments in immunosuppression developed in the last 20 years. Others have used donor bone marrow infusion with ex vivo graft irradiation as adjuvant therapies to improve small bowel survival.[219,221]

Preoperative screening and aggressive therapy for cytomegalovirus and Epstein-Barr virus are also important considerations for extending organ and patient survival.[222,223]

Gastrointestinal Bleeding GI bleeding often represents a major diagnostic and therapeutic challenge. Initial signs may be hematemesis, melena, hematochezia, or occult blood in the stool. A loss as little as 60 mL per day can result in a black stool, and less than 10 mL can result in a positive hemoccult test. Many patients with GI bleeding are elderly or debilitated, and symptomatic hemorrhage causes major stress to other organ systems (eg, cardiac, renal, central nervous).

Upper Tract Bleeding The list of potential etiologies for upper GI hemorrhage is lengthy, but the 4 most common causes appear to be peptic ulcer disease, erosive gastritis, esophageal varices, and Mallory-Weiss tears of the esophagus.[224] Other causes include malignancy, blood dyscrasias, hemostatic disorders, aortoenteric fistulas, Dieulafoy syndrome, and collagen vascular diseases. In 1 series, 12% of patients with upper GI bleeding had chronic renal failure and bled from angiodysplastic lesions of the stomach and duodenum. **It usually is stated that if the patient's systolic pressure is less than 100 mm Hg, with a pulse greater than 100 beats/min (ie, a loss of 2 or 3 units or more of blood) and red or maroon stools, then the mortality rate is greater than 20% and surgical intervention is necessary in more than 50% of patients.**[225] Chronic lung, renal, cardiac, and liver disease and age older than 60 years add to this burden.

Diagnosis is aided by esophagogastroduodenoscopy in the first 24 hours. Management includes volume replacement and attention to illness in other systems. Some patients may receive parenteral vasopressin, such as an arterial infusion after angiography locates a bleeding ulcer or Mallory-Weiss tear, or an IV infusion for variceal bleeding. Varices often can be controlled with a Sengstaken-Blakemore tube, usually in preparation for more definitive management, such as sclerotherapy. Vasopressin often is still infusing when patients arrive for surgery to control bleeding. Vasopressin increases splanchnic and hepatic arteriolar resistance while decreasing portal venous pressure and hepatic blood flow. After a bolus dose, effects may last for approximately 1 hour.[226] Worrisome side effects of vasopressin include coronary artery vasoconstriction with myocardial infarction, a potential complication of its use in patients with myocardial ischemia. Intestinal and extremity ischemia also can occur.[227,228]

Lower Tract Bleeding The more frequent causes of lower GI bleeding are anorectal polyps, colonic polyps, colorectal cancer, inflammatory bowel disease, submucosal angiodysplasia, and diverticular disease. In children, juvenile polyps, Meckel diverticulum, and arteriovenous malformations are additional causes. Because the bleeding often is intermittent, diagnostic evaluation may be frustratingly negative. Endoscopy, radiographic examinations, and selective angiography are among the diagnostic and therapeutic (eg, electrocoagulation, embolization) modalities. Technetium-99m–labeled erythrocyte scans appear to be useful for slow, recurrent lower GI bleeding. Surgical procedures are directed toward the suspected diagnosis. Infrequently, when troublesome and symptomatic bleeding persists without a diagnosis, laparotomy may be undertaken for intraoperative endoscopy. Video camera capsule endoscopy and balloon enteroscopy have revolutionized lower tract bleeding diagnosis. The entire small bowel, or nearly so, can be visualized with a double balloon enteroscope making it the nonsurgical gold standard for evaluation of the deep small bowel.[229]

GASTROINTESTINAL OBSTRUCTIVE DISEASE

Impaired GI transit results from various conditions causing pseudo-obstruction (ie, decreased motility) and paralytic ileus, and those producing varying degrees of mechanical obstruction (**Box 56-12**). Considerable variation exists within each of these broad categories, and associated illness can be extensive.

Pseudo-obstruction and paralytic ileus generally represent intestinal motility disorders, and the list of causes is long (**Box 56-13**).[303] Patients with pseudo-obstruction usually have an insidious clinical course that evolves over months and years for the primary disease and for any coexisting GI manifestations. In general, remissions and exacerbations often occur.

Paralytic ileus tends to be acute in onset and to develop in patients with no suspected predisposing disease process. Although probably caused by neurohumoral mechanisms, paralytic ileus is not well understood. **The most common ileus is that seen after intra-abdominal operations.** Length of hospitalization following abdominal surgery depends on several factors including pain control, presence of mechanical devices (drains, catheters, and intervenous tubes), and postoperative ileus. In 2000, the Health Care Financing Administration demonstrated that 161 000 Medicare patients underwent major intra-abdominal operative procedures costing more than $1 billion. Postoperative ileus has the potential to play a significant role in length of hospitalization, morbidity, mortality, and cost.

Normal gastrointestinal motility is an integration of smooth muscle contraction, neural input, hormonal signals, and an enteric nervous system. The digestive system has as many neurons (Auerbach and Meissner plexus) as the spinal cord. After an intra-abdominal operation, the electrical disorganization and ineffective coordination of propulsion characterizing an ileus usually resolves after 4 to 5 days.[231] **The small intestine usually recovers motility within a few hours. The stomach resumes its ability to empty after about 24 hours, but the colon may not regain effective motility for 48 hours or longer.**[232-234]

Physical manipulation of the abdominal viscera, opioids, catecholamines, and inhalational anesthesia decrease bowel motility.[235] To date, there is no specific treatment for postoperative ileus. Nasogastric tubes historically have been inserted to reduce pulmonary complication, hasten bowel function return, increase patient comfort, and shorten hospital stay. In fact, a Cochrane analysis (4194 patients, 2108 routine nasogastric tube, 2087 no or selective tubes) demonstrated that *not* having a nasogastric tube after a procedure hastened return of bowel function ($P < 0.001$) and marginally decreased pulmonary complications ($P = 0.07$).[236] Early ambulation is an inexpensive therapy that decreases risk of thromboembolism and may be psychologically helpful for patients, but does not appear to benefit patients in resolution of postoperative ileus.[237] In 1928 Steinbrok et al reported treatment of ileus by splanchnic epidural anesthesia. Although there have been suggestions that sympathectomy from epidural anesthesia will cause an increase in anastomotic leaks, an analysis of 12 trials with 562 patients failed to find an association between epidural anesthesia and anastomotic breakdown.[238] Furthermore, when compared with patients who were receiving patient-controlled parenteral opioids, epidural analgesia provided better postoperative pain control.[239]

BOX 56-12

Causes of Impaired Intestinal Transit

Impaired motility

Mechanical obstruction

Paralytic ileus

Pseudo-obstruction

BOX 56-13

Pseudo-obstruction Syndromes

- I. Primary idiopathic pseudo-obstruction
  - A. Familial syndromes
    - 1. Visceral myopathies
    - 2. Visceral neuropathies
  - B. Sporadic syndromes
    - 1. Visceral myopathies
    - 2. Visceral neuropathies
- II. Secondary pseudo-obstruction
  - A. Diseases of GI muscle
    - 1. Collagen disease
      - a. Scleroderma
      - b. Dermatomyositis and polymyositis
      - c. Systemic lupus erythematosus
    - 2. Amyloidosis
    - 3. Generalized muscle disease
      - a. Myotonic dystrophy
      - b. Progressive muscular dystrophy
  - B. Diseases of GI nerves
    - 1. Parkinson disease
    - 2. Hirschsprung disease
    - 3. Chagas disease
    - 4. Primary autonomic dysfunction
  - C. Endocrine diseases involving GI tract
    - 1. Myxedema ileus
    - 2. Diabetes mellitus
    - 3. Hypoparathyroidism
    - 4. Pheochromocytoma
  - D. Drug-induced syndromes
    - 1. Opiates
    - 2. Psychotropic drugs
    - 3. Antiparkinsonian drugs
    - 4. Cathartics
  - E. Miscellaneous
    - 1. Jejunoileal bypass
    - 2. Jejunal diverticulosis
    - 3. Inflammatory bowel disease
    - 4. Paraneoplastic neuropathy
- III. Paralytic ileus
  - A. Intra-abdominal disease
  - B. Extra-abdominal disease

Data from Christensen J. Intestinal pseudo-obstruction and paralytic ileus. In: Moody FG, ed. *Surgical Treatment of Digestive Disease.* 2nd ed. Chicago: Mosby-Year Book; 1990.

Although neostigmine, metoclopramide, cisapride, erythromycin, ceruletide, somatostatin, laxatives, and nonsteroidal anti-inflammatory agents have theoretical advantages for enhancing GI motility, investigations have not demonstrated useful effects in humans.[231] It is well established that opioids acutely and chronically slow gastrointestinal

TABLE 56-2 Fluids Entering Bowel Daily

Source	Volume (mL)
Diet	2000
Saliva	1000
Gastric juice	2000
Bile	1000
Pancreatic juice	2000
Succus entericus	1000

motility. Administration of peripheral opioid antagonists appears to lead to a faster return of bowel function and faster hospital discharge, without an increase in readmissions, and with *no difference* in pain scores.[239,240]

Other abdominal causes of paralytic ileus include blunt trauma, bowel perforation, bile peritonitis, and intra-abdominal sepsis. Nonabdominal causes include lobar pneumonia, myocardial infarction, massive trauma, generalized sepsis, and electrolyte abnormalities such as hypophosphatemia and hypokalemia.

Mechanical obstruction is a vexing diagnostic problem that generally requires surgical intervention. Simple obstruction implies adequate blood flow to the obstructed area, whereas strangulation connotes insufficient circulation to the area. Obturated obstruction is caused by an intraluminal foreign body. Mechanical obstruction tends to be acute, with fairly rapid progression to complete obstruction.

Approximately 60% to 80% of obstruction occurs in the small intestine.[241] Pain, distension, emesis, and obstipation typically are present. Volume loss, tachycardia, and electrolyte disturbances can occur from severe vomiting and the massive volumes that are sequestered in strangulated bowel.

Approximately 7 to 9 L of fluid are presented to the gut daily[242] from varied sources (**Table 56-2**). With obstruction, not only is reabsorption hindered, but intestinal fluid secretion may be increased.[243] In addition, rapid infusion of IV fluids, which may be necessary for hemodynamic support, has been reported to increase secretion.[244] Once intraluminal pressure exceeds approximately 20 cm H_2O, reabsorption fails.[245]

Because intestinal fluid has a tonicity and electrolyte composition similar to extracellular fluids, acid-base and electrolyte disturbances generally are not severe. Duodenal obstruction can lead to hypokalemic alkalosis resulting from severe emesis. In addition, once strangulation occurs (and no definitive criteria exist for this diagnosis), necrosis of bowel and bacterial proliferation contribute to rapid sequestration of fluid and colloid in the affected bowel and peritoneal cavity. Together with vomiting, this can produce marked depletion of intravascular volume and the potential for renal and cardiovascular instability.

Other conditions can mimic small bowel obstruction (**Box 56-14**), making the diagnosis difficult. This especially applies to elderly patients, who often have only minimal evidence of peritoneal irritation.

Acute large bowel obstruction is associated with pain, distension, vomiting, and obstipation, although large bowel obstruction can be more insidious than small bowel obstruction and may present without pain but with "overflow" diarrhea. Fifty percent or more of large bowel obstructions result from colorectal cancer, with much of the rest caused by diverticulitis, volvulus, and fecal impaction.[246] Small bowel obstruction may occur concurrently. An incompetent ileocecal valve may permit the eventual development of feculent vomiting.

Management includes decompression of the stomach, appropriate IV fluids, and attention to conditions in other systems (eg, infection, renal and cardiovascular problems). Depending on the patient's age and the severity of illness or suspected intervention, invasive hemodynamic monitoring may be warranted.

Patients with GI motility disorders and those with obvious obstruction are at risk for regurgitation and aspiration during the induction and maintenance of anesthesia and postoperatively. The anesthesiologist should be aware of the potential for such difficulty with this group of patients and treat appropriately. At the least, this would include the omission of oral premedication and the use of postoperative (and preoperative when indicated) nasogastric suctioning. Anesthesia should be induced using awake intubation or rapid sequence considerations.

BOX 56-14

Conditions Mimicking Small Bowel Obstruction

Diabetic ketoacidosis
Food poisoning
Pancreatitis
Porphyria
Pseudo-obstruction
Sickle crisis
Ureteral and biliary colic

THE SYSTEMIC INFLAMMATORY RESPONSE SYNDROME–MULTIPLE ORGAN FAILURE CONTINUUM

Many severely ill patients require emergency surgical intervention for life-threatening conditions such as abdominal trauma, resection of nonviable bowel, relief of obstruction or strangulation, drainage of an abscess, or removal of a severely inflamed gallbladder. In addition to their abdominal disorder, they may be intubated in an intensive care unit, may have evidence of organ system failure (eg, pulmonary, renal, central nervous system, and major metabolic changes), or may be older with serious cardiac and vascular disease. Many behave as if they have a severe infection whether or not one is eventually discovered. In the past, varying etiologies have been suggested, including gram-negative sepsis, endotoxemia, sepsis syndrome, and multiple system organ failure. Because of the many similarities among such patients, even for those whose clinical course falls outside these diagnoses (eg, patients with gram-positive sepsis, viral or fungal infection, or no infection at all), other explanations have been sought.

Common to many of these patients is evidence of major inflammatory mediator production and release by polymorphonuclear leukocytes, macrophages, monocytes, platelets, and the endothelium. The cyclooxygenase pathway has important effects. More than 30 such mediators have been identified, with cytokines such as tumor necrosis factor; interleukins-1, -6, and -8; substance P; granulocyte-macrophage colony-stimulating factor; interferon; and platelet-activating factor among the most studied.[247,248]

It has been suggested that the *systemic inflammatory response syndrome* (SIRS) represents the earliest, fairly nonspecific phase of a process that may lead to organ dysfunction and, ultimately, organ failure. Currently, the diagnosis of SIRS requires that 2 of the find ings in **Box 56-15** be present.[249] **Systemic inflammatory response syndrome and multiple organ failure appear to be the ends of a**

BOX 56-15

Diagnostic Findings in Systemic Inflammatory Response Syndrome[a]

Temperature >100.4°F (38°C), <96.8°F (36°C)
Heart rate >90 beats/min
Respiration rate >20 breaths/min or $Paco_2$ <32 mm Hg
Leukocyte >12.0 × 10^9/L or <4 × 10^9/L or >0.10 immature cells

[a]Two or more should be present for a diagnosis to be made.

hierarchical continuum with an increasing inflammatory response to infectious and noninfectious stimuli. Initially organ dysfunction is more functional than permanent, organ failure and mortality increase with increasing inflammatory response.[250-252]

The GI tract is a vulnerable organ system. Any insult to adequate core tissue perfusion (eg, hemorrhage, cardiac arrest, cardiopulmonary bypass) may result in severe or relative hypotension, with ensuing GI mucosal ischemia. Endogenous vasoconstrictors may be released[253] (**Box 56-16**), which may affect the splanchnic bed more consistently than others.[254-257] Reperfusion after shock may be associated with oxygen and free radical mucosal damage. In addition, so-called myocardial depressant factors can be released from the pancreas and possibly the small intestine, which further contribute to tissue hypoperfusion and low cardiac output syndrome. As much as 15% to 65% of the circulating volume can redistribute to damaged bowel during this process. Although inadequate perfusion limits delivery of oxygen for cellular processes, other mechanisms that directly affect mitochondria may have similar effects even with relatively adequate (or increased) perfusion. A host of factors affect the mitochondria, including reactive oxygen species, local Po_2, levels of adenosine triphosphate, and hormonal influences such as thyroid, catecholamines, corticosteroids, and leptins. Nitric oxide is a strong inhibitor of mitochondrial electron transport. If insufficient energy is available to fuel metabolism, critical thresholds of adenosine triphosphate result and cellular dysfunction and death ensue.

Although the systemic cardiovascular response demanded by these conditions usually is hyperdynamic, it often is inadequate, either because metabolic requirements are too high (or because of end-organ inability to use oxygen) or because of limitations imposed by evolving or underlying myocardial dysfunction. Management of these patients is beyond the scope of this chapter. When the anesthesiologist encounters these patients, they frequently are already receiving vasopressor and inotropic support. Intraoperative care includes intensive evaluation of oxygen delivery, optimization of volume and cardiovascular function, and avoidance of drugs and agents that will further compromise their already tenuous status.[258,259]

BOX 56-16

Vasoactive Substances Affecting Splanchnic Bed

Vasoconstrictors

Endogenous

Angiotensin II
Vasopressin
Catecholamines
Certain prostaglandins
- PGB_2
- PGD_2
- $PGF_{2\alpha}$

Certain leukotrienes
- C_4
- D_4
- E_4

Certain thromboxanes
- TxA_2

Serotonin

Exogenous

Digoxin
Atropine
Physostigmine

Vasodilators

Endogenous

Vasoactive intestinal peptide
Histamine
Glucagon
Cholecystokinin
Other eicosanoids
PGI_2 (prostacyclin)
PGE_2
Serotonin
Nitric oxide

SUMMARY

The complex physiologic and metabolic interactions of the GI tract and other organ system functions can present fascinating challenges for the anesthesiologist. Because GI surgery often can seem so benign, it is perhaps more difficult to remain "tuned in" to such concerns. The rewards of good patient care should be sufficient incentive to reexamine important issues in GI surgery and anesthesia from time to time.

KEY REFERENCES

- Block BM, Liu SS, Rowlingson AJ, Cowan AR, Cowan JA Jr, Wu CL. Efficacy of postoperative epidural analgesia: a meta-analysis. *JAMA*. 2003;290:2455-2463.
- Cash BD. Evidence-based medicine as it applies to acid suppression in the hospitalized patient. *Crit Care Med.* 2002;30: S373-S378.
- Goyal RK, Hirano I. The enteric nervous system. *N Engl J Med.* 1996;334:1106.
- Mokdad AH, Bowman BA, Ford ES, Vinicor F, Marks JS, Koplan JP. The continuing epidemics of obesity and diabetes in the United States. *JAMA*. 2001;286:1195-1200.
- Ng A, Smith G. Gastroesophageal reflux and aspiration of gastric contents in anesthetic practice. *Anesth Analg.* 2001;93:494-513.
- Rangel-Frausto MS, Pittet D, Costigan M, et al. The natural history of the systemic inflammatory response syndrome (SIRS): a prospective study. *JAMA*. 1995;273:117.
- Shah M, Simha V, Garg A. Long-term impact of bariatric surgery on body weight, comorbidities, and nutritional status [review]. *J Clin Endocrinol Metab.* 2006;91:4223-4231.
- Singer M, De Santis V, Vitale D, Jeffcoate W. Multiorgan failure is an adaptive, endocrine-mediated, metabolic response to overwhelming systemic inflammation. *Lancet.* 2004;363:545–548.
- Sollinger HW. Pancreas transplantation in humans. In: Moody FG, ed. *Surgical Treatment of Digestive Disease.* 2nd ed. Chicago, IL: Mosby-Year Book; 1990:577-598.

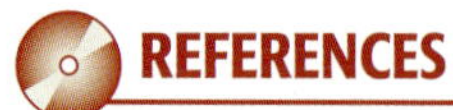

REFERENCES

Complete references available on DVD and online version at www.LongneckerAnesthesiology.com

CHAPTER 57

Anesthesia for Liver Surgery and Transplantation

Michael A. Pilla
Douglas E. Raines
Warren S. Sandberg

KEY POINTS

1. Patients with chronic liver dysfunction and cirrhosis have a hyperdynamic circulation with low peripheral vascular resistance and an increased cardiac index.
2. Coagulopathies, edema and ascites, renal dysfunction, portopulmonary hypertension, hepatopulmonary syndrome, and autonomic neuropathies are common in patients with liver disease.
3. The cause of hepatic encephalopathy is believed to be multifactorial. Hepatic encephalopathy resembles and must be differentiated from many other nonfocal neurologic conditions such as hypoglycemia, hyponatremia, intracranial hemorrhage or mass lesions, and meningitis.
4. Patients scheduled for a hepatic resection should be evaluated as any patient scheduled for major noncardiac surgery. Plans for monitoring, vascular access, induction and maintenance of anesthesia, postoperative pain control, and postoperative care should take into account a large subcostal incision and the potential for sudden massive hemorrhage and severe physiologic derangements during and after surgery.
5. The most common indication for liver transplantation is chronic hepatocellular disease due to alcohol and/or hepatitis. Hepatitis C is increasingly important, representing a unique and growing health risk for anesthesiologists.
6. Cardiac assessment of the patient being considered for liver transplantation focuses on functional and invasive tests of cardiac performance that assess ischemic potential and the search for cardiac structural anomalies that might compromise outcome from orthotopic liver transplantation.
7. Liver transplantation comprises 3 phases. During the preanhepatic phase, a complete hepatectomy is performed. During the anhepatic phase, vascular anastomoses between the donor liver and the recipient's vessels are constructed. During the neohepatic phase, the hepatic arterial and biliary anastomoses are constructed, and the wound is closed.
8. The 2 common techniques for liver transplantation are the en-bloc technique with interruption of vena caval flow and the piggyback technique with preservation of vena caval flow.
9. The goals of hemodynamic management are to provide sufficient circulating volume, vascular tone, and cardiac output to perfuse the vital organs. This is not guided by any single parameter but rather by a synthesis of all available data.
10. The effects of portal hypertension and ascites are alleviated by nonshunting and shunting procedures. Nonshunting procedures are aimed at controlling hemorrhage from portosystemic varices. Shunting procedures redirect the portal venous flow into the systemic venous circulation via a nonvariceal conduit, thus relieving portal hypertension, decompressing varices, and at the same time relieving ascites.
11. Most livers made available for transplantation come from heart-beating cadaveric donors. When caring for organ donors, the focus of care has shifted from preserving the patient to preserving the function of graft organs. Due to the shortage of cadaveric donors, the use of living donors is growing. In these cases, donor safety is a primary concern, as the donor derives no physical benefit from the surgery.

INTRODUCTION

Anesthesia for surgery of the hepatobiliary system is a challenging and rapidly evolving subspecialty of anesthesiology. The growth of this subspecialty has paralleled the evolution of hepatic surgery from a risky and heroic enterprise to a more routine undertaking over the past decades. Better understanding of hepatic anatomy, improved diagnostic imaging capabilities, enhanced patient selection and risk stratification, and technical advancements in surgical and anesthetic techniques have at once improved the morbidity and mortality profiles of liver surgery while extending the limits of what can safely be accomplished.

This chapter describes the anesthetic management of patients undergoing hepatic surgery, ranging from minimally invasive procedures, such as transjugular intrahepatic portosystemic shunting, to orthotopic liver transplantation (OLT). Patients presenting for hepatic surgery may generally be divided into 2 groups, each of whom provide unique challenges for the anesthesiologist:

1. Patients presenting for surgery on the liver who do not have significant liver disease—for example, the patient with isolated hepatocellular carcinoma. These patients can generally be evaluated and managed as patients presenting for other types of major intra-abdominal surgery.
2. Patients with significant liver disease presenting for hepatic surgery either to ameliorate the liver disease itself or, more rarely, for treatment of a distinct hepatobiliary problem. Hepatobiliary operations performed on patients with liver disease include portosystemic shunts, hepatic resection, and orthotopic liver transplantation.

Patients with liver disease who need nonhepatic surgery are a broader group unified by a common derangement. In these individuals, the liver disease must be taken into account and will shape the preoperative preparation, anesthetic technique, and postoperative care. For more details on the evaluation and general anesthetic management of the patient with liver disease presenting for nonhepatic surgery, the reader is referred to Chapter 15.

The general principles evinced in Chapter 15 apply as well to patients with liver disease presenting for hepatobiliary surgery. In this chapter, we first review the relevant anatomy, physiology, and hepatobiliary pathophysiology that affect the anesthetic management of patients presenting for hepatic surgery. Next, we describe at a high level the surgical considerations informing the various groups of hepatic operations, followed by detailed consideration of the consequent anesthetic management goals.

ANATOMY AND PHYSIOLOGY

ANATOMY OF THE LIVER

The liver contains lobes (right and left) that are separated on the anterior side by the falciform ligament and supplied by right and left branches of the portal vein and the hepatic artery. Two smaller additional lobes may be visualized on the posterior aspect of the liver, the caudate and quadrate lobes. The liver is further subdivided into 8 segments that are defined by secondary and tertiary branching of the blood supply. The caudate lobe contains segment 1, the left lobe contains segments 2 and 3, the quadrate contains segment 4, and the right lobe contains segments 5 through 8.

Blood flow to the liver is 1 $L/min^{-1}/kg^{-1}$ of hepatic tissue, or approximately 25% of the cardiac output. Most of this blood supply is via the portal vein (75%), which delivers about 45% to 50% of the hepatic oxygen supply, with the balance coming via the hepatic artery. Portal venous blood flow is controlled primarily by the arterioles within upstream splanchnic organs and to a more limited extent by resistance within the liver. Hepatic artery blood flow is controlled directly via arterial smooth muscle under autonomic regulation. In addition, metabolic factors such as blood pH and/or oxygen content can also modulate hepatic arterial resistance and hence blood flow. After coursing through the liver, blood drains via the hepatic veins and into the inferior vena cava.

OVERVIEW OF LIVER FUNCTIONS

The liver is among the most complex organs in the body and is responsible for a wide range of important synthetic and metabolic processes. A detailed review is beyond the scope of this chapter, but a brief overview is provided in the following.

Albumin Synthesis The liver synthesizes more albumin than any other protein, in the range of 10 to 20 g/d. As the most abundant plasma protein, it serves an important role in maintaining the normal oncotic pressure of plasma, and a decrease in albumin synthesis can allow transudation of fluids into extravascular spaces, producing edema and ascites. Albumin has a half-life of approximately 20 days and therefore is not a good indicator of liver function in patients with acute hepatic disease. Because many drugs, including barbiturates and benzodiazepines, are bound by albumin in the blood, the hypoalbuminemia frequently observed in patients with significant hepatic dysfunction can lead to an increase in their free or active concentrations. This may, in part, account for the increased sensitivity of patients with severe hepatic disease to sedatives and anesthetics.

Coagulation Factor Synthesis The liver is the major site of synthesis of most procoagulant and inhibitory clotting factors, including fibrinogen; factors II, V, VII, IX, XII, and XIII; plasminogen; antithrombin; and proteins C and S. Consequently, the loss of hepatic parenchymal cells can lead to clotting factor deficiencies with resultant coagulopathy. Systemic fibrinolysis, which is found in 30% of patients with end-stage liver disease, may also contribute to clotting factor deficiencies.[1,2] Although the pathogenesis of this fibrinolysis has not been clearly defined, studies suggest that it involves altered tissue plasminogen activator activity, impaired synthesis of the inhibitors of plasminogen and plasmin, α-2 antiplasmin, and histidine-rich glycoprotein.[3-7] Additionally, patients with advanced liver disease exhibit an exaggerated fibrinolytic response to major surgery, such as liver transplantation, predisposing them to significant perioperative hemorrhage.[2,8]

Carbohydrate Metabolism Regulation of blood glucose concentrations is largely controlled by the liver and is under hormonal control. In response to lowered concentrations of glucose in the portal vein, glycogen stored in the liver is broken down to glucose for use by other tissues (glycogenolysis). During periods of fasting when glycogen stores have been depleted, the liver can also generate glucose from noncarbohydrate sources such as lactate, amino acids, and glycerol (gluconeogenesis). Ingestion of carbohydrates replenishes glycogen stores and allows fatty acids to be synthesized by the liver.

Bile Acid Synthesis Bile acids are important compounds required for the elimination of cholesterol and the absorption of vitamins and fats. The liver converts approximately 500 mg/d of cholesterol into bile acids in processes that involve 17 different enzymes and are regulated by many factors, including nutrients and hormones.[9,10] Bile acids are stored in the gall bladder and released into the small intestine to emulsify lipids, cholesterol, and the fat-soluble vitamins A, D, E, and K. Most (90%-95%) of the secreted bile acids are reabsorbed by the liver and recycled.

Drug Metabolism Although there are a number of enzymatic pathways involved in the metabolism of drugs by the liver, each can be placed into 1 of 2 reaction categories. Phase 1 reactions use the chemical processes of oxidation, reduction, and hydrolysis; occur in the hepatocyte smooth endoplasmic reticulum; and are mediated primarily by the cytochrome P-450 family of enzymes. Phase 2 reactions increase the water solubility of drugs by coupling (conjugating) drugs with polar moieties, thereby facilitating biliary excretion. Often, phase 2 reactions follow phase 1 reactions because the products of phase 1 reactions may not be sufficiently water soluble to be readily excreted.

PATHOPHYSIOLOGY RELEVANT TO ANESTHESIA FOR LIVER SURGERY

In this section, we briefly review the disease entities leading to liver failure. For a more complete description, the reader is referred to Chapter 15. Also in Chapter 15, the reader will find a discussion of the Child-Turcotte-Pugh classification scheme for evaluating the surgical risk associated with progressive worsening of liver disease. Later in this section, we describe the pathogenesis and medical management of organ system derangements that are associated with acute and chronic liver disease.

CHRONIC LIVER DISEASE

Chronic liver disease may result from a variety of conditions, including infection, biliary obstruction, toxicity, and inborn errors of metabolism (**Box 57-1**). These conditions can progress to cirrhosis, which is characterized by hepatic cell death, fibrosis, and the formation of regenerative nodules. This process is essentially irreversible and leads to important physiologic disturbances. Elevation of the blood pressure within the portal venous system (ie, portal hypertension) is common in patients with significant chronic liver disease and results from increased portal blood flow and/or intrahepatic resistance. It is associated with the formation of ascites, esophageal varices, hepatic encephalopathy, and splenomegaly. Ascites is a hallmark of decompensated liver cirrhosis, and its cause is multifactorial. These factors include alterations in portal blood flow dynamics, activation of the renin-angiotensin-aldosterone system, and reduction in plasma oncotic pressure. The primary treatments for ascites are sodium and water restriction, administration of diuretics, and abdominal paracentesis, which can lead to intravascular fluid depletion.

Esophageal variceal bleeding is a potentially lethal complication of cirrhosis. Treatment options depend on the severity of the bleeding and include the administration of beta-blockers, variceal banding, sclerotherapy, and portosystemic shunting. As compared to variceal banding, carvedilol, a noncardioselective vasodilating beta-blocker, is more effective at preventing first bleeds in patients with high-risk varices.[11] However, an important potential complication of portosystemic shunting is that it may cause or worsen existing hepatic encephalopathy.[12,13]

BOX 57-1

Major Causes of Chronic Liver Disease

- Intraparenchymal disease
  - Viral infections
    - Chronic active hepatitis B
    - Chronic active hepatitis C
    - Hepatitis D
  - Toxins
    - Ethanol
  - Miscellaneous
    - Cystic fibrosis
    - Hemochromatosis
    - Wilson disease
    - α_1-Antitrypsin deficiency
    - Metabolic errors of carbohydrate, lipid, and proteins
  - Cholestatic disease
    - Primary biliary cirrhosis
    - Primary sclerosing cholangitis

FULMINANT HEPATIC FAILURE

Fulminant hepatic failure is generally defined as severe hepatic dysfunction that occurs either in the absence of preexisting liver disease or in the presence of well-compensated liver disease. Drug toxicity, most frequently by acetaminophen, is the most common cause of fulminant hepatic failure (**Box 57-2**), followed by viral hepatitis. However, not uncommonly (17%), no causative agent is identified.[14] Acute hepatic encephalopathy is a prominent clinical feature of fulminant hepatic failure and is associated with progressive brain swelling and an increase in intracranial pressure (ICP) that can result in brain herniation and death. In patients with fulminant hepatic failure, brain herniation is the most commonly identifiable cause of death found at autopsy.[15] Regular neurologic examinations can be used to exclude dangerous brain swelling in patients who are awake and responsive. However, neurologic examinations cannot detect dangerous increases in ICP in encephalopathic comatose patients or those undergoing general anesthesia. Therefore, some centers regularly institute ICP monitoring during major surgery. However, such monitoring is controversial because patients with fulminant hepatic failure are commonly coagulopathic, and the placement of ICP monitors is associated with a significant (10%-20%) risk of intracranial bleeding,[16,17] although recent studies suggest this can be done safely with the preadministration of recombinant activated factor VII (rFVIIa).[18]

Treatment of fulminant hepatic failure is supportive, and many patients recover. However, some patients do not recover and thus require liver transplantation. Regardless of the final path to resolution, supportive care aims to reduce the impact of severe encephalopathy and brain swelling. Mild hypothermia appears to be protective in patients with encephalopathy during acute liver failure awaiting liver transplantation, but this has not been unequivocally demonstrated by randomized studies.[19,20] Similarly, barbiturates may be used to lower brain oxygen consumption as an additional temporizing measure.

Bacterial infection develops in up to 80% of patients with fulminant hepatic failure.[21,22] These infections most commonly involve the respiratory and urinary systems.[22] Acute infection may prevent transplantation.

HEMODYNAMIC CHANGES IN LIVER DISEASE

Patients with chronic liver dysfunction and cirrhosis commonly have a hyperdynamic circulation (**Box 57-3**) with a low peripheral vascular resistance and an increased cardiac index.[23] It has been suggested that a low systemic vascular resistance results from an increase in circulating endogenous vasodilators, including nitric oxide, calcitonin gene-related peptide, and substance P, the metabolism of which is reduced by the presence of intrahepatic and extrahepatic arteriovenous shunts.[24-26] Cardiac output is frequently elevated in cirrhotic patients, attributable to increased sympathetic nervous system activity, increased blood volume and preload, and reduced systemic vascular resistance, and mimics hemodynamics seen in patients with extrahepatic portal vein obstruction.[27-29] However, even in the setting of increased cardiac output, patients with cirrhosis may have significant cardiac dysfunction. Typical features of "cirrhotic cardiomyopathy" include impaired cardiac contractility, conduction abnormalities, impaired excitation-contraction coupling, and decreased β-adrenergic receptor function.[30,31] Endogenous cannabinoids have been implicated in the progression of liver disease and subsequent development of cirrhotic cardiomyopathy, and the finding of CB receptor upregulation in liver disease patients suggests a role for targeting CB1 and CB2 receptors in the potential treatment of this disease.[31,32] Some patients with a hyperdynamic circulation develop significant left ventricular failure after liver transplantation. It has been suggested that this is due to increased peripheral vascular resistance after relief of vasodilation by transplantation. With inotropes, mechanical ventilation, and close monitoring, results from small series suggest that these patients will survive.[33]

BOX 57-2

Major Causes of Fulminant Hepatic Failure

Toxins
- Acetaminophen
- Ethanol
- *Amanita phalloides*
- Halothane
- Phosphorus

Viral infections
- Hepatitis A
- Hepatitis B
- Hepatitis C
- Hepatitis D

Miscellaneous
- Budd-Chiari syndrome
- Acute fatty liver of pregnancy
- Wilson disease

BOX 57-3

Hemodynamic Derangements in Cirrhotic Liver Disease

Decreased systemic vascular resistance due to:
- peripheral vasodilation
- arteriovenous shunting

Redirection of blood flow
- increased pulmonary, splanchnic, muscle, and skin blood flow
- decreased portal vein flow to liver
- normal or increased hepatic arterial flow
- normal to decreased renal blood flow

Increased blood volume
- decreased serum albumin
- decreased plasma oncotic pressure

Increased cardiac output
- apparent cardiomyopathy despite increased output

Decreased arteriovenous O_2 content difference
- increased venous O_2 content

Decreased responsiveness to catecholamines

RENAL FUNCTION IN PATIENTS WITH LIVER DISEASE

Renal dysfunction is common in patients with liver disease and has at least 3 major causes.[34] First, prerenal azotemia resulting from the overaggressive use of diuretics used to control ascites can result in rising BUN and creatinine concentrations, indicating worsening renal function. This usually responds to reducing the diuretic dose and gentle hydration. The second common cause of renal dysfunction in patients with liver disease is acute tubular necrosis in the setting of another acute, precipitating factor. In patients with liver disease, a common scenario is the development of a low-tone, sepsis syndrome in the setting of an infection, such as spontaneous bacterial peritonitis, followed by renal failure. Renal failure commonly develops in the setting of infection in patients with liver disease. For example, it has been reported that 27% of patients with cirrhosis and

BOX 57-4

Diagnostic Criteria for Hepatorenal Syndrome[a]

Major criteria

- Low glomerular filtration rate, as indicated by serum creatinine >1.5 mg/dL
- Exclusion of shock, ongoing bacterial infection, volume depletion, or use of nephrotoxic drugs
- No improvement in renal function after stopping diuretics and volume repletion with 1.5 L of normal saline
- No proteinuria or evidence of obstructive uropathy or parenchymal renal disease

Minor criteria

- Urine volume <500 mL/d
- Urine sodium <10 mEq/L
- Urine osmolality > plasma osmolality
- Urine RBC <50 per high-power field
- Serum sodium <130 mEq/L

[a]Only major criteria are needed to establish the diagnosis.

From Lee FY, Lin HC, Tsai YT, et al. Plasma substance P levels in patients with liver cirrhosis: relationship to systemic and portal hemodynamics. *Am J Gastroenterol.* 1997;92(11):2080-2084.

sepsis progressed to renal failure.[35] Of these patients, renal failure was reversible in 76%,[35] demonstrating that renal function tends to recover with the removal of the inciting insult. However, the mortality for patients with high Model for End-Stage Renal Disease (MELD) scores (ie, severe liver disease) was high.[35] The third most common cause of renal failure in the cirrhotic patient is hepatorenal syndrome.[36] The diagnostic criteria for hepatorenal syndrome are given in **Box 57-4**. Changes in serum sodium along with changes in creatinine and GFR indicate worsening renal function and decreased survival in this patient population.[37]

Hepatorenal syndrome is marked by a worsening of renal function as the liver disease progresses. Renal function will not recover unless there is an improvement in liver function.[34] Temporizing measures to treat hepatorenal syndrome are based on theories of its pathophysiology. One such theory is that the inciting factor is the peripheral vasodilation that characterizes late cirrhosis.[38] Serum levels of nitric oxide and L-arginine rise progressively in cirrhotic patients with worsening renal function.[39] Decreased peripheral vascular resistance activates vasoconstrictor systems (eg, renin-angiotensin-aldosterone, antidiuretic hormone, and sympathetics), leading to renal vasoconstriction. This in turn leads to sodium and water retention and the formation of ascites. Another theory is that portal hypertension reduces blood flow to hepatocytes,[40] which sense this as a manifestation of inadequate blood volume and activate a hepatorenal reflex to cause vasoconstriction and sodium and water retention. Thus the temporizing therapies for hepatorenal syndrome include both renal vasodilators and splanchnic vasoconstrictors. Splanchnic vasoconstrictors, such as vasopressin and its longer-lived relatives, are sometimes coadministered with a plasma expander such as albumin.[34,41] For patients with liver transplantation as an option, this is the preferred treatment, and renal function typically recovers after transplantation.[34,42] However, transplantation is complicated by the presence of renal failure, and renal replacement therapy for control of pH, serum potassium, and intravascular volume is frequently required for these patients. In patients who develop hepatorenal syndrome, cardiac dysfunction as indicated by low cardiac output precedes and may herald hepatorenal syndrome.[43]

THE PULMONARY SYSTEM IN LIVER DISEASE

Some patients with chronic liver disease and portal hypertension develop alterations in pulmonary physiology leading to 2 clinically distinct syndromes: portopulmonary hypertension and hepatopulmonary syndrome. Although these 2 syndromes can coexist in the same patient, management depends on appreciating the difference between portopulmonary hypertension and hepatopulmonary syndrome, and the therapeutic approaches to each.[44,45]

Portopulmonary Hypertension Portopulmonary hypertension occurs most frequently in patients with advanced liver disease. In 1 study of patients with cirrhosis and refractory ascites, the prevalence of portopulmonary hypertension was 16%.[46] Portopulmonary hypertension is characterized by a mean pulmonary artery pressure greater than 25 mm Hg with a normal pulmonary capillary wedge pressure (ie, <15 mm Hg) and an elevated pulmonary vascular resistance (ie, >120 dyne/s/cm^5) in the setting of portal hypertension.[45] Multiple factors have been implicated in the etiology of portopulmonary hypertension, including (1) increased pulmonary arterial blood flow secondary to the increase in cardiac index frequently observed in cirrhosis, (2) increased circulating blood volume, and (3) vasoconstriction and progressive pulmonary vascular remodeling due to a proliferation of endothelial and smooth muscle cells with or without thrombotic change.[45,47] The most common symptom of portopulmonary hypertension is dyspnea on exertion, with fatigue, palpitations, chest pain, and syncope being less frequent.[48,49]

Evidence of portopulmonary hypertension may be obtained noninvasively using transthoracic Doppler echocardiography. **Figure 57-1** outlines the diagnostic approach to pulmonary hypertension. Although transthoracic echocardiography is a useful screening tool for portopulmonary hypertension, it frequently overestimates right ventricular pressure,[50] producing a large number of false positives as determined by direct pressure measurements at subsequent cardiac catheterization.[50,51] For example, a right ventricular systolic pressure estimate from transthoracic echocardiography of 40 mm Hg or greater is associated with significant pulmonary hypertension (ie, mean pulmonary artery pressure >25 mm Hg) at right heart catheterization in only about 65% of cases.[51] Conversely, the sensitivity of Doppler echocardiography for detecting portopulmonary hypertension is high enough that a normal study rules out portopulmonary hypertension.[51] Because of the severe consequences of failing to diagnose and manage portopulmonary hypertension during later liver surgery or transplantation, the best current approach is to screen with transthoracic echocardiography and perform pulmonary artery catheterization to confirm or exclude portopulmonary hypertension in patients with high right ventricular systolic pressure estimates at transthoracic echocardiography. Although moderate to severe portopulmonary hypertension is often a contraindication to hepatic transplantation, there are case reports of such patients undergoing successful hepatic transplantation with resolution of the pulmonary component of their disease.[52]

The effective management of portopulmonary hypertension is important because reducing pulmonary artery pressures, unloading the right heart, and allowing time for pulmonary vascular remodeling may allow patients who are not liver transplant candidates to become potential recipients.[53] Pulmonary vasodilator treatment may also allow a marginal patient to receive a transplant with reduced mortality.[53] Vasodilators, such as epoprostenol, sildenafil, or nitric oxide, can reduce pulmonary vascular resistance[54,55] and are used for this purpose by programs that consider liver transplantation in patients whose pulmonary pressures can be satisfactorily lowered. However, it is unclear with the current level of evidence whether these interventions improve survival at liver transplantation. It is also unclear how long pulmonary artery pressures must be lowered to confer the benefit (if any) of the intervention at subsequent transplantation. Case reports of patients with good response to pulmonary vasodilators who subsequently have poor outcomes of transplantation temper enthusiasm about the prospects for such patients.[56]

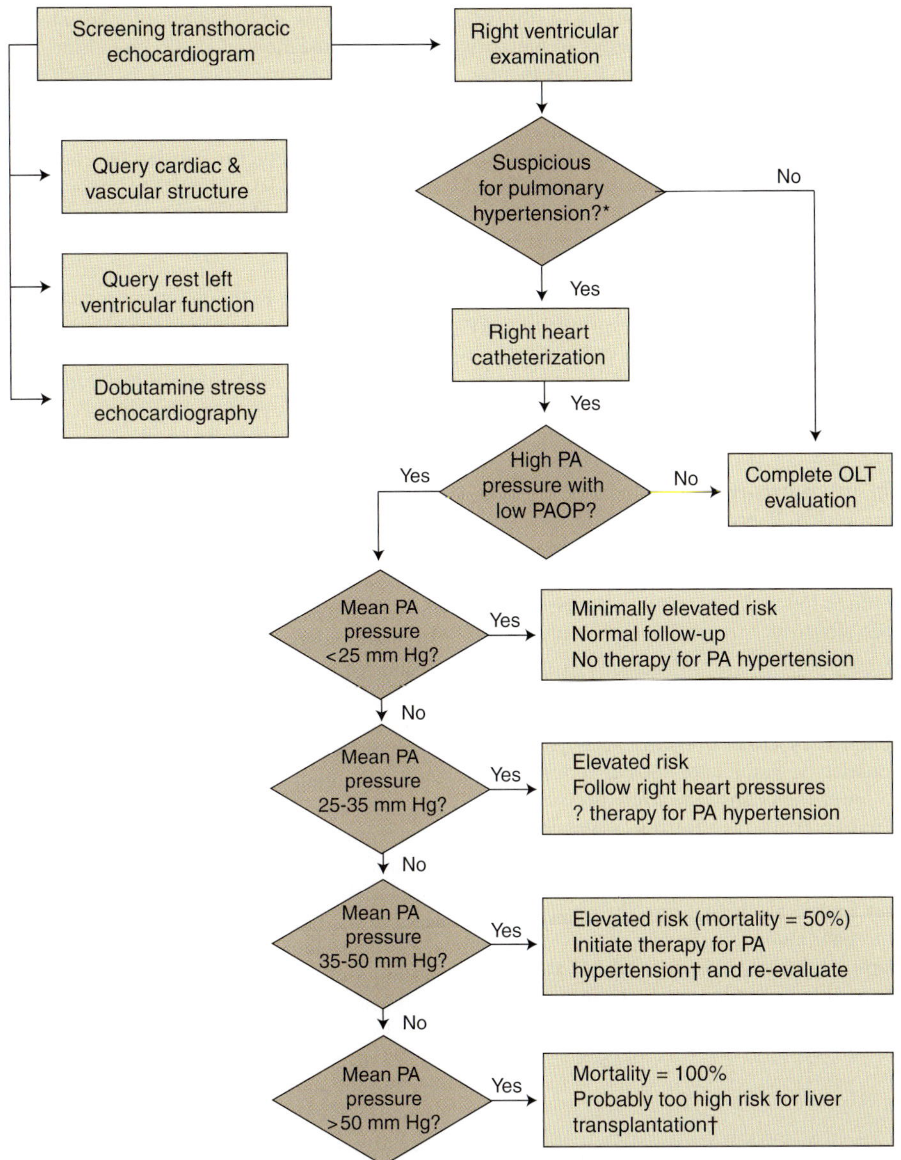

FIGURE 57-1. Suggested diagnostic paradigm to exclude or monitor pulmonary hypertension. Although there are many variations, it is important to complete the process with a detailed knowledge of the patient's pulmonary hemodynamics. Normal follow-up: repeat transthoracic echocardiogram or right heart catheterization 1 year after previous test. Elevated risk implies high risk of perioperative mortality (see text for details). OLT, orthotopic liver transplantation; PA, pulmonary artery; PAOP, pulmonary artery occlusion pressure.

Experience with pulmonary vasodilators is greatest with intravenous epoprostenol. Epoprostenol appears to be effective in reducing pulmonary artery pressures, although it can lead to splenomegaly.[57] Epoprostenol use was a more common feature of patients with pulmonary hypertension who survived liver transplantation than it was in nonsurvivors with the same degree of pulmonary hypertension, although the difference was not significant.[58] Unfortunately, intravenous epoprostenol requires continuous intravenous access for infusion, with all of the attendant complications of permanent venous access and pump failures.

The difficult logistics of continuous epoprostenol use have prompted a search for more convenient routes of administration and/or longer-lived prostaglandin analogues. For example, early reports indicate that continuous subcutaneous administration of treprostinil[59] reduces the symptoms of pulmonary hypertension and lowers pulmonary artery pressures. Oral beraprost[60] also reduces symptoms of pulmonary hypertension, but the reductions in pulmonary artery pressures were modest and did not achieve statistical significance despite a relatively large sample size. Inhaled iloprost reduces right heart pressures quickly and is easy to deploy (and should be pulmonary selective).[61-63] In a recent study looking at both acute and long-term effects of iloprost on hepatic and pulmonary function in patients with portopulmonary hypertension, pulmonary vasodilation was immediately improved in treated patients without altering hepatic hemodynamics. At 12 months of follow-up, patients were clinically improved with an increased exercise capacity.[64] It should be noted that none of the above-mentioned alternatives to intravenous epoprostenol produce more than a few millimeters of mercury reduction in the mean pulmonary artery pressure. Consequently, these drugs may have limited effectiveness in preparing patients with pulmonary hypertension for liver transplantation. Conversely, results from individual patients indicate that intravenous epoprostenol can lower the mean pulmonary artery pressure from approximately 50 to 25 mm Hg.[54,65]

The discovery that nitric oxide can induce pulmonary vasodilation has provided another approach to lowering pulmonary arterial pressures. Inhaled nitric oxide is a selective pulmonary vasodilator that lowers pulmonary artery pressures in patients with portopulmonary hypertension.[55] Nitric oxide administered by face mask can be used as a diagnostic tool to assess pulmonary artery pressure response to vasodilators during right heart catheterization.[66]

When pulmonary hypertension is discovered unexpectedly in the operating room (OR) at the beginning of a transplant, reversible causes of pulmonary hypertension, such as hypoventilation-induced hypercarbia, should be ruled out or reversed. **Figure 57-2** illustrates apparently severe pulmonary hypertension, with pulmonary pressures equal to the systemic pressure. Reversal of hypercarbia attributable to hypoventilation and lightening the anesthetic lowered the pulmonary pressures and raised the systemic pressures, after which the patient had an uneventful liver transplant.

When newly discovered apparent pulmonary hypertension does not respond to such simple maneuvers, inhaled nitric oxide may be very effective in lowering the pulmonary artery pressures acutely, without the systemic effects of a nonselective vasodilator such as epoprostenol. It is probably important to lower the pulmonary artery pressures (and consequently the central venous pressure) as effectively as possible, both to minimize hemorrhage and to avoid acute graft congestion that could cause early graft compromise in the OR.[45] It is also important to extend the treatment of pulmonary hypertension well into the postoperative period, as graft failure due to poor blood flow remains a concern. Thus as the patient moves toward extubation, it is necessary to transition from inhaled nitric oxide to an intravenous agent (eg, epoprostenol) or an oral agent (eg, sildenafil) as part of weaning from the ventilator, with the lowest achievable pulmonary artery pressure being the goal.

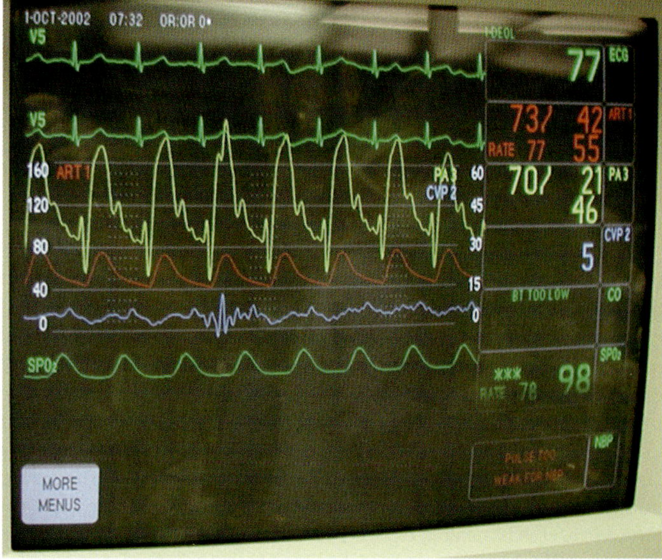

FIGURE 57-2. Pulmonary and systemic pressures immediately after pulmonary artery catheter placement during liver transplantation in a patient with pulmonary hypertension.

Sildenafil is an inhibitor of phosphodiesterase 5 (PDE5), which blocks degradation of cyclic guanosine monophosphate, the second messenger of nitric oxide. Sildenafil also produces selective pulmonary vasodilation.[67] There are early anecdotal reports of its use as a pulmonary vasodilator in pre–liver transplant patients.[68,69] Oral sildenafil is also a useful adjunct to inhaled iloprost, a prostacyclin analogue.[70] To date, there is far less evidence to support the efficacy of sildenafil, particularly as monotherapy, than there is for intravenous epoprostenol as therapy for portopulmonary hypertension, but early reports are encouraging.

In addition to PDE inhibitors, endothelin receptor antagonists have proven effective in treating pulmonary hypertension in patients with portopulmonary hypertension. Bosentan, an endothelin receptor antagonist, has been used successfully in lowering pulmonary artery (PA) pressures in this patient population.[71] Compared to iloprost, patients treated with bosentan had higher survival rates at 1, 2, and 3 years.[72] However, the use of bosentan in the treatment of pulmonary hypertension may not be effective in patients with concomitant heart failure.[73]

Hepatopulmonary Syndrome Hepatopulmonary syndrome is defined by the presence of hepatic dysfunction or portal hypertension, an elevated alveolar-arterial oxygen gradient, and intrapulmonary vasodilation.[74] Thus, although portopulmonary hypertension is associated with pulmonary vascular vasoconstriction, hepatopulmonary syndrome results from vasodilation and pulmonary vascular remodeling. Patients may present with digital clubbing, spider angiomata, arterial hypoxemia, and dyspnea that worsens upon moving from a recumbent to an upright position (orthodeoxia and platypnea).[74] Early diagnostic criteria required ruling out the presence of other cardiopulmonary abnormalities. However, it is now apparent that hepatopulmonary syndrome may contribute to hypoxemia even when other cardiopulmonary abnormalities are present.[75,76] Intrapulmonary vasodilation may reflect true anatomical shunt, physiologic shunt, and precapillary or capillary dilation, leading to alterations in oxygen diffusion.[77] Nitric oxide is elevated in the exhaled breath of patients with hepatopulmonary syndrome, suggesting a causative role.[78,79] Interestingly, there is a case report of normalization of exhaled nitric oxide accompanied by return to normoxia after liver transplantation.[79]

The diagnosis of hepatopulmonary syndrome depends on documenting the presence of arterial desaturation and pulmonary vasodilation in patients with liver disease. Other causes of hypoxia in patients with liver disease (**Box 57-5**) must be excluded. Pulse oximetry is a sensitive, noninvasive screening tool for detecting low arterial oxygen saturation, the results of which can be confirmed using arterial blood gas analysis and echocardiography.[80] Pulmonary vasodilation can be documented

BOX 57-5

Major Causes of Hypoxia in Patients With Liver Disease

- Ventilation–perfusion mismatching
  - Premature airway closure
  - Pulmonary vasodilation
  - Impaired hypoxic pulmonary vasoconstriction
  - Diffusion–perfusion deficit
  - Pulmonary emboli
- Compression of lung tissue
  - Impaired diaphragmatic function due to ascites
  - Pleural effusion
- Pulmonary edema
  - Pulmonary manifestations of specific liver disease (eg, α_1-antitrypsin deficiency)
- Acute exacerbations of intercurrent chronic lung disease

using a variety of modalities, including contrast echocardiography, lung perfusion scanning, or pulmonary artery catheterization.[45,81] During contrast echocardiography, late appearance (ie, 3-6 cardiac cycles) of contrast in the left heart suggests intrapulmonary shunting, whereas early appearance (immediate to 1 cardiac cycle) indicates intracardiac shunting.[45] Pulmonary angiography is rarely indicated but may be useful to exclude or embolize arteriovenous malformations causing large right-to-left shunts.[45] A flow chart outlining the assessment for hepatopulmonary syndrome is shown in **Fig. 57-3**.

There are no effective medical therapies for hepatopulmonary syndrome, although selective inhibition of nitric oxide production shows theoretical promise.[45,81] For patients with end-stage liver disease, liver transplantation frequently leads to reduced intrapulmonary shunting and improved oxygenation.[82] Transplantation in patients with hepatopulmonary syndrome is no riskier than transplantation in patients without hepatopulmonary syndrome, as the outcomes of transplantation are the same whether the recipients have the condition or not.[83,84] Among patients with hepatopulmonary syndrome, orthotopic liver transplantation leads to longer survival than medical management without transplantation.[85] Furthermore, cirrhotic patients with hepatopulmonary syndrome are more likely to die with medical therapy alone (as opposed to transplantation) than matched cirrhotic control patients without hepatopulmonary syndrome.[85,86] However, it is important to transplant hepatopulmonary syndrome patients early; delaying transplant until patients are profoundly hypoxemic is associated with mortality as high as 30%.[87,88]

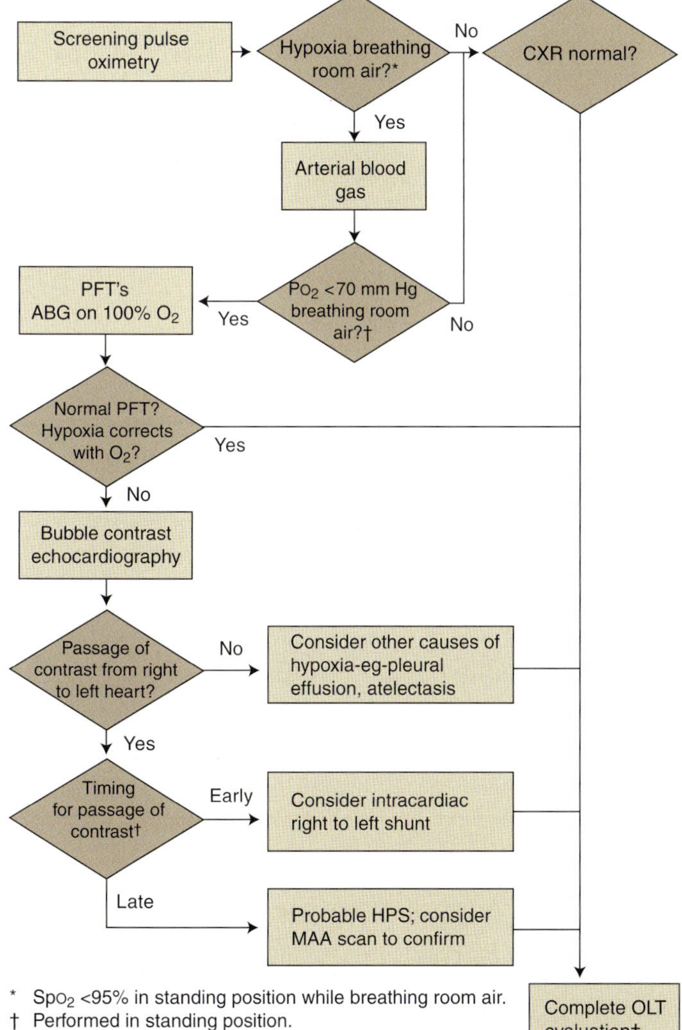

FIGURE 57-3. Diagnostic algorithm for hepatopulmonary syndrome. Some centers extend this algorithm by the routine performance of 99Tc macroaggregated albumin scanning, which is very sensitive to intrapulmonary shunts when other possible right-to-left shunts have been excluded. Screening pulse oximetry should be carried out at every clinic visit and at least annually, as development of hepatopulmonary syndrome shortens life expectancy and is accorded additional MELD points when discovered. ABG, arterial blood gas; CXR, chest x-ray; HPS, hepatopulmonary syndrome; MAA, 99Tc macroaggregated albumin; OLT, orthotopic liver transplantation; PFTs, pulmonary function tests.

THE NERVOUS SYSTEM IN LIVER DISEASE

Hepatic Encephalopathy It is generally believed that the cause of hepatic encephalopathy (HE) is multifactorial. Elevated ammonia levels are frequently but not always found in patients with HE, and it is traditionally believed that ammonemia plays a role in its development. Patients with higher gut-ammonia levels have an increased incidence of HE, and those patients with delayed gastric emptying secondary to diabetes mellitus have more severe HE as compared to nondiabetic cirrhotic patients.[89] Activation of γ-aminobutyric acid (GABA) receptors in the brain may also contribute to HE, as evidenced by the ability of the $GABA_A$-receptor-antagonist flumazenil to produce a short-term improvement in HE.[90,91] Interestingly, ammonia has been shown to enhance GABAergic currents, perhaps explaining its role in HE.[92] In animal models examining GABA modulation in hepatic encephalopathy, chronic hyperammonemia in rats is associated with increased GABAergic tone in the cerebellum with resultant cognitive impairment, and GABAergic tone in the cortex is decreased.[93] Hepatic encephalopathy resembles many other nonfocal neurologic conditions (**Box 57-6**) from which it must be differentiated. Many of these occur as comorbid conditions in patients with liver failure. The severity of encephalopathy contributes to the Child-Turcotte-Pugh system for stratifying the severity of hepatic disease, as described in Chapter 15.

Autonomic Neuropathy Autonomic neuropathies are found in up to 50% of patients with chronic liver disease.[94,95] This is most commonly manifested as impaired cardiovascular function[95] and gastric motility.[96] In addition, patients with autonomic neuropathies experience a higher incidence of hypotension during general anesthesia.[97] More importantly, autonomic neuropathy predicts increased mortality in cirrhotic patients relative to cirrhotic controls without autonomic neuropathy.[98] The development of autonomic neuropathies is not dependent on the etiology of the liver disease, and studies have not consistently found a correlation between the severity of liver disease and the incidence of autonomic neuropathies. Importantly, autonomic neuropathies resolve with the return of normal liver function after transplantation.[95,99]

BOX 57-6

Conditions Resembling Hepatic Encephalopathy

- Metabolic problems
  - Hypoglycemia
  - Hyponatremia
  - Hypernatremia
- Intracranial processes
  - Subdural hematoma
  - Intracranial hemorrhage
  - Intracranial mass lesion
- Infectious diseases
  - Meningitis

HEPATIC RESECTION

INDICATIONS AND PATIENT CHARACTERISTICS

Hepatic resection is performed to remove lesions in the liver by resecting either an entire hepatic lobe, 1 or more anatomic segments of the liver, or nonanatomic wedges of liver tissue. Such operations were first reported in the 1950s and for the next 30 years were considered to be high risk. For example, the rate of mortality from hepatic resection reported in 1977 was 13% to 20%, depending on the extent of the resection.[100] Many of these deaths were due to hemorrhage. However, during the 1990s improved surgical and anesthesia techniques, along with a growing operative experience and an increased ability to plan resections, have reduced perioperative mortality. The current perioperative mortality for hepatic resections performed in high-volume centers is estimated to be 1% to 7%.[101-105] In addition, multiple trends in morbidity and mortality are developing. In 1 center, the number of hepatic segments resected declined during the 1990s, and a concomitant decline in mortality has been demonstrated.[101] At the same time, high-volume centers performing hepatic resections are liberalizing their acceptance criteria for patients, operating on older patients with more comorbid illnesses, including liver dysfunction, all while sustaining reductions in morbidity and mortality.[105] Advanced age (ie, >70 years) is no longer a contraindication to hepatic resection for primary hepatocellular carcinoma or for metastases from other cancers.[106-108] Furthermore, even patients with significant cirrhosis and liver dysfunction tolerate hepatic resections, in part because operative approaches now allow shorter hepatic ischemic time and the removal of less liver tissue, all while achieving satisfactory surgical margins.[109] Even in patients with cirrhosis, morbidity from hepatic resections ranges from 20% to 50% (comparable with that reported in noncirrhotic cohorts), and mortality ranges from 0% to 10%.[109]

Long-term outcomes after hepatic resection are also reasonable: after resection of hepatocellular carcinoma, the 3-year survival ranges from 40% to 70%, whereas 5-year survival ranges from 40% to 50%.[109] Even hepatic resections for metastatic cancer (eg, colon) have 1-, 3-, and 5-year survival rates of 90%, 54%, and 34%, respectively.[110]

Most patients present for hepatic resection due to malignancy (**Box 57-7**). In the United States, approximately 90% of patients in 1 large series had a malignancy; 69% of these were metastatic lesions, and 80% of these were colorectal in origin, making metastatic colon cancer the leading cause for hepatic resection.[101] In Asia, the ratio of malignant to benign indications for hepatic resection is similar, but three-fourths of the malignancies are hepatocellular carcinoma,[105] reflecting the regional heterogeneity of the distribution of this cancer. Together, these 2 studies report on more than 3000 patients undergoing hepatic resection between roughly 1990 and 2000.[101,105] With such large numbers it was possible for the authors to conduct multivariate analyses to detect factors associated with increased risk of morbidity and mortality in the perioperative period after hepatic resection. Multivariate analysis yielded the following factors associated with elevated morbidity: blood loss, number of hepatic segments resected, added major biliary procedure, low preoperative albumin, presence of 1 or more comorbid conditions, male gender, elevated serum creatinine, added major vascular procedure, and thrombocytopenia.[101,105] Risk factors for elevated mortality include blood loss, number of segments resected, preoperative bilirubin, complex hepatic resection, preoperative platelet count, low preoperative albumin, and patient age.[101,105]

Currently, most hepatic resections are performed for cancer. However, the major modes of therapy are in flux. State-of-the-art therapy for hepatocellular carcinoma includes radiofrequency ablation, hepatic resection, or orthotopic liver transplantation, depending on the number, size, and location of the lesions. Thus minimally invasive destructive therapies may significantly reduce the need for major hepatectomy in future.[109]

BOX 57-7

Potentially Resectable Hepatic Lesions

- Benign lesions
  - Hemangioma
  - Focal nodular hyperplasia
  - Liver cell adenoma
  - Cysts
  - Hydatid disease
- Malignant lesions
  - Primary hepatobiliary cancers
    - Hepatocellular
    - Cholangiocarcinoma
    - Hepatoblastoma
    - Angiosarcoma
    - Lymphoma
  - Cancers with local invasion of liver
    - Gall bladder and extrahepatic bile ducts
    - Colon
    - Stomach
    - Duodenum
    - Adrenal
  - Metastatic cancers
    - From possibly "isolated hepatic" spread
      - Colorectal
      - Rectum
      - Pancreatic islet cell
      - Carcinoid
      - Sarcoma
    - From possibly widespread metastases
      - Lung
      - Breast
      - Esophagus
      - Stomach
      - Pancreas
      - Other GI tract
      - Melanoma

OPERATIVE CONSIDERATIONS FOR HEPATIC RESECTION

After the incision for hepatic resection, the abdomen is explored for metastases. If previously unsuspected widely metastatic disease is found, the operation ends quickly. Therefore, large doses of long-acting opioids and paralyzing agents should be avoided in the initial stage of surgery. If a large volume of ascites is drained immediately after the incision, hemodynamic instability may ensue due to sudden shifts of fluid out of the intravascular system with a resultant drop in central venous pressure (CVP). Often, treatment with crystalloid or colloid replacement may be warranted to correct profound hypotension.

After the initial exploration, a self-retaining retractor (Bookwalter or equivalent) is placed to ensure good exposure. The placement of the retractor itself can depress splanchnic venous return and compromise respiratory mechanics by compressing the lung and overlying ribs.

The liver is dissected free of its attachments as needed to gain exposure, first to establish control of the vasculature and then to complete

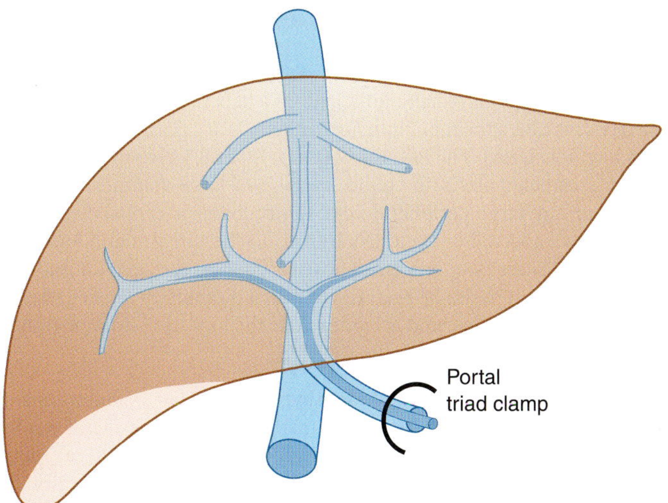

FIGURE 57-4. Location of vascular clamp for the classic "Pringle" maneuver, in which the portal vein (purple) and hepatic artery (red) inflows to the liver are temporarily occluded to reduce blood loss during hepatic resections. The liver is still exposed to the vascular system by the hepatic veins (blue) draining into the inferior vena cava. Thus bleeding is strongly influenced by the central venous pressure.

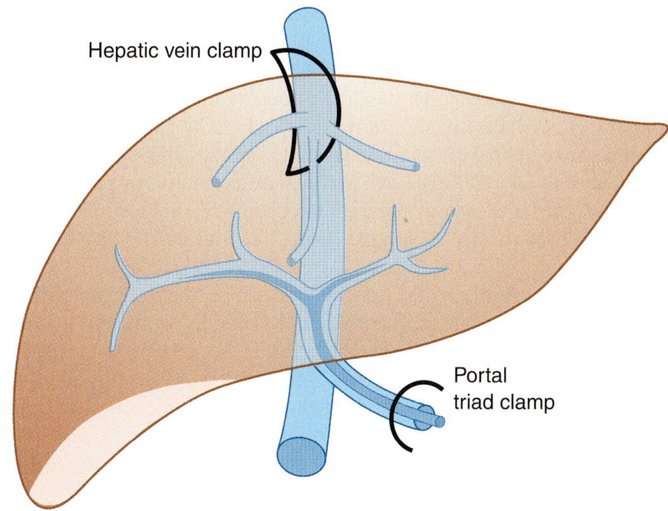

FIGURE 57-6. Total vascular exclusion of the liver with preservation of vena cava flow. The portal vein (purple) and hepatic artery (red) inflows to the liver are temporarily occluded. Additionally, the hepatic veins (blue) are clamped to exclude the liver from the central venous circulation. Hepatic venous clamping can involve the entire liver or only the territory to be resected.

the hepatic resection. This involves moving the liver to gain exposure to the vascular structures underneath, which may twist the liver on its vascular pedicle or compress the vena cava, both leading to sudden changes in venous return with consequent hemodynamic effects. Careful observation of the surgical field and good communication between surgeon and anesthesiologist are essential. After gaining vascular control, the surgeon usually attempts to create anatomic planes (ie, ones that will bleed relatively little) between liver segments, or a dissection for a formal hepatic lobectomy is performed. Again, discussion with the surgeon prior to incision as to whether an anatomic or nonanatomic resection is planned is an essential component of the anesthetic plan.

It is important to understand the techniques for hepatic vascular occlusion during hepatic resection, as uncontrolled and massive blood loss is still a major risk of the operation. There are multiple hepatic vascular occlusion techniques, each with implications for the anesthesiologist.[111] These are illustrated in **Figs. 57-4 through 57-6**. In one common

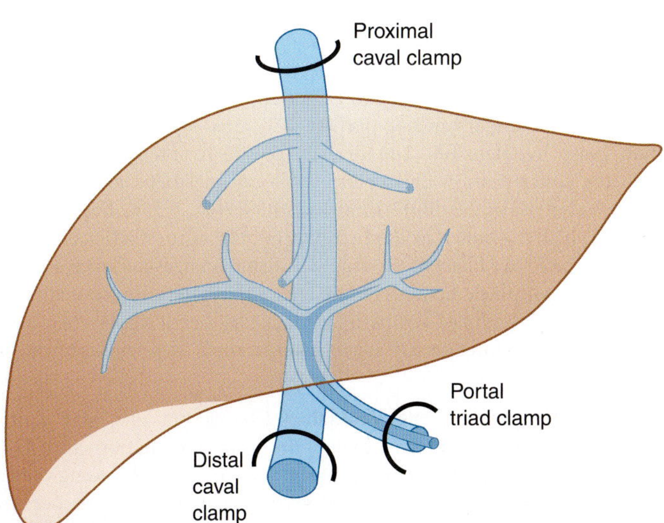

FIGURE 57-5. Total vascular exclusion of the liver. The portal vein (purple) and hepatic artery (red) inflows to the liver are temporarily occluded. Additionally, the inferior vena cava (blue) is cross-clamped above and below the hepatic veins to exclude the liver from the central venous circulation.

vascular exclusion maneuver, a clamp is placed on the portal triad. In this case, "portal triad" encompasses the hepatic artery, portal vein, and the common bile duct (Fig. 57-4).

Total vascular exclusion techniques allow "bloodless" surgery. In addition to clamping the portal triad, clamps are placed on the inferior vena cava above and below the liver (Fig. 57-5). This combination of clamps prevents both inflow of blood and backflow from the vena cava. In one report using total vascular exclusion, the average red cell transfusion was 2.2 units.[112] Selective techniques have been described for total vascular exclusion in which the hepatic veins are clamped rather than the inferior vena cava.[113] Portal triad clamping is accompanied by venous outflow clamping of either all of the hepatic veins or only those draining the resected territory (Fig. 57-6). In the report mentioned previously, most patients received no transfusion.[113] Vascular exclusion techniques were first described by Pringle and are collectively described as the "Pringle maneuver." During vascular exclusion, the liver is warm and ischemic, so great attention is paid to keeping track of and minimizing "Pringle time." In a study comparing the Pringle maneuver with hemihepatic vascular inflow occlusion and main portal vein occlusion techniques, the Pringle maneuver was performed in a significantly shorter period of time, but postoperative liver recovery was better in both the hemihepatic and main portal occlusion techniques.[114]

At the conclusion of the resection, hemostasis is obtained and the incision is closed. These portions of the procedure can be lengthy and deserve attention, as control of hemorrhage is the key to a successful early postoperative period. During the latter phases of the operation, the anesthesia team should make plans for postoperative disposition, either to the recovery room or to an intensive care unit (ICU) if the insult from surgery has been severe.

ANESTHESIA FOR HEPATIC RESECTION

Anesthesia for hepatic resection is appropriately changing over time and corresponds to the improvements in surgical technique and changes in patient selection.[115,116] In general, patients scheduled for a hepatic resection should be evaluated as any patient scheduled for major noncardiac surgery. Plans for monitoring, vascular access, induction and maintenance of anesthesia, postoperative pain control, and postoperative care should take into account a large subcostal incision and the potential for sudden massive hemorrhage and severe physiologic derangements during and after surgery.

The history and physical examination includes a typical preanesthetic history, including questions directed to assess hepatic synthetic function, as well as global and focal neurologic status. For example, evidence of hepatic encephalopathy should be sought, both from the patient and any escorts present. Significant encephalopathy predicts worsened postoperative neurologic status if a hepatic resection or portal diversion is planned. Focal neurologic deficits (ie, sensory, motor, or pain abnormalities localized to a body part) should be sought and documented, as the procedures require prolonged immobility and positioning injuries may occur.

The assessment of cardiac ischemia risk cannot be overemphasized, as hepatic resections are frequently characterized by significant hemorrhage, leading to hypotension and tachycardia that may persist for some time as the anesthesia team restores intravascular volume. In addition to derangements in myocardial oxygen supply and demand during the case, the surgical stress induces a proinflammatory state. Major liver resection also leads to a hyperdynamic state with increased cardiac output and decreased systemic vascular resistance in the postoperative period.[117,118] Thus the patient should be questioned in detail about risk factors pertaining to coronary artery disease as well as his or her level of physical activity and exercise tolerance. Symptoms of angina or anginal equivalents should be carefully sought.

The laboratory examination prior to hepatic resection includes an assessment of hepatic synthetic function (albumin, clotting factors as assessed by prothrombin time [PT], partial thromboplastin time [PTT], and fibrinogen measurement), metabolic function (aspartate aminotransferase [AST], alanine aminotransferase [ALT]), and excretory function (bilirubin). Assessment of coagulation function (PT, PTT, platelet count), oxygen-carrying capacity (hematocrit), and serum electrolytes completes the general picture of the patient. It is useful to obtain a chest x-ray to assess lung volumes and the status of the lung parenchyma and to search for preoperative pleural effusions (common in patients with significant liver disease, but rare in others).

Preoperatively, it may be useful to obtain a transthoracic echocardiogram to assess resting atrial and ventricular function and valve performance, and to exclude (within the power of this relatively noninvasive test) septal defects that might allow paradoxical embolization. As mentioned previously, cardiac risk stratification begins with careful history taking but should include functional testing indicated by the history and the guidelines of the American Heart Association.[119]

Preanesthetic Planning Hepatic resections are almost always performed in supine position through a right-sided subcostal incision, although smaller resections may be approached initially via mini laparotomies in conjunction with laparoscopic instrumentation. There may be extensions either into the left subcostal region, superiorly in the midline, or both. The area of the surgical prep usually includes the entire abdomen and the lower chest up to the nipples. Monitor placement, warming strategies, and pain management planning should account for this.

Typical monitoring consists of standard monitors and selected invasive monitors directed toward managing problems likely to arise during the case. An arterial catheter is useful for early recognition of hypotension and for obtaining blood samples. Central venous pressure measurement is useful to guide intravascular volume replacement and to assess right heart pressures when a large hepatic resection is planned or when the dissection is expected to be bloody. If a low CVP technique is planned, CVP monitoring is essential. Central venous access has the added benefit of providing a conduit for potent vasopressor administration. A pulmonary artery catheter is useful for measuring pulmonary artery pressures, assessing left heart filling pressures, and guiding pharmacologic therapy. Transesophageal echocardiography can also provide information regarding both intravascular volume status and cardiac performance, and may replace invasive pressure measurements if the potential need for central venous access as a conduit for vasopressors is judged to be low.

Peripheral vascular access with sufficiently large catheters (eg, 14 gauge or larger) is usually sufficient for a hepatic resection. One helpful device is called the rapid infusion catheter (RIC, Arrow International, Reading, PA, USA). The RIC is a 6.4 cm × 7.0 or 8.5 French peripherally inserted catheter useful for rapid infusion of large volumes. It can be placed in any large peripheral vein. Antecubital or cephalic veins are commonly chosen, but even distal veins on the forearm and hand can be used if they are large enough. The RIC alleviates the need for multiple central lines that might be required to pass a pulmonary artery catheter, run multiple infusions, and accommodate the high-flow administration of large volumes.

Induction and Maintenance of Anesthesia Induction of anesthesia is readily accomplished using standard methods. Major considerations for induction are directed toward comorbidities (gastroesophageal reflux disease, coronary artery disease, etc) rather than any unique feature of the liver disease. Patients with ascites should be considered to have a full stomach and receive a rapid-sequence induction with cricoid pressure, if not otherwise contraindicated.

Maintenance of anesthesia is also by standard methods, with attention to homeostatic control. Patient warming is important to maintain good clotting performance and to minimize the risk of surgical site infection.[120,121] A single forced-air warming unit applied to the upper chest, arms, and head is usually sufficient, although underbody warming may be preferred. Intravenous fluids should either be warm or be actively warmed during infusion.

As large hepatic resections may produce transient hepatic dysfunction, it may be preferable to choose drugs whose elimination is not completely dependent on hepatic metabolism. In general, all usual techniques for the maintenance of general anesthesia are acceptable, although there are some minor differences between drugs commonly chosen for maintenance. Compared with isoflurane, sevoflurane was associated with smaller elevations in liver enzymes after hepatic segmentectomy.[122] These were of uncertain clinical relevance, as no clinical liver damage was detected in either group. However, later comparison between sevoflurane and desflurane showed desflurane to be superior to sevoflurane in terms of postoperative hepatic and renal function at equipotent doses of 1 minimum alveolar concentration (MAC).[123] *Cis*-atracurium, atracurium, and remifentanyl might be more reliably eliminated than drugs that depend on hepatic hydrolysis and/or conjugation for termination of their effect. In practice, the dose-to-effect mode of administration is almost always sufficient to minimize the interaction between choice of anesthetic and the effect of liver resection.

If an epidural catheter has been inserted, it may be used intraoperatively with the understanding that the associated sympathetic blockade may cause hypotension. The severity of the hypotension correlates with the concentration and volume of local anesthetic administered. Conversely, relatively dilute local anesthetic (eg, 0.25% bupivacaine, 7-10 mL/h after a bolus) or dilute mixtures of local anesthetic combined with an opioid are likely to provide significant analgesia during general anesthesia, with little hemodynamic effect. If hypotension results from local anesthetic-induced sympathetic blockade, then it can be effectively treated with an infusion of a vasopressor such as phenylephrine or norepinephrine.

Goals for Oxygenation and Ventilation Changes in FIO_2 and ventilation predictably result in changes in liver oxygenation and CO_2 elimination.[124] Vascular exclusion techniques to reduce bleeding create periods of hepatic ischemia. Thus it seems prudent to provide normal systemic conditions by ventilating to keep the pH normal and the oxygen saturation high so that the liver is best prepared to tolerate these insults.

Hemodynamics Clamping the portal triad reduces venous return, and one would expect cardiac output and blood pressure to fall. Cardiac output does indeed fall, but the blood pressure increases due to an increase in systemic vascular resistance evoked by portal triad clamping. This appears to be a neurally mediated reflex, as the increase in systemic vascular resistance can be ablated by infiltrating the portal triad with lidocaine prior to clamping.[125] In contrast to portal triad clamping, total vascular exclusion of the liver via a vena cava cross clamp does reduce blood pressure concomitant with a fall in cardiac output because the loss of venous return is so much larger.

Bleeding and Coagulation Blood loss is affected by central venous pressure during surgery. When central venous pressure is maintained below 5 cm H_2O, blood loss is predictably lower than when central venous pressure is 6 cm H_2O or greater. In the original publication describing low central venous pressure approaches to hepatic resection, the median blood loss was only 200 mL, with most patients in the low central venous pressure study group avoiding transfusion.[126] In contrast, when the central venous pressure was 6 cm H_2O or greater, the median blood loss was 1 L, and half of the patients required transfusion.[126] Other centers practicing low central venous pressure techniques for hepatic resection report average estimated blood losses of about 1 L.[104]

Low central venous pressure approaches affect outcomes beyond transfusion and blood loss, as reflected in longer hospital stays for patients whose central venous pressure was greater than 6 cm H_2O during hepatic resection.[127] Blood loss (and the subsequent requirement for transfusion) is associated with longer hospitalization, greater perioperative morbidity, and a doubling of the perioperative mortality (from 1.2% to 2.5%).[110] Authors in the surgical literature caution that extreme care must be taken during the dissection of the liver so as not to make holes in the hepatic veins, which can lead to catastrophic hemorrhage or air embolism.[128] Obviously, the risk of severe air embolism is elevated under low central venous pressure conditions, and the anesthesia team must be highly vigilant for such an event.

Low central venous pressure anesthesia is apparently safe with respect to renal function, as only 3% of patients experience any degree of permanent renal dysfunction after hepatic resection using a low central venous pressure technique.[104] This was lower than the historical incidence of renal failure complicating hepatic resection without the use of low central venous pressure.[104] However, these favorable outcomes are predicated on maintaining good renal perfusion pressure (typically believed to be 60 mm Hg or more) and renal blood flow throughout surgery.[116] In a recent study evaluating the effects of β-adrenergic agents on liver oxygenation during hepatectomy, patients receiving low-dose dopamine (4 mcg/kg/min) had improved hepatic oxygen supply and uptake as compared to controls during hepatectomy with low CVP technique.[129]

Control of Clotting Multiple drugs that modify clotting are available to minimize blood loss during hepatic resection. Pharmacologic aids to minimize blood loss are attractive given the concerns regarding transfusion in cancer surgery, but they are no substitute for good surgical technique. A complete discussion of the use of procoagulants during liver surgery appears in the section Liver Transplantation. Briefly, 3 classes of agents are available: those that modify platelet and von Willebrand factor function (desmopressin and its analogues), the antifibrinolytics (aprotinin, ε-aminocaproic acid, and tranexamic acid), and direct replacement of specific clotting factors (eg, recombinant factor VII).

Desmopressin increases factor levels and improves laboratory measures of clotting during hepatectomy but has no effect on blood loss.[130] The antifibrinolytic drug aprotinin reduces blood loss during elective liver resection,[131] as demonstrated in a small prospective trial. However, a large multicenter outcome study comparing aprotinin with the other antifibrinolytics and placebo in cardiac surgery demonstrated that the drug is not superior to ε-aminocaproic acid or tranexamic acid for reducing blood loss.[132] Aprotinin is, however, associated with excess renal failure and mortality compared with the other alternatives in cardiac surgery.[132] Therefore, routine use of aprotinin during hepatic resection must be questioned until studies demonstrating its safety in large numbers of hepatectomy patients appear. Recombinant factor VII does not reduce blood loss or transfusion requirements in patients undergoing major hepatic resections,[133] but off-label use of this drug has been associated with unwanted thrombotic complications.[134]

Postoperative Planning Postoperative planning after hepatectomy addresses 3 major concerns: immediate postsurgical airway management, postoperative disposition, and pain management.

Assessment of the airway after surgery and planning for extubation are guided by the same considerations as applied to any major case with the potential for large volume shifts and with a high abdominal incision. First, the magnitude of the operation and the patient's preoperative functional status are inventoried, followed by the magnitude of hemorrhage and the adequacy of its replacement, manifested by hemodynamic stability and acid–base status. Factors within the anesthesiologist's control (ie, patient temperature, sedation, residual general anesthetics, and muscle strength) are considered. A physical examination of the face and upper airway assesses the degree of edema and swelling that might compromise the extubated airway. If all of these considerations are judged to be in satisfactory order, then it is reasonable to extubate the trachea at the end of a hepatic resection; otherwise, the prudent course is a period of postoperative airway protection and support with mechanical ventilation.

Postoperative disposition is dictated by the patient's clinical condition. The same considerations that bore upon the decision to extubate the trachea apply to planning for disposition. A patient who has had an uncomplicated operation and uneventful extubation may be managed in the recovery room and discharged to the hospital floor. Intubated patients and those with important postoperative concerns should be managed in an intensive care unit. Additionally, patients who have received large-bore central access for the hepatectomy may not be candidates for transfer to non-ICU settings, necessitating change or removal of the catheter used prior to discharge to the floor.

Analgesic requirements for patients after hepatic resection deserve careful consideration. Subcostal incisions are typically quite painful, and ineffective pain therapy will reduce the patient's ability to comply with postoperative pulmonary recruitment maneuvers and early ambulation. Regional anesthesia (eg, epidural catheter) added to general anesthesia provides superior early postoperative pain control.[135] This must be balanced against the potential for postoperative hepatic synthetic failure and coagulopathy complicating subsequent removal of the epidural catheter. In 2 separate studies evaluating the use of epidural catheters in patients undergoing hepatectomy, 727 total patients safely received epidurals for perioperative analgesia without increased complications, although the use of epidural analgesia was related to an increased use of red blood cells in 1 study.[136,137] Despite the potential risks, many practitioners opt to place the epidural catheter and monitor patients carefully for signs and symptoms of epidural hematoma.

COMPLICATIONS DURING HEPATIC RESECTION

Intraoperative complications of hepatic resection can almost always be ultimately traced to excessive blood loss. Bleeding can result either from poor hemostatic control or coagulopathy. Coagulopathy rarely ensues during hepatic resection unless the patient had tenuous liver function at the start, the hemorrhage is severe, or patient warming has been inadequate. Reversible causes of coagulopathy should be sought and corrected and the circulating blood volume supported by infusions of crystalloids, colloids, and transfusion as appropriate.

Air embolism is another common complication. Air embolism during hepatic resection (as well as transplantation) is problematic because it alters pulmonary vascular resistance, right heart performance, and left heart filling. The pathophysiology of venous air embolism has been studied in dogs.[138] Slow entrainment of air (ie, rates of

0.01-2.0 mL/kg/min), as might occur during surgery with small sites of venous opening, causes a progressive rise in central venous pressure, an early abrupt rise in pulmonary arterial pressure to a hypertensive plateau, and an unexplained decline in systemic vascular resistance. Air irritates the vascular endothelium, with resulting pulmonary edema, hypoxia, and reduced pulmonary compliance. Bolus infusion of air (ie, 1-13 mL/kg in a sudden bolus), as might occur with a major tear in the vena cava, causes increased central venous pressure. Because air fills the right ventricle, pulmonary and systemic pressures plummet, and cardiovascular collapse ensues.[138]

Air embolism is apparently a complication of many hepatic resections, although it is not always symptomatic. Some procedural approaches that may be advantageous from a surgical perspective may not be ideal from the anesthetist's viewpoint. For example, when comparing techniques for parenchymal dissection of the liver, the Cavitron ultrasonic aspirator (CUSA) is associated with less blood loss[139] than a clamp-and-crush method. However, all CUSA patients had air emboli during hepatectomy, and in 44% of these, the air filled more than half of the right ventricle. Air emboli occurred in 68% of patients having clamp-and-crush hepatic resection as well, but to a much smaller extent. None of these emboli had pulmonary or hemodynamic effects on the patients, but this study suggests that air embolism is so common as to be considered ubiquitous during hepatic resection. Gas embolism from other commonly used devices, such as argon beam coagulators, has been described, in this instance with a fatal outcome.[140]

Air embolism is also problematic during liver surgery and transplantation because of the risk of catastrophic paradoxical embolism.[141] Paradoxical embolism need not occur through an intracardiac right-to-left defect. Many patients presenting for hepatic resection (and certainly most liver transplant patients) have cirrhosis, and many cirrhotic patients have abnormal arteriovenous connections in the pulmonary circulation. Thus venous air embolism should be minimized to lower the risk of paradoxical embolus. Massive venous embolism and/or paradoxical embolus must be high on the differential diagnosis of unexplained cardiopulmonary performance problems during hepatic resection. **Figure 57-7** shows the hemodynamic consequences of a large venous air embolism during a liver transplant. The first indication is an abrupt fall in end-tidal CO_2 (black trace), followed a few moments later by rising pulmonary artery pressure (yellow trace). Systemic hypotension ensued (red trace). Inferior and lateral (see inset) ST-segment elevations accompanied systemic hypotension, caused either by coronary hypoperfusion or by air in the coronary circulation. The circuit gas composition (green trace) was changed to 100% oxygen to minimize the size of the gas bubbles. Cardiac output (orange rectangles) fell by 50% after the embolus.

Some practitioners recommend conducting hepatic surgery with the OR table in a 15-degree head-down tilt to prevent embolized air from migrating cephalad,[142] but this may interfere with surgical exposure and may contribute to head and neck edema. If air embolism occurs, ventilation with 100% oxygen should be instituted. In severe embolism, placing the patient in the left lateral decubitus position with the head down may shift the gas bubble away from the right ventricular outflow tract and restore cardiac output. A central line placed into the right atrium can be used to aspirate gas from the heart. These measures must be undertaken while other supportive measures, including cardiopulmonary resuscitation (CPR) and fluid/pressor administration, are being continued. Cardiopulmonary bypass has been used successfully in resuscitation from gas embolism and should be considered if initial measures are unsuccessful.[143]

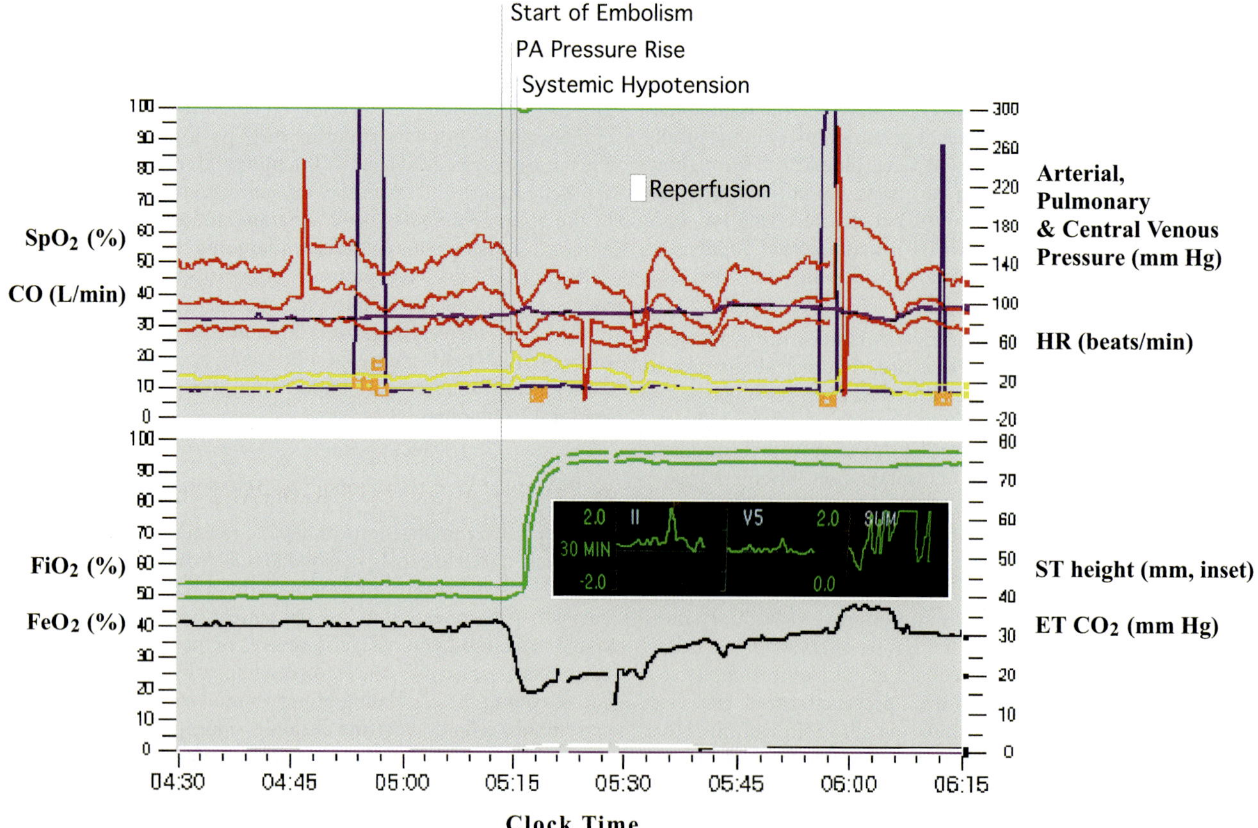

FIGURE 57-7. Screen shot of automated anesthesia information management system trend display marked by accidental venous air embolism. The inset (black) shows a trend display of the electrocardiographic ST segments, demonstrating inferior and lateral ST elevations.

LIVER TRANSPLANTATION

INDICATIONS, CONTRAINDICATIONS, AND PATIENT CHARACTERISTICS

The indications for liver transplantation are myriad in detail (**Box 57-8**) but all come down to liver failure sufficiently severe to preclude further survival without transplantation.

The most common indication for liver transplantation is chronic hepatocellular disease due to alcohol and/or hepatitis. Hepatitis C is an increasingly important indication for liver transplantation, representing a unique and growing health risk for anesthesiologists who provide care for these patients. There is currently no vaccine against hepatitis C, and medical therapy is suboptimal. Thus the most effective protection from the disease is to avoid exposure.

Hepatitis B and C both predispose patients to hepatocellular carcinoma. As the prevalence of hepatitis C in the population increases, so does the incidence of hepatocellular carcinoma. Thus this tumor is becoming increasingly common as an indication for liver transplantation.

As surgical techniques, risk stratification of potential recipients, and the management of intercurrent diseases (eg, HIV infection) all improve, the contraindications to liver transplantation are becoming more nuanced. For example, advanced age is not necessarily considered a contraindication to transplantation. Instead, elderly patients are assessed using sophisticated testing of cardiopulmonary performance and rigorous assessment of nutritional status, body mass index, and exercise tolerance. **Box 57-9** provides a general list of contraindications to liver transplantation, but each patient must be evaluated as an individual with many extenuating and complicating factors considered.

Patients with fulminant hepatic failure require particular attention, as their status with respect to contraindications to transplantation may change on a daily or even hourly basis. As mentioned previously, acute infection is common in patients with fulminant hepatic failure but should be actively sought (or at least there should be a high index of suspicion) in any candidate who is high on the recipient list because acute infection is a clear contraindication to transplantation. Brain herniation (portending brain death) is another clear contraindication to transplantation. In critically ill, comatose transplant candidates, herniation is always a possibility, yet transplantation may avert this disastrous outcome. Incipient brain herniation is commonly assessed by serial head computed tomography (CT) or, ideally, by intracranial

BOX 57-8

Indications for Liver Transplantation (Not Exhaustive)

- End-stage liver disease (chronic)
  - Hepatocellular disease
    - Chronic viral hepatitis (mostly hepatitis C)
    - Alcoholic liver disease
    - "Cryptogenic" cirrhosis
    - Chronic drug-induced liver disease
  - Cholestatic disease
    - Primary sclerosing cholangitis
    - Primary biliary cirrhosis
    - Biliary atresia (mostly children)
    - Other familial cholestatic syndromes
  - Vascular disease
    - Budd-Chiari syndrome
    - Venooclusive disease
  - Polycystic liver disease
- Hepatic malignancies not amenable to other therapy
  - Hepatocellular carcinoma (often in setting of hepatitis C)
  - Cholangiocarcinoma
  - Carcinoid tumor
  - Other cancers (eg, insulinoma)
- Fulminant hepatic failure
  - Drug induced
  - Acute viral hepatitis (A, B, C, delta)
  - Metabolic diseases
    - Wilson disease, organic acidurias, others
- Metabolic diseases affecting the liver
  - α_1-Antitrypsin deficiency
  - Wilson disease
  - Hemochromatosis
    - Other rare diseases (eg, Alagille syndrome, glycogen storage diseases, urea cycle deficiencies)

BOX 57-9

Contraindications to Liver Transplantation

- Absolute contraindications
  - Brain herniation/brain death
  - Sepsis outside the hepatobiliary tree (ie, peritonitis)
  - Metastatic hepatobiliary tumors
  - Current extrahepatic malignancy
  - Advanced cardiopulmonary disease
    - Unrevascularized ischemic coronary disease
    - Recent drug-eluting stent placement
    - Critical aortic stenosis
    - Severe pulmonary hypertension (mean PA pressure >45 mm Hg)
  - AIDS (but not HIV infection)
- Relative contraindications
  - Obesity (BMI >30)
  - Moderate pulmonary hypertension (mean PA pressure >35 mm Hg)
  - Mild or moderate aortic stenosis
  - Revascularized coronary artery disease with depressed cardiac function
  - Advanced chronic renal failure
  - Severe hyponatremia
  - Portal vein thrombosis
  - Hepatitis: HBsAg or HBeAg positive
  - Prior open vascular portosystemic shunt
  - Prior complex hepatobiliary surgery
  - Hypoxemia with intrapulmonary shunts
  - Hepatic coma with intracranial hypertension
  - Active alcohol abuse
  - Active drug abuse
  - Cholangiocarcinoma or other aggressive tumor
  - Advanced age (no consensus on definition of "advanced age")
  - Poor social supports to assist with post-transplant medical compliance
  - Advanced malnutrition

BMI, body mass index; PA, pulmonary artery.

pressure monitoring, so that donor organs are not mistakenly allocated to patients who can no longer benefit from them. However, many neurosurgeons are reluctant to place intracranial pressure monitors because of the risk of hemorrhage (see above).

Patient Selection for Liver Transplantation Liver transplantation is an arduous process before, during, and after the operation. Part of the evaluation aims to identify individuals who can comply with lifestyle requirements needed to maintain the health of the grafted organ. Recipients must be able to sustain lifelong abstinence from alcohol, illicit drugs, and diverted prescription narcotics. Lifelong immunosuppression is also a requirement, and patients must have the means to obtain these necessary drugs and the personal organization and/or social supports to follow the complex medication regime.

Evaluation seeks to identify individuals with sufficient psychologic resilience, insight, and social supports who will be able to benefit over the long term from a resource as scarce as donor livers. Thus liver transplant listing committees are made up not only of surgeons and hepatologists, and, ideally, anesthesiologists, but also psychiatrists, addictions specialists, social services specialists, family therapists, and financial assistance experts.

Potential liver transplant recipients must be willing to accept massive blood transfusion during and after surgery. This requirement, formerly absolute, is relaxing as some centers gain sufficient expertise to reliably perform liver transplantation with little or no requirement for transfused blood. For example, Jehovah's Witnesses were formerly excluded from orthotopic liver transplantation candidacy unless they were willing to accept blood product transfusion. The first case reports of successful transplants occurred in 1996,[144,145] and since that time, increasing numbers of these patients have undergone successful transplantation in multiple centers willing to offer transplantation to Jehovah's Witnesses who refuse transfusion.[146,147] It should also be noted that Jehovah's Witnesses are allowed some latitude regarding their choice to receive or refuse transfusion, although the ultimate choices are personal ones made by the patient.

Potential recipients must be in the best possible physical condition within the context of hepatic failure and end-stage liver disease. For example, many programs require obese potential candidates to lose weight because obesity (body mass index [BMI] >30) is associated with excess mortality in the perioperative period.[148] A BMI greater than 30 is considered a relative contraindication to transplantation.

MODEL FOR END-STAGE LIVER DISEASE (MELD) SCORING SYSTEM

The United Network for Organ Sharing (UNOS; www.unos.org) administers the allocation of donated organs in the United States. Liver transplant recipient candidates are priority ranked by application of the MELD scoring system. The MELD system ranks patients by expected mortality based on the severity of their liver disease. An analogous system for pediatric patients, the Pediatric End-Stage Liver Disease (PELD) scoring system, is applied for patients younger than 12 years of age. Thus the MELD and PELD scores provide a way to rank patients in descending order of severity of disease (as reported by the likelihood of death from untreated disease), with higher scores indicating more severe disease burden.

The MELD scoring system uses a multivariate regression model to calculate a risk of death from the patient's liver disease based on the prognostic factors (laboratory values reflecting hepatic synthetic and excretory function) and regression coefficients (**Table 57-1**). Patients are assigned a MELD score based on the following calculation:

$$\text{MELD Score} = [0.957 \times \log_e(\text{creatinine mg/dL}) + 0.378 \times \log_e(\text{bilirubin mg/dL}) + 1.120 \times \log_e(\text{international normalized ratio [INR]}) + 0.643] * 10$$

Scores are rounded to the nearest whole number. Thus the risk score of a hypothetical patient with cirrhosis who has a serum creatinine concentration of 1.9 mg/dL, a serum bilirubin concentration of 4.2 mg/dL, and an INR value of 1.2 would be calculated as follows:

$$\text{MELD Score} = [(0.957 \times \log_e 1.9) + (0.378 \times \log_e 4.2) + (1.120 \times \log_e 1.2) + 0.643] * 10 \approx 20$$

TABLE 57-1 Model for End-Stage Liver Disease (MELD) Scoring System

Prognostic Factor[a]	Regression Coefficient
Serum creatinine[b] ($\log_e$ value)	0.957
Serum bilirubin ($\log_e$ value)	0.378
INR ($\log_e$ value)	1.120

INR, international normalized ratio.

[a]Laboratory values less than 1.0 are set to 1.0 for the MELD score calculation.

[b]The maximum serum creatinine considered in the MELD score equation is 4.0 mg/dL (ie, for patients with a serum creatinine of greater than 4.0 mg/dL, the serum creatinine level is set to 4.0 mg/dL). Patients on dialysis have their serum creatinine level automatically set to 4.0 mg/dL.

Recognizing that the MELD score does not fully encompass the unique characteristics of patients needing liver transplantation, UNOS defines several exceptions and modifications to the MELD system. For example, patients with hepatocellular carcinoma receive additional MELD points, improving their likelihood of receiving a transplant. Similar adjustments are made for adult patients with hepatic metabolic syndromes. MELD exception points are also granted to patients with hepatopulmonary syndrome, with additional MELD points given to patients with documented Pao_2 less than 60 mm Hg and stratified by the degree of hypoxemia with increasing severity given increased MELD credit.[149] Finally, patients with acute liver failure can receive a special listing status—Status 1A—that puts them at the top of the waiting list. A candidate can be listed as Status 1A if he or she has fulminant liver failure with a life expectancy without a liver transplant of less than 7 days, as defined by these 4 categories:

1. Fulminant hepatic failure defined as the onset of hepatic encephalopathy within 8 weeks of the first symptoms of liver disease. The absence of preexisting liver disease is critical to the diagnosis. One of 3 criteria must be met to list an adult patient, who must be in the ICU, with fulminant liver failure: (1) ventilator dependence, (2) requiring dialysis or continuous venovenous hemofiltration (CVVH) or continuous venovenous hemodialysis (CVVD), or (3) INR greater than 2.0, or
2. Primary nonfunction of a transplanted liver within 7 days of implantation; as defined by (a) or (b):
   (a) AST of 5000 or greater and one or both of the following:
   - An INR of 2.5 or greater
   - Acidosis, defined as having a pH of 7.3 or lower and/or lactate greater than or equal to 2 times normal

   (b) Anhepatic patient, or
3. Hepatic artery thrombosis in a transplanted liver within 7 days of implantation, with evidence of graft failure as defined in 2(a) and 2(b) above; or
4. Acute decompensated Wilson disease

Status 1 patients accrue additional points for time spent waiting for an organ in that status. There are separate waiting lists for each major blood group. To ensure the fair allocation of livers, adhering to the system is mandatory throughout the United States. Similar systems are in place throughout the developed world.

When a donor organ becomes available it is offered to transplant programs in the following order of priority:

1. The organ is offered to Status 1 patients (in descending point order) in the same local area as the procuring center.
2. The organ is offered to transplant programs with Status 1 patients (in descending point order) in the same organ-sharing region as the procuring center.
3. The organ is offered to candidates with MELD/PELD Scores 15 or higher in descending order of MELD/PELD scores, first locally and then regionally.
4. The organ is offered to patients with MELD/PELD scores of less than 15, locally and then regionally.

If no transplant program has accepted the organ by the end of this list, then it is offered at the national level, first to the Status 1 patients in rank order and then down the MELD/PELD waiting list.

PREANESTHETIC EVALUATION OF THE LIVER TRANSPLANT CANDIDATE

Because of the prescreening process for listing a patient for liver transplantation, most patients are "well studied"—that is, they have had an extensive prior diagnostic and risk stratification assessment. Thus, on the day of surgery, the immediate preoperative evaluation of the patient for liver transplantation focuses on the history and physical examination relevant to the case immediately at hand and any changes that may have occurred since the patient's last evaluation. Furthermore, although technically elective surgery, liver transplantation is an unscheduled, urgent case with many surgical teams, recipient patients, and hospitals throughout the region preparing for synchronous receipt of donor organs. Thus efficient and effective immediate preoperative care of the potential liver recipient is beneficial, both to the patient and to the medical system in general.

A typical preanesthetic history is taken, with attention to a few key points. Specific questioning pertinent to liver transplantation covers a variety of topics:

- Because liver transplants are unscheduled, the patients are rarely fasted. However, the quality and quantity of recent oral intake helps define the risk and potential consequences of regurgitation and aspiration of gastric contents. This often does not affect the anesthetic induction plan, as these patients are usually considered as "full-stomachs" and as such, warrant rapid sequence induction of general endotracheal anesthesia.
- Liver transplantation requires ample vascular access for resuscitation and monitoring. A history of previous central venous and/or arterial catheter placement will alert the anesthesia team to possible difficulty with access due to occluded vessels, although in practice, ultrasonography used in catheter placement also shows vessel patency.
- Questions should also be directed to assess hepatic synthetic function, which may have deteriorated further since the patient's last reevaluation. A history of increasing abdominal girth or peripheral edema indicates failure to synthesize sufficient albumin and other plasma proteins to maintain plasma oncotic pressure. A history of easy bruising, bleeding during oral hygiene, or prolonged bleeding from minor injuries indicates insufficient hepatic function to maintain clotting factor levels at even a fraction of normal levels.
- The history should address neurologic status, searching for evidence of worsening encephalopathy, manifesting itself as loss of mental acuity, forgetfulness, fatigue, and somnolence. It is also important to characterize and document any preoperative focal neurologic deficits to establish the patient's status prior to the case. Positioning injuries with consequent neurologic deficits are not uncommon. It is useful to know, when a patient complains of a deficit in the postoperative period, whether that deficit was present prior to surgery.
- The anesthesia team should reassess cardiac risk during the history, as many orthotopic liver transplant candidates wait for months or years between rescreening tests of cardiac function and ischemic risk. It may be difficult to decide whether decreasing exercise tolerance is attributable to cardiac dysfunction or worsening liver disease, so symptoms or signs of angina should be sought. Additionally, documentation of portopulmonary hypertension or hepatopulmonary syndrome should be sought, and this information could alter the anesthetic plan or cancel the surgery if PA pressures are elevated, uncontrolled, and/or untreatable in the time frame of the perioperative period.
- Renal function should likewise be reviewed, as worsening renal function secondary to disease progression or concomitant hepatorenal syndrome may warrant intraoperative or postoperative hemodialysis.

The physical examination should be as complete as that conducted for any patient undergoing major intra-abdominal surgery. Special attention should be paid to the assessment of ascites. Ascites potentiates the possibility of regurgitation and aspiration. It also compromises pulmonary performance and may prevent the patient from being able to breathe while supine for central venous catheter placement. Finally, ascites pushes the diaphragm upward, causing atelectasis and diminishing the functional residual capacity. Thus ascites predisposes liver transplant patients to rapid and severe desaturation during induction of anesthesia, even after assiduous denitrogenation.

Attention should also be paid to sites for vascular access. Large-bore (ie, 14 gauge or 8.5 French) venous cannulae are essential for volume resuscitation during the case, and these must be above the diaphragm, as the inferior vena cava will be cross-clamped at times. A femoral arterial catheter for pressure monitoring may be useful (see below). Landmarks for internal and external jugular cannulation, as well as subclavian access, should be examined, as well as peripheral venous and arterial sites on both arms.

DIAGNOSTIC STUDIES IN THE LIVER TRANSPLANT CANDIDATE

Laboratory tests obtained in the immediate preoperative period should include measures of hepatic synthetic and excretory function, and should specifically include serum albumin and bilirubin. Routine coagulation studies (PT, PTT, fibrinogen, and platelet count) give a measure of how hepatic synthetic failure has affected clotting factor levels. The platelet count can be low in the case of portal hypertension, as platelets are sequestered in the enlarged spleen.

Preoperative measurement of serum electrolytes is essential to provide baseline data about possible hyponatremia, hypo- or hyperkalemia, hypocalcemia, and hypomagnesemia. BUN and creatinine concentrations should be measured to assess the patient's renal function, which may in turn presage poor platelet function if uremia is present. This assessment of renal function (and acid–base status; see below) guides the possible use of intraoperative renal replacement therapy. Although rarely required, intraoperative renal replacement therapy may be needed if significant renal failure, electrolyte abnormality, or acid–base problems are found in the immediate preoperative laboratory investigation.

Hemoglobin should be measured to establish the preoperative baseline oxygen-carrying capacity. The patient's blood type should be redetermined, and a sample sent to the blood bank for antibody screening in anticipation of allogeneic transfusion. An electrocardiogram should be obtained in the immediate preoperative period to search for new changes suggestive of coronary artery disease. Finally, a preoperative chest x-ray is obtained as a baseline for comparison of postoperative films.

Patients presenting for liver transplantation almost always have an extensive body of laboratory and diagnostic test results available to aid in perioperative risk assessment and anesthetic planning. Patients with acute liver failure may be exceptions to this generalization, being listed for transplantation and subsequently receiving grafts within a few days of their initial presentation.[14] This may also be true of patients previously evaluated as transplant candidates but moved up on the transplant list due to an abrupt worsening of their MELD score. However, in almost all cases, the following assessments are either repeated upon admission for transplantation or have been performed within the prior year.

Laboratory assessment of pulmonary function includes arterial blood gas measurement and pulmonary function testing. Blood gas measurement identifies patients with hypoxia, suggesting hepatopulmonary syndrome. Pulmonary function testing often reveals small lung volumes reflecting the effect of ascites. In patients with a long history of smoking, there may be a superimposed obstructive pattern on spirometry. These results are important, as the liver transplant patient is mechanically ventilated for a prolonged intraoperative period and perhaps for some time in the postoperative period.

Cardiac assessment of the patient being considered for liver transplantation focuses on functional and invasive tests of cardiac performance that assess ischemic potential and the search for cardiac structural anomalies that might compromise outcome from orthotopic liver transplantation.[150]

The incidence and severity of coronary artery disease increases with age and with well-known risk factors, many of which are commonly found in patients with liver failure such as diabetes, smoking, and obesity. Furthermore, better surgical and anesthetic techniques are allowing older patients—that is, patients with greater age-related risk of significant coronary disease—to be considered for liver transplantation. Flow-limiting coronary artery disease is of grave concern because liver transplantation is still a highly stressful operation. The potential for sudden, massive, and ongoing blood loss complicated by extreme electrolyte derangements is still present, so all potential liver transplant recipients must be evaluated as if they will be required to tolerate minutes to hours of a hypothetical state with a heart rate above 110 beats/min and a mean arterial pressure of less than 50 mm Hg, with a hemoglobin of 7 g/dL and a pH under 7.2. Only patients with ideal cardiac status are likely to survive this scenario unscathed.

To ensure that new and previously listed transplant candidates meet these criteria, the liver transplant anesthesia team periodically reviews the preoperative evaluation of individuals high on the liver transplant list. This task involves reviewing the echocardiogram, the results of functional stress testing, and, if performed, cardiac catheterization results. This is not an academic exercise, as a significant fraction of patients being evaluated for liver transplantation have coronary artery disease, and the coronary disease of many of these patients was unsuspected prior to pretransplantation evaluation. For example, in a study applying coronary angiography to all potential liver transplant recipients older than 50 years of age, there was a 27% incidence of moderate to severe coronary artery disease, with 13.3% of the cohort having clinically unsuspected moderate or severe coronary disease.[151] Another study showed an incidence of 5.6% for coronary artery disease in patients older than 40 years of age,[152] and the consensus seems to be that about 2.5% to 10% of patients have moderate to significant coronary artery disease.[153] Untreated significant coronary disease is potentially lethal in the setting of liver transplantation.[150] In 1 study, half of all patients with coronary artery disease who underwent liver transplantation died in the perioperative period, and the morbidity rate was 81%.[154]

It appears that dobutamine stress echocardiography or possibly exercise stress thallium imaging is the best screening test in patients with end-stage liver disease.[153,155-157] A recent meta-analysis indicates that dobutamine stress echocardiography has a superior negative predictive value in patients having elective noncardiac surgery.[158] Dobutamine stress is commonly used in pretransplant evaluation because it is considered to most closely mimic the state commonly found during liver transplantation and in end-stage liver disease.[155] A negative dobutamine stress echocardiogram with adequate stress appears to predict a favorable perioperative cardiac outcome.[156,159] It is important to achieve at least 85% of the predicted maximal heart rate so that the dobutamine stress echocardiogram is diagnostic. Otherwise the diagnostic value of the test is compromised.[160] However, a recent retrospective analysis of OLT patients who underwent both dobutamine stress echocardiography and coronary angiography prior to their transplants showed that in patients who did achieve target heart rates, dobutamine stress echocardiography had a low sensitivity (13%) and a low positive predictive value (22%), questioning the accuracy of stress echocardiography in this population and the possible need for an alternative method of cardiac risk stratification.[161]

In the hyperdynamic state produced by the dobutamine stress echocardiography protocol, a significant number of patients develop a dynamic left ventricular outflow tract obstruction. However, despite the fact that more patients with dynamic left ventricular outflow tract obstruction developed intraoperative hypotension at transplantation, the overall outcomes (mortality) were the same between patients with obstruction and those without.[162]

Most transplant programs use a cardiac risk stratification schema similar to that devised by Plevak[155]; the version used by our program, for example, is shown in **Fig. 57-8**.

The ideal management of potential liver transplant recipients with significant coronary disease is a difficult problem with little evidence to guide decision making. Patients with end-stage liver disease who undergo coronary artery bypass grafting have significant morbidity. For example, in 1 study, patients with cirrhosis who underwent coronary artery bypass grafting had a 58% incidence of morbidity and significant complications.[163] Even patients with relatively mild liver disease (Child class A and B liver disease) who underwent coronary artery bypass grafting had extremely high mortality and morbidity.[164] The benefit of an intervention, such as coronary angioplasty, stenting, or atherectomy, has not been formally studied on a large scale to show outcome compared with coronary artery bypass grafting.[153] Small series have reported good results with combined orthotopic liver transplantation and coronary artery bypass grafting,[152,165,166] but at present, such a combined procedure is considered heroic in most transplant centers.

Independent of ischemic coronary artery disease, many patients with end-stage liver disease have a poorly understood disorder known as cirrhotic cardiomyopathy (a different entity from alcoholic cardiomyopathy) despite supranormal cardiac outputs.[30] This condition is multifactorial, and its mechanisms may include impairment of the β-adrenergic system, nitric oxide (overproduced in liver failure), cytokines, and the prolonged hyperdynamic circulation.[167] Many patients with apparently normal ventricular function prior to surgery develop left ventricular failure in the postoperative period.[33,159] These patients, representing 1% to 6% of liver-transplanted individuals, may have had occult cirrhotic cardiomyopathy. Unfortunately, prospective diagnostic criteria for cirrhotic cardiomyopathy are lacking, although a recommendation made at the 2005 World Congress of Gastroenterology in Montreal suggested that a classification system of cirrhotic cardiomyopathy includes systolic and/or diastolic dysfunction in response to stress in the absence of any preexisting cardiac disease.[168]

All patients being considered for liver transplantation should undergo a screening transthoracic echocardiogram. This is a good screening test to search for cardiac structural abnormalities as well as anomalies of the surrounding vasculature. It is also an important test to exclude portopulmonary hypertension.

Cardiac structural anomalies can affect outcome by impairing cardiac performance intraoperatively (eg, functional or fixed valve stenoses) or by allowing passage of emboli from the right to the left side of the heart. Patent foramen ovale (PFO) and other septal defects may be a significant risk to orthotopic liver transplant patients and patients undergoing hepatic resection when fixed or transient right-to-left shunting occurs. Right-to-left shunt increases the possibility of paradoxical embolus of clot, air, or debris. Hepatic surgery can lead to large openings in the inferior vena cava, so the embolization problem can be severe. In fact, in 2 series, between 1% and 6% of all patients undergoing orthotopic liver transplantation had thrombus detected in the right heart.[169,170] Because roughly 25% of all hearts in unselected autopsy subjects have PFOs[171] the risk of injury due to paradoxical embolism may be greater than

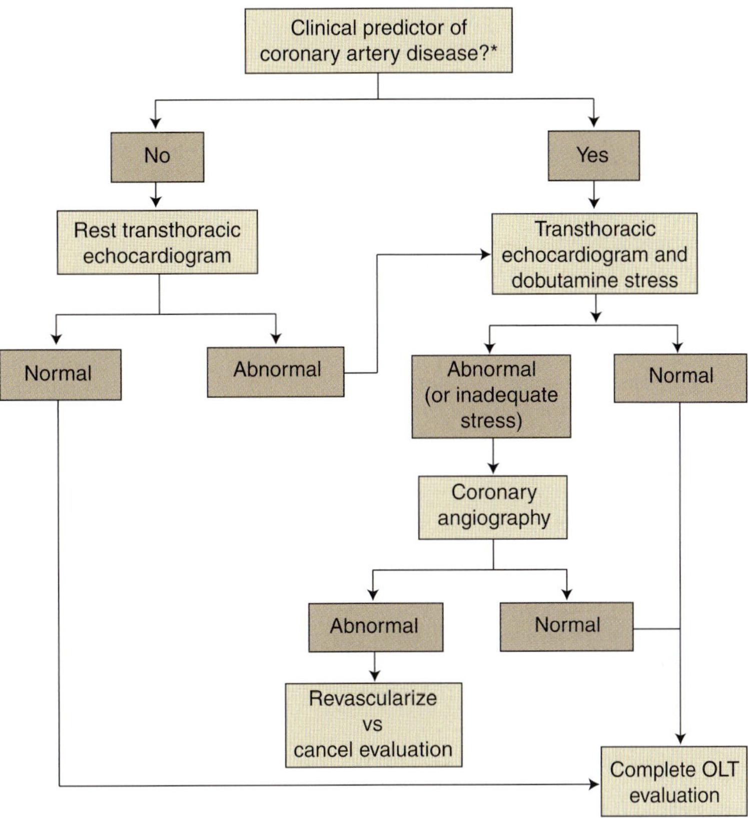

FIGURE 57-8. Suggested algorithm for assessment of inducible myocardial ischemia. OLT, orthotopic liver transplantation.

currently appreciated. On the other hand, in a recent study evaluating the risk of hepatic transplant patients with patent foramen ovales, 27 patients with patent PFOs were compared to 61 non-PFO transplant patients, and both perioperative outcomes and 30-day mortality rates were similar in both groups.[172] This does not prove that PFO patients are not at elevated risk. Their anesthesia and surgical teams might simply have avoided accidental emboli better. Therefore, in preparation for elective hepatic surgery and certainly in the evaluation for orthotopic liver transplantation, cardiac septal defects should be sought by echocardiography or magnetic resonance imaging (MRI).

Transthoracic echocardiography can be used to interrogate the intra-atrial septum using color-flow Doppler mode. Additionally, bubble contrast echocardiography is a highly sensitive test for septal defects. Early passage (within 1-2 beats) of air from the right to the left heart indicates a septal defect, whereas later arrival of air on the left side indicates intrapulmonary shunting. This latter finding cannot be remedied, but when atrial defects are detected, consideration should be given to closing them before transplantation.

Closure of patent foramen ovales prior to orthotopic liver transplantation is controversial, although it can now be accomplished percutaneously.[173] No controlled studies evaluating the usefulness of this intervention have appeared. Factors favoring closure are (1) embolism is common, particularly during the reperfusion period; (2) right heart dysfunction with right heart pressures greater than left heart pressures is common during reperfusion; and (3) paradoxical embolism occurs in this setting.[174] On the other hand, the relationship between the presence or size of a patent foramen ovale and the likelihood of paradoxical embolus has not been clearly established. Although there are case series of paradoxical embolism documented by transesophageal echocardiography during liver transplantation,[174] it is not clear whether these necessarily occur through a patent foramen ovale. Furthermore, closing a patent foramen ovale commits the coagulopathic patient with liver disease to months of antiplatelet agents.

Magnetic resonance imaging has recently been applied to the assessment of the intra-atrial septum. Small studies comparing this technique with color-flow Doppler echocardiography and bubble contrast studies indicate that MRI has similar sensitivity and specificity to these echocardiographic techniques.[175]

The final cardiopulmonary problem to be investigated in the prelisting evaluation is portopulmonary hypertension, the management of which has been described previously. Figure 57-1 outlines the diagnostic and therapeutic decision approach to portopulmonary hypertension. Portopulmonary hypertension occurs in 2% to 4% of patients with end-stage liver disease and 5% to 10% of patients being evaluated for orthotopic liver transplantation.[53] The clinical predictors of pulmonary hypertension in liver transplantation include systemic hypertension, right ventricular dilation by echocardiography, estimated pulmonary artery systolic pressure of 40 mm Hg or greater by transthoracic echocardiography, right ventricular hypertrophy by echocardiography, or a right ventricular heave.[176] The mortality associated with pulmonary hypertension during liver transplantation is significant. Half of the patients with mean pulmonary pressures between 35 and 50 mm Hg died in the peritransplant period, and mortality was 100% in those with mean pulmonary artery pressure greater than 50 mm Hg.[177] These results are similar in a multicenter retrospective review,[58] leading many centers to deny orthotopic liver transplantation to patients with more than mild portopulmonary hypertension. However, in some centers, mild portopulmonary hypertension (ie, mean pulmonary artery pressure <35 mm Hg with good ventricular function) is not associated with poor early or late outcomes.[178] A retrospective study examining outcomes in portopulmonary hypertensive patients demonstrated 5-year survivals of 14%, 45%, and 67% for patients in 3 subgroups, respectively, who had (1) no therapy or liver transplantation alone, (2) only therapy for portopulmonary hypertension, or (3) therapy for portopulmonary hypertension followed by liver transplantation.[179]

Transesophageal echocardiography is rarely indicated in the preoperative assessment of orthotopic liver transplantation candidates. The procedure may require sedation, which can be complicated in the patient with end-stage liver disease. Furthermore, there is the risk of disrupting esophageal varices during the examination.

OPERATIVE APPROACHES FOR LIVER TRANSPLANTATION

Liver transplantation is conveniently divided into 3 phases: the preanhepatic phase, the anhepatic phase, and the neohepatic or reperfusion phase. During the preanhepatic phase, a complete hepatectomy is performed. During the anhepatic phase, vascular anastomoses between the donor liver and the recipient's vessels are constructed. During the neohepatic phase, the hepatic arterial and biliary anastomoses are constructed, and the wound is closed.

A liver transplant begins like a hepatic resection, using the same incision and exposure and imposing the same hemodynamic consequences. The surgeon exposes and gains control of the hepatic vasculature. The hepatic artery, portal vein, and the common bile duct are clamped and divided. Two different techniques are commonly used for controlling hepatic venous outflow and constructing this anastomosis: (1) an en-bloc technique in which part of the recipient's vena cava is resected and replaced with a section of the donor vena cava, or (2) a "piggyback" technique in which the recipient vena cava is clamped with a side-biting clamp and a side-to-side anastomosis is constructed to the donor liver venous outflow. The choice of technique has important implications for anesthetic management and the expected course of the case, as described in the following.

In the en-block resection technique, the inferior vena cava must be clamped above and below the liver, with consequent severe reduction in venous return to the heart. Because both the portal vein and the inferior vena cava are clamped, the entire body below the caval cross-clamp, as well as the abdominal viscera, suffers venous congestion and ischemia unless an alternate route of venous return can be established. This massive loss of venous return, coupled with the insult of recirculating blood from such a large ischemic territory at the time of reperfusion, leads to profound hemodynamic instability requiring pharmacologic intervention, sudden hypothermia at reperfusion, and elevated potential for malignant cardiac arrhythmias. These difficulties have motivated the development and routine use of venovenous bypass techniques. This is commonly achieved via venovenous bypass from the lower half of the body to a great vein draining into the superior vena cava (**Fig. 57-9**).

Venovenous bypass may be used to decompress the lower systemic venous circulation, the portal circulation, or both. The advantages and disadvantages of venovenous bypass have been reviewed.[180] Without the

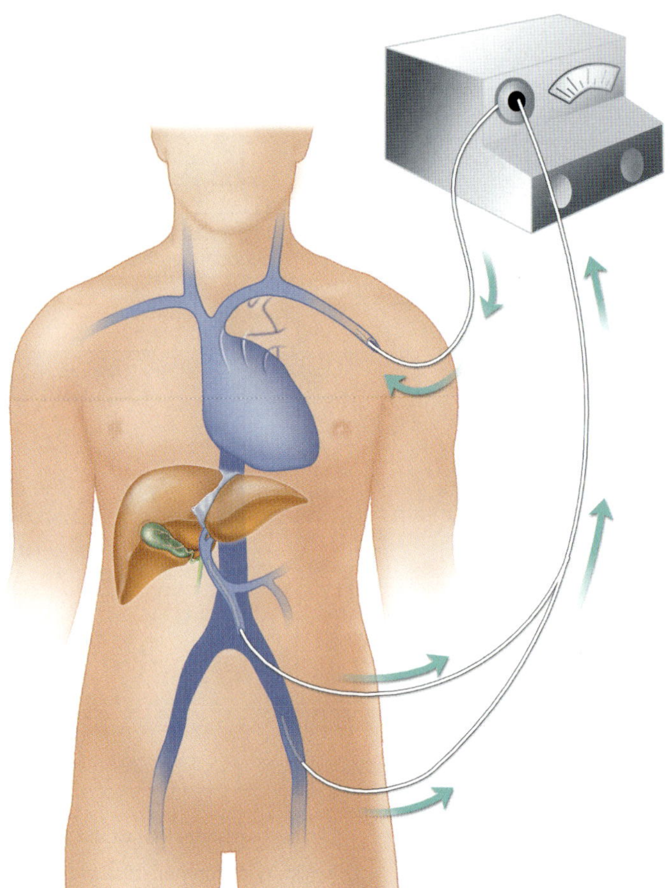

FIGURE 57-9. Schematic diagram of a venovenous bypass circuit.

preserved venous return afforded by venovenous bypass, the cardiac output and blood pressure may fall dramatically; often the cardiac output falls by more than 50%. Such falls in cardiac output are suggested to increase morbidity and mortality,[180] although primary research has failed to detect this association.[181,182]

Failure to decompress the lower systemic and portal venous systems leads to severe venous congestion below the caval cross-clamp. Above the clamp, reduced venous return reduces left ventricular preload and cardiac output, with a net result of reduced perfusion pressure for organs below the caval cross-clamp. Thus, without venovenous bypass, renal venous pressure is elevated, systemic arterial pressure is depressed, and renal perfusion pressure is degraded. Thus venovenous bypass might be expected to afford some protection from renal failure in the perioperative period, but the net effect on renal function is equivocal. For example, venovenous bypass is not associated with improved postoperative renal function relative to matched patients whose liver transplant was performed without bypass.[183]

First described in 1984,[184] venovenous bypass is a technique wherein blood is actively pumped using a centrifugal pump from large-bore drainage cannulae to a similarly large return line (**Fig. 57-10**). These can be inserted percutaneously or via a cut-down procedure. A common drainage site for the lower systemic venous circulation is the left femoral vein. The portal vein, if drained, is accessed from the surgical field. Common return sites are the right internal jugular and left subclavian veins via percutaneous access or the left axillary vein via a cut-down technique.

Percutaneous insertion of the bypass cannulae may be performed by the surgical team or by the anesthesia team at the beginning of the case. An alternative approach is to prep the left groin and axilla for possible

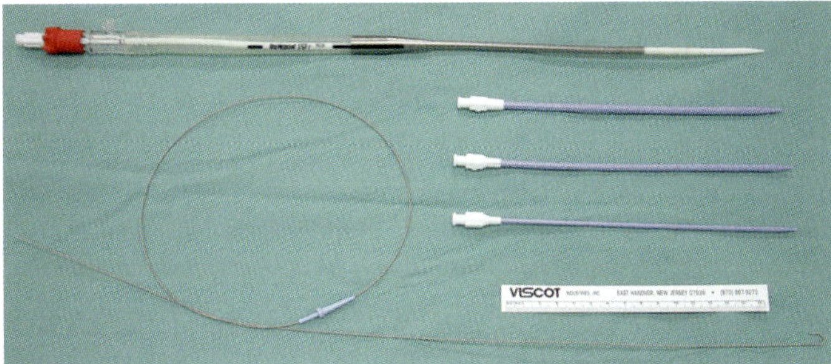

FIGURE 57-10. Large-bore venovenous bypass cannula with guidewire and dilators.

cut-down access and then defer access until it becomes clear that venovenous bypass is needed. Percutaneous access appears to be quicker and to provide better flows,[185,186] but the cut-down technique persists. The bypass cannulae are very large, and when placed percutaneously, require multiple passes with successively larger sharp, stiff dilators passed over a stiff guidewire to create a large enough skin entrance, as illustrated in **Fig. 57-11**.

Assiduous care should be taken to pass the dilators only deep enough to enlarge the skin punctures, and under no circumstance should the tip of any dilator be allowed to pass beyond the end of the guidewire. Exsanguinating hemorrhage into the chest and cardiac tamponade from cardiac puncture have occurred as mishaps of venovenous bypass cannula placement.[187] Extreme care should be taken to facilitate reliable cannulation of the target vein, including the possible use of ultrasonography to guide initial venous access and manometry to confirm venous placement using a small, temporary catheter prior to beginning dilation. A postinsertion chest x-ray to confirm vascular placement and correct insertion depth is mandatory prior to initiating venovenous bypass.

The bypass circuit should be carefully cleared of air as connections are made, and all connections should be secured prior to initiating bypass. Systemic heparinization is not performed, as the bypass circuit is heparin bonded.[188] Bypass flow rates of 1.5 to 5 L/min are typical. The initiation of bypass is a critical period, as malplacement of the return line becomes apparent with disastrous consequences almost immediately. For example, accidental placement of the tip of the return line through a cardiac chamber wall and into the pericardial sac will lead to near-instantaneous, severe cardiac tamponade with initiation of flow.

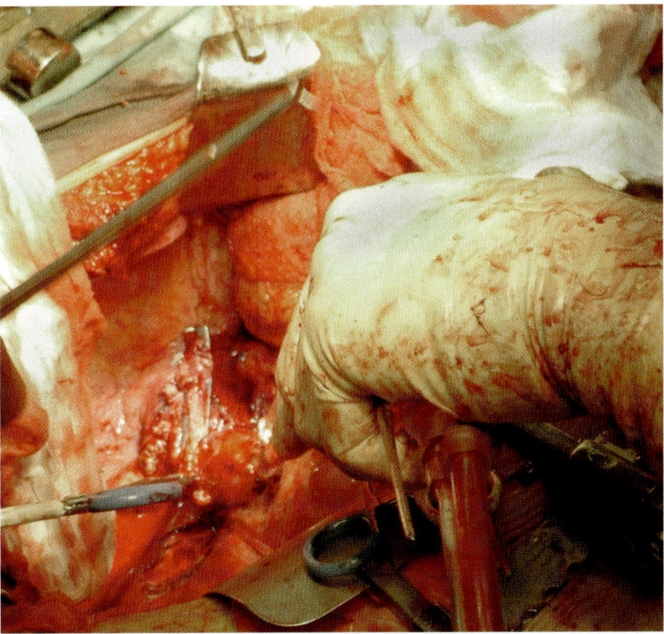

FIGURE 57-12. Photograph of a side-biting cross-clamp (lower left) on the inferior vena cava after removal of the liver. The patient's head is to the upper left.

Fatal air embolism has occurred due to connection failure during venovenous bypass, so the pump and its circuit require constant attention by dedicated, specialized personnel.

Despite the improved conditions afforded during surgery, it is not clear that venovenous bypass improves long-term outcomes. Because of the potential for complications, coupled with improvements in surgical techniques (see below) some have questioned the usefulness of routine venovenous bypass.[180]

The alternative approach to liver transplantation, the vena cava preservation (or "piggyback") technique,[189] is designed to preserve vena cava flow for all but a few minutes of the transplant procedure. Portal venous and hepatic arterial control is obtained as above. Instead of a cross-clamp, a "side-biter" clamp placed on the inferior vena cava isolates the liver from the systemic venous system. Figures 57-6 and 57-12 illustrate this clamping method. In **Fig. 57-12**, a button of vena cava with the

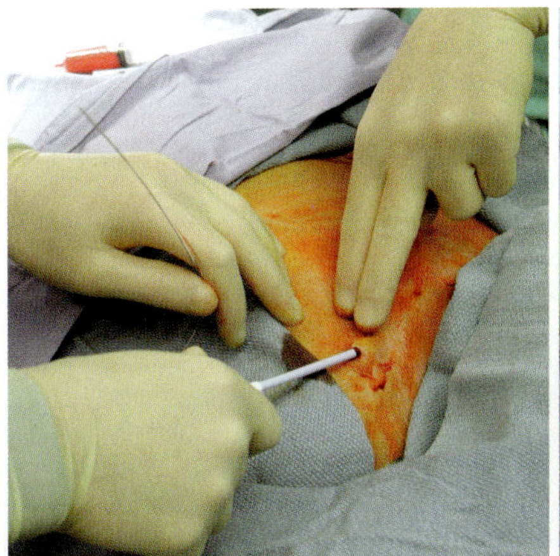

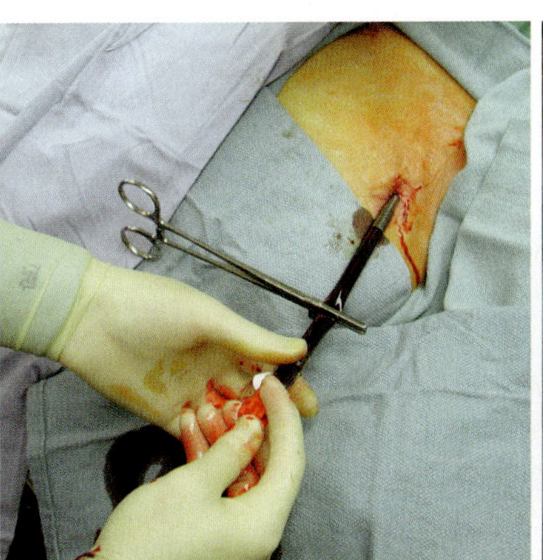

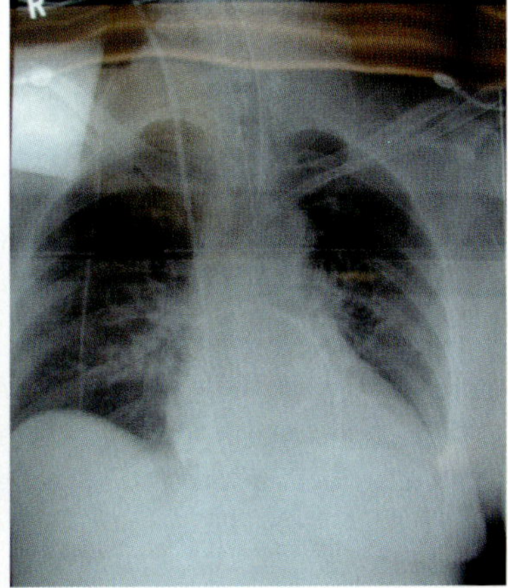

FIGURE 57-11. Subclavian placement of a percutaneous venovenous bypass cannula. The left panel demonstrates the use of a large-bore dilator after placement of the guidewire into the central circulation. The center panel shows the cannula in place and clamped prior to connecting to the venovenous bypass pump tubing. The right panel shows a portable chest x-ray confirming intravascular placement.

hepatic vein attachments has been removed, and the hole is held closed by the side-biter clamp at the bottom of the wound. The vena cava deep to this clamp is largely open to flow. This allows venous return from the lower systemic but not the portal venous system. Frequently, a brief period of total venous occlusion with a vena cava cross-clamp is needed to position the side-biter clamp. Vena cava distension due to overzealous volume replacement during the hepatectomy can make the piggyback technique more difficult for the surgeons. Because exposure for the hepatectomy is more difficult and the anastomosis is more complicated, the piggyback technique may take longer to perform. However, many programs now use this technique almost exclusively.[190]

Piggyback transplantation is associated with a lower incidence of renal failure,[191] better gas exchange, and better acid–base status at reperfusion,[192] as well as better intraoperative hemodynamic stability. A retrospective, 3-year analysis of 426 liver transplantations utilizing either retrohepatic caval resection with venovenous bypass, piggyback technique with venovenous bypass, or piggyback technique without venovenous bypass demonstrated that the piggyback-only technique utilized the smallest amount of blood products, had the lowest incidence of renal failure, and had overall better patient and graft survival when compared to the other 2 techniques.[193] Additionally, this technique results in little to no need for venovenous bypass, as demonstrated in a series of 500 liver transplantations in which the piggyback technique was utilized and no patients required venovenous bypass in order to maintain hemodynamic stability.[194]

Failure to decompress the portal system may lead to splanchnic congestion unless the recipient has large portosystemic shunts. Nevertheless, the piggyback technique reduces the transfusion requirement as well as the need for vasoactive drugs during the completion of the hepatectomy and construction of the venous anastomoses.[195] Temporary portocaval shunts have been described in association with the piggyback technique. The temporary shunt appears to improve intraoperative hemodynamics and reduce transfusion requirements,[196] but is not widely used. In general, use of the piggyback technique dramatically reduces the severity of problems during the anhepatic and reperfusion stages of the operation.

As the hepatectomy is being completed, a separate surgical team prepares the donor liver for implantation, working at a separate table. The graft vessels are trimmed to fit their counterparts in the recipient. Next, the graft is brought to the recipient surgical field, and the vascular anastomoses are constructed. The surgical goal during this phase of the operation is to construct patent, nonleaking anastomoses as efficiently as possible to minimize the warm ischemic time of the liver. Thrombosis of the recipient portal vein is a relatively common finding, either during the dissection or at the time of initial graft reperfusion. When discovered, portal venous thrombosis typically prompts an attempted thrombectomy using Fogarty catheters, a potentially bloody process. Typically, the donor hepatic to recipient vena cava and the donor portal to recipient portal venous anastomoses are constructed, flushed, and opened as quickly as possible to establish a circulation in the graft. Then the hepatic arterial anastomosis is constructed, flushed, and opened, completing the graft blood supply.

Finally, a biliary drainage is constructed. This may either be by direct anastomosis of the graft bile duct to the recipient common bile duct or via a Roux-en-Y construct using the jejunum.

ANESTHESIA FOR LIVER TRANSPLANTATION

Concerns and activities during anesthesia for liver transplantation mirror the major phases of the surgery. The anesthesia can thus be roughly divided into the following phases:

- Preinduction
- Induction, preparation for surgery, and maintenance
- Preanhepatic phase
- Anhepatic phase
- Venous reperfusion of the graft
- Neohepatic phase
- Emergence/transport to ICU

The anesthesia team attends to multiple homeostatic goals throughout the case (**Table 57-2**). Liver transplant anesthetics are some of the most complex currently performed because of the surgical and medical criticality of the patients and because of the complexity of the equipment required to perform the case.

Figure 57-13 is a panorama from the anesthesiologist's perspective during a liver transplant. Multiple user interfaces, cables, monitoring lines, and infusions must be well organized and systematically set up to make the cognitive load from the equipment acceptable and predictable so that the anesthesiologist can attend properly to the patient and the operation. Liver transplantation consumes tremendous resources. Most programs responding to a recent survey reported assigning at least 2 anesthesiology personnel and at least 2 additional professional personnel (ie, perfusionist, monitoring nurse, auto-transfusion nurse) to each case.[197] Thus, in addition to the complexity of the equipment, team leadership, communication, and delegation of responsibility must be considered and managed during the case.

During the preinduction phase, the final evaluation of the patient is performed. Although there is unlikely to be any doubt about the identity of the patient and the operation to be performed, the anesthesia team must independently confirm the patient's identity, the operation to be performed, the recipient's blood type, and any allergies. Last-minute laboratory results should be reviewed. It is always prudent for a member of the anesthesia team to personally consult with the blood bank about the upcoming liver transplant so that it may prepare for a possible heavy demand for blood products. This is particularly true if the patient has developed antibodies to allogeneic red blood cells from previous transfusions, presenting an added challenge to the blood bank.

Close communication with the graft harvest team is essential to best sequence the activities with the donor to minimize graft ischemic time while at the same time minimizing the recipient's exposure to risks of anesthesia and invasive monitoring. Thus one might obtain initial peripheral intravenous (IV) access and then wait to place any additional monitors or vascular access until confirmation that the graft is suitable. In most situations, graft suitability is known at least 1 hour before the need to start the recipient's surgery, leaving ample time for induction of anesthesia, placement of central venous or pulmonary artery catheters, positioning of the patient, application of warming devices, and the initial surgical prep and drape.

Most patients with end-stage liver disease have at least some encephalopathy. Thus it is prudent to dose sedative premedications, such as benzodiazepines and opioids, judiciously, giving small doses and monitoring closely for desired and undesired effects.

Monitoring for liver transplantation relies on standard monitors plus invasive monitors directed toward the likely areas of additional concern during the case. Central venous pressure monitoring is often needed to assess intravascular volume status, as well as to goal-direct low CVP technique when utilized. Additionally, central venous catheterization provides large-bore transfusion access, allows passage of a PA catheter if needed, and provides a conduit for central vasopressor administration. Thus placement of a central venous catheter for liver transplantation seems almost obligatory. However, central venous pressure monitoring gives much of the same information as provided by intraoperative transesophageal echocardiography (TEE), which could replace the intravascular monitor if another suitable route can be found for the drugs.

Pulmonary artery catheterization is carried out if left or right heart performance is in doubt, if problems with pulmonary hypertension are anticipated, and to distinguish hypotension due to hypovolemia or heart failure from that due to lack of peripheral vascular tone, especially if TEE is not utilized during the case. One type of pulmonary artery catheter also allows for A-V pacing. The pulmonary artery catheter

TABLE 57-2 Major Foci of Intraoperative Management During Anesthesia for Orthotopic Liver Transplantation

Major Focus (Problem or Organ System)	Subtopics	Perturbing Factors
Cardiac	Ischemic potential Dysrhythmias Right ventricular performance	Hemorrhage (demand and carrying capacity) Acid/base and electrolyte disturbances Emboli, hepatic washout
Portal-to-central venous gradient	Graft perfusion is tenuous	Need to keep CVP adequate to provide cardiac preload during vena cava cross-clamping Need to prevent venous air embolism Sudden hemorrhage
Renal performance	Urine output	Hypovolemia and hypotension Preexisting renal disease Need for intraoperative renal replacement therapy
Anesthesia	Hypnosis Analgesia Muscle relaxation	
Brain protection		
Immunosuppression		
Prophylaxis	Temperature management DVT prophylaxis Preemptive antibiotics	Large incision, large prepped area Dilution due to massive hemorrhage
Glucose management	Coexisting diabetes	Steroid administration Absent gluconeogenesis during anhepatic phase
Coagulation	Hypocoagulable state due to liver failure Platelet sequestration Platelet dysfunction due to uremia	Massive hemorrhage Acute fibrinolysis at graft reperfusion
Electrolytes	Potassium Sodium Calcium	Elevated by K load in blood products Hyponatremic patients at risk for central pontine myelinolysis with massive infusions of Na^+-rich fluids Citrate in blood products chelates Ca^{+2}
Pulmonary performance	Ventilation Oxygenation Pulmonary vascular resistance	May be impaired by pleural effusions May be impaired by intrapulmonary shunts Acutely elevates in the face of acid load at graft reperfusion
Hemodynamics	Vasodilated hyperdynamic circulation Massive hemorrhage Vena cava compression Possible venovenous bypass	

CVP, central venous pressure; DVT, deep vein thrombosis.

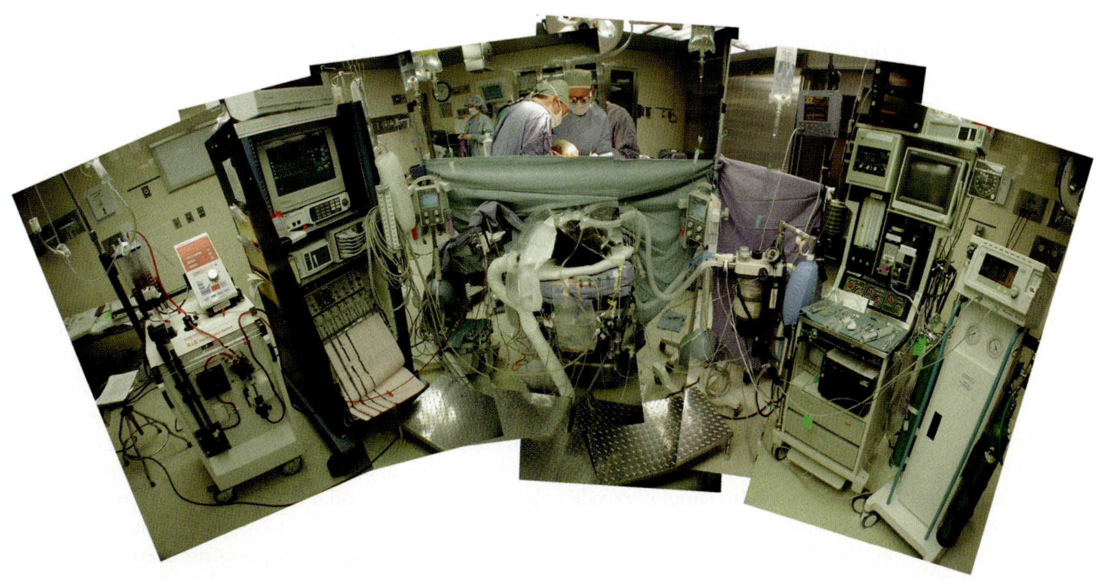

FIGURE 57-13. Panorama of anesthesia equipment for liver transplantation. The equipment (from left to right) includes rapid infusion system; 6-pressure physiologic monitor with 8-channel chart recorder; syringe microinfusion pumps for vasoactive drugs; forced-air warmer; syringe microinfusion pumps for anesthetics, muscle relaxants, etc; level-of-consciousness monitor; anesthesia machine; and delivery system for inhaled nitric oxide. Out of view to the right: blood recovery system.

allows one to follow cardiac output and stroke volume throughout the case. The initial cardiac output measurements typically confirm a hyperdynamic circulation, with cardiac outputs of 10 to 11 L/min frequently seen at rest in adult male patients with end-stage liver disease.

An arterial catheter is usually inserted to closely monitor blood pressure and to provide convenient access for frequent laboratory sampling. When compared with femoral arterial catheters, radial artery catheters may not reflect the true systolic pressure during the reperfusion phase of transplantation or during vasopressor administration.[198] However, mean pressures measured in the radial and femoral arteries correlate well regardless of the phase of the case or vasopressor administration.[198] Thus a radial arterial catheter is sufficient to guide the management of the mean pressure. In some centers, 2 arterial catheters are placed so that blood pressure monitoring may proceed without interruption during frequent arterial blood gas withdraws, or as backup in case of an arterial line failure.

Transesophageal echocardiography should be considered for assessment of cardiac performance during transplantation, either as an adjunct or in place of pulmonary artery catheterization, and for monitoring embolism of air or thrombus. Air embolism is common, and TEE frequently reveals such events. Transesophageal echocardiography is most useful for early detection of large embolic events, with the hope of minimizing their effect by virtue of early detection and removal of the source. It is also a useful tool to assess the effect both of embolic events and therapeutic interventions on cardiac performance.

It is also useful to consider level-of-consciousness monitoring (BIS® or similar). Liver transplant patients may be very sensitive to anesthetics, requiring smaller doses than typical patients. Level-of-consciousness monitoring can thus be used to minimize exposure to anesthetic agents and their potential deleterious effects on the circulatory system while providing some assurance that the patient will not recall the surgery.

Vascular access for rapid volume replacement can either be peripheral or in the central circulation. The patient likely requires central venous access for vasopressor administration, so it is tempting to use this route for volume as well. However, it is important to isolate vasopressors from the main volume cannula, as fluid for resuscitation may be delivered under pressure, effectively stopping the vasopressors. Multilumen large-bore central venous catheters or multiple catheters at separate central venous sites provide the necessary isolation. Alternatively, peripheral vascular access (eg, multiple 14-gauge IV catheters or a rapid infusion catheter as described previously) may be established. It is important to have at least 1 dedicated cannula that can carry the maximum flow rate of the available rapid infusion device (see below).

Anesthetic Induction, Preparation for Surgery, and Maintenance Because most patients with end-stage liver disease have ascites and/or have had sclerotherapy of lower esophageal varices, rapid-sequence induction is the norm, with cricoid pressure applied and with the patient in optimal position for laryngoscopy. Careful denitrogenation is important, as most end-stage liver disease patients have reduced functional residual capacity. In patients with poor cardiac function, a preinduction arterial line may be warranted. Vasodilation and encephalopathy make patients with end-stage liver disease sensitive to induction agents. Thus the induction dose of hypnotic drugs, such as propofol or thiopental sodium (Pentothal), should be reduced (eg, 1 mg/kg^{-1} of ideal body weight for propofol in a cachectic patient with encephalopathy). Some clinicians elect to sidestep this issue entirely by using an induction agent such as etomidate. Skeletal muscle paralysis is typically obtained with succinylcholine followed by a nondepolarizing agent, or with rocuronium at a dose sufficient for rapid-sequence induction.

Antibiotics targeted against skin flora (eg, cefazolin) should precede skin incision by no more than 60 minutes.[199] Antibiotics should be redosed throughout the case to account for elimination and loss due to hemorrhage.

During maintenance of anesthesia, hepatic encephalopathy reduces opioid and anesthetic requirements. Thus it is possible to inadvertently administer relative overdoses of anesthetics by overestimating the patient's needs. Similarly, opioids may have enhanced potency and prolonged duration of action due to hepatic failure. On the other hand, massive hemorrhage and resuscitation can diminish the circulating opioid concentration. Thus it is appropriate to titrate intermediate acting opioids, such as morphine, hydromorphone, or fentanyl, to the patient's needs throughout the case. The choice of paralyzing agent should also be guided by the clinical situation. For example, agents requiring hepatic degradation are probably not optimal if early extubation is contemplated.

Positioning the patient requires special attention. Liver transplants are long cases with the potential for hypotension and consequent extremity hypoperfusion. Furthermore, surgeons may lean heavily on the patient to perform parts of the operation. Thus positioning injuries are possible, and great care should be taken to protect the patient by generously supporting and padding all of the body, either with compressible foam or viscoelastic gel. As surgical needs may warrant frequent changes in table position throughout the case, all extremities should be carefully secured. Pneumatic compression stockings are applied, and a urinary catheter is inserted.

The case is performed with the patient in supine position. If required, the right arm may be tucked alongside the patient's body to allow access for several surgeons. If so, the right arm is out of reach of the anesthesiologist, and no critical monitors or access devices should be placed there unless no alternative sites are available. In addition to problems with accessibility, devices placed in the tucked right arm may cause patient injury due to compression. Accordingly, we typically limit devices in the right arm to a single large-bore peripheral IV and arterial line. The left arm is abducted to facilitate access for venovenous bypass. Therefore, the left arm is also an ideal site for arterial monitoring and peripheral venous access. Venous access in the left arm may be occluded if venovenous bypass is instituted via cut-down to the axillary vein, but the bypass circuit has a separate high-flow inlet into which this infusion can be attached. Other sites of access include both femoral regions. Venous access below a potential vena cava cross-clamp is of little utility, either for monitoring or volume administration. Furthermore, the left femoral vein is typically reserved for possible venovenous bypass access. However, cannulation of the right femoral artery may be useful if a complicated case is anticipated. Both internal jugular veins are available with the patient in supine position. If required, dual large-bore catheters may be placed in a single internal jugular vein. Care must be exercised to ensure that the catheters are sufficiently separated along the axis of the vein to prevent forming a larger, single connected hole.

The entire abdomen and chest are prepped for surgery. Additionally, the left groin and axilla are included in 1 large, contiguous prep if venovenous bypass via open access is contemplated.

Patient warming becomes a major issue due to the extensive use of alcohol-based skin prep solutions over a large surface, the size of the incision, the duration of the case, and reperfusion of a cold graft. Hypothermia should be avoided because it negatively affects coagulation,[121] resistance to infection,[120] and the potential for early extubation. Warming strategies commonly focus on IV fluids and forced-air warming devices.

Forced-air warming is effective, although the extensive area exposed and prepped during liver transplantation makes finding sufficient surface area on which to apply warmers a challenge. A procedure involving the entire abdomen, as well as the left groin and axilla for establishment of venovenous bypass, leaves the head, left arm, and lower legs for warming. Forced-air warming blankets for underbody use, which presumably function by forming a warmed-air plenum under the drapes, are available and should be considered. These appear to be effective to the extent that they are not compressed and deflated by the weight of drapes and surgeons pressing against them. In this instance, we place forced-air warming blankets on all available sites, including under the patient. In our experience, patient temperature drops to about 36°C during induction, prepping, and draping; increases to 37°C during the preanhepatic phase; and then falls by approximately 1°C at hepatic reperfusion. Subsequently, the temperature increases to 37°C during the neohepatic phase, prompting the gradual discontinuation of forced-air warming to maintain normothermia. If lower-extremity forced-air warming is used, anesthesiologists must remember to cease use of these if aortic cross-clamping occurs at any time during the case, or thermal injury may result.

Warming intravenous infusions is mandatory, given the volume of refrigerated banked-blood products that will likely be transfused. Fluid warming for liver transplantation is usually achieved with commercially available high-flow warming devices. The ideal transfusion device has a reservoir to allow the user to establish a reserve of blood for sustained rapid infusion in the face of uncontrolled hemorrhage. The infusion flow rate should be reported. The device must contain an air detector that stops the infusion when air is detected in the patient limb of the circuit. Ideally the device contains a debris filter between the reservoir and the patient.

Three devices are in common use, and each has unique advantages and weaknesses. The characteristics of the 3 major rapid infusion systems are listed in **Table 57-3**. The first, manufactured by Level-1 (Rockland, MA, USA) uses a counter-current heat exchanger to warm fluid administered under pressure from bags. The second device, formerly manufactured by Haemonetics (Braintree, MA, USA), is no longer commercially available but is still in common use. The final device is manufactured by Belmont Instrument Corp. (Billerica, MA, USA) and is called the Belmont Fluid Management System (FMS). The pumped devices are pressure limited at 300 mm Hg; that is, their maximum flow rates in actual clinical use are limited by the resistance characteristics of the infusion catheter or by the maximum rate of the pump if the back-pressure is less than 300 mm Hg when maximum pump flow is attained. Of the 3 devices listed in Table 57-3, the RIS most closely approaches the characteristics of the ideal transfusion device. It has a debris filter/air removal system downstream of the warmer and pump but proximal to the final air detector, thus providing maximal embolism exclusion. The RIS also has the highest flow rate, delivering 1500 mL/min, or roughly one-third of the normal adult cardiac output, exceeding the flow capacities of all but the largest catheters. However, the RIS disposable insert is bifurcated, allowing the pumped flow to be sent to 2 infusion catheters in parallel, increasing maximum flow and volume delivered as compared to a single set due to a decrease in resistance.

Of the 2 available devices, the FMS is preferable in that it satisfies more of the requirements listed above. Its maximum flow rate does not exceed the capacity of a RIC or a percutaneous introducer sheath, but it does exceed the capacity of a 14-gauge peripheral IV or the auxiliary lumen of a centrally inserted device such as the MAC (Multi-Access Catheter, Arrow International, Reading, PA, USA) or AVA (Advanced Vascular Access, Edwards Lifesciences, Irvine, CA, USA).

The Preanhepatic Phase As in a hepatic resection, clamping the portal triad reduces venous return. In the hepatic resection, as mentioned above, cardiac output and blood pressure do not necessarily fall. Liver transplantation almost always requires a vena cava cross-clamp, creating total vascular exclusion physiology for at least a brief duration. In contrast to portal triad clamping, total vascular exclusion of the liver via a vena cava cross-clamp reduces systemic blood pressure and cardiac output because the loss of venous return is quite large. The vena cava cross-clamp may be applied briefly to facilitate completion of the hepatectomy or for a longer time to allow construction of the hepatic venous anastomoses. Severe cardiovascular compromise during the vena cava cross-clamp may necessitate institution of venovenous bypass. Prior to committing to vena caval and portal resection, the surgeon will often "test clamp" the cava and portal vein to ensure that the patient will tolerate hepatectomy without venovenous bypass. However, more moderate decreases in cardiac output and blood pressure can be treated by vasopressor administration coupled with judicious intravascular volume expansion. Modest doses of a vasopressor during caval cross-clamp to construct caval anastomoses are apparently well tolerated, with graft and patient survival rates comparable with those obtained when venovenous bypass is used.[200]

Low central venous pressure does not seem advantageous during liver transplantation, in contrast to hepatic resection. For patients undergoing orthotopic liver transplantation, keeping central venous pressure less than 5 mm Hg may be associated with higher incidences of postoperative renal failure and 30-day mortality relative to patients whose central venous pressure was allowed to run between 7 and 10 mm Hg, although more recent studies indicate that it may in fact be beneficial in that it decreases intraoperative blood loss, protects graft function, and has no detrimental effects on renal function in patients undergoing OLT.[201,202]

As in partial hepatectomy, 2 major contributors to hemodynamic changes during liver transplantation are changes in cardiac performance due to episodic alterations in venous return (discussed above) and hemorrhage. However, these factors are only 2 of the many sources of cardiovascular instability during liver transplantation. Sepsis, acidemia, hypocalcemia due to citrate toxicity, embolism, and acute right ventricular failure are all major contributions to hemodynamic problems. The period of graft reperfusion (described below) is particularly unstable in many instances.

The goals of hemodynamic management are to provide sufficient circulating volume, vascular resistance, and cardiac output to perfuse the vital organs. This is not guided by any single parameter but rather by a synthesis of all available data, including urine output, central venous pressure (in relation to the preoperative central venous pressure and with a full appreciation of the factors that may artificially alter it), and the absence of a vasopressor requirement except during periods of inadequate venous return.

Choice of Vasopressor With adequate volume management, vasopressors are rarely required intraoperatively except during periods of inadequate venous return (ie, during inferior vena cava cross-clamping) and transiently at liver reperfusion. Patients with higher MELD scores (>30) are more likely than those with lower MELD scores to require vasopressors.[203] Administration of vasopressors is a choice between the global detrimental effects of untreated significant hypotension and the potential negative effect of vasoconstrictors on perfusion of the new graft. In animal models, both epinephrine and norepinephrine reduced graft macro- and microperfusion,[204] but the functional consequences of these effects on human allograft performance or survival are unclear.

Vasopressin is a tempting choice because it is effective regardless of the pH, it reduces norepinephrine requirements, and it is effective for managing hepatorenal syndrome before transplantation. Most studies of vasopressin to date are in patients with septic or postcardiotomy shock. Vasopressin is effective in these circumstances, reducing the

TABLE 57-3 Characteristics of Common Rapid Infusion Devices

Device	Reservoir	Pump	Air Detector	Postpump Filter	Measured Flow Rate	Max Flow Rate
Level 1	No	No	Yes	No	No	Catheter limited
Haemonetics RIS	Yes	Yes	Yes	Yes	Yes (from pump)	1500 mL/min
Belmont FMS	Yes	Yes	Yes	No	Yes (from pump)	750 mL/min

FMS, fluid management system; RIS, rapid infusion system.

requirement for catecholamine vasopressor support. Limited observational studies indicate that although vasopressin raises the blood pressure, it does not compromise the microvascular circulation.[205] In 1 study retrospectively reviewing the use of vasopressin in septic shock, vasopressin was associated with increased liver enzyme levels, bilirubin, or both.[206] However, a recent study utilizing vasopressin in 16 patients undergoing liver transplantation showed that an infusion of vasopressin started after hepatic artery clamping and before caval clamping yielded a significant decrease in both portal vein pressure and blood flow but without a concomitant decrease in either cardiac output or intestinal perfusion.[207]

Terlipressin, a vasopressin analogue available in Europe and Asia, has been used in patients with cirrhosis and portal hypertension, demonstrating decreases in both hepatic and renal arterial resistance and portal venous blood flow, but without changes in portal vascular resistance.[208]

Adjuvant drugs, such as aprotinin, reduce the requirement for vasopressors, presumably by improving clotting performance and minimizing blood loss.[209] However, these advantages must be balanced against the other potential risks of aprotinin infusion (see below).

Transfusion and Other Therapies to Maintain Intravascular Volume The goal of volume management and transfusion in liver transplantation is to maintain sufficient intravascular volume to support a well-functioning circulation. Additionally, in many instances, the hemorrhage is sufficiently large that the anesthesiologist must intervene directly to control the composition of the circulating intravascular volume. Thus, in addition to red cell mass and intravascular volume, the anesthesiologist attends to plasma oncotic pressure, electrolyte composition, serum glucose, clotting factor levels, platelets, etc. In many cases, maintaining intravascular volume and management of coagulopathy are intertwined, so these topics are treated together in this section. **Figure 57-14** gives a high-level overview of a strategy for volume and transfusion management as a function of blood loss during transplantation.

Plasma oncotic pressure is a function of the osmotically active species in the plasma (proteins and, to a very small degree, cells). Albumin and other plasma proteins, mostly synthesized by the liver, provide plasma oncotic pressure. During liver transplantation, colloids should be used to replace intravascular volume lost through hemorrhage, with the addition of formed blood components as needed to meet specific needs (eg, red blood cells for oxygen-carrying capacity).

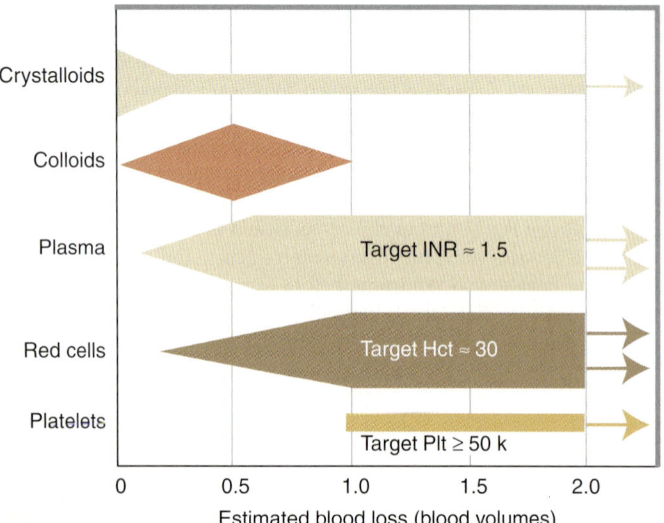

FIGURE 57-14. High-level overview of volume and blood component replacement strategy for liver transplantation requiring massive transfusion. All fluids are warmed (see text). The thickness of the bars represents the approximate relative proportions of each fluid in the replacement infusions.

One attractive approach to manage plasma oncotic pressure is to use fresh frozen plasma as a volume expander. This is particularly appropriate when the patient is coagulopathic due to hepatic synthetic failure, as fresh frozen plasma contains most of the proteins found in normal plasma. However, fresh frozen plasma also contains most of the citrate added to blood at the time of collection to prevent clotting. Thus rapid infusions (ie, >1 mL/kg/min) of fresh frozen plasma can chelate Ca^{+2}, causing acute hypocalcemia with consequent vasodilation and hypotension at inopportune times.[210] **Figure 57-15** illustrates the consequences of rapid infusion of citrated blood products during liver transplantation.

Fresh frozen plasma is a poor choice for volume expansion when the patient is not coagulopathic, as each unit of fresh frozen plasma carries with it the potential to trigger transfusion-related lung injury. Also, liver transplantation entails the construction of multiple low pressure, low flow anastomoses. Some practitioners believe that maintaining a slightly hypocoagulable state lessens the possibility of unwanted hepatic or portal venous thromboses. Thus, in the absence of significant coagulopathy, 5% albumin solution is probably a better choice for volume expansion. Synthetic colloids comprised of long-chain polysaccharides are available but are not popular because they can interfere with clot formation. Additionally, anesthesiologists must be cognizant of not volume overloading the patient, as excessive volume postreperfusion can add to liver congestion and swelling within the capsule, likely amplifying ischemic reperfusion injury.

Transfusion and Other Therapies to Maintain Coagulation Capacity Coagulation is monitored using standard laboratory tests, augmented in some cases by point-of-care functional tests, and ultimately by clinical correlation of the laboratory test results with direct observation of the surgical field. The basic tests to monitor coagulation status are the prothrombin time, the activated partial thromboplastin time, and the platelet count. D-dimer and fibrinogen levels provide information about the presence of clot lysis, and the latter, the ability to form clot. However, these tests provide a far-from-complete picture of a patient's coagulation performance. Many centers use thromboelastography to obtain near-patient diagnostics of clot initiation, formation, and lysis.[211,212] Thromboelastography is a mechanical test described in detail in Chapter 15. The test is sensitive to extraneous influences (including environmental disruption), and it is not well standardized. However, thromboelastography is useful in liver transplantation because, unlike other tests, it gives information about clot lysis.[212]

Coagulation performance during liver transplantation in the patient with end-stage liver disease tends to follow a predictable course.[213] Patients with hepatic synthetic failure start out hypocoagulable, and with appropriate transfusion of fresh frozen plasma as part of the volume replacement strategy, coagulation status tends not to get significantly worse during the preanhepatic and anhepatic phases of the operation. After reperfusion of the graft, a clot lysis syndrome develops, and some patients become hypercoagulable at the same time (ie, disseminated intravascular coagulation develops).[213] Even patients who present with normal hepatic synthetic function and no coagulopathy can develop a dilutional coagulopathy as well as the reperfusion clot lysis syndrome. A worsening coagulopathy postreperfusion despite adequate replacement of coagulation factors, platelets, and fibrinogen may herald a nonviable graft and the immediate need for a replacement organ.

Volume replacement therapy should attend to preserving or moving clotting potential toward a normal state as part of the effort to reduce blood loss. However, transfusion therapy and coagulation management are no substitute for good surgical technique. Successful transplantation requires attention to both. Typically, fresh frozen plasma is used to replace clotting factors. Liver transplant patients are frequently in a state of low-grade disseminated intravascular coagulation and thus consume fibrinogen and clotting factors even in the absence of massive hemorrhage. Fresh frozen plasma usually supplies sufficient fibrinogen, but cryoprecipitate may be helpful if the fibrinogen levels become unacceptably low.

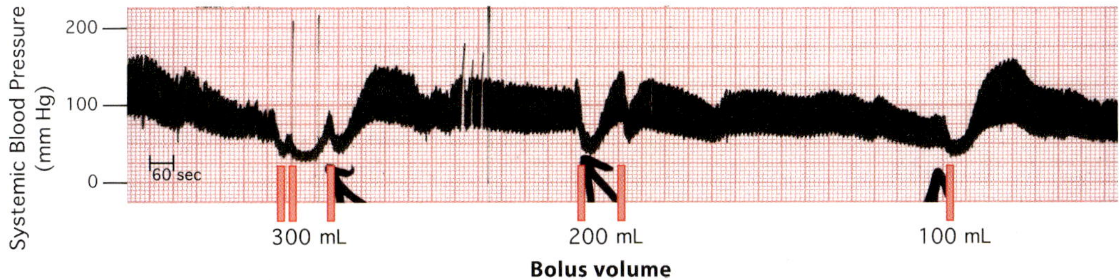

FIGURE 57-15. Acute systemic hypotension due to rapid transfusion of a citrate-containing 50:50 mixture of fresh frozen plasma and packed red blood cells. Boluses of 100 mL (vertical bars) were infused at 500 mL/min using a rapid infusion system (Haemonetics, Braintree, MA, USA). The hypotensive response is superimposed on acute hypotension due to sudden hemorrhage that was to be treated by the fluid challenge. The infusion-exacerbated hypotension was treated by infusion of norepinephrine.

Platelets are rarely needed prior to graft reperfusion, even in patients with low platelet counts (eg, 50 000/ml). Furthermore, many patients manifest splenic sequestration of platelets and have no response to transfusion, both exposing the patient to unnecessary risk of transfusion and wasting a valuable blood component.

Antifibrinolytic drugs and other procoagulants can be used prophylactically in the preanhepatic phase to minimize bleeding. These drugs are discussed in detail in the section on the postanhepatic phase of liver transplantation.

Anhepatic Phase The anhepatic phase of liver transplantation is frequently described as the time from explantation of the diseased liver to the reperfusion of the new liver. However, the anhepatic phase of the operation actually begins once the native liver is sufficiently compromised to have no further function. During liver transplantation, this is usually when the hepatic artery is clamped, which can precede portal and hepatic vein clamping by many minutes. During this time, especially in the setting of portal hypertension, the diseased liver receives no oxygenated inflow and begins to die, with a consequent effect on the patient's acid–base status. However, once the liver is completely excluded from the circulation, this problem ends. After this, the anhepatic phase is often a relatively quiet period in the case. Bleeding should be under control, and the surgeons are engaged in the delicate task of constructing the venous anastomoses. During the construction of the venous anastomoses, the liver is kept on ice (**Fig. 57-16**, left panel).

Any drugs dependent on hepatic metabolism begin to accumulate once the portal vein and hepatic artery are clamped. Thus infusions of drugs should be titrated to effect. Of course, drugs not dependent on hepatic metabolism (eg, inhaled agents, remifentanyl) are unaffected by this transition.

The anesthesia team should attend to immunosuppression during the early anhepatic phase. The patient will have received an induction dose of an immunosuppressant, such as mycophenylate mofetil, prior to coming to the operating room. Obviously, this should be confirmed prior to starting the case. Typically, a modest dose of steroid (eg, 100-500 mg methylprednisolone) is given in the operating room as the new liver is initially placed into the recipient (before opening of the anastomoses; Fig. 57-16, right panel). For patients with hepatitis C, alternative regimens may be used such as an infusion of rabbit antithymocyte globulin begun at the completion of the hepatectomy and 10 mg methylprednisolone when the liver is placed into the recipient. In practice, the immunosuppression regimen is chosen by the surgeon, and the anesthesia team should ascertain the drugs, doses, routes, and timing prior to starting surgery.

Hemodynamics frequently stabilize during the anhepatic phase, particularly if a piggyback technique is used. This period of stability may derive from the fact that the rapid alterations in venous return during gross manipulations of the liver are superceded by more delicate tasks. If an en-bloc resection has been used with a complete vena cava

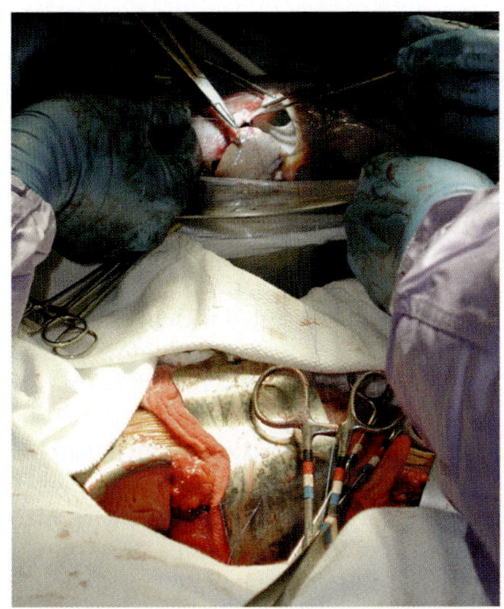
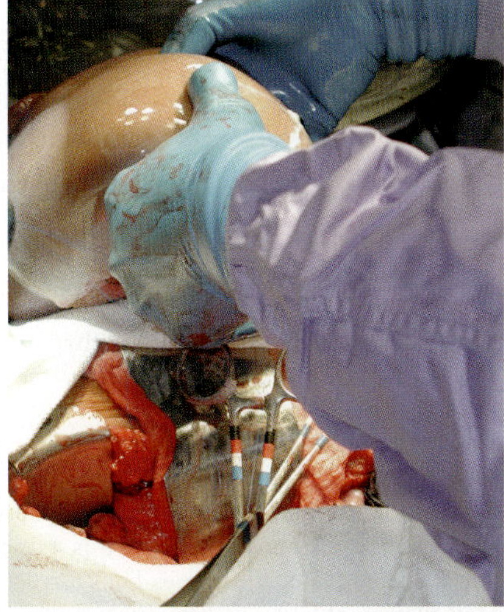

FIGURE 57-16. Liver transplantation surgery. Left panel illustrates construction of the initial anastomosis, with the liver kept on ice to minimize warm ischemic time. The right panel illustrates the liver being placed into the body cavity. At this point, immunosuppressants should be given. The anastomoses are partially tied, after which the liver is flushed and the anastomoses opened.

cross-clamp, the circulation may still be stable if venovenous bypass is also used. However, if the vena cava is clamped without a venous return conduit, it is often necessary to support the circulation with a potent vasoconstrictor, preferably an agent with some inotropic activity such as norepinephrine.

Hypotension with diminished central venous pressure may occur even with significant preservation of venous return during the anhepatic phase. Lower extremity and splanchnic congestion lowers the effective circulating volume and central venous pressure above the diaphragm, with attendant hypotension. However, it is important not to overtreat this condition with aggressive volume replacement, as it can lead to hypervolemia at the time of graft reperfusion. Instead, it is preferable to support the circulation with a low dose of a vasopressor, anticipating the mobilization of blood from below the diaphragm once the liver is reperfused.

Finally, some poorly understood physiologic feature of the anhepatic phase might directly affect left ventricular performance, contributing to hypotension. Echocardiographic studies of ventricular function demonstrate, for example, that left ventricular shortening fraction diminishes during the anhepatic phase, relative to the preanhepatic phase, then returns to normal[214] after reperfusion. Although this was a small study, a more recent and larger study revealed a decrease in right ventricular ejection fraction from baseline during the anhepatic phase of liver transplantation in 20 patients, but with a gradual return to baseline 30 minutes postreperfusion.[215]

Electrolyte Management Serum electrolytes and acid–base balance are subject to wide and rapid swings during liver transplantation, especially if the case is bloody and extensive transfusion is required. These are most severe during the anhepatic phase, when even the small residual function of the native liver has been removed. However, even during the preanhepatic phase, the patient's acid–base, electrolyte, red cell mass, and coagulation statuses are likely to change rapidly due to brisk hemorrhage, various cross-clamping maneuvers, and compression of abdominal vasculature, as well as potentially massive transfusion. Thus frequent monitoring of arterial blood gases, serum electrolytes, red cell mass, and laboratory measures of clotting is mandatory from the beginning of surgery.[216] During the active portion of the case, we interpret and respond to laboratory results as they are returned, allow for equilibration, and then recheck the laboratory values.

Metabolic acidosis may develop in the anhepatic phase due to portal cross-clamping, as well as partial or complete inferior vena cava (IVC) cross-clamping, creating imperfect lower extremity and splanchnic venous return. There is also loss of any residual ability to clear organic acids. At the time of reperfusion, the donor liver and underperfused tissues from the patient release acid loads. Ongoing transfusion of low-pH, citrated blood products also contributes to the acidemia.

Various maneuvers can mitigate acidemia during liver transplantation. Hyperventilation can be used to establish an acute respiratory compensation for metabolic acidosis. Sodium bicarbonate can be administered to correct acidemia, although the need to minimize sodium loads, particularly in patients who are hyponatremic, may limit the usefulness of bicarbonate. Sodium bicarbonate must not be coadministered in the same infusion as Ca^{+2} solutions, as the combination will precipitate. Tromethamine (THAM) can also be used to control acidemia.

Acidemia at the time of reperfusion should be corrected by hyperventilation and administration of bicarbonate. This minimizes the hemodynamic and cardiac effect of the acid load and metabolic waste products released by reperfusion of the allograft. However, overzealous correction of metabolic acidemia is undesirable, particularly in the setting of massive transfusion. This is because the new liver clears citrate and organic acids, resulting in a rebound metabolic alkalosis; this may be seen developing even during the late neohepatic phase. Thus a reasonable strategy is to use modest hyperventilation to keep the pH near normal, with the use of bicarbonate of THAM only as needed to keep the pH above approximately 7.35 after respiratory maneuvers have been fully implemented.

Patients presenting for liver transplantation may be either hyper- or hypokalemic, depending on whether potassium-sparing or potassium-wasting diuretics have been used to control ascites. Potassium balance is also influenced by the underlying renal function or compromise. Serum potassium is subject to strong influences favoring hyperkalemia during the anhepatic phase. This may lead to large swings in serum potassium, especially if renal function is compromised or if large volumes of blood products are required. Additionally, splanchnic ischemia during the case tends to elevate serum potassium. Metabolic acidosis tends to worsen hyperkalemia. Finally, the preservative solution in the donor liver is rich in potassium.

Dangerous levels of serum potassium should be treated to avoid myocardial irritability and cardiac dysrhythmias. In patients with preserved renal function, this is accomplished initially by controlling the pH, by the use of potassium-wasting diuretics if the volume status permits, and by avoidance of potassium-containing solutions. Bicarbonate to increase pH tends to drive potassium intracellularly, whereas Ca^{+2} administration to replete deficits stabilizes irritable myocardium. Rapid or persistent increases in serum potassium are treated with glucose and insulin to drive potassium intracellularly by glucose cotransport. The combination of insulin and glucose predictably reduces serum potassium even during the anhepatic phase.[217]

Inhaled β_2-agonists, including albuterol and levalbuterol, may be used to lower serum potassium by driving serum potassium intracellularly, and recently salbutamol was used to treat hyperkalemia resistant to other treatments during the anhepatic stage of a patient undergoing liver transplantation.[218]

If renal function is severely compromised, renal replacement therapy, either by continuous venovenous hemofiltration or by conventional dialysis, may be warranted to control serum potassium, sodium, and pH. Intraoperative renal replacement therapy can strain the resources of hospital dialysis services, so early consultation with a dialysis nephrologist is important once it appears that such therapy is needed.

Calcium is required for smooth muscle and myocardial contractility. Thus hypocalcemia during liver transplantation depresses inotropy (manifested as depressed cardiac index, reduced cardiac stroke index, and left ventricular work index[219]) and reduces vascular tone. In this setting, vasopressor activity is also compromised. Hypocalcemia may also interfere with clotting, as calcium is a required cofactor for many clotting factors. Thus it is important to monitor and correct abnormal serum calcium. During liver transplantation, serum ionized calcium tends to decrease due to vigorous administration of citrated blood products. As a rule of thumb, administration of 6 units or more of acid citrate dextrose (ACD)-preserved packed red blood cells requires supplementation of calcium.

Calcium can be repleted with calcium gluconate or calcium chloride. The positive inotropic effects of calcium administration are quick in onset but short lived. Again, overaggressive correction of ionized calcium intraoperatively precipitates a rebound hypercalcemia during the postoperative period as the liver metabolizes the citrate chelator. Thus the goal for intraoperative calcium management is to achieve the lowest ionized calcium concentration consistent with good cardiac performance and coagulation, typically 0.9 to 1.0 mmol/L. Postoperative hypercalcemia is treated with hydration and furosemide diuresis.

Serum sodium is frequently low in liver transplant patients due to the formation of ascites, the effects of renal failure, the use of diuretics, or combinations of all of these. It is important to avoid accidental aggressive overcorrection of hyponatremia, as too-rapid correction of hyponatremia can cause central pontine myelinolysis, an irreversible neurologic injury. Unfortunately, many useful replacement fluids contain sodium. For example, fresh frozen plasma, packed red blood cells, and 5% albumin all contain sodium at normal physiologic concentrations. To maintain intravascular volume while avoiding too-rapid correction of hyponatremia, a strategy of administering colloids along with 5% dextrose while inducing a diuresis of sodium and water with furosemide may be used. In patients with renal failure, dialysis or continuous venovenous hemofiltration against a low sodium bath can be used to remove the volume without increasing sodium too abruptly.

Glucose management during liver transplantation is usually fairly straightforward despite the liver's central role in glucose handling. The liver is the major site for gluconeogenesis, and this function is preserved to some degree in even the most severe cases of end-stage liver disease. Thus complete hepatectomy creates the possibility of intraoperative hypoglycemia during liver transplantation. This is particularly true if the anhepatic phase of the operation is prolonged.

Serum glucose during liver transplantation is also influenced by exogenous sources, including carrier infusions and the release of glucose from graft preservation solution. Thus intraoperative hypoglycemia is rarely a problem in practice, especially if some IV fluids (eg, drug-carrier infusions) contain 5% dextrose. Additionally, the use of methylprednisolone during the anhepatic stage often results in serum hyperglycemia. The liver is at once the major site of gluconeogenesis and insulin-mediated glucose uptake. Therefore, the anhepatic phase may be marked by hyper- or hypoglycemia, both of which should be avoided and treated. As in the case of other major surgeries, tight glycemic control is probably beneficial, and blood glucose should be measured frequently. Target blood glucose should be 150 to 200 mg/dL.

Renal Protection During Transplantation Renal failure requiring renal replacement therapy (eg, dialysis or continuous venovenous hemofiltration) is common after liver transplantation, with rates of approximately 5% to 10%.[220,221] Peritransplantation acute renal failure requiring renal replacement therapy is associated with higher mortality as compared with liver transplant patients not requiring dialysis.[222] It is not clear whether there is a cause-and-effect relationship between acute renal failure and death after liver transplantation, but renal failure is an unwelcome outcome.

Protection of renal function probably depends, among other things, on maintaining renal perfusion during the liver transplant procedure. Renal perfusion is subject to many insults during transplantation, including hypovolemia and increased resistance to venous outflow due to vena cava compression or cross-clamping. Maintaining an adequate circulating volume facilitates preserving renal function. However, this is at times difficult, and a selective medical therapy to protect the kidney in the peritransplant period would be useful.

Attention has focused on selective splanchnic vasodilators, such as low-dose dopamine or, more recently, fenoldopam, as protective agents during major surgery. Fenoldopam has recently been studied in liver transplant patients randomized to 1 of 3 groups (fenoldopam, low-dose dopamine, or placebo) prior to surgery. Neither fenoldopam nor dopamine was superior to placebo for preservation of any measure of renal function (urine output, serum creatinine, creatinine clearance, use of diuretics, or use of pressors) immediately after surgery. On the third and fourth day after transplantation, creatinine clearance was reduced in patients receiving placebo or low-dose dopamine, whereas it was preserved in patients receiving fenoldopam.[223] The authors concluded that fenoldopam might counteract the renal arterial constrictive effects of cyclosporine.[223]

In this small, unblinded study, neither low-dose dopamine nor fenoldopam demonstrated obvious renal protective effects in the early perioperative period.[223] Similarly, another small study by the same researchers demonstrated that fenoldopam led to better creatinine and blood urea nitrogen values at day 3 after liver transplant, but the functional effect of this result on the incidence of acute renal failure was not demonstrated.[224] Slightly lower (but not statistically significant) BUN and creatinine levels were observed in OLT patients who received continuous infusions of fenoldopam, although increased splanchnic perfusion was seen in the study group as compared to placebo.[225]

More conventional approaches to renal protection include maintaining adequate circulating volume and perfusion pressure. Urine output is commonly used to judge real function in the operating room, and "target" urine flows of 1 $mL/kg^{-1}/h^{-1}$ are frequently sought. When the urine output falls below this target and the circulating volume and perfusion pressure are judged to be adequate, furosemide or mannitol are sometimes used to increase the urine output.

Reperfusion of the Graft Preparation for reperfusion involves optimizing volume status and hemodynamic performance and preparing the operating room for a potentially chaotic reperfusion period. Potential distractions related to the anesthetic (eg, the need to redose drugs, change syringes, carrier infusions) should be addressed in advance. Laboratory studies should have been sent in time for the results to arrive 5 minutes prior to reperfusion. Constant communication between surgeon and anesthesiologist must be the rule rather than the exception, with each team informing the other well in advance of any major intervention or treatment.

Abnormalities in pH, serum potassium, or calcium should be corrected prior to reperfusion. Sodium bicarbonate, glucose and insulin, and calcium chloride should be prepared and ready for use. Some practitioners use combinations of these agents prophylactically prior to reperfusion.[174]

Vasopressors may be required at the time of reperfusion and should be available for immediate infusion. Among the commonly used vasopressors, there is no compelling or logical best choice, so institutional preferences prevail. Epinephrine, dopamine, and norepinephrine are all acceptable choices, although some practitioners may consider the use of phenylephrine or vasopressin. Vasopressors are also commonly used prophylactically at reperfusion, frequently as a small bolus such as epinephrine, 10 mcg.

Just prior to reperfusion, the new liver is flushed antegrade from the portal vein to the hepatic vein to wash out the preservative solution (which contains large doses of potassium and heparin). Flushing is accomplished with crystalloid, colloid (such as 5% albumin), or blood. A blood flush is performed by constructing the portal and hepatic venous anastomoses, after which the portal anastomosis is closed but the hepatic venous anastomosis is left open. The portal vein cross-clamp is removed, and blood is allowed to flush the liver and run out into the field where it is recovered by suction. Concomitant with this controlled hemorrhage, fluid should be rapidly transfused to maintain euvolemia.

Graft reperfusion has its most obvious effect on cardiac performance, and the anesthesia team should be prepared for pulmonary hypertension and acute right heart dysfunction. Liver transplantation in and of itself does not appear to cause right heart dysfunction.[226] However, release of preservative solution, air, clot, and debris (as well as acidemic blood from the reperfused splanchnic circulation) into the pulmonary vasculature can cause sudden and severe pulmonary hypertension, elevated right heart pressures, and right ventricular failure (as mentioned previously). Systemic pressure (and coronary perfusion pressure) decreases due to inadequate left ventricular preload. The elevated right heart pressures may open an occult patent foramen ovale, with risk of paradoxical embolism.[227] The central venous pressure frequently increases due to right heart and pulmonary congestion. Ordinarily this is desirable to a point to ensure right ventricular preload. However, in the immediate reperfusion period, elevated central venous pressure compromises graft perfusion and may contribute to early graft failure. Thus it becomes important to preserve or reestablish efficient right ventricular pumping and a low-resistance pulmonary circulation.

Pulmonary hypertension, right ventricular overload, and the resulting central venous congestion reduce the hepatic perfusion pressure, which is simply the difference between the portal and central venous pressure when only the venous anastomoses have been constructed. The portal venous pressure is not typically measured, so the hepatic perfusion pressure is not directly accessible. However, inadequate perfusion pressure can be deduced if the liver becomes engorged. This alarming appearance somewhat mimics that of hyperacute rejection. To avoid confusion, the hepatic perfusion pressure is ideally controlled by keeping the central venous pressure low at the time of reperfusion. This is not possible in the event of acute pulmonary hypertension unless inotropes and selective pulmonary vasodilators are used. Typically, the heart is supported with an inotrope, and the lungs are hyperventilated to raise the pH and induce vasodilation. Inhaled nitric oxide and/or a low-dose infusion of nitroglycerine may be useful at this point.

As stated previously, good communication between the surgical and anesthesia teams is also important to minimize the effect of reperfusion. Reperfusion should not occur until the anesthesia team has optimized the patient's physiology, and this should be accomplished in time to allow prompt reperfusion. In the event of severe problems at reperfusion, the surgeon can partially reclamp the portal vein to lessen the effect of the effluent from the new liver.

The combined effect of multiple insults on cardiac and pulmonary performance at reperfusion may lead to cardiovascular collapse. Advanced cardiac life support protocols directed at the presumptive major problem should be promptly initiated while the underlying insults are identified and corrected. In the event of cardiopulmonary arrest not responsive to pharmacologic support (or due to reversible causes such as pulmonary embolus), mechanical circulation and oxygenation can be provided by percutaneous femoral venoarterial cardiopulmonary bypass with acceptable survival.[228]

In the early postreperfusion period, severe volume overload from overaggressive fluid replacement during the period of poor venous return may compromise hepatic perfusion even with adequate cardiac performance. If the problem is slight, then it may be possible to administer furosemide to induce diuresis, or to wait for the blood volume to fall due to bleeding. In the case of severe volume overload and poor graft perfusion, phlebotomy from a large port on a central venous catheter is a logical option.

Neohepatic Phase The neohepatic phase begins with the initial reperfusion of the liver. Frequently, the next step is to construct the hepatic arterial anastomosis. The liver ultimately needs a high-pressure, oxygenated perfusion source, and the surgical team will turn its attention to this as soon as the immediate effects of venous reperfusion have passed. Opening of the hepatic arterial anastomosis usually has little or no hemodynamic effect.

An acute clot lysis syndrome frequently develops in the early neohepatic phase. This manifests clinically as diffuse bleeding from previously coagulated sites in the surgical field, new oozing from previously quiescent vascular catheter insertion sites, and ongoing transfusion requirements. Laboratory analysis shows a further elevation of the prothrombin time relative to baseline, and a sometimes profound elevation of the partial thromboplastin time (eg, to >150 seconds), as if the patient had received a large dose of heparin. Thromboelastography demonstrates poor clot initiation and rapid dissolution of clot. **Figure 57-17** shows sequential thromboelastograms obtained from a single patient during the course of transplantation.[229]

The cause of this clot lysis syndrome is not completely understood, which limits the ability to tailor treatment to specific causes. Multiple mechanisms have been proposed and may operate simultaneously, including release of heparin (from preservative solution) during reperfusion or release of endogenous activators of tissue plasminogen activator and/or endogenous heparinoids from the graft.[213]

A central goal in this phase of the transplant is to stop clot lysis. A key first step toward achieving this goal is to provide adequate levels of platelets and factors to support clotting in the face of ongoing consumption, with the expectation that a functioning graft will begin to provide appropriate clot lysis inhibitors and clotting factors on its own. One could consider administering a small (20-50 mg) dose of protamine[213] in the event that clot formation is suspected to be deficient, especially if the liver flush prior to reperfusion was not optimal and the patient might have received heparin from the graft.

Fibrinolytic activity is frequently increased during liver transplantation, reflecting reduced hepatic clearance of tissue plasminogen activating factor (tPA) during the anhepatic phase and release of tissue plasminogen activator from the epithelial cells of the reperfused graft.[230-232] In addition, plasminogen activator inhibitor-1 activity is reduced[231] during transplantation. Fibrinolysis probably contributes to the unwanted clot lysis syndrome after reperfusion.

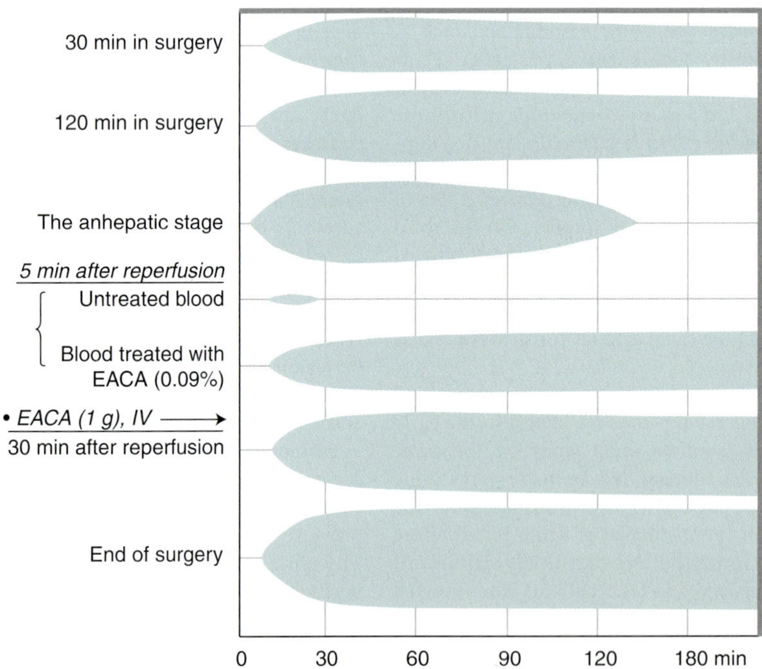

FIGURE 57-17. Sequential thromboelastograms from a single patient having liver transplantation. Marked fibrinolysis developed during the anhepatic phase. Note the development of severe coagulopathy in the "5 min after reperfusion" sample consisting of poor clotting and early fibrinolysis more severe than during the anhepatic phase. ε-Aminocaproic acid (EACA) was given, which arrested the clot lysis. [From Kang Y, Lewis JH, Navalgund A, et al. Epsilon-aminocaproic acid for treatment of fibrinolysis during liver transplantation. *Anesthesiology.* 1987;66:766-773. Reproduced with permission.]

Strategies for reducing fibrinolysis and transfusion requirements include the use of antifibrinolytic agents such as aprotinin,[233] tranexamic acid, and ε-aminocaproic acid.[234] However, the use of antifibrinolytics in liver transplantation is somewhat controversial because of concerns about unwanted thrombosis.

ε-Aminocaproic acid and tranexamic acid are both synthetic analogues of the amino acid lysine. ε-Aminocaproic acid and tranexamic acid competitively inhibit the binding of plasminogen (a lysine protease) to lysine residues on fibrin, thus inhibiting fibrinolysis. Both drugs also prevent the conversion of plasminogen to plasmin, again by virtue of acting as competitive antagonists of a lysine protease. ε-Aminocaproic acid is used during liver transplantation as a loading dose (typically a 1- to 2-g bolus over 1-10 minutes), followed by infusions of 1 to 2 g per hour. It reliably arrests fibrinolysis as assessed by thromboelastography (see Fig. 57-17).[229] The drug is eliminated by the kidney, with 65% of a dose appearing unchanged in the urine. The elimination half-life of ε-Aminocaproic acid is about 2 hours.

Tranexamic acid is 6 to 10 times more potent than ε-aminocaproic acid and has a longer elimination half-life. It is also renally eliminated, with 95% of the drug appearing unchanged in the urine. It is the least well studied of the 3 major antifibrinolytics.[234] Dose rates between 2 mg/kg/h and 40 mg/kg/h have been reported in small studies with either ε-aminocaproic acid or aprotinin as comparisons.

Aprotinin is a protease inhibitor isolated from the lungs of swine or cows. It inhibits a variety of human proteases, including plasmin, trypsin, kallikrein, chymotrypsin, activated protein C, and thrombin. These proteases are important in fibrinolysis and coagulation, as well as complement activation and inflammation. Each uses a serine residue for catalysis at the active site, and aprotinin acts by forming a specific aprotinin-active site serine complex with each protease. Aprotinin has an approximately 1-hour redistribution half-life after a bolus, and a 7- to 10-hour elimination half-life. It is given as a bolus, followed by an infusion. A typical bolus is 2 million kallikrein inactivator units (KIU), followed by an infusion of 500 000 to 1 million KIU per hour.[234]

The use of antifibrinolytic drugs may have deleterious effects. There is anecdotal evidence that antifibrinolytic therapy may increase the incidence of thrombotic events during liver transplantation, including fatal pulmonary thromboembolism.[235] Additionally, as mentioned previously, aprotinin is no more effective than the lysine analogues, but it is associated with excess morbidity and mortality relative to these other drugs when used in cardiac surgery.[132] This suggests that during liver transplantation, antifibrinolytic agents should be reserved for patients who have a relatively high risk of severe hemorrhage,[236] and aprotinin might best be avoided altogether. However, the clotting cascade in liver transplant patients is quite deranged, and cardiopulmonary thromboembolism, even in the absence of exogenous procoagulants, may be more common than is usually appreciated.[169]

Thus antifibrinolytics might be considered for rescue if bleeding becomes a problem in the postanhepatic phase,[234] as judged by the disappearance of clot from the surgical field, or as a prophylactic measure in patients expected to have severe bleeding problems (eg, multiorgan transplant in a patient with renal failure). Balanced against this cautious approach are some practices that advocate the use of antifibrinolytics prophylactically, in advance of any pathologic bleeding.[234] However, in addition to enhanced fibrinolysis, many other factors contribute to blood loss late in orthotopic liver transplantation, including coagulopathy due to synthetic failure, thrombocytopenia, platelet dysfunction, dysfibrinogenemia, dilutional coagulopathy, hypothermia, and bleeding from surgical technical problems. As postreperfusion fibrinolysis is largely a diagnosis of exclusion, all of these other factors must be ruled out before administration of potent procoagulants.

Procoagulant agents, such as purified specific clotting factors, can also be used, either prophylactically or as an attempted therapy for excessive bleeding. For example, in 1 study, recombinant factor 7 corrected coagulopathy when given as single bolus prior to transplant, but there was no effect on transfusion requirements.[237] In a different study, recombinant factor VII was used in a small number of patients without clear evidence of clinical harm or benefit.[238] Recombinant factor VII has the theoretical advantage of being selective only for areas that are bleeding—that is, those areas that have sustained tissue damage. This is because recombinant factor VII requires tissue factor for full activity, and tissue factor is only available in areas in which the subendothelial layers are exposed. Of course, the vascular anastomoses in the new graft would have exposed tissue factor, at least theoretically increasing the risk of thromboses of the anastomoses. Furthermore, recombinant factor VII is apparently not as selective as initially hoped. A recent report documents many episodes of arterial and venous thromboses distant from the hoped-for site of action (eg, cerebrovascular accident, myocardial infarction, pulmonary embolism, and deep venous thrombosis) when recombinant factor VII was used in various "off-label" applications.[134]

If the fibrinolysis reaction cannot be controlled, the patient will have an ongoing transfusion requirement. The anesthesia team should quantify the hourly transfusion needs in the neohepatic phase and make preparations to meet this during the end of the case, the move from OR table to ICU bed, transport to the ICU, and in the intensive care unit itself.

L-arginine, an essential component of the L-arginine/nitric oxide (NO) synthase pathway, is diminished in patients postreperfusion due to liberation of arginase from the donor graft, and may lead to hemodynamic changes in the reperfusion stage.[239,240] With a decrease in L-arginine and an increase in arginase, there is a concomitant increase in L-ornithine levels.[241] Blockade of the L-arginine/NO synthase pathway is implicated in hepatic apoptosis and liver transplant preservation injury, and blockade of arginase or administration of L-arginine protects against hepatic warm ischemia reperfusion injury and has demonstrated improvements in cardiac output and liver blood flow, while reducing pulmonary vascular resistance.[242-244]

During the neohepatic phase, the anesthesia team prepares for the postoperative disposition of the patient. Most liver transplant recipients are discharged from the operating room to an ICU bed. The anesthesia team seeks to manage this transition as smoothly as possible. The patient should be transported on an ICU bed, with all necessary infusions running and the patient fully monitored. Comprehensive communication between the operating room and the ICU team is essential to facilitate the smooth transition of care.

The anesthesia team also prepares for the early postoperative care of the patient. One large, multicenter study looking at early extubation in 391 patients demonstrated that early extubation is safe under specific conditions, with only 7.7% having adverse outcomes secondary to either pulmonary issues or need for additional surgery.[245] Suitability for extubation is influenced by many factors. Among these are the intraoperative transfusion requirement (as a warning of possible airway edema); the presence or development of pulmonary, cardiac, and renal compromise; and the presence and severity of encephalopathy.[246] Fluid administration and possible volume overload are some of the many factors that can interfere with the patient's readiness for extubation at end of case. Controlled fluid administration supported by adjuvant vasopressors led to reduced rates of reintubation in 1 study.[247] Intraabdominal hypertension is common after orthotopic liver transplantation and limits the potential for extubation. Intraabdominal hypertension (pressure >25 mm Hg in the bladder) developed in 32% of patients[248] in 1 series. It is expected that these patients are less likely to meet criteria for early extubation and are harder to wean from the ventilator.

If in doubt, it is always acceptable and prudent to leave the patient intubated for pulmonary support in the early postoperative period. Postoperative mechanical ventilation allows the team to focus on ongoing transfusion requirements, to exclude the possibility of intra-abdominal hypertension, and to gradually prepare the patient for extubation. Despite the concern about elevated intra-abdominal pressures on graft viability, postoperative application of positive end-expiratory pressure (PEEP) does not have a major effect on graft function, although in half of the patients the cardiac output declined with PEEP.[249] This is encouraging because PEEP may be needed to counteract the pulmonary consequences of intra-abdominal hypertension.

Pain management is relatively straightforward after liver transplantation. Many patients remain intubated and receive potent opioids as sedatives. Epidural analgesia is traditionally avoided due to the profound coagulopathy manifested by end-stage liver disease patients, both preoperatively and in the postoperative period, although some centers report successful use of thoracic epidural anesthesia for patients who meet strict criteria.[250] Furthermore, orthotopic liver transplant patients have less postoperative pain than hepatectomy patients.[251] The reason for this difference in pain threshold is unclear, although some have implicated the steroids used for immunosuppression. Steroids have analgesic properties in other patient populations.[252]

PERIOPERATIVE COMPLICATIONS OF LIVER TRANSPLANTATION

Complications of liver transplantation are frequent. Here we focus on the early complications of liver transplantation—that is, those that occur in the operating room or the intensive care unit within hours or days of the procedure.

Complications of massive transfusion should be mentioned at this juncture. Risks of massive transfusion consist of pulmonary edema, transfusion-related acute lung injury (TRALI),[253,254] and viral infection. Analysis of pulmonary edema from liver transplant recipients has demonstrated rich edema fluid/plasma protein levels, consistent with increased permeability pulmonary edema and TRALI.[255] Increased use of blood products, and more specifically plasma and platelets, is associated with an increased incidence of TRALI in liver transplantation.[256] Various strategies including volumetric diffusive respirator (VDR) ventilation, PEEP, and prone ventilation have been successfully used in the treatment of posthepatic transplantation patients with TRALI.[257]

Much attention has focused on the transmission of cytomegalovirus. The incidence of cytomegalovirus transmission is much higher with a cytomegalovirus-infected donor organ than with blood that has not been screened or reduced for cytomegalovirus.[258] Cytomegalovirus is an independent risk factor for mortality after liver transplantation, due in part to allograft rejection or chronic graft dysfunction.[259] Many centers now use routine pharmacoprophylaxis against cytomegalovirus infection, as leukoreduction of blood or the use of cytomegalovirus-negative donors has been deemed impractical by many blood banks.

Massive transfusion contributes to the development of intra-abdominal hypertension. Patients with intra-abdominal hypertension had a higher incidence of renal failure, more postoperative complications, and higher intensive care unit mortality than patients without this complication.[248]

Anastomotic leaks involving the vascular or bile duct connections can prompt reexploration and anastomotic revisions. Anastomotic bleeding tends to be most severe during the latter stages of the surgery and on the first postoperative day. An ongoing brisk transfusion requirement, an expanding abdomen, or falling hematocrit can prompt reexploration even before leaving the operating room. There should be a low threshold to reexplore for bleeding, as an abdomen full of blood or clot is a nidus for infection. In addition, the compressive effect of a large hematoma potentially compromises graft, pulmonary, and cardiac function. Reexploration in the early postoperative period should be handled with the same degree of preparation as the original transplant procedure. In particular, a disruption of one of the anastomoses without surgical control of the vessel can lead to massive hemorrhage.

Other vascular complications necessitating prompt reexploration include stenosis or thrombosis of the anastomoses of the liver vessels. This may occur intraoperatively or postoperatively. In the intraoperative and postoperative period, vascular patency is monitored by serial ultrasound examinations.[260] Hepatic artery thrombosis is the most common vascular complication in the postoperative period.[260] Radiologists must be vigilant and knowledgeable of locations of surgical anastomoses to help identify potential sites for complications in the immediate postoperative period.[261] If hepatic artery thrombosis is not diagnosed and treated promptly, severe graft dysfunction or total graft loss will occur. Treatment of hepatic artery thrombosis typically requires urgent reoperation to remove the obstruction, although endovascular treatment has been successfully used.[262] If flow cannot be restored, the patient probably needs to be relisted for liver transplantation as a Status I candidate. However, there is a small but growing experience of temporizing with hyperbaric oxygen therapy.[263]

Neurologic complications are relatively common after liver transplantation. Their causes are multifactorial, related both to intraoperative and early postoperative events, as well as the ongoing effects of toxic immunosuppressants. Of particular concern to anesthesiologists is central pontine myelinolysis,[264] which has been associated with rapid correction of hyponatremia in the peritransplant period. This syndrome is characterized by a general neurologic decline hours or days after a sudden correction of hyponatremia. Much attention focuses on central pontine myelinolysis because patients presenting for liver transplantation are frequently hyponatremic and because of the association between the syndrome and an inciting event (eg, rapid correction of hyponatremia). However, central pontine myelinolysis is a relatively rare neurologic complication of liver transplantation. For example, in a study of 463 patients having transplants performed at multiple centers,[265] 93 (20.1%) patients had peritransplant neurologic complications. Of these, 6 patients (1.2% of the starting cohort) were confirmed to have central pontine myelinolysis. Two of these patients had rapid increases in their serum sodium for a period of hours during transplant; the rest did not.[265] In another multicenter prospective cohort study involving 1730 liver transplant patients, there were 60 patients with radiologically confirmed central nervous system lesions. Of these, 5 patients (0.3% of the original cohort) had central pontine myelinolysis.[266]

SPECIAL OPERATIONS ON THE LIVER

PROCEDURES FOR PORTAL HYPERTENSION AND ASCITES

A variety of surgical and minimally invasive interventional procedures have been developed to ameliorate the problems associated with liver disease. Portal hypertension underlies most of these problems, leading to ascites or to varices that are the source of life-threatening hemorrhage. Procedures to alleviate portal hypertension and ascites are listed in **Box 57-10**. These are divided into nonshunting procedures (ie, those that do not seek to redirect portal venous flow) and shunting procedures. Nonshunting procedures are aimed at controlling hemorrhage from portosystemic varices. Varices at the gastroesophageal junction are the most troublesome of these, but they are amenable to endoscopic therapy. Shunting procedures redirect the portal venous flow into the systemic venous circulation via a nonvariceal conduit, thus relieving portal hypertension, decompressing varices, and at the same time relieving ascites. Because these shunts bypass the liver, they may create new problems due to encephalopathy. Shunting procedures have undergone a transformation from open surgical procedures on high-risk patients (high Child-Turcotte-Pugh scores predicting elevated perioperative morbidity and mortality) to a more minimally invasive approach.

NONSHUNTING PROCEDURES FOR PORTAL HYPERTENSION

These procedures (eg, ablation of esophageal varices or hemorrhoids) aim to reduce variceal hemorrhage. The procedures ligate decompressive alternate conduits for portal blood flow around the cirrhotic liver, so they are expected to worsen portal hypertension and ascites. Minimally

BOX 57-10

Procedures to Alleviate Portal Hypertension and/or Ascites

- Nonshunting procedures
  - Endoscopic therapy of esophageal varices
  - Percutaneous embolization of varices
  - Surgical ligation of varices, including hemorrhoids
  - Portal-azygous disconnection
- Surgical vascular shunting procedures
  - Nonselective
    - Portocaval shunts
    - Mesocaval shunts
    - Proximal splenorenal shunt
  - "Selective" vascular shunt:
    - Distal splenorenal shunt
- Percutaneous vascular shunting procedure:
  - Transjugular intrahepatic portosystemic shunt (TIPSS)
- Peritoneovenous shunts (nonvascular)
  - Denver
  - LaVeen

invasive procedures have largely replaced surgical approaches for managing varices. Minimally invasive approaches include endoscopic ligation or embolization (eg, endoscopic sclerotherapy of esophageal varices) and percutaneous embolization procedures. Many of the minimally invasive procedures to obliterate varices are performed outside of the operating room (ie, in remote procedure areas in the hospital), frequently with local or topical anesthesia and conscious sedation provided under the direction of the proceduralist. Thus anesthesiologists now encounter relatively few patients presenting for variceal ligation, and frequently these are only the most complex procedures, the sickest patients, or both. Anesthesia for these patients should follow the model for patients with severe decompensated liver disease as outlined in Chapter 15.

PORTOSYSTEMIC SHUNTS

Portosystemic shunts aim to reduce the hydrostatic pressure in the portal venous system by providing an alternate, nonvariceal conduit that bypasses the cirrhotic liver. A variety of approaches have been developed to shunt portal venous blood away from the liver and into the central venous circulation, first by open surgical procedures and now increasingly via percutaneous approaches. Again, there is a group of patients whose medical conditions or procedural needs preclude a minimally invasive approach, so a limited population of patients present for surgical portosystemic shunts.

Open Portosystemic Shunts Surgical or "open" portosystemic shunts are listed in Box 57-10. Each is designed to reduce portal hypertension, differing mostly in the topology of the vascular connection that is constructed. The surgery is in every case an open abdominal procedure in which venous vascular anastomoses are constructed. Anesthesia for open portosystemic shunts should follow the model described for patients with decompensated end-stage liver disease as described in Chapter 15.

Transjugular Intrahepatic Portosystemic Stent Shunts Transjugular intrahepatic portosystemic stent shunts (TIPSS) are indicated for patients with refractory ascites due to portal hypertension. Refractory ascites carries substantial morbidity (ie, spontaneous bacterial peritonitis, renal failure) and has a 1-year survival of less than 50%. Thus removal of ascites may benefit these patients, and TIPSS is successful in decompressing the portal system in about 90% of cases. Two meta-analyses of studies comparing TIPSS with conventional therapy (periodic large-volume paracentesis) indicates that TIPSS is superior for removing ascites but at the expense of a higher incidence of hepatic encephalopathy.[267,268] This comes as no surprise, as the shunt routes blood past the liver.

TIPSS has important implications for subsequent orthotopic liver transplantation. For example, TIPSS causes transient (ie, lasts for about 6 months) increases in cardiac volume load. Importantly, pulmonary systolic pressures (as estimated during transthoracic echocardiography) in 1 cohort increased from approximately 30 mm Hg prior to TIPSS to 44 mm Hg in the period immediately after the TIPSS,[269] potentially jeopardizing candidacy for transplantation. During transplantation, the shunt must be removed along with the diseased liver. As the shunt by design drains into the hepatic venous circulation, a piggyback technique may be precluded if the shunt protrudes into the proximal hepatic veins. The presence of a TIPSS frequently leads to a complicated and bloody dissection during the hepatectomy phase of liver transplantation. In extreme cases, the shunt can be dislodged and migrate into the right heart or the pulmonary circulation.[270]

TIPSS is frequently performed "off site" (ie, in a radiology procedure area, rather than an OR), so all of the special concerns for out-of-OR anesthesia apply. Patients presenting for TIPSS are usually severely debilitated and may be acutely ill, and this level of acuity coupled with the out-of-OR location magnifies the effort required to safely care for them.

Monitoring for TIPSS should be tailored to meet the needs of the patient and the anesthetic plan. Standard monitoring is usually sufficient for patients having TIPSS under sedation, monitored anesthesia care, or general anesthesia. TIPSS is usually performed under monitored anesthesia care or general anesthesia. This is because the procedure can require long periods of immobility, and it may be difficult or impossible for an awake patient with massive ascites to remain motionless and supine for the procedure.

The TIPSS procedure typically does not involve large fluid shifts, potential for massive hemorrhage, etc, so a reliable peripheral intravenous catheter is usually sufficient vascular access. The invasive radiologist establishes separate central venous access for the procedure, usually via the right internal jugular vein. The radiologist then tunnels a catheter from the inferior vena cava (actually a hepatic vein) through the liver parenchyma and into the portal circulation. The shunt is then placed via the catheter and dilated within the liver parenchyma.

Complications of TIPSS are relatively common but must be balanced against the complications of no therapy, frequent large-volume paracentesis, or surgical portosystemic shunts, none of which are benign. Complications of TIPSS include those of central venous cannulation in patients with coagulopathy. Complications related to central venous cannulation could be avoided or minimized by using an internal jugular site (which is compressible in the event of inadvertent arterial puncture) and ultrasound guidance to visualize the target vessel during the vascular access procedure. The procedure requires passing guidewires, catheters, and dilators from the superior vena cava, through the right atrium, and into the inferior vena cava. Cardiac perforation and tamponade[271] have occurred as rare complications. Acute volume overload[269] from the sudden outflow of portal blood into the systemic circulation is a much more frequent complication. Hepatic encephalopathy occurs frequently after TIPSS.[272] Encephalopathy is refractory to treatment or prophylaxis,[272] and acute onset of encephalopathy may make extubation impossible.

HEPATIC DONATION

Heart-Beating Cadaveric Donor Most livers made available for transplantation come from heart-beating cadaveric donors and are obtained in the course of harvesting other organs. Anesthesia care is often complicated by the numerous complex physiologic derangements that are manifested by these organ donors.[273] Such physiologic changes are responsible for the loss of up to 25% of potential organ donors.[274] Hemodynamic instability commonly develops and may occur in 2 phases. An initial phase may occur soon after brain death, which is characterized by excessive sympathetic activation leading to tachycardia, vasoconstriction, hypertension, and increased cardiac workload. This may be followed by a hypotensive phase in which sympathetic activity is reduced, leading to a loss of vascular tone, decreased cardiac output, and hypotension.[275] Hemodynamic stability may be further compromised by volume depletion resulting from the prior use of diuretics to manage elevated ICP, blood loss from injuries, insensible losses, and/or diabetes insipidus associated with damage to the neurohypophyseal-hypothalamic axis.

Sympathetic stimulation may be treated with short-acting beta-blockers and vasodilators that may be easily titrated such as nitroprusside and esmolol. As the brain-dead patient progresses into the hypotensive phase, it must be remembered that hypotension can have multiple causes. It is important to identify and appropriately treat the underlying etiology. Hypovolemic patients should receive volume resuscitation to achieve a hematocrit of 30%. Beyond that, crystalloid solutions are appropriate to replace free water as guided by central venous pressure measurements and to maintain or correct electrolyte and glucose concentrations. To reduce volume loss and electrolyte derangements associated with diabetes insipidus, desmopressin acetate (DDAVP) may be administered. Vasopressors and inotropic drugs are appropriate for donors with impaired vascular tone or myocardial function, respectively, to maintain adequate perfusion to organs. In such cases, therapy is most effectively guided by measurements of cardiac function and central filling pressures using a pulmonary artery catheter and/or echocardiography.

Organ donors can also present with significant pulmonary dysfunction.[276] Neurogenic pulmonary edema is most commonly observed in patients with increased ICP, and although the etiology is not entirely clear, it is likely related to excessive sympathetic stimulation. Excess pulmonary interstitial and alveolar fluid can be treated with fluid restriction and diuresis, but it should be recognized that a negative fluid balance may compromise the viability of other organs. Other common causes of pulmonary dysfunction in organ donors include pneumonia, pulmonary emboli, mucus plugging, and pulmonary contusions.

An important principle to recognize when caring for organ donors is that the focus of care has shifted from preserving the patient to preserving the function of graft organs. This can best be achieved by being well prepared, as organ harvesting is a major surgical procedure requiring full homeostatic support for the donor organs. In addition to routine intraoperative monitors, intra-arterial and central venous or pulmonary artery catheters are required. Because procurement may be accompanied by significant blood loss, it is important to be adequately prepared with large-gauge intravenous catheters and packed red blood cells for transfusion. Inotropic agents and vasopressors should be readily available to treat hypotension caused by myocardial dysfunction and reduced vascular tone. Nondepolarizing neuromuscular blockers should be used to facilitate surgical exposure and ablate reflex movements mediated by the spinal cord. General anesthesia is not necessary, but general anesthetic drugs may be useful for blunting the hemodynamic response to surgical stimulation associated with the dissection.

As the relative availability of heart-beating cadaveric donor organs has progressively decreased, other organs previously deemed unsuitable or high risk have been evaluated and used for hepatic transplantation. A large retrospective study looking at over 20000 liver transplants in a 4-year period identified 7 characteristics of donor grafts that significantly predicted an increased risk of graft failure and led to the development of the donor risk index (DRI).[277] It was initially thought that high-risk organs would confer increased risk in patients with higher MELD scores, relative to patients with lower MELD scores at transplant. This has not proven true, but still leads practitioners to evaluate the decision to proceed with transplantation of a higher DRI organ in a patient or wait until a better organ becomes available, weighing the risk of each.[278]

Living Donor The shortage of cadaveric livers has also led to the use of living donors to meet the growing need for liver grafts. Donor safety is a primary concern, as the donor derives no physical benefit from the surgery. Donor deaths have been reported during the perioperative period, and serious complications can occur. Like orthotopic liver transplantation itself, living donor hepatectomy has a steep and long learning curve with many opportunities for morbidity. For example, in 1 program, major complications were frequent in the first 50 living donor patients but declined significantly in the subsequent 50 patients.[279] In experienced centers, living donor hepatectomy can be performed with an average blood loss of 1 L and minimal requirements for transfusion.[280]

Most liver transplantations using living donors involve donor/recipient pairs who are ABO compatible. ABO-incompatible transplantations may be performed in some cases, and recent studies from Japan show that since portal graft infusion therapy has been used in ABO-incompatible living donor liver transplantation, outcomes are similar to those in ABO-compatible transplantations.[281] Potential donors should undergo thorough screening to assess their suitability. Such screening includes a detailed history along with a physical and psychologic examination, evaluation of routine laboratory values with particular attention to measurements of liver function, testing for transmissible viral illnesses, and, in some cases, percutaneous liver biopsy. Radiologic imaging studies are also a routine part of the donor evaluation. Doppler ultrasound can be used to detect gross pathologic conditions such as tumors or portal vein thrombosis. Computed tomography and magnetic resonance imaging are useful for defining a potential donor's vascular anatomy and hepatic volume, and to provide a roadmap for surgical planning.[282]

Typically, a right hepatic lobectomy from an average-sized adult living donor provides sufficient liver mass for an adult recipient. A left hepatic lobectomy from an adult donor provides enough liver mass for a pediatric recipient. This is advantageous for the donor, as the larger right hepatic lobectomy regularly leads to transient measurable compromise in liver synthetic function, with resultant coagulopathy.

General anesthesia for a living donor hepatectomy may be induced and maintained using a variety of techniques. Anesthetic concerns for living donor hepatectomy are similar to those of any major intra-abdominal surgical procedure and include the potential for significant hemorrhage and hemodynamic changes. In particular, systemic vascular resistance commonly decreases after donor hepatic resection, whereas cardiac output and heart rate increases.[117] The cause(s) of these changes is not known, but a role for splanchnic mediators, such as endotoxins, has been suggested.[283] It has been recommended that maintaining low central filling pressures is useful for reducing intraoperative blood loss and improving surgical exposure.[284] However, these benefits must be balanced against the potential increased risk of air embolism.

Because transient coagulopathies are commonly observed in the early postoperative period, the placement of epidural catheters for postoperative analgesia was initially the subject of controversy.[285-287] However, pain control requires careful consideration, and some programs use epidural catheters. In 1 study, donor hepatectomy patients had more pain than patients having equivalent-sized right hepatectomy for tumor resection, despite identical pain management regimes, including thoracic epidural use.[288] The authors suggested that this finding might be due to longer operative times required for donor hepatectomy.[288] Postoperatively, liver donors have significant coagulopathy, which can complicate the timing of discontinuation of epidural analgesia.[286,289] On the other hand, thromboelastography studies indicate that liver donors become hypercoagulable during the first postoperative week, despite conventional laboratory studies that indicate elevations of conventional coagulation parameters such as the partial thromboplastin time or the activated prothrombin time and thrombocytopenia.[290] This may give a protective effect against epidural hematoma, but this theory has not been tested. In 3 independent studies looking at complications due to epidural placement in donor hepatectomy patients, over 570 patients in 3 centers underwent donor hepatectomies without any episodes of epidural hematomas despite postoperative coagulation changes.[137,291,292]

Donation After Cardiac Death The number of livers from brain-dead donors has been relatively stagnant, and living donation is not a common option. The shortage of organs has resulted in renewed interest in a procedure for recovering organs known as donation after cardiac death. This term refers to a donation protocol for patients who have sustained a traumatic brain injury but do not meet the definition of brain death and thus cannot be declared brain dead. Nevertheless, families may realize that there is no hope for recovery and decide to withdraw invasive life support. Once such a decision has been made, the family may decide to donate the patient's organs after cardiac death has occurred.

Donations after cardiac death occur only after patients are declared dead after cardiac and respiratory arrest following the removal of life support. Donation after cardiac death is only considered after the family has decided to withdraw life support. The patient is taken to the operating room, usually with the family in attendance. There, the patient is extubated, vasoactive infusions may be discontinued, and the patient is allowed to die peacefully. The family leaves the room, and a surgical removal of organs for transplantation ensues.

Donation after cardiac death exposes the donor liver to a period of warm ischemia that does not occur in beating-heart donors. Liver viability declines as a function of the elapsed time after cardiac arrest in animals.[293] In humans, the immediate outcomes appear to be worse in recipients of donation-after-cardiac-death livers, relative to recipients of beating-heart donor organs, but the overall outcomes appear promising relative to no organ at all.[294]

Despite the fact that donation after cardiac death involves patients who are dead by every definition, and thus have no use for homeostatic support, there is much that the anesthesia team can contribute to these cases. Planned death in the operating room, with grieving family present in large numbers and in civilian dress, is an extraordinary event and flies in the face of many of the assumptions and mores of operating room personnel. Anesthesiologists can manage operating room access to allow donation to occur promptly and with respect to the deceased and his or her family, even to the point of mediating the cancellation of elective surgery to facilitate these singularly lifesaving events.

The anesthesia teams should sequence the preparation of recipient(s) to minimize donor organ ischemic time if possible. Anesthesiologists do not currently have any direct interaction with the donor, except possibly to perform the extubation. Extubation should be skillfully handled, both to protect the family members from unnecessary psychologic trauma and to minimize the risk of aspiration that spoils the lungs for donation. Anesthesiologists may become more involved in donation after cardiac death cases, as they may be asked to reintubate the trachea for lung protection (allowing lung donation) after asystole occurs. In many centers, however, no member of the anesthesia team may be present until after the death of the donor occurs.

KEY REFERENCES

- Abdalla EK, Noun R, Belghiti J. Hepatic vascular occlusion: which technique? *Surg Clin North Am.* 2004;84(2):563-585.
- Emond JC, Samstein B, Renz JF. A critical evaluation of hepatic resection in cirrhosis: optimizing patient selection and outcomes. *World J Surg.* 2005;29(2):124-130.
- Hoeper MM, Krowka MJ, Strassburg CP. Portopulmonary hypertension and hepatopulmonary syndrome. *Lancet.* 2004;363(9419):1461-1468.
- Jarnagin WR, Gonen M, Fong Y, et al. Improvement in perioperative outcome after hepatic resection: analysis of 1,803 consecutive cases over the past decade. *Ann Surg.* 2002;236(4):397-406; discussion 406-397.
- Keeffe BG, Valantine H, Keeffe EB. Detection and treatment of coronary artery disease in liver transplant candidates. *Liver Transpl.* 2001;7(9):755-761.
- Pham PT, Pham PC, Rastogi A, Wilkinson AH. Review article: current management of renal dysfunction in the cirrhotic patient. *Aliment Pharmacol Ther.* 2005;21(8):949-961.
- Reddy K, Mallett S, Peachey T. Venovenous bypass in orthotopic liver transplantation: time for a rethink? *Liver Transpl.* 2005;11(7):741-749.
- Xia VW, Steadman RH. Antifibrinolytics in orthotopic liver transplantation: current status and controversies. *Liver Transpl.* 2005;11(1):10-18.

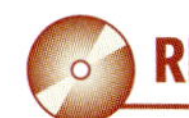

REFERENCES

Complete references available on DVD and online version at www.LongneckerAnesthesiology.com

CHAPTER 58 Anesthesia for Heart or Lung Transplantation

Benjamin A. Kohl
Joseph S. Savino

KEY POINTS

1. All heart and/or lung transplantations are considered emergency operations. As a result, the anesthetic preparation and management should reflect a consideration of the risks inherent in such a patient population.
2. The most common indications for adult cardiac transplantation are ischemic and idiopathic dilated cardiomyopathies, congenital heart disease, and viral myocarditis. The most common indications for adult lung transplantation are chronic obstructive pulmonary disease (particularly emphysema and α_1-antitrypsin disease) followed by idiopathic pulmonary fibrosis.
3. Acute rejection after lung transplantation occurs with greater frequency compared with transplantation of other solid organs, particularly during the first 6 months after surgery. Thus timely administration of immunosuppressants is believed to be of key importance in lung transplantation.
4. Although immunosuppressant agents have dramatically reduced the incidence of acute rejection after cardiac transplantation, these drugs have been implicated in cardiac allograft vasculopathy, which remains a leading cause of morbidity and mortality among heart transplant recipients.
5. Patients with primary pulmonary hypertension may have an exacerbation and incremental increase in pulmonary vascular resistance caused by anxiety

and agitation. Sedation with minimal respiratory depression is the goal in the lung transplantation population.

6. Typically, aortic cross-clamping of the donor coincides with induction of general anesthesia in the recipient. This coordinated event across centers is intended to achieve arrival of the donor organ at the recipient's operating room at the time when the recipient has been prepared for receiving the new organ. Delay in implantation of the transplanted organ leads to increased organ ischemia and may increase the risk for early postoperative allograft failure.
7. The anesthetic management of end-stage lung disease patients is aimed at minimizing further increases in pulmonary vascular resistance, as the patient is transitioned from awake and spontaneously breathing to anesthetized, paralyzed, and mechanically ventilated.
8. Familiarity and appreciation of pulmonary allograft physiology is imperative for ventilation of the new lung. Native lung explantation and subsequent allograft implantation results in denervated lungs and airways, loss of a functional pulmonary lymphatic system, and loss of bronchial artery blood flow.
9. Right heart failure can be precipitated by increased pulmonary vascular resistance in the cardiac recipient. Treatment includes inotropes and pulmonary vasodilators, as well as hyperventilation, increasing oxygen tension, decreasing positive end-expiratory pressure, and decreasing lung water.

INTRODUCTION

In patients with end-stage heart and/or lung disease, transplantation often represents the last resort for an improved quality of life. The perioperative care of patients undergoing lung and heart transplantation challenges even the most experienced anesthesiologists, surgeons, and intensivists, and dedicated teams are devoted to this high-risk procedure despite its relative low volume. Understanding the anesthetic implications and underlying pathophysiology is necessary for a successful outcome. This chapter reviews heart and lung transplantation, with an emphasis on intraoperative anesthetic management and postoperative care. The first section reviews the history of lung and heart transplantation. The following section discusses surgical alternatives to transplantation. The third section reviews the immunobiology of transplantation, an area in which much research has been devoted. The fourth section reviews methods of organ procurement and the concept of reperfusion and "washout" and discusses various methods used to protect the allograft. The remainder of the chapter is devoted to specific anesthetic concerns, management, recovery, and postoperative complications.

HISTORICAL ASPECTS

The history of heart and lung transplantation parallels the discovery and development of immunosuppressive drugs (**Table 58-1**). As is often the case, many of the pioneers in this field received little notoriety because their operations were performed on animals or on humans who survived only a short time. In 1946, Vladimir P. Demikhov was the first to perform intrathoracic transplantation of the heart alone, lung alone, and the heart and lungs combined in a warm-blooded animal.[1,2] Incidentally, these operations were performed without the use of hypothermia or extracorporeal oxygenation. Similarly, Alexis Carrel and Charles Guthrie first performed heart transplants in dogs in 1905.[3] However, attempts at human orthotopic heart transplantation were not made until the 1950s. Finally, although Reitz and Shumway are credited with the first heart–lung transplants in humans in 1981, Denton Cooley, in 1968, first replaced the heart and lungs of a 2-month-old infant who had an atrioventricular canal defect with those of an anencephalic donor. Although the recipient survived only 14 hours, precedent was certainly established for future endeavors.[4-6] These are the pioneers of modern-day transplantation. First-person accounts of their trials and tribulations abound in the literature and convey the frustrations many experienced to advance the field.[7-9]

EPIDEMIOLOGY

Lung Transplant The most common indications for lung transplantation in the United States are chronic obstructive pulmonary disease (COPD, particularly emphysema and α_1-antitrypsin deficiency) followed by idiopathic pulmonary fibrosis (IPF).[10] The most common indication for lung transplantation in children is cystic fibrosis. Since 2005, there has been a dramatic increase in the number of patients

TABLE 58-1 Key Time Points in the History of Heart and Lung Transplantation

Date	Event
1962	Introduction of antirejection drug azathioprine (Imuran).
1963	First single-lung transplant performed by Dr James D. Hardy (University of Mississippi, Oxford, Mississippi). The patient died on postoperative day 8. Immunosuppressive regimen included azathioprine and mediastinal irradiation.
1967	First successful heart transplant performed by Dr Christian Barnard (Groote Schur Hospital, Cape Town, South Africa). The patient died on postoperative day 18. Immunosuppressive regimen included azathioprine, prednisolone, and mediastinal irradiation.
1969	First artificial heart implantation (Liotta Total Artificial Heart) performed by Dr Denton A. Cooley (Texas Heart Institute, Houston, Texas). The patient survived for 64 hours, at which point she received a donor heart.
1978	Introduction of the immunosuppressant cyclosporine.
1981	First successful heart–lung transplant performed by Dr Bruce Reitz and Dr Norman Shumway (Stanford University, Stanford, California). Immunosuppressive regimen included cyclosporine.
1982	First permanent artificial heart (Jarvik 7) implanted by Dr William C. DeVries (University of Utah, Salt Lake City, Utah). The 61-year-old patient survived for 112 days.
1983	First successful long-term single-lung transplant performed by Dr Joel Cooper (Toronto General Hospital, Toronto, Ontario, Canada) in patient with pulmonary fibrosis. The patient survived 6 years (died of progressive renal failure).
1986	First successful double-lung transplant performed by Dr Joel Cooper (Toronto General Hospital, Toronto, Ontario, Canada) in patient with emphysema. The patient survived 15 years (died of brain aneurysm).
1990	Introduction of the immunosuppressant FK506 (tacrolimus).

transplanted for IPF, likely related to the new lung allocation system. Other indications include sarcoidosis and primary pulmonary hypertension. Less commonly, lung transplantation has been offered as a viable option for patients with bronchoalveolar carcinoma[11] and rejection of a previously transplanted lung (retransplant). The US Organ Procurement and Transplantation Network (OPTN) and the Scientific Registry of Transplant Recipients (SRTR) jointly publish an annual report (dating back to 1993) of organ-specific statistics.[12] Recipients are getting older and, as a result, have an increasing incidence of comorbidities. In 1993, patients older than 50 years comprised only 43% of registrants, whereas in 2005 this age group comprised almost 60% of registrants. The major limiting factor in the number of heart or lung transplantations is the lack of availability of donor organs. Despite low numbers of donors, beginning in 2005, there has been a significant reduction in the number of patients awaiting transplant (a trend that had been steady for 7 years prior) and an increase in the number of lung transplants performed. This can be attributed to the implementation of a new allocation policy (Lung Allocation Score) beginning in 2005.[12]

The suitability of lung donation is based on a number of criteria (**Table 58-2**).[13] Most donors do not meet all of these standards. Attention is given both to the viability of the graft as well as the urgency for the recipient. Because of the new allocation scheme, there has been a significant reduction in the median waiting time for transplantation (792 days in 2004, 141 days in 2007).[12] As experts continue to refine this system, there will have to be ongoing evaluation of the concomitant impact this has on the population. Although patient survival after lung transplantation continues to improve, both 1- and 5-year survival rates remain the lowest (86% and 56%, respectively) compared with all other solid organ transplants (excluding combined heart–lung). Early mortality rates (first year post–lung transplant) continue to decline from 296 per 1000 patient-years at risk in 1998 to 176 per 1000 patient-years at risk in 2007.[12]

Heart Transplant As a result of improvements in pharmacotherapy and advances in both surgical- and catheter-based management of acute coronary syndromes, many patients are presenting with heart failure later in life. Among industrialized countries, the incidence and prevalence of heart failure are 0.15% and 1%, respectively.[14] Concomitant with progress in medical management, heart transplantation and circulatory assist devices have become viable alternatives, particularly for patients with advanced heart failure.[15-17]

The number of heart transplants being performed annually in the United States ranges from 3000 to 3500.[18] The volume appears to have reached a plateau and is limited primarily by the availability of donors. The median time to transplant after being placed on the waiting list is between 200 and 300 days.[19] In general, older patients comprise a larger number of those listed for heart transplantation. By 2007 more than 15% of registrants were older than 65 years. The 2 most common reasons for transplantation are ischemic cardiomyopathy and idiopathic dilated cardiomyopathy, which together comprise approximately 90% of cases.[18] Although there is no absolute age limit to cardiac transplantation, in general the upper age limit in most centers is 65 years.[20] The premise of any therapeutic intervention is that survival and quality of life are better than those in the natural history of disease. The 1-year mortality of patients with symptomatic congestive heart failure is estimated to be 45%, and the 5-year survival is less than 30%.[21,22] In comparison, the 1-year survival after heart transplantation is approximately 85%, the 10-year survival is between 40% and 50%, and the 15-year survival is as high as 30% to 40%.[18]

TABLE 58-2 Ideal Donor Criteria for Lung Transplantation

Age <55 years
ABO compatibility
No radiographic anomalies
No history of tobacco use
No evidence of pulmonary contusion or other chest trauma
No evidence of aspiration
No evidence of sepsis
Pristine bronchoscopic appearance/no purulent secretions
$<10^5$ organisms on quantitative sputum sample
$Pa{O_2}$ >300 mm Hg on $F{IO_2}$ = 1.0, PEEP 5 cm H_2O
No prior thoracic surgery

$F{IO_2}$, fraction of inspired oxygen; PEEP, positive end-expiratory pressure.

Adapted from Orens JB, Boehler A, de Perrot M, et al. A review of lung transplant donor acceptability criteria. *J Heart Lung Transplant.* 2003;22:1183-1200. Copyright Elsevier 2003.

INDICATIONS

Lung Transplantation In 1998 a consensus statement was released that proposed indications and contraindications for lung transplantation.[23] Since that time, significant changes have been made in our understanding and management of end-stage pulmonary disease, with increasing evidence of improving posttransplant survival rates.[24] In 2005 the United Network for Organ Sharing/Organ Procurement and Transplantation Network Thoracic Organ Transplantation Committee established a revised allocation system for donor lungs. The revised system, which became effective in the summer of 2005, assigns a lung allocation score (0-100) to each potential recipient based on the patient's projected benefit received from transplantation, the patient's waiting list urgency, and the predicted 1-year posttransplant survival score (UNOS calculation). Practitioners can use disease-specific guidelines to classify patients with regard to eligibility (**Table 58-3**).[25,26] Additionally, indications for lung transplantation can be generally divided into those for single-lung transplantation and those for double-lung transplantation (**Table 58-4**). Single-lung transplantation is contraindicated and bilateral lung transplantation is necessary in patients in whom the donor lung would be cross-contaminated by the infections from the contralateral native lung (eg, cystic fibrosis, bronchiectasis). Single-lung transplantation has most commonly been used in the treatment of end-stage COPD, although more recently there is an increasing trend toward performing bilateral transplantation in this population as overall survival appears to be improved.[27] Such a survival advantage with bilateral lung transplantation has not yet been seen in patients with pulmonary fibrosis.[28,29] Single-lung transplantation also yields the opportunity of offering lungs to 2 recipients from 1 donor.

Heart Transplantation The most common indications for adult cardiac transplantation are ischemic and idiopathic dilated cardiomyopathies (**Fig. 58-1**).[18] The benefit of transplantation must outweigh the enhanced quality of life offered by maximal medical therapy without surgery. Patients in whom medical management may achieve similar survival outcomes to those with heart transplantation warrant reconsideration for the planned operation. Potential candidates must be significantly disabled despite optimal medical therapy.

The most widely used criteria for identifying potential heart transplant candidates are based on peak oxygen consumption ($V{O_2}$) and the Heart Failure Survival Score (HFSS).[30,31] Peak $V{O_2}$ below 14 cc/min/kg or medium- to high-risk HFSS is believed to be predictive of patients who will sustain a survival benefit with transplantation.[32] Other important factors that are considered before a patient is listed for cardiac transplantation are pulmonary vascular resistance (PVR), age, and comorbidities. Patients with severe heart failure frequently have elevated PVR as a consequence of chronically elevated left ventricular end-diastolic pressure. The concern with transplanting a heart in such patients is

TABLE 58-3 Disease-Specific Guidelines for Lung Transplant Eligibility

The following patient populations are considered to be in the transplant window if they meet the listed criteria:

Nonbronchiectatic chronic obstructive lung disease
- BODE index of 7-10 or *at least* 1 of the following:
- FEV_1 <20% and either DLCO <20% or homogeneous distribution of emphysema
- History of hospitalization for exacerbation associated with acute hypercapnia ($Paco_2$ >50 mm Hg)
- Pulmonary hypertension or cor pulmonale, or both, despite oxygen therapy

Cystic fibrosis and other bronchiectatic diseases
- FEV_1 <30% predicted or rapid deterioration of FEV_1
- Exacerbation of pulmonary disease requiring ICU admission
- Increasing frequency of exacerbations requiring antibiotic therapy
- Refractory and/or recurrent pneumothorax
- Recurrent hemoptysis not controlled by embolization

Idiopathic pulmonary fibrosis and nonspecific interstitial pneumonia
- Histologic or radiographic evidence of IPF and *any* of the following:
- DLCO <39% predicted
  - Decrease in FVC ≥10% during 6 months of follow-up
  - Decrease in pulse oximetry below 88% during a 6-minute walk test
  - Honeycombing on high-resolution computed tomography

Histologic evidence of nonspecific interstitial pneumonia (NSIP) and *any* of the following:
- DLCO <35% predicted
- Decrease in FVC ≥10% *or* a decrease in DLCO ≥15% during 6 months of follow-up

Pulmonary arterial hypertension
- Persistent NYHA class III or IV on maximal medical therapy
- Low (<350 m) or declining 6-minute walk test
- RAP >15 mm Hg
- CI <2 L/min/m²
- Failing therapy with intravenous epoprostenol, or equivalent

BODE, body mass index, obstruction, dyspnea, exercise capacity; CI, cardiac index; DLCO, diffusing capacity of carbon monoxide in lung; FEV_1, forced expiratory volume in 1 second; mPAP, mean pulmonary arterial pressure; NYHA, New York Heart Association; $Paco_2$, partial pressure of carbon dioxide in arterial blood; Pao_2, partial pressure of oxygen in arterial blood; PAP, pulmonary arterial pressure; RAP, right atrial pressure; VC, vital capacity.

Data from International Guidelines for the Selection of Lung Transplant Candidates: 2006 update–a consensus report from the Pulmonary Scientific Council of the International Society for Heart and Lung Transplantation. *J Heart Lung Transplant.* 2006;25:745-755.

TABLE 58-4 General Indications for Lung Transplantation

Single-lung transplant
- Chronic obstructive pulmonary disease with FEV_1 ≤25% predicted
- Pulmonary hypertension (mPAP ≥55 mm Hg)
- Connective tissue disorder (sarcoidosis, lymphangioleiomyomatosis, eosinophilic granulomas)
- Pulmonary fibrosis
- Interstitial lung disease
- Bronchoalveolar carcinoma

Double-lung transplant
- Emphysema
- Pulmonary hypertension
- Cystic fibrosis
- Bronchiectasis

FEV_1, forced expiratory volume in 1 second; mPAP, mean pulmonary arterial pressure.

Adapted from Rosenberg AL, Rao M, Benedict PE. Anesthetic implications for lung transplantation. *Anesthesiol Clin North Am.* 2004;22:767-788. Copyright Elsevier 2004.

the increased right ventricular afterload, which the donor heart is unaccustomed to generating. There is a linear correlation between PVR and 1- and 5-year mortality.[31] Most centers consider PVR above 3 to 4 Wood units (on maximal medical therapy) to be a contraindication to cardiac transplantation. Although the recipient's age historically was a common limiting factor, survival rates of selected recipients older than 60 years were found to be acceptable.[33] Finally, in addition to comorbidities of the recipient that may affect survival, the decision to list a patient for heart transplantation must be based on psychologic and social factors, and may even take into account ethical and religious beliefs.[34] In the end the decision is individualized and must be made by a designated transplantation team (including, but not limited to, physicians, nurses, and social workers) along with the patient and his or her family.

SURGICAL ALTERNATIVES TO TRANSPLANTATION

Transplantation of any organ frequently represents the penultimate rescue therapy for patients with end-organ disease. These patients typically, although not always, have undergone numerous attempts at alternate strategies to improve both organ function and quality of life. Both heart and lung transplantation represent decisive therapy that often follows 1 or more surgical alternative therapies. This section is not meant to be a comprehensive review of alternate therapies but rather introduces several strategies with which the anesthesiologist should be familiar, as a transplant recipient may have been exposed to 1 or more of these operations previously.

LUNG

Surgical options other than transplantation for treating advanced lung disease are few, and their efficacy is equivocal. The most common option for treating advanced emphysema is lung volume reduction surgery (LVRS). The procedure is often performed as a "bridge" to lung transplantation as a means for patients to survive the transplant waiting period.[35,36] Volume reduction surgery involves excision of as much as one-third of the emphysematous lung, thus increasing elastic recoil in the remaining lung. Although no randomized study has compared LVRS with lung transplantation, the latter carries higher perioperative mortality and predisposes the patient to infection as a result of immunosuppression. LVRS can be performed via median sternotomy or video-assisted thoracoscopic surgery. Patients presenting for lung transplantation status post-LVRS should be considered at high risk during thoracic entry and standard "redo" precautions should be taken. Although continuous intravenous prostacyclin is another alternative to transplantation, many use this therapy as a "bridge" to transplantation. Prostacyclin is a metabolite of arachidonic acid and is a potent vasodilator. Because it usually is administered by long-term continuous intravenous infusion, permanent central venous access is necessary. Significant risks associated with this therapy are central line infection and thrombosis.

HEART

A number of surgical and nonsurgical procedures are available for heart failure patients short of heart transplantation, including reduction ventriculoplasty, transmyocardial laser revascularization, cardiac resynchronization therapy, dynamic cardiomyoplasty, and insertion of partial or total heart assist devices.[37-39] Often 1 or more of these procedures has been performed on the patient presenting for heart transplantation. Reduction ventriculoplasty (also called the *Batista procedure*) has been used as an alternative to transplantation for patients with dilated cardiomyopathy.[40] By decreasing ventricular volume and excising dyskinetic myocardium, the ejection efficiency in patients with dilated cardiomyopathy is improved and cardiac output is maintained. Transmyocardial laser revascularization is an option in patients with small, diffusely diseased coronary arteries that are not amenable to other interventional therapies.[41] The procedure applies a laser to permeate

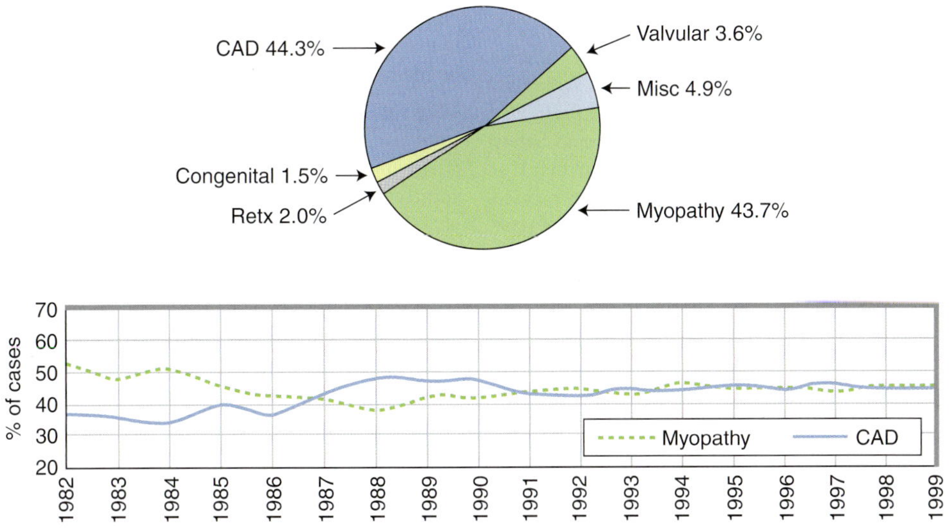

FIGURE 58-1. Indications for adult heart transplantation. CAD, coronary artery disease; Misc, miscellaneous; Retx, retransplantation. [Reprinted from Hosenpud JD, Bennett LE, Keck BM, et al. The Registry of the International Society for Heart and Lung Transplantation: seventeenth official report–2000. *J Heart Lung Transplant.* 2000;19:909-931. Copyright Elsevier 2000.]

the myocardium and incite an inflammatory reaction that, over time, promotes angiogenesis and neovascularization in the ischemic region. Heart function tends to deteriorate in the immediate postoperative period secondary to acute myocardial edema and the benefit is often not evident until months later. Transmyocardial laser revascularization typically is performed via a minithoracotomy. This procedure aims to optimize myocardial perfusion by creating a number of transmural channels within the ischemic myocardium.[41] Dynamic cardiomyoplasty involves encasing the heart with muscle, usually the latissimus dorsi, which subsequently is stimulated to contract in synchrony with cardiac systole. Stimuli are generated through an implantable cardiomyostimulator.[42] All of these procedures place the recipient for heart transplantation at greater risk as a result of adhesions, particularly during redo sternotomy. Type- and cross-matched blood in the operating room before incision is necessary.

One of the most invasive therapies for heart failure is insertion of a ventricular assist device (VAD). This involves removal of blood from the superior vena cava (SVC), right atrium, or right ventricle for a right VAD and removal of blood from the left atrium or left ventricle for a left VAD. The blood is returned distal to the affected ventricle: the pulmonary artery in a right VAD and the ascending or descending thoracic aorta in a left VAD. The design of VADs has improved, allowing patients who are not transplantation candidates to remain indefinitely on the device (so-called "destination therapy"). However, most devices continue to be used as a "bridge" to transplantation, sustaining the function of all other organs until heart transplantation.[43] The evolution/advancement of VAD technology has sacrificed pulsatile flow for miniaturization. Heart transplant recipients commonly arrive in the operating room with a VAD that may have been in place for months.[44]

IMMUNOBIOLOGY OF TRANSPLANTATION

Transplant immunology was borne from an observation by Karl Landsteiner in 1901 that the clumping of donor red blood cells was responsible for manifestations of the transfusion reaction. He went on to formally classify human blood into the A, B, AB, and O groups.[45] Blood group compatibility is a requirement not only for blood transfusion but also for organ transplantation. In the early 1950s Peter Medawar further advanced the field of transplant immunology by observing the viability of skin grafts on burns. The observation that first-time grafts from donors lasted approximately 10 days, whereas subsequent grafts were rejected immediately, suggested that the subsequent response was somehow affected by prior exposure. If, however, mouse embryos were inoculated with cells from another strain and then grafted after birth with skin from that strain, the grafts were not rejected. In 1958 Dausset described the first leukocyte antigen that allowed for tissue matching.[46,47] Human leukocyte antigens (HLAs) are encoded by a group of genes on chromosome 6 known as the human *major histocompatibility complex* (MHC). Because these genes are highly polymorphic (HLA-B has >50 alleles), 2 unrelated individuals likely will not have the same HLA type. Because HLA mismatch necessarily causes rejection (by antibodies, lymphocytes, or both), immunosuppressive drugs are required to ensure recipient tolerance of the allograft. Identical twins have identical HLA typing.

Three main types of rejection can occur in clinical transplantation: hyperacute, acute, and chronic. Hyperacute rejection typically occurs within minutes to days and is caused by preformed recipient IgG antibodies reacting against the allograft class I HLA. A profound and immediate decrement in organ function caused by complement activation and antibody deposition leads to vascular destruction. As cross-matching techniques have improved, hyperacute rejection is less commonly seen. The most common form of rejection is acute rejection, usually occurring within 6 months of transplantation. Acute rejection is caused by infiltration of allograft tissue with host T cells and subsequent clonal expansion. As these alloreactive lymphocytes enter the circulation, they react with allograft vascular endothelium (the primary target of the initial stages of acute rejection), leading to eventual tissue destruction. Immunosuppressive drugs are most effective in subjugating this phase of rejection. Chronic rejection is not well understood. It may occur as early as 6 to 12 months after transplantation but usually occurs much later. It is typified by a slow deterioration in allograft function and is identified histologically by intimal hypertrophy and fibrosis. In heart transplant patients, chronic rejection is accompanied by progressive atherosclerosis and coronary artery disease, whereas lung transplant recipients develop bronchiolitis obliterans. Currently there is no standard treatment of chronic rejection. Most heart transplant recipients average 1 to 2 episodes of rejection per year. Most of these episodes are minor, resolving with corticosteroids or small changes in the immunosuppressive regimen.

IMMUNOSUPPRESSION REGIMENS

Safety The anesthesiologist is frequently asked to prepare and/or administer an immunosuppressive agent intraoperatively. Although proper handling of all medications is always recommended, particular attention should be focused on these drugs. The Occupational Safety and Health Administration (OSHA) through the US Department of Labor has published a technical manual that includes a section entitled "Controlling Occupational Exposure to Hazardous Drugs."[48] The realization that many of these drugs are cytotoxic and genotoxic, and are potential carcinogens has prompted OSHA to continually revise these recommendations. Some specific recommendations to limit exposure include the following:

1. Clearing air from syringe before injection to avoid aerosolization
2. Careful attention to avoid leakage in syringe, tubing, or stopcock sites
3. Immediate disposal of contaminated materials (syringes, needles, bottles, etc)
4. Careful handling of excreta of patients because many drugs are excreted unchanged or are converted to mutagenic metabolites

Additionally, because many drugs must be reconstituted, particular recommendations to avoid aerosolization include attention when withdrawing a needle from a vial, attention when breaking open an ampule, and limiting the expulsion of air from a drug-filled syringe.

Drugs As stated before the preceding list, and as seen in the following Lung and Heart sections, a plethora of immunosuppressive regimens are available. The decision to administer a particular drug frequently is dictated by patient comorbidity, pharmacodynamics, and kinetics of the drug, as well as institutional preference. The purpose of this section is not to give a comprehensive review on the pharmacology of immunosuppressant agents, but rather to introduce several drugs commonly given by the anesthesiologist.

Before the discovery of cyclosporine in 1976, the most common pharmacologic regimen for immunosuppression was a combination of azathioprine and corticosteroids. Azathioprine is a derivative of 6-mercaptopurine. Its mechanism of action includes suppression of cell-mediated hypersensitivity and antibody production. Metabolism occurs in the liver and erythrocytes with very little renal accumulation. Because azathioprine inhibits cell proliferation in a nonselective manner, the major toxicity associated with this drug includes neutropenia and thrombocytopenia as a result of profound bone marrow suppression. With the discovery of cyclosporine, immunosuppression without significant bone marrow suppression became possible. Since 1983, when the drug was Food and Drug Administration (FDA) approved to prevent graft rejection in transplantation, cyclosporine has been limited by its nephrotoxicity and the inability to completely control chronic rejection. The incidence of nephrotoxicity with cyclosporine is 40% to 70%.[49] Newer classes of drugs have since been developed for use in heart and lung transplantation.

Tacrolimus (FK506) is a macrolide antibiotic that inhibits calcineurin and T-lymphocyte function with greater potency than cyclosporine.[50] Although the incidence of nephrotoxicity is similar to that of cyclosporine, less arterial hypertension and hyperlipidemia is seen with FK506. Deciding which calcineurin inhibitor to use usually is patient dependent and often institutionally biased.

Mycophenolate mofetil (MMF; CellCept, Roche Pharmaceutical, Nutley, NJ, USA) is a morpholinoethyl ester of mycophenolic acid. It acts as a reversible uncompetitive inhibitor of inosine monophosphate dehydrogenase and inhibits guanine nucleotide synthesis in lymphocytes. A comprehensive review of its proposed mechanism of action is available elsewhere.[51] Almost all studies in heart and lung transplantation have substituted MMF with azathioprine as a triple-drug regimen and have shown better graft survival and fewer episodes of rejection.[52]

Almost every transplant recipient receives a corticosteroid. Although methylprednisolone typically is started perioperatively, the patient can be maintained on oral prednisone.

Lung Acute rejection after lung transplantation occurs with greater frequency compared with transplantation of other solid organs, particularly during the first 6 months after surgery.[53] The lung is constantly exposed to the external environment (and its antigens) with each inhalation. There is also greater risk for chronic transplant dysfunction progressing to allograft loss. Although bronchiolitis obliterans syndrome is the major cause of morbidity and mortality among long-term survivors after lung transplantation, acute or early allograft rejection is a major risk factor for the development of bronchiolitis obliterans syndrome.[54] Thus timely administration of immunosuppressants is believed to be of key importance in lung transplantation. Immunosuppressive agents frequently are given to lung transplant recipients immediately before or during surgery. The most common agents administered are steroids, cyclosporine A, azathioprine, and tacrolimus. A typical regimen may include cyclosporine (2.5-5 mg/kg PO), azathioprine (2 mg/kg intravenously [IV]), or MMF (1000 mg IV) administered preoperatively. Methylprednisolone usually is administered just before lung reperfusion (500 mg to 1 g IV). Although the mainstay of therapy remains calcineurin inhibitors and corticosteroids, newer therapies are being investigated including total lymphoid irradiation, photopheresis, and other biological agents.[55] Anesthesiologists may be asked to administer an agent to induce immune tolerance at the time of transplantation (so-called "induction therapy"). The purpose of such agents is to globally suppress the recipient's immune system in the immediate posttransplant period to minimize acute rejection. Although theoretically this seems plausible, clinical trials have not yielded consistent results in the lung transplant population. Despite being controversial, this therapy has become more widespread in recent years. The most common immune tolerance induction agents are OKT3, antithymocyte globulin, basiliximab, daclizumab, and alemtuzumab. The most popular induction agents are daclizumab and basiliximab, both antibodies being targeted to the interleukin (IL)-2 receptor. Daclizumab dosing is 1 mg/kg administered within the first day after transplant and then every 2 weeks for 8 weeks. The half-life of this drug is 20 to 40 days. Basiliximab has a greater proportion of murine components compared with daclizumab and therefore has a shorter half-life (13 days). Dosing of basiliximab is 20 mg on the first and fourth day after transplantation.

Heart Most immunosuppressive regimens for heart transplantation currently include a calcineurin inhibitor, a corticosteroid, and some adjunct. Usually a postoperative triple-drug regimen of cyclosporine or tacrolimus (FK506), azathioprine or MMF, and prednisone is typical. With a combination of these 3 agents, acute rejection has been dramatically reduced.[56] Newer agents used in some institutions include sirolimus (rapamycin) and monoclonal antibody IL-2 receptor antagonists such as dacliximab (daclizumab) and basiliximab.[57] Cardiac allograft vasculopathy remains a leading cause of morbidity and mortality among heart transplant recipients.[58] Although this vasculopathy is multifactorial and has been shown to arise from both immune- and nonimmune-related mechanisms, immunosuppressants have been implicated as contributing factors.[59] For example, calcineurin inhibitors, such as cyclosporine and tacrolimus, in addition to having profound nephrotoxic effects, can alter vascular remodeling, contributing to graft vasculopathy. However, although several prospective studies have found similar efficacy of the 2 drugs in preventing acute rejection in heart transplant recipients, more centers are using tacrolimus in preference to cyclosporine as the primary calcineurin inhibitor.[60-63] Furthermore, mycophenolate appears to be replacing azathioprine as the antiproliferative drug of choice.[64] Thus a future challenge in heart transplant immunosuppressive regimens remains the prevention of cardiac allograft vasculopathy.

As in lung transplantation, induction chemotherapy in cardiac transplantation remains controversial. Although studies have shown a reduction in the risk of early acute rejection, substantial evidence has demonstrated an association between this therapy and post-transplant lymphoproliferative disorder. As a result, roughly half of all centers currently use induction therapy in their cardiac transplant recipients.[64]

DONOR SELECTION AND ORGAN PROCUREMENT

LUNG

Most potential multiorgan donors are not suitable candidates for donating lungs because lungs are common targets of end-of-life events. Chest trauma, pulmonary edema, aspiration, pulmonary infection, and pulmonary embolism often preclude the use of lungs for donation. A smoking history does not preclude the use of donor lungs for transplantation. Oxygen challenge tests are performed on the donor with administration of 100% oxygen with 5 cm H_2O positive end-expiratory pressure (PEEP). An acceptable oxygen response is an arterial partial pressure of oxygen greater than 300 mm Hg. Cytomegalovirus (CMV) serology of the donor affects the selection of the recipient. Regardless of the CMV status of the recipient, long-term outcomes in recipients receiving CMV-negative allografts are improved compared with those receiving CMV-positive allografts.[18]

Once a donor has been identified, all possible recipients for organ transplantation are evaluated for ABO compatibility and size matching.[65] In recipients with COPD, disparity in size between donor and recipient lungs is less important. Patients with COPD tend to have large barrel chests that can accommodate lungs that ordinarily come from larger donors. Donor lungs increase in size when implanted and partially fill an enlarged pleural space in patients with COPD. Recipients with restrictive lung disease, however, tend to have a normal or decreased thoracic cavity volume, and lung sizing is paramount. Too large a lung may preclude its implantation in a recipient. During procurement, the donor lungs are flushed in situ, and the harvest is completed. Bilateral lungs are excised in their entirety and separated from the native airway at the trachea. Single-lung harvests require separation with the main bronchus, pulmonary artery, and cuff of the left atrium. Total ischemic time is defined from aortic cross-clamp of the donor to reimplantation and reperfusion in the recipient.

Before 1984 lung procurement in close proximity to the recipient was deemed necessary because of unrefined preservation techniques. Since that time, however, improved understanding of ischemia–reperfusion injury has led to the development of novel solutions that have reduced the incidence of primary graft dysfunction after lung transplantation. Although ischemic time was traditionally kept to under 6 hours, newer preservation protocols now allow procurement at centers as far away as 6 to 10 hours from the recipient.[65-68]

Procurement of any solid organ involves confirmation of donor eligibility, dissection, and isolation of the specific organ, followed by preservation and transport. The sole principle of preservation is to minimize both ischemia and reperfusion injury to the allograft. Confirmation of donor eligibility includes review of pertinent consents, history, radiographs, laboratory values (including arterial blood gas), blood type, and bronchoscopy. Methods for minimizing injury include donor pretreatment, organ preservation, and recipient treatments. Although preservation techniques and solutions differ among transplantation centers, 1 commonality is the use of deliberate hypothermia, which is used universally during explantation, storage, and reimplantation. Hypothermia can reduce the tissue's metabolic demand by 99%. Before explantation, lungs are flushed with solution at 32°F to 50°F (0°C-10°C) and stored at a similar temperature. The lung is flushed most commonly with a low-potassium dextran (eg, Perfadex, Vitrolife AB, Gothenburg, Germany) or University of Wisconsin solution at the time of harvest and kept cold during transport to the recipient site and implantation and until reperfusion.[69] During implantation, the lungs are covered with gauze soaked in ice saline slush in an attempt to maintain a cold environment.

Potential lung transplant recipients require careful cardiovascular evaluation. Right-heart function is assessed to determine the ability of the recipient's right ventricle to tolerate acute increases in PVR associated with pulmonary artery clamping and pneumonectomy. Standard assessment modalities include echocardiography and right heart catheterization. Left heart catheterization and coronary arteriography are often used in older patients to detect coronary artery disease and left ventricular dysfunction. Intracardiac shunts, such as a patent foramen ovale, are detected preoperatively because they predispose to paradoxical embolization in patients with increased right-sided pressures.

Unlike many other transplanted organs, lungs and hearts must be functional immediately on reperfusion. Improvement in both donor management and procurement strategies has increased the likelihood of viability and remains an active area of investigation.[70,71]

HEART

Unlike lung transplantation, the recipient waiting list for heart transplantation continues to grow.[72] As a result, the criteria for heart donation are broad and continue to be liberalized (**Table 58-5**).[73,75] Absolute contraindications continue to include most malignancies and positive serologies for human immunodeficiency virus (HIV) and hepatitis B and C. Although low-dose vasopressor requirements are commonplace in the donor population, high doses of catecholamines may downregulate β receptors on cardiac myocytes and can cause intramyocardial hemorrhage and necrosis. Echocardiography may provide valuable information but frequently is unavailable in many hospitals.[76] Thus transplant surgeons frequently rely on direct inspection and palpation to assess for significant coronary artery disease, contractility, and/or myocardial hematoma suggestive of blunt thoracic injury. Height and weight of the donor preferably should match those of the recipient; however, differences of up to 20% to 30% are acceptable.[77]

Procurement of the heart begins with median sternotomy and pericardial incision. The procurement team (of which there may be more than 1 in the case of multiple donations) inspects and manually palpates the heart and coronary arteries to rule out blunt injury or significant cardiac disease. After administration of 30 000 units of heparin intravenously, the superior and inferior vena cavae and azygos vein are clamped and divided. The aortic cross-clamp is placed proximal to the takeoff of the innominate artery, and the heart is arrested with an infusion of 500 mL of cold cardioplegic solution injected proximal to the cross-clamp. The heart is cooled with topical ice slush, and the

TABLE 58-5 Donor Criteria for Heart Transplantation

Donor Criteria
Age ≤60 years
No evidence of prolonged shock causing
SBP <90 mm Hg or MAP <60 mm Hg
Profound inotropic support (>10 mcg/kg/min dopamine)
No evidence of prolonged hypoxemia
Normal electrocardiogram and/or echocardiogram
Preserved right ventricular/left ventricular function
No intrinsic myocardial disease
No history of severe chest trauma
No evidence of extracerebral malignancy

MAP, mean arterial pressure; SBP, systolic blood pressure.

Adapted from Harringer W, Haverich A. Heart and heart-lung transplantation: standards and improvements. *World J Surg.* 2002;26:218-225. With permission from Springer Science and Business Media.

remaining vessels (pulmonary veins and artery, ascending aorta) are transected. The allograft is placed in a sterile container and transported expeditiously to the recipient hospital. Allowable cardiac ischemic time is 4 to 6 hours. Most transplants proceed with transport of the heart after a single flush of cardioplegic solution followed by hypothermic storage. Commonly used solutions include University of Wisconsin, Euro-Collins, St Thomas, and HTK.[78] The optimal transport temperature likely is between 39°F (4°C) and 50°F (10°C) in order to minimize oxygen consumption.

PERIOPERATIVE CARE

LUNG TRANSPLANTATION

Preoperative Assessment Candidates for lung transplantation include patients with severe pulmonary vascular or parenchymal disease resulting in debilitating respiratory failure. Allocation of scarce resources (eg, donor lungs) to high-risk patients with serious comorbidities often precludes the eligibility of this patient population because of the high risk for death. However, lung transplantation in the less sick does not appear to significantly increase lifespan. In the end-stage emphysematous population, lung transplantation does not improve survival compared with aggressive pulmonary rehabilitation.[79] The Lung Allocation Score (LAS), which was first implemented in 2005, takes into account the waitlist urgency (the number of days expected to live while on the waiting list) as well as the posttransplant survival (the number of days expected to survive the first year posttransplant). These 2 factors are used to compute a score. As a result, many organ procurement organizations have liberalized the selection criteria for lung transplants to include patients with severe comorbidities and systemic disorders such as renal failure. These patients would have a very high mortality rate if they did not receive the benefit of a new lung. The long-term outcome of this new allocation strategy remains to be determined, but these high-risk patients are at increased risk of perioperative mortality and initial results appear to be promising.[80,81]

An efficient but comprehensive evaluation often is performed immediately before surgery. Many of these patients are on a waiting list for months, and their medical conditions may change rapidly during this time. Lung transplants are emergencies, and recipients should be considered at increased risk for aspiration. Full stomach precautions are warranted.

Operating Room Preparation The operating room is set up in typical fashion for cardiothoracic surgery. This includes fiberoptic bronchoscope equipment, a cardiopulmonary bypass machine, different-sized double-lumen tracheal tubes, and medications. A full complement of PEEP valves and the ability to provide continuous positive airway pressure may prove useful. On occasion, extremely ill patients require a "Surgical Intensive Care Unit (SICU) ventilator" to maintain adequate ventilation and oxygenation after induction of anesthesia. Prepared medications include heparin, diuretics, antiarrhythmics, inotropic and vasoactive agents, induction agents, muscle relaxants, and sedative–hypnotics. Immunosuppressive medications should be discussed with the transplant coordinator. Antibiotic administration usually is based on institutional protocol, although often it must be tailored to culture results from the donor and the recipient. This is especially true in the setting of chronic infections, such as patients with cystic fibrosis and bronchiectasis.

All lung transplant operations are emergency procedures and, for some yet-undetermined reason, typically occur during off hours. The cardiothoracic anesthesiologist usually is notified of the impending lung transplant procedure by the transplant coordinator and/or attending surgeon. This initial communication establishes the identification of the donor and the donor blood type and includes a brief synopsis of the primary and secondary diagnoses. In addition, this communication identifies the location and condition of the donor, including associated medical disorders, and anticipated cross-clamp time and arrival time of the donor organ to the transplanting center. From this information, the operating room team establishes the time the recipient is brought to the operating room. Often, the patient's arrival to the operating room is the first (and only) encounter with the anesthesiologist. In certain centers, a preoperative evaluation clinic provides a mechanism for the assessment and evaluation of lung transplant recipient candidates as part of the pretransplant evaluation. However, patients may wait for a lung transplant for many months, and conditions may change rapidly as patients are waiting for a transplant organ to become available. The lung transplant recipient is brought to the operating room in sufficient time to perform a comprehensive preoperative assessment, with acquisition of informed consent, placement of thoracic epidural, and invasive hemodynamic monitoring. These activities should be completed in advance of the anticipated time for induction of anesthesia and beginning of surgery. Anesthesia equipment and supplies are similar to those required for thoracic and cardiac surgery. Mechanisms for maintaining normothermia in patients undergoing lung transplantation without cardiopulmonary bypass are important adjuncts to intraoperative care. This is particularly important if the procedure is done without cardiopulmonary bypass (CPB) because typically ice is used to fill the thoracic cavity to keep the allograft cold until reperfusion. Options include fluid warmers, heated operating room table mattresses, warmed and humidified gases, increased room temperature, and body surface heating devices.

The operating room medications that should be readily available include antiarrhythmics, inotropic agents, vasodilators, and vasoconstrictors. Inhaled pulmonary vasodilators, such as nitric oxide and prostacyclin, typically are available via operating room pharmacy systems.

Patient Arrival The patient is greeted by the attending anesthesiologist immediately on arrival. A high level of anxiety and anticipation is to be expected from patients undergoing lung transplantation. These patients are afflicted with a life-threatening disorder and typically have a good understanding of the severity of their illness and the magnitude of the operative procedure for which they are being prepared to undergo. Indeed, many of these patients have reached this point, only to find out later that the donor lungs were unacceptable (after which time they are usually observed for 24 hours). The anesthesiologist informs the patient of the conduct of the planned anesthetic and associated risks and obtains consent for anesthesia and related procedures. The exchange of information between the anesthesiologist and the patient is designed to inform the patient of the upcoming events and risks without producing harmful levels of anxiety and fear. The patient's preoperative laboratory workup is reviewed before his or her arrival, typically through electronic computerized databases. The patient is questioned regarding changes in physical condition since his or her last evaluation.

Preinduction Activity The patient is brought into the operating room, routine monitors are applied once the patient is on the operating room table and large bore venous access is achieved. Placement of an intravenous catheter in the antecubital fossa is discouraged because many patients are positioned in a manner that may compromise patency of the catheter if the elbow is flexed.

Postoperative analgesia is planned before induction of anesthesia. Thoracic epidural catheters are routinely inserted for single or bilateral sequential single-lung transplants that do not require cardiopulmonary bypass.[82] Placement of an epidural catheter for administration of local anesthetics and/or narcotics provides effective postoperative analgesia and can be used intraoperatively to decrease the anesthetic requirement. A common analgesic regimen includes low-concentration local anesthetics and narcotics administered intraoperatively and continued into the postoperative course. In patients with significant pulmonary hypertension or other indications for the use of cardiopulmonary bypass, the benefit of placing an epidural catheter in a patient who is anticoagulated must be balanced against the risk of epidural hematoma.[83-85] The data supporting this contraindication are sparse, and this clinical judgment is based more on intuition and clinical impression rather than on evidence.[86] In many centers, if placement of an epidural needle produces a "bloody tap," surgery is postponed if anticoagulation is anticipated. Although this practice is acceptable for most operations, lung transplantation cancellation may result in loss of the donor organ. In addition, the recipient may not have another opportunity to receive a transplant.

Strict aseptic techniques are used throughout the surgical and anesthetic care of the patient because the patient receives large doses of immunosuppressants and is at very high risk for postoperative infections. Before insertion of intravascular catheters, the skin is prepared with either a chlorhexidine- or iodine-based solution that provides lasting antimicrobial effects.

The administration of anxiolytics is done judicially and with caution. Low doses of sedative–hypnotics or narcotics could render a patient with end-stage lung disease unstable because these medications may significantly blunt the patient's respiratory drive. Antisialagogue administration can be helpful in patients with increased secretions; however, care must be taken to avoid tachycardia with the administration of vagolytic agents. Patients with primary pulmonary hypertension may have an exacerbation and incremental increase in PVR caused by anxiety and agitation. Sedation with minimal respiratory depression is the goal in this cohort of patients. All sedated patients receive supplemental oxygen in addition to standard monitoring. All lung transplant patients receive a central venous catheter, although a pulmonary artery catheter is not absolutely indicated. A radial artery catheter is inserted for the continuous measurement of blood pressure and access to arterial sampling of blood for laboratory testing.

A central venous catheter usually is inserted before induction of general anesthesia. The pertinent information deemed from the pulmonary artery catheter includes assessment of pulmonary hypertension and an estimate of the risk of cross-clamping the right or left pulmonary artery. Induction of anesthesia can proceed safely without the information provided by a central venous or pulmonary artery catheter. However, the urgency of moving forward with the surgical procedure once the donor organ has been deemed suitable often precludes placement of the catheter after this notification. Typically, aortic cross-clamping of the donor coincides with induction of general anesthesia in the recipient. This coordinated event across centers is intended to achieve arrival of the donor organ at the recipient's operating room at the time when the recipient has been prepared for receiving the new organ. Delay in the implantation of the transplanted organ leads to increased organ ischemia and may increase the risk for early postoperative graft dysfunction.[87,88]

Confirmation of the laterality of the operation is critical in the early moments of the interaction between anesthesiologist and patient. The laterality is confirmed through repeated, redundant mechanisms set in place at each transplantation center. Typically, the right, left, or midline chest of the recipient undergoing a single-lung transplant is marked soon after arrival of the recipient to the operating room, indicating the site of incision. Confirmation of the proposed surgery and laterality by the patient requires participation by all members of the team: operating room nurse, anesthesiologist, transplant coordinator, and surgeon. Patients for planned double-lung transplant (eg, no laterality) also have the site of their incision marked. The patient's blood type is confirmed with data from the blood bank and posted in the operating room.

Antibiotics are administered according to institutional protocol and known organismal sensitivities soon after intravenous access is attained. Administration of vancomycin should be done over 30 to 60 minutes and administered within 120 minutes before incision to attain effective soft-tissue drug concentration levels.[89] Administration of immunosuppressants typically is delayed until the time when full commitment to proceed with the lung transplant has been made.

In the early management of lung transplant anesthesia and surgery, a "hurry-up-and-wait" approach is not uncommon. Typically, patients arrive to the operating room 90 minutes before the anticipated cross-clamp time in the donor and hence anticipated incision time in the recipient. However, delays at both donor and recipient sites are common. Delays at the donor site often are related to coordinating various transplant teams arriving from different institutions. The harvest of various organs for multiple institutions often leads to unanticipated delays resulting in the recipient waiting with anticipation in an otherwise quiet operating room. During this time of waiting and anticipation, low doses of sedatives, as well as warm blankets and comfort measures are appropriate. Information regarding the source of the donor organs should not be shared with the recipient.

Anesthesia Induction and Maintenance The commitment to proceed with surgery is intimately linked with the functional status of the donor organ. Deterioration in pulmonary function occurring at the donor site that precludes use of the lungs for transplantation is not uncommon. The harvest team reviews the laboratory data, including arterial blood gas measurements, chest radiographs, and visual inspection of the lungs through bronchoscopy and direct inspection. Oxygen challenge testing typically is undertaken in the donor to calculate alveolar–arterial oxygen gradients. Progressive increases in alveolar–arterial oxygen differences are a common reason for abandoning the donor lungs as a transplant organ. Other causes include pneumonia, infiltrate on radiograph, contusion, edema, and injury during harvest. Lack of recipient is an uncommon cause for not using a donor organ. If the donor organ is considered unsuitable, the recipient operating room is immediately notified, and the planned lung transplantation is canceled. Unfortunately, the cancellation of lung transplants occurs all too often, and potential recipients may become disappointed, discouraged, or die of their disease before being offered another opportunity for a transplant. The case provided to the anesthesiologist does not end when the procedure is canceled. The invasive monitoring is removed from the patient, taking care that sites of insertion are clean and without hematoma. The cancellation of a lung transplant procedure challenges many institutions as to appropriate accommodations for the patient. Typically, these patients have traveled long distances to the operating hospital. They have end-stage lung disease, have received sedatives and antibiotics, and have had intravenous, intra-arterial, and central venous catheters inserted. Many patients have received a thoracic epidural for postoperative analgesia. Canceled lung transplant procedures should not result in the immediate discharge of patients to home even if they were admitted from home. Instead, these patients are admitted to a postanesthesia care unit, where they are subject to the same discharge criteria as patients who have undergone surgery. The lung failure medical team is notified of the patient's condition and coordinates the patient's admission to the hospital, if necessary, or discharge to home.

If the donor lungs are deemed acceptable by the harvest team, the message usually arrives directly in the operating room: "The donor lungs are acceptable. We anticipate cross-clamp in [X] minutes and arrival time at recipient hospital in [Y] minutes." The mode of transportation and anticipated arrival time of the harvest team are critical to the timing of induction of general anesthesia. Ideally, the donor lungs arrive at the operating room with the chest open and native lungs excised or in the process of being excised. Minimizing ischemic time of the donor lungs is crucial because postoperative graft dysfunction appears to be related to the duration of organ ischemia.[90] Delays in induction and operation contribute to ischemic time and may lead to poor outcome.

A common trigger for induction of anesthesia in the recipient is cross-clamp in the donor. Induction of general anesthesia must always assume that the patient is at increased risk for aspiration because he or she is likely to have eaten in the previous hours. Mode of induction is dictated by the underlying disease process. Patients with severe COPD poorly tolerate positive-pressure ventilation. Air trapping and auto-PEEP are common, often producing circulatory instability. A severely decreased inspiratory:expiratory ratio with permissive hypercapnia is commonly necessary to maintain hemodynamic stability.

Patients are preoxygenated and denitrogenated with 100% oxygen applied by facemask, followed by intravenous induction of general anesthesia with application of cricoid pressure. Intravenous induction agents may include sodium thiopental, propofol, etomidate, and/or benzodiazepines. Narcotics are added for analgesic supplementation even if an epidural is inserted. Nondepolarizing muscle relaxants are administered to facilitate laryngoscopy and tracheal intubation. The administration of anesthetics, analgesics, and muscle relaxants should account for planned immediate postoperative extubation. Isolated lung ventilation during lung transplantation is vital to performing the operation without cardiopulmonary bypass. Techniques include the use of double-lumen endotracheal tubes or bronchial blockers. Procedures anticipated to be done using cardiopulmonary bypass may still require single-lung isolation for pneumonectomy and postcardiopulmonary bypass repair. On occasion, only 1 of the 2 donor lungs is implanted using cardiopulmonary bypass.

The trachea is intubated using an appropriately sized left-sided double-lumen endotracheal tube. Standard procedure dictates the insertion of a left-sided double-lumen tube in all patients having lung transplantation because of the variability of the position of the right upper lobe orifice and alignment of the Murphy eye of a right-sided double-lumen tube. Bronchial blockers can be used for single-lung isolation during lung transplantation, but they have the disadvantage of being more prone to dislodgement and are not as reliable for preventing contamination of the trachea and contralateral lung. Bronchial blockers do not permit selective suctioning. Bronchial blockers of the right lung do not reliably isolate the right upper lobe. Positioning of the double-lumen tube is confirmed using bronchoscopy and reconfirmed once the patient has been moved from the supine to the operating position.

Initiation of single-lung ventilation is associated with increased peak airway pressure and may produce rupture of bulla and cause pneumothorax or air trapping resulting in "pulmonary tamponade." To mitigate the sudden increase in airway pressures, the initial set title volume is decreased when instituting single-lung ventilation with a compensatory increase in respiratory rate in an attempt to maintain adequate minute ventilation. However, the relationships among tidal volumes, peak and mean airway pressures, and volume of air trapping and auto-PEEP are not linear. In many patients, only a nominal reduction in tidal volume is necessary. Persistent pulmonary blood flow through the nonventilated lung increases shunt fraction and may produce hypoxemia. Standard measures for treating hypoxia during single-lung ventilation include the use of 100% oxygen, application of PEEP to the dependent lung, and the use of conventional critical care ventilators that permit multiple ventilator modes (eg, pressure control ventilation, alternate ramp settings, wide variety of inspiratory:expiratory ratios). On occasion, circulatory deterioration during 1-lung ventilation may require partial cardiopulmonary bypass.

Anesthetic maintenance is achieved through the administration of oxygen and/or air mixed with a volatile anesthetic (eg, isoflurane, sevoflurane, desflurane). Volatile anesthetics may be contraindicated when alternate modalities of ventilation such as a jet ventilator are used. Decreasing inspired oxygen concentrations to decrease the risk of oxygen toxicity and reperfusion injury in the newly transplanted lung is controversial.[91] Epidural analgesia is often used to supplement intraoperative anesthesia, although epidural administration of dilute local anesthetics may produce significant sympatholysis and hypotension.

Patients undergoing lung transplantation have parenchymal, airway, and/or vascular disease. Patients with pulmonary vascular disease (eg, primary pulmonary hypertension) may have pulmonary arterial pressures equal to or exceeding systemic arterial pressures. The anesthetic management of these patients is aimed at minimizing further increases in PVR as the patient is transitioned from the awake, spontaneously breathing condition to the anesthetized, paralyzed, mechanically ventilated condition. Inhaled pulmonary vasodilators may decrease PVR to some degree. Typically, these patients do not tolerate right or left pulmonary artery clamping for pneumonectomy without the use of cardiopulmonary bypass. Inhaled prostacyclin or nitric oxide, intravenous prostaglandin E_1, hyperventilation, 100% oxygen, and mild hypovolemia may contribute to decreasing pulmonary arterial pressures in anticipation of pulmonary artery clamping. Poor tolerance of right or left pulmonary artery clamping in the setting of severe pulmonary hypertension is manifested by severe systemic hypotension, increasing pulmonary hypertension (initially), increased central venous pressure, and heart failure. If this condition persists, the pneumonectomy is delayed, the cross-clamp is removed, and the patient is anticoagulated and prepared for cardiopulmonary bypass. A cardiopulmonary bypass machine and perfusionist should be on standby for most lung transplant cases.

Patients with nonvascular lung disease have either parenchymal disease (eg, pulmonary fibrosis, sarcoidosis) or airway disease (eg, COPD, α_1-antitrypsin deficiency). COPD typically is characterized by normal or mildly elevated pulmonary arterial pressures. COPD patients usually tolerate clamping of 1 of the pulmonary arteries and pneumonectomy without the use of cardiopulmonary bypass.[92]

Intraoperative hemodynamic instability is not uncommon during lung transplant surgery. The loss of autonomic tone with induction of general anesthesia may be exaggerated in patients with end-stage lung disease in the setting of relative hypovolemia. Strategies for managing hypotension rely on information gained from central venous catheters (central venous pressure, pulmonary arterial pressure, and cardiac output). These strategies may include judicious expansion of intravascular volume and the administration of α-adrenergic and/or β-adrenergic agonists.

Pneumonectomy is performed upon confirmation of arrival of the donor lung. Appropriate sizing of the donor organ with the recipient is crucial, especially in patients with restrictive pulmonary disorders who often have a small thoracic cavity relative to total body mass. Patients with COPD typically have large, hyperinflated chest cavities that can accommodate donor lungs without difficulty.

During the pneumonectomy, a second surgeon at a separate operating table prepares the donor lung. Aggressive attempts are made to keep the donor organ cold before reperfusion. Completion of the pneumonectomy by clamping the pulmonary artery eliminates the source of venous admixture and improves oxygenation and ventilation. However, clamping of the pulmonary artery also produces a sudden increase in right ventricular afterload and increases the risk for right ventricular failure. The acute increase in pulmonary arterial pressure may cause acute right ventricular dilation and tricuspid regurgitation. Alterations in right ventricular geometry affect the contractility of the right ventricle and the ventricular septum, thus affecting left ventricular contractility. Inotropic agents may increase right (and left) ventricular contractility. Pulmonary vasodilators are administered in an attempt to decrease right ventricular afterload. Intravenous nitroglycerin, nitroprusside, and prostaglandin E_1 may produce systemic hypotension. Differential infusion of vasoconstrictive agents into the left side of the heart and vasodilating agents into the right side of the heart has been suggested.[93,94] Inhaled nitric oxide or inhaled prostacyclin may have a similar role in decreasing PVR and allowing the right ventricle to tolerate pulmonary artery clamping with minimal systemic effects.[95] Monitoring with transesophageal echocardiography provides continuous qualitative assessment of right ventricular function, although this modality is not standard in lung transplant surgery.

The donor lung is placed into the void created by the pneumonectomy, and the first anastomosis usually is donor bronchus to native bronchus. The competency of this anastomosis is assessed with the application of continuous positive airway pressure with the anastomosis submerged in saline. The surgeon inspects for air leaks and performs repairs to the anastomosis if necessary. Once the bronchial anastomosis has been completed, the surgeon performs the anastomosis between donor and recipient pulmonary arteries and pulmonary veins. The latter usually are included in a cuff of left atrium. As the pulmonary transplant is nearing completion, the clamps are gradually released to produce back-bleeding in an attempt to remove any residual air or debris from the left atrium and pulmonary vascular bed. Restoring circulation to the transplanted nonventilated lung results in shunting and potentially significant hypoxia. In addition, the acute blood loss associated with back-bleeding and the flushing out of the preservative solution and its metabolites into the systemic circulation may produce hypotension. Gradual unclamping and administration of intravenous fluids blunt the hypotensive effect. If anastomosis of the bronchus precedes revascularization and the lung is ventilated before reperfusion, the risk of hypoxemia is reduced. Ventilation of the reperfused allograft should be performed with oxygen concentrations sufficient to adequately oxygenate. Evidence is accruing that high oxygen levels in the early reperfusion period may be detrimental to the allograft, thus many transplant centers attempt to oxygenate with FIO_2 50% or less.[91] Corticosteroids typically are administered immediately prior to reperfusion of the new lung.

Patients for single-lung transplantation for end-stage lung disease typically have either chronic idiopathic pulmonary fibrosis or emphysema. Patients with end-stage emphysema pose a significant added challenge if they undergo single-lung transplantation. Posttransplant, hyperinflation and hyperventilation of the native emphysematous lung often produce severe ventilation–perfusion mismatch and compression of the newly transplanted lung. Avoidance of positive-pressure ventilation after single-lung transplantation in patients with preexisting emphysema appears to decrease this risk.[96]

The benefit of single-lung transplantation in patients with pulmonary hypertension *and* Eisenmenger syndrome remains controversial.[24,97] These procedures typically require the use of cardiopulmonary bypass to prevent acute right ventricular failure at the time of pulmonary artery clamping. Single-lung transplantation in this patient population may produce a functional pneumonectomy for the remaining native lung. Although both lungs are well ventilated posttransplant, blood flow is severely diverted to the transplanted lung from the native (high PVR) lung, with increasing risk of pulmonary infarction in the native lung. Thus it has been suggested that combined heart–lung transplantation might be best in this population.[98]

Bilateral and bilateral sequential single-lung transplantations are performed in patients with infection in 1 or both lungs or in patients with severe pulmonary hypertension. Historically, bilateral lung transplantation was performed using an en bloc procedure with a tracheal anastomosis and cardiopulmonary bypass. Disadvantages include the need for systemic anticoagulation, increased use of blood products, use of cardiac arrest, and increased risk of ischemia at the site of tracheal anastomosis. The advent of bilateral lung transplantation performed as sequential single-lung transplantation using bronchial anastomoses averted most of these disadvantages. Bilateral sequential single-lung transplantation has a number of advantages compared with en bloc double-lung transplantation. Single-lung transplantation is technically easier, and cardiopulmonary bypass is not necessary in most patients; thus ischemic arrest of the heart is not required. The en bloc transplantation of both lungs is performed through a median sternotomy and requires an abdominal laparotomy for access to the omental flap. In addition, double bronchial anastomoses appear to result in fewer ischemic complications compared with the single anastomosis of the trachea that is required in the en bloc technique.

The surgical approach for sequential bilateral lung transplantation is either through sequential right and left thoracotomies or through a median sternotomy.[99] The large transverse thoracosternotomy that extends from axillary line to axillary line producing the classic "clamshell" or "chevron" incision has fallen out of favor because of its effects on postoperative respiratory function. Bilateral sequential single-lung transplants can be performed through a muscle-sparing thoracotomy. The native lung with the more severe disease (poorer function) is transplanted first. After the first new lung is implanted, ventilation is switched to the newly transplanted lung, and the second lung is excised and transplanted. In patients with severe obstructive disease, the contralateral chest cavity is not open during the first single-lung transplant because the lung becomes severely hyperinflated when not confined to the pleural cavity. The resulting air trapping can create significant ventilatory and hemodynamic derangements.

In patients with primary pulmonary hypertension, lung disease may have been the primary disease process, with the patient having relatively normal underlying heart function. However, chronic pulmonary hypertension leads to progressive right ventricular hypertrophy and heart failure. Often, lung transplantation results in remodeling of the right ventricle, obviating the need for heart transplantation.[100]

Postoperative Management After completion of surgery while the patient is still in the operating room, either the patient is awakened from general anesthesia and extubated, or the double-lumen endotracheal tube is exchanged with a single-lumen endotracheal tube. In patients having lung transplantation with a single-lumen tracheal tube and bronchial blocker, only removal of the bronchial blocker is necessary because the existing tracheal tube suffices as the conduit supporting mechanical ventilation in the postoperative setting. Caution should be taken to ensure that the tracheal tube has an internal diameter of at least 8 mm to facilitate suctioning and bronchoscopy. The concentration of oxygen is decreased after surgery to avoid oxygen toxicity. Problems of postoperative ventilation–perfusion mismatch, shunting, and increased dead space are more pronounced in patients undergoing single-lung transplantation compared with bilateral lung transplantation. In patients who are not eligible for extubation at the completion of surgery or soon after arrival to the intensive care unit, a ventilator weaning protocol is instituted in the ICU.

The contribution of a "denervated" lung to pulmonary mechanics and physiology in the postoperative period is poorly understood. Familiarity and appreciation of allograft physiology are imperative for ventilation of the new lung. Native lung explantation and subsequent allograft implantation produce denervated lungs and airways, loss of a functional pulmonary system, and loss of bronchial artery blood flow. Normally, afferent input from the pulmonary stretch receptors via the vagus nerve is relayed to the medulla.[101] In lung transplant recipients, respiratory rate and tidal volumes cannot be dependent on the medulla via the vagus system. Instead, ventilatory information depends more on chest wall afferent signals.[102] Denervation of the vagus nerve input to the lungs includes blunting of the cough reflex and possible increased risk of aspiration in the early postoperative period, although patients appear to tolerate this denervation fairly well, with fewer than expected long-term sequelae. Patients undergoing left lung transplantation are at risk for injury to the recurrent laryngeal nerve. Disruption of the lymphatic system in the donor lung increases the risk of fluid accumulation and interstitial pulmonary edema. Judicious fluid administration and the use of diuretics to keep patients "relatively dry" are attempts to minimize this effect.[103] Hypoxic pulmonary vasoconstriction remains intact in the denervated allograft.[104] The newly transplanted lung is susceptible to fluid overload as a result of the disruption of pulmonary lymphatics. The incidence of early postoperative pulmonary edema with normal pulmonary artery occlusion pressure may be as high as 60%.[105] In this low-pressure pulmonary edema, the ratio of protein concentration of the edema fluid compared with that of the serum is greater than 0.5, suggesting increased permeability (so-called exudate) that could have resulted from endothelial damage.[106] An association exists between the occurrence of pulmonary edema and graft ischemic time.[105] In an attempt to minimize volume administration to minimize pulmonary edema, low-dose vasoconstrictors are often used to support blood pressure, especially in the setting of sympatholytic treatments such as epidurally administered local anesthetics.

Some degree of acute pulmonary rejection may occur in as many as 50% of patients after lung transplantation.[53] Clinical manifestations include cough, breathlessness, low-grade fever, and wheezing.

Decreases in the forced expiratory volume in 1 second (FEV_1) and forced vital capacity with characteristic abnormalities on the chest radiograph are common.[107] Differential diagnosis includes postoperative edema, infection, and bronchiolitis obliterans. A bronchial lavage is often sent for culture.

Bronchiolitis obliterans is a devastating complication of lung transplantation and is a leading cause of morbidity and mortality beyond the first year after transplantation.[108] It is characterized by decreased FEV_1 and obstruction and destruction of pulmonary airways, which lead to hypoxia. Diagnosis is established by transbronchial biopsy. Therapeutic options are limited because the condition is relatively refractory to increasing immunosuppressant therapy.[109,110] Retransplantation often is the only option, and these patients may present again to the operating room anesthesiologist.

Infectious complications after lung transplantation cause significant morbidity and mortality. Predisposing factors to bacterial infection include immunosuppressant therapy, ischemic injury to the lung, persistent pleural effusions, interruption of lymphatic drainage, and diminished cough reflex secondary to denervation. Donor-transmitted infections are associated with high mortality rates. Therefore, the airways of the donor lungs are routinely cultured, and antibiotics in the recipient are adjusted accordingly. Infection with CMV is associated with significant mortality in lung transplant recipients and is the most common viral infection in the recipient population (although the incidence has decreased since ganciclovir prophylaxis became routine practice).[111] Symptoms are nonspecific and include malaise and fever. Laboratory findings include leukopenia, thrombocytopenia, atypical lymphocytosis, and hepatitis.[112-114] The recipient may acquire primary infection from a CMV antibody–positive donor or from blood products. Therefore, blood transfused to a transplant recipient should be CMV negative. Even recipients who are CMV-antibody positive before transplantation can experience reactivation of previous infection or be infected with a different strain from the donor.[115,116] Fortunately, ganciclovir is an effective antiviral agent in the treatment of most CMV infections and pneumonitis, and often is administered prophylactically in the posttransplant period. Given the morbidity associated with CMV infection in this population, some have called for indefinite prophylaxis with ganciclovir.[117] Fungal infections are more common in the lung transplant recipient than in other solid-organ transplant recipients. The 2 most common species isolated are *Candida* and *Aspergillus*. Although treatment of invasive infection usually includes amphotericin, many transplant programs prophylactically administer an azole agent such as itraconazole.[118]

HEART TRANSPLANTATION

Heart transplants, similar to lung transplants, are always emergency operations. The most common disorders leading to heart transplantation include ischemic cardiomyopathy, idiopathic cardiomyopathy, congenital heart disease, and viral myocarditis. Patients are evaluated as candidates for heart transplantation through a heart failure clinic, which typically includes cardiac surgeons and cardiologists. A battery of preoperative tests aims to define the cause of heart failure and comorbidities. The workup usually is performed on an outpatient basis, and input from the department of anesthesiology can be gained if the institution has a preoperative clinic. However, in many sites in the United States, the first interaction between the anesthesiologist and the patient undergoing heart transplantation occurs a few moments before the heart transplant. The preoperative workup of patients for heart transplantation includes assessment of pulmonary vascular resistance (PVR). PVR is the difference between mean pulmonary arterial pressure and left atrial pressure divided by cardiac output. PVR is expressed in Wood units (normal = 1-2). Increased PVR that is irreversible and greater than 6 Wood units may preclude eligibility for heart transplantation. Donor hearts typically are harvested from patients who have normal or near-normal cardiopulmonary physiology. The donor right ventricle is accustomed to pumping blood through a low PVR bed. Once explanted, the donor heart undergoes a period of ischemia until reimplanted and reperfused. The donor right ventricle, in the setting of acute ischemia and reperfusion, is then exposed to an acute increase in PVR (afterload) from the chronically ill recipient who may have a PVR significantly greater than that of the donor. The clinical manifestations of acute increased PVR after a period of cross-clamp ischemia may include right ventricular failure and dilation. The right ventricle in these patients often requires pharmacologic support during this critical time.

DONOR

Organ harvests are conducted in large and small community hospitals. The quality of the donor organ often depends on the ability to maintain hemodynamic stability prior to and at the time of harvest. Criteria for heart donation are multifactorial and include age, preexisting cardiovascular disease, heart size, and echocardiographic, electrocardiographic, and cardiac catheterization data. The Organ Procurement Organization (OPO) is notified of potential organ donors. The list of eligible candidates is reviewed. The recipient is selected based on ABO blood typing compatibility, heart size, and acuity of illness. The recipient is notified and instructed to go to the hospital.

The timing of the recipient's transportation to the operating room and the donor harvest is dependent on multiple factors and, as in lung transplants, depends on what other organs are being harvested, the distance between the 2 sites, and the mode of transportation. In many organ harvests, procurement teams arrive from multiple institutions and from various locations across the country. Organ procurement is conducted under the auspices of the OPO, the harvest teams, and the on-site anesthesiologist and physician group. Most donors are patients with recently diagnosed brain death for whom the family has consented for organ donation. A small fraction of organ harvests originate from "nonbeating-heart donors." The latter group is not currently used for the donation of hearts. Nonbeating-heart donors are patients with terminal illness who do not meet the criteria for brain death but in whom prognosis is grim and discontinuation of life support has been selected by the patient and/or family. If the patient or family is willing to donate, these patients are transported to the operating room, comfort measures are emphasized, and discontinuation of support and end of life are followed by organ harvest.

The avoidance of significant hypotension, myocardial ischemia, and high vasopressor dependency is believed to be important in organ function after implantation. The heart is excised in its entirety, including significant portions of the superior and inferior vena cavae, pulmonary artery, and aorta. Before its excision, the heart is inspected by the harvest team as a final check for viability for transplantation. In many centers, induction of anesthesia in the recipient is linked to the final viability check of the donor heart.

RECIPIENT

Typically the recipient is notified by pager or cell phone that a heart transplant is available. The recipient arrives at the hospital, goes through the admission process, and is transported to the perioperative area. Clinical data pertinent to the preoperative workup typically are available through the heart failure clinic and ideally in a condensed packet format. These data are most readily accessible via an electronic database format.

The operating room is set up in a conventional format for cardiac surgery. Medications that are available but not necessarily open include isoproterenol, milrinone, epinephrine, systemic vasodilators, and inhaled pulmonary vasodilators (nitric oxide or prostacyclin).

PREOPERATIVE MANAGEMENT

The heart transplant recipient is often brought to the operating room directly from home. Admission processes, updated laboratory testing, and a blood sample to the blood bank for type and cross-match require time and should be considered when the sequence to heart transplantation is planned. Informed consent is obtained in the usual fashion, including placement of invasive monitors, postoperative ventilatory support, and transesophageal echocardiography. Intravenous access is followed by insertion of intra-arterial and central venous catheters. Large-bore intravenous access (eg, 2 large-bore catheters) is vital for redo sternotomy cases because bleeding can be abrupt and severe. Blood products should be immediately available in the operating room. A pulmonary artery catheter is not absolutely required but often is useful in the titration of pulmonary vasodilators in patients with increased PVR. Defibrillation pads are placed on all patients who have undergone prior heart surgery or sternotomy. Antibiotics should be administered 30 to 60 minutes before incision and should cover broadly both gram-positive and gram-negative organisms. Institutional sensitivities to particular antibiotics should be considered.[119] Sedation is administered judiciously. No epidural is inserted. Postoperative pain is controlled with parenteral narcotics. Toradol and other nonsteroidal anti-inflammatory drugs are avoided because of their risk for renal toxicity, particularly in patients who receive high doses of cyclosporine or tacrolimus.

INTRAOPERATIVE MANAGEMENT

Induction of general anesthesia often coincides with confirmation of a suitable donor organ. Induction is accomplished with intravenous sedative–hypnotics and narcotics accompanied by a muscle relaxant. Aspiration precautions are prudent because these emergency operations often occur in the setting of a full stomach. Preoperative inotropes (eg, intravenous milrinone) are titrated based on hemodynamics and often are continued until cardiopulmonary bypass. Immunosuppressive therapy begins after induction of anesthesia based on institution-specific protocols. The pre-bypass period is characterized by sternotomy, exposure of the heart, heparinization, and cannulation. Ventricular assist devices (VADs) are becoming more commonplace and have been shown to be a successful mechanism of sustaining these very sick patients prior to transplantation.[120] Patients with a VAD (inserted as a "bridge to transplantation") will require explantation before heart transplantation. These patients often are anticoagulated preoperatively and are at very high risk for bleeding.

Use of antifibrinolytic therapy is common during heart transplantation. In addition to avoiding the risk of transmission of infection, the avoidance of blood transfusion may decrease the risk of postoperative infection. The available antifibrinolytics are tranexamic acid and ε-aminocaproic acid (Amicar). Red blood cell replacement therapy is leukocyte depleted and CMV matched. Treatment of coagulopathy includes plasma, cryoprecipitate, platelets, and recombinant factor VIIa. Protamine is administered to reverse heparin after cardiopulmonary bypass. Point-of-care bedside testing of coagulation parameters and hemoglobin and platelet count, as well as viscoelastic tests (eg, thromboelastography) can guide "goal-directed" therapy of bleeding.

Vascular cannulation before cardiopulmonary bypass includes the insertion of bicaval cannulas and a standard aortic cannula. If effective drainage is not achieved through the SVC cannula, there is a risk of SVC hypertension. Monitoring the venous pressure proximal to the purse-string suture of the SVC is prudent. Initiation of cardiopulmonary bypass occurs when the donor heart has arrived. Systemic cooling is common, but cardioplegia of the native heart is not necessary. The explanted heart is excised in its entirety except for residual portions of left and right atria. The newly arrived donor heart is prepared cold on a separate table by a separate surgeon. The aorta, pulmonary artery, and left and right atria are anastomosed. A variation in the technique is to perform bicaval anastomosis. If a pulmonary catheter is inserted, it must be withdrawn out of the heart that will be excised. Some surgeons prefer to pull the pulmonary catheter out of the native heart but keep it clamped to the side on the surgical field and manually insert it into the donor heart before right atrial anastomosis.

Rewarming typically triggers a series of checks and balances in all cardiac operations, including heart transplants. Typically, a large dose of corticosteroids is administered before unclamping and reperfusion of the new heart. The preseparation from bypass checklist includes achieving normothermia; balanced acid–base and electrolyte status, especially potassium, calcium, and magnesium; pacing capability; adequate sedative hypnotic and analgesic drug concentrations; and availability of inotropes, vasodilators, and vasopressors. Adequate oxygen-carrying capacity is ensured. There is no predefined hemoglobin concentration below which red cell transfusion is indicated. These decisions are based on the individual patient and conditions, as well as institutional protocol. Use of selective pulmonary vasodilators is more common in heart transplants than in conventional coronary artery bypass graft (CABG) surgery. Inhaled prostacyclin or nitric oxide is frequently initiated when ventilation is resumed to decrease right ventricular afterload. Unclamping of the aorta results in reperfusion of the donor heart. Return of heart rhythm soon follows, and assistance with external pacing may be necessary. The duration of reperfusion before separation from bypass is controversial. It is desirable to minimize bypass time and its deleterious effects on blood and vital organs (inflammation, red cell destruction, dilution, emboli). However, the ischemic heart (from cross-clamp in the donor to unclamping in the recipient) is depleted of energy stores, such as glycogen, adenosine triphosphate, and other high-energy molecules. In addition, intracellular and extracellular acidosis is severe in the heart after a period of prolonged ischemia, even if the heart is kept cold with cardioplegia. The needed recovery time is somewhat arbitrary and institution dependent.

Separation from bypass often is performed slowly, with gradual loading of the right ventricle. Pharmacologic support is common and often includes isoproterenol. This pure β-agonist is a potent inotrope and pulmonary vasodilator. The increased heart rate often is well tolerated and many times desirable, as cardiac output from hearts from young donors is often heart-rate dependent with a relatively fixed or limited stroke volume. Left heart failure is less common in heart transplantation compared with other forms of heart surgery because presumably a normal or near-normal heart is retrieved. Difficulty with preservation of myocardium, prolonged ischemic time, occult coronary artery disease, and air emboli to the coronary circulation can contribute to left ventricular dysfunction. Right-heart failure can be precipitated by increased PVR in the recipient. Treatment of the latter includes inotropes and pulmonary vasodilators, as well as hyperventilation, increasing oxygen tension, decreasing PEEP, and decreasing lung water.[121]

Once separation from bypass has been achieved, circulatory stability is confirmed and heparin is reversed with protamine. The postbypass period is characterized by correction of coagulopathy (if present), maintaining circulatory stability and body homeostasis (temperature, electrolytes, acid–base balance), and closure of the incision. Point-of-care coagulation testing offers the opportunity to quickly diagnose a bleeding diathesis and its cause, thereby permitting a targeted blood product replacement strategy. On completion of surgery, the patient is transported to the intensive care unit with full monitoring.

SUMMARY

Although the long-term mortality remains high for heart and lung transplantation, advances in immunosuppressant regimens and other medical treatment will most certainly improve the viability of the allograft. The population of patients receiving intrathoracic transplantation continues to change, and with continual assessment of outcomes through agencies such as the United Network for Organ Sharing (UNOS) and the International Society for Heart and Lung Transplantation (ISHLT), investigators will hopefully have the needed data to use scientifically justifiable interventions. Much improvement has resulted from a better understanding of the immune mechanisms involved in allograft rejection, which has spurred the ongoing development of novel immunosuppressive regimens. The anesthesiologist plays a pivotal role in the management of the transplant recipient's physiology and, as a result, both the short- and long-term morbidity/mortality of these patients. Attention to detail, an understanding of the operation, and an appreciation of allograft physiology all contribute to patient outcome. Greater insight into mechanisms of ischemia–reperfusion injury and acute rejection will have a positive effect on the outcome of this high-risk population. Additionally, as anesthesiologists continue to increase their presence in intensive care units, postoperative management of this high-risk population, including, but not limited to, volume administration (colloid vs crystalloid), ventilatory strategies (low stretch vs open lung), and glycemic control, will be relegated to the domain of anesthesiology. It is incumbent on anesthesiologists to be leaders in this advancement and to act as vital members of the entire transplantation team.

KEY REFERENCES

- Baez B, Castillo M. Anesthetic considerations for lung transplantation. *Semin Cardiothorac Vasc Anesth.* 2008;12:122-127.
- Christie JD, Edwards LB, Aurora P, et al. The Registry of the International Society for Heart and Lung Transplantation: twenty-sixth official adult lung and heart-lung transplantation report—2009. *J Heart Lung Transplant.* 2009;28:1031-1049.
- Hunt SA, Haddad F. The changing face of heart transplantation. *J Am Coll Cardiol.* 2008;52:587-598.
- McIlroy DR, Pilcher DV, Snell GI. Does anaesthetic management affect early outcomes after lung transplant? An exploratory analysis. *Br J Anaesth.* 2009;102:506-514.
- Taylor DO, Stehlik J, Edwards LB, et al. Registry of the International Society for Heart and Lung Transplantation: twenty-sixth official adult heart transplant report—2009. *J Heart Lung Transplant.* 2009;28:1007-1022.

REFERENCES

Complete references available on DVD and online version at www.LongneckerAnesthesiology.com

CHAPTER 59 Anesthesia for Kidney, Pancreas, or Other Organ Transplantation

Mojca Remskar Konia
David S. Beebe
Kumar G. Belani

KEY POINTS

1. The 5-year survival of patients on chronic hemo- or peritoneal dialysis is only 30%. In contrast, the 5-year survival following transplantation for end-stage renal disease is 70%. Therefore, transplantation is considered the treatment of choice for patients with renal failure.
2. Living related kidney transplant is associated with fewer episodes of acute and chronic rejection than cadaveric organ transplant.
3. Cardiac events related to coronary artery disease and autonomic nervous system dysfunction are the most common causes of morbidity and mortality in the first year following kidney or pancreas transplant.
4. Significant hypotension upon induction of general anesthesia is common in recently hemodialyzed patients. Diabetics with autonomic neuropathy are at increased risk for severe hypotension and bradycardia during induction of general anesthesia.
5. According to the most recent ACC/AHA guidelines for those receiving β-blocker therapy, these drugs should be continued in patients preoperatively, or initiated in patients with a positive stress test. The evidence also favors perioperative β-blockers in high-risk patients (more than 3 risk factors: high-risk surgery, ischemic heart disease, congestive heart failure, cerebrovascular disease, insulin-dependent diabetes mellitus, renal failure—creatinine >2.0 mg/dL). Use of β-blockers in low- and intermediate-risk patients is not supported by current available data.
6. Patients with long-standing diabetes often develop stiff joints due to glycosylation of the connective tissue that results from elevated blood sugars. The inability to oppose the palms of the hands is 1 sign in a diabetic patient that stiff connective tissue may be present. Patients with stiff joints may be difficult to intubate and may require an awake, fiberoptic intubation.
7. Adults and children who receive hematopoietic stem cell transplantation (HSCT) are at risk for complications, including respiratory failure or acute graft versus host disease. Acute graft versus host disease is the most important complication that significantly influences clinical outcome. HSCT recipients are at risk for airway complications during the first 2 months of transplantation.
8. Due to the high incidence of venous thrombosis in patients on long-term hyperalimentation, all patients referred for intestinal transplantation should undergo preliminary mapping of their venous access by Doppler ultrasound, and patients with multiple thrombosed vessels should be considered for additional angiographic evaluation.
9. Small bowel transplantation is a long surgical procedure that can take up to 17 hours. It can be associated with large fluid shifts due to abdominal manipulation and significant intraoperative bleeding, dehydration, vascular clamping, long ischemia times, visceral exposure, and lymphatic interruption. Therefore, adequate vascular access is essential.

The kidneys were the first organs to be transplanted in humans. This led to the development of the field of immunobiology along with surgical and anesthesia advancement, allowing other organs to be transplanted. In this chapter we discuss the anesthesia care, perioperative considerations, and outcome in patients undergoing transplantation of the kidneys, pancreas, islet cells, hematopoietic stem cells, and small intestine.

KIDNEY TRANSPLANTATION

HISTORY AND INTRODUCTION

The first successful kidney transplant, performed in the mid 1950s, was between identical twins.[1] Transplantation between identical twins resulted in excellent long-term graft and patient survival. However, the growth of kidney transplantation began in earnest with the development of improved immunosuppressive agents, particularly cyclosporine in 1983. In the United States alone, approximately 16830 kidney transplants were performed in 2009.[2]

ORGAN MATCHING, AVAILABILITY, AND ALLOCATION

Kidney transplantation is now the preferred treatment for end-stage renal disease (ESRD) of almost any origin. There is evidence that patients may benefit from earlier transplantation even if the donor

TABLE 59-1 Types of Donor Kidneys

Cadaveric	Living
Standard criteria[a]	Related
Expanded donor criteria (EDC)[b]	Nonrelated
Dual kidney transplant with EDC	
Nonbeating-heart donor	

Both cadaveric and living donor kidneys are used for transplantation. Expanded criteria increases the availability of donor organs. Moreover, ABO and HLA compatibility has been deemphasized to further increase the donor pool.

[a]Standard criteria–donor <50 years of age without hypertension (HTN) or diabetes, who fulfills the criteria for brain death.

[b]Expanded donor criteria–age >60 years or 50-59 years with at least 2 comorbidities (HTN, creat >1.5 mg/dL, or death caused by cerebrovascular accident).

organ is not optimal because the high mortality of long-term dialysis favors the risk:benefit ratio toward transplantation.[3,4] The 5-year survival of patients on chronic hemo- or peritoneal dialysis is only 30%. In contrast, the 5-year survival following transplantation for ESRD is 70%. Therefore, except in rare instances, transplantation should be performed in all patients with renal failure where it is technically feasible.[5]

Several methods are used or being investigated to increase the number of kidneys available for transplantation (**Table 59-1**). Living kidney donation is becoming an important source of donor kidneys. **Approximately 6388 patients received a transplant from a living donor in the Unites States in 2009.[2] Recipients of living related kidney transplants generally suffer fewer episodes of acute and chronic rejection than those receiving cadaveric organs. Recipients also benefit because living related and unrelated transplantation is performed on an elective, nonemergent basis.[6]**

Voluntary organ donation from living related and unrelated donors has led to the establishment of "the living donor exchange."[7] Living donors may ask the anesthesia provider about the risks associated with kidney donation. A recent study[8] reported that short-term (90-d) mortality was significantly increased when compared to a matched cohort that did not undergo donor nephrectomy, but the difference disappeared over time and the long-term mortality was actually less in those that underwent donor nephrectomy (**Fig. 59-1**). The early mortality was greater for men, black individuals, and those with a history of hypertension. Obesity and age did not have an impact. The long-term survival may reflect their better preexisting health status that led to them being selected as living donors.

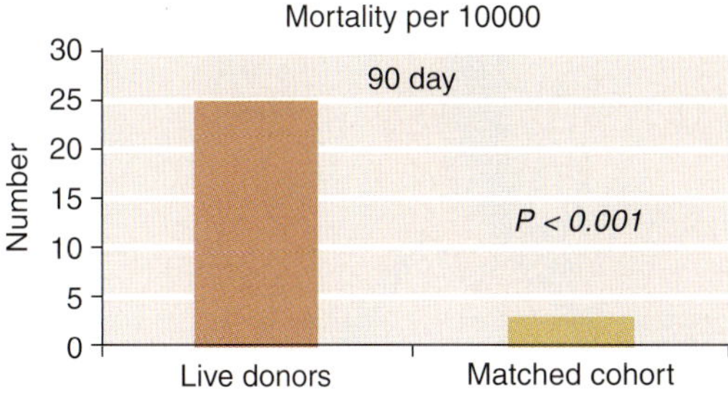

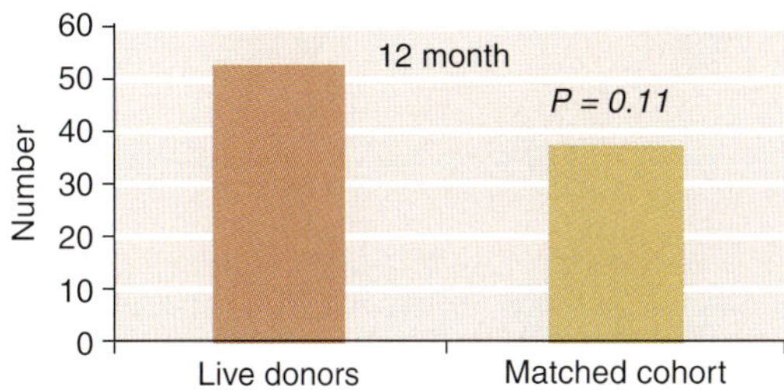

FIGURE 59-1. Perioperative and 12-month mortality following donor nephrectomy in live altruistic donors in the United States. There is a significantly higher mortality in the first 90 days following donor nephrectomy when compared to a matched cohort that did not undergo donor nephrectomy. However, this difference was not significant at 12 months. The authors of this study also found that beyond the 12-month period, those undergoing living donor nephrectomy actually had better survival when compared to their matched cohorts. [Data from Segev DL, Muzaale AD, Caffo BS, et al. Perioperative mortality and long-term survival following live kidney donation. *JAMA.* 2010;303:959-966.]

INDICATIONS AND CONTRAINDICATIONS

The most common causes of end-stage renal failure in adults are diabetes mellitus, systemic hypertension, glomerulonephritis, and polycystic kidney disease. In children and adolescents, the most common causes of ESRD are congenital malformations of the kidneys and urinary tract and focal segmental glomerulosclerosis.[5]

Ideally, patients with progressive renal failure should receive a kidney transplant before they begin dialysis.[5,9] Also, diabetic patients with marginal renal function who receive a pancreas transplant should receive a simultaneous kidney transplant because the immunosuppressive agents required for the pancreas transplant may cause further deterioration of renal function to the point of requiring dialysis.[9]

There are a decreasing number of absolute and relative contraindications to renal transplantation: Many conditions that were thought to be contraindications to transplantation previously, such as HIV, hepatitis C, age over 65, and advanced congestive heart failure, are now considered as acceptable.[10-13] Highly sensitized patients, T-cell positive cross-match, and ABO blood group–incompatible patients are now considered potential renal transplant candidates, albeit with an increased morbidity and mortality.[14]

Although the indications for kidney transplantation have been expanded significantly, some individuals with ESRD are not good candidates for this procedure. Active infection, active drug abuse, complete thrombosis of the vena cava and iliac veins, and disseminated malignancies are among the contraindications to transplantation. Sensitization by previous failed transplants, blood transfusions, or pregnancy will require individual assessment because in some the graft survival would be too poor to transplant.[15] Patients who have a history of noncompliance or mental retardation where it is unlikely that they will take their medications constitute relative contraindication to transplantation. However, patients with mental retardation can be transplanted successfully if they have a caregiver responsible for administering the medications.[16]

SURGICAL PROCEDURE

The surgical procedure of kidney transplantation is straightforward. In adults and older children (>20 kg), the transplanted kidney is usually placed in the extraperitoneal iliac fossa via a curvilinear incision along the lateral margin of the rectus muscle approximately 8 to 10 in from just above the pubic bone to just above the umbilicus (**Fig. 59-2**). The common and external iliac arteries and veins are exposed retroperitoneally. The renal vein is anastomosed before the renal artery, and an end-to-side or end-to-end anastomosis may be performed depending on the anatomy of the vessels and depth of the renal pelvis. The renal artery is then anastomosed to the internal or external iliac artery. Occasionally, donors have multiple renal arteries, and several arterial anastomoses are required. Renal revascularization involves clamping of the iliac artery and vein. This can result in ischemia to the lower extremity for as long as 60 minutes. After the vascular anastomoses are completed the clamps are released in a staged fashion, resulting in perfusion of the kidney graft and lower extremities. The final stage of the operation involves reconstruction of the urinary drainage by anastomosing the donor ureter to the patient's bladder.

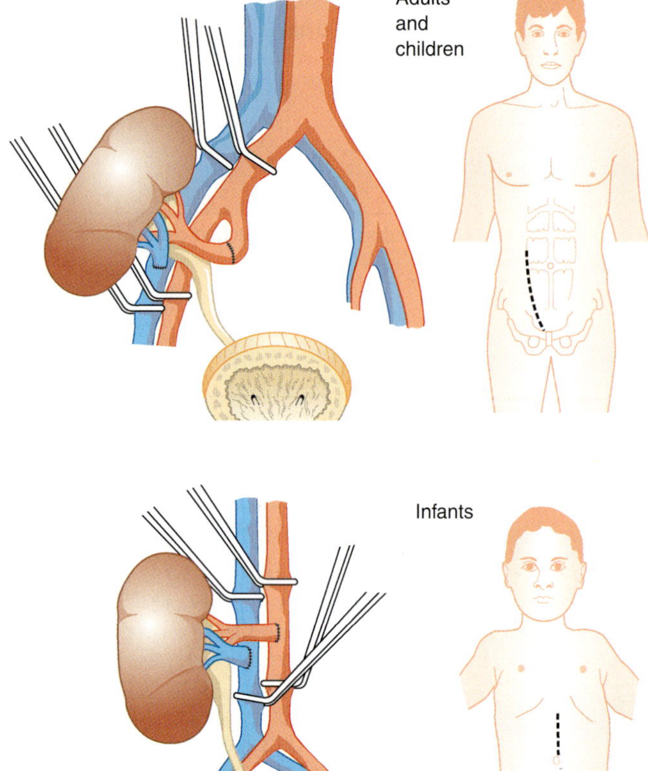

FIGURE 59-2. Surgical procedure for kidney transplantation in adults, children, and infants. (See text for details).

In infants and small children (<20 kg), a transperitoneal approach is used. An incision from the xiphoid process to the pubis is made (see Fig. 59-2). The bowel is mobilized and the aorta and vena cava are exposed. The donor artery and vein are then anastomosed to the aorta and vena cava end to side. Once the vascular anastomoses are complete, the clamps are released, resulting in reperfusion of both lower extremities and the donor kidney. The urinary drainage is then reconstructed.[17]

For living kidney donors, the laparoscopic and laparoscopy-assisted approach to nephrectomy is preferred due to a decreased need for pain medication, earlier discharge, and more rapid functional recovery.[18] The left kidney is preferred due to implantation advantages associated with a longer renal vein. The patient is positioned in the left lateral position with elevated kidney rest. Positioning of the patient requires great care to prevent positioning-related injuries (see Chapter 27).

PRETRANSPLANT EVALUATION

Patients undergoing kidney transplantation require a complete medical review and evaluation prior to surgery. (Preoperative evaluation of patients with renal disease is presented in Chapter 14; only brief comments that apply to transplantation will be provided here.) The evaluation is best done by the transplant surgery team prior to placing the patient on the transplant list. After the initial evaluation, cardiovascular surveillance is necessary. Frequency and type of surveillance, however, are a matter of discussion. In high-risk patients it may be prudent to do it annually or at least biannually.[19]

Comorbid Conditions **Table 59-2** lists medical conditions related to ESRD.

Cardiac Evaluation **Half of all deaths after renal transplantation are cardiac related, and cardiac disease is the leading cause of death in the first year posttransplant.[20] Besides severe coronary artery disease, sudden cardiac death of arrhythmic origin is also important.[21]**

Patients with diabetes, peripheral vascular disease, angina, or a longer duration of ESRD have a greater risk of mortality due to cardiovascular disease.[20] However, what constitutes the optimal pretransplant evaluation is still debated. Exercise stress testing, myocardial perfusion studies such as dobutamine stress echocardiography and thallium scintigraphy, and cardiac computed tomography (CT) or cardiac magnetic resonance imaging (MRI) can be used. Coronary angiogram remains the gold standard with the ability to predict cardiac events.[22] Data to strongly support preemptive myocardial revascularization in patients with stable coronary disease are lacking.

Special Considerations in Patients With ESRD

Diabetics Due to a high incidence of cardiac disease, some centers recommend coronary angiography in patients with ESRD associated with diabetes if they are older than 45 years of age, have a smoking history, have a body mass index above 25, have had diabetes for more than 25 years, or have electrocardiographic signs of ischemia.[23] Diabetic patients who have significant coronary disease with treatable lesions should have coronary artery surgery or an angioplasty prior to receiving

TABLE 59-2 Medical Problems in Patients With End-Stage Renal Disease

System	Complications Associated With Renal Failure
Cardiovascular	Hypertension, atherosclerosis, coronary artery disease, congestive heart failure, pulmonary edema, pulmonary hypertension, pericarditis, cardiomyopathy, arrhythmias
Hematologic	Anemia, platelet dysfunction, coagulopathies, increased capillary fragility
Immune	Impaired immunity
Neurologic	Peripheral neuropathy, autonomic neuropathy
Musculoskeletal	Myopathy
Gastrointestinal	Impaired gastric emptying, gastroparesis, nausea, vomiting, anorexia, peptic ulcer disease
Electrolyte and acid-base regulation	Potassium, sodium, calcium, magnesium, phosphate, bicarbonate imbalances, metabolic acid accumulation
Endocrine	Hyperparathyroidism, osteodystrophy, impaired growth and development (especially in children), glucose intolerance
Pulmonary	Pneumonia, pulmonary edema, pleuritis, atelectasis
Hepatic	Hypoalbuminemia, cytochrome P450 abnormality, hepatitis

Adapted from Koehntop DE, Beebe DS, Belani KG. *Kidney Transplantation*. In: Klinck JL, Lindop MJ eds. *Anesthesia and Intensive Care for Organ Transplantation*. London: Chapman and Hall; 1998:254-280.

a kidney transplant.[23] Some diabetics have significant but diffuse coronary disease (identified by angiography) that cannot be treated surgically or by angioplasty. These patients may still benefit from combined kidney and pancreas transplantation instead of chronic dialysis, but they are at higher risk for perioperative cardiac events.[24] Successful pancreas transplant in these patients slowed the progression of atherosclerotic lesions (mean segmental diameter loss 0.024 mm/y vs 0.044 mm/y) and caused regression of atherosclerotic lesions in 38% of patients with a functioning pancreas graft.

Furthermore, diabetic patients can suffer from a host of comorbidities that affect anesthetic care, including autonomic neuropathy, gastroparesis, peripheral neuropathy, and peripheral vascular disease. The time of insulin administration is important to note in diabetic patients because it can influence the plan for perioperative glucose management. Diabetic patients should also be asked about symptoms of gastroparesis, such as heartburn, bloating, and explosive diarrhea, because they may be at risk for aspiration of gastric contents upon induction of general anesthesia. These patients will benefit from a nonparticulate antacid, such as sodium citrate or related compounds, prior to induction of general anesthesia. (See Chapter 13 for a detailed review of the preoperative assessment of diabetics.)

Hypertension Hypertension is another common cause of renal failure that affects multiple organ systems. Patient's usual blood pressure, years of hypertension, and the type and last dose of antihypertensive medications that the patient receives should be recorded. In general, patients should receive their usual blood pressure medications prior to surgery.[25] However, angiotensin-system inhibitors administered immediately before operation have been associated with a greater incidence of hypotension upon induction of general anesthesia in hypertensive patients.[26]

β-Blocker therapy should be continued in those receiving treatment preoperatively, and started in those with a positive stress test, according to the most recent ACC/AHA guidelines. **The evidence also favors perioperative β-blockers in high-risk patients (more than 3 risk factors: high-risk surgery, ischemic heart disease, congestive heart failure (CHF), cerebrovascular disease, insulin-dependent diabetes mellitus, renal failure—creatinine >2.0 mg/dL).[27] The use of β-blockers in low- and intermediate-risk patients is not supported by current available data.**

Sleep-Related Breathing Disorders An increasing number of patients with ESRD are being recognized to have sleep-related breathing disorders (SRBDs).[28] Lee et al examined patients before and after kidney transplantation. Kidney transplantation was effective in improving sleep patterns and also improving the apnea/hypopnea index (**Fig. 59-3**). (See Chapter 11 for a more detailed discussion of sleep-related breathing disorders.)

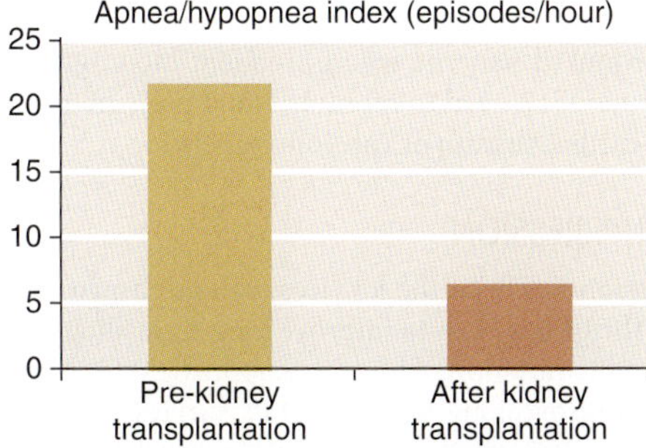

FIGURE 59-3. Patients with ESRD have a high likelihood of apnea/hypopnea during sleep. This sleep-related breathing disorder improves significantly after successful kidney transplantation. [Data in figure from Lee JJ, Kim GS, Kim JA, et al. Improvement of sleep-related breathing disorder in patients with end-stage renal disease after kidney transplantation. *Clin Transplant.* 2009;25:126-130.]

Physical Examination Several components of the physical examination deserve special consideration in the preanesthetic evaluation of the renal transplant patient. **The evaluation of the airway is particularly important for diabetics. Patients with long-standing diabetes often develop stiff joints due to glycosylation of the connective tissue that results from elevated blood sugars. The inability to oppose the palms of the hands is 1 sign in a diabetic patient that stiff connective tissue may be present. Patients with stiff joints may be difficult to intubate and may require an awake, fiberoptic intubation.[29]**

The arms of patients on chronic hemodialysis should be examined for the presence of both functioning and nonfunctioning dialysis shunts and fistulas. Upper-extremity fistulas may clot during transplantation surgery from reduced blood flow during surgery or the perioperative elevation of clotting factors. Care must be taken in padding the upper extremity with a forearm fistula so that no restriction of blood flow in the fistula occurs. The blood flow through the fistula during surgery can be monitored by palpation or a Doppler device. The arm with a functioning fistula should not be used for blood pressure monitoring, venipuncture, or the placement of intravascular catheters because each such a maneuver may cause the fistula to thrombose.[25] In the event of delayed graft function or even nonfunction following kidney transplantation, a functioning dialysis shunt is invaluable in the postoperative period.

Assessment of Fluid Balance **Fluid balance is often difficult to assess in patients on chronic dialysis.** One method to help evaluate the volume status of a patient on chronic dialysis is to review the patient's body weight before and after dialysis. The weight of the patient at the completion of dialysis, the "dry" weight, can be determined and compared to the weight when the patient presents for surgery.[17] **The type of dialysis, time of last dialysis, and frequency of dialysis are important to obtain as well.[25] Depending on the type of dialysis and the interval since last dialysis, the patient is rarely euvolemic and usually arrives in the operating room either hyper- or hypovolemic.** Significant hypotension upon induction of general anesthesia in recently hemodialyzed patients is therefore not uncommon.[17] Anesthesia care providers must be prepared to rapidly replace the intravascular volume in these patients. Depending on the extent of hypovolemia, either intravenous normal saline or 5% albumin may be used to provide a more rapid and sustainable cardiovascular response.

Laboratory Tests There are several laboratory tests that should be performed in all patients. Because electrolytes and blood glucose can change markedly over several days, particularly in patients on dialysis, most of these tests should be performed at or close to the time of operation. An electrocardiogram should be obtained in all patients at risk for cardiac disease, and the results compared to those of previous studies. The serum potassium may increase during surgery from the effects of drugs administered, blood transfusions, or from the infusion of hyperkalemic preservative solution from the new kidney. Therefore, surgery may have to be delayed and dialysis or other intervention performed if the patient is hyperkalemic (>6 mmol/L) preoperatively. Coagulation studies (international normalized ratio [INR], partial thromboplastin time [PTT], fibrinogen, platelet count) should be obtained if the patient has a prior history of bleeding or other evidence of a possible coagulopathy. Finally, the hemoglobin value should be determined and several units of blood made available preoperatively because patients with renal failure are often markedly anemic preoperatively.[25] Fluid loading to increase central venous pressure in preparation for reperfusion and surgical blood loss may further decrease blood hemoglobin values and thus warrant intraoperative packed red cell transfusion.

INDUCTION AND MAINTENANCE OF GENERAL ANESTHESIA

The choice of induction agent depends on the overall health of the patient, the volume status of the patient, the presence of autonomic neuropathy, and the presence of cardiovascular or other disease. **Relatively healthy renal transplant recipients tolerate induction of general**

anesthesia with propofol (2.0-3.0 mg/kg) or thiopental (2.5-3.0 mg/kg) without difficulty. However, etomidate (0.2 mg/kg) is better tolerated in hemodynamically compromised patients because it exerts minimal myocardial depression and preserves autonomic tone. This is particularly important in diabetic patients with autonomic neuropathy. Fentanyl (3-5 mcg/kg intravenously [IV]) can be administered during induction to blunt the hypertensive response to tracheal intubation. In patients who do not have a history of gastroparesis or acid reflux disease, intermediate-duration nondepolarizing muscle relaxants that do not depend on renal excretion for elimination, such as *cis*-atracurium (0.2 mg/kg), rocuronium (0.5 mg/kg), or vecuronium (0.1 mg/kg), can be administered to facilitate tracheal intubation.[25]

In patients with gastroparesis or acid reflux disease, a rapid sequence induction, including Sellick maneuver to prevent regurgitation of gastric contents, should be performed. The depolarizing agent succinylcholine (1.5 mg/kg IV) has classically been used in patients without renal failure to provide rapid skeletal muscle relaxation for immediate tracheal intubation. However, the serum potassium can increase 0.6 mmol/L with its administration, so it should be used with caution, if at all, in patients with renal failure who have an elevated preoperative potassium level (>5.5 mmol/L). Many anesthesia providers therefore prefer to use nondepolarizing agents even if a rapid sequence induction is required. Rocuronium is useful for this purpose because at high doses (1.2 mg/kg) it has an onset of action of 60 to 90 seconds and does not require renal function for elimination.[25]

The inhaled agents desflurane and isoflurane are both extremely useful for the maintenance of general anesthesia for kidney transplantation. Neither agent has nephrotoxic properties, and no deterioration of renal function has been noted with either agent in patients with or without renal disease.[5] Nitrous oxide may be used along with the potent inhaled agent. It has minimal side effects, no renal toxicity, and rapid elimination. However, it is associated with increased nausea and vomiting in the postoperative period.[30] As a result it may be used less frequently for these procedures in the future. Sevoflurane is rarely used for renal transplantation due to concerns of fluoride and compound A toxicity.[31] Most human studies have *not* demonstrated deleterious effects of sevoflurane on the kidney.[32] Many authors, however, feel that in the presence of other alternatives, there seems to be little reason to select sevoflurane for inhalation anesthesia in renal transplant patients. However, sevoflurane has been demonstrated to have anti-inflammatory and antinecrotic effects on renal tissue, which may be protective against ischemia-reperfusion injury.[33] Overall, uncertainty remains regarding the use of sevoflurane in renal transplantation.

During anesthesia care, opioids such as fentanyl (50-100 mcg/h) are often administered throughout the transplant procedure to reduce the amount of inhaled agent required and decrease the likelihood of the patient awakening in severe pain. The pharmacokinetics and pharmacodynamics of fentanyl, sufentanil, alfentanil, and remifentanil are not significantly altered by kidney disease, and all have been successfully used during renal transplantation.[34]

Ongoing skeletal muscle relaxation can be provided with nondepolarizing muscle relaxants that do not depend on the kidney for elimination, such as *cis*-atracurium, rocuronium, or vecuronium. All 3 have been used successfully in patients with marginal or no renal function, and have minimal effects on the heart rate or blood pressure. *Cis*-atracurium is broken down in the plasma by Hoffman elimination, which does not depend on renal or hepatic function. Its duration of action is not prolonged in renal failure. Although the liver is the primary metabolic site for both rocuronium and vecuronium, the duration of blockade may be prolonged with these drugs if large doses are used, due to accumulation of metabolites that are excreted by the kidney.[5,35] Pancuronium should not be used in kidney transplant recipients because it depends primarily on the kidney for elimination. If the new kidney does not function adequately initially, a prolonged neuromuscular block may result.[5]

Blood glucose determinations should be made every hour in renal transplant recipients who have insulin-dependent diabetes mellitus. Evidence suggests that the incidence of wound infections can be reduced in diabetic patients if the blood sugar is tightly controlled.[36] The extent of glucose lowering, however, is questionable. The NICE (Normoglycemia in Intensive Care Evaluation) study demonstrated a 2.5% increase in mortality for patients on intensive insulin therapy where blood glucose was kept in the 80 to 110 mg/dL range.[37] Middle-ground target glucose of between 140 and 180 mg/dL is suggested at this time.[38] Whenever the intraoperative blood sugar is between 90 and 110 gm/dL, a low-dose dextrose solution ($D_5$1/2 normal saline at 25 mL/h) should be administered concurrently throughout the procedure to provide for intraoperative nutrition and prevent hypoglycemia.[39]

Emergence From General Anesthesia Following the operation, most patients can be extubated in the operating or recovery room when they are alert, strong, and able to maintain adequate ventilation. Rarely is postoperative ventilation required.

Pain control can be achieved with neuraxial anesthesia, and the successful use of combined spinal-epidural anesthesia for both surgical anesthesia and postoperative pain relief has been described.[40] However, although rare, there is a small risk of an epidural hematoma.

Because most graft recipients receive heparin intraoperatively, and some in the postoperative period, intravenous opioids such as fentanyl, morphine, or hydromorphone are usually used for postoperative analgesia. These drugs may also be used for patient-controlled analgesia following discharge from the recovery room.[5]

All opioids must be used cautiously in renal transplant recipients, particularly if the graft is not functioning properly. For example, a metabolite of morphine, morphine-6-*B*-glucuronide, has opioid agonist activity and is excreted by the kidneys. It can accumulate in renal failure and cause respiratory depression with long-term use. The metabolism of hydromorphone produces a neuroexcitatory compound that can accumulate in renal failure. However, hydromorphone has been used extensively in renal failure patients with no adverse effects. In contrast, a metabolite of meperidine (Demerol), normeperidine, can accumulate in significant amounts in patients with renal failure, and this compound can cause seizures. Therefore, meperidine should not be used for postoperative analgesia in renal transplant recipients.[34]

MONITORING

Patients undergoing renal transplantation usually benefit from central venous access. It provides convenient vascular access to obtain blood samples and for administration of the immunosuppressive drugs that must be administered centrally. Measurement of the central venous pressure (CVP) has been used in the past to determine if the volume status of the recipient is adequate at the time of reperfusion of the allograft. Alternative newer technologies based on pulse pressure variation and stroke volume variation are currently being validated as tools to determine volume responsiveness. Rarely is transesophageal echocardiography or pulmonary artery catheterization necessary except in those patients with severe cardiac disease (cardiomyopathy) or pulmonary hypertension. Direct arterial catheters are also used infrequently except in compromised patients where frequent blood gases must be determined[25] or there is a need to monitor blood pressure more closely, as in those with cardiac disease or cardiomyopathy.

IMMUNOSUPPRESSION

Immunosuppression has been the key to success of organ transplantation. The major thrust has been to improve long-term allograft survival. There is considerable variation of immunosuppressant protocols among institutions. To improve long-term allograft survival, researchers are trying to minimize exposure to drugs that are used to prevent acute cellular rejection.[41] Commonly used agents for immunosuppression are calcineurin inhibitors (cyclosporine, tacrolimus), antiproliferative agents (mycophenolate mofetil), rapamycin (mTOR) inhibitors (sirolimus, everolimus), corticosteroids, and monoclonal and polyclonal antibodies. Occasionally, reactions to immunosuppressive drugs occur.[42]

For example, cyclosporine administration can result in hypomagnesemia, rhabdomyolysis, and other electrolyte disorders.[43] Reactions to antibody OKT_3 can be severe and result in hypotension and pulmonary edema. Treatment with diphenhydramine, vasopressors, steroids, diuresis, and postoperative ventilation may be required.[25]

ALLOGRAFT PERFUSION

Intraoperative volume expansion is widely used and is supported by studies that have shown increased renal blood flow and better immediate graft function with generous volume administration.[44] **Immediate graft function is associated with increased allograft and patient survival.**[5] One method to ensure adequate volume expansion in patients with good cardiac function is to raise the central venous pressure to 14 or 15 mm Hg with intravenous normal saline or 5% albumin prior to perfusion of the allograft. If the patient is relatively anemic (Hgb <10 g/dL), packed red blood cells may be used for this purpose as well. One needs to be aware that static measures of volume, such as CVP or pulmonary capillary wedge pressure, may not be reliable measures of volume responsiveness, especially in patients with decreased cardiac function. Dynamic measures such as pulse pressure variation, stroke volume variation, and changes in aortic flow velocity may be better but have not been extensively studied in this population.[45] Furthermore, new studies suggest that overly aggressive fluid administration may not be necessary.[46]

In spite of adequate volume expansion, hypotension can still result from products of ischemia from the graft or lower extremity when the vascular clamps are released. The microvasculature of the graft and lower extremity are maximally vasodilated with reperfusion after a period of ischemia and can result in a low peripheral resistance. Therefore, it is helpful to intentionally raise the systolic blood pressure to 130 or 140 mm Hg by reducing the concentration of inhaled anesthetic agents administered prior to reperfusing the allograft. A vasopressor such as ephedrine (5-10 mg), phenylephrine (100-200 mcg), or an infusion of dopamine (3-5 mcg/kg/min) is occasionally required to treat hypotension during and after reperfusion. One advantage dopamine has over the other vasopressors is that it can increase diuresis in the allograft. However, graft survival has not been shown to increase despite this increased diuresis.[5]

Mannitol administration (0.25-1 g/kg) prior to perfusion of the allograft, when combined with volume expansion, has been shown to decrease the incidence of acute tubular necrosis in the transplanted kidney. The mechanism by which it does this may be related to decreasing tubular swelling by its osmotic effect, its action as a free-radical scavenger, or by flushing away sloughed renal tubule cells before they can cause injury by secondary obstruction.[47] Other diuretics such as furosemide can be administered to enhance diuresis, but have not been shown to reduce the incidence of acute tubular necrosis or delayed graft function in the transplanted kidney.[5]

MONITORING URINE OUTPUT

After reperfusion of the allograft, the urine output, intravascular volume, and overall circulatory status should be followed carefully. Hypovolemia, hypotension, acute tubular necrosis, or acute rejection can result in diminished urine output. Evaluation of decreased urine output posttransplant usually begins with an assessment of the patient's volume status. A biopsy of the transplanted kidney may also be necessary to determine if the patient is suffering from acute tubular necrosis or graft rejection.[25]

Decreasing urine output may indicate a reversible surgical problem. Anuria may also be due to a mechanical factor. Vascular complications such as arterial thrombosis, arterial stenosis, or venous occlusion may result in oliguria. Distal obstruction of the ureter by a clot or kinking, or pressure on the kidney by a lymphocele or hematoma may compromise function of the new kidney as well. Fortunately, many of the mechanical causes of oliguria are correctible, if the diagnosis can be made in a timely fashion.[25]

POSTOPERATIVE CONSIDERATIONS AND COMPLICATIONS

Most patients do not require admission to the intensive care unit in the postoperative period provided the nursing unit is experienced in the care of transplant recipients. In addition to providing the standard postoperative care for a patient who has undergone major abdominal surgery, the function of the new kidney must be followed carefully in the transplant recipient. Rejection, viral infection, vascular thrombosis, and urinary obstruction are all complications that may occur in the perioperative period.[25]

However, the most common causes of death after transplantation are cardiovascular-related events, and studies estimate a 3-year cumulative incidence of myocardial infarction of 4.7% to 11%.[48] Up to 6% of patients with coronary artery disease experience a cardiac complication within 30 days of transplantation.[49] Providing perioperative β-blockade, normothermia, maintaining a hematocrit of greater than 30%, and ensuring that patients have optimum analgesia in the perioperative period are all measures that may help reduce the risk for patients with cardiac disease undergoing renal transplantation.[5]

ANESTHETIC CONSIDERATIONS FOR PATIENTS WITH PRIOR RENAL TRANSPLANTATION

Even with a functioning graft, the renal excretion of drugs in transplant recipients is usually decreased when compared to those with normal functioning native kidneys. Further, recipients may still suffer from their other systemic disease, such as diabetes or hypertension that resulted in their renal insufficiency initially. Therefore, the anesthetic care of patients with a prior renal transplant is similar to the transplant itself. Muscle relaxants that depend on renal excretion for their elimination, such as pancuronium, should be used only with the recognition that there may be delayed excretion. Adequate hydration should be ensured in the perioperative period and hypotension avoided to ensure adequate perfusion to the allograft.[50]

Long-term immunosuppression can result in significant morbidity in kidney transplant recipients.[51] The effect of immunosuppressive drugs should be considered when evaluating a kidney transplant recipient for nontransplant surgery. For example, cyclosporine use may cause hypertension and hyperlipidemia, and worsen atherosclerosis in kidney transplant recipients. Tacrolimus is associated with new-onset diabetes after transplant. Most patients have adrenal suppression to some degree because of long-term steroid use. Therefore, a stress dose of steroids may be necessary in renal transplant recipients who have received steroids for immunosuppression.[50]

SPECIAL CONSIDERATIONS IN PEDIATRIC PATIENTS

The anesthetic care of older children and adolescents is similar to adults. Infants and small children less than 2 years of age are more challenging. Infants and small children usually receive an adult kidney rather than one from a donor similar in age because there is a high incidence of vascular thrombosis with allografts from infants and small children. However, an adult kidney is so large compared to an infant that it must be anastomosed to the infant's aorta and vena cava rather than the iliac vessels (see Fig. 59-2) as in older children or adults.[52] Therefore, the aorta and vena cava both must be cross-clamped during performance of the vascular anastomoses. The adult kidney can sequester up to 300 mL of blood upon reperfusion. Reperfusion can also result in acidosis from the ischemic organ and lower extremities. Hyperkalemia may result from absorption of the standard hyperkalemic (University of Wisconsin) preservative solution. Hypothermia may result with reperfusion of the allograft. Ischemic vasodilatation upon reperfusion of the allograft can also result in a low peripheral vascular resistance and hypotension. In addition, the adult kidney can initially produce urine at a rate equal to the patient's blood volume every hour.[53] All this dictates that caregivers pay close attention to circulatory hemodynamics in young infants receiving an adult kidney allograft.

Allograft Perfusion The goals of the anesthetic management of kidney transplantation in infants and small children are the same as those for older children and adults. Adequate volume expansion must occur to prevent severe hypotension upon perfusion of the allograft. Often a permanent, large-bore (2-mm internal diameter) dialysis catheter is valuable for central vascular access and also provides a means for hemodialysis if the kidney does not function immediately. Direct arterial pressure monitoring is useful in infants and very small children because blood pressure changes can be rapid and profound. **In contrast to older children and adults, in infants the central venous pressure must be increased to 16 to 20 mm Hg before reperfusion of the allograft. Colloids such as 5% albumin as well as blood products are generally used for this purpose.** The amount of colloids and/or blood products administered can be profound. In 1 review of infants and small children receiving an adult kidney transplant, the amount of colloids and/or blood products administered averaged 90 ±41 mL/kg.[53]

Postoperative Admission to Intensive Care Unit Postoperatively, pediatric patients are at an increased risk for pulmonary edema. Most pediatric patients tolerate the volume administration without morbidity. In 1 review of 24 infants receiving an adult kidney transplant, 17 (71%) were extubated in the recovery room, and most of the others in the intensive care unit the following day. Only 2 patients (8.3%) required mechanical ventilation beyond 24 hours to aid in fluid management. However, 7 of the 24 patients (29%) had radiographic evidence of pulmonary edema on the postoperative chest x-ray. Therefore, the pulmonary status of pediatric patients should be monitored in an intensive care unit setting following surgery, and some may require postoperative ventilatory support.[53]

OUTCOME

Approximately 25 000 patients per year now receive a kidney transplant, either from a living or cadaver donor. The most recent 1-year graft survival is 92% from cadaveric nonextended criteria donors, 85% from extended criteria donors, and 96% from living related donors. At 5 years, the graft survival is 81% from living related donors, 72% from cadaveric nonextended criteria, and 57% from cadaveric extended criteria donors. The 5-year patient survival is 84% to 72% for recipients of cadaveric organs and 91% for recipients of living donors. In addition, comparison with earlier data shows improved survival of both patients and the allografts over time.[54] Renal transplantation has become one of the great success stories in medicine.

The future may give us a new understanding of transplant failure. Recent genetic research has identified a gene variant in the CAV1 gene of kidney donors that carries a higher risk of graft failure following transplantation. This finding may allow us to identify biomarkers that predict graft survival ahead of time.[55]

SUMMARY

Kidney transplantation offers both better survival and a better lifestyle to patients in renal failure. Patients with renal failure are a challenging group for the reasons discussed above. With careful anesthetic care, knowledge of the pathophysiology of renal failure and associated disease, and understanding of the physiology of perfusion of the renal allograft, satisfying outcomes can be obtained.

PANCREAS AND ISLET CELL TRANSPLANTATION

HISTORY AND INTRODUCTION

In 1967 Kelly et al reported the first combined transplantation of the pancreas and duodenum along with a kidney in a human with diabetic nephropathy.[56] Today this procedure is commonplace for the surgical treatment of Type 1 diabetes mellitus in patients with ESRD. Because renal failure often accompanies diabetes mellitus, and although pancreas transplantation can be done alone, it is most commonly done (as mentioned in the discussion on kidney transplantation) simultaneously with a kidney transplant procedure or following kidney transplantation.[57] Thus transplantation of the pancreas or islet cells constitutes surgical treatment for patients with Type 1 diabetes mellitus and now increasingly for those with Type 2 diabetes mellitus (**Fig. 59-4**).[58] Cadaveric donors provide whole pancreas grafts and islet cells, and living donors provide distal segments for transplantation. Autoislet transplantation is the method of choice to treat endocrine deficiency following total pancreatectomy.[59] **The most recent published data (2009) indicate that more than 30 000 pancreas transplants from approximately 140 centers in the United States were reported to the International Pancreas Transplant Registry.**[60] Most (>22 000) were performed in

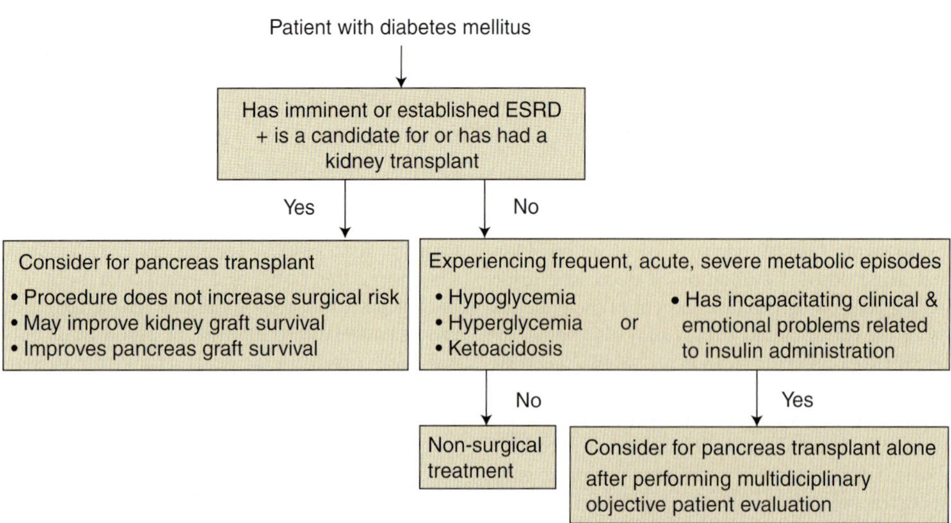

FIGURE 59-4. Flow diagram summarizing the indications for pancreas transplantation in patients with diabetes mellitus. Islet cell transplantation will be the procedure of choice in the future and will also require immunosuppression, but it is still in the developmental stages. [Adapted from Robertson RP, Davis C, Larsen J, Stratta R, Sutherland DE. Pancreas transplantation for patients with type 1 diabetes. *Diabetes Care.* 2003;26(Suppl 1):S120.]

the United States. Most transplants done are simultaneous pancreas-kidney transplants (73%), then pancreas-after-kidney transplants (19%), followed by pancreas transplants alone (9%).[60]

PATHOPHYSIOLOGY OF DIABETES MELLITUS

Diabetes mellitus is a multisystem disease characterized by hyperglycemia resulting from deficiency in insulin secretion or action. It is one of the leading causes of death and disability in the United States (see Chapter 13 for a detailed discussion of the pathophysiology of diabetes.)

Diabetes mellitus (DM) is classified based on the pathogenic process leading to hyperglycemia.[61] Type 1 diabetes occurs when there is an absolute insulin deficiency that is immune mediated or of idiopathic origin. This is usually the result of the synergistic effects of genetic, environmental, and immunologic factors leading to pancreatic beta-cell destruction. Approximately 5% to 15% of diagnosed cases of diabetes are Type 1 and affect individuals during childhood and adolescence.[62] The nonsurgical treatment of Type 1 diabetes involves life-long administration of exogenous insulin. The Diabetes Control and Complications study demonstrated that tight glucose control delays the onset and slows the progression of diabetic retinopathy, nephropathy, and neuropathy.[63,64] These studies have concluded that the risk of the 3-fold increase in severe hypoglycemia outweighs the benefits of delay in progression of diabetic end-organ damage. The surgical option of pancreas or islet cell transplantation offers patients with insulin-dependent diabetes mellitus (IDDM) an endogenous source of insulin. Even though sicker recipients are being transplanted, long-term insulin independence is achieved in 77% to 85% of pancreas transplant recipients.[57,65]

Insulin resistance with a relative insulin deficiency is classified as Type 2 diabetes.[61] It is the more common type of diabetes that is managed by diet, oral hypoglycemic agents, and/or exogenous insulin administration.[58] It is usually seen in adults over age 40 years, but the incidence of adolescent onset is increasing rapidly as is metabolic syndrome, which consists of obesity, hypertension, and diabetes mellitus.[66] In patients with metabolic syndrome, high amounts of visceral fat are influential in the development of diabetes-related complications, such as cardiovascular disease.

Patients with Type 1 DM develop progressive changes in almost every organ system due to microangiopathy. Chronically increased blood glucose concentration leads to glycosylation of proteins. Acute complications of diabetes include diabetic ketoacidosis, hyperglycemic hyperosmolar nonketotic coma, lactic acidosis, and hypoglycemia.[67] Chronic complications of Type 1 DM include coronary artery disease, peripheral vascular disease, cerebrovascular disease, nephropathy, autonomic and peripheral neuropathy, and retinopathy.[58,63,64,68] The cumulative prevalence and relative risk of these complications is 21% for myocardial infarction and 22% for renal failure, followed by blindness, amputation, and stroke of approximately 10% in patients with insulin-dependent diabetes mellitus.[69]

RATIONALE FOR PANCREAS TRANSPLANTATION

The goal of pancreas and islet cell transplantation is to restore normoglycemia and the glucagon response to hypoglycemia, allowing patients to be insulin-free and eat a regular diet.[58,70] Carbohydrate metabolism after pancreas transplant may stabilize and even improve macro- and microvascular disease.[71] A secondary benefit is the improved quality of life reported by patients.[72] Although most patients are insulin-free, some may still develop retinopathy and show progression of macrovascular disease despite successful kidney and/or pancreas transplantation.[73]

The current recommendations for pancreas transplantation are summarized in Fig. 59-4. The American Diabetes Association's position statement[74] on pancreas and islet transplant recommends pancreas transplant as an acceptable therapeutic alternative to insulin therapy in diabetic patients with imminent or established end-stage renal disease who will have a renal transplant. Survival is better if a pancreas transplant is also done in patients requiring a kidney transplant.[75] Diabetic patients with a history of frequent, acute, and severe metabolic complications; incapacitating clinical and emotional problems with exogenous insulin therapy; and consistent failure of insulin-based management to prevent complications should be considered for pancreas transplant in the absence of indications for kidney transplant. Islet cell transplantation is projected to be the method of choice for the future care of patients with Type 1 diabetes. Many centers are conducting research with both human cadaveric islets as well as pig-encapsulated islets. However, these technologies are still in an infancy stage and thus should be performed only in a controlled setting where facilities for doing this procedure are available.

SURGICAL OPTIONS

Several surgical techniques have been described but all require vascularization of the pancreas and a method to drain the pancreatic duct.[76] Exocrine secretions can be managed by either enteric or bladder drainage (**Fig. 59-5**). From 1987 to 1995 over 90% of pancreas transplants were done using bladder drainage (Fig. 59-5B), which allows serial measurements of urinary amylase to monitor for rejection.[57,77,78] Chronic loss of pancreatic secretions into the bladder can result in dehydration, electrolyte abnormalities, local bladder irritation, hematuria, urethritis, and allograft pancreatitis.[79] With improvement in surgical technique, enteric drainage (Fig. 59-5A) has now become the surgical procedure of choice.[77] Initially, it was associated with a high morbidity rate due to leakage and need for frequent reoperations. However, enteric drainage avoids the complications associated with bladder drainage[77].

Vascular management includes arterial anastomosis and venous drainage either systemically or into the portal venous system. Portal venous drainage has remained constant for patients undergoing simultaneous pancreas and kidney transplantation, but has been decreasing since 2002 for the other transplant categories.[57] Both portal and systemic drainage are associated with excellent glycemic control, but fasting serum insulin levels are significantly lower in portal drainage without an effect on graft survival rates at 1 year for simultaneous pancreas-kidney or pancreas-after-kidney transplantation.[80] Currently, vascular management strategies have little impact on graft survival rate.[57]

Because of technical problems, pancreas grafts are associated with the highest surgical complication rate of all routinely transplanted solid organs. Causes for technical failure of cadaveric primary pancreas transplants include pancreatitis, anastomotic leak, bleeding, and rejection.[81] Significant risk factors for graft loss include older donor age, donor obesity, retransplantation, relaparotomy for infection, leak, or bleeding, and the immunosuppression protocol.[82] The quality of a cadaveric donor graft can directly affect graft performance.[82] **Table 59-3** lists the inclusion criteria for a cadaveric pancreas donor.[58] As experience with pancreas transplant increases, the incidence of relaparotomy has decreased.[83] Risk factors for recipient death include older recipient, retransplantation, and relaparotomy for thrombosis, infection, leak, or bleeding.[57,58]

PREOPERATIVE EVALUATION

Cadaveric pancreas procurement is usually part of a multiple organ harvest, and for successful graft function, preservation time should preferably be limited to less than 24 hours. This requires that the anesthesia provider be able to perform a thorough evaluation of the recipient in an efficient manner. As emphasized in the discussion on kidney transplantation, for patient care efficiency it is imperative that pancreas transplant centers exercise a stringent policy with regard to evaluation and selection.[77] An advance evaluation should include coronary artery disease,[84] renal status, autonomic nervous system, systemic neuropathy, metabolic status, presence of gastroparesis, and the possibility of

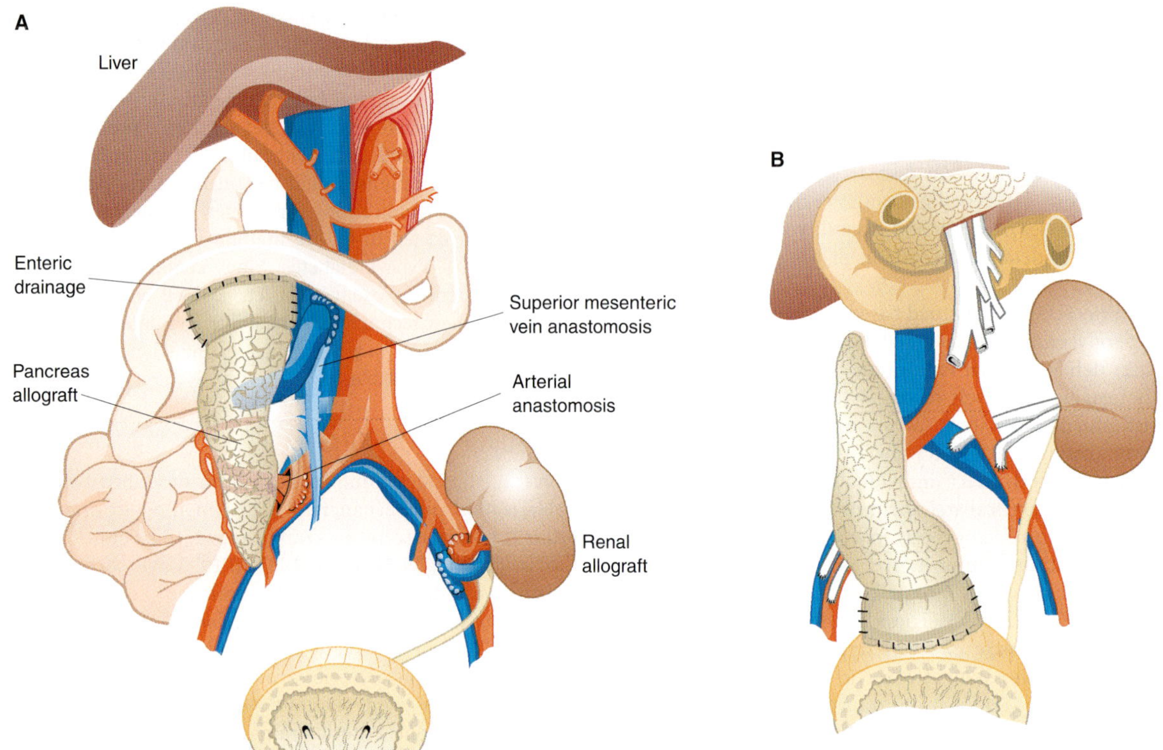

FIGURE 59-5. Surgical vascularization of the graft showing enteric drainage (**A**) and bladder drainage (**B**). [**A** and **B.** Courtesy of Sutherland DER. Modified from Bretzel RG, Eckhard M, Brendel MD. Pancreatic islet and stem cell transplantation: new strategies in cell therapy of diabetes mellitus. *Panminerva Med.* 2004;46:25-42.]

difficult intubation.[58] **Table 59-4** outlines areas that should be included during the preoperative assessment.

Coronary artery disease is responsible for most perioperative mortality in pancreas recipients.[23,85] Noninvasive screening tests or coronary angiography done preoperatively help plan intra- and postoperative care to decrease complications.[23,85,86] Pretransplantation coronary revascularization reduces the risk of subsequent cardiac events.[86] Because simultaneous pancreas-kidney transplants account for 78% of pancreas transplants, and pancreas-after-kidney account for 16% of transplants,[57] it is important to evaluate renal function, including determination of acid-base status, glucose levels, electrolyte concentrations, and time of last hemodialysis. ESRD is often associated with anemia, which can have a significant impact on morbidity and graft success.[58]

Autonomic nervous system dysfunction predisposes patients to severe hypotension during anesthesia. There also are reports of sudden death in patients not continuously monitored during the immediate postoperative period, possibly from an altered response to hypoxia.[87,88]

When gastroparesis is present, aspiration prophylaxis with nonparticulate antacids, H_2-antagonists, and metoclopramide are suitable options. Rapid sequence induction with cricoid pressure should be considered in patients with gastroparesis.

Careful evaluation of the airway is necessary in pancreas transplant recipients. As discussed earlier, patients with long-standing Type 1 diabetes have an increased incidence of intubation difficulty. The inability to oppose palms due to stiffness of the interphalangeal joints is predictive of difficult tracheal intubation.[29,89]

INTRAOPERATIVE CARE

General anesthesia is induced with agents appropriate for the patient's baseline medical condition followed by orotracheal intubation. A combination of anesthetic drugs is used to maintain general anesthesia.

TABLE 59-3 Inclusion Criteria for Cadaveric Pancreas Donors

10-50 years old
Ideally, death from trauma rather than intracerebral hemorrhage
Hemodynamic stability
No diabetes
No alcohol abuse
No hypertension
Normal renal function
No sepsis, hepatitis B surface antigen negativity, hepatitis C negativity, human immunodeficiency virus negativity
No malignancy
Donor surgeon macroscopic assessment for normalcy

TABLE 59-4 Preoperative Assessment for Pancreas Transplantation Recipients

Routine	Specific
Medications	End-stage renal disease
Allergies	Cardiomyopathy
History of smoking	Ischemic heart disease
Other	Hypertension
	Stroke/TIA
	Autonomic nervous system dysfunction:
	Neuropathy
	Gastroparesis
	Orthostatic hypotension
	Airway

In patients with renal dysfunction, isoflurane and desflurane appear to be virtually devoid of nephrotoxicity. As described earlier in the discussion on kidney transplantation, one may choose among the opioids fentanyl, sufentanil, alfentanil, and remifentanil if renal disease is present. Morphine and meperidine are best avoided for the reasons enumerated earlier. At our institution, fentanyl is the opioid of choice; it is also associated with minimal hemodynamic alterations. The choice of muscle relaxant should take into account the degree of renal impairment. Thus patients who are on dialysis should not receive pancuronium (see discussion on kidney transplantation); vecuronium and rocuronium are eliminated by both the hepatic and renal routes and may be used in those with chronic renal disease if neuromuscular junction monitoring (eg, train-of-four response) is used to guide repeat dosing after an initial bolus dose has been administered. At our institution, *cis*-atracurium is used most commonly because it is cleared by Hoffmann elimination rather than hepatic or renal function. In addition to standard anesthetic monitors, patients receiving a pancreas transplant need central venous access, which is useful in the assessment of intravascular volume status, to provide access for possible pressor support, immunosuppressive drugs, and as a means for frequent intraoperative blood sampling. In patients with significant cardiovascular disease, direct arterial pressure monitoring, and right heart monitoring with a pulmonary artery catheter and/or transesophageal echocardiography are available monitoring options to assist during surgery.[90]

Blood glucose levels must be checked at least hourly or more frequently during general anesthesia with the goal of keeping serum glucose levels between 100 and 150 mg/dL.[90] Animal studies have shown hyperglycemia to cause islet cell dysfunction.[91] Maintaining serum glucose levels in an acceptable range is accomplished by continuous infusion of regular insulin at a rate of 1 to 5 U/h with concurrent dextrose infusion when blood glucose levels are below 150 mg/dL (**Table 59-5**). The addition of dextrose ensures uninterrupted intracellular nutrition to avoid intraoperative ketosis.

Pancreatic beta cells can start releasing insulin as early as 5 minutes after reperfusion.[92] Delayed graft function may be treated postoperatively with an insulin infusion titrated to keep blood glucose levels less than 150 mg/dL.[93] Somatostatin may be administered to decrease pancreatic enzyme secretion.[94]

To ensure adequate perfusion and prevent hypotension upon allograft reperfusion, the patient's hemodynamic status must be optimal prior to release of the vascular clamps. Administration of intravenous fluids, either crystalloid or colloid, to achieve a CVP in the 12 to 14 mm Hg range and a systolic blood pressure of at least 140 mm Hg is recommended in patients without significant heart disease.[58] Alternatively, in those with a pulmonary artery catheter, careful titration of volume versus filling pressures and cardiac output can be used to optimize intravascular fluid status prior to vascular unclamping. In preparation for unclamping, potent inhalational agents may need to be reduced. Hypotension at unclamping may require administration of fluids, the use of pressors, and blood products as appropriate. It is important to maintain perfusion pressure and blood flow to the new allograft. Hetastarch is often preferred as a colloid in those who have functioning kidneys, as it not only improves preload but also improves graft vessel flow. This prevents graft vessel thrombosis, the most common cause of technical pancreatic graft failure.[57] The goals of successful intraoperative care are cardiovascular stability, maintaining graft perfusion pressure with mean arterial pressure (MAP) of greater than 70 mm Hg, metabolic control, normothermia, and electrolyte homeostasis.

Most patients can be extubated in the operating room after surgery provided they meet extubation criteria, that is, they are alert, normothermic, have recovered from neuromuscular blockade, and are hemodynamically stable. When the patient arrives in the postanesthesia care unit, blood glucose, hemoglobin, electrolytes, and troponin levels should be checked. Dehydration, electrolyte, and acid-base disorders, and hypoglycemia or hyperglycemia can develop quickly in the postoperative period. Patients with a bladder anastomosis may get dehydrated and develop frequent infections and often require supplemental sodium bicarbonate to treat the metabolic acidosis caused by the loss of pancreatic secretions into the bladder.[77,79,81,93,94] In our institution all diabetic patients undergoing solid-organ transplant are assessed for myocardial infarction (MI) with serial troponins and electrocardiogram (ECG) due to the incidence of silent MI in this patient population. Postoperatively, patients receive 5% dextrose in 0.45 N saline as maintenance fluid. Nasogastric and urine output losses are replaced in equivalent amounts with 0.45 N saline.

TABLE 59-5 Insulin and Dextrose Infusion Guidelines for Pancreas Recipients

Blood Glucose Concentration (mg/dL)	Insulin Infusion (U/h)	Dextrose[a] (mL/h)
>350	3-5 (after a bolus of 4 U)	0
250-350	2 (after a bolus of 3 U)	0
150-250	2 (after a bolus of 2 U)	0
100-150	2	20
70-100	1-2	20-100
<70	0	100

[a]As 5% dextrose in water with half normal saline.

IMMUNOSUPPRESSION

Pancreas transplant recipients have a higher incidence of acute rejection and immunologic graft loss than transplant recipients of any other solid organ. There were 4 main agents of initial maintenance immunosuppression from 1996 to 2002 for US cadaveric primary pancreas transplants: azathioprine, cyclosporine, mycophenolate mofetil, and tacrolimus. Sirolimus was also used.[57,95] In recent years in the United States, the most common induction protocol uses antithymocyte globulin, alemtuzumab, or interleukin-2 receptor antibody followed by tacrolimus, mycophenolate mofetil, and steroids.[54]

Pancreas transplant recipients are at risk of developing infection for numerous reasons, including immunosuppression, contamination from the duodenal segment of the graft, and blood glucose irregularity due to diabetes.[93] Infection prophylaxis with broad-spectrum antibiotics for community-prevalent bacterial infections, antivirals for CMV, and antifungals is routine in many centers.[77,83,94] Prophylaxis against vascular thrombosis consists of either low-dose intravenous heparin (300-500 U/h) or subcutaneous heparin followed by aspirin.[77,83]

ISLET CELL TRANSPLANTATION

The transplantation of pancreatic islet cells is a developing alternative treatment of diabetes mellitus. In 2000 Shapiro et al reported 7 patients who were rendered insulin independent after islet cell transplantation.[96] Recent reports suggest that 72% of recipients become insulin independent.[97] Further, an increasing number of recipients can become insulin independent with cells from a single donor.[98] Major drawbacks of islet cell transplantation are related to logistical problems of setting up an infrastructure to perform islet isolation on a large scale.[99,100] Advances in immunosuppression and isolation techniques have been shown to improve outcomes with islet cell transplantation.[101] Similarly, it has been found that recipients with a low body mass index (BMI) have a higher success rate with islet cell transplantation when the islets are obtained from a donor with a high BMI because of a higher yield of islets.[102] In spite of numerous advancements, islet cell transplantation is still hampered with lack of durability, and approximately 50% of patients require insulin treatment within 2 years.[103]

Islet isolation requires special processing of pancreas tissue to yield a maximum number of islets available for transplantation.[104] Pancreatic islet cell preparations with greater than 5000 islet equivalents and a volume of less than 5 to 10 mL are generally acceptable for transplant after proper dilution in Connaugh Medical Research Laboratories (CMRL) media supplemented with albumin or Hetastarch and heparin.[105,106] These harvested islet cells can be transplanted in diabetic recipients using local anesthesia and sedation.[107] At our institution we commonly use a mixture of propofol plus ketamine (1 mg of ketamine per 10 mg of propofol) and titrate to a level that provides sedation plus analgesia with spontaneous breathing and supplemental oxygen by nasal cannula. If required, one may also consider adding a low-dose infusion of dexmedetomidine (0.2-0.5 mcg/kg/h). For the surgical procedure, a cannula is placed either percutaneously directly into the portal vein via the liver or via a mini-laparotomy into a mesenteric vein draining into the portal vein. After final catheter position is confirmed (by ultrasound and fluoroscopy when the percutaneous approach is used), the portal vein pressure is measured and the islets are infused by gravity over 20 to 60 minutes.[108] Portal pressures are measured every 15 minutes to monitor for acute portal hypertension that commonly occurs if the islets are transfused rapidly. After the islets are transplanted, before removal of the percutaneously placed portal vein infusion catheter, heparin is administered directly into the portal vein.[106,107] As the infusion catheter is removed, thrombin-soaked gelfoam is embolized into the peripheral hepatic parenchymal catheter tract.[107,109]

Complications of islet cell transplant include posttransplant hemorrhage (requiring transfusion), intraparenchymal hemorrhage, subcapsular hemorrhage, portal vein thrombosis, hemothorax, pneumothorax, hemobilia, and inadvertent puncture of the neighboring structures.[107] Some patients require more than 1 islet transplant to achieve insulin independence.[109]

Due to a limited supply of islet cells, research has explored other possible sources of beta cells. Progress has been made with stem-cell biology, transdifferentiation, and xenotransplants, and there is evidence that beta-cell regeneration within the pancreas is possible.[110]

OUTCOME FOLLOWING TRANSPLANTATION

Analysis of the results reported in the International Pancreas Transplant Registry (IPTR) indicates that following transplantation, long-term insulin independence has improved over time.[57] The patient survival rates for all 3 categories (simultaneous pancreas-kidney, pancreas-after-kidney, pancreas transplant only) are over 90% at 3 years posttransplant.[57] Most deaths occur as a result of cardiovascular disease. Pancreas graft survival rates are better with simultaneous pancreas-kidney (85% vs 79% for pancreas-after-kidney, vs 77% for pancreas transplant only) transplantation. Chronic rejection continues to be a major challenge.[111]

CONCLUSIONS

Pancreas transplantation is now an established procedure for the surgical treatment of diabetes mellitus. It is most commonly done simultaneously during kidney transplantation because the patients will already be receiving immunosuppression, and individual graft survival is improved when both organs are transplanted. Islet cell transplantation will no doubt be the procedure of choice once it becomes a more routine procedure because of the minimal surgery involved. The perioperative care of patients for pancreas transplantation involves understanding the goals of the procedure and the pathophysiology of diabetes mellitus and renal failure.

HEMATOPOIETIC AND STEM CELL TRANSPLANTATION

INTRODUCTION

Anesthesia providers may encounter patients who have an illness requiring hematopoietic stem cell transplantation (HSCT), who are being prepared for HSCT, or who have undergone prior HSCT and are encountered because of a complication. The success of HSCT was recognized as early as 1968[112] when a 2-year-old boy with severe Wiskott-Aldrich syndrome was successfully treated with bone-marrow cells provided from his histocompatible, healthy sister, and he has been followed up for 15 years.[113] HSCT has since become quite popular for patients with severe combined immunodeficiency[114] and also many other diseases. Autologous HSCT as rescue therapy for the bone marrow is usually done following chemotherapy to treat malignancy (**Table 59-6**).[115] Hematopoietic stem cells (HSCs) may be used for autologous, syngeneic, and allogenic transplantation. Autologous HSCT involves stem cell transplant with the patient's own HSCs, whereas allogenic transplantation involves HSCs from another human; transplantation between genetically identical members of the same species is referred to as syngeneic transplantation (eg, identical twins). The most common source of HSCs is bone marrow harvest, and another is the peripheral blood compartment; mobilization protocols are often used to increase the efficiency of this source. Umbilical cord blood is another source of HSCs and has become a popular marrow source for both adults and pediatric patients.[116] There is minimal risk of viral exposure with cord blood, and the donor is not placed at risk. In addition, the incidence of graft versus host disease is markedly lower than that for standard bone marrow or peripheral stem cell transplants.[117] Although the death rate from graft failure, infection, and graft versus host disease is still high (approximately 40%), the success rate has improved over time

TABLE 59-6 Distribution of Diseases for Which HSCT Was Performed[a]

Disease	Allogeneic Transplants[b]	Autologous Transplants[c]
Acute lymphoblastic leukemia	27059	1549
Acute myelogenous leukemia	42594	7552
Chronic myelogenous leukemia	26996	730
Chronic lymphocytic leukemia	3067	607
Non-Hodgkin lymphoma	10650	37565
Hodgkin disease	1182	15733
Plasma cell disorders	3100	34791
Myelodysplastic syndromes	12871	251
Severe aplastic anemia	10143	17
Inherited erythrocyte abnormalities	4865	4
SCID and other immunodeficiencies	3768	6
Other leukemia	2085	394
Inherited disorders of metabolism	1884	4
Malignancies[d]	2497	36137
Nonmalignancies	380	333
Autoimmune diseases	69	388
Total	**153210**	**136061**

HSCT, hematopoietic stem cell transplantation.

[a]As reported in the Center for International Blood & Marrow Transplant Research (progress report January-December 2009 (http://www.cibmtr.org/).

[b]Since 1970.

[c]Since 1989.

[d]Malignancies include breast, ovarian, testicular, lung cancer, neuroblastoma, melanoma, sarcoma, Ewing sarcoma, Wilm tumor, medulloblastoma, germ-cell tumor, brain tumors, histiocytic disorders, and others.

with advances in immunosuppression, chemotherapy, antibiotics, and supportive care.[118] The number of children receiving HSCTs for various disorders is increasing approximately 10% to 15% per year[119] and has reached a steady number of between 4000 and 4500 per year.[120]

INDICATIONS FOR HSC TRANSPLANTATION

In a recent review, Gratwohl et al reported that 50 417 first HSCTs were performed globally (**Fig. 59-6**) in 2006 with the most frequent malignant disease being acute myeloid leukemia and the most frequent nonmalignant disease being bone marrow failure syndrome. A plasma cell disorder was the most frequent indication for an autologous HSCT.[120] HSC transplantation is also done to treat a variety of hematologic, metabolic, genetic, and oncologic disorders in adult and pediatric patients.[121-123] Table 59-6 is a summary of the annual report by the Center for International Blood and Marrow Transplant Research (CIBMTR; http://www.cibmtr.org/) that lists the diseases for which HSCT was performed. Most HSCTs are done for either acute or chronic myeloid leukemia, followed by acute lymphoblastic leukemia, myelodysplastic leukemia, and non-Hodgkin lymphoma. HSCT is also done for a variety of metabolic disorders and inborn errors of metabolism. Most recently, HSCT has also had initial success as definitive treatment for children with epidermolysis bullosa dystrophica.

PRECONDITIONING, ASSOCIATED RISKS, AND COMPLICATIONS

Adults and children who receive HSCT are at risk for complications.[124] Thus they may develop respiratory failure or acute graft versus host disease.[124,125] Acute graft versus host disease is the most important complication that significantly influences clinical outcome.

Almost all patients who receive HSCT undergo total body irradiation and/or myeloablative preconditioning to eradicate malignant disease if present, to suppress the recipients' immune system (to decrease the chance for graft rejection), and to create space in the bone marrow microenvironment to allow donor stem cell engraftment.[126] This predisposes them to hemorrhagic and infection risks as noted by Bacigalupo and others (**Figs. 59-7 and 59-8**).[125] Infection risks occur from the secondary immunodeficiency and neutropenia. Because neutropenia ensues as a result of the preparatory regimen prior to HSCT and lasts until full engraftment of transplanted stem cells occurs, patients are at risk for infection. This is another cause of morbidity and mortality for several weeks. T- and B-cell function may also be depressed for several months following bone marrow transplantation and cause recipients to be susceptible to viral and fungal infections.[118,127] Some patients may also require help from the anesthesia pain service due to calcineurin-inhibitor (tacrolimus)–induced pain syndrome after bone marrow transplantation.[128,129]

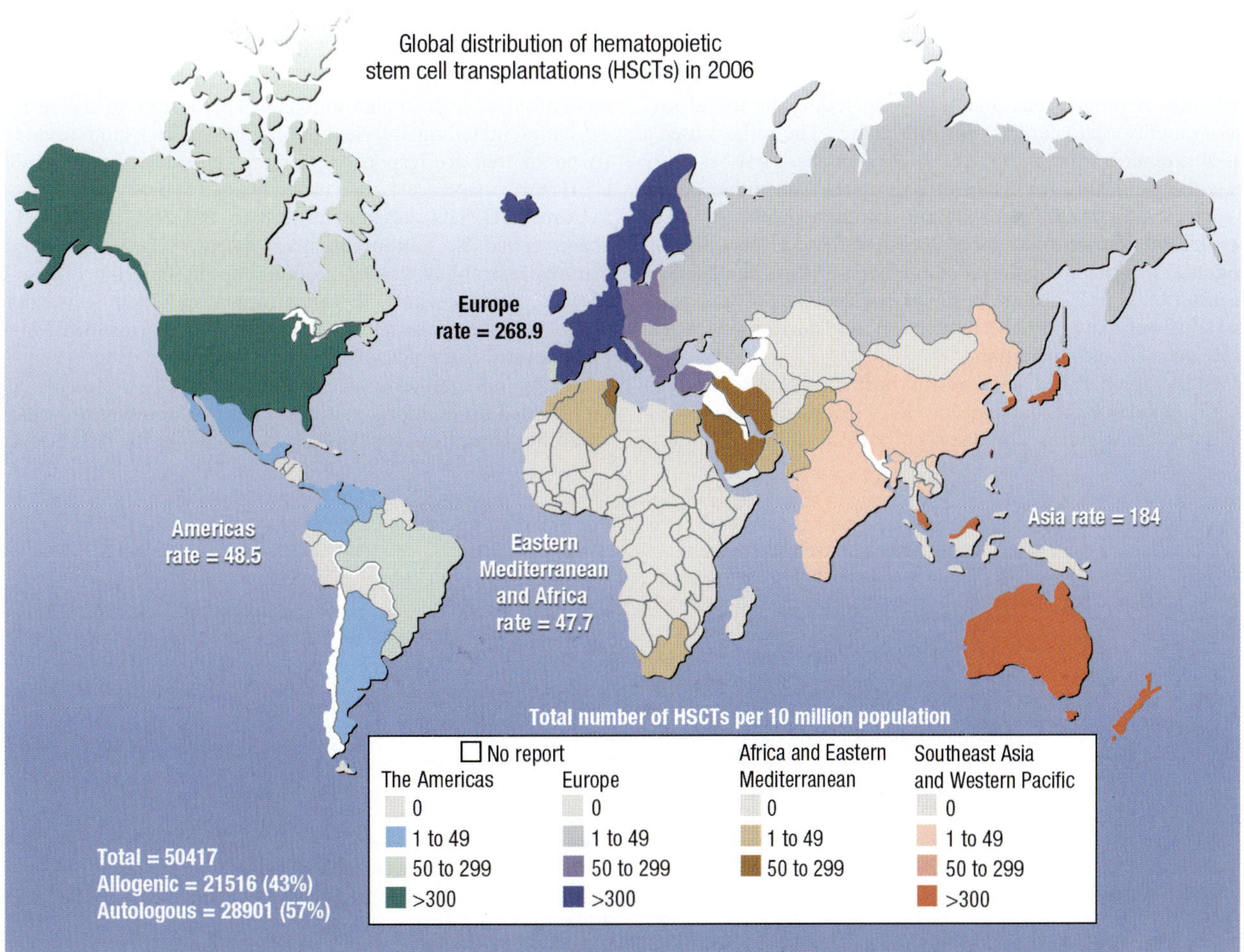

FIGURE 59-6. Hematopoietic stem cell transplantation (HSCT) is performed in many countries. The above figure provides data for different continents. The rate is the median value per 10 million people. No HSCTs were performed in countries with fewer than 300 000 inhabitants, that are smaller than 960 km^2, or that have a gross national per capita income less than US$680. [From Gratwohl A, Baldomero H, Aljurf M, et al. Hematopoietic stem cell transplantation: a global perspective. *JAMA*. 2010;303:1617-1624.]

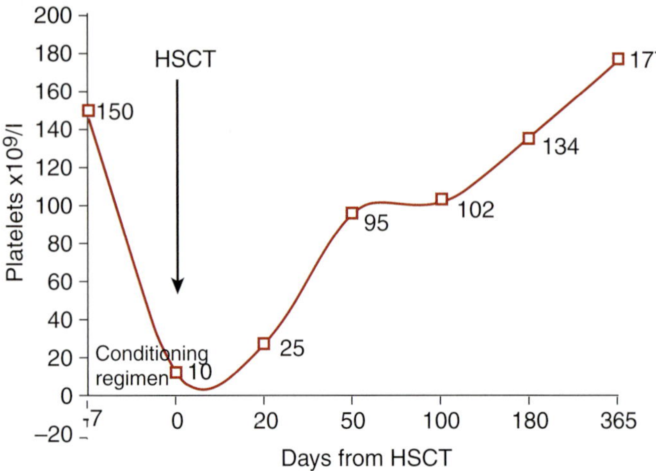

FIGURE 59-7. Prior to hematopoietic stem cell transplantation (HSCT), patients undergo preparation with myeloablative therapy. This results in significant thrombocytopenia predisposing them to hemorrhagic diathesis. At day 100 following HSCT, the platelet count stabilizes to clinically acceptable values. Because of this, HSCT recipients will often require blood and blood products perioperatively. [From Bacigalupo A. Haemopoietic stem cell transplants: the impact of haemorrhagic complications. *Blood Rev.* 2003;17(Suppl 1):S6-S10.]

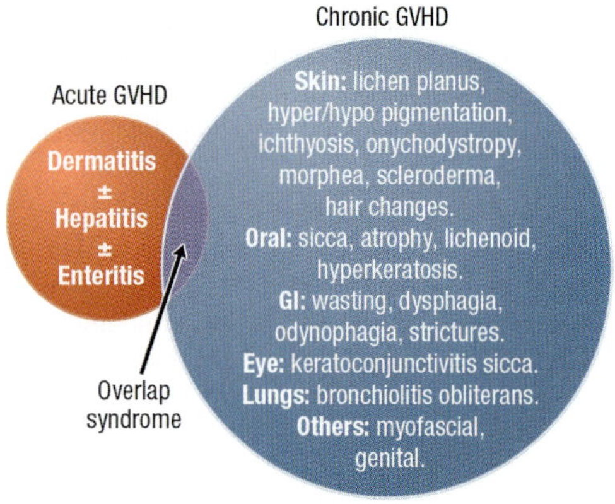

Chronic GVHD
Acute GVHD
Dermatitis ± Hepatitis ± Enteritis
Skin: lichen planus, hyper/hypo pigmentation, ichthyosis, onychodystropy, morphea, scleroderma, hair changes. Oral: sicca, atrophy, lichenoid, hyperkeratosis. GI: wasting, dysphagia, odynophagia, strictures. Eye: keratoconjunctivitis sicca. Lungs: bronchiolitis obliterans. Others: myofascial, genital.
Overlap syndrome

FIGURE 59-9. Acute GVHD (graft versus host disease) typically manifests as presence of a skin rash, nausea, vomiting and diarrhea, and elevation in liver enzymes, whereas chronic GVHD resembles an autoimmune phenomenon, involving multiple organs such as the skin, with lichen planus–like or sclerodermoid changes. Recently the National Institutes of Health consensus conference addressed several issues pertaining to the diagnosis and staging of chronic GVHD and published its guidelines, and defined a third syndrome known as overlap syndrome where features of both acute and chronic GVHD coexist. [Courtesy of Dr Mukta Arora, Department of Medicine, University of Minnesota.]

Total body irradiation as part of the HSCT preparation protocol may cause pneumonitis, restrictive cardiomyopathy, pulmonary fibrosis, and oral mucositis. Oral mucositis can be extremely painful and in addition to opioids may require special oral swishes including the use of ketamine as a mouthwash to control mucositis pain.[130] The authors used a solution of ketamine (20 mg/5 mL) for oral mouthwash swishes every 4 hours with significant oral mucositis pain relief. Chemotherapeutic agents such as adriamycin can result in cardiomyopathy or other toxicities. In addition, veno-occlusive disease of the liver may develop following intensive chemo- and irradiation therapy. This complication, which is most often fatal, occurs approximately 2 weeks posttransplant when the small hepatic venules become fibrotic and develop pericentral hepatocyte necrosis and congestion.[131]

Another condition called graft versus host disease (GVHD) can significantly influence the outcome of HSCT recipients (**Fig. 59-9**). GVHD starts off as an acute disorder but sometimes manifests as chronic GVHD. Acute GVHD may be mild or life threatening (**Table 59-7**).[132] In GVHD, immunologically competent donor T cells transplanted in the recipient react against host tissue cells that are recognized as host-foreign antigens. This results in the secretion of cytokines including interleukin-1, interleukin-2, and tumor necrosis factor that are responsible for the signs and symptoms of acute GVHD.[132]

Chronic GVHD develops more than 100 days after HSCT and is characterized by multiorgan involvement.[132] Patients present with features resembling naturally occurring autoimmune disease due to chronic cytokine effect, thymic atrophy, and lymphocyte depletion. Thus they may present with scleroderma, oral mucositis, interstitial pneumonitis, and polymyositis.[118,133-135]

During preanesthesia assessment for HSCT, recipients must be investigated for multiorgan involvement.[136] **Noninfectious pulmonary and other complications typically occur before the first 100 days fol-**

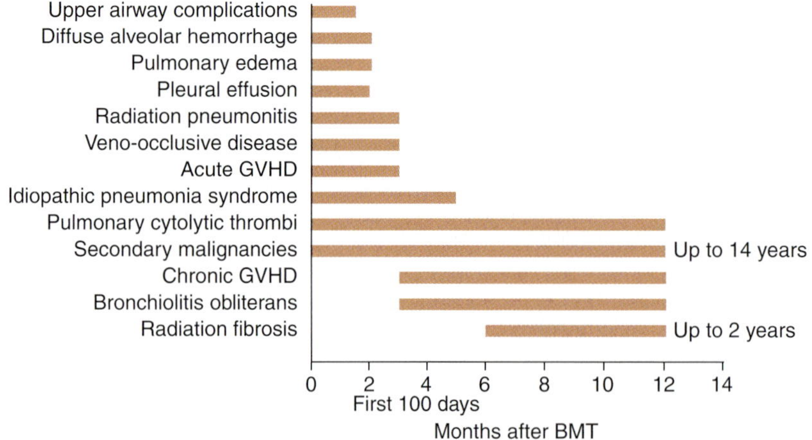

FIGURE 59-8. Upper airway and other nonpulmonary complications following hematopoietic stem cell transplantation. Note that most acute problems occur in the first 100 days following transplantation. [From Khurshid I, Anderson LC. Non-infectious pulmonary complications after bone marrow transplantation. *Postgrad Med J.* 2002;78:257-262.]

TABLE 59-7 Acute GVHD (Graft Versus Host Disease)—Clinical Grading

Overall Grade	Skin	Liver	Gut	Functional Impairment
0 (none)	0	0	0	0
1 (mild)	+ to ++	0	0	0
2 (moderate)	+ to +++	+	+	+
3 (severe)	+ to +++	+ to +++	+ to +++	++
4 (life threatening)	+ to ++++	+ to ++++	+ to ++++	+++

From Flowers ME, Kansu E, Sullivan KM. Pathophysiology and treatment of graft-versus-host disease. *Hematol Oncol Clin North Am.* 1999;13:1091-1112, viii-ix.

lowing HSCT (see Fig. 59-8).[137] **Thus HSCT recipients are at risk for airway complications during the first 2 months of transplantation.**

ANESTHESIA CONSIDERATIONS

Before receiving a bone marrow transplant, pediatric (and some adult) patients often require anesthesia for permanent central venous catheterization, biopsies, and total body irradiation. Following transplantation these same individuals often need anesthesia for (1) biopsies to evaluate the status of the bone marrow transplant and determine if GVHD has developed and (2) treatment of the surgical complications that may follow this procedure. Most patients undergoing HSCT tolerate anesthesia for these procedures without difficulty. However, complications can occur, particularly in those recipients less than 2 years of age. In these individuals, anesthesia providers must keep in mind the unique medical problems associated with children undergoing bone marrow transplantation.[118,127] **Children with inborn errors of metabolism may also require anesthesia for several procedures related to HSCT and may be anesthetic challenges because of their primary disease.**[138] **Thus some patients with metabolic disease may be difficult to intubate.** In addition, mucositis and upper airway edema can complicate anesthesia care. When endotracheal intubation is required either for complications related to HSCT or for anesthesia needs, the airway care must be provided in an environment equipped to handle a patient with a difficult airway. Clinical judgment also needs to be exercised to determine whether an otolaryngologist skilled in pediatric and adult upper airway care needs to be present during anesthesia induction and/or sedation and intubation, and for extubation in some instances.

Radiation and/or chemotherapy and GVHD can result in nausea and vomiting. Tracheal intubation and airway protection may therefore be required in some patients.

ANESTHETIC MANAGEMENT

There are a variety of anesthetic techniques that can safely be used to anesthetize children and adults receiving care for HSCT. No drug, agent, or technique is absolutely contraindicated.[118,135] Nitrous oxide suppresses methionine synthetase, and other anesthetics are myelosuppressive but are not contraindicated during anesthesia care.[139-141]

The concern that is unique to bone marrow recipients is the high incidence and potential morbidity from mucositis that occurs when patients are neutropenic. Pediatric anesthesia care providers must minimize airway manipulation if possible, and thus intravenous propofol has proved useful for sedation for total body irradiation using spontaneous ventilation without airway instrumentation. It is the preferred drug because of its rapid recovery and antiemetic profile. This allows earlier feeding and better nutrition in infants undergoing radiation therapy than other intravenous agents such as ketamine or thiopental.[118] Even in children with Hurler syndrome, proper neck and head positioning can allow safe propofol sedation, but in some instances the laryngeal mask airway has been used. Because of potential injury it must be used with caution in cases of mucositis.[142] When tracheal intubation is required for airway care, the preoperative airway examination may be difficult due to severe pain.[143] For the same reason, awake intubation may be impossible as well. Movement and struggling during the procedure may cause bleeding and edema, and obscure the laryngeal inlet. Therefore, one may have to resort to a rapid sequence induction technique to minimize the time with an unprotected airway while providing as optimal conditions as possible for rapid endotracheal intubation. However, when stridor or other signs of airway obstruction are evident, an inhaled induction of general anesthesia with sevoflurane and oxygen similar to that used in a child with epiglottitis may be required. In such patients, anesthesia providers must be prepared with adequate suction and several tracheal tube sizes because the laryngeal inlet may be narrowed due to edema and inflammation.[118]

Care must be taken with extubation as well. Most patients with mucositis can be extubated when fully awake. Often these patients develop croup in the postoperative period and may require treatment with dexamethasone (0.5-1 mg/kg) and 1 or more courses of racemic epinephrine. However, patients with mucositis and severe edema of the laryngeal inlet may require prolonged intubation until the edema resolves.[118]

Children may also require procedural sedation for follow-up after HSCT. In a recent study the authors found that a combination of propofol/ketamine was better than propofol/alfentanil to provide deep procedural sedation for lumbar puncture in children with acute lymphoblastic leukemia.[144] The use of ketamine instead of alfentanil prevented the need for respiratory assistance because respiratory depression was noted with alfentanil when used with propofol.

CONCLUSIONS

For the successful care of patients requiring HSCT, the anesthesia practitioner must be aware of the unique problems that accompany the process of patient preparation and those related to myeloablative therapy. Most acute problems occur in the first 100 days following transplantation. Children may require HSCT for metabolic diseases including some inborn errors of metabolism. The primary disease can be challenging for anesthesia providers. The outcome of HSCT depends on the indication and also the severity of the disease prior to HSCT.

SMALL BOWEL TRANSPLANTATION

HISTORY AND INTRODUCTION

Lillehei et al performed the first transplant of a small bowel in humans at the University of Minnesota when they performed a graft of the stomach, small bowel, and pancreas in a patient with a mesenteric venous thrombosis.[145] Further attempts were made over the years, but all were unsuccessful due to a very high mortality from uncontrolled graft rejection and patient sepsis. Grant et al reported the first long-term survivor from combined small bowel-liver graft using cyclosporine-based immunosuppression in 1990.[146] It was not until the introduction of tacrolimus for immunosuppression in 1991 that outcomes improved.[147]

The number of patients undergoing intestinal transplantation is still rather modest. For example, in 2009 only 180 patients underwent intestinal transplantation.[2] Graft survival rates by the end of 2008 were 86% at 1 year and 61% at 5 years.[2] These outcomes are markedly improved from earlier reports, and single centers have reported survival rates of 92% at 1 year and 70% at 5 years when antilymphoid pretreatment immunosuppressive strategies were used.[148] Living related bowel transplantation is also being developed.[149] The progress in the field of intestinal transplant is especially important due to the high mortality of patients on transplant lists (20%).[150]

INDICATIONS

The primary reason for intestinal transplant is intestinal failure, which is defined by the inability to maintain nutrition, fluid and electrolyte balance, or normal growth and development of the body. Conditions that lead to intestinal failure differ between children and adults (**Table 59-8**). In children gastroschisis, necrotizing enterocolitis, intestinal atresia, midgut volvulus, aganglionosis, and pseudoobstruction are most frequent. In adults ischemia, inflammatory bowel disease, volvulus, tumors, and trauma are most prevalent.[151] The Center for Medicare and Medicaid accepts the following indications for intestinal transplant when liver failure/injury due to parenteral nutrition has occurred: thrombosis of 2 or more central veins, 2 or more episodes of catheter-related sepsis or 1 episode of fungemia, septic shock ,or ARDS, and dehydration despite adequate fluid supplementation.

TABLE 59-8 Leading Causes of Intestinal Failure in Children and Adults

Children	Adults
Intestinal atresia	Crohn disease
Gastroschisis	Superior mesenteric artery disease
Crohn disease	Superior mesenteric vein thrombosis
Microvillus involution disease	Trauma
Necrotizing enterocolitis	Desmoid tumor
Midgut volvulus	Volvulus
Chronic intestinal pseudoobstruction	Pseudoobstruction
Massive resection secondary to tumor	Massive resection secondary to tumor
Hirschsprung disease	Radiation enteritis

Data from Greenstein SM, Friedmann JC, Prowse O. Intestinal transplantation. Available at: http://emedicine.medscape.com. Updated January 14, 2009. Accessed July 3, 2010.

SURGICAL PROCEDURE

Isolated Intestinal Transplantation Isolated intestinal transplantation is recommended for patients with irreversible intestinal failure without liver failure.[152] **Figure 59-10** demonstrates the isolated bowel transplant. Vascular continuity is established between the superior mesenteric artery bowel graft and the aorta, and superior mesenteric vein of the graft and the recipient vena cava.

Combined Liver and Small Bowel Transplant The presence of cirrhosis or advanced bridging fibrosis of liver is a well-known complication of total parenteral nutrition. For patients with irreversible intestinal failure and end-stage liver disease, a combined small bowel–liver transplant is

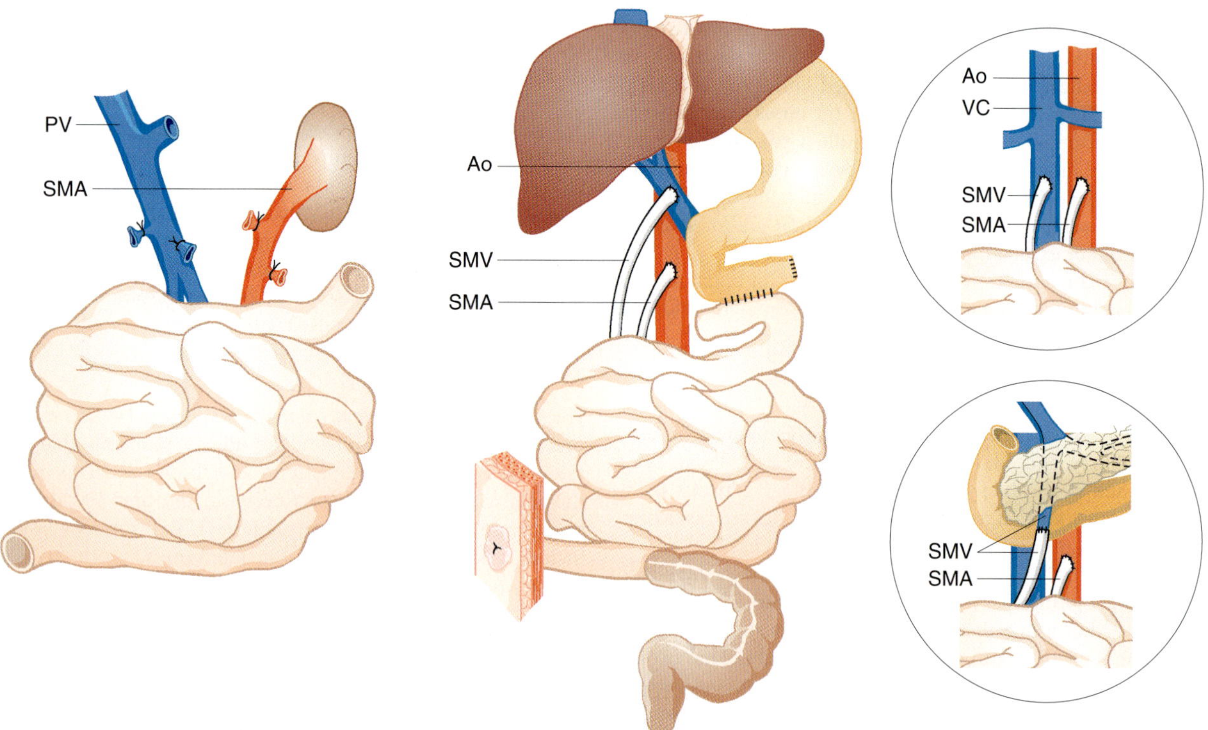

FIGURE 59-10. Isolated intestinal transplantation. This is the simplest form of intestinal transplantation. Ao, aorta; PV, pulmonary vein; SMA, superior mesenteric artery; SMV, superior mesenteric vein; VC, vena cava.

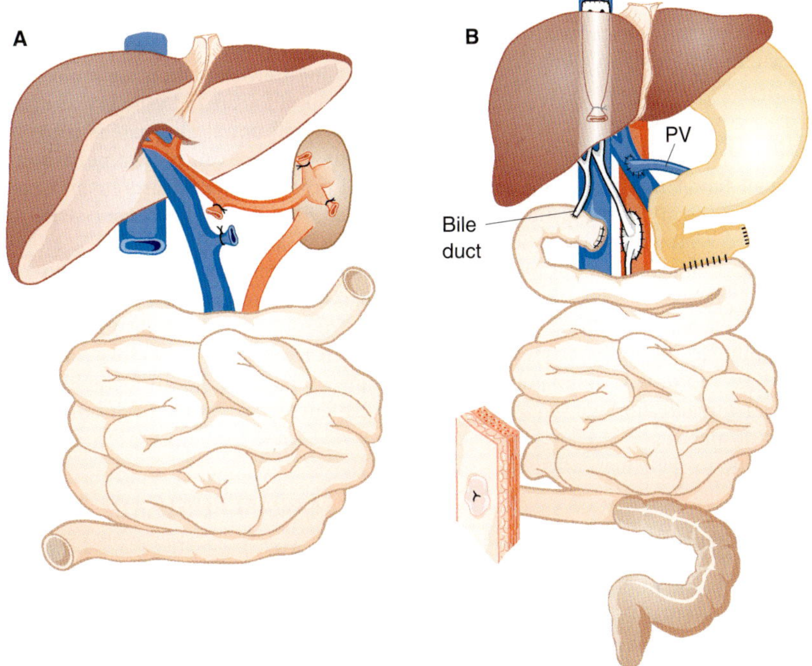

FIGURE 59-11. Liver–intestine en bloc graft. **A.** Graft. **B.** Graft after implantation. PV, pulmonary vein.

the recommended treatment.[152] In a combined liver-bowel transplant, the liver and bowel can each be transplanted separately. This is the method used if a living related combined liver-bowel transplant is performed. In certain circumstances en bloc combined liver-bowel transplants may be performed (**Fig. 59-11**).

Multivisceral Transplantation At the 2007 International Small Bowel Transplantation Symposium, a more descriptive anatomic nomenclature was proposed for multivisceral transplant. The procedure is performed in patients with debilitating trauma, massive resections, multiple surgeries with short-gut syndrome, dysmotility disorder, extensive mesenteric vascular thrombosis, multiple enterocutaneous fistulas, and irresectable tumor.[151] Complete evisceration of the native foregut and midgut followed by en bloc transplant of the stomach, pancreaticoduodenal complex, liver, and small bowel or different modifications of surgery are possible (**Fig. 59-12**).

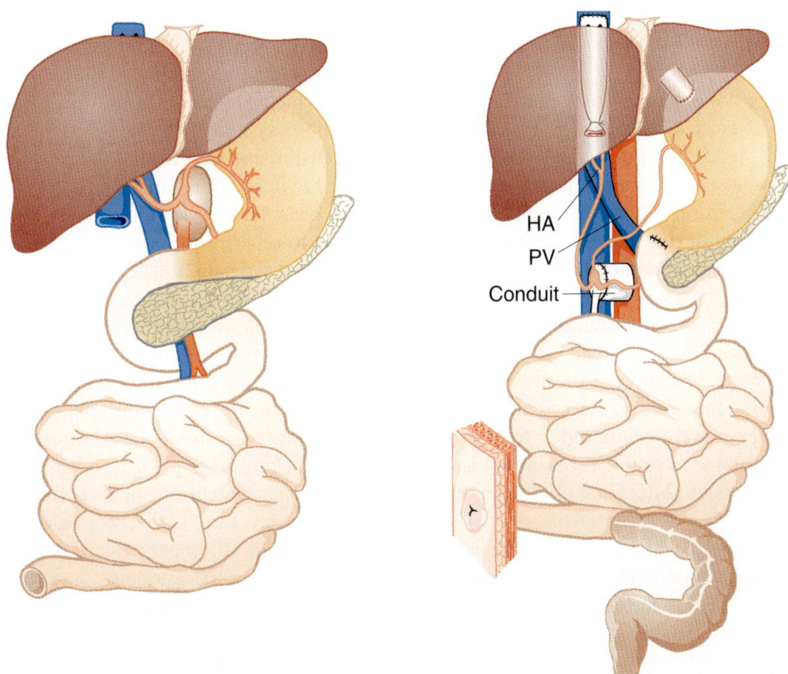

FIGURE 59-12. Multivisceral transplantation. Multivisceral transplantation involves en bloc transplantation of the stomach, pancreas, liver, and intestine. HA, hepatic artery; PV, pulmonary vein.

Living related intestinal transplantation is an option entertained especially in countries where the availability of cadaveric organs is limited. It has so far been successfully performed in a limited number of patients.[153]

PREOPERATIVE CONSIDERATIONS

Patients being considered for small bowel transplantation require a thorough evaluation of each organ system. If the patient is over 40 years of age or has a history of cardiac disease, tests such as an echocardiogram, dobutamine stress test, or assessment of the coronaries by angiography may be required. The patient's liver function must be evaluated because most patients have been on chronic intravenous hyperalimentation, which is hepatotoxic. Electrolyte and acid-base imbalance is common due to diarrhea and/or dehydration and should be checked preoperatively. Some patients with short gut syndrome have lost their intestines from vascular thrombosis. Therefore, a thorough investigation of the coagulation status of patients undergoing small bowel transplantation is required.[154]

EVALUATION OF PATENCY OF CENTRAL VESSELS

Due to the high incidence of venous thrombosis in patients on long-term hyperalimentation, it is recommended that all patients referred for intestinal transplantation undergo preliminary mapping of their venous access by Doppler ultrasound, and patients with multiple thrombosed vessels should be considered for additional angiographic evaluation.[155]

ANESTHETIC MANAGEMENT

Induction and Maintenance of Anesthesia Often patients presenting for bowel transplantation have delayed gastric emptying. Therefore, a rapid sequence induction of general anesthesia is indicated. In many instances, this may require intravenous induction of general anesthesia with attention to hemodynamic stability. Maintenance of general anesthesia is similar to that for liver or renal transplantation. Balanced anesthesia using desflurane or isoflurane for the potent inhaled agent along with opioids (fentanyl, sufentanil) and muscle relaxants (vecuronium, *cis*-atracurium, rocuronium) is commonly used.[154] Because many of these patients have impaired renal function, muscle relaxants such as pancuronium that are dependent on renal elimination are not utilized. Similarly, sevoflurane is generally not utilized because its safety in patients with impaired renal function has not been established.[25]

Small bowel transplantation is a long surgical procedure that can take up to 17 hours.[152] It can be associated with large fluid shifts due to abdominal manipulation and significant intraoperative bleeding, dehydration, vascular clamping, long ischemia times, visceral exposure, and lymphatic interruption.[156] Therefore, adequate vascular access must be established. **A rapid infusion device is often beneficial and should be available, and blood-salvaging devices should be used.** Frequent (hourly) determinations of laboratory values such as arterial blood gases, electrolytes, lactate levels, hemoglobin and platelet levels, and clotting studies are often necessary.[157] These patients can also be hypothermic due to the long, extensive dissection in the abdomen and exposure of the bowel to ambient temperature. **Forced air surface warming and application of other newer technologies to preserve core temperature are extremely valuable to prevent significant hypothermia in patients undergoing extensive abdominal operations such as bowel transplantation.**[158]

When bowel transplant surgery is completed it is rare that the patient can be extubated in the recovery room. Often patients require positive pressure ventilation for a period equivalent to the duration of surgery or longer because the edematous graft placed in the small abdominal cavity limits the descent of the diaphragm. Positive pressure ventilation may be needed until the edema resolves and the abdominal cavity stretches to accommodate the new bowel.[159] The peripheral edema also resolves after several days postoperatively.[156]

MONITORING

All patients need a large-bore central venous catheter placed prior to beginning transplantation for rapid volume administration and measurement of the central venous pressure. **Because the venous drainage of the small bowel allograft is into the vena cava, elevated central venous pressure can reduce perfusion of the allograft and increase small bowel edema.** Measurement of pulmonary artery pressures and cardiac output may be beneficial in patients where it is technically feasible.[154] Monitoring of cardiac output may help in the handling of the hypotension often seen with reperfusion of the small bowel allograft.[154] Direct arterial pressures should also be monitored, preferably from a catheter in an upper extremity artery because the aorta is partially or completely cross-clamped for some of the procedure.[159] Transesophageal echocardiography may also be helpful, particularly in patients with chronic occlusions of the central venous system that preclude access for pulmonary artery catheterization.[154]

ALLOGRAFT PERFUSION AND FLUID MANAGEMENT

In most cases of isolated small bowel transplantation, both the aorta and vena cava must be cross-clamped while the venous and arterial anastomoses are made. In some cases, the vascular anastomoses can be made with side-biting or partially occluding vascular clamps for either the aortic or venous anastomoses. With partial occlusion, the hemodynamic effects of cross-clamp release are usually diminished. Also in some cases, if technically feasible, the venous drainage of the intestinal allograft is made into the portal system of the recipient. The portal vein rather than the vena cava is completely or partially occluded.[154] This may result in less hemodynamic compromise because venous drainage from the lower extremities is maintained. Finally, in combined small bowel–liver transplants or multivisceral transplants, separate anastomoses for the small bowel may not be made. Instead, the small bowel is reperfused as the liver and other organs are reperfused. The hemodynamic changes with reperfusion are likely to be profound in these operations.[160,161] With the aid of a rapid infusion device one can ensure rapid fluid replacement during reperfusion. This diminishes the likelihood of hypovolemia-related hypotension and hypoperfusion of the newly anastomosed allografts.

Regardless of the type of anastomoses or operation, the small bowel prior to reperfusion is cold and filled with University of Wisconsin solution for preservation. University of Wisconsin solution is very high in potassium. Particularly if the venous drainage of the bowel is to the inferior vena cava, flushing of the cold preservative solution into the venous system with release of the aortic cross-clamp can result in hypotension and myocardial depression. With portal drainage, buffering by the liver occurs and the direct effect of the preservative solution on the heart is less profound.[159]

Prior to reperfusion of the allograft, the anesthesia provider should be sure that the patient has been adequately hydrated with blood products and/or colloid solution as guided by the central venous pressure and hemogram assessments. Excessive crystalloid solution beyond the maintenance rate should not be administered to minimize peripheral edema. If the urine output decreases below 1 mL/kg/min despite a central venous pressure of 10 mm Hg, mannitol, furosemide, or dopamine (2-3 mcg/kg/min) should be administered.[159]

Ten to 15 minutes prior to release of the vascular clamps, the volatile agent can be reduced to raise the systemic pressure to counter the fall commonly seen with reperfusion. The anesthesia provider must be prepared to administer calcium chloride (10 mg/kg) to counteract the hyperkalemia occasionally seen with wash out of the preservative solution, as well as vasopressors such as phenylepherine (50-100 mcg). Inotropes such as dopamine and/or epinephrine may also be required if the hypotension persists.

Reperfusion changes can occur several minutes after cross-clamp release as well. A recent review of 30 adults undergoing small bowel transplantation showed that reperfusion was associated with an increase in cardiac filling pressures, an increase in the cardiac output, a decrease in the mean arterial pressure to less than 60 mm Hg in 47% of the patients, and a decrease in the systemic vascular resistance, which persisted 5 minutes after release of the vascular clamps. Approximately one-half of the patients required inotropic support. However, the changes resolved by the end of surgery.[160]

IMMUNOSUPPRESSION

Intestinal transplant has been a challenge for scientists due to its immune and functional complexity. Immunosuppression developed through 3 phases.[152,162] Initially, high-dose tacrolimus in combination with steroids was used. In the second phase, induction therapy with cyclophosphamide was followed by multiple maintenance drugs with numerous side effects causing morbidity and mortality. Current immunosuppressive protocols use induction therapy with lymphoid ablating agents such as thymoglobulin or alemtuzumab and maintenance therapy with decreasing doses of tacrolimus. Some centers are attempting a steroid-free maintenance regimen to decrease the side effects of immunosuppressive therapy. Furthermore, immune modulation with single-dose bone marrow cell infusion and ex vivo allograft irradiation has been attempted.[152]

POSTOPERATIVE CONSIDERATIONS AND COMPLICATIONS

All patients undergoing small bowel transplantation require care in the intensive care unit in the immediate postoperative period. Many patients require postoperative positive pressure ventilation. Intravenous infusions of vasopressors may still be required. Close observation for early complications such as arterial or venous thrombosis, which require immediate action to correct, is needed.[159] Following the immediate postoperative period most patients still require a prolonged period of hospitalization. Small bowel function is impaired in the immediate postoperative period from denervation, dysmotility, and interruption of the lymphatics. High ileostomy output is also common in the perioperative period and may result in dehydration.[159]

Other complications are also serious and may result in mortality and graft loss.[163] Rejection is still a common cause of graft loss and mortality, although less so than during earlier time periods. Innate immunity plays a role in the development of graft rejection as suggested by a higher rate of rejection in patients with Crohn disease with nucleotide oligomerization domain 2 polymorphism.[164] Graft versus host disease where the lymphoid cells transplanted from the intestinal graft reacts against the host can occur after intestinal transplants in up to 5% of recipients.[159] It manifests itself with skin and gastrointestinal changes (rash, blisters, ulceration of oral mucosa, diarrhea), pancytopenia, pneumonitis, altered mental status, and native liver dysfunction. Unfortunately, bacterial, fungal, and viral infections still result in graft loss and/or mortality. The barrier to bacterial translocation is altered following ischemic injury to the bowel. Immunosuppression can further alter the bowel flora as well as the patient's ability to fight infection if bacterial translocation occurs.[165] Posttransplant lymphoproliferative disease also may develop in bowel transplant recipients and is more prevalent in children, after splenectomy, and was high prior to the use of tacrolimus. It still occurs, but less often, with tacrolimus as the immunosuppressive agent.[159]

ANESTHETIC CONSIDERATIONS FOR PATIENTS WITH PRIOR INTESTINAL TRANSPLANTS

A high level of multidisciplinary support is required for prior recipients of intestinal and multivisceral transplants. The nutritional status of the bowel transplant patient needs to be assessed prior to surgery. If the transplant is functioning poorly, the patient may be malnourished. Dehydration from diarrhea may also be a problem. These patients will benefit by consultation from those who specialize in the management of bowel transplantation whenever possible.[50]

Patients with prior intestinal or multivisceral transplants are also prone to infection for multiple reasons, including the chronic need for immunosuppressive medications to prevent rejection, altered intestinal permeability and absorption, and intestinal denervation and lymphatic dysfunction. Strict aseptic technique is mandatory. Stress-dose steroids may be necessary in the perioperative period if the patient is taking prednisone as part of the immunosuppression regimen.[50]

If the patient requires abdominal surgery, difficult dissection with the potential for massive bleeding and need for large-volume fluid resuscitation should be anticipated as these patients have usually undergone multiple previous laparotomies and adhesions can be extensive. Early on, patients may still have a long-term venous access device such as a Hickman catheter, which can be utilized. However, if the patient presents years later he or she may no longer have a venous access device. Venous access may be extremely challenging; previous studies should be reviewed and ultrasound guidance or assistance requested by interventional radiology.[50]

RESULTS AND OUTCOME FROM INTESTINAL TRANSPLANTATION

As noted earlier, the initial results for small-bowel transplantation were disappointing and resulted in few organs being transplanted. The results have improved since the late 1990s. Recently, a patient survival rate of 89% for intestine transplant was reported.[166] Eighty percent of the survivors had stopped total parenteral nutrition and resumed normal daily activities. Over 60% of grafts transplanted since 1998 are functioning 5 years or more. The longest survivor was on an oral diet 14 years following an intestinal transplant for volvulus.[167]

SUMMARY

Intestine transplantation has improved significantly over the past few years. As immunosuppression improves, it is likely that it will be used more often to prevent the complications from long-term hyperalimentation. The medical care of these patients can be challenging for the anesthesia provider. However, it can also be rewarding because many patients can benefit from this procedure who earlier could not be treated.

KEY REFERENCES

- Abu-Elmgad KM, Costa G, Bond GJ, et al. Five hundred intestinal and multivisceral transplantations at a single center. *Ann Surg.* 2009;250:567-581.
- Beebe DS, Urban M, Belani KG. Anaesthetic management of bone marrow transplant recipients less than two years of age. *Paediatr Anaesth.* 1995;5:107-114.
- Fleisher LA, Beckman JA, Brown KA, et al. ACC/AHA 2007 guidelines on perioperative cardiovascular evaluation and care for noncardiac surgery: a report of the American College of Cardiology/American Heart Association Task Force on Practice Guidelines: developed in collaboration with the American Society of Echocardiography, American Society of Nuclear Cardiology, Heart Rhythm Society, Society of Cardiovascular Anesthesiologists, Society for Cardiovascular Angiography and Intevention, Society for Vascular Medicine and Biology, and Society for Vascular Surgery. *Circulation.* 2007;116:e418-e499.
- Gratwohl A, Baldomero H, Aljurf M, et al. Hematopoietic stem cell transplantation: a global perspective. *JAMA.* 2010;303:1617-1624.
- Libby P, Nathan DM, Abraham K, et al. Report of the National Heart, Lung, and Blood Institute—National Institute of Diabetes and Digestive and Kidney Diseases Working Group on Cardiovascular Complications of Type 1 Diabetes Mellitus. *Circulation.* 2005;111:3489-3493.

- Khurshid I, Anderson LC. Non-infectious pulmonary complications after bone marrow transplantation. *Postgrad Med J.* 2002;78:257-262.
- Marcen R. Immunosuppressive drugs in kidney transplantation: impact on patient survival, and incidence of cardiovascular disease, malignancy and infection. *Drugs.* 2009;69:2227-2243.
- Segev DL, Muzaale AD, Caffo BS, et al. Perioperative mortality and long-term survival following live kidney donation. *JAMA.* 2010;303:959-966.
- Siniscalchi A, Spedicato S, Dante A, et al. Fluid management of patients undergoing intestinal and multivisceral transplantation. *Transplant Proc.* 2008;40:2031-2032.
- Tse W, Bunting KD, Laughlin MJ. New insights into cord blood stem cell transplantation. *Curr Opin Hematol.* 2008;15:279-284.
- Van Den Berghe G, Wonters P, Weckers F, et al. Intensive insulin therapy in mixed medical/surgical intensive care units: benefit versus harm. *Diabetes.* 2006;55:3151-3159.

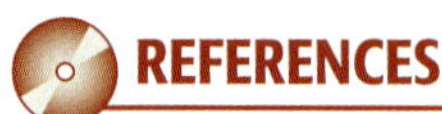

REFERENCES

Complete references available on DVD and online version at www.LongneckerAnesthesiology.com

CHAPTER 60 Endocrine Surgery and Intraoperative Management of Endocrine Conditions

Robert A. Peterfreund
Stephanie L. Lee

KEY POINTS

1. Endocrine diseases are common comorbid conditions in surgical patients.
2. The patient's type of diabetes mellitus must be known and the differing therapies of Types 1 and 2 appreciated.
3. Frequent monitoring of glucose levels is a mainstay in the management of the diabetic patient undergoing anesthesia and surgery.
4. **Tight perioperative glucose control is no longer generally recommended. Consider keeping glucose levels less than 150 to 180 mg/dL.**
5. Hypothyroid patients may exhibit sensitivity to sedative and hypnotic drugs used perioperatively. Hemodynamic instability should be anticipated.
6. Hyperthyroid patients may exhibit dehydration, hemodynamic instability and are at particular risk for tachydysrhythmias, metabolic or vascular decompensation, and thyroid storm.
7. The airway is a key consideration in patients undergoing thyroid surgery.
8. Pheochromocytoma patients require careful preoperative preparation, and plans must be made to manage hemodynamic extremes during surgery.
9. Glucocorticoid deficiency in patients at risk for adrenal suppression should be anticipated.
10. The implications of growth hormone excess (acromegaly) and adrenal steroid excess (Cushing disease) should be considered when preparing patients for pituitary surgery.

Endocrine diseases are common comorbid conditions in patients undergoing surgery. The consequences of a coexisting endocrine disorder may have an impact on anesthetic and immediate perioperative management. Diabetes mellitus (DM) is the most common comorbid endocrine condition, affecting as many as 20% of patients scheduled for surgery and requiring anesthesia.[1,2] The prevalence of thyroid disease is approximately 20% in the general population, so large numbers of patients who present for nonendocrine surgery have concomitant diagnoses of a thyroid disorder.

The surgical condition may result in part or entirely from the endocrine disorder, for example, vasoocclusive disease in the patient with DM requiring peripheral vascular surgery. Alternatively, the surgery may directly target endocrine tissue, either for biopsy or for excision. The pathophysiologic implications of the endocrine lesion and of surgical manipulation of the diseased tissue must be understood in the context of anesthetic and perioperative management.[3] The most common endocrine surgery involves the thyroid gland.

This chapter reviews the immediate perioperative implications of major endocrine disorders and addresses the specific issues encountered in surgery for common endocrine pathologies.

DIABETES MELLITUS

DM is a condition with an absolute (Type 1) or a relative (Type 2) deficiency of insulin. Chapter 13 discusses the complex physiology of DM. Recent comprehensive reviews discuss perioperative glucose management.[2,4,5] A fundamental concept is that the *Type 1 diabetic patient has an absolute requirement for continuous exogenous insulin.*[1] In the absence of insulin, despite a normal or low blood sugar concentration, the patient with Type 1 DM will develop *ketoacidosis*. The pharmacokinetic profiles of the various insulin preparations warrant careful consideration (**Table 60-1**).[6] Without a source of glucose in the perioperative period, a patient may develop hypoglycemia from the residual effects of a long-acting insulin preparation.

In the immediate perioperative period, it is generally recommended that patients receive regular insulin by intravenous (IV) bolus or IV infusion. The uptake of intramuscular or subcutaneous insulin may be unpredictable in the perioperative period because of changes in tissue perfusion.[2,4,5]

Patients with Type 2 DM can be managed with diet, an oral agent, insulin, or combinations of drugs including one of the newer medications (incretin mimetics, pramlintide). The pharmacokinetic and pharmacodynamic profiles of oral hypoglycemic agents differ markedly (**Table 60-2**). Some oral agents (eg, sulfonylureas) remain active for 24 hours, predisposing the patient to hypoglycemia during fasting. Other oral agents act as insulin sensitizers, improving the postreceptor action of insulin. Insulin sensitizers and incretin mimetics do not cause hypoglycemia when used in single-agent therapy. Some of these agents are newly introduced into clinical practice,[7,8,9] so experience with their use in surgical patients during the perioperative period is limited. Clinicians may soon encounter patients treated with bromocriptine, an old drug with a good safety profile. The metabolic control is likely achieved by a central mechanism, possibly in the hypothalamus.[10]

CLINICAL FEATURES OF DM

Although both major types of DM can share a number of clinical features, such as the presence of neuropathy, peripheral vascular, cardiovascular, and renal disease, and a predisposition to infection (see Chapter 13), an appreciation of the essential and distinctive features of each type is important.

Type 1 DM The patient with Type 1 DM usually is first diagnosed at a young age, but the disease may occur at any stage of life. Obesity is not a predisposing factor for Type 1 DM, unlike Type 2 DM. Conventional teaching holds that the patient with Type 1 DM is generally thin or of normal body habitus, but obesity may be present as a comorbid condition. The patient with Type 1 DM has an absolute requirement

TABLE 60-1 Insulin Preparations for the Management of Diabetes Mellitus

Agent	Time to Onset (h)	Peak (h)	Duration of Action (h)
Insulin (Subcutaneous Administration)			
Lispro (Humalog)	0.1-0.25	1-2	4-6
Aspart (NovoLog)	0.1-0.25	1-2	4-6
Glulisine (Apidra)	0.1-0.25	1-2	4-6
Regular	0.5-1	2-4	6-10
Semilente	0.5-3	2-10	12-16
NPH	2-4	6-12	12-18
Lente	1-3	6-15	22-28
Protamine zinc	1-6	14-24	≥36
Ultralente	2-8	10-30	≥36
Glargine (Lantus)	2-4	"Peakless"	20-24
Detemir (Levemir)	2-4	"Peakless"	20-24

Regular insulin can be administered intravenously. The biologic effect of receptor-bound insulin lasts approximately 1 hour. The circulating half-life of unbound insulin is a few minutes. Renal insufficiency prolongs the half-life of circulating insulin. An inhaled insulin preparation (Exubra) is no longer available.

for chronic insulin therapy to prevent diabetic ketoacidosis (DKA). As a general rule, patients with Type 1 DM are sensitive to the effects of insulin compared to patients with Type 2 DM, and therefore receive relatively small doses of insulin to both control blood sugar levels and prevent DKA. Acute medical or surgical conditions can precipitate DKA (diagnostic criteria are listed in **Table 60-3**). Consequently, these patients may arrive urgently in the operating room and require surgical intervention (ie, due to trauma, acute abdomen, abscess, ischemic limb, coronary artery bypass grafting [CABG]) but may have a concurrent metabolic derangement. Therefore, intraoperative anesthetic management of the patient with Type 1 DM may include treatment of DKA.

Diabetic Ketoacidosis Features of DKA (Table 60-3) include circulatory depression, as acidosis and metabolic derangements can reduce cardiac contractility and peripheral vascular tone.[11] Hyperglycemia with attendant hyperosmolarity produces osmotic diuresis, resulting in hypovolemia. Abnormalities often include hyperglycemia (although glucose usually is <500 mg/dL), intracellular dehydration, hyperkalemia, and hyponatremia. Dehydration frequently is severe because of poor oral intake due to the primary illness and is exacerbated by hyperglycemia-induced osmotic diuresis. Plasma potassium (K^+) levels can be elevated because metabolic acidosis drives K^+ from the intracellular space to extracellular fluids. Insulin concentrations are insufficient to maintain intracellular K^+ levels, so total body K^+ actually is depressed (reduced by 3-10 mEq per kilogram body weight). Measured sodium (Na^+) concentrations are artificially lowered approximately 1.6 mEq/L for every 100 mg/dL that the glucose level is elevated above 100 mg/dL. Thus the serum Na^+ level of a severely hyperglycemic patient may not reliably reflect the degree of dehydration. Plasma hypophosphatemia and hypomagnesemia commonly result from excessive urinary losses in DKA.

Management of DKA includes repletion of intravascular volume with electrolytes and water to resolve fluid deficits and help restore blood pressure, tissue perfusion, and glomerular filtration. Initial volume resuscitation usually is accomplished with normal saline even in the setting of hypernatremia. Vigorous hydration also decreases glucose levels by 20% to 40%. Insulin therapy (regular insulin by IV bolus and subsequent infusion) is crucial in treating DKA. Insulin inhibits gluconeogenesis and ketone production in the liver, and decreases lipolysis in adipose tissues. Insulin administration must be continued if acidosis or ketosis persists, even though glucose levels have normalized. During

TABLE 60-2 Other Agents Used for the Treatment of Type 2 Diabetes

Agent	Route of Administration	Mechanism of Action	Major Side Effects	Time to Onset (h)	Duration of Action (h)
Chlorpropamide	Oral	Increases insulin secretion	Hypoglycemia	1	60
Glimepiride				1	24
Tolbutamide				≤0.25	6-12
Tolazamide				1	10-24
Glyburide				1	6-12
Glipizide XL				1	3-4
Nateglinide				1	24
Repaglinide				1	3-4
Exenatide (Byetta)	Subcutaneous	GLP1 mimetic, increases insulin secretion only with hyperglycemia	Low risk for hypoglycemia as single agent, delays gastric emptying, nausea, anorexia	≤0.25	6-12
Liraglutide (Victoza)				Slow	12-24
Pramlintide (Symlin)		Suppresses postprandial glucagon secretion	Hypoglycemia when given with insulin, delays gastric emptying, nausea	≤0.25	2-4
Sitagliptin (Januvia)	Oral	DPP4 inhibitor increases GLP1		1	24
Saxagliptin (Onglyza)				1-2	24
Rosiglitazone	Oral	Insulin sensitizer	Peripheral edema, abdominal obesity congestive heart failure, anemia, hepatotoxicity	1	24
Pioglitazone	Oral	Insulin sensitizer		1	24
Metformin	Oral	Decreases hepatic glucose output, insulin sensitizer	Lactic acidosis, diarrhea	1	8-12
Acarbose	Oral	Decreases gastrointestinal glucose absorption	Malabsorption, flatulence, diarrhea	Immediate	<0.3
Miglitol				Immediate	<0.3

Incretin-mimetics and insulin sensitizers in single-agent therapy do not predispose to hypoglycemia, even in the fasting state.

DPP4, dipeptidyl peptidase 4; GLP1, glucagon.

TABLE 60-3 Typical Laboratory Findings During DKA and HONK

Laboratory Parameter	DKA	HONK	Mixed
Serum glucose (mg/dL)	>300	>600	>600
Serum bicarbonate (mEq/L)	<15	≥15	<15
Serum osmolarity (mOsm/L)	≤320	>320	>320
pH	<7.3	<7.3	
Urinary ketones	>3+	a	b
Serum ketones	+	a	b

DKA, diabetic ketoacidosis; HONK, hyperglycemic hyperosmolar nonketotic coma.

[a]Trace to small amounts of ketones may be present.

[b]Ketones may be present.

administration of insulin when plasma glucose concentrations decrease to less than 250 mg/dL, an infusion containing 5% dextrose (eg, D_5NS, 100 mL/h) will prevent hypoglycemia. Blood glucose levels should be monitored every hour, with frequent electrolyte determinations.

Potassium and phosphate replenishment are essential for insulin's action. These electrolytes should be replaced carefully, after first verifying that the patient has normal renal function and adequate urine output. Ensure proper function of the IV access as extravasation of potassium can cause tissue damage. Rapid potassium administration can precipitate dysrhythmias. Potassium can be replaced with an equal mixture of potassium chloride and potassium phosphate.

Serum K^+ <3 mEq/L, give K^+, 40 mEq/h

Serum K^+ <4 mEq/L, give K^+, 30 mEq/h

Serum K^+ <5 mEq/L, give K^+, 20 mEq/h

Serum K^+ ≥5 mEq/L, no replacement

Consideration should be given to bicarbonate therapy only for severe acidosis (eg, when arterial pH falls to <7.0) or hemodynamic instability, or for patients with cardiac rhythm disturbances. Following administration of bicarbonate, arterial pH levels should be monitored.

An emerging form of diabetes associated with obesity and presenting with ketoacidosis is called *Flatbush Type 2 DM.* Most or almost all of these patients can be treated with oral agents after initial management with intensive insulin therapy. Initial treatment of ketoacidosis in the patient with Flatbush Type 2 DM is the same as for the typical Type 1 DM patient.

Type 2 DM Patients with Type 2 DM generally are older, obese, and subject to metabolic syndrome, a complex pathophysiologic state characterized by hypercholesterolemia, hypertriglyceridemia, hyperglycemia, hypertension, and Type 2 DM.[12-14] In patients with metabolic syndrome, the cardiovascular risk of anesthesia and surgery may elevate markedly. Hypercoagulability is 1 feature of metabolic syndrome potentially relevant to these patients, who may be prone to thrombosis as a result of their surgical conditions or the consequences of surgery and anesthesia.[15] Of burgeoning clinical importance is the growing population of young, typically obese, patients with Type 2 DM. The practitioner encounters a juvenile or adolescent patient with the combined anesthetic management challenges of youth, obesity, and diabetes. Type 2 DM may occur in young, nonobese adolescents (maturity-onset diabetes of the young [MODY]) because of autosomal dominant inheritance of a mutation in the glucokinase gene that results in impaired hepatic glucose uptake and reduced insulin secretion.

A fundamental concept of Type 2 DM is that patients with the condition usually produce sufficient insulin to avoid DKA, the severe metabolic consequence of absolute insulin deficiency seen in patients with Type 1 DM. However, patients with Type 2 DM have reduced cellular responses when insulin binds to its receptor. Patients are described as being resistant to the hypoglycemic actions of insulin. To achieve normal glucose levels, patients with Type 2 DM may require doses of insulin that are large compared to doses required for Type 1 DM therapy.

Initial medical therapy in the ambulatory Type 2 DM patient includes administration of agents to increase endogenous insulin release, reduce intestinal uptake of carbohydrates, or increase peripheral sensitivity to insulin. When these measures are insufficient to normalize blood sugars, insulin therapy should be initiated, but patients may require very high insulin doses. New classes of therapeutic agents, currently represented by pramlintide and agents acting along the incretin pathway, increase insulin secretion, reduce postprandial glucagon secretion, and suppress hepatic glucose production.[8,8a,16]

Hyperglycemic Hyperosmolar Nonketotic Coma Hyperglycemic hyperosmolar nonketotic coma (HONK), also known as *hyperglycemic hyperosmolar syndrome,* is a clinical syndrome encountered in some Type 2 diabetic patients with decompensated DM.[11] Features include hyperglycemia, hyperosmolarity, and dehydration (typical water deficit 10-12 L). Severe ketosis is rare, but mild acidemia can be caused by starvation ketosis, inadequate circulation, and lactic acidosis (Table 60-3). The precipitating factors for HONK are similar to those of DKA **(Table 60-4)**. Patients presenting for surgery, especially urgent procedures, may have HONK as a comorbid condition requiring management during administration of their anesthetics. The classic presentation of patients with HONK includes fatigue, blurred vision, polydipsia, polyuria, leg cramps, and weight loss. The laboratory findings of HONK are related to dehydration and hypovolemia. Derangements in serum electrolyte levels occur, and hemoconcentration causes increases in blood levels of hemoglobin, protein, calcium, amylase, lactate dehydrogenase, and transaminases. Some patients present a mixed picture, with features of both DKA and HONK (Table 60-3).

Fluid administration in the setting of HONK is crucial. The rate of fluid administration depends on the patient's volume status, total body water deficit, serum osmolarity, and renal and cardiac function. Normal saline (2-3 L) is an appropriate fluid bolus in a patient with adequate cardiac and renal function, and serum osmolarity less than 320 mOsm/L. Even larger fluid boluses may be required if serum osmolarity is greater than 320 mOsm/L. In hypotensive patients who do not respond to aggressive crystalloid administration, colloidal or vasopressor infusions are additional treatments. Central venous pressure or pulmonary arterial monitoring may help guide therapy, especially in patients with HONK who are elderly and at significant risk for concomitant cardiovascular disease.

Medical therapy for HONK includes a low-dose, continuous IV infusion of insulin. If no decrease in glucose levels occurs over the first 2 to 4 hours, doubling the insulin infusion rate every hour until a response occurs is recommended. Potassium chloride usually is administered as part of the fluid regimen. The total body potassium deficits encountered in HONK are modest compared to DKA because of the absence of acidosis (see guidelines for potassium replacement in DKA). Potassium acetate and/or potassium phosphate can be used in order to avoid excessive chloride levels. Bicarbonate need not be given unless lactic acidosis causes arterial pH to decrease to less than 7.0. Thrombotic/embolic events are common complications of HONK. Prophylaxis

TABLE 60-4 Precipitating Factors for Hyperglycemic Hyperosmolar Nonketotic Coma

Precipitating Events	Pharmacologic Agents	
Infection (pneumonia, urinary tract infection, sepsis)	Amphetamines	Niacin
	β-Blockers	Pentamidine
Noncompliance with insulin regimen	β-Agonists	Protease inhibitors
First presentation of diabetes mellitus	Diuretics	Salicylates
Dehydration	Glucocorticoids	Sympathomimetics
Impaired renal function		

against thrombosis warrants consideration. Should thrombosis occur, an anticoagulating dose of IV heparin or low-molecular-weight heparin anticoagulation is indicated.

PERIOPERATIVE INSULIN/GLUCOSE MANAGEMENT

As a rule, long-acting oral hypoglycemic agents (sulfonylurea drugs) should not be given before surgery to reduce the risk of hypoglycemia, signs and symptoms of which may be masked by general anesthesia. It is unlikely that insulin sensitizers will produce hypoglycemia. Theoretically, inhibitors of glucagon secretion (eg, GLP-1 analogues) may lead to hypoglycemia in the fasting state. However, the actions of these drugs are glucose dependent; they should have no effects when blood sugars are low. Nevertheless, prudence suggests that agents acting along the incretin pathway and pramlintide should be held on the day of surgery. Patients with Type 2 DM treated with insulin are at risk for hyperglycemia if their insulin is withheld completely. Typically, these patients receive about half of their usual morning insulin dose in the form of long-acting insulin preparations, such as NPH insulin. Short-acting insulins are omitted. *Patients with Type 1 DM must receive some insulin.* In this population, half of the usual morning dose of long-acting insulin may be appropriate before surgery. One key to management is frequent monitoring of glucose levels in all patients with DM. As a general rule, diabetic patients should undergo their anesthetic and surgical procedures as early in the day as possible. This limits the perturbations caused by prolonged fasting and disruption of customary diabetes medical regimens.

Recently, more patients have been managed with their insulin requirements supplied by continuous and bolus infusions delivered by an insulin pump. Recommendations for the perioperative period for patients with pumps include (1) maintaining the basal infusion rate of insulin, (2) omitting any preprandial insulin boluses in the fasting patient, (3) monitoring of glucose levels at frequent intervals, and (4) resuming the usual diet and insulin therapy regimen as soon as possible.[16] However, the anesthesiologist must recognize that these pumps deliver the insulin dose subcutaneously. Uptake of the drug from this depot may be affected by alterations (usually reductions) in tissue perfusion that are commonly encountered during surgery or the perioperative period.[3] Consequently, depending on the surgical circumstances, it may be advantageous to interrupt the continuous subcutaneous administration of insulin by pump and to substitute carefully titrated IV infusions of insulin. To decide on the initial IV insulin infusion rate, first determine the total 24-hour basal insulin dose typically administered by the subcutaneous infusion. Divide this basal dose by 24. Start the IV infusion with this number of units of regular insulin per hour, again with close monitoring of blood glucose and serum potassium levels.

Intraoperative Insulin Therapy A variety of regimens exist for IV infusion of regular insulin in the operating room. For the routine surgical population, the "Vellore regimen" has been evaluated.[18] Other schemes also are acceptable[2,19] as long as glucose and potassium levels are closely monitored and treated when necessary. **Table 60-5** outlines 1 practical method of insulin administration in the operating room that is used at our institutions. Cardiac surgical patients[20] and pediatric surgical patients[11] may benefit from regimens tailored to the special needs of these particular populations.

Perioperative Glucose Target Range Several studies providing evidence for the clinical benefits of tight glucose control (eg, 80-110 mg/dL) in critically ill patients led to initially enthusiastic adoption of intensive insulin therapy (IIT) regimens. Later reports demonstrated adverse (eg, hypoglycemia) or neutral effects of IIT. Current expert opinion suggests keeping glucose below 180 mg/dL in the critically ill patient.[3,4,22-24] Few data exist to guide *intraoperative* glucose management practices. In some surgical situations (eg, neurovascular procedures or carotid endarterectomy) associated with significant risk for cerebral ischemia, it might be argued that blood glucose levels should be more tightly controlled to avoid hyperglycemia. For other procedures, the optimum insulin regimen and the ideal range of blood glucose levels for routine anesthetics remain undetermined.[23,25,26]

TABLE 60-5 A Perioperative Intravenous Regular Insulin Regimen

A. Initial regular insulin IV bolus: 0.05-0.1 U/kg

Dose additional boluses based on glucose levels.

B. Regular insulin infusions (1 U regular insulin/mL normal saline)

Initial Regular Insulin Infusion Rate (U/h)

Type 1 DM (female)	0.5
Type 1 DM (male)	1.0
Type 2 DM (male or female)	1.0

Notes on IV Regular Insulin Action

1. Onset is immediate.
2. Duration is ~1 h.
3. Duration of action is prolonged in renal insufficiency.

Adjustment of IV Regular Insulin Infusion Rate (U/h) based on hourly point of care glucose measurement

Glucose (mg/dL)	Rate Change	Other Rx
<70	Hold 30 min	Give D_{50}, 15-20 mL. Recheck blood glucose level after 30 min. Give more dextrose until blood glucose level >70 mg/dL.
70-120	↓ 0.3 U/h	
121-180	No change	
181-240	↑ 0.3 U/h	
241-300	↑ 0.6 U/h	
>300	↑ 1.0 U/h	

Notes on IV Regular Insulin Dosing

1. Insulin guidelines assume patient is fasting and is not in diabetic ketoacidosis.
2. *Dosing must be individually titrated based on frequent blood glucose monitoring.*

DM, diabetes mellitus.

Glucose Monitoring Glucose monitoring is the foundation for safe and effective glucose management and perioperative insulin therapy. Clinicians use point-of-care testing with various devices or send arterial or venous blood samples to a central laboratory for analysis.[3,4] The technology for glucose analysis is complex.[27] Unrecognized pitfalls exist with the convenient handheld devices, and clinicians must recognize that multiple factors have an impact on the accuracy of the result, upon which therapeutic decisions may be based.[28] Potential confounding factors include anemia, hypoxemia, hyperoxia, the presence of other sugars, elevated triglyceride, bilirubin, urea or uric acid levels, and perhaps also blood pH and body temperature.

Metformin Metformin is an oral hypoglycemic agent of the biguanide class with an important role in Type 2 diabetes therapy, particularly because of its favorable effects on cardiovascular mortality.[29] This drug, which has multiple pharmacologic effects, has also been associated with the serious side effect of lactic acidosis, which may become life threatening. Whether metformin causes lactic acidosis or exacerbates lactic acidosis resulting from other conditions remains undetermined.[30,31] When administered according to guidelines and avoiding contraindications including renal and hepatic insufficiency and a history of alcohol abuse, the incidence of lactic acidosis is very low.[29] In conditions where tissue hypoxia already exists (including circulatory failure) or circulatory insufficiency is anticipated (eg, major surgery), it is prudent to withhold metformin. In anticipation of IV radiologic contrast exposure, metformin should be stopped and not restarted until the creatinine level has been checked to confirm baseline renal function. Recognizing that conclusive data do not exist to support their suggested guidelines, Jones et al[32] and Vreven and De Kock[33] proposed that metformin be withdrawn 2 days before general anesthesia and reinstated when renal function is demonstrated to be stable. This is not universally practiced. Metformin should not produce hypoglycemia in the fasting preoperative patient.

STEROID (GLUCOCORTICOID) THERAPY: IMPLICATIONS FOR DM

Administration of pharmacologic doses of glucocorticoids increases resistance to insulin action by inhibiting glucose uptake into muscle and fat.[34] In many patients the effect is primarily postprandial hyperglycemia. Thus morning fasting glucose levels are only mildly elevated, but glucose levels rise substantially after meals in the afternoon and evening.

Glucose levels will increase in patients with known diabetes. Glucocorticoid therapy reveals previously undiagnosed insulin resistance in 25% of all patients receiving such treatment.[18] The hyperglycemia resulting from glucocorticoid therapy can be managed with insulin, oral hypoglycemic agents, or combination therapy. When glucocorticoid therapy is tapered, insulin resistance decreases with a lag of 1 to 3 days. Hyperglycemia therapies (eg, insulin infusions) must then be reduced to avoid hypoglycemia. The complexities of the patient's regimen for controlling hyperglycemia must be considered when managing medications and glucose in the perioperative period.

Postoperative stress usually leads to excess endogenous glucocorticoid production and consequent insulin resistance. This may result in hyperglycemia lasting 1 to 3 days after the procedure or for as long as significant infection or pain-related stress is present. Treatment of this manifestation of hyperglycemia is accomplished by administering a long-acting insulin plus a short-acting insulin at mealtime in the patient who is able to eat. Other patients may require regular insulin administered by IV infusion.

COUNTERREGULATORY HORMONES

Glucagon Alpha cells of the pancreatic islet secrete glucagon. Glucose is the most important regulator of glucagon secretion. Hyperglycemia decreases glucagon secretion. Hypoglycemia stimulates glucagon secretion via direct effects on islets and via central nervous system pathways activated by hypoglycemia. β-Adrenergic receptor activation stimulates glucagon secretion.[36] Glucagon acts primarily on the liver to increase both glycogenolysis and gluconeogenesis. Increased glucose output balances glucose utilization during the fasting state to maintain euglycemia.[37] Patients with hepatic or pancreatic insufficiency are theoretically at risk for hypoglycemia as a result of lack of glucagon effects. In addition, β-blocker therapy potentially reduces glucagon secretion, thereby potentially increasing the risk of hypoglycemia. The implication for anesthetic management is the need to monitor glucose levels frequently in patients at risk and to intervene as needed.

Epinephrine Epinephrine and glucagon are the most important hormones maintaining euglycemia during the fasting state.[38] The central nervous system reacts to hypoglycemia by stimulating the secretion of epinephrine. Activation of pancreatic α-adrenergic receptors by epinephrine inhibits insulin secretion. β-Adrenergic receptor activation stimulates the secretion of glucagon. Epinephrine, via β_2-adrenergic receptors, also acts directly on the liver to increase glycogenolysis and gluconeogenesis. Therefore, patients at risk for blunted sympathetic responses, either following neuraxial anesthesia or from receiving β-blocker therapy, may fail to react normally to hypoglycemia. The implication for anesthetic management is, again, a need to anticipate potential hypoglycemia, with close monitoring of glucose levels in patients at risk, and to treat as needed.

Glucocorticoids and Growth Hormone Growth hormone (GH) and cortisol play minor roles in the restoration of euglycemia after hypoglycemia. The prevention of cortisol secretion and GH deficiency does not inhibit restoration of euglycemia after hypoglycemia.[39] The hyperglycemic response to the combination of glucagon, epinephrine, and cortisol is larger than the response to each of these hormones given individually, suggesting that synergism contributes to normal physiologic responses to hypoglycemia.[40]

HYPOGLYCEMIC UNAWARENESS

Some patients with long-standing DM and frequent bouts of hypoglycemia lose their normal sympathetic response to low blood sugar levels. The failure to consciously recognize low blood sugar levels is known as "hypoglycemic unawareness." Fasting in the perioperative period, particularly in the setting of continued insulin therapy administered by infusion pump, may predispose these patients to potentially dangerous hypoglycemia. The anesthesiologist cannot rely on such patients to symptomatically monitor their own blood glucose levels and to respond appropriately, even when managed with regional anesthesia and minimal sedation. Blood glucose measurement, and appropriate therapy, is essential for these patients.

DM: IMPLICATIONS FOR ANESTHESIA

Although general anesthesia may be mandatory for some surgical procedures, other options (including regional anesthesia or neuraxial anesthesia) exist for some situations.[41] Neuraxial anesthesia may provide an advantage by blocking "stress responses" to surgery involving counterregulatory hormones such as epinephrine and glucocorticoids. Regional or neuraxial block anesthetic techniques may allow some diabetic patients to return to their customary diets earlier than they would if given general anesthesia, facilitating resumption of chronic diabetes regimens. Metabolic control in the diabetic patient may be improved by regional anesthetic techniques, at least in some patient populations.[42] Regional anesthesia or neuraxial techniques may also be useful for patients with diabetic gastroparesis who are at elevated risk for aspiration under general anesthesia, or who may be difficult to intubate because of stiff joints (including the temporomandibular joints and the cervical spine) associated with their disease. In addition, preexisting autonomic neuropathy may compound the effects of sympathectomy produced by neuraxial block. Data suggest that cerebrospinal fluid (CSF) composition differs between patients with DM and healthy patients, and that this difference correlates with enhanced sensitivity to neuraxial drugs.[43]

There is some concern that patients at risk for diabetic neuropathy may be more likely to develop peripheral nerve injury in association with regional or neuraxial techniques, either from local anesthetic toxicity or mechanical trauma from the block needle.[44] Only a small amount of published evidence addresses these issues. Blumenthal et al describes 1 patient with a preexisting, nondiabetic, asymptomatic polyneuropathy who developed symptomatic neuropathy after a peripheral nerve block.[45] Hebl et al reported 2 patients in a retrospective series who developed exacerbations of preexisting neuropathy after neuraxial anesthesia or analgesia. Both patients had Type 2 DM.[46] These authors suggest that local anesthesia toxicity is a possibility. Adjuvants (eg, clonidine) may prove beneficial in providing desired anesthetic effects with smaller doses of local anesthetics, thereby reducing toxicity risks.[47] McAnulty and Hall[48] conclude that there is no evidence to indicate that regional anesthesia alters overall surgical morbidity and mortality in the diabetic patient population. Consequently, a well-conducted anesthetic, regardless of specific technique, probably is the most important factor in the care of the diabetic patient. Of note, general anesthesia often masks the autonomic response to hypoglycemia, and changes in vital signs can easily be misinterpreted as a response to increased surgical stimulation rather than hypoglycemia. Consequently, close monitoring of glucose levels in patients at risk for hypoglycemia and appropriate therapy are essential.

SPECIFIC SURGICAL PROCEDURES AND GLUCOSE HOMEOSTASIS

Total pancreatectomy eliminates insulin-producing islet cells as well as cells secreting the counterregulatory hormone glucagon. This surgery renders the patient a Type 1 diabetic with an absolute requirement for insulin therapy. The biologic effect of insulin molecules bound to cellular receptors lasts for approximately 1 hour, but the chemical half-life of insulin in the circulation is just a few minutes. Consequently, following a total pancreatectomy, the need for insulin therapy to prevent DKA begins within 60 minutes of devascularizing the pancreatic islets.

Surgery for insulinoma or glucagonoma poses particular management challenges. Glucagonoma may cause elevations in glucose and resistance to insulin during surgery, so glucose levels should be monitored closely and managed as needed. Insulinomas may cause life-threatening, profound hypoglycemia. There can be wide swings of glucose levels perioperatively. Frequent measurements of glucose and therapeutic interventions (IV insulin or IV glucose administration) may be necessary.

THYROID DISEASE

Thyroid diseases comprise the second most common endocrine conditions appearing as comorbidities in patients presenting for surgery of any kind. Hypothyroidism and hyperthyroidism have significantly different implications for anesthetic management. Where possible, assessment of the current status of the patient's thyroid condition provides information useful for predicting sensitivity to drugs commonly administered in the perioperative period, hemodynamic responses during surgery and anesthesia, and physiologic perturbations potentially requiring investigation and treatment, such as electrolyte disorders and adrenal insufficiency.[49] Coagulation disorders (hypercoagulability with hyperthyroidism and coagulopathy with severe hypothyroidism) have recently drawn attention.[50] Medical treatment of altered thyroid function (hypothyroidism or hyperthyroidism) may require several weeks to achieve a new steady state. In general, mildly hypothyroid patients can proceed to elective surgery without delay. Postponement of elective surgery may be indicated to allow for the evaluation and treatment of hyperthyroidism and to allow for the medical management of hypothyroid patients with more than mild to moderate thyroid insufficiency.

TABLE 60-6 Clinical Features of Thyroid Disease Significant for the Perioperative Period

Hyperthyroidism/Thyrotoxicosis	
Volume depletion	Eyelid retraction, lid lag, stare
Tachycardia or atrial fibrillation	Vasodilation, decreased SVR
Systolic hypertension	Elevated liver function tests
Congestive heart failure	Decreased cholesterol
Hyperthermia and increased perspiration	Exophthalmos (Graves disease only)
Adrenocortical insufficiency	Warm, moist skin
Proximal muscle weakness	Hypercalcemia
Motor hyperkinesis	Tremor
Hypothyroidism	
Decreased spontaneous respiration	Hypothermia
Reduced plasma volume	Enlarged tongue
Hypoglycemia	Slow movement
Hyponatremia	Slow speech
Impaired hepatic drug metabolism	Hoarseness
Hypometabolic state	Elevated creatine phosphokinase
Adrenocortical insufficiency	Dry, sallow skin
Obesity	Periorbital edema
Enlarged cardiac silhouette on radiography	Nonpitting edema (myxedema)
Congestive heart failure	Delayed relaxation of deep tendon reflexes
Bradycardia	
Hypertension (especially diastolic)	Low-voltage electrocardiogram with inverted T waves
Depressed mental state	Elevated cholesterol
Vasocontriction, increased SVR	Ileus

SVR, systemic vascular resistance.

IMPLICATIONS OF HYPERTHYROIDISM

The clinical features of hyperthyroidism result from excess thyroid hormone and enhanced β-adrenergic activity.[49,51] Etiology, manifestations, and medical management of thyroid disorders are discussed in detail in Chapter 13. Endocrinologists distinguish *thyrotoxicosis*, which is a general term for excessively elevated thyroid hormone of any cause (including excessive exogenous thyroid hormone), from *hyperthyroidism*, in which thyroid gland hypersecretion is the reason for excessive thyroid hormone activity. **Table 60-6** summarizes the clinical features of hyperthyroidism and thyrotoxicosis that are particularly relevant to the anesthetic management of thyroid surgery, or of nonthyroid surgery that cannot be postponed until the patient is rendered euthyroid. Atrial dysrhythmias, including atrial fibrillation, and premature atrial contractions, tachycardia, systolic hypertension, ischemic cardiac disease, and congestive heart failure should be specifically considered when planning an anesthetic for the hyperthyroid patient.[52-54] Muscle weakness may impair perioperative respiratory reserve. β-Adrenergic blockade is the mainstay of anesthetic management. High doses of β-blockers may be required to control cardiac manifestations of hyperthyroidism in the immediate perioperative period.

IMPLICATIONS OF HYPOTHYROIDISM

The clinical features of hypothyroidism result from a deficiency of thyroid hormone action.[49,55,56] Etiology, manifestations, and medical management are discussed in detail in Chapter 13. The clinical features that are particularly relevant to the anesthetic management of thyroid or nonthyroid surgery that cannot be postponed until the patient is rendered euthyroid are summarized in Table 60-6. Bradycardia, diastolic hypertension, congestive heart failure (systolic and diastolic dysfunction), pericardial or pleural effusions, seizures, depressed mentation or frank coma, hypothermia, coagulopathy, and ileus should be specifically considered when evaluating for suspected hypothyroidism. The patient may have a blunted hypercapnic or hypoxic ventilatory drive. Adrenal cortical insufficiency may impair normal stress responses. Laboratory findings include hyponatremia and hypoglycemia.

PHARMACOLOGIC IMPLICATIONS

Minimum Alveolar Concentration Conventional anesthetic wisdom holds that thyroid status does not alter the minimum alveolar concentration. Data from studies of experimental animals using agents such as halothane and cyclopropane support this assertion.[57,58] Data from studies of humans or of any species on the interaction of thyroid status with minimum alveolar concentration for newer potent inhalational agents such as desflurane and sevoflurane have not been reported. As demonstrated in rats, thyroid status may alter the metabolism of the older potent inhalational anesthetics halothane, enflurane, and methoxyflurane,[59] but the clinical relevance of this finding for commonly used, newer agents is not reported.

Altered Drug Metabolism/Sensitivity Conventional wisdom holds that hypothyroidism increases the sensitivity to sedative, analgesic, and anesthetic medications.[55] Evidence supporting this concept is limited to older drugs without recent studies.[60] One case report cites the accumulation of midazolam in prolonged sedation of a critically ill patient with hypothyroidism as a comorbid condition.[61] Whether this observation can be generalized to all hypothyroid patients or to the use of other commonly administered sedative, hypnotic, and analgesic agents remains unproven.

Amiodarone Amiodarone is widely used for the management of atrial and ventricular dysrhythmias. The amiodarone molecule contains approximately 37% iodine by weight, resulting in the delivery of large amounts of iodine to patients receiving standard doses of the drug.

The effects of amiodarone therapy on thyroid function are complex, and patients may become either hypothyroid or hyperthyroid when their cardiac electrophysiologic disturbances are treated with amiodarone.[51,62,63] Consequently, patients presenting for surgery who are receiving chronic amiodarone therapy may warrant consideration of their risk for thyroid dysfunction in the perioperative period.

EXOPHTHALMOS: ANESTHETIC IMPLICATIONS

Exophthalmos, a clinical feature of Graves disease, results from the accumulation of retroorbital fat and swollen ocular muscles resulting in proptosis (**Fig. 60-1**). The eyelid may not cover the globe, and the exposed cornea and prominent globe are subject to mechanical trauma, including pressure injury. With significant proptosis, corneas are at risk for drying; consider the use of ointments or lubricants and ensure that the eyes are closed during surgery.

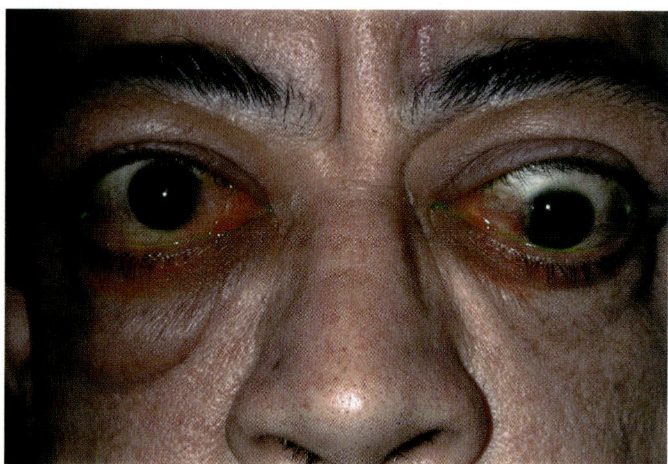

A

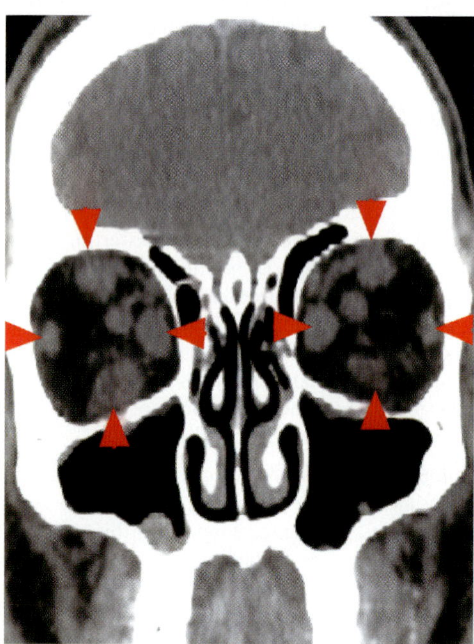

B

FIGURE 60-1. Graves ophthalmopathy with exophthalmos. **A.** Photograph of the face. Note the protuberant orbits and disconjugate gaze caused by accumulation of tissue in the retroorbital area, and edema and fibrosis of the extraocular muscles. **B.** CT scan through the orbits of a different patient showing extraocular muscle edema (*arrows*).

TABLE 60-7 Treatment of Severe Hyperthyroidism or Decompensated Hyperthyroidism (Thyroid Storm)

Therapy to Control the Thyroid
- Thionamides (PTU, methimazole)
- Iodinated medications (iopanoic acid, stable potassium iodide, Lugol solution), Graves disease only (administered at least 1 h after thionamide)
- Lithium carbonate

Therapy to Block Conversion of T_4 to T_3
- PTU
- Iopanoic acid
- Propranolol (High dose)
- Corticosteroids (High dose)

Therapy to Enhance Clearance of Thyroid Hormones
- Gastrointestinal clearance
  Cholestyramine
- Blood clearance
  Hemoperfusion
  Plasmapheresis

Therapy to Block the Effects of Thyroid Hormones
- β-Blockers to control heart rate
- Corticosteroids

Supportive Measures
- Antipyretics (acetaminophen)
- Cooling
- Meperidine (blocks shivering induced by cooling)
- Correction of dehydration
- Nutrition
- Oxygen
- Treatment of congestive heart failure

Therapy for the Precipitating Illness

PTU, propylthiouracil; T_3, triiodothyronine; T_4, L-thyroxine.

MANAGEMENT OF SEVERE HYPERTHYROIDISM OR THYROID STORM IN URGENT SURGERY

Severe hyperthyroidism is a relative contraindication to anesthesia and surgery. When extreme hyperthyroidism progresses to physiologic decompensation with circulatory collapse, altered mental status, and hyperthermia, the diagnosis is thyroid storm, a life-threatening condition that ideally should be medically controlled before a patient is brought to surgery (**Table 60-7**). If an operation cannot be delayed, the patient must be rapidly prepared in order to limit the effects of the endocrine disorder on the clinical course. Mainstays of therapy include medications to control thyroid gland production of thyroid hormone, β-adrenergic blockers to blunt sympathetic effects, glucocorticoids, and circulatory support.[64,65] Iopanoic acid is a valuable treatment option now available only in Europe. The drug may be particularly useful in the setting of amiodarone-induced thyrotoxicosis.[64,66] In the United States, saturated solution of potassium iodide (SSKI) may be used in combination with β-adrenergic blockers.[67,68]

THYROID SURGERY

Anesthetic Options General anesthesia is commonly administered for thyroid surgery. General anesthesia has the advantages of patient comfort, amnesia, and immobility, along with control of the airway. Airway control often is achieved by intubation with a cuffed endotracheal tube.[69] However, use of the laryngeal mask airway (LMA) has been considered an option for airway control because intraoperative inspection of vocal cord function and glottic structures can be accomplished with a fiberoptic scope.[70-75] Direct visualization may be particularly valuable if the surgical procedure places a recurrent laryngeal nerve (RLN) at significant risk. An advantage of the technique is that the RLN can be continuously monitored throughout the surgical procedure if the fiberoptic scope is left in place, allowing real-time identification of compromised RLN function. Because some patients may require endotracheal intubation but also benefit from continuous direct observation of glottic structures, Hillermann et al[75] proposed the use of a small-diameter (5.0-mm inner diameter) endotracheal tube together with an LMA through which a fiberoptic scope was positioned. This setup allows control of the airway with a cuffed endotracheal tube while permitting visual monitoring of RLN function.

Muscle relaxants facilitate endotracheal intubation and may constitute 1 component of anesthesia maintenance. Muscle relaxants may interfere with motor monitoring of the RLN or other nerves placed at risk by the surgical procedure. Partial pharmacologic paralysis may permit motor nerve monitoring in some situations[76] if the level of muscle relaxation is closely monitored.

An alternative to general anesthesia is regional anesthesia with supplemental local anesthetic infiltration as needed.[77-80] Advantages of regional anesthesia include the ability to assess spontaneous respiration and the voice as indicators of RLN integrity during the procedure. In addition, regional anesthesia provides the possibility of early postoperative pain control with little or no need for systemic analgesics and could be used in conjunction with general anesthesia.[81-83] However, recent clinical studies do not demonstrate particularly effective pain relief with regional blocks.[84,85] A consideration in planning a regional anesthetic is that systemic absorption of epinephrine, a common additive to local anesthetic solutions, may exacerbate tachycardia or other tachydysrhythmias encountered in hyperthyroid patients. Thus epinephrine should be given cautiously or avoided entirely.

Unilateral and bilateral *deep cervical plexus block* or superficial cervical plexus block with local supplementation has been described for thyroid surgery. Deep cervical plexus block carries the associated risk of anesthetizing the phrenic nerve with resulting diaphragm dysfunction. Unilateral or bilateral diaphragmatic dysfunction may precipitate respiratory distress, especially if the surgical procedure disturbs RLN function with airway compromise. However, little or no change of the forced vital capacity (FVC) measured by incentive spirometry was detected in 21 patients undergoing thyroid surgery with bilateral deep cervical plexus block, and no patient experienced subjective respiratory distress.[78] A study that focused on the analgesic efficacy of cervical plexus block administered in conjunction with general anesthesia for thyroid surgery reported no subjective respiratory complaints among the 39 subjects.[81] However, the study did not include any quantitative objective assessments of respiratory function. Deep cervical plexus block may impair RLN function when the anesthetic spreads to block the vagus nerve. Although this would not affect the direct stimulation of an RLN (as for electromyographic [EMG] monitoring) during surgery, the ability to assess spontaneous vocal cord function would be compromised by anesthetizing the vagus nerve with a deep cervical plexus block. *Superficial cervical plexus block* avoids the potential airway or respiratory problems of a deep cervical plexus block, but may not provide sufficient analgesia for the deeper structures of the neck that may be involved in the surgery.

Cervical epidural anesthesia has been used successfully for parathyroid surgery in patients maintained awake to evaluate their vocal cord function.[82] Significant decreases in FVC were encountered, but other measured respiratory variables remained stable, with minimal subjective respiratory compromise. Because the airway and respiratory considerations for thyroid and parathyroid surgery are comparable, the findings suggest that cervical epidural anesthesia may provide an anesthetic option for thyroid surgery where general anesthesia is not desirable.

Taken together, the findings of small clinical studies suggest that regional anesthesia may be suitable for appropriately selected patients, but more definitive investigation, particularly of the incidence of perioperative respiratory complications, is needed. Lack of airway control, in a situation where the location of the surgical site complicates establishing emergency airway control, is a disadvantage of regional anesthesia techniques.

Anatomic Concerns Situated at the base of the anterior neck, the thyroid gland lies in close proximity to major vascular structures, including the internal jugular veins and the carotid arteries (**Figs. 60-2** and **60-3**).[86] Distortion of normal anatomic relationships, as in the case of a large goiter or a thyroid cancer, can complicate the insertion of an internal jugular catheter (**Fig. 60-4**). The thyroid gland wraps around the trachea in a nearly circumferential fashion. Direct extension of thyroid cancers into the trachea may obstruct the lumen. Large thyroid masses sometimes compress the tracheal lumen (**Fig. 60-5**) or distort the subglottic or supraglottic airway (**Figs. 60-6** and **60-7**). Some thyroid masses penetrate or compress the esophagus with implications for the patient's nutritional status. Insertion of nasogastric or orogastric tubes also may be complicated.

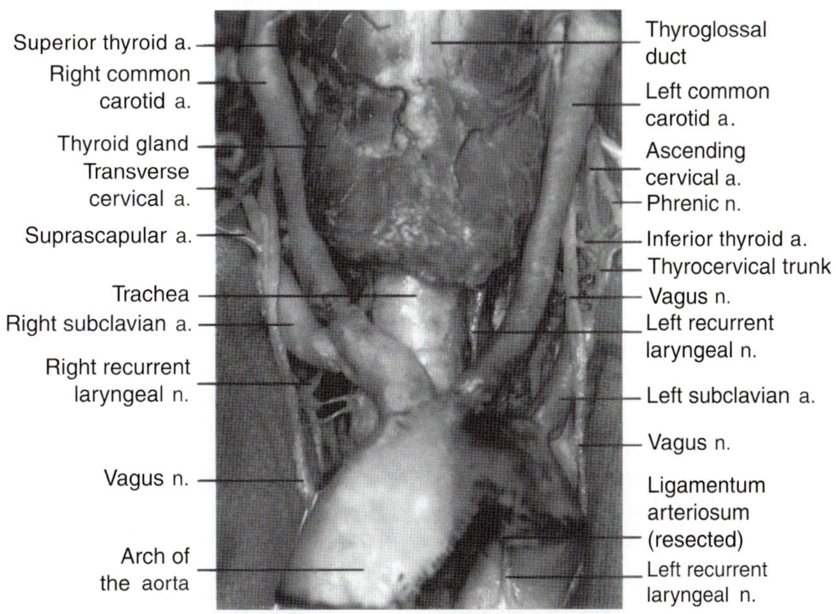

FIGURE 60-2. Anatomic relationships of the normal anterior neck. [From Monfared A, Gorti G, Kim D. Microsurgical anatomy of the laryngeal nerves as related to thyroid surgery. *Laryngoscope.* 2002;112:386-392, with permission.]

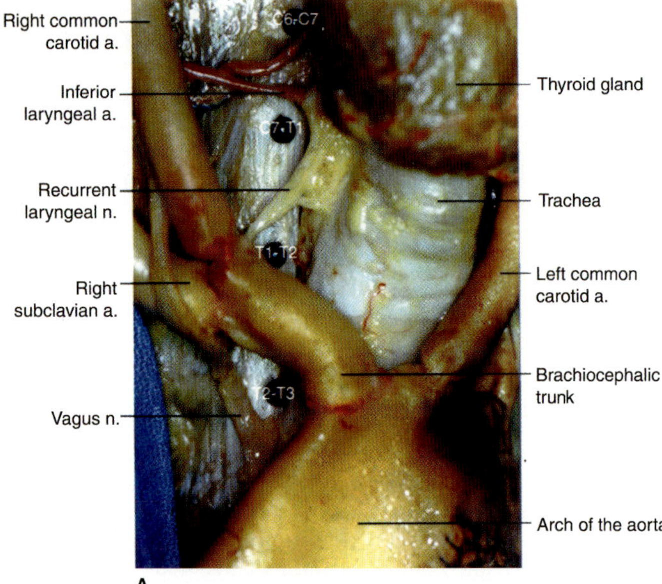

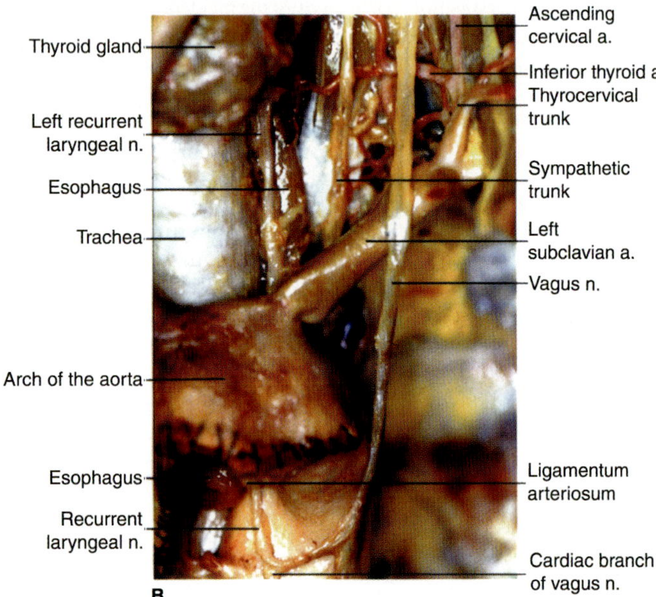

FIGURE 60-3. Anatomic relationships of the thyroid gland. The recurrent laryngeal nerve branches from the vagus and ascends in a groove between the trachea and the esophagus. **A.** Right exposure. **B.** Left exposure. [From Monfared A, Gorti G, Kim D. Microsurgical anatomy of the laryngeal nerves as related to thyroid surgery. *Laryngoscope.* 2002;112:386-392, with permission.]

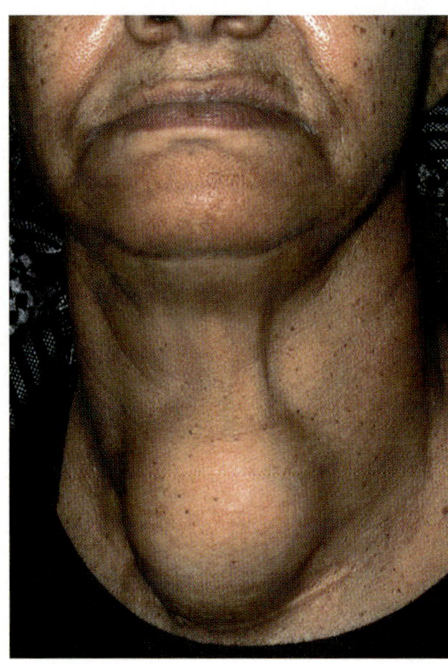

FIGURE 60-4. Large recurrent goiter overlying the anterior and right neck in a patient with a previous partial thyroidectomy.

Emergency airway algorithms contain a provision for establishing a surgical airway, either by cricothyrotomy or by tracheostomy. Extension of thyroid tissue rostrally over the cricothyroid membrane, or caudally toward the sternal notch, positions this highly vascular tissue directly in front of the airway. Thyroid isthmus tissue may be encountered even in routine tracheostomy placement.[87] A cadaver study reported a high incidence of percutaneous tracheostomy catheters malpositioned so as to puncture the thyroid isthmus.[88] Complications of surgical airway insertion related to thyroid tissue or vessels have been reported.[89] Hemorrhage can easily complicate attempts to establish a surgical airway.

Other structures in close proximity to the thyroid gland include the parathyroid glands, which are placed at risk during thyroid surgery, and the recurrent and superior laryngeal nerves, which supply the larynx.[90,91]

Airway Concerns Airway management is a principal anesthetic concern in thyroid surgery. Thyroid masses can affect the airway in the supraglottic region. Lingual thyroid tissue arising from the base of the tongue may obstruct the oropharynx, compromising spontaneous respiration,[92] mask ventilation, and direct laryngoscopy. Thyroid masses invading or compressing the glottis potentially compromise visualization of the glottic opening or passage of an endotracheal tube through the vocal cords. Bouaggad et al[93] studied 320 patients scheduled for thyroidectomy in an analysis of potential factors helpful for predicting difficult endotracheal intubation. Endotracheal intubation was found to be easy in 36.9% of patients, and the investigators encountered only minor difficulties in 57.8% of the study group. The study concluded that the presence of a large goiter is not itself predictive of a difficult endotracheal intubation. However, multivariate analysis identified the presence of Cormack grade III or IV view and the presence of a cancerous mass as independent predictors of a difficult oral intubation. Potential risk factors for difficult airway management include the body mass index, Mallampati class, thyromental distance, neck mobility, and airway compression.

Thyroid masses within the thorax compromise the airway in the subglottic region by external compression of the trachea or direct extension into the airway. Preoperative imaging studies[94] and flow–volume loops may provide information useful for planning the approach to the airway.

Laryngeal Nerve Monitoring: Anesthetic Implications Several methods have been described to monitor the function of the RLN, which controls the function of the vocal cords and other nerves at risk, such as the external branch of the superior laryngeal nerve, which supplies the cricothyroid muscle and therefore regulates voice pitch.[95,96] Most attention has been devoted to monitoring the RLN. Monitoring techniques generally require some form of direct RLN stimulation. Function following stimulation usually is detected by (1) direct visualization of the cords via a fiberoptic scope (see above), (2) palpation of the larynx during RLN stimulation,[97] (3) EMG monitoring using recording electrodes inserted directly into the laryngeal muscles,[98] or (4) EMG monitoring via endotracheal tubes fitted with external sensing electrodes.[99] Nerve monitoring often has an impact on anesthetic management by the need for a special method of airway control (eg, LMA vs cuffed endotracheal tube) or the need to avoid muscle relaxants as part of the anesthetic technique.

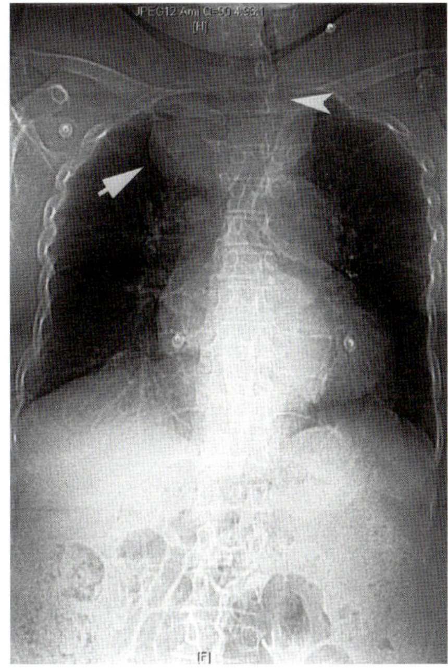
A

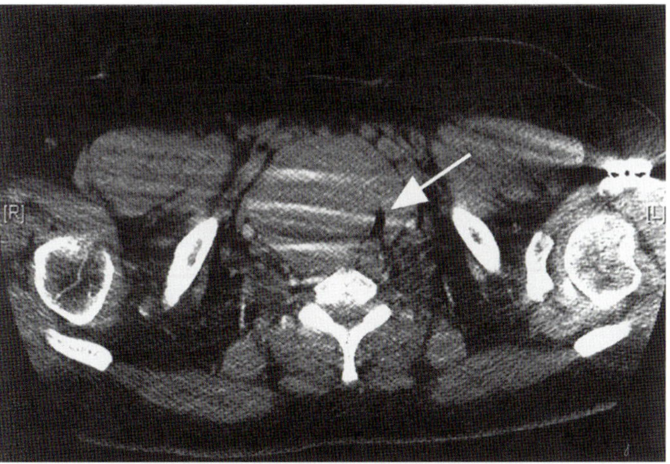
B

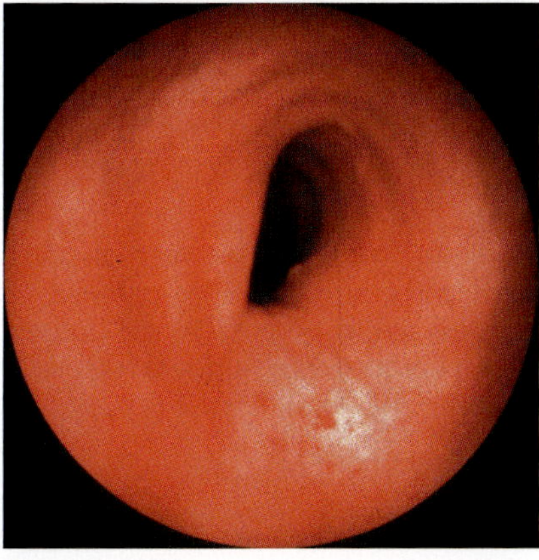
C

FIGURE 60-5. Mediastinal mass compressing and displacing the intrathoracic trachea. **A.** Chest radiograph. Arrow indicates mass. Arrowhead indicates deviated and distorted tracheal lumen. **B.** CT scan from the same patient shown in **A**. Arrow indicates distortion and compression of the tracheal lumen. **C.** Extrinsic tracheal compression by a papillary thyroid cancer demonstrated by rigid bronchoscopy in a different patient. [Fig. 60-5C courtesy of Dr Hermes C. Grillo.]

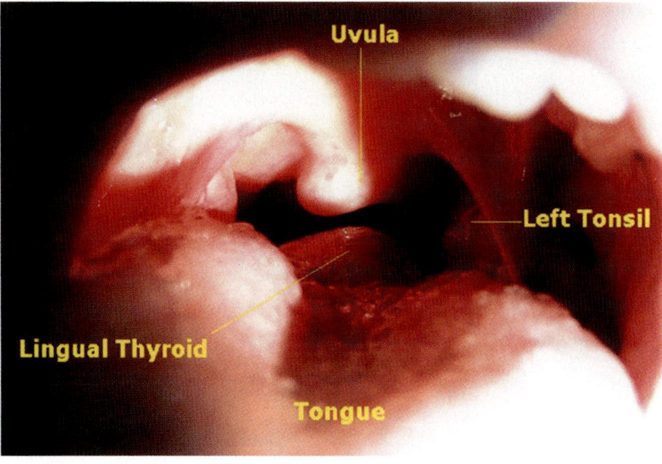

A

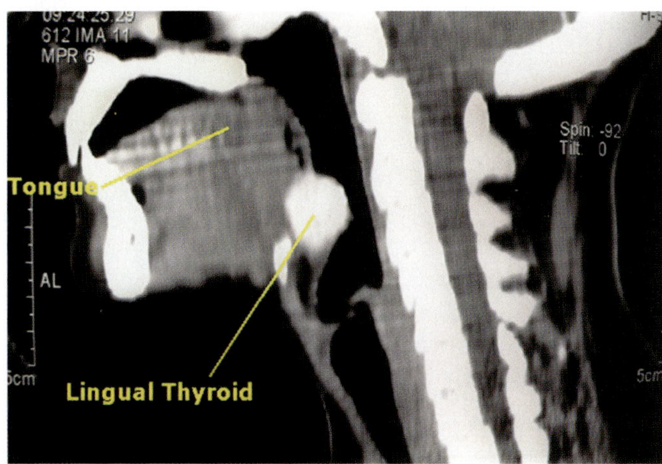

B

FIGURE 60-6. Lingual thyroid tissue obstructing the airway. **A.** Intraoral photograph showing a mass arising at the base of the tongue. The ectopic thyroid tissue may be friable and prone to bleed with manipulation or trauma. **B.** CT scan, midline sagittal image of the same patient shown in **A**. [Images courtesy of Dr B.Y. Ghorayeb, http://www.ghorayeb.com.]

PERIOPERATIVE COMPLICATIONS OF THYROID SURGERY

Laryngeal Nerve Injury A major complication of thyroid surgery that usually appears early (immediately or within hours) in the postoperative period is airway obstruction attributable to RLN injury with resultant narrowing of the glottic opening. A unilateral RLN palsy would not produce significant respiratory compromise if the contralateral nerve and vocal apparatus function normally. However, bilateral nerve palsy, as from a new unilateral RLN injury in the setting of a preexisting deficit on the other side, can produce complete closure of the glottis and respiratory obstruction. Prompt endotracheal intubation may be lifesaving.

Estimates of the overall incidence of unilateral temporary RLN palsy after major thyroid surgery range from 1.2% to 1.4%, to 5.1% to 8.7%.[100-104] Estimates of the incidence of permanent nerve palsies range from 0.4% to 0.6%, to 0.9% to 1.4%.[100-104] Factors associated with an increased likelihood of RLN injury include surgery for thyroid cancer or Graves disease, reoperation, and extensive neck and lymph node dissections. Positive identification of the RLN and documentation of its integrity during the course of surgery are associated with a reduced likelihood of palsies in the postoperative period. Despite extensive investigation, the question of whether intraoperative RLN monitoring confers protection against RLN injury after surgery remains without a definitive answer.[105-114] Monitoring may facilitate visual identification of the RLN,

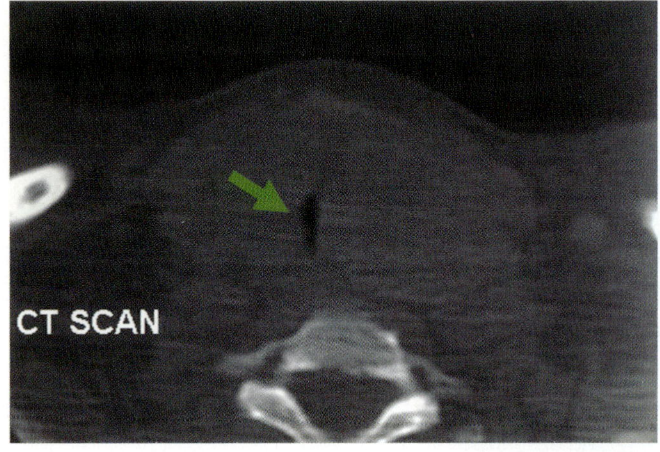

A

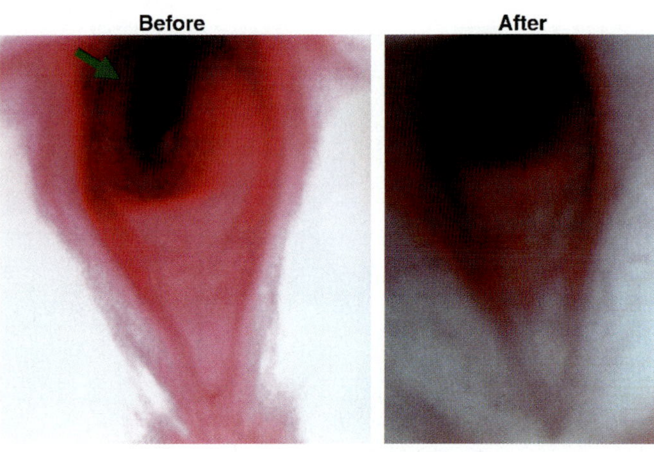

B

FIGURE 60-7. Airway obstruction by a thyroid mass. **A.** CT scan showing tracheal compression. Arrow indicates compressed tracheal lumen at the level of the clavicles. **B.** Endoscopic view of the same patient showing extrinsic narrowing and distortion of the glottis (*arrow*) before surgical resection (*left*) and relief of the obstruction resulting from surgical decompression (*right*).

as in cases of reoperation or anatomic variants of nerve position. Of note, endotracheal intubation alone may account for 7% to 11% of all RLN paralyses.[115]

Hypocalcemia Damage to parathyroid glands during thyroid surgery can cause reduced secretion of parathyroid hormone (PTH), resulting in hypocalcemia. Positive identification of the parathyroid glands at the time of surgical dissection can prevent postoperative hypocalcemia. Estimates of the prevalence of temporary hypocalcemia range from 8.3% to 27.5%, and estimates of permanent hypocalcemia range from 1.7% to 5.1%.[100,101] Patients with acute hypocalcemia can present with paresthesias, muscle cramps, stridor, dysrhythmias, or seizures. Some studies suggest that the circulating PTH level obtained during surgery or in the immediate postoperative period is predictive of laboratory or symptomatic evidence of hypocalcemia.[116,117]

Hemorrhage The thyroid bed is extremely vascular. Inadequate hemostasis may result in the formation of hematomas. Rapid onset of life-threatening airway obstruction is a known complication of thyroid (and parathyroid) surgery. Consideration should be given to prompt intubation to preserve airway patency, even before a return to the operating room for neck exploration. Decompression of the neck at the bedside by opening the wound is a potentially lifesaving option.[95] The use of surgical drains is advocated, at least in selected circumstances, to prevent the accumulation of blood or serous fluid in the closed potential space of the neck.[105]

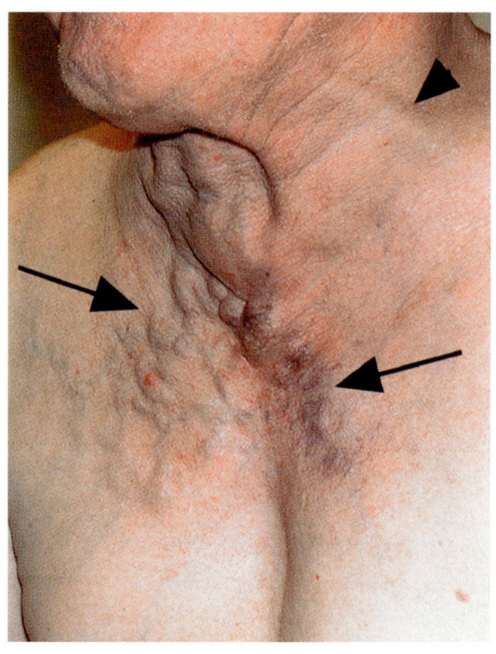

A

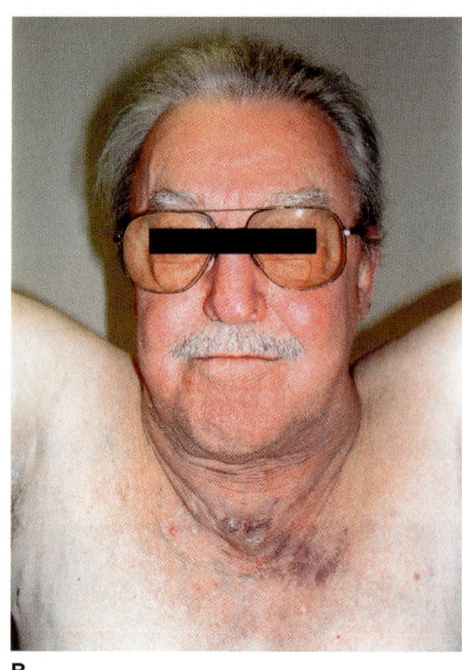

B

FIGURE 60-8. Large cervical and intrathoracic goiter obstructing venous drainage from the head. Note venous engorgement and cutaneous venous varicosities returning blood from the head to the chest (**A**) and facial erythema (**B**). This patient lost more than 5 L of blood during surgery to resect the thyroid mass.

Obstruction of venous drainage from the head by large intrathoracic thyroid masses sometimes results in superior vena cava syndrome (**Fig. 60-8**). Resection of such lesions may be compromised by substantial blood loss.

Positioning Injuries Thyroid surgery typically is accomplished with the patient in the supine position with the neck extended and the arms wrapped and supported at the patient's side (**Fig. 60-9**). Cervical spine conditions may limit the ability to extend the patient's neck safely

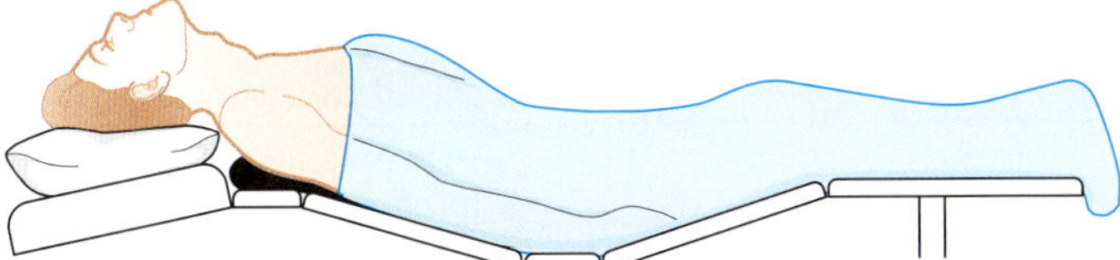

FIGURE 60-9. Patient positioning for thyroid and parathyroid surgery. The patient lies supine with the neck extended, usually by an inflatable pouch positioned under the scapulae ("thyroid bag"). The arms are tucked at the sides or rest on the abdomen. The anesthesiologist has little access to the patient once surgical drapes are placed.

or comfortably. A pressure injury to the occipital nerves has been described in a patient with the potential risk factors of obesity and DM undergoing thyroid surgery.[118] Risk of ulnar neuropathy related to positioning of the arms at the sides with the potential for pressure on the elbow should be considered. In addition, patients with proptosis from Graves ophthalmopathy may be at particular risk for corneal abrasions, drying of the cornea, or pressure injuries to the globe.

PARATHYROID DISEASE AND DISORDERS OF CALCIUM METABOLISM

Patients may present for surgery to treat parathyroid disease (parathyroidectomy) or require surgery in the setting of disorders of calcium homeostasis. Anesthetic considerations for parathyroidectomy substantially overlap with many of the issues encountered in thyroid surgery. These concerns include monitoring of RLN function, risks of postoperative hypocalcemia and postoperative neck hematoma, and positioning.[105,119] Manifestations of renal insufficiency are particularly important for patients presenting for parathyroidectomy to treat secondary or tertiary hyperparathyroidism.

Advanced preoperative imaging techniques facilitate the identification of abnormal parathyroid tissue, sometimes permitting less invasive surgery with achievement of therapeutic goals.[79,105,120] However, failed explorations persist as a surgical problem. Rapid intraoperative immunoassay for PTH can assist the surgeon in determining whether pathologic parathyroid tissue has been identified and removed.[121] In patients with secondary hyperparathyroidism, propofol does not affect PTH levels.[122] It is not known if propofol affects PTH levels in patients with primary or tertiary hyperparathyroidism.

Anesthesia options for parathyroid surgery include general anesthesia with or without endotracheal intubation, and regional anesthesia techniques.[78,82,105,123] One advantage of regional anesthesia is the avoidance of nausea and vomiting, which is common following parathyroid surgery.[124]

IMPLICATIONS OF HYPOCALCEMIA

Hypocalcemia is a feature of many medical conditions (**Table 60-8**). Of particular relevance to the anesthesiologist planning to take a hypocalcemic patient to the operating room are critical illness conditions, including pancreatitis or fat embolism syndrome, hepatic or renal failure, and rhabdomyolysis. Detection of hypocalcemia should provide an impetus to comprehensively evaluate the overall condition of a patient to ascertain whether other significant disorders are present.

Features of hypocalcemia of particular relevance to perioperative management include a predisposition to laryngospasm, cardiac dysrhythmias, muscle weakness, hypotension, congestive heart failure, altered mental status, and coagulopathy (see Chapter 13). Massive transfusion with attendant citrate intoxication, especially in the setting of hepatic insufficiency, is a commonly encountered clinical situation with a significant risk for hypocalcemia that may exacerbate the hemodynamic and metabolic disturbances of complicated surgery. Hypocalcemia should be considered in the differential diagnosis of altered mental status following emergence from a craniotomy.

TABLE 60-8 Causes of Hypocalcemia Significant for the Perioperative Period

Hypoparathyroidism	Critical illness
• Primary	• Alkalosis
• Surgical	• Burns
• Idiopathic	• Toxic shock
• Autoimmune	• Pancreatitis
• Hypomagnesemia	• Fat embolism
• Peripheral resistance (pseudohypoparathyroidism)	Anticonvulsant therapy
• Hemosiderosis	Hypoalbuminemia
• Amyloidosis	Osteoblastic metastases
Hyperphosphatemia	Loop diuretics
• Rhabdomyolysis	Contrast media containing EDTA
• Phosphate therapy	Intestinal malabsorption
• Renal failure	Massive transfusion (citrate intoxication with chelation of calcium)
• Chemotherapy/tumor lysis	
Vitamin D deficiency	
• Hepatic failure	
• Renal failure	
• Lack of sun exposure	
• Dietary deficiency	

EDTA, ethylenediaminetetraacetic acid.

Particularly when symptomatic, hypocalcemia should be treated if total calcium is less than 7.5 g/dL. Of note, alkalosis decreases ionized calcium 0.1 mg/dL (0.25 mEq/L) for every increase of 0.1 pH unit. Total calcium is not affected by pH changes.

Treatment of hypocalcemia in the perioperative setting is best accomplished with IV calcium chloride, although calcium gluconate is another option. Clinicians should recognize that 1 g of calcium chloride solution (13.5 mEq or 273 mg elemental calcium) provides 3 times the amount of elemental calcium present in 1 g of calcium gluconate (4.5 mEq or 93 mg elemental calcium). Serial blood ionized calcium measurements should guide therapy. Of note, concentrated calcium solutions may be caustic to peripheral veins and should be administered cautiously.

IMPLICATIONS OF HYPERCALCEMIA

Hypercalcemia is a feature of many medical conditions (**Table 60-9**). The detection of hypercalcemia warrants evaluation for the possible

TABLE 60-9 Causes of Hypercalcemia Significant for the Perioperative Period

Endocrine	Immobilization
• Hyperparathyroidism (primary, tertiary)	Granulomatous disease
• Hyperthyroidism	• Sarcoidosis
• MEN syndromes	• Histoplasmosis
• Acromegaly	• Coccidiomycosis
• Pheochromocytoma	• Tuberculosis
• Adrenal insufficiency	• Berylliosis
Malignancy	Drugs
• Squamous cell cancers (ie, lung)	• Iatrogenic administration
• Pancreatic cancer	• Theophylline
• Hypernephroma	• Lithium
• Myeloma	• Thiazides
• Breast cancer	• Vitamin D
• Lymphoma/leukemia (rare)	• Antacids (containing calcium)
AIDS	• Vitamin A Paget disease
Renal disease (various)	
Familial/genetic causes (various)	

AIDS, acquired immune deficiency syndrome; MEN, multiple endocrine neoplasia.

TABLE 60-10 Medical Management of Symptomatic and/or Severe Hypercalcemia

Mode of Action	Measure/Substance	Indication	Side Effects/Complications
Intravenous hydration	Isotonic saline administration at 200-300 mL/h (4-6 L/d)	Universal	Volume expansion, hypokalemia, hypomagnesemia
Loop diuretic	Furosemide 20-40 mg, q6-12h, up to 500 mg/d or continuous infusion 100 mg/h with saline infusion	Universal in cases of fluid retention	Hypokalemia, hypomagnesemia
Bisphosphonates	Pamidronate 60-90 mg IV over 4 h	Universal (preferred in HHM)	Fast administration → renal insufficiency
	Zoledronate 4 mg IV over 15 min Repeat every 2-3 wk[a]		Fever, myalgia
Calcitonin	200-500 IU/d subcutaneously	Universal (adjuvant)	Nausea, vomiting, tachyphylaxis
Steroids	Prednisone 40-100 mg/d for 3-5 d	Vitamin D intoxication, sarcoidosis (rarely HHM)	Iatrogenic Cushing syndrome
Hemodialysis (if renal failure)	Ca^{2+}-free dialysate	Hypercalcemic crisis and renal insufficiency	Dialysis related
Diet low in Ca^{2+}/vitamin D	<100 mg Ca^{2+}/d	Universal	None

HHM, humeral hypercalcemia of malignancy.

[a]Reduce bisphosphonate doses in renal insufficiency.

presence of other major physiologic disturbances, including pheochromocytoma, adrenal insufficiency, and acromegaly. Hypercalcemia should be considered in the differential diagnosis of altered mental status in the perioperative period.

Features of hypercalcemia of particular relevance to perioperative management include a predisposition to cardiovascular disturbances, such as dehydration, dysrhythmias, cardiac conduction disturbances, hypertension, catecholamine resistance, and sensitivity to digitalis.

Muscular weakness caused by hypercalcemia can exacerbate respiratory insufficiency. Nervous system manifestations can include seizures or altered sensorium. Positioning should take into account the risk of fracturing osteopenic bone. Urgent treatment of hypercalcemia may be required in the operating room or in the immediate perioperative period. First-line therapy includes IV hydration and diuresis. Treatment modalities are summarized in **Table 60-10**.

PHEOCHROMOCYTOMA AND PARAGANGLIOMA

Pheochromocytomas are neuroendocrine tumors arising from chromaffin cells in the adrenal medulla.[125] These tumors may be benign or malignant. The secretion of vasoactive substances, including the catecholamines (dopamine, norepinephrine, and epinephrine), leads to clinical manifestations of the tumors. Neuroendocrine chromaffin tumors that arise outside of the adrenal medulla are referred to as *paragangliomas.*[126,127] Because the clinical presentation and management issues are similar, the anesthetic implications of pheochromocytoma and paraganglioma are discussed together. Several excellent reviews of the pathophysiology, presentation, and perioperative management of pheochromocytoma appear in the literature.[125-131]

CLINICAL MANIFESTATIONS OF PHEOCHROMOCYTOMA

As reviewed in Chapter 13, the clinical manifestations of a pheochromocytoma in a patient depend on the profile of catecholamine secretion. Tumors secreting primarily norepinephrine are associated with sustained or episodic hypertension. If epinephrine is the major secreted catecholamine, tachycardia, tachydysrhythmias, and hypotension often result. Dopamine is the major catecholamine secreted by some tumors, and hypotension is the significant clinical feature. However, the overall manifestations of pheochromocytoma are variable, often paroxysmal or episodic, and sometimes similar to other conditions such as severe hyperthyroidism[126,127] or preeclampsia.[125] If a patient is diagnosed with pheochromocytoma, rapid, extreme perturbations in hemodynamics or other signs and symptoms can be anticipated and should be promptly and appropriately managed in the operating room, postanesthesia care unit (PACU), or intensive care unit (ICU). The undiagnosed patient poses a significant management challenge in the perioperative period because the differential diagnosis of extreme physiologic perturbations is so extensive and treatments differ markedly.

For the anesthesiologist, particularly salient clinical features of pheochromocytoma are hypertension, tachycardia and dysrhythmias, cardiac ischemia or myocardial dysfunction, insulin resistance with hyperglycemia, intravascular volume depletion, and lactic acidosis. Patients may present in shock, caused by either the secreted products of the tumor or some complication of the disease, such as myocardial infarction, cardiac failure, or dissected/ruptured aorta. Acute manifestations of an unsuspected pheochromocytoma must be considered in the differential diagnosis of many intraoperative clinical scenarios.

PREOPERATIVE PREPARATION

A patient with a known pheochromocytoma scheduled for tumor resection undergoes extensive preparation for the procedure. Preoperative medical management has been reviewed.[125,126,132] The major concerns are as follows:

1. Control of elevated blood pressure
2. Repletion of intravascular volume
3. Assessment of end-organ consequences of the disease (eg, cardiomyopathy)
4. Recognition of the potential impact of conditions associated with a pheochromocytoma (eg, multiple endocrine neoplasia type II, von Hippel-Lindau syndrome)
5. Normalization of glucose and electrolyte levels

A number of regimens have been reported to reduce blood pressure in the preoperative period in preparation for surgery to resect a pheochromocytoma. (See also Chapter 13.) α-Adrenergic blockade has been widely used. Phenoxybenzamine, a nonselective, noncompetitive, α-adrenergic blocker that covalently binds to α-adrenergic receptors, has been a mainstay of therapy.[125,129,130,133] Competitive blockers selective for the α_1 subtype of α-adrenergic receptors (eg, doxazosin) have been used to successfully prepare patients for surgery.[134]

A potential advantage of competitive, selective α_1-blockade is that once the tumor has been resected and excess catecholamine release eliminated, α-adrenergic receptors can return quickly to normal function, for example, in regulating vascular tone and blood pressure. A disadvantage of competitive α-adrenergic blockade is the possibility that massive concentrations of catechols released by the tumor can overwhelm the competitive receptor antagonist, resulting in clinical manifestations including hypertension. Covalent, noncompetitive deactivation of α-adrenergic receptors, as with phenoxybenzamine, can withstand a surge in circulating catechol levels. However, following resection of the tumor and removal of excess circulating catecholamines, permanent deactivation of α-adrenergic receptors by phenoxybenzamine may result in hypotension refractory to α-adrenergic agonists for days until new receptors are synthesized.[126,127,135]

Tachycardia is one consequence of elevated catecholamine levels. β-Adrenergic blockade is commonly used to control tachycardia. However, β-blockade must not be instituted before initiation of α-blockade so that α-adrenergic activation would be unopposed in the vasculature, resulting in dangerous elevation of blood pressure.[136] α-Adrenergic blockade is physiologically complex because activation of α_2-adrenergic receptors, which are presynaptic, reduces catecholamine secretion, whereas activation of α_1-adrenergic receptors, which are postsynaptic, causes vasoconstriction. A theoretical advantage of drugs such as doxazosin lies in their selectivity for α_1-adrenergic receptors so that the normal regulatory activities of presynaptic α_2-receptors are not impaired, as in the case with the nonselective agent phenoxybenzamine. Urapidil, another selective α_1-antagonist deliverable by IV infusion, provides similar advantages.[137]

Other approaches to preoperative control of blood pressure use calcium channel blockers such as nicardipine,[138] the mixed α- and β-receptor antagonist labetalol,[139] infusions of magnesium,[128,140-142] and treatment with metyrosine,[143] which inhibits catecholamine biosynthesis. The aims of preoperative preparation are to prevent an acute hypertensive crisis before entering the operating room and then to minimize catecholamine-induced hemodynamic changes during anesthesia and surgery. With adequate preoperative preparation, which has been defined as a systemic blood pressure stabilized below 160/90 mm Hg with only modest orthostatic hypotension, rare ventricular extrasystoles, and no electrocardiographic evidence of ischemia, perioperative mortality from pheochromocytoma has dropped to less than 3%.[127,133] However, intraoperative hemodynamic lability (both hypertension and hypotension) requiring treatment remains a persistent challenge.[133]

ANESTHESIA FOR PHEOCHROMOCYTOMA RESECTION

Laparoscopy is currently the favored surgical approach for abdominal pheochromocytoma resection.[125,127,144-146] However, open surgery may be required depending on the exact location of the lesion (eg, neck paraganglioma) or the anatomic features of an abdominal tumor. Epidural anesthesia provides one option for hemodynamic control.[140] Infusions of nitroprusside, nitroglycerin, magnesium sulfate, esmolol, fenoldopam, phentolamine, urapidil, dexmedetomidine, and nicardipine are reported to successfully control hemodynamics in a readily titratable fashion (**Table 60-11**).[135,137,138,142,147] Case reports suggest that remifentanil infusions fail to blunt episodes of hemodynamic lability.[148,149] Careful reading of various publications advocating the advantages of particular agents for controlling hemodynamics during pheochromocytoma surgery reveals that, in fact, multiple drugs of different classes often are administered in combination. Appropriate sedation contributes to hemodynamic control in the perioperative period.[125]

During administration of the anesthetic, the usual triggers for hemodynamic activation, such as laryngoscopy, may result in exaggerated hemodynamic responses in a patient with pheochromocytoma. Insufflation of the abdomen with CO_2 for laparoscopy may stimulate the release of catecholamines from tumors,[126] and direct manipulation of the tumor may precipitate the rapid secretion of vasoactive substances.[125,150] Once the major draining vein of the tumor is ligated, plasma catecholamine levels generally decline precipitously. Hypotension often ensues. Volume repletion, infusions of α-adrenergic agonists such as phenylephrine, and cessation of vasodilators can be used to support hemodynamics. However, as discussed in the section on preoperative preparation, phenoxybenzamine produces sustained deactivation of α-adrenergic receptors, which limits the response to phenylephrine. Vasopressin may circumvent this problem.[151] Hypoglycemia should be specifically anticipated and treated as needed.[125,127]

TABLE 60-11 Medications Used in the Perioperative Management of Pheochromocytoma

Drug	Dose	Indication
Phentolamine	2.5-5 mg IV at 1 mg/min, repeated every 5 min until blood pressure is controlled. Constant infusion, 100 mg/500 mL D_5W, infusion rate adjusted to targeted blood pressure	Treatment of acute hypertensive crisis
Nitroprusside	0.5-10 mcg/kg/min IV, infusion rate adjusted to targeted blood pressure	Treatment of acute hypertensive episodes
Nitroglycerin	0.5-10 mcg/kg/min IV, infusion rate adjusted to targeted blood pressure	Treatment of acute hypertensive episodes
Doxazosin	2-16 mg/d, orally	Preoperative preparation
β-Blockers	Atenolol, metoprolol, propranolol, esmolol, labetalol, dose titrated to effect	Used preoperatively only after complete α-adrenergic blockade is achieved. Used intraoperatively for treatment of acute hypertensive episodes or tachycardia
Phenoxybenzamine	20-30 mg/d initially, then can be increased to 60-250 mg/d (1 mg/kg/d in 3 divided doses) until blood pressure is controlled	Preoperative preparation may be achieved in 10-14 d Used for prevention of hypertensive crisis
Nicardipine	20-60 mg/d, 3 divided doses, orally 0.5-10.0 mcg/kg/min IV infusion rate adjusted to targeted blood pressure, or IV bolus 1-2 mg	Preoperative preparation and intraoperative hemodynamic control
$MgSO_4$	Bolus 2-4 g IV Infusion 1-2 g/h IV	Preoperative control of hypertensive crisis Control of intraoperative hemodynamics
Fenoldopam	0.02-0.1 mcg/kg/min IV infusion	Control of intraoperative hemodynamics
Urapidil	10-15 mg/h IV infusion	Preoperative preparation and intraoperative hemodynamic control
α-Methyl-para-tyrosine	Start at 250 mg orally, 4 times per day. Increase to maximum of 4 g/d	Preoperative depletion of catecholamine stores by inhibiting catecholamine synthesis at rate-limiting enzyme. Maximal effect in 2-3 d, start 7-14 d preoperatively

No particular anesthetic technique is specifically indicated, or contraindicated, for pheochromocytoma surgery. Agents known to cause the release of catecholamines, such as ketamine, ephedrine, meperidine, and desflurane, should be used with care or avoided entirely. Whereas neuraxial anesthesia produces sympathectomy (thereby blunting physiologic autonomic responses to surgical stimulation) and may be a useful adjunct to general anesthesia, especially for postoperative analgesia, the release of catecholamines from tumor cells is not prevented by spinal or epidural anesthetics.

The choice of monitors and vascular access should take into account the need to assess volume status and cardiac performance, and the utility of a central route for delivering vasoactive or inotropic drugs. An arterial line likely will be useful.[133] Central venous access and pulmonary arterial catheter insertion remain important considerations. Prys-Roberts[126] reported few pulmonary arterial catheter insertions in a large series of pheochromocytoma resections. Consider the use of intraoperative transesophageal echocardiography (TEE), particularly if there is concern for Takotsubo cardiomyopathy.[129] Volume loss due to surgical bleeding during pheochromocytoma or paraganglioma resection typically is on the order of a few hundred milliliters, although plans for volume access should take into account potential overall volume depletion, especially in the patient who has not been well prepared for surgery, and the location of the tumor. General preparations should include planning for postoperative care in a setting capable of monitoring and treating volume, hemodynamic, and metabolic concerns.

ADRENAL CORTEX AND PERIOPERATIVE MANAGEMENT OF GLUCOCORTICOIDS

Surgeons approach lesions of the adrenal cortex by both laparoscopic and open methods. Anesthetic considerations resemble those for other procedures in the abdomen or retroperitoneum. The physiology of adrenal cortical hormones and pathophysiologic conditions of the adrenal cortex are covered in Chapter 13. In general, an excess or deficiency of the mineralocorticoid aldosterone and of adrenal sex steroids has little impact on perioperative anesthetic management, as long as their existence is recognized and medical management is appropriate, including control of blood pressure and treatment of any electrolyte imbalances.

ADRENALECTOMY FOR PRIMARY ADRENAL HYPERCORTISOLISM

For the patient undergoing surgery on 1 adrenal cortex for primary hyperadrenal cortisolism, anesthesia considerations include the consequences of prolonged production of excess cortisol. Relevant features of this condition are summarized in **Table 60-12**. Hypertension may be particularly difficult to treat during surgery. Plasma glucose levels are likely to be high, requiring therapy. Prolonged excess cortisol levels affect body habitus and can potentially complicate airway management, positioning, and vascular access. Osteoporosis renders the patient at risk for fractures, even with minimal mechanical stress. In general, mineralocorticoid function is preserved in primary adrenal hypercortisolism. Following unilateral adrenalectomy, mineralocorticoid replacement probably is unnecessary. Because the function of the opposite normal adrenal cortex may be suppressed, glucocorticoid replacement will be required in the early postoperative period until the hypothalamic–pituitary–adrenal (HPA) axis recovers. This may take several weeks. Because the half-life of cortisol is several hours, an Addisonian crisis likely will not develop in the operating room. However, glucocorticoid replacement therapy must be started early in the postoperative period.

If the patient undergoes bilateral adrenal resection, replacement of both a glucocorticoid and a mineralocorticoid ultimately will be necessary.[152]

TABLE 60-12 Clinical Features of Glucocorticoid Excess or Deficiency Significant for the Perioperative Period

Glucocorticoid Excess	
Proximal myopathy	Osteoporosis
Muscle wasting	Truncal obesity
Glucose intolerance, diabetes mellitus	Inhibited wound healing
Hypertension	Immunosuppression
Coronary artery disease, peripheral vascular disease	Bowel perforation
Hypervolemia	Gastric ulcers
Hypernatremia	Pancreatitis
Hypokalemia	Behavioral disturbances
Hypercalciuria	Depression
Hypercoagulability	Easy bruising
Glucocorticoid Deficiency	
Postural hypotension	Anorexia
Weakness/fatigue	Nausea/vomiting
Depressed catechol responses	Abdominal pain
Fever	Diarrhea, constipation
Weight loss	Hyperpigmentation

ADRENAL INSUFFICIENCY

As reviewed in Chapter 13, native adrenal cortex function may be absent or suppressed by a variety of conditions. Administration of exogenous glucocorticoid is the most common reason for native adrenal suppression. Key features of adrenal insufficiency are summarized in Table 60-12. Of particular relevance in the perioperative period, adrenal insufficiency warrants consideration in the differential diagnosis of refractory hypotension.

In the 1950s, case reports described perioperative deaths of patients who were chronically treated with glucocorticoids and found to have adrenal atrophy.[153] The concept emerged that patients at risk for adrenal insufficiency should receive glucocorticoid supplementation in the perioperative period. Risk factors for adrenal suppression and perioperative adrenal insufficiency include prolonged glucocorticoid therapy and doses of steroids exceeding prednisone 5 to 7.5 mg/d or equivalent for 3 weeks or longer.[154] **Table 60-13** lists the relative potencies of a variety of common glucocorticoids and their mineralocorticoid activities. Recovery from adrenal cortical suppression is variable but may take up to 1 year. Thus patients treated with glucocorticoids within 12 months of surgery are considered to be at risk for adrenal suppression. Provocative testing with cosyntropin may help identify patients at risk for adrenal suppression, but such evaluation is expensive and cumbersome, and the biochemical results may not correspond to clinical events.[155]

An accepted regimen for perioperative patients that was developed without formal clinical trials calls for the administration of hydrocortisone in "stress" doses. Typically, at least 3 doses of hydrocortisone, 100 mg IV, are administered every 8 hours, followed by tapering of the dose over several days to the patient's baseline steroid regimen. However, this commonly accepted stress-dose steroid regimen has been questioned, based on an increased understanding of physiologic stress responses and glucocorticoid secretion.[155] Baseline normal cortisol production may be as low as 10 to 15 mg/d,[156-158] rather than 30 mg or more as once believed.[159] Thus, even if extreme surgical stresses result in a 10-fold increase in cortisol production,[160] 100 to 150 mg of exogenous cortisol or glucocorticoid equivalent should suffice to sustain hemodynamics and metabolism in the absence of any endogenous HPA axis activity. Of note, Leopold et al[161] did identify larger increases in glucocorticoid production in a group of joint replacement patients; however, these elevations were transient.

The requirement for exogenous glucocorticoid support has been tested in controlled clinical studies of patients chronically treated with steroids.[162-164] The chief end point in these studies was blood pressure or

TABLE 60-13 Relative Potencies of Glucocorticoid and Mineralocorticoid Hormones

Steroid	Glucocorticoid	Mineralocorticoid	Equivalent Dose (mg)	Duration (h)
Short-acting				
Cortisol	1.0	1.0	20	8-12
Cortisone	0.8	0.8	25	8-12
Aldosterone	0.3	3000	–	8-12
Intermediate-acting				
Prednisone	4.0	0.8	5	12-36
Prednisolone	4.0	0.8	5	12-36
Methylprednisolone	5.0	0.5	4	12-36
Fludrocortisone	10.0	125	–	12-36
Long-acting				
Dexamethasone	25-40	0	0.75	>24

heart rate. Withholding steroid supplementation resulted in minimal evidence of hemodynamic instability. Based on these results and the limited number of similar studies in animals and humans, a graded approach to steroid supplementation has been recommended for patients believed to be at risk for adrenal insufficiency in the perioperative period. Recommendations take into account the anticipated magnitude of surgical stress. **Table 60-14** combines the recommendations from several sources.[136,155,165] Of note, prolonged tapering of exogenous glucocorticoid therapy does not appear to be essential, as long as baseline therapy is resumed within a few days of surgery.[166] These recommendations should not necessarily be taken to apply to critically ill patients who come to the operating room from an ICU setting. Some evidence suggests that adrenal insufficiency occurs in at least some critically ill patients,[154] particularly those with sepsis. Such patients may require large doses of supplemental steroids for prolonged periods.

ETOMIDATE

The favorable hemodynamic properties of the IV induction agent etomidate give this drug an important place in the anesthesiologist's armamentarium. However, unique among all anesthetic agents, etomidate inhibits the mitochondrial enzyme 11β-hydroxylase, an essential enzyme in the biosynthetic pathway for steroids. An induction dose of etomidate reduces cortisol and aldosterone production for approximately 8 hours. Repeated doses or infusions of etomidate have more prolonged suppressant effects on steroid production, which may become clinically relevant. Consequently, the use of etomidate should be evaluated in the context of the patient's adrenal reserve. Interestingly, prolonged administration of etomidate has been used as a therapeutic strategy to control glucocorticoid levels in severe Cushing disease.[167]

PITUITARY DISEASES AND PITUITARY SURGERY

ANATOMY OF THE PITUITARY GLAND

The pituitary gland lies within a recess of the sphenoid bone, the sella turcica. The gland is composed of 2 major subdivisions, the anterior pituitary and the posterior pituitary. Magnetic resonance imaging (MRI) readily visualizes these structures because the posterior pituitary appears as a bright spot on T1 weighted images, as shown in the sagittal view in **Fig. 60-10**A. Structures next to the pituitary are shown in the coronal view in Fig. 60-10B.

The posterior pituitary contains axon terminals of specialized neurons arising within the supraoptic and paraventricular nuclei of the hypothalamus. These nerves secrete oxytocin and vasopressin (antidiuretic hormone [ADH]). Thus the posterior pituitary is a direct extension of the brain. In contrast, the anterior pituitary derives embryologically from the Rathke pouch; it is composed primarily of epithelial cells. It does not have direct neuronal connections to the brain. The anterior pituitary

TABLE 60-14 Suggested Perioperative Steroid Supplementation With Hydrocortisone in Patients With Chronic Adrenal Insufficiency

Anticipated Surgical Stress	Preoperative	Intraoperative	Postoperative
Minor[a]	25 mg or usual dose	None, unless complications	Resume usual replacement POD 1
Moderate[b]	50-75 mg or usual steroid dose, whichever is higher	50 mg IV	20 mg IV q8h on POD 1, then resume preoperative replacement dose on POD 2
Major[c]	100-150 mg or usual steroid dose, whichever is higher, within 2 h of start of procedure	50 mg IV q8h after initial dose	50 mg IV q8h, or 150 mg continuously over 24 h for 2-3 d, then reduce dose by 50% per day until preoperative regimen is reached

POD, postoperative day.

[a]Inguinal herniorrhaphy, minor urologic or gynecologic procedures, oral surgery, plastic surgery.

[b]Total joint replacement, open cholecystectomy, lower extremity revascularization.

[c]Thoracotomy, cardiac surgery, major abdominal surgery.

Note that these guidelines may not meet the requirements of all patients, and perioperative or stress steroid replacement should be individually tailored.

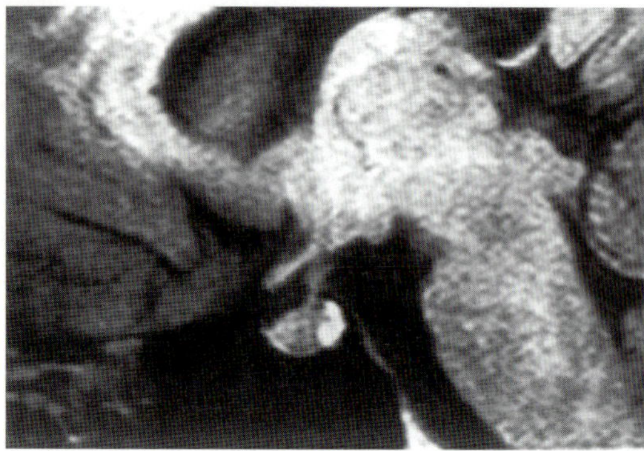

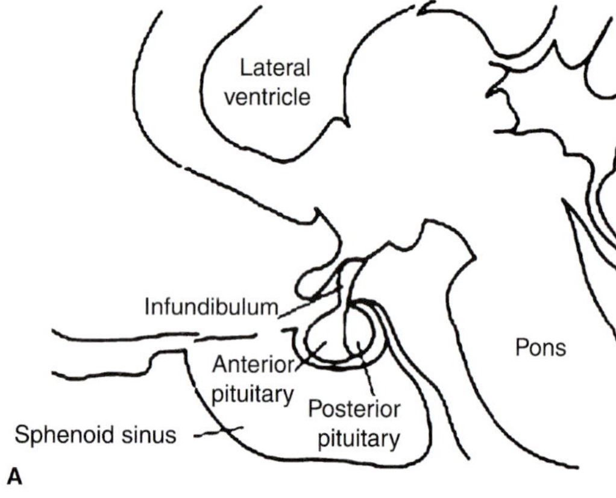

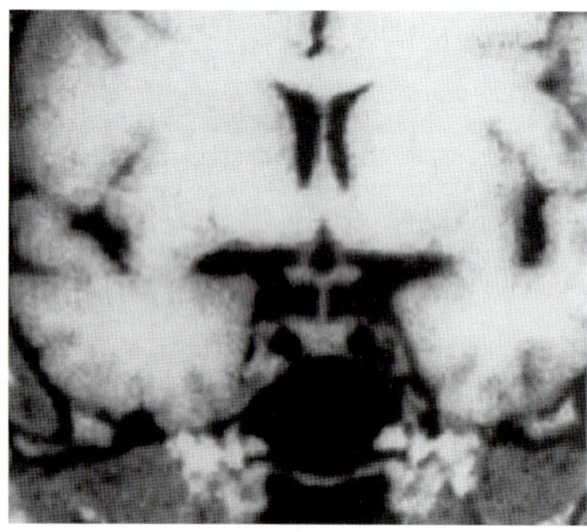

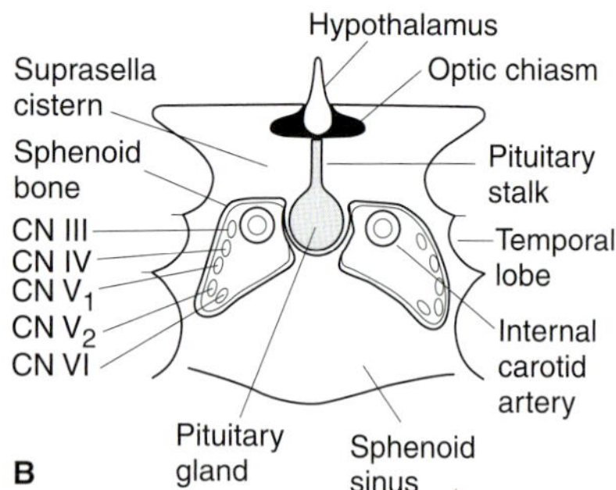

FIGURE 60-10. Anatomic relationships of the normal pituitary gland. **A.** Sagittal view. **B.** Coronal view.

is dependent on a vascular conduit, the pituitary portal plexus, which directly links the hypothalamus to the anterior pituitary gland. The portal plexus is a venous plexus and is the major source of blood flow to the anterior pituitary, which has little or no arterial blood supply.

PITUITARY LESIONS

Pituitary lesions can be placed in broad categories according to their functional effects. Lesions can cause mass effects, anterior pituitary hyperfunction, or anterior pituitary hypofunction.

Pituitary adenomas arise from anterior pituitary cells; therefore, they almost always are located in the sella turcica. They compose approximately 10% to 15% of all intracranial neoplasms. Adenomas less than 1 cm in diameter typically are referred to as *microadenomas*, whereas adenomas with diameters of 1 cm or greater are commonly referred to as *macroadenomas*.[168,169] Macroadenomas and some microadenomas can be visualized by MRI following IV infusion of gadolinium. Autopsy studies reveal that 25% of individuals have asymptomatic pituitary adenomas. Only adenomas with endocrine syndromes as a result of hyposecretion or hypersecretion, or that cause symptomatic mass effects on adjacent brain structures, come to medical attention. The prevalence of diagnosed pituitary adenomas is 8.9:100 000.[169]

In addition to pituitary tumors, many other masses appear in the sella or parasellar region.[168,170] Meningiomas, craniopharyngiomas, chordomas, and metastatic carcinomas occasionally appear as pituitary masses. Benign sellar cysts derive primarily from the Rathke cleft; they frequently are asymptomatic and are found incidentally. Infiltrative diseases mimicking masses in the pituitary include sarcoidosis, lymphocytic hypophysitis, histiocytosis X, and tuberculosis.

Classification of Pituitary Adenomas Pituitary adenomas are classified by either their hypersecretory product or their lack of hormonal secretion (nonsecretory pituitary adenomas).[168,170] Some tumors secrete more than 1 pituitary hormone (plurihormonal adenomas). The most common combination seen in these tumors is GH and prolactin.[171] Other pituitary adenomas do not secrete bioactive hormone but may secrete the α- or β-subunits of the glycoprotein hormones luteinizing hormone (LH), follicle-stimulating hormone (FSH), or thyroid-stimulating hormone (TSH).

Clinical Symptoms of Pituitary Masses Because the pituitary gland lies adjacent to the cavernous sinus, temporal lobes, and sphenoid sinus (**Figs. 60-10** and **60-11**), the presentation of pituitary lesions occasionally

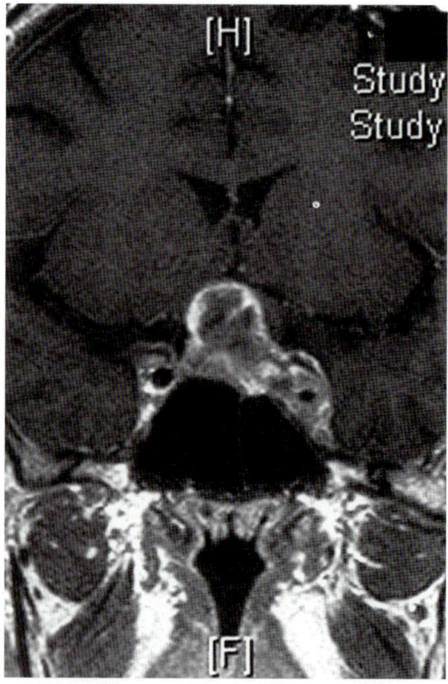

FIGURE 60-11. Pituitary mass encroaching on nearby structures. Coronal magnetic resonance imaging shows a large pituitary mass extending laterally, encasing and narrowing the left carotid artery within the cavernous sinus and abutting the left temporal lobe.

TABLE 60-15 Clinical Signs and Symptoms of Pituitary Lesions

Direction of Tumor Expansion	Neighboring Structures	Symptoms of Compression
Upward	Optic pathways	Visual field cuts, blindness
	Hypothalamus	Disturbed temperature autoregulation
	Olfactory nerve	Anosmia
Lateral	Cavernous sinus	Proptosis, eyelid edema
	Internal carotid	Hemiplegia, altered level of consciousness
	Oculomotor nerve	Ophthalmoplegia, ptosis, pupil defects
	Abducens, trochlear nerves	Ophthalmoplegia
	Ophthalmic nerve	Facial pain, corneal anesthesia
Downward	Sphenoid sinus	Epistaxis, cerebrospinal fluid rhinorrhea

includes other clinical symptoms (**Table 60-15**). Palsies of extraocular muscles, sensory disturbances in the first and second branches of the fifth cranial nerve, temporal lobe seizures, and cerebrospinal fluid (CSF) rhinorrhea may bring a patient to medical attention.[168] Disorders of both the hypothalamus and pituitary can compress or infiltrate the optic chiasm, resulting in a variety of visual field abnormalities affecting peripheral vision (superolateral visual field defect).

PITUITARY HYPOFUNCTION: CAUSES, PRESENTATION, AND TREATMENT OF HYPOPITUITARISM

Causes of Deficient Pituitary Hormone Secretion Many disorders cause hypopituitarism by affecting either the hypothalamus or the pituitary gland. Pituitary adenomas are the most common cause of hypopituitarism.[168,172] Other less common causes are listed in **Table 60-16**.

Diagnosis of Deficient Pituitary Hormone Secretion Although the diagnosis of some pituitary deficiencies can be inferred based on history and clinical findings, demonstrating hormone deficiencies by biochemical testing is essential to establishing the diagnosis of hypopituitarism. A more detailed description of hypothyroidism and cortisol insufficiency can be found in the thyroid and adrenal sections of Chapter 13. A variety of tests can be performed to evaluate the reserve of each of the pituitary hormones. It is extremely important to make the diagnosis of adrenocorticotropic hormone (ACTH) and/or TSH deficiency, because these anterior pituitary hormones are essential to surviving perioperative stress.[168,172] Destruction of the posterior pituitary, stalk compression, or stalk section results in a complete or relative lack of ADH. ADH causes the renal tubules to reabsorb water. Lack of ADH results in failure to concentrate urine, producing dilute urine (low specific gravity and low osmolality), despite dehydration with an elevated blood osmolality. Urine output can exceed 1 to 2 L/h, resulting in severe dehydration, hypernatremia, and vascular collapse.[172,173]

TABLE 60-16 Disorders That Can Cause Hypopituitarism

Benign Neoplasms	Malignant Neoplasms	Cysts
Pituitary adenoma Craniopharyngioma Meningioma Optic nerve glioma	Germ cell tumors (germinoma) Lymphoma Plasmacytoma Metastatic disease (breast, lung)	Arachnoid Dermoid Epidermoid Rathke cleft
Granulomatous Disease	**Vascular Disorders**	**Infections**
Eosinophilic granuloma Histiocytosis Sarcoidosis	Aneurysm Cavernous angioma Infarction (postpartum, diabetes mellitus)	Abscess Cysticercosis Tuberculosis
Autoimmune	**Traumatic**	**Other**
Lymphocytic hypophysitis Vasculitis	Pituitary stalk transection	Cerebral edema Pituitary apoplexy

Treatment of Deficient Pituitary Hormone Secretion The aim of treatment is to replace the hormonal deficiencies needed for normal function and to treat the underlying disease process.[168,173] In most instances, replacement of hormone deficiencies can be accomplished by oral, IV, cutaneous (skin patch), subcutaneous, or nasal administration of deficient hormones. The dose usually is the same from day to day, with the exception of glucocorticoid replacement, which must be increased during times of stress (see the section Adrenal Cortex and Perioperative Management of Glucocorticoids for a detailed discussion of baseline and stress doses of glucocorticoids). As a general rule, glucocorticoid replacement therapy should be given first. Thyroid hormone replacement therapy should never be given before glucocorticoids have been replaced in order to avoid precipitating an Addisonian crisis.[168,173]

PITUITARY HYPERSECRETION AND NEOPLASIA

Pathophysiologic causes of pituitary hormone hypersecretion include hyperplasia of 1 or more cell types in the anterior pituitary, driven by the excessive production of hypothalamic releasing factors. Tumors in the hypothalamus (hamartomas, gangliocytomas) or in the periphery (carcinoids, islet cell tumors) may secrete these factors. However, the most common cause for pathologic hypersecretion of anterior pituitary hormones is pituitary adenoma.[168,170] The most common pituitary adenoma is a prolactinoma.[174] The lesions with greatest significance for anesthetic management are corticotroph and somatotroph adenomas.

Prolactinomas The prolactinoma is the most common pituitary adenoma.[174] In women most tumors present as microadenomas, whereas in men macroadenomas predominate. Symptoms due to compression of local structures thus are generally found in men.[168] Signs and symptoms associated with hyperprolactinemia mainly relate to reproductive tissues and function, including amenorrhea and impotence.

Treatment of patients with a prolactinoma depends on the size of the adenoma and the degree of symptoms. If the adenoma is small and endocrine consequences are minor, management is conservative because most lesions will not enlarge. Adenomas requiring therapy generally respond to medical management with the dopamine agonists bromocriptine or cabergoline.[168,176] By stimulating D_2 receptors on the adenoma, these drugs cause a reduction in tumor size and inhibit prolactin synthesis and secretion. Most adenomas will regrow, however, if therapy is stopped. If tumors resist medical therapy, transsphenoidal (TSP) surgery is performed. Surgical success rates are high for microadenomas (>70%), but postoperative recurrence may reach 50% over 5 years.[176] Macroadenomas are difficult to cure by surgery, with success rates of approximately 30%. Conventional external radiation is not very effective and is used as a last resort.[168,176]

Somatotroph Adenomas GH hypersecretion is almost always due to a pituitary adenoma. GH hypersecretion causes gigantism in children and adolescents (before closure of the epiphyses) and acromegaly in adults. Acromegaly, largely a disorder of middle age, has a peak incidence between the ages of 40 and 50 years. If untreated, it is associated with a 2- to 3-fold increased mortality due to cardiovascular disease (hypertension, cardiomyopathy, arrhythmias, stroke), cancer (especially adenocarcinoma of the colon), and respiratory impairment.[170]

Acromegaly leads to profound physical deformity due to skeletal overgrowth (bone and cartilage) and fibroblast proliferation under the influence of insulin-like growth factor (IGF)-1. This is particularly manifested in the facial bones, where enlargement of the mandible results in

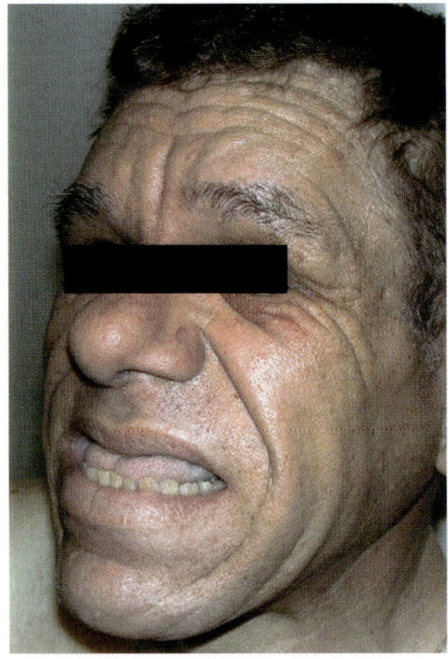

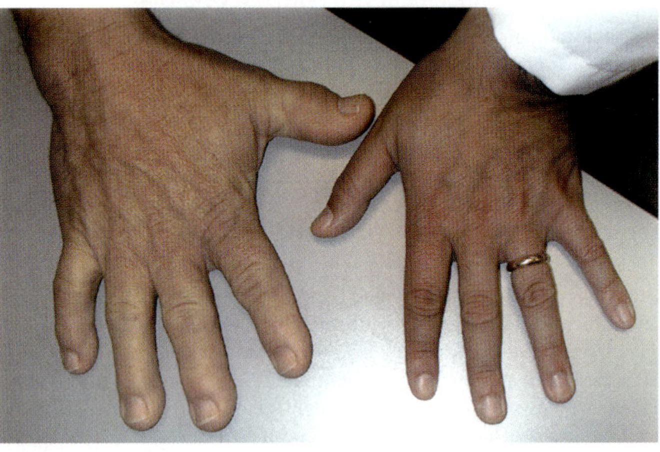

FIGURE 60-12. Patient with acromegaly: bony tissue changes. **A.** Face view. Note the coarsening of the features with jaw prominence and distortion of the tooth occlusion. Also note the large nose and tongue. **B.** Hand view of acromegalic patient (*left*) and normal adult (*right*).

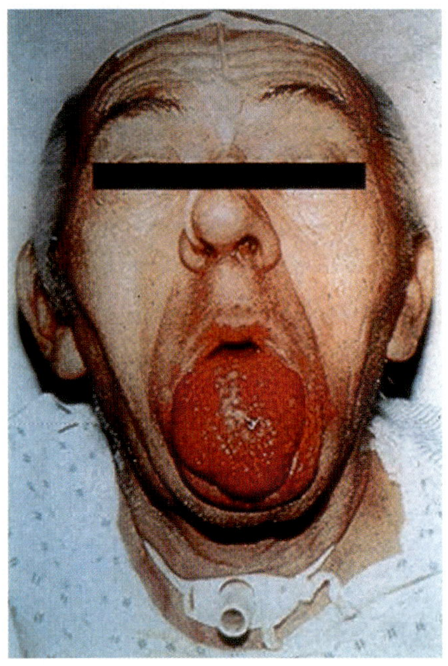

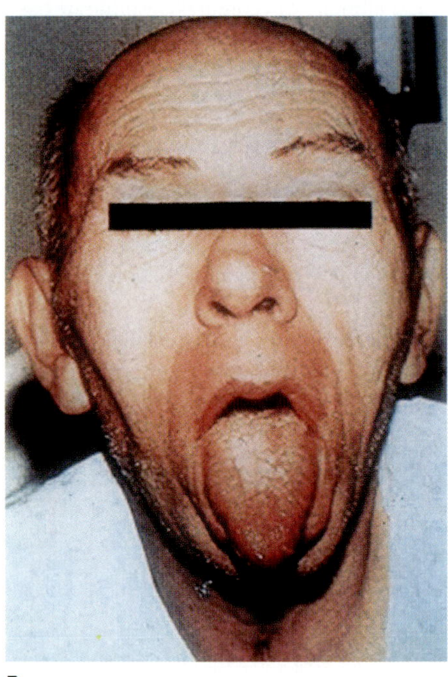

FIGURE 60-13. Soft tissue changes in a patient with acromegaly: tongue enlargement. **A.** Before treatment. The large tongue obstructs the airway. The patient received a tracheostomy. **B.** After treatment. Soft tissue changes have substantially reversed, allowing decannulation of the tracheostomy.

protrusion of the jaw (prognathism), dental malocclusion, and often an increased space between the teeth (**Fig. 60-12**). Facial features are thickened, coarsened, or swollen, making skin creases very pronounced, partly due to sodium and water retention and increased glycosaminoglycan accumulation in the skin. The lips, tongue, and tissue in the posterior pharynx become very large (**Fig. 60-13**). Increased cartilaginous growth contributes to the very prominent nose. Enlargement of the hands and feet result in the common complaint that ring, glove, and shoe sizes increase. Arthralgias are particularly common (75%) due to cartilaginous overgrowth in the joints, resulting in misalignment and destabilization of the joints and ultimately joint destruction. Other manifestations of acromegaly are listed in the **Table 60-17**. It is important to make the diagnosis of acromegaly early to prevent irreversible, devastating complications.[168]

Because of the insidious nature of the disease and delays in diagnosis, most individuals with acromegaly have macroadenomas when they come to medical attention. Approximately 30% have microadenomas. TSP surgery successfully removes approximately 80% of microadenomas. Only approximately 30% of individuals with macroadenomas have a surgical cure.[168] Radiation therapy is only partly successful in reducing GH hypersecretion to normal, although preliminary data using radiosurgery therapy suggest a 60% cure rate over 4 years. Several medical treatments have become available to control GH hypersecretion and, in some cases, tumor growth. These medications, which include somatostatin analogues and blockers of dopamine receptors, can be given singly or in combination.

Successful treatment of acromegaly results in the reduction of left ventricular hypertrophy and some improvement of diastolic function (increase in transmitral peak flow velocity and decreased isovolumic

TABLE 60-17 Manifestations of Acromegaly

General	Cardiovascular	Gastrointestinal
Soft tissue swelling Acral enlargement	Hypertension Cardiac enlargement Congestive heart failure Ischemic heart disease	Colonic polyps Enlarged colon Colon cancer
Musculoskeletal	**Respiratory**	**Neurologic**
Arthralgia Arthritis Prognathism	Tongue enlargement Sleep apnea Somnolence	Paresthesias Carpel tunnel syndrome
Cutaneous	**Psychological**	**Metabolic**
Increased sweating Acne Skin tags	Depression Decreased vigor	Diabetes mellitus Hyperlipidemia Hypercalcemia

Adapted from Harris AG. *Acromegaly and Its Management*. New York, NY: Lippincott-Raven; 1996.

TABLE 60-18 Medical Therapy for Cushing Disease

Drug	Mechanism of Action
Ketoconazole	Antifungal agent. Blocks cholesterol side-chain cleavage to reduce cortisol.
Metyrapone	Inhibits 11β-hydroxylase to reduce cortisol. May cause hypertension and hypokalemia due to increase in 11-deoxycorticosterone and hirsutism due to increased androgens.
Aminoglutethimide	Often used with metyrapone to reduce side effects. Inhibits cholesterol side-chain cleavage and 11-/18-hydroxylation.
Mitotane	Destructive to adrenal cortex. Frequent adverse reactions.
Mifepristone (RU-486)	Glucocorticoid antagonist (not available in the United States).

relaxation time).[177,178] However, skeletal and soft-tissue changes persist and may pose challenges when patients require surgery and anesthesia for conditions other than their pituitary disease.

Corticotroph Adenoma Cushing disease is the condition of excess ACTH secretion from the pituitary gland. The major cause is pituitary adenoma. Table 60-12 summarizes the clinical characteristics of glucocorticoid excess relevant to perioperative management.

Pituitary secretion of ACTH normally is under negative feedback inhibition by circulating cortisol. ACTH and cortisol can be suppressed in individuals with ACTH-secreting pituitary adenomas when they receive sufficiently large doses of exogenous glucocorticoids. Dexamethasone, a semisynthetic steroid, is often used for this purpose because it does not interfere with cortisol radioimmunoassays. By administering graded doses of dexamethasone (Liddle test) to individuals suspected of having Cushing syndrome and measuring ACTH and cortisol levels, it is possible to distinguish individuals having ACTH-secreting adenomas, adrenal adenomas, and ectopic ACTH secretion (eg, oat cell carcinoma, medullary thyroid carcinoma, islet cell tumors, pheochromocytoma) from individuals who simply are obese, stressed, or abuse alcohol.

Alternatively, measurement of a late-night plasma or salivary cortisol level can be used to distinguish individuals with Cushing disease from normal individuals. This discrimination is based on the normal physiologic diurnal variation of cortisol levels, which peak at around 8 AM and have their nadir at around midnight. Thus a normally suppressed midnight cortisol level excludes the diagnosis of Cushing disease. In some patients, midnight cortisol levels are elevated, but MRI fails to demonstrate a pituitary adenoma (60% of cases due to the small size of ACTH-secreting pituitary adenomas; macroadenomas are rare). In this situation, a corticotropin-releasing hormone (CRH) stimulation test can be performed with sampling of venous blood draining the pituitary gland.

Treatment of Cushing disease is primarily surgical, with removal of the pituitary adenoma by TSP surgery. For individuals not cured by surgery, treatment options include conventional radiation or radiosurgery therapy, with or without medical therapy. Medications used in the management of Cushing disease and their mechanisms of action are summarized in **Table 60-18**.

Thyrotroph Adenomas Thyrotroph adenomas are rare pituitary adenomas.[168,170] Most of these tumors are macroadenomas; therefore, they may be associated with mass effects. Their principal clinical presentation is thyrotoxicosis due to excessive TSH secretion. A goiter occurs in more than 90% of cases. Graves disease is often misdiagnosed in these patients. Inappropriately elevated TSH levels (for the levels of thyroid hormones) and the absence of ophthalmopathy allow differentiation between the 2 disorders. Surgery is the primary therapy for a thyrotroph adenoma, but complete removal often is difficult because of the large size of these tumors. Radiation therapy and/or medical therapy with octreotide are used for treating persistent disease. Octreotide is very effective in reducing TSH secretion to normal and reversing thyrotoxicosis, but is not very effective in shrinking tumors.

Nonsecreting Adenomas Most (90%) nonsecreting pituitary adenomas are actually glycoprotein hormone–producing adenomas, manufacturing various subunits of glycoprotein hormones including α-subunit, β-LH, and β-FSH.[171] Because these subunits are biologically inactive, clinical syndromes usually are not observed. As a result, most of these tumors come to medical attention because of mass effects and/or hypopituitarism.

Treatment depends on the size of the adenoma. Small adenomas do not necessarily require treatment if they do not compress local structures or cause hypopituitarism. Periodic MRI can assess their rate of growth. Large tumors are treated by TSP surgery. Bulky residual or recurrent tumor is treated by radiotherapy. Complete resection of the tumor is not necessary. Relief of compressive symptoms is adequate. If hypopituitarism persists following surgery or is caused by surgery, replacement therapy is given. Occasionally, anterior pituitary function recovers after decompression of the residual normal anterior pituitary cells.[168]

ANESTHETIC CONSIDERATIONS FOR PITUITARY SURGERY

Most sellar lesions are accessible by a TSP approach.[173,179-181] The nares is the preferred route for entering the sella (**Fig. 60-14**A). However, this approach may not be anatomically feasible, so the surgeon may achieve adequate exposure by dissecting over the palate with an incision above the maxillary teeth (sublabial approach; Fig. 60-14B). Consequently, the surgeon and anesthesiologist share the head during TSP surgery. General endotracheal anesthesia is indicated. To prevent the accumulation of secretions, blood, or CSF in the airway or stomach, a throat pack typically is inserted.

Preoperative assessment requires an understanding of the implications of the patient's endocrine condition. Nonsecreting adenomas, prolactinomas, and the rare adenomas secreting glycoprotein hormones generally have little impact on anesthetic management. Patients with Cushing disease may have all the features of sustained cortisol excess. Potential anesthetic concerns with these patients include airway management, positioning, glucose and electrolyte disturbances, and control of blood pressure. Some patients with Cushing disease have refractory hypertension that poses a significant treatment challenge.

Patients with acromegaly have a propensity for ischemic cardiac disease as well as myocardial dysfunction. Cardiac status should be specifically assessed before surgery. Because of the skeletal and soft tissue

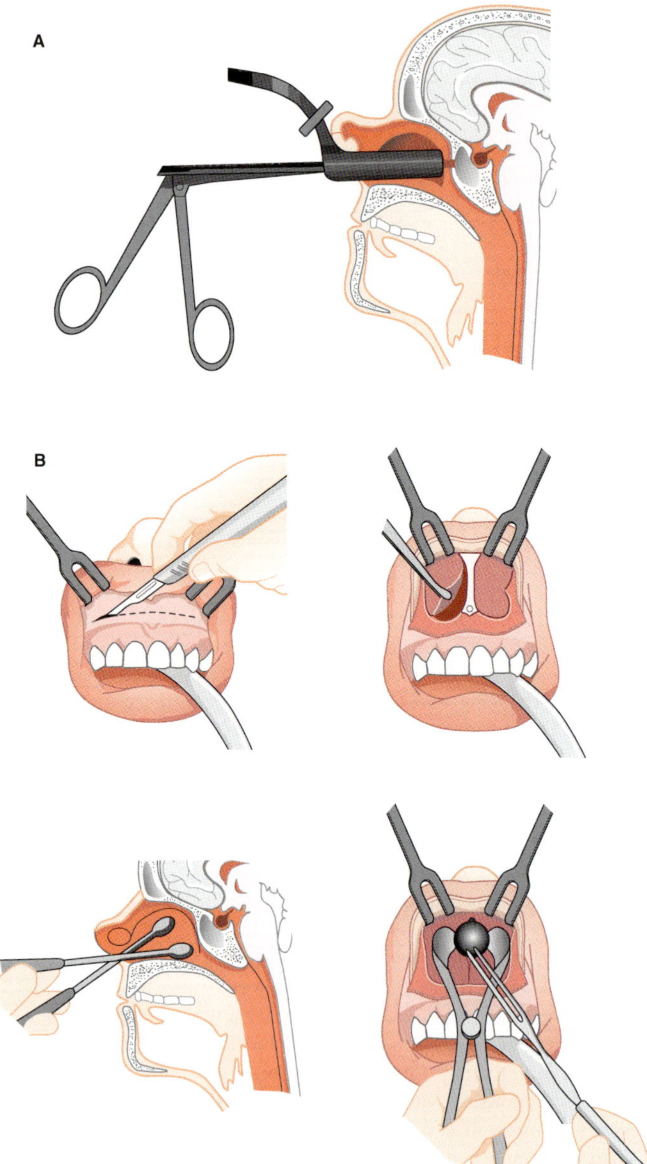

FIGURE 60-14. Transsphenoidal approach to the sella turcica for pituitary surgery. **A.** Following induction of general anesthesia, the surgeon inserts a speculum into the nares. Instruments are manipulated through the speculum. The sphenoid bone is breached to expose the sella and the pituitary gland within. **B.** If a nasal approach is not anatomically feasible, the sella can be accessed over the roof of the mouth (sublabial approach) following an incision above the maxillary teeth. [From Molitch M. Neuroendocrinology and pituitary disease. In: *Atlas of Clinical Endocrinology*. Vol. 4. Philadelphia, PA: Current Medicine; 2000, with permission.]

effects of sustained exposure to GH, patients with acromegaly may present substantial challenges in airway management. Mask ventilation and conventional direct laryngoscopy may be difficult or impossible (**Fig. 60-15**). Advanced airway management devices may be required. Consideration should be given to awake fiberoptic intubation in selected patients.

For most patients undergoing TSP surgery, standard monitoring and routine IV access suffice.[173] The addition of an arterial line may be indicated for patients with comorbidities, or Cushing disease or acromegalic patients with refractory hypertension or cardiac issues. Volume loss likely will be minimal, so large-bore IV access usually is unnecessary. However, the sella is situated near major vascular structures, and the need to augment IV access may develop during surgery.

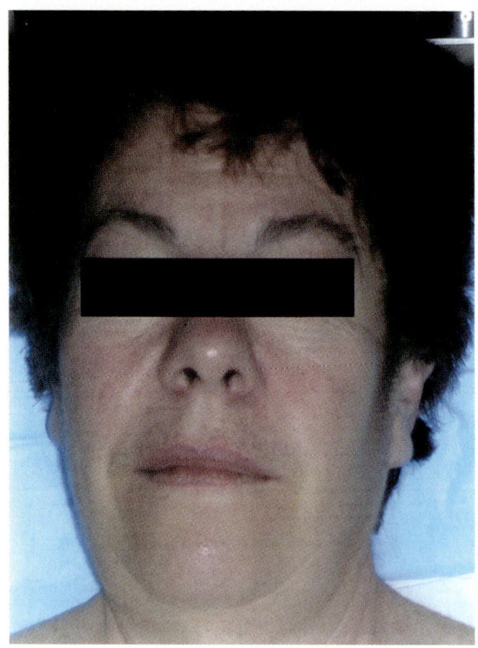

A

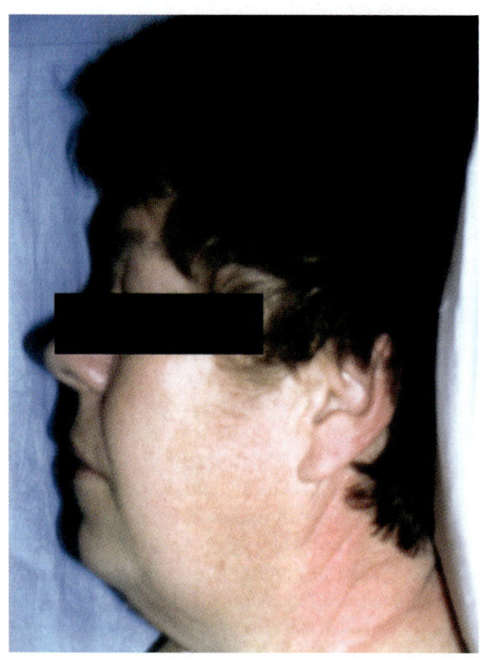

B

FIGURE 60-15. Patient with acromegaly who could not be intubated by conventional means. This woman lacked symptoms of airway obstruction. There was little external evidence of excessive airway soft tissue. With induction of general anesthesia, a mask airway was established with only moderate difficulty. Attempts at direct laryngoscopy by experienced anesthesiologists with different blades failed to produce any view of recognizable glottic structures. Excess soft tissue prevented the insertion of a fiberoptic scope into the trachea. The patient emerged from anesthesia without airway compromise; the planned surgery was cancelled. **A.** Frontal face photograph. **B.** Profile photograph.

The transnasal TSP surgical procedure is only moderately stimulating, and postoperative pain control requirements are modest.[172] Early hypertension during the surgical procedure may be a result of the application of vasoconstrictors to the nasal mucosa by the surgeon, with subsequent systemic effects. Watch for hypotension if the patient is positioned with the head elevated. Surgical procedures generally terminate abruptly, so the anesthesiologist must titrate drugs carefully to permit a prompt and smooth emergence. It is highly desirable for the patient to be able to maintain his or her own airway without support or the need for bag-mask positive-pressure ventilation following extubation. The dura has been opened at the surgical site, which now communicates with the nasal passages. Positive-pressure ventilation can, in theory, cause the introduction of air or infectious material through the dural opening into the CSF space.

Some centers use intraoperative MRI techniques to assist the surgeon in gauging the extent of dissection or resection. This poses some additional concerns for easy access to the patient's airway. In addition, preparations include ensuring the availability of MRI-compatible equipment (eg, monitoring devices and the anesthesia machine itself).

POSTOPERATIVE CARE AFTER PITUITARY SURGERY

Patients are at risk for diabetes insipidus immediately after surgery.[173,182] Monitoring includes frequent determinations of serum sodium levels and meticulous recording of daily weight and fluid balance, with hourly measurement of urine output and assessment of urine specific gravity every 4 hours. A triphasic course is often seen. Early ADH deficiency is attributed to immediate perioperative neuronal damage, followed a few days later by excess ADH release and associated hyponatremia from retrograde neuronal death and release of ADH stores. Finally, permanent deficiency of ADH develops with return of diabetes insipidus.

The vasopressin analogue desmopressin should be administered postoperatively when urine output exceeds fluid intake and the serum sodium level rises. Careful monitoring of body weight, fluid balance, urine specific gravity, and plasma sodium level should continue daily to avoid electrolyte abnormalities. Desmopressin therapy starts with a single dose at bedtime in a patient diagnosed with partial central diabetes insipidus to avoid hyponatremia. Patients with acromegaly can have salt and water diuresis after successful tumor removal. Such patients should not be immediately treated with vasopressin.

With the exception of patients with Cushing disease, all patients undergoing pituitary surgery should be placed on steroids appropriate for surgical stress. The rate of decrease in steroid dose should be guided by clinical and hemodynamic status after surgery. In an uncomplicated postoperative course, taper steroids to physiologic replacement doses over 2 to 3 days. Patients with Cushing disease should not be placed on glucocorticoid replacement immediately after surgery, but cortisol levels should be checked every 6 hours and replacement therapy initiated as needed.

KEY REFERENCES

- Brown CJ, Buie WD. Perioperative stress dose steroids: do they make a difference? *J Am Coll Surg.* 2001;193:678-686.
- Connery LE, Coursin DB. Assessment and therapy of selected endocrine disorders. *Anesthesiol Clin North America.* 2004;22:93-123.
- Cooper DS. Hyperthyroidism. *Lancet.* 2003;362:459-468.
- Coursin DB, Connery LE, Ketzler JT. Perioperative diabetic and hyperglycemic management issues. *Crit Care Med.* 2004;32 (4 Suppl):S116-S125.
- Eckel RH, Grundy SM, Zimmet PZ. The metabolic syndrome. *Lancet.* 2005;365:1415-1428.
- Hirsch IB. Insulin analogues. *N Engl J Med.* 2005;352:174-183.
- Jabbour SA. Steroids and the surgical patient. *Med Clin North Am.* 2001;85:1311-1317.
- Kinney MA, Narr BJ, Warner MA. Perioperative management of pheochromocytoma. *J Cardiothorac Vasc Anesth.* 2002;16: 359-369.
- Langley RW, Burch HB. Perioperative management of the thyrotoxic patient. *Endocrinol Metab Clin North Am.* 2003;32: 519-534.
- Lenders JW, Eisenhofer G, Mannelli M, Pacak K. Phaeochromocytoma. *Lancet.* 2005;366:665-675.
- Nemergut EC, Dumont AS, Barry UT, Laws ER. Perioperative management of patients undergoing transsphenoidal pituitary surgery. *Anesth Analg.* 2005;101:1170-1181.
- Roberts CG, Ladenson PW. Hypothyroidism. *Lancet.* 2004;363: 793-803.
- Van Braeckel P, Carlier S, Steelant P-J, Weyne L, Vanfleteren L. Perioperative management of phaeochromocytoma. *Acta Anaesth Belg.* 2009;60:55-66.

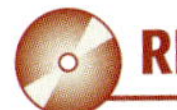

REFERENCES

Complete references available on DVD and online version at www.LongneckerAnesthesiology.com

CHAPTER 61 Anesthetic Considerations for Genitourinary and Renal Surgery

Maurizio Cereda
Sean Kennedy

KEY POINTS

1. Anesthetic management of urologic patients requires confidence with the management of elderly patients who typically have multiple comorbidities.
2. Surgical positioning is often complex and exposes the patient to the risk of severe complications.
3. Most endourologic procedures can be safely accomplished with either general or regional anesthesia. The anesthetic plan can be tailored to patient characteristics and individual preferences.
4. Urologic cancer requires highly invasive surgeries that have a high risk of complications. Patients undergoing these procedures require thorough physiologic monitoring and proactive hemodynamic, respiratory, and analgesic management.
5. Despite an unclear clinical benefit, the use of minimally invasive and robotic surgery in urology is increasing rapidly. These procedures may require prolonged pneumoperitoneum and head-down positioning, introducing a new set of clinical challenges to anesthesiologists.

INTRODUCTION

The perioperative management of urologic patients is often complicated by their advanced age and their multiple comorbidities. Urologic surgery includes procedures with broad complexity, ranging from endoscopies to major abdominal operations. In addition, recent years have seen the expansion of this specialty, which now incorporates minimally invasive, laparoscopic, and robotic techniques. Anesthesiologists must have background knowledge of the indications, technical aspects, and complications of the procedures used in urologic surgery in order to formulate a sound anesthetic plan.

MACROSCOPIC ANATOMY OF THE URINARY TRACT

KIDNEY

The kidneys are located in the retroperitoneal space between T12 and L4 along the medial borders of the psoas muscles. Positioned inferior to the liver, the right kidney lies slightly lower than the left. The kidneys are surrounded by the perirenal fat and enclosed in the perirenal or Gerota fascia. The adrenal glands lie on top of each kidney, also contained by Gerota fascia. Diaphragmatic movement transmits to the kidneys, causing a physiologic excursion of 4 to 5 cm with each respiration. Upon section, the kidney is composed of a cortex and a medullary section. The medulla is divided into several pyramids whose tips, named papillae, are indented with the minor calices. The latter converge in the major calices and then drain into the renal pelvis, which tapers into the ureter.

Each kidney receives its blood supply from a single renal artery, although occasional variants with multiple arteries are encountered. The renal arteries originate just inferior to the superior mesenteric vein and enter the kidney at its hilum. The right artery crosses the midline behind the vena cava. The renal veins run in front of the arteries, the left vein crossing the midline anterior to the aorta. The lymphatic circulation of the kidney drains into lymph nodes located in the lumbar region.

The kidneys receive vegetative innervation (**Fig. 61-1**) from the renal plexus, which receives fibers mainly from the celiac plexus and the vagus nerve. Sympathetic vasoconstrictor and afferent fibers originate from T8 to L1. For this reason, kidney pain is typically perceived in the costovertebral angle and below the 12th rib. Anesthesia for kidney surgery requires effective blockade of the nerve roots between T8 and L3 to allow incision through the overlying skin and abdominal wall.

URETERS

The ureters originate from the renal pelvis and run along the course of the psoas muscle. They cross the course of the common iliac arteries and swing laterally in the lower pelvis, entering the base of the bladder. The ureteral blood supply derives from the renal arteries in their upper tract, from the spermatic or ovarian arteries in their mid portion, and from hypogastric and vesical arteries in their terminal tract. Ureteral innervation originates from the renal, hypogastric, and pelvic plexuses. Sympathetic afferent fibers enter the spinal cord at T10-L2 for the upper ureteral portion, and parasympathetic afferents reach the S2-S4 levels. This distribution explains why pain from a ureteral stone is perceived in different locations depending on the position of the stone in the ureter.

BLADDER

The bladder is a hollow organ with a capacity of 400 to 500 mL and a wall mainly composed of smooth muscle tissue. When empty, it lies behind the pubic symphysis, anterior to the rectum in males and to the vagina in females. When the bladder is full, it rises significantly above the pubic bone and becomes palpable. The ureters enter the bladder posteriorly and emerge into the bladder cavity 2.5 cm apart, constituting the base of the vesical trigone. The dome of the bladder is covered by peritoneum, and the inferior portion lies on top of the prostate and seminal vesicles.

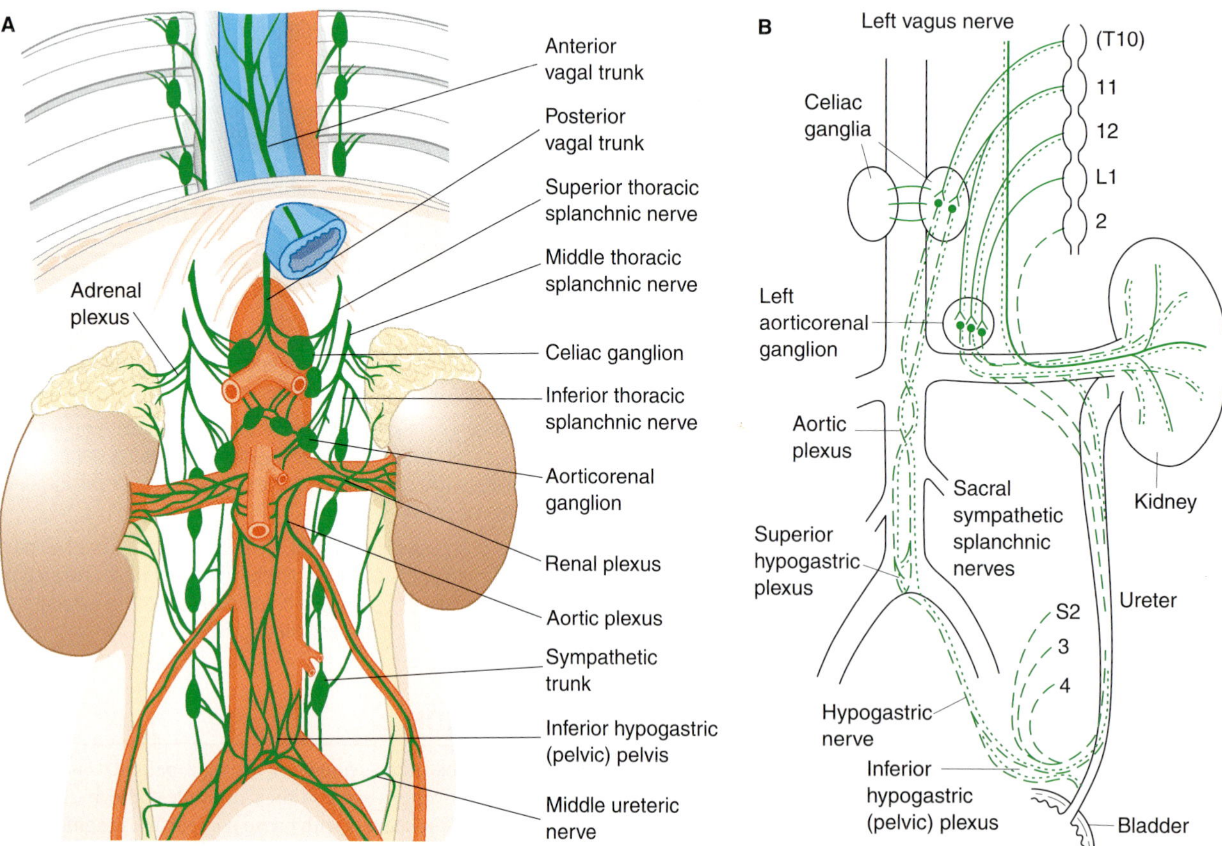

FIGURE 61-1. **A.** Gross anatomy of the kidneys. **B.** Autonomic and sensory nerve supply.

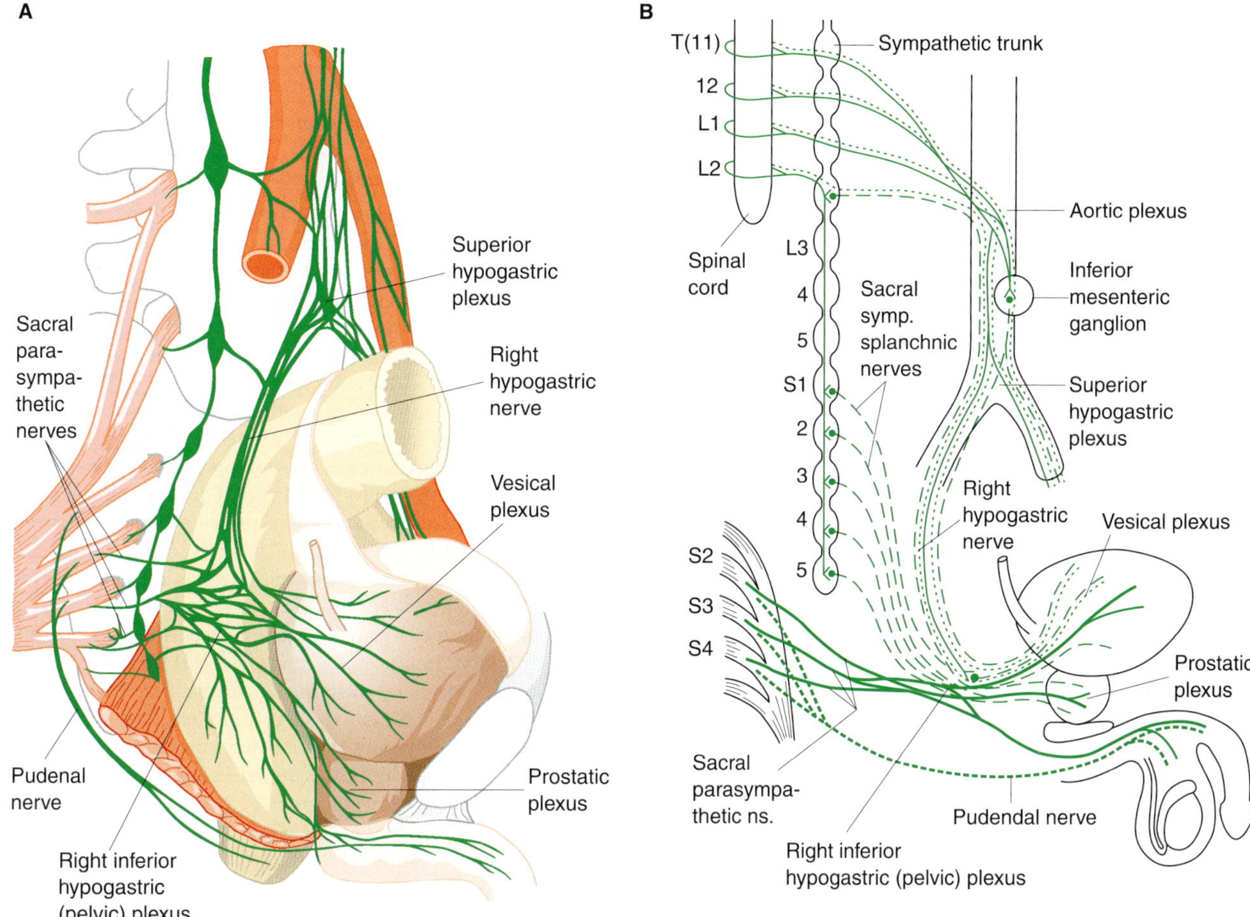

FIGURE 61-2. **A.** Gross anatomy of the bladder and the prostate. **B.** Autonomic and sensory nerve supply.

The blood supply of the bladder is provided mainly by the superior, middle, and inferior vesical arteries, arising from the hypogastric artery. The venous blood collects in a plexus located at the bladder neck, which drains into the hypogastric vein. This plexus is also joined by the prostatic venous plexus and by the deep dorsal vein of the penis, making this region prone to marked bleeding during surgical dissection. The lymphatics of the bladder drain in lymph nodes located near the iliac vessels.

The bladder receives its nerve supply from the hypogastric plexus (**Fig. 61-2**). Sympathetic fibers from lumbar splanchnic nerve fibers originate at T11-T12. Parasympathetic innervation originates at S2-S4 and is carried by the pudendal nerves. Afferent fibers follow both the sympathetic and the parasympathetic pathways. Somatic afferents are carried by the pudendal nerves to the sacral spinal cord. Efferent sympathetic stimulation relaxes the bladder muscle fibers and causes contraction of the involuntary internal bladder sphincter. Parasympathetic stimulation contracts the bladder muscle fibers and relaxes the internal sphincter. Additionally, the external (striated) bladder sphincter is under voluntary control through the somatic fibers of the pudendal nerves originating at S2-S3. Therefore, micturition and urine storage can be altered not only by spinal cord injury but also by cerebral lesions.

PROSTATE AND SEMINAL VESICLES

The prostate gland has a strong fibromuscular component and normally weighs about 20 g. It is surrounded by a thick, fibrous capsule and is located just beneath the bladder behind the pubic symphysis and anterior to the rectum. The prostate contains the prostatic portion of the urethra, which is about 2.5 cm long. The prostate can be seen as composed of five lobes (anterior, posterior, median, right lateral, and left lateral). An alternative classification divides the prostate into a peripheral zone, a central zone, a transitional zone, an anterior segment, and a preprostatic sphincteric zone. The transitional zone is the closest to the urethra and is also the zone where symptomatic prostatic adenomas are usually located.

Blood supply to the prostate derives from the inferior vesical arteries and drains into the prostatic venous plexus, which is in continuity with the vesical plexus and the dorsal vein of the penis. The prostate receives efferent sympathetic nerve supply from T11-L2 through the hypogastric plexus, and parasympathetic afferent fibers that run through the pelvic splanchnic nerves to reach S2-S4 (see Fig. 61-2). The lymphatic circulation of the prostate drains into the hypogastric, sacral, and external iliac lymph nodes.

The seminal vesicles are located under the base of the bladder immediately above the prostate and anterior to the rectum. They join the ipsilateral vas deferens, forming the ejaculatory duct, which then perforates the prostate to empty into the prostatic urethra. The blood, nerve, and lymphatic distribution are in common with the prostate.

TESTES

The testicle is separated by connective tissue into approximately 250 lobules. It is covered by a dense fascia called the tunica albuginea, which is invaginated posteriorly and forms the mediastinum testis. The testicle is capped by the epididymis, which is composed of a convoluted tubule connected to the testis through the efferent ducts and, at its other end, continues in the vas deferens. The latter continues its ascent within the spermatic cord together with spermatic arteries and the venous pampiniform plexus.

Because of its embryogenesis near the kidneys, the blood and nerve supply of the kidneys and testicles are closely associated. The arteries of the testicle originate from the aorta below the renal arteries and reach the testes after running near the ureters then through the spermatic cord. The venous blood ascends the spermatic cord through the pampiniform plexus, which forms the spermatic vein at the internal inguinal ring. The spermatic vein then drains into the vena cava on the right side and into the left renal vein on the left side.

The testicular nerve supply originates at T10 and reaches the testis after joining the aortic plexus, located near the kidney. The anterior scrotum is supplied by the ilioinguinal nerve and by the genital branch of the genitofemoral nerve, with fibers originating from T12 to L2. The posterior face of the scrotum is supplied by fibers that originate at S1-S4 and travel through branches of the perineal nerve and of the posterior femoral cutaneous nerve. Regional anesthesia for testicular surgery requires blockade up to the T10 level. The testicular lymphatic circulation drains into the lumbar nodes, which are connected with the mediastinal nodes. The scrotal lymph circulation drains into the superficial inguinal and subinguinal nodes.

URETHRA AND EXTERNAL GENITALIA

The penis is composed of the corpus spongiosum, which contains the urethra, and of two corpora cavernosa. Each of these elements is contained in the tunica albuginea. They are distally capped by the glans and proximally attached to the pelvic bone. Arterial blood supply to the penis is delivered by the two deep internal pudendal arteries, which divide in the deep artery of the penis, the dorsal artery and the bulbourethral artery. Venous blood runs through the superficial and deep dorsal vein of the penis, which reaches the internal pudendal vein through the pudendal plexus. The ilioinguinal nerve innervates the root of the penis, and the body and glans are supplied by the paired dorsal nerves of the penis, a continuation of the pudendal nerves (**Fig. 61-3**). Parasympathetic and sympathetic innervation originate from S2-S4 and from L1-L2, respectively. Erection is promoted by parasympathetic stimulation that causes arterial vasodilatation.

The female urethra is much shorter than the male's and is located between the pubic symphysis and the vagina. Its arterial supply derives from the inferior vesical, vaginal, and internal pudendal arteries; venous blood drains into the internal pudendal veins.

PATIENT POSITIONING IN UROLOGIC SURGERY

Patient positioning is often complex during urologic surgery, and some of the positions adopted may result in important complications (see Chapter 27 for a broader discussion of surgical positioning).

LITHOTOMY POSITION

The lithotomy position (**Fig. 61-4**) is used for patients undergoing transurethral procedures and transperineal prostatectomy. In the lithotomy position, the patient is supine, and the lower extremities are flexed at the hips and at the knees to a variable degree. In the standard position, the hips are flexed approximately 90 degrees, and the legs are parallel to the floor. In the low lithotomy position, the hips are flexed only 30 to 45 degrees, and in the extreme position, the legs are extended and the hips are flexed on the trunk with the goal of having the perineal floor almost parallel to the ground. A variety of leg and foot supports are used, including ankle straps, boot supports, and knee supports. The lithotomy positions have physiologic consequences on the respiratory system. The increased intra-abdominal pressure decreases lung volumes and respiratory system compliance, possibly causing atelectasis and hypoxemia. The head-down position, often used to increase perineal exposure, further enhances these effects.[1]

Lower extremity neuropathies have been reported after surgery in the lithotomy position. In a prospective study of 991 patients, Warner et al[2] reported a 1.5% incidence of sensory neuropathies. These became evident within 4 hours of the end of surgery and resolved within 6 months. Placement in the lithotomy position for longer than 2 hours was a risk factor for neuropathy in this study. In a retrospective analysis of 1170 patients, Gumus et al[3] reported 12 cases (1.02%) of neuropathy, of which only two were reversible. Older age and operative time were risk factors. Compression of the superficial peroneal nerve on leg support,[2] strain of the obturator and lateral femoral cutaneous nerves,[4] and stretching of the sciatic plexus probably contribute to the genesis of postoperative neuropathies in the lithotomy position. An American Society of Anesthesiologists (ASA) task force recommended that during lithotomy, hip flexion more than 90 degrees should be avoided to limit sciatic and femoral neuropathy.[5] Back pain is frequent after the lithotomy position, probably caused by the loss of lumbar lordosis. Finger injury from trapping in the operative bed is possible when the leg rest

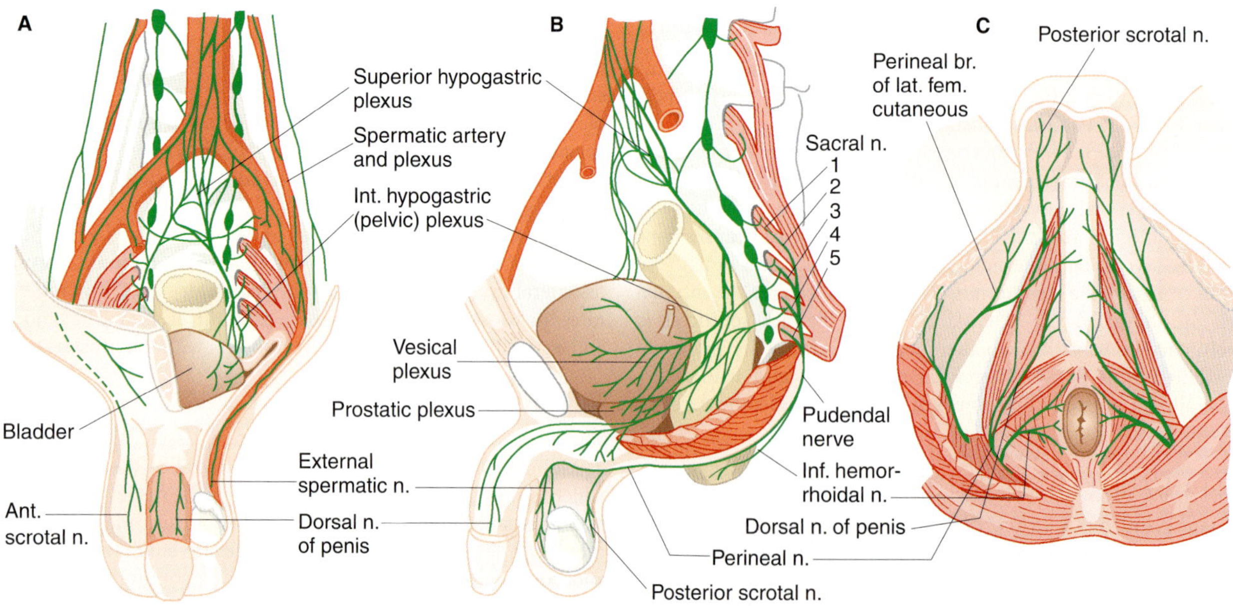

FIGURE 61-3. Gross anatomy and nerve supply of the male genitalia. **A.** Anterior view. **B.** Sagittal view. **C.** Transperineal view.

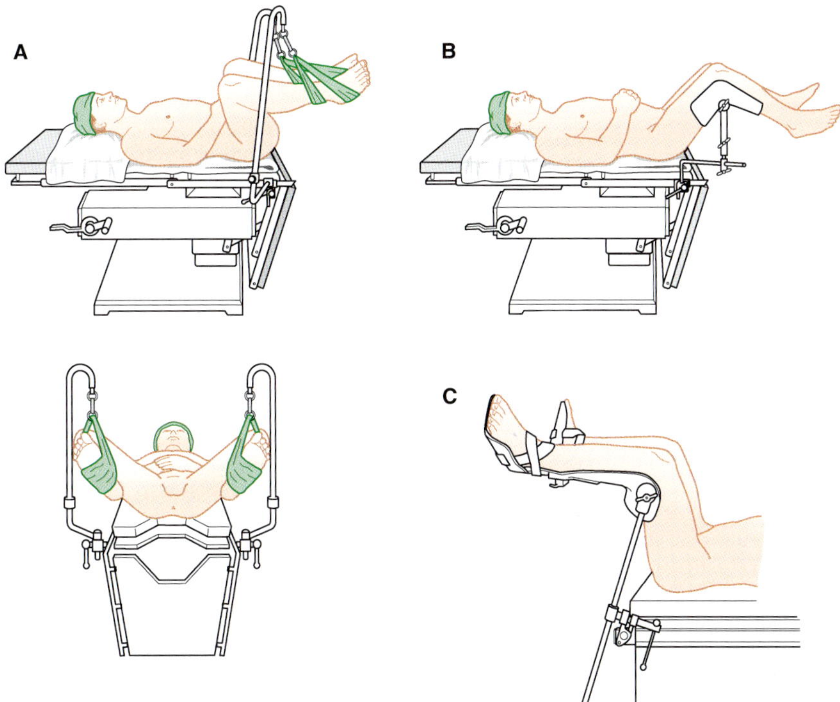

FIGURE 61-4. Lithotomy position. **A.** Strap stirrups. **B.** Bier-Hoff stirrups. **C.** Allen stirrups.

is lowered. "Well leg" compartment syndrome with rhabdomyolysis is a severe complication of the lithotomy position, and its incidence may not be as small as initially thought. In a survey of 261 urologists, 61 cases of compartment syndrome were reported, the majority after radical cystectomy and procedures longer than 4 hours.[6] In a series of 473 patients requiring prolonged lithotomy, eight cases of compartment syndrome requiring fasciotomies were recorded.[7] Prolonged surgery, extreme lithotomy, and compressive leg supports seem to predispose patients to the development of compartment syndrome. The genesis of this complication seems to be related to a decrease in arterial pressure in the lower extremity caused by leg elevation combined with an increased tissue pressure in the muscle compartments. The end result is muscle hypoperfusion, ischemia, and subsequent swelling, finally generating the compartment syndrome. The use of leg or calf supports increases muscle pressure significantly, as opposed to ankle supports, which do not increase it.[8,9] After surgery, patients should be observed for lower extremity swelling, hypoperfusion, and paresthesias because loss of peripheral pulse is a late sign of compartment syndrome. Acute renal failure may result if fasciotomies are not performed in a timely manner. Well-padded leg or ankle supports help prevent this complication during prolonged surgery.

HEAD-DOWN POSITION

The head-down, Trendelenburg position is often used in urologic surgery to improve perineal exposure or facilitate laparoscopic and robotic procedures, in which a steep position is often chosen. Among the physiologic consequences of this position are atelectasis caused by cephalad shifting of the diaphragm and increased intracranial pressure (ICP).[10] Although the head-down position has long been used to treat hypovolemia, no beneficial hemodynamic effects were demonstrated by Sibbald et al[11] in critically ill patients with hypotension. The head-down position may predispose patients to venous air embolism, a complication occasionally reported during urologic procedures.[12,13] With pronounced head-down positioning, shoulder braces are often used to avoid downward displacement of the patient. This practice may result in brachial plexus stretching and injuries,[14] particularly when the shoulder is simultaneously abducted.[15] Based on these considerations, the ASA has discouraged the use of these devices.[5] When a shoulder brace cannot be avoided, the arms should be left resting at the sides of the patient.

LATERAL POSITION, FLEXED POSITION, AND KIDNEY REST

To facilitate access to the kidney, a lateral position with flexion and kidney rest elevation is often used (**Fig. 61-5**). The patient is placed on the side with the dependent iliac crest on the break point of the table. The table top is angled approximately 30 degrees, and the kidney rest is then elevated to raise the lower iliac crest and enhance exposure of the nondependent flank. An "axillary roll" is placed between the upper chest and the table to prevent brachial plexus compression unless a "bean bag" is used. The dependent leg is flexed at the knee, and the other leg is left extended. Similar to other types of lateral positioning, this position may cause dependent atelectasis, maldistribution of perfusion, and an unfavorable ventilation/perfusion (V/Q) ratio. Hemodynamic consequences of this position include decreased systemic arterial pressure and decreased cardiac output. Although the exact mechanism of these hemodynamic effects is not clear, decreased blood flow in the vena cava

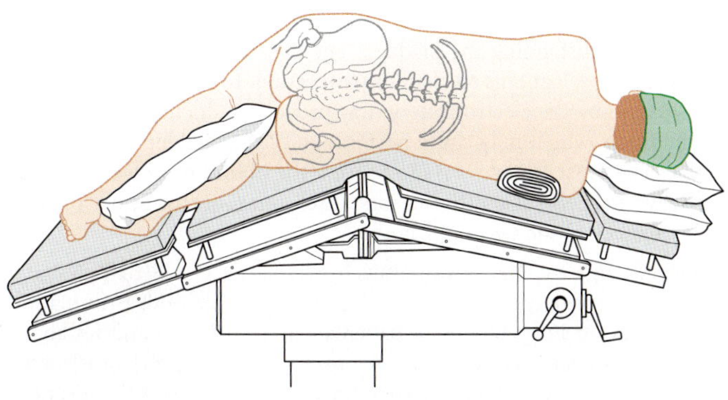

FIGURE 61-5. The kidney rest position, commonly used for renal surgery.

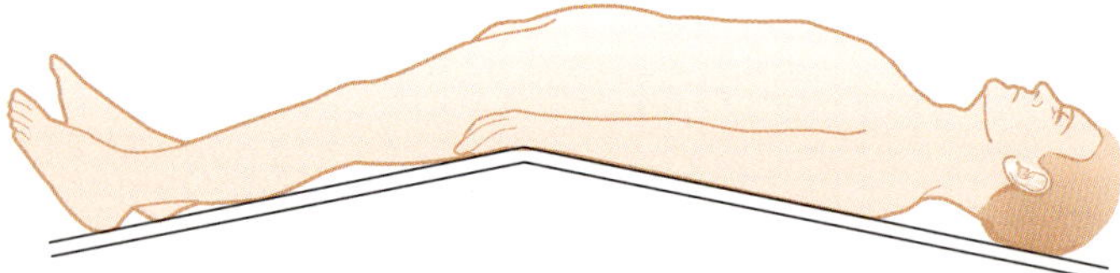

FIGURE 61-6. Hyperextended supine position, commonly used for prostate and bladder surgery to facilitate pelvic exposure.

caused by its compression and stretching is likely. Hypotension should be promptly treated with fluid and, if severe, with immediate decrease of flexion. Rhabdomyolysis has been reported also with the nephrectomy position, likely related to excessive compression of the gluteal compartment.[16]

HYPEREXTENDED SUPINE POSITION

This position is commonly used during retropubic prostatectomy to improve access to the pelvic organs (**Fig. 61-6**). The patient is supine with the iliac crests placed over the break of the operating table, which is then extended to increase the distance between the iliac crest and the ribs. The patient is usually placed in a head-down position, maintaining the operative field parallel to the floor. For thoracoabdominal incisions, the patient is placed in a semisupine position with the shoulder on the operative side raised to about 30 degrees by a roll, and the ipsilateral arm is placed on an armrest. The nonoperative leg is semiflexed, and the contralateral leg is kept extended. When the patient is placed in a hyperextended position, there is a possibility of nerve and back injuries. Similar to any head-down position, there is also the potential for venous air embolism, which should be considered in case of otherwise unexplained hemodynamic instability.[12,13]

ENDOUROLOGIC PROCEDURES

CYSTOSCOPY AND TRANSURETHRAL RESECTION OF BLADDER TUMORS

Cystoscopy and transurethral resection of bladder tumors (TURBT) are among the most common urologic procedures performed, particularly in the elderly population. These procedures are used to diagnose and resect bladder tumors, evaluate and treat other causes of urinary obstruction, place ureteral stents, and remove bladder and ureteral stones.

Complications

Bladder Perforation Perforation of the bladder is one of the most serious complications of cystoscopy. If the tear is extraperitoneal, conscious patients may complain of nausea and lower abdominal pain, and a poor return of irrigation fluid may be detected. When an intraperitoneal rupture occurs, alert patients may have diffuse abdominal pain. In unconscious patients, bladder perforation may present only as hemodynamic instability. High irrigation pressures can predispose to perforation by overdistending the bladder. The onset of obturator reflex can also predispose patients to bladder perforation. In fact, obturator nerve stimulation by the electrocautery may provoke adduction and rotation of the thigh, which may cause perforation of the bladder by the cystoscope. The most reliable ways to prevent the obturator reflex are either by delivering general anesthesia and muscle relaxation or by performing a nerve block of the obturator nerve.[17]

Autonomic Hyperreflexia Autonomic hyperreflexia is a life-threatening hypertensive emergency that is triggered by lower body stimulation and may occur in up to 85% of patients with spinal cord injuries above the sixth thoracic vertebra. Bladder overdistension is the most common trigger of autonomic hyperreflexia, explaining why this event is particularly frequent in patients with spinal cord injury who undergo cystoscopy. Afferent stimulation from the bladder, rectum, and lower extremities ascends to the brain through the spinothalamic tract and the dorsal columns. Interneurons project to sympathetic neurons between T5 and L2, causing reflex vasoconstriction, visceral contraction, and piloerection. Normally, these reflexes are inhibited by higher nervous centers and by control mechanisms originating in the carotid and aortic baroreceptors. However, in patients with high spinal cord injuries, inhibitory efferents cannot reach the thoracic sympathetic neurons, and the response to stimulation from the lower body cannot be modulated, resulting in an uncontrolled vasoconstriction that can have catastrophic consequences if not corrected in a timely manner (**Fig. 61-7**). Hypertension can be dramatic, although an increase in blood pressure of only 50 mm Hg is required to diagnose autonomic hyperreflexia.[18] The clinical manifestations of autonomic hyperreflexia are headache, chest tightness, and piloerection ("gooseflesh") in the body below the level of the lesion. Above the lesion, flushing, sweating, mucous membrane congestion, and conjunctival erythema are visible because of a parasympathetic response to the hypertension. For the same reason, bradycardia is usually observed.

Besides early recognition, there is no definitive recommendation guiding the management of autonomic hyperreflexia. When possible, sitting up the patient may provoke an orthostatic decrease in blood pressure. Antihypertensive drugs with rapid onset and short duration of action should be chosen. Calcium channel blockers such as nifedipine and nicardipine, hydralazine, nitroglycerine, alpha- and beta-blockers, and sodium nitroprusside usually achieve rapid blood pressure control.[18] Magnesium infusion has also been reported effective in controlling hypertension in autonomic hyperreflexia.[19]

Anesthetic Management The choice of anesthetic technique for cystoscopy depends on patient and procedural factors. Males require regional or general anesthesia more often than females, particularly for operative procedures. The patient population is older and has multiple comorbidities, which explains why spinal anesthesia is popular for endourologic procedures. Although some believe that regional anesthesia affords better cardiovascular protection than general anesthesia, no outcome studies have shown a significant difference in morbidity among anesthetic techniques during cystoscopy. There are only a few circumstances in which there is a clearer indication for either a general or a regional anesthetic. The former may be required for resections performed in the area of the obturator nerve unless an obturator nerve block is performed.[17] Patients who are prone to autonomic hyperreflexia may benefit from a neuraxial anesthetic, which can block the transmission of afferent impulses and prevent the triggering of uncontrolled reflex vasoconstriction. In all other populations, the choice of anesthetic technique should be directed at allowing rapid onset and emergence because most endourologic procedures are brief and are performed in an outpatient setting. With general anesthesia, avoidance of muscle relaxation and relatively rapid induction can be accomplished with a laryngeal mask airway (LMA). The choice of inhaled anesthetic agent may have a role in achieving rapid recovery times. In a randomized controlled study of elderly patients undergoing short urologic procedures, significantly more patients reached criteria for postanesthesia care unit bypass when desflurane was used as a maintenance agent compared with isoflurane.[20] When spinal anesthesia is chosen, the anesthetic agent should allow a rapid resolution of motor block with early ambulation and discharge. Lidocaine has been the drug of choice for these procedures for many years, but the association of this drug with transient neurologic symptoms (TNS) has decreased its appeal. TNS is defined as onset of pain and dysesthesia in the buttocks, thighs, and lower extremity, within 24 hours of the anesthetic.[21] Although this complication is transient and not associated with abnormal nerve function,[22] it causes significant patient discomfort and some functional impairment in a small percentage of patients.[23] TNS was initially observed after spinal anesthesia with 5% lidocaine, but the incidence of this complication is similar with other concentrations.[23] The use of a single-orifice versus multiple-orifice spinal needle increased the rate of TNS threefold.[24] Alternative drugs and doses

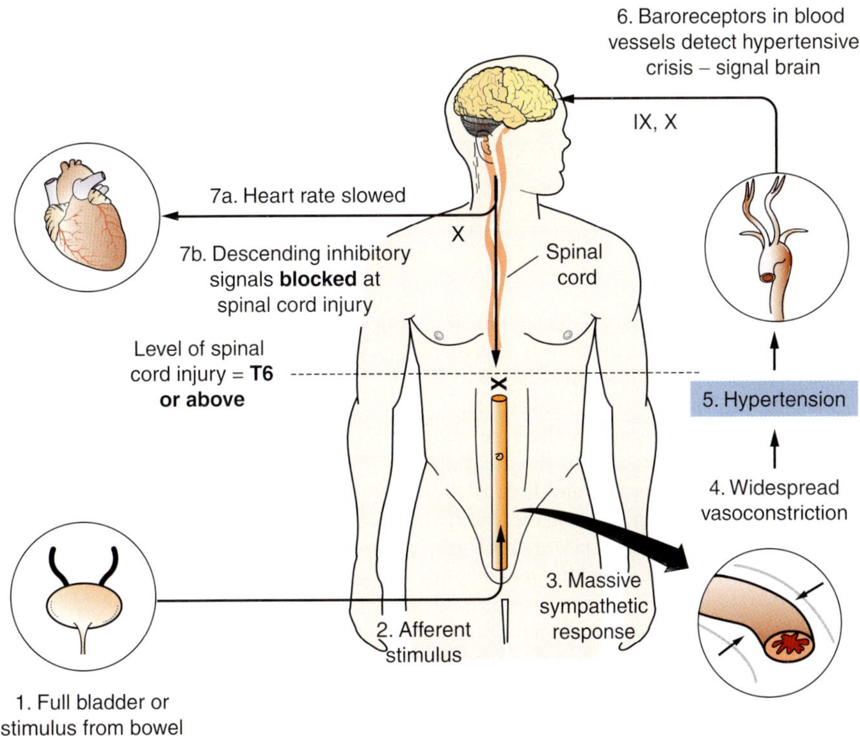

FIGURE 61-7. Mechanisms of autonomic hyperreflexia. In patients with spinal cord injury above T6, stimulation from the lower body triggers a sympathetic response that cannot be controlled by descending inhibitory efferents. Hypertension is accompanied by bradycardia caused by vagal response. [From Blackmer J. Rehabilitation medicine: 1. Autonomic dysreflexia. *CMAJ*. 2003;169:931-935.]

have been investigated to obtain rapid resolution of spinal anesthesia in urologic surgery.[25] In a randomized study, 80 patients undergoing various urologic procedures received bupivacaine at different doses with or without the addition of intrathecal fentanyl. Administration of 5 mg of bupivacaine with 25 mcg of fentanyl achieved a comparable block level (higher than T7) and similar anesthetic quality with shorter lasting motor block, compared with 10 mg of plain bupivacaine.[26] In elderly patients undergoing brief transurethral procedures, 4 mg of bupivacaine with 20 mcg of fentanyl achieved adequate anesthetic level with no need for either rescue therapy or hypotension treatment.[27]

TRANSURETHRAL RESECTION OF THE PROSTATE

Preoperative Considerations Benign prostatic hyperplasia (BPH) is the most common benign tumor in males. Its prevalence is age related and reaches 90% in men older than 80 years of age.[28] BPH develops in the transition zone, the part of the prostate that is closest to the urethra, and is histologically characterized by increased cellularity in a nodular pattern.[29] Not all patients with an enlarged prostate are symptomatic. The extent of symptoms is affected by the size of the gland, the degree of intrusion into the urethra, and the effect of alpha-adrenergic tone. The presence of symptomatic BPH significantly affects quality of life and, if left untreated, predisposes patients to frequent urinary tract infections (UTIs), the development of bladder diverticula, and hydronephrosis and may cause nonreversible renal damage.

Patients with mild symptoms can be managed with watchful waiting, because some patients may have spontaneous improvement. Pharmacologic treatment with selective and nonselective alpha-blockers and with 5-alpha-reductase blockers is effective in patients with more significant symptoms. Both classes of drugs are more effective than placebo in improving lower urinary tract symptoms and, when used in combination, slowed the progression of disease and reduced the need for surgery[30] Surgical treatment is chosen in patients who fail medical therapy. Open prostatectomy has the greatest success rate in increasing urinary flow, but it also has the highest rate of complications and is performed in a minority of patients.[29] Transurethral resection of the prostate (TURP) is currently considered the gold standard for prostate resection, reducing symptoms in 88% of cases. However, it has a risk of morbidity, including a 5% to 10% risk of sexual dysfunction. Minimally invasive therapies for BPH include transurethral needle ablation (TUNA), transurethral microwave therapy (TUMT), hot water–induced thermotherapy (WIT), and interstitial laser therapy (ILT).[31] Among these techniques, TUMT appears to be to a viable alternative to TURP because it can be performed without anesthesia on an outpatient basis.[32] Minimally invasive therapies are advantageous for patients who are sexually active. However, these techniques have a higher rate of obstruction recurrence than TURP, and they cannot replace it as the gold standard for surgical management of BPH.

Complications Mortality from TURP is estimated around 0.1%, with an overall early morbidity of 11.1%.[33] Postoperative morbidity is related to patient age, operative time, and the amount of tissue resected.[34]

TURP Syndrome TURP is performed by resecting prostatic tissue with a cautery loop introduced through a special cystoscope. During the resection, venous sinuses are opened, and the irrigation fluid can be absorbed into the systemic circulation. As a result, a complication known as TURP syndrome may develop. Advances in surgical techniques, including the introduction of bipolar electrocautery, laser ablation, and new irrigation fluids, have minimized the incidence of this adverse event,[35] which is now reported to be less than 1.5%.[33] However, TURP syndrome remains relevant because it is potentially fatal. It has multiple manifestations characterized by fluid overload, hypoosmolality, hyponatremia, and neurologic disturbances. Asymptomatic hyponatremia has been observed in 50% of patients undergoing TURP,[36] and its extent is related to the duration of the procedure.[37]

The onset of TURP syndrome may occur as early as 15 minutes after the beginning of the procedure, but later onset has been observed, likely because of bladder rupture and transperitoneal fluid absorption.[38] In patients under general anesthesia, signs of fluid overload may be the only hint that TURP syndrome is occurring.[39] These signs include

TABLE 61-1 Signs of Transurethral Resection of the Prostate Syndrome

Awake Patient	Anesthetized Patient
Confusion	Hypertension
Nausea	Bradycardia
Visual loss	Electrocardiographic changes
Coma	Desaturation
Seizures	Delayed emergence

hypertension, reflex bradycardia, and pulmonary edema, but for unclear reasons, hypotension can also be observed. In patients receiving regional anesthesia, neurologic symptoms may allow early diagnosis of TURP. Otherwise, they may be observed at emergence (**Table 61-1**).

The manifestations of TURP syndrome depend on the type and amount of fluid absorbed. Fluid absorption is related to the duration of the procedure, number of vascular spaces opened, and hydrostatic pressure in the bladder.[40] Regional anesthesia may increase the absorption of irrigation fluid compared with general anesthesia with mechanical ventilation because of lower bladder pressures with spontaneous breathing.[41]

The irrigation fluid used during TURP is chosen based on its electrical conductivity. Electrolyte solutions disperse cautery current and were not used for TURP, although they would be better tolerated in case of systemic absorption. However, new-generation bipolar electrocauteries allow use of isotonic saline, which should reduce the biochemical effects of irrigation fluid abosorption.[42] Distilled water was commonly used in the past and was associated with acute renal failure, intravascular hemolysis, and cerebral edema caused by pronounced serum hypoosmolality. Nausea, restlessness, confusion, coma, seizures, and hemispheric herniation may occur. It is commonly thought that hyponatremia is the main cause of the neurologic manifestations of TURP syndrome. However, low sodium levels do not cause cerebral edema if serum osmolality is maintained. Additionally, nerve conduction and transmembrane potentials are little altered even in the presence of significant hyponatremia.[43]

Since the adoption of alternative irrigation fluids, the incidence of TURP syndrome has decreased by 50%.[44] Solutions with near physiologic osmolality such as 1.5% glycine and 2.7% sorbitol with 0.54% mannitol are now routinely used. Plain sorbitol, mannitol, dextrose, and urea solutions are also available. The osmolality of these solutions ranges from 195 mOsm/L to isotonic. Because some of these fluids are relatively hypotonic, plasma hypoosmolality may still occur when irrigation fluid is absorbed in large amounts. Additionally, neurologic manifestations may still occur even when serum osmolality is not significantly affected. Direct toxic actions of some of the solutes used in irrigation fluids have been implicated. In a randomized study, a higher incidence of TURP syndrome was detected in patients who received 1.5% glycine irrigation fluid as opposed to dextrose and saline.[45] The rate of TURP was associated with the level of glycine. This amino acid, an inhibitory neurotransmitter in the cortex and retina, is likely the causative agent of postoperative blindness and seizures observed in some TURP patients. In patients with visual impairment after TURP, the pupillary reflexes are often sluggish or absent, unlike cortical blindness, in which reflexes are maintained. This suggests that the mechanism of blindness in these patients is direct inhibition of retinal potential transmission. Blindness resolves with decreasing blood levels of glycine.

Glycine metabolism in the liver produces ammonia. Hyperammonemia has been observed after TURP with glycine solutions and can be prevented by the intravenous (IV) administration of L-arginine. However, it is not clear whether hyperammonemia has a significant role in TURP syndrome. The absorption of sorbitol can result in the development of hyperglycemia and lactic acidosis related to the metabolism of sorbitol.[46] Metabolic acidosis has been reported during TURP and is attributable to a decrease of the strong ion difference caused by electrolyte dilution.[47]

TABLE 61-2 Management of TURP Syndrome

Inform surgeon Stop procedure Obtain electrolytes, arterial blood gases, hemoglobin, measured serum osmolality Support breathing and circulation Treat fluid overload	Consider ventilatory support if severe pulmonary edema Consider invasive hemodynamic monitoring if severe heart failure
If symptomatic hypoosmolality: Start 0.9% normal saline infusion Administer furosemide, mannitol, or both **In patients with convulsions or coma:** Give hypertonic saline	Monitor electrolytes q1h Limit sodium correction to <1.5 mEq/L/h Maintain negative fluid balance in patients with fluid overload Consider hemodialysis or ultrafiltration in symptomatic patients with poor urine output

Rapid diagnosis of TURP syndrome requires a high level of suspicion, especially when the patient is unconscious (**Table 61-2**). There are no clinically available monitors of irrigation fluid absorption. By adding ethanol to the fluid and measuring its expired concentration, it is possible to detect and quantify irrigation fluid absorption,[48] but this tool has not find wide use outside of clinical research. Hemodynamic changes that cannot be otherwise explained may be the only available clues.

When TURP syndrome is suspected, the procedure should be stopped. Serum sodium, potassium, and osmolality should be measured. The latter value is essential to distinguish between true hypoosmolality and hyponatremia in the presence of circulating solutes such as glycine. Hemoglobin should be measured, because it is an index of the extent of fluid absorption. Although rare, hemoglobinuria can occur even with glycine irrigant absorption and should be ruled out by urinalysis.

Hyponatremia does not need to be treated aggressively when it is not accompanied by hypoosmolality or in the absence of neurologic symptoms (see Chapter 35 for a full discussion of electrolyte and acid–base disturbances). If hyponatremia needs to be treated, rapid correction should be avoided because it can cause pontine myelinolysis.[49] Hypertonic saline should be used only in the presence of life-threatening manifestations such as coma and seizures. Otherwise, sodium levels can be increased by administration of normal saline in combination with a loop diuretic or mannitol. Sodium correction should never exceed 1 to 1.5 mEq/L/h. A diuretic is also used to treat fluid overload. Patients who had bladder perforation may have signs of hypovolemia caused by transperitoneal loss of sodium and may require volume resuscitation.[38]

Myocardial Ischemia A relatively high frequency of myocardial ischemic events has been observed in patients undergoing TURP, with a higher rate in patients with increased risk factors. Wong et al[50] reported an 18% rate of ST segment changes in the immediate postoperative period in patients undergoing TURP. Edwards et al[51] observed a 26% rate of ischemic electrocardiographic (ECG) changes in patients undergoing TURP. The onset of cardiac events seems to be related to blood loss and glycine absorption.[52]

Other Complications The risk of bleeding is related to prostate size and duration of resection.[53] It is hard to estimate intraoperative blood loss, but it has been reported between 3 and 5 mL/min.[54] Patients with very large prostates should have blood promptly available for possible transfusion. Coagulopathies have been observed in 6% of patients undergoing TURP.[55] Occasionally, disseminated intravascular coagulation may arise, probably caused by thromboplastin release by prostatic tissue.[54] Bladder perforation is also possible during TURP, with a reported rate of about 1%.[53]

Anesthetic Management Neuraxial anesthesia is probably the most commonly used anesthetic technique for TURP. However, no association between anesthetic technique and morbidity of TURP has been reported. Although patients undergoing TURP have an increased risk of myocardial ischemia by ECG changes, the choice of regional versus general anesthesia did not affect the rate of this complication in a randomized study.[51] Choosing a particular anesthetic technique may have an effect on patient satisfaction, postoperative pain and comfort, and discharge times, but no data suggest that anesthetic choice affects these variables. In a matched cohort study of 267 patients undergoing TURP, the choice of general or regional anesthesia had no effect on the length of stay in the recovery room or with patient satisfaction with analgesia.[56] However, there are several theoretical advantages to regional anesthesia that make it appealing for this procedure. The onset of TURP syndrome can be recognized from its neurologic symptoms,[57] and bladder perforation can present with abdominal or shoulder pain if the patient is allowed to remain awake. Regional anesthesia may be associated with less blood loss than general anesthesia.[58] This effect has been attributed to the fact that venous pressure is lower during spontaneous breathing than during mechanical ventilation. However, a similar reduction of venous pressure can be obtained during general anesthesia if spontaneous breathing is allowed. In patients undergoing TURP, a randomized controlled trial showed that spinal anesthesia and general anesthesia had opposite effects on T-helper lymphocyte populations, an effect that may suggest less immunosuppression with spinal anesthesia.[59] The clinical significance of these results is unclear.

When general anesthesia is chosen, avoidance of muscle relaxation and relatively fast induction can be accomplished with an LMA. Despite their age and comorbidities, a significant portion of TURP patients may have relatively rapid recovery times after general anesthesia, particularly if short-acting anesthetic agents are used.[20] Among regional techniques, subarachnoid anesthesia is usually preferred to epidural for TURP because it allows better relaxation of the pelvic floor and reliable anesthesia of the pelvic roots. Blocks higher than T9 are generally avoided because they do not allow the perception of the pain caused by rupture of the prostatic capsule; a T10 level of sensory loss is required to avoid the sensation resulting from bladder distension from the irrigation fluid. Bladder sensation is conducted by sympathetic afferent fibers of the hypogastric plexus, which originate from T11 to L2. Lower level blocks are possible as long as bladder pressure is monitored and maintained low. Beers et al[60] showed that a level higher than L1, obtained with intrathecal hyperbaric bupivacaine 7.5 mg, is acceptable as long as bladder pressure is monitored and maintained below 15 mm Hg. This level of block had the advantage of less decrease in blood pressure and may be considered in patients with significant hemodynamic compromise. Monitoring bladder pressure is cumbersome and may not be convenient. An alternative approach to a low block is the intrathecal administration of a small dose of local anesthetic together with a narcotic. When 4 mg of intrathecal tetracaine was administered with 10 mcg of fentanyl, the block level was comparable to 8 mg of plain tetracaine in a randomized study of 45 patients undergoing TURP,[61] but the number of hypotensive episodes was greater in the patients who had 8 mg of tetracaine. Five milligram of bupivacaine with 25 mcg of fentanyl achieved a sensory block higher than T7 in 50% of patients anesthetized with this dose.[25] Adequate anesthesia for TURP has been obtained also with only 4 mg of bupivacaine and 25 mcg of fentanyl.[62]

Prolonged postoperative analgesia may be beneficial after TURP because patients often complain of pain from detrusor muscle spasm. Intrathecal morphine along with a local anesthetic effectively provided postoperative pain in a trial on patients undergoing TURP.[63] In this study, 0.1 mg of intrathecal morphine was as effective as 0.2 mg but with a lower incidence of nausea and vomiting. Compared with other types of surgical procedures, relatively small doses of intrathecal morphine seem to be effective during TURP. In a randomized controlled trial, whereas 0.05 mg and 0.1 mg of intrathecal morphine had similar effect in controlling post-TURP pain, the incidence and intensity of pruritus were lower with the lower dose.[64] Alternative agents have been used in an attempt to avoid the side effects of intrathecal morphine, such as respiratory depression. Epidural tramadol provides postoperative analgesia,[65] but intrathecal tramadol with bupivacaine does not provide additional pain relief compared with plain bupivacaine after TURP.[66]

PROCEDURES FOR NEPHROLITHIASIS

EXTRACORPOREAL SHOCK-WAVE LITHOTRIPSY

Nephrolithiasis ranks third in frequency among the conditions affecting the urinary tract after infections and prostatic diseases.[28] The management of urinary stones has progressed greatly since the introduction of extracorporeal shock-wave lithotripsy (ESWL), and surgical stone extraction has become a very uncommon procedure.

Preoperative Considerations and Technical Aspects Extracorporeal shock wave lithotripsy uses acoustic shock waves to fragment stones. These waves generate high-amplitude pressure oscillations that transfer impressive amounts of energy when the density of the medium changes significantly, such as at the interface between tissue and stones or between tissue and air. Stones are fragmented through erosion by cavitational forces at the entry and exit sites of the waves and through shattering by energy absorption within the body of the stone. The application of this physical principle was developed by the German aeronautic company Dornier while studying supersonic aircraft. The Dornier HM3 lithotripter was the first commercially available machine.

Two types of shock-wave generators are used clinically. Supersonic generators release high energy in a small space using a spark gap electrode, creating a small underwater explosion. The shock waves are then focused on the target stone using an ellipsoid reflector. Finite amplitude generators create an acoustic wave by displacing a surface. This can be accomplished using piezoceramic emitters, in which thousands of ceramic components placed on a spheric surface are elongated by an electric discharge, or by using electromagnetic systems, in which an electric impulse displaces a metal membrane, similar to loudspeaker woofers. An acoustic lens then focuses the waves on the target stone.

A key element of all lithotripters is the coupling that allows shock waves to progress from the site of formation to the surface of the patient's body. In waterbath models, the patient sits on a chair and is immersed in a tub full of heated water. Newer models transmit waves through a water cushion placed against the patient's skin, often with the interposition of a layer of coupling gel. Inadequate coupling, particularly when air is entrapped between the skin and the coupling membrane, may result not only in insufficient wave transmission but also in skin ecchymosis and breakdown. Stone localization and aiming of the shock waves can be accomplished by fluoroscopic imaging or by ultrasonography. Successful stone fragmentation depends on stone size, location, and composition.

Complications

Cardiac Arrhythmias Shock waves have the potential to trigger ventricular arrhythmias when they coincide with the repolarization period of the cardiac cycle. For this reason, ECG synchronization and shock delivery 20 msec after the R wave has been used. The onset of significant arrhythmias is probably rare,[67] and many lithotripter models do not synchronize with ECG. Some machines synchronize with the respiratory cycle to avoid loss of aim with respiratory movement of the kidney.

Shock waves can occasionally inhibit or reprogram cardiac pacemakers. To avoid this complication, the patient should be positioned so the pacemaker is not in the path of the wave, and resuscitation equipment, including an external pacemaker, should be available.[68]

Hemodynamic and Respiratory Effects Immersion in a waterbath can have hemodynamic effects. Increased hydrostatic pressure on the lower extremities and the abdomen may shift blood to the intrathoracic vessels, precipitating congestive heart failure in susceptible individuals. Systemic vascular resistance may increase during immersion, which could increase left ventricular work and precipitate ischemia.[69]

Immersion in water causes upward shifting of the diaphragm, increased work of breathing, and decreased arterial oxygenation.

Renal Injury Gross hematuria is the rule after ESWL and should recover within 1 week. Severe abdominal pain should alert for the rare presence of perinephric hematoma. The management is generally conservative but may require laparotomy in case of hypotension. A bleeding diathesis is a relative contraindication to ESWL.

Other Complications Patients with a high stone burden are prone to obstruction by fragments after ESWL. "Steinstrasse," the columnation of fragments along the ureter, may require nephrostomy drainage or endoscopic stone extraction to relieve obstruction. Fever and sepsis are possible after ESWL and are more common in patients with an infected urinary tract before the procedure. Pneumothorax may occur if the wave path crosses the lung and is more likely in children.

Anesthetic Management ESWL causes pain at the skin, where the waves enter the body, and at the visceral level where they dissipate. Subjective pain reported by unanesthetized patients during ESWL is higher than during endoscopic urologic procedures.[70] The Dornier HM3 generates high-intensity waves and requires deeper levels of analgesia than newer models that generate waves with lower intensity and smaller entry area. The latter are ideal for the ambulatory setting, although stone fragmentation may be less effective and requires longer procedure times. The goals for anesthesia are not only to provide patient comfort during and after the procedure but also to achieve rapid recovery times because ESWL is performed as an outpatient procedure in the majority of cases. Additionally, postoperative pain is usually mild and, for these reasons, short-acting anesthetic and analgesic techniques are usually preferred.

Even after many years, the best anesthetic approach for ESWL is still a topic of debate. General anesthesia with muscle relaxation offers the advantage of optimizing stone targeting by avoiding patient movement and controlling respiration, but it prolongs recovery times. Epidural and spinal anesthesia have been widely used for ESWL. However, these techniques have longer induction times and may also prolong recovery times. A randomized comparison between epidural anesthesia with lidocaine and general anesthesia showed markedly longer recovery times in the group that received epidural anesthesia.[71] In this study, general anesthesia included the administration of propofol and N_2O and the use of an LMA; no narcotics were given. Safety concerns of intrathecal lidocaine have made the use of this drug for short procedures such as ESWL less appealing. A possible alternative approach is the injection of plain narcotics. In a randomized controlled study, intrathecal sufentanil was as effective as lidocaine in controlling pain, but it provided shorter recovery times during ESWL with the Dornier HM3.[72] In a subsequent study, intrathecal sufentanil doses of 15 to 17.5 mcg provided the best profile of effectiveness and safety.[73] IV analgesia and sedation with short-acting agents is widely used and presents several advantages in the ambulatory setting, particularly rapid recovery time. Deeper levels of sedation are required if high-intensity shock waves are used and, consequently, side effects such as respiratory depression are more likely. When compared with desflurane general anesthesia administered through a cuffed oropharyngeal airway, sedation with propofol and remifentanil infusion was associated with more episodes of desaturation and with greater narcotic requirement during ESWL with the Dornier HM3.[74] The success of a sedation regimen depends also on the type of medication used. Remifentanyl infusion is popular because of its rapid clearance with faster recovery times than fentanyl and its other derivatives.[75] Compared with sufentanil, remifentanil had similar analgesic properties but a lesser incidence of respiratory depression and nausea in a randomized controlled study.[76] The pharmacologic properties of remifentanil render this drug appealing also for patient-controlled sedation in the presence of varying levels of discomfort. A remifentanil infusion at 0.05 mcg/kg/min with patient-controlled supplementation of 10 mcg boluses has been effective in controlling pain during ESWL.[77] When patient-controlled sedation with remifentanil alone or with remifentanyl-propofol as compared, both techniques were highly effective, but the latter had a greater incidence of respiratory depression.[78] Remifentanyl alone had a higher incidence of nausea and vomiting, a common effect with this drug that is effectively prevented by 5HT3 antagonists.[79] Alternative anesthetic techniques such as EMLA cream,[80] skin infiltration with local anesthetics such as prilocaine,[81] and paravertebral blocks, have been proposed. Perioperative nonsteroidal anti-inflammatory drugs (NSAIDs) are often used and provide acceptable analgesia. The use of a combination of EMLA and preoperative diclofenac achieved better pain control than either medication alone.[80] In summary, the anesthetic choice for ESWL should be based on patient characteristics, machine type, and patient and local preferences. IV sedation provides adequate comfort in most patients, particularly if low-intensity waves are used. Inhalation anesthesia via LMA and without muscle relaxation also provides good operating conditions and rapid recovery in a predictable manner.

PERCUTANEOUS NEPHROLITHOTOMY

Percutaneous nephrolithotomy, used for management of large kidney stones, is typically performed in the prone position. For this reason, general anesthesia is often chosen for the procedure. However, neuraxial anesthesia is also a viable option. A recent matched case control study documented comparable surgical and an anesthetic results between combined spinal-epidural and general anesthesia in patients undergoing percutaneous nephrolithotomy.[82] The use of low-dose (7.5 mg of hyperbaric bupivacaine) unilateral subarachnoid anesthesia with the addition of intrathecal fentanyl (10 mcg) achieved satisfactory analgesia.[83]

CANCER SURGERY

SURGERY FOR PROSTATE CANCER

Preoperative Considerations

Epidemiology One of the most common major surgical procedures in the United States, approximately 60,000 radical prostatectomies are performed yearly. In fact, prostate cancer is the most common cancer and the second leading oncologic cause of death in men.[84] Its incidence increases progressively with age, has no definite peak age of incidence, and reaches 17% in men between 60 and 79 years old.[85] Probably as a result of screening by prostatic specific antigen and by rectal examination, the mortality rate from prostate cancer has decreased during the past few years.[84,86] The histologic diagnosis is adenocarcinoma in 95% of cases; most of the remaining ones are transitional cell carcinomas. The most popular grading system for prostate carcinoma is the Gleason score, which assigns a grade to the appearance of the glandular architecture based on its level of differentiation.

Therapeutic Choices Prostate cancer has a broad spectrum of activity that ranges from indolent to highly virulent; for this reason, management decisions are often difficult. It is still unclear what the best management should be, particularly for patients with early, localized disease. Older patients tend to have well-differentiated cancers with a slow progression. At the same time, they have significant comorbidities and increased surgical risk. Watchful waiting is therefore often offered to patients who are candidates for curative therapy with the goal of identifying those whose cancer progresses. In a recent randomized trial, radical prostatectomy was compared with watchful waiting in a group of 695 patients with early prostate cancer.[87] During a 10-year follow-up, prostatectomy resulted in a 26% decrease in mortality and in a 40% decrease in the rate of distant metastases compared with watchful waiting. However, the beneficial effects of surgery on mortality were limited to patients younger than 65 years. These results suggest that radical prostatectomy is probably the best option in this group of patients. Radical prostatectomy is often preceded by dissection of pelvic lymph nodes to stage the disease accurately. Patients with positive nodes are very likely to have distant metastases. These patients and patients with locally advanced disease are candidates for nonsurgical treatments. In patients with localized disease, external-beam radiotherapy[88] and brachytherapy are common alternatives. Brachytherapy involves implanting radioactive needles or "seeds" into the prostate, guided by transrectal ultrasonography, and has a rate of cancer control that is comparable to radical prostatectomy.

Traditionally, radical retropubic prostatectomy (RRP) has been the most common surgical treatment for prostate cancer; however, minimally invasive laparoscopic radical prostatectomy, including robotic surgery, is widely gaining favor (see section Minimally Invasive Urologic Surgery). During RRP, the prostate is approached through a low, midline abdominal incision. The whole prostate is removed together with the seminal vesicles, the ejaculatory ducts, and a section of the bladder neck. The bladder neck is then anastomosed to the urethra. At this stage, indigo carmine is often injected to identify the ureters. The injection of this drug can cause hypertension.[89] Among the long-term complications of RRP, the most frequent one is probably sexual dysfunction. A "nerve-sparing" prostatectomy is performed by approaching the prostate gland from the bladder side while preserving the neurovascular bundle, with the advantage of less postoperative sexual dysfunction. This procedure may result in a higher rate of cancer recurrence if there is extracapsular extension.[29]

Radical perineal prostatectomy is used more rarely because of the inability to simultaneously dissect the perineal lymph nodes and the requirement of extreme lithotomy position.[90] However, technical improvements have led to a reevaluation of this technique,[91] which is associated with decreased hemorrhage, reduced hospital stay, and less postoperative pain than RRP.[92]

Complications

Bleeding Hemorrhage is the most common complication and is more frequent with the retropubic approach. Various techniques have been proposed to limit the amount of bleeding or the need for blood transfusion, which is associated with an increased risk of nosocomial infections and cancer recurrence.[93] Preoperative autologous donation (PAD) is among the most popular transfusion-sparing techniques for radical prostatectomy. However, PAD has a high cost and does not eliminate the risk of transfusion errors. Acute normovolemic hemodilution (ANH) has been advocated as a more cost-effective technique because it is as effective as PAD in avoiding allogenic transfusion but avoids the cost of blood storage and the waste of unused blood.[94] In a randomized study of patients undergoing radical prostatectomy, PAD was compared with ANH and with ANH combined with preoperative recombinant human erythropoietin administration.[95] The latter technique was the most effective in avoiding postoperative anemia, but the elevated cost of erythropoietin eliminated the financial advantage of using ANH. Intraoperative cell salvage has been proposed as an alternative technique to PAD during radical prostatectomy because it has similar effectiveness but generally lower cost.[96] The concern of possibly spreading cancers cells in the circulation has limited the use of this technique, although there is no demonstrated link between cell salvage and cancer recurrence.[97] Another often proposed technique is induced hypotension, which can be achieved using IV antihypertensives[98] or epidural infusion of local anesthetic.[99]

Anesthetic Management

Monitoring As is the case for most major abdominal surgical procedures, the extent of hemodynamic monitoring should be based on patient characteristics. The management is complicated by the fact that urine output is not measurable while the continuity of the urethra is interrupted; thus, it cannot be used to assess renal perfusion. Invasive monitors are often used, although the accuracy of central venous pressures in estimating blood volume is questionable,[100] and the routine intraoperative use of pulmonary artery catheters has no documented outcome benefit.[101] Multiple alternative cardiac output monitors are now available, but their relative value versus pulmonary artery catheterization remains to be established.

Anesthetic Choice The choice of anesthesia may have a role in affecting the rates of cancer recurrence[102] and of venous thromboembolism after prostatectomy. In fact, epidural analgesia maintained for 24 hours postoperatively after prostatectomy significantly reduced the incidence of deep venous thrombosis compared with general anesthesia alone.[103] This effect could be related to intraoperatively increased venous blood flow in the lower extremities,[104] local anesthetic effects on the hemostatic system,[105] and attenuation of the stress response. Decreased blood loss was reported with the use of epidural anesthesia, alone or combined with general anesthesia.[106]

Regional analgesia appears to improve postoperative pain control. A randomized controlled study detected less pain in patients undergoing RRP with a combined general–epidural technique compared with general anesthesia alone.[92] Pain control achieved with the combined technique was comparable to that for patients undergoing a perineal approach. However, it is unclear whether the use of regional anesthetic or analgesic techniques significantly improves the perioperative outcomes of prostatectomy. In a retrospective review, the addition of paravertebral blocks to a multimodal analgesia strategy conferred advantages in terms of narcotic usage and duration of hospitalization.[107] According to a recent randomized trial, spinal anesthesia combined with conscious sedation offers advantages compared with general anesthesia, including shorter recovery times and decreased blood loss.[108] Other studies did not detect major outcome benefits. A blinded randomized trial on 60 RRP patients detected an improvement in pain control and expiratory flows in the group randomized to low-thoracic epidural analgesia compared with the control group receiving patient controlled IV analgesia. However, these benefits did not translate into earlier discharge or a reduced complication rate.[109] Similarly, in a small randomized study on patients undergoing RRP, the addition of epidural analgesia to general anesthesia did not confer any significant advantage compared with wound infiltration and systemic analgesics.[110] In this study, reported pain scores were relatively low in all groups.

A recently introduced technique, the transversus abdominis plane block, allows sensory blocking of the anterior abdominal wall[111] and appears to achieve adequate pain control in RRP patients.[112] The technique is simple to perform and of relatively low risk, but experience with this block is still limited.

SURGERY FOR BLADDER CANCER

Preoperative Considerations Bladder cancer is the fourth most common malignant tumor in men and the ninth among women in the United states, with a mortality rate that is strongly influenced by the stage at diagnosis and ethnicity.[84] For this reason, emphasis has been placed on early diagnosis and aggressive management of early-stage disease. The most important risk factors for cancer of the bladder are sex, age, smoking history, and exposure to arylamines. Fluid intake may influence the risk of bladder cancer, suggested by a prospective study in which the consumption of water or other beverages was inversely related to the odds of developing bladder cancer in a 10-year follow-up.[113]

The majority of patients with bladder cancer present with hematuria or voiding disturbances. The standard diagnostic method is cystoscopy and biopsy. Subsequent management depends on the degree of invasiveness. The majority of patients have superficial disease managed by transurethral resection, often followed by intravesical administration of adjuvant chemotherapy or of Bacille Calmette-Guerin instillation.[114] The surgical and anesthetic management of patients undergoing transurethral resections has been described in the above section.

Radical Cystectomy Patients who have high-risk superficial tumors or who have invasive tumors are candidates for radical cystectomy. This is the most common procedure for invasive cancer of the bladder; the use of partial cystectomy has decreased considerably given its high recurrence rate.[115] Radical cystectomy has a high rate of cure for patients with localized disease, with survival rates of about 70%.[114] A significant portion of patients will have distant recurrence even after radical cystectomy;

therefore, adjuvant or neoadjuvant chemotherapy is often given. A recent randomized study detected better survival rates in patients with locally advanced bladder cancer who received a course of chemotherapy before radical cystectomy as opposed to patients who received surgery alone.[116] During radical cystectomy, a low midline incision is performed followed by removal of the bladder; peritoneum; perivesical fat; lower ureters; prostate; seminal vesicles; and depending on tumor spread, the urethra. In women, the uterus, ovaries, tubes, urethra, and the anterior vaginal wall are removed. Pelvic lymph node dissection is usually performed during radical cystectomy because it provides important staging and prognostic information and may contribute to improved control of disease and survival rates.[117] Finally, a type of urinary diversion or bladder reconstruction is performed. Creation of an orthotopic neobladder using a segment of ileum or colon anastomosed to the native urethra is the first line choice because of improved quality of life. This approach may not be possible in patients who have urethral or prostatic involvement. Alternative approaches include continent cutaneous diversion, in which a reservoir is created from a bowel segment and open to the abdominal wall, and noncontinent diversions such as ileal loop or cutaneous urostomy. A continent diversion affords better quality of life compared with noncontinent ones, but requires intermittent self-catheterization. All patients with intestinal pouches have chronic bacteriuria and are subject to recurrent UTIs and pyelonephritis.[118]

Complications Radical cystectomy is a relatively high-risk procedure, although improvements in surgical and perioperative care have reduced the rate of major complications to an acceptable level (**Table 61-3**). Patients commonly are of advanced age and more often men. Additionally, they have significant risk factors for complications and comorbidities, such as history of smoking and chronic pulmonary and heart disease. In an observational study of more than 2500 veterans undergoing cystectomy, independent predictors of postoperative morbidity included age, preoperative renal failure, elevated ASA status, the use of general anesthesia, operative time, intraoperative transfusions, alcohol use, dyspnea, and dependent status.[119] Morbid obesity does not seem to confer an increase risk of morbidity.[120] According to a smaller observational study, surgical factors predisposing to complications include blood loss, operative time, type of diversion, and stage of cancer.[121] In this study, the overall rate of complications was reported to be around 30%. Postoperative ileus is the most common minor complication and results in increased hospital stays.[122] Unlike other types of major abdominal surgery, cystectomy is not associated with a particularly elevated risk of postoperative pulmonary complications, probably because the site of incision is far from the diaphragm.[123]

Anesthetic Management

Monitoring Despite improvements in surgical technique, radical cystectomy continues to be associated with significant blood loss. In a recent study, blood transfusion was required in 30% of the cases.[124] Female gender, preoperative anemia, and performance of ileal conduit were predictors of a higher need for transfusion. Controlled hypotensive anesthesia has been advocated to reduce transfusion requirements, but the advantages of this practice should be critically compared with its risk in a population with a significant cardiovascular risk.[125,126] The procedure is relatively lengthy depending on the type of urinary diversion performed. Thorough monitoring of blood loss and attempts at estimating intravascular volume are necessary during this procedure. Invasive arterial blood pressure monitoring has the additional advantage of allowing frequent measurement of hematocrit. Volume status monitoring is hindered by the fact that the urinary tract is interrupted during most of the operation. In patients with heart dysfunction or renal disease, measuring central venous pressure may be indicated, but the limitations of this variable should also be recognized (see Chapter 30 regarding hemodynamic monitoring). Alternatively, monitoring blood pressure variations provides an accurate estimate of the need for fluid administration, with a predictive power superior to central venous and left atrial pressure monitoring in critically ill patients.[100] Pulmonary artery catheters should not be used routinely but only in selected cases and to allow goal-directed hemodynamic management.

TABLE 61-3 Major Complications of Radical Cystectomy

Complications	Reported Rate (%)
Return to operating room	2
Cerebrovascular accident	1
Sepsis	1
Respiratory failure	1
Pulmonary embolus	1
Myocardial infarction	1
Death	1-3

Data from Carrion R, Seigne J. Surgical management of bladder carcinoma. *Cancer Control.* 2002;9:284-292.

Anesthetic Choices Radical cystectomy is usually performed under general anesthesia, although it is possible to use neuraxial block. Epidural anesthesia is more likely to be used in combination with general anesthesia because of the length of the procedure and patient discomfort during regional anesthesia alone. The use of epidural anesthesia together with general anesthesia has been reported to result in a decreased blood loss and transfusion rate compared with general anesthesia alone but with no effect on the overall rate of complication, similar to radical prostatectomy.[127] In this study, postoperative pain control was also improved in patients receiving epidural anesthesia. A large observational Veterans Health Administration study identified general anesthesia versus neuraxial block as a risk factor for complications after cystectomy.[119] To date, no randomized controlled study has demonstrated an outcome benefit. A large well-conducted study on the outcomes of anesthetic choices in urologic surgery is needed.

Sympathectomy from neuraxial blockade promotes intestinal muscle spasm caused by unopposed parasympathetic stimulation, which can render the fabrication of an ileal pouch technically difficult. Epidural infusion can be delayed until after pouch completion or, alternatively, IV glycopyrrolate or papaverine has been used to obviate this problem.[128]

SURGERY FOR TESTICULAR CANCER

Preoperative Considerations Malignant tumors of the testicle are relatively rare, with an incidence of 2 to 3 cases per 100,000 males each year. Histologically, 95% of testicular cancers are germ cell tumors, and 35% of them are seminomas. Nonseminomas such as embryonal cell carcinoma, teratoma, choriocarcinoma, and mixed cell type tumors are clinically more invasive and require more aggressive management.[129] The incidence of germ cell tumors is highest in the third and fourth decades of life and is heavily affected by ethnicity. In fact, germ cell tumors are significantly more frequent in whites than in people of Asian or African descent. The only known risk factors known to date are a history of cryptorchidism and of Klinefelter syndrome. Orchiopexy reduces the risk of testicular cancer if performed before puberty.[129]

Testicular tumors may present with a painless testicular mass or, more often, with testicular pain and swelling, which may be confused with orchitis or epididymitis. Only occasionally, patients may have germ cell tumors that do not originate in the testicle. The diagnosis of testicular cancer is confirmed by testicular ultrasonography. Abdominal computed tomography (CT) scans are usually obtained for clinical staging. Metastatic spread of testicular tumors follows a characteristic stepwise pattern along the retroperitoneal lymphatics.

Therapeutic Choices Radical orchiectomy is required for all patients with testicular tumor, and further management depends on the extent of metastatic spread and tumor histology. The curability of germ cell tumors, particularly seminomas, is more than 90% with current management protocols. The stage at presentation and the survival worsen with delay of recognition, which suggests the importance of early detection.[129] Patients with low-stage seminomas are treated with retroperitoneal radiation therapy after orchiectomy, although active surveillance is also practiced in select cases.[130] Nonseminomatous tumors are clinically more invasive and require a more aggressive management, but the curability is still greater than 90%. Retroperitoneal lymph node dissection (RPLND) is often used for these tumors, although observation may also be chosen because RPLND is often complicated by retrograde ejaculation and infertility. During RPLND, the lumbar sympathetic chain is ablated. Alternatively, a modified RPLND that spares the sympathetic nerves is often used.[29] The response to therapy and recurrence is evaluated after CT scan of the abdomen and the trend of biological markers such as alpha-fetoprotein, human chorionic gonadotropin (hCG), and lactate dehydrogenase. Combination chemotherapy is the standard protocol for recurrent or high-stage testicular cancer. It incorporates cisplatin, etoposide, and bleomycin. Chemotherapy may be complicated by nerve and renal toxicity and by pulmonary fibrosis caused by bleomycin.

Orchiectomy Radical orchiectomy is performed by inguinal exploration, cross-clamping, and ligation of the spermatic cord at the internal inguinal ring. Transscrotal orchiectomy is not used because it predisposes to local and pelvic lymph node metastasis. This procedure can be safely performed with either general or regional anesthesia, depending on patient preferences.

Retroperitoneal Lymph Node Dissection Performed through a midline abdominal or thoracoabdominal incision, the standard RPLND involves removal of all lymphatic tissue between the ureters and between the superior mesenteric artery and the iliac vessels. The modified RPLND limits the extent of lymph node dissection and spares the sympathetic chain and hypogastric plexus on the side contralateral to the involved testicle. This technique preserves ejaculatory function in 80% to 90% of cases. General anesthesia is commonly used for this procedure. Pain management is particularly important for thoracoabdominal incisions and can be achieved with epidural anesthesia or intercostal nerve blocks. Blood and fluid losses can be significant during this procedure and should be replaced carefully. Large-bore IV access is strongly recommended.

Patients undergoing surgery for testicular cancer are usually young without significant comorbidities; however, patients who have undergone combination chemotherapy before the procedure may experience the toxicities of the agents used. Bleomycin is associated with pulmonary toxicity. Patients at higher risk for this complication are those who received higher doses, those who are older, and those with renal insufficiency. Acute respiratory distress syndrome has been reported after surgery in patients who had been exposed to bleomycin. Exposure to high concentrations of oxygen seems to favor the onset of this complication, according to evidence from animal studies and a series of patients.[131,132] There is little evidence that a short exposure to high inspired oxygen results in acute pulmonary toxicity in patients with normal baseline pulmonary function.[133] The lowest inspired oxygen concentration that achieves acceptable oxygen saturation values is a reasonable choice in patients treated with bleomycin.[134]

During left-sided dissection, ligation of the intercostal arteries may lead to loss of circulation through the artery of Adamkewicz, with consequent ischemia of the spinal cord. It is therefore important to document motor function before and after surgery. When patients who received epidural anesthesia develop neurologic signs postoperatively, this complication should be included in the differential diagnosis.

SURGERY FOR RENAL CANCER

Preoperative Considerations Renal carcinoma accounts for 3% to 4% of all cancers in the United States.[84] A total of 85% of renal masses are renal cell carcinoma, and only 2% of these cancers are associated with inherited conditions such as von Hippel-Lindau disease.[135] However, defects in the von Hippel-Lindau suppressor gene, an important regulator of cellular response to hypoxemia, may be responsible for a significant fraction of sporadic renal cell carcinomas. Tobacco smoking is an important risk factor for this disease. The peak incidence of renal carcinoma is 60 years, and there is a 1.6 to 1 male-to-female ratio.[135]

About 50% of renal carcinomas are incidentally detected from abdominal imaging. A common presentation of this disease is hematuria, and its presence should always prompt further evaluation. The diagnostic and staging process includes contrast CT scan or gadolinium-enhanced magnetic resonance imaging of the abdomen. In 5% to 10% of patients, tumor extension to the renal vein or to the vena cava occurs, worsening survival and complicating surgical management. Its presence and extent should be investigated.

Some patients may present with paraneoplastic phenomena caused by secretion of hormones by cancer cells. These include erythrocytosis in 3% to 10% of patients, hypercalcemia in up to 20% of patients, and hypertension refractory to medical treatment in up to 40% of patients.[29] Determination of the prognosis of renal carcinoma in the individual patient is important in treatment and decision making. The survival rate worsens significantly with the stage of the disease. It goes from 95% at 5 years in tumors less than 7 cm and limited to the kidney to 20% in tumors that extend beyond Gerota fascia or with more than 1 lymph node involved.[135]

Nephrectomy Radical nephrectomy is the standard approach to renal cell carcinoma because this tumor is not responsive to chemotherapy. During a radical nephrectomy, the renal artery and then vein are ligated, and the kidney is removed along with the adrenal gland, perinephric fat, Gerota fascia, and regional lymph nodes. Nephron-sparing partial resections had been performed mainly in patients at high risk of postoperative renal failure because of preexisting chronic kidney disease, diabetes, or hypertension because there is concern that these limited resections may be associated with higher rates of tumor recurrence. Partial resection is becoming more popular and is now often chosen for smaller tumors.[136] In the past 10 to 15 years, minimally invasive laparoscopic nephrectomy has become increasingly popular. Chemotherapy, interferon, and interleukin therapy are sometimes used in metastatic disease or as adjuvant therapy, although their effectiveness is unclear.

Anesthetic Management The preoperative evaluation of nephrectomy candidates should follow the standard approach for patients receiving intermediate-risk surgery of the upper abdomen and should be focused on cardiovascular and pulmonary risk factors. A significant fraction of this patient population is composed of smokers and elderly persons at increased risk of cardiac and respiratory complications. Preexisting renal dysfunction should also be noted because its presence may influence intraoperative and anesthetic management. The majority of patients undergoing nephrectomy are anemic, so an adequate amount of red blood cells should be available before surgery, particularly when the renal mass is large.

During nephrectomy, the kidney is usually approached through a flank incision, although subcostal and thoracoabdominal incisions are also used. The thoracoabdominal incision is the most commonly used if vena caval infiltration is known because the flank incision allows adequate access only to the kidney and retroperitoneum but not to the vena cava. The most commonly used position for nephrectomy is lateral with kidney rest elevation. With the flank incision, the pleural space can be accidentally entered through a diaphragm tear, requiring chest tube placement. Routine postoperative chest radiographs should be obtained in the recovery room. With thoracoabdominal incision, a chest tube is placed routinely at the end of the procedure. Other intraoperative complications of radical nephrectomy are hollow viscus injuries and splenic lacerations.

Radical nephrectomy is usually performed under general endotracheal anesthesia. Both intraoperative and postoperative epidural analgesia are also used commonly, although there is little evidence suggesting outcome benefits. Intercostal nerve blocks may be used for thoracoabdominal incision and can contribute to reducing the rate of postoperative atelectasis.[137] Paravertebral nerve blocks are also effective for postoperative pain caused by flank incisions.[138]

Hemodynamic instability is common during open radical nephrectomy. As discussed in the section on positioning, the lateral kidney rest position can cause hypotension that may require reduced flexion of the operating table and treatment with fluid loading. Compression of the vena cava by retractors can cause the same phenomenon. More importantly, nephrectomy patients are prone to significant blood loss, particularly if the mass is large or very vascular, a common finding in renal cell carcinoma. Large-bore IV access is mandatory, and central venous cannulation with a large-bore catheter may be helpful. Pulmonary artery catheterization should not be used routinely but should be reserved for patients with significant cardiovascular comorbidities or used with the intent to reach and maintain specific hemodynamic goals. Arterial cannulation can also be helpful for blood pressure monitoring and for blood sampling. Hemodynamic monitoring and fluid management are particularly important in patients at significant risk of postoperative renal dysfunction to prevent or treat renal hypoperfusion. Controlled hypotension may limit intraoperative blood loss but may not be suitable in patients with preexisting chronic kidney disease. There is no evidence that any pharmacologic strategy effectively provides perioperative renal protection. In particular, loop diuretics, mannitol, and renal vasodilators are not protective in patients undergoing vascular and cardiothoracic surgery. There is currently no evidence supporting the use of these agents in patients undergoing nephrectomy and other high-risk urologic procedures.

In patients with vena cava invasion, nephrectomy is a very high-risk procedure. However, this operation is frequently undertaken because patients have very poor life expectancies without surgery. The complexity of the procedure increases with the extent of tumor invasion. Patients at highest risk for mortality are those with tumor invasion above the diaphragm and into the right atrium. The procedure has to be performed with cardiopulmonary bypass in these cases or when it is not possible to surgically control the vena cave above the level of tumor invasion. Additionally, detachment of tumor fragments with pulmonary embolization is possible during the operation. These patients require large-bore IV access because massive blood loss is a possibility. Additionally, tumors partially or totally occluding the vena cava lumen cause distal elevation of venous pressures and formation of venous collaterals that together increase the extent of blood loss. Invasive hemodynamic monitoring is desirable, but central access is complicated by the risk of detaching tumor emboli when tumor extends to the right atrium, particularly for pulmonary artery catheterization. Alternatively, transesophageal echocardiography (TEE) for hemodynamic monitoring may be useful. TEE allows intraoperative confirmation of the extent of tumor invasion and diagnosis of pulmonary embolization.[139] Patients undergoing nephrectomy should always receive perioperative thromboembolic prophylaxis. This and other major urologic procedures are associated with a high risk of venous thromboembolic complications, and this risk is probably not reduced with the use of laparoscopic techniques.[140]

MINIMALLY INVASIVE UROLOGIC SURGERY

Techniques The past 15 years have seen increasing interest in minimally invasive and laparoscopic urologic procedures. The first procedures accomplished through laparoscopy were procedures for undescended testis and varix ligation followed by retroperitoneal node dissection for testicular, prostate, and bladder cancer. Laparoscopic nephrectomy and prostatectomy are now currently performed in many centers. Laparoscopic urologic surgery offers the obvious advantages of decreased postoperative pain and reduced postoperative hospitalization.

More recently, minimally invasive surgery has been enhanced by the introduction of robotic techniques. These allow the operators to perform complex procedures in less time and with more reliability compared with nonrobotic laparoscopy, improving the learning curve

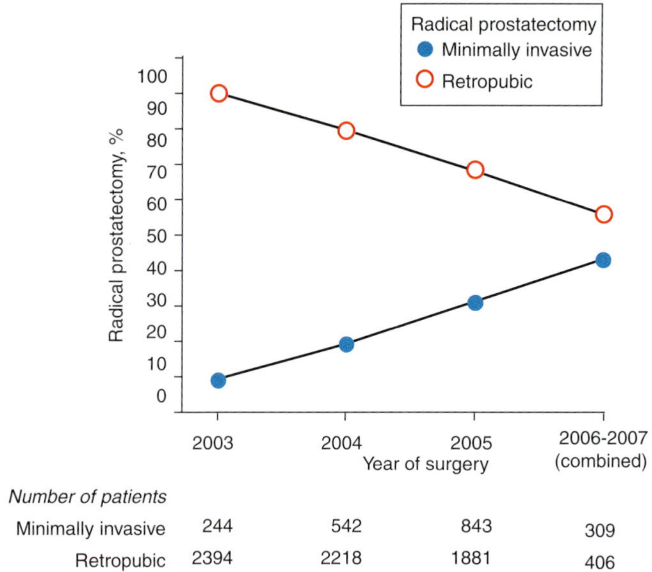

FIGURE 61-8. Relative use of minimally invasive and open retropubic radical prostatectomy between 2003 and 2007. [From Hu JC, Gu X, Lipsitz SR, et al. Comparative effectiveness of minimally invasive vs open radical prostatectomy. *JAMA*. 2009;302(14):1557-1564.]

of the surgeon. It is likely that the use of robotic techniques will become increasingly more common in urology.[141]

Robot-assisted radical cystectomy with neobladder construction seems to be associated with a lower rate of complications and faster postoperative recovery based on early reports.[142] Acceptable rates of complications have been reported.[143] Although this technique still requires prolonged operating time, it is likely this will improve as experience accumulates.[144] Robot-assisted pelvic lymphadenectomy[145] and intracorporeal neobladder construction[146] appear to be feasible and will probably be used more frequently.

Minimally invasive radical prostatectomy (MIRP), performed laparoscopically with and without the use of robots, has seen a rapidly increasing demand, reaching more than 40% of all prostatectomies in 2006[147] (**Fig. 61-8**). This technique reduces blood loss, postoperative pain, and hospital stays,[148-150] but its long-term benefits over conventional techniques are still unclear.[151] A recent retrospective epidemiologic review confirmed a decreased rate of blood transfusion, shorter hospitalization, and reduced incidence of postoperative respiratory complication and anastomotic strictures compared with open RRP.[147] However, MIRP was associated with a twofold increase in the rates of genitourinary complications. Therefore, MIRP cannot yet be recommended as the standard of care. A recent prospective study could not identify differences in pain scores and narcotic use between robot-assisted radical prostatectomy and standard RRP.[152]

Laparoscopic nephrectomy can be performed through a transperitoneal or retroperitoneal approach. With the latter, the patient is placed in a lateral or semilateral flexed position, and a working space is created in the retroperitoneum by inflation of a balloon inserted through a small incision. This space is then distended by CO_2 insufflation. The technique minimizes pain and reduces postoperative recovery time. It is particularly appealing for living donor nephrectomy because of reduced pain and disability.[153] Laparoscopic partial nephrectomy allows early discharge from the hospital when coupled with a multimodal pain management approach that includes narcotics, NSAIDS, and local anesthesia to the port sites.[154] Robot-assisted nephrectomy has been introduced more recently and will probably be used more often as the technique is perfected.[155]

It is still not entirely clear whether laparoscopic cancer surgery achieves the same degree of eradication as standard procedures such as retroperitoneal node dissection and radical nephrectomy. However, the use of minimally invasive and robotic procedures is likely to continue to increase. Although minimally invasive procedures may simplify anesthetic and perioperative management, these techniques will likely permit surgery on patients who, because of comorbidities, are not good candidates for traditional procedures. This will ultimately render the perioperative management of these patients more challenging for anesthesia providers.

Anesthetic Management[156] There is no standard anesthetic management of patients undergoing minimally invasive urologic procedures. The physiologic changes and problems encountered by patients undergoing laparoscopic operations are well known. Laparoscopy in urologic surgery poses additional challenges, such as those related to particular positions adopted in this specialty. Pneumoperitoneum combined with the head-down position is often used for a prolonged time to facilitate surgical access during laparoscopic and robotic prostatectomy. Pneumoperitoneum causes an upward shift of the diaphragm and decreased chest wall compliance, resulting in reduced lung volumes and increased airway pressures.[157] In the head-down position, the diaphragmatic shift is exaggerated, further decreasing lung volume.[1] Atelectasis may result, but it can be prevented by application of positive end-expiratory pressure or treated by inflation maneuvers. The increased airway pressure observed during pneumoperitoneum is the result of decreased chest wall compliance, not of lung hyperinflation, and it should not be considered as a factor predisposing to barotrauma. It is important to periodically reconfirm endotracheal tube position because both the head-down position and pneumoperitoneum cause the carina to migrate cephalad, predisposing patients to accidental bronchial intubation.[158] Transperitoneal absorption of CO_2 causes parallel increases in arterial and end-tidal P_{CO_2} that must be compensated by increased ventilation to avoid acidemia. This can be done by increasing the respiratory rate, tidal volume, or both. The retroperitoneal space is very vascular, which explains the increased CO_2 absorption observed in patients undergoing retroperitoneal laparoscopy compared with intraperitoneal insufflation.[159] However, not all studies have confirmed this difference.[160] The combination of pneumoperitoneum and the head-down position also causes increased systemic arterial resistance.[161] systolic heart volumes, and ventricular systolic work.[162] These changes may potentially lead to myocardial ischemia in patients at risk. Laparoscopy in the lateral, flexed position may significantly decrease venous return, causing low cardiac output and hypotension. During pneumoperitoneum in the head-down position, the resulting changes in venous pressures, together with hypercapnia, can lead to significant increases in ICP and, potentially, brain injury in selected patients.[163] In patients without space-occupying intracranial lesions, even prolonged pneumoperitoneum in the head-down position seems to be well tolerated as shown in a prospective study on patients undergoing robotic prostatectomy in the steep (40 degrees) head-down position. These patients had clinically acceptable changes in cerebral perfusion pressure and brain oxygenation.[164] A rare but devastating complication during minimally invasive prostatectomy is the occurrence of visual changes caused by ischemic neuropathy.[165] Although the risk factors of this complication are unclear, it may be related to the time-dependent increase in intraocular pressure observed during robotic laparoscopic prostatectomy in the steep head-down position.[166] Patients with glaucoma could be at increased risk for visual loss, but data supporting this statement are scanty. Other reported complications are postextubation respiratory distress caused by laryngeal edema and brachial plexus neurapraxia caused by shoulder braces in the head-down position.[156] In nephrectomy patients with pre-existing renal disease, laparoscopy may create additional kidney injury caused by elevated intra-abdominal pressure and kidney manipulation. Kidney injury may be limited by maintaining adequate blood volume and hemodynamic stability. To date, none of the existing "renal protection" pharmacologic strategies has proven effective.

Depending on the surgeon's experience with these procedures, the anesthetic plan should anticipate the possibility of conversion to open procedure or significant bleeding. Laparoscopy patients should have a preoperative evaluation identical to patients undergoing the equivalent open procedure. Cardiovascular monitoring should be appropriate for the planned procedure based on the patient's clinical status. Central venous and pulmonary artery wedge pressure measurements are biased during laparoscopy caused by transmission of intra-abdominal pressure to the mediastinal space. The use of transesophageal echocardiography in high-risk patients allows more accurate assessment of cardiac volumes and stroke volume.[161] Bladder catheterization and nasogastric intubation are usually performed for laparoscopic procedures.

When laparoscopic procedures are performed in an ambulatory setting, the choice of induction and maintenance anesthetic agents reflects the need for prompt awakening and rapid recovery. In laparoscopic surgery, nitrous oxide is often avoided to prevent bowel distension in case the procedure becomes prolonged. Intraoperative and postoperative analgesia is usually performed with a combination of opioids and NSAIDs.[154] Epidural analgesia is not routinely offered.

Among the complications of laparoscopic procedures are bleeding, subcutaneous emphysema, pneumothorax, diaphragmatic tears, and gas embolism.[167] Although the use of CO_2 for pneumoperitoneum reduces the probability of massive embolism, it is a potentially fatal complication and should be considered in case of intraoperative hemodynamic deterioration.

KEY REFERENCES

- Arozullah AM, Daley J, Henderson WG, Khuri SF. Multifactorial risk index for predicting postoperative respiratory failure in men after major noncardiac surgery. The national Veterans Administration Surgical Quality Improvement Program. *Ann Surg*. 2000;232:242-253.
- Gravenstein D. Transurethral resection of the prostate (TURP) syndrome: a review of the pathophysiology and management. *Anesth Analg*. 1997;84:438-446.
- Gupta A, Fant F, Axelsson K, et al. Postoperative analgesia after radical retropubic prostatectomy: a double-blind comparison between low thoracic epidural and patient-controlled intravenous analgesia. *Anesthesiology*. 2006;105:784-793.
- Hu JC, Gu X, Lipsitz SR, et al. Comparative effectiveness of minimally invasive vs open radical prostatectomy. *JAMA*. 2009; 302:1557-1564.
- McDonnell JG, O'Donnell B, Curley G, et al. The analgesic efficacy of transversus abdominis plane block after abdominal surgery: a prospective randomized controlled trial. *Anesth Analg*. 2007;104:193-197.
- Practice advisory for the prevention of perioperative peripheral neuropathies: a report by the American Society of Anesthesiologists Task Force on Prevention of Perioperative Peripheral Neuropathies. *Anesthesiology*. 2000;92:1168-1182.
- Zaric D, Pace NL. Transient neurologic symptoms (TNS) following spinal anaesthesia with lidocaine versus other local anaesthetics. *Cochrane Database Syst Rev*. 2009;(2):CD003006.

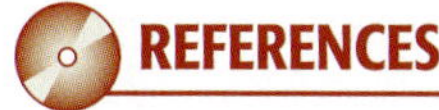

REFERENCES

Complete references available on DVD and online version at www.LongneckerAnesthesiology.com

CHAPTER 62 Anesthesia for Obstetric Care and Gynecologic Surgery

Lawrence C. Tsen

KEY POINTS

1. The use of epidural, spinal, combined spinal–epidural, and dural-puncture epidural techniques for obstetric care has increased dramatically because of the quality and safety of the analgesia and anesthesia produced, the ability to titrate the degree and duration of pain relief, and the expanding number of situations for which their use is appropriate.
2. Labor analgesia and obstetric anesthesia can have beneficial effects on the outcomes of external cephalic version, in utero fetal and placental surgery, and parturients with significant comorbid conditions.
3. Major fetal organogenesis occurs during weeks 3 to 10 of gestation. Teratogenicity is difficult to evaluate in prospective clinical trials because of the low incidence of occurrence and the number of confounding factors, but the list of proven human teratogens does not include the anesthetics commonly used in clinical practice.
4. Although important reductions in anesthesia-related maternal mortality have occurred in the past 5 decades, a greater risk (1.7 times) of maternal death is still witnessed with the use of general versus regional anesthesia. This finding can be partially explained by changes in the airway that occur over the course of pregnancy. Promotion of neuraxial techniques, skill with alternate airway devices, and review of difficult airway algorithms are strongly encouraged.
5. Antenatal and postpartum maternal hemorrhage can be masked until significant blood loss has occurred, but a cogent plan for diagnosis and response can significantly affect the outcome. Interventional radiologists may place occlusion balloons within the uterine or hypogastric arteries in high-risk parturients to allow timely control of bleeding.
6. Preeclampsia is a multisystem disease that raises numerous concerns for anesthesia care, but neuraxial techniques remain the preferred option unless contraindicated by coagulations disorders, severe hypovolemia, or patient preference.
7. Anesthetic care for gynecologic surgery requires an understanding of gender-related differences in physiology, including sensitivity to pain, and pharmacodynamics, including responses to anesthetic drugs; such differences ultimately may affect patient outcomes and satisfaction.
8. Both obstetric and gynecologic surgery involve positions, techniques, and organ systems that require special vigilance. The uterus and other female viscera are highly vascular. Blood loss can be sudden and profuse; air emboli can occur unexpectedly (especially in the Trendelenburg position); and in pregnancy-related procedures, amniotic fluid emboli can occur without provocation.
9. Hysteroscopic and laparoscopic procedures can result in significant adverse outcomes from absorption of carbon dioxide (CO_2) or the distending medium. CO_2 insufflation of the abdomen or pelvis may cause a number of disturbances in cardiac and respiratory physiology, which can be minimized if anticipated.
10. The Trendelenburg lithotomy position, which is commonly used for gynecologic procedures, may lead to a number of peripheral nerve injuries. Excessive hip flexion, abduction, and external rotation may cause femoral nerve, obturator, lateral femoral cutaneous, sciatic, and peroneal nerve injuries. Attention to positioning throughout the procedure, use of protective padding, and avoidance of contact with hard surfaces or supports are important elements of optimal care.

Just a few months separated the introduction of anesthetics for general surgical procedures and obstetric care. Ether, then believed to be the panacea to "cure all ills," was found to be efficacious but not optimal in both environments. Today, although the use of general volatile anesthetics remains popular, the advent of regional anesthetic techniques has greatly expanded the ability to provide analgesia and anesthesia for a wide spectrum of procedures and conditions. Selection of the optimal anesthetic technique for obstetric and gynecologic patients should consider the significant anatomic, hormonal, and physiologic adaptations that ultimately allow a female to conceive and carry a pregnancy. This chapter discusses the provision of analgesia and anesthesia for obstetric care and gynecologic surgery. Emphasis is placed on the three primary settings of care: provision of analgesia for labor and delivery, anesthesia for obstetric and nonobstetric surgery during pregnancy, and anesthesia for gynecologic surgery.

ANALGESIA AND ANESTHESIA ASSOCIATED WITH PREGNANCY

With the application of diethyl ether to aid in a vaginal delivery in 1847, James Young Simpson, an obstetrician, ushered in the use of anesthetics for obstetrics. The next half century was associated with increased acceptance and evolution of anesthetic drugs and techniques for labor and delivery. Regional anesthetic techniques, which deliver pain relief to a discrete region of the body, were introduced to obstetrics in 1900, when Oskar Kreis described the use of spinal anesthesia. Since that time, central neuraxial techniques have evolved from single, limited-duration injections into the intrathecal (subarachnoid) space to titratable, controlled infusions through flexible catheters most commonly placed into the epidural space. These techniques are often the optimal method for providing analgesia for labor, anesthesia for obstetric or nonobstetric surgery during pregnancy, and analgesia for postoperative care. Because these techniques are so fundamental to the practice of anesthesia for parturients, they are discussed initially and then the rationale and details for their use are expanded throughout the chapter.

NEURAXIAL TECHNIQUES

Regardless of which neuraxial technique is used for labor, delivery, or nonobstetric operations, a standardized approach is warranted. A preprocedure history and physical examination with notation of allergies; baseline vital signs; and assessment of the airway, body habitus, and hematologic system (eg, preeclampsia-induced thrombocytopenia; see Hypertensive Disorders of Pregnancy below and Chapter 21) are mandatory, even if the situation is urgent. An intravenous (IV) catheter and fluid administration should be started, especially because hypotension can abruptly follow neuraxial technique placement and affect both maternal and fetal welfare. Whether crystalloid or colloid solutions are administered to minimize hypotension is controversial. Colloids have been observed to minimize but not eliminate hypotension but can be associated with increased costs, risk of allergies, and coagulation disorders (when given in large doses eg, hetastarch in doses >20 mL/kg). IV fluids, regardless of the amount administered, do not reliably minimize hypotension. Thus, in urgent situations, waiting for an arbitrary amount of fluid to be infused before the neuraxial anesthesia or analgesia is not necessary. The seated position is often selected for the purportedly enhanced ability to palpate the vertebral spinous processes and identify the midline plane. However, these landmarks can also be achieved in the lateral recumbent position. In addition, in pregnant patients, the lateral recumbent position has the particular advantage of minimizing venous plexus engorgement, resulting in reductions in vessel trauma, vessel cannulation, and placement attempts.[1] In certain emergent situations, such as umbilical cord prolapse or fetal head entrapment, the seated position is not a viable option. As such, a general anesthetic would be the only available method for delivering anesthesia if the anesthesiologist is not comfortable instrumenting the back in the lateral position.

Selection of the optimal neuraxial technique depends principally on the desired onset, reliability, and titratability of the resulting analgesia

TABLE 62-1 Local Anesthetics for Epidural Analgesia and Anesthesia

Anesthetic	Usual Concentration (%)	Onset	Duration
Analgesia			
Lidocaine	1-1.5	Moderate	Intermediate
Bupivacaine	0.0625-0.25	Slow	Slow
L-Bupivacaine	0.0625-0.25	Slow	Slow
Ropivacaine	0.1-0.2	Slow	Long
Anesthesia			
2-Chloroprocaine	2-3	Fast	Short
Lidocaine	2-5	Moderate	Intermediate
Mepivacaine	2	Moderate	Intermediate
Bupivacaine	0.5	Slow	Long
L-Bupivacaine	0.5	Slow	Long
Ropivacaine	0.5-1	Slow	Long
Tetracaine	1	Slow	Long

or anesthesia, with catheter-based techniques offering the greatest flexibility. The spinal technique offers confirmation of the space via cerebrospinal fluid (CSF) flow, fast onset, and very reliable sensory and motor blockade; however, the duration of blockade is time limited and may be associated with abrupt hemodynamic alterations. By contrast, the epidural technique has a slower onset; does not intentionally create a dural puncture; and when used with a catheter, offers an almost unlimited duration of blockade; however, the resulting block may be patchy or one sided, and a large dural puncture may occur inadvertently. The dose, onset, and duration of various local anesthetics for epidural labor analgesia and anesthesia are well characterized (**Table 62-1**). The epidural technique may enable a lesser incidence and extent of maternal hypotension because of the ability to administer the dose of local anesthetic in a fractionated manner and allow compensatory cardiovascular mechanisms to respond to the more slowly developing sympathetic blockade. The combined spinal–epidural (CSE) technique, which consists of epidural needle placement, administration of subarachnoid medications via a spinal needle placed through the shaft of the epidural needle, and placement of an epidural catheter (**Fig. 62-1**),[2] appears to combine the best of both techniques with a blockade that is rapid in onset, is reliable, and can be prolonged. A variation of the CSE technique is the dural puncture epidural (DPE) technique, which includes all of the same steps except for the omission of direct medication dosing through the spinal needle. Instead, all medications are dosed into the epidural space, which allows transit through the dural puncture and provides faster onset and an improved sacral and bilateral blockade compared with a standard epidural technique.[3] With the CSE and DPE techniques, the spinal needle emerges 10 to 15 mm beyond the tip of the epidural needle,[2] the presence of CSF can confirm that the epidural needle is proximal to or in the epidural space. This information can be of value when multiple "losses of resistance" are encountered during epidural needle placement.

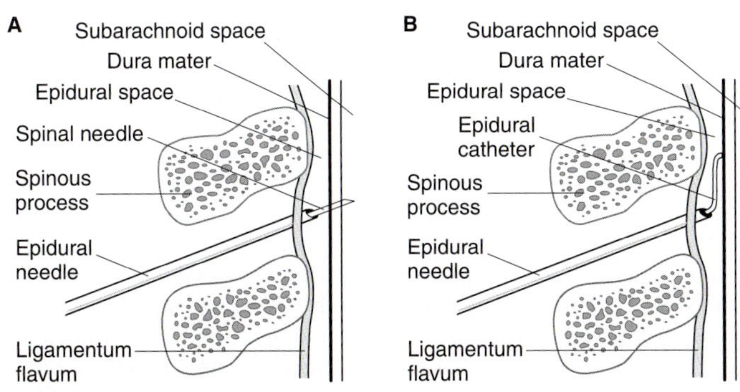

FIGURE 62-1. Combined spinal–epidural technique.

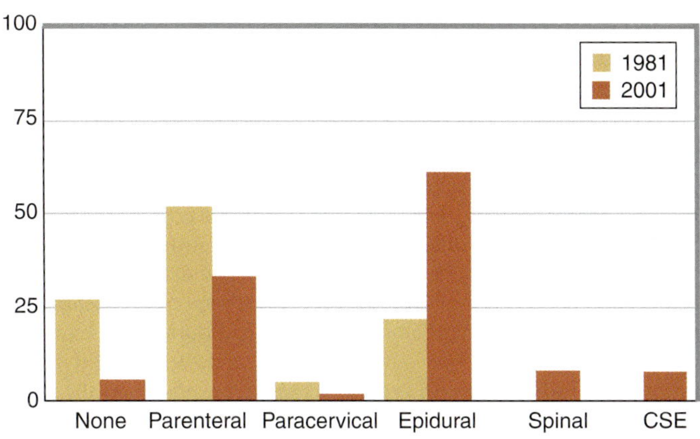

FIGURE 62-2. Types of analgesia provided for labor. Reported as percent of total cases in hospitals with more than 1500 births annually. CSE, combined spinal–epidural technique. [Based on data from Bucklin BA, Hawkins JL, Anderson JR, et al. Obstetric anesthesia workforce survey: twenty-year update. *Anesthesiology.* 2005;103:645-653.][9]

Intentional puncture of the dural ligament with an epidural needle and placement of a catheter into the subarachnoid space, called a "spinal catheter technique," is a viable option. Spinal catheter techniques have the benefit of CSF confirmation and the ability to provide a highly reliable and titratable blockade.[4] Such techniques are often used in parturients who are morbidly obese, in those with significant cardiac disease, and after an unintentional dural puncture with an attempted epidural catheter placement. Because placement of a spinal catheter depends on use of epidural equipment (eg, 17-gauge Tuohy needle and 20-gauge catheter), a significant postdural puncture headache risk exists. Smaller needles and catheters for labor and delivery are currently being used or evaluated in Europe and the United States, respectively, with the hope of avoiding the cauda equina syndrome observed during the earlier microcatheter trials. This complication most likely resulted from pooling of excessive amounts of local anesthetics.[5,6]

Use of epidural, spinal, and CSE techniques has increased dramatically, particularly for obstetric indications (**Fig. 62-2**). This increase has been driven in large part by the quality and safety of the analgesia and anesthesia produced, the ability to dictate the intensity and duration of pain relief as required by the circumstances, and an expanding number of situations in which their use is appropriate. Use of neuraxial opioids results in improved analgesia compared with IV opioid administration, likely because of actions on both supraspinal and spinal opioid receptors (**Table 62-2**).[7] Currently, in developed countries, central neuraxial techniques provide labor analgesia for 30% to 50% of all parturients and the anesthesia for the majority of instrumental and operative deliveries.[8,9]

TABLE 62-2 Opioids for Neuraxial Use in Obstetrics

Opioid	Epidural Dose	Spinal Dose	Duration (h)	Comments
Morphine	2.5-5 mg	0.1-0.2 mg	18-24	Useful primarily for post–cesarean section analgesia
Fentanyl	50-100 mcg	10-20 mcg	3-4	Useful as labor and operative adjuvant
Sufentanil	10-20 mcg	5-10 mcg	3-4	Useful as labor and operative adjuvant
Meperidine	25 mg		2-3	
Hydromorphone	1 mg		12	
Methadone	4-5 mg		5-6	
Diamorphine	2.5-5 mg		5-15	Not available in the United States

CONSIDERATIONS ON MATERNALLY ADMINISTERED ANESTHETICS

Although only a limited percentage of systemically or neuraxially administered anesthetics eventually reaches the fetus (see Chapter 21), an overlying concern during assisted reproductive technologies and pregnancy is the effect on fertilization and embryonic and fetal development. Teratogenicity, defined as any significant postnatal change in function or form in an offspring after prenatal treatment, is difficult to evaluate in prospective clinical trials given the low incidence of occurrence and the number of confounding factors; species susceptibility, genetic predisposition, and amount, timing, and duration of exposure all can affect reproductive outcome. The criteria for identifying an agent as a human teratogen require (1) proven exposure to the agent at the critical time of development; (2) consistent findings in two or more high-quality epidemiologic studies; (3) careful delineation of the clinical cases, ideally with identification of a specific defect or syndrome; and (4) an association that makes "biologic sense."[10] Of note, the list of agents or factors proven to be human teratogens does not include anesthetic agents used routinely in clinical practice (**Box 62-1**); however, readers are encouraged to refer to package inserts provided by drug manufacturers and standard teratology reference sources for more specific information.[10,11] The effect of anesthetics on early cellular division has been reviewed extensively.[12]

Early studies of neurotropic agents (eg, opioids, tricyclic antidepressants, phenothiazines, benzodiazepines, butyrophenones) demonstrated significant teratogenicity in rodents. Subsequent studies, however, questioned the relationship given the high doses of drugs administered and the resulting respiratory depression and impaired feeding. Using more elegant study designs at clinically relevant doses, often provided with chronically implanted osmotic minipumps, the absence of teratogenicity in the agents commonly used for induction (barbiturates, propofol, ketamine, benzodiazepines), analgesia (opioids), and muscle relaxation has been confirmed.[10,13-15] With the exception of the association of chronic cocaine exposure with congenital defects and adverse reproductive outcomes, local anesthetics per se are devoid of teratogenic effects in clinically used doses.[10,16] As described in section Considerations on Maternal Physiology, however, uncorrected maternal hypotension that may result from local anesthetics provided via neuraxial techniques may lead to decreased fetal perfusion, fetal acidosis, and fetal death. The effects of volatile agents demonstrate the importance of timing; exposure to nitrous oxide and halogenated agents during in vitro oocyte fertilization causes delays in division from the one- to two-cell stage and impaired spindle cell function during meiosis, respectively. In vivo, mice and rats exposed during pregnancy to 50% or 0.75 minimum alveolar concentration (MAC) halothane, isoflurane, or enflurane at various stages of pregnancy have resulted in increased fetal resorptions and altered body laterality with nitrous oxide but no teratogenic effects with the halogenated agents.[17] The teratogenicity with nitrous oxide initially was believed to result from rapid inhibition of methionine synthase in both animals and humans. However, this likely is not the only route of activity for several reasons: Maximal methionine synthase inhibition occurs at concentrations much lower than those required to produced teratogenic effects, use of folinic acid to bypass methionine synthase partially prevents minor skeletal defects, coadministration of isoflurane or halothane prevents almost all teratogenic effects without affecting methionine synthase activity, and replacement of methionine prevents malformations except for situs inversus defects.[18] As such, the weak teratogenic effects of nitrous oxide are multifactorial. Regardless, the threshold requirements for adverse effects with nitrous oxide (ie, >50% concentrations for 24 hours) are not likely to be encountered clinically.

The animal and human experience with all drugs suggests critical periods of susceptibility to teratogens. In general, exposure to known teratogens during the first 2 weeks of embryonic development is marked by either death or minor cellular damage and ongoing survival; highly sensitive periods for developmental effects are during fetal organogenesis when major morphologic changes are occurring. Of note, clinical estimates of gestational age originate from the first day of the last menstrual period; however, because fertilization does not occur until 2 weeks after this time, 14 days are added to actual fetal development to correct for the discrepancy. Thus, whereas the period of major fetal organogenesis is considered to occur between 5 and 55 days of gestation, within the clinically used schemas, this period occurs in weeks 3 to 10 of pregnancy. Overall, anesthetic agents have limited effects from their earliest applications in assisted reproduction throughout pregnancy. Despite their limited effects, it seems prudent to limit the dose of anesthetics by using drug combinations or regional techniques.

BOX 62-1

Teratogenic Drugs and Chemicals in Humans

Aminopterin
Androgenic hormones
Busulfan
Captopril
Chlorobiphenyls
Cocaine
Coumarin anticoagulants
Cyclophosphamide
Diethylstilbestrol
Diphenylhydantoin
Enalapril
Etretinate
Iodides
Lithium
Mercury
Methimazole
Methylaminopterin
Penicillamine
13-Cis-retinoic acid
Tetracycline
Thalidomide
Trimethadione
Valproic acid

CONSIDERATIONS ON MATERNAL PHYSIOLOGY

The maternal and fetal consequences of anesthesia and surgery may be altered by pregnancy or pregnancy-related comorbid conditions (see Chapter 21). Even transient hypoxia, hypercapnia, stress, hypotension, and abnormalities in temperature and metabolism may adversely affect maternal and fetal outcomes. Alterations such as engorgement of the respiratory mucosa, increased consumption of oxygen, and hemodynamic effects of the gravid uterus represent important sources of concern in the provision of anesthesia during pregnancy.

Anesthesia-related maternal mortality has been declining over the past few decades but still accounts for 3% to 12% of maternal deaths; the majority occur as a result of failed intubation, ventilation, and oxygenation, or pulmonary aspiration with general anesthesia. These statistics rank anesthesia as the sixth leading cause of peripartum maternal mortality in the United States, with a risk of maternal death 1.7 times greater with general versus regional anesthesia.[19] A comparison of maternal deaths caused by anesthesia in the Confidential Enquiries data of 2000 to 2002 with the data from 1964 to 1966 yields a 30-fold improvement associated with a reduction in general anesthesia use.[20] Maternal deaths associated with

BOX 62-2

Contraindications to Central Neuraxial Anesthesia

Absolute

- Patient refusal or inability to cooperate
- Localized infection at insertion site
- Sepsis
- Severe coagulopathy
- Uncorrected hypovolemia

Relative

- Mild coagulopathy
- Severe maternal cardiac disease (including congenital and acquired disorders)
- Neurologic disease (including intracranial and spinal cord pathologies)
- Severe fetal depression

general anesthesia can be partially explained by the significant airway changes that occur over the course of pregnancy and even during labor.[21] The ability to secure the airway emergently has been associated with even greater difficulty,[22] often requiring the use of alternative airway devices and techniques.[23] Moreover, data from the recent national maternal mortality database in the United Kingdom[20] and an epidemiologic analysis of maternal deaths in Michigan[24] reveal that issues with extubation and postoperative respiratory failure have emerged as leading critical sources of maternal morbidity and mortality, particularly in women of high body mass index (BMI). These maternal outcome data strongly support the use of neuraxial techniques in both elective and emergent delivery situations when no contraindications exist for their use (**Box 62-2**).

The gravid uterus leads to progressively increasing cardiac demand and compromise of venous return during gestation. The growing uterus ultimately receives 600 to 700 mL/min of blood flow, which is of major importance when uterine trauma, including surgery, occurs. Moreover, the association between hypotension and the supine position in pregnant women, particularly in the late gestational state, is well demonstrated.[25] Upon assuming the supine position, acute hypotension, with increased pulse rate, increased femoral venous pressure, pallor, and sweating, can occur within minutes, so use of left lateral displacement, even as little as 15 degrees, can reduce the incidence of hypotension and ultimately improve uterine blood flow and fetal health, as evidenced by improved blood gas values. This syndrome most likely is a manifestation of hormonal as well as mechanical changes. Hormonally, pregnancy-related alterations in renin, angiotensin II, cardiac natriuretic peptide, prostaglandins, progesterone, estrogen, and endothelin cause a relaxation in vascular tone, reduction in stroke volume, decrease in left ventricular compliance, and overall reduction in cardiovascular reserve. These changes ultimately make the cardiovascular system less able to compensate for any mechanical reductions in venous return by the gravid uterus, particularly when the patient is in the supine position. This difficulty in compensation is also observed after spinal anesthesia-induced hypotension.

Additional concerns witnessed only during pregnancy stem from the presence of trophoblastic tissue (ie, outermost layer of cells of the developing embryo that attaches to the uterine wall) and amniotic fluid. Intravascular systemic distribution of amniotic fluid may accompany uterine rupture or placental separation, leading to sudden cardiovascular collapse accompanied by coagulation disorders. More commonly, however, trophoblastic tissue from the maternal–fetal interface is implicated in the complications associated with preeclampsia, an entity for which delivery of the fetus or fetal tissues remains the only definitive therapy. Hypertensive crises, potential for seizures, intravascular depletion, and thrombocytopenia witnessed with preeclampsia are concerns relevant to anesthetic care (see section Hypertensive Disorders of Pregnancy).[26]

CONSIDERATIONS FOR SPECIFIC SITUATIONS

Concerns regarding the provision of analgesia and anesthesia for obstetric patients begin before pregnancy and continue through pregnancy, delivery, and the postpartum period. Throughout, anesthesia providers have the responsibility to consider the effects of their interventions during a variety of procedures, including assisted reproductive technologies, cerclage placement and removal, external cephalic version (ECV) attempts, nonobstetric surgery during pregnancy, in utero fetal surgery, labor and vaginal delivery, cesarean delivery, and tubal ligation. Anesthesia care during dilatation and evacuation procedures, which are performed for pregnancy termination, pregnancy loss and retained products, and procedures involving ectopic pregnancies, are discussed in Considerations for Specific Situations.

Assisted Reproductive Technologies Whereas most patients undergoing procedures related to assisted reproductive technologies are young and otherwise healthy, a growing percentage has significant comorbid states that are responsible for either infertility or the inability to carry a pregnancy. For these individuals, assisted reproduction represents a mechanism to preserve fertility or to obtain oocytes for later use or transfer to gestational carriers. Almost all interventions that require anesthesia are for the purposes of oocyte retrieval and gamete (ie, sperm or oocyte) or embryo transfer. Most of these procedures are performed transvaginally with ultrasound guidance; on occasion, a transabdominal approach is used.

The anesthetic options for these procedures include paracervical, conscious sedation, spinal, epidural, and general anesthetic techniques.[12] Paracervical anesthesia, which blocks sensation from vaginal but not ovarian pain fibers, often requires additional analgesia (**Fig. 62-3**). Conscious sedation techniques are the most commonly used mode of analgesia for oocyte retrievals; however, loss of consciousness, patient movement at critical times, and prolonged recovery room stays may result.[12] Total IV general anesthesia provided with IV propofol (titrated) and fentanyl (50-100 mcg) offers an optimal approach. Midazolam (1-2 mg) can be added if needed to allay patient anxiety. Most patients can be managed with spontaneous ventilation via a high-flow oxygen mask and continuous carbon dioxide (CO_2) analysis to monitor the adequacy of ventilation. On rare occasion, as in individuals with multiple risk factors for aspiration or the need for laparoscopy, an endotracheal tube is placed. Inhalational anesthesia with enflurane and 70% nitrous oxide has been shown to produce significantly greater rates of nausea and emesis and more unplanned admissions compared with an IV technique of propofol and alfentanil combined with an inhaled air–O_2 mixture.[12]

Neuraxial techniques provide excellent pain relief with minimal oocyte exposure to anesthetic agents. Compared with sedation with propofol and mask-assisted ventilation with nitrous oxide, neuraxial techniques have been associated with fewer complications, especially nausea and emesis. Spinal anesthesia may be preferable to epidural anesthesia because of the reduced failure rate, lower systemic and follicular levels of anesthesia, and faster recovery profile.[27] Short-acting local anesthetics (1.5% concentrations of lidocaine or mepivacaine 45 mg) or low-dose longer acting agents (0.75% bupivacaine 3.75 mg) can be used intrathecally for these procedures with good results. Use of low-dose bupivacaine may appeal to anesthesia providers hoping to reduce the incidence of transient radicular irritation associated with lidocaine or mepivacaine; however, a longer time to urination is witnessed, and greater amounts of intrathecal opioids (25 mcg) must be added.[27] The addition of small doses of intrathecal opioids (fentanyl 10 mcg) to local anesthetics for spinal anesthesia improves postoperative analgesia for oocyte retrieval for the first 24 hours, with no increase in time to urination, ambulation, or discharge compared with local anesthetic alone.[28]

Pronuclear stage tubal transfer, zygote intrafallopian transfer, tubal embryo transfer, and gamete intrafallopian transfer are procedures that involve the transfer of gametes (sperm and oocytes) or embryos into the fallopian tubes during laparoscopy and local, regional, or general anesthesia. A general anesthetic with propofol and succinylcholine induction, intubation, and maintenance with isoflurane–oxygen and a

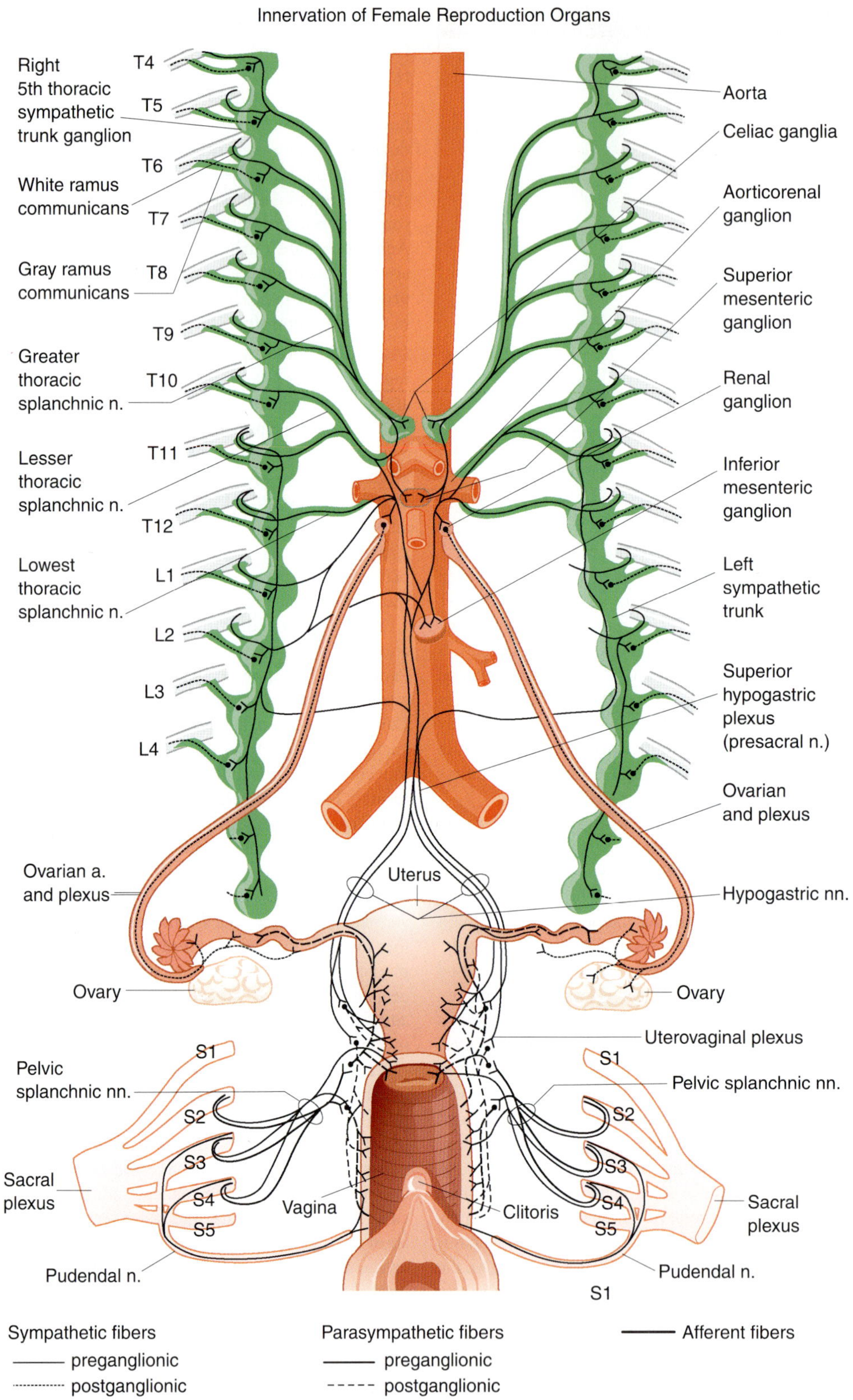

FIGURE 62-3. Innervation of the female reproductive organs.

short-acting muscle relaxant (eg, atracurium or vecuronium) or a succinylcholine infusion can be used. A propofol with nitrous technique also can be used and has been observed to cause less postoperative sedation, lower pain scores, and less emesis compared with an isoflurane with nitrous technique.[12] Most embryo transfers occur 3 to 5 days after oocyte retrieval through a transcervical catheter technique that does not require sedation, analgesia, or anesthesia.

Postoperatively, especially after laparoscopic techniques, patients experience abdominal pain, uterine cramping, shoulder pain, nausea, and emesis. Pain is best treated with small doses of fentanyl (50-100 mcg IV) because use of nonsteroidal anti-inflammatory drugs may affect the prostaglandin milieu associated with embryo implantation.[12] Droperidol and metoclopramide for treatment of nausea and emesis should be avoided when possible because of the associated high prolactin levels and the potential for adverse fertility effects.[29] As with other outpatient procedures, patients should be able to drink and retain oral liquids, ambulate, and void before being discharged from the ambulatory procedure facility.

Special Concerns Based on the presence of preexisting disease states, preoperative evaluations for patients requiring assisted reproductive technologies may range from simple, immediate preprocedural discussions to more complex investigations that require time to collect consultant reports, laboratory studies, electrocardiograms (ECGs), chest radiographs, and other testing results. All patients should be required to remain nil per os (nothing by mouth [NPO]) from solid foods for 8 hours before the time of retrieval, and if they have risk factors for aspiration (eg, obesity, history of reflux), a nonparticulate antacid should be administered orally before the procedure. Use of IV metoclopramide, as a gastric prokinetic agent or as prophylaxis for nausea, should be used sparingly because of potentially adverse fertility effects.[29] Occasionally, a patient may not adhere to NPO policies, and although delaying or cancelling the case is a viable option, the decision should consider the risks of not proceeding, particularly with an oocyte retrieval. If the window for maximal oocyte retrieval (34-36 hours after human chorionic gonadotropin [hCG] administration) is missed, spontaneous ovulation and loss of oocytes can occur, invalidating the considerable effort and expense leading to the retrieval procedure. More importantly, if follicle aspiration is not performed, the patient is at increased risk for ovarian hyperstimulation syndrome, with its potential for tension ascites, thromboembolic phenomena, renal and hepatic dysfunction, and mortality.[30] By contrast, the reduction in aspiration risk produced by delay or cancellation of the procedure is difficult to quantify, and a spinal anesthetic, instead of a technique that impairs airway reflexes, has an exceptional safety profile. As with all ambulatory surgical procedures, the ideal anesthetic results in effective pain relief with minimal postoperative nausea, sedation, pain, and psychomotor impairment.

Cerclage A cervical cerclage is a circumferential suture placed around the cervical os to prevent pregnancy loss because of an incompetent cervix. It can be placed transvaginally or transabdominally with a laparoscopic technique. The clinical management guidelines from the American College of Obstetricians and Gynecologists (ACOG) acknowledge the limited data available on the efficacy of cerclages, yet the ACOG suggests that an elective cerclage should be performed at weeks 13 to 16 of gestation in patients with a viable fetus and a history of three or more otherwise unexplained second-trimester pregnancy losses or preterm deliveries.[31] Urgent, or therapeutic, cerclages are often recommended for women with ultrasonographic changes consistent with a short cervix or evidence of funneling (ie, internal cervical os dilation).[31]

When the cerclage procedure is performed transvaginally, a hyperbaric subarachnoid anesthetic with a local anesthetic that produces approximately 30 to 45 minutes of anesthesia is a good option to avoid maternal airway manipulation and minimize fetal anesthetic exposure. By contrast, if the cerclage is performed transabdominally, a general anesthetic with endotracheal intubation is recommended.

Special Concerns Although cerclage procedures are performed before week 20 of gestation, when the uterus transitions from a pelvic to an abdominal organ, the implications of NPO status and aspiration prophylaxis should be considered. The risk of aspiration during pregnancy, particularly early pregnancy, is controversial (see Chapter 21). However, in most situations requiring a cerclage placement, time exists to allow for gastric clearance, administration of aspiration prophylaxis, or both.

External Cephalic Version Use of external abdominal pressure to turn a fetus from a breech to cephalic presentation is called ECV. Although the procedure is often performed in obstetric clinics without anesthetic intervention, improved maternal comfort, fetal safety, ECV success, and favorable cost-to-benefit analyses have been observed with neuraxial techniques.[32] Neuraxial techniques most likely improve ECV efficacy by relaxing the abdominal wall muscles, improving patient comfort during the attempt and allowing the obstetrician to make a more concerted effort.[32] In the more difficult setting of a repeat ECV after a previously failed attempt, a high success rate (83%) was reported with a spinal technique using 45 mg of lidocaine with 10 mcg of fentanyl.[33] A CSE technique with a short-acting local anesthetic (1.5% lidocaine 45 mg) is the optimal technique for an ECV attempt because it allows for timely discharge from the hospital in the event of a successful version without labor, and if a trial of labor or an operative delivery is warranted or precipitated, the epidural catheter can be used for additional analgesia or anesthesia.[33]

Special Concerns External cephalic version attempts may lead to maternal and fetal complications, including fetal heart decelerations, placental abruption, preterm labor, uterine rupture, amniotic fluid embolism, nausea, emesis, and fetal demise. These adverse outcomes should encourage an ECV attempt in the operating room with maternal and fetal monitoring and with anesthesia providers readily available. Even if neuraxial techniques are not used for the ECV attempt, rapid administration of anesthesia may be necessary for maternal or fetal intolerance. Moreover, although tocolytics (terbutaline, ritodrine) are frequently used to relax the uterus before ECV attempts, IV nitroglycerin (50-mcg bolus; wait 45 seconds before reattempt) has been reported to provide additional uterine relaxation.[33] Because nitroglycerin administration is often accompanied by hypotension, the anesthesia provider should encourage its use only with maternal and fetal monitoring and anesthesia provider presence.

In Utero Fetal and Placental Surgery A growing number of interventions are being used to correct placental abnormalities and fetal defects in utero. Laser photocoagulation of placental vessels responsible for twin-to-twin transfusion syndrome, percutaneous catheter dilation of fetal cardiac valvular defects, and open hysterotomy with fetal repair of diaphragmatic hernias or resection of tumors are a few currently available procedures.[34] Ex utero intrapartum therapy, most commonly performed for large fetal head and neck tumors or severe heart and lung disorders immediately before cesarean delivery, allows partial fetal surgical exposure while maintaining placental circulation until an airway or alternate circulatory arrangement, such as extracorporeal membrane oxygenation, is secured.

Minimally invasive approaches with laparoscopic or percutaneous catheter techniques can be performed under local field blocks or neuraxial techniques. By contrast, operations that involve partial fetal exteriorization are best performed under general anesthesia for uterine quiescence and fetal anesthesia.[35] Fetal anesthesia and immobility can be augmented through intramuscular administration of opioids, muscular relaxants, and atropine to the fetus. Maternal postoperative analgesia can be improved with neuraxial preservative-free morphine (3 mg epidural, 0.2 mg subarachnoid) even if a general anesthetic is planned. Occasionally, more invasive monitoring, as with an arterial or central venous catheter, is warranted to allow for more immediate blood pressure and central venous pressure (CVP) monitoring and vascular access for laboratory studies during the perioperative and intraoperative periods.

Special Concerns The ability and timing of sentience, the capacity to experience painful or unpleasant sensations, in fetuses is a subject of growing interest and controversy.[36] Because structural and behavioral maturation ultimately determine the capacity to feel pain, the presence of reflex responses and cortical connections may not necessarily represent the ability to experience nociception. Although synapses to and from the cortex are present as early as 8.5 weeks of gestation, structures believed necessary for conscious pain perception, such as thalamic projections, intracortex connections, and synchronous electroencephalographic activity, have not been observed until 20 to 30 weeks.[36] Fetal analgesia or anesthesia, however, should be considered to prevent hormonal stress responses that may be associated with poor neonatal surgical outcomes or long-term neurodevelopmental and behavioral responses to pain and to inhibit fetal movement during procedures.[37] Fetal analgesia and anesthesia can be achieved by passive analgesic administration via maternal general anesthesia or by direct intramuscular injection into the fetus. Injection of opioids directly into the amniotic fluid, which results in greater fetal than maternal concentrations in animal models, is a modality that may have application in the future.[38]

Labor and Vaginal Delivery The pain of labor and vaginal delivery evolves through the first and second stages of labor (see Fig. 62-3). The first stage of labor, defined as the onset of regular uterine contractions that result in progressive uterine cervical dilation, produces pain originating from both uterine and cervical stretching. Described as dull, aching, crampy, and poorly localized, the pain sensations are carried by visceral afferents entering the spinal cord at the T10 to L1 level. By contrast, the second stage of labor, defined as the time from complete cervical dilation to the delivery of the fetus, produces pain originating from vaginal and perineal stretching. More somatic in origin, the pain is sharp, is discrete in location, and is carried by the lower lumbar and sacral fibers. Of interest, the contemporary pattern and progress of labor appear slower than previously described a half a century earlier.[39] Attributed to the greater maternal age and weight, increased fetal size, and significantly higher use of induction of labor, these factors may contribute to labor pain of longer duration.

A variety of techniques are used to provide analgesia during labor and delivery (see **Box 62-3**). Neuraxial techniques have been demonstrated to be the most effective form for labor analgesia,[40] but there are some contraindications to their use (see Box 62-2). Moreover, other techniques have been found to be useful or comforting for parturients and may add to overall maternal satisfaction with the birth experience. Various techniques are often used sequentially as labor progresses; however, their simultaneous use may not offer advantages greater than an epidural technique. Transcutaneous nerve stimulation, for example, does not appear to augment either epidural or CSE techniques.[41,42] Clear communication between the patient and all members of the health care team is essential for the proper timing of anesthetic care. In some cases, such as morbid obesity or preexisting back pathology, early placement of an epidural catheter with activation later during labor may be an optimal approach for maternal and fetal outcomes.[43] The concern that neuraxial analgesia techniques could mask the pain of a uterine rupture in women with previous cesarean deliveries or uterine scars appears unfounded. Indeed, the presence of an epidural catheter in women undergoing vaginal birth after cesarean delivery may improve maternal and fetal outcomes by allowing for expedient cesarean delivery anesthesia if uterine rupture or fetal distress occurs. Overall, the use of epidural, spinal, CSE, and DPE techniques should be evaluated for each parturient because the duration of labor and the mode of delivery are not known a priori in most cases. If the patient desires or requires analgesia or anesthesia, a catheter-based technique allows for the most flexibility.

BOX 62-3

Analgesic Techniques During Labor and Delivery

- Nonpharmacologic techniques
  - Psychologic preparation
  - Emotional support
  - Touch and massage
  - Therapeutic heat and cold applications
  - Hydrotherapy
  - Biofeedback
  - Vertical or alternative positioning
  - Transcutaneous electrical nerve stimulation
  - Acupuncture and acupressure
  - Hypnosis
- Pharmacologic techniques
  - Parenteral agents
    - Opioids, opioids antagonist, and agonists
    - Nonsteroidal antiinflammatory drugs
    - Barbiturates
    - Phenothiazines
    - Hydroxyzine
    - Scopolamine
    - Benzodiazepines
    - Ketamine
  - Inhalation agents
    - Nitrous oxide
    - Volatile halogenated agents
  - Neuraxial agents
    - Opioids
    - Local anesthetics
    - α_2-Agonists

Epidural Analgesia The epidural technique is the most common neuraxial technique used for labor analgesia because of relatively rapid sensory analgesia with minimal motor blockade, uterine effects, and maternal or fetal toxicity (see Fig. 62-2).[9,40] Almost all local anesthetics can be used in low concentrations; however, the longer-acting agents allow for less variation in the quality of analgesia (see Table 62-1). Bupivacaine, which provides a high ratio of sensory to motor block, is the most commonly used agent for labor epidural analgesia worldwide. Ropivacaine and levobupivacaine are newer long-acting agents that, when given in equipotent concentrations to bupivacaine, may result in slightly less motor blockade and fewer cardiotoxic effects should intravascular absorption occur.[44,45] Epidural opioids alone provide sufficient analgesia for the first stage of labor (see Table 62-2),[46] but the combination of small doses of sufentanil (0.2-0.3 mcg/mL) or fentanyl (0.2 mcg/mL) with low doses of bupivacaine (0.0625-0.125%) is necessary for second-stage labor and vaginal delivery. An epidural bolus of 100 mcg of fentanyl with or without local anesthetic can improve maternal comfort during the second stage of labor when patchy analgesia or perineal sparing cannot be remedied with local anesthetics alone.[47]

After the initial sensory blockade has been established, epidural analgesia can be maintained by intermittent bolus injections, continuous infusion, or both techniques simultaneously. The development of inexpensive infusion pumps has offered perhaps the optimal method: continuous infusion coupled with patient-controlled intermittent bolus injections through the epidural catheter. This combined method reduces the total amount of medication used, decreases the amount of motor blockade, and increases patient satisfaction compared with continuous infusions or intermittent bolus methods alone.[48]

Is an instrumental or operative delivery, laceration repair, or postpartum tubal ligation occurs, labor epidural analgesia can be transitioned to anesthesia with a change in the concentration or type of local anesthetic used through the catheter (see Table 62-1). Vacuum or forceps deliveries often require denser perineal sensory anesthesia for placement of instruments than offered by contemporary labor analgesia infusion concentrations as noted earlier in this section. This can be accomplished using 6 to 7 mL of 1% lidocaine solution with 8.4% bicarbonate in a 10:1 ratio. Increasing the sensory level from the tenth to the seventh or eighth thoracic dermatome also allows for more rapid anesthetic extension to a fourth thoracic dermatome if the need for an emergent cesarean delivery develops.

Spinal Analgesia The limited duration of action of a single injection and the increased risk of PDPH with multiple injections limit the utility of spinal anesthesia for the management of labor. Spinal techniques, however, can be used successfully in the immediate peripartum period, especially in the event of a precipitous vaginal delivery, use of outlet forceps or vacuum extractions, or repair of extensive perineal lacerations. Short-acting, low-level spinal anesthesia can be used for many of these procedures; however, the range of likely obstetric outcomes should be evaluated carefully. A delivery by "trial of forceps," for example, can quickly transition to an urgent cesarean delivery. Spinal techniques that offer more flexibility include the CSE technique and a spinal catheter technique.

Combined Spinal Epidural Analgesia The CSE technique for labor analgesia has increased in popularity.[9] When placed early in labor and compared with parenteral opioid or standard epidural techniques, a CSE technique with opioids alone or in combination with local anesthetics may have beneficial effects on motor ability and the progress of labor.[49,50] Used later in labor, the CSE technique can provide quick onset of analgesia and the ability to extend the duration or level of the blockade in case delivery methods mandate such augmentation. The DPE technique is a variation of the CSE technique, in which a dural puncture is performed in the typical needle-through-needle method; however, medications are not directly dosed into the intrathecal space. Instead, all medications are administered into the epidural space and indirectly allowed to spread into the intrathecal space through the dural puncture. The technique provides faster onset, improved bilateral and sacral analgesia, and no alterations in motor or cephalad sensory spread compared with a conventional epidural technique.[3] When dilute labor analgesic concentrations (eg, <0.25% bupivacaine) are used, the effect appears to be present when a 25-gauge spinal needle is used[3] but not with a 27-gauge needle.[51]

Special Concerns: Progress of Labor Whether central neuraxial analgesia affects the progress and outcome of labor remains a controversial topic. The myriad of maternal and fetal variables and the differences in anesthetic and obstetric practices are confounding factors in such studies. Moreover, methodologic problems, such as difficulties in randomization and blinding, make an association difficult to evaluate. Overall, however, the use of epidural analgesia appears to have little effect on the progress and outcome of labor. A meta-analysis of 10 trials comparing parturients of mixed parity randomized to epidural analgesia or parenteral opioids noted a prolongation of the first and second stages of labor by 42 and 14 minutes, respectively, in association with the use of epidurals.[52] Despite the belief that an arbitrary threshold of 5 cm of cervical dilation should be achieved before epidural analgesia administration to prevent cesarean delivery,[53] early (<4 cm) placement of CSE labor analgesia versus parenteral opioids[49] or standard epidural techniques[50] has resulted in shorter times to achieve full cervical dilation with no alterations in the cesarean delivery rate. Overall, the risk of cesarean delivery does not appear to be increased with the use of neuraxial labor analgesia.[54]

Anesthetic Complications A number of complications may occur after neuraxial techniques (**Table 62-3**). Hypotension, defined as a 20% to 30% decrease in systolic blood pressure from baseline, can be observed in 20% to 100% of pregnant women as a result of the sympathetic vasomotor blockade associated with neuraxial analgesia and anesthesia.[55] Left uncorrected, hypotension may result in decreased uteroplacental perfusion, fetal hypoxia, and acidosis.[56] Preventive measures include maternal intravascular volume expansion with 500 mL of colloid (eg, hetastarch) or 1000 mL of crystalloid (eg, lactated Ringer solution) within 15 minutes of the neuraxial technique and positioning with a 15-degree left lateral tilt to avoid uterine aortocaval compression. Titrated doses of IV vasopressors, such as 5 to 10 mg of ephedrine or 40 to 100 mcg of phenylephrine, can be used prophylactically to minimize and treat hypotension. The nausea and vomiting after neuraxial techniques may be associated with reductions in sympathetic tone, blood pressure, and cerebral blood flow and can be reduced significantly with vasopressor use.[57] PDPH occurs in approximately 1% to 3% of the obstetric population after dural puncture and is related to needle size and tip design, with larger, cutting (beveled) needles associated with a greater incidence.[58] Typically, PDPH presents as a positional headache that worsens and improves in the upright and recumbent positions, respectively. The differential diagnosis should include other types of headaches, hypertensive disorders, infectious diseases, dural venous sinus thromboses, and other intracranial pathologies. If the diagnosis of PDPH is made, bed rest may aid in pain relief,[59] and conservative measures of hydration and oral intake of caffeinated and analgesic products (including Fioricet or Fiorinal) can be used for 24 to 48 hours. An epidural blood patch, with 10 to 20 mL of autologous blood placed in the epidural space, has been associated with a greater than 80% incidence of success in most trials.[58,60] Although significant complications (eg, cauda equina syndrome, transverse myelitis, arachnoiditis, spinal–epidural abscesses, and vascular trauma) after neuraxial analgesia and anesthesia in the obstetric population are extremely rare,[60] when signs and symptoms are unclear or rapidly progressing, consultation with a neurologist may assist in diagnosis and treatment. Finally, an unexpected high level of anesthesia can result in hypotension, dyspnea, an inability to speak, and loss of consciousness. Ventilatory and circulatory support should always be readily available when these techniques are provided.

Relatively few complications are inherent to the CSE or DPE techniques per se. The risks of a dural puncture with an epidural needle may actually be reduced because CSF within the smaller spinal needle can be used to confirm proximity to the epidural space and prevent inadvertent dural puncture by the larger epidural needle. The likelihood of the epidural catheter passing through the spinal needle dural puncture site is low in laboratory and clinical studies.[61] With the DPE technique, the timing and dose of the epidural bolus and the size of the dural puncture appear to be important. Labor analgesia medications placed in the epidural space after a 25-gauge dural puncture have salutary analgesic effects,[3] however, appear to have limited passage through a 27-gauge dural puncture.[51] The risk of a high spinal blockade as a result of a CSE or DPE technique appears negligible.[3] The failure of an "untested" epidural catheter after the spinal portion of a CSE technique is a potential concern, but epidemiologic evidence suggests that CSE epidural catheters have a lower failure rate than does the epidural technique alone.[62] In parturients with difficult airway access or those with a high probability of an instrumental or operative delivery, a standard epidural technique, which tests the function of the catheter at the time of placement, may be a safer alternative.

Cesarean Delivery With the advent of fetal heart rate and tocodynamometric monitoring, a reduction in breech and forceps-assisted deliveries, and the changing social and medicolegal environment, cesarean deliveries now account for 25% to 30% (range 1.8%-40.5%) of deliveries nationally and internationally.[63,64] Although anesthesia-related maternal mortality has been declining during the past few decades, it still accounts for 3% to 12% of maternal deaths, with the majority associated with general anesthesia secondary to failures in intubation, ventilation, and oxygenation.[20,24] As such, the use of neuraxial techniques has been strongly preferred. However, the urgency of the procedure, the health and comorbidities of the mother and fetus, and the desires of the mother and health care providers must be considered when deciding on the optimal anesthetic technique.

Cesarean delivery is performed most commonly through a low transverse abdominal incision (Pfannenstiel) above the pubic crest, with dissection of the fascia and separation of the rectus muscles. After opening of the peritoneum, a transverse uterine incision (hysterotomy) typically is used for delivery of the fetus. Advantages of the transverse incision include better cosmetic results, less pain, and a low incidence of hernia formation. Disadvantages include limited access to the upper abdomen, a greater incidence of subfascial hematomas from small perforating vessels through the rectus muscle, and increased nerve injury resulting in overlying skin paresthesias. In the setting of a preterm cesarean delivery, especially before elongation of the lower uterine segment in week 34 of gestation, the hysterotomy is sometimes performed with a vertical incision for greater surgical exposure. Because a vertical uterine incision is more prone to dehiscence or rupture with uterine contractions, all subsequent pregnancies must undergo a cesarean delivery.

Regardless of the type of incision, uterine tone may be compromised in preterm deliveries and with prolonged exposure to oxytocin (eg, induction and augmentation of labor) because of low or downregulated numbers of oxytocin receptors, respectively.[65] Uterine tone may be further limited in conditions that augment the size of the uterus, such as polyhydramnios,

TABLE 62-3 Major Complications of Neuraxial Analgesia and Anesthesia

	Transient Neurologic Syndrome	Cauda Equina Syndrome	Traverse Myelitis	Anterior Spinal Artery Syndrome	Arachnoiditis	Epidural Hematoma	Epidural Abscess
Signs and symptoms	Pain in lower back, buttocks, or both	Pain in low back with variable motor and sensory deficits	Pain in low back with motor weakness and sensory alterations	Painless loss of motor and sensory function	Pain in low back with variable motor and sensory deficits	Pain or pressure in low back with progressive motor or sensory blockade	Pain in low back that is tender on palpitation and accompanied by sensory or motor deficits and fever; may progress
	With or without unilateral or bilateral radicular pain described as aching, burning, or cramping	Unilateral or bilateral radicular pain, sensory loss, particularly in the saddle region	Allodynia (heightened sensitivity to touch)	Preservation of vibration and joint position	Unilateral or bilateral pain that increases with activity	Unilateral or bilateral radicular pain	Unilateral or bilateral radicular pain
		Bladder and bowel dysfunction	Bladder and bowel dysfunction			Bladder and bowel dysfunction	Bladder and bowel dysfunction
Cause	All contemporary local anesthetics	Ischemic compression by hematoma or abscess, or direct neurotoxicity, possibly caused by prolonged nerve exposure to high doses or concentrations of local anesthetics	Exact cause unknown; however, infections, abnormal immune reactions (eg, lupus), ischemia, and multifocal neurologic disease (eg, multiple sclerosis), and neuraxial techniques have been suggested	Hypotension, disruption of blood supply, vasoconstrictors or vasospasm	Disinfectants, local anesthetics, contrast media, blood, infections, vasoconstrictors, hemorrhage, multiple spinal surgeries	May occur spontaneously, after trauma, or after instrumentation; higher risk if abnormal coagulation status at time of instrumentation or catheter removal	Bacterial, immunocompromised patients are at higher risk; nonsterile techniques involving neuraxial technique
Testing	None	MRI	MRI or myelography	MRI and angiography	MRI or myelography	MRI	MRI
Consults	Anesthesiologist	Neurologist or neurosurgeon	Neurologist	Neurologist	Neurologist	Neurologist or neurosurgeon	Neurologist and/or neurosurgeon
Onset	12-24 h after surgery		Acutely (hours to days) or subacutely (1-2 wk)	After insult whether surgical or traumatic	May occur years after the precipitating cause	Spontaneously, or 0–2 d after insult	2–7 d after instrumentation
Treatment	NSAIDs	Corticosteroids (limited data)	Corticosteroids (no clinical data), pain management, physiotherapy, exercise, psychotherapy	Correction of any existing hypotension, correction of vasospasm, physiotherapy, exercise	Pain management, physiotherapy, exercise, psychotherapy	Surgical decompression usually is indicated within 6–12 h of symptom onset	Intravenous antibiotics, percutaneous drainage, laminotomy with washout of epidural space, laminectomy
	Opioids Heat Muscle relaxants Leg elevation				Steroid injections and electrical stimulation may be helpful		
Recovery	Full	Limited clinical data	Within 2-12 wk of symptom onset and continue for up to 2 y; if no improvement within 3-6 mo, significant recovery unlikely	Variable, may have full, partial, or no recovery	No significant improvement with treatment; usually a chronic pain disorder that is not progressive	Variable and dependent on extent of neurologic involvement and treatment	Variable, dependent on extent of neurologic involvement and treatment
Duration	Symptoms last for 6 h to 7 d	Variable	Variable	Variable	Incurable	Variable	Variable

MRI, magnetic resonance imaging; NSAID, nonsteroidal anti-inflammatory drug.

TABLE 62-4 Medications Used to Augment Uterine Tone in Obstetric and Gynecologic Surgery

Medication	Uses	Route of Administration	Risks
Oxytocin	Induces labor, increases uterine tone	IV infusion; initial and additional doses of 0.3 IU (3 IU if prior oxytocin exposure) administered over 15 sec	Uterine hyperactivity; hypotension; reflex tachycardia; ADH-like response if given in high doses with risk of water intoxication; should be given in electrolyte-containing solutions, not dextrose in water
Methylergonovine	Increases uterine tone	IM 0.2 mg	Acute hypertension, seizures, cerebrovascular accidents, retinal detachment if given IV; use with caution in patients with coronary artery disease, essential hypertension, preeclampsia, atherosclerotic disease; nausea and vomiting may reflect direct CNS effect
Prostaglandin E_2	Increases uterine tone	Oral, rectal, or vaginal; dose depends on desired effect	Nausea, vomiting, diarrhea, fever, tetanic uterine contractions, hypotension; hypertension
Prostaglandin $F_{2\alpha}$	Increases uterine tone	IM 0.25 mg	Nausea, vomiting, bronchospasm; tetanic uterine contractions; hypotension; hypertension

ADH, antidiuretic hormone; CNS, central nervous system; IM, intramuscular; IV, intravenous.

multiple gestation, and fibroids. Uterine atony accounts for 75% to 90% of postpartum hemorrhage and remains a leading cause of postpartum hysterectomy and blood transfusion. In an attempt to reduce the incidence of uterine atony and its sequelae, initial efforts at time of cesarean delivery include uterine massage and IV oxytocin, a uterotonic medication (**Table 62-4**). Only small doses of oxytocin (0.3 IU and 3 IU for parturients without and with prior exposure to oxytocin, respectively) appear necessary to produce adequate uterine tone after cesarean delivery.[65-67] Oxytocin bolus doses should be administered slowly (no faster than 15 sec) and followed with a maintenance dose of 3 IU/h for 5 to 8 hours after delivery.[65-67] Particularly when given as a rapid IV bolus, oxytocin has been associated with a high incidence of morbidity, including hypotension, nausea and vomiting, antidiuretic effects leading to fluid retention and pulmonary edema, and even death from cardiovascular collapse.[68,69] If oxytocin fails to provide sufficient uterine tone, other more powerful uterotonic agents, including prostaglandins (15-methylprostaglandin 250 mcg) and ergot preparations (methylergotamine 200 mcg) should be administered intramuscularly or directly into the myometrium at intervals of 15 to 20 minutes up to a total dose of 1 mg. These agents, however, are associated with significant side effects, including nausea, bronchospasm (especially with prostaglandins), hypertension, pulmonary edema, and cerebral hemorrhage.[70] If these medical therapies fail, uterine or hypogastric artery ligation, interventional arterial balloon catheterization, or hysterectomy may be necessary.

Spinal Anesthesia A simple and reliable technique with rapid onset, spinal (subarachnoid) anesthesia provides an awake and comfortable patient with minimal risks for pulmonary aspiration of gastric contents. Despite the lower abdominal incision, a T4 sensory dermatome level is required to prevent referred pain from traction on the peritoneum and uterus. The type and dose of local anesthetic used to provide the spinal anesthetic must include consideration of the level of anesthesia desired, duration of surgery, postoperative analgesia plan, and preferences of the anesthesiologist. Spinal administration of hyperbaric 0.75% bupivacaine with fentanyl and preservative-free morphine may be the optimal combination (**Box 62-4**). Whereas the almost immediate onset of fentanyl reduces visceral discomfort and even nausea during the procedure, the delayed onset and 18- to 20-hour duration of morphine provides prolonged relief following the procedure. Although ropivacaine and levobupivacaine can be used in similar concentrations and doses, the potential for reduced toxicity if intravascular absorption occurs seems limited given the extremely small doses of agents used. Adjuvant spinal medications, including epinephrine, may augment the quality and duration of the anesthesia and analgesia.[71,72]

After administration of a subarachnoid technique, the patient may complain of dyspnea. This can occur because of several factors, including blunting of thoracic proprioception, partial blockade of abdominal and intercostal muscles, and increased pressure of the abdominal contents against the diaphragm in the recumbent position. Despite these changes, significant respiratory compromise is unlikely because the blockade rarely affects the cervical nerves that control the diaphragm. If the patient loses the ability to vocalize, give a strong hand grip, or demonstrate oxygen desaturation by pulse oximetry, a rapid sequence induction of general anesthesia, with cricoid pressure and placement of an endotracheal tube, can be performed to maintain ventilation and prevent pulmonary soiling with gastrointestinal contents.

The most common complications of spinal anesthesia have been described earlier under Anesthetic Complications and include hypotension, nausea and vomiting, and risk of PDPH.

BOX 62-4

Recommended Neuraxial Medication Combinations for Cesarean Delivery

Medication	Spinal	Epidural
Local anesthetic	Bupivacaine 12 mg (range, 9-15)	Lidocaine 2%; chloroprocaine 3% if urgent; both added in 10:1 volume ratio to 8.4% bicarbonate
Fentanyl	15-35 mcg	50-100 mcg
Morphine	0.1 mg	3.75 mg

Epidural Anesthesia Use of epidural anesthesia for cesarean delivery has increased during the past 2 decades, primarily as a result of its use for labor analgesia. Although medications used in the spinal and epidural space are identical, epidural doses are 5 to 10 times greater and given in much larger volumes to encourage adequate blockade and spread of the drug. Overall, a greater sensitivity of nerves to local anesthetics during pregnancy has been observed clinically through decreased anesthetic requirements for epidural blockade,[73,74] For cesarean delivery, the most commonly used agents are 2% lidocaine with epinephrine 1:200,000 or 3% 2-chloroprocaine. Chloroprocaine is the agent of choice for emergency cesarean deliveries because of its rapid onset and rapid maternal and fetal metabolism; fetal accumulation, especially when acidosis is present, is minimized.[75] By contrast, chloroprocaine is avoided for routine nonurgent deliveries because the short duration requires multiple doses, and its use can adversely affect the efficacy of subsequent epidural opioid analgesia.[76] In addition, chloroprocaine used in higher total volumes (>40 mL) can increase the incidence of back pain.[77] Alkalinization with sodium bicarbonate hastens the onset time of local anesthetics significantly and is recommended for use in urgent cesarean deliveries with 1 mL of 8.4% bicarbonate for every 10 mL of lidocaine or chloroprocaine (**Fig. 62-4**).[78] By contrast, 10 mL of bupivacaine, levobupivacaine, or ropivacaine precipitates out of solution with less than 0.5 mL of bicarbonate, leading to an inability to inject the local anesthetic through a needle or catheter; therefore, bicarbonate should not be added to these longer-acting local anesthetics.[79]

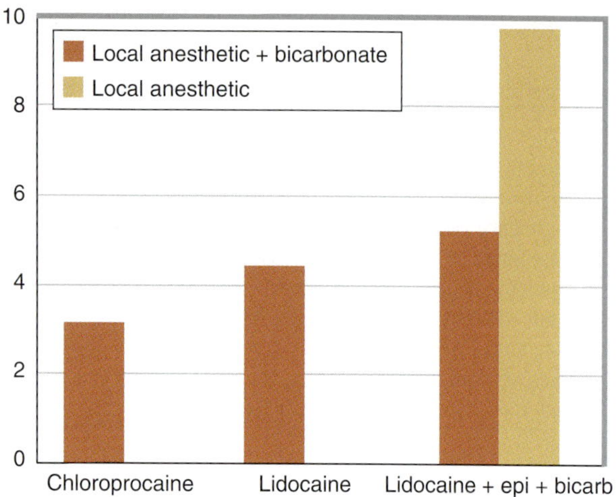

FIGURE 62-4. Extension of labor epidural analgesia for cesarean delivery. Onset (in minutes) for extension of T10 labor analgesia to T4 cesarean anesthesia. Note the values for chloroprocaine and bicarbonate (bicarb). [Based on data from Gaiser RR, Cheek TG, Adams HK, et al. Epidural lidocaine for cesarean delivery of the distressed fetus. *Int J Obstet Anesth.* 1998;7:27-31; Lam DT, Ngan Kee WD, Khaw KS. Extension of epidural blockade in labour for emergency caesarean section using 2% lidocaine with epinephrine and fentanyl, with or without alkalinisation. *Anaesthesia.* 2001;56:790-794.]

The complications of epidural anesthesia have been described previously under Anesthetic Complications and include hypotension, risk of PDPH, systemic toxic reactions, and (rarely) neurologic complications. Epidural techniques can provide patchy or inadequate blockade because of anatomic or technical reasons.[80] Often, these failures can be identified a priori through observation of the quality of labor epidural analgesia or quickly after partial augmentation of the blockade. Alternative techniques, such as supplementation with IV or inhalational agents, spinal anesthesia, or general anesthesia, must always be considered as options when analgesia is clearly inadequate.

Combined Spinal–Epidural Anesthesia The principal advantage of the CSE technique for cesarean delivery is the ability to augment the density or duration of the anesthesia administered via the epidural catheter. This is particularly useful in obstetrics when a trial of labor may be attempted before an operative delivery or the duration of the surgery may be prolonged (eg, possible placenta accreta, history of multiple abdominal surgeries, high index of suspicion for gravid hysterectomy).

Special Concerns During Cesarean Delivery Although neuraxial anesthesia is used whenever possible to avoid the potential airway complications associated with general anesthesia, certain conditions or time constraints may contraindicate its use (see Box 62-2).[81] Such comorbidities include localized infection or generalized sepsis, coagulation disorders, severe hypovolemia, and cardiac pathologies where hypotension may be especially detrimental. Severe obstetric hemorrhage in the antepartum period, including uterine rupture and acute and severe fetal distress, also may contraindicate the use of neuraxial anesthesia procedures because of the time necessary to establish a surgical anesthetic.

Patients with severe preeclampsia or hypertension may undergo rapid hemodynamic changes with neuraxial techniques; however, both epidural and spinal techniques have been used successfully in this setting with similar vasopressor requirements as nonpreeclamptic patients.[82,83] In addition, gravid hysterectomies can be performed safely with neuraxial techniques.[84] Overall, however, general anesthesia should be considered if questions exist regarding the ability of maternal compensatory mechanisms to react to the neuraxial anesthetic or surgery.

Hypotension presents the greatest risk to maternal and fetal comfort and health.[56] Prevention and prompt treatment with IV fluids and administration of vasopressors have been beneficial but may not be completely successful.[85,86] In terms of volume expansion, spinal anesthesia in the urgent setting should not be delayed until a fixed arbitrary volume has been infused. In addition, aggressive hydration with large fluid volumes (>20 mL/kg crystalloid) may increase the risk of edema with only limited reductions in hypotension.[85] Colloid solutions appear to be more effective than crystalloids in preventing the hemodynamic consequences of spinal anesthesia.[87] However, in most cases, the allergic, cost, and coagulation implications offset their benefit. Current investigations into the use of vasopressors for prevention and treatment of hypotension in this setting include use of phenylephrine, sometimes in combination with ephedrine, administered via bolus and infusion pump techniques.[88,89] Although most animal studies indicate combined α- and β-adrenergic agonists (eg, ephedrine) are more effective than α-adrenergic agonists (eg, metaraminol, phenylephrine) in terms of restoration of maternal blood pressure and fetal acid–base status, clinical investigations appear to favor the use of α-adrenergic agonists.[90] Because clinical and animal data do not support a single agent in all circumstances, a rational strategy is vigilance and a proactive response with both ephedrine and phenylephrine as guided by maternal blood pressure and heart rate.

Nausea and emesis during and after cesarean delivery can have a number of causes but are best prevented by controlling hypotension, optimizing the use of neuraxial and IV opioids, improving the quality of surgical blockade, minimizing surgical stimuli, and judiciously administering uterotonic agents.[91]

Although pruritus after neuraxial blockade is attributed to a number of postulated mechanisms and has several treatments,[92] a narcotic antagonist or partial antagonist (eg, nalbuphine 4 mg IV) appears more effective than some other modalities. Postoperative shivering also may have several etiologies and treatments. Administration of 25 mg of IV meperidine, 150 mcg of clonidine, 100 mg of doxapram, 10 mg of ketanserin, and 250 mcg of alfentanil all have been used with success, although meperidine appears to be the most consistently effective.[93]

General Anesthesia There are few, if any, absolute contraindications to general anesthesia. However, neuraxial anesthesia remains a preferred method to avoid the risks of airway management and allow the patient the ability to witness delivery of the fetus. General anesthesia, however, may offer advantages in cases in which uterine relaxation would be beneficial, such as extracting difficult breech presentations, removing retained placentas, restoring uterine inversions, and performing in utero fetal operations.

The importance of proper airway evaluation during the antenatal period or in early labor, if possible, cannot be overemphasized because failed intubation, failed ventilation and oxygenation, and pulmonary aspiration of gastric contents are the leading anesthetic causes of maternal death.[94,95] If the airway evaluation suggests a difficult intubation or risk factors for a difficult neuraxial placement (eg, morbid obesity, scoliosis, dropping platelet count), the establishment of a continuous neuraxial technique early in labor should be strongly encouraged.[43,96] If the parturient does not desire epidural analgesia during labor, the epidural catheter still can be placed, tested for a bilateral sensory distribution with 6 to 7 mL of 1% to 2% lidocaine with bicarbonate, and then allowed to wear off until such time that analgesia or anesthesia is desired.[43] If a difficult airway is discovered during a rapid sequence intubation attempt, options include allowing the patient to awaken, using alternate techniques (eg, fiberoptic- or light-guided intubation) to place an endotracheal tube, or using alternative airway devices (for a detailed review of airway management, see Chapter 35). Although the laryngeal mask airway (LMA) cannot prevent pulmonary soiling with gastric contents, it can be a lifesaving measure in failed intubation situations.[97] LMAs have been used without adverse sequelae with continuous cricoid pressure held for the duration of cesarean delivery.[98] Emergency airway equipment should be readily available in all obstetric operating rooms.

Attempts should be made to minimize the risk of maternal aspiration even when the need for intubation is not anticipated. With an elective cesarean delivery, adherence to a food and clear liquid NPO policy for

8 and 4 hours, respectively, before surgery is advised. A nonparticulate antacid is believed to decrease damage to the respiratory epithelium if aspiration occurs,[99] and H_2 antagonists (cimetidine, ranitidine) and promotility agents (metoclopramide) can reduce gastric acid secretion and facilitate emptying, respectively.[100,101]

The patient should be placed supine with left uterine displacement and optimal airway positioning. After the placement of routine monitors, including ECG, pulse oximetry, blood pressure, and capnography, preoxygenation and denitrogenation with 100% oxygen should be performed to delay the onset of hypoxemia stemming from the parturient's decreased functional residual capacity and increased oxygen consumption. In urgent situations, four maximal (ie, approaching vital capacity) breaths of 100% oxygen will provide adequate preoxygenation.[102] After the surgical drapes have been applied and the operating personnel are ready at the bedside, the surgeon should be instructed to delay the initial incision until the anesthesia provider confirms correct placement of the endotracheal tube and gives verbal confirmation to proceed with the operation. A rapid-sequence induction with full cricoid pressure after induction with 4 to 5 mg/kg of thiopental and 1 to 1.5 mg/kg of succinylcholine is performed. Ketamine 1 to 1.5 mg/kg should be substituted for thiopental if hemodynamic instability is present before induction. Cricoid pressure should be continued until correct positioning of the endotracheal tube is validated with auscultation and confirmation of carbon dioxide. A short-acting nondepolarizing agent or succinylcholine infusion can be used to maintain muscle relaxation.

In most instances, less than 50% fraction of inspired oxygen (FiO_2) is sufficient, but 100% FiO_2 oxygen should be used if fetal compromise exists. Some evidence suggests that greater than 60% FiO_2 may result in detrimental fetal oxygen-free radical formation in the fetus.[103] Maintenance of anesthesia can be provided with volatile anesthetics titrated as necessary; however, upon delivery, concentrations should be reduced to less than 1 to 1.5 MAC, the threshold above which relaxation of uterine tone cannot be attenuated with oxytocin. No advantage in minimizing uterine tone relaxation or fetal effects has been found with the selection of specific volatile anesthetic agents (isoflurane, sevoflurane, or desflurane). Overall, a 25% to 40% reduction in halogenated agent requirements is witnessed during pregnancy.[104] Comparison of neonatal outcomes after general versus epidural anesthesia for cesarean delivery suggests small, transient differences.[105] However, with both techniques, a uterine incision to delivery time longer than 180 seconds can result in lower Apgar scores and greater fetal acidosis (most likely reflecting the difficulty in delivering the baby rather than direct effects of the anesthetic agents).[106] General anesthetic agents can redistribute from the fetal fat to the fetal circulation and result in secondary depression of neonatal ventilatory effort. Thus, the presence of a pediatrician in such cases is advisable until a normal ventilatory pattern is observed.

Maternal oxygenation and ventilation should be carefully observed after extubation in both the immediate and later postoperative periods. In contrast to earlier reports that identified failures during intubation as the cause of inadequate airway management and ventilation, the majority of recent maternal deaths related to anesthesia have occurred in the postoperative period after general anesthesia administration.[20,24] Risk factors for maternal postoperative respiratory arrest include high BMI and the presence of highly pigmented skin (impairing the clinical observation of hypoxemia).[24]

Postoperative Pain Management By directly activating spinal and supraspinal opioid receptors, epidural and spinal opioids blunt nociceptive input and produce analgesia of greater intensity than doses administered parenterally or intramuscularly (see Chapter 74).[7] Morphine has emerged as the leading agent for post–cesarean delivery analgesia because of its long duration of action and low cost (see Table 62-2); optimal doses are 0.1 and 3.75 mg in the intrathecal and epidural spaces, respectively.[71,107] Because of its low lipid solubility, the peak analgesic effects of morphine are delayed 60 to 90 minutes but persist to provide reliable analgesia for up to 24 hours.[107] A sustained-release epidural morphine preparation that can provide up to 48 hours of post–cesarean delivery analgesia has been developed[108]; however, its use is limited by its immediate release when mixed with local anesthetics and the inability for its use in the intrathecal space. Thus, it is being used as a part of a CSE technique in which the local anesthetic is placed in the intrathecal space followed by administration of morphine in the epidural space.

The choice of local anesthetic for epidural anesthesia may influence the efficacy of epidural morphine. In parturients who received 2-chloroprocaine (a short-acting, rapid-onset local anesthetic used primarily for emergent cesarean deliveries) versus other local anesthetics, post–cesarean delivery analgesia was significantly reduced to less than 3 hours.[109] The mechanism by which chloroprocaine affects the duration of opioids, as well as other local anesthetics, is unknown. These interactions, coupled with the potential for neurotoxicity, especially when preserved with metabisulfite, limit the use of chloroprocaine to emergent situations where rapid augmentation is desired.[110] Patient-controlled epidural infusions of low-concentration local anesthetics with opioids (eg, bupivacaine 01.25% with 0.2 mg/mL of hydromorphone or 2 mcg/mL of fentanyl at 6 mL/h) may offer an analgesic option in patients in whom prolonged, nonsystemic analgesia is desired.[111]

Postoperative analgesia has been greatly improved through the use of central neuraxial techniques, most commonly provided through a single-dose administration of morphine. Given in the spinal and epidural compartments, opioids provide enhanced quality and duration, with a very acceptable side effect profile compared with oral and IV analgesics. Adequate management of postoperative cesarean delivery pain may decrease the low but notable occurrence of chronic pain.[112]

CONSIDERATIONS FOR HIGH-RISK PARTURIENTS

Antenatal and Postpartum Hemorrhage Vaginal bleeding occurs in up to 24% of clinically diagnosed pregnancies and most often is associated with minimal blood loss and limited pathology. However, major antepartum and postpartum bleeding may occur at any time and is a leading cause of maternal and perinatal morbidity and mortality. What constitutes "bleeding" versus "hemorrhage" is an issue of semantics. More important is recognizing that blood loss and physiologic deterioration can occur rapidly and that a cogent plan of investigation and response can significantly affect the outcome.

Divided by week 20 of gestation into early and late time periods, antepartum hemorrhage is associated with a number of etiologies. Early-pregnancy bleeding can result from implantation or miscarriage of the embryo, an ectopic pregnancy, gestational trophoblastic disease, dysfunctional uterine bleeding, and reproductive tract tumors. In first-trimester pregnancies complicated by bleeding, less than 50% will progress normally beyond 20 weeks of gestation, 10% to 15% will be an ectopic pregnancy, 0.2% will be a hydatidiform mole, and more than 30% will result in a miscarriage.[113] Bleeding during late pregnancy complicates 2% to 5% of pregnancies, with the most common causes being placental abruption (31%) and placenta previa (22%; **Table 62-5**).

Although obstetric hemorrhage can be masked by physiologic adaptations in blood volume and cardiac output (see Chapter 21), ultimately, the 600 to 700 mL of blood flow through the placental intervillous spaces each minute can result in signs of shock (**Table 62-6**).[113] Coagulopathy, initially dilutional from the ongoing loss of blood components and rapid volume replacement, may be accompanied by disseminated intravascular coagulation (DIC). Laboratory analysis of DIC includes a prolonged prothrombin time (PT), prolonged partial prothrombin time (PTT), hypofibrinogenemia, thrombocytopenia, and elevated fibrin degradation products.

Underestimation of blood loss and inadequate resuscitation are common problems in cases of antepartum hemorrhage resulting in maternal mortality. In a report on maternal deaths in the United Kingdom, substandard responses were noted to be a contributing factor in 79% of maternal deaths resulting from hemorrhage.[114] Rapid volume replacement is more important for tissue perfusion and oxygenation than is the type of fluid given. Large-bore IV access with pressurized transfusion equipment is essential during severe hypovolemia. Intravascular expansion with colloids

TABLE 62-5 Characteristics of Early and Late Antepartum Hemorrhage Diagnoses

Early Pregnancy	
Miscarriage	Vaginal bleeding (+/− pain) >8 wk after last menstrual period Slight tenderness to uterine examination No adnexal mass
Ectopic pregnancy	May not have vaginal bleeding Pain <8 wk after last menstrual period Unilateral tenderness May present as shock with normal-sized uterus
Late Pregnancy	
Placenta previa	Painless vaginal bleeding (although 10% may have coexisting, painful abruption) Malpresentation of fetus (35%) Difficulty palpating presenting part
Placenta abruption	Painful vaginal bleeding Uterine irritability or tetany Coagulopathy Fetal distress or death
Uterine rupture	Vaginal bleeding (+/− pain) Hypotension Cessation of labor Fetal distress
Vasa previa	Painless vaginal bleeding Presence of fetal hemoglobin in shed blood
Unclassified bleeding	Painless vaginal bleeding Mild bleeding that often resolves spontaneously Often >37 wk of gestation

versus crystalloid preparations during pregnancy has been observed to be longer in duration and more effective in augmenting cardiac output. These qualities are helpful in cases of peripartum hemorrhage and may be an effective bridge until blood products are available.[87] Although many institutions require a type and screen for parturients who are at high risk for hemorrhage and undergoing vaginal delivery or for all parturients undergoing cesarean delivery, a cross-match for 2 to 4 units of packed red blood cells (PRBCs) should be considered when the potential for significant blood loss appears eminent. Such cases often involve abnormalities with placentation, including low implantation (previa), partial abruption, adherence without a decidual layer, invasion into the myometrium, or penetration through the myometrium (placenta accreta, increta or percreta, respectively). Imaging tests, especially ultrasonography and magnetic resonance imaging, have dramatically altered the evaluation and outcome of these placental abnormalities. More recently, the use of interventional radiologic techniques for placement of prophylactic or treatment transcatheter occlusion balloons within the uterine or hypogastric arteries has allowed for timely control of bleeding.[115] When uterine bleeding occurs postpartum, use of an inflated balloon catheter placed in the uterine cavity and filled with 70 to 300 mL of warm saline has been demonstrated to tamponade and potentially treat intrauterine sources of bleeding and allow time to correct coagulopathies.[116]

When the need for emergent blood transfusion precedes the availability of cross-matched blood, then uncross-matched, type O, Rh-negative blood should be used. Continued blood loss and hemodynamic instability despite transfusion of PRBCs often is an indication for an arterial line and more invasive monitoring. However, restoration of circulating volume takes precedence. Urine output, heart rate, and blood pressure assessments can assist in rapid assessment of volume resuscitation. After the delivery of the fetus, when uterine perfusion and oxygenation become less relevant, parturients usually are able to tolerate low hemoglobin, coagulation proteins, and platelets. Although obstetric transfusion protocols are beginning to consider defined transfusion ratios of PRBCs, plasma, and other component therapy in the presence of major hemorrhage, there is no consensus on an optimal protocol. The task force on blood component therapy of the American Society of Anesthesiologists has stated that transfusion of PRBCs, platelets, and fibrinogen component therapy is rarely indicated unless the hemoglobin concentration is less than 6 g/dL, platelet count is less than 50×10^9/L (unless platelet dysfunction and microvascular bleeding is present), and fibrinogen concentration is less than 80 to 100 mg/dL in the presence of microvascular bleeding (for details of transfusion therapy, see Chapter 85).[117]

Simultaneously with fluid resuscitation, a hemorrhaging parturient should be prepared for an operative delivery, if not already accomplished, and a possible hysterectomy. Complete replacement of blood loss before or during surgery is frequently an unrealistic goal because bleeding often continues until the offending pathology is corrected or removed. Although a neuraxial anesthetic approach can be continued if the bleeding is modest and controllable, the case of a briskly bleeding, hemodynamically unstable patient requires induction of general anesthesia, controlled ventilation, and aggressive fluid resuscitation.

Hypertensive Disorders of Pregnancy Whether preexisting, gestational, or related to preeclampsia or eclampsia, hypertension is associated with a higher incidence of maternal, fetal, and neonatal mortality and morbidity. Preeclampsia, with its systemic vasoconstriction, intravascular volume and protein depletion, and simultaneous retention of extravascular sodium and water, is of particular concern to anesthesiologists. In addition to individual organ dysfunction, abnormalities in coagulation and edema of the brain, larynx, and lungs may occur. Medical management of blood pressure should be achieved before obstetric or anesthetic interventions if possible. Control of blood pressure with labetalol, hydralazine, or infusions of nitroglycerin or nitroprusside should be commenced with arterial and central venous monitoring in severe cases. Of note, use of magnesium for prevention of seizures and use of antihypertensive medications for control of severe hypertension (systolic pressure >160 mm Hg or diastolic pressure at least 110 mm Hg) may affect the duration of muscle relaxants and the response to induction medications, respectively.[118] Overall, the suggested goal of antihypertensive therapy is systolic pressure between 140 and 155 mm Hg and diastolic pressure between 90 and 105 mm Hg.[118]

Fluid management guided by CVP in severe cases has been demonstrated to improve urine output, maintain mean arterial pressure, and decrease diastolic pressure.[119] If oliguria persists after normalization of CVP (usually between 2 and 3 cm H_2O) or the physiologic state is complicated by pulmonary edema or cardiovascular decompensation, a pulmonary arterial (PA) catheter may be helpful. Emerging minimally or noninvasive technologies to assess cardiac output may also provide information during pregnancy[2]; however, their use should focus on identifying trends in hemodynamic parameters until further validation

TABLE 62-6 Assessment of Obstetric Hemorrhage

Severity of Shock	Findings	Blood Loss (%)
None	None	15-20
Mild	Tachycardia (<100 beats/min) Mild hypotension Peripheral vasoconstriction	20-25
Moderate	Tachycardia (100-120 beats/min) Hypotension (SBP 80-100 mm Hg) Restlessness Oliguria	25-35
Severe	Tachycardia (>120 beats/min) Hypotension (SBP <60 mm Hg) Altered consciousness Anuria	>35

SBP, systolic blood pressure.

of these methods during pregnancy occurs, particularly in the presence of comorbid states. A cardiology consultation and an assessment of cardiopulmonary function with a transthoracic echocardiogram may assist with the diagnosis and management. The course of preeclampsia can be complicated by mild to severe coagulopathy even in the presence of a normal platelet count.[120] For the benefit of both obstetric and anesthetic management, if the initial platelet count is less than an arbitrary 70 to $75/L^{-9}$, the clinical history and the results of additional studies, such as PT or PTT or thromboelastography, should be reviewed. If the low (>70-$75/L^{-9}$) platelet count has been stable or trending slowly downward for 2 to 3 weeks and the patient has no clinical history of bleeding gums, prolonged bleeding, or significant bruising with trauma, a neuraxial approach to analgesia or anesthesia appears reasonable. However, if the platelet count has rapidly fallen within the 2 to 3 weeks or the clinical signs noted are present, a few options exist. In patients who will undergo labor, the analgesia can be managed with a patient-controlled IV pump; 13 mcg of fentanyl every 6 minutes with a lockout of 300 mg per 4 hours has been used with some success. Of note, intramuscular administration of opioids, a common method of analgesia used for labor, is not recommended because of the possibility of hematoma formation. If an instrumented or operative delivery is planned, additional laboratory testing, such PT or PTT and thromboelastography, may provide information on the extent of coagulation dysfunction. If thrombocytopenia or prolonged PT or PTT indicates that pooled platelets or fresh-frozen plasma may reduce the risk of maternal hemorrhage with delivery, placement of neuraxial techniques should await the administration of these products.

During labor, epidural analgesia offers the advantage of limiting pain or stress, thus reducing catecholamine release, decreasing maternal blood pressure, and indirectly increasing placental perfusion.[119] Epidural anesthesia can also be a preferred technique for cesarean delivery because the dose of medications can be slowly titrated, resulting in more gradual blood pressure changes. Spinal anesthesia should not be avoided, particularly in urgent or emergent cases where rapid onset of anesthesia is important. Limited studies suggest that the incidence of hypotension is not significantly different compared with epidural anesthesia for cesarean delivery.[82,122] A CSE technique with a small initial spinal dose (7.5 mg of bupivacaine) followed by sequential epidural catheter dosing is another method that may produce rapid anesthetic onset with less profound hypotension; however, the value of this technique in limiting hypotension has not been validated in randomized controlled trials. Overall, neuraxial techniques represent an optimal approach to analgesia and anesthesia in the preeclamptic patient. This is particularly true when assessing awake, nonsedated patients during labor and delivery for the severity of disease and avoiding the risks of general anesthesia associated with airway narrowing that accompanies pregnancy, labor, and preeclampsia[123] and the increases in systemic and intracranial pressures that can occur during intubation and extubation.

Intravascular hypovolemia associated with preeclampsia, use of antihypertensive medications, and administration of magnesium for seizure prophylaxis may augment the hypotension produced by neuraxial techniques. When responding pharmacologically to hypotension, restraint is advocated because patients with hypertensive disorders may have an exuberant response. Small doses of vasopressors (ie, 5 mg of ephedrine or 20-40 mcg of phenylephrine) should be given initially. Similarly, the response to hypertension associated with the disease or reactive hypertension from labor pain, intubation, or emergence from general anesthesia should be treated judiciously. Labetalol (5-10 mg IV) is a popular first-line agent that has a relatively wide margin of safety and can be doubled every 20 minutes until an effect is observed or 150 to 200 mg has been reached. At these thresholds, other agents such as hydralazine or calcium channel blockers can be used. Infusions of nitroglycerine, nitroprusside, and trimethaphan can be initiated, but arterial monitoring should be used to more carefully titrate the effect (see section Invasive Monitoring in the Parturient).

Invasive Monitoring in the Parturient Whereas noninvasive measurement of blood pressure, heart rate, oxygen saturation, urinary output, and fetal cardiotocography is standard practice in most labor and delivery facilities, the use of invasive monitors is variable and controversial. Despite practice guidelines written by a number of professional organizations, including the joint task force of the American College of Physicians, the American College of Cardiology, and the American Heart Association,[124] poor collection and incorrect interpretation of hemodynamic data from invasive monitors remain the key problems with their use.[125,126]

In addition to correctly interpreting the data produced, knowing when to use invasive monitoring is a vital clinical skill. The indications for invasive arterial blood pressure monitoring during pregnancy include the desire to more carefully manage blood pressure, lack of reliable noninvasive cuff measurements, need for vascular access for blood studies, and planned use of certain hemodynamic agents (particularly drugs given by infusion, such as nitroglycerin and nitroprusside). By contrast, the indications for invasive central monitoring are not as clear or uniformly accepted. A CVP catheter is often placed to yield an approximation of volume status (or to follow a trend in blood loss or replacement therapy) and to give a greater understanding of the mechanical phases of the cardiac cycle. Management of oliguria unresponsive to a fluid challenge, pulmonary edema, and refractory hypertension are clinical situations in which some clinicians desire CVP monitoring.

Although a PA catheter can assist in determining the etiology of pulmonary edema, oliguria with normal CVP, or cardiovascular failure, its use is the most controversial. Advocates of PA catheter use suggest that it can provide information on left and right ventricular function, systemic vascular resistance, and cardiac output. Detractors question the validity of the data, noting that in the setting of preeclampsia, for example, the correlation between CVP and pulmonary capillary wedge pressure is unreliable for CVP readings greater than 6 cm H_2O.[127] In deciding between a PA versus CVP catheter, the clinician should recognize that although the insertion-related complications are similar,[128] the PA catheter is associated with more use-related complications, including balloon rupture, pulmonary infarction, valvular damage, and erosion of the PA. Thus, the benefits of PA catheter use should clearly outweigh its inherent risks before its use can be recommended. The 2007 practice guidelines of the American Society of Anesthesiologists Task Force on Obstetrical Anesthesia state that "the decision to perform invasive hemodynamic monitoring should be individualized and based on clinical indications that include the patient's medical history and cardiovascular risk factors."[43] To date, although PA catheter use has been reported in parturients (primarily with cardiac pathology or pulmonary hypertension), their use has been questioned.[129] No controlled trials are available that confirm the benefit of PA catheter monitoring on maternal or fetal outcome. PA pressures are observed with different etiologies of pulmonary edema and oliguria (**Boxes 62-5** and **62-6**).[130,131] Renal and postrenal etiologies of oliguria, such as renal artery vasospasm, acute tubular necrosis, and postrenal obstruction, are less commonly encountered in the obstetric population. Future modalities for hemodynamic monitoring, such as Doppler ultrasonography and three- and

BOX 62-5

Diagnosis of Pulmonary Edema by Pulmonary Arterial Wedge Pressure

Etiology	Pulmonary Arterial Wedge	Stroke Work Index
Left ventricular dysfunction	Increased	Decreased
Altered capillary permeability	Normal	Normal or increased
Low hydrostatic or oncotic pressure	Increased	Normal

BOX 62-6

Diagnosis of Prerenal Oliguria by Pulmonary Arterial Wedge Pressures

Etiology	Pulmonary Arterial Wedge Pressure	Left Ventricular Function	Systemic Vascular Resistance	Treatment
Hypovolemia	Low	Increased	Increased	IV fluids
Sepsis	Low	Increased	Decreased	IV fluids, vasopressors, inotropes
Congestive heart failure	Increased	Decreased	Increased	Fluid restriction, diuretics, inotropes

IV, intravenous.

even four-dimensional echocardiography, are able to provide detailed, dynamic information on cardiac structures and function and in the future may offer significant clinical advantages.[132]

ANESTHESIA FOR GYNECOLOGIC SURGERY

Although many of the procedures in gynecologic surgery are approached using standard surgical techniques, the care and anesthetic management should be provided with an understanding of gender-related differences that ultimately may affect patient outcomes and satisfaction. In addition to the many alterations discussed in the obstetric section of this chapter, gender-related changes in the sensitivity to pain and anesthetic agents are relevant to each case. Full appreciation should be given to the highly vascular uterus and other visceral structures found in women, which can result in sudden and profound blood loss; air emboli; and in pregnancy-related procedures involving the pregnant or peripartum state, amniotic fluid emboli.

PREOPERATIVE ASSESSMENT AND EVALUATION

A few elements in taking a gynecologic history deserve emphasis, particularly because a few weeks may have lapsed between the gynecologic surgeon's assessment and the surgical date. The menstrual cycle can serve as a guide to other pathology and rule out the possibility of pregnancy. Abnormal or prolonged uterine bleeding can be produced by a variety of endocrine and metabolic disorders, including hypothyroidism, hyperprolactemia, coagulopathies, and insulin metabolism disorders, which in turn may impact anesthetic care. Because pregnancy has implications on surgical interventions and anesthetic care, testing should be used in individuals with absent or irregular menses, unreliable knowledge of menstrual cycle or contraceptive use, and noncompliance with hormonal birth control regimens or if the report is desired. Algorithms for the use of serum and urine beta hCG pregnancy tests are helpful if applied appropriately (**Fig. 62-5**). The serum test uses a radioimmunoassay that can detect a pregnancy within 24 to 72 hours after conception at levels as low as 1 to 3 mIU/L.[133] By contrast, the urine test uses an antibody agglutination methodology that detects a level greater than 25 mIU/L, which is achieved only after 10 to 12 days.[133] A positive serum hCG combined with a positive uterine ultrasound result (demonstrating decidual thickening of the uterus) can diagnose pregnancy with 100% clinical accuracy.

The psychologic impact of the surgical condition should be considered and managed with sensitivity. Fear, anxiety, embarrassment, and even guilt may be associated with some procedures. Infertility patients may exhibit a number of emotions as they undergo an escalating series of tests, medications and procedures, including tubograms, laparoscopies, laparotomies, tubal reconstructions, and in vitro fertilization. Patients who have spontaneous, missed, or therapeutic abortions may have feelings of guilt or mourning. Patients with chronic pelvic pain may have concerns regarding complicated, multimodal pain therapies; such individuals often benefit from preoperative pain and psychiatric consultations. Patients with urinary or fecal incontinence may be acutely embarrassed by their condition. Patients with malignant breast or pelvic masses may have anxiety or fear of disfigurement and concern over loss of sexual function and desirability.

Patients who present for surgical management of gynecologic malignancies require additional considerations. The tumor mass may create anatomic and physiologic alterations, including aortocaval compression, respiratory embarrassment, changes in renal or hepatic function, and the potential for adhesions and scarring. The additional comorbidity of prior surgeries, chemotherapy, and radiation therapy must be considered as well. Chemotherapy may be associated with disruptions in hematopoiesis; infection resistance; nausea and emesis; and myocardial, renal, and hepatic function (**Table 62-7**). Anemia, coagulation disorders, and platelet dysfunction also may be present. Alternatively, malignancies may result in hypercoagulable states, and the impact of various regimens for prophylaxis and treatment should be considered in the perioperative period.[134,135]

INTRAOPERATIVE CONSIDERATIONS AND MANAGEMENT

Gender Differences in Sensitivity to Pain Gender differences in biologic, psychologic, and sociocultural factors are believed to be responsible for

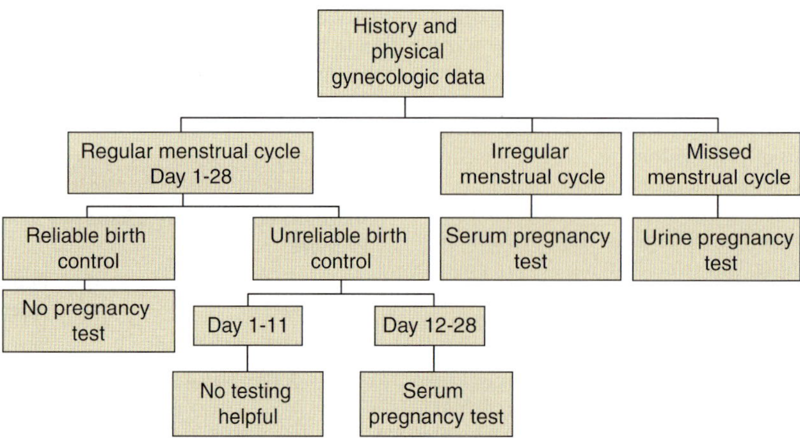

FIGURE 62-5. Preoperative pregnancy testing algorithm.

TABLE 62-7 Chemotherapeutic Agents with Unique Toxicities Affecting Anesthetic Management

Agent	Gynecologic Malignancy	Usual Dose	System Affected	Toxic Manifestation	Diagnostic Tests
Adriamycin (doxorubicin)	Endometrial carcinoma, ovarian carcinoma	500 mg/M²	Heart	Myocardial fibrosis, congestive heart failure	Echocardiogram, ejection fraction
Bleomycin (Blenoxane)	Cervical carcinoma, germ cell tumors of the ovary	400 U	Lung	Pulmonary fibrosis	Spirometry, diffusing capacity
cis-Platinum	Endometrial carcinoma, cervical carcinoma	50–75 mg/M²	Kidney	Renal tubular dysfunction	Creatinine clearance (dose related)

women reporting pain that is more severe, frequent, and of longer duration than that experienced by men.[136] Although gender role expectations may be partially responsible for these observations, female gonadal hormones have been associated with pain sensitivity, albeit contradictory to most expectations. Female hormonal increases, as occur during pregnancy, have been associated with decreases in response to noxious stimuli. By contrast, hormonal decreases, such as those witnessed in menopause, have been associated with increases in pain sensitivity.[137] Although progesterone previously was demonstrated in animal and human studies to be the female gonadal hormone most responsible for modulating pain,[138] the demonstration of an inverse relationship between estrogen and β-endorphins and estrogen receptors in the noxious stimuli processing areas of the brain and spinal cord suggests a greater role for estrogen. Acute estradiol exposure decreases the number of opioid binding sites; reduces the antinociception effect produced by morphine in ovariectomized rats; and diminishes the plasma, pituitary, and hypothalamic levels of β-endorphin.[138,139] In human clinical models, high estrogen levels alter noxious stimuli processing,[140] a finding that may be relevant to therapies that involve estrogen replacement or manipulation.

Gender-related differences in pain from the surgical exploration of abdominal and pelvic organs also may stem from the more complex anatomy and function of the female reproductive organs. The relative contributions of somatic and visceral sensory fibers to pain originating from the pelvic, uterine, cervical, and perineal structures have not been completely characterized. Investigations into visceral afferent contributions to pain have been particularly abbreviated because of the lack of suitable experimental models and noninvasive neurophysiologic techniques. Recent and future work, however, promises to more fully elucidate the contribution of female reproductive organs to gender-related pain.[141]

Gender Differences in Sensitivity to Anesthetic Agents Gender-related pharmacokinetic and pharmacodynamic alterations are produced by the greater percentage of body fat and the smaller body water content in females. In general, this results in a greater distribution per kilogram of body weight for lipophilic drugs, such as opioids and benzodiazepines, and a smaller distribution for water-soluble drugs, such as muscle relaxants.[142] Because the volume of distribution is the most important pharmacokinetic factor responsible for initial drug concentrations, the response to induction and bolus administration agents may be altered. Drug clearance, which is dependent on metabolism and excretion and is related to steady-state concentrations, also is affected by gender. Hepatic metabolism, which accounts for a major route of elimination of most IV anesthetic drugs, has gender-related alterations within the cytochrome P450 (CYP) and uridine diphosphate–glucuronosyltransferase systems (**Table 62-8**). Glomerular filtration rate, the most important renal parameter for excretion of nonactively secreted or reabsorbed drugs, is lower in females, but the impact of this change is not well characterized.[142]

Hormonal alterations from the use of contraceptive pills, in vitro stimulation regimens, pregnancy, menstrual cycles, and menopause may modify CYP enzyme activity. Although clearance of drugs may be higher in the middle of the menstrual cycle,[143] minimal to no menstrual phase variations have been noted with the disposition of certain anesthetic drugs, including alfentanil, alprazolam, and midazolam.[144,145] Menopause has been associated with decreases in midazolam and alfentanil clearance; however, this phenomenon is not entirely hormonally mediated because hormonal replacement does not return clearance to premenopausal levels.[146] Faster emergence from propofol anesthesia in women likely is related to a rapid decline in plasma levels[147]; whether this condition is attributable to elimination or intercompartmental distribution remains unclear. The analysis is further complicated by

TABLE 62-8 Gender Differences in Cytochrome Systems With Relevance to Anesthetic Drugs

Enzyme	Female Alteration	Drugs Affected
CYP 1A2	Decreased	Ropivacaine Theophylline
CYP 2C9	None	Propofol[a] NSAIDs
CYP 2C19	Contradictory	Hexobarbital Diazepam Propranolol
CYP 2D6	Contradictory	Codeine Tramadol Oxycodone Hydrocodone Metoprolol Propranolol
CYP 2E1	Contradictory	Halothane Enflurane Isoflurane Sevoflurane
CYP 3A4	Increased	Fentanyl Alfentanil Sufentanil[a] Methadone Buprenorphine Lidocaine Ropivacaine Bupivacaine Midazolam Diazepam[a] Verapamil Tirilazad Glucocorticoids
UGT	Decreased	

CYP, cytochrome P450; NSAID, nonsteroidal anti-inflammatory drug; UGT, UDP-glucuronosyltransferase.

[a]Studied in vitro.

Adapted from Pleym H, Spigset O, Kharasch ED, et al. Gender differences in drug effects: implications for anesthesiologists. *Acta Anaesthesiol Scand.* 2003;47:241-259.

the greater sensitivity of women to given plasma concentrations of propofol.[147] These changes demonstrate that the effect of gender on pharmacokinetics and pharmacodynamics is a multimodal issue for which more information is needed.

ANESTHETIC SELECTION AND CARE

Performing a history and physical examination; reviewing the chart, previous anesthetic records, and relevant testing; and discussing the overall plan with the surgeon are essential steps in selecting an appropriate anesthetic plan. This is particularly true given the variety of positioning requirements and surgical approaches for certain gynecologic procedures (eg, abdominal, laparoscopic, vaginal hysterectomy).

All patients, including those who received local anesthesia, should be monitored with ECG, blood pressure cuff, and pulse oximeter. Additional monitors include a capnography sampler, temperature probe, peripheral nerve stimulator, and Foley catheter as appropriate. Invasive monitors, such as an arterial catheter, central venous catheter, PA catheter, or transesophageal echocardiography probe, may be indicated in patients with serious medical problems or who are undergoing radical, prolonged procedures accompanied by extensive fluid shifts and volume replacement.

Monitored IV sedation, often used with a local anesthetic field block, is often appropriate for certain procedures, such as dilation and curettage (D&C), hymenotomy, and breast biopsy. IV sedative and analgesic medications may be beneficial before placement of the field block, particularly when the block is administered to the paracervical or perineal region. Because the cervix is highly vascular, field blocks in this region can result in high plasma local anesthetic concentrations, so vigilance should be given to signs of toxicity.

Neuraxial techniques are suitable for many operations, including conservative abdominal and pelvic procedures. However, the duration of the case, requirements for Trendelenburg position, and unanticipated need for extensive exploration may limit the use of spinal and epidural anesthesia. The selection of local anesthetics and the specific neuraxial technique depend on the magnitude and duration of the operation; however, a T4 to T6 level is advised for intra-abdominal surgery. Prophylactic antiemetic and supplementary opioid use may prevent the nausea and discomfort that result from peritoneal stimulation. Catheter-based techniques, as opposed to single-dose techniques, offer the most control and flexibility. When provided as part of a CSE technique, a short-acting spinal anesthetic can be given for procedures of potentially short but unknown duration. The catheter then can be used if the duration of the operative event is longer than anticipated or postoperatively for analgesia is appropriate. Whether these catheters should be placed intrathecally or epidurally is controversial. Microcatheters, which historically were passed through standard 25- to 32-gauge needles into the intrathecal space, were associated with cauda equina syndrome when used with 5% lidocaine in 7.5% dextrose. Speculation for this outcome has been placed on drug "pooling" by the nerve roots within the subarachnoid space. These outcomes were associated with clinical abandonment of these catheters in the United States but not in Europe. Since that time, slightly larger microcatheters, which pass through a 22- to 26-gauge spinal needle, have been evaluated. Microcatheters are believed to contribute to lesser risk for PDPH than standard macrocatheters (20-gauge) placed through a 17-gauge Tuohy or Weiss needle used in similar fashion. The combination of general anesthesia and an epidural catheter, whether used for intraoperative anesthesia or postoperative analgesia, can be advantageous for particularly large or painful procedures.

General anesthesia is best suited for procedures that require extensive abdominal dissection, steep Trendelenburg positioning, extended CO_2 insufflation for laparoscopy and pelviscopy, or deep levels of anesthesia for a short period of time. Although mask and LMA devices are often used, endotracheal intubation remains the conduit of choice for ventilation and anesthesia when pulmonary soiling is a risk. These cases include patients with suspected gastric contents (a "full stomach"), obesity, severe anxiety, nausea, or vomiting; surgical cases that will result in an aggressive Trendelenburg position or massive fluid shifts; and cases in which emergent exploration is required. Overweight or obese patients are increasingly prevalent even within younger age groups. The National Health and Nutrition Examination Survey found that obesity is becoming more common at younger ages and more prevalent with age.[148] Among nonpregnant women 20 to 39 years of age, the prevalence of obesity (BMI >30) is 34%.[148] If instrumentation of the airway presents a concern, alternative anesthetic options and the difficult airway algorithm should be invoked. An elective, awake fiberoptic intubation in a controlled environment with adequate assistance is often the optimal approach.

CONSIDERATIONS FOR SPECIFIC SITUATIONS

In general, gynecologic surgery can be divided into four major categories: perineal, transvaginal, intra-abdominal, and transabdominal (**Box 62-7**). Anesthetic management for these procedures depends on a number of factors specific to the procedure, patient, and health care providers.

Perineal and Urologic Surgery

Anatomy The vulva includes all of the structures visible externally from the pubis to the perineum, including the mons pubis, labia, clitoris, vestibule, urethra, and Skene and Bartholin glands. The primary blood

BOX 62-7

Common Gynecologic Procedures

- Transvaginal
  - Dilation and curettage
  - Dilation and evacuation
  - Cervical
  - Cone biopsy
  - Cerclage
  - Hysteroscopy
  - Vaginal reconstruction
- Perineal
  - Laser fulguration of condylomata
  - Hymenotomy
  - Marsupialization of Bartholin cyst
  - Anteroposterior repair
  - Vulvectomy
  - Stamey urethropexy (urologic)
- Intra-abdominal
  - Oophorectomy
  - Cystectomy
  - Salpingectomy
  - Salpingostomy
  - Myomectomy
  - Hysterectomy
  - Radical hysterectomy
  - Ruptured ectopic pregnancy
- Transabdominal
  - Laparoscopy
  - Pelviscopy

supply to the vulva is via the internal pudendal artery, a branch of the internal iliac artery. The nerve supply is via the pudendal nerve that arises from the sacral nerve roots (S2, S3, and S4; Fig. 62-3). The pudendal nerve, artery, and accompanying veins pass from the pelvis via the lesser sciatic foramen and along the lateral wall of the ischiorectal fossa. The pudendal nerve can be readily blocked through a transperineal or transvaginal approach with local anesthetic placed posterior and medial to the ischial tuberosity;[149] this block can be used in obstetrics to provide analgesia during a vaginal delivery or perineal repair. The lymphatic drainage of the vulva is principally through the superficial inguinal lymph nodes to the deep inguinal and pelvic nodal systems.

Specific Procedures Although a number of minor vulvar procedures are routinely performed under local anesthesia, most procedures performed in the operating room require regional or general anesthesia. Such procedures include biopsies, hymenectomies, drainage of Bartholin glands, and laser fulguration of intraepithelial neoplasia.

Surgical interventions to treat stress urinary incontinence in women include procedures to reestablish the posterior urethrovesical angle and resuspend the urethra. Traditional approaches include retropubic (eg, Marshall-Marchetti-Krantz or Burch procedures) and transvaginal approaches (eg, Kelly plication or Pereyra and Stamey urethropexy). Most of these procedures involve suturing the vaginal epithelium to the rectus fascia above the pubis. During placement of the paraurethral suture, the patient must not cough or strain. Neuraxial anesthesia, usually in the form of a spinal technique, provides a quiescent surgical field and good postoperative conditions. Prophylactic use of antiemetics (10 mg IV of metoclopramide, 4 mg IV of ondansetron, and 8 mg IV of dexamethasone) is recommended.

Major vulvar procedures, including operations for trauma or invasive carcinomas, often require extensive dissection into the tissues of the inferior fascia of the urogenital diaphragm, pelvis, and abdomen. These procedures frequently result in major blood loss from the vestibular bulbs, pudendal artery, and retropubic space of Retzius. Preparation for these cases should include use of large-bore IV catheters, immediate availability of resuscitation equipment and fluids, and use of invasive monitoring and blood products where appropriate. Anesthetic management that includes epidural catheter-based techniques allows for minimization of intraoperative general anesthetic agents and provision of superior postoperative analgesia. Patients with significant cardiac or pulmonary comorbid conditions, obesity, a potentially difficult airway, or an expectation for significant blood loss may benefit from induction of general anesthesia at the beginning of the case when the intubation can be achieved in a controlled, stable environment.

Special Considerations Use of operative lasers entails risks to the patient and the operating room staff through thermal and retinal injury from reflected light, ignition of operative drapes, and possible viral inoculation from inhalation of laser plume particulates. Human papilloma viral DNA has been found in laser plumes, but whether this represents an infectious risk is unclear.[150] Regardless, the smoke contains bioaerosols that can cause lung irritation and other potentially adverse effects.[150] Therefore, appropriate eye protection, occlusive laser masks, and properly functioning smoke evacuators are necessary. For patient safety, surgical site immobilization is of great importance. Dense regional anesthesia or general anesthesia with ventilation by mask, LMA, or endotracheal intubation are reasonable approaches.

TRANSVAGINAL SURGERY

Anatomy The vagina is an 8- to 10-cm compliant musculomembranous canal that extends from the external genitalia to the uterine cervix. Anteriorly and posteriorly related to the urethra and bladder, respectively, the vagina is in close proximity to the rectal ampulla, perineum, and cul-de-sac of Douglas. The primary blood supply to the vagina is derived from branches of the uterine and pudendal arteries. Whereas lymphatic drainage of the upper third of the vagina is predominately to the parametrial and pelvic lymph nodes, the lower two-thirds share the superficial inguinal lymph nodes with the vulva. The sensory nerve supply to the vagina arises from S2, S3, and S4 via the pudendal nerve. The sympathetic and parasympathetic nerve supplies originate from the hypogastric plexus (L1-L3) and sacral nerves, respectively (see Fig. 62-3).

The cervix enters the vagina at a variable angle through the anterosuperior wall and is composed of myometrial muscle and dense stroma. The blood supply is derived from the descending branch of the uterine artery, and lymphatic drainage is through the paracervical nodes. Innervated by the nerves arising in the hypogastric plexus, the exocervix is poorly supplied by sensory nerves and thus are relatively insensate. By contrast, the endocervix has an abundant nerve supply and is very sensitive to surgical manipulation.

Specific Procedures Dilation and curettage requires dilating the cervix and mechanically scraping or suctioning the uterine walls to obtain tissue for evaluation, perform an abortion, or investigate abnormal uterine bleeding. Frequently performed in an office setting, D&C procedures should be performed in an operative setting in patients with significant comorbid conditions, distorted anatomy, or an inability to tolerate an office procedure. The major surgical risk of the procedure is uterine perforation and subsequent hemorrhage, particularly when the perforation occurs through the lateral wall and involves the uterine artery. Preexisting acute or chronic anemia may exacerbate the patient's condition. If a perforation is suspected, gentle probing to localize the defect, observation, and laparoscopy or laparotomy may be needed for surgical repair.

Dilation and evacuation (D&E) and dilation and extraction (D&X) are similar to D&C but usually are performed to interrupt pregnancy. From gestational week 16, fetal size and structure dictate the mechanical disruption and then evacuation of fetal tissue. Extraction involves evacuation of intracranial contents after delivery of the fetal body through the dilated cervix to minimize uterine or cervical injury. Because these procedures disrupt fetal and placental tissue, amniotic fluid emboli, DIC, and uterine atony accompanied by maternal hemorrhage can follow.[151] Procedures being performed for an in utero fetal demise warrant coagulation studies, particularly if associated with an abruption or uterine dehiscence; however, a dead fetus per se does not result in coagulopathies for a period of days to weeks.[152,153] Complication rates correlate with the gestational age of the fetus and the experience of the surgeon. D&E procedures are also performed in patients with hydatidiform moles or persistent gestational trophoblastic tissues, which are neoplastic conditions resulting from deranged placental growth. Such pregnancies are associated with vaginal bleeding, anemia, and the need for subsequent chemotherapy.[154]

D&C, D&E, and D&X procedures often are performed with a paracervical block with the assumption that a uterine perforation would be accompanied by sudden, acute report of abdominal pain, but this has not been validated. Spinal and general anesthesia are viable options with the notation that volatile halogenated anesthetics, including sevoflurane and desflurane, have a dose-dependent association with uterine atony in in vitro experiments.[155] No clinical differences in blood loss with volatile agent administration in doses up to 1 MAC have been observed. Moreover, oxytocin appears to successfully diminish these volatile effects up to 1.5 MAC.[155] A number of uterotonic agents, such as methylergonovine and prostaglandin $F_2\alpha$, also can be used to augment uterine tone (see Table 62-4).

Diagnosis and therapy for preinvasive or invasive cervical lesions is often achieved with a cone biopsy, which provides concentric excision of both exocervical and endocervical stroma. Because the cervix is well vascularized, bleeding is common, especially in pregnant patients. Hemostatic sutures can be placed laterally in the descending cervical branches of the uterine artery. Dilute solutions of vasopressin (20 units in 20 mL of normal saline) or epinephrine (1:200,000) can be injected locally into the cervix to induce vasospasm; both of these agents may induce hypertension. Resulting hypertension that is severe and sustained may require a direct-acting vasodilator such as hydralazine; β-adrenergic blocking agents are less effective. Most cone biopsies are performed as day surgery procedures under spinal or general anesthesia. A mask or LMA technique can also be used with spontaneous or assisted ventilation.

Rigid or flexible hysteroscopic procedures are performed to evaluate the endocervix or endometrial cavity. The scope is inserted through the cervix into the uterine cavity. CO_2 or liquid then is used to distend the uterus for improved visibility and surgical access. Isoosmolar, nontoxic, nonconducting distending mediums, such as glycine, dextrose, sorbitol or mannitol, and saline, are used, and accurate accounting of the volume used and returned are essential to minimize water intoxication, hyponatremia, and ammonia toxicity. Diagnostic examinations for evaluation of unexplained fertility or abnormal uterine bleeding are performed with minimal cervical dilation using small-caliber devices that are placed under a paracervical block. By contrast, operative procedures, such as ablation or resection of intracavity uterine lesions, septae, or adhesions, are performed with larger-caliber devices capable of electrocautery, wire loop cutting, or lasering and necessitate a neuraxial or general anesthetic.

Vaginal hysterectomies are performed for benign conditions or early-stage malignancies of the uterus and cervix. They also are used in patients with loss of pelvic support associated with uterine prolapse. Excessive uterine size, prior abdominal surgery, and suspicion of intrapelvic malignancies all are contraindications to a vaginal approach. The procedure requires entry into the anterior and posterior culs-de-sac to expose the broad ligament containing the uterine artery and can be performed in association with cystocele or rectocele (bladder or rectal prolapse, respectively) repair or an urethropexy (see section Perineal and Urologic Surgery, Specific Procedures). The ovaries may be conserved or removed vaginally. These procedures can be performed under a hyperbaric spinal anesthetic at a T6 to T8 level to block the peritoneal sensation of uterine traction (see Fig. 62-3). If significant Trendelenburg positioning and laparoscopy-assisted techniques will be used, a general anesthetic with endotracheal intubation is recommended.[156]

Special Concerns The majority of transvaginal procedures are performed in the lithotomy position. Excessive hip flexion, abduction, and external rotation may allow the inguinal ligament to apply continuous pressure on the femoral nerve[157] or place the obturator and lateral femoral cutaneous nerves in a position where they are prone to stretch injury.[158] Extensive rotation of the thighs at the hip or extension of the legs without knee flexion may result in sciatic and peroneal nerves injury.[157] Compression of the lateral fibular head results in common peroneal nerve injury, which can result in foot drop and lateral lower extremity paresthesias.[157] Protective padding, avoidance of contact with hard surfaces or supports, and attention to positioning are important elements of optimal care.[159]

The Trendelenburg position is often used in transvaginal procedures to assist with surgical visualization. This position is associated with potentially severe consequences, including venous air emboli, alterations in circulation and respiration, and upper extremity peripheral nerve injuries.[156,159] When combined with laparoscopy, further hemodynamic and respiratory encroachment may occur.[156]

Use of distending mediums for hysteroscopy may result in absorption of large volumes of irrigating fluid, leading to hypervolemia, hyponatremia, and decreased osmolarity. Together, these alterations may produce hypertension, bradycardia, altered mental status, nausea, vomiting, headache, agitation, and lethargy. These symptoms are masked if general anesthesia is used. If the resulting "hypoosmolar hyponatremia" is not recognized, seizures, coma, and death may occur. Treatment includes halting or rapidly completing the surgery; sending blood for a complete blood count, electrolytes, and osmolality; and administering normal saline and furosemide. Although severe hyponatremia (<120 mEq/L) has a significant association with mortality, correction with hypertonic saline (3% NaCl) should occur no faster than 1 to 2 mEq/L/h with a goal of 125 to 130 mEq/L. Overly rapid correction can lead to central pontine myelinolysis, with paresis, mutism, pseudobulbar palsy, and other neurologic disorders.[160,161]

Intra-abdominal Operations

Anatomy Intra-abdominal operations relate mostly to the vagina, uterine cervix, uterus, fallopian tubes, and ovaries. On occasion, especially when associated with sepsis or tumor invasion, the rectum and bladder are involved through fistulous communications. The blood supply to the pelvis is largely derived from the internal iliac (hypogastric) artery, which in turn gives rise to the uterine arteries; the superior, middle, and inferior vesical arteries; the middle and inferior hemorrhoidal arteries; and the vaginal arteries. The extensive collateral circulation network to organs within the pelvic viscera alternatively allows extensive bleeding during pelvic dissection or obstetric hemorrhage as well as the possibility of ligating major arteries, including the internal iliac, with few untoward effects.

The pelvic organs are innervated by sympathetic fibers derived predominately from the first through fourth lumbar nerves (L1-L4) and enter the hypogastric or presacral plexus (see Fig. 62-3). The presacral sympathetic plexus serves the uterine fundus, cervix, vagina, and excretory organs, including the rectosigmoid region of the colon, anus, bladder, and urethra. Parasympathetic preganglionic fibers arise from the second through fourth sacral nerves (S2-S4). Sensory nerves from the pelvic viscera, including the uterus, arise from the T10 to L4 spinal cord segments. By contrast, the cervix is served by nerve fibers from the S2 to S4 spinal cord segments. Lymphatic drainage of the female reproductive organs is predominately through the pelvic and paraaortic lymph nodes in the retroperitoneum, although the superficial and deep inguinal lymph nodes may be involved as well.

Specific Procedures Ovarian surgery is performed for a variety of conditions, including removal of cystic masses, endometrial lesions, and neoplastic tissues. Ovarian carcinomas are the most lethal of all gynecologic malignancies because of their ability to grow silently until the disease is advanced and widespread.[162] With extensive ovarian cancer, subdiaphragmatic lymphatic obstruction often results in profound ascites that may impair diaphragmatic excursion, impede venous return, and delay gastric emptying. Cytoreductive procedures, which remove all visible tumor masses to improve the response to chemotherapy, can include extensive retroperitoneal dissections with bowel resections and bypasses.

Surgery of the fallopian tubes is performed most often for nonneoplastic processes; both benign and malignant neoplasias are rare. Salpingoscopies are becoming more common because of their association with infertility evaluations.[163] Tubal ectopic pregnancies, which occur in approximately 1 of 100 pregnancies, are associated with pelvic inflammatory disease, intrauterine device use, diethylstilbestrol exposure, and prior tubal procedures or pathology.[164] Ectopic pregnancies may be located throughout the fallopian tube, including the uterine anastomosis; the pregnancy is surrounded by myometrial uterine tissue at this site and may grow significantly before becoming symptomatic. Ectopic pregnancies may rupture without warning, leading to acute hemoperitoneum and massive exsanguination. Management should center on providing rapid fluid resuscitation, securing the airway, and preparing for massive blood transfusion and immediate surgery. Procedures for removing ectopic gestations are time consuming because hemostasis may be difficult to obtain. On occasion, particularly if the ectopic gestation is implanted near the uterus, a salpingectomy and hysterectomy may be required.

Tuboovarian abscesses are managed surgically when they are larger than 8 cm, nonresponsive to antibiotic therapy, or potentially ruptured. Ruptured tubo-ovarian abscesses may be accompanied by peritonitis, septic shock, respiratory distress, and coagulopathies. Surgical management of intact abscesses includes percutaneous or laparoscopic drainage. However, a laparotomy with a salpingo-oophorectomy and hysterectomy may be necessary, particularly when associated with a rupture or extensive pelvic inflammatory disease.

Uterine leiomyomas (fibroids) are the most common benign tumor in women and may be associated with menometrorrhagia; ureteral obstruction; pain; infertility; and, rarely, pregnancy loss. Usually well-circumscribed but nonencapsulated, fibroids occur in the submucosal, intramural, or subserosal layers (innermost to outermost layers, respectively) of the uterus. Patients often are placed preoperatively on leuprolide, a gonadotropin-releasing hormone agonist, in an attempt to reduce the size of the fibroids. Myomectomies can range from straightforward hysteroscopic procedures of pedunculated subserosal fibroids to prolonged dissections of intramural fibroids accompanied by extensive bleeding. Vasospastic solutions of vasopressin or epinephrine are sometimes injected directly into the myometrium to reduce blood loss. Myomectomies can be performed under regional or general anesthesia.

Uterine reconstructive surgeries are performed for congenital malformations of the uterus and include removal of uterine septa or reunification of duplicate uterine horns. Most are performed to enable fertility or gestation.

Abdominal hysterectomies, which include subtotal (supracervical), total, and radical types, are performed for a variety of benign and malignant diseases. Common indications include symptomatic uterine fibroids, pelvic pain, and endometriosis. Acute inflammatory disease, endometriosis, and malignancies may result in extensive adhesions, increased vascularity, and destruction of normal tissue planes. These alterations prolong surgery and increase blood loss. Because a steep Trendelenburg position is often required for these operations, general anesthesia with endotracheal intubation is used.

Special Considerations Although vertical and transverse approaches can be used for intra-abdominal surgeries, the low transverse incision is selected when possible for its cosmetic acceptability and strength of repair. The Pfannenstiel incision, the most common approach for cesarean delivery, often is modified to include dissection of the rectus abdominis (Maylard or Cherney incisions) for improved access to the lateral margins of the pelvis. When access to the upper abdomen is required, vertical midline or paramedian incisions are used. Such incisions are avoided, when possible, because the intrinsic strength and structural integrity of the repair are less robust, and respiratory splinting may occur.

Blood loss in gynecologic surgery may be precipitous and unexpected, although such cases often can be anticipated. Additional vascular access; invasive monitoring; and blood conservation techniques, such as erythropoietin-induced red cell production, autologous donation, and acute normovolemic hemodilution, should be considered in advance.[165,166] Because preoperative autologous donation is limited by the maximum life span of stored blood, collection must occur within 6 weeks of the planned operation, with an average unit collection interval of 3 to 7 days.[166] Although the use of blood cell salvage technologies remains controversial, particularly in the presence of malignancies, recovery of 2 to 3 units of blood has been deemed to be cost effective.[166] Moreover, the irradiation of blood cells retrieved intraoperatively has been demonstrated to eliminate cancer cells.[167] Most recently, the placement of prophylactic balloon catheters in major vessels by interventional radiologists may allow for timely control or embolization of intraoperative bleeding, particularly from the uterus.

The extent of surgery for gynecologic malignancies often depends on the clinical staging of the disease, the presence or absence of lymph node metastases, and an examination of involved tissues by a surgical pathologist. The gynecologic surgeon and the anesthesia provider should discuss the likelihood of progression to a more radical surgery before and during an operation. Such discussions help guide decisions about placement of invasive monitoring catheters, use of large doses of opioids and neuromuscular blocking agents, and selection of an anesthetic technique that is inappropriate for the duration and surgical exposure necessary for the case. On occasion, if the malignancy is confined to the pelvis without fixation to the pelvic sidewall, a pelvic exenteration is performed. This massive procedure involves radical hysterectomy, cystectomy with urinary diversion, and proctocolectomy with a permanent colostomy. Major fluid and electrolyte shifts, blood and heat loss, and coagulopathies can occur. Low-flow or closed-circuit volatile agent techniques and use of passive humidifiers, heating blankets, and fluid warmers are encouraged. A combined epidural–general anesthetic technique offers the benefits of a sympathetic blockade during the surgery and optimal analgesia postoperatively. Epidural analgesia is a particularly effective technique for reducing pain after intra-abdominal procedures. With the exception of a herniotomy, use of incisional local anesthesia is not consistently effective for reducing postoperative pain.[168]

Transabdominal Surgery In distinction to open surgical procedures, transabdominal surgery occurs through small incisions with rigid or flexible scopes and instrumentation; an increasing number of these procedures are performed with robot-assisted technologies. Advantages of these procedures include smaller incisional sites, lower risks of wound complications, reduced postoperative pain and complications, and improved recovery.[169] Disadvantages include poor visualization, injury to viscera and blood vessels, and complications from CO_2 insufflation. In some cases, such as hysterectomies, vaginal approaches may be superior to laparoscopic approaches; however, both have benefits over open laparotomy.[170]

Although initially developed as a means for diagnosis, laparoscopy and pelviscopy are used routinely for a variety of operative procedures, including tubal ligation and repair, endometriosis fulguration, ovarian cyst aspiration and resection, ectopic pregnancy removal, and fibroid excision. Laparoscopic-guided carcinoma staging and resection procedures have been demonstrated to result in improved short- and long-term outcomes compared with open laparotomies.[171] Most recently, "hand-assisted laparoscopy," which uses laparoscopy combined with a small incision for insertion of a hand, has shown increased utility and benefit over open laparotomy.[172]

Laparoscopy and pelviscopies are performed, often after catheterization of the bladder, with the surgeon placing a needle with a stopcock periumbilically through the fascial layers into the peritoneum. CO_2 is insufflated through this needle to a pressure of approximately 19 mm Hg. If the pressure increases rapidly, the needle may be inappropriately located between the fascial planes of the muscle layers and will need to be replaced. In the proper location and with the appropriate degree of abdominal distension achieved, the hollow needle is replaced with a trochar with a self-sealing opening for the laparoscope. The laparoscope then is placed and connected to an insufflator that provides gas (CO_2) flows at a rate of 200 mL/min to maintain pressure.

Special Considerations Although CO_2 is a biologically produced gas and is nonflammable and rapidly absorbed, a number of consequences and complications may result from CO_2 insufflation. During the routine practice of laparoscopy and pelviscopy, distension of the abdomen may cause a number of disturbances that have implications for the anesthesiologist (**Box 62-8**). Pressure on the diaphragm, coupled with the use of anesthetic agents, tends to impede respiration. If patients are breathing spontaneously, minimal to moderate respiratory acidosis and oxygen desaturation may occur. Use of controlled ventilation with increased minute volumes can compensate for increased CO_2, however, higher inspiratory pressures are frequently observed, particularly in obese patients in the Trendelenburg position. Because sustained high plateau pressures can lead to bronchoalveolar damage, several changes may be necessary, such as modification of ventilatory settings to lower tidal volumes, release of some gas from the abdomen by the surgeon, and reduction of the degree of Trendelenburg positioning. Tension pneumothorax related to excessive inspiratory pressures can occur and must be ruled out if a sudden increase in inspiratory pressure is accompanied by decreasing oxygen saturations.

BOX 62-8

Concerns and Complications from Laparoscopy and Pelviscopy

Concerns

- Cardiovascular alterations
  - Low-pressure (14-20 mm Hg) insufflation: increased central venous pressure, stroke volume, and blood pressure
  - High-pressure (40 mm Hg) insufflation: decreased venous return, hypotension
- Ventilatory alterations
  - Decreased functional residual capacity, increased airway pressures and closure, decreased lung compliance, right main stem intubation, hypoxemia
- Other alterations
  - Carbon dioxide absorption with possible increase in plasma catecholamines, tachycardia, arrhythmias, vasodilation
  - Increased intra-abdominal pressure

Complications

- Carbon dioxide gas embolism
- Hemorrhage
- Pneumothorax
- Pneumomediastinum
- Subcutaneous emphysema
- Perforated viscus
- Explosion
- Retroperitoneal emphysema
- Cardiovascular collapse
- Carbon monoxide accumulation
- Pulmonary edema

A massive CO_2 embolus, although rare, is rapidly fatal unless recognized and treated immediately. The usual sequence is the onset of sudden and severe hypotension, arterial desaturation, and cardiovascular collapse shortly after placement of the insufflation needle or laparoscope. A "mill wheel" murmur throughout the cardiac cycle from gas in the right heart and pulmonary outflow tract has been reported; however, this is an unreliable sign. Capnography most likely will reveal a sudden decrease in expired CO_2 because an acute increase in "physiologic" dead space, and fulminant pulmonary edema may occur. Treatment is largely supportive, with immediate discontinuance of CO_2 insufflation, intubation (if not already part of the anesthetic technique), provision of 100% oxygen, and cardiovascular support. Placing the patient in a left lateral head-down position to trap the gas in the apex of the right ventricle rather than the pulmonary outflow tract (ie, Durant maneuver) is controversial. Placement of a central venous catheter into the right atrium to remove gas or air acting as a mechanical obstruction is also controversial. Fortunately, CO_2 is highly soluble and rapidly cleared, and more favorable outcomes have been observed than with massive air emboli. If pulmonary edema develops, 5 to 10 cm H_2O of positive end-expiratory pressure and use of IV furosemide may be helpful. If significant CO_2 sequelae occur, the procedure should be rapidly terminated and the patient brought to an intensive care environment for continued observation and therapy.

Postoperatively, laparoscopy and pelviscopy have been significantly associated with postoperative nausea and vomiting. Moreover, laparoscopy may be a risk factor for superficial thrombophlebitis, deep venous thrombosis, and pulmonary embolism.[173]

CONCLUSION

The care and management of women undergoing obstetric and gynecologic surgery involves an appreciation of the physiologic, pharmacologic, and anatomic differences related to their gender or gravid state. Anesthesiologists should guide their practice according to these differences for optimal patient safety, outcomes, and satisfaction.

KEY REFERENCES

- Briggs GG, Freeman RK, Sumner JY. *Drugs in Pregnancy and Lactation*. Philadelphia, PA: Lippincott Williams & Wilkins; 2005.
- Esler MD, Douglas MJ. Planning for hemorrhage. Steps an anesthesiologist can take to limit and treat hemorrhage in the obstetric patient. *Anesthesiol Clin North Am*. 2003;21:127-144, vii.
- Hawkins JL, Chang J, Palmer S, Gibbs CP, Callaghan WM. Anesthesia-related maternal mortality in the United States: 1979-2002. *Obstet Gynecol* 2011;117(1):69-74.
- Lee SJ, Ralston HJ, Drey EA, et al. Fetal pain: a systematic multidisciplinary review of the evidence. *JAMA*. 2005;294:947-954.
- Marx GF. Aortocaval compression syndrome: its 50 year history. *Int J Obstet Anesth*. 1992;1:60-64.
- Mhyre JM, Riesner MN, Polley LS, Naughton NN. A series of anesthesia-related maternal deaths in Michigan, 1985–2003. *Anesthesiology*. 2007;106:1096-1104.
- Ngan Kee WD, Lee A, Khaw KS, Ng FF, Karmakar MK, Gin T. A randomized double-blinded comparison of phenylephrine and ephedrine infusion combinations to maintain blood pressure during spinal anesthesia for cesarean delivery: the effects on fetal acid-base status and hemodynamic control. *Anesth Analg*. 2008;107:1295-1302.
- Practice advisory for the prevention of perioperative peripheral neuropathies: a report by the American Society of Anesthesiologists Task Force on Prevention of Perioperative Peripheral Neuropathies. *Anesthesiology*. 2000;92:1168-1182.
- Practice guidelines for obstetric anesthesia: an updated report by the American Society of Anesthesiologists Task Force on Obstetric Anesthesia. *Anesthesiology*. 2007;106:843-863.
- Pleym H, Spigset O, Kharasch ED, et al. Gender differences in drug effects: implications for anesthesiologists. *Acta Anaesthesiol Scand*. 2003;47:241-259.
- Tsen LC. Neuraxial techniques for labor analgesia should be placed in the lateral position. *Int J Obstet Anesth*. 2008;17:146-149.
- Ueyama H, He YL, Tanigami H, et al. Effects of crystalloid and colloid preload on blood volume in the parturient undergoing spinal anesthesia for elective Cesarean section. *Anesthesiology*. 1999;91:1571-1576.
- Wong CA, Scavone BM, Peaceman AM, et al. The risk of cesarean delivery with neuraxial analgesia given early versus late in labor. *N Engl J Med*. 2005;352:655-665.

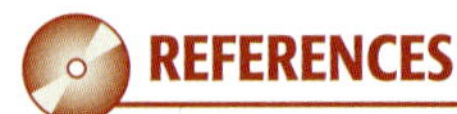

Complete references available on DVD and online version at www.LongneckerAnesthesiology.com

CHAPTER 63

Aesthesia for Newborn Surgical Emergencies

Myron Yaster
Mark I. Rossberg

KEY POINTS

1. Newborns require anesthesia for surgery. Newborns respond to noxious stimuli, and failure to provide analgesia and anesthesia increases perioperative morbidity and mortality
2. Pharmacokinetics and pharmacodynamics differ in newborns. Concentrations of albumin and alpha-1 acid glycoprotein are lower in newborns, and binding sites are fewer; thus, a greater proportion of active ("free") drug is available. Furthermore, the newborn cytochrome P450 system does not reach adult functionality until 1 to 2 months of life.
3. All potent inhalational anesthetics produce unacceptable hypotension in newborns. Thus, the risk of cardiovascular collapse during the induction of general anesthesia is much greater in newborn than in older children and adults.
4. Newborns have a fixed stroke volume and can increase cardiac output only by increasing heart rate. Atropine requirements in newborns (0.03-0.05 mg/kg intravenous [IV]) are almost three times greater than in adults, and total doses of less than 0.1 to 0.15 mg may produce paradoxical bradycardia, further contributing to hypotension.
5. Fentanyl (10-12.5 mcg/kg) produces insignificant hemodynamic changes and provides reliable anesthesia in newborns, provided the infants are preloaded with a balanced salt solution (20 mL/kg IV) and a vagolytic agent (eg, pancuronium or atropine) is administered.
6. Rapid-sequence induction with gentle cricoid pressure, rather than "awake" intubation, is usually the preferred method of securing the airway.
7. Newborns are at high risk for hypothermia during transport and in the operating room (OR). This is countered by wrapping the infant in plastic bags; using forced-air heating mattresses; increasing the OR temperature to or above 90°F, warming IV fluids; and using heated, humidified respiratory gases.
8. "Right-to-left" shunting of blood across the ductus arteriosus and the atrial septum is a catastrophic return to fetal circulation (ie, persistent fetal circulation or persistent pulmonary hypertension of the newborn); it occurs when pulmonary vascular resistance exceeds systemic vascular resistance. Treatment is directed at improving oxygenation and increasing pulmonary blood flow by the judicious use of muscle relaxants, analgesics (usually fentanyl), hyperventilation, ventilatory rates of greater than 100 breaths/min and low inflating pressures, preventing hypothermia, and correction of acidosis with IV bicarbonate therapy.
9. Accumulating data from animal studies suggest that some anesthetics, opioids, and related drugs (eg, benzodiazepines) may be neurotoxic in the developing brain, and there is some evidence of behavioral changes (eg, learning disabilities) in children who have had multiple anesthetic exposures. However, definitive evidence of neurotoxicity in newborns or children who have had single or limited exposures is lacking and is balanced by concerns about outcomes in newborns who are not anesthetized for painful procedures.

INTRODUCTION

Except for extraordinary circumstances, all newborns require anesthesia for surgery.[1-4] In the past, it had been assumed that newborn infants neither experienced nor perceived painful stimuli to the same degree that adults do. Indeed, it was thought that newborns did not have the neurologic substrate necessary for the perception of pain because of a lack of myelinization, incomplete pain pathways from the periphery to the cortex, or immaturity of the cerebral cortex. There is absolutely no evidence that any of this is true.[2-5] Indeed, by the 24th week of gestation, newborn respond to noxious stimuli with behavioral, physiologic, metabolic, and hormonal responses suggestive of substantial stress.[6] It is also clear that the neurophysiologic pathways for nociception from the peripheral receptors to the cerebral cortex are developed even in premature infants. Furthermore, the primary pathways of pain transmission involve unmyelinated C and A delta fibers, so postnatal myelination is not required for most pain perception.[7-10] Finally, failure to provide anesthesia is associated with an increased incidence of circulatory, respiratory, and metabolic complications in newborns.[11,12] Thus, the preponderance of evidence suggests that newborns not only respond to noxious stimuli but that the failure to provide analgesia and anesthesia significantly increases perioperative morbidity and mortality.

Newborns differ from adults and older children in the uptake, distribution, metabolism, and excretion of all drugs. During the first month of life (the "neonatal" period), newborns must function independently and adapt to extrauterine life. This involves anatomic, physiologic, and pharmacologic changes to maintain homeostasis and to ensure the infant's survival. Disease, congenital anomalies, surgery, and anesthesia may interfere with these adaptations and threaten survival. The important elements of the preoperative history and preanesthetic assessment, including review of systems, developmental physiology, and the transition from intra- to extrauterine life, are discussed in Chapter 18. This chapter discusses anesthetic pharmacology in neonates, an approach to intraoperative management, and the specific management of commonly encountered surgical problems. The general principles of pharmacokinetics and pharmacodynamics are discussed in detail in Chapter 40; the following focuses on the unique aspects that apply specifically to neonates.

ANESTHETIC PHARMACOLOGY IN NEONATES

When physicians administer drugs to patients of any age, they do so with the expectation that an anticipated therapeutic effect will occur. Unfortunately, other less desired results can also occur; the patient may derive inadequate or no therapeutic benefit from the administered drug, or worse yet, he or she may develop side effects or a toxic reaction. The aim of modern clinical pharmacology is to take the guesswork out of this process and to establish the relationship between the dose of a drug given and the response elicited. To attain this goal, clinicians need a working knowledge of the principles of drug absorption, distribution, and elimination and how these processes are related to intensity and duration of drug action. Additionally, they need a thorough understanding of the chemical and physical properties, physiologic effects, disposition, mechanisms of action, and therapeutic uses of the drugs that are used to provide anesthesia and analgesia in newborns.

An understanding of the factors that determine drug concentrations within the body is crucial to rational drug use in patients of any age and to achieving desirable plasma drug concentrations. *Pharmacokinetics* is the term used to describe the study of drug disposition within the body. It includes absorption, distribution, metabolism, and elimination of drug molecules from the body. *Pharmacodynamics* is the term used to describe the study of drug action within the body. It defines the relationship between the concentration of the drug at the site of action and the physiologic response. The relationship between pharmacokinetics and pharmacodynamics provides an understanding of the dose–response curves for the onset of action, magnitude of action, and duration of action of drugs used in treating patients.

DRUG DISTRIBUTION

How much drug reaches a receptor or effector site depends on the extent of protein binding, tissue volume, tissue solubility coefficients, and blood flow. Anatomic and maturational changes involving body composition, distribution of water, metabolism, protein binding, and organ function in health and in disease contribute to the unique responses of newborns to various drugs. In the blood, opioids (eg, fentanyl, morphine), amide local anesthetics (eg, bupivacaine, lidocaine), and muscle relaxants (eg, pancuronium, rocuronium) bind to albumin and other serum proteins, such as alpha-1 acid glycoprotein.[13,14] The unbound or "free" drug is available to cross biological membranes, bind to receptors, and initiate a pharmacologic effect. Concentrations of both albumin and alpha-1 acid glycoprotein are lower in newborns than at any other moment in life. Additionally, the number of binding sites on these proteins and their affinity for drugs is less than in later life. Thus, a greater proportion of active, unbound (or "free") drug is available to penetrate the brain, heart, and other viscera. Furthermore, the membranes that separate target receptors from the blood (ie, the "blood–brain barrier") may also be immature at birth and thereby allow agonists with limited lipid solubility, such as morphine, greater access to the brain. Kupferberg and Way[15] and Way et al[16] demonstrated that morphine concentrations were 2 to 4 times greater in the brains of younger than older rats despite equal blood concentrations. On the other hand, decreased protein binding may contribute to the larger apparent volume of distribution (Vd) of many drugs as well. A large apparent Vd, in effect, dilutes the plasma concentrations of parenterally administered drugs and explains, in part, why some drugs must be given in larger doses (mg/kg basis) to achieve a therapeutic effect.[17]

Body composition also changes with age. About 80% to 90% of a newborn's body mass is composed of water (**Table 63-1**).[18] In fact, in very-low-birth-weight premature infants (<2 kg), total body water can be estimated at 100% of body weight. This increase in total body water occurs primarily in the extracellular fluid (ECF) space, mostly in interstitial water, and explains the larger apparent Vd of most parenterally administered drugs in newborns. In newborns, interstitial water makes up 40% of the body weight but declines to10% to 15% in adults.

Blood flow determines how much drug reaches a target receptor. As in adults, a high proportion of cardiac output perfuses vessel-rich organs, such as the brain, kidney, and intestinal viscera. Very high brain concentrations are achieved after the administration of any lipophilic or inhalational anesthetic because the infant's brain receives almost 30% of the cardiac output versus only about 15% in adults. The very small muscle and fat mass of infants provides less of a reservoir to lower blood concentrations of drugs. Furthermore, the potent vapors are less soluble in neonatal blood than adults' blood. As a result, higher concentrations of an administered vapor anesthetic (eg, sevoflurane, isoflurane) are achieved more quickly than might be expected.[19,20] Finally, the perinatal adaptation to extrauterine life produces rapid changes in the circulation. This process may be inhibited by congenital heart disease or any other condition that increases pulmonary vascular resistance more than systemic vascular resistance, such as hypoxia, hypercarbia, and acid–base problems. Uptake, distribution, metabolism, and excretion may be drastically affected when cardiovascular function is abnormal.

TABLE 63-1

Body Compartment	Premature Infants (<2.5 kg)	Full-Term Infants (>2.5 kg)	Adults
Total body water (% body weight)	90-100	70-85	60
Extracellular fluid (% body weight)	40-60	40	20
Intracellular fluid (% body weight)	40	40	40
Blood volume (mL/kg)	90-105	80-95	50-65
Muscle mass (% body weight)	15	20	50
Fat (% body weight)	3	10	15-30

BIOTRANSFORMATION AND ELIMINATION

After administration, the disposition of a drug depends on distribution ($t_{1/2}\alpha$) and elimination. The terminal half-life of elimination ($t_{1/2}\beta$) is directly proportional to the Vd and inversely proportional to the total body clearance (Cl) by the following formula:

$$t_{1/2}\beta = 0.693 \times (\text{Vd/Cl})$$

Thus, prolongation of the $t_{1/2}\beta$ may be caused by either an increase in a drug's Vd or to a decrease in its clearance.

After redistribution, the major processes that lead to the termination of a drug's effect are biotransformation, metabolism, and excretion. Many anesthetic-related drugs (eg, opioids, muscle relaxants, hypnotics) are biotransformed in the liver before excretion. Many of these reactions are catalyzed in the liver by microsomal mixed-function oxidases that require the cytochrome P450 (CYP_{450}) system, NADPH (nicotinamide adenine dinucleotide phosphate), and oxygen. The CYP_{450} system is very immature at birth and does not reach adult functionality until the month 1 or 2 of life. This immaturity of this hepatic enzyme system may explain the prolonged clearance or elimination of some drugs in the first few days to weeks of life and the inability of the liver to convert a precursor into its active form (eg, codeine into morphine).[21,22] However, the CYP_{450} system can be induced by various drugs (eg, phenobarbital) and substrates, and this enzyme system matures regardless of gestational age. Thus, it is the age from birth, not the duration of gestation, that determines how premature or full-term infants metabolize many drugs. Greeley and de Bruijn[23] demonstrated that sufentanil is more rapidly metabolized and eliminated in 2- to 3-week-old infants than newborns less than 1 week of age. Elimination may be further prolonged by abnormal or decreased liver blood flow, which may occur after an acute illness or abdominal surgery. Certain conditions that may raise intra-abdominal pressure (eg, closure of an abdominal wall defect, such as an omphalocele or gastroschisis) may further decrease liver blood flow by shunting blood away from the liver via the still patent ductus venosus.[24,25] Finally, in all newborns, excretion may be reduced compared with in older children and adults because both glomerular and tubular renal function, which are responsible for active secretion and passive resorption, are reduced in newborns.[26]

CHOICE OF ANESTHETICS

INHALATIONAL ANESTHETICS

At equipotent doses, all of the potent inhalational anesthetics (eg, sevoflurane, desflurane, and isoflurane) produce unacceptable hypotension in newborns requiring emergency surgery. Thus, the risk of cardiovascular collapse during the induction of general anesthesia is much greater in newborns than in older children and adults.[27-32] This greater decrease in blood pressure is attributable to differences in uptake and distribution of the anesthetic, anesthetic dose requirements, vascular actions of the anesthetics, and sensitivity of the newborn's myocardium to these agents.[33-36] Newborns attain a greater absolute concentration of halothane (or any of the potent vapors) in the brain and heart and at a faster rate than adults do at the same inspired concentration. If the inspired concentration of an inhaled agent is kept constant, the ratio of the inspired to the alveolar concentration (F_A/F_I) is significantly greater in the newborn compared with adults because of differences in ventilation and anesthetic uptake. Infants have three to four times the minute ventilation of older children and adults but the same functional residual capacity on an mL/kg basis (**Table 63-2**). Thus, inhalational anesthetics wash in (and wash out) rapidly because the time constant of the lung is so markedly reduced compared with in adults (0.19 min in infants vs 0.73 min in adults). Controlled ventilation further exacerbates this phenomenon.

The uptake of a potent vapor is very rapid in newborns as well. Because the mass of vessel rich organs is so small, the uptake of inhalational agents by the tissues is rapid, and tissue concentrations saturate

TABLE 63-2 Selected Pulmonary Function Differences Between Newborns and Adults

Respiratory Variable	Newborns (mL/kg)	Adults (mL/kg)
Tidal volume	7	7
Respiratory rate	30-40	10-15
Vd/Vt	0.3	0.3
FRC	20-30	20-30
Vital capacity	50-70	50-70
Alveolar ventilation: FRC	5:1	1.5:1

FRC, functional residual capacity; Vd/Vt, dead space to tidal volume ratio.

quickly. Venous blood returning to the lung arrives at a relatively high anesthetic partial pressure compared with the case in adults, and this further reduces the F_A/F_I ratio and increases the amount of potent agent in the alveolus. This allows a higher concentration of inhalational agent to be taken up by the blood for delivery to the major organs. End-tidal gas monitoring may help prevent inadvertent overdosage. Finally, both left-to-right and right-to-left shunting occur in infants. A left-to-right shunt has little to no effect on anesthetic uptake, but a right-to-left shunt may slow the rate of rise of the arterial concentration of an inhaled anesthetic.

The minimum alveolar concentration (MAC) of all vapor anesthetics is also significantly lower in newborns than in infants 1 to 6 months of age. Furthermore, premature infants have lower MAC requirements than full-term infants. Thus, some of the hypotension associated with the inhalational agents may result from relative anesthetic overdose. Nevertheless, even at "true" MAC concentrations in newborns, heart rate and blood pressure decrease by 12% and 30%, respectively, with all vapor anesthetics . This can be partially attenuated by pretreating the infant with an intravenous (IV) anticholinergics such as atropine immediately before the induction of anesthesia.[37] Atropine requirements in newborns are greater than in adults (0.03-0.05 mg/kg vs 0.01-0.02 mg/kg, respectively). Additionally, IV doses of atropine less than 0.1 to 0.15 mg may produce paradoxical bradycardia.

Characteristics of the myocardium in newborns also contribute to hypotension; newborns' myocardium are less compliant than those of older children and adults.[38] Indeed, newborns have a fixed stroke volume and can increase cardiac output only by increasing heart rate. Additionally newborns' myocardium have decreased contractile mass and a decreased velocity of shortening. The negative inotropic and chronotropic effects associated with the inhaled anesthetics are therefore poorly tolerated. Furthermore, the baroreceptor reflexes are blunted or obliterated by these agents.[27,39] Reflex tachycardia, which is vital in supporting blood pressure and cardiac output, may not occur.

FENTANYL(S)

Fentanyl and its structurally related relatives, sufentanil, alfentanil, and remifentanil, are highly lipophilic drugs that rapidly penetrate all membranes, including the blood-brain barrier. After an IV bolus, fentanyl is rapidly eliminated from plasma as the result of its extensive uptake by body tissues. The fentanyls are highly bound to alpha-1 acid glycoproteins in the plasma, but these are reduced in newborns.[40,41] The fraction of free unbound sufentanil is significantly increased in neonates and children younger than 1 year of age (19.5% ± 2.7% and 11.5% ± 3.2%, respectively) compared with older children and adults (8.1% ± 1.4% and 7.8% ± 1.5%, respectively), and this correlates to levels of alpha-1 acid glycoproteins in the blood.[41,42]

Fentanyl pharmacokinetics differ among newborn infants, children, and adults. The total body clearance of fentanyl is greater in infants 3 to 12 months of age than in children older than 1 year of age or adults (18.1 ± 1.4, 11.5 ± 4.2, and 10.0 ± 1.7 mL/kg/min, respectively), and the half-life of elimination is longer (233 ± 137, 244 ± 79, and 129 ± 42 min, respectively).[41,42] The prolonged elimination half-life of fentanyl from plasma has important clinical implications. Repeated doses lead to accumulation of fentanyl and resulting ventilatory depressant effects. Very large doses (0.05-0.10 mg/kg) may be expected to induce long-lasting respiratory depression because plasma fentanyl levels will not fall below the threshold level at which spontaneous ventilation occurs during the distribution phases.[43]

Robinson and Gregory[44] reported the first use of fentanyl, 30 to 50 mcg/kg, as the principal anesthetic in neonates undergoing ductus ligation surgery. Using heart rate and blood pressure responses as an index of adequate anesthesia, they demonstrated that the combination of fentanyl, oxygen, and pancuronium could provide anesthesia with minimal hemodynamic consequences, and these findings have been confirmed by several other investigators.[11,45] In all reported studies, both hypotension and bradycardia are rare as long as the infant is preloaded with a fluid bolus of a balanced salt solution (20 mL/kg) and a vagolytic agent (either pancuronium or atropine) is administered concomitantly. Furthermore, in newborn lambs, fentanyl does not significantly affect heart rate, blood pressure, cardiac output, or the regional distribution of blood flow to the major organs (eg, the brain and gastrointestinal tract) when it was administered in doses ranging between 30 and 3000 mcg/kg.[46] However, the safety of "fentanyl" anesthesia may be diminished when other anesthetics, such as nitrous oxide, barbiturates, or benzodiazepines are administered concomitantly.[47,48]

Yaster[45] extended the observations of Robinson and Gregory[44] in a prospective study of premature and full-term infants younger than 7 days of age undergoing a variety of thoracic, abdominal, and genitourinary emergency operations. In Yaster's[45] study, fentanyl in doses of 10 to 12.5 mcg/kg produced insignificant hemodynamic changes and provided reliable anesthesia for at least 75 minutes. There are reasons for the discrepancies in fentanyl requirements in these studies. Whereas Robinson and Gregory[44] studied premature infants varying in age from 1 day to 6 weeks undergoing thoracic surgery, Yaster's[45] patients were younger (the majority were "newly born," ie, less than 24 hours old). Analgesic requirements reduced in the first few days of life, perhaps because endogenous opioids are released in response to birth or to fetal and neonatal distress. As mentioned, the blood–brain barrier is immature in the first few days of life, and this may allow more fentanyl to reach the μ-opioid receptors within the central nervous system, although this is more important for less lipid-soluble agonists such as morphine. Alternatively, the increased fraction of free, unbound fentanyl in newborns may allow more drug to penetrate into the brain. Additionally, fentanyl clearance increases markedly in the first weeks of life, probably as a result of increasing activity of the CYP450 system and increasing hepatic blood flow after closure of the ductus venosus. Thus, the increased fentanyl metabolism that occurs in older newborns may increase their anesthetic (fentanyl) requirements. Finally, many of the patients in Yaster's study underwent abdominal surgery or had significant abdominal pathology such as necrotizing enterocolitis (NEC). Fentanyl clearance as well as analgesic requirements may be significantly decreased in these situations, particularly if intra-abdominal pressure is increased. Increased intra-abdominal pressure (>15-20 mmHg) markedly reduces liver and splanchnic blood flow and has been documented to occur after closure of abdominal wall defects such as omphalocele or gastroschisis.[24,25] This decreased liver blood flow reduces fentanyl biotransformation and thereby anesthetic requirements. Thus fentanyl dose may depend on the neonate's postnatal age; on the type of surgery being performed; and on patient factors such as acidosis, hypoxia, and circulatory instability.

The use of fentanyl in newborns may result in the need for postoperative intubation and ventilation independent of the infant's medical or surgical condition. All opioids produce profound respiratory depression in newborns. A number of studies suggest that the respiratory depression and analgesia produced by μ-opioid agonists involve different receptor subtypes. These receptors change in number in an age-related fashion and can be blocked by naloxone. Zhang and Pasternak[49] and

Pasternak et al[50] showed that 14-day-old rats are 40 times more sensitive to morphine analgesia than 2-day-old rats and that morphine decreases the respiratory rate to a greater extent in the 2-day-old animals. Thus, newborns may be particularly sensitive to the respiratory depressant effects of the commonly administered opioids.

The need for early extubation and minimal residual respiratory depression has led to the increased use of remifentanil in newborn anesthesia practice.[51,52] Remifentanil is primarily metabolized by plasma esterases. The pharmacokinetics of remifentanil are characterized by small distribution volumes, rapid clearances, and low variability compared with other IV anesthetic drugs.[53,54] The drug has a rapid onset of action (half-time for equilibration between blood and the effect compartment, 1.3 min) and a short context-sensitive half-life (3-5 min). The latter property is attributable to hydrolytic metabolism of the compound by nonspecific tissue and plasma esterases. Virtually all (99.8%) of an administered remifentanil dose is eliminated during the “half-life (0.9 min) and $half-life (6.3 min). The pharmacokinetics of remifentanil suggest that it will reach nearly steady state within 10 minutes of starting an infusion, so changing its infusion rate will produce rapid changes in drug effect. The rapid metabolism and small Vd mean that remifentanil will not accumulate. Discontinuing the drug rapidly terminates its effects regardless of how long it was being administered.[43,55] Finally, the primary metabolite has little biologic activity, making it safe even in patients with renal disease. Collectively, these properties are especially advantageous for opioid administration in newborns.

MUSCLE RELAXANTS

The structural and functional development of the neuromuscular system is incomplete at birth.[56] In fact, newborns have decreased neuromuscular reserve compared with older children and adults. At a stimulation rate of 20 Hz, many neonates demonstrate tetanic fade, and premature infants demonstrate posttetanic exhaustion.[57,58] At a higher stimulation rate (50 Hz), all newborns demonstrate posttetanic exhaustion. The train-of-four ratio and the magnitude of posttetanic facilitation all increase with age. Based on these findings and on clinical criteria, it has been suggested that newborns are more “sensitive” to nondepolarizing muscle relaxants than older patients and should theoretically require less drug to produce neuromuscular blockade.[56]

However, this is counterbalanced by an increased ECF space and a larger apparent Vd.[17] Thus, a first dose of a paralytic agent may on a mg/kg basis have the same effect and duration of action in the newborn as it does in older children and adults. However, subsequent doses may have a prolonged duration of paralysis.

At appropriate doses, all of the nondepolarizing muscle relaxants are effective paralytics in newborns, and the choice of which to use is more often based on their duration, side effects, and elimination profiles. Because pancuronium is a potent vagolytic, it remains one of the most commonly used agents in newborns.[59] Unlike in adults, tachycardia is often a *desired* side effect because infants respond to a variety of stimuli, such as hypoxia, intubation, and fentanyl administration, with bradycardia. Because newborns' cardiac output is heart rate dependent, bradycardia can potentially be catastrophic. Occasionally, other relaxants (eg, cis-atracurium) are selected because end-organ pathology (liver or kidney) may interfere with drug elimination or because the onset or duration of paralysis is inappropriate for the surgery being performed.

Interestingly, newborns are relatively resistant to succinylcholine even though plasma cholinesterase levels are reduced after birth. IV doses of 1 to 2 mg/kg, rather than 0.5 mg/kg, are required for complete paralysis. IV succinylcholine produces myriad arrhythmias, including sinus bradycardia, sinus arrest, nodal rhythms, and ventricular ectopy, even with a first dose. Furthermore, several neonates have developed pulmonary edema and hemorrhage in the absence of upper airway obstruction after IV use of succinylcholine.[60] Other well-known complications of succinylcholine include malignant hyperthermia, hyperkalemia, myoglobinemia, and increased intraocular (?intracranial) pressure. Because of these effects, increasing numbers of pediatric anesthesiologists are discouraging the routine use of this drug. Nevertheless, succinylcholine “remains one of the most rapidly acting neuromuscular blocking agents available, and despite the problems associated with its use, there is no substitute for it when “full stomach” precautions are required or when laryngospasm occurs. Thus, the authors' practice is to “always have it; rarely use it.”

KETAMINE, GENERAL ANESTHETICS, SEDATIVES, AND THE DEVELOPING BRAIN

As pointed out in Chapter 25, most studies of anesthetic and analgetic drugs (in any age group) have been short-term evaluations, often tied to the perioperative interval only. However, 10 years of accruing data from animal studies suggest that almost all of the commonly used anesthetic and sedative agents used in general anesthesia can be neurotoxic and that young developing brains may be particularly vulnerable to such injury.[57] Furthermore, it is increasingly clear that many anesthetic and sedative agents are agonists at the gamma-aminobutyric acid_A (GABA_A) receptor and as antagonists at glutamic acid (glutamate) receptors such as the *N*-methyl-D-aspartate (NMDA) receptors.[58-65] When anesthetic or sedative drugs bind to these receptors in vulnerable periods in brain development, programmed cell death (apoptosis) may occur with potentially catastrophic consequences.

In brief, the GABA_A receptor is a ligand-gated ion channel that selectively conducts chloride ion through its pore, resulting in hyperpolarization of neurons.[66,67] This inhibits neurotransmission and diminishes the occurrence of action potentials. The active site of the GABA_A receptor is the binding site for GABA and several drugs such as bicuculline. The protein also contains a number of different allosteric binding sites that modulate the activity of the receptor indirectly and increase the efficiency of chloride conductance. These allosteric sites are the targets of various drugs, including the benzodiazepines, barbiturates, ethanol, neuroactive steroids, and the inhaled vapor general anesthetics, among others.[66-68] Mild inhibition of neuronal firing at the GABA_A receptor causes a reduction of anxiety or amnesia in patients, and more pronounced inhibition induces an anticonvulsant effect, sleep, and general anesthesia.

The NMDA receptor (NMDAR) is the predominant molecular device for controlling synaptic plasticity and memory function.[69-71] The NMDAR is a specific type of ionotropic glutamate receptor.[72,73] Activation of NMDA receptors results in the opening of an ion channel that is nonselective to cations. A unique property of the NMDA receptor is its voltage-dependent activation, a result of ion channel block by extracellular magnesium (Mg^{2+}) ions. This allows voltage-dependent flow of sodium (Na^+) and small amounts of calcium (Ca^{2+}) ions into the cell and potassium (K^+) out of the cell. A positive change in transmembrane potential will make it more likely that the ion channel in the NMDA receptor will open by expelling the Mg^{2+} ion. This allows more Ca^{2+} flux through NMDARs and is thought to play a critical role in synaptic plasticity, a cellular mechanism for learning and memory. The NMDAR is distinct in 2 ways: First, it is both ligand gated and voltage dependent; second, it requires coactivation by 2 excitatory ligands, glutamate and glycine.

NMDAR antagonists such as ketamine, phencyclidine (PCP), nitrous oxide, xenon, and ethanol have general anesthetic and analgesic properties.[67,69,74,75] In addition, some opioids, particularly methadone, are also NMDAR antagonists, and it is this property that makes methadone so effective in treating neuropathic pain. Of the NMDAR antagonists, ketamine is the most commonly used as a general anesthetic. It is a hallucinogen that produces an altered or “dissociative” level of consciousness. Ketamine has many salutary properties that make it an ideal anesthetic in patients with congenital heart disease, those who are hemodynamically unstable, and those who have asthma. It increases both systemic and pulmonary vascular resistance and is often used in newborns with known congenital heart disease and in newborns in whom the ductus arteriosus and the foramen ovale are still open.

Olney and colleagues have shown that even a brief exposure to NMDAR antagonists or $GABA_A$ receptor agonists during vulnerable developmental ages in rats can cause apoptotic neurodegeneration ("Olney lesions").[57,58,61,63,65,76-78] These studies in combination with a few epidemiologic studies in older children who were exposed to these agents as newborns and infants have fueled concern regarding the safety of general anesthesia in infants and young children.[79,80] Wilder and colleagues[79] performed a retrospective analysis based on the educational and medical records of all children who were born to mothers living in Olmsted County, Minnesota, from 1976 to 1982, and who remained in that community at age 5 years. They found that the risk of developing a learning disability increased with the number of exposures to anesthesia (greater than one exposure) before age 4 years. A single anesthetic exposure was not associated with increased risk. Furthermore, the longer the cumulative duration of anesthetic exposure, the greater the risk of learning disability. It is unclear if it is the anesthesia exposure that is the risk factor for the development of these learning disabilities or if multiple and prolonged anesthetic exposures are a marker of other comorbidities and causative factors. DiMaggio et al[81] retrospectively reviewed the New York State Medicaid program data from 1999 to 2002. They found that in children younger than age 3 years, there was an association between surgery and anesthesia for inguinal hernia and subsequent behavioral and developmental learning disorders in children. The extrapolation of the results from experimental animal studies combined with the newer epidemiologic studies in children has aroused concern regarding the safety of general anesthetics in children with developing brains. It is somewhat reassuring that the greatest risks for anesthetic-related neurodegeneration involve multiple anesthetic exposures,[82-86] the use of a combination of anesthetic drugs, high doses of specific drugs (higher than commonly used in clinical practice), and prolonged drug administration.[87]

Nonetheless, we are left with the dilemma: Are these and other drugs that we routinely use in newborns to provide anesthesia safe?[88] The animal studies showing deleterious neurologic effects of anesthetic drugs have been in the absence of surgery, but pain in newborn rats and young children has also been shown to cause neuroapoptosis and memory impairment. So, there may be serious consequences to developing brains when not providing analgesia and anesthesia for surgery as well. Further study in this area is needed and will likely influence future pediatric anesthesia practice.

LOCAL ANESTHETICS

All currently available local anesthetics work by blocking sodium ion flux through open, voltage-gated sodium channels and are of 2 classes: amino amides and amino esters.[89,90] The amino amides, lidocaine, bupivacaine, and ropivacaine, are metabolized in the liver by the CYP_{450} (CYP linked) isoenzymes. Details of local anesthetic pharmacology are provided in Chapter 45. These metabolic pathways are markedly diminished in function in the neonatal period and therefore clearance of these drugs will be greatly reduced.[91,92] As mentioned, these drugs are bound to plasma proteins, which are reduced in newborns. Thus, more unbound or free drug is available, and the potential for severe toxicity is increased. In contrast, the amino esters are metabolized by plasma esterases. These enzymes are also reduced in quantity and function in newborns, but the clearance of amino esters is much less impaired than that of amino amides.

MONITORING

Critically ill neonates undergoing emergency surgery require as much, if not more, monitoring than do critically ill adults because the margin of error is so small and because disaster can strike so quickly. Unfortunately, compromises are often made because of the technical difficulty in monitoring small children and because, after they are positioned and draped on the operating room (OR) table, observation, palpation, and even auscultation are often difficult, if not impossible. Meticulous attention to detail is absolutely necessary; no machine can replace a vigilant anesthesiologist who constantly evaluates analyzes, interprets, and acts on the patient's condition.

One of the simplest and most effective monitors in newborn anesthesia is the precordial or esophageal stethoscope. Stethoscopy provides beat-to-beat, breath-by-breath information on the patient's condition. For example, the first indication of cardiovascular deterioration in children may be a change in heart sounds, from brisk and close to muffled and distant. Loss of breath sounds may indicate a mechanical disconnection or an endobronchial intubation well before a mechanical alarm sounds. Despite its historical importance, this simple, effective, and inexpensive monitor is rapidly becoming as extinct as the slide rule and rotary dial telephone.

Only slightly less important than the precordial stethoscope is the pulse oximeter. This noninvasive, beat-to-beat monitor has revolutionized anesthesia monitoring and should be used not only in the OR but also in transport to and from the OR as well.[93] In neonates, the probe is preferentially placed to measure preductal oxygen saturation because in the presence of intracardiac shunting, it best reflects what the brain is "seeing." This is easily accomplished by placing the probe on the right hand, ear lobe, or buccal mucosa and is used to maintain an oxygen saturation between 90% and 95% (Pao_2 of 50-70 mm Hg). Higher oxygen saturations may produce retinopathy of the premature (ROP). Indeed, because of intracardiac shunting, many anesthesiologists use 2 pulse oximeters, one on the right hand and one on the lower extremity, to measure pre- and postductal flow. Preductal arterial oxygen saturation reflects coronary and cerebral oxygen saturation, and the cerebral oxygenation affects the eyes and is responsible for ROP. Nevertheless, in our zeal to protect the eyes, we must never compromise oxygen delivery to the neonate's brain!

The next most important monitor is blood pressure. Newborns, particularly premature newborns weighing less than 1.5 kg, may have normal systolic blood pressures of only 40 to 50 mm Hg. Blood pressure measurement and control become Herculean tasks. Indeed, this explains in part why many pediatric anesthesiologists prefer fentanyl-based anesthetics to inhalational agents when providing anesthesia for surgery in newborns. In most cases, blood pressure can be adequately measured with an appropriately sized blood pressure cuff and commonly available noninvasive automatic blood pressure devices. Occasionally, a Doppler ultrasonic transducer or a strategically placed oxygen saturation probe can help in blood pressure measurement. However, for most major operations, continuous intra-arterial monitoring is indicated for the safe conduct of anesthesia. Catheterization of preferably the radial artery is accomplished either percutaneously or by surgical access. The temporal arteries must be avoided for intra-arterial cannulation because catastrophic brain injury, presumably from embolization of clot and debris, has been associated with its use. Alternative catheterization sites include the dorsalis pedis, the posterior tibial, and the umbilical artery. The arterial catheter provides beat-to-beat monitoring and access to sample blood gases, hematocrit, and glucose, and it is an extremely sensitive guide of the intravascular volume status. Finally, meticulous attention to detail and technique is needed when flushing these catheters. We recommend high-pressure, low-volume tubing and after aspiration of blood for sampling flushing the tubing with 0.5 to 1 mL of saline to minimize the risk of embolization into the cerebral circulation.

Judging intravascular volume clinically is extremely difficult in neonates. During abdominal surgery (eg, NEC) third-space fluid losses may approach 100 to 200 mL/kg. Analysis of the arterial wave form from an indwelling intra-arterial catheter is one of the best methods of evaluating and detecting early intravascular volume losses (**Fig. 63-1**). One looks for either a change in the shape of the wave form (decreased area under the curve) or the development of respiratory variation in the wave form. During positive-pressure ventilation, decreased venous return causes a decease in the arterial wave form with each breath; this decrease is dramatically more evident when the intravascular volume has been depleted.

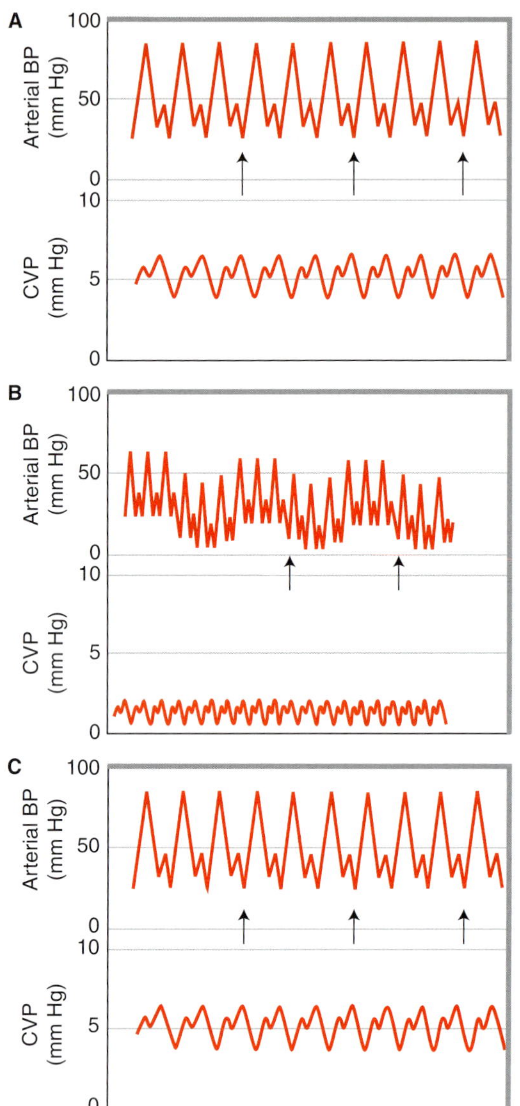

FIGURE 63-1. In normovolemia (**A**) arterial blood pressure (BP) and central venous pressures (CVP) are normal and there is little response to a positive pressure breath (*arrow*). In hypovolemia (**B**) arterial BP and CVP are reduced and a positive pressure breath (*arrow*) produces a pulsus paradoxus in the arterial wave form. Volume resuscitation (**C**) returns the tracing to normal.

In adults, the more commonly used monitors for measuring (or estimating) intravascular volume include either a central venous or a pulmonary artery catheter. Historically, central venous pressure (CVP) measurements in newborns have been considered both technically difficult and insensitive to volume status. Experiments done in the 1960s during exchange transfusions demonstrated little correlation between blood losses of as much as 20% of the estimated blood volume (EBV) and CVP as measured by umbilical central venous catheters.[94] Unfortunately, these experiments have never been repeated with central venous catheters placed in the internal or external jugular veins and pressure transduced with modern equipment. In our experience, measurement of the CVP is very useful, particularly in surgery involving major blood or third-space loss or shock or when intra-abdominal pressure is elevated.[24,25] Furthermore, because these are large-bore catheters securely inserted within the vascular tree, usually the internal jugular vein, they supply a reliable means of administering fluids and vasoactive drugs.

One of the mainstays in the assessment of volume status of the newborn is the measurement of urine output (or lack thereof). Bladder catheterization is easily accomplished using a 5-Fr feeding tube (not a balloon-tipped Foley catheter). The catheter is secured to the skin with tape and connected to a calibrated urinometer by low-volume tubing. Minimum acceptable urine outputs range between 0.5 and 1.0 mL/kg/h.[26,95] Unfortunately, in very small children, this small volume of urine may take hours to travel under the surgical drapes to the urinometer. Additionally, the drainage tubing is usually not easily accessible to the anesthesiologist, making identification of kinks and disconnects almost impossible. Because of this, measurement of urine output during surgery may be of marginal value.

Because neonatal anesthesia is virtually always performed with controlled mechanical ventilation, respiratory monitoring with capnography is essential. Despite the many technical problems involved in measuring end-tidal carbon dioxide concentrations through small uncuffed endotracheal tubes, it is a "standard of care" and is a mandatory monitor for the provision of safe anesthesia.[96,97]

Last, but not least, is temperature monitoring. All newborns are at extraordinarily high risk of becoming cold during transport to and from the OR and while in the OR. To minimize this risk, we routinely wrap children in plastic bags; use forced-air heating mattresses; increase the ambient temperature of the OR (usually above 90°F); and use warm IV fluids and heated, humidified respiratory gases.[98,99] Temperature is routinely monitored with either a rectal or a nasopharyngeal temperature probe. We strive to maintain core temperature at 36°C to avoid the consequences of hypothermia. These include hypoventilation or even apnea, relative anesthetic overdose (reduced MAC at lower temperatures), metabolic acidosis, norepinephrine secretion, and increased oxygen demand. Increased oxygen demand to maintain normal core temperature and increased norepinephrine secretion may cause pulmonary and peripheral vasoconstriction, right-to-left shunting, anaerobic metabolism, and increased acidosis and oxygen consumption, all of which may exacerbate preexisting cardiopulmonary insufficiency.

FLUIDS

Intraoperative IV fluid therapy provides infants with maintenance requirements of water, electrolytes, and glucose to replace preoperative deficits and ongoing intraoperative "third-space" and blood losses. Maintenance fluid requirements are calculated based on the assumption that 100 mL of water is required for every 100 calories consumed. The newborn's energy requirements are 100 calories/kg/24 h. Thus, fluid requirements are 100 mL/kg/24 h or approximately 4 mL/kg/h.[100] Although basal caloric requirements are significantly reduced under general anesthesia, we continue to provide maintenance fluid, usually with 5% to 10% (50-100 mg/mL) glucose, at a rate of 4 mL/kg/h delivered by an infusion pump.

Because the majority of newborns presenting for emergency surgery are in neonatal intensive care units (NICUs) and are receiving IV fluids before surgery, the logical presumption is that preoperative deficits are nonexistent. Unfortunately, this is rarely true. Most newborns are fluid restricted in the NICU despite the presence of a surgical emergency and third-space fluid losses. Furthermore, infants are rarely given solutions containing electrolytes even though the newborn's kidney cannot tolerate a water load and will waste sodium even when water overloaded. Indeed, the maximum urine osmolality achievable by the neonatal kidney is only 800 mOsm/L. When combined with anesthetic drugs, unsuspected hypovolemia can be catastrophic. Thus, before the induction of general anesthesia in neonates requiring emergency surgery, we routinely provide a fluid bolus of 20 mL/kg of Ringer lactate solution in an attempt to ensure an adequate preload. An additional 10 to 20 mL/kg may be necessary if there is evidence of hemodynamic instability (eg, tachycardia, hypotension).

Surgical trauma and manipulation or inflammation of the bowel results in internal sequestration of functional ECFs and is often referred to as "third-space" losses. The fluid and salt within the third space acts as sequestered fluid and is nonfunctional in terms of the duties of the ECF. Replenishment of this interstitial water and salt loss with balanced salt solutions ("isotonic crystalloid solutions"), such as Ringer lactate or normal saline, is essential. The magnitude of the third-space loss depends on the site and extent of injury. Abdominal surgery, particularly if there is extensive bowel pathology or manipulation, may require third-space replacement therapy of 10 to 20 (or more) mL/kg/h, whereas, peripheral or thoracic surgery may require only 3 to 5 mL/kg/h.

All blood loss must be replaced with a balanced salt solutions, 5% albumin, or blood. Normally, infants are born with high hematocrits (>50%), which decrease to 30% over the first 3 months of life. Additionally, these red blood cells (RBCs) are made primarily of hemoglobin F (HbF), which has a greater affinity for oxygen than adult hemoglobin (HbA). Indeed, the partial pressure at which 50% of hemoglobin is saturated (P_{50}) is 19 for HbF versus 27 for HbA. Because newborns have limited stores of iron and limited ability to replace lost RBCs, the hematocrit (Hct) should not be allowed to fall below 35% during surgery. The allowable blood loss before transfusing can be estimated at 20 mL/kg or can be calculated by the following formula:

$$\text{Weight (kg)} \times \text{EBV} \times (\text{Hct start} - \text{Hct}_{0.35})/\text{Hct average Hct}_{\text{average}} = (\text{Hct}_{\text{start}} + \text{Hct}_{0.35})/2$$

As an example, assume a 3-kg, full-term infant with a 45% (0.45) starting hematocrit is undergoing surgery. The EBV would be 90 mL/kg (see Table 63-1), or 270 mL, and we would allow a blood loss to a hematocrit of 35% (0.35). Because the hematocrit of the blood lost is not constant, we use an average to estimate it. In this example, it would be 40% (45 + 35 = 80/2 = 40). Thus, the allowable blood loss is 67.5 mL (3 × 90 × 0.1/0.4). Ideally, blood would be replaced with fresh whole blood because it contains platelets and clotting factors as well as RBCs. Unfortunately, this is rarely, if ever, available. Packed (PRBCs) are usually used instead. This blood product typically has a hematocrit of 60% to 70%; high potassium concentration; and little, if any, of factors V and VIII. Large blood losses and massive RBC cell transfusion (2-3 times the EBV) often produce a secondary coagulopathy and hyperkalemia.[97] This bleeding is often caused by either dilutional or consumptive thrombocytopenia. Platelets can be transfused based on the following formula:

$$\text{Platelet increment/mm}^3 = 30{,}000 \times (\text{number of units})/\text{EBV (L)}$$

Fresh-frozen plasma is rarely necessary and should be given only when a legitimate indication exists, such as a documented factor deficiency or intraoperative bleeding with massive blood transfusion. All blood products, including fresh-frozen plasma, may be contaminated with viruses. Additionally, newborns should be considered immune compromised hosts. Therefore, one should consider irradiating any blood product that may contain white blood cells before transfusion because of the possibility of producing a graft-versus-host reaction. Finally, all banked blood (especially older blood) contains significant amounts of potassium.[101] Life-threatening hyperkalemia has occurred after large-volume blood transfusions in newborns and may be prevented with washed RBCs or fresh whole blood.[102]

AIRWAY

Understanding the anatomic differences among infants, children, and adults is crucial for successful airway management in normal children and children with congenital anomalies (**Fig. 63-2**). Infants younger than 3 to 6 months of age are obligate nose breathers. Anatomic (eg, choanal atresia), physical (eg, nasogastric tube), or infectious obstruction of the nasopharynx rapidly causes respiratory distress or failure. The abundant and friable lymphoidal tissue of the nasopharynx also precludes the routine placement of nasopharyngeal airways in this age group when treating upper airway obstruction.

The tongue is relatively large in relation to the mandible in children younger than 2 years of age, making visualization of the larynx difficult. Indeed, the tongue most commonly obstructs the upper airway when consciousness is lost after the induction of anesthesia. The larynx is also difficult to visualize because it is anterior and more cephalad in the newborn. It is located at C2-C3 vertebrae in infants and C4-C5 in adults. The vocal cords are also different in their appearance. In infants, they are 40% ligament and 60% arytenoid cartilage. These ratios are reversed in adults.

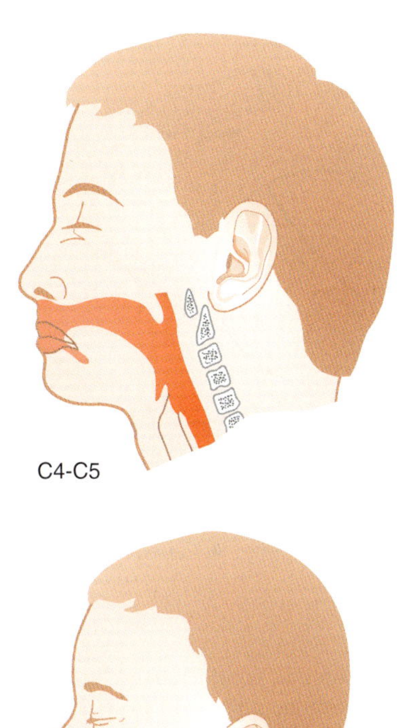

FIGURE 63-2. Comparative anatomy of the adult and infant airways.

In infants, the epiglottis is omega-shaped floppy, and has a 45-degree angle of entry into the pharyngeal wall. Visualization of the larynx requires lifting the epiglottis directly with an appropriately sized straight laryngoscope blade ("0" or "1" Miller blade). In contrast, in adults, the epiglottis is stiff, flat, and parallel to the tracheal wall. Visualization of the larynx can be made indirectly by placing the laryngoscope blade in the vallecula (**Fig. 63-3**). The trachea is different as well. The narrowest part of the airway in children younger than 8 to 10 years of age is the cricoid ring. Uncuffed endotracheal tubes, usually 2.5 to 3.5 mm in diameter, are used in neonates to prevent damage to the mucosa underlying this structure. Furthermore, the trachea in infants may be only 4 to 5 cm in total length. This makes inadvertent endobronchial intubation extremely likely even by very experienced practitioners. To minimize this risk, we use the "1-2-3 . . . 7-8-9" rule to assist in correct endotracheal tube positioning. The "1-2-3" refers to the patient's weight in kilograms, and the "7-8-9" refers to the position of the endotracheal tube in centimeters at the patient's lip. An alternative estimation is: "6 + weight in kg = Position of the endotracheal tube in centimeters at the patient's lip." Thus, a 1-kg infant would have the tip of the endotracheal tube taped at the 7-cm mark at the lip. Proper positioning of the endotracheal tube can be made by auscultation (return of breath sounds after a deliberate right main stem intubation), palpation of the tip of the endotracheal tube in the sternal notch, inspection of the distal line marker at the level of the vocal cords, and by chest radiography. After being positioned, the endotracheal tube must be secured in place with adhesive tape in a way that minimizes the likelihood of dislodgement or accidental extubation. The "fishmouth" technique is the authors' preferred technique (**Fig. 63-4**).

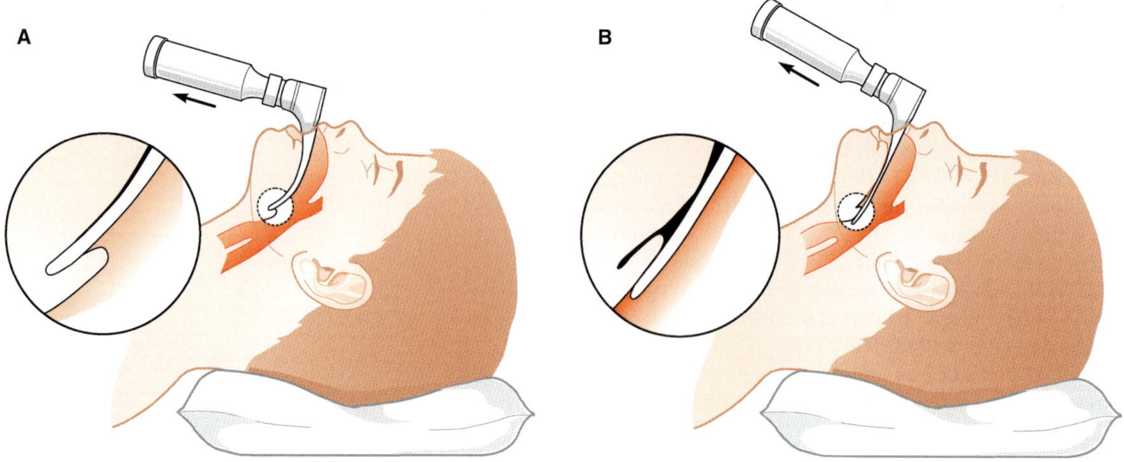

FIGURE 63-3. Laryngoscope blades. **A.** Curved (Macintosh) blade inserted in the vallecula only. **B.** Straight (Miller) blade inserted either under the epiglottis or in the vallecula.

Because of the anatomic considerations listed above and because newborns rapidly desaturate after only 15 to 20 seconds of apnea or breath holding, in the past, many anesthesiologists believed it was safer to intubate newborns' tracheas "awake." This is no longer true. Increasing evidence indicates that awake intubation may cause intraventricular hemorrhage in fragile, premature newborns.[103,104] Furthermore, awake intubations are technically more difficult to accomplish and often result in trauma to the vocal cords, hemorrhage, bradycardia, and desaturation secondary to breath holding. The authors prefer to use a "rapid sequence" induction in infants requiring "full stomach" precautions, that is, infants who are at risk of aspirating their gastric contents (eg, intestinal obstruction, NEC) and who on physical examination have a normal airway. After fluid volume resuscitation (10-40 mL/kg of Ringer lactate), preoxygenation, and pretreatment with atropine (0.15 mg), gentle cricoid pressure is applied to occlude the esophagus.[105,106] If cricoid pressure is applied too vigorously, the position of the larynx may be distorted or the trachea itself occluded. In hemodynamically stable patients, a rapid-sequence IV induction can be accomplished by bolus administration of 4 to 7 mg/kg of thiopental, 2 to 3 mg/kg of propofol, 2 to 4 mg/kg of ketamine, or 12.5 mcg/kg of fentanyl immediately followed by 2 mg/kg of succinylcholine or 0.9 to 1.2 mg/kg of rocuronium.[107,108] Newborns not requiring full-stomach precautions are in the minority (eg, myelomeningocele or bladder exstrophy), and in these patients, anesthesia can be induced by inhalational agents delivered by mask or IV without cricoid pressure.

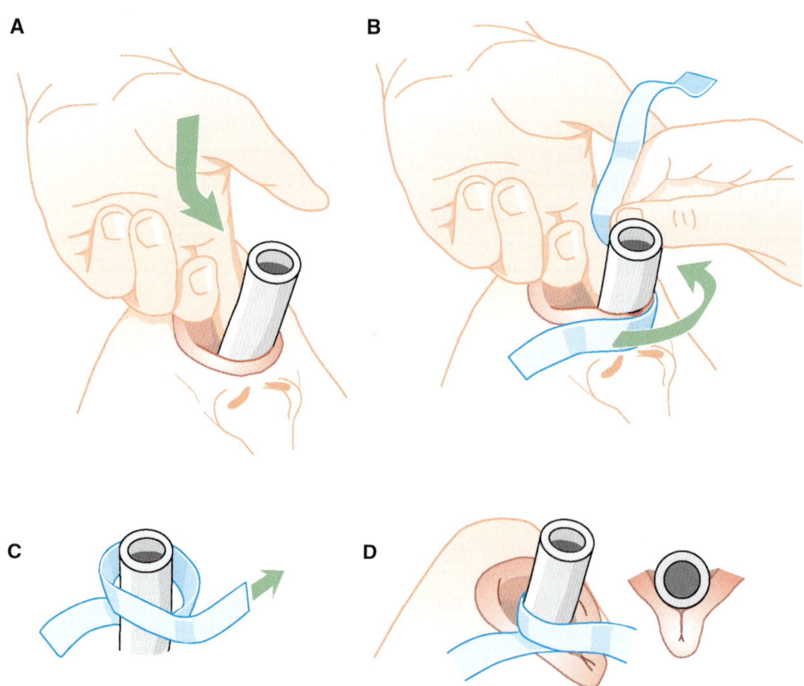

FIGURE 63-4. Using 1/2-inch adhesive tape, the endotracheal tube is secured with the "fishmouth technique." Starting at **A** zygoma, the tape is pulled (**B**), wrapped around the endotracheal tube (**C**), and then pulled to the opposite zygoma (**D**).

SURGICAL EMERGENCIES IN NEWBORNS

The spectrum of surgical emergencies that may occur in the first few weeks of life is extensive; the following discussion focuses on the most common ones, but the basic principles provided can be applied to conditions that are not specifically discussed.

CONGENITAL DIAPHRAGMATIC HERNIA

One of he most challenging of all neonatal surgical emergencies, this malformation involves herniation of the abdominal viscera into the thorax; it has a high (20%-50%) mortality rate regardless of the method of treatment.[109-111] Even early prenatal ultrasound diagnosis and attempts at in utero, fetal surgical correction, has done little, if anything, to affect outcome. The incidence of this devastating problem, which has significant short- and long-term morbidity, is reported to be 1 in 2000 to 5000 live births.[111,112]

In its most common presentation, the abdominal viscera, including the small bowel and colon, liver, and occasionally the kidneys, herniates into the left hemithorax during the first or second trimester of affected pregnancies and interferes with the development of both the lung parenchyma and its blood supply. Infants born with this anomaly present with the classic triad of dyspnea, cyanosis, and apparent dextrocardia. Physical examination reveals a scaphoid abdomen, bowel sounds in the chest, distant or displaced heart sounds, and absent breath sounds in the affected chest. Chest radiography demonstrates loops of gas-filled bowel or a gastric tube in the affected chest; mediastinal shift; absent lung markings in the affected chest; and most ominously, a contralateral pneumothorax. Pneumothorax is an iatrogenic complication that usually occurs as a result of vigorous attempts at ventilation, oxygenation, or resuscitation. The major differential diagnosis is a cystic adenomatoid malformation of the lung or congenital lobar emphysema. Approximately 20% of patients with congenital diaphragmatic hernia have associated congenital heart disease.

Surgical decompression of the herniated abdominal viscera (which may consist of midgut, stomach, colon, kidney, or liver) from the affected hemithorax and repair of the diaphragmatic defect, although essential in the management of this malformation, does not determine ultimate survival. Rather, outcome depends on the pulmonary vasculature and whether it will respond in an exaggerated, hyperreactive fashion to the stimuli that vasoconstrict and elevate pulmonary artery pressure.[113,114] Histologic studies of the lungs of children born with this anomaly reveal decreased number and size of the bronchi, lung saccules, and alveoli and abnormalities of the pulmonary vascular bed. The numbers of pulmonary blood vessels are reduced, and the arterial muscularis and media are hypertrophied. Hyperactive pulmonary arterial vasoconstriction caused by hypoxia, hypercarbia, acidosis, pain, or positive-pressure ventilation can set in motion a catastrophic cycle of events in which desaturated blood returning to the lung is preferentially shunted across the still patent ductus arteriosus and atrial septum into the systemic circulation. This "right-to-left" shunting of blood across the ductus and atrial septum is a return of the circulation to the pattern that existed in utero and is referred to as persistent fetal circulation (PFC) or persistent pulmonary hypertension of the newborn (PPHN). The goal of anesthetic management is to prevent this catastrophic cascade from occurring by maximizing arterial oxygenation and preventing pain and metabolic or respiratory acidosis.

The most severely affected infants require immediate intubation and decompression of the stomach as soon as the diagnosis is suspected. This usually takes place in the delivery room or in the NICU before surgery. Medical management is directed at improving oxygenation and increasing pulmonary blood flow. This may be accomplished by the judicious use of muscle relaxants, analgesics, usually fentanyl (1-10 mcg/kg as an initial bolus followed by a continuous infusion of 3-10 mcg/kg/h), hyperventilation using rapid rates (> 100 breaths/min) and low inflating pressures, preventing hypothermia, and correction of acidosis with IV bicarbonate therapy. Interestingly, this is also the basis of intraoperative anesthetic management. Nevertheless, aggressive proactive management may be harmful; barotrauma and volume trauma from too vigorous ventilation may induce alveolar and capillary damage and induce a catastrophic inflammatory cascade. Inhalational anesthetic agents are mostly avoided because of their hypotensive and cardiac depressant effects, and nitrous oxide is contraindicated because it can diffuse into the bowel and further compromise lung function. The importance of inadequate cardiac output in PFC should not be overlooked. Decreased cardiac output leads to decreased pulmonary perfusion and further hypoxemia. Blood returning to the heart from poorly perfused organs arrives with a lower oxygen content that potentiates the hypoxemia caused by right-to-left shunting.

Bohn et al[115] advocated the avoidance of the "mad dash" to the OR and recommend instead a 24- to 48-hour period of stabilization.[116] Furthermore, they contend that infants who do not respond to this therapy will fail to survive with surgery or any other therapy, including extracorporeal membrane oxygenation (ECMO). Bohn et al[117] also suggested a nomogram to predict the extent of pulmonary hypoplasia present in these infants and their chance of survival. They used the preoperative $Paco_2$ and correlated it and an index of ventilation that is determined by the mean airway pressure times the respiratory rate. If the $Paco_2$ could be reduced to less than 40 mm Hg and the ventilatory index was less than 1000, survival was almost universal. On the other hand, if $Paco_2$ and the ventilatory index were greater than 40 mm Hg and 1000, respectively, death was virtually inevitable. Interestingly, these latter infants were found at autopsy to have less than 10% of the normal number of alveoli bilaterally.

Others have approached newborns with congenital diaphragmatic hernia with a different perioperative management strategy.[118] They work to stabilize these newborns preoperatively and bring them through their period of PPHN with a strategy of "gentle ventilation." Using low peak inflating pressures and permissive hypercapnia, they are careful to avoid iatrogenic damage from barotrauma to the already hypoplastic lungs of these newborns. After a period of stabilization, during which pulmonary arterial pressure falls, the patient is electively taken to the OR for surgical repair.

Blood loss is minimal during the surgical repair of this problem, and third-space losses can be assumed to average 8 to 10 mL/kg/h. Aside from routine monitoring, these patients require an intravascular arterial and central venous catheter for continuous blood pressure monitoring and for blood gas, hemoglobin, and blood chemistry sampling. Central venous access is obtained either via an umbilical vein or from the jugular or subclavian veins. If the latter approach is attempted, it is essential to avoid a pneumo- or hemothorax in the normal lung. A precordial stethoscope placed in the unaffected right axilla may help alert the anesthesiologist to one of the most feared intraoperative catastrophes, namely, the development of a contralateral pneumothorax. This is heralded by sudden hypoxia, hypotension, or both. Placement of a chest tube when this occurs may be lifesaving. In fact, some authors have suggested the insertion of a prophylactic chest tube on the contralateral side because this complication is so catastrophic.

Vasodilator therapy has also been advocated for perioperative control of the increased pulmonary artery pressures. IV agents suggested include isoproterenol, nitroglycerin, tolazoline, adenosine, and adenosine triphosphate. These are rarely effective because the pulmonary vasodilation produced is matched by an equal decrease in systemic vascular resistance. These have been largely replaced by inhaled nitric oxide (NO).[119-121] NO diffuses across alveolar capillary membranes and stimulates cyclic guanylate cyclase, which increases cyclic GMP (cGMP). cGMP is a potent dilator of vascular smooth muscle. Because NO is rapidly metabolized by RBCs, it has a potent local effect and should preferentially dilate only the pulmonary vascular musculature. NO can be used anytime during the perioperative or intraoperative period as needed. Finally, the anesthesiologist should anticipate the possibility of a cardiac arrest during this operation, and vasopressors, including dopamine (4-10 mcg/kg/min) and epinephrine (0.1-1.0 mcg/kg/min) should always be available for emergency intraoperative administration.

The most recent and important innovation in the treatment of infants with congenital diaphragmatic hernia is the perioperative use of ECMO.[122,123] Infants who either would not survive by Bohn's criteria or who develop a PFC pattern after a "honeymoon" period may be placed on ECMO to allow the infant's lungs time to develop and restructure. Unfortunately, decisions pathways about when to initiate ECMO therapy (either before or after surgery), when to operate if an infant is on ECMO, and when to withdraw ECMO support are not well defined; they remain parochial decisions that may differ even among physicians within the same institution.

OMPHALOCELE OR GASTROSCHISIS

Abdominal wall defects are rare and although at first glance appear to be similar, they are in fact quite different. An omphalocele is a central, midline defect and is always associated with other congenital anomalies. It occurs because of failure of the gut to return to the abdominal cavity at the 10th week of gestation. The herniated bowel is covered by the amnion, which protects it from fluid loss; infection; and a chemical, amniotic fluid burn. The apex of the herniated sac is the umbilical cord. A gastroschisis, on the other hand, is not a midline defect and is therefore rarely associated with other defects. It results from an intrauterine vascular accident that results in the interruption of the abdominal wall and musculature. The herniated bowel is not covered by any membrane, is "burned" by the amniotic fluid, and is covered by an inflammatory coating or peel. It is subject to tremendous postnatal evaporative fluid losses as well as infection. In gastroschisis, the umbilical cord is found to the side of the herniated bowel.

The optimal method for operative management of infants with congenital abdominal wall defects remains controversial. Two options exist, either primary fascial closure with or without intra- and postoperative muscle paralysis or a staged repair using either a silicone elastomer silo or a primary skin closure. Primary fascial closure of omphalocele or gastroschisis carries the risk of placing the abdominal contents under pressure, which may produce a reduction in cardiac output, hypotension, bowel ischemia, venous stasis, and postoperative respiratory and renal failure.[24,25,124] When primary fascial closure cannot be achieved, either because of the large size of the defect or because it critically compromises respiratory or cardiovascular function, the alternative approach is a staged repair using either a silicone elastomer silo or a skin closure with secondary fascial closure. When using the silo, the defect is reduced over several days until a stable infant with a small defect can be taken to the OR for final repair. The staged silicone elastomer repair carries an increased risk of infection.

Traditional criteria for deciding on which course to choose have been based on the size of the defect; the presence of associated congenital anomalies; or clinical observations of the infant's respiratory rate, pulmonary compliance, blood pressure, skin color, and peripheral perfusion during fascial approximation. Unfortunately, these clinical observations may not be reliable, particularly in paralyzed, anesthetized infants.

Anesthetic Management Infants are transported to the OR by placing the exposed bowel in a bag designed for this purpose. It helps maintain normothermia and reduces evaporative fluid losses. Patients are fluid resuscitated with a balanced salt solution; preoxygenated; anesthetized with fentanyl (10-12.5 mcg/kg), pancuronium, and oxygen; and intubated. In addition to routine monitoring, we routinely place catheters in the right radial artery, an internal jugular vein, and in the stomach. An oral or nasal gastric tube both decompresses the abdomen and allows measurement of intragastric pressure by fluid filling the tube. Yaster et al[24,25] suggested that successful management of omphalocele or gastroschisis can be successfully and reliably determined by the intraoperative measurement of intragastric and CVPs (**Fig. 63-5**). In this treatment algorithm, primary repair is always attempted. However, if the intragastric pressure rises above 20 mm Hg or the CVP increases by 4 mm Hg or more after closure of the abdominal fascia, the primary

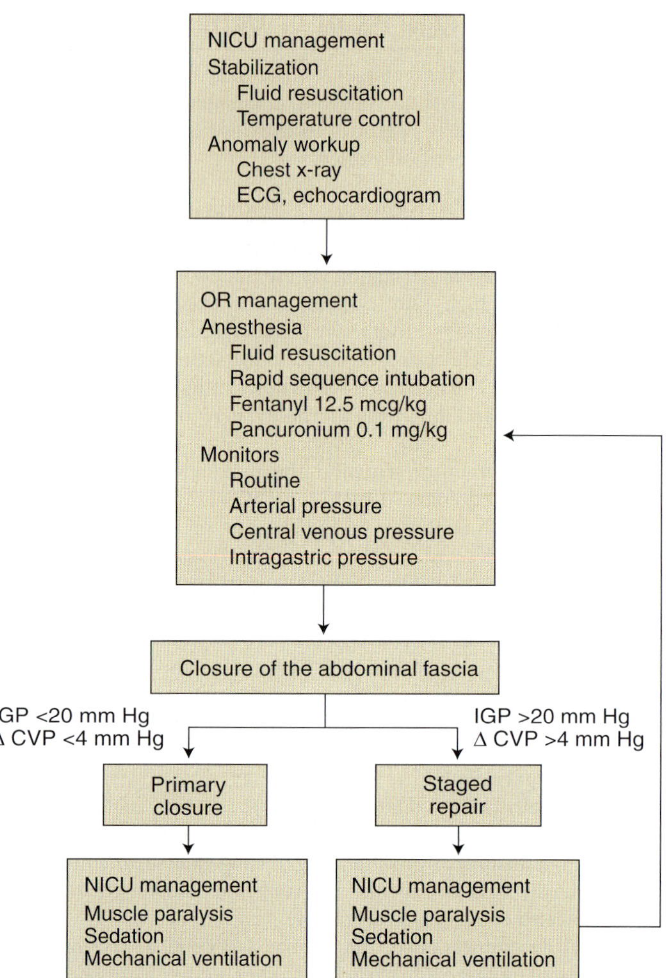

FIGURE 63-5. An algorithm for the intra- and postoperative management of children with congenital abdominal wall defects. Note that one measures intragastric pressures and changes in central venous pressure (CVP). ECG, electrocardiography; IGP, intragastric pressure; NICU, neonatal intensive care unit; OR, operating room.

repair is abandoned and a staged repair with a silicone elastomer chimney is performed. This algorithm avoids the consequences of acutely elevating intra-abdominal pressure. After surgery, the patient is taken to the NICU intubated and placed on controlled mechanical ventilation. Infants treated with a staged repair have their chimneys gradually reduced over 5 to 10 days. Central venous and intragastric pressure can be used to guide this therapy as well.

Newborn infants with abdominal wall defects have significantly increased fluid requirements because of the increase in insensible losses that occur when eviscerated bowel is exposed to the environment. Additionally, they have enormous "third-space" losses because of the traumatized, inflamed bowel and adynamic ileus that develops perioperatively. Fluid requirements are even greater in gastroschisis patients because the herniated viscera lack a protective covering, resulting in a chemical burn preoperatively.

INTESTINAL OBSTRUCTION, NECROTIZING ENTEROCOLITIS, AND PYLORIC STENOSIS

Intestinal obstruction is among the most common surgical emergencies encountered in newborns and is characterized by feeding intolerance, bilious or projectile vomiting, and abdominal distension. Common sites of obstruction include the pylorus; duodenum; jejunum–ileum, particularly the terminal ileum; and the anus. NEC, on the other hand, is caused by a bacterial invasion of previously injured or ischemic bowel wall.[125-127]

It is characterized by intestinal obstruction, gangrene, perforation, intramural air ("pneumatosis intestinalis"), and peritonitis. Patients are usually premature and are often septic, hypotensive, thrombocytopenic, and in respiratory failure. Metabolic and respiratory acidosis and electrolyte disturbances are also common. Although the initial management is nonoperative and supportive (eg, decompression, antibiotics, correction of hematologic abnormalities), evidence of intestinal gangrene (eg, positive results of paracentesis), pneumoperitoneum, and clinical deterioration results in the need for emergency exploratory laparotomy.

Duodenal obstruction typically presents within the first hours of life and is extremely common in children with trisomy 21 (Down syndrome). An abdominal radiograph will show the classic "double bubble" sign or a dilated, air-filled stomach and proximal duodenum. Because these children present so early in life, usually within the first 12 hours, they are rarely dehydrated or hypochloremic. Small and large bowel obstructions typically present later, usually 2 to 7 days after birth, and are often associated with hemodynamic compromise and metabolic disturbances. Jejunal or ileal atresias are thought to be caused by intrauterine vascular accidents. Meconium ileus is an obstruction of the small bowel caused by inspissated, abnormal meconium and is pathognomic of cystic fibrosis. At the time of presentation, these infants do not have the lung disease associated with this devastating disease. Malrotations of the bowel also present with obstruction and are very common in patients with congenital diaphragmatic hernia and omphalocele or gastroschisis. Infants with Hirschsprung disease have a functional distal obstruction caused by a lack of ganglia in the rectum and distal colon. Imperforate anus, which should be readily obvious in the delivery room, requires special attention because of the many anomalies associated with it. At one time called the VATER syndrome for vertebral, anal, tracheoesophageal fistula (TEF), esophageal atresia (see below), and renal anomalies, this syndrome also has a 20% incidence of significant congenital heart disease. Patients diagnosed with it should have an echocardiogram obtained before surgery.

Finally, despite being a congenital defect, pyloric stenosis usually does not present until 2 to 6 weeks of age. This is one of the most common surgical emergencies in newborns. Infants with pyloric stenosis have prolonged, repeated projectile nonbilious vomiting that results in a hypochloremic, hypokalemic metabolic alkalosis and profound dehydration. Interestingly, one would expect that the body's response to this alkalosis would be to eliminate bicarbonate in the urine. However, the sodium losses in pyloric stenosis are so great and the dehydration so profound that hydrogen ion is wasted in the urine in place of sodium with a resultant "paradoxical aciduria." Although it is considered to be an urgent surgical procedure, pyloric stenosis never requires immediate emergency surgical correction. Rather, patients require fluid resuscitation, restoration of an effective circulating volume, and correction of metabolic derangements. Only when this is done should surgery and anesthesia be performed. An easy way to assess successful resuscitation is to measure urine pH. When the urine pH is no longer acidotic (pH >6), it is usually safe to proceed with anesthesia and surgery.

Regardless of the underlying pathology, the major anesthetic challenge with this entire group of surgical patients is maintaining an adequate circulating blood volume and preventing the pulmonary aspiration of gastric contents. Virtually all newborns presenting for emergency abdominal surgery are intravascularly depleted secondary to the enormous ongoing third-space losses. Sepsis, bowel manipulation, peritonitis, the use of contrast agents, and the release of vasoactive peptides significantly deplete the circulating blood volume and ECF space of water and electrolytes. In the presence of NEC, third-space fluid replacement therapy in the perioperative period may exceed 100 to 200 mL/kg/h. Fresh-frozen plasma, platelets, and PRBCs are often needed and should be used early in surgery in response to clinical and laboratory evidence of coagulopathy. Additionally, critically ill, septic patients may not be able to tolerate these enormous fluid shifts, and 4 to 10 mcg/kg/min of dopamine should be infused to help maintain blood pressure and blood flow. Both arterial and CVP monitors are required to monitor intravascular volume in these situations.

All newborns presenting for emergency abdominal surgery may aspirate their abdominal contents at the induction of anesthesia. Therefore, methods that minimize these risks, such as an awake intubation or a rapid sequence induction with cricoid pressure, must be used. We prefer to maintain anesthesia with the fentanyl, pancuronium, and oxygen technique for this group of patients. Potent inhalational anesthetics are often poorly tolerated in this group of infants. Nitrous oxide is almost never used in these patients because it will further distend the bowel and complicate intestinal perfusion and fascial closure.

ESOPHAGEAL ATRESIA AND TRACHEOESOPHAGEAL FISTULA

Ninety percent of infants born with a TEF have a blind esophageal pouch and a fistula connecting the distal esophagus and the distal trachea, usually within 1 to 2 cm of the carina (**Fig. 63-6**).[128,129] About 30% to 50% of these infants have the associated anomalies of the VATER syndrome (see above). The most common associated defect is cardiac and necessitates an echocardiogram before surgery.[130] Often suspected prenatally by polyhydramnios, infants present with excessive salivation ("mucousy mouth"), choking, coughing, aspiration pneumonia, and cyanosis. Attempts at feeding are met with explosive vomiting,

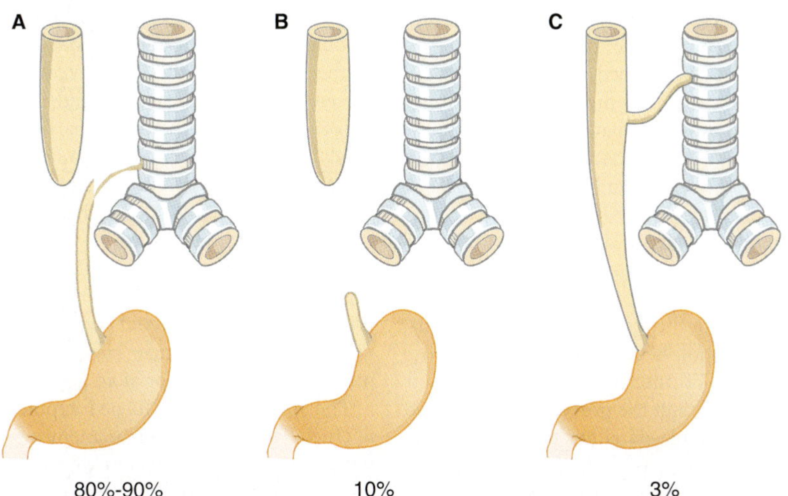

FIGURE 63-6. Three most common types of esophageal atresia and tracheoesophageal fistula (TEF). **A.** Proximal atresia and distal TEF account for 80%-90% of cases. **B.** Pure esophageal atresia with no TEF accounts for 10% of cases. **C.** H-type TEF accounts for 3% of cases.

and it is impossible to pass an oral (nasal) gastric tube. Indeed, a chest radiograph of a coiled oral gastric tube in the cervical esophageal pouch is diagnostic of TEF. Because of the potential for aspiration, contrast media should not be instilled to confirm this diagnosis.

The tracheal to distal esophageal fistula aerates the gastrointestinal tract and allows for regurgitation of gastric juice up the fistula into the lung. Thus, pulmonary aspiration occurs by 2 methods. The first involves aspiration of saliva or attempted feedings from the blind esophageal pouch and the second by gastric juice contamination via the fistula tract. If significant aspiration pneumonia occurs, definitive corrective surgery is deferred, and a decompressing gastrostomy is placed under local or caudal anesthesia.[131]

As soon as the diagnosis is confirmed, the child is placed in a head-up position, and the upper pouch is decompressed with a large-bore sump (Replogle) tube. After the diagnostic workup the child is transported to the OR for corrective repair, which has historically been performed through a right-sided thoracotomy. Increasingly, thoracoscopic surgical repair is being performed with excellent results.[132,133] Routine monitors are placed. The authors highly recommend the use of a strategically placed precordial stethoscope during this surgical repair. The precordial stethoscope is placed in the left axilla and carefully secured in place with both a "double-stick" and clear plastic adhesive dressing. This immediately alerts the anesthesiologist to a change in the endotracheal tube position from the juxtacarinal position to the right mainstem bronchus. Adequate IV access and a radial artery catheterization complete the preinduction preparation.

Immediately before intubation, the infant is given 0.15 mg IV of atropine, and the esophageal pouch is suctioned. Then with the infant in a semi-sitting position, the trachea is intubated while the patient is awake. This allows the appropriate positioning of the endotracheal tube without positive-pressure ventilation, which can cause gastric distension through the fistula. Then, in the classic technique, with the infant spontaneously breathing sevoflurane, the endotracheal tube is positioned below the fistula but above the carina by deliberately intubating the right mainstem bronchus and then slowly pulling back the tube until breath sounds are heard in the left axilla and not in the stomach. Isolation of the fistula is possible because in most cases, the fistula is approximately 0.5 to 1.0 cm above the carina on the posterior surface of the trachea. If the endotracheal tube has a side ("Murphy eye") hole, it should be turned to the left, opposite to its normal orientation, to maximize left lung ventilation. Even if the endotracheal tube does not have a side hole, it is helpful to turn the bevel of the tube 180 degrees, so that the curve of the tube faces forward. This will reduce ventilation into the fistula and stomach. After being positioned, the endotracheal tube is secured with the "fishmouth" technique to avoid displacement of the endotracheal tube down the right main stem bronchus or, more ominously, into the fistula tract itself (see Fig. 63-4). Indeed, this is why the precordial stethoscope is so securely placed in the left axilla.

After the endotracheal tube has been positioned, anesthetic management is based on the presence or absence of a decompressive gastrostomy and by the preferential flow of gases down the path of least resistance, namely through the fistula tract into the stomach. Positive-pressure ventilation may allow oxygen and other gasses to bypass the lungs and acutely dilate the stomach. This interferes with ventilation and venous return and can lead to cardiopulmonary arrest and gastric rupture; if this occurs, an emergency decompressive gastrostomy may be lifesaving. Unfortunately, the insertion of a gastrostomy may substitute one problem for another. Airflow resistance through the fistula–stomach–gastrostomy may be so low that ventilation of the lungs becomes impossible. The gastrostomy may need to be intermittently clamped and unclamped or left partially clamped through the procedure. Some have advocated the use of a Fogarty catheter placed either through a bronchoscope or through a gastric endoscope to occlude the fistula tract if this becomes a problem.[134] Great caution must be exercised when using a Fogarty catheter alongside an endotracheal tube; if the catheter slips out of the fistula tract into the trachea, it can completely occlude the end of the endotracheal tube. Thus, because of these myriad problems with positive-pressure ventilation, many anesthesiologists recommend an anesthetic technique that uses spontaneous ventilation with sevoflurane. Alternatively, others believe that paralysis may be a safe and effective alternative as long as the fistula can be effectively isolated by careful positioning of the endotracheal tube.

Unfortunately, in the authors' experience, it is rarely possible to have a spontaneously breathing newborn sufficiently anesthetized with sevoflurane without compromising blood pressure and oxygenation. This is particularly true in the repair of an esophageal atresia with TEF because this surgery is performed in the lateral position. An intriguing option, which is our preferred technique, is to supplement spontaneous ventilation with a potent vapor general anesthetic with a caudally placed thoracic epidural anesthetic.[135,136]

The caudal approach to the epidural space is remarkably easy to perform in newborns and does not require specialized equipment even though small-diameter Crawford needles (17-20 gauge) and catheters (19-24 Fr) are now commercially available. The epidural space of young children and infants is filled with loosely packed fat and blood vessels, making it possible to advance a caudally placed catheter as far as the thorax. Typically, either 0.5 to 1 mL/kg of 0.25% bupivacaine with epinephrine (5 mcg/mL) or 0.5 mL/kg of 3% chloroprocaine (15 mg/kg) with epinephrine is administered, and the inspired sevoflurane concentration is significantly reduced.[132] Using this combination technique, patients can be adequately anesthetized and hemodynamically stable even while breathing spontaneously. Analgesia can be maintained with this technique postoperatively as well.

Surgery is performed in the left lateral decubitus position. During the surgical repair, the right lung is compressed and packed away, which may result in hypoxia. Additionally, the infant may become hypoxemic if the trachea or endotracheal tube is compressed and occluded by the surgeon. Alternatively, the endotracheal tube can become obstructed by blood clots or may migrate into the fistula tract. Thus, to provide a greater margin of safety, the authors routinely use 100% oxygen during these anesthetics even in premature infants who are at risk of developing retinopathy of prematurity.

MENINGOMYELOCELE

Failure of neural tube closure early in intrauterine development results in a spectrum of abnormalities ranging from spina bifida occulta, a relatively benign process, to myelomeningocele, an abnormality involving vertebral bodies, the spinal cord, and the brainstem. The brainstem lesion (ie, Arnold-Chiari malformation) may be the cause of rather than the effect of the failure of neural tube closure. Ninety percent of infants with myelomeningocele have Arnold-Chiari malformation, which consists of downward displacement of the brainstem and cerebellar tonsils through the cervical spinal canal. This together with an obliteration of the foramina of the fourth ventricle blocks the normal circulation of cerebrospinal fluid (CSF) and leads to progressive hydrocephalus. Associated skeletal anomalies, particularly of the lower extremities, and urodynamic problems are common, and patients born with this defect undergo multiple corrective surgical procedures in their lifetimes.[137] Thus, fetal corrective surgery has been proposed and has shown some preliminary positive results.[138,139]

Infants with a meningomyelocele are transported to the OR in the prone position. The defect is covered with moist, sterile dressings, and great care is taken to avoid contamination and infection. If the meningocele is ruptured, Ringer lactate solution is used to replace CSF losses milliliter for milliliter or at an approximate rate of 4 to 6 mL/kg/h.

The infant must be turned supine for intubation, and positioning is crucial to facilitate this maneuver. A foam head ring or OR towels folded into a ring is covered with a sterile drape or towel. The baby is then turned to the supine position with the defect resting in the pocket of the ring. Towels are then placed under the child's back to build up a level platform for intubation (**Fig. 63-7**). Anesthesia is induced with

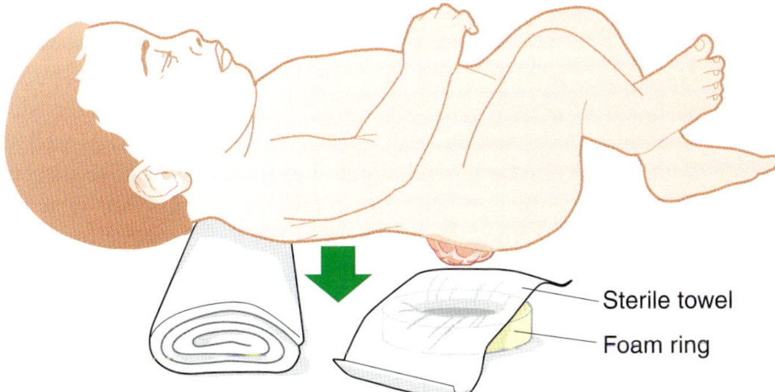

FIGURE 63-7. Positioning of newborn with myelomeningocele for endotracheal intubation.

either inhalational or IV agents (thiopental or propofol). Virtually any anesthetic technique is possible for this operation as long as it allows for rapid extubation after surgery. Succinylcholine does not cause catastrophic hyperkalemia in patients with this defect.[140] After the trachea has been intubated, the endotracheal tube is secured with a "fishmouth" technique (see Fig. 63-4), and the infant is turned to the prone position for surgery.

Spinal anesthesia may be used alone or in combination with general anesthesia for this surgery. When combined with a general anesthetic, the patient is induced as described above. After being turned prone and surgery starts, the surgeon drops 0.5 to 0.7 mg/kg of hyperbaric tetracaine (5 mg/mL) directly into the open meningomyelocele sac.[142] Within minutes, the concentration of inhaled general anesthetic is reduced to a level that provides immobility and allows the child to tolerate the endotracheal tube. Less commonly, spinal anesthesia may be used as the sole anesthetic for this repair. Using a small-gauge needle, 0.5 to 0.7 mg/kg of hyperbaric tetracaine (5 mg/mL) with epinephrine is injected into the most inferior region of the meningomyelocele sac. Supplemental doses are administered as described above for the combined approach.

The decision to place a ventricular-peritoneal (VP) shunt at the time of the initial surgery or several days later is a surgical one. Some surgeons defer placement of the VP shunt because they fear that the drain will become infected. Additionally, because 5% to 10% of these patients do not develop hydrocephalus, some surgeons prefer to wait until it develops rather than treating it expectantly.

PATENT DUCTUS ARTERIOSUS

After birth, the increase in arterial oxygen that occurs by breathing room air results in the closure of the ductus arteriosus. In premature infants, this may not occur and often results in a large left-to-right shunt, heart failure, pulmonary edema, and an inability to be weaned from mechanical ventilation. Medical management consists of fluid restriction, diuretic therapy, digoxin, and 0.2 mg/kg of the cyclooxygenase (COX) inhibitor indomethacin. Other COX inhibitors, such as ibuprofen, may also be effective.[142,143] When they are not effective, surgical correction becomes essential if the child is to be weaned from mechanical ventilation. Unfortunately, in the smallest of premature infants (<1000 g), indomethacin is often unsuccessful because it significantly impairs renal function.

Because these infants have been fluid restricted and are intravascularly volume depleted before surgery, volume expansion with Ringer lactate solution is essential to prevent profound hypotension during the induction of anesthesia even when a fentanyl anesthetic is used. Fentanyl (10-50 mcg/kg has become the most common anesthetic technique used.[8,46] Obviously, nitrous oxide must be avoided and 100% oxygen is often required to maintain oxyhemoglobin concentrations above 90%, especially after the chest is opened and the lung is retracted. Lung retraction, which is necessary to provide surgical exposure, may result in vagal stimulation, and if the infant has not been pretreated with atropine or pancuronium, bradycardia and hypotension results. During closure of the ductus, hemorrhage and exsanguination may occur if this fragile structure is inadvertently torn by the surgeon. Thus, typed and crossmatched blood should always be available before the start of surgery. Additionally, closure of the ductus is associated with an abrupt increase in diastolic blood pressure, which may contribute to the development of intraventricular hemorrhage in this patient population.

Recently, epidural anesthesia has been used to treat postoperative pain in these infants and to reduce intraoperative anesthetic requirements. Both local anesthetics and epidurally administered opioids are effective. Typically, opioids are administered via a caudal approach, and local anesthetics are administered via a caudally placed catheter that has been advanced to the thorax. Finally, because these infants are so fragile, many centers advocate the closure of a patent ductus in NICU rather than transporting the infant to the OR.[144]

SUMMARY

Except for extraordinary circumstances, all newborns require anesthesia and analgesia for surgery. During the first month of life, newborns must function independently and adapt to extrauterine life. This involves anatomic, physiologic, and pharmacologic changes to maintain homeostasis and to ensure the infant's survival. Disease, congenital anomalies, surgery, and anesthesia may interfere with these adaptations and threaten survival. This chapter has attempted to provide an in-depth review of developmental physiology, pathophysiology, and pharmacology and common management techniques that are essential to provide safe, effective anesthesia care to newborns.

KEY REFERENCES

- Anand KJ, Hickey PR. Pain and its effects in the human neonate and fetus. *N Engl J Med.* 1987;317:1321-1329.
- Berde CB, Jaksic T, Lynn AM, Maxwell LG, Soriano SG, Tibboel D. Anesthesia and analgesia during and after surgery in neonates. *Clin Ther.* 2005;27:900-921.
- Bosenberg AT, Bland BA, Schulte-Steinberg O, Downing JW. Thoracic epidural anesthesia via caudal route in infants. *Anesthesiology.* 1988;69:265-269.
- Goudsouzian NG, Standaert FG. The infant and the myoneural junction. *Anesth Analg.* 1986;65:1208-1217.
- Ikonomidou C, Bosch F, Miksa M, et al. Blockade of NMDA receptors and apoptotic neurodegeneration in the developing brain. *Science.* 1999;283:70-74.
- Morray JP. Anesthesia-related cardiac arrest in children. An update. *Anesthesiol Clin North Am.* 2002;20:1-28, v
- Wilder RT, Flick RP, Sprung J, et al. Early exposure to anesthesia and learning disabilities in a population-based birth cohort. *Anesthesiology.* 2009;110:796-804.
- Yaster M. The dose response of fentanyl in neonatal anesthesia. *Anesthesiology.* 1987;66:433-435.

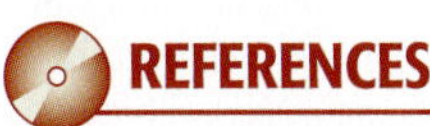

REFERENCES

Complete references available on DVD and online version at www.LongneckerAnesthesiology.com

CHAPTER 64

Anesthesia for Children

Lucinda L. Everett

KEY POINTS

1. Overall, pediatric anesthesia is extremely safe in the hands of experienced providers. Factors that may increase risk include age younger than 1 year and coexisting disease. Careful attention to maintenance of a patent airway is critical to the safe care of infants and children.
2. One of the challenges of pediatric anesthesia for trainees is selecting appropriately sized equipment and supplies. Endotracheal tubes are generally selected to yield a leak at 15 to 30 cm H_2O. Cuffed tubes are gaining wider use in young children as well as those older than 8 years. Straight blades are most commonly used for intubation in infants, with the usual choices being Miller 0 for neonates and Miller 1 for infants. A Wis-Hipple 1.5 blade is often used in toddlers, with progression to Macintosh size 2 for children 3 years and older.
3. The physiologic and psychological contexts must be considered in planning an anesthetic for any child. Premedication and parental presence may be appropriate for children. Induction of anesthesia for elective surgery in young children frequently is accomplished by inhalation of a volatile anesthetic. Sevoflurane is the most common choice in modern practice based on the drug's rapid effect, low degree of airway irritation, and cardiovascular stability.
4. Succinylcholine is no longer used routinely in children because of the potential for hyperkalemia in undiagnosed myopathy. Succinylcholine may still be used when indicated for rapid-sequence induction or treatment of laryngospasm.
5. Regional anesthesia is a useful adjunct to general anesthesia in children for a variety of procedures. Surgery with a regional anesthetic alone is uncommon in young children; one exception is the use of spinal anesthesia in premature infants at risk for postoperative apnea. For common outpatient surgery such as hernia repair or orchidopexy, caudal blockade with a local anesthetic such as ropivacaine provides good intraoperative and postoperative analgesia. Epidural catheters also may be placed in children for more major procedures and generally are placed after induction of general anesthesia in children who are too young to cooperate.
6. Selection of an appropriate plan for postoperative analgesia is important for both inpatient and outpatient situations. Adequate doses of acetaminophen, nonsteroidal anti-inflammatory drugs when not contraindicated, and regional anesthesia may be appropriate in addition to or in place of opioid analgesia, depending on the procedure. Postoperative vomiting is common in children and may occur more frequently during certain procedures, such as strabismus surgery, and in patients with a history of motion sickness or postoperative vomiting. Prophylaxis frequently includes use of a 5-hydroxytryptamine3 (5-HT_3) receptor antagonist or a steroid such as dexamethasone. Because of restrictions on the use of droperidol, 5-HT_3 receptor antagonists are generally used as first-line treatment of postoperative nausea and vomiting in children.
7. Emergence agitation occurs in a significant number of toddlers and young children, particularly after use of a volatile anesthetic. Appropriate analgesia and possibly supplemental sedation may be helpful. The results in the literature are mixed with regard to links with specific agents (eg, sevoflurane); patient and parental anxiety may contribute to the development of agitation.
8. Many of the procedures performed in children involve concepts similar to those used in parallel adult cases (eg, neurosurgery, thoracic surgery). The concepts related to the surgical subspecialty must be integrated with those specific to the anesthetic care of children. Procedures specific to the pediatric population are discussed.

HALLMARKS OF PEDIATRIC ANESTHESIA

Perioperative care of infants and children presents a number of special challenges. The anesthesia care team must evaluate and interface with both the child and parents and must consider psychological as well as physiologic factors. In the United States, anesthesia for elective surgery in children is frequently initiated with an inhalation induction, which is significantly different from the intravenous (IV) induction commonly performed in adults. Physiologic differences, such as an increased rate of oxygen consumption, create the potential for rapid arterial blood desaturation with apnea or hemodynamic compromise. Finally, specific technical skills are required in infants and children.

RISK AND OUTCOME IN PEDIATRIC ANESTHESIA

Overall, safety in pediatric anesthesia is excellent. Complications are uncommon, and improvements over the past several decades are attributed to better monitoring (pulse oximetry and capnography), safer anesthetic agents, and better understanding of specific areas of increased risk. Outcome studies dating from the late 1980s[1] to the current era[2] have identified increased rates of complications and cardiac arrest during anesthesia in children younger than 1 year, although in some studies, the risk appears to be explained by coexisting diseases. American Society of Anesthesiologists (ASA) classification and emergency status also have been predictors of increased risk in pediatric anesthesia outcome studies.

RESPIRATORY RISK

Respiratory complications are common in infants and children. These include laryngospasm, bronchospasm, airway obstruction, and decreased systemic oxygen saturation. Factors that may contribute to respiratory risk include younger age, concurrent disease (syndromes, airway anomalies, or obstructive sleep apnea), recent upper respiratory infection[3] (see Chapter 20), and airway procedures (tonsillectomy, airway surgery, cleft palate repair). Screening for potential airway abnormalities, a backup plan for managing airway difficulties, and rapid attention to respiratory changes are critical components of pediatric anesthetic care.

Pulmonary aspiration of gastric contents is reported in pediatric patients in a range similar to that seen in adults (1-10 cases per 10000 anesthetics).[4] Aspiration occurs more frequently in emergency cases and in "full-stomach" situations such as bowel obstruction. The majority of cases of aspiration occur during laryngoscopy, particularly with coughing or unexpected airway difficulties, but some cases occur during maintenance or emergence from anesthesia. Aspiration using a laryngeal mask has generally been related to a predisposing factor such as inadequate depth of anesthesia, gastrointestinal disease or full stomach, lithotomy position, movement of the laryngeal mask airway (LMA), or multiple insertion attempts.[5] If clinical signs develop (decreased oxygen saturation, coughing, wheezing), they usually occur in the first 2 hours after aspiration. The long-term outcome is generally good in healthy pediatric patients who aspirate gastric contents, but the acuity of perioperative care may be higher than would otherwise have been planned.

Infants born prematurely have an increased risk of apnea and bradycardia after general anesthesia; apnea risk is inversely proportional to both gestational and postconceptual age and increased by anemia.[6] Caffeine administration[7] or the use of spinal anesthesia without sedation[8] reduces the risk of postoperative apnea. Newer anesthetic agents, such as sevoflurane, are not free of the risk of apnea in infants born prematurely.[9] Many hospitals require postoperative overnight admission for monitoring until 50 to 60 weeks' postconceptual age in infants born before 37 weeks; they also may consider anemia, prior apnea, and coexisting disease. Little specific evidence about apnea risk in term infants is available. Some facilities restrict the lower age for day surgery procedures to older than 44 to 46 weeks' postconceptual age in term infants or require a longer observation period (eg, 4 h) before discharge.

CARDIAC RISK

An analysis of pediatric cases from the ASA Closed Claims Study found that claims in infants and children were more likely to be related to respiratory events, more often classified as "preventable" (eg, by better monitoring), and resulted in greater injury severity and mortality than adult claims.[10] The Pediatric Perioperative Cardiac Arrest (POCA) Registry analyzes anesthetic-related cardiac arrests. POCA data published in the year 2000 showed an overall incidence of anesthetic-related cardiac arrest of 1.4 per 10 000 anesthetics based on more than 1 million anesthetics from 63 institutions.[11] Cardiac arrest was most frequent in patients younger than 1 year (55% of cases) and in those with severe underlying disease (ASA classes 3, 4, and 5). Among healthy patients (ASA classes 1 and 2), the most common causes of cardiac arrest were respiratory (related primarily to either laryngospasm or anatomic airway obstruction) and medication related (primarily halothane). In the more recent period, cardiac arrests related to potent inhalational anesthetics have declined,[12] presumably related mainly to the use of the safer agent sevoflurane. Cardiac arrest in children with underlying congenital heart disease occurs most frequently in patients with aortic stenosis, cardiomyopathy, and single-ventricle physiology[13] and may occur in the setting of the general operating room (OR) as well as during cardiac surgery. Cardiac arrest related to succinylcholine administration was reported in the late 1980s[14]; the children were found to have unrecognized myopathy with the development of hyperkalemia after succinylcholine administration. Succinylcholine now is used with caution in pediatric patients but is considered an appropriate choice when rapid intubation is required and for treatment of laryngospasm.

RISK OF NEUROCOGNITIVE IMPAIRMENT

Concern over the possibility that anesthesia could cause impairment of neurodevelopment stems from animal studies showing apoptosis in the brain of immature laboratory animals. There is inadequate evidence to date to decide how relevant this is to clinical practice in human children, but it is an active area of research. Some of the limitations in applying laboratory research include a long duration of exposure, extremely high anesthetic doses, questionable correlation of the age of the experimental animals to human infants, possible species differences, and the anesthetic management in animal studies.[15] Adverse neurologic outcomes are more common in research animals when anesthesia is given without a painful stimulus. Certainly, large numbers of children receive anesthetic care without obvious neurologic or cognitive injury, but better epidemiologic evidence is needed in humans. Some preliminary and retrospective work suggests an association between anesthesia and markers of cognitive dysfunction, but others do not. A causal relationship has not been demonstrated, and it is possible that the need for anesthesia is simply a marker for other comorbidities that could contribute to neurocognitive dysfunction. A recent study using the Netherlands Twin Registry was reassuring in that exposed and unexposed co-twins did not differ in cognitive outcomes; the authors concluded that this suggests that anesthesia at an early age is a marker of vulnerability for later learning disabilities rather than a causal factor.[16] Several large prospective studies are in process to attempt to obtain more conclusive evidence.[17] Until these are available, we should provide parents with available information and reassurance and participate in risk-to-benefit discussions with surgeons and others who request anesthetized procedures.

FACILITY AND PROVIDER EXPERTISE

One of the complex administrative issues in pediatric anesthesia is determining which patients require care by an anesthesiologist who specializes in the care of children. In the United States, pediatric anesthesia fellowship programs are accredited by the Accreditation Council for Graduate Medical Education; subspecialty board certification in pediatric anesthesia is expected to be offered in 2013. Although the link between provider qualifications and outcomes has not been extensively studied, some evidence suggests that children have fewer adverse outcomes when cared for by anesthesiologists with frequent ongoing experience in anesthetizing children.[18,19] Several organizations have put forth guidelines for the care of pediatric patients. The American Academy of Pediatrics (AAP) recommends that anesthesiologists caring for children designated by the facility as being at increased risk either should be fellowship trained in pediatric anesthesiology or have equivalent experience.[20] The ASA and the Society for Pediatric Anesthesia have made similar recommendations. The AAP guidelines also recommend having airway and monitoring equipment in sizes suitable for pediatric patients, a separate preoperative area for children and their families, and OR and recovery staff with age-specific competencies and resuscitation skills.

EQUIPMENT FOR PEDIATRIC ANESTHESIA

BREATHING CIRCUITS AND VENTILATORS

Circuits such as the Mapleson D, a modification of a T-piece, were historically recommended for children because they are lightweight and flexible, have minimal resistance to gas flow, and were designed to prevent rebreathing. Potential disadvantages include rebreathing of carbon dioxide (CO_2) if fresh gas flow is inadequate to wash out exhaled gas and significant tidal volume lost to expanding the expiratory limb during controlled ventilation. The newer pediatric circle systems, which have a smaller diameter and lower compliance than adult circuits, are primarily used today. The minor resistance of the valves is generally not clinically significant with modern anesthesia machines, but avoidance of prolonged spontaneous respiration by small infants is prudent. Lower fresh gas flows can be used with resultant conservation of volatile anesthetic agents and airway moisture.

Circuit compliance does not significantly affect delivered tidal volume when a peak inspiratory pressure is chosen that provides good chest movement.[21] There may be a discrepancy between actual and measured tidal volume unless the machine measures and compensates for circuit compliance. Pressure mode ventilation may be best in infants, particularly if there is a leak around the endotracheal tube, and higher fresh gas flow may be needed in the presence of a leak. With pressure ventilation, changes in pulmonary and chest wall compliance can result in significant changes in delivered tidal volume. In some older anesthesia ventilators, fresh gas flow contributes to tidal volume, so a large increase in gas flow can cause barotrauma. A good understanding of the characteristics of the ventilator and circuit being used is essential to safe ventilation of a child's lungs.

MONITORING

Pulse oximetry has vastly improved the safety of pediatric anesthesia, but capnography, auscultation, movement in the rebreathing bag, and observation of chest motion all contribute to the clinical assessment of airway patency and should detect airway obstruction before desaturation. Electrocardiographic (ECG) monitoring in healthy children is primarily geared toward monitoring heart rate and rhythm. Ischemic changes are extremely rare except in pediatric cardiac surgery; however, if they occur, rapid assessment of the cause must be undertaken with efforts to improve coronary perfusion. Noninvasive blood pressure monitoring can be used on an upper or lower extremity in children. The decision to place arterial or central venous lines is based on the severity of illness or the extent and potential complications of the procedure. Temperature should be monitored for all but the shortest cases. Appropriate warming devices should be chosen to minimize the risk of hypothermia; these are discussed further in Chapter 20.

APPROACH TO PEDIATRIC PATIENTS: THE ANESTHETIC PLAN

Developing an anesthetic plan for a pediatric patient involves several decisions. Is the procedure elective or emergent? Does the child have significant coexisting disease, airway concerns, or behavioral challenges? Are there expectations of how the anesthetic will be conducted based on prior experiences of the child or the child's family or friends?

PREPARATION AND PREMEDICATION

Many children younger than 6 to 9 months of age will separate from their parents easily if kept engaged. Older children and those who seem anxious or fussy may benefit from premedication before entering the OR. Midazolam is commonly given orally as a premedication; other routes and doses are summarized in **Table 64-1**. Oral transmucosal fentanyl is infrequently used because of side effects of nausea or vomiting and pruritus, but it may be a reasonable option when other premedication is not well accepted or when an opioid is indicated for analgesia. Oral ketamine may be useful when analgesia is desired. Intramuscular ketamine is administered to patients who are combative or difficult to approach; a sedative dose usually will result in adequate cooperation to obtain IV access or complete induction by administering an inhalation agent. Finally, rectal administration of methohexital is really an induction rather than a premedication. If used, it should be given in a monitored setting with the anesthesiologist present and prepared to move the patient into the OR or procedure area.

Parental presence during induction can be used in addition to or in place of premedication.[22] The child's behavior and family dynamics should be considered; transmitted parental anxiety may limit the value of parental presence. Parents who are going to participate in induction should be appropriately instructed. Provider behavior may also have an impact on how the child responds; providing distraction appears to be more effective than reassuring behaviors.[23] OR personnel should have an understanding as to who will be interacting with the child so multiple people will not be competing for the child's attention.

ANESTHETIC INDUCTION

Induction of anesthesia in elective situations for children younger than 8 to 10 years of age frequently occurs by inhalation to avoid venipuncture until the child is asleep. Sevoflurane provides smooth, rapid inhalation induction with good cardiovascular stability; it has largely replaced halothane for inhalation induction. Desflurane and isoflurane should not be used for inhalation induction because both cause airway irritation. In a cooperative child, mask induction can be initiated with 50% to 70% nitrous oxide in oxygen (**Fig. 64-1**). After 1 to 2 minutes, sevoflurane is introduced either incrementally or at 8%. If the child is agitated initially or becomes combative during the initial stages of induction, a

TABLE 64-1 Premedication Options

Drug	Route	Dose	Onset (min)	Advantages	Disadvantages
Midazolam	PO	0.5-0.75 mg/kg Maximum, 15-20 mg	10-15	Effective Minimal effect on respiratory function in healthy patients	Bitter taste Possible contribution to postoperative delirium
Midazolam	Rectal	0.5-0.75 mg/kg	10-15	Effective Minimal effect on respiratory function in healthy patients	May not be an appropriate route for older children Possible contribution to postoperative delirium
Midazolam	Nasal	0.2-0.3 mg/kg	5-10	Effective Minimal effect on respiratory function in healthy patients	Burns on administration; bitter Reduced effectiveness if crying or copious nasal secretions Possible contribution to postoperative delirium
Midazolam	IV	0.05-mg/kg increments	1-2	Effective Minimal effect on respiratory function in healthy patients	Requires IV access
Fentanyl	PO transmucosal (Oralet or lozenge)	5-10 mcg/kg	10-20	Better taste than midazolam Analgesia	Pruritus Nausea and vomiting Potential for "stiff chest" with large doses Variable absorption
Ketamine	PO	6-9 mg/kg	15-20	Better taste than midazolam Analgesia	Nystagmus; possibility of hallucination Delayed emergence if combined with midazolam at this dose Increased salivation
Ketamine–midazolam combination	PO	2.5 mg/kg ketamine with 0.25 mg/kg midazolam	10	May have slightly better onset and recovery than midazolam alone	Need to combine drugs
Ketamine	IM	2-3 mg/kg	3-5	Useful for combative or uncooperative patients	Secretions, which may be diminished with antisialagogue
Ketamine	IM (induction)	10 mg/kg	3-5	Useful for combative or uncooperative patients Deeper sedation than smaller dose	Delayed emergence
Methohexital	Rectal (induction)	30 mg/kg	6	Smooth induction for frightened or uncooperative small children	Higher incidence of airway obstruction than with midazolam

IM, intramuscular; IV, intravenous; PO, oral.

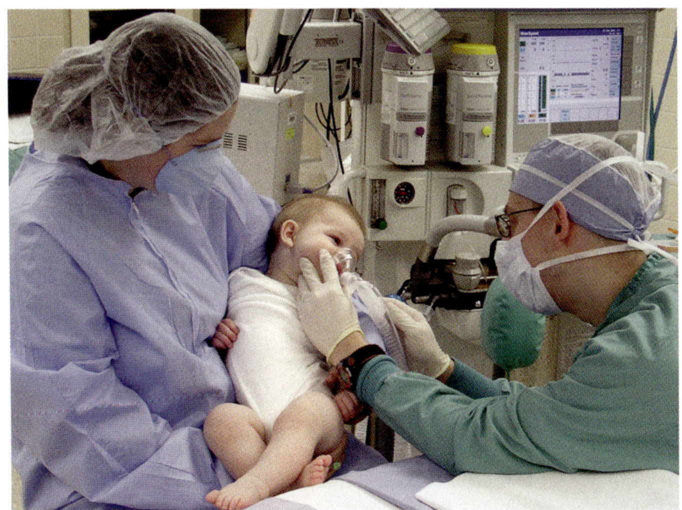

FIGURE 64-1. Mask induction of anesthesia. [Courtesy of Scott Tolle.]

rapid decision must be made either to stop and pursue premedication or to proceed with a high inspired concentration of sevoflurane. As soon as the child's eyes close, the parents (if present) are escorted out, and attention is turned to maintaining a patent airway. Nitrous oxide can be discontinued at this time to improve oxygen reserve. An "excitement phase" is frequently seen with inhalation induction and may include limb movement, rigidity, rapid respirations, and tachycardia, all of which usually resolve over several minutes as the anesthetic deepens. When the child has passed the excitement phase, IV access is established for all but very brief cases.

Children often develop some degree of airway obstruction during inhalation induction. Keeping one hand on the breathing bag to feel gas movement, auscultation by precordial stethoscope, and observation of the end-tidal CO_2 tracing and chest movement all provide useful information. Lack of gas exchange during inhalation induction should be assessed rapidly to differentiate central apnea (from high concentration of anesthetic agent) from airway obstruction by attempting a gentle positive-pressure breath. If the patient is easily ventilated, slow manual ventilation using a lower concentration of volatile agent should result in resumption of spontaneous respiration, which may in turn help avoid excessive anesthetic depth. If airway obstruction is present, further evaluation must attempt to distinguish upper airway obstruction from laryngospasm. Upper airway obstruction in a child often can be managed by opening the mouth slightly to displace the tongue from the roof of the mouth and lifting the jaw anteriorly; continuous positive airway pressure (CPAP) of 5 to 10 cm H_2O may be helpful. Pressure on the soft tissue beneath the chin may worsen airway obstruction. An oral airway can be inserted if anesthetic depth is sufficient or if the other maneuvers are unsuccessful. If these measures fail to open the airway, an LMA is inserted if upper airway obstruction is believed to be the cause of obstruction or treatment of laryngospasm can be pursued with 100% oxygen, CPAP, and succinylcholine when necessary.[24] Succinylcholine 4 mg/kg can be administered intramuscularly or sublingually if IV access has not been established.

IV induction is generally chosen for older children and adolescents, for children at risk for aspiration of gastric contents, and for any child with IV access already in place unless airway considerations make inhalation induction preferable. Preoxygenation is important in children but may be difficult to accomplish; judicious premedication may be helpful in gaining cooperation. Propofol is frequently used as an induction agent in pediatric anesthesia unless there are hemodynamic contraindications. Burning on injection of propofol into a peripheral IV can be minimized with prior injection of lidocaine, an opioid, or both; thiopental may cause less pain on injection. Ketamine or etomidate is used

TABLE 64-2 Induction Drugs for Children

Induction Drugs	Dose (mg/kg)	Indications	Potential Side Effects
Propofol	1-3	Routine induction, particularly for shorter procedures or to decrease the potential for postoperative nausea and vomiting	Burning on injection Occasional myoclonus
Thiopental sodium	3-6	Routine induction	Precipitation with other drugs, particularly steroidal nondepolarizing muscle relaxant
Etomidate	0.2-0.3	Cardiovascular instability	Mild discomfort on injection Myoclonus Adrenal suppression reported
Ketamine	1-2	Cardiovascular instability Bronchospasm	Increases cerebral blood flow Increases secretions Nystagmus Possible dysphoria

for induction for specific indications such as hemodynamic instability. Pediatric dosing for induction drugs is summarized in **Table 64-2**. Intubation can be accomplished with use of a muscle relaxant, with a volatile agent supplemented with propofol or a narcotic or with deep inhalation anesthesia alone. Intubation with a volatile agent alone, particularly sevoflurane, must be accomplished quickly while the patient is at an adequate depth of anesthesia.

Neuromuscular blockade can be used to facilitate endotracheal intubation or may be required to provide optimal surgical conditions. As noted earlier, succinylcholine is indicated in infants and children only when rapid control of the airway is required. Atropine should be given before succinylcholine in infants and young children to minimize the potential for bradycardia. The nondepolarizing muscle relaxants all can be used safely in pediatric practice. Rocuronium is the best alternative for rapid-sequence intubation, but the effective dose of 1 mg/kg has a duration longer than 1 hour. Pediatric doses for muscle relaxants are listed in **Table 64-3** and are generally similar to those used in adult practice. Infants appear to have a somewhat increased volume of distribution but also an increased sensitivity to relaxants, so the initial dose remains similar to that used for adults. Rocuronium may have a longer duration of action in infants compared with older children or adults when 0.6 mg/kg is given; a smaller dose (0.45 mg/kg) has been shown to produce good intubating conditions with a shorter duration.[25]

TABLE 64-3 Neuromuscular Blockade in Children

Drug	Dose	Duration
Succinylcholine	1.5-2.0 mg/kg	Short
Cisatracurium	0.1-0.2 mg/kg	Intermediate
Vecuronium	0.1 mg/kg	Intermediate
Rocuronium	0.45-0.6 mg/kg routine 1 mg/kg rapid sequence	Intermediate Long
Pancuronium	0.1 mg/kg	Long

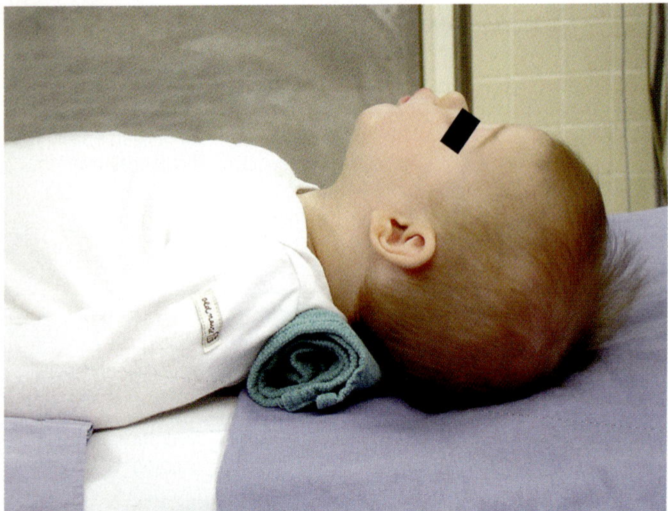

FIGURE 64-2. Positioning in infants and toddlers. Because of the relatively large head, a roll under the shoulders may avoid flexion at the neck and maintain a patent airway. [Courtesy of Scott Tolle.]

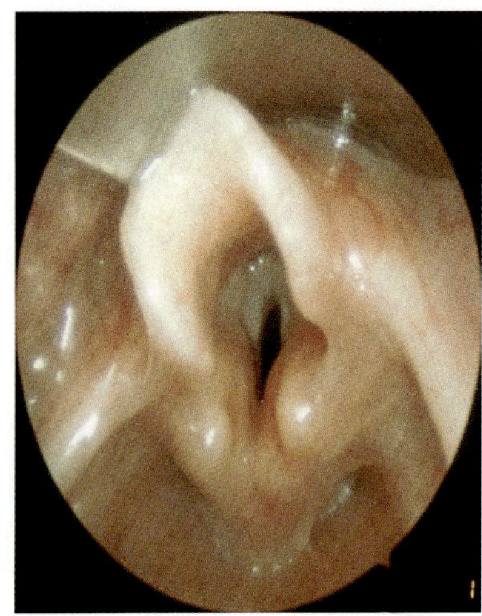

FIGURE 64-3. Infant glottis. [Courtesy of A. Inglis, MD.]

Reversal of nondepolarizing neuromuscular blockade is advisable unless significant time has elapsed (2 h after a routine intubating dose) or unless the patient clearly exhibits clinical signs of full neuromuscular function. Neostigmine in a dose of 0.05 to 0.075 mg/kg is most commonly administered for reversal. Alternatively, edrophonium can be given at 0.5 to 1.0 mg/kg, although it may be less effective for reversal of profound neuromuscular block. Atropine or glycopyrrolate is administered with reversal agents to prevent bradycardia. Edrophonium has a rapid onset and strong tendency to cause bradycardia; if it is used, atropine should be given first.

AIRWAY MANAGEMENT

Unique anatomic and physiologic aspects of the pediatric airway are discussed in Chapter 20. Because infants and younger children have a large occiput, a roll placed under their shoulders may help to maintain a neutral (and patent) airway (**Fig. 64-2**). If the mask airway is stable after inhalation induction, maintenance anesthesia can be administered by a face mask, as is commonly done for ear tubes and other minor surgical procedures. An oropharyngeal airway can be inserted when needed to maintain airway patency or if positioning of the mask airway requires frequent manipulation; it should reach from the lips to the angle of the jaw when held next to the child. If access to the face will be limited but intubation is not required, an LMA can be used. LMAs are generally well tolerated in children, but their use is not free from adverse airway events.[26,27] Appropriate LMA sizes for various patient weights are listed in **Table 64-4.** Newer laryngeal mask devices, such as those that afford the ability to vent the stomach, are now being produced in pediatric sizes.

Laryngoscopy in infants and young children has some unique technical aspects related to age-related anatomic changes (see Chapter 20). A child's epiglottis, although rigid, is "slippery" and may be difficult to control with the laryngoscope blade (**Fig. 64-3**). In the United States, a straight blade is most commonly used in patients younger than 2 years. When performing laryngoscopy with a straight blade, it is important to sweep the tongue to the patient's left; passing the tube down the flange of the blade will obscure the view. If the glottis is not seen after passing under the epiglottis, most likely the blade has already gone too deep and posteriorly; withdrawing the blade slowly with gentle cricoid pressure often brings the glottic opening into view. Choice of laryngoscope blade size by patient age is summarized in **Table 64-5**.

Traditionally, pediatric endotracheal tubes are selected to allow a small leak at 20 to 25 cm H_2O. Because the narrowest portion of a young child's airway is subglottic, the tube must not be forced if any resistance is felt. Approximate endotracheal tube sizes by age are listed in Table 64-5. Tube size can be selected based on age or height or by selecting a tube with an outer diameter similar in size to the child's fifth finger. Tubes are packaged according to internal diameter; specialized endotracheal tubes, such as reinforced tubes, may have a much larger outer diameter than a standard tube of the same internal diameter. Uncuffed endotracheal tubes were traditionally used in children younger than 8 to 10 years of age because of concerns of pressure injury to the tracheal mucosa. Modern tubes are made of less reactive materials and do not cause significant complications when appropriately sized (usually one-half size smaller than uncuffed). Use of a cuffed tube more often results in an appropriate fit[28]; specific indications include aspiration risk and poor pulmonary compliance. Cuffed tubes allow the use of lower fresh gas flow rates and a decrease in OR pollution from volatile anesthetics. Balloon inflation must be performed carefully, and ideally cuff pressure should be measured, particularly if nitrous oxide is used.

The small distance from vocal cords to carina leaves relatively little margin between correct placement and endobronchial location in small

TABLE 64-4 Laryngeal Mask Airway Sizes for Pediatric Patients

Weight (kg)	Laryngeal Mask Airway Size
<5	1
5-10	1.5
10-20	2
20-30	2.5
30-50	3

TABLE 64-5 Laryngoscope Blade and Endotracheal Tube Sizes

Age	Blade	Endotracheal Tube Size
Premature neonate	Miller 0	2.5-3.0
Term neonate	Miller 0 or 1	3.0-3.5
6-12 mo	Miller 1	3.5-4.0
1-2 y	Miller 1 or Wis-Hipple 1.5	4.0-4.5
2-8 y	Wis 1.5–Macintosh 2	4 + Age/4
>8 y	Miller 2, Macintosh 3	≥6.0

children. For cuffed tubes, the cuff should pass just a short distance below the vocal cords. With uncuffed tubes, options include positioning based on the line markings at the distal end of the tube, deliberate endobronchial intubation and withdrawal until bilateral breath sounds are heard, or use of the common formula

$$\text{Tracheal tube (TT) depth (cm)} = 3 \times \text{TT size [mm inner diameter (ID)]}$$

Auscultation of bilateral breath sounds does not guarantee proper TT position.[29]

A variety of options exist for dealing with the difficult pediatric airway; in contrast to adult practice, inhalation induction with spontaneous respiration is often used because children do not tolerate awake intubation. Insufflation of gas through a nasal airway or endotracheal tube advanced into the nasopharynx may provide a stable airway to allow fiberoptic intubation in an anesthetized child. The LMA can serve as a rescue device or a conduit for fiberoptic intubation. Flexible fiberoptic intubation is a mainstay for difficult intubation; video laryngoscopes and intubating stylets are also available. Skill with these options should be gained first in patients with normal airways. Awake or sedated intubation is possible in infants and children and should be considered when there is no obvious way to ventilate the patient, as in children with congenital abnormalities that preclude achieving a mask seal or when an LMA cannot be inserted. Topical anesthesia can be provided by allowing an infant to suck on a small amount of local anesthetic jelly or by nebulized administration.

ANESTHETIC MAINTENANCE

A variety of maintenance anesthetic techniques may be appropriate depending on the patient's status and type of surgery. Opinion varies as to whether one volatile agent has a significant advantage over another for pediatric anesthetic use (see Emergence Delirium later). Total IV anesthesia is being used more frequently for a variety of pediatric indications (minor procedures with spontaneous respiration; procedures requiring neurophysiologic monitoring). Metabolic acidosis related to prolonged propofol infusion has been of concern in pediatric intensive care patients.[30] Although propofol infusion is widely used in pediatric anesthesia, there is no clear cutoff regarding safe case duration.

EXTUBATION CHOICES

The endotracheal tube can be removed either when the patient awakens or while the child is deeply anesthetized. The choice depends partly on the preference and experience of the practitioner. Those who advocate "deep extubation" cite smoother emergence with less coughing. Risks include laryngospasm and airway obstruction as the child emerges. Deep extubation requires particular attention to detail and should not be undertaken by individuals inexperienced with the technique; in institutions without proper support for anesthetized pediatric patients in a recovery area; or in patients with full stomachs, oral blood or secretions, or the inability to protect their airway. If deep extubation is chosen, the patient should have a stable pattern of spontaneous respiration and no response to suctioning the oropharynx, stimulation such as jaw thrust, or slight in-and-out movement of the endotracheal tube. Moving the patient while he or she is still deeply anesthetized can prevent the need for stimulation after extubation. Close attention to gas exchange is required after extubation. Evidence supporting or refuting the safety of deep extubation is inconclusive; existing studies are small and cover variable patient populations. Smoother emergence, particularly decreased coughing, has also been suggested when an LMA is removed during deep anesthesia rather than in awake children.

FLUID THERAPY

Fluid therapy in pediatric anesthesia is based on calculation and replacement of the fasting deficit, maintenance fluid requirement, insensible and third-space losses, and blood loss. Maintenance fluid and fasting deficits are based on rates of 4 mL/kg/h for the first 10 kg, 2 mL/kg/h for the second 10 kg, and 1 mL/kg/h for weight above 20 kg. Insensible and third-space losses can be high in abdominal surgery, in which the starting replacement volume is 10 mL/kg/h with titration to normal heart rate, blood pressure, urine output, and clinical signs of perfusion. No evidence favors colloid over crystalloid as a generalization, but colloid replacement may have a role in maintaining oncotic pressure when large fluid volumes are given. Fluid boluses for volume-depleted children are given in increments of 10 to 20 mL/kg followed by assessment of clinical parameters. Fluids should be warmed if large volumes are given.

Most healthy children do not need supplemental dextrose to maintain plasma glucose levels unless they have undergone prolonged fasting,[31] and liberalization of fasting guidelines may have further reduced any risk of hypoglycemia in healthy children. Patients in whom IV dextrose administration should be strongly considered include neonates, critically ill children with limited metabolic reserve or hepatic failure, children who receive concentrated tube feedings or IV hyperalimentation, and children with inborn errors of metabolism characterized by hypoglycemia. If given, dextrose is preferably administered at a maintenance rate after replacement of the deficit or as a separate infusion. For neonates and high-risk patients, concentrated dextrose solutions may be appropriate; for healthy older children, 1% to 2.5% dextrose solutions are preferred to prevent hyperglycemia.

BLOOD AND BLOOD PRODUCTS

Calculation of circulating blood volume and allowable blood loss is covered in depth in Chapter 20. As a useful quick estimate, children who start at a relatively normal hematocrit can lose at least 20% of their blood volume before requiring transfusion if they are kept normovolemic. The patient's clinical condition as well as the rapidity of blood loss and expected further loss should be considered in deciding when to begin transfusion. If crystalloid is used for replacement, it should be given in a 3:1 ratio. Packed cells 10 mL/kg will raise the hematocrit by approximately 6 to 10 percentage points. The amount required to replace the estimated blood loss also can be calculated based on a hematocrit of 70% contained in packed cells:

$$\text{Transfusion volume} = \text{Patient's blood volume} \times [(\text{Desired} - \text{Current Hct})/\text{Hct of unit PRBCs}],$$

where Hct is hematocrit and PRBCs is packed red blood cells.

When total transfused volumes of packed cells approach the patient's blood volume, both thrombocytopenia and depletion of clotting factors may occur. Ideally, these parameters are measured to guide replacement therapy, but rapidly changing clinical circumstances may dictate empirical blood component therapy. Platelets are administered in a volume of 5 to 10 mL/kg; 10 mL/kg can be expected to raise the platelet concentration by 100 000/mm^3. Thawed fresh-frozen plasma when indicated is also started at 10 mL/kg. Infused packed cells or plasma may cause hypocalcemia if given too rapidly as a result of binding of ionized calcium by citrate. In the setting of large-volume transfusions, potassium release from banked blood may be significant; requesting fresh units or washing the cells may prevent hyperkalemia.

PEDIATRIC REGIONAL ANESTHESIA

OVERVIEW AND SAFETY

Regional anesthesia can provide a useful adjunct for a variety of procedures in pediatric patients, either as a single injection or with postoperative infusion of local anesthetic or other adjuncts. Advantages of regional anesthesia, such as postoperative analgesia, avoidance of narcotic therapy with decreased nausea and vomiting, and early discharge from the recovery area, apply to pediatric patients. This chapter presents particular applications in pediatric anesthesia; further details on standard regional techniques are found in Chapters 46 to 49.

Performing a regional anesthetic in children who are too young to cooperate may require that the block be done during general anesthesia. Using a nerve stimulator to perform "surface mapping" before placing the needle may improve accuracy and decrease the number of attempts required.[32] Ultrasound imaging is becoming more common for both neuraxial and peripheral blocks in children. Potential complications of regional techniques in anesthetized patients include intraneural injection, direct needle damage, and local anesthetic toxicity, although these complications are rare. Venous air embolism with hemodynamic consequences has been described during caudal or epidural placement in small children as has neurologic injury been believed to be caused by cerebrovascular air embolism or ischemic injury[33]; loss of resistance to air is not recommended in pediatric patients. The pediatric anesthesia community has endorsed epidural placement under anesthesia as appropriate practice when it is perceived that the patient will benefit from having the regional anesthetic and there is a risk that the patient might otherwise move during the block.[34] The risks and benefits must be weighed in each individual pediatric patient, especially if the procedure is technically difficult.

Local anesthetic toxicity may result from intravascular injection, rapid absorption of an inappropriately large dose, or intravascular accumulation of drug over time. If combinations of local anesthetic agents are used, the toxicity of the agents should be considered to be additive. Local anesthetic blood levels after caudal and peripheral blocks in pediatric patients are generally within acceptable limits. Several cases of toxicity caused by accumulation of high levels in blood occurred in the early 1990s in the setting of postoperative infusion of local anesthetics; these resulted in revision of the recommendations of doses for pediatric infusion, with a maximum dose of 0.4 to 0.5 mg/kg/h for bupivacaine.[35] Infants may be at higher risk for toxicity because of lower levels of plasma-binding proteins, diminished clearance, or both, particularly with redosing or catheter infusion techniques. The maximum recommended infusion rates of bupivacaine for patients 6 months and younger is 0.25 to 0.3 mg/kg/h.

Local anesthetic toxicity may not be obvious in the anesthetized patient; aspiration of blood may not reliably occur, and central nervous system signs are difficult to detect. The use of a test dose is recommended to detect inadvertent intravascular injection. Heart rate changes may be less sensitive in the pediatric population, particularly with volatile anesthetics; changes in T-wave morphology on the ECG are a useful indicator. Criteria for a positive test dose in an anesthetized child are heart rate increase greater than 10 beats/min, systolic blood pressure increase greater than 15 mm Hg, and change in T-wave amplitude greater than 25% in lead II. The recommended test dose in children is 0.5 mcg/kg epinephrine (0.1 mL/kg of local anesthetic containing 1:200 000 epinephrine),[36] up to the 15-mcg adult test dose. Use of a short-beveled needle or Angiocath may minimize the risk of intravascular injection. In addition, slow incremental injection of local anesthetic is recommended (after test dose, administer a total dose over 1-2 min). Because small veins may easily collapse, observing for passive blood return may be useful in addition to aspiration.

SPECIFIC TECHNIQUES FOR PEDIATRIC REGIONAL ANESTHESIA

Caudal Blocks and Alternatives The caudal approach to the epidural space is simple in young children, easy to learn, and has a good safety record (**Fig. 64-4**). Potential complications in anesthetized patients include intravascular injection of local anesthetic, which occurs in approximately 4 in 10 000 patients, and intrathecal injection with total spinal, with a reported incidence of 2.6 in 10 000 cases.[37] Children may not develop hypotension or bradycardia even in the presence of a total spinal, but apnea may still occur because of medullary blockade.

Caudal blocks provide excellent analgesia for lower extremity, lower abdominal, and penoscrotal surgery. A short-beveled needle is placed through the sacral hiatus until a typical "pop" is felt, and the needle is anchored in the sacrococcygeal ligament (**Fig. 64-5**). Aspiration and free drainage should be negative for blood and cerebrospinal fluid (CSF). With correct placement, injection will be easy and will not result in swelling of the subcutaneous tissue. After an epinephrine-containing test dose, the full dose is injected incrementally. Clinical signs of correct placement are generally adequate, but use of a nerve stimulator to confirm caudal needle placement has been described. Laxity of the anal sphincter after placement of a caudal block has been shown to predict success of the block.[38] If there is doubt as to efficacy, this sign may assist with the decision to provide additional analgesia. Although the time to first urination may be longer than that without a caudal block, urinary retention is generally not a significant clinical problem. Hemodynamic changes after a caudal block usually are minimal in normovolemic patients.

Bupivacaine in concentrations of 0.125% to 0.25% traditionally has been used for caudal blocks in children in a dose of 1 mL/kg. Freshly added epinephrine to a concentration of 1:200 000 (5 mcg/mL) may improve the duration of analgesia. Because the block will begin to regress after several hours, the more concentrated solution or redosing

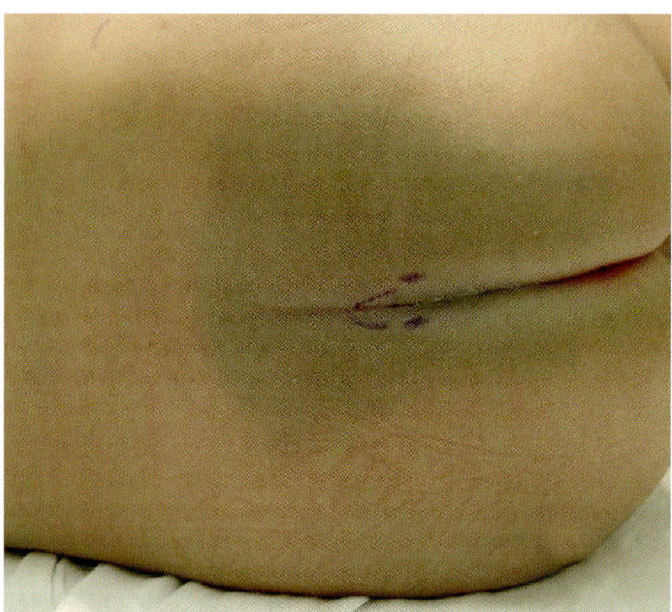

FIGURE 64-4. Surface landmarks for caudal block. Both sacral cornua and the lateral borders of the sacrococcygeal hiatus can be palpated and outlined. The needle is inserted at the midpoint of the triangle at an approximately 45-degree angle to start.

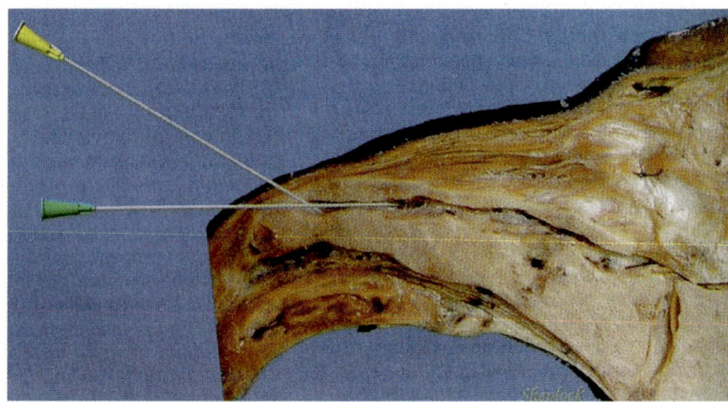

FIGURE 64-5. Caudal block. [Reprinted from Hahn MB, McQuillan PM, Sheplock GJ, eds. *Regional Anesthesia: An Atlas of Anatomy and Techniques*. St. Louis, MO: Mosby; 1996, with permission.]

the block at the end of the case is appropriate for longer procedures. Duration of analgesia from a single-shot caudal injection ranges from 4 to 12 hours. Use of a larger volume of local anesthetic to achieve a higher level may block stimulation from traction during procedures such as orchidopexy.[39] The newer local anesthetics ropivacaine and levobupivacaine offer the advantages of decreased cardiac toxicity[40] and reduced motor block. Ropivacaine and levobupivacaine have equivalent efficacy at either 0.2% or 0.25% compared with bupivacaine 0.25% (all given at 1 mL/kg); ropivacaine produced the least motor blockade.[41]

Caudally administered clonidine has shown good efficacy for augmenting and prolonging the analgesia produced by local anesthetics in a variety of procedures.[42] A few studies question the benefit.[43,44] Single doses of 1 to 2 mcg/kg provide analgesia with a lower incidence of nausea and vomiting than produced by opioids. Some sedation is seen at the higher dose of 5 mcg/kg. Most studies have not shown respiratory depression with epidural or caudal clonidine, although 2 case reports suggest apnea risk in premature infants. Use of epidural or caudal clonidine is fairly common in children in the United States, although a Food and Drug Administration (FDA) "black box" label warns of hypotension in adult patients after epidural clonidine administration. Ketamine has been shown to have good efficacy by the caudal route, but appropriate preparations of preservative-free *S*-ketamine are not available in the United States.[45]

Ilioinguinal or iliohypogastric nerve blocks can be performed preoperatively by the anesthesiologist or intraoperatively by the surgeon for procedures such as hernia repair and orchidopexy in children. Some surgeons believe that the injected local anesthetic distorts the surgical dissection planes and prefer to perform the block at the end of surgery. In this situation, a caudal block might be preferable to allow a contribution of the block during surgery. Ilioinguinal blocks generally have equivalent efficacy to caudal blocks, but this may be operator dependent. Cadaver dissection has shown that the optimal insertion site is more lateral than is generally taught and is located approximately 2.5 mm medial to the anterior superior iliac spine on both sides of a line drawn between the anterior superior iliac spine and the umbilicus.[46] Ultrasound guidance may improve success and allow use of a lower volume of local anesthetic.[47] Although quite safe, complications such as puncture of the bowel wall with hematoma formation have been reported after ilioinguinal block. Other techniques, such as paravertebral or lumbar plexus blockade, have been used in pediatric patients in select settings. Further experience with these techniques is needed before their use can be recommended outside of centers performing them frequently.

Penile block is commonly performed for circumcision and sometimes for simple hypospadias repair. Epinephrine should never be injected in a penile block because of the risk of vascular compromise. As with ilioinguinal blocks, many studies have compared caudal and penile blocks with variable results; most suggest that they are approximately equal. In the traditional dorsal penile block, the needle is passed from the base of the penis until the symphysis pubis is contacted and then withdrawn slightly and redirected to each side of the midline before local anesthetic is deposited. Because of the small risk of hematoma or damage to the dorsal penile vessels, some advocate a "ring block" or subcutaneous injection around the base of the penis. A combination of dorsal and ring blocks may provide the best analgesia. Simple application of topical anesthetic cream (eutectic mixture of local anesthetics [EMLA]) provided equivalent analgesia to dorsal penile block, but the duration of blockade was significantly longer with the injected nerve block.[48]

Spinal Anesthesia The primary use of spinal anesthesia in the pediatric population is for hernia repair or other relatively minor surgery in infants considered to be at risk for postoperative apnea. The dose requirement on a weight basis is significantly higher than in adults, and the duration is relatively shorter: 1 mg/kg hyperbaric bupivacaine has a duration of 1 to 2 hours. Levobupivacaine and ropivacaine also have been used. The decision to administer spinal anesthesia should depend on the patient's medical condition and the extent of the procedure. The perceived benefit of a reduced apnea frequency compared with general anesthesia in premature or former premature infants is valid only if no sedation is given. Spinal anesthesia may not be a good choice for a large or incarcerated hernia because of the limited duration and the fact that unsedated babies may fuss and strain.

Epidural Analgesia Either thoracic or lumbar epidural catheters can be placed in children. Postoperative epidural analgesia may be of benefit to pediatric patients after major thoracic, abdominal, urologic, and lower extremity surgery. For patients weighing between 10 and 25 kg, the approximate depth of the epidural space in millimeters will be predicted by the weight in kilograms. Postoperative infusions should be prescribed to optimize analgesia and minimize side effects. Patient-controlled epidural analgesia can be given to children as young as 5 years of age and may decrease total drug administration.[49] The pediatric orthopedic community has expressed concern that epidural analgesia may "mask" development of a compartment syndrome, but in the reported cases, pain was out of proportion to what was expected and was unrelieved by the epidural analgesia.[50] Nevertheless, complications other than inadequate epidural analgesia must always be considered and evaluated promptly.

An epidural catheter can be threaded via the caudal route either to allow redosing for longer infraumbilical surgery or for the purpose of threading the tip of the catheter to a higher thoracic or lumbar level.[51] In general, the ability to thread the catheter cephalad is best in infants because the epidural fat is not as dense as in older patients. The type of catheter may affect the success rate, and some recommend using a styletted catheter. Radiographic confirmation of tip placement[52] or stimulation of the trunk musculature[53] may be helpful in positioning the catheter.

Extremity Blocks Regional anesthesia of the upper extremity can be used in children for procedures performed on the arm and hand. Performing the entire surgical procedure under a regional technique is less common in children than in adults. In conjunction with general anesthesia, even distal blocks can provide excellent analgesia for hand procedures. Axillary blockade is the most common brachial plexus approach in children, although various infraclavicular approaches have been reported. Because of case reports of syrinx formation in adults after interscalene blocks placed under general anesthesia or deep sedation,[54] this approach has not been recommended unless the patient can cooperate with block placement with minimal sedation. Some consider that ultrasonography may improve the safety adequately to permit this block under anesthesia.

A number of regional techniques can be performed in children for lower extremity surgery. A psoas compartment approach to the lumbar plexus has been described in children using a nerve stimulator and can be used for unilateral surgery on the hip, thigh, or knee.[55] This block may require significant experience for the anesthesiologist to develop mastery,[56] and there is some potential for vascular puncture. Femoral nerve blocks are useful in managing pain from a femur fracture even preoperatively. The "fascia iliaca" block has a high rate of success in children when anesthesia of the obturator and lateral femoral cutaneous nerves is needed in addition to the femoral nerve. The sciatic nerve can be blocked by the traditional posterior approach, at the midthigh, or in the popliteal fossa.

POSTOPERATIVE PAIN MANAGEMENT

The anesthetic plan should include management of pain both in the immediate postoperative period and during later recovery, whether the patient is admitted to the hospital or sent home after surgery. Managing pain in children is a special challenge because our ability to evaluate their pain and their ability to communicate their needs may be limited. Pain scales based on behavior and facial expressions are available for younger children. The analgesic plan may include opioid or nonopioid analgesics, regional or local anesthesia, or a multimodal approach. When a regional anesthetic is used in the early postoperative period, the patient and parent should be told what to expect in terms of duration of effect, and plans for a transition to other types of analgesia should be formulated. Particularly for outpatients, parents should be instructed to begin administering oral analgesics before the child is in severe pain.

Acetaminophen and nonsteroidal anti-inflammatory drugs (NSAIDs) can provide significant postoperative pain relief and may have an opioid-sparing effect. A rectal loading dose of acetaminophen may be given intraoperatively, but onset is slow with peak plasma concentration at approximately 200 minutes. A rectal loading dose of 40 mg/kg of acetaminophen followed by 20 mg/kg every 6 hours does not appear to result in drug accumulation in the first 24 hours.[57] An oral loading dose has faster onset; 40 mg/kg (compared with the traditional dose of 15 mg/kg) resulted in plasma levels at 30 and 60 minutes in an effective range to treat pain (after tonsillectomy) and below levels considered to be toxic.[58] Although these higher doses are considered safe and effective in healthy children, parents of outpatients must understand the instructions regarding the concentration and amount to be administered postoperatively. Smaller doses may be appropriate in critically ill patients and those with impaired drug clearance. Injectable forms of acetaminophen may offer an advantage in eliminating the variability of onset time.

Nonsteroidal anti-inflammatory drugs have been used in a wide variety of pediatric procedures with good safety and efficacy; the usual contraindications are concern for bleeding and renal function. As with many drugs, detailed data are not available for infants, but in limited studies, ketorolac appears to be a safe and effective analgesic for infants. NSAIDs appear to be effective in treating pain after tonsillectomy, but studies are mixed as to whether this causes an increased bleeding risk because of inhibition of platelet aggregation.

Opioid analgesics are needed after many pediatric procedures. Side effects include somnolence, vomiting, pruritus, and a risk of respiratory depression. Codeine, which has commonly been prescribed to children after surgery, is dependent on conversion to morphine for its effect; genetic variability in metabolism makes dosing relatively unreliable.[59] Fentanyl is given IV at a dose of 1 to 2 mcg/kg for short procedures. For more major procedures, a loading dose of 5 mcg/kg is followed by hourly dosing of 1 to 3 mcg/kg as needed. Morphine can be administered as a sole analgesic in a total dose of 0.1 mg/kg or titrated in smaller increments (0.02 mg/kg) after the initial use of fentanyl or another opioid intraoperatively. Nasal administration of fentanyl is useful for minor procedures when IV access is not established, such as myringotomy with tubes.[60] Remifentanil can be infused as a component of a general anesthetic technique, allowing intraoperative titration and rapid emergence, but it provides no residual postoperative analgesia. Regardless of the drugs or technique chosen, frequent assessment of analgesic efficacy and side effects, as well as access to appropriate breakthrough pain medication, is important to providing postoperative pain relief for children.

RECOVERY PROBLEMS

POSTOPERATIVE NAUSEA AND VOMITING

Postoperative vomiting is distressing to children and their parents and may delay or prevent discharge of postsurgical patients from the recovery room. Because nausea may be difficult to quantify in children, most studies focus on the incidence of vomiting. Overall, the incidence of vomiting is higher in children than in adults; the incidence appears to increase with age up to puberty and then decrease.[61] Procedures with a high incidence of postoperative vomiting in children include strabismus surgery, adenotonsillectomy, orchidopexy, and laparoscopic surgery. Gender differences are not believed to be a major factor until puberty. Even in small doses, opioids may increase the incidence of postoperative vomiting in children. Adult risk scores for postoperative nausea and vomiting do not apply well to children.[62] A 4-component pediatric risk score has been proposed using: surgery 30 minutes or longer; age 3 years or older; strabismus surgery; and positive history of postoperative vomiting in the patient, parents, or siblings.[63] Value was demonstrated in giving prophylactic antiemetics to patients with 2 or more risk factors. For patients at risk for postoperative vomiting, tailoring the anesthetic technique may be of benefit, as well as using propofol rather than volatile anesthetics[64] and regional anesthesia, NSAIDs, and acetaminophen rather than opioids. The impact of nitrous oxide in pediatric patients is as controversial as in adults, but one comparison of sevoflurane-anesthetized children did not show an increase in postoperative vomiting when nitrous oxide was used.[65] Adequate hydration intraoperatively and avoiding early oral intake may help reduce postoperative vomiting.

TABLE 64-6 Predicted Depth of Epidural Space in Children

Weight (kg)	Predicted Depth of L4-L5 Epidural Space (cm)	
	0.8 + 0.05 × Weight (kg)	1.094 + 0.048 × Weight (kg)
5	1.05	1.33
10	1.3	1.57
15	1.55	1.81
20	1.8	2.05
25	2.05	2.29
30	2.3	2.53

Data from Hasan MA, Howard RF, Lloyd-Thomas AR. Depth of epidural space in children. *Anaesthesia.* 1994;49:1085; and Ozer Y, Ozer T, Altunkaya H, Savranlar A. The posterior lumbar dural depth: an ultrasonographic study in children. *Agri.* 2005;17:53.

Pediatric dosing for antiemetic agents is summarized in **Table 64-6**.

Ondansetron and the newer 5-hydroxytryptamine$_3$ (5-HT$_3$) receptor antagonists dolasetron and granisetron have excellent efficacy for prophylaxis and treatment of postoperative vomiting in children.[66] Some dose-related improvement in antiemetic efficacy is seen, but for most patients, the lack of a significantly important effect does not justify the added expense of a larger dose. Administering ondansetron early in a case appears to be of no "preemptive" value; effect duration relates to the half-life of the drug. Dexamethasone used in tonsillectomy to prevent edema also reduces postoperative vomiting and improves pain scores. Although frequently given at 0.5 mg/kg, the antiemetic effect appears not to have a significant dose–response relationship,[67] and doses as small as 0.05 mg/kg have been shown to be effective.[68] A combination of dexamethasone and ondansetron is frequently given for antiemetic prophylaxis and may be more effective than ondansetron alone.[69]

Droperidol has largely disappeared from routine use because of the FDA "black box" drug label warning related to case reports of torsades de pointes in adults. It may be used for refractory nausea and vomiting if administered with ECG monitoring. A meta-analysis suggested that droperidol was as effective as ondansetron in adults but not in children,[70] but several individual pediatric studies found equal efficacy at higher doses of droperidol. Side effects of sedation and dysphoria may be troubling. Metoclopramide, which has commonly been given for postoperative emesis, is no more effective than placebo.[71] Finally, there is interest in nonpharmacologic antiemetic therapy in children; acupuncture or electrostimulation may be as effective as the available medications.[72]

EMERGENCE DELIRIUM

Postanesthetic agitation is a common problem in toddlers and young children; the risk factors and mechanism remain incompletely understood. Pain is a contributing factor in postanesthetic agitation, but emergence agitation also is exhibited after anesthesia for nonpainful procedures, such as magnetic resonance imaging, in children.[73] Agents that provide analgesia as well as sedation have shown efficacy in reducing agitation; these include fentanyl, ketamine, clonidine, and dexmedetomidine. Results have been mixed as to whether residual postoperative sedation with benzodiazepines or propofol reduces agitation. One study found a higher incidence of emergence delirium in children who had received midazolam premedication.[74]

Agitation occurs with variable frequency after use of all volatile agents.[75] It occurs less frequently after propofol, and crossover studies between sevoflurane and propofol show a lower incidence with propofol in individual patients, but a small percentage of children receiving frequent anesthetics exhibit severe agitation after propofol use. The perceived prominence of agitation after sevoflurane may be attributed to a higher incidence in the very early postoperative period, but the overall postanesthesia care unit incidence may be similar among the inhalation agents.[76] The actual rate of emergence does not appear to be the cause of postanesthetic delirium; children emerging at the same rate from propofol or sevoflurane showed a significantly higher agitation rate in the sevoflurane group.[77] Delaying emergence by continuing the volatile anesthetic into the postoperative period does not appear to decrease the incidence of agitation,[78] although using nitrous oxide during the washout period may reduce the incidence.[79]

In addition to acute postoperative agitation, children may develop postoperative maladaptive behavioral changes, such as changes in sleep or eating patterns, separation anxiety, and withdrawn or aggressive behavior. No clear association has been established with a specific anesthetic agent.[80,81] Kain et al[82] identified an association between preoperative anxiety in both the child and the parent, emergence delirium, and maladaptive behaviors after discharge. They suggest that some children, based on their own personality traits and those of their parents, may be more susceptible to developing these changes after the experience of anesthesia and surgery. Negative behavioral changes are more common in younger children.

SELECTED CLINICAL AREAS IN PEDIATRIC ANESTHESIA

The remainder of this chapter is devoted to specific clinical scenarios that are unique to pediatric anesthesia; the basic concepts are discussed more thoroughly in other subspecialty chapters. Other cases in pediatric anesthesia are presented within specialty chapters in this text (eg, spine surgery in Chapter 65; tonsillectomy and pediatric airway surgery in Chapter 67)

PEDIATRIC GENERAL SURGERY AND UROLOGY

Elective surgery in healthy children typically involves inhalation induction; maintenance can be with a mask or LMA for shorter or simpler procedures. General anesthesia may be supplemented with a regional technique. Hernia surgery is common in infants and children. Surgical practice varies with regard to indications for exploration of the contralateral side if no clinical evidence of a hernia is seen; this also can be done laparoscopically. For boys with undescended testes, orchidopexy is performed through a groin incision when the patient has a palpable testis or may be combined with laparoscopy when the testis cannot be felt. Although orchidopexy is performed through a groin incision similar to herniorrhaphy, orchidopexy patients tend to have more severe pain of longer duration; multimodal analgesia, including a regional technique, may be helpful. During both of these procedures, the occurrence of sudden intraoperative stimulation because of traction on the spermatic cord should be anticipated.

Hypospadias repair may require from 30 minutes to several hours and can require skin grafting or staged repair, depending on the complexity of the lesion. A caudal or penile block is frequently performed; a urethral stent may be left in at the end of surgery. Ureteral reimplantation for vesicoureteral reflux is performed through a low transverse abdominal incision. Children are hospitalized for 2 to 3 days and may have a urinary catheter in place overnight. Advances in the operative management of ureteral reimplantation (eg, minimizing use of catheters) have shortened the postoperative course. Bladder spasm may occur and can be treated with ketorolac.[83] Caudal and epidural analgesia also are frequently used for this surgery. Congenital anomalies of the kidney and ureters may lead to infection; these usually are repaired either through a flank incision or by laparoscopy.

LAPAROSCOPY IN CHILDREN

Laparoscopic operations performed in children include transperitoneal procedures such as cholecystectomy, fundoplication, appendectomy, and exploration for undescended testes; retroperitoneal approaches to the kidney and urinary tract; and use of the laparoscope to visualize the contralateral side in inguinal hernia repair. Before or during laparoscopy, producing a pneumoperitoneum with CO_2 may cause systemic hypercarbia, and a higher peak airway pressure may be needed for adequate ventilation and oxygenation.[84] Hemodynamic compromise from impairment of venous return or from gas embolism during insufflation is possible. Another potential source of gas embolization is use of argon beam coagulation during laparoscopic procedures such as partial nephrectomy.[85] Although early studies suggested a decrease in aortic blood flow and stroke volume with a compensatory increase in systemic vascular resistance, other studies in healthy children having low-pressure insufflation for laparoscopic procedures showed that the cardiac index is preserved or minimally affected.[86] Transient oliguria or anuria may occur during laparoscopy, particularly in younger children. This appears to be a reversible phenomenon in brief procedures.[87]

Laparoscopy in children usually is performed with general anesthesia. Endotracheal intubation is usually used to control respiratory changes, although an LMA may be acceptable if low intra-abdominal inflation pressures are used. Analgesia is provided by some combination of local anesthetic infiltration, acetaminophen, and NSAIDs. Caudal or epidural analgesia can be used as a supplement but may not provide any benefit over simple local infiltration for uncomplicated laparoscopy.

THORACOTOMY AND THORACOSCOPY

Children present for thoracic procedures for primary lung processes, tumor, or drainage of empyema, as well as for access to tracheal structures or vascular anomalies. Systemic hypoxia may be a problem in small children because of their nonrigid rib cages and the potential for compression of the dependent lung.[88] Video-assisted thoracoscopic surgery (VATS) is used in pediatric patients for biopsy or limited resection of a tumor or infectious lesions and for drainage and decortication of empyema. Empyema may develop as a complication of community-acquired pneumonia even in otherwise healthy patients, and early VATS results in fewer postoperative complications and a shorter overall hospital stay compared with tube thoracostomy.[89]

Traditionally, thoracotomy in children was performed with the surgeon packing 1 lung out of the surgical field. However, thoracoscopy and advances in equipment and anesthetic techniques (bronchial blockers, fiberoptic bronchoscopes) have led to broader use of 1-lung ventilation in children. Double-lumen tubes, when available in appropriate sizes, allow suctioning of each lung and provision of oxygen and CPAP to the deflated lung. The outer diameter of available tubes must be compared with the expected tracheal and bronchial sizes.[90] The smallest available double-lumen tube is 26 Fr, which is slightly larger than a 6.5-mm ID endotracheal tube suitable for children as young as 8 years. The Univent tube is a single-lumen tube with a built-in bronchial blocker; a 3.5-mm ID Univent tube has an external diameter similar to a standard 6.0 endotracheal tube. In children younger than 6 years of age, options for 1-lung ventilation include use of a bronchial blocker (placed using a fiberoptic bronchoscope) or intentional mainstem bronchial intubation (blindly or with fiberoptic guidance). If mainstem intubation is planned, a smaller endotracheal tube must be used than would be chosen for tracheal placement; a small cuffed tube allows lung reinflation after the tube is withdrawn into the trachea. Options for 1-lung ventilation in children are summarized in **Table 64-7**.

Other considerations for pediatric thoracic surgery include adequate venous access and appropriate monitoring. Use of an arterial catheter

TABLE 64-7 Antiemetic Doses for Children

Drug	Dose
Ondansetron	50-100 mcg/kg up to 4 mg
Dolasetron	350 mcg/kg up to 12.5 mg
Dexamethasone	150 mcg/kg up to 8 mg
Droperidol	50-75 mcg/kg up to 1.25 mg (reserve for refractory vomiting and use under monitored conditions)
Dimenhydrinate	0.5 mg/kg
Perphenazine	70 mcg/kg

From Gan TJ, Meyer T, Apfel CC, et al. Consensus guidelines for managing postoperative nausea and vomiting. *Anesth Analg* 2003;97:62, with permission.

depends on the extent of the procedure and the underlying lung function. Most children can be extubated after a thoracotomy or VATS unless respiratory function is severely impaired. Appropriate analgesia is helpful in speeding recovery; for open procedures, this may include administration of a local anesthetic with or without an opioid through a thoracic epidural catheter or via a caudal catheter threaded to the thoracic region in small children.

PECTUS EXCAVATUM AND THE NUSS PROCEDURE

Pectus excavatum is the most common congenital chest wall deformity of children. Left uncorrected, it can result in respiratory and cardiac compromise. Traditionally, pectus excavatum was corrected during the teenage years by an open approach. More recently, a convex steel bar is inserted ("Nuss procedure") to mechanically raise the sternum. Cartilage remodels over time, and the bar is removed several years later. After bar removal, patients have a subjective improvement in functional status and a small but significant improvement in pulmonary function studies.[91] Preoperatively, most patients have some mild degree of exercise limitation, but significant dyspnea should prompt further evaluation. The mechanism of exercise limitation in pectus excavatum may reflect a combination of restrictive lung disease and impaired right ventricular function. Pulmonary function testing and echocardiography are frequently performed but probably are not essential except for patients with significant symptoms.

Early studies of the Nuss procedure reported a moderate intraoperative complication rate, including cardiac compression, disruption of great vessels with significant hemorrhage, and tension pneumothorax. A very low rate of complications occurs now because of improved surgeon experience and refinement of the surgical technique, particularly the use of thoracoscopy to guide bar placement.[92] Postoperative complications include dislodgement of the bar (which has been minimized through use of lateral stabilizers), pneumothorax, pneumonia, and significant pain. Outcomes appear better in younger patients, and the trend is toward correcting these deformities in the preteen years.

The Nuss procedure is performed with general anesthesia, often in conjunction with a thoracic epidural. Arterial lines (frequently placed in the early days of this procedure because of concern for hemodynamic compromise and blood loss) are rarely required. The duration of surgery is approximately 2 hours; patients can be extubated at the end of the procedure unless they experienced intraoperative difficulties. Although pectus bar placement is considered a minimally invasive procedure, the initial postoperative period can involve significant pain caused by the pressure of the bar. Thoracic epidural infusion of local anesthetic and opioid is commonly used for the first 2 to 3 days.

CANCER-RELATED PROCEDURES IN CHILDREN

Abdominal Tumors Neuroblastoma, the most common extracranial solid tumor of childhood, arises from neural crest cells. Risk varies depending on clinical stage and biologic features of the individual tumor. Children with neuroblastoma require biopsy for diagnosis and multiple imaging studies during treatment. Treatment may include limited or aggressive surgical resection, chemotherapy, and radiation therapy. High-risk patients may receive a bone marrow transplant. Considerations for resection include adequate venous access, arterial monitoring if extensive blood loss is expected, and a complete blood count if chemotherapy has been given before surgery. A subset of these tumors may produce significant catecholamine secretion, causing perioperative hemodynamic lability.

Wilms tumor (nephroblastoma) most commonly occurs in young children. If diagnosed in its early stages, it can be approached by laparoscopic nephrectomy. However, the tumor may remain asymptomatic until the mass is quite large, and resection may involve a more extensive procedure. If vascular and intracardiac extensions have occurred, then cardiopulmonary bypass may be required for resection. Renin production or renovascular compression may result in hypertension. Treatment and prognosis are stratified by surgical stage and histologic type.

Mediastinal Mass Tumors, particularly lymphoma, may develop rapidly and present with respiratory symptoms related to mediastinal involvement. Inducing general anesthesia may lead to compression of the airway or vascular structures when thoracic muscle tone is reduced, with catastrophic results. Exercise tolerance and tolerance of the supine position may give some idea of the severity of disease, but absence of symptoms does not eliminate the possibility of difficulties during anesthetic induction. Respiratory flow–volume loops can be helpful in delineating the extent of airway compression. Unless the possibility of airway and vascular compression can be ruled out with preoperative tests, serious consideration should be given to performing a minimal procedure with local anesthesia to obtain the diagnosis and deferring major interventions until initial treatment has reduced the tumor mass. If general anesthesia is required, maintenance of spontaneous respiration is preferred and can be accomplished with volatile or IV agents (propofol, opioids, ketamine). A head-up or lateral induction position may prove helpful. Emergency backup plans should be formulated before induction and may include rigid bronchoscopy and cardiopulmonary bypass.[93]

ANESTHESIA FOR PEDIATRIC NEUROSURGERY

Even in the absence of overt signs or symptoms of increased intracranial pressure (ICP), children presenting for ventriculoperitoneal shunt revision, resection of a brain tumor, or posterior fossa decompression may be near the point of decompensation and should be managed so that ICP does not increase. The history should address recent nausea and vomiting and the potential for volume depletion as well as aspiration risk. Preoperatively, oversedation should be avoided because of the risk for hypercarbia, but individual patients may benefit from judicious premedication in a monitored setting to minimize agitation. Intraoperatively, the various inhalational agents may cause a slight increase of ICP; maintenance of mean arterial pressure is critical to maintain the cerebral perfusion pressure.[94] Steroids, anticonvulsant medications, or both are usually continued perioperatively. If treatment of increased ICP is needed, hyperventilation, mannitol infusion (0.5-1 g/kg), increasing anesthetic depth, and drainage of CSF all may be appropriate.

VENTRICULOPERITONEAL SHUNT

Ventriculoperitoneal shunts in infants are discussed in detail in Chapter 63. Older children may require replacement or revision of shunts because of malfunction or growth, or they may require new shunts after tumor resection or discovery of other intracranial pathology. In some cases of cysts or other obstruction to CSF outflow, endoscopic ventriculostomy may restore normal flow patterns and obviate the need for shunting. Patients with multiple shunts may have an acquired latex allergy or may be receiving treatment in a latex-free environment to prevent sensitization.

CRANIOTOMY FOR TUMOR

A higher percentage of brain tumors are infratentorial in pediatric patients than in adults, with medulloblastoma and astrocytoma being the common posterior fossa lesions. Other common tumors include the supratentorial counterparts of medulloblastoma (pineoblastoma and primitive neuroectodermal tumor), glioma, and ependymoma. Anesthetic management for craniotomy is discussed in more depth in Chapter 51. In general for a pediatric craniotomy, adequate peripheral venous access and an arterial line are needed. Central lines are of limited use for aspirating air in the pediatric population and usually are not placed for this purpose in smaller children. If the anatomy and positioning suggest a risk of venous air embolus, then precordial Doppler monitoring should be used. Depending on the location of the tumor and the course of surgery, development of diabetes insipidus or other endocrine abnormalities may occur during or after surgery.

POSTERIOR FOSSA DECOMPRESSION

Chiari type I malformation, a caudal displacement of the cerebellar tonsils through the foramen magnum into the spinal canal, may result in a variety of symptoms, including headache or other pain, weakness, ataxia, and sensory loss. Patients may have brainstem and spinal cord dysfunction, the latter often as a result of syrinx formation. Surgical management consists of suboccipital craniectomy with posterior fossa decompression. Extreme flexion should be avoided to minimize the risk of brainstem compression. Postoperatively, these patients may have respiratory abnormalities, perhaps related to ischemia or edema of the brainstem respiratory centers.

CRANIOSYNOSTOSIS

Craniosynostosis represents premature closure of 1 or more cranial sutures. The incidence is approximately 1 in 2000 births, with more boys than girls affected. Uncorrected, craniosynostosis may lead to increased ICP. Correction may be performed for cosmetic reasons. Simple craniosynostoses usually are corrected between 3 and 6 months of age, with more complex craniofacial reconstruction after 9 months of age. Significant blood loss and venous air embolism are risks of the procedure; overall, morbidity and mortality are low. Adverse events are significantly associated with secondary versus primary operation and in patients with craniofacial syndromes.

Craniosynostosis may be an isolated defect or part of a craniofacial syndrome, such as Crouzon or Apert syndrome, which can include a difficult airway, cleft palate, syndactyly, and cardiac or other abnormalities. Children with uncorrected complex craniosynostosis may have increased ICP; decreased cerebral perfusion pressure; and obstructive respiratory symptoms, particularly during sleep.[95]

Preparation for the case includes consideration of positioning, access to the patient and lines, and avoidance of soft tissue or ischemic injury. Surgeons may request elevation of the head to enhance venous drainage; however, this advantage must be weighed against the risk of venous air entrainment. Goals of anesthetic management include minimizing severe increases in ICP. Hyperventilation, administration of mannitol, or both may be indicated if the craniectomy is technically difficult. Monitoring must include evaluation of circulating blood volume status, blood loss and associated metabolic changes, and maintenance of temperature. Adequate venous access and availability of blood and blood products are critical to safe management.

Craniosynostosis repair requires transfusion in almost 95% of patients; however, newer surgical techniques may result in reduced blood loss.[96] Techniques that have been used to minimize allogeneic blood transfusion include preoperative administration of erythropoietin, selection of an optimal age to achieve a favorable balance between fetal and adult hemoglobin, preoperative preparation of an autologous blood supply, and intraoperative and postoperative blood salvage and reinfusion. When massive transfusion is required, coagulopathy may develop.[97]

Several studies suggest that venous air embolism occurs frequently during craniosynostosis repair, although the majority of episodes are not hemodynamically significant.[98] Maintenance of adequate vascular volume, positive-pressure ventilation, and precordial Doppler or end-tidal nitrogen monitoring for early detection may all help to minimize the incidence and consequences. Management of venous air embolism includes putting the head down, flooding the field with saline, and using bone wax to attempt to limit the amount of entrained air. Compression of the jugular veins may increase venous pressure and prevent further air entrainment. Aspiration of air is technically difficult to achieve in small children.

After routine craniosynostosis repair, most patients with a normal airway can be extubated. Ideally, an anesthetic technique is chosen so that surgery is completed with adequate analgesia and a calm patient but with the ability to evaluate neurologic status. Ongoing blood loss from drains may require further transfusions during the next 24 hours. If the procedure was extensive or blood loss was very large, hemodynamic stability or swelling may suggest the need to leave the patient intubated and perhaps mechanically ventilated in the early postoperative period.

PEDIATRIC AMBULATORY SURGERY

Many pediatric procedures can be performed on an outpatient basis; this is frequently done in a mixed adult and pediatric setting, but facilities, equipment, and staff competencies must be suitable for children. The general concepts of ambulatory anesthesia discussed in Chapter 68 apply to children: the anesthetic should be tailored to rapid recovery with attention to pain management and control of postoperative vomiting. A qualified caregiver should be present at home for the remainder of the day and night, and parents must be given careful instructions about postoperative medications and any signs or symptoms that should prompt contact with or return to the hospital.

OUT-OF-OPERATING ROOM PROCEDURES IN CHILDREN

Children frequently require anesthesia for even nonpainful procedures simply because they are unable to hold still. Teaching about the procedure and distraction may help some older children to cooperate. Planning an appropriate anesthetic requires evaluation of the patient as well as understanding the logistics of the procedure. General considerations about safety in offsite anesthesia locations are presented in Chapter 69.

Magnetic resonance imaging scans can range from 15 minutes to several hours in length; some sequences are noisy, and some are associated with significant vibration of the table. Simple scans are often done with the child breathing spontaneously with a propofol infusion and supplemental oxygen. Certain abdominal and cardiac scans may require breath-holding to optimize the image; this as well as scan length may prompt a general anesthetic with controlled ventilation. Equipment safety in the magnetic environment is a prime concern; the child is monitored either directly or through a window with remote monitors.

Radiation therapy is often done with a similar propofol technique. For radiation of the head and neck area, the child is immobilized in a rigid face mask; ensuring an adequate area during construction of the mask is extremely important. If at all possible, airway instrumentation is avoided because children will come for sequential treatment over a prolonged period.

Endoscopy is performed frequently in pediatric patients for a variety of indications (eg, evaluation of bleeding, inflammatory bowel disease, esophagitis from a variety of etiologies, malabsorption or failure to thrive). Knowing the proceduralist and what to expect are key; these cases are often done with spontaneous respiration using propofol with or without an opioid.

Finally, brief diagnostic and therapeutic procedures such as lumbar puncture and bone marrow aspiration are often performed in oncology clinics and sedation rooms. Because these children usually have indwelling venous access, propofol with or without an opioid is again a frequent choice. Use of topical local anesthetic cream over the site can be useful in minimizing anesthetic requirements.

CONCLUSION

The practice of pediatric anesthesia encompasses a broad spectrum of surgery and patients and creates many challenges in terms of patient and family dynamics, technical skills, and anatomic and physiologic factors. Meticulous attention to detail and anticipation of common perioperative problems are essential, as are training and ongoing experience in the care of children.

KEY REFERENCES

- Birmingham PK, Tobin MJ, Fisher DM, et al. Initial and subsequent dosing of rectal acetaminophen in children: a 24-hour pharmacokinetic study of new dose recommendations. *Anesthesiology.* 2001;94:385.
- Cote CJ, Zaslavsky A, Downes JJ, et al. Postoperative apnea in former preterm infants after inguinal herniorrhaphy. *Anesthesiology.* 1995;82:809.
- Giaufre E, Dalens B, Gombert A. Epidemiology and morbidity of regional anesthesia in children: a one-year prospective survey of the French-Language Society of Pediatric Anesthesiologists. *Anesth Analg.* 1996;83:904.
- Hackel A, Badgwell JM, Binding RR, et al. Guidelines for the pediatric perioperative anesthesia environment. *Pediatrics.* 1999; 103:512.
- Kain ZN, Caldwell-Andrews AA, Weinberg ME, et al. Sevoflurane versus halothane: postoperative maladaptive behavioral changes: a randomized, controlled trial. *Anesthesiology.* 2005;102:720.
- Kain ZN, Mayes LC, Wang SM, et al. Parental presence and a sedative premedicant for children undergoing surgery: a hierarchical study. *Anesthesiology.* 2000;92:939.
- Krane E, Dalens B, Murat I, et al. Epidural catheters in anesthetized patients. *Reg Anesth Pain Med.* 1998;23:433.
- Mamie C, Habre W, Delhumeau C, et al. Incidence and risk factors of perioperative respiratory adverse events in children undergoing elective surgery. *Paediatr Anaesth.* 2004;14:218.
- Morray JP, Geiduschek JM, Caplan RA, et al. A comparison of pediatric and adult anesthesia closed malpractice claims. *Anesthesiology.* 1993;78:461.
- Murat I, Constant I, Maud'huy H. Perioperative anaesthetic morbidity in children: a database of 24,165 anaesthetics over a 30-month period. *Paediatr Anaesth.* 2004;14:158.
- Tait AR, Malviya S. Anesthesia for the child with an upper respiratory tract infection: still a dilemma? *Anesth Analg.* 2005;100:59.

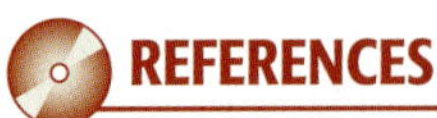

REFERENCES

Complete references available on DVD and online version at www.LongneckerAnesthesiology.com

CHAPTER 65

Anesthesia for Orthopedic Surgery

Joshua Dooley
Gavin Martin

KEY POINTS

1. Orthopedic surgery is associated with high incidences of deep venous thrombosis and pulmonary embolism.
2. The need for anticoagulation results in anesthesia issues specifically related to the potential for neuroaxial hematomas.
3. Unique complications in orthopedic surgery are related to tourniquet use and fat embolism.
4. Regional anesthesia is associated with lower morbidity and mortality than is general anesthesia.
5. Prone spinal surgery cases have unique complications related to patient positioning, such as nerve injuries, ventilation problems, and blindness.

Orthopedic anesthesia presents many challenges to anesthesiologists. Patients range in age from infant to centenarian. This patient population shows the full spectrum of comorbidities. Many of the procedures are associated with significant postoperative pain. Surgery on isolated extremities can be performed using a variety of regional anesthetic techniques for both anesthesia and postoperative analgesia. However, providing adequate analgesia using central neuraxial techniques can be challenging, especially when deep venous thrombosis (DVT) prophylaxis with low-molecular-weight heparin (LMWH) is needed. This challenge has led to the development of many peripheral nerve block techniques and advances in the equipment used for these techniques, including continuous nerve catheters and ultrasonography for identification of nerve plexuses. Recent literature has shown a benefit of regional anesthesia over general anesthesia with respect to mortality, morbidity, postoperative analgesia, and functional recovery. The use of ultrasonography to place nerve blocks may offer a significant advantage over peripheral nerve stimulation. A meta-analysis looking at the advantage of ultrasonography over nerve stimulation technique showed improved efficacy in respect to onset and quality of block.[1] It also appears that the minimum amount of local anesthetic required to successfully perform the nerve block may be greatly reduced by using ultrasonography instead of the traditional nerve stimulation technique.[2] This may be of great benefit in reducing the incidence of local anesthetic toxicity. This chapter considers the factors pertinent to anesthesia for orthopedic surgery and reviews the appropriate management.

SPECIFIC PROBLEMS IN ORTHOPEDIC PATIENTS

RHEUMATOID ARTHRITIS

Because of the nature of the disease, patients with rheumatoid arthritis present for many orthopedic procedures, ranging from joint replacement surgery to cervical spine surgery. These patients can be very challenging to treat for a variety of reasons. Deformities of the extremities are common, which may make arterial and intravenous (IV) access and positioning of the patient more difficult. Great care must be taken when positioning patients, with adequate padding needed to prevent pressure necrosis of the patient's skin. Positioning the patient while he or she is awake often is useful. Of major concern in any patient with rheumatoid arthritis is the possibility of cervical spine instability.[3] Cervical spine involvement occurs in more than half of patients with rheumatoid arthritis, with atlantoaxial dislocation the most common abnormality. Pain and evidence of spinal cord injury are the main symptoms and

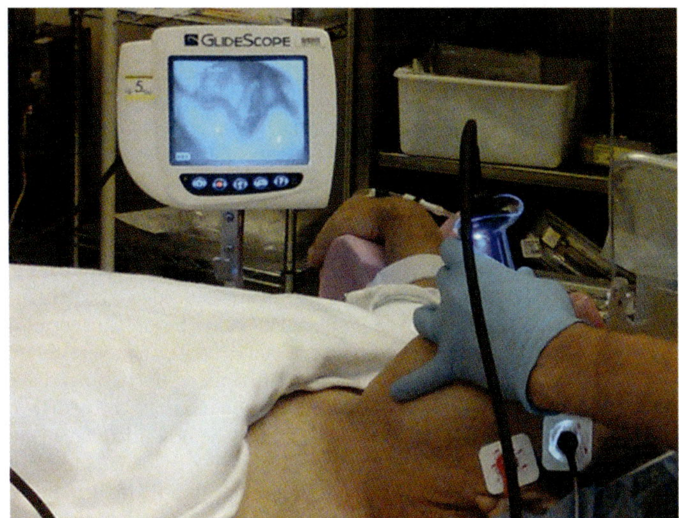

FIGURE 65-1. View of the vocal cords on a digital screen from a video laryngoscope.

signs of cervical spine involvement. However, the presence of symptoms may not correlate with the severity of radiologic abnormalities. Computed tomography and magnetic resonance imaging provide detailed images of the bone and spinal cord and should be considered in at-risk patients before anesthesia is provided. Flexion and extension cervical radiographic views may be required to exclude instability and are often done as first-line imaging of the cervical spine. Cervical spine instability may be overlooked in some patients based on clinical examination alone. Temporomandibular involvement may further restrict the anesthesiologist's ability to gain adequate access to the airway.[2] Both atlantoaxial instability and temporomandibular involvement may necessitate an awake fiberoptic intubation. The development of fiberoptic laryngoscopes has altered the management of rheumatoid patients when general anesthesia with intubation is considered necessary. These fiberoptic laryngoscopes allow the physician to proceed with induction in the usual fashion and use the optics of the device to navigate difficult airways (**Fig. 65-1**). However, patients with confirmed subluxation in the cervical segment should be intubated under appropriate sedation that allows for the assessment of neurologic symptoms in case of spinal cord trauma. Another airway problem is related to the potential for cricoarytenoid arthritis, which makes passage of an endotracheal tube extremely difficult.[4] Passing of an endotracheal tube in itself may cause dislocation of the laryngeal cartilages. Hoarseness and inspiratory stridor may indicate the presence of cricoarytenoid arthritis.

As a systemic disease, rheumatoid arthritis may result in a variety of organ dysfunctions (**Table 65-1**). Pulmonary, cardiac, renal, and hematologic changes are important to anesthesiologists. All of these systems must be thoroughly assessed before any surgical procedure. Patients with rheumatoid arthritis are commonly managed with a variety of drugs, including steroids and nonsteroidal anti-inflammatory drugs (NSAIDs). Thus, patients may require preoperative steroid supplementation to prevent acute adrenocortical insufficiency and cardiovascular collapse during anesthesia. However, use of NSAIDs is controversial because of implications with regard to their effects on gastric mucosa, renal toxicity, platelet dysfunction, and cardiovascular effects. Use of cyclooxygenase-2 (COX-2) inhibitors, such as celecoxib, may allow reduction in the prevalence of hemorrhage in the gastrointestinal tract as well as renal dysfunction. Recent studies have shown an increase in death from cardiovascular events in patients taking these drugs long term. The Food and Drug Administration (FDA) subsequently issued a warning that COX-2 inhibitors potentially increase the risk of heart attack and stroke.[5] The risk however, appears to be similar to that of other NSAIDs. It appears that all NSAIDs increase the risk of cardiovascular events. Methotrexate, also used in the management of rheumatoid arthritis, is responsible for hematologic and pulmonary side effects, including pancytopenia and irreversible pulmonary fibrosis. Etanercept, a tumor necrosis factor inhibitor used in the management of patients with aggressive rheumatoid arthritis, has also been suggested to be the cause of acute lung injury and polyneuropathy because of demyelinization of nerve fibers.

TABLE 65-1 Extra-articular Manifestations of Rheumatoid Arthritis

Cardiovascular	Pericardial inflammation and effusions, myocarditis, vasculitis, valvular fibrosis
Pulmonary	Pleural effusions, pulmonary fibrosis, pulmonary granulomata, fibrotic nodules (Caplan syndrome)
Hematopoietic	Normocytic normochromic anemia, Felty syndrome (enlarged spleen, leucopenia, and recurrent infections), platelet dysfunction (NSAID therapy)
Renal	Amyloidosis
Endocrine	Adrenal insufficiency (glucocorticoid therapy)

NSAID, nonsteroidal anti-inflammatory drug.

BLOOD LOSS

Orthopedic surgery can be associated with significant blood loss, particularly trauma surgery, multilevel back surgery, redo arthroplasty surgery, and surgery in which tourniquet use is precluded. Spinal and joint replacement surgeries offer a unique problem because of the large surface of cancellous bone that is exposed during surgery. Bleeding from cancellous bone is not easily controlled using standard techniques such as vessel ligation and cautery.

Despite improvement in the screening process for allogenic blood donations, there still exists the potential for transmission of infectious diseases and transfusion reactions. Bierbaum et al[6] investigated the need for blood transfusion in 9482 patients who had undergone total hip or total knee replacement surgery. Fifty-five percent of patients undergoing hip surgery and 39% of the knee replacement patients required some form of blood transfusion. Of these patients, 66% received autologous blood, and 34% received allogenic blood. Patients who receive a blood product transfusion are more likely to have infections and thus an increased hospital stay. Techniques regularly used in orthopedic surgery to reduce the need for allogenic blood transfusion include hypotensive anesthesia, preoperative hemoglobin optimization using iron and erythropoietin, preoperative autologous blood donation, acute normovolemic hemodilution, and intraoperative and postoperative red blood cell salvage techniques.[7-9] Hypotensive anesthesia has been shown to significantly reduce blood loss during surgery. A study by Sharrock et al[10] showed that intraoperative blood loss in 250 consecutive hip replacement patients was approximately 250 mL if the surgery was performed with hypotensive anesthesia. The lower arterial and central venous pressures and—importantly—lower peripheral venous blood pressure in the surgical wound may explain this difference. This study showed that hypotensive anesthesia produced by regional anesthesia is superior to general hypotensive anesthesia.[10] Of concern with any hypotensive technique is the potential for increasing ischemic cardiovascular and neurologic events, which was not seen in the study by Sharrock et al.[10] However, this technique should be used with caution in elderly adults and in patients with a significant cardiovascular history. The use of hypotensive techniques in the prone position should be cautioned because of the potential complication of postoperative blindness. The subject is discussed at a later stage in this chapter.

Preoperative autologous blood donation has been widely used in orthopedic patients but has many drawbacks, including iatrogenic anemia, high cost, clerical errors resulting in transfusion reactions, and wastage of blood products. Its main benefit is the potential to reduce the transmission of infectious diseases and the avoidance of immune-mediated transfusion reactions such as acute lung injury. A benefit of intraoperative normovolemic hemodilution over autologous blood donation is that the blood is taken off and replaced with crystalloid or colloid just before incision, and the blood remains with the patient at all times. This process reduces the potential for clerical errors that lead to transfusion reactions and substantially reduces cost. Downsides to this technique are that it is labor intensive and that excessive hemodilution may result in coagulation disturbances. Recombinant human erythropoietin used either in conjunction with autologous blood donation or normovolemic hemodilution or alone has the potential to ensure higher preoperative hematocrits and reduce the need for allogenic blood transfusion.[11] Use of procoagulants, such as tranexamic acid (proteinase inhibitor) and aminocaproic acid, is not routine but may reduce intraoperative blood loss.[12,13] These medications block proteolytic enzymes such as plasmin, the enzyme responsible for fibrinolysis. The concern with use of any procoagulant, especially in joint replacement surgery, is the possibility of an increased incidence of DVT, although studies have not shown this side effect.[14]

CEREBRAL PALSY AND PEDIATRIC ORTHOPEDIC SURGERY

Cerebral palsy (CP) is a nonprogressive neurologic disorder that results from a variety of insults that may occur perinatally and during the first 2 years of life. The incidence of CP is estimated at 2.4 per 1000 live births.[15] Most cases of CP are of unknown etiology. Known causes of CP include antenatal infections, thyroid disease, asphyxia, meningitis, and trauma. Premature infants have a greater incidence of CP because of periventricular hemorrhages. A variety of classification systems for CP are available, with the Swedish classification the most commonly used.[16] Spastic CP constitutes 70% of cases followed by dyskinetic CP (10%), ataxic CP (10%), and mixed CP (10%). Children with CP commonly present for orthopedic procedures, such as tenotomies and osteotomies, to improve their gait and posture. Another common orthopedic procedure is surgery for scoliosis correction. A number of anesthetic considerations must be considered when anesthetizing children with CP. These pediatric patients have a high incidence of chronic respiratory infections because of repeated aspiration and a restrictive lung pattern caused by the presence of a scoliotic spine. The high incidence of aspiration is related to gastroesophageal reflux and the presence of bulbar palsies, which limit the child's ability to cough and clear oropharyngeal secretions. In fact, the second most common cause for surgery after orthopedic procedures is Nissen fundoplication for gastroesophageal reflux. These children should be seen preoperatively with special assessment of their respiratory function. They may require antibiotics, bronchodilators, and physiotherapy to optimize their conditions before they undergo surgery. Approximately 30% of children with CP also have epilepsy, most commonly the spastic hemiplegia variety. Anticonvulsant medication should be continued up to the time of surgery and restarted as soon as possible after surgery. Latex allergy resulting from the number of procedures these children undergo is common and should be sought in all children with CP. A latex-free environment for all CP cases should be practiced. Benzodiazepines and baclofen all have been used in CP children to reduce muscle tone. Baclofen acts as an inhibitor of γ-aminobutyric acid, an inhibitory neurotransmitter, and has been shown to reduce pain and the development of contractures associated with increased muscle spasms.[17] Baclofen can be given orally, but an intrathecal pump is the preferred route of administration. Because abrupt withdrawal of baclofen can result in seizures and hallucinations, it should be continued in the perioperative period.[17] Baclofen has been implicated in delayed arousal, bradycardia, and hypotension during general anesthesia.[18] Premedication with sedatives should be considered, but care is necessary, especially in hypotonic children, because a sedative may easily compromise the child's airway. Antacids and prokinetics should be used because of the high incidence of gastroesophageal reflux. Antisialagogues, such as glycopyrrolate, also should be considered to reduce the oropharyngeal secretions. The presence of gastroesophageal reflux may necessitate a rapid-sequence induction, but the muscle relaxant of choice is controversial. Studies have shown an increased number of extrajunctional acetylcholine receptors at the neuromuscular junction in children with CP, making hyperkalemia a potential problem when succinylcholine is used for muscle relaxation.[19,20] In addition, use of succinylcholine in children is controversial because of the potential for anaphylactic reactions. Nondepolarizing agents show less potency in children with CP, so larger doses of nondepolarizing agents may be needed to maintain a neuromuscular block during surgery.[21] The mean alveolar concentrations of the inhalational agents are lower in children with CP compared with normal children.[22] Intraoperative hypothermia caused by hypothalamic dysfunction is often a problem, and extra care is needed to maintain normothermia. Postoperative pain management can be an issue because of the child's inability to communicate adequately. Regional anesthetic techniques, such as caudals, epidurals, and peripheral nerve blocks, are very useful in these situations. Because of the young age of pediatric patients, these regional techniques often must be administered while the children are under general anesthesia. However, evidence indicates that this can be performed safely.[23] Epidural combinations of local anesthetics, opioids, and clonidine may be useful for postoperative pain management but require adequate postoperative management to detect oversedation and respiratory depression.

ANTIBIOTIC PROPHYLAXIS

Surgical site infections remain a serious complication in surgery. A recent advisory statement from Medicare National Surgical Infection Prevention Project states that infusion of the first antimicrobial dose should begin within 60 minutes before surgical incision.[24] When a fluoroquinolone or vancomycin is indicated, infusion of the first antimicrobial dose should begin within 120 minutes before the incision because these drugs have significantly longer half-lives.[24] Adhering to this advisory statement is imperative not only to decrease the risk of surgical site infections but also to attain full reimbursement.

MAJOR ORTHOPEDIC PROCEDURES

ANESTHESIA FOR EXTREMITY SURGERY

A general anesthetic can be used as the anesthetic of choice for all orthopedic procedures. However, a regional anesthetic technique can be used to provide both anesthesia and postoperative analgesia for a variety of orthopedic procedures, including arthroscopic, fracture, and joint replacement surgery. For lower limb surgery, central neuroaxial techniques can be used in addition to peripheral nerve blocks.

UPPER EXTREMITY SURGERY

The variety of brachial plexus blocks available means that several options for block technique can be used for upper extremity procedures.[25] The most important factor in choosing a block is the anticipated location of the incision, although other variables can affect the decision. Patient factors, such as weight, degree of pulmonary dysfunction, and coagulation status, also play a role. Choice of local anesthetic depends on balancing the time of onset with the desired duration of block. For procedures on the shoulder, interscalene block using 30 to 40 mL of local anesthetic is the preferred technique. This dose should ensure block of the suprascapular nerve, which branches off from the plexus quite proximally. Superficial cervical plexus block also is important, although it usually is achieved as an effect of an interscalene block. To cover anterior incision sites, supplemental intercostobrachial nerve block is needed as well. The sensory distribution of this nerve is highly variable. To cover posterior incision sites, paravertebral blocks of the T1 and T2 nerve roots or skin infiltration by the surgeon are necessary. If paravertebral blocks are used, separate injection of the intercostobrachial nerve is unnecessary. Anesthesia from the midhumerus to the hand can be achieved with a supraclavicular, infraclavicular, or axillary block. Each of these techniques has unique advantages and drawbacks that may make that technique particularly useful in a given patient. Ultrasonography is playing

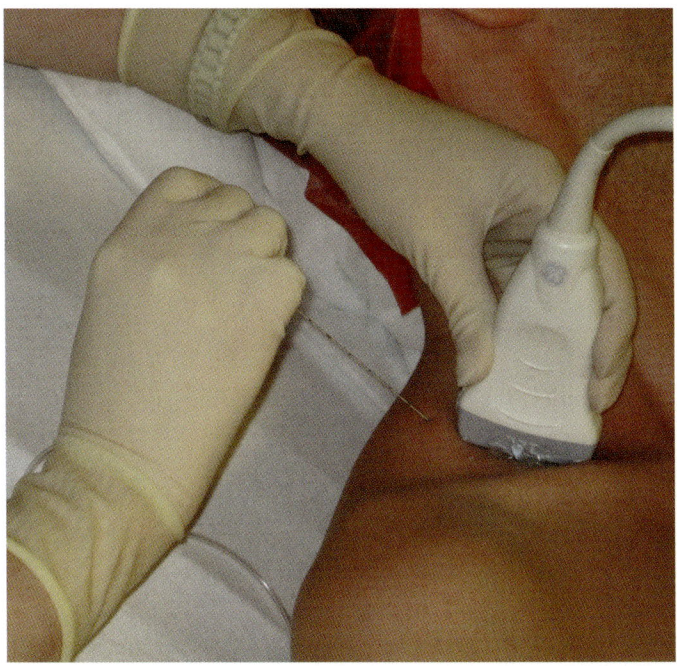

FIGURE 65-2. Supraclavicular nerve block using ultrasound.

an increasing role, particularly in more superficial upper extremity blocks (**Fig. 65-2**). Supplemental injection of the peripheral nerves more distally can be performed to salvage partially successful proximal blocks. Bier block can be used to perform short-duration forearm and hand surgery, but it does not provide postoperative analgesia. A description of the various peripheral nerve block techniques is given in Chapter 48.

Shoulder Replacement Surgery More than 80 000 shoulder arthroplasty procedures are performed annually in the United States. Shoulder replacement surgery, similar to knee and hip replacement surgery, can result in significant postoperative pain. Both general anesthesia and interscalene nerve blocks can be used for anesthesia, either alone or combination. Increasingly more shoulder procedures are performed on an outpatient basis, which has necessitated the use of a variety of techniques to improve postoperative pain. Use of interscalene nerve blocks alone for anesthesia and analgesia offers patients a significant advantage in terms of pain scores, time to ambulation, time to discharge, and need for unexpected admission compared with general anesthesia.[26] Other techniques used for postoperative pain include intra-articular infusions of local anesthetics and suprascapular nerve blocks. The continuous delivery of intra-articular local anesthetic via means of an indwelling-catheter has recently been discredited because of the erosion of the articular cartilage by the local anesthetic infusion. Suprascapular nerve blocks have been shown to be superior compared with patient-controlled IV analgesia.[27] Potential benefits of suprascapular nerve block compared with interscalene nerve block are ease of performance, lower volumes of local anesthetics needed, and fewer complications such as phrenic nerve paralysis and intrathecal injection. The major drawback of suprascapular block compared with interscalene nerve block is that suprascapular nerve block must be combined with general anesthesia, thus necessitating airway manipulation and exposing the patient to the deleterious physiologic changes associated with general anesthesia. In some studies, intra-articular infusion of bupivacaine has shown no benefit compared with placebo.[28] Many shoulder surgeries are undertaken with the patient placed in a 45-degree semirecumbent position (beach chair position). This position presents problems related to potential difficulties with airway access if a regional anesthetic is the sole anesthetic technique. It is essential to test whether the interscalene block is adequate for the surgical procedure before the procedure is started because access to the airway during the case can be difficult. Another problem with this position is reduced venous return to the right side of the heart, resulting in reduced preload and potential hypotension, especially with use of general anesthesia. This condition may result in the need for increased fluid resuscitation. Lower extremity noninvasive blood pressure measurements should be used with caution, if at all, because these measurements do not provide accurate information for determining cerebral perfusion pressure for the patient in a beach chair position. To ensure cerebral perfusion is adequate, continuous processed electroencephalogram or cerebral oximetry should be monitored on some patients in the beach chair position.[29] These considerations include patients with previous neurologic ischemic events, carotid stenosis, arterial vascular disease, and significant cardiovascular risk.

Patients with significant cardiovascular problems should be positioned slowly, and the anesthesiologist should always be aware of the potential for venous air embolism, particularly with patients in the sitting position.

The problems of embolic phenomenon, as seen in hip or knee replacement surgery, are generally not seen in shoulder replacement surgery. In general, use of invasive lines, such as central lines and arterial lines, is not required for these cases, depending on the presence of comorbidities.

LOWER EXTREMITY SURGERY

Many different regional anesthesia techniques are available for lower extremity orthopedic surgery.[30] Neuraxial techniques are appropriate for any lower extremity procedure in most patients, but aggressive use of postoperative anticoagulation for prevention of DVT and pulmonary embolism (PE) may limit the use of postoperative epidural analgesia. Peripheral nerve blocks with or without continuous catheter use offer an alternative to neuraxial techniques, which may be safer in the setting of perioperative anticoagulation with efficacy at least equal to that of epidural analgesia. For procedures on the hip and proximal femur, lumbar plexus block[30] in conjunction with a proximal sciatic nerve block[30,31] provides acceptable analgesia. A femoral nerve block can be used instead of a lumbar plexus block, although it is less likely to provide block of the obturator and lateral femoral cutaneous nerves.[32] Addition of paravertebral nerve blocks at the first and second lumbar levels may be needed to provide complete anesthesia. Alternatively, the procedure can be accomplished using a spinal anesthetic alone or a combination of spinal anesthesia with a lumbar plexus and sciatic blocks or catheters for postoperative analgesia. Epidural or combined spinal epidural anesthesia provides a simpler route of anesthesia and analgesia[33] and may be acceptable for postoperative use if the epidural is managed in accordance with the third consensus statement on neuraxial anesthesia and anticoagulation of the American Society of Regional Anesthesia and Pain Medicine (ASRA) (2010).[34] The main goal of these guidelines is to decrease the occurrence of neuraxial hematoma. In general, hip procedures are associated with less postoperative pain than are knee procedures, making prolonged regional analgesia less important. Anesthesia and analgesia for procedures involving the knee and distal femur can be accomplished with either neuraxial techniques or peripheral nerve blocks. Lumbar plexus block offers more complete anesthesia of the thigh than does femoral block but is deeper and may be more difficult in obese patients and those with a history of lumbar spine surgery.[32] Sciatic nerve block is crucial for coverage of the posterior cutaneous nerve of the thigh and for the knee joint itself.[35] Procedures involving the foot and ankle, as well as those involving the tibia and fibula, are primarily covered by a sciatic nerve block. This can be achieved by blockade of the sciatic nerve at the popliteal level. **Figure 65-3** shows an ultrasound scan of the popliteal nerve. Block of the saphenous nerve may be necessary, depending on the location of the incision and the need for tourniquet. The saphenous nerve can be blocked via either femoral nerve block or a distal dedicated saphenous nerve block. Blocking the saphenous nerve at the femoral nerve level results in weakness of the quadriceps femoris with an inability to extend knee. This may make mobilization more

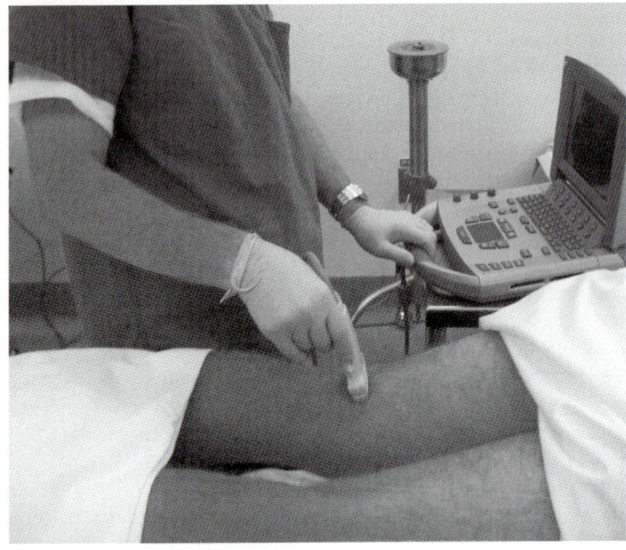

A

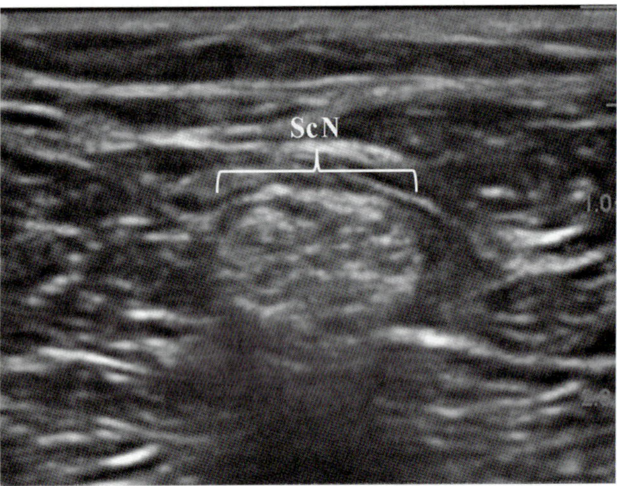

B

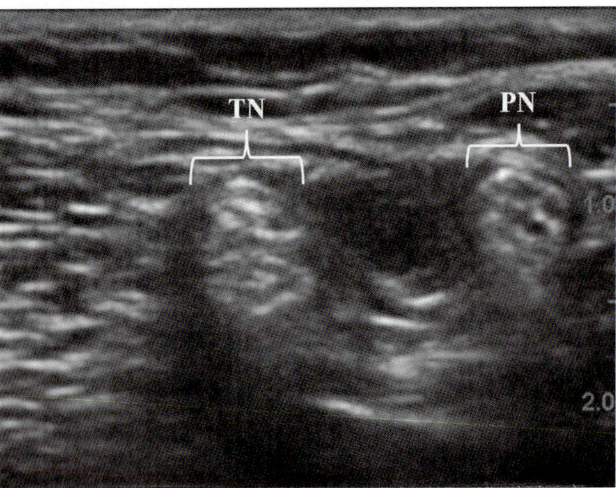

C

FIGURE 65-3. **A.** Popliteal nerve block performed with ultrasound in a patient in the prone position. **B.** Ultrasound scan of the sciatic nerve 7 cm above the popliteal crease. Note that the nerve lies 1.0 cm below the skin (centimeter markings on right side of figure). ScN, sciatic nerve. **C.** Ultrasound scan in the popliteal fossa showing the division of the nerve into the medial tibial branch and lateral peroneal branch. PN, peroneal nerve; TN, tibial nerve.

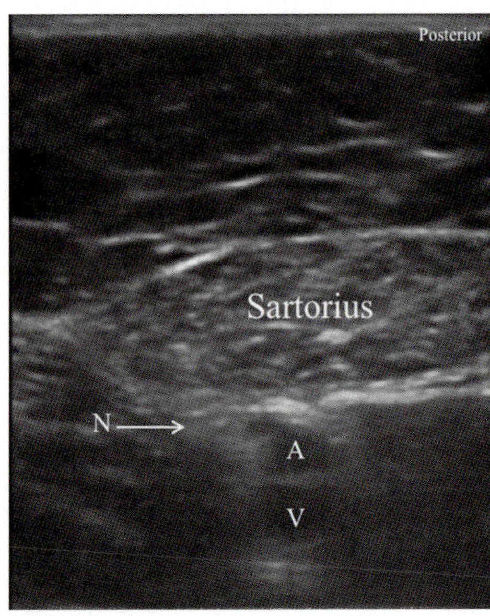

FIGURE 65-4. Ultrasound image of saphenous nerve in the adductor canal illustrating the relationship with the sartorius muscle, femoral artery, and femoral vein. A, artery; N, nerve; V, vein.

problematic compared with performing a dedicated saphenous block, which is purely sensory. Recently, ultrasound techniques have been described in which the saphenous nerve is blocked in the adductor canal just below the sartorius muscle[36] (**Fig. 65-4**). Ankle block without the use of epinephrine is adequate for procedures on the foot if no tourniquet use is expected.

The question as to whether general or regional anesthesia is superior with respect to outcome is controversial. A number of studies have shown no improvement in outcome with respect to mortality and morbidity.[37,38] However, other studies have shown that regional anesthesia and analgesia may reduce morbidity and mortality after surgery.[39-41] In a meta-analysis study, Rodgers et al[40] showed a 33% reduction in mortality. They also showed a significant decrease in the incidences of myocardial ischemic events, respiratory depression, rate of DVT formation, and blood loss. Wu et al[42] showed a death rate of 5.8 per 1000 (95% confidence interval [CI], 2.9-8.7) at 30 days postsurgery for cases using epidurals versus a death rate of 9.9 per 1000 (95% CI, 8.6-11.3) for cases using only general anesthesia. However, this benefit to patients must be considered in the context of the risk of epidural hematomas when neuroaxial anesthesia is given in the presence of anticoagulants such as LMWH. The risk, although small, has led to the publication of guidelines for use of regional anesthesia in patients receiving anticoagulants.[34] The 2010 guidelines depart from the 2003 guidelines by stating that LMWH should not be administered concomitantly with medications that affect hemostasis, such as antiplatelet drugs, standard heparin, or dextran. This has resulted in the reinvention and development of many peripheral nerve block techniques, including continuous peripheral nerve catheter techniques,[43] and use of ultrasonography to place these regional nerve blocks.[44,45]

Hip and Knee Joint Replacement Surgery With the population of the United States aging and the prospect of "baby boomers" reaching retirement age in the next couple of decades, the number of patients requiring joint replacement will increase greatly. It is estimated that more than 1 million joint replacement procedures per year will be performed in the United States during the next decade. A variety of anesthetic techniques, consisting of general, spinal, epidural, combined spinal and epidural, and peripheral nerve blocks, are available to anesthesiologists. These techniques have been shown to be superior to routine patient-controlled analgesia and as efficacious as epidural anesthesia but with fewer side effects.[46-48] Some evidence suggests that regional techniques may result in earlier discharge and improved functional outcome.[47,49] Knee replacement surgery is especially associated with significant postoperative pain, and patients undergoing this surgery benefit greatly from some form of postoperative regional analgesia. Use of epidurals in the joint replacement setting has been severely restricted by the widespread use of LMWH. The introduction of a new synthetic antithrombin III pentasaccharide sequence, fondaparinux, that has a half-life of 17 hours may have huge implications for the performance of regional techniques.[50] Normal practice is to wait at least 2 half-lives after discontinuation of such drugs before placing a neuraxial block or manipulating epidural catheters. Unfortunately, this means that with fondaparinux, there will be no window of opportunity to perform the regional anesthesia techniques or remove an epidural catheter.

A variety of peripheral nerve blocks have been used for analgesia in knee replacement surgery. They include psoas compartment blocks (lumbar plexus), femoral nerve blocks, and sciatic nerve blocks. The psoas compartment approach may be superior to the femoral approach because it is associated with greater success in blocking the 3 main components of the lumbar plexus: femoral, obturator, and lateral femoral cutaneous nerves. Capdevila et al[51] showed a 95% probability of blockade of all 3 nerves if the psoas compartment approach is used versus 33% if the femoral approach is used. A study by Macalou et al[52] showed that addition of an obturator nerve block to a 3:1 femoral nerve block resulted in superior postoperative pain relief compared with a 3:1 femoral nerve block alone. The addition of a sciatic nerve block for postoperative pain management is controversial. Studies have shown a significant improvement in postoperative pain management if the sciatic nerve block is also used.[53,54] Other studies have shown no improvement in postoperative opioid requirements if a sciatic nerve block is used.[55]

Whether the addition of peripheral nerve blocks to general anesthesia or spinal anesthesia offers any benefit to patients undergoing hip arthroplasty surgery is not as clear as in the case of knee replacement surgery. Biboulet et al[56] compared patient-controlled analgesia with morphine and a single injection of either a femoral or psoas compartment block. No difference in morphine consumption or pain scores was noted 4 hours after extubation. Other investigators have reported similar results using psoas compartment block for postoperative pain.[49] Thus, for hip replacement surgery, use of a spinal, epidural, or both may offer benefits to patients compared with general anesthesia in terms of mortality, morbidity, and pain control, but the addition of peripheral nerve blocks for postoperative pain appears to be of limited benefit. This may be in part because the pain after hip replacement surgery is of much shorter duration than in knee replacement surgery.[49,56]

The maximum duration of a single-shot nerve block depends on the local anesthetic used and the site of injection (lidocaine 2%, mepivacaine 1.5%, 4-6 h of analgesia vs ropivacaine 0.5%, bupivacaine 0.5%, 8-16 h of analgesia). Administration of additives, such as clonidine (50-150 mcg), may prolong the nerve block by another 2 or 3 hours. Use of continuous catheters in knee replacement surgery can extend the block indefinitely and can help patients avoid the severe pain experienced when the single-shot nerve block wears off. Evidence indicates that use of a stimulating nerve catheter improves the success rate of nerve catheters by avoiding subsequent failure of the catheter when the initial nerve block wears off (so-called "secondary block failure"). Salinas et al[43] showed a 100% success block rate when using a stimulating nerve catheter compared with an 85% success rate when using a nonstimulating nerve catheter. A recent semiquantitative systematic review including 11 randomized controlled studies has also shown improved analgesia with the use of stimulating catheters compared with nonstimulating catheters.[57]

Early mobilization and rehabilitation are important for the functional outcome of the patient. Use of a continuous catheter with local anesthetic causes motor weakness. Close collaboration among the anesthesia, orthopedic, and physiotherapy teams is needed to allow early mobilization with adequate analgesia. Lower concentrations of local anesthetic infusions produce less motor block but also may produce inferior analgesia. Starting patients on some form of oral analgesics before discontinuing the peripheral nerve catheters is essential to maintain adequate postoperative analgesia.

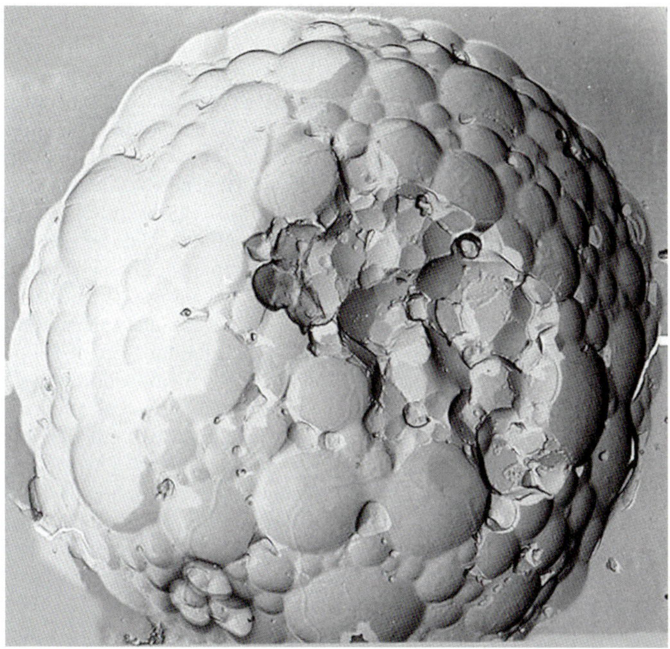

FIGURE 65-5. DepoFoam (SkyePharma, London, UK), an example of a liposomal delivery system used for epidural administration of 10 to 15 mg preservative-free morphine.

A new approach to postoperative pain management in patients undergoing lower limb joint replacement is the use of extended-release epidural morphine sulfate (DepoDur, SkyePharma, London, UK). This technology is based on liposomal products into which doses of 10 to 20 mg of morphine are incorporated (**Fig. 65-5**). This form allows the slow release of morphine into the epidural space over a 48-hour period without the need for an epidural catheter, thus avoiding anticoagulation issues. A study of hip replacement patients has shown a significant reduction in postoperative fentanyl requirements and pain scores.[58] The side effects are similar to those of other neuroaxial opioids. The most serious potential side effect is respiratory depression,[59] so patients must be monitored closely for 48 hours. Further developments of slow-release preparations of local anesthetics are awaited.

Invasive monitoring with arterial or central venous lines is generally not required except in patients with significant comorbidities or in patients undergoing revision of a previous joint replacement. Blood loss tends to be higher during revision joint replacement procedures. Methods used to reduce the requirement for blood transfusion are relevant to all patients undergoing joint replacement surgery (discussed earlier in this chapter in the section on blood loss).

Neck of Femur Fractures Repairing neck of femur fractures is a common surgical procedure at trauma institutions. Management is generally surgical and involves either internal fixation with screws or plates or a hemiarthroplasty. Hip arthroplasty for management of femoral neck fractures is associated with a nearly 10-fold increase in the rate of perioperative mortality compared with elective hip arthroplasty. The 30-day mortality is 10%, and 20% to 30% of patients die within 1 year of surgery.[60,61] The reasons for this high mortality rate probably are the age of this population group (>70 years of age), the presence of comorbidities, and the high incidence of DVTs and PEs. Optimization of patient medical conditions before surgery is generally but not always recommended because delay in surgery caused by the need for management of comorbidities may increase the mortality rate by 2.5 times.[62] Thus, appropriate and timely medical care is important before anesthesia and surgery.

Anesthesia involvement in the management of patients with neck of femur fractures can occur before the need for anesthesia for surgery and may involve the placement of a 3:1 femoral nerve block or fascia iliaca block in the emergency department for analgesia. Preoperative use of a femoral 3:1 block has been shown to be simple and to reduce the pain experienced, with few side effects.[63] The reduction in opioid doses required by patients can have substantial benefits. The question of whether general anesthesia or some form of regional anesthesia is best for these patients is controversial. The authors hold the opinion that regional anesthesia, including the use of spinal anesthesia, epidural anesthesia, combined spinal epidural anesthesia, or peripheral nerve blocks, is beneficial. Use of lumbar paravertebrals, lumbar plexus, and sciatic nerve block as the sole anesthetic technique for neck of femur fracture is a beneficial technique, especially in patients who, because of their comorbidities, cannot tolerate the drop in preload or afterload caused by spinal or epidural anesthesia.[31,64] An alternative method in this group of patients is the use of a continuous spinal catheter.[65] This method allows the anesthesiologist to titrate intrathecally the local anesthetic in small amounts while still obtaining the desired effect without the usual hemodynamic changes associated with a single large dose of intrathecal local anesthetic. Invasive line monitoring, such as arterial and central lines, may be needed, depending on the presence of comorbidities. The need for blood transfusion is uncommon, but adequate IV access and a blood cross-match should always be available. Keeping patients warm during the procedure is especially important in this elderly population. Finally, this group is at a much higher risk for development of DVT and subsequent PE. All patients must be adequately anticoagulated during the postoperative period to prevent this complication (see Deep Vein Thrombosis).

SPINAL SURGERY

Spinal surgery is frequently a challenge for anesthesiologists, involving a wide variety of procedures for treatment of different pathologies in the young to the very old patient population. It may involve surgery on the vertebrae of the spine in addition to the neural structures of the spinal cord.[66] Common pathologic reasons for surgery are listed in **Table 65-2**.

The required position of patients frequently is prone. The prone position requires extra care and attention because it may be associated with an increased incidence of complications. Major spinal surgery can be associated with extensive blood loss. Although the majority of spinal surgery is elective, urgent surgery may be required after trauma or when spinal cord viability is a concern. Some patients undergoing spinal procedures require repeat surgery and may have high requirements for analgesics in the postoperative period.

Positioning The majority of spinal surgery is performed with the patient in the prone position, although an anterior approach is sometimes used, particularly for cervical spine surgery. In addition, an anterior or lateral approach may be used for lumbar and thoracic spinal surgery. The ideal position allows easy access and maximal exposure to the site of surgery while allowing for a good operative field with minimal bleeding. Decompression of the stomach and bladder using an orogastric tube and a urinary catheter along with avoiding compression of the abdomen results in decreased pressure in the epidural veins and decreased blood loss. The site of surgery may be above the level of the heart, resulting in low venous pressure and decreased blood loss; however, it also is associated with a risk of venous air embolism. Hence, appropriate positioning of the patient is essential while being careful to avoid many of the potential complications. Although many different surgical tables and positions largely determined by surgeons' preference are available to improve exposure to the surgical site, many of the pertinent issues are common to all cases. First, extreme care must be taken when turning the patient, particularly patients at risk for spinal cord compromise. Particular attention should be paid to positioning of the head, neck, and arms. Complications associated with malpositioning of the arms, including vascular and brachial plexus injury, have been reported (**Table 65-3**).[67] Such injuries are least likely to occur when the arms are placed by the patient's side. However, this position may invade the surgeon's space and restricts the anesthesiologist's access to arterial and venous access. Therefore, the patient is frequently positioned with the arms resting on padded arm boards and flexed at the elbow (**Fig. 65-6**). The elbow should not be flexed more than 100 degrees because such a position is associated with increased pressure within the cubital tunnel.[68] The abdomen, genitalia, and breasts all should be checked because prolonged surgery in the prone position can result in injury to these areas. Adequate protection and padding of the eyes and head are essential. Blindness resulting from surgery performed with the patient in the prone position has been reported. Although its etiology probably is multifactorial but still is incompletely understood, prolonged surgery, anesthetic length greater than 6 hours, hypotension, large blood loss (>1 L), anemia, edema, and changes in intraocular perfusion pressure all may contribute to blindness.[69,70] Changes in ocular perfusion pressure resulting in decreased blood flow to the optic nerve may result in ischemic optic neuropathy. Increases in intraocular pressure or decreases in mean arterial pressure result in decreased ocular perfusion pressure.[71,72] Avoidance of prolonged periods of hypotension and perioperative anemia may reduce the risk of perioperative blindness in patients in the prone position.[73] In addition, direct pressure on the eye can result in injury to the eye. Tape marks and facial skin loss may result, especially in prone patients with significant facial edema and friable skin.

TABLE 65-2 Pathologic Reasons for Spine Surgery

Degenerative disease or arthritis
Congenital
Idiopathic
Trauma
Malignancy
Infection
Vascular abnormalities

TABLE 65-3 Complications of Positioning for Spine Surgery

Endotracheal tube dislodgement/kinking
Eye injury
Corneal abrasion
Ischemic optic neuropathy
Edema (facial, orbital, or airway)
Facial skin damage
Airway obstruction
Nerve damage (brachial/lumbar/sacral plexus)
Compression
Stretch
Compression of vessels
Ischemia
Thromboembolic complications
Compartment syndromes

The sitting position occasionally is used for surgery on the cervical spine. The risks and complications associated with surgery performed in the sitting position are described elsewhere in this textbook.

Anesthetic Technique A standard preoperative assessment is essential in patients undergoing spinal surgery. In addition to standard American Society of Anesthesiologists monitoring, use of invasive monitoring depends on patient comorbidities and the anticipated complexity of the surgical procedure and anticipated blood loss.[66] Surgeries involving multiple levels, repeat operations, and procedures for treatment of trauma and neoplasms typically are associated with increased blood loss.

A thorough airway examination should be performed. This assessment is critical, particularly in patients presenting for cervical spinal surgery and in patients with disease processes that affect the vertebral column, such as rheumatoid arthritis, ankylosing spondylitis, or generalized osteoarthritis.

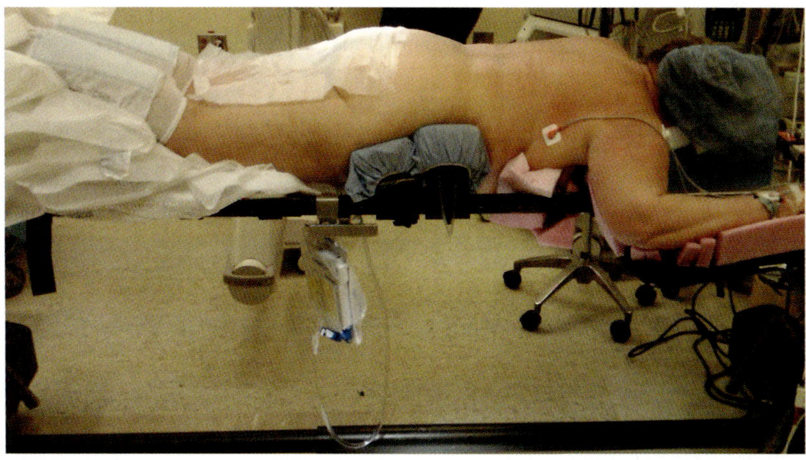

FIGURE 65-6. Proper positioning of the patient in the prone position.

In addition, patients who have undergone previous neck surgery may have increased difficulty at intubation. The aim is to safely secure the airway while avoiding any damage to the spinal cord. This can be achieved safely in both awake and anesthetized patients using a variety of techniques, such as standard laryngoscopy, intubating aids, manual inline stabilization, laryngeal mask airways (LMAs; LMA North America, Inc., San Diego, CA), and fiberoptic intubations. The precise technique depends on the clinical situation; management of the difficult airway is discussed in Chapter 36. The majority of movement in the cervical spine during intubation occurs at the atlantooccipital joint and between the first 2 cervical vertebrae.[74,75] Particular caution should be exercised in the airway management of patients with C1–C2 injury and at-risk patient populations (rheumatoid arthritis, Down syndrome) that are more prone to pathology of C1–C2. Use of rigid collars may increase the difficulty of intubation but does not affect the degree of cervical spine movement. After the airway is secured, the cervical collar alerts staff members that the patient may have a neck injury. Awake intubation allows neurologic examination after intubation and positioning of the patient, although this may be difficult in uncooperative patients. Thoracic spinal surgery may require use of a double-lumen tube or bronchial blocker if 1-lung ventilation is required with an anterior or lateral approach.

Anesthesia induction can be either IV or inhalational, with IV induction appropriate for the majority of patients. Intubation and muscle relaxation can be facilitated with either nondepolarizing muscle relaxants or succinylcholine. Use of succinylcholine should be avoided in patients with muscular dystrophies and in patients with spinal cord injuries in whom an exaggerated hyperkalemic response may be seen. Use of succinylcholine probably is safe in the 48 hours immediately after spinal injury and again 9 months after the injury.[76] Intraoperative use of muscle relaxants may be avoided depending on whether motor-evoked responses are monitored and surgeon preference. This is relevant in patients at risk for nerve root injury during surgery in which nerve root stimulation results in muscle movement. Anesthesia can be maintained using either a potent volatile anesthetic in a nitrous oxide–oxygen or air–oxygen mixture or IV anesthesia such as propofol infusions. Potent volatile agents may hinder the use of sensory and motor-evoked responses. If motor-evoked potentials are to be used by the surgeon, potent volatile agents are avoided completely, and a total IV infusion (TIVA) technique is used. Intubation can be accomplished with succinylcholine or under deep propofol-induced anesthesia. Nondepolarizing agents should not be used so as not to interfere with the motor-evoked potential. Many opioids have been used as part of a balanced anesthetic technique, with remifentanil having the advantage of providing potent analgesia and rapid offset of action. This may assist in the early assessment of the patient's neurologic status in the early postoperative period. Remember that all anesthetic agents may affect the use of somatosensory and motor-evoked potentials, which can be used to monitor spinal cord function (see Chapter 89). Changes in anesthetic concentrations and arterial blood pressure also affect the interpretation of evoked potentials. Spinal cord monitoring is discussed in Chapter 90.

Measures for minimizing intraoperative blood loss and reducing allogeneic blood transfusion in spinal surgery are particularly important. Careful positioning, avoidance of abdominal compression, surgical technique, hypotensive techniques, use of preoperative autologous donation, intraoperative normovolemic hemodilution, and use of intraoperative cell savers all may help avoid the use of allogeneic blood products. However, combinations of these techniques to reduce requirements for homologous blood products have not produced consistent results.[77,78] Use of antifibrinolytics may reduce intraoperative blood loss.[79] Hypotensive anesthesia is very effective at reducing blood loss, although it may be a contributory factor to the rare but devastating complication of posterior optic neuropathy. These techniques are particularly important in spinal surgeries associated with large blood loss. Minimally invasive spinal surgery has increased substantially. Primarily by using endoscopic, computer navigation and microsurgical techniques, surgeries to treat a wide variety of conditions ranging from spinal stenosis to tumor removal can be performed through much smaller incisions. These techniques allow for a quicker recovery time, reduced blood loss, and decreased opioid requirements with fewer postoperative complications.[80] Many of these new techniques use not only sensory-evoked potentials but also motor-evoked potentials. Many surgeons request the use of no muscle relaxants during the case as well as avoidance of potent inhalational agents to minimize disturbance on the motor-evoked potentials. To achieve this, a TIVA technique is required.

Postoperative Care Postoperative analgesia can be a challenge, particularly in patients who have experienced chronic back pain. Postoperative pain management has shifted from opioid-only patient-controlled analgesia to a multimodal approach. This multimodal approach uses drugs of various classes (e.g., NSAIDs, acetaminophen, gabapentenoids, antidepressants, ketamine) along with regional anesthesia to reduce or eliminate the amount of opioids required by the patient. Ketamine has made a resurgence of use in the management of some of our chronic pain patients undergoing orthopedic procedures. Ketamine is typically administered as an infusion during the case and occasionally continued postoperatively with great success. Perioperative infusion rates of ketamine range from 0.15 mg/kg/h to 0.35mg/kg/h. Use of NSAIDs is controversial. They may reduce opioid requirements by up to 40% and reduce the incidence of opioid-related side effects such as nausea, vomiting, sedation, and respiratory depression.[81] However, they may interfere with bone healing.[82] Initial studies using COX-2 inhibitors suggest minimal effect on bone healing, particularly when used for short durations.

In some cases, surgeons insert a catheter under direct vision into the epidural space. Either epidural opioids or opioids in addition to local anesthetics may be infused. Low concentrations of local anesthetics typically are used to avoid a motor block, which may delay accurate diagnosis of motor dysfunction as a complication of surgery.[83]

The majority of patients undergoing spinal surgery can be managed in the postsurgical unit postoperatively. Those who have undergone extensive surgery, experienced significant blood loss, received large fluid resuscitation, or experienced fluid shifts should be monitored postoperatively in an intensive care or stepdown unit. Patients with significant facial and airway edema may require ventilation postoperatively. In addition, patients who have undergone certain cervical and thoracic spinal procedures may require postoperative ventilation; those requiring extensive neurologic monitoring should be cared for in a monitored bed postoperatively.

Neurogenic shock is characterized by loss of sympathetic tone, resulting in hemodynamic instability, as evident from significant hypotension and bradycardia. This may be accentuated by hypovolemia. Shock tends to occur in injuries above the T6 level caused by disruption of sympathetic outflow and unopposed vagal tone. Arterial and central venous pressure monitoring is helpful in the management of these patients. Fluid administration in addition to vasopressors may be required to treat the hypotension along with appropriate management of the bradycardia. Autonomic dysreflexia is a syndrome of sympathetic imbalance that may occur after the phase of spinal shock. It occurs more commonly in males and may result in hypertension associated with myocardial ischemia, retinal or cerebral hemorrhage, and seizures.

AMBULATORY ORTHOPEDIC SURGERY

The 1990s saw a dramatic increase in the number of surgical cases performed in the ambulatory setting. Nearly 60% of all cases now occur as outpatient procedures, with orthopedic surgery accounting for a large number of cases. This trend has huge socioeconomic implications, such as reduced costs, more rapid return to daily activity, and lower risk of nosocomial infections. Shoulder and knee procedures, including shoulder arthroplasty and anterior cruciate ligament repair, occur routinely on an outpatient basis. All ambulatory orthopedic surgical procedures can be performed under general anesthesia. However, these procedures may be most suited for a regional anesthetic technique, and improved analgesia seen in the perioperative period can be safely and effectively extended to the postoperative period with the use of perineural catheters.[84] With more complicated procedures occurring on an outpatient basis, adoption of a multimodal approach to postoperative pain management is essential. This will allow better pain control with the need for less opioid medication, thus reducing the potential for side effects such as nausea and vomiting, which often can derail a timely discharge from the ambulatory center. The cornerstone of these techniques is frequently a peripheral nerve block. New disposable infusion devices allow patients to be discharged with peripheral nerve catheter infusions, further prolonging the effect of a single shot of peripheral nerve block.[85] When general anesthesia is required, the aim should be to provide adequate anesthesia and analgesia while minimizing perioperative-related side effects such as nausea and vomiting.

POSTOPERATIVE ANALGESIA IN ORTHOPEDICS

Limited evidence indicates that improvements in postoperative pain control result in better functional outcome and reduced morbidity and mortality.[40,47] The best approach to postoperative pain management is a multimodal approach of different agents and routes of administration used in a synergistic manner.[86-88] Using a multimodal approach, we have the potential to reduce or eliminate the amount of opioids required by patients and thus reduce side effects such as nausea and vomiting, respiratory depression, and oversedation.[87,89] The cornerstone of any multimodal approach is a regional technique, including epidural and peripheral nerve blocks (see Chapter 48). Subcutaneous injection of local anesthetics is also widely used. Use of intra-articular opioids, such as morphine, after joint surgery is controversial, with some evidence of benefit.[90-95] Use of intra-articular morphine is based on the presence of opioid receptors on peripheral nerve endings within the capsule of joints. Administration of intra-articular opioids produces analgesia only in the presence of inflammation, and it has been postulated that the inflammatory process is necessary for activation of the opioid receptors.[96] Morphine doses between 1 and 5 mg have been shown to have an analgesic effect until 24 hours after intra-articular administration.[97] The side effects normally seen with systemic opioids are not seen with these doses of intra-articular opioids. Cryotherapy devices have been used in both shoulder and knee surgery to further augment postoperative analgesia.[98,99] Nonsteroidal agents play an important role in reducing postoperative opioid requirements.[100] COX-2 inhibitors have largely displaced the nonselective COX inhibitors because of their improved side effect profile with regard to the potential for gastric bleeds and coagulation disturbance. The controversy regarding rofecoxib (Vioxx, Merck & Co., Whitehouse Station, NJ), which was found to result in an increased incidence of death because of myocardial infarcts when used at high doses and for long periods, has significantly reduced the use of other COX-2 inhibitors in the perioperative period.[101] Data are insufficient to recommend the use of other COX-2 inhibitors, such as celecoxib (Celebrex, Pfizer, New York, NY), which should be given with caution in the perioperative period.[102,103] Another important issue with COX-2 inhibitors is their potential to reduce bone healing in animal models. In vitro studies have shown that the presence of COX-2, but not COX-1, is essential for adequate bone healing.[104,105] However, no clinical evidence in humans shows the effect of reduced bone formation, particularly when COX-2 inhibitors are used for short-term treatment.[100]

FACTORS RELATED TO ORTHOPEDIC SURGERY

TOURNIQUETS

Tourniquets (derived from the French *tourner*, meaning "to turn") are routinely used in orthopedic surgery to provide a bloodless field. This practice is purported to improve visualization of critical structures and decrease operative blood loss.[106] However, tourniquets have significant risks, and these risks and the strategies to minimize them should be part of the knowledge base of all practicing anesthesiologists.[107]

By inflating a cuff around an extremity, arterial inflow to the extremity distal to the cuff is eliminated. Careful exsanguination of the limb distal to the cuff immediately before cuff inflation, either via application of an elastic Esmarch bandage or elevation of the extremity for 5 minutes, empties the vascular system. The distal limb is thus rendered ischemic, which may have significant physiologic and biochemical implications.

Limb exsanguination causes an increase in central blood volume that is reflected as a transient rise in central venous pressure.[108] This increase in preload can be significant if multiple tourniquets are used, as in simultaneous bilateral knee arthroplasties. Tourniquet inflation also causes an increase in afterload. Patients with diminished cardiac function may not be able to tolerate this combined insult of increased preload and afterload. After tourniquet deflation, preload decreases acutely as blood reenters the affected extremity, which undergoes a period of postischemic reactive hyperemia. This is accompanied by an acute decrease in afterload that often produces hypotension.[109] Reperfusion of an extremity typically is associated with a decrease in core temperature of up to 1.0°C.

During limb ischemia, oxygen and high-energy phosphate stores decrease progressively, and carbon dioxide and lactic acid levels increase as ischemic tissues convert to anaerobic metabolism.[110] The pH of the ischemic limb decreases as the duration of ischemia increases.[111] After tourniquet deflation, aerobic metabolism resumes, with marked increases in oxygen consumption and carbon dioxide production.[112] Systemic partial pressure of carbon dioxide increases in this interval, and pH transiently decreases as a result of combined metabolic and respiratory acidosis.[113] Spontaneously breathing patients increase minute ventilation markedly to compensate. The minute ventilation of mechanically ventilated patients must be increased to minimize the duration and magnitude of hypercapnia. The increase in carbon dioxide tension can produce a marked increase in cerebral blood flow, with potentially deleterious results in patients with increased intracranial pressure.[114] In this setting, it is especially critical to increase minute ventilation in patients who are unable to compensate effectively.

Ischemia of the affected limb causes significant changes on the cellular level. Tissue becomes progressively acidotic while the cuff is inflated.[110] Ultrastructural changes within the endothelium of the ischemic capillaries lead to diffuse capillary leak after reperfusion.[110] In conjunction with reactive hyperemia, significant edema can develop after tourniquet deflation. This can even lead to a compartment syndrome in the affected extremity. The coagulation system undergoes significant changes in the setting of tourniquet use. Platelet aggregation is increased by both tissue compression and pain caused by the surgical insult and the tourniquet.[115] Capillary obstruction by red blood cells and platelets that accumulate during the period of stasis and the concomitant release of inflammatory mediators can lead to microvascular thrombosis, causing no-reflow phenomena and further exacerbating tissue injury.[110] Tissue acidosis also leads to release of tissue plasminogen activator, which causes a brief period of fibrinolysis after tourniquet deflation.[115] This is postulated to play a role in posttourniquet bleeding. Muscle is most susceptible to injury secondary to ischemia, with the duration of ischemia correlating with the severity of injury. Injury is most severe under the cuff as a result of the combined effect of tissue compression and ischemia.[116] Fortunately, these injuries are generally reversible when tourniquet time is not excessive. Rhabdomyolysis has been reported after tourniquet use. A practical guideline is to limit tourniquet time to 2 hours if possible. Experiments have shown that a 10-minute period of reperfusion every hour allows for disposal of accumulated waste products and regeneration of adenosine triphosphate stores in the involved limb, facilitating tissue recovery after completion of surgery and minimizing the extent of muscle injury.[110]

Cuff pressure is the most significant risk factor for nerve injury after tourniquet use.[117] Use of a wider cuff allows arterial occlusion at lower cuff pressures. Conical rather than rectangular cuffs can produce the desired effect at lower inflation pressures.[118,119] Numerous methods for determining the inflation pressure to be used in a particular situation are recommended. Inflating the cuff 50 to 75 mm Hg above the systolic pressure for upper extremity procedures and 100 to 150 mm Hg above systolic pressure for lower extremity operations appears reasonable. Others have recommended empirically determining the appropriate inflation pressure by first ascertaining via Doppler ultrasonography the pressure at which arterial inflow is occluded and then setting the cuff pressure 50 mm Hg higher. Using the lowest pressure possible decreases the risk of nerve injury. The incidence of significant nerve injury in the upper extremity is estimated at 1 in 11 000, with radial nerve palsy representing the most common injury; lower extremity nerve injuries are believed to occur at a much lower rate. Most nerve injuries are not permanent and resolve with time.[120] A detailed neurologic examination should be obtained in a timely fashion if such an injury is suspected to document any preexisting dysfunction.

Careful padding of the limb under the cuff with cast padding, with care taken to avoid any wrinkles, decreases the risk of skin injury from compression or pinching. The tourniquet should not be manipulated after it is applied to avoid bunching up the padding underneath the tourniquet. Creating an impervious barrier with adhesive plastic drapes to prevent cleaning solutions from seeping under the tourniquet is helpful in minimizing the risk of skin injury. The vascular system is not immune to injury from tourniquet application. Patients with atherosclerosis appear to be at highest risk for this type of injury. Mechanical forces applied to these vessels are believed capable of fracturing calcified plaque within the vessel wall.[121] This can lead to vascular compromise and potentially to limb loss. Tourniquet use is relatively contraindicated in patients with risk factors for peripheral vascular disease, absent distal pulses, and previous vascular surgery on the operative extremity.[122]

Use of a tourniquet can affect the pharmacokinetics of other drugs given during an anesthetic procedure. Drugs administered before tourniquet inflation can become sequestered in the ischemic limb. When the tourniquet is deflated at the end of surgery, a bolus of that particular drug is delivered to the central circulation.[123] This effect can be significant in elderly patients who have received opioids or benzodiazepines before tourniquet inflation. The volume of distribution is decreased for drugs administered after the tourniquet is inflated. This can produce a greater-than-expected effect from a given dose. Antibiotic administration must be coordinated with tourniquet inflation to ensure that adequate tissue penetration occurs at the surgical site. For most antibiotics, a minimum interval of 5 minutes is recommended between completion of drug administration and tourniquet inflation.[124] Muscle relaxants sequestered in an ischemic limb have not proved to be as significant a problem upon tourniquet release as anticipated.

Tourniquet pain is the final major issue that complicates use of a tourniquet. In an unsedated patient, it presents as dull, aching pain that becomes intolerable within approximately 30 minutes. This time period can be extended somewhat by IV administration of sedatives and analgesics.[125] During a general anesthetic, tourniquet pain manifests as increases in heart rate and both systolic and diastolic blood pressures 45 to 60 minutes after tourniquet inflation.[126] This typically is treated with only limited success by increasing the depth of anesthesia or administering additional analgesics. Ultimately, tourniquet deflation is the only factor that eliminates tourniquet pain, with resolution within 30 minutes. This phenomenon also has been reported during spinal and epidural anesthetics, with an apparently adequate level of anesthesia to pinprick.[127] An adequate level of anesthesia to touch is more predictive of prevention of tourniquet pain. The postulated mechanism for tourniquet pain is a differential conduction block of large myelinated A-δ fibers and small unmyelinated C fibers.

FAT EMBOLISM SYNDROME

Fat embolism syndrome (FES) was first described by Zencker in an article published in 1862. Nearly all patients with long bone fractures or patients who have undergone hip or knee replacement surgery experience some degree of fat embolization.[128,129] However, the incidence of clinically significant FES is only 0.5% to 3%.[130,131] The incidence may be higher (30%) in patients with multiple long bone fractures. FES is much more likely to occur with long bone fractures of the lower limb than with fractures of the upper limb. Likewise, the incidence of FES in children is much lower than in adults. Changes in surgeons' preference for early operative reduction and fixation of fractures have led to a marked decreased in FES incidence.

Fracture of the long bone causes an increase in intramedullary pressure. This coupled with disruption of the venous sinusoids within the long bones results in fat and bone debris entering the venous circulation. Manipulation and surgical preparation of the long bones, such as reaming, also can cause an increase in intramedullary pressure and result in fat embolization. Careful attention by the surgeon in clearing the femoral canal with adequate lavage can reduce the incidence of fat embolization (see Methylmethacrylate). Commonly, fat globules lodge in the pulmonary vasculature, resulting in obstruction of pulmonary circulation. Fat globules are hydrolyzed into free fatty acids that are directly toxic to the pulmonary endothelium and pneumocytes, resulting in endothelial damage, platelet adhesion with clot formation, capillary leakage, and perivascular bleeding. Some evidence indicates that elevated C-reactive protein levels resulting from trauma may cause chylomicrons to coalesce and form fat globules. These fat particles may pass into the systemic circulation via intracardiac (foramen ovale) and pulmonary shunts, resulting in cerebral and cutaneous manifestations.

Fat embolism syndrome may present intraoperatively as cardiorespiratory collapse after femoral reaming, insertion of intramedullary cemented prosthesis, or tourniquet release. FES also may present postoperatively as a variety of clinical signs and symptoms. Gurd and

TABLE 65-4 Major and Minor Features of Fat Embolism Syndrome[a]

Major features
Respiratory distress
Cerebral changes
Petechial rash
Arterial blood gas[b]
Minor features
Fever
Renal damage
Retinal changes
Hemolysis
Lipuria
Jaundice

[a]As described by Gurd and Wilson.[132]

[b]Not an original major feature but added by Schonfeld et al[133] and Lindeque et al[134] in their classifications.

Wilson[132] described major and minor features of FES (**Table 65-4**). To make the diagnosis of FES, at least 1 major and 4 minor features must be present. The 3 major symptoms of FES are respiratory distress, cerebral manifestations, and petechial rash. The minor symptoms are fever, renal damage, retinal changes, hemolysis, lipuria, and jaundice. The Gurd and Wilson criteria were criticized for not including assessment of the patient's oxygenation with the use of an arterial blood gas, which may be a useful early indicator of FES. The criteria of both Schonfeld et al[133] and Lindeque et al[134] include the measurement of arterial blood gases to determine the presence of hypoxemia. Respiratory distress consists of tachypnea, hypoxia, and hyperventilation and is seen in 75% of patients with the syndrome.[135] The majority of patients present with Po_2 below 50 mm Hg. Chest radiographs classically show bilateral diffuse infiltrates, especially in the upper and middle lobes of the lung. Pulmonary function usually resolves in 7 days. Approximately 10% of patients require mechanical ventilation for respiratory failure. Cerebral involvement consists of a wide range of clinical symptoms, such as confusion, convulsions, drowsiness, and coma, and normally is present in 86% of presenting cases.[129] Petechial rash classically involves the conjunctiva, mucous membranes, and skin on the anterior aspect of the chest and neck and likewise is seen in 50% to 60% of cases.[132] Classically, these symptoms and signs do not present within the first 6 to 12 hours after the insult. Onset after 72 hours from the insult is unusual. The best treatment of this condition is prevention by early surgical reduction and immobilization of the fracture site. Management consists of supportive care that may include ventilation. Adequate fluid resuscitation is essential and may lessen the severity of the presentation. Steroids to reduce the inflammatory response caused by free fatty acids have long played an important role in the management of this condition, but studies that steroids are not as effective as previously believed.[136,137] There is no evidence supporting the use of heparin or IV alcohol in the management of FES. The overall mortality rate is high (7%-20%), and death normally is related to pulmonary involvement.[129]

METHYLMETHACRYLATE

Use of cement, with its main component of methylmethacrylate (MMA), has been linked to a clinical scenario consisting of hypotension, bronchoconstriction, hypoxia, cardiac arrest, and sudden death. The terms *bone implantation syndrome* and *bone cement implantation syndrome* have been coined to describe this phenomenon. A study has shown rates of death in hip arthroplasty procedures between 0.02% and 0.5%.[138] These rates initially were believed to be attributable to a hypersensitivity reaction to the MMA, resulting in acute vasodilatation and cardiac collapse. MMA given during in vitro studies has been shown to result in vasodilatation; however, plasma levels during use of MMA in clinical practice have been found to be 10- to 20-fold below the levels required to cause clinically significant vasodilatation and hypotension.[139] It has become clear that the phenomenon is caused by embolization of fat particles and debris from the intramedullary canal of long bones during their manipulation, reaming, and cementing. During these procedures, intramedullary pressures may exceed pressures within the medullary venous plexuses, resulting in fat and debris entering the venous system. Use of transesophageal echocardiography can clearly demonstrate the increased load of debris entering the right atrium during cementing of the long bones.[140] Intramedullary pressure peaks are 680 mm Hg in humans with cement use compared with peaks below 100 mm Hg with noncemented arthroplasties.[141] In an attempt to minimize increased intramedullary pressure, orthopedic surgeons have used various techniques, such as new cementing devices, drilling distal venting holes within the long bones, and aggressive lavage of the canal before insertion of the cement and prosthesis to reduce the amount of intramedullary debris. The technique of venting results in significant extravasation of cement, and none of the techniques has been found to reliably prevent this phenomenon. Some surgeons use uncemented techniques for joint replacement procedures. Cemented prosthesis and the need for revision procedures have made the use of uncemented devices more appealing to surgeons. Clinical signs of bone implantation syndrome or bone cement implantation syndrome are similar to those found in PE or fat embolism. They include fever, tachycardia, hypotension; hypoxemia, and, in spontaneously breathing patients, dyspnea and tachypnea; end-tidal carbon dioxide may decrease with a large embolus. Other signs of fat emboli also may be seen. The electrocardiogram may show right-axis deviation or right bundle branch block. These signs reflect increased pulmonary artery pressure and intrapulmonary shunt, potentially leading to right ventricular failure and cardiac arrest.

Management of this phenomenon is similar to that caused by fat emboli. It requires both support of the cardiovascular system with aggressive fluid management and inotropic and vasopressor support. Oxygen therapy and ventilation often are required, depending on the severity of the response.

DEEP VEIN THROMBOSIS

The incidence of DVT in unprotected patients can be extremely high, varying between 80% and 90%, with a 2% incidence of fatal PE in hip and knee replacement surgery.[142] Hip fractures have an even higher occurrence of fatal PE with an incidence of 4% to 7%.[143] Whereas hip replacement surgery typically results in thrombosis of vessels above the knee, knee replacement surgery commonly involves vessels below the knee. Fatal PEs are normally associated with thrombosis above the knee. The Virchow triad has classically been used to describe the etiology of DVT. The 3 main causes of DVT are prolonged stasis, damage to the intima of blood vessels, and increased viscosity of blood. All of these factors may play a role in causing DVT in joint replacement surgery, but the problem is increased greatly for 2 reasons: extended use of tourniquets in total knee replacements, and distortion of lower limb blood vessels during manipulation and preparation of both the femur and tibia. This increase has necessitated the use of a variety of pharmacologic drugs and pneumatic devices to reduce the high incidence of DVT. Different regimens are used at various of institutions, with no best way to manage this problem. Whether warfarin (Coumadin) is superior to LMWH or vice versa is controversial.[143-145] In a study by Freedman et al,[143] the risk of proximal DVT was lowest with warfarin (6.3%) compared with LMWH (7.7%), but no differences in the incidence of PE and mortality were noted. Miric et al[144] found that LMWH was better than warfarin in preventing DVT in total hip replacements (4% vs 12%, respectively). What is clear is that use of unfractionated heparin does not offer sufficient DVT prophylaxis in patients undergoing joint replacement procedures and that LMWH compared with warfarin is classically associated with an increased incidence of minor and major wound blood loss.[143,146] According to the latest recommendations from The Seventh American College of Chest Physicians Consensus Conference, only warfarin, fondaparinux, and LMWH are adequate forms of DVT prophylaxis when used alone for hip or knee replacement surgery.[147] Pharmacologic agents should always be combined with mechanical prophylaxis, which should begin intraoperatively if possible. Mechanical prophylaxis should be used alone only when there is a significant risk of bleeding. Use of the newer anticoagulants, particularly LMWH, has resulted in the need for anesthesiologists to modify their anesthetic plan. Vandermeulen[148] demonstrated a significant increase in the incidence of epidural hematomas if epidural anesthesia is used in conjunction with LMWH. This finding resulted in the addition of an FDA black box warning to LMWH prescribing information and a review of the current practice of regional anesthesia, particularly neuroaxial anesthesia and analgesia in the presence of certain anticoagulants.[149] The ASRA has developed guidelines for the use of regional techniques in the presence of a variety of anticoagulants.[34] The guidelines include not performing a neuroaxial technique within 12 hours after a dose of LMWH and waiting 2 hours after removal of an epidural catheter before initiating LMWH. This guideline has severely limited the use of epidural anesthesia for postoperative pain and resulted in the development of a number of new techniques (discussed earlier in this chapter in the section on anesthesia for extremity surgery and in the section on blood loss).

COMPARTMENT SYNDROME

Volkmann first described compartment syndrome in 1881. The disfigurement of the upper limb that may result from the condition is still called a Volkmann contracture. Compartment syndrome is one of the most litigated topics in orthopedic surgery. A variety of injuries and medical conditions may initiate an acute compartment syndrome, including fractures, contusions, bleeding disorders, reperfusion injuries, burns, and trauma. Fractures of the tibial shaft are the most common fractures associated with compartment syndrome, accounting for 40% of cases, followed by forearm fractures, which account for 18%.[150] However, many cases of compartment syndrome can occur in the absence of a fracture and are solely related to soft tissue damage (23%). Compartment syndrome occurs when the pressure within an osseofascial compartment increases to a level that decreases the perfusion gradient across tissue capillary beds, leading to cellular anoxia, muscle ischemia, and death, with eventual replacement of the muscle with fibrous tissue, leading to contractures and a nonfunctional limb. The normal compartmental pressure is less than 10 to 12 mm Hg, with compartmental perfusion pressures normally greater than 70 to 80 mm Hg. Compartmental perfusion pressures can be calculated by subtracting compartmental pressures from mean arterial pressures. Thus, increasing compartmental pressures and decreasing mean arterial pressures can lead to a situation in which the compartment perfusion pressure is inadequate. It is not possible to determine the compartmental pressure value critical to perfusion because compartmental pressure at which perfusion problems occur can vary greatly among individuals. Delta p (Δp), which is diastolic pressure minus intracompartmental pressure, is much more reliable in determining the need for fasciotomy.[151] Δp below 30 mm Hg in the presence of clinical signs of compartment syndrome requires a fasciotomy. Diagnosis is primarily clinical, supplemented by compartment pressure monitoring (**Fig. 65-7**). Signs include pain, especially with passive stretching of the involved muscle group, pallor of the limb, lack of a distal pulse, a cold limb, paresthesia, paralysis, and a swollen and tense compartment.[152] The presence of a distal arterial pulse does not exclude the presence of compartment syndrome. These signs can be reliably diagnosed only in fully conscious patients. Patients who are unconscious or sedated should be monitored with continuous compartment pressures, and sometimes a prophylactic fasciotomy is needed. Complete fasciotomy of all compartments involved is required to reliably normalize compartment pressures and restore perfusion to affected tissues. Recognizing compartment syndromes requires having and maintaining a high index of suspicion, performing serial examinations in patients at risk, and carefully documenting changes over time. The earlier the diagnosis, the better the outcome, with neural structures being much more at risk than muscle. Anesthesiologists must be aware of this condition to allow for early diagnosis. Compartment syndrome should be considered in any patient in whom the intensity of pain is out of proportion to the injury and in any patient with a long bone fracture who is not responding to normal amounts of analgesia. In choosing the anesthetic technique for cases that normally are associated with compartment syndrome, the anesthesiologist must avoid any postoperative technique, such as epidurals or peripheral nerve blocks, that may delay diagnosis of the syndrome. If these techniques are used and there is a potential for compartment syndrome, consideration should be given to continuously monitoring compartment pressures. The effect of anesthetic techniques, such as spinals and epidurals, that cause sympathectomy (and thus vasodilatation) is unclear. The increased blood flow to muscle compartments may cause a further increase in compartment pressures. What is clear is that in cases of suspected or potential compartment syndrome, the anesthesiologist should maintain a high mean arterial blood pressure during the case. Use of mannitol has been shown to reduce the occurrence of compartment syndromes in revascularization cases and may be of help in other patients with compartment syndrome.

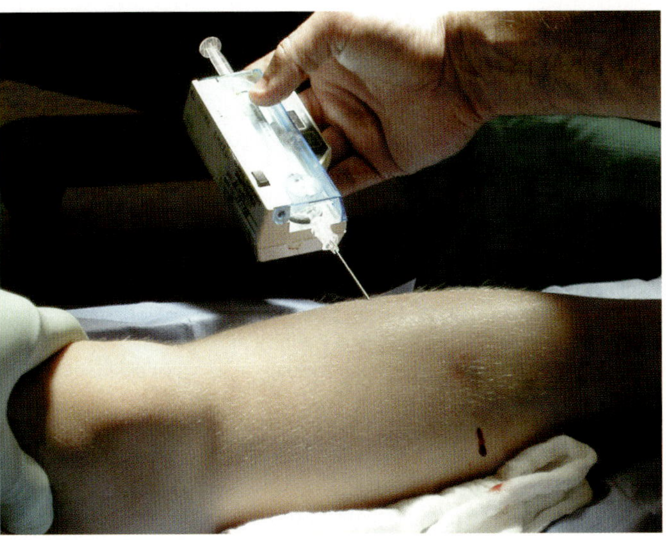

FIGURE 65-7. Compartment pressure monitoring.

KEY REFERENCES

- Enneking FK, Chan V, Greger J, et al. Lower-extremity peripheral nerve blockade: essentials of our current understanding. *Reg Anesth Pain Med.* 2005;30:4.
- Gurd AR, Wilson RI. The fat embolism syndrome. *J Bone Joint Surg Br.* 1974;56B:408.
- Horlocker TT, Wedel DJ, Rowlingson JC, et al. Regional anesthesia in the patient receiving antithrombotic or thrombolytic therapy: American Society of Regional Anesthesia and Pain Medicine Evidence-Based Guidelines (Third Edition). *Reg Anesth Pain Med.* 35:64 2010.
- Kam PC, Kavanagh R, Yoong FF. The arterial tourniquet: pathophysiological consequences and anaesthetic implications. *Anaesthesia.* 2001;56:534.
- Raw DA, Beattie JK, Hunter JM. Anaesthesia for spinal surgery in adults. *Br J Anaesth.* 2003;91:886.
- Rodgers A, Walker N, Schug S, et al. Reduction of postoperative mortality and morbidity with epidural or spinal anaesthesia. *BMJ.* 2000;321:1493.

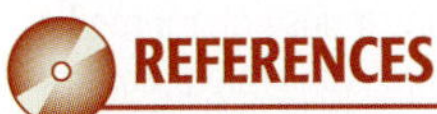

REFERENCES

Complete references available on DVD and online version at www.LongneckerAnesthesiology.com

CHAPTER 66

Anesthesia for Ophthalmic Surgery

Joseph Bayes
Salvatore J. Basta

KEY POINTS

1. Even patients with serious medical problems can often undergo eye surgery under regional anesthesia provided their medical condition(s) are well controlled, they can lie flat without moving for the length of the procedure, and they are able to communicate with their ophthalmologist and anesthesia staff.
2. True ophthalmic emergencies are rare. Central retinal artery occlusion and chemical burns require immediate treatment. Uncontrolled glaucoma, ruptured globe and threatened macula detachment are urgent conditions but can usually be delayed long enough to allow appropriate management of the patient's medical condition.
3. Cataract and other eye operations under regional anesthesia have a low risk of serious perioperative complications. Regional anesthesia greatly reduces the risk of pain, nausea, and vomiting occurring in the immediate post operative period.
4. General anesthesia increases the risk of minor complications (eg, nausea and vomiting) and in some instances (eg, patients with valvular heart disease or pulmonary hypertension) major perioperative complications. During general anesthesia, akinesis and hemodynamic stability must be maintained to avoid eye damage. A smooth emergence and control of pain and postoperative nausea and vomiting are important.
5. Safe performance of regional orbital blocks requires knowledge of orbital anatomy, instruction by a qualified practitioner, knowledge of possible complications, adequate patient monitoring, and immediate availability of resuscitation equipment. Patients should be mildly sedated but cooperative during needle placement for orbital blocks. Knowledge or estimation of the axial length of the eye before performing retrobulbar block may reduce the risk of globe perforation. Eyes 26 mm or longer in length, with previous scleral buckles, and with enophthalmos have greater potential for injury from retrobulbar blocks. Needles longer than 32 mm in the inferolateral orbit and longer than 25 mm in the medial orbit increase the risk of serious complications. Inserting a retrobulbar or peribulbar block needle below the lateral canthus ("modified" inferolateral insertion point) instead of the junction of the medial and lateral third of the lower eyelid may reduce extraocular muscle (EOMs) injury.
6. The oculocardiac reflex (OCR) can occur when pressure is applied to the globe or traction applied to the EOMs. It can present as sinus bradycardia, atrioventricular block, or asystole. OCR is more common during general than regional anesthesia and more common in children than adults. Prompt cessation of the inciting maneuver sometimes is sufficient therapy. Although it is often a fatigable reflex, OCR may require treatment with glycopyrrolate or atropine if severe or persistent. The reflex can often be prevented or abolished with an orbital block.
7. Coughing or "bucking" increases intraocular pressure (IOP) and the risk of intraoperative eye damage. The increase in IOP from laryngoscopy and intubation can be blunted by sufficient doses of propofol, a narcotic, lidocaine, and a muscle relaxant. If a rapid-sequence induction is considered with globe injury, the risk of difficulty in securing the airway and the viability of the eye should first be assessed. Rocuronium (0.6-1.2 mg/kg) is often a good choice for muscle relaxant if the intubation is anticipated to be easy. If succinylcholine is deemed necessary, a dose of 1.5 mg/kg preceded by a prefasciculating dose of rocuronium is indicated. Both of these regimens usually provide good intubating conditions with minimal rise of IOP within 60 to 90 seconds.
8. Nitrous oxide has caused bubble expansion and blindness in patients with recent intravitreal injections of gases. Nitrous oxide should not be used for patients who had an intravitreal injection of sulfur hexafluoride (SF6) within the last 30 days or octafluoropropane (C_3F_8) within the last 90 days.
9. To reduce the risk of fire during eye surgery under regional anesthesia, consider the use of compressed air at 10 L/min or an oxygen concentration of no more than 30%, instead of 100% oxygen. If 100% oxygen is required, the surgeon should be warned of its use and it should be discontinued for several minutes before any surgical heat source is used.
10. Pediatric ophthalmology requires knowledge of the comorbidities of prematurity as well as underlying congenital syndromes.

Patients undergoing ophthalmic surgery, despite having a low risk of serious perioperative complications, frequently present challenges to anesthesiologists because they tend to be at the extremes of age, they have a high incidence of systemic diseases, and intraoperative access to the head is limited. This chapter reviews orbital anatomy, the relationship between intraocular pressure (IOP) and anesthesia, the systemic effects of ophthalmic medications, preoperative medical preparation, regional and general anesthetic techniques, complications from orbital blocks, and the management of some commonly encountered pediatric and adult surgical procedures.

ORBITAL ANATOMY

Knowledge of orbital anatomy is required for safe, effective regional anesthesia. The eyes lie within 2 bony cavities of the skull termed *orbits*. The orbits are pyramidal in shape. Each eye or *globe* is positioned anteriorly in the orbit and occupies about one-third of the orbit (**Fig. 66-1**). Each orbit has a volume of approximately 30 mL. The anterior opening of the orbit is approximately 35 mm in height and 45 mm in width. The depth of the orbit varies with race and gender but averages slightly more than 40 mm.

The average adult globe diameter is 23.5 mm.[1] Normal adult globe diameter ranges between 21 and 26 mm. At birth, the diameter is approximately 16 mm but reaches approximately 23 mm by age 3 years. The globe reaches maximum size at puberty.

The transparent *cornea* occupies the center of the anterior pole of the globe and is approximately 11 to 12 mm in diameter. The cornea, lens, and aqueous humor form the main refractive elements of the eye. The curvature of the cornea contributes approximately one-third of the refractive power. The *limbus* is the edge of the cornea where it joins the sclera. The *sclera* is opaque and white, and covers the remaining 80% of the globe. Tendons of the rectus muscles insert into the superficial scleral collagen.

The conjunctiva is a mucous membrane that lines the inner surface of the eyelids and the anterior surface of the globe between the cornea and limbus. The bulbar (posterior) extension of the conjunctiva fuses with the underlying Tenon capsule near the limbus. Tenon capsule continues posteriorly as an incomplete fascial layer composed of collagen fibers and fibroblasts that surrounds the posterior globe and the extraocular muscles (EOMs). Tenon capsule is perforated by the optic nerve sheath and the posterior ciliary vessels and nerves.

The wall of the globe is composed of 3 layers: the sclera, uveal tract, and retina (**Fig. 66-2**). The middle layer is the *uveal tract*. It is composed of 3 specialized structures: the iris, ciliary body (located in the anterior uvea), and choroid (located in the posterior uvea). The *iris* contains dilator and sphincter muscle fibers that control the central aperture, the pupil. Parasympathetic stimulation originating from the cranial nerve (CN) III nucleus contracts iris sphincter fibers, causing pupillary constriction or *miosis*. Conversely, sympathetic fibers traveling with the ophthalmic division of CN V stimulate iris dilator fibers, dilating the pupil. Directly adjacent and behind the iris is the *ciliary body*. The ciliary body had 2 primary functions: production

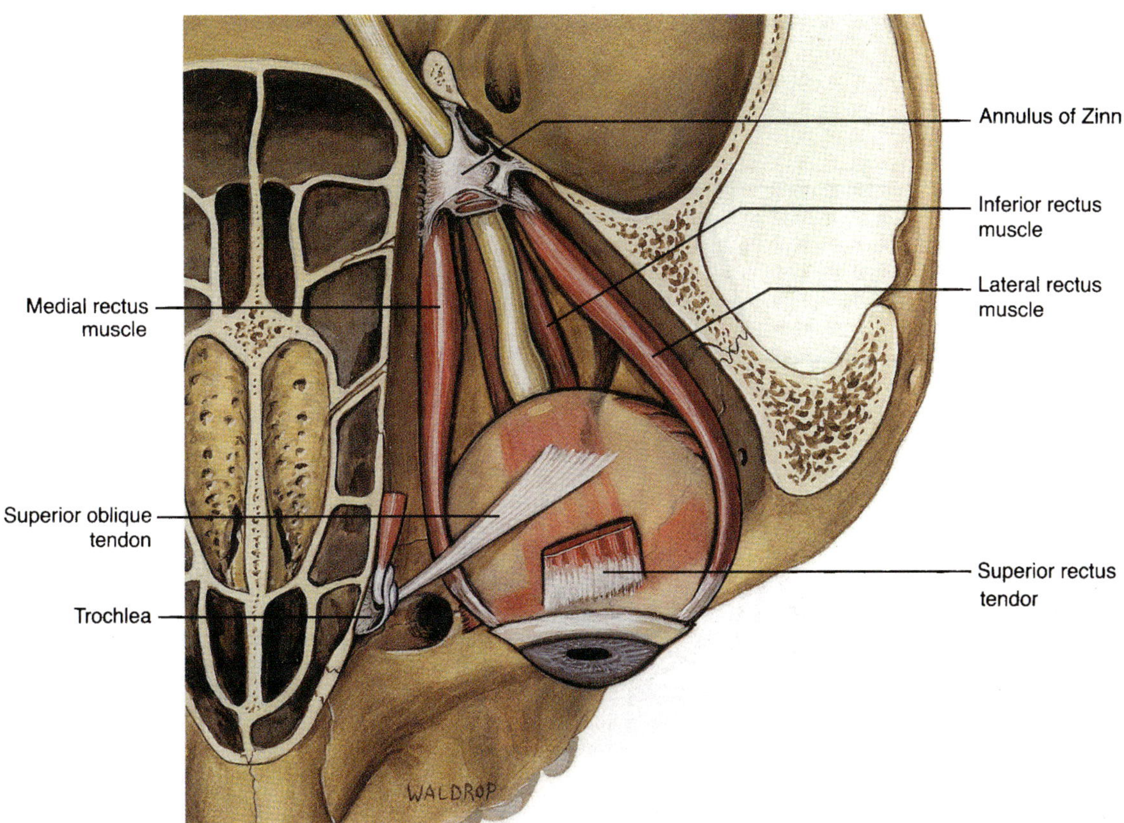

FIGURE 66-1. Eye and extraocular muscles, superior view, showing insertion of extraocular muscles. [Reprinted from Dutton JJ. *Atlas of Clinical Surgical Orbital Anatomy*. Philadelphia, PA: WB Saunders; 1994, with permission from Elsevier.]

of aqueous humor and accommodation. Ciliary muscles within the ciliary body are responsible for fine tuning visual focus by releasing tension on the suspensory fibers or zonules of the lens, increasing the refractive power of the lens. The contraction of ciliary muscles also opens space for increased aqueous drainage.

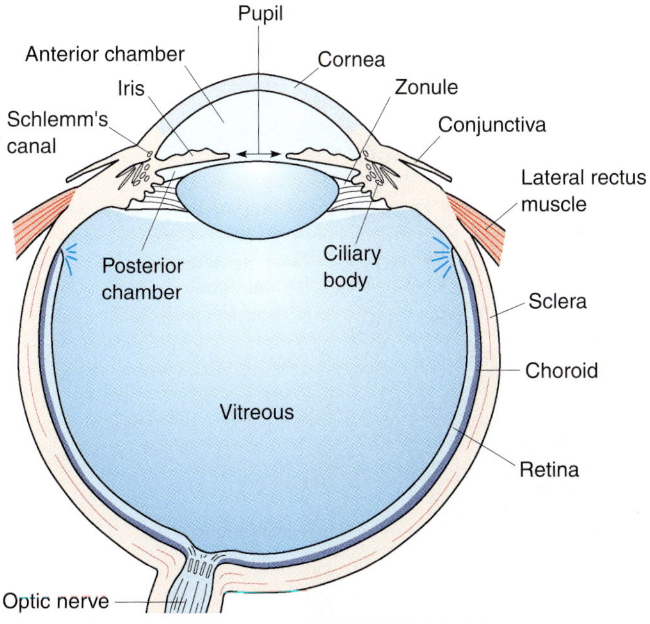

FIGURE 66-2. Anatomy of the eye. [Reprinted from Bruce RA Jr, McGoldrick KE, Oppenheimer P, eds. *Anesthesia for Ophthalmology*. Birmingham, AL: Aesculapius Publishing; 1982, with permission from Dr Kathryn McGoldrick.]

The posterior part of the uveal tract is a layer of blood vessels and capillaries called the *choroid*. These vessels nourish the outer portion of the retina, providing oxygen and nutrients. Bleeding from the choroid layer can cause catastrophic intraoperative expulsive hemorrhage.

The *retina* is a thin, transparent structure that differentiates from the optic cup and constitutes the inner layer of the medioposterior wall of the globe. Photoreceptors of the retinal layer convert light into neural signals, which are processed and carried to the brain via the optic nerve.

The *vitreous cavity* in the posterior portion of the globe occupies more than 80% of the volume of the globe. The transparent *vitreous humor* or *vitreous* contained within this cavity is important in the metabolism of the intraocular tissues; it provides a passageway for metabolites used by the lens, ciliary body, and retina. Although it has a gel-like structure, the vitreous is composed of 99% water. Vitreous adheres to the retina peripherally at the vitreous base, at the disk margin, and onto the posterior margin. Separation of the vitreous from the inner retina proceeds with age and sometimes causes small tears of the retina as it retracts. It is the most common event associated with retinal detachment. Scarring, bleeding, or opacification of the vitreous is treated by its removal, or vitrectomy.

The *eyelids* are composed of an outer layer of skin, a muscle layer, a cartilaginous tarsal plate, and an inner layer of conjunctiva. The upper eyelid can be raised 15 mm by the action of the levator palpebrae superioris muscle, which is innervated by CN III. The orbicularis oculi muscle, innervated by CN VII (facial), allows tight closure of the eyelids.

The *lacrimal gland* is located in a shallow depression within the orbital portion of the frontal bone. Tears are formed here by the serous secretion of acinar and myoepithelial cells. Under both reflex and psychogenic stimulation, tears pass from the surface of the eye via the puncta through either the upper or the lower canaliculi to the lacrimal sac and duct and drain into the nasopharynx below the inferior turbinate.

The blood supply to the ocular structures is primarily the *ophthalmic artery*. The ophthalmic artery is a branch of the internal carotid artery just before the circle of Willis. Venous drainage flows though the *superior and inferior ophthalmic veins* directly to the cavernous sinus.

The *ciliary ganglion* provides sensory innervation of the cornea, iris, and ciliary body. Parasympathetic motor fibers originating from the oculomotor nerve synapse in the ciliary ganglion before innervating the sphincter muscle of the iris and the ciliary muscle. Sympathetic motor fibers originating from the carotid plexus travel through the ciliary ganglion to innervate the dilator muscle of the iris.

The *CN* innervate ocular structures. The *optic nerve* (CN II) carries the sensory information from the retina. The optic nerve is a special sensory nerve, but it is not a true nerve. Developmentally speaking, both the retina and optic nerve are part of the brain. The optic nerve extends from the retina and enters the cranial cavity through the optic canal (optic foramen). The intraorbital part of the optic nerve is approximately 25 mm long. The optic nerve is enclosed by 3 sheaths that are continuous with the meninges of the brain. These sheaths extend as far as the back of the globe. The thick outer sheath is continuous with the dura mater of the brain and the sclera of the eye. The thin intermediate sheath is continuous with the arachnoid of the brain and is separated from the outer sheath by the subdural space and from the inner sheath by the subarachnoid space. The vascular inner sheath is continuous with the pia mater of the brain and closely invests the optic nerve. The inner sheath sends connective tissue partitions and blood vessels into the nerve. The ventral artery and vein of the retina pierce the dural and arachnoid coverings of the optic nerve approximately 1 cm behind the globe after a short course in the subarachnoid space, penetrate the optic nerve, and run within it to the inner aspect of the retina.

There are 6 *EOMs* that produce eye movement (**Fig. 66-3**). Four of these (superior rectus, inferior rectus, medial rectus, and lateral rectus) define the *intraorbital cone* (Figs. 66-1 and **66-4**). Structures within the cone (intraconal space) relevant to providing regional anesthesia include the posterior ciliary (sensory) nerves from the globe, ciliary ganglion, branches of CN III and VI, optic nerve, branches of ophthalmic artery and vein, parasympathetic and sympathetic fibers, adipose tissue, and septae.

The *oculomotor nerve* (CN III) is the somatic motor nerve to 4 of the 6 muscles that move the eye and to the levator palpebrae superioris, the muscle that raises the eyelid. The oculomotor nerve was so named because it supplies most of the muscles that move the eye. It also contains parasympathetic fibers to the involuntary muscles that constrict the pupil and change the curvature of the lens (*accommodation*).

The *trochlear nerve* (CN IV) has the fewest nerve fibers of any CN, but it has the longest intracranial course. The trochlear nerve enters the orbit through the superior orbital fissure. It then extends superiorly to innervate the superior oblique muscle. This location of the nerve, outside of the muscle cone, delays the abolition of depression and adduction of the globe after retrobulbar block.

The *trigeminal nerve* (CN V) provides sensory innervation to the skin and conjunctiva of the lower eyelid via that maxillary nerve and to the upper eyelid and conjunctiva via the frontal branch of the ophthalmic nerve. The nasociliary branch of the ophthalmic nerve provides sensory innervation to the medial canthus, lacrimal sac, and canaliculi and sends sensory fibers to the ciliary ganglion.

The *abducens nerve* (CN VI) passes through the superior orbital fissure to innervate the lateral rectus muscle on its ocular surface. No sympathetic or parasympathetic fibers appear to accompany the motor fibers.

A summary of the function and innervation of the EOMs is given in **Table 66-1**. A mnemonic that may aid in remembering the motor innervation of the EOM is *SO4-LR6*. (Superior oblique is innervated by CN IV, lateral rectus by CN VI, all others EOM by CN III.)

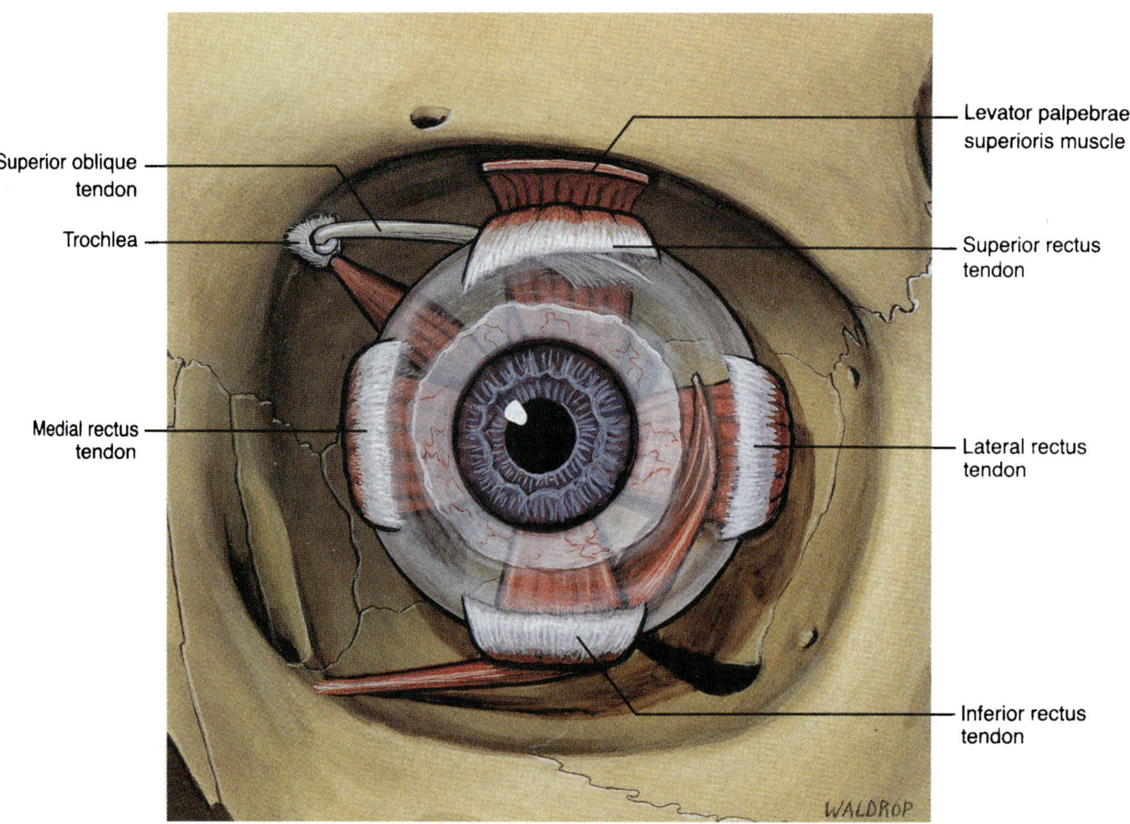

FIGURE 66-3. Eye and extraocular muscles, frontal view. [Reprinted from Dutton JJ. *Atlas of Clinical Surgical Orbital Anatomy*. Philadelphia, PA: WB Saunders; 1994, with permission from Elsevier.]

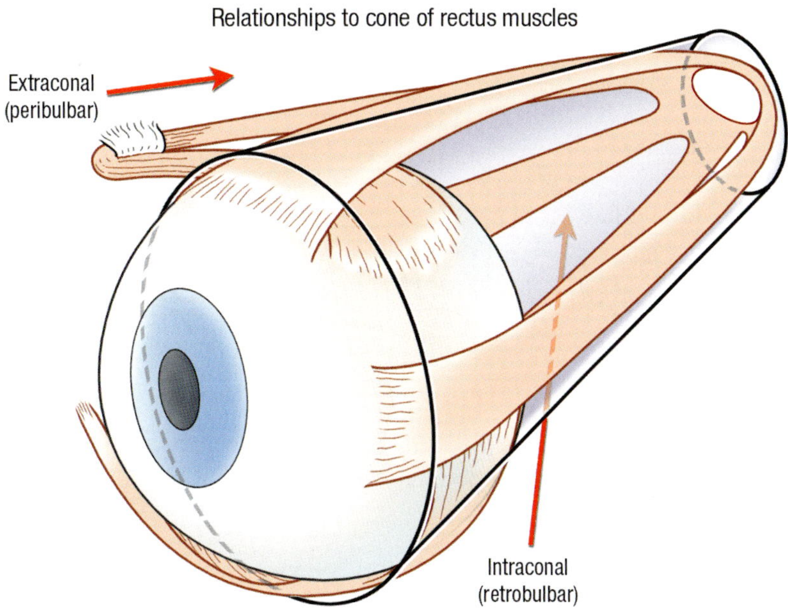

FIGURE 66-4. Illustration demonstrating intraconal (retrobulbar) and extraconal (peribulbar) block.

TABLE 66-1 Extraocular Muscles: Innervation and Function

Muscle	Innervation	Function
Superior rectus	III (oculomotor)	Elevation
Inferior rectus	III (oculomotor)	Depression
Medial rectus	III (oculomotor)	Adduction
Inferior oblique	III (oculomotor)	Elevation, abduction, and medial rotation (intorsion)
Superior oblique	IV (trochlear)	Depression, adduction, and external rotation (extorsion)
Lateral rectus	VI (abducens)	Abduction

Adapted from Snell RS, Lemp MA. *Clinical Anatomy of the Eye.* 2nd ed. Oxford, UK: Blackwell Science; 1998.[2]

The *facial nerve* (CN VII) is a mixed nerve, but it is predominantly motor in function. It was given its name because of large motor branches that spread across the face. The facial nerve exits the skull through the stylomastoid foramen (along with the internal carotid artery) and passes into the substance of the parotid gland, where it divides into 5 branches that supply the muscles of facial expression. The orbicularis oculi muscle, innervated by the zygomatic branch of the facial nerve, allows the patient to close the eyelids tightly. Local anesthetic blockade of the facial nerve can be important in intraocular surgery by eliminating squeezing caused by contraction of the orbicularis oculi.

In the posterior orbit, the optic nerve, ophthalmic artery, and sympathetic fibers from the carotid plexus pass through the optic foramen. Just lateral to the optic foramen is the superior orbital fissure. It is 22 mm long and conducts the lacrimal, frontal, and nasociliary branches of CN III (oculomotor), CN IV (trochlear), CN V (trigeminal), CN VI (abducens), the superior ophthalmic vein, and the sympathetic nerve plexus. The maxillary and pterygoid branches of CN V, a nerve from the pterygopalatine ganglion and the inferior ophthalmic vein, pass through the inferior orbital fissure, which is located just below the superior fissure and extends laterally.

INTRAOCULAR PRESSURE AND ANESTHESIA

Intraocular pressure is the pressure exerted by the contents of the eye upon the cornea and sclera. Normal IOP is 16 ± 5 mm Hg in the sitting position and is generally maintained within this narrow range. IOP undergoes normal minor fluctuations because of changes in body position (+1 mm Hg supine), diurnal rhythm (2-3 mm Hg), blood pressure oscillations (1-2 mm Hg), and respiration (deep inspiration decreases IOP by 5 mm Hg).

Aqueous humor is the major transport system in the eye for oxygen, glucose, proteins, medications, and inflammatory cells. It provides nourishment for the lens and the corneal endothelium. Approximately half of the cornea's oxygen supply comes from aqueous; the remainder comes from diffusion with the air. Drugs may enter the eye with aqueous humor via the cellular pumping action of the ciliary body, but a distinct blood–aqueous barrier prevents high-molecular-weight drugs from entering aqueous from the blood.

Aqueous humor volume is determined by the production and drainage of aqueous. Aqueous humor is formed by the ciliary body, which is the vascular component of the uveal tract located in front of the pars plana and behind the fibers of the suspensory ligament of the lens (**Fig. 66-5**). The ciliary body is folded over into a series of 80 folds, each 2 to 3 mm, termed processes, which extend to the posterior aspect of the iris. This structure is supplied by a vascular plexus and covered with epithelium that is impervious to proteins and high-molecular-weight substances.

The aqueous flows forward from the suspensory ligament of the lens and passes between the anterior capsule of the lens and posterior surface of the iris through the pupil to the anterior chamber. Flow then proceeds laterally to the meshwork of the trabecula and into the circular canal of Schlemm. This lateral drainage area is termed the *angle*. Episcleral veins drain aqueous to the venous system. Approximately one-third of the aqueous produced is reabsorbed through the veins in the iris and choroid. The blood vessels of the choroid constitute a large and variable volume in the eye. The sclera is inelastic, and this reduces compliance of the globe; thus, small changes in volume result in large changes in pressure. The volume of the globe is determined principally by the aqueous humor and the blood vessels of the eye, particularly of the choroid.

Clinical measurement of IOP is made indirectly. Commonly used measurement techniques include indentation (Schiotz) and applanation. Goldman applanati on is the "gold standard" for IOP measurement but requires a cooperative, sitting patient. Intraoperatively, a portable applanation tonometer (Tonopen, Reichert Inc., Depew, NY) is often used.

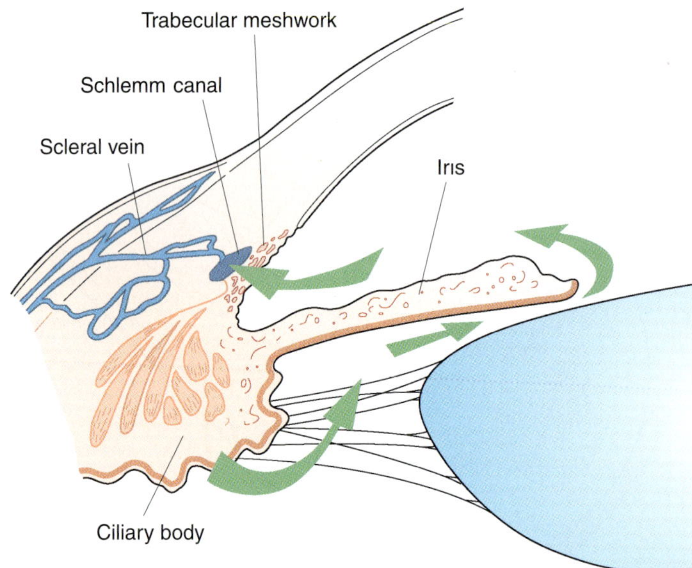

FIGURE 66-5. Anatomy of aqueous flow. [Reprinted from Bruce RA Jr, McGoldrick KE, Oppenheimer P, eds. *Anesthesia for Ophthalmology*. Birmingham, AL: Aesculapius Publishing; 1982, with permission from Dr Kathryn McGoldrick.]

The Schiotz technique uses a plunger activated by a small weight to indent the cornea. The plunger is connected to a lever that points to a number on an arbitrary scale. This number, along with the weight used in the measurement, allows determination of IOP from a nomogram. A small amount of aqueous is forced out of the eye with each indentation. Because of this action and because of the mechanical friction of the tonometer, Schiotz readings decrease as the measurements are repeated. The applanation method exerts graduated pressures to the cornea and results in a more reproducible IOP measurement. In the operating room (OR), the Schiotz tonometer or Tonopen is used. Invasive measurements of IOP are not common because of the risk of eye damage, danger of infection, and likelihood that the measurement itself may alter IOP.

Intraocular pressure should be maintained in as normal a range as possible during intraocular surgery. Increases in IOP interfere with choroidal and retinal blood supply as well as corneal metabolism, potentially causing retinal ischemia and corneal opacification. Severe increases in IOP can lead to choroidal hemorrhage, intraocular bleeding, and expulsion of intraocular contents. Large decreases in IOP (*hypotony*) increase the risk of retinal detachment, vitreous hemorrhage, and corneal edema.

Whereas hypotension, hyperventilation, and hypothermia all decrease IOP, hypoventilation, hypoxia, and venous obstruction increase IOP.[3] Hypertension may marginally increase IOP. Endotracheal intubation is another potent stimulus for increasing IOP. External pressure from a face mask, fingers, orbital tumors, contraction of the orbicularis oculi muscle, or retrobulbar hemorrhage also increase IOP.

Many drugs alter the production or drainage of aqueous humor and consequently IOP. Most medications exhibit a "dose–response" relationship with IOP. Initial dosing has minimal effect, a rapid linear response then occurs, leading to a plateau effect, in which increasing dosages have little or no effect on IOP. Most drugs used in anesthesia either have minimal effect on or decrease IOP. Inhalational and intravenous (IV) drugs have the most rapid and pronounced effect. Most sedatives and induction agents (eg, propofol and thiopental) reduce IOP in a dose-related manner.[3,4] Narcotics generally cause a small decrease in IOP.[3,4] Metoclopramide[5] and dexmedetomidine[6] do not increase IOP. Ketamine may slightly increase IOP.[7] Succinylcholine has been reported to increase IOP 6 to 12 mm Hg,[8-14] but straining or coughing raises IOP much more. (See discussion of the use of succinylcholine in the open globe, full stomach scenario in the General Anesthesia section of this chapter.)

The increase IOP observed from succinylcholine has been ascribed to contraction of the EOMs, leading to compression of the globe. But Katz et al[10] studied patients undergoing elective enucleation and compared the IOP between the normal eye and diseased eye in which all EOMs were detached. After administration of succinylcholine, both eyes exhibited a precipitous increase in IOP, leading the authors to conclude that EOM contraction does not contribute to the increase in IOP after succinylcholine administration.

SYSTEMIC EFFECTS OF OPHTHALMIC DRUGS

Some topical ophthalmic medications can have rapid systemic effects. Although topical medications are absorbed slowly from the conjunctival sac, much more rapid absorption can occur via the mucosal surfaces of the nasolacrimal duct. Systemic absorption may be altered in a diseased or postsurgical eye. Systemic absorption may be reduced if the lacrimal duct is compressed until topical absorption from the surface of the eye is complete.

Phenylephrine topical solution is commonly used as a mydriatic (dilates the pupil). There is little increase in mydriasis when solutions with concentrations greater than 5% are used.[15] This response is important because significant complications have been reported with 10% phenylephrine. A single drop of this high-concentration solution may contain 5 mg of phenylephrine (100 mg/mL ÷ 20 drops/mL). Complications seen include myocardial infarction, hypertension, reflex bradycardia, and cardiac dysrhythmias.[16] Only the 2.5% solution should be used in pediatric patients because excessive absorption can cause hypertension.

Epinephrine 2% topical solution causes a decrease in aqueous secretion and improves outflow, both of which act to reduce IOP in open-angle glaucoma. Complications include hypertension, tachycardia, dysrhythmias, and fainting. Because a single drop of 2% solution contains 0.5 to 1.0 mg of epinephrine, it is reasonable to expect systemic complications to occur. Intraocular epinephrine administered during halothane anesthesia is poorly absorbed and has no significant cardiac effects.[17]

β-Adrenergic antagonists (eg, timolol) topical solutions are used in the treatment of glaucoma. This class of medication acts to reduce aqueous humor secretion with minimal effects on aqueous outflow. Pupillary size is not affected. Patients may complain of light-headedness, fatigue, and disorientation and may exhibit a general depression of central nervous system (CNS) function. Excessive dosage of β-adrenergic antagonists may lead to cardiovascular dysfunction, including bradycardia, palpitations, syncope, an increase in heart block, and congestive heart failure.[18] Rare exacerbations of asthma have been reported.[19] Particular caution should be exercised with neonates receiving timolol eye drops because cases of apnea have been reported.[20]

Apraclonidine is a relatively new α_2-adrenergic agonist that has found a role as a topical antiglaucoma medication. Similar to epinephrine, it causes a decrease in aqueous formation and improves aqueous outflow. Systemic absorption may cause significant sedation and drowsiness. Hypotension is a possible complication but has not been reported. Acute withdrawal from long-term therapy may result in rebound hypertension.

Echothiophate iodide is a long-acting topical anticholinesterase drug now rarely used to treat glaucoma. Its duration of action is 4 to 6 weeks. Three weeks after cessation of treatment with echothiophate, plasma cholinesterase activity remains at 50% of normal.[21] If a patient receives succinylcholine, a relative overdose of succinylcholine leads to 2 to 3 times the usual duration of action. Careful titration of succinylcholine with use of a peripheral nerve stimulator will avoid prolonged paralysis. The effects of ester local anesthetics (procaine and chloroprocaine) may be significantly prolonged. Amide-type local anesthetics may be a better choice for regional anesthesia.

Topical muscarinic agonists are given to cause prolonged mydriasis. A drop of *atropine* 1% solution contains 0.2 to 0.5 mg of the drug. One drop of 0.5% *scopolamine* contains 0.2 mg of the drug. Systemic reactions have been seen in both young and elderly patients after administration of topical ocular atropine or scopolamine. These reactions are manifest by tachycardia, flushing, thirst, and dry skin. Elderly patients may show agitation. CNS excitement and agitation can be treated with incremental doses of 0.15 mg/kg IV of physostigmine.

Acetazolamide (given IV) causes carbonic anhydrase inhibition and interferes with the formation of aqueous humor and lowers IOP. Aside from a metabolic acidosis with depletion of sodium and potassium, long-term therapy may result in dyspepsia. When the drug is given rapidly IV, the patient may exhibit an acute decrease in blood pressure. Caution should be exercised in patients with renal disease, dehydration, and sodium or potassium depletion.

PREOPERATIVE EVALUATION (BOX 66-1)

Patients coming to the OR for ophthalmologic surgery tend to be very young or very old and have comorbid conditions. Infants often present with apnea of prematurity, bronchopulmonary dysplasia, and patent ductus arteriosus. Congenital glaucoma often is associated with other syndromes. Congenital strabismus may be associated with a myopathy, and if so, malignant hyperthermia precautions should be considered (see Chapter 87). Elderly adults are likely to present with coronary artery disease, valvular heart disease, hypertension, cerebrovascular disease, chronic obstructive pulmonary disease, diabetes, dementia, Parkinson's disease, renal disease, arthritis, osteoporosis, or cancer. Since 1990, the proportion of Medicare patients requiring surgical treatment of chronic eye diseases grew from 13.4% to 45.4%.[22] In a study by Kraushar and Turner[23] on medical litigation in cataract surgery, failure of proper coordination of preoperative care among anesthesiologists, surgeons, and internists resulted in indemnity findings in 16% of patients. Because most ophthalmic procedures are now performed in outpatients and in free-standing day surgery facilities, obtaining an adequate preoperative evaluation (sometimes requiring additional information from primary care physicians, ophthalmic surgeons, and consultant physicians) can be challenging.

Fortunately, most patients undergoing ophthalmologic procedures are at low risk for major perioperative complications. This may be because there are usually no major perioperative physiologic derangements or blood loss. When general anesthesia is required physiologic changes can occur during induction and emergence. Most of the risk associated with anesthesia relates to patient movement,[24] changes in IOP, and postoperative nausea and vomiting (PONV). If these potential problems can be controlled, the morbidity and mortality of ophthalmic surgery will be low[25] despite the high-risk population. The anesthesiologist can draw on several sources as guides when performing a preoperative evaluation,[26-30] and this topic is covered more extensively elsewhere in this text (see especially Chapters 6, 9, 11, and 13).

All patients should have a preoperative history and physical examination assessing their medical conditions, ensuring they are appropriately managed for surgery, and given instructions on what medications to take before and on the day of surgery (**Table 66-2**). For patients having eye surgery (low-risk surgery) with no other medical problems, routine laboratory tests and electrocardiography (ECG) have not been demonstrated to improve outcome,[31] and preoperative ECGs are not recommended for asymptomatic patients undergoing low-risk surgery.[26] Laboratory tests and ECGs are warranted only if indicated by history and physical examination[26,30,31] (**Table 66-3**; see Chapters 6 and 7). Some of the suggestions drawn from the American Society of Anesthesiologists Task Force on Preoperative Evaluation and Institute for Clinical Systems Improvement are listed in Table 66-2. Of note, for patients without changes in medical history, normal laboratory and

BOX 66-1

Special Concerns in Ophthalmic Anesthesiology

- Elderly patients with multiple systemic diseases
- Pediatric patients, often premature with congenital syndromes
- Patients anxious from loss of vision
- Limited access to the airway
- Oculocardiac reflex is common with general anesthesia and occasionally seen with blocks
- Potential for eye injury with intraoperative movement
- Intraocular pressure and anesthetic interactions
- Systemic effects of ophthalmic medications

TABLE 66-2 Preoperative Basic Health Assessment

General Medical History
Indications for surgery and proposed procedure, including documentation of which eye(s) being operated on
Allergies or other reactions to medications, latex, environmental allergens, or foods
Current medications, doses, timing, and reasons for taking
Prior surgical and anesthesia history
Focused Medical History and Physical Examination (concentrating on)
Functional status (can lie flat without moving, no acute cough)
Cardiac problems
Pulmonary problems
Neurologic problems
Hemostasis problems
Other medical problems
Smoking, alcohol, and illicit drug use
Possibility of pregnancy
Physical Examination (concentrating on)
Weight and height
Blood pressure
Pulse (rate and regularity)
Respiratory rate
Heart sounds
Breath sounds

TABLE 66-3 Examples of Laboratory Tests That May Be Indicated for Eye (Low-Risk) Surgery

Test	Possible Indication
Glucose	Diabetes
Potassium	Diuretic use
BUN, creatinine	Renal disease and general anesthesia anticipated
Coagulation studies	History of coagulopathy
	Anticoagulation as a medical treatment
ECG	Signs or symptoms of cardiac disease

BUN, blood urea nitrogen; ECG, electrocardiography.

ECG results do not need to be repeated if they were performed within the previous 6 months.[27]

Patients must meet the following criteria to undergo eye surgery under local anesthesia: able to lie flat for the duration of the procedure, have no symptomatic gastric reflex, have no condition that might preclude lying without movement during the procedure (eg, severe claustrophobia, head tremor, or dementia), have no uncontrollable cough, have sufficient command of English or other language understood by at least 1 member of the operative team so as to be able to communicate, be able follow commands, and comprehend that he or she will be awake or only mildly sedated during the procedure (**Table 66-4**).

An inability to achieve 4 metabolic equivalents (eg, climb 2 flights of stairs or walk 4 blocks without stopping) may be indicative of significant heart disease[32] but can also occur in pulmonary, neurologic, and orthopedic conditions or poor conditioning. It is common in elderly adults and is not a contraindication to proceeding with low-risk surgery if the patient can lie supine for the duration of the procedure and active cardiac conditions have been ruled out.[26]

A preoperative visit to the facility, or a phone call from OR staff can allay patient anxiety and educate the patient about the anesthesia plan and about the management of medications before and on the day of surgery. After obtaining informed consent, confirming patient identity, identifying any allergies, and confirming the correct eye to be operated on, one can proceed with the anesthesia and surgery

Historically, anticoagulants (eg, warfarin) and antiplatelet drugs (eg, aspirin and clopidogrel) were routinely held for 5 days or more before many eye operations to minimize the risk of bleeding. However recent studies suggest that the small risk of a bleeding complication should be balanced against the small (but potentially life-threatening) risk of thromboembolism or myocardial infarction if these medications are discontinued.[33,34]

Although the risk of minor bleeding (eg, conjunctival, eyelid, and mild hyphema) seems to be greater for patients taking clopidogrel or warfarin,[35,36] the risk of major (sight-threatening) bleeding complications from continuing therapeutic doses of aspirin or warfarin[37-39] or clopidogrel (Plavix)[35,36,40] alone or in combination for clear cornea cataract surgery is no greater than for patients not taking antithrombotic agents. Some authors advocate topical anesthesia or sub-Tenon block for patients taking antithrombotic agents[41,42] before cataract surgery. If a needle block is performed, peribulbar block may have a lower incidence of retrobulbar hemorrhage than retrobulbar block.[43]

TABLE 66-4 Basic Requirements for Cataract and Other Eye Surgery Under Local Anesthesia

- Can lie flat for length of procedure
- No symptomatic reflux
- No claustrophobia, head tremor, or dementia
- Ability to control cough
- Knowledge of English or other language understood by OR staff and can:
  - Communicate
  - Follow commands
  - Understand will be awake or only mildly sedated

OR, operating room.

Many internists and surgeons now continue therapeutic doses of aspirin, warfarin, and clopidogrel up to the day of surgery for patients having cataract surgery.[44] A few small studies have demonstrated an increased incidence of serious bleeding complications in patient taking warfarin immediately before glaucoma surgery,[45,46] but a survey of British glaucoma surgeons found most did not stop antithrombotic medications preoperatively before glaucoma surgery.[47]

There is more concern by retinal surgeons about the potential of antithrombotic drugs causing retinal bleeding. One study suggested warfarin (but not aspirin) caused a higher risk of bleeding complications and suggested that the drug may be stopped if the patient's thrombotic risk is low,[48] but several other studies suggest that the risk of significant bleeding complications from continuing anticoagulants up to the day of retinal surgery is low.[49-51] Although some retinal surgeons routinely request stopping antithrombotic drugs before retinal surgery, some continue these drugs for patients at high risk of thromboembolism.

If patients need to stop warfarin preoperatively, a recent review recommends using subcutaneous low-molecular-weight heparin preoperatively for several days before and after surgery for patients at high risk (and consider its use in patient at moderate risk) of thromboembolism (ie, heparin bridging therapy).[52] The intent is to minimize the interval when the patient is not receiving antithrombotic drugs. The decisions regarding management of oral anticoagulation therapy preoperatively, whether to institute heparin bridging therapy, and when to restart anticoagulation therapy postoperatively are best made by consultation among the surgical and medical management team to ensure that all factors are considered regarding the risks and benefits of these various treatment options.

Recently, it has been recommended aspirin and clopidogrel should be continued for at least 1 full year after a drug-eluting cardiac stent is placed and 6 weeks after a bare metal stent is placed.[53] Stopping these medications prematurely greatly increases the risk of cardiac stents clotting with potentially lethal results. If clopidogrel needs to be stopped prematurely in these situations, it is essential that aspirin be continued. The decision to stop aspirin or clopidogrel therapy in these patients is best made in consultation with the patient's cardiologist.

Adult patients presenting for eye surgery are more likely than the general population to be elderly, have cardiac disease, and have a pacemaker or implanted cardiac defibrillator (ICD). Several reviews on perioperative management of these devices exist.[54,55]

Implanted cardiac devices have high reliability, but it has been reported that about 5% of these devices will be at or near the end of battery life when these devices undergo routine interrogation.[56] To ensure that these devices have adequate battery life and are appropriately programmed for the patient's operation, measures should be taken to confirm that implanted cardiac devices are functioning appropriately before elective surgery.[54,55]

At the Massachusetts Eye and Ear Infirmary (MEEI) before elective surgery, we send a request form (**Fig. 66-6**) to the patient's cardiac electrophysiology laboratory or cardiologist to obtain the latest complete interrogation results. We require device interrogation within 3 months for ICDs and 6 months for pacemakers. We use this information to confirm that the device has adequate battery life and is functioning appropriately.

For most eye operations, no electrosurgical device or only battery-operated cautery or bipolar electrosurgical instruments are used. These instruments are very unlikely to interfere with pacemakers or ICDs. There is a very small risk of an active ICD delivering a shock and potentially causing patient movement and eye trauma during eye surgery. One author estimated the risk of a shock being delivered (if patient has never had ventricular tachycardia or fibrillation or recent ICD-delivered electrical therapy) of about 1 in 243 000 cataract cases.[57]

One author suggests temporarily inactivating all ICDs during eye surgery to eliminate this risk,[58] but we believe this risk must be balanced against the risk of inhibiting the device from delivering potentially

MEEI PREOPERATIVE INFORMATION FOR PATIENTS WITH PACEMAKERs, ICDs, and other IMPLANTED ELECTRONIC DEVICES.

Please fill out and returned this form ASAP or your patient's upcoming surgery may need to be delayed or cancelled.

Pacemaker/ICD Clinic______________________Phone____________________Fax_____________
Cardiologist or Responsible M.D. ______________Phone____________________Fax_____________

Dear Pacemaker/ICD Clinic or Doctor:

Your patient:
Patients' Name______________________________
Date of Birth______________________________
is coming to the Massachusetts Eye and Ear Infirmary on (Date) ________________ to have the following type of surgery_________________________with Dr. __________________ (Surgeon.)

Paragraph below to be completed by patient's Pacemaker/ICD Clinic or M.D.

Please provide us with the following information.

1. Type of implanted device (e.g. Pacemaker/ICD/Other) ______________________________
2. Manufacturer____
3. Model # ____
4. Most recent insertion date of generator____
5. Reason for insertion____
6. Date of most recent interrogation ____
7. Battery life estimate ____
8. Leads and Generator functioning appropriately Yes/No_______________________________
9. How device will respond to magnet placement and removal___________________________
10. Pacemaker dependent? Yes/No ____
11. Underlying rhythm (NSR? AF? Other?)____
12. What will happen to the device if it converts to noise reversion mode?______________
13. Manufacturer Recalls or Alerts ? Yes/No ____
14. PACEMAKER INFO: A. Rate Responsive? Yes/No B. Uses Bio Impedence Sensor to Determine Minute Ventilation? Yes/No C. Sleep Mode Active? Yes/No
15. ICD INFO: Within last 12 months has Tachy Rx been delivered, or NSVT/SVT/AFib recorded? Yes/No (If yes, brief description and date(s) of event(s)) ____________________

Any other pertinent information or management suggestions?_______________________________
Name, Title and Telephone # of Person Completing Form__________________________________
Today's date____

Please fax completed form to Preop Review MEEI 866 339 2791, or mail to Preop Review 8th Floor, MEEI, 243 Charles Street, Boston, MA 02114.

Thank you very much for taking the time to complete this form! It will greatly assist in caring for your patient.

Meeipacericdinforequest.10.14.10

FIGURE 66-6. Massachusetts Eye and Ear Infirmary (MEEI) preoperative information for patients with pacemakers, implanted cardiac defibrillators, and other implanted electronic devices.

lifesaving electrical therapy in a timely manner. In a survey of Ophthalmic Anesthesia Society members, 83% left ICDs active during eye surgery with no reports of ICD malfunction or ICD discharge.[59] Various device manufacturers report a 6- to 15-second interval between arrhythmia onset and the ICD delivering antiarrhythmic therapy.[57] We believe this interval is likely to allow enough time to warn the surgeon of an impending shock if the ECG monitor is vigilantly monitored. At the MEEI, unless there are contraindications (see the following text), we routinely leave ICDs active during eye operations.

If unipolar electrosurgery (eg, Bovie) is required, ICDs should be temporarily disabled (after ensuring a working external defibrillator is immediately available) to prevent inappropriate electrical discharge. These and additional perioperative management recommendations are given in reviews on this subject.[54,55] Transcutaneous electrical nerve stimulation units have been reported to cause ICDs to discharge inappropriately,[60] so it may be safest to temporarily inactivate ICDs during eye surgery if peripheral nerve stimulators are required. Interestingly, succinylcholine has not been reported to cause ICDs to discharge.[54] Temporary inactivation of ICDs should also be considered if within the previous 12 months an ICD delivered a shock or anti-tachycardia pacing (ATP) if the patient had nonsustained ventricular tachycardia, supraventricular tachycardia, or atrial fibrillation or if a "lead alert" is present. These conditions increase the possibility of an ICD delivering a shock during surgery.

Hypertension is a common problem in elderly patients. Although there is concern that moderate to severe hypertension may increase the risk of perioperative bleeding, CHF, and cerebrovascular events, numerous studies have shown that there is no increased cardiac morbidity for patients with systolic blood pressure below 180 mm Hg and diastolic blood pressure below 110 mm Hg.[26,61-63] One study showed no difference in outcome for patients with preoperative hypertension controlled on the day of surgery with medication versus patients whose surgery was cancelled and returned after control of hypertension with oral medications.[64]

Hypertension can be exacerbated by eye drops containing phenylephrine or epinephrine. At MEEI, we attempt to decrease systolic blood pressure to less than 180 mm Hg and diastolic blood pressure to less than 100 mm Hg before administering these eye drops. If patients with hypertension did not take their prescribed antihypertensive medications on the day of surgery, they are given preoperatively. If patients normally have well-controlled blood pressure but we suspect they are anxious in the hospital setting ("white coat syndrome"), a sedative (eg, midazolam 0.5-2 mg IV), and/or an antihypertensive (eg, labetalol 5-10 mg IV or hydralazine 5-10 mg IV), may be administered. Only if patients have untreated chronic hypertension or normally well-controlled blood pressure unresponsive to medications do we (after consultation with their surgeon) delay their surgery and refer them urgently to an internist.

REGIONAL ANESTHESIA TECHNIQUES

Technical advances in ophthalmologic surgery have made it possible for many adult patients, even those with multiple chronic conditions, to undergo outpatient eye surgery under regional anesthesia. Regional anesthesia has a lower perioperative morbidity than general anesthesia for ophthalmic surgery.[65] If heavy sedation is avoided during regional anesthesia, the already low risks of perioperative problems are reduced further.[66] More than 2 million people undergo cataract surgery in the United States every year. At MEEI, about 7000 ophthalmic procedures are performed every year. In adults, most ophthalmic procedures are performed under some form of regional anesthesia, and about 80% of the regional blocks at our institution are performed by anesthesiologists. Patients with a history of orthopnea should be kept upright before and after the procedure and kept supine intraoperatively for the minimum time necessary to reduce the risk of exacerbating congestive heart failure or chronic obstructive pulmonary disease. Patients with a history of mild claustrophobia can often tolerate brief periods of being covered with sterile drapes if they are reassured, lightly sedated, given supplementary air or oxygen, and using clear and suspended drapes if possible so room air and light can enter around the patient's head. Patients who cannot tolerate lying supine or covered for the anticipated duration of the procedure should have their procedure performed at a facility that can provide general anesthesia.

TOPICAL ANESTHESIA

Topical anesthesia involves instillation of local anesthesia eye drops or gel on the surface of the cornea and conjunctiva. Topical anesthesia is appropriate for some uncomplicated procedures in the anterior globe (eg, cataracts, pterygiums) in properly informed and cooperative patients and by surgeons comfortable with these techniques. Topical anesthesia has the lowest rate of eye complications compared with other regional techniques[67] and is currently the most popular anesthetic for cataract surgery in the United States.[68] The conjunctiva, cornea, iris, and sclera are rapidly anesthetized from absorption of local anesthesia. Tetracaine 0.5%, proparacaine 0.5%, lidocaine 4%, and lidocaine gel 2% to 4% are often used. The advantages of topical anesthesia are that no preprocedural sedation or injections are required, and visual improvement is immediate after lens placement. The duration of analgesia is brief and occasionally requires supplementation with additional topical instillation, or intracameral, subconjunctival, or sub-Tenon injection of local anesthetic.

Eyelid pressure, bright ophthalmic lights, and vision of surgical instruments can be bothersome to some patients. Potential concerns for some surgeons include lack of akinesia, the ability of patients to move their eyelids, a relative lack of IOP control compared with needle blocks or general anesthesia, and the potential requirement of heavy sedation if patients cannot cooperate intraoperatively. Intraoperative comfort may be more reliable with needle-based and sub-Tenon blocks. Interestingly, patients experiencing bilateral cataract extractions who were randomly assigned to topical for 1 eye and retrobulbar block for the other eye preferred the block technique by 71% to 10%.[69]

SEDATION FOR NERVE BLOCKS AND OPHTHALMIC SURGERY

Sedation before performing needle-based regional anesthesia has several benefits. It can reduce patient anxiety (and sometimes memory) relating to needle insertion near the eye, and it can reduce the pain that is otherwise common during needle blocks. By providing adequate analgesia and sedation, patient cooperation is enhanced, and the risk of movement during the block is reduced. Lastly, sedation and analgesia may keep the patient relax after the block has been placed. At MEEI, a combination of IV midazolam (0-2 mg) and remifentanil (20-60 mcg) appropriate for patient age, weight, and condition are used. Although there is debate over the most appropriate NPO (nothing by mouth) guidelines for patients undergoing eye surgery under regional anesthesia, at our hospital, we use the current ASA NPO guidelines (see Chapter 6).

Because of the risks of oversedation or possible local anesthesia spread to the brain, all patients undergoing sedation or orbital blocks require oximetry, ECG, and blood pressure monitoring. Resuscitation equipment and drugs must be immediately available. As in other situations, the decision to use sedation should be based on need, not routine protocol. For many anxious patients, holding their hands or reassuring words my provide a calming effect. Finally, no amount of sedation, short of general anesthesia, will compensate for inadequate analgesia. Therefore, it may be necessary to remind the surgeon to supplement local anesthesia if it is inadequate initially or decreasingly effective over time.

Supplementary oxygen can be useful in reducing hypoxemia during preprocedural sedation. But routine use of 100% oxygen by nasal prongs, masks, or other delivery systems during surgery under local anesthesia should be questioned. Although a rare event, there is an increased risk of fire during eye surgery whenever there is an enriched oxygen environment, a heat source (eg, bipolar or battery operated cautery), and a fuel source (eg, facial hair, oxygen tubing, drapes).[70-73]

Most patients do not require high concentrations of oxygen during eye surgery. Two studies showed that patients who received compressed air under the drapes during cataract surgery had the same oxygen saturation as patients who received 100% oxygen.[74,75] If supplementary oxygen is required during the procedure, it should be started at a concentration of 30% if possible[72] (ie, oxygen mixed with compressed air in a ratio of 1:8). If oxygen is used in higher concentrations, the surgeon should be alerted to its use and no heat source (eg, cautery) should be used until the oxygen is stopped for a few minutes to minimize the risk of supporting combustion.[71]

It is possible for CO_2 to accumulate under the drapes during eye surgery causing hypercarbia, tachycardia, tachypnea, and restlessness. However, 1 study showed that giving additional oxygen at 2 L/min did not prevent hypercarbia.[76] Insufflating fresh gas (eg, compressed air) under the drapes at 10 L/min and using paper drapes helped mitigate this increase in CO_2.[77] Use of a suction device to remove accumulated CO_2 under the drapes has also been successful in decreasing CO_2 levels when oxygen was insufflated under the drapes at 2 to 3 L/min.[78,79]

RETROBULBAR (INTRACONAL) BLOCK AND PERIBULBAR (EXTRACONAL) BLOCK

Retrobulbar block (more precisely defined anatomically as an intraconal block) was first described more than 120 years ago and has been the predominant technique of ophthalmologists and many anesthesiologists for providing regional anesthesia to the orbit during the 20th century and currently. The goal is to inject local anesthetic into (or near) the middle of the muscle cone formed by the 4 recti muscles (the intraconal space) (Figs. 66-1 and 66-4). The local anesthetic spreads from this location to anesthetize the ciliary ganglion (and the sensory nerves that run through it) and motor nerves to the eye. Patient requirements to undergo surgery with sedation and a retrobulbar block are similar to those of topical anesthesia.

Commonly used local anesthetics include lidocaine 2% mixed with bupivacaine 0.75% (in a 1:1 ratio), lidocaine 2% with epinephrine 1:200 000, and chloroprocaine 2%. Lidocaine 4% can be myotoxic and should be avoided.[80] Epinephrine in a concentration of 1:200 000 or less can be used if vasoconstriction is desired (eg, during enucleation) or to prolong the effects of lidocaine. Because of the concern that epinephrine could cause tachycardia and inadequate blood flow to the optic nerve in patients with vascular disease, it is best avoided unless specifically indicated. The bulk of evidence suggests that adding the enzyme hyaluronidase increases the speed of onset of ophthalmic blocks and reduces the chance of EOM injuries from local anesthesia.[81-83] Hyaluronidase is commonly used in concentrations between 2.5 and 15 U/mL; however, there is evidence that it has effect in concentrations as low as 0.5 to 0.75 U/mL.[1,84]

Unlike topical anesthesia, a retrobulbar block is effective in anesthetizing the posterior chamber of the eye and causing akinesis. In experienced hands, retrobulbar block has a success rate of more than 90%.[85] Retrobulbar block (especially if used with ≤5 mL local anesthesia) may require supplementation with a Van Lint block (a peripheral facial nerve block) if blinking interferes with surgery.

At our institution, before performing a needle block, we administer a topical anesthetic (proparacaine) and then swab a 10% povidone–iodine solution over the eyelids and around the eye. The solution is allowed to contact the skin for several minutes to provide optimal antibacterial effect. We request patients to look straight ahead during the block (primary gaze position). Looking up and in (the Atkinson position) brings the optic nerve closer to the midline and increases the risk of injury from the needle tip.[86]

A palpating finger identifies the lower part of the globe and orbital rim. This finger indents the skin and pushes the globe slightly up. The authors prefer a needle length of 7/8 in (23 mm) to reduce the risk of injuring structures that are tightly packed together deep in the orbit (**Figs. 66-7** and **66-8**). We use an Atkinson needle (blunter than the traditional hypodermic needle to help identify the sclera if inadvertently touched). The needle is inserted, bevel toward the globe, about 1/4 in (6-7 mm) directly below the lateral canthus and above the inferior orbital rim (**Fig. 66-9**). There is some evidence insertion at this "modified" insertion point instead of the "traditional" insertion point at the junction of the middle and lateral third of the lower eyelid reduces the risk of injury to the inferior rectus and the neurovascular bundle supplying the inferior oblique muscle (**Fig. 66-10**).[1,80]

The needle is initially directed perpendicular to all planes of the skin (**Figs. 66-11** and **66-12**). There may be slight resistance as the needle pierces the skin and a slight "pop" after penetration through the orbital septum (**Fig. 66-13**) several millimeters below the skin. The needle when correctly positioned is only 3 to 4 mm away from the globe, so great care must be taken not to perforate the globe. One of the authors (JB) wiggles the needle several millimeters (parallel to the globe) during insertion to ensure the globe is not encountered by the needle. (If so, the globe would move while wiggling the needle.) After the needle is judged to pass the lowest point of the globe called the *inferior equator* (for average axial length eyes, about 0.5 in [13 mm] posterior to the cornea), the needle is directed slightly more superiorly and medially, with the intent of entering the anterior intraconal space (**Fig. 66-14**). Kumar et al[1] recommend that the tip of the needle when fully inserted lie in the imaginary vertical plane starting at the limbus (the junction of the cornea and the sclera) and proceeding posteriorly into the orbit (**Fig. 66-15**). When the tip of the needle is thought to be in the intraconal space, aspirate for signs of blood. If blood is identified, withdraw the needle, apply intermittent digital pressure, and reevaluate the orbit for possible hematoma before attempting to proceed. When using a 7/8- to 1-in needle, 6 to 8 mL of local anesthesia is usually required to obtain a satisfactory block, although some authors use up to 10 mL. If a 1.25-in (32-mm) needle is used, 5 to 7 mL is usually required. Akinesia of EOMs after orbital block usually correlates with adequate analgesia for eye surgery.

Patients with long axial length globes are at significantly higher risk of posterior globe perforation if an intraconal block is attempted.[87-89] Patients having cataract surgery will have had their axial lengths measured during preoperative ultrasonography. If the axial length is greater than about 26 mm, the patient has a *scleral buckle* (a band placed around the globe to treat retinal detachment) or *enophthalmos* (globe recessed in orbit), and the risk is increased of perforating the posterior aspect of the elongated globe when attempting to enter the retrobulbar space. The presence of a *staphyloma* (an outpouching of the posterior or inferior sclera associated with long axial length eyes detected by ultrasonography) also increases the risk of globe perforation from retrobulbar block[90] (**Figs. 66-16** and **66-17**), For these conditions, other anesthetic techniques should be considered (eg, topical, extraconal block, sub-Tenon block, general anesthesia). If the length of the eye has not been measured, a longer than normal eye can be assumed if the patient wore glasses as a child or young adult to see distant objects (*myopia*).[1,91]

Unfortunately, the anatomic definition of a *peribulbar block* is imprecise. Some understand it to mean an extraconal block, but the term is sometimes used to denote an anterior retrobulbar block with a needle 1 in or less in length. For the purposes of this discussion, we will use *peribulbar* to mean *extraconal.* The goal of a peribulbar block is to insert a needle near and parallel to but not into the intraconal space and deposit enough local anesthesia so it diffuses into the intraconal space (**Fig. 66-18**). Because there are no discrete septal barriers separating the extraconal from retrobulbar space, adequate volume of local anesthesia injected near the retrobulbar space can diffuse through adipose tissue into the cone and anesthetize the intraconal structures[92] (**Fig. 66-19**). Because the needle tip is farther away from the globe and retrobulbar structures than with a retrobulbar block, an extraconal block may reduce the risk of injury to these structures but at the cost of a slightly lower success rate in providing analgesia and akinesia. Although the reported success rates of 83% to 84% with the extraconal block[93,94] are not quite as high as with the retrobulbar technique, it is sufficient to consider performance of this block.

The insertion site is similar to that of the retrobulbar block. (See the discussion of the retrobulbar technique above.) The needle perforates the skin in the same spot as with the retrobulbar block. It is directed perpendicular to all the planes of the skin and posteriorly below the globe and parallel to the intraconal space but not attempting to enter it. Needles between 7/8 and 1¼ in (23-32 mm) are commonly used for this block. Six to 10 mL of local anesthetic is injected. Extraconal block may be safer for patients with axial length 26 mm or larger, scleral buckle, or severe enophthalmos. When this block was initially described,[95] one needle was placed in the inferolateral orbit and a second one in the superior orbit. Most practitioners now routinely use a single inferolateral extraconal injection because evidence has shown that 1 injection is likely to be as effective as 2.[96,97]

If retrobulbar or peribulbar block does not produce global akinesia (and analgesia) after 5 to 10 minutes, it may be repeated once, preferably with a slightly lower volume of local anesthesia. Multiple repeat injection of local anesthesia should be avoided.

MEDIAN ORBITAL BLOCK AND SUPERIOR ORBITAL BLOCKS

If a retrobulbar or peribulbar block is inadequate in blocking the medial rectus or the superior oblique muscles, practitioners may supplement the block by performing a *median orbital* (extraconal)

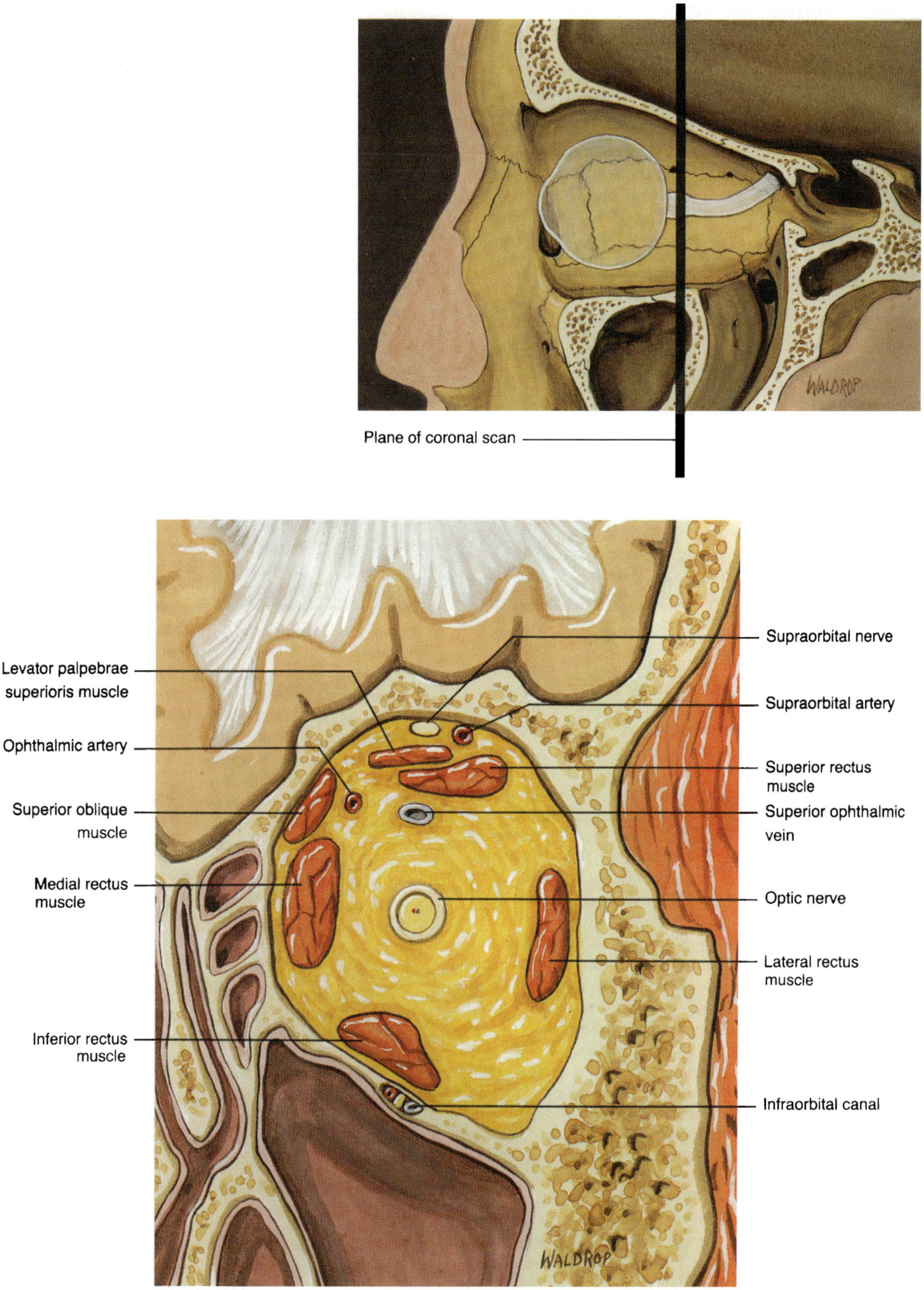

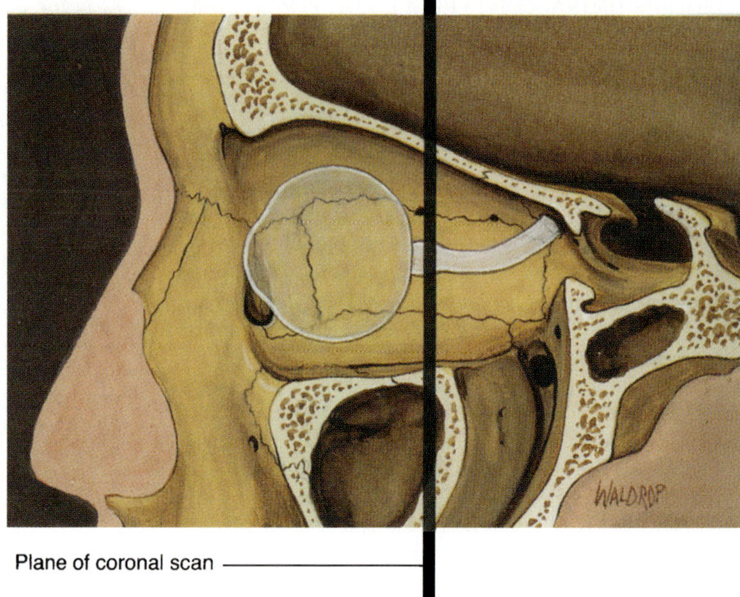

FIGURE 66-7. Coronal views of intraconal space just posterior to globe. Note most of inferior-lateral intraconal space just posterior to the globe is adipose tissue. This is a safe area for the tip of a sharp needle to be placed to provide local anesthesia. [Reprinted from Dutton JJ. *Atlas of Clinical Surgical Orbital Anatomy*. Philadelphia, PA: WB Saunders; 1994, with permission from Elsevier.]

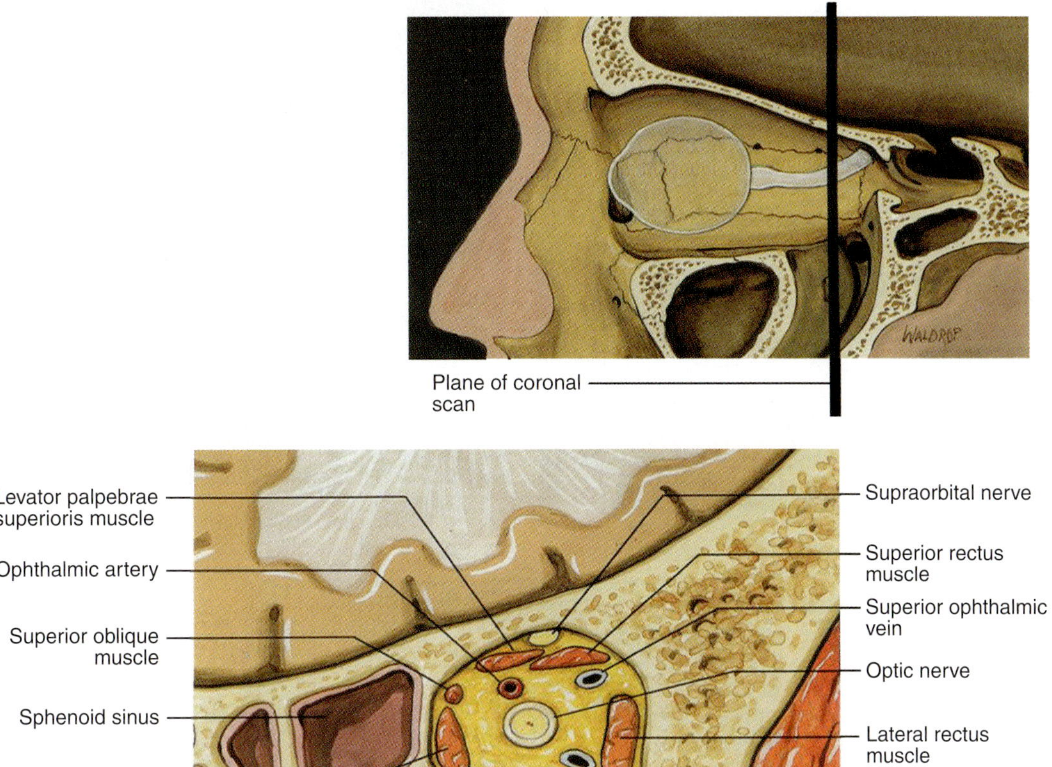

FIGURE 66-8. Coronal view of intraconal space in the posterior orbit at the level of the annulus of Zinn. Note how tightly packed the intraorbital contents are ("pickle jar" effect). Needles placed deep in the orbit are more likely to injure these vital structures. [Reprinted from Dutton JJ. *Atlas of Clinical Surgical Orbital Anatomy*. Philadelphia, PA: WB Saunders; 1994, with permission from Elsevier.]

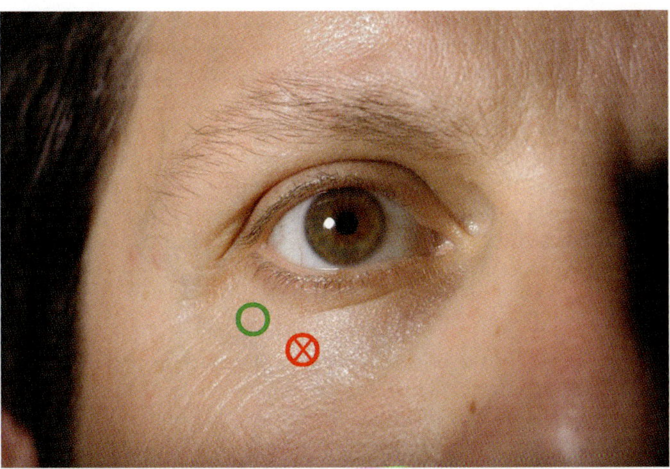

FIGURE 66-9. Photo of eye with a *green circle* denoting the recommended "modified" needle insertion point. The *red circle* denotes the "traditionally" taught insertion point (at the junction of the medial and lateral third of the lower eyelid).

block.[1,98] The space between the medial rectus muscle and the medial orbital wall is primarily filled with adipose tissue and is the target area for this block. After topical anesthesia and 5% Betadine ophthalmic solutions are applied, a ½- to 1-in (25- to 30-g) blunt needle is inserted between the caruncle and the medial canthus (**Fig. 66-20**). The needle is aimed at the medial orbital wall and gently advanced until the wall is just touched.

The wall here (*lamina papyracea*) is extremely thin and can be easily perforated if too much force is applied. After gently touching the wall, the needle is withdrawn 1 to 2 mm and redirected parallel to both the orbital wall and floor. To avoid injury to the medial rectus muscle, the needle must be close to the wall but not subperiosteal. To avoid injury to the optic nerve, the needle should be no longer than 1 in in length, and its shoulder should be no deeper than the plane of the iris. Two to 4 mL of local anesthesia and a compression device after the block are commonly used.

Although some practitioners perform a superior orbital block lateral to the supraorbital notch to anesthetize the superomedial orbit, the authors are concerned that in this location, the globe is close to the orbit, the superior orbit is more vascular than the inferior and medial orbit,

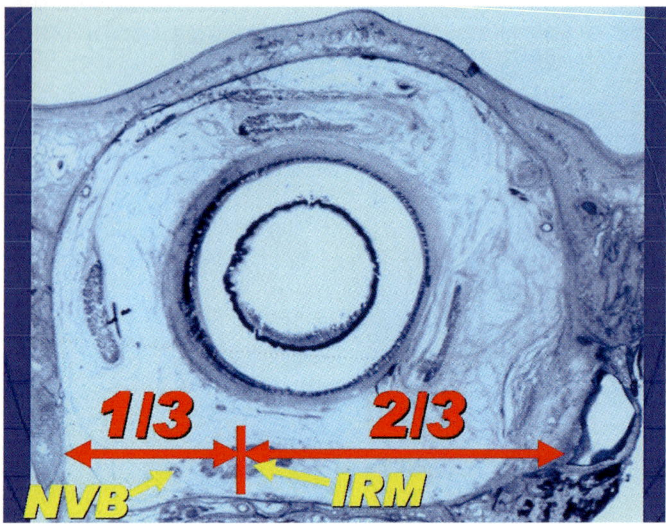

FIGURE 66-10. Anterior orbit through the posterior globe (histologic slide). Note how inferior rectus and neurovascular bundle to inferior oblique muscle are very near the junction of the inferolateral third of orbit. (This is the "traditionally" taught insertion point.) To reduce risk of injuring these structures, needles should be inserted further laterally in the orbit. IRM, Inferior rectus muscle NVB, Neurovascular bundle to the inferior oblique muscle. [Adapted by Dr Gary Fanning from photograph in Dutton JJ. *Atlas of Clinical Surgical Orbital Anatomy*. Philadelphia, PA: WB Saunders; 1994, with permission from Elsevier and Dr Gary Fanning.]

and the trochlear nerve and apparatus are in the vicinity. All of these structures are susceptible to needle injury.

SUB-TENON ANESTHESIA

Sub-Tenon block is accomplished by injecting local anesthetic into the *episcleral space* (the space between the sclera and the overlying sub-Tenon capsule) via needle or cannula.[1] The conjunctiva is fused several millimeters posterior to the limbus with the underlying sub-Tenon capsule.

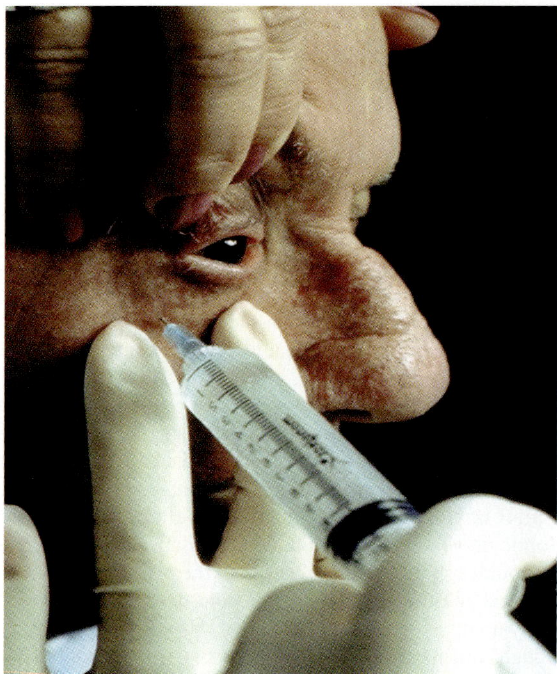

FIGURE 66-11. Photo demonstrating "modified" insertion site below lateral canthus. [Photo courtesy of Dr Gabriele Troll.]

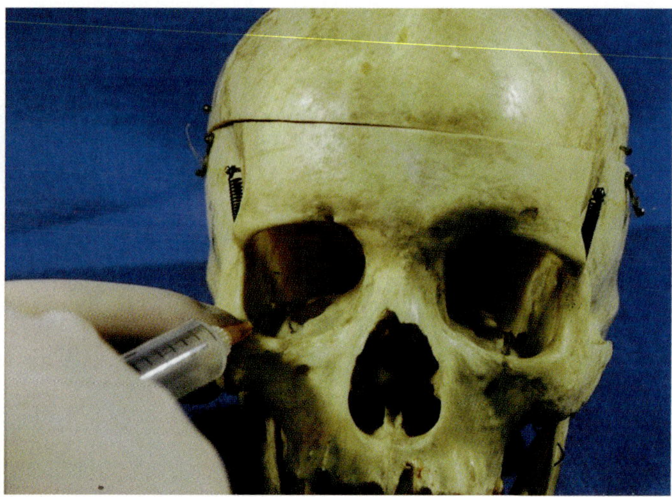

FIGURE 66-12. Photo demonstrating "modified" insertion site using skull. [Photo courtesy of Dr Gabriele Troll.]

If the conjunctiva is lifted off the sclera posterior to this fusion, the sub-Tenon capsule is also elevated, allowing insertion of local anesthesia between the scleral and the now exposed episcleral space (Fig. 66-20).

The principles of sub-Tenon block were described in the late 1800s. Modern cannula-based sub-Tenon block was developed as a method to potentially avoid complications of sharp needle blocks, including globe perforation, EOM injury, and retrobulbar hemorrhage. It has become very popular in Great Britain, and many European and Asian countries. Sub-Tenon block has been reported to have a lower rate of sight-threatening complications versus needle blocks, but it is important to be aware that most of the same complications that can occur with sharp needle blocks have also been reported with sub-Tenon block.[99-102]

The technique is most often performed in the inferomedial quadrant. After sterile preparation, application of topical anesthetic drops or gel to the surface of the globe, and topical application of 5% Betadine solution to the conjunctiva, the conjunctiva is grasped 3 to 5 mm from the limbus, and blunt Westcott scissors are used to create an opening in the conjunctiva and Tenon capsule to access the episcleral space. Specially designed blunt, often curved cannulas are advanced into the episcleral space, and the local anesthesia mixture is injected. Three to 5 mL of local anesthesia is commonly used. Three mL of local anesthesia provides analgesia to the globe and 5 mL will spread to the EOMs and provide akinesia.

Chemosis (subconjunctival spread of local anesthesia) and *conjunctival hemorrhage* are more common with sub-Tenon block than with needle blocks. Sub-Tenon block is contraindicated in patients with a prior scleral buckling (preventing posterior spread of anesthetic) or local infection and should be used with caution with glaucoma surgery (can interfere with lifting flap), highly myopic eyes (can perforate thin sclera or posterior staphyloma), previous pterygium repairs (can damage repair), or prior vitreoretinal surgery. Sub-Tenon block is also frequently used intraoperatively by ophthalmologists as a supplement to poor-quality or receding regional anesthesia blocks.[103]

Needle-based sub-Tenon block has been described by Ripart et al[104] and Mouvellon et al.[105]

MODIFIED VAN LINDT BLOCK

When paralysis of the orbicularis oculi is necessary to prevent squinting during eye surgery, a modified *Van Lindt block* can be performed.[106] The orbicularis oculi is innervated by the superior branch of the facial nerve. This nerve can be blocked by inserting a needle 1 cm lateral to the lateral junction of the superior and inferior orbital rims. Two to 4 mL of anesthetic is injected just lateral to both the superolateral and inferolateral orbital rim. One should avoid injections into the eyelids because this is painful and frequently causes a hematoma.

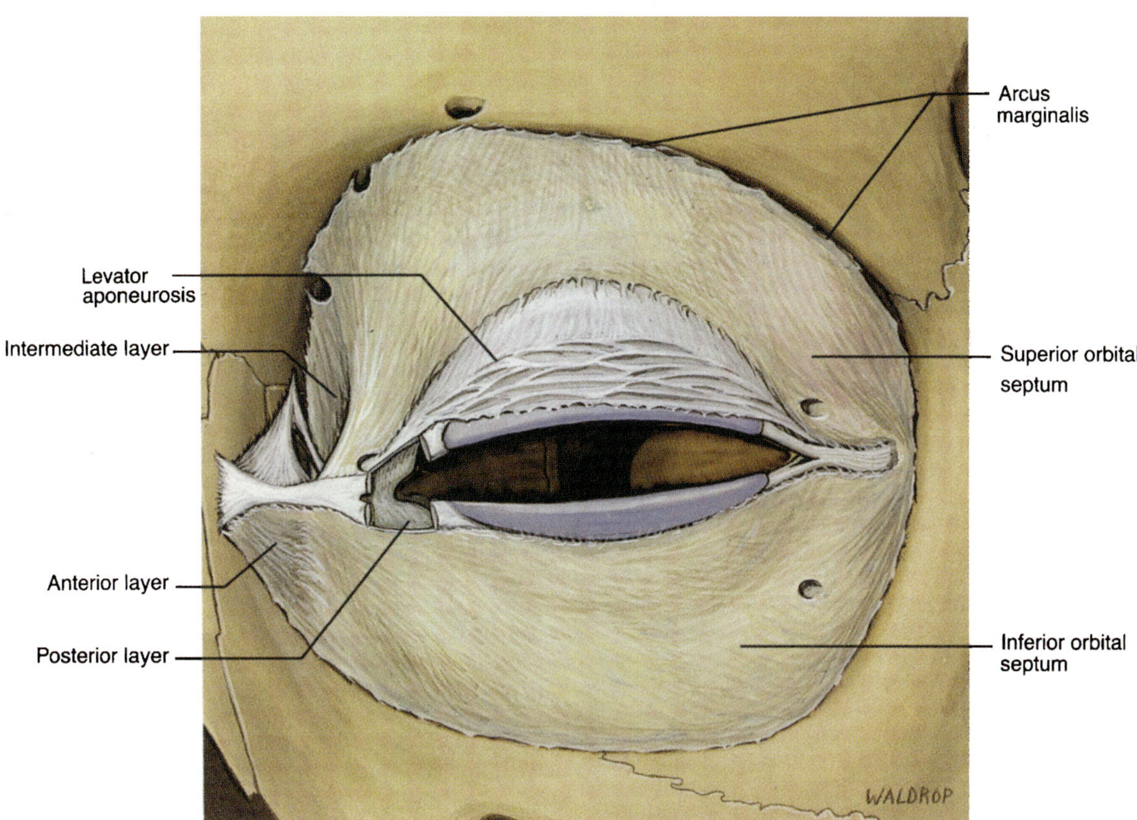

FIGURE 66-13. Illustration exposing extensive orbital fascia keeping the globe contained within the orbit. When dull needles pass this tissue, one frequently feels a mild "pop." [Reprinted from Dutton JJ. *Atlas of Clinical Surgical Orbital Anatomy*. Philadelphia, PA: WB Saunders; 1994, with permission from Elsevier.]

REGIONAL POSTOPERATIVE ANALGESIA

Postoperative pain is usually minimal after cataract surgery, and patients are usually instructed to take acetaminophen for postoperative analgesia. Severe pain after cataract surgery is abnormal and should prompt urgent consultation with an ophthalmologist because it may indicate infection or increased IOP. Postoperative pain is greater after posterior segment surgery. Inadequate pain relief can lead to nausea, vomiting, crying, and restlessness in children as well as hematoma formation, prolonged recovery, hospital admission, and reduced patient satisfaction. Use of opioids to treat pain also can lead to nausea and vomiting, resulting in admission or surgical complications. For these reasons, if general anesthesia is required, consideration should be given to administration of sub-Tenon, retrobulbar, or peribulbar anesthesia after induction or before emergence to provide analgesia in the immediate postoperative period. Some centers advocate the use of indwelling catheters to relieve postoperative pain,[107,108] but life-threatening complications have been

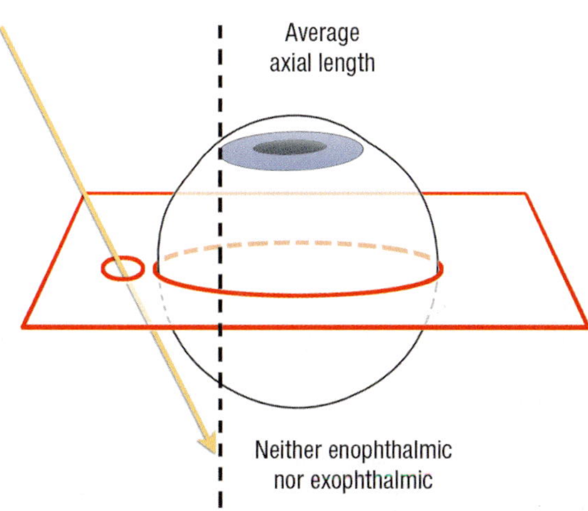

FIGURE 66-14. Illustration of normal globe showing needle angle required to enter the anterior interconal space.

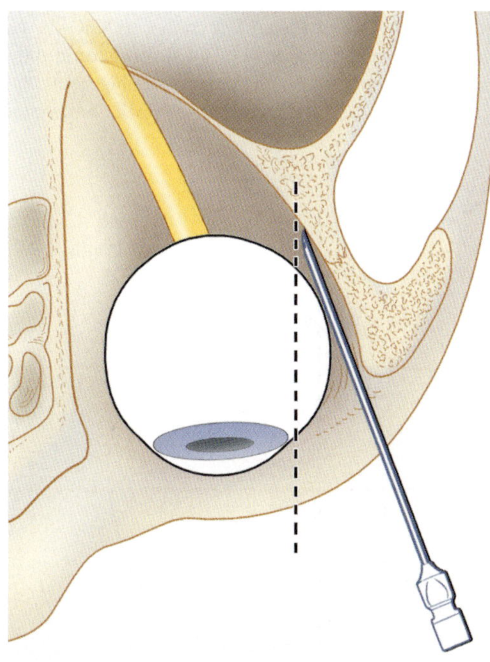

FIGURE 66-15. Illustration of the globe with the tip of the needle in plane projecting posteriorly from the limbus.

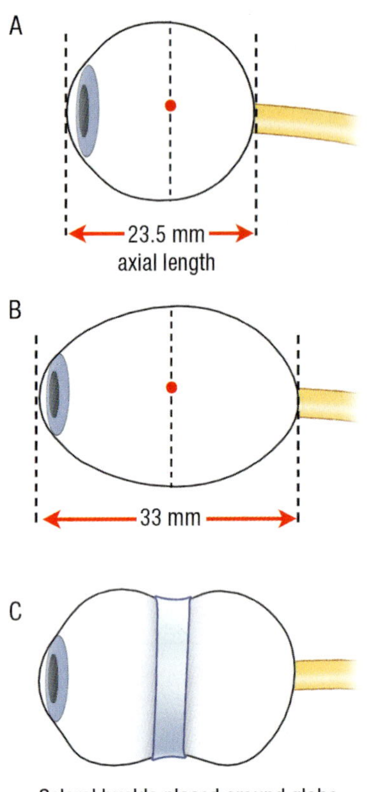

FIGURE 66-16. **A.** Normal axial length eye. **B.** Severely elongated (myopic) eye. **C.** Eye with a scleral buckle. Intraconal block in severe myopia and prior scleral buckle has an increased risk of globe perforation.

reported from this practice (usually related to catheter migration); for this reason, this technique has not gained wide acceptance.

COMPLICATIONS OF REGIONAL TECHNIQUES

MINOR COMPLICATIONS

Oculocardiac Reflex The *oculocardiac reflex* (OCR) is commonly observed during eye manipulation. The OCR most commonly presents as sinus bradycardia, but it also may appear as bigeminy, other ectopic beats, nodal rhythms, atrioventricular block, or asystole. These dysrhythmias may persist as long as the stimuli are present, but repeated stimuli often fatigue the reflex. It is more common during general anesthesia than regional anesthesia and more common in children than adults. Alexander[109] reported that 90% of patients experienced the OCR during traction of the EOMs.

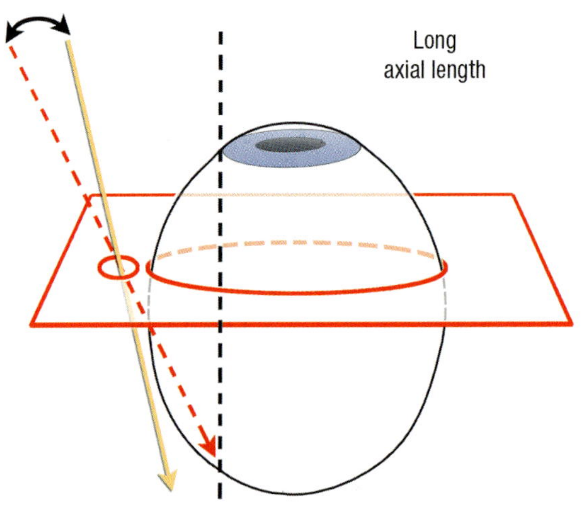

FIGURE 66-17. Illustration depicting a myopic eye and an altered angle of approach required to safely enter the anterior intraconal space.

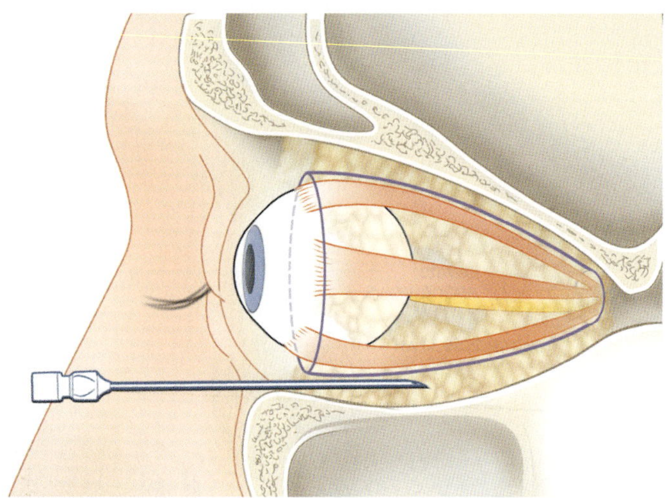

FIGURE 66-18. Drawing showing the needle entering the extraconal (peribulbar) space.

The afferent pathway of the OCR is via the ciliary ganglion to the ophthalmic division of the trigeminal nerve through the gasserian ganglion to the trigeminal nucleus in the fourth ventricle. The efferent pathway is exclusively through the vagus nerve. The vagus innervation to the abdominal viscera causes nausea and vomiting that can accompany the cardiac manifestations.

Diagnosis of the OCR relies on continuous monitoring of the ECG. Treatment varies based on the severity of the reflex. If the reflex manifests as mild sinus bradycardia or infrequent ectopic beats and the blood pressure remains stable, no treatment may be warranted. If the dysrhythmias become significant, cessation of the surgical stimuli is indicated. Often the procedure may resume after a brief pause. When the OCR is severe, treatment with anticholinergics (glycopyrrolate or atropine) is indicated. Caution must be exercised with large doses of atropine because more severe, prolonged tachydysrhythmias may result.[110] Regional block of the orbit is sometimes used to prevent or treat the OCR.

Other Minor Complications Chemosis is common with both needle blocks and sub-Tenon block. Eyelid bruising is common after needle blocks. Conjunctival hemorrhage is common after sub-Tenon block.

SERIOUS COMPLICATIONS

Serious complications of regional ophthalmic nerve blocks are rare but can be sight and life threatening.[111] **OPHTS** is a modified mnemonic[80] that may be useful to help remember serious complications. These complications are **o**ptic nerve injury, **p**erforation of the globe, **h**emorrhage (retrobulbar), **t**oxins (local anesthetics causing EOM dysfunction), and **s**ystemic complications (eg, CSF spread, seizures, cardiac arrest). Frequently, these complications are related to needle misplacement. Risk factors for these complications include inadequate knowledge of orbital anatomy, inadequate training, anatomic variations, and uncooperative patients (**Tables 66-5** and **66-6**).

Direct optic nerve injury secondary to needle trauma is rare, but when it occurs, it usually results in poor visual outcome or blindness. The usual cause is inadvertent needle insertion or injection into the optic nerve or its sheath with a 1½-in needle during retrobulbar block. It is estimated by Katsev et al[112] that up to 20% of the population (those with have short orbits) are at risk of this injury if a 1½-in (38-mm) needle is used in the inferolateral approach. In this study,

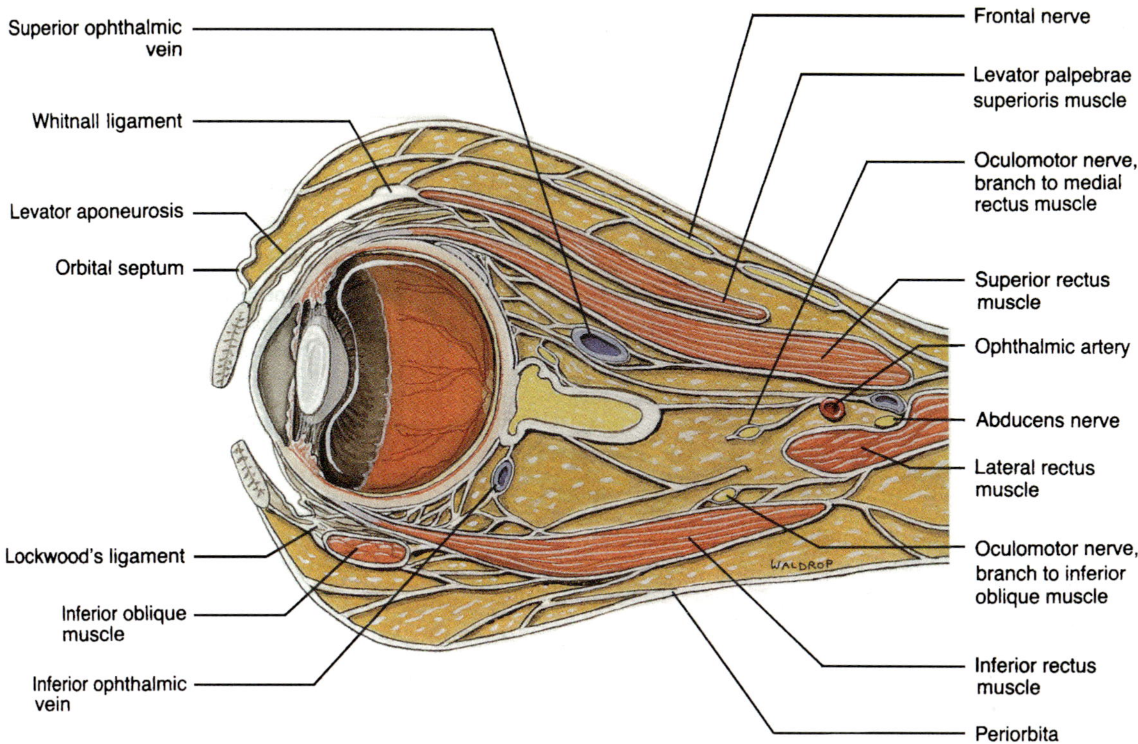

FIGURE 66-19. Lateral view of the central intraconal space. Mostly composed of adipose tissue in mid orbit, with only few thin septal barriers inhibiting diffusion of local anesthesia. [Reprinted from Dutton JJ. *Atlas of Clinical Surgical Orbital Anatomy*. Philadelphia, PA: WB Saunders; 1994, with permission from Elsevier.]

the optic nerve could not be reached from this approach with needles 1¼ in (32 mm) or less (**Fig. 66-21**).

Perforation of the globe has been estimated to occur between 1 in 1000[90] and 1 in 10 000[113,114] sharp needle eye blocks. Severe loss of vision or blindness usually results. A major risk factor is using a retrobulbar technique in patients with long axial length eyes. (See discussion about this subject in the Retrobulbar [Intraconal] Block and Peribulbar [Extraconal] Block section of this chapter.)

Retrobulbar hemorrhage can result from venous or arterial injury and can cause proptosis and periorbital hematoma. Intermittent manual compression should be instituted and the ophthalmologist consulted. Severe cases require surgical decompression. Visual outcome is usually good after retrobulbar hemorrhage. However, arterial bleeding is more likely to lead to a compressive hematoma sufficient to cause retinal ischemia.

Ocular and orbital muscle injuries are possible. Ptosis can be caused by surgical sutures on the eyelid speculum as well as disruption of the

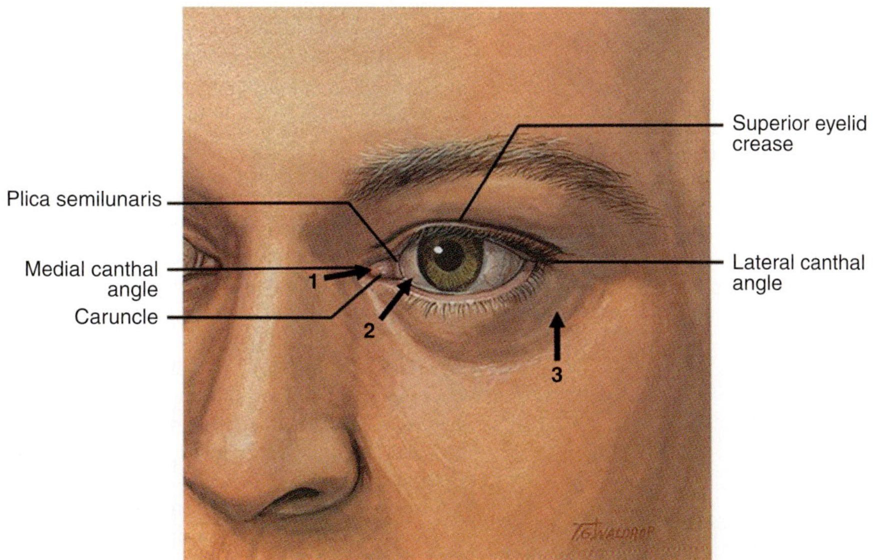

FIGURE 66-20. *Arrow 1* indicates the entry point for a median orbital block. *Arrow 2* indicates the site of dissection for a sub-Tenon (episcleral) block. *Arrow 3* indicates the entry point below the lateral canthus and above the inferior orbital rim for inferotemporal intraconal and extraconal block. [Modified from Dutton JJ. *Atlas of Clinical Surgical Orbital Anatomy*. Philadelphia, PA: WB Saunders; 1994, with permission from Elsevier.]

TABLE 66-5 Complications of Regional Blocks

Rare	
Sight Threatening	**Life Threatening**
Optic nerve injury or retinal vascular occlusion	Oversedation
Perforation of globe or detached retina	Brainstem anesthesia
Hemorrhage (retrobulbar)	Seizures
Toxins (myotoxin to EOM)	

EOM, extraocular muscle.

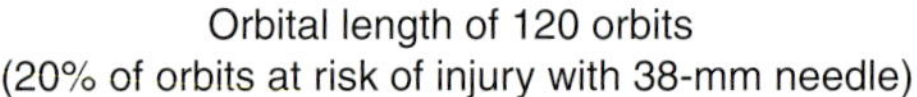
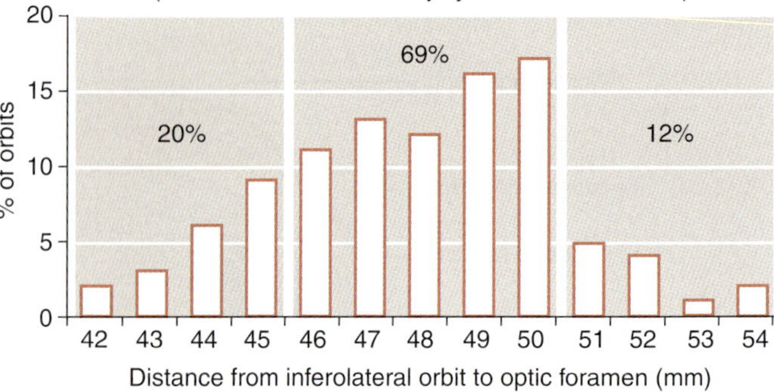

FIGURE 66-21. Up to 20% of optic nerves are at risk of being injured with 1½-in (38-mm) needles with the traditional inferolateral approach. (The optic nerve extends on average 7 mm anteriorly within the rigid annulus of Zinn and can be injured within this structure by a 38-mm needle if orbit ≤45 mm in an anteroposterior diameter.) [Data from Katsev Drews RC, Rose BT. Anatomic study of retrobulbar needle path length. *Ophthalmology.* 1989;96:1221.]

levator aponeurosis from trauma or stretching of the periorbital septum. Strabismus can be seen after injury to the rectus muscle by direct needle trauma, injection into other EOMs, or toxicity from local anesthetics. The risk of postoperative strabismus may be reduced if the lidocaine concentration in block solutions is 2% or less and hyaluronidase is used as an adjuvant for local anesthetics.

Spread of local anesthesia to the CNS can cause life-threatening problems. The reported incidence is 1 in 375 patients when practitioners use 1½-in needles and a retrobulbar injection.[115,116] We have not seen this complication at our institution in more than 30 000 patients when a 7/8-in needle was used for an anterior retrobulbar or extraconal block. However, this complication has been reported after peribulbar block.[117]

Subarachnoid spread of local anesthesia can cause partial or complete brainstem anesthesia.[115] Onset usually is within a few minutes but can occur as late as 20 minutes. Signs and symptoms may include restlessness, confusion, apnea, bradycardia, hypotension, sympathetic activation, and on occasion cardiac arrest. Oxygen with bag-mask ventilation to treat apnea may be all that is required to treat milder cases, but vasopressors, intubation, sedation, and prolonged ventilation may be necessary. The possibility of these complications occurring mandates oximetry, ECG, and blood pressure monitoring during and for about 20 minutes after orbital blocks and that resuscitation equipment and medications be immediately available.

Inadvertent intra-arterial injection is rare but can cause retrograde flow of local anesthesia from the ophthalmic artery into the brain. As little as 2 mL can produce seizures. This condition is usually associated with longer retrobulbar needle injections within the muscle cone. Blood should always be attempted to be aspirated before injecting local anesthetic to detect intravascular needle insertion.

GENERAL ANESTHESIA

General anesthesia is used in approximately 35% of the ophthalmic surgery cases at our institution; the most common indications are pediatric strabismus surgery and lengthy retinal surgery (eg, >2-3 h). Indications for general anesthesia also include an inability of the patient to cooperate with monitored anesthesia care (MAC), an inability to achieve ocular anesthesia or akinesia with local anesthesia (eg, patients with multiple previous eye operations with scar tissue), surgical procedure not amenable to regional anesthesia (eg, open globe, coagulopathy), and surgeon or patient preference.

Controversy exists regarding the relative safety of general anesthesia versus regional anesthesia in ophthalmic surgery. Studies reveal no differences between these techniques postoperatively with regard to memory,[118] cognitive function,[119] and oxygen saturation,[120] and the incidences of mortality and major complications are similar.[121] Regional anesthesia has been reported to be associated with fewer episodes of intraoperative oxygen desaturation, hemodynamic fluctuation, PONV, and less initial postoperative pain.[122] Regional anesthesia for ophthalmic surgery also has been shown to be free of the hormonal stress response associated with general anesthesia.[123,124] With these considerations in mind, it seems prudent to avoid general anesthesia if possible in patients with severe cardiovascular or pulmonary disease as well as those who are prone to PONV.

The goals of general anesthesia for ophthalmic surgery include a smooth induction with a stable IOP, avoidance or treatment of severe OCR, maintenance of a motionless field, a smooth emergence, and avoidance of PONV. These goals can be accomplished in a variety of ways using inhalation anesthesia, IV agents, or a combined technique. A remifentanil infusion is a popular adjuvant at our institution. Intermediate-acting muscle relaxants are also frequently used during intraocular surgery (and routinely used by the authors for intraocular surgery) when the slightest patient movement can be disastrous.

An orbital block should be considered intraoperatively during general anesthesia to reduce narcotic requirements perioperatively, reduce the incidence of OCR, reduce the incidence of PONV from narcotics, and control pain in the immediate postoperative period.

Extubation and emergence from general anesthesia require special attention after eye surgery. Deep extubation (deep enough to prevent straining when the endotracheal tube is removed) but ensuring adequate spontaneous ventilation after extubation is frequently used after eye surgery to reduce the of increased IOP or damage to delicate surgical repairs. There is a small possibility of aspiration from deep extubation because airway reflexes have not yet completely returned. Patients having recently ingested food or liquids and patients with compromised airways are not good candidates for deep extubation. When awake extubation is indicated, judicious use of adjuvant medications such as lidocaine and narcotics (eg, remifentanil infusion) may decrease straining on the endotracheal tube during emergence.

TABLE 66-6 Avoidance of Regional Complications

Knowledge of orbital anatomy
Training and supervision under qualified instructor of orbital regional anesthesia techniques
Knowledge of patient's ocular history, eg,
Myopia
Presence of scleral buckle
Multiple eye surgeries (scar tissue?)
Monitoring of oxygen saturation, ECG, and blood pressure
Appropriate peri-block sedation
Fastidious technique
Availability of emergency equipment and medication

ECG, electrocardiography.

OPEN GLOBE, FULL STOMACH

Succinylcholine causes an increase in IOP by 6 to 12 mm Hg within 1 to 4 minutes after its IV use; 7 to 10 minutes later, the IOP usually returns to baseline.[8,125] There has been concern that use of succinylcholine in patients with open globe injuries could further damage the globe because of this increase in IOP. The history of this controversy has been reviewed by Vachon et al.[126] Several large retrospective studies do not link the use of succinylcholine to further eye injury in this scenario.[127,128] Although the increase in IOP associated with succinylcholine is not insignificant, that associated with coughing and straining is 3 or 4 times greater (ie, to ~40 mm Hg), indicating that many other factors in addition to succinylcholine can influence the quality of anesthetic care. Direct pressure on the eye (from the mask or fingers) can also increase IOP and should be avoided. Efforts to quickly obtain good intubating conditions and prevent bucking and straining in the open globe scenario are much more important for reducing the risk of extrusion of eye contents than the avoidance of succinylcholine.

The most appropriate airway management of patients with an open globe and full stomach should be determined after assessing the likelihood of a difficult intubation and the viability of the eye. An algorithm has been proposed for this scenario.[129] If the intubation is judged to be difficult but the eye is viable, succinylcholine (after pretreatment with a small dose of a nondepolarizing muscle relaxant, eg, 0.3-0.5 mg of rocuronium in adults) is an appropriate option. If the patient is likely to be an easy intubation, a short- to intermediate-acting nondepolarizing agent, administered in greater-than-normal doses, such as 0.6 to 1.2 mg/kg of rocuronium, has proven effective.[130-132] The use of propofol has been shown to improve intubating conditions if rocuronium is used.[130] IV lidocaine and narcotic may also reduce the risk of straining and bucking. A fiberoptic intubation should be used if the eye is nonviable and the intubation is judged to be difficult.

Small "self-taming" doses of succinylcholine,[133,134] some nondepolarizing muscle relaxants,[135] and diazepam[14] have not been show to be effective in blocking the succinylcholine-induced increase in IOP. If small amounts of a nondepolarizing relaxant (eg, rocuronium) are used to block the succinylcholine-induced increase in IOP, 1.5 mg/kg of succinylcholine should then be used to achieve paralysis, waiting 60 to 90 seconds to ensure good-quality intubating conditions.

Potentially serious complications can occur if nitrous oxide (N_2O) is provided as part of the anesthetic regimen and the surgeon administers an intravitreal gas . Several cases of *blindness* have been reported from the use of N_2O in patients undergoing general anesthesia *weeks* after injection of 2 medical gases, sulfur hexafluoride (SF_6) and octafluoropropane (C_3F_8) into the vitreous cavity (eg, for the treatment of retinal detachment.)[136,137] N_2O enters the intraocular gas bubble much more rapidly than SF_6 and C_3F_8 exits. If N_2O is used after the injection of these gases, the injected gas bubble can expand up to 3 times its original volume. To prevent this complication, all patients undergoing general anesthesia should be asked about recent eye surgery. Small residual bubbles of SF6 and C3F8 have been observed in the vitreous as long as 3 and 10 weeks, respectively, after injection. *To provide a margin of safety, N_2O should not be used for patients who had intravitreal injections of SF6 within the last 30 days or C3F8 within the last 90 days.* If N_2O is used during retinal surgery, the ophthalmologist should be informed and the N_2O should be discontinued at least 15 to 20 minutes before the injection of a gas into the vitreous cavity.[138]

ANESTHESIA FOR PEDIATRIC OPHTHALMOLOGY

Anesthesia for pediatric ophthalmology encompasses a diverse group of patients and procedures. It has been said that pediatric ophthalmic anesthesiology can be considered a separate subspecialty.[139] Patients range from newborns with medical problems associated with prematurity to children with congenital syndromes to healthy adolescents. Many of the ophthalmic procedures performed in adults with MAC require general anesthesia in the pediatric population.

Measurement of IOP in awake children is difficult because of their lack of cooperation and frequently requires general anesthesia. IOP is affected by most anesthetic drugs and practices such as laryngoscopy and intubation. Therefore, most ophthalmologists prefer to measure IOP before a deep level of anesthesia has been reached and intubation has been performed. It is our practice to allow measurement of IOP soon after induction of anesthesia and before instrumentation of the airway has taken place. This is accomplished by positioning the mask and hand of the anesthesiologist so the ophthalmologist has unobstructed access to the eye. Instillation of topical anesthetic drops into the eye may allow earlier IOP measurement than otherwise possible. If necessary, the mask can be removed to allow IOP measurement and then replaced. If further examination is required (eg, ultrasonography, gonioscopy), either the trachea is intubated or an laryngeal mask airway (LMA) is inserted.

Measurement of IOP in the pediatric patient is performed to diagnose glaucoma or to follow the efficacy of therapy. Congenital glaucoma can be associated with several systemic syndromes (eg, rubella, oculocerebrorenal [Lowe] syndrome). In addition, Sturge-Weber syndrome or congenital capillary hemangioma may affect the skin of the face, neck, mucous membranes, meninges, and choroid plexus. These patients frequently have seizure disorders. If the affected areas include the distribution of the fifth CN, glaucoma is commonly found. Children with Sturge-Weber syndrome come to the OR for frequent examinations under anesthesia to follow the efficacy of surgical and medical interventions. Good rapport and appropriate use of premedicants allow a smooth induction of anesthesia and the most accurate measurement of IOP.

Strabismus surgery is the most common type of ophthalmic surgery performed in children. Several studies have reported the incidence of PONV as greater than 50%.[140,141] Several different anesthetic techniques and antiemetic regimens have been used in an attempt to decrease this high incidence of nausea and vomiting. Wachta et al[140] showed that patients anesthetized solely with propofol after halothane induction had an incidence of emesis in the first 24 hours of 23% compared with 50% in those who received halothane, N_2O, and droperidol. All patients in all groups received opioids for pain relief, a technique that undoubtedly contributed to the high incidence of PONV. The OCR is frequently elicited during strabismus surgery by traction on the EOMs.[109]

At MEEI, patients at moderate to high risk of PONV receive a $5HT_3$ antagonist (eg, ondansetron) and dexamethasone (Decadron) unless contraindicated. For strabismus surgery, pain is minimized with nonopiate analgesics, most commonly 0.5 to 1 mg/kg IV of ketorolac (maximum pediatric dose, 15 mg IV). Patients with congenital strabismus may have a higher risk than the general population of developing malignant hyperthermia, and this risk should be factored into anesthetic management. (See Chapter 87 for a full discussion of malignant hyperthermia.)

Nasolacrimal duct probing for obstruction is another common procedure performed in pediatric ophthalmic patients. Successful relief of obstruction diminishes after the first year of life, so many of these patients are infants. Use of an LMA provides the surgeon with unobstructed access to the patient and protects the airway from the fluorescein dye that is injected into the nasolacrimal duct.

When an infant or young child presents with poor vision but normal ocular structures, electroretinography can help differentiate among retinal disorders. This procedure is generally performed in a completely dark laboratory and requires a period of approximately 20 minutes for the retina to dark-adapt. General anesthesia or sedation is required because the child usually is not able to cooperate for the examination. Before beginning the procedure, the anesthesiologist must become familiar with the location of the various pieces of equipment and power outlets and be completely satisfied with the setup.

Retinopathy of prematurity, previously called *retrolental fibroplasia*, is a condition usually associated with prematurity. Although a disease of complex etiologies, it is believed to be primarily related to hyperoxic periods during neonatal intensive care. Nonetheless, full-term infants can have this condition, as can premature infants who have never received oxygen therapy. After initial examination in the intensive care unit, the child may come to the OR for multiple examinations under anesthesia and vitreoretinal procedures such as scleral buckling or vitrectomy. The care of ex–premature infants is complex and must start with a thorough history and physical examination. Important historical data include gestational age at birth, birth weight, duration of intubation and ventilation, history of apneic episodes and other breathing disorders, and history of heart and other congenital anomalies.[142] Hyaline membrane disease occurs in 60% to 80% of infants born at less than 28 weeks of gestation. Hyaline membrane disease may progress to the chronic pulmonary disease of prematurity called *bronchopulmonary dysplasia.* Although bronchopulmonary dysplasia improves with growth and development, these children should be considered at risk for increased airway reactivity.

If an inhalation induction is chosen, IV or inhalation anesthesia can be used for maintenance. Intravenous access is rapidly secured so the amount of inhalational agent can be decreased and muscle relaxant administered. For intraocular surgery, a motionless field is critical. For this reason, the authors believe it is prudent to supplement an adequate depth of anesthesia with muscle paralysis during the intraocular portion of the procedure. Conservative amounts of opioids, most commonly fentanyl, are administered. Although extubation should be the goal at the conclusion of surgery, the endotracheal tube should be left in place until the child meets criteria for extubation.

In 1982, anesthesiologists were alerted to the occurrence of postoperative apnea in ex–premature infants recovering from minor surgical procedures after general anesthesia.[143] When these infants are no longer at risk is not always adequately defined[144]; however, the incidence of apnea is known to be strongly related to gestational age and postconceptual age. Most hospitals have guidelines to admit infants younger than 54 to 60 weeks postconceptual age for overnight monitoring. It is especially important in pediatric patients to calculate the maximum amount of local anesthetic allowable to avoid toxicity, to know if local anesthesia solutions contain epinephrine, and to remind the surgeon of these dosages. The recommended safe maximal doses of commonly used local anesthetics in ophthalmology are as follows: lidocaine: 7 mg/kg with epinephrine (maximum dose, 500 mg) or 4.5 mg/kg without epinephrine (maximum dose, 300 mg) and bupivacaine: 2.5 mg/kg (maximum dose, 175 mg). When isoflurane is used, up to 3 mcg/kg epinephrine is acceptable. These dosages of epinephrine are conservative and can be repeated after 10 minutes if no untoward effects are observed.

OPHTHALMIC PROCEDURES

STRABISMUS

Strabismus means ocular misalignment or deviation of one eye relative to the visual axis of the other. Although most strabismus is caused by refractive errors or muscle imbalance, rare causes include retinoblastoma or other serious ocular defects and neurologic disease. Left untreated, about 50% of children with strabismus have some visual loss because of amblyopia. A detailed nomenclature has evolved to describe the various patterns of strabismus. Whereas the prefix *eso-* denotes deviation nasally, *exo-* denotes temporal deviation. The suffix *-phoria* describes the tendency of one eye to turn inward or outward when covered, and *-tropia* describes manifest inward or outward deviation of the eye.

The surgical correction of strabismus is a repositioning of the EOMs. To strengthen a muscle, a resection is performed. To weaken a muscle, a recession is performed. In severe cases, a resection may be performed on one muscle and a recession on the opposing muscle. Because visual maturation occurs by age 5 years, strabismus correction usually is attempted early in childhood. If left uncorrected, *amblyopia* (partial or complete loss of vision in 1 eye caused by conditions that affects normal development) can occur. Adjustable sutures are sometimes used to improve the chances of alignment with a single operation. The adjustment is performed in the immediate postoperative period when the patient is fully awake and able to focus.

Pediatric patients undergoing strabismus surgery require general anesthesia. Some adult patients do well with a regional technique and IV sedation. Most patients prefer general anesthesia and have a satisfactory result with propofol, remifentanil, $5HT_3$ antagonists, or dexamethasone and nonopiates for pain.

CORNEA

Keratoplasty *Penetrating keratoplasty* refers to surgical replacement of the entire cornea with donor tissue. Donor tissue that comes from the patient is called an *autograft.* Tissue that comes from another person is called an *allograft.* The indications for this procedure are many; corneal opacity, keratoconus, infection, and scarring are a few. Lamellar keratoplasty replaces only a portion of the cornea. *Endothelial keratoplasty* replaces Descemet membrane and endothelium, and *deep anterior keratoplasty* replaces the top 90% of the cornea. Either regional or general anesthesia may be appropriate for these procedures. The importance of suppressing coughing when the anterior chamber is open cannot be overemphasized.

Pterygium A *pterygium* is a benign growth of conjunctiva and fibrovascular tissue that has invaded the superficial cornea. Excision is indicated when vision becomes impaired, the lesion causes irritation, or the lesion becomes cosmetically significant. Topical or injection anesthesia, with or without IV sedation, is satisfactory for removal.

Radial Keratotomy *Radical keratotomy* is the surgical procedure used to correct myopia. Recall that the cornea contributes approximately 30% of the refractive element of vision. Under topical anesthesia, a series of incisions is made in the cornea in a spoke-like manner, causing a positive diopter change in vision. The indications and rationale for radical keratotomy remain controversial. Typically, these procedures are performed with topical anesthesia only.

Cataracts *Cataracts* are a common cause of visual impairment in older individuals. The pathogenesis of cataracts is multifactorial but results in opacity of the lens. Small incision *extracapsular cataract extraction,* also known as phacoemulsification, is the preferred method of modern cataract extraction. The procedure is performed through a small (3-4 mm) incision and is usually less traumatic to the corneal endothelium than older techniques. The nucleus of the lens is fragmented by an ultrasonic needle and then aspirated. Residual cortical material is then removed. Removal of the lens with an intact posterior capsule provides for better positioning of an intraocular lens implant. *Intracapsular cataract extraction* (ICCE) is an older technique that completely removes the lens with the capsule through a much larger (12 mm) incision. ICCE is sometimes required with very dense cataracts and in areas of the world where modern ophthalmology equipment is not available. Cataract extraction can be performed with topical anesthesia or with retrobulbar, peribulbar, or sub-Tenon block.

Glaucoma Altered circulation of aqueous humor can produce an increase in IOP, termed *ocular hypertension. Glaucoma* refers to ocular hypertension with associated optic neuropathy and visual field loss. Glaucoma is commonly associated with an increase in outflow resistance.

Acute angle-closure glaucoma is one of the leading causes of blindness in the United States. It occurs when there is a sudden occlusion of the drainage angle because of papillary block. This occlusion often is associated with a patient with a narrow anatomic angle hyperopic, a pupil dilated by atropinergic compounds, or an iris propelled anteriorly. Often the patient has a history of an episode of coughing or straining.

The onset of *chronic open-angle glaucoma* is insidious. Although peripheral vision is gradually lost in the early stages of the disease, the angle is found open and the trabecula appears to operate normally. Chronic open-angle glaucoma may be congenital or associated with a familial diathesis or increasing age.

Goniotomy is a procedure performed to treat infantile glaucoma. A superficial incision is made in the trabecular meshwork to improve outflow of aqueous humor from the anterior chamber. Infants and children require general anesthesia for this procedure.

Trabeculectomy is the most commonly performed filtering procedure in adults. A block of limbal tissue is removed beneath a scleral flap, permitting outflow of aqueous. Antimetabolites, such as mitomycin, can be injected intraoperatively to help prevent surgical failures secondary to scarring.

Many different tubes or shunts have been used to divert aqueous (eg, Molteno valve). These implants are generally reserved for patients who have not responded to other management. Implants in current use have a plastic tube placed in the anterior chamber connected to a plate placed posterior to the limbus.

Iridectomy usually is performed with an yttrium-aluminum-garnet laser at 1064 nm; however, an incisional iridectomy occasionally is required. Iridectomy is the definitive treatment for angle-closure glaucoma.

Anesthesia for glaucoma surgery in adults usually is performed with a retrobulbar or peribulbar injection and, if needed, a facial nerve block.

VITREORETINAL SURGERY

Vitrectomy refers to surgical extraction of the contents of the vitreous chamber and replacement with a physiologic solution. An anterior segment vitrectomy is performed for vitreous loss during cataract surgery and for late anterior segment vitreous complications. A posterior segment vitrectomy is indicated for removal of an intraocular foreign body, management of complicated retinal detachments with intraocular membranes, removal of media opacities, and alleviation of vitreous traction on the retina.

General anesthesia was traditionally used for vitreoretinal surgery. However, using regional anesthesia with MAC is now common and has many advantages over general anesthesia.[145] After a regional block, the OCR usually is absent. The rapid recovery associated with MAC allows early prone positioning in the recovery room after posterior chamber gas injection. Patient comfort is increased because of less nausea and vomiting and diminution of postoperative pain. Unfortunately, MAC is not suitable for long procedures. Procedures lasting longer than 2 or 3 hours exceed the tolerance of most patients to lie supine and motionless. If necessary, a retrobulbar or peribulbar block can be supplemented during surgery with a sub-Tenon injection using a blunt, 19-gauge needle.

General anesthesia is appropriate for longer cases. It is a useful technique when communication with the patient is difficult or for patients who cannot lie supine or motionless. General anesthesia has some disadvantages. An increase in IOP from straining risks retinal repairs and expulsion of intraocular contents when the globe is open. The OCR is much more common during general anesthesia than regional anesthesia, frequently requiring anticholinergic treatment. After general anesthesia, patients require more systemic postoperative analgesics and antiemetics. Somnolence, pain, and nausea may delay the proper positioning of patients postoperatively.

After general anesthesia is administered, use of long-acting retrobulbar blockade has significant advantages. Retrobulbar block with 0.75% bupivacaine greatly reduces the need for parenteral analgesics within the first 24 hours after surgery.[146] In a prospective double-blinded study of patients receiving general anesthesia with or without retrobulbar block with 0.5% bupivacaine, the group receiving the bupivacaine had significantly less pain and nausea postoperatively.[147] Alternatively, under direct vision, a blunt 19-gauge cannula can be used to directly inject the anesthetic agent into the episcleral space via a sub-Tenon approach. This technique minimizes the risk of scleral perforation.

The dangers of N_2O use during surgery when intravitreal gas is administered and for several weeks to months thereafter are reviewed in the General Anesthesia section of this chapter. A similar hazard exists with air transport of patients. Because the aircraft cabin is pressurized to an altitude of approximately 2000 m above sea level, the gas bubble will expand, resulting in elevated IOP. Therefore, patients should avoid air travel for similar periods of time after injection of these intravitreal gases.[148]

OCULOPLASTIC SURGERY

All of the following oculoplastic procedures can be performed with regional anesthesia on adult patients.

Ectropion Repair An *ectropion* results from excess, loose eyelid tissue or scarring that causes the margin of the eyelid to turn outward away from the globe (eversion). Repair consists of excising excess tissue and tightening the remaining eyelid or releasing the related scar tissue.

Entropion Repair An *entropion* usually is caused by senile or involutional changes, primarily in the lower eyelids, resulting in weakening of the eyelid retractor muscles and horizontal laxity. The eyelid margin is turned inward toward the globe (inversion). The goal of surgical repair is to increase the tension of the retractor muscles (eg, by reattaching them) and tighten any horizontal laxity.

Ptosis Repair *Ptosis* is a congenital or acquired drooping of the eyelid. Most often it is repaired by shortening or reattaching the levator palpebrae aponeurosis. When levator function is inadequate, the upper eyelid can be suspended from the frontalis by a sling of fascia lata.

Blepharoplasty *Blepharoplasty* is any plastic surgery of the eyelids, usually to remove redundant tissue. The procedure is performed to remove visual field obstruction and for cosmesis.

Dacryocystorhinostomy *Dacryocystorhinostomy* is the creation of a communication between the lacrimal sac and the nasal cavity to allow for tear drainage. A Jones tube is sometimes used to bypass the canaliculi and form a conjunctivorhinostomy. Nasolacrimal duct probing is performed in children with congenital nasolacrimal duct obstruction. The duct is probed with a wire, then dye is injected into the duct and aspirated from the nasal cavity to test the patency of the duct. Silicon tubes can be inserted to act as stents.

ORBITAL SURGERY

Most orbital surgery requires general anesthesia unless the procedure is limited to the anterior orbit and does not involve the bones of the orbit.

Orbitotomy An *orbitotomy* is performed to gain surgical access to the orbit. Approaches include transconjunctival, transseptal, and transperiosteal. Indications for orbitotomy include tumor, abscess, foreign body, and orbital fractures.

Orbital Decompression *Orbital decompression* is indicated for correction of exophthalmos resulting from Graves disease. Access to the orbit is obtained by either a transconjunctival or transperiosteal approach. Some surgeons use a coronal incision with reflection of the scalp anteriorly to the level of the orbit. Cases can be long (≥4 h), and blood loss can be large enough to require transfusion.

Acknowledgments: The authors would like to thank Dr Roberto Pineda for his assistance in reviewing and updating information about ophthalmic procedures; Dr Gary Fanning, Dr Jonathan Dutton, and Dr Gabriele Troll for their generous lending of personal photographs and drawings; Mr Peter Goldberg for assistance with photographic material; and Ms Elizabeth Kiernan and Ms Viviana Silva-Kong for their assistance with the preparation of figures used in this chapter.

KEY REFERENCES

- Hamilton RC. A discourse on the complications of retrobulbar and peribulbar blockade. *Can J Ophthalmol.* 2000;35:363.
- Katsev DA, Drews RC, Rose BT. Anatomic study of retrobulbar needle path length. *Ophthalmology.* 1989;96:1221.
- Kumar C, Dodds C, Fanning G. Pharmocolgy for regional ophthalmic anaesthesia. In: Kumar C, Dodds C, Fanning G, eds. *Ophthalmic Anaesthesia.* Lisse, The Netherlands: Swets & Zeitlinger; 2002.
- Schein OD, Katz, J, Bass EB, et al. The value of routine preoperative medical testing before cataract surgery. *N Engl J Med.* 2000;342:168.
- Snell RS, Lemp MA. *Clinical Anatomy of the Eye.* 2nd ed. Oxford, UK: Blackwell Science; 1998.

REFERENCES

Complete references available on DVD and online version at www.LongneckerAnesthesiology.com

CHAPTER 67

Anesthesia for Otorhinolaryngologic (Ear, Nose, and Throat) Surgery

Bil Ragan

KEY POINTS

1. Successful middle ear surgery depends on controlled hypotension to minimize blood loss and maintain a clear surgical field, use of short-acting muscle relaxants to promote facial nerve monitoring, avoidance of nitrous oxide to prevent graft disruption, and smooth extubations to prevent prosthesis displacement.
2. Middle ear surgery can result in profound postoperative nausea and vomiting, requiring an aggressive, multimodal, pharmacologic approach for prevention and treatment.
3. Complications of sinus surgery include hemorrhage, eye injury, vision loss, venous air embolism, cerebrospinal fluid leak, permanent neurologic injury, and death.
4. Pediatric patients with obstructive sleep apnea syndrome may present with altered right ventricular diastolic function, pulmonary hypertension, arrhythmias, and silent carditis.
5. Posttonsillectomy hemorrhage is a surgical emergency. Patients may be profoundly hypovolemic and tachycardic before the complication is recognized, and anesthetic care includes both fluid resuscitation and meticulous airway management.
6. Careful preoperative planning will prevent the conversion of a partial airway obstruction into a complete airway obstruction when managing patients with foreign body aspiration.
7. After radiation therapy to the head and neck, tissues become fixed, firm, and fibrotic. Despite a normal appearance, direct laryngoscopy may be extraordinarily difficult, if not impossible. Fiberoptic laryngoscopy is often the preferred approach for tracheal intubation.
8. Lasers can produce thermal injury, cause photochemical reactions, have mechanical effects, and release toxins, including viable microorganisms. Most laser injuries result from reflected beams, with the eye being the most vulnerable organ.
9. No laser tube is perfect, and airway fires can occur under any condition. Precautions can reduce the risk of a surgical fire but cannot eliminate the risk.
10. Use of a Nerve Integrity Monitor (NIM) endotracheal tube can greatly reduce the risk of recurrent laryngeal nerve injury during thyroid and parathyroid surgery.

INTRODUCTION

It is accepted that the first anesthetic was provided to James Venable for the removal of a neck tumor. Therefore, it is only fitting that all subsequent anesthetic techniques have descended from the care of an ear, nose, and throat (ENT) patient. These procedures challenge the creativity and skills of the finest anesthesiologist. On a routine basis, anesthesiologists provide mask anesthetics, spontaneous or jet ventilation, controlled hypotension, and extubations during deep levels of anesthesia. Most of these cases are performed with little or no muscle relaxation. Moreover, in the contemporary surgical environment, the majority of these cases are performed in an outpatient setting. This presents its own challenges in the areas of analgesia and the prevention of postoperative nausea and vomiting (PONV). The patient population varies from neonates to elderly adults, with a significant number of pediatric cases.

As a unique feature of this subspecialty, anesthesiologists work with physician colleagues who have an understanding and appreciation of the airway. This is unlike most other surgical experience. The complicated nature of these procedures demands nothing less than complete cooperation between these 2 specialties. Frequently, the airway will be shared, and commonly, one practitioner will assist the other in times of difficulty. When a compromised airway is involved, any pretensions of ego are best removed from the setting.

For purposes of clarity and ease of use, this chapter is organized by anatomic regions. When anesthesia is being provided for a particular procedure, the performance of an additional, different procedure at the same time is unlikely. Furthermore, from an anesthesia point of view, the concerns for a particular anatomic region differ from those of other regions and should be discussed separately.

ANESTHESIA FOR EAR SURGERY

As in other subspecialties, a broad range of interventional surgical techniques can be performed for the patient's benefit. For these procedures, patient positioning, facial nerve preservation, hemostasis, smooth emergence, prevention of PONV, and use of nitrous oxide (N_2O) become primary concerns of the anesthesiologist.

EAR CANAL AND TYMPANIC MEMBRANE DISORDERS

Disorders of the ear canal and tympanic membrane all involve processes that interfere with the reception and transmission of sound from an external source to the middle ear. These cases are routinely performed under general anesthesia, but some patients can tolerate local anesthesia with sedation. After induction of anesthesia and with the airway secured, the patient's head is turned and fixed with the operative ear. These cases are not necessarily lengthy. Some practitioners use a laryngeal mask airway (LMA), but most prefer endotracheal intubation. With canalplasties, use of N_2O is permitted but not encouraged. However, with tympanoplasties, use of N_2O is best avoided to prevent expansion and dislocation of the surgical graft.

MIDDLE EAR DISORDERS

Disorders of the middle ear manifest as a decline in hearing caused by compromised sound conduction. Commonly, they are caused by either infectious or inflammatory processes.

Myringotomy is among the most frequently performed pediatric surgeries. In the hands of an experienced surgeon, bilateral myringotomies can be performed in as few as 3 minutes. Because of this, both induction and maintenance usually are performed with mask anesthesia using sevoflurane. Postoperative discomfort can be addressed by acetaminophen given as a 40-mg/kg dose.[1] The use of intranasal fentanyl at a dose of 2 mcg/kg has also been used with good effect as demonstrated by Galinkin et al.[2] More recently, similar results were obtained when using a nerve block of the auricular branch of the vagus (nerve of Arnold).[3] In certain patients, chronic otitis media can result in temporomandibular joint ankylosis,[4] which can make laryngoscopy difficult, if not impossible. Although instrumentation of the airway is not expected with this procedure, it is prudent to be aware of this possibility and to evaluate accordingly.

Stapedectomy is the removal or freeing of the stapes superstructure and replacement with a prosthesis. In most cases, this condition is caused by otosclerosis. Typically, this procedure is performed under general anesthesia, although local anesthesia with sedation can be done. Lasers are frequently used to free the stapes, and appropriate precautions must be taken (see Lasers later). These cases usually last between 1 and 2 hours, and facial nerve monitoring may be done. Hence, a short-acting muscle relaxant, if any, should be used. Ho et al[5] found that facial nerve twitch was quite vigorous when the ulnar train of four began to return, suggesting that the surgeon should be able to identify the facial nerve by electrical stimulation even in the presence of some neuromuscular relaxation. Despite this, most practitioners limit the use of longer acting relaxants to ensure that neuromuscular blockade does not contribute to potential surgical complications.

Another goal is to reduce bleeding during this procedure. This is accomplished by injecting a mixed local anesthetic and epinephrine solution, elevating the patient's head to improve venous drainage, and often applying deliberate hypotension. Several volatile agents and intravenous (IV) combinations have been used successfully to provide mild hypotension and reduce blood loss. In a study by Marchal et al[6] they found that preoperative clonidine reduced blood loss, blunted the response to intubation, and reduced isoflurane and fentanyl requirements. A recent study by Ryu et al[7] demonstrated less pain and less PONV when using IV magnesium rather than remifentanil.

While the surgeon is placing the prosthesis, it is absolutely essential that the patient be motionless. This requires a deeper plane of anesthesia using volatile anesthetics alone or in combination with a remifentanil infusion. Although N_2O can be used for earlier portions of the procedure, it should be avoided in the last portion to prevent tympanic membrane graft disruption and possible nausea and vomiting. Extubation must be smooth without any bucking or violent motions, thus preventing displacement of the prosthesis. The success of the procedure may depend on these details. It is best to have the patient breathing spontaneously and extubated during a deep plane of anesthesia.

The anesthesia concerns for ossiculoplasty are similar to those for stapedectomy. However, this procedure may last longer because these patients typically have long-standing disease that requires a lengthy dissection. PONV is a risk of all middle ear surgery and requires multiple agents to treat. The addition of dexamethasone with granisetron gave excellent results in a recent study by Gombar et al.[8]

Looking to the future, it has been suggested that total IV anesthesia (TIVA) may allow better control and smoother emergence for these procedures. The results in a comparison trial by Mukherjee et al[9] are promising. This investigation found that TIVA (ie, via propofol and remifentanil infusions) provided better conditions for surgery and significantly less PONV in the early postoperative interval. However, patients who received TIVA had higher pain scores during recovery. Those who received balanced anesthesia had been given fentanyl and experienced less discomfort.

NITROUS OXIDE CONCERNS

Although N_2O has been used as an anesthetic in millions of patients for more than 150 years, there are serious concerns with its use in middle ear surgery.

The healthy middle ear contains air spaces that are intermittently ventilated and thus decompressed via the eustachian tube. If disease or trauma interferes with this venting, middle ear pressure can rise rapidly. When N_2O is used in any concentration, it can enter these airspaces much faster than nitrogen can exit. Likewise, after N_2O is discontinued, rapid absorption can result in profound negative pressure within the middle ear. Both of these processes reflect the 34-fold difference between the blood–gas partition coefficients of N_2O and nitrogen[10] (**Fig. 67-1**).

These sudden changes in middle ear pressure can result in impaired middle ear function with a decline in hearing, tympanic membrane rupture, graft disruption, or nausea and vomiting. Patients who are especially susceptible include those with concurrent upper airway infections, enlarged adenoids, otitis media, and a history of otologic surgery. Thus, N_2O should be used judiciously during middle ear surgery. If used at all, concentrations should be less than 50%. It should be discontinued a minimum of 20 minutes before expected closure of the middle ear. It is helpful if the surgeon flushes the ear with air before closing the surgical incision. Given all of these factors, prudent practice implies that N_2O should be used only with considerable caution and for clear indications that cannot be met with other approaches.

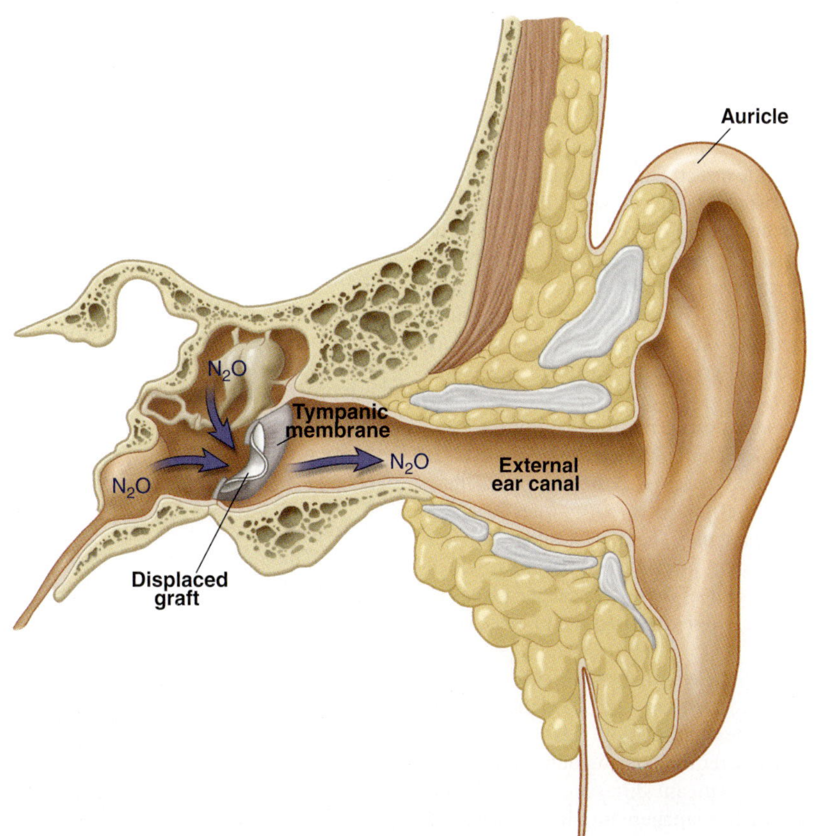

FIGURE 67-1. Disruption of the tympanic membrane graft by nitrous oxide. [Illustration by Daniel Muller, Haderer & Muller Biomedical Art, LLC.]

SENSORINEURAL HEARING LOSS DISORDERS

Cochlear Implant Patients who are profoundly deaf may have sufficient spiral ganglion cells for stimulation and thus possible recovery of hearing. With advances in electrode and processing technology, placement of cochlear implants has become a common procedure. These are lengthy cases that last anywhere from 4 to 6 hours. The surgeon must perform a mastoidotomy to place the signal coupler. Surgeons prefer the use of controlled hypotension, if appropriate and tolerated by the patient, to minimize blood loss. N_2O is not contraindicated from the surgical perspective but should be avoided to decrease PONV. Placement of electrodes must be precise, and a smooth, motionless extubation is expected. Any untoward movement can compromise the entire procedure.

PERILYMPHATIC FISTULA AND PONV

Perilymph leakage has been implicated in sudden hearing loss, tinnitus, aural fullness, and both episodic and positional vertigo. Surgical treatment usually involves an exploratory tympanotomy, which is performed under general anesthesia with endotracheal tube intubation.

These patients may have profound PONV. The approaches to prevention and treatment of PONV are considered in detail in Chapters 68 and 72. The association between middle ear surgery and this undesired complication should be prominent in the planning and management of anesthesia. In addition to avoiding N_2O use, limiting opioids, and administering aggressive hydration, prevention requires a multimodal pharmacologic approach,[11] including preoperative use of metoclopramide and postinduction gastric suctioning. For these and other reasons, our preferred anesthesia technique includes a volatile agent, oxygen, and air supplemented with a propofol infusion.

MASTOID DISORDERS AND OTHER EAR DISORDERS

The introduction of antibiotics has greatly reduced the incidence of mastoiditis. However, it remains a disease with significant morbidity and even mortality. Untreated chronic otitis media remains the most common cause. Patients with failed antibiotic response require surgical intervention.

These procedures are performed under general anesthesia with endotracheal tube intubation. The surgeon's goal is to reestablish ventilation of the middle ear, debride infected material, and drain subperiosteal abscesses. Removal of osteitic bone can result in substantial blood loss. Controlled hypotension is helpful for the majority of the procedure. Facial nerve exposure is a possibility, and frequently the surgeon will seek to identify the nerve using a nerve stimulator. Short-acting muscle relaxants should be used. The return of neuromuscular responses should be documented and reported to the surgeon before attempted identification of the facial nerve and subsequent aggressive dissection.

Depending on the clinical presentation, a mastoidectomy may last anywhere from 3 to 6 hours. N_2O is permitted but must be removed at least 20 minutes before tympanoplasty begins. Postoperatively, these patients have large head dressings that take 5 to 10 minutes to place. As with other anesthetics, if the patient is lightly anesthetized, this head movement can result in significant bucking and bleeding, which contribute to postoperative complications. Therefore, deeper planes of anesthesia should be maintained until these dressings are in place, even at the cost of prolonged emergence.

Effort has been made to determine whether these cases can be performed as outpatient procedures. A study by Rowlands et al[12] determined that the need for inpatient admission was significantly related to the extent of surgery. However, comparing outpatient complications and overall success, no significant differences were found between outpatient versus inpatient management. It is suggested that mastoidectomy can be done safely as outpatient procedures in selected patients.

PATULOUS EUSTACHIAN TUBE

Classically, a patulous eustachian tube will result in autophony ("rushing air" sound) that disappears in the supine position. Occasionally, this experience is disturbing enough for the patient to seek surgical intervention. This is a rarely performed and challenging procedure for any otologist. Essentially, a stent is placed to partially occlude the eustachian tube. With the patient in a supine position, this correction is accomplished by an intraoral approach. All of the concerns and precautions of oral surgery (discussed later under Anesthesia for Throat Surgery) apply to this technique.

MICROTIA

Auricular malformations, either congenital or acquired, can be severe. A normal appearing ear is important to all patients, young and old. The Centers for Disease Control and Prevention estimates the incidence of microtia to be 1 in 10 000. Although it may occur as an isolated finding, microtia can occur with a variety of syndromes, including Goldenhar and Treacher Collins syndromes. A study by Uezono et al[13] noted that 42% of patients with bilateral microtia were likely to pose significant intubation challenges (ie, probable "difficult intubation"). Any associated dysmorphic features should prompt a thorough evaluation of the patient before reconstruction.

Depending on its extent, microtia usually is managed as a multistage repair. Initially, a rib graft is obtained and carved to resemble a matching template. This is then placed subcutaneously and allowed to heal. The patient then returns for additional skin grafts and refinement to the superior auricle. General anesthesia is necessary, and postoperative pain relief frequently requires patient controlled analgesia after the rib harvest. Typically, the surgeon infiltrates the donor site with local anesthetic, but it will remain a source of significant discomfort in the postoperative period.

Reconstruction in adults usually is done after traumatic injury or excision of neoplastic disease; thus, the airway concerns associated with congenital microtia usually are not present. Depending on the presentation and the patient, this operation can be accomplished with either general anesthesia or local anesthesia with sedation.

TEMPORAL BONE DISORDERS

Within the temporal bone lies the facial nerve. Of the cranial motor nerves, it has the longest intraosseous course and is threatened by any disruption of the temporal bone. Tumors are relatively rare but can result in significant morbidity upon resection. Blunt trauma with fractures is far more common. Approximately 80% are longitudinal fractures caused by a blow to the front or side of the head. A blow to the occiput results in a transverse fracture, accounting for another 15%. The remaining types consist of complex or combination fractures. Before the operation, the patient must be fully evaluated for any other injuries, such as cervical instability, other fractures, and cerebrospinal fluid (CSF) leaks. Besides hemostasis, the major postoperative concern with these procedures is persistent CSF leak with infection. Neurosurgeons are commonly involved with the repair.

ANESTHESIA FOR NOSE SURGERY

Procedures described in this section include those of the nose and sinuses. These structures are important components of the airway, and disorders can have a significant impact on a patient's well-being. Nasal and sinus surgery is conducted with the airway secured by endotracheal intubation and general anesthesia. Recently, the use of LMAs has become more common, but potential pulmonary aspiration remains a concern. If the patient is debilitated and at increased risk for complications with general anesthesia, these procedures can be performed under local anesthesia with sedation.

EXTERNAL AND INTERNAL NASAL DEFORMITY

Rhinoplasty is reconstruction of the external nose. Indications include trauma, neoplastic excision, deformity, and perceived malformation. Typically, these patients are young and healthy. After induction of anesthesia and intubation, the surgeon requests that the endotracheal tube be secured to the mandible in the midline position. This neutral position prevents any soft tissue distortion of the nose and allows the surgeon a more accurate reconstruction. Lubricant ("artificial tears") is placed in the eyes or the eyes are taped at the lateral margins. This minimizes the risk of corneal abrasion and provides access to the bridge of the nose. Slight elevation of the head is common to provide better surgical access and to promote venous drainage.

Despite the use of local anesthetics with vasoconstrictors, bleeding can be brisk. Suction of the gastric and oral cavities before emergence and extubation decreases the likelihood of PONV. Swallowed blood on an empty stomach is a well-known emetic. From an analgesia point of view, this procedure is relatively benign, with 1 exception. Toward the latter part of the procedure, the surgeon will do an osteotomy, which depends on the patient's specific anatomy and what the surgeon wishes to accomplish. If the patient's anesthetic depth is inadequate, patient movement or bucking may occur, both of which are undesired. Topical lidocaine may be useful here: Granier et al[14] demonstrated that intranasal topical lidocaine combined with naphazoline decreased both intra- and postoperative pain and reduced the need for rescue opioids.

At the end of the procedure, nasal packs or stents are placed, and a small plastic or fiberglass cast is fitted. Nasal stents are preferred because they allow ventilation through the nasal passages postoperatively. Care must be taken not to press upon the nasal bridge with the face mask. The mask is gently placed on the mandible with the superior portion free. The seal will not be good, but when combined with a jaw thrust, sufficient gas exchange should occur. As an alternative, Erbay et al[15] reported the beneficial use of a pediatric mask as a mouth mask in this scenario.

Rarely, neoplastic lesions require wide excision involving the entire nose and possible underlying structures. These patients will subsequently present for total reconstruction. Each patient's airway must be fully examined. Depending on their initial disease, the majority of patients have patent posterior nasal passages. Other patients may present after partial reconstruction and have a completely obstructed nasal airway, or a maxillary prosthesis may obstruct the nasal passages. It is wise to discuss these cases well in advance with the surgeon to understand the surgical plan and the patient's pathology. The anesthetic arrangements and concerns are as previously described. Reconstructions usually involve a forehead flap and are performed as multistage repairs.

Septoplasty is a functional procedure intended to correct a deviated septum. This condition may have occurred because of trauma, deformity, or malformation. A malpositioned septum can lead to complete airway obstruction on the affected side. It also can lead to poor sinus drainage and result in chronic sinusitis. The anesthesia arrangements and concerns are the same for a septoplasty, open nasal fracture reduction, and rhinoplasty. These are usually brief cases lasting anywhere from 30 minutes to 1 hour.

Closed reduction of a nasal fracture is a very brief procedure that requires the surgeon to apply vigorous pressure to realign structures. The definitive procedure literally takes seconds. To the awake patient, those seconds can be frightening and quite painful. An intense but brief general anesthetic usually is preferred. The author prefers to have the patient in a semi-sitting position and premedicated with midazolam and fentanyl. When the surgeon is in position with instrument ready, a single bolus of lidocaine and propofol is administered. Upon loss of consciousness, the reduction is accomplished. Typically, emergence occurs as the cast is being fitted. This technique works very well as long as blood loss is minimal. If the reduction is expected to be more complicated or if blood loss is a concern, then the airway should be protected by LMA or preferably an endotracheal tube.

CHOANAL ATRESIA

This is an uncommon anomaly that presents often as unilateral obstruction but bilateral obstruction can also occur. Other congenital anomalies are present in 20% to 50% of these patients.

Bilateral choanal atresia classically presents as a newborn who experiences complete airway obstruction that is relieved by crying. Gujrathi et al[16] have written a series review of the surgical techniques involved in these repairs. Recently, an endoscopic approach has been promoted, but the "puncture, dilation, and stent" technique remains the standard. Specific to this repair, the anesthesiologist must be vigilant that the stents are secured postoperatively. If one or both stents become dislodged, complete airway obstruction can occur as with any other foreign body (FB). These stents will remain in the patient for several weeks.

Lim et al[17] described a case of unilateral atresia repair complicated by a persistent buccopharyngeal membrane. One should be wary for other sources of airway obstruction. These patients may return to the operating room (OR) multiple times for stent cleaning and granuloma debridement.

SINUS DISORDERS

Contemporary sinus surgery is performed almost entirely by fiberoptic endoscopy (fiberoptic endoscopic sinus surgery [FESS]). An exception is open maxillary sinusotomy (Caldwell-Luc procedure). Indications for surgery include persistent sinusitis, recurrent nasal polyps, obstructed nasal ventilation, and CSF leak.

The anesthetic approach is similar to that used with other nasal procedures, but the surgeon may desire the endotracheal tube to be secured on the left margin of the oral cavity. It is common for the surgeon to stand (or sit) on the patient's right with the patient's head turned slightly toward the operator. The surgeon also will request that the patient's eyes be lubricated and left open or taped on the lateral borders. The operator should observe the patient's eyes throughout the procedure because some conditions require activity in close proximity to the orbit. Unfortunately, intraorbital eye injury has occurred in some cases, including vision loss secondary to intraorbital hematomas, eye muscle injury, and proptosis. Other complications include venous air embolism,[18] CSF leak, excessive bleeding, and permanent neurologic injury. Superficially, FESS appears to be a benign procedure, but the complications can be devastating. The advent of image-guided endoscopy (eg, StealthStation, Medtronic, Inc., Minneapolis, MN) has reduced some of the risks (**Fig. 67-2**). This is another procedure in which controlled hypotension may be helpful. The sinuses are well vascularized, and blood losses of 300 to 500 mL are common.

Surgeons will attempt to minimize bleeding by using local vasoconstriction, but such approaches are not without consequences. Yang et al[19] noted that low-dose epinephrine and lidocaine solutions caused a brief but marked decrease in blood pressure. As an alternative, Durmus et al[20] and Goksu et al[21] demonstrated the benefits of using infusions of dexmedetomidine to obtain stable, controlled hypotension and analgesia. Often, 4% topical cocaine is used as the vasoconstrictor; it is rapidly absorbed from the mucous membranes, and brief tachycardia and hypertension may occur. The effects of cocaine and other ester-linked local anesthetics can be prolonged in a patient who has pseudocholinesterase deficiency or one using pseudocholinesterase inhibitors (ie, echothiophate). Systemic toxicity can result in seizures, coronary vasospasm, myocardial ischemia, and arrhythmias. Aggressive treatment with short-acting mixed α- and β-blockers, oxygen, and deeper anesthesia may be necessary.

At the end, the surgeon will desire a smooth extubation with minimal movement or bucking of the patient. This can be a challenge when the oral cavity is filled with secretions and blood. A deep extubation can be performed, but this will place the patient at risk for laryngospasm as the anesthesia lightens. Deep extubations can be achieved with confidence if complete hemostasis has been obtained and if oral

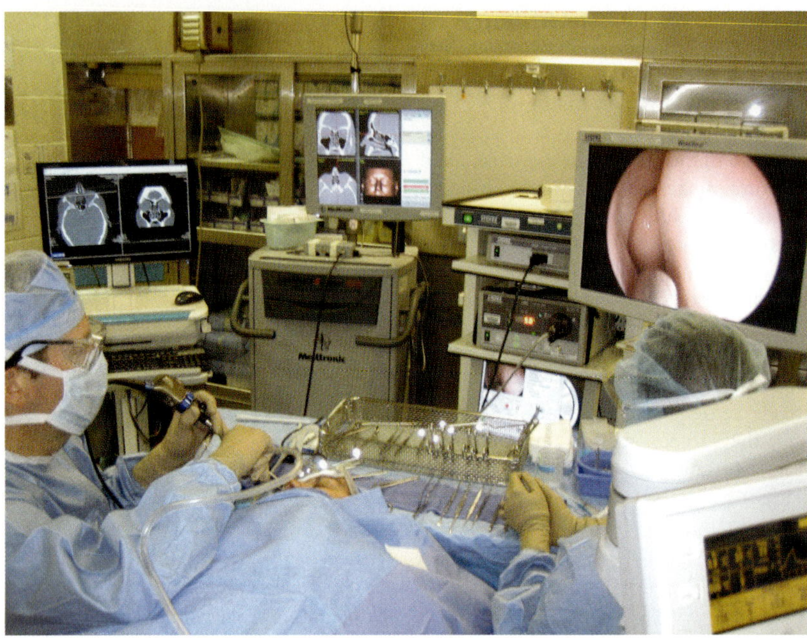

FIGURE 67-2. Contemporary sinus surgery. Note the real-time 3-dimensional positioning images in the upper center and the endoscopic view on the right. [Courtesy of Ralph Metson, MD, and Bil Ragan, MD, Massachusetts Eye and Ear Infirmary.]

and gastric suctioning have been extensive. Stents or packing may be placed, and the mouth remains the most reliable airway.

In addition to PONV, analgesia must be provided. Although FESS procedures are not particularly painful and local anesthetics will have been used, minimal amounts of narcotics can be added. Other analgesics such as dexmedetomidine may be helpful; Turan et al[22] found gabapentin to be useful for postoperative pain control, but patient dizziness was a limiting side effect.

FRONTAL SINUS OBLITERATION

Frontal sinus obliteration is a procedure for patients who have frontal sinusitis not responsive to other therapies. An internal approach can be used, or the scalp can be lowered and a bone flap raised over the frontal sinus. After complete and meticulous debridement of the sinuses, they are packed or obliterated with donor adipose tissue harvested from the abdomen. Typically, blood loss is not as severe as with a FESS procedure. Other concerns and anesthetic approaches are similar to those described for sinus disorders.

CEREBROSPINAL FLUID LEAK

For various reasons, including trauma, neoplastic disease, and prior surgery, a patient may present with a persistent sinus CSF leak. A successful repair requires locating the precise source of the drainage. While in the preoperative holding area, the patient is prepped and draped for subarachnoid access. After a spinal needle is placed successfully, 0.5 mL of a 10% fluorescein dye is diluted with 9.5 mL of CSF and injected slowly. The patient then proceeds to the OR and undergoes induction of general anesthesia. The fluorescein dye is expected to emerge in the sinuses approximately 20 minutes after injection, thus indicating the source of the leak. Other anesthetic considerations are similar to those for sinus disorders.

ANESTHESIA FOR THROAT SURGERY

The word "shared airway" evokes a subtle anxiety in the most experienced anesthesiologist. As a specialty, we are known for our skills to secure, maintain, and control the airway. Any activity that threatens a secure airway is a source of concern, if not annoyance. All aspects of throat surgery involve sharing the airway with another airway expert. Like any relationship, it requires communication, understanding, and trust.

ABNORMAL AIRWAY DISORDERS

Surgery to correct the abnormal airway will exercise all of the anesthesiologist's skills. Myriad disorders affect the airway, and patients can be of any age and present under any circumstances. The potential combinations of patient and airway are too numerous to allow detailed consideration of each possible scenario. This overview focuses on the most common disorders associated directly with the supraglottic, glottic, and subglottic structures.

As a conceptual approach, consider that the abnormal airway is any airway compromised by an acquired disorder, such as an infection, mass lesion, FB, and therapy (radiation), or by an anatomic disorder, such as congenital malformations, the malacias, and stenoses. These definitions are not strict because it is apparent that some lesions share features of both disorders. They are characterized in this manner only for ease of understanding. Yellon[23] has summarized an excellent approach to management of pediatric patients with abnormal airways. The guiding principles include a thorough preoperative evaluation of the patient and careful planning between the surgical and anesthesia teams. Physical examination may include endoscopy, laryngoscopy, and bronchoscopy to identify both dynamic and fixed lesions before performing any definitive surgical procedure. Safe, successful surgical and anesthetic outcomes depend on these efforts. Many of the same considerations apply to adult patients as well (**Fig. 67-3**).

ACQUIRED AIRWAY DISORDERS

Infections Epiglottitis is an acute bacterial infection that untreated can become a life-threatening disease. Most commonly, it affects pediatric patients in the 2- to 7-year age range. *Haemophilus influenzae* (type B) usually is the causative organism. With the use of *H. influenzae* vaccine in children, epiglottitis is becoming a disease of adults. Age notwithstanding, epiglottitis is a serious condition that must be treated aggressively.

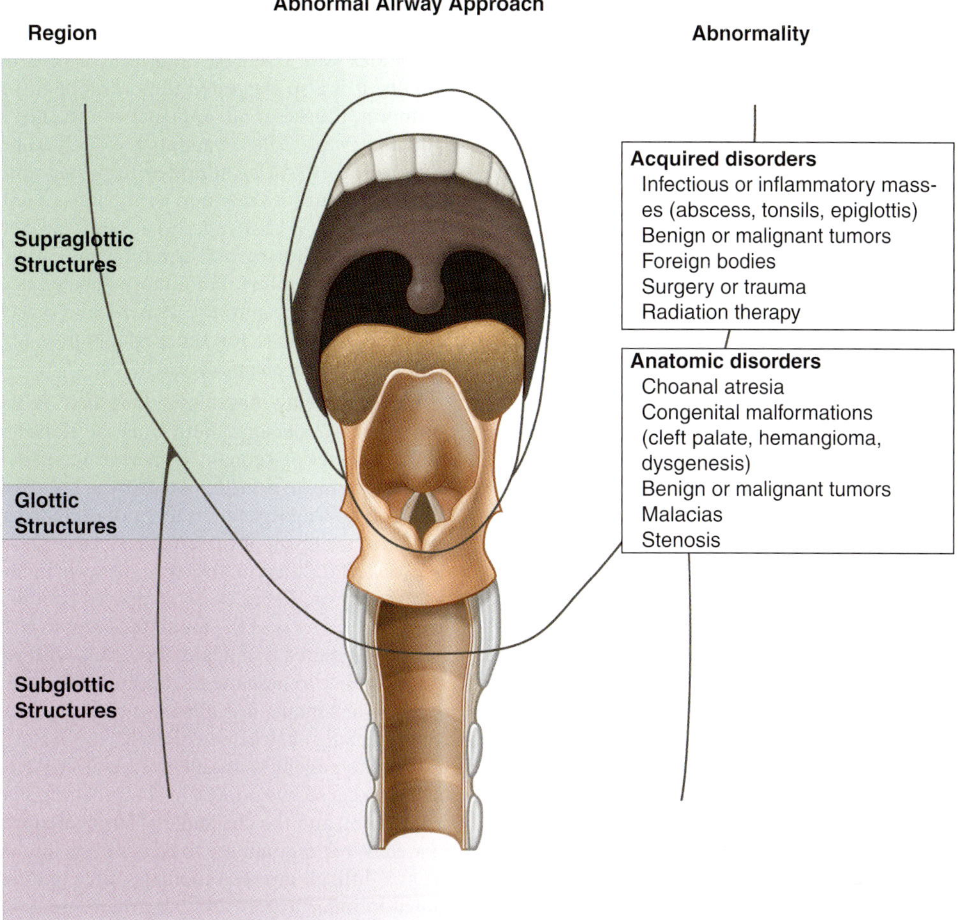

FIGURE 67-3. Conceptual approach to the abnormal airway. [Illustration by Daniel Muller, Haderer & Muller Biomedical Art, LLC.]

In the classic presentation, the patient arrives with an abrupt high fever, sore throat, stridor, dysphagia, and drooling. Physical examination reveals an anxious, pale patient sitting in the sniffing position. Epiglottitis can be distinguished from croup by the lack of a spontaneous cough. A lateral neck film will show a thickened, flat epiglottitis akin to a "thumbprint." *Supraglottitis* is a newer term suggested for this condition because the inflammation involves all supraglottic structures.

Adult patients are admitted and treated conservatively. Rarely do they require intubation. In the pediatric population, total airway obstruction can occur at any time. These patients cannot be left unattended until the airway is secured. In a controlled setting with an ENT surgeon and anesthesiologist present, an inhalational induction is done in the sitting position. Muscle relaxation is to be avoided. Laryngoscopy confirms the diagnosis, and endotracheal intubation immediately follows. It is suggested that the endotracheal tube be 0.5 to 1 size smaller than usual. If the airway obstructs and intubation becomes impossible, rigid bronchoscopy or tracheotomy must be performed immediately. Patients with epiglottitis usually respond to cephalosporin therapy after several days.

Croup is a benign disease typically affecting pediatric patients in the 3-month to 3-year-age range. It follows 2 to 3 days after a respiratory tract infection (RTI), and parainfluenza virus is the most common cause. The subglottic structures are involved, and the patient presents with stridor, dyspnea, and the classic "barking cough." Croup can be distinguished from epiglottitis on clinical grounds, and lateral neck radiographs are rarely needed. If obtained, they should reveal a normal epiglottis. Treatment is conservative with oxygen, nebulized racemic epinephrine, and IV dexamethasone. Endotracheal intubation is indicated only for respiratory fatigue, progressive intercostals retractions, and cyanosis. As with epiglottis, endotracheal intubation should be done in the OR under similar controlled conditions and with surgical expertise immediately available.

ADENOTONSILLAR HYPERTROPHY

Pediatric and Preoperative Concerns A tonsillectomy probably is the most frequently performed airway surgical procedure. It is estimated that more than 300 000 tonsillectomies are done annually in North America alone. Indications for surgery include obstructive tonsillar hyperplasia, recurrent or chronic tonsillitis, and peritonsillar abscess. Often, a combined procedure including the adenoids is performed. Adenoidectomy is done to relieve nasopharyngeal obstruction caused by adenoid hyperplasia. Frequently, these patients also have reflux.

The majority (but not all) of these patients are in the pediatric age range, and children have unique physiologic responses and psychological needs. The anesthetist's primary focus is the child, but one must address the concerns of the parents as well.

The relationship between the parent and child in the perioperative setting has been the subject of much research. Not surprisingly, Kain et al[24] confirmed that whereas a relaxed parental presence at induction had a calming effect on an anxious child, a stressed parent was of no benefit to an anxious child. Arai et al[25] found that induction and emergence behavior of children closely correlated with the maternal serum amylase activity during the preoperative period. The children of mothers who were experiencing more stress exhibited more anxiety than the children of calm mothers. These factors can contribute greatly to an uneventful anesthetic.

On the day of operation, parents should be queried regarding a current or recent RTI. These infections are frequent in this population, and a concurrent illness can affect the anesthetic management. In the past, the presence of an RTI would result in immediate cancellation of an elective procedure. In current practice, a decision is determined on a case-by-case basis. Most practitioners agree that children with a concurrent RTI have more respiratory complications. Most studies suggest that factors associated with these adverse events include endotracheal intubations, age younger than 6 years, and an RTI within 2 weeks before planned surgery.[26] According to Tait and Malviya,[27] children with RTIs have more respiratory complications, but they are not associated with serious morbidity. The child who presents with an uncomplicated RTI can be managed safely as long as the practitioner understands and anticipates likely adverse events, such as laryngospasm or bronchospasm. This view is further maintained in a review article by Mamie et al.[28]

Another preoperative issue is the anxiety or agitation level of the child. Although a thorough preoperative consultation can relieve much concern, some patients are still inconsolable. Should the child be premedicated? Any premedication will sedate the patient and can contribute to both preoperative and postoperative respiratory complications. Premedication also will delay emergence and the return of protective airway reflexes. It can also delay discharge from the recovery unit. Conversely, any child who has a very frightening experience will be difficult to bring back to the OR, and this may contribute to a lifelong fear of the health care profession. Sedative premedication should not be given on a routine basis. Only very anxious and agitated children should be treated. When required, orally administered midazolam (0.5 mg/kg; maximum, 10 mg) given at least 20 minutes before operation is the most common sedative. Alternatives include rectal ketamine, oral fentanyl, nasal fentanyl, clonidine, diazepam with midazolam, and dexmedetomidine. Oral dexmedetomidine was found to be especially effective in patients with neurobehavioral disorders resistant to previous sedative attempts.

Obstructive Sleep Apnea Syndrome Pediatric patients with obstructive sleep apnea syndrome (OSAS) present additional challenges because these obese children have a greater incidence of perioperative complications than normal-weight children.[29] Furthermore, these patients may have cardiovascular involvement, with altered right ventricular diastolic function, pulmonary hypertension, arrhythmias, and silent carditis. This diagnosis increases the risk of postoperative respiratory complications from approximately 1% to 20%. Granzotto et al[30] found a correlation between the palatine tonsil size and pulmonary artery pressure. This may prove to be a useful predictor of cardiac complications in children with OSAS. It is suggested that a polysomnography (PSG) be obtained in these patients before operation. Yellon[31] reported that preoperative PSG is indicated for patients younger than 3 years of age, with medical comorbidities, small tonsils and adenoids, and physical findings inconsistent with the extent of obstruction. Other significant risk factors include carbon dioxide (CO_2) tension greater than 50 mm Hg during rest while awake, witnessed severe upper airway obstruction, and nocturnal oxygen desaturation (<90%). These patients are not candidates for outpatient procedures and should be admitted for overnight observation.

Tonsillectomy can be performed in adults with obstructive sleep apnea, but the more common procedure for treatment of adult OSAS is uvulopalatopharyngoplasty (UPPP). This is a partial resection of the soft palate and is not a lengthy procedure. Extensive preoperative evaluation of the patient's airway is required. If the patient reports that nightly continuous positive airway pressure (CPAP) use relieves the symptoms, it is a good indication that the patient will be able to be ventilated with a face mask. However, when in doubt, awake fiberoptic intubation remains the technique of choice for airway management. Of interest, Kim and Lee[32] found that the preoperative apnea-hypopnea index was a reliable indicator of difficult intubation in UPPP patients. It is also suggested that intraoperative narcotics be kept to a minimum, if used at all, and that the trachea be extubated when the patient is awake. These patients are likely to be sensitive to sedatives. Moreover, they will be admitted for observation. Postoperatively, the UPPP procedure is known to be the most painful of ENT procedures. Pain control is a challenge because of the desire to limit the use of narcotics. Monitoring and careful observation are required to manage patient discomfort. For a more detailed discussion, see the review article by Isono[33] and the American Society of Anesthesiologists "Practice Guidelines for the Perioperative Management of Patients With Obstructive Sleep Apnea."[34]

Adenotonsillectomy Anesthesia Induction Pediatric anesthesia induction requires 2 persons. Both must be skilled in airway management and IV catheter placement. To perform a mask induction in a child by oneself is to invite disaster. Apart from the usual concerns of pediatric induction (laryngospasm, bradycardia-hypotension, lack of IV access), significant numbers of these patients have OSAS. Several investigators have looked at different airway maneuvers to improve mask ventilation in this situation. Reber et al[35] compared chin lift with CPAP versus jaw thrust with CPAP and the found the latter to be superior. Young-Chang et al demonstrated that a lateral position with jaw thrust returned heart rate variability to baseline in children with OSAS.[36] Regardless of one's preferred technique, it is apparent that jaw thrust and CPAP are effective in partially obstructed children.

After the patient is anesthetized and IV access obtained, the airway must be secured by endotracheal intubation. Tonsillar hypertrophy can be extensive, and the challenge of laryngoscopy should not be underestimated. What may appear to be a routine intubation can quickly manifest as a difficult airway. Another source of difficulty is the presence of lingual tonsillar hypertrophy. Furthermore, trauma to fragile inflamed tonsils during laryngoscopy can cause bleeding.

There is no uniformity of opinion regarding the use of muscle relaxants during these procedures. An uncomplicated tonsillectomy will last anywhere from 15 to 30 minutes with an experienced surgeon. Relaxants, if used, should be of the short-acting type. These patients also require narcotics for postoperative analgesia, and these drugs affect the child's ability to breathe. In a related issue, Khan and Memon[37] compared spontaneous with controlled ventilation for tonsillectomy. Their results suggest that controlled ventilation offers more hemodynamic stability and rapid recovery. It is the author's practice to give morphine immediately after IV access has been obtained and to intubate the trachea under the effects of both morphine and the inhaled anesthetic sevoflurane, thus avoiding muscle relaxants altogether.

Several techniques and drugs have been evaluated to facilitate tracheal intubation without the use of neuromuscular blockade. Woods and Allam[38] have provided an excellent review. Of the inhaled anesthetics, sevoflurane has emerged as the best choice, especially when combined with remifentanil. Of the IV agents, remifentanil followed by propofol seems to provide the best intubating conditions. Whatever approach is used, the avoidance of muscle relaxants allows the rapid return of spontaneous ventilation and protective airway reflexes (**Fig. 67-4**).

As an alternative, LMAs have been used successfully on healthy patients having ambulatory procedures. Although by definition an endotracheal tube provides a more secure airway than an LMA, adverse events have been quite rare. In a study Gravningsbraten et al[39] used LMAs in 1126 patients and converted 6 patients from an LMA to an endotracheal tube (0.5%). A concern with the use of a classic LMA in this setting is its displacement by the mouth gag. On occasion, the straight, solid blade of a traditional mouth gag will compress the tube of an LMA and move the tip posterior. To alleviate this problem, a new open channel mouth gag is being investigated and it

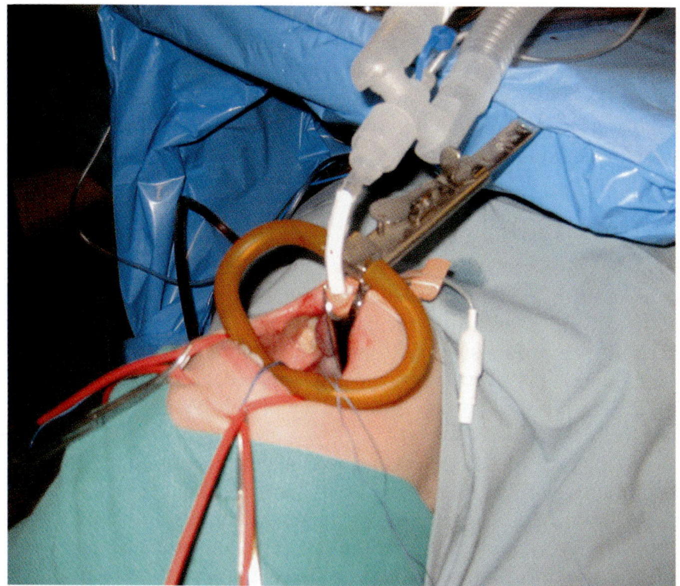

FIGURE 67-4. Twelve-year-old girl prepared for tonsillectomy. The endotracheal tube is secured midline on the mandible, and the mouth gag is in position with the handle placed on the operating room tray. [Courtesy of Michael Cunningham, MD, and Bil Ragan, MD, Massachusetts Eye and Ear Infirmary).]

appears promising (**Fig. 67-5**). By not compressing the LMA tube, it allows it to maintain its normal curvature and glottic seal. Use of an LMA is less invasive and easier and requires less recovery time than endotracheal tubes.

Intraoperative Management After the airway is secured, the surgeon places a mouth gag in the oral cavity to better expose the tonsils. This is a stimulating event with the potential for complications. Some surgeons disconnect the anesthesia circuit before placing the mouth gag. Others work around the endotracheal tube. During this manipulation, the endotracheal tube can be compressed, kinked, or displaced. Rarely, an unexpected extubation occurs. After the mouth gag is in place, one should recheck to verify bilateral breath sounds. The endotracheal tube is secured to the midline mandible; any extension can result in the tube moving several centimeters. When the mouth gag is in position, the surgeon places the inferior handle of the mouth gag on the OR instrument tray. If the child is lightly anesthetized and moves, potential cervical injury can occur. The other option is to place the handle on a stack of towels placed on the patient's sternum. This places pressure on the patient's chest, which can affect spontaneous ventilation. Before incision, the surgeon usually requests that an antibiotic and anti-inflammatory steroid be given.

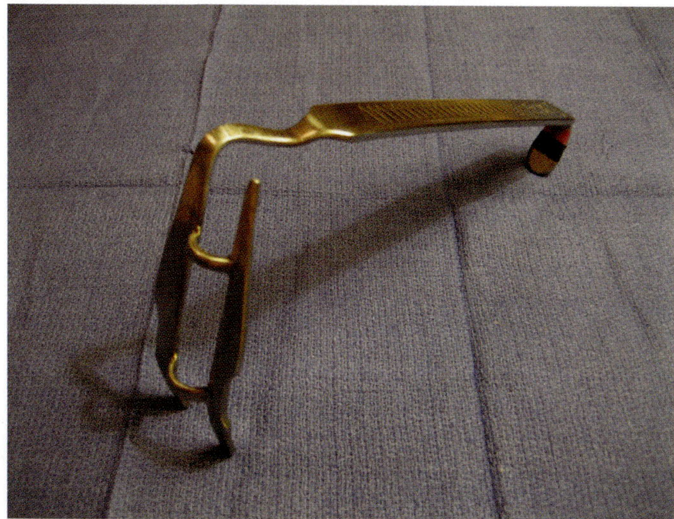

FIGURE 67-5. The open channel mouth gag, which allows the laryngeal mask airway to maintain its curve without displacement. [Courtesy of Samir Bhatt, MD, and Bil Ragan, MD, Massachusetts Eye and Ear Infirmary.]

Surgical techniques for tonsillectomy include guillotine resection (rare), cold dissection, bipolar dissection, and cold ablation (coblation) dissection. Each has its particular merits. Blood loss is greater, but pain is less with the first 2 techniques. Bipolar dissection allows immediate coagulation and less blood loss. However, thermal injury to the surrounding healthy tissue is responsible for greater postoperative discomfort. Coblation passes a radiofrequency bipolar current through a saline medium to produce a plasma field of sodium ions. Using a much lower frequency than standard bipolar diathermy, these ions essentially vaporize soft tissue at only 140°F (60°C). It also requires no electrical ground, and irrigating saline reduces thermal injury to adjacent tissue. Coblation offers the advantages of both cold dissection and bipolar diathermy with less postoperative pain and blood loss.

Postoperative Management At the end of the procedure, the patient should be breathing spontaneously. In addition to morphine, the author also gives ondansetron for emesis control. After hemostasis has been achieved, the patient's stomach and oral cavity are suctioned. An awake extubation can be performed to ensure that the protective airway reflexes have returned. These children are at high risk for laryngospasm secondary to blood and secretions in the oral cavity. Tsui et al[40] explored a "no touch" extubation technique. The patients were turned to a head-down lateral recovery position while still anesthetized. If the nondependent hip is flexed, the patient will easily stay in this position. The importance of the head-down position cannot be overemphasized. This arrangement allows pooling of blood and secretions to occur on the side of the mouth rather than midline. In addition, the upper airway of a child widens in the lateral position and is less likely to obstruct. Aside from oximetry monitoring, no additional stimulation was allowed with the technique. After the patient emerged from anesthesia, confirmed by eye opening, extubation of the trachea was performed. No incidences of laryngospasm, oxygen desaturation, or coughing were observed.

Complications of tonsillectomy include hemorrhage (discussed in Posttonsillectomy Hemorrhage), postoperative airway obstruction secondary to laryngeal edema, and dental trauma. In a study of 864 children, Isaacson[41] was able to reduce postoperative airway obstructive events by using a protocol that included (1) rapid bloodless tonsillectomy, (2) repeated release of the tonsillar retractor, (3) avoidance of uvular edema, (4) intranasal oxymetazoline with nasal airway placement, and (5) extended postanesthesia care unit stay. Raghavendran et al[42] have shown a reduction in respiratory events by the administration of dexamethasone and reduced need for opioids.

Analgesia and Antiemesis Postoperative analgesia of some type is required after this procedure. Local anesthetic infiltration before incision has provided satisfactory results. However, bupivacaine infiltration has been implicated in short-term vocal cord paralysis, and large quantities of local anesthetic can suppress protective airway reflexes for several hours. As an alternative, peritonsillar infiltration with ketamine[43,44] or tramadol[45] has produced good results.

Of the IV agents, ketamine, morphine, and meperidine all are proven potent analgesics. However, each has its own undesired side effects. Ketamine can cause an extreme dysphoric reaction if the patient is not pretreated with a benzodiazepine. It can also cause increased oral secretions, which is undesired in this patient group. The narcotics morphine and meperidine are very effective, but they provoke nausea. They also have sedative effects, can cause pruritus, and are respiratory depressants. Alhashemi and Daghistani[46] found IV acetaminophen as effective as intramuscular meperidine in the treatment of posttonsillectomy pain. White and Nolan[47] used fentanyl but not morphine and noted a significant decrease in the incidence of PONV; analgesia remained excellent.

Tramadol is a synthetic codeine derivative that behaves as a centrally acting atypical opioid. It lacks many of the opioid side effects while exhibiting both opioid and monoaminergic mechanisms of action. For adenotonsillectomy procedures, tramadol has been favorably compared with ketamine, morphine, and meperidine. Tramadol has been shown to have analgesic properties that are similar to those of morphine but without the associated respiratory depression. It is well tolerated with less nausea. Good results have been obtained when tramadol was combined with acetaminophen. However, a study by Arcioni et al[48] noted that ondansetron has an inhibitory effect when used simultaneously with tramadol. Despite this concern, tramadol remains a promising analgesic agent.

Nonsteroidal anti-inflammatory drugs (NSAIDs) have also been considered for postoperative analgesia. They provide excellent pain relief without the side effects of narcotics. NSAIDs also cause platelet dysfunction and prolonged bleeding time. Their use in adenotonsillectomies remains controversial. Moiniche et al[49] did a quantitative review of 25 studies to examine the relationship between NSAID use and postoperative bleeding. They concluded that NSAIDs offer similar analgesia and significantly less emesis than opioids, but they also contribute to more reoperations for hemostasis. A review by Marret et al[50] went even further and suggested that NSAIDs should not be used after tonsillectomy. Both of these reports contrast with a review by Cardwell et al,[51] which found no increase in bleeding requiring a return to the OR. Overall, the weight of the evidence appears to support avoidance of NSAIDs in adenotonsillectomy patients.

In addition to pain, PONV must be expected and treated. Even if narcotics are not used, swallowed blood can cause nausea. Several studies demonstrated the antiemetic effects of dexamethasone and it is often requested by the surgeon to reduce postoperative swelling and pain. Aouad et al[52] found dexamethasone significantly better than placebo for both decreasing vomiting and promoting postoperative oral intake. Elhakim et al[53] confirmed these findings and noted an analgesic benefit as well. Dexamethasone was also found to act synergistically when combined with serotonin (5-HT$_3$) antagonists.[54] Karaman et al[55] found that a dexamethasone dose of 0.7 mg/kg was optimal in preventing PONV. In a systematic review and meta-analysis, Bolton et al[56] determined that the most effective antiemetics were a serotonergic antagonist and dexamethasone.

Posttonsillectomy Hemorrhage Posttonsillectomy hemorrhage remains the most serious complication of this procedure. Posttonsillectomy hemorrhage occurs in about 5% of all cases and most often within 24 hours (primary hemorrhage). Secondary hemorrhage can occur anytime thereafter. A study by Brown et al[57] noted that nearly half of posttonsillectomy hemorrhage cases occurred in patients with previously undiagnosed coagulation disorders. Typically, posttonsillectomy hemorrhage is characterized by slow oozing. These patients can be hypovolemic and tachycardic before the complication is recognized. Bleeding can be quite brisk; a clot may dislodge upon intubation, and in a matter of seconds, the entire oral cavity can be filled with blood. These patients also may demonstrate orthostatic hypotension and may have swallowed a large volume of blood. They should be considered as having a "full stomach" regardless of their actual NPO (nothing by mouth) status.

Posttonsillectomy hemorrhage is a surgical emergency that requires immediate treatment. Windfuhr[58,59] has concluded that immediate surgical intervention prevented mortality in most cases. Before anesthesia induction, intravascular fluid expansion should be accomplished using either crystalloids or blood products if indicated. Failure to do so can result in fatal outcomes. As already mentioned, these patients should be considered as having full stomachs, and the airway should be secured immediately after a rapid-sequence induction. Large-bore, high-volume suction should be available, and the patient's stomach should be emptied after the airway is secured.

Windfuhr[60] also described treatment of excessive posttonsillectomy hemorrhage by ligature of the external carotid artery. He reported in follow-up studies that an age younger than 8 years and repeated episodes of secondary bleeding were risk factors for massive hemorrhage.

MASS LESIONS

Pharyngeal Abscesses (Peritonsillar, Retropharyngeal) Patients who present with a pharyngeal abscess can have significant coexisting morbidity. For example, the author treated an elderly man who arrived with progressive quadriplegia and somnolence. The underlying etiology was a retropharyngeal abscess compressing the patient's brainstem. Thus, although of infectious origin, pharyngeal abscesses are "mass lesions."

The majority of these cases occur in children or young adults. Incision and drainage of the abscess usually are performed under general anesthesia, with the airway secured by endotracheal intubation. Conversely, if the abscess is relatively small and not compressing the airway, some surgeons perform the procedure in the emergency department under local anesthesia alone. This requires a cooperative patient with a high pain tolerance. Under this condition, the patient is at risk for aspiration and additional complications. For patient care and comfort reasons, these cases are best handled in the OR.

After a general anesthetic has been decided upon, a thorough examination of the airway is required. This includes reviewing the relevant computed tomographic (CT) scans with the surgeon. Airway obstruction can occur, and intubation can be difficult. Depending on its extent, a retropharyngeal abscess can cause atlantoaxial subluxation. Furthermore, the underlying tissue may be quite friable, and the goal is to prevent any abscess contents from entering the trachea before securing the airway. This step should be a gentle intubation, attempting to not disturb the abscess. After the abscess is drained, the surgeon irrigates and suctions the oral cavity multiple times. These cases are not lengthy, and an awake extubation is indicated.

In a related scenario, patients with deep neck infections should be considered to have compromised airways despite their appearance. The classic example is Ludwig angina, which is a severe cellulitis involving the sublingual and submental spaces. Symptoms include tongue elevation, rapid breathing, difficulty swallowing, glottic edema, leukocytosis, and fever. Airway assessment is similar to that described above. An analysis and review by Ovassapian et al[61] concluded that an awake fiberoptic intubation is the safest approach. If an awake fiberoptic intubation is not feasible, an awake tracheostomy under local anesthesia should be pursued.

Benign or Malignant Tumors In addition to infectious masses, a wide variety of benign or malignant tumors may affect the throat and related structures. Hemangiomas can be found anywhere in the oral cavity. They are not treated unless they compromise the airway or interfere with function. Lasers are frequently used in the surgical management of these hemangiomas. Other benign masses include lymphangiomas of cavernous or cystic hygroma origin and papillomas. Malignant tumors are no less diverse and can be ulcerative, exophytic, or infiltrative lesions. Patients may present before diagnosis or after multiple excisions and chemotherapy or radiation therapy.

These cases must be thoroughly reviewed with the surgeon before bringing the patient to the OR. This includes discussing the surgical plan, the airway issues and a review of relevant CT and magnetic resonance imaging (MRI) scans. Previous anesthesia records should be located and reviewed, especially if prior diagnostic or therapeutic procedures have been performed, because the experience of others can be helpful in guiding the anesthetic plan.

Finally, careful evaluation of the patient is mandatory. One must determine the extent of mouth opening and attempt to visualize the mass lesion. An awake fiberoptic intubation is suggested if any sign of obstruction, limited neck extension, or any other factor is encountered that can interfere with direct laryngoscopy. Conversely, a small lesion in an otherwise normal appearing airway is reassuring. When managing a mass lesion, regardless of origin, one must be prepared with multiple approaches that can be invoked to secure the airway, including emergent surgical intervention, and the spectrum of options must be well rehearsed to prevent serious consequences.

FOREIGN BODY ASPIRATION

Foreign body aspiration is a life-threatening emergency and a leading cause of death in 1- to 3-year-old children. The variety of possible FBs is limited only by the imagination and seemingly, local culture. If an object can be picked up and placed in the mouth, it will be by some children. Where it may travel becomes the challenge for the ENT surgeon and anesthesiologist. Most commonly, FB ingestion or aspiration is encountered in pediatric patients in the age range from 6 months to 5 years. Occasionally, one meets the young adult attempting to do a "party trick" while under the influence of alcohol or drugs. Alternatively, trauma to the neck can result in bone, cartilage, or soft tissue occupying previously open space akin to a FB. Whatever, the source, airway assessment and management are similar.

Complete airway obstruction is rarely seen by the tertiary care team. Primary intervention by a Heimlich maneuver is the therapy of first choice, followed by digital extraction. Be aware that digital manipulation can push an obstructing FB further into the airway. If the patient has become hypoxic, cyanotic, and moribund, the only lifesaving option is emergent tracheotomy.

Partial airway obstruction is the clinical entity most frequently encountered. The guiding principle of management should be, "Do not convert a partial airway obstruction into a complete airway obstruction." The patient and family will arrive in an emotionally charged state. The child may be dyspneic, drooling, sitting forward, and frightened. Prominent, stridorous breathing may be noted and is indicative of supraglottic or glottic involvement. Wheezing is heard more often with subglottic obstruction. The nature of the FB and the context of its ingestion must be determined. Nonmetallic objects are difficult to visualize on plain radiographs. Secondary radiographic findings, such as a hyperinflated lung or lobe, can help localize the object. If the patient is stable and the FB is fixed in position, one can wait and allow the stomach to empty before going to the OR. However, this is not often the case.

Bronchoscopy and Foreign Body Management After the FB has been identified and located, a definitive management plan can be made. If the object lies near or within the trachea, the patient will require a laryngoscopy and bronchoscopy. If the patient is cooperative, it is possible to perform a bronchoscopy under topical anesthesia, but most patients require general anesthesia. Most practitioners advocate an inhalation induction for the patient with a partially obstructed airway to avoid positive pressure that might displace the FB and convert a partial obstruction to a total obstruction or cause the FB to migrate more distally in the airway. After induction, a rigid ventilating bronchoscope allows maintenance gases and oxygenation to continue, but hypoxemia remains a risk. Chen et al[62] identified the following risk factors for hypoxemia: patient age (younger more likely), FB type (plant seed), surgical duration, preexisting pneumonia, and spontaneous ventilation (jet ventilation or JV, decreased risk). Be aware that there is a significant leak around the end of the bronchoscope, and the entrained air often dilutes the inhaled anesthetic gases. Inhalation anesthesia may be supplemented by IV drugs given as a continuous infusion or intermittent boluses. Either alone or in combination, propofol, remifentanil, and fentanyl have been studied in this scenario. It appears that remifentanil provides greater hemodynamic stability and rapid recovery.

Bronchoscopy under general anesthesia is a delicate procedure. Complications arise from poor ventilation (hypercapnia, hypoxemia) and inadequate anesthesia (bronchospasm, bucking).

Bronchoscopy and Foreign Body Management Any FB ingestion posterior to the glottis is managed by esophagoscopy. If the airway is not compromised, a rapid-sequence induction with cricoid pressure can be performed. After the airway has been secured, there is no fear of aspiration. Rigid esophagoscopy is used for diagnostic purposes, FB removal, and tumor localization. The most serious complication is esophageal perforation, which frequently occurs in the hypopharynx. The consequences are significant; resulting mortality can range from 34% to 84%. Appropriate muscle relaxation can reduce the incidence by preventing unwanted movement or "bucking" during the procedure. In addition to perforation, other complications are compression of the endotracheal tube, dysrhythmias, and aspiration.

Flexible esophagoscopy is more of a diagnostic procedure and can be done as a monitored anesthesia care (MAC) anesthetic with sedation. It is not indicated for FB management.

IATROGENIC CAUSES

Surgery and Radiation Therapy Acquired airway disorders may result from other therapeutic activities that permanently alter the airway. Many otolaryngologic malignancies are treatable, and patients do survive. They will return to the OR for additional biopsies and surveillance endoscopies, but their airways may be significantly deformed.

Common surgical procedures include wide intraoral excisions, laryngectomies, and radical neck dissections with free flap reconstruction. Many of these patients present with a preexisting tracheotomy that makes their management straightforward. Others present with an intact airway that is greatly altered. As emphasized earlier, these cases must be discussed well in advance with the surgeon, previous anesthesia records must be reviewed, and the patient must be examined carefully.

These patients understand their postsurgical condition. Most are cooperative after the anesthesia concerns are explained. Unless the patient has a near-normal airway (unlikely), an awake fiberoptic intubation is the approach of choice. During laryngoscopy, the glottis is rarely found in the midline position; it is typically displaced laterally and the surrounding structures may be unrecognizable.

Radiation therapy often results in airway abnormalities. Radiation, which can be imagined as a form of burn, leads to fibrosis and shrinkage of the affected tissues. Schmitt et al[63] described factors that better identify potential difficult fiberoptic intubations in patients after radiotherapy. These include laryngeal edema, hoarseness, and stridor. The patient may appear to have a normal neck and mouth, but the difficulty of laryngoscopy should not be underestimated. After radiation, muscle tissue becomes very firm and fixed. The patient likely will not be able to extend the neck and may not be able to open the mouth more than a few millimeters. Muscle relaxants are of little or no benefit in this scenario. Similar to scar contractures caused by burn injuries, these patients have small, fixed upper airways. Laryngoscopies are extraordinarily difficult, if not impossible. Awake fiberoptic intubation is frequently the technique of choice.

VOCAL CORD DISORDERS

Disorders of the vocal cords can be of infectious origin, such as papillomas; they can be benign masses, such as hemangiomas and granulomas; or they can be neoplastic masses. Besides mechanical mass effects, mobility can be affected by fibrosis, inflammation, and nerve injury. Whereas some diagnostic procedures can be accomplished by flexible endoscopy, most surgical procedures are done by laryngoscopy and microlaryngoscopy. Medialization or voice restoration operations (phonosurgery) typically are conducted under MAC. The patient must be able to phonate (eg, say "EEE . . .") to guide the repair. If the lesion is well defined, general anesthesia can be used. Special techniques, such as apneic oxygenation and jet ventilation, may be necessary. Frequently, the surgeon requests profound muscle relaxation for a relatively brief procedure. Vocal cord surgery often uses lasers as the primary surgical instrument.

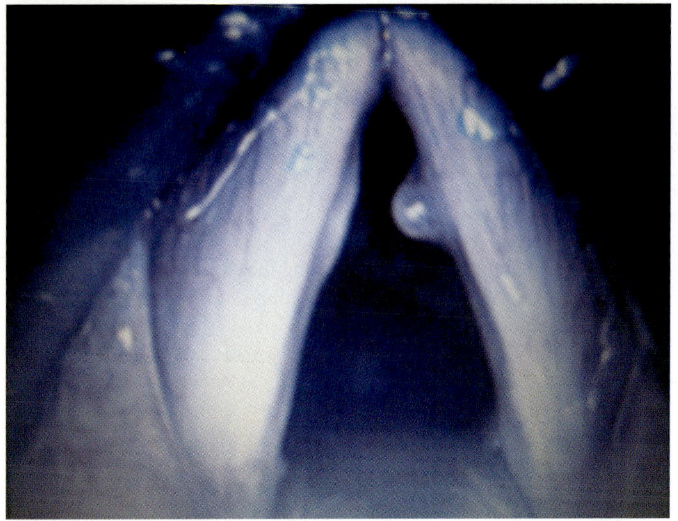

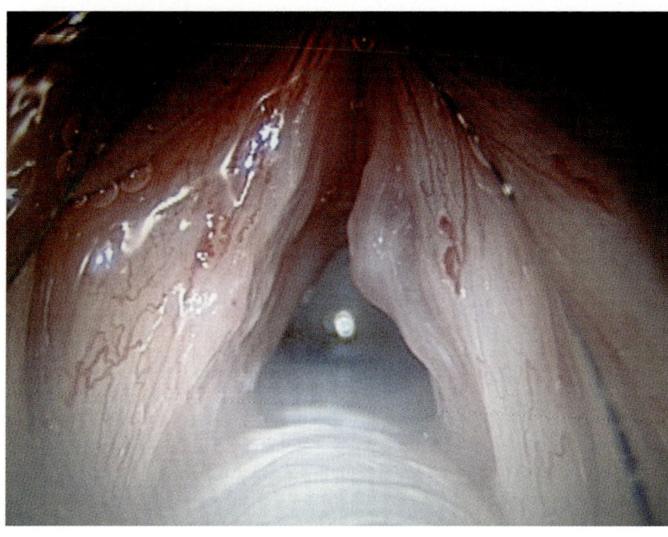

FIGURE 67-6. **A.** Vocal cord cyst. **B.** Bilateral vocal cord hemangiomas. [Courtesy of Christopher Hartnick, MD, Massachusetts Eye and Ear Infirmary.]

Using a combination of local and topical anesthesia can prepare the airway for laryngoscopy and some minor procedures. This requires blocking both superior laryngeal nerves and the glossopharyngeal nerves and injecting the trachea with local anesthetic. More commonly, these procedures are done under general anesthesia. Laryngoscopy is a stimulating event. It can elicit hypertension and tachycardia, which can lead to myocardial ischemia or even infarction in vulnerable patients. Conversely, laryngeal stimulation in a lightly anesthetized patient can cause bradycardia and dysrhythmias. The mechanism is a reflex pathway between the superior laryngeal nerve afferent fibers and vagal cardioinhibitory fibers. As with any general anesthetic, the patient must be sufficiently anesthetized before laryngoscopy begins. Giving β-blockers or opioids (ie, remifentanil) may blunt the hemodynamic effects (**Fig. 67-6**).

Microlaryngoscopy Microlaryngoscopy with suspension is a technique that uses both a surgical laryngoscope and an OR microscope. The surgical laryngoscope is attached to either an instrument tray or the OR table by extension, and the patient's upper torso is practically suspended for the duration of the procedure. A small-diameter, laser-compatible endotracheal tube with a large cuff volume is used. The head and neck are padded and braced; if the patient moves, injury can occur. Muscle relaxation is required for these procedures. The arrangement provides excellent exposure of the vocal cords, and the combination of microscope and laser allows the surgeon to make precise excisions. Prolonged suspension can cause glottic edema, resulting in airway obstruction in the recovery room. IV steroids can reduce this risk (**Fig. 67-7**).

Ventilation Ventilation during this procedure is a challenge. Unless a cuffed endotracheal tube is used, all volatile anesthetics will be diluted by entrainment of air. Pollution of the OR also may occur. Induction and maintenance of anesthesia are best accomplished using IV techniques. Some anesthesiologists have used apneic oxygenation for brief procedures. Others have advocated an intermittent ventilation technique whereby an endotracheal tube is placed and removed multiple times until the operation is complete. This places the airway at risk and prolongs the time needed to finish the procedure. It can also lead to additional vocal cord irritation and trauma.

Jet Ventilation Other practitioners have used jet ventilation to good effect. Essentially, a volume of gas is compressed and delivered under high pressure through a small tube or catheter. In a tubeless technique, this gas can be given through a side port in the laryngoscope. Depending on the situation, jet ventilation may be administered above, at, or below the glottis. Various devices are available to provide jet ventilation, and all have at least 3 common components. A compressor provides a blend of oxygen and N_2O (or nitrogen, helium, and so on) under high pressure. This mixture then passes through a pressure regulator before patient exposure. For adults, the initial jet pressure should be 20 pounds per square inch (psi) or less and for children should be 10 psi or less. Actual gas delivery is controlled by a hand-operated valve.

Jet ventilation is advantageous because it provides an unobstructed operating field to the surgeon and increases safety during laser procedures. However, there are some significant concerns. Jet ventilation requires additional time, effort, and skill to set up and operate. Because ambient air is being entrained along with high-pressure gas via the Venturi principle, the patient receives a diluted mixture that results in

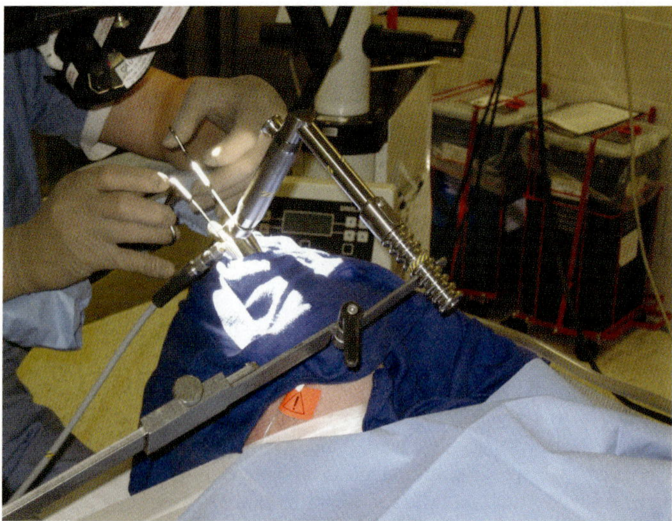

FIGURE 67-7. Patient positioned for microlaryngoscopy under suspension. Note that the patient's head is covered in a damp cloth. The microscope and laser are in the upper left, and the suspension laryngoscope is in the center. [Courtesy of Phillip Song, MD, and Bil Ragan, MD, Massachusetts Eye and Ear Infirmary.]

inadequate anesthetic depth. Furthermore, in the absence of a sealed airway, this can lead to OR pollution. Furthermore, Buczkowski et al[64] have shown that when using high-frequency jet ventilation (HFJV) above the stenosis, air entrainment occurs resulting in higher distal airway pressures. This complication is avoided if HFJV is given below the stenotic lesion. General anesthesia must be supplemented or maintained by IV agents when jet ventilation is used. Respiratory gas monitoring is inaccurate, and one must rely upon chest movement and pulse oximetry to assess ventilation. Air trapping can lead to barotrauma if a mass blocks expiration in a "ball-valve" phenomenon. Carbon dioxide can accumulate, leading to respiratory acidosis and its unwanted effects (tachycardia, arrhythmias). Moreover, the exit opening for the high-pressure gas, whether it is a needle, tube, or catheter, should not lie near the mucosa. The Hunsaker tube has extensions to keep it away from the airway surface and is a proven device in microlaryngeal surgery.[65] Barotrauma associated with jet ventilation can result in subcutaneous emphysema, pneumothorax, and pneumomediastinum. Jet ventilation is a sophisticated technique and complications are related to practitioner experience.[66]

Most recent research on jet ventilation has focused on ventilatory frequency. Whereas hand-operated valves allow delivery of low-frequency jet ventilation, newer, automated devices allow delivery of up to 600-Hz, HFJV. First described in 1976, this mode of jet ventilation is advantageous with certain types of airway pathology and in patients with severe pulmonary failure. High-frequency jet ventilation allows easy positioning in airway stenosis, decreases risks in laser surgery (no tube), decreases aspiration risk because of continuous outflow of gas, provides continuous ventilation, and allows cricothyroid rescue ventilation (see Unzueta et al[67]). In the latest variation, superimposed HFJV (SHFJV) has been shown to be quite useful in cases of severe stenosis.[68] This technique simultaneously uses 2 jet streams of different frequencies.

High-frequency jet ventilation has disadvantages. Hautman et al[69] identified that complications of HFJV included hypertension, hypotension, bronchospasm, hypercarbia, and hypoxia. Insufficient humidification is another concern. Histologic injury correlates with frequency of jet pulses and manifests as mucosal edema, congestion, and epithelial cell flattening, all of which can contribute to necrotizing tracheobronchitis. In addition to barotraumas, other complications include dysrhythmias, pneumoperitoneum, and gastric rupture secondary to misdirected gas flows. Some studies have suggested that preterm infants receiving HFJV have a greater incidence of necrotizing enterocolitis. With these concerns in mind, other investigators have examined the benefits of using combined-frequency jet ventilation. These techniques use both low-frequency jet ventilation and HFJV in differing ratios and have given satisfactory results. Regardless of the approach used, jet ventilation remains a useful but specialized anesthetic technique. It requires experience and should not be attempted by unaccompanied novices.

Lasers Schawlow and Townes first theoretically proposed lasers (light amplification by stimulated emission of radiation) in 1958, and development followed rapidly. In 1960, Maimon produced a laser, and since that time, lasers have become common in multiple applications, including medical and surgical practice. Anesthesia providers should have a basic understanding of how lasers function and of the benefits and hazards associated with their use.

A laser beam can be described as monochromatic (same wavelength), coherent (in phase), and collimated (parallel waves) light. Most lasers are 1 of 4 types. *Dye lasers* use an active material (usually an organic dye) in a liquid suspension as the lasing medium. By changing the chemical composition of the dye, the laser can be "tuned" to different wavelengths. *Diode lasers* use an optical cavity to amplify light emitted from the energy-based gap that exists in semiconductors. *Gas lasers* consist of a gas-filled tube upon which a voltage is applied to excite molecules to a state of population inversion. *Free electron lasers* function by having an electron beam in an optical cavity pass through a magnetic undulator. Free electron lasers can produce a wide variety of wavelengths (**Fig. 67-8**).

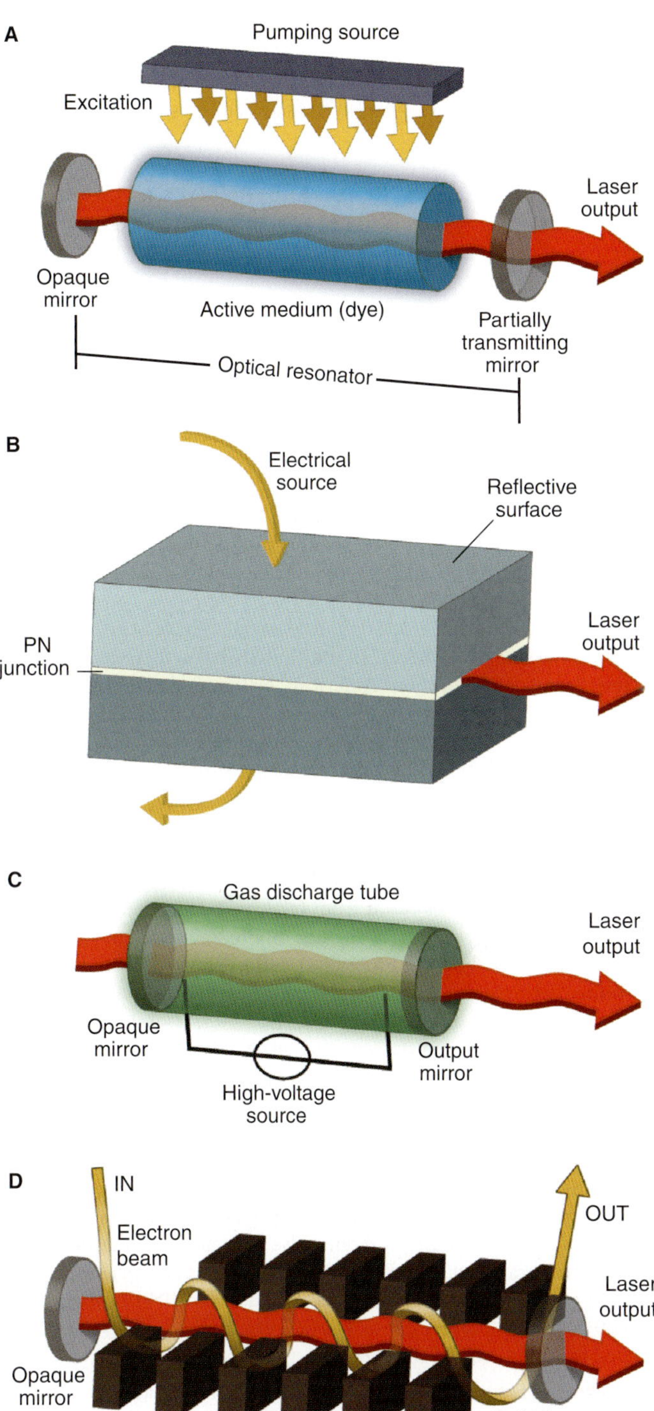

FIGURE 67-8. Schematic diagrams illustrating the components and types of common medical lasers. **A.** Dye laser. **B.** Diode laser. **C.** Gas laser. **D.** Free electron laser. [Illustration by Daniel Muller, Haderer & Muller Biomedical Art, LLC.]

Laser Effects and Safety Lasers focus a large amount of energy on a discrete area to exert their effects. In biologic tissue, this can manifest as thermal effects via energy absorption, photochemical effects by the reaction of radiant energy with specific molecules, and mechanical effects by disruption secondary to propagation of photo acoustic shock waves. In

TABLE 67-1 Laser Effects

Thermal injury: Burns secondary to energy absorption
Photochemical reactions: Secondary to interaction between specific molecules and radiant energy
Mechanical effects: Tissue disruption secondary to photoacoustic shock waves
Toxin release: Toxic gases, carcinogens, and viable microorganisms within the laser "plume"

TABLE 67-3 Commonly Used Medical Lasers (Pulse Mode)

Type of Laser	Wavelength (nm)	Primary Effect	Protective Eyewear
CO_2	10,600	Thermal	Clear
Nd:YAG	1,064	Thermal	Clear
Dye	583-587	Thermal/Mechanical	Blue (dye specific)
KTP-diode	532	Thermal	Orange
Argon	514	Thermal	Orange (argon specific)

KTP, potassium titanyl phosphate; Nd:YAG, argon, neodymium:yttrium-aluminum-garnet.

addition, the smoke, or laser "plume" can contain known carcinogens, toxic gases, and viable microorganisms (**Table 67-1**).[70]

Every facility that uses medical lasers should have a laser safety officer or committee. The responsibilities should include education of health care providers, protocol formulation, and implementation of safety policies. When a laser is in use, signs and appropriate safety glasses must be available at all entrances. All persons in the OR should wear safety glasses, and the patient's eyes should be taped closed and covered with soaked gauze.

As with any medical device, national standards have been established to ensure the safe use of lasers. In the United States, these can be found in the industry publication American National Standards Institute (ANSI) Z136.3-2005, *Safe Use of Lasers in Health Care Facilities*.[71] Two important concepts are emphasized in this handbook. One is the *nominal hazard zone*. This is the minimal distance in which lasers beams can have effects. For the majority of medical lasers, this distance varies between 0.46 and 178 m. The other concept is borrowed from radiation safety studies and is the *maximum permissible exposure*. This represents the maximal laser energy that can be absorbed without resulting in harm. Most laser injuries result from reflected beams, and the eyes are most vulnerable. Eye injuries include photokeratitis, photochemical cataracts, thermal retinal injuries, and corneal burns. Within the eye, the retina is vulnerable to laser wavelengths of 400 to 1400 nm (argon, neodymium:yttrium-aluminum-garnet [Nd:YAG] lasers). Wavelengths of 1400 nm or above can damage the cornea. Aside from wavelength, the extent of eye injury is determined by pupil size, degree of pigmentation, size of retinal image, pulse duration, and pulse repetition rate (**Table 67-2**).

The safety glasses needed are wavelength specific and depend on the laser being used. Argon (514-nm) pulse lasers exhibit a green beam and cause thermal effects. They require orange glasses. The potassium titanyl phosphate (KTP; 532 nm) diode pulse laser also has thermal effects and requires orange glasses. Dye pulse lasers have both mechanical and thermal effects and require blue glasses. Nd:YAG (1064 nm) and CO_2 (10600 nm) pulse lasers cause thermal effects, and clear glasses are needed for protection (**Table 67-3**).

Laser Fire and Laser Endotracheal Tubes The greatest danger caused by a laser is an endotracheal tube airway fire. Although rare, the results of an endotracheal tube airway fire can be catastrophic and fatal. If the endotracheal tube is penetrated by the laser beam, the oxygen-rich environment within the tube can produce a vivid, intense flame. Every practitioner should have the image of a "blow torch" in his or her mind to appreciate the danger. All of the elements to support a fire are found in this setting: oxygen (supports combustion along with N_2O), combustible material (endotracheal tube), and an ignition source (laser). Much effort has been expended to develop a laser-safe endotracheal tube, but as of yet, there are no "perfect" laser endotracheal tubes.

TABLE 67-2 Determinants of Eye Injury

1. Pupil size
2. Degree of pigmentation
3. Size of retinal image
4. Pulse duration
5. Pulse repetition rate
6. Wavelength

Metal endotracheal tubes are laser resistant but have other disadvantages. They are not as pliable or as easy to handle as conventional polyvinyl chloride (PVC) tubes. This characteristic can lead to unnecessary manipulation and potential vocal cord trauma. Metal endotracheal tubes do not have a cuff, and one cannot seal the trachea. Furthermore, the laser beam can reflect off the tube and damage healthy adjacent tissue. Metal tubes can transmit heat to surrounding tissue. A Mallinckrodt Laser-Flex is a metal tube containing an inner PVC endotracheal tube fitted with tandem cuffs. If one cuff is damaged, the remaining cuff can still maintain a seal. Despite its other advantages, the PVC cuff still conveys a risk of laser ignition.

The Xomed Laser Shield II is a silicone endotracheal tube covered with metallic particles. Its cuff also has a metallic covering to improve its survivability. This is the endotracheal tube used at the author's institution, with safe, reliable results obtained. However, under certain circumstances, this tube can burn. Typically, a cool saline-blue dye mixture is used to inflate the cuff. This allows easy visualization of any cuff damage and provides a "heat sink" to slow potential ignition of the cuff. (**Fig. 67-9**)

A Sheridan 2 is a polyvinyl acetate (Merocel), copper foil–wrapped endotracheal tube. Red rubber tubes wrapped with a metallic tape have been used safely for many years. One advantage is that ignited rubber tends to char rather than melt. In addition, more energy is required to ignite rubber than PVC. Great care must be taken when applying the metallic tape. Any exposed areas are liable to ignition. Rough or loose edges can injure the patient's airway. Similar to a metal tube, certain metallic tapes can reflect the metal beam onto healthy tissue.

Airway Fire Precautions and Management To reduce the risk of an airway fire, certain precautions should be observed:

1. Consider a tubeless technique using spontaneous ventilation, apneic techniques, or jet ventilation.
2. Use an appropriate laser endotracheal tube, such as metal, Mallinckrodt, Xomed, Sheridan, or Red Rusch.
3. Reduce inspired oxygen as tolerated by the patient to less than 30% but ideally 21%.
4. Use either air or helium to dilute the oxygen; N_2O supports combustion.
5. Fill the endotracheal tube cuff with a saline–dye mixture or lidocaine jelly.
6. Completely soaked gauze should be placed within and around the airway to reduce ignition risk.
7. Use H_2O-based ointments; petroleum-based ointments are flammable.

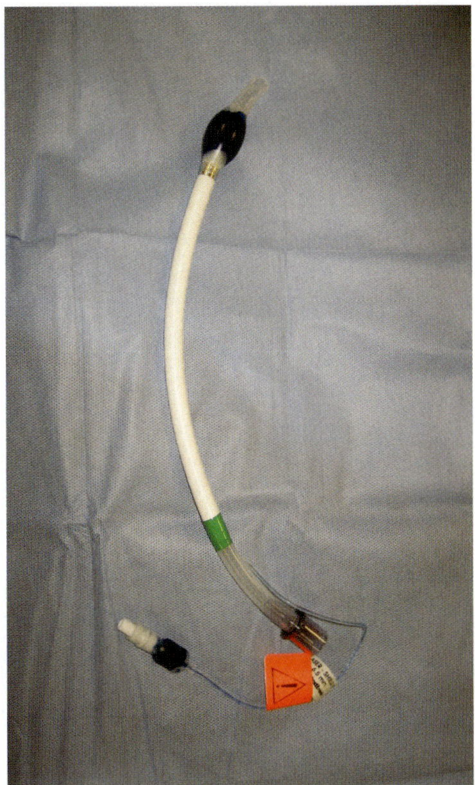

FIGURE 67-9. A Xomed Laser Shield II endotracheal tube. Note that the cuff has been test filled with saline and blue dye. [Courtesy of Bil Ragan, MD, Massachusetts Eye and Ear Infirmary.]

8. Limit the duration and intensity of laser exposure; continuous mode allows heat buildup.
9. Maintain a ready source of water in case of fire (multiple 60-mL filled syringes).

These steps will not eliminate the risk of an airway fire, but they will reduce it.

Despite these precautions, what should the anesthesiologist do in the event of an airway fire? The ANSI has developed the following protocol:

1. Stop ventilation.
2. Disconnect the oxygen source and flood the airway with water.
3. Remove the burned endotracheal tube and examine the airway.
4. Mask ventilate the patient and reintubate.
5. Survey the extent of injury using a flexible bronchoscope.
6. Monitor the patient for 24 hours.
7. Administer steroids to reduce inflammation and edema.
8. Provide antibiotics and ventilatory support if indicated.

It is common practice at the author's institution not to tape or secure the endotracheal tube to the patient's face. This will allow rapid removal of the tube in the event of an airway fire; however, this raises a controversial point. In the author's own research (unpublished observations), it appears that the first step is to remove the endotracheal tube as rapidly as possible even if gas flows and ventilation are still occurring. After being ignited, even without gas flow, the endotracheal tube will continue to burn and cause injury. By the time an endotracheal tube fire is recognized, approximately 3 to 4 seconds have passed. It will take another 3 to 4 seconds to stop ventilation, stop gas flows, and flood the airway before removing the endotracheal tube. In contrast, simply removing an untaped endotracheal tube will take approximately 1 second, thus potentially reducing the amount of injury to the patient.

TABLE 67-4 Airway Fire Precautions

1. Use a laser endotracheal tube or consider tubeless technique, apnea, or jet ventilation.
2. Reduce inspired O_2 to less than 30%.
3. Avoid N_2O; use air or helium.
4. Fill the endotracheal tube cuff with saline dye or lidocaine jelly.
5. Place a soaked gauze around the airway.
6. Use only H_2O-based solvents.
7. Limit laser exposure.
8. Maintain a ready source of H_2O.

Besides endotracheal tubes, lasers can ignite surgical drapes and other flammable items within the OR. Electrocautery can be a source of surgical fires. Under the right conditions, drapes, towels, ointments, and gowns can be combustible. Only by taking all possible precautions and practicing due diligence are surgical fires prevented. Every member of the OR team must be aware and prepared to intervene if necessary (**Tables 67-4** and **67-5**).

ANATOMIC AIRWAY DISORDERS

Congenital Malformations These malformations were alluded to in the discussion of choanal atresia. In contemporary obstetric practice, it is now possible to identify and diagnose many airway lesions in the prenatal period. Polyhydramnios can be associated with atresia, webs, gastrointestinal obstruction, and neurologic disorders. Mass lesions include teratomas, cystic hygromas, and hemangiomas. If an airway lesion is undetected and the delivery unexpected, securing the airway may be difficult or impossible. Fatal outcomes can be prevented with advance planning.

Farrell[72] examined this problem. After a diagnosis has been established, elective cesarean section is the preferred technique for delivering the fetus; it is usually scheduled early enough to avoid spontaneous labor and yet late enough to allow pulmonary maturation to occur. Such a complicated delivery requires 2 surgical teams, an obstetric team and a neonatal team. The neonatal team should include a pediatrician, pediatric anesthesiologist, and pediatric otorhinolaryngologist. Each team will have its own setup and equipment. Careful planning and practice are necessary before delivery. When the infant's head emerges, the neonatal team secures the airway as planned. This often occurs before umbilical separation.

Craniofacial abnormalities range from an incomplete cleft lip to complete centrofacial dysgenesia. Congenital malformations include Beckwith-Wiedemann syndrome; cleft lip and palate; craniocarpotarsal dysplasia/Freeman-Sheldon/whistling face syndrome; craniofacial dyostosis; fibrodysplasia ossificans progressive; hemifacial microsomia; Klippel-Feil syndrome; mandibulofacial dyostosis or Treacher-Collins syndrome; mucopolysaccharidosis; Pierre-Robin

TABLE 67-5 Airway Fire Protocol

1. Stop ventilation.
2. Stop O_2 flow and flood the airway with water.
3. Remove the endotracheal tube and examine the airway.
4. Mask ventilate the patient and reintubate.
5. Determine injury via bronchoscopy.
6. Monitor the patient for 24 h
7. Consider steroid administration.
8. Provide antibiotics and ventilator support as needed (**Fig. 67-10**).

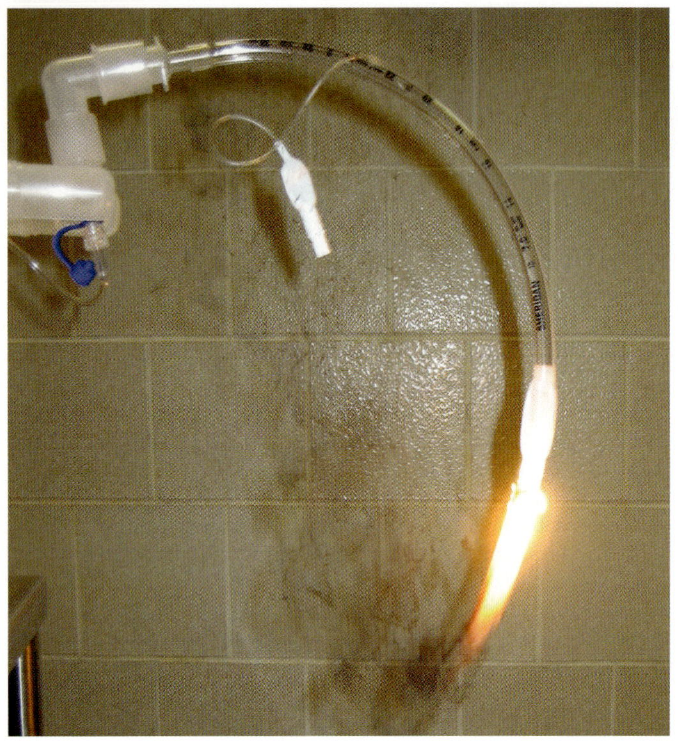

A

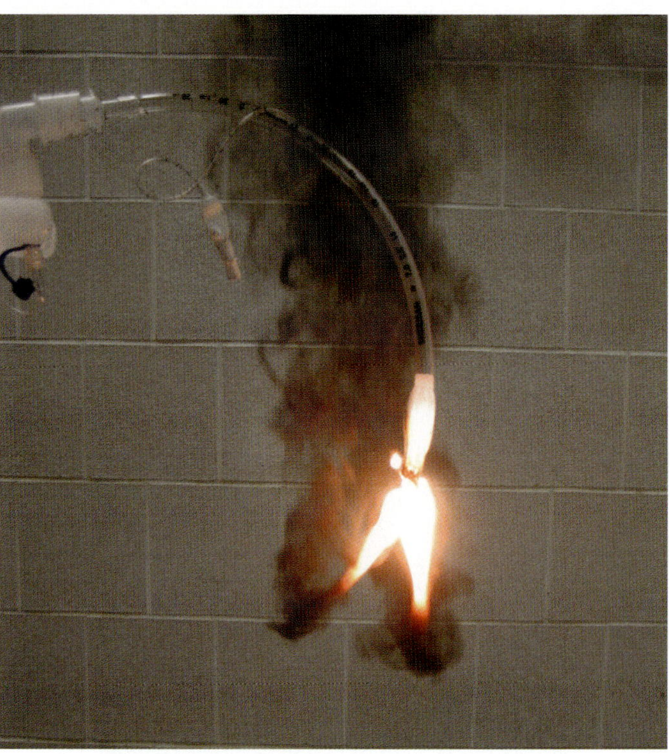

B

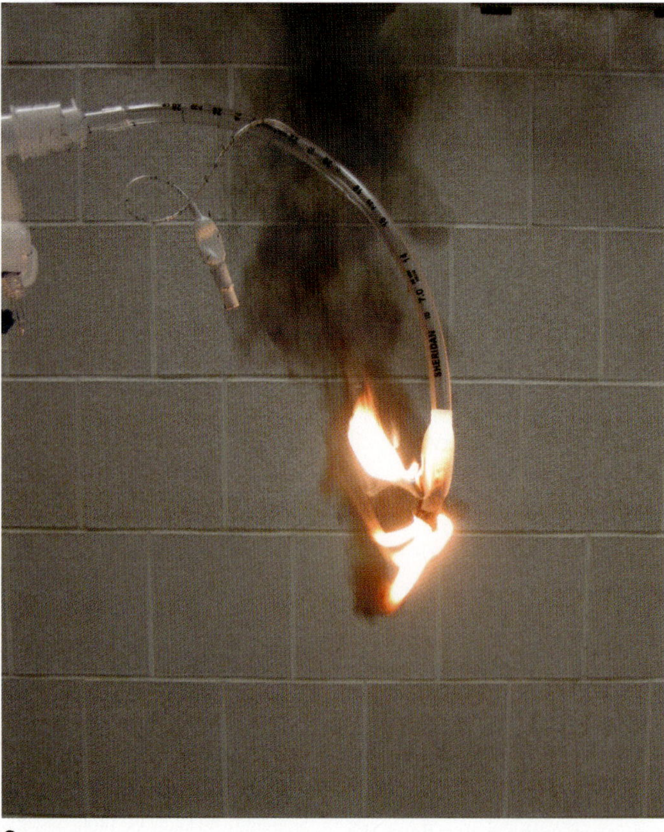

C

FIGURE 67-10. A standard polyvinyl chloride 7.0 endotracheal tube on fire. **A.** Approximately 3 seconds after ignition while receiving 1 L of oxygen and 2 L of nitrous oxide, note the "blow torch." **B.** Approximately 10 seconds after ignition; the flame intensifies and is accompanied by a large volume of combustible products. **C.** Gas flows have been stopped, but the tube continues to burn vigorously. [Courtesy of Bil Ragan, MD, and Artem Grush, MD, Massachusetts Eye and Ear Infirmary.]

syndrome; trisomy 21 or Down syndrome; and vascular malformations. Nargozian[73] has described an approach to airway management in these special patients. *Pediatric Anesthesia* published a special supplement in July 2009 titled "The Pediatric Airway."[74] It contains a series of comprehensive review articles covering all aspects of the pediatric airway. This overview briefly discusses cleft lip and palate repair.

CLEFT LIP AND PALATE

Cleft malformations may be an isolated finding or associated with other syndromes. These infants have difficulty feeding and fail to gain weight. Aspiration may lead to pulmonary problems. Aside from feeding issues, cleft malformations are associated with chronic serous otitis, which can lead to hearing deficits and speech delay. Parents will desire a timely repair for functional as well as cosmetic reasons. Initial lip repair may be done as a "lip adhesion" at approximately 6 weeks of age. This is simply a sutured approximation of the cleft edges that will promote better feeding and weight gain before later procedures. The definitive repair is done at approximately 12 weeks of age, with revisions after that as needed.

Similar to lips, cleft palates may be unilateral or bilateral, and they may be complete or incomplete (only soft palate involved). There is a strong association between an incomplete cleft palate, micrognathia, and various syndromes. A submucous cleft only involves the muscles beneath the mucous membranes and cannot be seen on visual examination. Some surgeons repair the soft palate with the lip at 12 weeks of age. Hard palate repair is accomplished between 9 and 18 months; most surgeons prefer approximately 1 year of age. The maxillae have better growth with later repair, but the infant will develop better speech with early repair. These procedures are managed with general anesthesia and endotracheal tube intubation. Securing the airway is not difficult if no other syndromic abnormalities are present. Mesnil et al[75] have shown that bilateral suprazygomatic maxillary nerve blocks provide excellent analgesia and decrease opioid use after repair.

MALACIAS

Malacias refer to conditions caused by cartilage softness that leads to airway collapse and obstruction. With the exception of reactive airway disease, the malacias are unique among the airway disorders in exerting their effects by dynamic processes. These disorders can lead to significant morbidity and mortality and are a rare condition characterized by softness of the airway structures. A review article by Austin and Ali[76] fully describes the assessment, treatment, and management of tracheomalacia and bronchomalacia in children. Laryngomalacia can produce similar symptoms.

Excessive intrathoracic pressure during expiration creates narrowing and airway collapse. The patient will have wheezing unresponsive to bronchodilators. Less commonly, extrathoracic pressure causes produce collapse during inspiration demonstrated by stridor. Most patients with airway malacia are neonates who have aortopulmonary malformations, bronchopulmonary dysplasia, or tracheoesophageal malformations. Congenital airway malacia may be an isolated finding or part of a syndrome. Acquired airway malacia results from chronic compression that limits cartilage growth. Thus, even after a "pexy procedure," airway collapse may still occur.

Being a dynamic airway disorder, malacia assessment is best accomplished by flexible bronchoscopy in a spontaneous breathing patient. Typically, this is accomplished by performing a mask induction on the neonate. After the patient is under anesthesia, a bronchoscope is introduced to observe and record airway structures while the child is breathing. The patient receives 100% oxygen under insufflation and supplemental IV anesthesia during the study. Combinations of propofol and remifentanil, when titrated to effect, work very well. The goal of the anesthetic is to prevent airway collapse by using positive end-expiratory pressure or CPAP and to avert coughing. Videofluoroscopy with or without contrast can be useful. CT and MRI scans cannot show the dynamic processes but can reveal which anatomic structures may be compressing the airway. Spirometry data allow one to assess the functional impact of the disorder. As discussed by Austin and Ali, treatment can be (1) long-term ventilation or CPAP, (2) resection of the affected segment, (3) external splinting, (4) pexy procedures, and (5) stenting. At present, the last 2 modalities appear to offer the most promising results (**Figs. 67-11** and **67-12**).

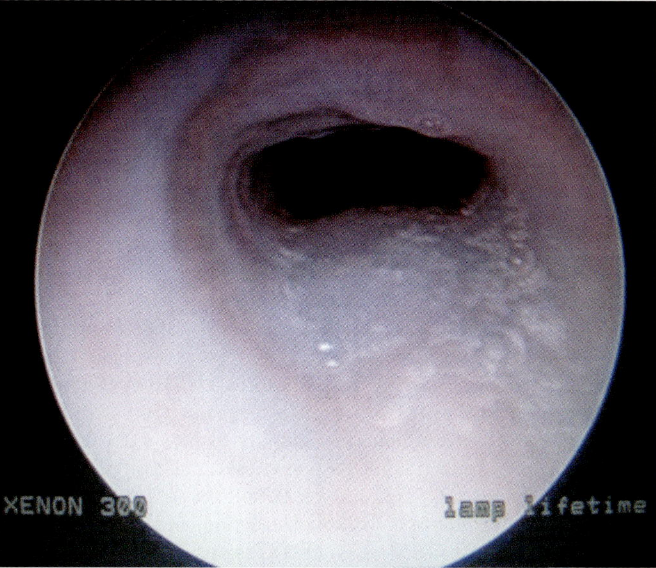

FIGURE 67-11. Tracheomalacia as seen in an 11-month-old girl. Note that the posterior wall has collapsed into the tracheal lumen. [Courtesy of Christopher Hartnick, MD, Massachusetts Eye and Ear Infirmary.]

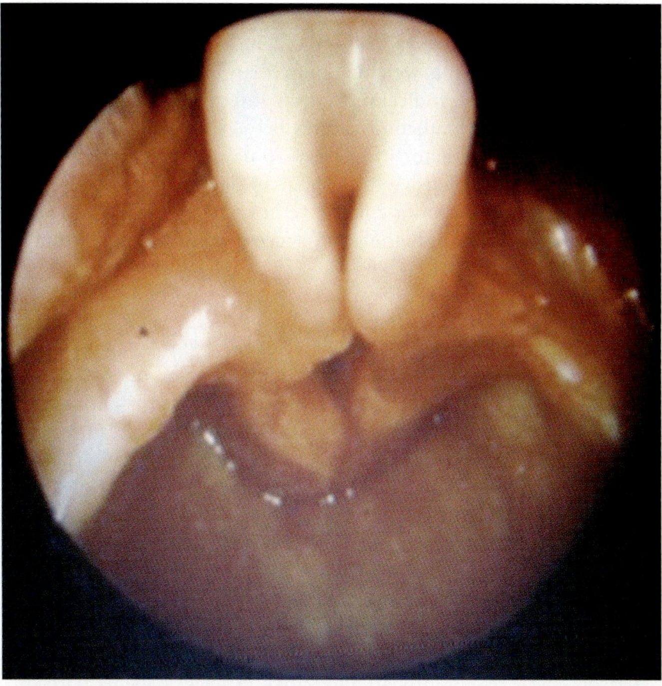

FIGURE 67-12. Laryngomalacia as seen in a 1-day-old neonate presenting with stridor. [Courtesy of Christopher Hartnick, MD, Massachusetts Eye and Ear Infirmary.]

SUBGLOTTIC STENOSIS

Subglottic stenosis refers to any condition in which the trachea is narrowed by a fixed lesion that compromises air flow. Pediatric subglottic stenosis can result from congenital causes, such as abnormal cartilage, or acquired causes, such as prolonged intubation, trauma, burns (thermal and chemical), gastroesophageal reflux disease, and mass compression. Adult subglottic stenosis is almost entirely of the acquired variety. There are few experiences as frustrating to the anesthesiologist as an inability to advance an endotracheal tube beyond the vocal cords following what appeared to be a routine laryngoscopy.

A full-term infant has a subglottic diameter of approximately 5 to 6 mm. Congenital subglottic stenosis is defined as a subglottic diameter smaller than 4 mm or the inability to pass a 3-mm endotracheal tube. For premature neonates weighing less than 1500 g, consider a smaller diameter, for example, the inability to pass a 2.5-mm endotracheal tube. A simple grading system is used to classify the severity of subglottic stenosis. Grade I lesions exhibit 0% to 50% obstruction. Grade II lesions exhibit 51% to 70% obstruction, and grade III lesions exhibit 71% to 99% obstruction. Grade IV lesions exhibit no detectable lumen and are incompatible with life unless a fistula or cleft is present, permitting air exchange. Typically, grade I and II lesions are mildly symptomatic. Patients with grade III and IV lesions require surgical repair (**Fig. 67-13**).

The short-term solution is to intubate the patient's trachea. Long-term treatment options include observation (only for grade I and II lesions), endoscopic dilation, CO_2 laser ablation, tracheostomy, an anterior cricoid split, laryngotracheal reconstruction, and cricotracheal resection. Endoscopic dilation may be of benefit in early stenosis but is ineffective in treating firm stenosis. CO_2 laser has been used for circumferential soft stenosis but is limited in other conditions. A tracheostomy often is the initial step in management. It provides a safe airway, allows the infant to grow, optimizes the patient's pulmonary status, and allows for treatment of gastroesophageal reflux disease. Tracheostomy is not a benign procedure. Aside from quality-of-life issues, complications can result in significant morbidity and mortality. For these reasons, early airway reconstruction is desired.

The anterior cricoid split is a procedure that can be used with or without a cartilage graft. Duration of stenting is based on the infant's weight. If the infant weighs less than 2000 g, the stent will remain in place for at least 2 weeks. For infants weighing more than 2000 g, the stent will be removed after 1 week. Indications for an anterior cricoid split include 2 or more previous extubation failures because of subglottic stenosis, weaned from the ventilator for at least 10 days, supplemental oxygen less than 30%, normotensive for at least 10 days, and no acute upper respiratory tract infection or congestive heart failure within the previous month. Ultimate decannulation success rates are approximately 75% to 80%.

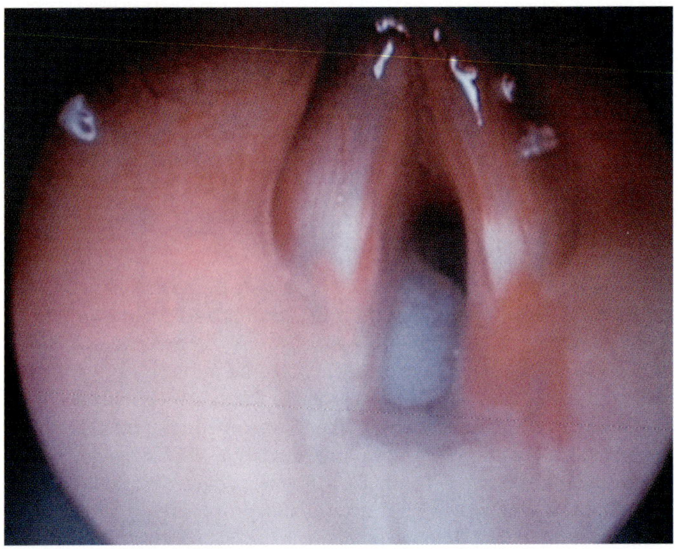

A

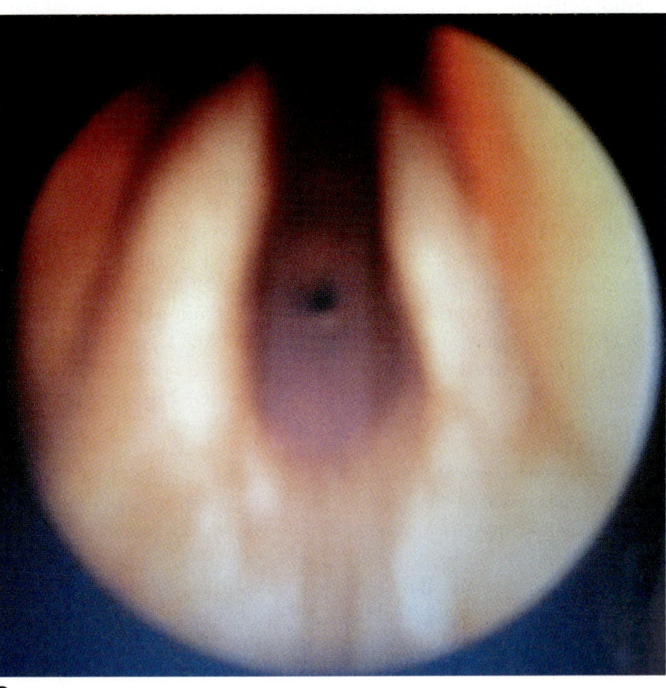

B

FIGURE 67-13. A. Type II subglottic stenosis in a neonate caused by a hemangioma. **B.** Type III subglottic stenosis secondary to trauma in an otherwise healthy 4-year-old boy. [Courtesy of Christopher Hartnick, MD, Massachusetts Eye and Ear Infirmary.]

TRACHEAL RECONSTRUCTION OR RESECTION

Laryngotracheal reconstruction is considered when an infant reaches a weight of 10 kg. A laryngotracheal reconstruction can be an anterior, posterior, or lateral repair, and the graft may be of rib, thyroid ala, or auricular origin. Single-stage laryngotracheal reconstruction procedures are indicated for older children with minimal glottic involvement and no pulmonary pathology. Usually only a single graft is involved. Indications for 2-stage laryngotracheal reconstruction procedures include extensive grafting, concomitant glottic pathology, and significant tracheomalacia. Decannulation rates for grade II and III lesions vary from 91% to 97%. For grade IV lesions, the rate declines to 71% (see Walner[77]).

Cricotracheal resection is an alternative in select patients with discrete grade III or IV lesions. The stenosis should be at least 4 mm distal to the vocal cords. This location will ensure later voice quality. Some investigators suggest that these patients have less speech pathology compared with laryngotracheal reconstruction patients. Triglia et al[78] have provided an extensive review of the technique. The duration of postoperative stenting remains controversial, and there is a greater risk of recurrent laryngeal nerve injury with this procedure. Various studies have demonstrated decannulation rates of 85% to 100% for grade III and IV lesions.

At the author's institution, anterior cricoids split, single-stage, and 2-stage laryngotracheal reconstructions are frequently performed. The patient typically arrives with a tracheostomy. After an inhalation induction and establishment of IV access, the tracheostomy cannula is removed and replaced with an appropriately size reinforced endotracheal tube. The graft is harvested next; this is the source of most postoperative discomfort. After the graft is obtained and shaped, the resection and reconstruction begin. Depending on the location of the lesion, the endotracheal tube may be advanced or withdrawn small distances to provide better surgical access. After the reconstruction is complete, a nasal intubation is performed. The patient is then taken to the intensive care unit and kept intubated for 7 to 10 days. The entire operation takes 4 to 6 hours to complete.

TRACHEOTOMY AND TRACHEOSTOMY

A tracheotomy is an incision or opening into the trachea. A tracheostomy is the creation of a permanent opening in the trachea such that the mucous membrane becomes continuous with the external epithelium. Tracheostomies are common surgical procedures that are performed for a variety of reasons, ranging from emergent care to chronic care. Anesthesia care varies depending on the specific condition. For example, if urgent surgical airway access is required, tracheostomy can be performed using only local anesthesia with sedation.

Most patients who require tracheostomy are brought to the OR and placed in the supine position with the back slightly elevated. This position promotes respiratory effort and provides better surgical access. An inflatable shoulder roll or stack of towels is placed under the shoulders to extend the head and further expose the neck. If the patient is already intubated, the surgeon proceeds directly to the tracheotomy. This procedure is not without its complications. Rarely, the surgeon pierces the endotracheal tube cuff and produces a large leak. If ventilation becomes compromised, a throat pack can be placed or the endotracheal tube replaced. The surgeon can also approximate the wound to reduce the leak. Airway fires are known to occur, particularly if 100% oxygen or high concentrations of N_2O are used in the presence of electrocautery. After the trachea is fully exposed, the surgeon requests that the endotracheal cuff be deflated and the tube slowly retracted cephalad but with the tube tip still below the glottis so it can be advanced again if necessary. After electrocautery is completed, ventilation with 100% oxygen is performed for at least 60 seconds before withdrawal of the endotracheal tube and insertion of the tracheostomy cannula. After the tube is withdrawn cephalad, the surgeon inserts the tracheostomy cannula and passes the new circuit to the anesthesiologist. Great resistance to ventilation should immediately alert the practitioner to incorrect cannula placement. The presence of CO_2 via capnography, the presence of bilateral breath sounds, and the ability to ventilate the patient all indicate a successful tracheostomy. Only after ventilation is verified should the endotracheal tube be removed entirely.

The approach to pediatric tracheostomy is similar to that for adults except that children will not cooperate for this procedure under local anesthesia. Indications for pediatric tracheostomy include prolonged ventilation, laryngotracheal malacia, subglottic stenosis, respiratory papillomatosis, alkali ingestion, and craniofacial syndromes. Pediatric tracheostomy may present airway challenges for anesthetists; Wrightson et al[79] reviewed 100 pediatric tracheostomies and noted that 26% were difficult to intubate. When intubation proved impossible, ventilation was accomplished by LMA or facemask until the surgical airway was established. A common surgical technique is the percutaneous dilational tracheostomy first described by Ciaglia in 1985. Used both in adult and pediatric patients, it is associated with a low complication rate.[80] A modified percutaneous dilational tracheostomy set called the Ciaglia Blue Rhino® has been introduced and used with good results. Other tracheostomy sets include the Percu-Twist®, Fanconi translaryngeal tracheostomy, and the Portex Ultraperc®. Pediatric tracheostomies frequently are accomplished using bronchoscopic guidance.

MAXILLOFACIAL RECONSTRUCTION

Maxillofacial surgery is performed to repair facial trauma or correct facial deformity. Midface fractures are described using the Le Fort classification. Class I involves the lower third of the nasal septum and maxilla above the nasal floor and mobilizes the maxillary alveolar process, palate, part of the palatine bone, and lower third of the pterygoid plates. Oral or nasal intubation can be established, and the airway usually is intact. Nasal intubation is contraindicated in a Le Fort class II fracture, which involves the upper nasal bone, under the zygomaticomaxillary suture and through the pterygoid plate. A Le Fort class III fracture separates the base of the skull from the midface, and nasal intubation is contraindicated here as well. Before surgery, the patient must be fully evaluated for any airway compromise, other traumatic injury, and other preexisting medical problems. Depending on the nature of the injuries, a facial fracture repair may be delayed to stabilize the patient's condition.

Often, a nasal intubation is requested to provide better surgical access. As mentioned, nasal intubations are contraindicated in Le Fort class II and class III fractures and in the presence of a CSF leak. Nasal intubations are not entirely benign. They can lead to bleeding, damage turbinates, increase the risk of sinusitis and otitis, and may be difficult to perform in the presence of a traumatized airway. It is unwise to blindly pass a nasal endotracheal tube into a potentially disrupted nasopharynx. The tube can be directed into a sinus, the orbit, the hypopharynx, and even intracranially. Nasal intubations are discussed in a separate section. A tracheostomy can be performed if facial trauma is too severe or in the presence of a basal skull fracture.

Other options for securing the airway are available. Kannan et al[81] described using an intubating LMA to facilitate an awake fiberoptic intubation in a severe facial trauma case. In another approach, Altemir described placing a submental intubation (SMI). An SMI is a secure surgical airway that gives open access to the oral cavity and does not elicit the complications of a nasal intubation or tracheostomy. Essentially, an SMI is an oral intubation with the proximal end of the endotracheal tube passing through an incision in the floor of the mouth and connected externally to the anesthesia circuit. It is a useful airway technique for maxillofacial surgery in patients with severe oral, nasal, and neck trauma. In a study of 13 patients with panfacial fractures, Anwer et al[82] found SMIs safe and effective. In a modification of this technique, Biswas et al[83] have used a percutaneous dilational tracheostomy set to create the passage for the endotracheal tube. SMI is also appropriate for patients undergoing elective procedures who are not expected to need prolonged postoperative ventilation. SMIs are used in European practice but have yet to be fully accepted in North American practice (**Fig. 67-14**).

An uncommon surgical procedure is facial bipartition. This is done to correct severe deformities or malformations. Mallory et al[84] reviewed a series of 22 cases and noted that the most significant complication was hemorrhage. Every patient required an intraoperative blood transfusion. Four of the 22 patients required postoperative ventilation, which was associated with younger age and major blood loss. Recently, Stricker et al[85] reviewed 159 cases, and it was noted that the intraoperative administration of fresh-frozen plasma resulted in fewer postoperative coagulation disorders and complications.

ORAL AND DENTAL SURGERY

Orthognathic reconstructions are elective procedures to correct malocclusion or facial deformity. These cases are performed by oral or maxillofacial surgeons. Typically, a sagittal split osteotomy of the mandible is done to advance or retract the lower jaw. The maxilla can also be moved forward or in a transverse direction. Care must be taken with the intubation. These patients may present with semi-permanent orthodontic devices in place. In addition, they may have anatomic abnormalities, such as prominent incisors, retrognathia, or small mouths.

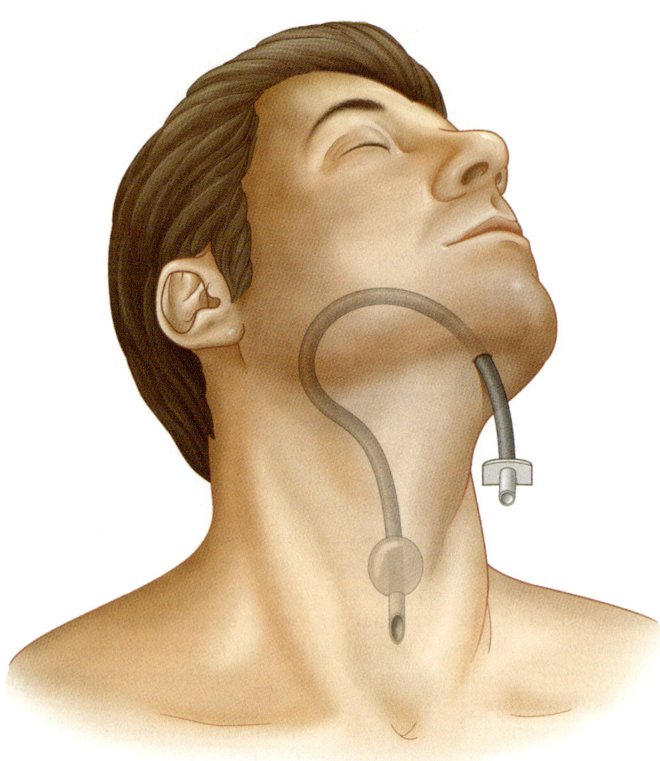

FIGURE 67-14. Submental intubation. Note that the proximal end of the endotracheal tube emerges just medial to the mandible. [Illustration by Daniel Muller, Haderer & Muller Biomedical Art, LLC.]

NASAL INTUBATIONS

Orthognathic surgery is an oral procedure, and the patient requires a nasotracheal intubation. As mentioned in the Maxillofacial Reconstruction section, nasal intubations are more traumatic than oral intubations and have their own complications. Hall and Shutt[86] have provided a complete and excellent review of nasotracheal intubations. Epistaxis, bacteremia, and possible posterior pharyngeal wall laceration are possible. It is also possible to enter the hypopharynx and create a false passage. Rarely, the tube becomes obstructed with avulsed tissue from the inferior turbinate. Other problems include maxillary sinusitis, otitis, and possible cuff rupture from passage through the turbinates or by use of the MacGill forceps.

Contraindications to nasal intubation include the presence of a CSF leak, basal skull fracture (Le Fort III), Le Fort II fracture, the presence of a nasal FB, or a traumatized nasopharynx. Relative contraindications include bleeding coagulopathy, cardiac valve disease, and an immunocompromised condition.

Before anesthesia and nasotracheal intubation, the patient should assist the practitioner by identifying the more patent nasal passage. If the patient is uncooperative, a steel blade or mirror can be placed beneath the nostrils, and the side that steams greater is more open. It is helpful to administer vasoconstrictors to both sides and to use a local anesthetic lubricant. Other techniques are available to assist the anesthesiologist. Use of a soft red rubber nasal tube to expand the nostril and spread the lubricant is helpful.

After induction and before laryngoscopy, the anesthesiologist should gently place the endotracheal tube in the selected nostril and advance the tube parallel to the palate. Ideally, one advances the tube along the floor of the nose under the inferior turbinate. This is referred to as the "lower pathway."[87] The endotracheal tube should not be advanced in a superior direction toward the nasal bridge. There will be resistance in the nasal passage until deep posterior, where a sudden "give" is felt as the nasotracheal tube passes the inferior turbinate. If laryngoscopy is planned, advancement should stop when the tube is in the pharynx.

Upon laryngoscopy, bloody secretions may be present in the oral cavity. Various devices, agents, and techniques have been used to reduce epistaxis. Among the newer endotracheal tubes, both the Parker Flex-Tip and the Endoflex endotracheal tubes have shown good results with reduced trauma to the nasal mucosa. If the tube bevel is inserted on the turbinate mucosa, it is likely to cause more bleeding.

Suctioning should reveal the tip of the endotracheal tube lying on the posterior pharyngeal wall. Examination of its location and the glottis will determine if the tube can be advanced into the trachea without the MacGill forceps. This will lessen the chances of a torn cuff or more trauma from airway instruments. After the trachea has been intubated, the practitioner should inflate the cuff, ventilate, and observe for CO_2 and condensation, and listen for bilateral breath sounds. When the tube is being secured, it should not pull on the nose or pressure necrosis may occur. The author prefers to place a band of tape completely around the patient's head just above the ears. This becomes the foundation on which the tube tape is secured. The circuit is brought down from the forehead and underneath the OR table. The endotracheal tube and circuit should be secured in a manner that will allow flexion and extension of the head without jeopardizing their position.

Other problems may arise after surgery begins. During maxillary osteotomy, the osteotome may slice through the endotracheal tube and pilot tube. When this occurs, a secure airway must be quickly reestablished to prevent a life-threatening event. In a brief communication, Davies and Dyer[88] reported the successful use of an Obwegieser nasal septal osteotome. This instrument has 2 blunt horns that prevent direct contact with the endotracheal tube. The author is familiar with a case in which extubation of a trachea became impossible after a palate expansion. CT scan revealed surgical wires passing through the nasotracheal tube, preventing its removal. These complications do occur, and one should be prepared.

ORTHOGNATHIC SURGERY

Hemorrhage may be significant with orthognathic surgery, especially when maxillary procedures are involved. Blood loss can vary between 300 and greater than 2000 mL. Depending on the procedure, autologous blood transfusion may be considered. Moreover, controlled hypotension with isoflurane or other agents may be helpful. These patients are generally young and otherwise healthy and will tolerate such techniques.

At the conclusion of surgery, the pharyngeal packs are removed and the stomach suctioned. As with nasal or sinus procedures, swallowed blood can provoke nausea. Appropriate antiemetics should be administered well in advance of the expected extubation. Only after the patient is fully awake with airway reflexes intact should the endotracheal tube be removed. Rigid internal fixation is beginning to replace intermaxillary fixation and provides more postoperative comfort. Intermaxillary fixation will still be encountered and will result in the patient's jaws being "wired shut" using elastic bands or wires. This obviously blocks access to the airway, restricts suctioning, and makes reintubation practically impossible until the mandible is free. When intermaxillary fixation is used, without exception, the patient must be fully awake before extubation. As long as the patient has intermaxillary fixation in place, cutting instruments to free the airway must be immediately available at the bedside.

Pain management begins early. Narcotics are supplemented by the surgeon providing local anesthetic infiltration directly into the wound. Besides the usual narcotics, other analgesic classes have been investigated. Moller et al[89] obtained good results with IV propacetamol. These results were supported by Van Aken et al,[90] who found the analgesic qualities of propacetamol similar to those of morphine and better tolerated.

DENTAL SURGERY

In recent years, dentists have reduced the use of N_2O in the office setting. This was prompted by a number of unfortunate events resulting in patient harm and subsequent increased legal liability. Most office procedures are now performed using topical anesthetic supplemented by local anesthetic injections. If needed, a preoperative oral sedative (usually a benzodiazepam) can be prescribed.[91]

Because of this trend, it is becoming more common to provide general anesthesia to certain dental patients in an OR. The vast majority are pediatric patients who are uncooperative and have behavioral problems or who need an extensive amount of repair that is easier to accomplish in one OR visit than multiple office visits.

All of the concerns regarding pediatric anesthesia and oral surgery apply here. Some have used flexible LMAs for these cases, but the dentist may request a nasal intubation to provide better access to a small oral cavity. These patients may not have seen a pediatrician before arrival, and the preoperative physical examination may yield unexpected findings.[92] As noted earlier, preoperative anxiety may be an issue with any pediatric patient. Appropriate doses of midazolam can be quite effective in this situation.

In older patients, these procedures are possible with conscious sedation as MAC anesthetics. Certainly the elderly patient needing total extractions before a cardiac valve replacement is a candidate for MAC. (See Chapter 69 for a description of monitored anesthetic care.)

PLASTIC SURGERY

Plastic surgery is a broad surgical field; this brief discussion focuses only on rhytidoplasty, commonly known as a "facelift." One may encounter both young and healthy patients as well as older patients who present for this procedure. Whereas some procedures can be done under local anesthesia with sedation, rhytidoplasty is often performed using general anesthesia with endotracheal intubation. When the procedure is complete, the surgeon will be especially concerned about bleeding and edema in the subcutaneous tissues. The anesthetic goals include prevention of patient "coughing" and "bucking" during tracheal extubation and avoidance of retching associated with PONV. Both coughing and vomiting contribute to facial and orbital ecchymoses. Rama-Maceiras et al[93] reported less PONV using propofol with remifentanil compared with propofol and fentanyl. Pretreatment with metoclopramide and ondansetron can decrease this risk. Others have successfully used combinations of haloperidol and dexamethasone.[94] In addition, the patient should be fluid loaded and carefully suctioned before extubation. When ventilation has been well established and with the patient's upper torso slightly elevated, the trachea should be extubated during a moderately deep plane of anesthesia. The face is commonly wrapped in soft gauze, and the eyes are covered with ice packs. Occasionally, the dressing may be wrapped tight enough to constrict the patient's airway, a matter that should receive special attention from the anesthesia provider.

ANESTHESIA FOR HEAD AND NECK SURGERY

Patients who present for head and neck surgery may undergo many of the procedures discussed previously as separate operations. The parotid gland, thyroid, and parathyroid glands and a variety of head and neck masses are included under this heading. Various macrosurgical and microsurgical techniques involving both soft tissue and bone may be used. Furthermore, reconstruction may include adjacent tissue or free tissue transfer. These cases can be complex and lengthy, lasting from a few hours to longer than 30 hours on occasion. For the anesthesiologist, airway management, tissue preservation, and nerve monitoring become primary concerns.

PAROTID SURGERY

Patients may have inflammatory disorders or, more commonly, mass lesions of the parotid gland. Parotid tumors may be classified as of epithelial origin or mesenchymal origin and the majority of patients arrive in the OR with a presumptive diagnosis. Occasionally anesthesiologists have managed the airway with an LMA for some of these procedures. However, considering the length of the operation (2-4 h) and a non-neutral head position, most anesthesiologists prefer endotracheal intubation to ensure a secure airway, especially when subsequent access is compromised by the sterile surgical field. After the airway is secured, the patient is positioned with the operative side exposed and the back slightly elevated.

Facial Nerve Concerns For the anesthesiologist and surgeon, preservation of the facial nerve is of utmost importance. Early in the dissection, the surgeon seeks to identify the facial nerve by electrical stimulation. With this in mind, it is essential to use a short-acting muscle relaxant or none at all. The surgeon should not begin dissection until a demonstrated train of four has returned. If for any reason the patient must be paralyzed, the surgeon should be informed of the patient's neuromuscular status.

THYROID SURGERY

Patients with thyroid disease are managed medically in the majority of cases. Surgical intervention is indicated for malignancy, obstructive symptoms, retrosternal goiter, unresponsive or recurrent hyperthyroidism, or cosmetic reasons. Thyroid surgery is reviewed extensively in Chapter 60, and preoperative evaluation is presented in detail in Chapter 13; only key highlights are addressed here.

Preoperative assessment of patients undergoing thyroidectomy should include evaluation of coexisting disease.[94] (For example, medullary carcinoma is rarely associated with pheochromocytoma, and cardiovascular disease can be exacerbated by untreated or poorly treated hyperthyroidism.) The patient should be euthyroid before operation. Apart from the routine concerns, the major focus of preoperative assessment is determining airway status. One should examine the patient and review radiographic images to look for any signs of tracheal compression or deviation. The surgeon should inform the anesthesiologist if airway difficulties are suspected. If so, more sophisticated imagings, such as CT or MRI scans, are indicated. If the patient experiences airway obstruction while supine, an awake fiberoptic intubation in the partially recumbent ("beach chair") position may be indicated. It is potentially catastrophic to perform a rapid sequence induction and fail to intubate or ventilate and then expect the surgeon to obtain an emergent tracheostomy through a large goiter.

Recurrent Laryngeal Nerve and the Nerve Integrity Monitor Endotracheal Tube Recurrent laryngeal nerve injury is a preventable surgical complication in most circumstances. In a study by Yumoto et al,[96] 40% of surgically related recurrent laryngeal nerve palsies were caused by thyroid procedures. The exceptions were patients in whom the malignancy had completely invested the nerve. With meticulous dissection and current monitoring techniques, one should not encounter a recurrent laryngeal nerve palsy after extubation, provided the palsy does not result from the tumor itself. For monitoring purposes, a short-acting muscle relaxant should be used, if at all. Most anesthesiologists advocate recurrent laryngeal nerve monitoring without any evidence of neuromuscular paralysis. This will ensure that neuromuscular blockade is eliminated as an etiologic factor if nerve palsy occurs. At the author's institution, a "nerve integrity monitor" (NIM) endotracheal tube is routinely used for thyroid surgery[97] (NIM EMG Endotracheal Tube, Medtronic Xomed Surgical Products, Jacksonville, FL). This particular endotracheal tube has

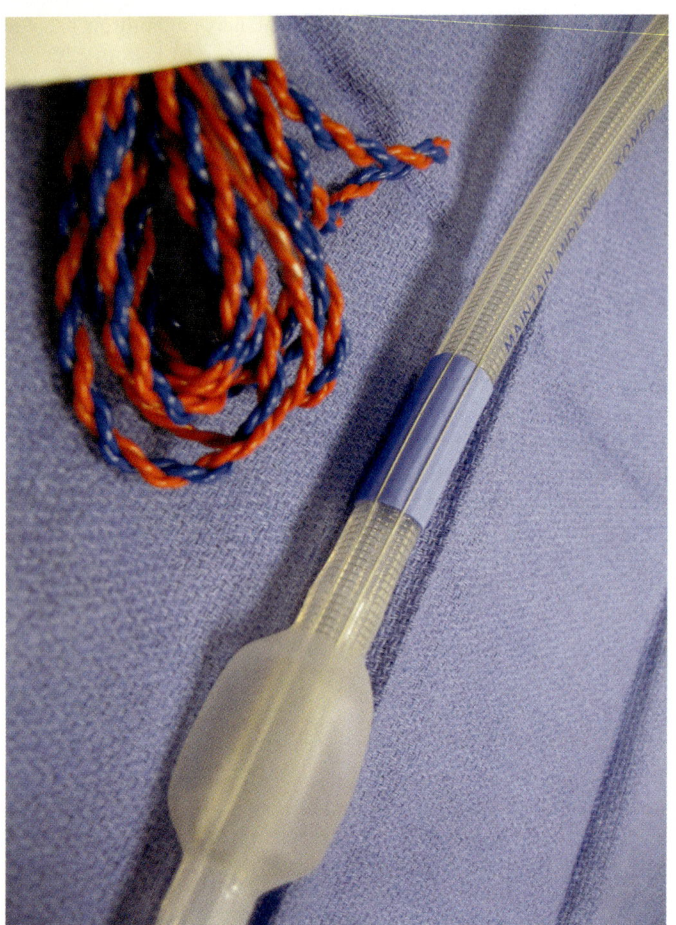

FIGURE 67-15. The Nerve Integrity Monitor (NIM) endotracheal tube (Medtronic Xomed Surgical Products, Jacksonville, FL). Note the 2 electrodes running the length of the tube and the blue band that is to be in contact with the vocal cords. [Courtesy of Bil Ragan, MD, Massachusetts Eye and Ear Infirmary.]

electrodes embedded within a band located just superior to the cuff. Under direct visualization, these electrodes are placed in contact with the vocal cords during intubation. The NIM tube is softer than standard endotracheal tubes, making it more difficult to handle. It is also slightly larger than a standard endotracheal tube, and it is the author's practice to use a size smaller than that usually indicated for the individual patient (eg, if inner diameter = 6.0 mm, then outer diameter = 8.8 mm, which is still large for an adult female). Just after induction and intubation, the patient's anesthetic is lightened and spontaneous ventilation is allowed to return. After the patient is positioned and before the first incision, the nerve signal strength is confirmed and measured by the monitoring technician. Although reliable, the NIM tube is expensive (**Fig. 67-15**).

Complications of Thyroid Surgery Complications of thyroid surgery can be life threatening. Postoperative hemorrhage can result in a rapidly expanding hematoma, which can directly compress the trachea. Venous and lymphatic obstruction by the hematoma also can produce laryngeal and pharyngeal edema. Recurrent laryngeal nerve injury can cause unilateral vocal cord paralysis, which manifests as hoarseness, breathlessness, glottic incompetence, poor cough, and aspiration. Bilateral recurrent laryngeal nerve injury producing bilateral vocal cord paralysis will lead to immediate stridor and require reintubation and probable tracheostomy. Chronic compression by a large goiter can lead to tracheomalacia. This condition leads to tracheal collapse, resulting in partial or complete obstruction. Unintentional parathyroidectomy can result in hypocalcemia. This may reveal itself several hours postoperatively. Hypocalcemia is suggested by a positive Chvostek sign (painful facial twitching after tapping the facial nerve) or Trousseau sign (carpopedal spasm after tourniquet inflation above systolic blood pressure for 3 minutes) and is confirmed by laboratory testing. Treatment involves IV administration of calcium chloride.

PARATHYROID SURGERY

Again, see Chapters 13 and 60 and the review by Mihai and Farndon[98] for detailed discussions of evaluation and anesthetic care of patients with endocrine disease; only key issues of parathyroid surgery are discussed briefly here.

The anesthesia concerns are similar to those encountered in thyroid surgery. A NIM endotracheal tube or similar device should be used to assess recurrent laryngeal nerve function. Before anesthetic induction, the patient's volume status should be normalized. The greatest danger is cardiac dysrhythmias caused by increased calcium levels. Use of normal saline and furosemide can decrease calcium concentrations to reasonable levels. If this method is not effective, IV bisphosphates, plicamycin, glucocorticoids, calcitonin, or even dialysis can be used. Acidosis increases serum calcium, so hypoventilation should be avoided. Muscle relaxants should be used judiciously in the presence of hypercalcemia. Chronic hyperparathyroidism can result in weakened bones. Care must be taken during patient positioning, movement, and laryngoscopy.

Parathyroid surgery can be tedious, and even experienced surgeons can have difficulty identifying the glands. Before incision, a PTH level is drawn. After the suspected gland is removed, a second PTH level is obtained. A significant decrease in PTH levels while the patient is still in the OR indicates that the offending source has been removed.

HEAD AND NECK CANCERS

Malignant disease of the head and neck represents approximately 5% of all human cancers. Surgical intervention includes laryngectomy, pharyngectomy, glossectomy, hemimandibulectomy, and neck dissection. Neck dissections are further described as "radical" or "modified radical"; the latter is intended to spare one or more of the nonlymphatic structures within the neck. This may include the sternocleidomastoid muscle, spinal accessory nerve, and jugular vein. Reconstruction follows dissection, and some of these cases may last anywhere from 12 to greater than 30 hours.

Most patients who present for surgery are between 50 and 80 years old, with men exceeding women by a 2:1 margin. Frequently, these patients have significant coexisting illness, including cardiovascular disease, chronic obstructive pulmonary disease, and renal disease. They often are heavy smokers and likely abuse alcohol. Consistent with this profile is poor nutrition; the patient may appear wasted and cachectic. If the patient appears to be an unreliable or devious historian, he or she should be observed closely for delirium tremens postoperatively. An extensive medical evaluation, including possible diagnosis and treatment of malnutrition, is indicated in an unusual number of these patients. (See Chapter 17 for details regarding the preoperative evaluation of patients with malnutrition.)

Patients may exhibit mass lesions that complicate their management. Mason and Fielder[99] have given a practical approach to the assessment and management of these patients. A key point is that if a patient presents with severe stridor and gross anatomic distortion limiting endoscopic views, then the airway should be secured by a tracheostomy performed under local anesthesia. An awake fiberoptic intubation can be attempted if the airway permits, and this requires proper preparation and sedation. Besides the usual agents, other medications have been examined in this setting, with remifentanil, dexmedetomidine, and low-dose ketamine showing promise. Well before surgery, the anesthesiologist should be prepared with multiple plans for securing the airway.

Free Flap Reconstruction If a reconstruction is planned, it is necessary to know the donor site before placing any IV or arterial cannulas. Donor tissue (flap) is used to reconstruct defects of the oral cavity, mandible, laryngopharynx, craniofacial region, and facial skin. Common pedicle flaps include cervicothoracic skin, pectoralis major myocutaneous, sternocleidomastoid myocutaneous, temporoparietal fascial, and pericranial. A free flap is donor tissue removed entirely from a distant site, with loss of prior blood supply, and transplanted to the area of defect. Microsurgery techniques are used to reconstruct the vascular supply to ensure flap survival. Typical free flaps include the radial forearm, rectus abdominus, and latissimus dorsi. Composite free flaps contain both soft tissue and bone and are used for oromandibular reconstruction. These complex flaps include the scapular osteocutaneous, iliac crest osteomyocutaneous, and, most useful, the fibular osteocutaneous. The fibular flap contains up to 25 cm of bone, making total mandibular reconstruction possible.

Because these cases are often lengthy, temperature maintenance and fluid management are just 2 of many concerns. In addition to the standard monitors, one may wish to place central venous and arterial catheters if indicated by the patient's condition. Early in the procedure, a tracheostomy is performed to secure the airway and provide unrestricted access to the oropharyngeal cavity and neck. Blood loss can be substantial and rapid. Slight elevation of the head may decrease venous bleeding but increases the risk of venous air embolism. A Foley catheter is needed to assess urine output and guide fluid replacement. Anesthesia is maintained by a combination of narcotics and volatile agents. Nerve stimulation is performed by the surgeon, so short-acting muscle relaxants should be used at least until the surgeon determines that nerve stimulation at the surgical site is no longer necessary.

The anesthesiologist's efforts should include a focus on factors that will promote flap survival. Success of the operation depends partially on maintaining intravascular volume and adequate blood pressure to enhance perfusion in the donor tissue. This can be a challenge in unhealthy patients who do not tolerate anesthesia well. Scholz et al[100] demonstrated improved flap perfusion by using a dobutamine infusion. This was a small study, but the encouraging results warrant further research. Fluid management and perfusion pressure should be mainstays of cardiovascular management; however, overloading runs the risk of pulmonary edema and flap congestion. Vasoconstrictors should be used only rarely, if at all, to prevent vasoconstriction in the flap microcirculation. Use of fluids, lighter levels of anesthesia, and, briefly, a slight head-down position, all contribute to donor graft circulation. To minimize microthrombosis, blood transfusions should be limited.

Complications of Neck Dissection Both medical and surgical complications are common in these patients. Hemorrhage can be acute or delayed. It may warrant surgical exploration for a hematoma, which can compromise the airway as well as the vascular supply to the flap. If a tracheostomy has not been performed, laryngeal edema can produce rapid airway obstruction. Pneumothorax can occur by air entering at the apex of the lung or rupture of the mediastinal pleura. Because the head and neck are commonly elevated above the heart, venous air embolism can occur with potentially fatal results. Other complications can include postoperative neurocognitive deficits from carotid microemboli.[101] Furthermore, the author has witnessed asystole in a patient when cold irrigation was used on exposed carotid sinuses. Immediate administration of warm irrigation restored sinus rhythm within several seconds. Other cardiac abnormalities can occur.[102] Neck dissection can result in injury to the superior laryngeal, facial, vagus, phrenic, hypoglossal, cervical sympathetic, spinal accessory, lingual, and brachial plexus nerves. Rarer complications include a chylous fistula, subcutaneous emphysema, increased intracranial pressure, salivary fistula, wound infection, and gangrenous flap tissue. Despite these issues, neck dissection with flap reconstruction has a success rate of greater than 90% (flap survival).

SUMMARY

Anesthesia for ENT surgery provides an extensive range of challenges for anesthesiologists. It is essential to develop an open working relationship with one's surgical colleague. There are perhaps few other anesthesia subspecialties in which intraoperative communication is so crucial.

Many of the skills used on a routine basis have applications in other areas. One can use mask, spontaneous, controlled, and jet ventilation in a single procedure. Likewise, it is common in one's daily practice to use controlled hypotension, perform deep extubations, assist in nerve monitoring, and treat seemingly intractable PONV. The challenges are great, as are the rewards. When a patient is safely and successfully discharged home, you may be the only one who knows the difficulties encountered. That itself can be immensely satisfying.

KEY REFERENCES

- American National Standards Institute. *Safe Use of Lasers in Health Care Facilities.* ANSI Z136.3-2005. Washington, DC: ANSI. 2005.
- American Society of Anesthesiologists. Practice Guidelines for the Perioperative Management of Patients With Obstructive Sleep Apnea Syndrome. *Anesthesiology.* 2006;104:1081-1093.
- Austin J, Ali T. Tracheomalacia and bronchomalacia in children: pathophysiology, assessment, treatment, and anesthesia management. *Pediatr Anesth.* 2003;13:3-11.
- Farling PA. Thyroid disease. *Br J Anaesth.* 2000;85:15-28.
- Gan TJ, Meyer T, Apfel CC, et al. Consensus guidelines for managing postoperative nausea and vomiting. *Anesth Analg.* 2003;97:62-71.
- Hall CEJ, Shutt LE. Nasotracheal intubation for head and neck surgery. *Anaesthesia.* 2003;58:249-256.
- Hammer GB, Holzki J, Morton NS, eds. The pediatric airway. *Pediatr Anesth.* 2009;19(Suppl):1-197.
- Mihai R, Farndon JR. Parathyroid disease and calcium metabolism. *Br J Anaesth.* 2000;85:29-43.
- Nargozian C. The airway in patients with craniofacial abnormalities. *Pediatr Anesth.* 2004;14:48-52.
- Randolph GW, Dralle H, et al. Electrophysiologic Recurrent Laryngeal Nerve Monitoring During Thyroid and Parathyroid Surgery: International Standards Guideline Statement. *Laryngoscope* 2011;121:S1-S16.
- Schmitt HJ, Mang H, Schmitt J. Fiberoptic intubation in patients after radiotherapy for carcinoma of the head and neck: difficulty and predictability. *Eur J Anaesth.* 2004;21:914-927.
- Tait AR, Malviya S. Anesthesia for the child with an upper respiratory tract infection: still a dilemma? *Anesth Analg.* 2005;100:59-65.
- Yellon RF. Prevention and management of complications of airway surgery in children. *Pediatr Anesth.* 2004;14:107-111.

REFERENCES

Complete references available on DVD and online version at www.LongneckerAnesthesiology.com

CHAPTER 68

Outpatient Anesthesia

Douglas B. Mayers
Judith Haas
Ellen Convery

KEY POINTS

1. The location for an outpatient surgical procedure can be either in a hospital or in a freestanding outpatient surgery center. The organizational structure for outpatient surgery centers is determined by their location in relation to a hospital and their governance model.
2. Evaluation of patients in preparation for outpatient surgery involves the usual standards plus the added issue that the patient is expecting to go home the same day. Thus, the patient must be undergoing a procedure appropriate for same-day discharge and must be physiologically able to go home.
3. There is no standard "best anesthetic" for outpatient surgery. An anesthetic plan must consider the planned procedure and the patient's physiology in addition to surgeon, anesthesiologist, and patient preferences. The drugs and modalities are chosen for effectiveness and speed of emergence in addition to safety.
4. Although major morbidity and mortality are rare and hospital admissions and readmissions uncommon, minor morbidities, especially of pain and postdischarge nausea and vomiting, continue to pose significant challenges.
5. Combination prophylaxis and treatment of postoperative nausea and vomiting is probably the most effective approach combined with adequate hydration and the least emetogenic anesthetic possible for a given procedure.
6. Multimodal opioid sparing pain management is most effective and enhances patient satisfaction and well being. Widespread use of ultrasound technology has led to improved efficiencies in the performance of peripheral nerve blocks and should remove as a barrier to their performance the belief that an outpatient surgery unit cannot afford their inefficiencies.
7. The pediatric patient population has special needs requiring family-centered education about the entire perioperative practice. A quiet area for recovery benefits not only the child but also the recovering adult patients.
8. Although obese patients and patients with obstructive sleep apnea are challenging, with appropriate selection of patient and procedure as well as careful management, these patients once thought unsuitable for outpatient surgery are now safely enjoying its benefits.

A BRIEF HISTORY OF AMBULATORY ANESTHESIA

Ambulatory anesthesia in 2010, with its extensive range of surgical interventions, anesthetic techniques, and patient characteristics, is unrecognizable from its historical antecedents, although the reasons for its continued growth are similar to the reasons for its birth: convenience, cost effectiveness, efficiency, and patient and physician satisfaction.[1]

Beginning in the 1840s, with neither the thought nor the ability to mix nitrous oxide (N_2O) with oxygen, dentists began using 100% N_2O for the painless and necessarily expeditious extraction of teeth. Although a practical delivery system for N_2O–oxygen mixture was available by the 1880s, the practice of hypoxic anesthesia with N_2O continued until the 1950s. In the early 20th century, the entrepreneurial anesthesiologist Ralph Waters began an enterprise that is the prototype of ambulatory surgery centers (ASCs) and office-based anesthesia. In 1915, he took the occasional request for anesthesia services from a dentist with a difficult extraction and turned it into The Downtown Anesthesia Clinic in Sioux City, Iowa, where dental and minor surgical services were performed in a large medical office building, catering to both the surgeons' and patients' desires for more convenient and lower cost care than hospitals were providing. Anesthesia was provided with N_2O, occasionally scopolamine and morphine, and rarely ether. By the 1930s, intermittent boluses of thiopental were part of outpatient anesthesia practices.[2]

It was not until the 1950s and 1960s that ambulatory surgery began to grow exponentially, driven in Canada by the lack of hospital beds and in the United States by the need to provide surgery less expensively than inpatient surgery. The hospital based ambulatory surgery units, pioneered at the University of California, Los Angeles, and quickly developed by hospitals across the country, in turn inspired John Ford and Wallace Reed to reach for even greater efficiencies and patient and surgeon satisfaction with the development of the Phoenix Surgicenter, the prototype of today's freestanding ASCs. During the 1990s, changes in reimbursement patterns encouraged the expansion of office-based anesthesia from the traditional dental, oral, and minor plastic surgery to include procedures in many surgical specialties using all kinds of anesthetic techniques.[2]

The explosion in outpatient surgeries, from 30% of all surgeries in 1985 to greater than 60% currently and projected rates of greater than 70%, would not have been possible without the concomitant development of newer anesthetic agents (propofol, rocuronium, remifentanil, sevoflurane, and desflurane), and anesthetic adjuncts such as non-opioid analgesics and low side effect antiemetics, as well as demonstrated safety. The development of the Society for Ambulatory Anesthesia (SAMBA)[3] in 1985 followed by the International Association for Ambulatory Surgery (IAAS)[4] in 1995 has done much to drive research, education, and quality in the subspecialty.

GOALS

In 2010, the goals of outpatient surgery remain remarkably similar to the century-old goals of decreasing health care costs with improved efficiencies, providing patients with a safe surgery as minimally disruptive to home life as possible, an early return to function, and hospital avoidance. It is the context of the goals that has changed. The 1915 dental extraction has been replaced by the minimally invasive computed tomography–guided endoscopic sinus surgery and even craniotomies[5]; the American Society of Anesthesiologists (ASA) class 1 and 2 patients have been replaced by patients with such challenging comorbidities as morbid obesity, obstructive sleep apnea (OSA), coronary artery disease (CAD), and diabetic patients on insulin pumps; the N_2O, morphine, and scopolamine of Dr Waters have been expanded to include modern general anesthetics, difficult airway algorithms and equipment, and ultrasound-guided nerve blocks. The economic landscape of affordable insurance and affordable self-pay has changed to a mix of expensive private and government insurance; no pay masquerading as self-pay; and an alphabet soup of regulators, quality initiatives, and pay for performance mandates. Continued growth in ambulatory procedures, if it reflects a shift from hospital care, may help to contain costs by minimizing actual costs of procedures as well as potential savings in reduced infection and thromboembolic rates and reduction in health care personnel costs. Continued shifting of care and costs must not be done at the expense of patient safety but instead should go along with the development of appropriate oversight in all patient care settings.[6]

ORGANIZATION OF THE OUTPATIENT SURGERY CENTER

Outpatient surgery facilities are typically divided into 4 types[7] based on their proximity with a hospital. These are:

- Hospital—integrated
- Hospital—dedicated
- Freestanding—hospital connected (physically attached)
- Freestanding— isolated from the hospital

In the hospital integrated model, the patients are usually admitted through a separate area of the hospital that only takes care of the outpatients, but the surgeries are done in the same operating rooms (ORs) and often commingled with in-house patients. Sometimes a separate postanesthesia care unit (PACU) is used, but usually the same PACU for phase I recovery of in-house and outpatients is used. Then in phase II recovery, the outpatients are transferred to the dedicated area. This model is simple and provides outpatient services with the simplest staffing and facility space utilization model. It is advantageous for a surgeon who works with a mixture of in- and outpatients on the same day. Unless care is taken to segregate the outpatients in the PACU from the most critically ill patients, the more aware recovering outpatients may endure more stress while in the PACU. In this model, outpatients are probably billed using the same charge structure as inpatients,[8] and the expected cost savings from other outpatient facility models are not realized.

The structure of the hospital-dedicated model is similar to the hospital-integrated one except that specific ORs are used for the outpatient procedures. These ORs may be prohibited from being used for inpatient cases or if unused for outpatients may be used for other cases. The OR staff may be completely separate from the inpatient staff or may be completely integrated with assignments changing on a daily or even partial day time period. Similarly, the PACU may be part of the main PACU or completely separate. In this model, if the staff and facility are separately managed, many of the efficiencies of a freestanding unit can be realized with the advantages of having ORs that can be used for inpatients or outpatients depending on need.

A freestanding but physically attached to the hospital facility has completely separate admission, ORs, PACU, and discharge areas from the hospital even though it is attached to the hospital. If administered properly, this kind of facility can take advantage of all the efficiencies of a freestanding, isolated facility while still maintaining the possibility of sharing staff and equipment when appropriate. If a patient requires hospital admission, the process usually only involves a hospital cart and appropriate transport personnel. A laboratory and blood bank are available if needed. Unfortunately, the converse could also happen, that is, the inefficiencies of a large, in-house OR could become the culture of the attached outpatient facility.[8]

Finally, the freestanding facility that is isolated from the hospital has now become a common entity. They come in many styles and sizes from single subspecialty to facilities that offer such a wide range of clinical services that their schedules look like those of small hospitals. Whereas the single-subspecialty facilities tend to be smaller and owned by a single physician or a small group of physicians, the multispecialty facilities are often owned or co-owned by a hospital with physician partners. In the three previous examples, the management of a facility integrated into the hospital or physically attached and typically owned and run by the hospital will be naturally controlled by the owner hospital entity, perhaps with input from key physicians. On the other hand, governance of a freestanding isolated outpatient facility depends on the ownership, which varies greatly from single physician to group of physicians to hospital and physician(s) joint enterprise to hospital alone to large national holding company that owns many health care facilities. The facility should have one physician named as the medical director and a director of nursing who will jointly make day-to-day decisions. The governance of a facility must coordinate decisions on what types of procedures will be done with appropriate equipment needed and appropriate staffing required. With proper planning, coordination of resources, and cooperation of all personnel (nursing, anesthesia, surgeon, and ancillary), a very efficient patient flow is possible that yields high satisfaction ratings from both patients and the rest of the staff.

In any outpatient facility, the governance must decide what procedures can be performed in the facility. The list of allowed procedures is negotiated among the various constituents. For freestanding, isolated facilities no blood or blood products can be given because no blood bank is typically on site. Procedures in which blood might be needed are therefore not done.

A very wide range of procedures are now done on an outpatient basis that historically required overnight stay in the hospital. Two examples, hysterectomy and cholecystectomy, illustrate procedural advances in laparoscopy that have changed historically in-hospital procedures to typically outpatient procedures.[9,10] Similarly, there are no absolute rules related to the length of a procedure because many facilities are providing 6-hour or longer plastic surgery procedures on an outpatient basis in appropriately selected patients. The guideline is that the patients who have a given procedure and encounter no complications are home ready in a reasonable amount of time postoperatively. Exactly what the term "reasonable amount of time" means depends on the facility but is typically as short as 1 hour but up to several hours.

OFFICE-BASED OUTPATIENT SURGERY

Office-based outpatient surgery is the next inevitable extension of procedures out of the classic in-hospital surgical care model. Estimates of 8 to 10 million surgical procedures are now done yearly in an office.[11,12] Historically, these procedures were minor and could be accomplished with minimal anesthesia, usually local and possibly some oral sedation. In recent years, more complex, invasive procedures are being performed in the office.

Although there is no standard classification system for office-based surgery, many states divide surgeries into three distinct levels based on anesthetic technique.

Level I: a minor surgical procedure requiring topical, local, or infiltration block and minimal oral sedation

Level II: a minor or major surgical procedure with oral or intravenous (IV) sedation during which analgesic or dissociative drugs are used

Level III: any surgical procedure that requires major conduction block, general anesthesia, or deep sedation during which the anesthesia provider is supporting bodily functions[13]

There have been questions of anesthetic safety issues in the office setting.[11] As of 2001 the ASA Closed Claims Database contained 14 closed claims related to office based anesthesia. Due to the low number of claims it is difficult to draw conclusions related to risk or safety from the database; however, the office based claims had a higher severity of injury (most often respiratory, cardiovascular, or equipment related) and 46% of the claims were deemed to be preventable (versus 13% of ambulatory claims). Concordantly, the claims resulted in payment greater in both frequency and amount, as the anesthesia care was more often deemed substandard.[14]

In response to safety concerns, an increasing number of states (although not all) require licensure of office based surgery practices. In addition, practices in states that do not require licensure may require accreditation by an outside organization. Currently there are three organizations with the ability to accredit office based surgery practices as deemed by Medicare.[13] In the dental office, permits are obtained from the state dental board allowing dentists to provide either unrestricted or restricted sedation/anesthesia. Only dentists who have completed an advanced education program accredited by the Commission on Dental Accreditation (CODA) that provides training in deep sedation and general anesthesia are considered educationally qualified to administer deep sedation and general anesthesia.[15]

In the office based anesthesia practice, the minimal standard of care should be that a surgeon should not perform any procedure in the office that he does not have privileges to do in a hospital. Offices that plan to perform procedures requiring MAC or general anesthesia should obtain certification from the appropriate organization.[16] The practice should have a medical director or governing body to establish and review policy. The practice must adhere to the standard of care as set forth by the ASA.

FACILITY CERTIFICATION

Some of the major differences between ambulatory surgical centers and office-based surgical practices are the certification and licensure requirements. All ambulatory surgical facilities are subject to state and local licensure and must adhere to the standards dictated by the state. As previously noted, not all states require licensure for office-based surgical practices. Most facilities are subject to certification by organizations that set national or international standards for a facility's physical structure, policies, and procedures. For ambulatory surgical centers, certifications come from The Joint Commission (formerly the Joint Commission for Accreditation of Health Care Organizations, [JCAHO]),[17] Centers for Medicare and Medicaid Services,[18] and American Association for Accreditation of Ambulatory Surgery Facilities (AAAASF).[19] For office-based surgical practices, certification can be given by The Joint Commission, the AAAASF, and the Accreditation Association for Ambulatory Health Care. These organizations' websites have detailed lists of standards that must be met for certification by each type of health care facility.

PREOPERATIVE PROCESS AND PATIENT SELECTION

The preoperative evaluation and selection for suitability of patients for outpatient surgery is similar to the evaluation process for any patient. "Is the patient adequately prepared for the scheduled surgical procedure?" is the overriding question. For ambulatory procedures, the "suitability for outpatient surgery and anesthesia" includes:

- Optimizing the patient's physical status
- Properly equipping and staffing the center for the planned surgical procedure
- Ensuring that the patient is an appropriate candidate for type of facility planned

For example, a patient may be in optimal clinical condition, but because of the nature of his or her comorbidities may not be a candidate for surgery at an outpatient facility. This is especially important if the location is away from a hospital such as a freestanding ASC or office. Several excellent reviews on preoperative evaluation exist; one of the more recent is edited by Jaffer.[20] This section deals with the process of evaluating patients with special attention to the differences between a routine preoperative evaluation and one for an outpatient surgical procedure.

The process for evaluation of patients is best accomplished with a preoperative clinic. This clinic has different names in different places such as Pre-Admission Testing (PAT), Preoperative Anesthesia Consultation and Evaluation (PACE), and many others. Some, such as the PACE clinic at the Cleveland Clinic, are designed to fully evaluate patients, including history, physical examination, needed laboratory studies, and referral to any medical consultant.[21] Other preoperative clinics are less elaborate and rely on the resources of the local hospital(s) and physician offices for much of the needed information and expertise. As long as there is a staff of nurses, physician's assistants, and administrative assistants who are adequately trained and adequate in numbers to handle the clinical responsibilities, many formats can be used.

Laboratory testing is indicated only if the surgical procedure or the patient's history and physical examination dictate their use.[22] Standard batteries of tests (eg, blood chemistry, blood counts, electrocardiography) based on age alone have not statistically or economically been shown to be warranted.[22,23]

The main difference between assessment of patients for any surgical procedure versus specifically outpatient surgery is the need for the patient to go home on the day of surgery. Thus, the combination of the surgical procedure requirements and the patient's physical status combined with the anesthetic management are expected to provide a recovery that will be short and uneventful enough to allow the patient to be discharged on the day of surgery. Historically, ASA class 1 and 2 patients were the standard for acceptability for outpatient surgery. However, over the years, this restriction has been dramatically loosened. Currently, most outpatient surgery centers accept ASA class 3 or even class 4 patients if they are stable and the nature of their disability will not impact their suitability for going home on the day of surgery. Studies have shown that with appropriate care and evaluation, ASA class 3 patients have an acceptably low incidence of postoperative complications and unplanned admission.[24,25]

SPECIFIC CLINICAL ISSUES

OBESITY

Obese patients are challenging because they add a level of complexity to every procedure. In addition to issues of comorbidities and the potential for difficult airway management, massively obese patients (body mass index [BMI] >50) may exceed the limits of the OR tables and the staff. Moving the patient from a cart to the OR table requires more staff than usual, which may not be readily available in an outpatient facility. These patients have increased respiratory complications compared with nonobese patients.[26] Thus, for practical reasons, an outpatient facility often defines a patient BMI or weight above which patients are excluded. However, no studies exist that define the upper limit for a BMI for outpatient surgery.

AGE

Infants younger than 60 weeks' gestational age, especially if they were born prematurely, should not be in an outpatient setting. The risk of apnea in this group can be as high as 25%.[27,28] From a practical standpoint, facilities often define a lower limit age (eg, 60 weeks' gestational age or 6 months old) below which patients are excluded. On the other end of the spectrum, elderly patients should not be excluded simply based on an arbitrary age limit. The comorbidities that become more common with increasing age (hypertension, CAD, chronic obstructive pulmonary disease [COPD], and others) are the true predictors of increased risk for postoperative problems after outpatient surgery.[29]

CHRONIC OBSTRUCTIVE PULMONARY DISEASE

Patients with well-compensated COPD have an increased incidence of postoperative pulmonary problems,[26] but these are usually easy to treat and do not often lead to postoperative morbidity or unplanned hospital admission after outpatient surgery. Although not necessarily delineated in the literature, a good rule of thumb is that a COPD patient who can do normal activities of daily living (ADLs) and is not oxygen dependent at home can safely have outpatient surgery.

ASTHMA

Reactive airway disease is very common, especially in children. If a patient with asthma presents to the outpatient surgery unit without symptoms or wheezing on auscultation, he or she may be more likely to develop perioperative complications, but these are typically easily treatable and only rarely lead to an unplanned hospital admission because of serious respiratory problems. Thus, these patients can routinely undergo surgery in an outpatient surgery setting. A patient who presents with wheezing that clears with routine clinical management (inhaled albuterol and perhaps steroids) should also be considered appropriate for the outpatient setting. In general, a patient who is actively wheezing and does not respond to routine management should not be electively anesthetized.[30,31]

UPPER RESPIRATORY INFECTION

Upper respiratory infection (URI) is a very common clinical issue, especially in outpatient surgery centers that have a high volume of children undergoing ear, nose, and throat (ENT) procedures. A patient with symptoms such as fever, lethargy, or significant productive cough is not a candidate for elective surgery. Many patients will present with recent URI (within 2-4 weeks) that has resolved or is resolving. The risk in these patients of developing mild perioperative events such as oxygen desaturation, coughing, or laryngospasm is 2 to 11 times that of control participants. Generally, these issues are treatable with the incidence of serious complication and unplanned hospital admission still being low.[32,33] In the ENT patient population, many children never have a significant period of time free of URI symptoms. Thus, it is probably acceptable to anesthetize a patient with a recent URI if the symptoms are minimal or resolved.[29]

OBSTRUCTIVE SLEEP APNEA

Obstructive sleep apnea is discussed in detail later in this chapter. Many patients with OSA are undiagnosed, so a suspicion of OSA in patients with increased risk factors (see below) should promote treating a patient as if he or she had the diagnosis. When care is taken to minimize these potential complications, patients with OSA have minimal perioperative and postoperative complications.[24,34]

CORONARY ARTERY DISEASE

Patients with known but stable and adequately treated CAD typically tolerate outpatient surgery well. The two most important factors are no new or escalating clinical symptoms and adequate cardiac function. In two large retrospective clinical studies, the rate of severe complications (myocardial infarction [MI] or death) was very low.[26,30] Patients who are on a stable medical regimen should be encouraged to continue it in the perioperative period. This includes β-adrenergic blockers even though the generalized use of this class of drug has recently been called into question.[35] Patients with recent coronary stent insertion who are taking platelet-inhibiting drugs (aspirin, clopidogrel, and others) may need to wait until 1 year after the stent placement to be allowed to come off the antiplatelet drugs and thus may need to delay elective surgery.[36]

CONGESTIVE HEART FAILURE

Congestive heart failure (CHF) has been shown to be an independent predictor of postoperative adverse cardiac outcomes in many studies.[24,37,38] Thus, a patient who is in CHF is not a candidate for outpatient anesthesia. Patients with a recent history of CHF need to have a cardiac evaluation that documents the resolution of the CHF and the patient's adequate functional status for the planned surgery before they are scheduled for an outpatient procedure.

AORTIC VALVE STENOSIS

Patients with aortic valve stenosis (AS), especially if severe (aortic valve area <1 cm^2), are at high risk for postoperative cardiac and pulmonary complications.[37] A patient with a typical systolic murmur of AS or other reason to suspect it by history or physical examination should have a cardiac evaluation with an echocardiogram. If the diagnosis is confirmed and the valve is severely stenotic, the patient may not be a candidate for outpatient surgery, especially in a freestanding setting.

MALIGNANT HYPERTHERMIA

It is now generally considered low risk to administer anesthesia to a patient with a history of malignant hyperthermia (MH) or a strong family history in an outpatient setting. The widespread and popular availability of nontriggering anesthetic regimens makes this possible. Some authors have suggested observing an MH patient at least 4 hours after surgery.[29]

DIABETES MELLITUS

Patients with diabetes offer a significant challenge whenever surgery and anesthesia are contemplated. Preoperative evaluation involves evaluation of the patient's degree of blood sugar control, which is measured by the hemoglobin A1c (HbA1c). In general, a patient with HbA1c greater than 8.6 is considered to have poorly controlled diabetes[39] and should be referred to an appropriate physician for evaluation and control. Complications of diabetes include cardiac, vascular, and renal disease. These should be evaluated and controlled as needed in addition to the diabetes before the patient is ready for surgery. Some institutions prefer that the patient take no hypoglycemic medications, including insulin or oral medications, on the morning of surgery. Others ask patients to take half of their long-acting insulin on the morning of surgery. Upon arrival for surgery, a blood sugar level should be taken and appropriate therapy instituted based on the measured value. In 2010, the Society for Ambulatory Anesthesia published consensus guidelines on perioperative glucose management, which are available on its website (sambahq.org)[3].

PATIENTS WITH CARDIAC RHYTHM MANAGEMENT DEVICES

As part of the outpatient preoperative evaluation, there should be documentation for patients with cardiac rhythm management device delineating the type of device, verifying its proper working order, and the management of such device during the perioperative period. If such management includes the disabling or reprogramming of any function, the outpatient setting must have the capabilities for reprogramming to the preoperative settings.[40]

PATIENT PREPARATION

In addition to a full evaluation of the patient, a process to educate the patient about the perioperative process is essential. Every person who has interaction with the patient should be able to explain to the patient what he or she will experience. In addition, a process that ensures adequate education of the patient must be designed and implemented. It is the job of the surgeons and their staff members to describe the surgical procedure, the reasons why the procedure is necessary, and the recovery process and expectations. The PAT staff members describe the preadmission evaluation process, give the patient NPO (nothing by mouth) instructions, and tell the patient what medications to take or discontinue.

Preoperative issues requiring detailed instructions include:

- **Diabetes:** What medications should or should not be taken on the morning of surgery? What to do for a hypoglycemic episode while a patient is NPO.
- **Blood thinners,** including aspirin, other antiplatelet drugs, and warfarin. For most surgical procedures, warfarin must be stopped 5 days before surgery. Some patients will need to be "bridged" with low-molecular-weight heparin.[20]
- **Hypertensive medications:** In general, β-blockers should be taken, and angiotensin-converting enzyme inhibitors should not be taken the day of surgery.
- **Asthma:** Inhalers and oral medications should be taken on their regular schedule as much as possible.

Whenever possible, patients should be encouraged to maintain their usual regimen of medications except when specifically told not to do so as noted.[20]

Many outpatient surgery centers have a booklet or folder with appropriate information for preoperative patients. The information should include details about NPO status, notification of timing of surgery, what patients should and should not bring with them, a map, and a general description of the perioperative process. Patient NPO status before an anesthetic is generally recognized to be adequate based on the following time periods of minimum fasting periods.[41]

- Clear liquids: 2 hours
- Breast milk: 4 hours
- Infant formula: 6 hours
- Non-human milk: 6 hours
- Light meal: 6 hours
- Heavy meal: 8 hours

At the end of the surgical process, all patients should be sent home with detailed written instructions that are procedure and surgeon specific. The instructions should describe the normal course of events for the first few days after surgery, common and serious complications to look for and what to do if they happen, and contact information if there are any questions or concerns.

ANESTHETIC MANAGEMENT

Many factors contribute to the choice of anesthetic technique. The principles involved are no different than for anesthesia choice for patients in the hospital. The patient's physiologic status must be maintained to the best possible extent. The patient must be rendered insensible to the painful stimulus of the procedure. Finally, the surgeon must be given adequate conditions to do the best procedure possible. In addition to these three principles, the expectations of patients at an outpatient or an office-based facility are that they will be discharged home on the same day in a condition allowing them to do basic ADLs in their home setting. No single anesthetic technique satisfies these requirements for all surgical procedures. There is no single anesthetic technique or drug combination that has been shown to be superior to all others. Almost any technique (sedation or MAC, regional anesthesia with or without sedation, general anesthesia) that allows for a rapid return to consciousness and mobility in addition to minimizing side effects will be an adequate technique.[42-44]

Many procedures can be performed with local anesthetic infiltration with or without sedation. The level of sedation can be varied from mild to deep depending on the degree of surgical stimulation. Deep sedation is often called monitored anesthesia care or MAC. The success of this technique requires that the surgeon is willing and able to inject an adequate amount of local anesthetic in the surgical field to block sensation. A MAC anesthetic will not be successful if the patient is unwilling to accept some sensation of touch or pressure. While discussing this issue with patients, it is important to reassure them that they will feel no pain because any discomfort will prompt an injection of more local or deepening of the level of sedation. The MAC anesthetic is successful when the patient is adequately sedated for the procedure but still spontaneously breathing. Occasionally, oral or nasal airways are inserted to promote adequate breathing status. The anesthetic relies on a continuous infusion of propofol with supplementation of a short acting opioid and midazolam or other benzodiazepine. Sometimes small doses of ketamine are used to supplement the sedation and add more analgesic effect without adding the potential for respiratory depression associated with opioids. Other supplemental drugs often used include antiemetics and antihistamines. A relatively recent variation on local anesthetic techniques is the tumescent technique.[45] Tumescent local anesthetic uses a dilute solution of lidocaine ($\leq$0.1%) with dilute epinephrine (1:600,000 or 1:1,000,000) infiltrated in large volumes over a wide area of skin and subcutaneous fat tissue. It is used to enhance the success of liposuction plastic surgery procedures and can be supplemented with MAC or general anesthesia to make a complete anesthetic.

Regional anesthesia is a routine component of anesthetics at outpatient surgery centers. Spinal and epidural anesthesia are commonly used. The drawback of these techniques is that patients cannot be discharged until fully recovered from the neuraxial block; otherwise, they are not stable enough to walk out of the facility. However, spinal anesthesia with a low dose of local anesthetic mixed with a lipid-soluble opioid (fentanyl) provides an excellent block and an acceptably short recovery period for procedures below the waist.[46] Similarly, an epidural with appropriate drug choice and dosing may be a reasonable choice.

Peripheral nerve blocks are frequently used for outpatient procedures.[47,48] Some of the reason for the increasing frequency of nerve blocks is the emerging technology of ultrasound-guided nerve blocks.[49,50] Another reason for the increased popularity of nerve blocks is the use of catheter placement at the nerve for continuous infusion of local anesthetic.[51] Nerve blocks offer profound sensory block without heavy sedation or general anesthesia. For a patient amenable to the block being performed, this can allow rapid recovery to "home readiness" even for relatively complicated procedures.

General anesthesia is often still the best or only choice for a given surgical procedure. When general anesthesia is chosen, a regimen of short-acting drugs with the fastest recovery profile should be chosen. The concept of a "fast track anesthesia protocol"[44] has become popular in which the anesthetic management is chosen to optimize recovery from the general anesthesia in the outpatient setting. The use of short-acting anesthetic drugs with other ancillary drugs to reduce the incidence of nausea and emesis and minimize pain (nonsteroidal anti-inflammatory drugs, small doses of narcotics, local anesthetic in the incision) are the hallmark of these protocols. Propofol is the universally accepted induction agent of choice.[52] Many drug regimens have been shown to be effective as the maintenance anesthetic for use in the outpatient population. None has been shown to be clearly superior, although some have advantages and disadvantages compared with other choices. Total IV anesthesia (TIVA) in which a continuous infusion of propofol supplemented with short-acting narcotics and other drugs as needed has become popular.[53] This technique offers an easily adjustable depth of general anesthesia with rapid recovery and good recovery profile. In most studies, but not all, comparing TIVA with inhalation technique (usually sevoflurane or desflurane), the recovery times were similar, but the nausea and emesis rate was lower for TIVA.[54] The common use of antiemetic medication prophylactically (ie, administered before anesthesia emergence) can significantly reduce the incidence of postoperative nausea and emesis and therefore minimize any advantage that the TIVA might have from that standpoint.[55,56] Several studies and systematic reviews have directly compared TIVA with inhalation techniques and compared various inhalation anesthetics (sevoflurane, desflurane, isoflurane) with each other[57-59] and with propofol-based TIVA. All are reasonable choices for anesthetic management in outpatients. The differences in emergence times and other markers of recovery were sometimes statistically significant but not different enough to make a clinical difference. Differences in recovery profile were not reproducible in multiple studies.

In recent years, the laryngeal mask airway and other supraglottic airway devices have become popular and useful alternatives to endotracheal intubation for general anesthetic procedures that do not require significant muscle relaxation for the surgical procedure. The reported advantages include ease of insertion even when a laryngoscopy will be difficult, less coughing and bucking upon emergence, no need for muscle relaxant reversal, and others.[60] They can be used as an airway rescue device and have been included in difficult airway protocols.[61]

The use of N_2O combined with either a propofol-based infusion technique or potent inhalation technique has been questioned in recent years. When comparing similar anesthetic techniques with or without N_2O, usage reduces emergence time and lowers the amount of other drugs required for a complete anesthetic. However, the use of N_2O also is usually associated with increased nausea and emesis. Although its use is not as ubiquitous as in the past, generally reviews on the use of N_2O find no reason that it should not be used in outpatient general anesthesia.[62] The nausea and emesis issue is dealt with easily by administering antiemetic drugs as discussed later in this chapter.

POSTANESTHESIA CARE

PHASES OF RECOVERY

Recovery from anesthesia is a process that begins with the termination of intraoperative care and ends with the return of the patient to his or her preoperative homeostasis. Phase I or early recovery begins with the cessation of intraoperative anesthetic management and ends with recovery of vital reflexes. This takes place in the PACU. A patient may bypass phase I at the determination of the anesthesiologist (fast tracking). Phase II (intermediate recovery) is terminated when the patient is "home ready"; this may occur in a part of the facility separate from the PACU. Phase III recovery (late recovery) is complete when the patient is "street ready" or has returned to his or her preoperative physiologic function.[63,64] This phase occurs after discharge. The challenge of ambulatory anesthesia is to minimize the amount of time spent in phase I and II without putting the patient at undue risk of readmission. Fast tracking has been shown to reduce the time to discharge but requires more nursing interventions in phase II. Whether or not fast tracking reduces costs depends largely on whether personnel costs are reduced.

TABLE 68-1 American Society of Anesthesiologists Standards for Postanesthesia Care

Standard	Language of the Standards	Comments
I	All patients who have received general anesthesia, regional anesthesia, or monitored anesthesia care shall receive appropriate postanesthesia management.	Recovery is to be in a PACU except by explicit order of a responsible anesthesiologist.
II	A patients transported to the PACU shall be accompanied by a member of the anesthesia care team who is knowledgeable about the patient's condition. The patient shall be continually evaluated and treated during transport with monitoring and support appropriate to the patient's condition.	
III	Upon arrival in the PACU, the patient shall be reevaluated and a verbal report provided to the responsible PACU nurse by the member of the anesthesia care team who accompanies the patient.	This standard requires communication of all pertinent patient information between teams before the anesthesia team member leaves the patient.
IV	The patient's condition shall be evaluated continually in the PACU.	Monitoring must include quantitative oxygenation assessments during phase I. A physician must be available in the facility to respond to emergencies. Nurses are encouraged to use PACU scoring systems at admission, discharge, and intervals appropriate to patient's condition.
V	A physician is responsible for the discharge of the patient from the PACU.	The PACU may discharge a patient based on written criteria.

PACU, postanesthesia care unit.

Adapted from American Society of Anesthesiologists. *Standards for Postanesthesia Care.* Approved October 27, 2004, amended October 21, 2009. Available at: https://www.asahq.org/For-Members/Clinical-Information/~/media/For%20Members/documents/Standards%20Guidelines%20Stmts/Postanesthesia%20Care%20Standards%20For.ashx. Parkridge, IL. Accessed June 11, 2011.

DISCHARGE

The American Society of Anesthesiologists has adopted five Standards for Post Anesthesia Care (**Table 68-1**) that broadly delineate the responsibility of the anesthesiologist in postanesthetic management. In essence, the anesthesiologist has the ultimate responsibility for the recovery and discharge of patients from the PACU to home. In practical terms in accordance with the standards, nurses recover and discharge the patients according to policies, procedures, and discharge criteria approved by the anesthesia department, with particular attention to monitoring oxygenation, ventilation, circulation, level of consciousness, and temperature. The only monitoring mandate by the ASA standards is a quantitative evaluation of oxygenation during early recovery. Although not required by the ASA Standards, the use of PACU scoring systems to monitor recovery is encouraged.[65]

POSTANESTHESIA CARE UNIT SCORING SYSTEMS

Patients may be discharged according to outcome-based clinical discharge criteria (**Table 68-2**) or by score in a numerical scoring system.

TABLE 68-2 Outcome-Based Clinical Discharge Criteria

Mental status	Alert and oriented
Vital signs	Stable
Pain	Controlled with oral analgesics
PONV	Controlled
Ambulation	Without dizziness
Bleeding	No unexpected
Discharge instructions	Written and verbal
Patient	Willing to be discharged
Responsible adult	Accepts instructions and responsibility for patient

PONV, postoperative nausea and vomiting.

Adapted from Awad I, Chung F. Factors affecting recovery and discharge following ambulatory surgery. *Can J Anesth.* 2006;53(9):858-872.

Although clinical discharge criteria address appropriate outcomes in discharge readiness, they lack the objectivity of a numerical scoring system. Numerical scoring systems are easy to administer, show a patient's objective progress through time, and can function as a useful quality tool in follow-up chart audits. Those in widespread use (Modified Aldrete, Postanesthesia Discharge Scoring System [PADS]; **Table 68-3**) provide consistency and common language across health care. The disadvantage of numerical scoring systems is that they fail to account for unique patient factors such as a patient's long distance to a hospital or MH susceptibility. The scoring systems must not be used without application of appropriate judgment.[63,66]

Attempts have also been made to use psychomotor tests, such as the Trieger dot test and reaction time tests, to assess discharge readiness. Their shortcomings include their complexity and hence impracticality for routine use and their narrow focus on one aspect of recovery. They remain a research tool.[67]

FROM PHASE I TO PHASE II

The original Aldrete Scoring System described in the 1970s assessed five parameters (color, respiration, circulation, consciousness, and motor function) with a score of 0, 1, or 2 in each category for a total of 10. A score of 9 or greater was required for discharge to phase II. This scoring system was modified in 1995 to replace color with the objective measurement of oxygenation through pulse oximetry. The modified Aldrete scoring system is in widespread international use.[63,64,67]

FAST TRACK CRITERIA

Which patients are candidates for fast tracking to phase II? With short- and ultra-short-acting anesthetics, it is possible for the majority of outpatients to achieve a modified Aldrete score of 9 or greater in the OR.[42,43,68,69] This score, however, does not consider the two most common reasons requiring phase I nursing interventions: pain and nausea or vomiting. White and Song[70] further modified the Aldrete scoring system to include the two additional factors of *pain and emetic symptoms*, suggesting a score of 12 or above with no individual parameter of zero necessary for phase I bypass (**Table 68-4**). Fast tracking to phase II has gained favor as a way of

TABLE 68-3 Common Numerical Scoring Systems

Modified Aldrete Score		PADS	
Maximum score	10	Maximum score	10
Respiration		Vital signs	
Deep breath or cough	2	Within 20% preoperative baseline	2
Shallow breath or dyspnea	1	Within 20%-40% preoperative baseline	1
Apnea	0	>40% preoperative baseline	0
Oxygenation		Activity	
>92% on room air	2	Steady or preoperative baseline	2
>90% with supplemental O_2	1	Needs assistance	1
<90% with/without O_2	0	Unable to ambulate	0
Consciousness		Nausea and vomiting	
Fully awake	2	Minimal: no treatment	2
Arousable on calling	1	Moderate: treatment effective	1
Not responsive	0	Severe: treatment ineffective	0
Circulation		Pain	
BP +/– 20 mm Hg preoperative level	2	VAS 0-3	2
BP +/– 20-50 mm Hg preoperative level	1	VAS 4-6	1
BP >/<50 mm Hg preoperative level	0	VAS 7-10	0
Activity		Surgical bleeding	
Four extremities	2	Minimal: no dressing changes	2
Two extremities	1	Moderate: up to 2 dressing changes	1
0 extremities	0	Severe: continued bleeding after 3 or more dressing changes	0
Score to discharge patients from phase I	9	Score to discharge patients from phase II	9

BP, blood pressure; PADS, Postanesthesia Discharge Scoring System VAS, Visual Analog Scale.

Data from Gan TJ, Meyer TA, Apfel CC et al. Society for Ambulatory Anesthesia guidelines for the management of postoperative nausea and vomiting. *Anesth Analg*. 2007;105(6):1615-1628; and Skledar, SJ, Williams BA, Vallejo MC et al. Eliminating postoperative nausea and vomiting in outpatient surgery with multimodal strategies including low doses of nonsedating, off patent antiemetics: is "zero tolerance" achievable? *Sci World J*. 2007;7:959-977.

reducing costs by minimizing recovery stays in ASCs but without sacrificing safety. Indeed, fast-tracked patients do have shorter stays and do not experience negative changes in outcomes.[42,43,68,69] Substantiating the initial premise of cost reduction remains elusive. The number of nursing interventions and active nursing time are not reduced, suggesting that in ambulatory surgery, the majority of postanesthesia nursing activity lies in getting the patients home ready, including conversion to oral medications, discharge instructions, ambulation, and follow-up care arrangements. Facilities may or may not be able to flex nurses from phase I to a separate phase II facility; case mix may not allow the time saved in recovery to be filled by additional cases.[63] The theoretical advantages of fast tracking will no doubt continue to inspire the search for real cost savings in the process.

TABLE 68-4 Phase I Bypass (Fast Track) Criteria

Criteria	Score
Consciousness[a]	0-2
Physical activity[a]	0-2
Hemodynamic stability[a]	0-2
Respiratory stability[a]	0-2
Oxygen saturation status[a]	0-2
Postoperative pain assessment	0-2
Postoperative emetic symptoms	0-2
Score for fast tracking	≥12 No individual score of 0

[a]Adapted from modified Aldrete Score.

Adapted from White PF, Song D. New criteria for fast-tracking after outpatient anesthesia: a comparison with the modified Aldrete's scoring system. *Anesth Analg.* 1999;88:1069-1072.

FROM PHASE II TO PHASE III

Safe discharge of patients to home requires that postanesthesia nurses follow discharge protocols adopted by the anesthesia department, which include validated criteria that are easily applied to all ambulatory patients. These may be outcome-based discharge criteria, scoring system based, or a combination. The IAAS recommends an outcome-based process with medical—both invariable (eg, stable vital signs) and variable (eg, micturition in a spinal anesthetic patient)—and nonmedical criteria (eg, access to a telephone after discharge).[64] Awad and Chung[63] developed the PADS, which addresses activity level, vital signs, nausea and vomiting, pain and surgical bleeding, assessment of which leads to a score of up to 2 in each parameter with at least a 9 necessary for discharge. The original PADS scoring included necessity for voiding and drinking fluids, but these two requirements have been dropped as being unsupported by the literature.[63,64,66] The ASA's Practice Guidelines for Postanesthetic Care recommend that each patient care facility should develop its own suitable discharge criteria that must be met before discharge, that a scoring system may assist in assessment and documentation, and that outpatients should be discharged to an adult who is responsible for accompanying the patient home and assisting with reporting and follow-up of any postoperative complications.[71]

DISCHARGE INSTRUCTIONS

The ASA's Practice Guidelines recommend that outpatients be provided with written instructions on diet, activity limitations (particularly important in patients with an insensate limb from a peripheral nerve block), medications, and an emergency phone number.[71] The importance of clear instructions cannot be underestimated. As ambulatory procedures continue to grow, so too does the shift in phase III recovery from a medical facility with trained personnel to a home with laypersons. Because the discharging nurse devotes much time to the education process with the patient and responsible escort, facilities must have plans in place for effective discharge instructions. If English is not the patient's primary language, the discharge process must accommodate the patient's translation needs. Also, the instructions must be in lay language to target the health literacy of the typical layperson so that compliance can be high.[63] In addition to safety concerns, clear communication with the patient is what patients may most highly prize. Fung and Cohen[72] asked patients to prioritize the importance of various aspects of their ambulatory surgery experience, including preoperative, intraoperative, predischarge, and postdischarge. The questionnaire included items from previous work that patients had identified as important and ones that anesthesiologists thought important. Most important to patients was that clear discharge instructions were given; next most important was that they were told of minor and major things to expect. Important but not as important as clear communication was avoidance of side effects.

Finally, because of psychomotor and cognitive impairments in the postoperative period, patients should not be discharged home unescorted.[71] Although several authors have found no impairment after 2 to 3 hours in healthy volunteers, Chung et al[73] demonstrated that even with the newer shorter acting anesthetics, surgical patients' driving performance is impaired both preoperatively and postoperatively, returning to normal within 24 hours. Driving performance is most impacted 2 hours postoperatively when many ambulatory patients are being discharged home. Although ambulatory surgery units can and must control discharge to a responsible driver, surveillance is lost postdischarge, making clear instructions on psychomotor and cognitive dysfunction mandatory.[74]

FUNCTIONAL RECOVERY

Most ambulatory practices have a system for following up on patients. Typical practice in the United States is a follow-up phone call the day after surgery. This practice serves the dual purpose of continuing patient care and education, possibly helping the patient avoid a trip to the physician's office or emergency department (ED), and data collection for quality reviews. However, by placing the phone calls within 24 hours of surgery and then "closing the book" on the patient, it is possible to miss issues that arise later and interfere with the patient's resumption of normal activities. Also, as the limits of ambulatory care are continually pushed, a valid assessment tool would assist in the evaluation of new surgical and anesthetic techniques and allow for appropriate adjustments in care. Postdischarge tools have not been developed and used to the extent of the predischarge scoring systems. The Quality of Recovery (QoR) 9 score is the most frequently cited in ambulatory anesthesia but has only moderate validity and reliability and was not developed for use in outpatients. A new tool, developed by Wong et al[75] is the Functional Recovery Index (FRI), which has 14 items covering three parameters (pain and social activity, lower limb activity, and general physical activity). The FRI was demonstrated to have excellent reliability, good validity, responsiveness, and acceptability, which may make this a useful tool for assessing patient outcomes and functional recovery in the future.

DISCHARGE DELAYS

Postoperative Nausea and Vomiting Postoperative nausea and vomiting (PONV) is the leading cause of unplanned admissions, either from PACU or from home after ambulatory procedures, and one of the two leading causes of delayed discharge from ambulatory surgery. A search of PONV literature reveals tens of thousands of articles, highlighting the importance of this topic for both patients and ambulatory anesthesiologists. It is the responsibility of the anesthesiologist to prevent or expeditiously treat PONV to both reduce hospital admission rates after ambulatory procedures and to enhance throughput in high-volume facilities.

The following is the current approach to PONV recommended by SAMBA in its 2007 Guidelines for the Management of Postoperative Nausea and Vomiting:

1. Identify a patient's risk for PONV.
2. Reduce baseline risk factors.
3. Administer PONV prophylaxis using one or two interventions in adults with moderate risk for PONV.
4. Use more than 2 interventions in adults with high risk for PONV.
5. Administer prophylactic antiemetic combination therapy in children at risk for PONV.
6. Provide antiemetic treatment to patients who did not receive or who fail prophylaxis.[76]

Apfel et al[77] predicted a patient's risk for PONV based on the independent predictors of female gender, nonsmoking, history of PONV or motion sickness, and need for postoperative opioids, as 10% with no risk factors, 20% with 1, 40% with 2, 60% with 3, and 80% with 4 risk factors. The guidelines do not include a recommendation for prophylaxis of patients with low risk (ie, 10%) for PONV. In a study that analyzed the statistical effect of 6 interventions to prevent PONV in patients with at least 2 risk factors (40% risk of PONV), the authors found that four interventions (ondansetron, droperidol, dexamethasone, propofol, and nitrogen-oxygen) each reduced the relative risk of PONV by 26%; thus, giving dexamethasone prophylactically to a patient with an 80% risk results in a risk of 59% (21% absolute risk reduction) with number needed to treat (NNT) of 5 to prevent 1 case of PONV; giving a second drug to the person with an 80% risk results in a reduction of risk to 45%. Giving that same drug to a person with a low risk of PONV (10%) results in the same 26% relative risk reduction to a risk of 7% but only a 3% absolute risk reduction, with an NNT of 40, calling into question whether it is cost effective to prophylactically treat patients without risk factors.[78] Unfortunately, studies of cost effectiveness are lacking in methodology; SAMBA recommends future studies in the area that properly measure resource use against value of health consequences.[76] Because of the importance of PONV in the outpatient setting, the relatively high risk of PONV in patients without risk factors other than having anesthesia, and the availability of off-patent nonsedating treatments, a group from the University of Pittsburgh is recommending a "zero tolerance" approach that includes prophylaxis for all patients.[79]

After the decision is made on which (or all) patients will receive interventions to avoid PONV, the approach should be multimodal. Techniques that decrease baseline risks include the use regional or local anesthesia whenever possible, propofol anesthetic induction and maintenance, avoidance of N_2O and volatile anesthetics, minimal use of opioids both intraoperatively and postoperatively, minimal use of neostigmine (especially in doses >2.5 mg), and adequate hydration.[76,79] The emetic effects of both opioids and volatile agents are dose related.

Pharmacologic intervention for prophylaxis may include serotonin (5-HT_3) receptor antagonists, steroids, phenothiazines, ephedrine, butyrophenones, antihistamines, and anticholinergics. (See **Table 68-5** for recommendations on dosing and time of dosing of specific drugs.) Because each class of antiemetic works in different ways, each successive drug used should be from an untried class for maximum efficacy. Stimulation of the P6 acupressure point has also been demonstrated to be effective at reducing PONV.[25] What do not seem effective are metoclopramide in standard clinical doses,[80], ginger,[81] and cannabinoids.[82] In the pediatric population, 5-HT_3 antagonists appear to be superior to other classes of drugs and are therefore viewed as the first-line prophylaxis. Ondansetron is approved for use from 1 month of age at doses of 50 to 100 mcg/kg.[76]

TABLE 68-5 Pharmacologic Prophylaxis Against Postoperative Nausea and Vomiting

Drug Class	Representative	Effect	Dosing	Timing	Comments
Anticholinergic	Scopolamine (effective PD)	Antagonism of muscarinic and histaminic receptors in vestibular and vomiting centers	1.5 mg td patch ≤72 h	Prior evening or 4 h before end of surgery	Patients should be advised of possible anticholinergic and CNS effects, especially elderly patients
Steroid	Dexamethasone (effective PD)	Antiprostaglandin; appetite stimulant; endorphin release	4-5 mg IV	At induction	Consider risks and benefit in patients with diabetes; causes perineal pruritus; use after sedation
Butyrophenone	Droperidol	Anti-dopaminergic in CTZ	0.625-1.25 mg IV	End of surgery	Black box warning because of torsades de pointes and QT_c prolongation; not likely at low antiemetic doses
Phenothiazine	Perphenazine	Anticholinergic, antidopaminergic, antihistaminergic	8 mg PO	On admission	Avoids risk of tissue necrosis with IV promethazine
5-HT_3 RA	Ondansetron (effective PD) Dolasetron	Serotonin blocker in CTZ	4 mg IV 12.5 mg IV	End of surgery rescue	Repeat dosing ineffective but alternative 5-HT_3 RA may be effective
Antihistamine	Cyclizine	Anticholinergic; antidopaminergic; antihistaminergic	50 mg PO	On admission	IV form not available in the United States
NK-1 antagonist	Aprepitant	Vomiting center	40 mg PO	Within 3 h of anesthesia induction	Only extended-duration FDA-approved PONV prophylaxis; cost limits routine use

CNS, central nervous system; CTZ, chemoreceptor trigger zone; FDA, Food and Drug Administration; 5-HT_3, serotonin; IV, intravenous; NK, neurokinin; PD, postdischarge; PO, oral; PONV, postoperative nausea and vomiting; RA, receptor antagonist; td, transdermal.

Data from Gan TJ, Meyer TA, Apfel CC et al. Society for Ambulatory Anesthesia guidelines for the management of postoperative nausea and vomiting. *Anesth Analg*. 2007;105(6):1615-1628; and Skledar, SJ, Williams BA, Vallejo MC et al. Eliminating postoperative nausea and vomiting in outpatient surgery with multimodal strategies including low doses of nonsedating, off patent antiemetics: is "zero tolerance" achievable? *Sci World J*. 2007;7:959-977.

For patients who failed prophylaxis, the chosen antiemetic should be from a pharmacologic category not previously used. If no prophylaxis was used, a 5-HT_3 antagonist should be the first-line treatment; this class has been adequately studied and shown superior efficacy against existing PONV.[76]

Postdischarge nausea and vomiting (PDNV), which occurs in as many as one-third of ambulatory patients, can lead to a delay in resumption of normal activities, including return to work, and inadequate treatment of postoperative pain for fear of aggravating PDNV.[83] Although much literature is devoted to PONV, scant literature exists on PDNV. Gupta et al[55] reviewed the literature that does exist to determine if PONV prophylaxis contributes to risk reduction of PDNV. Interestingly, both 4 mg of ondansetron, with its half-life of 3.5 hours, and 4 mg of dexamethasone, but not droperidol, were indeed effective in reducing risk of PDNV; combination therapy was most effective. Small randomized controlled studies suggest the efficacy of orally disintegrating ondansetron tablets, stimulation of P6, and transdermal scopolamine.[84-86]

In summary, based on the existing literature, a reasonable approach to this vexing problem is:

1. Identify a patient's PONV and PDNV risk factors (few have zero).
2. Plan the least emetic anesthetic possible for a surgery (eg, TIVA, regional, local).
3. Provide multimodal prophylaxis to include at least ondansetron and dexamethasone because these are effective after discharge as well as immediately after surgery.
4. Adequately hydrate the patient.
5. Discharge patients home with a prescription for an antiemetic.

Pain Pain, along with PONV, is one of the two most common complications of outpatient surgery, outpatient discharge delays and unplanned admissions, and postdischarge symptoms. Pain is the most common cause of readmission to the hospital after ambulatory discharge followed by PONV, a common consequence of opioid-centered pain management.[87] Although much is known about the superiority of a multimodal approach to pain management,[87,88] clinical practice lags far behind.[89] Minimizing pain and its consequences requires careful anesthetic and surgical planning and a multimodal treatment approach. Generous use of local anesthetic by the surgeon and nerve blocks by the anesthesiologist when indicated has been shown to reduce PACU stays, improve patient satisfaction, and improve the quality of pain control. Additionally, nonopioid analgesics have been shown to enhance pain control without the side effects of increased nausea or respiratory depression. In addition to nonsteroidal anti-inflammatory drugs and acetaminophen, gabapentin and pregabalin show promise in reducing opioid consumption and side effects as well as pain, although they do have side effects of sedation and dizziness.[90]

Voiding Historically, requiring all patients to void before discharge was a widespread practice. The main effect of the practice was delayed discharge without any improvement in patient care. Current practice, endorsed by the ASA, does not require delay of discharge until voiding; rather, the patient's risk for complications from failure to void must be assessed. Patients at high risk of urinary retention (genitourinary and colorectal surgery, high residual volumes, or neuraxial anesthesia) may be kept until voiding occurs or bladder catheterization may be required. Patients should be discharged with instructions on what to do if they remain unable to void after discharge (6-8 hours).[71]

Oral Intake Requiring patients to drink and eat is another historical practice that has been revisited. Not only has mandatory consumption been shown to not be necessary to prevent occurrence of adverse outcomes, but it can cause them. Forcing oral intake has been shown to contribute to nausea and thus delay discharge. Permissive oral intake, especially of liquids only, results in earlier discharge and less PONV.[71]

EXTENDED RECOVERY

Many ambulatory surgery units offer outpatient surgery with extended (23-h) stay capabilities, either in a nursing ward–type setting or a hotel-type setting. Several reasons exist for the practice. Freestanding surgery centers have been able to expand the types of surgery performed and, at least in the private sector, enjoy a greater return on investment; busy academic hospital centers have been able to decompress their surgical schedules and improve waiting times for patients in need of inpatient care by sending less complex surgeries and patients offsite, and patients who live alone are able to enjoy the many benefits of same-day surgery and recover with a surrogate relative at a hospital hotel at one quarter of the cost of an inpatient stay.[91] Additionally, 23-hour stay facilities have allowed the expansion of cases acceptable for outpatient surgery (admission and discharge within a normal working day). Laparoscopic cholecystectomies and anterior cruciate ligament repairs have moved from the 23-hour stay arena to be routinely performed as outpatient surgeries as surgeons and anesthesiologists have gained confidence in the feasibility and safety of the patient's recovery at home; undoubtedly, more procedures being done using extended stay will transition to outpatient surgery.[12]

Although there may be many benefits of having 23-hour stay capabilities, cost considerations are complex. If the patient is transferred from the ambulatory surgery area to a hospital ward, all of the costs of inpatient care apply, including the transfer costs if from a freestanding facility. If the patient remains at the ambulatory surgery unit for extended stay, staffing costs may even exceed those of overnight hospital stays because 2 nurses are required whether for 20 patients (hospital) or 2. A much less expensive alternative to a 23-hour stay for patients living alone is the use of a home companion service.

UNANTICIPATED ADMISSIONS

MINOR MORBIDITY

Reported unanticipated admission rates after ambulatory surgery range 0.28% to 1.5%.[92] After discharge, readmission rates within 30-days of discharge from ambulatory surgery are up to 3%. The most common causes for unanticipated admission and readmission include pain, surgical complications and bleeding, medical complications, and anesthetic complications such as PONV.[92,93] Coley et al[92] reported their experience at a major teaching hospital: Two-thirds of the readmissions occurred during the first week after discharge, and of those readmitted, 80% were treated and released from the ED and 20% were admitted for inpatient care. Total patient charges for 303 returning patients approximated $2.5 million, with 92% of the charges being for inpatient care and 8% ED care. It is critical for each ambulatory site to analyze its rates and causes for admission and readmission to elucidate opportunities for improvement in care, such as improvement in pain management, and to ensure that the considerable health care dollars saved by outpatient care are only minimally offset by the costs of unanticipated admissions and readmissions.[92]

MAJOR MORBIDITY AND MORTALITY

Warner et al[94] prospectively studied the 30-day postoperative courses of more than 38,000 patients receiving 45,000 anesthetics over a 2-year period for the occurrence of death, MI, central nervous system (CNS) deficit, pulmonary embolism (PE), and respiratory failure. There were 4 deaths (2 from car accidents in which the patient was a passenger and 2 from MIs), 14 MIs, 7 CNS deficits, 5 PEs, and 5 patients with respiratory failure. Of these 31 major morbidities, 27 appeared unrelated to the ambulatory procedure. Using population-based epidemiologic data, the authors found that similar morbidity and mortality rates would have occurred randomly in a population not undergoing surgery.[94] A Danish retrospective study of less than half the anesthetics in the Warner study confirms that serious morbidity in outpatient anesthesia is rare: No major morbidity or mortality events occurred.[95]

TRANSFER PROCESS

All freestanding ASCs and office-based surgery sites must have in place a protocol for transfer of patients requiring direct admission to a hospital for further management. Different levels of transport care need to be considered, including critical care transport. In addition, freestanding surgery sites may have to contract with private ambulance or transport services. As soon as it is determined that a patient requires critical care, such as stroke management or possible coronary intervention, the plan needs to be activated to expedite the patient's transfer for definitive care. Transfer should not be delayed, but care should continue on site until the transport team arrives. A special case is when the critical event is an MH episode. Definitive therapy with dantrolene cannot wait for transfer, nor can the treatment of hyperkalemia. At a minimum, 2.5 mg/kg of dantrolene should be given. One individual should be assigned the time-consuming task of mixing the dantrolene. The dantrolene treatment goal should be resolution of tachycardia, normal minute ventilation and end-tidal carbon dioxide, and temperature below 38°C. Because of recrudescence of MH, it is difficult to know how stable the patient will be on transport and arrival at the receiving hospital. Both the transport team and the hospital must be prepared to continue management of an MH crisis. Guidelines about transfer of care in this circumstance are currently being developed.[96]

SPECIAL ISSUES

OBSTRUCTIVE SLEEP APNEA

As the epidemic of obesity has skyrocketed in this country, so too have associated disorders, including OSA. The prevalence of the disorder depends on the population studied: In the general population, women have a rate of 4.7% of moderately severe OSA (apnea/hypopnea index [AHI] >15), and men have a rate of 11.4%; in patients having bariatric surgery, 70% have OSA. It is estimated that the disorder affects millions of men and women and that 80% to 90%, including those presenting for surgery, are undiagnosed and therefore untreated at the time of presentation.[34] OSA occurs as a result of partial or complete airway obstruction during sleep. The obstruction is attributable to a combination of airway craniofacial and soft tissue malproportion as well as complex neurohumoral mechanisms[97]; OSA leads to hypoxemia and an increased risk of cardiac arrhythmias, MI, stroke, and sudden death in the general population not having surgery. Patients with OSA are particularly susceptible to the effects of sedatives, anesthetics, and opioid analgesics, and given the high prevalence of the disorder, they pose a challenge in the daily practice of any anesthesiologist.[98] The particular challenges for the ambulatory anesthesiologist include the appropriate preoperative evaluation of the outpatient for OSA to minimize delays while ensuring safe management and deciding which patients with OSA are candidates for ambulatory surgery. The gold standard for diagnosing OSA is an overnight polysomnogram that yields an AHI as an index of severity of OSA. The waiting time for a formal sleep study ranges from 2 to 10 months in the United States[99]; furthermore, a requirement of a sleep study in all patients suspected of OSA would overwhelm available resources. A screening tool with high sensitivity can be the surrogate for a sleep study.

The ASA's 2006 Practice Guidelines for the Perioperative Management of Patients with Obstructive Sleep Apnea included a risk-assessment screening tool of 14 items based on predisposing physical characteristics, history of apparent airway obstruction during sleep, and daytime somnolence, absent a polysomnogram.[100] The false-negative rate for the ASA screening tool is unacceptably high at 38% for mild OSA and 12% for moderate to severe OSA.[96] Chung et al[101] developed the STOP questionnaire (**s**noring, daytime **t**iredness, **o**bserved apnea, high blood **p**ressure), but this sacrificed accuracy for simplicity with similarly high false-negative rates. STOP was modified to STOP-BANG (adding **B**MI >35, **a**ge >50 y, **n**eck circumference >40 cm,

TABLE 68-6 Perioperative Sleep Apnea Prediction (P-SAP) Predictors of Obstructive Sleep Apnea

Demographic variables	Age >43 years Male gender Obesity
History variables	Snoring DM II Hypertension
Airway measures	Thick neck Mallampati 3 or 4 Reduced TMD

DM, diabetes mellitus; TMD, thyromental distance.

Adapted from Ramachandran SK, Kheterpal S, Consens F, et al. Derivation and validation of a simple perioperative sleep apnea prediction score. *Anesth Analg.* 2010;110(4):1007-1015.

male gender), which improved the false-negative rate in severe OSA to zero and less than 10% in moderate OSA. Because the underlying prevalence of OSA in the STOP-BANG study was high, the diagnostic accuracy of the tool could be overestimated.[99] Ramachandran et al[99] developed the P-SAP (Perioperative Sleep Apnea Prediction) scale to avoid this by studying the general surgical population with a lower prevalence of OSA and developed a scale with nine independent clinical predictors. Six of the 9 are also in STOP-BANG. The information was obtained from standard preoperative history and physical examination information obtained found in the electronic medical record (**Table 68-6**). The P-SAP does not include observed apnea or daytime somnolence.[99]

Which of the OSA patients as identified by an appropriate screening tool (STOP-BANG or P-SAP) should have surgery on an outpatient basis? The ASA guidelines consider the severity of OSA taken together with the invasiveness of surgery and anesthesia and requirement for postoperative opioids to yield a numeric score that may suggest no increased risk, increased risk, or significantly increased risk for perioperative complications. Additional considerations include anatomic and physiologic abnormalities; coexisting disease; patient age; adequacy of postoperative observation; and capabilities of the outpatient facility, including availability of difficult airway and respiratory care equipment, radiology and laboratory facilities, and a transfer agreement with an inpatient care facility.[100] These guidelines are expert opinion and do not reflect evidence-based conclusions because the literature was and continues to be generally insufficient to support conclusions about OSA management in the perioperative setting. In the end, the judgment of the anesthesiologist prevails.

If a patient is deemed suitable for outpatient anesthesia, management techniques recommended to minimize risk include use of local anesthetics and regional anesthesia where possible, only light to moderate sedation with CO_2 monitoring and continuous positive airway pressure (CPAP) if feasible, general anesthesia with a secure airway preferred over deep sedation, and awake extubation after full reversal of neuromuscular blockade in a semi-sitting position. During recovery, the patient should be in a nonsupine position, oxygen should be used as needed until the patient maintains baseline saturation, CPAP should be used for patients used to it, and opioid-sparing analgesic techniques and continuous pulse oximetry should be used until the patient maintains room air saturation above 90% during sleep. At that point, the OSA patient may be discharged home.[100]

PEDIATRICS

Several concerns must be addressed in pediatric ambulatory anesthesia.

Will this ambulatory surgery unit anesthetize children? Many common pediatric surgical procedures, such as tympanostomy tubes, tonsillectomy and adenoidectomy, and herniorrhaphy, are ideal for outpatient surgery and indeed are routinely performed in freestanding ASCs and hospital-based units. Although some ASCs are limited by choice to adult patients, this model does not serve a large patient base and may be an inefficient model for community surgeons with a mixed adult and pediatric population. If the unit decides to perform pediatric surgeries, there must be adequate pediatric experience not only in the surgeons, anesthesiologists, and anesthetists but also in the perioperative nursing. Preoperative teaching and preparation is critical to management of patient and family anxiety, and consideration should be given to the use of child life specialists. The physical environment should ideally address the need for privacy and provide quiet areas for admission and recovery of children, not only for their benefit but also for that of adult patients sharing the unit.

How young is too young? Anesthetic risk decreases with increasing age; generally, age eligibility is determined by the experience and expertise of the staff. Besides the exclusion of children less than 60 weeks postconceptual age,[27] children for tonsillectomy younger than the age of 3 years because of the risk of OSA are also excluded.[102]

How will parents be involved? It is common practice for parents to be present for induction of anesthesia and to be reunited as quickly as possible with the pediatric patient in the PACU. In general, parental presence during induction is less effective than sedative premedication in reducing a child's preoperative anxiety and postoperative behavioral disturbances.[103] Parental maladaptive behaviors that increase a child's anxiety include parental anxiety, excessive reassurance, granting of inappropriate control to the child, and criticism of the child.[104] In certain groups of children, however, parental presence is a benefit; these include older children, less active children, children with calmer parents, and children with parents who value preoperative preparation.[103] Family-oriented behavioral preparation has been shown to improve parental and child anxiety and postoperative outcomes.[105] If parental presence at induction is allowed, preoperative teaching of exactly what is to be expected during induction and recovery must be done, and there must be enough staffing to allow the accompaniment of the parent to the waiting room without interfering with the care of the patient in the OR. Parental presence in the PACU may not reduce the incidence of crying, but it has been shown to reduce the incidence of postdischarge maladaptive behaviors,[104] and it most certainly assists the PACU nursing staff.

What to do with emergence delirium? Emergence delirium is as troublesome today as it was when first described in association with ether, cyclopropane, and ketamine anesthesia.[106] It is distressing to the parents and may cause danger to the thrashing child and inadvertent loss of IV catheters and surgical dressings, it requires extra nursing staff, and it is disruptive to the other patients' recovery. The busy pace of an ambulatory surgery unit, from admission to discharge, may even exacerbate the problem. As surely as an ambulatory anesthesia practice devotes time and resources to the prevention and treatment of pain and PONV, it will also devote itself to emergence delirium.

The incidence in the literature ranges from 10% to 80%, depending on criteria used and populations studied, and prevention and treatment strategies are varied because the exact etiology of the disorder is not understood, although several associated factors have been identified, including preschool age, rapid time to awakening (particularly with sevoflurane and desflurane as opposed to halothane and propofol), preoperative anxiety of child and parent, poor tolerance of induction, the child's underlying temperament (more emotional and impulsive), and some adjunctive medications (including benzodiazepines).[107-109] Untreated pain is a confounding factor in the diagnosis, but lack of fentanyl in an anesthetic even for nonpainful procedures has been shown to increase the risk of emergence delirium.[108]

Preventive pharmacologic strategies based on randomized controlled studies include midazolam (0.5 mg/kg orally), the α_2-agonists clonidine (1-3 mcg/kg IV or caudally) and dexmedetomidine (0.2 mcg/kg/h IV or 0.15-0.3 mcg/kg), fentanyl (1 mcg/kg IV or 2 mcg/kg intranasally), and ketorolac (1 mg/kg IV). Even with these strategies, the rate of emergence delirium ranged from 5% to 39% except for 0% with clonidine 3 mcg/kg caudally.[107] Additional strategies may include IV propofol induction and maintenance, although the benefits of avoiding sevoflurane induction may be offset by the distress caused by securing IV access and after a sevoflurane induction switching to propofol, although this is not evidence-based practice. Finally, enhanced parent and child preparation may help in the reduction of perioperative anxiety, but parents who display anxiety-provoking behaviors may also be discouraged from being present during induction with the assurance that their presence is not necessary.

Management of emergence delirium in the PACU may include watchful waiting while keeping the child safe because the typical incident is self-limiting within a short period of time. Pharmacologic interventions used with some success include doses of fentanyl (1-2 mcg/kg IV), propofol (0.5-1 mg/kg IV), midazolam (0.02-0.1 mg/kg IV), and dexmedetomidine (0.5 mcg/kg IV). Voepel-Lewis and colleagues found that the most effective intervention is early reuniting with the parents.[110] Recovering the child in the least stimulating environment in the PACU is also helpful.

HOME-GOING PERIPHERAL NERVE BLOCK CATHETERS

The benefits of peripheral nerve blocks are well substantiated and include reduced PONV, reduced pain, potential for shorter stays in ambulatory units, improved postdischarge sleep, improved compliance with physical therapy, and improved patient satisfaction and cost savings.[47,111] This has led to a gradual increase in interest over the past decade in extending the benefits of single-shot peripheral nerve blocks longer into the postdischarge period with continuous peripheral nerve blocks (CPNB) or perineural infusions, with similarly improved outcomes. Tempering enthusiasm for outpatient CPNBs are concerns about both potential complications and logistics. The expanding literature is beginning to offer some reassurances with respect to low rates of complications, such as catheter or pump malfunction, catheter dislodgement, infection and local anesthetic toxicity, as well as guidance on the logistics of developing a home-going CPNB program.[112] A review of the literature on placement technique, dosing regimens, and complications is beyond the scope of this chapter, but several concerns for the outpatient anesthesiologists are addressed.

Patient Selection The patient or caretaker must first be willing to learn about and manage the pump and catheter system and should be deemed a good historian for purposes of eliciting the earliest signs of complications. Secondly, the procedure should be something that would otherwise require postoperative opioid analgesia for a length of time comparable to the intended duration of the CPNB to maximize the risk-to-benefit balance. Finally, a conservative inclusion approach should be considered when deciding on patients with systemic diseases who may be more compromised than healthy patients by potential at-home complications such as higher than programmed infusion rates until more research is available from study of hospitalized patients.[113]

Infusion Pump Selection Two basic types of devices are commonly used, electronic and elastomeric.[114-116] Both types have advocates and detractors and, both types are enjoying high success rates in clinical practice.[111] For home use, the ideal pump should be simple to use, reliably deliver an accurate and consistent infusion, provide for an adjustable basal rate to avoid injuries caused by an insensate limb, and have the capacity to deliver a bolus dose. Use of a pump with both adjustable basal rate and bolus dose capabilities results in often superior analgesia with lower consumption of local anesthetic, prolonging the local anesthetic reservoir life while reducing risks from motor blocks.[117,118] Not all pumps provide all features. If a bolus dose feature is absent, alternatives must be available for management of breakthrough pain.

Discharge Instructions Both the patient and accompanying caretaker should be given oral and written instructions covering the infusion pump management, what to expect as the surgical block wears off, how to manage breakthrough pain, how to care for the catheter and protect an insensate body part, what to look for as signs or symptoms of complications, and the catheter removal plan.[119] Because it is difficult to predict who will need an oral opioid pain reliever, a prescription should be provided. Finally, contact numbers for the health care providers responsible for the duration of the infusion should be provided.

Follow-up The amount and type of follow-up varies from one or more telephone calls per day from nurses or anesthesiologists to one or more home nursing visits per day. The optimal regimen has not been determined, but it is important whatever method of oversight is used to explore with the patient the possibility of complications and to assess the quality of analgesia and verify that the patient is adjusting the basal rate and bolusing appropriately (if available).[119] The catheter is to be removed by the patient at home, and patients prefer telephone coaching (98% comfortable) to relying only on written instructions (43% comfortable) for this task.[120]

FUTURE DIRECTIONS

OUTCOMES RESEARCH

Traditional outcomes used for assessing the quality of ambulatory anesthesia include death; major morbidities of organ dysfunction; and minor morbidities such as pain, nausea, and dizziness, as reflected in delayed discharge, unplanned admissions, and readmissions. As Warner et al[94] so clearly demonstrated, outpatient surgery is remarkably safe with mortality and major morbidity rare events. It is appropriate to view these traditional statistics as a benchmark for what should continue to be rare events, but these are not the sine qua non of quality care. Outcomes research includes the study of the effects that people experience and care about, such as changes in the ability to function. Future outcomes research will address patient-oriented outcomes such as quality of recovery (eg, fatigue, pain, physical and social functioning), quality of life, and patient satisfaction.[121,122] To be able to compare clinical trials with better guide practice, a standardized instrument to assess quality of recovery in ambulatory patients still needs to be developed according to rigid statistical guidelines and adopted in widespread use.[122] The Society for Ambulatory Anesthesia is developing a clinical outcomes registry (SCOR), which will provide benchmarks and root cause analysis,[123] similar to the Pediatric Perioperative Cardiac Arrest (POCA) and Perioperative Visual Loss (POVL) registries.[124]

THE CHALLENGES

As surgical techniques continue to advance, leading to more expansion of outpatient health care, anesthesia must keep pace as it has in the past. The not infrequent postdischarge symptoms of pain and PDNV must be better managed. Anesthesiologists should consistently use techniques of multimodal pain control and multimodal PONV prophylaxis that are well known today. Future studies need to further elucidate the most effective treatments for PDNV, including the role of aprepitant, and the optimum dosing, both concentration and volume, of local anesthetics for home-going peripheral nerve block catheters and the best follow-up protocols.

The obesity epidemic, if not reversed, will continue to impact outpatient anesthesia in very practical ways, including facility design or costly redesign to accommodate unique demands.

Most challenging of all may be the practice of high-quality yet cost-effective ambulatory anesthesia in an era of legislative health care reform in which access to care has been greatly expanded. Cost savings cannot be assumed but should be demonstrated to be true savings and not merely shifting of costs to EDs or home nursing care.

As always, continued expansion of outpatient care to more complex problems and patients demands unwavering vigilance both toward each patient and any unwelcome evolving trends in morbidity and mortality.

KEY REFERENCES

- American Society of Anesthesiologists. Practice guidelines for the perioperative management of patients with obstructive sleep apnea. A report by the American Society of Anesthesiologists task force on the perioperative management of patients with obstructive sleep apnea. *Anesthesiology.* 2006;104(5):1081-1093.
- American Society of Anesthesiologists. *Standards for Post-anesthesia Care, Approved October 27, 2004, Amended October 21, 2009.* Available at: http://asahq.org/publicationsAndServices/standards/36.pdf. Accessed June 8, 2010.
- Apfelbaum JL, Walawander CA, Grasela TH, et al. Eliminating intensive postoperative care in same-day surgery patients using short-acting anesthetics. *Anesthesiology.* 2002;97:66-74.
- Awad I, Chung F. Factors affecting recovery and discharge following ambulatory surgery. *Can J Anesth.* 2006;53(9):858-872.
- Chung F, Mezei G, Tong D. Pre-existing medical conditions as predictors of adverse events in day-case surgery. *Br J Anaesth.* 1999;83:262-270.
- Gan TJ, Meyer TA, Apfel CC et al. Society for Ambulatory Anesthesia guidelines for the management of postoperative nausea and vomiting. *Anesth Analg.* 2007;105(6):1615-1628.
- Gupta A, Stierer T, Zuckerman R, et al. Comparison of recovery profile after ambulatory anesthesia with propofol, sevoflurane, and desflurane: a systematic review. *Anesth Analg.* 2004;98: 632-641.
- Ilfield BM. *Lecture: Outpatient Perineural Catheters: Who, When and How?* Given at the American Society of Regional Anesthesia meeting, April 2010.
- Ring WH, Wong HC. Designing and administering an outpatient facility. *Problems Anesthes.* 1988;2(1):1-8.
- Roizen MF, Kaplan EB, Schreider BD, et al. The Relative roles of history and physical examination, and laboratory testing in preoperative evaluation for outpatient surgery: the "Starling" curve of preoperative laboratory testing. *Anesth Clin North America* 1987;5(1):15-34.
- Skledar, SJ, Williams BA, Vallejo MC et al. Eliminating postoperative nausa and vomiting in outpatient surgery with multimodal strategies including low doses of nonsedating, off patent antiemetics: is "zero tolerance" achievable? *Sci World J.* 2007;7:959-977.
- Warner MA, Shields SE, Chute CG. Major morbidity and mortality within 1 month of ambulatory surgery and anesthesia. *JAMA* 1993;270(12):1437-1441.
- White PF, Song D. New criteria for fast-tracking after outpatient anesthesia: a comparison with the modified Aldrete's scoring system. *Anesth Analg.* 1999;88:1069-1072.

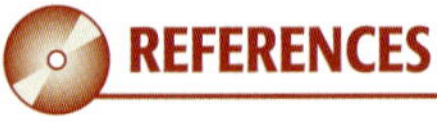

REFERENCES

Complete references available on DVD and online version at www.LongneckerAnesthesiology.com

CHAPTER 69 Monitored Anesthesia Care and Anesthesia Outside the Operating Room

Basem Abdelmalak
Ihab Riad

KEY POINTS

1. Many patients who are scheduled for monitored anesthesia care (MAC) are considered high risk for general anesthesia, and MAC is mistakenly presumed to be safer than general anesthesia.
2. MAC does not describe the continuum of depth of sedation; rather, it describes a specific anesthesia service in which an anesthesiologist has been requested to participate in the care of a patient undergoing a diagnostic or therapeutic procedure.
3. Many patients who are considered for minimally invasive procedures out of the operating room (OR) are considered high risk for traditional surgical procedures.
4. For deep sedation/MAC, proper choice of sedatives and their dosing can optimize patient safety, recovery, and discharge times.
5. The same monitoring and equipment, preprocedure evaluation, NPO (nothing by mouth) status, and recovery room standards used in the OR apply to remote locations.
6. The length and type of procedure, airway considerations, and remoteness of the location should all be considered when choosing the anesthetic technique.
7. Patient safety should supersede any other considerations in remote location anesthesia.
8. Open communication between the anesthesiologist and the proceduralist is key to safety and favorable outcomes.
9. Propofol sedation is classified as deep sedation in many circumstances. It may result in significant changes in airway anatomy and cardiopulmonary physiology. Therefore, propofol should be administered only by clinicians qualified to rescue patients from any level of sedation, including general anesthesia.
10. Involvement of the anesthesiologists in institutional sedation policy and in planning and developing remote anesthesia locations is essential.

INTRODUCTION

Recent advances in medical practices such as imaging and minimally invasive diagnostic and therapeutic procedures have led to an exponential growth in the need for anesthesia services outside of the operating room (OR); so-called remote anesthesia. Each area presents unique challenges for the anesthesia care team (eg, the patient population served, the nature of the location, the procedures performed). The trend of expanding the range of procedures outside of the OR will continue, and the demand for anesthesia services in these locations will grow. For these reasons, anesthesia care teams must become involved in the care of patients and in the details of the procedural area into which they are called to provide their services. This includes ensuring that the same standards and codes that govern the OR and the recovery of patients from anesthesia are present in these remote locations before administration of an anesthetic.[1]

A variety of anesthetics have been successfully used for these procedures. A very commonly used technique is monitored anesthesia care (MAC). This chapter reviews the concept, definitions, and details of the MAC technique; the common procedures performed out of the OR, which often require the expertise of trained anesthesia personnel; and the specific challenges faced by the anesthesia care team in remote areas. Because these issues have been of great interest to anesthesia providers in general and anesthesiologists in particular, the American Society of Anesthesiologists (ASA) has issued many relevant and useful position statements and practice guidelines related to MAC and remote anesthesia care; this chapter also reviews these.

MONITORED ANESTHESIA CARE AND CONSCIOUS SEDATION

DEFINITIONS

Monitored Anesthesia Care *Monitored anesthesia care* does not describe the continuum of depth of sedation; rather, it describes a specific anesthesia service in which an anesthesiologist has been requested to participate in the care of a patient undergoing a diagnostic or therapeutic procedure.[2]

Monitored anesthesia care was defined by the ASA in 2008 as a specific anesthesia service for a diagnostic or therapeutic procedure.[3]

Indications for MAC include the nature of the procedure, the patient's clinical condition, or the potential need to convert to a general or regional anesthetic. MAC includes all aspects of anesthesia care: a preprocedure evaluation, intraprocedure care, and postprocedure anesthesia management. During MAC, the anesthesiologist provides or medically directs a number of specific services, including but not limited to:

- Diagnosis and treatment of clinical problems that occur during the procedure
- Support of vital functions
- Administration of sedatives, analgesics, hypnotics, anesthetic agents, or other medications as necessary for patient safety
- Psychologic support and physical comfort
- Provision of other medical services as needed to complete the procedure safely

Monitored anesthesia care may include varying levels of sedation (**Table 69-1**), analgesia, and anxiolysis as necessary. The provider of MAC must be prepared and qualified to convert to general anesthesia when necessary. For instance, if the patient loses consciousness and the ability to respond purposefully, anesthesia care must then convert to a general anesthetic, regardless of whether airway instrumentation is used or not.

Moderate Sedation (Conscious Sedation) Moderate sedation is a drug-induced depression of consciousness during which patients respond purposefully to verbal commands, either alone or accompanied by light tactile stimulation. No interventions are required to maintain a patent airway, and spontaneous ventilation is adequate. Cardiovascular function is usually maintained.[2]

Deep Sedation Deep sedation/analgesia is a drug-induced depression of consciousness during which patients cannot be easily aroused but respond purposefully after repeated or painful stimulation. The ability to independently maintain ventilatory function may be impaired. Patients may require assistance in maintaining a patent airway, and spontaneous ventilation may be inadequate. Cardiovascular function is usually maintained.[2]

General Anesthesia General anesthesia is a drug-induced loss of consciousness during which patients are not arousable, even by painful stimulation. The ability to independently maintain ventilatory function is often impaired. Patients often require assistance in maintaining a patent airway, and positive-pressure ventilation may be required because of depressed spontaneous ventilation or drug-induced depression of neuromuscular function. Cardiovascular function may be impaired.[2]

GUIDELINES AND STATEMENTS

The ASA issued a statement on granting privileges to a non-anesthesiologist practitioner for personally administering deep sedation or for supervising deep sedation by individuals who are not anesthesia professionals.[4] It should be noted that because of the significant risk that patients who receive deep sedation may enter a state of general anesthesia, privileges to administer deep sedation should be granted only to practitioners who are qualified to administer general anesthesia or to appropriately supervised anesthesia professionals.

Another important ASA statement issued on granting privileges to a non-anesthesiologist practitioner for administering moderate sedation[5] expressed genuine concern that individuals, however well intentioned, who are not anesthesia professionals may not recognize that sedation and general anesthesia lie on a continuum and thus deliver levels of sedation that in fact represent general anesthesia; however, they lack the training and experience to recognize this state and respond appropriately. Because of this concern, the ASA suggested a framework for granting privileges that would help ensure competence of individuals who administer or supervise the administration of moderate sedation. The aim of this statement is to assist health care organizations develop a program for granting privileges for providing moderate sedation.

Additional important points from the statement:

Only physicians, dentists, or pediatrists who are qualified by education, training, and licensure to administer moderate sedation should supervise the administration of moderate sedation. These practitioners should have completed formal training in the safe administration of sedative and analgesic drugs and in rescuing patients who exhibit adverse physiologic consequences of a deeper-than-intended level of sedation. Additional stipulations are that practitioners:

- Have the skills necessary for obtaining the patient's medical history and performing a physical examination to assess risks and comorbidities.
- Be able to assess the patient's risk for aspiration of gastric contents.
- Understand the pharmacology of all sedative and analgesic drugs the practitioner requests privileges to administer and their pharmacologic antagonists, vasoactive drugs, and antiarrhythmics.
- Understand the benefits and risks of supplemental oxygen.

TABLE 69-1 American Society of Anesthesiologists Definitions of General Anesthesia and Levels of Sedation and Analgesia

	Minimal Sedation (Anxiolysis)	Moderate Sedation/Analgesia (Conscious Sedation)	Deep Sedation/Analgesia	General Anesthesia
Responsiveness	Normal response to verbal stimulation	Purposeful response to verbal or tactile stimulation	Purposeful response after repeated or painful stimulation	Unarousable even with painful stimulation
Airway	Unaffected	No intervention required	Intervention may be required	Intervention often required
Spontaneous ventilation	Unaffected	Adequate	May be inadequate	Frequently inadequate
Cardiovascular function	Unaffected	Usually maintained	Usually maintained	May be impaired

Adapted with permission from American Society of Anesthesiologists. *Continuum of Depth of Sedation: Definition of General Anesthesia and Levels of Sedation/Analgesia.* Approved by ASA House of Delegates on October 13, 1999, and last amended on October 21, 2009.

- Be proficient in airway management with facemask and positive-pressure ventilation.
- Monitor physiologic variables.
- Document the drugs administered and at regular intervals monitor the patient's level of sedation and physiologic condition.

Fasting Guidelines Because it is frequently not easy to predict the level of a patient's responsiveness to sedatives and because the sedation is a continuum, in which deeper levels of sedation might end up with a state of general anesthesia, it is recommended that the same NPO (nothing per os) guidelines for general anesthesia be followed in MAC cases. In urgent or emergent cases, the risk of pulmonary aspiration should be considered when determining the required level of sedation.

Preprocedure Evaluation Preprocedure evaluation of the patient is crucial in determining the risk factors related to the patient's condition and also to anesthesia.

Some MAC cases are treated outside ORs; therefore, preprocedural evaluation of the place where the planned procedure will be performed is also of great importance. In many instances, patients undergoing interventional procedures are deemed to be at high risk for surgery because of multiple comorbid conditions or a specific life-threatening condition. Nevertheless, regardless of the anesthetic technique planned, these patients should receive the same level of attention given to patients being prepared for a surgical procedure in the main OR (MOR) pavilion. Focused history (major illnesses, medication allergies, NPO status, and previous anesthesia complications) and physical examination (mainly cardiovascular, respiratory, and airway) are mandatory. Relevant laboratory studies and other investigations (eg, electrocardiography [ECG], chest radiographs) should be reviewed. Patient counseling before the start of the procedure is vital to the success of the planned procedure and the anesthesia care. A patient who is well informed of the entire plan regarding MAC and who knows what to expect regarding the level of consciousness and awareness during the procedure is a more satisfied patient. Not all patients are candidates for MAC. The preprocedure visit is also important to determine candidacy for MAC.

Candidacy for Monitored Anesthesia Care Procedures performed under MAC primarily depend on the patient's cooperation and motivation, as well as on the nature of the procedure being performed.

Mild to moderate sedation can actually disinhibit a patient's response to painful stimulation; therefore, if adequate local or regional anesthesia is unavailable for a patient who must undergo a painful procedure, MAC cannot be implemented successfully.

Although MAC carries no absolute contraindications, it may be unsuitable for the following patients and under the following conditions:

- Pediatric patients
- Patients without full mental capacity
- Intoxicated patients
- Patients with a condition that inhibits them from lying still for the period of time needed for the procedure
- Language barrier between the patient and the provider
- Psychotic or uncooperative patients
- Medically unstable patient, such as a patient with congestive heart failure, who is scheduled for an emergency procedure that requires supine position and the patient has orthopnea and cannot lie supine, although the procedure requires a supine position
- Patient with a suspected or known difficult airway; for instance, the airway may be difficult to monitor because of the position required or the nature of the procedure
- Excessively long procedures
- Procedures performed in an uncomfortable position. (eg, prone, lithotomy, kidney rest, and kneeling positions)
- Procedures in which a large volume blood loss or cardiorespiratory instability is expected
- Procedures in which even minor movement could be hazardous to the patient.

Intraoperative Monitoring Standards for intraoperative monitoring of cases performed under MAC should be identical to those performed under general or regional anesthesia. These standards would naturally extend to providing anesthesia in settings outside the ORs as well.

Monitoring Depth of Sedation During Monitored Anesthesia Care Accurate assessment of sedation depth is important in minimizing the risks of MAC and procedural sedation both inside and outside the OR. Many patients, particularly the elderly and very ill patients, may rapidly move from a plane of light sedation to obtundation. Practitioners should have the means to effectively monitor depth of sedation. Because the direct effect of sedatives and hypnotics on the brain cannot be measured, clinicians usually rely on indirect measures of the level of sedation, such as frequent patient stimulation (eg, Observer's Assessment of Alertness/Sedation Scale (OAA/S), **Table 69-2**) to measure the depth of sedation. These techniques, however, require persistent patient cooperation and are subject to testing fatigue. Additionally, there are procedures and cases during which periodical patient movement and speech might preclude the successful completion of the procedure. Also, clinicians traditionally have relied on subjective measures or autonomic signs of patient responsiveness to judge depth of sedation and analgesia. However, changes in autonomic signs (eg, hypertension and tachycardia) do not reliably predict awareness and discomfort during general anesthesia.[6-8]

An objective measure of sedation depth theoretically could decrease the incidence of patients being undersedated and oversedated, reduce anesthetic wastage, and shorten recovery and discharge times. Because the brain is the target of anesthetic action, and electrical activity of the cerebral cortex can be measured via electroencephalography (EEG), most depth-of-anesthesia monitors have focused on measuring changes in the EEG. The Bispectral Index Scale (BIS) was the first clinically

TABLE 69-2 Observer's Assessment of Alertness and Sedation Scale

Assessment Categories

Responsiveness	Speech	Facial Expression	Eyes	Composite Score Level
Responds readily to name spoken in normal tone	Normal	Normal	Clear, no ptosis	5
Lethargic response to name spoken in normal tone	Mild slowing or thickening	Mild relaxation	Glazed or mild ptosis (less than half the eye)	4
Responds only after name is called loudly or repeatedly	Slurring or prominent slowing	Marked relaxation	Glazed and marked ptosis (half the eye or more)	3
Responds only after mild prodding or shaking	Few recognizable words			2
Does not respond to mild prodding or shaking				1

available depth-of-anesthesia monitoring device. The BIS is a proprietary algorithm (Aspect Medical Systems, Newton, MA) that generates a linear dimensionless number ranging from 0 to 100 that decreases in proportion to increased anesthetic depth. The BIS does not correlate with movement, heart rate, or blood pressure. Although the BIS has been used more commonly during general anesthesia, it has been evaluated measuring the depth of sedation with propofol,[9,10] midazolam,[8] and even sevoflurane.[11] During propofol-induced sedation, the BIS was shown to correlate with OAA/S scores,[10,12] loss of response to verbal commands,[9] suppression of learning,[13] and propofol blood concentrations.[13] Gan and colleagues[14] demonstrated faster recovery times and decreased propofol usage with the addition of the BIS monitor, although formal cost-effectiveness studies during MAC or regional anesthesia have not been undertaken. Furthermore, BIS monitoring accurately and objectively measures patient sedation level during endoscopy[15] and during procedural sedation in the emergency department (ED).[16] In contrast to the targeted BIS readings for patients undergoing general anesthesia (BIS values 40-60), BIS readings of 60 to 80 are targeted during MAC. BIS values approaching 60 are associated with a low probability of recall.[9,10,17] However, recall is impaired at much higher BIS values than is response to command.[18] It is important to realize that BIS measurements are slightly dependent on the type of anesthetic agents used. Several authors have shown higher BIS values for loss of consciousness when opioids were added to an anesthetic.[11,18,19] This phenomenon, which extends to other agents (eg, ketamine, nitrous oxide), exists because noncortical structures underrepresented in the EEG contribute to the mechanism of hypnosis and sedation with opioids.[20] It should be noted that ketamine can cause loss of response to verbal command in doses as low as 0.25 mg/kg without altering BIS measurements.[21] It also has been suggested that spinal and epidural anesthesia may affect BIS measurements independently of other anesthetics.[22,23] Morley and colleagues[22] demonstrated a small but detectable EEG suppression in patients receiving spinal anesthesia without concomitant intravenous (IV) sedation. The mechanism appears to be related to decreased afferent stimulation of the reticular activating system and is independent of block level.

A priori, the authors believe there is a selective subset of patients undergoing MAC in whom BIS monitoring is a valuable adjunctive clinical monitor to standard clinical evaluation. BIS monitoring would probably be particularly beneficial during procedures in which patients should not move or speak, procedures of prolonged duration, and procedures involving patients of advanced age or ill health. Whenever possible, patients should be monitored via behavioral methods (eg, continual assessment of response to commands) in addition to the BIS. Because both the general public and many non-anesthesiologists have difficulty distinguishing between deep levels of sedation and general anesthesia, it is advisable to discuss patient concerns about "awareness" or "being awake" during the patient's preanesthetic assessment and interview. Patients insisting on guaranteed amnesia and hypnosis for procedures under MAC should be offered general anesthesia if feasible.

MINIMAL REQUIREMENTS FOR ANESTHESIA IN REMOTE LOCATIONS

SPACE ALLOCATION AND EQUIPMENT NEEDS

The ASA has published a statement that includes the following[24]:

- Availability of a reliable oxygen source and delivery method (nasal cannulas, face masks), along with backup supply of oxygen in the form of a full E cylinder
- Availability of adequate suction
- Ability to scavenge waste gases when inhaled anesthetic agents are required
- Presence of a self-inflating resuscitator bag that can administer at least 90% oxygen and deliver positive-pressure ventilation in the event of respiratory distress
- Adequate anesthetic drugs, monitoring equipment, and supplies for the duration of the case
- Adequate lighting and electrical outlets for proper visualization and operation of anesthesia equipment
- Availability of sufficient space for the anesthesia provider and any other necessary personnel, as well as unobstructed access to the patient, anesthesia equipment, and emergency supplies
- Emergency cart with a defibrillator and emergency drugs for cardiopulmonary resuscitation
- Observance of all applicable building codes and facility standards
- Availability of adequately trained staff for immediate assistance of the anesthesia provider, as well as reliable two-way communication with which to request additional assistance
- Provision of adequate postanesthesia care, which should include appropriately trained staff and equipment that ensures safe transport of the patient to the designated recovery area

After these conditions have been met, the anesthesia caregiver can focus on the actual care of the patient undergoing the proposed procedure.

COMMONLY USED PHARMACOLOGIC AGENTS

An ideal sedative should have the following properties:

- Easy titration
- Potent sedative and amnestic agent with analgesic properties
- Rapid onset with predictable pharmacodynamics and pharmacokinetics
- Rapid recovery with no residual effect
- High safety profile with cardiorespiratory stability
- Painless injection

Unfortunately, this sedative has yet to be discovered, although the commonly used sedatives posses some but not all of these properties.

PROPOFOL

Propofol is the most commonly used agent for IV induction of general anesthesia in the United States. It is also commonly used for maintenance of general anesthesia, for sedation in MAC cases, and for sedation of critically ill patients in intensive care units (ICUs). Because sedation is a continuum, it is not always possible to predict how an individual patient will respond. Accordingly, agents such as propofol require special attention because of the potential for rapid, profound changes in sedative and anesthetic depth, and the lack of antagonist medications. Even if moderate sedation is intended, patients receiving propofol should receive care consistent with that required for deep sedation. Propofol has the advantages of rapid onset and short recovery time,[25-27] easy titration, and antiemetic action. However, it may inhibit hypoxic ventilatory drive and depress the normal response to hypercarbia; moreover, at higher doses, it can cause apnea and inhibit airway protective reflexes. Additionally, it has a hypotensive effect and may induce pain on injection, and prolonged infusion may result in propofol infusion syndrome.[28] This syndrome is of greater concern in the ICU than in the procedural sedation setting.

BENZODIAZEPINES

Midazolam, diazepam, and lorazepam are the three benzodiazepines commonly used in anesthesia. The benzodiazepines are used primarily for anxiolysis and amnesia as well as for moderate sedation in MAC cases. Midazolam can be administered orally, intranasally, intramuscularly, or intravenously. It can be used as a bolus IV dose or continuous IV infusion. The onset of action as well as duration of action of midazolam depend on its route of administration as well as the dose given; it is also affected by concurrent administration of other medications. Several studies pointed out the effectiveness of midazolam in the prevention of nausea and vomiting.[29-31] However, midazolam has no analgesic properties, so it is generally used with other opioids during MAC cases.

After a single dose of IV midazolam, the peak effect is reached in 2 to 3 minutes, and the duration varies depending on the dose and on the age and condition of the patient. Incremental doses of 0.5 to 1 mg of IV midazolam are usually given every 2 to 3 minutes to reach the desired level of sedation. The oral dose is 5 to 15 mg for adults and 0.5 to 0.75 mg/kg for pediatric patients. Midazolam can be used as a continuous infusion with a dose 1 to 2 mcg/kg/min.

Among midazolam's many advantages are that it causes less respiratory depression than with other sedatives at the desired levels of sedation; has a reliable anxiolysis and amnestic action; prevents nausea and vomiting; and elevates seizure threshold, which increases the safety of local anesthetics used.

OPIOIDS

Opioid analgesics have been the mainstay of pain control for thousands of years; they mimic the effects of endogenous substances known as endorphins. Because of the unreliable amnestic effect of opioids, they are usually used in conjunction with other sedatives such as benzodiazepines in MAC cases. In MAC cases, opioids play an important role in providing analgesia in conjunction with local anesthetics. Opioids exert their analgesic action at the brain 32 as well as at the spinal cord levels.[33] The peripheral analgesic effects of opioids have also been described (**Table 69-3**).[34,35] Opioids may cause pruritus, nausea and vomiting, and respiratory depression even in doses too small to disturb the level of consciousness. More importantly, they can induce chest wall rigidity that is severe enough to compromise respiration; however, this can be treated by induction of general anesthesia and muscle relaxation.

TABLE 69-3 Classification of Opioid Receptor Subtypes and Actions From Animal Models

	Receptor Subtype	Actions of: Agonist	Antagonist
Analgesia			
Supraspinal	μ, κ, δ	Analgesic	No effect
Spinal	μ, κ, δ	Analgesic	No effect
Respiratory function	μ	Decrease	No effect
Gastrointestinal tract	μ, κ	Decrease transit	No effect
Psychotomimesis	κ	Increase	No effect
Feeding	μ, κ, δ	Increase feeding	Decrease feeding
Sedation	μ, κ	Increase	No effect
Diuresis	κ	Increase	
Hormone regulation			
Prolactin	μ	Increase release	Decrease release
Growth hormone	μ and/or δ	Increase release	Decrease release
Neurotransmitter release			
Acetylcholine	μ	Inhibit	
Dopamine	μ, δ	Inhibit	
Isolated organ bioassays			
Guinea pig ileum	μ	Decrease contraction	No effect
Mouse vas deferens	δ	Decrease contraction	No effect

From Gutstein HB, Akil H. Opioid analgesics. In Brunton LL, Lazo JS, Parker KL, eds. *Goodman and Gilman's The Pharmacological Basis of Therapeutics*. 11th ed. New York, NY: McGraw-Hill; 2005.

Individual Opioids

Morphine Morphine has a delayed onset and prolonged duration of analgesia. These two properties may render morphine a poor choice for MAC cases in which rapid titration to effect is desired. Morphine in small doses intraoperatively administered may be suitable to provide prolonged postprocedure analgesia if significant pain is anticipated postoperatively.

Meperidine Meperidine 50 to 100 mg IV together with diazepam were commonly used agents in procedure sedation in the early days of gastrointestinal (GI) endoscopies when sedation was ordered by the endoscopist and administered by the nurse.[36] Meperidine was the most commonly used medication in the GI suite about 20 years ago.[37] However, in today's practice, when anesthesiologists are more involved in the care of these patients and the number of MAC cases has increased, meperidine is used less often, and other opioids with faster onsets and shorter durations of action (eg, fentanyl, remifentanil, alfentanil, and sufentanil) are being used more often. Meperidine has an atropine-like action, inducing tachycardia, which can confuse the picture during sedation because it might be interpreted as patient discomfort. Also, its central cholinergic actions are undesirable. On the other hand, the advantage of meperidine lies in its anti-shivering action, which can be beneficial in MAC cases. Meperidine in a dose of 12.5 to 25 mg IV is effective for the relief of shivering.

Fentanyl Fentanyl is still one of the most commonly used analgesics in MAC cases. Fentanyl can be used as a bolus dose or as a continuous infusion. Fentanyl's safety and potency as an analgesic and as a sedative rendered it an attractive choice for anesthesiologists as well as non-anesthesiologists for procedural sedation in the ED,[38-40] radiology, and endoscopy suites. Fentanyl has the advantage of easy titration if given in repeated boluses (0.5-1 mcg/kg) or as a continuous infusion (0.01-0.05 mcg/kg/min).

Remifentanil, Alfentanil, and Sufentanil Relatively newer rapid-onset, short-acting synthetic opioids have gained a place in modern anesthesia in general anesthesia as well as MAC cases. These newer agents have the advantage of easy titration as well as potency. The relative potency ratios for fentanyl, sufentanil, alfentanil, and remifentanil, to each other are approximately 1:12:0.0625:1.2, respectively.[41]

Usually, these potent short-acting opioids are used as continuous infusion with or without an initial bolus dose. Remifentanil was evaluated as a sole agent for procedural sedation and resulted in good patient and practitioner satisfaction,[42] but patients' recall of the procedure was high, although not usually unpleasant, and respiratory depression was common. Remifentanil usually is used in combination with other sedatives such as propofol or midazolam, and much experience has been documented with these combinations.[43,44] Remifentanil is usually given in a bolus dose of 0.5 to 1 mcg/kg, a dose that can be repeated, and the continuous infusion rate is usually 0.05 to 0.1 mcg/kg/min.

Alfentanil is significantly less potent than fentanyl or remifentanil and has been successfully used for sedation when combined with propofol. It is another rapid-onset, short-acting medication that can be administered in bolus doses or continuous infusion. The usual bolus dose of alfentanil is 5 to 10 μ/kg, which can be repeated in 1.5-μ/kg increments. The infusion rate for alfentanil sedation is usually 0.25 to 1.0 μ/kg/min.

Both remifentanil and alfentanil are associated with significant postprocedure pain because of their short durations of action, so traditionally, another longer-acting analgesic is recommended to be given during the procedure, especially when significant postoperative pain is anticipated.[45]

Sufentanil is the most potent synthetic opioid. It is approximately 5 to 15 times more potent than fentanyl and has a similar onset of action. Both sufentanil and fentanyl are formulated with the same concentration (50 mcg/mL), and an overdose resulting in severe respiratory depression could occur if sufentanil were mistaken for fentanyl. Sufentanil can be given as a bolus (0.1-0.5 mcg/kg) or infusion (0.005-0.01 mcg/kg/min) during MAC. Bailey and colleagues[46] compared the effects of sufentanil and fentanyl on volunteers and showed that sufentanil produced longer lasting analgesia but less depression of ventilation than did fentanyl. Few other studies have focused on sufentanil in the setting of MAC, particularly since the advent of alfentanil and remifentanil. One possible reason for the dearth of studies lies in the unpredictable cardiovascular depression associated with sufentanil use, including bradycardia and hypotension, especially because these effects do not appear to be dose dependent.[47]

KETAMINE

Ketamine is a phencyclidine derivative that produces profound analgesia, amnesia and sedation, and bronchodilatation. It usually preserves spontaneous breathing, cardiovascular stability, and airway reflexes. However, in larger doses, ketamine can produce hypoventilation and even a short period of apnea.[48] When added to N_2O and fentanyl, ketamine produces a state of dissociative anesthesia, a form of general anesthesia characterized by catalepsy, catatonia, and amnesia but not necessarily involving complete unconsciousness.

In low doses, ketamine elevates the pain threshold, causing analgesia. Ketamine's analgesic action lasts through the postprocedure period. The IV induction dose of ketamine is 2 mg/kg; below this dose (0.2-0.8 mg/kg), ketamine has a sedative and analgesic effect. After a single IV dose of ketamine, its onset of action is 30 to 60 seconds, and its peak effect occurs in 1 minute, with a 15-minute duration of action. The use of ketamine was limited because of the high incidence of emergence phenomena (10%-20%)[49] in which there is postoperative disorientation, sensory and perceptual illusions, and vivid dreams. Emergence reactions can be prevented or attenuated by the coadministration of a benzodiazepine, barbiturate, or propofol with ketamine during sedation.[50-52] In addition, ketamine increases salivation, intracranial pressure, intraocular pressure, and myocardial oxygen consumption.

NEWER SEDATIVES

Dexmedetomidine Dexmedetomidine is a highly selective α_2-adrenergic agonist with sedative and analgesic properties. The Food and Drug Administration (FDA) approved dexmedetomidine in 1999 for short-term use (<24 h) for mechanically ventilated patients in the ICU, but since then, it has gained popularity in procedural sedation and MAC cases. Dexmedetomidine is used as a continuous infusion at a rate of 0.2 to 1 mcg/kg/h with or without an initial loading dose of 0.5 to 1 mcg/kg over 10 to 20 minutes.

After a bolus dose of dexmedetomidine, the onset of action is within 5 to 10 minutes with a peak effect in 15 to 30 minutes and a duration of action 60 to 120 minutes that is dose dependent.

Dexmedetomidine has the unique property of maintaining respiratory stability.[53,54]

Patients sedated with dexmedetomidine are easily arousable and maintain their ability to cooperate with the anesthesia provider, especially during airway instrumentation and awake fiberoptic intubation.[55] It also has moderate analgesic,[56] limited amnestic,[57,58] and antisialagogue properties.[59]

Bradycardia after administration of α_2-agonists is well documented.[60,61] Blood pressure response to dexmedetomidine infusion is reported to be biphasic, with initial brief hypertension followed by more prolonged hypotension.[57] Cardiovascular side effects are more profound in elderly patients, especially with bolus doses and higher infusion rates. A slower onset and delayed recovery compared with propofol were also reported.[62,63]

Fospropofol Fospropofol is a water-soluble prodrug of propofol. Fospropofol liberates propofol by the enzyme alkaline phosphatase. One milligram of fospropofol liberates 0.54 mg of propofol. Because of the conversion of the prodrug to propofol, the time to peak of propofol concentration after a bolus and the elimination of propofol after infusion is longer than for propofol formulated in a lipid emulsion. The recommended fospropofol dose is 4.9 to 6.5 mg/kg IV bolus for individuals who weigh between 60 and 90 kg followed by supplemental doses of 0.25 of the initial dose administered no more frequently than every 4 minutes as needed to achieve desired level of sedation. Patients who weigh less than 60 kg are dosed as if they weigh 60 kg, and those who weigh more than 90 kg are dosed as if they weigh 90 kg. Fospropofol has the advantage over the traditional propofol preparation by being less painful with IV injection as well as no lipid load when prolonged infusion is required.

Side Effects of Fospropofol Side effects of fospropofol include:

- Pruritus (incidence, 8%-28%), including genital, perineal, and generalized pruritus
- Paresthesia (incidence, 52%-74% percent), including perineal discomfort or a burning sensation
- Mild risk of hypoxemia, headache, and hypotension

Clinical experience with fospropofol remains limited, but the safety margin is apparently good.

The FDA-approved package insert of fospropofol states as follows [64]: "Lusedra [fospropofol disodium] should be administered only by persons trained in the administration of general anesthesia and not involved in the conduct of the diagnostic or therapeutic procedure. Minimal requirement for MAC applies here as well."

ADJUVANT MEDICATIONS DURING MONITORED ANESTHESIA CARE

ANTIEMETICS AND ANTINAUSEA MEDICATIONS

Postprocedure nausea and vomiting are less likely to occur with MAC cases because the effects of inhalational anesthetics are absent. However, nausea and vomiting may occur because of the stress of the procedure, the procedure itself (such as GI endoscopies and ophthalmic procedures), or the sedatives or analgesics (opioids) used. Postprocedure nausea and vomiting might explain patient dissatisfaction as well as a delayed discharge.

Commonly used medications for the prevention and treatment of postprocedure nausea and vomiting are dopamine antagonists, histamine antagonists, serotonin antagonists, anticholinergics, neurokinin antagonists, and dexamethasone. These medications can be used before, during, or after the procedure, depending on the relative risk of a patient to develop postoperative nausea and vomiting. Care should be taken with the sedative properties of some of these agents, especially in elderly patients.

ANALGESICS

A postprocedure pain control plan should be considered during MAC cases to provide analgesic coverage when the effect of the local anesthetic used for the procedure, as well as the sedatives and analgesics used during the procedure, wear off. Opioids as well as nonsteroidal anti-inflammatory drugs are good agents for controlling postprocedure pain.

COMMON MONITORED ANESTHESIA CARE TECHNIQUES

INTERMITTENT BOLUS TECHNIQUE

Different techniques have been used in MAC to administer sedatives and analgesics. Of these, the simplest and most commonly used is the intermittent bolus technique in which the medications are intermittently administered by the anesthesia provider to titrate to a desired level of sedation.

The advantage of this technique lies in its simplicity; however, that might not be the case with the newer agents with higher potencies and short durations of action, which can result in over- or undersedation. This technique is suitable for minor procedures of short duration when relatively longer-acting sedatives such as benzodiazepines and opioids are used; it is also suitable for use in younger healthy patients for whom the safety margins with medications are wider than for chronically debilitated elderly patients who may be oversensitive to the load of a bolus medication.

CONTINUOUS INFUSION TECHNIQUE

Conventionally, IV anesthetics have been administered as a large bolus or by multiple intermittent doses during a procedure. However, clinical studies have demonstrated that IV anesthetics given by variable-rate continuous infusion provide certain advantages over intermittent bolus techniques. They include (1) improved cardiopulmonary stability, (2) more predictable plasma drug concentrations, (3) reduced need for supplemental anesthetics or vasoactive drugs, (4) faster recovery times, and (5) lower total drug doses used.[65,66]

TARGET-CONTROLLED INFUSIONS

In 1983, Schuttler and colleagues[67] used a computer-assisted infusion system to administer a constant plasma concentration of alfentanil and etomidate for surgical anesthesia. At the time, the concept was novel because drugs usually were dosed at a constant infusion rate regardless of expected changes in plasma concentrations over time. Many research groups have since developed their own systems for a variety of anesthetics. By delivering a target concentration of a drug rather than a target infusion rate, these target-controlled infusion (TCI) systems can effectively and rapidly achieve, maintain, and adapt plasma concentrations of drugs to changing patient and surgical needs.

A TCI device is a computerized infusion pump in which the selected drug is administered according to its known therapeutic window, the patient response, and the predicted (via computer modeling) drug concentration. The computer is programmed with a pharmacokinetic model as well as pharmacokinetic data. The computer automatically controls the infusion pump to maintain the target plasma concentration. Target concentrations can be increased or decreased over time based on clinical need.[68]

Pharmacokinetic data used in TCI systems have generally been derived from the literature, and the effectiveness and accuracy of TCI systems depend on such data. Most of these pharmacokinetic parameters are derived from small sample sizes of healthy individuals.[69]

There is considerable interpatient variability in both pharmacokinetics and pharmacodynamics. Compared with standard infusion pumps, TCI systems allow the incorporation of patient covariates (eg, weight, age, hepatic function, cardiac output) into dosing models that would otherwise be impossible to replicate without TCI systems.

RECOVERY AND DISCHARGE CRITERIA AFTER MONITORED ANESTHESIA CARE

Anesthetics used during MAC should permit rapid recovery with minimal or no residual cognitive or psychomotor impairment. At the same time, each patient care facility should develop recovery and discharge criteria that are suitable for its specific patients and procedures. Recovery and discharge criteria for MAC should be no different from those for general or regional anesthesia.[70]

Physicians should be able to assess home readiness in a simple, clear, reproducible manner. Medicolegal considerations mandate that physicians have evidence that the patient's discharge criteria were met (**Tables 69-4** and **69-5**) and that all discharge instructions have been signed by the patient and documented in the medical record. Patients should be duly informed that home readiness does not confer the ability to drive a car or return to work.

MISPERCEPTION OF MONITORED ANESTHESIA CARE SAFETY

Although MAC is generally believed to be much simpler and safer than general anesthesia or regional anesthesia, this perception is unfounded, according to the ASA Closed Claims study published in 2006.[71] The study was based on 7000 claims obtained from 35 professional liability insurance companies in the United States over a period of almost 20 years. Of 1952 claims for surgical anesthesia in the analysis, 121 claims (6%) were associated with MAC, 1519 (78%) were associated with general anesthesia, and 312 (16%) were

TABLE 69-4 Aldrete Postanesthetic Recovery Score

Activity: Able to Move Voluntarily or on Command	
4 extremities	2
2 extremities	1
0 extremities	0
Respiration	
Able to deep breathe and cough freely	2
Dyspnea; shallow or limited breathing	1
Apneic	0
Circulation	
BP ± 20 mm of preanesthesia level	2
BP ± 20-50 mm of preanesthesia level	1
BP ± 50 mm of preanesthesia level	0
Consciousness	
Fully awake	2
Arousable on calling	1
Not responding	0
Color	
Normal	2
Pale, dusky, blotchy	1
Cyanotic	0

BP, blood pressure.

Adapted with permission from, Aldrete JA, Kroulik D. A postanesthetic recovery score. *Anesth Analg.* 1970;49;924-934.

TABLE 69-5 Postanesthesia Discharge Scoring System[a]

Vital Signs	
2	Within 20% of preoperative value
1	20%-40% of preoperative value
0	40% of preoperative value
Activity, Mental Status	
2	Oriented and steady gait
1	Oriented or steady gait
0	Neither
Pain, Nausea, Vomiting	
2	Minimal
1	Moderate
0	Severe
Surgical Bleeding	
2	Minimal
1	Moderate
0	Severe
Intake and Output	
2	PO fluids and voided
1	PO fluids or voided
0	Neither

PO, per os (by mouth).

[a]The total score is 10; patients scoring ≥9 are considered fit for discharge to home.

Reprinted from Chung F, Chan VW, Ong D. A post-anesthetic discharge scoring system for home readiness after ambulatory surgery. *J Clin Anesth.* 1995;7:500-506, with permission from Elsevier.

TABLE 69-6 Patient and Case Characteristics in the American Society of Anesthesiologists Closed Claims Study

	MAC (n = 121), n (%)	GA (n = 1519), n (%)	RA (n = 312), n (%)
Age, y			
Mean age ± SD	55 ± 19	44 ± 20	55 ± 17
>70 y	31 (26%)	150 (10%)	71 (23%)
<16 y	1 (1%)	140 (9%)	2 (1%)
Sex			
Female	76 (63%)	776 (52%)	150 (48%)
Male	44 (37%)	730 (48%)	161 (52%)
ASA Physical Status			
I, II	48 (48%)	735 (59%)	164 (67%)
III-V	53 (52%)	504 (41%)	79 (33%)
Emergent Procedure			
Emergent	9 (8%)	228 (17%)	26 (9%)
Elective	99 (92%)	1145 (83%)	258 (91%)
Outpatient or Inpatient			
Outpatient	83 (74%)	377 (27%)	142 (51%)
Inpatient	29 (26%)	1004 (73%)	137 (49%)
Surgical Procedure			
Eye surgery	25 (21%)	25 (2%)	45 (14%)
Head, neck, or face repair or superficial biopsy	23 (19%)	69 (5%)	4 (1%)
Endoscopy	9 (7%)	20 (1%)	10 (3%)

ASA, American Society of Anesthesiologists; GA, general anesthesia; MAC, monitored anesthesia care; RA, regional anesthesia; SD, standard deviation.

Adapted with permission from Bhananker SM, Posner KL, Cheney FW, et al. Injury and liability associated with monitored anesthesia care: a closed claims analysis. *Anesthesiology.* 2006;104:228-234.

associated with regional anesthesia. Patients who had undergone procedures under MAC were older and sicker (**Table 69-6**) compared with those who had undergone procedures under general anesthesia or regional anesthesia.

Interestingly, the proportion of claims for death and permanent brain damage was less in regional anesthesia compared with MAC (14% vs 33% for death and 8% vs 7% for brain damage, respectively). In contrast, the severity of injury was similar between MAC claims and those associated with general anesthesia (27% death and 10% brain damage; **Fig. 69-1**). Respiratory events were in similar proportions for MAC (41%) and general anesthesia (44%) claims but were much smaller for regional anesthesia claims (6%) (**Table 69-7**). Of these events, inadequate ventilation or oxygenation was the most common respiratory event in MAC cases, in which the patients were heavily sedated with a combination of sedative, hypnotic, and analgesic agents; the most common combination was propofol, midazolam, and fentanyl. About 50% of the cases involved procedures performed around the head and neck, which deprived the anesthesiologist of direct access to the patient's airway. Contributing factors entailed inattention to monitors, poorly functioning monitors, or inactive alarms, which caused delay in the recognition of problems and thus failure to intervene in adverse respiratory events. The standard of care was judged by reviewers to be appropriate in only 59% of the MAC claims, which was thus no different from general anesthesia claims. Payment frequency and amounts were similar for all types of anesthesia.

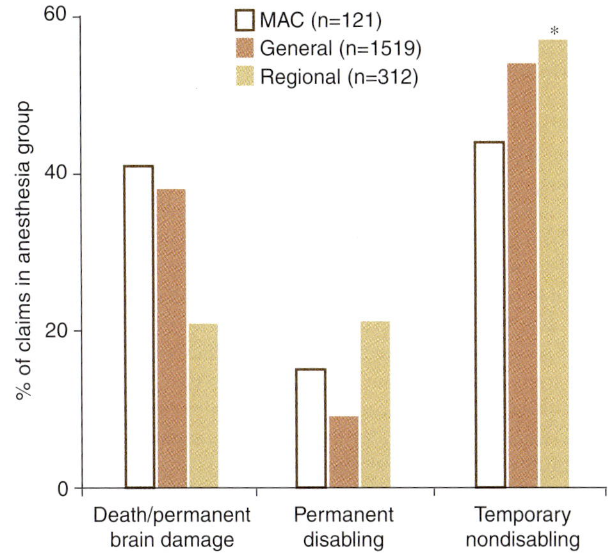

FIGURE 69-1. Severity of injury in monitored anesthesia care (MAC), general anesthesia, and regional anesthesia claims.

COMMON REMOTE PROCEDURAL AREAS

ELECTROCONVULSIVE THERAPY

Electroconvulsive therapy (ECT) is used for treatment of bipolar affective disorder, major depressive episodes, and schizoaffective disorders, which are resistant to medical therapies. Overall, ECT is a relatively safe procedure with a very low incidence of major cardiovascular complications. It involves the induction of generalized seizure activity by introduction of an electrical stimulus through electrodes placed along the temporal area, either unilaterally or bilaterally. Often these procedures are performed in the morning in the postanesthesia care unit (PACU) because this area lies close to the OR, is well equipped, has monitored

TABLE 69-7 Mechanisms of Injury in the American Society of Anesthesiologist Closed Claims Study in Different Anesthetic Techniques

	MAC (n = 121), n (%)	GA (n = 1519), n (%)	RA (n = 312), n (%)
Respiratory event	29 (24%)	337 (22%)	11 (4%)
Inadequate oxygenation or ventilation	22 (18%)	33 (2%)	5 (2%)
Cardiovascular event	17 (14%)	253 (17%)	23 (7%)
Equipment failure or malfunction	25 (21%)	199 (13%)	8 (3%)
Cautery fires	20 (17%)	10 (1%)	1 (0%)
Related to regional block	2 (2%)	7 (0%)	168 (54%)
Inadequate anesthesia/ patient movement	13 (11%)	42 (3%)	7 (2%)
Medication related	11 (9%)	95 (6%)	11 (4%)
Other events	24 (20%)	586 (39%)	84 (27%)

GA, general anesthesia; MAC, monitored anesthesia care; RA, regional anesthesia.

Adapted with permission from Bhananker SM, Posner KL, Cheney FW, et al. Injury and liability associated with monitored anesthesia care: a closed claims analysis. *Anesthesiology.* 2006;104:228-234.

beds, and is staffed with nurses who are very familiar with anesthesia procedures and recovery from it.

Because of the nature of the therapy and the associated physiologic responses to generalized seizures, general anesthesia is required. Many patients have comorbid illnesses in addition to their psychiatric disorders. Although the overall number of procedures performed in the United States is large, morbidity and mortality associated with ECT are surprisingly low. These low rates result primarily from the use of standard monitors during the course of treatments as well as recent advances in pharmacologic agents used for anesthetic management and control of hypertensive and cardiac responses to seizure activity. A large retrospective review by Nuttall and colleagues[72] reported a low incidence of complications associated with anesthesia for ECT. The most notable complications associated with ECT were prolonged seizures, which in this study were successfully treated with benzodiazepines. The goal of the anesthesia provider in the anesthetic management for ECT is to institute adequate airway support, suppress any recall or awareness of the session, and attenuate the physiologic responses to the stimulus. When the patient is ready to begin the session, the appropriate monitors are placed, and oxygen is delivered to the patient via face mask. General anesthesia is induced via an IV induction agent. When the patient loses consciousness, a muscle relaxant, generally succinylcholine, is administered in preparation for the induced seizure. For patients with a pseudocholinesterase deficiency or any contraindications to succinylcholine, a suitable nondepolarizing muscle relaxant is used in place of succinylcholine. When general anesthesia has commenced, the patient's airway and breathing are supported via face mask and positive-pressure ventilation.

The anesthesia provider continues to support respiratory function until the return of spontaneous ventilatory effort by the patient. In some instances, other forms of airway intervention may be necessary, such as endotracheal intubation for patients with severe gastroesophageal reflux disease. Because the ECT treatment course can last from several days to several weeks, any difficulties with the airway should be duly noted for any subsequent sessions and appropriate arrangements made.

Methohexital has been the most widely used induction agent in recent times. All hypnotic agents cause some reduction in seizure activity, but methohexital affects such activity to a lesser degree than the other agents. However, methohexital alone fails to prevent the resulting tachycardia and hypertension associated with ECT. The hemodynamic effects of ECT have been well studied in animal models with brief initial parasympathetic stimulation followed by sympathetic stimulation. Similar cardiovascular effects have been reported with humans. In ECT patients, brief episodes of bradycardia followed by significant tachycardia associated with hypertension may occur. Whereas the parasympathetic response is mediated by the vagus nerve, the sympathetic response reflects hippocampal activity as well as circulating catecholamines. The increase in systolic blood pressure and heart rate immediately after the stimulus may be as much as 30% to 40% and 20%, respectively.[73] In patients with known cardiovascular disease or significant risk factors, these responses should be kept to a minimum to prevent any untoward cardiac events during the course of treatment. Several studies have been performed to determine which agents or combinations of agents best suppress this hyperdynamic response to ECT stimulation. A study by Gazdag and colleagues[74] examined the difference in duration of seizure activity and hemodynamic response to ECT between methohexital and propofol. Although propofol significantly lowered the duration of seizure activity compared with methohexital, the clinical efficacy of the treatment was not diminished, and the resultant lower mean arterial pressure associated with propofol could be beneficial to patients who demonstrate a higher cardiovascular risk profile. Other studies investigated anesthetic regimens that included methohexital with adjuvant therapies. Locala and colleagues[75] performed a prospective, randomized, double-blind study on the use of methohexital alone and remifentanil supplemented with a dose of methohexital sufficient to suppress recall. Patients who received remifentanil demonstrated a significant reduction in systolic blood pressure and heart rate associated with ECT. In addition to the ability of remifentanil to suppress the sympathetic response to seizure activity, some reports in the literature have indicated that it may increase the duration of seizure activity, making it an attractive agent in the anesthesia provider's arsenal.[76]

Other means of attenuating the hemodynamic response to ECT in patients with cardiovascular disease include the use of antihypertensive medications, most notably β-blockers. A study by Zhang and colleagues[77] examined the effect of different doses of nicardipine administered before induction of seizure activity. They discovered that a dose of 40 mcg/kg IV of nicardipine in addition to 0.15 mcg/kg of labetalol sufficiently blunted the hyperdynamic response without a significant decrease in seizure duration or postprocedural hypotensive effects.

On the other hand, asystole is very rarely reported in association with ECT. It has been suggested that asystole results from multiple factors, including the use of bilateral versus unilateral electrode placement, history of atrioventricular blockade, higher doses of succinylcholine, the use of thiopentone as an anesthetic agent, history of significant coronary artery disease, administration of β-blockers as a premedication, and subconvulsive electroshock.[78] These factors alone or in combination may increase the risk of bradydysrhythmias and asystole. Premedication with glycopyrrolate has been proposed to prevent bradyarrhythmias; however, it has not gained popularity because of its side effects and the fact that sympathetic response is more commonly seen than parasympathetic response.

In the authors' clinical practice, they have found that this postseizure hemodynamic turbulence is very short lived, and in most patients, no treatment is necessary and one need only to "wait it out." However, for cardiac patients, especially those who exhibit symptoms of ischemia on their ECG, the use of short-acting agents such as esmolol to treat tachycardia or nitroglycerine IV boluses to treat hypertension may be of value.

Most patients who present for ECT either are currently taking or have taken antidepressants or other psychiatric agents. Historically, the agents of most concern with regard to anesthesia have been the monoamine oxidase (MAO) inhibitors. According to previous recommendations, these medications were to be discontinued 2 weeks before any elective procedure.[79] However, in a series of case reports presented by Dolenc and colleagues,[80] patients experienced no adverse effects from general anesthesia with concurrent use of an MAO inhibitor.[19] Furthermore, no difference in hemodynamic response to ECT sessions was noted in patients either currently receiving or not receiving an MAO inhibitor. Perhaps then, more important that discontinuation of MAO inhibitors is avoidance of any known contraindicated drugs, such as indirect-acting sympathomimetics and meperidine.

GASTROENTEROLOGY ENDOSCOPY SUITE

The number of diagnostic and therapeutic procedures performed in gastroenterology suites has increased greatly as the benefit of early screening for and treatment of both benign and malignant conditions have been established. The majority of cases use some form of anesthesia, either moderate sedation administered by the gastroenterologist or deep sedation and general anesthesia administered by the anesthesia provider. The anesthesia team usually becomes involved in the more complicated or emergent cases. To that effect, most patients who present to an anesthesia provider for periprocedural care often are elderly or tend to have multiple comorbid conditions that should be addressed before commencement of the anesthetic.

The most common procedures performed in the gastroenterology suite are upper endoscopy, colonoscopy, sigmoidoscopy, and endoscopic retrograde cholangiopancreatography. Each of these

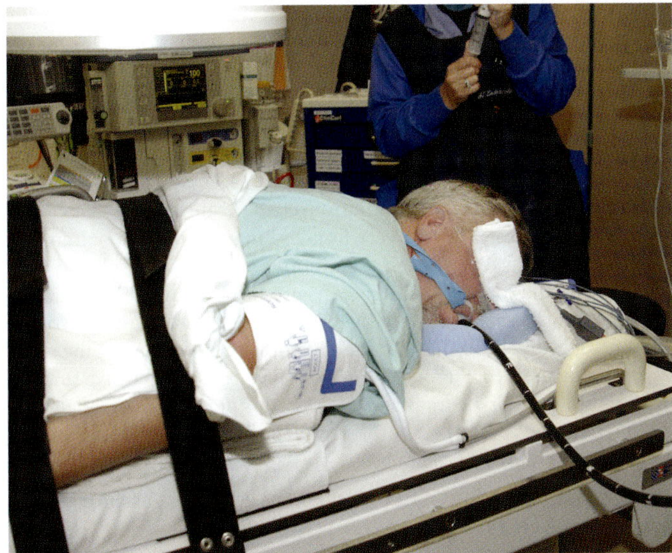

FIGURE 69-2. Patient in a prone position for endoscopic retrograde cholangiopancreatography under monitored anesthesia care deep sedation with spontaneous ventilation.

procedures carries its own unique challenges for anesthesia providers. Colonoscopy traditionally is performed either without sedation or under moderate sedation administered by the endoscopist. A deeper lever of anesthesia is required in some patients because of their increased apprehension or severe discomfort experienced during the procedure. Important considerations for the anesthesiologist during colonoscopy include hemodynamic instability caused by dehydration from a preparatory bowel regimen and uncompensated anemia from severe GI bleeding. During upper endoscopy procedures, patients usually are placed in the extreme lateral or prone position (**Figs. 69-2** and **69-3**). The combination of patient positioning and the nature of the procedure itself limit access to the head and consequently the airway. Airway obstruction and apnea during sedation may develop, so the endoscopist and the anesthesia provider must have a clear understanding between them that emergency management of the airway supersedes continuation of the procedure until the situation has been safely controlled. Bradycardia or other arrhythmias can result from distension of the GI tract or from probe insertion.[81] Other complications include bleeding, perforation, aspiration, and infection.[82] To block the gag reflex during gastroscope insertion, a topical anesthetic spray is usually used. Most GI physicians use IV sedation, usually midazolam and an opioid (meperidine or fentanyl), for the patient's comfort. Some procedures require the use of more potent agents because the procedures are longer and more complex and necessitate a high degree of patient cooperation.[83] Propofol, with its potent amnestic properties and rapid recovery time, has become an ideal choice for these procedures. It can be titrated to produce any level of anesthesia, from anxiolysis to general anesthesia. Its tendency to produce deep sedation with subsequent loss of protective airway reflexes at standard doses has limited its use to anesthesiologists and other individuals trained in airway management.[84] The level of sedation needed to successfully complete endoscopic procedures varies among populations. In general, elderly patients tolerated these procedures well at propofol concentrations associated with moderate sedation, but younger patients typically required larger doses (deep sedation) to suppress the somatic response to endoscopy.[85]Although most GI procedures can be completed successfully under MAC (see Fig. 69-2), general anesthesia with endotracheal intubation (see Fig. 69-3) may be necessary, for example, in patients who have a difficult airway, undergoing a relatively long procedure, or are at high risk for aspiration. The need for intubation should be addressed with the endoscopist because the presence of an endotracheal tube may make the procedure difficult to perform.

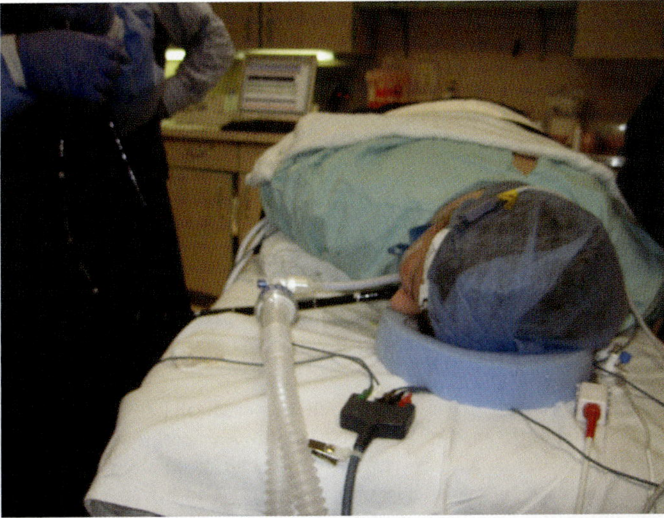

FIGURE 69-3. Patient is in a prone position with an endotracheal tube in place under general anesthesia for endoscopic retrograde cholangiopancreatography.

BRONCHOSCOPY SUITE

There has been exponential growth in procedures for interventional pulmonology as a result of the proliferation of these procedures and the new indications for them (**Table 69-8**). Many traditional thoracic surgical procedures (eg, mediastinal staging) are now minimally invasive and can be performed as outpatient procedures.[86] Increased demand has led to the establishment of specialized interventional pulmonology centers outside of the ORs.

TABLE 69-8 Bronchoscopic Surgery Procedures

Common Traditional Procedures	New Procedures	Procedures Under Investigation
Endotracheobronchial stenting	Endobronchial ultrasound-guided transbronchial needle aspiration (EBUS-TBNA)	Bronchoscopic lung volume reduction (BLVR)
Endobronchial biopsy	Complete mediastinal staging using EBUS-TBNA	Bronchial thermoplasty for treatment of poorly controlled asthma
Endotracheobronchial laser	Electromagnetic navigational bronchoscopy (ENB)	
Bronchoscopic balloon dilation	Fiducial implantation	
Bronchoscopic cryotherapy		
Endotracheal-bronchial electrocautery		

Adapted with permission from Abdelmalak B. Anesthesia outside of the operating room. In Urman R, Gross W, Phillip B, eds. *Anesthesia Care for Interventional Pulmonology.* Oxford, UK: Oxford University Press; 167-174.

NEW PROCEDURES

Endobronchial Ultrasound-Guided Transbronchial Needle Aspiration Through endobronchial ultrasound-guided transbronchial needle aspiration (EBUS-TBNA), the structure of the tracheobronchial wall and adjacent structures can be well visualized. This is an accurate, safe, and cost-effective technique that allows biopsy of mediastinal lymph nodes and peribronchial lesions.[87,88]

Complete Mediastinal Staging Using Endobronchial Ultrasound-Guided Transbronchial Needle Aspiration EBUS-TBNA has proved valuable for mediastinal lymph node staging of lung cancer.[89]

Electromagnetic Navigational Bronchoscopy Electromagnetic navigational bronchoscopy is designed to enable the pulmonologist to biopsy lesions within the periphery of the bronchial tree. The system uses computer software that converts computed tomography (CT) scan images into three-dimensional virtual lung reconstruction. This setup allows navigational guidance within the lungs to endobronchially invisible targets and subsequent biopsy, almost in the same fashion as stereotactic brain biopsy or brain surgery.[9]

Procedures Under Investigation **Bronchoscopic lung volume reduction** is a technique by which unidirectional endobronchial valves are inserted through a flexible bronchoscope aimed at deflating existing bullae. This procedure is indicated in managing terminal chronic obstructive lung disease as an alternative technique for surgically removing diseased lung tissue, the so-called "lung-volume reduction surgery."

Bronchial thermoplasty includes heat that is applied endobronchially to reduce the mass of the airway smooth muscle as a treatment for patients with poorly controlled asthma.[90]

ANESTHETIC CARE

Preoperative Evaluation The extent of preoperative evaluation depends on whether the procedure is elective or emergent and how stable or critical the airway is. Preoperative assessment is usually conducted in the customary fashion with special attention to the following:

- Airway evaluation and symptoms of compromise
- Review of the pulmonologist's evaluation of the size of the lesion or tumor, its location with the bronchial tree, and its extent
- CT scans of the neck and chest to rule out airway abnormalities and mediastinal masses

Judicious use of premedication sedatives and anxiolytics is advised because of the compromised respiratory status of these patients. The majority of uncomplicated and routine diagnostic bronchoscopic procedures can be performed under light sedation. However, when the lung is compromised or when the procedure entails more than a simple diagnostic bronchoscopy, deep sedation MAC and general anesthesia by an anesthesiologist is needed. In these situations, many sedatives (eg, midazolam, fentanyl, morphine, remifentanil, alfentanil, or propofol) have been traditionally and successfully used. More recently, dexmedetomidine and fospropofol have become acceptable choices.[55,91,92]

A total IV anesthetic technique (TIVA), usually an infusion of propofol, is preferred over an inhalational anesthetic technique for the following reasons:

1. It ensures continuous delivery of anesthesia compared with an inhalational anesthetic technique because the integrity of the airway conduit for delivering inhalation anesthetic to the patient is not guaranteed for the whole duration of the operation because of the nature of the procedure.[93]

2. It prevents pollution of the OR by inhalational anesthetic agents when leaks occur during airway instrumentation, thereby avoiding the risk of sedating OR personnel.

Muscle relaxants are commonly used in these procedures to facilitate endotracheal tube insertion. Relaxation of the jaw muscles makes it easier and safer for the rigid bronchoscope to be inserted. Muscle relaxants also improve overall lung compliance by eliminating the chest wall component. Finally, they provide a motionless patient, which is advantageous because unexpected patient movement can have serious consequences, as in lasering airway lesions. It is wise to restrict all administered fluids to the minimum needed for these patients because many of them present with a very limited lung reserve, and pulmonary congestion may aggravate their condition.

Many anesthesiologists and surgeons use corticosteroids, in particular dexamethasone, as a prophylactic measure to decrease airway edema after airway surgery so that residual postoperative swelling of the vocal cords can be avoided. Steroids are also used in cases of extensive surgical tracheobronchial tissue trauma. However, this practice is defended only on the basis of its putative clinical advantage because evidence of its real advantage is controversial at best.[94-97]

Management of the Fraction of Inspired Oxygen Administering a fraction of inspired oxygen (FIO_2) of 1.0 in such procedures is very common. However, it is usually necessary to maintain FIO_2 at the lowest tolerable level (<0.4) during airway laser usage or electrocautery. Periods of extended apnea and complete airway obstruction can be expected during more challenging cases. Complete airway occlusion frequently occurs during the critical phase of removing the stent or stent fragments or the inflated balloon dilators used for tracheobronchial dilation. Therefore, it is always advisable to return to ventilation with 100% oxygen before extraction of the stent before exchange of airways and before extubation. Finally, during any part of the procedure, if the patient cannot tolerate lower oxygen levels it may be necessary to defer treatment temporarily and ventilate with higher oxygen concentrations.

Airway Management Choices

No Airway This is a popular technique because relatively short procedures are performed in a remote bronchoscopy suite where an anesthesia machine and capnography are unavailable. Great emphasis should be placed on airway topicalization to ensure that a patient can tolerate the bronchoscope without needing deeper planes of sedation, that may add to their concurrent risks.

Endotracheal Tube Intubation with a large-diameter endotracheal tube (eg, size 8.5) facilitates ventilation around the relatively large-diameter flexible bronchoscope, and when it is cut short, it facilitates navigation of the fiberoptic bronchoscope. A short large-bore endotracheal tube could be used via an existing tracheotomy with flexible bronchoscopic instruments. Use of a fiberoptic swivel adaptor will allow continuous ventilation, thereby avoiding circuit disconnection during flexible bronchoscopy.

Rigid Bronchoscope (Figure 69-4) Because of the size and noncompressible material in silicon stents, a rigid bronchoscope is preferred for insertion and removal of silicon stents, for removal of granulation tissue and large tumors invading the tracheobronchial tree, and in some instances to support airway patency in the face of a large mediastinal mass compressing the airway. When a rigid bronchoscope is used, ventilation could be accomplished through either attaching the anesthetic circuit to the bronchoscope side port or through jet ventilation where the jetting device is attached through a special adaptor to the bronchoscope side port. Leaks around the rigid bronchoscope are common but can be easily remedied by maximizing the fresh gas flow and packing the mouth with saline-soaked gauze.

Supraglottic Airway In cases in which the tracheal lesion is subglottic, a supraglottic airway (SGA) (eg, a laryngeal mask airway) can be effective[98,99] because it allows access to the subglottic lesion with the flexible bronchoscope, and offers a means of ventilation as well. However, it does not guarantee reliable protection against aspiration.

The techniques described above require clear communication between the anesthesiologist and the pulmonologist. Most of the procedures

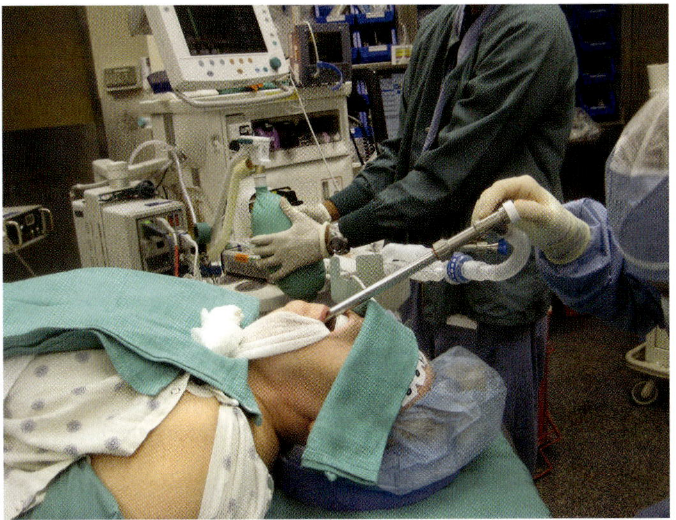

FIGURE 69-4. Positive-pressure ventilation through connecting the anesthesia circuit to the side port of a rigid bronchoscope. Note the wet gauze packing around the rigid bronchoscope barrel to minimize leakage around the scope.

described above are performed as outpatient procedures; patients are discharged the same day. However, extremely sick patients undergoing a complicated resection or lasering of endotracheobronchial lesions may benefit from overnight admission. This compares favorably with that of invasive thoracic surgery, which requires postoperative ICU admission and a prolonged hospital stay.

Potential complications of bronchoscopic surgery are numerous, ranging from hypercarbia and minor levels of hypoxemia on the one hand to major bleeding, tracheal rupture, and loss of airway integrity on the other.

Stent removal provides an example of a risky pulmonologic intervention. Potential complications include retention of stent pieces, mucosal tears with bleeding, reobstruction, the need for postoperative mechanical ventilation, pneumothorax, damage to the pulmonary artery, and death.[93] The jet ventilation technique can lead to barotrauma, including pneumothorax, necessitating chest tube insertion. Laser airway fire, although rare, is also a very serious complication.

The key to favorable outcomes lies in deep understanding of the underlying lung pathology; open two-way communication between the anesthesiologist and pulmonologist; understanding the nature of the procedure; and above all, vigilance and preparedness.

CARDIAC/ELECTROPHYSIOLOGY LABORATORY

An increasing number of patients are undergoing invasive cardiology procedures that require the presence of trained anesthesia providers. In the past, certain procedures, such as placement of pacemakers/defibrillators, were performed in the OR by a cardiothoracic surgeon with a cardiac anesthesiologist in attendance.[100] Recently, however, implantation of these devices is being performed by the interventional cardiologist in the cardiac/electrophysiology laboratory with the assistance of a noncardiac anesthesiologist. The physiologic status of patients presenting for placement of implantable cardioverter-defibrillators (ICDs) varies from young, otherwise healthy individuals with supraventricular dysrhythmias (Wolff-Parkinson-White syndrome) to elderly patients with significant coronary artery disease or congestive heart failure who have survived a life-threatening arrhythmia (ventricular tachycardia, ventricular fibrillation). Many have severe ventricular dysfunction. The extent of their cardiac disease should be assessed preoperatively by the anesthetist, and appropriate consultations should be obtained from the cardiologist responsible for the patient's care.

Anesthetic management for these cases ranges from sedation to general anesthesia with an endotracheal tube. Complicated cases of pacemaker or ICD wire extraction are typically performed under general anesthesia. In the case of automatic ICD implantation, after the device has been implanted, a device check is performed, consisting of induction of ventricular tachycardia or ventricular fibrillation, recording detection of the arrhythmia by the device, and treatment of the arrhythmia. This process can be quite uncomfortable to the patient, especially if multiple cycles are necessary. When sedation is used, the anesthesia provider must be prepared for a brief period of general anesthesia to allow for such device testing.[101] Antiarrhythmic drugs and an external defibrillator should be present at all times in case the device fails to restore normal sinus rhythm. Along with standard monitors, an arterial line is usually used for this purpose. However, central venous catheters, providing ideal access for injecting vasoactive drugs, are reserved for sicker patients scheduled for more invasive procedures. A postprocedural chest radiograph should be obtained to rule out pneumothorax or pericardial effusion and to confirm lead placement. Patients may recover in the cardiac laboratory recovery room if the nurses are trained and qualified to recover patients from anesthesia; otherwise, they should recover in the main hospital PACU.

Electrical cardioversion is used to convert patients to normal sinus rhythm. The usual indications are atrial fibrillation, atrial flutter, and supraventricular tachycardia. Cardioversion can be performed either emergently (hemodynamically unstable arrhythmias) or electively (failed medical therapy). Because of the physical discomfort and psychologic distress caused by the procedure, electrical cardioversion is performed either under deep sedation or general anesthesia. For emergent cases, patients should be treated as having "full stomach" and appropriate aspiration precautions taken. In elective cases, a brief period of general anesthesia using an induction dose of etomidate, propofol, or methohexital for the actual delivery of the stimulus is sufficient. It is usually so brief that ventilatory support is generally unnecessary.[102] However, patients with difficult airway may require a SGA or endotracheal tube for ventilatory management during the procedure. The induction dose should be adjusted cautiously; sedatives received by the patient should be considered if the procedure is to follow a transesophageal echocardiography, so as to avert atrial thrombus before the cardioversion. The postprocedural recovery time is generally brief.

INTERVENTIONAL RADIOLOGY

Interventional radiology is currently exhibiting unprecedented growth, from state-of-the-art imaging studies to placement of vascular stents. As interventional radiologists continue to expand their scope of practice to the limits of modern medicine, the role of anesthesiologists in this medical odyssey has become increasingly prominent. Initially, the majority of interventional procedures were performed with local anesthesia and minimal sedation administered by a radiologist. However, as the nature of the procedures became increasingly complex and the need for total patient compliance became necessary, the level of sedation required to successfully perform these interventions gradually began to rise. The frequent need for deeper sedation coupled with the increasing number of high-risk patients presenting for these "minimally invasive" procedures has led to the growing involvement of trained anesthesia personnel in perioperative management in the radiology suite. The radiology community generally believes that the presence of a separate anesthesia provider responsible for sedation/anesthesia, pain control and continuous resuscitation during technically challenging procedures, especially in critically ill patients, should be mandatory.[103] A wide variety of cases are performed in the radiology suite, many of which involve the services of an anesthesiologist. This section focuses on the most common and clinically demanding procedures and their complications as they relate to the anesthetic management.

RADIOFREQUENCY ABLATION

Radiofrequency ablation (RFA) is a widely used noninvasive treatment for primary and metastatic tumors and painful bone and neural lesions. One limitation of this form of therapy has been the relatively small area of tumor destruction achieved in a single treatment. However, recent technologic advances in this modality have allowed for destruction of larger lesions (>5 cm in diameter) during a given session.[104] This improvement has led to the expanded use of RFA in the treatment of many malignant tumors, including pulmonary, hepatic, bone, and renal cancers.

Radiofrequency ablation entails placement of either a single electrode or multiple electrodes contained in a single needle into the lesion targeted for ablation. Once in place, tissue coagulation is induced through an electromagnetic source within the electrode.[105] Correct positioning of the electrode into the lesion of interest is accomplished through guidance from imaging techniques, which include ultrasonography, CT, CT with fluoroscopy, or magnetic resonance imaging (MRI). Although CT is the preferred modality, the choice of imaging depends on the availability of the technology at a particular center and on the technical expertise of the interventionalist performing the procedure.[42] Anesthetic management of RFA depends on the size and location of the tumor. For most cases, MAC is sufficient and is generally well tolerated by patients. For larger lesions or lesions near vascular structures, general anesthesia with placement of endotracheal tube may be required to prevent patient movement during critical portions of the procedure. Complications of RFA include hemorrhage, pneumothorax, hemothorax, thermal injury, electrical shock, and hyperthermia because the patient may exhibit significant increases in body temperature in response to direct heating of large masses.[106] Patients can recover in the hospital PACU or in the recovery area of the interventional suite, if appropriate.

CRYOABLATION

Cryoablation is a minimally invasive technique for treating lung, liver, breast, kidney, and prostate masses. It uses liquid nitrogen or gaseous argon for cooling, which results in tissue destruction through direct freezing and in denaturation of tissue. Both MAC and general anesthesia have been used successfully for these procedures, depending on patient characteristics and the size and location of the mass.

INTERVENTIONAL NEURORADIOLOGY

Perhaps one of the most challenging and exciting fields of interventional medicine is the area of interventional neuroradiology. Noninvasive treatment of neurovascular disease has evolved significantly. The most common treatments are embolization or sclerotherapy of tumors and arteriovenous malformations (AVMs), angioplasty for cerebral vasospasm, embolectomy for acute stroke, and coil embolization of cerebral aneurysms. In most of these cases, general anesthesia is the preferred method of anesthetic management because patients are often required to remain motionless for extended periods. Each of these procedures carries its own patient and risk profiles, which the anesthesia provider should consider in formulating a management plan. Common complications of interventional neuroradiologic procedures include cerebral ischemia, hemorrhage, catheter displacement, and pulmonary embolism.[107] The goals of perioperative management in these procedures are no different from those set for any neurosurgical case: maintenance of hemodynamic stability, preservation of cerebral blood flow and cerebral perfusion pressure, and rapid emergence after completion of the procedure to assess the patient's neurologic status.[108]

Arteriovenous malformations are vascular structures in which one or more aberrant arteries feed into a nidus that is then drained by coexisting aberrant veins. In the past, embolization of AVMs was performed before surgical resection of the abnormality. However, many of these lesions are now being treated by embolization alone in light of the availability of experienced neuroradiologists.[109] Embolization is accomplished by deploying thrombosing coils or permanent balloons or by injecting sclerosing agents, glues, or particulate material. Complications after embolization include cerebral hemorrhage or edema resulting from sudden reperfusion into areas that previously were underperfused.[110]

Careful management of arterial blood pressure and thus cerebral perfusion pressure is important. This is best accomplished under general anesthesia with the use of muscle relaxation to avoid the sudden increase in blood pressure and intracranial pressure associated with coughing or involuntary paroxysmal movement. Some patients may require preoperative and intraoperative pharmacologic agents to assist in controlling blood pressure during the procedure. Propranolol, in addition to its known hemodynamic effects, has been shown to possibly reduce cerebral metabolic rate and cerebral blood flow without significant impairment of metabolism–flow coupling.[111] Invasive blood pressure monitoring is recommended for patients for whom deliberate hypotension is planned. Placement of other invasive monitors will depend on the current physical status of the patient and on the need for postprocedural hemodynamic monitoring.

The endovascular approach via coil placement is gaining popularity in the treatment of unruptured aneurysms.[112] The basic goal of this approach is obliteration of the aneurysm sac through the placement of coils.[113] Possible complications associated with coil embolization include hemorrhage, thromboembolism, and vasospasm, which is most notably problematic in the case of aneurysm rupture. Nimodipine remains the agent of choice for prevention or continued treatment of vasospasm. Additionally, hypervolemia–hypertension–hemodilution (triple H) therapy remains popular for treating cerebral arterial spasm. Patients who undergo these procedures are admitted to the ICU for postprocedural monitoring of their neurologic status.

Carotid artery stenting is another minimally invasive procedure that is being performed in place of the traditional carotid endarterectomy because it is believed to improve outcomes.[114] Although it could be performed under MAC or general anesthesia, MAC has the advantage of allowing the assessment of neurologic status and the detection of changes in mental status.[115]

TRANSJUGULAR INTRAHEPATIC PORTOSYSTEMIC SHUNTING

Transjugular intrahepatic portosystemic shunting (TIPS) is a technique that involves the creation of a shunt through the liver between one of the hepatic veins and either the right or left portal vein.[116] TIPS traditionally has been used to treat esophageal varices, but its uses have been expanded to include the treatment of several other hepatic conditions, such as portal vein thrombosis and Budd-Chiari syndrome. TIPS can be performed under MAC or general anesthesia, depending on the patient's physical and mental status and the practitioner's familiarity and experience with the technique. Patients who present for TIPS may have a large amount of ascites or other complications of hepatic disease, pleural effusions, intrapulmonary shunting (which can restrict ventilatory effort and decrease oxygenation),[117] cirrhotic cardiomyopathy, encephalopathy, coagulopathy, and hepatorenal syndrome. Patients who have a significant amount of ascites or who have experienced a recent episode of GI bleeding are at increased risk for aspiration. The procedure itself may require several hours to perform, which requires a cooperative and stable patient. Often, TIPS is preceded by paracentesis to relieve some of the increased intra-abdominal pressure. All of these factors must be taken into consideration when choosing an appropriate anesthetic method. Standard monitors usually are sufficient, but more invasive monitors may be required in emergent cases and in hemodynamically unstable patients (exhibiting active bleeding, severe cardiomyopathy, and acid–base disturbances). Adequate IV access in the form of a large-bore catheter should be established because hemorrhage is one of the complications of the procedure, and the patient may experience hemodynamic instability. Recovery usually takes place in the PACU or ICU.

DIAGNOSTIC IMAGING

The previous section discussed therapies in the radiology suite that involve some type of invasive technique. For many of these procedures, the need for sedation or anesthesia is self-explanatory. However, the services of the anesthesia providers may also be required for various noninvasive diagnostic modalities. This section discusses the most frequently performed examinations, MRI and CT scan.

MAGNETIC RESONANCE IMAGING

Magnetic resonance imaging is a diagnostic imaging tool that uses both static and magnetic field gradients, the strength of which ranges from 0.15 to 3.0 Tesla. MRI entails certain risks, the most serious of which stem from ferromagnetic objects or equipment near the magnetic field. Many of the reports of injury or fatality are related to these objects, which become projectiles when exposed to the strong magnetic field. Furthermore, patients who have any indwelling metallic device, such as a pacemaker, ICD, aneurysm clip, or infusion pump, are generally contraindicated for MRI.[118] However, MRI can be performed on a limited bases for patients who have implanted devices such as a deep-brain stimulator or vagal and phrenic nerve stimulators. Monitors should be attached to patients with care; MRI-compatible ECG pads should be used, and the monitor wires should be prevented from coiling because coiling may result in patient burns.[119] Finally, risks may occur that are associated with contrast material, such as the increased risk of nephrogenic systemic fibrosis when gadolinium is administered to patients with acute or severe renal insufficiency.[119]

Quenching Anesthesiologists should become familiar with this process, which entails rapid helium evaporation and the loss of superconductivity of the current-carrying coil. The loss may occur unintentionally from accidentally pressing the emergency button or intentionally turning off the scanner to release a ferromagnetic object that became attached to it in a superconducting magnet. As the superconductive magnet becomes resistive, heat is released that can lead to the boiling of liquid helium in the cryostat. This event may pose a hazard if it has not been expected and properly planned for. The evaporated coolant requires emergency venting systems to protect patients and operators. Cryogenic liquids and their associated cold vapors can produce effects on the skin similar to those of a thermal burn and can cause frostbite. In addition, prolonged breathing of extremely cold gases may damage the lungs. Finally, unprotected skin can stick to very cold metal (eg, metal cooled by liquid helium) and then tear when pulled away.

Quenching can cause total magnet failure, which cannot be reversed. MRI systems are designed so that all of the escaping cryogenic gas is directed out of the building. If pipes are blocked, helium gas will be released into the scanner room, creating a large white cloud of chilled gas and displacing oxygen. Under such circumstances, it is essential that the scanner room be evacuated because displacement of oxygen under such extreme conditions could lead to asphyxiation and death. The force of quenching can be strong enough to destroy the walls of the scanner room or the MRI equipment. Access to the scanner room during quench may prove to be impossible because the high pressure created by escaping gas may make it difficult to open the doors. In addition, magnetic fields may persist after a quench, necessitating continued caution in approaching the area with ferromagnetic materials or equipment.[120]

ANESTHESIA FOR MRI

Because of the need for absolute immobility and the length of some types of scans, some patients, most notably pediatric patients, require deep sedation or general anesthesia for successful completion of the study (discussed further in Chapter 63). In the adult population, claustrophobia, chronic back pain (which precludes lying still within the scanner, a condition that allows good image quality), and movement disorders are the most common reasons that call for anesthesia services. Studies have shown that a fairly large percentage of adults (14%-20%) require some anesthesia in order to tolerate MRI.[121] In these cases, anesthetic techniques range from moderate sedation for adults with mild claustrophobia or anxiety to general anesthesia for patients in whom airway issues are expected (eg, patients with obstructive sleep apnea). One of the more effective and popular techniques is TIVA with propofol as the drug of choice or inhalational anesthetic when an MRI-compatible anesthesia machine is available. Whatever the preferred method, the presence of MRI-compatible airway equipment is essential during any anesthetic in this location. Ideally, an MRI-compatible anesthesia machine and monitors should also be available. Additional anesthetic considerations for MRI include limited access to the patient and decreased visibility.[122] Most institutions have a window or video equipment with which to view the patient throughout the examination, as well as an intercom with which to talk to the patient who is mildly sedated. Technicians or other personnel in the area should clearly understand that the scan should be halted if any issue arises. If designated space and trained personnel are available, patients may recover in the radiology area.

The ASA issued a practice advisory in 2009 regarding the MRI and practice safety in that environment; this is a very useful resource for clinicians who care for MRI patients.[120]

SURGICAL MAGNETIC RESONANCE IMAGING SUITE

This is a fully equipped OR with an integrated imaging system that includes both MRI and a C-arm for pre-, intra- and postoperative imaging for diagnosis, intervention, and postoperative follow-up. It is typically used for cranial and spine surgery. This complex system requires special OR and anesthesia equipment that is MRI compatible, and the same precautions and practices that apply to MRI are valid here as well. General anesthesia is the modality of choice in these cases, and the anesthesia team should receive formal in-service training on how to manage cases in such an environment before they embark on taking care of patients there.

COMPUTED TOMOGRAPHY SCANS

Computed tomography scans are generally of shorter duration than MRI scans and rarely require the presence of an anesthesia provider. Access to the patient undergoing a CT scan is limited because of the ionizing radiation being used to produce the required images. However, use of specialized anesthesia equipment is unnecessary, and the patient is much more visible to the anesthesia provider because the patient is not completely enclosed in a cylinder. Propofol is the drug of choice because the procedures often are short, and lingering sedative effects are undesirable. Patients who receive oral contrast should be intubated and the contents of their GI tract suctioned before extubation. The recovery time usually is short, depending on the agent used. Many patients can bypass the PACU and recover on site if they are stable.

FINANCIAL ASPECTS OF MONITORED ANESTHESIA CARE AND REMOTE ANESTHESIA SERVICES

In this era of rapid medical changes, more complex procedures are being performed outside the ORs, especially in endoscopy, radiology, and electrophysiology suites and in cardiovascular catheterization laboratories. A significant number of these procedures are being performed under MAC. One report estimates that charges to Medicare for anesthesia for colonoscopy increased by 86% (to $80,000,000)[123] between 2001 and 2003. These numbers are probably even greater now. In response to the rapid increase in anesthesia services, payment for anesthesia in these cases has been thoroughly examined. Most payors distinguish between high- and average-risk cases. In general, payors have allowed charges for anesthesia in high-risk patients. Payment policies for average-risk patients are evolving; however, there are differences among Medicare contractors.[36]

Monitored anesthesia care cases take place in surgical/ambulatory centers, radiology suites, endoscopy suites, or even physicians' offices. Because of the broad range of cases, the availability of a dedicated anesthesia team to provide MAC is generally considered a financial challenge for anesthesia providers. Scheduling plays a major role in the financial success of providing these services, especially when they are provided outside OR complexes. Cases requiring the service of an anesthesiologist should be grouped together when possible to increase the likelihood of financial viability for that provider. If the volume of sedation cases is large enough, an anesthesiologist may dedicate the entire day to a specific location. Otherwise, the anesthesia provider probably will spend part of the day providing sedation in one location and the other part of the day providing anesthesia in another location.

CONCLUSION

As more minimally invasive procedures replace conventional surgeries, the demand for MAC will increase, and anesthesiologists' role outside the OR will expand. Accelerating this trend are new developments in the field of natural orifice transluminal endoscopic surgery (NOTES) in which access is gained through the mouth, rectum, vagina, and possibly urethra, and no incision is needed. As a result, anesthesiologists must leave the familiar environment of the operating room pavilion and venture into the unfamiliar territory of hospital policy and procedures to ensure that our non-OR patients receive the same high standard of care that is available to them in the OR. Successful safe delivery of remote anesthesia care requires a well-thought-out plan and organization (**Table 69-9**). Anesthesiologists' specialized training, airway management skills, and thorough knowledge of the physiologic effects of anesthetic agents in various disease processes give us a distinct advantage over many of the personnel who currently provide sedation services in these remote areas. Although an increasing amount of literature regarding our role and current practices in non-OR locations is available, even more studies are necessary if we are to maximize patient safety through better training and better use of technology and pharmacology. Enhanced knowledge will enable us to strengthen our efficiency in this field and accommodate the growing number of patients and specialists requiring our services.

TABLE 69-9 The Eight Effective Habits for Successful Remote Location Anesthesia

1	Improvement in preprocedure evaluation
2	Improvement in remote location PACUs
3	Adequate anesthesia equipment and reliable support
4	Development of database for clinical outcomes
5	Improved billing for anesthesia services
6	Identification and formalization of leadership (anesthesiologists, proceduralists, nurses)
7	Involvement of anesthesia in moderate sedation
8	Improvements in scheduling

PACU, postanesthesia care unit.

Adapted with permission from Dr. Walter Maurer, MD, Emeritus President of the Society for Ambulatory Anesthesia (SAMBA) and Chair of the Committee on Anesthesia for Remote Locations, Anesthesiology Institute, Cleveland Clinic, Cleveland, OH (personal communication).

KEY REFERENCES

- Abdelmalak B, Makary L, Hoban J, Doyle DJ. Dexmedetomidine as sole sedative for awake intubation in management of the critical airway. *J Clin Anesth.* 2007;19:370-373.
- Alspach D, Falleroni M. Monitoring patients during procedures conducted outside the operating room. *Int Anesthesiol Clin.* 2004; 42:95-111.
- American Society of Anesthesiologists. *Continuum of Depth of Sedation: Definition of General Anesthesia and Levels of Sedation/Analgesia.* Approved by the ASA House of Delegates on October 27, 2004, and amended on October 21, 2009.
- American Society of Anesthesiologists. Practice advisory on anesthetic care for magnetic resonance imaging: a report by the American Society of Anesthesiologists Task Force on Anesthetic Care for Magnetic Resonance Imaging. *Anesthesiology.* 2009;110: 459-479.
- American Society of Anesthesiologists. *Statement on Nonoperating Room Anesthetizing Locations.* Approved by the ASA House of Delegates on October 15, 2003 and amended on October 22, 2008.
- American Society of Anesthesiologists Task Force on Postanesthetic Care. Practice guidelines for postanesthetic care: a report by the American Society of Anesthesiologists Task Force on Postanesthetic Care. *Anesthesiology.* 2002;96:742-752.
- Doyle DJ, Abdelmalak B, Machuzak M, Gildea TR. Anesthesia and airway management for removing pulmonary self-expanding metallic stents. *J Clin Anesth.* 2009;21:529-532.
- Kelhoffer ER, Osborn IP. The gastroenterology suite and TIPS. *Int Anesthesiol Clin.* 2003;41:51-61.
- Osborn IP. Anesthetic considerations for interventional neuroradiology. *Int Anesthesiol Clin.* 2003;41:69-77.

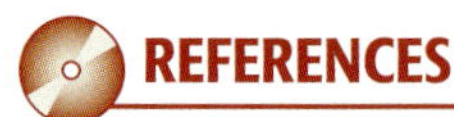

REFERENCES

Complete references available on DVD and online version at www.LongneckerAnesthesiology.com

PART 5

Postoperative Care of the Anesthesia Patient

CHAPTER 70

Recovery of the Healthy Patient

Loreta Grecu
Edward A. Bittner
Edward George

KEY POINTS

1. The postanesthesia care unit (PACU) requires specially trained personnel to recognize and respond to clinical problems of patient care in the immediate postoperative period.
2. The PACU should be located in close proximity to the operating rooms to access key personnel in a timely manner.
3. The majority of patients admitted to the PACU experience an unremarkable recovery and are discharged from the PACU without problems.
4. Prophylaxis for postoperative nausea and vomiting is far more effective than rescue therapy.
5. Effective postoperative analgesia should be initiated during the surgical procedure.
6. Hypoxia is most often the result of residual effects of anesthetic agents.
7. Hypotension unresponsive to fluid resuscitation in a postoperative patient is most likely attributable to bleeding (unless proven otherwise).

Recovery of patients after procedures requiring anesthesia or sedation is most commonly performed in the postanesthesia care unit (PACU) or recovery room. These are specialized areas designed for the observation, treatment, and discharge of postoperative patients. Optimally, the PACU is located near the operating room (OR), thereby minimizing transport time for the patient and affording quick access to anesthesiologists and surgeons who have cared for the patient. The PACU is staffed by nurses specially trained in the care of patients recovering after surgical and other invasive procedures. Under the supervision of an anesthesiologist, the PACU provides care to a broad cross section of postprocedural patients, with the majority subsequently transferred from the PACU to a general care floor of the hospital, or in the case of an ambulatory care facility, discharged home. The diversity of patients and their surgical procedures admitted to the PACU is quite varied. Many postoperative patients are healthy and have an uneventful hospital course, but some patients experience a perioperative course influenced by their preexisting medical conditions or a complicated intraoperative course.

Patients are usually admitted to the PACU at the conclusion of procedures requiring anesthesia or sedation. With some exceptions, such as healthy patients receiving only local anesthetics and carefully selected patients capable of bypassing the PACU (see later discussion), most patients undergoing surgical procedures require a period of postprocedural close observation. Although most patients are admitted to the PACU after surgical procedures in the OR, patients may also undergo procedures under anesthesia that take place outside of the OR in departments such as radiology, cardiology, or gastroenterology. These patients may also receive postprocedural care in remote areas from the hospital's main recovery areas. Regardless of the procedure and its location, personnel trained and experienced in postprocedural recovery of patients must be present to monitor and oversee the recovery phase and must be able to treat or obtain immediate help in the event of an urgent or acute deleterious change in a patient's condition.

Given the wide range of patients recovering in the PACU, the potential postoperative issues are quite varied. Being able to anticipate the common issues in advance facilitates the initiation of appropriate action(s) in a timely manner and may even avoid postoperative complications.

There are many common aspects in the recovery of healthy patients whether they are to be discharged home on the day of surgery or to be admitted to the hospital. However, viewing these two patient groups as identical may represent an oversimplification of the recovery process.

Healthy patients may undergo procedures as either inpatients or outpatients, depending on the extent of the surgical intervention. Some complex surgical procedures, even in otherwise healthy subjects, may require prolonged postoperative care in the hospital. In such cases, the planned length of the hospital stay is influenced by the duration required for functional recovery, as well as possible postoperative complications. An uncomplicated recovery in the PACU is generally anticipated in most patients. However, patients often present to the PACU with comorbid conditions that may impair their postoperative course, both in the immediate recovery period and during the subsequent hospital stay. Although numerous patients with multiple medical conditions are often discharged home on the day of surgery, a patient's comorbidities are a major factor in deciding whether to admit the patient to the hospital after surgery. This chapter reviews clinical scenarios most commonly encountered during routine postoperative recovery of surgical patients.[1] Less common and more clinically demanding issues associated with the recovery of the postoperative patient are discussed in Chapter 71. The recovery of pediatric patients is discussed in Chapter 64.

ORGANIZATION OF THE POSTANESTHESIA CARE UNIT

The PACU is usually staffed by anesthesiologists, specially trained recovery room nursing staff,[2] and support personnel. In addition to providing the ability to appropriately monitor patients and provide routine postoperative care, the PACU also affords the capability to provide mechanical ventilation, invasive monitoring, emergency equipment, and a team able to smoothly conduct emergency resuscitation and provide advanced care.

The staff assigned to the PACU must have a thorough understanding of the surgeries performed and be familiar with potential postoperative complications[3] associated with the anesthetic provided and the surgical procedure. The American Society of Anesthesiologists (ASA) Standards for Postanesthesia Care specifically identify five principles intended to encourage quality patient care (**Table 70-1**). These standards for PACU operations were approved by the ASA's House of Delegates in 2004 and amended in 2009.[4] They include standards for admission, patient transport, and transfer of care from the OR team to the patient care team in the PACU, as well as discharge procedures.

Specialized nurses, certified by the American Society of Peri-Anesthesia Nurses (ASPAN), are essential in providing care for postoperative patients. Standards for recovery established by ASPAN[5] are similar to those developed by the ASA for physicians, therefore underlining the significant convergence of these work groups in providing optimum postoperative care.

Standard monitors capable of displaying vital signs are used to monitor patients arriving in the PACU. An oxygen supply and a method for providing suction are also required for each recovering patient. In addition, supplies used for postsurgical patient care (eg, dressings, intravenous [IV] fluids, drains) as well as a method for providing emergency positive-pressure ventilation (ie, self-inflating bag-valve-mask or "Ambu bag") must be provided for each bed. Emergency equipment and medications must be readily accessible, and a team trained in emergency resuscitation must be immediately available.

POSTANESTHESIA CARE UNIT OPERATIONS

Patients receiving general anesthesia, moderate or deep sedation, or regional anesthesia should be admitted into the PACU at the completion of their procedures. Patients are monitored in the PACU until they are free from the depressant effects of the administered anesthetic and are clinically stable, at which time they are transferred to a general care

TABLE 70-1 Standards for Postanesthesia Care[a]

I.	All patients who have received general anesthesia, regional anesthesia, or monitored anesthesia care shall receive appropriate postanesthesia management.
II.	A patient transported to the PACU shall be accompanied by a member of the anesthesia care team who is knowledgeable about the patient's condition. The patient shall be continually evaluated and treated during transport with monitoring and support appropriate to the patient's condition.
III.	Upon arrival in the PACU, the patient shall be reevaluated and a verbal report provided to the responsible PACU nurse by a member of the anesthesia team who accompanies the patient.
IV.	The patient's condition shall be evaluated continually in the PACU.
V.	A physician is responsible for the discharge of the patient from the PACU.

PACU, postanesthesia care unit.

[a]These standards apply to postanesthesia care in all locations. The standards may be exceeded based on the judgment of the responsible anesthesiologist. They are intended to encourage quality of patient care but cannot guarantee a specific patient outcome. They are subject to revision from time to time as warranted by the evolution of technology and practice. Under extenuating circumstances, the responsible anesthesiologist may waive requirements, and it is recommended that it should be so stated and a note be placed in the patient's medical record to that effect.[4]

floor in the hospital or discharged home. Patients undergoing surgical procedures without receiving sedation (ie, local anesthetics) may not require admission to the PACU as determined by institutional policy.

In many institutions, recovery may be conducted in several specialized PACU facilities, including a main PACU for inpatients, a separate recovery facility for children, and an ambulatory PACU specifically designed for patients who will be discharged home. The focus of these units may be slightly different, but there is a large degree of overlap in clinical operations and patient care. This is particularly important because patients may be recovered in multiple sites, depending on the characteristics of the case, operational tempo, and institutional practices.

Early recovery (phase I) takes place in the PACU, lasting from the initial admission to the PACU until protective airway reflexes and adequate motor function have recovered. Phase I mimics the immediate postemergence phase of recovery conducted in the OR. Fully monitored during this stage, treatment of clinical issues such as nausea and vomiting, pain, respiratory compromise, and hemodynamic lability may be required. Phase II of recovery is composed of patient education and preparation for home discharge. Ambulatory patients may be recovered in the PACU (phase I), or may bypass the PACU and go directly into phase II of recovery (see discussion of fast tracking below) facility. Phase II recovery of a patient being admitted to the hospital constitutes a period during which the patient returns to an appropriate level of consciousness, vital signs remain stable, pain is effectively managed, and nausea and vomiting are adequately controlled.

Fast tracking refers to the recovery of patients in areas other than a formal PACU, such as by direct transfer from the OR to a postrecovery lounge.[6] This system can be used for patients undergoing ambulatory anesthesia. With the marked increase in numbers of surgical procedures performed on an outpatient basis, fast tracking is more commonly used. This process can offer faster recovery without admission to the PACU. Fast tracking can provide safe and appropriate recovery of postoperative patients in an efficient and resource-sensitive manner.[7]

The personnel required for the various phases of recovery may differ based on the acuity of the patient after surgery and are defined by standards established by the ASPAN practice. In phase I recovery, staffing may range from one nurse per two patients to two nurses for one unstable or complex patient. In phase II of recovery, the staffing ratio can similarly vary. Phase III of recovery is designated for patients requiring continued observation in preparation for discharge from the hospital or transfer to a general care ward. A ratio of 1 nurse per 3 to 5 patients can be used in this final stage of recovery before discharge.

ADMISSION TO THE POSTANESTHESIA CARE UNIT

TRANSFER TO THE POSTANESTHESIA CARE UNIT

Transport from the OR is carried out under the direct supervision of an anesthetist. If possible, the head of the bed is elevated to augment respiration or the semiconscious patient is placed in the lateral decubitus position to maximize airway patency and minimize aspiration risk. Oxygen delivered via facemask or nasal cannula is indicated for most patients to prevent hypoxemia caused by hypoventilation or diffusion hypoxia. Unstable patients, such as those receiving vasoactive medications, usually require careful monitoring of vital signs during transport. In such complex patients, the transport may require additional proximate resources such as airway management devices, a self-inflating bag-valve mask (Ambu bag), blood pressure and electrocardiographic (ECG) monitoring, and emergency medications. This level of monitoring and transport is similar to that required by a critically ill patient and is discussed in detail in Chapter 78. The anesthetist transporting the patient to the PACU must remain in charge of the care of the patient until the PACU team is ready to assume responsibility for his or her own care. After vital signs are obtained, a full status report is given to the PACU staff, and the patient is deemed stable for care by the PACU staff.

STATUS REPORTING TO THE POSTANESTHESIA CARE UNIT STAFF

A patient status report is most often provided to the nurse in the PACU who will assume first-line responsibility for providing care to the patient. The PACU nurse, depending on institutional guidelines, may accept responsibility for care of the patient on behalf of the physician overseeing the PACU or as a representative to the surgical team. In the event of an intraoperative complication or in the setting of a complex procedure, the patient status report should also be provided directly to the physician in charge of the PACU. The information included in the report to PACU staff may include, but is not limited to, the guidelines listed in **Table 70-2**. This table is a

TABLE 70-2 Report to Postanesthesia Care Unit Staff[a]

Significant Preoperative Issues	Intraoperative Issues
Patient's demographics	Access and invasive monitoring
Diagnosis	Special catheters (epidural, cooling)
Surgical procedure and urgency	Airway management issues
Past medical history	Induction medications
Allergies and medications	Maintenance medications
Social history	Paralytics and reversal agents
Past medical history relevant to anesthetic complications (personal or familial)	Vasoactive agents
	Anticoagulants
	Antibiotics
Last meal	Analgesics and anxiolytics
Preoperative medications	Ventilatory parameters
	Events of note
	Hemodynamic instability
	Hemorrhage
	Emergence (pain, consciousness level)
	EBL and urine output
	Fluids and blood products
	Tubes, lines, and drains
	Precautions

[a]A concise report must be provided to the postanesthesia care unit team accepting responsibility for the care of the patient. The suggested information should be used as a framework to report pertinent information. The nature and extent of the information provided will be influenced by multiple factors, including the patient's overall medical condition, the surgical procedure, and any intraoperative factors that could influence postoperative recovery.

suggested template for the transfer of information and may be modified as dictated by institutional practice. Upon arrival in the PACU, the staff measures vital signs, and the anesthetist provides a complete status report to the PACU team. At Massachusetts General Hospital, a member of the surgical team also accompanies the patient from the OR to the PACU and provides pertinent details of the surgical procedure to the PACU staff.

The formal status report is an essential component of the process of transferring responsibility for care of the patient from the OR team to the team in the PACU. This report is often the sole formal account of intraoperative events exchanged between the team providing care in the operating team and those personnel who will carry out immediate postoperative care.[8]

The patient's status report should include:

1. Patient identification number, age, surgical procedure, diagnosis, a summary of prior medical history, medications, allergies, and preoperative vital signs. Specific features of the patient such as deafness, poor vision, psychiatric issues, language barriers, or necessary precautions for infection control should be mentioned.
2. Location and size of intravascular catheters and monitoring devices; presence of cardiac pacemakers or defibrillator (manufacturer and model)
3. Premedication, antibiotics, anesthetic drugs for induction and maintenance, use of regional anesthetic techniques, opioids, muscle relaxants, and reversal agents; vasoactive drugs, bronchodilators, and other relevant drugs administered should also be listed
4. Exact nature of the surgical procedure. If relevant surgical issues exist (eg, adequacy of hemostasis, care of drains, restrictions on positioning), the PACU staff should be informed.
5. Anesthetic course, with emphasis on problems that may impact on the immediate postoperative course, including difficult IV access, difficult airway management, intraoperative hemodynamic instability, ECG changes, and abnormal laboratory values
6. Fluid balance, including amount, type, and rationale of fluid replacement, urine output, and estimated fluid and blood loss.

COMPLEX PATIENTS OR MAJOR PROCEDURES

As dictated by the clinical situation, the accompanying anesthetist may elect to speak directly to the anesthesiologist in charge of the PACU or a consultant regarding issues of particular importance for the patient. Issues commonly communicated directly to the anesthesiologist responsible for the patients in the PACU or a consultant can include intraoperative instability, pertinent comorbidities, excessive blood loss or airway difficulties, and as the need for continued mechanical ventilation.[9] The surgical team must be kept apprised of any clinical issues that may impact the postoperative course of the patient.

MONITORING IN THE POSTANESTHESIA CARE UNIT

The ASA's Standards for Postanesthesia Care require periodic monitoring of multiple parameters during the recovery phase, including respiratory and cardiovascular function, neuromuscular function, mental status, temperature, pain, nausea and vomiting, drainage and bleeding, and urine output. The frequency and duration of monitoring is dictated by the clinical status of the patient.[4]

COMMON POSTOPERATIVE ISSUES

Clinical issues encountered in the postoperative patient may range from very common events, such as inadequate analgesia, to less frequently experienced clinical problems such as negative pressure pulmonary edema. This section reviews the more commonly occurring postoperative clinical events. For detailed discussion of less frequently encountered issues, please see Chapter 71.

POSTOPERATIVE NAUSEA AND VOMITING

Postoperative nausea and vomiting (PONV) is one of the most common complications of general anesthesia, and although less frequent, PONV can also occur after regional anesthesia techniques.[10] Patients are commonly stratified preoperatively (see Chapter 6) with regard to their risk for PONV, with the incidence of PONV higher in women, nonsmokers, and patients with a history of PONV or motion sickness.[11,12] Additional risk factors involve the administration of narcotics, nitrous oxide, volatile anesthetics, and neostigmine as components of the anesthetic.[13] Certain types of surgery such as abdominal; breast; ear, nose, and throat; neurosurgery; and correction of strabismus may also increase the risk for PONV. Prolonged surgeries are associated with an increased incidence of PONV. A more careful implementation of the guidelines would improve the patients' outcomes.[14] Apfel et al[15] showed that a general anesthetic composed of a volatile anesthetic, nitrous oxide, and fentanyl without giving prophylactic antiemetics has an incidence of PONV as high as 59% in contrast with an anesthetic technique using propofol and avoiding nitrous oxide in combination with remifentanil, ondansetron, dexamethasone, and droperidol, in which the incidence for PONV was 17%. The same group showed that the overall incidence of PONV is about 34%, with a reduction of postoperative risk by 26% with administration of ondansetron, dexamethasone, or droperidol. Prevention of PONV is more effective than treatment after symptoms occur because the later options are much more limited.[16,17]

If PONV occurs in a patient who did not receive prophylaxis, therapy should be initiated with a serotonin antagonist and supplemented, if necessary, with other classes of drugs. In patients who received prophylaxis, subsequent therapy should consist of drugs from classes other than those already administered.[18,19] Administration of drugs from the same class within the first 6 hours after the surgery is not effective in the treatment of PONV (**Table 70-3**). Tramèr[20] suggests that treatment of nausea and vomiting may be more cost effective than prophylaxis. This view is, in part, based on the poor results associated with prophylaxis using a single agent.[21] Common agents for the treatment of PONV include:

1. **Serotonin antagonists** are effective as prophylactic antiemetics when administered before the use of narcotics or before the completion of

TABLE 70-3 Antiemetic Treatment for Patients With Postoperative Nausea and Vomiting[a]

Initial Therapy	Failed Prophylaxis
No prophylaxis or dexamethasone	Small dose of a serotonin antagonist
Small dose of a serotonin antagonist plus a second agent	Use a drug from a different class
Triple therapy with serotonin antagonist plus two other agents when PONV occurs <6 h after surgery (V)	Do not repeat initial therapy Use drug from different class or propofol, 20 mg as needed, in the PACU (adults)
Triple therapy with serotonin antagonist plus two other agents when PONV occurs > 6 h after surgery (V)	Repeat serotonin antagonist and droperidol (not dexamethasone or transdermal scopolamine) Use drug from a different class (V)

PACU, postanesthesia care unit; PONV, postoperative nausea and vomiting.

[a]Escalation of antiemetic therapy, as required, is based on the introduction of additional agents from categories of medications not previously employed. Repeated dosing of a previously ineffective agent will yield little success in the treatment of postoperative nausea and vomiting.[63]

surgery. About one quarter of the dose used for prophylaxis can be used for rescue therapy.

2. **Phenothiazines** (eg, Compazine) have been used both for prevention and treatment of PONV. This class of antiemetics can be associated with significant sedation.
3. **Dexamethasone** is most effective for prophylaxis if administered before the induction of anesthesia. It can also be used as a rescue drug.
4. **Transdermal scopolamine**, often used in the ambulatory care setting, is effective in prophylaxis when applied at least 4 hours before the end of surgery. Potential side effects include changes in vision, dry mucous membranes, and sedation.
5. **Droperidol** is no longer used as a first-line drug for the prevention and treatment of PONV. A "black box" warning issued in 2001 by the Food and Drug Administration associated droperidol with QT segment prolongation and producing torsades de pointes in some patients. Documentation of a normal QT segment before droperidol administration and continuous ECG monitoring for 2 to 3 hours after administration are currently recommended. Droperidol can be used for the treatment of PONV that has been refractory to other drugs. Charbit et al[22] demonstrated that patients with PONV have a high incidence of a prolonged QTc interval because of a variety of factors associated with anesthesia even before the administration of an antiemetic such as low-dose droperidol or ondansetron. And both classes of agents may increase the QTc interval after administration for treatment of PONV. Given this concern for producing cardiac arrhythmias, clinicians have sought alternatives to droperidol and have given **haloperidol** at low doses. In a recent meta-analysis, Büttner et al[23] demonstrated that low-dose IV haloperidol is an effective drug for PONV with minimal side effects.

A generalized approach to the perioperative evaluation, prophylaxis, and treatment of PONV is provided in **Figure 70-1**.

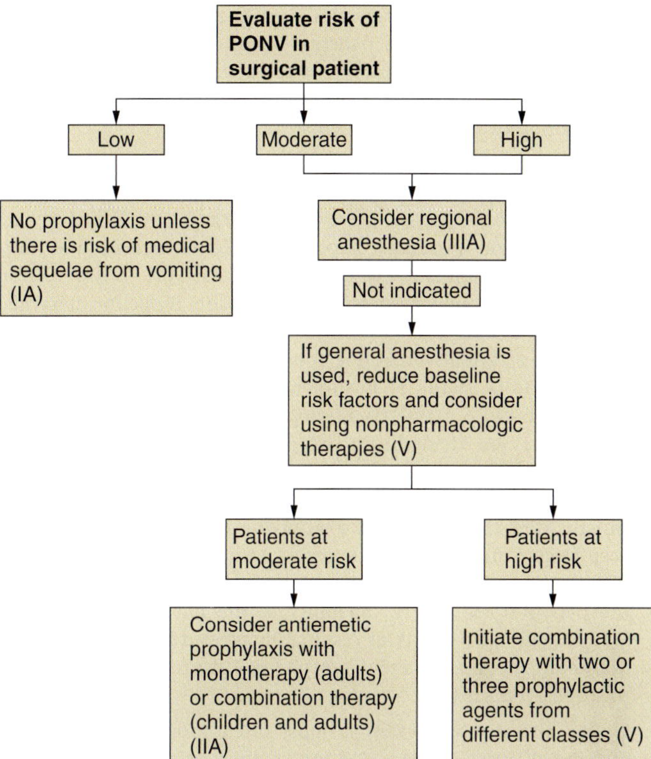

FIGURE 70-1. Algorithm for the treatment of postoperative nausea and vomiting (PONV). The algorithm is a suggested approach for the prophylaxis of patients at moderate to high risk for PONV. Prophylaxis of patients at minimal risk for PONV appears relatively ineffective. However, in the setting of patients undergoing procedures in which the potential risk for damage caused by postoperative emesis is unacceptable, prophylaxis should be initiated. The characters IA to V noted in the boxes of the diagram reflect the strength of evidence supporting the therapeutic intervention as explained by Sessler.[63]

RESPIRATORY AND AIRWAY COMPLICATIONS

Most surgical patients arrive in the PACU after extubation in the OR with supplemental oxygen provided. Supplemental oxygen is delivered by nasal cannula or a face mask during transport of the patient from the OR and is generally well tolerated by the patient. Most patients wean from the supplementary oxygen soon after arrival in the PACU. However, some patients may have a continued requirement for supplemental oxygen in the PACU or may require escalation of therapy such as a high-flow mask, noninvasive mechanical ventilation, or reintubation. For hypoxia not responsive to oxygen therapy and management of intubated patients, please refer to Chapters 71 and 79.

Respiratory and airway complications are some of the most common perioperative problems occurring in the immediate postoperative period. Risk factors for postoperative pulmonary complications include preexisting patient conditions such as chronic obstructive pulmonary disease (COPD), obstructive sleep apnea (OSA), extreme age, tobacco use, high ASA status, and malnutrition as well as surgical factors such as the proximity of the surgical site to the diaphragm. Thoracic; neurosurgical; upper abdominal; peripheral vascular surgery; and ear, nose, and throat procedures as well as emergency surgery all increase the risk for postoperative pulmonary complications.[24] The predominant issues include inadequate oxygenation or ventilation, upper airway obstruction, laryngospasm, and aspiration.[25]

General anesthesia is associated with inhibition of hypoxic and hypercapnic ventilatory drive and a reduction of functional residual capacity (FRC). These changes may persist for a variable period of time postoperatively and predispose the patient to hypoventilation and hypoxemia. In the immediate postoperative period, hypoxia is commonly caused by the presence of residual anesthetic agents. After sufficient time for recovery from anesthetic depressant effects, hypoxia may be attributable to the side effects of other medications prescribed for the patient. Analgesia and the degree of respiratory depression can differ based on the route of administration. The effects may range from a slight decrease in oxygen saturation (Spo_2) requiring supplemental oxygen to severe hypoventilation requiring administration of the opioid antagonist naloxone to reverse the respiratory depression.[26] The present standard of care suggests that all patients should receive supplemental oxygen in the immediate postoperative period.[4] Although supplemental oxygen may mask and delay the detection of hypoventilation by pulse oximetry,[27] evidence suggests that the use of supplemental oxygen in the immediate postoperative period may be associated with a reduced rate of wound infection.[28-30] Therefore, the decision to administer supplemental oxygen should be individualized for each patient. Clinical signs of hypoxemia include dyspnea, cyanosis, altered mental status, agitation, obtundation, tachycardia, hypertension, and arrhythmias. Causes of hypoxemia include the following:

1. **Atelectasis,** with increased intrapulmonary shunting, is a predictable effect of a decreased FRC caused by general anesthesia. An additional reduction in the FRC that occurs in obese patients and after thoracic or upper abdominal procedures can further potentiate the impact of atelectasis in postoperative patients. Patients undergoing procedures with epidural anesthesia without general anesthesia usually have little or no atelectasis.[31] Deep breathing and incentive spirometry are equally effective in reexpanding small areas of alveolar collapse.

Noninvasive ventilation can reinflate atelectasis and improve oxygenation in postoperative patients. Occasionally, hypoxemia may persist and a chest radiograph may reveal a segmental or lobar collapse. Chest physiotherapy or fiberoptic bronchoscopy may facilitate the inflation of atelectatic segments.

2. **Hypoventilation** is characterized by a low minute ventilation and causes hypoxemia by promoting alveolar collapse despite increasing the CO_2 partial pressure in arterial blood. When severe, hypoventilation produces hypoxemia, CO_2 narcosis, and ultimately apnea. Supplemental oxygen may mask the early detection of hypoventilation by preventing desaturation. A decline in oxygen saturation, as a sign of hypoventilation, has been found to be accurate only in patients breathing room air.[27] Therefore, monitoring the ventilatory status of postoperative patients should not rely entirely on pulse oximetry. Etiologies of postoperative hypoventilation may be divided into two groups. **Decreased ventilatory drive**, resulting from medications and agents administered during the intraoperative course, is normally short lived and resolves shortly after the patient's arrival in the PACU. **Pulmonary and respiratory muscle insufficiency** or compromise caused by conditions such as COPD, obesity, or surgical manipulation can limit the patient's ventilatory capability in the postoperative setting. Additionally, the effects of residual neuromuscular blockade can markedly impair the patient's respiratory efforts in the immediate postoperative setting.
3. **Upper airway obstruction** is most often caused by inadequate recovery of airway reflexes and muscle tone. Principal signs are the lack of adequate air movement, intercostal and suprasternal retractions, and discoordinate abdominal and chest wall motion during inspiration. Whereas complete upper airway obstruction is silent, partial obstruction is often accompanied by snoring (if the obstruction is above the larynx) or inspiratory stridor (if perilaryngeal). Obstruction is commonly seen in patients with OSA, obesity, or nasal obstruction caused by tonsillar or adenoidal hypertrophy.[32] To treat this, 100% oxygen is delivered by mask, and rapid airway management is required. A chin lift, with or without a jaw thrust, often reduces the obstruction, but some patients (eg, patients with OSA) may benefit from applying continuous positive airway pressure (CPAP). This is especially true in patients using CPAP at home. Additional conditions with the potential to impact respiratory function in the postoperative patient include laryngospasm, bronchospasm, pulmonary edema, and aspiration of gastric contents. For a detailed discussion of postoperative respiratory complications, please refer to Chapter 71.

HYPOTENSION

The differential diagnosis of hypotension is aided by a review of the patient's history and intraoperative management. Preoperative dehydration in the setting of a bowel preparation or inadequate intraoperative fluid resuscitation is a common cause of hypotension in the immediate postoperative patient. Review of the patient's intraoperative course by a review of the anesthetic record and a discussion with the intraoperative team often yield insights to the nature of postoperative hypotension. Common causes of postoperative hypotension include:

1. **Hypovolemia** is the most common cause of hypotension in the PACU, and **bleeding** must be considered to be the proximate cause until proven otherwise. Inadequate fluid replacement, osmotic polyuria, and fluid sequestration (intestinal obstruction, ascites) are other common causes of hypovolemia in the postoperative patient. Nonspecific signs of hypovolemia include hypotension, tachycardia, decreased skin turgor, dry mucous membranes, oliguria, and thirst. An IV volume challenge (250-1000 mL of crystalloid or an equivalent volume of a colloidal solution) should be considered in the setting of a patient suspected of hypovolemia after surgery. Persistent hypotension after adequate volume replacement mandates further assessment, including placement of a urinary bladder catheter and, if necessary, invasive monitoring.
2. **Impaired venous return** can occur when mechanical forces decrease venous return to the heart. Common causes include **positive-pressure ventilation** and an increased intra-abdominal compartment pressure caused by edema or a fluid collection. Signs of obstruction to venous return may be differentiated from true hypovolemia by the presence or absence of jugular vein distension. Volume administration is the mainstay of symptomatic therapy, but treatment of the cause is the ultimate intervention.
3. **Vasodilation**. Neuraxial anesthesia, residual inhalation agents, rewarming after hypothermia, transfusion reactions, adrenal insufficiency, anaphylaxis, systemic inflammation, sepsis, liver failure, and the administration of vasodilators can induce vasodilation, resulting in hypotension. Hypovolemia accentuates the hypotension secondary to vasodilation, and volume replacement alone may not fully restore the systemic blood pressure. Pharmacologic treatment may include α-adrenergic receptor agonists such as phenylephrine or norepinephrine. The use of such agents mandates close monitoring of blood pressure. Diagnosis and treatment of the specific etiology must be concurrent with such symptomatic treatment.
4. Additional causes of hypotension can be the result of cardiac dysfunction, sepsis, and chronic antihypertensive therapy. For a detailed discussion of the causes of postoperative hypotension, please refer to Chapter 71.

CARDIAC DYSRHYTHMIAS

Increased sympathetic outflow, hypoxemia, hypercarbia, electrolyte and acid–base imbalance, myocardial ischemia, increased intracranial pressure (ICP), drug toxicity, thyrotoxicosis, pericardial irritation, and malignant hyperthermia (MH) are possible causes of perioperative dysrhythmias. Premature atrial contractions and unifocal premature ventricular contractions (PVCs) generally do not require treatment.[33] Assessment and definitive therapies are presented in Chapters 9 and 71.

Commonly occurring cardiac dysrhythmias seen in the immediate postoperative setting include:

1. **Supraventricular dysrhythmias**
   a. **Sinus tachycardia** may be secondary to pain, agitation, hypovolemia, fever, hyperthermia, hypoxemia, hypercarbia, congestive heart failure, or pulmonary embolism. The symptomatic treatment of tachycardia with β-blockers should be instituted only after the underlying etiology is sought. However, a high risk for myocardial ischemia may dictate early drug intervention.
   b. **Sinus bradycardia** may result from a high neuraxial anesthetic block, opioid administration (with the exception of meperidine), vagal stimulation, α-adrenergic blockade, and increased ICP. Symptomatic treatment with anticholinergic muscarinic agents is indicated when hypotension is present or for severe bradycardia compromising cardiac output.
2. **Stable ventricular dysrhythmias**. Patients with PVCs and stable nonsustained ventricular tachycardia do not routinely require intervention. However, reversible causes, such as hypoxemia, myocardial ischemia, acidosis, hypokalemia, and hypomagnesemia, should be treated. PVCs resulting from ventricular irritation in the setting of a central venous catheter generally resolve after withdrawal of the catheter.

For further discussion and therapy, refer to Chapters 9, 71, and 76

OTHER CARDIAC-RELATED EVENTS

Postoperative pain, respiratory distress, hypovolemia, and anemia are common clinical conditions that may result in excess stress on the cardiovascular system and can result in myocardial ischemia or infarction in the PACU. Changes in the ECG may provide the earliest indication of cardiac compromise. Common abnormal findings on the ECG include:

1. **T-wave changes** (inversion, flattening, pseudonormalization) may be associated with myocardial ischemia and infarction, electrolyte imbalance, hypothermia, surgical manipulation of the mediastinum, or incorrect lead placement. Isolated T-wave changes must be considered within the clinical context of the individual patient because these changes may be benign in the postoperative setting. It is essential that postoperative changes in the ECG be compared with preoperative ECGs.[34]
2. **ST-segment** elevation or depressions are generally indicative of myocardial infarction (MI) and ischemia, respectively. ST-segment elevation can be a normal variant or may occur in other conditions such as left ventricular hypertrophy, left bundle-branch block, pericarditis, or hyperkalemia.[35] Unlike MIs in the nonsurgical setting, in the postoperative period, most MIs are associated with ST-segment depression and have a non–Q-wave pattern. While initiating standard therapy for myocardial ischemia, including supplemental oxygen, narcotics for pain, and heart rate and blood pressure control, potential precipitating factors for the ST-segment changes must be sought and corrected.

   Common causes of myocardial ischemia in the immediate postoperative period include hypoxemia, anemia, tachycardia, hypotension, and hypertension. Cardiac enzymes should be monitored in patients with persistent ECG changes. If clinically appropriate, aspirin, **β-blockade**, and IV nitroglycerin should be considered, particularly in the setting of patients with ST-segment elevation. Consultation with the cardiology service is indicated in the setting of hemodynamic instability and transfer to a cardiac intensive care unit (ICU) may be required. Ongoing ischemia mandates the institution of invasive monitoring or specialized treatment (eg, thrombolysis, percutaneous angioplasty).
3. In patients at high risk for cardiac events (patients with ischemic heart disease, cerebrovascular disease, renal insufficiency, diabetes mellitus and patients undergoing intrathoracic, intraperitoneal, or suprainguinal vascular procedures), β-blockade has been found to decrease the risk of perioperative cardiac events.[36-38] An institutional perioperative β-blockade protocol may be useful to standardize care. For patients receiving vasoactive agents for hemodynamic support, the use of β-blockade should be initiated on an individual basis. The patient with a **permanent pacemaker (PPM)** or an **implantable cardioverter defibrillator (ICD)** requires special consideration in the perioperative setting.[38] Information regarding the patient's pacemaker dependency state and the features of the device (model, manufacturer) must be obtained from the OR team. Continuous ECG monitoring is essential with particular attention to the patient's rhythm, rate, and hemodynamic status. Electrocautery used during surgery can electrically reset pacemakers, with older models likely more susceptible. Placement of a magnet over the PPM or ICD during surgery can temporarily or permanently deactivate or reset it, depending on the age and specifics of the device. Newer pacemakers may have rate-adaptive capabilities, requiring intervention by the pacemaker service before surgery. Given the potential for inadvertent program modification in the perioperative setting, interrogation of the device and communication with the electrophysiology service before and after the surgery is generally recommended. Although the ASA recommends that all patients with ICDs should have their devices interrogated in the PACU, this practice appears to be controversial because many cardiologists and manufacturers support follow-up after discharge for many patients. Interrogation of the ICDs before discharge is recommended in situations in which diathermy was used within 15 cm of the device or its leads or if there were perioperative problems with the device.[39] For a detailed discussion of patients with cardiac pacemakers and ICDs, please refer to Chapter 9.

HYPERTENSION

Postoperative hypertension is commonly observed in patients not receiving scheduled antihypertensives preoperatively in patients having undergone vascular, head and neck, thoracic, or neurosurgical procedures. Additional postoperative causes of hypertension include pain, bladder distension, fluid overload, hypoxemia, hypercarbia, hypothermia, increased ICP, and overzealous administration of vasoconstrictors. Hypertension is usually asymptomatic but may present as a headache, visual disturbances, dyspnea, restlessness, or chest pain. The initial assessment should include a review of the patient's history and operative course and verification of the accuracy of the blood pressure measurement. The management of hypertension is targeted to restoring blood pressure to within 20% of the patient's baseline. When appropriate, resumption of the patient's chronic antihypertensive oral therapy is ideal. If necessary, this can be supplemented or substituted with parenteral medication. Commonly used medications include:

1. **β-Adrenergic antagonists.** Labetalol (an α- and a β-blocker), metoprolol, esmolol, and propranolol are effective in controlling heart rate and blood pressure.
2. **Calcium channel blockers**. Verapamil or diltiazem can be used as a bolus or an infusion, and nicardipine can be administered enterally. Sublingual nifedipine is no longer recommended because it can be associated with rapid and severe hypotension, resulting in myocardial ischemia. Clevidipine, a novel third-generation dihydropyridine calcium channel blocker, is a very short-acting agent approved for use in the management of acute perioperative hypertension. Acting primarily as an arterial vasodilator, its half-life of only 2 minutes combined with metabolism by esterases in the blood and extravascular tissues makes it an appealing drug for use in the perioperative period.[40]
3. **Hydralazine** is a potent vasodilator that may induce reflex tachycardia.
4. **Nitrates.** Nitroglycerin is preferentially a venodilator that is particularly useful in patients with known myocardial ischemia. Sodium nitroprusside is a potent arterial and venodilator and requires invasive blood pressure monitoring.
5. **Fenoldopam,** a selective peripheral dopaminergic receptor agonist, may be administered as an IV infusion. Side effects include tachycardia, headache, and increased intraocular pressure.
6. **Enalaprilat,** a parenterally administered angiotensin-converting enzyme (ACE) inhibitor, is of particular value in patients routinely treated with ACE inhibitors or angiotensin receptor blockers in a setting where enteral medications are not clinically appropriate.

NEUROLOGIC COMPLICATIONS

Neurologic complications include:

1. Residual paralysis after general anesthesia, described as residual neuromuscular blockade or residual curarization, has a prevalence between 4% and 50%.[41] This phenomenon is most often observed in the PACU, making it an important consideration in the postoperative recovery period. Residual paralysis usually results in mild muscle weakness, but it can also result in serious complications such as hypoxia, pulmonary collapse, and acute respiratory failure. Supportive therapy and reversal of neuromuscular blockade with an acetylcholinesterase inhibitor may be indicated in the immediate postoperative period. The selective binding relaxant sugammadex, a γ-cyclodextrin, which binds rocuronium and to a lesser extent vecuronium and pancuronium, may soon be available for rapid reversal of residual blockade.[42]
2. **Delayed awakening** is most often the result of persistent **cerebral depression by anesthetic and analgesic** agents.[43] **Metabolic causes** of delayed awakening include hypothermia, sepsis, preexisting encephalopathies, hypoglycemia, and electrolyte or acid–base derangements. Additional causes of delayed awakening include

decreased cerebral perfusion during or after surgery that may cause diffuse or localized injury to the brain. In patients with cerebrovascular disease, short periods of hypotension may cause a critical reduction of cerebral perfusion and stroke. If such an event is suspected, immediate consultation with a neurologist should be obtained together with radiologic imaging (eg, computed tomography, magnetic resonance imaging, or angiography). If a seizure is suspected as the cause of delayed awakening, then treatment should be started immediately (see Chapter 51). Neurologic damage may range in severity and be as benign as diplopia after cataract surgery or as severe peripheral nerve injury or may be caused by a stroke.[44] Strokes have an incidence of 0.08% to 2.9%, even as high as 5.2%, depending on patient risk factors and the type of surgery and may be ischemic or hemorrhagic.[45,46] Early diagnosis of a stroke may be difficult because symptoms such as slurred speech, visual changes, dizziness, agitation, confusion, psychosis, numbness, muscular weakness, or paralysis may overlap with residual anesthetic effects.

a. **Ischemic strokes** are more common in patients with cerebrovascular disease, hypercoagulable states, or atrial fibrillation and may be associated with intraoperative hypotension. Fat emboli secondary to long bone fractures can also produce strokes.
b. **Hemorrhagic strokes** are more common in patients with coagulopathies, uncontrolled hypertension, and cerebral aneurysms or arteriovenous malformations and head trauma. Hemorrhagic strokes are more frequent after intracranial surgery, carotid endarterectomy, cardiac surgery, or multiple traumas. Neurologic consultation in conjunction with appropriate imaging techniques is mandatory to guide the possible choice of immediate and possibly lifesaving treatment options.

3. **Emergence delirium** is characterized by excitement alternating with lethargy, disorientation, and inappropriate behavior. Delirium can vary from hyperactive **delirium**, characterized by a state of agitation, hyperarousal, or hyperalertness, or **hypoactive delirium**, in which patients present with a flat affect and are poorly responsive or lethargic. Delirium may occur in any patient but more frequently occurs in elderly patients and in those with a history of drug dependency, dementia, or other psychiatric disorders. Many perioperative agents, such as ketamine, opioids, benzodiazepines, metoclopramide, anticholinergics (atropine or scopolamine), and droperidol, may precipitate delirium. Delirium may be symptomatic of a wide variety of clinical abnormalities, including hypoxemia, acidemia, hyponatremia, hypoglycemia, intracranial injury, sepsis, severe pain, and alcohol withdrawal and as such mandates investigation to exclude these causes.[47] The mainstay of treatment of patients with postoperative delirium is reassurance and reorientation while identifying and reversing treatable causes. Antipsychotic medications such as **haloperidol** can be used for management of agitation in patients with hyperactive delirium. **Physostigmine** may reverse delirium caused by anticholinergic agents. Other strategies used with some success are using different classes of medication in smaller doses, such as mood stabilizers (Depakote or Tegretol) with benzodiazepines and antipsychotics and even the use of dexmedetomidine.
4. **Peripheral nerve injury** may result from improper intraoperative positioning, direct surgical damage, or as a complication of regional anesthetic techniques. In the ASA closed claim analysis, ulnar nerve injury accounted for approximately one-third of the cases of nerve injury followed by damage to the brachial plexus and the common peroneal nerve.[48] Risk factors for nerve injury after surgery include a slender body habitus, a previous history of neuropathy, smoking, and diabetes. Additional information on perioperative nerve injury is discussed in Chapter 49.
5. **Intraoperative awareness and recall** are rare complications of general anesthesia (0.13% in a large multicenter trial) that may initially be detected in the PACU.[49,50] Awareness and recall are most commonly associated with trauma, cardiac, and obstetric surgery.[51] Risk factors include young age, history of substance abuse, ASA physical status III to V, a history of recall, light anesthesia, and the use of muscle relaxants.[52] The modified Brice Questionnaire (**Box 70-1**) may be used as a screening tool in the PACU to identify patients at risk for recall. Patients with evidence of recall should receive reassurance, sympathetic care, and referral for psychologic counseling as required.[53]

BOX 70-1

Brice Questionnaire for Awareness[a]

What is the last thing you remember before going to sleep for the operation?

What is the first thing you remember on waking after the operation?

Do you remember anything between going to sleep and waking up?

Did you have any dreams?

What was the most unpleasant thing you remember from the operation and anesthesia?

[a]The Brice questionnaire can be used in the immediate postoperative period to determine any issues that may suggest the possibility of intraoperative awareness. Although the first indications that intraoperative recall may have occurred can be noted in the PACU, it is important to ensure that the patient has recovered adequately from the effects of anesthesia to be able to appropriately cooperate with the examination.

PRINCIPLES OF PAIN MANAGEMENT

Adequate analgesia begins in the OR and continues in the PACU.[54] In the postoperative period, incisional pain is the most common discomfort experienced by patients.[55,56] A detailed discussion of the management of postoperative pain is presented in Chapter 72. A general overview of some common therapeutic modalities is described below:

1. **Opioids** (IV or epidural) are the mainstay of postoperative analgesia. **Fentanyl**, a potent synthetic opioid with a rapid onset of action, is commonly limited to the intraoperative setting. However, small parenteral doses can be titrated postoperatively to establish rapid analgesia. **Morphine, hydromorphone,** and **meperidine** are effective longer acting analgesic agents.

   Meperidine must be avoided in patients taking monoamine oxidase inhibitors.
2. **Nonsteroidal** anti-inflammatory drugs (NSAIDs) and **acetaminophen** are used in combination with other analgesics to provide more effective analgesia compared with either drug alone.[57] **Ketorolac** is a potent IV NSAID commonly given for postoperative analgesia. Potential toxicities of all NSAIDs include decreased platelet aggregation, gastrointestinal bleeding, and nephrotoxicity.[58] Additional **adjuvant analgesics** include spasmolytics (**cyclobenzaprine**) and small doses of benzodiazepines.
3. **IV patient-controlled analgesia** has been shown to be superior in patient satisfaction compared with intermittent analgesia administered by the medical staff. **Continuous epidural analgesia**, when appropriate, should be continued postoperatively or promptly initiated in the PACU if not used in the OR.[59]

Neuraxial and **regional sensory blocks**, discussed in Chapter 47, are attractive alternatives for postoperative analgesia, especially for patients in whom opioids may be contraindicated.[60] Although the use of ultrasonography for placement is widespread because it seems to be associated with an increased success rate of regional blocks, any role for acupuncture or transcutaneous electrical nerve stimulation for postoperative pain control is uncertain.[61]

TEMPERATURE CONTROL

Hypothermia is a common occurrence in the PACU, resulting from the cold environment in the OR combined with anesthesia-induced impairment of effective thermoregulation. Even mild hypothermia (a body temperature between 34°C and 36°C) can be perceived as uncomfortable by a conscious patient. Additional side effects associated with hypothermia include shivering,[62] increased duration of residual paralysis, coagulopathy, cardiac dysrhythmias, surgical site infections, and an increased duration of postanesthetic recovery.[63] Treatment with warm blankets or with forced-air warming systems is generally effective.[64] If fluid administration or transfusion is required, fluid warming should be used to avoid further cooling of the patient.

Hyperthermia is less common than hypothermia in the immediate postoperative period. Fever in the PACU may be associated with postoperative atelectasis or a normal inflammatory response related to surgery. However, the presence of an elevated temperature in the immediate postoperative patient can also be associated with conditions such as sepsis or reactions to medications and requires appropriate investigation. Fever should not be automatically assumed to be a sign of infection, and suppressing fever may be harmful in some patients.[65] Although relatively uncommon, hypermetabolic states such as **MH** and **thyrotoxicosis** may present as a fever in the PACU. Hypothermia and hyperthermia are discussed in Chapter 87.

FLUID ADMINISTRATION AND HEMORRHAGE

All patients in the PACU must be evaluated for the adequacy of the intraoperative fluid resuscitation. Parameters that may indicate that the patient requires additional fluid administration include hypotension, tachycardia, and low urine output. **Hypovolemia** is the most common cause of postoperative hypotension. And until proven otherwise, **bleeding** must be the primary concern in postoperative hypotension. Gan et al[66] demonstrated that intraoperative goal-directed fluid administration can decrease postoperative complications and is associated with an earlier return of the gastrointestinal function and a shorter hospital stay. The approach to fluid resuscitation can vary according to the clinical situation and institutional protocol.

There is significant debate in the literature regarding the appropriate fluid for resuscitation of postoperative patients. Some clinicians advocate the use of colloid solutions for resuscitation because they may ensure a more rapid and effective expansion of the intravascular volume and do not cross capillary membranes into the interstitial space as readily as crystalloids. Investigators in the Saline Versus Albumin Fluid Evaluation (SAFE) trial demonstrated that albumin and saline are both safe and clinically equivalent, rendering the same 28-day outcome for resuscitation of critically ill patients in the ICU.[67]

Blood transfusion carries specific risks, including viral infections, bacterial contamination, parasites, prions, hemolytic transfusion reactions, alloimmunization, autoimmunization, immunosuppression, and transfusion-related lung injury. Hebert et al[68] showed that critically ill patients who receive a restrictive approach to blood transfusion have a better outcome than patients who receive liberal blood transfusions, thereby motivating a trend to limit phlebotomies, decrease transfusion thresholds, and ultimately reduce the number of blood transfusions in critically ill patients. Ultimately, clinicians must consider the risks and benefits for the individual patient in developing a volume replacement strategy that may involve blood component therapy.[69]

Unrecognized or ongoing **hemorrhage**, although uncommon in the immediate postoperative patient, is an emergency requiring immediate treatment and can rapidly overwhelm PACU resources. Coordination with the blood bank, surgery and anesthesia team members, and the ORs is necessary in a timely manner. Personnel assigned to the PACU must have a plan established to address the requirements of rapidly hemorrhaging postoperative patients.

Hemorrhage may present in an obvious manner, such as the rapid saturation of a dressing or an increase in drainage or chest tube output. However, the presentation may be more subtle, with signs of hypovolemia such as hypotension or tachycardia, abdominal distension, a decrease in urine output, or a downward trend of hematocrit or hemoglobin values.

In laparoscopic procedures involving the abdomen and thorax, signs of bleeding may not be apparent in the OR and may only later be identified in the PACU.[70] This bleeding of a delayed nature may be associated with procedures requiring the insertion of tracers.[71]

Patients receiving chronic anticoagulation therapy may be at greater risk for postoperative complications associated with bleeding. In a study of 600 surgical patients chronically anticoagulated with Coumadin when anticoagulation was either discontinued or reversed before surgery, Torn and Rosendaal[72] demonstrated an increased incidence of hemorrhage-related complications. A detailed discussion regarding the management of fluid and blood component replacement therapy is presented in Chapters 71 and 83.

POSTANESTHESIA CARE UNIT DISCHARGE

As described in the ASA's Standards for Postanesthesia Care, a physician should be responsible for the discharge of each patient from the PACU.[4] A variety of discharge criteria and systems for the evaluation of a patient for discharge from the PACU are used and should be approved by the local anesthesia department and the medical staff. The criteria may also require modification to address the specifics of discharge (ie, criteria for a patient being discharged to a surgical floor in the hospital vary to some extent from those used for a patient to be discharged from the hospital).[73] In the absence of a physician in the PACU, the nurse may determine that the patient meets discharge criteria and should note the physician accepting responsibility for the discharge.

Discharge criteria may be based on length of stay in the PACU (time based) or can use a clinical scoring system. In commonly used scoring systems, vital signs, level of consciousness, pain control, resolution of nausea, and other parameters are assigned scores in a manner that will set a minimum composite score for discharge eligibility. In the 1970s, a scoring system was developed to assess the appropriateness of discharge to an ambulatory unit, or phase II recovery. Later modified to condense discharge criteria into a more effective scoring system, use of the **Aldrete recovery score** (**Table 70-4**) appears to decrease the PACU length of stay.[74,75]

Although no set of criteria or system has been shown to be superior, evidence suggests that a clinical-based system may reduce overall length of stay in the PACU without risk to the patient. Predictors of increased length of stay include the length of the surgical procedure and the use of opioids, intubation, and antiemetics. Surprisingly, age, gender, ASA classification, and urgency of surgery did not predict the PACU length of stay.[76]

The decision to admit a patient to the hospital or to discharge the patient to home is based upon a number of factors, including the nature of the surgical procedure, complications encountered, and the patient's comorbidities and living situation. In most hospitals, patients who will be admitted to the ICU after surgical procedures are transferred to those units directly from the OR. However, these patients may be initially transferred to the PACU awaiting ICU bed availability. Occasionally, patients may require a period of observation in the PACU for airway monitoring before ICU transfer where staff may be less skilled in acute airway management.

Given the ever-increasing operational tempo in hospitals, there is often a shortage of ICU beds. As such, hospitals often use the PACU as a short-term ICU for patients who are expected to recover within a 24- to 36-hour period to permit safe transfer to a general care hospital floor.[76,77]

Although controversial, ambulatory patients are expected to void before discharge home. New evidence suggests that some patients who are having general anesthesia and nonpelvic procedures are considered to be at low risk and can be safely discharged home without voiding.[78] Patients with a history of voiding difficulties or who underwent pelvic surgery (eg, hernia, anal surgery, or transurethral resection of the prostate) or underwent spinal or epidural anesthesia should void before discharge. If difficulty with voiding occurs, then they should be evaluated

TABLE 70-4 Post-Anesthesia Recovery (PAR) Scoring Criteria: Modified Aldrete Recovery Score[a]

PAR Score	Admission	15 Min	30 Min	60 Min	Discharge
Activity					
Able to move voluntary					
4 extremities: 2					
2 extremities: 1					
0 extremities: 0					
Respiration					
Breathes deeply, coughs freely: 2					
Dyspnea, shallow or limited: 1					
Apneic: 0					
Circulation					
BP ± 20% of preoperative: 2					
BP ± 20%-49% of preoperative: 1					
BP ± 50% of preoperative: 0					
Consciousness					
Fully awake: 2					
Arousable with minimal stimulation: 1					
Not responding: 0					
O_2 Saturation					
>92% on room air: 2					
Needs O_2 to maintain >90%: 1					
<90% even with O_2: 0					
TOTAL 0-10					

BP, blood pressure.

[a]The primary shortfall of the Aldrete scoring system is that it does not consider pain, nausea, or emesis common occurrences in the postanesthesia care unit (PACU). Institutions may create individual systems with similar parameters for evaluation. The goal of any system is to reliably predict a point where a patient can be safely transferred from observation in the PACU, either for transfer to a general care ward or for accompaniment to home. A minimum composite score of 8 is required for discharge consideration.

for possible urinary retention.[78] In this era of progress in medicine, with use of da Vinci–assisted procedures, as well as minimally invasive surgical procedures, PACU clinicians face new and unexplored challenges. These issues require collaboration from the anesthesiologist, whose role is extending toward being a coordinator and in charge of planning the entire perioperative period. The emphasis should be on minimally invasive surgery complemented by multimodal nonopioid analgesia, use of regional anesthesia when indicated, fluid optimization, early nutrition, and ambulation. The ultimate goals are not to decrease hospital stay but to enhance recovery, decrease intraoperative organ dysfunction, and ultimately decrease morbidity. After undergoing sedation or general anesthesia for a surgical procedure, a patient's memory and judgment are often impaired. Therefore, a responsible person should be present to assist the patient upon discharge from the hospital.[79]

KEY REFERENCES

- American Society of Anesthesiologists. *American Society of Anesthesiologists Standards for Postanesthesia Care.* Available at: http://www.asahq.org/publicationsAndServices/standards/36.pdf. Accessed September 25, 2010.
- Cashman JN, Dolin SJ. Respiratory and haemodynamic effects of acute postoperative pain management: evidence from published data. *Br J Anaesth.* 2004;93:212-223.
- Gan TJ. Risk factors for postoperative nausea and vomiting. *Anesth Analg.* 2006;102:1884-1898.
- Hines R, Barash PG, Watrous G, O'Connor T. Complications occurring in the postanesthesia care unit: a survey. *Anesth Analg.* 1992;74:503-509.

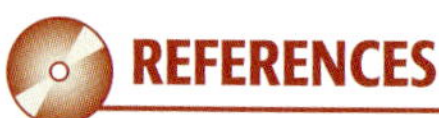

REFERENCES

Complete references available on DVD and online version at www.LongneckerAnesthesiology.com

CHAPTER 71 Postoperative Complications

Edward A. Bittner
Loreta Grecu
Edward George

KEY POINTS

1. Complications in the postanesthesia care unit (PACU) are common. Despite pharmacologic and medical advances over the last 10 years, the incidence of postoperative complications appears largely unchanged. Even minor postoperative complications are important to patients, and greater efforts at preventing and treating such complications should lead to improved postoperative recovery and patient satisfaction.
2. Knowledge of the expected postoperative course for a given operation is essential to identifying and managing problems when they occur. Awareness of the temporal patterns of complications is important to anticipating periods of increased perioperative risk.
3. Airway obstruction is common in the postoperative period. Upper airway obstruction arises in the pharynx (posterior tongue displacement, soft tissue collapse), larynx (laryngeal edema, laryngospasm, vocal cord paralysis), or trachea due to extrinsic compression. Anesthetics, and even minimal residual neuromuscular blockade, may lead to upper airway obstruction.
4. Hypoxemia is common in postoperative patients not receiving supplemental oxygen (O_2). Following general anesthesia or sedation, all patients should receive supplemental O_2 during their transport from the operating room and during their initial PACU stay. Continuous monitoring of O_2 saturation with pulse oximetry is essential for early detection of hypoxemia.
5. Several conditions may necessitate continued intubation after surgery. They include delayed emergence from general anesthesia, inadequate reversal of neuromuscular blockade, potential for airway obstruction, inadequate gas exchange, and hemodynamic instability.
6. Hypotension is a common postoperative complication that results from hypovolemia (most common), decreased vascular tone, and/or reduced cardiac output. Causes of hypovolemia in the PACU include inadequate fluid replacement, ongoing hemorrhage, and fluid sequestration ("third spacing"). Clinical evaluation of a patient's intravascular volume status requires consideration of preoperative status, type and duration of surgery, estimated blood loss, fluid replacement, and evidence of hemostasis.
7. Cardiac dysrhythmias are common during the perioperative period, and most dysrhythmias are benign. The precipitating factor is usually a transient imbalance such as hypoxia, ischemia, increased catecholamines, altered acid–base status, or electrolyte abnormalities. The management strategy for a new dysrhythmia is focused on stabilizing hemodynamics and treating the underlying problem.

8. Hypertension is a very common problem in the postoperative period. Sympathetic nervous system activation resulting from noxious stimuli, such as pain, anxiety, bladder distension, fluid overload, hypoxemia, hypercarbia, and hypothermia, are common precipitants. The decision to treat hypertension should take into consideration the patient's baseline blood pressure, coexisting diseases, and perceived risk of complications.
9. Urinary retention and oliguria are common problems in the PACU. Oliguria is most commonly caused by hypovolemia (prerenal) in the immediate postoperative period, but postrenal and intrinsic renal causes should also be considered.
10. Patients who develop bleeding postoperatively require rapid evaluation to differentiate poor surgical hemostasis (which may require immediate reoperation) or from a diffuse coagulopathy. It is important to appreciate that surgical and nonsurgical bleeding often coexist. If there is evidence of significant bleeding, diagnosis and treatment usually occur simultaneously. Adequate intravenous (IV) access should be established, availability of appropriate blood products ensured, and a diagnostic evaluation performed.
11. Hypothermia remains a common PACU problem. Even mild hypothermia (core temperature between 34°C and 36°C) has been associated with adverse outcomes, including myocardial ischemia, arrhythmias, coagulopathy, wound infection, decreased drug metabolism, and poor patient satisfaction.
12. The major causes of delayed awakening after general anesthesia can be divided into 3 groups: (1) prolonged pharmacologic effects, (2) metabolic abnormalities, and (3) neurologic injury.
13. Awareness with recall of intraoperative events is an infrequent but recognized complication of general anesthesia that can result in significant distress to patients and long-term psychological sequelae. In cases of possible awareness, the patient should be offered counseling and psychological support.

Complications in the PACU are common. In a study of 18473 patients entering the PACU at a university teaching hospital, Hines et al[1] reported a complication rate of 23%, with nausea and vomiting (9.8%), need for upper airway support (6.9%), and hypotension (2.7%) the most frequently encountered problems (**Fig. 71-1**). Despite pharmacologic and medical advances over the last 10 years, the incidence of postoperative complications appears largely unchanged.[2] Even minor postoperative complications are important to patients (**Table 71-1**), and greater efforts at preventing and treating complications should lead to improved postoperative recovery and patient satisfaction.[3,4]

TABLE 71-1 Ranking of Patient's Preferences for Postoperative Anesthesia Outcomes

Outcome	Rank (Mean)[a]
Vomiting	2.56
Gagging on endotracheal tube	2.97
Pain	3.46
Nausea	4.02
Recall without pain	4.85
Residual weakness	5.34
Shivering	5.36
Sore throat	8.02
Somnolence	8.28

[a]Outcomes are ranked in relation to each other on a scale from 1 (most undesirable) to 10 (most desirable).

Modified from Macario A, Weinger M, Carney S, et al. Which clinical anesthesia outcomes are important to avoid? The perspective of patients. *Anesth Analg.* 1999;89:652-658. With permission.

This chapter focuses on postoperative complications commonly encountered in the PACU setting, with emphasis on early diagnosis and treatment. Naturally there is some overlap with events that occur during routine recovery (see Chapter 70). Many of the specific details of diagnosis and management are covered in other chapters of this book and are not repeated here.

As with intraoperative anesthetic care, knowledge of the expected postoperative course for a given operation is essential for identifying and managing problems when they occur including awareness of the perioperative risk (**Table 71-2**).[5] When complications do occur, early communication with the surgical team is essential.

AIRWAY COMPLICATIONS

UPPER AIRWAY OBSTRUCTION

Upper airway obstruction can arise in the pharynx from posterior tongue displacement or soft tissue collapse; the larynx from laryngeal edema, laryngospasm, or vocal cord paralysis; or the large airways from

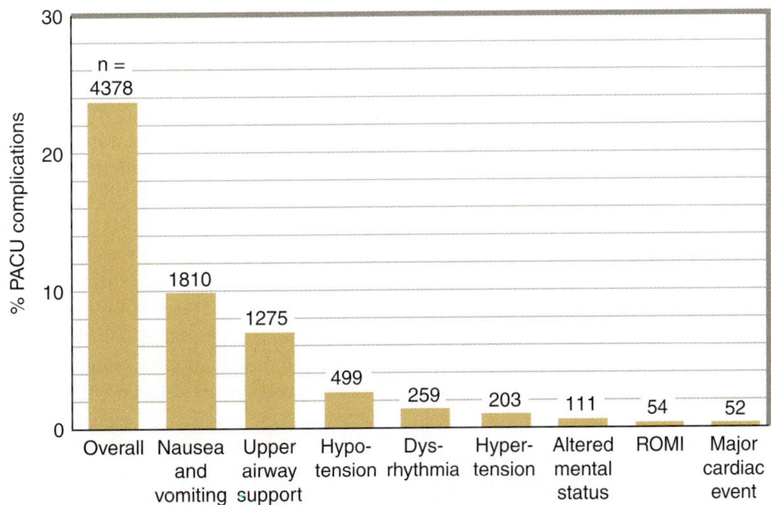

FIGURE 71-1. Major postanesthesia care unit complications by percentage of occurrence from a prospective study of 18473 patients. PACU, postanesthesia care unit; ROMI, rule out myocardial infarction. [From Hines R, Barash PG, Watrous G, et al. Complications occurring in the postoperative care unit: a survey. *Anesth Analg.* 1992;74:503-509. With permission.]

TABLE 71-2 Temporal Patterns of Postoperative Complications

Complications	Time/Interval of Greatest Risk
Hypotension	Day 1
Myocardial infarction	
Respiratory depression	
Congestive heart failure	Days 1-3
Pulmonary embolism	
Respiratory failure	
Pneumonia	Days 4-7
Cerebrovascular accident	Days 8-30
Sepsis	
Renal failure	Days 1-3, 8-30

Results of 1021 patients undergoing intra-abdominal operations in Veterans Administration (VA) medical centers.

Data from Thompson JS, Baxter BT, Allison JG, et al. Temporal patterns of postoperative complications. *Arch Surg.* 2003;138:596-603.

extrinsic compression. Anesthetics, and even minimal residual neuromuscular blockade, may lead to upper airway obstruction.[6] Principal signs are lack of adequate air movement, intercostal and suprasternal retractions, and discoordinate abdominal and chest wall movements during inspiration.

Pharyngeal Obstruction Usually simple maneuvers such as a chin lift, jaw thrust, and lateral decubitus positioning, as well as decreasing the level of sedation, are successful in relieving pharyngeal obstruction. Oropharyngeal or nasopharyngeal airways are useful adjuncts. Nasopharyngeal airways are better tolerated than oral airways at light levels of sedation because they are less likely to provoke a gag reflex. Careful insertion of nasal airways is necessary to avoid creating a nosebleed.

Laryngeal Obstruction

Laryngeal Edema Laryngeal or subglottic edema can create airway obstruction. This is particularly true in children because of the smaller airway diameter and in patients recovering from neck surgery. Treatment of partial airway obstruction resulting from airway edema includes head-up positioning to promote venous drainage and administration of steroids and nebulized epinephrine. Treatment of severe airway edema may require emergency reintubation or tracheostomy.

Prolonged surgery in a head-down position can result in significant swelling of the airway. The common practice of listening for an air leak with a positive pressure breath after deflation of the endotracheal cuff is a reliable method to determine that extubation will likely be successful if a leak is present.[7] However, a failed leak test does not preclude uneventful extubation.[8] Patients at risk for significant swelling should be evaluated (using direct or fiberoptic laryngoscopy) before extubation because they are at risk for complete airway obstruction. Patients with significant obstruction should remain intubated until airway edema resolves.

Laryngospasm Laryngospasm is a reflex resulting from prolonged glottic closure. Although the cords are adducted, the primary obstruction is caused by tonic contraction of the laryngeal muscles and descent of the epiglottis over the laryngeal inlet. Laryngospasm may be precipitated by light anesthesia and the presence of an airway irritant such as secretions, blood, or a foreign body. It also can be caused by stimulation from an elongated uvula, may be sleep related, or may be stimulated by distal esophageal afferents.[9] Partial laryngospasm allows for some air movement and may be difficult to distinguish from other causes of upper airway obstruction. Complete laryngospasm prevents all air movement and is a prominent cause of negative pressure pulmonary edema (see later section on pulmonary edema). Management of laryngospasm consists of jaw thrust, positive pressure ventilation, and possibly administration of intravenous propofol or a small dose of succinylcholine (0.1 mg/kg).

Vocal Cord Paralysis Vocal cord paralysis can be due to either nerve injury or mechanical injury and may be unilateral or bilateral. Injury to the recurrent laryngeal nerve prevents abduction of the ipsilateral vocal cord, which becomes fixed in a paramedian position because of the unopposed action of the cricothyroid muscle. An inflated endotracheal tube cuff in the subglottic larynx can compress the anterior branch of the recurrent laryngeal nerve as it enters between the cricoid and thyroid cartilage, resulting in nerve injury. Recurrent laryngeal nerve injury may occur after operations such as a rigid bronchoscopy, thyroid and parathyroid surgery, or laryngeal and thoracic surgery. Arytenoid avulsion can result in vocal cord immobility.[10]

Hoarseness usually is noted immediately after extubation. Healthy patients generally tolerate the resulting increased airway resistance, but it may become a problem in patients with preexisting pulmonary compromise. Bilateral recurrent laryngeal nerve injuries result in inadequate glottic opening and require emergent reintubation or tracheostomy. Vocal cord paralysis usually is associated with spontaneous recovery, but it may take a period of days to months. Otolaryngologic evaluation in the acute setting is generally warranted.

Extrinsic Airway Compression Acute extrinsic neck compression from an expanding neck hematoma can be life threatening. Neck hematomas can develop after carotid endarterectomy, thyroid or parathyroid surgery, or other neck surgery. Although many neck hematomas can be treated conservatively, they should be closely monitored for progression and signs of airway compromise. A rapidly expanding hematoma can cause marked tracheal deviation and make emergency reintubation extremely difficult. If possible, subcutaneous clot should be decompressed by removing surgical sutures. Definitive treatment usually requires returning to the operating room for hematoma evacuation and exploration.[11,12]

PULMONARY DYSFUNCTION

General anesthesia inhibits hypoxic and hypercapnic ventilatory drive and reduces the lung's functional residual capacity. These changes may persist for variable periods of time postoperatively and predispose to hypoventilation and hypoxemia. Additional causes of hypoxemia and hypercapnia encountered in the PACU include aspiration, pulmonary edema, pulmonary embolism (PE), and pneumothorax.

HYPOXEMIA

Hypoxemia is common in postoperative patients not receiving supplemental O_2. In a study of patients undergoing transfer from the operating room to the PACU, Tyler et al[13] found that 30% of patients had O_2 saturations (Spo_2) less than 90% while breathing air. The most common causes of hypoxemia in the early postoperative period include hypoventilation and atelectasis. Patients with preexisting lung disease or obesity and those recovering from thoracic and upper abdominal surgery are at increased risk (**Fig. 71-2**).[14]

Following general anesthesia or sedation, all patients should receive supplemental O_2 during transport from the operating room and during their initial PACU stay. Continuous monitoring of O_2 saturation with pulse oximetry is essential to early detection of hypoxemia. It is important to remember that supplemental O_2 can prolong the time to desaturation, which may delay the detection of hypoventilation. Hypoxemia is treated by increasing the inspired O_2, elevating the head of the bed, performing lung expansion maneuvers, and eliminating other reversible causes (eg, bronchospasm, secretions, and mucus plugs). Continuous positive airway pressure may be effective in treating more severe hypoxemia in some patients and decrease the need for endotracheal intubation (**Fig. 71-3**).[15,16]

Hypoventilation Hypoventilation is characterized by an inappropriately low minute ventilation with resulting hypercapnia and respiratory

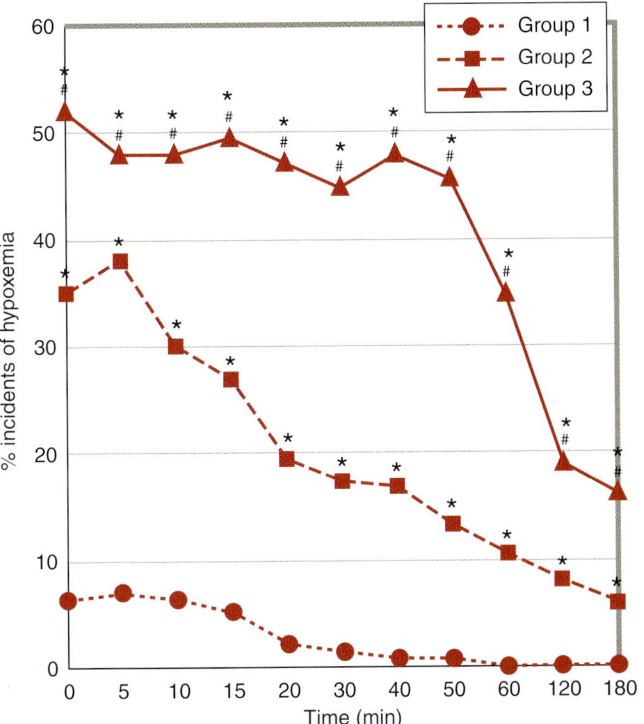

FIGURE 71-2. Incidence of hypoxemia in the first 180 minutes after surgery while patients were breathing room air. Group 1, superficial plastic surgery; group 2, upper abdominal surgery; group 3, thoracoabdominal surgery. Points are incidence of hypoxemia (Sp_{O_2} 85%-90%). **p* < 0.01 versus group 1. #*p* < 0.05 vs group 2. [From Xue FS, Li BW, Zhang GS, et al. The influence of surgical sites on early postoperative hypoxemia in adults undergoing elective surgery. *Anesth Analg*. 1999;88:213-219. With permission.]

acidosis. Severe hypoventilation results in hypoxemia, carbon dioxide (CO_2) narcosis, and ultimately apnea. Causes of postoperative hypoventilation include decreased ventilatory drive, respiratory muscle insufficiency, increased CO_2 production, and acute or chronic lung disease.

Decreased Ventilatory Drive The typical combination of inhaled anesthetics, opioids, and benzodiazepines can depress both the hypercarbic and hypoxic drive, resulting in hypoventilation. Development of postoperative hypercarbia can be deceptive because patients may appear awake and even complain of pain while experiencing significant hypoventilation. Ventilatory depression from opioids and sedatives will become significantly worse, however, if the patient falls asleep (see Chapter 41). A balance must be achieved between adequate analgesia and an acceptable level of respiratory depression. Opioid-induced hypoventilation can be reversed by small incremental doses of naloxone (0.04-0.08 mg) while preserving some analgesia. Reversal of narcosis usually occurs within 1 to 2 minutes and lasts for 30 to 60 minutes. Caution should be exercised because the duration of action of naloxone is shorter than that of most opioids, and repeated doses of naloxone or an infusion may be required. Flumazenil can reverse the sedative effects of benzodiazepines, but it does not reverse the depression of hypoxic drive (see Chapter 40). Flumazenil does not reverse opioid-induced respiratory depression.

Respiratory Muscle Insufficiency Incomplete reversal of neuromuscular blockade can result in airway obstruction and hypoventilation. The patient may exhibit discoordinated movements, generalized weakness, hypoxemia, or shallow breathing. The frequency of residual blockade ranges between 4% and 50% is more common in patients who receive long-acting muscle relaxants such as pancuronium and those not treated with reversal agents (**Fig. 71-4**).[17-19] Residual blockade is associated with muscle weakness, O_2 desaturation, atelectasis, and respiratory failure.

Limited chest expansion may be caused by pain (splinting) after thoracic and upper abdominal surgery, resulting in atelectasis and consequently right-to-left shunting. Better analgesia (particularly that produced by neuraxial and intercostal blocks) facilitates deep breathing and significantly reduces hypercapnia and hypoxemia.

Many factors increase the work of breathing for postoperative patients. For example, functional residual capacity can be reduced by airway closure and collapse; significant muscular effort is required to reexpand the lung. Other intrathoracic factors, such as pulmonary edema, pneumothorax, restrictive lung diseases, and skeletal abnormalities, can reduce lung compliance and increase energy expenditure for breathing. Obesity, gastric distension, and restrictive dressings on the chest or abdomen are extrathoracic factors that result in increased work of breathing and the potential for inadequate ventilation. Incentive

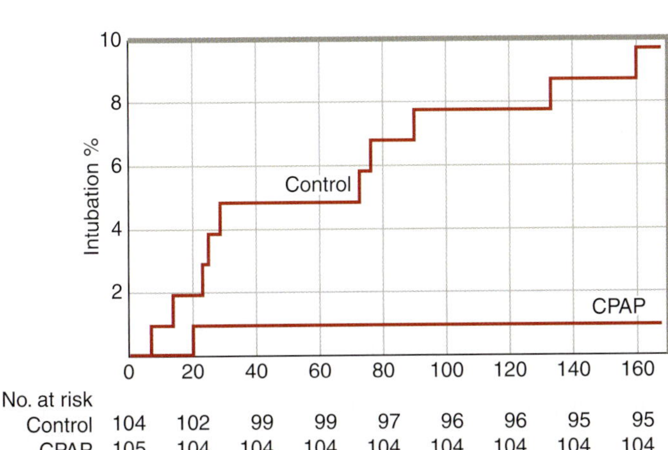

FIGURE 71-3. Intubation rates: continuous positive airway pressure plus oxygen (CPAP) versus oxygen alone (control) for treatment of postoperative hypoxemia. The CPAP group had a significantly lower intubation rate (*p* = 0.005, log-rank test) than the group treated with oxygen alone. [From Squadrone V, Coha M, Cerutti E, et al. Continuous positive airway pressure for treatment of postoperative hypoxemia. *JAMA*. 2005;293:589-595. With permission.]

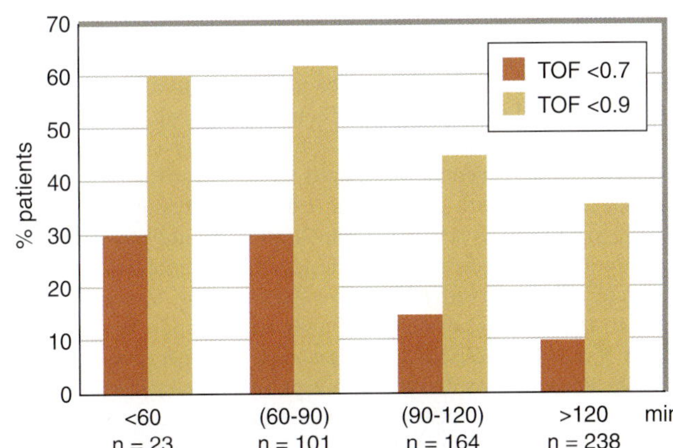

FIGURE 71-4. Residual paralysis rate. Partial paralysis rate (percent) according to delay between administration of an intermediate-duration muscle relaxant (atracurium, vecuronium, rocuronium) and arrival in the postanesthesia care unit. Train-of-four (TOF) ratios less than 0.7 and less than 0.9 were examined as criteria for partial paralysis. Neuromuscular blockade was not reversed at the end of the procedure. [From Debaene B, Plaud B, Dilly MP. Residual paralysis in the PACU after a single intubating dose of nondepolarizing muscle relaxant with an intermediate duration of action. *Anesthesiology*. 2003;98:1042-1048. With permission.]

spirometry, chest physiotherapy, upright positioning, and continuous positive airway pressure may be effective therapeutic maneuvers for these patients.

Acute or Chronic Lung Disease Preexisting pulmonary disease is an important risk factor for developing postoperative pulmonary complications.[20] Respiratory diseases usually are categorized according to the manner in which they alter pulmonary mechanics, producing either a limitation of expiratory airflow (obstructive disease) or a limitation of lung expansion (restrictive disease). Exacerbations of obstructive diseases, such as asthma and chronic obstructive pulmonary disease (COPD), are frequently accompanied by increasing hypercapnia and worsening hypoxemia. The key management issues are similar in both acute asthma and COPD exacerbations. They include treating bronchospasm and airway inflammation, correcting hypoxemia and respiratory acidosis, clearing secretions, and removing/treating precipitating factors. The concern for CO_2 retention and respiratory depression resulting from administration of supplemental O_2 to patients with COPD has been overemphasized.[21] In all cases, correction of hypoxemia should take precedence over concerns for CO_2 retention.

Restrictive pulmonary disorders are characterized by decreased lung compliance resulting from intrinsic disease of the lungs (eg, pulmonary fibrosis, pulmonary edema) or extrinsic disorders (eg, pleural effusions, obesity, scoliosis, abdominal distension, massive ascites) that impair normal lung expansion. Management is directed at treating the underlying disease process (eg, steroids for pulmonary fibrosis, draining the pleural space, etc) and supportive respiratory care.

ASPIRATION

General anesthesia and surgery depress airway protective reflexes and predispose patients to aspiration. Gastric contents or objects such as dislodged teeth can enter the trachea during induction or emergence and even after PACU admission. Perioperative pulmonary aspiration is an infrequent event (1 in 2000-3000 general anesthetics), but it can result in severe morbidity and mortality.[22] Signs of significant aspiration include bronchospasm, hypoxemia, atelectasis, tachypnea, tachycardia, and hypotension. Radiographic evidence of aspiration (usually infiltrates in the upper lobes of supine patients) may take some time to appear.

The severity of symptoms depends on the type and volume of material aspirated. *Aspiration pneumonitis* (Mendelson syndrome) is a chemical injury to the lungs caused by inhalation of sterile acidic gastric contents, whereas *aspiration pneumonia* refers to inhalation of contents colonized by pathogenic bacteria.[23] Initial treatment of a significant aspiration consists of oropharyngeal suctioning, administration of bronchodilators for bronchospasm, and supplemental O_2. Plans should be made for transfer of the patient to an intensive care unit (ICU). Bronchoscopy may be of benefit to remove particulate matter from the tracheobronchial tree, but pulmonary lavage with large volumes of saline is generally believed to be detrimental. Mechanical ventilatory support with positive end-expiratory pressure may be necessary if hypoxemia is severe. Administration of empirical antibiotics for aspiration is not recommended unless the material aspirated has a high bacterial load, as with a small bowel obstruction. Steroids are of no benefit in treatment if administered after an aspiration has occurred.[24] In cases of mild or uncertain aspiration, close postoperative observation should be undertaken with continuous pulse oximetry monitoring and chest radiography. Patients with clinical evidence of aspiration who do not develop signs or symptoms (cough, wheeze, hypoxia on room air, or radiologic abnormalities) within 2 hours of aspiration are unlikely to develop pulmonary complications (**Fig. 71-5**).[25,26]

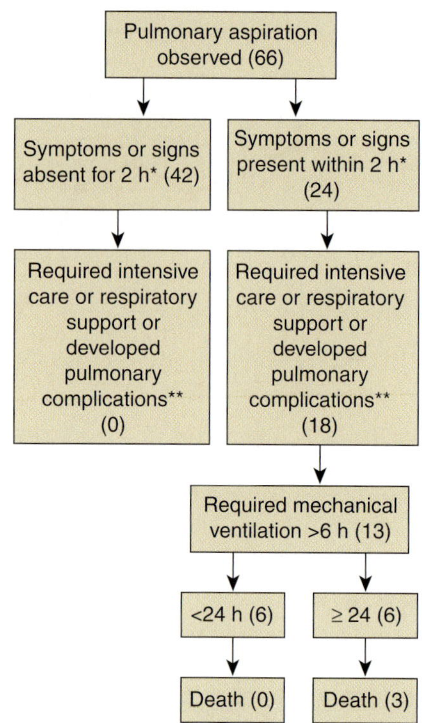

FIGURE 71-5. Relationship of symptoms or signs of perioperative pulmonary aspiration that develop within 2 hours of aspiration to pulmonary outcomes. *Symptoms or signs of pulmonary aspiration include development of a new cough or wheeze, decrease in Spo_2 while breathing room air 10% or more preoperative value, alveolar-arterial oxygen tension 300 mm Hg or more, and radiologic evidence of pulmonary aspiration. **Pulmonary complications included development of radiologic evidence of acute respiratory distress syndrome, pneumonitis, or pneumonia. [From Warner MA, Warner ME, Weber JG. Clinical significance of pulmonary aspiration during the perioperative period. *Anesthesiology*. 1993;78:56-62. With permission.]

PULMONARY EDEMA

Pulmonary edema is the accumulation of fluid in the interstitium and alveoli of the lungs that can hinder gas exchange. Cardiogenic pulmonary edema results from increased pulmonary capillary pressure secondary to elevated left atrial pressure that may be precipitated by fluid overload, left ventricular dysfunction, or mitral valve disease. A careful physical examination, chest x-ray film, electrocardiography (ECG), and arterial blood gas analysis are useful for diagnosis. Evaluation by a cardiologist may be indicated when myocardial ischemia or acute valvular disease is considered the cause of the pulmonary edema. Noncardiac pulmonary edema usually is due to increased pulmonary capillary permeability. Mainstays of treatment include supplemental O_2, diuretics, vasodilators, and mechanical ventilatory support with positive end-expiratory pressure.

Pulmonary edema can occur in the operating room or PACU most commonly secondary to acute upper airway obstruction (*negative-pressure pulmonary edema*). During upper airway obstruction, forceful inspiratory efforts against a closed glottis can result in large negative intrathoracic pressures with an increased left ventricular preload and afterload. In addition, hypoxia and increased circulating catecholamine levels may elevate pulmonary and systemic vascular resistance, shift the intraventricular septum to the left, and cause left ventricular diastolic dysfunction. These result in negative-pressure pulmonary edema, a rapid onset of copious pink fluid with bubbles due to acute fluid filtration into the lung, and capillary failure resulting in alveolar hemorrhage and hemoptysis.[27,28] Negative pressure pulmonary edema generally resolves within 12 to 48 hours when recognized early and respiratory support and diuresis are instituted promptly.[29]

PULMONARY EMBOLISM

Pulmonary embolism (PE) contributes to 50 000 to 200 000 deaths annually.[30] The mortality rate exceeds 15% in the first 3 months after the diagnosis is made, and in nearly 25% of patients with PE, the initial clinical sign is sudden death.[31] Under pathologic conditions, thrombi escape the normal fibrinolytic system, propagate in the deep veins of the lower extremities and pelvis, and then dislodge and embolize, blocking pulmonary vessels. Thrombosis is triggered by venous stasis, hypercoagulability, and vessel wall inflammation (Virchow triad). The diagnosis of PE can be challenging because the clinical presentation can vary substantially. Dyspnea is the most frequent symptom, although patients may be asymptomatic. A patient with a massive PE may present with hypotension, severe hypoxemia, cardiogenic shock, or cardiac arrest. ECG may reveal signs of right ventricular strain but may be entirely normal in previously healthy patients, and the chest x-ray film is often normal. Chest computed tomography (CT) has become the primary diagnostic imaging modality to evaluate suspected PE. Alternative imaging modalities include a ventilation-perfusion lung scan, magnetic resonance angiography, echocardiography, and pulmonary angiography. Treatment of PE is supportive (volume infusion, vasopressors, and mechanical ventilation) because anticoagulation or thrombolytic therapy often is not an option in the immediate postoperative period. Inhaled nitric oxide has been given experimentally to reverse pulmonary vasospasm following pulmonary embolism.[32] Insertion of an inferior vena cava filter may be beneficial to prevent further embolism in patients in whom anticoagulation is contraindicated. In patients with severe hypoxemia and/or hypotension, emergency pulmonary embolectomy may be required.

PNEUMOTHORAX

Pneumothorax is the accumulation of gas within the pleural space. It can result from surgical entrance into the pleural space during thoracic, upper abdominal, or retroperitoneal surgery, tracheostomy, or surgery on the chest wall or neck. Other causes include blunt or penetrating trauma, rupture of blebs or bullae, barotrauma from positive pressure ventilation, and as a complication of procedures such as central line placement, thoracentesis, or upper extremity neural blockade.[33]

A *tension pneumothorax* occurs when the site of pulmonary air leak forms a 1-way valve, allowing airflow into the pleural space during inspiration but preventing its elimination during expiration. The rapid unilateral increase in intrathoracic pressure can be life threatening because it can produce a contralateral mediastinal shift with a rapid deterioration in gas exchange, diminished cardiac output, and marked hemodynamic instability. Diminished or absent chest sounds on auscultation may be present over 1 hemithorax. If a tension pneumothorax is suspected and hemodynamic or respiratory status is compromised, then decompression should be performed immediately, without waiting for confirmation of the diagnosis by chest radiography. A 14-gauge Angiocath can be placed through the chest wall in the second intercostal space at the midclavicular line or the fourth intercostal space at the midaxillary line. The needle is removed, and the catheter is held securely in position until a tube thoracostomy can be performed. A rush of released air and immediate improvement in respiratory and hemodynamic status should occur when decompression is successful.

A disposable 1-piece suction device (eg, Pleurovac) is commonly used for chest tube drainage. The underlying principle of drainage is the same as the original 3-bottle system, but the apparatus is more compact with fewer connections. The proximal compartment collects drainage, the middle prevents flow of air back into the thorax by forming a water seal, and the distal compartment regulates the amount of suction that is applied to the pleural cavity (**Fig. 71-6**). Generally, the chest tube initially is given active suction of 20-cm water. If no bubbles are observed in the water seal (ie, no air leak is detected), active suction may not be necessary.

Chest tubes should be monitored continuously to ensure that they are functioning properly and achieving the desired therapeutic effect. The position of the chest tube, lung expansion, and fluid content of the pleural space should be evaluated by chest radiography.

PROLONGED INTUBATION

Several conditions may require continued intubation after surgery. These include delayed emergence from general anesthesia, inadequate reversal of neuromuscular blockade, potential for airway obstruction, inadequate gas exchange, and hemodynamic instability.

Delayed emergence from general anesthesia due to volatile or IV agents is an indication to delay extubation (see later section on delayed awakening). Although reversal of narcosis may be facilitated with naloxone, it is prudent to provide support with controlled or assisted ventilation until the patient emerges spontaneously. Spontaneous ventilation of the intubated patient through a T-piece may be sufficient when prolonged emergence is not expected. To minimize the risk of aspiration, the presence of a full stomach mandates that laryngeal reflexes and consciousness are fully recovered before extubation.

The potential for airway obstruction is highest after surgical procedures of the head and neck, drainage of pharyngeal abscesses, or when the jaws are wired closed following facial trauma. As stated previously, obstruction from glottic edema can occur after prolonged surgery, especially in the prone or head-down position. Hemodynamic instability, when severe, may be associated with a variable degree of impaired gas exchange or impaired consciousness that requires continuation of mechanical ventilation. Marginal oxygenation or ventilation provides additional stresses to a cardiovascular system subjected to hypovolemia, hypothermia, or myocardial ischemia. Early admission to an ICU should be considered for patients who are not anticipated to improve after a few hours in the PACU.

CARDIOVASCULAR DYSFUNCTION

HYPOTENSION

Hypotension is a common postoperative complication that can result from hypovolemia, decreased systemic vascular tone, and/or reduced cardiac output. Hypotension can result in myocardial ischemia or infarction, stroke, acute renal failure, and bowel ischemia. During hypotension, the body attempts to redirect blood flow toward the brain, heart, and kidneys: Signs of hypoperfusion of these organs suggest that compensatory mechanisms have failed. Hypotension may be defined as a more than 20% decline of blood pressure from baseline or evidence of end-organ hypoperfusion.

Accurate measurement of blood pressure is essential to making a correct diagnosis of hypotension. An inappropriately large blood pressure cuff or an arterial transducer that is improperly zeroed, positioned, or dampened will provide falsely low blood pressure readings.

HYPOVOLEMIA

Causes of hypovolemia in the PACU include inadequate fluid replacement, ongoing hemorrhage, and fluid sequestration ("third spacing"). Clinical evaluation of a patient's intravascular volume status requires consideration of preoperative status and comorbid conditions, type and duration of surgery, estimated blood loss, fluid replacement, and evidence of hemostasis. Signs of hypovolemia include hypotension, tachycardia, orthostasis, decreased skin turgor, oliguria, and dry mucous membranes. Administration of a fluid bolus during the initial assessment is generally a safe maneuver. Persistent hypotension despite seemingly adequate fluid replacement requires further assessment and may require monitoring of central venous and pulmonary artery pressures or echocardiography.

SYSTEMIC VASODILATATION

Neuraxial anesthesia, residual inhalation agents, administration of vasodilators, rewarming after hypothermia, transfusion reactions, systemic inflammation, and sepsis can cause hypotension by decreasing systemic vascular resistance and impairing venous return. Hypovolemia increases systemic hypotension due to vasodilatation, but fluid resuscitation often does not fully restore the blood pressure.

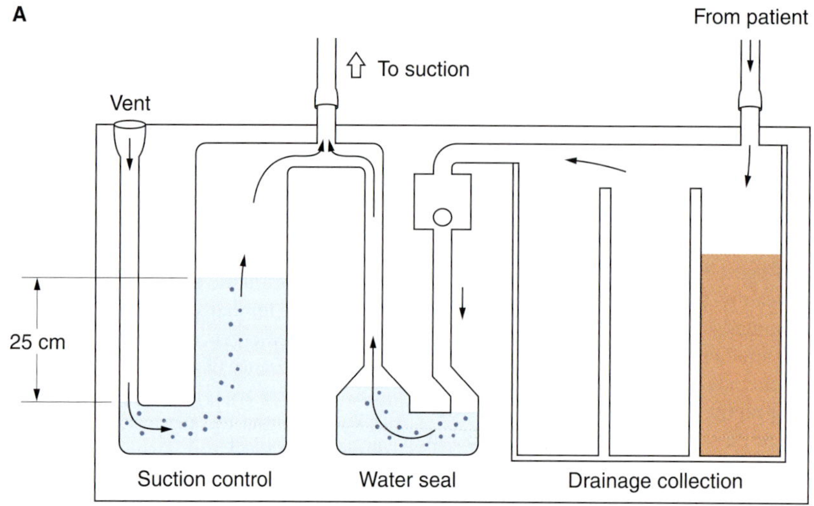

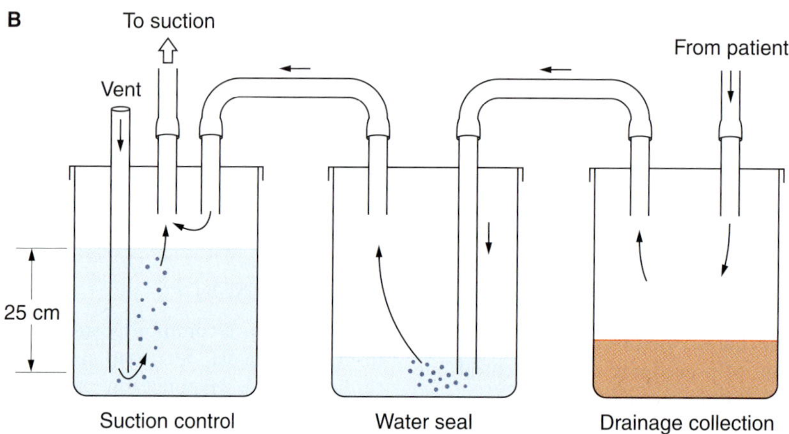

FIGURE 71-6. Chest tube drainage system. **A.** Commercial apparatus. The proximal chamber is for pleural drainage, the middle chamber (water seal) prevents air of fluid from being driven in to the thorax, and the distal chamber regulates the level of suction. **B.** Traditional 3-bottle system for comparison. [From Davignon K, Haspel KL. Thoracic surgery. In: Bigatello LM, ed. *Critical Care Handbook of the Massachusetts General Hospital*. 4th ed. Philadelphia, PA: Lippincott Williams & Wilkins; 2006. With permission.]

Pharmacologic treatment includes administration of a peripheral vasoconstrictor. A pure α_1-agonist, such as phenylephrine, often is chosen because it is unlikely to cause dysrhythmias and can be administered through a peripheral intravenous line. More potent pressor agonists, such as norepinephrine, usually require central venous access for administration. Diagnosis and treatment of the specific etiology of the vasodilatation should be concurrent with symptomatic treatment.

MYOCARDIAL ISCHEMIA AND INFARCTION

A variety of factors in the perioperative period may alter the balance between myocardial O_2 supply and demand. The body's physiologic response to surgery is an increase circulating catecholamines; these increase myocardial demand by increasing heart rate, myocardial contractility, and peripheral vascular resistance. Myocardial O_2 supply may be decreased by perioperative factors such as hypoxemia and hypotension. Patients with coronary artery disease or those at risk for coronary disease have significantly higher rates of perioperative myocardial ischemia, infarction, and cardiac death.[34] Mangano et al[35] reported that the incidence and severity of perioperative myocardial ischemia was greatest during the first 48 hours after surgery. Badner et al[36] reported the peak incidence of perioperative myocardial infarction (MI) occurred during the first 24 hours following surgery.

The diagnosis of perioperative ischemia can be difficult because often the condition is silent. Postoperative chest pain may be masked by residual anesthesia or analgesics, and pain perception may be altered by the competing stimulus of incisional pain. The patient at high risk for perioperative myocardial ischemia and infarction should be assessed by ECG preoperatively, immediately after surgery, and on the first 2 postoperative days.[37] In patients with ECG changes or chest pain typical of an acute coronary syndrome, serial markers of myocardial injury (troponin, creatine phosphokinase) should be followed. Therapy for perioperative ischemia or MI is similar to that for other medical patients with MI and includes aggressive pain control, β-blockade, aspirin, and nitrates. Administration of anticoagulants is generally reserved for cases of acute coronary stent thrombosis or ST elevation MI and requires weighing the risks of surgical bleeding with the benefits of anticoagulation.

DYSRHYTHMIAS

Cardiac dysrhythmias are common during the perioperative period; transient dysrhythmias reportedly occur in 62% to 84% of patients.[38] Most perioperative dysrhythmias are benign. They are most likely to occur in patients with underlying structural heart disease; however, the precipitating factor is usually a transient event such as hypoxia, ischemia, increased circulating catecholamine levels, altered acid–base status, or electrolyte abnormalities. The clinical significance of a dysrhythmia depends on the patient's underlying cardiac function. Bradycardia may cause a clinically significant reduction in cardiac output in a patient with relatively fixed stroke volume. Tachycardia may reduce cardiac output by decreasing diastolic filling time and increasing myocardial O_2 consumption, resulting in myocardial ischemia. Loss of atrial contraction in atrial fibrillation may decrease cardiac output by decreasing diastolic filling. The management strategy for a new dysrhythmia is focused on stabilizing hemodynamics and treating the underlying problem. Significant hemodynamic instability that results from dysrhythmia is an indication for emergent cardioversion.

Specific antiarrhythmic therapy in the postoperative setting is similar to that in the nonoperative setting, but generally therapy will not be effective unless the precipitating factors are identified and treated.

Tachycardia Tachyarrhythmias usually are classified according to their anatomic origin as either supraventricular or ventricular. Supraventricular arrhythmias include sinus tachycardia, atrial fibrillation and flutter, ectopic atrial tachycardia, multifocal atrial tachycardia, junctional tachycardia, atrioventricular nodal reentrant tachycardia, and accessory pathway reciprocating tachycardias. Ventricular arrhythmias consist of ventricular premature beats, ventricular tachycardia, and ventricular fibrillation. For a comprehensive discussion of cardiac arrhythmias, see Chapters 44 and 51.

Sinus tachycardia is the most common dysrhythmia in the immediate postoperative period. Increased sympathetic discharge resulting from pain, hypovolemia, anemia, anxiety, hypoxia, and hypercarbia are common causes. Sinus tachycardia usually is benign; however, it may precipitate myocardial ischemia in a patient with coronary artery disease. Treatment of the underlying cause(s) (eg, analgesics for pain, intravenous fluids for hypovolemia, sedatives for anxiety) usually is adequate for resolution. In patients at risk for myocardial ischemia, β-blockade usually is effective in reducing the heart rate.

Supraventricular tachyarrhythmias are more common after thoracic surgery than after other types of noncardiac surgery with a reported incidence of 15% or more.[39] In these patients, prophylaxis with calcium channel blockers or β-blockers significantly reduces the occurrence of atrial fibrillation.[39]

Atrial fibrillation is the most common supraventricular dysrhythmia after both cardiac and noncardiac surgery and has the greatest potential for serious consequences.[40,41] For unstable patients with atrial fibrillation and a rapid ventricular rate, urgent cardioversion is indicated. In hemodynamically stable patients, β-blockers, calcium channel blockers, or amiodarone are alternatives for rate control. In most patients, atrial fibrillation resolves within 36 to 48 hours. New-onset atrial fibrillation raises increased risk of stroke from cerebral embolism; anticoagulation may not be possible in a postoperative patient at risk for bleeding.

Bradycardia Bradycardia usually is associated with sinus node or atrioventricular node dysfunction. The various possible presentations are sinus bradycardia, sinus pause, sinoatrial block, sinus arrest, junctional rhythms, and varying degrees of heart block. At sufficiently slow heart rates, ventricular escape beats may be seen. In the postoperative setting, bradycardia is often due to increased vagal tone as a result of hypoxemia, pain, nausea, drugs (eg, neostigmine, β-blockers, or opioids) or the effects of neuraxial anesthesia. Sinus bradycardia can be a normal rhythm in a young healthy patient. Bradycardia without hypotension usually is benign and no treatment is necessary. If bradycardia is associated with hemodynamic compromise (hypotension, low cardiac output), treatment with antimuscarinic agents (glycopyrrolate or atropine) or β-agonists (ephedrine) can restore normal sinus rhythm.

Development of complete heart block can occur in patients with preexisting conduction disorders, and the resulting idioventricular bradycardia often compromises systemic hemodynamics. Treatment includes atropine to improve atrioventricular nodal conduction and permit supraventricular impulse transmission, or epinephrine, isoproterenol, or ventricular pacing to increase ventricular rate. In the setting of complete heart block, the need to provide either external or internal pacing must be anticipated; consultation with a cardiologist in anticipation of requirement for pacing is recommended.

Ectopy Ectopic beats, whether atrial or ventricular, are common and by themselves do not necessarily imply underlying cardiac disease. In the postoperative period, ectopic beats often are associated with electrolyte imbalances, hypoxia, acid–base abnormalities, and hypertension. They may result from drug therapy (eg, digitalis toxicity) or cardiac irritation from central venous catheters. Hypokalemia and hypomagnesemia are the most common electrolyte abnormalities associated with ectopy. Care should be taken when correcting these abnormalities because rapid administration of large quantities of either potassium or magnesium can produce hemodynamic and rhythm disturbances more deleterious than simple ectopy.

Frequent premature atrial contractions are usually of minor hemodynamic significance but may be harbingers of supraventricular tachycardia or atrial fibrillation. Medical therapy is generally not needed, but patients should be monitored closely.

Similarly, premature ventricular contractions in an asymptomatic patient generally do not require treatment. Preoperative ventricular ectopy usually reoccurs postoperatively and does not predict an adverse outcome.[42]

POSTOPERATIVE ECG CHANGES

ECG changes are common after anesthesia and surgery. Changes in P- or T-wave morphology, intraventricular conduction, or ST segments may occur in the absence of a cardiac abnormality or ischemia. These changes can result from cardiac effects of anesthetics and other drugs, increased sympathetic tone, hypothermia, and electrolyte imbalances. Breslow et al[43] reported an 18% incidence of T-wave changes in a postoperative population; changes occurred with equal frequency in all age groups and were not more common in patients with preexisting coronary artery disease. These patients did not demonstrate any evidence of postoperative myocardial ischemia or injury, and most of the ECG changes resolved with 24 hours. If there is a suspicion of perioperative ischemia, T-wave changes should be treated as a potential MI; therapeutic control of heart rate and blood pressure, serial ECGs and cardiac enzyme levels, as well as a cardiology consultation are indicated.

HYPERTENSION

Hypertension is a very common problem in the postoperative period. Typical onset is early, usually within 2 hours after surgery, and generally requires treatment for 6 hours or less. It occurs most commonly after vascular, head and neck, and neurosurgical procedures (**Table 71-3**).[44] Patients with preexisting hypertensive disease are more likely to develop postoperative hypertension, especially if antihypertensive medications

TABLE 71-3 Frequency of Acute Postoperative Hypertension by Surgical Procedure

Procedure	Frequency (%)
Carotid endarterectomy	9-64
Cardiac surgery	22-54
Abdominal aortic surgery	33-75
Radical neck dissection	10-20
Intracranial surgery	57-91
Elective general surgery	3-20
Flexion contracture release	46

Adapted from Haas CE, LeBlanc JM. Acute postoperative hypertension: a review of therapeutic options. *Am J Health Syst Pharm*. 2004;61:1661-1673.

are withheld preoperatively. Noxious stimuli, including pain, anxiety, bladder distension, fluid overload, hypoxemia, hypercarbia, and hypothermia, activate the sympathetic nervous system producing hypertension. Complications of severe postoperative hypertension include myocardial ischemia/infarction, dysrhythmias, congestive heart failure, stroke, and increased surgical bleeding.

The decision to treat hypertension requires consideration of the patient's baseline blood pressure, coexisting diseases, and perceived risk of complications: systolic or diastolic blood pressure more than 20% above baseline, signs or symptoms of complications such as chest pain or dysrhythmias, or a perceived increased risk of complications are indications for treatment.[45] Reversible causes of hypertension (eg, pain, anxiety, bladder distension) should be ruled out before initiation of antihypertensive therapy. For patients with preexisting hypertension, resumption of chronic antihypertensive therapy is a sensible option. Short-term control of blood pressure in the PACU is best accomplished with drugs that have a rapid onset and possess a short to intermediate duration of action. Intravenous agents such as labetalol, esmolol, propranolol, and hydralazine are commonly used for short-term control of blood pressure. For persistent or refractory hypertension, continuous infusions of vasodilators such as nitroprusside, nitroglycerin, nicardipine, or fenoldopam may be required.

URINARY AND RENAL DYSFUNCTION

Postoperative bladder distension with associated urinary retention may induce pain, restlessness, and delirium and may delay PACU discharge. Furthermore, severe or prolonged bladder distension may cause permanent damage to the detrusor muscle.[46] The prevalence of postoperative bladder distension ranges from 1% to more than 50% of patients and depends on the population, type of surgery, and method of estimating bladder distension.[47] A study of predictive factors for early postoperative urinary retention in the PACU found older age (≥50 y), bladder volume on entry to PACU (≥270 mL), and quantity of intraoperative fluids administered (>750 mL) each independently increased risk of urinary retention.[48] Based on these results, regular evaluation of bladder volume with ultrasound in the PACU was suggested, especially in patients with the enumerated risk factors.

Oliguria, defined as a urine output less than<0.5 mL/kg/h, is a frequent postoperative occurrence. Oliguria may be a sign of acute kidney injury (AKI), a condition associated with a markedly increased morbidity and mortality in the postoperative patient.[49,50]

- Prerenal AKI is caused by decreased renal perfusion due to decreased effective circulating blood volume or impaired renal hemodynamics. Hypovolemia is the most common prerenal cause of oliguria in this setting. Administration of a 250- to 500-mL IV fluid bolus helps to rule out hypovolemia. Maintenance of adequate systemic blood pressure (based on preoperative values) is essential for sufficient renal perfusion. If urine output does not improve despite what appears to be adequate fluid resuscitation and blood pressure, a more extensive investigation is warranted. Central venous pressure monitoring and/or echocardiography may provide better assessment of intravascular volume status and cardiac function.
- Postrenal AKI is caused by obstruction of urinary flow. In patients without a bladder catheter, it is important to determine the time since last voiding. Placement of a urinary catheter helps differentiate insufficient urine production from the inability to void. Irrigation of the urinary catheter to assess for kinking, obstruction, or migration is important to exclude these common postrenal causes of oliguria.
- Intrinsic AKI is divided into tubular (acute tubular necrosis), interstitial, glomerular, and vascular etiologies. Analysis of urine electrolytes, osmolality, and cast formation may be helpful in this assessment. Diuretics should be given sparingly because they may worsen preexisting renal injury, and forced diuresis does not improve the prognosis of AKI. Intraoperative events that may cause AKI (eg, extended aortic crossclamping, prolonged systemic hypotension, possible ureteral ligature, or trauma) should be investigated. Imaging studies such as ultrasonography, CT, angiography, or radionuclide scanning may be indicated to clarify renal status and exclude reversible causes of injury. Early consultation with a nephrologist is indicated.

Absorption of irrigation fluid into the intravascular space during cystoscopy may lead to substantial fluid overload and electrolyte shifts. This condition is referred to as *transurethral resection of the prostate (TURP) syndrome*.[51] A similar syndrome has been described in women undergoing transcervical endometrial ablation.[52] In both cases, irrigation is performed with an isotonic nonconductive glycine-containing solution that permits use of electrocautery for the procedure. Signs and symptoms result from acute increase in intravascular volume, increased levels of plasma glycine, and rapid decreases in plasma sodium concentration. At the extreme, hyponatremia may produce convulsions, coma, and death. Cardiovascular findings can include hypertension (from hypervolemia) or hypotension (from congestive heart failure), dysrhythmias, pulmonary edema, and cardiac arrest. The diagnosis is confirmed by measuring plasma sodium and osmolality. Management involves providing supportive care, including diuretics for volume overload and administration of isotonic saline. Hypertonic saline therapy may be necessary when plasma sodium decreases below 120 mmol/L or in the event of acute neurologic deterioration.[53] Caution should be exercised when infusing hypertonic saline because rapid correction of sodium has been linked to central pontine myelinolysis.

CENTRAL NERVOUS SYSTEM DYSFUNCTION

DELIRIUM

Delirium is a transient, fluctuating disturbance of consciousness, attention, cognition, and perception. Postoperative delirium is a common problem in the PACU with a reported incidence in adults of 3% to 5%.[54,55] The delirious patient often is hypertensive and tachycardic, and the accompanying agitation can have serious consequences, including trauma, disruption of suture lines or surgical repairs, and accidental removal of catheters, tubes, and drains. Health care providers are also at risk for injury. Postoperative delirium is more common in the elderly and may delay recovery and prolong hospital stay.[56,57] Other preoperative risk factors include organic brain disease, withdrawal from alcohol and sedatives, anxiety, and depression. Intraoperative risk factors include specific types of surgery (eg, cardiac, orthopedic, ophthalmologic) and administration of certain drugs (eg, anticholinergics, barbiturates, benzodiazepines). Perioperative hypoxemia, hypotension, and sepsis are believed to be risk factors. There appears to be no difference in the incidence of postoperative delirium with either neuraxial or general anesthesia.[58]

The first priority in management of postoperative delirium is to rule out physiologic causes, including hypoxemia, hypotension, and acidemia. Postoperative pain often plays a significant role and should be treated adequately.[59] Other treatable causes include hypoglycemia, electrolyte disturbances, sepsis, and sensory overload. Bladder or gastric distension, or other nonsurgical pain sources (eg, corneal abrasion, infiltrated IV, poor positioning) should be excluded. Delirium should be treated supportively with verbal reassurance that the surgery is over and that the patient is doing well. Medications may be indicated in some circumstances; physostigmine is helpful when delirium is believed to be the result of central anticholinergic drugs such as scopolamine. Haloperidol is the most widely used agent to treat delirium; benefits include reducing severity and duration of delirium episodes.[60]

DELAYED AWAKENING

The major causes of delayed awakening after general anesthesia can be divided into 3 groups: (1) prolonged pharmacologic effects, (2) metabolic abnormalities, and (3) neurologic injury.[61] The residual effects of anesthetic drugs are the most common cause of delayed awakening. It is important to obtain information on the patient's preoperative level of consciousness, the timing and dosage of administered sedatives and opioids, and use of volatile anesthetics and muscle relaxants. Volatile anesthetics, especially those with high solubility, are more likely to result in delayed awakening after longer procedures or in obese patients. If residual sedative effects of opioids or benzodiazepines are suspected, then pharmacologic reversal with naloxone or flumazenil, respectively, can be used for evaluation as well as treatment. Administration of physostigmine (1.25 mg IV) nonspecifically reverses the anesthetic effects of some sedative and inhalational agents.[62,63] The effects of profound neuromuscular blockade can mimic unconsciousness by preventing a motor response to stimuli. In this situation, spontaneous ventilation and movement will be absent and autonomic responses may remain. Possible causes of prolonged paralysis include an overdosage of neuromuscular blocking agents, impaired clearance, drug interaction (eg, with certain antibiotics), or a failure to reverse. The possibility that the patient has pseudocholinesterase deficiency or an unrecognized neuromuscular disease also should be considered. Evaluation with a train-of-four nerve stimulation is recommended.

Metabolic causes of delayed awakening include hypoxemia, hypercapnia, hepatic, renal or endocrine dysfunction, and glucose and electrolyte abnormalities. Hypoglycemia should be considered early, and 50% dextrose should be administered immediately if hypoglycemia is suspected. Hyperglycemia, resulting in hyperosmolar coma or diabetic ketoacidosis, can reduce level of consciousness. Obtaining arterial blood gas and plasma chemistries are the first steps to identify a metabolic etiology.

Sleep deprivation and disruption of normal sleeping patterns in children can result in difficult arousal (see Chapter 64). Profound hypothermia (<33°C) can cause unconsciousness and increase the sedative effects of anesthetics. Extreme hypothermia can cause fixed dilated pupils and areflexia. Overdosage with local anesthetics or inadvertent subarachnoid injection during retrobulbar block can cause unconsciousness.

If the diagnosis remains uncertain, neurologic consultation should be sought. Urgent radiologic imaging (eg, CT, magnetic resonance imaging [MRI]) can be performed to rule out an intracranial process, including stroke, hemorrhage, or hypoxic injury. Trauma patients may be found to have unrecognized intracranial injury. Cerebral vascular accidents, although uncommon after general surgery, can occur in the perioperative period.[64,65] Subclinical generalized seizures are an uncommon cause of postoperative unconsciousness. Patients often are slow to awaken after long intracranial procedures; however, consideration should be given to the occurrence of complications such as intracranial hemorrhage or increased intracranial pressure. Rarely, psychiatric causes can result in impaired consciousness.[66]

STROKE

The incidence of perioperative stroke varies with the type and complexity of the surgical procedure with the reported incidence ranging from as low as 0.08% after general surgical procedures to more than 9% in complicated cardiac and vascular surgery.[65,67] Perioperative strokes are predominately embolic and ischemic. Approximately half of perioperative strokes are identified within the first postoperative day.[65] These early strokes generally result from emboli generated by manipulations of the heart, aorta, or the carotid, or from particulate matter emanating from cardiopulmonary bypass. Strokes occurring after the first postoperative day generally are caused by emboli resulting from atrial fibrillation, MI, or cerebral hypoperfusion and coagulopathy. Preexisting renal disease, history of stroke, and cardiac valvular disease are additional risk factors for stroke in patients undergoing noncardiac, nonvascular surgery.[67] Surgery-induced hypercoagulopathy, general anesthesia, dehydration, bed rest, and perioperative withholding of antiplatelet and anticoagulant medications may also contribute to thrombogenic events such as stroke. Early diagnosis and management is essential to improving outcome after stroke. However, diagnosis may be difficult because symptoms such as somnolence, slurred speech, visual changes, agitation, confusion, numbness, and muscular weakness or paralysis may overlap with the effects of residual anesthetics. Neurologic consultation in conjunction with radiologic imaging is mandatory to guide therapy. Administration of IV thrombolytics may be contraindicated in patients who have recently undergone major surgery. However, intra-arterial administration of tissue plasminogen activator and endovascular mechanical clot disruption are potentially safer options in the postoperative period.[68,69]

INTRAOPERATIVE AWARENESS

Awareness with recall of intraoperative events is an infrequent but recognized complication of general anesthesia, with a reported incidence of 0.1% to 0.2%.[70] Awareness can result in significant distress to patients and long-term psychological sequelae, including symptoms associated with posttraumatic stress disorder.[71] Certain patient characteristics (eg, younger age, higher American Society of Anesthesiologists [ASA] physical status, history of alcohol or drug tolerance, history of difficult intubation), types of procedures (eg, cesarean delivery, cardiac surgery, trauma surgery), and anesthetic techniques (eg, rapid sequence induction, reduced anesthetic doses) are associated with an increased risk of intraoperative awareness.[72] A questionnaire such as proposed by Brice et al[73] is a useful screen for intraoperative awareness in the PACU and during the postoperative visit.

For the patient indicating possible awareness, the clinician should speak with the patient to obtain specific details of the event and to ascertain potential causes.[74] A structured interview instrument may be useful to obtain a detailed account of the patient's experience.[75] An occurrence report regarding the event should be completed for the purpose of quality management. The patient should be offered counseling and psychological support.

COMPLICATED ACUTE PAIN MANAGEMENT

Despite increased knowledge of the mechanisms of acute pain and increased emphasis on pain management programs, postoperative pain continues to be undermanaged (**Fig. 71-7**).[76,77] Inadequate pain

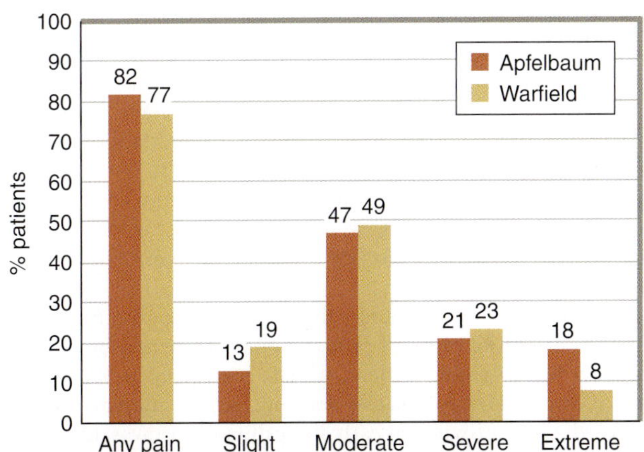

FIGURE 71-7. Severity of postoperative pain. Results from a national survey of patients who had recently undergone surgical procedures. Patients reported intense pain after surgery, and the incidence of reported pain did not decrease compared with a similar survey reported 8 years earlier. [From Apfelbaum JL, Chen C, Mehta SS, et al. Postoperative pain experience: results from a national survey suggest postoperative pain continues to be undermanaged. *Anesth Analg.* 2003;97:534-540. With permission.]

relief may have harmful physiologic and psychologic consequences, resulting in increased postoperative morbidity. In addition, inadequate, pain control delays PACU recovery and discharge to home, may result in development of a chronic pain syndrome, and increases resource utilization and health care costs.[78,79]

For patients to function well postoperatively, they must have adequate pain relief at rest and with movement. Multimodal analgesic approaches that combine regional techniques, nonsteroidal anti-inflammatory drug (NSAID), and opioid therapies are recommended to provide pain relief during movement while producing a low incidence of side effects.[80,81] Procedure-specific guidelines for pain therapy may be helpful because pain intensity, as well as the risks and benefits of different analgesics, clearly are procedure related.[82,83] Chapter 72 provides a thorough discussion of acute postoperative pain management.

Patients who are opioid tolerant (either from substance abuse or legitimate medical therapy) often present a management challenge in the immediate postoperative period. These patients may be receiving large doses of long-acting oral opioid agonists or even high doses of the opioid partial agonist buprenorphine (see Chapters 23 and 41). When possible, regional anesthetic techniques and nonopioid adjuncts (eg, NSAIDs, clonidine) should be used to provide multimodal therapy. If a regional technique is used as the primary anesthetic in a patient known to be physically dependent on opioids, it is important to provide a supplemental opioid to prevent the symptoms of withdrawal.

Frequently opioid-tolerant patients require parenteral opioids as a primary mode of analgesia after surgery. Tolerant and nontolerant patients are at similar risk for opioid-induced respiratory depression if comparable levels of pain relief are achieved (see Chapter 48). Unfortunately, assessing pain relief in opioid-tolerant patients can be difficult and sometimes inaccurate. Relying on a "pain score" as an analgesic end point may be unwise because these individuals report higher pain scores even when quite sedated.[84] For this reason, patients requiring very large doses of opioids should undergo careful monitoring of O_2 saturation and respiratory rate for signs of respiratory depression. Patients with coexisting respiratory diseases such as sleep apnea may be best managed in an ICU during the early postoperative period.[85] In addition, consultation with a specialist in addiction medicine may assist with acute management as well as follow-up during or after patient hospitalization.

HEMORRHAGE

Patients who develop bleeding postoperatively require rapid evaluation to differentiate poor surgical hemostasis (perhaps requiring immediate reoperation) from a diffuse coagulopathy. It is important to appreciate that surgical and nonsurgical bleeding often coexist. Visible bleeding from wounds or drains makes the diagnosis easier, whereas bleeding into the chest, pelvis, thigh, or retroperitoneum can be difficult to detect. Drains can become blocked, kinked, or malpositioned, resulting in a false sense of security.

The patient should be examined for tachycardia, diminished urine output, and delayed capillary refill. Blood pressure may be preserved, especially in the young patient, despite loss of up to 40% of total blood volume.[86] Orthostatic hypotension, narrow pulse pressure, and tachycardia may provide an early indication of intravascular volume depletion. Hemoglobin levels may remain stable for a time, and initial declines may be attributed to hemodilution despite significant hemorrhage.

If there is evidence of significant bleeding, diagnosis and treatment usually occur simultaneously. Adequate IV access should be established and the availability of appropriate blood products ensured. Diagnostic studies include measurement of filling pressures (ie, central venous pressure or pulmonary capillary wedge pressure) and imaging (ultrasound, CT) of body cavities. Angiography eventually may be required for definitive diagnosis, localization, and therapy by embolization.

The diagnosis of a coagulopathy in the surgical setting commonly occurs with a dilutional thrombocytopenia and decline in clotting factors. Coagulation tests should be guided by knowledge of preexisting medical illnesses (eg, hepatic disease, bone marrow suppression) or specific surgical factors (eg, sepsis leading to disseminated intravascular coagulation). Hypothermia if present should be corrected because it can cause platelet dysfunction. Laboratory test results can change rapidly, and serial measurements are often required.

TEMPERATURE ABNORMALITIES

HYPOTHERMIA

Hypothermia remains a common postoperative problem despite the ASA requirement for the "availability" of intraoperative temperature monitoring and the improved technology for patient warming in the operating room. Multiple sources of heat loss, decreased heat production, and impairment of thermoregulatory control all contribute to intraoperative hypothermia. Even mild hypothermia (core temperature between 34°C and 36°C) has been associated with adverse outcomes, including myocardial ischemia, arrhythmias, coagulopathy, wound infection, and decreased drug metabolism.[87] Furthermore, hypothermia can result in substantial discomfort, rated by some patients as worse than their surgical pain.[88] Mild hypothermia may increase the duration of PACU stay by 40 minutes or more.[89] Violent shivering may increase the risk of trauma or subcutaneous bleeding. It also may dislodge medical devices and interfere with ECG and pulse oximetry monitoring.

Restoration of normothermia is an important goal during the postoperative period. For patients with mild hypothermia, warm blankets and verbal reassurance usually are adequate treatment. Forced-air warming devices are more efficient, if available. Shivering can be rapidly suppressed with small doses of meperidine, which acts by stimulating α_{2B} receptors (see Chapter 41). This will decrease heat production but will make the patient more comfortable. Clonidine, dexmedetomidine, and doxapram also have been used successfully to treat shivering.[90]

HYPERTHERMIA

Although fever is common during the first few days after surgery, significant hyperthermia is relatively uncommon in the PACU. Most early postoperative fever is caused by cytokine release in response to surgery and resolves spontaneously.[91] A 1.4°C average increase in core temperature set point occurs in patients undergoing major surgical procedures (**Fig. 71-8**).[92] Brief periods of hyperthermia also can occur when patients are closely draped and subjected to aggressive warming techniques in the operating room. Infection is always a concern; this is less likely in the PACU unless the patient had a preexisting infection or bacteremia was provoked by the surgical procedure. A febrile reaction to a medication or blood product given during surgery can occur. Less common etiologies include hyperthyroidism, malignant hyperthermia, and the neuroleptic malignant syndrome. Fever can be associated with other adverse events, including PE, adrenal insufficiency, and ethanol withdrawal.

Evaluation of fever in the early postoperative period begins with a careful review of the and physical examination. Preoperative fever or leukocytosis, preoperative and intraoperative medications, and surgery that involves abscess drainage or fecal spillage can all contribute to postoperative fever. Routine use of blood and urine cultures, urinalysis, and chest radiography is costly, and these tests should be ordered only when indicated by the history and physical examination. The decision to administer antibiotics depends on the perceived

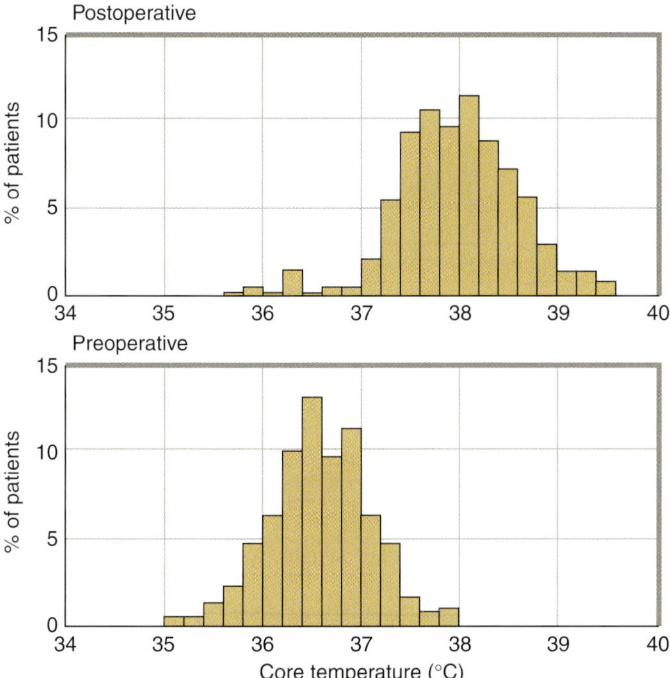

FIGURE 71-8. Histograms illustrating preoperative and maximum postoperative core temperature in the first 24 hours after surgery in 271 patients. Data indicate a postoperative shift in the set point to a higher core temperature. [From Frank SM, Kluger MJ, Kunkel SL. Elevated thermostatic setpoint in postoperative patients. *Anesthesiology*. 2000;93:1426-1431. With permission.]

urgency of treatment and the level of clinical suspicion of infection. Symptomatic treatment with rectal or oral acetaminophen is useful for patient comfort and minimizes increased metabolic demands of fever.

HYPERGLYCEMIA

Hyperglycemia due to diabetes, impaired glucose tolerance/fasting glucose or "stress induced" is common in the adult population.[93] Hyperglycemia in perioperative patients has been identified as a risk factor for morbidity and mortality. Whether tight glycemic control improves mortality in the perioperative period remains controversial. Several studies suggest that intensive insulin therapy may have a favorable impact on outcome in specific subpopulations, including improved survival after cardiac surgery, decreased infection rates, improved outcome after neurologic injury, and decreased rejection in cadaveric renal transplantation.[94] However, recent evidence of severe hypoglycemia and adverse events associated with intensive insulin therapy calls into question both safety and efficacy. Concerns have been raised over the optimal glucose level, accuracy of measurements, the resources required to achieve tight glycemic control, and the impact of tight glycemic control across the heterogeneous surgical population of diabetic and nondiabetic patients.[95] There is currently insufficient evidence to support the routine use of tight glycemic control in the perioperative period. However, maintaining blood glucose less than 150 mg/dL and reducing blood glucose variability may be effective.[94] Other strategies to maintain glycemic control in the perioperative period include avoiding oral hypoglycemic agents when not on a regular diet, providing basal insulin doses for patients who are insulin deficient, and implementing a program to prevent and manage hypoglycemia.[96] These issues are covered more extensively in Chapters 12 and 59.

INJURIES

OCULAR

Visual changes after anesthesia for nonocular surgery are relatively infrequent, with an incidence of 0.0008% after all noncardiac surgery and 0.2% following spine surgery.[97, 98] Severity ranges from transient blurring of vision to irreversible blindness. Transient blurring of vision can be due attributed to cycloplegia from anticholinergic medications, use of ocular lubricants, excessive corneal drying, or a corneal abrasion.[99] Corneal abrasion is suggested by symptoms of tearing, miosis, photophobia, and the sensation of a foreign body in the eye. The diagnosis is confirmed by fluorescein staining of the cornea. Ophthalmologic consultation is recommended, and management usually consists of patching and administration of topical antibiotics, anesthetics, and cycloplegics.

Prolonged or permanent visual loss is a recognized complication after head/neck, neurovascular, cardiopulmonary bypass, and spine surgery.[100] Impairment of retinal perfusion may result from direct ocular compression, but it also is associated with acute anemia, hypotension, emboli, and large-volume crystalloid administration in the absence of direct compression.[101] The risk is higher in patients with preexisting vascular disease and in those receiving long anesthetics and surgery in the prone position.[102]

If there is a postoperative concern regarding potential visual loss, urgent ophthalmologic consultation should be obtained to determine its cause. Optimizing hemodynamics, hemoglobin levels, and arterial oxygenation may improve recovery, but this has not been confirmed prospectively. MRI may be needed to detect intracranial causes of vision loss.[103]

OROPHARYNGEAL

Sore throat, hoarseness, and dysphagia are common postoperative complaints following tracheal intubation and laryngeal mask airway (LMA) insertion. In most cases, the laryngeal or pharyngeal trauma is minor, and symptoms resolve without treatment. Gargling with viscous lidocaine may provide symptomatic relief but increases the risk of aspiration during recovery. Severe or persistent pain, dysphagia, or hoarseness may suggest more significant pathology warranting otolaryngologic consultation. Pathologic changes from laryngoscopy and intubation include epithelial loss, glottic hematoma and edema, submucosal tears, and granuloma formation. Oropharyngeal injuries resulting from LMA insertion include pharyngeal abrasion, nerve palsy, arytenoid dislocation, epiglottitis, and uvular bruising.[104]

DENTAL

Perioperative dental injury has a reported incidence of 1 in 4500 general anesthetics.[105] Risk factors include preexisting poor dentition and a difficult laryngoscopy/intubation.[106,107] The upper incisors are most often involved. Damage to teeth should be carefully documented and a dental consultation obtained. If a tooth is missing and cannot be found, a chest x-ray should be obtained to rule out a pulmonary aspiration.

NERVE

Sixteen percent of claims in the ASA closed claims project database were for anesthesia-related nerve injuries.[108] Nerve injury may result from improper intraoperative positioning, direct surgical damage, or as a complication of needles and drugs used in regional anesthesia. Preexisting nerve abnormalities also may play a role.[109] Many perioperative neuropathies have no identifiable cause. Examination of the patient in the PACU may lead to earlier recognition of a peripheral neuropathy.[110] The patient should be positioned in a manner to prevent further compression or stretch of the involved nerve. Evaluation for potentially treatable sources of injury, such as constrictive dressings or improperly applied casts, is important. Prompt neurologic consultation should be obtained when a new deficit is identified to document the patient's status, arrange additional testing or intervention, and provide follow-up. Neurophysiologic assessment, such as nerve conduction studies, evoked potentials, and electromyography, may be helpful in localizing the injury and establishing the diagnosis and prognosis. This information may be helpful in directing a treatment plan.

Major neurologic complications after spinal or epidural anesthesia are rare but can be devastating. The etiology may be traumatic injury to the spinal cord or nerve roots during needle or catheter placement, spinal hematoma or abscess, or a direct toxic effect of injected medications or contaminants.[111] Several of these possibilities require urgent MRI and neurologic evaluation. Lack of recovery from spinal or epidural anesthesia may indicate spinal cord compression from a hematoma. Persistent motor blockade after recovery of sensory anesthesia may be due to spinal artery occlusion or spasm. In both cases, prompt diagnosis with MRI and early intervention greatly increase the likelihood of a successful outcome.

HEARING

Hearing loss has been reported after general and neuraxial anesthesia, but it is often subclinical and goes unnoticed unless audiometry is performed. Hearing loss after spinal anesthesia or lumbar puncture is reported most frequently, with 10% to 50% of patients experiencing an audiometrically measurable low-frequency hearing loss.[112] The etiology appears to be related to cerebrospinal fluid leak; likelihood of impairment is increased with use of larger-gauge and cutting-tip needles. Hearing loss after dural puncture generally resolves completely within days to weeks. In severe cases, an epidural blood patch may hasten recovery.[113]

Hearing loss after general anesthesia has been reported after both cardiac and noncardiac surgery. The etiology often is unclear but may be related to changes in middle ear pressure, injury to the inner ear microcirculation, embolism, or the effects of ototoxic drugs. Some patients who received nitrous oxide may actually have developed hyperacusis (increased sensitivity to sound), presumably from changes in middle ear pressure.

EXTRAVASATION INJURY

Extravasation injury can result from unintentional injection or leakage of IV fluids or medications into the perivascular or subcutaneous space. The amount of injury depends on the specific drug and concentration, the site of injury, the infusion pressure, and the duration of tissue exposure.[114] Extravasation of vasoconstrictors, alkaline solutions such as thiopental, and hyperosmolar or concentrated electrolyte solutions may cause significant tissue necrosis. Pain, swelling, and local hyperthermia are not reliable predictors of the degree of tissue damage. The IV infusion should be stopped immediately. Conservative measures such as elevating the involved extremity or applying heat or cold have not been shown to be beneficial, although early aspiration of the intravenous cannula and flushing with saline may be useful. In the case of extravasation of vasopressors, early infiltration with phentolamine may be effective. Surgical consultation and radiologic imaging (eg, MRI) may be helpful if there is concern regarding tissue damage (**Fig. 71-9**).

A compartment syndrome may result from extravasation of fluid into an extremity. If the amount of extravasated fluid is sufficiently large, blood flow to the distal portion of the extremity may be compromised with resulting tissue ischemia. Untreated ischemia may result in reversible changes in nerve function within 30 minutes and irreversible changes after 12 to 24 hours.[115] Impairment in muscle function can be seen during the first 4 hours with irreversible impairment thereafter. Measurement of elevated compartment pressures in conjunction with the clinical examination is used to make the diagnosis of compartment syndrome. Fasciotomy may be required for perfusion to the compromised extremity.

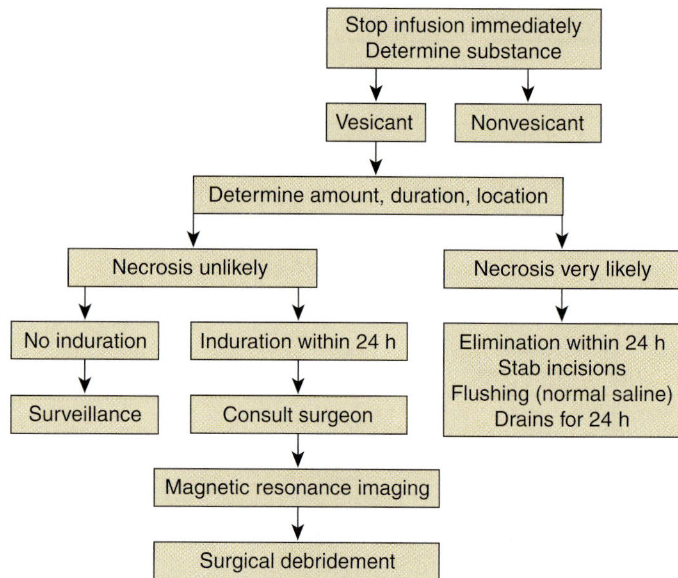

FIGURE 71-9. Algorithm for managing extravasation injury in the perioperative setting. Vesicants refer to drugs that can cause tissue destruction. Common vesicants used in the perioperative setting include vasoconstrictors (eg, epinephrine, dopamine, norepinephrine), concentrated electrolyte solutions (eg, calcium chloride, potassium chloride, sodium bicarbonate), and hyperosmolar solutions (eg, glucose 20%, mannitol, phenytoin [Dilantin]). [From Schummer W, Schummer C, Bayer O, et al. Extravasation injury in the perioperative setting. *Anesth Analg.* 2005;100:722-727. With permission.]

KEY REFERENCES

- Breslow MJ, Miller CF, Parker SD, et al. Changes in T-wave morphology following anesthesia and surgery: a common recovery room phenomenon. *Anesthesiology.* 1986;64:398-402.
- Hines R, Barash PG, Watrous G, et al. Complications occurring in the postoperative care unit: a survey. *Anesth Analg.* 1992;74:503-509.
- Hollenberg SM, Dellinger RP. Noncardiac surgery: postoperative arrhythmias. *Crit Care Med.* 2000;28:N145-N150.
- Macario A, Weinger M, Carney S, et al. Which clinical anesthesia outcomes are important to avoid? The perspective of patients. *Anesth Analg.* 1999;89:652-658.
- Practice advisory for intraoperative awareness and brain function monitoring. *Anesthesiology.* 2006;104:847-864.
- Practice advisory for the prevention of perioperative peripheral neuropathies: a report by the American Society of Anesthesiologists task force on prevention of perioperative peripheral neuropathies. *Anesthesiology.* 2000;92:1168-1182.
- Selim M. Perioperative stroke. *N Engl J Med.* 2007;356:706-713.
- Sessler DI. Complications and treatment of mild hypothermia. *Anesthesiology.* 2001;95:531-543.
- Thompson JS, Baxter BT, Allison JG, et al. Temporal patterns of postoperative complications. *Arch Surg.* 2003;138:596-603.
- Warner MA, Warner ME, Weber JG. Clinical significance of pulmonary aspiration during the perioperative period. *Anesthesiology.* 1993;78:56-62.

REFERENCES

Complete references available on DVD and online version at www.LongneckerAnesthesiology.com

CHAPTER 72

Management of Acute Postoperative Pain

Kieran A. Slevin
Jane C. Ballantyne

KEY POINTS

1. Analgesia, as distinct from hypnosis, is a vital and integral component of anesthesia.
2. Anesthesiologists must plan for the continuum of intra- and postoperative pain.
3. The principles of "opioid sparing" or "multimodal analgesia" are central to the goal of rapid recovery because opioid side effects delay recovery.
4. Patient-controlled analgesia (PCA) has greatly facilitated acute pain management at both provider and institutional levels.
5. Epidural analgesia continues to play an important role in the treatment of pain after major intra-abdominal and thoracic surgery, although the benefit versus risk should be reexamined in an era of potent thrombosis prophylaxis.
6. Chronic opioid use and abuse are emerging as prominent challenges during acute pain treatment.

INTRODUCTION

After the first public demonstration of ether anesthesia at the Massachusetts General Hospital in 1846, the news that "We have conquered pain" spread around the world. What was not understood at the time is that the potent hypnotics merely suspend pain perception but do little to change pain transmission. The addition of neural blockade or strong analgesics (notably opioids) is needed to halt the pain processes that excite the nervous system, trigger neuroendocrine stress responses, and produce pain once it can be perceived. The provision of analgesia, during and after surgery, is now considered a vital and integral part of anesthesia, and its central goal to reduce the stress and derangements of surgery. Anesthesiologists apply their knowledge of pharmacology, anatomy, physiology, pathophysiology, surgery, and medicine toward optimizing pain relief. Whether by means of an informal relationship with surgical colleagues or a more structured service—an acute pain service—they play a key role in managing postoperative pain.[1] As experts, they help educate others in the tools of pain management and teach the importance of pain control in terms of postoperative recovery.

BACKGROUND

INSTITUTIONAL CONSIDERATIONS

The Role of the Acute Pain Service The idea of the acute pain service arose during the 1980s when "walking" epidurals made epidural analgesia suddenly more feasible for postoperative patients and when the microchip made patient-controlled analgesia (PCA) pumps small enough to have wide applicability. Initially, pain services ran both these modalities, developed treatment protocols, and taught nurses and others how to manage these new therapies. Soon, surgeons and nurses became familiar with the use of PCA, so that this component of postoperative management, at least for routine cases, is largely being managed by them. Epidurals remain the province of anesthesiologists, and the core function of the acute pain service is to manage postoperative epidural analgesia. The acute pain service is also available to help with complex cases, notably cases that cannot be managed using routine measures. Naturally, each institution will structure its pain service differently, according to institutional and local factors. Smaller hospitals and ambulatory facilities may not have a service as such.

Acute pain services are usually staffed by a mixture of attending physicians (sometimes pain trained and commonly anesthesiologists), nurses, physician assistants, pain fellows, and anesthesia residents. Rotation to the acute pain service is a valuable component of residency training because this is likely the only point during training that anesthesia residents have the opportunity to follow patients postoperatively on a daily basis. The allocation of roles on the service will depend to a large extent on factors such as reimbursement, hospital policies, the relationship between anesthesia and surgery, and the expectations and support of both the hospital and the department of surgery. For example, funding for nursing on the service varies according to institution, and the provision of nonbillable services, such as daily follow-up of PCA, may only be feasible if nurses are available and funded. Epidural management remains the most favorably reimbursed of acute pain services. Unfortunately, as pain management becomes increasingly challenging because of rising numbers of opioid-tolerant patients (both substance abusers and opioid-treated chronic pain patients), and because of mandated pain management, reimbursement often fails to cover the realistic costs of ideal pain management.

Pain Management and Quality Assurance Pain management has become an important metric by which standards of medical care are measured, and there are sound reasons for this. First, experience tells us that despite the extensive efforts of advocates,[2-4] pain is easy to neglect, it being "silent" unless it is sought. It becomes necessary, then, to find mechanisms for encouraging active pain management, knowing that educational efforts alone have limited impact. Although it is easy for busy practitioners to skirt over pain issues, pain is not something patients easily forget, and it is now recognized that there is a clear correlation between patients' satisfaction with pain management and their satisfaction with medical care overall.[5,6] In a competitive health care milieu, pain management thus becomes important to hospital administrations.

The Joint Commission on Accreditation of Healthcare Organizations (JCAHO), known as The Joint Commission, became involved in pain management when it was recognized that published guidelines, including an acute pain guidelines published by government and professional bodies, had a limited impact on hospital practice.[7,8] JCAHO evaluates and accredits more than 19000 health care organizations in the United States and its status as an accreditation body is such that it serves as an alternative to state and federal inspection mechanisms. Because of its wide reach, it was chosen for collaboration when various bodies seeking to improve pain management—including the American Pain Society, the Agency for Healthcare Policy and Research (now the Agency for Healthcare Research and Quality), and the University of Wisconsin Medical School (supported by a grant from the Robert Wood Johnson Foundation)—determined that the accreditation body could potentially improve pain's visibility by mandating the development of processes that increase provider accountability for the assessment and treatment of pain. Five elements were established that were considered essential for establishing institutional responsibility for making pain management a priority[9]:

- Pain must be recognized and treated promptly.
- Information about analgesics should be readily available to clinicians in a way that facilitates order writing and interpretation of orders.
- Patients must be assured of attentive pain care.
- Explicit policies should be developed for the use of advanced analgesic technologies.
- Processes and outcomes should be examined for continued improvement.

The idea was to make pain management a priority in the health care system and to establish systems to support, reinforce, and reward good pain management practice. The standards were approved in 1999 and formally introduced into the accreditation process in 2001.[10] Perhaps the most obvious manifestation of the mandate was the introduction of "pain as a fifth vital sign," part of the effort to "make pain visible." Many hospitals have now introduced a requirement to record a pain score on the vital signs chart. Although it was never the intention of JCAHO or the pain advocates that this should become the focus of the pain mandate, and indeed there is no written requirement for the "fifth vital sign" in current JCAHO documentation, nevertheless it has become the hallmark of the JCAHO mandate.

Measurement of patient satisfaction with medical care has become an essential part of hospital management in the competitive health care environment, and satisfaction with pain care is an integral component. Yet curiously, patients often express satisfaction with pain management even if conventional goals of pain care such as pain relief or improved mobility are not achieved.[11,12] This paradox can probably be explained at least in part by the high patient satisfaction that arises by simply addressing pain.[13] Pain relief scores per se seem less important than do the patient-clinician interactions, validation of the pain complaint, and confidence that relief is available.[12] One must question also the validity of patient satisfaction measures. Patient satisfaction instruments have limitations that include lack of psychometric standards and reliance on surveys that tend to have poor reliability and validity.[14,15] Patient satisfaction is a complex concept with sociodemographic, cognitive, and affective dimensions, in their turn influencing the expectation that underpins satisfaction.[16] All in all, what seems important is that pain is addressed because the mere addressing of pain can result in less distress for patients, translated into improved satisfaction.

Although the efforts of accreditation bodies and hospital management systems toward improving pain care have undoubtedly had positive effects, there have also been unexpected adverse consequences, most related to opioid prescribing. Mandated pain management, even if it does not specify opioid use per se, inevitably encourages opioid prescribing. In the case of acute pain, the introduction of hospital-wide protocols that link pain scores to opioid dosing have resulted in a rash of opioid overdosing, sometimes with disastrous consequences.[17] Clearly, opioids must always be prescribed on a case-by-case basis, and what is learned is that there is no easy substitute for patient-clinician interactions and continuous assessment and dose adjustments. Mandated pain management can sometimes bring clinicians into conflict with their patients when demands for opioid are seen as irrational or due to addiction. Patients have a stated right to receive opioids,[2-4] yet experience shows that indiscriminate use of opioids can have disastrous consequences.[18,19] Clinicians may feel pressured into prescribing against their best judgment not only because of mandates, but also because they may need to meet patient satisfaction metrics. Opioid prescribing must always be balanced, and because opioids can be dangerous if not prescribed judiciously, it is important that mandates and efforts to meet quality metrics do not interfere with sensible opioid use.

PREPARATION

Patient Education Patients who are informed about their likely postoperative experience are much better able to cope with pain and the other discomforts of the postoperative state than those who enter the experience uninformed.[20] Whether it is the surgeon, the anesthesiologist, or the nurse who talks to the patient about the postoperative course, the message should always be that the team will use all methods available to make the experience tolerable but that a goal of total pain abolition is unrealistic. This approach makes patients less fearful when they find that pain has not been completely removed. Anxious and fearful patients do not handle pain well, patients become fearful very quickly if they experience unexpected pain, and telling patients that the methods we have available are good enough to remove all pain is unhelpful. How often do we hear enthusiastic residents or nurses tell patients that if they accept an epidural, they will not have any pain?

Patients should be informed of their options with regard to pain management, preferably early in the preoperative course. The use of brochures or pamphlets describing analgesic options is helpful. A description of risks as well as benefits is necessary. Some patients expect to be informed and to take an active role in decisions regarding their care; others prefer that decisions be made by their medical team. In either case, informed patients are better prepared psychologically than those who have not received the benefit of being informed.

The preoperative visit is also an opportunity to teach patients how to communicate their pain. For example, if they are likely to be asked to relate pain using a verbal pain score, they should be taught about this. They should be encouraged to express pain and not try to be stoical. They should learn that uncontrolled pain may have undesirable consequences such as splinting of the diaphragm, atelectasis, and possible chest infection. They should learn how to use a PCA pump if they are likely to receive one. In particular, they should be aware that early on, they will need supplementary analgesia and should not expect that pressing the button will necessarily remove the severe pain that can occur in the immediate postoperative period. They should also be aware of the inherent safety of PCA and that overdose is unlikely.

Anesthesia Planning Anesthesiologists can have a significant impact on patients' postoperative pain experience, even if they are only involved in intraoperative care. This is not only by means of sustainable analgesia (epidurals and other catheter treatments), but also by anesthesia planning that results in a pain-free or near pain-free emergence. The importance of a pain-free emergence cannot be overemphasized; patients who wake from anesthesia in severe pain, especially those who are not expecting pain, are already disadvantaged in terms of being able to control their pain—again, fear and anxiety intervene to make pain control difficult.

Every anesthetic plan should incorporate planning for postoperative analgesia. The first question is whether a nerve block, a spinal, an epidural, or a plexus catheter treatment would help. This decision must also involve whether these treatments can additionally be used intraoperatively to provide analgesia or even anesthesia. How does the risk weigh against the benefit of these procedures when considering their role for both intraoperative and postoperative use? When one of these techniques is chosen, it becomes necessary to plan the exact injection regime. Will a nerve block last into the postoperative period or need to be supplemented by systemic analgesics? Can spinal analgesia be prolonged by using an opioid in the injectate? How will an epidural or other catheter treatment be used so that both its intra- and postoperative effects are optimized?

Despite the usefulness of neural blockade and catheter treatments, the vast majority of cases are managed without these. Planning for intraoperative and postoperative analgesia remains important. The basic principles of opioid-sparing and preemptive analgesia, described later, are incorporated into the analgesia plan. Opioids are the only strong analgesics capable of controlling severe pain with systemic use, and they are the mainstay of both intra- and postoperative pain relief. Opioids can be used liberally during anesthesia but less liberally postoperatively because of side effects. Individual practices vary, but the goal of a pain-free emergence should always be incorporated into the plan. Provided they are not contraindicated, nonsteroidal anti-inflammatory drugs (NSAIDs), including injectable ketorolac or other adjuncts, can be used when predicted pain is mild or as an adjunct to opioids for moderate to severe pain.

PAIN ASSESSMENT

Pain is a complex, multidimensional symptom resulting from a combination of tissue damage and nociception, previous pain experience, personal beliefs, culture, and mood. This explains why patients with the same degree of tissue damage can differ widely in their pain reports. Because there is no objective measure of pain, we must trust that patients' report of pain reflects their pain experience or distress. Acute pain is relatively straightforward to assess because, unlike chronic pain, it generally bears a predictable relationship to obvious tissue damage. The level of postoperative pain tends to change rapidly throughout the postoperative course, especially early after surgery; therefore, a policy of regular assessment of pain using simple measurement tools is the best way to ensure that pain treatment can be appropriately titrated. Side effects and recovery milestones are also measured to optimize analgesia and recovery.

Many institutions record pain as a "fifth vital sign" on the vital signs chart, especially since the introduction of the JCAHO mandate; others have a policy of recording a pain level in the medical record. Wherever it is documented, the recorded level is useful for communication between medical professionals and for assessing trends in an individual's pain level.

Verbal numeric rating scales are most commonly chosen to measure acute pain. The patient is asked to rate pain on a numeric scale, usually 0-10, where 0 is no pain and 10 is the worst pain imaginable. Verbal descriptive scales could also be used, but they are difficult for postoperative patients to cope with. Examples would be "mild, moderate, or severe" or "mild, discomforting, distressing, horrible, or excruciating." Visual analog scales are used in research, and unlike verbal numeric rating scales, they are validated for this purpose. The patient marks on a measured line labeled "no pain" at one end and "worst pain imaginable" at the other. Visual analog scales are rarely used in clinical practice, again because compliance is difficult for postoperative patients. Although the use of pain scales is necessary for documentation purposes, the clinical assessment of pain should always include asking patients to describe their pain and their pain experience since the last assessment. This is likely to reveal more information than the simple level. At the same time, the clinician should assess pain location, radiation, quality, and etiology. It is always important to expand the assessment to identify or exclude sources of pain not accounted for by the primary and expected source.

Assessment of pain in children, especially young children, is much more difficult. Although developmentally normal children older than 6 to 7 years of age will respond to adult assessment tools, younger children than this need a different approach. Infants, neonates, and very young children (0-4 years) are the most challenging. Children as young as 3 years old may be able to express pain and point to a painful area, but they are unlikely to be able to rate their pain. Children younger than this are unable to express pain other than by crying or screaming, posturing, grimacing, palmar sweating, and respiratory and heart rate changes—signs that are not specific to pain. Older children (4-7 years) are usually able to rate their pain, but it is helpful to use a scale designed for children, such as the Wong-Baker faces pain scale (**Fig. 72-1**). Parents are usually better able to recognize the presence of pain in their children than any of the other caregivers, and they should always be asked to contribute to the assessment process.

BASIC PRINCIPLES

Two important principles influence our choice of drug, dose, route of delivery, and timing for the treatment of acute pain. These are the principles of preemptive analgesia and opioid sparing.

Preemptive Analgesia Preemptive analgesia is described by Igor Kissin as "an anti-nociceptive therapy that prevents establishment of altered processing of afferent input, which amplifies postoperative pain."[21,22] In simpler terms, a preemptive analgesic intervention is one that stops or alters pain transmission so that pain will not become amplified by the nervous system. Kissin's definition embraces the fundamental principles necessary for understanding the concept of preemptive analgesia: (1) that the central nervous system is capable of changing so that pain becomes either improved and worsened via central processes such as desensitization and sensitization, and (2) that alterations in sensory and pain transmission can effect such changes. The idea that pain treated early in its course is easier to control than established pain is not new; in fact, it is a truism passed down through generations. The new idea is that in addition to psychologic factors, which remain important especially in humans, a central process—central sensitization—can be altered by altering afferent input using analgesic drugs or neural blockade. Animal studies showed strong and convincing effects after preemptive interventions including nerve blocks and systemic analgesics.[23] Human studies have been less convincing.[24,25] But the idea that our interventions before, during, and after surgery could attenuate pain responses is too attractive to lay to rest. Studies are still being conducted, and the clinical role of preemptive analgesia is still uncertain and much debated.

A systematic review published by Møiniche et al in 2002[24] found no support for preemptive analgesia when 80 trials assessing preemptive administration of epidural analgesia, systemic opioids, NSAIDs, local infiltration, and *N*-methyl-D-aspartate (NMDA) antagonists were grouped and analyzed, finding no overall benefit to any of the preemptive treatments. (The last intervention may have a special effect in that central sensitization is mediated by NMDA receptor activity).[26,27] In all 80 trials selected here, preincision treatment was compared with postincision treatment. Despite this disappointing result, Ong et al went on to conduct a new meta-analysis, which included 10 newly published RCTs.[25] Their methods differed from those of Møiniche et al in several respects: They included trials that compared the preemptive intervention with no intervention as well as the comparison with postincision interventions,[28] they used a different approach for analyzing pain scores, and they used different exclusion criteria (fewer studies met the inclusion criteria). And in this case, several preemptive treatments—epidural analgesia, NSAIDs, and wound infiltration—were strongly effective. Preemptive opioid and NMDA antagonists were not effective. Note that Ong's analysis of NSAID preemptive effects needs reexamination after Reuben's studies were found to be fraudulent (see section Prevention of Chronic Postsurgical Pain).

The preemptive analgesia concept may seem simple: Stop central sensitization and pain will improve. But it is far from simple. Central sensitization itself is a complex process; NMDA antagonists may alter central sensitization but not necessarily because they are given prior to versus after an incision; opioids may actually cause central sensitization under some circumstances;[29-31] neural blockade does not always succeed in preventing all afferent input from a surgical process.[21,28] It is no surprise, then, that study results seem conflicting, and meta-analyses do not provide clear answers to the question of whether preemptive analgesia has an important clinical role. We have a lot to learn about how preemptive analgesia studies should be designed and how to combine them rationally in meta-analyses. Until we have better answers,

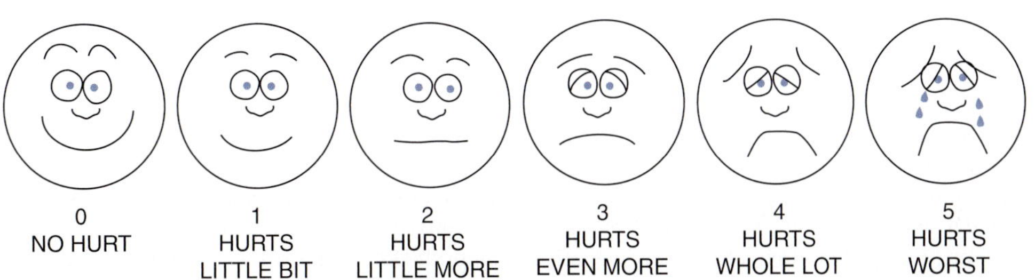

FIGURE 72-1. Wong-Baker FACES Pain Rating Scale. [Reproduced with permission from Hockenberry MJ, Wilson D, Winkelstein ML, eds. *Wong's Essentials of Pediatric Nursing*. 7th ed. St. Louis, MO: Mosby; 2005. Used with permission. Copyright, Mosby.]

we should be guided by preliminary data that suggest there is little to lose and possibly much to gain, from early use of neural blockade and NSAIDs, although the benefit of early NSAIDs may have as much to do with the pharmacology of NSAIDs (particularly delayed peak effects), as with any effect on central sensitization, the core mechanism proposed for true preemptive analgesia.[32]

Opioid-Sparing and Multimodal Analgesia Opioid drugs mimic endogenous analgesic responses, so it is not surprising that they are our most powerful analgesics. Centuries of opioid (opium) use have provided humans with relief from pain and suffering. Yet, throughout this long history, there have been concerns about the opioids' toxic effects, particularly their addictive effects and the potentially fatal side effect of respiratory depression. The extent to which opioids have been used for the relief of pain has fluctuated, not only throughout history, but also between cultures. In the United States and other industrialized nations, opioid use for severe pain has been strongly encouraged, especially since the 1980s when it was recognized that antidrug regulations had severely inhibited opioid use to the detriment of pain control. Current teaching states that good pain relief during and after surgery, using opioids whenever necessary, can improve surgical recovery.[33] Pain relief is an important component of accelerated recovery programs that aim to achieve early return of mobility, coughing, and bowel and bladder function, and to restore normal physiologic functioning as rapidly as possible thereby reducing complication rates.[34-36] Yet herein lies a paradox: Opioids are our most effective analgesics; but they can delay recovery because of their sedative effects, their nauseating effects, and most importantly, by slowing bowel activity. Opioid-sparing interventions reduce opioid requirements, and in some cases they obviate the use of opioids altogether. Such interventions include the use of adjunctive medications, epidurals, and other nerve blocks, as well as nondrug interventions. The concept of "multimodal analgesia,"[37,38] using several analgesic modes together, is similar to the concept of opioid sparing. It allows for administration of a combination of opioid and nonopioid analgesic drugs to be given that act at a variety of receptor sites within the central and peripheral nervous systems in an effort to minimize potent opioid use and therefore decrease opioid-induced adverse effects. The ability of nonopioid medications, such as gabapentin, to minimize the opioid analgesic requirements and associated side effects confers an opioid-sparing effect on these agents. Most published clinical data focus on the effects of adding a single therapeutic agent to an already established therapeutic analgesic regimen. More recently, data have begun to emerge using combination approaches to manage acute and postoperative pain such as local anesthetic infiltration of the surgical site, NSAIDs, NMDA antagonists, and α_2-Δ-receptor modulators such as gabapentin and pregabalin. NSAIDs and selective cyclooxygenase (COX)-2 inhibitors consistently reduce opioid consumption postoperatively.[39] Studies of NMDA antagonists have produced variable results, but there is evidence that low-dose ketamine has an important role as an adjunct to opioids in multimodal analgesia.[40] Recent studies have shown an opioid-sparing effect by pregabalin in both hip arthroplasty and laparoscopic cholecystectomy patients, making it a useful adjunct in both same-day and short stay surgical procedures.[41,42] Pregabalin has some advantages over gabapentin in that it has higher bioavailability and more linear pharmacokinetics that allow it to have more rapid onset. Local anesthetic infiltration into the surgical site has also shown to be clinically effective in a combination regimen for multimodal analgesia when treating acute postoperative pain.

Prevention of Chronic Postsurgical Pain Apart from their role in reducing perioperative pain and analgesic requirements, a role in reducing chronic postsurgical (incisional) pain has been proposed for both preemptive and multimodal analgesic protocols.[43,44] The hypothesis that postsurgical pain can be prevented or attenuated by perioperative analgesic interventions is appealing, yet the scientific evidence supporting the hypothesis remains inconclusive at present.[45] Most convincing is the evidence that conduction blockade (paravertebral and epidural) is helpful for reducing persistent pain after breast surgery and thoracotomy. Evidence also suggests that surgical technique has an important role in minimizing persistent pain after surgery, not simply careful technique, but specific modifications such as use of minimally invasive and muscle- or nerve-sparing techniques and lightweight mesh (for hernia repairs).[43,45]

The present discussion would not be complete without mentioning the case of Reuben, a formerly respected and much published clinical investigator who fabricated data for 21 of his published studies in respected anesthesia journals. The studies all concerned perioperative analgesic interventions, and several supported the claim that adjunct and multimodal analgesia is capable of reducing postsurgical pain. The fraud is believed to be one of the largest known cases of academic misconduct, and the story was reported in the lay press as well as the scientific literature. The collateral damage was enormous because every paper, systematic review, and meta-analysis incorporating Reuben's studies had to be reexamined. Despite the enormity of this task, the greatest damage was, of course, to the credibility of the academic endeavor.

Although the damage the Reuben fraud has caused to the broader concept of multimodal analgesia is minimal, except in loss of credibility, the fraud has actually forced a reexamination of the concept that preemptive or multimodal approaches can reduce late pain. Countless studies and meta-analyses, many of which do not include Reuben's studies, support the opioid-sparing effect of epidural, regional anesthesia, NSAIDs, and other adjuncts. However with respect specifically to the concept that immediate or late pain can be prevented through the timely administration of nonopioid analgesics, Reuben's studies did have some influence so that reexamination became necessary. White et al, in an editorial in *Anesthesia and Analgesia* published in May 2009, examined each of the discredited studies and their potential influence.[46] They concluded that the area where reexamination is necessary concerns the ability of NSAIDs (notably the selective COX-2 NSAIDs), and neuropathic pain medications (notably venlafaxine and pregabalin) in multimodal regimes to provide preemptive or long-term benefit after orthopedic surgery.

TREATMENT OPTIONS

SYSTEMIC TREATMENTS

Opioids Opioids remain the mainstay of acute pain treatment, despite concerns about their side effects. Systemic opioids are used alone or in combination with other analgesics.[47,48] Generally, higher doses of parenteral opioids are given during the first 24 to 48 hours after surgery when pain tends to be severe and patients are not able to tolerate oral medications. The intravenous (IV) route is the preferred parenteral route because most hospitalized patients already have IV catheters in place. Later, oral opioids, often in combination preparations such as Percocet (oxycodone with acetaminophen), replace the parenteral opioid. Side effects may limit opioid use, but there are few absolute contraindications, and true allergy to opioids is rare. Meperidine should not be used with monoamine oxidase inhibitors (MAOIs).

Choice of Opioid **Morphine** is the main constituent of opium, it was the first opioid alkaloid to be identified, and it is the standard opioid to which other opioids are often compared. Codeine is the only other naturally occurring opioid in common use. The other familiar opioids are *semisynthetic*, derived from opium constituents (hydromorphone, hydrocodone, and oxycodone) or *synthetic*, synthesized de novo (meperidine, methadone, fentanyl, and fentanyl derivatives). These drugs are all opioid agonists, chiefly at the μ-opioid receptor. Other opioids are mixed agonists/antagonists or partial agonists (buprenorphine, butorphanol, pentazocine, nalbuphine) and are generally used for treating chronic rather than acute pain (or addiction), at least in the United States. They are not described in detail here. Naloxone is a pure opioid antagonist and can be useful to treat opioid overdose. The

TABLE 72-1 Standard Doses of Commonly Used Opioids

		Equianalgesic Doses		Typical First Dose	
Generic Name	Trade Name	Oral	Parenteral	Oral	Parenteral
Codeine		200 mg	120 mg	30 mg q3-4h	10 mg q3-4h
Fentanyl patch	Duragesic	N/A	N/A	N/A	25 μg/h patch q72h[a]
Fentanyl Oralet	Actiq	N/A	N/A	N/A	200 μg[b]
Hydrocodone	Vicodin[c], Lorcet[c], Lortab[c], Norco[c]	N/A	N/A	10 mg q3-4h	N/A
Hydromorphone	Dilaudid	7.5 mg	1.5 mg	2-4 mg q3-4h	1.5 mg q3-4h
Levorphanol	Levo-Dromoran	4 mg	2 mg	4 mg q6-8h	2 mg q6-8h
Meperidine	Demerol	300 mg	100 mg	100 mg q3h	100 mg q3h
Methadone[d]	Dolophine	2-4 mg	10 mg (acute) 2-4 mg (chronic)	5 mg q8-12h	5 mg q8-12h
Morphine		30 mg	10 mg	15 mg q3-4h	10 mg q3-4h
Morphine SR	MS Contin	N/A	N/A	15 mg q8-12h	N/A
Oxycodone	Percocet[c], Percodan[c]	N/A	N/A	5 mg q3-4h	N/A
Oxycodone CR	OxyContin	N/A	N/A	10 mg q8-12h	N/A

[a]Lowest available dose. Risk of overdose in opioid-naive patients. 25 μg/h patch = 50-75 mg oral morphine per 24-h period. Conversions should be made conservatively (consult product literature) and titrated slowly.

[b]Lowest available dose. Contraindicated in opioid-naive patients, especially children. Not for use in children less than 10 kg. 200 μg Oralet = 2 mg IV morphine; 800 μg Oralet = 10 mg IV morphine.

[c]Combination formulations, with either acetaminophen or aspirin.

[d]The equianalgesic conversion dose for methadone decreases significantly with increasing dose of previous opioid. Caution guided by experience is mandatory.

From Black DR, Brenner GJ, Abdi S, Gill J. Drugs commonly used in pain practice (Appendix VII). In: Ballantyne JC, ed. *The Massachusetts General Hospital Handbook of Pain Management.* 3rd ed. Philadelphia, PA: Lippincott, Williams & Wilkins; 2006.

commonly used opioid-agonists are listed, with recommended doses, in **Table 72-1**. Opioid effects are summarized in **Table 72-2**. The opioids described next are μ-agonists with essentially similar effects. Choice of opioid depends as much on the familiarity and preference of the treating physician as on the generally subtle differences in pharmacology between these drugs.

Morphine is the standard, most widely used of the opioids, and in some countries, it is the only available opioid. It is the least lipophilic opioid, which delays its peak effect (occurs at 20 min after IV injection) but makes it a good choice for epidural administration when a widespread effect is desirable. Morphine is highly metabolized and has at least 2 active metabolites (morphine-6-glucuronide and morphine-3-glucuronide), which can delay normalization after morphine administration, especially during renal compromise and continuous administration. (Morphine metabolites may also contribute to morphine toxicity and morphine-induced hyperalgesia in the special circumstance of sustained use.) Morphine induces histamine release, and rapid bolus injection may produce local erythema, hypotension, or rarely, bronchospasm. The normal duration of a standard dose (10 mg) is 3 to 4 hours. Morphine has poor oral bioavailability, and the oral dose is 3 times the parenteral dose. Morphine may cause biliary and urinary tract spasm, and a different opioid is often substituted (meperidine or fentanyl) during treatment for gallstones and renal stones or during biliary tract and urinary tract surgery, although recent studies suggest that the effect is an opioid effect, not specifically a morphine effect.[49,50]

TABLE 72-2 Opioid Effects

Analgesia
Respiratory depression
Nausea and vomiting
Sedation
Direct bowel effects
Dizziness
Pruritus
Meiosis
Euphoria
Dysphoria
(Biliary spasm: typically morphine)
(Urinary retention: uncertain)

Codeine is less potent, although more constipating, than morphine. Constipation limits the recommended dose to 30 mg, which has only mild analgesic (and respiratory depressant) effects. Codeine is available for oral use only and is commonly found in combination analgesics such as Tylenol 3 (acetaminophen with codeine). In many countries, codeine is available over the counter because it is considered to have low abuse potential and a good safety record. Its main use is for pain of moderate severity, especially for children.

Hydromorphone (Dilaudid) is a useful alternative to morphine. For ill-defined reasons, many patients seem to prefer hydromorphone and claim they feel more clear headed, less dizzy, and less nauseated. At present, these can only be considered anecdotal observations. There are no active metabolites; therefore hydromorphone is a good choice for continuous administration, especially in patients with renal compromise.

Hydrocodone is used for mild to moderate pain, most commonly in the oral combination formulation Vicodin (hydrocodone with acetaminophen).

Oxycodone is not available for parenteral use in the United States, although it is elsewhere. It is a familiar opioid in the United States in the form of Percocet (oxycodone with acetaminophen) and widely used for the treatment of moderately severe acute pain, including home treatment. More recently, oxycodone was formulated as a long-acting preparation (OxyContin), which has become a useful alternative to morphine and MS Contin (long-acting morphine) for the treatment of cancer and selected chronic pain. OxyContin and other long-acting oxycodone preparations have also been used for the treatment of acute pain, to aid sleep at night and function during the day. OxyContin availability has been limited by constraints associated with its popularity as a drug of abuse.

Meperidine (Demerol) was widely used for sedation and analgesia during procedural treatments, particularly in the office setting, as well as for hospital treatment of intra- and postoperative pain, until in the early 1980s several problems with the drug became clear. The first was normeperidine toxicity. Normeperidine is a toxic metabolite capable of inducing central nervous system excitation and seizures, and liable to accumulate in the elderly and those with impaired renal function. The second was the propensity of meperidine to cause addiction, probably related to its lipophilicity and rapid onset of both analgesia and euphoria. Published guidelines began to state that meperidine should not be used routinely,[7,8] and many hospitals withdrew it from their formularies. When it is available, meperidine remains a useful drug, and its ability to produce fast-onset analgesia and euphoria is its great advantage, especially during the treatment of postoperative pain. It also has an idiosyncratic and little understood advantage for treating postoperative shivering. It must, however, be used cautiously, being particularly mindful of normeperidine toxicity that can occur with repeated or continuous use. Meperidine has mild anticholinergic, antihistaminic, and local anesthetic effects. There may be a dangerous interaction (serotonin syndrome) with MAOIs producing seizures, coma, and possibly death, even after a single meperidine dose.

Methadone is a complex drug, rarely used for acute pain, except in patients already treated with this drug. Important considerations are its multiple interactions with other drugs, especially with antibiotics and antifungals, and its propensity to prolong the QT_c interval, especially at high doses.[51,52] Refer to more detailed texts if you are faced with a patient requiring high-dose methadone or receiving methadone as part of a complex drug treatment regime.

Fentanyl use in the postoperative setting is largely confined to PCA and epidurals, where its high lipophilicity and short duration can be used to advantage.

Tramadol (Ultram) is an interesting drug with weak opioid activity and additional norepinephrine and serotonin reuptake inhibition. It has low abuse potential and is not a controlled substance. It is widely used in Europe to treat acute and postoperative pain but is less favored in the United States, where it is only available for oral use. Its use for severe pain is limited by the fact that it has a ceiling effect, but it may be useful for mild to moderate pain, particularly in patients who refuse opioids or tolerate them badly.

Adverse Effects Respiratory depression is the most feared of the opioid side effects, and rightly so, because this is a potentially fatal side effect. The possibility of respiratory depression produces a real conflict when trying to balance effective analgesia with safety. A key issue is to understand the likelihood of the event, and therefore the risk, and to provide adequate monitoring in high-risk situations. The immediate postoperative period is a period of high risk: The patient is often opioid naive, has been given multiple sedating drugs during surgery, may be weak, and may have a high analgesic requirement. Neonates and infants are always at high risk because of their immature nervous systems, propensity to apnea, and poor ability to metabolize opioid drugs. The elderly display similar risks. Patients established on a stable opioid regime are at lower risk. The level of monitoring required is a matter of judgment, whether this consists of frequent checks by a nurse or the application of a monitor such as an apnea monitor or pulse oximetry.

Other side effects are less catastrophic but can significantly compromise the success of opioid therapy. Patients may prefer to be in pain than feel disorientated, dizzy, or nauseated; physicians may undertreat pain rather than delay hospital discharge because of ileus or nausea. Secondary treatments such as antiemetics may help, but it is the principles of opioid sparing that play a key role in minimizing opioid side effects and optimizing pain control.

Tolerance, Dependence, and Addiction It is important to understand tolerance, dependence, and addiction, and the differences between these 3 phenomena. Drug **tolerance** arises when an increase in dose is required to achieve the effect of an initial dose. Opioid tolerance arises through a combination of receptor desensitization (nonassociative tolerance) and psychologic factors (associative tolerance).[53,54] Apparent tolerance could also result from opioid-induced hyperalgesia (OIH).[31,55,56] Patients receiving chronic opioid therapy could manifest either or both pharmacologic tolerance and OIH, and in fact, the 2 may be difficult to distinguish clinically because both are manifest as increased opioid dose requirement, and both result from biologic adaptations to continued opioid use.[57,58] The phenomenon of OIH becomes increasingly important during acute and postoperative pain management as more and more patients present for surgery with opioid refractoriness caused by the neuroadaptations to it.[59] The management of these patients is described in the section Special Populations. The development of tolerance and hyperalgesia during acute treatment is rare but can occur, especially when opioid infusions are used (eg, remifentanil during surgery or opioid infusions on an intensive care unit).[60-62] NMDA antagonists such as ketamine may have an increasingly important role in the treatment of acute and postoperative pain because they seem to be effective for attenuating hyperalgesia, OIH, and opioid tolerance.[63-65]

Dependence, also known as **physical dependence,** arises after chronic opioid use, is thought to reside in norepinephrine pathways of the locus ceruleus, and results in a typical withdrawal syndrome when an opioid-dependent patient is deprived of opioid. The typical opioid withdrawal syndrome comprises central neurologic arousal and sleeplessness, irritability, psychomotor agitation, diarrhea, rhinorrhea, and piloerection. In the management of acute pain, withdrawal may occur if habitual doses are not maintained during acute pain treatment. Patients who use opioids illicitly are not typically honest about their use, so physicians must be watchful for the signs of withdrawal when there is any suspicion of illicit use. Treatment consists of reestablishing previous opioid levels, before a gradual taper. Clonidine can be a useful adjunct and effectively treats many of the manifestations of opioid withdrawal.

Addiction, a behavioral syndrome with a neurobiologic basis, virtually never arises out of hospital treatment of pain with opioids. Patients who are worried about the addiction risk can be assured of this.[66] However, addicted patients present for surgery and with acute trauma-related pain, and they require skillful pain management. The management of these patients is described in the section Special Populations.

Nonsteroidal Anti-Inflammatory Drugs and Acetaminophen The NSAIDs are a group of drugs that inhibit cyclooxygenase (COX) (an enzyme in the arachidonic acid pathway), thereby inhibiting prostaglandin and thromboxane production (**Fig. 72-2**). Prostaglandin and thromboxane actions are summarized in **Table 72-3**. Inhibition of prostaglandin and thromboxane accounts for the analgesic and anti-inflammatory effects of NSAIDs, as well as for their adverse effects. Acetaminophen is not strictly an anti-inflammatory drug but is included here because it shares many of the properties of the NSAIDs. In contrast to the true NSAIDs, which are polarized and therefore do not readily cross the blood-brain barrier, acetaminophen is nonacidic and crosses the blood-brain barrier. Its action resides mainly in the central nervous system where prostaglandin inhibition produces analgesia and antipyresis. Its peripheral and anti-inflammatory effects are weak. Commonly used NSAIDs and their doses are listed in **Table 72-4**.

The NSAIDs and acetaminophen are commonly used over-the-counter analgesics, and have a long history of use for mild to moderate surgical pain, especially during home treatment. They are also used with opioids in oral combination formulations. The advent of ketorolac, the first injectable NSAID with Federal Drug Administration (FDA) approval for use in surgical patients, triggered a surge in interest in the use of NSAIDs as sole analgesics and as adjuncts for the treatment of moderate to severe acute and surgical pain. Ketorolac is a potent NSAID, unfortunately with a side-effect profile that reflects its potency, which can be used as a sole analgesic, even for severe pain. The NSAIDs and acetaminophen have emerged as useful adjuncts in multimodal analgesic regimes.

A new subclass of NSAIDs was recently released for clinical use: the selective COX-2 inhibitors. COX-2 is an inducible isoenzyme and

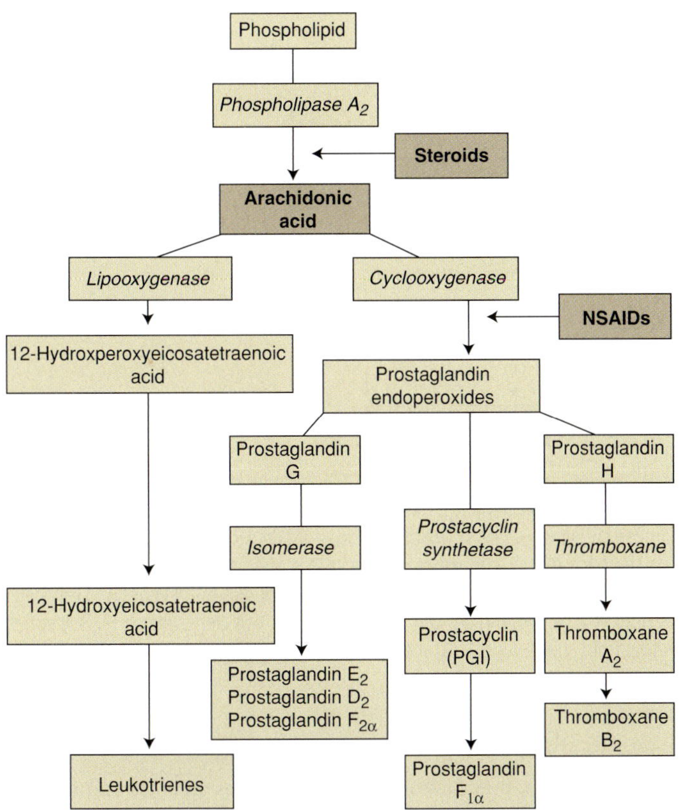

FIGURE 72–2. A schematic diagram showing the metabolism of phospholipid and arachidonic acid. Nonsteroidal anti-inflammatory drugs (NSAIDs) inhibit cyclooxygenase and thereby suppress the synthesis of prostaglandin E, prostacyclin, and thromboxane, and alter the balance between these eicosanoids and the leukotrienes. [Reproduced with permission from Ballantyne JC, Barna SB. Non-steroidal anti-inflammatory drugs. In: Ballantyne JC, ed. *The Massachusetts General Hospital Handbook of Pain Management*. 3rd ed. Philadelphia, PA: Lippincott, Williams & Wilkins; 2006.]

a source of prostaglandins during inflammatory processes. COX-1, in contrast, is a constitutive isoenzyme and has protective effects on the stomach where it mediates the production of cytoprotective prostaglandins (**Fig. 72-3**).[67] The selective COX-2 inhibitors were developed in the hope of being able to reduce NSAID side effects, particularly the damaging gastrointestinal (GI) effects. Early clinical trials and clinical experience confirmed the analgesic efficacy and favorable side-effect profile of these drugs with regard to their effect on the gastric mucosa and their platelet effects, although some of the early trial results have now been brought into question. The great hope for these drugs was that they would replace standard NSAIDs and reduce complications, particularly NSAID-induced GI bleeding, which is thought to account for up to 100 000 hospitalizations and 20 000 deaths per year in the United States. However, these hopes have been crushed by the steady emergence of evidence that deleterious cardiovascular and thrombotic effects preclude the use of these drugs in many patients.[68,69] In fact, most are now withdrawn, and the only selective COX-2 inhibitor on the market in the United States at the time of writing is celecoxib (Celebrex).

TABLE 72-3 Prostaglandin and Thromboxane Actions

Fever vascular smooth muscle relaxation (predominant action)
(PGI_1 and PGE) and contraction (PGF_1 and TXA)
Increased capillary permeability (LTB)
Uterine smooth muscle contraction (PGE, PGF_2)
Bronchial smooth muscle relaxation (PGE) and contraction (PGF_2, TXA, LTC, LTD)
Increased GI contraction and motility (PGE_1, PGI)
Protection of GI tract by inhibiting gastric acid secretion and enhancing gastric mucous secretion (PGE_1, PGI)
Regulation of renal blood flow and sodium/potassium exchange (PGE_1, PGI)
Marked potentiation of the effects of other mediators of inflammation and pain (serotonin, bradykinin, histamine) (PGE_1, PGI)
Sensitization of nociceptors (PGE_1, PGI)
Inhibition of platelet aggregation (PGI)
Increased platelet aggregation (TXA)
Constriction of vascular smooth muscle (TXA)

PGI, prostacyclin; PGE and PGF, prostaglandin E and F; TXA, thromboxane A; LTB, LTC, and LTD, leukotriene B, C, and D.

TABLE 72-4 Standard Doses of Commonly Used Oral NSAIDs

Generic Name	Trade Name	Adult Oral Dosage
Acetaminophen	Tylenol	650-975 mg q4-6h
Acetylsalicylic acid	Aspirin	650-975 mg q4-6h
Celecoxib	Celebrex	100-200 mg bid
Diclofenac sodium	Voltaren	25-75 mg q8-12h
Diflunisal	Dolobid	250-500 mg q8-12h
Etodolac	Lodine	200-400 mg q6-8h
Fenoprofen calcium	Nalfon	200 mg q4-6h
Flurbiprofen	Ansaid	100 mg q8-12h
Ibuprofen	Motrin	400-800 mg q6-8h
Indomethacin	Indocin	25-50 mg q8-12h
Ketoprofen	Orudis	25-75 mg q6-8h
Ketorolac	Toradol	10-50 mg q6-8h
Meclofenamate sodium	Meclomen	50 mg q4-6h
Meloxicam	Mobic	7.5-15 mg qd
Naproxen	Naprosyn	250-500 mg q8-12h
Naproxen sodium	Anaprox	250-550 mg q6-8h
Phenylbutazone	Butazolidin	100 mg q6-8h
Piroxicam	Feldene	10-20 mg qd
Sulindac	Clinoril	150-200 mg q12h
Tolmetin	Tolectin	200-600 mg q8h

From Black DR, Brenner GJ, Abdi S, Gill J. Drugs commonly used in pain practice (Appendix VII). In: Ballantyne JC, ed. *The Massachusetts General Hospital Handbook of Pain Management.* 3rd ed. Philadelphia, PA: Lippincott, Williams & Wilkins; 2006.

Adverse Effects and Limitations on Perioperative Use Adverse effects of NSAIDs in surgical patients are listed in **Table 72-5**. Contraindications arise out of these adverse effects, listed in **Table 72-6**. Acetaminophen is relatively safe and not associated with the adverse effects listed for standard NSAIDs. The COX-2 inhibitors are less likely to cause bleeding (platelet effects), particularly GI bleeding (unprotected GI mucosa), but they carry the same risk as standard NSAIDs with the other listed adverse effects and additional cardiovascular and thrombotic risks. These drugs therefore have similar contraindications to the standard NSAIDs.

Patients should be advised to stop taking NSAIDs before surgery, chiefly because of their platelet effects and their propensity to increase surgical bleeding. Aspirin, whose platelet effects are not reversible, should be stopped for up to 10 days before elective surgery. Other NSAIDs have rapidly reversible platelet effects, and 24-hour cessation is probably sufficient, although 2 to 3 days cessation is usual. Acetaminophen and COX-2 inhibitors can be continued because they do not have platelet effects.

A factor that makes perioperative NSAID use relatively safe is the fact that they are used for a short period, and most adverse effect are associated with prolonged use. This is true of platelet, GI, and renal effects. Thus even in patients chronically treated with NSAIDs who

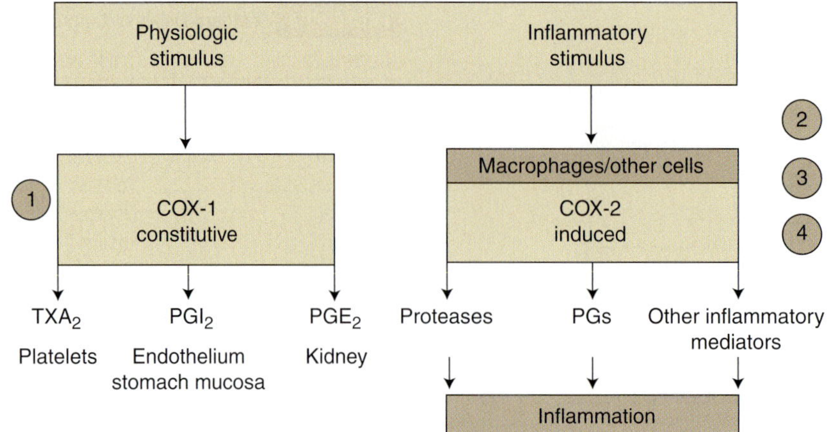

FIGURE 72-3. Relationships between the pathways leading to the generation of eicosanoids by cyclooxygenase (COX)-1 and COX-2. Under physiologic conditions, activation of COX-1 (eg, in platelets, endothelium, stomach mucosa, or kidney) results in the release of thromboxane A_2 (TXA_2), prostacyclin (PGI_2), or prostaglandin E_2 (PGE_2). The release of these eicosanoids is selectively inhibited by drugs such as aspirin (1). Inflammatory stimuli release cytokines, such as interleukin-1, that induce the synthesis of COX-2 in cells such as macrophages, resulting in the release of prostaglandins (PGs). The release of PGs together with proteases and other inflammatory mediators (such as reactive oxygen radicals) results in inflammation. The COX-2 pathway can be interrupted at several levels by antagonists or antibodies to cytokines and mitogens (2), inhibitors of the induction of COX-2 (eg, glucocorticoids) (3), or selective inhibitors of COX-2 (4). [Reprinted with permission from Van Der Ouderaa FJ, Buytenhek M, Nugteren DH. Purification and characterization of prostaglandin endoperoxide synthetase from sheep vesicular glands. *Biochim Biophys Acta*. 1977;487:315-331, with permission from Elsevier.]

have stopped the treatment to minimize surgical bleeding, short-term perioperative use may be appropriate. This brings into question the issue of timing of NSAID administration, which is linked to the drugs' liabilities. There are theoretical advantages to giving NSAIDs early in the surgical course, even preoperatively. These include the drugs' pharmacokinetics—for example, the peak effect of ketorolac may occur as late as 4 hours after administration—and the consideration that the drugs may have preemptive effects. However, for major surgery, where there is a likelihood of bleeding and/or hypotension with deleterious effects on clotting and renal function, it is probably better to wait until the extent of any derangement is clear. Surgical considerations are also important when deciding whether to use an NSAID. These include possible postoperative bleeding, especially into closed cavities such as the knee joint, as well as retardation of bone remodeling, a consideration after bone fusion especially of the spine.

Use of NSAIDs and Acetaminophen for Postoperative and Acute Pain For mild postoperative or acute pain, NSAIDs or acetaminophen can be used as sole analgesics. In addition, even though they are considered weak analgesics, they have an important role as adjuncts and in multimodal analgesic regimes. Their mechanism of action (prostaglandin inhibition) means that they are synergistic with many other analgesic interventions, particularly with opioid analgesia. Multiple studies and meta-analyses confirm an average 30% to 50% opioid-sparing effect of NSAIDs.[68,70-74] Whether this reduction in opioid dose with NSAIDs translates into improved recovery and morbidity is less clear. The most recent meta-analysis of 22 RCTs by Marret et al affirmed a reduction in nausea (30% reduction) and sedation (29% reduction), but effects on urinary retention and respiratory complications were inconclusive. Overall, studies assessing the effects on adjunctive NSAID use on recovery have had mixed results.[70,71] The availability of the injectable NSAID ketorolac has extended perioperative use to the many patients who cannot tolerate oral medications after surgery. Initially, the side effects of this drug seemed unacceptable, but this was an effect of an initial recommendation to use a 60 mg first dose with 30 mg repeat doses. Now that the recommended dose has been halved (30 mg first dose, 15 mg repeat doses) and a 5-day limit has been placed on ketorolac use, the early problems of catastrophic bleeding (GI, surgical, and joint) seem

TABLE 72-5 Adverse Effects of NSAIDs in Surgical Patients

Gastrointestinal hemorrhage *(occasionally catastrophic)*
Renal dysfunction or failure
Decreased hemostasis and hematoma formation
Asthma in susceptible individuals *(due to blockade of the cyclooxygenase pathway, leading to exaggerated effects of the metabolites of the lipooxygenase pathway (ie, leukotrienes)*
Anaphylaxis *(risk of immune-related anaphylactoid reactions is small, although some individuals suffer anaphylaxis-like symptoms that are unrelated to an immune process)*
Decreased healing of gastrointestinal anastomoses *(proposed)*
Delayed fracture healing *(not established in humans but demonstrated in animals)*

From Ballantyne JC, Barna SB. Non-steroidal anti-inflammatory drugs. In: Ballantyne JC, ed. *The Massachusetts General Hospital Handbook of Pain Management.* 3rd ed. Philadelphia, PA: Lippincott, Williams & Wilkins; 2006.

TABLE 72-6 Contraindications to NSAID Use

History of peptic ulcer disease or intolerance to NSAIDs
Bleeding, bleeding diatheses, or anticoagulant therapy
Renal failure, renal dysfunction, or risk factors for renal dysfunction *(ie, hypovolemia, sodium depletion, congestive heart failure, hepatic cirrhosis, concurrent use of nephrotoxic drugs including aminoglycosides)*
Old age, particularly in the presence of any of the above[a]
Prophylactic use in major surgery *(ie, preoperative or intraoperative use, particularly if there is a potential for bleeding)*

[a]The elderly (>60 y of age) appear to be especially vulnerable to the effects of prostaglandin inhibition by NSAIDs.

From Ballantyne JC, Barna SB. Non-steroidal anti-inflammatory drugs. In: Ballantyne JC, ed. *The Massachusetts General Hospital Handbook of Pain Management.* 3rd ed. Philadelphia, PA: Lippincott, Williams & Wilkins; 2006.

to be resolved. Injectable acetaminophen is available and widely used perioperatively in Europe, but it is not available in the United States.

Novel Adjuncts Although the NSAIDs are the most widely used and useful systemic analgesic adjuncts in postoperative pain regimes, there has recently been interest in testing other possible adjuncts.

NMDA receptor antagonists are known to reduce central sensitization, hyperalgesia, and opioid tolerance.[27,31,55] This makes them theoretically an attractive option for treating acute pain: By reducing central sensitization they might reduce postoperative pain and possibly reduce the likelihood of developing chronic pain; they could also reduce opioid requirements and opioid tolerance. Ketamine is the most widely tested of currently available NMDA receptor antagonists (ketamine, dextromethorphan, and amantadine), but use has been limited by this drug's side effects (psychomimetic effects, including nightmares and hallucinations). These side effects can be reduced by concomitant use of benzodiazepines and by dose restriction; efforts to study the possible usefulness of ketamine as an adjunct analgesic for postoperative pain have centered on dose-finding and regime modeling. A recent detailed study suggests that although ketamine has demonstrable antihyperalgesic effects (as shown by skin measurements around the surgical incision), this may not translate into a useful opioid-sparing effect.[35,75] A 2005 systematic review by Elia and Tramer incorporating 53 trials (2839 patients) found a small difference (<1 cm on a 0-10 cm visual analog scale) in postoperative pain level, a significant difference in opioid use during the first 24 hours after surgery, and no difference in opioid side effects.[76] The highest risk of hallucinations occurred in awake or sedated patients receiving ketamine without a benzodiazepine. The role of ketamine and other NMDA receptor antagonists remains uncertain at present, although ketamine is being used increasingly as evidence is accumulating that it may have a useful adjunctive role in reversing hyperalgesia, OIH and opioid tolerance.[63-65]

Neuropathic pain medications such as anticonvulsants and antidepressants, as their name suggests, have their chief pain indication for the treatment of chronic neuropathic pain. Gabapentin has long been a useful adjuvant medication for chronic neuropathic pain, and its use for perioperative and acute postoperative pain is increasing. A more recent addition to this class of agent, pregabalin, also has antiallodynic and antihyperalgesic properties useful for treating neuropathic pain, which appear to make them beneficial agents in acute postoperative pain.

Gabapentin and pregabalin are inhibitors of the α_2-Δ-subunit of the high-voltage-activated calcium channel. Their use reduces both neurotransmitter release as well as postsynaptic excitability. Data increasingly suggest that both of these agents have a role to play in the attenuation of postoperative pain. A systematic review of randomized controlled trials (RCTs) by Ho et al in 2006 demonstrated that a single preoperative dose of 1200 mg of gabapentin was associated with significantly decreased cumulative opioid consumption at 24 hours after surgery. Even when gabapentin was administered at doses less than 1200 mg, pain intensity was lower at both 6 and 24 hours, and 24-hour cumulative opioid consumption was less, although these findings did not reach statistical significance. In all cases, gabapentin was associated with an increased risk of sedation with less opioid-induced adverse effects such as pruritus and postoperative nausea and vomiting (PONV).[77] A systematic review by Tiippana et al in 2007 supports that gabapentinoids effectively decrease acute postoperative opioid consumption and opioid-induced adverse events following surgery.[78]

A more recent systematic review by Dauri et al in 2009 analyzed the evidence supporting gabapentin and pregabalin use for postoperative pain. When administered solely as a preemptive analgesic, gabapentin provided better postoperative analgesia and decreased opioid use postoperatively than placebo in 6 of 10 RCTs. However, gabapentin did not reduce PONV compared with placebo in 14 RCTs.[79] Although studies support the role of gabapentin and pregabalin versus placebo in reducing pain and opioid consumption, comparisons with other postoperative regimens are lacking. More refined data delineating the optimal dose and duration of therapy, including when to begin, do not exist as yet.

PATIENT-CONTROLLED ANALGESIA

Simple although it seems, PCA technology represents a huge advance in acute pain management. Computer-controlled pumps allow patients to control their own injections and to do this safely, and microchips have made controllable pumps easily portable. PCA satisfies the needs of patients to receive pain medication easily and quickly when needed. Nursing time spent obtaining, checking, documenting, drawing up, giving, and monitoring frequent doses is minimized. The hospital's need to comply with JCAHO's pain mandate is greatly aided. Most moderate to severe postoperative pain in hospitalized patients can be managed satisfactorily using routine IV opioid PCA for 24 to 48 hours after surgery, with or without adjuncts. A proviso is that pain in the immediate postoperative period is controlled by nurse bolus injections until it is under adequate control; patient-triggered boluses using standard settings may be inadequate for treating immediate postoperative pain, and early failed analgesia can prove difficult to overcome. Ideally, patients should be educated in the use of PCA before surgery.

The Inherent Safety of PCA Because of the ease with which each PCA bolus dose can be given, PCA dosing regimes were devised using small frequent doses. For example, a standard regime for morphine is 1 mg every 6 minutes. A maximum hourly limit can be used, as can a background infusion if desired (the latter is particularly useful at night so that the patient can sleep). Part of the logic was to avoid the large swings between high peaks and low troughs associated with less frequent and larger doses (**Fig. 72-4**) but another was to improve safety. Small patient-controlled doses are inherently safe because a single dose is too small to produce overt sedation or respiratory depression, and an obtunded patient will stop pushing the button so there will be no further dosing beyond this early warning stage. The inherent safety of PCA also means there is less need for monitoring and no need to use the intramuscular route (with its slower absorption) for the sake of safety. Naturally, no method of delivery of opioids is completely safe, so a degree of vigilance is always required. The inherent safety of PCA is lost if persons other than the patient are permitted to push the button.

Benefits of PCA Many studies have been conducted since PCA became popular in the 1980s to assess whether the use of PCA results in better analgesia, lower opioid requirements, fewer side effects, better surgical outcome, or superior patient satisfaction. Two meta-analyses of PCA versus "conventional analgesia" (intermittent large-dose opioid injection) have been published, the first in 1993[80] and the second in 2001.[81] The second analysis added 17 new trials to the first, but its results were essentially similar to those of the first. There was slightly better analgesia associated with PCA use (difference 5.6 on a 0-100 scale, $p = 0.006$, debatably not a clinically important difference) and a large difference in patient satisfaction favoring PCA (42% improvement; $p = 0.02$). There was no difference in opioid usage, side effects, or surgical outcome. Thus the overriding benefit of PCA seems to be that patients like it. It has, in fact, become a standard of care in most US hospitals.

Cost of PCA The issue of cost of PCA is frequently analyzed and debated.[82-84] It has proven difficult to come up with a global assessment of PCA costs and the cost savings associated with reduced nursing involvement, improved safety, and other factors. This is because all related costs, including the initial outlay or rental of the PCA systems and their hardware, and including nursing costs, vary from location to location. Overall, it seems that the literal costs to a hospital are slightly higher for PCA versus "conventional analgesia," but imponderables such as increased safety and greater patient satisfaction are hard to translate into cost benefits.

Patient-Controlled Epidural Analgesia PCA technology can also be used for epidural analgesia. As with IV PCA, the main advantage is that patients like the sense of control offered by the patient-triggered pump.

Novel PCA Technologies Using iontophoretic transdermal and intranasal delivery systems, new methods of providing PCA are now in development.[85,86] The most advanced of these is the fentanyl

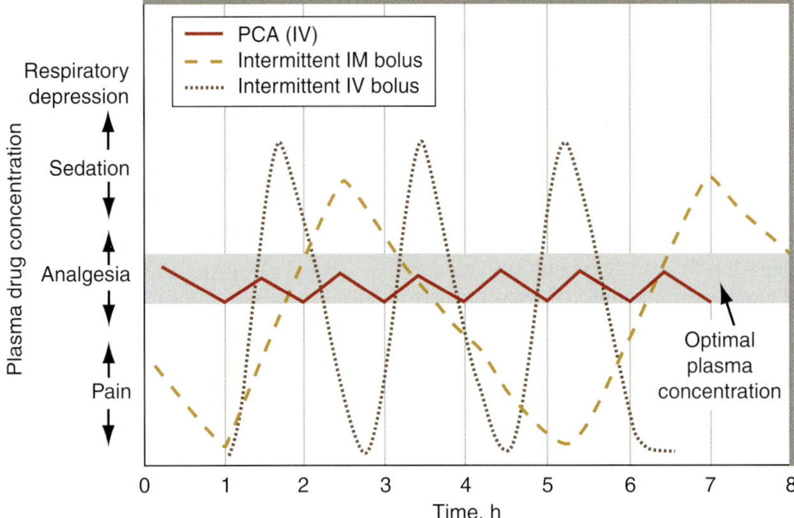

FIGURE 72-4. Serum drug levels from frequent small dosing using patient-controlled analgesia (PCA) compared with 2- to 4-h large intramuscular (IM) or intravenous (IV) dosing. Ideally, serum drugs levels are kept within the "analgesic" range, avoiding the high peaks associated with oversedation and respiratory depression and the low troughs associated with inadequate analgesia. Frequent small dosing would not be practicable without PCA. [Reprinted with permission from Ballantyne JC. Systemic opioids and patient controlled analgesia. In: Neal JM, Rathmell JP, eds. *Complications in Regional Anesthesia and Pain Management.* Philadelphia, PA: Elsevier; 2006:1667-1675. Copyright 2006, with permission from Elsevier.)]

patient-controlled transdermal system (PCTS), which is a noninvasive, needle-free, credit card size, self-contained drug delivery system. A small imperceptible electric current drives ionized drug across the normally impenetrable stratum corneum (outer layer of skin). The adhesive system can be placed on any patch of hairless skin, and for convenience, the upper arm is usually chosen. The system is preprogrammed to deliver 40 μg fentanyl per dose and can deliver up to 6 doses per hour for 24 hours, or 80 doses, whichever comes first. Each dose is triggered by the patient pushing a button on the system twice (twice so it is not triggered accidentally). Cost is likely to play a large part in whether this type of system is adopted for hospital versus home use, or acute versus cancer/chronic pain.

EPIDURAL ANALGESIA

The provision of epidural analgesia is probably the single most important contribution that anesthesiologists currently make to postoperative pain management for individual patients. There are 2 reasons for this: (1) after major surgical procedures, particularly abdominal and thoracic, epidural analgesia has proven analgesic superiority,[87] an effective opioid-sparing effect, and probably a beneficial effect on surgical outcome,[34,88,89] and (2) the ease with which the alternative (systemic opioid) can be provided using PCA has diminished the role of anesthesiologists in the provision of standard treatment. A perplexing thought, however, is how much we truly understand the risk versus benefit of epidural analgesia, especially in an era of potent thrombosis prophylaxis and seemingly increasing numbers of epidural hematomas. How do we weigh rare but catastrophic outcomes against common benefits of debatable value? This is one of the most important issues we face as we continue to teach and encourage the use of epidural analgesia.

Indications A review of indications for intraoperative epidural use is outside the scope of this chapter, but there are also independent indications for postoperative epidural analgesia. These include patients having thoracic or abdominal surgery, patients having lower limb surgery in whom early mobilization is important, patients having lower body vascular procedures in whom a sympathetic block is desirable, and patients with compromised cardiac or pulmonary function.

Contraindications Epidural placement is always contraindicated in patients who refuse this option. It is also contraindicated in patients with coagulopathy, concurrent or planned treatment with low-molecular-weight heparin or with potent antiplatelet agents, and in patients with bacteremia or local infection at the insertion site. The presence of spine pathology is a relative contraindication: The placement may be technically challenging and the treatment may fail if distorted anatomy prevents good distribution of the epidural medications. Neurologic disease is also considered a relative contraindication because if there is a change in neurologic status, which is not uncommon after the stress of surgery, diagnosis of the deterioration can be confused in the presence of an epidural.

Drug Choices and Drug Effects Drugs injected or infused into the epidural space diffuse and spread according to their pharmacokinetics. The epidural space is complex because it contains arteries, veins, and lymphatics that are capable of absorbing drugs into the systemic circulation, nerve roots on which drugs can act directly, and fat in which drugs can form a reservoir (**Fig. 72-5**). The intrathecal space is a close neighbor

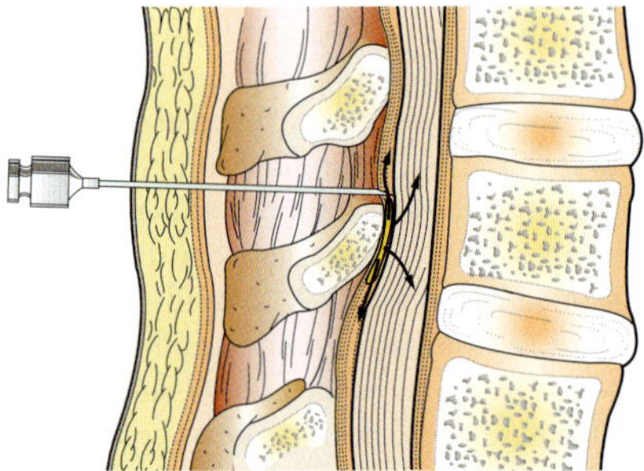

FIGURE 72-5. The epidural space. The space is always approached via the elastic and resistant ligamentum flavum. The space itself contains fat, veins, arteries, lymphatics, and nerve roots. Drugs injected or infused into the space will diffuse into all the tissues and structures within the epidural space, as well as to neighboring structures. Thus local anesthetics will have a direct effect on nerve roots within the space, as well as diffusing through the dura and arachnoid membranes to cerebrospinal fluid and intrathecal nerve roots. Opioids have little activity in the epidural space itself but will diffuse into the systemic circulation (the more lipophilic the opioid, the more the systemic uptake), and across to the opioid receptors in the substantia gelatinosa of the dorsal horn.

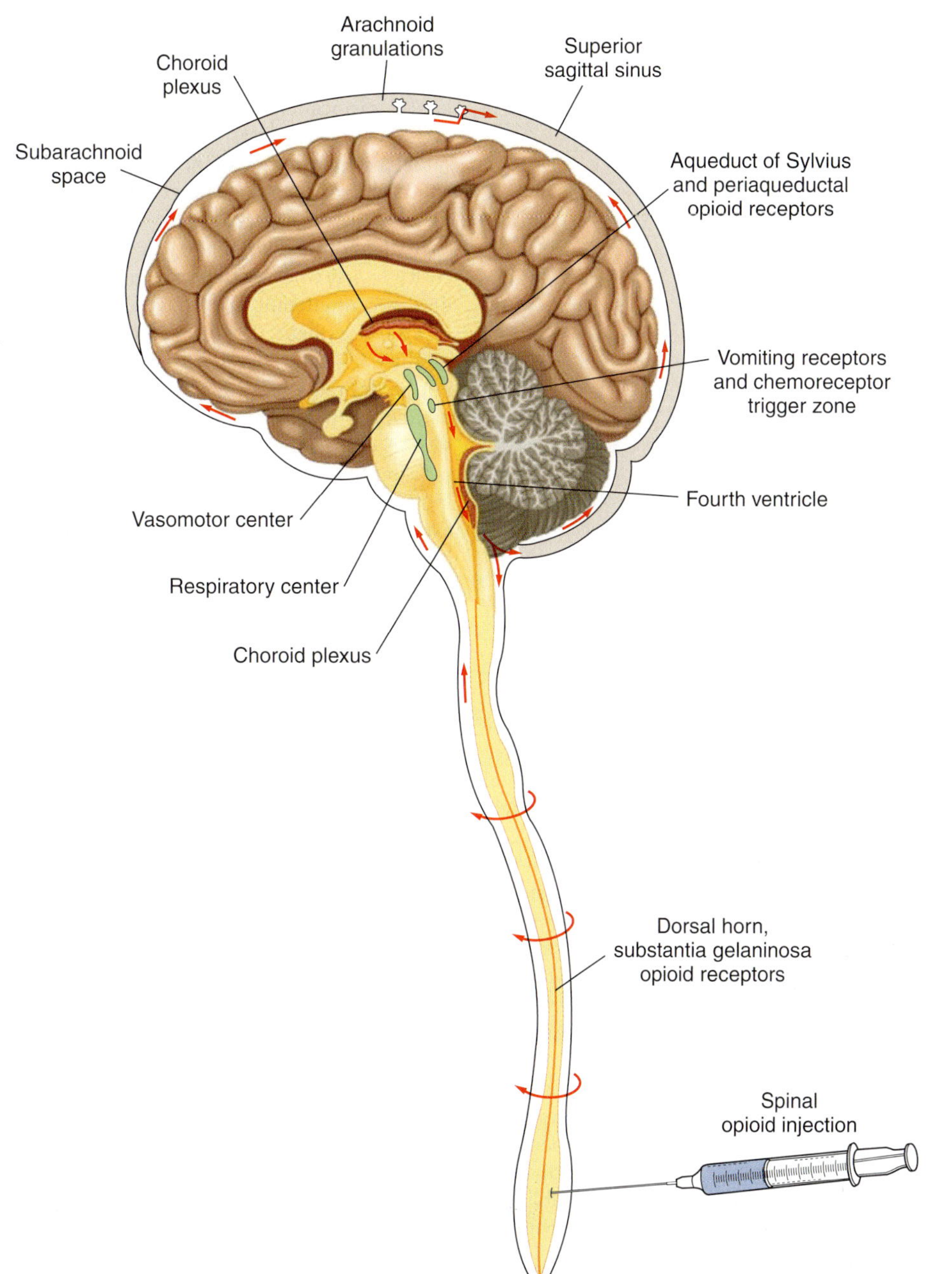

FIGURE 72-6. Cerebrospinal fluid (CSF) flow. Drugs injected into the epidural space or intrathecal space tend to accumulate in CSF at the level of injection. The accumulation of hydrophilic drugs such as morphine will tend to be greater than that of more lipophilic drugs such as fentanyl. Slowly diffusing drugs such as morphine are subject to the bulk flow of CSF and tend to move cephalically toward the ventricular system in the brain. Bulk CSF flow varies markedly from patient to patient. If drug does reach the ventricular system, notably the fourth ventricle, it is likely to cause respiratory depression, and possibly nausea, because the respiratory center and chemoreceptor trigger zone are at the base of the fourth ventricle. Slowly diffusing drugs will likely provide a good spread of analgesia because drug will spread widely to the opioid receptors concentrated in the substantia gelatinosa of the dorsal horn.

of the epidural space, and diffusion into this space brings the epidural drugs across to more nerve roots, to the spinal cord, and, if spread is extensive enough, into the ventricular system of the brain (**Fig. 72-6**). When planning epidural infusion regimes, one has to consider not only local effects but also distant effects, as related to the individual drug's epidural pharmacokinetics.

Local anesthetics act directly on nerve axons to block sodium channels and thus block saltatory conduction. They can block nerves in the epidural space itself, or more widely once they cross into the intrathecal space. Because of the arrangement of nerve fibers within the nerve roots, with small fibers lying outside larger fibers, small fibers are the first to be blocked and the most sensitive to local anesthetics. This characteristic of the spinal nerve roots means that differential blockade can be achieved using low-dose local anesthetics to block only small fibers (C-fibers: sympathetic, pain, and temperature fibers) and high-dose local anesthetics to achieve total sensory blockade, often accompanied by motor blockade (α and β fibers). To achieve analgesia without sensory decrement, a low-dose local anesthetic (eg, 0.1% bupivacaine) is chosen for postoperative use. Epidurals with low-dose local anesthetic infusion are sometimes termed *walking epidurals*, a useful term because it emphasizes that patients can and should be walking around to hasten recovery and minimize complications.

TABLE 72-7 Opioid Lipophilicities

Opioid	Octanol/Buffer Coefficients	Meningeal Permeability Coefficient (cm/min × 1/1000)	MEAC (ng/mL)
Morphine	1	0.6	30
Meperidine	525	NA	455
Hydromorphone	525	NA	4
Fentanyl	955	0.9	0.6
Sufentanil	1737	0.75	0.04
Alfentanil	129	2.3	41
Bupivacaine	560	1.6	NA

MEAC represents a range of plasma levels, not a specific value. MEAC plasma levels may vary up to 5-fold between different patients and with time and activity in specific patients.

From de Leon-Casasola OA, Lema MJ. Postoperative epidural opioid analgesia: what are the choices? *Anesth Analg.* 1996;83(4):867-875.

Opioids have a completely different target: the opioid receptors in the dorsal horn of the spinal cord. Epidural opioid analgesia is also more likely to be complicated by systemic effects because, in contrast to the local anesthetics, which also undergo a degree of systemic absorption, there are clinically relevant systemic effects, especially when highly lipophilic opioids such as fentanyl are used. The degree to which opioids are absorbed systemically versus into cerebrospinal fluid (CSF) versus onto spinal cord receptors depends almost entirely on their lipophilicity (**Table 72-7**). As can be seen from Table 72-7, morphine is several times less lipophilic than all the other commonly used opioids. So it tends to be less readily absorbed into the systemic circulation and therefore provides a better selective spinal effect, and it also tends to spread more within the intrathecal space because it will favor staying in the watery medium of the CSF. This has advantages (more widespread spinal analgesia) and disadvantages (a higher risk that the drug will reach the ventricular system and cause respiratory depression; see Fig. 72-6). However, more lipophilic opioids such as fentanyl tend to have much greater systemic absorption (less selective spinal analgesia), and absorption onto spinal cord receptors tends to be localized, with poor spread. There is a great deal of experience using morphine and other opioids safely and effectively, and individual institutions must choose suitable regimes on the basis of the published experience and their ability to adequately follow and monitor patients receiving epidural analgesia.

The addition of **clonidine** to the local anesthetic and opioid has been found to significantly improve the quality and duration of neuraxial analgesia.[90] The effect is mediated by descending modulatory pathways to the spinal dorsal horn. Despite the low doses used for neuraxial administration, systemic side effects (hypotension, bradycardia, and sedation) can occur. Dose-finding studies are still underway, and the therapeutic window for useful analgesia without side effects seems to be narrow. A reasonable regime uses a 1 to 2 μg/kg bolus followed by 0.4 μg/kg per hour.

Management Principles The management of epidural catheters should always be under the direct supervision of anesthesiologists. Patients should be seen daily to ensure that catheters and medications are working effectively and possible complications are recognized, and recognized early. Pain reports should be satisfactory, and side effects such as pruritus, sedation, and changes in sensation or motor function should be carefully evaluated. Medication charts should be checked, especially for unintentional anticoagulant administration. Catheters and their insertion sites should be inspected for migration, integrity of the dressing, and for inflammation or back tenderness. Anesthesia personnel should make changes to the analgesic regime and administer specific medication as necessary. At the end of treatment, the anesthesia team should be responsible for pulling the catheter and ensuring it is removed intact. Nurses should be properly educated before they care for patients with epidural catheters. Important teaching points include typical medication doses and concentrations, anticoagulation issues, assessment parameters, the normal appearance of the catheter and catheter site, operation of the infusion pumps, common medication side effects that can be treated by them, and side effects requiring a call to the physician in charge.

If an epidural does not appear to be functioning well, it is first necessary to test whether the catheter is well positioned. The ideal way to do this is to attempt to produce a discernable level using a bolus dose of local anesthetic. However, the dose of local anesthetic needed to produce a sensory level may also induce hypotension, which would not be desirable in an unmonitored situation such as a regular floor, particularly if there are no means readily available to treat the hypotension. A surprisingly helpful test is to inject 5 to 7 mL of the analgesic infusion (low-dose local anesthetic), in which case no special monitoring is needed because the low-dose anesthetic is unlikely to produce extreme hypotension. If the catheter is well positioned, analgesia should be noticeably improved by the injection.

Once good catheter function is established, several approaches to improve analgesia can be taken. Bolus injections can be continued until good analgesia is achieved. The infusion rate can be titrated upward as tolerated. Epidural medication can also usefully be administered through a patient controllable pump, termed *patient-controlled epidural analgesia.* Systemic analgesic can be added to the regime. NSAIDs are useful adjuncts to epidural analgesia, especially when the epidural level does not cover the entire area of surgical pain, for example when the incision is high or when pain is referred outside the epidural area as occurs when chest tubes irritate the diaphragm and produce shoulder pain via the phrenic nerve. Systemic opioids (including PCA) can also be added, in which case it is preferable to remove the opioid from the epidural infusate, if used.

Managing Side Effects Hypotension, mild sensory and/or motor changes, and urinary retention are the most common side effects of epidural local anesthetics, whereas pruritus, sedation, dizziness, and urinary retention are the most common side effects of epidural opioids. Most side effects are alleviated by either lowering the infusion rate or changing the drug or dose. Hypotension can become a considerable nuisance during epidural analgesia, even though the sympathectomy from low-dose local anesthetics is theoretically minimal. Some patients are particularly sensitive to the local anesthetic and manifest hypotension that does not respond to the primary measure of fluid replacement. For these patients, the local anesthetic can be removed from the epidural mix, or the epidural treatment may have to be abandoned altogether. Pruritus is a common side effect and usually responds well to antihistamine treatment. The mixed agonist/antagonist nalbuphine (Nubain) (5-10 mg IV, 4-6 mg hourly) also works well, as does low-dose naloxone infusion. Contrary to popular belief, nausea rarely occurs because opioid doses are low. Gut mobility is in fact improved by epidural therapy because of opioid sparing and the favorable effects of neuraxial local anesthetic on bowel motility. Urinary retention is common, and it is common practice to keep a Foley catheter in place until epidural therapy is discontinued.

Unilateral lower extremity numbness with occasional weakness or motor block occurs fairly frequently. It is often a result of the epidural catheter tip migrating along a nerve root so that the local anesthetic is concentrated in one area. Pulling the catheter back, or lowering the infusion rate, often rectifies the problem. However, one should always remain vigilant and continue to watch for more serious complications.

Complications The most common complications are failed block/analgesia and postdural puncture headache (PDPH). Both are considered benign, although they may be devastating to patients who have committed to an epidural to optimize their surgical recovery. The exact incidence of these common complications is difficult to establish because reports vary, and the occurrences likely vary according to reporting and practice habits. Recent reports suggest that failed analgesia occurs in as many as 15% of cases.[91-93] PDPH may occur in up to 86% of patients after accidental dural puncture (rate: 0.16%-1.3%).[94] The incidence of other self-limiting neurologic complications such as radicular pain and peripheral nerve lesions is difficult to determine because these occurrences are rarely reported.

PDPH is thought to result from a small CSF leak secondary to accidental dural puncture. Typically, there is a delay in onset of the headache of up to 24 hours, so that the complication tends to manifest on the first postoperative day. Because PDPH tends to worsen on sitting up, and particularly on walking, it may not present itself until the patient gets out of bed for the first time after surgery. Other characteristics of the headache are that it tends to occur at the back of the head (occiput) and neck, and it produces a tight, pulling, and throbbing sensation. Conservative management consists of bed rest (up to bathroom only), plenty of fluids (IV or oral), and headache medication (NSAIDs, acetaminophen, Fioricet, caffeine, and theophylline all work well). If there is no resolution, or if conservative measures are contraindicated, a blood patch is recommended. This consists of an epidural injection of 20 mL of the patient's own blood (drawn under aseptic conditions). The exact mechanism by which an epidural blood patch works is uncertain but is probably either a pressure effect or a laying down of clot or fibrosis onto the puncture site.

Epidural hematoma with consequent paraplegia is extremely rare but a catastrophic complication of epidural therapy. Permanent paraplegia can occur even when a hematoma is diagnosed and treated in a timely manner, although early intervention usually reverses the neurologic injury. Persistent lower extremity neurologic changes or cauda equina syndrome (loss of bowel and bladder control) should always be taken seriously, especially if there is accompanying back pain and tenderness, which are cardinal signs of epidural hematoma and abscess although not necessarily present. Neurology can be consulted, but early imaging, preferably with magnetic resonance imaging (second choice computed tomography), should always be instituted. The presence of a space-occupying intracanal spinal lesion should always herald immediate transfer to the operating room for surgical decompression.

The incidence of epidural hematoma after neuraxial injection, catheter placement, or catheter removal has been estimated to be 1 in 190 000, with many of the reported cases associated with anticoagulant use.[95-97] A rash of reports of epidural hematoma occurring after neuraxial interventions in patients receiving low-molecular-weight heparin alerted us to the dangers of epidural injections and catheters in patients receiving highly effective thrombosis prophylaxis. More problems followed when chronic treatment with potent and long-acting antiplatelet agents such as clopidogrel became more widespread.[96] In view of the rapidity with which new agents are being introduced and the time lag before the extent of a problem can be assessed, we are left with a great deal of uncertainty about the safety of neuraxial procedures. **Table 72-8** summarizes guidelines for managing epidurals in patients receiving anticoagulants. These recommendations are based on the consensus guidelines published by the American Society of Regional Anesthesia and Pain Medicine (ASRA). The guidelines are updated periodically and published on ASRA's Web site. Epidural bleeding is known to occur secondary to single-shot neuraxial techniques as well as neuraxial catheter insertion and removal, so recommendations are needed for the start and end of neuraxial therapy, as well as for starting anticoagulant therapy after neuraxial instrumentation or catheter removal.

Epidural abscess occurs less often than epidural hematoma, but it can be equally catastrophic and may cause permanent and serious neurologic injury, even death.[98] Fever is a likely accompaniment to epidural abscess; otherwise it presents much as epidural hematoma. In fact, it may not be clear whether the mass is blood or pus until it is exposed during surgery. The mortality of spinal abscess can be as high as 18% (from case report).[99] The incidence of epidural abscess secondary to neuraxial blockade is estimated at 1 in 250 000 in healthy patients, but 1 in 2000 in diabetic or immunocompromised patients.[100,101] Other serious complications such as anterior spinal artery syndrome, transverse myelitis, and meningitis have been reported but are extremely rare.

Epidurals and Surgical Outcomes In terms of truly understanding the benefit versus the risk of epidural analgesia in any individual patient, it is important to understand whether or not the benefit extends beyond that of the simple provision of excellent analgesia. Is mortality

TABLE 72-8 Guidelines for Epidural Placement and Removal During Anticoagulant Therapy

Drug	Monitoring	Time After Last Dose Before Placing or Removing Catheter	Time After Placing or Removing Catheter Before Restarting Medication
Warfarin	INR (<1.5)	Check INR if treatment >24 h	Same day
NSAID, ASA	No significant risk		
Thrombolytics	None	10 d	10 d
SC heparin	No significant risk		
IV heparin	PTT	2-4 h	1 h
LMWH	Anti-Xa (however, not predictive of risk of bleeding)	12 h	2 h
Low Dose			
Dalteparin (Fragmin) (<5000 U qd)			
Enoxaparin (Lovenox) (<60 mg qd)			
High Dose		>24 h	2 h
Twice-daily dosing			
Ticlopidine (Ticlid)	None	14 d	24 h
Clopidogrel (Plavix)	None	7 d[a]	24 h
Abciximab (ReoPro)	None	48 h	12 h
Tirofiban (Aggrastat)	None	8 h	4 h
Eptifibatide (Integrilin)	None	8 h	4 h

[a]After a single dose, catheter can be removed within 24-48 hours. If this window is missed, it is necessary to wait 7 days before catheter removal. Note: Regional anesthesia is contraindicated in patients receiving fondaparinux (Arixtra).

From Ballantyne JC, Ryder E. Postoperative pain in adults. In: Ballantyne JC, ed. *The Massachusetts General Hospital Handbook of Pain Management.* 3rd ed. Philadelphia, PA: Lippincott, Williams & Wilkins; 2006.

improved? Is recovery hastened? Are high-risk patients such as those with serious cardiac disease less susceptible to cardiac morbidity? Do the bowels recover quicker? Do epidurals reduce thromboembolism? Is postoperative pulmonary function improved? These are all questions that have been asked in countless trials often with conflicting results.[74,89] Perhaps the clearest result is that epidural analgesia (particularly that from thoracic epidurals) does improve bowel mobility and reduce the period of ileus, with consequent earlier hospital discharge.[102] There is also considerable support for improved pulmonary function.[103-107] But support for a beneficial effect on other outcomes, particularly catastrophic outcomes, seems to be elusive. Large multicenter studies published relatively recently found no advantage to epidural analgesia in terms of mortality or major morbidity.[105,107] Yet earlier trials and meta-analyses had suggested significant improvements in mortality and serious morbidity.[103,104,106,108,109] Has some of the earlier advantage of neuraxial anesthesia and analgesia dissipated because they no longer provide the benefit of reduced thromboembolism in this era of improved thromboprophylaxis? And could general improvements in perioperative care such as better preoperative optimization, shorter acting anesthetic drugs, improved standards of vigilance and monitoring, and accelerated recovery programs have diminished the role of neuraxial anesthesia and analgesia?[89]

Epidural or No? Despite all the blows against epidurals—incompatibility with modern thromboprophylaxis and dwindling returns in terms of improvements in mortality and major morbidity—they remain a beneficial and helpful intervention for selected patients undergoing invasive surgical procedures. For patients who accept the risks because of a promise of good postoperative pain relief, that promise is usually fulfilled. Patients with serious respiratory disease and those undergoing extensive lung resection benefit from opioid sparing and the favorable effects of epidural analgesia on pulmonary mechanics. Recovery can be hastened after bowel surgery because of favorable effects on bowel mobility. And patients with cardiac ischemia or failure can benefit from the moderate reductions in afterload and the negative inotropy and chronotropy of a well-managed thoracic epidural.

NERVE BLOCKS

The primary indication for nerve blocks is for the provision of surgical anesthesia. But there are secondary benefits in terms of pain relief in the postoperative period, and in some cases analgesic effects can be prolonged using plexus catheters. As nerve blocks wear off, there remains some degree of analgesia (probably from residual small fiber blockade), and surprisingly, these effects appear prolonged beyond the known half-life of the local anesthetic, especially in the case of distal peripheral blocks such as hand and ankle blocks. Certain nerves are accessible enough to be injected intermittently should the need arise: Femoral nerve blocks provide good but incomplete analgesia after knee surgery, and intercostal nerve blocks can be useful after thoracic surgery or chest trauma when epidural analgesia is contraindicated. The analgesia from single-shot neuraxial blocks can be prolonged by injecting an opioid at the time of placing the block. Injection or infiltration of local anesthetic into the wound by the surgeon can provide helpful analgesia during the early postoperative phase. These techniques are particularly useful for postoperative pain control: (1) prolongation of neural blockade using catheters, (2) neuraxial opioid injections, and (3) prolongation of neural blockade using catheters.

With the increasing number of procedures being performed in the ambulatory setting in the United States and elsewhere, it becomes especially important to ensure adequate postoperative analgesia. In fact, ambulatory surgical procedures now account for at least 50% to 70% of all surgical procedures performed throughout the United States.[110] Regional anesthesia has several benefits in the ambulatory setting, and has grown in popularity among physicians and patients alike.[36] The ability to provide an alternative to general anesthesia with associated rapid recovery, early analgesia, decreases in consumption of postoperative opioids, nausea, and sedation as well as improved mobility of the operative extremity make regional techniques a welcome and attractive addition to our armamentarium. A recent meta-analysis by Liu et al confirms that peripheral nerve blocks are associated with reduced pain, decreased postanesthesia care unit time, less postoperative nausea, and a decreased analgesic requirement.[111] Reduction of patients' overall time in the ambulatory surgery setting was not demonstrated, but patient satisfaction was improved.

The type of regional technique chosen depends on the site and anticipated length of the surgery, any postoperative mobilization requirements, as well as a review of patients' comorbidities and possible contraindications to specific regional techniques (eg, peripheral techniques may be safer than neuraxial in patients with a coagulopathy).

Brachial plexus blocks are commonly used for upper extremity surgery. In general, these blocks are well tolerated and have few contraindications. Interscalene blocks produce ipsilateral phrenic nerve paresis for the duration of the blockade and should be avoided in patients who cannot tolerate a modest (25%) decrease in pulmonary function. The supraclavicular approach carries with it the risk of pneumothorax, and the infraclavicular approach may be useful particularly in the ambulatory setting. Regional techniques have transformed both total elbow and total shoulder arthroplasties from procedures commonly requiring several days of hospitalization into ambulatory procedures with the further option of continued analgesia via a perineural catheter.[112,113]

For the lower extremity, spinal anesthesia has largely been superseded by peripheral blocks in the ambulatory setting to minimize side effects such as urinary retention and inability to ambulate, all of which can delay discharge. Femoral, sciatic, and ankle blocks all provide excellent conditions for surgery as well as analgesia extended well into the postoperative period. As with the upper extremity blocks, plexus catheters can be placed at the time of block placement and used to prolong analgesia.

Intercostal nerve blocks can be useful when in the case of chest trauma; regional anesthesia helps improve pulmonary mechanics but epidural is contraindicated. Intercostal bupivacaine has been used successfully in patients with severe chest pain following rib fractures to provide sustained analgesia and a significant increase in both pulse oximetry saturation and peak expiratory flow rates.[114,115]

When a perineural catheter is placed, a PCA pump can be used to infuse via the catheter so that patients can control and adjust their own demand dosage of medication on the background of a preprogrammed continuous basal infusion. More recently, the development of new disposable pumps allows for patients to experience at home the type of analgesia that was recently available only as an inpatient. Recent data suggest that disposable pumps are as successful as battery-operated mechanical pumps, with fewer technical problems and higher patient satisfaction scores.[116]

Whatever peripheral nerve block is used to control postoperative pain, it is important to realize that a plan for either supplemental coverage of noncovered surgical areas or provision of breakthrough pain coverage is necessary and should be provided in addition.

Neuraxial Opioid Injections Neuraxial morphine is safe provided dosing is reasonable and patients are appropriately monitored. A single shot of morphine into the epidural space (1-4 mg) or intrathecal space (0.1-0.4 mg) can provide prolonged analgesia (up to 24 h), but it carries a risk of delayed respiratory depression. Morphine is poorly lipophilic, tends to stay in CSF once there, and is subject to CSF bulk flow with passage to higher centers including the respiratory center (see Fig. 72-6). At the same time, the fact that morphine tends to remain in CSF is the reason that it produces excellent selective spinal analgesia (ie, good spread to spinal cord receptors). Single-shot neuraxial morphine is an excellent means of providing analgesia when there is no epidural catheter. Patients should be monitored in the same way as those receiving epidural opioid infusions. PCA can be used to provide supplementary analgesia if necessary, but for safety, only demand doses should be used, and continuous background infusions should be avoided.

SPECIAL POPULATIONS

NEONATES, INFANTS, AND CHILDREN

Throughout childhood, the management of pain presents special challenges. Very young children (neonates and infants) tolerate opioids poorly because they are prone to apnea, and their handling of this and other groups of drugs is altered by several factors, including slow conjugation by the liver. It is no longer acceptable to avoid giving opioids to neonates on the basis that they do not feel pain because there is now a great deal of evidence that they feel pain just as adults do and that untreated pain can produce an imprint that may have psychologic and even physical consequences later in life.[117-120] Older children can also be scarred by traumatic and painful experiences, and it is sometimes difficult for adult caregivers to understand childhood and adolescent psychology and to communicate effectively so as to optimize pain management. Pain assessment is challenging, particularly in preverbal children (see the section Pain Assessment). Good pediatric pain management requires a great deal of time and patience and is therefore labor intensive; unlike adults, children, especially young children, cannot simply be left with a PCA pump. Unfortunately, the resources for providing excellent and safe pain care for children, which often must be done at the bedside, may be lacking other than in specialty hospitals and centers of excellence.

Planning for the Postoperative Experience Anesthesiologists play a key role in preparing children and their parents for the postoperative period and the pain the children are likely to experience. First, they can explain what is going to happen and how pain will be managed and assessed. They can explain treatment options and help parents (and older children) select the right approach. Often an intervention such as an epidural, a single-shot caudal or a nerve block is helpful, and these options can be discussed. For children who are old enough for PCA (generally ≥6 years of age), this should certainly be discussed, and the children should understand how to use the pump. Parents should understand that the inherent safety of PCA will be bypassed if they press the button themselves and that it is better if they do not intervene other than to encourage the children to take doses. If the child has had past surgery, it is helpful to know what pain treatments worked well.

Treatment Choices Essentially the treatment options available to adults are available to children. However, there are differences in the way neonates and infants metabolize drugs, particularly opioids, and these must be understood. In general, smaller, more frequent dosing is needed in the very young, but there is no substitute for referring to pediatric dosing guidelines. As in adults, opioids are the mainstay for treating severe pain, but given the safety issues, especially in young children, it is always preferable to reduce opioid requirements whenever possible by using adjunctive treatments such as NSAIDs and acetaminophen that are generally well tolerated. Epidurals, caudals, and other nerve blocks, even single shots, can be extremely helpful and are usually successful because the anatomy is straightforward. However, catheters can be difficult to maintain, especially if they are small-diameter catheters (when they have a tendency to block) and especially if the insertion site is within the diaper area (when the skin can become macerated and the catheter tends to slip out). Opioids can be given as a low-dose infusion in neonates and infants, which obviates the need for intermittent injections and is generally safe and effective, provided breakthrough pain is controlled by bedside bolus injections and the temptation to try and overcome uncontrolled pain by repeatedly increasing an infusion rate is resisted.

Safety Maintaining safety while providing good pain relief is an especial challenge in children, chiefly because of their sensitivity to opioids. Young children require extra vigilance and great care with dosing. Dosing is calculated on a per kilogram basis, and because children's weights and sizes vary considerably, it always warrants careful calculation. Frequent checking of vital signs is mandatory in neonates and infants receiving opioids, and the use of respiratory rate and oxygen saturation monitors improves safety and is a standard of care for this population in many institutions.

THE ELDERLY AND INFIRM

Just as children present a special challenge, so do the elderly and infirm. Again, this is a group of patients that is particularly sensitive to opioids. They are prone not only to opioids' respiratory depressant effects but also to their central dysphoric and euphoric effects. Opioid-induced confusion is common in this age group. The elderly are liable to become confused with other psychotropic drugs such as benzodiazepines, and they are sensitive to NSAID side effects, particularly GI bleeding and renal dysfunction. They can also develop a confusional state simply because they are moved from familiar surroundings. These factors combined make good pain control hard to achieve. Pain control may become a low priority because it is hard to assess pain in confused patients, and drugs are blamed for the confusional state and therefore withdrawn.

The elderly tend to appear stoical, and it is not clear whether they have a different threshold for pain, whether past experience has altered their attitude toward pain, or whether they truly do not feel pain to the same extent as younger adults. It is probably best to treat pain according to the patients' demands and not to project pain on them because of a preconceived notion that their pain must be worse than they say it is. PCA is not a suitable choice for confused patients, and it may not work well even in nonconfused elderly patients because they tend to undermedicate. A simple approach such as nurse-determined intermittent low-dose opioid with acetaminophen as an adjunct is often the best approach. Epidurals and nerve blocks are useful for reducing reliance on poorly tolerated systemic medications.

OPIOID-TOLERANT PATIENTS

Pain specialists and acute pain services are increasingly preoccupied treating patients who are opioid tolerant and who get into difficulty when an episode of acute pain, notably due to surgery or trauma, proves refractory to standard treatments.[56,58,121] Nonspecialists are often uncomfortable prescribing the high doses of opioid that may be needed to overcome acute pain in opioid-tolerant patients. There are several reasons that the numbers of patients presenting with opioid tolerance is increasing, some related to societal factors, others to changes in medical practice. (1) All efforts to control drug and heroin abuse by means of regulation have failed, and illicit drug trading, distribution, and use steadily increase as high illicit drugs prices and profits are maintained. (2) Prescription drug abuse increased exponentially during the 5 years before 2001,[122] largely because opioid use for chronic pain was liberalized during the late 1900s, resulting in a greater availability of prescription opioids in homes, pharmacies, and on the streets. Addicts choose prescription drugs over illicit drugs because of their greater reliability and safety. (3) In the 1980s and 1990s, pain advocates, carrying the success of their much needed lobbying for the use of opioids for acute and cancer pain, extended the principle to the treatment of chronic noncancer pain. Thus today there are many more patients with chronic pain conditions treated with opioids than there were just 20 years ago. (4) Cancer is now a curable disease for many patients, and others experience long remissions. They often need treatment for pain associated with their primary disease, or with its treatments, and they may need this treatment for years. Because of a tradition of opioid use for cancer pain, opioids are being used for long-term treatment of cancer-related pain.

Managing pain in opioid-treated patients, whether they are substance abusers or chronic pain patients, can be extremely challenging.[56,59,121] There are issues related to opioid tolerance and pain refractoriness, and a withdrawal syndrome could further complicate the clinical picture. In addition, there may be difficult behavioral issues in both groups of patients, so that the dedication and professionalism, particularly of the nursing staff, can be severely tested. The possibility that drugs are being diverted complicates matters even further. Prejudices set in about the veracity of pain complaints, there is a breakdown in trust, and the simplicity of treating pain according to the patient's report is lost.

Substance Abusers Substance abusers are notorious deceivers, but they recognize that they put themselves at risk if they deny use and are usually honest about whether or not they are currently using drugs, including opioids. They are less honest about past use and unreliable in terms of reporting doses. The treating physician must be cognizant that opioid requirements for pain are unknown and can only be learned by titration; that a withdrawal syndrome may arise if doses are underestimated; and that manifestations of other abused drugs (cocaine, amphetamines, alcohol, etc) or withdrawal from these may also require treatment. Treatment for withdrawal syndromes is generally supportive, but in the surgical setting, opioid withdrawal should be treated with opioid. An α_2-agonist such as clonidine may help reduce norepinephrine effects.

The period of hospitalization for surgery or trauma is not the time for tackling an entrenched addiction problem. Nevertheless, if the patient agrees (and often the person does not), the involvement of a psychiatrist or addictionologist during the hospitalization can be helpful. The surgical and pain teams should focus on optimizing pain management and direct the patient to the appropriate resource after discharge, assuming he or she wants treatment. An opioid-abusing patient may have an inadequate response to the opioids given for pain, and it is helpful to make maximum use of alternatives such as epidurals, nerve blocks, and NSAIDs. At the same time, opioids should not be withheld, particularly if there has been recent use.

Chronic Opioid-Treated Pain Opioid tolerant chronic and cancer pain patients are among the most difficult patients to treat for pain after surgery, particularly if they are being treated with high doses of opioids and have become hyperalgesic or refractory.[55,123] Despite the fact that there is now convincing evidence that the analgesic efficacy of high-dose opioid therapy may diminish over time and has unacceptable side effects such as gonadal suppression, there are still patients admitted to hospital on doses exceeding the common upper limit of 180 mg morphine or morphine equivalent per day.[31] The addition of chronic intrathecal opioid treatment may further complicate and compromise the treatment of acute pain.

Principles of treatment are similar to those for substance abusers. The normal regime should be continued if possible, and if not, it should be converted to an IV regime. Nonopioid treatments should be used to as great an extent as possible, to minimize reliance on opioids. Neuraxial interventions should be avoided in patients with implanted stimulators or pumps, unless the position of the implanted system is clear, because the needle can cut or damage electrodes, leads, or catheters. PCA is again a useful mode of delivery for opioids because a background infusion can be used to whatever level is needed, and the ability to get extra bolus doses reassures the patients. High-dose boluses are likely to be needed.

The period of hospitalization is not a good time to change the chronic pain regime, and most efforts should focus on treating the acute pain. However, if the surgical or pain team is having difficulty managing a patient, it may be very helpful to talk to the patient's pain physician or whoever normally manages their pain. Sometimes issues are revealed that are relevant to the management of pain in the hospital but not necessarily clear from the patient or the patient's chart. It is also helpful to have a plan for treating pain after discharge, which could involve the patient's normal physician or could involve rehabilitation or a pain program.

Behavioral problems can arise in opioid-treated chronic pain patients, although these will be different from those in substance abusers. Chronic pain patients tend to have difficulty coping, and when they are faced with uncontrolled and excruciating pain, which they have not necessarily predicted, they can be angry, mistrustful, demanding, or uncooperative. They may display typical opioid-seeking behaviors (frequent demands for pain medication, refusal of all but opioid treatments, accusations against the medical staff for undertreating pain), and these behaviors appear much like addictive behaviors. Yet it will be difficult to determine whether the behaviors have arisen because of undertreated pain (pseudoaddiction) or because there is, in fact, an underlying addiction problem.

PAIN MANAGEMENT IN THE INTENSIVE CARE UNIT

Several challenges are associated with managing postoperative pain in patients requiring care in the ICU. In many cases, these patients are unable to communicate because of severe illness, extensive surgical trauma, or because they are ventilated and sedated. Continuous infusion is the most frequently chosen means of delivery for opioids, but prolonged use of opioid infusions may lead to rapid development of tolerance or opioid-induced hyperalgesia, making pain control and weaning from opioids difficult.[30] One of the most obvious manifestations of opioid-induced hyperalgesia is the ICU patient treated with high-dose opioid infusion who cannot tolerate touch or even the sheets. Patients with compromised renal function may accumulate opioid metabolites, notably the active metabolite morphine-6-glucuronide and the toxic metabolite normeperidine. Meperidine is not a good choice for prolonged infusions; if morphine is used, the possible accumulation of active metabolites must be considered in the weaning protocol. Epidural analgesia is an extremely useful option that is opioid sparing and can help during weaning from ventilation.[106,124-126] However, epidurals are often contraindicated in ICU patients because of a need to treat with anticoagulant therapy. Use of activated protein C, our current best agent for severe sepsis, also precludes the use of epidurals.

It is important to treat pain in ICU patients to reduce the anxiety associated with pain and the inability to communicate pain. When it is impossible to assess pain, as in heavily sedated or unconscious patients, it is reasonable to assess analgesic requirements on the basis of the amount of surgical or other trauma the patient has undergone. Ventilated patients can be treated with higher than normal doses of opioids (if desired) because there is no risk of respiratory depression. However, it is important to remember that prolonged infusions may lose their efficacy if tolerance or hyperalgesia develop, and all opioid-sparing strategies are helpful. Methadone may also be useful for prolonged ICU stays because there is less development of tolerance. It has recently been found beneficial to use the α_2-agonist dexmedetomidine for ICU sedation, not only because of its hypnotic effects, but also because of its analgesic synergy with opioids (opioid sparing), and possibly a contribution to minimizing opioid withdrawal at the time of weaning.[127,128] Dexmedetomidine (often in combination with remifentanil or other opioids) is gaining increasing popularity also as a sedating agent during airway and other relatively noninvasive procedures.[129,130]

CONCLUSION

Advances in surgery, anesthesia, drugs, and technology have combined to markedly reduce the trauma and morbidity of surgery. Part of this success can be attributed to improvements in pain management, both during and after surgery. In the 1980s, several changes revolutionized postoperative pain management. Portable PCA pumps became available, and gradually the use of PCA was adopted widely. Clinical use of neuraxial opioids began after endogenous opioids and opioid receptors were identified in the 1970s. It was soon recognized that neuraxially administered opioids could provide excellent targeted analgesia at low doses without the need for larger systemic doses and associated side effects, or the sensory and motor blockade from the high-dose local anesthetics previously needed for adequate epidural pain relief when local anesthetics were used alone. So-called walking epidurals began to be widely used for postoperative pain control. Several professional and political bodies, recognizing that good pain control was an important component of perioperative care, developed guidelines to propagate good evidence-based practice (Agency for Healthcare Policy and Research). Insurers, spearheaded by Medicare, also recognized the importance of good pain control and began to reimburse pain management services, allowing for the development of acute pain services. Later, pain advocates succeeded in enlisting JCAHO in the war on pain, and their 2001 mandate requires all accredited hospitals to have a systematic means of recognizing and assessing pain, and treating it appropriately. Postsurgical pain may not be fully conquered, and there is certainly room for more research and further improvement. But tremendous progress has been made since the not so distant days when uncontrolled pain meant that patients routinely remained motionless in bed for days after surgery, prone to complications of immobility such as thromboembolism, atelectasis, and protein wasting.

KEY REFERENCES

- Angst MS, Clark JD. Opioid-induced hyperalgesia: a qualitative systematic review. *Anesthesiology.* 2006;104(3):570-587.
- Ballantyne JC. Does epidural analgesia improve surgical outcome? *Br J Anaesth.* 2004;92(1):4-6.
- Brennan TJ, Kehlet H. Preventive analgesia to reduce wound hyperalgesia and persistent postsurgical pain. Not an easy path. *Anesthesiology.* 2005;103:681-683.
- Kehlet H. Postoperative opioid sparing to hasten recovery: what are the issues? *Anesthesiology.* 2005;102(6):1083-1085.
- Kissin I. Preemptive analgesia at the crossroad. *Anesth Analg.* 2005;100(3):754-756.
- Perkins FM, Ballantyne JC. Post-surgical pain syndromes. In: Stannard C, Kalso E, Ballantyne JC, eds. *Evidence-based Chronic Pain Management.* Oxford, UK: Blackwell; 2010.
- Practice guidelines for acute pain management in the perioperative setting: an updated report by the American Society of Anesthesiologists Task Force on Acute Pain Management. *Anesthesiology.* 2004;100(6):1573-1581.
- White PF, Kehlet H, Liu S. Perioperative analgesia: what do we still know? *Anesth Analg.* 2009;108(5):1364-1367.

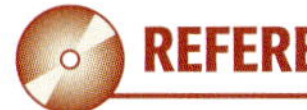

REFERENCES

Complete references available on DVD and online version at www.LongneckerAnesthesiology.com

PART 6

The Critically Ill Patient

CHAPTER 73

The Pathophysiology of Critical Illness

Luca M. Bigatello
Judith Hellman
Sascha Beutler
Warren M. Zapol

KEY POINTS

1. Acute injuries of various etiologies (eg, trauma, infection, shock, etc) cause immediate local and systemic physiologic responses involving all major organ systems.
2. The timing and intensity of the physiologic response to injury is affected by the severity of the injury as well as host factors. An initial activation of the proinflammatory immune responses may be followed by late immunosuppression.
3. Nosocomial infections are a major cause of death of critically ill patients and can be reduced by adopting best practices of infection control.
4. The vascular endothelium is a major organ target of the initial response to injury that activates vasomotor, inflammatory, and procoagulant cascades.
5. Our increased understanding of the molecular biology of the immune response to injury will hopefully lead to new and effective therapies that may include oxygen or nitrogen free-radical scavenging, mitochondrial protection, prevention of apoptosis, and enhancement of the immune response.

The term *critical illness* defines a variety of clinical situations that are cared for primarily in intensive care units (ICUs) and have in common varying degrees of dysfunction of single or multiple organ systems and a guarded immediate prognosis. Anesthesiologists care for critically ill patients in the operating room, in the ICU, and during procedures in areas outside of the operating room, such as radiologic, endoscopic, and cardiac electrophysiology suites. Thus it is crucial that anesthesiologists have an in-depth understanding of the pathophysiologic processes encountered during critical illness to contribute effectively to the perioperative management of critically ill patients.

This chapter focuses on a number of basic elements of critical illness, including inciting factors, the transition to organ dysfunction, the role of the immune system, and current as well as potential future therapies for various aspects of critical illness. We analyze the progression of critical illness examining common types of primary injuries, the body's response to them, and the progression of the response either toward healing and recovery or to deterioration and death. Epidemiologic and therapeutic considerations are also reviewed. The chapter begins with a case report of a critically ill patient through different stages of her illness that are referred to in subsequent sections of the chapter.

CASE REPORT

A 77-year-old woman with a history of severe chronic obstructive pulmonary disease and hypertension was admitted to the surgical ICU from a general ward with acute respiratory distress. She had been recovering uneventfully from a pancreatic resection for cancer until that morning when she experienced nausea and malaise, then vomited a large amount of dark fluid, and immediately complained of shortness of breath.

Upon arrival at the surgical ICU, she was in obvious respiratory distress, with a marginal (87%-89%) arterial oxygen saturation (Spo_2) on a nonrebreathing oxygen mask. Following a rapid-sequence tracheal intubation, a large amount of dark green material was suctioned from her airways, similar in appearance to that suctioned from her stomach. A bronchoscopy revealed diffuse staining of the tracheobronchial mucosa with biliary material, down to the lobar bronchi bilaterally. Over the next 4 to 6 hours, the patient's condition deteriorated. She required high levels of ventilatory support and large doses of intravenous (IV) infusions of vasopressors to maintain an adequate systemic arterial blood pressure. A pulmonary artery catheter revealed moderate to severe pulmonary artery hypertension and a low cardiac output, primarily a result of right ventricular dysfunction, which was confirmed by transthoracic echocardiography. She was treated with broad-spectrum antibiotics, recombinant human activated protein C, and inhaled nitric oxide (NO), and was ventilated using a "lung-protective" strategy of low tidal volumes at a moderate level of positive end-expiratory pressure (7-10 cm H_2O). Over the next few days, she was extremely unstable from the cardiovascular and pulmonary standpoints: She had three episodes of pulseless electrical activity requiring cardiopulmonary resuscitation and developed severe hypoxemia with minimal stimulation, which greatly impeded basic care.

By day 10 her cardiovascular and respiratory function began to stabilize, and a computed tomogram of her chest was obtained (**Fig. 73-1**). Subsequently, hemodynamic and ventilatory support was tapered, and she was transitioned to assisted ventilation; vasopressors were discontinued, and she started to interact with ICU personnel. On ICU day 13, she had a bedside percutaneous dilatational tracheostomy. On ICU day 15 her bronchial secretions became purulent; she developed a fever and leukocytosis, and required increased ventilatory support. She was diagnosed with ventilator-associated pneumonia (VAP) from *Pseudomonas aeruginosa* based on clinical and bacteriologic criteria. She was again treated with antibiotics, and she gradually improved. She was discharged from the surgical ICU on day 24 and transferred to a semi-intensive (step-down) respiratory unit to complete the process of weaning from mechanical ventilation.

Thirty-eight days after ICU admission, and 45 days after her surgery, she was transferred to a rehabilitation facility. Although she was sustaining unassisted breathing, she was still extremely debilitated: she could not stand for more than a few minutes or walk more than a few steps and was unable to feed herself. In addition, she continued to require narcotic-based analgesics and antipsychotic medications to allow sleep at night and diminish her recurring episodes of delirium.

PATHWAYS OF INJURY: THE STRESSES LEADING TO CRITICAL ILLNESS

A variety of acute injuries can result in critical illness and the need for ICU care. In the following material, we classify these "stresses" as related to a few main categories: surgery and trauma, metabolic disorders, and infection. In many patients, as in the patient just described, multiple stresses (eg, surgery, inflammation, and infection) coexist.

DIRECT TISSUE INJURY DURING SURGERY AND TRAUMA

Direct tissue injury during surgery and trauma can produce major perturbations of the body's homeostasis, including hemodynamic instability, respiratory abnormalities, and marked fluid shifts. Pain, immobility, and prolonged bed rest can contribute to perioperative morbidity. Only a few decades ago, these phenomena constituted a formidable challenge for surgeons and anesthesiologists, and they made many surgical procedures complex and dangerous for the patient. Today, the physiologic changes associated with so-called "routine" surgery can be flawlessly managed by the proper administration of perioperative anesthesia care. However, certain situations still carry a significant risk of perioperative complications, including complex elective procedures (eg, pneumonectomy, thoracoabdominal aneurysm repair), major trauma, emergency surgery, and procedures performed in patients with significant comorbidity. These patients constitute most of the population admitted to a surgical ICU.

Trauma is the primary cause of death in individuals younger than 40 years in the United States.[1] In underdeveloped countries, trauma victims may have limited or no access to the type of structured intensive care that could save thousands of lives every year. Traumatic injuries are

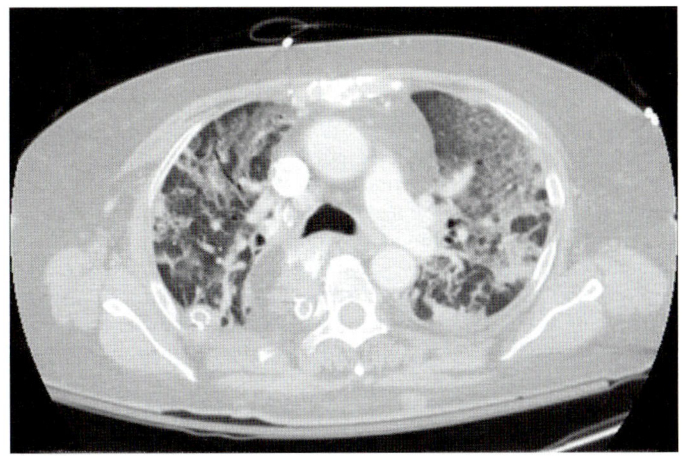

FIGURE 73-1. Computed tomography of the chest at the level of the upper thorax shows diffuse bilateral ground-glass parenchymal opacities consistent with acute lung injury/acute respiratory distress syndrome.

TABLE 73-1 Values of Oxygen Delivery at Different Levels of Anemia

	Hgb (g/dL)	CO (L/min)	$\dot{D}O_2$ (mL/min)
Normal	14	5	900
Anemia	9	6	700
Severe anemia	5	7	450

$\dot{D}O_2$ = arterial O_2 content (CaO_2) × cardiac output (CO)

CaO_2 = Hg × 1.34 × oxygen saturation (Spo_2) + Pao_2 × 0.003.

Normal CaO_2 = 14 g/dL × 1.34 × 0.98 + negligible dissolved O_2 = 19 mL O_2 per dL of blood; × CO of 5 L/min, $\dot{D}O_2$ = 900 mL/min.

With severe anemia: Hgb 5 g/dL, normal Spo_2, and a CO of 7 L/min, $\dot{D}O_2$ is ≥350 mL/min, still above the resting average oxygen demand of tissues of 250 mL/min. We assumed a moderate increase of CO for each level of anemia.

classified as penetrating and blunt injuries (see Chapter 76). *Penetrating injuries* (stab and gunshot wounds) require immediate control of hemorrhage, drainage of blood or air under pressure, and rapid transfer to a trauma center. Immediate appropriate care increases survival and can reduce the need for intensive care.[2] *Blunt trauma* (eg, motor vehicle accidents, falls) can produce a combination of injuries that may require immediate treatment, such as a ruptured spleen or an open bone fracture, and others that are best treated conservatively. A *damage control* approach minimizes the time of surgical intervention and emphasizes perioperative surgical ICU care, including volume resuscitation, temperature control, hemodynamic monitoring, nutrition, and protocols for the prevention of nosocomial infectious complications. The injuries associated with major surgery and trauma derive from three main mechanisms: hemorrhage, tissue injury, and hypoperfusion.

Hemorrhage causes an immediate physiologic response to preserve oxygen delivery to vital organs. Using the large venous reservoir of the splanchnic and cutaneous circulation, the body maintains venous return and thus cardiac output to a certain extent.[3] In healthy individuals, symptoms of shock develop when acute blood loss exceeds 20% of the blood volume (approximately 1 L of blood in a 70-kg adult). Immediate resuscitation is necessary to prevent cardiovascular collapse and death. Even at the low hemoglobin (Hgb) levels that accompany this degree of bleeding, what limits the tolerability of hemorrhage is the reduced blood volume and cardiac output, not the decreased oxygen-carrying capacity of the blood. For example, a 30% to 40% blood loss would eventually reduce the plasma Hgb concentration to a level that still produces ample delivery of oxygen to the tissues. With an adequate cardiac output and arterial oxygen tension (Pao_2), a Hgb concentration as low as 5 g/dL still provides ample oxygen delivery to tissues supplied by normal vessels (**Table 73-1**).

Implementing early and effective therapies carry great importance in determining the subsequent clinical course. Despite a long-standing belief that aggressive volume resuscitation should be included in the initial care of the bleeding patient, this approach is now being revised for several reasons. First, the infusion of large volumes of crystalloids can cause a dilutional coagulopathy, characterized by thrombocytopenia and decreased concentrations of circulating clotting factors.[4] Counteracting these defects by infusing platelets and fresh-frozen plasma, in conjunction with massive crystalloid resuscitation,[5] results in intravascular volume overload and in edema of organs. Second, there is evidence that massive volume resuscitation for penetrating trauma of the torso may exacerbate bleeding from the site of injury and actually increase mortality.[6] Third, transfusion of blood products may have immunosuppressive effects leading to an increased risk of infection, cause acute lung injury/acute respiratory distress syndrome (ALI/ARDS), and death.[7,8]

Tissue injury produces local and systemic perturbations that are minimized during elective surgery by using proper anesthetic and surgical techniques but can produce major damage in the random, unprotected situation of a traumatic injury. Tissue damage, loss of perfusion, and cell necrosis result in the immediate release of tissue factors into the bloodstream, which trigger a systemic inflammatory response characterized by the synthesis and release of cytokines. Tumor necrosis factor (TNF)-α and interleukin (IL)-6 are among the earliest cytokines to appear in the systemic circulation immediately after tissue trauma, and they amplify the complex inflammatory response that is an integral part of critical illness.[9]

Tissue trauma of different types can produce both direct and systemic effects leading to critical illness. One well-documented example occurs in injuries to the lung. In our case report, the initial cause of the patient's complex critical illness was a chemical injury to the alveolar epithelium caused by the aspiration of gastric contents. A similar evolution to critical illness can occur with other lung injuries, such as a lung contusion from blunt chest trauma or a pneumonia. Despite the variety of inciting factors, the lung responds to acute injury in a stereotypical fashion, leading to the pathologic picture of *diffuse alveolar damange*[10] and the clinical picture of ALI/ARDS, which is a syndrome combining local and systemic inflammation.[11] Although not as well studied, a similar sequence of events appears to follow major acute injury to the kidneys[12,13] and the gut.[14]

Hypoperfusion and *ischemia* may result from direct tissue trauma, impaired regional blood flow, or a generalized decrease of blood flow: a *low-flow state*. A severe reduction of oxygen supplied to the tissues is marked by the local production of lactate from anaerobic glycolysis and may cause or exacerbate metabolic acidosis. However, even when profound ischemia occurs, tissue viability can be reestablished. The effects of restoration of blood flow after ischemic injury has been best characterized in the heart, where reversal of arterial occlusion is common with advanced techniques of coronary revascularization.[15] Myocardial *stunning* describes the acute ischemic dysfunction caused by acute cessation of regional coronary circulation and can be reversed by rapid restoration of blood flow.[16] Myocardial *hibernation*, a chronic state of dysfunction caused by insufficient coronary perfusion, can also, but less predictably, be improved with coronary revascularization procedures.[17] However, global hypoperfusion is often irreversible: In the "postresuscitation syndrome" that occurs following prolonged cardiopulmonary resuscitation, stunning of the cardiac muscle (*stony heart*)[15] is largely responsible for the high fatality rate observed early after cardiopulmonary resuscitation, and it is characterized by severely depressed contractility and malignant arrhythmias.

Although restoration of tissue oxygen supply may prevent cell death and reestablish function, acute reperfusion of ischemic tissues can cause significant cellular injury, known as *ischemia-reperfusion injury*. In the absence of adequate oxygen supply, mitochondrial production of adenosine triphosphate (ATP) decreases, causing an increase in adenosine monophosphate and its by-product hypoxanthine, and the conversion of the enzyme xanthine dehydrogenase to xanthine oxidase. Upon reperfusion with oxygen-rich blood, hypoxanthine is oxidized by xanthine oxidase at a high rate, producing large quantities of cytotoxic oxygen free radicals, including molecular oxygen, superoxide, and hydrogen peroxide ions.[18] Ischemia-reperfusion injury has been described in patients with the crush syndrome,[19] organ transplantation,[20] restoration of blood flow to limbs or splanchnic organs,[21] and during experimental alterations of ventilation and perfusion of the lung.[22,23]

METABOLIC FAILURE

Metabolic failure is a less common reason for admission to a surgical ICU. The most representative metabolic derangements include the consequences of severe malnutrition, such as extreme weight loss, kwashiorkor, and avitaminosis. These diseases are rarely seen in industrialized societies.

A different metabolic derangement, morbid obesity, has become more prevalent in the United States and other industrialized countries.[24] Morbid obesity (defined as weight 30% in excess of ideal body weight, or a body mass index >40 [body mass index = weight in kg ÷ height in m^2]) increases the risk of complications related to surgery and anesthesia. Morbidly obese patients are increasingly admitted to the ICU because of complications following bariatric surgery or unrelated events, such as trauma. Prevalent comorbidities of obesity include hypertension, diabetes mellitus, obstructive sleep apnea, chronic lung disease, and heart failure, which increase the rate of postoperative cardiovascular and respiratory complications. In addition, morbid obesity often presents logistical problems, such as the need for a special bed, a limited ability to perform important diagnostic tests such as magnetic resonance imaging and computed tomography scans, difficulty of vascular access and monitoring,[25,26] and complex issues of proper drug dosing.[27]

Common metabolic derangements requiring ICU care include those related to chronic diseases such as diabetes mellitus, diabetic ketoacidosis, and hyperosmolar nonketotic coma. See Chapter 13 for management recommendations for diabetes mellitus and its complications.

INFECTION

Infection contributes importantly to both the onset and the progression of critical illness. In a survey of 198 European ICUs, sepsis was responsible for 25% of the ICU admissions, and 37% of ICU patients experienced sepsis and septic shock at some time during their stay.[28] Infection is the leading cause of death in ICU patients. It is estimated that approximately 750 000 people develop sepsis annually in the United States, and 30% to 40% of these patients will die.[29] The specific entity of severe sepsis following elective surgery has recently been reported to have an incidence of 0.5% to 1%, and a mortality rate that has decreased from 44% to 34% over the present decade.[30] The presence of a proven infection in patients with ICU length of stays of more than 48 hours increases the mortality rate from 22% to 35%.[31] The terms *sepsis, severe sepsis, septic shock*, and *refractory septic shock* describe the spectrum of severity of sepsis. Multiorgan dysfunction syndrome (MODS) is a common complication of sepsis and other inflammation-driven critical illnesses. MODS is associated with a high mortality. These terms were reviewed in a consensus conference of the Society of Critical Care Medicine and the American College of Chest Physicians[32] and are thoroughly discussed in Chapter 72.

The most common *community-acquired* infections that require ICU admission include pneumonia, urosepsis, and peritonitis. Microorganisms involved in these infections are highly susceptible to antibiotic therapy when used properly. However, recent spread of multiresistant microorganisms outside health care institutions into the community has occurred, as exemplified by the case of *methicillin-resistant staphylococcus aureus* (MRSA). Community-acquired MRSA pneumonia is emerging as a particularly virulent infection due to the production of bacterial toxins, which is not well treated by vancomycin.[33] Infections are also important because of their enormous impact on public health, current (tuberculosis, malaria, and AIDS) or potential (severe acute respiratory syndrome, avian influenza, and H1N1 influenza), and are summarized in **Table 73-2**.

Health-care-acquired, or "*nosocomial*" infections (**Table 73-3**), are prevalent in the ICU and increase the mortality rate of critically ill patients.[34-39] In our case report, the development of a *Pseudomonas aeruginosa* pneumonia acquired in the ICU halted the course of recovery from ARDS and prolonged the patient's time on the ventilator and in the ICU. Nosocomial infections are often caused by multiresistant bacteria such as *P. aeruginosa*, MRSA, vancomycin-resistant *Enterococcus*, and various enteric gram-negative bacteria, many of which have become difficult to eradicate. Independent risk factors for developing nosocomial infections such as VAP include the severity of the patient's underlying illness, its endogenous microflora, and the performance of invasive procedures. In turn, the patient's own microflora is affected by general practices of antibiotic therapy and by the transmission of nosocomial bacteria from patient to patient through breaches in

TABLE 73-2 Infections That Constitute a Public Health Threat

Disease	Spread	Current Status	Treatment
TB (bacterial)	Person-to-person droplets	14 000 cases in the United States in 2003; enormous public health problem in Africa, Asia; on the rise in Europe; association with HIV	Antibacterial combinations are effective, but induced resistance develops
Malaria (parasite)	Anopheles (mosquito) bites	Widespread to warm and humid areas; sub-Saharan Africa has highest prevalence	Prevention and treatment with oral chloroquine and IV quinine; resistance is a problem
AIDS (virus)	Blood and body fluids, sexual	Relatively contained in United States; enormous public health problem in Africa, Asia, South America	Antiretroviral therapy slows progression but is not universally available
SARS (virus)	Person-to-person droplets	Worldwide outbreak in 2003; little in United States, now quiescent	Supportive
Avian flu	Birds to humans; sporadically person to person	Isolated cases; small outbreaks in Asia and Eastern Europe	Supportive
H1N1 flu	Person-to-person droplets	Worldwide outbreak in 2009, 2010	Supportive; antiviral therapy for high-risk group; prophylaxis: vaccination

SARS, severe acute respiratory syndrome; TB, tuberculosis.

Data from http://www.cdc.gov/nchstp/tb/faqs/qa_introduction.htm#Introl; http://www.cdc.gove/ncidod/sars/factsheet.htm; http://www.cdc.gov/malaria/faq.htm; http://www.cdc.gov/hiv/topics/surveillance/index.htm; http://www.cdc.gov/flu/avian/outbreaks/current.htm; http://www.cdc.gov/h1n1flu/. Accessed June 5, 2010.

TABLE 73-3 Nosocomial Infections

	Estimated Incidence	Estimated Mortality	Suggested Interventions
Ventilator-associated pneumonia[34,35]	5-10 per 1000 ventilator days[36,39]	10%-50%[37]	Semirecumbent position Continuous aspiration of subglottic secretions[40] Prophylactic "bundled" interventions[41]
Central line–associated bloodstream infection[35]	1-5 per 1000 central line days[36,39,42]	30%-35%[42]	Hand wash, full sterile attire, alcohol-based prep, full-body sterile draping, discontinuing the line as soon as possible[42]
Catheter-associated urinary tract infection[35]	2-8 per 1000 catheter days[36,39]	Unknown; very low	Discontinuing the catheter as soon as possible

proper infection-control measures.[38,39] The most frequent ports of entry of nosocomial bacteria are indwelling devices such as central venous lines and urinary catheters. It has been clearly demonstrated that the incidence and related morbidity of nosocomial infections can be significantly curtailed by adopting simple procedures of sterile insertion and maintenance, and by removing devices as soon as they are no longer necessary.[42]

SHOCK: THE ULTIMATE STRESS

The term *shock* describes the pathophysiologic manifestations of a catastrophic event that causes a profound, protracted reduction of perfusion to vital organs. Originally used to describe refractory hypotension, a more modern definition of shock indicates a state of tissue hypoperfusion caused by low blood flow, toxic agents, or both, where the circulation fails to meet the metabolic requirements of the cell. Initially, neurohumoral compensatory mechanisms maintain perfusion to vital organs. However, if appropriate supportive treatment is not promptly instituted, these compensatory mechanisms are overwhelmed, and progressive tissue ischemia leads to organ failure. Clinically, signs and symptoms of end-organ hypoperfusion include mental status changes, loss of skin turgor, cool extremities, oliguria, acidemia, a high serum lactate concentration, and a reduced mixed or central venous oxygen saturation.

HOST RESPONSES DURING CRITICAL ILLNESS

The body responds to an acute injury—such as the aspiration of gastric contents into the lungs as in our case report, or a bacterial infection, or a surgical wound—in a reproducible way. The initial local inflammatory response aims to control the immediate effects of the injury and generates signals from various cells at the site of injury that activate a systemic response. Hence an injury of sufficient severity triggers a complex response involving multiple cell types, including leukocytes, endothelial cells, and even cells within the nervous system.[43] When these homeostatic responses are coupled with appropriate interventions, they enable us to maintain or restore the function of vital organs and to expedite repair, which leads to healing and rehabilitation. When the injury hampers the host's regulatory processes or when our intervention is inadequate or delayed, the attempt to preserve the body's integrity is overwhelmed by the injury and organ dysfunction, and death ensues.

TIMING

The complexity of the body's response to injury over time constitutes a major challenge to our ability to develop effective treatments that will inhibit the progression of traumatic, inflammatory, and infectious injuries to MODS and death. The classical view of an initial hypodynamic and a subsequent hyperdynamic phase of the cardiovascular and metabolic responses to injury was overly simplistic.[44] The timing and intensity of this complex response appears to vary widely among patients and is influenced by multiple factors, including the magnitude of the injury, the patient's physiologic status, and therapeutic interventions. **Figure 73-2** illustrates three hypothetical time sequences of the evolution of critical illness, showing different patterns of activation and suppression of the immune system following an infectious injury. Although studied thoroughly in the case of sepsis, this sequence of events is likely to be applicable to other noxious events, such as after major surgery, trauma, inflammation, and shock.[45,46]

Physical examination following a serious injury may reveal changes of skin color and turgor, body temperature, arterial blood pressure, breathing pattern, and mental function. Other easily measured parameters, including urine output, base deficit, and serum lactate level, may also be abnormal. Although we separately describe the characteristic responses of various organ systems, in the body these systems are highly interconnected and have certain similar characteristic responses, such as upregulation of inflammatory mediators. Dysfunction of one

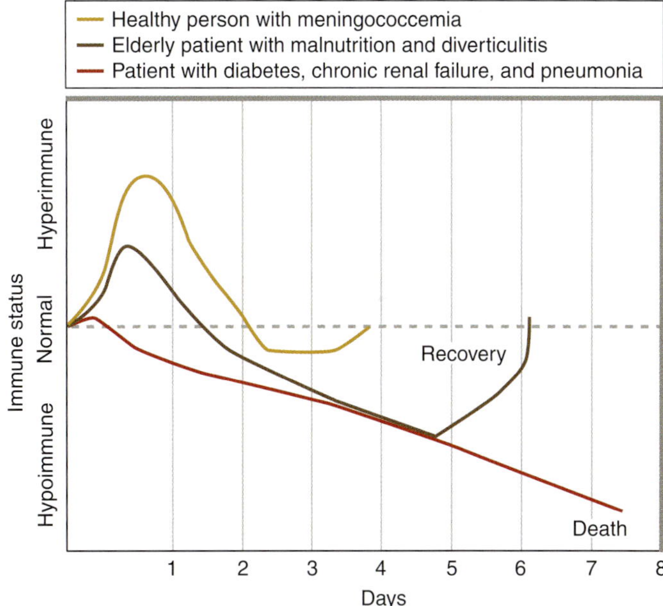

FIGURE 73-2. The immune-inflammatory response to injury: hypothetical time course of three representative patients. The healthy individual with a severe infection (eg, meningococcemia, *top line*) shows a robust inflammatory response; if this patient survives the initial phase, there will be only a short hypoimmune period, and the patient will progress along the path of recovery. For an elderly, malnourished patient with a moderate infection (eg, acute diverticulitis, *middle line*), the initial inflammatory response is limited, and if the infection is not promptly eradicated, a prolonged hypoimmune state ensues, and death can occur from further infectious complications. For a patient with significant comorbidity (eg, diabetes, obesity, chronic obstructive pulmonary disease, and a pneumonia, *bottom line*) the initial inflammatory response may be completely blunted, and the clinical course is dominated by a hypoimmune state, where the risk of death from persistent or new infection is high. [From Hotchkiss RS, Karl IE. The pathophysiology and treatment of sepsis. *N Engl J Med.* 2003;348:138-150. Copyright 2003, Massachusetts Medical Society. All rights reserved.]

system often impairs the functions of other organs; a classic example is the development of functional renal failure because of decompensated hepatic failure (hepatorenal syndrome) as can arise in a cirrhotic patient with an intra-abdominal infection.

THE IMMUNE-INFLAMMATORY RESPONSE

Over the last decade and a half, numerous advances have been made in the understanding of how the host recognizes and responds to threats, be they exogenous (infectious) or endogenous (tissue injury). It is clear that the immune-inflammatory response plays a central role in the evolution of critical illness. Both the *innate* immune system and the *adaptive* immune system are activated by injury and infection. The innate immune system is designed to recognize and initiate inflammatory responses to exogenous (ie, parts of microorganisms) or endogenous (ie, released by damaged tissues) factors. The innate immune system is also involved in the development of adaptive responses during infection and other inflammation-driven processes.[47] The innate immune system uses a family of receptors, known as pattern recognition receptors (PRRs), to recognize conserved molecular motifs on microorganisms and on endogenous factors that seem to be released when there is damage to tissues. Thus far a number of PRRs have been identified, including toll-like receptors (TLRs), NODs, scavenger receptors and mannose binding lectins. The TLRs have been most extensively studied since their initial discovery in the late 1990s, and TLRs and innate immune pathways are being extensively examined as potential targets for sepsis. In particular, antagonism of TLR4, the host receptor for endotoxin (lipopolysaccharide), has undergone multiple clinical trials.

Activation of innate immune pathways leads to the upregulation of the inflammatory mediators that contribute to the pathophysiology of sepsis, including cytokines, chemokines, arachidonic acid metabolites, complement factors, acute-phase reactants, reactive oxygen species, coagulation pathway intermediaries, and so on. Although leukocytes, in particular monocytes and macrophages, have been most extensively studied as contributors to the so-called cytokine storm and other effects of sepsis, multiple other cell types express innate immune receptors/pathways and participate in inflammatory responses during sepsis and other inflammation-driven disorders. These include endothelial and epithelial cells, and fibroblasts. The downstream effects of innate immune activation are complex, involving multiple cell types, systemic cascades (inflammation, complement, coagulation), and multiple intracellular pathways. The complexity of the system and the fact that the components of the system are important in clearing infection likely explain the failure of anticytokine strategies in larger clinical sepsis trials. More recently, some degree of success has been achieved by supplementing individual substances or pathways that seem deficient during certain phases of critical illness, and treating these "relative insufficiencies" with natural or synthetic equivalents of the undersupplied substance. Examples of such strategies are described in the following sections.

Immediately following acute tissue injury, a variety of inflammatory mediators is released by activated leukocytes, endothelial cells and fibroblasts. These mediators include cytokines, arachidonic acid metabolites, complement fractions, various acute-phase proteins, and oxygen and nitrogen free radicals.[46] Cytokines are polypeptide messengers of this huge cascade of reactions that have been extensively studied and identified as critical mediators of physiologic and laboratory manifestations of inflammation. Unlike hormones, which are produced by specialized endocrine tissues, cytokines are not stored, and their acute increase following tissue injury reflects upregulated gene transcription, translation, and synthesis by activated immune and/or endothelial cells. A characteristic of this type of response is that it tends to modulate itself by upregulating the expression of both pro- and anti-inflammatory cytokines and acute-phase reactants.

Over the past 3 decades there has been a prevailing view that the pathogenesis of traumatic and infectious injury is based on an excessive and uncontrolled response to the initial insult ("cytokine storm") that turns a beneficial defense system into the actual offender, and, ultimately, causes critical illness. This appealing view, brought forward by Lewis Thomas in the 1970s[48] and further championed by Roger Bone in the 1990s,[49] led to the development and testing of many therapies that targeted or modulated inflammatory mediators, including high-dose corticosteroids, ibuprofen, antibodies against bacterial endotoxin (lipopolysaccharide [LPS]), TNF-α, and IL-1 receptor antagonists.[50-52] However, human trials with these agents were largely unsuccessful. Given the complexity of the inflammatory response, it is not surprising that inhibiting the activity of a single mediator may not provide sufficient benefit.

THE CENTRAL NERVOUS SYSTEM

The central nervous system response to major injury and stress involves activation of the autonomic system, as well as interactions with the endocrine and the immune systems. The classical neurohumoral response to acute injury includes early activation of the autonomic sympathetic system resulting in tachycardia, increased myocardial contractility, tachypnea, splanchnic and cutaneous vasoconstriction, and increased availability of metabolic substrates. This "fight-or-flight" response is closely linked to activation of the hormonal pathways of the adrenal medulla, the pituitary-adrenal axis, antidiuretic hormone (ADH), and angiotensin-aldosterone (see "The Hormonal Response"); all these physiologic pathways, in various ways, tend to preserve perfusion to vital organs.[53]

The brain also interacts with the immune system, and recent experimental observations have identified a vagal-mediated neural pathway that participates in the regulation of inflammation. **Figure 73-3** shows a schematic of this "cholinergic anti-inflammatory pathway."[54] Inflammatory stimuli including LPS, TNF-α, and IL-1 activate visceral vagal afferents that reach multiple vagal nuclei in the medulla and hypothalamus. This neural input elicits an immediate anti-inflammatory response mediated by the same autonomic parasympathetic system. Experimental activation of the cholinergic/anti-inflammatory pathway inhibits function and reduces the expression of TNF during endotoxemia through the binding of nicotinic receptors on macrophages.[55] Knowledge of this cholinergic/anti-inflammatory pathway has possible therapeutic implications: Experimental activation of vagal output by electrical, as well as pharmacologic, vagal stimulation has inhibited macrophage activation and cytokine release.[54]

THE HORMONAL RESPONSE

The hormonal response to acute injury tends to increase vascular pressures, preserve circulating blood volume, and provide substrates for tissue metabolism and regeneration. These hormonal pathways include the synthesis and release of adrenal corticosteroids and catecholamines, ADH and aldosterone-angiotensin, prolactin, growth hormone, and other anti-insulin hormones. The role of these hormones in the acute response is complex, and significant understanding of their role has been gained over the past several decades.[56] Recent evidence reveals that some of these pathways may be key determinants of survival for critically ill patients and suggests they may be successfully modulated pharmacologically.[57]

The output of the *pituitary-adrenal axis* increases several-fold as a normal response to acute illness.[58] Any malfunction of this axis, whether at the level of the precursors, the end product (cortisol) or the cellular receptors, leads to an ineffective response and may be associated with a reduced chance of survival. The term *relative adrenal insufficiency* refers to a state in which the pituitary-adrenal axis fails to mount a sufficient response in the presence of an acute and severe stress, despite functioning adequately in health.[59] Based on this concept, patients who fail to mount an appropriate increase in the activity of the pituitary-adrenal axis in response to a severe stress like sepsis may benefit from exogenous replacement of corticosteroid hormones. However, clinical data concerning the effectiveness of physiologic doses of corticosteroids for the treatment of severe sepsis and septic shock remain controversial.[60,61] Although a physiologic benefit (increased arterial blood pressure, earlier

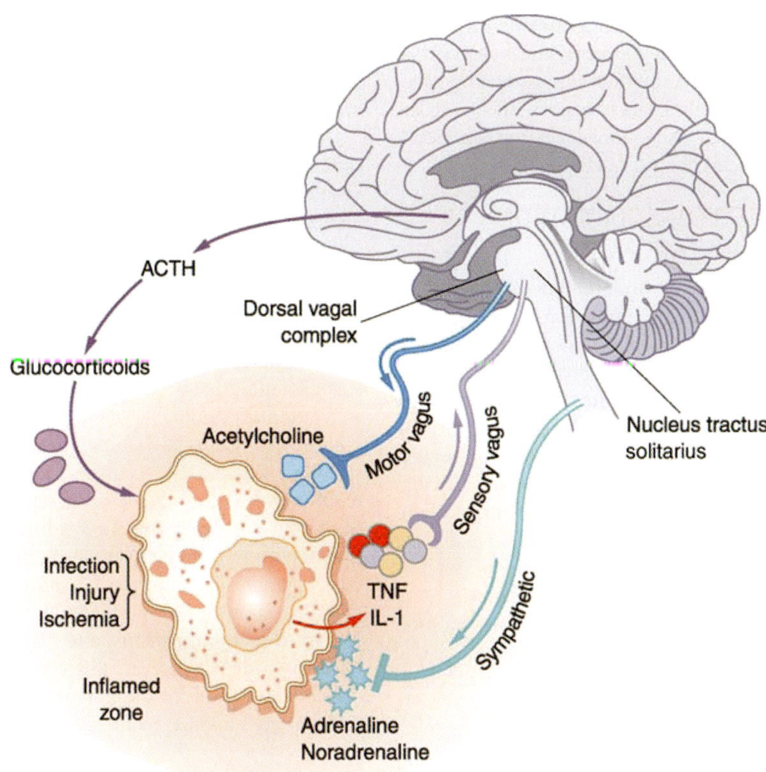

FIGURE 73-3. The cholinergic–anti-inflammatory pathway. Inflammatory products produced at the site of injury activate neural signals that are relayed to the nucleus of the tractus solitarius. From there, efferent vagal activity (the cholinergic–anti-inflammatory pathway) inhibits cytokines expression. In addition, vagal afferents can also be relayed to the hypothalamus and stimulate adrenocorticotropic hormone (ACTH) release. IL, interleukin; TNF, tumor necrosis factor. [From Tracey K. The inflammatory reflex. *Nature.* 2002;420:853-859. Reprinted by permission from Macmillan Publishers Ltd.]

resolution of shock) has been shown consistently, the most recent and largest controlled trial to date[61] failed to find any effect on survival. It is possible that corticosteroids may be beneficial in selected patients that we are still unable to identify and/or treat properly. In particular, our standard clinical evaluation of the function of the *pituitary-adrenal axis* in critically ill patients through the administration of adrenocorticotropic hormone (ACTH) and subsequent dosage of circulating cortisol is probably insensitive.[62]

Similarly, ADH is insufficiently synthesized in a significant fraction of critically ill patients, particularly those suffering from vasodilatory shock.[63] The administration of a low dose of vasopressin, a synthetic analog of ADH, appears to improve general systemic hemodynamics and reduce the need for infusing other vasopressor medications such as norepinephrine. However, a recent trial in vasodilatory shock patients did not demonstrate a benefit of adding vasopressin to norepinephrine when compared with increasing the dose of epinephrine alone.[64] As in the case of corticosteroids, it is clear that this therapy does not benefit all patients, and we still do not have adequate means to evaluate the complex physiologic response to stress and injury at the bedside. Further post hoc analyses of this large study may reveal possible benefits of vasopressin administration in subgroups of critically ill patients with vasodilatory shock, such as those with concomitant adrenal insufficiency[64] or acute renal insufficiency.[65]

The hormonal response to acute stress includes a surge in the synthesis and release of anti-insulin hormones such as epinephrine, glucocorticoids, glucagon, and growth hormone. This proglycemic response increases the availability of glucose as a ready source of energy for vital organs during a time of starvation and massive catabolism. However, the resulting *hyperglycemia of critical illness*, which is independent of any coexisting diabetic state, may affect the course of critical illness in a number of ways, including an increased susceptibility to infections, immunosuppression, and neurologic damage.[66] A provocative clinical trial from a single surgical ICU suggested that a morbidity and mortality benefit occurs if the blood sugar level is maintained between the very narrow range of 80 and 110 mg/dL. Such an effect seemed to be mediated through a decrease in the incidence of bacteremia, critical illness polyneuropathy, and the need for blood transfusions.[67] Over the ensuing years, the strength of this finding was significantly mitigated by the repeated observation that the intensive insulin therapy required to achieve this goal often resulted in severe hypoglycemia, which in turn was independently associated with an increased mortality.[68,69]

THE HEMODYNAMIC RESPONSE

The hemodynamic response to injury has been extensively investigated by monitoring central vascular pressures, cardiac output, and indices of oxygen delivery and consumption.[70] Systemic vasoconstriction commonly predominates in the immediate period following an acute injury, most likely as a reflex response to intravascular hypovolemia from hemorrhage or sequestration of body fluids outside the vascular compartment. After normovolemia is restored, a hyperdynamic pattern of high cardiac output and normal-to-low blood pressure ensues. The extent of this hyperdynamic response varies with the type and magnitude of the injury. It is important to note that hyperdynamic states occur in other conditions, such as hyperthyroidism, liver cirrhosis, and with large arteriovenous fistulae, even if acute injury and/or inflammation are not present.

This hyperdynamic response may be part of a *systemic inflammatory response syndrome* (SIRS) that is associated with acute injury of various etiologies and caused by the release of cytokines and other inflammatory mediators such as prostaglandins, bradykinins, and complement fractions.[71] The cardinal manifestations of SIRS include hyper- or hypothermia, tachycardia, leukocytosis or leukopenia, and hyperventilation. In addition, a number of other signs and symptoms, such as hypotension, platelet and coagulation abnormalities, and changes in mental status, are characteristic of SIRS, although each taken individually lacks specificity both as a diagnostic sign and as an end point for defining therapy.

THE ENDOTHELIUM: SYSTEMIC VASODILATATION, INFLAMMATION, AND COAGULATION

The endothelium, through its effects on inflammation, coagulation pathways, blood flow, and vascular barrier function, contributes to the pathophysiology of organ dysfunction in sepsis and other inflammation-driven disorders.[72-75] The endothelium produces proinflammatory cytokines such as IL-6 and IL-8, and participates in leukocyte recruitment to organs. It is also involved in modulating the coagulation pathways. Endothelial activation is a critical contributor to vascular leak during sepsis.[76] Endothelial activation, coagulopathy, and vascular leak occur at locations removed from sites of infection, causing inflammation, edema, and ultimately to "bystander organ injury." Finally, the endothelium participates in the cardiovascular response to systemic inflammation, including decreased systemic vascular resistance.

Immediately following injury there is upregulation of adhesion molecule expression on endothelial cells and leukocytes leading to increased endothelial cell–leukocyte interactions and eventual migration of leukocytes across the vessel wall into the adjacent tissues (**Fig. 73-4**).[77,78]

Direct injuries and inflammatory mediators cause the endothelium to lose its anticoagulant properties. Plasminogen activator inhibitor (PAI)-1 is produced by endothelium and is the principal inhibitor of tissue plasmin activator and urokinase. When PAI-1 is released in increased amounts into the bloodstream, fibrinolysis is severely suppressed. This mechanism is postulated to contribute to sepsis-induced disseminated intravascular coagulation (DIC).[79-81] The imbalance between thrombin and plasmin and the increased platelet stickiness result ultimately in clot formation on the endothelial surface. Thus widespread activation of the coagulation system in response to stress may lead to DIC, intravascular formation of fibrin, decreased fibrinolytic activity, and widespread thrombosis.[82] Although the full syndrome of diffuse vascular thrombosis is rare, DIC often presents a considerable clinical challenge because of the concomitant presence of a consumptive coagulopathy and thrombosis. The coagulation system has been targeted therapeutically in patients with sepsis and septic shock. Antithrombin III and protein C are both anticoagulants maintained in an active state by endothelial activity, and they are decreased in conditions of stress such as SIRS and sepsis. Although a clinical trial of the therapeutic administration of antithrombin III was unsuccessful,[83] the infusion of recombinant human activated protein C (drotrecogin-α) modestly increased the survival rate of critically ill patients with severe sepsis at high risk of death.[84]

The endothelium produces multiple mediators that have diverse functions. Some mediators have multiple effects, such as protein C, vasodilator mediators like NO and prostacyclin (both also inhibit platelet aggregation), and the vasoconstrictor endothelins, and all have potent vasoactive and immunologic properties. NO is produced constitutively in endothelial cells by the isozyme nitric oxide synthase (NOS-3, endothelial nitric oxide synthase [eNOS]). Following stimulation of various kinds, there is upregulation of the inducible form of NOS (NOS-2, iNOS), which results in increased production of NO and contributes to the profound vasodilatation that occurs with severe systemic inflammatory processes.[85] Activation of endothelial cells also results in the production of mediators with opposing effects, such as the endothelins, which can cause vasoconstriction, whereas NO causes vasodilatation.[86] When the induction of iNOS is overwhelming, such as in septic shock, the massive vasodilatation of the extreme hyperdynamic syndrome results in profound hypotension that may compromise vital tissue perfusion and lead to MODS and death (see Chapter 74). NO-induced vasodilatation has been reversed by the administration of nonspecific NOS inhibitors such as methylene blue,[87] NG-nitro-L-arginine methyl ester (L-NAME),[88] and *N*-methyl-L-arginine hydrochloride.[89] However, this clinical strategy has been unsuccessful, possibly as a result of the importance of the constitutive isoenzymes of NO that are inhibited by these nonselective compounds.

THE METABOLIC RESPONSE

The metabolic response to traumatic injury is characterized by hypercatabolism and increased urinary nitrogen excretion. Once initial hemodynamic resuscitation and stabilization are achieved, substrates are used to enhance tissue repair and preserve vital organ function. Tissues that do not have a high resting energy requirement, such as fat and skeletal muscle, release nutrients from storage (glucose and fatty acids) or proceed to break down their structural proteins to provide fuel for visceral organs. High levels (3- to 4-fold increase) of circulating catecholamines coexist with this metabolic response. Epinephrine, in particular, promotes glycogenolysis in muscle and liver, lipolysis and ketogenesis in adipose tissue, and hepatic gluconeogenesis.[90,91] These processes provide energy for the high metabolic requirements during recovery and repair. In addition, epinephrine induces insulin resistance in skeletal muscle, which contributes to the development of hyperglycemia. Like many homeostatic responses, the high catecholaminergic

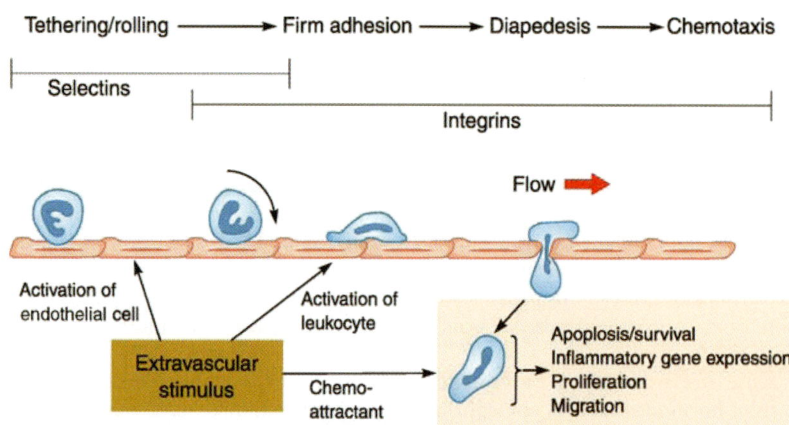

FIGURE 73-4. Schematic of leukocyte adhesion to the activated endothelium during inflammation. Leukocytes are initially tethered and roll along the endothelium predominantly via interactions with selectins. Once on the endothelium, leukocytes' integrin receptors are activated and bind to ligands on the extracellular matrix, favoring migration of leukocytes between endothelial cells. Signaling from integrin receptors also modulates the survival or apoptosis of leukocytes and gene expression and proliferation. [Reproduced with permission from Harlan J, Winn R. Leukocyte-endothelial interactions: clinical trials of anti-adhesion therapy. *Crit Care Med.* 2002;30:S214-S219.]

state has dual and opposing effects; although catecholamines promote healing and repair, high catecholamine levels may cause excessive catabolism, hyperglycemia, muscle wasting, and reduced host defenses. One clinical study of children with acute burn injuries has shown the benefits of blocking the catecholaminergic response to acute burn injury. Because children with burns have a particularly high metabolic demand,[92] it remains uncertain whether this benefit can be extrapolated to critically ill adults without burns.

THE CELLULAR RESPONSE TO INJURY

At the tissue level, the ability to live or die can be reduced to the ability of the body to supply adequate amounts of oxygen and nutrients (eg, glucose) for cellular respiration and to remove metabolic by-products (carbon dioxide [CO_2] and toxins). These two seemingly simple end points are reached through enormously complex phenomena. This section reviews several aspects of this process that are relevant to acute injury, whether traumatic, inflammatory, or infectious.

THE CELLULAR RESPONSE TO TRAUMATIC INJURY

The extent of the damage caused by a traumatic injury (eg, amount of energy received on impact, size of the wound) often determines the immediate outcome of a patient. An uncontrollable hemorrhage will result in early death, with the possible salvage strategy being very simple: a tourniquet and immediate transport, not ICU care. A complex but not immediately lethal injury will then evolve over time, and the outcome will depend on the adequacy of the endogenous response to injury and the ability to support it successfully.

The body's immediate response to traumatic injury requires the generation of signals that communicate the presence of a threat to the rest of the body. These danger signals, which may include necrotic tissue by-products and local changes in pH and temperature, activate endothelial cells, monocytes, and macrophages to produce and release inflammatory mediators. Production and release of cytokines begins within a few minutes of injury and facilitates a systemic response that has protean clinical manifestations. Early measurements of plasma cytokine levels in trauma and surgical patients indicate that the degree of increase in IL-6, one of the earliest responders, correlates with the degree of injury.[92,93] In addition to the immediate synthesis and release of cytokines, soluble receptors and antagonist mediators are released following trauma, further modulating the effects of the cytokines and initiating a competitive anti-inflammatory, immunosuppressive response.[94,95] This balance between the activation and suppression of inflammation continues throughout the course of critical illness, and it likely affects the ultimate evolution toward recovery or death.[96] Better understanding of the determinants of this balance between the pro- and anti-inflammatory responses could guide the generation of more effective therapeutic strategies. A state of immunosuppression or anergy is well described after severe trauma and surgery and may increase susceptibility to nosocomial infections, a common determinant of further morbidity and a longer ICU stay.[97]

INNATE IMMUNE RECEPTORS IN INFECTION

Like traumatic injury, in which the extent of damage determines the bodily response, a sufficient inoculum of pathogenic microorganisms triggers the host's systemic inflammatory response, manifesting in its most severe form as septic shock. The host response to infection is initiated by interactions between structural components of the invading organism (pathogen-associated molecular patterns [PAMPs]) and the immune cells of the host. All classes of microbes, including gram-positive and gram-negative bacteria, fungi, viruses, and parasites, have PAMPs, although their exact PAMPs vary. For instance, gram-negative bacteria have endotoxin (LPS) in the outer membrane of their cell walls. LPS is a potent bacterial toxin that is thought to play an important role in gram-negative sepsis. Gram-positive bacteria do not have LPS, but they have other PAMPs that have inflammatory effects, such as lipoproteins, peptidoglycan, and lipoteichoic acid.

LPS is the best characterized and most extensively studied PAMP. A variety of host mediators, including soluble mediators in the blood, cell surface receptors, and intracellular signaling pathways, are involved in PAMP-induced activation of inflammation. For instance, both LPS-binding protein and the monocyte surface antigen CD14[98] bind LPS, and they are involved in initiating inflammatory responses to LPS. CD14 is vital for LPS-induced activation of immune cells and has both membrane-bound and soluble forms. Soluble CD14 is required for LPS-induced activation of CD14-negative cells.[99] CD14 also seems to play a role in cell signaling by gram-positive bacterial PAMPs, such as peptidoglycan.[95]

Over the last decade, a great deal has been discovered about the mechanisms of inflammation induced by microorganisms. Despite considerable structural heterogeneity, inflammatory responses to different microbial components are mediated through common receptors and intracellular pathways. TLRs recognize various classes of PAMPs and are critical proximal mediators of inflammation during infection. TLRs are evolutionarily conserved innate immune receptors that are present in both insects and mammals. They sense common motifs in components of microorganisms (PAMPs). Mammalian TLRs were discovered in 1998 when TLR4 was identified as the LPS receptor.[100] The same year, human TLRs 1-5 were cloned.[101] Since that time, multiple mammalian TLRs have been identified, each recognizing a different PAMP.

As with all biologic systems, intercellular signaling in early inflammation and infection has an intrinsic redundancy. In addition to the TLRs, other innate immune receptors and signaling pathways seem to be important in the recognition of and response to infection, including NOD receptors, scavenger receptors, mannose binding lectins, and dectin. Refer to recent reviews for a more inclusive discussion.[102-105]

FROM INFLAMMATORY RESPONSE TO IMMUNOSUPPRESSION

Within the first 30-90 minutes after exposure to endotoxin, mononuclear cells release proinflammatory cytokines such as TNF-α, IL-6, and IL-1β. This activates inflammatory cascades that stimulate further production and release of cytokines, chemokines (chemoattractant cytokines), lipid mediators, and free radicals, which are involved in leukocyte migration and adhesion and in tissue injury.[77,78] A similar inflammatory response can be triggered by all of the stressors or insults described in earlier sections of this chapter. The failure of early therapies aimed at blocking isolated aspects of the inflammatory response, such as infusing high-dose corticosteroids, TNF antagonists, IL-1 receptor antagonists, and non–isozyme-specific inhibitors of NO synthesis, has led investigators to search for a deeper understanding of this extraordinarily complex and redundant system.

There is mounting evidence to support the concept of *immunomodulation*, that is, an equilibrium between activation and suppression of the immune system, during critical illness. It is postulated that a state of immunoparalysis can occur, whereby the host has inadequate immune responses to microorganisms and plays an important role in subsequent morbidity and mortality following injury or infection. Anti-inflammatory mediators and altered cellular responses are believed to predispose patients to the development of nosocomial infections and subsequent MODS.[106,107] At various times after the initial proinflammatory state of traumatic and infectious injury, counterregulatory cytokines, soluble decoy receptors for cytokines, and antagonists of proinflammatory cytokines are secreted. Immunosuppression is believed to occur when this response supersedes its function of restoring immunologic balance. This is exemplified by studies that indicate that blood from septic patients has reduced endotoxin-induced cytokine production, unlike blood from control patients.[108] Anergy, or the inability of T cells to proliferate and secrete lymphokines upon stimulation, is often observed in severe trauma and septic patients.[109-111] In trauma, a decrease in the number of T cells probably results from interactions between T cells and immunosuppressive mediators such as IL-10.[112,113] Regulator T cells (T-reg), which are important elements of the normal immunologic equilibrium, may play a role in the immunosuppression resulting from burn injury.[112,114]

In acute infection, adaptive immunity may be impaired because of apoptosis of T lymphocytes[115] rather than cell necrosis. The term *necrosis* refers to *accidental* cell death, whereas the term *apoptosis* refers to *programmed* cell death. In contrast to necrosis, which generally has a stimulating effect on the innate immune system, apoptosis can induce secretion of anti-inflammatory cytokines leading to immunosuppression and anergy. It has been shown that the B lymphocytes, CD4 T lymphocytes, and dendritic cells undergo apoptosis but that CD8 T lymphocytes or natural killer cells do not undergo apoptosis.[115] After the initial decrease in the number of CD4 T cells, the subset of these cells that recovers are selectively T-reg and not T-helper (Th) cells.[116] T-reg cells have multiple negative regulatory effects on immune function and can contribute to immunosuppression.[112] The importance of immune cell apoptosis in sepsis has also been demonstrated in animal models. Strains of mice that produce the antiapoptotic protein Bcl-2 are protected from death after intra-abdominal sepsis induced by cecal ligation and puncture.[117] With late immunosuppression as the predominating state after the initial injury, critically ill patients become a target for nosocomial infections, which can lead to vital organ failure and death.

METABOLIC DISTURBANCES

Critically ill patients may develop metabolic disturbances that hinder the ability to generate sufficient energy to maintain body homeostasis. ATP is the primary fuel source for cellular respiration. The mitochondria are the principal sites of aerobic ATP production. Here, pyruvate, a product of glucose metabolism, is used in the citric acid cycle to generate the reduced forms of nicotinamide adenine dinucleotide (NADH) or flavin adenine dinucleotide (FADH) and provide the flow of electrons necessary to synthesize ATP by oxidative phosphorylation. Ultimately, 36 or 38 mol of ATP are generated from the oxidation of 1 mol of glucose. Conversely, anaerobic glycolysis occurs in the cytoplasm, and generates only 2 mol of ATP per mole of glucose, with the production of lactate or ethanol as end products. During critical illness, the failure to generate adequate amounts of ATP can lead to cellular and organ dysfunction.

Several studies describe a decrease in ATP production in septic patients[118-120] and lower ATP levels in the tissues of critically ill septic patients who died when compared with tissues of those who survived.[121] One reason for the failure to generate ATP during critical illness is inadequate delivery of oxygen to vital tissues, secondary to impaired oxygenation and perfusion. During SIRS and septic shock, multiple factors may decrease tissue perfusion, including inadequate cardiocirculatory performance, hypoxemia from acute lung injury, mediator- or vasopressor-induced vasoconstriction, and/or coagulation derangements causing microvascular obstruction.

CYTOPATHIC HYPOXIA

Cytopathic hypoxia is postulated to contribute to the failure to generate adequate ATP because of the inability of cells to consume available oxygen.[122] Experimental and clinical studies show that tissue oxygen tension during sepsis is often higher than in nonseptic states.[123-125] Mitochondrial dysfunction is hypothesized to underlie the apparent disconnection between cellular oxygen tension and the low ATP levels. Mitochondrial dysfunction is reported in cells exposed to macrophages, inflammatory cytokines, LPS, and infection.[126-128] Multiple factors may contribute to mitochondrial dysfunction in acute injury, including the production of NO and reactive oxygen species. Low doses of LPS can increase iNOS messenger RNA activity in the intestinal tissues of experimental animals,[127] and physiologic concentrations of NO can reversibly inhibit the activity of cytochrome oxidase by competition with oxygen.[129,130] In addition, NO can damage mitochondria by generating peroxynitrite when reacting with the molecular oxygen of the superoxide radical anion. Peroxynitrite is a potent oxidizing and nitrating that can inhibit multiple mitochondrial functions.[131] The presence of peroxynitrite is associated with mitochondrial inhibition, DNA breakage, and activation of poly ADP-ribose polymerase (PARP), an enzyme responsible for repair of single-strand DNA breaks.[132] PARP activation can lead to energetic failure by causing a decrease in the oxidized form of nicotinamide adenine dinucleotide (NAD^+) and NADH, an important electron donor in mitochondrial oxidative phosphorylation (see earlier).[133]

ORGAN FAILURE, SURVIVAL, AND DEATH

The transition from organ failure to recovery or to further damage and death is still incompletely understood. An autopsy study of patients who died from sepsis showed discordance between the clinical manifestations and histologic findings in various organs.[117] In the heart, there was no histologic evidence of injury to myocytes despite reduced contractility. In the kidneys, there was only focal injury with preservation of normal glomerular and tubular architecture despite the acute impairment of renal function. Furthermore, it is a common observation that most patients who survive septic shock recover the baseline function of their heart, lungs, and kidneys, suggesting that reversible factors, rather than cell death, are responsible for organ dysfunction.[134] What is known about the mechanisms of the organ failure of critical illness is discussed in Chapter 74. Here we provide a schema of pathophysiologic events occurring in the progression of critical illness. At successive steps, different therapeutic approaches may be useful for influencing the progression of illness toward survival and away from death (**Fig. 73-5**).

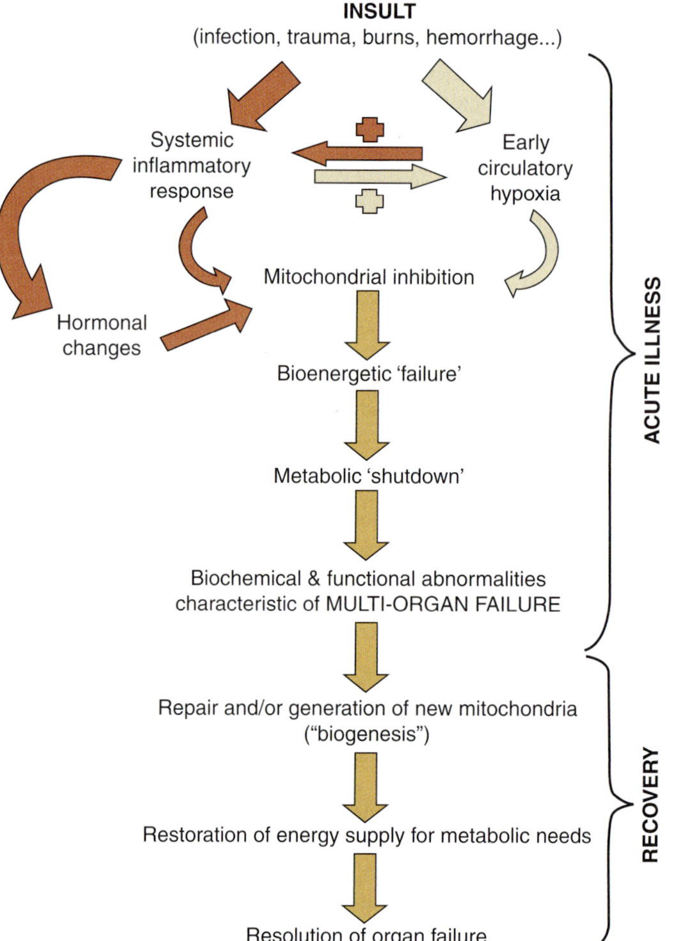

FIGURE 73-5. A proposed paradigm of the evolution of critical illness (see text).

Initially, the inciting "stress" should be countered with early and appropriate etiologic therapy (eg, antimicrobials for sepsis) and early resuscitation directed to the physiologic goals that we use as surrogates of adequate tissue perfusion (eg, arterial blood pressure, central venous pressure, urine output, and mixed venous oxygen saturation or Pao_2, lactate).[135] Intervening the cascade of tissue hypoperfusion, systemic inflammation and dysregulation of the immune response may prevent subsequent organ damage. However, even this principle is not universal, as exemplified by the successful use of limited fluid resuscitation in selected trauma patients.[2] In our case report, the presence of pulmonary hypertension and right ventricular insufficiency further complicated the management of resuscitation via goal-directed therapy, prompting the use of invasive monitoring with a pulmonary artery catheter, which may not be indicated routinely for the management of ALI/ARDS.[136]

Subsequently, therapies supporting the natural response to acute stress, such as an infusion of activated protein C (as was done in our case report), may improve survival of the most critically ill patients. In the future, therapies targeting mitochondrial protection, such as the administration of PARP inhibitors, superoxide and peroxynitrite scavengers, or selective NOS-2 inhibitors, can attenuate the cytopathic effects of oxygen and nitrogen free radicals, and decrease mitochondrial dysfunction. Immunosuppression, a persistent catabolic state, and poor nutritional status can all decrease host defenses and cause increased susceptibility to infectious complications. Inappropriate use of antibiotics and lack of adequate attention to basic procedures to prevent transmission of antibiotic-resistant bacteria may further increase the chances of nosocomial infections at this stage. In our case report, *Pseudomonas* pneumonia hindered the progression of our patient's course toward recovery, although ultimately our patient survived. Future therapies may target various aspects of immunosuppression, including apoptotic mechanisms (eg, by manipulation of Bcl-2), and may provide an appropriate balance of nutrients that can stimulate immune function. In addition, stimuli to increase mitochondrial energy generation can potentially play a role, so that cellular energy production regains baseline levels.

As the basic mechanisms of critical illness are further defined through basic and clinical research, it is likely that the therapeutic algorithms for treating critical illness will evolve, from a gross physiologic approach supporting respiration and circulation to a more targeted mechanistic approach.

CONCLUSION

Acute injuries of various etiologies, such as the aspiration of gastric contents into the lungs (our case report), cause immediate local and systemic physiologic responses that are mediated by well-characterized inflammatory and humoral phenomena. Despite the complexity of these phenomena, our understanding of the evolution of critical illness has greatly increased in recent years as investigators have begun to elucidate the cellular and molecular mechanisms of the host's response to injury. The interaction between the initial "stress" (usually trauma, surgery, or infection) and the response of the host determines the evolution of a critical illness toward either healing and recovery or complications and death. Although a robust inflammatory response is necessary to fend off the most severe injuries, a subsequent decrease in its intensity and the onset of a hypoimmune state favor the onset of late infections that may lead to dysfunction of organs and death.

Critically ill patients undergo complex therapies and invasive interventions. The effectiveness of our therapies depends on a number of factors, including our ability to intervene properly and at the optimal time. Recent therapeutic interventions have improved the probability of survival of many critically ill patients. As knowledge of the basic mechanisms that underlie critical illness evolves, additional effective therapeutic strategies should emerge that will improve the care and outcome of critically ill patients.

KEY REFERENCES

- Fink MP. Bench-to-bedside review: cytopathic hypoxia. *Crit Care.* 2002;6:491-499.
- Gelman S. Venous function and central venous pressure. *Anesthesiology.* 2008;108:735-738.
- Hotchkiss RS, Karl IE. The pathophysiology and treatment of sepsis. *N Engl J Med.* 2003;348:138-150.
- Lipshutz AKM, Gropper MA. Perioperative glycemic control. *Anesthesiology.* 2009;110:408-421.
- Ochoa JB, Makarenkova V. T lymphocytes. *Crit Care Med.* 2005;33:S510-513.
- Peleg AY, Hooper DC. Hospital- acquired infections due to gram-negative bacteria. *N Engl J Med.* 2010;362:1804-1813.
- Rittirsch D, Flierl MA, Ward PA. Harmful molecular mechanisms in sepsis. *Nat Rev Immunol.* 2008; 8:776-787.
- Russell J, Phang P. The oxygen delivery/consumption controversy. Approaches to management of the critically ill patient. *Am J Respir Crit Care Med.* 1994;149:533-537.
- Tracey K. The inflammatory reflex. *Nature.* 2002;420:853-859.

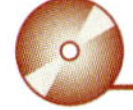

REFERENCES

Complete references available on DVD and online version at www.LongneckerAnesthesiology.com

CHAPTER 74 Evaluation of the Patient With Multiple Organ Dysfunction Syndrome

Binbin Wang
Jean Kwo
Judith Hellman

KEY POINTS

1. Multiple organ dysfunction syndrome (MODS) is common in critically ill patients and associated with a high mortality rate.
2. There are many underlying etiologies of MODS. In the overall intensive care unit (ICU) population, sepsis is the most common cause of MODS.
3. MODS is characterized by dysfunction of 2 or more organs or systems.
4. Inflammation and microvascular abnormalities are involved in the development of MODS.
5. Therapies for MODS should target the underlying cause, supporting the patient and correcting the physiologic and metabolic derangements caused by dysfunction of the organs and systems.
6. Patients with MODS often require surgery and other invasive procedures.
7. Whenever possible, optimize MODS patients preoperatively.
8. Methods of optimization are dictated by the affected organs and the severity of physiologic and metabolic derangements.

INTRODUCTION

Progress in life support therapies has led to the recognition of pathophysiologic states that are unique to critically ill patients. Diverse disease states can cause progressive dysfunction and ultimately complete failure of various organs and systems. This condition is commonly referred to as the multiple organ dysfunction syndrome (MODS). High-grade organ failure that necessitates life-sustaining therapies is often referred to as *multiorgan system failure.* The development of MODS portends a poor outcome. In fact, MODS is one of the leading causes of death for ICU patients.[1,2] This chapter reviews basic aspects of MODS, surgical and nonsurgical procedures that are commonly performed in patients with MODS, and the preoperative preparation and optimization of MODS patients for surgery.

MULTIORGAN DYSFUNCTION SYNDROME

The development of organ dysfunction as a separate disease process from the initial injury was first appreciated during World War II. Wounded soldiers were rapidly and aggressively resuscitated with blood products to normalize blood pressure, and they were more promptly evacuated to medical facilities than in previous wars. Although initial survival was improved, many soldiers who survived the initial trauma subsequently died of renal failure.[3,4] This led to changes in fluid resuscitation practices in subsequent wars, including the rapid infusion of crystalloids and more aggressive resuscitation. During the Vietnam War, many soldiers who survived their initial trauma developed "shock lung" (acute respiratory failure). At the same time, acute lung injury (ALI) and acute respiratory distress syndrome (ARDS) were increasingly being described in civilian ICUs.[5] During the 1970s, advances in critical care medicine led to improved initial survival from many injuries. However, many patients who survived initial resuscitation went on to develop progressive failure of various organs and systems.[6,7]

Various terms have been used to describe the spectrum of dysfunction of different organs and systems (reviewed in Bone et al[8]), including *multiple organ failure,*[9] *multiple-organ-failure-syndrome,*[1] *multiple system organ failure,*[10] *progressive or sequential organ failure,*[6] or MODS.[8,11] The term MODS is most widely used and encompasses the spectrum from mild organ dysfunction to complete organ failure. In addition, scoring systems have been devised to assess patients and to predict outcome.[4,12-16] In this chapter the term MODS is used as an inclusive definition for all the studies and articles that have used all of these terms over the past several decades.

DEFINITIONS

In 1992, recommendations for the definitions of sepsis, systemic inflammatory responses, and organ dysfunction were published based on a consensus conference of the American College of Chest Physicians and Society of Critical Care Medicine.[8] The acronyms SIRS (the systemic inflammatory response syndrome) and MODS were coined at the consensus conference, and they are widely used in patient care and in clinical study design.

SIRS The term SIRS describes a complex inflammatory process that is driven by many differing disease states. Underlying etiologies of SIRS include, but are not limited to, infection, trauma, burns, aspiration, pancreatitis, vascular compromise with resultant ischemia and/or necrosis, malignancy, and multiple blood transfusions. **Table 74-1** lists the criteria for SIRS.

Sepsis Sepsis was defined as the systemic inflammatory response to infection. Sepsis was further stratified based on its severity, with severe sepsis and septic shock representing the spectrum of progressively worsening status.

MODS MODS was used to describe a pattern of progressive dysfunction of organs that is related pathogenically regardless of the inciting process and requires intervention to maintain homeostasis.

TABLE 74-1 Systemic Inflammatory Response Syndrome Criteria

Diagnosis of systemic inflammatory response syndrome (SIRS) requires at least 2 of these criteria:

1. Tachycardia: heart rate >90 beats/min
2. Leukocytosis (white blood cell count >12 000), leucopenia (white blood cell count <4000), or high band count (>10%)
3. Fever (temperature >100.4°F [38°C]) or hypothermia (temperature <96.8°F [36°C])
4. Tachypnea (respiratory rate >20 breaths/min), low $Paco_2$ (<32 mm Hg), or mechanically ventilated

Data from Bone RC, Balk RA, Cerra FB, et al. Definitions for sepsis and organ failure and guidelines for the use of innovative therapies in sepsis. The ACCP/SCCM Consensus Conference Committee. American College of Chest Physicians/Society of Critical Care Medicine. *Chest.* 1992;101(6):1644-1655. Levy MM, Fink MP, Marshall JC, et al. 2001 SCCM/ESICM/ACCP/ATS/SIS International Sepsis Definitions Conference. *Crit Care Med.* 2003;31(4):1250-1256.

ETIOLOGIES

There are 2 broad categories of MODS.[17] Primary MODS results from direct organ injury, such as from trauma, and occurs early after the injury. Secondary MODS occurs later and results from the systemic host response to an injury. For the remainder of the chapter, the term MODS is used to describe secondary MODS, which occurs far more frequently than primary MODS.

MODS is caused by inflammatory processes. Common etiologies are infection, trauma, aspiration pneumonitis, pancreatitis, surgery, blood product transfusions, ischemia-reperfusion, necrosis, and burns.[18] Other etiologies include cardiac arrest, malignancy, and vasculitis.

Surgical and nonsurgical patients can develop MODS. In patients with nonoperative MODS, the most frequent ICU admission diagnoses are cardiac arrest, sepsis, pneumonia, congestive heart failure, upper gastrointestinal (GI) bleeding, and nonoperative head trauma.[19] Postoperative MODS occurs most frequently following surgery for head trauma, elective abdominal aneurysm repairs, aortic dissection or rupture, GI perforation, GI inflammatory diseases, and GI malignancy. Other risk factors for the development of MODS include preexisting organ dysfunction, delayed or inadequate resuscitation, an ongoing infection or focus of inflammation, major hematoma, age 65 years or older, surgical complications, seriously deranged physiologic parameters on admission to the ICU, and chronic health problems.[12,13,18-21]

Sepsis is the most common cause of MODS. In septic shock, systemic inflammation triggers pathophysiologic processes that cause vasodilatation, relative or absolute hypovolemia, myocardial dysfunction, and an altered systemic blood flow distribution.[22] About half of the patients who succumb to septic shock die of multiple organ failure.

EPIDEMIOLOGY

MODS occurs in approximately 15% of ICU admissions[23] and is associated with up to 80% of ICU deaths.[2,19,24] MODS occurs more frequently and has a higher mortality in patients admitted to the ICU with medical as compared with those admitted with surgical diagnoses.[2,19,25] In addition, high Acute Physiology and Chronic Health Evaluation III scores on the first day of admission to the ICU are associated with MODS.[19]

For the general ICU population, the risk of MODS is related to age older than 65 years, severity of coexisting diseases, and a nonoperative ICU admission diagnosis.[2,19] However, trauma patients who develop MODS do not seem to fit this profile. A prospective study of multiple organ failure (MOF) following major trauma showed that age, a large red blood cell transfusion requirement, a high Injury Severity Score, a large base deficit, and elevated lactate levels are risk factors for the subsequent development of MOF.[26]

MODS SCORING SYSTEMS

Many scoring systems have been devised to assist with the diagnosis and quantification of the severity of MODS. The sepsis-related or sequential organ failure assessment (SOFA) score[14] and the MODS score[15] are widely used systems that take into account the number of dysfunctional organs or systems and the degree of dysfunction of each organ.

The SOFA *score* was created to describe organ dysfunction in individual patients and groups of patients over time.[14] It is calculated based on the degree of dysfunction of 6 organ systems (respiratory, renal, cardiovascular [CV], central nervous system [CNS], hepatic, and coagulation) and is commonly used to follow the progression of organ dysfunction rather than to predict outcome.

The MODS *score* was developed to provide a "reliable and meaningful index of the severity" of MODS in individual ICU patients and to quantify the association between the degree of dysfunction and the risk of mortality.[15] The MODS score incorporates 6 organ system evaluations (respiratory, renal, cardiovascular, CNS, hepatic, and hematologic). Data are collected repeatedly during the ICU stay. The highest possible score is 24, which indicates the most severe MODS.

The Denver Multi Organ Failure (MOF) *score* is widely used in outcome studies of trauma patients.[4] The revised Denver MOF score takes into account 4 organ systems: pulmonary, cardiac, renal, and hepatic. Each is assigned a grade based on the degree of dysfunction.

PROGNOSIS OF MODS

The mortality of MODS is in excess of 50%.[4,16,26,27] Studies consistently show that across all ICU populations, mortality in MODS is proportional to the number of failing organs. Single-organ failure is associated with a low mortality, whereas 3 failing organs is associated with 80% to 90% mortality, and mortality approaches 100% with 4 failing organs.[2,17,19,23] Mortality is higher in MODS patients older than 65 years.[2,28] The prognosis of MODS differs depending on the inciting process. For example, the mortality associated with MODS due to trauma was reported to be lower than that associated with MODS due to sepsis or cardiac arrest (45% vs 75%-80%, respectively).[19] Finally, the degree of physiologic derangement on the first day of failure of the organ is an important determinant of mortality.[19]

PATHOGENESIS

The combination of systemic inflammation (SIRS), microcirculatory abnormalities, and impaired oxygen delivery and/or use can all contribute to the development of MODS.[18,29,30] SIRS is initiated by mediators that are released into the circulation by inflammatory cells in response to infection and other inflammatory stimuli. Leukocytes, platelets, and endothelial cells participate in SIRS. Endothelial cells help to maintain homeostasis in the coagulation system and participate in leukocyte recruitment to sites of infection and inflammation.[31-34] Imbalances in the coagulation system can result in disseminated intravascular coagulopathy (DIC) and are believed to be important in the development of microvascular thrombosis.[35,36]

The GI tract has been postulated to contribute to MODS through the failure of mucosal integrity brought on by stresses such as trauma, burns, or septic shock. This is believed to result in translocation of bacteria and their products out of the GI tract lumen and/or to increased production of inflammatory mediators by the gut.[29,37,38] Thus far clinical studies have neither proven nor disproven this hypothesis.[29,39,40]

MODS: MANIFESTATIONS, COMPLICATIONS, PREVENTION, AND THERAPIES

MANIFESTATIONS

MODS can affect any organ or system (**Table 74-2**). Dysfunction may be mild or total. The lungs and circulatory system are most often involved.[2] Trauma patients often exhibit a biphasic pattern of organ failure.[26,41] Early organ failure (within 3 d of trauma) results from the initial shock, resuscitation, and tissue injury, whereas later organ failure (defined as >3 d after trauma) frequently results from infection.[41]

TABLE 74-2 Organs and Systems Affected by Multiple Organ Dysfunction Syndrome

Organ or System	Manifestations
Lung	Acute lung injury, acute respiratory distress syndrome, ventilator dependence
Cardiovascular	Arterial hypotension, hyperdynamic physiology, vasodilatation, myocardial dysfunction, pulmonary hypertension, shunting
Kidneys	Oliguria, anuria, renal failure, acute tubular necrosis, renal tubular acidoses, acid-base abnormalities, electrolyte abnormalities
Neurologic	Confusion, lethargy, agitation, coma
Liver	Elevated liver enzymes, hyperbilirubinemia, coagulopathy, hepatic encephalopathy
Hematologic	Anemia, thrombocytopenia, coagulation abnormalities, disseminated intravascular coagulopathy
Endocrine	Hyperglycemia, inappropriate adrenal response to stress ("relative adrenal insufficiency")
Metabolic	Electrolyte and glucose abnormalities, hyper- and hypokalemia, hyper- and hyponatremia, hypomagnesemia, hyper- and hypophosphatemia, hypocalcemia
Gastrointestinal (GI) tract	Hypomotility, inability to tolerate enteral nutrition, GI hemorrhage, stress ulcers

Acute Respiratory Failure Respiratory failure occurs in approximately 70% of patients with MODS.[42] Risk factors for ARDS include pneumonia, sepsis, aspiration, trauma, and pancreatitis. MODS patients with respiratory failure have a high mortality rate.[2] ALI and ARDS occur most frequently in patients with sepsis, particularly when the source of the sepsis is pulmonary.[43-45] Moreover, mortality is highest when ARDS is caused by sepsis.[46] A large study reported a 99% incidence of respiratory failure in trauma patients with MODS.[47] However, they also found that the presence of respiratory failure did not correlate with mortality.

Cardiovascular CV dysfunction occurs in approximately 87% of MODS cases and carries a high in-hospital mortality rate.[2] Patients may manifest CV instability secondary to hypovolemia, vasodilatation, and/or myocardial dysfunction. Septic patients who have been volume resuscitated are often described as "hyperdynamic"; that is, they have an elevated cardiac output associated with decreased systemic vascular tone. These classic CV manifestations of sepsis also occur in patients with MODS caused by other systemic inflammatory processes. Septic patients can also develop myocardial dysfunction, manifested as a decreased left ventricular ejection fraction, ventricular dilation, and an impaired contractile response to volume loading.

Dysrhythmias Patients with MODS may develop dysrhythmias on the basis of metabolic abnormalities, intravascular volume disturbances, hypoxemia, or myocardial ischemia. Atrial dysrhythmias are common. Although immediate interventions, such as cardioversion, may be required for hemodynamically unstable dysrhythmias, correction of the underlying stimulus is usually required to prevent further occurrences.

Renal Renal disturbances are common in MODS patients and range from mild renal dysfunction with an elevated blood urea nitrogen (BUN) and creatinine (Cr), to frank anuric renal failure.[48] The introduction of the RIFLE classification, which stands for "risk of renal failure: injury to the kidney, failure of kidney function, loss of kidney function, and end-stage renal failure," has greatly aided both in defining the severity of acute kidney injury and in the risk stratification and prognosis of ICU patients with kidney injury.[49,50] Based on stringent criteria for serum Cr levels and urine output, this classification system also allows early recognition of kidney injury and thus earlier institution of renal protective measures.

Renal dysfunction usually results from acute tubular necrosis (ATN). The urine sediment in ATN contains granular or "muddy" casts. Other causes of acute kidney injury include endogenous toxins such as myoglobin in patients with rhabdomyolysis, nephrotoxic drugs such as aminoglycosides or amphotericin B, intravenous (IV) contrast agents for imaging procedures, and cholesterol emboli caused by manipulation of the diseased aorta. The mortality in MODS patients with renal failure is high, particularly in the context of CV or respiratory failure.[2,28]

Hepatic A variety of hepatic disturbances may occur in noncirrhotic patients with MODS. These include elevation of liver enzymes, hyperbilirubinemia, hypoglycemia, and impaired synthesis of proteins, including clotting factors. Preexisting hepatic dysfunction may complicate MODS in several ways. First, patients with cirrhosis fare poorly when they develop MODS. Mortality rates in excess of 80% have been reported in cirrhotic patients with either coma, renal failure, CV instability, or acute respiratory failure.[51] Second, liver failure can further worsen in critically ill patients. Third, a coagulopathy and a propensity for bleeding may result from DIC and/or from decreased liver synthesis of clotting factors. Lastly, new acute liver failure can cause MODS, a situation that carries a particularly poor prognosis.[52]

Hematologic Multiple hematologic abnormalities occur in MODS patients. Patients commonly exhibit either leukocytosis or leukopenia. Coagulation problems may arise from impaired synthesis and/or from increased coagulation factor consumption. Thrombocytopenia occurs in DIC but may also result from decreased production or increased destruction from other causes.

Anemia Anemia results from acute blood loss from trauma, GI bleeding, surgery, and frequent phlebotomy. Cytokines may contribute by decreasing endogenous erythropoietin production, by directly hindering bone marrow production of red blood cells (RBCs), and by altering iron metabolism. These observations have led to development of the term *anemia of critical illness*.

Coagulopathy Coagulopathy is evaluated by measuring coagulation times (prothrombin time [PT] and activated partial thromboplastin time [aPTT]) and fibrinogen levels. A prolonged PT or aPTT can be caused by either an absence of coagulation factors or the presence of factor inhibitors. Transfusion with normal plasma should correct a factor deficiency. Factor inhibitors should be suspected when the prolonged PT or aPTT does not correct with administration of normal plasma. Antiphospholipid antibodies such as lupus anticoagulant can also produce a prolonged aPTT. Paradoxically, lupus anticoagulants and the antiphospholipid antibody syndrome are associated with thrombosis, not bleeding.

Platelet Abnormalities Platelets are vital in hemostasis. Three basic mechanisms are responsible for thrombocytopenia in ICU patients: decreased platelet production, increased platelet destruction or sequestration, or dilution. Transfusion of blood for massive blood loss causes dilutional thrombocytopenia. Thrombocytopenia also results from sequestration of platelets in the liver, spleen, and, in patients with acute respiratory failure, lungs.[53]

Drug-induced thrombocytopenias may be hard to diagnose because many drugs can impair platelet production rates. Heparin-induced thrombocytopenia (HIT) is often considered as the cause of thrombocytopenia in critically ill patients.[54] Treatment of HIT involves discontinuation of heparin administration, including both unfractionated heparin and low molecular weight heparins, and the use of alternative anticoagulants. Anticoagulant alternatives for patients with HIT include lepirudin, argatroban, and fondaparinux.[55] Lepirudin is cleared by the kidneys, whereas argatroban is cleared by the liver. Thus the choice of one agent over another depends on the patient's renal and hepatic function. Both agents have short plasma half-lives (80 min for lepirudin and 40 min for argatroban) allowing rapid reversal of anticoagulation after administration is stopped. Platelets should never be given to patients with type 2 HIT because of an increased risk of thrombosis after platelet transfusions.

Disseminated Intravascular Coagulation DIC is common in sepsis, occurring in up to 70% of patients with septic shock.[56] In DIC, there is simultaneous activation of both the coagulation and fibrinolytic systems. Activation of the fibrinolytic portion of the clotting system can lead to hemorrhage including widespread oozing of blood, and bleeding from wounds and procedure site. The activation of coagulation can result in thrombosis. One dramatic manifestation of thrombosis is digital necrosis, which can be severe enough to require amputation. It is believed that microvascular thrombosis causes impaired oxygen delivery to tissues and resultant ischemia and organ dysfunction. The diagnosis of DIC is suggested by prolongation of the PT and/or the aPTT, and a reduction in the platelet concentration. Elevated D-dimer and reduced plasma fibrinogen levels provide useful supplemental diagnostic tests but are not diagnostic of DIC and may be abnormal in other disorders.

Neurologic CNS manifestations range in severity from mild confusion and lethargy or agitation to frank coma. It is estimated that CNS disturbances occur in 70% of patients with sepsis.[57] The presence of severe neurologic impairment, as manifested by a Glasgow Coma Scale score higher than 6 in the context of MODS, is associated with a high mortality rate (≥70%).[2]

Patients with MODS may also develop profound neuromuscular weakness from deconditioning and/or critical illness polyneuropathy. This can be exacerbated by the use of corticosteroids and neuromuscular blocking agents.[58] Complications of weakness include difficulty weaning from mechanical ventilation and a prolonged rehabilitation period.[59]

Critically ill patients frequently require sedative = hypnotic agents and analgesics to treat anxiety and pain. Unfortunately, these very agents can significantly increase morbidity and mortality. Sedative-hypnotics are routinely titrated based on protocols that incorporate regular reassessment of the patient's level of pain and sedation, and daily interruptions of sedation. Both measures have been shown to reduce the complications of oversedation, including delirium and prolonged mechanical ventilation.[60,61] Typical regimens include analgesic agents such as opioids and ketamine, and hypnotic agents such as benzodiazepines and propofol.[62] Dexmedetomidine is also commonly used to facilitate sedation based on studies that suggest that as compared with benzodiazepines, this newer sedative allows patients to be more interactive with less delirium and to spend less time on mechanical ventilation.[63-65] Further studies are necessary to assess the merits dexmedetomidine in comparison with agents such as propofol. Agents commonly used to treat delirium in the ICU include haloperidol, and atypical antipsychotic agents such as olanzapine, risperidone, and quetiapine.

Metabolic/Endocrine Patients with MODS may have electrolyte abnormalities, including hyperkalemia, hypokalemia, hypernatremia, hyponatremia, hypocalcemia, hypomagnesemia, hyperphosphatemia, and/or hypophosphatemia. Glucose disturbances are common. Current evidence suggests that a moderate level of glycemic control using insulin infusions is sufficient to improve outcome in critically ill patients while avoiding the complication of hypoglycemia associated with tight glycemic control.[66]

Adrenal dysfunction is believed to complicate the course of many patients with septic shock. Although frank adrenal insufficiency is uncommon, there is evidence that critically ill patients experience a state of "relative adrenal insufficiency."[67] Although controversy exists over whether or not to use corticosteroids to treat septic shock, corticosteroids should still be considered in patients with refractory septic shock despite volume resuscitation and maximal inotropic support.[68,69] However the current data do not support using cosyntropin stimulation tests to identify patients to treat with corticosteroids.[69]

Gastrointestinal Common gastrointestinal disturbances in MODS patients include GI hypomotility and GI bleeding. GI dysmotility may lead to gastric distension, which increases the chance of regurgitation and aspiration. Critically ill patients often require nasogastric decompression. GI dysmotility may lead to intolerance of enteral nutrition. GI hemorrhage may result from stress ulceration. Critically ill patients who are at risk of stress ulceration should be treated with prophylactic agents (H_2 blockers, proton pump inhibitors, or sucralfate). Patients may also develop low-grade GI bleeding from mucosal breakdown from nasogastric tubes.

MODS AND PREDISPOSITION TO INFECTIONS

Patients with MODS have a propensity to develop infections,[4] which is believed to result from a state of immunosuppression.

PREVENTIVE STRATEGIES

Prevention of MODS is a major goal in managing critically ill patients. Preventive strategies include prompt therapy targeting the underlying source of inflammation, optimizing oxygen delivery to balance the increased demands that accompany SIRS, maintaining adequate tissue perfusion, and providing physiologic support to maintain homeostasis when required. Other strategies include prevention of the loss of gut integrity and ICU-related complications such as ventilator-associated pneumonia and catheter-related bloodstream infections. GI tract integrity may be supported with early enteral nutrition,[4,70,71] VAP may be reduced by diligent head-of-bed elevation and oral hygiene,[72] and central line infections may be reduced by improved sterile insertion techniques and careful line maintenance.[73]

MANAGING PATIENTS WITH ESTABLISHED MODS

The management of MODS involves a combination of locating and reversing the condition(s) that are driving the MODS, and supportive therapies that target specific organs and systems.

SUPPORTIVE THERAPIES

Respiratory failure is managed with mechanical ventilation, the CV system is supported with volume, vasopressors, and inotropes, and renal failure is managed with renal replacement therapies. Management of specific organs and systems is discussed later in "Preoperative Preparation of Patients with MODS."

ADJUNCTIVE THERAPIES

Numerous studies have tested the effects of agents that interfere with inflammatory responses. Most of these studies focused on SIRS caused by sepsis.

Antimediator Therapies Experimental therapies that have targeted specific inflammatory mediators including cytokines such as tumor necrosis factor or interleukin-1, have not improved patient outcomes in large clinical trials.[74]

Activated Protein C Activated protein C (APC) is currently approved by the US Food and Drug Administration for the treatment of patients with severe sepsis in the appropriate clinical setting. APC is postulated to exert its effects by preventing microvascular thrombosis and by modulating inflammation. Although initial studies showed a significant mortality reduction in patients with severe sepsis,[36] concerns about the efficacy and potential complications of APC have reduced its widespread use. Therefore, another large multicenter trial of APC is currently underway.

Insulin Therapy Based on recent studies and concerns for deleterious hypoglycemia, tight glycemic control, targeting plasma glucose concentrations between 80 and 108 mg/dL has given way to moderate glycemic control targeting plasma glucose concentrations of more than 180 mg/dL.[66] Protocols to regulate insulin infusions for effective glycemic control are commonly used.

Nutritional Support Patients with MODS are often profoundly malnourished. The GI tract is the preferred route of nutrition, both for the benefits of maintaining GI mucosal integrity and for decreasing the infectious complications associated with parenteral nutrition. Studies suggest that early enteral nutrition may modulate the systemic stress and immune response to reduce infections in ICU patients.[71] MODS patients often do not tolerate high-rate enteral feedings, but many practitioners advocate continuing tube feeds at a low rate for these patients to prevent mucosal atrophy. For those patients who cannot be fed enterally, total parenteral nutrition (TPN) can be used. Enteral or parenteral supplementation with arginine, glutamine, and ω-3 fatty acids are being studied for their immune-modulating properties in certain illnesses, such as ARDS, and may be useful in specific critically ill populations.[71]

SURGICAL AND NONSURGICAL PROCEDURES IN PATIENTS WITH MODS

Patients with MODS require a variety of procedures. Some may be necessary to correct the underlying cause of the MODS, whereas other procedures may be necessary to deal with the complications of MODS. The timing of procedures should be based on the urgency of the intervention balanced against the precariousness of the patient's physiologic status.

COMMON SURGICAL PROCEDURES IN PATIENTS WITH MODS BASED ON ETIOLOGY

Infection Infection is the most common cause of MODS. Although some infections may be treated with antibiotics alone, many require either surgical debridement or drainage. Immediate debridement for necrotizing fasciitis and infectious myonecrosis is of paramount importance. Similarly, exploratory laparotomies are performed immediately on patients with sepsis due to intestinal perforation. Other infections that may require surgery include toxic megacolon caused by *Clostridium difficile* colitis, empyema that has failed thoracostomy drainage as a result of a pleural peel or adhesions, and mediastinitis. Abscesses located in the thorax, abdomen, and pelvis may be treated with drainage, either with surgery or using percutaneous catheters.

Pancreatitis Patients with pancreatitis may require surgery for pancreatic necrosis, pancreatic hemorrhage, or drainage of pancreatic abscesses or infected pseudocysts.[75]

Trauma Often surgery is performed early in the trauma patient's course. However, in some situations, surgery may be delayed while the patient is stabilized. Some of these patients develop MODS before definitive procedures for their traumatic injuries, for instance, before pinning of hip fractures or before definitive procedures for spine stabilization.

Limb Ischemia-Necrosis Patients with limb ischemia-necrosis may require fasciotomies, vessel exploration with revascularization (embolectomy or bypass procedures), or amputation.

Burns Patients may require excision and grafting, and other treatments.

SURGICAL PROCEDURES STEMMING FROM MODS

Common procedures in MODS patients include tracheostomy tube placement for ventilator dependence or the inability to handle secretions, and placement of feeding tubes for nutritional support and drug administration. Other procedures that are sometimes required include amputations of digits or distal limbs and debridement of secondarily infected wounds.

NONSURGICAL PROCEDURES IN PATIENTS WITH MODS

Sometimes nonsurgical procedures are required to treat the underlying etiology of MODS, such as catheter drainage of intra-abdominal fluid collections. Other nonsurgical procedures include placement of central venous, peripheral arterial, and hemodialysis catheters, and bronchoscopy.

PREOPERATIVE ASSESSMENT AND CONSENT

A thorough preoperative evaluation with prioritization of the importance of the various physiologic derangements is essential in anticipating the needs for every phase of the perioperative period (**Table 74-3**).

TABLE 74-3 Preoperative Assessment and Optimization

Organ System	Questions to Answer
Cardiovascular	• Is the patient adequately volume resuscitated? • Does the patient require pressors or inotropic agents? • Is there any clinical evidence of hypoperfusion
Respiratory	• What are the ventilator settings? • Does the patient need a critical care ventilator in the OR?
Neurologic	• What is the patient's baseline neurologic status? • What sedatives is the patient receiving, and will they be continued intraoperatively?
Renal	• Does the patient have renal dysfunction? • If the patient is on renal replacement therapy, what is the volume status, electrolyte balance, and acid-base status?
Endocrine	• Is there any evidence of adrenal insufficiency? • How is the patient's glycemic control?
Hematologic	• What is the patient's hemoglobin/hematocrit? • What is the patient's coagulation status? • Is the patient receiving anticoagulants? Type?

Based on a comprehensive preoperative evaluation, the anesthesiologist should (1) determine whether or not additional therapies should be initiated preoperatively to optimize the patient's condition, (2) anticipate and arrange for appropriate transportation to the operating room, (3) prepare an anesthetic plan, (4) prepare the operating room in advance for the arrival of the patient, and (5) set up tentative plans for postoperative care. Several of these issues are discussed in more detail in other chapters.

The preoperative assessment should include a review of past and present medical problems, a targeted physical examination, a complete review of the medications and available laboratory and radiographic data, assessment of the ventilator settings, a review of in situ tubes and lines, and, in some cases, a clarification of the plans for resuscitation in the operating room.

REVIEW OF PAST MEDICAL HISTORY

The basic aspects of the past medical history that are important in planning any anesthetic should be reviewed. Preexisting vascular disease, cardiac dysfunction, dysrhythmias, the presence of pacemakers or an implantable cardioverter-defibrillator, preexisting respiratory disease, and cirrhosis may all profoundly impair the response of MODS patients to anesthesia and surgery.

REVIEW OF RECENT HISTORY

A thorough knowledge of the inciting event(s) and all of the organs and systems that are involved is a crucial part of the preoperative assessment.

Respiratory Information about the degree and nature of respiratory dysfunction and past responses to different ventilation strategies should be actively sought. The chart should be reviewed for information on the airway, including anatomic issues with intubation, difficulties with the endotracheal tube or cuff, quantity and frequency of suctioning of respiratory secretions, and any need for cervical spine immobilization.

Circulation Critically ill patients have a myriad of cardiovascular problems. The patient's current hemodynamic status, including intravascular volume status, myocardial function, and peripheral vascular tone, should be ascertained. Bedside clinical assessment can provide useful information about global perfusion. Indications of decreased perfusion include oliguria, clouded sensorium, delayed capillary refill, and cool skin. However, organ dysfunction and regional hypoperfusion can occur in the absence of overt signs of global hypoperfusion.[76] Elevated serum lactate may reflect anaerobic metabolism caused by hypoperfusion, and a rising lactate may be an indicator of septic shock. Arterial waveform analyses have been shown to be beneficial in predicting the patient's fluid responsiveness.[77] The central venous pressure may reflect intravascular volume status in some patients but may be an unreliable estimate of the patient's volume status in the context of cardiac dysfunction, pulmonary hypertension, or elevated intra-abdominal or intrathoracic pressures. Patients with these problems may benefit from echocardiography or pulmonary artery catheterization to help estimate volume status, ventricular filling, myocardial function, and vasomotor tone.

In addition to perfusion and volume assessment, the preoperative evaluation should note the degree of hemodynamic instability, electrocardiographic evidence of dysrhythmias or ischemia, and the hemodynamic responses to vasopressors, inotropes, and fluids.

Renal Renal dysfunction along with its consequent metabolic and intravascular volume disturbances should be identified. Evaluation should focus on volume status, electrolyte balance, and acid-base status. Physical examination may reveal the presence of a pericardial friction rub secondary to significant uremia or rales secondary to pulmonary edema. Patients can be hyper-, hypo-, or euvolemic. In fact, these patients are often total-body-volume overloaded but intravascularly depleted. Data such as BUN, Cr, plasma potassium, arterial blood pH, and urine output rate should be obtained.

In patients receiving renal replacement therapy (RRT), the type of therapy—continuous venovenous hemofiltration (CVVH), continuous venovenous hemodialysis, or intermittent HD (hemodialysis)—should be noted. If the patient is on HD, the frequency and timing of the last dialysis should be noted. The ability of the patient to tolerate being without a continuous form of RRT should be assessed. In patients on RRT, electrolyte levels should be measured often. Either hyperkalemia from inadequate clearance or hypokalemia from aggressive preoperative dialysis can lead to life-threatening dysrhythmias. Profound hypophosphatemia from excessive clearance can lead to muscle weakness, increased susceptibility to muscle relaxants, and respiratory insufficiency. A compensated mild metabolic acidosis is common in patients with chronic renal failure. Profound acidemia can occur quickly in the context of shock because of a diminished serum buffering capacity. In this setting, hemofiltration may be performed with the explicit goal of bicarbonate repletion to increase the serum buffering capacity. Uremia can cause platelet dysfunction that improves with dialysis or with the infusion of cryoprecipitate, 1-deamino-8-D-arginine-vasopressin (DDAVP), or estrogen conjugates.

Hepatic The presence of hepatic dysfunction can have important effects on a patient's response to surgery. Hepatic failure can cause hypoglycemia, coagulation disturbances, and impaired processing of drugs and toxins. Blood studies that should be considered preoperatively include coagulation profile (PT/PTT), platelet count, glucose, bilirubin, albumin, lactate, and transaminase levels to assess the degree of liver injury and synthetic dysfunction.

Hematologic Anemia, thrombocytopenia, and coagulation dysfunction should be identified, and in some cases corrected, preoperatively. It may be necessary to assess the hemoglobin, platelet concentration, and coagulation studies immediately before surgery. The patient's medication record should be reviewed for anticoagulants such as heparin, Coumadin (warfarin), thrombolytic agents, and antiplatelet drugs.

Metabolic/Endocrine Major metabolic and endocrine disturbances and recent use of steroids should be identified. The acid-base status should be analyzed. Appropriate preoperative chemical studies in MODS patients include measuring plasma potassium, sodium, chloride, bicarbonate, calcium, magnesium, phosphate, glucose, and arterial blood gases (pH, $Paco_2$, Pao_2).

The insulin infusion rate should be noted as well as how frequently the rate requires adjustment.

Neurologic Baseline neurologic function should be ascertained. Dosages and rates of infusions of sedative-hypnotic and analgesic agents should be noted, and a decision made whether or not these agents should be continued intraoperatively. Opioids, benzodiazepine, and hypnotic infusions used in the ICU may be titrated intraoperatively as part of the anesthetic or alternative agents can be given.

Infection The sites and severity of infection should be noted. Patients who are actively infected often have more pronounced hemodynamic depression with anesthetic administration. In addition, if the purpose of the surgery is source control, manipulation of the infected site may precipitate or worsen existing instability, including producing hypotension, metabolic acidosis, DIC, and/or worsening respiratory dysfunction.

PHYSICAL EXAMINATION

The respiratory system should be evaluated by visual assessment of the airway and the respiratory pattern, and auscultation of breath sounds. Signs of respiratory distress such as tachypnea, labored breathing, accessory respiratory muscle use, and inability to clear respiratory secretions should be noted. In addition to assessing the patient's anatomy for the ease of direct laryngoscopy, the airway examination should note the position and fixation of a preexisting endotracheal tube, the presence of tracheal deviation, and the degree of airway edema. The chest should be auscultated and abnormalities noted. Positions of arterial, peripheral venous, and central venous catheters, and other drainage tubes should be noted. Pressure sores and areas of skin breakdown should be identified to plan for appropriate padding in the operating room.

REVIEW OF MONITORS

A review of the monitors and lines already present and any technical issues associated with these monitors is crucial. Trends of hemodynamic parameters and peak airway pressures should be noted. In addition to standard ICU monitors, including pulse oximetry, electrocardiogram (ECG), and noninvasive blood pressure, monitors that are commonly used in patients with MODS include intra-arterial catheters, central venous catheters, and intracranial pressure monitors.

REVIEW OF SCHEDULED MEDICATIONS AND INFUSIONS

All medications should be reviewed. There should be close attention to continuous drug infusions, including rates of infusions, the lines being used for infusions, and their compatibility with drugs that will be infused in the operating room. Because abrupt cessation of TPN can cause hypoglycemia, plans should be made to either continue the TPN infusion in the operating room or to provide another continuous source of sugar, such as 10% aqueous dextrose solution ($D_{10}W$).

LABORATORY AND RADIOGRAPHIC DATA

The basic laboratory data to review should include recent values of electrolytes (Na^+, K^+, Cl^-, HCO_3^-, ionized Ca^{2+}, Mg^{2+}), BUN and Cr, hemoglobin or hematocrit, coagulation studies, and an ECG. Liver function studies, including transaminases and bilirubin levels, also may be useful. All pertinent radiographic data should be reviewed, and the chest radiograph should be visualized to assess endotracheal tube positioning and seek evidence of infiltrates, pulmonary edema, pneumothorax, and pleural fluid.

VENTILATOR SETTINGS

Most patients with MODS require mechanical ventilation. The details of the ventilator settings should be noted, including the mode of ventilation (controlled vs spontaneous ventilation, pressure vs volume ventilation), the ventilator rate, the Fio_2, the level of positive end-expiratory pressure (PEEP), tidal volume and airway pressures, and inspiratory-to-expiratory (I:E) ratios or inspiratory time. Often the standard operating room ventilators are inadequate for patients with low compliance and severe respiratory failure and an ICU ventilator may need to be used for transport and intraoperative management. Generally, patients receiving high levels of PEEP should travel with a PEEP valve. In patients with severe respiratory failure, it may be helpful to perform a trial of manual ventilation in the ICU before transporting to the operating room. In some critical situations it may be appropriate to perform the procedure in the ICU.

CONSENT FOR ANESTHESIA

Unless the surgery is emergent, informed consent must be obtained from either the patient or from a designated surrogate if the patient is unable to give consent.

RESUSCITATION STATUS

Occasionally, critically ill patients who have a do not resuscitate (DNR) order require surgical procedures. In some cases, based on the wishes of the patient or their surrogate decision maker, the DNR status is suspended for the intraoperative and immediate postoperative period. This is based on the notion that acute, but reversible intra- and postoperative events, as opposed to the underlying process, may precipitate a cardiac arrest during and immediately after surgery. It is important to clarify whether or not the ICU DNR status will remain in effect or will be suspended in the operating room.

PREOPERATIVE PREPARATION OF PATIENTS WITH MODS

Whenever possible, efforts should be made to correct physiologic derangements and optimize the patient's condition before surgery. Examples of situations that may require preoperative optimization include CV instability, respiratory failure, bronchospasm, renal failure, coagulopathy, thrombocytopenia, electrolyte imbalances, and hyperglycemia or hypoglycemia.

IMMEDIATE VERSUS DELAYED SURGERY

The risk-to-benefit ratio of doing immediate surgery versus delaying surgery for optimization must be carefully assessed. The extremes are usually obvious: Totally elective surgery should not be performed until the patient's physiologic/metabolic situation has been fully optimized, whereas emergency surgery, such as for a ruptured aortic aneurysm or necrotizing fasciitis, needs to be performed before or during optimization. For urgent surgery, there may be sufficient time available to improve physiologic and metabolic parameters. Decisions about the timing of surgery are made by close communication between the anesthesiologist, the surgeon, and the intensivist.

RESPIRATORY

Preoperative optimization of respiratory status may include treatment of bronchospasm with bronchodilators and steroids, pulmonary suctioning for copious secretions, and antibiotics if the clinical scenario is consistent with a respiratory infection. Patients with a tenuous respiratory status may need to be intubated before they are moved to the operating room. A chest tube should be placed if a pneumothorax is present and the patient is to receive positive pressure ventilation.

Mechanical ventilation with positive pressure can cause ventilator-associated lung injury[78] and may play a role in causing or worsening MODS.[79] A lung protective strategy of mechanical ventilation in ARDS has been shown to decrease mortality, improve respiratory function, and decrease MODS.[80] The ARDS Network strategy of limiting tidal volumes and airway pressures has changed the approach to ARDS. The current standards for mechanical ventilation of patients with ARDS are reviewed in **Table 74-4**.[81] With the ARDS network strategy, permissive hypercapnia is used as long as an acceptable arterial pH can be maintained. Recent studies suggest that permissive hypercapnia and acidosis may be protective in early ARDS and sepsis.[82-84] However, the degree of hypercapnia should be limited in patients with preexisting metabolic acidosis, and hypercapnia is contraindicated in patients with increased intracranial pressure.

Several other therapies have been investigated in patients with refractory hypoxemia. Inhaled nitric oxide, prone positioning, high-frequency oscillatory ventilation, and extracorporeal membrane oxygenation have all been shown to improve hypoxemia in the short term, but thus far, none have demonstrated a long-term mortality benefit.[15,85,86] The

TABLE 74-4 Recommended Ventilator Settings for Patients With Acute Lung Injury or Acute Respiratory Distress Syndrome

Ventilator Mode	Volume Assist Control
Tidal volume	6 mL/kg of predicted body weight
Plateau pressure	≥30 cm H_2O
Ventilator rate	6-35 breaths/min to achieve pH goal of 7.3-7.45
I:E ration	1:1-1:3
Oxygenation	Pao_2 55-80 mm Hg
	Spo_2 88-95%
Fio_2/PEEP combinations	0.3 and 5
	0.4 and 5
	0.4 and 8
	0.5 and 8
	0.5 and 10
	0.6 and 10
	0.7 and 10
	0.7 and 12
	0.7 and 14
	0.8 and 14
	0.9 and 14
	0.9 and 16
	0.9 and 18
	1.0 and 18
	1.0 and 20
	1.0 and 22
	1.0 and 24
	PEEP could be increased up to 34 cm H_2O

Fio_2, fraction of inspired oxygen; I:E, inspiration-to-expiration ratio; PEEP, positive end-expiratory pressure; Spo_2, oxygen saturation as measured by pulse oximetry.

From Brower RG, Matthay MA, Morris A, et al. Ventilation with lower tidal volumes as compared with traditional tidal volumes for acute lung injury and the acute respiratory distress syndrome. The Acute Respiratory Distress Syndrome Network. *N Engl J Med.* 2000;342:1301.

worldwide clinical experience with severe ARDS caused by the H1N1 influenza virus that emerged in 2009 has renewed interest in many of these rescue modalities.[87] If these adjunctive therapies have been implemented in the ICU preoperatively, consideration should be given to the necessity and urgency of the planned surgical procedure, and efforts should be made to wean patients off these modalities before transport to the operating room.

CARDIOVASCULAR

Patients with MODS may have hemodynamic instability as a result of impaired myocardial function, decreased systemic vascular tone, hypovolemia, and/or restrictive and obstructive processes that impair ventricular filling. Anesthesia and surgery may further complicate the hemodynamic issues. Poor cardiac contractility and low vascular tone may be exacerbated by inhaled or IV anesthetics, and hemodynamic instability may be worsened by blood loss and third space fluid losses.

Before volume repletion, patients with septic shock may have a combination of low peripheral vascular tone, reduced cardiac filling pressures, and decreased stroke volume. A hyperdynamic picture can emerge after volume resuscitation. Hypovolemia should be corrected with balanced electrolyte solutions and/or blood products, depending on the etiology and associated issues (such as a coagulopathy). Fluid infusion alone will reverse the hypotension and restore hemodynamic stability in roughly half of the septic patients who present with hypotension.[76] If fluid resuscitation fails to restore adequate systemic blood pressure and organ perfusion promptly, infusion of vasopressor agents should be initiated.[76] The choice of vasopressors in sepsis has been the subject of debate. Norepinephrine and dopamine have both emerged as acceptable first-line agents, whereas phenylephrine and epinephrine are not currently recommended as first-line agents.[69] In addition, recent evidence suggests there is a relative "vasopressin-depleted" state in sepsis,[88] which has prompted an evaluation of the early addition of vasopressin for the treatment of septic shock.[89] Most recently, dopamine and norepinephrine have been compared with each other in the treatment of shock.[90] Although no difference was observed in 28-day mortality between the 2 groups, those receiving dopamine experienced more dysrhythmias, and the subgroup of patients with cardiogenic shock receiving dopamine had a higher mortality rate.[90]

In some patients pulmonary artery catheters (PACs) may be used to facilitate preoperative optimization and/or for intraoperative and postoperative care. In recent years, PAC use has fallen out of favor in ICU patients and in the intraoperative setting based on multiple studies that failed to show a survival benefit of the PAC.[91] Transesophageal echocardiography has replaced the PAC for intraoperative monitoring in many surgical situations. However, the PAC may still be useful for patients undergoing major surgery who have significant myocardial dysfunction, pulmonary hypertension, or constrictive or restrictive cardiac processes.

RENAL

Goals for renal optimization before surgery include correction of metabolic and physiologic derangements, and protecting the kidneys from further damage. Whenever possible metabolic disturbances should be corrected before surgery. Some patients with renal failure may require preoperative RRT to treat metabolic acidosis, electrolyte imbalances, uremic pericarditis, or volume overload. Hyperkalemia should be corrected, either with binding agents such as sodium polystyrene sulfonate or with RRT. Consideration should be given to infusing DDAVP to correct uremic platelet dysfunction.

Both CVVH and intermittent hemodialysis are used in critically ill patients who require RRT. However, CVVH is often preferred because it is better tolerated hemodynamically and allows continuous control of fluid balance and toxin removal. In hemofiltration, blood under pressure passes along one side of a highly permeable membrane that allows transfer of both water and substances below a molecular weight of approximately 20 000 Da.[92] Urea, Cr, and phosphate are cleared from the blood at similar rates. Larger molecules, such as heparin, insulin, and vancomycin, are also cleared. The filtrate is discarded and the patient receives a replacement fluid composed of physiologic levels of the major crystalloid components of plasma. Total-body-fluid balance is regulated by varying the volume of replacement fluid.

A variety of factors may have a negative impact on kidney function. Intravascular hypovolemia, systemic inflammation, and the infusion of nephrotoxins such as IV contrast agents can all contribute to perioperative renal failure. Preventive measures include optimization of intravascular volume and avoidance of nephrotoxins. In patients who are to receive an IV contrast agent, preemptive strategies should be considered, including volume loading, alkalinization using IV $NaHCO_3$, and/or administration of *N*-acetylcysteine.[93]

HEPATIC

Patients with liver dysfunction have a variety of issues. Hypoglycemia should be identified and plasma glucose levels should be maintained in a normal range using a dextrose infusion. Severe coagulopathy should be corrected. Hepatic encephalopathy should be treated with lactulose.

HEMATOLOGIC

Critically ill patients often have anemia, coagulopathy, and thrombocytopenia. Their preoperative management will depend on the cause and severity of the disturbance, and the nature of the surgery. The anesthetic plan should take into account the anticipated blood loss for the procedure and the risks and benefits of stopping anticoagulant therapy preoperatively. If transfusion of blood products is anticipated, an adequate recipient sample should be available in the blood bank and the availability of sufficient supplies of blood products should be confirmed preoperatively. Patients who have had multiple transfusions may have developed circulating antibodies to non-ABO antigens. A consultation with a blood bank physician may be needed to select appropriate blood components for transfusion.

Anemia RBC transfusions are given to augment oxygen delivery and to avoid the deleterious effects of oxygen debt. ICU patients are at increased risk for complications of transfusion therapy. Current recommendations are that in the absence of active coronary artery disease, RBC transfusions should only be given for hemoglobin levels of 7.0 g/dL or lower.[94,95]

Coagulopathy Coagulopathy may result from consumptive processes such as DIC or from decreased factor production, as occurs in hepatic failure. Prophylactic administration of plasma products may be indicated to correct a coagulopathy before invasive procedures. If there is active bleeding, plasma products should be administered until the bleeding stops or the coagulopathy is reversed.[94,96] Vitamin K administration is indicated if vitamin K deficiency is present to raise the levels of vitamin K-dependent clotting factors (II, VII, IX, and X).

In the absence of coagulation inhibitors (including heparin) and in the presence of adequate fibrinogen levels (>100 mg/dL), hemostasis can usually be achieved when the activity of coagulation factors is at least 25% to 30% of normal. Fresh-frozen plasma (FFP) contains all of the plasma clotting factors and is used to correct coagulopathies that result from a factor deficiency or from anticoagulation with warfarin. Cryoprecipitate is rich in von Willebrand factor, factor VIII, factor XIII, and fibrinogen, and it is used to treat deficiencies of fibrinogen and factor XIII, and to manage von Willebrand disease.

Some patients may be receiving anticoagulation therapy because of deep vein thrombosis, atrial fibrillation or atrial flutter, the presence of prosthetic valves, or HIT. If possible, time should be allowed for Coumadin anticoagulation to reverse before, which may require several days. For emergent or urgent procedures, the PT can be rapidly corrected with FFP. If vitamin K is used to reverse the effects of Coumadin, very low doses should be administered (about 1 mg) because larger doses may make it difficult to re-anticoagulate the patient after the procedure. Patients with severe vascular disease or with coronary artery stents may be receiving antiplatelet agents such as Plavix (clopidogrel) and aspirin. When possible, surgery should be delayed in patients who are on Plavix until 7 days after the last dose. Consideration should be given to continuing aspirin in patients who have drug-eluting stents because they may be at risk for perioperative stent thrombosis.

Thrombocytopenia Platelet transfusions are used to manage patients who are bleeding or who are at risk of bleeding as a consequence of thrombocytopenia or impaired platelet function. Surgical bleeding solely caused by thrombocytopenia usually occurs when platelet concentrations are below 50 000/μL, and spontaneous bleeding occurs when platelet levels drop below 10 000/μL. However, additional factors, such as a concomitant coagulopathy, fever, renal failure, or treatment with nonsteroidal anti-inflammatory drugs, may increase the bleeding risk from severe thrombocytopenia. Consequently, the threshold platelet concentration for triggering a prophylactic platelet transfusion should take into account these clinical considerations.[94,96]

METABOLIC/ENDOCRINE

Acid-Base Status Acid-base disturbances may complicate intraoperative management and/or be exacerbated by major surgery. For instance, metabolic acidosis may worsen during and after a surgery in which there is hemorrhage. Metabolic acidosis may also result from ischemia-reperfusion events, such as relief of vascular occlusion, opening an aortic cross clamp, or releasing a tourniquet on a limb at the conclusion of a peripheral orthopedic procedure.

In the preoperative period, acid-base disturbances should be identified, classified, corrected, if severe. Common causes of metabolic acidosis in MODS patients include impaired tissue perfusion from hypovolemia and/or hypotension, limb or GI vascular occlusion, renal failure, and administration of large volumes of normal saline.

Respiratory acidosis may be managed by increasing the minute ventilation. Some patients with severe hypercapnic respiratory failure do not augment carbon dioxide exchange with increased minute ventilation due to a very high dead space fraction.[97] Moreover, currently used lung protective ventilation strategies often require patients to have a high $Paco_2$. Perioperatively, the acidosis of permissive hypercapnia may be more problematic because of the propensity to develop a superimposed metabolic acidosis.

Electrolytes If time permits, electrolyte abnormalities should be corrected before surgery. CVVH or hemodialysis may be required to correct hyperkalemia. Hypokalemia and hypomagnesemia can generally be corrected using IV supplementation. If surgery is emergent, IV treatment with insulin and glucose, and rectal or oral administration of sodium polystyrene sulfonate may be required to treat hyperkalemia.

Glucose Hyperglycemia and hypoglycemia should be corrected with insulin and glucose infusions, respectively. All patients who are receiving an insulin infusion should also receive an infusion of glucose to prevent hypoglycemia. Consideration should be given to continuing insulin infusions intraoperatively and measuring frequent blood sugar levels.

Adrenal Dysfunction Adrenal insufficiency should be considered in patients with persistent vasopressor requirements despite adequate volume repletion and other appropriate therapies. In addition, patients who have been receiving steroids for sustained periods of time may have suppressed adrenal function, and they may require perioperative "stress-dose" steroids.

PLANNING THE ANESTHETIC AND PREPARING THE OPERATING ROOM FOR PATIENTS WITH MODS

PLANNING THE ANESTHETIC

As is the case for all procedures, the anesthetic should be carefully planned and tailored to the individual patient's constellation of problems/issues. Specifics of developing the anesthetic plan in critically ill patients with MODS is reviewed elsewhere in this text.

DECISIONS REGARDING CONTINUATION OF INTENSIVE CARE UNIT THERAPIES IN THE OPERATING ROOM

During the preoperative visit, the anesthesiologist will decide whether or not to continue various therapies that are ongoing in the ICU. Some therapies may be too cumbersome to implement in the operating room. For instance, because CVVH requires extra equipment and extensive education for proper use, if it is continued in the operating room, the presence of additional personnel with CVVH expertise will be necessary. The anesthesiologist will also assess the need to continue infusions such as TPN, sedative-hypnotics, opioids, vasoactive agents, and insulin. If the patient requires high levels of ventilatory support or a complicated mode of ventilation, arrangements should be made to use an ICU ventilator in the operating room and to have someone who is skilled in its use immediately available to assist with ventilatory changes in the operating room.

PREPARING THE OPERATING ROOM

The operating room should be completely ready to receive the patient before leaving the ICU. The operating room should be equipped with an ICU ventilator, if appropriate, and should be stocked with the same vasopressors and inotropic agents that the patient is receiving in the ICU.

TRANSPORTING PATIENTS WITH MODS TO THE OPERATING ROOM

Transportation to the operating room can be risky. This topic is reviewed in detail in Chapter 78. Briefly, the anesthetist should plan to personally accompany the patient from the ICU to the operating room. Arrangements should be made to continue monitoring appropriate parameters, such as systemic arterial, central venous, pulmonary arterial, and intracranial pressures. It may be necessary to transport the patient with severe respiratory failure with an ICU ventilator. Transport with a PEEP valve may be appropriate in patients who are PEEP dependent and who can tolerate short periods of manual ventilation. An early trial of manual ventilation in the ICU may be helpful in determining if a respiratory failure patient can tolerate traveling from the ICU to the operating room.

SUMMARY

As technologies and therapies for basic diseases and acute processes such as shock and respiratory failure advance, a modern syndrome has evolved. MODS is an enigmatic process that is caused by generalized inflammation and microvascular circulatory abnormalities. The similarity of MODS resulting from either infectious or noninfectious diseases suggests that common pathways are involved.

Anesthesiologists are frequently involved in the care of patients with MODS, either in the ICU or in the operating room. MODS patients require surgery to treat the primary processes that have caused MODS or to deal with complications. The anesthesiologist will be involved in decisions regarding the timing of surgery and in optimizing the patient for surgery. Communication between the anesthesiologist, the ICU team, and the surgeon is crucial as part of preoperative preparation.

Before transport to the operating room, a comprehensive plan tailored to each patient's individual constellation of abnormalities should be in place. Preoperative planning should include making informed decisions regarding continuation of therapies such as CVVH, TPN, and insulin; arrangements for the patient's ventilator to accompany the patient to the operating room if appropriate; sedation and analgesia; availability of appropriate fluids, drugs, blood products and monitoring equipment; and a clear understanding of the plan regarding perioperative resuscitation for unexpected cardiac arrest or catastrophic events. Preoperative and intraoperative interventions will be dictated by the pattern and intensity of organ failure.

KEY REFERENCES

- Beal AL, Cerra FB. Multiple organ failure syndrome in the 1990s. Systemic inflammatory response and organ dysfunction. *JAMA.* 1994;271(3):226-233.
- Bone RC, Balk RA, Cerra FB, et al. Definitions for sepsis and organ failure and guidelines for the use of innovative therapies in sepsis. The ACCP/SCCM Consensus Conference Committee. American College of Chest Physicians/Society of Critical Care Medicine. *Chest.* 1992;101(6):1644-1655.
- Dellinger RP, Levy MM, Carlet JM. Surviving Sepsis Campaign: international guidelines for management of severe sepsis and septic shock: 2008. *Intensive Care Med.* 2008;34(1):17-60.
- NICE-SUGAR Study Investigators, Finfer S, Chittock DR, et al. Intensive versus conventional glucose control in critically ill patients. *N Engl J Med.* 2009;360(13):1283-1297.
- Levy MM, Fink MP, Marshall JC, et al. 2001 SCCM/ESICM/ACCP/ATS/SIS International Sepsis Definitions Conference. *Crit Care Med.* 2003;31(4):1250-1256.
- Sprung CL, Annane D, Keh D. Hydrocortisone therapy for patients with septic shock. *N Engl J Med.* 2008;358(2):111-124.

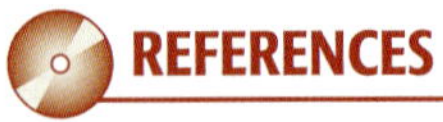

REFERENCES

Complete references available on DVD and online version at www.LongneckerAnesthesiology.com

CHAPTER 75 Evaluation and Anesthetic Management of the Burn-Injured Patient

Edward A. Bittner
J. A. Jeevendra Martyn

KEY POINTS

1. Hemodynamics in the early phase of severe burn injury are characterized by a reduction in cardiac output and increased systemic and pulmonary vascular resistance with or without pulmonary edema. Approximately 3 to 5 days after major burn injury, a hyperdynamic and hypermetabolic state begins with tachycardia, increased stroke volume, hyperthermia, and increased protein catabolism.
2. Patients with severe burn injury often suffer from nonthermal traumatic injuries. Failure to diagnose these associated injuries during initial evaluation can lead to serious morbidity and mortality. All burn patients should be approached initially as multiple-trauma patients.
3. Inhalation injury is a major source of mortality in burn patients. If the history and physical examination suggest inhalation injury, one should have a low threshold for early intubation.
4. Multiple fluid resuscitation formulas exist for estimating fluid needs and differ somewhat in their recommendations for the amount of crystalloid and colloid replacement. The Parkland formula, one of the most popular resuscitation regimens, recommends using 4 mL per percentage total body surface area (%TBSA) burn per kilogram administered over the first 24 hours, with half of this calculated volume administered during the first 8 postinjury hours. The remaining half is administered over the next 16 hours.
5. The magnitude of burns is classified according to percentage of total body surface area (TBSA) involved, depth of the burn, and the presence or absence of inhalational injury. TBSA burned in adults can be estimated using the "rule of 9s," an age-specific diagram, or by estimation using the palmar surface of the hand.
6. Electrical burns can have acute and chronic effects not occurring with other types of burn injury, and with morbidity far higher than expected based on burn size estimation alone. High-voltage injuries are typically associated with loss of consciousness, arrhythmias, myoglobinuria, and extensive deep tissue damage that can result in compartment syndromes. However, significant injury can also result from low- and midrange voltage burns.
7. Major burn injury results in pathophysiologic changes in virtually all organ systems. The perioperative care of burn patients requires knowledge of these changes from the initial period of injury through the period when wounds are covered and healed.
8. In patients with severe burn injury, massive heat loss can occur through the open wounds, making the maintenance of normothermia challenging. Multiple strategies are used to maintain body temperature in the operating room, including high ambient room temperatures, use of warming blankets, radiant warmers, blood/fluid warmers, and wrapping the head and extremities with plastic or thermal insulation.
9. Securing the endotracheal tube in a patient with facial burns can be difficult. It is essential to secure the endotracheal tube with a carefully secured harness to avoid the potential catastrophe of accidental extubation.
10. Transport of a burned patient to and from the operating room can be a high-risk event. A systematic approach to maintenance of the patient's respiratory, hemodynamic, and general support helps ensure patient safety. The need for continuous observation by the anesthesia team during patient transport cannot be overemphasized.

11. Burn patients develop tolerance to most narcotics and sedatives, thereby requiring higher doses than patients without thermal injury. Sedatives and narcotics should be titrated to effect while the patient is carefully monitored.
12. In burn patients, exposure to succinylcholine can result in an exaggerated hyperkalemic response that can induce cardiac arrest. The general recommendation is to avoid succinylcholine administration in patients beginning 24 to 72 hours after burn injury. The duration of this dangerous response to succinylcholine after burn injury is unknown.
13. Blood loss during burn wound excision can be deceptively large. It is not difficult for the surgical team to remove eschar so rapidly that the patient becomes hypovolemic and unstable. Good communication between the surgical and anesthesia teams as well as limiting the operative duration and extent of excision can prevent such problems.
14. Burn injury leads to increased susceptibility to infection through multiple mechanisms including loss of the physical barrier of an intact skin, damage to lining of the respiratory tract from inhalation, and altered gut permeability and function. Maintaining strict aseptic techniques both in the operating room and during transport is essential.
15. Nearly every aspect in the treatment of burn injury is associated with pain. Poorly controlled pain and anxiety can have significant adverse physiologic and psychological effects. Standardized pain and anxiety guidelines are used to provide appropriate, consistent patient comfort.

EPIDEMIOLOGY

In the United States, approximately 500 000 people seek treatment for burn injury each year, of whom 40 000 are hospitalized and 4000 die.[1] The natural history of serious burns is characterized by burn shock, which can be fatal within the first hours to days, particularly in those with untreated large burns. Burn wound sepsis is the major cause of mortality among those who survive burn shock. After recovery from the acute inflammatory phase, postburn deformities can delay full functional recovery.[2] In-hospital fatality rates are approximately 4% for burn patients with major injuries even when treated in specialized burn units. Survival and outcome after major burn injury have improved over the last 20 years because of a greater understanding of the pathophysiology of burn injury, improved early resuscitation, development of multidisciplinary burn-treatment teams, and advances in control of postburn sepsis including early, aggressive surgical treatment and improved perioperative care.[2]

BURN INJURY PATHOPHYSIOLOGY

RAPID EDEMA FORMATION AND HYPOVOLEMIA

Severe burn injury results in significant tissue trauma and hypovolemic shock. Intravascular volume loss is related to the formation and release of local and systemic inflammatory mediators. In addition, the pathophysiologic changes occur at local and distant sites even when the hypovolemia is corrected. Increases of pulmonary and systemic vascular resistance (SVR) in association with myocardial depression often occurs despite adequate fluid resuscitation.[3-6]

A generalized capillary leak syndrome leads to decreased plasma volume, cardiac output, and urine output, and increased systemic vascular resistance. In contrast to nonburn trauma, the fluid loss associated with burn injury, in the absence of marked cell volume loss, leads to hemoconcentration. Thus the initial therapeutic goal is restoration of intravascular volume so as to preserve tissue perfusion and minimize the inflammatory response. The fluid loss of burns occurs not only in the area of the burn wound but also at distant nonburned sites. Continued loss of plasma volume secondary to edema formation can occur up to 48 hours—or even longer—after major burn injury, prolonging the risk of hypovolemia. The immediate and rapid increase of edema in burn tissue is followed by a more gradual loss of fluid by extravasation in both burned and nonburned tissues. Edema in noninjured tissues usually occurs when the injury exceeds 25% of TBSA and the fluid loss in distant nonburned tissues is accompanied by plasma protein loss.[7,8]

Burn injury causes direct and indirect mediator-modulated changes of capillary integrity leading to increases in protein and water permeability.[8,9] Circulating endogenous mediators play pivotal roles in the pathogenesis of edema formation and the cardiovascular abnormalities associated with burn injury. These mediators alter vascular permeability directly and/or indirectly by increasing microvascular hydrostatic pressure or surface area via arteriolar vasodilatation. Because of the multiplicity of mediators released by burns, therapy to antagonize a single mediator (eg, histamine) has not proven successful.

HEMODYNAMIC RESPONSE TO BURNS

Hemodynamic function in the early burn period is characterized by a reduced cardiac output and an increase in systemic and pulmonary vascular resistance, with the possibility of pulmonary edema.

ALTERED CARDIAC OUTPUT

There is an immediate depression of cardiac output even before any detectable reduction in plasma volume. This rapid depression suggests a neurogenic response and/or increased circulating mediators. Soon thereafter, hypovolemia contributes to the depressed cardiac output. The persistence of reduced cardiac output after repletion of fluid volume has been attributed to circulating myocardial depressant factors.[10-13] In addition, decreased adrenoreceptor affinity and second-messenger function may result in an attenuated response to catecholamine infusion when vasoactive therapy is initiated.[14,15] Approximately 3 to 5 days after major burn injury, a supranormal cardiac output (sometimes more than double) is seen. This correlates with the onset of a hypermetabolic state.

INCREASED SYSTEMIC VASCULAR RESISTANCE

Sympathetic stimulation and hypovolemia related to burn injury result in release of catecholamines, vasopressin, angiotensin II, and neuropeptide Y, leading to increased vasoconstriction and SVR.[16] Increased SVR immediately after burn injury is also partly the result of increased blood viscosity secondary to hemoconcentration. Organs particularly susceptible to ischemia and dysfunction secondary to inadequate resuscitation and vasoconstriction are the kidneys and gastrointestinal (GI) tract. Myoglobinemia as a consequence of muscle destruction can also contribute to renal injury.[17,18] Sustained vasoconstriction of the GI tract can occur despite adequate resuscitation leading to ischemia and bacterial translocation.[19,20]

PULMONARY EDEMA

There is an increase in pulmonary vascular resistance (PVR) following major burns. Pulmonary edema may occur, especially after the fluid resuscitation phase and restoration of capillary integrity (48-72 hours after burn injury) when extravascular edema fluid is reabsorbed leading to hypervolemia. Initially the edema results mainly from an increased capillary pressure secondary to increased PVR. Pulmonary capillary wedge pressure is increased greater than left atrial pressure after experimental burn injury and appears caused by postcapillary venoconstriction.[21] It is likely that some left-heart failure also contributes to pulmonary edema. Developing hypoproteinemia may be an important contributing factor to postburn pulmonary edema.[21] Pulmonary dysfunction from inhalation injury may also occur as a consequence of direct alveolar injury, sloughing of bronchial mucosa, impaired clearance of secretions, and development of pneumonia.

INITIAL EVALUATION

Successful management of the patient with burn injury begins with a thorough assessment soon after the time of injury. This requires a combined strategy of airway assessment and protection, initiation of resuscitation, and evaluation for coexisting injuries. The initial management proceeds in a stepwise process as outlined in the Advanced Burn Life Support course sponsored by the American Burn Association.[22]

PRIMARY SURVEY

Between 5% and 7% of patients admitted to burn centers suffer from nonthermal traumatic injuries.[23] Failure to diagnose associated injuries during the initial evaluation can lead to unnecessary morbidity and mortality. Therefore, all burned patients should be approached initially as multiple-trauma patients.

Securing the airway is the first priority during initial evaluation; safe airway management begins by its assessment. The presence of airway injury, signs of airway obstruction, and presence of a preexisting airway abnormality should be assessed as soon as the patient arrives at the hospital. Airway injuries may not be evident initially, but with massive fluid resuscitation airway edema may result. As a general rule it is safer to intubate the patient early rather than risk a difficult intubation after airway swelling has occurred. With injuries to the face or neck, direct laryngoscopy may be difficult or impossible. When the upper airway is severely damaged and laryngoscopy and endotracheal intubation are anticipated to be difficult, a direct surgical approach to the airway may be indicated. Options include a cricothyroidotomy or tracheostomy.

INHALATION INJURY

Inhalation injury increases the resuscitation fluid requirements by up to 50% and is a major source of mortality in burn patients.[24,25] A history of exposure to fire in a closed space, loss of consciousness, and presence of chemical irritants in combination with the physical examination revealing carbonaceous sputum and singed nasal or facial hair are all suggestive of inhalational injury. Chest radiographs are usually normal until secondary complications occur, such as atelectasis, pulmonary edema, or pneumonia. Fiberoptic bronchoscopy may be used to support the diagnosis, which may reveal carbonaceous debris, erythema, or ulceration.[26] The mechanisms of inhalation injury consist of a combination of (1) direct thermal injury to the upper airway from inhalation of hot gases, (2) damage to the cellular and oxygen transport processes by inhalation of carbon monoxide and cyanide, and (3) chemical injury to the lower airways and lung caused by inhalation of toxic products from the fire.[27]

DIRECT INJURY TO THE UPPER AIRWAY

Direct heat injury to the airway usually only occurs to the depth of the carina because of efficient dissipation of heat by the upper airway, the low specific heat of air, and reflex closure of the glottis as a result of the irritant. Direct heat injury to the upper airway can lead to marked swelling of the tongue, epiglottis, and glottic opening, resulting in airway obstruction.[27] Because airway swelling may not occur immediately but may develop over a period of hours (especially with concurrent fluid resuscitation), a high index of suspicion and frequent reevaluations are essential. Upper airway edema can have severe consequences in small children. Signs of impending upper airway obstruction include hoarseness, retractions, and stridor. If the history and physical examination suggest inhalational injury, one should have a low threshold for early intubation, particularly in children. If intubation is delayed and significant swelling occurs, intubation can become difficult or impossible. Upper airway edema usually resolves in 3 to 6 days and is facilitated by elevation of the head of the bed and avoiding of excessive fluid administration.

CARBON MONOXIDE POISONING

Carbon monoxide (CO) can cause tissue hypoxia. The oxygen-carrying capacity of blood is decreased because both CO and oxygen compete for the same binding site on hemoglobin (Hgb). Because CO binds to Hgb 200 times more readily than oxygen, it can significantly reduce the oxygen-carrying capacity of blood.[28] Binding of CO to Hgb also shifts the oxyhemoglobin dissociation curve to the left, increasing the affinity of Hgb for oxygen and reducing oxygen release to tissues (**Fig. 75-1**). In addition, CO interferes with peripheral oxygen use by binding to molecules such as myoglobin, nicotinamide adenine dinucleotide phosphate reductase, and cytochrome oxidase, resulting in impaired oxidative phosphorylation at the mitochondrial level.[29] The mitochondrial dysfunction caused by CO is best documented in the heart where it can produce myocardial stunning.[30] The consequence of these changes is decreased oxygen delivery to the tissues, impaired release of the available oxygen at the capillaries, and a reduced ability to consume the delivered oxygen resulting in tissue hypoxia and metabolic acidosis.

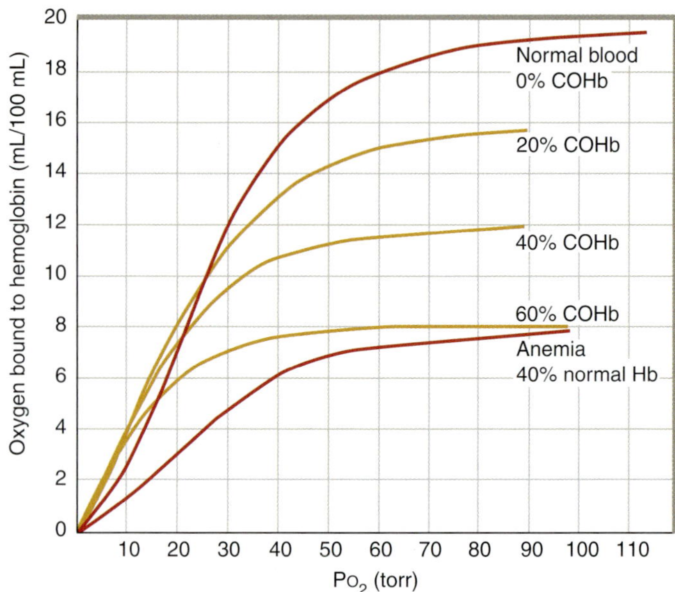

FIGURE 75-1. Carboxyhemoglobin dissociation curve. The changes in the oxygen-hemoglobin (Hb) dissociation curve that occur with carbon monoxide (CO) poisoning. The oxygen bound to hemoglobin is decreased depending on the CO concentration, and the oxygen-hemoglobin dissociation curve is shifted to the left, resulting in less oxygen being delivered to tissues and the oxygen carried by hemoglobin being more tightly bound. Po_2, partial pressure of oxygen. [Reproduced with permission from McCall J, Cahill T. Respiratory care of the burn patient. *J Burn Care Rehabil*. 2005;26:200-206.]

CO poisoning can be difficult to detect. CO is an odorless, tasteless, nonirritating gas. The clinical findings of CO poisoning are variable and largely nonspecific. Clinical signs and symptoms of tissue hypoxia as a result of CO poisoning include headache, nausea, shortness of breath, tachypnea, angina, and changes in mental status.[31] The half-life of carboxyhemoglobin is 4 hours for patients breathing air. This can be reduced to 40 to 60 minutes when breathing 100% oxygen. Hyperbaric oxygen delivery can further reduce the half-life of carboxyhemoglobin to 23 minutes.[32] In those patients with more severe exposures (a carboxyhemoglobin level >30% or evidence of neurologic changes), hyperbaric oxygen has been suggested to diminish the incidence of long-term neurologic sequelae.[33,34] Unfortunately, hyperbaric oxygen chambers are often unavailable.

The absorbance spectrum of carboxyhemoglobin and oxyhemoglobin are similar; therefore, standard pulse oximeters cannot distinguish between these 2 forms of hemoglobin. Consequently, oximeter readings can be normal even when lethal amounts of carboxyhemoglobin are present in blood.[35] The Pao_2 measured from the arterial blood gas sample often reflects the amount of oxygen dissolved in blood and does not indicate the quantity of oxygen bound to hemoglobin (saturation).

Thus the Pa_{O_2} can be normal even with high levels of carboxyhemoglobin. The diagnosis of CO poisoning is made by measuring the carboxyhemoglobin level in arterial blood, expressed as a percentage saturation of hemoglobin. Carboxyhemoglobin levels higher than 15% are toxic; those exceeding 50% are lethal.[36] Because of the inevitable time delay between exposure and testing, the levels of carboxyhemoglobin measured in the hospital may not reflect the true extent of poisoning, especially when the patient has been breathing a high concentration of oxygen during transport.

CYANIDE POISONING

Hydrogen cyanide is a toxic gas produced in fires by the burning of nitrogenous materials, including natural fibers (wool and silk) and synthetic polymers (polyurethane, polyacrylonitrile, and acrocyanate). Cyanide binds to mitochondrial cytochrome oxidase, which catalyzes the last step of oxidative phosphorylation (adenosine triphosphate [ATP] formation), preventing the use of oxygen by mitochondria. The pathophysiologic sequel of cyanide poisoning is that cells can only generate ATP via anaerobic metabolism, which results in a metabolic acidosis from lactic acid production.

As with CO poisoning, cyanide toxicity can be difficult to diagnose. Cyanide toxicity should be suspected in any patient with a history of inhalation injury. Concentrations greater than 20 ppm are considered dangerous. Early symptoms include headache, dizziness, tachypnea, and tachycardia. Cardiac toxicity may manifest as ST-segment elevation on the electrocardiogram (ECG), which can mimic an acute myocardial infarction. Cyanide increases minute ventilation by stimulating the carotid body and peripheral chemoreceptors. Concentrations of 100 ppm can lead to seizures, coma, respiratory failure, and death.[37] Laboratory findings include an anion gap metabolic acidosis that does not respond to oxygen administration. The mixed venous oxygen saturation in cyanide poisoning is often elevated, suggesting an inability to consume oxygen.[38,39] Direct detection of cyanide poisoning in blood is difficult. Cyanide has a short half-life in blood and measurement is not universally available.

The treatment of cyanide toxicity has generated controversy because treatment itself may be hazardous. The deleterious effects of cyanide are normally neutralized by the conversion of cyanide to thiocyanate, which is excreted in the urine. This can be enhanced by the administering of exogenous thiosulfate.[40] Cyanide can also combine with hydroxocobalamin (vitamin B_{12}), to form cyanocobalamin. Nitrate administration results in the oxidation of hemoglobin to methemoglobin, which can combine with cyanide to form cyanomethemoglobin. Methemoglobin, however, does not transport oxygen and may be harmful to a patient whose oxygen-carrying capacity is already compromised because of carboxyhemoglobin.[41]

CHEMICAL INJURY TO THE LOWER AIRWAYS

The burning of many materials in a house fire can release combustion products that are toxic and damaging to the lower airways, including respiratory mucosal epithelium and capillary endothelium of the airway and alveoli. The damage to epithelium results in destruction of mucociliary transport, impairing clearance of bacteria and mucosal debris. Alveolar collapse and atelectasis can occur because of loss of surfactant production or from plugging because of mucus debris.[42] Chemical damage to alveoli and lung capillaries will lead to extravasation of plasma protein. Activation of injury-induced alveolar macrophages will enhance the inflammatory response and damage. Bronchial swelling and bronchospasm can lead to obstruction of both large and small airways. The end result can be acute respiratory failure from increased ventilation-perfusion mismatch, decreased lung compliance, and increased dead-space ventilation, generally occurring 12 to 48 hours after the inhalation event.[27] The respiratory failure may worsen several days later from continued airway mucosal sloughing, barotrauma, bacterial invasion, and pneumonia.[43,44]

INDIRECT RESPIRATORY INJURY

Injury to the lung can occur in patients with severe cutaneous burns in the absence of an inhalational injury.[45,46] Mechanisms include release of inflammatory mediators from the burn-injured area, effects of fluid resuscitation, and infection. Pulmonary edema often occurs after a large burn injury as a result of decreased oncotic pressure and pulmonary hypertension. After restoration of capillary integrity, the edema fluid present throughout the body is resorbed and can lead to hypervolemic pulmonary edema.

MANAGEMENT OF INHALATION INJURY

The treatment of inhalation injury is supportive care with airway management, mechanical ventilation, and aggressive pulmonary toilet. Nebulization of bronchodilators, anticoagulants, and antioxidants have a role in management[25,47] Close surveillance for infection is important, although prophylactic administration of antibiotics is not recommended because of the potential for developing resistant organisms.[25]

FLUID RESUSCITATION

In 1930, Underhill first described "burn shock" that results from intravascular fluid loss as a cause of early death.[48] An appreciation of the exaggerated fluid requirements of burn patients and formulas for their estimation subsequently evolved. Multiple fluid resuscitation formulas exist for estimating fluid needs (**Table 75-1**). As a general rule, burns of less than 15% TBSA are not associated with extensive capillary leak and can be managed with intravenous fluid administered at 1.5 times the maintenance rate with careful attention to hydration status.

The commonly used resuscitation formulas differ somewhat in their recommendations of the amount of infused crystalloid and colloid. Most formulas recommend giving isotonic crystalloid initially and later use of colloids.[9,49] The times at which colloid administration is initiated varies from institution to institution, on the size of the burn, patient age, and other cardiorespiratory parameters. Lactated Ringer solution is often the crystalloid chosen because it contains physiologic concentrations of major electrolytes, and lactate replaces some of the chloride in the solution, resulting in less hyperchloremic metabolic acidosis. In younger children and in patients where hypoglycemia is a concern, 5% dextrose solution can be added to the lactated Ringer solution.

Once capillary integrity returns, generally within 24 to 48 hours, most resuscitation formulas recommend administration of colloid. Most authorities advocate 5% albumin in isotonic crystalloid, which is ideally administered by continuous infusion at a dose adjusted to burn size. Some clinicians advocate infusion of fresh-frozen plasma, but it is better used to correct significant coagulopathy because it incurs the added risks of transfusion. Side effects of large-volume crystalloid resuscitation include pleural and pericardial effusions and intestinal ileus with an abdominal compartment syndrome.[50] Thus more burn units are advocating the early use of colloids.

TABLE 75-1 Formulas for Estimating Burn Resuscitation Fluid Needs

Crystalloid formulas		
Parkland	Lactated Ringer	4 mL/kg/%TBSA burn
Modified Brooke	Lactated Ringer	2 mL/kg/%TBSA burn
Colloid formulas		
Evans	Normal saline	4 mL/kg/%TBSA burn
	Colloid	1 mL/kg/%TBSA burn
	5% dextrose	2000 mL/24 h
Brooke	Lactated Ringer	1.5 mL/kg/%TBSA burn
	Colloid	0.5 mL/kg/%TBSA burn
	5% dextrose	2000 mL/24 h

TBSA, total body surface area.

Hypertonic saline has been advocated for resuscitation in burn injury, especially for patients with large burns, inhalational injury, or circumferential burns, because the administered fluid volume is smaller and tissue edema can be reduced.[51] However, in one study comparing hypertonic saline to lactated Ringer solution for burn resuscitation, there was a significant increase in renal failure and deaths in the hypertonic saline group.[52] Consequently, resuscitation with hypertonic saline is not a common practice.

The Parkland formula remains the most widely used resuscitation formula for burn injury in the United States. The Parkland formula, 4 mL per %TBSA burn/kg, is administered over the first 24 hours with half of the calculated volume administered during the first 8 postinjury hours.[53] The remaining half is administered over the next 16 hours. If resuscitation is delayed, this volume is administered so that infusion is completed by the 8th postinjury hour. No matter which formula is used, it should serve as a guideline with fluid resuscitation titrated to physiologic end points (see Table 75-4). Actual fluid requirements will vary, depending on size and depth of the burn, patient's weight, interval from injury to start of resuscitation, presence of associated injuries, and presence of inhalational injury.

Cardiac index and oxygen delivery have been investigated as end points to guide fluid resuscitation.[54,55] Bernard et al showed that patients who survived large burns had a higher cardiac index and better oxygen delivery than did nonsurvivors.[56] Subsequently, some investigators proposed supranormal oxygen delivery as a means of ensuring adequate tissue delivery. Schiller et al demonstrated improved survival in burn patients by maintaining a hyperdynamic circulation by infusing fluids and inotropes.[57] However, studies of achieving supranormal cardiac output and oxygen delivery have failed to demonstrate an improvement of survival rates or decrease in organ failure. One study, examining the infusion of dobutamine to augment cardiac output and oxygen delivery, demonstrated an increased mortality.[58]

Blood lactate and base deficit have been proposed as global markers of systemic oxygen delivery and the adequacy of tissue perfusion in burn patients.[59,60] Lactic acid is produced during anaerobic metabolism and indicates inadequate oxygen delivery or use. Holm et al reported the lactate level to be the most predictive index of tissue perfusion. Lactate levels less than 2 mmol/L in the first 24 to 48 hours after burn injury correlated with improved survival rates.[61] Base deficit is another indicator of global tissue perfusion and is calculated from an arterial blood gas using normograms. In a retrospective study in burn patients, Kaups et al reported the base deficit predicted fluid replacement requirements and survival.[62]

In burn injury, when tissue perfusion is not uniform throughout the body, an indirect measure of less well-perfused tissues may prove useful. One such measure is the intramucosal gastric pH, as measured by gastric tonometry. After burn injury, blood flow to the heart, brain, and kidneys is maintained at the expense of splanchnic blood flow. Several studies report that a lower intramucosal pH predicts organ failure and increased mortality and have suggested the use of mucosal pH as a guide to resuscitation.[63-65] This technique has not become routine in clinical practice, however.

A small percentage of patients fail to respond to conventional fluid resuscitation. These patients frequently have large deep burns, are at extremes of age, and have inhalational injury or coexisting medical conditions.[66] If the total fluid requirement exceeds 6 mL/kg/%TBSA per 24 hours, it is advisable to obtain more information regarding intravascular volume and cardiac function. This information can be obtained by a physical examination or by measurement of central venous pressure and/or pulmonary artery pressure. Based on the information, inotropic support may be required. Echocardiographic evaluation of ventricular volume and function has been used in burns.[67] After 24 to 48 hours, capillary integrity returns to normal in nonburned areas, especially with repletion of circulating volume. At this stage, fluid requirements dramatically decrease; it is important to decrease fluid administration promptly because overzealous administration of fluid can be associated with substantial morbidity.

A great deal of recent interest has focused on administering antioxidants as adjuncts to fluid resuscitation. Reactive oxygen species generated by thermal injury are involved in edema formation associated with burns. In particular, high-dose vitamin C infusion during resuscitation has been studied in animals and shown to reduce total fluid requirements significantly.[68] Tanaka et al demonstrated a 45% reduction in fluid resuscitation volumes using a vitamin C infusion in a small group of patients.[69] Antioxidant use is not yet a standard adjunct to clinical resuscitation.

Recent studies have reported that excessive volumes of resuscitation fluids are administered with increasing frequency in many burn centers. This trend toward excessive fluid resuscitation is termed "fluid creep."[70] There is concern for the deleterious effects of excessive fluid administration including extremity, orbital, and abdominal compartment syndromes, acute respiratory distress syndrome (ARDS), prolonged ventilator dependence, and increased mortality.[71]

ESTIMATION OF SIZE/DEPTH OF BURN

The magnitude of burns is classified according to the TBSA involved, depth of the burn, and the presence or absence of inhalational injury. TBSA burned in adults can be estimated using the "rule of 9s" (**Fig. 75-2**). The Lund-Browder chart is an age-specific diagram that accounts for changes of body surface area with age (**Fig. 75-3**).[72,71] Estimation by palmar surface of the hand (without the fingers, 0.5% TBSA) is age invariant and can also provide a quick estimate.[72,73] The depth of skin destruction is characterized as first, second , or third degree, based on whether there is superficial, partial-thickness, or full-thickness destruction of the skin (**Table 75-2**). *Fourth degree* is used to describe burns that have injured deeper structures such as muscle, fascia, and bone. Deep second- and third-degree burns require surgical debridement and grafting, whereas more superficial burns do not. Revisions of burn-depth estimates are often necessary after the first

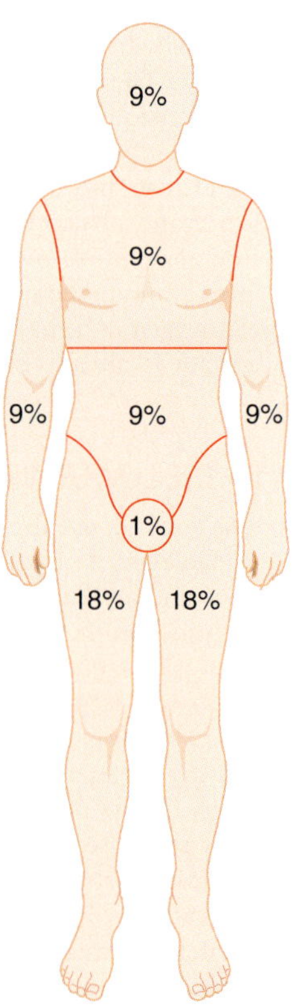

FIGURE 75-2. The rule of 9s for estimating the percentage of body surface area burned in adults.

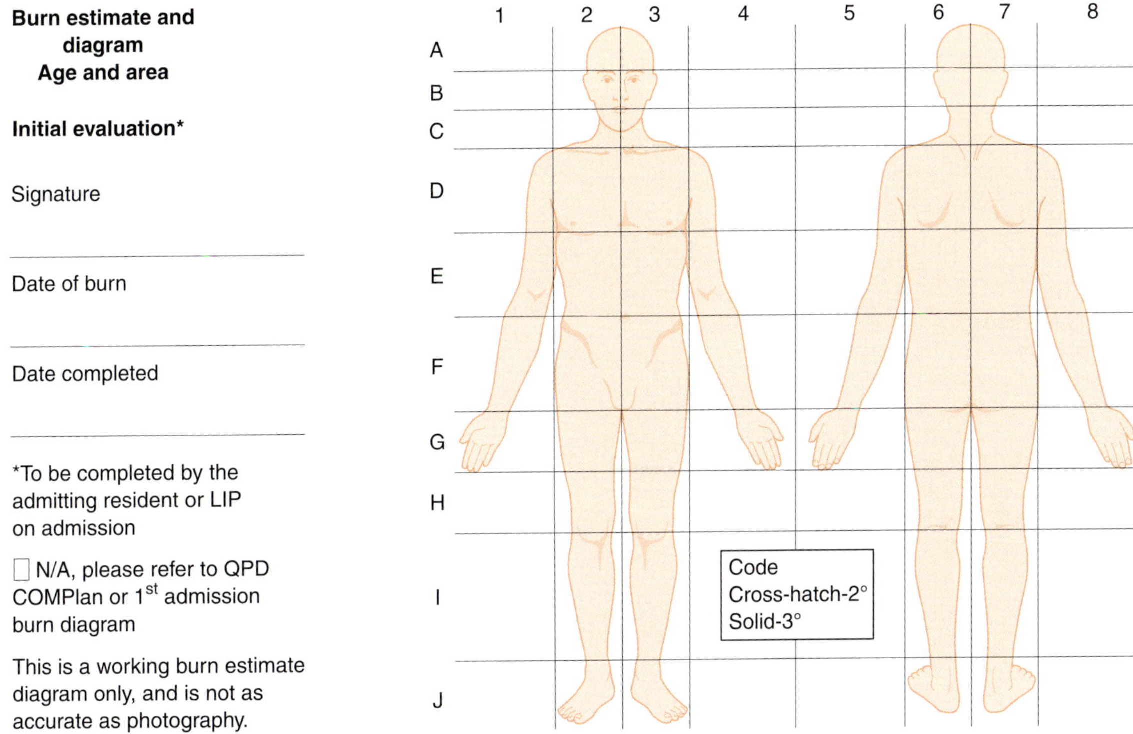

Area	Birth-1 yr.	1-4 yrs.	5-9 yrs.	10-14 yrs.	15 yrs.	Adult	2°	3°	Total
Head	19	17	13	11	9	7			
Neck	2	2	2	2	2	2			
Anterior trunk	13	13	13	13	13	13			
Posterior trunk	13	13	13	13	13	13			
Right buttock	2.5	2.5	2.5	2.5	2.5	2.5			
Left buttock	2.5	2.5	2.5	2.5	2.5	2.5			
Genitalia	1	1	1	1	1	1			
Right upper arm	4	4	4	4	4	4			
Left upper arm	4	4	4	4	4	4			
Right lower arm	3	3	3	3	3	3			
Left lower arm	3	3	3	3	3	3			
Right hand	2.5	2.5	2.5	2.5	2.5	2.5			
Left hand	2.5	2.5	2.5	2.5	2.5	2.5			
Right thigh	5.5	6.5	8	8.5	9	9.5			
Left thigh	5.5	6.5	8	8.5	9	9.5			
Right lower leg	5	5	5.5	6	6.5	7			
Left lower leg	5	5	5.5	6	6.5	7			
Right foot	3.5	3.5	3.5	3.5	3.5	3.5			
Left foot	3.5	3.5	3.5	3.5	3.5	3.5			
**Only 2° and 3° burns are included in the total TBSA burn percent						Total			

FIGURE 75-3. Burn diagram. A careful burn diagram should be completed at the time of initial evaluation including wound size, location, and estimated burn depth.

TABLE 75-2 Classification of Burn Depth

Depth	Level of Injury	Clinical Features	Result/Treatment
Superficial	Epidermis	Dry, red; blanches; painful	Healing time: 3-6 d
Superficial partial thickness	Papillary dermis	Blisters; moist, red, weeping; blanches; painful	Cleaning; topical agent; sterile dressing; healing time: 7-12 d; hypertrophic scar rare; return of full function
Deep partial thickness	Reticular dermis	Blisters; wet or waxy dry; does not blanch; absent pain sensation	Treatment as for superficial partial-thickness burns; possible surgical excision and grafting; hypertrophic scar common; earlier return of function with surgery
Full thickness	Subcutaneous fat, fascia, muscle, or bone	Waxy white to leathery dry and inelastic; does not blanch; absent pain sensation	Treatment as for superficial partial-thickness burns plus surgical excision and grafting at earliest possible time; functional limitation more common

TABLE 75-3 American Burn Association Burn Center Transfer Criteria

Second- and third-degree burns on >10% of total body surface area (TBSA) in patients <10 or >50 y of age
Second- and third-degree burns on >20% of TBSA in other age groups
Second- and third-degree burns that involve the face, hands, feet, genitalia, perineum, and major joints
Third-degree burns on >5% TBSA in any age group
Electrical burns including lightning injury
Chemical burns
Inhalation injury
Burn injury in patients with preexisting medical disorders that could complicate management, prolong recovery, or affect mortality
Any patients with burns and concomitant trauma (such as fractures) in which the burn injury poses the greatest risk of morbidity or mortality; in such cases, if the trauma poses the greater immediate risk, the patient may be treated initially in a trauma center until stable before being transferred to a burn center; physician judgment will be necessary in such situations and should be in concert with the regional medical control plan and triage protocols
Hospitals without qualified personnel or equipment for the care of children with burns should transfer the patient to a burn center with these capabilities
Burn injury in patients who will require special social/emotional and/or long-term rehabilitative support, including cases involving suspected child abuse and substance abuse

24 to 72 hours. This is especially true in patients with thin skin, who can sustain deeper burn injuries than may be evident on the initial examination of the wound. Skin can be presumed to be thin in young children and the elderly. Mortality from burn injury is related to the TBSA of deep second-degree or third-degree burns. A large analysis has revealed 3 risk factors that predict of death after burns: age older than 60 years, burn size greater than 40% of body surface area, and inhalation injury. Mortality is a function of the number of risk factors present. The mortality was 0.3%, 3%, 33%, or 90% depending on whether 0, 1, 2, or 3 risk factors were present, respectively.[74]

BURN CENTER REFERRAL

Data analysis demonstrates improved outcomes from major burns with early referral to a burn center.[75] It is well recognized that burn care requires specialized expertise, personnel, and equipment that are not cost effectively maintained in low-volume centers. **Table 75-3** lists criteria for referral to a regional burn center.

SECONDARY SURVEY

The burn-specific secondary survey complements the trauma secondary survey and focuses on aspects of the neurologic, otolaryngologic, ophthalmic, thoracic, cardiac, abdomen, genitourinary, and extremity issues as related to patients with acute burn injury.

NEUROLOGIC

Central nervous system function (CNS) can be altered by inhalation of neurotoxic chemicals, the effects of hypoxia and hypotension, and from the effects of anxiety and pain or their treatment. Signs of CNS dysfunction in burn patients include delirium, hallucinations, personality changes, seizures, and coma. It is essential to rule out coexisting intracranial injury by history, clinical examination, and radiologic imaging. Patients with serious burn injuries commonly become obtunded because of hemodynamic instability as well as following administration of drugs for sedation and analgesia, making it important to know that this change does not represent a missed intracranial injury. The need for radiologic evaluation of the neck is based on the mechanism of injury. In rare instances, patients with deep neck burns may need escharotomies at that site to facilitate cerebral venous drainage.

EAR, NOSE, THROAT, AND EYE

The primary otolaryngologic and ophthalmic evaluation includes assessment and initial treatment of burns to the airway, corneal epithelium, and the external ear. Signs of airway involvement include perioral and oropharyngeal burns, presence of carbonaceous sputum, and signs of hoarseness. Hot liquid can be aspirated in conjunction with a scald injury to the face and can result in rapid airway compromise. One should have a low threshold for intubation when airway involvement exists. The globes of the eye should be examined early because adnexal swelling can make the examination difficult. Severe corneal burns are usually obvious by the cloudy appearance they impart, but less severe injury to the cornea is more often subtle requiring fluorescein staining. Topical antibiotics are the initial treatment if the cornea is burned. Burns to the external ear can be complicated by suppurative chondritis. Treatment with topical mafenide acetate cream may decrease its development.[76]

CHEST

The focus of the initial evaluation of the chest is to ensure sufficient chest wall excursion for both hemithoraces. Impaired chest wall compliance can be caused by a deep circumferential eschar impairing chest wall motion and/or bronchospasm resulting from inhalation of airway irritants. The inhalation of toxic fumes may precipitate a bronchospastic attack in a patient with a previous history of asthma. A patient with decreased chest wall compliance because of a circumferential eschar exhibits rapid shallow respirations. A patient requiring mechanical ventilation then exhibits increased peak airway pressures. Escharotomy is the treatment of choice for the latter condition, whereas bronchodilators, pulmonary toilet, and ventilation strategies to minimize breath stacking are used to treat bronchospasm. Severe inhalational injury may result in thick secretions and the sloughing of airway mucosa, which can occlude the endotracheal tube or distant bronchi resulting in atelectasis. In such instances, suctioning and bronchoscopy may be required.

CARDIAC

If adequate intravascular volume and oxygenation are maintained and electrolyte abnormalities corrected, significant arrhythmias are unusual in otherwise healthy burn patients. Coexisting cardiac disease can result in the resuscitation and acute care being less well tolerated. Direct myocardial injury and arrhythmias resulting from electrical injury are discussed later in the section "Special Situations: Electrical Injuries."

ABDOMEN

Primary objectives in the evaluation of the abdomen are to exclude associated injuries, ensure adequate compliance to permit ventilation, and decrease the risk of gastric dilation and gastrointestinal ulceration. Coincident abdominal trauma should be evaluated with imaging studies or diagnostic peritoneal lavage if indicated. Occult abdominal trauma can explain excessive fluid resuscitation requirements or a paradoxical fall in hematocrit in the early phase of burn injury. In some cases, escharotomies of the torso may be necessary to facilitate spontaneous respiration or mechanical ventilation of patients with deep circumferential eschars. Circumferential abdominal eschar, accumulation of intraperitoneal fluid, or bowel edema can lead to the abdominal compartment syndrome, which can cause diminished urine output, decreased pulmonary compliance, and hemodynamic instability.[77] Obtaining bladder pressure measurements can be useful to make this diagnosis.[78] In some cases, abdominal decompression may be necessary.

Patients with severe burns often develop a paralytic ileus and require nasogastric decompression for varying lengths of time. Gastroduodenal ulceration, likely due to reduced splanchnic blood flow, is a risk of severe burn injury, and ulcer prophylaxis with H_2 receptor antagonists or proton pump inhibitors should be initiated as early as possible.

GENITOURINARY

Catheterization of the bladder is important for patients with moderate to severe burns who require intravenous fluid resuscitation because it facilitates the use of urine volume as an indicator of the adequacy of resuscitation. Soft tissue swelling in the genital area can be significant with severe burn injury whether or not the burn involves the genital region. This can make urinary catheterization more difficult as time passes in the acute resuscitation phase. For this reason an appropriate-size Foley catheter should be inserted as early as possible. In males it is important to ensure that the foreskin is reduced over the urinary catheter after its insertion to prevent the development of paraphimosis if soft tissue edema develops.[79]

EXTREMITIES

Exclusion of associated (nonburn) injuries and monitoring of peripheral perfusion are the initial priorities in an evaluation of the extremities. Careful clinical examination and radiologic imaging, if necessary, should be preformed. Extremity perfusion can be compromised by soft tissue swelling in the noncompliant fascial compartments or by a circumferential eschar.

Extremities that are at risk for ischemia, especially in those with circumferential burns or with electrical injury, should be monitored closely for tense fascial compartments and signs of impaired perfusion. Frequent checks of pulses, capillary filling, venous congestion, and blood flow by Doppler analysis are important. Dressings should be loosely applied to facilitate frequent examination. Tense extremities should be decompressed by escharotomy and/or fasciotomy when clinical examination reveals signs of impaired perfusion. Escharotomies can be performed at the bedside using electrocautery to minimize blood loss. The need for escharotomy usually becomes apparent in the early hours of acute resuscitation. Fasciotomies are generally performed in the operating room to minimize damage to underlying structures that can be obscured by tissue edema.

ANTIBIOTICS

Prophylactic antibiotics have no proven role in burn care and are not routinely given.[80] All burn injuries are potentially contaminated soft tissue wounds, and therefore tetanus toxoid should be given to all burned patients.[81,82] If the patient has not been previously immunized, tetanus immunoglobulin as well as tetanus toxoid should be administered.

PEDIATRIC CONSIDERATIONS

Children suffering burn injuries have unique physiologic, medical, surgical, and psychosocial issues requiring additional considerations. Younger children are at higher risk of burn injury, and up to 20% of their burn injuries are a result of abuse or neglect.[83] Approximately 70% of pediatric burns are caused by hot liquid, whereas flame burns are more common in working-age adults.[84]

Airway and respiratory considerations in children include their smaller airway, which can rapidly occlude with airway edema and swelling. In pediatric patients with scald injury, respiratory failure can occur during and after fluid resuscitation, even in the absence of inhalational injury.[85] Stridor and retractions should be taken as signs of airway compromise and a need for intubation. The trachea in children is shorter, and small changes in endotracheal tube positioning are more likely to lead to mainstream bronchial intubation. Bronchospasm, common in children suffering inhalational injury, should be treated early and aggressively. Fluid considerations include greater susceptibility to fluid overload, especially in younger children, particularly if all the administered fluids (flush solutions, medications, carrier fluids) are not taken into account. The kidneys of young infants have less concentrating ability. The children are particularly susceptible to cerebral edema if they become hyponatremic, which can result in seizures or brain herniation.[86]

GERIATRIC CONSIDERATIONS

Caring for geriatric patients with burn injuries requires consideration of their unique issues and needs. Burn injury in elderly patients is more likely the result of impaired dexterity or mobility and may indicate an inability to live independently.[87] Older patients do not have the physiologic reserve of the young. Coexisting cardiac and pulmonary disease can result in complications related to resuscitation and acute burn care itself. Preexisting renal disease can result in greater sensitivity to nephrotoxic drugs and hypotensive episodes. Resuscitation should be carefully weighed in elderly patients with large burn injuries, especially in the presence of inhalation injury, because mortality rates can reach 90%.[74] Advanced directives, health care proxies, and families should be consulted as early as possible. Nutritional requirements are less well predicted by standard equations.[88] The skin of elderly patients is thinner and therefore more susceptible to deeper burn injury. In addition, harvesting of donor skin repeatedly may not be possible because of poor healing. Finally, elderly patients may live alone or have a spouse who is unable to provide the care needed after discharge, including wound care, transportation, and support.

SPECIAL SITUATIONS

ELECTRICAL INJURIES

Electrical burns can have acute and chronic effects not produced by other types of burn injury and with morbidity much higher than expected based on burn size analysis alone.[89]

Electrical burns are classified as high-voltage (>1000 V) or low-voltage (<1000 V) injuries. High-voltage injuries are typically associated with loss of consciousness, arrhythmias, myoglobinuria, and extensive deep tissue damage that can result in compartment syndromes. However, significant injury can also result with low- and midrange voltage sources.

Approximately 15% of patients who sustain an electrical injury suffer other traumatic injury in addition to their burn.[90] These injuries often involve falls, being thrown against an object, or result from tetanic muscle contractions.

Both arrhythmias and direct myocardial injury can result from electrical injury. Creatine kinase and creatine kinase myocardial band enzymes are poor indicators of myocardial injury in the absence of ECG findings, particularly if muscle injury is present.[91] The diagnostic value of cardiac troponin levels has not been evaluated in this setting. The myocardial injury behaves more like a cardiac contusion than a myocardial infarction, with minimal hemodynamic consequences. This may be related to the fact that the heart, unlike the skeletal muscle, cannot sustain tetanic contractions. Virtually any cardiac arrhythmia may be associated with electrical injury. Ventricular fibrillation is the most common cause of death at the scene of the injury. Arrhythmias from electrical injury are managed using the same medical therapies as those resulting from any other cause. Patients with electrical injury should have ECG monitoring during transport to the hospital, in the emergency department, and afterward. Indications for more prolonged cardiac monitoring include documented cardiac arrest, cardiac arrhythmia on transport or in the emergency department, and an abnormal ECG.[92,93]

The hidden (deeper) injury associated with an electrical burn makes standard fluid resuscitation formulas inaccurate. Adequate fluid resuscitation is achieved by reaching the standard resuscitation end points (**Table 75-4**).

Myoglobinuria as a result of muscle damage manifests as pigmented urine and usually indicates more severe muscular damage. Myoglobin and hemoglobin pigments pose a risk of acute renal failure and require prompt treatment with crystalloid loading to a target urine output of 2 mL/kg/h. Addition of sodium bicarbonate to intravenous fluids may facilitate pigment clearance and minimize renal injury. Mannitol and furosemide are also effective in promoting a prompt diuresis, but

TABLE 75-4 Burn Resuscitation End Points

Arousable and comfortable
Warm extremities
Systolic blood pressure: for infants 60 mm Hg; for older children, 70 + 2 × age (in years) mm Hg; for adults, mean arterial pressure >65 or within 20% of baseline
Heart rate 80-150 beats/min (age dependent)
Urine output 0.5-2 mL/kg/h (glucose negative)
Base deficit <2 mEq/L

they compromise the value of measuring urine output as an indicator of the adequacy of resuscitation.

CHEMICAL BURNS

Although only 3% of all burns are caused by chemical exposures, approximately 30% of burn deaths are a consequence of chemical injuries.[94] The range of chemical injuries is vast. However, an understanding of the general principles of treatment is essential to those caring for patients with these injuries. First aid begins by removing the offending agent from contact with the patient. This involves removing all clothing and removal (dusting off) of any powder. It is important for health care personnel to protect themselves from injury by wearing masks, gloves, and aprons. Copious irrigations with tap water should be performed for at least 30 minutes. Because alkaline substances are less soluble in water, longer irrigation times may be required.

The large-volume lavage required to dilute chemical exposures can lead to hypothermia because of conductive and evaporative cooling, particularly from unwarmed irrigation fluid. Recognition of this potential complication is essential to avoid it.

Litmus paper can be used to verify the completeness of irrigation of acid or alkali. There is no role for neutralization of acid or alkali burns because such reactions generate heat that can further exacerbate the injury. Because of the wide range of chemicals involved in chemical injuries, consultation with a poison control center should be initiated early because there may be systemic toxicities in addition to the burn injury.

COLD INJURIES

Frostbite is a traumatic injury caused by failure of the normal protective mechanisms to protect against an environment that results in tissue temperatures falling below freezing. Terminology to describe cold injuries is not standardized. A number of factors have been associated with the development of frostbite, including ethanol consumption, psychiatric disease, smoking, diabetes, fatigue, and extremes of age.[95] Cold injuries are initially managed by rewarming in water warmed to 104°F (40°C).[96] Injured parts are then elevated and protected from further injury. Topical wound care is performed until an area of necrotic tissue is demarcated. Nonviable tissue is excised and reconstruction performed with primary closure, grafting, or flaps.[97]

TOXIC EPIDERMAL NECROLYSIS

Toxic epidermal necrolysis syndrome (TENS) and Stevens-Johnson syndrome (SJS) are severe exfoliative diseases of the skin and underlying structures caused by immunologic reactions, usually triggered by a medication or a viral syndrome. Most authorities consider TENS and SJS to be the same disease entity, differing only in total body surface area involved. Cases with less than 10% TBSA involved are labeled as SJS; those with more than 30% TBSA involvement are labeled as TENS; and cases between 10% and 30% involvement are labeled as overlap SJS-TENS.[98] The disease consists of cutaneous exfoliation together with varying degrees of mucosal and conjunctival involvement. Mortality for TENS is reported in the range of 25% to 80%.[99,100,101] Because of their expertise in management of patients suffering skin loss from thermal injury, burn centers often provide care for patients with TENS. Treatment consists of airway protection if needed, fluid resuscitation, nutritional support, close monitoring for septic complications, and eye care.[102,103]

ANESTHETIC MANAGEMENT

Major burn injury results in pathophysiologic changes in most organ systems (**Table 75-5**). The perioperative care of burn patients requires knowledge of these changes from the initial injury until wounds have been covered with skin and healed. Patients suffering from burn injuries often require surgical treatment for years following their initial injury.

PREOPERATIVE EVALUATION

Patients are often brought to the operating room in the early phase of burn injury when they are undergoing significant fluid shifts, with cardiovascular instability and/or respiratory insufficiency. The most frequently performed surgical procedure is excision and grafting of the burned area. Other procedures that may be required during their hospital stay include escharotomies, tracheostomy, and exploratory procedures related to accompanying trauma. During the early phase of burn injury, the patient's physiology is not optimal to maintain normal homeostasis. Nevertheless, attempts should be made to optimize organ function. The physiologic and psychological changes resulting from burn injury must be taken into account in addition to the usual considerations for a patient undergoing anesthesia and surgery. Useful and important preoperative information includes the time and extent of burn injury, coexisting medical problems, medications, drug allergies, previous problems with anesthetics and a family anesthetic history, and nothing by mouth status (**Table 75-6**). In addition, the anesthesiologist must be cognizant of the problems unique to burn patients including altered responses to anesthetics and muscle relaxants, difficulties with airway management, altered ventilatory status, difficult intravascular access and monitoring, positioning, potentially significant transfusion requirements, the marked potential for hypothermia, and methods of safe transport to and from the operating room.

THERMOREGULATION

In addition to conductive and convective heat loss, considerable evaporative heat loss can occur through open burn wounds, making maintenance of normothermia challenging. This is especially true during transport to and from the operating room. Patients should be covered with warm blankets during transport. Children have greater surface-area-to-body-weight ratios, resulting in more rapid heat loss. The ambient temperature of the preinduction area and operating room should be maintained at above-normal levels.

Burn patients, when given a thermostat, will set their environmental temperature higher than normal.[104] Multiple strategies are used to maintain body temperature in the operating room, including increasing ambient room temperature, using warming blankets, radiant warmers, blood/fluid warmers, and wrapping the head and extremities with plastic or thermal insulation. Temperature in the operating room is commonly maintained at 90°F to 100°F (32.2°C to 37.8°C), depending on the age and severity of the burn. Although a hot operating room can be uncomfortable for the medical staff, maintaining the patient's temperature is essential to minimize metabolic demand, maintain normal coagulation, and prevent shivering on emergence. Shivering can dislodge recently placed grafts.

INTRAOPERATIVE MANAGEMENT

AIRWAY MANAGEMENT

If injuries allow standard airway management (mask fit, mouth opening, and neck extension), direct laryngoscopy and intubation can be performed. Gastric emptying may or may not be delayed in burn patients.[105]

TABLE 75-5 Systemic Effects of Burn Injury

System	Early	Late
Cardiovascular	Hypovolemia Impaired cardiac contractility Decreased cardiac output	Increased cardiac output Hypertension
Pulmonary	Upper/lower airway obstruction Bronchospasm Decreased pulmonary/chest wall compliance Complications of resuscitation (pulmonary edema)	Complications of ventilation (pneumonia, barotrauma) Tracheal stenosis Dysphonia Dysphagia
Renal	Decreased renal blood flow/function Myoglobinuria	Increased renal blood flow
Hepatic	Impaired function as a result of decreased circulation, blood volume, hypoxia, hepatotoxins	Altered function as a result of hypermetabolism, increased cardiac output, enzyme induction Hepatic steatosis
Hematologic	Hemoconcentration Hemolysis Activation of fibrinolytic and thrombotic systems	Anemia Low platelets or clotting factors
Neurologic	Encephalopathy Seizures Acute pain	Encephalopathy Delirium Chronic pain
Metabolic	Increased metabolic rate Impaired thermoregulation Hypocalcemia	Increased O_2 consumption and CO_2 production
Skin	Increased heat and fluid losses	Contractures, scar formation
Gastrointestinal	Stress ulceration (Curling ulcers) Impaired intestinal barrier function	Stress ulceration (Curling ulcers) Impaired intestinal barrier function
Pharmacologic	Altered volume of distribution Altered protein binding Altered pharmacokinetics and pharmacodynamics	Increased tolerance to sedatives, narcotics Enzyme induction, alteration of receptors Drug interactions

If bowel sounds are present and there is no ileus, rapid sequence induction may not be necessary. Infection/sepsis, intestinal edema, and opioids may slow gastric emptying, increasing the risk of aspiration. Laryngeal mask airways (LMAs) have been used successfully in burn patients.[106] Use of the LMA for airway management may avoid laryngeal injury associated with tracheal intubation. It can also serve as an aid to fiberoptic intubation. The use of the LMA in the presence of decreased chest or abdominal compliance can redirect ventilated volume from the lungs into the stomach. Regurgitation of gastric contents has been observed in these instances.

Securing the endotracheal tube in a patient with facial burns can be difficult. Tape or ties crossing burned areas can irritate the wound or cause graft injury. It is essential to secure the endotracheal tube with a carefully secured tie harness (**Fig. 75-4**) to avoid unintentional extubation. Placement of a circumferential tie around the patient's head, using

TABLE 75-6 Major Preoperative Concerns for Burn Patients

Age of patient
Extent of burn injury (total body surface area, depth, and location)
Mechanism of injury
Presence of inhalational injury
Airway patency
Adequacy of resuscitation
Presence of organ dysfunction
Elapsed time from injury
Associated injuries
Presence of infection
Coexisting diseases
Surgical plan

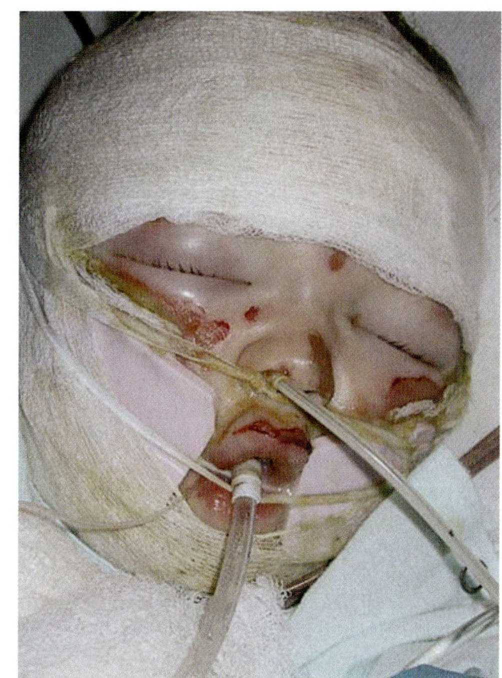

FIGURE 75-4. Photo of secured endotracheal tube. It is essential to stabilize the endotracheal tube with a carefully secured tied harness to avoid accidental extubation.

wire to secure the tube to a tooth, or the use of arch bars can provide safe fixation.[107,108]

Use of cuffed endotracheal tubes (ETTs) in pediatric patients with significant burn injury is now the norm. Use of cuffed ETTs in the pediatric population, both in the operating room and in the intensive care unit (ICU), is safe and recommended regardless of the child's age.[109-111] In the younger age group, considerable fluctuations in airway diameter can occur throughout the patient's hospital course, with narrowing of the airway during the acute resuscitation phase because of laryngeal and bronchial tissue edema. With fluctuations in airway diameter, the ETT cuff volume should be adjusted to facilitate mechanical ventilation without a leak. The proper timing and indication of tracheostomy in burn patients remains controversial. Early studies of tracheostomy reported complications to be more frequent and severe in burn patients.[112-116] Several factors contribute to the complications, particularly when tracheostomies are performed through burned tissue or in the presence of edema. The tracheal stoma can allow the passage of secretions from wound areas to the lungs leading to pneumonia. Tracheostomy, however, can be helpful, particularly when weaning from mechanical ventilation is difficult or when thick secretions require frequent pulmonary toilet. Ideally, the tracheostomy is performed under controlled conditions with the patient adequately anesthetized and positioned. Resolution of neck edema and absence of burns over the planned tracheostomy site are preferable. Recent reports examining the use of tracheostomy in severely burned children indicate that tracheostomy is appropriate.[117,118] Palmieri et al, in a case series of 38 severely burned pediatric patients undergoing early tracheostomy, found no tracheal site infections, tracheostomy-related deaths, or tracheal stenoses.[119] Patients with severe burn injury who have prolonged tracheostomy are at risk of dysphagia, dysphonia, and laryngotracheal pathology.[120]

VASCULAR ACCESS

Managing vascular access in burn patients can be difficult. In the setting of acute burn injury, patients can be hypovolemic, making venous access technically difficult to obtain. In addition, the typical vascular access sites can be involved in the burn injury. In pediatric patients, the task can be even more difficult. Central venous access is usually necessary in patients with large burn injuries. Because burn patients undergo multiple surgical procedures during their hospitalization, access is required multiple times. Furthermore, frequent catheter changes are often performed to minimize the risk of catheter-related sepsis. The sites of these lines can be rotated. Localization of vessels using ultrasonographic guidance can be useful in placing peripheral and central catheters in patients when access is difficult.[121] For excision and grafting procedures, securing adequate vascular access before the surgical procedure begins is necessary because blood loss can be rapid, substantial, and difficult to quantify.

VENTILATORY MANAGEMENT

Respiratory failure is common after serious burns caused by inhalation injury, due to inflammatory mediators from the burn, effects of fluid resuscitation, and infection. In providing mechanical ventilation, care must be exercised to provide adequate oxygenation and ventilation without inducing further morbidity from oxygen toxicity, hemodynamic compromise, barotrauma, or alveolar overdistension. A growing appreciation of the effects of ventilator-related morbidity has triggered a search for the optimum strategy for mechanical ventilation for critically ill patients with respiratory failure. The ARDS Net trial was the first large randomized study demonstrating a reduction in mortality with the use of lower tidal volumes in patients with ARDS.[122] The strength of their findings has changed ventilatory strategies and is becoming the standard of care for burn patients with acute lung injury. The empirical use of a tidal volume of 6 mL/kg ideal body weight and plateau airway pressure below 30 cm H_2O are recommended in all patients with acute lung injury. Furthermore, lower tidal volume ventilation may decrease the incidence of the development of acute lung injury that develops after the initiation of mechanical ventilation.[123] In the ARDS Network trial, positive end-expiratory pressure (PEEP) was assigned on the basis of the requirement for an elevated inspired oxygen concentration (Fio_2); in the low-tidal-volume group, the average PEEP was 9 cm H_2O. Although the assessment of optimal PEEP is still a topic of ongoing investigation, in patients with refractory hypoxemia, a trial of higher PEEP levels may be useful.

Permissive hypercapnia is a common consequence of low-tidal-volume ventilation because of the decreased minute ventilation and an increased dead-space-to-tidal-volume ratio. Permissive hypercapnia is an acceptable side effect of lung-protective ventilation and associated with excellent outcomes in burn patients.[124,125] Contraindications to permissive hypercapnia include a predisposition to an increased intracranial pressure and hemodynamic instability.

Because of their hypermetabolic state, oxygen consumption and carbon dioxide production can be significantly increased in patients with major burns. Consequently, the minute ventilation can exceed 20 L/min in an adult patient with a large burn. Such a large minute volume requirement may exceed the capacity of some anesthesia machine ventilators; an ICU ventilator may be needed in the operating room.

Extensive excision and grafting procedures may cause such great physiologic compromises that postoperative mechanical ventilation is needed. The decision to wean from mechanical ventilation and extubate after burn surgery is based on the same considerations as in the nonburn patient. Weaning is not performed in the presence of hemodynamic instability, significant metabolic derangement, hypothermia, sepsis, or worsening pulmonary function. In addition, in these patients assessment of the status of airway edema is essential before extubation.

MONITORING

As with any patient suffering from multiorgan system dysfunction, monitoring the burn patient depends on the patient's physiologic status and extent of planned surgery.

Difficulty may be encountered in the adherence of standard ECG electrodes to the skin of burn patients as a result of exudation of fluid from the injured sites or the presence of topical antibiotic ointment. Use of needle electrodes or surgical staples over skin to fix the electrodes can be effective. Alternatively, placing the electrodes on the back or dependent sites may hold them in place.

Application of pulse oximetry probes can also be difficult when standard sites are burned or within the surgical field. Alternative sites, such as the ear, nose, or tongue, can be used in such circumstances. Reflectance oximetry has been suggested as an alternative if skin sites for monitoring are limited.[126]

In an extensively burned patient, a blood pressure cuff may have to be placed directly over injured or recently grafted tissue. In these cases, great care should be taken to protect the underlying area, and the cuff should be sterilized before application. If blood loss is expected to be rapid and extensive, an arterial line should be placed for continuous direct measurement of blood pressure and blood sampling. An arterial catheter provides easy access for repeated measurements of blood gases, electrolytes, and hemoglobin. In addition, the arterial pressure waveform and its alterations in relation to respiration provide continuous hemodynamic information about preload and cardiac output and can be used to guide volume and vasoactive therapy.[127] Insertion of invasive monitors through burned tissue is sometimes necessary. Temperature monitoring is imperative because burned patients are prone to hypothermia, which carries its own morbidity.

Neuromuscular function monitoring in patients receiving neuromuscular blocking drugs is required because dose requirements can be significantly altered in burn patients.

In patients with more severe burns, a central venous catheter may be helpful for administering blood and fluids, vasoactive medications, and for pressure monitoring. Although blood sampled from a central venous catheter provides central venous and not mixed venous oxygen content, this value may be helpful in assessing the adequacy of tissue perfusion. Furthermore, central venous pressure may provide additional information on the status of intravascular volume. Central pressures should be interpreted carefully because PEEP, pleural, or pericardial fluid and abdominal distension can affect the measured pressures. More recently esophageal Doppler monitoring has been used to monitor cardiac output in burn patients undergoing early burn wound excision.[128,129] However its use is not routine.

PATIENT TRANSPORT

Transport of a burn patient to and from the operating room can be a time of increased risk. A systematic approach to maintenance of the patient's respiratory, hemodynamic, and general support will optimize patient safety. Continuous close observation by the anesthesia team during patient transport is required. In patients with major burns who require mechanical ventilation, at least 2 anesthesia personnel are required to manage ventilation, observe the monitors, and administer medications during transport.

Providing adequate sedation and analgesia is essential before moving patients to or from the bed or operating room. Intravenous narcotics and benzodiazepines are often used in combination to provide analgesia and sedation. Burn patients develop tolerance to most narcotics and sedatives, thus requiring higher doses than patients without thermal injury. Sedatives and narcotics should be titrated to optimize effect while the patient is monitored.

PHARMACOLOGIC CONSIDERATIONS

CLINICAL PHARMACOLOGY

Burn injury causes pathophysiologic changes of the cardiovascular, pulmonary, renal, and hepatic systems, as well as altered concentrations of circulating plasma proteins. These changes result in altered pharmacokinetic and pharmacodynamic responses to drugs. Consequently, changes in the usual dosages of drugs may be necessary to ensure efficacy or avoid toxicity.

There are two distinct phases of metabolic response to burn injury that affect pharmacokinetics in different ways. During the acute injury phase (0-72 h) there is rapid loss of fluid from the intravascular space, resulting in decreased cardiac output and blood flow to organs and tissues. Fluid resuscitation during this phase dilutes plasma proteins and expands the intravascular volume. Despite adequate resuscitation, patients may continue to have a decreased cardiac output. Decreased renal and hepatic blood flow reduces drug elimination by these organs. Following the resuscitation phase, the hypermetabolic-hyperdynamic phase begins, characterized by an increased cardiac output, oxygen consumption, and temperature. Because increased blood flow to the kidneys and liver may increase drug clearance, drug doses may need to be adjusted.

Plasma protein concentrations are altered in the resuscitation and hypermetabolic phases of burn injury. The 2 major drug-binding proteins, albumin and α_1-acid glycoprotein (AAG), have different responses to burn injury. The concentration of albumin that binds mostly acidic and neutral drugs is decreased in burn injury.[130] AAG is an acute-phase reactant, and its concentration may double after an acute burn. Cationic drugs (lidocaine, propranolol, muscle relaxants, and some opioids) bind to AAG, resulting in decreases of free fractions.

Hepatic clearance of drugs highly extracted by the liver depends primarily on hepatic blood flow and is relatively insensitive to alterations in protein binding. Clearance of drugs may decrease during the early postburn phase as a result of hypoperfusion from hypovolemia and hypotension. Similarly, clearance of drugs may increase during the hyperdynamic phase when hepatic blood flow increases (eg, methohexital, fentanyl).[131] In contrast, clearance of drugs that have a low hepatic extraction coefficient is unaffected by changes in hepatic blood flow but is sensitive to alterations in plasma protein levels because it is the unbound fraction of drug that is metabolized. Hepatic clearance of drugs with low extraction coefficients is also sensitive to alterations in hepatic enzyme activity. Hepatic enzyme activity appears to be altered in patients with burns.[132] Phase 1 reactions, which include oxidation, reduction, hydroxylation, and demethylation, are impaired in burn patients. Phase 2 reactions involve conjugation, glucuronidation, and sulfation and seem to be relatively unaffected.[133] Other excretion pathways may result in altered drug clearance. Thus some antibiotics and H_2-receptor antagonists will undergo enhanced clearance because of increased renal blood flow and glomerular filtration rate.[134,135] Additionally, systemically administered drugs may diffuse out through the burn wound, and blood loss during surgery can potentially exaggerate the elimination of drugs from the skin.

MUSCLE RELAXANTS

Muscle relaxant pharmacology is significantly altered after burn injury.[136] In burn patients, exposure to succinylcholine can result in an exaggerated hyperkalemic response, which can induce cardiac arrest. The general recommendation is to avoid succinylcholine administration in patients from 24 to 72 hours after burn injury.[137,138] An increase in the number of extrajunctional acetylcholine receptors has been suggested as the mechanism for increased hyperkalemia after succinylcholine administration and decreased sensitivity to the effects of nondepolarizing muscle relaxants. The duration of this response to succinylcholine is unknown. However resistance to nondepolarizing relaxants was reported in a pediatric patient 463 days after burn injury, suggesting that the hyperkalemic response to succinylcholine can persist for more than a year.[139] Although a hyperkalemic response to succinylcholine may be seen, whether lethal levels would be reached is unknown after such a long period. Consequently, even in the treatment of laryngospasm, succinylcholine should be avoided. Whether extremely small doses (0.1 mg/kg) of succinylcholine will result in less hyperkalemia has been inadequately studied. Martyn and Richtsfeld have reviewed this subject.[140] Nondepolarizing muscle relaxants are the relaxants of choice in burn patients.

Rocuronium or high doses of other nondepolarizing muscle relaxants can be used if rapid intubation is needed and one is confident that the patient can be ventilated. It must be remembered, however, that even with a dose of 1.2 mg/kg of rocuronium, the onset time to effective paralysis approximates 90 seconds in burn patients as compared with less than 60 seconds in nonburned patients.[141]

The dose of nondepolarizing muscle relaxant necessary to achieve paralysis in burn patients can be substantially elevated in a patient with burn injury. Studies with nondepolarizing muscle relaxants have demonstrated that resistance to the muscle relaxants is highly correlated with the magnitude of the burn (**Fig. 75-5**). One study demonstrated the dose of *d*-tubocurarine and the serum concentration necessary to achieve a given degree of twitch depression was 3 to 5 times greater in patients with burn injury than in nonburn patients.[142] Studies with intermediate-and short-acting muscle relaxants have also shown resistance to the neuromuscular effects of the drugs, but it is less pronounced than with long-acting relaxants. Pharmacologic reversal of neuromuscular blockade poses no special problems in patients with burn injury. Complete recovery from neuromuscular blockade has been observed at serum concentrations that would cause 100% twitch depression in nonburned patients.[142]

ANESTHETIC AGENTS

Many anesthetic agents have been used successfully for the induction and maintenance of anesthesia in burn patients. Choice of agent should be based on the patient's hemodynamic and pulmonary status and the potential difficulty in securing the patient's airway. Because of its rapid onset and lack of pungency, sevoflurane offers advantages for smooth inhalational induction in children or adults with abnormal airways. The choice of volatile aesthetic does not appear to influence the outcome

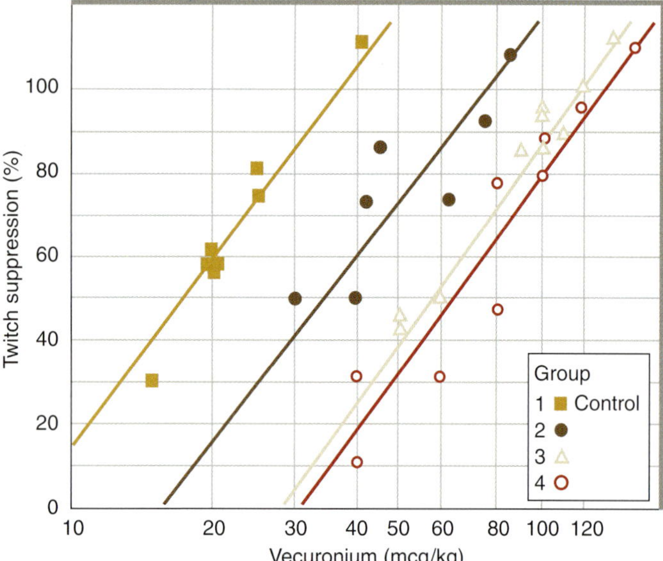

FIGURE 75-5. Dose-response curves for vecuronium in normal and burned children. Logarithm of dose versus twitch suppression for vecuronium in control subjects and burned children. With acute injury, the vecuronium-effective dose values increased with increasing burn size. *Solid squares*, children without burn injury; *solid circles*, children with less than 40% burn injury; *open triangle*, children with 40% to 60% burn injury; *open circles*, children with more than 60% burn injury. [Reproduced with permission from Mills AK, Martyn JAJ. Neuromuscular blockade with vecuronium in paediatric patients with burn injury. *Br J Clin Pharmacol.* 1989;28:155-159.]

in burn patients. All anesthetics cause dose-dependent depression of cardiac output.

Ketamine has many potential advantages for the induction and maintenance of anesthesia in burn patients and is used by some centers as the primary anesthetic. Ketamine can be associated with hemodynamic stability, preserving hypoxic and hypercapnic responses, and decreasing airway resistance. Ketamine occasionally causes a hypotensive response, particularly in patients with major burns who have desensitized adrenocepters.[143] Ketamine may be the agent of choice if one wishes to avoid manipulation of the airway (eg, after placement of fresh facial grafts, for brief procedures such as dressing changes, or for patients with TENS).[144] Ketamine can also be used to supplement other anesthetics because of its effects as an analgesic acting via the *N*-methyl-D-aspartate (NMDA) receptor.[145] The major disadvantage of ketamine is production of dysphoria. The addition of benzodiazepines is often recommended to reduce the incidence of dysphoria. Because of the increased secretions associated with ketamine, glycopyrrolate is frequently coadministered.[145]

Regional anesthesia may have a role in burn surgery, either alone or in combination with general anesthesia, but it is usually limited to patients with small burns. An epidural catheter offers the advantage of prolonged postoperative analgesia. Lumbar paravertebral blocks have been used successfully to manage postoperative pain from skin donor sites.[146] Patients with major burns may have multiple areas of injury or donor sites that cannot be easily blocked with a regional technique.

METABOLIC AND NUTRITIONAL MANAGEMENT

Severe burn injury results in a hypermetabolic response that is more severe and sustained than any other form of trauma.[147] The resting metabolic rate ranges from near normal with burns less than 10% TBSA, to twice normal in burns more than 40% TBSA.[148,149] The early phase of burn injury (first 1-2 d) is characterized by a decreased cardiac output and metabolic rate. Cardiac output and metabolic rate increase over time plateauing around postburn day 5. This increase in metabolism in association with muscle catabolism lasts through the convalescent period—and can last 12 months or more postinjury in patients with major burns.[150] As a result, lean muscle mass continues to decrease with a negative nitrogen balance despite aggressive nutritional support. This is concerning as loss of a quarter of total body nitrogen can be fatal, and this limit can easily be reached within 3 to 4 weeks in burn patients who are not receiving maximal nutritional support.[151] Nutritional support, even with exogenous insulin, cannot, in isolation, prevent or reverse the catabolic response to burn injury.

A number of strategies are used to minimize this catabolic response, including early wound excision and grafting, prompt treatment of sepsis, maintenance of high environmental temperature, early institution of feeding, and exercise programs.[152]

Early excision and grafting is the treatment that has the greatest impact on decreasing the hypermetabolic response to burn injury. If a large burn (>50%) is excised and covered within 2 to 3 days of injury, the metabolic rate is decreased by 40% as compared with a burn that is not covered with skin until 1 week postinjury.[153]

Sepsis in burn patients can be difficult to diagnose because even in the absence of sepsis, burn patients are hypermetabolic with hyperdynamic physiology. Septic patients can have an additional 40% increase in metabolic rate and catabolism as compared with nonseptic patients.[153] Thus prevention, early diagnosis, and treatment of infection are essential to reducing hypermetabolism.

Burn patients can have substantial water loss (4 L H_2O/m^2 TBSA per day in adults) from unhealed wounds.[154] The hypermetabolic response is further increased by the body's effort to generate heat to offset the inevitable temperature loss that occurs with evaporation. Consequently, maintaining the environmental temperature with high humidity is important to minimize the hypermetabolism.

Continuous enteral or parenteral nutrition partially abates the hypermetabolic response to burns and maintains the body weight. A high-carbohydrate, high-protein diet (82% carbohydrate, 15% protein, 3% fat) stimulates protein synthesis, increases endogenous insulin production, and improves lean body mass.[155] Enteral feeding is preferable to parenteral feeding because it maintains GI motility and reduces bacterial translocation and sepsis. Parenteral feeding is associated with impaired liver function, hepatic steatosis, reduced immune function, and increased mortality.[156,157] Consequently, parenteral nutrition is reserved for patients with intolerance of enteral feeding or a prolonged ileus.

Children have higher energy needs per unit body weight than adults and tolerate periods of inadequate nutrition poorly. Consequently, early nutritional support of children is essential.

Because metabolic rate can rise significantly with pain or anxiety, optimal use of analgesics and anxiolytics, together with psychological support during burn care, are of great importance. A number of pharmacologic adjuncts have been proposed to minimize loss of lean body mass after burn injury, including administration of anabolic agents, recombinant human growth hormone, insulin, oxandrolone, and propranolol.[158,159]

GLYCEMIC CONTROL

Hyperglycemia is a common metabolic response after major burn injury. Levels of gluconeogenic hormones such as glucagon, cortisol, and catecholamines are elevated postinjury and contribute to increased plasma glucose levels. In addition, insulin resistance of skeletal muscle results in decreased glucose uptake and increased hepatic glucose production and release. Hyperglycemia and insulin resistance are associated with increased morbidity and mortality in severely burned patients.[160] Furthermore, intensive insulin therapy has been shown to decrease infectious complications and mortality in critically ill burned children and adults.[161-163] Although the mechanism is not well understood, reductions of resting energy expenditure and mitochondrial oxidative capacity associated with intensive insulin therapy may partially explain the benefit.[164] Although the optimal level of glucose control is unclear, targeting blood glucose levels less than 150 mg/dL during the perioperative period seems warranted.

FLUID MANAGEMENT AND BLOOD LOSS DURING BURN WOUND EXCISION

The goal of surgical management is to remove layers of burned eschar until the bleeding dermis is reached. Blood loss during burn wound excision can be deceptively large. It is not uncommon for the surgical team to remove eschar so rapidly that the patient becomes hypovolemic and unstable. Children have thinner skin than adults, making burns relatively deeper. This may result in relatively greater bleeding during excision and grafting procedures. Correction of intravascular volume before induction of anesthesia is essential. Good communication between the surgical and anesthesia team, as well as limiting the operative duration and extent of excision, can prevent such problems. Blood should be readily available before extensive burn excision is initiated. Published estimates of the amount of blood loss during burn excision operations are in the range of 3.5% to 5% of the blood volume for every 1% TBSA excised.[165,166] This amount of blood loss results because diffuse bleeding is used as an end point for excision, informing the surgeon that the tissue is viable. However, diffuse bleeding is not the only sign of tissue viability. The experienced surgeon can identify viability with other signs, including the presence of moist yellow fat, patent small blood vessels, and the absence of extravascular hemoglobin.[167] Blood loss during these procedures can be minimized by the use of an intraoperative tourniquet for limb surgery, injection of dilute epinephrine (1 mg/L), and a brisk operative pace. Injection of higher-than-usual doses of epinephrine is permissible because the adrenoreceptors of burn patients are desensitized.[143] The dose limitation of epinephrine in normal patients is approximately 15 to 20 mcg/kg. In burn patients, even with twice this dose, no arrhythmias and a mild rise (15%) in blood pressure have been observed. If blood loss appears significant, it is prudent to assess the patient's hematologic and coagulation status regularly.

CALCIUM HOMEOSTASIS

Depression of plasma ionized calcium levels is common with acute burn injury, and abnormalities in calcium metabolism may persist for several weeks after injury, depending on the burn size.[168] These levels can be further diminished by the administration of citrate containing blood products that bind calcium. Normal calcium levels are necessary for optimal myocardial and smooth muscle contraction. Severe hypocalcemia can lead to dysrhythmias, hypotension, and/or electromechanical dissociation. Consequently, the administration of supplemental calcium is important for severely burned patients, particularly during rapid administration of (citrated) fresh-frozen plasma or albumin, both of which bind calcium.[169]

TEMPERATURE MANAGEMENT

Intraoperative consequences of hypothermia include a decreased cardiac output, arrhythmias including ventricular fibrillation if severe enough, abolition of hypoxic pulmonary vasoconstriction, left shift of the hemoglobin dissociation curve, release of catabolic hormones, interference with the normal blood clotting mechanism, and reduction of hepatic and renal function. Postoperative consequences include shivering, impairment of drug clearance, and masking of hypovolemia.[170] Furthermore, shivering can dislodge grafts and increase oxygen consumption by 400% to 500%, resulting in increased stress to the cardiopulmonary system, which already has increased demands.[171]

INFECTION CONTROL

Infection in burn patients is a leading cause of morbidity and mortality. Patients are immunocompromised and therefore susceptible to colonization and infection by organisms in the environment. Sources of organisms that can cause infection include the patient's own (endogenous) flora, exogenous environmental sources, and transmission by health care personnel. Burn injury leads to increased susceptibility to infection through multiple mechanisms, including loss of the physical barrier of an intact skin, damage to lining of the respiratory tract from inhalation, and altered gut permeability and function. Using invasive devices, including endotracheal tubes, intravascular catheters, and urinary catheters, bypass the body's normal defense mechanisms and therefore require meticulous attention to aseptic techniques during insertion, and continuing care is essential.

Central line–related infection may be associated with significant morbidity and mortality in burn patients. One large study of 1183 burn patients and 1346 central venous catheters reported an incidence of catheter-related infection of 19.5% with a mortality of 14%.[172] Adherence to multifaceted evidence-based guidelines for prevention of catheter-related bloodstream infections (CR-BSIs) has been shown to reduce (CR-BSIs) dramatically in ICU patients.[173,174] The guidelines recommend hand hygiene, maximal barrier precautions, chlorhexidine skin antisepsis, optimal catheter site selection, and removing unnecessary catheters. Although there is limited evidence regarding the efficacy of these interventions in preventing CR-BSIs of burn patients in particular, it seems prudent to adhere to the guidelines for burn patients.[175,176]

Microorganisms causing infection in burn patients include gram-positive and gram-negative bacteria, as well as yeast and fungi. The typical burn wound is colonized early with gram-positive organisms, which are rapidly replaced by antibiotic-susceptible gram-negative organisms. With persistence of open wounds, these flora are replaced by resistant bacteria, yeast, and fungi. Strategies to prevent infection include strict aseptic techniques, including use of sterile gloves and dressings, wearing masks, and spatial separation of patients.[177,178] Maintaining sterile technique both in the operating room and during transport is essential.

The diagnosis of sepsis and infection can be particularly challenging in patients with extensive burns because these patients are chronically exposed to inflammatory mediators. This exposure can result in baseline temperature elevation, persistent tachycardia and tachypnea, and an altered white blood cell count that are the standard criteria for the diagnosis of sepsis and infection. Consequently, other clues of infection or sepsis are often used such as increased fluid requirements, altered mental status, worsening pulmonary or renal status, and dropping platelet counts. Burn experts have recently developed standardized definitions for sepsis and infection-related diagnoses in burn patients.[179]

SURGICAL CONSIDERATIONS AND BURN WOUND MANAGEMENT

Early excision of dead tissue and closure of burn wounds are important advances that have been made in the management of patients with severe burns during the last 3 decades. Early excision and closure results in a decreased metabolic rate, reduced incidence of sepsis, and improved pain control. In addition, early surgical therapy before extensive bacterial colonization may decrease operative bleeding and transfusion requirements.[180]

At present, most full-thickness burn wounds are closed with split-thickness autografts. Nonetheless, the split-thickness autograft is an imperfect replacement for full-thickness skin, and harvesting normal skin is associated with pain and donor-site morbidity.[181] Skin substitutes, either temporary or permanent, may be needed. Temporary skin substitutes provide transient physiologic wound closure giving protection from mechanical trauma, minimizing evaporative water and heat losses, and acting as a physical barrier to bacteria. These skin substitutes can also be used as a dressing on donor sites to decrease pain, enhance epithelialization, and provide temporary closure while awaiting the healing of underlying, widely meshed autografts. These skin substitutes can also be used as a "test" graft in questionable wound beds. No ideal permanent skin substitute exists at present, although a number of techniques are in use, including cultured epithelial cells and dermal analogs.[181-183]

CONSIDERATIONS OF TOPICAL AGENTS

Microorganisms grow rapidly in burn wounds as a result of damage to the normal skin barrier, as well as from impaired immunologic

TABLE 75-7 Topical Antimicrobial Agents and Their Toxicities

	Effectiveness	Side Effects	Ease of Use	Pain
Silver nitrate ($AgNO_3$) 0.5% aqueous solution	Broad spectrum Inhibits cell wall growth Penetrates 2-4 mm into wound	Hypoallergenic Leeches plasma electrolytes	0.5-inch-thick wet dressings Change daily and soak q2h to keep damp Stains tissue and environment black	Stings briefly
Mafenide acetate (Sulfamylon aqueous solution)	Broad spectrum	Causes dose-related metabolic acidosis as a result of HCO_3 wasting	0.5-in-thick wet dressings	Stings briefly
	Effective for resistant organisms (ie, *Pseudomonas*)	Sensitivity rash	Change daily and soak q6h to keep damp	
Silver sulfadiazine (Silvadene 1% cream)	Broad spectrum Chemical debriding agent	Dose-related neutropenia Contains sulfur Sensitivity rash	Change daily To prevent buildup, remove residue with each dressing change	Stings briefly
Bacitracin ointment	Broad-spectrum antibiotic ointment for partial-thickness wounds	Hypoallergenic (does not contain sulfur compounds)	Daily dressing change Apply and cover with dressing	No pain

function. Because burn eschar is often distant from patent microvasculature, systemically administered antimicrobial agents may be ineffective in preventing colonization or treating infection at the wound surface. Topical antimicrobials, however, provide high concentrations of drug at the wound surface and penetrate the eschar to varying degrees, depending on the agent. Topical antimicrobials delay the interval between injury and colonization and can reduce levels of wound flora. Considerations in choice of topical agents include antimicrobial spectrum, degree of eschar penetration, patient comfort, and toxicity.[184] Topical agents commonly used in the treatment of major burns are mafenide acetate (Sulfamylon), silver nitrate, and silver sulfadiazine (Silvadene) (**Table 75-7**).

METHEMOGLOBINEMIA

Some strains of gram-negative bacteria can reduce nitrates from silver nitrate to nitrites. Nitrites can diffuse into the bloodstream, converting hemoglobin to methemoglobin.[185] Methemoglobin decreases the oxygen-carrying capacity of hemoglobin and shifts the oxyhemoglobin dissociation curve to the left, resulting in decreased oxygen delivery to tissues. Therefore, methemoglobin should be considered in the differential diagnosis of cyanosis in this setting. Blood that contains more than 10% methemoglobin usually appears dark red or brown despite a high Pao_2. Pulse oximetry, although showing a decreased saturation, will be falsely elevated. Treatment of methemoglobinemia consists of removing the silver nitrate, breathing supplemental oxygen, and administration of methylene blue (2 mg/kg).[186]

POSTOPERATIVE CARE

A phone call to the burn unit should be made at least 30 minutes before completion of the procedure in the operating room to allow the care team adequate time to warm the room and obtain necessary supplies and equipment (eg, infusions, ventilator) that will be needed on the patient's arrival in the burn unit.

Ensuring adequate sedation and analgesia is essential in the immediate postoperative period. The presence of newly excised tissue and harvested donor sites can be very painful, requiring large doses of analgesics and sedatives. As indicated previously, it is common for burn patients to become quite tolerant to sedatives over time and thus doses substantially larger than normal may be required.

Patients should be recovered in a prewarmed room because considerable heat loss can develop during transport. Radiant heaters, fluid warmers, and warming blankets are useful in maintaining normothermia.

PAIN MANAGEMENT

Nearly every aspect of the treatment of burn injury (eg, dressing changes, excision and grafting procedures, physical therapy) produces pain. Pain results from direct treatment itself and is exacerbated by anxiety. Poorly controlled pain and anxiety can have significant adverse physiologic and psychological effects. Posttraumatic stress disorder has been reported to occur in up to 30% of patients with severe burn injury, often developing in the setting of inadequate treatment of anxiety and pain.[187,188] The amount of pain associated with burn injury has been reported to be directly proportional to the size of the thermal injury. Early concerns over fear of addiction to opioids were unwarranted. No studies of pediatric patients have documented opiate addiction, and the addiction rate in adult patients is very low.[189] Patient-controlled analgesia has been shown to be a safe and effective method of opioid delivery for acute or procedure-related pain in both children and adults with burn injury.[190-192]

In the early stages of burn injury there may be an increased potency of analgesic medications, but over time marked increases in analgesic requirements can occur. Continuous administration of analgesics by itself can result in opioid-induced hyperalgesia. This will accentuate the need for higher opioid levels.[193]

To provide appropriate, consistent patient comfort, standardized pain and anxiety guidelines are used in many burn centers. The ideal characteristics of such a guideline include (1) safety and efficacy over a

TABLE 75-8 Pain Treatment Guidelines

Stage of Injury	Background Anxiety	Background Pain	Procedural Anxiety	Procedural Pain
Acute burn mechanically ventilated	Midazolam infusion Dexmedetomidine	Morphine infusion	Midazolam bolus	Morphine bolus Ketamine
Acute burn not mechanically ventilated	Scheduled lorazepam PO or IV	Scheduled morphine PO or IV	Lorazepam PO or IV	Morphine PO or IV Ketamine
Chronic acute burn	Scheduled lorazepam PO	Scheduled morphine or methadone PO	Lorazepam PO	Morphine PO
Reconstructive burn surgery	Scheduled lorazepam PO	Scheduled morphine PO	Lorazepam PO	Morphine PO

PO, by mouth; IV, intravenous.

broad range of ages and burn injury severities, (2) explicit recommendations for drug selection, dosing, and increases of dose, (3) a limited formulary to promote staff familiarity with the drugs used, and (4) regular assessment of pain and anxiety levels with guidance for intervention through adjusted drug dosing.[194,195] **Table 75-8** gives one example of a pain treatment guideline. Adjustments to treatment of opioid tolerance include switching of opioids (morphine to fentanyl to methadone) and coadministration of drugs acting on nonopioid receptors (ketamine, an NMDA antagonist; dexmedetomidine, an α_2-agonist).

Acetaminophen is a useful first-line analgesic for minor burns. Nonsteroidal anti-inflammatory drugs and benzodiazepines are commonly combined with opioids to relieve procedural pain. Pain is exacerbated by anxiety that may be reduced by benzodiazepines. Antidepressants appear to enhance opiate-induced analgesia, especially in patients with chronic (neuropathic) pain. Antidepressants have potential cardiovascular effects and for this reason are contraindicated in the early stages of burn treatment. Anticonvulsants may be useful to treat pain following burns. Clonidine, an α_2-agonist, may be a useful adjunct in reducing pain without causing pruritus or respiratory depression. However, it can cause hypotension in high doses and therefore should not be given to hemodynamically unstable patients.[196] Dexmedetomidine has been used to provide sedation-analgesia for burned patients and to decrease opioid requirements.[197,198] Its usefulness and side effects in burn patients have not been thoroughly studied.

As the patient recovers, the painful stimuli decrease and opioid dosing is gradually reduced. Prompt, definitive wound closure is the most effective treatment for minimizing pain and narcotic requirements. When a patient is being weaned, opioid and benzodiazepine dosages are decreased to allow an awake sensorium for airway protection yet still produce adequate analgesia and anxiolysis. Patients may be safely extubated while receiving opioid infusions.[199]

Pruritus is a common problem during the healing process. The causes of pruritus are multifactorial, often being triggered or worsened by heat, physical activity, and stress. Pruritus usually diminishes gradually with time but sometimes persists even after complete wound healing. A variety of approaches can control itching including systemic antihistamines, moisturizing lotions, and wearing loose-fitting clothing.

Children have unique developmental and psychosocial needs that must be considered. Pain and anxiety may be more difficult to assess but should be anticipated and treated. Support and involvement of parents and family members are important adjuncts to care and recovery.

SUMMARY

The anesthetic and intensive care management of burn patients requires a detailed knowledge of the pathophysiologic effects of burn injury on multiple organ systems. Optimal treatment of the burn patient requires cooperation and care from anesthesiologists, surgeons, nurses, psychiatrists, and family members. Awareness of the alterations of pharmacokinetics and pharmacodynamics in patients with burn injury is essential. Safe care can be provided by understanding, appreciating, and anticipating the unique preoperative, intraoperative, and postoperative issues and problems of the burned patient.

KEY REFERENCES

- Alvarado R, Chung KK, Cancio LC, Wolf SE. Burn resuscitation. *Burns.* 2009;35(1):4-14.
- Arnoldo BD, Purdue GF, Kowalske K, Helm PA, Burris A, Hunt JL. Electrical injuries: a 20-year review. *J Burn Care Rehabil.* 2004;25:479-484.
- Budny P, Regan P, Roberts A. The estimation of blood loss during burns surgery. *Burns.* 1993;19:134-137.
- Demling R. The burn edema process: current concepts. *J Burn Care Rehabil.* 2005;26:207-227.
- Faucher LD, Furukawa K. Practice guidelines for the management of pain. *J Burn Care Rehabil.* 2006; 27:659-668.
- Housinger T, Lang D, Warden G. A prospective study of blood loss with excisional therapy in pediatric burn patients. *J Trauma.* 1993;34:262-263.
- Latenser BA. Critical care of the burn patient: the first 48 hours. *Crit Care Med.* 2009;37:2819-2826.
- MacLennan N, Heimbach DM, Cullen BF. Anesthesia for major thermal injury. *Anesthesiology.* 1998;89:749-770.
- Martyn J, Richtsfeld M. Succinylcholine-induced hyperkalemia in acquired pathologic states. *Anesthesiology.* 2006;104:158-169.
- McCall J, Cahill T. Respiratory care of the burn patient. *J Burn Care Rehabil.* 2005;26:200-206.
- Pereira CT, Murphy KD, Herndon DN. Altering metabolism. *J Burn Care Rehabil.* 2005;26:194-199.
- Sheridan R. Burns. *Crit Care Med.* 2002;30(Suppl):S500-S514.
- Weber J, McManus A. Infection control in burn patients. *Burns.* 2004;30:A16-A24.

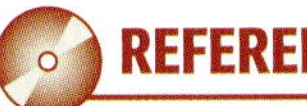

REFERENCES

Complete references available on DVD and online version at www.LongneckerAnesthesiology.com

CHAPTER 76 Evaluation and Anesthetic Management of the Trauma Patient

Edward George
John Benjamin

KEY POINTS

1. Anesthesiologists, offering airway expertise and experience in resuscitation, are uniquely qualified to be involved in both the initial evaluation and subsequent management of trauma patients.
2. Due to rising global geopolitical instability in the form of natural disasters and terrorism, anesthesiologists not normally involved in trauma care may be called on to participate in large-scale casualty events outside the operating room.
3. Acute trauma life support (ATLS) provides a systematic approach to the evaluation and emergent treatment of the trauma patient, and a vital framework for the care of the trauma patient.
4. Trauma research is accelerated during times of military conflict.
5. The effects of pain and the attendant stress response are most often detrimental to the trauma patient. Methods of pain relief range from simple continuous or on-demand intravenous (IV) opioids to more sophisticated techniques such as regional or neuraxial blocks. Use of adjuvant drugs, such as dexmedetomidine, gabapentin, or celecoxib, may decrease opioid dose and improve analgesia.

Providing care to the trauma patient can be one of the most challenging situations encountered by an anesthesiologist. The urgency of the event, often in a setting with little or no advance notice, places special burdens on the care team. Given the unpredictable nature of trauma, the anesthesiologist may be faced with caring for these patients in settings ranging from a level 1 academic hospital center with a complete array of specialists and capabilities, to a small rural hospital with limited resources, where the anesthesiologist may be the only physician present. Adding to these complexities is the emerging awareness of the special burdens imposed by the scenario of mass casualties. Prior to September 11, 2001, medical centers planned for large traumatic events on the scale of an airline crash at the airport or an industrial accident involving dozens of injured patients arriving over a brief period of time. Now with heightened awareness as a result of events such as the World Trade Tower attacks and natural disasters such as Hurricane Katrina and the more recent earthquake in Haiti, it is critical that all medical personnel including anesthesiologists become familiar with the evaluation and care of the trauma patient.

To better understand the challenges of evaluating the trauma patient, it is important to appreciate the evolution of trauma care over the history of modern medicine. Although trauma has been a major cause of morbidity throughout history, until quite recently, most progress in the area of trauma care was closely tied to the experience and expertise gained by providing care to the casualties of war. By examining the progress made in these arenas, coupled with the insights gained over the past few decades by investigators in the evaluation and care of the trauma patient, the anesthesiologist will be better positioned to contribute as a member of the trauma team.

HISTORICAL EVOLUTION OF TRAUMA CARE

Trauma remains one of the most common causes of death in modern society.[1] In the history of modern medicine, research and advancement in the care of the trauma patient has lagged well behind developments in other areas of science and technology. To better appreciate the issues underlying this discrepancy in comparison with the great strides made over the past 2 centuries in other areas of medicine, it is important to understand the context under which a large component of trauma research has been conducted.

Many of the significant advances in the care of the trauma patient have evolved from experience gained in the care of the military casualty. The Mexican-American War and the Civil War marked the first major experiences of US military surgeons operating on patients receiving a general anesthetic. The advent of surgical anesthesia using ether and chloroform, discovered less than 2 decades before the Civil War, offered a new opportunity for surgical intervention in the treatment of casualties. Surgery could be undertaken, not in the quickest way possible to minimize the agony inflicted on the unanesthetized patient, but rather in a manner permitting the surgeon time and an opportunity to perform a more detailed and delicate procedure.[2] This period also marked the development of a casualty evacuation system using ambulances to deliver casualties from the battlefield to the field hospital, the integration of nursing care into the field hospitals, and the use of antiseptics such as bromine to reduce the risk of wound infection.

With the advent of trench warfare in World War I, further advances in trauma care were developed. Typed blood transfusions were administered in field hospitals. Rapid evacuation of the casualty to treatment facilities to initiate care as soon as possible after injury and the dawn of the specialty of reconstructive surgery were a few of the major advances in trauma care that evolved from this conflict.

Advances after World War I, such as the discovery of penicillin and the development of the specialties of hand surgery and blood banking, had a further impact on the care of the combat casualty. Despite these major advances, the inability to treat shock adequately in the field during World War II remained a major cause of mortality in the battlefield casualty. During the Korean War deployment of surgical facilities in forward areas, closer to the front lines, along with the more widespread use of casualty evacuation by helicopter, reduced the delay in the treatment of casualties. New techniques in vascular surgery helped reduce the number of amputated limbs. The concept of the Mobile Army Surgical Hospital unit, now known as Forward Surgical Teams and Forward Resuscitative Surgical Sites, still remains as the entrance to modern-day battlefield surgical care. The Vietnam War saw greater improvements in the evacuation systems and a new understanding of the need for early resuscitation of the trauma patient. However the underlying physiology regarding acute respiratory distress syndrome (Da Nang lung) and hemorrhagic shock and resuscitation were still not well understood, and these problems remained a major cause of mortality.[3,4]

The period leading up to and including the conflicts in Iraq and Afghanistan resulted in greater appreciation of issues that have an impact on the trauma patient. Investigations of resuscitation and pharmacologic treatment for the hemorrhaging patient and understanding the underlying pathophysiology became areas of active investigation. These investigations herald a new era of collaboration between military and civilian academic centers, perhaps even more robust than those seen during previous major conflicts.[5]

NATURE OF TRAUMA

Trauma, both accidental and intentional, is the fourth leading cause of death in the United States.[1] Over the past several decades, death from trauma has been described by a trimodal pattern of distribution (**Fig. 76-1**), with peaks corresponding to deaths occurring at the time of injury (immediate), within several hours after injury (early), and finally those that occur days to weeks (late) after injury.[6] Deaths in the immediate group are most likely a result of severe injury to the central nervous system, the heart, or a major blood vessel. Early victims have often suffered injuries resulting in internal hemorrhage into the brain, the lungs, or other internal organs. These injuries may be amenable to treatment if the patient arrives in an appropriate facility in a timely manner, where ongoing resuscitation may later transition into more definitive therapy. It is during this golden hour, the first hour after injury, that these patients are most vulnerable to delays in treatment. The late group is composed of those patients with multiple injuries, often progressing to multiorgan system failure or death as a result of systemic infection, often occurring over the ensuing several days to weeks. The nature of the treatment facility and the degree of experience of the staff in dealing with victims of major trauma may well have an impact on the survival rate of these patients.[7]

Recent analysis suggests that the original trimodal pattern of trauma deaths may not be uniformly applicable.[8] In the setting of modern-day urban trauma centers, the distribution of death appears bimodal, with late-occurring deaths far less common. This may in part be a result of this pattern being described in an era before the widespread development of major centers focusing on care of the trauma patient. This bimodal pattern suggests that experienced and accessible centers may have a marked positive impact on the survival of the trauma victim.

Although a trauma patient often presents to the hospital with multiple injuries, it is important to appreciate that the nature of these injuries may be diverse and present different challenges to the urgent and emergent management of the patient. Injuries caused by trauma are broadly categorized into 3 main types, as a function of the mechanism of injury. Injuries are penetrating, blunt, caused by burns, or produced by a combination of these modalities. Injuries can be further subdivided, as in the case of penetrating trauma, along the lines of high energy, such as a gunshot wound, versus lower energy, as in a stabbing. Burn injuries can be subdivided into those caused by chemical agents, flames, or electrical injury. Injuries are often complex, and it may be vital to learn that a patient presenting with several fractures from a motor vehicle accident, in the setting of a prolonged extraction from a burning vehicle, may have inhaled a great deal of smoke during the rescue.

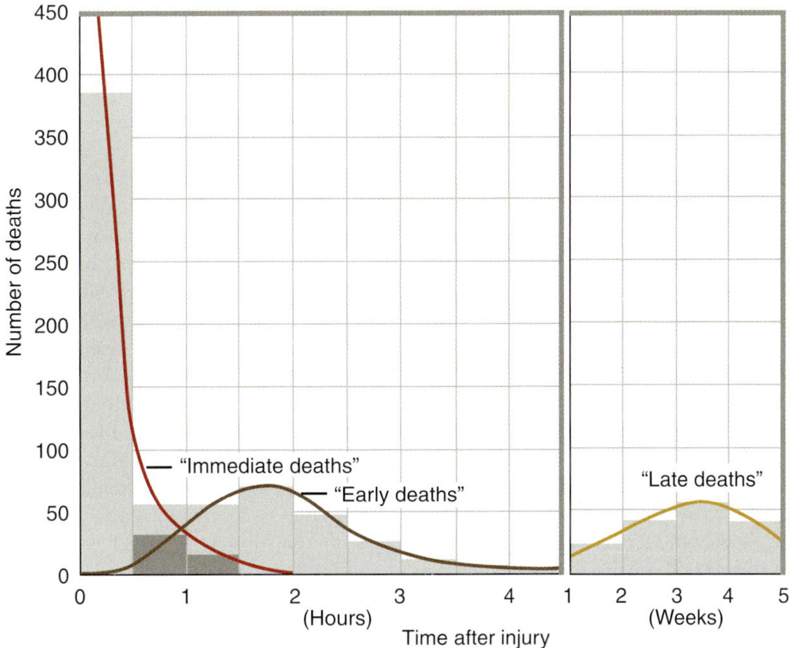

FIGURE 76-1. Trimodal distribution of trauma deaths is observed when the death rate for a large enough sample of such deaths is plotted as a function of time after injury. The first peak (*immediate deaths*) corresponds to people who die very soon after an injury; the deaths in this category are typically caused by lacerations of the brain, the brainstem, the upper spinal cord, the heart, or one of the major blood vessels. The second peak (*early deaths*) corresponds to people who die within the first few hours after an injury; most of these deaths are attributable to major internal hemorrhage or to multiple lesser injuries resulting in severe blood loss. The third peak (*late deaths*) corresponds to people who die days or weeks after an injury; these deaths are usually caused by infection or multiple organ failure. The graph is based on a sample of 862 trauma deaths recorded over a 2-year period by the author's group at San Francisco General Hospital. [Trunkey DD. Trauma. *Sci Am.* 1983;249(2):28-35.]

A detailed and systematic method for the evaluation of the trauma patient is discussed in subsequent sections of this chapter. However a generalized description of the various types of injuries aids in the appreciation of the mechanism and forces involved in the traumatic insult. It is also important to appreciate that any categorization is only partially helpful in understanding the underlying forces associated with the various injuries. Trauma patients often present with multiple injuries inflicted by diverse mechanisms, and, as a result may be far more complex in their management than apparent on initial arrival.

BLUNT TRAUMA

A common scenario involving blunt trauma or circumstances where blunt trauma should be suspected is a motor vehicle accident. The unrestrained occupants in a vehicle, particularly individuals not afforded protection by an air bag system, may present with blunt injuries to the chest, thorax, abdomen, or any other part of the body. The outward appearance of the injury, such as a seemingly minor bruise on the abdomen or thorax, may belie the severity of the underlying injury. A minor bruise on the abdomen could signal a lacerated spleen or liver, and the faint impression of a steering wheel on the anterior chest wall may signal underlying pulmonary contusions or a deceleration injury of the great vessels. A small contusion on the flank of a blast victim may not at first glance appear to be a serious injury. However in the setting of an attendant tympanic membrane injury or pneumothorax,[9] this injury may suggest a significant degree of force associated with the mechanism of injury and may signal the presence of severe and potentially life-threatening injuries. Additionally, blunt trauma can be complicated by problems such as rhabdomyolysis, which are often associated with crushing injuries to the thorax and extremities.

PENETRATING TRAUMA

Whether caused by a high-velocity projectile, such as a rifle bullet, or lower-energy insult such as a knife wound, it is vital to appreciate that the external appearance may mask the extent of the internal injury. In the case of knife wound to the left flank, a small wound with little visible bleeding may mask a trajectory that injures the bowel, spleen, diaphragm, and heart. Similarly, a small entry wound caused by a gunshot, with no apparent exit wound and scant visible bleeding, may be associated with multiple internal injuries because of internal fragmentation of the projectile.

BURNS

Although the care of the burn patient is addressed in detail in other chapters (eg, Chapter 75), basic issues regarding the challenges of evaluating and caring for the burn victim are briefly addressed here. Thermal injury can result in a severe physiologic impact on the patient, despite the minor outward appearance. Evaluation and care of burn patients require a thorough understanding of the insult caused by the burn; the disruption of the body's ability to maintain a normal fluid balance and an enhanced risk of infection are 2 areas of major importance. Chemical burns, often requiring specialized debridement, present special risks to the patient and the care team. Inhalation injury caused by smoke or toxic or high-temperature gases can be life threatening in a patient who may otherwise appear unhurt. These patients may be the most challenging to support with mechanical ventilation. Patients with an electrical burn may appear to have a small injury at the sites of contact and exit, yet they may have experienced severe damage to internal structures and organs.[10]

PATHOPHYSIOLOGY OF TRAUMA

The physiologic response to trauma is complex and tightly regulated. An understanding of the range and nature of the involved mechanisms is critical in the evaluation of the trauma patient.

Multiple injuries (polytrauma) in the trauma patient have long been associated with an increased morbidity and mortality. Patients who survive the initial insult are subject to a number of physiologic challenges that can induce immunologic and/or host defense responses. Both the initial physiologic challenges, such as hypoxemia, hypotension, fractures, and soft tissue injuries, as well as subsequent insults because of reperfusion injury, a compartment syndrome, multiple operations, and infections, all play a role in this response. The systemic inflammatory response (SIRS) is associated with the release of proinflammatory cytokines, arachidonic acid metabolites, proteins of the contact phase and coagulation systems, hormonal mediators, complement factors, and acute-phase proteins.[11] However, in the body's attempts to maintain homeostasis, a parallel mechanism of anti-inflammatory mediators is released. This compensatory anti-inflammatory response syndrome involves the release of anti-inflammatory mediators that serve to quench the initial inflammatory response. T-cell cytokines, such as interleukin (IL)-4, IL-10, and IL-13 are known to modulate monocyte activity. However, defective T cells, released after trauma, may synergize with activated monocytes and contribute to a further deterioration of the patient's clinical condition, impairing the body's ability to fight infection.[12] An imbalance of these 2 response systems may be an underlying element producing the organ dysfunction and increased susceptibility to infections seen after trauma. Over time, endothelial damage, leukocyte accumulation, disruption of the microcirculation, and disseminated intravascular coagulation (DIC) can lead to widespread apoptosis and necrosis. This can result in multiorgan dysfunction syndrome or multiple organ failure (MOF). Although the early use of anti-inflammatory agents in the trauma patient has not been encouraging, research into the detailed understanding of the immune response to trauma is providing new insight into the complexities of response with great interest in specific inhibitors of key steps in the cascade.[13] This may also serve to identify individuals at risk for posttraumatic complications and assist in creating early and specific interventions. This cascade of events can be characterized by 2 distinct mechanisms of cell death: apoptosis and necrosis.

COAGULATION SYSTEM

There is a marked physiologic reserve of the factors associated with the coagulation system in the healthy individual. Several issues common to the trauma patient can dramatically compromise coagulation and have a negative impact on the survival of the victim. Although the reserve of coagulation factors in the healthy individual provides a significant buffer in the capacity of the system to correct for hemorrhage, the patient suffering from large-scale blood loss as a result of injury is faced with a rapid exhaustion of the factors associated with coagulation. In the setting of aggressive crystalloid resuscitation, the resulting dilution of available coagulation factors can limit the ability of the patient to achieve hemostasis. An environmental factor with a further impact on the function of the coagulation system in the trauma patient is that of hypothermia. Trauma victims are often hypothermic because of factors associated with prolonged exposure, massive blood loss, and resuscitation with fluids well below 98.6°F (37°C). Conditions for enzymatic pathways associated with coagulation are then less than optimal, resulting in further compromise of function. The combination of such events can result in DIC and is often associated with a dismal prognosis for the trauma patient.[14] This "lethal trauma triad" of hypothermia, acidosis, and coagulopathy is a known risk factor for trauma-associated morbidity and mortality.

TRAUMA MANAGEMENT

Improvements in both prehospital and emergency department care have resulted in a reduction in morbidity and mortality, as well as the identification of critical areas of vulnerability in the care of the trauma patient.

PREHOSPITAL CARE

The scope of care in the prehospital setting ranges from ambulances in more rural areas, often staffed by local volunteers, to the more extensive emergency services systems seen in large metropolitan areas. These may be run under the direction of state or regional agencies, often in close coordination with major trauma centers. Although there is diversity in the nature of assets available in any specific setting, there has been a major effort over the past few decades to improve standards of care, methods of delivery, and the training available to the care providers across the United States. The evolution of air evacuation systems using helicopters has further extended our ability to respond rapidly to the challenges of the trauma patient.

First responders trained in basic cardiopulmonary resuscitation and first aid are often local law enforcement and fire department personnel. With the arrival of one or more emergency medical technicians (EMTs), a more detailed evaluation of the patient's condition takes place, integrating the mechanism of injury with the physical findings, making diagnoses, and initiating treatment. Although the level of training and certification of the EMT ranges from a basic EMT to a paramedic capable of providing advanced cardiac life support (ACLS), the EMT provides early treatment, often guided by the treatment facility designated to receive the patient. In addition to airway, breathing, and circulation support, the EMT is able to address issues related to wounds and fractures, supplementing the basics of securing an airway, obtaining IV access, initiating resuscitation, and administering medications as indicated.

At the scene the overall process undertaken by emergency medical personnel is focused on assessment and management. An initial assessment for site safety is performed to ensure that any potential risks to cause further injury to the patient or to emergency personnel are identified. Requirements for additional personnel or specialized equipment may be identified at this point. An appreciation of the nature of the incident resulting in the trauma also provides the EMT insight into potential patterns of injury. At this point, a primary survey of the patient is performed to identify and treat life-threatening injuries. In critically injured patients, minimizing delay in transport is critical. As such, treatment and resuscitation are instituted as quickly as possible, with transport measures often being instituted in a parallel process.[15]

Intuitively, the ability to provide more advanced care in the prehospital setting would be expected to have a positive impact on patient outcome. However, studies suggest that the ability to provide more advanced care, such as tracheal intubation and ACLS, has little impact on survival, whereas minimal resuscitation and rapid transport to a trauma center appears to make a positive effect improving outcome.[16,17] Certain interventions, such as tracheal intubation of the patient with a severe head injury and IV resuscitation of the hypotensive patient in shock caused by penetrating trauma, may represent special categories of patients who will benefit from field interventions.[18] However, the survival of severely head-injured patients who are intubated in the field may be higher when compared with a similarly injured group of patients who are not intubated in the field only when variables such and hyper- and hypocapnia are controlled.[19] It would appear that in the setting of improved capabilities for the delivery of prehospital care, the apparent lack of benefit to the patient suggests there are underlying issues contributing to the morbidity and mortality of the trauma patient that are, as yet, not well understood.[20]

HOSPITAL CARE

The nature and setting of care for the trauma patient in the hospital can vary. Although a markedly unstable patient may be brought directly from the ambulance entrance of the hospital to the operating room, the more commonly encountered sequence involves the arrival of the patient to the emergency department for a detailed evaluation, resuscitation, and development of a course of treatment. The effective organization of the emergency department is vital to the delivery of appropriate care to the patient. **Figure 76-2** depicts the typical configuration of a trauma bay. Often a near-chaotic environment, a team of key personnel, with appropriate equipment and support services, is

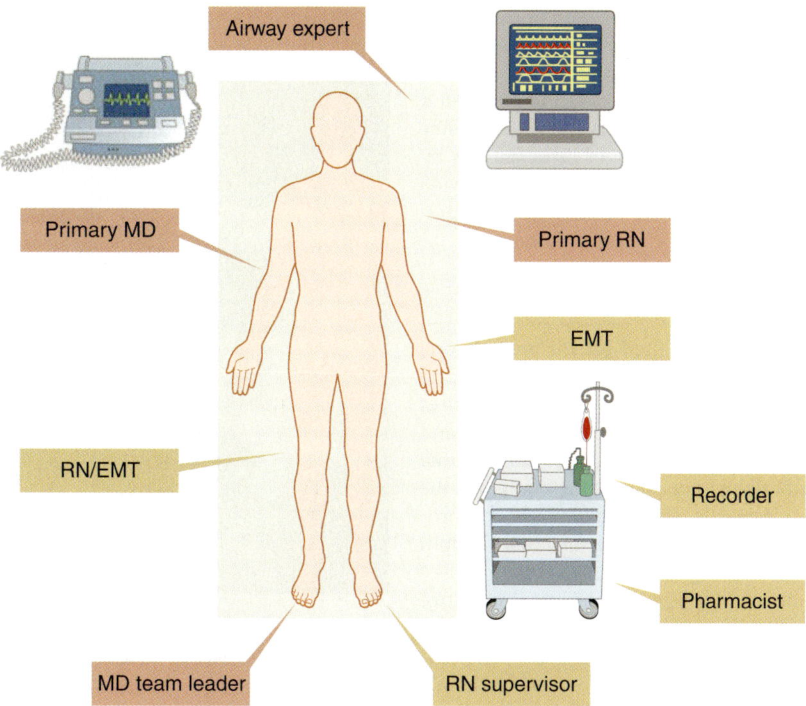

FIGURE 76-2. Configuration of a typical trauma bay. Designed to maximize efficiency of multiple key personnel and associated equipment for the care of an acutely injured patient. Specific roles and coordination are critical in effectively functioning in an often chaotic environment. EMT, emergency medical technician; MD, medical doctor; RN, registered nurse.

required to ensure the most expeditious assessment and treatment of the patient.

Organized around a team leader, the emergency team requires designated personnel with specific skills. Task organized in a manner to provide critical expertise and capabilities, this group often draws on personnel from services throughout the institution. The team leader, often an emergency medicine physician, is responsible for directing all components of patient care, as well as obtaining pertinent information from the prehospital phase of care regarding patient information and mechanisms of traumatic injury. The team leader is also responsible for the conduct of the primary and secondary surveys of the patient. An airway expert from the department of anesthesia, respiratory therapy, emergency medicine, or surgery is tasked with securing the airway and regulating mechanical ventilation as required. The team leader may often function as the airway expert as well. In the setting of a trauma patient with obvious requirements for surgical intervention, the trauma surgeon will assume the role of the team leader. Procedural personnel may be used for placing IV access, obtaining lab samples, coordinating with the blood bank, the placing of monitors, and performing additional tasks as determined by the team leader. Depending on the extent of the trauma, multiple personnel may play a role in performing procedures in the emergency department. Nurses comprise an integral portion of the trauma team. Responsibilities run from direct involvement in resuscitation to key roles in the interaction with supporting services as well as with patient families. Additional personnel involved in the trauma team may include a radiography technician, recorder, family and patient care support personnel, mental health providers, pharmacist, specialty surgeon(s), and clergy.

One of the most important aspects of the trauma team is the ability to respond immediately to an injured patient in a timely, efficient, and reliable manner. This response capability is born of a specific training plan, with clearly identified roles and requirements for each team member.[21] This facilitates a coordinated approach to a trauma patient, in a setting that often requires multiple parallel tracks of assessment and intervention (**Fig. 76-3**).

The disposition of the trauma patient in the emergency department varies. A patient injured in a motor vehicle collision who is stable on arrival in the emergency department may be sent to the radiology department for studies and then taken immediately to the operating room or admitted to the hospital for further treatment and/or evaluation. These patients must be carefully observed for acute changes in clinical conditions while being transferred from the emergency department to other sites within the hospital (eg, computed tomography [CT]

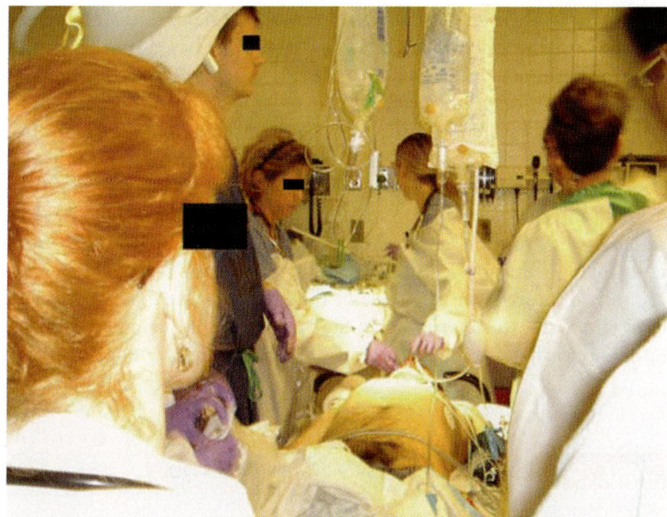

FIGURE 76-3. Trauma team caring for an acutely injured patient in the emergency department. Clockwise from left foreground: team leader (emergency department attending), primary physician. Respiratory therapist at the head of the stretcher, with assistance provided by an emergency department nurse at the patient's right and primary nurse at the patient's left.

scanner, interventional radiology). A similar patient, with unstable vital signs, may require resuscitation in the emergency department before proceeding to additional studies or the operating room. Some patients arrive emergently and are brought directly to the operating room for a lifesaving intervention or undergo emergency surgery in the emergency department. This serves to illustrate the diversity of presentations by a trauma patient and the need for emergency departments to provide experienced and well-trained personnel capable of immediate adaptation of therapeutic plans to rapidly changing clinical conditions.

PATIENT ASSESSMENT

The emergent presentation of an acutely injured patient presents one of the greatest clinical challenges for the anesthesiologist. The need to perform a critical assessment rapidly, often in a chaotic setting, requires that the anesthesiologist approach the situation in an efficient and focused manner. Additionally, the uncertainty associated with a trauma patient mandates that the anesthesiologist be vigilant for changes in the clinical situation (**Table 76-1**). Typically, the most severely compromised patients offer the least amount of time to perform an in-depth survey.

Since the late 1960s, the American College of Surgeons Committee on Trauma has developed a systematic and stylized approach to the trauma patient. The advanced trauma life support system (ATLS) evolved from the experience of an orthopedic surgeon and his family involved in a private plane crash. The evaluation and treatment provided to this family in a small community hospital was disorganized and haphazard. The efforts precipitated by this experience have led to a system that facilitates a prioritized approach to the trauma patient. This has resulted in a standardized and widely accepted protocol to initially address potentially life-threatening issues, using the principles of airway, breathing, and circulation (ABCs), followed by a more extensive survey to better determine the extent and nature of the injuries. This process also facilitates communication within an institution, as well as between institutions in the case of patient transfer requirements, providing assistance in the subsequent disposition.[22] Even if ATLS is not required by the hospital's credentialing office, any anesthesiologists who have even a remote chance of dealing with trauma patients should be familiar with the ATLS principles so they understand the modern approach to trauma.

PRIMARY SURVEY AND RESUSCITATION

The well-established approach to the ABCs remains the standard of approaching the trauma patient. Prioritization is based on the immediacy of the threat to life. The need to support and/or secure the airway remains the highest priority. The inability to oxygenate a patient can result in irreversible damage to the brain in as little as 4 minutes. Supporting the airway may be as simple as opening the mouth and clearing away debris, to as complicated as securing the airway in a patient with severe trauma to the head and neck requiring the need of an emergency surgical airway. Managing the airway in a trauma patient often involves the physical constraints of maintaining cervical spine precautions. Protocols for clearance of the cervical spine may vary across institutions. However it is likely that most trauma patients requiring intubation will also require cervical spine stabilization.[23] Specific issues regarding the approach to the difficult airway in the trauma patient are addressed in the airway management section of the chapter. Even in the setting of a protected airway, the respiratory drive may be impaired from an injury to the head, metabolic compromise, or depressant drug administration, and the anesthesiologist must ensure that adequate oxygenation and ventilation are maintained (**Fig. 76-4**). Issues affecting circulation are also addressed in this initial survey. Although the sequence of emergency treatment prioritizes airway and breathing, in the setting of the trauma bay, parallel efforts are often directed toward circulatory issues at the same time the airway issues are being addressed. The threat to life by hemorrhage can also occur as rapidly as a few minutes to a few hours after injury and, as such, occupies a priority following oxygenation (**Table 76-2**). The most commonly encountered issue in the hypotensive trauma patient is hypovolemia. In the setting of a stable cardiac rhythm a fluid challenge of 1 to 2 L of warm crystalloid is administered. A plan to treat ongoing hemorrhage needs to be developed and is roughly delineated along the lines of compressible versus noncompressible hemorrhage. Controlling or temporizing bleeding from an extremity may provide adequate time to obtain necessary studies (radiography, angiography), whereas an incompressible hemorrhage (torso, cranium) may require emergent treatment in the operating room or the emergency department.

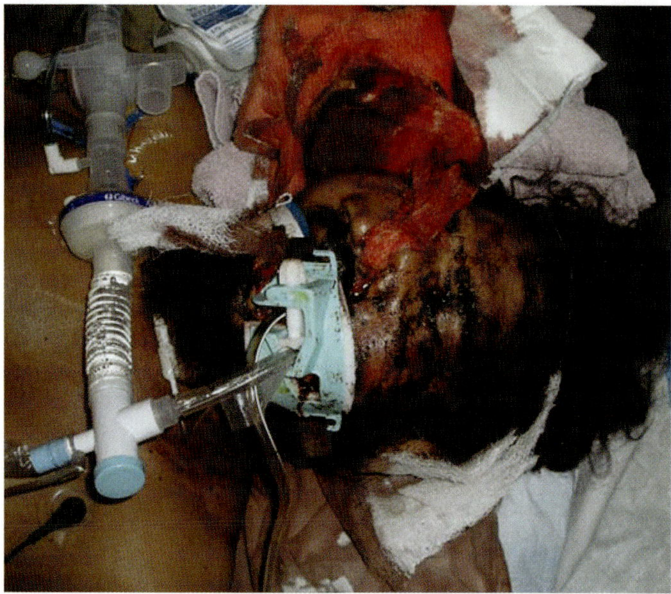

FIGURE 76-4. Massive facial injury. High-energy injury resulting in multiple fractures of the mandible, maxilla, tongue, hard palette, sinus, and nose, and enucleation of the right eye. Patient was awake and alert immediately prior to intubation.

TABLE 76-1 Trauma Team Roles for the Anesthesiologist
Anesthesiologist
Team leader
Critical care specialist
Transport coordinator
Pain management
Mass casualty coordinator

This initial assessment phase requires that personnel be able to recognize immediately and treat issues that present an imminent threat to survival. The mechanism of injury, if known during this phase, may provide some insight to the team; however the primary issues in a systematic approach are as follows:

Airway

- Inadequacy
- Obstruction

Breathing

- Pneumothorax
- Hemothorax
- Tension pneumothorax
- Flail chest

TABLE 76-2 Physiologic Effects of Hemorrhage for 70-kg Male

	Class I	Class II	Class II	Class IV
Blood loss (mL)	<750	750-1500	1500-2000	>2000
Blood loss (% blood volume)	<15%	15%-30%	30%-40%	>40%
Pulse rate	<100	>100	>120	>140
Blood pressure	Normal	Normal	Decreased	Decreased
Pulse pressure	Normal or increased	Decreased	Decreased	Decreased
Respiratory rate	14-20	20-30	30-40	>35
Urine output (mL/h)	>30	20-30	5-15	Negligible
Mental status	Slightly anxious	Mildly anxious	Anxious/confused	Confused/lethargic
Fluid replacement	Crystalloid	Crystalloid	Crystalloid/blood	Crystalloid/blood

Circulation

- Hemorrhage
- Cardiac tamponade
- Shock
- Cardiogenic
- Neurogenic
- Obstructive
- Septic

Recognition and timely treatment of these conditions usually requires urgent intervention. It is imperative that the trauma team have the personnel, equipment, and supplies immediately available to intervene as needed.[24] The initial assessment then continues to address issues with regard to the extent of neurologic compromise, commonly referred to as D for disability, in the conventionally accepted ABCDE format. A brief examination, using the Glasgow Coma Scale (GCS) can coarsely evaluate the patient's neurologic condition with regard to verbal and gross motor function (**Table 76-3**). Pupillary response is also determined at this phase. A GCS score less than 8 usually requires immediate tracheal intubation to protect the airway.[25] The final component of the initial assessment is termed as E for exposure and environment. Clothing is removed while attention is directed toward preventing hypothermia by ensuring that the patient's environment is adequately warmed.

TABLE 76-3 Glasgow Coma Score

Eye-opening response	
4	Spontaneous
3	To speech
2	To pain
1	None
Verbal response	
5	Oriented to name
4	Confused
3	Inappropriate speech
2	Incomprehensible sounds
1	None
Motor response	
6	Follows commands
5	Localizes to painful stimuli
4	Withdraws to painful stimuli
3	Abnormal flexion (decorticate)
2	Abnormal extension (decerebrate)
1	None

The Glasgow Coma Score is the sum of the highest score in all categories.

During this initial phase, resuscitation is initiated, monitoring is established, to include a Foley catheter and an orogastric tube for the intubated patient, and any available history is obtained (often referred to as F, G, and H of the ABC mnemonic). Information regarding the nature of the events resulting in the patient's injury and transport is obtained in coordination with the prehospital care team. At this point, samples for critical lab values, such as arterial blood gas tensions and pH, blood glucose, and hematocrit, if not obtained during the earlier establishment of IV access, are sent with additional lab tests. Plans for radiographs and/or additional studies are formulated. Throughout the primary survey, the evaluating physician is obtaining information and may determine there is a need to transfer the patient to another facility. Support personnel, after direction by the team leader, may initiate the process of transfer. Physician-to-physician direct communication remains a critical factor in transferring a patient between institutions.[26]

A common error in management during the primary survey involves delay in securing the patient's airway. Trauma team leaders may be hesitant to secure the airway because of distraction or inexperience. It is important for the anesthesiologist to be appropriately aggressive in this arena.[27-29] An unrecognized pneumothorax is another common error. Excessive fluid resuscitation often occurs to the trauma patient. Once again, the anesthesiologist can guide the fluid management of the trauma patient. As discussed in the section on resuscitation, the area of hypotensive resuscitation is being examined as a more appropriate management strategy in the trauma patient.[30] Failure to establish adequate IV access and failure to involve a surgeon early may also become problematic in situations such as a difficult or lost airway, as well as in the case of a patient with a noncompressible hemorrhage.

Focused Assessment Sonography for Trauma is a rapid ultrasound examination directed solely at identifying the presence of free intraperitoneal or pericardial fluid. It is considered an adjunct to the primary survey in the ATLS guidelines.

RESUSCITATION

Prehospital guidelines suggest the placement of 2 large-bore (14- to 16-gauge) IV cannulas and the infusion of warmed lactated Ringer solution for the resuscitation of the trauma patient. When IV access is limited, consideration should be given to the placement of an intraosseous access device. Because field conditions can limit the ability to treat many of the conditions underlying hypotension, emergency medical personnel are encouraged to avoid delays in transport, continuing fluid resuscitation as clinically indicated. Currently, the goal for resuscitation of the trauma patient on arrival to the hospital is the restoration or optimization of oxygen delivery to the tissues in the face of hemorrhagic shock. Warmed crystalloids (normal saline, lactated Ringer solution), with the addition of specific blood products as clinically indicated, are the rule. Initiated in what may be a chaotic field environment, resuscitation is often carried out without any laboratory values. Although crystalloid infusion may be the only means initially available for the treating of systemic hypotension, the hemodilution associated with massive crystalloid resuscitation is often accompanied by hypothermia, coagulopathy, and acidosis. An additional concern is the inflammatory cascade initiated by trauma that is believed to be an underlying issue in the subsequent multiorgan failure of the trauma patient. In the face of ongoing uncontrolled hemorrhage, blood flow to tissue may be markedly reduced. Avoidance of tissue ischemia is likely to limit the impact of ischemic reperfusion. As such a goal of resuscitation to less than the normal physiologic state may offer some protection from the sequelae of ischemia. The impact of resuscitation to less than optimal physiologic parameters may prove beneficial to the long-term survival of the trauma patient. Resuscitation targeted to lower mean arterial pressures may provide a greater margin of safety in the early attempts to locate and control hemorrhage. And permissive hypercapnia may help limit the negative hemodynamic impact of positive pressure ventilation on the hypovolemic/hemorrhaging patient. Current investigations may suggest a role for the targeted use of anti-inflammatory therapies in early resuscitation.[31] During resuscitation, the limitation of crystalloid solution, a known activator of neutrophils, may also serve to attenuate the early inflammatory response. The use of hypertonic saline is beneficial, particularly in the setting of trauma patients with closed-head injuries.[32]

The manner of resuscitation has been a major topic for debate over the entire history of research into the care of the trauma patient. Knowledge gained through the care of the combat casualty and more recent investigations suggest that the tradition of resuscitation to normal physiologic values using isotonic fluids may be detrimental to the long-term survival of the trauma patient.[33]

During the past decade, controversy over the appropriate end points of IV fluid resuscitation in the trauma patient has led to investigations regarding optimal resuscitation strategies. From the Vietnam War era, it was appreciated that systemic perfusion pressures needed to be maintained in the hemorrhaging patient. However, there was a concern that in the setting of uncontrolled hemorrhage, aggressive fluid administration could interfere with thrombus formation and decrease the survival rate.[34] The National Institutes of Health has established the establishment of the Post-Resuscitative and Initial Utility of Life-Saving Efforts Workshop. A Trauma Work Group has undertaken to endorse strategies and priorities for research into trauma resuscitation.[35]

SHOCK

Current understanding of shock describes inadequate cellular oxygenation from hemorrhage (hypovolemic shock), cardiac failure (cardiogenic shock), and massive vasodilatation (distributive shock), although no precise pathophysiologic definition exists.

Traumatic hemorrhage causes shock principally through loss of circulating blood volume. Early physiologists described the tachycardia, hypotension, ashen complexion, and cool moist skin of the injured patient suffering from hemorrhagic shock.[36] Walter Cannon, with service as a US Army surgeon in World War I before becoming a professor of physiology at Harvard, recognized that loss of blood reduced cardiac output and caused traumatic shock. Cannon[37] proposed that the term *shock* be replaced by the term *exemia* to emphasize that blood loss was the cause of shock following wounding. A mechanical model developed by Henderson[38] advanced the understanding of the role of blood loss in hemorrhagic shock. Arthur Guyton et al refined this concept with the venous return curve, which was severely depressed following hemorrhage with a reduction in the mean filling pressure of the circulation, thus limiting maximum cardiac output.[39] Most of a person's blood volume resides in the venules as the "unstressed volume" (blood that fills the anatomic space of the veins and venules without stretching the vascular structures and, therefore, does not generate pressure).[40] A trauma patient can lose as much as 25% to 30% of his or her blood volume before developing systolic hypotension because the available vascular space contracts to reduce the unstressed volume (**Box 76-1**).

BOX 76-1

Pathophysiology of Shock

- Loss of circulating blood volume causes decreases in venous return and cardiac output.
- Arterial pressure decreases.
- Sympathetic nervous system is activated by reduced cardiac output and reduced arterial pressure at aortic and carotid baroreceptors.
- Catecholamines are released from the adrenal medulla.
- Heart rate increases in response to circulating and intramyocardial catecholamines.
- Stroke volume decreases in response to decreased venous return and increased heart rate.
- Available blood volume stores are mobilized from unstressed blood volume because of arterial inflow diverted by vasoconstriction from vascular beds with large venous capacitance such as cutaneous and splanchnic vascular beds.
- Clinical picture consists of increasing heart rate and decreasing pulse pressure; diastolic pressure rises before further hemorrhage causes systolic pressure to fall. Renal vasoconstriction and secretion of antidiuretic hormone decrease urinary output.
- Increasing hemorrhage leads to progressive increases in heart rate. Heart rates >140 beats/min are common with ≤40% loss of blood volume.
- Loss of >30% blood volume is required to cause systolic hypotension consistently in the supine position.
- Mental status changes to confusion and then lethargy with >30% loss of blood volume.
- Urinary output decreases with increasing blood loss and becomes negligible with 40% loss of blood volume.

In addition to hypotension, loss of a significant portion of the unstressed blood volume will result in decreased cardiac output and thereby restrict oxygen delivery to various organs. This in turn causes anaerobic metabolism and metabolic acidosis and eventually triggers a series of characteristic neurohumoral responses to the insult.[41-43] These neurohumoral responses range from increases in circulating levels of epinephrine, norepinephrine, growth hormone, glucagon, adrenocorticotropic hormone, and cortisol (and a reduction in insulin) to activation of various cytokines and white blood cells, modulation of coagulation, and more. Tachycardia, hyperglycemia, increased white blood cell count, and hypokalemia all result from these neurohumoral responses to trauma.

Decreased tissue blood flow following hemorrhage causes decreased oxygen delivery to the cells and mitochondria.[44,45] As the mitochondria become starved for oxygen, aerobic production of adenosine triphosphate (ATP) ceases, and cells become dependent on their small stores of ATP and phosphocreatine for energy. Anaerobic glycolysis replaces some of the lost ATP as long as an adequate supply of glucose can be maintained by the reduced blood flow. Initial changes in cellular structure and function occur when the cells no longer have the energy stores to maintain transmembrane ion gradients. Under optimum conditions, these changes are reversible for up to 1 hour, and then the cells proceed to irreversible changes and cell death, thus the origins of the concept of the so-called golden hour. Inability to restore adequate circulating supplies of oxygen and glucose within a relatively short time leads to massive cell death and irreversible shock, followed by death of the patient.

TREATMENT OF SHOCK

An appreciation of the relationships among these issues is important for the anesthesiologist managing an injured patient because restoration of circulating blood volume is critical to restoring tissue oxygen delivery. Restoration of tissue oxygenation is required to first arrest and then reverse impending organ death. World War I era surgeons realized that blood loss reduced venous return, cardiac filling, and ultimately cardiac output, but it was not until work during the 1950s of replacing interstitial and intracellular fluid losses that IV fluids were routinely administered to restore circulating blood volume. Cellular dehydration following traumatic blood loss was a significant issue, and administration of excess electrolyte solutions after traumatic hemorrhage was required to restore interstitial and cellular hydration.[46] Rapid replenishment of shed blood volume restored sufficient tissue oxygen delivery and improved organ function.[47-49] The concept of a golden hour, which seeks to establish a limited time frame in which to restore hemodynamic and metabolic homeostasis to prevent irreversible shock, promoted a concerted improvement in trauma resuscitation and survival.

DELAYED FLUID AND SMALL VOLUME RESUSCITATION

The anesthesiologist caring for a severely injured trauma victim faces a dilemma regarding blood pressure management. Hypotensive patients frequently respond to fluid boluses; however, evidence suggests that large-volume crystalloid resuscitation significantly increases postoperative complication rates.[50] The concept of delayed fluid resuscitation originated from animal data evaluating hemorrhagic shock models. Large-volume crystalloid use in the early phases of bleeding is thought to "wash off" fragile early clots.[51] Similar studies show complications from aggressive fluid resuscitation are related to severity of blood loss. Large-volume resuscitation is associated with improved survival in rapidly hemorrhaging patients but worse outcomes in patients experiencing less severe bleeding.[52] Although this information is intuitive to most clinicians, the dilemma for anesthesiologists is to determine where their patient falls in this spectrum of hemorrhage.

In some ways, this concept is intuitive and actually represents a renaissance or rediscovery of a similar idea presented almost a century ago. Thus current dogma is that, based on the mechanisms of injury, rapid replacement of some of the shed blood volume (within the golden hour) is critical to assuring survival of an injured patient with hemorrhagic shock. However, fluid resuscitation must be used judiciously before surgical hemostasis to minimize ongoing hemorrhage and avoid compounding the adverse development of dilutional coagulopathy with anemia, hypothermia, and other iatrogenic sequelae.[53-55]

In the operating room, initial evidence in both animal models and in retrospective analysis of trauma patients demonstrates evidence that tolerating a lower blood pressure is beneficial to hemorrhaging patients. This concept is not new to anesthesiologists who practice deliberate hypotension for surgical cases involving large blood loss. The data in trauma patients have certain limitations. Caution applying lower blood pressure tolerance to the elderly or patients with significant comorbidities should be exercised. In addition, lower pressures can be catastrophic in head injury patients.[56]

Management strategies in the operating room clearly must be tailored to the individual patient with continued reassessment and modification of the resuscitation. Choosing a marker of resuscitation, such as lactate, base deficit, or mixed venous oxygen saturation, can guide therapy. However, clinicians must be aware that these markers may reflect the type of resuscitation per se and not the actual status of the patient (ie, acidosis associated with large-volume saline administration). Data supporting other modalities (stroke volume variation, echocardiography, esophageal Doppler) are available, and these may be helpful but require both familiarity with the technology and interpretation of the data. Early use of blood products to prevent coagulopathy and maintain oxygen-carrying capacity may be beneficial. Although the data on hyperoncotic fluid administration is still indeterminate, there is promise associated with small-volume resuscitation.

OTHER SHOCK THERAPIES

Blood gas analysis of the "typical" major trauma patient in shock admitted to the emergency department reveals a metabolic acidosis (the extent of which often correlates with the amount of blood loss), a mild degree of hypocarbia, and a moderate hypoxic state. Because of decreased tissue oxygen delivery, respiratory muscles perform very poorly during shock. Moreover, there are myriad reasons for compromise of the entire respiratory system, ranging from mechanical (eg, rib fracture, flail chest) to central drive (eg, head injury, narcotics) to parenchymal (eg, pulmonary contusion) to physiologic (ie, ventilation-perfusion mismatching due to lung and/or heart trauma).

Characteristically the injured patient with hemorrhage develops a marked increase in pulmonary dead space and must mount an increased minute ventilation to effectively excrete additional carbon dioxide (CO_2) produced. Further influencing the patient's "optimum minute ventilation" is the need to buffer the metabolic acidosis with hypocarbia. The poorly perfused ventilatory muscles soon fatigue and further contribute to a feedback situation that compounds ventilatory failure, with worsening hypoxia and eventually death.

It is therefore prudent that the anesthesiologist view traumatic hemorrhagic shock as an indication for urgent endotracheal intubation and mechanical ventilation. Mechanical ventilation supports the patient's gas exchange needs while "unloading" the ventilatory muscles and not diverting precious supplies of blood from other vital organs.

Hemostasis is critical for survival from traumatic injury; however, patients who lose large volumes of blood exhibit coagulopathy.[57] Part of the neurohumoral response to trauma may lead to DIC, which is a combination of blood hypercoagulability causing clot formation that leads to depletion of fibrin and coagulopathy from clot lysis in the small arteries. Thus trauma patients may exhibit the paradoxic state of systemic anticoagulation but local thrombus formation, possibly causing a variety of thromboembolic phenomena. Hypothermia adds to the coagulopathic component because the various clotting factors have temperature-dependent kinetics.[58] Therefore, the goals for management of the trauma patient during both resuscitation and emergency surgery include restoration and/or maintenance of normothermia as well as replacement of depleted coagulation factors.[59,60]

A number of strategies for rewarming the hypothermic trauma patient have been studied. Arteriovenous perfusion through a hot water heat exchanger has been used successfully to rewarm cold trauma patients.[59] The less invasive technique of applying a vacuum to dilate cutaneous veins of a limb surrounded by a hot water heat exchanger has worked well in experimental settings but has not yet achieved clinical application, partially because of the lack of commercial practicality.[60]

The classic therapy for posttraumatic coagulopathy has been monitoring of prothrombin time, international normalized ratio, partial thromboplastin time, and platelet count. Replacement therapy with fresh-frozen plasma (FFP), platelet concentrates, and/or cryoprecipitate is used in an attempt to restore normal coagulation states.

"WHOLE BLOOD" RESUSCITATION

Anecdotal evidence from trauma teams resuscitating combat trauma patients supports the value of whole blood utilization.[61] This practice in not practical in a civilian system due to the short shelf life of whole blood, the extensive financial benefits of component therapy ("give the patient only the component needed"), and the infection risks of whole blood. Recent trends in the treatment of hemorrhaging patients involve earlier use of plasma and platelets.[62,63] In the words of one trauma surgeon, "It's not just red blood cells and saline on the floor and in the suction container." Research is ongoing to determine whether rapidly exsanguinating patients actually benefit from a 1:1:1 ratio of packed red blood cells (PRBCs), FFP, and platelets. Plasma is the blood component most associated with transfusion-related acute lung injury

(TRALI). To further complicate the issue, a recent study evaluating early plasma administration to trauma patients who did not require a massive transfusion (<10 units of PRBCs) did worse than patients receiving less plasma.[64] In the light of this evidence, it is still critical to consider that a massively transfused patient will develop a dilutional coagulopathy if only crystalloid and red cells are administered. Vigilance concerning resuscitation fluids must be maintained foremost to prevent coagulopathy rather than attempting to restore clotting function. Each hospital should maintain a multidisciplinary team to develop a massive transfusion protocol. The protocol should address both when and who may initiate it and what is delivered; for example, some institutions stock prethawed plasma, and often type AB (universal donor) plasma is in critical supply.

SECONDARY SURVEY

The secondary survey only takes place after the primary survey has been completed; resuscitation is then underway and the patient's vital signs should demonstrate a trend toward normalization/stabilization. In the setting of treating a trauma patient, it is critical to review the vital signs continually for any indication of change or deterioration in the patient's condition. The secondary survey is a thorough head-to-toe examination of the patient in conjunction with a more detailed history of the patient's general health in the context of the mechanism(s) of traumatic injury. This purposeful and systematic evaluation reduces the likelihood of a serious injury being overlooked, particularly in the unresponsive patient.[65]

A comprehensive description of the secondary survey is provided in the advanced trauma life support manual.[22] However an overview of the systematic approach with the most common issues of concern for the preoperative patient is presented here to sensitize the anesthesiologist to critical issues that can have an impact on the preoperative trauma patient.

Head The head requires a complete neurologic examination. An examination of the eyes (to include visual acuity), if possible, should be assessed because facial swelling may later preclude an eye examination. The possibility of fractures to the head must be considered.

Face Assess for bony and soft tissue injury. Continue to reassess the airway for patency and security of any airway appliances and sources of supplemental oxygen.

Neck Blunt trauma to the neck region may result in injuries that are not immediately appreciated, such as certain nerve and vascular injuries. Patients with distracting injuries, including intoxicated patients, are presumed to have an unstable neck, and cervical spine precautions against injury must be maintained.

Chest Recheck the chest for rib fractures. A pneumothorax may not be clinically significant until the patient is intubated and being maintained on positive pressure ventilation. Also injuries to the great vessels may not become evident during the primary survey.

Abdomen Special attention must be directed to the retroperitoneum as well as the genitalia. A diagnostic peritoneal lavage or a focused abdominal ultrasound for trauma may be performed in the emergency department.

Spine The patient must be log-rolled for a complete examination of the spine. This process also facilitates examination of the back for evidence of injuries not appreciated during the primary survey.

Soft Tissues Abrasions and contusions, often a consequence of the mechanism of injury, may provide insight into the presence of an occult injury.

It is also during the secondary survey that further investigation is considered. Additional imaging, CT, angiography, bronchoscopy, and transesophageal echocardiography may be indicated. It is critical that the patient's hemodynamic status is stabilized before any attempt at further testing occurs. At the conclusion of the secondary survey, the plans for further care of the trauma patient should be well-formulated.

As the patient is being prepared for additional tests or transfer to the operating room, the tertiary phase is entered. This phase is designed to ensure regular reevaluation of the patient in recognition of the dynamic clinical situation of the trauma patient.[66]

TRAUMA SCORING

Since the 1950s, attempts have been made to develop a scoring system to characterize traumatic injury effectively. In the 1970s, with the development of trauma centers and the appreciation of the epidemic nature of trauma, the need for a more effective means to quantify the severity of trauma was identified. Used as part of a field triage system, the scoring system can help the clinician decide the appropriate evacuation of a patient, or while in the hospital, it may be used to evaluate the impact of therapy and the appropriateness of intervention. It may also be used to determine the patient's inclusion into a research study.

There are 3 major categories of trauma scoring systems (**Table 76-4**). These are divided into physiologic or anatomic groups, with a third group being a combined or specialized group.[67]

ANATOMIC SCORES

The anatomic-based systems are based on the anatomic sites of injury. These scoring systems have evolved to correlate reasonably with in-hospital morbidity and mortality data. A disadvantage to using these systems is the relative complexity involved in the calculation process.[68]

PHYSIOLOGIC SCORES

Using data that can be obtained noninvasively in the field, such as systemic blood pressure and heart rate, the physiologic scoring systems are often used by prehospital personnel in triage decisions (**Table 76-5**). Disadvantages are associated with the issue that physiologic patterns often change rapidly and the scoring system requires the conversion of measured values into standardized scores.[69]

COMBINED SCORES

By combining assessment of both anatomic and physiologic compromise after an injury, these scoring systems have been used as predictors of mortality. Although the most common of the systems is used to predict outcome in trauma patients, the combined systems require more complex calculations and bear the same limitations as the anatomic- and physiologic-based systems.[70,71]

TABLE 76-4 Trauma Scoring Systems

Anatomic
Abbreviated Injury Score (AIS)
Injury Severity Score (ISS)
New Injury Severity Code (NISS)
Anatomic Profile (AF)
Penetrating Abdominal Trauma Index (PATI)
ICD-based Injury Severity Code (ICES)
Physiologic
Glasgow Coma Scale (GCS)
Trauma Score (TS)
Revised Trauma Score (RTS)
Acute Physiological and Chronic Health Evaluation (APACHE)
Systemic Inflammatory Response System (SIRS) Score
Combined
Trauma and Injury Severity Score (TRISS)
A Severity Characterization of Trauma (ASCOT)
Harborview Assessment to Risk of Mortality (HARM)

TABLE 76-5 Revised Trauma Score

Parameter	Range	Score
A. Respiratory rate (breaths/min)	10-29	4
	>29	3
	6-9	2
	1-5	1
	0	0
B. Systolic blood pressure (mm Hg)	>89	4
	76-89	3
	50-75	2
	1-49	1
	0	0
C. Glasgow Coma Scale Score	13-15	4
	9-12	3
	6-8	2
	4-5	0
		1
	<4	0

The Revised Trauma Score is the summation of the 3 categories above: RTS = A + B + C.

CRITICAL ISSUES IN TRAUMA MANAGEMENT

A myriad of issues may have an impact on the trauma patient, during both the prehospital and in-hospital phases of care. Although the algorithm of the ABCs remains the primary focus of any approach to the trauma patient, the risks imposed by hypothermia and the consequences of resuscitation merit special consideration in any discussion of the approach to or evaluation of the trauma patient.

AIRWAY MANAGEMENT

Airway management in trauma patients is frequently challenging, and often a secured airway must be obtained rapidly. Barriers to intubation included impaired mobility (cervical collars and spine injuries), impaired anatomy (facial fractures, soft tissue trauma), or impaired visualization (blood, emesis, debris). All trauma patients are assumed to have a full stomach; moreover, all head injury patients have cervical spine injury until proven otherwise. Generally, the approach to securing the airway of a trauma patient does not differ significantly from other emergency patients, and the techniques discussed in Chapter 10 on the difficult airway will apply. Similarly to the chaos frequently seen in "code blue" situation, the trauma bay is often a loud environment, mandating end-tidal CO_2 presence as a method of proper endotracheal tube placement.

HYPOTHERMIA

Trauma patients are often hypothermic by the time emergency medical personnel assume care for the individual. Exposure to the extremes of environmental cold, as well as the physiologic effects of blood loss and changes in mental status, can lead to a marked reduction in core body temperature.[72] Coupled with cold fluid resuscitation in the field, this can place the patient at risk for the multiple physiologic effects of low body temperature (**Table 76-6**).

TABLE 76-6 Effects of Hypothermia

Coagulopathy
Cardiac dysrhythmias
Peripheral vasoconstriction
Increased metabolic demand (shivering)
Decreased metabolic demand (attenuated metabolic rate)

ANESTHETIC DRUGS IN TRAUMA

Anesthesia induction in the trauma patient must always be viewed as occurring in the setting of a full stomach, associated head, neck, thoracic, or abdominal injuries, and hypovolemia. The more hemodynamically unstable the trauma patient, the more careful the anesthesiologist must be with titrating the induction drugs to effect (**Table 76-7**). Some investigators suggest that the combination of only oxygen and a neuromuscular blocking drug was adequate for the severely hypovolemic trauma patient, but that viewpoint has been replaced by the judicious use of IV anesthetics because of the high incidence of intraoperative awareness.[73]

Ketamine is recommended because of its perceived property of stimulating or at least stabilizing the sympathetic nervous system. Although ketamine usually causes hypertension and tachycardia secondary to increased sympathetic nervous system activity in unstressed patients, it can cause hypotension by direct myocardial depression in patients with maximally stimulated sympathetic responses secondary to shock. Thus even ketamine must be used in small, preferably titrated, doses.

Etomidate similarly should be titrated to effect. Many clinicians believe that etomidate does not cause hypotension, but we have observed that etomidate may decrease blood pressure when administered to hypovolemic and maximally sympathetically stressed patients, similar to the clinical scenario noted with ketamine. There is conflicting data regarding etomidate's effect on the adrenal system. Although most evidence supports the safe use of a single induction dose of etomidate, communication with the clinician taking care of the patient postoperatively is warranted should the patient develop refractory hypotension.

Thiopental or propofol can be titrated to effect without causing excessive hypotension. Often the doses needed to induce anesthesia in the patient with reduced blood volume and cardiac output (and possibly other abnormal pharmacodynamic and pharmacokinetic derangements) are so small that profound hypotension can be avoided. Overall, the operating principle should be small titrated doses of any utilized induction agent. Given current evidence, this is perhaps more important than the specific choice of drug.

The combination of ketamine and propofol is gaining popularity for induction of trauma anesthesia and as an IV infusion to supplement regional anesthesia for the trauma patient. Ketamine and propofol appear to be somewhat synergistic in inducing anesthesia, and the sympathetic stimulation associated with ketamine is thought to counteract the cardiovascular depression associated with propofol.

TABLE 76-7 Anesthetic Drugs for Trauma Patient

Function	Drugs	Trauma Dose (mg/kg)
Hypnosis (induction of anesthesia)	Etomidate	0.1-0.2
	Thiopental	0.5-2.0
	Propofol	0.5-1.0
	Ketamine	0.5-1.0
Analgesia	Fentanyl	0.001-0.003
	Morphine	0.05-0.1
	Sufentanil	0.1-0.5 μg/kg
Muscle relaxation	Vecuronium	0.15-0.3
	Rocuronium	0.9-1.2
	Succinylcholine	1.0-1.5
	Cisatracurium	0.10
Anesthesia maintenance	Isoflurane	Titrate to blood pressure
	Total intravenous anesthesia (propofol, fentanyl, dexmedetomidine)	50-100 μg/kg/min, 1-2 μg/kg/h, 0.5 μg/kg/h
	Ketamine, propofol	50-100 μg/kg/min propofol, 10-20 μg/kg/min ketamine

Careful attention to both adequacy of ventilation and protection of the airway is required when inducing anesthesia in the trauma patient, especially when incremental doses are administered while "titrating" to effect, an approach that minimizes the potential cardiovascular instability that commonly results with use of typical doses of induction agents. The patient's gas exchange should be supplemented by hand ventilation through a face mask while an assistant administers effective cricoid pressure. Cricoid pressure (ie, the Sellick maneuver) has been used for many years to prevent both insufflation of ventilatory gases into the stomach during mask ventilation and regurgitation and aspiration of gastric contents from the hypopharynx.[74,75] Control of ventilation while titrating induction drugs to effect will cause a loss of consciousness at the lowest efficacious dose, with less drug-induced hypotension. An additional benefit is an increase in alveolar oxygen and decrease in alveolar CO_2 immediately preceding the obligatory apneic period during intubation of the trachea. Some of the disadvantages of "classic" rapid sequence induction include the hypoxia hypercarbia that may occur during the 60- to 90-second apneic interval associated with endotracheal intubation. This often is further complicated in trauma patients by poor visualization (eg, blood in the hypopharynx) or the need for special protection of the cervical spine in patients with head or neck injuries. Modified rapid sequence induction using cricoid pressure and sustained mask ventilation avoids this substantial insult.

The choice of muscle relaxant remains controversial. Succinylcholine delivers a rapid onset, whereas nondepolarizing neuromuscular blocking drugs avoid the undesirable side effects of succinylcholine, such as hyperkalemia, cardiac arrest ("black box" warning in package insert), and malignant hyperthermia. Because many trauma patients present for anesthesia without a complete medical/anesthetic history, the side effects of succinylcholine must be taken seriously and balanced against the benefits of that drug.

The possibility that a patient who cannot be ventilated or intubated would recover to spontaneous ventilation before sustaining neurologic injury secondary to cerebral hypoxia probably is not one of the benefits of succinylcholine. The 1 to 1.5 mg/kg dose of succinylcholine needed to achieve relatively rapid onset will require at least 5 minutes before recovery to produce meaningful spontaneous ventilation. In the trauma patient in shock with increased pulmonary shunt, dead space, as well as the various hemodynamic and metabolic issues previously noted, this interval is long enough to result in profound hypoxia. Rapid onset of neuromuscular blockade can be achieved with nondepolarizing relaxants by increasing the dose administered to multiples of the effective dose (ED_{95}). The most commonly used nondepolarizing neuromuscular blockers are vecuronium, rocuronium, and cis-atracurium.

Opioid analgesics are an important component of trauma anesthesia practice, not only for critically injured patients who require immediate anesthesia induction for a variety of urgent imaging studies and/or surgery but also for less critically injured patients who may only require analgesia, sedation, and monitoring of vital signs but need appropriate opioid analgesics for pain management. Fentanyl is an opioid useful for trauma care because its high lipophilicity, potency, and rapid redistribution make it easy to titrate to effect without causing hemodynamic deterioration. Morphine has a long history of use in trauma care, but its relatively slow onset makes it difficult to titrate and avoid subsequent overdose. Hydromorphone may be a more attractive option.

PAIN MANAGEMENT IN TRAUMA PATIENTS

Analgesia in trauma patients is often neglected because they are deemed too unstable for significant systemic analgesia. The growing popularity of regional anesthesia has yet to become widely accepted in trauma pain management largely due to a fear that many trauma patients become coagulopathic at some point in their clinical course. The anesthesiologist faced with caring for a trauma patient needs to embrace a multimodal approach to pain management including regional techniques, opioids, nonsteroidal anti-inflammatory drugs (NSAIDs), and a variety of adjunct medications.

Pain is a significant contributor to the considerable stress response seen in trauma patients. Hemodynamic stability, ventilatory mechanics, and renal and gastrointestinal function may all be compromised when pain is not controlled. In particular, recently literature supports the use of regional anesthesia to reduce perioperative complications. The incidence of deep venous thrombosis, pulmonary embolism, perioperative blood loss, pneumonia, respiratory depression, and renal failure is reduced when neuraxial blockade was compared with patient-controlled opioid analgesia.[76] Long-term disability in the form of chronic pain, complex regional pain syndrome (CRPS), and phantom limb pain is associated with poorly controlled pain after trauma. Early regional intervention in combat casualties can both prevent and treat CRPS in addition to phantom limb pain. The US military is currently placing continuous regional nerve catheters in casualties on postinjury day 0 or 1.[77]

Trauma patients often present additional barriers to regional anesthesia. Spinal fractures may precluded proper positioning or prevent needle placement. Often the spine is not "cleared" until several days postinjury. Consent is also an important consideration. Although several instances may merit consideration for placement without consent (epidural or paravertebral catheters for multiple rib fractures), most would not initiate a procedure primarily for pain control without informed consent. Current guidelines do not consider neuraxial techniques contraindicated in head injury patients unless the injury is accompanied with elevated intracranial pressure.

Thoracic trauma merits consideration for regional techniques. The pain coupled with multiple rib fractures is associated with the development of atelectasis and pneumonia and may lead to intubation and subsequent prolonged mechanical ventilation. In a review of multiple rib fractures, Flagel et al reported epidural analgesia was associated with a reduction in mortality for all patients sustaining rib fractures; in particular, those sustaining greater than 4 fractures.[78] Although most anesthesiologists are most comfortable placing epidurals for rib fractures, paravertebral catheters have equal efficacy and may have less associated hypotension. The potentially devastating complication of epidural hematoma is likely avoided with paravertebral nerve blocks, but current American Society of Regional Anesthesia (ASRA) guidelines extend anticoagulation restrictions to all regional anesthesia.

The dynamic nature of the critically injured trauma patient requires continuous reevaluation and assessment. The multimodal approach to pain management is no different. Intravenous opioids and regional techniques commonly dominate the initial phase. As the patient stabilizes, several medications such as clonidine, ketamine, and NSAIDs can be added. Anticonvulsants and antidepressants may be initiated once enteral medications are tolerated. Continuous peripheral nerve catheters are an excellent technique for both acute pain needs and for patients requiring frequent trips to the operating room for wound washouts and vacuum changes. If placed sterilely and the site is evaluated daily by personnel familiar with regional anesthesia, peripheral nerve catheters and epidurals may be left in place for extended periods. Tunneling the catheter beneath the skin at the insertion site may extend this interval.

SPECIFIC INJURY PATTERNS

HEAD INJURIES

Head injuries lead to increased mortality and morbidity in victims of both blunt and penetrating trauma. Therapeutic goals for patients with central nervous system (CNS) injuries are designed to minimize the amount of injured tissue, prevent secondary CNS injury, and facilitate rehabilitation and recovery. Maintaining adequate perfusion pressure and preventing hypoxia and hyperglycemia are critical during the resuscitation of a head injury patient. Cerebral perfusion pressure (CPP), which is the mean arterial pressure (MAP) minus the intracranial pressure (ICP), is recognized as a more important parameter to monitor than ICP alone due to the role of increased ICP reducing nutrient blood flow to the brain.[79] With elevated ICP obstructing cerebral perfusion, ischemia develops and regions of the brain may suffer necrosis.[80,81] Maintaining CPP at higher than 70 mm Hg provides sufficient pressure for perfusion through arteries partially obstructed by elevated ICP and prevents ischemia. Evidence indicates that even CPP higher than 60 mm Hg may be adequate to prevent secondary brain injury. Loss of adequate CPP, usually resulting from arterial hypotension, is one of the more ominous events in the early treatment of head injury. Thus anesthesia induction should be planned and implemented to minimize hypotension. Ketamine, an antagonist of the *N*-methyl-D-aspartate (NMDA) receptors associated with secondary brain injury, is being investigated as a potential neuroprotective anesthetic for head injury.[82] Some investigations have shown that the *S*-isomer has neuroregenerative properties,[83] although this form remains unavailable for clinical use in the United States. Ketamine tends to elevate ICP in normovolemic patients, but this effect is unlikely in hypovolemic patients (studies in animals confirm this concept). Thus ketamine is being reevaluated as an induction agent for patients with traumatic brain injury. The combination of NMDA antagonism produced by ketamine and γ-aminobutyric acid agonism produced by propofol may be beneficial in the anesthetic management of traumatic brain injury.

Hypoxia is deleterious to all organs and tissues, although the brain is relatively resistant to arterial hypoxia if perfusion is well maintained to clear the toxic by-products of anaerobic metabolism from the brain.[84] The patient with traumatic brain injury and multisystem trauma may become hypoxic because of chest trauma or ventilation-perfusion ($\dot{V}/\dot{Q}$) mismatch; therefore, it is imperative to prevent hypotension and maintain CPP to allow the brain to tolerate the period of hypoxia. Hypotension is treated with pressors and fluid loading because hypovolemia rapidly leads to hypotension and loss of adequate CPP, leaving the injured brain starved for blood flow. In the past, treatment of traumatic brain injury (TBI) emphasized induced dehydration through aggressive diuresis in an attempt to extract water from edematous regions of the injured brain. However, little was achieved except the resultant cerebral ischemia leading to higher ICP, followed by further diuresis with the subsequent dehydration of the patient, which led to worsening ischemia and further increases in ICP.

The concept of reducing ICP as another method of enhancing cerebral perfusion remains viable. Reduction of ICP usually involves draining cerebrospinal fluid through a ventriculostomy catheter. Other methods for reducing ICP, such as diuretics or barbiturates to reduce intracerebral blood volume, may be poorly tolerated or minimally effective in trauma patients and must be used with caution. Hyperventilation to reduce $Pa{CO_2}$ was once considered a mainstay in the treatment of increased ICP. Current guidelines recommend normal to low-normal arterial levels of CO_2 to prevent cerebral ischemia due to vasoconstriction. Moreover, patients with traumatic brain injuries are at high risk for focal cerebral ischemia due to vasospasm.[85] Mannitol is used to reduce ICP and is well-tolerated in moderate doses. Drugs that increase MAP can help restore perfusion to the uninjured brain and possibly help reduce the size of the injury. The future will see the development of anesthesia strategies for reducing secondary brain injury from excitatory neurotransmitters; the earlier discussion regarding ketamine and propofol is an example of these potential strategies.

SPINAL CORD INJURIES

The general principles of anesthetic management described for patients with TBI also apply to the care of patients with spinal cord injury. However, in addition there are significant concerns regarding the potential for mechanical injury from movement of the cervical, thoracic, or lumbar spine, depending on the site of injury. Stabilizing the spine is essential to prevent additional injury to the spinal cord and to foster healing of spinal cord lesions. There is no evidence-based standard that supports the use of high-dose steroid in the care of blunt spinal cord injuries.

Anesthesia management of patients with potential spinal cord injury can be challenging because of the critical need to prevent motion of the spine. Airway management has perhaps the highest probability of extending the injury. Most maneuvers used to secure a patent airway with either an oral airway or an endotracheal tube are associated with some motion of the cervical vertebrae.[86] There are several recommendations for stabilizing the cervical spine during anesthesia induction and endotracheal intubation. These maneuvers vary from awake fiberoptic intubation to direct laryngoscopy controlled by manual inline axial stabilization (**Box 76-2**). The anesthesiologist's choice of technique depends on the stability of the fracture and the urgency of airway management.[86] (Details of airway management are presented in Chapters 10 and 36.)

Unstable fractures with disruption of both anterior and posterior elements of the spine require more caution in choice of intubation method, especially in patients with fractures but no spinal cord injury or in those with incomplete injury. A flexible fiberoptic bronchoscope can be used to direct the endotracheal tube through the larynx with minimal movement of the cervical spine. However, the fiberoptic bronchoscope is vulnerable to blood or secretions that obscure the operator's vision and render intubation very difficult. Direct laryngoscopy provides better vision in patients with copious bloody secretions but frequently causes an obligatory extension of the upper cervical vertebrae, even with application of manual inline axial stabilization. Video laryngoscopes often can expose the larynx with little to no motion of the cervical vertebrae. Other techniques, such as the intubating laryngeal mask airway and the transtracheal retrograde wire technique, have been used with generally good results. It is of paramount importance to become proficient in these techniques before attempting to intubate a patient with an unstable cervical spine.

BOX 76-2

Modified Rapid Sequence Induction and Intubation for Trauma Patients

1. Be familiar with evaluation of the difficult airway and the American Society of Anesthesiologists practice guidelines for management of the difficult airway.
2. Be familiar with noninvasive and invasive techniques of airway management.
3. Evaluate the airway and be prepared to execute multiple contingency plans.
4. Preoxygenate the patient with 100% oxygen (O_2) by face mask.
5. Remove anterior portion of the cervical spine collar and apply manual inline axial stabilization of the head and neck if suspected cervical spine injury.
6. Give appropriate medications intravenously, as indicated by the clinical setting and hemodynamic status:
   Lidocaine 1.5 mg/kg if suspected head injury
   Sedative-hypnotics (see Table 76-6)
   Muscle relaxants (see Table 76-6)
7. Apply cricoid pressure until intubation is completed.
8. Manually ventilate the patients' lungs with 100% O_2 using inflation pressures <20 cm H_2O to prevent (or treat) hypoxemia and hypercarbia before (or between) intubation attempt(s). Continue cricoid pressure during bag-mask ventilation.
9. Confirm correct position of endotracheal tube by visualizing tube passing through cords, sustained presence of end-tidal carbon dioxide, auscultation of breath sounds, and self-inflating bulb.
10. After successful intubation, administer additional increments of sedative-hypnotics and analgesics or begin a potent volatile agent, as dictated by clinical need. Consider using a longer-acting relaxant once the effects of succinylcholine, if used, have worn off.

Although blind nasal intubation once was the technique of choice for injured patients with cervical spine fracture, it has several drawbacks in patients with acute trauma. Achievement of blind nasal intubation requires a spontaneously breathing patient, and adequate sedation for this procedure is difficult to achieve without depressing respiration and thus adding to the potential for hypoxemia or hypotension. In contrast, inadequate sedation or analgesia may result in excess cervical motion in a patient who actively resists the painful procedure. Acute head injury associated with blunt trauma presents additional risks for blind nasal intubation, with the potential for introduction of a foreign body (endotracheal tube) through a basilar skull fracture that extends into the nasopharynx as well as increased risks of a serious sinus infection that may result in meningitis. For these reasons, nasal tracheal intubation is reserved for patients who require intraoral surgery and postoperative intramaxillary fixation. In these cases, a controlled nasotracheal intubation guided by a fiberoptic bronchoscope is preferable to a blind nasal intubation. The patient with maxillofacial fractures and TBI who will require prolonged ventilatory support will be best served by a preoperative controlled tracheostomy for ongoing airway management.

DAMAGE CONTROL SURGERY

Patients with profound hemodynamic instability and intra-abdominal hemorrhage may benefit from "damage control surgery," an operative strategy designed to rapidly achieve hemostasis without attempting definitive repair of solid organ injury.[87] For example, a patient with a grade 5 liver laceration (involving hepatic veins) would undergo an exploratory celiotomy for repair of the hepatic venous laceration and packing of the liver wound for hemostasis. The patient then would be transferred to the intensive care unit (ICU). After rewarming the patient and completing hemodynamic resuscitation in the ICU, the trauma team returns the patient to the operating room 24 to 48 hours later for a "second look." Here packs are removed and the wound in the liver is judiciously debrided. The patient may require several more trips to the operating room to complete repairs of all the intra-abdominal injuries.

This approach to resuscitating the injured patient with major intra-abdominal hemorrhage is consistent with the ATLS guidelines of delivering simultaneous emergency lifesaving treatment with definitive diagnosis of injuries. Thus uncontrolled hemorrhage is contained, and the patient is allowed to stabilize and return to the operating room for definitive correction of major injuries when sufficiently stable to undergo more lengthy surgical repair(s). This avoids the often fatal triad of ongoing massive transfusion—hypothermia, coagulopathy, and persistent metabolic acidosis—while the surgeon struggles to debride and repair massive liver lacerations or other extensive intra-abdominal organ injury during the initial operation.[57,87]

The anesthesia team must continually monitor fluid replacement and the efficacy of resuscitation efforts by following trends in metabolic acidosis during damage control surgery. General anesthesia, including neuromuscular blockade to facilitate surgery, and judicious use of analgesic and hypnotic drugs (either inhalation or IV), as tolerated by the patient, are required for damage control surgery. These patients require controlled ventilation, large-bore IV access (infusion into both the superior and inferior vena cavae systems is recommended), and direct monitoring of blood pressure (with an intra-arterial catheter used also for blood sampling), core temperature, and urinary output. Maintenance of body temperature and/or rewarming requires keeping the room temperature high as well as use of hot air convective body warmers and fluid-warming devices. Following initial damage control surgery, patients may be managed with heavy sedation and/or neuromuscular blockade in the postoperative ICU phase. The anesthetic plan should incorporate transportation from operating room to ICU, with the patient remaining intubated and fully monitored during transport.

After anesthesia induction, the fractured spine must be carefully immobilized during all patient movements (such as transfer to the operating table). Patients who must be placed in the prone position require special care to prevent flexing or extending the spine during turning, and a neurosurgeon or orthopedic surgeon should supervise this procedure. Following stabilization surgery, patients are less vulnerable to spine motion when being transferred out of the operating room. However, external stabilization is still required for all movements throughout the period of bone fracture healing.

AIRWAY INJURIES

The true incidence of airway injury is unknown because many patients with such injuries presumably die at the accident scene or during transport. However, airway injuries present one of the greatest of challenges for trauma anesthesia care. Airway injuries may dramatically complicate the preoperative preparation and anesthetic induction of trauma patients. These injuries often require extreme measures of ingenuity and innovation on the part of the anesthesiologist to safely manage a patient with an airway injury for emergency surgery; the situation represents a continuous high risk until the airway is secured. Although in most cases intubation via the mouth or nose is recommended, upper airway injuries associated with disruption of laryngeal cartilage may be best treated with primary tracheostomy. However, in the emergent setting of ventilatory distress, translaryngeal intubation with a small endotracheal tube can be lifesaving and support the patient's ventilation during subsequent tracheostomy.

An initial triage assessment that assigns patients with airway injuries into relative categories of "stable" or "unstable" is important because it facilitates subsequent evaluation and management planning. In stable patients, obtaining imaging studies that elucidate the site (ie, tracheobronchial level) and extent of injury to the airway permit more comprehensive anesthetic management and formulation of a treatment plan in collaboration with surgical colleagues.

In urgent situations that include suspected injuries to the trachea, intubation with a fiberoptic bronchoscope may allow inspection of tracheal integrity as well as assist in guiding an endotracheal tube into position. Most blunt tracheobronchial lacerations (approximately 80%) occur within 1 cm of the carina, and fiberoptic bronchoscopy can easily view most of these lacerations. Clinical signs of tracheal or bronchial lacerations include pneumomediastinum, subcutaneous emphysema, pneumothorax, and persistent air leak.

In less urgent presentations, consideration should be given to full bronchoscopic examination of the tracheal bronchial tree of patients who suffered blunt chest trauma and have a persistent air leak.

Although chest trauma can potentially compromise a patient's ventilatory and hemodynamic status, most chest injuries are managed outside of the operating room. However, the anesthesiologist must be familiar with devices used for chest tube drainage and management because patients with chest trauma and hemothorax or pneumothorax often require operative care of other injuries.

LONG BONE AND PELVIC FRACTURES

Fat embolism is a potential cause of respiratory compromise in patients with major lower extremity or pelvic fractures. The fat embolism syndrome starts with respiratory compromise and then proceeds to a diffuse distribution of petechia and neurologic dysfunction. Release of bone marrow from long bone and pelvic fractures initially affects pulmonary gas exchange and then leads to systemic manifestations, multiple cutaneous hemorrhages, and cerebral dysfunction. Fat globules can be found in the urine and observed in retinal blood vessels. Early fracture fixation with hardware combined with intubation and mechanical ventilation prevents continued leaching of marrow fat into the venous and pulmonary circulation and reverses pulmonary dysfunction from fat emboli before the full syndrome develops.[88] Fat released into the venous circulation from fractures through the marrow compartments of long bones also releases mediators that react with pulmonary blood vessels, leading to $\dot{V}/\dot{Q}$ mismatching and hypoxia. These injuries, especially pelvic fractures, cause major hemorrhage and ongoing blood loss. Although closed fractures can be stabilized and treated with bed rest, open fractures require prompt operative intervention, preferably within 6 hours of injury. Patients with blunt trauma often require multiple trips to the operating room for debriding of contaminated open fractures as well as operative stabilization of complex highly comminuted fractures, so their management commonly involves multiple frequent anesthetics.

Patients with blunt trauma and multiple systems injuries have improved outcomes with early operative fixation of fractures. Prolonged bed rest with femur traction is associated with increased risk of both pneumonia and venous thromboembolic disease. Additionally, stabilizing long bone fractures may reduce the risk of fat embolization by minimizing motion of the fracture site. Although the incidence of fat embolism varies based on multiple considerations (location, extent of injury, comorbidities, medications, etc), mortality from fat embolism remains high and is a serious threat that must be guarded against and managed aggressively.

Arterial blood gases of patients with long bone fractures should be measured following hospital admission. Patients with hypoxia (low Pao_2-to-Fio_2 ratio) should be intubated and mechanically ventilated. These patients should be monitored with an arterial catheter ("a-line") during anesthesia and surgery to facilitate measurements of blood gases. Patients with a low Pao_2-to-Fio_2 ratio should remain intubated and ventilated in the ICU postoperatively.

ABDOMINAL COMPARTMENT SYNDROME

Critical care observation has demonstrated the importance of increased intra-abdominal pressure in the genesis of multiorgan failure, including acute respiratory distress syndrome. Intra-abdominal pressure can be monitored by measuring the pressure in the urinary bladder after instillation of 25 mL of saline. Classically, sustained intra-abdominal pressure greater than 20 mm Hg with organ failure has been called *abdominal compartment syndrome.* This syndrome is associated with increased ventilatory pressure to expand the lungs adequately and with oliguria because the high pressure compresses the renal veins (thus decreasing renal perfusion) and possibly the ureters as well. Evidence indicates that intra-abdominal pressures greater than 12 mm Hg may be associated with the SIRS and multiorgan failure.[89] Left unchecked, high intra-abdominal pressure is associated with release of inflammatory mediators from the relatively ischemic intestines and subsequent development of MOF.

Patients with abdominal compartment syndrome require urgent surgical decompression to relieve the tension and to allow improved parenchymal blood flow and restoration of renal function. Continuous neuromuscular blockade can relax the abdominal wall and reduce mild increases in intra-abdominal pressure. More persistent and serious increases require surgical intervention. Relief of increased intra-abdominal pressure also facilitates ventilation because motion of the diaphragm is no longer impeded.

THE PREGNANT TRAUMA PATIENT

Motor vehicle accidents are responsible for most maternal-fetal trauma and are associated with the greatest incidence of trauma-related fetal death. Less common causes include falls and assault/domestic violence. The fetus completely depends on the mother for life and is particularly vulnerable after trauma. In major trauma, the incidence of fetal death approaches 50%. Even in minor trauma, the fetal death rate is 1% to 5%, mandating hospital admission for observation and monitoring.

A detailed description of the anatomic and physiologic alterations that occur during pregnancy is addressed in the chapter on evaluation of the pregnant patient. Although the "2-patient" view of the pregnant trauma victim is important to remember, in almost all circumstances, prompt treatment of the mother is the best way to improve fetal outcome. Radiologic evaluation of the mother must not be delayed. Any study deemed necessary for the mother should be performed and not omitted due to concerns over fetal radiation exposure. A missed injury due to an incomplete evaluation could be much more devastating to the fetus than a brief radiation exposure. Early involvement of an obstetrician is recommended.

Initial assessment and treatment should follow standard ATLS guidelines. The patient should be placed left-side down to displace the gravid uterus off the inferior vena cava (IVC). IV access is generally obtained above the diaphragm if possible due to possible IVC compression. Unless contraindicated, the relative hypervolemic state of pregnancy should be maintained. Prompt treatment of hypotension to preserve placental circulation is essential. If the mother is Rh negative, Rh immunoglobulin therapy should be initiated unless the injury is isolated and remote from the uterus.

Injuries specific to the pregnant patient include uterine rupture, placental abruption, and amniotic fluid embolization. The gravid uterus makes differentiating abdominal pathology difficult. Vaginal bleeding is not always present, but in almost all cases abdominal pain and cramping exists. Ultrasound, CT, and occasionally surgical exploration may be required to properly diagnose and differentiate injury. Patients with amniotic fluid embolism or significant placental separation are at particular risk for DIC. A patient with falling platelets or fibrinogen and elevated fibrin split products in the setting of trauma is likely experiencing DIC.

FUTURE TRENDS

The care of the trauma patient has become a major subject of analysis and investigation over the past several decades. Areas of opportunity to improve care for the trauma patient, as well as the training of personnel involved in the care of these patients, have emerged over the past 15 years. Some of these topics offer the potential to have a marked impact on the care of the trauma patient.

BLOOD SUBSTITUTES

Acute hemorrhage remains one of the most challenging factors in the care of the trauma patient. In the setting of massive blood loss, resuscitation with crystalloid solutions is ineffective for the treatment of shock. Although the use of blood products is the standard of care, the nature and lack of availability of these products in the field presents cause for concern. An inherent risk of infection with transfusion, although small, is present and the potential for blood incompatibility must also be considered. Also, evidence suggests that reductions in morbidity and mortality over the past decade are associated with a decreased use of blood transfusion during resuscitation.[90] In circumstances where blood products are not readily available, such as in rural settings, there is a need for the development of effective blood substitutes with the ability to transport oxygen to tissues.

Particularly in the area of trauma care, blood substitutes offer obvious advantages over conventional blood products. Availability would be markedly improved because these agents would require minimum storage requirements, offer extended shelf life, and would eliminate compatibility issues. Infectious risk and immunologic concerns would be eliminated and the potential for enhanced oxygen-carrying capability and improved rheologic properties would be beneficial.[91] Although this is obviously an exciting and needed area of development, investigation into blood substitutes is not without controversy. No synthetic blood substitute has been approved by the Food and Drug Administration. A current clinical trial in the United States is examining the use of a blood substitute during prehospital resuscitation and transport. Ethical concerns remain in the area of community, rather than individual, consent for the procedure, and the possibility that minority and socioeconomically disadvantaged groups may be unfairly targeted.[92]

HEMORRHAGE CONTROL

Uncontrolled bleeding remains a primary cause of mortality in both the prehospital and early in-hospital course of the trauma patient. Although surgical control of bleeding is the paramount approach to the exsanguinating patient, attendant conditions, such as coagulopathy, anemia, and acidosis, further complicate the timely resolution of hemorrhage. Recent data support the use of antifibrinolytic therapy in trauma patients with significant hemorrhage.[93] The infusion of recombinant activated factor VII (rFVIIa), initially developed for the treatment of patients with hemophilia, has been a subject of interest for the control of hemorrhage in the trauma patient.[94] Infusion of rFVIIa has been used as an off-label therapy of last resort in trauma patients with active hemorrhage and clinical coagulopathy in which surgically accessible hemorrhage has been controlled.[95] Although there is considerable literature consisting of case reports, observational trials, and surveillance, it was not until the publication of the CONTROL trial that significant prospective data was available for review.[96] In this study, Hauser et al found that administration of rFVIIa to patients with refractory traumatic hemorrhage reduced blood product use but had no significant affect on mortality. More recently, a review conducted by Levi et al found that patients receiving rFVIIa for hemorrhage control had a significantly increased risk of arterial thromboembolic (coronary or cerebrovascular) events.[97] There appears to be an age-related risk for these events as well. The use of activated factor VII in the care of trauma patients with uncontrolled bleeding appears to be a valuable therapeutic modality and continues to be an area of active investigation. Clearly the off-label administration of this drug warrants careful consideration of the risks and benefits before its use.

HYPOTHERMIC RESUSCITATION

Hypothermia and the associated physiologic changes of homeostatic mechanisms are critical factors in the acute care of the trauma patient. As a result of prolonged exposure, extrication and transport times, and resuscitation with cold fluids in the field, the severity of injuries in the trauma patient is further complicated by this physiologic compromise. However, controlled hypothermia has been effectively used in the treatment of refractory intracranial hypertension and TBI.[98] Hypothermia reduces morbidity and mortality in infants with hypoxic-ischemic encephalopathy.[99] Profound hypothermia is associated with intact survival after prolonged lethal hemorrhage and trauma in animal models. This approach of emergency preservation and resuscitation may offer the ability to extend the time from severe injury in the field to definitive therapy after evacuation to a hospital.[100]

SIMULATION TRAINING

The past decade has seen a marked increase in interest regarding the use of simulation in many areas of medicine. Evolving in part from military applications, the use of simulation training using computer-controlled mannequins has been shown to be an effective means for trauma assessment and trauma team training.[101] The ability to reproducibly evaluate team performance also has been demonstrated using a human patient simulator. Additionally, using human performance-assessment tools, resuscitation training has been shown to improve after a focused refresher course in a simulator.[102] Although continued investigation is needed to further develop and validate the use of simulation training, the potential to improve behavior and performance by trauma team members suggests the possibility of improved refinement of simulation as a critical component for team training in trauma care.[103]

MASS CASUALTIES

The events of the last decade have brought a new interest in the management of incidents involving multiple casualties. Mass casualties may be the result of natural disasters, acts of terrorism, as well as result from industrial accidents.[104] Although victims of a hurricane may have different medical needs than victims of a terrorist act using a chemical or biologic agent, the demands placed on public health assets can be very similar. Augmenting the training of emergency health care providers and increasing their logistical support, as well as increasing the capacity and numbers of health care facilities, can maximize the emergency health care system's ability to rapidly expand capacity and capability, and it can help reduce the severe strains being placed on medical resources.[105,106] The need to develop new strategies in anticipation of the large-scale burdens imposed by mass casualties remains an area of major concern to public health sector and hospital managers.

CONCLUSIONS

Trauma patients present the anesthesiologist with many clinical challenges because of the varied nature of traumatic injury. Although no 2 injuries are exactly alike, traumatic injury causes a characteristic physiologic and metabolic response usually recognized as hemorrhagic shock. Without resuscitation within the golden hour, posttraumatic hemorrhagic shock leads to cellular hypoxia and irreversible organ ischemia. Because excess fluid administration before surgical hemostasis can lead to further uncontrolled hemorrhage, administering some fluid resuscitation in the golden hour is critical. Head-injured patients require somewhat higher blood pressure than do patients who are not head injured. Because a CPP of 60 mm Hg may be adequate to maintain perfusion following head injuries, a target mean arterial pressure of 80 mm Hg before surgical hemostasis should provide adequate cerebral perfusion, assuming an ICP of 20 mm Hg.

Airway management presents special challenges in trauma patients, especially in those with potential cervical spine injury and/or airway injury. Modified rapid sequence intubation with cricoid pressure, gentle mask ventilation before oral intubation, and manual inline spine stabilization is the technique of choice for most trauma patients.

Metabolic management of the trauma patient includes aggressive rewarming and maintenance of normothermia, maintenance of a euglycemic state, and correcting acidosis.

KEY REFERENCES

- Holcomb JB, Niles SE, Miller CC, Hinds D, Duke JH, Moore FA. Prehospital physiologic data and lifesaving interventions in trauma patients. *Mil Med.* 2005;170(1):7-13.
- Kaufmann C. Advanced Trauma Life Support for Doctors. 7th ed. Chicago, IL: American College of Surgeons; 2004:391.
- Keel M, Trentz O. Pathophysiology of polytrauma. *Injury.* 2005;36(6):691-709.
- Kunisaki SA, McCabe CJ. Initial evaluation and resuscitation: primary survey and immediate resuscitation. In: Sheridan RL, ed. *The Trauma Handbook of the Massachusetts General Hospital.* Philadelphia, PA: Lippincott, Williams & Wilkins; 2004:71-88.
- Trunkey DD. Trauma. *Sci Am.* 1983;249(2):28-35.

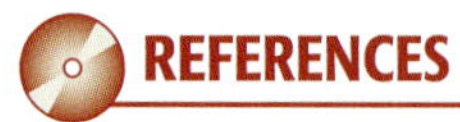

REFERENCES

Complete references available on DVD and online version at www.LongneckerAnesthesiology.com

CHAPTER 77 Developing an Anesthetic Plan for a Critically Ill Patient

Jean Kwo

KEY POINTS

1. Critically ill patients often need surgery to correct the underlying cause of their illness or to deal with the complications of their illness.
2. Advanced planning and open communication between the anesthesiologists, surgeons, the critical care team, and the patient and the patient's family is crucial to understanding the goals and priorities of treatment.
3. Critically ill patients may have impaired function of multiple organ systems. Preoperative evaluation of the degree of organ dysfunction and optimization of the patient's condition ensures that the patient is in the best possible condition to undergo the additional stresses associated with surgery and anesthesia.
4. The simplest surgical procedure resulting in the least physiologic upset is generally the best option for the critically ill patient.
5. Planning for transport to the operating room is essential because patients are at high risk for adverse events during transport.
6. The anesthesiologist must decide which monitors are needed to assess the assessment of the patient's condition.
7. Although general anesthesia is most often necessary for surgery in the critically ill patient, regional anesthesia can play a valuable role helping achieve patient comfort and reduce physiologic stress.
8. There should be specific goals and end points defined in the management of the critically ill patient to optimize hemodynamics and minimize further end-organ damage.

More than 5 million patients are admitted annually to intensive care units (ICUs) across the United States. Many of these patients undergo a surgical procedure during their hospitalization either to correct the underlying cause of their illness or to deal with its complications. Similar to the healthy patient, the anesthesia plan for the critically ill patient should include a clear delineation of the goals of management, an assessment of the priorities of care, and a consideration of alternative strategies to avoid or treat complications.

Many studies indicate that the patient's outcome depends on the interaction of several factors, including the type and extent of the procedure, the physiologic reserves of the patient, the presence of chronic health problems, and the nature of the acute physiologic derangements.[1] The number of complications attributable to anesthesia is 8 times greater for patients with American Society of Anesthesiologists (ASA) Physical Status grades P3 and P4 rather than for patients with ASA grade P1 or P2.[2] One study reports that the presence of an anesthesiologist intraoperatively and certain characteristics of intraoperative and postoperative care were associated with a decreased risk of severe postoperative morbidity and mortality.[2] Thus the plan for a critically ill patient should include preoperative optimization of the patient's condition, a chronological plan for intraoperative management, a plan to ensure that adequate support personnel and equipment are available, and a plan for postoperative care.

The critically ill patient often has many caregivers from various medical and surgical specialties. There should be open communication regarding the likely outcomes and realistic goals of treatment between the anesthesiologists, surgeons, critical care team, and the patient and the patient's family. Preoperatively, one person or team should be designated as the coordinator of the patient's care and should ensure that everyone taking care of the patient in the perioperative period understands the goals and priorities of treatment. Because these goals often change with time, frequent communication to update all is vital.

This chapter focuses on the key points for preoperative planning and some considerations for intraoperative management and optimization to ensure safe delivery of anesthetic care to the critically ill patient.

PREOPERATIVE ASSESSMENT AND OPTIMIZATION

Critically ill patients may have impaired function of some or all their organ systems. An assessment of the degree of organ dysfunction and, whenever possible, optimization of the patient's condition should be undertaken before surgery to ensure that the patient is in the best possible condition to undergo the additional stresses associated with surgery and anesthesia.

HEMODYNAMIC CONSIDERATIONS

A variety of cardiovascular abnormalities may be present in critically ill patients, including hemodynamic instability and dysrhythmias. Patients may manifest shock secondary to hypovolemia, vasodilatation, and/or myocardial dysfunction. Because shock represents the failure of the circulatory system to maintain adequate delivery of oxygen and other nutrients to tissues, cellular and organ dysfunction often ensues. Thus the ultimate goals of hemodynamic therapy in shock are to maintain or restore adequate tissue perfusion and organ function. Evaluation of the hemodynamic status of the critically ill patient should include the following: assessing the patient's volume status, determining whether pressors or inotropic agents are needed to maintain an adequate blood pressure and cardiac output (CO), and learning whether there are any clinical or laboratory indicators of hypoperfusion.

RESPIRATORY FAILURE AND VENTILATOR MANAGEMENT

Critically ill patients often have respiratory failure and require mechanical ventilation. A review of the ventilator's settings preoperatively should include the mode of ventilation, the ventilator rate, the fraction of inspired oxygen, the level of positive end-expiratory pressure (PEEP), and the tidal volume and airway pressures. Arterial blood gas values should be reviewed for adequacy of oxygenation and ventilation. Arrangements should be made to transport the ICU ventilator to the operating room if the patient's ventilation cannot be supported by the similar operating room ventilator.

NEUROLOGIC ASSESSMENT

The critically ill patient often has compromised neurologic function due to a myriad of causes including drugs, infection, metabolic derangements, trauma, and cerebrovascular accidents. Their preoperative evaluation should include an assessment of baseline neurologic function. Dosages and rates of infusions of sedative hypnotic and analgesic agents should be noted, and decisions should be made whether or not infusions of these agents should be continued intraoperatively.

Neuromuscular blocking agents are associated with critical illness polymyopathy/neuropathy, and in general they should be avoided in the septic patient.[3,4] However, because neuromuscular blocking agents are often needed to facilitate surgery, monitoring the depth of blockade with a train-of-four monitor is advised.

Critical illness is associated with prolonged immobilization and a severe myopathy. Thus the use of succinylcholine in critically ill patients can precipitate severe hyperkalemia and/or rhabdomyolysis and should be avoided.

EVALUATION OF RENAL FUNCTION

Critically ill patients often have renal dysfunction. Evaluation of the patient with renal failure should include an assessment of volume status, electrolyte balance, and acid-base status. Because renal ischemia is the primary cause of acute renal failure in the perioperative setting, intraoperative maintenance of adequate intravascular volume, mean arterial pressure, and CO are important measures to preserve renal perfusion. Furthermore, nephrotoxic drugs should be avoided to prevent further renal injury in these patients. Although the measurement of urine output is usually the primary means of evaluating renal function, invasive monitoring may be required to assure adequate volume repletion in the critically ill patient who is at risk for postoperative renal dysfunction.

ENDOCRINE ABNORMALITIES IN THE CRITICALLY ILL PATIENT

Recent clinical trials have examined 2 particular endocrine abnormalities in critically ill patients: adrenal insufficiency and glycemic control (see Chapter 13).

Adrenal Insufficiency Patients with septic shock may have relative adrenal insufficiency. Thus intravenous (IV) corticosteroids may be administered to patients with septic shock who are poorly responsive to fluid replacement and vasopressor therapy. The dose of corticosteroids should equivalent to less than 300 mg hydrocortisone daily,[5]

Glucose Control Critically ill patients are frequently hyperglycemic. Whereas a previous study showed that "intensive glucose control" (maintaining plasma glucose concentration between 80 and 100 mg/dL) was associated with decreased ICU mortality,[6] a more recent study found that maintaining plasma glucose concentrations less than 180 mg/dL resulted in lower mortality and less risk of severe hypoglycemia.[7] Because ICU patients often receive insulin infusions to achieve these goals, consideration should be given to continuing insulin infusions intraoperatively. Patients receiving insulin infusions must be given an external source of glucose to prevent hypoglycemia, and blood sugar levels should be checked frequently intraoperatively.

COAGULATION DYSFUNCTION AND ANEMIA

Evaluation of the critically ill patient should include an assessment of their circulating hemoglobin levels and coagulation status.

Anemia is often present in patients with critical illness. Although current recommendations for critically ill patients state that packed red cell transfusions should be given only when the hemoglobin level decreases to 7.0 mg/dL or less,[8,9] these recommendations should not be applied to individuals who are undergoing short-term resuscitation. In the operating room, the decision to transfuse must be based on how the patient responds to other interventions, including early, aggressive fluid resuscitation. In patients with evidence of hypoperfusion (eg, a low central venous oxygen saturation or lactic acidosis), a target hemoglobin of 10 g/dL has been suggested to maximize tissue oxygen delivery.[10]

Thrombocytopenia can occur in critically ill patients and may be a result of sepsis, drug therapy (**Table 77-1**), or hemodilution caused by massive transfusion. Platelet transfusions are given to patients who are bleeding or at risk of bleeding as a consequence of thrombocytopenia or impaired platelet function. Surgical bleeding may occur when platelet counts are less than 50,000/μL. Additional factors such as a coagulopathy, fever, and renal failure may increase the bleeding risk from severe thrombocytopenia. Therefore, the threshold platelet concentrations for triggering a prophylactic platelet transfusion must take all these considerations into account.[8,11] Platelets should never be given to patients with type 2 heparin-induced thrombocytopenia because of the increased risk of thrombosis after platelet transfusions.

Coagulopathies can occur in the critically ill patient and are initially evaluated by measuring the prothrombin time, activated partial thromboplastin time, and fibrinogen levels. Fresh-frozen plasma or cryoprecipitate are infused to stop active bleeding associated with a coagulopathy or to correct a coagulopathy before surgical procedures. Vitamin K is administered to raise the levels of vitamin K–dependent clotting factors (II, VII, IX, and X).

Recombinant human coagulation factor VIIa (rFVIIa*)* is used to treat bleeding and promotes hemostasis by activating the extrinsic pathway of the coagulation cascade (**Table 77-2**). rFVIIa bypasses inhibitors of factors VIII and IX in patients with hemophilia A and B, and treats patients who have severe von Willebrand factor (vWF) deficiency caused by antibodies to vWF. Other uses of rFVIIa include the treatment of

TABLE 77-1 Drugs That Can Cause Thrombocytopenia

Acetaminophen	Antimicrobials/Antivirals	Antineoplastic drugs	Heparin
Antidepressants	Acyclovir	Benzodiazepines	Unfractionated heparin
Amitriptyline	Cephalosporins	Diazepam	Low molecular weight heparin
Desipramine	Cefamandole	Cardiac medications	Illicit drugs
Doxepin	Cefotetan	Amiodarone	Cocaine
Imipramine	Ceftazidime	Diltiazem	Heroin
Antiepileptic drugs	Cephalothin	Digoxin	Iodinate contrast agents
Carbamazepine	Ciprofloxacin	Procainamide	Quinine/quinidine
Phenytoin	Clarithromycin	Enalapril	Miscellaneous drugs
Valproic acid	Fluconazole	Captopril	Tamoxifen
Anti-inflammatory drugs	Ganciclovir	Diazoxide	Desmopressin
Diclofenac	Gentamicin	α-Methyldopa	Cyclosporine
Fenoprofen	Penicillins	Diuretics	Levamisole
Ibuprofen	Ampicillin	Acetazolamide	Lidocaine
Indomethacin	Methicillin	Chlorothiazide	Morphine
Meclofenamate	Penicillin	Furosemide	Papaverine
Mefenamic acid	Piperacillin	Hydrochlorothiazide	Ticlopidine
Naproxen	Rifampin	Spironolactone	Octreotide
Piroxicam	Sulfa group	H_2-antagonists	Ondansetron
Salicylates	Sulfamethoxazole	Cimetidine	
Aspirin	Sulfamethoxypyridazine	Famotidine	
Diflunisal	Sulfisoxazole	Ranitidine	
Sulfasalazine	Vancomycin		
Sulindac			
Tolmetin			

TABLE 77-2 Uses of Recombinant Factor VIIa

- Hemophilia
- Hemophilia with inhibitors and acquired inhibitors of factors VIII and X
- Other conditions
  - Liver failure
  - Liver transplantation
  - Drug-induced coagulopathies
  - Platelet disorders (thrombocytopenia and thrombasthenia)
  - After bone marrow transplantation
  - Renal failure
  - Factor VII deficiency
  - Factor XI deficiency
  - Severe von Willebrand disease
  - Amyloidosis with factor X deficiency
  - Postsurgical bleeding or bleeding as a result of trauma
  - Disseminated intravascular coagulation

congenital or acquired factor VII deficiency, congenital factor XI or V deficiency, the coagulopathy of severe liver dysfunction, hemostatic changes that arise from extensive surgery, trauma, and bleeding, reversal of warfarin-induced excessive anticoagulation, certain inherited disorders of platelet function (eg, Glanzmann and Bernard-Soulier thrombasthenias), and bleeding from thrombocytopenia that is a result of antiplatelet glycoprotein antibodies that thwart the effects of platelet transfusion.[12] The minimum effective rFVIIa dose for managing these hemorrhagic disorders is uncertain. The rFVIIa dose depends on the specific hemorrhagic disorder being treated; in various clinical studies the dose has ranged from 3 to 320 μg/kg.

Recombinant activated protein C (drotrecogin alfa) is a critical protein that reduces excessive thrombosis in the microcirculation and appears to reduce the mortality from severe sepsis associated with organ dysfunction in adult patients who are at high risk of dying (Acute Physiology and Chronic Health Evaluation II scores ≥25).[13,14] Because of its anticoagulant effects, bleeding is the most common serious adverse effect associated with drotrecogin alfa therapy. Drotrecogin alfa should be discontinued 2 hours prior to undergoing an invasive surgical procedure or performing procedures with an inherent risk of bleeding. Once adequate hemostasis has been achieved, initiation of drotrecogin alfa may be considered 12 hours after major invasive procedures or surgery, or therapy may be restarted immediately following uncomplicated minor procedures.

THE ELDERLY CRITICALLY ILL PATIENT

Advancing age is associated with an increased incidence of intercurrent diseases and declining physiologic reserve. Before the age of 60 years, both basal organ function and physiologic reserve (the difference between basal and maximal organ function) are generally well maintained. Subsequently, physiologic reserve diminishes. Both aging and a higher American Society of Anesthesiologists (ASA) Physical Status classification score are associated with an increased incidence of postoperative complications. In the healthiest patients, for example, those who are classified as ASA class P1 (free of systemic disease) and P2 (mild systemic disease), the frequency of major complications increases gradually with age until about 70 years of age. For ASA class P3 patients, an increasing incidence of major postoperative complications begins at an earlier age and increases rapidly with age. For ASA class P4 patients (a patient with disease that is a constant threat to the patient's life), the complication rate rises even more steeply. Many studies show that age and comorbidity are independent predictors of mortality in both the general surgical population and in the critically ill patient.[15-17]

Mortality and complication rates have been well-studied in the elderly (age ≥65 years) general surgical population.[18-20] Characteristics of the elderly population include a reduced functional status, more emergency operations, a higher ASA classification (20% of patients ≥80 years of age were ASA P4), and more frequent do-not-resuscitate orders. Mortality rates vary widely across many types of operations but are higher for those 80 years and older. Postoperative complications were also more common in patients 80 years and older (20% had one or more complications), and mortality was higher in those who suffered complications postoperatively. One study reported a 5% increase in perioperative mortality risk for every year after age 80.[19]

Morbidity and mortality rates in elderly patients admitted to the ICU are higher than in younger patients. Compared with younger patients, elderly patients are more severely ill on admission, and they are more likely to have shock and renal dysfunction. One study reported that hospital mortality was more than doubled for patients 75 years and older in comparison with patients younger than 65 years.[21-24]

CONSIDERATIONS FOR THE SELECTING AND TIMING OF THE SURGICAL PROCEDURE

Critically ill patients undergo a myriad of surgical procedures, including a tracheostomy for respiratory failure, surgery to remove a septic focus, or procedures for traumatic injuries. Whether definitive surgery should be undertaken or whether it should be delayed and performed electively when the patient has recovered depends on the stability of the patient and the nature and complexity of the intervention that is needed. In general, the simplest intervention resulting in the least physiologic upset is the best option for the critically ill patient. The decision to proceed to surgery and the extent of the surgical procedure must weigh the benefits and risks of the specific intervention to cause complications, such as bleeding or inadvertent injury to other organs or tissues. Ideally, surgery should be undertaken following adequate resuscitation. However, timely and emergent intervention may be vital and lifesaving in certain conditions, for example, patients with necrotizing soft tissue infection or intestinal ischemia.

INTRAOPERATIVE MANAGEMENT

TRANSPORTING THE CRITICALLY ILL PATIENT

Unless the surgical procedure will occur in the ICU, the critically ill patient must be transported from the ICU to the operating room. These patients are at high risk for complications en route. Adverse events during transport include both minor and serious mishaps such as the loss of IV access, accidental tracheal extubation, occlusion of the endotracheal tube, and exhaustion of the oxygen supply, as well as physiologic deterioration of the patient's state (eg, worsening hypotension or hypoxemia). Studies report adverse events rates in 5.9% to 66% of the transports of critically ill patients.[25,26] One study reported a high incidence of hemodynamic changes requiring therapeutic intervention during and after transport from the operating room to the ICU.[27] Guidelines for the transport of critically ill patients have been published.[28] Having a plan for transport to minimize potential complications is an important area of patient safety (**Table 77-3**).

The patients should be hemodynamically stable before transport. All critically ill patients undergoing transport should receive the same level of basic physiologic monitoring during transport as they had in the ICU and should include, at a minimum, continuous electrocardiographic monitoring, continuous pulse oximetry, and periodic measurement of blood pressure, pulse rate, and respiratory rate. Selected patients may benefit from capnography, continuous intra-arterial blood pressure, or intracranial pressure monitoring.

The patient should have a secured airway to allow safe transport. Patients should be assessed for their need for intubation before transport. Intubated patients are usually taken off mechanical ventilation and switched to manual ventilation with a self-inflating Ambu bag during transport. Adequate PEEP should be applied during manual ventilation.

TABLE 77-3 Transport Checklist

Intravenous access	• Check size and placement • Check patency
Monitors	• Same level of basic physiologic monitoring during transport as in the intensive care unit • Should include Continuous electrocardiogram monitoring Continuous pulse oximetry monitoring Periodic blood pressure, pulse rate, and respiratory rate monitoring
Infusions	• Note infusion rate of medications • Is there an adequate volume to last during transportation? • Are infusions pumps securely attached to bed or transport unit? • If total parenteral nutrition is stopped, check that glucose infusion is running • Ensure battery-operated equipment has enough charge to last during transport
Drugs for transport	• Have basic resuscitation drugs available • Consider Sedatives Pressors Antihypertensive agents
Airway	• Assess airway; consider need for intubation before transport • Have self-inflating bag for ventilation available • Assess need for positive end-expiratory pressure • Oxygen: ensure adequate supply for transport • Have mask, laryngoscope, extra endotracheal tubes available for transport
Assess need for sedatives/ muscle relaxant	• If needed, administer and monitor for side effects before transport
Ensure adequate help to transport patient	• At least 2 people should be present during transport
Ensure operating room is ready to receive patient	

The oxygen tank should be checked to ensure an adequate supply at the required flow rate for transport.

Before transport the anesthesiologist should check the size and placement of the patient's IV access. Patency of the IV routes should be assessed. All drug infusions (eg, sedatives, pressors, insulin), their rates, and their IV routes should be noted. There should be an adequate volume of drug to last during transport. If total parenteral nutrition is stopped, an alternative source of glucose must be provided. If a sedative and/or muscle relaxant is needed for transport, it should be administered in the ICU and the patient monitored for hemodynamic and respiratory side effects (eg, hypotension) before transport. The anesthesiologist should have common drugs needed for resuscitation, such as epinephrine and atropine, readily available in the event of cardiac arrest or arrhythmia. As well, a mask, laryngoscope, and extra endotracheal tubes should be available should an accidental extubation occur during transport. Standardized transport kits can ensure that the necessary drugs and equipment are always present and available (**Fig. 77-1**).

All infusion pumps should be securely attached to the bed or to specialized transfer devices. Battery-operated equipment should be fully charged and capable of functioning for the duration of the transport. There should be adequate assistance to transport the patient and treat minor problems. The operating room should be ready to receive the patient prior to leaving the ICU.

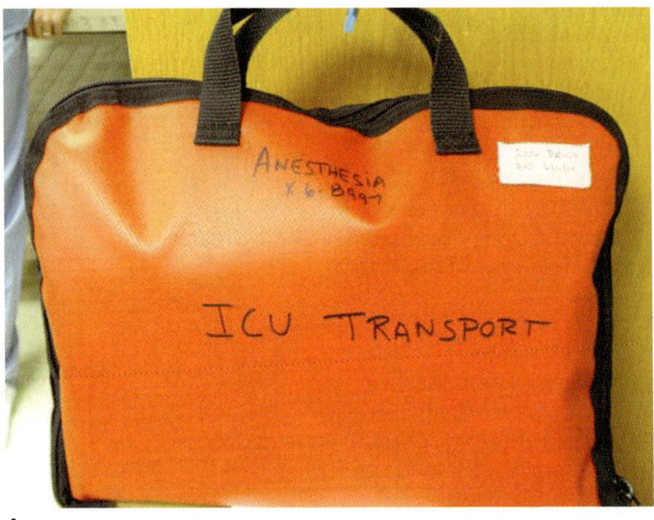

A

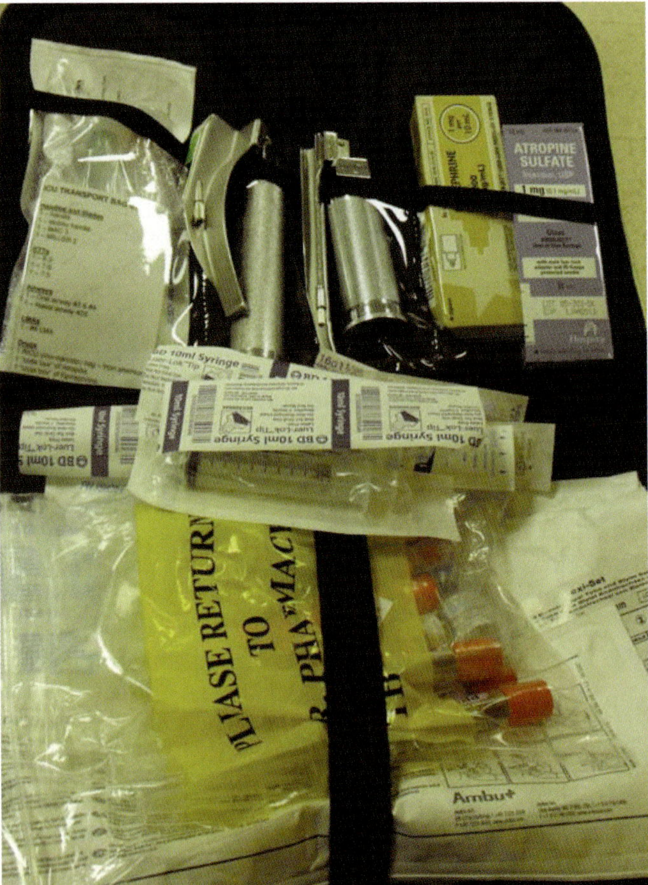

B

FIGURE 77-1. A, B. Example of standardized transport kit containing equipment for emergency airway management and resuscitation drugs.

MONITORING OPTIONS

STANDARD MONITORS

Basic standards for monitoring have been established by the ASA (**Table 77-4**) and should be used for the critically ill patient.[29] The patient's systemic oxygenation (Spo_2), ventilation ($ETCO_2$), circulation (blood pressure and heart rate), and core temperature should be continuously monitored and evaluated during each anesthetic procedure.

TABLE 77-4 American Society of Anesthesiologists Standard Monitors

Parameter	Recommendation
Oxygenation	• Oxygen analyzer • Pulse oximetry
Ventilation	• Clinical signs Chest excursion Auscultation of breath sounds • Exhaled carbon dioxide monitoring • Notification of breathing system disconnection with audible alarm
Electrocardiogram	• Continuous display
Blood pressure	• Evaluation every 5 min
Heart rate	• Evaluation every 5 min
Circulatory function	• Assess adequacy Palpate pulse Auscultate heart sounds Monitor intraarterial pressure trace Pulse plethysmography or oximetry
Core temperature	• Use when clinically significant changes in body temperature is anticipated
Personnel	• Qualified anesthesia personnel should monitor conduct of all general anesthetics, regional anesthetics, and monitored anesthesia care

Excerpted from ASA Standards for Basic Anesthetic Monitoring: www.asahq.org/publicationsAndServices/standards/02.pdf of the American Society of Anesthesiologists. A copy of the full text can be obtained from ASA, 520 N. Northwest Highway, Park Ridge, IL 60068-2573.

An oxygen analyzer to measure the oxygen concentration in the patient breathing system and a quantitative assessment of systemic blood oxygenation (eg, Spo_2 via pulse oximetry) should be used to monitor adequate oxygenation. Ventilation should also be evaluated by clinical signs (eg, chest or abdominal excursion and auscultation of breath sounds) as well as quantitative continuous monitoring of the level of expired carbon dioxide. Monitoring the tidal volume of expired gas is strongly encouraged. There should be a rapid audible alarm if any of the components of the breathing system are disconnected.

Each critically ill patient should have their electrocardiogram (ECG) continuously displayed, and blood pressure and heart rate should be determined and assessed every 5 minutes at a minimum. To ensure the adequacy of the patient's circulatory function, the patient should be continuously evaluated by either palpation of an arterial pulse (at a minimum), auscultation of heart sounds, observing the trace of intraarterial systemic pressure, ultrasound peripheral pulse velocity monitoring, pulse plethysmography, or oximetry.

Core temperature monitoring should be used when clinically significant changes of body temperature are likely.

Because of possibly rapid changes of hemodynamic status occurring during anesthesia, there must be qualified anesthesia personnel to monitor the patient and provide care throughout all general and/or regional anesthetics and during monitored anesthesia care.

INVASIVE MONITORS

Additional monitors may be needed to provide an accurate picture of the patient's hemodynamic status and to guide therapy to optimize the patient's condition. However, there are limitations to each monitor and some risk to the patient when using invasive monitors. Thus the anesthesiologist must be cognizant of these limitations and weigh the risks and benefits of invasive monitoring to choose appropriate monitors for each critically ill patient (**Table 77-5**).

Invasive Arterial Pressure Monitoring Because shock represents failure of the circulatory system to maintain adequate delivery of blood flow to tissues, and the goal of hemodynamic therapy is to restore adequate tissue perfusion, systemic pressure measurement is the most frequently used parameter to indirectly assess perfusion.

In healthy individuals, blood pressure as determined by noninvasive blood pressure (NIBP) monitors is, on average, within 5 mm Hg of measurements obtained by direct arterial pressure monitoring. Sources of error in NIBP measurements include using the incorrect cuff size or highly irregular or rapid cardiac rhythms. However, in shock states, NIBP measurements are often inaccurate. Therefore, inserting an arterial catheter provides a more accurate and reproducible measurement of systemic arterial pressure. Invasive arterial monitoring allows beat-to-beat display so decisions regarding therapy can be based on continuous blood pressure analysis.

Blood pressure does not directly equate to tissue blood flow, and the level of mean arterial pressure (MAP) to aim for is not necessarily the same in all patients. Below a MAP of 60 mm Hg, autoregulation of the coronary, renal, and central nervous system vascular beds is compromised and organ flow becomes linearly dependent on pressure. Thus in adults, maintenance of a MAP 65 mm Hg or higher is recommended to maintain and optimize flow.[4] However, because the loss of autoregulation may occur at different levels in different organs, some patients require higher blood pressures to maintain adequate tissue perfusion. Furthermore, the degree to which flow autoregulation remains intact in septic patients is uncertain. Thus it may be necessary at times to supplement blood pressure measurement with other means of assessing regional and global perfusion (eg, urine output; see section on downstream monitoring).

The invasive arterial pressure waveform can also be used to estimate blood volume status and assess fluid responsiveness in mechanically

TABLE 77-5 Comparison of Monitors Used in Critically Ill Patients

Monitor	Indications	Limitations
Central venous pressure (CVP)	• Reflects intravascular volume	• Depends on right-heart function, venous return, right-heart compliance, intrathoracic pressure, patient positioning
Pulmonary artery catheter (PAC)	• Measures pulmonary artery pressure, cardiac output, and pulmonary artery occlusion pressure, which reflects left ventricular end-diastolic volume	• Depends on right- and left-heart compliance, intrathoracic pressures, valvular lesions
Transesophageal echocardiography (TEE)	• Qualitative measurement of ventricular function, ventricular volume, and valvular abnormalities	• Requires training to perform procedure and correctly interpret images • Can consume anesthesiologist's time and attention
Gastric tonometry	• Indication of regional hypoperfusion	• pH_{im} calculation affected by both systemic and respiratory alterations
	• Reflects blood flow-to-demand ratio	• Unproven utility to guide therapy

ventilated patients. A positive pressure breath reduces venous return and decreases left ventricular filling resulting in a decreased stroke volume, CO, and blood pressure. This effect can be especially marked in hypovolemic patients. Marked variations in pulse pressure, which is proportional to stroke volume, and systolic pressure tracing variations usually predict that an increase in CO will occur with volume loading.[30,31]

Central Venous Pressure Catheter Systemic hypotension is the most common reason to initiate invasive central hemodynamic monitoring in the critically ill patient. The central venous pressure (CVP) reflects pressure in the large systemic veins. Although the CVP also reflects intravascular volume, it does not measure blood volume directly and is influenced by right-heart function, venous return, right-heart compliance, intrathoracic pressure, and the patient's positioning. Consequently, the CVP level should be interpreted with other measures of cardiac function and circulating volume (eg, pulse, blood pressure, urine output). A single CVP value may not be as important as serial CVP measurements or their change with therapy.

Measurement of the CVP may provide useful information in patients with normal cardiac function who are hypotensive because of blood loss or widespread vasodilatation because a decreased venous return will result in a falling right atrial pressure and CVP. A central venous catheter (CVC) should be inserted when an infusion of vasopressors or inotropes is planned.

Pulmonary Artery Catheter In addition to the CVP, a flow-directed pulmonary artery catheter (PAC) allows measurement of the pulmonary artery pressure, the pulmonary artery occlusion pressure (PAOP), the CO, and the mixed-venous oxygen saturation (SvO_2). The PAOP reflects the pulmonary venous pressure and the left atrial and left ventricular end-diastolic pressure and therefore can provide a crude indirect estimate of left ventricular end-diastolic volume (LVEDV). Indications for placing a pulmonary artery catheter are related to the planned procedure and the patient's state of health (**Table 77-6**). The pulmonary artery catheter may provide useful information in any procedure associated with acute, severe changes of preload, afterload, or myocardial contractile state. For example, procedures where blood loss may be massive or where partial or complete caval occlusion might occur can cause acute changes of cardiac preload. Similarly, proximal aortic cross-clamping can cause a rapid increase of left ventricular afterload. Patient factors that can lead to the insertion of a PAC include septic shock or other significant cardiac, respiratory, or renal disease. In septic shock, both hypovolemia and myocardial dysfunction may contribute to impaired tissue perfusion. Pulmonary artery catheter placement can be used both to monitor CO and assess ventricular stroke volume.

Unjustified use of the pulmonary artery catheter has been suppressed by the publication of an observational study demonstrating an increased mortality associated with the use of the pulmonary artery catheter in critically ill patients during the first 24 hours of intensive care as compared with case-matched controls.[32] Multiple randomized controlled trials evaluating the use of the PAC in many different patient populations have not demonstrated a decreased overall mortality or obvious benefit.[33-35] In all of these studies, the PAC has proven primarily to be a diagnostic tool. The studies also highlight our lack of consensus and data about our therapeutic interventions that will improve the outcome of the critically ill patient in shock.

A major pitfall of central pressure monitoring occurs when pressure alone is used to estimate volume. Important variables in addition to the volume of the systemic and pulmonary circulations can affect the central pressure measurement. The relationship between pressure and volume is controlled by the compliance of the chamber. In patients with an abnormal left ventricular compliance, the PAOP may over- or underestimate the LVEDV. Right ventricular (RV) dysfunction is common in critically ill patients and can result from pulmonary embolism, severe acute respiratory distress syndrome (ARDS), or other conditions that increase RV afterload, such as high levels of PEEP or an increased pulmonary vascular resistance as a consequence of other vascular, cardiac, metabolic, or pulmonary causes. Because the right and left ventricles are both enclosed within the relatively stiff pericardium, pressure and volume overload of the RV can lead to abnormal motion of the interventricular septum and will impair left ventricular (LV) relaxation. In this situation, the pressure–volume relationship of the left ventricle is altered, and information obtained from the PAC may be misleading. Other factors that can affect the ability of central pressures to reflect ventricular filling volumes include increased intrathoracic pressures and valvular lesions. Increased intrathoracic pressure caused by positive pressure ventilation or increased intra-abdominal pressures can also elevate central vascular pressures. Stenotic lesions of the atrioventricular valves can also elevate central vascular pressures.

Other potential pitfalls include problems with the transducer system (eg, improper transducer placement or reference level zeroing), improper interpretation of waveforms, and erroneous thermodilution CO measurements due to errors of injectate volume or temperature. The presence of marked tricuspid valve regurgitation, which can occur in the critically ill patient as a consequence of high pulmonary artery pressures, can also produce erroneous CO measurements. Mixed venous blood gas tensions and saturation measurements may be invalid if the blood gas analysis is inaccurate or if the pulmonary artery specimen is "arterialized" by being withdrawn from a wedged or partially wedged PAC.

There are major but uncommon complications associated with the presence of a PAC. Rupture of the pulmonary artery is a rare occurrence (<1%) but a potentially catastrophic one with a mortality rate approaching 50%. Patients who have pulmonary hypertension, are older than 60 years, or are receiving anticoagulation therapy are at greater risk. The sudden onset of hemoptysis (especially after inflation of the pulmonary artery catheter balloon) is a sign of possible pulmonary artery rupture. Immediate management includes lateral decubitus positioning the bleeding side down, intubation with a double-lumen endotracheal tube, and increasing PEEP. Embolization via angiography, or even a lobectomy, may become necessary if pulmonary bleeding continues or is massive. The incidence of pulmonary infarction associated with the use of the pulmonary artery catheter is less than 7% and usually caused by unintentional distal migration of the PAC tip. Catheter-related thrombi may also cause pulmonary infarction. Infection related to the PAC is

TABLE 77-6 Indications for Use of Pulmonary Artery Catheter

- Determination of cause of shock
  - Cardiogenic
  - Hypovolemic
  - Distributive (sepsis)
  - Obstructive (massive pulmonary embolism)
- Determination of cause of pulmonary edema
  - Cardiogenic
  - Capillary leak
- Evaluation of pulmonary hypertension
- Diagnosis of pericardial tamponade
- Management of complicated myocardial infarction
- Guide to pharmacologic therapy
  - Vasopressors
  - Inotropes
  - Vasodilators (for patients with pulmonary hypertension)
- Guide to fluid management
- Guide to management of patients with burns
- Guide to management of patients with sepsis
- Guide to management of patients with renal failure
- Guide to management of patients with heart failure
- Guide to management of patients with decompensated cirrhosis

fairly common with a risk for clinical sepsis of less than 0.5% per day of catheter use.

Thus hemodynamic measurements obtained from a PAC should be interpreted with the full knowledge of possible confounding factors. It may often be more appropriate to respond to trends of change in central hemodynamic measurement (eg, a slowly falling pulmonary capillary wedge pressure or CVP) rather than to the absolute values themselves.

ECHOCARDIOGRAPHY

In view of the risks and benefits of pulmonary artery catheterization, other noninvasive methods for improving monitoring and resuscitation have been developed and evaluated. Echocardiography has been used in the operating room since the 1970s. Transesophageal echocardiography (TEE) is preferred in the operating room because the acoustic images of transthoracic echocardiography (TTE) are generally poorer than those of TEE.[36] Furthermore, factors such as patient positioning, the surgical field, and surgical equipment, drapes, or other monitors may block access to the chest, limiting the usefulness of TTE.

There are some important limitations to TEE.[36] Some regions of the heart and great vessels cannot be well visualized. Insertion and manipulation of the TEE probe can produce pharyngeal and/or laryngeal trauma, dental injuries, esophageal trauma, arrhythmias, and hemodynamic effects. The inaccurate interpretation of TEE images may result in improper clinical decisions by the anesthesiologist or surgeon. The performance of TEE will require the anesthesiologists' time and attention and may thus detract from other intraoperative responsibilities or delay other important interventions.

Nevertheless, the role of TEE is expanding both in the operating room and the ICU. Current indications for the use of intraoperative TEE include the diagnosis of myocardial ischemia, confirmation of the adequacy of valve reconstruction and other surgical repairs, and determining the causes of hemodynamic instability and other intraoperative complications.[36] TEE can readily provide information on biventricular volumes and contractility, and valvular and wall-motion abnormalities.

The perioperative period is a time of increased risk of myocardial ischemia as a result of hemodynamic and other physiologic stresses associated with anesthesia and surgery. Wall-motion abnormalities generally precede ECG changes during myocardial ischemia[37] and may allow earlier detection of ischemia. The incidence of regional ventricular dysfunction detected by TEE ranges from 10% to 60% in various surgical populations.[36] Intraoperative TEE detection of ischemia may permit corrective interventions such as altering surgery and/or anesthetic management, initiating infusions, and postoperative triage, which may prevent perioperative complications. There is a lack of studies demonstrating that the detection and treatment of regional ventricular dysfunction or other TEE evidence of ischemia can improve perioperative clinical outcome or increase long-term survival.

Perioperative TEE is often used emergently to determine the cause of acute persistent, life-threatening hemodynamic disturbances. However, elective use of the TEE should be considered in the care of the critically ill surgical patient. TEE has become a useful tool for assessing hemodynamic function qualitatively and for imaging the heart (eg, to diagnose a hemopericardium or cardiac tamponade). It provides an assessment of LV function and an indirect measurement of CO, contractility, and left, and often right, ventricular volume. Because of the limitations in using catheter-derived pressure data to estimate LVEDV, TEE may determine the precise causes of hemodynamic instability (eg, a low CO) in patients with left ventricular dysfunction in a more useful fashion than the PAC.

ESOPHAGEAL DOPPLER

Esophageal Doppler monitoring measures aortic flow velocity in the thoracic aorta. A fixed relationship between aortic blood flow and CO is assumed, and thus CO can be calculated using this relationship. The esophageal Doppler is smaller than an ordinary transesophageal echocardiographic probe and thus less invasive. There have been no case reports of esophageal perforation and only reports of minor complications such as mucosal trauma and endobronchial placement. However, proper positioning of the probe is necessary to get an optimal waveform. Although the correlation between CO measured by esophageal Doppler and PAC is modest, there is an excellent correlation with the change in CO with therapeutic interventions.[38] One meta-analysis found that use of the esophageal Doppler to guide intraoperative fluid management resulted in an increase of the amount of fluid administered and a reduced length of hospital stay, time to resume full oral diet, and postoperative morbidity or complications.[39]

DOWNSTREAM MARKERS OF ORGAN PERFUSION

Derangement of blood flow at the capillary and tissue level is one of the critical pathogenic events in sepsis and is associated with multiorgan failure and mortality.[40] The relationship between global hemodynamics as measured by blood pressure, CVP, and CO and microcirculatory blood flow is incompletely understood. Thus, although practice parameters suggest maintaining a MAP of 65 mm Hg or more,[4] it is unclear this pressure ensures adequate tissue perfusion. In practice, indices of organ function, such as ECG evidence of myocardial ischemia, urine output, chemical measurements of blood urea nitrogen and creatinine, and liver function tests, are used to indirectly assess the adequacy of regional perfusion.

Blood lactate levels are a product of anaerobic metabolism and an indirect marker of tissue perfusion and the adequacy of resuscitation. An elevated blood lactate concentration (>4 mEq/L) is associated with a high risk of death, and the rate of blood lactate clearance is a good marker of outcome.[38] Because lactate clearance lags therapeutic interventions, lactate levels are not suited for immediate assessment of resuscitation. A recent multi-institutional study reported no survival difference in patients with severe sepsis who were resuscitated to normalize CVP, MAP, and either a lactate clearance of 10% or a normalized central venous oxygen saturation ($S_{cv}O_2$).[41]

Gastric tonometry is a method used to assess regional perfusion of the gut. A balloon is placed in the stomach to measure the intramucosal partial pressure of carbon dioxide ($P{CO_2}$). This in turn is used to indirectly determine gastrointestinal mucosal pH (pH_{im}). Hypoperfusion causes mucosal carbon dioxide (CO_2) to increase and produces gut tissue acidosis. Because CO_2 readily diffuses across membranes, the $P{CO_2}$ in the gut lumen leads to an increase in the gradient between arterial and luminal $P{CO_2}$. Tonometry provides an indicator of the gut's blood flow-to-CO_2 production ratio because a decreased pH_{im} may arise as a result of either decreased blood flow or increased CO_2 production. A low gastric pH_{im} and increased gastric luminal $P{CO_2}$ are highly predictive of postoperative complications.[42] Although tonometry is a reasonably good predictor of mortality in critically ill patients,[43] its usefulness as a therapeutic guide in patients with sepsis and septic shock has not been proven.

Mixed venous oxygen saturation (SvO_2) is measured either in the pulmonary artery with a PAC or estimated via the right atrium with a CVC. It can be used as an end point for therapeutic interventions.[10] A low SvO_2 may be due to increased oxygen consumption or a decreased hemoglobin, CO, or arterial oxygen saturation. Its major disadvantage is that it is a global measurement, and thus blood from vital organs with low tissue Po_2 will be diluted by blood from organs with lower metabolic requirements and a higher Po_2. Furthermore, in sepsis, there may be organ or tissue shunting at the microcirculatory level resulting in a higher SvO_2.

AIRWAY EVALUATION AND MANAGEMENT

There are myriad indications for endotracheal intubation of the critically ill patient. These patients may lose their airway, potentially develop an inadequate respiratory drive because of central nervous system disease or the administration of sedative drugs, suffer disruption of their rib cage as a consequence of trauma, develop lung parenchymal disease secondary to ARDS or aspiration, or have an impaired ability to cough or protect their airway against the aspiration of gastric or pharyngeal contents.

As in the healthy patient, preparation for endotracheal intubation should begin with an assessment of airway anatomy. If a difficult intubation is anticipated, fiberoptic intubation should be considered. Airway adjuncts such as a laryngeal mask airway and oral and nasal airways of various sizes should be immediately available. Additional personnel should be on hand and a surgeon should be available to perform a cricothyrotomy or tracheostomy should endotracheal intubation be unsuccessful and ventilation inadequate via mask or laryngeal mask airway.

Studies show that an increased ASA classification and emergency surgery are associated with an increased risk of aspiration.[44] Information such as recent vomiting, bowel obstruction, morbid obesity, diabetes mellitus, or a depressed mental status should be factored into the assessment of aspiration risk in the critically ill patient. Prior to intubation, nothing by mouth status should be confirmed if possible. Consider placing a nasogastric tube to empty liquid gastric contents. In the conscious patient, an awake intubation is preferred, although a rapid sequence intubation may also be considered.

Direct laryngoscopy to facilitate tracheal intubation produces a marked stress response.[45] Although these responses are short lived, they may produce detrimental effects on the coronary or cerebral circulation of high-risk patients.[46] Thus patients should first be assessed for the presence of angina or ischemia, dysrhythmias, and congestive heart failure. The patient's neurologic status including the presence of an increased intracranial pressure, intracranial aneurysms, and hemorrhage should be determined. In these patients, hypertension should be avoided and heart rate and blood pressure should be maintained within a narrow range during laryngoscopy and intubation. Before intubation, adjuncts such as airway blocks with local anesthetics, use of adequate β-adrenergic blockade, and deep anesthesia with opioids or barbiturates should be considered.

In trauma patients, the presence of cervical and mandibular fractures and instability should be sought. All patients with multiple trauma, head, or facial injury should be presumed to have a cervical spine injury unless it has been excluded by a thorough radiographic and physical evaluation. A second skilled person should be present during intubation to provide inline stabilization to maintain the head and neck in a neutral position. Nasotracheal intubation is relatively contraindicated in patients with oropharyngeal and facial trauma because of the possibility of cranial vault disruption.

Patients with spinal cord denervation injuries, crush injuries, or burns should not be given depolarizing muscle relaxants because of the risk of life-threatening hyperkalemia. The patient's coagulation status should be evaluated because mucosal trauma and bleeding associated with laryngoscopy can impair visualization of the airway and increase the risk of aspiration.

ANESTHETIC CHOICES

General anesthesia is most often used for surgery in the critically ill patient because of multiple factors, among them surgical and hemodynamic considerations. However, a regional anesthetic can be a valuable adjunct to general anesthesia and in the management of postoperative pain in the critically ill patient to enhance patient comfort and to reduce physiologic stress.[47]

Epidural analgesia is a regional analgesic technique commonly used in the ICU. It is used to manage pain after chest trauma, thoracic and abdominal surgery, major orthopedic surgery, and intractable anginal pain. Studies show that to manage patients after chest trauma, thoracic epidural analgesia provides superior analgesia and improves lung function.[48] High levels of thoracic epidural analgesia (T1-T4) can provide effective treatment of myocardial ischemia refractory to conventional medical therapy.[49] Benefit probably occurs through both increased myocardial oxygen delivery as a result of coronary artery vasodilatation and decreased myocardial oxygen demand because of a reduced heart rate and blood pressure. Issues such as local or systemic infection and coagulopathy can limit or prevent the use of epidural analgesia. Furthermore, there remains a controversy over the safety of placing epidural catheters in sedated patients, and confirmation of catheter position can be difficult when sensory-level testing is unreliable.

The use of peripheral nerve blocks to produce anesthesia in the critically ill patient has not been evaluated by randomized controlled trials. Continuous interscalene, infraclavicular, and axillary catheters may provide excellent postoperative analgesia after shoulder or upper extremity surgery. Similarly, a femoral nerve catheter in combination with a sciatic block can provide pain relief for the entire leg. These techniques can be used to provide surgical anesthesia for procedures such as external fixation, painful dressing changes, or debridement of burns and large soft tissue wounds. Regional analgesia may be particularly advantageous in the patient with brain injury where opioid analgesic agents might mask their neurologic examination.[47] Although there are concerns about placing regional blocks in patients with an impaired mental status because of neurologic injury or sedation, using ultrasonography and nerve stimulation to guide the placement of the needle or catheter may minimize the risk of complications.

INTRAOPERATIVE MANAGEMENT

Specific goals and end points should be defined for the hemodynamic management of the critically ill patient. Therapies such as fluid administration and vasopressor and inotropic support should be titrated to reach those end points. The results of these interventions should be evaluated on an ongoing basis by monitoring a combination of variables reflecting both global and regional tissue perfusion.

HEMODYNAMIC MANAGEMENT

Early Goal-Directed Therapy The care of the critically ill patient is largely supportive. Based on the old observation that improved survival was associated with the ability to sustain a hypermetabolic state by increasing CO and oxygen delivery, the hypothesis was proposed that by proactively increasing the systemic oxygen delivery rate, oxygen debt could be reversed and mortality from multiple organ failure might be reduced. Unfortunately, a large randomized controlled trial investigating the effect of increasing oxygen transport on the outcome of the critically ill patient found no overall benefits.[50] However, some studies have found that the perioperative hemodynamic optimization of high-risk surgical patients appears to be associated with a reduction in morbidity and mortality.[51,52] These studies are consistent with a report that early goal-directed therapy in patients with septic shock reduced in-hospital mortality.[10]

Studies on the intraoperative use of goal-directed fluid therapy have focused on patients who are not critically ill. Goal-directed fluid administration in this less severely ill population has been shown to decrease hospital length of stay, reduce complication rates, and shorten the time to recovery of gut function.[53,54]

One of the challenges is to define the precise goal in goal-directed therapy. Some studies have targeted a systemic oxygen delivery rate of 600 mL/min per m^2 body surface area.[52] Others have used a central venous oxygen saturation greater than 70% as the goal.[10] More recently, an *individualized* approach to fluid resuscitation using each patient's response to fluid administration to guide resuscitation has been advocated.[53-55]

Another challenge is determining the best therapeutic maneuvers to achieve the targeted goal. Most studies have used fluid (either crystalloid or colloid) infusion and inotropic agents (dobutamine and dopexamine). One study required blood transfusions to a hematocrit of 30% or more to help achieve the goal of achieving a central venous oxygen saturation greater than 70% (**Fig. 77-2**).[10]

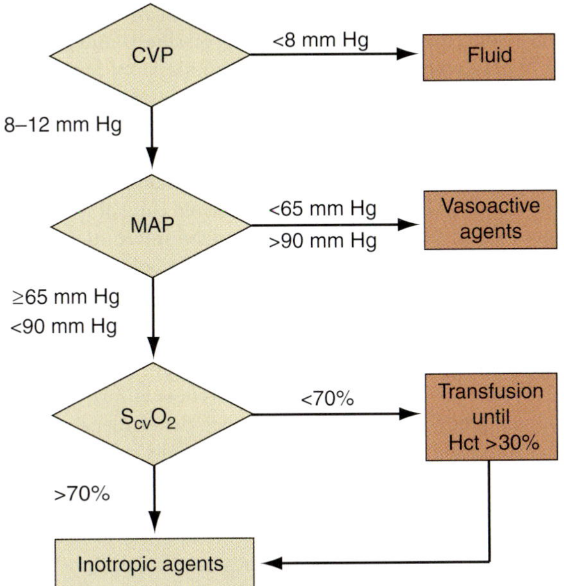

FIGURE 77-2. Goal-directed therapy. CVP, central venous pressure; Hct, hematocrit; MAP, mean arterial pressure; $S_{cv}O_2$, central venous oxygen saturation. [From Rivers E, Nguyen B, Havstad S, et al. Early goal-directed therapy in the treatment of severe sepsis and septic shock. *N Engl J Med.* 2001;345:1368. Copyright 2001, Massachusetts Medical Society. All rights reserved.]

Although the goals of treatment in the critically ill and the ideal therapy needed to achieve those goals remain uncertain, it seems clear that early optimization of hemodynamic status will provide a significant benefit in reducing the mortality rate in patients with severe sepsis and septic shock.

FLUID MANAGEMENT

Fluid resuscitation consists of infusing natural or artificial colloids or crystalloids. Meta-analyses of clinical studies comparing crystalloid and colloid resuscitation in surgical patient populations show no difference of clinical outcome between infusing colloids or crystalloids.[56] This has also been demonstrated in the critically ill patient.[57] Although no human studies have been done, a goal-directed colloid therapy resulted in increased tissue oxygen in animals suggesting that one benefit of colloid use could be an improved microcirculatory blood flow.[58] Resuscitation with crystalloids also results in more edema because the volume of distribution is much larger for crystalloids than for colloids thus requiring more fluid to achieve the same end points.

PHARMACOLOGIC MANAGEMENT

Although hypovolemia is the most common factor contributing to shock in the patient with sepsis, below some mean systemic arterial pressure, perfusion becomes linearly dependent on pressure because of the loss of autoregulation. Therefore, it is frequently necessary to infuse vasopressors to maintain an adequate blood pressure in patients with severe shock. Patients with a low CO despite adequate fluid resuscitation (eg, too high CVP or pulmonary capillary wedge pressure) may require an inotropic agent to increase their CO.

Pressor Support Norepinephrine and dopamine are the first-choice vasopressor agents to reverse the hypotension of septic shock.[4] Both human and animal studies suggest some advantages for norepinephrine over epinephrine and phenylephrine. Epinephrine can produce a tachycardia and may have disadvantageous effects on the splanchnic circulation because of vasoconstriction. Use of phenylephrine may result in a decreased stroke volume because it is a pure α-agonist, but it is least likely to cause tachycardia. Norepinephrine increases mean systemic arterial pressure due to its vasoconstrictor effects with little change of heart rate and stroke volume, and it has only weak β-adrenergic effects. Dopamine increases the mean arterial pressure and CO primarily as a consequence of an increased stroke volume and heart rate. Its use may be limited because it produces tachycardia and can be arrhythmogenic. Norepinephrine is more potent than dopamine and may be more effective at reversing the hypotension of patients suffering septic shock. A multicenter randomized trial comparing norepinephrine with dopamine in patients with shock demonstrated no significant difference between the 2 groups in mortality at 28 days although subgroup analysis showed that dopamine was associated with an increased rate of death in patients with cardiogenic shock. Dopamine was also associated with more arrhythmic events than norepinephrine.[59]

Vasopressin infusion should be considered in patients with refractory shock after infusing adequate fluid volumes and administering high doses of conventional vasopressors.[4] Its vasoconstrictor effects are mediated by stimulating peripheral vasopressin receptors. In contrast to catecholamine-mediated vasoconstriction, the effects of vasopressin are preserved despite hypoxia and severe acidosis. Exogenous infusion of vasopressin can reverse the natural arginine vasopressin deficiency that occurs in prolonged shock.[60] However, whether this is important to its mechanism of action is unclear. Additional vasopressin mechanisms that might be helpful in septic shock include facilitation of myocyte depolarization and vasoconstriction of vascular smooth muscle, attenuation of nitric oxide generation by cytokines and inflammatory mediators, enhanced adrenergic responsiveness, and stimulation of synthesis of endothelin-1, a potent endogenous vasoconstrictor.[61] When infused into adults, vasopressin should be administered at infusion rates of 0.01 to 0.04 units/min. Doses of vasopressin greater than 0.04 units/min are associated with myocardial ischemia, significant decreases of CO, and splanchnic hypoperfusion.

Inotropic Support Dobutamine is the first-choice inotropic agent for critically ill patients with a measured or suspected low CO in the presence of an adequate left ventricular filling pressure and adequate fluid resuscitation.[4] Because a low arterial blood pressure may be produced by both a low CO as well as systemic vasodilatation, infusion of both an inotropic agent such as dobutamine to augment CO and a vasopressor such as norepinephrine to achieve an adequate MAP may be needed.

Dopexamine is a dopamine receptor agonist developed to treat heart failure and low CO states. It is not available for clinical use in the United States. Dopexamine increases splanchnic blood flow and may possess intrinsic anti-inflammatory properties. These additional actions may contribute to the reported reduction in sepsis-related mortality associated with the infusion of dopexamine. Additional controlled trials are needed to demonstrate these clinical effects of dopexamine.

PRESERVATION OF RENAL FUNCTION

Patients with sepsis, cirrhosis, jaundice, hepatorenal syndrome, congestive heart failure, malignant hypertension, preeclampsia and toxemia, hypotension as a consequence of hemorrhage, or recent exposure to IV radiocontrast agents are predisposed to develop acute renal failure when exposed to a subsequent intraoperative ischemic insult. A 2008 meta-analysis found no evidence that pharmacologic or other interventions used to protect the kidneys during surgery are of benefit to patients. However, the authors noted that there is a lack of high-quality studies on this topic and further research is needed to establish the usefulness of interventions during surgery to protect the kidneys from adverse effects.[62]

Sodium Bicarbonate and *N*-Acetylcysteine The most extensive literature on renal failure protection comes from studies of radiocontrast nephropathy. Radiocontrast dye can induce severe changes of intrarenal hemodynamics leading to ischemic injury. Studies show that hydration before the administration of contrast is effective in lowering the rate of acute renal injury.[63-65] Furthermore, hydration with sodium bicarbonate has been shown to be more effective than hydration with sodium chloride for the prophylaxis of contrast-induced renal failure.[66] The purported mechanism is by inhibition of free radical formation at the higher pH. The prophylactic administration of *N*-acetylcysteine, an antioxidant, improves renal outcome after radiocontrast administration.[67] Although there is no evidence that these maneuvers improve the outcome of patients at risk for other types of acute renal injuries, these studies are often extrapolated to high-risk surgical procedures.

Dopamine Many studies demonstrate that "renal dose" dopamine infusion (1-2 μg/kg/min) has no beneficial effect on renal outcome perioperatively.[68] Urine flow rate frequently increases during dopamine administration. However, urine output may not correlate with adequate oxygenation of the renal medulla. Dopamine infusion causes an increase in renal cortical blood flow, leading to increased glomerular filtration, solute excretion, and urine output. These actions increase renal oxygen consumption. Dopamine also has a diuretic and natriuretic effect, believed to be a result of inhibition of sodium-potassium adenosine triphosphatase in the proximal tubule and medullary thick ascending limb. This inhibitory effect would decrease tubular energy requirements and medullary oxygen requirements. Thus the net effect of a dopamine infusion on renal medullary oxygenation is unclear.

Mannitol Mannitol has traditionally been given IV to patients considered at high risk for acute renal failure. It increases tubular diameter and decreases tubular resistance to fluid flow by decreasing endothelial cell swelling by dehydration. The enhanced urine flow is believed to help prevent tubular obstruction and further renal injury. Mannitol is a weak free radical scavenger. Although mannitol is beneficial in animal studies and small clinical trials,[69] there are no large prospective controlled trials demonstrating any benefit in surgical patients who are at high risk of renal damage.

Mannitol is usually administered as a single IV dose (0.5-1.0 g/kg) intraoperatively before the application of the cross-clamp in aortic surgery patients, or it is included in the cardiopulmonary bypass prime solution for cardiac surgery. Volume status and electrolyte balance, especially plasma potassium shifts, should be monitored after the administration of mannitol.

Furosemide Furosemide inhibits energy-dependent reabsorptive work in the medullary thick ascending limb and thus ameliorates hypoxia in the renal medulla. Because it can cause cortical vasodilatation resulting in medullary hypoperfusion, prolonged administration of furosemide may be more deleterious than protective to renal function. Thus it may be prudent to only administer furosemide as a single large-bolus dose shortly before the anticipated ischemic stress. There are no randomized studies evaluating furosemide as a sole renal protective agent in surgical patients.

Fenoldopam Mesylate Fenoldopam is a selective dopamine-1 (DA1) receptor agonist used to treat hypertension.[70] Unlike dopamine, it has no activity at dopamine-2 (DA2) or at α- or β-adrenergic receptors, and thus it does not cause either tachycardia or hypertension. Fenoldopam reduces blood pressure in a dose-dependent manner while preserving renal perfusion and glomerular filtration rate.[71] It inhibits sodium reabsorption and thus may attenuate medullary oxygen demand while enhancing its supply. Large prospective trials evaluating fenoldopam as a renal protectant in humans have not yet been published.

Dopexamine Dopexamine, a dopaminergic (DA1 and DA2) agonist with β_2-adrenergic activity, has generated interest as a renal protectant based on the hypothesis that it could improve renal perfusion without causing α-adrenergic stimulation.[72] Dopexamine lacks the myocardial side effects of dopamine, although it may cause hypotension. Large well-designed trials are needed to assess its usefulness as a renal protectant.

INTRAOPERATIVE GLUCOSE MANAGEMENT

Anesthesia and surgery are associated with increased catecholamine levels resulting in increased glycogenolysis, gluconeogenesis, and lipogenesis. Furthermore, glucagon levels increase and insulin secretion decreases. Thus patients undergoing anesthesia and surgery are at risk for hyperglycemia caused by the combination of increased insulin resistance and decreased insulin secretion. Data regarding the outcome of intraoperative glucose control in noncardiac surgery are lacking. Based on evidence in cardiac surgery patients, the Society of Thoracic Surgeons recommended maintaining intraoperative blood glucose less than 180 mg/dL. They also note that glycemic control is best achieved with continuous insulin infusions rather than intermittent subcutaneous insulin injections or intermittent IV insulin boluses.[73]

AWARENESS

Awareness is the postoperative recollection of events occurring during general anesthesia. The incidence of awareness is rare in the general surgical population (0.1%-0.2%).[74] However, the incidence of awareness is greater in certain at-risk populations, especially patients who receive light anesthesia, usually because of hemodynamic instability. For example, the incidence of awareness in patients undergoing surgery for major trauma is reported to be as high as 43%. Awareness can be difficult to detect clinically because the typical indicators of "light" anesthesia such as an increased heart rate, hypertension, or movement may be masked by drugs or the patient's overall status. More than half of the patients who report experiencing intraoperative awareness have postoperative mental distress, including posttraumatic stress syndrome. If light anesthesia is required because of hemodynamic considerations, then amnestic drugs such as midazolam, scopolamine, or subanesthetic doses of ketamine should be administered. When available, neuromonitoring technologies to detect the presence of awareness should be considered. One randomized controlled study found that Bispectral Index Sensor monitoring of the electroencephalogram (EEG) of high-risk patients (defined as patients undergoing caesarian delivery or high-risk surgery, patients with a history of chronic benzodiazepine, opioid, or heavy alcohol use, and patients with acute trauma and hypovolemia) reduced their risk of awareness by 82%.[75]

POSTOPERATIVE CARE AND HANDOFF TO THE ICU TEAM

Ideally, the critically ill patient should be transported to the ICU from the operating room by an anesthesiologist. The considerations for transport to the ICU should be similar to those for transport to the operating room. The patient should be hemodynamically stable and have a secure airway before transportation. Emergency medications, ample oxygen, and supplies for airway management must be available. There should be functional IV access. All infusions should be running well and sufficient medications to last the time needed for transportation to and restabilization in the ICU should be available.

The anesthesia team is responsible for the care of the patient until a full verbal report is given to the ICU team and the ICU team accepts caring for the patient. At this time, the anesthesiologist is the caregiver who is most aware of the patient's status and therefore should be available to assist with any problems that arise. A full report, including the patient's medical history, location of monitors and lines, anesthesia technique, including the amounts and types of drugs administered, surgical procedure, other medications administered, estimated fluid and blood volume loss and replacement, anesthetic and surgical complications, and any special issues (eg, allergies, isolation precautions) should be provided to the nurses and physicians who will be caring for the patient in the ICU. The report should include specific problems (eg, oxygenation, ventilation, hemodynamic instability) that were encountered intraoperatively, the maneuvers, whether successful or unsuccessful, made to resolve the problems, and the rationale behind these maneuvers. A well-considered plan for postoperative pain management should be conveyed. The ICU team should be informed of any special care plans for the postoperative period as well as any potential postoperative problems.

SUMMARY

Anesthesiologists are involved in the care of critically ill patients in the operating room because they often need surgery to correct the underlying cause of their illness or to deal with the complications of their illness. Planning for the anesthetic management of the critically ill patient begins with a careful preoperative evaluation because the patient may have impaired function of multiple organ systems. Ideally, optimization of the patient's condition should occur preoperatively to ensure that the patient is in the best possible condition to undergo the additional stresses associated with surgery and anesthesia.

Preoperative planning should include a well-considered plan for transport to the operating room because patients are at high risk of adverse events during transport. The anesthesiologist must decide which monitors are necessary to assess the patient's condition, taking into account the advantages and pitfalls of the various options. General anesthesia is most often planned for surgery in the critically ill patient. The anesthesiologist may need to plan a total IV anesthetic technique if the patient has severe respiratory failure and will require an ICU ventilator intraoperatively for adequate oxygenation and ventilation. Regional anesthesia should be given due consideration because it can play a valuable adjunctive role to achieve optimum patient comfort and reduce physiologic stress both intraoperatively and postoperatively.

There should be specific goals and end points defined in the intraoperative management of the critically ill patient to optimize hemodynamics and minimize further end-organ damage. Advanced planning and communication between the anesthesiologists, surgeons, critical care team, and the patient and the patient's family are vital to understanding the goals and priorities of treatment.

KEY REFERENCES

- Arbous MS, Meursing AE, van Kleef JW, et al. Impact of anesthesia management characteristics on severe morbidity and mortality. *Anesthesiology.* 2005;102:257.
- Bundgaard-Nielsen M, Holte K, Secher NH, et al. Monitoring of peri-operative fluid administration by individualized goal-directed therapy. *Acta Anaesthesiol Scand.* 2007;51:331.
- Dellinger RP, Levy MM, Carlet JL, et al. Surviving Sepsis Campaign: international guidelines for management of severe sepsis and septic shock: 2008. *Intensive Care Med.* 2008;34:17.
- Perel P, Roberts I, Pearson M. Colloids versus crystalloids for fluid resuscitation in critically ill patients. *Cochrane Database Syst Rev.* 2009:CD000567.
- Rivers E, Nguyen B, Havstad S, et al. Early goal-directed therapy in the treatment of severe sepsis and septic shock. *N Engl J Med.* 2001;345:1368.
- The NICE-SUGAR Study Investigators. Intensive versus conventional glucose control in critically ill Patients. *N Engl J Med.* 2009;360:1283.
- Zacharias M, Conlon NP, Herbison GP, et al. Interventions for protecting renal function in the perioperative period. *Cochrane Database Syst Rev.* 2008:CD003590.

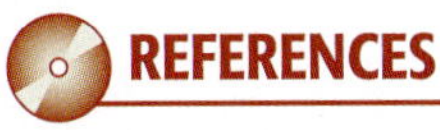

REFERENCES

Complete references available on DVD and online version at www.LongneckerAnesthesiology.com

CHAPTER 78 Monitoring and Transport of the Critically Ill Patient

Michael G. Fitzsimons
Nathaniel Sims

KEY POINTS

1. Intrahospital transport is performed within the same hospital to different sites for diagnostic and therapeutic interventions. Interhospital transport involves the movement of a critically ill patient from one treatment facility to another.
2. Subsequent clinical management will be altered in approximately 40% of patients after transport out of the intensive care unit for diagnostic procedures and facilitated interventions. Abdominal computed tomography and angiography results are most likely to result in a change of management; thus transport is often well-justified.
3. Hemodynamic changes commonly encountered in transport include systemic hypertension, hypotension, and tachycardia. No clear factors predict hemodynamic deterioration during transport have been identified, except the level of overall pretransport morbidity, instability, or the presence of a recent myocardial infarction.
4. Respiratory deterioration including hypercarbia, hypocarbia, and hypoxemia may occur in a significant fraction of transported patients. Factors that predict changes include the need for positive end-expiratory pressure, an Fio_2 greater than 50%, and age older than 43 years.
5. Appropriate assessment and management of the patient's airway is paramount in safe movement. Intubation during transport can be highly successful when performed by trained personnel, although patients with potentially difficult-to-manage airways are best intubated before transport.
6. Mechanical ventilation may maintain respiratory stability better than manual ventilation. Individuals trained in optimum manual ventilation (eg, respiratory therapists and anesthesiologists) and those with excellent patient assessment skills tend to maintain satisfactory respiratory parameters in patients undergoing transport. However, transport ventilatory systems may lack optimum alarms and may require constant surveillance for malfunction.
7. The US Emergency Medical Treatment and Active Labor Act (EMTALA, 1986) was established to mitigate financially motivated transport and requires that hospitals with emergency medical departments provide appropriate medical screening examinations within the capability of that hospital's emergency department, including ancillary services, to any individual who enters the department. If an acute medical condition is found, the department must either provide care or stabilize the patient before transfer to another facility.
8. Current regulations and good medical practice require that the competent patient or a legally authorized representative give informed consent before transfer to another hospital.
9. Physiologic monitoring of patients during transport should be maintained at the current level of care in the interest of patient's safety.
10. The advantages of air transport include reduced transport time over long distances and the ability to transfer many patients at one time. The primary disadvantages include a need for dedicated landing space, vibration, and expense. Potential insults related to transport by air include hypoxemia, decreases in ambient pressure, and hypothermia. "Altitude restrictions" are commonly ordered for patients with eye trauma, pneumothorax, intracerebral air, and sinusitis.
11. Pediatric patients (newborns and older children) are transferred most commonly for pulmonary insufficiency, cardiovascular compromise and congenital heart disease, or neurologic injury. This population benefits from dedicated specialty transport teams with specialized equipment.

12. Transport system design must involve integration of space, monitors, and support equipment that is compatible among the various sites to which a patient will be moved. Equipment engineering teams must design systems that minimize discontinuation of monitoring and disconnection of infused medications and mechanical ventilation. They must also prevent loss of continuous hemodynamic measurements.

Transport is assuming a more important role in the medical and surgical management of critically ill adult and pediatric patients. Patients with severe injuries today are transported over long distances, between countries and continents, and across time zones for advanced care. Advances in medical technology and treatment options have resulted in the need to move critically ill patients within and between hospitals for specialty care.

Intrahospital transfer may be performed to the operating room urgently for surgery, the radiology suite for diagnostic and therapeutic procedures, and from the emergency department throughout the hospital for additional care. Interhospital transfer involves the movement of a critically ill patient from one treatment facility to another. Transport exposes the patient to multiple stresses that may result in alterations of blood pressure, hypoxemia, arrhythmias, and potential airway compromise. These and other adverse events of transport can occur far from the skilled personnel, equipment, and monitoring of the intensive care unit (ICU) or operating room. Effective and safe transport of a patient does not simply involve movement but also the creation of compatible systems to minimize transport time, eliminate monitoring and medication interruptions, and reduce distractions that take the focus away from the patient.[1]

INTERHOSPITAL TRANSPORT

Transfer of a patient to a referral center occurs when the perceived benefit exceeds the risks associated with moving the patient. The Society of Critical Care Medicine convened a task force to examine the benefits of regionalization of medical care based on benefits demonstrated in neonatal and perinatal medicine,[2] trauma,[3,4] and burn care. Such a transfer is commonly referred to as *secondary transport*.[5] The reasons for transport vary among individual hospitals, within medical systems, and across countries. Indications vary over time as technologic advances result in better care.

INTRAHOSPITAL TRANSPORT

Intrahospital transport involves the movement of a patient throughout the same hospital for additional care that cannot be performed safely or adequately at the patient's bedside. Certain technology has brought procedures that previously required transport (eg, right-heart catheterization, certain computed tomography [CT] studies, echocardiography, ultrasonography, closure of patent ductus arteriosus, tracheostomy, and inferior vena cava filter placement) to the patient. Other studies and treatment may require movement of the critically ill patient to distant and more isolated areas of the hospital (**Table 78-1**). The duration of the trip may be long because of complicated diagnostic and therapeutic procedures. Patients who are "too ill" for a procedure in the operating room are frequently taken to radiology or other sites by a single nurse and respiratory therapist.

The overall benefit of transporting a patient out of the safety of the ICU for studies or procedures has been studied. The necessary "travel" results a change in patient management in 24% to 39% of cases.[6,7] Abdominal CT and angiography most commonly result in changes.

TABLE 78-1 Intrahospital Destinations

Operating suite
Radiology
Angiography
Computed tomography
Magnetic resonance imaging
Interventional radiology
Cardiac catheterization
Gastroenterology
Intensive care unit
Nuclear medicine

RISKS OF PATIENT TRANSFER

Knowledge of the risks of patient transfer within a hospital or between facilities is imperative for informed decision making. Relative contraindications to transport may include the inability to oxygenate or ventilate a patient, uncontrolled hemodynamic instability, inadequate monitoring, inability to maintain an airway, and inadequate personnel. Despite these complicating circumstances, the life-threatening condition may still necessitate transfer to other facilities or sites of treatment. Morbidity and mortality are primarily related to hemodynamic and respiratory deterioration but also include interruption of medication administration, disconnection of intravenous (IV) access, loss of airway support, and human error (**Table 78-2**).

Patients transported within a particular hospital commonly experience hemodynamic and respiratory changes that can be associated with adverse outcomes or unexpected morbidity. These "complications" may be defined as inconsequential such as minor hemodynamic perturbations or may include major events resulting in death. In previously reported studies, the incidence of hemodynamic and respiratory changes varies widely from 5% to 68%.[6-10] Most mishaps occur at the destination (**Table 78-3**). Many complications occur in radiology where the physical isolation, need to move the patient from the stretcher to the imaging table and back, duration of the procedure, and delay at the site may contribute to the occurrence of a mishap.[9] There appears to be no correlation of the mishap rate with severity of illness as defined by the Acute Physiology and Chronic Health Evaluation score, number of escorts, number of lines, monitoring, or time spent out of the ICU.[9] Szem et al found an overall mortality rate of 28.6% for patients requiring transport out of the ICU that was significantly higher than the control group (11.4%).[10] There were no deaths directly related to transport, although patients who required transport out of the ICU may have been sicker.

TABLE 78-2 Hazards and Complications of In-Hospital Transport

Cardiovascular	Pulmonary	Other Physiologic	Equipment
Hypotension Hypertension	Hypercarbia Hypocardia	Hyperthermia Hypothermia	Power failure Oxygen supply failure
Arrhythmias	Aspiration	Pain	Dislodgement of vascular access
Cardiac arrest	Extubation Hypoxemia Pneumonia Airway obstruction Increased risk of pneumonia	Anxiety Intracranial hypertension Physical injury	

TABLE 78-3 Distribution of Locations in the Hospital When Mishaps Occur

Location	% Mishaps
In ICU, preparing for transport	2
On transport to the destination	19
At destination before procedure	29
During the procedure	41
At destination, preparing to return to ICU	5
During return transport	2
Arrival in ICU	2

ICU, intensive care unit.

Reproduced with permission from Smith I, Flemming S, Cernaianu A. Mishaps during transport from the intensive care unit. *Crit Care Med.* 1990;18:278-281.

The Australian Incident Monitoring Study in Intensive Care evaluated all reports from 91 units submitted in relation to incidents occurring during transport within the hospital between 1993 and 1999. Of 7525 submitted reports, 176 described 191 incidents during intrahospital transport. Analysis revealed that 39% of the incidents were equipment related and 61% were patient/staff management issues. System-based and human-based problems occurred equally.[11] Significant adverse outcomes to the patients occurred in nearly a third of the events. The high incidence of system-based problems may have arisen from a need to disconnect a patient from ventilation, interrupt the delivery of vital infusions while changing to pumps and monitors specific to the transport process, and the limited battery life of transport devices. Often another monitoring system was in place at the site of treatment or destination, requiring further interruptions.

Patient movement between hospitals may be associated with longer transport times, greater isolation from advanced care, and stresses related to vibration, noise, and gravitational forces if transport is accomplished by air. In addition these patients may be more ill and transfer undertaken with more limited monitoring than usual within a hospital. Adverse events occurred in at least a third of interhospital transports with 30% of these attributable to technical problems.[12] An analysis of incidents during out-of hospital patient transportation demonstrated that most errors are due to equipment failure, patient problems, transport operations, and interpersonal communications (**Table 78-4**).[13] Review indicated that more than 90% are considered preventable.[13]

TABLE 78-4 Nature of Incidents During Out-of Hospital Transport

Equipment Problems
- Equipment failure
- Equipment unavailable
- Breathing circuit disconnection
- Oxygen not available
- Inadequate or inappropriate equipment

Patient Care Problems
- Condition more severe than expected
- Inappropriate or inadequate preparation at referring site
- Hospital not prepared to receive patient
- Deterioration of patient condition
- Medication, dose/drug error

Transport Operations
- Difficulty with patient transferring or loading
- Problem with vehicle configuration for patient transport
- Other problems related to vehicle
- Delay in arrival/no ambulance to meet patient
- Retrieval aborted or postponed due to weather

Interpersonal Communication Problems
- Receiving hospital not made aware of patient's condition
- Problem with staff communication
- Inaccurate patient information from site
- Staff unhelpful or uncooperative
- Unprepared or incomplete referral documentation

Adapted from Flabouris A, Runciman WB, Levings B. Incidents during out-of-hospital transportation. *Anaesth Intensive Care.* 2006;34:228-236.

HEMODYNAMIC CHANGES

Adverse hemodynamic alterations are among the most common events during both intrahospital and interhospital transport. The cause of the instability may be interruption of vasopressor infusions, stress and anxiety, pain, inadequacy of sedation, or fluid redistribution with patient movement.

Hypotension or hypertension occurs in 25% to 50% of intrahospital transports.[7,14,15] Factors demonstrated to contribute include emergence from the effects of anesthetic agents, manual ventilation, and spinal anesthesia in the obstetric patient.[14,16,17] Arrhythmias requiring treatment may occur in up to half of patients transported for "high-risk" cardiovascular conditions.[18] The care provider is often confronted with these changes while dealing with unfamiliar drug delivery systems, the need to disconnect and reconnect to a new monitor, and the need to search for therapeutic medications in an unfamiliar area or while maneuvering a stretcher through halls or elevators.

Hemodynamic changes are at least as common with secondary transport between hospitals. Unless blood pressure is monitored by invasive means, these changes may be missed with noninvasive means as a consequence of vibration and noise.

High-risk cardiac patients, including those with recent myocardial infarctions, may demonstrate instability when transferred to higher levels of care, often manifested as arrhythmias, pump failure, or cardiogenic shock.[19] The intubated patient may be "safer" from an "airway management" point of view, but pretransport intubation in this group of patients tends to be a marker for precarious and unstable hemodynamics. The era of thrombolysis means that many patients will have had some degree of reperfusion before transport to a center capable of definitive management and actually a lower incidence of difficulties than in earlier years.[20] Rubenstein's study of 755 acutely ill cardiac patients, most with class III or class IV New York Heart Association heart failure, transported from community hospitals to tertiary care centers showed no complications. However, half required urgent intervention (coronary artery bypass graft or percutaneous transluminal coronary angioplasty) upon arrival. Studies show, however, that even the most tenuous patients can be safely transported including those on extracorporeal life support.[21]

RESPIRATORY IMPAIRMENT

Respiratory compromises encountered in patient transport include hypoxemia, hypercarbia with respiratory acidosis, hypocarbia with respiratory alkalosis, drying of secretions, plugging or displacement of the endotracheal tube, unexpected extubation, and an increased risk of ventilator-associated pneumonia.[22] The incidence of respiratory changes during transport varies widely in reported studies. Factors potentially responsible for these changes include changes in the pattern of ventilation, mode of ventilation (manual versus mechanical), loss or absence of positive end-expiratory pressure (PEEP) with disconnection, endotracheal tube displacement, and equipment failure.

Hypoxemia (defined as a decreased Pao_2-to-Fio_2 ratio) occurs in up to 86% of transports involving patients artificially ventilated.[23] The need for PEEP and higher Fio_2 before transport correlates with a higher risk of deterioration.[23,24] Even brief interruptions of PEEP for connection and disconnection can be detrimental to systemic oxygenation. Decreases in measured Pa_{O_2} end points of oxygenation may be less frequent with manual ventilation as the F_{IO_2} is more commonly increased to 100%, whereas transport ventilators may maintain the pretransport F_{IO_2}.[25]

Hypercarbia may have detrimental effects on patient populations including those with increased intracranial pressure, pulmonary hypertension, or an existing acidosis. Hypercarbia and a resulting acidosis do occur in a very high percentage of critically ill intubated patients transported within and between hospitals.[16,26,27] The incidence of respiratory acidosis and alkalosis appears to be less with mechanical as compared with manual ventilation during transport. Hypocarbia may result from overly aggressive ventilation and may be detrimental in patients with neurologic injury. Hyperventilation may also result in air trapping or dynamic hyperinflation, which is especially dangerous in the setting of hypovolemia. Failure of a ventilator during transport may be catastrophic, and yet transport ventilator alarms may be less sophisticated and not well heard in a noisy transport environment, hence a need for heightened team vigilance.

Drying of secretions and damage to the tracheobronchial tree as a result of prolonged exposure to desaturated air has been demonstrated.[28] Dried secretions may result in occlusion of the airways or endotracheal tube. Efforts should be made to humidify the air that intubated patients receive, especially those subject to the very dry dehumidified environment during flight at altitude (tank gas is always dry unless actively humidified).

Extubation can be a major catastrophe during transportation. Up to 15% of all extubations in the critically ill patient are accidental.[29] Patient transport is among the factors responsible. Difficulty is encountered in 20% of reintubations.[29] Moving the head or repositioning of the patient commonly results in accidental extubation even in the presence of sedation or restraints.[30] Transport of a patient with a new tracheostomy needs to be considered an especially dangerous event if extubation occurs.

Either manual or mechanical ventilation can be effective and safe in transport. One disadvantage to manual ventilation is that a care provider must focus on management of ventilation and the airway while potentially neglecting hemodynamic monitoring and other support activities. Other disadvantages include the need for 2 hands, management of decreased lung compliance, and fatigue with long transport.

TEMPERATURE AND INJURY

Patient transport removes the individual from the controlled setting of the ICU or operating room with both inter-and intrahospital movement. Use of fluid warmers is generally interrupted, warming blankets are disconnected, transport oxygen is commonly inhaled dry, and patients may require exposure for procedures in settings where room temperature cannot be optimally adjusted to protect the patient from hypothermia. Higher death rates are reported among those individuals who develop hypothermia in transport between hospitals or from the scene of an accident to the hospital. The reduction of temperature does not necessarily correlate with gender, age, flight time, outside air temperature, or type of patient.[31] Hypothermia precautions are especially important in patients who are prone to hypothermia, including children and the elderly, burn patients, and victims of spinal cord injury. Shivering in an attempt to maintain body temperature increases oxygen consumption, which may prove detrimental in patients with myocardial ischemia.

Other risks of transport include exacerbation of injury by displacement of fractures, movement of an unstable cervical spine, and dislodgement of tubes or drains. Finally, pressure injuries to limbs, eyes, and skin may result from contact with equipment or accidental trauma.

PATIENT ASSESSMENT AND PREPARATION

Appropriate assessment and preparation is imperative before transporting the patient within or between hospitals. Research has shown that even the sickest patients can be transported when appropriate interventions are established early. General assessment for transport between hospitals includes a review of the medical history, current condition, recent interventions, hemodynamic and respiratory status and stability, current monitors and therapeutic device settings and function, and any changes prompting transfer. Consent for transport from the family or guardian must be obtained for the critically ill, and communication with the receiving physician, nurse, or hospital must be established. Assessment also includes planning for possible deterioration and establishing a course of action to deal with physiologic compromise. Wallace and Ridley identified 9 principles of safe patient transfer, which are listed in **Table 78-5**.[32]

TABLE 78-5 Principles of Safe Transfer

Experienced staff
Appropriate equipment and vehicle
Full assessment and investigation
Extensive monitoring
Careful stabilization of patient
Reassessment
Continuing care during transfer
Direct handover
Documentation and audit

Adapted from Wallace PG, Ridley SA. ABC of intensive care: transport of critically ill patients. *BMJ.* 1999;319:368-371. With permission from BMJ Publishing Group.

Much effort has been expended to predict the physiologic deterioration and mortality associated with patient transport. Some studies examined hemodynamics, respiratory status, monitoring, pharmacologic support, and laboratory analysis but failed to predict which patient will do poorly.[33,34] Other studies looked at PEEP, Injury Severity Score, and Therapeutic Intervention Score before transport and demonstrated that the more ill a patient is, the more likely the patient is to demonstrate instability with transport.[35,36] Generally speaking, there is no accurate and reproducible method to predict accurately which patients will experience difficulty with transport. Those patients who demonstrate hemodynamic and respiratory instability before transport are more likely to manifest these changes during movement. The difficulty in predicting instability may be a result of a bias that results in sicker patients being transported by specialized transport teams, whereas those thought to be more stable may be subject to less vigilant care and treated by more inexperienced personnel. Logically the more ill a patient and the more interventions required to maintain that patient, the more at risk the patient is for complications during transport.

The need for stabilization before transport within and between hospitals cannot be sufficiently stressed. There is no evidence that a "scoop-and-run" approach to interhospital transport of critically ill patients is beneficial. Stabilization before transport is similar to any resuscitation and follows the traditional ABCs (airway, breathing, and circulation). Checklists can prove invaluable in assuring that appropriate steps have been taken (**Table 78-6**).

AIRWAY AND INTUBATION

The benefits of appropriately securing a patient's airway prior to transport include avoiding the potentially difficult conditions for intubation found during ground transport, aeromedical evacuation, and in remote sites within the hospital. A patient whose airway is judged to be stable should receive supplemental oxygen in nearly all circumstances. Patients intubated before transport should be assessed for endotracheal tube (ETT) position and adequacy of tube function, along with making sure it is appropriately secured. Auscultation of lung fields, exhalation fogging of the ETT, rise and fall of the chest, nail bed or lip color, and pulse oximetry help to confirm effective intubation. Chest radiography

TABLE 78-6 Pretransport Assessment Checklist

Risk management
- Correct identification of patient
- Correct destination for correct therapy

Airway/breathing
- Endotracheal tube if present secured appropriately
- Assesses need for intubation if not secure
- Current ventilator settings (mode/V_T/RR/Fio_2/PEEP)
- Current status (ABG/CXR)
- Trends in stability
- Airway supplies available
- Plan for manual versus mechanical ventilation
- Definitive plan for management of compromise
- Adequate oxygen
- Backup airway supplies present and functioning

Circulation
- Current monitoring
- "Zero" reference established for all monitors
- Current hemodynamic status (blood pressure, pulmonary artery, pressure, CVP, rhythm)
- Intravenous access functioning properly
- Current and recently used vasopressors
- Blood available if indicated
- Resuscitation drugs available
- Adequate electrical supply for monitors
- Definitive plan for compromise

Neurologic status
- Current function/Glasgow Coma Score
- Cervical stability if indicated
- Assessment of level of sedation
- ICP monitor functioning is present
- Appropriate "zero" reference on ICP monitors
- Pain control/adequacy of sedation
- Definitive plan for treatment of increases in ICP, hypotension, changes in mental status

Extra
- Assessment of stability of traction/fractures
- Tubes, lines, and drains all functioning properly, secure
- Precautions?

Investigations
- Radiography
- Medical records
- Operative reports/discharges summary
- Most recent labs, radiography, studies
- Consent

Communication
- Receiving team made aware of receiving time
- Contact numbers
- Alternative destination known

ABG, arterial blood gas; CVP, central venous pressure; CXR, chest radiography; ICP, intracranial pressure; PEEP, positive end-expiratory pressure; RR, respiratory rate; VT, end-tidal volume.

confirms not only the ETT position but also may define underlying lung pathology. Colorimetric or infrared end-tidal carbon dioxide (CO_2) detection serves as an additional confirmation of appropriate tube position.

Certain patients may be successfully managed without intubation but are at risk for airway compromise during movement. These patients may benefit from intubation before transfer. Common indications for "elective intubation" in anticipation of transport include a Glasgow Coma Score less than 9, respiratory acidosis or impending respiratory failure, status asthmaticus, severe hypoperfusion, or shock. Patients with anatomic airway compromise arising from burns, epiglottitis, angioedema, anaphylaxis, or tracheolaryngeal trauma can benefit from intubation because the course subsequent to injury may be downhill. Certain stable but combative patients may require airway intubation and paralysis or sedation to assure safety.

Emergency medical personnel are particularly skilled in management of the airway, and their advanced training includes intubation.[37,38] The 97% success rate for intubation during transport by emergency medical services (EMS) personnel is the same as intubation before transport. Experienced and highly trained care providers are more likely to intubate those patients whose airway appeared to be difficult to manage before transport. This may account for the high rate of success and neglect the true difficulty that would be encountered if the same patients were transported without prior intubation.

The laryngeal mask airway (LMA) serves as a valuable alternative or "backup option" to the ETT in the setting of difficult intubation. The LMA is not a definitive airway and does not protect against aspiration nor does it allow prolonged positive pressure ventilation. Routine suctioning of the airway is not possible. Generally the LMA does not depend on facial and tracheal anatomy, and placement can be successful from almost any position.[39] Emergency medical personnel have used the LMA successfully in managing the airway in 89% of failed intubations.[40]

The American College of Critical Care Medicine and the Society of Critical Care Medicine recommend certain airway supplies be transported with patients (**Table 78-7**).[41] These supplies must be available even with a so-called secured airway because inadvertent dislodgement and loss of an airway can occur. Appropriate-size bag-valve systems with an oxygen reservoir are imperative for transport in addition to a variety of masks, laryngoscope blades, endotracheal tubes, oral and nasal airways, and a portable oxygen supply.

BREATHING AND VENTILATION

Adequacy of breathing and ventilation should be assessed before transport. It is imperative that tidal volume, respiratory rate, inspired oxygen

TABLE 78-7 Recommended Airway Supplies for Transport

- Appropriate adult or pediatric bag-valve systems with oxygen reservoir
- Appropriate variety of masks
- Flexible adaptors
- End-tidal carbon dioxide detector
- Variety of sizes of MacIntosh and Miller laryngoscope blades and handles
- Appropriate endotracheal tubes (cuffed and uncuffed)
- Magill forceps
- Nasopharyngeal and oral airways
- Scalpel blade for cricothyroidotomy
- Nasal cannula
- Oxygen tubing
- Positive end-expiratory pressure

Adapted from Warren J, Fromm RE, Orr RA, Rotello LC, Horst M; American College of Critical Care Medicine. Guidelines for the inter- and intrahospital transport of critically ill patients. *Crit Care Med.* 2004;32:256-262.

concentration, PEEP, and mode of ventilation be noted and recorded. The respiratory trend may actually be more important that the actual current status of the patient. Increases in $Paco_2$ may indicate pending ventilatory failure, whereas decreases in arterial oxygen saturation or Pao_2 may herald further failure of oxygenation. Sedation or deepening of sedation should be considered to facilitate oxygenation and ventilation. Transfer at altitude by reducing alveolar oxygen concentration can contribute to hypoxemia.

The risks of positive pressure ventilation include barotrauma, hypercarbia and hypocarbia, and dynamic hyperinflation (auto-PEEP), resulting in a reduced venous return and hypotension. The benefits of manual ventilation versus mechanical ventilation during transport are commonly debated. Traditional volume-controlled ventilators used for transport cannot deliver the specialized modes, such as pressure support and inverse ratio ventilation that may be required for critically ill patients. Comparisons between mechanical and manual ventilation for pediatric transport found greater variation in parameters with manual ventilation.[42] These changes may be more significant for longer than shorter duration transport and more important in patients who are subject to compromise of pulmonary or cerebral blood flow, such as newborns with persistent pulmonary hypertension or victims of traumatic brain injury. Weg and Haas compared manual and mechanical ventilation and concluded that manual ventilation can be both safe and effective if the inspired oxygen concentration and minute ventilation are known before transport and ventilation performed by skilled care providers.[25] Most transport services use a combination of manual and mechanical ventilation. Some use mechanical ventilation exclusively. Only a small number of services use only manual support.[43] Austin et al have identified the ideal characteristics of a transport ventilator (**Table 78-8**).[44]

Both manual and mechanical ventilation are satisfactory for most patients. Those requiring complicated modes of ventilation or high PEEP, or who are subject to long transport times, should be transported with mechanical ventilatory support.

Transport within the hospital is commonly done on a stretcher with the patient in a supine position. The benefits of a slightly head-up position in the ICU may be lost for several hours during transport, increasing the risk of aspiration and pneumonia.[45] The supine position may need to be maintained for minutes to hours while a procedure is performed within the hospital. Patients transported between hospitals by ground or air may encounter turbulence that may exacerbate pain and interfere with the ability to cough. Precautions to protect the airway from aspiration must be taken, especially when sedatives are administered.

Continuous monitoring of saturation by pulse oximetry is imperative during transport for all patients. End-tidal CO_2 monitors are recommended for all intubated patients. Capnography may serve 2 purposes: to confirm appropriate placement of an ETT and to monitor respiration in an environment in which direct auscultation is difficult. Quantitative capnography may especially benefit head trauma victims who are at risk from either hyper- or hypocarbia.[46] Less physiologic variability occurs when end-tidal CO_2 is continuously monitored during manual ventilation.[47] Continuous capnography is associated with a lower incidence of false alerts and malfunction as compared with pulse oximetry and is not as subject to motion artifact or loss of signal due to vasoconstriction.[48]

The options for treatment of a respiratory/airway complication during transport must be considered. Elevation of Fio_2 to 100% during brief periods of transport may avoid hypoxemia. Increasing PEEP levels to compensate for hypoxemia may be necessary, but decreased venous return and barotrauma must be avoided. Administration of skeletal muscle relaxation may increase chest wall compliance and facilitate ventilation.

TABLE 78-8 Ideal Characteristics of a Transport Ventilator

Ideal Characteristics of a Transport Ventilator
Person portable (4-6 kg)
Durable
Pneumatically powered or electrically powered
Low oxygen consumption
Easy-to-read controls that are not easy to adjust accidentally
Safety features, including a high-pressure relief valve and functional high-visibility alarms
Cost-efficient

Data from Austin PN, Campbell RS, Johannigman JA, Branson RD. Transport ventilators. *Respir Care Clin.* 2002;8:119-150.

CARDIOVASCULAR

The hemodynamic stability of a patient before transport is imperative. Many of the hemodynamic changes seen with patient transport are reflections of the course prior to movement. Monitors of hemodynamic function should include displays of the electrocardiogram and blood pressure by either invasive or noninvasive means. Monitors must have visible and audible alarms, a long battery life, and illuminated displays. Transport defibrillators are essential for transport between hospitals and for patients within the hospital who are at a high risk of an arrhythmia (myocardial infarction, cardiac surgery). If transcutaneous pacing is possible (and likely to be needed), adequate capture should be confirmed.

Oscillotonometric or noninvasive measurement of blood pressure facilitates monitoring in the operating theater, postanesthesia care unit, and treatment wards. This form of monitoring may be subject to error during the movement of patients. Although this might not be important in hemodynamically stable, nonventilated patients, it may be critical for others. If invasive arterial monitoring is expected, it should be secured before movement. Invasive monitors must be calibrated to a "zero" reference point. Zero points change with patient positioning. Reestablishing the appropriate "zero" reference upon patient transfer or at altitude during flight is imperative.

Adequate IV access for delivery of fluids, continuous medication delivery, and intermittent treatment must be established. The confines and motion of any transport vehicle or stretcher can make placement en route difficult (**Fig. 78-1**). Adequate function and placement of backup or secondary lines should be considered. If transfusion is anticipated during transport, blood should be brought with the patient.

Hemodynamic compromise may result from inadequate preload, afterload, impaired myocardial contractility, or disturbances of cardiac rate and rhythm. Assessment must include a strategy for addressing the hemodynamic instability by assessment, volume resuscitation, and infusion of inotropic or vasopressor support as needed. The resources needed to provide these therapies must be provided during transport.

NEUROLOGIC STATUS AND SEDATION

Secondary insults during transport of head-injured patients are common and may include hypoxemia, hypotension, and intracranial hypertension, each of which worsens neurologic outcome. Although physiologic instability during transport is correlated with instability before movement, anticipation of problems and preparation for the management of problems is imperative.[49] Appropriate physiologic monitoring of oxygenation and ventilation is necessary. Transport patients may benefit from continuous end-tidal CO_2 analysis to avoid detrimental periods of hyper- and hypocarbia. In the patients with significant head trauma and cerebral swelling, invasive arterial access is necessary because even brief episodes of hypotension are detrimental to the brain. If an intracranial bolt or catheter drain is placed, an appropriate "zero" level must be established. Protection of the device must be assured to avoid dislocation. Increases of intracranial pressure (ICP) are detrimental in head injury. ICP is a dynamic

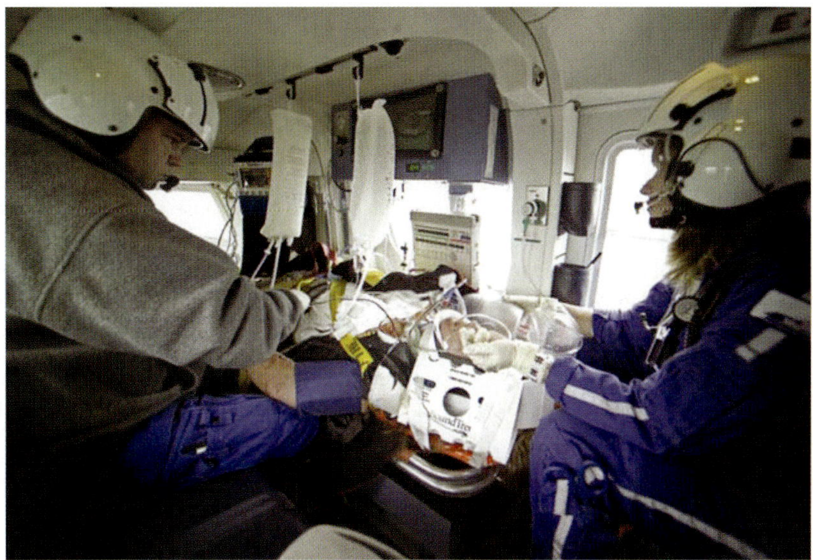

FIGURE 78-1. Confines of rotor-wing transport. [Courtesy of Boston MedFlight.]

measurement, and the importance of a single measurement is unclear. A plan and resources for addressing an increase in ICP are necessary. Interventions include head elevation, hyperventilation, mannitol and/or Lasix infusions, and cerebrospinal fluid drainage. The effects of these interventions on other parameters (eg, cardiovascular) must be considered. The effects of sedation on the neurologic assessment must be taken into consideration.

Sedation and pain control are rarely addressed in the transport literature despite the fact that transport subjects a patient to significant stress. The levels of epinephrine and norepinephrine in healthy male volunteers subject to EMS protocols are increased without sedatives as compared with individuals receiving midazolam during the same protocol.[50] Increased catecholamine levels can increase myocardial oxygen consumption, cardiac ischemia, and infarction. Planning for transport involves an assessment of pain before movement because ground or air vehicles often impair the ability to communicate effectively with the patient. Short-acting benzodiazepines are generally chosen as sedatives because of their ease of titration and historical success. Devellis et al studied the use of small doses of fentanyl (0.33-5.0 μg/kg) in pediatric trauma victims. There was a statistically significant decrease in systolic blood pressure but no other major complications.[51] Small doses of fentanyl (25-200 μg per administration) with a total dose of 1.0 to 5.0 μg/kg were well tolerated in patients transported by air.[52] Complications associated with prehospital sedation seemed to occur more often in patients receiving both sedation and analgesia and are more common in patients who received sedation for endotracheal intubation.[53] Sedation during patient transport within the hospital has not been well-studied. Planning must take into account the side effects of the medication and the potential pain and anxiety that the patient will experience during a procedure.

CONSENT

Many care providers do not consider transport of the critically ill patient a high-risk procedure despite its high complication rate. Although consent is commonly implied when a patient must be moved, good medical care requires that the patient or a proxy be aware of the risks. Current guidelines suggest that a competent patient or legally authorized representative of a patient give informed consent before transfer to another hospital.[41] Despite these recommendations a minority of patients actually give consent for a hospital transfer.[54] Unfortunately, at the time of the study, transfer of patients from private to public hospitals of minorities, the unemployed, and those without insurance was a common practice. The Emergency Medical Treatment and Active Labor Law (EMTALA, 1986) required that hospitals appropriately screen patients and provide treatment. If transfer is necessary the hospital is liable to ensure that within medical probability, no worsening of the patient's condition occurs during transfer.[55] Three principles result in compliance with EMTALA: avoidance of financially motivated transfer, transfer only in the best interest of the patient, and maintenance of standards of care during all transport.

COMMUNICATION

Communication between those initiating patient transfer and those ultimately receiving the patient is imperative. The referring physician should identify and contact an admitting physician at the receiving hospital to accept the patient in transfer and confirm before the transfer occurs that appropriate higher level resources are available.[41] The patient remains the responsibility of the transferring team until a formal nursing and medical handover has occurred in the receiving department.[5] Continual communication to provide guidance for transport personnel must be established.

Communication not only refers to the verbal transfer of information but also that appropriate records, images, and consent accompany the patient. Duplication of records and studies is often needed and should be done early to avoid delaying transfer. The advent of regional health information systems may mitigate the problem of difficulty with transfer of information.

EQUIPMENT AND MONITORING

No specific national standards exist for monitoring or required equipment for the transport of patients. Guidelines for transport have been published by several organizations including the American College of Critical Care Medicine and the Society of Critical Care Medicine.[41] In general, the equipment for transport must be similar to that used in the ICU, yet it must be portable, small, lightweight, and rugged.[56] Additionally, equipment intended for aeromedical transport must be low in weight, compact, and should not interfere with navigation, communication, or control mechanisms. The electrical load must not overwhelm the aircraft's system. Incompatibility of monitors and medication infusion systems creates time delays and results in periods of inadequate monitoring in critical situations. Transport personnel are frequently required to disconnect and reconnect cables and reestablish zero references for invasive pressures. Medical infusion pumps may need to be discontinued briefly as a device capable of transport is prepared. Upon arrival at the receiving site another change in patient care technology may again be necessary.

Equipment used for transport within a hospital should be compatible in different locations ideally avoiding the need to change pressure transducers, electrocardiogram (ECG), and pulse oximeter probes. Care providers receiving a patient should also be comfortable with the equipment that arrives with the patient.

INFUSION TECHNOLOGY

Critically ill patients are often transferred while receiving continual infusions of medications. Medications to control hemodynamics, total parenteral nutrition, anticoagulation, and antibiotics are the most common agents. These medications often have a very narrow therapeutic window separating benefit from potential adverse events. Infusion devices allow the uninterrupted delivery of medications to patients based on the specific drug, concentration, and desired rate of delivery.

Care providers involved in the transfer of patients must be familiar and proficient with the mode or modes of infusion technology used for the delivery of medications. A misprogrammed decimal point may result in the death of a patient.[57] New "smart pumps" have many of the safety features of older devices including dose calculations, free-flow protection, and occlusion alerts. The "smart pumps" also have programmable drug libraries with standardized concentrations and both "soft" and "hard" delivery limits based on the ability to override the delivery rate or not. When "smart" pump technology was applied to patients in the cardiac surgery perioperative period, though, a reduction in the number of errors did not occur. Most adverse drug events occurred because care providers bypassed the drug library in programming or elected to override limits.

Hospital systems must be configured so drug infusion devices and drug concentrations are standardized between units. These devices have become increasingly sophisticated. The US Food and Drug Administration (FDA) has declared infusion pumps as a critical technology in response to a number of deaths, recalls, and other incidents.[58] This decision changed the way that devices are designed, tested, and assessed by the FDA before approval.[58] Modern drug infusion systems must possess certain characteristics to assure patient safety and clinical function (**Table 78-9**).

TABLE 78-9 Characteristics of Ideal Infusion Devices
Low cost
Small
Easy to use
Easy-to-read alarms
"Free-flow" prevention
Alarms that respond to interruption of delivery
Precise infusion rate
Wide range of flow rates
Suitability for various fluids
Drug library that reflects practice
Durable
Disposable tubing
Connectivity to clinical information
Method of identifying a medication with a patient
"Soft" and "hard" lockout
Bar-coded medication system
Ability to interface with computerized order entry

TRANSPORT PERSONNEL

Personnel accompanying a patient in transport within the hospital and between hospitals must at a minimum possess all the skills of basic life support. Potential transport personnel include physicians, nurses, respiratory therapists, paramedics, and emergency medical technicians. Guidelines published by the Society of Critical Care Medicine for interhospital transport state that a minimum of 2 people in addition to the vehicle operator must accompany the patient, and at least one should be a registered nurse, physician, or advanced medical technician skilled in airway management, IV therapy, and dysrhythmia interpretation and management.[41] Recently revised guidelines recommend that a physician with advanced skills in airway management and advanced cardiac life support accompany all unstable patients.[45] The safety of transport of routine patients without a physician has been demonstrated.[60] Of note, transport mandating that a physician be in attendance may remove an essential health care provider from the transporting facility, so backup coverage should be provided.[19]

The efficacy of specially trained teams responsible for transport has also been demonstrated for adult[8] and pediatric patients.[61] Use of specialty teams allows continual training, development of specialized skills, and the ability to cross-train in the skills of others.

SAFETY OF HEALTH CARE PROVIDERS

Maintaining the safety of the health care provider responsible for patient transport is vital. Back injuries are frequently cited as a reason nurses transfer to less physically demanding jobs or leave nursing entirely.[62] Tasks such as transferring, lifting, moving, and turning patients comprise a major part of the nurse's daily activities. In 2003, the Occupational Safety and Health Administration published guidelines regarding ergonomics for the prevention of musculoskeletal injuries in the medical workplace. This document called for the manual lifting of patients to be eliminated whenever possible. Texas was the first state to adopt safe patient handling legislation and requires that hospitals and nursing homes adopt a policy to identify, assess, and develop strategies to control the risk of injury to both patients and nurses associated with lifting, transferring, repositioning, or moving.[63] Few other states have adopted such legislation.

The movement of a patient from the bed to a stretcher and then from the stretcher to the operating table or radiology scanner has traditionally been accomplished with a draw sheet placed under the patient. The draw-sheet method requires the greatest amount of physical force as compared with methods such as a plastic bag placed under the patient or a friction-reducing device.[64] The least amount of force is required when a mattress inflated with a blower is used. Small holes release air on the underside of the mattress providing a smooth surface over which to move the patient. A study recently completed showed a substantial decrease in the number of claims related to back injury when a lateral transfer system was used in a hospital-wide initiative.[65] An understanding of the appropriate ergonomics of lifting is important as well as ready availability of air mattresses, friction-reducing devices, lifts, and hoists.

MODES OF TRANSPORT

The risks and benefits of ground versus air transport must be considered when transporting a patient between hospitals. Gray et al suggested 7 factors that should influence the choice of the mode of transport (**Table 78-10**).[5] Staff responsible for initiating and performing evacuation should be familiar with the physiologic factors that may potentially affect the patient in transport, especially when considering air transport. The special needs of neonates and pediatric patients must be understood. The American College of Emergency Physicians endorsed the following principle regarding patient transfer: "The health and well-being of the patient must be the overriding concern

TABLE 78-10 Influencing Factors on Choice of Transport

The nature of illness
Urgency of transfer
Availability of transport
Mobilization times
Geographic factors
Traffic and weather conditions
Cost

From Gray A, Bush S, Whitley S. Secondary transport of the critically ill and injured adult. *Emerg Med J.* 2004;21:28:281-285. With permission from the BMJ Publishing Group.

when any patient transfer is considered. The patient should be transferred in a vehicle that is staffed by qualified personnel and contains appropriate equipment."[66]

AIR TRANSPORT

Air transport can be divided into the fixed-wing type (aircraft) and the rotor-wing type (helicopter). Fixed-wing transport tends to cover distances greater than 250 miles, whereas rotor-wing transport covers distances less than 250 miles.[67] Helicopter transport is primarily beneficial for distances greater than 45 miles when compared with ground transport.[68] Specific advantages of transport by airplane include long-distance capabilities, larger areas for patient care, space for more care providers, the ability to transport and care for many patients, less vibration, and generally less noise than rotor-wing transport. Disadvantages include the need to transport the patient by ground to and from the aircraft and the need for dedicated landing facilities. Advantages of transport by helicopter include the capability for rapid mobilization, vertical takeoff and landing, ease of transport at lower altitudes, and the ability to transfer patients at speeds of up to 150 miles per hour.[67] The disadvantages include limited space for patient care, vibration, and noise, as well as greater dependence on good weather for flying (Fig. 78-1). Awareness of altitude-sensitive conditions and specific preparation for transport by air decrease complications (**Table 78-11**; see also Table 78-14).

Hypoxemia is a risk to any patient in transport but especially those with coronary ischemia, pulmonary compromise (acute respiratory distress syndrome [ARDS]), or neurologic injury. Hypoxemia commonly results in tachycardia and hypertension that may increase myocardial oxygen consumption. The barometric pressure of ambient air declines as altitude increases, although oxygen concentration remains at a constant 21%.[69] At sea level, barometric pressure is 760 mm Hg with a partial pressure of oxygen of 160 mm Hg. Most aircraft cabins are usually pressurized to a pressure equivalent to 5000 to 8000 feet, giving an atmospheric partial pressure of oxygen of 118 mm Hg.[70] This accounts for the fact that the oxygen requirement (FiO_2) of a patient on mechanical ventilation may increase at altitude. Lawless and colleagues demonstrated that animals with chemically induced ARDS were resistant to increases of FiO_2 yet responded to increased PEEP during transport.[71] Benumof suggests that hypoxemia, even at low altitudes (3281-9843 feet), may contribute to global hypoxic pulmonary vasoconstriction and pulmonary edema.[72] Helicopter transport may allow a patient to be transported at lower altitudes so as to minimize this effect.

The decrease in ambient pressure at altitude contributes to the expansion of air within a cavity in accordance with Boyle law.[67] This effect may result in hemodynamic compromise (tension pneumothorax), barotrauma (sinuses), equipment malfunction (blood pressure cuffs), and possible patient injury or compromised monitoring.[67] Conditions such as pneumopericardium, subcutaneous emphysema, gas gangrene, systemic air emboli, decompression sickness, and gastric distension may be worsened at altitude. Equipment considered "altitude sensitive" includes endotracheal and tracheostomy cuffs, pneumatic antishock garments (eg, medical antishock trousers), air splints, colostomy bags, Foley catheters, orogastric and nasogastric tubes, ventilators, invasive monitors, and intra-aortic balloon pumps. Additionally patients with a closed head injury may experience increases in ICP. An experimental model showed an increase in intracranial air volume by 30% at the usual maximum cabin altitude of 8000 feet.[73] "Altitude restrictions" are commonly ordered for patients with eye trauma, pneumothorax, intracerebral air, and sinusitis.[74] These restrictions and flying at low levels may result in more turbulence and longer transport times.

Temperature decreases with altitude. Cold air holds far less moisture than warm air. This contributes to the drying of secretions, potential occlusion of endotracheal tubes, and dehydration during transport at altitude.

The flight environment subjects the patient to other unique physiologic challenges. Acceleration and deceleration may induce hemodynamic changes, stress, and injury. These may be exacerbated in patients suffering from hypovolemia and spinal cord injury. Aircraft vibrations contribute to fatigue and discomfort along with interference with the appropriate function of equipment.[68]

TABLE 78-11 Preparation for Transport by Air Checklist

Patient appropriate for air transport
Critically ill
Benefit justifies risk
No contraindications to air transport (weather, hostile environment, dangerous patient, contaminated area)
Airway
Airway secure
Endotracheal tube cuff pressure adequate for transport but unlikely to cause mucosal injury
Ability to humidify gases if long transport time or high-altitude transport
End-tidal carbon dioxide monitor present
Breathing
Consideration of chest tube in setting of simple pneumothorax
Impact of altitude on respiratory dynamics (increases FiO_2 requirement, positive end-expiratory pressure, increased minute ventilation)
Circulation
Hemodynamics at risk with altitude (pneumothorax/pneumopericardium, gas embolism)
Monitors calibrated with plan to reestablish "zero" reference at altitude
Volume status optimized to prevent drastic changes with acceleration/deceleration
Neurologic
Condition at risk with altitude (pneumocephali/decompression sickness/middle eustachian tube dysfunction)?
Risk of secondary brain injury from hypoxemia
Others
Fractures stabilized?
Gastric decompression (nasogastric tube) for intubated patients

GROUND TRANSPORT

The advantages of ground transfer are primarily related to lower cost, rapid mobilization of resources, less dependency on weather conditions, and easier patient monitoring. The disadvantages include limited space to perform interventions and procedures, potential for delays because of traffic, and vehicle accidents with further injury to the patient and care providers (**Fig. 78-2**).

Modes of ground transport are not equivalent, and optimization of ground transport depends in part on equipment availability and to a larger extent on care provider skill levels available. Skills range from simple basic life support to advanced cardiac life support, to specialized transport teams. The skills of the transport team must be known

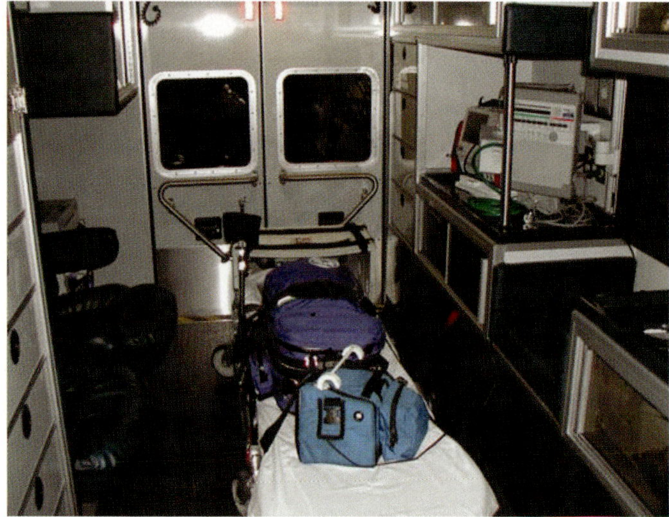

FIGURE 78-2. Limited space of ground transport vehicle. [Courtesy of Boston MedFlight.]

when transfer is arranged, and there must be optimum matching of patient acuity and type of illness with the transport team's skills and resources.[75] The critically ill patient with conditions requiring care at the level of a physician or specially trained nurse should be transported by a specifically trained physician or Critical Care Transport Team. The Commission on Accreditation of Medical Transport Systems defines a critical care mission as "the transport of a patient, from a scene or a clinical setting, whose condition warrants care commensurate with the scope of practice of critical care professionals (ie, physician or registered nurse)."[76] The Association of Air Medical Services defines 6 conditions appropriate for transport by a specially trained critical care ground team:

1. Patient in critical condition.
2. Potential for deterioration into critical condition during transport.
3. Unstable vital signs.
4. Patient is intubated and ventilated for an acute medical condition.
5. Patient is receiving continuous infusion pharmacologic blood pressure support.
6. Conditions require time-sensitive treatment.

Before ground transport it is imperative that the transferring physician be aware of the strengths and limitations of the team with respect to personnel, equipment, and training.

SPECIAL CONSIDERATIONS

Certain patient disease categories deserve discussion including neurologic injury, obstetric patients, chemical injuries and toxic agent exposure, pediatric patients, and transport for mass casualty.

NEUROLOGIC CONDITIONS

Three populations of neurologic patients are commonly transferred: traumatic brain injury, spinal injury, and stroke.

Patients transported with traumatic brain injury are commonly subject to secondary insults that can potentially worsen the injury, including systemic hypertension, hypotension, raised ICP, reduced cerebral perfusion pressure, hypoxemia, and hyperthermia. The most common of these are hypertension and raised intracranial pressure. In a study by Andrews et al, complications occurred in about half of transfers for neurologic injury.[77] The number of insults

TABLE 78-12 Pretransport Stabilization of the Head-Injured Patient

Pulse oximetry >95%
End-tidal $Paco_2$ 35 mm Hg
Mean arterial blood pressure >90 (adults) and systolic blood pressure >120 mm Hg
Intracranial pressure ≤20 mm Hg
Cerebral perfusion pressure >70 mm Hg (adults)
Central body temperature 96.8°F (36°C)

Data from Ferdinande P. Recommendation for intra-hospital transport of the severely head injured patient. *Intensive Care Med.* 1999;25:1441-1443.

during transport mimics the number of insults both before and after the move. The higher an individual's injury score (based on systemic and mean blood pressure, intracranial pressure and cerebral perfusion pressure, temperature, heart rate, oxygenation, and ventilation) before transport, the more likely the occurrence of a transport complication. The Working Group on Neurosurgical Intensive Care of the European Society of Intensive Care Medicine has recommended guidelines for pretransport stabilization of the head injury patient (**Table 78-12**).[78]

Benefits of transport for the patient with acute spinal cord injury to centers skilled in this type of specialized care have been reported.[79] The earlier the transfer, the greater the benefit.[80] Outcome is best for patients transported within 12 hours. Benefits are less certain for those transferred more than 48 hours after a cord injury. The Congress of Neurologic Surgeons recommends that patients with acute spinal cord injury be expeditiously and carefully transferred from the site of injury to the nearest capable definitive medical care facility. The mode of transport should be chosen based on the clinical characteristics of the patient, distance to the receiving facility, and geography.[81] Despite the best efforts of health care providers, additional movement of the spine-injured patient is associated with risk of further cord injury. Del Rossi et al demonstrated that both a log roll and lift-and-slide technique of movement can cause additional injury at the site of cord damage.[82]

Patients with acute stroke are commonly transferred for specialized medical care to provide diagnostic angiography and intra-arterial thrombolysis after a hemorrhagic stroke has been ruled out.[83] Studies demonstrate that thrombolysis delivered within 3 hours after the onset of an occlusive stroke significantly improves outcome. Benefit may be seen with treatment up to 6 hours after occlusion, but these are inconsistent. Delays in transport commonly occur because of geographic characteristics, delayed patient/physician awareness of stroke symptoms, slow referral pathways, and in-hospital factors. Nedeltchev et al note that patients with symptoms consistent with stroke may benefit from direct referral to a tertiary care center equipped to provide thrombolysis without delaying them at a community hospital for CT imaging.[83]

HIGH-RISK OBSTETRICS

Obstetric patient transfers comprise only a small percentage of transports between hospitals, approximately 5% in one study.[84] Common indications include premature labor, premature rupture of membranes, eclampsia, preeclampsia, and multiple gestations. The greatest concerns of those transferring these patients include in-flight delivery of the fetus, inadequate fetal monitoring, and inexperience with this type of transport. General crew configuration is frequently a nurse and paramedic. A physician is directly involved in only 5% of transfers. Complicating factors include systemic hypertension, hypotension, increased contractions, and decreased maternal respiratory drive.[85] Nausea and vomiting occur often. The potential for a difficult airway to be managed must be recognized. Placenta previa and placenta accreta have the potential for sudden deterioration, and such patients

TABLE 78-13 Consensus Statement on Transport for Chemical Incidents

Transportation requirements depend on the number of casualties
Once decontaminated, priority for transport is determined as for nonchemical incidents
Chemical casualties should only be transported to hospitals with chemical personal protective equipment and decontamination facilities
Vehicles should be reused at the incident
Helicopters are not acceptable as a mode of transport

Adapted from Crawford IW, Mackway-Jones K, Russel DR, Carley SD. Delphi-based consensus study into planning for chemical incidents. *Emerg Med J.* 2004;21:24-28. With permission from the BMJ Publishing Group.

should be transported rapidly with appropriate volume line access. Outcome is improved if the mother is transferred before delivery of the fetus.[86]

CHEMICAL INJURY AND DISASTER TRANSPORT

Exposure to toxic chemical substances occurs in a variety of ways including industrial accidents and the deliberate release of toxic substances by terrorists. The health service must assure that appropriate care is provided to the injured without endangering the lives of health care providers. The Department of Health Emergency Planning Coordination Unit of the United Kingdom released a series of consensus statements addressing transfer and transport of chemical casualties (**Table 78-13**).[87] According to a study in Washington state, most victims of hazardous material events are transported to a hospital (70%) yet only a small percentage are admitted for further care (5%).[88] Victims of trauma, thermal burns, dizziness, or central nervous system symptoms such as headache are most likely to require admission. It is imperative that physicians involved in the care of critically ill patients be familiar with the hospital's plan for evacuation and transport of such patients.

PEDIATRIC TRANSPORT

The development of neonatal transport systems in the 1970s preceded the focus on pediatric transport programs in the 1980s and 1990s.[89] The primary indications for pediatric transport to referral centers are respiratory failure and cardiovascular insufficiency followed by neurologic compromise.[90] Today improved care at centers of excellence in the management of pediatric conditions such as congenital heart disease results in more transfers.[91] Common complications encountered during transport in the pediatric population include hypotension, decreased arterial oxygen saturation, and hyperthermia.[92] Adverse technical events such as loss of IV access, failure of monitors, and dislodgement or malposition of the ETT occur in nearly 36% of transfers. Clinically adverse events such as hypotension, hypoxia, or hypoglycemia occurred in 27% of transfers reported by Hatherill et al.[93]

Pediatric transport is highly specialized. Interviews with pediatricians reveal that nearly half report insufficient knowledge of sophisticated transport equipment.[90] Transport complication frequencies are higher in children transported by a referring physician compared with children transported by a specialized pediatric transport team. The higher rate of complications is believed due to a lower rate of appropriate pretransport interventions, lack of expertise with equipment, insufficient specialized equipment, materials, and lack of medications usually available to specialized teams and indeed all transport teams. The complexity of neonatal and pediatric transport and improved outcomes at tertiary care centers has resulted in the creation of specialist retrieval teams composed of physicians and nurses. Bellingan et al compared transport by a pediatric specialist retrieval team to standard practice. Patients transported by standard support teams commonly led by a trainee physician were more acidotic and demonstrated more hypotension than those moved by specialist teams.[94] Patients transported by standard teams also had a higher mortality within the first 12 hours. Transport of the complicated pediatric patient is an area where clear benefit is demonstrated by specialized teams.

The key to safe pediatric transport is adequate preparation. A high percentage of patients require some preparatory intervention prior to transport.[92] Those who receive these interventions have a lower rate of decompensation during transport or upon arrival at the receiving center. Routine resuscitation priorities take precedence. Preparation requires appropriately securing the airway and assuring correct ventilation. More than a third of pediatric transport patients require a change of the mode of ventilation before departure, whereas intubation is required by the transport team in 16.1% of patients.[92] Fluid resuscitation is initiated in nearly a third of transports, and approximately a quarter require the IV infusion of vasoactive drugs.[92]

Several factors increase a child's susceptibility to hypoxemia and respiratory compromise, including a more compliant lung cage, reduced diameter of the airways, increased pulmonary vascular reactivity to hypoxia (infancy), a predisposition to a decreased respiratory drive in the setting of hypoxia (up to 1-2 months of age), and reduced surfactant production (neonates).[68]

TRANSPORT OF PATIENTS WITH ACUTE CORONARY SYNDROME

Myocardial infarction continues to be a leading cause of morbidity and mortality in industrialized nations.[95] The timely treatment of patients with an acute coronary syndrome (unstable angina, ST segment elevation myocardial infarction (STEMI), and non-ST segment elevation myocardial infarction) contributes significantly to improving outcome. Survival is directly related to the rapidity of reperfusion therapy.

Once a patient with a myocardial infarction arrives at a hospital, the role of timely transport for treatment is imperative. The American College of Cardiology has established an initiative that all patients with STEMI receive an acute coronary intervention within 90 minutes of arrival at the hospital.[96] The 90-minute time frame is only a guideline. Work has shown that even greater reduction in mortality occurs when "door-to-balloon" time is reduced even further.[97]

COORDINATION, INTEGRATION, DATA COLLECTION, AND QUALITY ASSURANCE

Changes in the system of patient transport over the years have resulted in many improvements, including an ability to transport sicker patients over long distances for specialized care. This need for transport will continue and will likely expand as technology results in increasingly sophisticated treatment. Smaller hospitals and medical centers may not be able to support the financial burden of expensive technology and teams, resulting in the expanded regionalization of services. Improvements have been made, but an apparent threshold of morbidity has been reached that will not be reduced unless systemwide changes are implemented. These changes should include the integration of technology and transport system design, generalized use of critical care transport teams for certain categories of patients that can benefit from advanced care, establishment of key protocols and guidelines, establishment of Internet-based electronic medical records for efficient transfer of information, collection of data and analysis of the metrics that indicate a satisfactory or unsatisfactory transfer, and critical care reporting systems that track the outcome of inter- and intrahospital transfer.

TECHNOLOGY AND TRANSPORT SYSTEM DESIGN

Safe movement of a critically ill patient requires the coordinated effort of numerous trained individuals. Often the patient, monitors, and infusion pumps must be changed several times during one movement.

Poorly designed or antiquated systems may even require the disconnection of medications and monitors and reconnection to completely different infusion systems and monitoring systems even within the same hospital, increasing transport time as well as subjecting the patient to periods without observation of vital signs or infusion of vital drugs. Systems that are not efficient, compact, and uncluttered can harm patients. Current work is being done on mobile ICU models that have integrated monitoring and support systems including ventilators, defibrillators, suction, point-of-care blood chemistry analysis, invasive monitoring of blood pressures, pulse oximetry, temperature, oxygen flow, and ECG. The benefits of such compact, contained systems include the need for fewer transport personnel, shorter preparation time, reduced periods of manual ventilation, and the potential to provide continuity of care and monitoring from the site of injury, transport to the hospital, emergency department admission, studies and transport to the ICU.[98,99] Not only must equipment be compact and standardized for transport, ideally it should be compatible among and between the emergency department, operating room, intensive care unit, and common sites of patient treatment (eg, cardiac catheterization, radiology). It is recognized that a system of universal compatibility among different hospitals may be too costly and difficult, but within a single transport system and hospital it is not only feasible but should be imperative.

The Cleveland Clinic Foundation and the Massachusetts General Hospital have established systems that allow the easy transfer of support equipment without interruptions in therapy or the flow of vital information.[1] The same monitors and infusion pumps used in the operating room are used during transfer and upon arrival in the ICU. Transport monitoring merely becomes an extension of the familiar bedside monitor. The benefits seen include more rapid preparation of the patient for movement, fewer personnel needed for transfer, and improved patient care.[100]

A multidisciplinary approach to ICU, operating room, and transport is imperative when hospitals upgrade their systems. Representatives from critical care, anesthesiology, surgery, respiratory therapy, nursing, and administration have vested stakes in safe, efficient patient movement.

CRITICAL CARE TRANSPORT TEAMS

Teams specialized in the transport of distinct categories of patients have proven to be beneficial by decreasing morbidity and mortality while increasing provider satisfaction. Specialist retrieval teams were initially developed to transport critically ill pediatric patients. Such studies suggest that specialized transport teams are needed to provide consistent safe care with a low rate of transport-associated complications and morbidity. Other populations best served by specialized teams include patients with ARDS or who require extracorporeal oxygenation or left ventricular assist devices, and perhaps those with head injuries. Factors to consider in the creation of these teams include the quality and scope of patient care, costs, medical justification, medicolegal issues, and return on investment based on the analysis of patient volume, overhead, and logistics.[101]

PROTOCOLS AND GUIDELINES

Multiple organizations have developed and published guidelines for the transfer of critically ill patients.[41,59] These guidelines are general and have not been adopted as standards. Four critical elements are required for the development of transfer plans: a multidisciplinary planning team, a medical needs assessment, a written standardized transfer plan, and continual evaluation and refinement as needed.[41]

Emergency medical services have established protocols. Transfer protocols are detailed and address not only common populations (pediatric patients, traumatic brain injury, asthma, myocardial infarction) but also specialized conditions and devices (intra-aortic balloon pumps, ventricular assist devices, inhaled nitric oxide).

TABLE 78-14 Protocol Outline

1. Planning prior to arrival
   a. Specialized equipment
   b. Vehicle type or configuration
   c. Changes in disposition, destination, weather
2. Preparation of patient for transport
   a. Full assessment
   b. Monitoring
   c. Pretransport interventions
3. Intratransport care
   a. Issues specific to condition prompting transfer
   b. Medical/procedural interventions during the transfer
4. Arrival at the receiving facility
   a. Communication
   b. Transfer of care
5. Documentation issues
   a. Medications administered and side effects
   b. Deviation from established protocols
6. Education/quality improvement

Courtesy of Boston MedFlight.

Boston MedFlight has developed complete protocols for both air and ground transport of patients. All protocols have 6 "organizing principles" (**Table 78-14**). Protocols may lead to improved outcomes when conditions are repeatedly encountered. Protocols also allow the stocking of standardized medications and acquisition of equipment based on these plans. Over time care providers develop comfort working within a common framework, and systematic "reiteration" of the protocols leads to improved quality and efficiency.

TRANSFER OF MEDICAL INFORMATION

Transfer involves not only the efficient movement of the patient but the exchange of vital information from the transferring physician to the care provider en route, and their final receiving care provider. A significant number of errors occur during a handoff when care is transferred from one individual or service to another. The Joint Commission National Patient Safety Goals now require that hospitals implement a standardized approach to "handoff" communications.[102] Direct verbal communication between the transferring and receiving physicians along with nurse-to-nurse reporting before patient movement ensures that the receiving facility is appropriate for current patient needs or condition and is prepared for receipt of the patient (medications, ventilation, studies, surgery if necessary). Clinical course may dictate that transfer be delayed or changed to another facility. Other factors important to communicate include directions to the receiving station or unit within a facility.

Electronic medical records and teleradiology should allow easier exchange of complete vital information. Internet-based record systems facilitate the receiving physician's ability to fully assess whether a transfer is appropriate.

REPORTING AND CRITICAL INCIDENT EVALUATION

Reporting of unsafe practices, complications during patient transport, and critical analysis of patient safety practices is imperative if the etiology of adverse events and errors are to be determined and rectified. The Australian Incident Monitoring Study in Intensive Care was developed in 1993 as an anonymous voluntary reporting system to identify critical incidents and determine their underlying causes and contributing factors.[11] A review of events related to patient transfer was carried out in 2004. The study revealed a high rate of serious outcomes (nearly a third of the incidents had significant adverse outcomes) almost evenly

TABLE 78-15 Recommendations from the Australian Incident Monitoring Study in Intensive Care

Recommendations for transportation

a. The decision to move a critically ill patient within the hospital should be made by a senior medical practitioner after careful consideration of the benefits to be gained weighed against possible risks.
b. A dedicated team should be available for the entire duration of the transport. The team members need to be familiar with the critically ill patients, skilled in airway management and resuscitation, patient monitoring and moving, and be familiar with all equipment.
c. Adequate monitoring of the critically ill patient should include electrocardiogram, blood pressure, oxygen saturation, and, if ventilated, end-tidal carbon dioxide monitoring.
d. Careful preparation for transport is essential, including patient and equipment checks and liaison with staff at the destination. A checklist should be used to assist in preparation. Oxygen supply, including the amount of oxygen in cylinders, and battery-life assessments are imperative. Transferring the patient to or from his/her bed must be carefully planned and appropriate equipment used by trained staff. All lines and tubes should be checked and simplified if possible.
e. All battery-operated transport equipment should have charge indicators and backup batteries. Regular servicing and checking of transport equipment is essential. The use of specialized transport trolleys, which include improved power supply, has been advocated.
f. Patient observations should be documented during transport.
g. Guidelines by professional bodies need to be updated in line with recommendations. Guidelines should develop a pretransport checklist.

Recommendations for monitoring outcomes

Local units need to be able to monitor compliance with these standards, including adequate in-servicing/training of staff, enhanced communication between destination sites, as well as monitoring the occurrence of incidents and their contributing factors.

Other recommendations

Because of the documented hazards and the expense of intrahospital transport, it is important to continue to develop the technology with which to perform diagnostic and therapeutic procedures at the bedside.

Reproduced with permission from Beckman U, Gillies DM, Berenholtz SM, Wu AW, Pronovost P. Incidents relating to the intrahospital transfer of critically ill patients. An analysis of the reports submitted to the Australian Incident Monitoring Study in Intensive Care. *Intensive Care Med.* 2004;30:1579-1585.

divided between system-based and human-based factors. Most events occurred between the ICU and operating room or radiology. Failure of equipment was primarily related to either battery or drug infusion pump failure. Other significant events included insufficient oxygen reserve within canisters. The most common patient/staff management issues were problems related to communication between the ICU and site of destination or origin. The value of incident monitoring lies not only in the systematic gathering of information but in the detailed analysis of the root causes of the events.[11] Several key recommendations arose from this important study (**Table 78-15**). These recommendations primarily emphasize careful consideration of the risks, careful preparation, dedicated transport teams, checklists, careful documentation of events in transport, and monitoring of compliance with established standards.

Incident reporting systems in health care arose from examinations of the benefits of safety reporting systems in the aviation industry. The aviation systems have been characterized by an organized process for collecting, analyzing, and dissemination of events, sentinel events, and near-miss events in a "no-fault" environment that focuses on fixing "systems" rather than identifying and blaming individual operators. The Institute of Medicine of the National Academy of Science has emphasized this strategy, reporting that system failures rather than individual incompetence are the primary cause of health care errors.[101] A reporting system optimized for the area of patient transport should be voluntary, nonpunitive, easy to carry out, and capable of providing feedback to participants.[103] Holzmueller et al developed an Internet-based reporting system to deal with common barriers to success in reporting systems including underreporting, fear of reprisal, patient confidentiality, time pressure, duplication, and a generalized opinion that efforts were wasted because of little feedback.[101] Their work, although preliminary, has demonstrated that an Internet-based system that collects data from multiple different ICUs across the United States is possible. Internet-based reporting systems may allow collection of data easily at multiple centers and facilitate sharing the findings. Although a single event at a particular reporting center may not lead to prompt action, the discovery of several similar events at various locations may acquire significance and require action.

Critical incident reporting and review results in better training of staff, implementation of guidelines for the maintenance and readiness of equipment, and a reduction in the number of adverse events.[104]

KEY REFERENCES

- Beckmann U, Gillies DM, Berenholtz SM, et al. Incidents relating to the intra-hospital transfer of critically ill patients. Analysis of the reports submitted to the Australian Incident Monitoring Study in Intensive Care. *Intensive Care Med.* 2004;30:1579-1585.
- Indeck M, Peterson S, Smith J, et al. Risk, cost, and benefit of transporting ICU patients for special studies. *J Trauma.* 1988;28:1020-1025.
- Smith I, Fleming S, Cernaianu A. Mishaps during transport from the intensive care unit. *Crit Care Med.* 1990;18:278-281.
- Szem JW, Hydo LJ, Fischer E, et al. High-risk intrahospital transport of critically ill patients: safety and outcome of the necessary "road trip." *Crit Care Med.* 1995;23:1660-1666.
- Warren J, Fromm RE, Orr RA, et al. Guidelines for the inter- and intrahospital transport of critically ill patients. *Crit Care Med.* 2004;32:256-262.
- Waydhas C. Intrahospital transport of critically ill patients. *Crit Care.* 1999;3:R83-R89.
- Woodward GA, Insoft RM, Pearson-Shaver AL, et al. The state of pediatric interfacility transport: consensus of the Second National Pediatric and Neonatal Interfacility Transport Medicine Leadership Conference. *Pediatr Emerg Care.* 2002;18:38-43.

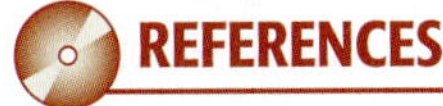

REFERENCES

Complete references available on DVD and online version at www.LongneckerAnesthesiology.com

CHAPTER 79

Postoperative Care of the Noncardiac Surgical Intensive Care Unit Patient

Michael C. Banks
C. William Hanson, III

KEY POINTS

1. Demand is growing for postoperative intensive care services due to advances in surgical techniques and the aging of the population. Anesthesiologists and surgical intensivists play a major role in ensuring responsible use of this costly resource.
2. Advances in neuraxial pain management have revolutionized certain types of surgery (eg, thoracic and major vascular), permitting patients to undergo major procedures without the need for prolonged intensive care following surgery.
3. Critical illness *polyneuropathy* and *myopathy* are acute illnesses that result in prolonged weakness or paralysis in subsets of intensive care patients.
4. Critically ill patients are at risk for a variety of pulmonary complications including aspiration, ventilator-associated pneumonia and acute lung injury. Intensive care management is directed at minimizing the risk factors predisposing patients to these complications.
5. Pulmonary artery catheter (PAC) guided therapy has not been shown to improve outcomes in critically ill patients with acute lung injury.
6. Conservative fluid management results in improved lung function and shortens the duration of both mechanical ventilation and intensive care stay without altering the rate of extrapulmonary organ failure.
7. The stress response after major surgery or injury is often accompanied by a period of endothelial cell dysfunction and capillary leak with loss of plasma volume into the extracellular "third space." The stress response may be initiated by tissue hypoperfusion due to inadequate fluid resuscitation, ischemia-reperfusion injury, cytokine release, or exposure of the circulating blood volume to an extracorporeal circuit (ie, blood salvage circuits, cardiopulmonary bypass).
8. Renal replacement therapy is a field that has evolved significantly over the past decade, and venovenous diafiltration and hemodialysis have displaced techniques such as arteriovenous hemodialysis.

INTRODUCTION

The surgical intensive care unit (SICU), or a combined medical-surgical ICU, is a specialized patient care floor designed to accommodate and treat critically ill surgical patients in the perioperative period, which may include preoperative, postoperative, and posttrauma injury management. As critical care techniques have evolved, it has become possible to both save the lives of some who might previously have died and prolong the lives of others who will nevertheless still not survive. The percentage of critical care beds has grown in many hospitals, and it is still an increasingly expensive and constrained resource due in part to shortages of qualified physicians, nurses, and ancillary personnel. It is vital, therefore, to find models of efficient and appropriately targeted intensive care.

The types of patients admitted to ICUs have changed considerably over the past several decades. The evolution of trauma systems, with rapid transportation of critically injured patients, has resulted in the concentration of complex multitrauma patients in trauma centers. The evolution of ventricular assist devices, thoracic aortic surgery, and heart and lung transplantation has revolutionized cardiothoracic surgery and changed the nature of perioperative cardiac intensive care. New approaches to the management of head injury and advanced neurosurgical techniques require increased technological sophistication in cerebral monitoring. Advances in the treatment of acute lung injury have resulted from research collaboratives such as the National Institutes of Health ARDS Network and been facilitated by improvements in mechanical ventilation technology. Perhaps the most important component of improvements in critical care has been the increased expertise of physician, nursing, and ancillary personnel in critical care management.

Although many innovations have increased the demands for critical care, endoscopic approaches to thoracic surgery and the use of postoperative epidural analgesia have allowed many patients to go directly to a hospital ward after surgery rather than the ICU. Aortic stents have had similar implications for vascular surgical patients who might once have undergone a laparotomy and several-day ICU stay. Many now go directly to a routine hospital ward.

As our ability to prolong life has improved, so has the complexity of ethical questions arising in the course of ICU care. The fact that we can temporarily or permanently replace the function of the failing heart, kidney, or lung increases the frequency with which we are confronted with questions as to whether it is appropriate to do so.

ICU TRIAGE

Critical care bed occupancy can have a major effect on the flow of patients through operating rooms (ORs). OR exit delays often result when ICUs are at a high census level. It is essential to make optimal use of these often scarce and invariably expensive resources. The criteria for admission to an ICU following surgery should be equitable and transparent, and they should prioritize those patients most likely to benefit from unit care.[1,2] Ideally, this prevents ICU admission for those who are "too well" or "too sick."

SCREENING TOOLS AND RESOURCE ALLOCATION

A Task Force of the American College of Critical Medicine and the Society of Critical Care Medicine developed ICU admission screening tools based on 3 different approaches: prioritization, diagnosis, and objective parameters.

- The *prioritization* approach classifies patients into 4 priorities (**Table 79-1**).
- The *diagnosis* approach (**Table 79-2**) identifies 8 diagnostic criteria: cardiac, pulmonary, neurological, drug ingestion and drug overdose, gastrointestinal disorders, endocrine, surgical, and miscellaneous, and divides them into admissible disease states.
- The *objective* approach (**Table 79-3**) is based on 5 objective criteria for admission into the ICU. These 5 categories are vital signs, laboratory values, radiology, electrocardiogram (ECG), and physical findings.

These admission criteria are widely used by health care organizations in the United States and abroad.[3,4] Health care organizations also benefit from the development of a triage plan by an internal ICU committee designed to optimally place patients when the demand for ICU beds is greater than the supply.[5] An institution-specific ICU committee is typically composed of health care professionals, ethics advisors, and legal advisors. An institutional triage officer can then direct patient triage based on institutional priorities. The principles outlined in the plan should be available to the public and to patients and/or their surrogates.[5] The triage plan should not be arbitrary or prejudicial.

The triage officer should also evaluate patients in the ICU to determine which patients are receiving the greatest benefit from ICU care. An example of a patient who might be deemed inappropriate for ICU admission is the patient with an advanced directive directing that cardiopulmonary resuscitation and/or mechanical ventilation not be initiated. In contrast, a brain-dead organ donor patient, although legally dead, might be kept in an ICU until organ harvest to maximize the

TABLE 79-1 Prioritization Model

Priority 1	Patient requires vasopressors, ventilatory support, and/or invasive monitoring.
Priority 2	Patient with acute disease complicating a chronic condition; patient needs monitoring.
Priority 3	Patient with acute disease complicating a severe chronic condition.
Priority 4	Too well or too ill to benefit from intensive care unit care.

benefit to potential recipients. The creation and distribution of explicit guidelines for ICU admission, discharge, and triage facilitate bed management when a family or physician wishes to admit a patient to an ICU bed for inappropriate reasons.

The triage plan should outline how to best prioritize admissions to the ICU. Although a hospital has an obligation to treat patients who are already admitted to the institution, a level-1 trauma center has additional obligations to the state and community to admit critically injured patients. These priorities may clash when beds are tight. Floor-based patients who suffer an acute decompensation should be transferred to the ICU as soon as feasible as should emergency department patients who are acutely ill. A hospital may also choose to prioritize admissions of certain patients for specialty care, for example, cardiac transplantation. These competing agendas may lead to the deferral or cancellation of elective surgical cases needing a postoperative ICU bed on rare occasions.

TABLE 79-2 Diagnosis Model

System	Disease State
Cardiac	Acute myocardial infection with complications; cardiogenic shock; complex dysrhythmias requiring monitoring or intervention; acute congestive heart failure with respiratory failure; hypertensive emergencies, unstable angina; cardiac arrest; cardiac tamponade; complete heart block
Pulmonary	Acute respiratory failure requiring mechanical ventilation; pulmonary emboli with hemodynamic instability; massive hemoptysis
Neurologic	Acute stroke with mental status change; coma; intracranial hemorrhage with possible herniation; acute subarachnoid hemorrhage; meningitis with altered mental status; central or peripheral nervous system disorder with deteriorating function; status epileptics; vasospasm; traumatic head injury; brain death with organ donation potential
Gastrointestinal	Gastrointestinal bleed with hypotension, angina, or continued bleeding; fulminant hepatic failure, severe pancreatitis; esophageal perforation
Endocrine	Diabetic ketoacidosis; thyroid storm, myxedema coma with hemodynamic instability; hyperosmolar state with coma or hemodynamic instability; adrenal crisis with hemodynamic instability; severe hypercalcemia with altered mental status; hypo- or hypernatremia with seizures and altered mental status; hypo- or hyperkalemia with dysrhythmias or hemodynamic instability; hypophosphatemia with muscular weakness
Surgical	Postoperative patients requiring hemodynamic monitoring, ventilatory support, and/or extensive nursing care
Drug ingestion or overdose	Seizures; hemodynamic instability; altered mental status with inadequate airway protection
Miscellaneous	Septic shock; hemodynamic monitoring; environmental injuries (lightning strike, near drowning, hyper-/hypothermia); experimental therapies with potential complications; conditions requiring extensive nursing care

Data from Egol A, Fromm R, et al. Guidelines for intensive care unit admission discharge and triage. *Crit Care Med.* 1999;27:633-638.

TABLE 79-3 Objective Parameter Model

Objective Parameter	Value/Limit
Vital signs	Pulse <40 or >150 beats/min; systolic arterial pressure <80 mm Hg or 20 mm Hg below baseline; mean arterial pressure <60 mm Hg; diastolic arterial pressure >120 mm Hg; respiratory rate >35 breaths/min
Laboratory values	Serum sodium <110 mEq/L or >170 mEq/L; serum potassium <2.0 mEq/L or >7.0 mEq/L, Pao_2 <50 torr; pH <7.1 or >7.7; serum glucose >800 mg/dL; serum calcium >15 mg/dL
Radiologic findings	Cerebral vascular hemorrhage, contusion, or subarachnoid hemorrhage with altered mental status or focal signs; ruptured viscera, bladder, liver, esophageal varices, or uterus with hemodynamic instability; dissecting aortic aneurysm
Electrocardiogram	Myocardial infection with complex dysrhythmia, congestive heart failure, or hemodynamic compromise; sustained ventricular tachycardia or fibrillation; complete heart block
Acute-onset physical findings	Unequal pupils in an unconscious patient; burns covering >10% of body surface area; anuria; airway obstruction; coma; continuous seizures; cyanosis; cardiac tamponade

Data from Egol A, Fromm R, et al. Guidelines for intensive care unit admission discharge and triage. *Crit Care Med.* 1999;27:633-638.

INTRAOPERATIVE EVALUATION FOR ICU CARE

Certain operations such as cardiac surgical procedures and certain neurosurgical procedures routinely require postoperative ICU care for the patients. These patients have predictable postoperative periods of instability during which intensive nursing and physician care are required, and they typically go to the ICU following surgery. However, some patients initially scheduled for ICU admission to the SICU may no longer be considered appropriate for ICU care because the planned procedure was aborted or the surgical course went better than expected. In other circumstances, unanticipated intraoperative events such as airway management problems, intraoperative aspiration of gastric contents, major blood loss, drug reactions, and cardiac events may necessitate unplanned admission to the SICU.

MANAGEMENT OF THE POSTOPERATIVE ICU PATIENT

TRANSPORT BETWEEN THE OR AND THE ICU

Intrahospital transport of critically ill patients is well-recognized as a possibly hazardous period potentially associated with complications such as hypoxia, hypotension, cardiac arrest, or ventilator-associated pneumonia.[6-8] See Chapter 78 on transport. Studies have shown that most transport-related complications occur during transit between the ICU and the OR or the radiology suite.[8] Before transporting a patient, it is imperative that the risk transport be weighed against its goal to see if it is possible to bring the study or procedure to the patient rather than the other way around. A review by Braxton et al summarizes 3 studies assessing the risks and benefits of transporting a patient from the ICU for the purposes of diagnostic testing. In 2 of the studies, the care plans changed within 48 hours of the transport in 24% and 39%, respectively, of the patients transported, and two-thirds of the patients experienced physiologic deterioration during transport. In the third study, only 30% of the diagnostic studies contributed to patient management.[9]

After determining the requirement for patient transport to or from the ICU, a comprehensive transfer plan should be designed including patient preparation, required personnel, and necessary monitoring. Pretransport preparation is a crucial step for safe patient transport. A checklist is recommended and should include oxygen supply, emergency resuscitation drugs, intravenous (IV) fluids and infusions (if needed). The monitor should be checked for function and level of battery charge. Arrangements should be made to ensure that any special mechanical ventilatory requirements (eg, bilevel ventilation) can be met with the portable ventilator; and all of the foregoing should be documented on a pretransport checklist.

It is essential that the appropriate personnel are available for transport. The team may include a critical care nurse and respiratory therapist or specially trained transport technicians. Some hospitals have developed specialized transport teams trained to care for critically ill patients. Studies have shown that a major cause of transport complications is failure to follow protocol and failure to recognize that a problem has occurred during transport.[9] If the patient is physiologically unstable at the time of transport, as during movement to and from the OR, a physician should also be present.

Efficient communication is another important aspect to providing safe transport. The transport team must notify the receiving unit or location at the time of transport to ensure adequate preparation at the receiving end and communicate details about the patient's history and present status. The receiving site should be ready with appropriate monitors, equipment, and drugs.

The last essential to safe patient transport is appropriate monitoring, which should include continuous ECG, blood pressure (BP) (invasive or noninvasive, as appropriate), oxygen saturation, and end-tidal carbon dioxide (CO_2) if the patient is ventilated. All portable monitoring devices should have fully charged batteries and working charge indicators.

Each patient care unit should have written transport policies as recommended by the American College of Critical Care Medicine, Society of Critical Care Medicine, and the American Association of Critical Nurses.[10] A review of the literature and recommendations for intrahospital transportation has been published by Fanara et al.[11] These policies should be modified for each health care institution.

POSTOPERATIVE LABORATORY TESTS AND VITAL SIGNS

Standard monitors for the intensive care patient include ECG, BP, pulse oximetry, and respiratory rate (often obtained by impedance analysis through the electrocardiographic leads). Laboratory assays that are obtained routinely include complete blood count (CBC), electrolytes, blood urea nitrogen and creatinine, coagulation panel, and arterial blood gas. Capnography is used in some ICUs for mechanically ventilated patients to assess respiratory dead space in acute and chronic diseases of the critically ill such as adult respiratory distress syndrome (ARDS), chronic obstructive pulmonary disease (COPD), and pulmonary embolism. Serial plasma lactate levels may be followed to assess the adequacy of systemic perfusion and resuscitation or as a marker of ischemia in large tissue beds such as the gastrointestinal tract. Serum calcium (ionized or total) and magnesium are important physiologic cations that may be included in intensive care laboratory panels. The absolute levels of these values as well as their trends can provide useful information during the course of resuscitation and treatment.

MANAGEMENT OF POSTOPERATIVE ANALGESIA, SEDATION, AND DELIRIUM IN THE ICU

Pain and sedation management in the ICU is important both for patient comfort and satisfaction, as well as an increasingly recognized contributor to patient outcome. Patients in the ICU routinely report pain and discomfort during routine nursing care (eg, airway care, dressing changes, and physical therapy), and resulting from the presence of catheters, drains, and endotracheal tubes (ETTs).[12,13] The potential complications of poorly managed analgesia may include prolonged intubation, ICU delirium, myocardial injury due to increased stress, and increased ICU and hospital length of stay with resulting increased cost. Effective pain management varies from patient to patient and involves an appreciation of the considerable variation in the population in pain tolerance and willingness to acknowledge suffering.

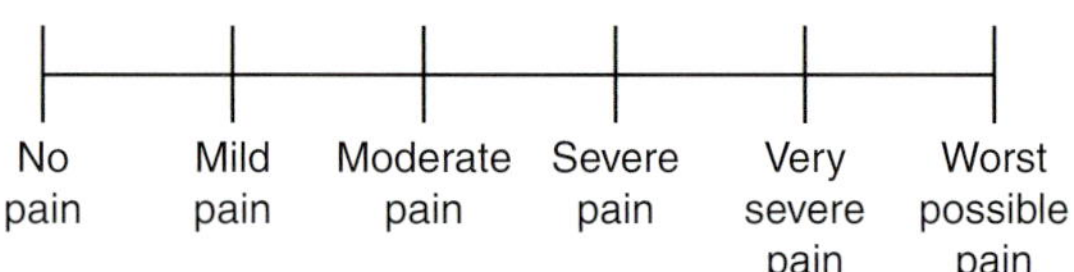

FIGURE 79-1. Visual Analogue Scale. [From Warfield CA, Bajwa ZH. *Principles and Practice of Pain Medicine.* 2nd ed. New York, NY: McGraw-Hill; 2004.]

Pain assessment tools have been developed to make measurement as objective as possible and include the Visual Analog Scale (**Fig. 79-1**) and Numerical Rating Scale (NRS) (**Fig. 79-2**). The Society of Critical Care Medicine published a practice guideline in 2002 for sedation and analgesia in critically ill patients that recommends assessing pain at regular intervals, using the NRS or a behavioral pain assessment scale in conjunction with physiologic parameters (BP and heart rate) in patients who cannot communicate.

There are many pharmacologic alternatives for the management of postoperative pain including patient-controlled epidural analgesia (PCEA) and IV patient-controlled analgesia (PCA). The patient must be awake, alert, and oriented to use these pumps effectively. PCA can result in somnolence and narcotization, but this is rare if the basal and bolus limits are set appropriately. PCEA is extremely effective after certain surgical procedures, particularly those involving the chest and upper abdomen; but hypotension and bradycardia may result from sympathectomy even at low infusion levels. These physiologic responses to pain control must be differentiated from pathophysiologic problems (ie, evolving myocardial infarction, bleeding, or sepsis). Hypotension and bradycardia do not mandate discontinuation of an epidural infusion; rather the level of the block should be evaluated and the infusion rate adjusted accordingly. The concentration of local anesthetic can be decreased or the BP can be supported with fluid boluses or pressors if the benefits of pain control outweigh manageable complications of the analgesic regimen. In a recent meta-analysis by Wu et al, epidural analgesia provided better analgesia than IV PCA.[14]

If a patient is unable to use a PCA or PCEA, continuous infusion or intermittent boluses of opioids can be administered as needed. Continuous infusions are usually reserved for patients with a controlled and stable airway (ie, ETT or tracheostomy tube). However, in patients with chronic pain issues or high opioid tolerance, continuous infusions may be used as long as appropriate respiratory monitoring tools are in place.

Agitation is common in the ICU patient and may result from the unfamiliar setting or the inability to communicate (eg, due to the presence of an ETT). Agitation resulting from delirium is a significant and common problem in the intensive care setting. Delirium is defined in the *Diagnostic and Statistical Manual of Mental Disorders, 4th Edition* as a disturbance of consciousness or cognition that has developed over a short period of time and is caused by direct physiologic consequences of a general medical condition. The incidence of delirium in the ICU is

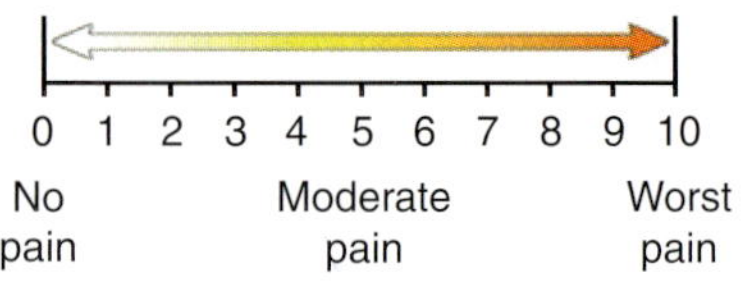

FIGURE 79-2. Numerical Rating Scale.

TABLE 79-4 The Ramsey Sedation Scale

Level	Characteristics
1	Patient awake, anxious, agitated or restless
2	Patient awake, cooperative, oriented and tranquil
3	Patient drowsy, with response to commands
4	Patient asleep, brisk response to glabella tap or loud auditory stimulus
5	Patient asleep, sluggish response to stimulus
6	Patient has no response to firm nail-bed pressure or other noxious stimuli

Reproduced with permission from Carrasco G. Instruments for monitoring intensive care unit sedation. *Crit Care.* 2000;4(4):217-225.

reported to be from 16% to 80%, depending on the assessor and assessment tool used.[15,16]

To evaluate a patient's degree of anxiety and discomfort objectively and reproducibly, intensive care providers typically use a sedation/analgesia scale. Plasma concentration levels of sedatives, frontalis electromyogram, and Bispectral Index Sensor (BIS) electroencephalographic analysis are more objective but less reliable alternatives. Plasma drug levels are not sufficient because the concentration of drug needed for analgesia varies from patient to patient. Frontalis electromyography (EMG) is not sensitive for monitoring sedation. The BIS analysis method has been studied as a monitor for level of sedation, but its results have not been confirmed in critically ill patients.

The measures in common ICU use include the Ramsay, the Richmond Agitation Sedation Scale (RASS), modified Glasgow Coma, visual analog pain, and sedation-agitation scales. The Ramsay scale is the most widely used scale for sedation monitoring (**Table 79-4**).[17]

The Ramsay scale has been found to have strong interobserver agreement and reliability as has the Richmond Analgesia and Sedation Scale (**Table 79-5**). The Glasgow Coma Scale modified by Cook and Palma (**Table 79-6**) provides a numerical score to evaluate neurologically impaired patients who are mechanically ventilated. Sedation tools are not appropriate for the evaluation of delirium in the ICU. Instruments currently available and validated to detect delirium in the ICU are the Confusion Assessment Method-ICU (CAM-ICU) and the Intensive Care Delirium Screening Checklist (ICDSC).

The γ-aminobutyric acid (GABA) receptor agonists such as propofol and benzodiazepines are frequently used to sedate agitated patients, although the latter may also be a cause of delirium. Alternative sedatives for delirious patients include haloperidol and dexmedetomidine. Dexmedetomidine is a centrally acting α-2 agonist that is more potent than clonidine with a faster onset and shorter length of action. It is also a potent analgesic and anxiolytic.

The potential complications of poorly managed analgesia and sedation include prolonged intubation, ICU delirium, and myocardial ischemia. Overly sedated patients may require longer periods of ventilator support, with a consequently longer ICU and hospital stay. Prolonged ventilation also increases the patient's risk of ventilator-associated pneumonia, and studies have also shown that inadequate pain control can cause increased morbidity and hospital stay.

TABLE 79-5 Richmond Analgesia and Sedation Scale

Score	Description
+4	Overly combative. Immediate danger to staff (Combative)
+3	Pulls on invasive devices or has aggressive behavior to staff (Very Agitated)
+2	Frequent nonpurposeful movements (Agitated)
+1	Anxious or apprehensive (Restless)
0	Alert and calm
−1	Not fully alert but has sustained awakening to voice (Drowsy)
−2	Briefly awakens to voice (Light Sedation)
−3	Any movement to voice (Moderate Sedation)
−4	No response to voice, but movement to physical stimulation (Deep Sedation)
−5	No response to voice or physical stimulation (Unarousable)

TABLE 79-6 The Glasgow Coma Scale as Modified by Cook and Palma

Characteristic	Score
Eyes open	
Spontaneously	4
In response to speech	3
In response to pain	2
None	1
Response to nursing procedures	
Obeys commands	5
Purposeful movements	4
Nonpurposeful flexion	3
Nonpurposeful extension	2
None	1
Cough	
Spontaneous strong	4
Spontaneous weak	3
On suction only	2
None	1
Respiration	
Obeys commands	5
Spontaneous intubated	4
Spontaneous intermittent mandatory ventilator triggering	3
Respiration against ventilator	2
No respiratory effects	1

Reproduced with permission from Carrasco G. Instruments for monitoring intensive care unit sedation. *Crit Care.* 2000;4(4):217-225.

MANAGEMENT OF ORGAN-SPECIFIC ISSUES AND SYSTEMS IN POSTOPERATIVE ICU PATIENTS

NEUROLOGIC ISSUES

Management of the postoperative neurosurgical patient is beyond the scope of this chapter. This section addresses the management of common neurologic disorders seen in other postoperative ICU patients.

New-onset seizures are a major postoperative complication in ICU patients with a reported incidence of 12% in ICU patients without a primary neurologic diagnosis.[18] The causes of postoperative seizures include medications, metabolic disorders, primary neurologic disorders, infection, hypoxia, and drug withdrawal (**Table 79-7**).

Accurate identification of new-onset seizures is important. Seizures must be differentiated from myoclonus and other rhythmic movement disorders (ie, tremor). Electroencephalographic testing is the standard test used to identify seizure activity. Once a new-onset seizure has been diagnosed, laboratory tests, computed tomography or magnetic resonance imaging of the brain and, in patients suspected of an infectious etiology, lumbar puncture are often performed to elucidate the etiology. The most common causes of new-onset seizures in ICU patients are metabolic disturbances with an incidence of 28.6%.[14]

TABLE 79-7 Causes of New-Onset Seizures in Postoperative Patients

Hypoxia/ischemia	
Metabolic disorders	Eclampsia, hyponatremia, hypophosphatemia, renal dysfunction, hepatic dysfunction
Medications	Antibiotics, antidepressants, antipsychotics, local anesthetics, cocaine, amphetamines, phencyclidine
Traumatic head injury	Contusion, hemorrhage
Infection	Febrile seizures, abscess, encephalitis
Drug withdrawal	Barbiturates, benzodiazepines, opioids, alcohol
Surgical injury	Craniotomy

Adapted from Mirski MA, Varelas PA. Diagnosis and treatment of seizures in the adult intensive care unit. *Contemp Crit Care.* 2003;1(4):1-12.

The initial treatment for new-onset seizures is typically an IV sedative-anticonvulsant such as a benzodiazepine, barbiturates, or propofol.[19] The patient is then started on a primary anticonvulsant medication. First-line anticonvulsants include phenytoin, levetiracetam, and carbamazepine.

Critical illness neuromuscular diseases are a relatively rare but important complication in ICU patients. These abnormalities are divided into polyneuropathies and myopathies of critical illness. Critical illness *polyneuropathy* is an acute degenerative disorder of motor and sensory nerve axons. Symptoms are flaccid tetraparesis and failure to wean from the ventilator. Critical illness *myopathy* is an acute degenerative illness of the myocyte that results in weakness and paralysis. There are 3 histologic types of myopathy: diffuse necrotizing, necrotizing, and myosin thick filament loss. The risk factors for development of critical illness neuromuscular abnormalities include sepsis, multiorgan dysfunction, hyperglycemia, and treatment with corticosteroids, nondepolarizing neuromuscular blocking agents, and aminoglycosides. The mechanisms by which these risk factors contribute to neuromuscular abnormalities are unknown. Bolton et al suggests that cytokines, free radicals, and activated complement fragments released during sepsis cause axonal injury.[20]

The incidence of critical illness polyneuropathy varies substantially depending on the diagnostic method used, the patient population, and the timing of the diagnosis. In septic patients, the incidence has been stated to be as high as 70% to 80%.[21] Studies have shown an association between corticosteroids and critical illness myopathy in patients with severe asthma;[22] however, no specific mechanism has been identified. Neuromuscular blocking agents (NMBAs) are also associated with acute myopathies. Concurrent administration of NMBA with steroids or aminoglycosides increases the incidence of myopathies. High blood glucose levels were associated with critical illness polyneuropathy in one study of septic patients with multiorgan dysfunction, and van den Berghe et al reported that axonal injuries were decreased by 50% in patients who received intensive insulin therapy.[23] It is not clear if catecholamines and hyperglycemia lead to polyneuropathy or if insulin or euglycemia protect neuronal axons.

Encephalopathy or sedation can mask critical illness neuromuscular diseases, complicating diagnosis. Objective studies, such as nerve and/or muscle biopsies, in conjunction with EMG, can facilitate diagnosis. Nerve and muscle biopsies can provide pathologic evidence of disease. Nerve biopsies, however, can lead to permanent neurologic deficits. Electrophysiologic studies including nerve conduction studies and EMG are the current gold standard for diagnosis of critical illness neuromuscular abnormalities. Nerve conduction studies measure the latency and amplitude of the conduction and the muscle's electrical response measured with EMG: the compound muscle action potential (CMAP). In critical illness polyneuropathy CMAPs are reduced and abnormal spontaneous activity is present, indicative of axonal neuropathy. EMG records the electrical activity of active and resting muscle.

In patients affected by critical illness neuromuscular abnormalities, abnormal muscle fibrillation occurs. To differentiate between a neuropathy and a myopathy, motor unit action potentials are evaluated using EMG. If a motor unit shows increased amplitude and latency, critical illness polyneuropathy is diagnosed. If the motor unit shows decreased amplitude and latency, critical illness myopathy is diagnosed.

The treatment alternatives for critical illness neuromuscular abnormalities are limited. Intensive physical therapy with discontinuation of steroids and NMBAs and tight glucose control are the mainstays. The long-term outcome is not well studied, and recovery depends on the severity of the disease. Many patients with critical illness neuromuscular abnormalities may regain normal strength after weeks to months; however, some patients never recover.

PULMONARY ISSUES IN THE POSTOPERATIVE ICU PATIENT

Postoperative critically ill patients often undergo a period of relative hypoxemia due to the effects of anesthetics and/or surgery superimposed on any primary disease process. Respiratory management in the ICU is often focused on the initiation, termination, or prevention of complications of mechanical ventilation.

Postoperative patients may be admitted to the ICU following surgery with an ETT in place. The newly arrived patient in the ICU should undergo a chest radiograph (CXR) to determine the location of any central lines placed in the OR, the position of the ETT, and identify pulmonary complications that may have occurred in the OR such as pneumothorax or aspiration. The ETT may need to be advanced (if the tip is above the level of the clavicle on CXR) or withdrawn (in the event of mainstem intubation).

So-called fast-track weaning, in which ventilatory support is weaned automatically by respiratory therapists as the patient meets certain milestones has become prevalent, and it has been shown to reduce the duration of mechanical ventilation in patients.[24] New approaches to noninvasive ventilation and their application in a variety of patient populations have reduced the threshold for early extubation. Continuous positive airway pressure and bilevel positive airway pressure (BiPAP) are effective in reducing the need for reintubation of patients who develop respiratory insufficiency after extubation. BiPAP can be administered by face or nasal mask and is used to treat patients with marked obesity, COPD, sleep apnea, or respiratory muscle weakness by allowing them to be extubated and then rested with periods of noninvasive positive pressure ventilatory support.[25]

Nosocomial pneumonias include ventilator-associated and other hospital-acquired pneumonias, such as in-hospital aspiration pneumonia. The definition of the former is an infection occurring greater than 48 hours after hospital admission that is radiographically consistent with pneumonia. Aspiration pneumonia can develop as a complication of endotracheal intubation in patients who regurgitate gastric contents, and it is more likely to occur when the pH of the aspirated material is low and the volume greater than 0.3 mL/kg of body weight. Critically ill patients are at risk for the development of both of these conditions, and predisposing factors include inadequate endotracheal cuff seal, the supine position, increased gastric contents, and bacterial colonization of the oropharynx.

Acute lung injury (ALI) and ARDS can occur in the postoperative patient. These diseases represent points on a continuum of acute lung disease and result from a multitude of etiologies including trauma, transfusion reactions, and sepsis. Although a variety of approaches have been investigated for the prevention and treatment of these diseases, the standard therapy is "protective ventilation," in which low tidal volumes are given to prevent overdistension of injured as well as healthy alveoli. The ARDS network funded by the National Institute of Health published the results of a landmark study of ALI/ARDS in 1999,[26] which showed that the use of low (6 mL/kg) tidal volume breaths conferred a mortality benefit when compared with the then more traditional (12 mL/kg) tidal volume ventilation. The same group recently published data from a factorially designed study comparing

ARDS patients managed with a pulmonary arterial catheter (PAC) versus a central venous line and patients with a conservative versus liberal approach to fluid management.[27] The results of this study showed that PAC-guided therapy did not improve outcomes and was associated with more complications, specifically those associated with placement of the PAC. The study also showed that a conservative fluid management approach resulted in improved lung function and shortened the duration of both mechanical ventilation and the ICU stay (when compared to liberal fluid management) without altering the rate of nonpulmonary organ failures.

CARDIOVASCULAR ISSUES IN THE POSTOPERATIVE ICU PATIENT

Postoperative cardiac management is directly comparable with intraoperative management in the indications for and methods of treating abnormalities such as intravascular volume depletion, hemorrhage, bradycardia, and tachydysrhythmias. As in the OR, intensive care monitoring invariably includes noninvasive or invasive BP measurement, continuous ECG, and pulse oximetry. The stress response after major surgery or injury is often manifested by a period of impaired endothelial cell function and the resulting loss of plasma volume into the "third space," or extravascular space. Precipitating factors include tissue hypoperfusion due to inadequate fluid therapy, ischemia-reperfusion injury, and cytokine and complement activation.

Postoperative patients require ongoing fluid resuscitation commensurate with the magnitude of the surgical or traumatic injury, and in some cases that requirement may exceed 10 mL/kg/h. In healthy patients, the need for fluid resuscitation typically ends after a period of 24 to 48 hours, and the accumulated excess volume and solute load is then eliminated through the kidneys spontaneously over the succeeding several days. The time courses of these phases may be altered in patients with underlying illnesses such as hepatic or renal failure. As distinct from a pure volume requirement, a progressive decrease in the blood hemoglobin concentration or hematocrit level necessitates a search for a bleeding source.

Patients with labile BP may require an intra-arterial, central venous, or pulmonary arterial catheter to better assess and manage their intravascular volume status and cardiac performance. The utility and safety of the pulmonary artery catheter has been the subject of much recent debate,[28] but current-generation catheters provide advanced functions such as continuous measurement of cardiac output, right ventricular performance, and mixed venous oxygen saturation, all of which can be used to guide short-term fluid resuscitation. Monitors such as the central line (venous pressure), pulmonary artery catheter (pulmonary pressure, occluded wedge pressure, mixed venous oximetry, cardiac output) or echocardiography (to assess ventricular filling and performance, valve abnormalities) can be used to guide resuscitation and the initiation and titration of inotropes or vasopressors.

Cardiac dysrhythmias are relatively frequent in the OR and ICU, where metabolic, ischemic, and neurohormonal stresses may cause premature atrial and ventricular contractions, conduction block, or atrial fibrillation. Cardiac rhythm abnormalities are more prevalent in patients with structural heart disease[29] and can be caused by surgical stress, electrolyte abnormalities, sympathetic stimulation, direct mechanical irritation of the heart (as by intracardiac catheters), or device malfunction.[30] Dysrhythmias can be separated into narrow and wide-complex QRS rhythms. Narrow QRS rhythm abnormalities typically originate in the atria and include sinus tachycardia, premature atrial complexes, atrial flutter/fibrillation, accessory pathway tachycardias, and sinus bradyarrhythmias.

In patients with wide complex QRS rhythms, it is may be difficult to differentiate between supraventricular dysrhythmias and ventricular dysrhythmias. Premature ventricular complexes (PVCs) are common and caused by structural heart disease, electrolyte imbalances, acidosis, and hypoxia. PVCs are usually benign and do not require antiarrhythmic treatment in patients without structural heart disease.[31] However, studies have shown that when PVCs have a frequency of 10 or more per hour or multifocal origins, there is an increased risk of developing a life-threatening dysrhythmia, especially in patients with structural heart disease.[32,33]

Atrial fibrillation is the most common perioperative dysrhythmia.[34] The differential diagnosis for postoperative atrial fibrillation is extensive and includes increased catecholamine levels due to stress response, electrolyte disorders, hypo- and hypervolemia, and hypoxia. The incidence in postoperative cardiac surgical patients is as high as 30% to 40%, and 3% to 4% of routine perioperative patients may develop the problem. Electrolyte and ventilatory abnormalities should be identified and corrected. Pharmacologic treatments include β-blockers, calcium channel blockers, and amiodarone. In most instances the atrial fibrillation is benign and self-limited, but for some patients in whom the arrhythmia persists, anticoagulation may be appropriate; and when accompanied by hemodynamic instability, electrical cardioversion is indicated.

Myocardial ischemia and infarction can occur in the postoperative period due to anemia, underresuscitation, tachycardia, volume overload, or the relatively hypercoagulable state that occurs 2 to 3 days after surgery. Proactive management of cardiac stressors including hyper- or hypovolemia and tachydysrhythmias improves the myocardial oxygen demand-to-supply ratio.

GASTROINTESTINAL ISSUES IN THE POSTOPERATIVE ICU PATIENT

Postoperative and traumatically injured patients have increased metabolic demand related to energy consumption by tissues during the repair process. Patients enter an inflammatory phase following surgery or trauma proportionate to the magnitude of the injury and become hypermetabolic as the reparative process proceeds. In the absence of adequate glucose, glycogen-based energy stores are rapidly depleted, forcing the body to break down protein from muscle to meet energy demands. Supplemental nutritional therapy is designed to meet daily energy requirements in critically ill postsurgical patients and thereby prevent protein loss. Several questions typically arise when discussing nutrition, including when to begin, how to assess nutritional requirements, and by what route to administer the feeds.

The timing of initiation of supplemental nutrition depends on both the baseline nutritional status of the patient and the disease process. Patients with disease states such as burns, sepsis, and cancer, and malnourished patients have higher caloric requirements than most other ICU patients. They require higher than standard nutritional support to heal and prevent infection. Laboratory parameters are often used to guide nutritional supplementation. Albumin, prealbumin, and transferrin levels are typically measured to guide the patient's nutritional status; however, the inflammatory response may alter the reliability of these laboratory values. Serum albumin levels often drop precipitously following surgery.

Depending on the route of delivery, nutritional support has differing complications. Enteral feeding may be complicated by pulmonary aspiration in patients who are unable to cough or gag. Additional complications include enteral anastomotic leak after gut anastomosis or intestinal ischemia in patients on vasopressors. Enteral nutrition should not be given to patients with intestinal obstruction. Supplemental feeds are typically started 3 to 5 days following surgery in patients who are unable to take adequate nutrition by mouth.

Enteral feeding is preferred over IV feeds when possible because it is physiologic and preserves gut mucosal barrier function and thereby reduces translocation of bacteria from the intestinal lumen into the vasculature. Gut feeding also preserves the immunologic function of gut-associated lymphoid tissue.

Parenteral nutrition can be administered through a peripheral or central vein. Central delivery of nutrition permits delivery of a high concentration of carbohydrates and protein, one that would irritate and sclerose peripheral veins. The disadvantages of parenteral nutrition include higher risks of infection and sepsis, intestinal atrophy, and complications associated with central venous access.

Abdominal compartment syndrome (ACS) has become an increasingly recognized gastrointestinal problem in critically ill patients. The abdominal compartment is a potential space that can fill with fluid or blood, compressing the organs and vessels within. In mechanically ventilated patients, elevated abdominal pressure can interfere with breathing by impeding downward excursion of the diaphragm. Unintubated patients may become dyspneic due to the same mechanism. Intra-abdominal pressure is assessed by measuring bladder pressure. The pressure of a column of fluid (typically urine) in continuity with the bladder can be measured using a urinary catheter, and the diagnosis of ACS should be considered when pressures exceed 20 mm Hg.

The increased intra-abdominal pressure resulting from ACS can also impair perfusion to any of the visceral organs as well as venous return to the heart. Abdominal compartment syndrome causes decreased venous return due to compression of the inferior vena cava, decreased ventricular compliance, and increased peripheral vascular resistance, all of which result in decreased cardiac output.

Renal function can be compromised as a secondary effect of impaired cardiac performance or due to direct compression of the kidneys, and it is indicated by decreased urine output. This is due to decreased renal blood flow glomerular filtration rate. Compression of the renal parenchymal and vessels can result in renin, aldosterone, and antidiuretic hormone release, leading to free-water retention that may exacerbate the primary problem.

Successful management of ACS requires that clinicians be aware of which patients are at greater risk for this complication of surgery and trauma, attentive monitoring, and early intervention. Trauma patients who have undergoing large-volume resuscitations, even in the absence of intra-abdominal injury, and surgical patients with edematous bowel following gastrointestinal surgery are at increased risk for the development of ACS. Pancreatitis, septic shock, acidosis, hypothermia, ileus, hemo- and pneumoperitoneum can predispose a critically ill patient to the development of intra-abdominal hypertension. The differential for ACS also includes a variety of medical, surgical, and traumatic conditions.

The detrimental effects of ACS can be treated in the ICU with fluids, vasopressors, and pharmacologic muscle relaxation to relax the abdominal wall. Definitive therapy is a decompressive laparotomy, although there is some controversy as to the appropriate threshold for this invasive procedure. Opening the abdomen incurs many risks including infection, sepsis, dehydration from large insensible fluid losses, and fistula formation.. A grading system has been proposed to guide the evaluation and treatment of ACS (**Table 79-8**).

Following laparotomy in patients with ACS, there is often a dramatic improvement in cardiac output and organ perfusion. The fascia may then be secured and the viscera covered with mesh, which can be drained with a VAC dressing, or a Bogota bag. The VAC dressing helps to quantify abdominal fluid losses, protects the abdominal contents from infection, and helps prevent the abdominal wall musculature from contracting laterally, thus preventing future closure. After the ACS has resolved, the abdomen can be closed primarily or with mesh.

TABLE 79-8 Diagnosis and Treatment of Abdominal Compartment Syndrome

Grade	IAP (mm Hg)	Associated Signs	Treatment
I	10-15	No signs of ACS	Normovolemia
II	16-25	May have increased PAP and oliguria	Hypervolemic resuscitation with caution
III	26-35	Anuria, decreased CO, increased PAP	Consider abdominal decompression
IV	>35	Anuria, decreased CO, increased PAP	Abdominal decompression

ACS, abdominal compartment syndrome; CO, carbon monoxide; IAP, intra-abdominal pressure; PAP, positive airway pressure.

HEMATOLOGIC ISSUES IN THE POSTOPERATIVE ICU PATIENT

Anemia is a common problem in the SICU, but transfusion can be associated with complications. Blood product administration can result in transmission of viruses, transfusion reactions, graft-versus-host disease, and depression of the recipient's natural killer cell function. Poor wound healing, risk of anastomotic leak, and postoperative infections have also been associated with perioperative blood transfusion. However, although treatment thresholds have risen as new research has shown that critically ill patients tolerate hemoglobin levels much lower than the traditionally treated trigger of 10 mg/dL with few adverse consequences, transfusion may be necessary to prevent end-organ ischemia.

In 1999, Hébert et al[35] conducted a randomized multicenter clinically controlled trial of transfusion requirements in critical care patients (the TRICC trial). The purpose of this study was to determine if a restrictive transfusion protocol that maintained circulating levels at 7.0 to 9.0 g/dL had an equivalent risk of morbidity and 30-day mortality as a liberal alternative that maintained hemoglobin (Hgb) levels of 10 to 12 g/dL. The results showed that there was no mortality difference between the 2 groups; however, in a subgroup of patients who were younger than 55 years with a low predicted mortality risk, the 30-day mortality was decreased and survival rate increased in the restrictive transfusion group.

In 2001,[36] the same group published a post hoc subgroup analysis of the TRICC trial to compare the morbidity and mortality in critically ill patients with cardiovascular disease comparing the restrictive transfusion strategy group with the more liberal transfusion strategy group. Cardiovascular disease was defined as patients with a primary or secondary diagnosis of myocardial infarction, angina, congestive heart failure, dysrhythmias, cardiogenic and "other forms of shock, vascular procedures, and cardiac procedures (except open heart surgery). The study results showed that there was no statistical difference with respect to survival, ICU mortality, and 30- and 60-day mortality, suggesting that lower Hgb levels did not produce additional harm in the subpopulation with cardiovascular disease.

Several other groups have subsequently examined transfusion strategies in patients with acute coronary syndrome (ACS). Patients with ACS suffer myocardial ischemia, angina, or myocardial infarction and it was believed this was due to the imbalance of oxygen supply and demand, perhaps attributable to anemia. In 2001, Wu et al[37] conducted a retrospective study of 78 974 Medicare patients older than 65 years with a confirmed acute myocardial infarction to determine the risk associated with anemia in these patients and the effect of blood transfusion on mortality. The results showed that 3680 patients (4.7%) received blood transfusions. It also showed that transfusion was associated with a lower 30-day mortality in patients who had an admission hematocrit 33% or lower and an increased mortality in patients with hematocrits 36.1% or greater.

In a 2005 study, Rao et al[38] examined the association between blood transfusions and mortality among patient with ACS who developed bleeding, anemia, or both during their hospital course. This retrospective analysis of 24 112 patients used data from 3 separate glycoprotein IIb/IIIa inhibitor trials: GUSTO IIb, PURSUIT, and PARAGON B. The study showed that 2401 of the patients (10%) had received transfusions and that these patients had a significantly higher unadjusted risk of 30-day mortality and 30-day myocardial infarction. Patients transfused to a hematocrit of 30% or greater were found to have a significantly higher risk of 30-day mortality.

In 2009, a task force consisting of representatives from the Society of Critical Care Medicine, the American College of Critical Care Medicine, and the Eastern Association for Surgery for Trauma developed clinical practice guidelines for the transfusion of red blood cells in adult trauma and critically ill patients.[39] Their recommendations included the following:

1. Transfusion of red blood cells in patients with hemorrhagic shock (level 1)
2. Red blood cells may be administered to patients with acute hemorrhage, hemodynamic instability, or a low SvO_2 (level 1)
3. Avoidance of the use of a numerical hemoglobin threshold for transfusion: Transfusion should be based on the patient's intravascular volume, hemodynamic parameters and cardiopulmonary status (level 2)
4. Red blood cells treatment with single units unless the patient is actively bleeding (level 2)
5. Avoidance of transfusion in patients with acute lung injury (ALI) or acute respiratory distress syndrome (ARDS) because transfusions can exacerbate ALI and ARDS (level 2)
6. The analysis concluded that there is no benefit in transfusing stable patients with moderate to severe traumatic brain injury who have a hemoglobin less than 10g/dL (level 2)

More clinical studies are still needed to clarify the roles for transfusion in patients with ACS and subarachnoid bleeding.

Coagulopathies are another common problem in postoperative ICU patients and include dilutional coagulopathy, heparin-induced thrombocytopenia (HIT), and disseminated intravascular coagulation (DIC). Dilutional coagulopathy may complicate massive transfusion in patients with large-volume blood loss. The transfusion of packed red blood cells may result in dilution of clotting factors, platelets, and consequent prolongation of the prothrombin and partial thromboplastin times. Clinical findings include diffuse oozing of blood from mucosal and serosal surfaces, as well as from wounds and vascular access sites.[40] A study by Cosgriff[41] described several risk factors for severe coagulopathy. In a 2-year prospective study that evaluated patients who received more than 10 units of transfusion of packed red blood cells, a multiple logistic regression analysis revealed 4 significant risk factors: (1) blood pH higher than 7.10; (2) rectal temperature lower than 34°C; (3) injury severity score higher than 25; and (4) systolic BP lower than 70 mm Hg. Patients with no risk factors had a 1% chance of a life-threatening coagulopathy, whereas patients with 1 risk factor had a 10% to 40% chance, and patients with all 4 risk factors had a 100% incidence of a life-threatening coagulopathy.

DIC is a consumptive coagulopathy that can occur in the postoperative ICU setting. Triggers for DIC include sepsis, bone marrow and fat emboli, amniotic fluid emboli, and brain tissue embolization after traumatic injury. These tissues contain hematologically active factors and thromboplastins that trigger the clotting cascade and subsequent consumption of clotting and anticlotting factors. There is a resulting inhibition of localized clot formation and simultaneous intravascular thromboembolism. DIC is treated by addressing the precipitating problem (eg, treating sepsis when possible). Replacement blood components may be administered if the patient is actively bleeding.

Hemodilutional thrombocytopenia resulting from crystalloid administration paradoxically causes increased coagulation, as measured by thromboelastogram.[42-44] The mechanism responsible for this hypercoagulability is not known.

Thrombocytopenia is common in critically ill patients. Although sepsis and hemodilution are the most common etiologies, HIT is a relatively unusual but significant platelet-based problem. There are 2 types of HIT. Type 1 has an incidence of 10% to 20% in heparin-treated patients, a nonimmune mechanism, and is not associated with thrombosis. Type 2 HIT has a 30% to 80% incidence and is an autoimmune-mediated thrombocytopenia that *is* associated with thrombosis. Treatment for HIT mandates the discontinuation of all forms of heparin and treatment with alternative anticoagulants such as argatroban or lepirudin.

Therapeutic anticoagulation with oral agents (as for the patient with atrial fibrillation) is typically interrupted during the perioperative period, when the risks of bleeding outweigh those of clotting. Patients at high risk for thrombosis or embolism may be started on IV heparin concurrently with discontinuation of oral anticoagulation. Heparin is then discontinued during the immediate operative and perioperative period and resumed as soon as the risk of bleeding from operative sites has abated, typically 12 hours following surgery. Oral anticoagulation can be resumed at the same time and heparin is discontinued when the prothrombin time international normalized ratio has reached the desired target level.

RENAL ISSUES IN THE POSTOPERATIVE ICU PATIENT

Acute renal failure (ARF) can increase the morbidity, mortality, and length of hospital stay in affected patients. In critically ill patients, the mortality associated with ARF ranges from 23% to 64% depending on the criteria used to define ARF. The incidence can range from 17.2%[45] to 24.7%[46] in critically ill patients. There are many precipitants for ARF in ICU patients, but in postoperative patients the most common are sepsis, ischemic acute tubular necrosis, drug-induced acute tubular necrosis, and pigment nephropathy, all of which are subgroups of acute tubular necrosis (ATN). ATN results from the injury and death of tubular epithelial cells that then slough off and obstruct the tubule, prompting the renal vasculature to constrict.

Common causes of ischemic ATN are cardiac arrest, hypotension from shock, and hypovolemia. The latter can occur postoperatively after large abdominal procedures with third space losses or vascular procedures with large fluid shifts. The treatment of ischemic ATN is to improve renal perfusion by increasing mean arterial BP with fluid administration for hypovolemic patients, the addition of vasoactive pressors to increase vascular tone in shock patients, or inotropes to improve cardiac function in patients with cardiac insufficiency.

- Drug-induced ATN is commonly caused by radiocontrast agents. Although the exact mechanism of injury is unknown, it is believed that contrast induces the production of free radicals that injure the nephron. Several studies have looked at ways to prevent ATN from radiocontrast agents. Tepel et al in 2000[47] showed that oral administration (pretreatment) of the antioxidant n-acetylcysteine actually decreased the serum creatinine in patients with chronic renal insufficiency. A 2004 study by Merten et al[48] showed that treatment with sodium bicarbonate before and after exposure to IV radiocontrast decreased the incidence of contrast-induced nephropathy when compared with a placebo infusion. Merten's hypothesis was that free radical production is increased in an acidic environment and that by raising the pH, the production of free radicals would be decreased. Other treatments such as mannitol and furosemide have been shown to be ineffective in preventing ATN.
- Dopamine has also been used to treat various causes of acute renal failure. Extensive research has shown that dopamine increases renal blood flow, glomerular filtration, and urine output. The rationale for the use of "renal dose" dopamine (1-3 μg/kg/min) stems from the hypothesis that increasing blood flow results in improved oxygen delivery to hypoxic areas of the kidney to help treat or prevent ATN. In 2001, Kellum and Decker[48] published a meta-analysis to determine whether low-dose dopamine decreased the incidence of acute renal failure, the need for dialysis, or the mortality in critically ill patients. They showed that dopamine did not significantly decrease the risk of mortality (relative risk [RR]: 0.83 [0.39-1.77]), development of acute renal failure (RR: 0.79 [0.54-1.13]), or the requirement for dialysis (RR: 0.89 [0.66-1.21]).

- Patients dependent on renal replacement therapy are defined as having acute renal failure or end-stage renal disease (ESRD). The ICU mortality of ESRD ranges from 11% to 40% in various studies.[40,50] It is interesting to note the ICU mortality associated with ESRD is less than the mortality associated with ARF. In a study by Clermont et al, ICU mortality was 5% for patients with no renal failure, 20.4% for patients with ARF without renal replacement therapy (RRT), 57% for patients with ARF requiring RRT, and 11% for patients with ESRD.[51]
- There is no consensus regarding the appropriate timing for initiation of RRT in the ICU. There are, however, some common indications for starting RRT: (1) excessive intravascular volume in a patient with ventilatory or hemodynamic compromise, (2) electrolyte abnormalities (ie, hyperkalemia), (3) metabolic acidosis, (4) hyperuremia, and (5) treatment for an overdose of a dialyzable toxin or drug. The dialysis techniques used most frequently in the ICU are intermittent hemodialysis (IHD) and continuous venovenous hemodialysis (CVVHD). Continuous arteriovenous dialysis and peritoneal dialysis were once prevalent but are no longer standard therapies. There are conflicting opinions concerning the comparative survival advantage of CVVHD versus IHD in acutely ill patients, and studies have shown no definitive advantage for either technique in critically ill patients. A retrospective study by Gangji, in 2005,[52] demonstrated that the use of CVVHD was associated with decreased mortality in the subgroup of patients with multiple organ dysfunction syndrome.

ENDOCRINE ISSUES IN THE POSTOPERATIVE ICU PATIENT

Postoperative patients have a complex endocrine response to surgical stress. The normal sympathetic response to surgery results in the release of epinephrine, glucagon, and cortisol to help repair injured tissue and fight off infection. However, critically ill postoperative patients often have an abnormal response to stress that leads to increased morbidity and mortality in the ICU. Tight glucose control and steroid replacement therapy have been used in the ICU to help decrease morbidity and mortality.

In 2001, van Den Berghe et al[53] studied the effects of intensive insulin therapy on critically ill postsurgical patients. The authors hypothesized that hyperglycemia during critical illness would increase the risk of severe infections, multiple organ failure, and death. They found that by maintaining glucose levels between 80 and 100 mg/dL, the risk of mortality in the ICU decreased by 32%. This observed risk reduction occurred in patients who stayed longer than 5 days in the ICU. A large subsequent meta-analysis, however, showed that "tight glucose control is not associated with significantly reduced hospital mortality but is associated with an increased risk of hypoglycemia."

Corticosteroid replacement therapy was first studied in 1952 when Fraser et al[54] described a patient with perioperative shock secondary to adrenal insufficiency. Cortisol is an endogenous corticosteroid that is produced by the adrenal glands. It is integral to the maintenance of vascular tone, vascular integrity, distribution of total body water, glucose metabolism, electrolyte homeostasis, catecholamine production and immunity, and many others In healthy patients during nonstress periods, plasma cortisol levels follow a circadian rhythm, increasing in the early morning and decreasing in the evening. After an operation, cortisol levels increase and the circadian rhythm disappears. Plasma cortisol concentrations normally reach their highest level during periods of severe stress (following burns, trauma, and sepsis).

When cortisol production is insufficient (eg, in patients suffering from Addison disease), the body appears to develop signs of shock (decreased SVR, decreased myocardial contractility, and decreased cardiac output) under the stresses of illness, surgery, or injury. In the postsurgical patient, as well as the critically ill patient, the incidence of total adrenal insufficiency is rare (2%-3%).[55] However, functional or relative adrenal insufficiency is common with an incidence of 30%.[56] The serum cortisol level fails to increase appropriately during stress states in patients with relative adrenal insufficiency. Steroid supplementation may be necessary for patients with functional adrenal insufficiency who develop shock that does not respond to volume resuscitation or vasopressors. A corticotrophin stimulation test can be used to determine the adrenal reserve, in which 250 µg of cosyntropin, a synthetic derivative of adrenocorticotrophic hormone, is given IV. Cortisol levels are then drawn at t_0, t_{30}, and t_{60} minutes. If the cortisol level 1 hour following "stimulation" is 9 µg/dL or less, the patient is considered a nonresponder.

Annane et al[57] published data showing that nonresponders have a decreased risk of death when given 50 mg of hydrocortisone every 6 hours and 50 µg of fludrocortisone daily for 7 days. However, in 2008, Sprung et al published a multicenter randomized, double-blinded, placebo-controlled trial to evaluate the safety and efficacy of hydrocortisone in patients who had a response to cosyntropin (The CORTICUS[58] [Corticosteroid Therapy of Septic Shock] trial). A total of 499 septic shock patients were randomized to receive 50 mg of hydrocortisone or a placebo. The study showed that there was no difference in mortality at 28 days between the 2 study groups or between cosyntropin responders and nonresponders. There was a subpopulation of patients with persistent hypotension unresponsive to vasopressors and fluids for whom hydrocortisone treatment was associated with decreased mortality.

Vasopressin, an endogenous endocrine hormone, is frequently used as an adjunct to catecholamines in the treatment of shock due to the evidence of its relative deficiency in septic patients.[59] The Vasopressin and Septic Shock trial (VASST)[61] was a multicenter randomized, double-blinded trial designed to compare low-dose vasopressin with norepinephrine to see if vasopressin conferred a mortality benefit in septic shock patients. A total of 778 septic shock patients were randomized to receive either low-dose vasopressin or norepinephrine titrated to a mean arterial pressure of 65 to 75 mm Hg. The study showed that there was no significant difference in 28- or 90-day mortality in either group. However, in patients with less severe septic shock (requiring 5-14 µg/kg/min of norepinephrine or its equivalent before randomization), the 28-day mortality was lower in the group treated with vasopressin.

PROPHYLAXIS AND PREVENTION BEST PRACTICES IN POSTOPERATIVE ICU PATIENTS

Nosocomial infections are major sources of morbidity and mortality in the ICU. Hospital-acquired infections result in increased ICU length of stay and health care costs. In a report from the Centers for Disease Control and Prevention (CDC) on nosocomial infection control, a third of all such complications may be preventable through rigorous infection control practices.[60] As this data has emerged, a series of best practice infection control measures have been developed including handwashing before and after examining patients, periodic surveillance of patients for antibiotic resistant organisms, co-location of patients infected with or colonized with antibiotic resistant organisms, and gowning and gloving when caring for patients with antibiotic-resistant organisms. In addition, the CDC recommends wearing a sterile gown, gloves and fully draping a patient when placing any invasive monitoring devices. Finally, the development of institutional antibiotic guidelines is important, and the guidelines will vary depending on the bacterial flora of a given institution.

The handwashing and barrier guidelines are designed to decrease the horizontal transmission of infections from health care worker to patient. Antibiotic guidelines are designed to help physicians choose the appropriate antibiotic therapy and length of therapy for a particular infectious disease and thereby decrease the inappropriate use of antibiotics and decrease the risk of developing antibiotic-resistant organisms. Other prophylactic measures that help decrease nosocomial

TABLE 79-9 Deep Venous Thrombosis Prophylaxis in At-Risk Populations

Level of Risk	Risk of DVT %	Risk of PE %	Antithrombotic Therapy
Low (eg, minor surgery in patients <40 y with no risk factors)	0.4-2	0.2	Ambulation only
Moderate (eg, minor surgery in patients with risk factors or age 40-60 y)	2-20	1-2	UH BID, LMWH daily, or ECS
High (eg, surgery in patients >60 y, major surgery in patients 40-60 y with risk factors)	8-40	2-4	UH TID, LMWH daily, IPC if anticoagulant contraindicated
Very high (eg, major surgery in patients >40 y with risk factors, major orthopedic surgery, neurosurgery, major trauma, or spinal cord injury)	20-80	4-10	LMWH daily plus ECS/IPC, or warfarin (INR 2-3)

DVT, deep venous thrombosis; ECS, elastic compression stockings; INR, international normalized ratio; IPC, intermittent pneumatic compression; LMWH, low molecular weight heparin; PE, pulmonary embolism; UH, unfractionated heparin.

Risk factors: prior venous thromboembolus, cancer, metabolic hypercoagulable state.

infection rates relate to central line placement and maintenance. The following measures have been shown to decrease catheter-related bloodstream infections: full barrier precautions during central line insertions, preparation of the insertion site with chlorhexidine,[62] and the use of single-lumen catheters rather than multilumen catheters when possible.[63]

Stress-related gastrointestinal mucosal damage occurs in many critically ill patients and may develop within 24 hours of ICU admission The incidence of clinically significant gastrointestinal bleeding with hemodynamic changes and a decreasing Hgb level due to stress ulceration has been estimated to be 1.5% in the ICU population. ICU stays are prolonged by an average of 8 days due to clinically significant bleeding, and mortality is increased 4-fold. Gastric hypoperfusion plays a major role in the pathogenesis of stress ulcers. Reduced gastric blood flow impairs the ability of gastric mucosal cells to regenerate and the consequent development of ulcers in the acid milieu of the stomach, but whereas gastric acidity may exacerbate stress ulcers, it does not cause them. Risk factors for stress ulcers in critically ill patients include major trauma, burns, respiratory failure, coagulopathy, hypotension, sepsis, hepatic failure, renal failure, and surgery. Prophylaxis is the preferred option for ICU patients at risk for stress ulcers. Therapies that have been shown to decrease the risk of stress ulceration include antacids, sucralfate, H2 blockers, and proton pump inhibitors. The goal of the therapies that alter gastric pH is maintenance of a gastric pH of 4.0 or greater,[64] whereas sucralfate binds to and protects ulcerated gastric tissue in the presence of acid and should not be used in combination with antacids.

Deep venous thrombosis (DVT) is a common complication in hospitalized patients, especially the critically ill. The risk of developing DVT in general surgery patients is 15% to 40%. Patients who have sustained major trauma, spinal cord injury, or who are critically ill have a risk as high as 80%. DVTs occur more frequently with increasing age, with an incidence of 200 per 100 000 in persons older than 70 years.[65] Clots formed in the deep venous system of the lower extremities may break away and migrate into the venous circuit, so prevention of DVTs decreases the risk of fatal pulmonary embolism. Prophylactic treatment also prevents the long-term sequelae of DVT including leg swelling, dermatitis, leg ulcers, and a decreased quality of life. Therapy for the prevention of DVT varies and has been stratified based on risk of acquiring a DVT. **Table 79-9** describes the thrombotic risk stratification for surgical patients and evidence-based guidelines for the use of antithrombotic prophylaxis.

CONCLUSIONS

Intensive care is a rapidly evolving specialty, particularly in the perioperative population. As new surgical procedures are developed, and as anesthesiologists are increasingly able to safely anesthetize patients at high risk such as the elderly, morbidly obese, and those with respiratory disease or severe heart failure, the demand for critical care services has escalated. Critical care specialists include anesthesia and surgery-based intensivists focusing on the care of patients in SICUs. Areas of subspecialization have emerged such as cardiothoracic critical care, neurocritical care transplant, burns, and trauma. As the promise of, and the demand for critical care services have increased, so has its expense. Modern intensivists must act as responsible stewards of these life-supporting, and sometimes merely life-prolonging, but highly expensive and in-demand ICU resources.

KEY REFERENCES

- Annane D, Sebille V, Charpentier C, et al. Effect of treatment with low doses of hydrocortisone and fludrocortisone on mortality in patients with septic shock.[see comment]. *JAMA.* 2002;288(7):862-871.
- Clearmont G. Renal failure in the ICU: comparison of the impact of acute renal failure and end-stage renal disease on ICU outcomes. *Kidney Int.* 2002;62:986-996.
- Hébert PC, Wells G, et al. A multicenter, randomized, controlled clinical trial of transfusion requirements in critical care. *N Engl J Med.* 1999;340(6):409-417.
- Hébert PC, Yetisir E, et al. Is low transfusion threshold safe in critically ill patients with cardiovascular diseases? *Crit Care Med.* 2001;29(2): 227-234.
- Mirski MA, Varelas PA. Diagnosis and treatment of seizures in the adult intensive care unit. *Cont Crit Care.* 2003;1(4):1-12.
- Society of Critical Care Medicine Ethics Committee. Consensus statement on the triage of critically ill patients. *JAMA.* 1994;271(15):1200-1203.
- van den Berghe G, Wouters P, et al. Intensive insulin therapy in the critically ill patients. *N Engl J Med.* 2001;345:1359-1367.

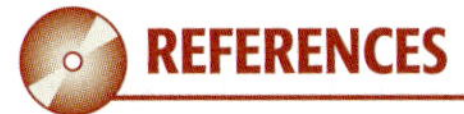

REFERENCES

Complete references available on DVD and online version at www.LongneckerAnesthesiology.com

CHAPTER 80 Hemodynamic Support of the Critically Ill Patient

Jean-Louis Vincent

KEY POINTS

1. Early and adequate resuscitation of patients with acute circulatory failure is important to restore the balance between oxygen needs and delivery. Effective resuscitation can result in improved outcomes.
2. Fluid resuscitation should be guided by repeated fluid challenges.
3. If fluid administration is insufficient to restore an adequate tissue perfusion pressure, vasopressors may be required; norepinephrine is currently considered the best first-line choice.
4. Inotropes or vasodilator drugs may be needed to improve myocardial contractility and cardiac output. Dobutamine remains the inotropic agent of choice.
5. Hemodynamic support should be titrated to the individual patient according to global parameters of hemodynamic and oxygenation status, supported by regional parameters when available.

INTRODUCTION

The most common cause of organ failure in the critically ill patient is inadequate tissue perfusion related to acute circulatory failure. This may result from persistent fluid deficits and/or alterations in regional blood flow or tissue oxygen utilization. Whatever the cause, early and adequate hemodynamic support of these patients is crucial if organ function is to be preserved and multiple organ failure, a common cause of death in critically ill patients, prevented. In this chapter, we briefly review the main causes and symptoms of acute circulatory failure before focusing on the hemodynamic support of such patients.

ACUTE CIRCULATORY FAILURE (SHOCK)

CLINICAL SIGNS OF SHOCK

Circulatory shock can be considered as a state of generalized circulatory failure resulting in tissue hypoxia. It is a major cause of organ failure. A diagnosis of shock can be based on a combination of various clinical, hemodynamic, and biochemical signs, which can broadly be summarized as follows:

1. *Arterial hypotension*: Hypotension is perhaps the hallmark of acute circulatory failure, but may be only moderate, especially in patients with chronic hypertension. Usually the systolic arterial pressure is less than 90 mm Hg or the mean arterial pressure is less than 70 mm Hg.
2. *Signs of tissue hypoperfusion*: These are usually recognized at 3 levels: (a) cutaneous: the skin is usually vasoconstricted, cold, and clammy; (b) renal: a reduction in renal perfusion is manifested in adults by a fall in urine output below 0.5 mL/kg/h and, in more severe cases, below 20 mL/kg/h; (c) neurologic: This can of course be appreciated only in the unanesthetized, unsedated patient. Decreased cerebral perfusion is demonstrated by an altered intellect, with disorientation and confusion, and lack of collaboration; there is often obtundation, but coma develops only in advanced stages of multiple organ failure.
3. *Biologic signs of altered cellular oxygen availability*: The development of anaerobic metabolism is manifest by the development of hyperlactatemia. The normal blood lactate level is around 1 mEq/L (or 1 mMol/L) but is usually increased above 1.5 mEq/L in acute circulatory failure.

PATHOPHYSIOLOGIC CLASSIFICATION OF SHOCK

Shock can essentially be classified according to 4 pathophysiologic mechanisms[1]: hypovolemic, cardiogenic, obstructive, or distributive. Many patients with acute circulatory failure have a combination of 2 or more of the 4 mechanisms. For example, a patient with severe pancreatitis may have characteristics of hypovolemic, distributive, and even cardiogenic shock. Similarly, patients with severe sepsis or anaphylaxis often have elements of hypovolemic and cardiogenic shock in addition to the baseline distributive mechanism.

Whatever the specific type of acute circulatory failure, the result is an imbalance between oxygen requirements and tissue oxygen availability, resulting in regional tissue hypoxia, an important contributor to the development of organ dysfunction and multiple organ failure. In hypovolemic, cardiogenic, and obstructive types of shock, the primary abnormality is the reduced cardiac output and hence inadequate oxygen transport. However, in septic shock, the main fault is increased oxygen requirements, due to the inflammatory response, in addition to altered oxygen extraction capabilities and myocardial contractility. Hence although cardiac output may be normal or even increased in such patients, it may still be inadequate to provide sufficient oxygen for the cells' increased requirements.

Hypovolemic Shock This form of shock occurs when the intravascular volume is depleted as a result of internal or external fluid loss. Hypovolemic shock is the most common form of circulatory shock. The most obvious cause of hypovolemic shock is acute hemorrhage, but it can also occur as a result of severe dehydration due to severe vomiting or diarrhea, particularly in children and the elderly. The hemodynamic pattern is characteristically one of a low cardiac output (due to reduced venous return), associated with decreased cardiac filling pressures and increased systemic vascular resistance (SVR).

Cardiogenic Shock This form of shock is characterized by primary failure of the cardiac pump. Cardiogenic shock is most commonly the result of acute myocardial infarction (MI), but other causes include severe cardiac valvular disease, severe myocarditis, end-stage cardiomyopathy, and severe cardiac arrhythmia. Cardiogenic shock is associated with mortality rates in the region of 75%, the highest of the 4 types of shock. Cardiogenic shock is characterized by a low cardiac output, increased cardiac filling pressures, and increased SVR.

Obstructive Shock This form of shock is the result of an impediment to the normal flow of blood, either due to an obstruction to the outflow of blood from the heart, such as in massive pulmonary embolism, severe aortic coarctation, or severe aortic stenosis, or due to an increased resistance to cardiac filling during diastole, such as in cardiac tamponade or tension pneumothorax. Obstructive shock is typically characterized by a low cardiac output and increased SVR. Right cardiac filling pressures are increased in pulmonary embolism, and right and left pressures are increased in tamponade. Pulmonary arterial hypertension is also present in cardiogenic shock associated with pulmonary embolism.

Distributive Shock This type of shock is characterized by an increase in the vascular capacity. It is most commonly due to sepsis, secondary to the release of inflammatory mediators. Other causes include anaphylactic shock, neurogenic shock, and acute adrenal insufficiency. The typical hemodynamic pattern is a normal or high cardiac output, reduced SVR (as vascular tone is reduced), and reduced cardiac filling pressures.

RESUSCITATION OF THE PATIENT WITH SHOCK

Intensive early resuscitation is essential to restore the imbalance between oxygen requirements and supply in the patient with acute circulatory failure, and therapy should be initiated while investigations are ongoing to determine and correct the underlying cause of the shock. Early resuscitation of patients with severe sepsis and septic shock has been shown to be associated with improved outcomes.[2]

A useful aid to describe the important steps of hemodynamic resuscitation is the VIP (ventilation, infusion, pump) rule introduced by Weil and Shubin in 1969.[3]

VENTILATORY SUPPORT

Oxygen should be started immediately with the aim of increasing oxygen delivery and reducing pulmonary vasoconstriction due to hypoxia. Importantly, oxygen should be administered even if the patient is not very hypoxemic. Although prolonged administration of high inspired oxygen fractions (Fio_2) can be toxic, this is not a problem in the acute situation, and once blood gas results are available, oxygen therapy can be adjusted accordingly. If mask ventilation is not possible (eg, due to facial trauma) or provides inadequate oxygenation, mechanical ventilation should be started. In addition to ensuring adequate oxygenation, mechanical ventilation has the additional benefit of reducing left ventricular afterload by increasing intrathoracic pressures, and resting the respiratory muscles, hence reducing oxygen requirements. The aim of oxygen administration should be to maintain Pao_2 above 8 kPa (60 mm Hg), and Sao_2 above 90%. Although hypoxia should be avoided, hyperoxia can also be harmful, causing peripheral vasoconstriction with reduced regional perfusion and oxygenation.

FLUID RESUSCITATION

Fluid therapy is an essential part of the treatment of any form of shock.[4] The rationale is to improve microvascular blood flow by increasing plasma volume, and to increase cardiac output by the Frank-Starling effect. However, too much fluid also carries risks, principally of pulmonary edema.

Which Fluid? Many fluids are available for use in resuscitation, and which, if any, is optimal remains controversial.[5] Crystalloid solutions (eg, normal saline, Ringer lactate) are inexpensive and well-tolerated, but these can have adverse effects when large volumes are infused. Infusion of large amounts of saline solutions typically results in hypernatremia and, notably, in hyperchloremic acidosis associated with a reduction in the strong ion difference.[6] Similarly, infusions of large amounts of the so-called balanced solutions (Ringer lactate, Hartmann solution) can influence electrolyte balance. Moreover, crystalloid solutions leak more into the interstitial space than colloid solutions, thus causing more tissue edema. Increased edema is associated with compromised lung function, reduced systemic oxygen availability, and impaired wound healing, myocardial function, and gut function (**Fig. 80-1**).[7,8] As colloids persist longer in the intravascular space, less colloid solution (eg, albumin, gelatin, hydroxyethyl starch [HES]) than crystalloid is needed to achieve the same hemodynamic goal, and colloids, therefore, have theoretical advantages over crystalloids. However, the clinical relevance of this potential advantage has not been clearly demonstrated, with no study convincingly demonstrating that one fluid type is superior to another. In addition, colloid solutions are more expensive, especially human albumin.

Although there has been some controversy surrounding the use of albumin in intensive care unit (ICU) patients,[9] the large randomized controlled Saline versus Albumin for Fluid Resuscitation in the Critically Ill (SAFE) study[10] showed no differences in mortality rates for ICU patients who received 4% albumin compared with those who received crystalloid solution as the initial resuscitation fluid. However, hypoalbuminemia is known to be associated with increased morbidity,[11] and albumin administration may reduce complications in critically ill patients.[12] In the SAFE study, there was a slight, but not significant, decrease in mortality in patients with hypoalbuminemia on admission who received albumin compared with those who received saline (23.7% vs 26.2%, odds ratio: 0.87; 95% confidence interval, 0.73-1.05; $p = 0.14$).[13] Clearly further studies assessing the role of albumin, particularly in certain subgroups of patients (eg, those with hypoalbuminemia) are needed to clarify this issue.

The 3 main types of artificial colloid are gelatin solutions, dextran solutions, and HES solutions. Gelatin solutions are not available in the United States but are still used elsewhere, largely because of their low costs. They have limited oncotic effects and relatively short intravascular persistence. These solutions can induce anaphylactic reactions, and adverse renal effects have been reported. Dextran solutions carry a substantial risk of anaphylactic reaction, so hapten prophylaxis must be given simultaneously. Dextrans also have antihemostatic effects, can cause formation

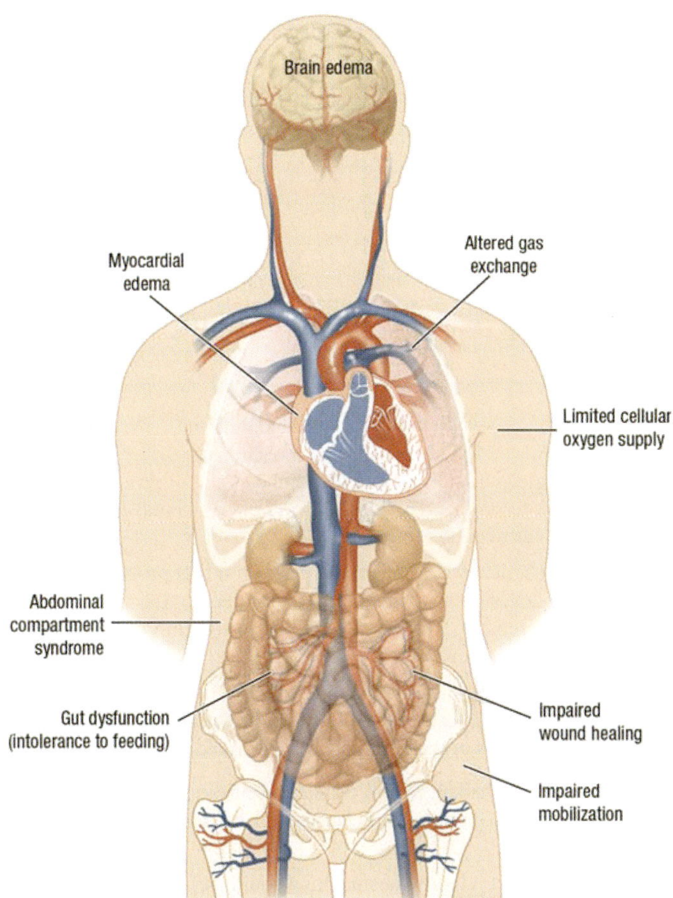

FIGURE 80-1. Some adverse effects of fluid overload and edema.

of "rouleaux," which may complicate the type and crossmatch in case of blood transfusions, and may precipitate renal failure. HES solutions have been promoted as having particularly beneficial effects on oxygen delivery to the tissues[7] and potentially reducing endothelial activation and inflammation in critically ill patients.[14] However, HES solutions have been associated with an increased incidence of acute renal failure in critically ill patients, particularly in those with severe sepsis.[15,16]

Further study is necessary to clearly define optimal fluid choices because all available fluids have advantages and disadvantages (**Table 80-1**). Until the results of such studies become available, the choice is best made according to the severity of the circulatory failure, the underlying disease, the type of fluid that has been lost, the serum albumin concentration of the patient, and the risk of bleeding. Using a combination of several fluids rather than excessive amounts of any one will help limit adverse effects.

How Much Fluid? Having selected the fluid, the physician must then decide how much to give. Precise end points for fluid resuscitation are difficult to define because sensitive tools for monitoring the regional microcirculation and oxygenation are not yet available, and, although systemic parameters may appear to have stabilized, regional tissue perfusion may still be inadequate.[17] In addition, the quantity of fluid needed varies among patients and in the same patient over time. A fluid challenge technique[18] is the best method of determining a patient's ongoing need for fluids. An example of the fluid challenge technique is provided in **Figure 80-2**. The fluid challenge approach incorporates 4 phases[18]:

- The type of fluid: As previously discussed, the optimal fluid remains controversial and either crystalloid or colloid can be used; the selection is determined on an individual patient basis.
- The rate of fluid administration: It is important to define the amount of fluid to be administered over a defined interval. The Surviving

TABLE 80-1 Comparative Effects of Different Fluid Types

	Crystalloids	Gelatins	Dextrans	Albumin	HES
Blood volume effect	+	++	+++	++++	++++
Edema formation	+++	++	+	+	+
Anti-inflammatory effect	–	–	–	++	+
Anaphylaxis	–	+	+++	–	+
Coagulopathy	–	–	++	+	+++
Renal failure	–	+	++	–	+++
Pruritus	–	–	–	–	++
Costs	–	+	++	++++	+++

Sepsis Campaign Guidelines for the management of severe sepsis and septic shock recommend at least 1000 mL of crystalloids or 300 to 500 mL of colloids over 30 minutes.[19]

- The goal to be achieved: The primary defect(s) that prompts the fluid challenge should be identified and quantitated so that a goal can be determined; most commonly this will be restoration of an adequate mean arterial pressure.
- Safety limits: Pulmonary edema due to congestive heart failure is the most serious complication of fluid infusion. A safety limit, generally the central venous pressure, must be set to avoid this complication.

Repeated fluid challenges will enable the physician to continuously reassess a patient's ongoing fluid needs and limit the risks of adverse effects.

Blood Transfusions Blood transfusions should be given as necessary, although there is again some debate as to what triggers should be used to determine the need for a blood transfusion. The aim of transfusion is to improve oxygen delivery and thereby to limit tissue hypoxia. However, although oxygen delivery is improved, tissue oxygenation or oxygen use do not necessarily increase.[20-22] In addition, risks are associated with blood transfusions including transmission of microorganisms and prions, transfusion-related acute lung injury (TRALI), transfusion-related immunomodulation, which may increase the risk of infections, and

EXAMPLE

Central venous catheter in situ
Problem = hypotension

Fluid challenge
1 – RL solution
2 – 1000 mL/30 min
3 – goal = MAP 75 mm Hg
4 – limit = CVP 15 mm Hg

	Baseline	+ 10 min	+ 20 min
MAP	65	70	75
CVP	12	13	14
Successful fluid challenge			
MAP	65	67	70
CVP	12	14	15
No need for further fluid administration		Continue	Stop

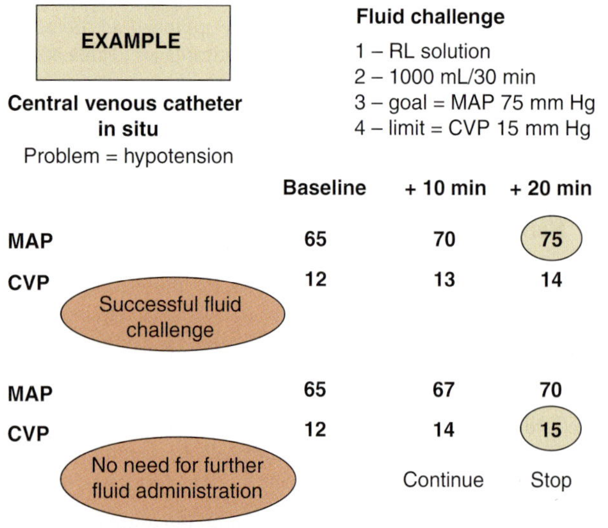

FIGURE 80-2. Example of a fluid challenge in a hypotensive patient. The figure gives an example of orders and 2 theoretical responses. In the first case, the patient benefited from fluid administration; in the second the patient did not. CVP, central venous pressure; MAP, mean arterial pressure; RL, Ringer lactate.

administration errors, including wrong type and crossmatch and incorrect patient identification, which can cause hemolytic reactions.

In 1999, Hebert et al[23] published the results of the Transfusion Requirements in Critical Care trial, which encouraged many to rethink their transfusion practice. This landmark study enrolled 838 critically ill patients with euvolemia who had hemoglobin concentrations of less than 9.0 g/dL and randomly assigned them to a restrictive strategy of transfusion, in which red cells were transfused if the hemoglobin concentration decreased below 7.0 g/dL, or a liberal strategy, in which transfusions were given when the hemoglobin concentration fell below 10.0 g/dL. The results suggested that the restrictive strategy, maintaining a hemoglobin of 7 to 9 g/dL, was adequate for most critically ill patients,[23] with the possible exception of patients with acute MI and unstable angina.[24]

Since that study, several epidemiologic studies have shown that patients who receive blood transfusions in the ICU have increased mortality rates.[25,26] In addition, studies in human volunteers have shown that isovolemic hemodilution to a hemoglobin of 5 g/dL or less does not result in biochemical evidence of anaerobic metabolism[27] and studies in Jehovah's Witness patients have shown that survival is possible with markedly decreased hemoglobin concentrations; one case study reported survival of a patient with a hemoglobin concentration of only 1.8 g/dL.[28]

Current recommendations for the management of patients with severe sepsis support a transfusion trigger of 7 g/dL.[19] However, the Sepsis Occurrence in Acutely ill Patients (SOAP) study, which evaluated data on 3147 patients in 198 ICUs across Europe in May 2002, reported that, unlike earlier studies, blood transfusion was not associated with an increased mortality in multivariate analysis or by propensity case matching.[29] In addition, the study by Rivers et al[2] on early goal-directed therapy (EGDT), showed that patients managed according to the EGDT protocol, who had lower mortality rates than patients receiving standard therapy, received more transfusions, suggesting that at least some patients may benefit from receiving more blood transfusions.

The pendulum would therefore seem to be swinging in favor of blood transfusions once again, and this apparent change may be related to the widespread introduction of leukoreduction in recent years. This technique is a process in which the white cells in blood units are intentionally reduced in number using centrifugation or filtration, with the aim of reducing some of the inflammatory response to transfusion and the transmission of infections. Leukocyte counts can be reduced by more than 99%, and the technique is effective in reducing the transmission of cell-associated viruses, especially cytomegalovirus, herpes viruses, and Epstein-Barr virus.[30] It may also reduce parasite and prion transmission, transfusion-related febrile reactions, and TRALI. In a before-after cohort study of 14 786 patients who received red blood cell transfusions following cardiac surgery or repair of hip fracture, or who required intensive care following a surgical intervention or multiple trauma, transfusion of leukoreduced blood was associated with fewer febrile reactions and reduced posttransfusion antibiotic use.[31] However, the evidence supporting the benefits of leukoreduction is not yet completely clear cut. In a meta-analysis of 14 randomized controlled trials comparing standard blood with leukoreduced or autologous blood, Vamvakas[32] reported no consistent effect of leukoreduction on long-term mortality, whereas in another meta-analysis of 10 randomized controlled trials, the authors concluded that "patients who were transfused leukoreduced red blood cells might benefit from a decrease in post-operative infections."[33] More recently, in a meta-analysis restricted to patients who received transfusions, Blumberg et al reported that leukoreduced blood significantly reduced the odds of postoperative infection by about 50%.[34] Many countries have now adopted leukoreduction as routine, although leukoreduced blood is more expensive, and it is not clear whether it is necessary in all patients.[35] (See Chapter 83 for a detailed discussion of blood transfusion.)

VASOPRESSORS

If hypotension persists despite fluid administration, the use of vasopressors will be required. In severe conditions, a vasopressor could be administered early in combination with fluids, but it should be discontinued as soon as the hypovolemia has been corrected.

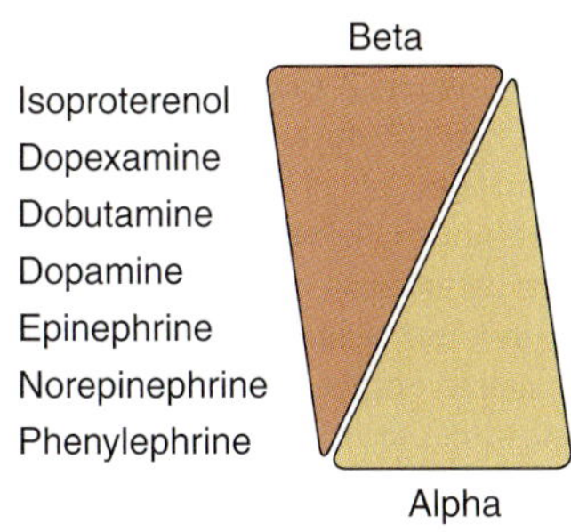

FIGURE 80-3. Various adrenergic agents available today, with schematic representation of their predominant effects on β- and α-adrenergic receptors.

Adrenergic agonists represent the first type of drug to be considered because of their potency and their short half-life, which allows easy titration. A range of drugs is available and can be considered for this purpose (**Fig. 80-3**). The specific effects of the various agonists are largely determined by the extent to which they act on α, β, and dopaminergic receptors (**Table 80-2**), although the precise action of any catecholamine varies among individuals. In addition, chronic sympathetic stimulation and the presence of inflammatory mediators, such as those that occur in sepsis, can reduce receptor response to stimulation.

There are 2 forms of α receptor: α_1, found primarily on the smooth muscle cells of arterioles and veins, and α_2, found at the presynaptic terminals of adrenergic nerves Stimulation of α_1 receptors usually causes smooth muscle contraction with vasoconstriction. Stimulation of α_2 receptors decreases the subsequent release of adrenergic transmitter.

There are 3 major forms of β receptor: β_1 found in heart muscle and in the kidney, β_2, found in smooth muscle and metabolic tissue, and β_3, found in adipose tissue. Stimulation of β_1 receptors results in increased heart rate and contractility, whereas β_2 receptor stimulation causes vasodilation in skeletal and cardiac muscle, bronchodilation, and decreased gastrointestinal motility. β_3 activation stimulates lipolysis.

Stimulation of each group of receptors therefore has potentially beneficial and potentially harmful effects. For example, β-adrenergic stimulation increases blood flow but can also increase heart rate and carry a risk of ischemia, whereas α-adrenergic stimulation increases blood pressure but may decrease cardiac output and cause peripheral vasoconstriction, with decreased renal and hepatosplanchnic blood flow.

Phenylephrine Although not a catecholamine, phenylephrine is an almost pure α-adrenergic agent, except at very high doses where some β activity is seen. Phenylephrine is a very powerful vasoconstrictor, but this carries the risk of decreasing blood flow and reducing tissue perfusion. In patients with septic shock, phenylephrine was associated with reduced splanchnic blood flow and oxygen delivery.[36] However, a small randomized controlled trial reported no differences in terms of cardiopulmonary performance, global oxygen transport, or regional hemodynamics when phenylephrine was administered instead of norepinephrine in the initial hemodynamic support of septic shock.[37]

TABLE 80-2 Comparative Effects of the Common Adrenergic Agents on α, β, and Dopaminergic Receptors

	α	β_1	β_2	Dopaminergic
Phenylephrine	+++	0	0	0
Epinephrine	+++	+++	++	0
Norepinephrine	+++	++	+	0
Dopamine	++	++	+	+++
Dobutamine	+	+++	+	0
Isoproterenol	0	+++	+++	0
Dopexamine	0	+	+++	++

Nevertheless, in the ICU, this drug is currently reserved for the occasional management of severe refractory hypotension.

Epinephrine Epinephrine is an endogenous catecholamine secreted by the adrenal medulla with potent α and β_1 activity and moderate β_2 effects. At lower doses, β effects predominate with α effects becoming more significant at higher doses. In acute hypotension, epinephrine is sometimes preferred to norepinephrine due to its stronger β-adrenergic effects that are useful to maintain or increase cardiac output. It is also the drug of choice in cardiac arrest, where it can be administered via the endotracheal tube if intravenous (IV) access is difficult, and in acute anaphylaxis (0.1-0.5 mg subcutaneously). However, epinephrine is associated with a decrease in splanchnic blood flow or gastric intramucosal pH (pHi).[38,39] Epinephrine treatment is also associated with an increase in cellular metabolism mediated by the increase in intracellular cyclic adenosine monophosphate (cyclic AMP) and leading to increased blood lactate levels.[38,40] A study comparing epinephrine with norepinephrine in patients with shock reported no differences in outcomes between the 2 groups, although epinephrine was associated with the development of significant tachycardia, lactic acidosis, and increased insulin requirements for the first 24 hours of the study, which resulted in withdrawal of 13% of the patients from the study.[40] Epinephrine is therefore best avoided in critically ill patients except in the specific circumstances mentioned here, but in countries where more expensive vasopressors are not available, epinephrine represents a reasonable alternative.

Norepinephrine Norepinephrine is an endogenous amine secreted by the adrenal medulla and the terminal endings of postganglionic nerve fibers. Norepinephrine has predominantly α-adrenergic properties, although its weak β-adrenergic effects can help to maintain cardiac output. Norepinephrine administration thus generally results in a clinically significant increase in mean arterial pressure, with little change in heart rate or cardiac output. The normal dose-range is 0.05 to 2 μg/kg/min IV. The increased afterload due to the vasoconstriction caused by norepinephrine can increase myocardial workload, and norepinephrine can precipitate cardiac failure, myocardial ischemia, and pulmonary edema. Although there have been concerns that excessive vasoconstriction with norepinephrine may have negative effects on blood flow, particularly in the hepatosplanchnic and renal circulations, studies have suggested that it can successfully increase blood pressure without causing any deterioration in organ function, particularly in the presence of decreased vascular tone, as in septic shock.[39,41]

Dopamine Dopamine is another naturally occurring compound (the precursor of norepinephrine) which also combines α- and β-adrenergic properties, but it has several specific features. First, dopamine also has dopaminergic effects, which predominate at very low doses (<3 mcg/kg/min IV), and may dilate the hepatosplanchnic and renal circulations, thereby selectively increasing flow in these important regions. Second, the adrenergic effects of dopamine vary with the dose; at lower doses (3-10 mcg/kg/min IV), β-adrenergic effects predominate, so that blood flow may increase together with blood pressure. At higher doses, α-adrenergic effects become increasingly powerful, which may be necessary in more severe cases of hypotension. Importantly, these dose ranges are not cutoff values at which one set of receptors are activated at the expense of another, but are ranges in which the effects of one group of receptors predominate over another. Dopamine increases arterial pressure primarily by increasing cardiac index, due to an increase in stroke volume and, to a lesser extent, to increased heart rate, with minimal effects on SVR. However, dopamine also has drawbacks. First, it is a relatively weak agent, so that norepinephrine or epinephrine must often be added to control hypotensive states. Second, although dopamine may increase blood flow more effectively than other vasopressors, it also increases heart rate. A study in patients undergoing coronary artery bypass grafting with cardiopulmonary bypass suggested that dopamine, even at low doses, is associated with an increased risk of developing atrial fibrillation.[42] Third, the advantage of the dopaminergic effects may be more theoretical than practical. Thus the routine administration of low dose dopamine to prevent renal failure is not recommended.[43] Finally, dopaminergic stimulation may have undesired endocrine effects on the hypothalamopituitary axis, resulting in immunosuppressant effects, primarily by a reduction in prolactin release.[44]

In a recent randomized trial, there were no overall significant differences in mortality rates between patients in shock who were treated with dopamine or norepinephrine as the first-line vasopressor agent, but the use of dopamine was associated with a greater number of adverse events, notably arrhythmias.[45] In subgroup analyses, dopamine administration was associated with increased 28-day mortality rates in patients with cardiogenic shock. It would thus seem reasonable to recommend norepinephrine rather than dopamine as the first-line vasopressor in patients with shock.

Vasopressin and Terlipressin Vasopressin is an endogenous stress hormone with a wide range of functions including effects on blood osmolality and volume, body temperature, insulin release, corticotropin release, memory, and social behavior; as a vasoconstrictor of vascular smooth muscle, it also has an important role in regulating blood pressure.[46,47] Patients with septic shock appear to develop relative vasopressin deficiency, with lower vasopressin levels than patients with cardiogenic shock for the same degree of hypotension.[48] This deficiency may be due, in part, to decreased central stores of vasopressin,[49] and administration of low-dose vasopressin to restore normal vasopressin levels can result in substantial increases in arterial pressure and reduced requirements for other catecholamines.[48,50-55] The 2008 VASST study showed that a combination of low-dose vasopressin and norepinephrine was as safe as norepinephrine alone in the treatment of patients with septic shock.[55] Further, the benefit of vasopressin compared with norepinephrine was greater in a subgroup of patients at risk of renal dysfunction, with a 28-day mortality reduction of 43.7% ($p = 0.01$), but not in those with more advanced renal dysfunction. These results suggest that vasopressin administration should perhaps be administered early in hyperkinetic states of septic shock.[56] Interestingly, in a post hoc analysis of this study, patients who received corticosteroids and vasopressin had reduced mortality rates compared with those who received norepinephrine, whereas in patients who did not receive corticosteroids, vasopressin was associated with increased mortality compared with norepinephrine.[57]

Vasopressin has also been assessed in patients with other forms of vasodilatory shock (eg, after cardiopulmonary bypass). In such patients, administration of low doses of vasopressin increased arterial blood pressure and reduced vasopressor requirements.[58,59] Interestingly, Morales et al[60] found that giving vasopressin (0.03 U/min IV) prophylactically before cardiopulmonary bypass to avoid vasopressin deficiency resulted in reduced requirements for norepinephrine and a shorter ICU length of stay, again suggesting that early use may be beneficial.

Vasopressin has also been investigated as a potential alternative to epinephrine for use in cardiorespiratory arrest. A randomized controlled study of vasopressin versus epinephrine in in-hospital cardiac arrest reported no advantage of vasopressin over epinephrine,[61] although a later, larger study comparing the 2 agonists in out-of-hospital cardiac arrest suggested improved outcomes for patients with asystole who received vasopressin.[62] Although a cohort study suggested that a combination of epinephrine and vasopressin may be better, providing the beneficial effects of both drugs but avoiding the harmful effects of excessive doses of either,[63] a randomized study in 2894 patients showed that the combination of vasopressin (40 units) and epinephrine (1 mg) was no better than epinephrine alone.[64] The risk with vasopressin is a reduction in cardiac output due to excessive vasoconstriction and a selective reduction in hepatosplanchnic blood flow. Studies are in progress to further evaluate the role of vasopressin in various shock states.

Terlipressin is an analog of vasopressin that has been available in Europe for more than 20 years. Terlipressin has a half-life of 6 hours and a duration of action of 2 to 10 hours, whereas the half-life of vasopressin is 6 minutes and its duration of action is 30 to 60 minutes. Terlipressin has been compared with norepinephrine in patients with hyperdynamic septic shock. Both drugs increased mean arterial blood pressure and improved renal function, but terlipressin administration was associated with a decrease in cardiac output.[65] The DOBUPRESS study reported that dobutamine administration could reverse terlipressin-induced reductions in cardiac output and SvO_2 but high doses of dobutamine were needed; nevertheless, no adverse effects associated with the high doses were reported.[66] The 2009 TERLIVAP study, which tested the efficacy and safety of continuous infusions of terlipressin, vasopressin, or norepinephrine in septic shock patients, suggested that terlipressin may be more efficient than vasopressin for shock reversal with no increased incidence of undesirable effects.[67] The ongoing TESST-1 (TErlipressin in Septic Shock Trial) is comparing terlipressin at low (2 mcg/kg/min) and ultralow dose (1 mcg/kg/min) to norepinephrine as a first-line agent in septic shock. Terlipressin may also be useful for the treatment of hypotension occurring after induction of anesthesia in patients who have received long-term treatment with renin-angiotensin system inhibitors.[68]

RESTORING AND MAINTAINING CARDIAC OUTPUT

An adequate cardiac output is essential to ensure sufficient tissue perfusion and oxygen delivery. However, a normal cardiac output is difficult to define, and the adequacy of cardiac output varies among individuals and in the same individual over time. To increase cardiac output, one must remember its 4 determinants (**Fig. 80-4**).[69]

- Heart rate: Bradycardia can limit cardiac output, but only when severe, and this is therefore easily recognized at the bedside. The management of bradycardia is beyond the scope of this chapter, but the principles of treatment consist primarily of a pacemaker, possibly with isoproterenol as a temporary measure. Outside these extreme situations, increasing heart rate by changing the rate of an in situ pacemaker usually does not increase cardiac output because stroke volume decreases concurrently. It may even be the opposite: Cardiac output may decrease if cardiac filling is impaired by a too short diastolic time, especially in cases of diastolic dysfunction.
- Preload: Fluid administration should be considered in all cases of inadequate cardiac output, and if uncertain of the need for fluid, a fluid challenge technique must be used as described earlier, in which a given amount of fluids is given rapidly under control of cardiac filling pressures.[18]

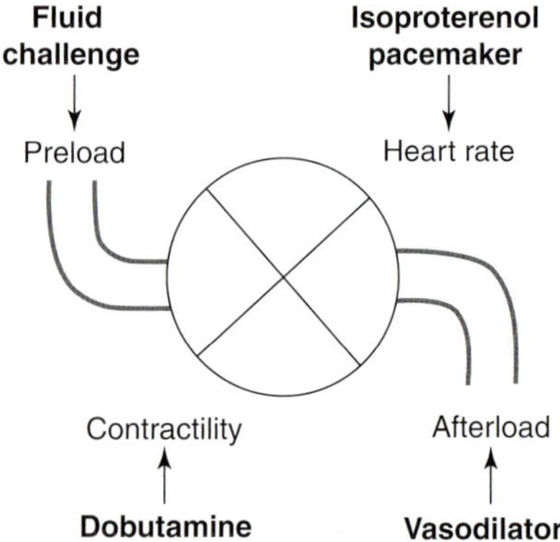

FIGURE 80-4. Various options to increase cardiac output, based on its 4 determinants.

- Contractility: If the increase in cardiac output is limited by impaired contractility, the use of inotropes may be considered. The major risk is increased oxygen demand due to the increased work of the myocardium, which may precipitate myocardial ischemia.
- Afterload: By reducing the factors that oppose ejection of blood by the ventricles, principally using vasodilators, cardiac output may be increased without increasing myocardial oxygen demand. The major limitation of this approach is the risk of decreasing arterial pressure to levels that may compromise tissue perfusion in the peripheral organs as well as in the myocardium, and vasodilators should be avoided in hypotensive states. In addition, all vasodilators may induce some increase in heart rate, especially in the presence of underlying hypovolemia. Such an increase in heart rate should raise the possibility of underlying hypovolemia and suggest the need for a fluid challenge.

Dobutamine Dobutamine is the first choice of inotropic agent for patients with low cardiac output who have received adequate fluid resuscitation. A decrease in arterial pressure during dobutamine administration should raise the possibility of underlying fluid deficits requiring another fluid challenge trial. With predominant β-adrenergic properties, dobutamine also possesses some α-adrenergic effects that limit the increase in heart rate seen with pure β-adrenergic stimulation using isoproterenol. An initial dose of just a few mcg/kg/min may increase cardiac output significantly. Doses in excess of 20 mcg/kg/min IV are seldom used because they add little benefit and may lead to excessive tachycardia. Dobutamine has limited effects on arterial pressure, although arterial pressure may increase slightly if heart failure is the primary abnormality. Dobutamine formed part of the EGDT protocol used by Rivers et al in their study of emergency department patients presenting with septic shock.[2] Dobutamine was used in addition to fluids and red cell transfusion to increase central venous oxygen saturation ($ScvO_2$) to more than 70%, and this protocol was associated with improved outcomes compared with standard care.[2] However, dobutamine should not routinely be used to increase oxygen delivery to supranormal levels because this approach has been associated with worse outcomes.[70] Rather it should be titrated on an individual basis to achieve acceptable oxygenation parameters. Interestingly, using orthogonal polarization spectral imaging, DeBacker et al showed that dobutamine improved capillary perfusion in patients with septic shock, independent of its systemic effects,[17] suggesting that it may have additional specific effects on regional blood flow.

Dopexamine Dopexamine hydrochloride is a newer synthetic catecholamine, structurally similar to dopamine. It has marked β_2-adrenergic agonist activity, some dopaminergic receptor activity, weak β_1-adrenergic activity, and no direct α-adrenergic effects. It also inhibits the neuronal uptake of endogenous catecholamines. Dopexamine's positive inotropic effects combined with its vasodilating effects make it useful in acute exacerbations of chronic heart failure and in heart failure associated with cardiac surgery. However, its use is limited by the development of marked tachycardia, particularly at higher doses. Although it was suggested that because of its dopaminergic effects it may have beneficial effects on renal and splanchnic blood flow, a meta-analysis of 21 randomized controlled studies found no evidence to support the use of dopexamine to improve hepatosplanchnic or renal blood flow in critically ill patients.[71]

Phosphodiesterase Inhibitors The phosphodiesterase inhibitors (PDEs) are a group of enzymes that degrade the cyclic nucleotides cAMP and cGMP. PDE inhibitors can thus prolong or enhance the effects of physiologic processes mediated by cAMP or cGMP. PDE3 inhibitors, such as enoximone and milrinone, have inotropic and vasodilating properties. These drugs may be poorly tolerated by patients with arterial hypotension, and their administration can be difficult due to their long half-life. Intermittent administration may be preferable to continuous infusion. The administration of very small doses of PDEIII inhibitors may reinforce the effects of dobutamine.[72] Short-term administration of PDEIII inhibitors has been associated with a high incidence of complications, including arrhythmias, especially in patients with ischemic heart disease, likely related to their effects on cAMP and Ca^{2+} levels. Dobutamine and milrinone provided equally effective inotropic support in patients awaiting cardiac transplantation with no differences in right heart hemodynamics, death, need for additional vasodilator/inotropic therapy, need for mechanical cardiac support before transplantation, or occurrence of ventricular arrhythmias requiring increased antiarrhythmic therapy. In critically ill patients with catecholamine-dependent heart failure, milrinone improved central hemodynamics and was associated with a reduction in dobutamine dose, although there was a tendency for milrinone-treated patients to require higher doses of vasopressors and more fluids.[73] Some studies have suggested that milrinone may have additional anti-inflammatory effects and beneficial effects on hepatosplanchnic perfusion.[74,75] Further studies are clearly needed to determine the exact place of these drugs in the management of patients with severe heart failure and shock.

Levosimendan Levosimendan is a relatively new agent that provides inotropic effects by increasing calcium sensitivity of myocytes by binding to cardiac troponin-C, and vasodilator effects by opening ATP-sensitive potassium channels in vascular smooth muscle.[76] Levosimendan has a long half-life that may limit the practicality of its use. Levosimendan may be useful in patients with severe heart failure, where it has been shown to improve hemodynamic performance more effectively than dobutamine and to reduce mortality.[77,78] It may also be of use for inotropic support after myocardial ischemia, after myocardial stunning, during and after cardiac surgery, and in patients with right ventricular dysfunction.[76,79] However, its place in acutely ill patients has not been well studied and remains poorly defined. In addition, the high costs of the drug limit its use. Several large phase 3 studies are ongoing to assess the use of levosimendan in various conditions.

Sodium Nitroprusside Sodium nitroprusside has a direct, short-acting relaxing effect on vascular smooth muscle and has been used primarily to reduce afterload, although by reducing venous return it also reduces preload. It has significant effects on arterial pressure, so that it is also used in the management of hypertensive crises. Sodium nitroprusside has the advantage of a short half-life, allowing easy titration. Administration should start at 20 mcg/min IV, and the dose can be progressively increased to 150 to 200 mcg/min. The administration of nitroprusside is complicated by the fact that it is very light sensitive, so that infusion sets must be opaque. Nitroprusside is rapidly metabolized to cyanide and thiocyanate, and accumulation of these metabolites can lead to cyanide or thiocyanate toxicity during prolonged administration, especially in patients with renal failure.

Nitrates Nitrate products include nitroglycerin or isosorbide dinitrate. They again cause relaxation of vascular smooth muscle and hence reduce afterload. Low doses (30-40 mcg/min IV) predominantly produce venodilatation; high doses (150-500 mcg/min) lead to arteriolar dilatation as well. These drugs are widely used IV in the treatment of recurrent ischemia, hypertensive emergencies, and congestive heart failure associated with MI. Nitroglycerin is the preferred vasodilator in acute MI, especially when infarction is complicated by congestive heart failure.[80] Nitrates are also indicated in patients with cardiogenic pulmonary edema for their strong relieving effects on venous congestion. Their dose is similar to that of nitroprusside.

Angiotensin-Converting Enzyme Inhibitors Angiotensin-converting enzyme (ACE) catalyses the conversion of angiotensin I to angiotensin II, a potent vasoconstrictor, and it is also involved in the inactivation of bradykinin, a potent vasodilator. ACE inhibitors therefore cause reduced formation of angiotensin II and increased levels of bradykinin, thus reducing vascular resistance. ACE inhibitors are widely used in the treatment of chronic heart failure and may be helpful in the acute care setting as well. However, they have 2 limitations in the acute setting. One is the risk of renal failure that can be precipitated by ACE inhibition especially in the presence of fluid shifts that may result in relative hypovolemia. The second is the lack of availability of an IV preparation. Enalapril is available as the only parenteral preparation, but its administration results in marked decreases in arterial pressure, so its use is very limited.

Hydralazine In contrast to nitrates, hydralazine has greater effects on the arteriolar side of the vasculature and is therefore more likely to increase cardiac output by decreasing SVR. It also increases heart rate, so may be useful in patients with a relatively slow heart rate. Its use requires close cardiovascular monitoring. Long-term administration may be complicated by the development of iatrogenic lupus. Hence hydralazine is not often prescribed today for prolonged therapy of heart failure because there are other drugs with a better benefit-to-risk ratio. However, it can still be considered as an alternative to ACE inhibitors in patients with heart failure.

END POINTS AND GOALS OF HEMODYNAMIC SUPPORT

INDICES OF GLOBAL PERFUSION

Mean Arterial Pressure Arterial hypotension represents a marker of serious disease, and a systolic pressure of less than 90 mm Hg (or a mean arterial pressure less than 70 mm Hg) or a decrease in mean arterial pressure greater than 30 mm Hg are indications of acute circulatory failure. Noninvasive measurement of blood pressure with the sphygmomanometer is perhaps one of the most widely used procedures in clinical medicine. However, in critically ill patients, especially those with significant hypotension, invasive intra-arterial monitoring of pressure is more accurate and continuous,[81] allowing rapid assessment of response to treatments.

Cardiac Output A so-called normal cardiac output is difficult to define because what is normal or adequate may vary widely among patients and even in the same patient over time.[69] For example, one cardiac output value may be perfectly adequate for an anesthetized, mechanically ventilated patient but inadequate should that same patient develop severe sepsis with increased oxygen requirements. The measurement of cardiac output provides an assessment of global systemic blood flow but provides no information on regional flow. Cardiac output can be judged inadequate when tissue perfusion is altered, as shown clinically by cutaneous vasoconstriction, decreased urine output attributed to kidney underperfusion, or altered mental status. Biochemical signs of reduced tissue perfusion include decreased SvO_2 or its surrogate, $ScvO_2$, or increased blood lactate concentrations (see later).

Cardiac output can be measured using various techniques, each of which has its own benefits and drawbacks. For many years, the thermodilution cardiac output measured using a pulmonary artery catheter (PAC) was the gold standard, but with concerns about the safety and overall benefits with PAC insertion and use,[82] less invasive techniques, including echocardiography and Doppler measurements, pulse contour analysis, partial carbon dioxide rebreathing, and electrical bioimpedance, are being used more commonly. Nevertheless, although the PAC is not indicated in all patients, it remains valuable in more complex cases, allowing almost continuous measurement not only of cardiac output, but also of other important parameters including cardiac filling pressures and SvO_2. Accurate absolute measures of cardiac output are perhaps less important than monitoring the trends in cardiac output in response to treatment and time, and if one wants to define the adequacy of cardiac output accurately, measures of SvO_2 are essential.[83] Importantly, targeting predefined cardiac output values for all patients or even for groups of patients is not advisable because adequacy of cardiac output varies among patients and in the same patient over time.

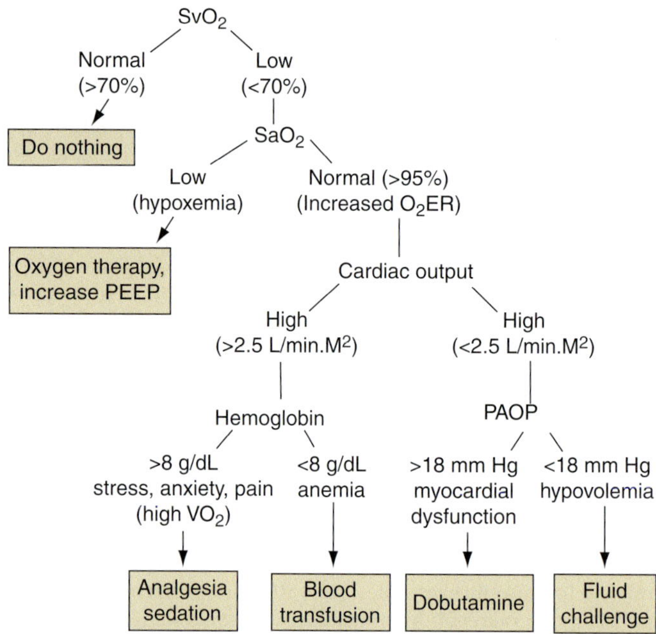

FIGURE 80-5. Diagnostic algorithm based on mixed venous oxygen saturation (SvO_2) measurements: Potential therapeutic options to be considered are presented in the rectangles. SaO_2, arterial oxygen saturation; O_2ER, oxygen extraction ratio; PEEP, positive end-expiratory pressure; PAOP, pulmonary artery occlusion pressure; VO_2, oxygen consumption. [Reproduced from Pinsky MR, Vincent JL. Let us use the PAC correctly and only when we need it. *Crit Care Med.* 2005;33: 1119-1122. With permission.]

Mixed Venous Oxygen Saturation SvO_2 can be measured using a PAC. The normal value is 70% to 75%. SvO_2 depends on cardiac output, oxygen demand, hemoglobin, and arterial oxygen saturation. Measurements of SvO_2 are very useful for the correct interpretation of cardiac output (**Fig. 80-5**). SvO_2 is typically decreased in low flow states, but normal or high in inflammatory conditions.

$ScvO_2$, measured in the superior vena cava using a central venous catheter, may represent a useful surrogate for patients who do not require a PAC. However, it must be remembered that as $ScvO_2$ reflects the oxygenation of the venous blood from the upper half of the body and not of the lower half of the body, it is an estimate of the true SvO_2, which measures whole body venous oxygen saturation. Physiologically, $ScvO_2$ is slightly less than SvO_2, but in critically ill patients it is often greater. This effect is explained by increased oxygen extraction in the kidneys (where blood flow is often reduced) and in the gut (where oxygen consumption is often increased), whereas oxygen extraction in the liver is more constant. A study has suggested that early therapy in patients with severe sepsis or septic shock targeting an $ScvO_2$ of 70% or higher may be associated with improved outcomes.[2] As with many other parameters, trends in $ScvO_2$ over time are of more use than individual values, and values must be interpreted in the light of clinical assessment and other hemodynamic and oxygenation parameters.

Blood Lactate Levels Blood lactate levels provide a useful indication of the presence of anaerobic metabolism due to hypoperfusion, and, although changes in blood lactate levels occur too slowly to guide therapy, nevertheless repeating measurements every hour or so can provide useful information on the ongoing adequacy of global tissue oxygenation. In patients with sepsis, the interpretation of blood lactate levels is not always straightforward, in that increased lactate levels may result from cellular metabolic failure as well as global hypoperfusion. However, the prognostic value of increased blood lactate levels is well established in septic shock patients, particularly if the high levels persist.[84]

INDICES OF REGIONAL PERFUSION

Although measurement and monitoring of cardiac output, SvO_2, and blood lactate levels provide valuable information regarding global adequacy or perfusion and oxygenation, they do not provide detail on the adequacy of regional microcirculatory blood flow or oxygen delivery and utilization, which is believed to be a crucial factor in the development of multiple organ failure in patients with shock. Measuring regional parameters is of particular importance because they can remain inadequate even when global parameters have returned to normal. However, although considerable progress is being made in this field, there is as yet no ideal technique that can be used in critically ill patients to assess regional blood flow or oxygenation.

Gut Tonometry The measurement of regional perfusion initially focused on the hepatosplanchnic circulation because this is particularly sensitive to changes in blood flow and oxygenation, and it may have a higher critical oxygen delivery threshold than other organs. Gastric tonometry was introduced to monitor gastric pHi, but this technique is limited by measurement errors and can be unreliable during patient feeding.[85] Calculations of pHi were replaced by gastric mucosal Pco_2 because this measure is not confounded by arterial bicarbonate, but because gastric mucosal Pco_2 is influenced by systemic arterial Pco_2, the gastric-arterial Pco_2 difference may be of more interest.[86] An early trial suggested that tonometry-derived parameters may be useful in guiding therapy,[87] but these findings were not confirmed in a later study,[88] and many investigators have emphasized the limited sensitivity, and especially specificity, of these measurements. Different vasoactive agents have been shown to have divergent effects on Pco_2 and pHi that are neither consistent nor predictable.[89]

Sublingual Capnography The methodological limitations of gastric tonometry encouraged researchers to look elsewhere for another easily accessible tissue where local Pco_2 could be measured, and the sublingual circulation has been suggested for this purpose. Several clinical studies have suggested that sublingual Pco_2 ($Pslco_2$) is a reliable marker of tissue hypoperfusion. However, as with gut Pco_2, $Pslco_2$ may also be influenced by arterial carbon dioxide and the gradient (ie, gap) between $Pslco_2$ and $Paco_2$ may be more specific for tissue hypoperfusion.[90] In a recent study, the sublingual Pco_2 gap was found to correlate with the alterations in microcirculatory blood flow seen in patients with severe sepsis.[91] Further work is clearly needed to define normal and pathologic sublingual Pco_2 levels and to establish whether targeting treatments to restore a normal sublingual Pco_2 can improve outcomes.

Microcirculatory Imaging The development of handheld orthogonal polarization spectral (OPS)/sidestream dark field (SDF) imaging techniques is providing a new means of directly visualizing the microcirculation and evaluating the effects of interventions on microcirculatory flow in easily accessible epithelial surfaces, such as the sublingual area.[92] Microcirculatory changes have been identified in various disease processes including sepsis, cardiogenic shock, heart failure, and after cardiac surgery.[93,94] The observed alterations include decreased capillary density and a reduced proportion of perfused capillaries, and increased heterogeneity of blood flow; persistent alterations are associated with worse outcomes.[95] Various therapeutic interventions have been shown to have an impact on the microcirculatory changes, but further studies are needed to determine whether therapy guided by OPS/SDF monitoring can improve outcomes.

Near-infrared Spectroscopy Near-infrared spectroscopy (NIRS) is a technique that uses near-infrared light to measure chromophores (oxy- and deoxyhemoglobin, myoglobin, and cytochrome aa3) in tissues. The tissue oxygen saturation (StO_2) is calculated from the fractions of oxy- and deoxyhemoglobin. However, the StO_2 represents the sum of oxygen saturations in the volume under the probe and can be unreliable in conditions of heterogeneous flow. Analysis of the changes in StO_2 during a brief episode of forearm ischemia enables quantification of microvascular dysfunction.[96] Again, recent studies have shown that patients with severe sepsis frequently have profound alterations in NIRS-derived dynamic variables and that these alterations are associated with a poor outcome.[97] Further studies are again needed to determine whether therapy guided by NIRS can improve outcomes.

CONCLUSION: THE GLOBAL PICTURE

Multiple organ failure is a serious problem in ICU patients, resulting in high morbidity and mortality and associated resource use and costs. Multiple organ failure can arise from many causes, but a key factor in its development appears to be an imbalance between tissue oxygen requirements and uptake. Tissue oxygen uptake can be limited by inadequate oxygen delivery and availability, and also by altered oxygen extraction ability. Appropriate hemodynamic support can improve both global and regional blood flow, and hence oxygen delivery. Early studies suggested that those patients with greater cardiac index and oxygen delivery values were more likely to survive conditions associated with the development of multiple organ failure.[98,99] This observation was the rationale behind several studies in the early 1990s, which assessed the benefits of increasing oxygen delivery to supranormal values using inotropes and fluids. Although this approach was shown to improve outcomes in some groups of critically ill patients, notably surgical and trauma patients,[100,101] routine application to all critically ill patients does not confer a uniform survival benefit and may worsen outcomes in some patients.[70,102] However, a protocol targeting adequate oxygen transport as reflected by the $ScvO_2$, in patients at risk of multiple organ failure, has been shown to result in improved survival,[2] and adequate oxygenation clearly remains an important parameter to target. Unfortunately, at present there is no clear marker of adequate tissue oxygenation, and we must therefore rely on surrogate markers of tissue perfusion and oxygenation as discussed earlier. Adequate oxygen delivery is likely to vary among patients and in the same patient over time, so that hemodynamic support must be titrated and adjusted carefully based on each individual's response to the therapy.

KEY REFERENCES

- Dellinger RP, Levy MM, Carlet JM, et al. Surviving Sepsis Campaign: international guidelines for management of severe sepsis and septic shock: 2008. *Crit Care Med.* 2008;36: 296-327.
- Hollenberg SM, Ahrens TS, Annane D, et al. Practice parameters for hemodynamic support of sepsis in adult patients: 2004 update. *Crit Care Med.* 2004;32(9):1928-1948.
- Vincent JL, Weil MH. Fluid challenge revisited. *Crit Care Med.* 2006;34:1333-1337.

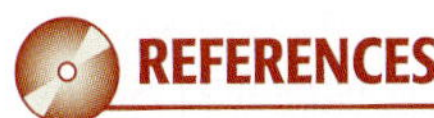

REFERENCES

Complete references available on DVD and online version at www.LongneckerAnesthesiology.com

CHAPTER 81

Mechanical Ventilation for the Surgical Patient

Robert M. Kacmarek
Dean R. Hess

KEY POINTS

1. Patients require mechanical ventilation because of apnea, acute or impending acute respiratory failure, or severe refractory hypoxemia.
2. The 2 basic forms of mechanical ventilation are pressure ventilation (peak airway pressure constant, tidal volume variable) and volume ventilation (tidal volume constant, peak airway pressure variable).
3. Although numerous modes of ventilation exist, few data are available to differentiate the benefits of one mode over another, and no mode has been shown to improve patient outcome.
4. A major concern during assisted ventilation is patient–ventilator synchrony—the ventilator should be set to match the patient's ventilatory demands.
5. Auto positive end-expiratory pressure (PEEP) is a common cause of patient–ventilator dyssynchrony; in patients with obstructive lung disease, properly set applied PEEP can improve synchrony and decrease patient efforts to ventilate.
6. It is unnecessary to achieve normal Pao_2 and $Paco_2$. In most critically ill patients, a Pao_2 of 60 mm Hg or higher is acceptable, and permissive hypercapnia may be useful in treating some patients.
7. Ventilator-induced lung injury is primarily caused by localized overdistension and the opening and closing of unstable lung units.
8. In most patients who are ventilated, the tidal volume should be 4 to 8 mL/kg predicted body weight (PBW) and the plateau pressure should be less than 30 cm H_2O, and PEEP should be set to avoid the collapse of unstable lung units.
9. High-frequency ventilation and airway pressure release ventilation, although useful in managing patients with acute respiratory distress syndrome (ARDS), show no outcome benefits over conventional pressure or volume ventilation.
10. Noninvasive positive-pressure ventilation is useful to transition patients who are at high risk of extubation failure from invasive ventilation to spontaneous breathing.

Most surgical patients do not require support of the respiratory system beyond the immediate postoperative period. However, others with preexistent chronic respiratory diseases, trauma patients, and patients who require extensive surgical procedures may require more lengthy periods of respiratory support. This chapter focuses on mechanical ventilation of the postoperative patient. It primarily discusses invasive ventilation but also reviews selected data for noninvasive respiratory support and the application of noninvasive positive-pressure ventilation (NPPV) and continuous positive airway pressure (CPAP) by mask.

INDICATIONS FOR INTUBATION AND MECHANICAL VENTILATION

The main objectives of mechanical ventilation in the postoperative patient are to decrease the work of breathing and the load on the cardiovascular system, and to reverse life-threatening hypoxemia or respiratory acidosis. **Table 81-1** summarizes some of the specific indications for mechanical ventilation.[1,2] In an international survey of 1638 patients requiring mechanical ventilation reported by Esteban et al, acute respiratory failure was the indication for mechanical ventilation in most patients (66%), followed by coma (15%), an acute exacerbation of chronic obstructive pulmonary disease (13%), and neuromuscular disorders (5%).[3] Included under the heading of respiratory failure were postoperative respiratory failure, acute respiratory distress syndrome (ARDS), heart failure, pneumonia, sepsis, and complications of trauma.[3]

MECHANICAL VENTILATION TARGETS

PRESSURE VERSUS VOLUME VENTILATION

During all forms of mechanical ventilation the ventilator must be programmed to deliver gas to achieve specific target values. The format for gas delivery in most ventilator modes is to target either pressure or volume (**Table 81-2**).[1] In volume-targeted ventilation (the original approach to ventilatory support), a specific tidal volume is set by the clinician and the ventilator ensures that the volume is delivered regardless of inspiratory pressure (up to a clinician-set limit). In addition to tidal volume, the flow waveform and peak flow or inspiratory time must be set. With this approach to ventilatory support the focus is on ensuring that ventilation is maintained at a targeted level.

Pressure ventilation is essentially an opposite approach to ventilatory gas delivery. A peak airway pressure is set, with the aim of limiting the peak alveolar pressure. That is, with each breath pressure increases to the set level before the breath terminates. However, the tidal volume and gas flow are allowed to vary from breath to breath. During pressure ventilation the clinician must set the targeted pressure, and in some modes the inspiratory time. Flow is provided rapidly at first, then in an exponentially decelerating pattern where the rate of deceleration is dependent upon the patient's inspiratory demand and lung mechanics.[4] Essentially, the ventilator rapidly delivers gas flow to establish the targeted pressure, but once the pressure target is met, the flow must decrease to avoid exceeding the set pressure. This approach to ventilatory support focuses on ensuring that a targeted pressure is met and never exceeded.

As noted in **Table 81-3**, pressure and volume ventilation respond differently to changes in the impedance to gas delivery. With volume ventilation, pressure increases if the patient becomes more difficult to ventilate, whereas with pressure ventilation the tidal volume is decreased. Most modes of ventilation currently available essentially function based on one of these 2 formats.

COMBINED PRESSURE AND VOLUME TARGETED MODES

Some of the newer modes of ventilation (see New Modes of Ventilation section) attempt to combine the beneficial effects of volume ventilation (delivering a target tidal volume) and pressure ventilation (the maximum airway pressure is limited).[4] With these modes both volume and pressure are targeted. Their gas delivery algorithms are designed to ensure that on average the set tidal volume is delivered, but also that the peak airway pressure does not exceed the set level.[4] In other novel ventilatory modes, gas may be delivered initially in a volume ventilation format, but if the patient's demand is increased, the gas delivery mode changes to a pressure format to ensure that ventilatory demand is met.[4]

CLASSIC MODES OF VENTILATION

The classic modes of ventilation include control, assist/control, assist (pressure support), and synchronized intermittent mandatory ventilation (**Table 81-4**). All of these modes have been available on mechanical ventilators for more than 25 years and generally can provide the basic approaches to ventilatory support for most surgical patients.

CONTROL MODE

This is the original mode of mechanical ventilation. Controlled ventilation is available in both pressure and volume ventilation formats (**Figs. 81-1 and 81-2**). In this mode, the ventilator controls *all* aspects of gas delivery. That is, the patient is assumed to be a passive recipient

TABLE 81-1 Indications and Select Specific Clinical Causes for the Need of Mechanical Ventilation

Pathophysiologic Indications	Specific Clinical Cause
Apnea	Anesthesia, head trauma, drug overdose
Acute or impending ventilatory failure; $Paco_2$ >50 mm Hg and pH <7.30	Anesthesia, asthma, acute exacerbation of chronic obstructive pulmonary disease, flail chest, postoperative respiratory failure
Severe refractory hypoxemia; Pao_2 <60 mm Hg (Sao_2 90%) with Fio_2 >0.8	Postoperative respiratory failure, acute respiratory distress syndrome, severe pneumonia, sepsis, pulmonary edema

of mechanical ventilation.[5] With the earliest generation of mechanical ventilators, patients were not able to trigger the ventilator to produce an inspiration. However, with today's modern ventilators, even when the airway sensitivity is set at the most insensitive setting, patients with a strong ventilatory drive can still trigger the ventilator. The control mode of ventilation is achieved today by sedating the patient to apnea.

ASSIST/CONTROL MODE

This mode is essentially the control mode with the sensitivity level set to trigger gas delivery by a spontaneous negative airway pressure. That is, the patient initiates gas delivery (**Fig. 81-3**). The sensitivity control adjusts the level of patient effort (spontaneous negative airway pressure) required to trigger the mechanical breath. Although the patient determines the ventilatory rate, a "backup" rate is set to ensure a minimum rate of ventilation.[5] Worldwide this is the most commonly used mode of ventilation.[3] During volume assist/control the following variables are usually set: tidal volume, flow waveform, backup rate, peak inspiratory flow rate or inspiratory time, inspiratory trigger sensitivity, Fio_2, and positive end-expiratory pressure (PEEP). With the pressure assist/control mode the peak pressure, inspiratory time, backup rate, inspiratory trigger sensitivity, Fio_2, PEEP, and rise time must be set.

PRESSURE SUPPORT

The closest classical mode to true assist ventilation available on all modern intensive care unit (ICU) ventilators is pressure support (**Fig. 81-4**). With assist ventilation there is no backup rate. In pressure support, backup safety modes of ventilation take over if patients become apneic for 20 seconds or longer, but no true backup rate is available.[5] Pressure support is very similar to pressure assist/control.[6] The major feature of gas delivery that differs in this mode is the mechanism that terminates inspiration. With pressure assist/control, inspiration is always terminated by time, whereas with pressure support, inspiration is usually terminated by decreasing gas flow. That is, when tracheal flow decreases to a specific level (usually 25% of the peak flow for that breath) the breath is terminated. There are, however, 2 alternate methods of terminating inspiration in pressure support: pressure exceeding the set level after about 300 milliseconds of inspiration or the inspiratory time exceeding the manufacturer's set level, usually 2 to 3 seconds. However, some newer ventilators allow the clinician to set the maximum inspiratory time during pressure support ventilation. Both of these secondary termination criteria are valuable for patient safety and prevent lengthy inspiratory times and prolonged elevation of airway pressures, which can reduce the cardiac output.

Of the classic modes of ventilation, pressure support allows the patient the greatest control over the process of ventilation. Not only does the patient trigger each breath, but the ending of the breath is based on the patient's demand. As with all pressure-targeted approaches to ventilation, the pressure support mode allows the patient to vary the tidal volume of each delivered breath. The only gas delivery variable set other than sensitivity is the pressure level. Pressure support may be used to ventilate any patient with a stable ventilatory drive.

Inspiratory Termination Criteria Inspiratory termination criteria, also referred to as E-sens or expiratory sensitivity, is an adjunct to pressure support available on many ventilators as a method of ensuring that the patient and ventilator end their inspiration simultaneously. As **Figure 81-5** illustrates, an increase in pressure at the end of a pressure support breath is abnormal and usually indicates that the patient has begun exhalation before the ventilator has allowed exhalation to occur.[7]

TABLE 81-2 Pressure- Versus Volume-Targeted Ventilation

	Pressure	Volume
Peak airway pressure	Constant	Variable
Peak alveolar pressure	Constant	Variable
Tidal volume	Variable	Constant
Peak flow	Variable	Constant
Flow pattern	Decelerating	Preset
Inspiratory time	Preset	Preset
Minimum rate	Preset	Preset

Reprinted from Kacmarek RM, Dimas S, Mack C. *Essentials of Respiratory Care*. 4th ed. St. Louis: Elsevier; 2005:690-714, with permission from Elsevier.

TABLE 81-3 Effect of Changing Compliance and Resistance During Pressure and Volume Ventilation

	Pressure	Volume
Decreased compliance	↓ Volume	↑ Pressure
Increased compliance	↑ Volume	↓ Pressure
Increased auto-PEEP	↓ Volume	↑ Pressure
Decreased auto-PEEP	↑ Volume	↓ Pressure
Pneumothorax	↓ Volume	↑ Pressure
Bronchospasm	↓ Volume	↑ Pressure
Mucosal edema	↓ Volume	↑ Pressure
Secretions	↓ Volume	↑ Pressure
Pleural effusion	↓ Volume	↑ Pressure
Increased patient effort	↑ Volume	↓ Pressure
Decreased patient effort	↓ Volume	↑ Pressure

PEEP, positive end-expiratory pressure.

Reprinted from Kacmarek RM, Dimas S, Mack C. *Essentials of Respiratory Care*. 4th ed. St. Louis: Elsevier; 2005:690-714, with permission from Elsevier.

TABLE 81-4 Available Modes of Mechanical Ventilation

Classic Modes of Ventilation
Control
Assist/control
Assist/pressure support
Synchronized intermittent mandatory ventilation

New Modes of Ventilation

Within Breath Adjustments	Between Breath Adjustments	Pressure Targeted
Automatic tube compensation	Pressure-regulated volume control	Airway pressure release ventilation
Proportional assist ventilation	Volume support	Bilevel pressure ventilation
Volume-assured pressure support	Adaptive support ventilation	
Neurally adjusted ventilatory assist		

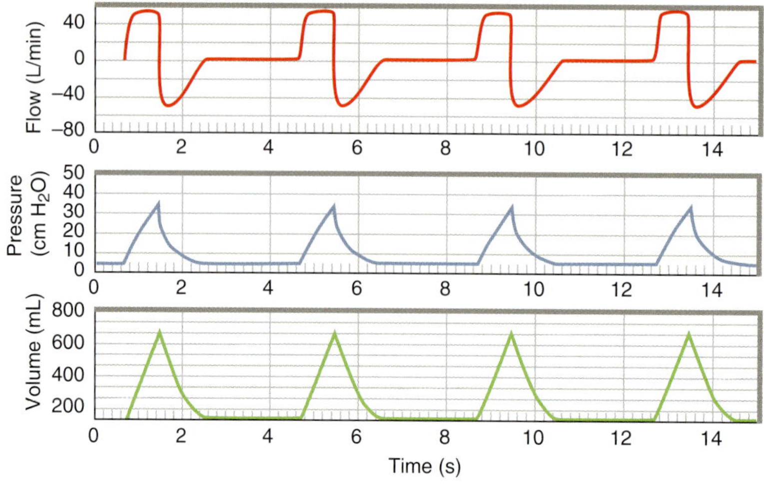

FIGURE 81-1. Volume-targeted square-wave flow-controlled mode ventilation. Note there is no negative deflection in airway pressure at the start of the breath. [Reprinted from Hess DR, MacIntyre NR, Mishoe SC, et al. *Respiratory Care: Principles and Practice*. Philadelphia: WB Saunders; 2002:786-791, with permission from Elsevier.]

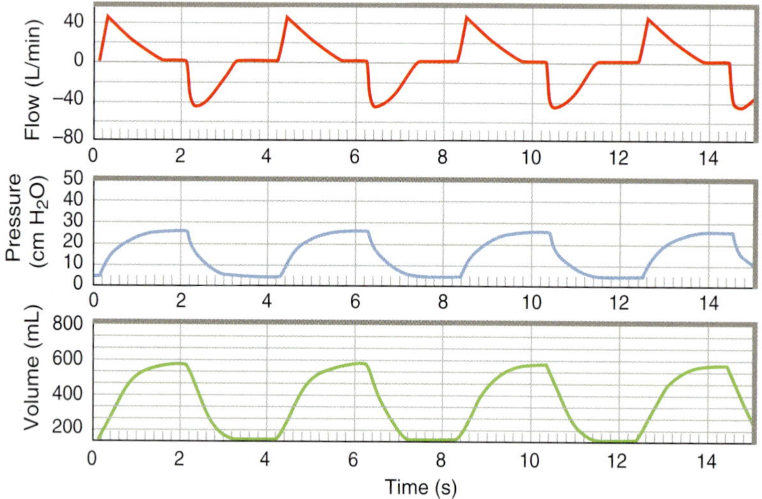

FIGURE 81-2. Pressure-targeted controlled-mode ventilation. Note there is no negative deflection in airway pressure at the start of the breath. [Reprinted from Hess DR, MacIntyre NR, Mishoe SC, et al. *Respiratory Care: Principles and Practice*. Philadelphia: WB Saunders; 2002:786-791, with permission from Elsevier.]

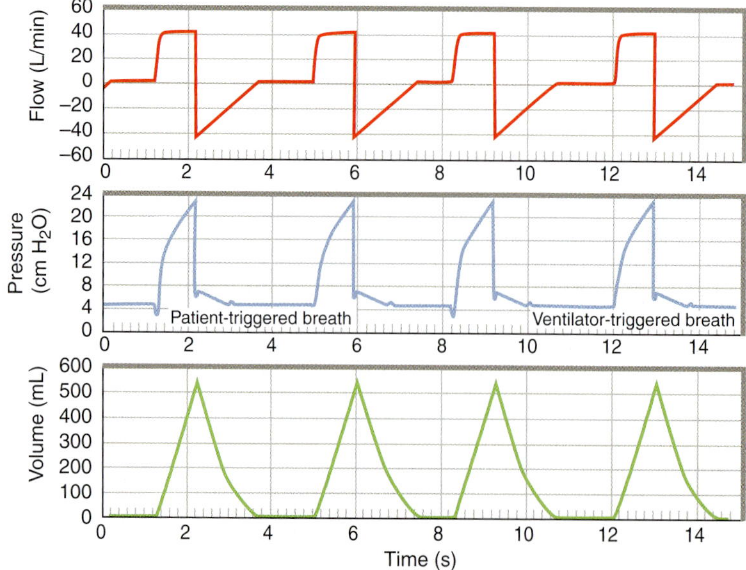

FIGURE 81-3. Volume-targeted assist/control mode ventilation. Note each breath is patient triggered as observed by the deflection in airway pressure at the onset of each breath. [Reprinted from Hess DR, MacIntyre NR, Mishoe SC, et al. *Respiratory Care: Principles and Practice*. Philadelphia: WB Saunders; 2002:786-791, with permission from Elsevier.]

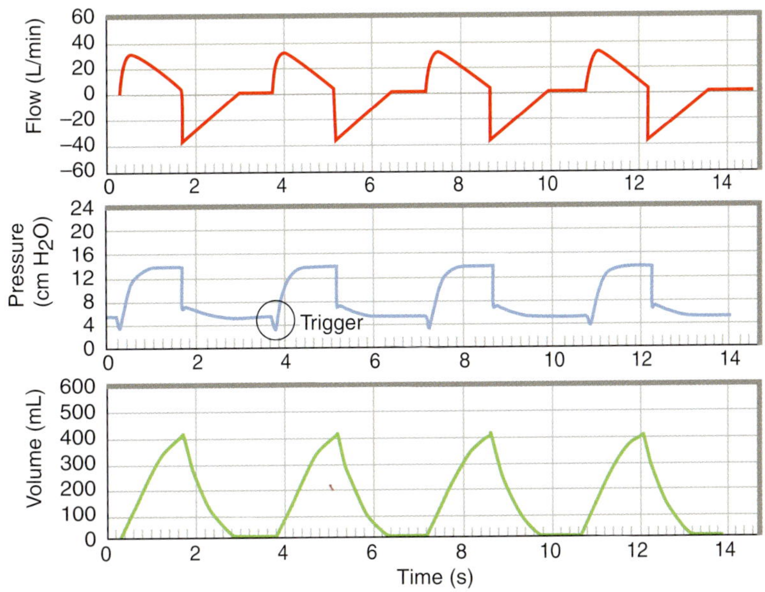

FIGURE 81-4. Pressure support mode ventilation. [Reprinted from Hess DR, MacIntyre NR, Mishoe SC, et al. *Respiratory Care: Principles and Practice*. Philadelphia: WB Saunders; 2002:786-791, with permission from Elsevier.]

When this increase in inspiratory pressure is observed, the patient is contracting accessory muscles of exhalation during the terminal aspect of the ventilator's inspiratory phase.[8] This results in an increased ventilatory drive and ventilatory rate, and the development of patient–ventilator dyssynchrony. E-sens allows adjustment of the percentage of peak flow terminating the breath. Whenever a spike at the end of a pressure support breath is present, a greater percentage of the peak flow should be set to terminate the breath. In this setting the E-sens percentage should be slowly increased until there is a smooth transition from inspiration to expiration.[9]

Rise Time Patient–ventilator synchrony at the onset of a pressure-targeted breath (eg, pressure assist/control, pressure support, pressure-regulated volume control) can be improved by adjusting the rise time. As noted in **Figure 81-6**, the flow rise time varies the slope of the pressure increase at the onset of a breath by varying the time it takes gas flow to increase from zero to peak.[7] Rise time should be adjusted to ensure that airway pressure rises rapidly to the peak level without any concavity during the initial airway pressure waveform. If the airway pressure waveform is concave the rise time should be increased (made more rapid); however, if peak pressure exceeds the set level at the onset of inspiration the rise time should be decreased. An increase in rise time generally results in an increase of peak flow and a decreased inspiratory time (with pressure support ventilation). In most patients with a strong ventilatory drive the rise time should be set between the mid and most rapid level. Proper setting of rise time usually results in a decreased mechanical ventilatory rate.

SYNCHRONIZED INTERMITTENT MANDATORY VENTILATION

This mode of ventilation combines spontaneous unsupported breathing with the assist/control mode. As with the assist/control mode, the mandatory positive-pressure breaths can be either pressure or volume targeted. **Figure 81-7** illustrates the typical volume-targeted synchronized intermittent mandatory ventilation (SIMV). A mandatory respiration rate is set, and between the mandatory breaths the patient can breathe spontaneously.[5] As noted in **Figure 81-8**, an assist/control window is open at specific intervals based on the selected mandatory respiration rate.[10] Within each window the patient is able to trigger positive-pressure breaths; if the ventilator does not sense the patient's

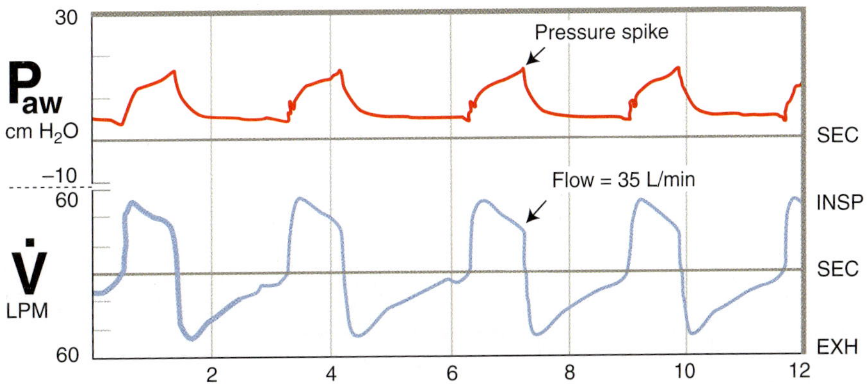

FIGURE 81-5. Pressure and flow tracings during pressure support ventilation with the Nellcor Puritan Bennett 7200ae demonstrating pressure cycling in pressure support. The pressure spike at the end of inspiration indicates that the patient desires to end the breath before the ventilator will allow exhalation. [Reproduced with permission from Branson RD, Campbell RS, Davis K, et al. Altering flow rate during maximum pressure support ventilation (PSV_{max}): effects on cardiorespiratory function. *Respir Care.* 1990;35:1056-1064.]

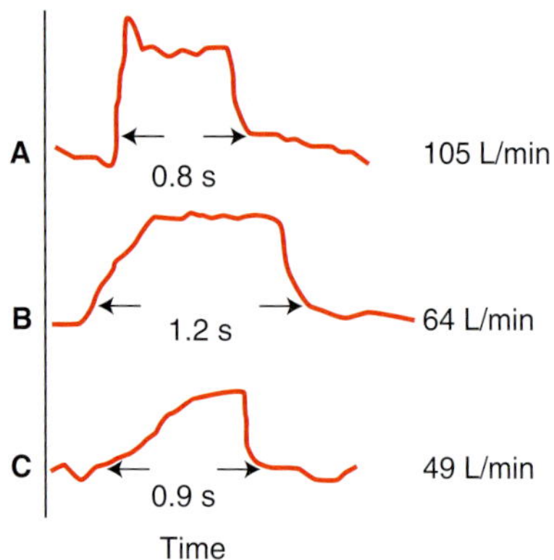

FIGURE 81-6. Effect of changing rise time in a lung model preferring a midrange rise time. **A.** Flow is in excess of demand, and a pressure spike is seen. **B.** As flow rate is decreased, inspiratory time (T_I) lengthens, and the pressure spike is absent—machine output matches patient demand. **C.** When flow rate is further reduced, patient demand exceeds machine flow rate, and T_I decreases. Peak flow is inadequate to establish the expected pressure waveform. [Reproduced with permission from Branson RD, Campbell RS. Pressure support ventilation, patient–ventilator synchrony, and ventilator algorithms. *Respir Care.* 1998;43:1045.]

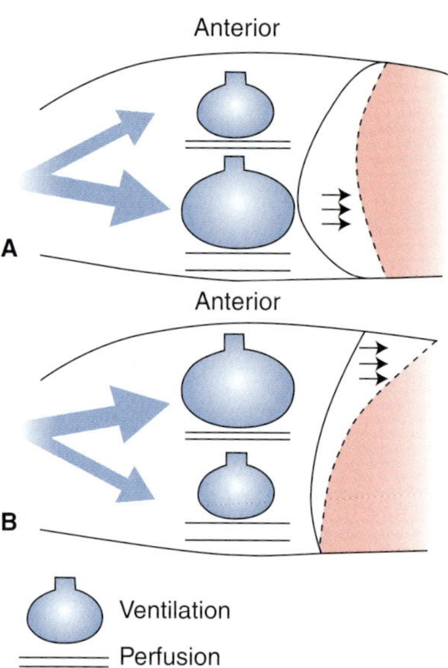

FIGURE 81-8. Effect of spontaneous ventilation and positive-pressure ventilation on gas distribution in a supine subject. During spontaneous ventilation (**A**) diaphragmatic action distributes most ventilation to the dependent zones of the lungs, where perfusion is greatest. The result is good matching of ventilation to perfusion. During positive-pressure ventilation (**B**) because the diaphragm is doing little to no contraction, ventilation is primarily distributed to nondependent lung, increasing the level of ventilation to perfusion mismatch. [Reprinted from Wilkens RL, Stoller JK, Scamlon CC. *Egan's Fundamentals of Respiratory Care*. 8th ed. St. Louis, MO: Mosby; 2003:972, with permission from Elsevier.]

efforts during this time period a controlled positive-pressure breath is delivered. Ventilator adjustment is the same as that with the control mode except that the sensitivity must also be properly set.

Advocates of SIMV emphasize the benefits of spontaneous breathing between mandatory breaths. As shown in Figure 81-8, spontaneous breathing can improve ventilation/perfusion (V/Q) matching by improving the distribution of ventilation to dependent lung regions.[10] In addition, the negative intrathoracic pressure generated during spontaneous breathing decreases the mean intrathoracic pressure, thereby improving cardiac output. However, the work of breathing during SIMV can be excessive. As noted in **Figure 81-9**, as the mandatory rate is reduced the work of breathing for both mandatory and spontaneous breaths increases.[11] The surprising reason for this is that the patient's respiratory center has a difficult time rapidly changing its output based on ventilatory load as the mandatory rate decreases. Essentially, each breath is interpreted as being at the higher load and requiring the higher muscular work output. This is nicely illustrated in **Figure 81-10**; note that the electromyelogram (EMG) activity of the diaphragm and the sternocleidomastoid muscles, as well as the esophageal pressure

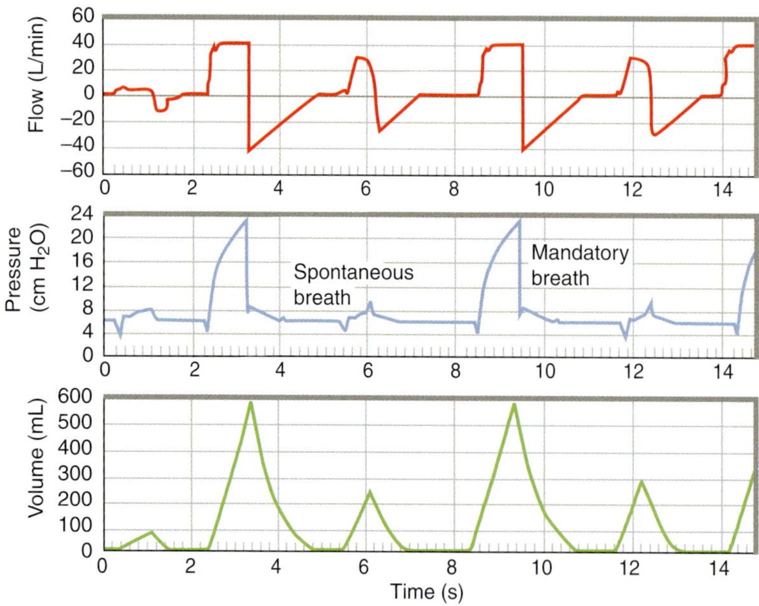

FIGURE 81-7. Volume-targeted synchronized intermittent mandatory ventilation (SIMV), showing spontaneous unsupported and mandatory (assist/control) breaths. [Reprinted from Hess DR, MacIntyre NR, Mishoe SC, et al. *Respiratory Care: Principles and Practice*. Philadelphia: WB Saunders; 2002:786-791, with permission from Elsevier.]

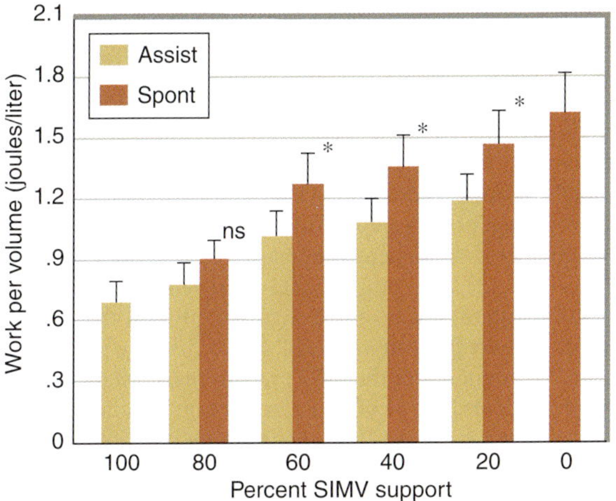

FIGURE 81-9. Inspiratory work per unit volume (work per liter [Wp/L]) done by the patient during assisted cycles (open bars) and spontaneous cycles (reverse cross-hatched bars). Wp/L increased with decreasing synchronized intermittent mandatory ventilation percentage for both types of breath. Wp/L for spontaneous breaths tended to exceed Wp/L for machine-assisted breaths. [From Marini JJ, Smith TC, Lamb VJ. External work output and force generation during synchronized intermittent mechanical ventilation. *Am Rev Respir Dis.* 1988;138:1169. © American Thoracic Society.]

changes, are the same for both mandatory and spontaneous breaths.[12] In other words, the patient's effort is the same regardless of breath type, although the efficiency of gas delivery may be better during the mandatory breaths. Unfortunately, this set of circumstances increases the patient's ventilatory drive and increases the level of patient–ventilatory dyssynchrony.

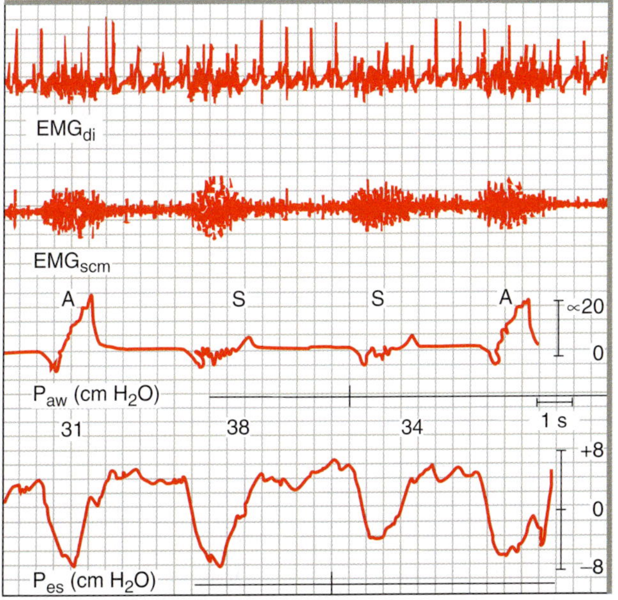

FIGURE 81-10. Electromyograms of the diaphragm (EMG_{di}) and of the sternocleidomastoid muscles (EMG_{scm}) in a representative patient, showing similar intensity and the duration of electrical activity in successive assisted (A) and spontaneous (S) breaths during synchronized intermittent mandatory ventilation. Also, note that esophageal (P_{es}) pressure changes are equal (equal effort) during A and S breaths. P_{aw}, airway pressure. [Reproduced with permission from Imsand C, Feihl F, Perret C, et al. Regulation of inspiratory neuromuscular output during synchronized intermittent mechanical ventilation. *Anesthesiology.* 1994;80:13-22.]

With most modern ventilators, the pressure support mode can be applied during spontaneous patient breaths; however, this negates the benefits of unassisted spontaneous breathing and increases the complexity of weaning patients from ventilatory support. In general, the lower the mandatory rate during SIMV the greater the likelihood that the patient's effort will be excessive and dyssynchrony will be present.

NEW MODES OF VENTILATION

Table 81-4 lists the latest modes of ventilation currently available on the newest generation of mechanical ventilators. These modes are designed to take advantage of the beneficial aspects of both volume and pressure ventilation. As noted in Table 81-4, they are divided into modes that adjust gas delivery during a given breath and those that adjust gas delivery on the subsequent breath. In this latter group, adjustment is based on the ability of current settings to achieve gas delivery targets.

PRESSURE-REGULATED VOLUME CONTROL

This mode of ventilatory support targets both a maximum airway pressure and a tidal volume and is a variation of the pressure assist/control mode. This same mode is referred to on some ventilators as autoflow, volume control plus, or possibly another term.[4,5] It accomplishes its goals by varying the pressure applied on the subsequent breath based on the tidal volume achieved on the current breath. All of the ventilators providing this mode of ventilation first deliver a test breath at some low level of pressure and from the volume delivered calculate the pressure required to deliver the targeted tidal volume. The ventilator then automatically adjusts the pressure in 1 or 2 steps to the pressure level needed to deliver the targeted tidal volume. During every subsequent breath, the tidal volume that is delivered is reassessed, and based on this assessment the pressure on the subsequent breath is adjusted ±3 cm H_2O to ensure that the targeted volume is delivered on the next breath.[4,5] Pressure during pressure-regulated volume control (PRVC) can be increased to a maximum level selected by the clinician and can be decreased with some ventilators all the way to the CPAP/PEEP level, thereby allowing unassisted spontaneous breathing. Herein lies our major concern with PRVC: If a patient has a strong ventilatory drive and the additional stimulus of, for example, hypoxemia, fever, or sepsis, the level of ventilatory support could decrease inappropriately to either a very low level or to no support. As a result, be cautious when using this mode with patients who have a strong ventilatory drive.[13] Marked improvement in the operation of this mode could be made by adding a minimum pressure limit, that is, setting a low pressure limit.[4] As a result, this mode is most useful in those patients who are receiving control mode ventilation or for those patients who have limited ventilatory demand. To use PRVC, first set all variables used during pressure assist/control, then add the target tidal volume and maximum pressure limit.

VOLUME SUPPORT

The volume support mode operates similarly to PRVC, but is based on the pressure-support mode and not the pressure assist/control format.[4,5] Ventilator software must assess the pressure needed to deliver the tidal volume and provide breath-to-breath pressure adjustment to ensure the targeted tidal volume. The same safety concern regarding a patient with a strong ventilatory demand exists with volume support (as with PRVC). The adjustments made to the ventilator during setup are the same as those with pressure support, with the addition of setting the target volume and maximum airway pressure.

Two randomized controlled studies of PRVC and/or volume support have been conducted—one in neonates[14] and the other in pediatric patients.[15] In the study of newborns,[14] PRVC was compared to intermittent mandatory ventilation (without synchronization of the mandatory breath). In this study, neonates who were studied weaned faster with PRVC. In the second,[15] volume support was compared to pressure support with and without a protocol for weaning children from mechanical ventilation. No difference in the rate of weaning was observed regardless of the mode of ventilation. As a result, there is little enthusiasm for the use of either of these new modes of ventilation for weaning.

ADAPTIVE-SUPPORT VENTILATION

This is a very unique new mode of ventilatory support. It attempts to adjust ventilator settings to ensure that an ideal ventilatory pattern is achieved,[16] with *ideal* being defined as the pattern requiring the least patient and ventilator work based on the patient's measured mechanical lung characteristics and breathing effort. The goal of adaptive-support ventilation (ASV) is to provide a preset level of minute ventilation while minimizing the total work of breathing expended by both the ventilator and the patient. It can be applied to both patients who require controlled ventilation and to those who are actively breathing.

During set up the clinician must indicate the patient's ideal body weight (males: predicted body weight [PBW] (kg) = 50 + 2.3 [height (in) (60)]; females: PBW (kg) = 45.5 + 2.3 [height (in) (60)])[17] and the percentage of minimal minute volume (% min MV) to be delivered. The % min MV can be adjusted between 25% and 350% of predicted body weight.[16] From the PBW and % min MV the maximum rate is calculated as

$$22 \times \%\ \text{min MV}/100 \text{ if PBW} > 15 \text{ kg}$$

or

$$45 \times \%\ \text{min MV}/100 \text{ if PBW} < 15 \text{ kg}$$

whereas the maximum tidal volume delivered is the targeted MV/5.[16] With this information the ventilator determines the optimal breathing pattern that will minimize the work of breathing, that is, a ventilatory pattern that results in minimum work of breathing based on the lung and chest wall mechanics of the patient.

With the initial application of ASV the ventilator provides a series of 5 pressure-limited test breaths at a rate of about 10 breaths/min with a maximum pressure of 15 cm H_2O. During these breaths, the ventilator measures dynamic compliance, the respiratory time constant, tidal volume, and the patient's respiratory rate.[16] These measurements are used to determine the initial targets for breathing rate and tidal volume. As ventilation continues the ventilator software recalculates the above variables from each breath and determines the new rate and tidal volume targets. Targets are based on the original work by Otis for estimating the patient's minimal ventilatory work.[18] If the patient's ventilatory pattern is not that determined to be ideal, the ventilator adjusts pressure level or rate to try to ensure that the ideal pattern is established.

This mode of ventilation is designed to ensure that an ideal ventilatory pattern is maintained and can be used in all phases of ventilatory support. It continually adjusts mechanical ventilation characteristics as the patient's status changes because it monitors the patient's lung mechanics on a breath-to-breath basis. Recently published data indicate that ASV works well in postoperative cardiac surgical patients[19,20] and in patients under controlled ventilation.[21] Recent lung model data indicate that during controlled ventilation ASV may provide better lung protection than a fixed tidal volume of 6 mL/kg.[22] More data during assisted ventilation of patients with lung injury are needed to determine if spontaneously breathing patients will accept the ideal ventilatory pattern this mode tries to impose.

AUTOMATIC TUBE COMPENSATION

This mode of ventilation has been referred to as electronic extubation. Automatic tube compensation (ATC) is designed to provide sufficient mechanical ventilatory support during inspiration and sufficient decompression of the ventilatory circuit during expiration to maintain the tracheal pressure equal to the set PEEP level. The ventilator software accomplishes this by having the resistance properties of various endotracheal and tracheostomy tube sizes programmed into its memory and continually measuring gas flow. From these data, the pressure needed to overcome the resistance (resistance = change in pressure ÷ flow) of the endotracheal tube is continually calculated and applied.[23]

Upon activation of the ATC mode, the clinician must indicate the type and size of artificial airway and the desired percentage of automatic tube compensation (20%-100% on most ventilators).[4,5] In addition, some ventilators only apply the ATC correction during inspiration, others during both inspiration and expiration. The precise clinical indications for ATC are still unclear. Because this mode responds only to the patient's demand, if demand is low, ventilatory support is low; that is, if the patient generates a low inspiratory effort then little pressure is applied, whereas if the patient generates great effort, the applied pressure is greater.[24] ATC, like proportional-assist ventilation, does not force a ventilatory pattern, but is only designed to unload the flow-resistive properties of the artificial airway. ATC may be used on patients ready to wean from the ventilator. If the ATC pressure level is stable and remains at a low pressure (5-7 cm H_2O), then extubation is indicated.

The use of expiratory ATC does raise some concerns when used in patients with airways obstruction. The decompression of the airway during early exhalation may precipitate greater airways collapse and obstruction. As with many of these newer modes of ventilation, additional research is required before clinical indications and contraindications can be clearly defined.

PROPORTIONAL-ASSIST VENTILATION

This mode of ventilation is similar to ATC but the software response is based on both the mechanics of the total respiratory system plus the resistive properties of the artificial airway; that is, the ventilator delivers a pressure assist in proportion to the patient's desired tidal volume (volume assist) and to the patient's instantaneous inspired flow (flow assist).[25] The response of these 2 aspects of ventilatory assistance are automatically adjusted to meet changes in the patient's ongoing ventilatory demand. This algorithm is based on the law of motion as it applies to the respiratory system:

$$P_{mus} + P_{appl} = (\text{volume} \times E) + (\text{flow} \times R)$$

where P_{mus} is pressure generated by the respiratory muscles,[25] P_{appl} is pressure applied by the ventilator, and *E* and *R* are elastic and resistance properties of the respiratory system. Assuming that E and R are linear during inspiration, the instantaneous flow and volume to be delivered are proportional to the resistive and elastic work of breathing, respectively. The ventilator continuously measures the instantaneous flow and volume, and periodically measures the E and R. Utilizing this information the ventilator software adjusts gas delivery accordingly by estimating P_{mus} and assisting P_{mus} in a proportional manner.[26] Thus the patient is the determinant of the ventilatory pattern. Patients are given the freedom to select a ventilatory pattern that is rapid and shallow or slow and deep.[26] If the patient desires a small tidal volume a low level of pressure is applied, and if a large tidal volume is desired a high pressure is applied. The ventilator does not force any control variable except the unloading of E and R in a proportional manner.

Proportional-assist ventilation (PAV) is only useful in patients with a stable ventilatory drive who choose an acceptable ventilatory pattern. Of concern is the inability of some mechanical ventilators to reassess E and R on an ongoing basis. With these ventilators the level of unloading may be inappropriate if respiratory system mechanics are dynamically changing. There are a number of clinical reports that compare the effects of PAV with those of pressure support.[27-30] In most of these studies PAV is able to minimize patient effort when lung mechanics or demand changes because of the ventilator's ability to assess lung mechanics and the proportional unloading provided. PAV improves patient ventilator synchrony when compared to pressure support.[30] PAV is also capable of reducing the sleep disturbances noted in the ICU. This occurs because PAV does not force a ventilatory pattern on the patient, allowing the patient to vary his or her minute volume and $Paco_2$ during sleep and decreasing the number of periodic apneas as compared with other modes of ventilatory support.[31] In addition, the PAV mode has been shown to be useful during noninvasive ventilation.[32,33]

NEURALLY ADJUSTED VENTILATORY SUPPORT

From a conceptual perspective, neurally adjusted ventilatory support (NAVA) is essentially the same as PAV except that PAV responds to changes in airway pressure and flow, whereas NAVA responds to changes in diaphragmatic EMG activity.[34] However, in order for NAVA to function properly a specially designed nasogastric catheter with a 10-cm length of EMG electrodes must be in place.[34] Both PAV and NAVA respond to patient effort, providing ventilatory support in a proportional manner. In either mode the clinician does not set pressure, volume, flow, or time. The only setting is the proportion of effort unloaded by the ventilator. In NAVA this is set as the number of centimeters of water applied per microvolt of diaphragmatic EMG activity.

NAVA, when compared to pressure support or pressure assist/control, results in a lower peak airway pressure and generally a smaller tidal volume and more rapid rate.[35] NAVA also markedly reduces the level of dyssynchrony.[36] NAVA is not affected by the size of the system leak or the presence of auto-PEEP because its response level is only affected by the level of EMG activity.

AIRWAY PRESSURE RELEASE VENTILATION

This mode of ventilation is a combination of pressure-targeted SIMV and inverse-ratio pressure-control ventilation.[37] As illustrated in **Figure 81-11**, airway pressure release ventilation (APRV) applies 2 levels of CPAP and allows spontaneous unassisted breathing at each CPAP level. There are 2 approaches to setting APRV based on the belief that spontaneous breathing should only occur at the high CPAP level[38] or at both CPAP levels.[39] If the clinician desires spontaneous breaths only at the high CPAP level, the time spent at the low CPAP level is kept brief to prevent complete exhalation, hence an inverse ratio between high and low CPAP levels. In this setting, the high CPAP level is set to maintain oxygenation and the lower level assists ventilation by periodically decreasing the lung volume.

The alternate approach is to set the low CPAP level to maintain oxygenation (as if setting a PEEP level) and the high CPAP level to provide ventilatory assistance, as in SIMV.[39] In the latter approach, the time spent at low CPAP levels is sufficient to allow complete exhalation and spontaneous breathing at the lower CPAP levels. Proponents of APRV cite the salutary benefits of spontaneous unsupported breathing to improve ventilation/perfusion matching, increase cardiac output, and reduce the need for sedation.[37-39] However, as noted in **Figure 81-12**, the effort associated with spontaneous breathing under these conditions can result in very high esophageal pressure swings and a high work of breathing for the patient, accounting in part for the greater cardiac output.[40] In addition, dyssynchrony is common with APRV. Dyssynchrony occurs at the mandatory transition from high-to-low or low-to-high CPAP levels. If the patient is exhaling when the ventilator increases airway pressure or inhaling when the ventilator decreases airway pressure, dyssynchrony results. Although this mode of ventilation is most commonly used in the management of acute lung injury or the acute respiratory distress syndrome, it has not been shown to be more beneficial than the assist/control mode.[39]

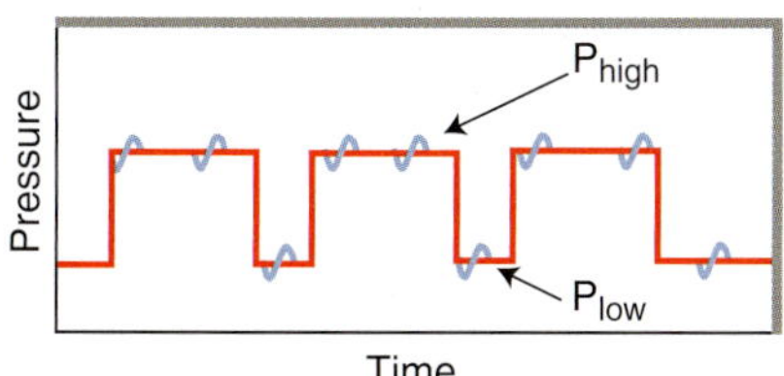

FIGURE 81-11. Airway pressure release ventilation (APRV). P_{high}, high continuous positive airway pressure (CPAP) level; P_{low}, low CPAP level. Note spontaneous breaths at both levels of CPAP. [Reprinted from Kacmarek RM, Dimas S, Mack C. *Essentials of Respiratory Care*. 4th ed. St. Louis, MO: Elsevier; 2005:690-714, with permission from Elsevier.]

BILEVEL PRESSURE VENTILATION

This is a modification of APRV. As noted in **Figure 81-13**, pressure support can be added to spontaneous breaths at either the high or low CPAP level or both.[4] This reduces the patient's effort and esophageal pressure swings, but it also increases the mean intrathoracic pressure, negating somewhat the increased cardiac output and beneficial augmentation of ventilation/perfusion matching. In addition, the transition from high-to-low and low-to-high CPAP levels is coordinated with the patient's muscular effort (as in SIMV), markedly decreasing dyssynchrony. Like APRV, the bilevel ventilation mode is primarily used in the management of acute lung injury and the acute respiratory distress syndrome.

VENTILATOR SETTINGS AND PATIENT–VENTILATOR SYNCHRONY

Patient–ventilator synchrony is a critical issue for every patient triggering the ventilator for a mechanically supported inspiration. A lack of synchrony increases ventilatory effort, respiratory rate, and the patient's work of breathing as the ventilator is not providing flow to match the patient's inspiratory demand. Pressure-targeted modes of ventilation are generally better than volume-targeted modes at reducing the likelihood of dyssynchrony, as pressure ventilation allows the ventilator to deliver a variable flow with each breath based on the patient's inspiratory demand.[41] In addition, most ventilators now allow adjusting the slope of the increase of flow delivery (rise time) to ensure that gas delivery is matched to patient's inspiratory flow demand.[5,42] Patient–ventilator synchrony is also affected by the inspiratory time. The ventilator's inspiratory time and the patient's inspiratory time should be equal. Trigger sensitivity should always be set to be as sensitive as possible without causing spontaneous autotriggering. In general, flow triggering is to be recommended over pressure triggering.[43] A final factor affecting patient–ventilator synchrony is auto-PEEP,[44] which normally is only a problem in patients with airways obstruction, although it is a potential concern in all patients. If the patient's inspiratory efforts fail to trigger the ventilator, the problem is usually auto-PEEP.[45]

PEAK FLOW AND FLOW WAVEFORM

If a patient is spontaneously triggering the ventilator, peak flow delivery during volume ventilation should match the patient's inspiratory flow demand.[46] Most adult patients with moderate to strong ventilatory demands require a peak flow of 80 L/min or greater. As clearly demonstrated by Marini et al (**Fig. 81-14**), if the peak flow does not meet the patient's inspiratory demand the work of breathing performed by the patient increases. In this setting the efficiency of the work may be greater than during spontaneous breathing, but the overall patient work may be similar.[46] In volume ventilation there is always an indirect relationship between the work provided by the ventilator and the patient's work of breathing.

It is important to remember that if the patient is triggering the positive-pressure breaths, the work of breathing is shared between the patient and the ventilator. It is for this reason that patients originally receiving assisted ventilation demonstrate altered gas-delivery patterns after they are sedated to apnea. With the transition to controlled ventilation, the peak airway pressures usually increase during volume ventilation, and tidal volumes decrease in pressure ventilation.[47] Because the patient is no longer performing a portion of the work of breathing, the work performed by the ventilator must increase.

Most ventilators during volume ventilation mode can deliver gas flow in a decelerating or square wave flow pattern. If the patient is triggering inspiration, we recommend a decelerating flow pattern, especially when a small tidal volume (V_T) is being delivered.[4,47] A decelerating flow pattern allows a high peak flow to be delivered, but also ensures that the inspiratory time can be adequately set.

In patients who are sedated and who are not triggering the ventilator, the choice of flow waveform is unimportant, and the setting of peak flow is dependent on the predetermined inspiratory time and tidal volume.

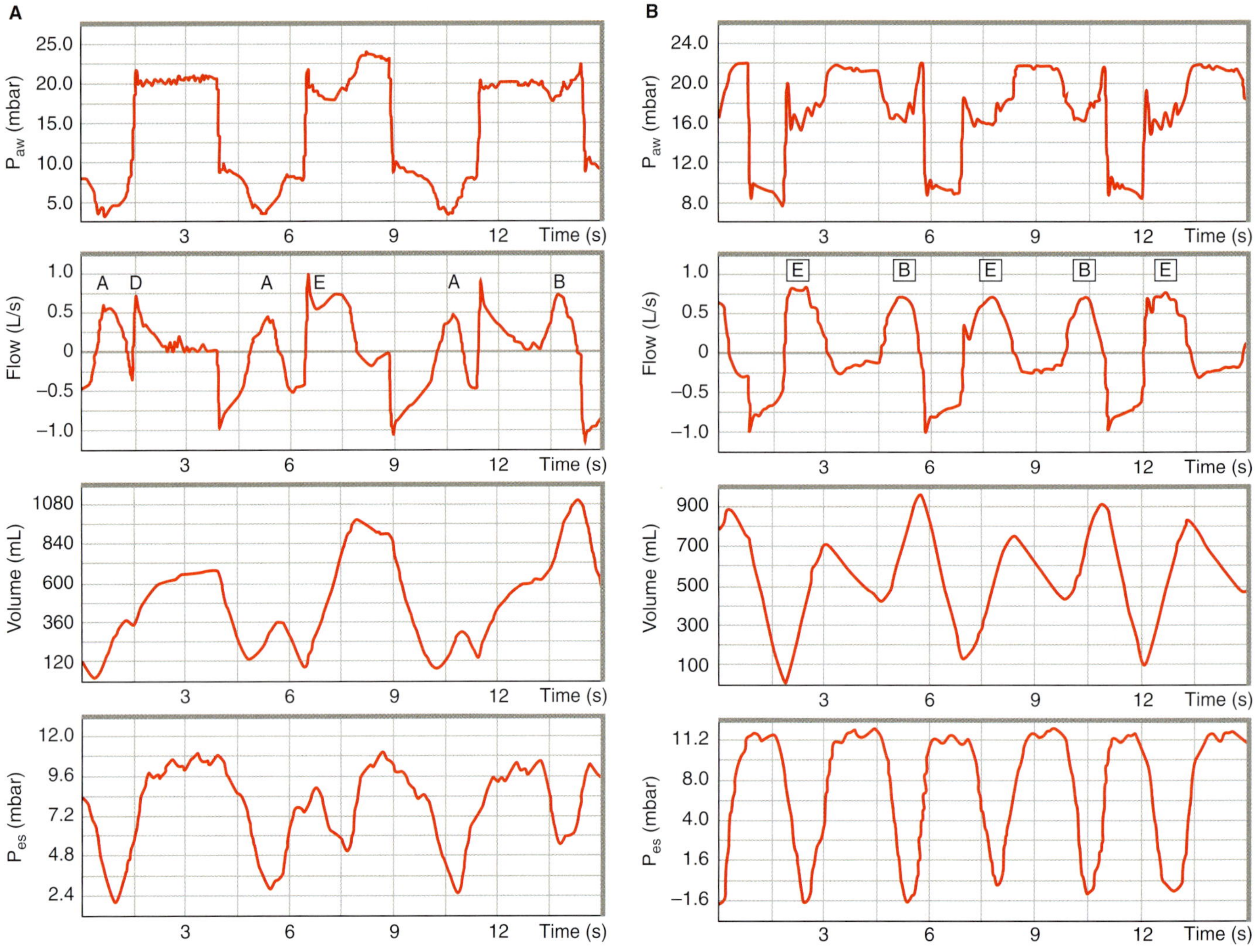

FIGURE 81-12. Airway pressure release ventilation actual patient tracings. A synopsis of airway pressure (P_{aw}), flow, volume, and esophageal pressure (P_{es}) is shown. **A.** Time intervals of the upper (P_{high}) and lower airway pressure (P_{low}) set to 2.5 seconds each. **B.** Time intervals of P_{high} = 4.0 seconds and P_{low} = 1.0 second in the same patient. Note that spontaneous breathing occurs on the upper and lower CPAP levels in (**A**) and that tidal volumes varied considerably, depending on the pressure level from which an inspiration started. When P_{low} was decreased to 1.0 second, as shown in (**B**), spontaneous breaths occurred almost exclusively during P_{high}. This results in a more regular breathing pattern as compared with (**A**). Note, however, the large esophageal pressure swings (10-12 mbar or cm H_2O) per breath, indicating high patient effort on each spontaneous breath. Breaths are classified as type A, spontaneous breath at the lower CPAP level; type B, spontaneous breath on the upper CPAP level; type C, the pressure increase from the lower to the upper CPAP level triggered by an inspiratory effort of the patient; type D, mechanical breath; and type E, combined mechanical and spontaneous inspiration without a triggered pressure increase from P_{low} to P_{high}. [From Neumann P, Golisch J, Strohmeyer A, et al. Influence of different release times on spontaneous breathing pattern during airway pressure release ventilation. *Intensive Care Med.* 2002;28:1742, with kind permission of Springer Science and Business Media.]

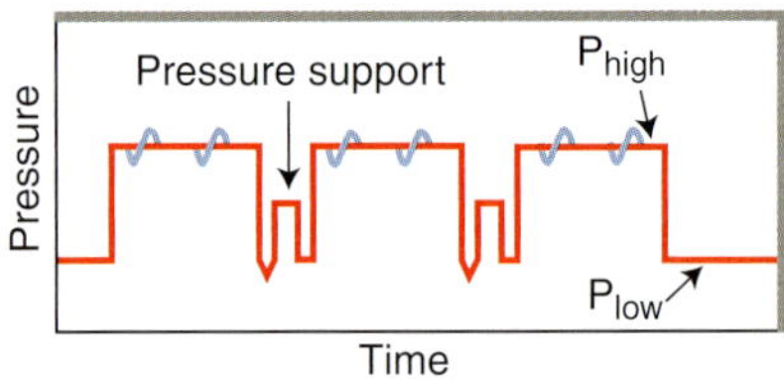

FIGURE 81-13. Bilevel ventilation upper airway pressure (P_{high}). High continuous positive airway pressure (CPAP) level and lower airway pressure (P_{low}) low CPAP level. Note spontaneous breaths at both levels of CPAP, but in this case pressure support is applied to the breaths at the P_{low}. Pressure support could also be applied to P_{high}. [Reprinted from Kacmarek RM, Dimas S, Mack C. *Essentials of Respiratory Care*. 4th ed. St. Louis, MO: Elsevier; 2005:690-714, with permission from Elsevier.]

INSPIRATORY TIME

In patients self-triggering every breath, the set inspiratory time should equal the patient's neuroinspiratory time.[48] As illustrated in **Figure 81-15**, when the inspiratory time is decreased to equal the patient's desired inspiratory time and peak flow is increased to match the patient's demand, then the patient's work of breathing and effort correspondingly decrease. It is rare that a patient with a moderate to high ventilatory demand desires an inspiratory time greater than 1 second.[48] In fact, many adults with moderate or high ventilatory demands desire an inspiratory time of between 0.6 and 0.9 seconds.[47] Carefully matching the patient's inspiratory time with the ventilator's inspiratory time generally markedly improves patient–ventilator synchrony.

In patients who are receiving controlled mechanical ventilation, inspiratory time is set based on the tidal volume and the clinician's perceived optimal time of inspiration. In most settings, an inspiratory time of about 1.0 second is ideal. Some clinicians prefer to lengthen the

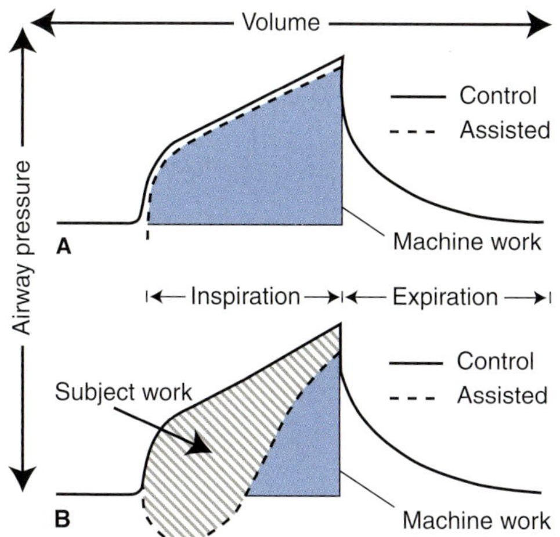

FIGURE 81-14. A. Depiction of an actual pressure-time curve (dotted line) during volume control ventilation superimposed on the ideal curve reflecting total work of breathing (solid line). **B.** Note the scooped-out actual pressure waveform when patient demand increases. The hatched area reflects the work performed by the patient during assisted volume-targeted ventilation. [From Marini JJ, Rodrigues RM, Lamb V. The inspiratory workload of patient-initiated mechanical ventilation. *Am Rev Respir Dis.* 1986;134:902-909. © American Thoracic Society.]

inspiratory time in ARDS/acute lung injury (ALI), thereby inversing the usual inspiratory-to-expiratory (I:E) time ratio; however, there are no data to indicate that longer inspiratory times result in better oxygenation or better outcomes in these syndromes than an appropriately set PEEP level.[49,50] Prolongation of the inspiratory time can have a minor positive effect of increasing CO_2 elimination by allowing time for inspired gas to transfer from fast time constant lung units to adjacent slower time constant units ("pendelluft"). In patients with severe asthma, the inspiratory time may need to be increased to 1.2 to 1.5 seconds to ensure that ventilation passes beyond markedly obstructed airways.[37] Note that in asthma the airways resistance is not only increased during exhalation but also during inspiration.

TIDAL VOLUME

Over the past 15 years, emphasis has been placed on the relationship between elevated tidal volumes and ventilator-induced lung injury (VILI; see Ventilator-Induced Lung Injury section).[51] Recent epidemiologic studies indicate that the most common tidal volume used to manage patients in acute respiratory failure is about 10 mL/kg PBW.[52] However, it is also important to emphasize that normal, healthy relaxed mammals breathe at a tidal volume of about 6 to 7 mL/kg of PBW.[53] There is no evidence indicating that tidal volumes above 10 mL/kg PBW are useful in the management of critically ill patients. In fact, evidence from a recent retrospective review indicates that the development of ALI is linked to large tidal volume ventilation (>10 mL/kg PBW).[52,54] As a general rule, all critically ill patients should be ventilated with tidal volumes below 10 mL/kg PBW regardless of the cause of their acute ventilatory failure. Patients with ALI/ARDS ideally should be ventilated with a V_T 4 to 8 mL/kg of PBW.[55]

PLATEAU PRESSURE

The plateau pressure (end-inspiratory equilibration pressure) is a function of the mean peak alveolar pressure and is a reflection of the transpulmonary pressure. Similar to V_T, it is unknown if there is a specific plateau pressure that is safe. Because of the high shear forces associated with the ventilation of heterogeneously diseased lung, mechanical lung injury is theoretically possible, even with transpulmonary pressures below 30 cm H_2O. However, most clinicians would agree that a plateau pressure less than 25 cm H_2O is unlikely to produce an injurious level of alveolar overdistension, and that a plateau pressure in this range and a tidal volume below 10 mL/kg PBW will not produce VILI regardless of the cause of respiratory failure. However, as plateau pressure increases, the delivered tidal volume should be decreased, regardless of the cause of respiratory failure. V_T should be kept at about 6 mL/kg PBW if the plateau pressure is 25 to 30 cm H_2O and V_T should be 4 to 6 mL/kg PBW if plateau pressures are greater than 30 cm H_2O. Ideally, all patients should be managed with a plateau pressure of less than 30 cm H_2O unless there is a marked decrease of their chest wall compliance (eg, burns, abdominal distension). If the chest wall compliance is decreased, the transpulmonary pressure is decreased and the risk of overdistension

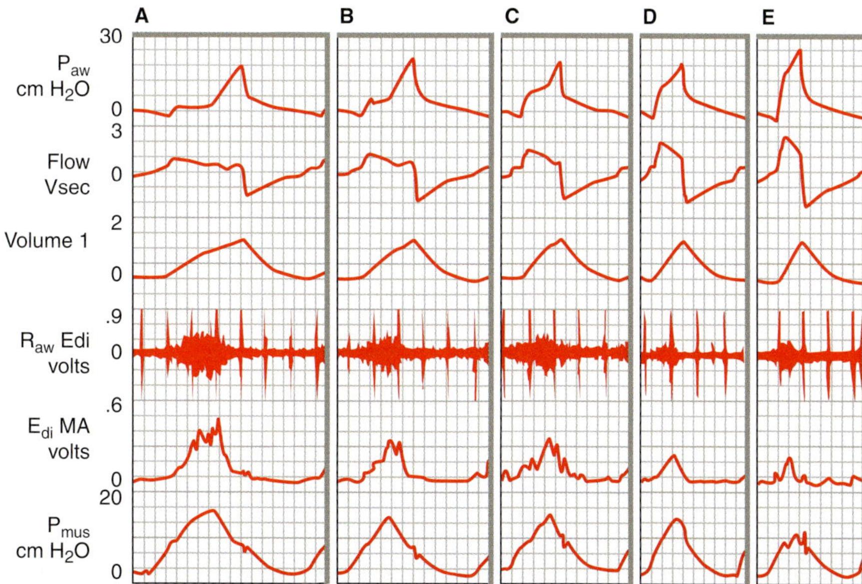

FIGURE 81-15. Representative example of the effect of alternations in peak flow and inspiratory time on airway pressure (P_{aw}), the raw diaphragmatic electromyography (EMG) signal (R_{aw} Edi), the diaphragmatic EMG signal after removal of the electrocardiographic interference and rectification, and the calculated pressure output of the inspiratory muscles (P_{mus}). Note the reduction in EMG activity and muscle output as flow increases. [From Fernandez R, Mendez M, Younes M. Effect of ventilatory flow rates on respiratory timing in normal humans. *Am J Respir Crit Care Med.* 1999;159:710-719. © American Thoracic Society.]

is reduced. In patients with stiff, noncompliant chest walls and abdomens because of sepsis, abdominal distension, fluid resuscitation, and the like, a plateau pressure greater than 30 cm H_2O may be required and would not be associated with an increased risk of VILI.[56] However, in all patients the plateau pressure should ideally be maintained below 40 cm H_2O. Alternatively, some have advocated the use of an esophageal balloon to estimate pleural pressure and guide mechanical ventilation strategies to limit transpulmonary pressure.[57]

AUTO-PEEP

Auto-PEEP, also known as *occult PEEP*, is defined as an alveolar pressure above the airway opening pressure. Auto-PEEP can be caused by flow limitation, dynamic hyperinflation, a high minute ventilation, expiratory muscle activity, and/or a high intra-abdominal pressure (**Fig. 81-16**).[44,58] *Occult auto-PEEP* is a term that is used to describe those lung units with trapped gas that do not communicate with the airway following a prolonged end-expiratory pause.[59] Occult auto-PEEP is likely a function of airway closure or occlusion secondary to mucous plugging, and can be difficult to clinically diagnose. The performance of an end-expiratory occlusion maneuver can be helpful in estimating auto-PEEP levels if the patient is not making expiratory muscle efforts (passive-controlled ventilation). However, the absence of auto-PEEP by this technique should not be completely reassuring, because occult auto-PEEP may still be present. In severe asthma, it is frequently better to monitor the level of plateau pressure, as the plateau pressure will increase or decrease as total auto-PEEP increases or decreases.[59]

Auto-PEEP is a major cause of dyssynchrony. As noted in **Figure 81-17**, when auto-PEEP is present, patients frequently cannot generate a sufficient inspiratory effort to decompress the auto-PEEP and trigger a breath.[45,60] Whenever the patient's respiratory rate exceeds the ventilator's response rate, this problem is almost always caused by auto-PEEP.

When auto-PEEP is caused by dynamic airflow limitation of exhalation volume, as in chronic obstructive pulmonary disease, the application of applied PEEP reduces the patient's effort to trigger the ventilator[45]; that is, applied PEEP can be titrated up to approximately 80% of the measured auto-PEEP without increasing the overall level of air trapping. Applying PEEP in the presence of auto-PEEP caused by dynamic airflow limitation increases central airway pressure without increasing auto-PEEP, so that the pressure change needed to trigger the ventilator is reduced, thereby increasing patient–ventilator synchrony, that is, decreasing the pressure difference across the obstruction. From a practical perspective, because auto-PEEP is difficult to measure in the spontaneously breathing patient, the applied PEEP is increased in 1 to 2 cm H_2O steps until every inspiratory effort made by the patient triggers the ventilator. In some patients, this may require more than

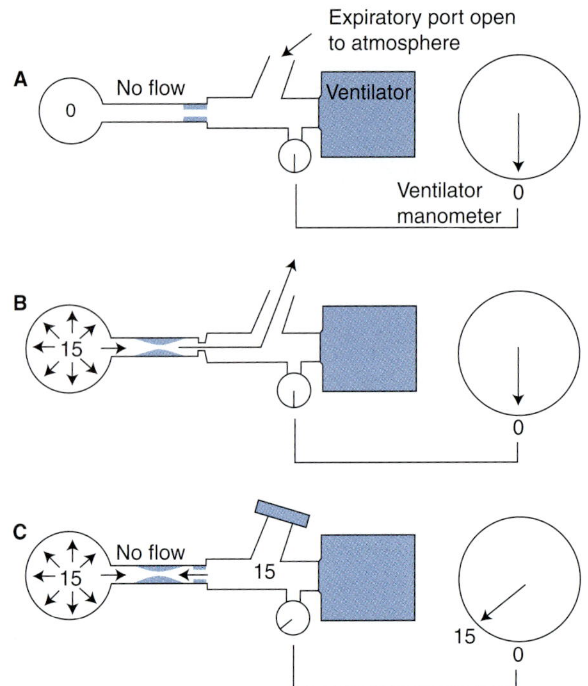

FIGURE 81-16. Relationship between alveolar, central airway, and ventilator circuit pressure under (**A**) normal conditions and (**B** and **C**) in the presence of severe dynamic airway obstruction, (**B**) with expiratory port open, and (**C**) with expiratory port occluded. Autopositive end-expiratory pressure (PEEP) level is identified by creating an end-expiratory hold, allowing alveolar, central airway, and ventilator circuit pressure to equilibrate. Note that during equilibration, auto-PEEP level can be read on the system manometer. [From Pepe PE, Marini JJ. Occult positive end-expiratory pressure in mechanically ventilated patients with airflow obstruction: the auto-PEEP effect. *Am Rev Respir Dis.* 1982;126:166-170. © American Thoracic Society.]

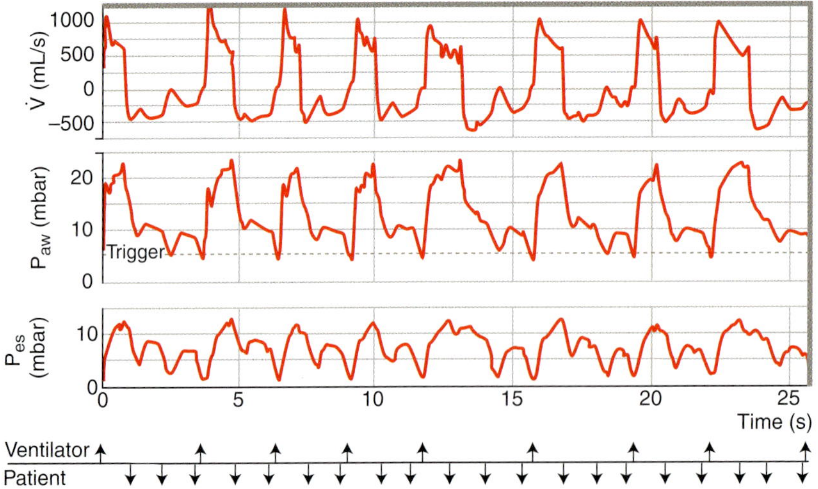

FIGURE 81-17. Gas flow, airway pressure, and esophageal pressure during pressure-supported ventilation with marked patient–ventilator dyssynchrony. Pressure spikes at the onset and termination of the breath indicate dyssynchrony, as well as the difference between patient inspiratory efforts (arrows) and the ventilator response (arrows). [Reproduced with permission from Fabry BE, Guttmann J, Eberhard LE, et al. An analysis of dyssynchrony between the spontaneously breathing patient and ventilator during inspiratory pressure support. *Chest.* 1995;107:1387-1384.]

10 cm H_2O of applied PEEP. During controlled ventilation, a controversy exists over the benefit of applying PEEP to balance the auto-PEEP, because no spontaneous ventilatory efforts are present.

GAS EXCHANGE TARGETS

Target blood gas tensions during mechanical ventilation are theoretically the normal range for the individual patient. This is usually a $Paco_2$ of about 35 to 45 mm Hg for all patients except those with chronic CO_2 retention. In patients with chronically elevated CO_2 levels, the $Paco_2$ should be maintained at the patient's normal level up to 90 mm Hg.[1] If the arterial pH and Pco_2 are reset in these patients to "normal" values, the patients may become impossible to wean from ventilatory support, because during spontaneous unassisted breathing they will maintain CO_2 levels at their baseline, which now results in an acute acidosis. In patients with ARDS, permissive hypercapnia may be unavoidable, as the effect of increasing the level of ventilation to reduce CO_2 levels may produce lung injury.

One factor limiting an increase in $Paco_2$ with a permissive hypercapnic ventilatory strategy is the acidosis induced by the elevated CO_2.[61] Most healthy young adults can tolerate a pH as low as 7.20 without adverse effect.[62] In fact, in acute lung injury or asthma, the increased cardiac output induced by the acidosis may be beneficial. Some clinicians have proposed that the acidosis associated with permissive hypercapnia protects the cell from hypoxemic injury.[63] In older or cardiovascularly unstable patients, the level of acceptable acidosis must be individually gauged based on the response of the patient's cardiovascular system. In all patients the more gradual the permissive hypercapnia is allowed to develop, the greater the likelihood it will be well tolerated.

Tissue oxygenation is dependent on appropriate blood levels of oxygen and cardiac output. Assuming a normal cardiac output, Pao_2 values in critically ill patients need only to be maintained higher than 60 mm Hg, whereas for some patients, because of a lack of alternatives, a PO_2 of higher than 50 mm Hg may be acceptable.[1] There is no value in most patients to maintaining a Pao_2 of 100 mm Hg or higher.

VENTILATOR-INDUCED LUNG INJURY

Although the application of mechanical ventilation can be lifesaving, it has become increasingly clear that the mechanical ventilator can induce lung injury. Laboratory data have defined 2 primary settings in which the mechanical ventilator can induce lung injury, by producing overdistension of the lung at end inspiration and by collapse and reexpansion of unstable lung regions during ventilation.

OVERDISTENSION

Figure 81-18 depicts the impact of a large tidal volume without PEEP on a rat lung as compared to a rat lung ventilated with a small tidal volume and one with 10 cm H_2O PEEP and a large tidal volume.[64] One hour of ventilation with a large tidal volume at zero PEEP caused marked hemorrhagic edema of the lung. This type of injury was termed *volutrauma* by Dreyfuss and Saumon because it is believed that the injury is primarily caused by an excessive tidal volume.[65] However, as described above, an excessive tidal volume is accompanied by an excessive transpulmonary pressure, making the distinctions between pressure and volume injury somewhat semantic. VILI is defined as an increase in the permeability of the alveolar capillary membrane, the development of pulmonary edema, the accumulation of neutrophils and protein within the lung parenchyma and airway, the disruption of surfactant production, and a decreased lung compliance.[65] VILI is indistinguishable from human ARDS and can be produced in rats within minutes by large tidal volume ventilation.[66] Indeed, VILI caused by inflation with large tidal volumes has been demonstrated in many small- and large-animal models. Parker et al,[67] in isolated perfused dog lungs, demonstrated that ventilatory pressures greater than 30 cm H_2O peak alveolar pressure resulted in VILI. Hernandez et al,[68] Egan,[69] and Kolobow et al[70] also demonstrated

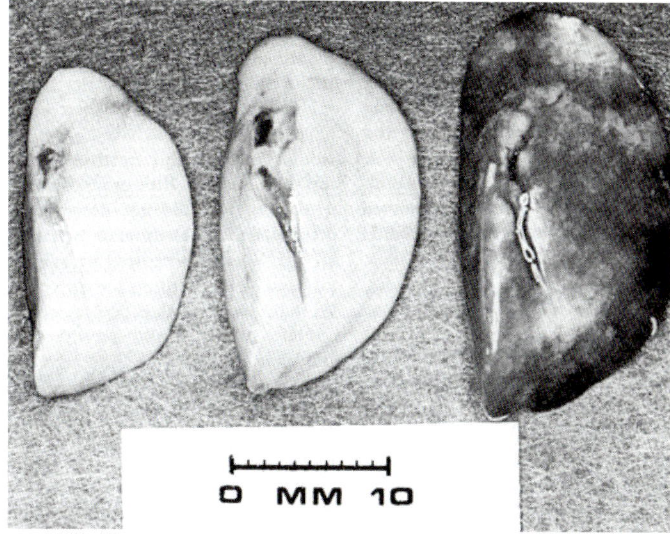

FIGURE 81-18. Comparison of lungs excised from rats ventilated with peak pressure of 14 cm H_2O, zero positive end-expiratory pressure (PEEP); peak pressure 45 cm H_2O, 10 cm H_2O PEEP; and peak pressure 45 cm H_2O, zero PEEP (left to right). The perivascular groove is distended with edema in the lungs from rats ventilated with peak pressures of 45 cm H_2O, 10 cm H_2O PEEP. The lung ventilated at 45 cm H_2O peak pressure zero PEEP is grossly hemorrhaged. [From Webb HH, Tierney D. Experimental pulmonary edema due to intermittent positive-pressure ventilation, with high inflation pressure protection by positive end-expiratory pressure. *Am Rev Respir Dis.* 1974;110:556-565. © American Thoracic Society.]

similar injuries in large-animal models. Ventilation of many species with large tidal volumes results in the development of VILI and an increase in the severity of preexisting lung injury.

The single factor most responsible for the development of VILI appears to be the transpulmonary pressure (pressure inside minus pressure outside the lung or alveolar minus pleural pressure).[66] In a now classic experiment, Dreyfuss et al[66] demonstrated that rats with strapped chest walls were protected from VILI as compared with those ventilated with the same peak pressure but without chest wall binding. In fact the lung injury was similar regardless of the use of positive- or negative-pressure ventilation, provided high transpulmonary pressures were established. As a result, we reason that higher ventilating pressures can be used in the presence of a decreased chest wall compliance without the development of VILI, as the reduced chest wall compliance decreases transpulmonary pressure at peak airway pressure and results in a lower delivered tidal volume.

RECRUITMENT/DERECRUITMENT INJURY: "ATELECTRAUMA"

As noted in Figure 81-18, the application of 10 cm H_2O PEEP in spite of a peak airway pressure of 45 cm H_2O decreased the level of VILI as compared with similar animals ventilated with the same peak pressure but at zero PEEP.[64] Only mild interstitial edema developed in animals ventilated at 10 cm H_2O PEEP. Similar findings have been reported by Corbridge et al in dogs with hydrochloric acid–induced lung injury.[71] Dogs ventilated with 12.5 cm H_2O PEEP and a V_T of 15 mL/kg after lung injury had far less pulmonary edema at autopsy than dogs ventilated with 3.2 cm H_2O PEEP and 30 mL/kg tidal volumes, in spite of the fact that peak alveolar pressure (33 cm H_2O) was the same for both groups during the 5 hours of ventilation.

BIOTRAUMA

Slutsky and Tremblay[72] have referred to the activation of pulmonary and systemic inflammatory mediators by an inappropriate ventilatory pattern as *biotrauma*. Increasing data from both animal and clinical studies indicate that a traumatic ventilatory strategy can augment the level of the pulmonary and systemic inflammatory response. Tremblay et al,[73] in an ex vivo healthy and injured rat lung model, demonstrated that both pro- and anti-inflammatory mediators are activated by ventilatory patterns associated with high peak alveolar pressure and zero PEEP. For ventilated animals in which PEEP was set greater than P_{flex} (lower inflection point on the respiratory system pressure-volume curve) and overdistension was avoided, minimal mediator activation was observed. Similar data were reported by Bethmann et al in an ex vivo perfused mouse lung model.[74] Hyperventilation at 2.5 times the normal transpulmonary pressure using either positive- or negative-pressure ventilation resulted in a 1.75-fold increased expression of tumor necrosis factor α (TNF-α) and interleukin-6 messenger RNA (mRNA). Imai et al[75] and Takata et al,[76] studying rats, noted greater TNF-α mRNA expression with conventional ventilation at low peak pressure (30 cm H_2O) and low PEEP (5 cm H_2O) as compared to high-frequency oscillation at a mean airway pressure of 15 cm H_2O (same as with conventional ventilation). Ranieri et al showed the same effect of ventilatory pattern on pulmonary lavage and plasma TNF-α level in ARDS patients.[77] In a randomized comparison, patients ventilated with PEEP set greater than P_{flex} and peak alveolar pressure kept below the upper inflection point of the pressure-volume curve had reduced TNF-α levels in both plasma and lung lavage fluid after 36 hours. Patients randomized to PEEP based on oxygenation with V_T set to produce eucapnia increased their TNF-α levels after 36 hours. In addition, the ARDSnet[45] demonstrated a lower systemic proinflammatory mediator response in a low tidal volume group of patients as compared to a high tidal volume group. Most recently, Chu et al[78] demonstrated that lung maintained at a high lung volume either by CPAP or ventilated at the same high peak pressure resulted in the same marked activation of inflammatory mediators.

Based on these data both Slutsky and Tremblay[72] and Dreyfuss and Saumon[79] proposed that the lung is the "engine" that drives the development of multisystem organ failure in ARDS patients. The additional lung injury resulting from inappropriate mechanical ventilation causes the movement of inflammatory mediators into the systemic circulation, increasing the systemic production of mediators influencing and damaging the function of distal organs and tissues.

As a result, it seems reasonable to conclude, as discussed by Marini,[56] that "excessive mechanical forces produce lung damage by at least three mechanisms: (a) the signaling of proinflammatory mediator release by mechanical stress, (b) trauma to the epithelium of the lung parenchyma by repetitive opening at high pressures and subsequent closing with each breath, and (c) physical stress on the parenchyma by high peak alveolar pressures." Marini also points out that there is some evidence that high ventilatory frequency[80] (higher frequency, greater injury), high pre- and postalveolar microvascular pressures,[81] decreased surfactant production,[82] supine body position,[83] high body temperature,[84] and immune suppression[85] all enhance the development and severity of VILI.

LUNG-PROTECTIVE VENTILATION

As already discussed, a primary aim of ventilatory support of the surgical patient is to achieve "lung protection," that is, to ensure that the process of mechanical ventilation does not amplify the extent of lung injury. Care should always be exercised to ensure that the plateau pressure and tidal volume do not result in overdistension. In general, based on current information the tidal volume should be maintained less than 10 mL/kg in all acutely ill patients or patients undergoing anesthesia. In ARDS, as presented in the previous section, it is certain that smaller tidal volumes are required. At least 3 clinical trials have demonstrated a benefit of ventilating at 6 to 7 mL/kg (PBW) tidal volumes in ARDS.[55,86,87] In conjunction with these small tidal volumes, the plateau pressures should be maintained below 30 cm H_2O unless the chest wall is stiff.[56] However, the lower the plateau pressure, the less likely tidal volumes of 8 to 9 mL/kg will present concern.

Outside of the clinical setting of ARDS the data are less clear; however, Hubmayr et al performed a retrospective analysis of data on mechanical ventilation in the ICU[44] and intraoperatively[88] at the Mayo Clinic, and on data from an international ventilation survey[89] indicate that small tidal volume (<10 mL/kg) ventilation should be the norm used in most critically ill patients. In 2 of these analyses[54,89] they found that patients in the ICU had a greater probability of developing acute lung injury when ventilated with large tidal volumes (≥10 mL/kg). In their most recent review[88] they demonstrated that patients undergoing pneumonectomy at the Mayo Clinic who were ventilated intraoperatively with larger tidal volumes (median: 8.3 mL/kg) versus smaller tidal volumes (median: 6.7 mL/kg, $P < 0.001$ groups differ) were more likely to develop postoperative respiratory failure and require ventilatory support for longer than 48 hours postoperatively.

In general, rapid respiratory rates (20-40 breaths/min) are needed to maintain gas exchange at low tidal volumes. The smaller the tidal volume and the more severe the lung injury, the greater the probability that patients will require permissive hypercapnia.[54,89,90]

The most appropriate method of setting PEEP in ARDS is still highly controversial.[55,76,77,90] However, there is no question that PEEP is necessary in lung injury to prevent derecruitment. The ARDSnet[55,90] recommends the use of a PEEP/FIO_2 table for setting PEEP, but these tables do not take into consideration the patient's lung mechanics. Incremental PEEP trials have been used for years to provide a reasonable estimate of the necessary PEEP for many patients[91] but may not be the best approach to setting PEEP in lung injury. Three prospective randomized trials have demonstrated positive outcomes when PEEP was set at P_{flex} + 2 cm H_2O.[77,86,87] In 2 studies,[86,87] mortality was decreased in the group ventilated with PEEP at P_{flex} + 2 cm H_2O along with a small delivered tidal volume, and in one, pulmonary and systemic inflammatory mediators were attenuated when this ventilatory strategy was used.[77] Most recently, a number of meta-analyses of the 6 trials[77,86,87,90,92,93] that evaluated different approaches to setting PEEP indicated that high PEEP in ARDS does reduce mortality.[94,95] In general, in ARDS patients a medium PEEP of about 15 cm H_2O is needed with the usual range from 10 to 20 cm H_2O of PEEP. However, some patients require greater than 20 cm H_2O PEEP.

In severe lung injury, the method of setting PEEP that appears best is a decremental PEEP trial following a lung recruitment maneuver.[96] That is, PEEP is titrated downward from a level higher than is needed to determine the minimum level that maintains the benefit of the lung recruitment maneuver.

A number of groups have demonstrated the ability of a lung recruitment maneuver to open the lung in ARDS/ALI patients and the ability of a decremental PEEP trial to keep the lung open.[97-99] However, no outcome benefit has been attributed to lung recruitment maneuvers. The 2 lung recruitment approaches that have received the most study are the use of a sustained CPAP level of 40 to 50 cm H_2O for 30 to 40 seconds[97,99] and the use of pressure-controlled ventilation at a peak pressure of 40 to 50 cm H_2O along with PEEP of 20 to 30 cm H_2O for 1 to 3 minutes.[98] Lung recruitment maneuvers can open the lung of patients with lung injury and should be applied in the first few days after lung injury, but only in patients who are hemodynamically stable with appropriate fluid resuscitation without the presence of, or an increased likelihood of developing, barotrauma.

An alternate approach to setting PEEP in patients with severe lung injury was recently reported by Talmor et al.[57] They randomized patients to be managed with the ARDSnet protocol PEEP table[55] or a table based on esophageal pressure. Their goal when setting PEEP was based on esophageal pressure. PEEP was increased to ensure that end-expiratory esophageal pressure was not negative and as a result reducing lung collapse at end expiration. They demonstrated marked physiologic improvement and a trend toward improved mortality; however, the study was underpowered to identify a mortality benefit. Additional data from multicenter studies are needed before this approach can be recommended.

HIGH-FREQUENCY VENTILATION

Various approaches to high-frequency ventilation (HFV) have been used over the last 30 years to manage patients intraoperatively, as well as to ventilate critically ill ICU patients. Although these techniques have demonstrated their ability to ventilate in both of these settings, limited beneficial outcome data regarding any of these techniques are available. The 3 common methods reported are high-frequency jet ventilation (HFJV), high-frequency percussive ventilation (HFPV), and high-frequency oscillatory ventilation (HFOV).

HIGH-FREQUENCY JET VENTILATION

HFJV is the approach to HFV that has been used most commonly intraoperatively.[100,101] With this technique, gas under high pressure is injected via a small-bore nozzle placed within the endotracheal tube or in the airway itself. The velocity of the gas delivery stream creates a "jet drag effect" entraining secondary gases. This technique can provide ventilatory support with or without a sealed or closed airway. As a result, it has been used successfully during upper-airway surgery, tracheal reconstruction, unilateral surgical procedures, and other procedures in which the airway is not sealed.[100,101] In addition, simple HFJV systems have been used to provide emergency ventilatory support in settings where immediate access to the airway via the pharynx is impossible.[102] This is accomplished by placing the injector through the cricothyroid membrane; however, an escape pathway for injected gases via the upper airway must be present.

HIGH-FREQUENCY OSCILLATORY VENTILATION

HFOV is the most commonly used high-frequency technique in the ICU. However, most of the successful applications of this ventilatory mode have been in neonates.[103] Randomized controlled trials evaluating the use of HFOV during ARDS/ALI in pediatric[104] and adult[105-107] populations have been negative, and HFOV is considered equivalent to conventional ventilation in these settings. With HFOV a high mean airway pressure is established because gas delivery is achieved by oscillating about the mean airway pressure. Tidal volumes as low as 1 mL/kg are delivered at high frequencies (8-12 Hz) in neonates. In adults, generally larger tidal volumes (2-4 mL/kg) are delivered at lower frequencies of 4 to 8 Hz. All clinical approaches to HFV require the use of ventilators specially designed to provide HFV.

A recent meta-analysis of the adult and pediatric randomized controlled trials indicates a mortality benefit from the use of HFO.[108] However, this meta-analysis failed to recognize and discuss the conventional ventilation arm in all of the studies that were evaluated. In none of these studies was conventional ventilation provided in what is considered an ideal lung-protective approach.

HIGH-FREQUENCY PERCUSSIVE VENTILATION

HFPV is a unique form of ventilation that combines the effects of conventional mechanical ventilation with HFO.[91] That is, a typical pressure-targeted breath is delivered but during the breath, oscillations are provided. Oscillations can also occur during the expiratory phase. The goal is to increase the distribution of ventilation and mobilization of secretions by adding the oscillations to conventional ventilation. Most of the data on HFPV have been accumulated in burn or trauma patients.[109,110] As with HFO this approach to managing critically ill patients is effective, but thus far no benefit over conventional mechanical ventilation has been demonstrated.[111]

PRONE POSITIONING

Prone positioning of critically ill patients has been shown to improve oxygenation in a number of case series.[112] The reasons indicated for this improvement are lung recruitment by removing the weight of the heart from the lungs and the positioning of two-thirds of the lung in nondependent regions, drainage of secretions, and better ventilation/perfusion matching. However, the primary concern with proning patients is the need to routinely reposition patients to the supine position. With turning the patient a number of adverse events have been identified including tracheal extubation, loss of vascular access, hemodynamic instability, and arrhythmias. A number of randomized controlled trials have compared prone positioning to continued supine positioning.[113-115] None of these trials were positive; overall mortality is almost exactly similar regardless of position. However, a recent meta-analysis indicates a mortality benefit for the sickest of patients. Prone positioning seems to benefit those patients with a Pao_2/Fio_2 of less than 100 mm Hg.[116] As a result it is considered a last line of therapy for treating severe hypoxemia.

MECHANICAL VENTILATION OF THE POSTOPERATIVE PATIENT

NORMAL PREOPERATIVE PULMONARY FUNCTION

Surgical procedures that require general anesthesia and invade the thorax or abdominal cavity can result in impaired ventilatory function. As a result, well over 50% of cardiac and thoracic surgical patients show postoperative radiographic evidence of atelectasis.[94] In patients with normal preoperative pulmonary function, this normally does not result in any compromise. But in patients with preexisting pulmonary disease, acute respiratory failure is more common.[117]

INITIAL MANAGEMENT

In patients without prior pulmonary disease, ventilatory management is normally uneventful. Pressure or volume assist/control is preferred with tidal volumes as large as the patient desires (6-10 mL/kg PBW) because lung function is normal and the period of total mechanical ventilation time is usually brief.[37] Five cm H_2O PEEP is applied to maintain the functional residual capacity, and the Fio_2 and rate are adjusted to maintain adequate gas exchange.

MAINTENANCE

Ventilatory management is short term in most patients. The Fio_2 is titrated to maintain Pao_2 above 70 mm Hg, and the rate or tidal volume is adjusted to maintain baseline $Paco_2$. Patients can frequently be rapidly transitioned to pressure support and extubated quickly.

CHRONIC OBSTRUCTIVE PULMONARY DISEASE

Pathophysiology Postoperative chronic obstructive pulmonary disease (COPD) patients are commonly encountered in the ICU and are challenging to ventilate. Of primary concern is patient–ventilator synchrony.[1] The single most significant factor affecting synchrony in these patients is air trapping and auto-PEEP.[58,60] In COPD patients, auto-PEEP is caused by dynamic airway compression; that is, unstable airways dilate during positive-pressure inspiration but are compressed by the increased intrathoracic pressure during exhalation. Because auto-PEEP occurs distal to airways obstruction, the airway pressure proximal to the obstruction at end exhalation is normally equal to baseline ventilator circuit pressure. This means that during spontaneous inspiration the patient must first decompress the auto-PEEP level, and then trigger the ventilator. This results in a marked increase in patient effort to trigger the ventilator and dyssynchrony. Many of the patient's inspiratory efforts may not produce sufficient negative force to trigger the ventilator. The patient's actual respiratory rate is then greater than the ventilator's response rate. This increases ventilatory drive, patient respiratory rate, and the patient's overall ventilatory effort. The dyssynchrony associated with auto-PEEP can best be managed at the bedside by applying PEEP as discussed earlier (see Ventilation Settings and Patient–Ventilator Synchrony—Auto-PEEP section).[45]

A second major concern is ensuring that the ventilator's gas delivery rate meets the patient's inspiratory demand. COPD patients who are spontaneously triggering the ventilator have their ventilatory demands best supplied with pressure, as opposed to volume ventilation.[47] However, in either case gas delivery (rise time during pressure ventilation, and peak flow and flow waveform during volume ventilation) should be set to match inspiratory demand. Inspiratory time should coincide with the patient's desired inspiratory time. In assist/control ventilation, the inspiratory time is generally set from 0.6 to 1.0 seconds, and with pressure-support ventilation, the inspiratory termination criteria should be adjusted to ensure a synchronous ending of inspiration.[48]

COPD patients require ventilatory support because of their inability to perform the work needed to maintain normal ("for them") gas exchange. As a result, the ventilator should ensure adequate rest but should always allow the patient to trigger the ventilator. In general, it is advisable not to use ventilatory modes that do not support every inspiratory effort, because they do not provide sufficient rest for the patient. Thus synchronized intermittent mandatory ventilation, airway pressure-release ventilation, and bilevel ventilation should not be used in COPD.

Initial Setting Initially, intubated, mechanically ventilated COPD patients should be managed with pressure support or assist/control (volume or pressure with pressure preferred). The delivered tidal volume should be 6 to 10 mL/kg PBW, dependent on plateau pressure and patient demand. Most COPD patients can be ventilated with a plateau pressure of 25 cm H_2O or less. The respiratory rate is patient determined; however, in assist/control, a backup rate sufficient to maintain the appropriate $Paco_2$ should be set. In volume ventilation, the peak flow should be set at 80 L/min or higher with a decelerating waveform. With pressure ventilation, the rise time and inspiratory termination criteria (pressure support only) should be properly set. Inspiratory time is set equal to the patient's neuroinspiratory time (0.6-1.0 s) and the PEEP level adjusted to ensure that all of the patient's inspiratory efforts trigger the ventilator.[48]

Maintenance In many COPD patients the key medical management issue is to provide rest for the patient. After 48 to 72 hours of ventilatory support, many patients are ready for ventilator discontinuation. In all cases, the focus should be on providing a level of ventilatory support consistent with minimal overall ventilatory effort to ensure recovery from ventilatory muscle dysfunction. As patients recover their PEEP level, pressure support or pressure assist/control level and Fio_2 can be decreased, provided that ventilation targets can be met without markedly increasing the patient's work of breathing.

Patients requiring long-term ventilation should be considered for extensive rehabilitation, including generalized muscle retraining. Patients should be weaned with a spontaneous breathing trial, and most COPD patients can be extubated after a successful 30- to 120-minute trial. However, those requiring long-term ventilatory support (2-4 wk) should be given a tracheotomy and normally require successful 12- to 16-hour spontaneous breathing periods before being allowed to breathe without ventilatory support during the night.

For COPD patients who are ventilated for short periods, who meet all the criteria for weaning, and who clinically seem ready for ventilator discontinuation but continue to fail spontaneous breathing trials, carefully consider extubation to NPPV.[118-120] Some COPD patients can be successfully transitioned to ventilator independence using NPPV. (See Weaning and Noninvasive Positive Pressure section.)

ACUTE RESPIRATORY DISTRESS SYNDROME

Pathophysiologic Issues ARDS and ALI are acute lung diseases characterized by atelectasis, edema, decreased compliance, and severe arterial hypoxemia. As a result, an important issue during mechanical ventilation is to avoid inducing greater lung injury either by end-inspiratory overdistension or by the repetitive opening and closing of unstable lung units. Other important issues are the recruitment of lung, the reversal of atelectasis, and the assurance of adequate systemic oxygenation and CO_2 exchange while avoiding pulmonary oxygen toxicity.

The end-inspiratory plateau pressure should be less than 30 cm H_2O to avoid lung injury unless chest wall compliance is decreased. This

TABLE 81-5 Initial Management of ARDS/ALI

Mode–assist/control (volume or pressure)
Plateau pressure–<30 cm H_2O
Tidal volume–4-8 mL/kg ideal body weight
Inspiratory time–0.6-1.0 s, if triggering equal to neuroinspiratory time
Rate–≤40/min to manage $Paco_2$
PEEP–10-12 cm H_2O
Fio_2–1.0 once stabilized
Lung recruitment–pressure control peak pressure 40-50 cm H_2O,
PEEP 20-30 cm H_2O for 1-3 min or 35-45 cm H_2O CPAP for 30-40 s
Fio_2–to maintain Pao_2 >60 mm Hg
PEEP–set by decremental trial to minimal level maintaining benefits of lung recruitment
ARDS–usually 10-20 cm H_2O
ALI–usually 8-15 cm H_2O

ALI, acute lung injury; ARDS, acute respiratory distress syndrome; CPAP, continuous positive airway pressure; PEEP, positive end-expiratory pressure.

means that for most ARDS/ALI patients the tidal volume should be set to 4 to 8 mL/kg PBW.[55,86,87] However, if the plateau pressure can be maintained below 25 cm H_2O and the patient desires a tidal volume up to 10 mL/kg PBW, it may be more acceptable to meet the patient's ventilatory demands than to force the patient to receive a low tidal volume (which may require intravenous [IV] sedation to apnea).

Some of the atelectasis in ARDS/ALI patients is recruitable by the use of short-term application of a "high" airway pressure (a recruitment maneuver).[97-99] These maneuvers work best on the initial day of identification of ARDS/ALI. The longer the patient has ARDS/ALI, the less likely that recruitment maneuvers will succeed and the greater the likelihood of hemodynamic compromise. Following a recruitment maneuver, sufficient levels of PEEP should be applied to maintain the benefits of lung recruitment.

Initial Settings Assist/control mode (**Table 81-5**), either pressure or volume, can be used with pressure targeting recommended if the patient is triggering each breath and has a variable ventilatory demand. A maximum plateau pressure of 30 cm H_2O should be set at a tidal volume of 4 to 8 mL/kg PBW unless the plateau pressure is less than 25 cm H_2O. The rate should be set to ensure adequate CO_2 elimination. Respiratory rates can be set as high as 40 breaths/min. The rate-limiting factor is the development of auto-PEEP. In most patients, a normal $Paco_2$ of 35 to 50 mm Hg can be established by adjusting the rate. In some patients with a low compliance, permissive hypercapnia may be necessary. Tolerance of hypercapnia depends on the pH; it is better to allow the $Paco_2$ to gradually increase over a day or 2 to prevent the development of a marked respiratory acidosis.

Fio_2 should initially be set at 1.0 and PEEP at 10 to 12 cm H_2O until hemodynamic stability is achieved. Once the patient is hemodynamically stable, a lung recruitment maneuver should be considered, using either a CPAP or pressure-assist/control approach as discussed earlier (in the section Lung-Protective Ventilation). Before recruitment the patient should be stable hemodynamically, sedated to near apnea, and breathing 100% oxygen. Careful monitoring of the hemodynamic response and oxygenation level during the recruitment maneuver should be performed, and the maneuver should be stopped if hemodynamic compromise or desaturation is observed. Following the maneuver, the minimum PEEP level maintaining the oxygenation benefit of the recruitment maneuver should be applied. This is best determined by a decremental PEEP trial.[96] First, the PEEP level is set at 20 cm H_2O and the dynamic compliance determined. Then the PEEP level is decreased by 2 cm H_2O and after the compliance has stabilized, the PEEP is decreased again by 2 cm H_2O. In general it takes about 3 to 5 minutes for the compliance to stabilize. The decremental trail is stopped once the PEEP level associated with the best compliance can be identified. The PEEP is then set

2 cm H_2O above this level because the best compliance PEEP underestimates the best oxygenation PEEP by about 2 cm H_2O. At this point another recruitment maneuver is performed, after which PEEP is set at the identified level plus 2 cm H_2O. If another method of setting PEEP is used and the oxygenation benefit of the recruitment maneuver is lost over a brief period, the PEEP level is set too low and should be increased. Many ARDS patients will require a PEEP level of 10 to 20 cm H_2O and ALI patients often require a PEEP level of 8 to 15 cm H_2O.

Regardless of the use of pressure or volume mode ventilation, the inspiratory time should be set at about 0.6 to 1.0 seconds, depending on the patient's ventilatory demand. In patients who are breathing spontaneously, the inspiratory time should be set equal to the patient's neuroinspiratory time. In volume ventilation, adequate peak flow should be provided to meet the patient's ventilatory demand (≥80 L/min) using a decelerating waveform.

A recently published report by Papazian et al[121] demonstrated that paralysis as compared to standard care for the first 48 hours of ventilation in severe ARDS patients resulted in decreased mortality. It has been speculated that this was a result of decreased oxygen consumption and lack of fighting the ventilator that may have precipitated atelectasis and increased the likelihood of developing ventilator-associated pneumonia.[122] In addition, paralysis was obtained with *cis*-atracurium, which has been shown to have anti-inflammatory properties.[123] However, before this approach can be universally recommended additional studies are needed.

Maintenance The FIO_2 should be decreased before PEEP when oxygenation improves. PEEP generally should not be decreased until the FIO_2 is less than 0.50. If the PaO_2 decreases as PEEP is lowered, the prior PEEP level should be reestablished, and the FIO_2 should not be increased. When this occurs, decreasing PEEP resulted in derecruitment of lung, indicating that the higher PEEP level is needed.

Once the patient's ventilatory drive has normalized and spontaneous triggering of the ventilator can be maintained, patients with ARDS/ALI can usually be maintained with pressure-support ventilation. As with assist/control, the peak pressure should be maintained as low as possible and always less than 30 cm H_2O.

In patients with reduced chest wall compliances as a result of abdominal sepsis, ascites, obesity, thoracic deformity, or massive fluid resuscitation following trauma, a plateau pressure greater than 30 cm H_2O may be necessary for adequate ventilation. This is acceptable, as the transpulmonary pressure is lower with the stiff chest wall preventing overdistension of the lung. However, when the plateau pressure is greater than 30 cm H_2O, the tidal volume should be reduced to less than 6 mL/kg PBW.

In ARDS/ALI, care should be exercised to never disconnect the ventilator circuit. Whenever the circuit is disconnected from the airway, lung derecruitment occurs within seconds. Inline suction catheters should always be used, and the use of manual resuscitators (Ambu bags) should be avoided. Suctioning should only occur when the presence of secretions is observed, and when performed, the suction pressure should be regulated to 120 mm Hg and performed gently to avoid lung derecruitment.

If lung recruitment and an appropriate PEEP setting are achieved but the FIO_2 remains greater than 0.60 to achieve adequate oxygenation, then consider prone positioning (if the PaO_2/FIO_2 is <100 mm Hg) of the patient. Although neither prone positioning nor lung recruitment have been shown to improve survival rates, both can recruit lung and may improve oxygenation. The recruitment of regions of atelectasis reduces the plateau pressure and FIO_2, improves surfactant function, and decreases the risk of pneumonia. At this time, the use of high-frequency oscillation or airway pressure-release ventilation does not appear to improve outcome in ARDS, but both modes can provide adequate management of ARDS/ALI patients. Neither mode has been shown to be superior to conventional assist/control ventilation.

UNILATERAL LUNG DISEASE

Patients with unilateral lung disease present a particularly difficult challenge for mechanical ventilation. The postoperative patient after single-lung transplantation illustrates these problems. One lung has relatively normal pulmonary mechanics (the transplanted lung), whereas the native lung has mechanics reflecting either obstructive or restrictive disease. In these patients, the ventilator should be set to ensure maximum function of the native lung, as this lung will present the greatest ventilatory challenge. If the native lung has chronic obstruction, ventilate with moderate volume and slow rates. With pulmonary fibrosis of the native lung, a smaller V_T and more rapid rate are indicated. In the case of pulmonary fibrosis, there is less concern about air trapping. However, peak alveolar pressure may be high because of the reduced lung compliance.

The greatest ventilatory challenge is the patient with a single-lung transplant where the native lung is obstructed and the transplanted lung has become stiff (low compliance) as a consequence of infection, rejection, or acute lung injury. In this setting, it is difficult to determine the ideal ventilator settings because of the differing pathology of each lung. Careful attention needs to be paid to 2 variables as adjustments are made: first, concern about peak alveolar pressure because of ventilator-imposed lung injury, damaging the transplanted lung and its bronchial anastomosis, and second, air trapping in the obstructed lung resulting in grossly compromised ventilation/perfusion ratios, overdistension, and the like. In this setting, permissive hypercapnia is often necessary with the final ventilator settings being a compromise between the conflicting needs of each lung.

TABLE 81-6 Criteria for Conducting a Spontaneous Breathing Trial

Partial reversal of factors contributing to ventilator dependence
Assessment of oxygenation
• PaO_2/FIO_2 ≥150 mm Hg
• Positive end-expiratory pressure ≤8 cm H_2O
• FIO_2 ≤0.5
• pH ≥7.25
Hemodynamic stability—only low-dose vasopressors required
Spontaneous inspiratory efforts present

Adapted from Evidence-based guidelines for weaning and discontinuing ventilatory support: a collective task force facilitated by the American College of Chest Physicians; the American Association for Respiratory Care; and the American College of Critical Care Medicine. *Chest.* 2001;120:375S-395S.

WEANING

Recent guidelines recommend the use of spontaneous breathing trials for weaning all patients from ventilatory support.[124] These guidelines also recommend that protocols be developed to allow assessment for weaning from the first day of ventilatory support. **Table 81-6** lists the criteria for initiation of a spontaneous breathing trial for any patient requiring ventilatory support. **Table 81-7** lists guidelines to identify those patients having failed a trial of spontaneous breathing.

If a patient meets the guidelines in Table 81-6 by midnight, sedation should be adjusted to ensure spontaneous breathing by early morning. A 30- to 120-minute spontaneous breathing trial is performed, and if the patient does not fail the trial based on the criteria in Table 81-7, consider the patient for extubation.[124] After short-term ventilatory

TABLE 81-7 Criteria Defining Failure of a Spontaneous Breathing Trial

Respiratory rate >35 breaths/min
SaO_2 <90%
Pulse >140 beats/min or sustained increase of 20%
Systolic blood pressure >180 mm Hg or diastolic blood pressure >90 mm Hg
Increased anxiety
Increased diaphoresis

Adapted from Evidence-based guidelines for weaning and discontinuing ventilatory support: a collective task force facilitated by the American College of Chest Physicians; the American Association for Respiratory Care; and the American College of Critical Care Medicine. *Chest.* 2001;120:375S-395S.

TABLE 81-8 Factors Contributing to Ventilator Dependence in Difficult-to-Wean Patients

WHEANS NOT
Wheezes
Heart disease
Electrolyte imbalance
Anxiety, aspiration, alkalosis
Neuromuscular weakness
Sepsis, sustained sedation
Nutritional deficits
Opiates not reversed, obesity
Thyroid disease

Adapted from Ely WE. The utility of weaning protocols to expedite liberation from mechanical ventilation. *Respir Care Clin N Am.* 2000;6:303-319.

support, most clinicians do not recommend measuring lung mechanics. Even the rapid shallow breathing index has not proven universally useful in identifying those patients who are ready for weaning. All of the current data indicate that the use of other approaches to weaning simply results in prolongation of the ventilatory support period.[95] Patients failing weaning trials should be carefully assessed for the specific factors causing failure. **Table 81-8** from Ely lists areas of concern that should be assessed in the patient falling multiple weaning trials.[125] Finally, in some patients the use of NPPV may facilitate the process of transition to unsupported spontaneous breathing.[118-120]

NONINVASIVE POSITIVE PRESSURE

Over the last 20 years increasing emphasis has been placed on the use of noninvasive (without tracheal intubation) positive pressure to support patients developing respiratory failure.[126] Although much of the emphasis in such studies has focused on the patient with COPD in an acute exacerbation,[127] a number of trials over the years have focused on the use of NPPV[128] or CPAP for the management of postoperative patients.[103-107,129-133]

The primary mechanism producing arterial hypoxemia after surgery is impaired ventilation/perfusion matching as a result of the development of atelectasis.[107] Atelectasis in this setting is a result of recumbent positioning, ventilation with high oxygen concentrations, diaphragmatic dysfunction, and incisional pain producing impaired secretion clearance.[129] Several studies show that mask CPAP ventilation in this setting improves gas exchange, minimizes the development of atelectasis, and increases functional residual capacity.[129-133] Most of these studies were case series[129-132]; the most recent study, however, was a randomized controlled trial.[133] Squadrone et al[133] demonstrated that mask CPAP at 7.5 cm H_2O at 0.5 FIO_2 for 6 hours in all patients following major elective abdominal surgery with a PO_2/FIO_2 less than 300 mm Hg prevented intubation compared to those receiving 50% oxygen by a Venturi mask (1% vs 10% intubation rate; $P < 0.005$). In addition, significant decreases in subsequent pneumonia and sepsis rates were observed.

In postoperative lung resection patients with hypoxemic respiratory failure, Auriant et al[128] demonstrated that the use of NPPV versus standard care prevented intubation ($P = 0.030$) and decreased hospital mortality ($P = 0.045$). Although CPAP and NPPV are useful in treating postoperative respiratory failure, they should be cautiously applied, and tracheal intubation for patients not responding to these therapies should not be delayed.[108] These concerns were recently illustrated by Delclaux et al.[134] They randomized patients with hypoxemic respiratory failure to either CPAP or standard therapy. They found no difference in the subsequent intubation rate or the mortality rate, but a greater incidence of cardiac arrest and stress ulcers in those managed with CPAP.

A number of recent studies have focused on the use of NPPV in the weaning process. The most commonly studied patients are those with COPD. At least 2 groups have shown beneficial results with COPD patients who were failing weaning trials and who were extubated and ventilated with NPPV; that is, NPPV provided a bridge from invasive ventilation to spontaneous breathing in these patients failing weaning trials.[118,119] However, it must be emphasized that these COPD patients were not postoperative patients.

The most encouraging use of NPPV during weaning are the results reported by Nava[135] and Ferrer.[110,136,137] In these studies patients passing their weaning trials and who were then extubated but at risk for failing extubation were studied. Those managed postextubation for 24 to 48 hours with NPPV had a significant decrease in the likelihood of their needing reintubation. The increased risks were defined as COPD, congestive heart failure, an Acute Physiology and Chronic Health Evaluation (APACHE) score above 12, age above 65 years, ineffective cough, and excessive secretions, 1 or more weaning failures, upper airway obstruction, or more than 1 comorbid condition. Of note, however, very few of these patients were postoperative patients.

There is considerable concern over the use of NPPV for the patient developing postextubation hypoxemic respiratory failure. Keenan et al[138] demonstrated no benefit from the use of NPPV as compared to standard therapy in about 160 randomized patients. No differences were observed in the length of mechanical ventilation, hospital stay, or hospital mortality. Of even more concern was the increased mortality reported by Esteban et al[139] in patients with postextubation hypoxemic respiratory failure who were managed with NPPV. These authors argue that the primary reason for the increased mortality was the delay in intubating those who were treated with NPPV (12 vs 2 h).

Based on the current data from these randomized controlled trials, NPPV is best used for patients passing weaning trials who are at an increased risk of developing respiratory failure as described by Nava[135] and Ferrer.[136,137]

KEY REFERENCES

- Smith TC, Marini JJ. Impact of PEEP on lung mechanics and work of breathing in severe airflow obstruction. *J Appl Phys.* 1988;64:1488-1496.
- Dreyfuss D, Saumon G. Ventilator-induced lung injury: lessons from experimental studies. *Am J Respir Crit Care Med.* 1998;157: 294-323.
- The Acute Respiratory Distress Syndrome Network. Ventilation with lower tidal volumes as compared with traditional tidal volumes for acute lung injury and the acute respiratory distress syndrome. *N Engl J Med.* 2000;342:1301-1308.
- Villar J, Kacmarek RM, Perez-Mendez L, Aguirre-Jaime A, for the ARIES Network. A high positive end-expiratory pressure, low tidal volume ventilatory strategy improves outcome in persistent acute respiratory distress syndrome: a randomized, controlled trial. *Crit Care Med.* 2006;34:1311-1318.
- Fernandez-Perez ER, Keegan MT, Brown DR, Hubmayr RD, Gajic O. Intraoperative tidal volume as a risk factor for respiratory failure after pneumonectomy. *Anesthesiology.* 2006;105:14-18.
- Borges JB, Okamoto V, Gustavo M, et al. Reversibility of lung collapse and hypoxemia in early acute respiratory distress syndrome. *Am J Respir Crit Care Med.* 2006;174:268-278.
- Ferrer M, Esquinas A, Arancibia F, et al. Noninvasive ventilation during persistent weaning failure. *Am J Respir Crit Care Med.* 2003;168:70-76.

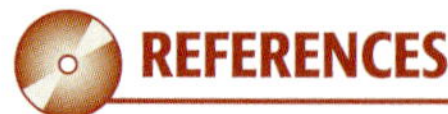

REFERENCES

Complete references available on DVD and online version at www.LongneckerAnesthesiology.com

CHAPTER 82

Cardiopulmonary Resuscitation

Charles W. Otto

KEY POINTS

1. During many in- and out-of-hospital resuscitation attempts less than half the time is devoted to chest compressions. Interrupting compressions reduces myocardial perfusion and is detrimental to the ultimate success of resuscitation. Maintaining uninterrupted chest compressions must be the first priority during cardiopulmonary resuscitation.
2. The relative importance of chest compressions, ventilation, and defibrillation during resuscitation must be adjusted for the context of the rescue situation and the personnel available.
3. When an arrest is witnessed, the arrest is likely to be of cardiac (rather than respiratory) cause, and advanced care will be available within a short time, closed chest compressions alone may be as efficacious as compressions and mouth-to-mouth ventilation.
4. Fluctuations in intrathoracic pressure play a significant role in blood flow during most resuscitations, and the cardiac pump mechanism contributes under some circumstances.
5. The critical myocardial blood flow is associated with aortic "diastolic" pressure exceeding 40 mm Hg.
6. Cardiac output is severely depressed during cardiopulmonary resuscitation (CPR), ranging from 10% to 33% of prearrest values in experimental animals. Nearly all of the cardiac output is directed to organs above the diaphragm.
7. During CPR, measurement of blood gases reveals an arterial respiratory alkalosis and a venous respiratory acidosis because the arterial P_{CO_2} is reduced and the venous P_{CO_2} is elevated.
8. Exhaled end-tidal CO_2 is an excellent noninvasive guide to the effectiveness of standard CPR.
9. Immediate defibrillation is most effective if applied within 4 to 5 minutes of collapse. Otherwise, a brief period of 2 to 3 minutes of chest compressions before defibrillation may improve survival.
10. Amiodarone and lidocaine are used during cardiac arrest to aid defibrillation when ventricular fibrillation is refractory to electrical countershock therapy or when fibrillation recurs following successful conversion.
11. Outcome studies prospectively comparing standard and high-dose epinephrine have not demonstrated conclusively that higher doses will improve survival.
12. Evidence currently suggests that, like other potent vasopressors, vasopressin is equivalent to but not better than epinephrine for use during CPR.
13. In contrast to pharmacologic therapy, 2 studies demonstrate improved neurologic outcomes when mild therapeutic hypothermia (89.6°F-93.2°F [32°C-34°C]) is induced for 12 to 24 hours in cardiac arrest survivors who remained comatose after hospital admission.

In the hospital, resuscitation from cardiac arrest depends on the rapid response of a well-trained cardiopulmonary resuscitation (CPR) team that usually includes physicians, nurses, respiratory care providers, and pharmacists. The anesthesiologist is usually a team member and frequently is expected to be the team leader. The team must be coordinated and communicate readily. The goals of published CPR guidelines and widely taught courses in basic life support (BLS), advanced cardiac life support (ACLS), and pediatric advanced life support (PALS) are to provide the knowledge base and framework for effective teamwork.[1] To function within the team, the anesthesiologist must be thoroughly familiar with ACLS protocols. Team leadership requires in-depth, current knowledge of physiology, pharmacology, and alternative CPR techniques. This chapter provides the scientific background on which current CPR practice is based. It focuses exclusively on cardiac arrest. Other circumstances requiring cardiovascular support, such as shock and dysrhythmias, are discussed in other chapters.

Approximately 50% of patients suffering in-hospital cardiac arrest are resuscitated, and 18% of adults and 27% of children survive to discharge.[2] The operating room is the location where CPR has the highest rate of success. Cardiac arrest occurs approximately 7 times for every 10 000 anesthesia events.[3] The cause for the arrest is anesthesia related approximately 4.5 times out of every 10 000 anesthesia events, but mortality from these arrests is only 0.4 per 10 000 anesthesia events. Resuscitation is successful approximately 90% of the time in anesthesia-related cardiac arrests. Excluding the operating room, the best initial resuscitation rates are in reports from the intensive care unit (ICU), and the best survival rates are shown in patients arresting in the emergency department. The in-hospital success is similar to resuscitation and survival rates from out-of-hospital arrest in cities with rapid response emergency medical systems.[4] In out-of-hospital arrests, poor outcomes are associated with (a) long arrest times before CPR is begun, (b) prolonged ventricular fibrillation (VF) without definitive therapy, and (c) inadequate coronary and cerebral perfusion during CPR.[5] Therefore, optimum survival is obtained only if uninterrupted chest compressions are started immediately and the emergency system is activated so that defibrillation can be applied within 8 minutes.[4] Rapid response times and expert personnel factor into better outcomes for in-hospital arrests. Intercurrent illnesses in hospitalized patients reduce the likelihood of survival and the arrest victim is more likely to be elderly, a factor that may reduce survival. The cause of arrest associated with the best outcome is ventricular fibrillation secondary to myocardial ischemia. This initiating event is less common in hospitalized patients. When applying CPR, attention to the details of effective resuscitation is important. However, CPR is only symptomatic therapy, thus attention should not only be paid to the mechanics of CPR but to a search for a treatable cause of the arrest.

HISTORY

Discoveries contributing to modern CPR have a long history recorded in many famous works.[6,7] These discoveries begin with the Bible story of Elisha breathing life back into the son of a Shunammite woman (II *Kings* 4:34) and continue with Andreas Vesalius's description of tracheotomy and artificial ventilation, William Harvey's manual manipulation of the heart, and the teachings of the Society for the Recovery of Persons Apparently Drowned, founded in London in 1774. Nevertheless, the combined techniques of modern CPR are just 50 years old. Although there were significant contributions from other centers in the United States and Europe, modern CPR developed primarily from the fortuitous assemblage of innovative clinicians and researchers in Baltimore in the 1950s and early 1960s. In the late 1950s Elam, Safar, and Gordon established mouth-to-mouth ventilation as the only effective means of artificial ventilation.[8-11] The internal defibrillator was developed in 1933 but was not applied successfully until 1947.[12,13] It was another decade before its general use was made possible by the development of external transthoracic defibrillation.[14,15] Despite these advances, widespread resuscitation from cardiac arrest was not possible until Kouwenhoven, Jude, and Knickerbocker described success with closed chest cardiac massage in a series of patients.[16] The final major component of modern CPR was added in 1963 when Redding and Pearson described the improved success obtained by administering epinephrine or other vasopressor drugs.[17]

CONTEXT-SENSITIVE APPROACH TO RESUSCITATION

The process of cardiopulmonary resuscitation consists of multiple elements including recognition of arrest; activation of an emergency response system; attention to airway, breathing, circulation, drugs, electrical therapy (ABCDEs); and postresuscitation care. Traditionally, basic life support (BLS) included the ABCs and was considered appropriate for the lay rescuer as well as the health care provider, without the use of additional equipment. Advanced life support (ALS) included BLS plus all other available modalities. The distinction between BLS and ALS has become blurred with the addition of public access defibrillators, more individuals trained in CPR, and the recognition that optimum performance of BLS provides better outcomes than the addition of any advanced therapies.

Physiologically, the objective of performing CPR is to provide oxygen to the vital organs—the brain and especially the heart—until normal circulation is restored. Cardiac arrest caused by ventricular fibrillation can be characterized in 3 phases (**Table 82-1**).[18] The *electrical* phase occurs during the first 4 to 5 minutes of the arrest, and early defibrillation is critical for success during this time. The *hemodynamic* phase follows for the next 10 to 15 minutes when perfusing the myocardium with oxygenated blood is critical. This is followed by what has been called the *metabolic* phase, when the ischemic injury to the heart is so great that it is not clear what interventions will be successful. This mechanism of cardiac arrest (that caused by VF) is most common in adults and obviously requires primary attention to defibrillation and perfusing the myocardium. Because arrest occurs with normal oxygenation of the blood and a reservoir of oxygen in the lung, ventilation is relatively less important. Cardiac arrest in children and certain adult situations, such as drowning, is more likely to be caused by hypoxia. In this circumstance, although restoring circulation with chest compressions remains important, providing adequate ventilation to reoxygenate the blood is also necessary. Consequently, rescuers are encouraged to take the context of resuscitation into account when applying the elements of CPR, adjusting the priorities to the situation at hand. These 2 different circumstances account for the slightly different approach to the airway-breathing-compression sequence in adults and children (**Boxes 82-1 and 82-2**).

Traditionally, CPR has been presented as a sequence of distinct steps (algorithm) to help a single rescuer prioritize actions or decisions. This approach has been continued in Boxes 82-1 and 82-2. However, it is common for multiple providers to be present at resuscitation and each should take responsibility for simultaneously instituting a critical action (eg, one to activate the emergency response, one to begin chest compressions, and one to retrieve a defibrillator). The actual priority of actions may vary depending on the context of the cardiac arrest.

THE IMPORTANCE OF THE TIMING OF INTERVENTIONS DURING CPR

It has been repeatedly demonstrated that early intervention is necessary for resuscitation attempts to be successful. CPR has had the most dramatic effect when prompt defibrillation is applied during the electrical phase of ventricular fibrillation, and the circumstance in which public-access automated external defibrillation has proven beneficial. The high oxygen consumption of the fibrillating heart causes the rapid depletion of myocardial high-energy phosphates. Myocardial adenosine-5′-triphosphate (ATP) levels during VF correlate with the success of defibrillation and, by about 4 minutes, the ATP levels in the heart have fallen to levels that make restoration of normal contractile function problematic. Effective chest compressions help replete or delay reductions in ATP by restoring myocardial blood flow. Therefore, the most important intervention during the hemodynamic phase of cardiac arrest is producing coronary perfusion by means of chest compressions. In the absence of prompt defibrillation, the most important intervention for neurologically normal survival from cardiac arrest is restoration and maintenance of cerebral and myocardial blood flow. Because perfusion pressures generated by chest compressions are quite low compared to the intact circulation, any interruption of chest compressions markedly reduces the chances for neurologically normal survival. Therefore, any intervention that interrupts chest compressions is strongly discouraged.

Early intervention in cardiac arrest requires not only rapid response emergency medical systems for out-of-hospital arrests and appropriate code teams for in-hospital arrests, but also immediate intervention by bystanders when cardiac arrest victims collapse. Unfortunately, the incidence of bystander CPR has been falling for 3 decades. The reasons for this reluctance to intervene are multiple but primarily seem to be (a) a lack of training, (b) the complexity of the task, and (c) a fear of

TABLE 82-1 Phases of Cardiac Arrest

Phase	Time From Collapse	Intervention
Electrical	4-5 min	Defibrillation
Hemodynamic	15-20 min	Myocardial perfusion
Metabolic	>20 min	Unknown

BOX 82-1

Sequence of Resuscitation Events in Children for the Lone Rescuer Proficient in Rescue Breathing

Recognition of Arrest

Unresponsive to aggressive stimulation

Absent or abnormal (gasps) breathing

	Teen	Child	Infant
Pulse check (<10 s)	Carotid	Carotid	Brachial or Femoral

Activate Emergency Response System

Call for help

Call 911 or activate facility's emergency response system

Airway

Position

Open airway

- Head tilt/chin lift
- Jaw thrust

Breathing

Perform rescue breathing

- Two breaths (1 second each)

Chest Compressions	**Teen**	**Child**	**Infant**
Placement	Two hands	One hand	Two or 3 fingers or encircling method
Depth of compression	2 in	$\frac{1}{3}$-$\frac{1}{2}$ depth of chest	
Rate/min	100	100	100
Compression/ventilation ratio	30:2	30:2	30:2

(Actions when additional providers available)

Drugs

Administer supplemental oxygen

Obtain intravenous/intraosseous access

Administer epinephrine or vasopressin

Electrical Therapy

Assess rhythm and defibrillate, if appropriate

Assess adequacy of CPR efforts

Secure airway

Additional drug therapy

BOX 82-2

Sequence of Resuscitation Events in Adults for the Lone Rescuer Proficient in Rescue Breathing

Recognition of Arrest

Unresponsive to aggressive stimulation

Absent or abnormal (gasps) breathing

Pulse Check (<10 s)	Carotid

Activate Emergency Response System

Call for help

Call 911 or activate facility's emergency response system

Electrical Therapy

Attach automatic external defibrillator (AED) or defibrillator as soon as available

Assess rhythm and defibrillate, if appropriate

Chest compressions

Placement	Two hands
Depth of compression	2 in
Rate/min	100
Compression/ventilation ratio	30:2

Airway

Position

Open airway

- Head tilt/chin lift
- Jaw thrust

Breathing

Perform rescue breathing

- Two breaths (1 s each)

(Actions when additional providers available)

Drugs

Administer supplemental oxygen

Obtain intravenous/intraosseous access

Administer epinephrine or vasopressin

Assess adequacy of CPR efforts

Secure airway

Additional drug therapy

doing harm. Many of these concerns focus on the mouth-to-mouth ventilation part of the CPR intervention and many experts are now stressing the importance of continuous chest compressions, even at the expense of ventilation, by bystanders and early rescuers. There is no doubt that chest-compression-only CPR given by bystanders is more acceptable for most, easier to learn and retain, and provides better hemodynamic support.

Early studies in anesthetized humans suggested that the airway would not remain open in the unconscious, leading to the teaching that airway control and artificial ventilation must accompany chest compressions.[8-11] However, there are now considerable data to suggest that eliminating mouth-to-mouth ventilation early in the resuscitation of witnessed fibrillatory cardiac arrest is not detrimental to outcome and may improve survival. Data from the Belgian Cardiopulmonary Cerebral Resuscitation (CPCR) Registry demonstrates that 14-day survival and neurologic outcome are the same regardless of whether bystanders initiate full basic life support or only do chest compressions. Both are significantly better than if the bystanders only do mouth-to-mouth ventilation or attempt no CPR.[19,20]

The necessity for ventilation during basic life support has been studied in animal models. Multiple studies have reported that in prolonged fibrillatory cardiac arrest, neurologically intact survival is the same with chest-compression-only resuscitation as with idealized standard CPR (as recommended by the 2000 American Heart Association [AHA] Guidelines), with a 15:2 compression-to-ventilation ratio and when compressions are only interrupted for 4 seconds to provide ventilation.[21-23] However, it has been demonstrated that a single lay rescuer interrupts chest compressions for an average of 16 seconds to deliver the 2 recommended mouth-to-mouth ventilations.[24] When the 16-second pause for 2 ventilations is incorporated, the 24-hour neurologically intact survival rate in the animal model is reduced. Survival is 13% with a 15:2 compression-to-ventilation ratio and 42% with a 30:2 ratio compared to approximately 70% survival with continuous chest compressions.[25,26] The animal studies are supported by a study of CPR technique instructions given by telephone dispatchers to inexperienced bystanders. Instruction in chest compressions alone resulted in the same survival as that of instruction in both compressions and ventilation.[27]

These observations suggest that when arrest is witnessed and likely to be of cardiac (rather than respiratory) cause, and when intubation will be available within a short time, closed chest compressions alone may be as efficacious as compressions and mouth-to-mouth ventilation. In many venues, basic life support teaching for the lay rescuer is being simplified to eliminate mouth-to-mouth ventilation. Yet the recognition that interrupting chest compressions is harmful and occurs frequently may be more important to the efficacy of intervention than dispensing with mouth-to-mouth. Compressions are interrupted during repeated patient assessment, ventilations, intubation, central line placement, change of rescuers, and defibrillation (especially with automatic external defibrillators [AEDs]). In many resuscitation efforts both in and out of hospital, chest compressions are performed during less than 50% of the attempt. Interrupting compressions is significantly detrimental to maintaining myocardial perfusion, and therefore to the ultimate success of the resuscitation attempt.

AIRWAY MANAGEMENT

The goal of airway management during cardiorespiratory arrest is the same as that during general anesthesia: to provide a clear path for respiratory gas exchange while minimizing gastric insufflation and the risk of pulmonary aspiration. Airway maintenance in an unconscious patient is a basic part of anesthesia practice, and all the techniques learned for its use during anesthesia are applicable for use in the cardiac arrest victim. Just as in the operating room, the most commonly used technique for opening the airway is the "head tilt–chin lift" method. If this is ineffective, the "jaw thrust" maneuver is frequently helpful. Oropharyngeal and nasopharyngeal airways are useful for helping maintain an open airway in patients who are not intubated. Care must be taken to ensure that airways are inserted correctly and do not worsen airway obstruction. Insertion in the semiconscious patient can induce vomiting or laryngospasm.

Effective airway management during CPR is a major problem, even for medical professionals. Many individuals cannot effectively manage a self-inflating resuscitation bag and mask. Larger tidal volumes at lower pressures are delivered by mouth-to-mouth or mouth-to-mask ventilation.[28] The bag and mask apparatus is more effective if 2 individuals manage the airway: 1 to hold the mask and maintain the airway and 1 to squeeze the bag.[29] A number of advanced airway devices designed for blind placement have been described for use by individuals who are not skilled laryngoscopists. The combination esophageal-tracheal tube (Combitube) and the laryngeal mask airway (LMA) have been studied for use during CPR. Neither of these methods allows the degree of airway control that is obtained with an endotracheal tube. However, intubation has not proven to be superior to the others in promoting successful resuscitation.[30] Intubation may be performed in prolonged

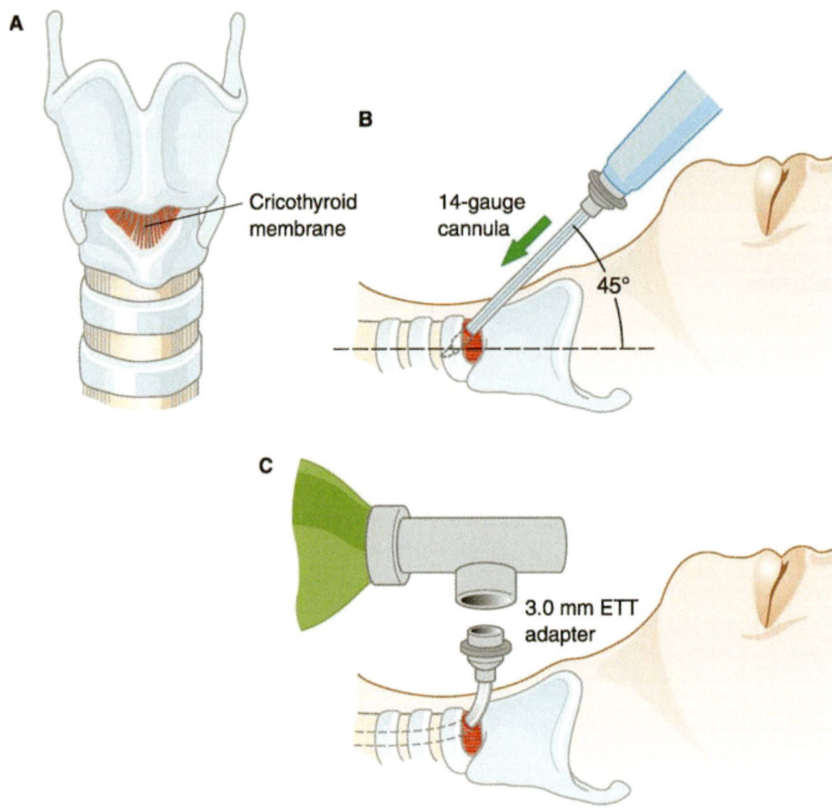

FIGURE 82-1. Cricothyroidotomy. **A.** Anatomic view. **B.** Insertion of 14-gauge IV cannula. **C.** Bag attached to 3.0 endotracheal tube (ETT) adaptor connected to IV cannula.

resuscitations if a skilled laryngoscopist is available. It should not be performed, however, until adequate ventilation by other means (preferably with supplemental oxygen) and circulation by chest compressions have been established and defibrillation performed, if appropriate. When other methods of establishing an airway are unsuccessful, translaryngeal ventilation or tracheotomy by cricothyroid puncture may be lifesaving (**Fig. 82-1**).

VENTILATION

Mouth-to-mouth or mouth-to-nose ventilation is the most expeditious and effective method of immediately available rescue ventilation. Although inspired gas with this method contains approximately 4% carbon dioxide and only approximately 17% oxygen (composition of exhaled air), it is sufficient to maintain viability. Mouth-to-mask ventilation using a simple anesthesia face mask is also very effective. If the mask is fitted with a nipple adapter, a flow of oxygen can also supplement inspired oxygen concentration. The self-inflating resuscitation bag with mask can also be used with or without supplemental oxygen. Recommendations for ventilation are 30 chest compressions followed by 2 breaths during basic life support, as summarized in **Box 82-3**. Once an advanced airway (endotracheal tube, LMA, Combitube) is in place, ventilation should proceed at 8 to 10 breaths/min without pauses in chest compressions. Do not hyperventilate. Blood flow during CPR slows rapidly when chest compressions are stopped and recovers slowly when they are restarted. Consequently, unless the cause of arrest is hypoxia, emphasis should be placed on maintaining chest compressions with as little interruption as possible.

PHYSIOLOGY OF VENTILATION DURING CPR

In the absence of an endotracheal tube, the distribution of gas between the lungs and stomach during mouth-to-mouth or mask ventilation will be determined by the relative impedance to flow into each: to the stomach, by the opening pressure of the esophagus; to the lungs, by lung-thorax compliance. It is likely that during cardiac arrest, esophageal opening pressure is no greater than that found in anesthetized individuals (~20 cm H_2O) and lung-thorax compliance is likely reduced.

Insufflation of air into the stomach during resuscitation leads to gastric distension, impeding ventilation and increasing the danger of regurgitation and gastric rupture. If gastric insufflation is to be avoided, inspiratory airway pressures must be kept low. Partial airway obstruction by the tongue and pharyngeal tissues often leads to increased airway pressures and gastric insufflation. During rescue breathing meticulous attention is necessary to maintain an open airway. To cause a rise in the chest of most adults, a tidal volume of 0.5 to 0.6 L will be needed. Rescue breaths should be given as quickly as possible without causing gastric insufflation.

BOX 82-3

Ventilation During CPR

A. Health care provider(s) without advanced airway
  1. 6-8 breaths/min, each delivered over 1 s
  2. Pause 2.0 s for 2 breaths after every 30 chest compressions
  3. Tidal volume adequate to cause chest rise (~0.5-0.6 L)

B. Health care provider(s) with advanced airway
  1. 8-10 breaths/min adequate to make chest rise (~0.5-0.6 L)
  2. Do not pause chest compressions for ventilation
  3. Avoid hyperventilation

CIRCULATION

PHYSIOLOGY OF CIRCULATION DURING CLOSED CHEST COMPRESSIONS

Two mechanisms of blood flow during closed chest compression have been described.[15,31] In the cardiac pump mechanism, the heart is compressed between the sternum and spine, resulting in ejection of blood from the heart into the aorta with the atrioventricular valves preventing backward blood flow. In the thoracic pump mechanism, chest compression raises intrathoracic pressure, forcing blood out of the chest; the venous valves and dynamic venous compression prevent backward flow and the heart acts as a passive conduit. The 2 mechanisms are not mutually exclusive (**Fig. 82-2**). Fluctuations in intrathoracic pressure play a significant role in blood flow during most resuscitations and the cardiac pump mechanism contributes to blood flow under some circumstances. The predominant mechanism probably varies from victim to victim and even during the course of resuscitating a single victim.

Successful resuscitation in experimental models is associated with myocardial blood flows of 15 to 20 mL/min/100 g (**Table 82-2**).[32] Obtaining such flows requires that closed chest compressions generate adequate cardiac output and coronary perfusion pressure. During CPR, coronary perfusion occurs primarily during the relaxation phase (diastole) of chest compression. In animal models the critical myocardial blood flow is associated with aortic "diastolic" pressure exceeding 40 mm Hg and coronary perfusion pressure (aortic diastolic minus right atrial diastolic pressure) exceeding 25 mm Hg.[32-42] One report has confirmed similar findings in humans, noting that all patients with successful return of spontaneous circulation had coronary perfusion pressures higher than 15 mm Hg.[42] Critical coronary perfusion pressure develops slowly when chest compressions are begun and is lost quickly when compressions are paused (**Fig. 82-3**). Again, for successful resuscitation, interruptions of chest compressions must be avoided whenever possible.

During CPR, cardiac output is severely depressed, ranging from 10% to 33% of prearrest values in experimental animals. Nearly all of the cardiac output is directed to organs above the diaphragm. Brain blood flow is 50% to 90% of normal and myocardial blood flow 20% to 50% of normal, and lower extremity and abdominal visceral flow is reduced to less than 5% of normal. Total blood flow tends to decrease with time, but the relative distribution of flow does not change. Flow to the brain and heart are improved by the administration of vasopressors, and flow to organs below the diaphragm is unchanged or further reduced.

TABLE 82-2 Physiological Variables Associated With Successful Resuscitation

Variables	Amount
Myocardial blood flow	15-20 mL/min/100 g
Arterial diastolic pressure	40 mm Hg
Coronary perfusion pressure	15-25 mm Hg
End-tidal carbon dioxide	>10 mm Hg

PHYSIOLOGY OF GAS TRANSPORT DURING CPR

During CPR, measurement of blood gases reveals an arterial respiratory alkalosis and a venous respiratory acidosis because the arterial Pco_2 is reduced and the venous Pco_2 is elevated. The cause is not respiratory in origin. Rather, these changes result from reduced cardiac output. During the low-flow condition of CPR, excretion of CO_2 (milliliters of CO_2 per minute in exhaled gas) is decreased to approximately the same extent as is cardiac output. This reduced CO_2 excretion is primarily a result of shunting of blood flow away from the lower half of the body. The exhaled CO_2 reflects only the metabolism of the part of the body that is being perfused. In the nonperfused areas, CO_2 accumulates during CPR. When normal circulation is restored, the accumulated CO_2 is washed out and a temporary increase in CO_2 excretion is seen.

Although CO_2 excretion is reduced during CPR, the mixed venous partial pressure of CO_2 ($Pvco_2$) is usually increased.[43] Two factors account for this elevation. Buffering acid causes a reduction in serum bicarbonate so that the same blood CO_2 content results in a higher $Pvco_2$. In addition, the mixed venous CO_2 content is elevated. When flow to a tissue is reduced, not all the produced CO_2 is removed, and CO_2 accumulates, increasing the tissue partial pressure of CO_2. This allows more CO_2 to be carried in each aliquot of blood, and mixed venous CO_2 content increases. If flow remains constant, a new equilibrium is established where all CO_2 produced in the tissue is removed but at a higher venous CO_2 content and partial pressure. In contrast to the venous blood, arterial CO_2 content and partial pressure ($Paco_2$) are decreased during CPR. This accounts for most of the observed increase in the arterial–venous CO_2 content difference. Although venous blood may have an increased CO_2, the marked reduction in cardiac output with maintained ventilation results in very efficient CO_2 removal.

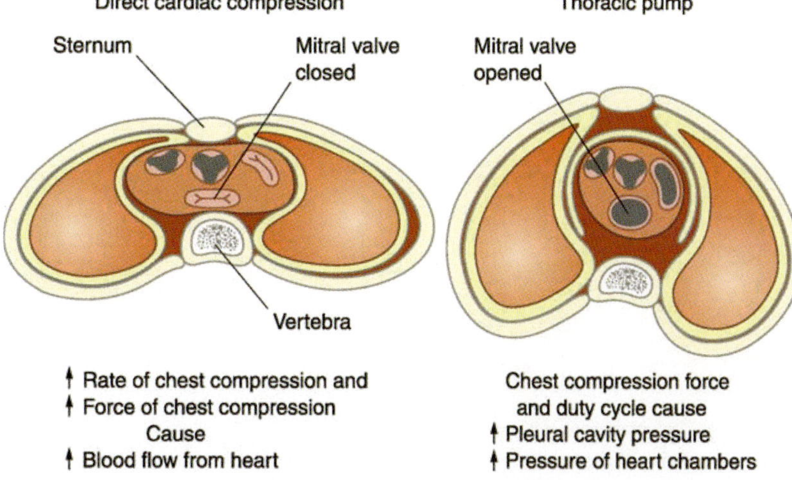

FIGURE 82-2. Possible mechanisms for blood flow during CPR include direct cardiac compression and the thoracic pump. With direct cardiac compression, an increase in chest compression rate causes an increase in blood flow by squeezing the heart between the vertebral column and sternum. With the thoracic pump mechanism, factors that increase pleural pressure cause an increase in pressure within the heart chambers and, ultimately, an increase in blood flow.

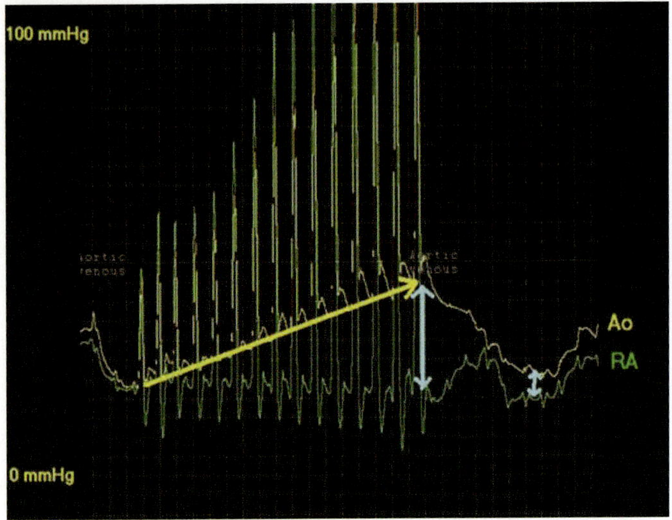

FIGURE 82-3. Aortic (Ao) and right atrial (RA) pressure tracings during single rescuer CPR providing 15 compressions followed by 2 breaths. There is little difference in Ao and RA pressure during chest compression ("systole"). When chest compressions are begun, Ao pressure during relaxation ("diastole") increases slowly (yellow arrow), providing the pressure difference for coronary perfusion (blue arrows), but is lost quickly during the pause for ventilations.

Decreased pulmonary blood flow during CPR causes lack of perfusion to many nondependent alveoli. The alveolar gas of these lung units has no CO_2. Consequently, the level of mixed alveolar CO_2 (ie, end-tidal CO_2) will be very low and will correlate poorly with arterial CO_2. However, end-tidal CO_2 does correlate well with cardiac output during CPR. As flow increases, more alveoli become perfused, there is less alveolar dead space, and end-tidal CO_2 measurements rise.

TECHNIQUE OF CLOSED CHEST COMPRESSION

Cardiac arrest should be presumed in a patient unresponsive to vigorous stimulation with absent or gasping (agonal) respirations. Even experienced health care providers take too long and have difficulty detecting the presence or absence of a pulse in arrest victims. Therefore, if a pulse check is done before or during rescue efforts, it should not take more than 10 seconds and should not be relied upon to determine successful resuscitation. After that time, if the patient remains unresponsive and apneic, the emergency response system should be activated and CPR begun (Boxes 82-1 and 82-2).

Standard chest compression technique consists of the rhythmic application of pressure over the lower half of the sternum. For compressions to be effective in providing blood flow to the brain and heart, the patient must be on a firm surface with the head level with the heart. The rescuer should stand or kneel at the side of the patient so that the hips are level with the victim's chest. Using the weight of the entire upper body, the compression is delivered straight down with enough force to depress the sternum at least 2 in (5.0 cm) in adults and teens, and to one-third to one-half the depth of the chest in children and infants. **Figure 82-4** illustrates the technique of chest compressions in infants. Following maximal compression, pressure is released completely from the chest. Chest compressions should be performed at a rate of 100 per minute. They are most effective if the compression and relaxation phases of the cycle are equal in length. This 50% compression time (compressions to relaxation) is easier to achieve at faster compression rates.

ALTERNATIVE TECHNIQUES OF CIRCULATORY SUPPORT

In recent years, better understanding of circulatory physiology during CPR, especially involving the thoracic pump mechanism, has resulted in several proposals for alternative techniques or adjunct devices. Most are intended to provide better hemodynamics and extend the duration during which CPR can support viability. Unfortunately, none has proven reliably superior to the standard technique, and no improvement in survival from cardiac arrest has been demonstrated consistently. Initial studies suggested hemodynamic advantages for techniques that raised intrathoracic pressure (such as simultaneous ventilation/compression, abdominal binding with compression, pneumatic antishock garment). Further investigations found that these techniques raised right atrial pressure and intracranial pressure, often more than aortic pressure. Consequently, there was no improvement in cerebral or myocardial blood flow. Outcome studies found no improvement in resuscitation success compared to standard CPR. These techniques are currently not recommended for support of the cardiac arrest victim.

Interposed Abdominal Compression CPR Interposed abdominal counterpulsation (IAC)-CPR consists of a dedicated rescuer providing manual abdominal compression between the xiphoid and umbilicus during the relaxation phase of conventional CPR.[44] IAC-CPR increases venous return and compresses the abdominal aorta to produce retrograde aortic flow, closing the aortic valve and augmenting diastolic pressure. Although initial hemodynamic studies were encouraging, a

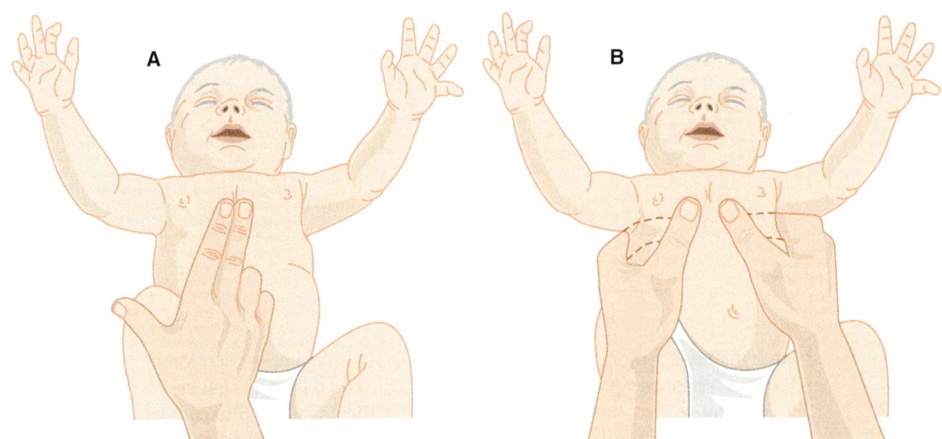

FIGURE 82-4. **A.** Two-finger method of external chest compression in infants. Rescuer places 2 fingers on the sternum and 1 fingerbreadth below the line intersecting the nipples and compresses 0.5 to 1 in at a rate of 100 compressions per minute. For the sake of clarity, ventilation is not shown. **B.** Encircling method of external chest compression in infants. Rescuer places thumbs over sternum 1 fingerbreadth below the line intersecting the nipples and clasps hands behind infant's back.

large randomized study of out-of-hospital arrest found no improvement in survival compared to standard CPR.[45] Two subsequent in-hospital studies using trained providers found improved return of spontaneous circulation (ROSC) and short-term survival with IAC-CPR compared to the standard technique.[46,47] In general, there has not been improvement in long-term survival with the use of this technique. Reports of human studies demonstrate that the frequency of complications, including laceration of abdominal viscera or esophageal regurgitation, is not increased with IAC-CPR. During in-hospital resuscitation, IAC-CPR may be considered when there are sufficient personnel trained in its use. Its use for out-of-hospital arrest remains experimental.

Active Compression–Decompression CPR Active compression–decompression (ACD)-CPR developed from the anecdotal report of CPR performed with a plumber's helper applied to the anterior chest wall.[48] This suggested that active decompression of the chest wall might reduce intrathoracic pressure during the relaxation phase of chest compressions, leading to improved venous return, increased stroke volume with compression, and better blood flow. Devices that can be applied to the chest wall in order to enable active compression and decompression have been developed, but none is currently approved by the Food and Drug Administration for sale in the United States. Hemodynamic studies in animals and humans show that coronary and cerebral perfusion may be somewhat improved with this method compared to standard CPR, although when epinephrine is used, there is no difference between techniques.[49,50] Clinical trials have found mixed results, with some showing short-term benefit but none showing long-term improvement in neurologically intact survival. A meta-analysis of 4162 patients in 10 out-of-hospital trials and 826 patients in 2 in-hospital trials found no difference in early or late survival with ACD-CPR compared to standard CPR.[51]

The Lund University Cardiac Arrest System (LUCAS) is a gas (oxygen or air) or electric powered piston-type device that produces a consistent chest compression rate of 100/min and a maximum compression depth of 5 cm, and incorporates a suction cup attached to the sternum to return the sternum to the starting position or to cause active decompression.[52] Case series have reported variable success with the device.

Impedance Threshold Device The impedance threshold device (ITD) is a valve that limits the flow of air into the lungs during the relaxation phase of chest compressions, reducing intrathoracic pressure during chest recoil and enhancing venous return.[53] Originally designed for use with an endotracheal tube, it has been adapted for use with a face mask, assuming the maintenance of a tight seal with the face. It has frequently been studied in association with ACD-CPR in the belief that the 2 techniques would act synergistically to improve venous return. One meta-analysis using data from randomized trials of both standard CPR and ACD-CPR found an improved short-term outcome with the use of an ITD but no significant improvement in survival to discharge.[54] Recently, a randomized trial (ROC PRIMED) involving 11 500 patients was stopped for futility because "researchers found that ITD use did not significantly improve or worsen survival rates for cardiac arrest patients" (https://roc.uwctc.org/tiki/tiki-index.php; statement released Nov. 6, 2009).

Pneumatic Vest CPR and Load-Distributing Band CPR Pneumatic vest CPR is a method of increasing intrathoracic pressure by phasically inflating a bladder around the chest (with or without simultaneous ventilation) yet without significantly changing the dimensions of the chest.[55,56] Experimental animal studies show excellent hemodynamics and the ability to maintain viability for prolonged periods. The technique continues to be investigated with a number of modifications from the original method. One modification of this technique is the load-distributing band (LDB) device consisting of a pneumatically or electrically actuated constricting band and backboard.[57] A multicenter randomized controlled trial comparing this device against manual CPR demonstrated no improvement in 4-hour survival.[58]

Invasive Techniques In contrast to the closed chest techniques, invasive methods have been able to maintain cardiac and cerebral viability during long periods of cardiac arrest. In animal models, open-chest cardiac massage can provide better hemodynamics and myocardial and cerebral perfusion than closed chest techniques.[59,60] When performed after 15 minutes of closed-chest CPR, open-chest CPR significantly improves coronary perfusion pressure and the rate of successful resuscitation.[61] Furthermore, when initiated early (probably within 20-30 min of arrest) following failure of closed-chest CPR, open-chest CPR may improve resuscitation.[62-64] However, if open-chest massage is begun after 30 minutes of ineffective closed-chest compressions, there is no better survival even though hemodynamics are improved.[65] This may be a useful technique when the chest or abdomen is already open in the operating room or early in the postoperative period after cardiothoracic surgery.

Preliminary trials of percutaneous cardiopulmonary bypass (through the femoral artery and vein using a membrane oxygenator) for refractory human cardiac arrest have been reported[66] and this is a technique available in some institutions. In canines, prompt restoration of blood flow and perfusion pressure with cardiopulmonary bypass can provide resuscitation with minimal neurologic deficit after 20 minutes of fibrillatory cardiac arrest.[67]

MONITORING DURING CPR

Assessment of the patient during CPR is similar to that in other clinical situations; **Box 82-4** lists the major points. A basic clinical examination and adherence to basic principles, including inspection, palpation, and auscultation of the patient, are performed. The chest is carefully observed for adequacy of expansion with artificial ventilation and for equal and normal breath sounds. In addition, the depth of compression and the position of the rescuer's hands in performing chest compressions should be reevaluated constantly.

Physiologic variables associated with successful resuscitation are listed in Table 82-2. When they are available, these variables should be used to guide resuscitation efforts. The use of an indwelling arterial catheter is an invaluable monitor in assessing the arterial blood pressure and estimating these critical perfusion pressures. In addition, an arterial line allows for the determination of arterial blood gases. If pressures are below the critical levels, adjustments should be made to improve chest

BOX 82-4

Assessment of Patient During Cardiopulmonary Resuscitation

A. Inspection
   - Chest rise
   - Depth of compression
   - Position of rescuer's hands

B. Palpation
   - Establish pulselessness
   - Assess peripheral pulses
   - Locate landmarks

C. Auscultation
   - Breath sounds
   - Heart sounds

D. Monitoring
   - Electrocardiogram
   - Arterial catheter
   - Central venous catheter
   - Pulse oximeter
   - End-tidal CO_2
   - Temperature

compressions and/or additional epinephrine should be administered. Greater pressures do not ensure success. Damage to the myocardium from underlying disease may preclude survival no matter how effective the CPR efforts. However, inadequate vascular pressures consistently result in poor outcomes.

Although invasive pressure monitoring may be the ideal, exhaled end-tidal CO_2 is an excellent noninvasive guide to the effectiveness of standard CPR.[68] Carbon dioxide excretion during CPR with an endotracheal tube in place is dependent primarily on flow rather than ventilation. Because alveolar dead space is large during low-flow conditions, end-tidal CO_2 is very low (frequently <10 mm Hg). If cardiac output increases, more alveoli are perfused and end-tidal CO_2 rises (usually to >20 mm Hg during successful CPR). When spontaneous circulation resumes, the earliest sign is a sudden increase in end-tidal CO_2 to greater than 40 mm Hg. Within a wide range of cardiac outputs, end-tidal CO_2 during CPR correlates with coronary perfusion pressure,[69] cardiac output,[70] initial resuscitation,[71,72] and survival.[73] End-tidal CO_2 measured during human CPR has been used to predict outcome. No patient with an end-tidal CO_2 of less than 10 mm Hg could be successfully resuscitated.[73] In the absence of invasive pressure monitoring, end-tidal CO_2 monitoring can be used to judge the effectiveness of chest compressions, and quantitative waveform capnography is encouraged for use during all resuscitations. Attempts should be made to maximize the value by alterations in technique or drug therapy. Sodium bicarbonate administration results in the liberation of CO_2 in the venous blood and a temporary rise in end-tidal CO_2. Therefore, end-tidal CO_2 monitoring will not be useful for judging the effectiveness of chest compressions for 3 to 5 minutes following bicarbonate administration.

DEFIBRILLATION

DURATION AND ELECTRICAL PATTERN OF FIBRILLATION

Ventricular fibrillation is a common rhythm disturbance in cardiac arrest. The only consistently effective treatment is electrical defibrillation. The fibrillating heart consumes considerable oxygen, which increases myocardial ischemia and decreases the time to irreversible cell damage. The longer that fibrillation continues, the more difficult it is to defibrillate and the less likely is successful resuscitation.[5,62,74-77] During the electrical phase of arrest (within 5 minutes of collapse), defibrillation should be the first priority of resuscitation (Box 82-2). The earlier that defibrillation is accomplished, the better the success of initial resuscitation following out-of-hospital fibrillation and the better the survival to hospital discharge.[5,76]

The application of defibrillation during the electrical phase has been facilitated by the development of AEDs that can recognize ventricular fibrillation, charge automatically, and give a defibrillatory shock. Minimally trained individuals can incorporate defibrillation into BLS skills using an AED, thus improving survival in out-of-hospital arrest by reducing the time to delivery of the first shock.[5,77-80] The value of public access defibrillation was dramatically demonstrated by early data after AEDs were installed in Las Vegas casinos and in Chicago airports.[78,79] Results included a 53% survival to hospital discharge[78] and a 55% 1-year neurologically intact survival rate over the first 2 years,[79] respectively. Early defibrillation is the paramount intervention during the electrical phase of cardiac arrest. However, in the usual out-of-hospital rescue, in which emergency medical technicians (EMTs) or paramedics perform the defibrillation, and in many in-hospital arrests, the first shock frequently is delayed until 6 to 10 minutes following collapse, well into the hemodynamic phase of arrest. A retrospective analysis in Seattle found that when response time was greater than 4 minutes, survival was improved if CPR was provided before defibrillation.[81] In a randomized trial of 200 out-of-hospital cardiac arrests in Oslo, a highly significant improvement in outcome resulted if CPR was provided before defibrillation when the response time was greater than 5 minutes.[82] Consequently, it now appears that immediate defibrillation is most effective if applied within 4 to 5 minutes of collapse. Otherwise, a brief period of 2 to 3 minutes of chest compressions before defibrillation may improve survival.

The coarseness of the fibrillatory waves on the electrocardiogram (ECG) may reflect the severity and duration of the myocardial insult, and thus have prognostic significance.[83] Increasing myocardial ischemia results in less-vigorous fibrillation, reduced-amplitude electrical activity, and more difficult defibrillation. Low-*amplitude* and low-*frequency* fibrillatory waveforms are associated with poor outcome.[83] Retrospective analysis of VF waveforms suggests that the probability of success of defibrillation can be predicted from the fibrillation waveform and that the shorter the time interval between the last chest compression and shock delivery, the more likely the shock will be successful.[84] A reduction of even a few seconds in the interval from pausing compressions to shock delivery can increase the probability of shock success. Catecholamines with β-adrenergic activity, such as epinephrine, increase the amplitude of the electrical activity but have no influence on the ability to defibrillate.[75,85] Consequently, defibrillation should not be delayed for drug therapy.

DEFIBRILLATORS

The modern defibrillator is a variable transformer that stores a direct current in a capacitor until discharged through the electrodes. Until recently, the current waveform of most defibrillators used for transthoracic defibrillation was a monophasic (single direction of current flow between paddle electrodes), damped sinusoid, although some delivered truncated exponential waves. Nearly all AEDs and defibrillators sold today deliver a biphasic current (direction of flow reverses during the shock) in either a truncated, exponential, or rectilinear waveform.[86] The output of most defibrillators is indicated in *energy* units (joules or watt-seconds). At a constant stored energy, the energy delivered to the patient will be inversely related to the impedance (resistance) between the paddle electrodes. For consistency, the energy level indicated on most commercially available defibrillators is the output when discharged into a 50-ohm load.

TRANSTHORACIC IMPEDANCE

Defibrillation is accomplished by the *current* passing through a critical mass of myocardium causing simultaneous depolarization of the myofibrils. Even at a constant delivered energy, delivered current will be reduced as impedance increases. At high impedance and relatively low energy levels, current could be too low for defibrillation.

Transthoracic impedance has been measured at 15 to 143 ohms in human defibrillation.[87] The major determinants of transthoracic impedance are known, and many are under the control of rescuers (**Box 82-5**). Impedance decreases with increasing electrode size, but too large a paddle size may diffuse the current over too great an area for effective defibrillation. Handheld paddles and self-adhesive pad electrodes of 8- to 12-cm diameter work well for adults and children and a 4.5-cm diameter is best for infants. The high impedance between metal electrode and skin requires the use of carefully applied self-adhesive pads or electrode paste/gel specifically designed to conduct electricity in the defibrillation setting. Transthoracic impedance decreases with

BOX 82-5

Factors Reducing Transthoracic Impedance During Defibrillation

Large paddle size (≥8-cm diameter)

Defibrillation paste or self-adhesive pads

Firm pressure on paddles (≥11 kg)

Defibrillation during exhalation

Successive shocks

successive shocks, a partial explanation for why an additional shock of the same energy can cause defibrillation when previous shocks have failed. Transthoracic impedance is slightly but significantly higher during inspiration than during exhalation. Air is a poor electrical conductor. Firm paddle pressure of at least 11 kg reduces resistance by improving paddle–skin contact and by expelling air from the lungs.[87]

Optimum success of defibrillation is obtained by keeping impedance as low as possible. The average transthoracic impedance in human defibrillation is 70 to 80 ohms. Impedance is probably of little clinical significance when reasonably proper technique and high-energy shocks are used. For lower-energy shocks, great care should be taken to minimize resistance. Some defibrillators measure transthoracic impedance during the charge cycle, allowing the use of low-energy shocks in appropriate patients and identification of victims needing higher energy.[88] Although not clinically available, current-based defibrillation may be a better way to describe defibrillation dose and may be superior to energy-based defibrillation.[89,90]

ENERGY REQUIREMENTS AND ADVERSE EFFECTS

The incidence and severity of myocardial damage from defibrillation in humans is not clear. In animal studies using the traditional monophasic defibrillator, repeated high-level shocks result in dysrhythmias, ECG changes, and myocardial necrosis.[91,92] In humans, dysrhythmia frequency and the degree of ST-segment depression is greater with increased energy doses.[93] Although there is no definitive evidence demonstrating myocardial damage within the range of clinically used doses, it would seem prudent to keep energy levels as low as possible during defibrillation attempts. However, if energy is too low, the delivered current may be insufficient for defibrillation, especially when transthoracic impedance is high.

With monophasic defibrillation, there is a general relationship between body size and energy requirements for defibrillation.[94] Children need lower energies than adults, perhaps as low as 0.5 J/kg.[95] However, over the size range of adults, body size does not seem to be a clinically important variable.[96] Multiple studies have demonstrated high rates of successful defibrillation using relatively low levels (160-200 J) of delivered energy. Studies of out-of-hospital and in-hospital arrests have demonstrated equal success when using 200 J or less initial energy compared to administering monophasic shocks at energies of 300 J or greater.[93,97]

Biphasic defibrillators with different waveforms have been demonstrated to be effective over specific dose ranges. AEDs have the shock energy preselected within the defibrillator algorithm. For manual biphasic defibrillation, most manufacturers display the effective dose range on the defibrillator. For biphasic truncated exponential waveforms, initial energies of 150 to 200 J have been shown to be successful more than 90% of the time.[1] For rectilinear biphasic waveforms, initial energy of 120 J has had similar success. Escalating doses of biphasic shocks have not clearly been shown to improve the success of defibrillation. Second and subsequent energy levels should be at least equivalent, and higher energy levels may be considered if available.

The current recommendation in adult patients using a monophasic defibrillator is to give a single shock of 360 J followed by immediate resumption of CPR for 2 minutes before rechecking rhythm and pulse (**Box 82-6**).[1] Because most defibrillations result in asystole or pulseless electrical activity (PEA), a period of CPR will be necessary; beginning compressions immediately following the shock minimizes interruption of critical blood flow. With an AED or biphasic defibrillator, use the preset or manufacturer's recommended energy. If that is unknown or unclear, a dose of 200 J may be selected. In children, with a manual defibrillator (monophasic or biphasic), an initial dose of 2 J/kg is used. As with adults, CPR is immediately restarted after a shock for 2 minutes before repeat rhythm and pulse check. If the first shock is unsuccessful, additional shocks of 4 J/kg are given separated by at least 2 minutes of CPR and appropriate drug and other therapy. If defibrillation attempts are unsuccessful, attention should be directed to the oxygenation, acid-base status, and administration of CPR and drugs such as epinephrine. In addition, factors that may increase transthoracic impedance should be evaluated, including pneumothorax, inadequate paddle–chest wall interface, improper paddle position, excessive distance between paddles, and inadequate paddle pressure on the chest.

Open-chest defibrillation can be used in the operating room when the thorax is already opened during surgery. Appropriate internal paddle size includes a diameter of 6 cm for adults, 4 cm for children, and 2 cm for infants. The paddles are applied with saline-soaked pads, one placed behind the left ventricle and the other over the right ventricle. When defibrillation is performed in this manner, 5 J should be used on the first attempt. If unsuccessful, repeated doses can be used with energy levels of up to 50 J.

BOX 82-6

Defibrillation Recommendations

Adults
- 2 minutes CPR if >5 min since collapse
- Countershock:
  - Monophasic: 360 J
  - AED: Preset
  - Biphasic: Device recommended (if unknown, 200 J)
- Immediately restart CPR for 2 min
- Recheck rhythm and pulse
- Repeat countershock
- Immediately restart CPR, oxygen, drugs
- Repeat sequence

Children
- 2 min CPR if >5 min since collapse
- First countershock: 2.0 J/kg monophasic or biphasic
- Immediately restart CPR for 2 min
- Recheck rhythm and pulse
- Repeat countershock with 4.0 J/kg
- Immediately restart CPR, oxygen, drugs
- Repeat sequence, all subsequent shocks: 4.0 J/kg

AED, automatic external defibrillators.

SUPPLEMENTAL THERAPY

Amiodarone and lidocaine are used during cardiac arrest to aid defibrillation when ventricular fibrillation is refractory to electrical countershock therapy or when fibrillation recurs following successful conversion. However, no antiarrhythmic agent has been shown to be superior to electrical defibrillation or more effective than placebo in the treatment of ventricular fibrillation. Consequently, defibrillation should not be withheld or delayed for drug therapy, but should be applied at the earliest possible time when treating ventricular fibrillation (Box 82-2).

Amiodarone and Lidocaine Amiodarone is a pharmacologically complex drug with sodium, potassium, calcium, and α- and β-adrenergic blocking properties that is useful for treatment of atrial and ventricular arrhythmias. Amiodarone can cause hypotension and bradycardia when infused too rapidly in patients with an intact circulation. This can usually be prevented by slowing the rate of drug infusion, or treating with fluids, vasopressors, chronotropic agents, or temporary pacing. Lidocaine is primarily an antiectopic agent with few hemodynamic effects. It depresses automaticity by reducing the slope of phase 4 depolarization and the heterogeneity of ventricular refractoriness. Lidocaine tends to restore the ventricular fibrillation threshold reduced

BOX 82-7

Indications for Use of Lidocaine

Frequent ventricular premature beats (>10 beats/min)

Coupled VPBs

Multiform VPBs

Ventricular tachycardia

Prophylaxis during cardiac catheterization

VPBs, ventricular premature beats.

BOX 82-8

Pulseless Electrical Activity

Pulseless electrical activity (PEA) includes:

- Electromechanical dissociation (EMD)
- Pseudoelectromechanical dissociation
- Idioventricular rhythms
- Ventricular escape rhythms
- Bradyasystolic rhythms
- Postdefibrillation idioventricular rhythms

by ischemia or infarction. It has no effect on conduction times through the atrioventricular node or on intraventricular conduction time.

Amiodarone is effective in treating multiple types of supraventricular and ventricular dysrhythmias. In contrast, lidocaine is effective in terminating ventricular premature beats (VPBs) and ventricular tachycardia associated with cardiac surgery, acute myocardial infarction, and digitalis intoxication. It is also effective in preventing and treating ventricular dysrhythmias during cardiac catheterization. Lidocaine is not effective in the treatment of atrial or atrioventricular junctional dysrhythmias (**Box 82-7**).

In cardiac arrest, antiarrhythmic drugs are administered when ventricular tachycardia or ventricular fibrillation have not responded to or have recurred following epinephrine and defibrillation. Two randomized, blinded clinical trials of shock-resistant cardiac arrest victims demonstrated improved admission alive to hospital with amiodarone treatment compared to placebo or lidocaine, although there was no difference in survival to discharge.[98,99] Amiodarone is initially administered as a 300-mg rapid infusion. Supplemental infusions of 150 mg can be repeated as necessary for recurrent or resistant arrhythmias to a maximum total daily dose of 2 g.

Lidocaine is an alternative therapy in refractory fibrillation when amiodarone is unavailable, but it has no proven short- or long-term benefits when used during cardiac arrest. To rapidly achieve and maintain therapeutic blood levels during CPR, relatively large doses are necessary. An initial bolus of 1 to 1.5 mg/kg should be given and additional boluses of 0.5 to 0.75 mg/kg can be given every 5 to 10 minutes during CPR up to a total dose of 3 mg/kg. Only bolus dosing should be used during CPR, but an infusion of 2 to 4 mg/min can be started after successful resuscitation.

TEMPORARY PACEMAKER THERAPY

When emergency pacing is indicated, intravenous or transthoracic pacing can be initiated. Temporary pacing can usually be quickly instituted using external, noninvasive, temporary pacemakers that use large, high-impedance electrodes, allowing relatively nonpainful stimuli.[100]

Temporary pacing is indicated for patients with preserved myocardial function whose primary problem is impulse formation or conduction, such as patients with severe bradycardia or high-grade heart block who have a palpable pulse. Studies of temporary pacing during cardiac arrest (out-of-hospital or in the emergency department) have found no improvement in admission to hospital or survival. Consequently, withholding chest compressions in patients with asystole to attempt pacing is not recommended.[1]

PULSELESS ELECTRICAL ACTIVITY AND ASYSTOLE

Pulseless electrical activity (PEA) and asystole are increasingly seen as the presenting rhythm in cardiac arrest and commonly follow defibrillation. They are seen more often in children and are associated with a poor outcome. PEA is the circumstance where no palpable pulse is present but an ECG rhythm is detectable. This includes a number of different rhythms, most commonly electromechanical dissociation (EMD; **Box 82-8**). Asystole is the absence of electrical activity on the ECG. Fine ventricular fibrillation can masquerade as asystole if the ECG lead being monitored is located at right angles to the fibrillatory wave.[101] For this reason, the trace from a second lead or from a different position of paddle electrodes should always be inspected before a decision is made not to defibrillate.

The predominant cause of primary PEA and asystole is severe myocardial ischemia. These rhythms may represent a failure of myocardial contractility caused by a depletion of intracellular energy stores and they carry a very poor prognosis. However, these ECG patterns also may be secondary, caused by a variety of noncardiac mechanisms that may be amenable to treatment. Therapy directed at the underlying disorder may result in a successful outcome. Consequently, consideration of a noncardiac cause for arrest (frequently referred to as the 5 H's and T's) should always be part of the resuscitation sequence when these rhythms are detected (**Box 82-9**).

DRUG THERAPY

During cardiac arrest, drug therapy is secondary to more fundamental interventions (Box 82-2). Chest compressions and defibrillation (if appropriate) should take precedence over medications. Establishing intravenous (IV) access and administering drugs, although important, should not interrupt sustained chest compressions and ventilation.

OXYGEN

Patients in cardiac arrest or low cardiac output states should receive 100% oxygen as soon as possible. Oxygen will increase arterial oxygen tension and hemoglobin saturation if ventilation is supported and will improve tissue oxygenation when circulation is supported. Although exposure to 100% inspired oxygen ($FIO_2 = 1.0$) during CPR and after resuscitation has potential toxicity, there is insufficient evidence to indicate that this occurs during adult CPR.[102-104]

VASOPRESSOR AGENTS

Mechanism of Action Epinephrine has been used in resuscitation since the 1890s and has been the vasopressor of choice in modern CPR since the studies of Redding and Pearson in the 1960s.[17,105] Its efficacy lies entirely in its α-adrenergic properties.[39] When epinephrine is administered during CPR, peripheral vasoconstriction results in higher

BOX 82-9

Possible Causes of Cardiac Arrest (H's and T's)

Hypo-/hyperkalemia	Tamponade (cardiac)
Hypovolemia	Tension pneumothorax
Hypothermia	Toxins (overdose)
Hydrogen ion (acidosis)	Thrombosis, pulmonary
Hypoxia	Thrombosis, coronary

aortic pressure, which causes an increase in coronary and cerebral perfusion pressures and myocardial and brain blood flows.[38,106,107] Flow to other organs either does not improve or diminishes further when epinephrine is given, despite the increase in aortic pressure. Animal studies demonstrate that all strong α-adrenergic drugs (epinephrine, phenylephrine, methoxamine, dopamine, norepinephrine) and nonadrenergic vasopressors (vasopressin) are equally successful in aiding resuscitation regardless of the β-adrenergic potency. β-Adrenergic agonists without α activity (isoproterenol, dobutamine) are no better than placebo.[17,34,105,108,109] α-Adrenergic blockade precludes resuscitation, whereas β-adrenergic blockade has no effect on the ability to restore spontaneous circulation.[36,37] Although it has been suggested that the ability of epinephrine to increase the amplitude of ventricular fibrillation (a β-adrenergic effect) makes defibrillation easier, animal studies show that epinephrine does not improve the success of, nor decrease the energy necessary for, defibrillation.[75,85] Retrospective clinical studies show no effect of epinephrine on defibrillation success.[83]

β-Adrenergic stimulation during cardiac arrest is potentially deleterious. In the fibrillating heart, epinephrine increases oxygen consumption. Large doses of epinephrine increase deaths in swine early after resuscitation as a consequence of tachyarrhythmias and hypertension, an effect partially offset by metoprolol treatment.[110] Despite these theoretical considerations, survival and neurologic outcome studies show no difference when epinephrine is compared to a pure α-agonist (methoxamine or phenylephrine) or to a nonadrenergic vasopressor (vasopressin) during CPR in animals or humans.[111-114] Recently, it has been questioned whether any drug therapy improves outcome from cardiac arrest. One study, comparing various outcomes after out-of-hospital cardiac arrest, was not able to demonstrate any improvements after introduction of advanced life support (epinephrine, atropine, lidocaine).[115] Another study demonstrated improvement in short-term outcomes (ROSC and survival to hospital admission) but no difference in survival to discharge, comparing placebo with the use of all drugs (epinephrine, amiodarone, atropine, vasopressin).[116] However, this study was not powered to detect clinically meaningful differences in long-term outcome. Neither of the studies was able to isolate outcomes specifically related to individual drug administration. If any effect was found, most drug trials demonstrated only short-term outcome advantage.

Epinephrine When added to chest compressions, epinephrine helps to develop the critical coronary perfusion pressure necessary to provide enough myocardial blood flow for restoration of spontaneous circulation. If invasive monitoring is present during CPR, an arterial diastolic pressure of 40 mm Hg or coronary perfusion pressure of 20 mm Hg must be obtained with good chest compression technique and/or epinephrine therapy (Table 82-2). In the absence of such monitoring, the dose of epinephrine must be chosen empirically. The standard dose used in animals and humans for many years has been 0.5 to 1.0 mg intravenously. On a weight basis, this dose is approximately 0.1 mg/kg in animals but only 0.015 mg/kg in humans. Animal studies in the 1980s suggested that higher doses of epinephrine in human CPR might improve myocardial and cerebral perfusion and improve success of resuscitation.

Outcome studies prospectively comparing standard and high-dose epinephrine do not demonstrate conclusively that higher doses improve survival. Two randomized, blinded animal studies (1 with fibrillatory arrest and 1 with asphyxial arrest) comparing standard and high-dose epinephrine found no difference in 24-hour survival or neurologic outcome, but more of the high-dose epinephrine animals died in the early postresuscitation period as a result of a hyperdynamic state.[110,117] Eight adult prospective randomized clinical trials involving more than 9000 cardiac arrest patients found no improvement in survival to hospital discharge or neurologic outcome, even in subgroups, when initial high-dose epinephrine (5-18 mg) was compared to standard doses (1-2 mg). Some of the studies and a meta-analysis suggest that there may be an improvement in immediate resuscitation with high-dose epinephrine.[118]

Because of the long experience with epinephrine, it remains the vasopressor of choice in CPR. It should be administered whenever resuscitation has not occurred after adequate chest compressions and ventilation have been started and defibrillation (if appropriate) attempted (Boxes 82-1 and 82-2). High doses of epinephrine apparently are not needed as initial therapy for most cardiac arrests and potentially could be deleterious under some circumstances. Current recommendations are to give intravenous epinephrine, 1 mg in the adult or 0.01 mg/kg in children, every 3 to 5 minutes. Higher doses, given as "rescue" therapy, may be indicated in specific circumstances, or if treatment has been delayed and the standard dose seems ineffective.

Vasopressin The newest addition to the pharmacologic armamentarium in CPR is arginine vasopressin. It is currently recommended as an alternative to either the first or second dose of epinephrine in a dose of 40 units IV. If additional vasopressor doses are needed, epinephrine should be used. Vasopressin is a naturally occurring (antidiuretic) hormone that, when administered in high doses, is a potent nonadrenergic vasoconstrictor, acting by stimulation of smooth muscle V1 receptors. The half-life in the intact circulation is 10 to 20 minutes and longer than epinephrine during CPR. Animal studies demonstrate that vasopressin is as effective as, or more effective than, epinephrine in maintaining vital organ blood flow during CPR.[119-121] Postresuscitation myocardial depression and splanchnic blood flow reduction are more marked with vasopressin than epinephrine, but they are transient and can be treated with low doses of dopamine.[122] Three randomized controlled trials and a meta-analysis have found no difference in short- or long-term outcomes with vasopressin compared to epinephrine as a first-line vasopressor in cardiac arrest.[114,123-125] Overall, evidence currently suggests that, like other potent vasopressors, vasopressin is equivalent to, but not better than, epinephrine for use during CPR.

ATROPINE

Atropine sulfate enhances sinus node automaticity and atrioventricular conduction by its vagolytic effects. Atropine is indicated when bradycardia coexists with hypotension, ventricular ectopy, or symptoms associated with myocardial ischemia. The drug can also be used to treat second- and third-degree heart block, and slow idioventricular rates. Although atropine is frequently given during cardiac arrest associated with an ECG pattern of asystole or slow PEA, no studies provide evidence that it actually improves outcome from asystolic or bradysystolic arrest.[126,127] The predominant cause of asystole and EMD is severe myocardial ischemia. Excessive parasympathetic tone probably contributes little to these rhythms during cardiac arrest in adults. Even in children, the significance of autonomic tone during arrest is doubtful. The most effective treatment for asystole or PEA is improvement in coronary perfusion and myocardial oxygenation with chest compressions, ventilation, and epinephrine. However, cardiac arrest with these rhythms has a very poor prognosis. Because atropine has few adverse effects, it can be tried in arrest refractory to epinephrine and oxygenation, but its routine use is not recommended. The recommended dose for bradycardia in adults is 0.5 mg IV every 3 to 5 minutes to a total dose of 3.0 mg. The pediatric dose for treating bradycardia is 0.02 mg/kg with a minimum dose of 0.1 mg and a maximum total dose of 1.0 mg in a child and 3.0 mg in an adolescent. The dose may be repeated every 3 to 5 minutes. When treating pulseless arrest in the adult, the dose is 1.0 mg IV every 3 to 5 minutes to a total dose of 3.0 mg. Occasionally, the use of atropine during CPR may cause a sinus tachycardia postresuscitation.

CALCIUM SALTS

With normal cardiovascular physiology, calcium increases myocardial contractility and enhances ventricular automaticity. For many years, consequently, calcium salts have been administered during attempted resuscitation of asystole and EMD. However, multiple clinical studies have found that calcium is no better than placebo in promoting resuscitation and survival from asystole or EMD.[128,129] Calcium is not indicated

BOX 82-10

Side Effects From Excessive Use of Sodium Bicarbonate

Hyperosmolality

Hypernatremia

Metabolic alkalosis

Hypercapnia

Decreased unloading of oxygen from hemoglobin

Paradoxical intracellular acidosis

for use during cardiac arrest in adults or children. It may be useful for treatment of hyperkalemia, ionized hypocalcemia, hypermagnesemia, or calcium channel blocker toxicity. If calcium is administered, the chloride salt (2-4 mg/kg) is recommended because it produces higher and more consistent levels of ionized calcium than other salts.

SODIUM BICARBONATE

Although in the past sodium bicarbonate was used commonly during CPR, there is little evidence to support its efficacy. Its use during resuscitation was predicated on the adverse cardiovascular consequences of acidosis, including impaired myocardial function, decreased catecholamine responsiveness, and peripheral vasodilatation. However, most studies have been unable to demonstrate improvement in the success of defibrillation or resuscitation with the use of bicarbonate.[130,131] The observation that metabolic acidosis develops very slowly during CPR may explain the absence of effect of buffer therapy. Acidosis does not become severe until 15 to 20 minutes of cardiac arrest have passed.[43,132,133]

Sodium bicarbonate use during CPR should be restricted, not only because of its lack of efficacy, but because of the documented complications from excessive use, including hyperosmolality, hypernatremia, metabolic alkalosis, and hypercapnia from CO_2 liberation (**Box 82-10**).[132,134] These abnormalities are associated with low resuscitation rates and poor survival.

Theoretically, sodium bicarbonate could cause a paradoxical worsening of intracellular and intracerebral acidosis as the CO_2 liberated during the reaction with acid readily diffuses across cell membranes and the blood-brain barrier, whereas bicarbonate diffuses much more slowly. Direct evidence for this effect has not been found. Animal studies have found no change in spinal fluid acid-base status with clinically relevant doses of sodium bicarbonate[135] and no worsening of myocardial intracellular acidosis during bicarbonate administration.[136] Consequently, paradoxical acidosis from sodium bicarbonate remains a concern primarily on theoretical grounds.

Current practice suggests that sodium bicarbonate should be considered for use during CPR only in arrests associated with hyperkalemia, severe preexisting metabolic acidosis, and tricyclic or phenobarbital overdose. It may be considered for use in protracted resuscitation attempts after other modalities have been instituted. These recommendations stem from its unproven efficacy in increasing patient survival and its known side effects. When bicarbonate is used, 1 mEq/kg should be given as the initial dose and no more than half this dose given every 10 minutes thereafter. However, dosing of sodium bicarbonate should be guided by blood gas determination, whenever possible.

ROUTES OF ADMINISTRATION AND VASCULAR ACCESS

The preferred route of administration of all drugs during CPR is intravenous or intraosseous. If one of these routes cannot be established rapidly because of technical difficulties, one of the other alternatives—endotracheal or intracardiac—can be used.

Intravenous Access The most rapidly reached and highest drug levels occur with administration into a central vein. Therefore, when a central venous catheter is available during CPR, as is often the case in the operating room, it should be used for drug therapy. However, peripheral intravenous administration is also effective. The antecubital or external jugular vein should be the site of first choice for starting an infusion during resuscitation because starting a central line usually necessitates stopping CPR. Sites in the upper extremity and neck are preferred because of the paucity of blood flow below the diaphragm during CPR. Drugs administered in the lower extremity may be extremely delayed or not reach the sites of action. Even in the upper extremity, drugs may require 1 to 2 minutes to reach the central circulation.[137] Onset of action may be speeded if a peripheral drug bolus is followed by a 20 to 30-mL bolus of intravenous fluid.

Intraosseous Administration The intraosseous route of fluid and medication administration, originally described in 1934,[138] has regained popularity recently for emergency vascular access. During CPR, all medications and fluids used, including whole blood, have been given by the intraosseous route. This technique should be considered a temporary measure during emergencies when other vascular sites are not available.

The technique of placing an intraosseous line is straightforward. A standard 16- or 18-gauge needle, spinal needle with stylet, or bone marrow needle is inserted into the anterior surface of the tibia, 1 to 3 cm below the tibial tuberosity. Commercially available kits can facilitate access in adults. The needle is directed to a 90° angle to the medial surface of the bone or slightly inferior to avoid the epiphyseal plate. There is a loss of resistance after the needle passes through the bony cortex of the tibia. Placement is successful if the needle is in the marrow cavity, as evidenced by its standing upright without support, and bone marrow can be aspirated into a syringe connected to the needle. The needle will lose the upright position if it has slipped into the subcutaneous tissue. Free flow of the drug or fluid infusion without significant subcutaneous infiltration also should be demonstrated (**Fig. 82-5**).[139] There are a number of reports of successful intraosseous infusions in children, with minimal complications. Animal models have demonstrated successful reversal of hemorrhagic shock,[140] effective buffering with sodium bicarbonate,[141] and equal hemodynamic response to epinephrine with intraosseous and central intravenous administration.[142]

Endotracheal Administration Drugs that can be absorbed from tracheal mucosa include lidocaine, atropine, naloxone, epinephrine, and vasopressin (**Box 82-11**). During CPR the rapid establishment of vascular access can be difficult, especially in the obese or in infants and small children. The endotracheal route can be used as an alternative following intubation in these settings. However, intravenous or intraosseous drug administration is the preferred route because the time to effect and the drug levels achieved are inconsistent using the endotracheal route.[143-145] Better results may be obtained by administering 5- to 10-mL volumes. It is unclear whether deep injection is better than simple instillation into the endotracheal tube.[32] Doses 2 to 2.5 times higher than the recommended IV dose should be administered when this route is used.

POSTRESUSCITATION CARE

In the past, the lack of optimal postresuscitation care has contributed significantly to the poor outcome from cardiac arrest. There is growing awareness that aggressive postresuscitation care can significantly improve survival. Out-of-hospital cardiac arrest victims should be transported to a facility with a comprehensive postresuscitation system of care that includes acute coronary interventions, neurologic care, goal-directed critical care, and the institution of therapeutic hypothermia. In-hospital victims should be moved to a critical care unit that provides comprehensive postresuscitation care. The precipitating cause for the arrest should be sought (review the 5 H's and T's; Box 82-9). Because cardiovascular disease and coronary ischemia are the most common causes of cardiac arrest, the search for acute coronary syndromes with possible coronary reperfusion should be a

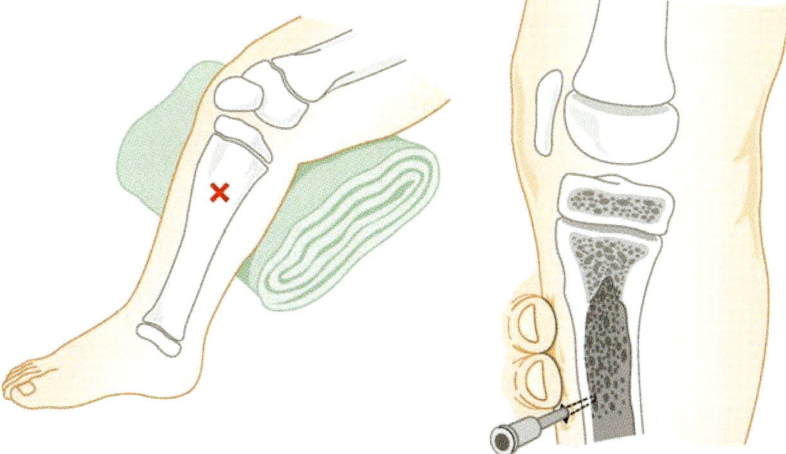

FIGURE 82-5. Intraosseous needle placement. Insert needle at the level of tibial tubercle on the medial portion of the tibia. The needle is aimed carefully and laterally.

high priority. Coronary interventions can be performed while efforts to stabilize hemodynamics and institute therapeutic hypothermia are ongoing.

The major factors contributing to mortality following successful resuscitation are progression of the primary disease and cerebral damage suffered as a result of the arrest. Any cardiac arrest, even of brief duration, causes a generalized decrease in myocardial function similar to the regional hypokinesis seen following periods of regional ischemia. This is usually referred to as global myocardial stunning and can be mitigated with inotropic agents, if necessary. Active management following resuscitation appears to mitigate postischemic brain damage and improve neurologic outcome without increasing the number of patients surviving in a vegetative state.[146] When flow is restored following a period of global brain ischemia, 3 stages of cerebral reperfusion are seen in the ensuing 12 hours. Immediately following resuscitation there are multifocal areas of the brain with no-reflow. Within an hour there is global hyperemia followed quickly by prolonged global hypoperfusion.

Postresuscitation support is focused on providing stable oxygenation and hemodynamics so as to minimize any further cerebral insult and to detect and treat any other organ failure. A comatose patient should have hypothermia instituted and be maintained on mechanical ventilation for 24 hours to ensure adequate oxygenation and ventilation. Restlessness, coughing, or seizure activity should be aggressively treated with appropriate medications including neuromuscular blockers, if necessary. Oxygen free radicals contribute significantly to brain reperfusion injury, which may be worsened by hyperoxia.[102-104] Although 100% oxygen is appropriate for use during initial resuscitation, postresuscitation oxygen therapy should be titrated to the lowest level to maintain arterial oxygen saturation above 94%. Hyperventilation should be avoided ($Paco_2$ 35-40 mm Hg). Blood volume should be maintained at normal, and moderate hemodilution to a hematocrit of 30% to 35% may be helpful. A brief 5-minute period of hypertension to mean arterial pressure of 120 to 140 mm Hg may help overcome the initial cerebral no-reflow. This frequently occurs secondary to the effects of epinephrine given during CPR. However, both prolonged hypertension (>110 mm Hg) and hypotension are associated with a worsened outcome. Hyperglycemia during cerebral ischemia is known to result in increased neurologic damage. Thus it seems prudent to control glucose in the 100 to 180 mg/dL range. Specific pharmacologic therapy directed at brain preservation has not been shown to have further benefit. Although animal trials of barbiturates and calcium channel blockers were promising, large, multicenter trials found no improvement in neurologic status when drugs were given following cardiac arrest.[146,147]

In contrast to pharmacologic therapy, 2 studies have demonstrated improved neurologic outcome when mild therapeutic hypothermia (89.6°F-93.2°F [32°C-34°C]) was induced for 12 to 24 hours in cardiac arrest survivors who remained comatose after admission to the hospital.[148,149] Both investigations studied only patients whose initial rhythm was ventricular fibrillation, and the larger of the trials included only witnessed arrests. Nevertheless, these are the first studies to document improved neurologic outcome with a specific postarrest intervention. The International Liaison Committee on Resuscitation (ILCOR) now recommends that "unconscious adult patients with return of spontaneous circulation after out-of-hospital cardiac arrest should be cooled to 32°C to 34°C for 12 to 24 hours when the initial rhythm was ventricular fibrillation. Such cooling may also be beneficial for other rhythms or in-hospital cardiac arrest."

BOX 82-11

Endotracheal Administration of Drugs

Administer:	**Do not administer:**
Lidocaine	Sodium bicarbonate
Atropine	Calcium chloride
Naloxone	
Epinephrine	
Vasopressin	

PROGNOSIS

For the comatose survivor of CPR, the question of ultimate prognosis is important. Neurologic prognosis may be difficult to determine during the first 72 hours in patients not undergoing hypothermia, and this time frame is likely extended in patients being cooled.[150] Many initially comatose survivors of cardiac arrest have the potential for full recovery. A neurologic exam for prognosis must not be undertaken if confounding factors (hypothermia, sedatives, neuromuscular blockers, seizures) exist. Even in patients not treated with hypothermia, no clinical signs reliably predict poor outcome less than 24 hours after cardiac arrest. Most patients who completely recover show rapid improvement in the first 48 hours. One older study found that if a patient is not awake by 4 days following arrest, the chance of ever awakening is less than 20%, and all those patients awakening had marked neurologic deficits.[151] Summarized in **Box 82-12** are the clinical signs that strongly predict death or poor neurologic outcome in comatose patients not treated with hypothermia.[152-154] The time frame for similar assessment in patients treated with hypothermia is unknown.

BOX 82-12

Prognosis of Comatose Survivors of Cardiac Arrest

Signs predicting death or poor neurologic outcome in patients not treated with hypothermia

Most Reliable

Absent corneal reflex at ≥72 h

Absent pupillary response at ≥72 h

Less Reliable

Absent vestibuloocular reflexes at ≥24 h

No motor response at ≥72 h

KEY REFERENCES

- Emergency Cardiac Care Committee, Subcommittees and Task Forces, American Heart Association: 2010 American Heart Association guidelines for cardiopulmonary resuscitation and emergency cardiovascular care. *Circulation.* 2010;122:S640-S946.
- Weisfeldt ML, Becker LB. Resuscitation after cardiac arrest: a 3-phase time-sensitive model. *JAMA.* 2002;288:3035.
- Berg RA, Kern KB, Sanders AB, et al. Bystander cardiopulmonary resuscitation: is ventilation necessary? *Circulation.* 1993;88:1907.
- Ewy GA, Zuercher M, Hilwig RW, et al. Improved neurological outcome with continuous chest compressions compared with 30:2 compressions-to-ventilations cardiopulmonary resuscitation in a realistic swine model of out-of-hospital cardiac arrest. *Circulation.* 2007;116:2525.
- Ralston SH, Voorhees WD, Babbs CF. Intrapulmonary epinephrine during prolonged CPR. Improved regional blood flow and resuscitation in dogs. *Ann Emerg Med.* 1984;13:79.
- Otto CW, Yakaitis RW, Blitt CD. Mechanism of action of epinephrine in resuscitation from asphyxial arrest. *Crit Care Med.* 1981;9:321.
- Sanders AB, Kern KB, Otto CW, et al. End-tidal carbon dioxide monitoring during cardiopulmonary resuscitation: a prognostic indicator for survival. *JAMA.* 1989;262:1347.
- Valenzulea TD, Roe DJ, Nichol G, et al. Outcomes of rapid defibrillation by security officers after cardiac arrest in casinos. *N Engl J Med.* 2000;343:1206.
- Wik L, Hansen TB, Fylling F, et al. Delaying defibrillation to give basic cardiopulmonary resuscitation to patients with out-of-hospital ventricular fibrillation. *JAMA.* 2003;289:1389.
- Kudenchuk PJ, Cobb LA, Copass MK, et al. Amiodarone for resuscitation after out of hospital cardiac arrest due to ventricular fibrillation. *N Engl J Med.* 1999;341:871.
- Wenzel V, Krismer AC, Arntz HR, et al. A comparison of vasopressin and epinephrine for out-of-hospital cardiopulmonary resuscitation. *N Engl J Med.* 2004;350:105.
- Olasveengen TM, Sunde K, Brunborg C, et al. Intravenous drug administration during out-of-hospital cardiac arrest: a randomized trial. *JAMA.* 2009;302:2222.
- Holzer M, The Hypothermia After Cardiac Arrest Study Group. Mild therapeutic hypothermia to improve the neurologic outcome after cardiac arrest. *N Engl J Med.* 2002;346:549.
- Booth CM, Boone RH, Tomlinson G, et al. Is this patient dead, vegetative, or severely neurologically impaired? Assessing outcome for comatose survivors of cardiac arrest. *JAMA.* 2004;291:870.

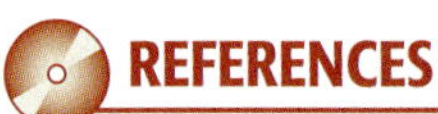

REFERENCES

Complete references available on DVD and online version at www.LongneckerAnesthesiology.com

PART 7

Special Considerations in Anesthesia Care

CHAPTER 83 Blood and Blood Component Therapy

Ian J. Welsby
Jessica A. Hathaway

KEY POINTS

1. ABO compatibility remains the major safety consideration for blood transfusion. Clerical errors of patient identification and sample labeling remain the primary cause of mistransfusion of ABO-incompatible units.
2. Prestorage leukoreduction of cellular blood products has greatly reduced, but not eliminated, the incidence of febrile reactions, transfusion-related immunosuppression, and cytomegalovirus transmission, and has led to improved outcomes in surgical patients compared to the use of nonleukoreduced products.
3. Redirecting blood from female donors away from transfusable plasma products appears to have reduced the incidence of TRALI mediated by leucocyte reactive antibodies. However, some plasma from female donors remains in platelet and red blood cell products.
4. International travel and associated exposure to pathogens not addressed by existing screening mechanisms will increasingly limit suitable blood donors. These and other pressures on the blood supply make imperative strategies all the more important for blood conservation and promotion of bloodless surgical techniques.

HISTORY OF BLOOD TRANSFUSION

Practical, safe transfusion derives from centuries of experimentation and discovery. Although the first known animal transfusion experiments took place in both England and France in the 17th century, early efforts to translate the technique to humans failed with such spectacular flair that the learned societies on both sides of the English Channel flatly banned the practice.

The first "modern" transfusion is attributed to John Syng Physick in Philadelphia in 1795. English physician James Blundell claimed success for 5 of 10 transfused patients during his professional career (1820-1840).

The 19th century saw the rapid expansion of bacteriology and a growing understanding of antisera. In 1900 Karl Landsteiner significantly advanced the cause of blood compatibility with his landmark discovery of the ABO blood groups, with O being derived from the German "ohne" or without, for which he received the 1930 Nobel Prize in Medicine and Physiology. Four decades later, in collaboration with Alex Weiner, Philip Levine, and R.E. Stetson, Landsteiner played an instrumental role in the recognition of Rh(D), a major cause of hemolytic disease of the newborn (HDN) and non–ABO-related hemolytic transfusion reactions.

Prior to effective schemes for anticoagulation, Alexis Carrel explored vascular anastomosis as a possible strategy for moving blood from donor to recipient. Although eclipsed by other approaches, this pioneering technique formed the basis of contemporary vascular anastomoses in solid-organ transplantation and won Carrel the 1912 Nobel Prize.

The use of citrate to anticoagulate stored blood by means of calcium chelation was a landmark, as heparin was unsuitable to transfuse into bleeding patients and citrate's rapid metabolic elimination in vivo proved ideal for purposes of transfusion. Its adoption paved the way for transition from direct to indirect transfusion. By 1916 Rous and Turner introduced glucose in addition to sodium citrate, extending ex vivo storage by several days.

The first blood depots were established during the First World War by the British and were stocked prior to major campaigns. The Soviets established the first permanent blood bank in a Leningrad hospital in 1932, and 5 years later Bernard Fantus established the first US blood bank at the Cook County Hospital in Chicago.

Although clinical efforts had focused largely on transfusion of whole blood, Professor Edwin Cohn at Harvard explored fractionation of plasma proteins using cold ethanol treatment and centrifugation. By 1940 these techniques yielded concentrated fractions of albumin, immunoglobulins, and fibrinogen. With the outbreak of war in Europe, the US War Department and American Red Cross launched Plasma for Britain, under the direction of Dr Charles Drew.

Despite highly successful initial resuscitation, casualties with significant blood loss treated exclusively with plasma developed "air hunger" from anemia. Improved logistics enabled a shift to the use of whole blood. With this transition, volume tolerance emerged as the next constraint to adequate replacement of oxygen-carrying capacity. The large-scale availability of red blood cell concentrates (and more general exploitation of blood component therapy) awaited development of the plastic, integrated blood-collection systems of the 1950s and 1960s.

Success was tempered by the identification of transfusion-borne infections. "Serum" hepatitis followed approximately 10% of transfusions. Worse, in some communities posttransfusion hepatitis reached rates of 30%, an observation that was explained by reliance on monetarily compensated donors. In parallel with these epidemiologic discoveries, advances in virology and radioimmunochemistry brought to market by 1969 limited supplies of tests for the detection of hepatitis B surface antigen (HBsAg, the "Australia Antigen"). With transition in the United States to an all-volunteer blood supply, rates of hepatitis B virus (HBV) transmission fell dramatically, and with full deployment of HBsAg testing in 1972, rates of transfusion-transmitted hepatitis B fell to between 0.3% and 0.9%. Although remarkably high by today's standards, this represented risk reduction by an order of magnitude.

Following the emergence of human immunodeficiency virus (HIV)/acquired immunodeficiency syndrome (AIDS), an epidemic that transformed public perceptions of blood safety occurred. Lessons learned for dealing with hepatitis led to rapid progress toward securing the safety of the blood supply. The answer to a patient's question, "Will this transfusion give me AIDS?" is, "No."

Although infectious risks of blood transfusion have diminished enormously in developed nations, high rates of endemic disease and limited testing resources in developing countries paint a variegated global picture of blood product safety. Today's tools include effective donor screening and testing. Tomorrow holds the promise of pathogen inactivation and improved controls of bedside transfusion practice as further steps on the long path toward safe transfusion.

CLINICALLY AVAILABLE BLOOD PRODUCTS

WHOLE BLOOD

Despite some clinicians' desires for fresh whole blood, especially for use in pediatric cardiac anesthesiology, the optimal use for a limited resource demands the use of red cells for oxygen-carrying capacity, plasma for coagulation proteins, and platelets for thrombocytopenia or platelet dysfunction. The component therapy approach maximizes the number of recipients benefiting from transfusion and optimally preserves the function of essential blood elements. Colloid replacement can be provided by synthetic colloids, such as gelatins and starches, or albumin products fractionated from plasma. The time required to perform federally mandated testing makes fresh whole blood practically unavailable to most clinicians; consequently, discussion is primarily focused on blood components.

A unit of whole blood is collected in citrate-phosphate-dextrose-adenine 1 (CPDA-1) anticoagulant, giving it a shelf life of 35 days and a volume of approximately 510 mL (450 mL of blood plus 63 mL of CPDA-1). Within 24 hours of collection, the platelets are dysfunctional[1] and several plasma coagulation factors are below optimal levels,[2] emphasizing the importance of the component products despite the disadvantage of increased donor exposure.

RED CELL CONCENTRATES

Red cell concentrates, or packed red blood cells (PRBCs), are obtained from CPDA-1–anticoagulated whole blood after centrifugation of most of the plasma and platelets. At most blood centers, the red cells are then mixed with 100 mL of an additive nutrient containing an additional dextrose and adenine (NutriCell or AS-3) or dextrose, adenine, and mannitol (Adsol or AS-1) solution that extends the storage period to 42 days[3] and results in flow properties similar to those of whole blood. PRBCs from CPDA-1–anticoagulated blood are stored for up to 35 days. Loss of viability during storage is caused by cellular adenosine triphosphate (ATP) depletion, which leads to loss of membrane phospholipids, increased rigidity, and reduced life span, with current standards requiring 75% of transfused cells to survive in the circulation for 24 hours.[2] At 35 days, 70% of cells survive in CPDA-1 versus 88% in Adsol, with a pH of 6.7 in both solutions; intracellular ATP is 45% baseline in CPDA-1 versus 75% in Adsol, whereas 2,3-diphosphoglycerate (2,3-DPG) levels are at 10% baseline in both. In vivo, 2,3-DPG levels rapidly normalize over 24 hours and recover to more than 50% within 1 or 2 hours.[4] PRBCs are the product of choice for the correction of an isolated defect in oxygen-carrying capacity, as in chronic anemia, with the advantage of lower volume load in this setting. During acute perioperative blood loss, however, attention must be paid to volume status as well as restoring oxygen-carrying capacity using crystalloid or colloid volume expanders.

LEUKOCYTE-REDUCED RED CELLS

Leukocyte-reduced red cells (LRRCs) can be prepared by a variety of methods, with varying efficiency of white cell removal. The minimum standard, established by the American Association of Blood Banks (AABB), is a leukocyte number in the final component of less than 5×10^6.[8] Early techniques involved centrifugation and washing with saline, repeatedly removing the buffy coat. Next the "spin-cool-filter" method was introduced, using 1-week-old red cells that were centrifuged and then cooled for 4 hours to enhance microaggregate formation, then were passed through a microaggregate filter. Currently, the most widely used method of leukoreduction is filtration, which can be performed either in the laboratory or at the bedside. The various filters on the market result in greater than 99% leukocyte reduction while depleting less than 10% of the red cells. Most recently, blood bags with in-line filters that allow prestorage leukoreduction have become available. Simple removal of the buffy coat from red cells (a routine procedure during component preparation in Europe) may provide a sufficient degree of leukoreduction.[5] Because component preparation in the United States does not include buffy coat removal and because soluble white cell fragments may be capable of mediating immunosuppression, a prestorage leukoreduction method might be required to abrogate this adverse effect in transfusion recipients in the United States. Introduction of leukoreduction in the United States began around 1998. Confirmation with individual blood banks is necessary to determine their policies, as there are often regional differences.

The major indication for the use of LRRCs has been prevention of the nonhemolytic febrile transfusion reaction, which is the most common adverse effect of transfusion, particularly in multiply transfused patients or multiparous females. It is believed to be a result of preexisting antihuman leukocyte antigen (anti-HLA) antibodies. The use of LRRCs reduces the incidence of such reactions.[6] Cytokines may cause these reactions, suggesting that prestorage leukodepletion may be more helpful.

A second important indication for LRRCs is the prevention of alloimmunization to HLA antigens that can adversely affect posttransfusion platelet increments.[7] Platelet components also require leukodepletion. The current AABB standards mandate less 5×10^6 leukocytes for this indication, possibly with third-generation leukoreduction filters for both red cells and platelets.[8] A large, multicenter study (TRAP, Trial to Reduce Alloimmunization to Platelets) confirmed that the use of leukoreduction filters significantly decreased but did not eliminate alloimmunization.[9]

WASHED RED CELLS

Red cells are washed using isotonic saline solutions with some degree of red cell loss with each wash cycle. This open system requires the resulting product to be transfused within 24 hours. The primary aim of washing is to remove plasma proteins (with some leukocytes and platelets also removed) to prevent severe allergic transfusion reactions mediated by recipient antibodies (most likely IgE) to donor plasma proteins or preformed antibodies to IgA in donor plasma, which can cause anaphylaxis in IgA-deficient patients.[10] Washed cells may also be indicated in paroxysmal nocturnal hemoglobinuria.

FROZEN RED CELLS

Red cells can be frozen (with glycerol used as a cryoprotective agent) and stored in liquid nitrogen or mechanical freezers.[11] Thawing and washing away the glycerol using a series of progressively less hypertonic saline solutions allows glycerol to diffuse gradually from the cells to prevent hemolysis before transfusion. This process removes most of the plasma, and any debris and red cells can be frozen for more than 10 years with good viability.[12] As with washed cells, frozen red cells need to be transfused within 24 hours; the posttransfusion survival rate is 85% to 90%.[11] Freezing, ideally using fresh blood, maintains ATP and 2,3-DPG levels, but solutions containing pyruvate, glucose, phosphate, and adenine can restore older blood.[12] The major use of frozen cells is to store units of a rare phenotype. In addition, the military can transport large volumes of frozen units.

INDICATIONS FOR RBC TRANSFUSION

A unit of PRBCs should increase the hemoglobin (Hgb) level by 1 g/dL or the hematocrit level by approximately 3%. However, continued blood loss causes a suboptimal response to transfusion. More chronically, hemolysis caused by either immune red cell damage or mechanical trauma shortens the survival of transfused cells, and hypersplenism can lead to sequestration and increased destruction of red cells. Also, transfusion suppresses erythropoiesis, thus sustained results of transfusion may be less than expected.

CHRONIC ANEMIA

Generally, the signs and symptoms of anemia develop at an Hgb level of less than 7 to 8 g/dL. With gradual onset, the body's compensatory mechanisms for maintaining oxygen delivery to the tissues are effective. Cardiac output and intracellular 2,3-DPG are increased, thus oxygen unloads at a lower pO_2 of the tissues. When chronic anemia is a result of red cell destruction, the healthy bone marrow can respond by increasing production by up to 6-fold, provided sufficient dietary iron, folate, and vitamin B_{12} is ingested. The decision to transfuse depends on how a given individual manifests the signs and symptoms of anemia, determined by underlying health status, cardiorespiratory reserve, and activity level. In the perioperative setting, it is important to cross-match sufficient units to compensate for the lower initial Hgb, particularly in a multiply transfused patient with alloantibodies that may be difficult to match.

PERIOPERATIVE PERIOD

Much of the dogma surrounding perioperative transfusion has few supporting data. One example is the use of 10 g/dL of Hgb as the gold standard for the red cell transfusion trigger during the perioperative period.[13] A rule of thumb is that, assuming no preoperative anemia, blood losses of 5% to 10% of total blood volume require minimal replacement therapy; losses of up to 20% can be replaced exclusively with volume expansion, whereas losses of greater than 25% generally require red cell transfusion to restore oxygen-carrying capacity, along with volume expansion to restore intravascular volume and maintain perfusion.

The availability of hemoglobin measurement, acid-base status, and central venous and mixed venous oximetry, combined with tools to assess intravascular volume in most hospital environments, supersedes such rules, allowing more individually tailored, closely monitored transfusion therapy designed to provide sufficient tissue oxygenation. This is still vague and subjective, therefore when to transfuse remains a clinical decision. The American Society of Anesthesiologists provides extensive guidelines, available at http://www.asahq.org. Societies, such as the Society for the Advancement of Blood Management (http://www.sabm.org), champion blood conservation techniques and appropriate safe but lower transfusion triggers aimed at minimizing allogeneic blood product usage in the perioperative period. The National Institutes of Health suggest that most surgical patients who are not actively bleeding do not need transfusion unless the Hgb level decreases to less than 7 g/dL, and such levels of Hgb may not interfere with wound healing or automatically make general anesthesia a risk.

Nonetheless, questions concerning an objective measurement to determine a safe transfusion trigger still arise. Animal models of acute normovolemic anemia can be helpful and describe the whole body oxygen extraction ratio (OER) as an indicator of when to transfuse.[14] These studies make the seemingly valid assumption that the heart is the major organ at risk. With progressive hemodilution, healthy animals with normal coronary trees were able to maintain normal levels of oxygen consumption (200-250 mL/min) through a moderate increase in cardiac output, an increase in coronary blood flow, and a linear increase in the OER up to a ratio of 50%. As the hematocrit decreased to less than 10%, however, oxygen consumption began to decrease, and the animals were no longer able to increase the OER. An OER of 50% was the critical point at which the myocardium converted from aerobic to anaerobic metabolism, reflected in net lactate production. At that point, metabolic acidosis developed, resulting in hemodynamic instability. Dogs with critical coronary stenosis converted to anaerobic metabolism and went into congestive heart failure at an OER of greater than 50%, but that an OER of greater than 50% occurred at a hematocrit of 17.0% in the dogs with critical stenosis, compared with a hematocrit of 8.6% in the healthy group, is consistent with the 10% above.[15,16] Dog hearts with normal coronary arteries developed subendocardial ischemia then cardiac failure at a hematocrit less than 10%; hypertrophied hearts, at higher risk of subendocardial ischemia, may fail at higher hematocrits, although this was not studied.[15] OER can be calculated whenever a pulmonary artery catheter is being used, and therefore mixed venous oximetry can be performed and thus used to help assess transfusion need. An OER of 50% can be used as a red cell transfusion trigger because it appears to be a valid indicator of marginal myocardial oxygen reserve in both healthy people and individuals with coronary artery disease if it is reasonable to directly extrapolate the above animal data to humans. Given the complexity that this adds to clinical practice, most clinicians follow published guidelines based on Hgb levels.

The controversies surrounding transfusion triggers in neonates are beyond the scope of this chapter and are complicated by uncertainties concerning the diagnosis of symptomatic anemia in this group. Similarly, there are fewer data addressing transfusion in pediatric patients compared with adults. Of interest, the humoral and cellular immune systems of the neonate are immature, particularly with prematurity. This introduces a small but real risk of transfusion-induced graft versus host disease or thrombocytopenia after transfusion of leukocytes (present to some degree in PRBCs or platelet transfusions) in premature infants or in a fetus undergoing intrauterine transfusion.[17] Irradiated cells are indicated in these settings. Another risk in premature infants is the development of clinical cytomegalovirus (CMV) infection in infants of CMV-seronegative mothers.[18] CMV-seronegative blood is now routinely used in these neonates. The only setting in which there may be some data to support the use of CMV-seronegative units is in severe combined immune deficiency infants undergoing bone marrow transplantation. Otherwise, contemporary leukoreduced products are considered "CMV safe," equivalent to seronegative products. Leukoreduction by filtration reduces but does not eliminate the risk of these complications.[19]

SAFETY OF BLOOD TRANSFUSION

Transfusion safety relies on the avoidance of transfusion reactions, as classified in **Table 83-1**, that have multiple etiologies. Immune-mediated reactions are a result of transfusion of an incompatible blood product, as described below. The single most important contribution to transfusion safety is uncompromising attention to all details of patient, sample, and blood product identification.

RED BLOOD CELL COMPATIBILITY

Compatibility relies on the recipient not recognizing the allogeneic blood transfusion as foreign. Sensitization to alloantigens, with formation of the alloantibodies that determine incompatibility, can occur after transfusion, transplantation, or pregnancy. The most clinically important antibodies, or isohemagglutinins, react with antigens of the ABO system; are naturally occurring, complement-fixing antibodies that require no prior sensitization; and typically result in immediate intravascular hemolysis of transfused erythrocytes and a severe hemolytic transfusion reaction (HTR). The chance of ABO incompatibility with an unmatched transfusion is 1 in 3, leading to a life-threatening HTR with approximately 10% mortality.[20] Anti-A and anti-B antibodies are classically associated with severe HTRs, but reactions to anti-Rh (D, C, E, c, e, f, or ce), Kell, Duffy, or Kidd system antibodies are actually more common.[21] **Table 83-2** details the ABO compatibility of blood products.

ALLOIMMUNIZATION

The likelihood of sensitization to other antigens depends on both the variable immunogenicity of the particular red cell antigen and the immune response of the host; HTRs are 3 times more common in females.[21] Such alloimmunization is best understood for the Rhesus (Rh) D antigen, studied extensively because of the important role it plays in hemolytic disease of the newborn. It is a highly immunogenic and clinically important antigen associated with severe HTRs. Up to 80% of Rh(D)-negative individuals, and up to 95% after massive transfusion, produce anti-D antibodies after exposure.[22] Those who generate anti-D after an exposure are more likely to develop other red

TABLE 83-1 Classification of Transfusion Reactions

Acute
Immune mediated
Acute hemolytic transfusion reaction (AHTR)
Transfusion-related acute lung injury
Febrile nonhemolytic transfusion reaction
Urticarial reaction
Anaphylactic
Nonimmune mediated
Nonimmune hemolysis
Bacterial contamination
Volume overload
Metabolic
Embolic
Delayed
Immune mediated
Delayed hemolytic transfusion reaction (DHTR)
Posttransfusion purpura
Graft versus host disease
Nonimmune mediated
Transfusion-transmitted infection
Iron overload

TABLE 83-2 ABO Compatibility of Blood Products[a]

		ABO-Compatible Blood Products				
Recipient Blood Group	Recipient Alloantibodies	Whole Blood	Packed Red Cells	FFP	Cryoprecipitate	Platelets
A	Anti-B	A	A or O	A or AB	Any	Any
B	Anti-A	B	B or O	B or AB	Any	Any
AB	Nil	AB	O, A, B, or AB	AB	Any	Any
O	Anti-A and anti-B	O	O	A, B, AB, or O	Any	Any

FFP, fresh-frozen plasma.

[a]Compatibility differs with components, as whole blood contains all components and packed red cells contain minimal plasma and antibodies. Donor antibodies are present in FFP, which is a component of platelet products; cryoprecipitate contains fewer alloantibodies than plasma and pediatric patients require ABO matched cryoprecipitate. ABO compatibility may, however, increase the lifespan of transfused platelets, and platelet units with high plasma volume should be ABO matched like FFP to avoid hemolysis of recipient native red cells. Patients with blood group O express the H antigen on the red cell surface but anti-H is very rare.

cell alloantibodies, whereas those not generating anti-D rarely develop other alloantibodies.[23] Other antigen systems are less immunogenic; Kell (K) antigens stimulate anti-K in 10% of cases, followed in order of magnitude by Rh c and E, Duffy (Fya), and Kidd (Jka). Antibodies recognizing antigens from the Kell, Duffy, Kidd, Lutheran, and MNSU systems can cause HTRs, typically delayed, although in many patients they only result in reduced red cell survival.

In terms of alloantibodies detected by blood banks, the most commonly recognized antigens are in the ABO blood group system followed by anti-D, anti-K, anti-E, anti-K, anti-c, anti-Fya, anti-C, anti-Jka, anti-S, and anti-Jkb. The incidence of others is less than 1%.[23] Studies of alloimmunization after transfusion have focused on chronically transfused patients with hemoglobinopathies (such as thalassemia or sickle cell disease), and an approximately 1% risk of alloimmunization has been attributed to every unit transfused.[24] The incidence of red blood cell (RBC) alloimmunization is up to 50% in adults with sickle cell disease,[25] increasing the likelihood of delayed HTRs, which can present as sickle crises.[26]

HLA ALLOIMMUNIZATION

Alloimmunization to antigens in the human leukocyte antigen (HLA) system occurs in multiply transfused or multiparous individuals and can be detected in 30% to 70% of patients given nonleukoreduced RBC or platelet transfusions.[27] The almost ubiquitous adoption of leukoreduction techniques for RBCs and platelets during the 1990s can reduce the incidence of HLA alloimmunization, which can cause febrile nonhemolytic transfusion reactions, platelet transfusion refractoriness, and increased risk of subsequent transplant rejection.[27] Alloantibodies to the human platelet antigen systems (HPA-1 to HPA-5) cause neonatal alloimmune thrombocytopenia and posttransfusion purpura; they may also lead to platelet transfusion refractoriness, but are clinically far less important than HLA alloantibodies.

HEMOLYTIC TRANSFUSION REACTIONS

Immune-mediated HTRs result from recipient alloantibodies reacting to transfused RBC surface alloantigens. HTRs can be classified as acute (within hours of transfusion), delayed (within days or weeks of transfusion), intravascular, and extravascular.

Acute HTRs Acute HTRs are a result of existing, circulating alloantibodies to alloantigens on transfused RBCs. If the alloantibody fixes complement (such as anti-A or anti-B), acute, intravascular hemolysis occurs, which is a medical emergency. Acute HTRs have an estimated frequency of 1 per 25 000 RBC units.[28] The mortality of 1 in 600 000 RBC units[29] is primarily caused by ABO incompatibility.[30]

Signs and symptoms of an acute HTR can be nonspecific and confounded by the patient's clinical condition; consequently, a high index of suspicion and meticulous identification of patients and blood products is essential. Although chills; infusion site, abdominal, chest, or back pain; nausea; anxiety; and dyspnea may be reported by a conscious patient, fever, hypo- or hypertension, hemoglobinuria, anuria, shock, or coagulopathic bleeding may be the first sign of an acute HTR in anesthetized patients. The etiology of profound shock is the activation of the complement cascade with bradykinin production from factor XII activation, C3a- and C5a-induced histamine and serotonin release from mast cells leading to increased vascular permeability, bronchial and intestinal smooth muscle contraction and neutrophil degranulation, and C5a-mediated capillary vasodilatation. Numerous cytokines (tumor necrosis factor, interleukin [IL]-1, IL-6, IL-8) also play a role.[31] Disseminated intravascular coagulation (DIC) results from complement-mediated activation of factor XII and extrinsic pathway activation by stromal thromboplastins from lysed erythrocytes.

Free hemoglobin does not appear to have direct toxic effects,[32] and shock-induced renal failure and DIC convey most of the morbidity and mortality.[33] Therefore, prompt supportive therapy with fluids, inotropes, and vasopressors as indicated is crucial, and corticosteroids may be considered in the setting of resistant vasoplegic shock. DIC can be managed with hemostatic blood products as required; the efficacy of heparin or activated protein C in this setting is not established.[34]

Immediate notification of the blood bank is essential, as another patient is likely to erroneously receive the unit intended for the patient experiencing the acute HTR. An anticoagulated ethylenediaminetetraacetic acid (EDTA) and a serum specimen, as well as a posttransfusion urine sample, should be sent with all suspected blood units and infusion tubing. **Table 83-3** details laboratory testing for suspected HTRs.

Delayed HTRs Delayed HTRs require a secondary or anamnestic antibody response to a transfused RBC alloantigen in a recipient previously sensitized by transfusion or pregnancy. Detectable antibody levels are not present at the time of pretransfusion serologic testing or transfusion, but appear within days of the transfusion, which is why transfused patients need to have serologic testing repeated after 4 to 5 days.[35]

The frequency of delayed HTRs is estimated to be 1 per 1500 units. Although fatalities have been associated with delayed HTRs, they were not believed to be causative.[30] Alloantibodies are typically against antigens in the Rhesus, MNS, Kell, Kid, or Duffy systems, but rarer antigens may also be involved.

Opsonized RBCs are cleared by the reticuloendothelial system, resulting in a slower and less severe extravascular hemolysis. A history of fever, anemia, and recent blood transfusion may be the only clue to

TABLE 83-3 Diagnosis of Hemolytic Transfusion Reactions

	Onset	Duration
Plasma free hemoglobin	Immediate	5-12 h
Methemalbumin[a]	1 h	24 h
Direct antiglobulin test (DAT)[b]	Immediate	Hours
Indirect antiglobulin (IAT)	Days	Weeks
Bilirubin[c]	1 h	12 h
LDH[c]	1 h	24 h
Haptoglobin[c]	Hours	Days
Urine free hemoglobin	1 h	24 h

HTR, hemolytic transfusion reaction.

[a]Primarily for acute hemolytic transfusion reactions.

[b]The DAT will only be positive until all incompatible cells have been destroyed; frank hemolysis (free hemoglobin >50 mg/dL) is visible as "pink" plasma. ABO incompatibility causes a positive DAT, whereas other alloantibodies (eg, anti-Kell) cause a positive IAT.

[c]May be seen in acute HTRs but more useful for confirming delayed hemolysis. When testing urine for free hemoglobin, distinguish from hematuria or myoglobinuria. The time course of urine hemoglobin is dependent on plasma hemolysis and bladder clearance (ie, urine output).

a delayed HTR, and many pass undetected.[21] Rarely, a delayed HTR causes intravascular hemolysis with the clinical picture described for acute HTRs. Erythrocyte destruction is maximal 4 to 13 days post-transfusion; a positive direct antiglobulin test is found after 2 to 3 days, followed by spherocytes in peripheral blood (3-4 days) and antibodies detectable by indirect antiglobulin test, anemia, jaundice, and possible hemoglobinuria (5-7 days).

Pseudo HTRs Poor transfusion practices, such as transfusion of aged, overheated, or frozen cells; osmotic hemolysis by hypotonic solutions; mechanical hemolysis from inappropriate administration equipment; hemolysis from bacterial or parasitic contamination; or coincidental presentation of congenital hemolytic conditions (eg, sickle trait or glucose-6-phosphate dehydrogenase deficiency) presenting at the time of transfusion (eg, surgery) all lead to a nonimmune-mediated or "pseudo" HTR. Nonimmune hemolysis can be induced by mishandling of blood, overheating, and mixing with nonisotonic solutions.

PLASMA COMPONENT DERIVATIVES

Plasma is separated from PRBCs through centrifugation of whole blood at the time of collection, or collected by apheresis as a single product or as a byproduct of platelet or red blood cell apheresis. Plasma can be further processed into its derivatives through the cold ethanol fractionation method of Cohn. This chapter discusses features and uses of fresh-frozen plasma (FFP), cryoprecipitate, and other products derived from pooled plasma.

FRESH-FROZEN PLASMA

Plasma is the fluid compartment of blood and consists of 90% water, 7% protein and colloids, and 2% to 3% nutrients, crystalloids, hormones, and vitamins. The protein fraction also contains the soluble clotting factors. Plasma frozen at −35°C (−22°F) or colder within 6 hours of donation is labeled FFP. This product may be stored up to 1 year before use, at which time it is thawed over 20 to 30 minutes. The activities of the labile coagulation factors (V and VIII) decrease after thawing but remain adequate for at least 24 hours. Plasma that is not immediately frozen as FFP becomes either "liquid plasma" (stored at 33.8°F-42.8°F [1°C-6°C]) or "source plasma" (stored at −35°C [−22°F] or colder) and is used for the preparation of plasma derivatives: albumin, clotting-factor concentrates, and immunoglobulin preparations. When FFP is thawed at 39.2°F (4°C), a precipitate separated by centrifugation forms, resulting in cryoprecipitate and cryo-poor supernatant.

Solvent detergent (SD) plasma is an alternative to FFP. SD plasma is a pooled product (2500 donor units per pool) and subjected to a solvent detergent treatment process combining the organic solvent tri(n-butyl)phosphate with a nonionic detergent, Triton X. This inactivates lipid-enveloped viruses, including HIV types 1 and 2, HBV, hepatitis C virus (HCV), human T-cell lymphotropic virus (HTLV) types 1 and 2, hepatitis G virus (HGV), vesicular stomatitis virus, and Sendai virus, while preserving the structural and functional integrity of most plasma proteins. However, it does not inactivate nonenveloped viruses, such as parvovirus B19 and hepatitis A virus (HAV), or prions, the causative agents of various rare encephalopathies including Creutzfeldt-Jakob disease. The increased prevalence of parvovirus B19 and HAV makes transmission by transfusion of pooled blood components a potential concern, although pooled SD plasma also contains significant amounts of neutralizing antibody to both parvovirus B19 and HAV. It is unclear what the real value and risk of SD plasma is compared with FFP, but, at present, the cost of SD plasma is much more than FFP.

Indications for FFP Audits of transfusion practices have consistently demonstrated that FFP is commonly used inappropriately.[36] Such inappropriate use includes reconstituting "whole blood" by coadministration with RBCs, volume expansion, and as a source of nutrients. Acceptable indications are discussed below.

Liver Disease and Transplantations Patients with severe liver disease have low levels of the vitamin K–dependent clotting factors (II, VII, IX, and X) in addition to thrombocytopenia associated with hypersplenism and a hyperfibrinolytic state. These patients develop a prolonged prothrombin time (PT) and partial thromboplastin time (PTT). In addition, the thrombin time (TT) may be prolonged, fibrin split products may be elevated, and in later stages the fibrinogen level decreases. Hemorrhage from portosystemic varices is complicated by this multifactorial coagulopathy.

Infusion of FFP is indicated during bleeding episodes to normalize the PT or PTT. In the absence of anatomic lesions, bleeding does not usually occur until the PT is longer than 16 to 18 seconds or the PTT is longer than 55 to 60 seconds, and prophylactic FFP (eg, before a liver biopsy) is not indicated at lower values. The PT and PTT are poor predictors of surgical bleeding, and mild abnormalities in these coagulation tests may not correct despite large volumes of FFP; platelet transfusion, cryoprecipitate, antifibrinolytic drugs, and even recombinant-activated factor VII may be required. This scenario is exaggerated in the setting of orthotopic liver transplantation complicated by an anhepatic stage, massive PRBC transfusion, and DIC. Large volumes of FFP are typically used, ideally guided by clinical assessment of bleeding and coagulation test results.[38]

Massive Transfusion This is the most common situation during which anesthesiologists administer combinations of blood products. FFP is often required after large quantities of PRBC (>1 blood volume in 24 hours) because of the dilutional coagulopathy arising from the PRBC and crystalloid solutions, both of which lack coagulation factors. A predetermined algorithm for FFP transfusion per units of PRBCs is often unreliable, as dilutional thrombocytopenia also complicates the coagulopathy after massive transfusion.[39,40] As recommended in the transfusion guidelines published by the American Society of Anesthesiologists, FFP transfusion should ideally be guided by abnormal PT and PTT results when available as the degree of coagulopathy can be unpredictable. Current trauma practices favor a 1:1 or 2:1 RBC-to-FFP ratio. Some studies appear to show a survival advantage but the evidence is not yet conclusive.[41,42]

Disseminated intravascular coagulation may be secondary to sepsis, liver disease, hypotension, perioperative hypoperfusion, trauma, obstetric complications, leukemia, or underlying malignancy. Successful treatment of the underlying cause is paramount. Patients with DIC leading to coagulopathic bleeding should be given FFP to correct PT and PTT abnormalities, but as in severe liver disease, FFP alone may fail to normalize PT and PTT.[43] The need for cryoprecipitate or platelet transfusion should also be evaluated.

Rapid Reversal of Vitamin K Antagonists Warfarin (Coumadin) inhibits the hepatic synthesis of vitamin K–dependent clotting factors (II, VII, IX, and X), inducing functional deficiencies of these factors that can correct within 48 hours after drug discontinuation if diet and vitamin K absorption are normal. Vitamin K administration corrects the coagulopathy in 12 to 18 hours. In an emergency, the deficiency of clotting factors can immediately be corrected by FFP transfusion. However, a large volume of FFP may be required, and if unlikely to be tolerated, smaller volumes of FFP can be augmented with a bypassing agent such as prothrombin complex concentrates or more commonly recombinant activated factor VII.[44] In the absence of bleeding, the potential danger of excessively prolonged PTs must be weighed against the risks of FFP infusion, and FFP is rarely indicated.[45]

Thrombotic Thrombocytopenic Purpura and Hemolytic Uremic Syndrome In some patients with thrombotic thrombocytopenic purpura (TTP); hemolytic uremic syndrome (HUS); or the syndrome of hemolysis, elevated liver enzymes, and low platelets associated with preeclampsia (HELLP), FFP exchange transfusion has been clinically therapeutic; plasmapheresis is preferred if there is concern for fluid overload.[46,47] The mechanism of the therapeutic effect of FFP is likely to involve transfused anticoagulant proteins such as protein C and antithrombin III, which may restore endothelial prostaglandin I2 (prostacyclin) production and inhibit the agglutinating activity of the abnormal plasma.[48] Alternatively, it may inhibit the release of large-molecular-weight von Willebrand factor (vWF) multimers or restore their normal processing in the circulation by deficient ADAMTS13 enzyme.[49] The use of cryo-poor supernatant for refractory TTP has been suggested, but the advantage is unestablished.[50]

Dosage One unit of FFP derived from a unit of whole blood contains 200 to 280 mL; apheresis may contain as much as 800 mL. On average, there are 0.7 to 1 unit/mL of activity of each coagulation factor per milliliter of FFP and 1 to 2 mg/mL fibrinogen. For perioperative use, the FFP dose may be estimated at 8 to 10 mL/kg and should be ordered as the number of milliliters to be infused for pediatric patients or units for adults. Laboratory measurements and clinical response determine the need for additional doses.

Compatibility and Side Effects Fresh-frozen plasma is screened for unexpected RBC antibodies and should be ABO-type compatible as it contains anti-A (groups O and B) and anti-B (groups O and A). Crossmatching is not performed. The Rh(D) type is not always matched because immunization to Rh(D) antigen has rarely been reported as a result of transfusion of Rh(D)-positive plasma to Rh(D)-negative individuals. Hemolytic reactions as a consequence of infusion of an undetected antibody directed toward recipient RBC antigens are rarely seen, as is alloimmunization to RBC antigens.[51]

Fever, chills, and allergic reactions may occur and are treated symptomatically. Typical urticarial reactions are believed to result from recipient antibodies interacting with donor plasma protein antigens. Rarely, severe allergic reactions occur. Some are believed to be caused by donor antibodies reacting with recipient leukocytes or protein antigens. Anaphylactic reactions may occur after infusion of plasma (containing IgA) into patients with IgA deficiency and antibodies to IgA.[52] IgA-deficient plasma from donors in the national registry can be obtained for these occasional patients. Transmission of infectious disease by FFP has been significantly reduced but not eliminated. Cell-associated CMV is not transmitted by FFP.[53]

IMMUNOGLOBULIN PREPARATIONS

Intravenous immunoglobulin (IVIg) is prepared by fractionation of large pools of human plasma. Indications for IVIg use include primary congenital immunodeficiency syndromes, children with HIV infection,[54] chronic lymphocytic leukemia complicated by hypogammaglobulinemia, CMV pneumonia complicating bone marrow transplantation (in combination with ganciclovir),[55] a possible role in preventing severe graft versus host disease after bone marrow transplantation, acute and chronic idiopathic thrombocytopenic purpura, and mucocutaneous lymph node syndrome (Kawasaki disease).[56]

Hyperimmune immunoglobulin (HIg) is prepared from large pools of plasma known to contain elevated antibody titers against specific infectious agents. Specifically, CMV HIg is indicated in transplantation recipients seronegative for CMV who receive a seropositive donor organ or in bone marrow transplantation patients with CMV interstitial pneumonia.[55] Hepatitis B HIg is used to provide passive immunity to hepatitis B virus associated with inoculation by or a liver transplantation in HBsAg-positive individuals.

Rhesus HIg is used when fetal Rh(D)-positive RBCs may have entered the maternal circulation of an Rh(D)-negative mother. Rhesus HIg is given to Rh(D)-negative mothers after abortion or amniocentesis, as well as before delivery and again postpartum if the child proves to be Rh(D) positive.[57,58] The therapeutic effect is believed to be caused by antibody feedback with T-cell suppression of the B-cell clone responsible for the formation of anti-Rh antibody. Its routine use in obstetrical practice has virtually eliminated alloimmunization of Rh-negative mothers.

Antithymocyte globulin (ATG) is purified from the hyperimmune serum of horses immunized with human T lymphocytes. ATG is used in transplant patients as an adjunct therapy in the treatment of graft rejection.

CRYOPRECIPITATE

Cryoprecipitate is prepared from 1 unit of FFP thawed at 39.2°F (4°C). The precipitate is then refrozen in 10 to 15 mL of plasma and stored at −35°C (−22°F) or colder for up to 1 year. Cryoprecipitate contains 80 to 100 units of factor VIII, 100 to 250 mg of fibrinogen, 50 to 60 mg of fibronectin, 40% to 70% of normal vWF levels, and anti-A and anti-B antibodies.

Cryoprecipitate is effectively the blood component containing the highest concentration of factor VIII, vWF, factor XIII, fibrinogen, and fibronectin. Cryoprecipitate may be used to treat bleeding associated with hypo- or dysfibrinogenemia or factor XIII deficiency states, although an equivalent amount of fibrinogen to the usual adult dose of 100 mL is also found in 4 units of FFP. Its use in vWF and factor VIII deficiency has been superseded by individual factor replacement therapy.

INDICATIONS

Fibrinogen Deficiency Fibrinogen deficiency may be a result of rare congenital afibrinogenemias or dysfibrinogenemias, or more commonly as a result of severe liver disease, DIC, or massive transfusion.[45] These patients often have multifactorial coagulopathies and may require the coadministration of FFP, platelets, and antifibrinolytic agents. Fibrinogen measurements are an important component of a coagulation screen because levels less than 100 mg/dL can cause prolongation of both the PT and PTT despite adequate levels of other clotting factors. Low levels of fibrinogen occur during liver transplantation, necessitating cryoprecipitate transfusion.[38]

von Willebrand Disease Initial platelet adhesion to disrupted endothelium is mediated by von Willebrand factor (vWF) interacting with the platelet surface GP1b complex; vWF is low or dysfunctional in the various types of von Willebrand disease. DDAVP (desmopressin acetate; 1-deamino-8-D-arginine vasopressin), which releases stored vWF from platelet granules and endothelial cells, is the initial treatment, but severe bleeding requires cryoprecipitate or vWF concentrate.[59]

Fibrin Glue Fibrin glue results from the mixture of a fibrinogen source (FFP; platelet-rich plasma; heterologous, or more recently autologous, cryoprecipitate) with bovine thrombin, which leads to fibrin formation and enhanced local hemostasis. It has been used for diffuse local bleeding during cardiac surgery[60] and to reduce blood loss and the factor concentrate requirement in surgical patients with von Willebrand disease.[61] Other uses include meniscal tear repair and sealing postoperative neonatal chylothorax.[62] Autologous cryoprecipitate avoids any infectious risks; bovine thrombin can cause anaphylaxis, formation of antibodies to factor V, or activation of coagulation.[63]

Uremic Bleeding Uremia causes coagulopathy, and historically, cryoprecipitate or DDAVP has been used to treat bleeding associated with this.[64] There are no data to support this, although cryoprecipitate could be considered if the bleeding is unresponsive to other therapies.[65]

DOSAGE

The dosage of cryoprecipitate is calculated on the basis of the amount of fibrinogen present in 1 unit of cryoprecipitate, the plasma volume, and the desired increment. The fibrinogen content of cryoprecipitate is variable, but even if relatively low, sufficient response is seen with transfusion of 2 to 4 U/10 kg. In practice, most adults are given a pooled 10-unit or 100-mL dose that is repeated if the desired response is not seen.

COMPATIBILTY AND SIDE EFFECTS

Cryoprecipitate can contain anti-A or anti-B antibodies; therefore, infused units should be ABO plasma compatible. The risks of fevers, chills, allergic reactions, and infectious disease transmission are similar to those of FFP.

THE DEVELOPMENT OF AND INDICATIONS FOR FACTOR CONCENTRATES

In the 1940s Dr Edwin Cohn developed an ethanol fractionation procedure (the Cohn fractionation procedure) that allowed the fractionation of human plasma into various components, greatly expanding this limited resource by deriving more products from each unit of donated plasma. Sufficient amounts of factor concentrates, however, require pooling of plasma. Present pathogen inactivation technologies have virtually eliminated infectious risks associated with plasma derivatives.

The development of recombinant products has been fueled by concerns of infectious disease risks, but recombinant expression processes are complex and expensive. Mammalian cell culture is most commonly used to optimize posttranslational modifications required for biologic activity, with transgenic recombinant technology being developed to decrease or eliminate reliance on donated human plasma resources or mammalian cell-culture–based recombinant production methods. Recombinant transgenic human antithrombin expressed in goat milk and human 1-antitrypsin produced in sheep's milk are currently clinically available.

The most common congenital deficiencies of coagulation proteins are hemophilia A (classic hemophilia or factor VIII deficiency) or hemophilia B (Christmas disease or factor IX deficiency). The genes for these coagulation factors are located in close proximity on the long arm of the X chromosome. Limited to males, hemophilia A affects 1 in 10 000 males, whereas hemophilia B affects 1 in 30 000. Familial cases predominate, but more than 30% of cases arise from spontaneous mutations.

Arthropathy is the major morbidity of the hemophiliac secondary to recurrent spontaneous joint bleeding, and such patients are frequently encountered for orthopedic surgery. The major cause of mortality (other than transfusion-related infection) is bleeding, with central nervous system (CNS) hemorrhage occurring in 3% to 14% of patients, conferring a mortality of 20% to 50%. CNS hemorrhage occurs predominantly in patients with severe disease (<1% factor level).

Citrated plasma was first used in 1923 for the treatment of hemophilia by Feissly in Paris, and the development of modern blood banking in the 1930s and expansion of transfusion during and after World War II allowed for more widespread use of whole blood and, subsequently, frozen plasma in the treatment of these fatal hemophilias. The advent of cryoprecipitate revolutionized hemophilia therapy. Cryoprecipitate derived from a single whole-blood collection contains approximately 125 Units of factor VIII, and it quickly replaced frozen plasma to treat hemophilia.

The fractionation of plasma using ethanol, glycine, polyethylene glycol, or a combination of glycine and polyethylene glycol, and calcium or barium to precipitate plasma proteins led to the production of factor VIII and factor IX concentrates for clinical use.[66] This enabled high concentration, low volume, intensive infusion therapy for serious and life-threatening bleeding complications, such as intracranial, retroperitoneal, and retropharyngeal hemorrhages, and major surgery. From an infectious standpoint, these large pools of more than 1000 donations were universally contaminated with viral pathogens, such as hepatitis B or C, and between 1978 and 1985 most hemophiliacs were tragically infected with HIV from concentrates. Pasteurization and dry heat inactivate HIV and limit hepatitis B transmission; other strategies to limit infection include screening of potential donors for risk factors, surveillance of the blood supply for new pathogens, screening for markers of infectious agents, and other purification steps, including physical and chemical viral inactivation methods. After cloning of the genes factor VIII and factor IX, recombinant factor VIII and factor IX products were made available that are effective and free from pathogens.[67]

TREATMENT REGIMENS

The use of prophylactic regimens to maintain trough factor levels at more than 1% of normal reduces the incidence of arthropathy and CNS hemorrhage but requires dosing every 2 to 3 days with attendant problems and complications associated with long-term venous access.[68]

For the treatment of bleeding, the goal of therapy is to achieve a plasma factor VIII or IX level of between 30% and 50% for non–life-threatening bleeding episodes and a level of 100% for life-threatening bleeds or prophylaxis for surgical procedures using repeated boluses or continuous infusion for a duration of 10 to 14 days or longer, depending on the severity of the bleed or surgical intervention.

Adjunctive therapy includes DDAVP, a vasopressin analogue used for the treatment of patients with mild or moderate hemophilia A. This synthetic octapeptide causes a release of factor VIII (and von Willebrand factor) from endothelial cells, raising plasma factor VIII by approximately 3-fold (range, 2- to 12-fold) in patients with hemophilia in whom the disease is caused by decreased production or secretion of a functional protein or a protein that has decreased activity. Patients with severe hemophilia do not benefit from its use, as the mutation results in no synthesis or secretion, or a protein with no activity. The DDAVP response is unpredictable but reproducible in a given individual and should be documented by measuring factor VIII levels. The recommended intravenous dose is 0.3 g/kg infused slowly, as vasodilatation may occur. There have been reports of myocardial infarction and cerebral thrombosis with its use in patients at risk of arterial thrombosis; therefore, it should only be used in the setting of a documented coagulopathy.[69]

Dosing of factor VIII concentrates assumes an increase in plasma factor VIII activity of 2% for every 1 IU/kg infused. Cryoprecipitate replacement assumes approximately 80 to 150 IU per bag of factor VIII per bag of cryoprecipitate (derived from a 450-mL single whole-blood donor collection unit). Thus a typical 1750-IU dose (50% correction for a 70-kg patient) requires between 10 and 21 units.

Highly purified plasma-derived factor VIII concentrates or recombinant factor VIII concentrates have been available in North America, Europe, and Japan since 1992. These are either full-length or B-domain deleted molecules (the B domain is not required for activity in coagulation) that are expressed in mammalian cell culture (Chinese hamster ovary or baby hamster kidney cell lines) and are purified using immunoaffinity techniques. These products are formulated with added albumin as a stabilizer, but some have been developed that stabilize the factor VIII molecule with nonprotein molecules; despite no reliance on donated blood, the supply of these products is not abundant because of the complex manufacturing process.

FACTOR IX CONCENTRATES

Intermediate- and high-purity plasma products and a recombinant factor IX product are available for the treatment of hemophilia B, all of which undergo at least 1 viral inactivation or exclusion step in manufacture. Recovery of factor IX after infusion is therefore approximately 1%/IU/kg. The recovery observed with recombinant factor IX is approximately 20% lower than that observed with plasma-derived factor IX, likely because of differences in posttranslational modifications between the recombinant and plasma-derived factor proteins.

Intermediate-purity factor IX products use anion exchange chromatography-selecting proteins containing highly negatively charged epitopes such as the vitamin K–dependent coagulation factors with γ-carboxyglutamic acid–rich domains. Therefore, the other vitamin K–dependent coagulation factors, factor VII, factor X, and prothrombin, are copurified with factor IX and referred to as "prothrombin complex concentrates" (PCCs). PCCs are contaminated with trace amounts of activated forms of these factors, which is the likely explanation for thromboses complicating their use.[70] To minimize the risk of thrombosis with the use of PCCs, it is advisable to achieve a peak factor IX level no higher than 50%; some manufacturers have formulated PCCs with heparin or antithrombin III.[70]

High-purity factor IX products are produced from plasma using techniques of ligand affinity or immunoaffinity chromatography, and typically have specific activities greater than 150 IU/mg. A single high-purity recombinant factor IX product has been marketed. Thrombotic complications have not been reported with these high-purity products.

HEMOPHILIA WITH CIRCULATING INHIBITORS

Replacement therapy may be complicated by the development of inhibitory antibodies against the infused factors that interfere with factor activity. The incidence of factor VIII inhibitors is approximately 30%, although titers and inhibitory activity vary.[72]

Treatment of acute bleeding episodes can be accomplished by 2 methods. For patients with low titer inhibitors, hemostasis can be accomplished with large doses of factor VIII or factor IX (eg, as high as 200 IU/kg given at frequent intervals) in an effort to neutralize, or "override," the circulating inhibitor. Porcine factor VIII can be used to treat an actively bleeding patient with inhibitors to human replacement factors, but problems include inhibitors cross-reacting with porcine factor VIII, allergic reactions, anaphylaxis, and thrombocytopenia caused by binding of porcine von Willebrand factor present in the concentrate to human platelets.

Alternatively, a bypassing agent is required. These bypass agents include PCCs in which contaminant-activated forms of these proteins, factors VIIa, Xa, IXa, and IIa (thrombin), likely enhance the production of a fibrin clot by activating the coagulation pathway later than the level of action of factors VIII and IX. Activated PCCs (aPCCs) have been treated to increase the levels of these activated factors and may be more effective in the treatment of bleeding episodes in patients with inhibitors. They were used as first-line therapy for patients with inhibitors, but because of the risk of thrombotic complications with aPCCs,[73] recombinant activated factor VII (rFVIIa) has been licensed as an alternative bypass agent in the treatment of hemophiliacs with inhibitors.[71] The dosage of rFVIIa is 90 g/kg every 2 hours as necessary, compared with 50 to 75 IU/kg every 8 to 12 hours for PCCs or aPCCs. Thrombosis has also been reported with the use of rFVIIa.[77] Coadministration of antifibrinolytic agents, such as ε-aminocaproic acid, is often used as an adjunct to replacement or bypass therapy.

VON WILLEBRAND DISEASE

von Willebrand disease (vWD) is an autosomal dominant mucosal, platelet-type bleeding disorder first described by Erik von Willebrand in 1926, which has a prevalence of up to 2% of the general population. The penetrance and severity of the disease vary depending on the type of vWD (type 1, 2, or 3), the specific mutation, the number of affected genes, the patient's blood type, and numerous drug, hormonal, and other parameters. The type of vWD and the patient's response to DDAVP influence the recommended treatment for acute bleeding episodes or for prophylaxis against bleeding.[66] DDAVP releases stored vWF as well as factor VIII from platelets and endothelium, and is often effective for type 1 disease and may be useful in certain patients with type 2 disease. It is not appropriate for use in patients with type 3 disease in whom no stores of vWF exist.

As described for hemophilia A, antifibrinolytic agents are useful adjuncts for replacement therapy for vWD such as in the setting of dental surgery to inhibit fibrinolysis. Estrogens upregulate vWF synthesis and may be useful especially in women, and may ameliorate menorrhagia.

PLASMA PROTEIN–BASED THERAPY: FACTOR VIII CONCENTRATES

Some intermediate-purity factor VIII concentrates are manufactured from plasma using methods that copurify significant amounts of vWF, but no product has the pattern of multimers that is present in normal plasma.

VON WILLEBRAND FACTOR CONCENTRATES (PLASMA-DERIVED AND RECOMBINANT)

Several chromatography-purified plasma-derived concentrates enriched in vWF have been studied and may be effective and amenable to viral inactivation steps. Recombinant vWF has been successfully isolated and partially characterized; it is being developed clinically.

Cryoprecipitate was the mainstay of plasma-based therapy for bleeding in patients with vWD until the availability of virally inactivated intermediate-purity factor VIII concentrates that retained functional vWF protein. The factor VIII concentrates are the products of choice for the treatment of bleeding in patients with types 1 and 2 vWD that are unresponsive to DDAVP, and for bleeding in patients with type 3 vWD, as they have a lower risk of transfusion-associated infection than cryoprecipitate.

OTHER FACTOR DEFICIENCIES

Approximately 15% of inherited bleeding disorders are caused by deficiencies of fibrinogen and factors II, V, VII, X, XI, and XIII.[66] As the genes for these factors are not located on the X chromosome, homozygous defects are typically required for symptomatic disease. Hereditary deficiencies of factor XII, prekallikrein, and high-molecular-weight kininogen do not result in bleeding diatheses. The mainstays of therapy for these disorders are cryoprecipitate (for fibrinogen and factor XIII deficiencies) and plasma. Bypass therapy with PCCs, aPCCs, or rFVIIa can be considered for refractory bleeding, and adjunctive therapy with antifibrinolytics may be useful.

ACQUIRED DISEASE

Antibodies that inhibit the activity of factor VIII can develop in previously normal patients. Most of these patients have no underlying disease; however, factor VIII antibodies can arise in the setting of autoimmune disorders or in the postpartum period. One-third of these inhibitors resolve spontaneously, but supportive therapy is required while they persist.

Acquired vWD is a rare autoimmune disorder that can occur in association with other autoimmune disorders or lymphoproliferative disease. Antibodies may interact with functional epitopes, and the immune complexes increase the clearance of vWF. Plasmapheresis or immunoadsorption can reduce the circulating levels of inhibitors. Immunosuppressive agents and intravenous immunoglobulin (IgG) are useful adjuncts to abrogate production of the autoantibody. Otherwise, the treatment of these conditions is as for congenital disease with associated circulating inhibitors.

Dilutional coagulopathy develops following resuscitation during trauma and major surgery or following hemodilution and cell salvage during cardiac surgery. It is a multifactorial deficiency and treatment should be guided by laboratory tests as recommended in the American Society of Anesthesiologists (ASA) guidelines for blood product usage.[74] In Europe there is increasing interest in using factor concentrates in these settings to instantly boost certain factor levels,[75,76] although this is preliminary and thrombotic complications may be similar to those plaguing the use of rFVIIa.[77]

ANTICOAGULANT PROTEINS

Plasma-derived concentrates enriched in protein C and antithrombin III are available for the treatment of congenital deficiencies that result in thrombosis, and FFP contains normal levels of these circulating anticoagulants. Recombinant-activated protein C (Xigris, Eli Lilly and Company, Indianapolis, IN) is now licensed for the treatment of severe sepsis, and recombinant, transgenic antithrombin III is also available for the treatment of venoocclusive disease in patients who are undergoing bone marrow transplantation, heparin resistance in patients who are undergoing cardiopulmonary bypass, and sepsis.[78]

PLATELETS

PREPARATIONS

In 1910 W.W. Duke described the Duke bleeding time, the importance of platelets in hemorrhagic disease, and the value of platelet transfusion. However, it was not until the 1970s before certain specialized centers could reliably offer platelet transfusions because of the preparation and storage problems resulting in loss of platelet viability. Platelets are prepared by centrifuging whole blood then separating the buffy coat (in Europe) or platelet-rich plasma (United States) for a second centrifugation to produce platelet concentrates (~50 mL/U). A typical adult dose pools units from 6 donors. Apheresis platelets are collected from single donors using various pheresis devices and reduce donor exposure and thus infection risk. Leukocyte counts are less in apheresis or buffy coat–derived units than in US concentrates (106 rather than 108), but the introduction of leukoreduction techniques makes this distinction obsolete. Similarly, the risk of alloimmunization to HLA antigens is equal for concentrates or apheresis platelets undergoing leukoreduction.[9] Platelets are stored at room temperature in plastic containers porous to the atmosphere to avoid anaerobic metabolism and acidosis, and are licensed for only 5 days of storage.[79] Beyond this time, a storage lesion develops that limits platelet viability.

Platelet preparations contain appreciable volumes of plasma. If inventory constraints or HLA compatibility considerations lead to transfusion of plasma-incompatible products, mild recipient hemolysis may result. This is rarely clinically important unless large volumes are transfused in small patients. Crystalloid-based preservation solutions may allow the removal of plasma; such processes could also facilitate viral inactivation by photosensitive dyes. Cryopreserved and lyophilized platelets are areas of future development, with lyophilized platelets being close to clinical trials.[80]

TRANSFUSION TRIGGERS

Anesthesiologists encounter the need for platelet transfusions in intensive care and operative settings. Most (86%) platelets are given to patients with hematologic malignancies; 68% are given prophylactically, and 32% to treat bleeding episodes.[81] Other indications include dilutional thrombocytopenia after massive transfusion-, autoimmune-, or drug-induced thrombocytopenia. Use may be relatively contraindicated in microangiopathic platelet destruction because of TTP, HUS, or DIC. Certain qualitative platelet disorders, either rare congenital conditions (Glanzmann thrombasthenia, Bernard-Soulier syndrome) or drug-induced dysfunction (aspirin, clopidogrel, Persantine, abciximab), respond to platelet transfusion. In contrast, high circulating plasma levels of eptifibatide or clopidogrel also render transfused platelets dysfunctional.

The current transfusion trigger for the most common indication of prophylaxis in oncology patients is 10 000/mm^3;[82] in patients who are bleeding or undergoing invasive procedures the trigger is typically higher.[83] A platelet count less than 50 000/mm^3 is quoted from the American Society of Anesthesiologists' guidelines. The use of recombinant activated factor VII has been used to augment or replace platelet transfusion, especially in patients refractory to transfusion.[84,85]

REFRACTORINESS TO PLATELET TRANSFUSION

Refractoriness to platelet transfusion can be caused by immune or nonimmune mechanisms.[86] In immune mechanisms, alloantibodies, autoantibodies, drug-associated antibodies, or immune complexes can be responsible. Platelet membrane–associated anti-class I HLA-A and -B antibodies are responsible for most platelet refractoriness, and matching of so-called "public" HLA antigens, such as Bw4 or Bw6, forms the mainstay of compatibility testing. Importantly, ABO incompatibility can reduce platelet survival by up to 20%. Other rarer antibodies are HPA or human platelet antigens (polymorphic platelet surface glycoproteins) or platelet surface glycoproteins absent in the recipient (such as GP1b in Bernard-Soulier syndrome or GPIIb/IIIa in Glanzmann thrombasthenia). An antibody does not guarantee refractoriness, and underlying disease processes or immunosuppressive therapy may modulate the clinical picture.[9] Nonimmune mechanisms include microangiopathic destruction (HUS or TTP), sepsis, or fever, especially in the presence of DIC, splenic sequestration, hepatic dysfunction, and certain drugs (such as vancomycin and amphotericin).

Posttransfusion purpura is a rare complication occurring 7 to 10 days after an immunogenic blood transfusion. It most often affects previously nontransfused, multiparous women. As with neonatal alloimmune thrombocytopenia, the risk for developing posttransfusion purpura is increased among HLA-DR3–positive individuals, and HPA-1a is the antigen most often implicated (in Western populations). At this time, there is no clear understanding of the exact pathology of posttransfusion purpura.

COMPATIBILITY TESTING

Human error is the root cause of almost all fatal acute HTRs, with transfusion of a unit into the wrong patient occurring in 50% of cases. Mislabeling of patient specimens sent to the blood bank and clerical errors in the blood bank occur more often than serologic testing errors, thus attention to design and implementation of safe transfusion practice is of paramount importance, more so than technological advances in serotyping. The aim of compatibility testing is to avoid immune-mediated HTRs resulting from recipient alloantibodies reacting to transfused RBC surface alloantigens. The direct (**Fig. 83-1**) and indirect (**Fig. 83-2**) agglutination tests are the mainstay of laboratory compatibility testing.

Pretransfusion testing assures ABO and Rh(D) compatibility, and screens recipient plasma for antibodies to less common but clinically important antigens. **Figure 83-3** describes the laboratory testing involved in grouping, typing, and cross-matching blood prior to transfusion. When performed in the setting of appropriate controls to prevent clerical error, compatibility determination effectively eliminates risk of acute intravascular hemolytic transfusion reactions. However, it does not eliminate the risk of alloimmunization to non-ABO/Rh antigens, nor does it afford complete protection against delayed hemolytic reactions.

INFECTION RISKS

In 2009 the AABB's Transfusion-Transmitted Diseases Committee made up of volunteer members with expertise in infectious disease, including representation from the Food and Drug Administration,

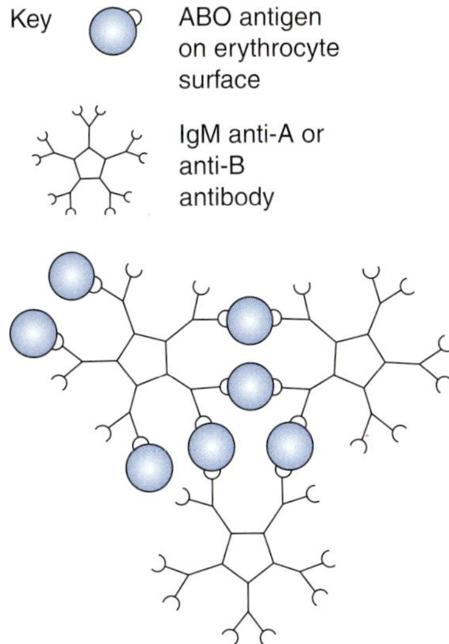

FIGURE 83-1. IgM alloantibodies cross-link via surface antigens leading to direct agglutination. Occasionally, IgG antibodies will cause a positive DAT if there is high antigen density.

Centers for Disease Control and Prevention, the US Department of Defense, the American Society of Hematology, and the Association of Public Health Laboratories, convened to publish a supplement to the journal *Transfusion* on the threat of emerging infectious diseases (EIDs).[87] They prioritized specific agents into categories: red agents had the highest priority, followed by orange and yellow. White agents have not yet been given a priority status. The prioritization was based on several features of the organism including scientific/epidemiological evidence regarding blood safety, public perception and/or regulatory concern regarding blood safety, and public concern regarding the disease agent. Curious readers are directed to the reference for further understanding of the classification system.[87]

Red agents include human variant Creutzfeldt-Jacob disease, dengue viruses, and *Babesia* species. Orange agents include Chikungunya virus, St Louis encephalitis virus, *Leishmania* species, *Plasmonium* species, and *Trypanosoma cruzi*. Yellow agents include chronic wasting disease

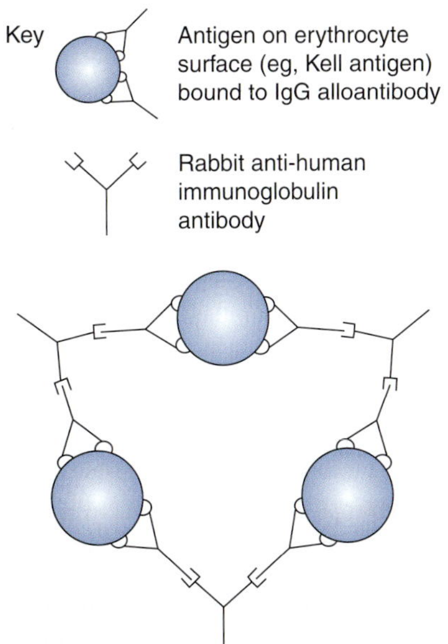

FIGURE 83-2. Antibodies only cross-link after addition of rabbit antihuman IgG, causing indirect agglutination.

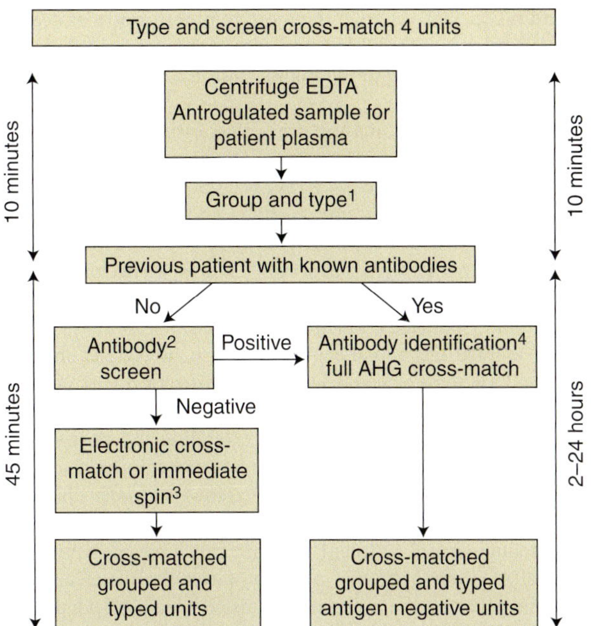

FIGURE 83-3. This schematic depicts the steps taken to type, screen, and cross-match blood. [1]To determine ABO group and rhesus type, commercial anti-A, anti-B, anti-Rh(D) agglutinate patient cells. This direct agglutination test and hemolysis is visible. [2]"Antibody Screening Test." A panel of commercial red cells of known antigen type (each cell carries numerous antigens) are incubated with patient plasma. In North America, a typical panel of 3 cells (eg, Immunor Gamma, Immunocor Inc, Norcross, GA) will detect alloantibodies to rhesus (C, c, E, e, f, V, CW), Kell (K, k, Kpa, Kpb, Jsa, Jsb), Kidd (Jka, Jkb), Duffy (Fya, Fyb), Lewis (Lea, Leb), MN (M, N, S, s), Lutheran (Lua, Lub), P1, and Xga antigens. The mostly IgG alloantibodies that bind cells then need rabbit antihuman IgG (antiglobulin reagent or Coombs serum) to agglutinate (indirect agglutination test). [3]Electronic or computer cross-match requires no history of a positive antibody screen; a previous group, type, and negative antibody screen from blood bank records; a current group, type, and negative antibody screen. An immediate spin is a final check of ABO compatibility, looking for direct agglutination (visible clumping or hemolysis) on mixing patient plasma with donor cells. [4]"Antibody identification." A more extensive panel of up to 8 commercial red cells of known antigen type (eg, Ortho Clinical Diagnostics Inc, Raritan, NJ) are tested against patient plasma to identify which antigens are responsible for the agglutination. This process may need to be extended to panels expressing rarer antigens not listed above (such as anti-U seen in some sickle cell patients) to identify alloantibodies. Occasionally, this process may take days for multiply transfused patients such as those with sickle cell disease. However, current US practice is to antigen-match patients needing repeat transfusions for all Rhesus and Kell antigens to prevent common alloantibody formation, and to reduce the development of subsequent "rarer" alloantibodies and the need for difficult cross-matching.

prions, human herpes virus 8, HIV variants, human parvovirus B19, influenza A virus subtype H5N1, simian foamy virus, *Borrelia burgdorferi*, and hepatitis A virus. White agents include hepatitis E and *Anaplasma phagocytophilum*.[87]

BACTERIAL CONTAMINATION

Bacterial contamination of blood components can be asymptomatic or induce sepsis with a high mortality. It occurs in random donor-pooled platelets (5-30 in 10 000 units) and apheresis platelets (0.5-23 in 10 000 units) stored at room temperature, PRBCs (0.25 in 10 000 units) stored at 39.2°F (4°C), and, rarely, in FFP or cryoprecipitate contaminated during thawing in water baths.[88,89] Bacterial contamination of platelet products is acknowledged as the most frequent infectious risk from transfusion, occurring in approximately 1 of 2000 to 3000 platelet units, and is considered one of the most common causes of death from transfusion (along with TRALI and clerical errors resulting in ABO mismatch) with mortality rates ranging from 1:20 000 to 1:85 000 donor exposures.[88]

Although bacterial contamination rate estimates vary, they are generally approximately 0.2% to 0.3%.[89,90] Clinically recognized septic reactions have been reported at a rate of 1:2500 to 1:11 400 for whole-blood–derived platelet concentrate pools and 1:15 400 for apheresis platelets. Symptoms occurred after 17% to 42% of contaminated platelet transfusions, with a 17% mortality rate.[90] The incidence of severe septic episodes has not been clearly established but is probably approximately 200 per million platelet units transfused (50% sensitivity).[28,91] Given the 5-day storage life and the persistent risk of platelet shortage, in September 2005 the Food and Drug Administration (FDA) approved the use of 7-day apheresis platelets under the surveillance program PASSPORT to determine the safety of extending the storage life. The study was discontinued early after 2 true positive cultures were detected in 2571 day-8 platelets (778/million).[92] However, after discontinuation, a group was convened to conduct a risk assessment. Based on their modeling, overall recipient risk may not have been improved by withdrawal of 7-day apheresis platelets, given the platelet pools that would have replaced them (surrogate-tested whole-blood platelets vs culture-tested apheresis or whole-blood platelets) and risk of delaying a TRALI risk reduction strategy, which could not be implemented without the additional platelet stores provided by the use of 7-day apheresis platelets.[93]

Bacteria can enter the blood bag during venipuncture as a result of inadequate skin preparation; during component preparation, transient bacteremia concurrent with the blood donation, or a break in technique during pooling or sealing; or through disruption of container integrity. Bacterial proliferation occurs more rapidly in platelet concentrates stored for up to 5 days at room temperature than in red cells refrigerated for up to 42 days.

The clinical response may include fever, rigors, skin flushing, abdominal cramps, myalgia, DIC, renal failure, cardiovascular collapse, and cardiac arrest; reactions may be immediate or delayed by several hours. This may be clinically indistinguishable from a febrile nonhemolytic transfusion reaction (FNHTR). If this picture presents, blood samples must be sent to rule out incompatible transfusion, and simultaneously the blood unit must be sent for culture. Patient evaluation includes blood culture; treatment includes stopping the transfusion, supportive measures for developing shock, and broad-spectrum antibiotics.

Gram-negative bacteria, including *Pseudomonas*, *Yersinia*, *Enterobacter*, and *Flavobacterium*, are organisms commonly associated with a contaminated unit of refrigerated blood. In contrast, platelet concentrates contaminated with *Bacillus*, *Escherichia coli*, *Klebsiella*, *Staphylococcus aureus*, *Staphylococcus epidermidis*, *Serratia marcescens*, and *Streptococcus* account for 85% of fatal reactions.[90,94] Bacterial contamination may be masked clinically by concomitant antibiotic administration.

SYPHILIS

Screening for syphilis was mandated in 1958, but the last reported case of transfusion-related disease was in 1966. Any risk of transmission is reduced by sensitivity to most penicillin or cephalosporin antibiotics. *Treponema pallidum* is not currently a threat to the US blood supply.

VIRAL CONTAMINATION

The risk for infection by HIV and hepatitis C viruses is extremely rare in the United States (<1 case per 2 million units transfused) after implementation of nucleic acid testing (NAT) in 1999.[95,96] Contrast this blood safety record to the risk of morbidity or mortality in people with indications for transfusion for which blood products are withheld, and HIV or HCV should not affect transfusion decisions. However, a rare but real risk exists, so inappropriate transfusion should be avoided.

OTHER VIRAL PATHOGENS

Hepatitis A The HAV, a nonenveloped RNA virus in the Picornaviridae family, is transmitted predominantly through the fecal–oral route. Because acute HAV infection is generally symptomatic, infected prospective donors are typically eliminated before donation.

Hepatitis B The HBV is a DNA virus in the Hepadnaviridae family. The infective virion is known as the Dane particle and has surface and core components: HBsAg and hepatitis B core antigen (HBcAg). Among blood donors, the prevalence of new HBV infections declined from 1.97 per 100 000 person years to 1.27 between 1998 and 2001. Most current HBV transfusion transmission cases correspond to blood donations by asymptomatic donors during acute infections before HBsAg appearance and therefore detection (a "window period" of 37-87 days). With current screening, the risk of HBV transmission per unit is approximately 1:205 000 units, with likely reduction in risk with the introduction of NAT testing.[95,96]

Hepatitis C The HCV is an RNA virus in the Flaviviridae family that has 6 genotypes. In the United States, genotypes 1, 2, and 3 cause 75%, 10%, and 10% of infections, respectively, and have similar replication and transmission rates and natural history. The risk of HCV transmission by transfusion declined after the introduction of serologic testing for HCV antibody in May 1990, and NAT testing for the HCV viral genome in 1999 reduced the test-negative window period to 40 days. Combined NAT and serologic testing reduced the risk from an estimated 1:276 000 units to 1:1 935 000 units.

Hepatitis D Originally called the delta agent, hepatitis D virus is a defective RNA-containing passenger virus that requires HBV to act as a "helper" for assembly of envelope proteins. Screening for hepatitis B therefore helps prevent transfusion-associated hepatitis D.

Hepatitis E The hepatitis E virus (HEV) is an RNA calicivirus associated with fecally contaminated water supplies, which usually causes a self-limited illness; it is not a known transfusion-related pathogen.

Human Immunodeficiency Virus-1 The Centers for Disease Control and Prevention (CDC) report 9352 AIDS cases in the United States linked to transfusion through December 31, 2001, including 41 adults or adolescents and 2 children who received blood from HIV-seronegative donors. In addition, during the 1980s, 4799 hemophiliacs and other patients with coagulation deficiencies acquired AIDS as a result of therapy with plasma derivatives.

Among 37 million donations screened for HIV-1 RNA by NAT between 1999 and 2002, only 12 were NAT positive and antibody negative.[96] The risk with plasma derivatives, such as coagulation factor concentrates and albumin and immunoglobulin preparations, can be expected to be even lower because of additional viral inactivation processes, including heat (pasteurization), physicochemical processes (SD treatment), and nanofiltration, that have been implemented since the mid-1980s; since then, no new HIV infections have been attributed to manufactured blood products.

Human Immunodeficiency Virus-2 Human immunodeficiency virus-2, a retrovirus linked more closely to the simian immunodeficiency virus than to HIV-l, was recognized initially in West Africa. In 1998, the CDC reported 79 cases of HIV-2 infection in the United States, mostly in natives of West African countries. Transmissibility of HIV-2 appears to be lower, the course of infection milder, and the interval between infection and AIDS longer than that associated with HIV-1, presenting a lower risk for HIV-2 transmission by transfusion.

Human T-Cell Lymphotropic Virus-I and -II HTLV-I and -II are closely related retroviruses in the Oncovirinae group. In contrast with HIV, HTLV is rarely present in cell-free plasma and shows little active replication in infected humans. HTLV is found around the globe, with endemic foci in southern Japan, the Caribbean, South America, and the Middle East. A sensitive HTLV-I/II combination assay was introduced in 1998, and the threat of acquiring HTLV infection from screened blood is currently minimal.

Human Herpesvirus Human herpesviruses (HHVs) are enveloped, structurally complex, double-stranded DNA viruses that cause common infectious diseases, usually associated with lifelong carrier states and the possibility of recurrent reactivation infections. However, the common alpha herpesviruses, herpes simplex and varicella zoster, are not linked to transfusion-transmitted infections.

Cytomegalovirus Infection CMV, a beta herpesvirus (HHV-5), can infect a wide range of cell types, primarily leukocytes; cell-depleted blood components (plasma, cryoprecipitate) do not transmit CMV. In immunocompetent people, this community-acquired infection is either asymptomatic or associated with a mild, self-limited infectious mononucleosis-like syndrome. However, latent virus persists permanently intracellularly, allowing lifelong potential for reactivation of infections or viral transmission by transfusion of cellular blood products or transplanted donor organs.

In immunosuppressed patients, CMV infection leads to morbid and occasionally lethal pneumonitis, hepatitis, gastroenteritis, retinitis, and other inflammatory conditions requiring treatment with ganciclovir and other antiviral agents. Primary infection in pregnancy may be associated with severe fetal malformations and congenital infections complicated by jaundice, hepatosplenomegaly, microencephaly, and thrombocytopenia with significant mortality. Screening for CMV status is essential for neonates, bone marrow transplant recipients, and transplant recipients. A CMV-seronegative transplant recipient is not denied an organ from a seropositive donor but is treated prophylactically and tested for infection. If leukoreduced blood components are not available, transfusion from CMV seropositive donors is avoided to reduce viral load.

At least 50% of blood donors have antibodies against CMV, thereby indicating previous CMV infection. CMV infection develops in 2% of CMV-seronegative transplant recipients given CMV-seronegative blood, compared with 30% to 60% historically seen after infusion of CMV-unscreened blood components.[66] Additional safety is conferred by prestorage leukocyte reduction and apheresis platelet collection.

Epstein-Barr Virus Epstein-Barr virus (EBV), a gamma herpesvirus (HHV-4), causes infectious mononucleosis and is closely associated with Burkitt lymphoma, nasopharyngeal carcinoma, and posttransplantation lymphoproliferative disease. More than 90% of the adult population has evidence of previous exposure, and virus-specific cytotoxic T lymphocytes lyse EBV-infected B lymphocytes, so transfusion-transmitted EBV infection is rare in both immunocompetent and immunosuppressed recipients.

Parvovirus Patients with sickle cell anemia, thalassemia, and other conditions associated with shortened red blood cell survival are at risk for developing acute aplastic or hypoplastic anemia after infection. Others at risk for aplasia after parvovirus infection include immunodeficient patients, HIV-infected patients, solid-organ transplant recipients, and children with malignancies. Persistent parvovirus infection may cause severe chronic anemia in immunocompromised patients. Acute parvovirus infection during pregnancy may result in fetal loss, neurologic abnormalities, and congenital infection. Red blood cell aplasia and chronic anemia caused by parvovirus infection often respond to infusion with immunoglobulin preparations.

Parvovirus can be expected to be present in 1:20 000 to 1:50 000 blood donors or a higher incidence during epidemic periods. Reactive antibodies may be present in the donor or the recipient, and only 3 cases of transfusion-related transmission have been reported. Pooled plasma products theoretically pose a greater threat, and factor VIII concentrates demonstrated a 40% risk of parvovirus infection.[97] The pasteurization process inactivates virus in albumin-based products.

West Nile Virus West Nile virus (WNV) is a member of the Flaviviridae family, the genus *Flavivirus*, and the Japanese encephalitis virus serocomplex that includes Japanese encephalitis virus and St Louis encephalitis virus. Viruses in this complex are arthropod-borne viruses, or arboviruses (ie, transmitted by mosquitoes and other arthropod vectors), with the potential to cause meningoencephalitis. WNV was first isolated in 1937 in the West Nile district of northern Uganda and derives its name from that region. The natural life cycle of the virus includes female mosquitoes as vectors, with birds serving as the primary vertebrate hosts. Humans are incidental hosts, with transmission occurring through bites of infected mosquitoes. Peak transmission occurs in the late summer and early fall.

Since 1999 there have been sporadic outbreaks in the United States, with more than 4000 cases—277 attributed to a 2002 epidemic. In 2002, 23 cases of transfusion (any blood component) or transplant-related transmission were reported; 12 patients developed meningoencephalitis and more severe outcomes were seen in immunocompromised patients.[98]

Currently, donors are asked about fevers or exposure to endemic areas, and recommendations exclude donors with suspected or confirmed diagnosis of WNV within 120 days of donation. Since June 2003 NAT was instituted on pooled donor samples, and 800 of 6 million US blood donations were WNV NAT positive. Despite this, 6 cases of transfusion-transmitted WNV infection occurred in susceptible individuals.[99] The risk of WNV infection depends on the immune status of the recipient, the presence of donor antibodies, and the rate of endemic disease prevalence.

Dengue Virus Dengue virus was prioritized in the red category based on scientific/epidemiological evidence regarding blood safety, specifically related to the asymptomatic viremia that poses a significant transfusion risk.[87] It is a mosquito-borne disease. Asia, Oceania, Africa, Australia, and the Americas contain at-risk populations. Transmission through blood transfusion has been documented. The clinical disease most commonly is limited to dengue fever with fever and rash, conjunctivitis, myalgia, nausea/vomiting, and prostration. Other more severe forms including dengue hemorrhagic fever and dengue shock syndrome are more rare and occur primarily in children. The mortality in this group is high, 10% to 20%. There is currently no FDA-licensed screening test.[87]

LYME DISEASE AND OTHER TICK-BORNE ILLNESSES

Borrelia burgdorferi, the agent responsible for Lyme disease, is transmitted to humans by deer tick bites. Spirochetemia probably occurs after infection and may be present in asymptomatic individuals, but again, only rarely documented transfusion-related transmissions have been reported for this or other tick-borne pathogens: *Babesia* species (babesiosis) and *Rickettsia rickettsii* (Rocky Mountain spotted fever).

MALARIA

Malaria in the United States is typically limited to travelers, military personnel, and immigrants from endemic countries. Prevention of transfusion-transmitted malaria relies on deferral of blood donors immigrating or returning from malaria-endemic regions; there are no available screening tests. Approximately 3 transfusion-associated malaria cases occur per year in the United States, with a reported incidence of 0 to 0.2 cases per million units.

BABESIOSIS

Babesia was placed in the red category based on scientific/epidemiologic evidence regarding blood safety.[87] Babesiosis is a malaria-like zoonosis in which humans are infected incidentally, usually through the bite of an infected tick. Blood transfusion has been documented. Babesia infections are usually asymptomatic or cause mild flu-like symptoms but can be fatal in the immunocompromised. Endemic throughout the United States, more than 40 cases of cellular transfusion-transmitted babesiosis have occurred since 1980. A history of babesiosis precludes blood donation, but no screening test is available.

TOXOPLASMOSIS

Toxoplasmosis is caused by the intracellular protozoal parasite *Toxoplasma gondii*, whose usual host is the domestic cat. Transmission is via cats or from undercooked pork, goat, lamb, beef, or wild game. There is evidence of infection in 20% to 25% of the US population, but transfusion-associated disease has only been described in immunocompromised patients.

CHAGAS DISEASE

Chagas was assigned category orange with primary concern with public perception and/or regulatory concern regarding blood safety.[87]

The flagellate protozoan parasite *Trypanosoma cruzi* causes Chagas disease. The disorder is widespread in South America, but *T. cruzi* is also found in North and Central America. Infection is not endemic in the United States, but it is considered emergent in the United States and Canada based on increased immigration. Routes of infection include exposure to feces from infected vectors (largely insects), blood transfusion and organ transplantation, and congenital transmission and breast-feeding. Severe complications include myocarditis, meningoencephalitis, cardiomyopathy, megacolon, or achalasia. Transfusion-associated cases of Chagas disease are more common in immunocompromised patients. In North America, testing is available but is not required by the FDA, and even testing of donors with risk factors or those from endemic areas has not been implemented.[87]

HUMAN VARIANT CREUTZFELDT-JAKOB DISEASE

Human variant Creutzfeldt-Jakob disease (vCJD) is a prion disease given red priority based on public perception and/or regulatory concern regarding blood safety.[87] Exposure is through consumption of bovine spongiform encephalopathy–infected neural beef products. Current to October 2008, 206 cases and 203 deaths had occurred in the United Kingdom or secondary to UK beef products. Blood transmissibility of the disease has been documented and a potentially long incubation period increases the theoretical possibility of transfusion-related transmission. The likelihood of clinical disease after transmission is hypothesized to be high, with mortality estimated to be 100% for those who are symptomatic. There are no screening tests available and there is no treatment. Screening questions that eliminate US donors with UK travel history, leukoreduction, and filtration methods may reduce prion content in US blood stores.[87]

New molecular assays, such as NAT, can enhance safety but at a high cost compared with the serologic screening that was effective for virtually negating the HBV, HIV, and HCV risk of transfusion. The advent of newer infectious agents, such as vCJD, WNV, severe acute respiratory syndrome (SARS), and potentially Avian influenza A (H5N1) virus, may lead to the deferral of increasing numbers of potential blood donors, with implications for blood supply.

The discussion of infectious agents is mostly based on North American data, but additional challenges exist for ensuring a safe blood supply in developing countries. With global travel and immigration, proactive and collaborative surveillance on an international level is essential to protect any country's blood supply.[100]

FEBRILE NONHEMOLYTIC TRANSFUSION REACTIONS

An FNHTR occurs when temperature increases above 1.8°F (1°C) during or after transfusion when no other cause can be found. These reactions are caused either by cytotoxic or agglutinating antibodies in the patient's plasma reacting against antigens present on transfused donor lymphocytes, granulocytes, or platelets, or by donor plasma containing antibodies against the recipient's cellular antigens. These antigens are typically, but not always, HLA antigens.[101] The febrile reaction results from antibody–leukocyte or antibody–platelet interactions leading to the release of inflammatory cytokines and pyrogens.

These cytokines are released from recipient leukocytes or donor leukocytes in response to antigen–antibody interaction, but could also be in the supernatant of the transfused unit, derived from the donor leukocytes during storage before transfusion.[102] Such generation of cytokines, mostly from mononuclear leukocytes, occurs during storage and is proportional to the leukocyte count of the unit and the duration of storage.[103] Febrile reactions to platelet transfusions are more likely caused by proinflammatory cytokines in the supernatant than by cellular elements.[104] Use of prestorage leukocyte reduction lowers, but not eliminates, the incidence of febrile reactions, as leukoreduction filters do not remove cytokines.[105]

The frequency of febrile reactions is approximately 0.5% per unit transfused, most commonly in recipients exposed to multiple white cell or platelet antigens such as oncology patients or multiparous women.[28] Previous alloimmunization leads to anti-HLA, granulocyte, or platelet-specific antibodies that react with white cells or platelets on subsequent exposure.

Clinically, an FNHTR is characterized by fever and chills occurring shortly after the transfusion begins. FNHTRs are usually self-limited, with fever persisting for no more than 8 to 10 hours. Elderly patients with a tenuous cardiovascular status and critically ill patients may develop respiratory complications, hypotension, or shock. With any transfusion reaction, the transfusion must be stopped, antipyretics and supportive measures instituted as necessary, and laboratory evaluation initiated.

A febrile reaction may be the first sign of an acute hemolytic reaction or infusion of a unit of red cells or platelets contaminated with bacteria. Repeat cross-matching is performed to confirm patient–donor ABO compatibility, examining the results of pre- and posttransfusion direct antiglobulin tests (DATs), evaluating the serum for hemolysis, and confirming the accuracy of paperwork. The posttransfusion DAT should yield negative findings, as an FNHTR does not involve red cell alloantibodies. Sending blood cultures from the patient and the blood product, and administration of broad-spectrum antibiotics can be considered depending on the severity of the reaction.

The diagnosis of FNHTR is one of exclusion after ruling out a hemolytic reaction, a septic transfusion, or other miscellaneous causes of fever. Routine premedication is not indicated, but antipyretics and corticosteroids can be reserved for patients with a prior history of FNHTR. The use of leukocyte-depleted blood components is not universal, but as discussed earlier, this practice reduces the incidence of FNHTRs and should be mandated for patients with a previous history of FNHTRs.[106]

ALLERGIC TRANSFUSION REACTIONS

Allergic transfusion reactions are most commonly caused by the infusion of plasma proteins. Manifestations include skin erythema with associated mild urticaria and pruritus, a confluent rash that is intensely pruritic, extensive urticaria, severe vasomotor instability, bronchospasm, and anaphylaxis. The severity of these reactions may not be dose related, so a patient developing hives or a mild allergic reaction during a blood transfusion may not necessarily progress to severe anaphylaxis by completing the transfusion.

Causative antibodies have not been conclusively demonstrated, but milder allergic reactions are usually IgG or IgE mediated; anaphylactic reactions are most often IgG mediated. Allergic transfusion reactions are quite common, occurring in approximately 1% of all transfusions and typically leading to pruritus followed by hives. Treatment involves holding the transfusion, administering antihistamines, and assessing the wisdom of continuing the transfusion based on improvement of symptoms and no progression to more serious symptoms such as fever, chills, bronchospasm, dyspnea, or hemodynamic instability.

Such mild urticarial reactions rarely progress to serious reactions and often do not recur with subsequent transfusions. The pathogenesis is believed to be recipient-antibody directed against donor plasma proteins, although the etiologic antibody is rarely detected, making the diagnosis of an allergic transfusion reaction a diagnosis of exclusion. Leukocyte depletion filters do not remove plasma proteins, so washed red cells are required to prevent reactions.[107] However, washed cells are reserved for patients with severe or recurrent reactions.

ANAPHYLACTIC REACTIONS

Other anaphylactic reactions can occur when plasma containing IgA is transfused to patients with IgG anti-IgA antibodies or after transfusion of red cells or, more commonly, platelets administered through certain bedside leukoreduction filters.[108] The latter scenario is believed to be a consequence of contact activation by the negatively charged surface of the filter converting prekallikrein to kallikrein, in turn converting high-molecular-weight kininogen to bradykinin. Bradykinin causes pain, cutaneous flushing, and hypotension without fever or chills, and its effects are exaggerated in patients taking angiotensin-converting enzyme (ACE) inhibitors, as ACE is identical to kininase II, which is responsible for degrading bradykinin. A common theme throughout this chapter is that prestorage leukoreduction avoids this problem.

OTHER ADVERSE EFFECTS OF TRANSFUSION

MICROAGGREGATE DEBRIS AND ADULT RESPIRATORY DISTRESS SYNDROME

Microaggregate debris consists of dead platelets, granulocytes, and fibrin strands that form in blood during storage. Theoretically, this debris (20-120 micron) passes through standard 170-m pore filters, infusing these microaggregates into the pulmonary vasculature, obstructing pulmonary capillaries, and causing pulmonary failure. Microaggregate filters have been suggested to prevent adult respiratory distress syndrome (ARDS) after massive transfusion, but they may reduce transfusion flow rates and do not appear to alter the onset of ARDS.[109] Hypotension and sepsis are postulated to trigger ARDS rather than microaggregate debris, and improvements in the general care of the critically ill treating shock and sepsis have likely decreased the incidence of postperfusion respiratory distress syndrome more than the use of microaggregate filters.

TRANSFUSION-ASSOCIATED CIRCULATORY OVERLOAD (TACO)

It is obvious to any practicing anesthesiologist that rapidly transfusing a patient who is euvolemic and not actively bleeding is unlikely to be of benefit and may cause harm. Infants, patients with cardiovascular disease, and the elderly are especially at risk. Importantly, transfusion-induced hypervolemia may be initially difficult to distinguish from hemolytic transfusion reaction, a febrile nonhemolytic transfusion reaction, transfusion-related acute lung injury (TRALI), or allergic reactions. Hypervolemia results in headache, dyspnea, tachycardia, tachypnea, and congestive heart failure. The absence of hemoglobinuria and hemoglobinemia or a positive posttransfusion DAT distinguishes hypervolemia from immune hemolysis, and the absence of fever, chills, or urticaria from febrile or allergic reactions.

Treatment involves stopping transfusion until the diagnosis is determined, administering diuretics and supportive therapy as indicated, and resuming the transfusion at a slower rate while monitoring for recurrence of symptoms and signs of hypervolemia.

TRANSFUSION-RELATED ACUTE LUNG INJURY

As TRALI recognition has grown there has been an international effort to formalize a definition, identify current etiologic theories, and provide insight into methods of prevention. In 2004 the Canadian Blood Services convened a consensus conference on TRALI, and in 2005 published their proceedings where they reviewed TRALI and proposed a definition.[110] Additionally, in 2005 the US National Heart, Lung, and Blood Institute offered insights from their work group.[111] It is clinically indistinguishable from acute lung injury (ALI)/ARDS and hence the definition includes this diagnosis,[112] noncardiogenic pulmonary edema and hypoxemia, but with the addition of a temporal association with transfusion.[110,111,113,114] The symptoms of TRALI include fever, chills, cyanosis, dyspnea, tachypnea, and hypotension or hypertension, and copious amounts of pulmonary edema fluid.[110] If a patient shows signs of pulmonary insufficiency, as with all other reactions, transfusion should be stopped, diagnosis sought, and supportive measures (including mechanical ventilation) initiated as indicated.

The incidence of TRALI in the United States is 1 in 1300 to 1 in 5000, and although mortality estimates range widely between 5% and 25%, it is the most common fatal transfusion-related reaction.[110,113,115] All blood products have been associated with TRALI; however, plasma-containing products are associated with a higher incidence.[110,116]

The pathophysiology is likely multifactorial. Two well-described mechanisms involve the transfusion of antileukocyte antibodies and/or the transfusion of older stored cellular products. Anti-HLA I, anti-HLA II, or antigranulocyte (antileukocyte) antibodies recognize recipient leukocytes, leading to complement activation and leukocyte aggregation.[113,117] Activated leukocytes express adhesive molecules on their surfaces, permitting attachment to pulmonary endothelial cells and entry into the interstitial space by diapedesis, with degranulation leading to pulmonary edema as a result of microvascular leukostasis/occlusion and capillary leakage.[118] These alloantibodies result from pregnancy, transfusion, and transplantation. Their prevalence has been reported to be less than 2% among women with no pregnancies, and nontransfused and transfused men, but 24.4% in previously pregnant women.[119] Although many studies are able to find a clear antibody–antigen link, this theory is troubled by the lack of consistent measureable specificity of the donor antibody–recipient antigen interaction. It appears that this antibody–antigen interaction is neither necessary nor reliably sufficient to cause TRALI; it has been reported to occur without a clear antigen–antibody interaction, and in cases where there is an antibody and a cognate antigen, TRALI is not assured. Nonetheless, female donors have been implicated in many TRALI cases,[116] and avoidance of transfusion of female plasma may decrease the incidence of TRALI, leading to the diversion of female plasma donation in Europe and the United States.[120,121] This does not have an impact on all female blood donations, however, as female donors only increased the risk of TRALI in plasma-rich products, not RBCs.[122]

A complementary theory, and one that may explain antibody-negative TRALI, is the idea of a 2-event model proposed by Silliman et al.[115,123,124] The first event is a systemic illness or the condition of the patient responsible for the priming of neutrophils and the activation of the pulmonary endothelium with neutrophil sequestration. The second event is the transfusion of biologic response modifiers (BRMs), which include lipids, and/or soluble CD40 ligand (a platelet-derived proinflammatory mediator),[115,123-125] both of which accumulate during the storage of blood. The BRMs activate the sequestered neutrophils and lead to the damage of pulmonary endothelial cells, the accumulation of lung water, and the clinical syndrome of ALI, temporally associated with the transfusion of blood product.[110,115,116,124-129] Therefore, based on this mechanism, avoidance of female donation is unlikely to eliminate TRALI.

In addition to multiparous females, exclusion policies include the deferral of donors with known antileukocyte antibodies or those who have been linked to 1 or more TRALI events. Future product management policies may include washing of cellular components to eliminate plasma or using fresher blood products to decrease BRMs; current policies do not address the controversy surrounding the storage age of RBCs.[130] More research is needed to clarify the benefits of each of these actions weighed against their cost to the blood inventory by reducing the donor pool.

HYPOTHERMIA

Hypothermia can occur with rapid infusion of large quantities of cold blood. Rapid infusion of cold blood (~5 min/U) may lower the temperature of the sinoatrial node to below 86°F (30°C), leading to serious arrhythmias. Numerous in-line blood-warming devices are available for clinically indicated rapid transfusion, as in major trauma, and may reduce the incidence of hypothermia-induced coagulopathy and platelet dysfunction that occurs with temperatures below 95°F (35°C).

Only approved blood warmers should be used for this purpose. Such devices monitor and regulate temperature to below 107.6°F (42°C) to avoid causing hemolysis. The use of hot water or microwave devices is unacceptable, as hot spots develop that can cause hemolysis.

ELECTROLYTE TOXICITY

Citrate is used for anticoagulation during storage, acting by chelating calcium and interfering with the coagulation cascade. Rapid transfusion of citrated blood thus can be associated with a decrease in ionized calcium levels. Typically, citrate is rapidly metabolized in the liver to bicarbonate, but mild to severe citrate toxicity can be seen after infusion of large volumes of citrated products or in the setting of transient or established liver dysfunction.

The effects of hypocalcemia range from mild circumoral paresthesia to frank tetany. If prolonged Q-T intervals or signs of tetany are seen, calcium can be administered. In practice, the routine availability of arterial blood gas analysis with ionized calcium measurement allows the close monitoring and guided treatment of developing hypocalcemia. Calcium should never be added to a unit of blood, as it recalcifies the unit and leads to clot formation; similarly, the use of calcium-containing solutions, such as Ringer lactate, should not be coadministered with blood products.

Hypomagnesemia, presumably caused by chelation of magnesium by citrate, has also been reported, but its clinical relevance has not been determined. In practice, administration of magnesium can accompany calcium administration in response to a large citrate load.

Hyperkalemia caused by infusion of stored blood is rare, and hypokalemia may be more common. With storage, leakage of potassium from red cells to the extracellular fluid occurs. However, after infusion into a recipient, the red cells reverse the biochemical storage lesion, and intracellular potassium levels are restored. In addition, citrate is metabolized to bicarbonate, causing alkalosis contributing to hypokalemia. In massive transfusion, this may not uncommonly result in the need for administration of potassium. Extracellular potassium increases at the rate of approximately 1 mEq/d during the first few weeks of storage. However, hyperkalemia is still a concern for neonates or patients with renal failure, and washed or fresher units can be requested. Potassium leakage from red cells is increased after exposure to 25-Gy irradiation to prevent posttransfusion graft versus host disease; the shelf life of irradiated units is a maximum of 28 days.

PLASTICIZERS

Plasticizers are chemicals used to make the rigid polyvinyl chloride plastic used in blood bags more malleable; traditionally, diethylhexyl phthalate (DEHP) is used. After concerns about carcinogenic properties and the possible production of peroxisomes by the metabolite monoethylhexyl phthalate, DEHP is being replaced with a citrate-based plasticizer.[131]

GRAFT VERSUS HOST DISEASE

Graft versus host disease (GVHD) occurs when immunologically competent lymphocytes are introduced into an immunoincompetent host who cannot destroy the donor lymphocytes. The immunocompetent donor lymphocytes engraft, recognize the host as foreign, and then attack host tissues. GVHD occurs after allogeneic bone marrow transplantation and less often after transfusion of nonirradiated cellular blood components, especially when the blood donor and recipient share some HLA antigens. There is an increased danger from posttransfusion GVHD in part because of the frequent failure of physicians to recognize and treat the reaction promptly. Another major factor, however, is the propensity of the donor's lymphocytes to attack and produce recipient bone marrow aplasia in contrast to after bone marrow transplantation GVHD, in which the bone marrow is of donor origin, and bone marrow aplasia does not occur.

Posttransfusion GVHD is fatal in more than 90% of cases, primarily because of aplasia of the recipient's bone marrow. Reports have shown that haploidentical-directed donor units of blood may produce fatal posttransfusion GVHD even in immunocompetent recipients. The use of irradiated blood (>2500 cGy) is now recommended in clinical situations in which transfusion poses a risk of GVHD such as when patients receive blood transfusions from their relatives or HLA-matched donors. Leukocyte reduction is not adequate prophylaxis against GVHD, as the exact number of leukocytes needed to produce the disease is unknown.[132]

HEMOSIDEROSIS

A unit of red cells contains approximately 250 mg of iron, and 1 g of iron is roughly the amount stored in the bone marrow; men and nonmenstruating women lose only approximately 1 mg of iron per day. Consequently, repeated transfusion in individuals with an extravascular hemolytic anemia, such as thalassemia or sickle cell anemia, in which iron is recycled rather than excreted, can result in the accumulation of excessive tissue stores of iron. Chronically, iron stored in parenchymal cells results in cell death and eventual organ failure. Iron chelation therapy, such as deferoxamine, is the mainstay of therapy to avoid predictable iron overload and maintain patients with chronic hemolytic anemias in negative iron balance.

AIR EMBOLI

Air is currently expelled from plastic blood bags but still may be pumped into patients by pressurized transfusion devices, especially after apheresis and intraoperative salvage. All such devices currently manufactured, however, contain air in-line sensors. Regardless, clinicians must remain alert to the potential risk of air embolization at all times while the patient is being treated. Patients suffering large air emboli (boluses of 3-8 mL/kg) can experience acute cyanosis, pain, cough, arrhythmia, acute right ventricular outflow obstruction, cardiogenic shock, and circulatory arrest. Infusions should be stopped and checked for air, and the patient should be placed head-down on the left side. This usually displaces the air bubble from the pulmonary valve and may be amenable to aspiration via a central venous catheter.

TRANSFUSION-RELATED IMMUNOMODULATION

Deleterious effects of transfusion can be caused by a reaction to or incompatibility with a component of the transfused blood product or by the subtler transfusion-related immunomodulation (TRIM). TRIM has been linked to 2 different forms of immunosuppression, one believed to predispose patients to infectious complications and the other pertaining to tolerance of allogeneic transplants. TRIM has a number of postulated immunosuppressive mechanisms related to leukocytes and cytokines present in blood components limiting the potential effect to transfused red cell concentrates and platelets. Leukocytes and leukocyte-derived bioactive substances, such as histamine, myeloperoxidase (MPO), eosinophil cationic protein (ECP), eosinophil protein X, plasminogen activator inhibitor 1 (PAI-1), and IL-6 are known to contaminate PRBCs[133] and platelet units,[134] accumulating in a storage time–dependent manner. Suppression of lymphocyte proliferation has been induced by these mediators, providing a mechanism for TRIM. Length of storage of transfused allogeneic PRBCs, but not plasma, is associated with pneumonia after coronary artery bypass graft surgery.[135]

In addition, phosphatidylserine is expressed on the surface of apoptotic leukocytes in PRBCs and platelets and erythrocytes, mediating phagocytosis of apoptotic cells. This induces transforming growth factor (TGF-α) secretion, resulting in an anti-inflammatory effect and suppression of proinflammatory mediators[136]; enhanced production of the anti-inflammatory cytokines IL-4, IL-10, and transforming growth factor is observed after blood transfusion. Anti-inflammatory cytokine release and decreased cellular immune function occur after allogeneic, but not autologous, transfusions.

Prestorage leukofiltration appears to reduce storage time–dependent immunosuppression after blood transfusion and the incidence of febrile transfusion reactions.[137] Indeed, leukoreducing PRBCs decrease postoperative mortality after cardiac surgery and the incidence of multiorgan failure after major surgery.[138] However, leukoreduction is not a panacea, as leukocytes are not eliminated. Leukoreduced PRBCs can still cause hypotensive transfusion reactions and HLA alloimmunization, and express surface phospholipids. It may be that a greater volume of leukoreduced products is required to produce the deleterious effects of transfusion compared with nonleukoreduced products.

CONCLUSION

In summary, the safety of the US blood supply is exemplary, with the chance of a fatal reaction to transfusion in the realm of 1 in every 100 000 patients transfused. Such risk is acceptable should there be definite benefit, which emphasizes the responsibility placed on the physician to use appropriate triggers for blood component therapy with physiologic evidence of a deficiency in oxygen-carrying capacity for red cell transfusion and an accurately defined coagulopathy for hemostatic blood product transfusion. Second only to hematology nurses, anesthesiologists transfuse more blood products than any physician group, and it is incumbent on them to lead blood conservation strategies, including research into safe and effective blood substitutes, and reinforce surgical philosophies that avoid unnecessary blood loss at all costs. Such approaches provide the best possible care for patients and prepare anesthesiologists well for practice in areas with less safe blood supplies or during unforeseen safety concerns with the US blood supply.

In 2008 the United States launched the Hemovigilance Module of the US Biovigilance initiative from the National Healthcare Safety Network (NHSN), jointly developed by the CDC and AABB, charged with data collection and analysis of transfusion practices and outcomes. In the coming years, this centralized database designed to report and monitor recipient adverse reactions and quality control incidents related to blood transfusion will undoubtedly provide important insight and direction in transfusion medicine.

KEY REFERENCES

- Leukocyte reduction and ultraviolet B irradiation of platelets to prevent alloimmunization and refractoriness to platelet transfusions. The Trial to Reduce Alloimmunization to Platelets Study Group. *N Engl J Med.* 1997;337:1861-1869.
- Hoeltge GA, Domen RE, Rybicki LA, Schaffer PA. Multiple red cell transfusions and alloimmunization. Experience with 6996 antibodies detected in a total of 159,262 patients from 1985 to 1993. *Arch Pathol Lab Med.* 1995;119:42-45.
- American Society of Anesthesiologists Practice Guidelines for Perioperative Blood Transfusion and Adjuvant Therapies. http://www.asahq.org/publicationsAndServices/practiceparam.htm#blood (accessed).
- Stramer SL, Hollinger FB, Katz LM, et al. Emerging infectious disease agents and their potential threat to transfusion safety. *Transfusion.* 2009;49(Suppl 2):1S-29S.
- Kleinman S, Chan P, Robillard P. Risks associated with transfusion of cellular blood components in Canada. *Transfus Med Rev.* 2003;17:120-162.
- Allain JP, Bianco C, Blajchman MA, et al. Protecting the blood supply from emerging pathogens: the role of pathogen inactivation. *Transfus Med Rev.* 2005;19:110-126.
- Silliman CC, Kelher M. The role of endothelial activation in the pathogenesis of transfusion-related acute lung injury. *Transfusion.* 2005;45:109S-116S.
- Vamvakas EC. Possible mechanisms of allogeneic blood transfusion-associated postoperative infection. *Transfus Med Rev.* 2002;16:144-160.
- Hebert PC, Fergusson D, Blajchman MA, et al. Clinical outcomes following institution of the Canadian universal leukoreduction program for red blood cell transfusions. *JAMA.* 2003;289:1941-1949.

REFERENCES

Complete references available on DVD and online version at www.LongneckerAnesthesiology.com

CHAPTER 84 Cognitive Dysfunction After Anesthesia and Surgery

Jessica A. Hathaway
Mark F. Newman
Joseph P. Mathew

KEY POINTS

1. Cognition represents key processes of memory, attention, perception, problem solving, and mental imagery that define who we are as individuals.
2. Cognitive functioning is key to the activities of daily living and our overall quality of life.
3. Cognitive assessment occurs by a number of well-validated measurements outlined in the field of neuropsychology. Assessment of cognitive functioning in the perioperative period is often less complete than normal; however, understanding what is measured by each individual test and how these values change over time is essential in understanding the implications to our patients of perioperative cognitive decline.
4. The incidence of postoperative cognitive dysfunction varies based on the sensitivity of the tests used and the time frame for evaluation. Correlation with appropriate control groups gives the best idea of the relative impact of surgery and anesthesia on changes in cognition and quality of life.
5. The etiology of cognitive function and/or cognitive dysfunction is complex and is associated with the severity of diseases including atherosclerosis and diabetes, as well as with surgery and anesthesia. The effect of anesthetic agents on short- and long-term cognition is controversial.
6. New studies indicate an association between patient factors including disease severity and genetic predisposition, and perioperative cognitive decline.
7. Determining the risks of perioperative cognitive decline enhances the probability of developing interventions to reduce cognitive decline and thus improve quality of life after surgery.

The brain is often a window to changes in blood flow, tissue perfusion, and early neural damage manifested by decline in higher cortical functions, including recall memory and cognitive processing. The elderly population in particular is at risk for cognitive deterioration as a consequence of reduced cognitive reserve seen with aging. These changes in cognitive function are associated with impaired activities of daily living, which substantially reduce the quality of life of the elderly. This can be magnified by physical or emotional stress in high-risk individuals.

The safety of anesthesia and surgery has progressed over several decades to the point that elderly and debilitated patients may safely undergo increasingly complex procedures with low risk of major morbidity or mortality. However, anesthesia and surgery appear to be associated with changes in cognitive functioning that outlast the effects of anesthesia or pain medications, inflammation, and the healing response. Several excellent studies have investigated changes in cognitive functioning associated with cardiac and noncardiac surgery.[1-3]

Understanding this decline and its etiology is complicated by the realization that anesthesia and surgery are rarely separated. This indicates that the differences may be caused by either the stress response associated with surgery or the administration of anesthetics. This chapter discusses the complex field of cognitive neurosciences and the intricate process of measuring and defining change in the perioperative period. Different types of surgery and implications for quality of life, as well as etiologic factors and how they relate to treatment are outlined.

POSTOPERATIVE CENTRAL NERVOUS SYSTEM DYSFUNCTION

Emergence delirium or emergence agitation, postoperative delirium (POD), postoperative cognitive dysfunction (POCD), and postoperative maladaptive behaviors complete the broad categorization of postoperative central nervous system (CNS) dysfunction. Although similarities exist, these diagnoses are distinct and can be differentiated, among other ways, by timing of presentation (**Fig. 84-1**).[4] This chapter focuses mainly on postoperative cognitive dysfunction because this entity seems to have the most significant long-term impact; however, it is important to recognize the other forms of postoperative impairment, as they can severely affect function, length of stay, and ability to return to independent living.[2,5] In addition, there is significant overlap in risk factors and suspected etiology between POD and POCD, and POD appears to affect the development of postoperative cognitive dysfunction.[6,7] Emergence delirium, which is seen predominantly in children, and postoperative maladaptive behaviors, a diagnosis reserved for children, is discussed in other chapters. Importantly, though, it is likely that these forms of CNS dysfunction also share some features and etiologies with POD and POCD.

POSTOPERATIVE DELIRIUM

Delirium is defined as an acute confusional state, marked by a disorder of attention and cognition that fluctuates throughout the day. It involves cortical dysfunction and the electroencephalogram (EEG) can show diffuse slowing. POD generally develops 24 to 72 hours postoperatively after a lucid interval. Its incidence is reported anywhere from 5% to 15% in noncardiac surgery,[8] 21% in cardiac surgery,[9] and as high as 62% in high-risk hip fracture groups.[10] Risk factors for POD include age greater than 70 years, history of delirium, history of dementia, history of alcohol abuse, increased comorbidities, perioperative use of narcotics, preoperative depression, greater intraoperative blood loss, more blood transfusions, postoperative hematocrit less than 30%, severe postoperative pain, and specific drugs, including narcotics, sedatives, and anticholinergics.[11-15] Recently, Smith et al found poorer executive function and higher levels of depressive symptoms to be associated with an increased incidence of postoperative delirium, reaffirming previous findings by other investigators.[16]

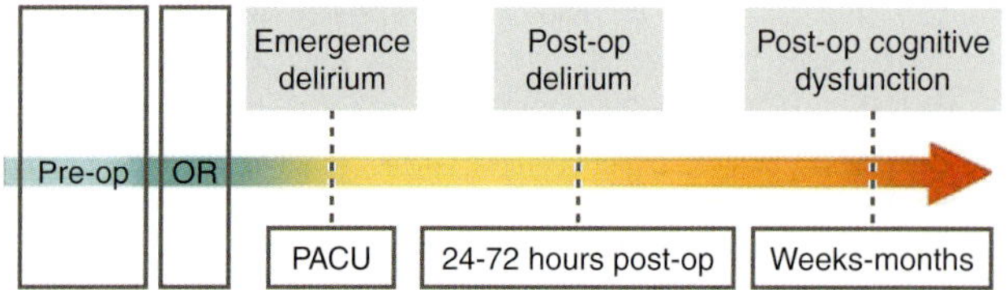

FIGURE 84-1. One of the principal distinctions between postoperative (Post-Op) delirium and postoperative cognitive dysfunction (POCD) is the time frame in which they are found. Emergence delirium occurs in the operating room (OR) or immediately after in the postanesthesia care unit (PACU). Postoperative delirium occurs 24 to 72 hours after surgery. POCD is measured at weeks to months after surgery and anesthesia. Pre-Op, preoperative. [Reprinted with permission from Silverstein JH, Timberger M, Reich DL et al. Central nervous system dysfunction after noncardiac surgery and anesthesia in the elderly. *Anesthesiology*. 2007;106(3):622-628.]

The appearance of POD in a patient can have significant implications. POD has been associated with increased morbidity, mortality, duration of hospital stay, nursing home placement, and technical, consult, and nursing costs.[17] Monk et al found POD to be a risk factor for the development of POCD at hospital discharge.[18] Koster et al found in delirious patients nonsignificant trends toward increased readmissions, dysfunction in memory, concentration problems, and a significant increase in sleep disturbance.[9]

POSTOPERATIVE COGNITIVE DYSFUNCTION

POCD refers to a deterioration in cognition temporally associated with surgery. Its diagnosis requires both preoperative and postoperative testing and it is the topic of this chapter.

COGNITIVE FUNCTION

The field of cognition is greatly expanding with ongoing research to define the key elements of intellectual functioning that allow us to learn, reason, and plan. The increasing body of literature typically defines cognition as a processing of information that applies both knowledge and preference. These processes include such dimensions as memory, attention, perception, problem solving, and mental imagery. Cognitive functioning is key to activities of daily living and quality of life; cognitive dysfunction is an impairment of these processes that leads to a decline in an individual's activities.[2,19,20] The patient or the family often defines a decline in activity as the inability to perform or a delayed ability to perform cognitive tasks. In many cases, the changes are more notable to family members than to patients. Thus studies describing the importance of cognitive change to quality of life are essential in defining the importance of POCD to the patient and family. Studies show significant associations between quality of life and perioperative cognitive decline, even when other physical or emotional factors are taken into consideration.[2,20]

In addition to aging and surgery, many disease entities alter cognitive function, especially in high-risk elderly populations.[21,22] **Figure 84-2** shows the complex interaction proposed for the development of mild cognitive impairment.[23]

Diabetes is associated with an increased incidence of mild cognitive dysfunction.[22] Increasingly the literature points to the impact of chronic elevations in blood sugar on the brain. However, it is difficult to differentiate this effect from the increased probability of atherosclerosis that is also associated with progression of aging-related cognitive decline.[24,25] Even at ages at which atherosclerosis is less likely, however, diabetes is associated with acceleration in cognitive decline (**Fig. 84-3**).[22]

Understanding susceptibility to aging-related decline has been a key area of investigation and overlaps substantially with the investigation of Alzheimer disease development and progression. Although the association between the occurrence of apolipoprotein E ε-4 (Apo E4) and the development of late-onset Alzheimer disease has been clearly demonstrated,[26,27] the association between the presence of the E4 allele and the progression of aging-related cognitive decline in the normal aging population is more controversial. The preponderance of data point to poorer learning and memory and other impairments in cognitive functioning associated with the presence of the allele.[28-33]

As has been noted in most investigations of biologic function, both genetic and environmental factors alter the progression of cognitive

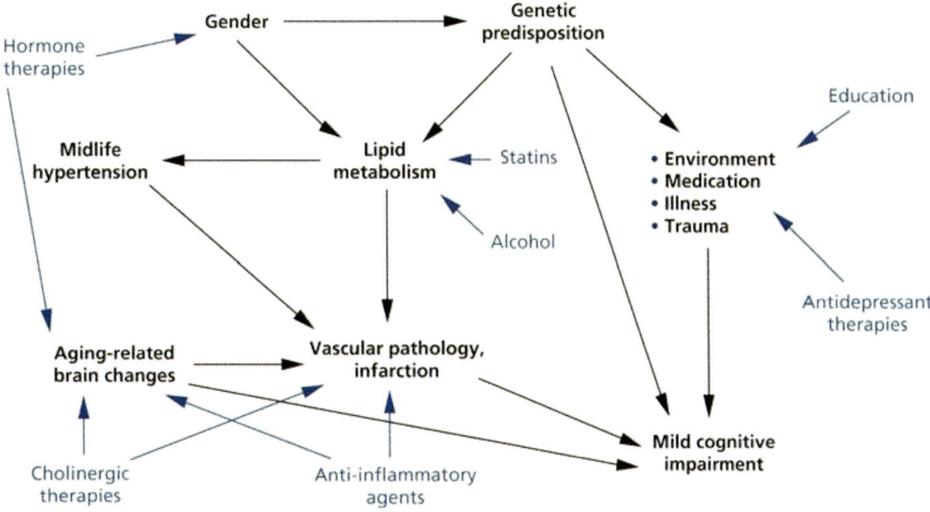

FIGURE 84-2. Hypothetical etiological model of mild cognitive impairment (MCI) in black, and possible treatment or lifestyle intervention points in blue. [Adapted from Ritchie K. Mild cognitive impairment: an epidemiological perspective. *Dialogues Clin Neurosc.* 2004;6(4):401-408.]

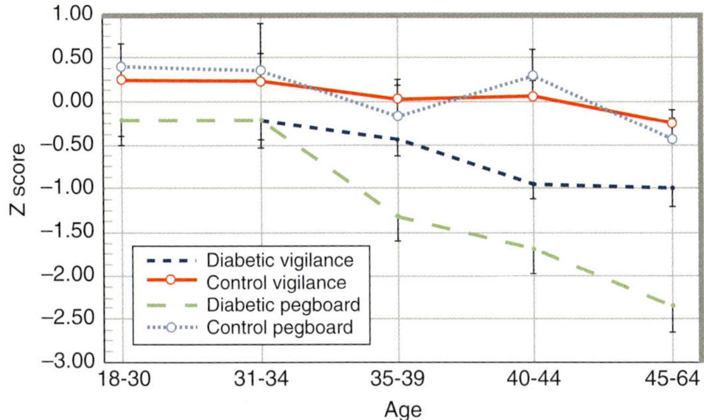

FIGURE 84-3. Performance (mean ± stand error of mean [SEM]) of diabetic and nondiabetic adults, stratified into 5 age bands, on 2 measures of psychomotor efficiency: the mean time taken by the dominant and nondominant hand to complete the Grooved Pegboard, and the total time taken to complete 2 pages of the Digit Vigilance Test. [Reprinted with permission from Ryan CM. Diabetes, aging, and cognitive decline. *Neurobiol Aging.* 2005;26:21-25. Copyright 2005 Elsevier.]

decline. In some studies, atherosclerosis and vascular disease are highly correlated factors associated with cognitive decline.[34] The influence of cardiovascular diseases and their inherent risks on cognitive decline is of substantial importance in our attempts to prevent cognitive deterioration and dementia. Haan et al as well as Slooter et al in the Rotterdam study assessed these interactions by measuring cognitive function with the Mini Mental Status Examination (MMSE) as well as other cognitive measures.[35,36] Following a group of 5888 randomly selected Medicare-eligible patients for 5 to 7 years, Haan et al demonstrated that 70% of the population showed no significant cognitive decline.[35] However, in the 30% of patients who did, the severity of atherosclerosis, diabetes, and peripheral vascular disease was associated with the extent of cognitive decline. The rate of this disease-related cognitive decline was increased by the presence of the Apo E4 allele.[35] The authors note that although many elderly individuals did not experience cognitive decline over the course of the longitudinal study, cardiovascular disease and the presence of the Apo E4 allele increased both the likelihood and severity of cognitive functional decline (**Fig. 84-4**).[35]

The results of Slooter et al, although from a smaller sample size of 838 patients, are similar.[36] These authors investigated the association of atherosclerosis and Apo E4, and their interaction on cognitive change

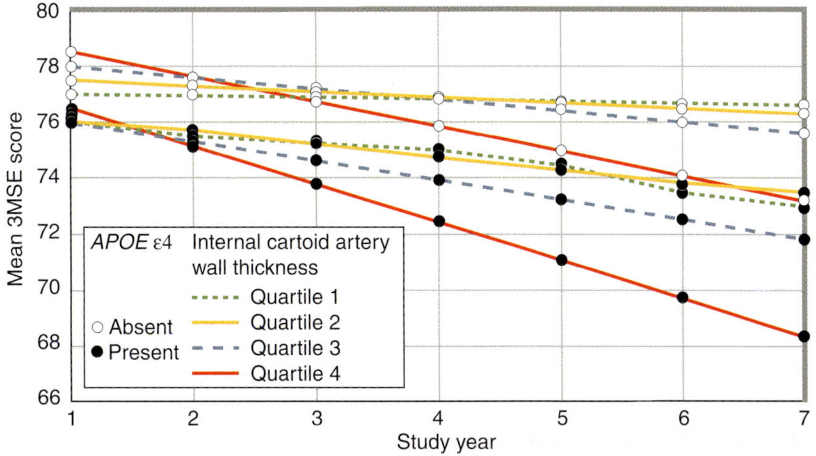

FIGURE 84-4. Change in modified Mini Mental State Examination scores by presence of Apo E4 alleles and the quartile of carotid atherosclerosis. [Data from Haan MN, Shemanski L, Jagust WJ, Manolio TA, Kuller L. The role of APOE epsilon4 in modulating effects of other risk factors for cognitive decline in elderly persons. *JAMA.* 1999;282(1):40-46.]

over 3 years in a group of patients 55 years of age and older. Their work suggests that the effects of Apo E4 and atherosclerosis are not independent, but that Apo E4 carriers with atherosclerosis are at increased risk for progressive cognitive decline.[36]

Although an initial association between the presence of Apo E4 and perioperative decline in cognitive function had been seen, larger trials have been unable to relate this association with acute perioperative changes.[37] Furthermore, identification of this allele did not help to predict postoperative cognitive dysfunction.[38,39]

Cognitive enrichment is a broad term that defines tasks or practices that, when undertaken, appear to enhance measures of crystallized intelligence and cognitive reserve. Cognitive enrichment is often broadly defined as the amount of education or the complexity of the work environment or leisure activities. Several studies show the value of education and an increased intensity of cognitive activity at work as significant factors in the delay of aging-related cognitive decline and dementia.[40] This protection against decline has also been demonstrated in multiple perioperative studies defining educational level as a protective factor in perioperative cognitive decline.[18,41,42] Education differs from intelligence level, which does not appear to provide protection from perioperative cognitive decline.[43]

ASSESSMENT OF COGNITIVE FUNCTIONING

The measurement of cognitive dysfunction is made via a large group of well-validated tests of a broad range of cognitive domains. One of the difficulties in interpreting the results of studies to date is that different tests with different scales or criteria are often used within the same populations to define outcome.[44,45] Several consensus statements and reviews have described these issues and put forward recommendations to allow consistent comparisons and sharing of data that would help in the drawing of accurate conclusions. The consensus statements[46-48] suggest minimum batteries of tests, as well as the use of individual change scores versus group mean, to define postoperative cognitive dysfunction. The difficulty arises in that the "cutoff" (the number of tests used) and the domains assessed can change the overall incidence of decline.[44,45] Furthermore, recent reviews strongly suggest the use of age-matched controls to better define the significance of this change to a similar population.[45] This is especially true when conclusions are to be drawn regarding the incidence of decline in a similar population. When interventions are compared, the value of this control or repeated control groups is lessened.

Cognitive dysfunction is often identified by the family's recognition of a patient's inability to perform what would previously have been normal activities. These include complex tasks, evoking memories, and other daily activities that are often part of a patient's overall life enjoyment. Thus, in the perioperative period, detecting changes in cognitive function becomes more challenging. Difficulties include a lack of suitable control groups to define practice effects, variable degrees of sensitivity in tests that detect change, lack of adequate time for assessment, and the lack of potential disease-matched controls to understand the importance of disease, as well as the effects of anesthesia and surgery.

In addition to the difficulties defined in the different types of tests utilized and the definition of decline,[1] other difficulties for detecting changes in cognitive function include lack of correlation between cognitive testing and both the patient's and family's assessments of the patient's status. This may indicate other behavioral factors that could define a patient's assessment of his or her current state or quality of life, such as anxiety, depression, or other factors that must be taken into account in assessing perioperative cognitive decline.

INCIDENCE AND SIGNIFICANCE OF POSTOPERATIVE COGNITIVE DYSFUNCTION

Many factors outlined in the previous sections alter the measured incidence of cognitive decline. Our group investigated the affect of different definitions of cognitive decline on the incidence of postoperative cognitive decline and found that event rates differed greatly depending on the definition used.[44] The relative rates as previously defined vary based on the sensitivity of the test used and the degree of representation of the more sensitive and time-specific domains assessed.[3,44] Concern has been expressed that early dysfunction within the immediate perioperative period may be related to the use of narcotics, benzodiazepines, or other related anesthetics. Therefore, many researchers have decreased the degree of testing conducted early postoperatively. However, this practice is criticized by some investigators, as later decline may be associated with factors other than perioperative neurologic injuries, such as sleep deprivation, depression, or other issues that may not indicate neurologic injury associated with cardiac surgery. Given these limitations, and a multitude of studies reporting their own populations' incidence, we identified an incidence of POCD in our cardiac surgery population to be 53% at discharge, and 36%, 24%, and 42%, respectively, at 6 weeks, 6 months, and 5 years follow-up. In studies of the noncardiac surgery population published from our institution, we found the incidence to be 41% at discharge and 12.7% at 3 months postdischarge in patients greater than 60 years old; in patients aged 40 to 59 years old, the incidence was 30% at discharge and 5.6% at 3 months postdischarge.[2,18] These percentages do not vary widely from those of other studies.

Defining decline based on different cognitive domains helps us to begin sorting out the areas of function more sensitive to perioperative neurologic injury. Visuospatial orientation and other aspects of visual construction seem to be some of the hardest hit domains, as well as aspects of executive function requiring multitasking or involving multiple areas of the brain for completion of an overall task. Although assessment of different domains may point to an area of the brain most affected, logistical limitations in the perioperative period and patient burden at a stressful time will limit the ability to investigate decline as thoroughly as most neuropsychologists would like.

Although few would question the significance of a stroke in the perioperative period, the importance of cognitive decline after surgery has long been debated. Despite the many studies showing cognitive decline after cardiac surgery, its effects are frequently minimized or dismissed because of the transient nature of cognitive decline in most patients. To address the importance of perioperative cognitive dysfunction, we investigated a broad range of quality-of-life measures in tandem with cognition at 5-year follow-up.[2]

Using a number of standardized, validated assessments[2] in patients undergoing cardiac surgery, significant univariate and multivariate correlations between cognitive function and multiple quality-of-life measures were detected. Furthermore, multivariable logistic regression on a 2-way classification of employment status adjusted for age, gender, educational level, and a history of diabetes revealed the 5-year overall cognitive function score to be a significant predictor of the likelihood of being productively working (**Fig. 84-5**). Finally, perception of general health also varied directly with cognitive functioning where patients with lower cognitive function score at 5 years self-reported a lower quality of general health. Postoperative cognitive decline has also been shown to affect daily activities such as driving.[49,50] Clearly, cognitive impairment following cardiac surgery has long-term consequences.

More recent studies have confirmed a similar impact of POCD showing that cognitive dysfunction after noncardiac surgery was associated with increased mortality, risk of leaving the labor market prematurely, and dependency on social transfer payments.[5]

POSTOPERATIVE COGNITIVE DYSFUNCTION IN CARDIAC SURGERY

Stroke and incapacitating CNS dysfunction after cardiac surgery with cardiopulmonary bypass (CPB) remain devastating complications, highlighted by a significant increase in overall cardiac morbidity and mortality.[51] Recent studies suggest that elderly patients with greater comorbidities and advanced cardiovascular disease benefit most from

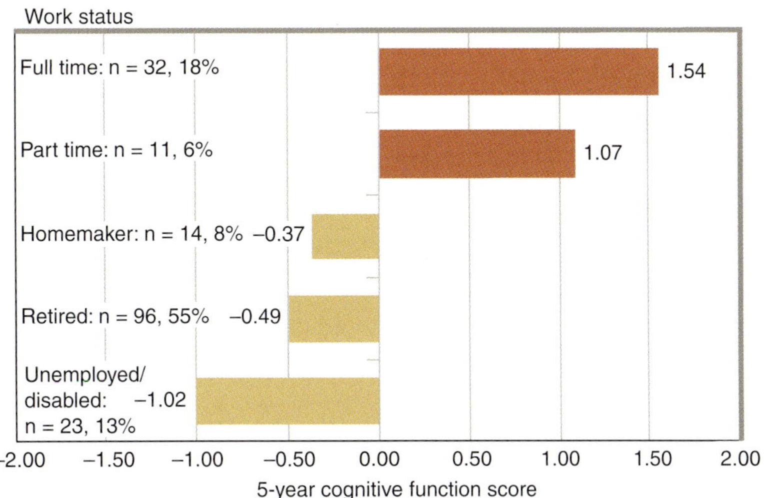

FIGURE 84-5. Patient's work status and 5-year composite cognitive index. The 5-year cognitive function score is the sum of the 4 domain scores, including cognitive decline and learning effects. [Data from Newman MF, Grocott HP, Mathew JP, et al. Report of the substudy assessing the impact of neurocognitive function on quality of life five years after cardiac surgery. Neurologic Outcome Research Group and Cardiothoracic Anesthesia Research Endeavors (CARE) Investigators of the Duke Heart Center. *Stroke.* 2001;32(12):2874-2881.]

cardiac surgery compared with medical therapy,[52,53] yet they have greater morbidity and mortality after cardiac surgery, specifically neurologic dysfunction.[51,54-56]

Neurologic injury associated with cardiac surgery ranges from severely incapacitating or life-ending stroke and coma, to encephalopathy or delirium and cognitive decline. Although stroke after cardiac surgery, with or without cardiopulmonary bypass, continues to represent a substantial concern for both short- and long-term disability, more subtle neurologic deficits, such as encephalopathy and cognitive dysfunction, are associated with increased medical costs and decreases in short- and long-term cognitive function and quality of life.[2] In fact, following an apparently successful operation, nothing may be more disappointing to the physician team, the patient, and the patient's family than for the patient to subsequently exhibit substantial neurologic or cognitive deficits that limit the ability to function independently.

As mentioned, when we evaluated the importance of cognitive dysfunction to long-term outcome in our 2001 study, approximately 50% of our cardiac surgery patients exhibited cognitive deficits at discharge in 1 or more domains: at 6 weeks, the proportion of patients who again showed a deficit dropped to 36%; at 6 months, 24%; and at 5 years, the proportion rose to 42%. Therefore, the pattern is one of early improvements followed by later decline. Cognitive deficit at discharge predicted long-term outcome, even if short-term gains occurred in the meantime. At 6 weeks, patients who initially had a deficit improved to a level similar to those who never deviated from baseline levels. But after 5 years, patients who had deficits at discharge had significantly worse outcomes than did those patients without initial deficits. In addition to cognitive deficit at discharge, predictors of cognitive dysfunction at 5 years included baseline cognitive level, age, and years of education. Ejection fraction, a history of hypertension and/or diabetes, and surgical variables were not found to be significant factors. As the population ages, patients are more fearful of mental disability and loss of independence than they are of death, which gives more weight to the importance of further efforts to improve perioperative CNS outcomes.

However, some researchers question whether cognitive decline after coronary artery bypass graft (CABG) is related to surgery or only to disease state. A consensus panel from the Outcomes Key West Meeting addressed this issue as a group and made a number of suggestions outlined in a consensus publication.[47]

VARIATION IN CNS INJURY AFTER CARDIAC SURGERY

The importance of different cardiac surgical procedures on cognitive decline is a controversial topic. Initial studies point to a higher degree of cognitive injury in valve procedure patients; however, more recent trials do not show a substantial difference. Patients who are undergoing combined procedures (CABG and valve) typically have a higher incidence of cognitive decline and overall neurologic injury compared to patients who are undergoing other procedures.[57] Institution of cardiopulmonary bypass, with its myriad systemic effects, including inflammatory and hematologic consequences, seems a likely contributor to cognitive decline. Microembolic load is also a logical contributor, and the effects of manipulation of the aorta, although still possible, are less with off-pump CABG. In an early study by Cleveland et al, off-pump coronary artery bypass grafting was associated with fewer neurologic complications; data from the Society of Thoracic Surgeons National Adult Cardiac Surgery Database showed a substantial reduction in stroke.[58] However, despite attempts to use controls for demographic and perioperative differences, the patient demographics of on- and off-pump techniques were not similar. The Octopus trial was not able to demonstrate a substantial difference in neurologic or cognitive injury between on- and off-pump CABG at 5 years.[59] In 2008, Jensen at al was again unable to identify cognitive protection from an off-pump strategy.[60] Liu et al recently compared on- and off-pump CABG for POCD, but also measured with bilateral transcranial Doppler the development of microemboli. They found a significant difference in the numbers of microemboli between the 2 groups: 430 versus 2 for on- and off-pump CABG, respectively ($p = .001$). However, they found no difference in the incidence of POCD at 1 week or 3 months.[61]

POSTOPERATIVE COGNITIVE DYSFUNCTION IN NONCARDIAC SURGERY

Postoperative cognitive dysfunction, an accepted complication of cardiac surgery, has been, until recently, less appreciated or defined after noncardiac surgery. In 1998 the International Study of Postoperative Cognitive Dysfunction (ISPOCD-1) evaluated cognitive decline in 1218 elderly patients who underwent major noncardiac surgery and found that cognitive dysfunction was present in 25% of patients 1 week after surgery and in 10% of patients 3 months after surgery.[1] Unfortunately, there were significant differences in the incidence of POCD at the

13 hospitals participating in the study. This variability makes generalization of the results to any single medical institution ill advised. In addition, in a letter to the editor, Bonke[62] pointed out numerous errors in the data reported in this manuscript. This combination of poor reliability and errors raises questions about this study's validity.

To further investigate the findings of the ISPOCD in noncardiac surgery, Monk et al completed a prospective assessment of 1064 patients undergoing elective noncardiac surgery. This assessment was divided among young (18-39 years of age), middle-aged (40-59 years of age), and elderly (60 years and older) patients. A group of 210 primary family members were used as controls to provide a change score similar to that used in the ISPOCD. For our study, inclusion criteria included age 18 years and older, history of major abdominal thoracic or orthopedic surgery, general anesthesia greater than 2 hours, and an MMSE score of 24 or greater at baseline. Exclusion criteria included cardiac or neurosurgical procedures, history of CNS disease with persistent deficits, history of alcoholism or drug dependence, history of major depression requiring treatment, and patients who were not expected to live 3 months or longer.[18]

The patients completed a battery of cognitive tests at baseline (preoperatively), and at both 1 week and 3 months postoperatively. To quantify the practice effect, we compared for each measure the changes in performance for control subjects in each age group at baseline, and at 1 week and 3 months later.

Figure 84-6 presents the incidence of POCD at the hospital-discharge and 3-month postoperative neuropsychological evaluations. At hospital discharge, the incidence of POCD was 36% in the young, 30.4% in the middle-aged, and 41.4% in the elderly patients. The incidence of cognitive decline was significantly lower in middle-aged patients compared to elderly patients ($p = .01$), but was not different for young versus elderly or young versus middle-aged patients. The incidence of cognitive decline was similar for control subjects of all age groups at the first postoperative testing session: 4.1% in young, 2.8% in middle-aged, and 5.1% in elderly patients. However, the differences in cognitive decline between age-matched controls and patients were significant for all age groups ($p < .001$).

At 3 months after surgery, POCD was identified in 5.7% of young, 5.6% of middle-aged, and 12.7% of elderly patients. POCD was significantly higher in elderly compared to young or middle-aged patients ($p = .001$). The incidence of cognitive decline in the control subjects was similar for all age groups at the 3-month testing interval and was

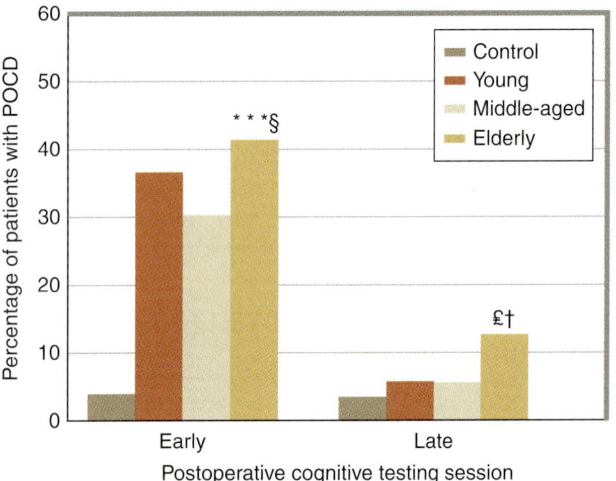

FIGURE 84-6. Incidence of POCD in adult patients after noncardiac surgery: Z score definition. [Data from Monk TG, Weldon BC, Garvan CW, et al. Predictors of cognitive dysfunction after major noncardiac surgery. *Anesthesiology*. 2008;108(1):18-30.]

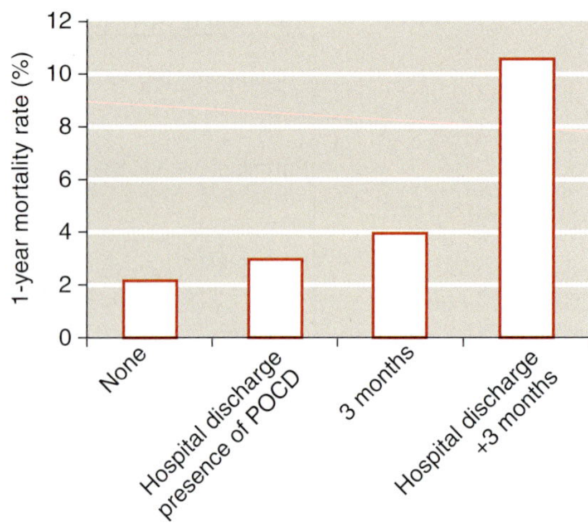

FIGURE 84-7. Relation between the presence of postoperative cognitive dysfunction (POCD) and the percentage of patients who died in the first year after surgery. This figure includes only patients who survived to test at the 3-month (late) test time. The figure includes the following 4 groups: none (patients who did not experience POCD at either of the testing times), hospital discharge (patients who had POCD only at hospital discharge), 3 months (patients who had POCD only at the late [3 months postoperative] testing session), and hospital discharge + 3 months (patients who had POCD at both hospital discharge and the late testing sessions). Hospital discharge + 3 months group was significantly different than the other 3 groups, $p = .02$. [Reprinted with permission from Monk TG, Weldon BC, Garvan CW, et al. Predictors of cognitive dysfunction after major noncardiac surgery. *Anesthesiology*. 2008;108(1):18-30.]

6.3%, 4.8%, and 1.8% in young, middle-aged, and elderly patients, respectively. At this testing interval, there was no difference in the incidence of POCD between age-matched control subjects and patients in the young and middle-aged groups. However, elderly patients exhibited a significantly greater incidence of cognitive decline at 3 months after surgery compared to elderly control subjects ($p < .001$). Of the significant univariate predictive factors for POCD at 3 months after surgery, only increasing age, lower educational level, and POCD at hospital discharge remained significant in the multiple logistic regression analysis.

Postoperative cognitive dysfunction after noncardiac surgery demonstrated a significant increase in the elderly, especially at 3 months postoperatively. The results of this trial indicate that postoperative cognitive dysfunction is common in all age groups at 1 week. However, at 3 months after surgery it is more common in the elderly with lower educational achievement. Monk et al not only reported on the incidence of POCD, but also reevaluated patients at 1 year to collect mortality data. They found an increase in 3-month mortality associated with POCD at discharge compared with those without POCD at discharge ($P = .02$). They also found that patients with POCD at both discharge and 3 months have a significantly higher 1-year mortality rate than any other group (**Fig. 84-7**).[18]

Following up on the work of Steinmetz et al. confirmed that POCD after noncardiac surgery is associated with increased employment status changes and increased requirement for government support.[5]

COMPARISON OF POSTOPERATIVE COGNITIVE DECLINE IN CARDIAC AND NONCARDIAC SURGERY

Historically, cardiac surgery compared with noncardiac surgery was performed on a more elderly population with progressive cardiovascular disease. These elderly patients were at higher risk for cerebrovascular complications including stroke and cognitive decline. With advances in the safety of anesthesia and surgery, the general

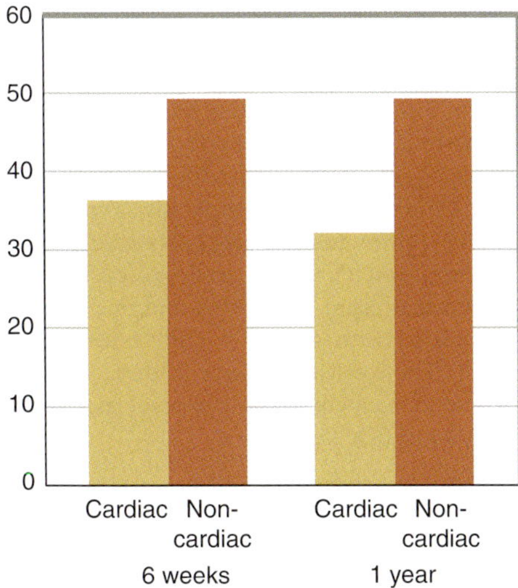

FIGURE 84-8. Comparison of the incidence of cognitive decline between cardiac and noncardiac surgery at 6 weeks and 1 year. [Data from personal communication between M.F. Newman and colleagues.]

population now receiving vascular, orthopedic, and general surgery is progressively older with increasing comorbidities. The result has been a greater recognition of the presence of POCD after noncardiac surgery as outlined in the previous section. However, direct comparisons in studies using similar testing, same institution, and same age range have been limited. We investigated 675 patients undergoing cardiac surgery and 342 patients undergoing noncardiac surgery during a 5-year period from 2000 to 2005 at our institution; institutional review board approval and patient informed consent were obtained beforehand.

Cognitive testing was accomplished at baseline (before surgery), as well as 6 weeks and 1 year postoperatively. We used a previously published battery of neuropsychological tests, with 4 independent domains established in a factor analysis of the 9 measures used.[41,44] Factor analysis provided for no substantial overlap between domains, and therefore a standard deviation decline in any 1 of 4 unique domains was identified as cognitive decline. A single factor analysis was used for comparison of the 2 groups.

Although demographic composition of the 2 groups was similar, the cardiac surgical population had lower cognitive scores at baseline, possibly because of the risk of cerebrovascular disease. Despite expectations for a higher incidence of cognitive decline after cardiac versus noncardiac surgery, the results were actually reversed: 49.1% of noncardiac surgical patients experienced cognitive decline at 6 weeks compared to 36% of cardiac patients. This trend continued through 1-year testing, with 42.0% of noncardiac patients showing decline compared to only 32.2% of cardiac surgical patients. The differences were not statistically significant (**Fig. 84-8**).

Contrary to our previous assumptions, the incidence of cognitive decline after noncardiac surgery appears to approximate that seen after cardiac surgery, possibly a result of the 2 samples being normalized for age. Because baseline scores were different in the 2 groups, the implications of a similar change may be different and requires further investigation to define the relative importance of the measured change to quality of life.

ETIOLOGY OF NEUROLOGIC DYSFUNCTION AND POSTOPERATIVE COGNITIVE DYSFUNCTION

Understanding patient risk factors associated with perioperative CNS injury is an important first step in understanding the etiology of this disease continuum.

AORTIC ATHEROSCLEROSIS AND CEREBRAL EMBOLIZATION

Multiple investigators have identified proximal aortic atherosclerosis, as identified by cardiac surgical palpation or, more importantly, by transesophageal and epiaortic scanning, as a risk factor associated with a manyfold increase in stroke risk.[63-65] There is little doubt that embolization of aortic atheroma or other debris from the surgical field is an important etiologic factor in stroke and major neurologic injury after cardiac surgery. In studies conducted by Roach and others before the widespread use of transesophageal echocardiography, those patients with surgical palpated aortic atherosclerosis were found to have a 5-times greater risk of overall stroke.[64] Further pathologic diagnoses have also defined small capillary arterial dilatations in the brains of patients or animals having recently undergone cardiac surgery with CPB.[66] Most of these presumed embolic changes disappear over time, and they are not typically seen in patients or animals who are investigated or who die weeks to months after the surgery. A number of investigators, using transesophageal echocardiography as well as epiaortic scanning, have defined an association between neurologic injury and the degree of aortic atherosclerosis, especially in the ascending and transverse aorta, whereas the degree of atherosclerosis in the descending aorta has been used more as a factor predictive of a need to use epiaortic scanning. Further support for identifying embolization as a major factor in neurologic injury comes from the use of transcranial Doppler and carotid ultrasound studies that show substantial numbers of cerebral emboli occurring, especially during aortic interventions such as cannulation, aortic cross-clamping or unclamping, use of partial side-biting clamps, and other cardiac nonaortic manipulations. However, as might be expected, the correlation with neurologic injury and the number of emboli is not as robust as the correlation we previously defined for transesophageal- or epiaortic-determined aortic atherosclerosis. This difference probably relates to our inability to differentiate between air and particulate emboli, and thus demonstrates the importance of these factors in defining overall injury.

The last and most definitive evidence for embolization, an important aspect in neurologic injury, are recent studies using new diffusion-weighted imaging (DWI) and perfusion-weighted imaging (PWI) techniques, which have demonstrated that after coronary artery bypass or aortic valve surgery, up to 45% of patients have new DWI-detected lesions postoperatively.[67] This demonstrates that ongoing neurologic injury is occurring, but the ability to better define the clinical implication for stroke or cognitive decline may relate to the location of the injury. That is, a small injury occurring in the internal capsule may produce a profound stroke, in comparison to large frontal or cerebellar infarcts that remain silent and therefore receive no extensive functional investigation.

Several investigators have associated increased cerebral emboli with degree of cognitive decline, although this has recently been challenged by Liu et al.[61] Despite the significant correlation between aortic atherosclerosis and stroke, the association with POCD has been tenuous at best (see elsewhere in this chapter). Many studies have failed to demonstrate a clear relationship between the severity of aortic atherosclerosis and the incidence of POCD.[68] Evered et al found that atheroma burden predicted POCD at 1 week ($p = .0002$), but that effect diminished over ensuing 3-month and 1-year evaluations.[69]

HYPOPERFUSION AND TEMPERATURE

Since the time of Gilman's classic study in 1965, the presence of nonpulsatile perfusion and lower perfusion pressure during cardiac surgery has been blamed for much of the neurologic injury that we have previously described.[70] Watershed infarcts in older individuals, especially those with carotid disease, have been an important factor in this association.[70] Furthermore, Caplan determined that lower perfusion pressure may be associated with a reduced washout of smaller emboli from the watershed areas, thus increasing the probability that hypoperfusion would play a role in causing watershed infarcts that we may see in cardiac surgery.[71,72]

Gold et al performed a randomized prospective trial of high (mean arterial pressure [MAP]: 80-100 mm Hg) versus lower perfusion pressure (50-70 mm Hg) during CPB for patients undergoing CABG.[72] This trial of 240 patients, comparing myocardial and neurologic outcomes between the 2 CABG groups, was unable to reach statistical significance when the individual outcomes were assessed. The combined cardiovascular outcome (myocardial and neurologic) shows a benefit for higher pressure, indicating that, at least in part, cardiovascular injury was increased with lower perfusion pressure.[72] However, looking at a subset of 188 of these patients and comparing the transesophageal assessment of aortic atherosclerosis severity, Hartman showed that atherosclerotic grade was an independent predictor of neurologic injury.[73] He further determined that for individuals with severe aortic atherosclerosis, higher perfusion pressure is associated with a reduced incidence of neurologic injury. This indicates that in individuals who are at high risk for embolization, perfusion pressure may determine the extent of measurable injury and the severity of that injury.[73] Although there appears to be a relationship between stroke and MAP in situations of severe aortic atherosclerosis, the association between reduced perfusion pressure and cognitive decline has not been well defined. Using new and more sophisticated recordings of blood pressure, we examined the relationship between MAP during hypothermic CPB and postoperative cognitive function. Moreover, because advanced age is an important predisposing variable,[74,75] we analyzed the interaction of age with MAP.

After institutional review board approval and written informed consent, 260 patients requiring elective cardiac surgery with CPB were enrolled. All patients were 21 years of age or older without a history of cerebral vascular disease (previous stroke, symptomatic carotid bruit, or documented transient ischemic attacks), alcohol or substance abuse, psychiatric illness (previous hospitalization or requirement of medication at the present hospitalization), uncontrolled hypertension (diastolic pressure >110 mm Hg or requiring interventions while hospitalized to reduce blood pressure), renal disease (creatinine >1.8), active liver disease (abnormal liver function tests if they were performed), or literacy at the seventh-grade level or above. A neuropsychological test battery, including mood and cognitive function, was administered the day prior to surgery and the day prior to hospital discharge (approximately 7-10 days after surgery).[76]

Of the 260 patients enrolled, 237 completed pre- and postoperative neuropsychological tests and had MAP and temperature data to allow analysis (19 patients refused postoperative testing, and data retrieval for intraoperative MAP and temperature was inadequate for analysis in 4 patients). The charts of the 237 patients were reviewed for temperature and MAP data at 1-minute resolution. A total of 26642 minute points were evaluated, with 0.5% of the points (136 points) discarded as artifactual. MAP and temperature data including initial MAP, MAPavg, AREA50, T5AREA50, minimum temperature, maximum temperature, maximum rate of rewarming over 5 minutes, and temperature area above 98.6°F (37°C) were measured for all patients.

Multivariable regression analysis for all 7 cognitive measures showed no significant associations between MAP or rewarming rate and cognitive decline. Similar to previously published reports on a portion of this database, consistently significant associations were found between preoperative score (all 7 measures), age (5 of 7), years of education (5 of 7), and maximum arterial-venous oxygen content difference [C(a-v)o_2], (2 of 7).[76] Despite the lack of primary effects of MAP and rewarming rate on cognitive decline, the interaction of age with these variables showed significant associations ($p < .05$) on 2 tests. With increasing age, AREA50 predicted increased decline in the Digit Symbol Test at discharge ($p = .005$). Characterization of MAP based on 5-minute or greater hypotension episodes presented no additional primary effects or interactions. These interactions without significant primary effects would indicate a differential effect of these variables on cognitive function as an effect of age. In elderly individuals who are at increased risk of cognitive decline, hypoperfusion may be associated with an increased risk of cognitive decline.

In 2008 Grocott evaluated temperature in a rat model in which 4 groups were created: A, normothermia (37.5°C) throughout; B, hypothermia (32°C) on bypass followed by complete rewarming (37.5°C); C, hypothermia (32°C) on bypass followed by limited rewarming (35°C); and D, normothermia (37.5°C) on bypass followed by hypothermia (35°C). The researchers found that hypothermia on bypass followed by limited rewarming and prolonged postoperative hypothermia decreased POCD in rats.[77] In addition to the animal data suggesting the beneficial effect of hypothermia on POCD, several prospective human studies have demonstrated that rapid rewarming and/or postoperative hyperthermia are associated with greater cognitive decline 6 weeks after cardiac surgery.[78,79] The consistent theme in these studies is that intraoperative or postoperative hyperthermia is associated with an increased incidence or severity of POCD.

SYSTEMIC INFLAMMATORY RESPONSE

Cardiac surgery is known to be associated with a profound systemic inflammatory response, especially when cardiopulmonary bypass is used. Although it is likely that systemic inflammatory response may play a role in the overall severity of injury, there are very little data to support that it alone is the causative factor. Westaby studied a group of patients undergoing CABG and found no significant association between inflammatory markers and cognitive injury, and we also were unable to find this.[80,81] However, it is likely that these factors were contributory and not causal. Thus, as we better understand the severity of injury and other susceptibility factors, we may be able to further determine the importance of these factors in neurologic and cognitive injury. Two recent trials evaluating the use of complement inhibitors in cardiac surgery have defined a small but measurable positive effect on cognitive decline with the use of the C-5 complement inhibitor continued for the surgical period and 24 hours postoperatively. However, in neither case was the overall decline in neurologic or cognitive function statistically altered.[82]

DEPRESSION

Our group and others have studied depression as it relates to cardiac surgery and found that depression is an important factor in defining long-term survival postoperatively.[20] However, when we have investigated depression as a factor in short-term cognitive change, we've been unable to demonstrate a significant association between a low-level of depression and acute changes in cognitive function. On the other hand, many groups, including our own, have been able to show an association between depression and long-term cognitive decline.[83] Whether cognitive decline leads to a greater degree of depression or depression defines cognitive function over time is a phenomenon that requires longitudinal studies to ascertain.

GENETIC FACTORS

An intriguing development in the field of neuroprotection is in the area of genetic predisposition or susceptibility in cardiac surgery–associated cerebral injuries. Expanding discoveries in this relatively new field of perioperative genetics and neurologic outcomes include our recent study of 1635 patients by the PEGASUS investigative group, in which patients undergoing cardiac surgery using cardiopulmonary bypass surgery were studied. DNA was isolated from preoperative blood and analyzed for 26 different single-nucleotide polymorphisms.[2] Multivariable logistic regression modeling was used to determine the association of clinical and genetic characteristics with stroke.

Permutation analysis was used to adjust for multiple comparisons inherent in genetic association studies. Of the 1635 patients, 28 patients (1.7%) suffered stroke and were included in the final genetic model. The combination of the 2 minor alleles of C-reactive protein (CRP; 3′UTR 1846C/T) and interleukin-6 (IL-6; −174G/C) polymorphisms, occurring in 583 (35.7%) patients, was significantly associated with stroke (odds ratio [OR]: 3.3; 95% confidence interval [CI]: 1.4-8.1; $p = .0023$). In a multivariable logistic model adjusting for age, the CRP and IL-6 single-nucleotide polymorphism combination remained significantly associated with stroke ($p = .002$). Genetic factors associated with inflammation predicted a 3-fold increase in stroke rate over and above other clinical risk factors, indicating the possibility of future risk stratification to focus neuroprotective strategies.

The possibility that one's genetic makeup might alter cognitive outcome after cardiac surgery was first delineated in a 1997 study.[37] In that study, the apolipoprotein E hypothesis was born, that is, that patients possessing the Apo E4 allele had worse cognitive outcomes after CPB. Although somewhat controversial,[84] this hypothesis may likely represent the beginning of our understanding of the complex role of individual genetic variations, represented by single nucleotide polymorphisms (SNPs), in moderating cerebral responses to surgery. Despite this initial positive association, others have been unable to replicate it in primarily white populations, making these findings "controversial."[84]

Mathew et al[85] characterized phospholipase A_2 (PLA_2), a polymorphism of the glycoprotein (GP) IIIa constituent of the platelet integrin receptor GP IIb/IIIa, and examined its influence on cognitive outcome after cardiac surgery. In their study, a multivariate analysis revealed that the PLA_2 genotype was significantly associated with greater decline on the Mini Mental State Examination ($p = .036$). The mechanism may be related to is an increased prothrombotic role, which has been shown in investigations of coronary artery thrombosis and myocardial infarction.[86,87] The progression of genetic predictors of perioperative cognitive decline have mimicked the progression of the field of genetic association moving from the investigation of single candidate genes to multiple candidate genes and then to genome-wide scans as technology advances.

Mathew et al have also hypothesized that candidate gene polymorphisms in biological pathways regulating inflammation, cell matrix adhesion/interaction, coagulation-thrombosis, lipid metabolism, and vascular reactivity are associated with postoperative cognitive deficit (POCD).[85] In a prospective cohort study of 513 patients (86% European American) undergoing CABG surgery with cardiopulmonary bypass, a panel of 37 SNPs was genotyped by mass spectrometry.[39] The association between these SNPs and cognitive deficit at 6 weeks after surgery was tested using multiple logistic regression accounting for age, level of education, baseline cognition, and population structure. Permutation analysis was used to account for multiple testing.

We found that in European Americans (n = 443), minor alleles of the *CRP* 1059G/C SNP (OR: 0.37; 95% CI: 0.16-0.78; $p = .013$) and the *SELP* 1087G/A SNP (OR: 0.51; 95% CI: 0.30-0.85; $p = .011$) were associated with a reduction in cognitive deficit. The absolute risk reduction in the observed incidence of POCD was 20.6% for carriers of the *CRP* 1059C allele and 15.2% for carriers of the *SELP* 1087A allele. This compared to a greater than 40% incidence of decline in those patients who did not possess either allele (**Fig. 84-9**).[39]

Perioperative serum CRP and degree of platelet activation were also significantly lower in patients with a copy of the minor alleles, providing biologic support for the observed allelic association. These results suggest a contribution of P-selectin and CRP genes in modulating susceptibility to cognitive decline following cardiac surgery, with potential implications for identifying populations at risk who might benefit from targeted perioperative anti-inflammatory strategies. Identifying genetic and mechanistic factors associated with lower rates of injury and sequelae help us define pathways to protection as well as provide the opportunity for preoperative genetic screening to identify patients who are at risk for cerebral injury and who will most likely benefit from interventional protective strategies.

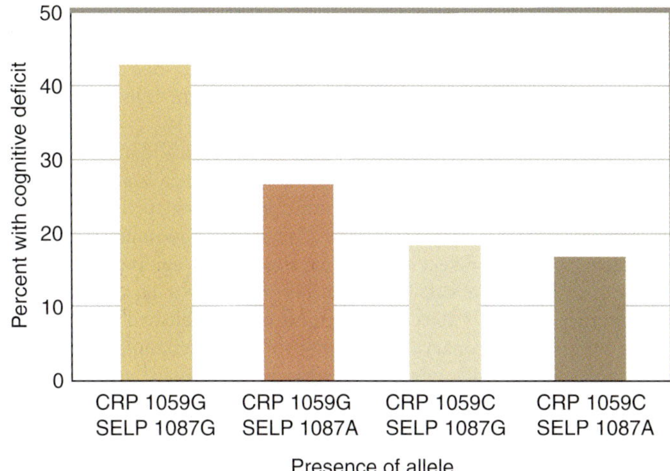

FIGURE 84-9. Incidence of postoperative cognitive deficit by *CRP* 1059G/C and *SELP* 1087G/A genotypes. The incidence of cognitive deficit was 16.7% in carriers of minor alleles at both of these loci, compared to 42.9% in patients homozygous for the major allele (n = 386). [Reprinted from Mathew J, Podgoreanu MD, Grocott GP, et al, Genetic variants in P-selectin and C-reactive protein influence susceptibility to cognitive decline after cardiac surgery. *J Am Coll Cardiol.* 2007;49: 1934-1942. Copyright 2007 American College of Cardiology.]

ANESTHESIA

Cognitive impairment occurring up to 6 weeks after cardiac surgery has been likened to the cognitive decline seen after noncardiac surgery by the ISPOCD group and Monk et al.[1,88] The incidence in noncardiac surgery originally appeared lower than that seen in cardiac surgery, as defined by our group and others, and is comparable to a group younger than 60 years old. However, as the noncardiac population has aged, there has been increased recognition of the cognitive decline occurring in elderly surgical patients, demonstrating that cognitive decline is observed in major noncardiac surgery after general anesthesia.[88]

Because POCD shares the features of Alzheimer-type dementia, much research has been done in an attempt to link cellular pathogenesis from one to the other. Alzheimer disease is associated with the degeneration of basal forebrain cholinergic neurons innervating the cortex, amygdala, and hippocampus. This degeneration is the consequence of amyloid β-protein production and accumulation from proteolysis of amyloid β (Aβ) precursor protein, and the creation of neurotoxic fibrillar Aβ, which increase apoptosis. Two basic theories for this degenerative process have arisen from our understanding of Alzheimer dementia: first, that anesthesia has an anticholinergic mechanism, and second, that anesthesia can enhance the Aβ generation, accumulation, and aggregation leading to neuronal apoptosis. Both of these processes could clinically manifest as dementia, or POCD.

Central anticholinergic syndrome (CAS) has been extensively reported in the literature, mostly as case reports. Physostigmine, a centrally acting anticholinesterase once commonly used in the recovery room, has largely been abandoned, most likely secondary to limited efficacy. The incidence of CAS has been reported to be between 1% and 9%, although authors suggest it is likely underidentified.[89]

The anticholinergic theory is convenient as the cholinergic system is responsible for a wide variety of cellular responses, including regulation of consciousness and cognitive functioning, thus suggesting a link not only between lack of acetylcholine and POCD, but also between lack of acetylcholine and POD.[90-92] Importantly, Alzheimer dementia can also have a delirium component (*DSM-IV*). Although the use of atropine as a premedication is less prevalent now, several anesthetics have been found to have significant anticholinergic properties, among them volatile anesthetics, barbiturates, propofol, morphine and fentanyl.[93-96]

General anesthesia agents, especially inhaled agents, may cause amyloid deposition or protein folding differences that could alter either short-term or long-term cognitive function.[97-102] In addition to the described ability of isoflurane to enhance Aβ-protein oligomerization and generation, and to potentiate the cytotoxicity of Aβ, it has also been shown in a recent investigation to induce apoptosis. Xie et al, in a neuroglioma cell culture model exposed to 2% isoflurane for 6 hours, found that isoflurane induces cellular apoptosis in a dose-dependent manner, and that Congo red inhibits isoflurane-induced apoptosis in H4 human neuroglioma cells.[99] The authors conclude that isoflurane contributes to well-described mechanisms of

Alzheimer neuropathogenesis and provides a plausible link between the acute effects of anesthesia, a well-described risk factor for delirium, and the more long-term sequelae of dementia. Despite evidence of similar cellular pathology, anesthetic exposure and the risk of Alzheimer Disease remains controversial.

Despite the cellular evidence, there are little clinical data to support the claim that repeated exposure to general anesthesia markedly alters cognitive function. Furthermore, studies attempting to find a difference in POCD in patients exposed to general versus regional anesthesia have been unable to detect a protective effect from regional anesthesia, suggesting that the effects of anesthesia may play a lesser role than that of surgery.[43,103,104] Recently, Everend et al. published results of a study comparing coronary angiography with light sedation to total hip joint replacement with general anesthesia, to coronary artery bypass surgery under general anesthesia. Although the incidence of POCD in the CABG groups was significantly higher than the total hip group at 7 days, by three months, they did not find a significant difference between the three groups, further suggesting that POCD is likely independent of type of surgery and anesthesia.[105] Further longitudinal trials as well as animal studies are needed to define whether any of the changes that have been identified to date are associated with true clinical sequelae.

PREEXISTING CEREBROVASCULAR DISEASE OR DOCUMENTED BRAIN ABNORMALITIES

A number of researchers have performed preoperative investigations on patients scheduled for cardiac surgery, including magnetic resonance imaging (MRI) or computed tomography (CT) scans in asymptomatic elderly individuals. The presence of silent infarcts in this population is not uncommon and may be associated with later decline in cognition or dementia.[67] Goto et al have conducted the largest study. Of 421 candidates scheduled for coronary artery bypass grafting, 126 (30%) had small brain infarctions preoperatively and 83 (20%) had multiple infarctions.[106] A surprising 50% of the sample had evidence of brain abnormalities before surgery. Thus it is likely that patient characteristics have a significant role in determining the probability of a patient exhibiting neurologic injury after surgery, both by defining the degree of atherosclerotic disease as well as potentially defining individuals with less cognitive or neurologic reserve who will express symptoms of injury to a much greater extent. This association between preoperative MRI lesions and risk of new postoperative lesions was confirmed by Floyd et al.[67] In their study of 34 patients, 6 patients had evidence of new lesions as defined by MRI. The severity of preexisting white matter disease was associated with a higher probability of new lesion occurrence. They concluded that preoperative MRI lesions were one of the best predictors of new postoperative lesions.[67]

CONCLUSIONS

Although controversies exist around the incidence and the significance of POCD after cardiac and noncardiac surgery, those patients who experience cognitive decline have measurable reductions in quality of life that offset the benefits provided by surgery. This chapter discusses a number of possible etiologies, including anesthesia and surgery; however, until we have better understanding of how all these factors interact to define outcome, aggressive intervention is difficult unless the intervention is of low risk. Understanding individuals at risk, reproducing the biochemical or physiologic responses in low-risk individuals, and effectively intervening in those who are at high risk for long-term decline are measures that hold the greatest potential for benefit.

KEY REFERENCES

- Eckenhoff RG, Johansson JS, Wei H, et al. Inhaled anesthetic enhancement of amyloid-beta oligomerization and cytotoxicity. *Anesthesiology.* 2004;101(3):703-709.
- Mathew JP, Podgoreanu MV, Grocott HP, et al. Genetic variants in P-selectin and C-reactive protein influence susceptibility to cognitive decline after cardiac surgery. *J Am Coll Cardiol.* 2007;49(19):1934-1942.
- Moller JT, Cluitmans P, Rasmussen LS, et al. Long-term postoperative cognitive dysfunction in the elderly ISPOCD1 study. ISPOCD investigators. International Study of Post-Operative Cognitive Dysfunction. *Lancet.* 1998;351(9106):857-861.
- Newman MF, Grocott HP, Mathew JP, et al. Report of the substudy assessing the impact of neurocognitive function on quality of life five years after cardiac surgery. Neurologic Outcome Research Group and Cardiothoracic Anesthesia Research Endeavors (CARE) Investigators of the Duke Heart Center. *Stroke.* 2001;32(12):2874-2881.
- Rasmussen LS. Defining postoperative cognitive dysfunction. *Eur J Anaesthesiol.* 1998;15(6):761-764.
- Roach GW, Kanchuger M, Mora Mangano C, et al. Adverse cerebral outcomes after coronary bypass surgery. *N Engl J Med.* 1996;335(25):1857-1863.

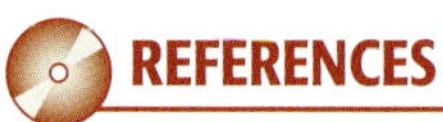

REFERENCES

Complete references available on DVD and online version at www.LongneckerAnesthesiology.com

CHAPTER 85 Protection of the Central Nervous System in Surgical Patients

W. Andrew Kofke

KEY POINTS

1. The incidence of perioperative stroke without predisposing factors is approximately 0.1%, but specific risk factors and procedures can increase the risk by 10-fold or more.
2. Cerebrovascular reserve refers to the capability of the brain's vasculature to dilate in order to compensate for perioperative physiologic stresses.
3. Attention to the maintenance of a normal physiologic milieu is the first principle of brain-oriented perioperative care.
4. Fever kills vulnerable neurons, and hypothermia is protective in cases of cardiac arrest and possibly traumatic brain injury.
5. Glycemic control improves outcome after severe critical illness and probably optimizes neurologic outcome.
6. Some anesthetics are neuroprotective, but some anesthetic drugs may have neurotoxic potential.

Neural function is the essence of human existence. Thus loss of any neural element in the course of a critical illness represents a major loss to a given individual. Neurons or supporting elements may be lost in a small, virtually unnoticeable manner, or they may perhaps manifest as cognitive or behavioral deficit, or there may be widespread selective neuronal loss or tissue infarction with more apparent and disabling deficits. Based on the notion that neural function is essential for acceptable survival from critical illness, it is crucial for perioperative management to include considerations of neural viability and the impact and interactions of the primary diseases and therapeutics on the nervous system.

There are numerous perioperative scenarios wherein a patient may be at risk for neurologic damage. These scenarios often involve ischemia, trauma, or neuroexcitation. Each of these, as they progressively worsen, involve a period of decreased cerebral perfusion pressure (CPP), either regionally or globally, the latter of which is usually associated with elevated intracranial pressure. The eventual result is a compromise in global or regional cerebral blood flow (rCBF) sufficient to produce permanent neuronal loss, infarction, and possibly brain death. A variety of biochemical pathways play a major role in this potential damage. This chapter reviews the important pathophysiologic factors and intracranial pressure (ICP) considerations and neuroprotective therapeutic options critical to contemporary perioperative care of the surgical patient at risk for central nervous system (CNS) injury.

PERIOPERATIVE STROKE

TYPES OF STROKE

Stroke is the third leading cause of death in the United States. For every patient who dies of a stroke, there are about 13 survivors who carry on with the effects of their loss of neural tissue.[1] The 2-year incidence of stroke is 10 per 1000 people and the incidence due to atherothrombotic brain infarction is 4.4 per 1000.[1]

Strokes are either ischemic or hemorrhagic. Hemorrhagic strokes are caused by subarachnoid hemorrhage (SAH), intraparencyhymal (intracerebral) hemorrhage, or subdural/epidural hemorrhage. Eighty-four percent of strokes are ischemic and 16% are hemorrhagic (6% SAH; 10% intracerebral hemorrhage, ICH). Ischemic strokes are caused by embolism, thrombosis, or hemodynamic factors such as anemia or hypotension in the setting of proximal stenosis or brain edema. Atrial fibrillation is a major risk factor for embolic ischemic stroke, comprising about 18% of first strokes. Notably, the 3-month mortality with atrial fibrillation–associated strokes is about 33% compared with 20% in patients without atrial fibrillation.[2] Genomic polymorphisms are also being identified as important in the risk of stroke.[3]

Another important risk factor in the predisposition to stroke is the capacity of cerebrovascular reserve. Reduced cerebrovascular reserve in the nonsurgical setting has been related to increased risk of stroke[4] and in the perioperative context to the inability to generate vasodilation to compensate for common stresses such as hypoxemia, hypotension, hypoglycemia, fever, and anemia. This attenuated vasodilative response increases the risk for developing a so-called *hemodynamic* stroke.

EPIDEMIOLOGY OF PERIOPERATIVE STROKE

Perioperative stroke incidence is related to the patient's underlying risk factors (**Table 85-1**) and the relative risk of the specific procedures (**Table 85-2**). Cardiac surgery, thoracic aortic surgery, and vascular neurosurgery have the highest risk of perioperative stroke. An increased risk is reported with procedures on the neck, with the lowest risk associated with general surgery.

TABLE 85-1 Patient-Specific Risk Factors for Stroke After Cardiac Surgery

Aortic arch atheroma
Renal insufficiency
Recent myocardial infarction
Prior stroke
Carotid disease
Hypertension
Age >75 y
Left ventricular dysfunction
Low cardiac output
Atrial fibrillation

TABLE 85-2 Possible Mechanisms of Perioperative Stroke

Intraoperative	Postoperative
Hypotension	Hypotension
Anemia	Emboli: myocardial infarction, subacute bacterial endocarditis, patent foramen ovale
Hypoxemia	Hypercoagulable
Hypocapnia	Atrial fibrillation
Hypercapnia	Anemia
Hypoglycemia	Iatrogenic polycythemia
Hypercoagulable	Hypoxemia
Head position	Hypertension
Hypertension	

Cardiac surgery is associated with a 1% to 5% stroke rate, which in the elderly is increased to 7% or higher. Several patient-specific risk factors that further worsen the risk are listed in Table 85-1.[5-7] Stroke rates after thoracic aortic surgery were reported by Goldstein et al.[8] Clearly the incidence increases when the procedure is done emergently.

After carotid endarterectomy (CEA) an accepted stroke rate is within the 3% to 5% range.[9,10] Data from the 2 major multi-institutional studies examining the efficacy of CEA in preventing stroke versus the operative risk were reviewed and summarized by Naylor et al.[11] Factors that increase stroke rate after CEA include female gender,[12-14] age greater than 75 years, global ischemia symptoms,[12,14] systolic hypertension,[12,14] and peripheral vascular disease.[12,14] A recent comparison between CEA and carotid stenting in 1713 patients revealed that patients allocated to stenting had a 3.3% higher risk of stroke, death, or procedural myocardial infarction within 120 days of randomization; disabling stroke or death in the stent and CEA groups was 4.0% and 3.2%, respectively.[15,16] Heyer et al[17] reported an association of post-CEA cognitive deficits with apolipoprotein E (ApoE) single nucleotide polymorphism, suggesting a significant role for genetic polymorphisms in ischemic injury after CEA.

Lanska and Kryscio[18] reported a stroke rate of 0.01% occurring in the puerperium. Strokes in this context tend to be due to venous thrombosis. Risk factors include caesarean section, fluid and electrolyte abnormalities, hypertension, and infections.

Ogilvy et al[19] reported cerebral aneurysm surgery to be associated with a perioperative stroke rate of 5% to 25% (overall rate 5.2%). However, the rate increases to 38% if the aneurysm ruptures intraoperatively. Increases in stroke risk also are associated with longer periods of temporary proximal occlusion of the artery feeding the aneurysm.

General surgery is not a high-risk procedure for stroke as long as the patient does not have any risk factors. Parikh and Cohen,[20] reviewing the data of almost 25 000 general surgery procedures, found a stroke rate of 0.08%; 84% of the strokes arose within 7 days postoperatively and a 26% mortality was associated with perioperative stroke. The authors suggest that most of these strokes were likely embolic in origin. Identified risk factors were preexisting hypertension, prior neurologic symptoms, smoking, and an abnormal rhythm on electrocardiogram, especially atrial fibrillation. Notably, they were unable to identify a relationship between preoperative carotid bruit and the development of a perioperative stroke. A recent very large comprehensive evaluation by Bateman et al[21] revealed an overall occurrence of acute ischemic stroke in 0.7% of 131 067 hemicolectomy patients, 0.2% of 201 235 total hip replacement patients, and 0.6% of 39 339 lobectomy/segmental lung resection patients. In patients older than age 65, stroke rates in these 3 groups rose to 1.0%, 0.3%, and 0.8%, respectively. Multivariate logistic regression analysis revealed renal disease (odds ratio, 3.0), atrial fibrillation (odds ratio, 2.0), history of stroke (odds ratio, 1.6), and cardiac valvular disease (odds ratio, 1.5) to be the most significant risk factors for perioperative acute ischemic stroke in this sample of noncardiac, nonneurological surgery patients. Beta-blocker use, initially surmised to contribute to perioperative stroke risk,[22] could not be linked to increased perioperative stroke risk when it was examined in a more detailed case-control study by van Lier et al.[23]

The importance of previous neurologic symptoms for the occurrence of stroke was underscored in a report by Landercasper et al[24] and another by Larsen et al.[25] Both groups found about a 2% stroke incidence in such patients after general surgery. This roughly 10-fold increase in risk was supported in the study by Bateman et al.[21] Limburg and Wijdicks,[26] comparing 61 strokes after general surgery with a group of matched general surgery patients who did not have a perioperative stroke, also identify previous neurovascular disease as an important risk factor. These observations underscore the importance of ascertaining the anatomy and circulatory pathology of any patient giving a history of prior stroke or transient ischemic attack. As such, this practice is analogous to that which arises in any patient complaining of angina or past evidence of coronary artery disease.

In addition, Limburg and Wijdicks[26] identified peripheral vascular disease and chronic obstructive lung disease as important risk factors for stroke. They could not correlate the occurrence of stroke with perioperative hypotension. Unfortunately, although extensive recommendations exist for perioperative evaluation of patients with coronary artery disease[27] a corresponding series of reports or recommendations for cerebrovascular disease is lacking.

PATHOPHYSIOLOGY OF PERIOPERATIVE STROKE

The mechanisms of perioperative stroke have not been firmly elucidated in any large prospective studies. Kam and Calcroft[28] suggest that the most likely mechanisms include perioperative hypotension, cardiogenic embolism especially with atrial fibrillation (or cardiac wall motion abnormalities), in situ atheromatous plaques leading to thrombosis or emboli (or hemodynamic strokes related to impaired cerebrovascular reserve), and increased perioperative coagulability.

Perioperative stroke tends to occur in the days after the surgery. Presumably the sequelae of the surgical intervention are important in the genesis of the stroke. Most ischemic strokes arise from emboli or thromboses, although some arise from problems with insufficient cerebrovascular reserve in the context of a perioperative physiologic challenge.

A hypercoagulable state is one consequence of the perioperative stress response.[29] This combines with patient factors and surgical factors to increase the propensity to create emboli or thromboses that can produce an ischemic stroke. Patients with anatomic pathways from the veins to the great arteries (eg, patent formen ovale) may be at particular risk. In addition, there may be local low-flow conditions related to the surgical manipulations, inflowing stenotic cerebral or carotid arteries, or positioning or low cardiac output states with ventricular hypo- or dyskinesis that may transiently occur. In particular, as described above, head position may put the vertebrobasilar system at particular risk. Cardiac arrhythmias, most notably atrial fibrillation, are also important factors for emboli or thromboses, and atrial fibrillation is relatively common postoperatively. Although unusual, perioperative polycythemia, either from an endogenous disease, dehydration, or iatrogenic factors, can increase viscosity to add another low-flow state that can lead to thrombosis.

Procedures that entail work on or near the carotid arteries are at particular risk for embolic phenomena. One example from the author's practice is illustrated in **Figure 85-1**.

CEREBROVASCULAR RESERVE

Central to physiologic considerations in the management of the acutely injured brain are considerations of cerebrovascular reserve. Simply stated, cerebrovascular reserve is the brain's capacity to successfully compensate for physiologic stresses such as hypoxemia, hypotension, hypoglycemia, fever, and anemia. In all these situations, vasodilatation occurs to provide a compensatory increase in cerebral blood flow (CBF). Inability to sustain vasodilatation in response to such physiologic stresses can result in brain damage.

Animal experiments indicate that it is possible to produce a condition in which cerebrovascular reserve is compromised, increasing the tendency for cerebral infarction.[30] For example, the occlusion of 1 carotid artery or the production of moderate hypoxemia each individually do not produce symptoms, as cerebral vasodilatation occurs to compensate. Indeed some contend that arterial hypoxemia, occurring

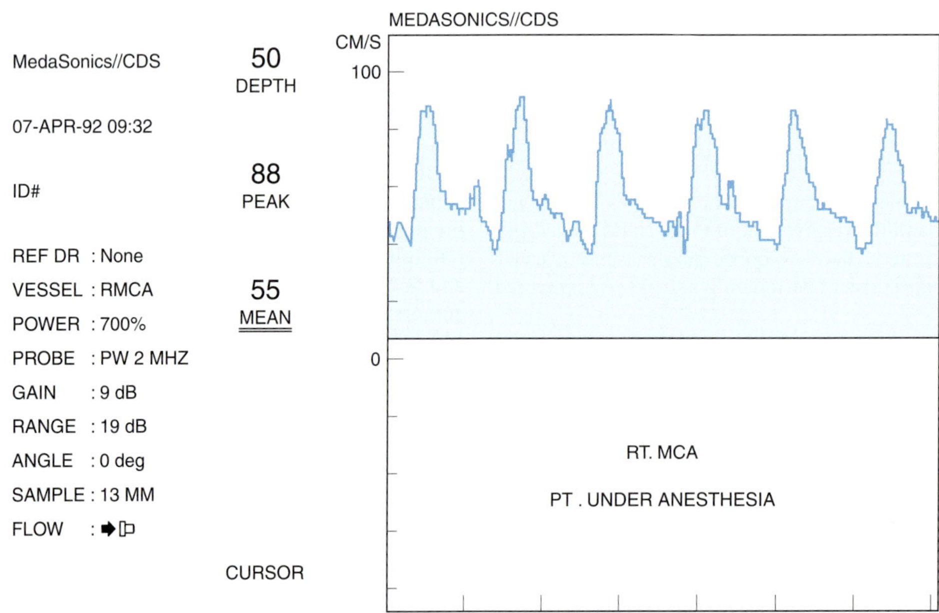

FIGURE 85-1. Transcranial Doppler ultrasonography of the middle cerebral artery during carotid endarterectomy. Flow velocity decrement after internal carotid clamping was transient, with flow restored by a shunt. Unclamping initially was associated with a shower of debris, followed by a transient period of hyperemia.

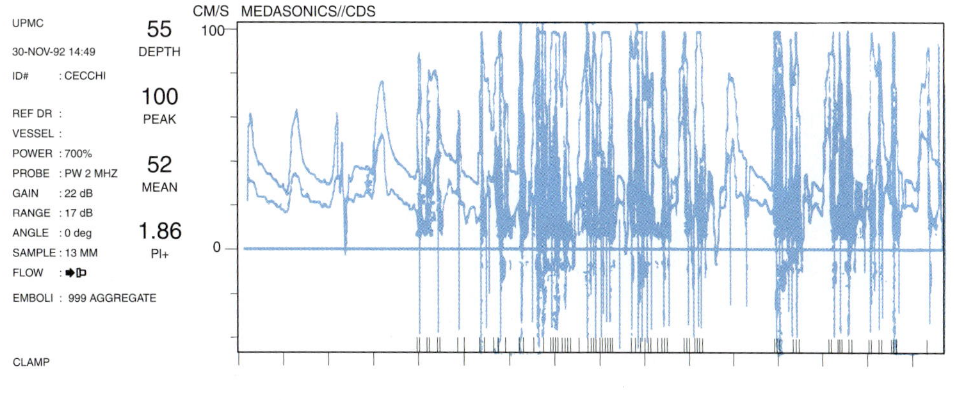

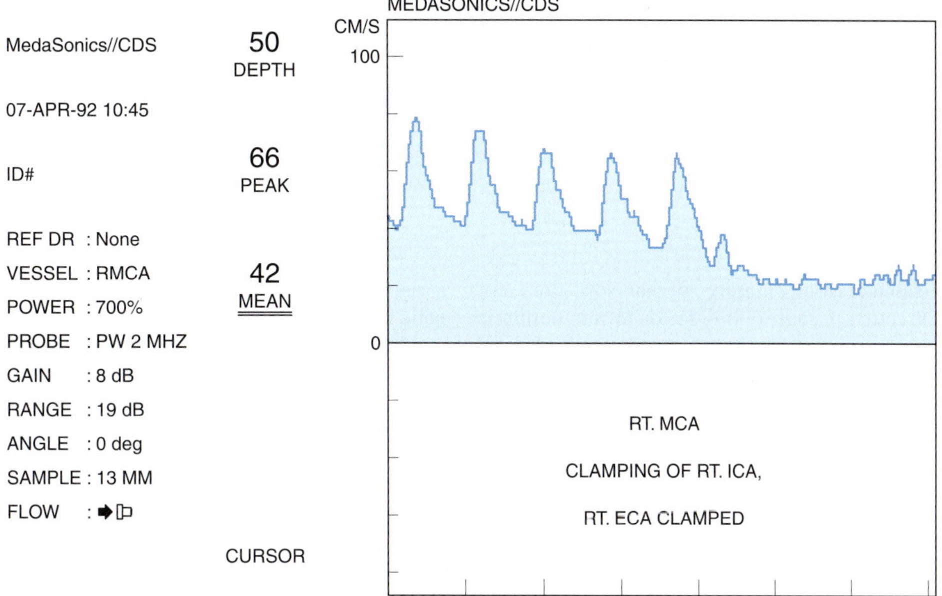

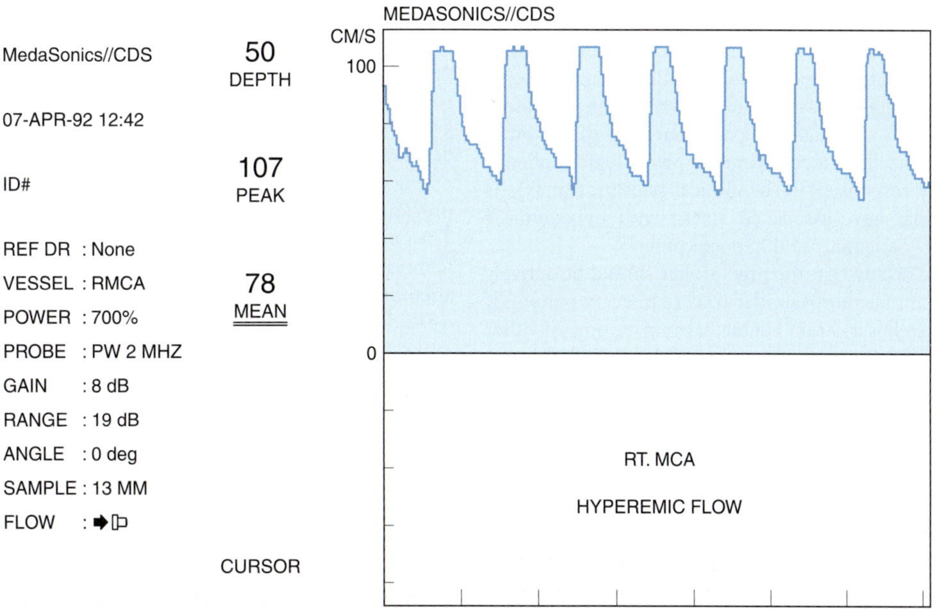

FIGURE 85-1. *(Continued)*

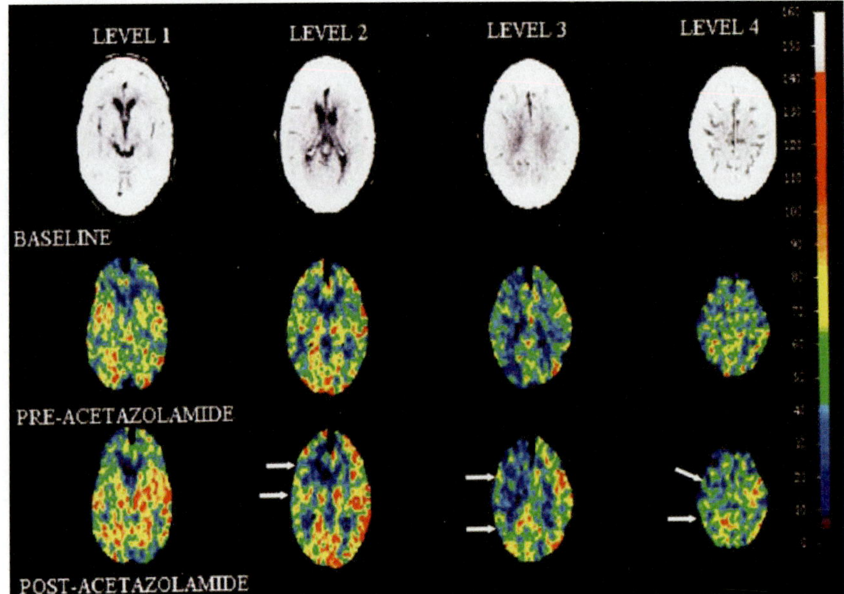

FIGURE 85-2. Stable xenon CT cerebral blood flow was performed before and after administration of intravenous acetazolamide. Areas of the brain with a suboptimal increase in flow in response to the vasodilatory stimulus (arrows) have impaired cerebrovascular reserve. [Courtesy of Howard Yonas, MD, University of New Mexico.]

with normal cerebral vascular compensatory mechanisms, does not cause brain damage. Of course 1 contributing factor to this notion is that hypoxic myocardial dysfunction produces organismic death such that isolated neuronal injury cannot occur. However, add hypoxemia to carotid occlusion, or vice versa, and a stroke occurs because compensatory mechanisms, already fully utilized, cannot accommodate the further decrease in oxygen supply.[30] Examples of variants of this situation abound clinically.[31] Such examples of attenuated cerebrovascular reserve include cerebral edema, hypoxemia, anemia, carotid stenosis, peri-infarct penumbra, and so on. In each of these situations, although not easy to quantitate, it is clear that added compromise of oxygen or nutrient supply to the brain increases risk of neuronal injury.[32] The phenomenon is illustrated in **Figure 85-2**.

As shown in Figure 85-2, one way to evaluate the extent of cerebrovascular reserve is through administration of acetazolamide with pre- and postacetazolamide CBF assessment. The acetazolamide produces a local brain tissue respiratory acidosis, which in turn, if the capability of cerebrovascular reserve is present, produces local vasodilatation. If reserve is impaired then, even though the baseline flow is normal, the impaired regional vasodilatation indicates that that particular area of the brain may be susceptible to injury from a perioperative physiologic challenge requiring a vasodilatory response.[33-35] The clinical relevance of this is supported by studies that have associated stroke with hypoxemia,[30] hypotension,[36-39] fever,[40,41] anemia,[42] and hypoglycemia.[42a]

This then leads to the notion that the practitioner should be actively thinking about the extent of cerebrovascular reserve in every patient. If the patient has arterial stenoses, brain edema, a brain tumor, or other factors that may impair the ability to vasodilate in response to hypoxemia, hypotension, hypoglycemia, fever, and anemia, then a so-called hemodynamic stroke with no emboli or thrombosis may arise. A more complete discussion of these physiologic factors follows later in this chapter.

ROLE OF HEAD POSITION

Thompson et al[43] reported from a review of the literature that surgery on the neck is an important risk factor for stroke, identifying a rate as high as 4.8% for these patients. However, in their own patients they could only identify a rate of 0.2%. Several reviews and reports have led to the suggestion that extreme turning or extension of the head may introduce a vascular risk factor for perioperative stroke. This is supported by magnetic resonance imaging (MRI) studies of the anatomic consequences of such head positions,[44] transcranial Doppler studies showing the potential for flow decrements with head extension,[45] a brainstem evoked potential case report,[46] and the beauty parlor stroke syndrome wherein vertebrobasilar ischemic symptoms were associated with head extension during head shampoo in a hair salon.[47] Another graphic demonstration of this effect was published by Grundy et al.[46] Her group showed a loss of brainstem evoked response that was clearly related to head turning for a posterior fossa procedure and was thought to have a vascular cause.

PERIOPERATIVE INTRACRANIAL HEMORRHAGE

Definitive studies on the pathogenesis of perioperative intracranial hemorrhage have not been published outside of the neurosurgical context.

Intracranial hemorrhage in postcraniotomy patients has been studied by Basali et al.[48] In a retrospective review of over 11 000 craniotomy patients, their group found an ICH incidence of 0.77%. Evaluating the role of hypertension, they determined that a systolic blood pressure greater than 160 mm Hg after intracranial surgery is a risk factor for the development of ICH.

Eng et al.[49] published an example of intraoperative re-rupture of a previously ruptured cerebral aneurysm during induction of anesthesia. This patient was already intubated and they report no significant hemodynamic changes with induction of anesthesia. Nonetheless, aneurysmal rupture was observed and cerebrovascular consequences were documented with concurrent transcranial Doppler ultrasonography. They observed a temporary transient intracranial circulatory arrest. Although these authors did not observe an association between high blood pressure and this event, there is enough correlation of SAH with chronic hypertension as a risk factor to suggest that it is similarly a perioperative risk factor. Ohkuma et al[50] reported an association between hypertension and early aneurysmal rebleeding. This supports the practice of vigorously preventing hypertension in patients with cerebral aneurysms.

PERIOPERATIVE STROKE PREVENTION AND TREATMENT

Extensive recommendations or research reports for the perioperative evaluation of patients with cerebrovascular disease are lacking.

In the absence of such research the above-noted factors regarding the pathophysiology of perioperative stroke can probably be used as a reasonable guide for stroke prevention. First and perhaps most important, the anesthesiologist and surgeon should have information regarding previous incidents of cerebral ischemia. Such information should prompt a search for prior evaluations that may include computed tomography (CT), angiography, ultrasound, and other types of assessments of the intracranial circulation. This information can then be used to decide whether to proceed or whether to adjust anesthetic management to try to deal with the risk factors.

In the process of making such determinations, cerebrovascular reserve should be considered. Any patient with carotid or intracranial atherosclerotic lesions can be assumed to have impaired cerebrovascular reserve, as can anyone with a history of transient ischemic attacks not followed by an evaluation. Any patient with intracranial edema should also be considered to have impaired reserve. Any patient judged to have impaired cerebrovascular reserve requires special attention by the anesthesiologist to ensure that stroke-causing physiologic stresses are avoided, even though they may be tolerated in the routine management of otherwise healthy patients. Examples of this include hemoglobin (Hb) concentration less than 10 gm%, or a mean arterial pressure (MAP) less than that of the awake baseline. The use of additional monitors such as encephalography (EEG), evoked potentials, or transcranial Doppler to confirm intraoperative flow should be considered a reasonable course, although such monitoring is unproven to affect outcome in any prospective study. Newer blood flow[51] and autoregulation[52,53] continuous monitoring techniques are under development and are discussed in more detail subsequently.

Arrhythmias, particularly atrial fibrillation, as aforementioned, put a patient at particulary high risk of perioperative stroke. Perhaps there is an adverse synergistic interaction between the hypercoagulable state and this arrhythmia. Nonetheless, it is prudent to consider the possibility that a patient with perioperative atrial fibrillation could have an atrial thrombus ready to become a perioperative embolus. Moreover, if atrial fibrillation arises in the perioperative context it is imperative that it be addressed with every effort made to produce a rapid cardioversion back to sinus rhythm.[54]

Perioperative intracranial hemorrhage is most likely related to hypertensive episodes in the context of individual risk factors. Thus, in patients with known cerebral aneurysm, hypertension, which might otherwise be tolerated, should be aggressively treated. Intracerebral hemorrhage, also, is likely related to perioperative hypertension. As previously mentioned, in the context of intracranial surgery, a systolic blood pressure greater than 160 mm Hg has been linked to postoperative intracranial hermorrhage.[48] Certainly in this specific context, then, this should be held as a reasonable goal to prevent ICH. There have been no other studies like this in the non-neurosurgical setting. Nonetheless, in general, it is better to err on the side of not contributing to a hypertensive-induced ICH, Therefore, 160 mm Hg seems like a reasonable maximal blood pressure to accept in other settings.

PRINCIPLES OF BRAIN-ORIENTED PHYSIOLOGIC MANAGEMENT

The essence of satisfactory perioperative neurologic care is to provide a physiologic and biochemical milieu that will promote a good recovery. Topics addressed here pertaining to perioperative neurologic care include oxygenation, positive end-expiratory pressure, ventilation, temperature, glycemic control, and cardiovascular issues.

OXYGENATION

Pao_2 Physiology Hypoxemia, usually defined as a state when the partial pressure of oxygen in arterial blood (Pao_2) is less than approximately 50 to 60 mm Hg, is associated with cerebral vasodilation.[55] Conversely, hyperoxemia and its accompanying hypocapnea have a vasonstrictive effect, as demonstrated by Floyd et al,[56] in a group of healthy volunteers, Nakajima et al[57] evaluated this phenomenon in patients with cerebrovascular disease, finding that areas of the brain with impaired cerebrovascular reserve were not adversely affected by hyperoxia.

The optimal Pao_2 in a brain-injured patient is presently unclear. There are data to support hyperoxic therapy, as well as data to suggest that such an approach is deleterious.[58] Furthermore, the bedside decision about Pao_2 management is coupled to cerebrovascular reserve issues, previously discussed. Thus a low Pao_2 that would normally be tolerated through vasodilation may be less well tolerated if vasodilatory reserve is compromised with, for example, carotid occlusion, brain edema, or anemia.

Fiskum et al,[59] among, others have reported in laboratory studies that hyperoxic therapy promotes the generation of free radicals and that such oxidative stress causes mitochondrial injury, which will act to impair neurologic recovery. This notion from in vitro considerations is supported by in vivo studies in rodents and dogs that demonstrate worse neurologic outcomes when hyperoxia is used before or after an ischemic insult.[60-62] Empirical support for the notion of hyperoxic toxicity has been provided through a study by Kilgannon et al,[58] who reported that hyperoxia was independently associated with increased in-hospital mortality after resuscitation for cardiac arrest.

Conversely, with the advent of reports supporting the feasibility and reliability of brain tissue partial pressure of oxygen (Po_2) monitoring,[63] data are accumulating to suggest that normoxemic therapy, in the context of cerebral tissue hypoxia, may promote ischemic injury.[63-65] Many recent reports from a nonrandomized retrospective and prospective series of both traumatic and SAH patients have described that a partial pressure of oxygen (Po_2) in brain tissue equaling less than 20 to 30 mm Hg is associated with worsened neurologic outcome (**Fig. 85-3**).[63,66-72] Notably, however, these studies did not examine for the effects of hyperoxia, which is the negative situation identified by Fiskum et al (described previously)[59]; rather, these studies point out the value of avoiding tissue hypoxia, perhaps at the cost of developing systemic hyperoxia but not intracranial hyperoxia. However, one side observation that falls out of these studies is the potential (theoretical) impact of avoiding hyperoxia; brain tissue oxygen monitoring allows one to provide that minimal fraction of inspired oxygen (Fio_2) which permits the optimal (not too high or too low) oxygen level in brain tissue. Moreover, the results of Jaeger et al[73] suggest the notion that an alternate way to use brain tissue Po_2 data is to help identify the autoregulatory optimum for a given patient.

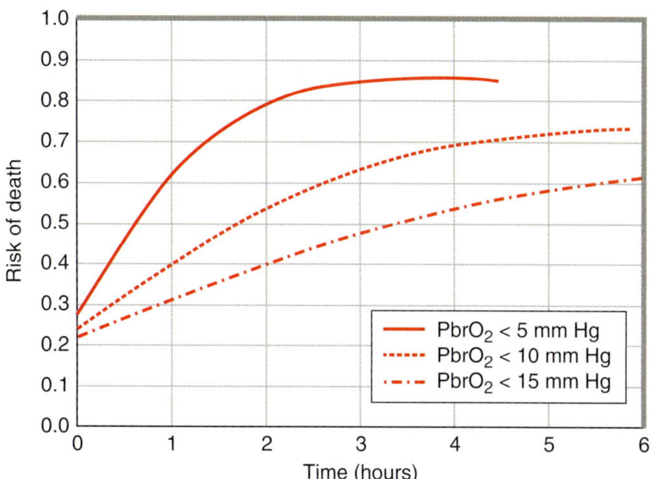

FIGURE 85-3. Relative risk of death as related to initial low brain Po_2 values categorized into groups <5, <10, and <15 mm Hg. Characterization follows from layering the curves, where <5 worse <10 worse <15. Note that the curves stabilize at long durations of hypoxia. [From van den Brink W, van Santbrink H, Steyerberg E, et al. Brain oxygen tension in severe head injury. *Neurosurgery.* 2000;46:868-878, with permission.]

Given these potentially conflicting therapeutic priorities, it seems that the most sensible approach at this time is as follows: In the presence of a brain tissue Po_2 monitor, adjust physiologic parameters to keep oxygen tension in brain tissue ($Pbro_2$) at greater than 20 mm Hg. This may entail the use of Fio_2 at greater than 60% with concomitant risk of pulmonary oxygen toxicity.[74] It seems that this risk can be incurred for 1 to 2 days; however, continued dependence on toxic pulmonary oxygen concentrations should produce a time-dependent imperative for caregivers to decrease Fio_2, even if this means using higher airway pressure or allowing $Pbro_2$ to decrease after a few days. As bedside computing technology improves, the added benefit of measuring ORx, as described by Jaeger et al,[73] to optimize blood pressure may be an added use of brain tissue Po_2 monitoring.

In the absence of a $Pbro_2$ monitor, the clinician is left to base therapy on assumptions about brain oxygenation. If the clinician believes that many brain areas are well perfused and at risk for hyperoxia, then pulmonary management should aim for a Pao_2 just sufficient to produce oxygen saturation (Sao_2) greater than 95%. Conversely, if there is elevated ICP and/or areas of brain hypoperfusion, then a reasonable empiric approach would be to utilize an Fio_2 of 0.60. This will maximize Pao_2 and $Pbro_2$ without a significant risk of acute pulmonary injury.

POSITIVE END-EXPIRATORY PRESSURE

Positive end-expiratory pressure (PEEP) is a modality commonly used to control Pao_2, and it is known to have important effects on ICP. The mechanism is cardiovascular and is discussed in greater detail in the section Cardiovascular Issues later.

VENTILATION

$Paco_2$ Physiology The partial pressure of carbon dioxide in arterial blood ($Paco_2$) is determined by the balance between CO_2 production and elimination. CO_2 production is determined by use of the metabolic rate and respiratory quotient (ie, CO_2 production divided by O_2 consumption, which is ordinarily 0.8). Factors that may increase CO_2 production are hyperthyroidism, fever, elevated catecholamine levels, exercise, sepsis, and some pharmacologic stimulants. The respiratory quotient is affected by energy metabolism; intake of calories in excess of needs results in lipogenesis, a CO_2-producing process. The net effect is that more CO_2 is produced than oxygen is consumed.[75]

Carbon dioxide elimination is determined by use of minute ventilation and dead space measurements. There is a linear relationship between minute ventilation and $Paco_2$ such that one can describe a simple proportion to predict the $Paco_2$ that will result with a given change in minute ventilation. Dead space effects are more complex. There are 2 types of dead space: anatomic and physiologic. Anatomic dead space is that portion of the airways that do not participate in gas exchange because they are not proximate to pulmonary capillaries. Such structures include the mouth, trachea, bronchi, and other large airways. Notably, anatomic dead space is roughly halved via endotracheal intubation and halved again by conversion from translaryngeal intubation to tracheostomy. In contrast, physiologic dead space is that portion of non–gas-exchanging ventilation that occurs in alveoli that are suboptimally perfused. Thus physiologic dead space will be increased in 2 ways: by anything that increases the amount of gas in alveoli without a commensurate increase in alveolar perfusion, or by anything that may decrease perfusion to alveoli without a commensurate decrease in ventilation. Physiologic situations associated with elevated physiologic dead space include use of PEEP in compliant lungs, pulmonary emboli, or shock. A more detailed overview of this physiology can be found in West.[75]

In the healthy brain CBF varies linearly with a $Paco_2$ between about 20 and 60 mm Hg.[76] The mechanism of effect is thought to be related to the effects of $Paco_2$ on cerebrospinal fluid (CSF) pH.[77] Thus patients who are chronically hypercapneic and sustain pH adjustment in the CSF may not be hyperemic. These patients, of course, may be expected

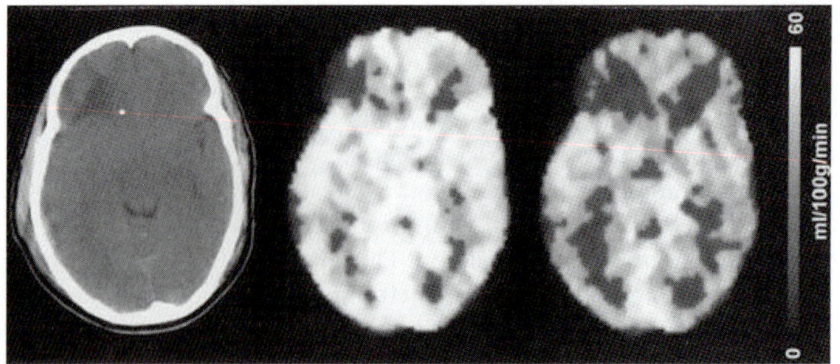

FIGURE 85-4. Effect of hyperventilation on the burden of hypoperfusion. Radiographic computed tomography (left) and grayscale positron emission tomographic imaging of cerebral blood flow obtained from a 31-year-old man 7 days after injury at relative normocapnia (middle), $Paco_2$ 35 torr (4.7 kPa), and hypocapnia (right) 26 torr (3.5 kPa). Voxels with cerebral blood flow less than 10 mL/100 g/min are shaded in black. Note right frontal contusion and small parietal subdural hematoma. Baseline intracranial pressure (ICP) was 21 mm Hg, and baseline cerebral perfusion pressure (CPP) was 74 mm Hg. Baseline jugular venous oxygen saturation ($Sjvo_2$) values of 70% and arteriovenous oxygen content difference ($AVDO_2$) of 3.7 mL/dL are consistent with hyperemia and support the use of hyperventilation for ICP control. Hyperventilation resulted in decrease of ICP to 17 mm Hg and increase of CPP to 76 mm Hg, with maintenance of $Sjvo_2$ and $AVDO_2$ within desirable ranges (58% and 5.5 mL/dL, respectively). Despite these values of $Sjvo_2$ and $AVDO_2$, however, baseline critically hypoperfused brain volume was 141 mL and increased to 428 mL with hyperventilation. These increases were observed in both perilesional and normal regions of brain tissue. [From Coles J, Minhas P, Fryer T, et al. Effect of hyperventilation on cerebral blood flow in traumatic head injury: clinical relevance and monitoring correlates. *Crit Care Med.* 2002;30:1950-1959, with permission.]

to sustain even more profound decreases in CBF with decrements in $Paco_2$ to equivalent levels.

Generally, the $Paco_2$-mediated changes in CBF have no neurologic import in health. However, in the context of head injury or other causes of ICP elevation, the effects can be profound because the changes in CBF induce changes in intracranial blood volume. In a brain with little capacitance for such a change in intracranial contents, the change in $Paco_2$ can have a significant impact on the intracranial pressure.

Thus for many years hyperventilation was embraced as a mainstay of the treatment of intracranial hypertension.[78] However, such therapy was observed to produce a significant cerebral oligemia; the lowered ICP[79] often developed from a low CBF baseline and a hyperventilation-induced ischemic burden developed (**Fig. 85-4**).[79] Conversely, in patients with brain injury, elevated $Paco_2$ was noted at times to lead to both high ICP and high CBF, producing a therapeutic quandary. Moreover, adding to the dilemma were observations from the basic science literature of some neuroprotective side effects associated with hypercapnic cerebral acidosis.[80]

Optimal $Paco_2$ Relatively recent studies debunked the previously accepted theory that hyperventilation is an automatic and necessary element of treatment for head injury. Muizelaar et al[81] conducted a prospective randomized study of the efficacy of hyperventilation in traumatic brain injury (TBI). Their outcome data showed a persuasively negative impact of hyperventilation (**Fig. 85-5**) such that it has been abandoned as a routine therapy in traumatic brain injury. However, there are some situations where it is still accepted. Some authors suggest that brain oxygen monitoring by either jugular oximetry or tissue $Pbro_2$ can be used to guide the use of hyperventiliation.[82] Direct CBF measuring techniques could also be used. Notably, such information can allow the clinician to identify whether the patient has an element of hyperemia contributing to the elevated ICP. Logically, this situation seems an appropriate use for hyperventilation therapy, but this notion has not undergone rigorous scrutiny.

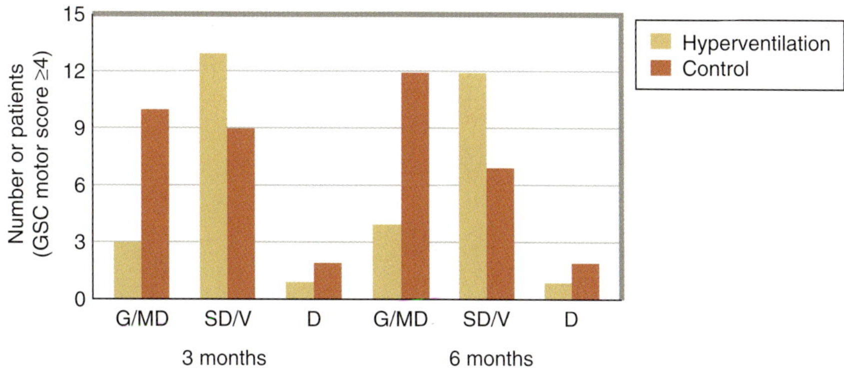

FIGURE 85-5. Head trauma patients were randomized to receive hyperventilation or normoventilation. Outcome was worse in hyperventilated patients. Outcomes: G, good; MD, moderate disability; SD, severe disability; V, vegetative; D, dead. [Data from Muizelaar J, Marmarou A, Ward J, et al. Adverse effects of prolonged hyperventilation in patients with severe head injury: a randomized clinical trial. *J Neurosurg.* 1991;75:731-739.]

TEMPERATURE

Temperature has a profound effect on the brain. Fever is convincingly associated with worsened outcomes including greater release and toxicity of neurotoxic amino acids, mismatch between flow and metabolism, oxidative stress, and many other likely unknown processes.[83,84] In normal brain, with every 1°C reduction in brain temperature, hypothermia produces a 7% reduction in the cerebral metabolic rate for oxygen.[85] The consequent result is a decrease in the consumption of energy metabolites and an increase in time until an hypoxic stress produces high-energy phosphate depletion, thus increasing the time that the hypoxia can be tolerated.[86] This reduction in cerebral metabolic rate for oxygen cannot explain the neuroprotective effect of mild hypothermia, which must be due to synergism of many physicochemical mechanisms. If one compares the neuroprotective efficacy of hypothermia with that produced by an anesthetic producing an equivalent decrement in cerebral metabolic rate, one always observes greater protection by hypothermia. This is thought to be somehow related to the differential effects of hypothermia and anesthetics on the compartments of brain energy metabolism.[87] Anesthetics reduce metabolic processes related to the work of the neuron (ie, neurotransmitter synthesis and metabolism), whereas hypothermia also affects the compartment responsible for constitutive activities of the cell (ie, membrane integrity, ionic concentration homeostasis, and so on). In addition, there are other biochemical processes that contribute to hypothermic protection. For example, with mild hypothermia there is a substantial blunting of the release of neurotoxic dicarboxylic amino acids such as glutamate and aspartate.[88]

It is thus not surprising that there are countless case reports and basic science studies showing the neuroprotective potential of hypothermia across a broad range of neurologic insults. It is of interest that clinical studies do not uniformly show comparable efficacy.

Hypothermia has been studied and clinically used for much of the 20th century. This interest arose from anecdotes describing miraculous recovery from drowning and other brain ischemia situations in cold environments. Deep hypothermic conditions have been used for many years for neuroprotection during cardiac surgery and during therapeutically induced deep hypothermic cardiac arrest for a variety of procedures.[89,90]

Used at less extreme levels, hypothermia has also been reported to be neuroprotective, although not uniformly so in recent studies. This discussion will focus on moderate hypothermia (30°C-34°C).

There are many reports of neuroprotection with hypothermia in traumatic brain injury. However, all these reports are single-institution studies. When hypothermia was examined in multi-institutional studies, protection could not be demonstrated.[91] However, notably, in a study by Clifton et al, neuroprotection was reported if the patient arrived already hypothermic, and rapid rewarming may have contributed to some of the negative findings.[92,93] This supports the notion that speed of induction and suspension of hypothermia may not have been uniformly applied across the participating institutions in the multi-institutional studies. Clifton et al[93] make a persuasive argument in this regard, asserting that significant degradation of the signal-to-noise ratio may have made detection of hypothermic neuroprotection very difficult. The variables contributing to this, which they documented, are the extensive practice variation that occurs across the United States in the approach to management of head trauma, many of which likely have an impact on outcome, and differences in admission temperature. This latter factor may have important geographic and climactic origins. Moreover, hypothermia requires an attentive multidisciplinary approach in order for it to be rapidly and safely induced. (The problem of clinical heterogeneity in the context of failed neuroprotection studies has been discussed in an editorial by Kofke.[94]) Hypothermia is associated with coagulopathy, immune suppression, and worsened pneumonia, among other effects.

Induction of moderate hypothermia (28°C-32°C) before cardiac arrest has been used successfully since the 1950s to protect the brain against the global ischemia that occurs during some open-heart surgeries. Data from Cheung et al provide recent biochemical support for this with their suggestion that about 30 minutes is a neurophysiologically identified safe limit for deep hypothermic arrest.[95] In additional unpublished studies at the University of Pennsylvania, Cheung's group has further correlated this 30-minute time limit for deep hypothermic arrest with retrograde perfusion of the brain between evoked potentials and biomarkers for brain injury taken from blood flowing from the ischemic human brain. Induction of hypothermia after return of spontaneous circulation (ROSC) following cardiac arrest has been associated with improved functional recovery and reduced cerebral histologic deficits in various animal models of cardiac arrest.[96-99] These and similar studies led to concurrent publication in the *New England Journal of Medicine* of 2 single-institution studies showing a neuroprotective effect of moderate hypothermia applied to patients sustaining out-of-hospital cardiac arrest.[100,101] These patients sustained a return of spontaneous circulation, but on initial examination were not responsive and thus were randomized to the protocol. The protection was observed when the target hypothermic temperature was successfully achieved up to 6 hours after the return of spontaneous circulation (**Fig. 85-6**). A summary of these 2 studies is presented in **Table 85-3**.

On the basis of the published evidence to date, the Advanced Life Support (ALS) Task Force of the International Liaison Committee on Resuscitation (ILCOR) made the following recommendations in October 2002[102]:

- Unconscious adult patients with spontaneous circulation after out-of-hospital cardiac arrest should be cooled to 32°C to 34°C for 12 to 24 hours when the initial rhythm was ventricular fibrillation.
- Such cooling may also be beneficial for other rhythms or in-hospital cardiac arrest.

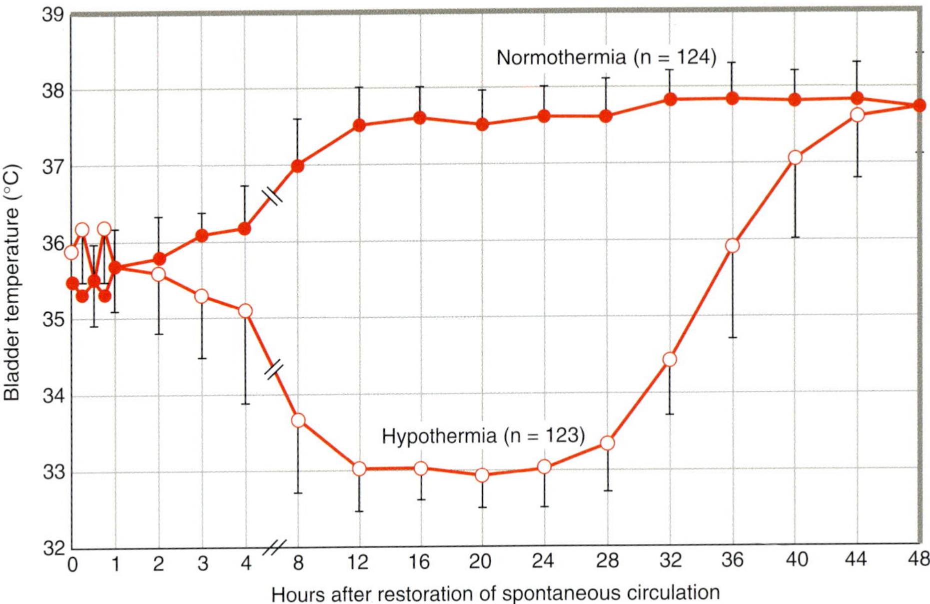

FIGURE 85-6. Time course for temperature in control and hypothermic patients after cardiac arrest. [From Hypothermia after Cardiac Arrest Study Group. Mild therapeutic hypothermia to improve the neurologic outcome after cardiac arrest. *N Engl J Med*. 2002;346:549-556.]

Although these data seem compelling in support of the use of hypothermia after global brain ischemia in various contexts, there are some potential issues to consider in applying these observations to the perioperative situation. These studies were very selective in their entry criteria. Thus up to 92% of cardiac arrests were excluded. Moreover, the 2 studies were not blinded, a practice that is thought to be essential to such investigations; this was clearly impossible for this specific therapy. In addition, Darby[103] suggests that nonuniform neurologic entry criteria were used. There has been some doubt as to whether they studied normothermia or simply prevention of fever, as the normothermia group had an increase in core temperature of up to 38°C, as is often seen after cardiac arrest. It is also important to note that the therapy is not trivial to implement and is associated with some morbidity. Hypothermia was associated with higher systemic vascular resistance, lower cardiac output, and higher blood glucose, and 22% of hypothermic patients developed complications, especially pneumonia, although statistical significance was not achieved.

TABLE 85-3 Summary of Postcardiac Arrest Hypothermia Studies

	Europe[100]		Australia[101]	
Study	Cold	Warm	Cold	Warm
Percentage dead	41	55	51	68
Percentage with good neurologic outcome	55	39	49	26
Time of assessment	6 months		Discharge	
N	136	137	43	34
Target temperature (°C)	32-34	Normal	33	
How cooled/warmed	Custom cold air mattress; ice	Nothing	Cold packs	
Time to target temperature (h)	4		2	
Duration of cold (h)	24		12	
Mode of rewarm	Passive		Active at 18 h	

One controversial issue is whether findings from animal experiments and published clinical studies are enough to extend the use of therapeutic mild hypothermia to patients who remain comatose after cardiac arrest from any rhythm, after in-hospital or perioperative cardiac arrest, and after cardiac arrest in children. Moreover, many perioperative cardiac arrests have noncardiac causes (eg, hemorrhage, anesthesia), and because the use of therapeutic hypothermia has not been studied to a significant extent in this population, its relative risks and benefits are unknown. Kofke suggests in an editorial that in cases like this, the value of the potential benefit, preservation of neural function, is so important as to merit the risk from uncertainty.[104] Further research is needed to determine the optimal duration of therapeutic hypothermia, optimum target temperature, and rates of cooling and rewarming. Animal data suggest that the sooner cooling is initiated after reperfusion from cardiac arrest, the better the outcome, although an impressive therapeutic benefit was seen in clinical studies when cooling was delayed for several hours. One important finding from these studies and from those investigating traumatic brain injury is that normothermia should be restored only slowly, as rebound hyperthermia is common and should be avoided.

Focal ischemia can be categorized as temporary or permanent. Temporary ischemia occurs often during aneurysm clipping surgery when a large cerebral artery may be temporarily occluded to facilitate clipping of the aneurysm. Typically this lasts only a few minutes, but occasionally it can last longer than 15 minutes such that risks arise for the development of ischemic injury. Ample animal data support the potential value of hypothermia in this context[105-107] and was the reason that most neuroanesthesiologists in the United States routinely used it prophylactically in patients undergoing cerebral aneurysm clipping up until 2005. At that time, another multi-institutional study, the Intraoperative Hypothermia for Aneurysm Surgery Trial (IHAST)[108] in over 1000 patients randomized to moderate hypothermia or normothermia, was unable to detect a difference in either stroke rate or cognitive deficits. Thus the use of prophylactic moderate hypothermia for this clinical context has been largely abandoned.

However, 1 criticism, similar to some of the issues with the Clifton TBI study,[91] is that the IHAST study, by examining all aneurysm patients without measuring the degree of intraoperative ischemia, may also have had a signal-to-noise problem. Only a small subset of the study group may actually have had a risk of stroke-inducing ischemia. Arguing against this in this case was the scrupulous oversight given to the physiologic support of all of the patients at the various sites and the power analysis that was done on the pilot data patients who were presumably reflective of the entire group. Notably, the pilot data came from a single institution study that showed a protective effect.[109] Nonetheless, this negative study supports not using prophylactically applied moderate hypothermia in unselected cases.

So, left unresolved in my opinion are 2 issues: whether it would be useful to apply hypothermia in a case that is expected to be complex with a high likelihood of significant focal ischemia, and whether rapid induction of moderate hypothermia could be of value in the patient in whom significant focal ischemia is actively occurring. I believe that a neuroprotective effect in this specific situation may have been missed in the IHAST study. Taking into account the data from many neuroprotective animal studies, and the possible therapeutic gain versus expected outcome and risks of the intervention, hypothermia seems a reasonable approach in cases where temporary focal ischemia is thought to be very likely.[104]

An opposite situation is that of fever, which, in both animal and clinical studies, has been convincingly associated with exacerbation of neurologic outcome in the injured brain. Many neuroscience intensive care unit (NeuroICU) patients have recurrent problems with significant fever in excess of 39°C in the absence of identifiable sepsis. Indeed, in a prospective quantification of 428 consecutive patients admitted to neurovascular or neurotrauma ICUs, 46.7% of patients had at least 1 febrile episode.[110] This is most likely a sequela of the neurologic process, thought by 1 group of authors to at times reflect autonomic dysfunction[111] induced by the neurologic injury.[112] SAH is an independent risk factor for development of fever without identifiable cause.[113] The notion that fever kills neurons is gaining widespread acceptance and is based on many clinical studies showing the improvement in neurologic outcome associated with prevention of fever. Normalization of fever in SAH patients with microdialysis probes was observed to improve the interstitial metabolic profile.[114]

In a study by Castillo et al,[114a] the mortality rate in patients who were hyperthermic within the first 72 hours after stroke was 15.8%, compared to a 1% mortality rate in patients who were normothermic during that time. Hyperthermia that occurred within the first 24 hours after stroke, without respect to infectious or noninfectious origin, was independently related to a larger infarct volume, and worse neurologic deficits and dependency 3 months postinjury.[114a] Azzimondi and Bassein[115] reported that fever of 37.9°C or above proved to be an independent risk factor predicting a worse outcome, and patients with high fever were far more likely to die within the first 10 days than those with lower temperatures. A prospective study by Reith et al[116] of 390 consecutive cases of acute stroke classified patients into 3 admission-temperature groups: hypothermic (36.5°C or less), normothermic (36.6°C-37.5°C) and hyperthermic (above 37.5°C). They showed that admission body temperature was highly correlated with initial stroke severity, size of the infarct, mortality rate, and poor outcome. For a 1°C difference in body temperature, the relative risk of poor outcome was more than doubled. This was supported by Ginsberg and Busto,[117] who reported that in stroke patients, fever that occurs soon after stroke onset is most strongly associated with poor outcome. Body temperature was significantly higher in patients who died within 3 days after admission compared with the rest of the study population. Moreover, in ICH patients surviving the first 72 hours after hospital admission, the duration of fever is associated with poor outcome and seems to be a prognostic factor in these patients.[118] In SAH fever is associated with vasospasm and poor outcome independent of hemorrhage severity or the presence of infection.

Pharmacologic methods can be used to control fever. Such modalities include acetaminophen[119] and ibuprofen,[120] although there is some evidence suggesting that ibuprofen is not efficacious in the context of ischemic stroke.[121] Acetaminophen's value can be limited by hepatotoxicity. It is also of theoretical concern that acetaminophen is an oxidizing agent that even at subhepatotoxic levels may decrease glutathione to lessen potentially helpful free-radical scavenging processes.[122] Ibuprofen is associated with gastric ulceration and bleeding.[123]

An alternate method is to use a hypothermia blanket or an indwelling hypothermia catheter.[124] Both techniques are based on a servo-controlled system wherein the cooling bath temperature decreases when the patient's temperature starts to rise. In our NeuroICU we have generated illustrations of temperature curves indicating that it is possible to virtually eliminate fever from the pathophysiology of severe brain injury. Notably, this has created a new vital sign, $T_{bathmin}$, which indicates the minimum bath temperature that was needed to prevent fever in a given patient. Ascertaining a low $T_{bathmin}$ may indicate a need to initiate an investigation for infection.

GLYCEMIC CONTROL

In non-neurologic critical care populations, recent randomized trials have yielded conflicting results regarding the importance of glycemic control. The initial "Leuven" study[125] in postcardiac surgery patients indicated a mortality improvement with tight glucose control in the 80 to 110 gm% range. This was a single-center study of a homogeneous patient population with specially trained nursing staff. However, subsequent studies in medical and more heterogeneous groups and muticenter studies have been unable to demonstrate a beneficial effect from tight glucose control.[126-128] Van den Berghe et al have nicely reviewed the issues in interpreting these conflicting studies with speculation as to contributing factors.[129] To date, none of the studies of tight glucose control have focused on patients with cerebral ischemia and, due to considerations reviewed elsewhere in this chapter, glucose management with neurologic disease is somewhat enigmatic.[130]

Hyperglycemia has been associated with exacerbation of brain damage with both head trauma and cerebral ischemia.[131-134] This is not a straightforward issue, however, because of the aforementioned conflicting clinical studies as well as pathophysiology considerations. Clearly, neuronal damage after global cerebral ischemia is exacerbated with hyperglycemia.[132,135-138] Some studies have suggested that a blood glucose greater than 120 gm% is deleterious in stroke patients.[131] However, subsequent studies with subhuman primates subjected to global ischemia have suggested a threshold of around 180 gm%.[138] It is apparent that blood glucose greater than 400 gm% causes striking worsening of neurologic outcome with global ischemia.[132,137]

With focal cerebral ischemia, the role of blood glucose is a good deal less clear. Animal and human studies have shown that hyperglycemia either worsens, does not affect, or lessens brain damage.[131,139-156] One report by Prado et al[153] in rats suggested that the discriminating factor in whether or not brain damage is worsened with hyperglycemia is the presence of collateral flow. Areas of the brain with minimal collaterals were not affected or were improved with hyperglycemia. Brain areas with a continued trickle of anaerobic hyperglycemic flow sustained worsened brain damage. Presumably the continued substrate supply in oligemic (not ischemic) areas allowed greater accumulation of organic acids in the cells, leading to worsening of brain damage.[133,144] Unfortunately, these observations are difficult to apply clinically to specific patients with focal ischemia.

Even if low levels of hyperglycemia were deleterious, it would not be straightforward to treat. Aggressive therapy of hyperglycemia would impose a risk of producing hypoglycemia, with deleterious effects arising therefrom.[157] Moroever, Oddo et al[158] report a paradoxical increase in interstitial lactate on microdialysis monitoring associated with tight glucose control, suggesting a direct deleterious effect of tight glucose control. The genesis of this increased lactate in the context of low precursor glucose is enigmatic, and thus the interpretation of these microdialysis data is unsettled. Therefore, given the data in the general critical care literature, it seems that a reasonable approach is to aim for a blood glucose of approximately 150 to 180 gm% in all acutely ill hyperglycemic patients at risk of cerebral ischemia, but to be less stringent in blood glucose control in less acutely ill patients who are expected to be in the ICU for less than 3 days. In any event, to avoid having the blood glucose swing to less than 80 gm% or greater than 400 gm%, it should not be allowed to undergo wide variations in concentration. Thus an insulin infusion should be used in acutely ill patients at risk of cerebral anaerobic metabolism who develop hyperglycemia greater than 200 gm%. In these patients, assess glucose levels frequently and titrate to maintain blood glucose at about 150 to 180 gm%. Once the hyperacute phase has resolved, the intensity of glucose monitoring can be lessened somewhat to match the lowered acuity. A sliding-scale insulin paradigm can be used; apply somewhat less stringent goals as the patient is readied for discharge from the ICU setting.

Hyperglycemia has not been shown to have deleterious or protective effects in 2 animal models of status epilepticus.[159,160] The model used in the report by Swan and Meldrum[160] produced limbic system damage whereas the report by Kofke et al[159] used a model producing substantia nigra damage. Nigral damage in this model is associated with hypermetabolic lactic acidosis,[161] which should have been exacerbated with hyperglycemia. The fact that hyperglycemia did not exacerbate nigral damage suggests one of the following: either metabolic acidosis may not be an important factor in the development of brain damage after seizure, or the lactic acidosis associated with hyperglycemic exacerbation of ischemic brain damage is not the true pathogenetic culprit but is, rather, an epiphenomenon.

CARDIOVASCULAR ISSUES

Blood Pressure Effects on ICP–Plateau Waves and Determination of Blood Pressure Optimum Lundberg in 1960[162] monitored ICP in hundreds of patients, identifying characteristic patterns of pressure waves. One of these patterns is that of plateau waves, known to be associated with increased cerebral blood volume (CBV).[163] Such waves occur when the ICP abruptly increases to nearly systemic levels for about 15 to 30 minutes, occasionally accompanied by neurologic deterioration. Rosner and Becker[164] provided observations and a synthesis of the data, which convincingly suggest that intracranial blood volume dysautoregulation is responsible for plateau waves. These investigators induced mild heterogeneous head trauma in cats and intensively monitored the animals after the insult. In normally fluctuating blood pressure, the development of plateau waves is preceded by decrements of mean-arterial blood pressure to a range of approximately 70 to 80 mm Hg. In normal brain tissue, cerebral blood volume increases due to autoregulatory vasodilation and blood pressure decreases. Moreover, the increase in CBV is nonlinear; as blood pressure decreases to below 80 mm Hg, CBV increases exponentially.[165] In a setting of abnormal intracranial compliance with the ICP, a small reduction in blood pressure, although in the normotensive range, produces an exponential rise in CBV. This phenomenon is represented by the "elbow" of the classical curve of the intracranial pressure–intracranial volume relationship. Thus a small decrease in blood pressure introduces an exponential change in CBV upon a dramatically increased ICP such that ICP will increase abruptly and to a significant extent. Plateau waves spontaneously resolve with a hypertensive response or with hyperventilation, which acts to oppose the increase in CBV. Clearly, to develop a plateau wave, some portion of the brain must have normally reactive vasculature in some other brain areas with a mass effect and elevated ICP, a situation of heterogeneous autoregulation. Such data suggest that in patients with an elevated ICP in the 80 to 100 mm Hg range, not only should plateau waves be prevented and treated, but also it is probably important to maintain MAP. However, this may be an overly simplistic conclusion based on more recent investigations into the notion of a CPP optimum; this issue is detailed below.

Conversely, systemic hypertension can also increase ICP. Ordinarily, in cases where blood pressure is within the normal autoregulatory range and there is a normal intracranical pressure, changes in blood pressure have no effect on ICP. However, with brain injury and associated vasoparalysis, blood pressure increases are presumed to mechanically produce autoregulatory cerebral vasodilation, which will increase ICP.[166] This observation forms the basis for the notion, detailed below, of using such ICP variations to quantitate autoregulation.[167]

Any consideration of hemodynamics and ICP also has to account for the veins. Blood coursing through the brain runs through arteries, capillaries, veins, the sagittal and other dural sinuses, and then on to the internal jugular and other extracranial veins. In the context of a closed intracranial space, the relationship of these vessels to the tissue and CSF surrounding them becomes important. Notably, several investigators, in laboratory preparations, have observed a distinct drop-off in intraluminal pressure for blood moving from cerebral cortical veins to the sagittal sinus. This phenomenon is most evident when ICP is elevated, and indicates the presence of a vascular waterfall at a point just proximal to the sagittal sinus, whereby the extraluminal high-pressure CSF is acting to impede flow from cortical veins to the sagittal sinus.[168-171] In fact, Nemoto[169] and Nakagawa et al[168] have further observed that the cerebral venous pressure (CVP) tends to be consistently higher than the ICP. The implications of these observations are the following: the elevated ICP begets increased CVP; the increased CVP promotes and exacerbates brain edema, which may have been the initial cause of the intracranial hypertension; and this then leads to a positive feedback cycle wherein increased ICP increases CVP, which increases ICP.[169,172] Thus any other factors that may promote brain edema or otherwise increase ICP in this tenuous situation (eg, high extraventricular drain, systemic hypertension[173] or hypo osmolarity) may initiate such a positive feedback process.

Notably, the Lund group[172] incorporates consideration of these issues of cerebral venous pathophysiology into its treatment approach and suggests that hypertension-induced exacerbation of brain edema increases ICP. The increase in ICP then acts to occlude venous outflow, increasing venous pressure, which in turn acts to further worsen the brain edema, constituting a positive feedback cycle initially started by arterial hypertension.

It thus appears that both increasing and decreasing blood pressure can increase ICP, suggesting the presence of a CPP optimum for ICP. In the absence of any patient-specific physiologic information, this optimum is probably about 80 to 100 mm Hg.

These considerations underlie a current controversy with respect to blood pressure management in the context of elevated ICP. One argument is that blood pressure should be maintained at high levels to ensure adequate CBF and minimize the probability of developing plateau waves. The contrary argument is to use ample fluids and consequent low blood pressure to primarily promote CBF rather than perfusion pressure. It is this author's opinion that the preferred approach would be to induce the lowest blood pressure that allows sufficient CBF as indicated by repeated (preferably bedside) measurements. Recent investigations indicate that such bedside assessment capability should soon be widely available.[51]

Recent advances in transcranial Doppler ultrasonograpy have allowed insights into the dynamic, nearly instantaneous assessment of cerebral autoregulation in critically ill patients. This approach uses the correlation coefficient, determined in real time at the bedside, to make inferences regarding autoregulation. A high correlation of blood flow velocity with ICP suggests poor autoregulation; a lack of correlation is normal. Czosnyka et al[174] observed in TBI patients a U-shaped curvilinear relationship in flow velocity versus arterial blood pressure (ABP), with worse autoregulation (ie, high correlation) at ABP readings of less than 75 mm Hg and greater than 125 mm Hg. The authors noted that increasing ABP also increased ICP, further indicating a correlation-based marker of dysautoregulation, the so-called pressure reactivity index, or PRx.[52,167,175] Dynamic time domain analysis of cerebrovascular autoregulation using transcranial Doppler (TCD) sonography, ICP, brain tissue oxygen partial pressure (Pbo_2), or near-infrared spectroscopy

(NIRS) is a current topic of investigation with promising reports of potential efficacious and valid bedside use.[51,167,176-178] For example, Joshi et al,[52] using the TCD-based autoregulation assessment mean velocity index (Mx) in cardiac surgery patients, reported an association of disturbed Mx with postoperative stroke; autoregulation feasibility in this context was demonstrated with NIRS.[179,180]

The ICP pressure-reactivity index (PRx) is another way to dynamically evaluate autoregulation in a number of conditions.[167,175,181] PRx is a quantitation of the aforementioned description of abnormal dynamic correlation of ICP changes and ABP changes. Reports indicate that PRx correlates well with other autoregulation indices.[52,175,182,183] Steiner et al[167] reported on the use of PRx monitoring in TBI patients to determine the optimal CPP in this population. Patients with better autoregulation in the optimal range as defined by PRx had better outcomes. Moreover, patients with dysautoregulation related to higher ABP with corresponding ICP elevation also had worse outcomes, suggesting that autoregulation monitoring, to ensure adherence to an individual's optimal CPP, may be an outcome-altering ICU measure. Zweifel et al[175] report congruent observations. Notably, PRx, as with TCD-based autoregulation studies, also appears to undergo a U-shaped curvilinear relationship with variations in CPP; in TBI patients it is abnormally high (ie, ICP varies with ABP) at both low (ischemic) and high (hyperemic) CPP. Moreover, further complementing this information are observations of abnormally high oxygen extraction fraction (OEF) and low OEF at these respective ABP extremes. This is underscored by reports of a significant ischemic burden in TBI patients,[79,184-186] suggesting a delicate balance between hypotension-associated hypoperfusion and hypertension-associated edema/ICP exacerbation, both of which will worsen regional ischemia. Taken together, these autoregulation studies introduce the hypothesis that there is an individualized ABP optimum in TBI patients,[175] which should be a therapeutic goal. Autoregulation monitoring is also being reported using a brain tissue oxygen pressure reactivity index (ORx)[73] and an NIRS-rendered cerebral oximetry index (COx), suggesting that noninvasive autoregulation assessment will be a feasible bedside modality that can be used to deliver the optimal CPP.

Blood Pressure Management Blood pressure management is an important issue in most NeuroICU patients and a matter of some concern. Systemic hypertension may exacerbate cerebral edema or intracranial hemorrhage, or have deleterious cardiopulmonary effects such as pulmonary edema or myocardial ischemia. Conversely, blood pressure reduction can lead to insufficient perfusion even at a pressure in the normal range of autoregulation. Moreover, mild blood pressure decreases have been implicated in the genesis of plateau waves. Several important principles apply to the management of blood pressure in NeuroICU patients. These principles are discussed below.

Hypertension When blood pressure is high, a fundamental initial question must be whether or not the pressure is elevated due to normal homeostatic mechanisms that are acting to maintain adequate perfusion. For example, in conditions with inadequate brainstem perfusion, a compensatory hyperadrenergic state may occur, leading to increased blood pressure, which acts to supply sufficient perfusion to maintain aerobic metabolism in the brainstem. If a decision is made to decrease blood pressure, brainstem failure and death may ensue.

Animal data with cerebral ischemia models provide strong support for the notion that sympatholytic drugs should be used to decrease blood pressure if cerebral ischemia is a possibility. When compared to hemorrhage-induced hypotension, ischemic damage occurred to a lesser extent with the use of ganglionic blockade with hexamethonium,[36] central adrenergic blockade with α_2 agonists,[37] and angiotensin-converting enzyme inhibition.[38] Hemorrhaged controls were noted to sustain an increase in exogenous catecholamine concentrations. To test the hypothesis that these catecholamines contributed to brain damage, some of the animals treated with hexamethonium also received

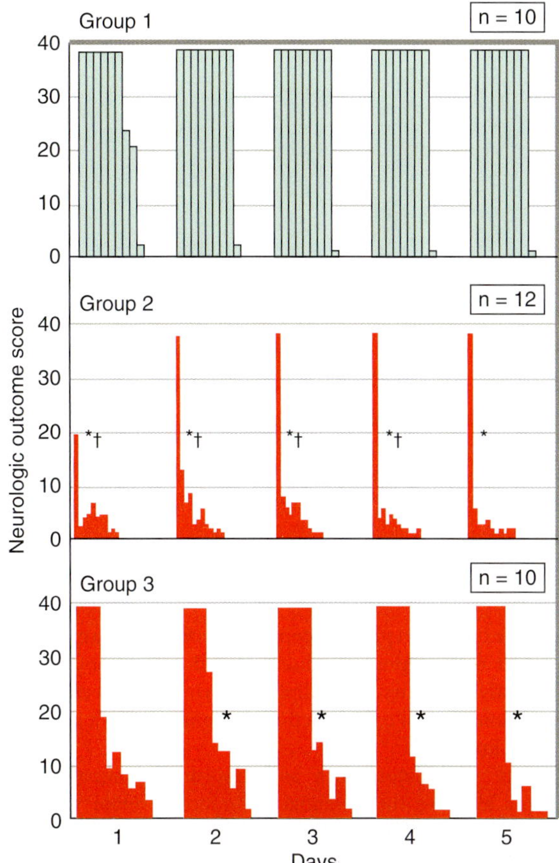

FIGURE 85-7. Neurologic deficit scores after incomplete focal cerebral ischemia in rats over a 5-day examination period. Each bar represents the neurologic score for one rat. $*P < .05$ versus group 1; = $\dagger P < .05$ versus group 3. Rats are ranked according to total outcome score in descending order (0 = normal). Cerebral ischemia was induced with occlusion of 1 carotid artery with hemorrhagic hypotension. Group 1 rats received no vasoactive drugs; group 2 rats received preischemic hexamethonium; group 3 rats received hexamethonium plus intravenous epinephrine and norepinephrine. Protection was conferred by hexamethonium in a catecholamine-reversible manner. [From Werner C, Hoffman W, Thomas C, et al. Ganglionic blockade improves neurologic outcome from incomplete ischemia in rats: partial reversal by exogenous catecholamines. *Anesthesiology.* 1990;73:923, with permission.]

intravenous (IV) catecholamine infusions. Reversal of hexamethonium brain-protective effect was observed in these animals (**Fig. 85-7**).[36] Similarly, brain protection has been observed in laboratory studies with preischemic[188] and preseizure[189] treatment with reserpine, a drug that depletes presynaptic catecholamine stores. Finally, there is a report by Neil-Dwyer et al[190] regarding subarachnoid hemorrhage patients given therapy with phentolamine and/or propranolol or with no sympatholytic agents (**Fig. 85-8**). Subjects who received sympatholytic therapy had significantly better neurologic outcome than controls. In addition, β-adrenergic blocking drugs have not been reported to produce cerebral vasodilatation or increased ICP.[191-193]

Other drugs that may have brain-protective effects are the calcium channel antagonists, also available for antihypertensive therapy. Nimodipine and nicardipine, developed specifically for brain-protection purposes, have been assessed in numerous studies, with several reports of their having conferred protection versus vasospasm and ischemic brain damage.[194-200] Based solely on these observations, these drugs thus become reasonable choices for antihypertensive therapy. Nimodipine and nicardipine are vasodilators; they can modestly increase ICP[201,202]

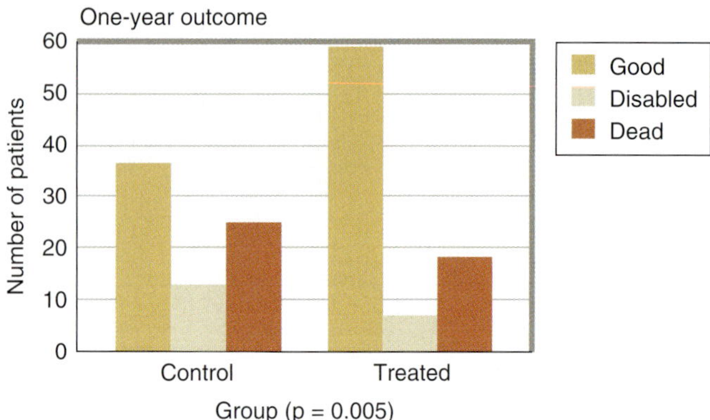

FIGURE 85-8. Subarachnoid hemorrhage patients were randomly treated with propranolol or placebo. Neurologic outcome was better in patients receiving β-blockade. Graph generated from data of Neil-Dwyer et al.[190] [Reprinted from Kofke WA. Critical neuropathophysiology. In: Fink MP, Abraham E, Vincent J-L, et al, eds. *Textbook of Critical Care*. 5th ed. Philadelphia: Elsevier, 2005:285, with permission from Elsevier.]

and may be expected to produce compensatory catecholamine release.[203] Thus, based on the previous discussion, this may obviate some of their protective qualities. Nimodipine moreover has been observed to decrease brain tissue Po_2.[204] Whether this phenomenon can alter outcome is not known.

Peripheral vasodilators such as nitroprusside, nitroglycerin, and hydralazine all have the potential to induce cerebral vasodilatation and thus cause hyperemic intracranial hypertension.[205-208] Moreover, they are associated with a compensatory increase in peripheral catecholamines and renin,[203] factors which theoretically may worsen ischemic brain damage.[36,188] However, the lack of bradycardia and bronchoconstriction associated with the use of these agents may make them the optimal treatment choice in some patients with these conditions. If one of these drugs is selected to treat a patient at risk of neurologic deterioration from ischemia or high ICP, close clinical observation is indicated. Any deterioration would mandate discontinuation of the drug. Such concerns are important for deciding among these 3 drugs. Although hydralazine is convenient to use, it cannot be reversed at the receptor, and its effects can last hours. Thus it may be preferable to use nitroprusside in such situations, as adverse effects can be treated quickly simply by discontinuing the infusion.

It should be clear that the choice of antihypertensive agent in a patient at risk of cerebral ischemia is not straightforward. Therapeutic urgency, sympatholytic and brain-protective side effects, and potential to increase ICP are all important considerations in the choice of an antihypertensive drug.

If it is deemed that blood pressure has to be decreased very quickly, (eg, within minutes), nicardipine in 100- to 500-µg boluses is very effective and safely titratable.[209,210] Once the blood pressure is reduced, a maintenance regimen of nicardipine or another drug can then be started. Alternatively, sodium nitroprusside can be started, although it has a variety of deleterious side effects (elaborated on previously) that might move it down the preference list for an antihypertensive agent in a neurologic patient. Sodium nitroprusside, however, may be the most potent and reliable antihypertensive drug available.

Plateau waves, first reported by Lundberg[162] and associated with neurologic deterioration, were demonstrated by Risberg et al to be associated with cerebral vasodilatation.[163] Rosner and Becker reported that mild reduction in mean arterial blood pressure to the 60 to 80 mm Hg range can be associated with plateau waves.[164] As mentioned previously, the decrease in blood pressure presumably prompts vasodilatation in normally autoregulating tissue. The increase in cerebral blood volume, which is an exponential function as compared with cerebral perfusion pressure,[164] superimposed on the exponential ICP (versus the intracranial volume relationship), then is associated with an explosive hyperemic increase in ICP: a plateau wave. This dynamic then introduces a concern for using any antihypertensive agent (aside from specific, direct cerebrovascular effects): When CPP falls to about 80 mm Hg or less, normal autoregulatoy mechanisms may also increase ICP.

Clearly, any time hypotensive therapy is used in a patient with altered intracranial compliance, edema, or ischemia, very close and recurrent observation of the patient is mandatory. Deterioration should prompt consideration that one of the above processes is occurring. Introduction of corrective therapy should be accompanied by a reconsideration of the need to decrease blood pressure.

Hypotension and Induced Hypertension Hypotensive patients require treatment for their low blood pressure as well as ongoing effort to ascertain the cause of the hypotension. In head trauma patients, consider other injuries that might result in hemorrhage or spinal shock. For instance, loss of blood flow to the brainstem can be associated with hypotension that can be quite difficult to treat. In addition, usual nonneurologic causes of hypotension in an ICU, such as pneumothorax, sepsis, and cardiogenic causes, should also be considered.

When contemplating therapy to increase blood pressure, as may be done with a patient with vasospasm, seriously consider the cost-benefit. Excessive increases in blood pressure can exacerbate cerebral edema.[211-215] This presumably occurs in brain areas with dysautoregulation and blood–brain barrier (BBB)–disruption, such that increasing blood pressure, rather than producing vasoconstriction with no change in rCBF, causes vascular distention, increased rCBF, and transudation of fluid across the damaged BBB. In addition, increases in blood pressure impose a risk for producing or exacerbating intracranial hemorrhage.

Catecholamines used to increase blood pressure are neurotransmitters or are chemically similar to neurotransmitters. It is thus to be expected that if they cross the BBB, neural effects will arise secondary to their use. Normally, exogenously administered catecholamines do not cross the BBB and have no effect on CBF or metabolism.[216] However, catecholamine infusion in the presence of BBB disruption has been shown to lead to increases in blood flow and metabolism.[217] In subarachnoid hemorrhage patients, catecholamine infusions produce a variety of disparate and unpredictable effects on CBF[218] and adrenergic blockade confers neurologic protection.[190] Finally, catecholamines have direct neurotoxic potential, as indicated by data showing neurotoxicity with application directly to the cortex in vivo.[219] Unfortunately, catecholamines are the only clinically accepted routine means to pharmacologically increase blood pressure in NeuroICU patients.

Increasing preload to the heart is one nonpharmacologic method of increasing blood pressure. The use of crystalloid or colloid infusion is generally associated with hemodilution. When this type of infusion is contemplated, consider the effects on a given patient's status. The hemodilution may improve flow to areas where microcirculation is compromised. However, it may be associated with increased CBV and hyperemic intracranial hypertension if hematocrit decreases excessively with compensatory vasodilatation.

Whether to use crystalloid or colloid for this purpose remains controversial. The BBB is functionally an osmometer.[220-225] Thus the added trivial increase in osmolarity with colloid is not a sufficient reason to use it. It makes sense, and is supported by animal studies, that iso-osmolar or slightly hyperosmolar fluids should be used to reduce the possibility of increasing brain edema secondary to fluid administration.

Some advocate the use of induced systemic hypertension with high ICP to prevent plateau waves. As blood pressure increases, incremental increases in vasoconstriction occur in normally reactive tissue and consequently decrease CBV and thus ICP. However, the advantage of this therapy may be offset by increased edema in injured brain regions.

Subarachnoid hemorrhage is an entity particularly notable for catecholamine effects, some of which will be described. However, catecholamine effects also occur with other intracranial processes including increased ICP, stroke, head trauma, or any situation of compromised midbrain-hindbrain oxygen delivery.

Serum catecholamine levels increase dramatically after SAH. Notably, levels peak at the same time as the peak incidence of post-SAH vasospasm, with symptom development corresponding to serum catecholamine levels.[226-229] This phenomenon has led to the notion that hypothalamic injury with excess catecholamine release may be an important factor in the genesis of post-SAH spasm and stroke,[229,230] observations that may be relevant to other intracranial processes previously elaborated. Several lines of evidence further support this hypothesis:

1. The cerebral vasculature is invested somewhat with adrenergic nerves. With SAH, the number of adrenergic receptors in the cerebral vessels decreases.[230] This suggests that denervation hypersensitivity may be occurring such that the increase in humoral catecholamines with SAH produces spasm in hyperreacting vessels.
2. Catecholamine release after SAH is sufficient to produce electrocardiographic changes[226] with ventricular wall motion abnormalities[227] and myocardial injury.[228]
3. Treatment of humans with SAH with β- and α-adrenergic antagonists is associated with an improvement in neurologic outcome[190] (Fig. 85-8) and electrocardiographic abnormalities.[226]
4. In animal models, selective destruction of hindbrain adrenergic nuclei with cephalad projections prevents the development of vasospasm.[229] Moreover, laboratory studies indicate an important role for vasopressin in vasospasm, as vasospasm cannot be produced in vasopressin-deficient rats.[230]
5. As discussed previously, animal data with cerebral ischemia models provide strong support for the notion that catecholamines can exacerbate cerebral ischemia. When compared to hemorrhage-induced hypotension, ischemic damage was decreased with hypotension induced through the use of ganglionic blockade with hexamethonium,[36] central adrenergic blockade with α_2 agonists,[37] and angiotension-converting enzyme inhibition.[38] Hemorrhaged controls were noted to sustain an increase in exogenous catecholamine concentrations. To test the hypothesis that these catecholamines contributed to brain damage some of the animals treated with hexamethonium also received IV catecholamine infusions. Reversal of the hexamethonium brain protective effect was observed in these animals (Fig. 85-7).[36]
6. Brain protection has been observed in laboratory studies with preischemic[188] and preseizure[189] treatment using reserpine, a drug that depletes presynaptic catecholamine stores.
7. Application of catecholamines directly to nonischemic cortical tissue has also been observed to have neurotoxic potential.[240] In addition, intravenous administration can exacerbate brain swelling after head trauma, although this is most likely a direct effect of blood pressure on a dysautoregulating brain (Fig. 85-8) rather than a manifestation of biochemical neurotoxicity.[213]

PEEP and Intracranial Hypertension Positive end-expiratory pressure (PEEP) can increase ICP.[242] Two mechanisms for this can be posited. The first is through impedance of cerebral venous return, which will increase cerebral venous pressure and ICP. The second mechanism is through decreased blood pressure with a reflex increase in cerebral blood volume, which will increase ICP. The data of Huseby et al[243] suggest that cerebral venous effects only occur with very high PEEP.

Shapiro[244] demonstrated increases in ICP in head-injured humans with intracranial hypertension with application of PEEP. Examination of Shapiro's data indicates that the most profound decreases in CPP occurred in patients with PEEP-induced decrements in mean arterial pressure consistent with the notion put forth by Rosner and Becker[164] that decreases in blood pressure increase CBV, which in turn increase ICP. Aidinis et al,[245] in studies with cats, confirmed these observations in a more controlled setting. In addition, they assessed the role of pulmonary compliance, finding that decreased pulmonary compliance with oleic acid injections lessens the effect of PEEP to increase ICP. Such observations indicate that in situations where PEEP is likely to be needed—situations that are often accompanied by decrements in pulmonary compliance—any adverse effects on ICP are less likely to manifest. This phenomenon may be related to observations that hemodynamic effects of PEEP are less apparent with noncompliant lungs[246] such that hypotensive-mediated increases in CBV do not occur.

The intuitive notion that PEEP increases cerebral venous pressure to increase ICP is not as straightforward as some may indicate. In order for PEEP to increase CVP to levels that will increase ICP, the cerebral venous pressure must be equal to at least the ICP (based on previously described notions of a cerebral venous vascular waterfall). Thus the higher the ICP, the higher PEEP must be in order to have such a direct hydraulic effect on ICP. This concept was nicely proved by Huseby et al[243] in dog studies in which PEEP was increased progressively along with different starting levels of ICP (**Fig. 85-9**A). It is important to note that the investigators prevented the development of PEEP-induced decrements in blood pressure, thus avoiding any reflex-mediated increases in cerebral blood volume. They suggested a hydraulic model to better demonstrate this concept (Fig. 85-9B). Thus, for example, if all of a 10 cm H_2O PEEP application was transmitted to the cerebral vasculature (which is unlikely given the decreased pulmonary compliance associated with the need for such PEEP), then ICP will only be affected if it is 10 cm H_2O (7.7 mm Hg) or less and does not increase to a level higher than the applied PEEP. Such observations are consistent with the notion that there is a Starling resistor regulating cerebral venous outflow.[247]

Optimal Hemoglobin Level Anemia is generally well tolerated neurologically except at extreme levels. This indicates the enormous cerebrovascular reserve that, in health, is in place to compensate for blood loss and similar physiologic stresses. The observations of Borgstrom et al[248] in rodents indicate that decreasing Hb levels produce an increase in CBF. This is initially due primarily to decreased viscosity, but as Hb continues to decrease to below 10 gm%, active vasodilatation arises (**Fig. 85-10**). If the brain vasculature is already maximally vasodilated because of other stresses, such as hypoxemia or low cerebral perfusion pressure, then the anemic stress may not be well tolerated and may produce hypoxic/ischemic brain damage.

Supporting observations of anemia-associated cerebral vasodilatation have been noted in a number of studies. Floyd et al noted this phenomenon in humans after cardiac surgery (**Fig. 85-11**).[249] Dexter modeled the competing issues of anemia and cerebral vasodilatation mathematically.[249a] His data approximated those of laboratory[249] and empiric observations that an Hb less than 10 gm% associated with vasodilatation can be expected to be deleterious in conditions of altered cerebrovascular reserve. Kim and Kang's[250] observations of post-gastrointestinal (GI) hemorrhage anemia-associated stroke support Dexter and Hindman's calculations. Other supporting data for the relationship of anemia and vasodilatation come from observations in brain-injured and SAH patients: low $Pbro_2$ was associated with anemia,[251] and after transfusion, brain tissue Po_2 increased to exceed an Hb of 10.[252] One of the approaches to managing low $Pbro_2$ is to transfuse to an Hb greater than 10 gm%, based on observations that such therapy can significantly improve brain oxygenation in the context of severe brain injury.

Notwithstanding reports that 7 gm% is optimal in a general critical care population,[253] these above-mentioned observations taken altogether suggest that transfusion to a goal of 10 gm% is reasonable in the context of impaired cerebrovascular reserve.

It should be noted, however, that considerable controversy continues as evidence accumulates of either no improvement or deleterious general[254-257] and neurologic[258-260] effects associated with transfusion, especially if older blood is used.[261] Thus a balance must be sought between risks and benefits such that transfusion is only used when there is good empiric evidence supporting its use or, lacking that, which is the usual situation, when a strong physiologic rationale exists to support the optimal decision.

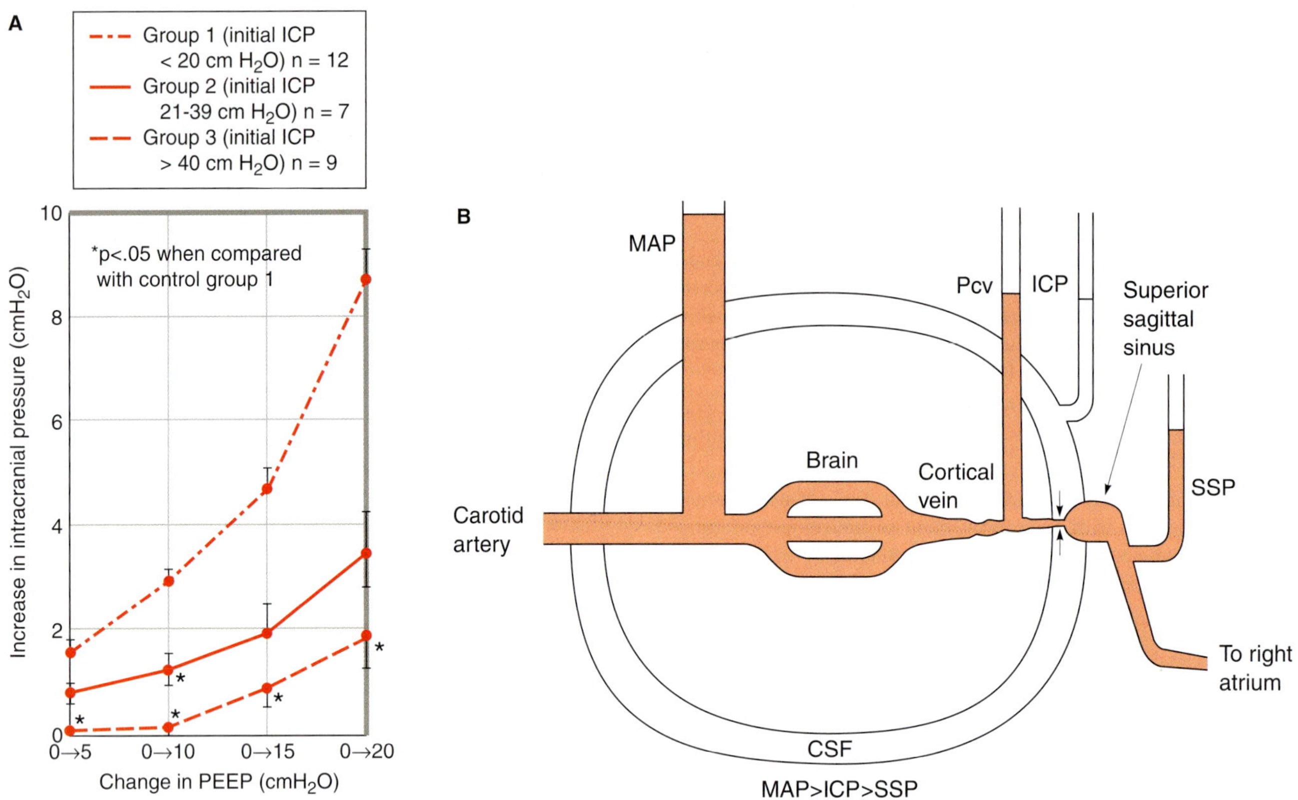

FIGURE 85-9. A. Increases in intracranial pressure (ICP) with positive end-expiratory pressure (PEEP) in dogs. Values are given as mean ± SEM. Group 1 included 12 animals with initial ICP <20 cm H_2O; group 2 included 7 animals with initial ICP 21-39 cm H_2O; group 3 included 9 animals with initial ICP >40 cm H_2O. Blood pressure was maintained constant in all animals. Note that when blood pressure was maintained constant, the most significant increases in PEEP occurred in the animals with the lowest starting PEEP level. **B.** Schematic illustration of the intracranial space during increased ICP. Arrows indicate the position of the hypothesized Starling resistor. Here, mean arterial pressure (MAP) is greater than ICP, which is greater than sagittal sinus pressure (SSP). Cortical vein pressure (Pcv) cannot fall below ICP; thus flow is dependent on MAP ICP and independent of small changes in SSP. [From Huseby J, Luce J, Cary J, et al. Effects of positive end-expiratory pressure on intracranial pressure in dogs with intracranial hypertension. *J Neurosurg.* 1981;55:704, with permission.]

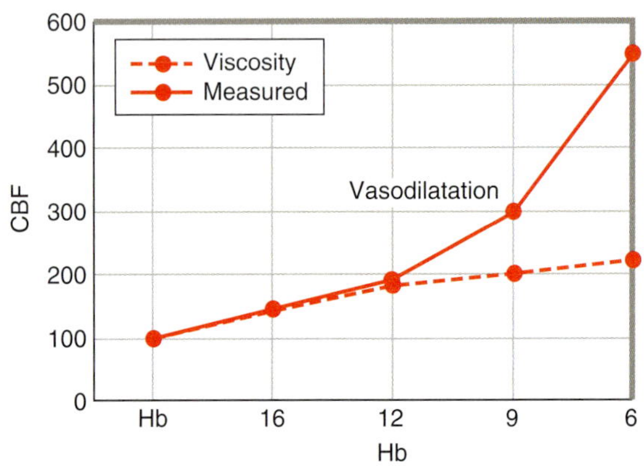

FIGURE 85-10. Rats underwent isovolemic anemia with measurement of per change in global cerebral blood flow (CBF). The theoretic CBF that arises solely from changes in viscosity is indicated by the viscosity curve. Measurement of CBF follows this line until the hemoglobin level falls to less than 10, below which active vasodilatation was observed. [Adapted from Borgström L, Jóhannsson H, Siesjö BK. The influence of acute normovolemic anemia on cerebral blood flow and oxygen consumption of anesthetized rats. *Acta Physiol Scand.* 1975;93:505-514.]

NEUROPROTECTIVE/NEUROTOXIC EFFECTS OF ANESTHETICS

Anesthetics for neuroprotection have been studied at least since the 1960s. Goldstein et al[262] were initially interested in the potential protective effects of barbiturates for global ischemia. A variety of studies eventually were published on the efficacy of barbiturates. A review of these many studies makes clear that the genesis of much of the confusion as to their efficacy was related to the timing of the barbiturate therapy, and the duration of and type of (focal vs global) ischemia. The studies, all in animals, suggest that barbiturates may have a protective effect when given before or shortly after the onset of focal temporary ischemia, as may occur during aneurysm surgery. The studies are conflicting regarding the efficacy of barbiturates in focal permanent ischemia. For global ischemia, there were some initial encouraging canine studies by Goldstein et al[262] and subhuman primate studies by Bleyaert et al.[263] However, the subhuman primate studies were criticized for the more intense care given to the treated animals, which may have accounted for their improved outcome. Indeed, this study could not be reproduced by Gisvold et al.[264] Moreover, an attempt some 13 years later to reproduce the original study by Goldstein et al was similarly unsuccessful.[265] Notably, in the original Goldstein et al study,[262] the control group had only a local anesthetic infiltration for thoracic surgery; the dog had received neuromuscular blockade and was ventilated at the time of the onset of ischemia. Subsequently, the effects of the barbiturates were compared to the effects produced in what was probably a highly sympathetically activated animal. Without such activation in the controls,

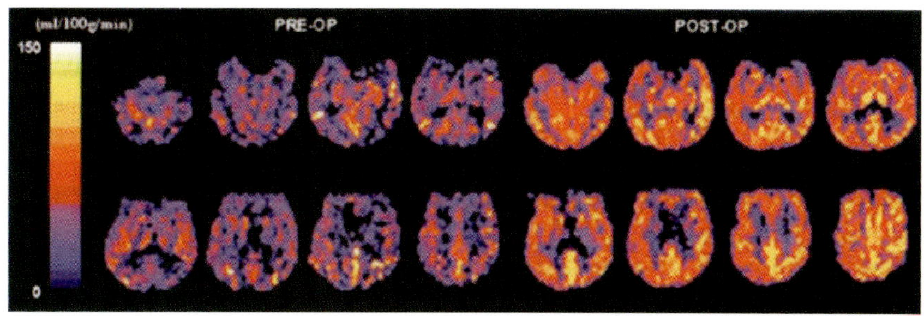

FIGURE 85-11. Preoperative (PRE-OP) and postoperative (POST-OP) (cardiac surgery) continuous arterial spin labeling perfusion magnetic resonance images show cerebral blood flow with color scale for subject 5, an 81-year-old man. Global cerebral blood flow has increased from baseline of 36 to 62 mL/100 g/min on the fifth day after surgery. Multiple regression over all subjects revealed a significant and inverse relationship between cerebral blood flow and hematocrit. [Reprinted from Floyd T, McGarvey M, Ochroch E, et al. Perioperative changes in cerebral blood flow after cardiac surgery: influence of anemia and aging. *Ann Thorac Surg.* 2003;76:2037-2042, with permission from Society of Thoracic Surgeons.]

Steen et al[265] were unable to reproduce this seminal study. Nonetheless, the Brain Resuscitation Clinical Trial Group evaluated the efficacy of thiopental loading immediately after the return of spontaneous circulation following cardiac arrest in humans.[266] They were unable to demonstrate a protective effect in this multi-institutional study. It was suggested that there may have been some subsets of patients in whom a protective effect may have been lost due to the signal-to-noise ratio inherent in the design of such studies. Nonetheless, at this time the data do not provide sufficient support for the general use of barbiturates for global brain ischemia.

If barbiturates are to be used, there are data regarding a suggested range of doses. Initial studies examined only high-dose barbiturates associated with an isoelectric electroencephalogram (EEG). Selman et al[267,268] published studies showing neuroprotection for focal temporary ischemia in subhuman primates. The investigators used very high-dose barbiturates given over at least 24 hours, enough to suppress any edema-mediated ICP elevations. However, Warner et al[269] found similar protective efficacy for a focal temporary ischemic insult in rats. Drug doses were sufficient to produce an isoelectric EEG; doses of about half that level were associated with significant EEG change but not an isoelectric state.

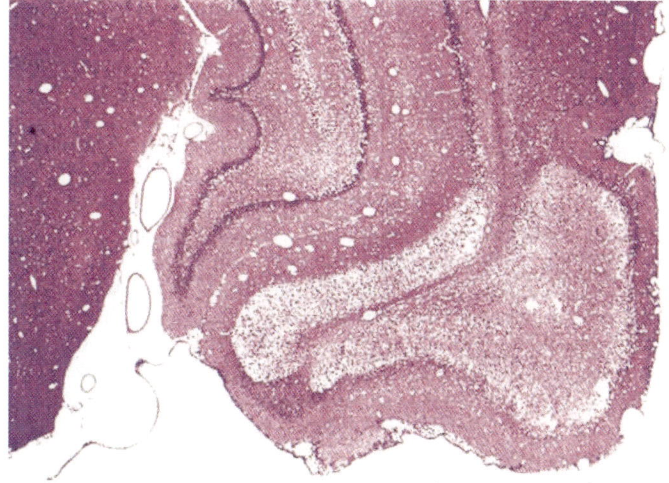

FIGURE 85-13. Histologic slide from a paralyzed ventilated rat that received high-dose alfentanil. Infarction of the amygdala is evident. [Unpublished slide from experiments by Kofke et al.[294]]

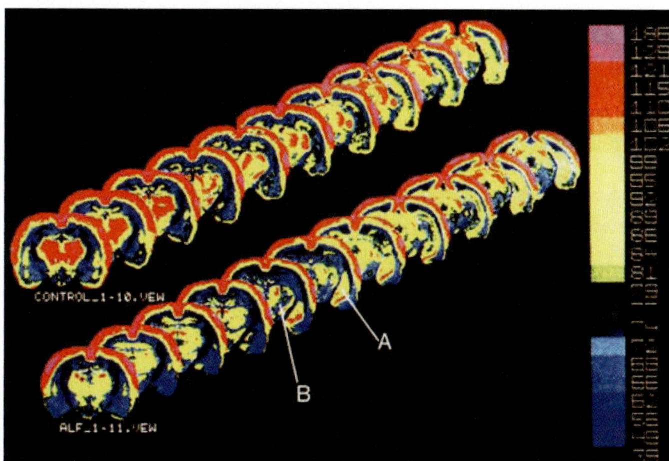

FIGURE 85-12. Glucose autoradiography during administration of high-dose alfentanil with epileptiform activity of paralyzed ventilated rats. Ventral hippocampal (**A**) activation and thalamic depression (**B**) were produced by alfentanil. [From Kofke W, Garman R, Tom W, et al. Alfentanil-induced hypermetabolism, seizure, and neuropathology in rats. *Anesth Analg.* 1992;75:953, with permission.]

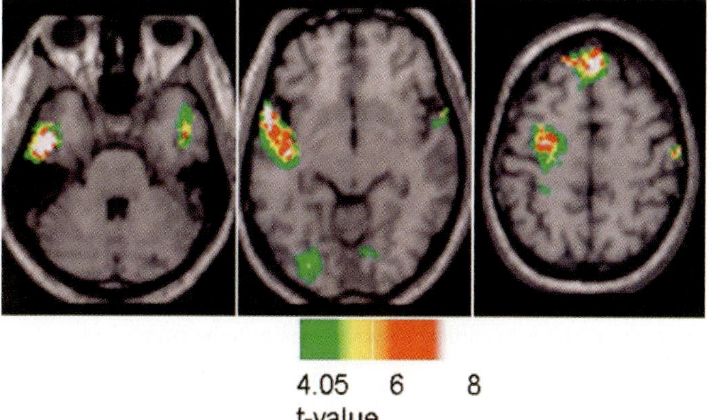

FIGURE 85-14. Fluorodeoxyglucose positron emission tomographic functional brain mapping statistical parametric map images from 4 ventilated healthy individuals who received brief high-dose remifentanil. Baseline awake scans were subtracted from scans acquired during remifentanil infusion. Areas with significant increases in cerebral metabolic rate for glucose ($t > 4.05$, $P < .05$) are displayed in lighter shades overlaid on a normalized magnetic resonance image. Scale for t values also is shown. Hippocampal and cingulate activation occurred. [Adapted from Kofke W, Attaallah A, Kuwabara H, et al. Neuropathologic effects in rats and neurometabolic effects in humans of high-dose remifentanil. *Anesth Analg.* 2002;94:1229-1236.]

These data would suggest that there may be value in occasionally using barbiturates as neuroprotection for focal temporary ischemia. If the amount of ischemic tissue is large and may be associated with elevated ICP, then higher isoelectric EEG–producing doses seem appropriate; if the ischemic insult is less severe, then lower doses may be appropriate. These recommendations are not based on any proper randomized human studies but rather on theoretical gain. In the prevention of stroke, this is a significant variable; this should be compared with the possible therapeutic risk, which may or may not be significant.[104]

Other γ-aminobutyric acid (GABA)ergic drugs, such as etomidate,[270,271] benzodiazepines,[272-274] and propofol,[274-277] have generally shown similar equivocal results as to their neuroprotective effects. The number and breadth of studies with GABAergic agents are not at all comparable to studies of barbiturates. Indeed, etomidate in some reports has been suggested as deleterious when given for cerebral ischemia,[278] and propofol worsened injury in 1 in vitro model[272] but not in another in vitro report.[279] In the context of seizure-induced injury, Kofke et al[280] reported that midazolam reduced substantia nigra injury, whereas thiopental and isoflurane, although stopping the seizure, conferred no neuroprotection. Ketamine was intermediate in its effect, and any other neuroprotective effect may have been missed due to small sample size.

Using isoflurane as a prototype, the volatile anesthetics have been demonstrated to clearly prolong the time that an animal's brain can tolerate an anaerobic condition.[281] Other reports in animals also have reported a capability of volatile anesthetics to confer early histologic protection against a variety of types of ischemic insults.[282-288] However, when the evaluations are extended to 2 weeks post–focal ischemia, the protective efficacy is no longer able to be demonstrated.[289] These data seem to suggest that initial damaging processes can be favorably altered by a volatile anesthetic, but that other deleterious postischemic processes, such as apoptosis, are not altered by isoflurane.[290] This temporary protection was not observed in a global ischemia model, however.[291] At this time the capability of isoflurane and other volatile anesthetics to contribute to permanent perioperative neuroprotection must remain unsettled.

Opioids have not been shown to have any neuroprotective effects. Indeed, several studies by Kofke et al have demonstrated the capability of high-dose fentanyl and congeners to produce limbic system activation (**Fig. 85-12**) and damage (**Fig. 85-13**).[292-295] Comparable limbic activation was demonstrated when humans were given brief high-dose remifentanil (**Fig. 85-14**),[295] and cingulate activation was noted with sedative dose–remifentanil in volunteers.[296] Notably, the cingulate activation did not occur in humans with the ApoE genotype, although hippocampal activation did arise in subjects with this single-nucleotide polymorphism. Moreover, in humans, μ opioids have been reported to have proconvulsant properties[297] that would be expected to be deleterious in the context of cerebral ischemia, as was demonstrated in 1 laboratory report of opioids used with cerebral ischemia[298] and another where they were used with traumatic brain injury.[299] These studies' designs incorporated isolated opioid use. The negative effects from μ opioids appear to be attenuated with concomitant hypnotic drug administration.[300] Although provocative, at this time the relevance of these observations to clinical practice remains to be established.

KEY REFERENCES

- Yonas H, Pindzola R. Physiological determination of cerebrovascular reserves and its use in clinical management. *Cerebrovasc Brain Metab Rev.* 1994;6(4):325-340.
- Kim J, Kang S. Bleeding and subsequent anemia: a precipitant for cerebral infarction. *Eur Neurol.* 2000;43(4):201-208.
- Muizelaar J, Marmarou A, Ward J, et al. Adverse effects of prolonged hyperventilation in patients with severe head injury: a randomized clinical trial. *J Neurosurg.* 1991;75:731.
- Marion D. Moderate hypothermia in severe head injuries: the present and the future. *Curr Opin Crit Care.* 2002;8(2):111-114.
- Nolan J, Morley PT, Vanden Hoek TL, et al. Therapeutic hypothermia after cardiac arrest an advisory statement by the Advanced Life Support Task Force of the International Liaison Committee on Resuscitation Writing Group. *Circulation.* 2003;108:118-121.
- Castillo J, Davalos A, Marrugat J, et al. Timing for fever-related brain damage in acute ischemic stroke. *Stroke.* 1998;29: 2455–2460.
- Diringer M, Neurocritical Care Fever Reduction Trial Group. Treatment of fever in the neurologic intensive care unit with a catheter-based heat exchange system. *Crit Care Clin.* 2004;32(2):559-564.
- Rosner M, Becker D. Origin and evolution of plateau waves. Experimental observations and a theoretical model. *J Neurosurg.* 1984;50:312.
- Steiner LA, Czosnyka M, Piechnik SK, et al. Continuous monitoring of cerebrovascular pressure reactivity allows determination of optimal cerebral perfusion pressure in patients with traumatic brain injury. *Crit Care Med.* 2002;30:733-738.
- Neil-Dwyer G, Walter P, Cruickshank J. Beta-blockade benefits patients following a subarachnoid hemorrhage. *Eur J Clin Pharmacol.* 1985;28:25.
- Koch CG, Li L, Sessler DI, et al. Duration of red-cell storage and complications after cardiac surgery. *N Engl J Med.* 2008;358: 1229-1239.
- Selman W, Spetzler R, Roessmann U, Rosenblatt J, Crumrine R. Barbiturate-induced coma therapy for focal cerebral ischemia. Effect after temporary and permanent MCA occlusion. *J Neurosurg.* 1981;55:220.

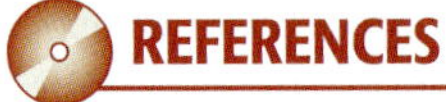

REFERENCES

Complete references available on DVD and online version at www.LongneckerAnesthesiology.com

CHAPTER 86 Anaphylactic Reactions and Anesthesia

Robert S. Holzman

KEY POINTS

1. Anaphylaxis is an acute reaction leading to severe physiologic derangements of multiple systems. True anaphylaxis denotes an IgE antibody–mediated reaction.
2. Non–IgE-mediated reactions resembling true anaphylaxis occur and are commonly called anaphylactoid reactions. These reactions can be of identical severity to anaphylactic reactions, may be clinically indistinguishable during the time of occurrence, and should be treated in an identical manner to anaphylactic reactions.
3. Clinical symptoms include urticaria, flushing, nausea, vomiting, abdominal pain, laryngeal edema, bronchospasm, and cardiovascular collapse. Under anesthesia, cardiovascular collapse and respiratory distress are the most common clinical signs.

4. Treatment consists of discontinuing the suspected initiating agent, securing the compromised airway, and establishing intravenous access. Bronchospasm and laryngeal edema are treated with epinephrine. Hypotension and cardiovascular collapse are treated with volume, epinephrine, and cardiopulmonary resuscitation if needed.
5. Evaluation of an anaphylactic reaction starts with a detailed history and may include skin testing, radioallergosorbent testing, and/or provocative challenge. Such efforts should be coordinated with the primary physician and an allergy specialist. The anesthesiologist's information about the timing and administration of the various medications and the signs and symptoms observed will be invaluable for the ultimate diagnosis of specific allergy.
6. Most serious and fatal allergic reactions to penicillin and β-lactam antibiotics occur in individuals who have never had a previous allergic reaction.
7. Many commonly used anesthetic agents and other drugs administered during anesthesia, including neuromuscular blocking agents, hypnotics, opiates, and antibiotics, lead to nonimmunologic histamine release.
8. True allergic reactions to local anesthetics are exceedingly rare, and cases labeled as such usually are due to other causes (vasovagal response, intravenous injection) or possibly metabolites (para-aminobenzoic acid), preservatives (methylparaben), or antioxidant additives (metabisulfite). If the previous drug is unknown, an amide-type local anesthetic should be chosen.
9. Diabetics exposed to protamine-containing insulin have a 40- to 50-fold increased risk for life-threatening reactions to protamine. Fish-allergic individuals and vasectomized men also may be at increased risk.
10. Health care workers regularly exposed to latex have a substantially increased risk of latex-specific IgE positivity (up to 18%), and 28% to 67% of children with spina bifida have a positive skin test result to latex proteins. Life-threatening anaphylaxis can occur intraoperatively in highly sensitive patients because of mucosal absorption of latex protein allergens from surgical gloves.

Anaphylaxis is an acute, severe, potentially life-threatening allergic reaction. The word "allergy," introduced by Baron Dr Clemens von Pirquet in 1906, was meant to describe the uncommitted biologic response that may lead to immunity *or* allergic disease. This concept is very much in keeping with our evolving understanding a century later. Preceding von Pirquet's neologism, Portier and Richet in 1902 reported that the second injection of sea anemone extract into dogs resulted in a fatal systemic reaction after the first injection had no directly observable effect, a finding totally unexpected at the time. Richet fashioned the word "anaphylaxis" by combining the Greek *ana* ("contrary to") and *phylaxis* ("protection") to describe an adverse reaction following repeated exposure to a foreign protein rather than the intended immunization, or prophylaxis.

This chapter takes the view of the anesthesiologist as perioperative specialist, focusing on the sequence of preoperative evaluation of the patient with a possible history of allergy, pathophysiologically based intra- and perioperative management, and as a consultant to the patient's further care by primary and specialist physicians.

BIOLOGY OF MAST CELL ACTIVATION

Why are some of us destined for a life of allergy and others not? We now know that our immune systems can choose from 2 pathways to express reactions to antigens, either a low-grade or high-grade immunologic response (**Table 86-1**). *Low-grade responders* produce allergen-specific IgG_1 and IgG_4 antibodies and their T cells respond to the allergen with a moderate proliferation and production of interferon-γ by type 1 T-helper (Th_1) cells. *High-grade responders*, however, have an exaggerated response, with increased production of allergen-specific IgE antibodies, as well as increased serum levels of IgE-specific antibodies to common allergens. In this group, cytokines produced by Th_2 cells, including interleukin (IL)-4, IL-5, and IL-13, are produced rather than cytokines such as interferon-γ and IL-2 from Th_1 cells.[1]

TABLE 86-1 Characteristics of Immunological Responses to Allergens

Phenotype	
Low-Grade Responders	**High-Grade Responders**
Th_1 Expression	**Th_2 Expression**
Small amount of antigen or low-affinity interaction between T cells and antigen-presenting cells	Large amount of antigen or high-affinity interaction between T cells and antigen-presenting cells
Mediated by IL-12	Mediated by IL-4
Presence of cytidine-phosphate-guanosine (CpG) repeats from bacteria favor Th_1 phenotype	Presence of transcription factors such as GATA-3, c-maf, and PGE2 favor Th_2 phenotype
	Nitric oxide favors Th_2 expression by being less inhibitory to Th_2 cells than to Th_1 cells
IL-10 and transforming growth factor-β inhibit responses of Th_1 and Th_2	
	Interferon-γ inhibits Th_2 expression
	IL-12 and IL-18 both release interferon-γ from T cells
IL-4 inhibits expression of Th_1 cells	IL-4 promotes expression of Th_2 cells

IL, interleukin; Th_1, type 1 T-helper cells; Th_2, type 2 T-helper cells.

Th_2 cells mediate atopy and allergic inflammation. In view of the reciprocity of the relationship, 1 theory about the rising incidence of allergy in Western countries is the cleanliness of the environment and the ubiquitous presence of antibiotics.

IgE-MEDIATED MAST CELL ACTIVATION

Antigenic molecules (usually proteins) capable of stimulating IgE antibody production may cause IgE-mediated anaphylaxis after initial sensitization and subsequent reexposure. Haptens, molecules too small to stimulate immune responses themselves, may bind to endogenous proteins such as albumin and become antigenic. Once produced, IgE antibodies to these antigens become fixed to tissue mast cells and/or circulating basophils, both of which contain high-affinity IgE receptors (**Fig. 86-1**).[2,3] Reexposure to antigens or haptens, with subsequent cross-linking of cell surface IgE antibody, induces activation of membrane-associated enzymes, causing biochemical cascades that lead to an influx of extracellular calcium and mobilization of intracellular calcium with the subsequent release of preformed granule-associated mediators and generation of new mediators from cell membrane phospholipids.

Cytokines are low-molecular-weight chemicals that modulate cell function locally. The cytokines that promote IgE isotype switching (IL-4 and IL-13) are generated by T-lymphocytes with a Th_2 cytokine profile. T cells that generate a Th_1 cytokine profile—by secreting interferon-γ—inhibit B-cell isotype switching for IgE synthesis. Th_1 and Th_2 cells reciprocally inhibit each other's development. When IgE production is increased, such as in atopy (from the Greek *atopos* or "out of place"), an imbalance in the Th_2/Th_1 ratio control is likely. Th_2-associated cytokines, such as IL-4, IL-5, IL-9, and IL-13, are associated with many stigmata of chronic allergic inflammation. IL-4 and IL-13 stimulate the production of IgE and vascular cell adhesion molecule (VCAM)-1. IL-5 and IL-9 are

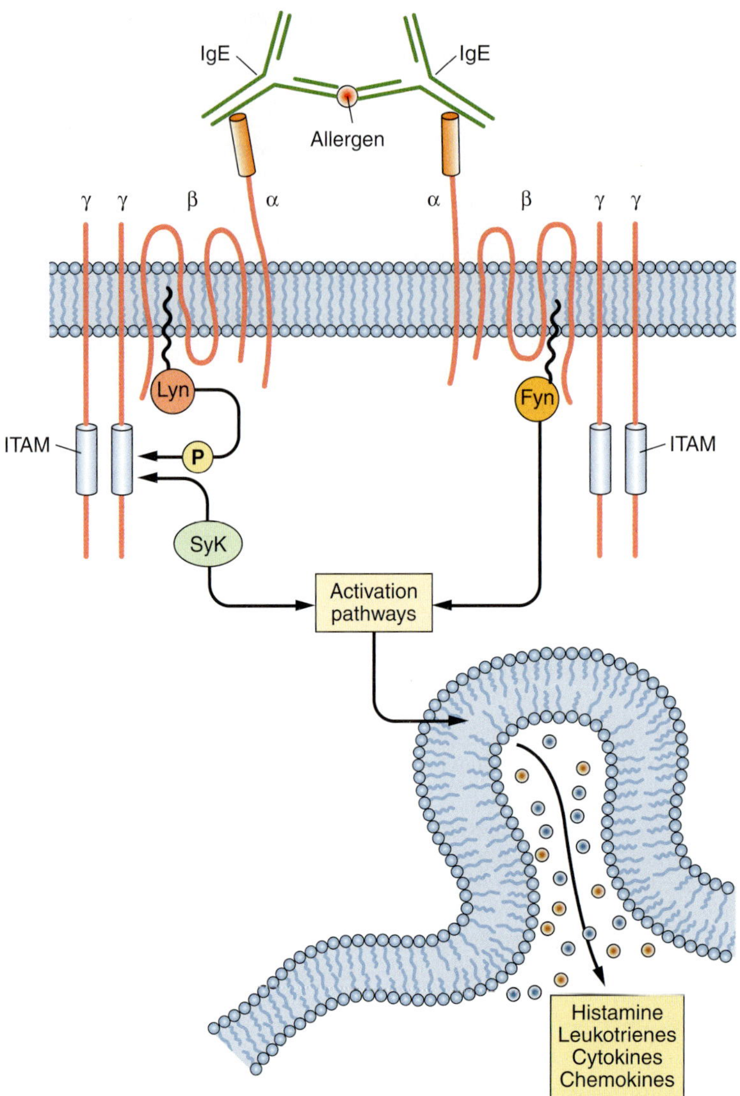

FIGURE 86-1. Mast cell activation. IgE binding unit (a chain); signaling unit (b and g chains). ITAM, immunoreceptor tyrosine-based activation motif; SyK, (spleen) tyrosine kinase; Lyn, Fyn, protein tyrosine kinases; P, phosphorylation. [From Kinet J. A new strategy to counter allergy. *N Engl J Med.* 2005;353:310-312. © 2005 Massachusetts Medical Society. Used with permission.]

involved in the development of eosinophils. IL-4 and IL-9 promote the development of mast cells. IL-9 and IL-13 promote airway hyperresponsiveness. IL-4, IL-9, and IL-13 promote the overproduction of mucus. In their turn, eosinophils injure mucosal surfaces by releasing toxic basic proteins, cysteinyl leukotrienes, and platelet-activating factor. They also damage inhibitory MK2 muscarinic receptors, ultimately leading to airway hyperresponsiveness. IL-5 also releases mature and immature eosinophils from bone marrow.

IgE molecules then bind to high-affinity receptors for IgE (Fc epsilon receptor I [FcεRI]) on circulating basophils and mast cells. This binding itself does not induce the allergic reactions; a second step is required. The allergens, because of their multivalency, express multiple epitopes recognized by specific IgEs and IgGs. Simultaneous multivalent binding of allergens to several membrane-bound IgEs induces receptor aggregation, triggering a signaling cascade that leads to the production and release of allergic and inflammatory mediators (histamine, leukotrienes, chemokines, and cytokines).[2] Release of these mediators is rapid (in minutes) and produces immediate symptoms.

There is a balance of activating and inhibitory cell-surface receptors, but how is the signaling cascade generated? FcεRI has an IgE-binding unit (the α-chain) and a signaling unit (1 β-chain and 2 γ-chains). Aggregation of FcεRI induces activation of a tyrosine kinase bound to the β-chain; the tyrosine kinase then phosphorylates 2 tyrosine residues in the γ-chains. These tyrosine residues are a central feature of the immunoreceptor tyrosine-based activation motif (ITAM), a feature of many receptors throughout the immune system. After phosphorylation, the ITAMs of the γ-chains activate spleen tyrosine kinase (SyK), which, through activation of downstream pathways, induces the release of allergic mediators.

Modulation of these FcεRI pathways occurs via inhibition mediated by the IgG receptor Fcg receptor IIb (FcgRIIb). Allergen-specific IgGs form complexes with allergens that can, in turn, form a bridge between FcεRI and FcgRIIb. This bridge induces the aggregation of activating FcεRI with inhibitory FcgRIIb, which inhibits the activation pathways activated by FcεRI. *This delicate balance of IgG counteracting IgE is putatively the central mechanism behind successful allergen desensitization.* In its inhibition of ITAM, FcgRIIb contains an immunoreceptor tyrosine-based inhibitory motif (ITIM), a modified version of ITAM present in FcεRI.

Making use of this membrane architecture, a chimeric molecule designed to bind both FcgRIIb and a specific IgE bound to FcεRI has been shown to create a bridge and *inhibit* allergic reactions, including allergen-mediated activation of basophils and mast cells in vitro as well as in a mouse model.[4] Such a strategy not only could provide prophylaxis for specific allergic reactions, but in addition could displace allergens already bound to IgE, in which case it would help terminate ongoing anaphylactic reactions following initial exposure.

COMPLEMENT-MEDIATED MAST CELL ACTIVATION

Complement was first identified as a heat-labile "principle" in serum that "complemented" antibodies in the killing of bacteria. Complement consists of a series of plasma and cell membrane proteins that lyse susceptible targets, promote phagocytosis, and generate peptide mediators of the inflammatory response. These anaphylotoxins cause mast cell and basophil mediator release, directly increase vascular permeability, make smooth muscles contract, cause platelet activation, and stimulate macrophages to produce thromboxane, effects almost identical to IgE-mediated mast cell activation. The job of the complement system is challenging: it provides host defense through opsonization, chemotaxis and activation of leukocytes, and lysis of bacteria and cells. It also acts to augment the antibody response and enhance immunologic memory. Finally, it must dispose of waste through clearance of immune complexes from tissues and clearance of apoptotic cells.

The complement cascade may be activated through the classical, alternative, or the mannose-binding lectin pathway (**Fig. 86-2**).[5] Complement activation through the *classical pathway* is initiated through IgG or IgM antibody binding to antigens, as in hemolytic ABO-incompatible blood transfusion reactions. Heparin–protamine complexes have been shown in vivo[6] and in vitro[7] to activate complement via the classical pathway. Injection of preformed immune complexes or IgG aggregates can activate complement and mimic clinical anaphylaxis. Patients with selective IgA antibody deficiency may develop IgG anti-IgA antibodies after receiving multiple transfusions, which may result in complement activation and anaphylactic reactions.[8]

Complement activation via the *alternative pathway* may be stimulated by lipopolysaccharides (endotoxin),[9] althesin,[10] radiocontrast media, and membranes used for cardiopulmonary bypass and dialysis.

The initiators of the *mannose-binding lectin pathway* are microbes with terminal mannose groups. Young children with recurrent infections may have low levels of mannose-binding lectin, suggesting the importance of the mannose-binding lectin pathway in the loss of passively acquired maternal antibody and the acquisition of a mature immunologic repertoire.[5]

The 3 pathways converge at the point of cleavage of C3, leading to formation of the membrane attack complex that directly affects the integrity of mast cell and basophile cell membranes. In addition, complement activation has an adjunctive role in amplifying the antibody response.

NONIMMUNOLOGIC MAST CELL ACTIVATION

Certain drugs can cause mast cell mediator release by nonimmunologic means, the exact mechanism of which is poorly understood but may be differentiated from immunologically mediated mast cell activation in certain ways. Nonimmunologic stimulation relies heavily on cellular Ca^{++}, is unaffected by neuraminidase treatment, shows rapid inactivation, and elicits no increase in the incorporation of 3H-methyl groups into the lipid fraction. In contrast, stimulation by immunologic agents relies primarily on extracellular Ca^{++}, is inhibited by neuraminidase treatment, shows a comparatively slow rate of inactivation, and causes a significant increase in the incorporation of 3H-methyl groups into the lipid fraction. The clinical implication of differentiating the 2 mechanisms is that prophylactic intervention may be affected; experimentally, pretreatment of mast cells with neurotensin desensitizes them to subsequent stimulation by compound 48/80.[11] Moreover, there are different mast cell phenotypes (eg, connective tissue mast cells, airway mast cells) that may vary in expression following activation.[12] Drugs that induce nonimmunologic mast cell activation include opiates, especially morphine and codeine,[13,14] and neuromuscular blocking agents such as atracurium and D-tubocurarine.[12] Intriguingly, there seems to be a disparity between a higher incidence of reaction to rocuronium in Europe and in the United States.[15]

MEDIATORS OF ANAPHYLAXIS

Once the mast cell, basophil, or eosinophil is activated by any of the mechanisms, release of mediators results in the attraction, accumulation, and activation of other cellular elements. Mediators released include those preformed and stored in granules and those newly generated upon appropriate stimulation. Release of these mediators causes various pathophysiologic responses that result in acute or chronic reactions. The complex of allergen, IgE, and high-affinity receptor for IgE on the surface of the mast cell triggers noncytotoxic, energy-dependent release of preformed, granule-associated histamine and tryptase, and the membrane-derived lipid mediators leukotrienes, prostaglandins, and platelet-activating factor. Mast cells produce the 3 cysteinyl leukotrienes C4, D4, and E4, which cause contraction of smooth muscles, vasodilatation, increased vascular permeability, and hypersecretion of mucus. Collateral sources of cysteinyl leukotrienes are eosinophils, macrophages, and monocytes. Mast cell tryptase activates receptors on endothelial and epithelial cells, which causes the upregulation of adhesion molecules that selectively attract eosinophils and basophils.

EPIDEMIOLOGY OF ANAPHYLAXIS DURING ANESTHESIA

Allergic disease is on the increase in Western countries. Environment may have a great deal to do with this increase; allergic disease was less common in East Germany than West Germany prior to reunification.[16] This finding supports the so-called "hygiene hypothesis," the notion that when the developing immune system is deprived of microbial antigens that stimulate Th_1 cells, the opportunity to prolong sensitization of Th_2 cells ensues. By promoting a Th_1 response, infection downregulates the tendency for development of Th_2-related disease.[17,18] Other factors that may favor a greater Th_2 response in infants include diet, birth dates during high pollen counts, viral infections, allergen exposure, tobacco smoke, and air pollutants.

The incidence of anaphylaxis during anesthesia is variable within an order of magnitude, but ranges between 0.5:10 000 and 16.3:10 000 in adults[19-23] and 5:10 000 in children.[24] Anaphylaxis during anesthesia has been attributed primarily to muscle relaxants, although there is an intriguing geographical variability. For example, muscle relaxants are the most commonly reported allergenic agents in France (~50%) with latex (~20%) and antibiotics (~15%) following.[25] A review of 826 patients referred to an anesthetic allergy clinic in Australia over a 17-year period revealed severe immediate anaphylactic reactions in 54%; in 59% a muscle relaxant was involved.[20] In a single center in Norway, muscle relaxants were the most common cause (93.2%) of IgE-mediated reactions, with latex approximately 3.6%. In 2 Spanish centers, antibiotics were the main etiology (44% of the 56% of patients with confirmed IgE-mediated reactions), and muscle relaxants were determined to be the cause in 37% and latex in 4%.[26] Local/cultural patterns of sensitization as well as underlying genetic factors likely play an important role in these variations. Gender differences are often found in allergic reactions; rodent studies have confirmed an estrogen effect on mast cell activation and allergic sensitization, and progesterone is shown to suppress histamine release but potentiate IgE induction.[27]

Patients who react have a greater incidence of allergy, atopy, asthma, and previous reactions than do nonreactors, suggesting that these are significant comorbidities. However, although a history of drug allergy was found in 37% of cases and atopy in 38%,[28] most patients do not have such a history, and most patients with such a history do not react.[29] In patients with suspected or unexplained hypersensitivity reactions

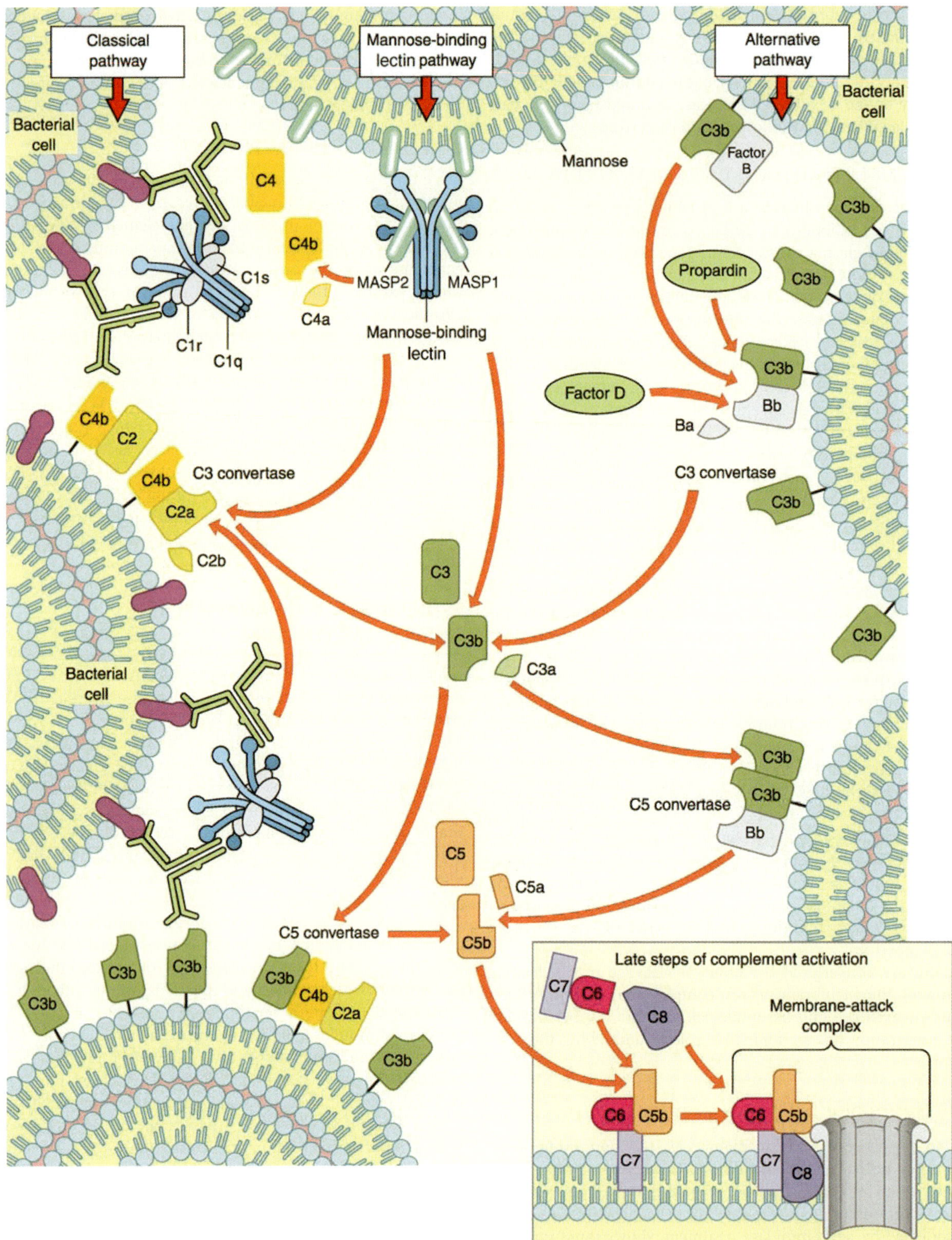

FIGURE 86-2. Three activation pathways of complement. MASP1 and 2, mannose-binding lectin-associated proteases; Factor B, D, binding/cleavage proteins; C5a and C5b, anaphylotoxins resulting from cleavage of C5, initiating the formation of the membrane-attack complex. From Walport M. Complement: first of two parts. *N Engl J Med*. 2001;344(14):1058-1066. © 2001 Massachusetts Medical Society. Used with permission.]

during anesthesia, follow-up evaluation strongly suggests anaphylaxis as a possible etiology, with an increase in estimated incidence from 2.1:10 000 to 3.1:10 000,[30] underscoring the importance of allergy evaluation following such an event. A multicenter survey carried out in France in 1990 and 1991 revealed a 3:1 ratio of females to males in a series of 1585 patients. The reactions occurred mostly in adults (80%); 9% occurred in children.[23] Cardiovascular collapse has consistently been described as the most common presenting problem, and evidence indicates that this form of shock is substantially different at the cellular level and potentially more harmful than other causes of shock.[31]

CLINICAL MANIFESTATIONS OF ANAPHYLAXIS

The evaluation and treatment of patients who develop anaphylaxis in the operating room is challenging even for the experienced clinician. In the perioperative period, multiple medications are frequently given in close proximity, making causative factors more difficult to interpret. Patients usually are unconscious, draped, and cold—situations that often hide early signs and symptoms of anaphylaxis. Anesthetics themselves alter mediator release, possibly delaying early recognition.[32]

In general, symptoms begin soon (within minutes) after introduction of the causative agent, but may be delayed for 1 to 2 hours. Along with other symptoms, conscious patients frequently describe a sense of impending doom. The primary anaphylactic target organs in humans are the cutaneous, gastrointestinal, respiratory, and cardiovascular systems (**Box 86-1**). *During general and regional anesthesia or during deep sedation, cardiovascular signs predominate.*[20,33] The speed and scope of initial intervention should be guided by the speed and severity of the reaction, which can be graded in a standard fashion (**Table 86-2**).

BOX 86-1

Target Organs of Anaphylaxis

System	Signs and Symptoms
Cutaneous	Pruritus
	Flushing[a]
	Erythema[a]
	Urticaria/angioedema[a]
Gastrointestinal	Nausea
	Abdominal pain
	Diarrhea
	Vomiting
Respiratory	Laryngeal edema
	Hoarseness
	Dysphonia
	"Lump" in throat
	Chest tightness
	Dyspnea
	Cough
	Wheezing[a]
	Cyanosis[a]
	Increase in peak airway pressure[a]
	Nasal itching
	Sneezing
	Rhinorrhea
	Nasal obstruction
	Hypersecretion of mucus
Cardiovascular	Light-headedness
	Faintness
	Syncope
	Tachycardia[a]
	Bradycardia[b]
	Hypotension[a]
	Dysrhythmias[a]

[a]Most likely to occur in patients during anesthesia.

[b]Paradoxical bradycardia due to extreme hypovolemia.

TABLE 86-2 Clinical Severity Scale of Immediate Hypersensitivity Reactions

Class	Clinical Manifestations
I	Generalized cutaneous signs: erythema, urticaria with or without angioedema
II	Moderate multiorgan involvement with cutaneous signs, hypotension and tachycardia, bronchial hyperreactivity (cough, ventilatory impairment)
III	Severe life-threatening multiorgan involvement that requires specific treatment: collapse, tachycardia or bradycardia, cardiac arrhythmias, bronchospasm; the cutaneous signs may be absent or occur only after the arterial blood pressure recovers
IV	Circulatory or respiratory arrest
V	Death due to a lack of response to cardiorespiratory resuscitation

From Kroigaard M, Garvey L, Gillberg L, et al. Scandinavian clinical practice guidelines on the diagnosis, management and follow-up of anaphylaxis during anaesthesia. *Acta Anaesthesiol Scand*. 2007;51:655-670. Used with permission.

DIFFERENTIAL DIAGNOSIS

In a conscious patient, anaphylaxis is most easily confused with a vasovagal reaction, which may occur when a patient collapses after an injection or painful procedure (**Box 86-2**). However, respiratory distress does not occur, and symptoms are relieved almost immediately once the patient is supine. Vasovagal reactions are often also accompanied by profuse diaphoresis and bradycardia, without flushing, urticaria, angioedema, prorates, or wheezing. The differential diagnosis of sudden collapse includes dysrhythmias, myocardial infarction, aspiration of food or foreign body, pulmonary embolism, seizure disorder, hypoglycemia, and stroke. In the presence of laryngeal edema, especially when accompanied by abdominal pain, the diagnosis of hereditary angioedema should be considered. *Globes hysterics* and factitious asthma must be considered when respiratory symptoms are present. Other conditions that can mimic anaphylaxis are overdose of medication, cold urticaria (especially if generalized), idiopathic urticaria, carcinoid tumors, and systemic mastocytosis.

BOX 86-2

Differential Diagnosis of Anaphylaxis

Vasovagal reaction
Dysrhythmia
Myocardial infarction
Overdose of medication or illicit drugs
Pulmonary embolism
Seizure disorder
Cerebral vascular accident
Aspiration
Globus hystericus
Fictitious asthma
Hereditary angioedema
Physical or idiopathic urticaria
Serum sickness
Carcinoid tumors
Systemic mastocytosis

TREATMENT OF ANAPHYLAXIS[34-38]

Anaphylactic reactions must be recognized and treated early because death may occur within minutes. Treatment of anaphylactic reactions can be divided into initial and secondary therapies (**Box 86-3**).

INITIAL TREATMENT

When possible, steps should be taken to interrupt further exposure to and absorption of the offending agent. Intravenous infusions of suspected allergens should be stopped immediately. Airway maintenance with 100% oxygen should be administered; continuous monitoring via pulse oximetry and arterial blood gas levels should ensure adequate oxygenation. If there is any suggestion of airway compromise due to laryngeal edema, the trachea should be intubated immediately. If laryngeal edema is present, aerosolized epinephrine (3 inhalations of 0.16- to 0.20-mg epinephrine per inhalation from a metered dose inhaler) or epinephrine by nebulizer (8-15 drops of 2.25% epinephrine in 2 mL normal saline) may be useful. If laryngeal edema is refractory to these measures or progresses too rapidly, a needle catheter cricothyrotomy, emergency surgical cricothyrotomy, or tracheostomy may be necessary.

Upon suspicion of a severe reaction, intravenous access should be established (if not already present), and intravascular volume should be maintained with administration of isotonic crystalloid (normal saline) or colloidal solutions. Potent volatile anesthetic agents should be discontinued in order to minimize negative inotropic effects, decreases in systemic vascular resistance, and interference with the reflex compensatory response to hypotension. Halothane specifically sensitizes the heart to circulating catecholamines, which are required for treatment of severe anaphylactic reactions; therefore, change of agents to an ether anesthetic such as isoflurane, sevoflurane, or desflurane is recommended if continued inhalation anesthesia is required.

Epinephrine is the cornerstone of initial pharmacologic treatment. In adults with *severe hypotension or airway obstruction*, 100-μg increments (typically 0.1 mL of a 1:1000 dilution) of epinephrine should be given intravenously, usually not exceeding 0.5 mg total, but dosage may be varied depending on severity, response, and patient factors (age, weight, etc). Risks of epinephrine include cardiac dysrhythmias (particularly if halothane is used), myocardial infarction, and stroke. In the rare instance when an intravenous access is not present, 300 μg of epinephrine can be given subcutaneously or intramuscularly, or 1 mg (10 mL of 1:10 000 epinephrine) can be administered through the endotracheal tube. However, when a patient is in shock, the absorption of intramuscular or subcutaneous epinephrine is unreliable. For persistent hypotension, catecholamine infusions can be used. Epinephrine also will be useful if hypotension and bronchospasm persist. Suggested starting doses of epinephrine are given in Box 86-3, based on recommendations made by the Australian Patient Safety Foundation from their review of allergic adverse events during the Australian Incident Monitoring Study (AIMS).[39] The *timing* of epinephrine therapy also contributes significantly to effective treatment. In a review of fatal anaphylaxis, Pumphrey determined that epinephrine was used in the treatment of 62% of fatal anaphylactic reactions, but before arrest in only 14%. Ironically juxtaposed, adrenaline overdose caused at least 3 deaths in this review[40] and has been the subject of warning in a case report of treatment of nonanaphylactic allergic reactions.[41]

If more than 8 to 10 μg/min of epinephrine is required, tachycardia may be a significant side effect and norepinephrine may be more effective. The suggested starting dose for norepinephrine is 0.05 μg/kg/min (2-4 μg/min in adults) and should be titrated to maintain tissue perfusion. Dopamine can also be used to maintain blood pressure and perfusion. A dose of 5 to 20 μg/kg/min may help maintain cardiac output, thereby improving coronary, cerebral, renal, and mesenteric blood flow. There is an emerging role for vasopressin as an adjunct to (but not a replacement for) epinephrine. In a rat model as well as case reports of refractory anaphylactic shock, there is evidence for improved survival with epinephrine-vasopressin combination therapy over epinephrine alone.[42,43]

SECONDARY TREATMENT

Once the patient's condition begins to stabilize, administration of additional drugs may be warranted. An antihistamine such as diphenhydramine will be helpful for symptomatic relief of itching. Although no evidence has demonstrated the effectiveness of H_2-receptor antagonists in the treatment of anaphylaxis, ranitidine (1 mg/kg intravenously [IV]) may be useful[44] when hypotension is persistent because the effects of histamine on endothelial H_2 receptors may exacerbate peripheral vasodilatation.

Glucocorticoids are useful for preventing potential late-phase reactions and treating persistent bronchospasm. Traditional teaching suggested that steroids provided no immediate effect, but there is an emerging understanding that membrane transactivation pathways are more rapid than previously recognized and therapeutic effects of

BOX 86-3

Recognition and Management of Anaphylaxis/Allergy for Allergic Reactions to Drugs, Colloids, Blood Products, Latex

Symptoms/Signs	Emergency Management	Further Care
Cardiovascular changes	Inform the surgeon.	The patient may relapse.
Hypotension, circulatory collapse	Request immediate assistance.	Continue the epinephrine infusion, for days if necessary.
Tachy-/bradycardia	Cease all drugs/plasma expanders/blood products.	Consider other drugs.
Respiratory changes	Immediate and aggressive volume expansion.	Admit to ICU.
Bronchospasm	Maintain ventilation with 100% oxygen.	Obtain bloodwork for testing as soon as possible.
Pulmonary edema	Elevate the legs, if practical.	Counsel the patient/relatives.
Erythema/skin rash/pruritus	Give epinephrine bolus IV 0.1-1 μg/kg (adult dose 1 mL of 1:10 000).	Arrange for allergy testing at 1 month.
Edema of the face and lips	Start epinephrine infusion at 0.1-0.15 μg/kg/min (adult dose 1 mL/min of 1 mg in 100 mL of diluent) and increase as necessary.	
Nausea and vomiting in awake patients	Titrate against heart rate and blood pressure.	

This algorithm is readily available online at http://www.apsf.com.au/crisis_management/crisisframe1_frame1.htm.

From Currie M, Kerridge R, Bacon A, Williamson J. Crisis management during anaesthesia: anaphylaxis and allergy. *Qual Saf Health Care*. 2005;14:e19. Used with permission.

steroid administration can occur within minutes.[45] Hydrocortisone 5 mg/kg (up to 200 mg initial dose) and then 2.5 mg/kg every 6 hours or methylprednisolone 1 mg/kg initially and every 6 hours may be given as indicated. Treatment with bicarbonate is controversial and probably should be reserved for profound acidosis, preexisting hyperkalemia, or use immediately after intubation following prolonged cardiac arrest. Acid-base status must be monitored using arterial blood gas levels to guide further therapeutic interventions.

The response to therapy usually is prompt, but despite all of the measures mentioned previously, some patients do not respond quickly, particularly in the form of shock known as refractory anaphylactic shock, for which evidence is emerging that arginine vasopressin in combination with epinephrine and intravascular volume administration is more effective in rat models and humans than epinephrine or vasopressin alone.[42,43] The treatment of anaphylaxis may be complicated by the use of β-adrenergic blocking agents, particularly in older patients. Beta-blocker therapy is associated with an increase in the severity and, possibly, the incidence of acute anaphylaxis during acute antigen exposure, as well as during immunotherapy. Anaphylaxis under these conditions may be severe, protracted, and resistant to conventional treatment because of the β-adrenergic blockade.[46,47]

ROLE OF TEST DOSES AND PRETREATMENT TO PREVENT ANAPHYLAXIS

Many clinicians choose to routinely administer a small amount of drug ("test dose"), such as an antibiotic, prior to administering the balance of the calculated dose. For IgE-mediated reactions, the test dose may or may not cause anaphylaxis; the lack of an immediate response does not guarantee absence of anaphylaxis with subsequent dosing,[48] but probably is a reflection of the antigen load, the IgE phenotype of the patient, and the elapsed time since the previous reaction.

Pretreatment regimens are particularly effective when used for repeat exposure to radiocontrast media in patients with previous reactions; these are discussed below. Desensitization as a form of pretreatment can be used for patients who must be reexposed to a medication known to have caused a previous reaction; however, the clinician must evaluate the risks, benefits, and alternatives to the readministration of the specific medication. This situation is discussed below as well.

DETERMINING THE CAUSE OF ANAPHYLACTIC REACTIONS

Patients who have had anaphylactic reactions require proper evaluation to identify the causal agents and to guide the selection and use of future medications; without rigorous investigation, some patients will be labeled with an incorrect allergy and some will be put at risk for subsequent reexposure to a real allergen.[49] The evaluation starts with a detailed history, including concurrent illness and earlier allergic and anesthetic encounters—it is here where the anesthesiologist can shine as a perioperative expert. It is helpful to prepare a flow diagram of the patient's reaction, temporally depicting the clinical manifestations of the reaction and the medications received, including indications, when initiated, doses, and duration of therapy. Equally important information includes previous exposure to the same or structurally related medications, effect of drug discontinuation, response to treatment, and any previous diagnostic testing or rechallenge. Medications should be considered with regard to their known propensity for causing anaphylaxis. The proximity of drug administration to the onset of acute reactions should be documented. In general, agents that have been used for long, continuous periods before the onset of an acute reaction are less likely to be implicated than are agents recently introduced or reintroduced. However, in the perioperative period, patients commonly receive many medications in close temporal proximity, making a diagnosis by history alone difficult.

IMMUNODIAGNOSTIC TESTS

Skin Testing for Immediate Hypersensitivity Reactions Skin testing is commonly used by allergists in the diagnosis of immediate hypersensitivity to aeroallergens and Hymenoptera, but the evaluation of drug allergy is hampered by the unavailability of relevant drug metabolites or appropriate multivalent testing reagents. Yet intradermal skin tests are still the most readily available and generally useful diagnostic tests for drug allergy. Skin testing clearly has an established role in the evaluation of IgE-mediated penicillin allergy.[34] Skin testing also is useful in the evaluation of allergy to muscle relaxants,[35,36] barbiturates,[35,37] chymopapain,[38] streptokinase,[39] insulin,[40] latex,[41,42] and miscellaneous drugs. Specific protocols for skin testing are well documented. Skin testing must be performed in the absence of medications that will affect the skin test response (especially H_1 antihistamines, tricyclic antidepressants, and sympathomimetic agents). Appropriate positive (histamine) and negative (diluent) controls should be used. Anesthesiologists should seek consultation with allergists for such evaluations; they should avoid informal and uncontrolled allergy evaluations using dilute intradermal solutions or patch tests performed without proper controls.

Other In Vivo Tests Delayed (tuberculin-like) skin tests have little, if any, place in the evaluation of drug allergy. Patch tests may be of value in cases of contact dermatitis.

IN VITRO TESTS

Total Serum IgE Levels Although increases in total serum IgE levels have been reported after allergic reactions,[43] the level of antigen-specific IgE is rarely, if ever, helpful in establishing the diagnosis of an allergic drug reaction.

Assays to Measure Complement Activation Assessment of complement activation includes measurement of the decrease in complement components (C4, C3, or total hemolytic complement [C_H50]) and increase in the generation of products of complement activation (C3a, C4a, C5a, and so on). If positive, these assays may implicate complement activation in specific reactions.

Release of Histamine and Other Mediators Washed leukocytes containing basophils with IgE antibody on their cell surfaces release histamine and other mediators when incubated with relevant antigens. Although this in vitro basophil–histamine release assay avoids drug exposure to the patient, the assay is clinically impractical because it requires whole blood drawn immediately before the test; presently the test is limited to research laboratories.

During or shortly after allergic reactions, blood can be obtained and analyzed for the release of various mediators. Urine also can be analyzed for metabolites of histamine or prostaglandin D_2 (PGD_2). Plasma histamine and PGD_2 levels remain increased only briefly, limiting their clinical use. Measurement of serum tryptase, a protease released specifically from mast cells, is useful for the assessment of mast cell–mediated allergic reactions.[25,33,37,50] Two forms of tryptase have been identified; b-tryptases appear to be the main isoenzymes expressed in mast cells and are a marker for mast cell mass, whereas in basophils, a-tryptases predominate and tend to be more of a marker for systemic mastocytosis. Serum tryptase (total tryptase, the sum of a and b) may remain elevated for hours after mast cell activation due to anaphylaxis. With nonallergenic histamine release, although histamine levels are elevated, tryptase typically remains normal.

Radioallergosorbent Testing The radioallergosorbent test (RAST) was first introduced in 1967. It measures circulating allergen-specific IgE antibody. The basic principle of the RAST is simple: the allergen is attached to a solid-phase (carbohydrate particle, paper disk, or wall of polystyrene test tubes or plastic microtiter wells) and incubated with the serum under study, during which time a specific antibody of all immunoglobulin classes is bound. The particles are washed, and a second incubation is undertaken with a radiolabeled, highly specific anti-IgE antibody. After washes, the bound radioactivity is directly related to the allergen-specific IgE antibody content in the original serum. When performed appropriately, the RAST correlates well with skin test end point titration, basophil–histamine release, and provocation tests. Results from the serum under study are compared with a positive reference serum and a negative control serum. False-positive tests may occur because of high nonspecific binding, high total serum IgE levels, or poor technique. False-negative tests may occur because of interference of high levels of IgG "blocking antibodies" or inability to maximize assay sensitivity.

REQUIREMENTS FOR SUBSEQUENT ADMINISTRATION OF AN ALLERGENIC OF DRUG IN THE FUTURE AND SPECIFIC IMMUNOTHERAPY

If a patient has experienced an allergic reaction to a medication in the past but must receive that medication again, the physician must evaluate the risks and benefits of readministration of the medication in question. If equally effective and non–cross-reacting alternative drugs are available, they should be used. If alternative drugs fail, induce unacceptable side effects, or are clearly less effective, then cautious administration of the drug using a premedication regimen or a desensitization protocol (prescribed by an expert allergist) may be considered. Premedication regimens (**Box 86-4**) have been tested, validated, and used most often in patients with previous reactions to radiocontrast media (RCM) who again require readministration of radiocontrast.[51-53]

Specific immunotherapy, consisting of the administration of increasing concentrations of allergen, has 3 mechanisms of action: downregulation of the cytokines produced by Th_2 cells, upregulation of the cytokines produced by Th_1 cells, and upregulation of regulatory T cells. As a result, allergic inflammation is inhibited, cytokines that control the production of IgE (interferon-γ and IL-12) are increased, IgG-blocking antibodies are enhanced, and cytokines involved in allergen-specific hyporesponsiveness (IL-10 and transforming growth factor-β) are increased. Specific immunotherapy is not without its risks, with anaphylaxis being the most prominent because of the relative crudeness of the allergen extracts. As recombinant technology becomes more available and precise, hypoallergenic isoforms of immunotherapy may minimize the risk of anaphylaxis. Additional strategies include naturally occurring hypoallergenic isoforms, DNA vaccines, blockade of IgE or its synthesis, and interruption of the Th_2-dependent allergic cascade. In addition, several ways of specifically inhibiting IL-4 and IL-5 currently are being investigated.[17] This basic understanding informs our targeting of new approaches to treatment.

BOX 86-4

Efficacy of Premedication for Patients With Previous Radiocontrast Media Reactions

Premedication With	Repeat Reaction Rate
A. No premedication	A: 33% (range 17%-60%)
B. Prednisone (50 mg PO) 13, 7, and 1 h before	
C. Diphenhydramine (50 mg IM or PO) 1 h before	B and C: 9% (mild reactions)
D. Ephedrine (25 mg PO) 1 h before	B, C, and D: 3.1% (historical controls)
E. Low osmolar ionic contrast media	B, C, D, and E: <0.5%

From Greenberger P, Patterson R. The prevention of immediate generalized reactions to radiocontrast media in high-risk patients. *J Allergy Clin Immunol.* 1991;87:867-872, with permission from the American Academy of Allergy, Asthma, and Immunology.

SPECIFIC ANAPHYLACTIC REACTIONS SEEN IN THE PERIOPERATIVE ENVIRONMENT

NEUROMUSCULAR BLOCKING DRUGS

Muscle relaxants are a common cause of anaphylactic reactions during anesthesia, with IgE-mediated mechanisms including positive Prausnitz-Kustner tests, basophil–histamine release studies, inhibition of basophil–histamine release after desensitization to anti-IgE, and demonstration of drug-specific IgE antibodies are observed in sera from patients with adverse reactions to muscle relaxants.[20,54-58]

Extensive in vitro cross-reactivity has been reported between muscle relaxants and other compounds that contain quaternary and tertiary ammonium ions.[59-61] Insofar as these compounds are found in many drugs, foods, cosmetics, disinfectants, and industrial materials, patients may become sensitized through environmental contact. Sensitization to ammonium ion epitopes in cosmetics has been postulated to explain the predominance of reactions in women.[61] Although the exact incidence of allergic reactions caused by muscle relaxants is unknown, reactions to muscle relaxants are less common in the United States than in France and Australia.

HYPNOTICS

Acute allergic reactions have been reported after administration of thiobarbiturates, especially thiopental. Proposed mechanisms for thiobarbiturate reactions include nonimmunologically induced mediator release and IgE-mediated reactions. A thiopental RAST has been developed,[62] and mast cell histamine release to thiopental in vitro has been described.[63,64]

Anaphylaxis to propofol *with laboratory confirmation* has been reported in only 2 patients,[65,66] without laboratory confirmation (therefore a presumptive diagnosis) in an infant with egg and peanut allergy,[67] and in 2 adult patients, one of whom had a pruritic maculopapular rash around the eyes (for 3 months)[68] and one of whom died from cardiovascular collapse with increased serum tryptase and methylhistamine levels at postmortem.[69] Although warnings about administration of propofol to patients with egg allergy can be strident, the lecithin in the propofol emulsion containing ethylenediaminetetraacetic acid (EDTA) as a preservative is derived from egg yolk, not egg albumin found in egg white. In most patients with egg allergies, egg albumin is the sensitizing protein. In the propofol emulsion using metabisulfite as the preservative, metabisulfite may be the allergenic component. Because the propofol emulsion also contains soybean oil, patients with soybean oil allergy should not receive propofol.

LOCAL ANESTHETICS

Despite patients commonly reporting "allergic reactions" to local anesthetics, true allergic reactions to injected local anesthetics are exceedingly rare. Adverse reactions to local anesthetics often are the result of vasovagal reactions, toxic reactions (probably caused by accidental intravenous injection), side effects from epinephrine, or psychomotor responses such as hyperventilation. *Toxic symptoms* often involve the central nervous and cardiovascular systems and may produce slurred speech, euphoria, dizziness, excitement, nausea, emesis, disorientation, or convulsions. *Vasovagal reactions* are usually associated with bradycardia, sweating, pallor, and rapid improvement in symptoms when the patient is supine. *Sympathetic stimulation*, either from epinephrine or anxiety, may result in tremors, diaphoresis, tachycardia, and hypertension. Rarely, signs of reactions to local anesthetics are consistent with IgE-mediated mechanisms such as urticaria, bronchospasm, and anaphylactic shock.[70] IgE-mediated sensitivity has, on rare occasions, been reported to parabens, preservatives used in local anesthetics.

Local anesthetics are divided into 2 general chemical classes, the esters and the amide compounds (**Box 86-5**). Ester local anesthetics are metabolized to para-aminobenzoic acid (PABA); therefore, ester local

BOX 86-5

Classification of Local Anesthetics

Amino Esters	Amino Amides
Benzocaine	Bupivacaine
Chloroprocaine	Etidocaine
Cocaine	Lidocaine
Procaine	Mepivacaine
Tetracaine	Prilocaine
	Ropivacaine

anesthetics cross-react and patients may present with allergic or hypersensitivity reactions. In addition, individuals allergic to other drugs metabolized to PABA, such as sunscreens and methylparaben preservatives, may experience a cross-reaction. There is no cross-reaction with the amide compounds. Epinephrine-containing local anesthetics with the antioxidant metabisulfite may be allergenic because of the metabisulfite component.[71,72]

Evaluation of the patient with a history of adverse reactions to local anesthetics should include a complete history of the episode, skin testing, and incremental drug challenge. The local anesthetic tested should be appropriate for the proposed procedure and not expected to cross-react with the drug implicated in the previous reaction. If the previous drug is unknown, an amide-type local anesthetic should be chosen. In a patient with a history suggestive of an IgE-mediated reaction or possible paraben sensitivity, preparations without paraben should be used for testing, challenge, and treatment. Preparations with epinephrine should not be used for skin testing because they may mask a positive skin test and induce toxic effects.

NARCOTICS

Narcotics typically cause nonimmunologically mediated histamine release from skin mast cells rather than anaphylaxis. In vitro studies suggest that skin mast cells are uniquely sensitive to narcotics, whereas gastrointestinal and lung mast cells and circulating basophils do not release histamine when exposed to narcotics.[13,14,73] Most opiate-induced reactions are self-limited, cutaneous, and restricted to hives and pruritus or mild hypotension treated by fluid administration. This nonimmunologic release of mediators is a far more common clinical occurrence than are the rare reactions induced by morphine-specific IgE antibody.

ANTIBIOTICS[74,75]

Penicillin Antibiotics Outside of the operating room, but also within our sphere of responsibility during resuscitation or perioperative care, penicillin antibiotics are the most common medications causing allergic drug reactions (0.7%-8% of treatment cases).[76,77] From 0.004% to 0.015% of penicillin treatment courses end in anaphylaxis, resulting in 400 to 800 deaths per year in the United States. Only 10% to 20% of patients who claim an allergy to penicillin react to skin testing with the major and minor determinants.

A low-molecular-weight chemical, penicillin must covalently combine with tissue macromolecules to produce multivalent hapten–protein complexes. The β-lactam ring, which opens spontaneously under physiologic conditions, forms the penicilloyl group. Other metabolic pathways result in additional antigenic determinants, known as the "minor determinants." Anaphylactic reactions to penicillin usually are mediated by IgE antibodies directed against minor determinants, although some anaphylactic reactions have occurred in patients with only penicilloyl-specific IgE antibodies.

Individuals with a history of penicillin reactions have a 4- to 6-fold increased risk for subsequent reactions to penicillin compared to those without previous reactions.[78] *However, most serious and fatal allergic reactions to penicillin and β-lactam antibiotics occur in individuals who have never had a previous allergic reaction.* Sensitization of these individuals may have occurred from their last therapeutic course of penicillin or (less likely) by occult environmental exposures. Approximately 10% to 20% of hospitalized patients claim a history of penicillin allergy; however, many of these patients either have been incorrectly labeled as allergic to penicillin or have lost their sensitivity. The most useful single piece of information in assessing an individual's potential for an immediate IgE-mediated reaction is the skin test response to major and minor penicillin determinants.

Negative skin tests indicate that penicillin antibiotics can be given safely. A limited number of patients with positive skin tests have been treated with therapeutic doses of penicillin. The risk of an anaphylactic or accelerated allergic reaction ranges from 50% to 70% in such patients.[79] Therefore, if skin tests are positive, equally effective non–cross-reacting antibiotics should be substituted when available. If alternative drugs fail, induce unacceptable side effects, or clearly are less effective, then administration of penicillin using a desensitization protocol to reduce the risk of anaphylaxis should be considered.

Cephalosporins Like penicillins, cephalosporins possess a β-lactam ring (**Box 86-6**), and allergic reactions were reported shortly after

BOX 86-6

β-Lactam Antibiotics

Penicillins	
β-Lactamase susceptible	
Narrow-spectrum	Penicillin G
Enteric-active	Ampicillin
Enteric-active and antipseudomonal	Ticarcillin
β-Lactamase resistant	
Antistaphylococcal	Methicillin, oxacillin, nafcillin
Combined with β-lactamase inhibitors	Ticarcillin plus clavulanic acid, ampicillin plus sulbactam, piperacillin plus tazobactam
Cephalosporins	
First generation	Cefacetrile, cefadroxil, **cephalexin,** cefaloglycin, cefalonium, cefaloridine, cefalotin, cefapirin, cefatrizine, cefazaflur, cefazedone, **cefazolin,** cefradine, cefroxadine, ceftezole
Second generation	**Cefaclor,** cefonicid, cefprozil, **cefuroxime,** biofuroksym, cefuzonam, cefmetazole
Carbapenems	Loracarbef
Cephamycins	Cefbuperazone, cefmetazole, cefminox, **cefotetan, cefoxitin**
Third generation	Cefcapene, cefdaloxime, cefdinir, cefditoren, cefetamet, cefixime, cefmenoxime, cefodizime, cefotaxime, cefovecin, cefpimizole, cefpodoxime, cefteram, ceftibute, ceftiofur, ceftiolene, ceftizoxime, **ceftriaxone,** cefoperazone, ceftazidime
Oxacephems	Latamoxef
Fourth generation	Cefclidine, cefepime, cefluprenam, cefoselis, cefozopran, cefpirome, cefquinome
Oxacephems	Flomoxef
Fifth generation	Ceftobiprole[a]
Monobactams	Aztreonam

[a]Currently under Food and Drug Administration fast-track review.

cephalosporins came into clinical use. Cross-reactivity between penicillins and cephalosporins is about 10% because of this common β-lactam ring structure,[80] and standard teaching was to avoid treatment with cephalosporins for those with possible penicillin anaphylaxis. However, evidence has accumulated that the side chain rather than the β-lactam ring is the antigen in cephalosporin allergic reactions. Because first-generation cephalosporins as well as cefamandole have similarities in their side chains, in general, patients with positive skin tests to any penicillin reagent or a history compatible with immediate hypersensitivity should not receive *first-generation cephalosporin* antibiotics unless alternative drugs are clearly less desirable.[37] For the most part, later-generation cephalosporins have significantly greater gram-negative antimicrobial properties, with decreased activity against gram-positive organisms. The fourth-generation cephalosporins have broad-spectrum activity.

The carbapenems and monobactams (aztreonam) are 2 additional classes of β-lactam antibiotics. Cross-reactivity between penicillin and carbapenems would be expected on the basis of the structure of the drugs. There are no published data on allergy to meropenem in patients who are allergic to carbapenem or penicillins. Allergic reactions to the monobactam aztreonam are thought to involve the side chain, so cross-reactivity with other β-lactams should be rare.

Vancomycin Although anaphylaxis to vancomycin is rare, hypotension is a serious immediate adverse effect associated with intravenous administration. Direct myocardial depression[81] and nonimmunologically mediated histamine release[82] have been reported as mechanisms of vancomycin-induced hypotension, and not IgE-mediated anaphylaxis. The hypotension occurs most commonly when the drug is rapidly infused or is administered in a concentrated solution. Vancomycin-associated hypotension may be exacerbated by the concurrent use of other drugs (eg, anesthetics) that cause vasodilatation and/or have a negative inotropic effect.[81] In addition to hypotension, vancomycin can produce the "red neck" or "red man" syndrome, an intense erythematous discoloration of the upper trunk, arms, and neck that may be associated with pruritus in conscious patients. Vancomycin also has been associated with the sudden development of throbbing pain or spasm in the chest or parasternal muscles in conscious patients, without evidence of myocardial ischemia. To minimize the risk of reactions, vancomycin should be infused over a period of at least 60 minutes and in a dilute solution (500 mg/100 mL). Reactions should be treated by discontinuation of the infusion, administration of an antihistamine for pruritus, and the use of vasopressors and other interventions (eg, fluids) that counteract the hypotension.

Sulfonamides and Trimethoprim Sulfonamides are generally safe and are often used for chronic prophylaxis. Occasionally, they cause allergic reactions such as minor skin rashes after approximately 1 week of therapy. Life-threatening reactions have been described in HIV-infected infants reexposed to sulfamethoxazole-trimethoprim (SMX-TMP). Stevens-Johnson syndrome and toxic epidermal necrolysis have been associated with SMX-TMP treatment, presumably mediated by an immune reaction similar to graft versus host disease.[83] Despite concerns having been raised about other sulfonamide-containing drugs such as diuretics, sulfonylureas, and celecoxib, these antimicrobial agents have an aromatic amine group and a substituted ring not found in the nonantibiotic sulfonamide-containing drugs, so cross-reactivity seems unlikely.[84,85]

Other Classes of Antibiotics Development of a serious allergic reaction to non–β-lactam antibiotics, such as the aminoglycosides, is rare. Nonurticarial rashes can be treated with antihistamines.

Multiple Antibiotic Allergy Syndrome The multiple antibiotic allergy syndrome, wherein certain individuals are recognized as making "generic" allergic antibody to unrelated antibiotics, is an evolving entity.[86] Female gender, a history of multiple antibiotic reactions, and reactions to nonsteroidal anti-inflammatory drugs appear to be the main risk factors.[87]

RADIOCONTRAST MEDIA

Adverse, allergic-type reactions induced by radiocontrast media (RCM) injections may occur immediately or have a delayed presentation. Most immediate reactions, the event for which an anesthesiologist would likely be summoned, begin 1 to 3 minutes after intravascular administration. Fatal reactions after radiocontrast administration result in an estimated 500 deaths annually in the United States. Patients with a previous reaction to RCM have an approximately 33% (range 17%-60%) chance of a repeat reaction on reexposure.[52] Depending on the chemistry of the RCM (**Table 86-3**), if ionic RCM was administered previously, the use of nonionic RCM will result in a 10-fold decrease in a severe immediate repeat reaction.[88]

The exact mechanism of adverse reactions to RCM is unknown. Intravascular injection activates complement, either by the classic or the alternative pathway[89]; therefore, production of anaphylatoxins with subsequent mast cell and basophil mediator release has been suggested as the cause of these reactions. However, RCM are capable of inducing nonimmunologic histamine release from mast cells and basophils in the absence of complement activation; hypertonicity has been suggested as the cause, as has an IgE-mediated cause based on elevated tryptase levels, particularly with severe or fatal reactions.[90-93]

Pretreatment of high-risk patients with oral prednisone (50 mg) and diphenhydramine (50 mg) 1 hour before radiocontrast administration reduces the risk of reactions to 9% (Box 86-4).[94] Almost all reactions in pretreated patients are of no clinical importance (eg, mild urticaria). The addition of oral ephedrine (25 mg) 1 hour before radiocontrast administration (in patients without angina, dysrhythmias, or other contraindications for ephedrine administration) further reduces the reaction rate to 3.1%.[53] Combining premedication with nonhyperosmolar contrast

TABLE 86-3 Reactions to Different Types of Radiocontrast Media

		Hypersensitivity Reactions			
	Chemistry	Mild Immediate	Severe Immediate	Fatal	Nonimmediate
Ionic monomers[a]	Highly water soluble	3.8%-12.7%	0.1%-0.4%	0.1-0.3:10 000	0.5%-23%
Nonionic monomers[b]	Rendered water soluble by introducing long-side chains of hydroxyl groups	0.7%-3.1%	0.02%-0.04%	0.1-0.3:10 000	
Ionic dimers[a]	Highly water soluble				
Nonionic dimers	Rendered water soluble by introducing long-side chains of hydroxyl groups				(Incidence on the higher side)

[a]Have been withdrawn in most countries.

[b]Most RCM marketed.

media may be of additional benefit in preventing reactions in high-risk individuals.[51]

PROTAMINE

Protamine sulfate, a polycationic protein extracted from salmon milt, is used to reverse heparin anticoagulation and slow the absorption of certain insulins (Neutral Protamine Hagedorn, or NPH, and protamine zinc insulin, or PZI). The use of intravenous protamine following cardiopulmonary bypass, cardiac catheterization, hemodialysis, or pheresis has resulted in increasing reports of life-threatening adverse reactions.

Diabetic patients receiving daily subcutaneous injections of insulins containing protamine have a greatly increased risk for life-threatening reactions when given protamine intravenously.[95-97] Another group that may be at increased risk for protamine reactions are men who have undergone vasectomies. After vasectomy, 55% to 73% of men will develop antibodies to sperm antigens, and of this group, 20% to 33% develop autoantibodies to protamine.[98] In addition, because protamine is produced from the matured testis of salmon or related species of fish belonging to the family *Salmonidae* or *Clupeidae,* it has been suggested that individuals allergic to fish may have serum antibodies directed against protamine.[99] Finally, prior exposure to intravenous protamine given for the reversal of heparin anticoagulation may increase the risk for a reaction with subsequent protamine administration.[100,101] Following cardiopulmonary bypass, risk factors found to correlate with adverse events following protamine administration included NPH insulin use (odds ratio = 8.18; 95% confidence interval [CI] 2.08-32.2), fish allergy (odds ratio = 24.5; CI 1.24-482.3), and a history of nonprotamine medication allergy (odds ratio = 2.97; CI 1.25-7.07).[91]

The exact mechanisms by which acute protamine reactions occur are incompletely understood. Some protamine reactions may be associated with complement activation, either through protamine–heparin complexes or through the interaction of protamine and complement fixing, antiprotamine IgG antibody, leading to pulmonary artery pressure elevation through the generation of thromboxane.[102,103]

TOPICAL PREPARATIONS

Cutaneous hypersensitivity and eczema may occur from chronic exposure to topical preparations. Of 50 case reports of chlorhexidine anaphylaxis, one-third occurred during surgery[104]; however, the risk of development of type I and type IV allergy to chlorhexidine, even with daily occupational exposure of health care workers, is extremely rare.[104] The intriguing explanation for allergic reactions lies in the fact that its molecular structure is symmetrical, with 2 identical epitopes. Therefore, it is capable of cross-linking mast and basophil cell surface IgE antibodies, thereby promoting degranulation and allergic reactions in sensitized individuals. This mechanism is similar to other divalent drugs such as succinylcholine. Moreover, sensitization to chlorhexidine is likely because of its presence in numerous consumer products such as cleaning fluids, toothpastes, mouth rinses, etc.

Concerns are often expressed about allergy to iodine in the context of povidone iodine preparation solutions or in patients with a history of seafood allergy. Similar concerns are voiced about patients with allergy to RCM because of the iodine component. The reaction to povidone iodine is typically allergic contact dermatitis or local irritation. There is, however, 1 case report of anaphylaxis to povidone-iodine applied intravaginally, but because of the lack of follow-up allergy testing, it is unclear if this reaction was caused by the iodine or the povidone.[105] Povidone is the carrier molecule for iodine atoms. A 9-year-old child has been confirmed to have eosinophilia, elevated specific IgE level, and a positive skin prick test for povidone iodine.[106] Fish allergy is due to protein M and tropomyosin, neither of which contain iodine.[107,108]

TRANSFUSION-RELATED ANAPHYLAXIS

Transfusion-related anaphylaxis, a serious, life-threatening condition, is discussed in Chapter 83.

NATURAL RUBBER LATEX

Natural rubber latex present in various materials, especially surgical gloves, is responsible for a dramatic change in the etiology of intraoperative anaphylactic shock, increasing in 1 series from 0.5% of cases in 1989 to 22.3% in 2002.

Natural rubber latex is a complex suspension of polyisoprene, lipids, phospholipids, and proteins. The proteins are found in 3 physical states: water soluble, starch bound, or latex bound, and there are at least 240 potentially allergenic proteins in the processed latex product. The protein content of latex gloves can vary up to 1000-fold among different lots marketed by the same manufacturer and 3000-fold between gloves from different manufacturers.[109] A number of chemicals, including preservatives, accelerators, antioxidants, and vulcanizing compounds, are added during the manufacturing process to yield the final product. Although the chemicals added to latex have long been associated with contact dermatitis and type IV reactions, it was only after the embracing of universal precautions that reports from around the world describing generalized urticaria, angioedema, upper and lower respiratory obstructions, and cardiovascular collapse first appeared. Patients who have suffered severe systemic reactions often have a history of contact urticaria or angioedema to rubber products such as gloves or rubber balloons, or atopy.

Certain populations are at significantly increased risk for latex allergy. These include health care workers, who have had increased exposure to latex usually in the form of gloves; patients with prolonged or frequent exposure to latex products such as urinary catheters; and latex factory workers.[110] A health care worker who is atopic is at increased risk, and the risk is increased if he or she had prior surgery.[111] Anesthesiologists have a 12.5% and 2.4% prevalence of latex sensitization and allergy, respectively.[112] Patients with meningomyelocele or congenital urologic anomalies seem particularly susceptible, with an estimated incidence of latex allergy averaging 50%.

IgE antibodies play a major role in the immunopathogenesis of latex-induced allergy and anaphylaxis. The diagnosis of latex allergy is made by a combination of medical history, physical examination, and reliable in vivo or in vitro tests. Although skin prick testing is both sensitive (100%) and specific (99%), this method should be restricted to patients with a compelling history and an inconclusive serologic test result because of possible systemic reactions. The RAST for latex-specific IgE is recommended, although it is less sensitive than skin prick testing.

Serum tryptase levels in the immediate postanaphylaxis period may be helpful in confirming the diagnosis following a clinical episode. The positive predictive value of tryptase for the diagnosis of anaphylaxis is 92.6%, and the negative predictive value is 54.3%.[113] Multiple allergies are often found in latex allergic patients. Cross-reactivity of latex with tropical fruits is not uncommon,[114] and such findings in the history can be used to heighten suspicion about a patient's potential for latex allergy.

Patients who have had serious allergic reactions to latex and patients at high risk (eg, patients with meningomyelocele) should avoid contact with latex products. Because prophylactic drug protocols have proven ineffective, a latex-safe environment is advocated.[115,116] **Box 86-7** provides a checklist for dealing with the latex-allergic patient. Moreover, patients in high-risk pediatric groups, such as children with urologic birth defects and myelomeningocele, should be offered latex-free exposure in the operating room from birth to avoid subsequent sensitization. The American Society of Anesthesiologists has a brochure available on its website summarizing current recommendations for anesthesiologists caring for latex-allergic patients.[117]

BOX 86-7

Checklist for Latex-Allergic Patients

Preoperative

History of:

Chronic care with latex-based products

Spina bifida, urologic reconstructive surgery

Multiple surgical procedures (eg, >9)

Intolerance to latex-based products: balloons, rubber gloves, condoms, dental dams, etc

Allergy to tropical fruits

Intraoperative anaphylaxis of uncertain etiology

Health care workers, especially with atopy or hand eczema

Consider referral for allergy consultation and in vitro or in vivo testing

Day of Surgery

Notify and coordinate care among surgical, anesthesia, and nursing teams.

Have lists available of nonlatex product alternatives.

First case of the day is preferable to decrease aeroallergen concentration.

Display "Latex Allergy" or "Latex Alert" signs inside and outside the operating room.

Minimize latex exposure for at-risk patients.

Latex alert: Patients with significant risk factors for latex allergy but no overt signs or symptoms

Latex allergy: Patients with or without significant risk factors for latex allergy and positive history, signs, symptoms, and confirmatory laboratory test

Anesthesia equipment

Latex-free gloves, airways, endotracheal tubes

Masks (polyvinylchloride if available, or old, well-washed black rubber masks)

Rebreathing bags and bellows (neoprene if available, or well-washed black rubber bags)

Breathing circuit (disposable, polyvinylchloride, packaged separately from latex rebreathing bag)

Blood pressure cuffs (if new latex, cover with soft cotton)

Ambu-type bag (ensure that bag and valve do not have latex components); alternative is silicone self-inflating bag

Dilute concentration of epinephrine (0.01 mg/mL or 1:100 000) readily available

Surgical equipment–avoid:

Latex surgical gloves; drains (eg, Penrose); urinary catheters; instrument mats; vascular tags; bulb syringes; rubber bands; rubber-shod clamps

Postoperative

Medical Alert tag

Warning sign posted on chart and on bed

From Holzman RS. Latex allergy: an emerging operating room problem. *Anesth Analg.* 1993;76:635-641, with permission.

CONCLUSIONS AND THERAPEUTIC IMPLICATIONS

1. **Once an allergen is identified, the most important clinical strategy is avoidance of that allergen.** As perioperative specialists, anesthesiologists have a critical role in understanding the etiology, treatment, and evaluation of patients' allergic reactions.
2. **Epinephrine is the most important medication to have available and to provide in the setting of anaphylaxis.** Early administration of the appropriate dose is crucial for optimum outcome because the outcome of shock due to anaphylaxis may be far worse than other forms of shock. For prophylaxis or attenuation of an anticipated allergic response, effective protocols exist that reduce the risk of anaphylaxis to less than 0.5%. Following primary treatment, adjunctive, or secondary, treatment (antihistamines, anticholinergics, β- and α-agonists) is important for patient comfort and reduction of symptoms of anaphylaxis.
3. **Specific immunotherapy strategies are emerging** for a variety of allergens to which patients and health care workers have become exposed. Chronic as well as acute desensitization strategies exist that reorganize an individual's profile from primarily a Th_2 to a Th_1 type of response. Because of the increasing understanding of the immune response, strategies now can be developed for therapeutically interfering with the interaction of IgE and allergen, inhibiting cytokine function and T-cell activation, or modifying allergy cell responsiveness.
4. There is an important epidemiologic challenge in explicating the reasons for the **increasing incidence of allergic disease**, particularly in Western countries.

KEY REFERENCES

- Brockow K. Immediate and delayed reactions to radiocontrast media: is there an allergic mechanism? *Immunol Allergy Clin N Am.* 2009;29:453-468.
- deShazo R, Nelson H. An approach to the patient with a history of local anesthetic hypersensitivity: experience with 90 patients. *J Allergy Clin Immunol.* 1989;63:387.
- Dewachter P, Jouan-Hureaux V, Franck P, et al. Anaphylactic shock: a form of distributive shock without inhibition of oxygen consumption. *Anesthesiology.* 2005;103:40-49.
- Gruchalla R, Pirmohamed M. Antibiotic allergy. *New Engl J Med.* 2006;354(6):601-609.
- Harper N, Dixon T, Dugue P, et al. Guidelines: suspected anaphylactic reactions associated with anaesthesia. *Anaesthesia.* 2009;64:199-211.
- Howarth P. ABC of allergies: Pathogenic mechanisms: a rational basis for treatment. *Brit Med J.* 1998;316:758-761.
- Kroigaard M, Garvey L, Gillberg L, et al. Scandinavian clinical practice guidelines on the diagnosis, management and follow-up of anaphylaxis during anaesthesia. *Acta Anaesthesiol Scand.* 2007;51:655-670.
- Lieberman P, Kemp S, Oppenheimer J, Lang D, Bernstein I, Nicklas R. The diagnosis and management of anaphylaxis: an updated practice parameter. *J Allergy Clin Immunol.* 2005;115:S483-S523.
- Mertes P, Laxenaire M, Lienhart A, et al. Reducing the risk of anaphylaxis during anaesthesia: guidelines for clinical practice. *J Invest Allergol Clin Immunol.* 2005;15(2):91-101.
- Soetens F. Anaphylaxis during anaesthesia: diagnosis and treatment. *Acta Anaesth Belg.* 2004;55(3):229-237.

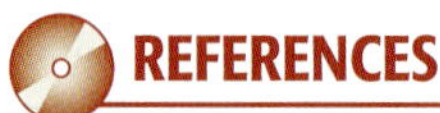

REFERENCES

Complete references available on DVD and online version at www.LongneckerAnesthesiology.com

CHAPTER 87

Malignant Hyperthermia

John Capacchione
Marilyn Green Larach
Nyamkhishig Sambuughin
Maria Voelkel
Sheila Muldoon

KEY POINTS

1. Malignant hyperthermia (MH) was first described in 1962 in a case report that also suggested an inherited basis for the syndrome.
2. Skeletal muscle is the primary target tissue in MH. A laboratory diagnostic test for MH was developed using the enhanced contracture response to caffeine and halothane in muscle strips from MH patients. Studies using these tests suggest that the cellular mechanism responsible for MH is a derangement in calcium regulation.
3. No convenient minimally invasive laboratory test for MH susceptibility is yet available. Halothane and caffeine contracture assays remain the most reliable tests.
4. Molecular genetic tests based on identification of mutations in the *RYR1* and *CACNA1S* genes can confirm the diagnosis of MH susceptibility.
5. A negative screen of the *RYR1* and *CACNA1S* genes does not rule out MH susceptibility.
6. The immediate cause of an MH crisis appears to be a sudden increase in the concentration of myoplasmic calcium, thought to be triggered by inhalational anesthetic or depolarizing muscle relaxant interactions with the sarcoplasmic reticulum (SR).
7. All potent halogenated anesthetics and depolarizing muscle relaxants are capable of triggering an MH reaction, but an MH event does not always occur with each exposure to triggering anesthetic agents, even in persons subsequently found to be MH susceptible. This situation reflects the variable expression and penetrance of the gene mutations.
8. Time of onset of a fulminant episode of MH is unpredictable, varying from minutes to within several hours of induction; it may even occur in the recovery room.
9. The earliest signs of MH are hypercarbia, sinus tachycardia, and masseter muscle rigidity (MMR).
10. Laboratory signs of MH may include increased $Paco_2$, metabolic and/or respiratory acidosis, hyperkalemia, increased creatine kinase (CK), myoglobinemia, and myoglobinuria.
11. In 1979, dantrolene, a drug that decreases skeletal myoplasmic Ca^{2+}, was approved for clinical use by the Food and Drug Administration; this was a major advance in the treatment and management of MH.
12. A very low mortality rate from MH can be achieved by prompt recognition of the clinical situation, ready access to supplies necessary for treatment, and initiation of appropriate therapeutic measures starting with dantrolene 2.5 mg/kg intravenously.

INTRODUCTION

Malignant hyperthermia (MH) is a dominantly inherited skeletal muscle disorder that predisposes susceptible individuals to a potentially fatal reaction upon exposure to potent volatile anesthetics and/or succinylcholine. In some individuals, MH-like reactions can also be triggered by high environmental temperatures and stress in the absence of anesthetics.[1] Fulminant MH episodes apparently result from dysregulation of intracellular Ca^{2+}, causing a rapid and sustained rise in myoplasmic Ca^{2+}. Molecular genetic studies have identified mutations in the ryanodine receptor type 1 gene (*RYR1*), encoding the skeletal muscle Ca^{2+} release channel, to be a major cause for MH. However, MH is known to be a heterogeneous disorder, as mutations in *RYR1* account for only 70% of all MH cases. There are also a few cases attributed to abnormalities in the *CACNA1S* gene, encoding the α_1-subunit of the L-type calcium channel of the dihydropyridine receptor (DHPR).[2]

An acute MH event may cause a hypermetabolic state with some or all of the following abnormalities: hypercarbia, tachypnea, tachycardia, generalized muscular rigidity, masseter muscle rigidity (MMR), respiratory acidosis, metabolic acidosis, and hyperthermia. Muscle membrane damage leads to the release of intracellular muscle constituents such as myoglobin, creatine kinase (CK), potassium, and lactate dehydrogenase. Hyperthermia, for which the syndrome is named, is most likely of metabolic origin caused by the maximum turnover of muscle adenosine triphosphate (ATP).[3,4] The formerly high mortality rate (70%) has decreased to approximately 1% to 5% since the introduction of dantrolene, a drug that decreases myoplasmic calcium and usually stops the crisis if administered when early symptoms are recognized.

There are still numerous aspects of MH that are not understood. First, fulminant MH remains unpredictable, with deaths still occurring in otherwise healthy people. Second, there is no convenient and rapid test to identify MH-susceptible (MHS) patients prior to surgery. Third, estimates of MH prevalence in the general population are, at best, uncertain. Fourth, many patients are labeled MHS without adequate laboratory confirmation of their susceptibility. This leads to a lifelong burden for many patients and their families with limitations in the kinds of anesthesia they can receive, the locations they can be anesthetized, and their entry into the military and police force. When appropriate, it is important that patients experiencing possible MH be referred for definitive diagnostic testing. This chapter discusses the history, epidemiology, pathophysiology, genetics, diagnosis, treatment, management, and evaluation of MH.

HISTORICAL PERSPECTIVE

The first link between inhalational anesthetics as etiologic agents and the inherited nature of a disorder called malignant hyperpyrexia or malignant hyperthermia was made in the early 1960s. Denborough and Lovell reported a case of a 21-year-old man reluctant to undergo surgical repair of his leg because 10 members of his family had died without explanation during or shortly after general anesthesia with ether-type anesthetics.[5] The patient was reassured, and surgery proceeded with caution. However, within 10 minutes of induction of anesthesia with halothane, the patient developed tachycardia, hypotension, cyanosis, and hot, sweaty skin. The anesthetic was discontinued, vigorous cooling was initiated, and the patient survived. When Denborough investigated the family history, he correctly surmised that they exhibited an inherited disorder that caused life-threatening hyperthermia when administered general anesthetic agents.[6] Subsequently, a large affected family from Wisconsin was identified in which 20 episodes of MH with 8 fatalities confirmed the dominant inheritance pattern of the disorder. This was an important step in spreading awareness of the syndrome in North America.[7]

Studies by Kalow and Britt reported that freshly biopsied skeletal muscle from MHS survivors had abnormally strong muscle contracture responses to caffeine in vitro.[8] Because caffeine in high doses had been previously reported to release Ca^{2+} from the sarcoplasmic reticulum (SR), their observations were important in linking MH contracture response to Ca^{2+} released from the SR. Also, the contractile responses to caffeine were potentiated by halothane, which suggested that halothane might also affect Ca^{2+} release and handling in skeletal muscle. Later, it was reported that halothane alone could cause abnormal contracture in human MH skeletal muscle.[9] These observations by Kalow, Britt, and Ellis led to the development of an MH diagnostic bioassay using freshly excised skeletal muscle samples, which later became the in vitro contracture test (IVCT) in Europe, Australia, and New Zealand, and the caffeine halothane contracture test (CHCT) in North America.

Susceptibility to MH is not confined to humans, but occurs in several animal species, including pigs, dogs, and horses. The porcine model has been studied most extensively, and the pharmacologic properties of MHS swine muscle appear to be similar to MHS human muscle.[10] The breeds of swine (Landrace, Poland China, and Pietrain) in which MH has been characterized are those in which there is a high incidence of porcine stress syndrome. Porcine stress syndrome is a condition associated with lean, heavily muscled pigs that develop acute shock-like episodes in response to stress, mild exercise, sudden increases in ambient temperature, fighting, coitus, and transportation. The porcine and human MH syndromes were bridged when it was discovered that administering halothane to pigs caused a metabolic and muscular syndrome similar to human MH. Subsequently, a single homozygous mutation in the *RYR1* was identified in all MHS and porcine stress syndrome–prone swine.[11,12]

In the 1970s, even as progress in understanding the pathophysiology was being made and human MH was recognized to be an inherited disorder, patient mortality from MH remained high because there was no effective pharmacologic treatment. In 1975 Harrison described the efficacy of dantrolene in preventing and treating porcine MH.[13] These results were confirmed by Kolb et al in humans,[14] and in 1979 the Food and Drug Administration approved intravenous dantrolene as an antidote for MH. The advent of dantrolene dramatically decreased the mortality rate.

Major advances in the past 3 decades involved elucidating the subcellular site of the MH defect in skeletal muscle, standardization of the diagnostic contracture tests, and identification of the SR Ca^{2+} release channel encoded by the *RYR1* on chromosome 19q as the major candidate gene for MH susceptibility and for central core disease (CCD), a human slowly progressive myopathy.[11,12] In 2005 investigators used stem cell technology to create "knock-in" mice and reported that mice harboring a specific *RYR1* mutation (Y522S) could be triggered to develop an MH syndrome by exposure to either volatile anesthetics or heat.[15] Transgenic "knock-in" mice will likely permit detailed analysis of how different mutations give rise to altered muscle calcium handling and function.

EPIDEMIOLOGY

The prevalence of MH susceptibility in the population is unknown, and estimates of the frequency of acute fulminant episodes vary widely. In a survey of a mixed surgical population of all ages in Denmark, Ørding found that fulminant MH occurred once in 250 000 anesthetics when all types of anesthesia were included, and once in 62 000 anesthetics when a combination of potent inhalation agents and succinylcholine was used.[16]

Recently, an International Classification of Diseases (ICD) code for MH was created, permitting studies utilizing administrative and clinical databases to estimate MH prevalence and mortality rates. Using these databases, Brady et al found an estimated prevalence for MH of 1.08 per 100 000 New York state hospital discharges in which there was any indication of exposure to anesthesia.[17] Using US multiple cause of death files of the National Center for Health Statistics and national estimates of hospital surgical discharges, Li et al estimated that 1% (n = 22/2211) of all anesthesia-related deaths were complicated by MH for the years 1999 to 2005. The estimated risk of MH-related mortality was 0.0082 per 100 000 surgical inpatients.[18] However, neither of these database studies had access to the clinical details of the actual MH events, so they were unable to verify the MH diagnoses.

In 1987 the North American Malignant Hyperthermia Registry (NAMHR) was created to acquire, analyze, and disseminate patient-specific clinical and laboratory information on MH. It currently contains data on nearly 3000 individuals with a possible history of MH susceptibility and has proven to be a valuable resource once a clinical grading scale (CGS) was created by international MH experts to provide a clinical case definition of MH.[19] The CGS scale permits comparisons between groups that are defined by similar characteristics because it ranks the qualitative likelihood that an adverse event represents MH and that, with further investigation of family history, an individual patient will be diagnosed as MHS. CGS ranks are assigned independently of any other MH diagnostic test. The CGS has been used extensively to validate the MH diagnostic contracture tests and to study the manner in which MH presents.

MH has been reported worldwide in all races. Although MH is inherited in an autosomal dominant pattern, North American MH Registry studies and multiple other observers[20] have found that MH is expressed primarily in males (75%) and in the young. In a recent NAMHR study, the median age at presentation was 22 years (range 116 days to 78 years) with 45% of 286 MH cases occurring in those who were 19 years or younger. Most patients were asymptomatic prior to their MH events, although 29% were noted to have a muscular build, 7% had a history of increased muscle tone, and 4% had a history of muscle cramps. Although MH is inherited, only 7% were found to have had a positive MH family history at the time of their triggering anesthetic.[21] These findings illustrate the importance of both obtaining a careful preoperative history and maintaining perioperative vigilance for signs of MH.

In the last decade, 2 independent epidemiologic studies estimated the incidence of *RYR1* variants in the general population at 1 in 2000 to 3000.[22,23] These data, coupled with the fact that MH is characterized by variable expression and penetrance, suggest that MH susceptibility may be more common than what is detected solely by experience of a clinical episode.

PATHOPHYSIOLOGY

SUBCELLULAR SITES OF DEFECT IN SKELETAL MUSCLE

It is now generally accepted that MH is a syndrome characterized by abnormal excitation–contraction (EC) coupling in skeletal muscle.[1] During EC coupling, muscle membrane depolarization induces a conformational change in the DHPR or voltage-gated L-type Ca^{2+} channels. This leads to activation of the ryanodine receptor type 1 protein (RYR1) and the rapid release of Ca^{2+} from its stores in the SR. Ca^{2+} travels down its concentration gradient from the lumen of the SR (Ca^{2+} concentration approximately 1 mM) to the cytosol (Ca^{2+} concentration approximately 100 nM) where it binds to troponin C, causing movement of tropomyosin away from the myosin-binding sites on the thin filament and triggering muscle contractions. Muscle contraction is terminated when Ca^{2+} is actively pumped back into the SR by the ATP-dependent calcium pump (sarco/endoplasmic reticulum $Ca2^{+}$ –ATPase or SERCA; see **Fig. 87-1** for a representation of the membrane systems involved in EC coupling).[24] The DHPR/RYR1 interaction underlies all voluntary movements, including respiration, and is therefore essential for life.[24] Major defects in either the DHPR or RYR1 proteins can result in poor development in utero and death at or before birth. A mutation in either protein will potentially cause Ca^{2+} dysregulation and muscle disease. For a more detailed discussion of EC coupling, see reviews by Dulhunty et al[24] and Franzini-Armstrong.[25]

PROPERTIES OF DHPR AND RYRs

The DHPR is a major component of the transverse tubular membrane. It contains α_1-, α_2/δ-, β-, and γ-subunits, forming an L-type channel protein that is the receptor for certain Ca^{2+} channel blockers such as dihydropyridines. The α_1-subunit of the DHPR is a pore-forming subunit of the Ca^{2+} ion channel. It is comprised of 4 repeat domains connected by large cytoplasmic loops (see **Fig. 87-2A**)[26,27]. The functions of the other subunits are not well defined, although it is known that the β-subunit is required for targeting the DHPR to the tubular membrane.

Electron microscopic studies reveal that the RYR1 and α_1-subunit of the DHPR have a highly specific spatial association in skeletal muscle.

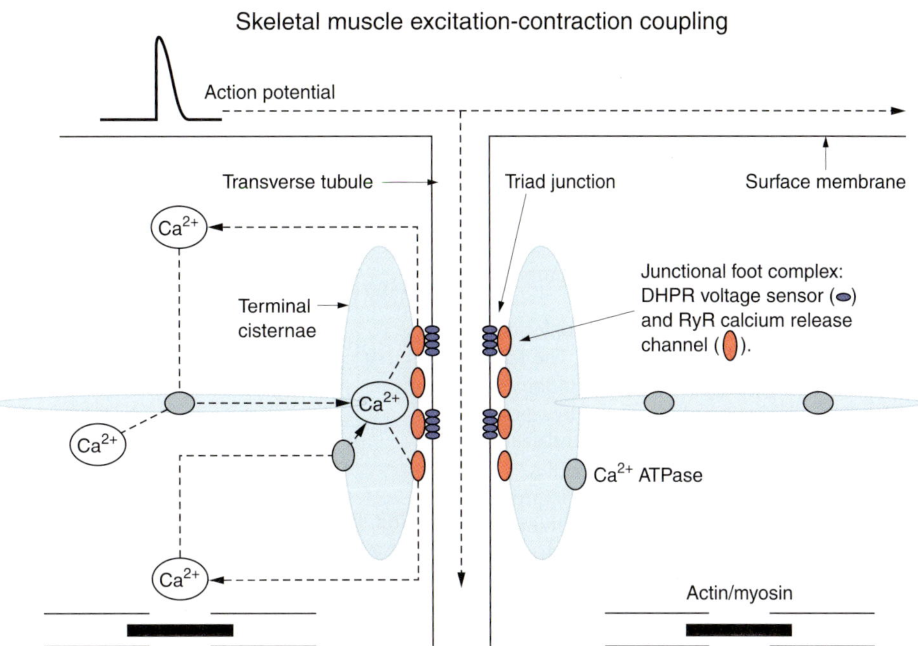

FIGURE 87-1. Membrane systems and membrane proteins involved in excitation–contraction coupling. The action potential propagates along the surface and transverse tubule membranes. The signal resulting from depolarization is transmitted across the triad junction that is formed between the transverse tubule membrane and the terminal cisternae membrane of the sarcoplasmic reticulum Ca^{2+} store. A triad is the usual junction between the transverse tubule membrane and sarcoplasmic reticulum in skeletal muscle, and is so named because it consists of a central transverse tubule membrane with a terminal cisternae of the sarcoplasmic reticulum on either side. The voltage sensor for excitation–contraction coupling is the dihydropyridine receptor (DHPR) in the transverse tubule membrane. The Ca^{2+} release channel in the sarcoplasmic reticulum is the ryanodine receptor (RYR). A tetrad of DHPRs opposes every second RYR. The contraction is terminated when Ca^{2+} is actively pumped back into the sarcoplasmic reticulum by the adenosine triphosphate (ATP)-dependant Ca^{2+} pump (Ca^{2+}-ATPase). [From Dulhunty AF, Haarmann CS, Green D, Laver DR, Board PG, Casarotto MG. Interactions between dihydropyridine receptors and ryanodine receptors in striated muscle. *Prog Biophys Mol Biol.* 2002;79(1-3):45-75.]

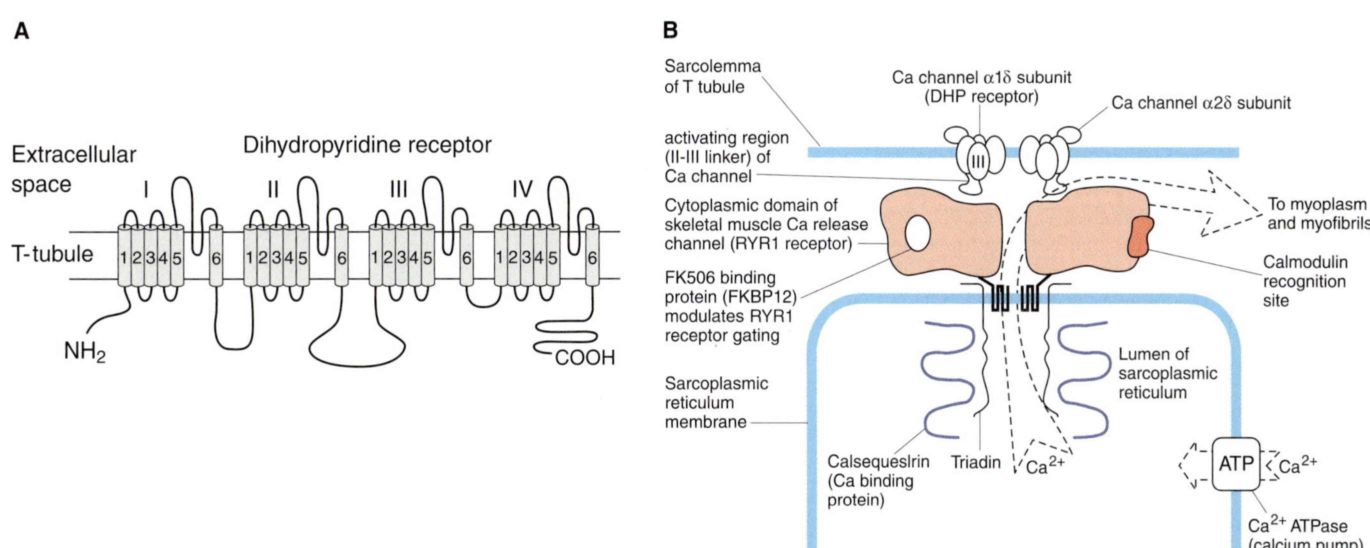

FIGURE 87-2. **A.** Voltage-gated Ca^{2+} channel dihydropyridine receptor (DHPR). The α_1-subunit of the DHPR consists of 4 repeat domains (I-IV), each with 6 transmembrane segments (1-6). Segment 5 and 6 loops form the ion channel pore, and segment 4 contains positively charged residues that confer voltage dependence to the protein. The II and III intracellular loop of the DHPR interacts with the ryanodine receptor to mediate excitation contraction coupling, as shown in (**B**). [Figure and legend adapted from Loke J, MacLennan DH. Malignant hyperthermia and central core disease: disorders of Ca^{2+} release channels. *Am J Med.* 1998;104:472, Fig. 2, and Jurkat-Rott K, McCarthy T, Lehmann-Horn F. Genetics and pathogenesis of malignant hyperthermia. *Muscle Nerve.* 2000;23:10, Fig. 2.]

B. Schematic representation of the triad junction of skeletal muscle shows the junctional foot protein (ryanodine receptor [RYR1]) and its associated proteins. In skeletal muscle, the α_{1s}-subunit of the dihydropyridine receptor (DHPR) participates in excitation-contraction coupling. These physical links transmit essential signals across the narrow gap of the triadic junction that activate RYR1 and release Ca^{2+} from the sarcoplasmic reticulum. [RYR and its interaction with DHPR are as adapted from Pessah IN, Lynch C 3rd, Gronert GA. Complex pharmacology of malignant hyperthermia. *Anesthesiology.* 1996;84(6):1275-1279.]

Clusters of 4 evenly spaced particles (tetrads) representing DHPRs are positioned in the muscle membrane such that each particle is located immediately above one of the 4 RYR1 subunits.[1] However, DHPR tetrads are associated with only every second subunit of RYR1, suggesting that not all release channels are directly coupled to DHPRs. Release channels that are not opposed by tetrads are most likely activated by Ca^{2+} via Ca^{2+}-induced Ca^{2+} release (CICR; see Fig. 87-2B).[28] Current evidence suggests that there is a direct physical coupling between the II and III loops of the α_1-subunit of the DHPR and cytoplasmic regions of the RYR1 that allows for communication between the 2 membranes during EC coupling.

The RYRs are extremely well-studied proteins, but the complexity of their function and regulation leaves much to be understood. The name ryanodine comes from the plant alkaloid that has a binding affinity for these receptors. There are 3 isoforms (RYR1, 2, and 3) encoded by separate genes on chromosomes 19, 1, and 15. The isoforms are differentially distributed and regulated, and have different pharmacologic properties.

RYR1 expressed in skeletal muscle is a very large tetrameric protein composed of 4 identical subunits that assemble into a homotetramer to form functional Ca^{2+} release channels. RYR1 has also been identified in human B-lymphocytes and in immature dendritic immune cells. RYR2 is expressed predominantly in cardiac tissue. RYR3 is expressed in skeletal muscle at relatively low levels, in smooth muscle, gut, and the brain. Each subunit (monomer) of RYR1 consists of a large cytoplasmic N-terminal, constituting approximately 80% of the protein called "the foot structure." The C-terminal region comprises one-fifth of the protein and contains a number of important structural features, including the transmembrane complex, the Ca^{2+} permeability pore, and the interaction sites for Ca^{2+}, caffeine, 4-chloro-*m*-cresol, ATP, and ryanodine.

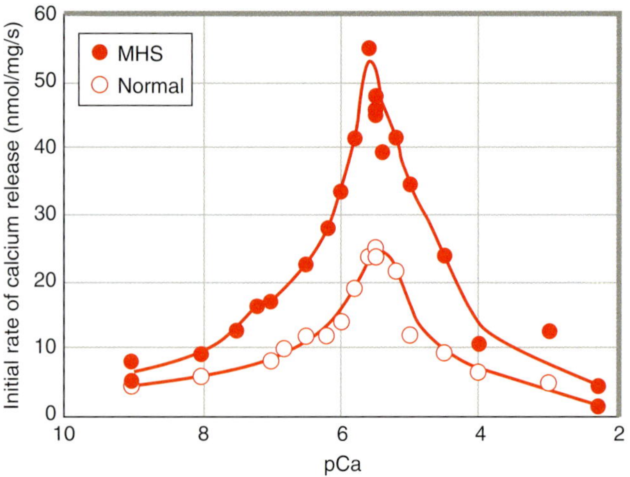

FIGURE 87-3. Ca^{2+} dependence of rate of Ca^{2+}-induced Ca^{2+} release from MH-susceptible and normal pig sarcoplasmic reticulum (SR) vesicles. SR vesicles were passively loaded with Ca^{2+}, and Ca^{2+} release was initiated by rapid filtration with a solution containing ionized Ca^{2+}. Under these conditions, the rate constant for Ca^{2+} release from MH-susceptible SR was significantly greater than that from normal SR. [From Carrier L, Villa M, Dupont Y. Abnormal rapid Ca^{2+} release from sarcoplasmic reticulum of malignant hyperthermia susceptible pigs. *Biochim Biophys Acta.* 1991;1064:179, Fig. 4, as reviewed in Mickelson JR, Louis CF. Malignant hyperthermia: excitation-contraction coupling, Ca^{2+} release channel, and cell Ca^{2+} regulation defects. *Physiol Rev.* 1996;76:548, Fig. 6.]

RYR1 MODULATORS

RYR1 binds to an accessory protein, calstabin 1 (FK506 binding protein or FKBP12), which stabilizes the channel and helps coordinate gating. RYR1 interacts with numerous proteins localized within the triad junction including calmodulin, triadin, junctin, junctophilin 1 and 2, calsequestrin, and many other accessory and regulatory proteins.[10] The principal endogenous modulator of RYR1 is Ca^{2+}, which has a biphasic effect. At micromolar concentration, Ca^{2+} activates the RYR1 channel, and at higher millimolar concentrations, Ca^{2+} inhibits channel activity.[29] Mg^{2+} is an important inhibitor of RYR1 either by competing with Ca^{2+} for its binding site or by binding to an inhibitory site. In addition, exogenous modulators can alter RYR1 activity. One of the most extensively studied is ryanodine. Ryanodine modulates RYR1 activity in a biphasic manner; low (nanomolar) concentrations activate RYR1; whereas concentrations greater than 100 μM inhibit channel activity. Caffeine is a channel activator that has complex effects on RYR1. Its primary effect is to increase the release of Ca^{2+} from the SR, but some of caffeine's effects appear to be dependent on the Ca^{2+} concentration. Thus caffeine-induced Ca^{2+} release may further influence the effects of caffeine itself.

One of the most important inhibitors of RYR1 channel activity is dantrolene. Dantrolene lowers myoplasmic Ca^{2+} and is used to treat clinical MH episodes. A binding site for dantrolene had been proposed within the N-terminal region of the RYR1, but independent confirmation is still required. Halothane and other volatile anesthetics activate the RYR1 channel, but their site of action is unknown.

EFFECT OF MUTATIONS ON CA^{2+} HOMEOSTASIS

The RYR1 Ca^{2+} release channel exists in 2 functional states, opened and closed. The gating mechanism for the channel integrates many complex protein–protein interactions that may be modified by soluble factors in the cytoplasm of the muscle cell and in the lumen of the SR.[1] As mentioned previously, the alkaloid ryanodine has dual actions on the RYR1 channels; at low concentrations, it can open the channel, and at higher concentrations, it irreversibly binds to the channel inhibiting channel activity.[29] Ryanodine has been used extensively to define the properties of the RYR1 channel and how genetic and physiologic factors can alter its activity. Mickelson et al first demonstrated that skeletal muscle samples from MHS swine exhibit higher *specific* radiolabeled ryanodine binding as well as increased sensitivity to micromolar Ca^{2+}. Because *specific* ryanodine binding is proportional to the open state of the Ca^{2+} channel, these results suggest that calcium release is linked to MH and that the channel has a higher probability of being in the open state.[1] In SR vesicle preparations isolated from MHS swine muscle, the initial rate of Ca^{2+} release examined over a range of Ca^{2+} concentrations (submicromolar to millimolar) showed a 2- to 3-fold increase compared to SR vesicles prepared from normal swine (**Fig. 87-3**).[10] At the single-channel level, RYR1 channels from MHS swine and humans have normal conductance and selectivity, but show increased open probability. The RYR1 channels in MHS species also appear to be less sensitive to inactivation by high Ca^{2+} concentrations (**Fig. 87-4**A and B).

Ca^{2+} and Mg^{2+} are both critical to the proper functioning of the RYR1 channel, and both cations shape the kinetics and the magnitude of the channel's response. Normally, the RYR1 channel responds to Ca^{2+} in a concentration-dependent biphasic manner. The biphasic effect is thought to occur via binding of Ca^{2+} to a high affinity stimulatory site and a low infinity inhibitory site. It is likely that Mg^{2+} acts by competing with Ca^{2+} at the activator sites and/or binding to its low affinity inhibitory sites. MHS-related RYR1 Ca^{2+} release channels are (1) more likely to open and (2) unable to close promptly with appropriate physiologic stimuli (high intracellular Ca^{2+} ($[Ca^{2+}]_i$), low pH, and/or high Mg^{2+}). The net effect is a sustained and large increase in myoplasmic Ca^{2+} concentration.[10] The gating properties are also altered by certain chemical substances. This is seen as a heightened sensitivity to volatile anesthetics, caffeine, 4 chloro-*m*–cresol, and potassium depolarization. RYR1 activities are also modulated by post-translation modifications such as phosphorylation, oxidation, and S-nitrosylation.[30]

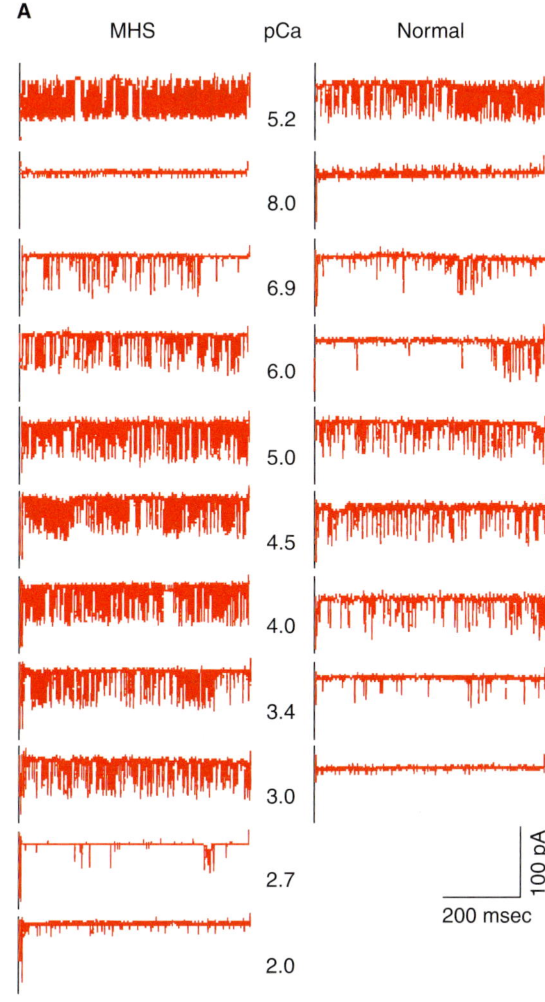

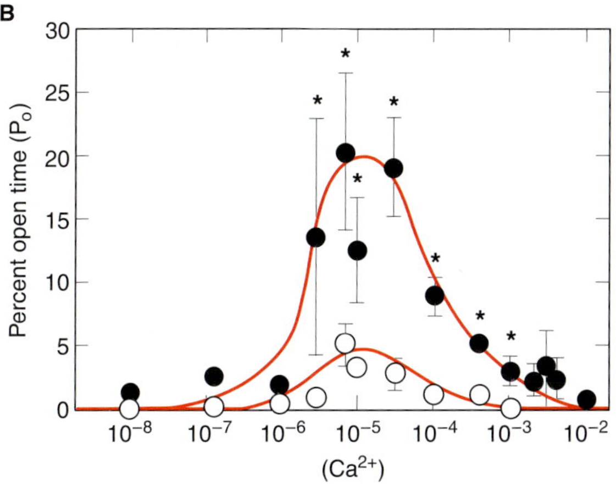

FIGURE 87-4. Ca^{2+} dependence of MH susceptibility and normal Ca^{2+} release channel P_0 at pH 6.8. **A.** Representative single-channel recordings of MH susceptibility and normal Ca^{2+} release channels recorded at a holding potential of −70 mV in 200 mM KCl-20 mM MOPS (pH 6.8) −7 μM *trans*-Ca^{2+} and indicated concentrations of *cis*-Ca^{2+}. **B.** Ca^{2+} dependence of MH susceptible (•) and normal (0) Ca^{2+} release channel P_0. Data points represent + standard error of 4 MH-susceptible and 6 normal channels; *P_0 significantly greater than that of normal channels, $p < .05$ (Student's *t*-test). [From Shomer NH, Mickelson JR, Louis CF. Caffeine stimulation of malignant hyperthermia-susceptible sarcoplasmic reticulum Ca^{2+} release channel. *Am J Physiol.* 1994;267:1256, Fig. 3B, as reviewed in Mickelson JR, Louis CF. Malignant hyperthermia: excitation-contraction coupling, Ca^{2+} release channel, and cell Ca^{2+} regulation defects. *Physiol Rev.* 1996;76:553, Fig. 12.]

ANIMAL MODELS

The porcine model of MH has been an invaluable tool for linking the *RYR1* to MH susceptibility. Functional studies from this model showed unambiguously that a single homozygous mutation in the *RYR1* was responsible for porcine stress syndrome, as well as for anesthetic-induced MH episodes. Studies confirming the linkage between MH and the gene encoding the SR Ca^{2+} release channel in skeletal muscle were independently established by 2 different groups in 1990.[11,12] Following these discoveries, an important role for ryanodine receptors as causal agents for MH was accepted. Studies by a number of investigators confirmed that the R615C amino acid substitution was both necessary and sufficient to alter the biochemical and physiologic properties of the RYR1 protein in the MHS animal model.[10]

Compared to the human MH syndrome, the porcine model has a number of limitations. The human analog of the porcine mutation, Arg614Cys, accounts for only 2% to 5% of MH susceptibility. The inheritance pattern also differs. The porcine model is homozygous for the trait, but in humans the disorder is heterozygous with variable expression. As a consequence, occurrence in humans is unpredictable. Although *RYR1* is located on chromosome 19 in humans, it is located on chromosome 6 in swine. Also, heat-, exercise-, and stress-induced MH-like reactions are observed more frequently in the MHS swine.

Recently, transgenic mice with specific *RYR1* mutations have been created, although those with homozygous mutations die at birth. Heterozygous mice, which correspond to the human mutations in R163C,[31] Y522S,[15] and I4898T,[32] have been created. The R163C mice develop fulminant MH episodes and die after exposure to volatile anesthetics. They also develop MH-like reactions and die after exposure to ambient temperatures of 42°C without anesthesia. The T522S mice also experience whole-body contractures and elevated core body temperatures in response to isoflurane or heat stress. Furthermore, they exhibit increased sensitivity to caffeine, which is an important tool for the clinical CHCT. In contrast, the I4898T mouse develops a severe form of CCD and exhibits a slowly progressive myopathy. The availability of these new animal models will permit detailed analysis of how mutations causative for MH relate to altered muscle function and other myopathies in vivo and in vitro.

GENETICS

INHERITANCE

Absence of apparent clinical symptoms in MHS individuals as well as variability in clinical presentations of MH caused by triggering agents present a challenge in assessing the inheritance of this condition in humans. Susceptibility to MH (MHS) is a genetic predisposition to MH and most commonly is inherited as an autosomal dominant trait.

GENES MUTATED IN MH

The first human MH susceptibility locus was linked to the *RYR1* on chromosome 19q12-13 in the early 1990s.[11,12] Soon after linking the porcine MH syndrome to the R615C mutation, the first human mutation in the *RYR1* (R614C) was linked to the MHS phenotype as defined by a highly suspicious clinical episode and/or positive CHCT or IVCT. The *RYR1* was proposed as a candidate gene for MH, and numerous *RYR1* mutations were found in many affected families. Molecular genetic studies showed that MHS is genetically heterogeneous with involvement of more than 1 gene.[27,34] The only gene other than *RYR1* where mutations have been identified in MH families is the gene coding for the α_1-subunit of the DHPR, or the *CACNA1S*.[2] Three causative mutations have been identified in the *CACNA1S*, but screening studies indicate that these mutations are linked to less than 1% of MHS families worldwide.[35]

Mutations in the *RYR1* are thought to account for approximately 70% of MHS subjects, but are found in almost 100% of families with CCD.[36] The *RYR1* is a complex gene containing 106 exons encoding a 15-kilobase messenger RNA molecule that is transcribed mostly in

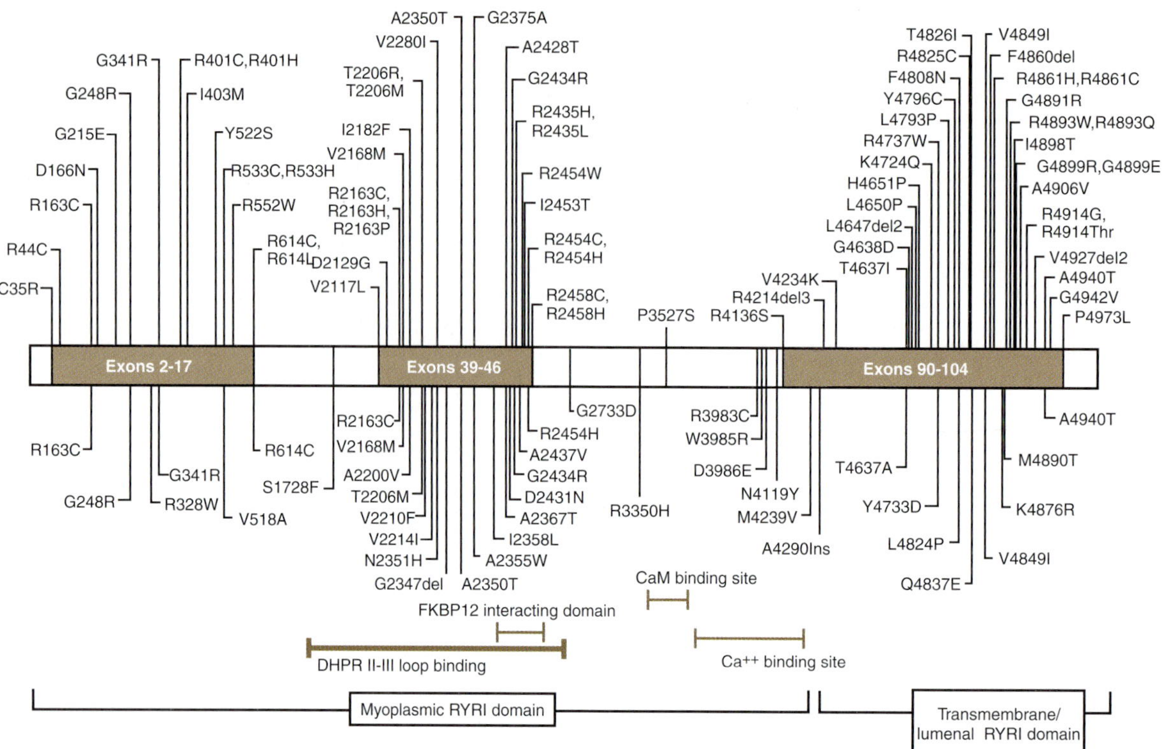

FIGURE 87-5. Location of ryanodine receptor type 1 (*RYR1*) mutations associated with malignant hyperthermia susceptibility and central core disease. Mutations found in European and Australian malignant hyperthermia–susceptible/central core disease families are shown at the top; mutations found in North American malignant hyperthermia–susceptible/central core disease families are shown at the bottom of the diagram. The mutations reported only in North American MHS families and new *RYR1* variants identified in North American MHS subjects are shown in *bold*. The 3 mutational hot spot areas are shadowed. CaM, calmodulin; DHPR, dihydropyridine receptor; FKBP12, FK506 binding protein 12. [Modified from Sambuughin N, Holley H, Muldoon S, et al. Screening of the entire ryanodine receptor type 1 coding region for sequence variants associated with malignant hyperthermia susceptibility in the North American population. *Anesthesiology.* 2005;102(3):515-521.]

skeletal muscle.[29] About 200 different variants have been identified in the *RYR1*.[34] Most of the variants are missense, that is, changes in single amino acids with preferential localization to 3 regions: the N-terminal region between codons 34 and 614; the central region between codons 2163 and 2458; and the C-terminal region between codons 3916 and 4973 (**Fig. 87-5**).[37] The central region of the gene is proximal to the region where the protein (RYR1) would interact with the regulatory protein, FKBP12, and the α_1-subunit of the DHPR, the voltage sensor of RYR1. The C-terminal region corresponds to the transmembrane domain of the protein.[34] Most of the mutations in this domain are associated with CCD (see Chapter 12).

Functional studies by a number of investigators confirmed that *RYR1* mutations associated with MH alter the biochemical and physiologic properties of the protein. The pathogenic character of many *RYR1* mutations have been studied experimentally by kinetic measurements of intracellular Ca^{2+} release in response to caffeine, 4-chloro-*m*-cresol, or halothane in different cell lines.[1] Other methodologies include analysis of the biophysical properties of channels incorporated into lipid bilayers, ryanodine-binding experiments, and patch-clamp experiments. Expression analyses of a series of *RYR1* mutations in HEK-293, COS7, and muscle cells have demonstrated that cells expressing a mutated protein were more sensitive to caffeine, halothane, and 4-chloro-*m*-cresol than the wild type. These studies suggested that most MH-linked mutations cause the RYR1 channels to become hypersensitive to stimuli, permitting greater amounts of Ca^{2+} release as compared to normal channels. Effects of mutations causing more severe phenotypes including CCD are more complex (see Chapter 12).

Phenotype–genotype correlations in MH susceptibility are difficult to study because fulminant MH episodes are now rare as a consequence of early dantrolene intervention in suspected cases, the large number of *RYR1* variants that have been identified, and the variability of CHCT results among diagnostic laboratories. Nevertheless, phenotype and genotype correlation studies show that different phenotypic expressions exist according to the nature and the location of the mutation. Analyses of a series of *RYR1* mutations associated with MH show good correlation with caffeine threshold and muscle tension values. In North America, contracture responses to halothane appear to provide a better correlation than caffeine.[38] The *RYR1* mutations associated with both MH and CCD (R163C, R2163H, and R2435H) exhibit more severe caffeine and halothane responses than those associated with MH alone.[34]

The widespread European practice of contracture testing both parents of MHS patients has allowed the identification of patients homozygous for the MH susceptibility trait. Surprisingly, these patients differ neither from a symptomatic point of view nor in their response to the contracture test from patients heterozygous for the same mutations. Also, there are a number of families in which 2 different mutations have been identified.[23,34,39]

CLINICAL SYNDROME: DIAGNOSIS AND TREATMENT

Box 87-1 contains all currently known anesthetics that are capable of triggering an acute MH reaction in humans, as well as a list of anesthetic drugs that are safe (nontriggering) for use in MHS individuals. All potent inhalational anesthetics and the depolarizing muscle relaxant succinylcholine may trigger MH events in susceptible individuals. An analysis of 284 MH cases reported to the North American MH Registry over a 19-year period found that 54% received an inhalational agent and succinylcholine, 45% received an inhalation agent but no succinylcholine, 0.7% (2 cases) received succinylcholine but no inhalational agent, and 1 case received no inhalational agents or succinylcholine.[21]

BOX 87-1

MH Trigger and Safe Anesthetic Agents

Trigger Agents	Safe Agents
Inhaled Anesthetics	*Inhaled Anesthetics*
Halothane	N_2O
Isoflurane	Xenon
Enflurane	*IV Anesthetics*
Sevoflurane	Barbiturates
Desflurane	Propofol
Muscle Relaxants	Ketamine
Depolarizing	Etomidate
(succinylcholine)	*Muscle Relaxants*
	Nondepolarizing (all)
	Local Anesthetics (all)
	Narcotics (all)
	Benzodiazepines (all)

The inhalational trigger agents included isoflurane (58%), sevoflurane (21%), halothane (16%), desflurane (12%), and enflurane (3%). Succinylcholine is known to enhance the severity of an MH episode induced by volatile anesthetics. Succinylcholine can also cause contracture of muscle that is myotonic or denervated, resulting in increased muscle membrane permeability. Thus succinlycholine can cause increases in serum potassium, myoglobin, and CK, even in non-MHS patients.[1]

Frequent first signs of MH include hypercarbia (92%), sinus tachycardia (73%), and masseter muscle rigidity (27%). In 64% of cases, elevated or rapidly increasing temperature was the first to third sign. **Box 87-2** lists the clinical and laboratory signs associated with MH. The clinical presentation and first signs of MH are highly variable.[3,40] In 89 of 268 cases reviewed from the MH Registry, the first clinical sign appeared within 30 minutes of induction; for all 268 cases, the median time was 60 minutes. In some reported cases, anesthesia was uncomplicated for 6 hours or more before the first clinical signs of MH appeared.[41]

The underlying events that trigger an MH episode and determine its severity are poorly understood. For example, many MHS individuals are known to have had prior uneventful exposure to triggering anesthetics before developing an MH episode. Also, differing intensities in clinical expression have developed with the same triggering agents in patients from the same family. Some patients may trigger without a clear family lineage, and occasionally, patients may trigger with exposure to high environmental temperatures and certain noxious chemicals. This suggests that environmental and genetic factors affect the responsiveness of patients carrying MH mutations. This may be a result of incomplete penetrance of the mutations, the influence of 1 or more modifying genes, and/or complex interactions between genes and the environment.

BOX 87-2

Clinical and Laboratory Signs Associated With MH

Clinical Signs	Laboratory Findings
Increased end-tidal CO_2 (with normal minute ventilation)	Increased Pa_{CO_2}
Increased minute ventilation (if spontaneously breathing)	Acidosis (may be mixed respiratory/metabolic)
Tachycardia, hypertension	Increased O_2 consumption
Dysrhythmia	Hyperkalemia
Cyanosis/mottling	Hypercalcemia
Generalized muscular rigidity, MMR[a], or both	Serum lactate elevation
Hyperthermia[b]	Creatine kinase elevation
Dark brown urine	Myoglobinuria
	Abnormal coagulation tests

[a]MMR, masseter muscle rigidity.

[b]During acute MH, body temperature may increase at a rate of 1.8°F to 3.6°F (1°C-2°C) every 5 minutes.

BOX 87-3

Differential Diagnosis of Increased $ETCO_2$

I. Equipment
   A. Machine: leak, disconnect, decreased fresh gas flow
   B. Breathing circuit: leak, disconnect, decreased fresh gas flow, obstruction, valve malfunction, depletion or channeling of CO_2 absorbent, improper attachment of circuit to machine
   C. Ventilator: leak, disconnect, improper settings, malfunction, decreased driving pressure
   D. Monitor: leak, disconnect, inaccurate calibration, moisture, baseline drift

II. Metabolic: increased production of CO_2
   A. Fever: iatrogenic, sepsis, thyrotoxicosis, pheochromocytoma, central nervous system injury
   B. Light anesthesia
   C. Release of aortic cross-clamp
   D. Release of tourniquet
   E. Malignant hyperthermia

III. Mechanical: decreased elimination of CO_2
   A. Pulmonary: airway obstruction, bronchial intubation, secretions, aspiration, pulmonary edema, asthma, pneumonia, acute respiratory distress syndrome, pneumothorax, hemothorax
   B. Extrathoracic: pressure on chest, retractors, increased abdominal muscle tone, ascites, Trendelenburg position
   C. Central: decreased ventilatory drive in spontaneously ventilating patients (narcotics or inhalational agents) via noninstrumented airway, laryngeal mask airway, or endotracheal tube
   D. CO_2 insufflation for pneumoperitoneum during laparoscopic abdominal surgery

An unexplained rise in end-tidal CO_2 ($ETCO_2$) may be the earliest and/or most common sign of an MH episode and underscores the importance of continuous monitoring. There is an extensive differential diagnosis for increased $ETCO_2$ (**Box 87-3**). Whenever there is an unexplained increase in $ETCO_2$ (>10%-20% above baseline) that does not respond to appropriate measures such as increased ventilation, the clinician should consider MH and obtain arterial blood gases and electrolyte analysis.

Multifocal ventricular dysrhythmias frequently occur in conjunction with tachycardia. If the syndrome is not recognized and treated, ventricular tachycardia, major conduction defects, and cardiac arrest, probably as a consequence of hyperkalemia, may occur.

The high intracellular Ca^{2+} levels activate Ca^{2+} pumps at the SR and the sarcolemma to reuptake calcium into the SR or to transport it into the extracellular space, respectively. The energetic cost to regain cellular calcium control is associated with large decreases in phosphorylation (ATP/[ADP × Pi]).[42] **Figure 87-6** and its legend provide an in-depth discussion of the cell biologic processes and bioenergetics related to cellular Ca^{2+} overload. The maximum temperature attained in MH episodes is variable with a range from 34.6°C to 45.0°C. The increase in temperature depends on the rate of rise of the metabolic rate, skin perfusion, patient size, site of surgery, ambient temperature, ongoing

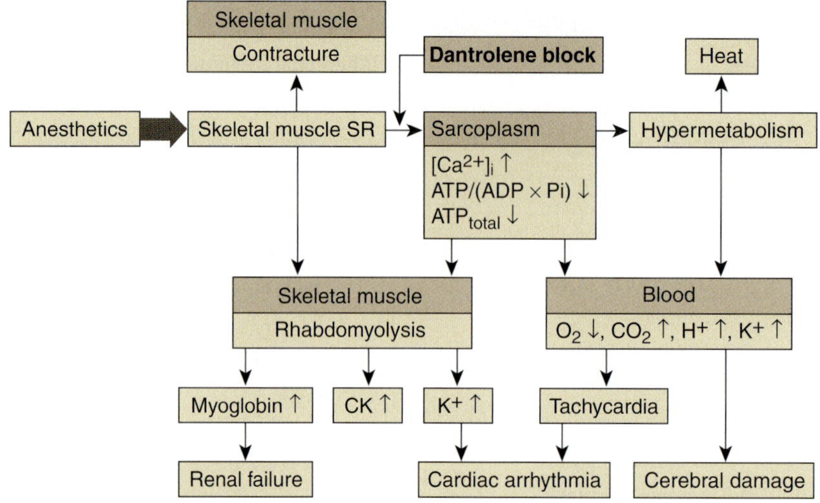

FIGURE 87-6. Current understanding of clinical and cell biologic processes in a malignant hyperthermia crisis. Volatile anesthetics like halothane sensitize skeletal muscle sarcoplasmic reticulum (SR) in MH-susceptible patients, leading to increased open probability of the RYR1 channel protein with simultaneously impaired ability to close the channel; channel closure is required to terminate SR Ca^{2+} release and allow muscle relaxation. Uncontrolled SR Ca^{2+} release produces calcium overload, that is, large increases in $[Ca^{2+}]_i$. The Ca^{2+} pumps at SR and the sarcolemma are activated to reuptake Ca^{2+} into the SR or to transport it into the extracellular space, respectively. The energetic costs to regain cellular calcium control is associated with large decreases in the phosphorylation potential (ATP/[ADP × Pi]). Because ATP/(ADP × Pi) also determines the Na^+-K^+ pump activity, cellular deenergization is associated with myocyte K^+ release (contributing to hyperkalemia) and Na^+ uptake. The muscle spasm greatly increases the extravascular resistance to perfusion, resulting in myocyte ischemia, lactate formation, and ATP breakdown, which releases free Mg^{2+} and large amounts of protons (H^+) resulting in acidosis. High $[Ca^{2+}]_i$ stimulates numerous metabolic pathways, enzymes, and oxidative phosphorylation (see text), so long as muscle oxygen supply remains sufficient. This hypermetabolic state produces heat (hyperthermia) and increased O_2 uptake and CO_2 production, along with hyperkalemia, and acidosis with hyperlactemia. Severe hyperkalemia is associated with cardiac arrhythmias and, if serum K^+ levels rise significantly, there is a risk of hyperkalemic cardiac arrest. The poor perfusion state during cardiac arrest or during hypotension leads to cerebral ischemia and cell death. Prolonged muscle ischemia will cause myocyte death due to necrosis resulting in rhabdomyolysis, which exacerbates systemic hyperkalemia and leads to excessive myoglobin and creatine kinase (CK) serum levels. Myoglobinemia can result in renal tubular failure. All of the above processes may lead to multiorgan failure. The main drug of choice to date is IV dantrolene, because it can block the uncontrolled SR Ca^{2+} release and, if given early in an episode, it can enable the skeletal muscle cells to regain calcium control. [Modified from Melzer W, Dietze B. Malignant hyperthermia and excitation-contraction coupling. *Acta Physiol Scand*. Mar 2001;171(3):367-378.]

infection, and use of other drugs (eg, atropine). High temperature directly induces tissue injury, and procedures to cool the body should be instituted quickly. The goal is to reduce muscle metabolism and avoid exposure to a critical core temperature of greater than 104°F (40°C).[43] Survival of MH has been reported in at least 1 case with temperatures as high as 111.2°F to 113°F (44°C-45°C).

Muscular rigidity may be either localized to the masseter muscles or generalized. The rigidity is due to a sustained increase in $[Ca^{2+}]_i$, which leads to muscle contraction without relaxation, that is, spasm, which, if prolonged, develops into severe contracture. The muscle contracture greatly increases the extravascular resistance to muscle perfusion, resulting in ischemia initially locally and eventually systemically. The overall higher metabolic activity and ATP consumption is reflected as an increase in metabolism with increased CO_2 production, increased O_2 consumption, lactate formation, and heat production. Also, hypercarbia, acidosis, hyperkalemia, and hyperthermia are produced. If the MH syndrome is not treated by withdrawing triggering anesthetic agents and administering dantrolene to decrease SR Ca^{2+} release, metabolic exhaustion will occur with resulting skeletal muscle edema, rhabdomyolysis (skeletal muscle breakdown), renal dysfunction, cardiac dysfunction, pulmonary edema, cerebral edema, and disseminated intravascular coagulation (see Fig. 87-6).[42]

Laboratory signs of MH, detailed in Box 87-2, include elevated $Paco_2$, acidosis, hyperkalemia, hypercalcemia, elevated CK, elevated lactate dehydrogenase, myoglobinemia, and myoglobinuria. As muscle metabolism increases, CO_2, lactate, and potassium are released into the blood. In the physiologic exercising state the body responds by increasing cardiac output and minute ventilation, but in MH, these compensatory mechanisms are soon overpowered, as reflected by continually rising $Paco_2$ combined with metabolic acidosis. The acidosis is associated with K^+ release into the blood. As the muscle membranes become more permeable, the hyperkalemia is exacerbated and there are further elevations in serum levels of inorganic phosphate (Pi), Ca^{2+}, myoglobin, CK, and lactate dehydrogenase. The muscle edema can result in excessive release of myoglobin, resulting in gross myoglobinuria, which can cause tubular renal failure. In humans, once the skeletal muscle membrane permeability is increased, myoglobin is lost before CK because myoglobin crosses the cell membrane more readily than CK. Thus drawing blood for baseline serum CK and myoglobin levels early in the episode will provide valuable information for monitoring clinical progress, although myoglobin measurements may not be rapidly available.

Box 87-4 outlines the differential diagnosis of MH.

MANAGEMENT OF MH

Successful treatment of MH relies on prompt recognition of the clinical signs (see Box 87-2), stopping the triggering anesthetics, rapid access to supplies necessary for treatment (**Box 87-5**), and initiation of appropriate therapeutic measures. This combination can result in a mortality rate that is very low. The Malignant Hyperthermia Association of the United States (MHAUS) MH Hotline (800-644-9737) is available 24 hours a day and is a valuable resource for all practitioners for the management of suspected MH. It is assumed that routine noninvasive monitors (ie, electrocardiography, blood pressure, pulse oximetry, capnography, and core temperature monitoring) will be used.

PATIENTS WITH HIGHLY SUSPICIOUS EPISODES OF MH

Box 87-6 outlines the management of the patient with a clinical episode highly suspicious for MH. In addition to these measures, providers should obtain assistance from operative personnel because many of the

BOX 87-4

Differential Diagnosis of MH

I. Iatrogenic
   A. Excessive warming measures
   B. Surgical drapes and coverings
II. Fever
   A. Infection
   B. Bacteremia
   C. Sepsis
   D. Transfusion reactions (acute hemolytic and nonhemolytic)
   E. Central nervous system dysfunction
   F. Allergic reactions
III. Endocrine abnormalities
   A. Pheochromocytoma
   B. Thyrotoxicosis (thyroid storm)
IV. Drug induced
   A. Neuroleptic malignant syndrome
   B. Cocaine overdose
   C. Tricyclic antidepressants
   D. Monoamine oxidase inhibitors (MAOIs)
   E. Anticholinergics (atropine, glycopyrrolate scopolamine)
   F. Amphetamines (methylenedioxymethamphetamine [MDMA])
   G. Alcohol withdrawal
   H. Drug interactions (MAOI and meperidine)
   I. Ecstasy
   J. Serotoninergic drugs
V. Rhabdomyolysis
   A. Dystrophinopathies
   B. Myotonias

actions should occur simultaneously. Prioritizing tasks is critical in the management of the acute MH episode. Additional anesthesia-trained personnel, as well as the professional skills and assistance of the operating room nurse, the operating room technicians, and the surgeon are invaluable. A telephone call to the MH Hotline should be placed. The tasks should be prioritized as outlined in Box 87-6.

The initial dose of dantrolene is 2.5 mg/kg and should be given as an intravenous bolus into a large vein. If elevated, a decrease in $ETCO_2$ is often the first sign that the therapy is effective and is followed by a decrease in heart rate and a reduction in the severity of muscle rigidity. If a decrease in $ETCO_2$ is not seen within minutes, the acid-base status should be monitored and dantrolene administration intravenously (IV) continued until the hypermetabolic state is controlled. A total of 10 mg/kg of dantrolene is recommended on the MHAUS website, but higher doses may be necessary. In a study of 229 MH events, the total dantrolene dose required was 5.9 (first quartile 3.0, third quartile 10.0, range 0.02-100.00) mg/kg.[21] Heart rate may remain elevated despite a decrease in $ETCO_2$ and temperature; this is usually an indication that the hypermetabolic state persists and more dantrolene may be needed. Additional sedation may also be required to treat tachycardia. Continuation of respiratory support is determined on a case-by-case basis. If the patient is ventilated via laryngeal mask airway, conversion to endotracheal intubation without the use of succinylcholine should be performed. After the episode is controlled, dantrolene should be continued at 1 mg/kg every 4 to 6 hours and continued for at least 24 hours postepisode until all signs of a hypermetabolic state are resolved and creatine kinase

BOX 87-5

Supplies Necessary for the Treatment of MH

The MH treatment cart must contain the following supplies:

1. Dantrolene, at least 36 vials
2. Sterile water for injection, 3 L (for reconstitution of dantrolene, 60 mL per vial)
3. 5-10 syringes (60 mL) and 16-gauge needles or spikes to mix the dantrolene
4. Sodium bicarbonate, 10 ampoules
5. Dextrose 50%, 4 ampoules
6. Furosemide, 200 mg
7. Regular insulin, 100 U/mL × 1 (refrigerated)
8. Calcium chloride 10%, two 10-mL vials
9. New, fresh gas hose; carbon dioxide absorbent canister; circuit; ventilator bellows; and ambu bag

Plan for rapid access to the following:

1. Refrigerated normal saline solution for irrigation
2. Ice maker or crushed ice
3. Central pressure and pulmonary artery catheters with transducers
4. Blood collection tubes/syringes for blood gas analysis, electrolytes, glucose, and creatine kinase
5. Cooling blanket
6. Freestanding ventilator
7. IV infusion pumps

is decreasing. During this time, clinical signs and laboratory results should be used to monitor the hypermetabolic state of the patient and to decide whether further dantrolene is necessary. Strict vigilance must be maintained at all times, for recrudescence of MH signs can occur in up to 20% of patients.[44] Recrudescence may be fatal and has to be managed with the urgency of a new episode of MH.

BOX 87-6

Management of Patient With Highly Suspicious Episode of MH

I. Discontinue all potent inhalational agents and succinylcholine. Maintain anesthesia with total intravenous, nontriggering anesthetics.
II. Increase minute ventilation to at least 10 L/min to flush out volatile anesthetics and to lower $ETCO_2$. Administer 100% oxygen. Insert activated charcoal filters into the inspiratory and expiratory limbs of the breathing circuit. Consider switching to a freestanding ventilator as soon as possible.
III. Inform the surgeon to expedite or abort the procedure, if possible, and obtain assistance from MHAUS Hotline (1-800-644-9737) for acute crisis.
IV. Administer IV dantrolene, 2.5 mg/kg. Be prepared to repeat this dose until the patient responds with a decrease in $ETCO_2$, rigidity, or heart rate.
V. Obtain blood gas analysis to determine if bicarbonate therapy is indicated. Place central or arterial catheter for serial blood gas and CK measurements.
VI. Begin cooling measures if the patient is hyperthermic. Efforts to cool the patient must correspond with the extent of temperature elevation. Patients can be cooled by decreasing room temperature, surface cooling with ice, or using cold solutions for gastric, bladder, and rectal lavage.
VII. Hyperkalemia is common and is treated with insulin and glucose. In adults use 10 units of regular insulin in 1000 mL of $D_{10}W$ (10% aqueous dextrose solution). Serum potassium and glucose levels must be monitored.
VIII. Measure baseline CK and serial CKs every 6 hours until CK plateaus.

Although the precise mechanism of action remains unclear, dantrolene lowers myoplasmic Ca^{2+}. Dantrolene's efficacy in the treatment of acute MH, however, is not in doubt. Dantrolene is packaged in a lyophilized form at 20 mg/vial and is dissolved with 60 mL of sterile water, in which it is relatively insoluble. The manufacturers add sodium hydroxide and 3 g of mannitol to the vial to allow the dantrolene to dissolve in 2 to 3 minutes. The resulting pH of the solution is 9.5, so care must be taken to prevent extravasation and to monitor for thrombophlebitis. Mannitol is an osmotic diuretic, and therefore central venous pressure monitoring may be necessary to manage volume status. Possible side effects of dantrolene include muscle weakness, phlebitis, and respiratory failure.

Cooling the patient is an important aspect of treatment to decrease core body temperature and thereby lower oxygen consumption. Core cooling is superior to surface cooling and is accomplished by cold gastric, bladder, and rectal lavage, and cold wound irrigation. Ice packs to the groin and axilla can be helpful in lowering core temperature. Decreasing the room temperature or packing the patient in ice may induce shivering and hence increase oxygen consumption, which is considered counterproductive. The patient's temperature needs to be continuously monitored to measure progress in treating the hyperthermia and to detect hypothermia from overaggressive cooling.

Treatment of the primary condition of MH should control dysrhythmias, but if they persist or become life threatening, providers should measure serum K^+ and arterial blood gases, and follow Advanced Cardiac Life Support (ACLS) guidelines. Arterial blood gas analysis is a useful laboratory evaluation to assess the effectiveness of therapy. Capnography does not eliminate the need for arterial blood gases for several reasons. First, rapid ventilation may underestimate the true $ETCO_2$. Second, metabolic acidosis, another MH marker in assessing the effectiveness of therapy, may still be present even when $ETCO_2$ has returned to baseline. Third, bicarbonate therapy for the correction of metabolic acidosis cannot be managed effectively without serial arterial blood gas analyses. Empiric bicarbonate therapy risks severe alkalosis and has the potential to exacerbate the intracellular acidosis. Fourth, arterial blood gases assess the adequacy of oxygen delivery more precisely than pulse oximetry. If central venous access is present, mixed venous oxygen measurements provide additional information to calculate oxygen consumption.

Electrolyte abnormalities include changes in serum potassium, calcium, and glucose; therefore, serial measurements are required. Hyperkalemia is generally considered to result from acidosis that shifts K^+ ions out of the cell in exchange for H^+ ions combined with the leakage of K^+ out of the damaged muscle cells. The most effective therapy for hyperkalemia is treatment of the underlying MH with dantrolene. If hyperkalemia persists or results in cardiac dysrhythmias, intravenous glucose and insulin (10 units of regular insulin in 1000 mL 10% aqueous dextrose solution [$D_{10}W$]), and bicarbonate should be administered slowly. Rarely, hemodialysis may be required. Calcium therapy is reserved for life-threatening dysrhythmias or inotropic support. Sodium values can be increased as a result of the large sodium load contained in mannitol or decreased because of a dilutional effect from fluid therapy. Serum glucose should be monitored if insulin and glucose therapy are used to treat hyperkalemia.

In addition to serum electrolyte and arterial blood gas analyses, laboratory evaluations should include CK, myoglobin, and coagulation studies. In cases resistant to dantrolene therapy, catecholamine levels, thyroid function tests, and drug screening should also be pursued. Serum CK and myoglobin should be followed every 6 hours until CK plateaus and the urine color has cleared. CK values may rise to very high levels (>100 000 IU/L). The elevated CK indicates the at-risk period for myoglobinuric renal failure and the need for renal protective measures; it may also signify an increased risk of compartment syndrome and renal failure. Disseminated intravascular coagulation (DIC) is not uncommon and is associated with an increased risk of death following a fulminant episode of MH.[45] Factors contributing to DIC include hemolysis, cellular edema with increased release of tissue thromboplastins, and inadequate tissue perfusion. A high level of suspicion combined with serial laboratory evaluation of the coagulation system aids in this diagnosis. There are no special considerations for treating DIC in this setting. As with DIC due to other diseases, treatment of the inciting cause is most effective.

When the episode has been reversed and the patient's status has stabilized, arrangements should be made for intensive care unit (ICU) care for at least 24 hours. The major areas of concern include MH recrudescence, myoglobinuric renal failure, DIC, compartment syndrome, delayed awakening, prolonged requirements for mechanical ventilation, and the patient's underlying medical condition.

PATIENTS WITH MASSETER MUSCLE RIGIDITY

Masseter muscle rigidity (MMR) is almost always triggered by the administration of succinylcholine regardless of whether volatile anesthetic agents are also given. Management of a patient with MMR depends on the degree of rigidity (**Fig. 87-7**)[1]. If a patient develops moderate or severe MMR, surgery may be aborted if it is elective, and the patient should be promptly awakened and closely monitored for other signs of MH. Urine should be tested for myoglobinuria. Serum CK should be measured initially and at 6-hour intervals over the next 24 hours. If there is no evidence of myoglobinuria and if the increases in CK are modest, many centers allow the patient to be discharged that day. Surgery may be rescheduled when CK has returned to normal, but succinylcholine should be avoided. See **Box 87-7** for the management of the patient with MMR.

AWAKE TRIGGERING: EXERCISE AND HEAT ILLNESS

Pigs homozygous for MH reproducibly develop fulminant MH episodes with each administration of potent inhalation anesthetics. They are also known to develop MH in response to heat, stress, and exercise. Interestingly, pigs that are heterozygous for MH have milder reactions to the same drugs and stresses. In humans, clinical reports have noted that acute MH syndromes may occur more readily after the stress of physical exercise. There are also a number of *awake episodes*[42] reported in which no anesthetics are given, but patients experience unusual stress and become symptomatic with myalgia, fatigue, heat stroke, and uncommonly, sudden and unexplained death. There is also a subset of patients who survive fulminant MH episodes, but then develop chronic muscle pain that is often severe and debilitating with exercise.[46]

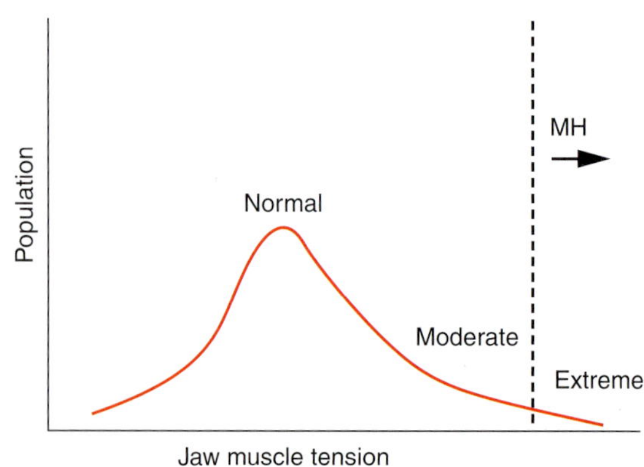

FIGURE 87-7. Succinylcholine usually increases jaw muscle tone slightly. In some patients the increase is moderate, and in very few, the effect is extreme (ie, "jaws of steel"). As much as 50% of this latter group may be susceptible to malignant hyperthermia (MH). Somewhere in the area of the declining curve is the boundary for the MH population. [From Zhou J, Pessah IN, Allen PD, Naguib M. Neuromuscular disorders and malignant hyperthermia. In: Miller R, ed. *Miller's Anesthesia*. Vol. 1. Philadelphia, PA: Churchill-Livingstone; 2010:1171-1195.]

BOX 87-7

Management of the Patient With MMR

I. When MMR is diagnosed during an anesthetic:

A. Discontinue any potent inhalation agent.

B. Continue to ventilate by mask with 100% oxygen.

C. Do not give a second dose of succinylcholine.

D. Call for assistance and the MH cart.

E. Continue to monitor $ETCO_2$, minute ventilation, electrocardiogram, blood pressure, and core temperature.

F. Obtain blood gases and electrolyte analysis if the situation does not rapidly improve.

G. Is the patient stable?[a]

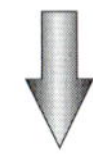

Yes

1. In elective surgery, cancel the procedure and observe the patient in the operating room until awake.
2. In emergency surgery, convert to a nontriggering technique and observe for changes in the patient's condition over 15-20 minutes; then proceed with surgery.

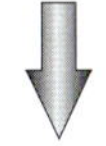

No

1. In elective surgery, cancel the procedure and treat as fulminant MH.
2. In emergency surgery, treat as fulminant MH and proceed with surgery using nontriggering anesthetics after the patient is stable.

II. Postprocedure management

A. Consider ICU/overnight recovery room observation for 24 hours to monitor urine output and signs of increased metabolism (increased heart rate, blood pressure, respiration, acidosis, and temperature).

B. Obtain serial serum CK measurements every 6 hours for 24 hours or until the CK plateaus.

C. Test urine for the presence of myoglobin:

1. If positive, maintain alkaline urine output at 1-2 mL/kg/h until clear.
2. If negative, continue to monitor until CK levels have reached a plateau.

[a]After the airway is secured, the patient may be considered stable if minute ventilation less than 1.5 times expected produces normal $ETCO_2$ levels and circulatory parameters and core temperature are normal or slightly low.

Strong evidence for a relationship between heat stroke and MH comes from a case report by Tobin et al.[47] This case concerned a 12-year-old boy who died following exercise. He had a previous clinical MH episode and was found to harbor one of the *RYR1* mutations established as causative for MH. In addition, Wappler et al studied 12 young men with exercise-induced rhabdomyolysis.[48] Ten were diagnosed as MH susceptible based on IVCT results, and 3 were identified with *RYR1* mutations strongly associated with MH susceptibility.

In the future, genetic testing will likely help to clarify the relationship between heat illness and MH susceptibility. From a clinical perspective, patients who have a personal or family history of MH have a greater likelihood of developing heat-related illness or rhabdomyolysis; they are advised to avoid exercise in extremes of heat. However, it is unlikely that all cases of rhabdomyolysis or heat-related illness are due to MH susceptibility.

PATIENTS PRESENTING WITH HISTORY OF MH

Patients must be managed as MH susceptible if they have a personal or family history of any of the following: evidence of a clinical MH event, positive CHCT, or the presence of an MH causative mutation in the *RYR1* or *CACNA1S* genes. If the patient's or relative's MH susceptibility status is unclear and difficult to verify, then the patient must be treated as though he or she is MHS (**Box 87-8**) until either a chart review or a negative contracture test proves otherwise. The North American MH Registry (www.mhreg.org) should be contacted to determine if the patient's or family's MH history is documented. Elective surgery can proceed as scheduled (follow the guidelines in Box 87-8) without the results of a contracture test as long as the anesthetizing location has adequate resources, including dantrolene, staffing, and laboratory availability. If CHCT is required, it should be scheduled at an MH diagnostic testing center. Although the goal is to avoid the unnecessary labeling of patients as MH susceptible, all family members must wear an MH identification tag (see Resources below) stating that they are MH susceptible while the review is in progress. When suspicion of MH susceptibility exists in a family member of a patient, the patient should not be given triggering anesthetic agents.

Anesthesia workstation preparation is variable according to the anesthesia machine manufacturer and model. Due to retained volatile anesthetic agents within the workstation, at least 10 L/min of gas flow must be used during the anesthetic (Box 87-8).[49] Regardless of the surgical procedure or anesthetic technique, additional time is required to prepare the anesthesia workstation or alternative setup, check the monitors, and inspect the MH cart.

Whenever possible, the North American MH Group recommends scheduling the surgical procedure as the first case of the day to allow time for preparation and to avoid contamination of the operating room by waste anesthetic gases. In most cases, pretreatment with dantrolene is not necessary, but if the patient is very anxious, anxiolysis is desirable. Anxiety and stress have been implicated in triggering MH.[50] If a patient has a history of repeated episodes of awake MH, anxiolysis and dantrolene pretreatment is recommended. In emergency cases, the infrastructure and the operating support services can also be factors in making a decision about whether pretreatment with dantrolene is needed. MHAUS and the North American MH Registry staff can be of assistance in making this decision.

When possible, MHS parturients should be evaluated prior to delivery and consent should be obtained for labor analgesia using a regional technique. If a patient is going to labor, the anesthesiologist should

BOX 87-8

Anesthetic Management of Patient With a History of MH

I. Equipment
   A. Prepare a "clean" anesthesia workstation by
      1. Removing vaporizers and replacing accessible internal components with new or autoclaved parts
      2. Flushing the workstation using the ventilator and an artificial lung (2-L rebreathing bag) with a fresh gas flow of at least 10 L/min for 2 hours
      3. Replacing the CO_2 absorbent, patient breathing circuit, the rebreathing bag, and insert activated charcoal filters into the inspiratory and expiratory limbs of the breathing circuit
      4. During the actual anesthetic, maintaining a fresh gas flow of at least 10 L/min
      5. Preparing the anesthetic workstation even if a regional technique or monitored anesthesia care is planned, in case of failed technique or emergency
      6. An alternative would be removing the anesthesia workstation and replacing it with IV pumps, a stand-alone ambu bag connected to an oxygen source, a backup ventilator that has never been exposed to anesthetics, and freestanding monitors (see B below).
   B. Capnography with real-time display, electrocardiogram, blood pressure, and electronic temperature monitoring are required.
   C. MH cart must be checked to make sure medications are current and dantrolene with sterile water diluent is present.

II. Scheduling
   A. First case of the day.
   B. Observation in the PACU for at least 3 hours.
   C. Outpatient surgery is acceptable if laboratory facilities are available, the patient can be observed in a PACU or a step-down unit for 3 hours, and intensive care support is readily available.

III. Premedication
   A. Dantrolene prophylaxis is not routinely recommended.
   B. Sedation is at the discretion of the anesthesiologist unless the patient has a history of triggering under stress.

IV. Technique
   A. Monitored anesthesia care
   B. Regional anesthesia (peripheral or neuroaxial) with sedation
   C. General anesthesia with nontriggering agents (no volatile anesthetics or succinylcholine)

V. Postoperative course
   A. Monitoring: respiratory rate, blood pressure, heart rate, and temperature.
   B. Laboratory: if clinical course remains uneventful, tests are not necessary.
   C. Health care providers in the PACU, step-down units, and hospital floors should always be alerted to the patient's MH status.

consider placing an epidural early in case an emergency C-section should be required. If the patient is undergoing an elective C-section, either spinal or epidural anesthesia may be used. In all cases, a clean anesthesia workstation or IV pumps with a freestanding ventilator must be prepared as a backup.

Extended postoperative monitoring of all patients suspected of possible MH susceptibility is required to ensure that late development of MH is diagnosed and treated promptly. In the postoperative period, the patient with a documented history of MH should be monitored for signs of MH for at least 3 hours. To ensure the early detection of postoperative MH, all staff must be alerted and educated regarding MH.

EVALUATION OF MH SUSCEPTIBILITY

Because MH is often apparent only after exposure to potent volatile anesthetics and/or succinylcholine, identifying MHS individuals prior to exposure is difficult and is usually made after an adverse response to anesthesia. Most MH episodes present as completely unexpected events, and there is no simple screening test that can predict the onset or severity of an MH episode prior to the administration of the triggering anesthetics. Evaluation of MH susceptibility starts with a history and physical examination of the patient. The history (personal and family) provides the most useful information, particularly if anesthetic or surgical records of an adverse response to anesthetics are available. The MH clinical grading scale (CGS) may be used as a guide (see above). This information is crucial in deciding what the appropriate testing is for an individual patient and related family. Patients who do not want to undergo diagnostic testing should be counseled about obtaining MH bracelets and wallet cards (see Resources below). Physical examination is generally not very helpful in the preoperative diagnosis of MH susceptibility. Nevertheless, examination of the musculoskeletal system can provide some clues that suggest MH susceptibility. In the past, it was suggested that MHS patients had a higher incidence of muscle cramps, increased muscle bulk, hyperextensible joints, strabismus, and scoliosis. However, the documented incidence of such musculoskeletal problems in MHS individuals appears to be no higher than that in the general population.

IN VITRO TESTING

Since the mid-1970s the standard diagnostic test for diagnosing susceptibility to MH has been the measurement of contracture response of biopsied skeletal muscle to graded concentrations of caffeine and the anesthetic halothane in vitro. This test is referred to as either the CHCT or the IVCT. In Japan, MH testing is performed on human skinned muscle fibers using the calcium-induced calcium release test.[51] Muscle histology and histochemistry are not diagnostic for MH susceptibility.[3] **Box 87-9** lists the indications for muscle biopsy and CHCT testing.[52]

LIMITATIONS OF THE CHCT

The limitations of the CHCT include several factors. It is invasive, requiring a surgical biopsy of the vastus lateralis to obtain the muscle specimen. The test cannot be performed on children with a lean mass less than 20 kg. The entire test must be completed within 5 hours of tissue removal. This requires the patient to travel to 1 of 5 North American MH diagnostic testing centers, and the cost is only partially covered by insurance.

The North American CHCT and the European IVCT are widely used to diagnose patients as MH susceptible (MHS) or MH negative (MHN). Both tests are highly sensitive (93%-97%), but the North American CHCT is less specific (78%).[53,54] Caffeine causes contracture in any skeletal muscle, but a contracture response will occur at a lower concentration in MHS individuals (**Fig. 87-8**)[55].

Patients requiring muscle biopsy for diagnostic CHCT can be safely anesthetized with general anesthesia using nontriggering agents (see Box 87-1) or with a femoral nerve block or one of its variants. The muscle bundles obtained during the surgical biopsy are exposed to various pharmacologic agents, such as halothane and caffeine, and the change in muscle tension is measured.[52] The protocols for the performance of the CHCT and IVCT are slightly different. The North American and European protocols both use incremental caffeine concentrations of 0.5, 1, 1.5, 2, 4, 8, and 32 mM, but it is the response to 2 mM of caffeine that is used for the evaluation of MH susceptibility in both protocols.

BOX 87-9

Indications for Muscle Biopsy and CHCT Testing

Definite Indications	***Possible Indications***	***Probably Not Indicated***
Suspicious clinical history of MH	Unexplained severe rhabdomyolysis during or after surgery in a patient	Sudden, unexpected cardiac arrest during anesthesia or early postoperative period that is not associated with rhabdomyolysis or hypermetabolism
First-degree relative of an index case with a suspicious history of MH if the index case cannot be tested (eg, too young, too old, MH death, index patient unwilling to undergo the muscle biopsy, no test center available)	Moderate to mild MMR with evidence of rhabdomyolysis	Neuroleptic malignant syndrome
Severe MMR during anesthesia with MH-triggering agents	Severe or recurring exercise-induced rhabdomyolysis	
Military service–the military requires determination of MH susceptibility by contracture testing in persons with a suspicion of MH susceptibility, as individuals with MH susceptibility are not eligible for military service.		

In testing with halothane, the North American protocol uses a single bolus dose of 3% halothane, whereas the European protocol uses incremental doses of halothane (0.5%, 1%, 2%, and 3%).[54] Additionally, the testing protocols for MH vary slightly in interpretation of the results. The North American protocol only requires that 1 muscle strip be positive to either caffeine or halothane for the patient to be diagnosed MHS, whereas the European MH Group's protocol requires that muscle samples must be positive to both halothane and caffeine for the patient to be called MHS. For the European MH Group protocol, if a patient is positive to only caffeine or only halothane, he or she is considered MH equivocal (MHE). This classification is not used in the North American protocol.

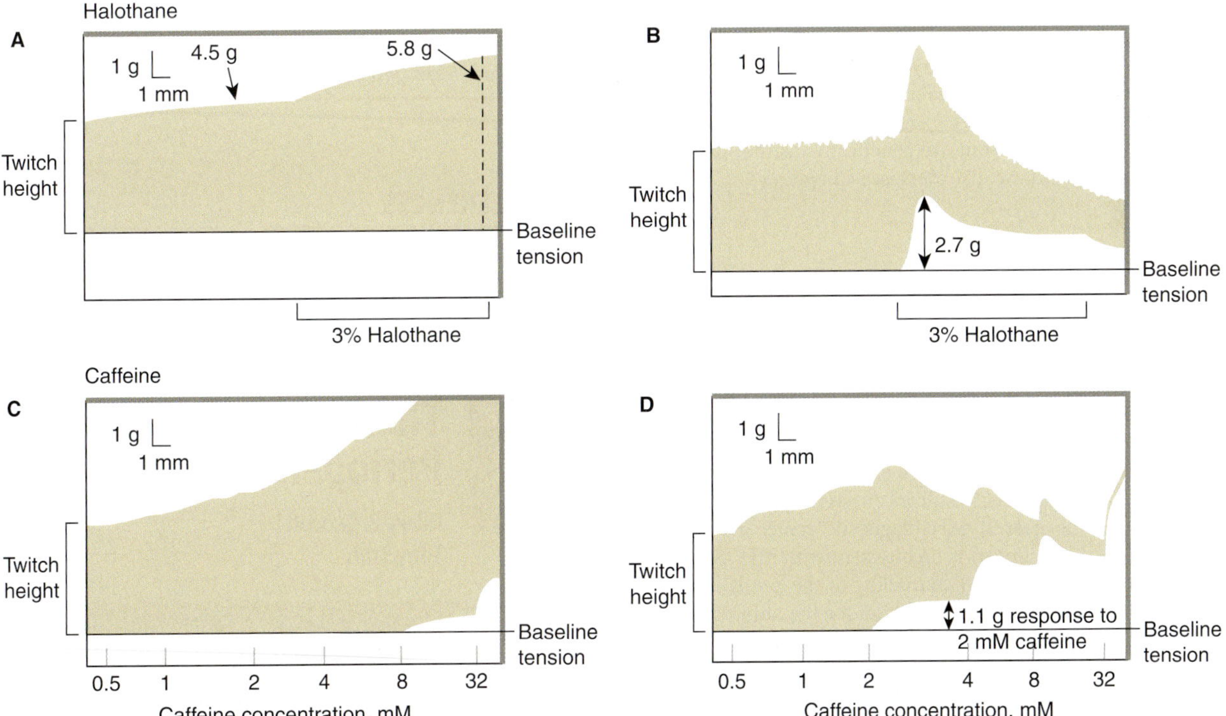

FIGURE 87-8. Halothane response (North American protocol). **A.** Normal halothane response. Halothane potentiates twitch height in all muscle strips similar to caffeine. The twitch height in this strip increases from 4.5 to 5.8 g of tension. However, there is no change in baseline tension in response to 3% halothane. A positive response to 3% halothane is an increase in baseline tension of 0.7 g or greater. **B.** Abnormal halothane response. The muscle strip has a 2.7-g increase in baseline tension in response to 3% halothane. Caffeine response (North American protocol). **C.** Normal caffeine response. Caffeine potentiates twitch height in all muscle strips. However, baseline tension remains unaffected until the bath concentration of caffeine is increased to 8 mM (0.6-g increase in tension). A caffeine contracture test result is considered positive when the muscle strip exhibits an increase in baseline tension of 0.2 g or more in response to a caffeine concentration of 2 mM or less. **D.** Abnormal caffeine response. The muscle strip has a 1.1-g increase in baseline tension in response to a caffeine concentration of 2 mM. [From Karan S, Lojeski EW, Muldoon SM. Malignant hyperthermia. In: Tremper K, ed. *Principles of Anesthetic Techinques and Anesthetic Emergencies.* Vol. 4. Philadelphia, PA: Churchill-Livingstone; 1998:9.10-19.13.]

OTHER TESTS

Molecular Genetic Testing Molecular genetic analysis has been proposed and incorporated in limited capacity as a diagnostic test for MH in Europe and North America.[56,57] The MHS patient or at-risk family members are referred for genetic testing based on CHCT results and clinical assessments. If MH susceptibility is diagnosed in a family member or index case by CHCT and a causative mutation is identified, then detection of mutations becomes valuable for other members of the family, reducing the number of relatives requiring contracture tests. However, a muscle biopsy for CHCT is currently recommended for cases in which a familial mutation is not detected because of the genetic heterogeneity of MH and because a negative genetic screen does not yet rule out MH susceptibility.[57] For more information, please contact MHAUS (see Resources below).

Ca^{2+} in Human B Cells An intracellular Ca^{2+} assay reflecting RYR1 function using human B-lymphocytes is an experimental method for diagnosing MH susceptibility. Sei et al reported that *RYR1* is expressed in human lymphocytes (B cells) and initial reports indicated a correlation between increased Ca^{2+} responses to caffeine and 4-chloro-*m*-cresol and the MH phenotype.[58] Several other laboratories have independently confirmed these observations and reported that RYR1-mediated intracellular Ca^{2+} release can be used as an end point to distinguish MHS patients from normal controls.[59] Thus measurements of RYR1-mediated Ca^{2+} release have the potential to diagnose MH susceptibility, but require further technical development and diagnostic validation before their clinical use.

OTHER DISORDERS ASSOCIATED WITH MH

Muscle disorders such as central core disease (CCD), multi-minicore disease (MmD), congenital fiber type disproportion, nemaline myopathy, and King Denborough myopathy are all associated with *RYR1* mutations. Patients with these myopathies are considered MHS. Separate from this group are muscular dystrophies and myotonias, which can exhibit "MH-like" crises in response to inhalational anesthetics and/or succinylcholine, but are genetically distinct from MH. For more information on these disorders, see Chapter 12.

RESOURCES

The North American MH Registry was established to collect and disseminate information regarding MH and the families involved. When evaluating a patient with a potential history of MH, a chart review is unnecessary if the patient or family member in question has been evaluated and entered into the registry by one of the MH diagnostic centers. If the new patient is not registered, a chart review of the initial episode is necessary to rule out alternative explanations for the episode (see Box 87-4). If the diagnosis is still in question, providers should contact MHAUS for the nearest MH diagnostic center available for consultation. Even if the diagnosis is inconsistent with MH, physicians should provide documentation and counseling to the family regarding the findings; this helps to eliminate confusion for the family and their future health care providers.

Public education is available through the Malignant Hyperthermia Association of the United States (MHAUS, 11 E. State Street, P.O. Box 1069, Sherburne, NY 13460-1069; telephone: 1-607-674-7901; fax: 1-607-674-7910; website: www.mhaus.org). The MH Hotline is a 24-hour, 7-day emergency telephone service available to medical professionals for consultation (1-800-MH-HYPER [644-9737]). The North American MH Registry of MHAUS may be contacted for registered patient-specific information (North American MH Registry of MHAUS, Ermire Building, 8th Floor (B), Rm. 8522-3, 1400 Locust Street, Pittsburgh, PA 15219; telephone: 1-888-274-7899; fax: 1-412-692-8658; website www.mhreg.org).

KEY REFERENCES

- Denborough MA, Lovell RR. Anesthesia deaths in a family. *Lancet.* 1960;2(45).
- Hopkins PM. Malignant hyperthermia: advances in clinical management and diagnosis. *Br J Anaesth.* 2000;85(1):118-128.
- Kalow W, Britt BA, Terreau ME, Haist C. Metabolic error of muscle metabolism after recovery from malignant hyperthermia. *Lancet.* 1970;2(7679):895-898.
- Larach MG, Gronert GA, Allen GC, Brandom BW, Lehman EB. Clinical presentation, treatment, and complications of malignant hyperthermia in North America from 1987 to 2006. *Anesth Analg.* 2010;110(2):498-507.
- Larach MG, Localio AR, Allen GC, et al. A clinical grading scale to predict malignant hyperthermia susceptibility. *Anesthesiology.* 1994;80(4):771-779.
- MacLennan DH, Duff C, Zorzato F, et al. Ryanodine receptor gene is a candidate for predisposition to malignant hyperthermia. *Nature.* 1990;343(6258):559-561.
- McCarthy TV, Healy JM, Heffron JJ, et al. Localization of the malignant hyperthermia susceptibility locus to human chromosome 19q12-13.2. *Nature.* 1990;343(6258):562-564.
- Mickelson JR, Louis CF. Malignant hyperthermia: excitation-contraction coupling, Ca^{2+} release channel, and cell Ca^{2+} regulation defects. *Physiol Rev.* 1996;76(2):537-592.
- Rosenberg H, Antognini JF, Muldoon S. Testing for malignant hyperthermia. *Anesthesiology.* 2002;96(1):232-237.
- Sambuughin N, Holley H, Muldoon S, et al. Screening of the entire ryanodine receptor type 1 coding region for sequence variants associated with malignant hyperthermia susceptibility in the north american population. *Anesthesiology.* 2005;102(3):515-521.

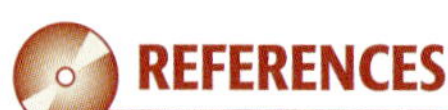

REFERENCES

Complete references available on DVD and online version at www.LongneckerAnesthesiology.com

CHAPTER 88 Thermoregulation and Perioperative Hypothermia

Hilary P. Grocott
Tony Tran

KEY POINTS

1. Adults thermoregulate with their environment by cutaneous vasomotor adjustments, sweating, shivering, and environmental behavioral adaptation (dressing appropriately, modifying environmental temperature).
2. Neonates do not shiver but can generate heat via nonshivering thermogenesis.
3. Heat loss occurs via sweating and cutaneous vasodilation. Heat conservation results from cutaneous vasoconstriction and behavioral adaptation.
4. Although not precisely defined, core temperature reflects mean temperature of the well-perfused organs (eg, brain, heart, kidney, and lungs).

5. Hypothermia that develops during general anesthesia typically follows a predictable pattern: (1) an initial rapid decrease in core temperature of between 0.5°C and 1.5°C during the first hour after induction, believed to be the result of internal redistribution of heat; (2) a more gradual linear decline in core temperature, usually lasting 2 to 3 hours, that results from cutaneous heat loss exceeding metabolic heat production (typically 0.5°C/h to 1°C/h); and (3) a plateau phase when core temperature stabilizes after 3 to 4 hours that results from the thermoregulatory balance of continual heat production and loss.
6. Following redistribution-mediated decreases in temperature, body heat loss occurs via radiation (60% of heat loss) and convection (30%), with less than 10% occurring via evaporation, and a negligible amount via conduction.
7. Postanesthesia shivering is most likely mediated via a normal thermoregulatory response to hypothermia.
8. Hypothermia during regional anesthesia is caused by the depression of regional thermal afferent input and efferent responses, such as vasoconstriction and shivering, loss of heat to the operating room environment, and redistribution of heat within the body.
9. Hypothermia during anesthesia may be prevented or treated by prewarming, the control of ambient temperature, skin insulation, warm intravenous solutions, heating and humidifying inspired gases, the application of a forced-air convective heating system, and the use of new-generation circulating-water convective heating systems.
10. There is an abundance of experimental evidence for the neuroprotective effects of hypothermia; clinical applications include deep hypothermic circulatory arrest for cardiac surgery, patients having suffered from witnessed cardiac arrest from ventricular fibrillation, and possibly perinatal asphyxia.

INTRODUCTION

Hypothermia is a common perioperative occurrence resulting in a number of clinical consequences that range in significance from mild to serious (**Table 88-1**).[1] With normal body temperature being 37°C, and taking into account a 1°C diurnal variation with an additional variation of 0.5°C in females depending on the menstrual cycle, perioperative hypothermia can be defined as a core temperature of less than 36°C.[2] As with other mammals, humans require a nearly constant internal body temperature to maintain optimal homeostatic function. Significant deviation in this internal temperature can result in alterations in numerous metabolic and physiologic functions that, if not reversed, may contribute to significant morbidity and eventually mortality. The human body has evolved a sophisticated thermoregulatory control system by which to maintain core temperature (usually to within 0.2°C of its ideal target temperature). Anesthetics profoundly affect these control mechanisms, and when coupled with adverse environmental conditions (such as a cool operating room) and other heat-losing perioperative events, the risk of developing hypothermia easily becomes apparent. An understanding of both normal and anesthetic-modulated thermoregulation is essential for the prevention and management of perioperative hypothermia.

NORMAL THERMOREGULATION

The body produces heat as a direct result of its metabolic activities. The major organs, and in particular the brain, generate the greatest proportion of this heat. In addition, muscle can significantly contribute to this, but usually only during relatively brief periods of intense use.[3,4] Thermal energy within the body is distributed between central (core) and peripheral compartments. The core compartment consists of the trunk (including the major organs) and the head. The skin (including superficial tissues of the trunk) as well as the arms and legs represent

TABLE 88-1 Major Consequences of Mild Perioperative Hypothermia in Humans[a]

Consequence	Reference	N	ΔT_{core} (°C)	Value in Normothermic Patients	Value in Hypothermic Patients	P Value
Surgical-wound infection	Kurz et al.[102]	200	1.9	6%	19%	<.01
Duration of hospitalization	Kurz et al.[102]	200	1.9	12.1 ± 4.4 d	14.7 ± 6.5 d	<.01
Intraoperative blood loss	Schmied et al.[94]	60	1.6	1.7 ± 0.3 L	2.2 ± 0.5 L	<.001
Allogeneic transfusion requirement	Schmied et al.[94]	60	1.6	1 unit	8 units	<.05
Morbid cardiac events	Frank et al.[166]	300	1.3	1%	6%	<.05
Postoperative ventricular tachycardia	Frank et al.[166]	300	1.3	2%	8%	<.05
Urinary excretion of nitrogen	Carli et al.[109]	12	1.5	982 mmol/d	1798 mmol/d	<.05
Duration of action of vecuronium	Heier et al.[112]	20	2.0	28 ± 4 min	62 ± 8 min	<.001
Duration of action of atracurium	Leslie et al.[167]	6	3.0	44 ± 4 min	68 ± 7 min	<.05
Postoperative shivering	Just et al.[29]	14	2.3	141 ± 9 $mL \cdot min^{-1} \cdot m^2$	258 ± 60 $mL \cdot min^{-1} \cdot m^2$	<.001
Duration of postanesthesia recovery	Lenhardt et al.[165]	150	1.9	53 ± 36 min	94 ± 65 min	<.001
Plasma (norepinephrine)	Frank et al.[168]	74	1.5	330 ± 30 pg/mL	480 ± 70 pg/mL	<.05
Thermal discomfort (VAS)[b]	Kurz et al.[169]	74	2.6	50 ± 10 mm	18 ± 9 mm	<.001

N, total number of subjects; ΔT_{core}, difference in core temperature between the treatment groups.

[a]Only prospective, randomized human trials are included; subjective responses were evaluated by observers blinded to treatment group and core temperature. Different outcomes of the first 3 studies are shown on separate lines.

[b]VAS is a 100-mm long visual analog scale (0 mm = intense cold, 100 mm = intense heat).

Used with permission from Sessler DI. Mild perioperative hypothermia. *N Engl J Med.* 1997;336(24):1730-1737.

the peripheral compartment.[5] Temperature in this peripheral compartment is usually 2°C to 4°C lower than the core—a gradient that becomes highly relevant when anesthesia is induced and vasodilation occurs.[3,5]

Just as defining terms for what comprises normothermia and hypothermia is important, choosing an appropriate site for monitoring is equally so. Wide discrepancies exist between different body sites and for different operative situations.[6,7] The skin is a peripheral temperature monitoring site and correlates poorly to core temperature.[8] Core temperature, a term widely used by anesthesiologists, is somewhat nebulously defined, but is generally accepted to reflect mean temperature of the well-perfused organs (ie, brain, heart, kidney, and lungs). Acceptable sites for measurement of core temperature include the tympanic membrane, nasopharynx, esophagus, and bladder.

Similar to many other physiologic systems, the thermoregulatory system has at least 3 major components: (1) sensory receptors (an afferent limb), (2) a central integrator or controller, and (3) an effector organ system (an efferent limb). The sensory receptors provide information from thermosensitive sites in the skin and other body structures (spinal cord and viscera) to a central controller that then integrates this information and compares it with a standard reference or set-point (**Fig. 88-1**).[2,9] The skin, deep tissues (viscera), spinal cord, hypothalamus, and other brain structures each contribute approximately 20% of the input to the autonomic thermoregulatory control center. On the basis of the difference between the afferent input and the target set-point, the controller provides information to effector systems that then initiate changes to regulate heat production or loss.

There is general agreement that the anterior hypothalamus is the central controller for body temperature, comparing the afferent input with the central set-point, and instituting an appropriate autonomic neural response. Investigations by neuroanatomists and neurophysiologists have greatly increased understanding of how the 3 components of the thermoregulatory system function to maintain a thermal balance; details concerning these experimental studies are the subject of numerous books and review articles.[2,5,10-15]

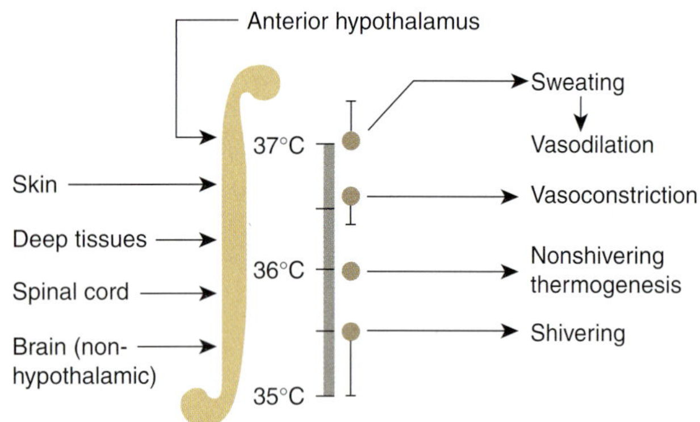

FIGURE 88-1. Hypothalamic thermoregulatory control. The hypothalamus, the primary thermoregulatory control center, is displayed as a large square. The skin, deep visceral and thoracic tissue, spinal cord, and nonhypothalamic brain areas each contribute approximately 20% of the input that is integrated by the hypothalamus in the control of autonomic thermoregulatory defenses (this input is shown entering the hypothalamus from the left of the figure). The temperature of the hypothalamus itself also contributes 20% of the efferent information used in thermoregulatory control. The hypothalamus integrates body temperature, comparing it with threshold temperatures that then trigger specific thermoregulatory responses. Values higher than the threshold for responses to warmth (ie, sweating) or lower than the threshold for responses to cold (ie, vasoconstriction and shivering) initiate the appropriate defense. Values between the thresholds for sweating and vasoconstriction lie in the interthreshold range (defined as the range of temperatures that do not trigger any thermoregulatory defenses, which is normally 0.2°C). The thresholds for sweating, vasoconstriction, and shivering are from Lopez et al[9] and are shown as means ± SD. The threshold for nonshivering thermogenesis is an estimated value. [Used with permission from Sessler DI. Mild perioperative hypothermia. *N Engl J Med.* 1997;336(24):1730-1737.]

An important concept to consider in the control of temperature is the inter-threshold range. This is defined as the range between which thermoregulatory responses to cold versus those for warmth are activated. That is, if body temperature is in this range, no autonomic thermoregulatory defenses are triggered. In the normal adult, this range is typically 0.2°C but may be wider in the elderly.[9,16]

Anesthesia significantly widens the inter-threshold range to as much as 4°C.[17-20] With a range this wide, it becomes easy to understand that under anesthesia, body temperature is greatly influenced by the surrounding environment and trends toward equilibrating with ambient temperature, thus defining the anesthetized patient as poikilothermic. Thermoregulatory responses are diminished in the elderly and may also be attenuated in persons with poor general health. An impairment of the skin sympathetic nerve traffic responses to thermal challenge has been demonstrated in the elderly.[21] This impairment of thermoregulation and vasoconstrictor response has been seen even in mild thermal (cold) challenges.[22] In contrast to the elderly, premature infants appear to have an intact central thermoregulatory control.

NORMAL THERMOREGULATORY EFFERENT RESPONSES

In normal, unanesthetized humans, behavioral regulation (dressing appropriately and/or modifying environmental temperature) is one of the most important mechanisms contributing to heat regulation. After this behavioral adjustment is made, humans further regulate heat exchange with their environment by balancing several thermoregulatory effects: (1) cutaneous vasomotor tone adjustments (vasodilation, vasoconstriction), (2) sweating, (3) shivering, and (4) nonshivering thermogenesis.

In hypothermic situations where the hypothalamus activates heat conservation and production mechanisms, thermoregulatory vasoconstriction occurs via the activation of arteriovenous shunts in the periphery.[23] Arteriovenous shunts (approximately 100 μm in diameter, roughly 10 times the size of a capillary) are located primarily in the fingers, toes, and nose. Cutaneous vasoconstriction can reduce heat loss by modulating convection and radiation from the skin surface. Shunt vasoconstriction initially halves the heat loss from the fingers and toes via a reduction of peripheral blood flow. This ultimately leads to a gradual cooling of the arms and legs.[24] These shunts are controlled by centrally mediated α-adrenergic receptors in response to the release of norepinephrine from presynaptic adrenergic nerve terminals.[25] In addition to the centrally mediated vasoconstriction, there is also a component of nonadrenergic vasoconstriction that can occur in response to local cooling.[26]

Cutaneous vasoconstriction is usually the first and most consistent thermoregulatory response to hypothermia. This vasoconstriction raises thermal insulation provided by the skin and can decrease whole body heat loss by 25% to 50%.[27,28] If heat loss continues and core temperature continues to fall, shivering, with its metabolically driven increases in heat production, is initiated.

The shivering response is the primary mechanism activated to increase heat production when hypothermic conditions persist in the presence of thermoregulatory constriction; it is dependent on central neuronal coordination and normal neuromuscular function. Shivering is initiated only after the failure of maximal vasoconstriction, nonshivering thermogenesis (in neonates), and behavioral adjustments have proven to be inadequate to maintain target body temperature (see Fig. 88-1). Shivering is an energy-inefficient means of heat production and can cause a 2- to 3-fold increase in whole-body oxygen consumption.[29] Cardiac output is directly dependent on metabolic rate. As a result, patients who shiver have a higher cardiac index and heart rate during maximal muscular activity.[30] This metabolic effect of shivering on oxygen consumption depends on its intensity and the affected muscle mass.[31] The actual increase reported in the literature has been widely variable (from as low as 7% to >700%), depending on the clinical situation, selected sample, and measuring technique.[32] More often, it is considered in the 200% to 400% range.[4,8]

Intermediate between the efferent vasoconstrictive and shivering thermoregulatory responses to cold is nonshivering thermogenesis. This response, occurring in both normal and premature infants, increases metabolic heat production without inducing any mechanical work.[33] Brown adipose tissue is an important site of nonshivering heat production in the neonate. The brown fat is rich in mitochondria (which gives it its brownish macroscopic hue) and is distributed over the neck, back, viscera, and great vessels. The metabolism of brown fat is initiated by β_3-adrenergic effects on terminal nerves within it.[34] Although the exact mechanism of heat production is not clearly understood, it is thought that it is either related to an uncoupling of oxidative phosphorylation within the mitochondria in the presence of fatty acids or results from lipolysis-lipogenesis coupled with ATP utilization.[2] It is generally agreed that nonshivering thermogenesis does not occur in adult humans.[35]

Under static conditions, heat produced by the body's metabolic process must eventually be dissipated to the environment. Close to 95% of this heat traverses the skin, with the remainder occurring via the respiratory tract. As a result, factors that modulate heat loss must involve the skin itself, either directly via sweating or indirectly via modifying cutaneous blood flow. Sweating is the most effective method of heat loss. Evaporation of sweat is an energy-absorbing process. In a dry environment, sweating alone can easily dissipate the heat generated at basal levels. Furthermore, an increase in temperature of 0.5°C can produce a 7-fold increase in sweat rate and body conductivity.[10,36,37] Sweating is mediated by cholinergic sympathetic fibers and can be nearly abolished by even small doses of atropine—something to consider in the perioperative state. Vasodilation is important for the transfer of heat from the core to the periphery. Sweating and vasodilation responses work synchronously to counter any increases in core temperature, with vasodilation increasing cutaneous blood flow and heat delivery for the evaporative sweating heat loss mechanism.[38]

GENERAL ANESTHESIA AND THERMOREGULATION

Hypothermia is a well-studied complication in anesthetized patients with numerous studies having documented its incidence and severity.[39-42] Hypothermia that develops during general anesthesia typically follows a predictable pattern. Following an initial rapid decrease in core temperature (0.5°C-1.5°C) during the first hour after anesthesia induction, a more gradual linear decline in core temperature, usually lasting 2 to 3 hours, occurs. A plateau in temperature, resulting from an equilibrium in heat loss and production, is then seen, usually after 3 to 4 hours.[41,43] This pattern is described in **Figure 88-2**. The rapid temperature decline phase is believed to be the result of internal redistribution of heat.[44] The linear second phase of the hypothermia curve is characterized by continual cutaneous heat loss that exceeds metabolic heat production (typically 0.5°C/h-1°C/h; **Fig. 88-3**).[45]

Most of the heat is lost through the skin, with radiation and convection resulting in most of the loss—far greater than losses from evaporation or conduction (**Fig. 88-4**).[2] About 90% of heat loss in the operating room (OR) is through the skin, with radiation and convection playing a more dominant role than evaporation or conduction.[2] Radiation accounts for the largest source of heat loss (representing ~60% of heat loss) and depends on the difference in temperature between the patient and the environment. The next significant source of heat loss is convection (leading to 30% of the heat loss), which is influenced by the temperature gradient between the body and the surrounding fluid or air. Evaporation can vary depending on the patient's current volume status and room humidity. Finally, conductive heat loss depends on the temperature difference between surfaces and any material that is in direct contact with them.[46]

In the unanesthetized patient, tonic thermoregulatory vasoconstriction maintains a significant core to peripheral temperature gradient. Induction of general anesthesia causes vasodilation, which results in

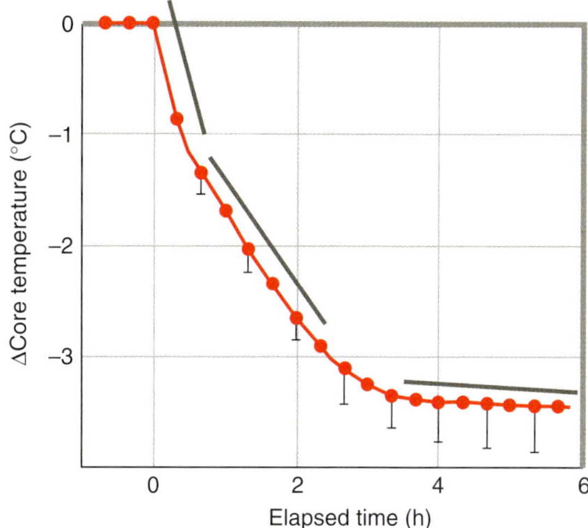

FIGURE 88-2. Typical pattern of hypothermia during general anesthesia. Hypothermia during anesthesia follows a predictable pattern. During the first hour, core temperature usually decreases rapidly by about 1°C to 1.5°C. This is followed by a slower, nearly linear decrease in core temperature. Eventually, core temperature reaches a plateau. Each phase of hypothermia development has a different cause. [Used with permission from Sessler DI. Perioperative heat balance. *Anesthesiology.* 2000;92(2):578-596.]

redistribution of heat from the warm core to the relatively cool periphery. The result is a markedly decreased core temperature, but mean (ie, the weighted average) body temperature and heat content remain unchanged (**Fig. 88-5**).[44] Although internal redistribution of heat is the major reason core body temperature decreases shortly after the induction of general anesthesia, several other factors continue to exert an affect on the patient's thermoregulatory balance. These factors include (1) decreased metabolic heat production under general anesthesia, (2) heat loss from the patient to the environment, and (3) the effects of anesthetic agents on thermoregulatory thresholds. Induction of anesthesia decreases metabolic heat production by approximately 20% by limiting muscular activity, reducing the metabolic rate, and diminishing the work of breathing.[47,48] Evaporation of surgical skin-preparation solutions,[49] anesthetic-induced vasodilation and impairment of central thermoregulatory control,[44,50] and cold operating room temperatures all increase cutaneous heat loss, although not enough to be the major cause of this initial hypothermia seen during surgery.

Behavioral regulation is not relevant during general anesthesia, and shivering is frequently prevented because of muscle relaxants. Therefore, vasoconstriction is the principal thermoregulatory response available to anesthetized, paralyzed, hypothermic adult patients. However, this response is profoundly affected by anesthetics. Clinically relevant doses of general anesthetics decrease the activation threshold (the temperature triggering a response) for hypothermia by 2°C to 4°C.[41,50,51] Interestingly, activation thresholds for responses to hyperthermia are also affected, but to a lesser degree than those for hypothermia.[3] The result is an increase in the inter-threshold range, with core temperature changes passively determined by redistribution of heat within the body combined with environmental heat loss.

The exact central temperature that triggers thermoregulatory vasoconstriction is both anesthetic agent and dose dependent, and may vary depending on the age of the patient and the intensity of surgical stimulation. Patients who become sufficiently hypothermic during surgery eventually reach the vasoconstriction threshold and trigger the response. Once triggered, the actual gain and maximum intensity of the thermoregulatory response remains near normal.[52-54] In summary, markedly altered thermoregulatory thresholds with preserved gain and maximal intensities characterize the effect of general anesthetics on the thermoregulatory system.[55]

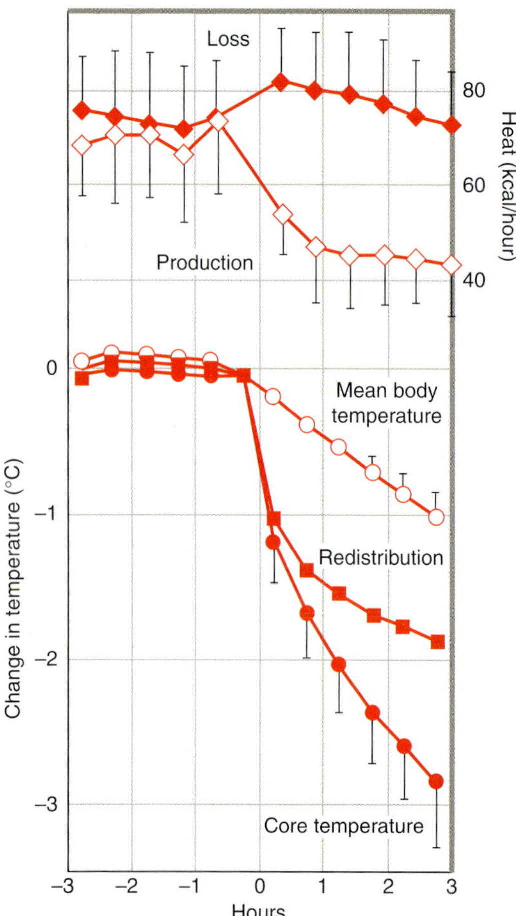

FIGURE 88-3. Changes in heat content and heat distribution in the body before and after the induction of general anesthesia. Hour zero denotes the induction of anesthesia in normal volunteers exposed to a typical operating room environment. The change in mean body temperature has been subtracted from the change in core temperature (tympanic membrane); the remainder represents the amount of core hypothermia specifically resulting from the redistribution of heat from the core to the periphery. Therefore, redistribution hypothermia is not directly measured, but instead is represented by the portion of the decrease in core temperature not attributable to the relatively small decrease in systemic heat content. After 1 hour of anesthesia, the core temperature had decreased by 1.6 ± 0.3°C, with redistribution accounting for 81% of the decrease. Even after 3 hours of anesthesia, redistribution accounted for 65% of the entire decrease (2.8 ± 0.5°C) in core temperature. [Used with permission from Sessler DI. Mild perioperative hypothermia. *N Engl J Med.* 1997;336(24):1730-1737.]

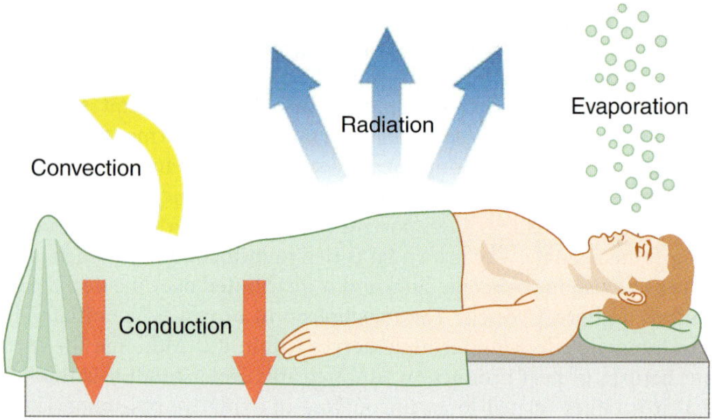

FIGURE 88-4. Mechanisms of heat loss. The linear second phase of the perioperative hypothermia curve results from heat loss exceeding metabolic heat production (approximately 1 kcal · kg^{-1} · h^{-1}). During anesthesia, heat loss is usually greater, with losses caused principally by radiation accounting for roughly 60% of the total. The remaining loss is largely convective with respiratory evaporative loss contributing to only approximately 10% of the total. Cutaneous evaporative loss is relatively small except during sweating, although evaporative loss from the surgical incisions can be substantial. Conductive loss is negligible during anesthesia. [Used with permission from Sessler DI. Perioperative heat balance. *Anesthesiology.* 2000;92(2):578-596.]

REGIONAL ANESTHESIA AND THERMOREGULATION

Regional anesthesia (in the form of spinal and epidural anesthesia) impairs thermoregulation via inhibition of both thermal afferents and efferents. As the usual thermoregulatory efferent responses are neuronally mediated, it is no surprise that central neuroaxial blockade would interfere with these responses (sweating, vasoconstriction, and shivering). Compounding these efferent abnormalities, blockade of thermoregulatory afferents results in the hypothalamic control centers incorrectly interpreting peripheral temperature to be normal (or high).[56,57] This explains the development of the warming sensation that patients report following the injection of neuroaxial local anesthetics.[58] Regional anesthesia affects the inter-threshold range, increasing it by 3 to 4 times its normal value. With the impairment in thermoregulatory efferents, the warm sensation reported by patients, and the general lack of temperature monitoring in the awake patient, hypothermia is common and frequently goes undetected in the patient undergoing regional anesthesia.

Traditionally, hypothermia during regional anesthesia was believed to primarily result from increased heat loss to the environment secondary to sympathetic blockade-induced vasodilation. However, Hynson et al[59] investigated the importance of different etiologic factors in causing hypothermia during epidural blockade. In healthy, nonpregnant, normal volunteers, core and skin temperature, heat loss, and oxygen consumption were measured before and after epidural blockade to an approximate T4 level was induced. They found that during epidural anesthesia, skin temperature increased, core temperature decreased, and heat loss to the environment increased only slightly. Most subjects shivered during the epidural block, so heat production actually increased somewhat during the study. These data suggest that heat loss to the environment cannot account for the fall in core temperature seen during regional anesthesia. Indeed, the authors concluded that redistribution of heat within the body is the primary factor responsible for the development of central hypothermia during epidural blockade. A subsequent study by Glosten et al confirmed this hypothesis.[60]

In summary, during regional anesthesia hypothermia occurs because (1) regional anesthetics depress regional thermal afferent input and efferent responses, such as vasoconstriction and shivering; (2) patients lose some heat to the operating room environment; but most importantly, (3) redistribution of heat within the body occurs.[61,62] Interestingly, rewarming from hypothermia can be accelerated in the patient with residual spinal anesthesia (if using active heating modalities) due to the relatively vasodilated state of the patient (**Fig. 88-6**).[63]

Hypothermia during regional anesthesia is often accompanied by shivering with an incidence of up to 70% being reported.[64] There is some variability in clinical studies being able to demonstrate a consistent relationship between core temperature and shivering during major regional anesthesia raising the question of whether this response is thermoregulatory or of some other etiology. As a result, shivering that occurs with regional anesthesia can often be prevented if normothermia is maintained, although this is not always the case.[65] Cutaneous warming of patients for 2 hours prior to inducing epidural anesthesia can help in preventing hypothermia and reduces shivering.[60] The same pharmacologic therapies used to treat shivering in patients recovering from general anesthesia can also be used in regional anesthesia patients.

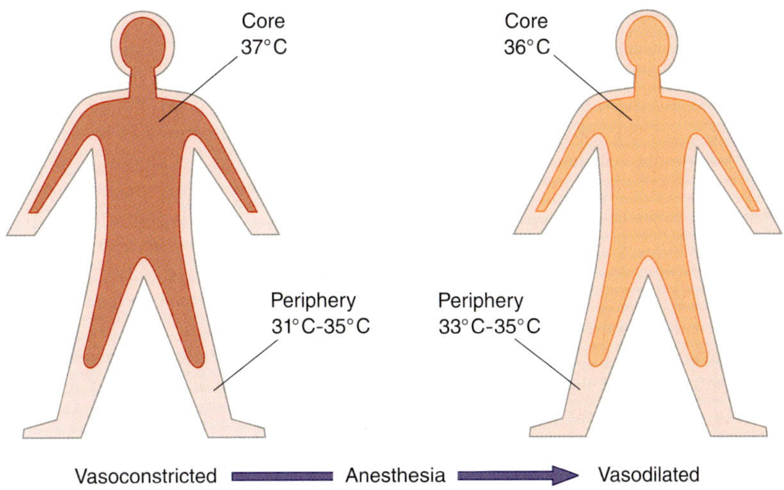

FIGURE 88-5. Redistribution hypothermia after induction of general anesthesia. Tonic thermoregulatory vasoconstriction usually maintains a core-to-peripheral temperature gradient. With the induction of general anesthesia, this vasoconstriction is inhibited, allowing a core-to-peripheral redistribution of body heat. [Used with permission from Sessler DI. Temperature monitoring. In: Miller RD, ed. *Anesthesia*. 4th ed. New York, NY: Churchill Livingstone; 1994:1363-1382.]

Interestingly, the tremor seen in pregnant patients undergoing regional anesthesia may have a different nonthermoregulatory etiology. A number of studies have shown an increased incidence of shivering in pregnant patients when cold solutions are injected epidurally.[66,67] This response is not seen in nonpregnant volunteers or patients, suggesting that thermosensitive tissue within the spinal canal contributes to the shivering observed with epidural anesthesia in parturients.[64]

POSTANESTHESIA SHIVERING

In the anesthetized patient, it is unusual to reach temperatures where shivering is induced. However, in the postanesthetic period, shivering is common and has been reported to occur in up to 40% of patients.[68,69] This common perioperative problem is both uncomfortable to the patient and problematic for the caregiver, but more importantly it may also increase perioperative morbidity. In addition to cold sensations that accompany shivering, postanesthesia tremor can itself lead to an increase in perioperative pain by stretching within surgical incisions. It can also lead to increases in intracranial and intraocular pressure in addition to its increases in metabolic demand.[29,70-72]

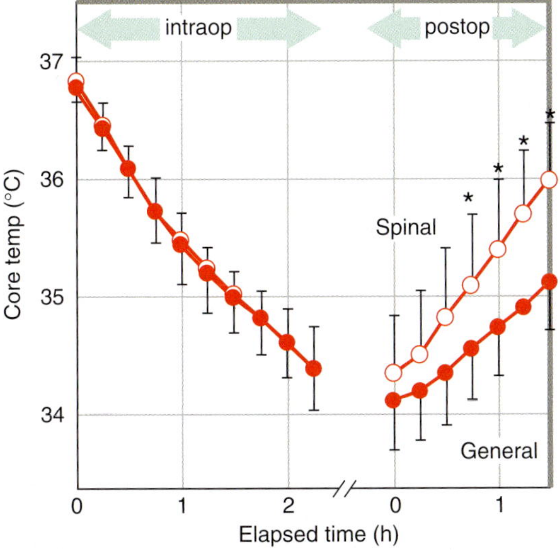

FIGURE 88-6. Residual spinal anesthesia can increase postoperative core rewarming as demonstrated in this study of intraoperative and postoperative core temperatures in patients assigned to general anesthesia (n = 20) and spinal anesthesia (n = 20). All patients were actively warmed during the postoperative period. Core temperature did not differ significantly during surgery, but increased significantly faster postoperatively in patients given spinal anesthesia: 1.2 ± 0.1°C/h *versus* 0.7 ± 0.2°C/h. Data are presented as mean ± SD. [Used with permission from Szmuk P, Ezri T, Sessler DI, et al. Spinal anesthesia speeds active postoperative rewarming. *Anesthesiology.* 1997;87(5):1050-1054.]

The etiology of this troublesome perioperative occurrence has been considerably debated.[15] General agreement suggests that the most likely explanation for this postanesthetic tremor relates to an abrupt change in anesthetic-induced thermoregulatory inhibition, thus increasing the threshold for shivering toward normal. That is, the residual low body temperature (resulting from the dysregulation of thermoregulation by anesthetic state itself) seen upon discontinuing of anesthesia is usually well below the near-normal threshold to activate thermoregulatory shivering.[73,74]

Despite this normal thermoregulatory response to intraoperative heat loss, there are alternative explanations for postanesthetic shivering that may partly explain some unusual observations. For example, postanesthesia shivering does not universally occur in the markedly hypothermic patient,[75] and shivering frequently occurs in normothermic postanesthetic patients.[73] As a result, there may be some other mitigating factors that influence whether or not a patient shivers after anesthesia. It has been suggested that surgery itself, due to the stress response or associated pain, can contribute to postoperative tremor.[76] For example, the surgical stress itself may abnormally increase the thermoregulatory set-point.[77] There is also evidence that residual volatile anesthetics (isoflurane) may cause a nonthermoregulatory shivering pattern.[59,78] The exact mechanism by which anesthesia may interact directly in causing the shivering pattern is not known. However, this tremor pattern that is observed at low concentrations of isoflurane (0.2%-0.4%) is very similar to the electromyographic (EMG) pattern that is seen after spinal cord transection, suggesting that the isoflurane may cause some inhibition of spinal cord reflexes resulting in this troublesome tremor.[79]

Postanesthetic shivering can be prevented in most patients by maintaining normothermia. Skin-surface warming may be effective therapy.[80] Pharmacologic treatments include meperidine (25 mg intravenously [IV]),[80-82] clonidine (75 μg IV),[82,83] and ketanserin (10 mg IV).[84-86] Most recently, dexmedetomidine has also been used.[81,87,88] The exact mechanism(s) by which these drugs abolish shivering is not completely understood, but the antishivering action is thought to involve the κ receptors on the spinal cord and μ receptors on the hypothalamus.

Unique among opioids, meperidine decreases the shivering threshold significantly more (twice as much) than the vasoconstriction threshold.[89] It is thought that meperidine reduces the vasoconstriction threshold through its μ effect in the hypothalamus, and the shivering threshold is reduced by both its hypothalamic μ effect and its κ activity at level of the spinal cord.[90,91] Another possible explanation is via the activation of α_{2b} adrenoreceptors.[92]

α_2-Adrenoceptor agonists have been shown to have anesthetic and analgesic sparing effects. Dexmedetomidine, an α_2-agonist with an 8 times higher affinity compared to clonidine, has been demonstrated to reduce both the vasoconstriction and shivering thresholds.[87] As postoperative surgical pain can promote nonthermoregulatory shivering, dexmedetomidine, with its analgesic sparing effect, may also play another role in decreasing incidence of postoperative shivering.[93] Tramadol and nefopam have also been used to treat postoperative shivering.[92]

COMPLICATIONS OF HYPOTHERMIA

Perioperative hypothermia is associated with a number of adverse consequences (see Table 88-1). Although the mechanisms linking hypothermia to these events are known for some, it is unclear for others. For example, although myocardial ischemia is a serious postoperative problem, and postoperative shivering can adversely affect oxygen consumption (increasing it by 200%-400%),[4,8] there are few actual data linking shivering to the occurrence of ischemic events.[16,23,27] Despite this, there is a strong link in high-risk patients between mild postoperative hypothermia (1°C-3°C) and overall adverse myocardial outcomes.[27] The mechanism by which this hypothermia leads to these adverse events is not clear, however. Potential mechanisms for the adverse myocardial events (other than shivering) includes cold-induced hypertension.[29] In addition, the increase in circulating catecholamines accompanying this hypertension can augment cardiac irritability and lead to ventricular arrhythmias.[28]

Although long considered to be a factor in increasing perioperative blood loss, the effects of mild hypothermia in studies designed to examine blood loss and transfusion have produced variable results. Schmied et al showed that just 1.6°C of hypothermia increased blood loss by 30%, which in this study of hip surgery, amounted to 500 mL.[94] Overall, the data suggest that there is an increase in both blood loss and transfusion requirements,[94] although there are certainly other studies discounting this association.[95] The surgical setting itself likely plays a role. For example, cardiac surgery, with a hemostatic system already stressed by the bleeding perturbations of cardiopulmonary bypass, may increase the risk of hypothermia-mediated hemostatic abnormalities. Boodhwani et al recently reported significantly increased bleeding in patients randomized to hypothermia (vs normothermia) during cardiopulmonary bypass.[96] This bleeding tendency was also seen in a trial of intraoperative hypothermia during intracranial aneurysm clipping.[97] Despite some conflicting results, there are clearly effects of hypothermia on platelet function and clotting factor function, as well as fibrinolytic activity. For example, Valeri et al demonstrated that platelet function can be impaired by mild degrees of perioperative hypothermia.[98] This has subsequently been demonstrated by others to be potentially related to a defect in the release of thromboxane-A2.[99-101] The effects of hypothermia on in vivo clotting factor function is not clear (due to most laboratory tests being performed at 37°C), although most in vitro clotting tests, if performed at hypothermic temperatures, will show some impairment. There are few data outlining the effects of hypothermia on the fibrinolytic response. Paradoxically, one can theorize that fibrinolysis may actually be inhibited by mild hypothermia (thus decreasing bleeding) because of the temperature-related impairment of the enzyme responsible for the conversion of plasminogen to plasmin, which is fundamental to the fibrinolytic process.

Infection is one of the most serious consequences of hypothermia. Trials investigating warming interventions to treat postoperative hypothermia have been successful in reducing postoperative wound infection. A pivotal trial by Kurz et al investigated 200 patients undergoing gastrointestinal (colorectal) surgery, assigning them to either conventional treatment (hypothermia group) or additional warming (normothermia group).[102] The normothermia group had significantly fewer wound infections (6%) compared to the hypothermia group (19%) and also had evidence for improved wound healing and shorter hospitalization.[102] The mechanisms behind these adverse affects of hypothermia on perioperative wound infection and healing are likely related to the vasoconstriction induced by the thermoregulatory responses[41,103] that lead to decreased subcutaneous oxygen tension (tissue hypoxia),[104] as well as direct hypothermia-mediated impairments in immune function.[105-108] In addition to the direct immune function impairment, the reduced oxygen tension in subcutaneous tissues also impairs wound healing. Duration of hospitalization, although clearly made worse by postoperative wound infection, has also been shown to be prolonged in hypothermic patients irrespective of the occurrence of any infection.[102] The mechanism behind this noninfection-related prolongation of hospitalization is not clear but is certainly consistent with evidence of impaired wound healing or potential metabolic disturbances such as protein wasting.[109]

Although the best evidence linking hypothermia to perioperative infection was seen in colorectal surgery, similar effects on infection risk have also been outlined in relatively clean surgery. A retrospective study analyzed infection in pediatric cardiothoracic surgery patients subjected to deep hypothermia, finding that the most significant risk factor for operative site infection was deep hypothermia. In spinal surgery, a recent study demonstrated that brief periods of mild hypothermia are not related to an increased rate of complications, but wound infection risk may be increased with longer periods of hypothermia.[110] A study by Melling et al[111] examined the impact of preoperative systemic and local surgical site warming on infection rates in clean operations (breast, hernia, or varicose vein procedures). A total of 416 patients were followed for 6 weeks postoperatively. Infections were found in 19 out of 139 control (unwarmed) patients presumed to have a higher risk of perioperative hypothermia. In comparison, only 5 of the 138 local warming patients and 8 of the 139 systemically warmed group developed infections. These statistically significant results stress the importance of preventing perioperative hypothermia, even in relatively clean surgery.

Although not necessarily a complication of hypothermia, there are several pharmacokinetic and pharmacodynamic effects of hypothermia that are relevant to anesthesia. For example, hypothermia has a significant impact on the duration of action of muscle relaxants. This is thought principally to be related to a pharmacokinetic effect (as opposed to a pharmacodynamic effect), although there is some evidence for a direct hypothermia effect on skeletal muscle responsiveness.[112-114] Another direct pharmacodynamic effect of hypothermia is its impact on minimal alveolar concentration (MAC). There is approximately a 5% reduction in MAC per degree in core body temperature.[115] This can be seen most dramatically in the cardiac surgical patient undergoing hypothermic circulatory arrest where, as the temperature drops to more moderate to severe ranges (20°C), significant changes (slowing) can be seen in the EEG, with the bispectral index significantly decreasing consistent with a significant reduction in the requirement of inhaled or intravenous anesthetics.[116] The principal hypothermic effects on intravenous anesthetics relate to changes in their pharmacokinetic profile with alterations in clearance from central and peripheral compartments. Some of these pharmacokinetic and pharmacodynamic effects may partly explain the prolonged recovery profiles in hypothermic patients in the postanesthesia period.[117]

Relatively minor (in terms of serious consequences) complications of hypothermia include thermal discomfort[118] as well as mild hypothermia-induced hypokalemia.[119,120] Finally, monitoring the hypothermic patient can be a problem at times because shivering may lead to artifacts in electrocardiogram monitoring, as well as vasoconstriction-induced reductions in cutaneous blood flow that may impair pulse oximetry measurements.[121]

PREVENTION AND TREATMENT OF PERIOPERATIVE HYPOTHERMIA

A number of strategies have been used to prevent and treat hypothermia. These are summarized in **Table 88-2**. Most therapies target the linear phase of the hypothermic curve where heat is lost cutaneously. As a result, these modalities attempt to either minimize this cutaneous heat loss or to deliver heat via skin-mediated mechanisms. However, as redistribution from the core to the periphery results in the initial and sharpest drop in temperature, minimizing the redistributive decrease in temperature can also be addressed.

Prewarming the patient prior to induction of either general or regional anesthesia has been successful,[60,122] but due to logistical and other time constraints, this is not as frequently practiced as it could be. It works through reducing the core-peripheral temperature gradient and in doing so, increasing the overall body heat content. As a result of the reduced core-peripheral temperature gradient, there are fewer redistributive-mediated decreases in temperature occurring with a much-reduced anesthetic vasodilation. The overall effectiveness of prewarming has been investigated in a study of spinal surgery under general anesthesia. Patients were prewarmed for 60 minutes at 38°C, which resulted in an attenuated decrease in core temperature and a reduction in perioperative hypothermia. In another study of total hip arthroplasty, a small subset of patients demonstrated that preanesthetic warming for at least 90 minutes reduced the incidence of hypothermia and subsequent postoperative shivering.[122] An additional study reported that 2 hours of prewarming before an epidural increased skin temperature and also prevented hypothermia during initiation of the epidural.[60]

Increasing ambient operating room temperature has also been shown to be an effective method of preventing heat loss in surgical patients, made most effective if the operating room temperature is increased to at least 24°C. This modality also relies on reducing the gradient between the body and the ambient environment decreasing the heat that is lost across this gradient. However, this temperature is generally considered to be too warm for the comfort of others in the operating room.[11] Relying solely on this modality will not be effective in maintaining normothermia.

Insulation of the skin has been demonstrated to reduce heat loss by approximately 30% mainly by reducing radiation losses.[1] Blankets, however, work principally via the insulating layer of air trapped between the skin and the external environment such that regardless of whether blankets are heated or not, they are equally effective at preventing further heat loss. Despite the thermal comfort they provide to patients by providing a perception of warmth, they do little to actively warm patients. A study by Sessler and Schroeder compared patients who were covered with either unwarmed or warmed blankets for 60 minutes. In addition, the use of a single or 3 blankets was also studied.[123] The results showed that the use of a single blanket, either warmed or unwarmed, reduced heat loss by 33 ± 5%, and the use of 3 warmed or unwarmed blankets had an additional 18 ± 6% reduction in heat loss. Compared to unwarmed blankets, the benefit of using warm blankets was found to be brief (dissipating within 10 minutes).

Heat loss is directly proportional to surface area. As a result, no skin surface is either more or less likely to lose heat. The head, for example, frequently thought to lose more heat than other parts of the body, does not lose any more heat than one would predict its 10% surface to do.[1] *Radiant heaters* have also been used to reduce surface heat loss and actively warm patients, but they have little benefit with the exception of situations where significant skin contact is limited, such as in the neonate.

Heating and humidification of inspired gases address the less than 10% of metabolic heat that can be lost from the respiratory tract.[124] Although heating and humidifying inspired gases can prevent all of this heat loss, it has a negligible effect on improving core temperature.[45] Inspired gases can be passively warmed and humidified by artificial devices to a similar degree to that induced by the nasopharynx. Although these types of devices are good at maintaining humidity and minimizing heat loss, such devices cannot deliver significant heat energy.[124,125] However, they do have other advantages including reducing the drying of pulmonary secretions.

Heated mattresses that usually circulate warmed water (up to 42°C) have not been demonstrated to be effective in the prevention or treatment of hypothermia. When placed under the patient, they make poor contact with the body surface and therefore cannot provide significant conductive transfer of heat. In addition, very little heat is lost via the posterior body surface because of the relatively good insulation provided by foam that is usually integrated into operating table surfaces. It is the anterior surface of the body that loses 90% of the body heat.[45] In addition, these devices have significant limitations related to safety. Due to body pressure points (with subsequent poor circulation) being unable to dissipate heat, they can increase the risks of localized burns to the skin.[45] Other non–water-heated mattresses would be expected to have similar limitations and subsequent poor efficiency.

Forced-air convective warming systems are one of the most effective active warming systems.[126,127] These systems work via 2 principal mechanisms. They first reduce radiant heat loss (by increasing the temperature of the surfaces surrounding the patient), and they also increase heat gain via convection. Lennon et al studied the efficiency of a forced-air heating system compared to covering patients only with cotton blankets warmed to 37°C.[128] With activation of the forced-air convective warming system, patients were warmer at all measured time intervals. Numerous other studies have evaluated forced-air systems and found them to maintain normothermia, even during prolonged and extensive procedures.[45,118,119] As this modality of warming has grown in acceptance and wide-scale use, multiple devices have emerged on the market. Although the various systems differ somewhat in their capabilities, in the hypothermic patient, all convective forced-air warming systems provide excellent warming.[129]

Despite the failure of conventional heated water mattresses to efficiently warm patients via conduction, a new generation of *circulating-water conductive heating systems* are now available (such as the Kimberly Clark Patient Warming System, Kimberly Clark, Roswell, GA; and Allon MTRE 3365, MTRE Advanced Technologies, Akiva, Israel). These devices differ from their predecessors by using markedly improved skin contact that optimizes conduction of heat through the skin. These devices have been particularly studied in cardiac surgery, both in on- and off-pump procedures, and have considerable efficiency.[118,120,130,131] They have significant advantages by heating the posterior body, which is otherwise not accessible in the supine patient. In addition, in surgery where there is large skin exposure (such as cardiac surgery) where forced-air warmers have limited skin surface contact, these devices excel.

When rapid infusion of large volumes of either cold IV fluids or blood products is required, significant hypothermia can result. For example, 1 unit of refrigerated blood, or 1 L of room-temperature crystalloid can decrease core temperature in adults by approximately 0.25°C.[132] *Fluid*

TABLE 88-2 Strategies to Prevent and Treat Perioperative Hypothermia
Prewarming patient
Increase ambient operating room temperature
Skin insulation (cover patient)
Connective forced-air warmers
Circulating water-heating devices
Fluid warmers
Heating and humidification of inspired gases
Warm prep solutions

warmers are effective methods to warm both blood products and other IV fluids prior to administration. Although fluid warming can reduce the degree of hypothermia, it cannot add any significant heat to patients. Warming skin preparation solutions and irrigation fluids can also help prevent evaporative heat loss.

Intravascular warming utilizing invasive intravascular catheters has also been applied to both warm patients and, in an opposite thermodynamic fashion, intentionally cool patients. These systems are less widely available. They are also limited by the technical need for large-bore (up to 14 Fr or more) vascular cannulation, with all its associated risks.[133-135] Their role in perioperative hypothermia treatment has not been directly examined. The CoolGard™ catheter heat exchange system (Alsius Corp, Irving, CA) is a multilumen central venous catheter that contains inflatable balloons that allow for the closed-loop recirculation of fluid that can be heated (or cooled). It is relatively new and can be used in conjunction with standard warming methods, although it is more frequently used to cool patients (such as after cardiac arrest). A case report demonstrated its effectiveness in warming a patient with severe hypothermia (27.9°C) to a temperature of 37.5°C within 12 hours.[136] A retrospective study examining 11 critically injured patients using the system demonstrated feasibility in warming in acute care settings.[137] Its safety and efficacy have not specifically been examined in the perioperative setting. Indeed, there is a case report of 2 catheter-related thromboses, so it is important to be cognizant of this possibility and to follow the manufacturer's recommended maximum period of use for each catheter.[138]

POTENTIAL ADVANTAGES OF HYPOTHERMIA: NEUROPROTECTION

Although much of the previous discussion outlined the spectrum of disadvantages of perioperative hypothermia, providing extensive reasons why it should at all costs be avoided, there are situations where, without its use, catastrophic consequences would result. This is no more apparent than the setting of the ischemic brain. A classic example of this is when deep hypothermia is used to protect the brain during circulatory arrest for surgery on the aorta[139,140] or cerebral aneurysms.[141] In these situations, the circulation to the brain and the rest of the body organs can be stopped for up to an hour with few (if any) significant long-term effects. This period of "suspended animation" makes possible lifesaving procedures that would have otherwise been impossible. This is not dissimilar to some of the anecdotal reports of accidental near-drowning whereby cold-water immersion and the ensuing hypothermia that followed allowed for dramatic survival despite long periods without oxygen.[142]

Although these extremes of temperature are clearly protective in that type of surgery, lesser degrees of hypothermia in other settings, such as cardiac surgery, are less obviously protective[121,143-145] and are also tightly linked to optimizing how rewarming is performed.[146] Interestingly, cardiac surgery is rather unique in its consideration of temperature. In addition to its use of hypothermic benefits, it is also a setting that has had little evaluation and description of hypothermic complications. Indeed, most of the studies outlining the adverse effects of hypothermia in the perioperative patient have not been performed in the setting of cardiac surgery. Therefore, extrapolating all the potential adverse effects to cardiac surgical patients would be erroneous. However, common sense dictates that some of the effects of temperature (possibly the effects of wound healing, infection, and coagulopathy) would also apply to the cardiac surgery patient.

The salutary effects of hypothermia on the brain are due to the numerous enzymatic and metabolic pathways modulated by temperature. In addition to depressing cerebral metabolism (~6%-7% decline per degree Celsius),[147] its other putative neuroprotective effects of hypothermia are likely mediated by nonmetabolic pathways. In the ischemic brain, moderate hypothermia blocks the release of glutamate,[148] reduces calcium influx,[149] hastens recovery of protein synthesis,[150] diminishes membrane-bound protein kinase C activity,[151] can slow the time of onset of depolarization,[152] suppresses nitric oxide synthase activity,[153] and reduces the formation of reactive oxygen species.[154] Protection from hypothermia likely results from a summation of all these mechanisms. Although experimental demonstrations of the neuroprotective benefits of hypothermia have been well characterized for decades,[155-158] it is only recently that clinical examples of its benefits have been described.[97,159-161]

Outside the surgical setting, hypothermia has been evaluated as a direct neuroprotective strategy. In patients suffering from cardiac arrest, 2 large, well-controlled trials demonstrated that comatose survivors of out-of-hospital cardiac arrest significantly benefit from prolonged (>24-h) periods of postarrest induced hypothermia. Bernard et al studied 77 patients following witnessed cardiac arrest who, within 2 hours of return of spontaneous circulation, had their core body temperature reduced to 33°C for 12 hours.[159] Both the numbers of surviving patients as well as those having either minimal or moderate disability were significantly greater in the hypothermic group. In a similar larger multicenter trial of 275 patients, induced hypothermia (32°C-34°C) for a period of 24 hours was associated with an increased number of patients with favorable neurologic outcomes, as well as a significant reduction in 6-month mortality.[160]

Subsequent to these 2 studies, guidelines have been instituted that have recommended the use of therapeutic hypothermia after cardiac arrest as part of an overall resuscitation strategy.[162] Although there were few adverse affects reported in these studies, there were some interesting trends that emerged that support some of the perioperative hypothermia studies highlighting the complications of hypothermia. For example, in the large multicenter trial,[160] there were trends toward an increase in bleeding as well as pneumonia and sepsis, although the study was not sufficiently powered to look at these complications. In general, however, for the nonsurgical patient suffering cardiac arrest, the weight of the evidence suggests that there is a significant advantage to the induction of a period of postcardiac arrest hypothermia.

Mid to moderate hypothermia has also been investigated as a neuroprotective strategy in the setting of neonatal hypoxic-ischemic encephalopathy.[163] Although hypothermia had been demonstrated to be protective against brain injury in animal models of asphyxia, only recently has this been demonstrated in 2 well-conducted, randomized trials. The first trial evaluated 238 infants who presented with perinatal asphyxia; hypothermia (33.5°C) was instituted within 6 hours of birth and was maintained for 72 hours followed by slow rewarming. Neurodevelopmental outcomes were assessed at 18 to 22 months of age. Whole-body hypothermia was shown to reduce the combined end point of death or moderate/severe disability compared to conventional therapy (maintaining these patients at a normothermic temperature). Importantly, the hypothermia did not increase severe disability in the survivors, a clinical situation that would be clearly disadvantageous.

A second study was the TOBY (Total Body Hypothermia for Neonatal Encephalopathy) trial. It was a multicenter, randomized trial that also examined term infants suffering from asphyxial encephalopathy. In this study, 325 infants were randomized to either cooling for 72 hours or to controls that did not receive cooling.[164] Although there was no significant difference in the primary outcome, the combined rates of death or severe disability, the assessment of survivors at 18 months showed a reliable improvement in neurologic outcomes. It is not known whether this improvement could be preserved in the long term. Studies continue in this field.

Considerable caution and balance should always be used when using these clinical applications of hypothermia. Extrapolating these 2 beneficial situations (cardiac arrest and possibly neonatal asphyxia) to other surgical settings of potential brain injury has, as yet, no foundation. Although there is a wealth of beneficial experimental studies outlining both the mechanisms and the degree to which hypothermia can protect the brain, other clinical applications apart from those discussed above are lacking. For example, hypothermia has been explored in patients undergoing cerebral aneurysm clipping, clearly a setting where the brain is at risk of ischemia. However, in a trial of 1001 patients by Todd et al,[97] there was no benefit to the use of mild degrees (33°C) of hypothermia induced intraoperatively using convective forced-air devices for cooling. Again, some cautious findings were also identified, including a higher incidence of bacteremia in the hypothermic group.

Overall, one's enthusiasm for doing everything to reduce hypothermia must be tempered with the realization that there are likely situations where hypothermia can have a benefit. As in many areas of medicine, there is clearly no right or wrong answer, only a balance of risk *versus* benefit.

KEY REFERENCES

- De Witte J, Sessler DI. Perioperative shivering: physiology and pharmacology. *Anesthesiology.* 2002;96(2):467-484.
- The Hypothermia after Cardiac Arrest Study Group. Mild therapeutic hypothermia to improve the neurologic outcome after cardiac arrest. *N Engl J Med.* 2002;346(8):549-556.
- Sessler DI. Complications and treatment of mild hypothermia. *Anesthesiology.* 2001;95(2):531-543.
- Sessler DI. Mild perioperative hypothermia. *N Engl J Med.* 1997;336(24):1730-1737.
- Sessler DI. Perioperative heat balance. *Anesthesiology.* 2000;92(2):578-596.
- Shankaran S, Laptook AR, Ehrenkranz RA, et al. Whole-body hypothermia for neonates with hypoxic-ischemic encephalopathy. *N Engl J Med.* 2005;353(15):1574-1584.

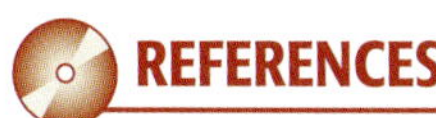

REFERENCES

Complete references available on DVD and online version at www.LongneckerAnesthesiology.com

PART 8

Care of the Chronic Pain Patient

CHAPTER 89

Mechanisms of Chronic Pain

Brian J. Wainger
Gary J. Brenner

KEY POINTS

1. Understanding the mechanisms underlying chronic pain requires knowledge of the neuroanatomy, neurochemistry, and neurophysiology of nociception and central pain processing.
2. Generation of pain hypersensitivity results from changes in the function, chemistry, and structure of both the peripheral and central nervous systems.
3. Pain can be categorized into the following broad etiologic groups: nociceptive pain is associated with an ongoing nociceptive stimulus and reflects minimal central modulation of the painful stimulus; inflammatory pain describes pain due to tissue inflammation; neuropathic pain results from injury of the peripheral or central nervous system; dysfunctional pain refers to pain due to abnormal functioning of the nervous system, despite the absence of an identified insult.
4. Nociception serves a protective function that is important from an evolutionary perspective. However, chronic pain—especially neuropathic pain and dysfunctional pain—do not serve such a protective role and result instead from a pathologic condition of the nervous system. In these circumstances, chronic pain is a disease.
5. As an injury heals, pain can dissipate with resolution of tissue injury and inflammation; alternatively, pain can persist and become independent of peripheral stimulation. The independence of ongoing stimulus reflects the marked pathologic changes that persistent pain effects on the nervous system.
6. Different mechanisms are responsible for different types of pain, and therefore the rational and successful treatment of pain requires diagnostic and therapeutic modalities that reflect the specific molecular mechanisms.

INTRODUCTION: TAXONOMY OF PAIN

The major function of the pain system is to protect the body from injury. Its evolutionary importance is underscored by the disfiguring injuries and frequent early death of people who have the rare recessive condition congenital insensitivity to pain. The importance of pain from a clinical perspective led the Joint Commission on Accreditation of Healthcare Organizations to declare that pain level constitutes a fifth vital sign. Unlike other diagnostic signs, the pain score is subjective, thus making pain difficult to study clinically. The initial step in pain signaling, *nociception*, was defined by Sir Charles Sherrington a century ago as the sensory detection of a noxious event or a potentially harmful environmental stimulus.[1] However, pain represents the integration of a wide range of inputs and modulations that span the neuraxis, from nociception in the distal periphery to complex processing of pain in the brain (**Fig. 89-1**). Consistent with this, psychologic trauma can cause pain that is perceived much in the same way as that associated with an injured extremity. And yet despite the similar experience of pain, the mechanisms underlying these 2 conditions must be different, at least in all but the highest-level representations of the pain. Indeed, we now know that virtually all chronic pain is fundamentally different from "nociception" in the sense of the simple detection of an acute noxious stimulus and its unmodulated transmission to the brain. Rather, chronic pain is the result of amplified and broadened inputs into a sensitized central system. This chapter focuses on mechanisms that generate and maintain pain.

In studying pain, clinicians and scientists have established taxonomies based on clinical presentation and animal models (**Fig. 89-2**). *Nociceptive pain* refers to pain in response to an ongoing high-threshold, noxious stimulus. Nociceptive pain ends when the stimulus ends, and does not involve additional short- or long-term changes in the pain receptors, higher-order signaling neurons, or other modulators. *Inflammatory pain* results from tissue damage and the associated release of inflammatory mediators that activate and sensitize nociceptors, and subsequently effect central changes that enhance pain transmission. Because of the sensitization of nociceptors, stimuli that are normally innocuous can elicit pain. The International Association for the Study of Pain (IASP) defines *neuropathic pain* as "pain initiated or caused by a primary lesion or dysfunction in the nervous system." We prefer to restrict the definition of neuropathic pain to a specific lesion in the nervous system that produces a sensitized pain state *and* loss of function, most often decreased sensation. As in inflammatory pain, neuropathic pain involves the sensitization of the afferent signaling machinery so that non-noxious stimuli elicit pain. However, despite the facilitated or enhanced nature of both nociceptive and neuropathic pain, as we will see, the mechanisms of the sensitization processes are different.[2]

Although inflammatory pain can play beneficial physiologic roles by preventing further tissue injury during healing, and neuropathic pain is associated with injury to the nervous system, *dysfunctional pain* refers to pain without a benefit to the organism and without a precipitant. Examples of dysfunctional pain conditions include fibromyalgia, interstitial cystitis, and irritable bowel syndrome. Although properties such as hyperalgesia may be present, there is no noxious stimulus that initiates the condition. Rather, the process is thought to result from a primary dysfunction of the nervous system.

One confounding issue arises from how the words that categorize pain conditions are used in the clinical and research arenas. Clinically, neuropathic pain refers to pain that has certain characteristic features (**Table 89-1**): allodynia, hyperalgesia, stimulus-independence (spontaneous pain), and evidence of sensory loss.[3] Patients report *allodynia*, pain upon non-noxious stimulation such as light stroking of the skin or wind blowing on the face. *Hyperalgesia*, an increased response to a normally painful stimulus, is also often present. In many cases, the "revving up" of the central pain signaling machinery occurs to such an extent so as to produce *spontaneous pain*, that is, pain that occurs without any stimulus. There is also often evidence of a sensory deficit, and frequently the painful area extends beyond any region for which pain might be expected, based on the region of tissue damage or distribution innervated by an injured or severed nerve. Neuropathic pain can result from nerve injury in the periphery or central nervous system. The most common peripheral causes of neuropathic pain include metabolic disease such as diabetic neuropathy, infectious or postinfectious processes such as postherpetic neuropathy or human immunodeficiency virus (HIV) neuropathy, toxic neuropathy such as in chemotherapy-induced neuropathy, and paraprotein-related processes such as in monogammopathy of unknown significance, paraneoplastic neuropathy, or cryoglobulin-related neuropathy most often seen in hepatitis C.[4,5] Central causes of neuropathic pain include spinal cord injury, ischemic or hemorrhagic stroke, multiple sclerosis and other causes of myelitis, tumors and abscesses, and structural abnormalities such as vascular malformations, syringomyelia, and syringobulbia.

In basic science research using animal models, neuropathic pain refers to pain due to an inflicted nerve injury, and inflammatory pain has been defined as pain resulting from an inflammatory stimulus. The benefit of such a distinction is that fundamentally different molecular mechanisms have been identified in each of the animal models of these 2 major forms of pain sensitization. However, the translation of this animal research to the clinical setting has been problematic: the degree to which mechanisms of nociceptive sensitization in animal models translate to mechanisms underlying chronic pain in

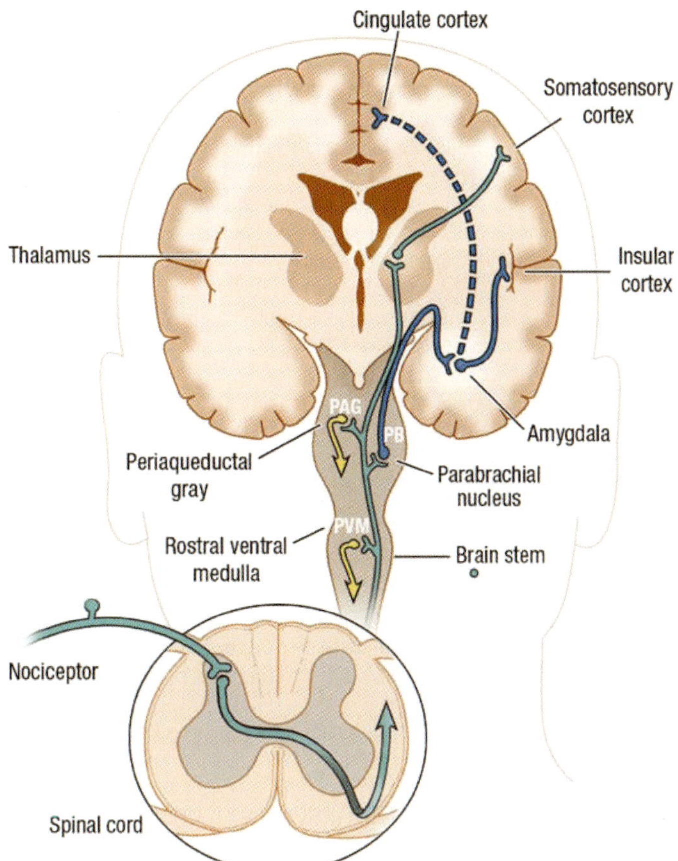

FIGURE 89-1. Primary afferent nociceptors convey noxious information to projection neurons within the dorsal horn of the spinal cord. A subset of these projection neurons transmits information to the somatosensory cortex via the thalamus, providing information about the location and intensity of painful stimulus. Other projection neurons engage the cingulate and insular cortices via connections in the brainstem (parabrachial nucleus) and amygdala, contributing to the affective component of the pain experience. This ascending information also accesses the neurons of the rostral ventral medulla and midbrain periaqueductal gray to engage descending feedback systems that regulate the output from the spinal cord. [Redrawn from Basbaum AI, Bautista DM, Scherrer G, Julius D. Cellular and molecular mechanisms of pain. *Cell*. 2009;139(2):267-284.]

humans remains unclear. This is highlighted by the virtual absence of novel human therapeutics for pain that have been derived from fundamental animal research.[6] In addition, the clinical classification of a chronic pain condition into inflammatory or neuropathic is often ambiguous. For example, should a painful inflammatory neuropathy be considered neuropathic pain or inflammatory pain? At least some overlap exists among taxonomical categories, reflecting a degree of common underlying mechanisms of pain sensitization (although we focus on the distinctions) as well as an incomplete understanding of disease processes. For example, although the pathologic process

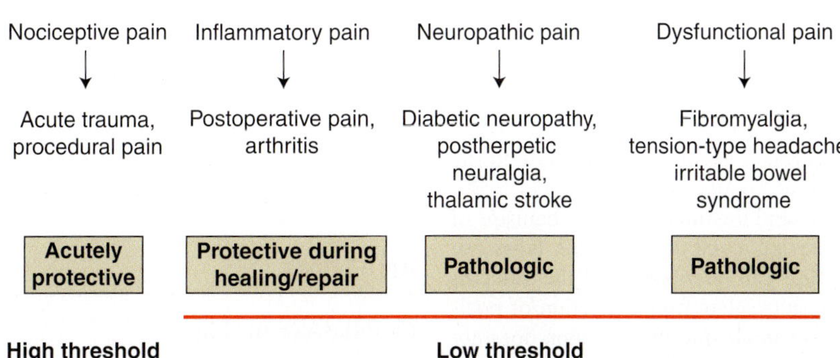

FIGURE 89-2. Four basic categories of pain. There are multiple types of pain, each with different causes and underlying mechanisms. Pain can be roughly categorized as nociceptive, inflammatory, neuropathic, and dysfunctional. Whereas nociceptive and inflammatory pain can have a protective function, both neuropathic and dysfunctional pain represent pathologic functioning of the nociceptive system. Nociceptive pain involves nociceptor activation by high-threshold stimuli only. With inflammatory, neuropathic, and dysfunctional pain, the nociceptive system can be stimulated by both high-threshold and low-threshold stimuli, and pain hypersensitivity (hyperalgesia and allodynia) occurs. Examples of each type of pain are listed beneath the arrows. (Note: the list is not exhaustive.)

TABLE 89-1 Definition and Assessment of Negative and Positive Sensory Symptoms and Signs in Patients With Neuropathic Pain

	Definition	Bedside Assessment	Expected Pathologic Response
Negative symptoms and signs			
Hypoaesthesia	Reduced sensation to non-painful stimuli	Touch skin with painter's brush cotton swab, or gauze	Reduced perception, numbness
Pall-hypoaesthesia	Reduced sensation to vibration	Apply tuning fork on bone or joint	Reduced perception threshold
Hypoalgesia	Reduced sensation to painful stimuli	Prick skin with single pin stimulus	Reduced perception, numbness
Thermal hypoaesthesia	Reduced sensation to cold or warm stimuli	Contact skin with objects of 10°C (metal roller, glass with water, coolants such as acetone); contact skin with objects of 45°C (metal roller, glass with water)	Reduced perception
Spontaneous sensations or pain			
Paraesthesia	Non-painful ongoing sensation (skin crawling sensation)	Grade intensity (0-10); area in cm^2	NA
Paroxysmal pain	Shooting electrical attacks for seconds	Number per time; grade intensity (0-10); threshold for evocation	NA
Superficial pain	Painful ongoing sensation, often a burning sensation	Grade intensity (0-10); area in cm^2	NA
Evoked pain			
Mechanical dynamic allodynia	Pain from normally non-painful light moving stimuli on skin	Stroke skin with painter's brush, cotton swab, or gauze	Sharp burning superficial pain; present in the primary affected zone but spreads beyond into unaffected skin areas (secondary zone)
Mechanical static hyperalgesia	Pain from normally non-painful gentle static pressure stimuli on skin	Apply manual gentle mechanical pressure to skin	Dull pain; present in the area of affected (damaged or sensitised) primary afferent nerve endings (primary zone)
Mechanical punctate, pin-prick hyperalgesia	Pain from normally stinging but non-painful stimuli	Prick skin with a safety pin, sharp stick, or stiff von Frey hair	Sharp superficial pain; present in the primary affected zone but spreads beyond into unaffected skin areas (secondary zone)
Temporal summation	Increasing pain sensation (wind-up-like pain) from repetitive application of identical single noxious stimuli	Prick skin with safety pin at intervals of <3 s for 30 s	Sharp superficial pain of increasing intensity
Cold hyperalgesia	Pain from normally non-painful cold stimuli	Contact skin with objects of 20°C (metal roller, glass with water, coolants such as acetone); control: contact skin with objects of skin temperature	Painful, often burning, temperature sensation; present in the area of affected (damaged or sensitised) primary afferent nerve endings (primary zone)
Heat hyperalgesia	Pain from normally non-painful heat stimuli	Contact skin with objects of 40°C (metal roller, glass with water); control: contact skin with objects of skin temperature	Painful burning temperature sensation; present in the area of affected (damaged or sensitised) primary afferent nerve endings (primary zone)
Mechanical deep somatic hyperalgesia	Pain from normally non-painful pressure on deep somatic tissues	Apply manual light pressure at joints or muscles	Deep pain at joints or muscles

NA, not applicable.

Reproduced with permission from Baron R, Binder A, Wasner G. Neuropathic pain: diagnosis, pathophysiological mechanisms, and treatment. *Lancet Neurol.* 2010;9(8):807-819.

in dysfunctional pain conditions such as fibromyalgia is presumed to reside in the central nervous system, a currently unidentified abnormality in the peripheral nervous system may contribute to the syndrome.

Although it is essential to understand the underlying mechanisms of basal and sensitized pain states, having a taxonomy of pain types can be helpful (**Fig. 89-3**). Several points can be made about the different types of pain. Nociceptive pain results solely from activation of nociceptors by high-threshold, noxious stimuli, and the sensation does not continue beyond the duration of the stimulus. No short- or long-term changes in the pain signaling machinery persist beyond the termination of the painful stimulus. In contrast, facilitated pain, whether due to inflammation associated with tissue damage (inflammatory pain), nerve injury (neuropathic pain), or primary nervous system dysfunction (dysfunctional pain), is enhanced; that is, the extent of the pain, whether with regard to intensity, duration, quality, or location, is heightened and expanded. As we will see, different molecular mechanisms underlie the facilitation in the different pain states.

We begin with a review of the anatomy of the nociceptive system.

ANATOMY

PRIMARY AFFERENTS

Primary afferent neurons have peripheral terminals that detect external stimuli, cell bodies located in the dorsal root ganglia for perception from the body, and central terminals in the spinal cord. Aside from the unusual exception of trigeminal proprioceptive neurons, which have their cell bodies in the central nervous system, primary afferent neurons have their cell bodies in the peripheral nervous system: first-order

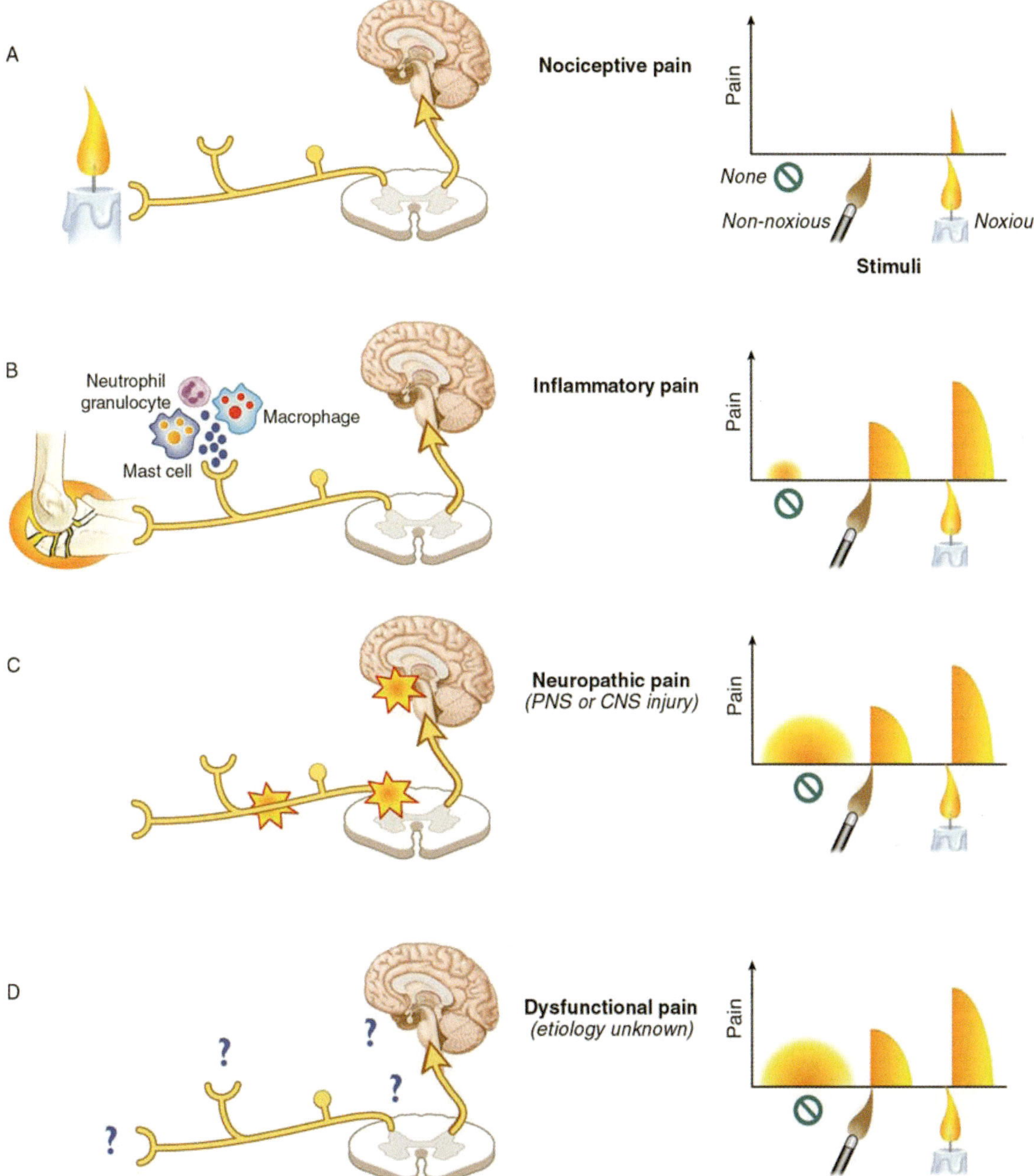

FIGURE 89-3. Underlying mechanisms of pain. Different types of pain (nociceptive, inflammatory, neuropathic, and dysfunctional) have different etiologies and are associated with different, but overlapping, mechanisms. They also have different properties with regard to the presence and duration of pain in the setting of no stimulus, a non-noxious stimulus, and a noxious stimulus.

neurons conveying perception from the face have cell bodies in the trigeminal ganglia and project to the brainstem, and first-order neurons carrying information from the body have cell bodies in the dorsal root ganglia and project to the spinal cord.

Nociceptors are high-threshold stimulus detectors and include the thinly myelinated A-δ fibers and unmyelinated C-fibers.[7] Nociceptors represent one of several functional groups of sensory fibers in peripheral nerves (**Table 89-2**), including those fibers involved in mediating proprioception, low-threshold mechanoreception, vibration sense, and innocuous thermal stimuli (**Table 89-3**). For both A-δ fibers and C-fibers, the distal dendritic inputs are simply bare nerve endings, as opposed to, for example, the more elaborate pacinian corpuscles and muscle spindles used to detect vibration and proprioception. The A-δ fibers mediate acute, precisely localized initial pain. A-δ fibers fall into 2 groups based on electrophysiological studies of the stimuli required for their activation: Type 1 or high-threshold mechanical A-δ nociceptors have high heat thresholds (>50°C) and respond to mechanical stimuli as well. Type 2 or low-threshold mechanical A-δ fibers have a much lower heat threshold but a very high mechanical threshold. Type 1 A-δ fibers most likely mediate pain due to pinprick, and Type 2 A-δ fibers convey the initial response to noxious heat.

C-fibers convey poorly localized, delayed pain. Most C-fibers are also polymodal, although a subset of mechanically insensitive, heat-responsive neurons develops mechanical sensitivity following tissue

TABLE 89-2 Classification of Fibers Found in Peripheral Nerves

Fiber Type	Innervation	Mean Diameter (μm)	Mean Conduction Velocity (m/s)
Sensory			
A-β	Cutaneous touch and pressure afferent fibers	8	50
A-δ	Mechanoreceptors, nociceptors, thermoreceptors	2-3	15
C	Mechanoreceptors, nociceptors, thermoreceptors, sympathetic preganglionic	1	1
Motor			
A-α	Primary muscle spindle, motor to skeletal muscle	15	100
A-γ	Motor to muscle spindle	6	20
Sympathetic			
B	Sympathetic postganglionic	3	7

injury. These neurons are known as "silent nociceptors" and are thought to be particularly important in the development of facilitated pain states.[8] Interestingly, distinct sets of C-fibers appear to be involved in itch[9] as well as pleasant touch.[10]

C-fibers can be divided into nonpeptidergic and peptidergic neurons. The nonpeptidergic population uses only the traditional excitatory neurotransmitter glutamate and expresses the c-Ret neurotrophin receptor, which binds the ligand glial-derived neurotrophic factor (GDNF).[11] Peptidergic C-fibers use both glutamate and neuropeptides, such as substance P and calcitonin gene-related peptide (CGRP), as neurotransmitters. They express the TrkA neurotrophin receptor, which binds the ligand nerve growth factor (NGF).

Knowledge about peripheral fibers involved in nociception allows us to formulate key concepts that relate not only to the encoding and transmission in the periphery but to the entire afferent system. First, there is a high degree of segregation of afferent information. This is reflected in the *labeled lines* hypothesis,[12] in which different receptors on different types of neurons encode information specific to different stimuli, such as cold, hot, or high-threshold mechanosensation. We see that this spatial segregation of the structures responsible for particular types or components of the painful experience is preserved in the spinal cord, thalamus, and higher brain regions as well.

Second, and in contrast, many nociceptors and other higher-order neurons are polymodal; the convergence and integration of particular types of inputs determine the properties of a response. Thunberg's thermal grill illusion in 1896 demonstrates an interesting example of the complexity of convergence: the combination of innocuous cool and warm stimuli applied in a grid produces a noxious sensation of heat,[13] despite the fact that neither component was noxious. The proposed explanation is that first-order neurons sensitive to innocuous cool converge on the same higher-order neurons as those activated by noxious cold; however, there is basal inhibition of the innocuous signal. The simultaneous warm stimulus in the grid removes that inhibition, allowing innocuous cool stimuli to cause pain.

SPINAL CORD

The central axons of nociceptors enter the gray matter of the spinal cord via the dorsal roots and synapse on second-order neurons in the dorsal horn of the spinal cord (**Fig. 89-4**). Some primary afferent fibers traverse caudally or rostrally 1 to 2 segments in the tract of Lissauer prior to synapsing. The gray matter of the spinal cord is organized into 10 laminae (of Rexed). Laminae I to V compose the dorsal horn of the spinal cord (**Fig. 89-5**). Terminals of different afferent fiber types are separated spatially in the spinal cord. C-fibers terminate superficially within laminae I and II of the dorsal horn (lamina II is termed the substantia gelatinosa, based on its appearance); however, the segregation of fiber type is even more detailed. Most peptidergic C-fibers project to lamina I and the dorsal or outer part of lamina II, and nonpeptidergic C-fibers tend to project more ventrally to the midregion of lamina II. A-δ fibers project to lamina I as well as to lamina V. The large myelinated A-β fibers that mediate light touch project to the deeper

TABLE 89-3 Functional Classification of Primary Afferent Nociceptors

Type of Fiber	Nociceptor Type	Noxious Stimuli Detected
A-δ (2-30 m/s)	AM	Mechanical
	AMC	Mechanical and cold
	AH	Heat
	AMH type I	Mechanical, heat >53°C
	AMH type II	Mechanical, heat <51°C
	A-Chem	Chemical
C-fiber (0.5-2 m/s)	CM	Mechanical
	CH	Heat
	CMH[a]	Mechanical, heat
	CMC	Mechanical, cold
	C-Chem	Chemical (algesic and pruritic)
	CMi[b]	None in resting state, mechanical (after activation)

[a]Many CMH nociceptors are also stimulated by algesic chemicals and are denoted "polymodal" nociceptors.

[b]CMi nociceptors are known as either C "mechanoinsensitive" or "silent" nociceptors and are sensitive to mechanical stimuli only in the presence of inflammation or other activating stimuli.

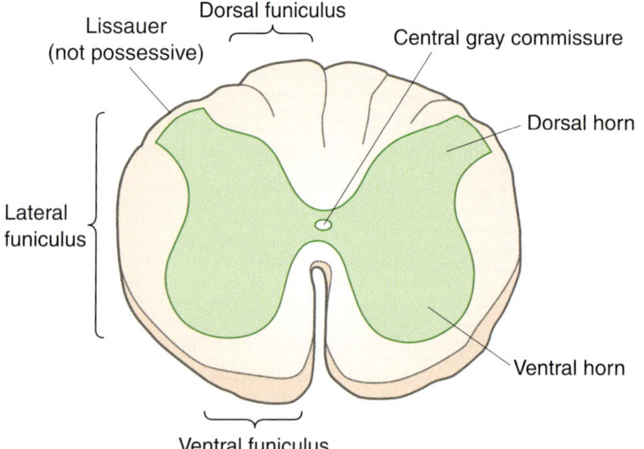

FIGURE 89-4. Cross-section of the spinal cord. Schematic of the spinal cord displays basic anatomic features. Cell bodies of second-order sensory neurons are located predominantly in the dorsal horn. Cell bodies of motor neurons are localized to the ventral horn. Nociceptive primary afferents may ascend or descend, covering as many as 6 spinal levels in the Lissauer tract prior to synapsing on second-order projection neurons and interneurons. Ascending and descending tracts in the white matter are not shown.

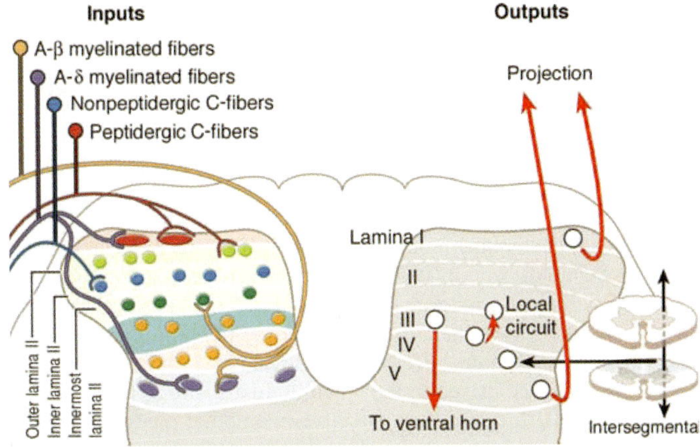

FIGURE 89-5. There is a very precise laminar organization of the dorsal horn of the spinal cord; subsets of primary afferent fibers target spinal neurons within discrete laminae. The unmyelinated, peptidergic C (red), and myelinated A-δ nociceptors (purple) terminate most superficially, synapsing upon large projection neurons (red) located in lamina I and interneurons (green) located in outer lamina II. The unmyelinated, nonpeptidergic nociceptors (blue) target interneurons (blue) in the inner part of lamina II. By contrast, innocuous input carried by myelinated A-β fibers (orange) terminates on PKC-γ expressing interneurons in the ventral half of the inner lamina II. A second set of projection neurons within lamina V (purple) receive convergent input from A-δ and A-β fibers.

laminae (III, IV, and V) as well as to a group of neurons in the ventral-most area of lamina II that express the γ isoform of protein kinase C (PKC-γ).

Thus neurons in lamina I generally respond to noxious stimulation and neurons in layers III and IV respond to innocuous stimuli. Layer V neurons receive dual noxious and non-noxious stimuli and are therefore known as wide dynamic range (WDR) neurons.

Recall that large A-α and A-β sensory fibers that mediate vibration, proprioception, and touch ascend ipsilaterally in the dorsal columns after sending branches that synapse within the deep laminae of the spinal cord. Indeed, some evidence suggests a role for the dorsal columns as well in pain signaling. Inputs from the large fibers may reduce the ascending transmission of nociceptive inputs.[14] Indeed, the dorsal columns themselves may transmit pain signals, as suggested by the reduction in visceral pain after dorsal column lesions.[15]

It is important to point out that most neurons in the dorsal horn of the spinal cord are interneurons, both inhibitory and excitatory, rather than the second-order projection neurons mentioned previously. Equally important is the recognition of the role of non-neuronal cells in the dorsal horn, such as microglia, in modulating neurotransmission. Thus the dorsal horn plays a primary role in sensory integration and modulation, as well as in transmission of nociceptive information. As will be covered, these functions are critical in modulating the gain of the nociceptive system and generating states of sensory sensitization.

Ascending Pathways The major projection neurons conveying the output from the dorsal horn reside in laminae I and V. These cells comprise the second-order neurons in the spinothalamic (anterolateral) tract, which carries sensory and discriminative information about painful stimuli to the thalamus. Projections to the posterolateral thalamus, near the terminals from the dorsal column/medial lemniscus pathway, transmit discriminative information about the nature of a noxious stimulus. In contrast, connections to the medial thalamic nuclei convey information associated with the affective component of pain. Separation of information from the superficial and deep layers of the spinal cord appears to be preserved in the thalamus.

Substantial nociceptive information passes from the dorsal horn to the brainstem via the spinobulbar tracts. This projection system terminates in 4 areas of the brainstem: the parabrachial region of the dorsolateral pons, the periaqueductal gray, regions of catecholamine cell groups, and the brainstem reticular formation. The parabrachial region of the pons provides a rapid connection to the amygdala, which mediates the aversive properties of pain; the periaqueductal gray balances ascending noxious inputs with descending pain-suppressing signals.

THE BRAIN

The integration and processing of nociceptive information (ie, pain) in the brain is perhaps the most difficult to study—largely due to its high degree of complexity. Indeed, much debate has transpired with regard to pain as a discriminative sense as opposed to an emotional experience.[16] Pain has not only a sensory dimension but an affective one as well. The affective component of pain is comprised of the unpleasant emotional feelings generated by pain and the associated desires to end or reduce pain.[17] Thus the intensity of perceived pain depends not only on the nature of a painful stimulus, but also on several other independent factors: emotional state—what emotions will a painful stimulus evoke in an individual person, and how will these additional emotions balance against the current emotional state; cognitive state—has the person learned to anticipate the pain itself or a reward associated with the pain; and level of arousal—how does the overall responsiveness of the person modulate a painful stimulus? In this sense, even the simplest pain, nociceptive pain, undergoes modulation by the brain. Perhaps the clearest demonstrations of modulation of pain are the suppression of pain by strong emotional stimuli. For example, intense emotions surrounding battle and athletics have been shown to suppress the response to pain. The soldier needs to focus on surviving and the athlete on performance.[18] Indeed, soldiers injured in battle "entirely denied pain,"[19] at least to some extent due to the positive experience associated with survival and perhaps also due to the positive expectation of returning home. Similar responses occur in animals, in which expectation of a reward completely suppressed response to pain, known as the *nocifensive* response, in dogs.[20] Such mechanisms can also clearly serve an evolutionary purpose, in that an animal's response to pain or injury can be suppressed in the presence of a predator or other danger.

Much has been learned about the different components of pain, suggesting that different regions of the brain are responsible for different aspects of pain processing, and that there are complex interactions between these different centers.[21] Moreover, pain is tightly linked to the reward pathways. Indeed, there is substantial overlap between regions of the brain activated by reward signals and those activated by pain signals.[22]

The ascending tracts terminate in both the lateral and medial thalamic nuclei. The lateral nuclei and their projections to primary sensory cortex transmit discriminatory pain, the perceptual identification of a precisely specified location, nature, and intensity of a noxious stimulus. The projections to the medial thalamus, in contrast, and the wide projections to limbic and frontal brain regions mediate the affective components of the pain experience.

One of the most expansive tools for studying pain has been functional imaging, including positron emission tomography (PET) and functional magnetic resonance imaging (fMRI). The assumption underlying these 2 techniques is that visualized blood flow and metabolic changes localized to precise regions reflect neuronal activity in the same locations. Although the metabolic effects of inhibitory neurons need to be considered in interpreting the imaging studies on a cellular level, brain imaging has consistently demonstrated regional effects of pain on the brain and has supported a structural segregation of discriminatory and affective pain processing.[21] For example, heat pain in patients with somatoform pain disorder was associated with a hyperactive state of several limbic structures including the parahippocampal gyrus, amygdala, and anterior insula.[23] Similar results were obtained in fibromyalgia patients during pain catastrophizing and inflammatory bowel patients during rectal distention. Additionally, the anterior insula and rostral anterior cingulate cortices were activated by both painful stimuli to volunteers and by observation of painful stimuli in their loved ones; in contrast, the posterior insula, sensorimotor cortex, and caudal anterior cingulated cortex were only activated by direct painful stimulation.[24]

Furthermore, these identified regions have been consistent with what might be expected, given prior neurologic knowledge from lesion-based studies. Thus pain asymbolia, the absence of the emotional or affective component of pain with preserved discriminative pain sensation, has been shown to occur after insular lesions.[25]

In conditioned place aversion tests, an animal associates a particular location with a noxious stimulus and subsequently learns to avoid that location. This anticipatory component of the affective pain response occurs in regions of the brain that are becoming more and more well defined. Indeed, animals with a lesion in the anterior cingulate do not undergo conditioned place aversion learning; that is, the rats do not avoid the place associated with a noxious stimulus.[26] Furthermore, microinjection of an excitatory neurotransmitter into the anterior cingulate provided a substitute for the noxious stimulus and an antagonist blocked the development of the process.[27] Thus excitatory stimulation of the anterior cingulate was sufficient to produce aversion to a particular location. Importantly, in all of these experiments, the nocifensive response was unaffected, suggesting that the affective dimension of pain—but not the sensory one—was selectively modulated.

The widespread changes in brain function associated with chronic pain conditions revealed by functional imaging studies support the presence of major effects of pain on cognition and mood, especially with changes in the frontal and limbic regions, respectively. In fact, degree of depression in patients with fibromyalgia has been correlated with amygdala and anterior insular activity. Although such studies do not "prove" that pain causes depression, they do highlight the connection and support a careful regard for a patient's mood in treating pain.

Chronic low back pain has been associated with reduced gray matter mass in the thalamus and the lateral prefrontal cortex.[28] The effects of pain itself are difficult to separate from secondary effects due to drug use or lack of normal activity and use-dependent structural reinforcements or changes; nonetheless, similar imaging studies have documented decreased gray matter among patients with chronic headache, fibromyalgia, irritable bowel syndrome, and chronic regional pain syndrome. Although the regions identified in the different studies are not identical, they tend to involve regions used during learning and during painful stimulation applied to healthy subjects.

On the cellular level, animal data also support changes in the brain associated with chronic pain, in particular with neuropathic pain. Investigation of cortical neurons after nerve injury shows increased length and branching of layer II/III pyramidal neurons in the contralateral motor cortex.[29]

Another important but confounding consideration in studying pain is the placebo effect.[30] Just as intense emotional experiences such as battle can suppress the sensation of painful stimuli, the anticipation of reward also can increase the pain threshold, suggesting that affective modulation of pain and the placebo response—pain relief due to the expectation of pain relief—operate via a common mechanism.[31] The widespread influence of the placebo effect is indeed extraordinary; placebo analgesia has even been shown to correlate with changes in fMRI signals within the dorsal horn of the spinal cord.[32] Similar brain regions are involved in the placebo effect and in opioid analgesia.[33] Opioid antagonists can block the placebo effect,[34] and opioid agonists can prevent increases in fMRI signal in response to a noxious stimulus.[35] Thus the placebo mechanism may involve activation of the descending pain modulatory system, to which we will now turn our attention.

DESCENDING PATHWAYS

The power of descending modulation of the pain system was first recognized by Reynolds, who in 1969 found that electrical stimulation of the midbrain periaqueductal grey (PAG) produced analgesia sufficient for surgery in rats.[36] Since then, the multiple descending projections from several brainstem centers have been investigated.

The best-characterized system originates in the periaqueductal grey and sends fibers to the rostral ventromedial medulla (RVM), which in turn projects via the dorsal part of the lateral funiculus to both superficial and deep laminae of the dorsal horn (see Fig. 89-1). The RVM is comprised of the serotonergic nucleus raphe magnus and adjacent reticular formation that are located in the midline near the pontomedullary junction. Within the RVM, cells are grouped as on-cells, off-cells, or neutral-cells, with regard to their firing pattern during a nocifensive withdrawal.[37] Although the initial emphasis was on the inhibition of pain transmission, recent studies have led to a greater appreciation of both inhibition and enhancement of pain pathways by descending fibers. The inhibitory descending fibers primarily target and blunt the nociceptive inputs of C-fibers.[38]

The descending pathways of the PAG and RVM receive extensive inputs from higher brain centers, including the hypothalamus, amygdala, and prefrontal cortex. Inputs from the amygdala are associated with intense fear-behaviors, and opioid injection into the basolateral nucleus of the amygdala activates off-cells in the RVM, presumably reducing pain during times of extreme fear.[39] In contrast, stimulation of the ventrolateral orbital cortex and anterior cingulate cortex mediates hyperalgesia by stimulating on-cells in the RVM.

In addition to the PAG-RVM pathways, the dorsal reticular nucleus and caudal ventrolateral medulla have also been demonstrated to mediate descending pain signal modulation that occurs at the level of the spinal cord.

Descending inputs can also be categorized by transmitter type. The major transmitters involved in the descending pain modulatory pathways are the endogenous opioids, noradrenalin, and serotonin (5-hydroxytryptamine, 5-HT). The 3 classes of endogenous opioids are enkephalins, β-endorphin, and dynorphins, and are found within neurons of different regions of the central nervous system. Enkephalins and dynorphins are found predominantly in the PAG, RVM, and dorsal horn of the spinal cord, and β-endorphin is found primarily in neurons within the hypothalamus. There are 3 major classes of opioid receptors, μ, δ, and κ, and a less well-understood orphan-type receptor. The role of the μ-opioid has been most securely established: knockout of the μ-opioid receptor abolishes the analgesic effect of morphine.[40] The contributions of the other receptor types have not been as clearly documented. The δ-receptor agonists may produce analgesia, with fewer side effects than the μ-receptor agonists. The δ-receptor seems to be involved in the development of opioid tolerance, as well as in anxiety. The κ-receptor may be involved in stress-induced dysphoria. The G-protein–coupled opioid receptors exert inhibitory effects by 2 major mechanisms: they decrease calcium conductances and increase potassium conductance, which can act either presynaptically to decrease transmitter release or postsynaptically to inhibit signal propagation.

Noradrenergic bulbospinal fibers that originate in the locus ceruleus mediate antinociceptive properties[41] and act through the G-protein–coupled adrenoceptors. α_1-Adrenoceptors are coupled to Gq, leading to an activation of phospholipase C, increased intracellular calcium, and

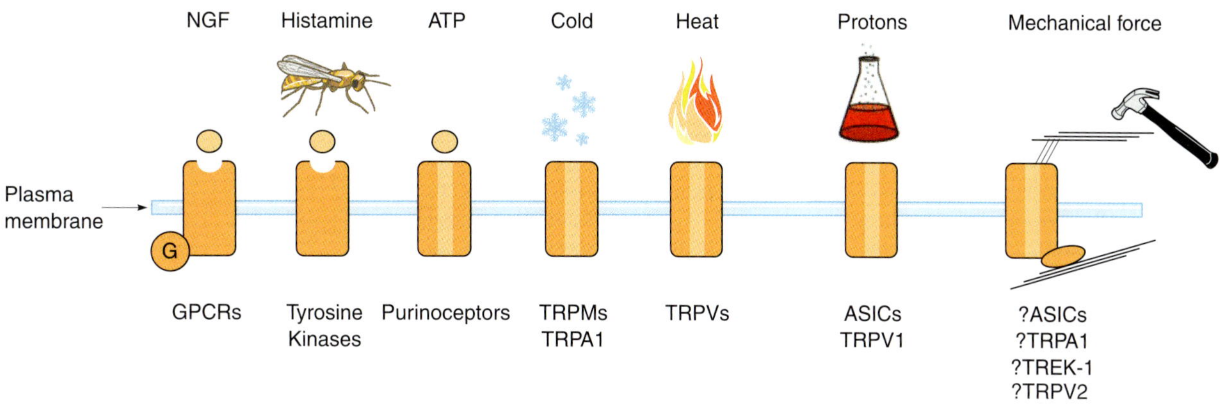

FIGURE 89-6. Transduction of nociceptive stimuli. The first step in the sensation of physiologic or "nociceptive" pain is the transduction of high-intensity stimuli by primary sensory afferents. These afferents, A-δ and C-fibers, transduce mechanical-, chemical-, and temperature-related stimuli. The gain of the primary nociceptive afferents can be increased by translational and post-translational modification, leading to pain hypersensitivity in a process termed *peripheral sensitization.* GPCRs, G-protein–coupled receptors; TRP, transient receptor protein; ASICs, acid-sensing ion channels; TREK, a member of the 2-pore-domain K+ channels.

transmitter release; α_2-adrenoceptors are coupled to Gi/o, which causes an increased potassium conductance and therefore membrane hyperpolarization and decreased transmitter release. The descending noradrenergic effects occur through the inhibitory α_2-adrenoceptor effects on nociceptive terminals and through the activation of presynaptic α_1-adrenoceptors on inhibitory interneurons.[42,43] Thus noradrenergic inhibition of the nociceptive pathway occurs either through inhibition of the nociceptors or stimulation of the antinociceptive inhibitory interneurons.

Serotonergic descending fibers from the RVM can mediate both antinociceptive and pronociceptive effects, depending on the receptor types activated.[42] Of the 14 subtypes of serotonin receptors, most of which are coupled to G-proteins, predominantly the 5-HT_{1A}, 5-HT_{1B}, 5-HT_{1D}, and 5-HT_3 receptor subtypes are found in the spinal cord. Serotonin hyperpolarizes second-order neurons in the dorsal horn via Gi/o-coupled 5-HT_{1A} receptors, which act by opening potassium channels and closing calcium channels. Unlike other serotonin receptors, the 5-HT_3 receptor is ionotropic, and the binding of serotonin leads to the opening of a nonselective, cation-permeable channel also found in the superficial layers of the dorsal horn. It is located on the afferent fibers of nociceptors and functions to enhance transmitter release from these neurons.

MOLECULES AND MECHANISMS OF ACUTE PAIN

DETECTION

Acute pain refers to pain due to the detection and transmission of an ongoing noxious stimulus, which can be due to heat, cold, or pressure (mechanical) (**Fig. 89-6**). Different receptors are involved not only in detecting different stimulus modalities, but also different stimulus intensities (**Table 89-4**). As mentioned earlier, this baseline, unenhanced pain is termed **nociceptive pain.**

We perceive temperatures greater than around 43°C as painful. This corresponds to temperature necessary to activate most C-fibers and Type 2 A-δ fibers, whereas minorities of these neurons have a threshold of 50°C. Nociceptors respond to heat through activation of a group of nonselective cation channels called *transient receptor potential (TRP) channels.* Among the earliest and best characterized of the thermoreceptors is TRPV1, which was identified as the molecular

TABLE 89-4 Ion Channel and Metabotropic Receptors (Found on Primary Afferent Peripheral Terminals) Involved in Noxious Stimulus Transduction

Ion Channel Receptors	Permeable To	Activated By
Transient Receptor Potential (TRP) Channels		
TRPV1	Cations, especially Ca^{2+}	Heat (>109°F [>43°C]), low pH, capsaicin
TRPV2	Cations, especially Ca^{2+}	Heat (>126°F [>52°C])
TRPV3	Cations, especially Ca^{2+}	Warm (88°F-102°F [31°C-39°C])
TRPV4	Cations, especially Ca^{2+}	Warm (>81°F [27°C])
TRPM8	Cations, especially Ca^{2+}	Cold (~46°F-79°F [~8°C-26°C]), menthol
TRPA1	Cations, especially Ca^{2+}	Cold (<63°F [17°C]), mustard oil
Acid-Sensing Ion Channels		
ASIC1, ASIC2, ASIC3	Na^+	Low pH, ? mechanical
Purine receptor, P2X3	Ca^{2+}	ATP
Metabotropic Receptors	**Second Messenger**	**Activated By**
Purine receptor, P2XY	G-protein–coupled receptor	ATP
Bradykinin receptor, B1 and B2	G_q-protein–coupled receptor	Bradykinin

ATP, adenosine triphosphate.

target of capsaicin, the primary pungent component of hot peppers. In support of a primary role for TRPV1 in sensing hot temperatures, TRPV1-deficient animals have a significant impairment in their ability to react to noxious thermal stimuli.[44,45] Indeed, TRPV1 activation occurs at temperatures above 42°C, correlating well with the onset of a painful sensation.

A number of other TRPV channels may transduce other heat signals. TRPV2 channels have an activation threshold of about 52°C, and TRPV3 and TRPV4 activate at mildly elevated temperatures (between 25°C and 35°C). Mice that lack TRPV3 and TRPV4 display changes in temperature preference when placed on a surface with graded temperatures.[46] Thus the receptors present on a particular C-fiber determine the temperature range to which it is sensitive.

TRP channels were also suspected as possible cold detectors after their role in heat detection was identified. Just as most temperature-sensing neurons respond to capsaicin, most cold-detecting neurons respond to menthol. TRPM8 activates in response to both menthol and cooling to about 28°C. Mice that lack TRPM8 show dual deficiencies in their responses to menthol and cold. Remaining cold sensation may be due to TRPA1, which is activated by higher concentrations of menthol and icillin, as well as a wide range of other stimuli discussed below.

The identity of receptors responsible for detecting noxious mechanical stimuli is not clear. Based on studies in the worm *Caenorhabditis elegans*, a group of epithelial sodium channels known as acid-sensing ion channels (ASICs) have been hypothesized to be involved. Deletion of 1 or even 2 of the 3 isoforms, however, has not revealed marked deficits, thus raising questions regarding their importance in mechanotransduction. TRP channels may also play a role in mechanotransduction, as TRPV2 responds to osmotic stretch (in addition to heat). Some studies of TRPA1-deficient mice have found changes in the response to mechanical stimulation,[47] and others have not.[48,49]

Receptors for a number of other noxious stimuli have been identified. For example, the TRPV1 receptor responds to protons (ie, acid). TRPA1 has been found to a wide range of agonists that share the structural property of forming covalent adducts with cysteines in the N-terminal region of the receptor. Activating molecules include the pungent ingredients in wasabi (allyl isothiocyanate) and garlic (allicin), as well as environmental toxins such as acrolein, an irritant found in tear gas and smoke.

The active pungent agent in Szechuan pepper, hydroxy-α-sanshool, produces a sensation "akin to the experience of touching one's tongue to the terminals of a 9-V battery."[50] This compound has been shown to exert its effect by closing the 2-pore potassium channels, KCNK3, KNCK9, and KCNK18. Interestingly, hydroxy-α-sanshool closes these channels, thereby producing an excitatory effect, in subgroups of both C-fibers and large-diameter myelinated fibers.

CONDUCTION

Like all neurons, electrical signals are transmitted through action potentials formed by tight regulation of the opening and closing of different ion channels. However, nociceptors have a number of unique properties in their assembly of ion channels (**Table 89-5**). *Voltage-gated sodium channels* are major determinants of the firing pattern of neurons. The pore of a sodium channel is encoded by a single gene that contains 4 subunits connected by intracellular linkers. Each subunit has 6 transmembrane segments, of which the fourth contains a series of positively charged residues that function as a voltage sensor, and a helix between the fifth and sixth segments forms the pore. Of the 9 voltage-gated sodium channels, nociceptors express $Na_V1.1$, 1.6, and 1.7, which are sensitive to very low concentrations of the pufferfish toxin tetrodotoxin (TTX), and $Na_V1.8$ and 1.9, which are tetrodotoxin resistant. Although $Na_V1.1$ and $Na_V1.6$ are expressed in a wide range of cells, $Na_V1.7$ is found predominantly in nociceptors and sympathetic neurons, but also in other sensory neurons and neuroendocrine cells. $Na_V1.8$ is expressed only in nociceptors, whereas $Na_V1.9$ is expressed predominantly in nociceptors.[51]

TABLE 89-5 Ion Channels (Found on Primary Afferent Nociceptors) Involved in Membrane Excitation/Conduction and Synaptic Transmission

Channel	Permeable To	Activated By
Tetrodotoxin-sensitive sodium channels $Na_V1.1$, $Na_V1.6$, $Na_V1.7$	Na^+	Depolarization
Tetrodotoxin-resistant sodium channels $Na_V1.8$, $Na_V1.9$	Na^+	Depolarization
Inward-rectifying potassium channels (multiple subtypes)	K^+	Depolarization, Ca^{2+}
Voltage-gated calcium channels, esp. the N-type Ca^{2+} channel ($Ca_V2.2$)	Ca^{2+}	Depolarization

Although the development of TTX-resistant sodium channel expression in the muscles of snakes that pray on TTX-producing newts provides an evolutionary advantage,[52] the explanation for the expression of toxin-resistant sodium channels in sensory neurons in humans is less clear. The TTX-resistant sodium channels have unusual gating properties that shape the nociceptive signal. $Na_V1.8$ produces the most current during the action potential upstroke and supports repetitive firing, a key property of nociceptors. $Na_V1.9$ has a much lower activation threshold and therefore amplifies and prolongs small depolarizations.

Nociceptors also have an array of *calcium channels* involved in modulating and conducting the electrical signal and in releasing transmitter.[53] The pore of voltage-gated calcium channels is formed by a tetramer of 4 α_1-subunits, each of which is analogous to 1 of 4 subunits encoded by a sodium channel protein, as well as modulatory $\alpha_2\delta$-, β-, and γ-subunits. The gabapentinoids, gabapentin and pregabalin, are thought to act by blocking calcium channels containing the $\alpha_2\delta$-subunit.[54] Subtypes of calcium channels can be identified pharmacologically as well as by their voltage-dependence and kinetics of gating. L-type, or low-voltage activated, calcium channels are expressed in many types of cells including muscle, neurons, and osteoblasts. T-type, transient, channels are most often found in neurons and osteocytes. N-type, neuronal, channels are found predominantly in neuronal tissue. P/Q-type channels are expressed at synaptic terminals in the superficial dorsal horn and other central nervous system synapses where they mediate transmitter release. R-type channels were first identified in cerebellar granule cells and are found predominantly in neurons, including dorsal root ganglion neurons.

TRANSMISSION

The dorsal horn is a critical region for the processing, modulation, and projection of nociceptive information to the brain (**Tables 89-6 and 89-7**). Invasion of the central terminals of nociceptors in the spinal cord by action potentials arriving from the periphery results in activation of voltage-dependent calcium channels and calcium entry, which lead to transmitter release. Enough transmitter may be released to produce depolarization of the postsynaptic cell sufficient to initiate an action potential in the second-order neuron. Alternatively, the invading action potential may result in minimal release of transmitter. Between these extremes lies a range of graded synaptic efficacies from strong to almost ineffective.

Although the dorsal horn is the site of primary afferent transmission, it is also the site of modulation by an extensive network

TABLE 89-6 Synaptic Mediators of Dorsal Horn Nociceptive Processing

Excitatory	Inhibitory
Amino acids: glutamate and aspartate	Endogenous opioids: enkephalin and β-endorphin
Neuropeptides: substance P (SP), calcitonin gene-related peptide (CGRP), vasoactive intestinal peptide (VIP)	Amino acids: glycine and γ-aminobutyric acid (GABA)
Growth factors: brain-derived neurotropic factor (BDNF)	Norepinephrine (NE)
Bradykinin	Serotonin (5-HT)
Somatostatin	Endogenous cannabinoids
Prostaglandin E_2 (PGE_2)	

of interneurons, as well as descending axonal projections. Indeed, primary connections between first-order neurons and projection neurons comprise only a small percentage of spinal cord neurons. Numerous transmitters and synaptic neuromodulators are involved in the transmission and modulation of nociceptive information in the dorsal horn (**Fig. 89-7**).

Synaptic transmission between primary afferent nociceptors (predominantly C-fibers) and second-order neurons has both fast and slow components. As in the case of the nervous system in general, the excitatory amino acid glutamate is the primary fast excitatory neurotransmitter used by nociceptors. Glutamate activates α-amino-3-hydroxy-5-methylisoxazole-4-propionic acid (AMPA)/kainate ionotropic glutamate receptors, leading to a short-lasting depolarization in second-order neurons (a few milliseconds), the fast excitatory postsynaptic potential. As discussed in more detail later on, the *N*-methyl-D-aspartate (NMDA) ionotropic glutamate receptor is another ionotropic glutamate receptor that is normally blocked by magnesium at resting membrane potentials and requires prolonged depolarization to relieve that block. The NMDA ion channel allows both calcium and sodium ion influx into the cell; calcium then can act as a second messenger and produce long-lasting changes in the cell.

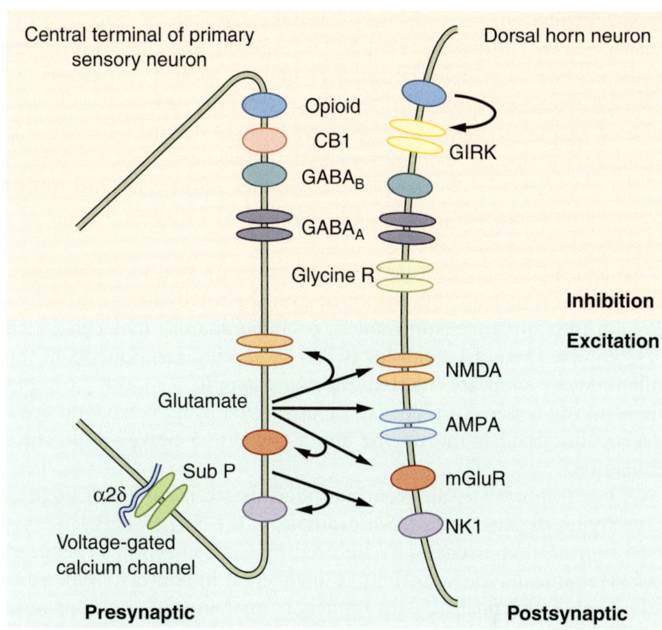

FIGURE 89-7. Inhibitory and excitatory influences of primary afferents in the spinal cord dorsal horn. Second-order neurons in the dorsal horn of the spinal cord are subject to both inhibitory and excitatory presynaptic influences by primary sensory afferents. This is one of several mechanisms through which excitability of dorsal horn neurons is controlled. Dorsal horn neurons also are subject to inhibitory and excitatory influences from local interneurons and descending brainstem pathways.

In addition to glutamate, peptidergic C-fibers have a variety of other cotransmitters (eg, substance P, calcitonin gene-related peptide [CGRP], neuropeptide Y [NPY], and brain-derived neurotropic factor [BDNF]). Whereas glutamate activates ionotropic AMPA/kainate receptors to produce a fast synaptic potential, the coreleased neuropeptides activate G-protein–coupled receptors, resulting in a delayed and longer-lasting slow postsynaptic potential that persists for several seconds.

Glycine and γ-aminobutyric acid (GABA) are the predominant mediators of *inhibitory* neurotransmission in the dorsal horn. Glycine and GABA activate glycine and $GABA_A$ ionotropic receptors to produce inward chloride currents that hyperpolarize and therefore inhibit neuronal activity. Several inhibitory metabotropic (ie, G-protein–coupled) receptors are present on afferent central terminals and dorsal horn neurons, including $GABA_B$, opioid, and cannabinoid receptors.

Control of synaptic efficacy is one of the major driving forces of neuronal plasticity in general and of pain hypersensitivity in particular. As we will see in the next section, changes in the synaptic efficacy comprise major mechanisms for pain facilitation.

TABLE 89-7 Dorsal Horn Neuronal Receptors Involved in the Processing of Nociceptive Information

Receptor	Major Ligand(s)
Excitatory Ionotropic	
NMDA receptor	Glutamate (glycine is a coligand)
AMPA receptor	Glutamate
Kainate receptor	Glutamate
Excitatory Metabotropic	
Neurokinin receptors, NK1	Substance P
Metabotropic glutamate receptor, mGluR5	Glutamate
Prostaglandin receptors	Prostaglandin E_2, prostaglandin $F_2α$
Tyrosine kinase B (TrkB) receptor	Brain-derived neurotrophic factor (BDNF) Neurotrophin 4/5 (NT4/5)
Inhibitory Metabotropic	
Opioid receptors	Endomorphins, enkephalins, dynorphin
$α_2$-Adrenergic receptor	Norepinephrine
Serotonin receptors, $5\text{-HT}_{1B/D}$ and $5HT_3$[a]	Serotonin
$GABA_B$ receptor	γ-aminobutyric acid (GABA)
Cannabinoid receptor, CB1	Endocannabinoids
Inhibitory Ionotropic	
Glycine receptor	Glycine

[a]Serotonin may have facilitatory effects in the dorsal horn via activation of $5HT_3$ receptors.

FACILITATED PAIN: MECHANISMS OF INFLAMMATORY AND NEUROPATHIC PAIN

In acute nociceptive pain, noxious stimuli produce pain that is restricted temporally to the stimulus duration and geographically to the site of the stimulus, with minimal change exerted on the nociceptive system. Other types of pain involve profound modulation of the receptive, synaptic transmissive, and transductive pathways.

Persistent noxious stimuli cause tissue damage, which results in the release and accumulation of a wide range of molecules, known as "inflammatory soup" released from the injured tissue. These factors are released from immune cells, neurons, and non-neuronal cells and include peptides (substance P, CGRP, bradykinin), eicosanoids (products of the cyclo-oxygenase and lipoxygenase pathways such as thromboxane, leukotrienes, and prostaglandins), neurotrophins (such as nerve growth factor and brain-derived neurotrophic factor), cytokines, and chemokines.

Animal models of persistent pain are often divided into inflammatory pain and neuropathic pain based on the method of pain induction. In inflammatory pain models, proinflammatory molecules such as Complete Freund's Adjuvant (CFA) or specific components of the inflammatory soup are injected into, for example, a mouse paw, and the resulting hypersensitivity can be quantified using behavioral tests. Neuropathic models involve the direct injury to a nerve via pressure or ligation.

Of key importance, different mechanisms are involved in the different types of pain models. For example, in the Na_V1.9-deficient animals thermal hypersensitivity induced by CFA injection is reduced and mechanical hypersensitivity is unaffected. In contrast, hypersensitivity in 2 neuropathic pain models is unchanged.[55] In a separate study, ablation of the population of nociceptors that express Na_V1.8 eliminates pain due to inflammatory stimuli but maintains pain due to nerve injury.[56]

Interestingly, C-fibers expressing the VGLUT3 type of glutamate transporter seem to be important in the facilitation of mechanosensitivity in both inflammatory and neuropathic pain models. These neurons are activated by light touch and cold but not heat under normal conditions. However, in models of persistent pain using inflammatory substance or nerve injury, mice lacking this type of C-fiber exhibit sensitization to heat but not mechanical stimuli.[57]

Thus there is a clear separation in mechanisms effecting different types of hypersensitivity, thermal or mechanical, and different pain models, inflammatory or neuropathic. This thesis forms the basis of the labeled-line study of pain mechanisms.

PERIPHERAL SENSITIZATION

Peripheral sensitization refers to a decrease in nociceptor threshold and an increase in output, and many inflammatory mediators promote such changes. The initial sensitization process occurs by direct or indirect activation of the detectors that respond to noxious stimuli and the transmitters that conduct the signal (**Figure 89-8** and

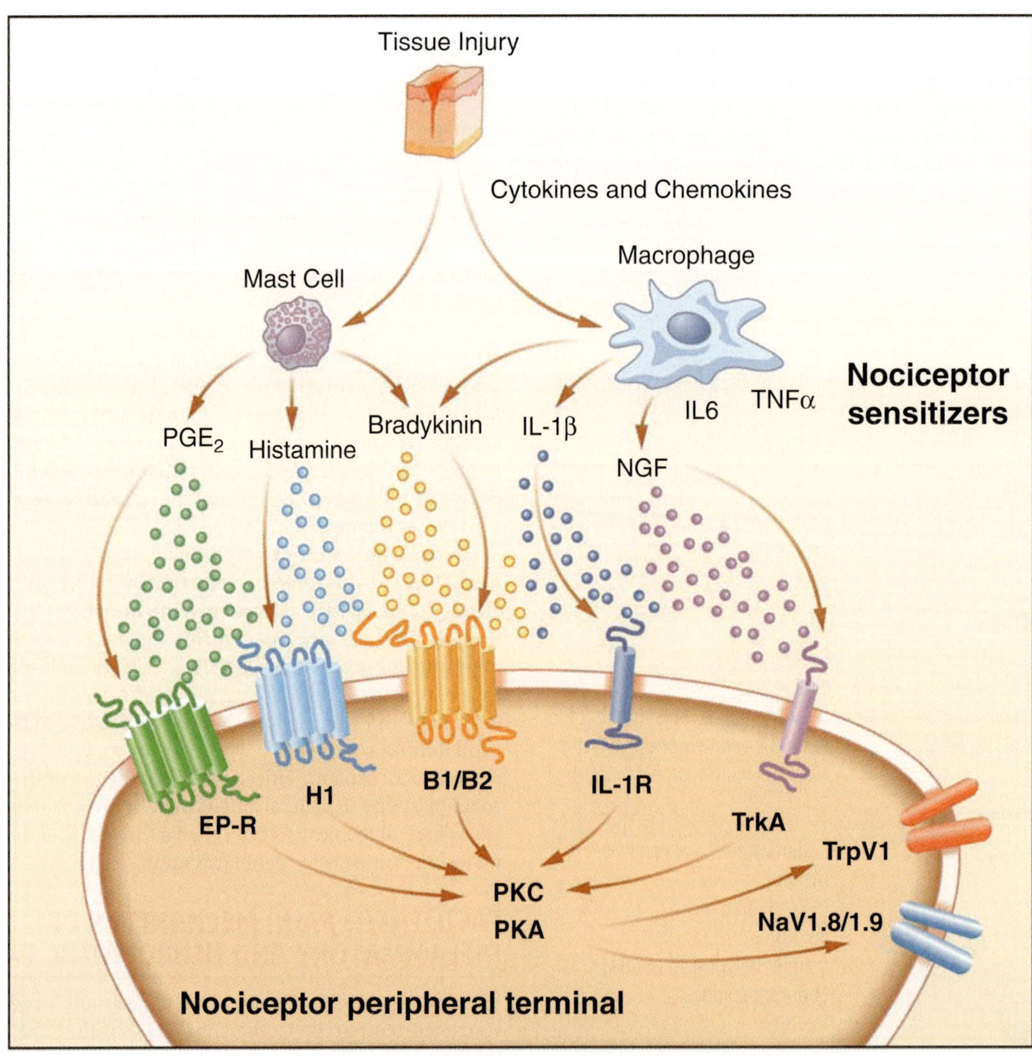

FIGURE 89-8. Primary afferent nociceptor sensitization. Following peripheral injury, a variety of inflammatory mediators are generated that are capable of sensitizing primary afferent nociceptors. These mediators bind to cell-surface receptors, activating a variety of second-messenger pathways that in turn can alter the transduction properties of both the receptors and ion channels involved in action potential generation and conduction.

TABLE 89-8 Some Receptors Involved in Nociceptor Sensitization

Metabotropic Receptors	Intracellular Transduction Mechanism
Serotonin receptors, $5HT_1$ and $5HT_2$	$G_{i/o}$-mediated inhibition of adenylate cyclase
Prostanoid receptors, EP, DP, IP	G-protein–mediated effects
ATP receptor, P2Y	G-protein–mediated effects, including TRPV1 sensitization
Histamine receptors, H_1, H_2, H_3, H_4[a]	G-protein–mediated effects
Growth Factor Receptors	**Major Ligand**
Tyrosine kinase (Trk) receptor, TrkA	Nerve growth factor (NGF)
Cytokine Receptors	**Ligand**
Tumor necrosis factor-α (TNF-α) receptor	TNF-α
Interleukin-1 (IL-1) receptor	IL-1α, IL-1β

[a]Activation of histamine receptors on cutaneous C-fibers causes itch under physiologic conditions. When neuropathic pain is present, application of histamine generates pain rather than itch.

Table 89-8). These modulatory effects occur early by mechanisms such as phosphorylation and ion channel insertion, and later through gene modulation by transcription factors activated at the end of the various pathways.

The signaling pathways that lie between the inflammatory mediators and their modulatory targets are complicated. Most of the pathways start with activation of a G-protein–coupled receptor (GPCR) or serine/threonine receptor kinase. For example, in the protein kinase A pathway, activation of adenyl cyclase by a GPCR produces increased levels of adenosine 3′,5′-cyclic monophosphate (cAMP), which heightens the activity of protein kinase A (PKA) and facilitates phosphorylation of targets. Another G-protein–coupled receptor activates phospholipase C, which hydrolyzes phosphatidylinositol into inositol triphosphate (IP3) and diacylglycerol (DAG), the latter pairing with increased calcium to activate protein kinase C (PKC). Other factors work by activating receptor tyrosine kinases that have their own signaling cascades.

Injection of the inflammatory mediators into animals and the subsequent demonstration of reduced threshold to noxious stimuli have formed the basis for inflammatory pain models. A number of key modulatory targets have been identified. Heat hypersensitivity follows treatment with several inflammatory factors such as bradykinin, ATP, or NGF. In TRPV1-deficient animals, heat hypersensitivity does not develop, supporting the role of TRPV1 in thermal hyperalgesia.[44,45] Prostaglandin E_2 causes an enhancement of the capsaicin-induced current.[58] This sensitization of the channel and resulting increased current has been shown to result from phosphorylation of the TRPV1 receptor, as mutation of the phosphorylation site abrogates the modulatory effect of PKC, which is a downstream effecter of prostaglandin E_2.[59] Activators of the PKA pathway have been shown to cause insertion of TRPV1 channels into the plasma membrane.[60,61]

Modulation of TTX-resistant sodium channels provides another mechanism for sensitization. Indeed, prostaglandin E_2 has also been shown to increase the amplitude of TTX-resistant sodium channels and decrease the voltage necessary for activating the channels.[62] The inflammatory cytokine interleukin-1β also increases TTX-resistant currents by relieving slow inactivation of these channels.[63] Furthermore, in $Na_V1.9$-deficient mice there is a reduction in pain hypersensitivity in response to a number of inflammatory mediators including prostaglandin E_2, interleukin-1β, bradykinin, and capsaicin.

More subtle sensitization may occur through "priming" of the primary afferent nociceptor. In this case, nociceptive thresholds are unchanged. Rather, the cell has an increased sensitivity to inflammatory mediators. Entry into and maintenance of the primed state depends on PKC.[64] In the primed state, cross-activation among pathways increases, so that, for example, protein kinase C, which is normally activated by calcium and DAG, can be activated by cAMP.

CENTRAL SENSITIZATION

Central sensitization refers to changes in the spinal cord and brain that result in an increase in the gain of the system with subsequent increased pain perception.[65] In contrast to peripheral sensitization, in which nociceptive signals to the brain still depend on continuous peripheral stimuli, albeit weaker ones, central sensitization can render pain stimulus-independent by uncoupling the pain response from the presence and duration of nociceptive inputs (see Fig. 89-3). Instead, the pathologic state of the central nervous system is sufficient in itself to cause pain. Central sensitization is thought to be critical to spontaneous pain, a key feature of clinical neuropathic pain. There are several major components to central sensitization: augmentation of existing inputs, recruitment of new inputs, loss of normal inhibitory signals, and changes in the glial and inflammatory milieu that affect neuronal signaling.

One feature of central sensitization, or perhaps more accurately the process that leads to central sensitization, is temporal windup, the progressive increases in the responses elicited by repeated identical stimuli. Repeated low-frequency stimulation of C-fiber stimulation leads to increased action potential firing in the second-order spinal cord neuron.[66] This electrophysiological phenomenon correlates with the development of pain reported by patients upon repeated stimulation with what is initially an innocuous stimulus, but one that becomes noxious on repeated stimulation and results in a prolonged pain following the end of the stimulation. In humans this clinical finding is termed "summation."

The initial experimental observations leading to the understanding of a central component to pain hypersensitivity took place in 1983.[67,68] Under normal conditions, a noxious mechanical or thermal stimulus to the skin of the paw is required to stimulate the biceps femoris α-motor neurons and thereby elicit the flexor withdrawal reflex. Non-noxious stimuli produce only subthreshold activity in the motor neurons. However, after repeated noxious stimuli, pain sensation is enhanced so that previously innocuous low-threshold stimuli such as light touch became sufficient to activate the reflex. Electrophysiological evidence supported a central as opposed to a peripheral mechanism. First, after noxious heat application, electrical stimulus of A-β sensory fibers becomes capable of eliciting responses in the α-motor neurons, whereas prior to the noxious heat the electrical stimulation was insufficient. Second, the receptive fields for the A-β sensory fibers are expanded, and local anesthetic block of afferents from the initial peripheral noxious stimulus do not decrease the enlarged receptive fields. Third, repeated low-frequency electrical stimulation, which is sufficient to stimulate only C-fibers, recapitulates the key findings of expanded receptor fields and the ability of previously non-noxious stimuli to activate the nociceptive system. Subsequent experiments clarified the findings by recording from the sensory neurons themselves (**Fig. 89-9**).

Having established that sustained peripheral nociceptor activation, whether through selective temperature or chemical stimulation, produces central sensitization, we now turn to the mechanisms that underlie the different components of central sensitization. As with peripheral sensitization, the mechanisms fall into 2 groups: early changes involve transcription-independent processes such as phosphorylation (termed *post-translational modification*); later, more persistent changes result from changes in gene expression (ie, *post-transcriptional modification*) and synaptic structure. However, in comparison to peripheral sensitization, the changes due to central sensitization tend to be much larger in magnitude and longer in duration.

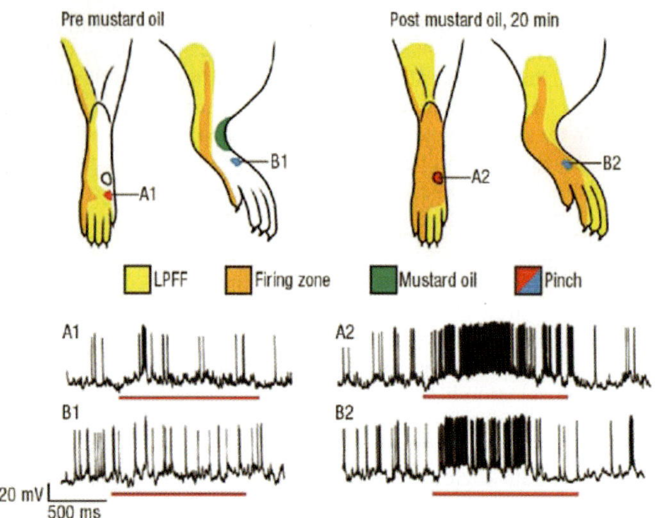

FIGURE 89-9. Expansion of receptor fields during central sensitization. Recruiting subthreshold synaptic inputs to the output of a nociceptive-specific neuron can markedly alter its receptive field properties, producing changes in receptive field threshold and spatial extent. When neurons in the dorsal horn spinal cord are subject to activity-dependent central sensitization, they exhibit some or all the following: development of or increases in spontaneous activity, a reduction in threshold for activation by peripheral stimuli, increased responses to suprathreshold stimulation, and enlargement of their receptive fields. The examples in this figure of intracellular recordings of rat dorsal horn neurons show the cutaneous receptive fields before central sensitization (pre–mustard oil) and after the induction of central sensitization (post–mustard oil) and indicate how subthreshold nociceptive (pinch, top) and low-threshold (brush, bottom) inputs in the low-probability firing fringe (LPFF) are recruited by central sensitization. Central sensitization was produced by topical application of mustard oil, which generates a brief burst of activity in TRPA1-expressing nociceptors and resulted in the neural equivalent of secondary hyperalgesia and tactile allodynia. [From Latremoliere A, Woolf CJ. Central sensitization: a generator of pain hypersensitivity by central neural plasticity. *J Pain*. 2009;10(9):895-926.][69]

SYNAPTIC PLASTICITY

Glutamate, the fast excitatory neurotransmitter at the primary afferent synapse, binds to several types of ionotropic and metabotropic receptors. The ionotropic receptors are tetramers and include those of the amino-3-hydroxy-5-methyl-4-isoxazole propionate (AMPA), *N*-methyl-D-aspartate (NMDA), and kainate types. Under basal conditions, AMPA receptors in excitatory neurons tend to be calcium impermeable, due to their inclusion of the GluR2 subunit. In contrast, inhibitory interneurons preferentially express the GluR1 subunit and not the GluR2 subunit, and thus are mostly calcium permeable. The distinguishing property of the NMDA receptor is that at rest the receptor is blocked by external magnesium ions. However, persistent and strong depolarization, such as those produced by inflammation or injury, relieves the block and allows the channels to open and conduct calcium into the cell. Thus the NMDA receptor is an "incident" receptor as it is only activated when there is both the presence of ligand (glutamate) and cellular depolarization. This quality of the NMDA receptor is essential for central sensitization: when a nociceptive signal is sufficiently strong and long acting, NMDA receptor activation effects a marked amplification, and prolongation of the afferent signal occurs.

Activation of the NMDA receptor is critical for central sensitization, as conditional deletion of an essential NMDA receptor subunit abrogates the development of central sensitization.[70] The key initial step downstream of NMDA receptor activation is calcium entry, and other signaling molecules and receptors that contribute to central sensitization also depend on calcium entry.

The 6 different metabotropic glutamate receptors act through 2 different types of G-proteins and are arranged in a lamina-specific manner. Group I metabotropic glutamate receptors (mGluR1 and mGluR5) are coupled to Gq-proteins, whose activation causes an increase in intracellular calcium. Increase in the intracellular calcium concentration appears to be the key initiating step in the development of acute central sensitization and occurs through calcium-dependent phosphorylation of transporters and receptors. The effect is amplification of the pain signal. Phosphorylation of AMPA and NMDA receptors increases the conducted currents and affect channel trafficking so that more channels are delivered to the membrane and fewer are removed.

The augmented inputs stimulate the signaling pathways that sustain central sensitization (**Fig. 89-10**). This process involves multiple signaling pathways including those of map kinase (MAPK), PKA, PKC, and Src. Many of the pathways have multiple downstream targets, and multiple pathways can activate the same target molecules.

A key target of many of the pathways is activation of the extracellular signal-related kinases (ERKs). ERK phosphorylates NMDA receptors, leading to increased activity. Phosphorylation of AMPA receptors by ERK increases trafficking of the receptors to the membrane. Additionally, ERK phosphorylation of the voltage-gated potassium channel Kv4.2 decreases the activity of that channel and thus leads to an increase in neuronal excitability.

Src interacts directly with the NMDA receptor. Injection of a peptide fragment of Src disrupts this interaction and thereby decreases hypersensitivity following injury. In contrast, the response to acute pain is unchanged, illustrating the mechanistic separation between acute and facilitated pain.[71]

The post-translational modifications lead to transcriptional changes, due to activity of the cAMP responsive element binding (CREB) protein and other transcription factors. These transcription factors increase the expression of several genes, including c-Fos and Cox-2, and receptors such as NK1 and TrkB.

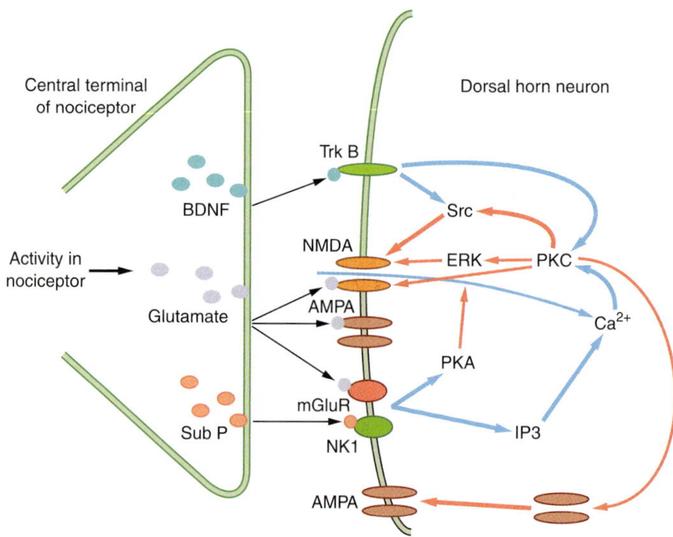

FIGURE 89-10. Activity-dependent central sensitization. Persistent or intense activation of central transmission can lead to postsynaptic calcium influx, primarily through *N*-methyl-D-aspartate (NMDA) and α-amino-3-hydroxy-5-methylisoxazole-4-propionic acid (AMPA) receptors. In conjunction with a variety of neuromodulatory signals, calcium influx activates signal transduction cascades that can facilitate both short-term and long-term excitability of the dorsal horn synapse.

Peripheral inflammation leads to a variety of changes in nociceptive neurons that underlie their sensitization. Large DRG neurons, which normally do not express the neuropeptides substance P and BDNF, begin to express these inflammatory mediators. Thus, nonnociceptive afferents develop the ability to release nociceptive signaling peptides.[72]

Cox-2 activation leads to the production of prostaglandin E_2 (PGE2), which binds to G-protein–coupled receptors on neurons to potentiate excitatory glutamatergic signaling[73] and reduce inhibitory glycinergic neurotransmission.[74] Elimination of Cox-2 from neurons does not affect pain due to peripheral inflammation and heat hyperalgesia, but almost completely eliminates mechanical hypersensitivity, thus again confirming the role of central sensitization in mechanical pain hypersensitivity.[75]

Nerve injury, the sine qua non for neuropathic pain, produces massive changes in the genes expressed in dorsal root ganglia neurons. Whereas peripheral inflammation affects only a small number of transcripts, nerve injury affects the expression of approximately 1000 transcripts, including ion channels, receptors, transmitters, and structural proteins involved in axonal regeneration.[76] Peripheral injury results in a degeneration of C-fiber terminals in lamina II. The combination of the loss of afferent stimuli together with the proregenerative environment after injury produces sprouting of myelinated A-β fibers, which normally only synapse into deeper laminae II to IV, into laminae I to II and the formation of new nociceptive inputs. Although there is some controversy in the interpretation of axonal labeling experiments, immunostaining and electrophysiological experiments have been convincing.[77,78] c-Fos activation in the superficial dorsal horn occurs only following noxious stimuli in noninjured animals; and A-β fiber stimulation is sufficient to induce c-Fos activation after nerve injury. The importance of A-β fibers in the development of nerve injury pain is underscored by the finding that ablation of most nociceptive inputs does not affect neuropathic pain,[79] and selective block of the large A-β fibers eliminates dynamic allodynia, a key component of neuropathic pain.[80] Furthermore, the elimination of PKC-γ–expressing neurons, which lie in the ventral-most part of lamina II and receive input only from A-β fibers, decreases pain in response to nerve injury.[81]

An additional component of pain enhancement is suggested by the observation that although norepinephrine administration to the skin of healthy subjects does not cause pain, norepinephrine administration does cause pain in the setting of preexisting nerve injury or inflammation. α_2-Adrenoreceptors have been found to be upregulated following nerve injury in both large- and small-fiber primary. That sympathetic fibers sprout onto primarily large non-nociceptive neurons in the DRG after nerve injury suggests that sympathetic pain modulation may occur through the nocicepive actions acquired by these large fibers as part of central sensitization.[82,83]

DISINHIBITION

Inhibitory neurons, which are densely distributed in the superficial layers of the dorsal spinal cord, use the neurotransmitters GABA and glycine to inhibit their postsynaptic targets. Application of blockers of these transmitters enhances the electrophysiological responses to activation of primary nociceptors[84] and produces behavioral sensitivity similar to that seen following peripheral nerve injury.[85,86]

Indeed, the very ability of inhibitory neurons to decrease activity is disturbed. BDNF is increased after nerve injury, and following BDNF treatment, the K-Cl transporter KCC2 is downregulated.[87] The decreased transporter expression disrupts the normal potassium and chloride gradient such that the internal chloride concentration in cells is increased. Consequently, after nerve injury, opening of chloride channels by the inhibitory neuropeptides then causes an outward flux of chloride, leading to cell depolarization and increased excitatory activity.[88] Thus normally inhibitory inputs are transformed into excitatory ones during the development of persistent pain.

IMMUNE AND GLIAL MODULATION

Under basal conditions, microglia are the only immunocompetent cells of the central nervous system. After peripheral nerve injury, microglia migrate to the superficial dorsal horn and undergo activation: they change their shape and gene expression. P38 MAPK upregulation leads to the production and release of several proinflammatory cytokines, including IL-1β and tumor necrosis factor α (TNF-α). As these require nerve injury and not just prolonged nerve activity, the activation of the microglia must be able to detect damage to the neuron. One potential signaling molecule for this role is adenosine triphosphate (ATP). Injection of ATP is sufficient to reproduce the pain behavioral phenotype produced by nerve injury. ATP receptors are divided into 2 types, ionotropic P2X receptors and metabotropic P2Y receptors.[89] Each of the 7 types of P2X genes encodes a single subunit of a nonselective cation channel, with a presumed stoichiometry of 3 subunits per channel. There is also coassembly of certain isomers. In immune cells, the most commonly expressed P2X genes include P2X1, P2X4, and P2X7. Indeed, in macrophages and microglia, P2X7 activation leads to caspase-1 activation and the release of IL-1β. In contrast, BDNF release seems to be due to P2X4 receptors. When microglia release BDNF, as discussed above, the result is a local reversal of the chloride gradient, thus shifting the hyperpolarizing effect of inhibitory neurons to a depolarizing and activating one. The 8 P2Y isoforms are coupled to heterotrimeric G-proteins. The P2Y12 isoform seems particularly important for microglial activation.[90]

A number of other ligands and receptors appear to be involved in the activation of microglia following nerve injury. Fractalkine is expressed by both primary afferent and spinal cord neurons, and its receptor, CX3CR1L, is upregulated on microglia following nerve injury.[91] Interfering with fractalkine signaling has been shown to reduce injury-induced pain. Additionally, interfering with signaling through the toll-like receptors affects both microglial activation and nerve injury–induced pain.

Although the activation of microglial cells is perhaps best characterized, these cells are not the only types of cells recruited and activated during peripheral nerve injury. T cells infiltrate the dorsal horn after nerve injury, and cytokines produced by T cells, such as interferon (IFN)-γ, are involved in pain following nerve injury.[92] Both Schwann cells in the periphery and astrocytes in the central nervous system are also activated by peripheral nerve injury.

Notably, the glial activation changes occur not only at the level of the spinal cord, but also at the level of the brainstem, where they are thought to interfere with the descending pain inhibitory systems.[93]

EVIDENCE FOR CENTRAL MECHANISMS OF PAIN IN HUMANS

Several studies in humans suggest that prolonged pain does indeed involve central sensitization. Injection of capsaicin in human volunteers produces nested circles of hypersensitivity of different sizes and types: in the center is a small circle of hyperalgesia to heat stimulus. Outside that is a circle of allodynia to light touch, and the outermost region shows hyperalgesia to noxious punctate stimuli. The innermost region exemplifies primary hyperalgesia, in that the symptoms are mediated by C-fibers with decreased thresholds. However, allodynia in the middle region and mechanical hyperalgesia in the outer area involve pain resulting from non-nociceptive fibers, thus requiring central changes that enable non-nociceptive afferents to cause pain. Thus these hypersensitivities mediated by A-β fibers are secondary in contrast to the nociceptor-mediated primary hyperalgesia.

In an elegant experiment, injection of capsaicin into anesthetized skin fails to produce hyperalgesia and mechanical allodynia in the surrounding unanesthetized skin.[94] Electrical intraneural stimulation that initially produces a non-noxious tactilelike sensation produces a noxious sensitization after capsaicin is injected adjacent into the adjacent skin region.[95]

Consistent with a mechanistic separation for peripheral and central pain enhancement, NDMA-receptor antagonists such as ketamine block secondary hyperalgesia but not primary hyperalgesia. Thus peripheral changes are insufficient to account for findings of allodynia; instead, central changes allow the activation of large mechanical fibers, normally unable to cause pain, to do so. As we discussed, this effect is neatly explained by the sprouting of afferents from these fibers into the superficial dorsal horn. Although some effects of central sensitization appear relatively local, other effects are impressively global. Indeed, capsaicin has been found to cause some degree of contralateral hyperalgesia and allodynia,[96] and this has been termed "tertiary hyperalgesia."

Not only does central sensitization underlie the development of allodynia in experiments on human volunteers, but it also is important in human diseases and their treatment.[63] Patients with chronic pain due to a wide range of diseases, including rheumatoid and osteoarthritis, fibromyalgia, headache, visceral pain syndromes such as inflammatory bowel syndrome, and headache, exhibit decreased thresholds to noxious stimuli, increased temporal summation, and increased pain. The changes in threshold and pain can be documented not only by patient report, but also by increased fMRI signal.[97] Both NMDA antagonists and the gabapentinoids block secondary allodynia and mechanical hyperalgesia induced by intradermal capsaicin. The importance of controlling postoperative pain in the healing process and the benefits of treatments that block central sensitization underscore the clinical relevance of central sensitization.

PAIN GENETICS

Research in human pain genetics has used 2 approaches. The first strategy requires the identification of rare single-gene mutations. Although very rare, these conditions can provide insights into pain pathways and suggest novel therapeutic possibilities. The second approach involves analysis of more common pain phenotypes or experimental models using genetic association.

The study and understanding of rare disorders has highlighted the importance of a number of molecules in the pain sensory transduction. Perhaps the best example of this involves mutations in the $Na_V1.7$ ion channel, which is preferentially expressed in nociceptors, but is also found in other dorsal root ganglion neurons, sympathetic neurons, and Schwann cells (**Table 89-9**). A striking phenotype known as *congenital insensitivity to pain* was identified in members of 2 cosanguineous families who carry mutations in both copies of the gene.[98] Despite completely intact sensation and transmission of all sensory modalities as demonstrated on quantitative sensory testing and nerve conduction tests, these people remarkably do not feel pain. In fact, they perform "stunts" such as driving knives through their arms. The disfiguring effects on the jaws and limbs underscore the importance of pain from a self-preservation point of view and explain why pain is so well enforced by evolution. One can only wonder about how the inability to experience physical pain affects the psyche of such people.

Affected family members were found to have homozygous nonfunctioning mutations in the $Na_V1.7$ ion channel. This study is extremely encouraging from a research perspective, because it shows that pain is not essential to the human condition, and that there is no a priori reason why pain cannot be blocked in the greater population.

Interestingly, mutations in the same ion channel, $Na_V1.7$, have been associated with 2 rare dominant familial conditions characterized by increased levels of pain.[99] In the first, *primary erythromelalgia*, affected individuals suffer from episodic redness and severe burning pain in the extremities. The age of disease onset can be as early as 1 year. Genetic linkage analysis of these patients also implicated the $Na_V1.7$ gene. Nearly 10 different point mutations have been identified in such families, and these mutations have been shown to facilitate opening of the channel and slow deactivation of the channel. These mutations lower the threshold necessary for the generation of action potentials (**Fig. 89-11**).

The second disease, *paroxysmal extreme pain disorder*, has a distinct phenotype with pain in the rectal, ocular, and mandibular areas. Again, genetic studies identified $Na_V1.7$ as the responsible gene, and over 5 distinct point mutations have been identified in affected families. Like those that cause inherited erythromelalgia, mutations responsible for paroxysmal extreme pain disorder also cause increased excitability in nociceptors. However, they do so by inhibiting channel inactivation, the process by which the channels rapidly close milliseconds after opening. This effect is quantified as a depolarizing shift in the voltage dependence of inactivation.

Another rare monogenic dominant pain syndrome has been associated with mutation in TRPA1.[100] Episodes of severe pain primarily localized to the upper body are triggered by conditions of fatigue, decreased food intake, and decreased temperature. The responsible mutation was showed to have an enhancing effect on TRPA1 currents.

Despite the meticulous detail in which researchers now understand the mutations responsible for these conditions, much still remains unknown. In particular, the reasons for the episodic nature of the diseases, as well as the restriction of symptoms to particular locations in the body remain mysteries.

In addition to the $Na_V1.7$-associated channelopathies, a number of other mutations have been associated with striking pain-related phenotypes. Another cause of congenital insensitivity to pain is hereditary sensory and autonomic neuropathy (HSAN), which is distinguished by the presence of peripheral neuropathy. Two of 5 types are due to mutations in genes encoding the NGF β protein and the NGF receptor (TRKA).[101]

Gene association studies have identified several genes that may modulate pain. For example, polymorphisms in catechol-O-methyltransferase (COMT) have been found to be associated with pain on injection of hypertonic saline and in pain originating from the

TABLE 89-9 Channelopathic Pain Syndromes

Disorder	Inheritance	Channel	Mutation	Effects on Channel	Clinical Phenotype
Inherited erythromelalgia (IEM)	autosomal dominant	$Na_V1.7$	missense	lower threshold for activation; enhanced response to subthreshold stimuli	attacks of burning pain and rediness in distal extremities; triggered by mild warmth and exercise
Paroxysmal extreme pain disorder (PEPD)	autosomal dominant	$Na_V1.7$	missense	impaired inactivation; enhanced persistent current	episodic lower body, ocular, and jaw pain accompanied by flushing and other autonomic abnormalities
Channelopathy-associated insensitivity to pain (CIP)	autosomal recessive	Na_V 1.7	nonsense	loss of function of $Na_V1.7$	inability to sense pain
Familial episodic pain syndrome (FEPS)	autosomal dominant	TRPA1	missense	enhanced inward current on activation	episodic upper body pain, triggered by fasting, cold, or stress

From Waxman SG. Channelopathic pain: a growing but still small list of model disorders. *Neuron*. 2010;66(5):622-624.

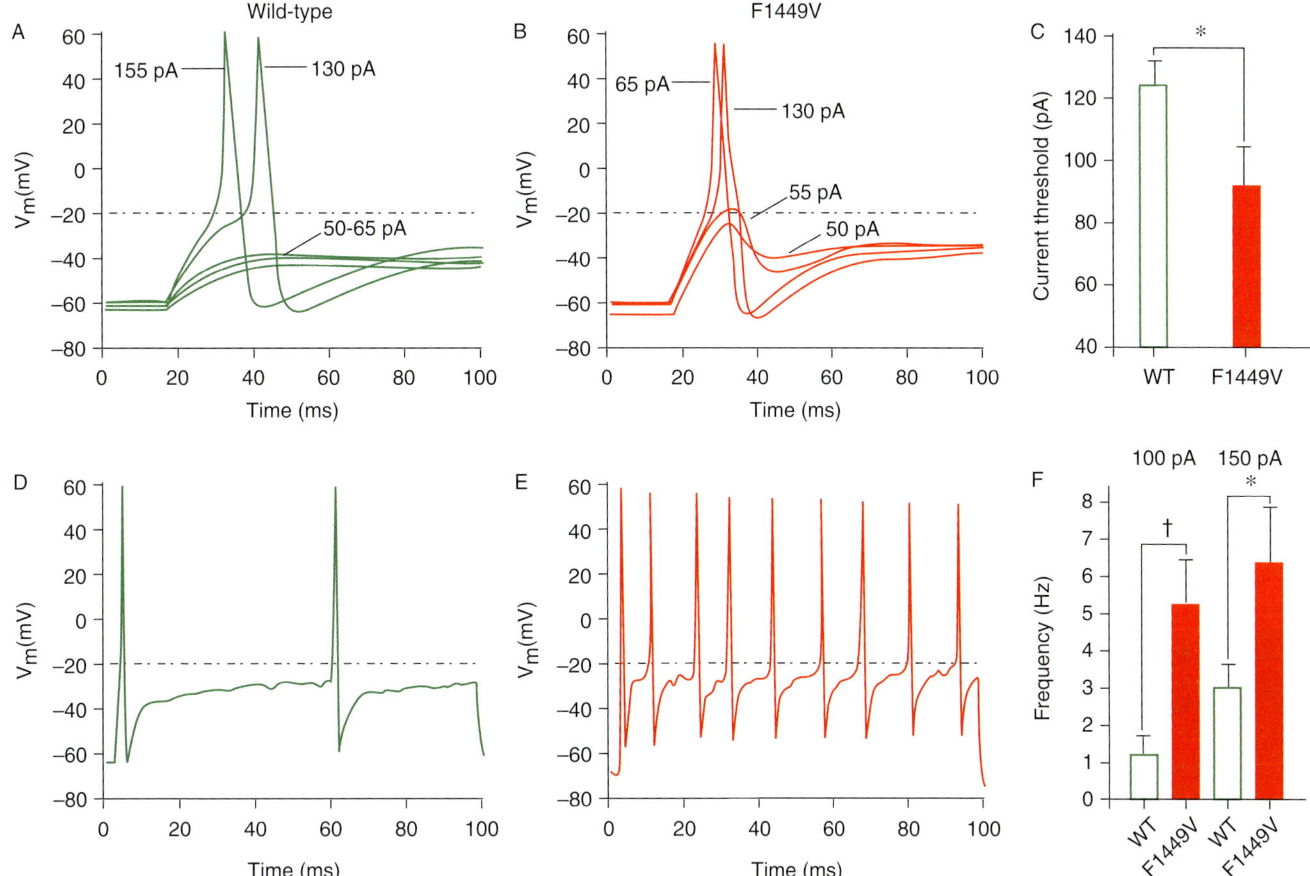

FIGURE 89-11. The effect of the F1449V mutation on the firing properties of dorsal root ganglion neurons. The current threshold for generation of single action potentials is reduced (**A**, **B**, **C**), and the frequency of firing in response to graded stimuli is increased (**D**, **E**, **F**) as a result of expression of mutant channels. V_m, membrane potential; WT, wild-type. *$P < .05$; †$P < .01$. [From Dib-Hajj SD, Rush AM, Cummins TR, et al. Gain-of-function mutation in $Na_v1.7$ in familial erythromelalgia induces bursting of sensory neurons. *Brain*. 2005;128:1847-1854.]

temporomandibular joint.[102,103] Other such studies have linked polymorphisms in the melanocortin-1 receptor (MCR1) to μ-opioid–induced analgesia[104] and in the κ-opioid receptor 1 (OPRM1) to morphine sensitivity (**Table 89-10**).[105-108] Given the known importance of $Na_v1.7$ in pain insensitivity and hypersensitivity, a search for polymorphisms in $Na_v1.7$ revealed an allele with a frequency of approximately 10% that was associated with increased pain perception and was found to impede sodium channel slow inactivation.[109] Such polymorphisms in $Na_v1.7$ may underlie common variation in pain thresholds.[110]

TABLE 89-10 Genes With Minor Alleles Shown to Contribute to Differences in Pain

Gene	Reference
GCH1	Tegeder et al, 2006
COMT (catechol-O-methyl transferase)	Zubieta et al, 2003
MC1R (melanocortin-1 receptor)	Mogil et al, 2003
TRPV1 (transient receptor potential cation channel, subfamily V, member 1)	Kim et al 2004
TRPA1 (transient receptor potential cation channel, subfamily A, member 1)	Kim et al 2006
OPRM1 (μ-opioid receptor)	Fillingim et al 2005
ORRD1 (δ-opioid receptor)	Kim et al 2004
FAAH (fatty acid amide hydrolase)	Kim et al 2006
$Na_v1.7$ (voltage-gated sodium channel 1.7)	Reiman et al 2010

Other approaches have used animal models to identify genes. Utilizing single nucleotide polymorphism analysis, the enzyme guanosine triphosphate cyclohydrolase (GCH1) was found to be increased in peripheral sensory neurons following axonal injury in mice.[111] By investigating haplotypes in humans, researchers identified a pain protective haplotype (frequency 15.4%), for which homozygotes have reduced postsurgical pain and lower pain thresholds.

CONCLUSION AND FUTURE DIRECTIONS

Nociception and pain perception are critical components of the nervous system that when functioning properly serve to protect an organism from injury. Multiple types of nociceptive inputs are processed through both segregated and convergent pathways, and are amplified and expanded during periods of prolonged pain. We now understand that chronic pain results from changes in gene expression and in neuronal and supporting cell architecture primarily within the central nervous system. Simply put, chronic pain results from changes in the spinal cord and brain that promote both sensitization of the nociceptive system and the continued and augmented sensation of pain. Through better understanding of the precise molecular mechanisms of how chronic pain develops and the genetic factors that predispose particular individuals to pain, tantalizing new targets for analgesics have been identified. In the future, pain treatments will be tailored to the specific underlying mechanisms responsible for pain in particular diseases and in individual patients.

KEY REFERENCES

- Basbaum AI, Bautista DM, Scherrer G, Julius D. Cellular and molecular mechanisms of pain. *Cell.* 2009;139(2):267-284.
- Costigan M, Scholz J, Woolf CJ. Neuropathic pain: a maladaptive response of the nervous system to damage. *Annu Rev Neurosci.* 2009;32:1-32.
- Perl ER. Ideas about pain, a historical view. *Nat Rev Neurosci.* 2007;8(1):71-80.
- Woolf CJ. Central sensitization: implications for the diagnosis and treatment of pain. *Pain.* 2011;152(3 Suppl):S2-S15.

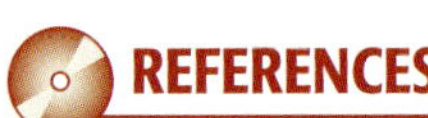

REFERENCES

Complete references available on DVD and online version at www.LongneckerAnesthesiology.com

CHAPTER 90 Common Pain Syndromes

Basem Hamid

KEY POINTS

1. Central sensitization is a cardinal element of chronic pain syndromes. Targeting factors contributing to this process is the cornerstone of managing chronic pain.
2. Chronic pain has a complex pathophysiology. Treatment should be multidisciplinary and aim for functional restoration.
3. Myofascial pain syndromes are characterized by the presence of trigger points, which have distinctive features that differentiate them from tender points.
4. Fibromyalgia is increasingly diagnosed. It is characterized by widespread pain and the presence of specific tender points. Multiple effective pharmacologic agents are now available.
5. Osteoarthritis (OA) is the most common joint disorder, is one of the most common chronic diseases in the elderly, and is a leading cause of disability. Certain measures may help prevent or slow the progression of OA. Conservative management options may delay or eliminate the need for surgery.
6. Tricyclic antidepressants, serotonin reuptake inhibitors, and antiepileptic drugs, especially calcium channel modulators, are considered good first-line options for treatment of most neuropathic pain syndromes.
7. Treatment of complex regional pain syndrome remains controversial but should start early and focus on mobility of the affected limb. Sympathetic blocks and multimodality analgesia help facilitate this. In advanced cases, more invasive options may be needed such as spinal cord stimulation or intrathecal analgesia.
8. Neck and back pain can be generated by a variety of different anatomic structures, which are targeted in the treatment plan. A careful history and physical examination along with imaging data will help reach the most specific pain generator, which should be targeted in the treatment plan instead of following a blind approach to target all potential generators.
9. Headache syndromes are numerous. The International Headache Society guidelines make the diagnosis of different headache syndromes easy and simple.
10. Tension and migraine headache are the most common primary headache. Preventative therapy is essential to their management.

Many pain conditions are encountered in clinical practice. This chapter provides a concise, practical, updated review of the most common pain syndromes. Along with the other chapters in this book on pain, a comprehensive review of pain is given.

MECHANISMS OF CHRONIC PAIN

Knowing the pathophysiology of chronic pain is essential for understanding the clinical features of different pain and the rationale of different treatment options used in the field. Chapter 89 covers this topic in detail. This chapter briefly summarizes the mechanisms of pain.

Pain sense starts by detecting noxious stimuli at the level of nociceptors, which are specialized receptors in the peripheral nervous system. An electrical signal is generated (transduction) and transmitted by the afferent fibers, A-δ fibers (slow, thin myelinated fibers), and C-fibers (the unmyelinated slowest fibers) of the spinal and cranial nerves. The first-order neurons of these fibers are located in the dorsal root ganglia or cranial nerve ganglia. Visceral afferent nociceptive fibers (A-δ and C) travel with sympathetic and parasympathetic fibers; their cell bodies also are found in the dorsal root ganglia. Muscles are also innervated by both A-δ and C-fibers. The pain signal then is transmitted to the sensory (second-order) neurons of the dorsal horn of the spinal cord. The ascending nociceptive tracts convey nociceptive stimuli from the dorsal horn of the spinal cord to higher centers in the central nervous system (CNS). These tracts include the spinothalamic, spinohypothalamic, spinoreticular, and spinopontoamygdala tracts. Multiple cortical and subcortical neural structures contribute to processing the pain signal, leading to pain perception. Pain is modified by the CNS via inhibitory descending tracts. Many inhibitory and excitatory neurotransmitters and other biochemical mediators mediate the physiologic process of pain perception.

Repeated peripheral tissue injury may result in a maladaptive phenomenon—*peripheral sensitization*—which refers to a decreased threshold and an increased response to stimulation, and is maintained by various endogenous biochemicals. Moreover, sensitization of the entire nociceptive pathway can arise secondary to chronic neuroplastic changes in the CNS, resulting in a phenomenon called *central sensitization.* As a result, multiple clinical features may arise and produce neuropathic pain (see Chapter 89). Once sensitization is established, it may be impossible to separate central contributions from peripheral contributions to the process of sensitization. Because of sensitization, pain may persist or may partially respond to therapy even when the primary injury is no longer active.

Treatment of chronic pain targets the different components contributing to the sense of pain by blocking the signal before it travels to the CNS, potentiating the inhibitory descending tracts, modifying the process of sensitization, or a combination of 1 or more of these mechanisms.

MUSCULOSKELETAL PAIN SYNDROMES

MYOFASCIAL PAIN SYNDROMES

Myofascial pain originates from active trigger points (TPs) within muscle structures and/or surrounding connective tissue. A typical TP is characterized by the presence of a taut band in the muscle, tenderness to palpation, and a reference pain zone distant from the TP center. Myofascial pain syndrome (MPS) can be primary or secondary to other painful conditions.

Although no clear mechanism has been defined, TPs are believed to begin after an initial macro or micro injury, which in vulnerable individuals evolves into a chronic MPS through the cascade of peripheral and central sensitizations.

Patients with myofascial pain usually present with muscle ache that is well localized to certain muscles with distinct radiating patterns or is of vague location and radiation. The pain usually is persistent but may fluctuate in intensity. It usually is associated with other symptoms such

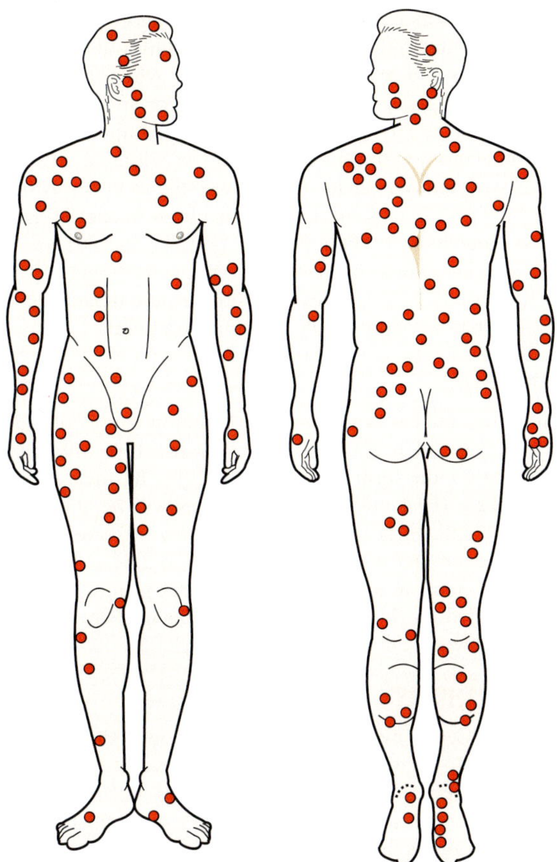

FIGURE 90-1. Common trigger points.

as joint ache, stiffness, paresthesias, decreased range of motion, fatigue, poor sleep, or headache. When the pain is chronic, autonomic features such as edema and hyperemia may appear.

Diagnosis of MPS is established by identifying TPs. TPs should be sought in a systematic manner. **Figure 90-1** illustrates some of the common TPs. TPs are best identified by palpation with the fingertips and application of steady incremental pressure over different areas until hypersensitive points are found and the patient's pain is reproduced. Tight bands are felt by rubbing the fingers across the muscle fibers. When the applied pressure is altered quickly, a brief local muscle twitch response can be observed.[1]

Treatment of MPS should focus on eliminating TPs to break the cycle enhancing chronic pain and to restore normal tone and function of the affected muscles. TP injections have been widely used to facilitate this process. Although clinicians use different solutions and medications for TP injections, no specific solution has been shown to be superior to others. Repeated steroid injection is associated with a risk for local muscle atrophy.

An alternative to injections is spraying of TPs with a vapocoolant such as chlorofluoromethane or ethyl chloride, with simultaneous stretching of the muscle. In combination with these treatments, muscle rehabilitation with exercises and thermal modalities is also useful. If analgesia is required, nonsteroidal anti-inflammatory drugs (NSAIDs) usually are given. Despite the wide use and acceptance of these therapies, no clear evidence supports their efficacy. Chronic MPS can be complex and refractory to treatment.

FIBROMYALGIA

Fibromyalgia (FM) is a multisymptomatic syndrome defined by the core feature of chronic, widespread pain. FM is a common entity that affects women more than men and increases steadily with age.[2]

Although a definitive causal relation has not been established, FM usually is precipitated by trauma, stress, infections, or other factors. It commonly accompanies a wide range of medical conditions, including rheumatoid arthritis (RA), low back pain, systemic lupus erythematosus, Sjögren syndrome, osteoarthritis (OA), inflammatory bowel disease, irritable bowel syndrome, headache, mood disorders, restless legs syndrome, and sleep disturbance, particularly stage 4. Research shows that certain individuals might have vulnerability to FM because of past life events or a complex genetic component interacting with environmental insults.[2,3]

Patients typically present with chronic, widespread stiffness and pain that is described as a constant dull ache worsened by muscle overactivity. FM is usually associated with a constellation of symptoms such as easy fatigability, nonrestorative sleep, cognitive dysfunction, depression, and somatic complaints other than musculoskeletal pain.[2]

The diagnosis of FM is usually based on the 1990 recommendations of the American College of Rheumatology (ACR) classification criteria, which comprise 1 historical feature (widespread pain of at least 3 months' duration) and 1 physical finding (the presence of tender points over at least 11 of 18 specified tender point sites on palpation at a force of 4 kg—the amount of pressure required to blanch a thumbnail).[2] The locations of the 18 tender points are shown in **Figure 90-2**. Palpation of control sites that typically are not tender is recommended. Some of these sites are the forehead, the medial third of the clavicle, the dorsum of the middle phalanx of the third digit, and the medial malleolus. If tenderness is present in these sites, the diagnosis of FM is questionable. Tenderness points are different from TPs in that they lack the other associated features. FM is distinguished from MPS by the absence of true TPs.

Treatment of FM is multidisciplinary and should consist of psychological intervention; physical therapy, especially aquatic-based

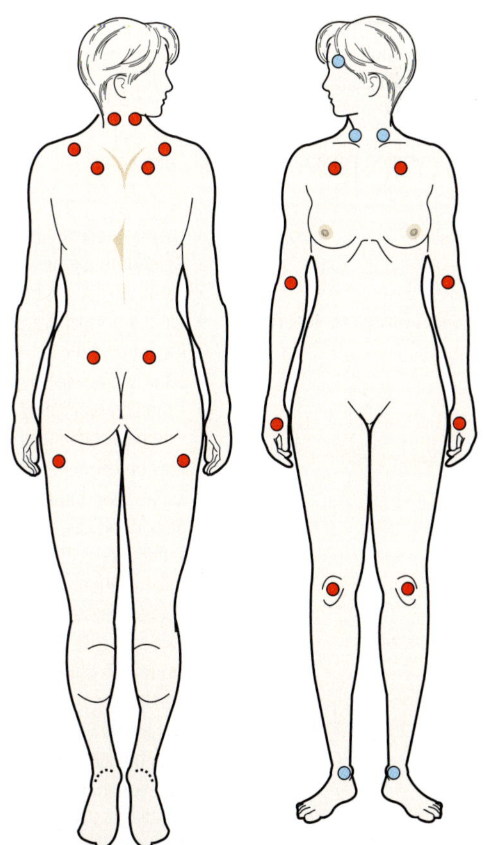

FIGURE 90-2. Recommended tender (red) and control (blue) point locations in fibromyalgia.

exercises; treatment of comorbid mental disorders and associated sleep disorders; and pharmacologic therapies. Multiple medications have proven effective for the management of pain in FM and are now approved by the Food and Drug Administration (FDA). These are Pregabalin,[4] Duloxetine,[5] and Milnacipran.[6] Tricyclic antidepressants (TCAs) have also been shown effective in FM and have the added benefit improving sleep. NSAIDs have varying degrees of success. Tramadol, a dual reuptake inhibitor of norepinephrine and serotonin with weak μ-receptor affinity, is proving useful. Pramipexole, an antiparkinsonian dopamine agonist, at a dose of 4.5 mg also appears to be a promising option for treatment of FM.[7,8]

Opioids have not been shown to be effective. Most FM patients tend to have a chronic course, with exacerbations, remissions, and fluctuating symptoms.

BURSITIS AND TENDINITIS

Tendinitis, bursitis, and other periarticular painful conditions are common causes of regional pain. Understanding of the musculoskeletal anatomy and a careful clinical examination are essential in determining the true cause of pain. Whereas arthritis (or synovitis) causes effusions in the synovial space or diffuse swelling of the synovium, producing global joint swelling, bursitis causes an effusion or swelling limited to the bursa only, and tendinitis causes little, if any, swelling limited to the tenosynovial structure. In synovitis, direct palpation of the synovium elicits diffuse tenderness over the entire synovial surface area. In bursitis, tenderness is localized to the bursal structure and spares the synovium. The tenderness in tendinitis is elicited best by active range of motion and active isometric loading against resistance, but can be detected by direct palpation. Tendinitis is painful with active or passive range of motion as the inflamed tendon experiences loading. Passive range of motion elicits tenderness only if the inflamed tendon is stretched and passively loaded, and active range of motion or isometric testing elicits tenderness by actively loading the tendon.

Table 90-1 lists each anatomic region and the more common periarticular conditions for each region.

In general, treatment of bursitis, tendinitis, and other periarticular conditions is similar and usually conservative. Physical therapy is helpful in most cases and may be more successful when therapy includes a combination of passive modalities, such as ice and heat, and active modalities, such as strengthening exercises to improve any biomechanical imbalances. Ultrasound is sometimes helpful and is of proven benefit for symptomatic calcific tendinitis of the shoulder. NSAIDs are helpful as analgesics but are of limited usefulness in alleviating chronic conditions. Judicious intralesional injections of steroids are helpful. However, caution should be exercised when considering intralesional steroids for bicipital and Achilles tendinitis because tendon rupture is a risk. Surgery may be required for refractory conditions.

ARTHRITIDES

Arthritides and related syndromes are common causes of pain, with a steady increase of prevalence. An estimated 15% (40 million) of Americans had some form of arthritis in 1995. By the year 2020, an estimated 18.2% (59.4 million) of Americans will be affected.[9] Thus, although pain specialists may not be the primary treating physicians, they should be familiar with these syndromes and be able to recognize them and participate in the overall management plan to help in reducing the associated morbidity and disability. Detailed coverage of these syndromes is beyond the scope of this chapter.

OSTEOARTHRITIS

Osteoarthritis (OA) is by far the most common joint disorder, is one of the most common chronic diseases in the elderly, and is a leading cause of disability. Increased weight is the most significant independent predictor of both incidence and progression of OA in weight-bearing joints. The risk for development of OA is increased by high-impact repetitive activities. Smoking and osteoporosis increase the frequency of OA.

The joints most commonly involved in OA are the metatarsophalangeal (MTP) joint of the great toe (hallux valgus or "bunion"), proximal interphalangeal (PIP) and distal interphalangeal (DIP) joints of the fingers, and carpometacarpal (CMC) joint of the thumb, hips, knees, and both lumbar and cervical spines. Other joints, even major

TABLE 90-1 Common Periarticular Painful Conditions

Shoulder	
Glenohumeral arthritis	• Usually preceded by trauma • Anterior tenderness below the coracoid process with passive range of motion, especially rotation • Swelling may not be easily appreciated because this joint lies deep beneath the deltoid muscle
Adhesive capsulitis (frozen shoulder)	• Loss of normal distensibility of the glenohumeral joint capsule and subsequent adhesions between the capsule and the humeral head • Usually preceded by joint-limiting states, such as rotator cuff, strokes, fractures • Gradually worsening pain and progressive loss of passive and active range of motion in all directions, especially external rotation and abduction • May be complicated by complex regional pain syndrome
Subacromial bursitis	• Largest and most frequently inflamed shoulder bursa • Pain in the lateral aspect of the shoulder, worsening with movement • Differs from rotator cuff tendonitis by the presence of tenderness on direct palpation beneath the acromion process
Rotator cuff	• Inflammation of supraspinatus and infraspinatus tendons lying between the humeral head and the acromial process • Pain aggravated by overhead reaching • Pain on active abduction of the shoulder focused over the lateral aspect • Normal passive range of motion • Tenderness on active resisted abduction or external rotation rather than on passive abduction or external rotation • Passive forward flexion to 90° impinges on the inflamed rotator cuff and confirms the diagnosis
Biceps tendinitis	• Inflammation of the long head of the biceps tendon as it traverses the humeral bicipital groove • Anterior shoulder pain aggravated by lifting or overhead reaching • Tenderness over the bicipital groove • Positive arc maneuver • Complete rupture may occur in chronic cases and presents as bulging in the antecubital fossa

(*Continued*)

TABLE 90-1 Common Periarticular Painful Conditions (*Continued*)

Elbow	
Olecranon bursitis	• Inflammation of the bursal sac located on the dorsal surface of the olecranon process of the ulna • Tenderness and swelling over the olecranon bursa (just below the elbow) • Can be differentiated from elbow arthritis, as the latter causes swelling and tenderness in the paraolecranon grooves
Lateral epicondylitis (tennis elbow)	• Injury of the common extensor tendon at the lateral epicondyle due to overuse • Pain and local tenderness at the lateral epicondyle • Pain aggravated by resisting wrist extension and radical deviation • Weak grip
Medical epicondylitis (golfer's elbow)	• Injury of the common extensor tendon at the medial epicondyle due to overuse • Pain and tenderness just distal to the medial epicondyle • Pain aggravated by resisting wrist extension and radial deviation • Weak grip
Wrist and Hand	
de Quervain tenosynovitis	• Inflammation of the tendons of abductor pollicis longus and extensor pollicis brevis within the first dorsal extensor compartment • Typically affects middle-aged women • Pain and swelling along the radial aspect of the wrist worsened by gripping • Finkelstein test confirms the diagnosis: thumb is held within the fist and the hand is deviated passively in an ulnar direction, eliciting exquisite tenderness
Trigger finger	• Inflammation of the flexor tendons of the finger at the metacarpophalangeal head • Caused by repetitive activity over the palm of the hand • Pain, swelling, and "locking" of the finger
Hip	
Trochanteric bursitis	• Inflammation of the bursa between the gluteus maximus muscle and the trochanteric process • Pain over the outer thigh, worsened by walking • Local tenderness over the trochanteric process
Iliopsoas tendonitis/bursitis	• Inflammation of the iliopsoas tendon and/or bursa anterior to the true hip joint • Tenderness in the anterior groin or anterior hip joint • Local enlargement in the groin with bursitis
Knee	
Prepatellar bursitis	• Inflammation of the bursa overlying the patella due to injury or infection • Pain, swelling, and tenderness in the prepatellar area overlying the patella • May become chronic
Pes anserine	• Inflammation of pes anserine bursa, which lies medial to the anterior tibial tuberosity and inferior to the medial joint line • Pain along the medial aspect of the knee below the medial tibial plateau • Swelling not often observed • Localized tenderness to the bursa unaffected by passive range of motion of the knee
Patellar tendonitis	• Inflammation of the patellar tendon due to overuse injury • Anterior knee pain exacerbated by active use of the quadriceps • Localized tenderness to palpation to the patellar tendon
Iliotibial band bursitis	• Caused by tight iliotibial band • Pain over the lateral aspect of the knee • Clicking as the band passes over the lateral femoral condyle • Tenderness confined to the lateral area of the knee with absence of knee effusion
Ankle	
Retrocalcaneal bursitis	• Inflammation of the retrocalcaneal bursa lying between the calcaneus and the Achilles tendon • Posterior ankle pain reproduced by active loading of the Achilles tendon (as occurs with walking) • Local tenderness and swelling in the space between the Achilles tendon and the ankle, aggravated by plantar flexion
Achilles tendinitis	• Inflammation of the musculotendinous junction due to repetitive irritation of overuse • Posterior ankle pain with tendon loading • Local tenderness aggravated by dorsiflexion • Paratendinous thickening above the calcaneus • May be complicated by tendon rupture or chronic tendinitis
Foot	
Plantar fasciitis	• Inflammation of the origin of the longitudinal ligament • Many biomechanical abnormalities of the foot predispose to this condition, such as pes cavus deformities, pes planus deformities, and Achilles tendon tightness • Pain along the plantar surface of the medial heel • Tenderness to calcaneal compression

weight-bearing joints such as the ankle, are regularly spared unless they are involved in secondary forms of OA. Pain is the main symptom leading to the diagnosis of OA. The pain is most often described as a deep ache, accompanied frequently by joint stiffness that follows periods of inactivity (on arising in the morning or after sitting). Pain is aggravated by using the involved joints, may radiate, or may be referred to surrounding structures. In the early stages of the disease, pain is commonly relieved by rest. With more severe disease, pain may be persistent, interfering with normal function and preventing sleep, even with medical management.

On physical examination, the joints may demonstrate tenderness, crepitus, and a limited range of motion. Joint swelling may be due to an accompanying synovial effusion or to bony enlargement and the presence of osteophytes. Radiographic findings help confirm the diagnosis. Joint space narrowing, subchondral bone sclerosis, subchondral cysts, and osteophytosis are characteristic.[2]

Nonpharmacologic management of OA includes correction of body mechanics and posture, weight loss, and physical therapy. Analgesia can be achieved by using acetaminophen and NSAIDs as first-line therapy. Intraarticular corticosteroid injections might have a positive role but should be judiciously implemented and not repeated more than 3 times per year because of possible secondary cartilage damage. The structure-modifying effects of drugs are being evaluated, and both glucosamine sulfate and diacerein have shown different results in treating pain.[10-12] Doxycycline has been proved to slow the rate of joint space narrowing in knees with established OA.[13]

Intraarticular injection of a viscosupplement such as Hylan has been shown to be effective in reducing pain in knee OA.[14] When conservative therapy fails, joint replacement surgery might be the only option to help with analgesia.

RHEUMATOID ARTHRITIS

Rheumatoid arthritis (RA) is a chronic multisystem disease with inflammatory polyarthritis of symmetric distribution affecting the peripheral joints of the hands (sparing DIP joints), feet, wrists, elbows, shoulders, hips, knees, and ankles. The cervical spine is generally the only axial skeleton affected by RA.

RA manifests in constitutional symptoms of fatigue, low-grade fever, weight loss, and morning stiffness. Synovitis (inflammation of the synovium) is the hallmark of RA. It produces pain, swelling, and tenderness of the joints. RA is characterized by a waxing-and-waning course with relapses and remissions. Pain in RA is multifactorial. In the early stages, it is secondary to inflammation. At later stages, the damaging effects of erosion of cartilage and bone also cause pain. RA can be accompanied by FM. RA complications can also result in pain such as vertebral body fractures, compression of the median nerves by synovial tissue in the carpel tunnel, rheumatoid vasculitis, cervical spine instability at the C1-2 level, and septic arthritis.[15]

Diagnosis is based on the history and physical examination and is supported by the presence of rheumatoid factor, which is present in 80% of patients with RA. Radiographically, soft-tissue swelling, juxtaarticular osteopenia, symmetric space narrowing, and bony erosions are seen.

Pharmacologic treatment of RA relies on NSAIDs, corticosteroids, analgesics, and disease-modifying antirheumatic drugs (DMARDs). Early and aggressive use of DMARDs is essential once the diagnosis is confirmed. Anti–tumor necrosis factor α agents, such as infliximab, etanercept, and adalimumab, have very potent anti-inflammatory properties and provide dramatic improvements in symptoms and signs. Interleukin-1 receptor antagonists such as anakinra also have been shown to be effective in slowing the damage of cartilage and progression of arthritis.

When pain is unresponsive to treatment, surgical options should be pursued, including synovectomy, arthroplasty, and joint replacement. Opioids might be the only option to provide adequate analgesia in advanced cases refractory to treatment or when contraindications to other analgesics exist.

OTHER ARTHRITIDES

Multiple other arthritic syndromes may have pain as a cardinal feature. They include spondyloarthropathies, gout, and pseudogout. Arthritis can also accompany other systemic diseases, such as systemic lupus erythematosus, scleroderma, polymyalgia rheumatica, giant cell arteritis, Reiter syndrome, and inflammatory bowel disease.

Treatment should always focus on treating the underlying condition. NSAIDs usually provide acceptable analgesia. Often, opioids are required for more severe cases.

NEUROPATHIC PAIN SYNDROMES

Neuropathic pain is a pathologic pain that results from sustained transmission of pain signals in the absence of ongoing tissue injury or activation of pain-sensitive afferent peripheral nerves. Neural injury or dysfunction at any point along the somatosensory system from the peripheral nerve endings to the brain can cause neuropathic pain. Multiple mechanisms (peripheral and central) are responsible for sustaining neuropathic pain. Although its role is less identified than in nociceptive pain conditions, primary sensitization of nociceptive nerve endings might be a contributing factor to sustaining neuropathic pain. Damaged nerve fibers, especially neuromas, may generate ectopic action potentials, which contribute to neuropathic pain. When input from peripheral nociceptors into the dorsal horn of the spinal cord decreases, as encountered in deafferentation conditions such as shingles and after amputation, the dorsal horn neurons become hyperexcitable and may even develop spontaneous activity. In addition, the reduction of peripheral sensory input leads to ephaptic sprouting of the neurons neighboring the affected central neurons, resulting in magnification of the perceived pain field. Central sensitization, as outlined, also plays a major role in neuropathic pain. Because the inhibitory interneurons normally are excited by peripheral input, attenuation of this input will decrease inhibition and amplify the pain signal. In general, the inhibitory circuits of pain signal are downregulated at the level of both the spinal cord and the brain. At the level of the brain, different sites are involved in the processing of pain signal, and the somatosensory-pain homunculus is not quite preserved. The initial neural injury and subsequent evolving mechanisms explain the complexity of clinical features encountered in neuropathic pain syndromes.

Some clinical features are common among neuropathic syndromes, whereas others are unique to specific syndromes. Patients usually have different types of pain. A stimulus-independent pain is a spontaneous pain experienced by patients without sensory stimulation. It consists of a background constant pain, intermittent exacerbations, and brief episodes of other symptoms. The pain usually is burning, aching, crushing, gnawing, lancinating, shooting, electrical, or lightning in quality, and associated with painful numbness and paresthesias (dysesthesias). The stimulus-evoked pain includes a variety of signs, such as hyperalgesia, mechanical and thermal allodynia, and hyperpathia. **Table 90-2** summarizes some features of neuropathic pain.

TABLE 90-2 Clinical Features of Neuropathic Pain
Hypesthesia: Decreased sensation or increased threshold for sensation
Hyperesthesia: Increased sensitivity to stimulus
Parethesia: Abnormal (but not painful) sensation (like pins-and-needles sensation), spontaneous or evoked
Dysesthesia: Unpleasant (painful) sensation, spontaneous or evoked
Hyperalgesia: Increased response to painful stimulus
Allodynia: Pain due to a stimulus that does not normally provoke pain
• Mechanical (tactile): Mechanical stimulus is the cause
• Thermal: Thermal stimulus is the cause
Hyperpathia: Abnormally painful and exaggerated reaction to stimulus, especially repetitive, where the stimulus is perceived initially less intense
Causalgia: Constant burning pain accompanied by allodynia and hyperpathia following nerve injury[99]

TABLE 90-3 Common Neuropathic Pain Syndrome

Peripheral Neuropathic Pain
Acute and chronic inflammatory demyelinating polyradiculoneuropathy (Guillain-Barré syndrome)
Alcoholic polyneuropathy
Chemotherapy-induced polyneuropathy
Complex regional pain syndrome (CRPS)
Congenital painful neuropathies
Entrapment neuropathies (eg, carpel tunnel syndrome)
Hereditary painful neuropathies
HIV neuropathy
Iatrogenic neuralgias (eg, postmastectomy or postthoracotomy pain)
Idiopathic sensory neuropathy
Compression neuropathy (ie, by tumor)
Nutritional deficiency–related neuropathies
Painful diabetic neuropathy
Paraneoplastic neuropathy
Phantom limb pain
Postherpetic neuralgia
Postradiation myelopathy/plexopathy
Radiculopathy syndromes (cervical, thoracic, lumbosacral)
Toxic exposure–related neuropathies
Cranial neuralgias (eg, trigeminal, glossopharyngeal)
Posttraumatic neuralgias
Central Neuropathic Pain
Compressive myelopathy (eg, spinal stenosis, tumor)
HIV myelopathy
Multiple sclerosis–related pain
Parkinson disease–related pain
Postischemic myelopathy
Postradiation myelopathy
Poststroke pain
Posttraumatic spinal cord injury pain
Syringomyelia

Modified from Dworkin RH, Backonja M, Rowbotham MC, et al. Advances in neuropathic pain: diagnosis, mechanisms, and treatment recommendations. *Arch Neurol.* 2003;60: 1524-1534, with permission.

Associated clinical features include abnormalities of reflexes and muscle function. Increased reflexes and tone are indicative of an upper motor neuron disease and suggest a central lesion such as stroke, whereas reduced reflexes or tone suggest peripheral origin as in compressive radiculopathies or neuropathies. Secondary motor changes could be a result of disuse and abnormal position. Autonomic abnormalities can be seen and include changes in color and temperature in the affected tissues, swelling due to abnormal leakage of intravascular fluid, and growth of skin, hair, nails, and other cutaneous structures. Other systemic features of autonomic dysfunction that could be seen include orthostatic hypotension, impotence, delayed gastric emptying, abnormal sweating and/or thermoregulation, difficulties with elimination, and occasionally cardiac arrhythmias. The management of specific neuropathic pain syndromes will be discussed in this chapter, but in general a common management algorithm may be followed for all neuropathic pain syndromes.[16]

Table 90-3 lists the most common neuropathic pain syndromes.[17] The following is a brief discussion of common neuropathic pain conditions.

PAINFUL PERIPHERAL NEUROPATHIES

A wide variety of etiologies lead to peripheral neuropathies. It is important to realize that not all neuropathies are painful, as is the case with most of the inherited neuropathies. Some patients with neuropathy have chronic pain due to other conditions, and their pain should not be immediately attributed to the concomitant nonpainful neuropathy. The distribution of neuropathy can be generalized and symmetric (polyneuropathy), such as diabetic and alcoholic polyneuropathy; multifocal (mononeuropathy multiplex), such as collagen vascular disease–related neuropathies; or focal (mononeuropathy), as seen in trauma and entrapment neuropathies. Polyneuropathy usually is symmetric and starts in a distal-to-proximal gradient in a "glove and stocking" distribution. Mononeuropathy multiplex affects multiple peripheral nerves arbitrarily and sometimes can be difficult to differentiate from polyneuropathy. Mononeuropathy follows the distribution of the affected nerve. Neuropathies may result from injury to the axons (axonal neuropathies), to myelin (demyelinating neuropathies), or mixed lesions. Most of the neuropathies encountered in pain medicine practice are axonal neuropathy types. Acute (AIDP) and chronic inflammatory demyelinating polyradiculoneuropathy (CIDP) are examples of demyelinating neuropathies usually seen in pain practice. **Table 90-4** highlights most of the painful neuropathies a pain physician might encounter.

Although the evaluation of neuropathy usually is conducted by neurologists, it is important for the pain medicine practitioner to be familiar with the diagnostic workup. **Figure 90-3** shows a simple diagnostic approach that leads to the diagnosis of most neuropathies.[18]

SMALL-FIBER NEUROPATHY

Small-fiber neuropathy (SFN) is the most common type of painful neuropathy. The smaller axons A-δ (small myelinated) and C (unmyelinated) are affected. The larger fibers usually are preserved but could be involved at a later stage. SFN is a disease of late middle age, but symptoms could start as early as the third decade or as late as the ninth decade.[19] SFN is vastly under recognized, and most cases are "idiopathic." SFN may predate diabetes mellitus[20] and neoplastic conditions by many years. Although SFN is more common in men, patients presenting with pain of SFN are more likely to be women.[21]

Pain and decreased temperature sensation are the predominant features. Proprioception, vibratory sensation, and muscle-stretch reflexes usually are intact because they are mediated by the larger nerve fibers A-β and A-α, which are not involved in the pathologic process.

Injury of affected fibers cannot be detected by standard nerve conduction studies (NCS) and electromyography (EMG), so these tests usually are unrevealing. Therefore, the diagnosis usually is clinical and relies on ruling out other possibilities. A definite diagnosis of SFN could be reached by autonomic testing or a skin biopsy if warranted. When fasting blood glucose or glycosylated hemoglobin (HgA_{1C}) levels are diagnostic of diabetes mellitus, obtaining an oral glucose tolerance test may unveil impaired glucose tolerance or early diabetes mellitus.[22-24]

The distinction between SFN and "large-fiber" neuropathies is important because the underlying cause is more likely to be identifiable when both large and small fibers are affected.

DIABETIC PERIPHERAL NEUROPATHIC PAIN

Current estimates suggest that more than 22 million Americans have diabetes.[25] Peripheral neuropathy is one of the most common complications of diabetes,[26] and conversely diabetes is the most common cause of peripheral neuropathy in developed countries.[27] Studies suggest that 30% to 60% of all diabetics have signs and/or symptoms of peripheral neuropathy.[25,28-30] The risk is greater than 50% in individuals who have had diabetes for more than 20 years. The prevalence of any neuropathy is 66% for patients with Type 1 diabetes mellitus and 59% for those with Type 2.[26] Neuropathy can be seen at any stage of diabetes progression, and approximately 10% of newly diagnosed Type 2 diabetics may have neuropathy.[26] Neuropathic symptoms may be the presenting complaint leading to the diagnosis of diabetes. Neuropathy also has been reported in patients with impaired glucose tolerance, or "prediabetes."[26] Multiple risk factors contribute to the

TABLE 90-4 Common Painful Neuropathies

Type of Neuropathy	Predisposing Factors	Features on Examination	Laboratory Findings
Idiopathic small-fiber painful sensory neuropathy	Age >50 y	Normal muscle-stretch reflexes Normal muscle strength Normal sensation of position and vibration Reduced pinprick sensation in lower extremities	Normal EMG and NCS Reduced sudomotor function Abnormal skin biopsy Normal blood tests
Diabetic peripheral neuropathy	Family history	Reduced muscle-stretch reflexes	Abnormal EMG and NCS (rarely, normal EMG and NCS)
	Obesity	Reduced distal sensation May have orthostatic hypotension (rarely, may have findings similar to those in idiopathic small-fiber painful sensory neuropathy)	2-h glucose-tolerance test ≥200 mg/dL Fasting blood glucose concentration ≥126 mg/dL
Inherited neuropathies	Family history	Per cavus or hammer toe Usually reduced muscle-stretch reflexes Reduced distal sensation	Abnormal EMG and NCS Normal blood tests
Peripheral neuropathy with connective tissue disease	History of rheumatoid arthritis, systemic lupus erythematosus, mixed connective tissue disease, Sjögren syndrome, or symptoms of sicca syndrome	Reduced muscle-stretch reflexes Reduced distal sensation	Abnormal EMG and NCS Positive for antinuclear antibodies, extractable nuclear antigens, or rheumatoid factor
Peripheral nerve vasculitis	Known systemic vasculitis (nonsystemic vasculitis may occur without systemic features)	Multifocal examination findings (may mimic polyneuropathy)	Abnormal EMG and NCS Blood test abnormalities may include antineutrophilic cytoplasmic antibodies, antinuclear antibodies, rheumatoid factor, hepatitis C, cryoglobulins
MGUS neuropathy	Age >50 y	Variable findings Reduced or normal reflexes Reduced distal sensation	Abnormal EMG and NCS (may be normal in rare cases) Monoclonal gammopathy
Paraneoplastic sensory neuropathy	Tobacco smoking, family history, asbestos exposure, occupational exposure to dyes, paints, printing rubber, textiles, or leather	Reduced muscle-stretch reflexes Reduced distal sensation	Abnormal EMG and NCS Anti-Hu antibodies
Familial amyloid polyneuropathy	Family history	Reduced muscle-stretch reflexes Sensory loss preferentially small fiber Postural hypotension	Abnormal EMG and NCS NCS may show carpal tunnel syndrome
Acquired amyloid polyneuropathy	Known plasma cell dyscrasia or monoclonal gammopathy	Reduced muscle-stretch reflexes Sensory loss preferentially small fiber Postural hypotension	Abnormal EMG and NCS NCS may show carpal tunnel syndrome Monoclonal gammopathy
Neuropathy with renal failure	Known renal disease	Reduced muscle-stretch reflexes Variable sensory examination	Abnormal EMG and NCS Abnormal renal function
Hereditary sensory autonomic neuropathy	Family history, foot ulcers, painless injuries	Reduced muscle-stretch reflexes Variable sensory examination Pes cavus and hammer toe Foot ulcers	Abnormal EMG and NCS
Sarcoid polyneuropathy	Pulmonary sarcoidosis	Multiple mononeuropathy or features of polyneuropathy	Abnormal EMG and NCS Elevated angiotensin-converting enzyme Abnormal chest radiography
Arsenic neuropathy	Industrial exposure to pesticides, wood preservatives, copper smelting	Reduced muscle-stretch reflexes Loss of all types of sensation Usually some distal weakness Mees lines	Abnormal EMG and NCS Elevated arsenic levels (in plasma, urine, nails, hair)
Fabry disease	Onset before age 20 y Renal failure, stroke	Normal muscle-stretch reflexes Normal muscle strength Normal sensation of position and vibration Normal or reduced pinprick sensation in feet	Normal EMG and NCS Reduced levels of α-galactosidase A in serum, leukocytes, or tears
Celiac disease	Gastrointestinal symptoms	Variable features may be normal except for loss of distal pinprick sensation or loss of all types of sensation Reduced muscle-stretch reflexes	EMG and NCS usually normal Positive serologic test for celiac disease (IgA antigliadin and IgA endomysial antibodies)
HIV-related neuropathy	Homosexual activity, drug abuse, blood transfusions, treatment with antinucleosides	Variable features may be normal except for loss of distal pinprick sensation or loss of all types of sensation Reduced muscle-stretch reflexes	EMG and NCS usually abnormal HIV antibody sensation

EMG, electromyography; HIV, human immunodeficiency virus, MGUS, monoclonal gammopathy of undetermined significance, NCS, nerve conduction studies.

From Mendell JR, Sahenk Z. Clinical practice. Painful sensory neuropathy. *N Engl J Med.* 2003;348:1243-1255, with permission.

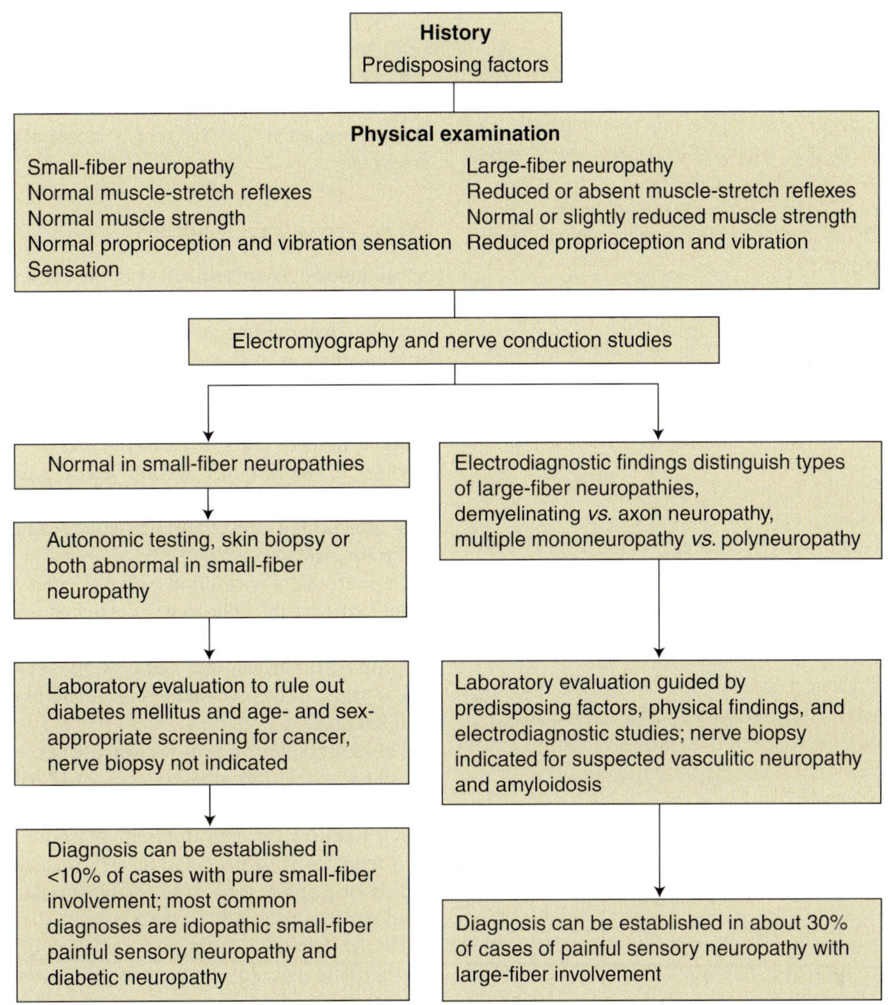

FIGURE 90-3. Algorithm for evaluation of painful peripheral neuropathy. [From Mendell JR, Sahenk Z. Clinical practice. Painful sensory neuropathy. *N Engl J Med.* 2003;348:1243-1255, with permission.]

risk of diabetic neuropathy, including duration of diabetes, age, male gender, increased height, hypertension, and smoking.[28] Poor glycemic control is a major modifiable risk factor for neuropathy, as demonstrated by the reduction in risk of neuropathy with intensive glucose lowering. This is demonstrated by a decrease of approximately 60% in Type 1 diabetic patients treated with intensive insulin therapy compared to those who received conventional therapy.[31]

The clinical manifestations of diabetic peripheral neuropathy depend on the specific nerves affected. Because all branches of the peripheral nervous system are susceptible to damage from diabetes, patients can exhibit abnormalities of sensory, motor, or autonomic function. Deficits frequently overlap or coexist.

Diabetic peripheral neuropathy is a heterogeneous condition that can manifest clinically as several types,[26] which can exist individually or overlap. **Table 90-5** lists the different types of diabetic peripheral neuropathy.

NCS and quantitative sensory testing (eg, quantitative vibration threshold testing) can be used to confirm neuropathy suggested by the physical examination or to confirm the diagnosis in patients with symptoms but no abnormalities on physical examination. Normal NCS do not necessarily rule out neuropathy as a cause of pain because neuropathic symptoms may be due to SFN.

Multiple pharmacologic agents have been used for treatment of diabetic peripheral neuropathic pain. Duloxetine[32,33] and pregabalin[34-37] are the only FDA-approved drugs for diabetic peripheral neuropathic pain. Multiple other medications have been shown to be effective, such as TCAs,[38,39] gabapentin,[27,40] venlafaxine,[41-43] tramadol, capsaicin,[29,44-48] opioids,[49-51] and a combination of more than one of these medications.[50,52] Zonisamide[53] also appears to be promising. Antiepilepsy drugs (AEDs)[54] and many other drugs have been used extensively, with varying degrees of success.[17,18,55] In a small case series, spinal cord stimulation was successful in the treatment of diabetic peripheral neuropathic pain refractory to conventional therapies, including opioids.[56,57]

TABLE 90-5 Common Diabetic Peripheral Neuropathies

1. Diffuse Neuropathies
   A. Distal symmetric sensorimotor polyneuropathy (peripheral polyneuropathy). This is the most common form of diabetic peripheral neuropathy. The small fibers, the large fibers, or a combination of both could be affected. It typically starts in the feet but may progress to a "stocking glove" distribution in all of the extremities. Sensory symptoms predominate.
   B. Autonomic neuropathy.
   C. Symmetric proximal lower limb motor neuropathy (amyotrophy).
2. Focal Neuropathies
   A. Mononeuropathies involving any of the peripheral or cranial nerves.
   B. Entrapment neuropathies such as carpal tunnel syndrome.

TABLE 90-6 HIV/AIDS-Related Neuropathies

1. Acute (AIDP) and chronic inflammatory demyelinating polyradiculoneuropathy (CIPD). AIDP (Guillain-Barré syndrome) occurs in the early stages of HIV infection. Symptoms usually peak in 4 weeks after onset and improve gradually to variable degrees. In CIDP, symptoms evolve over several weeks or months and have periods of remissions and relapses.
2. Distal sensory polyneuropathy (DSPN). DSPN is the most common HIV-associated neuropathy. It has similar presentation to the other distal symmetrical sensory neuropathies.
3. Drug-induced neuropathies. Several drugs used for treatment of HIV infection or AIDS complications can cause neuropathy that is identical to DSPN. Antiretroviral medications include didanosine (ddI; Videx), stavudine (d4T; Zerit), and particularly zalcitabine (ddC).
   Chemotherapeutic agents such as vincristine and paclitaxel used for Kaposi sarcoma and lymphoma also cause neuropathy. DSPN is a common side effect of thalidomide used for treatment of aphthous ulcers and isoniazid, an antituberculosis agent. Typically, drug-induced neuropathies improve after the neurotoxic agent is withdrawn.
4. Mononeuropathy multiplex (MM). MM can occur early or late in the disease. Individual nerves are affected, resulting in isolated symptoms as seen in cranial neuropathies, hand or foot drop.
5. Cytomegalovirus (CMV) polyradiculopathy. This entity occurs in severely immunosuppressed HIV patients. It initially presents with pain and paresthesias in the saddle distribution due to involvement of the sacral roots, in association with or followed by severe symptoms that progress distally down both lower extremities. If this condition is left untreated, flaccid paraparesis, areflexia, and sphincter function impairment follow. CMV infection must be aggressively treated.

HIV/AIDS-RELATED NEUROPATHY

Neuropathic pain occurs in approximately one-third of patients with human immunodeficiency virus (HIV) and acquired immunodeficiency syndrome (AIDS).[58] A variety of disorders can result in neuropathic pain in HIV and AIDS patients. The different types of HIV/AIDS-related neuropathies are summarized in **Table 90-6**.[59,60]

Treatment of HIV/AIDS-related neuropathic pain relies on treatment of the underlying infection(s) and removal of toxic agent if possible. Neuropathic agents have been used, with variable results. Lamotrigine[61,62] and probably ziconotide[63] have documented efficacy.

CARPAL TUNNEL SYNDROME

Carpal tunnel syndrome (CTS) is the most common painful mononeuropathy of the upper limb. It results from compression (entrapment) of the median nerve as it passes under the ligamentous canal in the wrist. Multiple factors predispose to or precipitate CTS, such as fractures, ganglions, synovial disorders, wrist arthritides, ergonomic stressors, repetitive use, pregnancy, obesity, chronic renal insufficiency, and other systemic disorders such as diabetes and acromegaly.

CTS is characterized by paresthesias and dysesthesias over the median nerve sensory area of the hand, which includes the thumb, index, and median half of the middle fingers. Weakness of the thenar muscles can occur. Symptoms are most pronounced upon awakening.

Physical examination shows decreased sensation over the palmer aspect of the thumb through the lateral half of the middle finger. At later stages, the thenar muscles are weak and could be atrophied. Tinel sign and Phalen test are not sensitive but help support the diagnosis when they are present.[64,65] Tinel sign is the elicitation of distal paresthesias by percussion on the wrist or at the base of the palm. Phalen test attempts to elicit paresthesias by applying pressure (inflating a tourniquet to 60 mm Hg) on the arm or holding the wrist in a flexed position. The diagnosis of CTS can be confirmed by NCS and EMG.

Most patients respond well to conservative treatment, which includes wrist splinting, NSAIDs, or steroid injections. If treatment fails, surgical decompression at the wrist may be necessary, especially when weakness progresses.

ACUTE HERPES ZOSTER

Acute herpes zoster (shingles) is the most common cause of sensory neuropathy. It results from infection reactivation of the dormant varicella-zoster virus in the ganglionic neurons or satellite cells, followed by transmission of the virus particles to the nerve endings proximally and distally. The incidence of herpes zoster varies with age and immune status, ranging from 0.4 to 1.6 cases per 1000 among healthy people younger than 20 years to 4.5 to 11 cases per 1000 among those 80 years or older.[66] The risk of a second attack is as high as the risk of a first attack.[67] The risk of acute herpes zoster is higher among patients with HIV infection or cancer and particularly among children with leukemia and transplant recipients.[66,68-71]

Dermatomal distribution and vesicular rash are the hallmarks of acute herpes zoster. The most affected nerves follow this order: thoracic spinal roots, ophthalmic division of the trigeminal nerve (V1), maxillary division of the trigeminal nerve (V2), cervical spinal roots, and sacral spinal roots.[72] The involvement is unilateral in most cases but can rarely be bilateral.

The earliest clinical features of acute herpes zoster noticed by patients are dermatomal dysesthesias associated with pruritus. This could be accompanied or followed shortly by the appearance of the typical rash, which matures through different stages until it crusts and heals. The pain worsens with progression and consists of dysesthesias, burning, and shooting pain. It tends to resolve spontaneously as the crust falls off, a process that takes 4 to 5 weeks.

Treatment of acute herpes zoster is discussed in the section on postherpetic neuralgia because of the close therapeutic strategies.

POSTHERPETIC NEURALGIA

Many definitions have arbitrarily been used for postherpetic neuralgia (PHN). Results of recent research distinguishes among 3 phases of pain: acute pain (which occurs within 30 days after rash onset; described earlier), PHN (pain that persists ≥120 days after rash onset), and subacute herpetic neuralgia (pain that persists beyond the acute phase but resolves before the diagnosis of PHN is made).[73,74] PHN may develop after a pain-free interval. Nearly all patients have pain in association with acute herpes zoster, and 10% to 70% of these patients go on to have PHN.[66,67,75] Not only does the risk of PHN increase with age, but so does the intractability of the pain.[66] The presence of prodrome, female gender, greater rash severity, and greater acute herpes zoster pain severity have been associated with increased risk for PHN.[74] The risk of PHN is not increased in immunocompromised patients.[69,75] Symptoms consist of a background dermatomal burning pain and dysesthesias with superimposed intermittent lancinating pain. Hypoesthesia, hyperalgesia, allodynia, and hyperpathia may be present.

Treatment The goal of treatment of acute herpes zoster is to alleviate the symptoms, shorten its course, and prevent the evolution of PHN. Antiviral drugs (famciclovir, valacyclovir, acyclovir) started within 72 hours after the rash appears reduce acute pain in immunocompetent patients, thus providing relief in the greatest number of patients and possibly reducing the likelihood of evolution of PHN.[66,76,77] Although corticosteroids do not alter the course of PHN, they improve the quality of life after zoster, thus justifying their administration in combination with an antiviral drug in high-risk patients 50 years or older with moderate to severe pain in whom corticosteroids are not contraindicated.[66]

Some reports suggest the efficacy of infiltration of the skin, peripheral nerves, sympathetic nerve blockade, or paravertebral or epidural spaces with local anesthetic drugs with or without steroids in patients with acute herpes zoster.[66,78-80]

A large retrospective study suggested that any benefits of somatic nerve blocks are limited to the first 2 months of pain.[66]

Treatment of pain associated with established PHN can be challenging. In general, drugs used for neuropathic pain are used for treatment of PHN. TCAs have well-documented efficacy.[39] Anticonvulsants are widely used.[81] Gabapentin[82-84] and pregabalin[85-87] have documented efficacy and are FDA approved. Opioids may be required for more severe cases. Topical lidocaine patches have been shown to be effective for PHN, especially in alleviating allodynia.[43,88,89] Data suggest the possible efficacy of epidural or intrathecal steroid injections in chronic PHN.[90-92]

Numerous other treatment modalities have been attempted, such as the transcutaneous electrical nerve stimulation unit,[93] topical agents, acupuncture, and hypnosis, with various results. In refractory PHN, more invasive surgical options have been implemented, including dorsal root entry zone lesions, cordotomy, rhizotomy, spinal cord stimulation, and sympathectomy.

MERALGIA PARESTHETICA

Meralgia paresthetica is an entrapment mononeuropathy of the lateral femoral cutaneous nerve as it passes under the inguinal ligament. It is associated with a number of conditions and factors, such as increased pressure on the nerves, as occurs with tight belts, pregnancy, CTS, regional operations, obesity, or after rapid weight changes.[94,95]

Meralgia paresthetica is characterized by a patch of dysesthesias and decreased sensation over the anterolateral thigh. Diagnosis can be easily confirmed by blocking the nerve. Management is conservative. Corticosteroid injections also can be used. The prognosis is very good, with most patients experiencing spontaneous remission in 6 to 12 months. Surgery might be helpful in refractory cases.[96]

TRIGEMINAL NEURALGIA

Trigeminal neuralgia, previously called *tic douloureux,* is a disorder of the trigeminal nerve. It is characterized by brief electric shock–like pain that is abrupt in onset and termination and is limited in distribution to 1 or more divisions of the trigeminal nerve. Pain is commonly evoked by trivial trigger factors such as washing, shaving, talking, and/or brushing the teeth. Small areas in the nasolabial fold and/or chin may be particularly susceptible to the precipitation of pain (trigger areas). The pain usually remits for variable periods.

Trigeminal neuralgia classically starts in the second or third division and affects the cheek or chin. The first division is involved in less than 5% of patients. Trigeminal neuralgia is a unilateral disorder but in rare cases is bilateral, in which case a central lesion such as multiple sclerosis should be excluded. Between paroxysms, patients usually are asymptomatic but may have a persistent dull background pain. In some cases, the trigeminal root in the posterior fossa is compressed by tortuous or aberrant vessels. Classic trigeminal neuralgia usually is responsive, at least initially, to pharmacotherapy.

Table 90-7 lists the International Headache Society (IHS) diagnostic criteria for trigeminal neuralgia.[97]

Carbamazepine is still the first-line treatment. Other AEDs, such as gabapentin, also have been shown to be effective.[98] TCAs are effective.[99] In refractory cases, invasive procedures (eg, ablative lesioning or decompression of the trigeminal ganglion) may be required.[100]

TABLE 90-7 International Headache Society Diagnostic Criteria for Trigeminal Neuralgia

A. Paroxysmal attacks of pain lasting from a fraction of a second to 2 minutes, affecting 1 or more divisions of the trigeminal nerve and fulfilling criteria B and C
B. Pain has at least 1 of the following characteristics:
   1. Intense, sharp, superficial, or stabbing
   2. Precipitated from trigger areas by trigger factors
C. Attacks are stereotyped in the individual patient
D. No clinically evident neurologic deficit
E. Not attributed to another disorder

GLOSSOPHARYNGEAL NEURALGIA

Glossopharyngeal (cranial nerve IX) neuralgia is a severe transient stabbing pain experienced in the distribution of this nerve and the distribution of the auricular and pharyngeal branches of the vagus nerves. The pain is felt in the ear, base of the tongue, tonsillar fossa, or beneath the angle of the jaw. The pain is commonly provoked by swallowing, talking, or coughing and may remit and relapse as in trigeminal neuralgia. **Table 90-8** lists the IHS diagnostic criteria for glossopharyngeal neuralgia.[97]

In Eagle syndrome, the nerve is compressed by a calcified or ossified stylohyoid ligament, which is visible on x-ray or computed tomography (CT) scan.[101] Pharmacologic treatment of glossopharyngeal neuralgia is similar to that of trigeminal neuralgia. In Eagle syndrome, resection of the stylohyoid ligament is effective.

TABLE 90-8 International Headache Society Diagnostic Criteria for Glossopharyngeal Neuralgia

A. Paroxysmal attacks of facial pain lasting from a fraction of a second to 2 min and fulfilling criteria B and C
B. Pain has all of the following characteristics:
   1. Unilateral location
   2. Distribution within the posterior part of the tongue, tonsillar fossa, pharynx, or beneath the angle of the lower jaw and/or in the ear
   3. Sharp, stabbing, and severe
   4. Precipitated by swallowing, chewing, talking, coughing, and/or yawning
C. Attacks are stereotyped in the individual patient
D. No clinically evident neurologic deficit
E. Not attributed to another disorder

OCCIPITAL NEURALGIA

Occipital neuralgia is a paroxysmal stabbing jabbing pain in the distribution of the greater or lesser occipital nerves or the third occipital nerve, sometimes accompanied by diminished sensation or dysesthesias in the affected area. It is associated with tenderness over the affected nerve. **Table 90-9** lists the IHS diagnostic criteria for occipital neuralgia.[97]

Treatment can be conservative using different analgesics, including TCAs and AEDs, or application of nerve blocks. For refractory cases, neuroablative measures can be used.[102]

TABLE 90-9 International Headache Society Diagnostic Criteria for Occipital Neuralgia

A. Paroxysmal stabbing pain, with or without persistent aching between paroxysms, in the distribution(s) of the greater, lesser, and/or third occipital nerves.
B. Tenderness over the affected nerve.
C. Pain is eased temporarily by local anesthetic block of the nerve.

CENTRAL PAIN SYNDROMES

Central pain is a "deafferentation" pain that can result from any lesion found in the CNS.[103] Virtually any type of lesion can produce this type of pain, including demyelinating, vascular, infectious, inflammatory, and traumatic. Pain onset may be delayed by several months after the initial insult, reflecting the slow degeneration process within the CNS. Pain usually correlates to the anatomic site of the causative lesion. The pain features are those of neuropathic pain.

Brain central pain results from a variety of etiologies. Thalamic pain (Dejerine-Roussy syndrome) is the prototype of central pain, but lesions in the brainstem and other sites also can produce central pain. Strokes are the most common cause, with pain reported to occur in up to 8% of poststroke patients.[104] Other etiologies include multiple sclerosis, brain abscess, encephalitis, and tumors.

Spinal cord central pain is a common complication of spinal cord injuries. Trauma is the most common etiology.[105] Iatrogenic, inflammatory, demyelinating, vascular, neoplastic, and congenital lesions are other possible causes. The most common level of injury associated with pain is cauda equina followed by the central cord injuries. Syringomyelia and syringobulbia can occur as delayed consequences of trauma or congenital malformations and produce neuropathic pain of segmental pattern.

Central pain is one of the most difficult pain states to effectively treat. Pregabalin[106] and lamotrigine[107,108] show encouraging results. Some evidence exists for the benefit of TCAs.[39] Other agents used for neuropathic pain, such as AEDs and opioids, have been used, but no sound evidence supports their efficacy.

SYMPATHETICALLY MAINTAINED PAIN AND COMPLEX REGIONAL PAIN SYNDROMES

Sympathetically maintained pain (SMP) is defined as "pain that is maintained by sympathetic efferent innervation or by circulating catecholamines."[109] Thus SMP is not a clinical diagnosis but rather a pathophysiologic mechanism in chronic pain marked by improvement of pain when sympathetic blockade is performed. When the pain does not respond to sympathetic blockade, it is called *sympathetically independent pain* (SIP). SMP is thought to be a major culprit in many chronic pain states, such as peripheral and central neuropathic pain syndromes.[110-112]

Complex regional pain syndrome (CRPS) is considered to be a neuropathic SMP syndrome. The 2 types of CRPS are type I (previously called reflex sympathetic dystrophy) and type II (previously called causalgia). CRPS is more common in women than in men, and the incidence reaches its peak in the fifth decade.[113,114] It involves 1 limb in most cases,[115] and there is a history of noxious traumatic injury with or without nerve involvement.[114] There is no correlation between the severity of injury and the severity of the ensuing pain syndrome. Direct injuries to CNS structures have been reported as causative, including spinal cord[116] and brain[117] injuries. In CRPS type II particularly, there may be a stretch injury to the nerve, without interruption of the nerve. Multiple risk factors have been postulated to predispose to CRPS, including immobilization,[118] smoking,[119] genetic predisposition,[120] and psychological factors.[121]

The exact mechanism of CRPS is not known, but it appears to be a disease of both the CNS and the peripheral nervous system[122,123] Peripherally, α-adrenergic sensitization of the nociceptive afferent fibers occurs. As a result, nociceptors are activated by release of norepinephrine by sympathetic postganglionic fibers. Release of certain mediators, such as prostaglandins, by sympathetic fibers can further sensitize the nociceptive afferents. If the injury results in myelin loss of the fibers, artificial synapses develop between the affected sensory afferents and sympathetic efferents, a process called *ephaptic transmission*. The dorsal root ganglion is thought to be another site for ephaptic transmission resulting from sprouting of sympathetic postganglionic fibers around sensory neurons. At the level of the dorsal horn of the spinal cord, the wide dynamic range neurons, which are second-order neurons, are activated and sensitized by the active injured C-fibers. Sensitized wide dynamic range cells are thought to be activated by other stimuli, such as light touch, explaining the phenomenon of allodynia. At the level of the brain, there is altered sensorimotor processing and increased hyperexcitability.[124,125] Thus CRPS results from interaction between the CNS and the periphery. Central changes are reflected as alterations in somatic sensation (including pain), the motor system, and the peripheral autonomically regulated effector systems (vasculature, sweat glands, inflammatory cells).[122]

In most cases the presenting symptom of CRPS is pain, which most often is burning and does not follow a dermatomal pattern.[113,126] Other common symptoms and signs include decreased range of motion, weakness, hyperpathia, allodynia, hyperalgesia, color change, altered skin temperature, edema, hyperesthesia, hypoesthesia, sweating change, nail or hair changes, and dystonia.[113,126]Although symptoms typically start in a distal limb, CRPS has been reported to start in other regions of the body, such as the head, proximal limbs, and genitalia.[127] Spread of CRPS features proximally or to other regions of the body has been well described.

The diagnosis of CRPS can be made only in the absence of any other diagnosis explaining the findings. **Table 90-10** summarizes the International Association for the Study of Pain (IASP) diagnostic criteria for CRPS.[128-131] These criteria are very sensitive and less specific. Criteria with improved specificity are proposed and summarized in **Table 90-11**.[129,131]

TABLE 90-10 International Association for the Study of Pain Diagnostic Criteria for Complex Regional Pain Syndrome

1. Presence of an initiating noxious event or cause of immobilization.
2. Continuing pain, allodynia, or hyperalgesia, with pain disproportionate to any inciting event.
3. Evidence at some time of edema, changes in skin blood flow, or abnormal sudomotor activity in the region of pain.
4. Diagnosis is excluded by the existence of conditions that would otherwise account for the degree of pain and dysfunction.

Type I: Without evidence of major nerve damage
Type II: With evidence of major nerve damage

From Wilson PR, Stanton-Hicks M, Harden RN, eds. *CRPS: Current Diagnosis and Therapy*. Seattle: IASP Press; 2005:47, with permission from the International Association for the Study of Pain.

TABLE 90-11 Proposed Modified Clinical Diagnostic Criteria for Complex Regional Pain Syndrome

1. Continuing pain that is disproportionate to any inciting event.
2. Must report at least 1 symptom in 3 of the 4 following categories:
   Sensory: Reports of hyperesthesia and/or allodynia
   Vasomotor: Reports of temperature asymmetry and/or skin color changes and/or skin color asymmetry
   Sudomotor/Edema: Reports of edema and/or sweating changes and/or sweating asymmetry
   Motor/Trophic: Reports of decreased range of motion and/or motor dysfunction (weakness, tremor, dystonia) and or trophic changes (hair, nails, skin)
3. Must display at least 1 sign at the time of evaluation in 2 or more of the following categories:
   Sensory: Evidence of hyperalgesia (to pinprick) and/or allodynia (to light touch and/or deep somatic pressure and/or joint movement)
   Vasomotor: Evidence of temperature asymmetry and/or skin color changes and/or asymmetry
   Sudomotor/Edema: Evidence of edema and/or sweating changes and/or sweating asymmetry
   Motor/Trophic: Evidence of decreased range of motion and/or motor dysfunction (weakness, tremor, dystonia) and/or trophic changes (hair, nails, skin)
4. No other diagnosis better explains the signs and symptoms.

No specific diagnostic test is available for CRPS.[132] Several tests can help confirm the diagnosis or rule out other conditions. Blood tests, including erythrocyte sedimentation rate, blood cell count, and rheumatologic testing, may be necessary to help rule out infection or a rheumatologic condition.[132] When vasomotor features are present, vascular studies can exclude a vascular etiology. NCS and EMG may clarify the presence of nerve injury necessary for the diagnosis of CRPS type II. An important distinction between CRPS type II and peripheral mononeuropathy is that the somatosensory symptoms in CRPS extend beyond the distribution of the affected nerve.[132] Radiographic studies including magnetic resonance imaging (MRI) often are necessary to exclude bone or soft-tissue pathology as the source of pain. Plain radiographic studies may show findings of bony demineralization, which is not specific to CRPS and could be the result of disuse.[133] A 3-phase bone scan of the affected extremity has variable sensitivity and is relatively nonspecific in the diagnosis of CRPS. Classic findings include increased periarticular uptake throughout the 3 phases (blood pool, blood phase, scan phase).[132] Thermography can assist in confirming thermal dysregulation. Simple measures also can provide this information, using infrared thermometer or skin temperature probes that document the temperature of the normal and the affected limbs. A temperature difference of 0.6°C between limbs is considered significant.[134] Quantitative sudomotor axonal reflex testing evaluates autonomic function by measuring sweat output in response to a cholinergic agent. Although a positive response to a sympathetic block can help in establishing the diagnosis, it is not required to diagnose CRPS.[132] A pharmacologic sympathetic block can be performed with intravenous infusion of phentolamine. However, the more common approach is performance of a local anesthetic sympathetic trunk block. A lumbar paravertebral sympathetic block is performed for lower limbs, and a cervicothoracic block (stellate ganglion block) or upper thoracic sympathetic block is performed for upper limbs. Evidence of a satisfactory sympathetic block (eg, thermography) in the absence of a somatic nerve block should be demonstrated.[132] If favorable results are achieved by sympathetic blocks, then their continued administration may be useful.

Treatment of CRPS remains controversial because of the lack of adequate evidence on most therapies implemented in clinical practice. A consensus statement released in 2002 by an interdisciplinary expert panel produced a reasonable treatment approach[135,136] Rapid initiation of multidisciplinary treatment is recommended, with advancement to higher levels of intervention if initial therapy shows no benefit in 2 weeks. Simultaneous physical rehabilitation, psychological therapy, and provision of adequate analgesia are key elements in the treatment plan. The primary goal of treatment is functional restoration of the affected region. In some studies, physical therapy has shown to be effective and thus should be started as soon as possible while effective analgesia is provided. Multiple physical and occupational therapy measures can be used in the process of rehabilitation, starting with desensitization and stress loading, then gentle active range of motion and stretching to increase flexibility, and eventually normalization of use and general conditioning.[137]

Psychological therapy should focus on educating patients that pain sensations in CRPS type I do not indicate tissue damage, and that reactivation of the affected limb is important. With persistent symptoms, clinical psychological assessment is recommended, eventually followed by cognitive behavioral therapy. Comorbid conditions such as depression, sleep disturbance, anxiety, and generalized physical deconditioning should be treated.

Analgesia is achieved using oral or topical neuropathic pain agents, including TCAs, AEDs, NSAIDs, opioids, and other agents.[138] Corticosteroids may be effective, especially if the inflammatory component is profound.[139] Calcitonin, topical dimethylsulfoxide (DMSO), and α_1-adrenoceptor antagonists (eg, terazosin, phenoxybenzamine) may be helpful. Many other drugs have been anecdotally used, with varied results (including prazosin, clonidine, mexiletine, ketamine, baclofen, bisphosphonates, muscle relaxants, and calcium channel blockers).[140]

When symptoms are persistent, patients who had favorable results with diagnostic sympathetic blockade are often offered intravenous regional sympathetic blocks (IRSBs). IRSBs using phentolamine, guanethidine, reserpine, droperidol, and atropine have been shown to be ineffective.[121] Patients who have not had good results with sympathetic blockade may require a combined somatic/sympathetic block using indwelling catheters to allow adequate physical therapy and rehabilitation. Epidural catheters also have been used in this fashion.[135] If sympathetic blocks are effective in producing analgesia but duration is limited, neurolysis with either neurolytic injections or radiofrequency-lesioning techniques can be considered.[141] Spinal cord stimulation appears to be an effective treatment, especially for CRPS type I.[142,143] Spinal analgesia may be an effective treatment of CRPS when other modalities fail.[135,144,145]

POSTAMPUTATION PAIN

Stump Pain Stump pain is a chronic sensation of pain at the site of amputation. It also is referred to as residual limb pain.[146] It may occur with phantom limb pain or alone. Several factors may account for stump pain and should be evaluated, including surgical trauma, ischemia, local infection, ill-fitting prostheses, or a painful neuroma formation.

Treatment should focus on treating the underlying etiology. Treatment of painful neuromas ranges from simple injections to surgical interventions, with varying degrees of success.[147]

Phantom Pain Phantom sensation is the perception of the amputated part and occurs in almost all amputees. Phantom pain is the perception of pain distal to the amputation site. It has unclear etiology, but deafferentation of central neurons seems to play a major role in the development of phantom pain. Its incidence peaks approximately 1 month after amputation and gradually improves as the pain "telescopes" toward the stump. The pain results in paroxysms of burning and twisting sensation in the amputated part. Phantom pain should be differentiated from stump pain.

Treatment of phantom pain is challenging. Pharmacologic agents for neuropathic pain should be attempted. TCAs, tramadol, and gabapentin have been shown to be effective.[148,149] Nerve blocks can be tried for more difficult cases. In refractory cases, surgical options (eg, dorsal root entry zone lesions) and more invasive procedures might be the only effective methods for treating the pain. Preemptive analgesia may prevent phantom pain, although this remains controversial.[150]

BACK AND NECK PAIN

Low back pain is one of the most common symptoms that prompt patients to seek medical care and is the leading cause of disability among workers younger than 45 years. Current data suggest that more than three-fourths of people will have back pain at one point in their life, with an annual prevalence up to 45%.[151,152]

Neck pain is a less common complaint but still has a point prevalence of approximately 10% to 35% and a lifetime prevalence of approximately 15% to 50%. It is more common in women.[153]

Pain can originate due to pathology in a variety of neuraxial structures, including vertebral bodies, intervertebral disks, ligaments, muscle structures, joints (facet, sacroiliac), nerve roots, meninges, and epidural space. A combination of etiologies is common and may be difficult to delineate. **Table 90-12** summarizes the most common etiologies of back and neck pain.

Obtaining an adequate history and physical examination is crucial for reaching the correct diagnosis and implementing a successful treatment plan. Special attention should be given to excluding emergency situations, such as epidural infection, epidural hemorrhage, cauda equine syndrome, spinal cord compression, spine metastasis, and

TABLE 90-12 Common Causes of Back and Neck Pain

Vertebral bodies • Fractures • Neoplastic lesions - Primary - Metastatic • Metabolic derangements - Osteoporosis - Paget disease - Osteitis fibrosa - Hyperthyroidism - Hyperparathyroidism - Cushing syndrome • Infections - Osteomyelitis Intravertebral disks • Structural lesions - Degeneration and herniation - Chondromalacia • Infections - Diskitis Ligaments • Acute strain • Involvement with other conditions Muscle structures • Primary myofascial pain • Secondary myofascial pain Joints • Facets joints (zygapophysial or "Z" joints) - Osteoarthritis - Mechanical arthropathy - Synovial impingement - Meniscoid entrapment	Sacroiliac joints • Mechanical arthropathy - Pregnancy • Degenerative and inflammatory - Osteoarthritis - Ankylosing spondylitis - Psoriatic arthritis - Reiter syndrome - Chronic inflammatory bowel disease Nerve roots (and dorsal root ganglia) • Compressive lesions • Neuroradiculopathies Meninges • Arachnoiditis • Scar tissue Epidural space • Hematoma • Infection (abscess) Multifactorial • Structural - Spine instability - Kyphosis - Scoliosis - Spondylolithiasis • Degenerative - Spinal stenosis - Spondylosis - Trauma - Infection • Psychosocial • Referred pain

aortic aneurysm. This chapter discusses only the more common pain syndromes.

DISCOGENIC PAIN

Discogenic pain is believed to occur as a result of damage to the annular lamellae by the disrupted inner internal disk and the resultant decreased pain threshold to mechanical loading. Usually a deep axial ache radiates to shoulders and scapular areas from cervical disks and to buttocks and posterior thighs from lumbar disks. The pain is worsened by mechanical loading maneuvers such as sitting, standing, and particularly bending forward.

Although CT scanning and MRI of the spine may show signs of disk degeneration, establishing clinical correlation with imaging findings is difficult.[154] A provocative discography test that consists of dye injection into the disk material followed by CT imaging has been advocated to confirm discogenic pain.[155]

Treatment is conservative, consisting of physical therapy, weight reduction, and NSAIDs. Patients with 1 or 2 diseased disks who are refractory to conservative therapy may benefit from intradiscal electrothermal therapy (see Chapter 92).[156-158]

RADICULAR PAIN

Radicular pain originates as a result of irritation of a nerve root due to a herniated nucleus pulposus or degenerative neuroforaminal narrowing. The most commonly affected levels in the lower back are L5-S1 and L4-5. In the neck, the affected levels are C5-6 and C6-7. Typically, the pain radiates from the neck or back in a dermatomal pattern (Fig. 90-3). Usually the patient has associated sensory disturbance and reflex decrease in the distribution of the affected root. A positive straight-leg raising (SLR) test while the patient is in a supine or sitting position indicates nerve root irritation. SLR test is considered positive when pain is reproduced in a dermatomal distribution. However, nerve root irritation is not always present in patients with low back pain or posterior thigh discomfort. MRI is helpful in identifying anatomy and changes near the nerve roots. NCS/EMG can help confirm the diagnosis and assess the severity of injury.

Conservative treatment, including NSAIDs and PT, is sufficient for most cases. Epidural steroid injections can provide symptomatic management.[159,160] Transforaminal steroid injections might be superior and prevent from surgery but may result in more complications, especially at the cervical spine level.[161-164] Surgical intervention may be required for refractory pain, especially if neurologic deficits are present. Microdiscectomy is the gold standard treatment for uncomplicated herniated nucleus pulposus.

Facet Arthropathy The facet joints (zygapophysial or Z joints) are true synovial joints whose main function is to limit rotation and resist compression during lordosis. Facet joint pain results from conditions that increase the load on them, such as arthritis, decreased disk space, and increased lordosis (as in obesity).

Pain usually is a gradual-onset deep axial ache that radiates to the scapular regions in the neck or to the buttocks and posterior thighs. It is associated with morning stiffness. The pain is reproduced by facet loading maneuvers by hyperextension and lateral rotation, which provokes pain ipsilaterally. Paraspinal tenderness often is present.[165-166]

MRI or CT can reveal arthritic changes in the facet joints, such as hypertrophy and joint space narrowing. The diagnosis can be confirmed by diagnostic block of the joints or of the medial branches innervating them.

Treatment is conservative, consisting of oral analgesics, weight loss, and physical therapy (PT). Intrajoint steroid injection can be attempted. Radiofrequency ablation of the medial branches appears to be promising.[167,168]

Sacroiliac Arthropathy The sacroiliac joint connects the sacrum to the iliac bones. It is subject to degenerative and inflammatory arthritides as well as mechanical dysfunction. The pain usually is precipitated by an injury, such as falling, lifting, or turning. The pain is a unilateral ache that radiates to the buttock, groin, and thigh area. It rarely goes below the knee. The pain is worsened by loading the joint, as occurs during prolonged sitting, standing, or bending. There is tenderness over the joint area, and the pain typically is reproduced by the Patrick test, in which the hip is forced into external rotation by placing the ankle on the opposite knee or thigh and pushing down on the knee. Intraarticular local anesthetic block can help confirm the diagnosis.

Treatment with NSAIDs and PT can be helpful. Fluoroscopy-guided intraarticular steroid injection has been the mainstay of treatment in clinical practice. Lateral branch block and radiofrequency ablation have been reported useful in advanced cases.[169]

SPINAL STENOSIS

Spinal stenosis results from narrowing of the central canal, lateral recesses, or neuroforamina due to age-related degenerative changes, including osteophyte formation, facet hypertrophy, ligamentum flavum hypertrophy, and diffuse broad-based disk bulge. Its occurrence in the cervical spine is referred to as cervical "spondylosis." When spinal stenosis occurs in people younger than 60 years, other comorbidities, such as diabetes or congenital stenosis due to short pedicles, scoliosis, and spondylolisthesis, should be ruled out.

Pain manifests as radicular when the narrowing occurs in the lateral recesses or neuroforamina. In the case of lumbosacral spinal canal stenosis, axial low back pain and neurogenic claudication are the predominant features.[170] Neurogenic claudication worsens with walking (especially downhill) and with extension of the spine. Rest and flexion of the spine usually provide temporary relief.

Cervical spondylosis can progress and cause cervical spondylotic myelopathy (CMS) and cord compression of varying severity. Motor weakness, spasticity, hyperreflexia, Babinski sign, Hoffman sign, paresthesias, imbalance, bowel and bladder function, and other features of spinal cord compression should be carefully assessed. Acute cervical spondylotic myelopathy can occur as a result of abrupt hyperextension of the neck. Radiographic changes reflecting degeneration associated with stenosis are common with aging; thus clinical correlation is critical in the assessment and management of related symptom complexes.[170]

Treatment of spinal stenosis should start with conservative measures, including oral analgesics, translaminar or transforaminal epidural steroid injections, and PT. Surgical options should be preserved for cases with rapid neurologic progression, CMS, or cauda equina syndrome, or for patients who remain symptomatic despite a course of nonsurgical therapy and who have advanced imaging studies that correspond to existing symptoms. Surgical management of lumbar and cervical stenosis includes discectomy, neural decompression, and spinal arthrodesis. Several studies report that surgical treatment produces better outcomes than nonsurgical treatment in the short term; however, improved results tend to regress over time.[171-175]

FAILED BACK SURGERY SYNDROME

Failed back surgery syndrome refers to the persistence or recurrence of low back pain after surgical intervention on the lumbosacral spine. Potential causes of surgical intervention failure include the following[60]: (1) poor patient selection, (2) unindicated surgery, (3) inadequate surgical decompression, (4) recurrence of lesions, (5) established neural injury, (6) complications of diagnostic and/or surgical intervention, and (7) secondary instability or degeneration. One study found that the predominant specific diagnoses in patients with failed back surgery syndrome were (in order) foraminal stenosis, painful disk(s), pseudarthrosis, neuropathic pain, instability, and psychological problems. Recurrent disk herniation is seen less often than in the past.[176]

Physical examination and imaging studies are essential to confirm the diagnosis and rule out other emerging etiologies. Treatment should be focused on the specific underlying etiology and may include repeated surgical intervention. Epidurolysis of adhesions via epiduroscopy or by catheter technique has limited evidence of efficacy.[177,178] Spinal cord stimulation was found to be both more effective and less costly than conservative medical management over the lifetime of a patient.[179-181]

WHIPLASH INJURY

Whiplash injury refers to neck injury caused by abrupt hyperextension due to indirect force, as occurs with acceleration–deceleration mechanisms. Whiplash injury is estimated to occur in 1% of the general population and to become chronic in up to 25% of these patients. Up to 60% of car accident victims evaluated in emergency departments have neck pain and up to 26% of them have persistent symptoms after 1 year.[177] Cervical facet joint pain is the most common source of pain after whiplash injury. The most common cervical segments involved are C2-3 and C5-6.[182,183]

Physical examination is nonspecific and may reveal tenderness and limited range of motion. Patients who have normal plain radiographic findings and no evidence of a neurologic deficit do not require additional MRI.[184]

Diagnostic medial branch block is helpful in delineating etiologies and differentiating between facet arthropathy and other causes of neck pain. Treatment of acute whiplash injury is conservative and includes oral NSAIDs, PT, and transcutaneous electrical nerve stimulation unit.[185] In chronic conditions where facet arthropathy is confirmed with diagnostic blocks, radiofrequency ablation appears to be promising.[183,186]

HEAD PAIN

Headache is one of the most common symptoms encountered in clinical practice. A pain medicine physician should be familiar with the common types of syndromes and be able to provide appropriate management. The IHS provides valuable sources for the classification and diagnosis of different syndromes.[97]

The prevalence of headache in the United States is estimated to be 78% in women and 68% in men. In general, headache is classified as primary or secondary. Primary headaches are diseases by themselves, as seen with migraine, tension-type, and cluster headaches. Secondary headaches are caused by an underlying condition. Most headaches seen in clinical practice are primary headaches (~90% or more).[187] The most common headache is tension headache, with a prevalence of 78%. Migraine also is very common, with an estimated prevalence of 16%. Among secondary headaches, the most common cause is attributable to fasting. Nasal- and sinus-related headaches and head trauma are less common. Many fear that headaches are caused by intracranial disease such as tumors; however, this actually occurs in a very small percentage of the population (0.5%).[188]

Evaluation of headache requires thorough history and physical examination. Special attention should be given to any "red flags" that may point to a secondary disorder. In the absence of warning signs, most likely the headache is of a primary disorder, with most headaches being either tension-type or migraine. Even in the absence of warning signs, possible secondary headache disorder may exist in patients presenting with "atypical features," such as migraine with prolonged aura lasting more than 60 minutes, migraine that lacks characteristic features (eg, no nausea, photophobia, or phonophobia), and migraine that does not quite meet all the diagnostic criteria, especially if they do not respond to normal therapy. These are the signals that are frequently elicited in a headache evaluation.

The most important feature is the temporal profile of the headache, specifically the mode of onset. Headache with a rapid time to peak intensity should always suggest an underlying cause of secondary headache. Not only the mode of onset but also the age at onset is important, as headache onset after age 50 years should raise concern of secondary headache. Other "red flags" include association with systemic signs or symptoms; the presence of a new or different headache, particularly in those with systemic malignancy, which may signify intracranial disease (eg, metastases); a change in headache pattern, such as progressive headache with loss of headache-free period; and a change in frequency or severity of a previously existing headache disorder (because underlying secondary causes in patients with a history of migraine can mimic normal headache patterns). Any, even subtle, abnormal neurologic findings also should raise suspicion.[189]

Electroencephalography is not useful in the routine evaluation of patients with headache. However, electroencephalography may be useful in patients with headache who have an alteration of consciousness, encephalopathy, or focal neurologic deficits and atypical symptoms.[190] Lumbar puncture (LP) is indicated in the evaluation of thunderclap or sudden headache to exclude the possibility of subarachnoid hemorrhage. CT can be negative in up to 25% of patients within 24 hours of occurrence of subarachnoid hemorrhage and can be negative in up to 50% of patients 1 week after initial presentation of headache resembling thunderclap. LP is indicated in any patient with subacute and progressive headache in order to exclude infections, an inflammatory condition, or carcinomatous meningitis. Any patient who presents with headache and fever, confusion, or seizure should be suspected of having acute intracranial infection. LP should be performed in patients with high or low intracranial pressure syndrome (idiopathic intracranial hypertension), even in the absence of papilledema. LP should be performed to confirm low-pressure states, as occurs with cerebrospinal fluid (CSF) leaks. In the absence of "red flags," CT or MRI typically is not performed unless a change in headache pattern occurs or the patient experiences changes in

TABLE 90-13 International Headache Society Diagnostic Criteria for Migraine Without Aura

A. At least 5 attacks fulfilling criteria B-D
B. Headache attacks lasting 4-72 h (untreated or unsuccessfully treated)
C. Headache has at least 2 of the following characteristics:
   1. Unilateral location
   2. Pulsating quality
   3. Moderate or severe pain intensity
   4. Aggravation by or causing avoidance of routine physical activity
D. During headache at least 1 of the following:
   1. Nausea and/or vomiting
   2. Photophobia and phonophobia
E. Not attributed to another disorder

TABLE 90-14 International Headache Society Diagnostic Criteria for Cluster Headache

A. At least 5 attacks fulfilling criteria B-D
B. Severe or very severe unilateral orbital, supraorbital, and/or temporal pain lasting 15-180 min if untreated
C. Headache is accompanied by at least 1 of the following:
   1. Ipsilateral conjunctival injection and/or lacrimation
   2. Ipsilateral nasal congestion and/or rhinorrhea
   3. Ipsilateral eyelid edema
   4. Ipsilateral forehead and facial sweating
   5. Ipsilateral miosis and/or ptosis
   6. Sense of restlessness and agitation
D. Attacks have a frequency ranging from 1 every other day to 8 per day
E. Not attributed to another disorder

neurologic status as evidenced by seizures or focal neurologic signs or symptoms.[191]

Following is a discussion of IHS criteria for common headaches and a brief review of major treatment options.

Migraine Multiple types of migraine exist. The more common types are discussed here.

Migraine Without Aura Migraine without aura previously was called *common migraine*. **Table 90-13** lists the IHS diagnostic criteria[97] for migraine without aura.

Migraine With Aura This type of headache previously was called classic migraine. It fulfills the criteria of migraine as described earlier and is associated with aura. The aura is a complex of neurologic symptoms that occurs just before or at the onset of migraine headache. A typical aura consists of visual and/or sensory and/or speech symptoms. It has gradual development, duration no longer than 1 hour, and complete reversibility.[97] Some patients have typical aura without having a typical migrainous headache.

Treatment of migraine headaches is abortive and preventive. Abortive treatment is directed toward the acute attacks as they occur. Many drugs have been shown to be effective abortive medications. Nonspecific treatments, such as acetaminophen, aspirin and caffeine combination (Excedrin), and NSAIDs, are effective for simple and less severe migraines. Other nonspecific migraine agents include corticosteroids, antiemetics, and opioid analgesics. The migraine-specific agents are considered the mainstay abortive treatment of migraine. They include ergotamine, dihydroergotamine, and the more selective serotonin antagonists (triptans). Multiple triptans are available in different forms, half-lives, and potencies. Preventive treatment of migraine should focus on modifying and/or eliminating the triggering factors, such as sleep disturbance, caffeine intake, analgesics overuse, and stressors. Pharmacologic preventive treatment is indicated when migraine intensity, duration, or frequency is severe enough to warrant chronic use of a daily medication. Preventive treatment also is indicated for more serious forms of migraine, such as basilar-type migraine (migraine with neurologic signs of posterior circulation dysfunction), migraine with complications (focal neurologic features), and hemiplegic migraine. TCAs (eg, amitriptyline), nonselective beta-blockers (eg, propranolol), and AEDs (eg, topiramate and divalproex sodium) are effective preventive agents.

Tension-Type Headache Tension-type headaches are the most common primary headache. Many features distinguish them from migraines. Each attack of tension-type headache can be much shorter or much longer than migraine. The pain generally is bilateral, is of mild to moderate intensity, is constant, and is not aggravated by movement or activity. Photophobia or phonophobia may be present but usually not both, and the patient experiences no nausea or vomiting. Tension-type headaches have a wide spectrum of frequency that varies from sporadic episodes to chronic forms.[97]

Infrequent episodes of tension-type headaches can be treated with simple analgesics. For more frequent and chronic forms, preventive treatment is essential.

Cluster Headache Cluster headaches are much less common than tension-type and migraine headaches but are excruciatingly painful and devastating. **Table 90-14** lists the IHS diagnostic criteria for cluster headaches.[97]

As for treatment of migraine headaches, treatment of cluster headaches is abortive and preventive. Abortive treatment consists of inhaled oxygen; triptans, especially the injectable form (sumatriptan); or dihydroergotamine. Multiple preventive agents can be tried. They include corticosteroids, hypertension medications (beta-blockers and calcium channel blockers), and lithium. In refractory cases, invasive treatments might be required. They include sphenopalatine ganglion blockade, trigeminal nerve and/or ganglion blockade, or deep brain stimulation.

Postdural Puncture Headache Low-CSF pressure headache results from a dural tear and subsequent CSF leak. Postdural puncture headache is the more common type of low-CSF headache. The IHS diagnostic criteria for postdural puncture headache are listed in **Table 90-15**.[97]

Epidural blood patch at the expected site of leak remains the mainstay treatment. Conservative therapy includes bedrest, aggressive hydration, caffeine, and analgesics.

TABLE 90-15 International Headache Society Diagnostic Criteria for Postdural Puncture Headache

A. Headache that worsens within 15 min after sitting or standing and improves within 15 min after lying down, with at least 1 of the following and fulfilling criteria C and D:
   1. Neck stiffness
   2. Tinnitus
   3. Hypacusia
   4. Photophobia
   5. Nausea
B. Dural puncture has been performed.
C. Headache develops within 5 days after dural puncture.
D. Headache resolves (in 95% of cases) either
   1. Spontaneously within 1 week
   2. Within 48 hours after effective treatment of the spinal fluid leak (usually by epidural blood patch)

KEY REFERENCES

- Graff-Radford SB. Myofascial pain: diagnosis and management. *Curr Pain Headache Rep.* 2004;8:463-467.
- Dworkin RH, O'Connor AB, Audette J, et al. Recommendations for the pharmacological management of neuropathic pain: an overview and literature update. *Mayo Clin Proc.* 2010;85(3 Suppl):S3-S14.
- Dyck PJ, Thomas PK. *Peripheral Neuropathy.* 4th ed. Philadelphia: WB Saunders; 2005.
- Warfield CA, Bajwa ZH. *Principles and Practice of Pain Medicine.* 2nd ed. New York: McGraw-Hill; 2004:386-389.

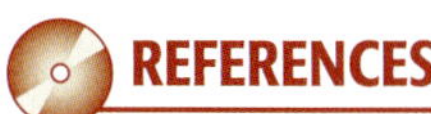

REFERENCES

Complete references available on DVD and online version at www.LongneckerAnesthesiology.com

CHAPTER 91 Medical Management of Chronic Pain

Teresa E. Dews
Riad Laham
Lokesh Ningegowda
Marc A. Huntoon

KEY POINTS

1. Patients with chronic pain usually require multimodal (pharmacologic, behavioral, physical modalities, and procedural) therapies for pain that are chosen based on the underlying mechanism and the impact of the pain on function and suffering.
2. Fear of reinjury, catastrophizing, and poor coping skills may undermine the success of any mode of therapy. Secondary gain (litigation, ongoing workers' compensation) may also undermine successful treatment.
3. The success of opioid therapies in acute pain must be tempered by the realization that for chronic pain treatment, opioid-induced hyperalgesia, pharmacologic tolerance, drug diversion, patient outcomes, and legal issues must be balanced appropriately for optimal care. Continuous monitoring and attention to the physician-patient relationship is vital.
4. Multiple new agents targeting ion channels and neurotransmitters are being developed, with improving efficacy. Optimal use of these agents requires a thorough understanding of their pharmacology as well as the ability to compare their effects through standardized study (allowing meta-analysis) and measures such as "number needed to treat" analysis.
5. New studies examining combination therapy (eg, an opioid plus anticonvulsant agent) are likely to represent future practice because of the complexity of pain treatment and the realization that one agent is rarely sufficient.
6. Several studies suggesting that physical modalities plus cognitive-behavioral interventions are equivalent to large surgical procedures are interesting. These studies point to a future blending of traditionally separate pain clinic and pain rehabilitative programs to include even more comprehensive approaches.

The approach to the patient with chronic pain shares some similarities with the treatment of acute pain, with several notable differences. Whereas acute pain involves a specific tissue injury and an often easily identifiable initiating event, chronic pain may not have a definable source, tissue injury may not always be apparent, and treatment may be ineffective (**Fig. 91-1**). Unlike acute pain where the course of the disease process may be self-limited and the treatment duration is generally brief, chronic pain often requires extended and multimodal treatment. Additionally, if pharmacologic therapy is the mainstay of treatment, then the long-term implications of popular drugs used for treatment of acute pain, such as opioids and nonsteroidal anti-inflammatory agents (NSAIDs), must be considered. Acute pain is caused by a short-term event (trauma, surgery, burn, etc) and has the chance of improvement or cure with treatment or elimination of the inciting event. It is appropriately managed with opioids, regional/neuraxial local anesthetics, numerous adjuvant drugs, and corticosteroids or NSAIDS. Long-term issues of drug-induced toxicities, such as opioid-induced endocrine abnormalities or hyperalgesia and cardiovascular or gastrointestinal side effects of NSAIDs, must be considered relevant to patients with chronic medical problems. In general, there is little evidence of long-term efficacy (ie, >2 years) of medications historically used for short-term analgesia.[1]

When acute pain becomes chronic, the physician must understand the mechanism of the pain in order to choose treatments based on validated outcome studies. This mechanism-based approach to pain therapy[2] or biomedical model likely will continue to dominate chronic pain treatment strategies and medication development for many years.[3] Realizing that all pain is not initiated and maintained by similar mechanisms, treatments must be tailored to the specific individual. The pain problem also must be considered within the fabric of the patient's health profile and the context of the patient's current psychosocial situation. This evaluation and management model of treating the patient with pain as a whole person often is characterized as the *biopsychosocial model* of care.[4,5] The chronic pain, after beginning with some acute process, gradually is supplanted by increasing layers of complexity as the patient's psychosocial environment and internal suffering interacts with the pain, sometimes amplifying its perception and magnitude (**Fig. 91-2**). Because most anesthesiologists currently do not possess significant training in physical medicine and rehabilitation, neurology, neurosurgery, and psychiatry (among many related pain medicine fields), the optimal care of patients nearly always requires a multidisciplinary approach. In today's health systems approach, with its multiple regulatory and managed care cost containment barriers, getting several specialists together at one time has become increasingly difficult and inefficient. Thus new models of care must be found, likely those in which the pain specialist interacts in parallel with multiple disciplines to find the cause and appropriate treatment of the pain, with ongoing primary care physician involvement. Pain evaluation and treatment can be intensified for episodes of pain relapse or exacerbation. These patients often are therapeutically challenging, and cognitive-behavioral, physical, and group therapies may be best administered in a controlled structured environment, such as a pain rehabilitation and management program. These programs are characterized by concomitant management by multiple physician and allied health therapists to effect changes in the patient's cognition regarding the pain and an emphasis on functional status improvement and behavioral change in addition to medication optimization.

EVALUATION OF THE CHRONIC PAIN PATIENT (FIG. 91-3)

HISTORY

The initial evaluation of any patient presenting with chronic pain begins with a comprehensive medical history. The *chief complaint* should be noted. The pain history should include a screen for descriptive features of the pain: *what*—the descriptors that best characterize the pain, such as burning, stabbing, pricking, aching, shooting, lancinating, dull,

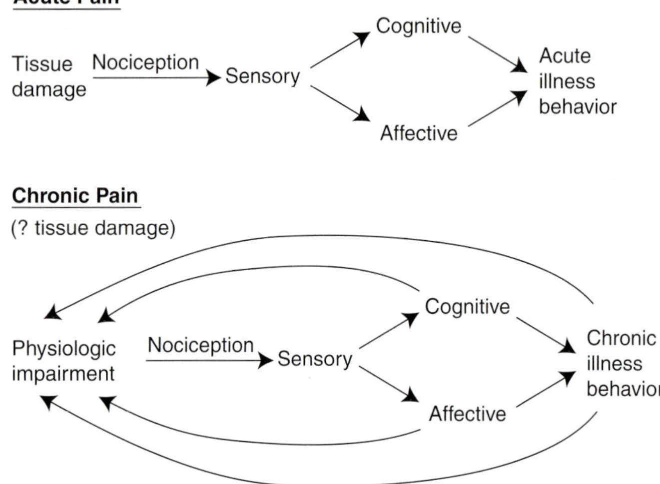

FIGURE 91-1. Top: In acute pain, tissue damage leads to a predominantly sensory phenomenon of pain, with some superimposed cognitive, affective response. Bottom: In chronic pain, tissue damage may not be apparent, and symptom magnification, affective distress, and illness behavior may be the primary identifiable manifestation of pain. [Reprinted from Waddell G, Newton M, Henderson I, et al. A fear-avoidance beliefs questionnaire (FABQ) and the role of fear-avoidance beliefs in chronic low back pain and disability. *Pain.* 1993;52:157-168. With permission from the International Association for the Study of Pain.]

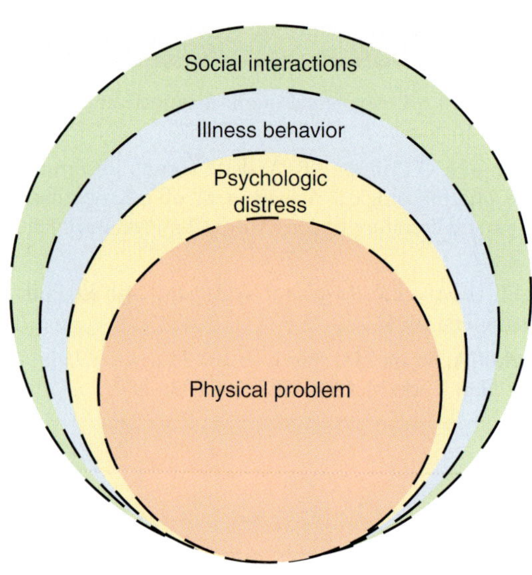

FIGURE 91-2. Pain, initially caused by an underlying physical problem, is increasingly magnified by psychosocial stressors. [From Waddell G, Main CJ, Morris EW, et al. Chronic low-back pain, psychologic distress, and illness behavior. *Spine.* 1984;9:209-213. With permission.]

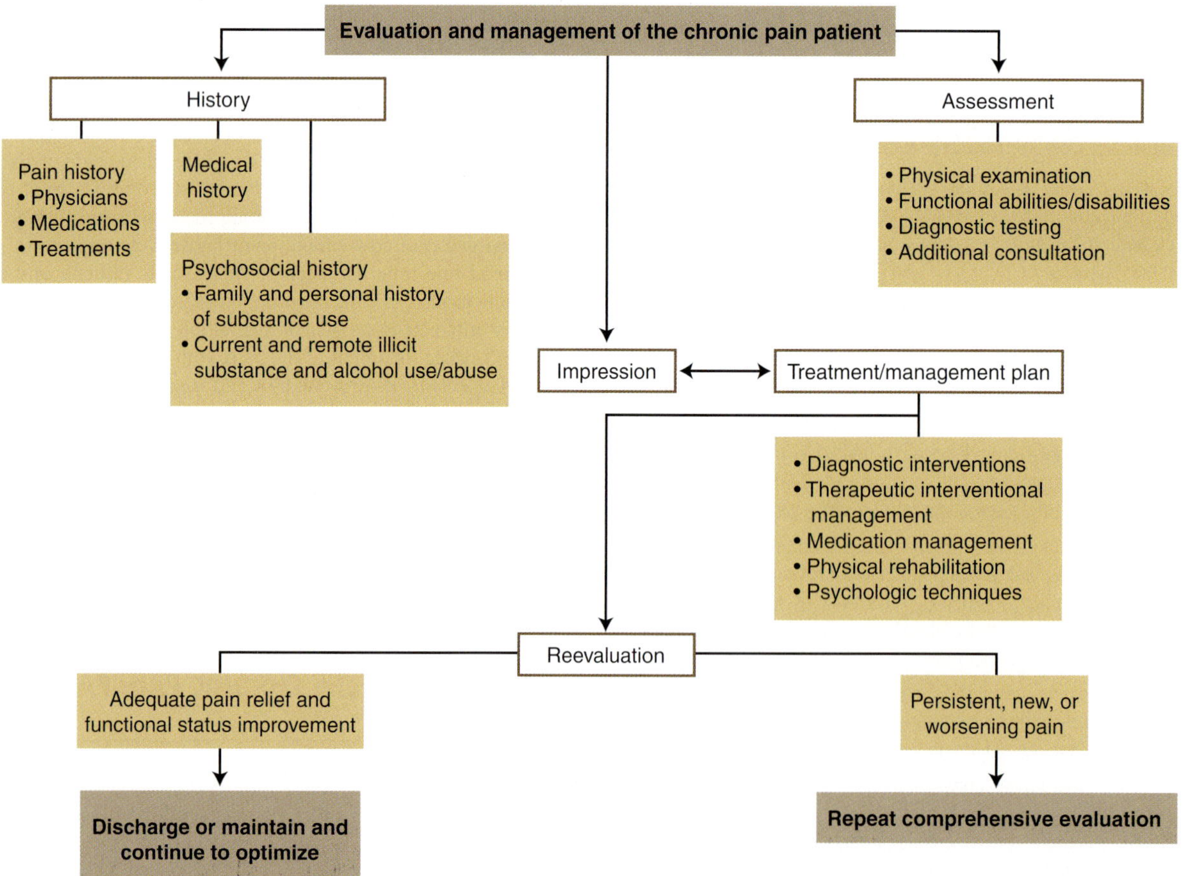

FIGURE 91-3. Evaluation and management of the chronic pain patient.

boring, etc; *where*—the current location of the pain and any radiation or referral, or the specific pattern that the pain takes going from one area to another (sometimes they follow known dermatomal patterns or are specific for a certain myofascial trigger point syndrome); *when*—the time that the pain occurs and what activities it may be associated with (eg, an arthritic patient with most pronounced pain on awakening and attempting to get up in the morning); *how much* (ie, the score the patient assigns the pain on an 11-point numerical scale from 0 to 10, or the impact on a measurable function such as walking distance).

The *history of present illness* should describe the origin *(the why)* of the pain, to the extent that it is discernible, and what has transpired up to the patient's presentation. *Past treatment history* should completely describe all previous attempts to diagnose and treat the current condition. The patient's response (eg, impact on intensity of pain and function as well as duration of effect) are important clues to the mechanism of pain and additional treatment options. All pain patients should have a *numerical pain scale* assessed for each visit and at appropriate follow-up times after new interventions or medications are started. Because pain is typically a variable experience, noting the range of pain ("worst and best" pain) may be more helpful than the snapshot at the time of the office visit. This allows a chronology of any improvement or worsening. Often, a pain diary can be kept by the patient and may be useful in identifying trends. All *therapeutic trials* should detail past pharmacologic treatments (maximum dosage reached and reason for cessation) as well as previous procedural, physical, and behavioral therapies (to understand exactly what was done and why). The *current medications* should list drug, dosage, and what the agent is treating. This list should include traditional pharmaceuticals as well as herbal and over-the-counter agents. *A substance use history* is critical, including not only prescribed opioids and benzodiazepines but also illicit substances used and a history of their use, including remote history (ie, high school/college exposure). Many pain patients have extremely long and detailed lists of "allergies" secondary to numerous previous failed drug trials, with cessation secondary to side effects. Thus *allergies* should document the specific nature of the reaction (true anaphylaxis vs side effect).

The remainder of the history should look specifically at the *functional impact* of the pain on the person's activities of daily living, work/physical activities, regularity of exercise, leisure/hobbies, yard work/housework, sexual function, and social activities or evidence of withdrawal and isolation from activities. *Goals of care* should be discussed so that both patient and provider have an understanding of what is potentially and realistically achievable. A complete *review of systems, past medical and surgical histories, and social and family histories* should be documented. Careful review of family chemical dependency history including alcoholism is important as well as patient history of physical, sexual, or emotional abuse (past or current). Finally, the presence of *fear-avoidance beliefs* should be evaluated, and, if present, a behavioral intervention should be instituted. Psychosocial pain-reinforcing mechanisms, such as patient beliefs, perceptions, and expectations about the impact of work, exercise, and disability, are important to treating persistent pain.[4,5]

PHYSICAL EXAMINATION

The chronic pain patient should undergo a complete physical examination, not only looking at the areas relevant to his or her chief complaint but also evaluating major systems (eg, cardiovascular, renal, hepatic, pulmonary) that may interact with or potentially limit therapeutic pharmaceutical trials or participation in an exercise-based program. A complete examination may include specific tests of joint movement/range of motion, for example, as well as correlation of examination findings with imaging modalities.

A thorough *mental status* examination should focus on the following areas: presence of confounding *personality disorders*; *affective* state, presence of alterations in mood, flattened/depressed affect, or hypomania/mania; *cognitive* state, orientation to person, place, and time, intelligence, judgment, insight; *speech*, fluidity, goal driven, presence of word-finding difficulties, comprehensibility; *attention*, concentration, abstract thinking, perception; and *emotionality*, anxiety, hopefulness, anger, frustration, fear. For example, the presence of a personality disorder may be a specific contraindication to ongoing opioid therapies because patients may experience worsening of behavioral manifestations while taking opioids.[6] Because the most prevalent types of pain commonly seen in pain clinics may include back/spine, extremity pain, and head pain, thorough examination of the musculoskeletal and neurologic systems should be emphasized. The neurologic examination should grade motor strength in major muscle groups (**Table 91-1**) and other examination findings (**Table 91-2; Fig. 91-4**). In addition, *Waddell signs* (**Table 91-3**) should be sought for patients whose neurologic and

TABLE 91-1 Muscle Grading System

Muscle Grading	Activity
5: Normal	Full ROM against gravity with full resistance
4: Good	Full ROM against gravity with some resistance
3: Fair	Active ROM gravity eliminated
2: Poor	Active ROM gravity eliminated
1: Trace	Slight contraction only
0: Zero	No contraction

ROM, range of motion.

TABLE 91-2 Summary of Reflexes

Reflexes	Afferent Nerve	Center	Efferent Nerve
Superficial Reflexes			
Corneal	Cranial V	Pons	Cranial VII
Nasal (sneeze)	Cranial V	Brainstem and upper cord	Cranials V, VII, IX, and X, and spinal nerves of expiration
Pharyngeal and uvular	Cranial IX	Medulla	Cranial X
Upper abdominal	T7-T10	T7-T10	T7-T10
Lower abdominal	T10-T12	T10-T12	T10-T12
Cremasteric	Femoral	L1	Genitofemoral
Plantar	Tibial	S1, S2	Tibial
Anal	Pudendal	S4, S5	Pudendal
Tendon Reflexes			
Jaw	Cranial V	Pons	Cranial V
Biceps	Musculocutaneous	C5, C6	Musculocutaneous
Triceps	Radial	C7, C8	Radial
Brachioradialis	Radial	C5, C6	Radial
Patellar	Femoral	L3, L4	Femoral
Achilles	Tibial	S1, S2	Tibial
Visceral Reflexes			
Light	Cranial II	Midbrain	Cranial III
Accommodation	Cranial II	Occipital cortex	Cranial III
Ciliospinal	A sensory nerve	T1, T2	Cervical sympathetics
Oculocardiac	Cranial V	Medulla	Cranial X
Carotid sinus	Cranial IX	Medulla	Cranial X
Bulbocavernosus	Pudendal	S2-S4	Pelvic autonomic
Bladder and rectal	Pudendal	S2-S4	Pudendal and autonomics
Abnormal Reflexes			
Extensor plantar (Babinski)	Plantar	L3-L5, S1	Extensor hallucis longus

Reprinted with permission from Waxman SG. *Clinical Neuroanatomy.* 26th ed. New York, NY: McGraw-Hill; 2010.

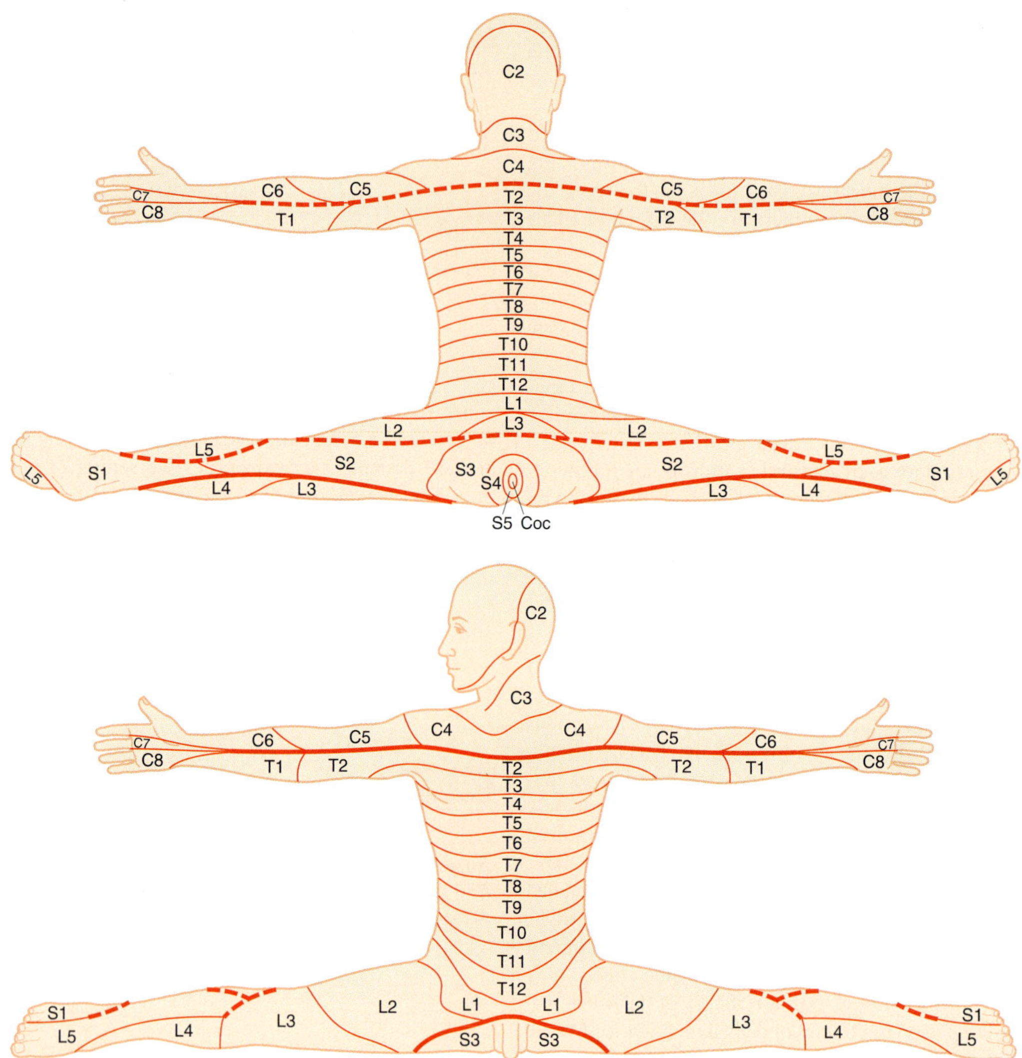

FIGURE 91-4. Sensory dermatomes. [From Tintinalli JE, Stapczynski JS, Cline DM, et al. *Tintinalli's Emergency Medicine: A Comprehensive Study Guide.* 7th ed. New York, NY: McGraw-Hill; 2010. With permission.]

musculoskeletal examinations diverge from expectations. For example, a patient may present with positive straight-leg raising sign in the supine position that changes with distraction. An understanding of the presence of these nonorganic physical signs may prevent the misapplication of pointless therapies and redirection to more appropriate treatment such as pain rehabilitation.

The presence of *spasticity* (upper motor neuron, corticospinal tract; increased resistance when the examiner moves a joint briskly or forcefully) versus *rigidity* (basal ganglia, eg, parkinsonism; enhanced resistance to movement throughout the range of a specific muscle-joint system) should be noted. Presence of *myopathy*, such as corticosteroid-induced or statin-induced muscle weakness (symmetric weakness without atrophy and normal sensation), should be documented. Evidence of true *atrophy* may signify a radiculopathy caused by spinal nerve irritation involving a specific muscle (**Table 91-4**); a more diffuse lumbosacral radiculoplexopathy, as occurs in diabetic patients; or peripheral neuropathy with distal weakness, atrophy, sensory loss, and possibly even fasciculations. Sensory examination, generally performed with a safety pin, light touch, temperature source, and 2-point discrimination and tuning fork, can help discriminate abnormalities. Knowledge of tender points (**Fig. 91-5**) in fibromyalgia can aid musculoskeletal examination of pain at these sites, and tenderness at 11 of the 18 sites meets diagnostic criteria. Referral zones for various regional myofascial syndromes also may help discriminate discomfort in various areas. For example, temporomandibular joint pain may radiate to the temple, face, and head.

TABLE 91-3 Waddell Signs

Nonanatomic	Widespread Tenderness
Simulation tests	Axial loading Stimulated rotation
Distraction	Straight-leg raise (ie, positive supine but not when distracted)
Regional	Weakness: atypical Sensory: nondermatomal
Overreaction	Exaggerated pain behaviors

From Waddell G, McCulloch JA, Kummel E, et al. Non organic physical signs in low back pain. *Spine.* 1980;5:117-125. With permission.

Nonorganic Physical Signs As previously discussed, patients who are being evaluated for chronic pain disorders may demonstrate confusing physical examination findings that confound the clinician's ability to categorize and treat their condition. Waddell and Main[7] described 7 inappropriate symptoms that seemed to be best characterized as magnifiers of physical illness: (1) pain at the tip of the

TABLE 91-4 Muscle Innervation: Shoulder and Upper Extremity

Nerve	Action to Test	Muscle
Long thoracic	Forward shoulder thrust	Serratus anterior
Dorsal scapular	Elevate scapula	Levator scapulae
Suprascapular	Arm extension rotation	Infraspinatus; C5, C6
Axillary	Abduct arm (>90 degree)	Deltoid; C5
Musculocutaneous	Flex and supinate arm	Biceps brachii
Ulnar	Ulnar flexion of hand	Flexor carpi ulnaris; C7, C8
	Flex DIP of fingers 4 and 5	Flexor digitorum profundus
	Thumb adduction	Adductor pollicis; C7, C8b, T1
	Abduction of finger 5	Abductor digitorum minimi
	Opposition of finger 5	Opponens digitorum minimi
	Flexion of finger 5	Flexor digitorum minimi brevis
	Finger abduction and adduction	Interossi; C8, T1b
	Flex PIP and extend DIP of fingers 4 and 5	Lumbricals 3 and 4
Median	Forearm pronation	Pronator teres
	Radial hand flexion	Flexor carpi radialis; C7, C8, T1
	Hand flexion	Palmaris longus
	PIP flexion of fingers 2-5	Flexor digitorum superficialis
	Abduct thumb at he MCP	Abductor pollicis brevis
	Flex proximal phalanx thumb	Flexor pollicis brevis; C7, C8b
Anterior interosseous	Flex DIP fingers 2-5	Flexor digitorum profundus (radial)
	Flex thumb IP	Flexor pollicis longus
	Oppose thumb	Opponens pollicis; C8, T1b
	Flex PIP and extend DIP of fingers 2 and 3	Lumbricals 1 and 2
Posterior interosseous	Extension of digits 2-5	Extensor digitorum
	Ulnar hand extension	Extensor carpi ulnaris
	Thumb abduction	Abductor pollicis longus
	Index finger extension	Extensor indicis proprius
Radial	Forearm extension	Triceps brachii; C6, C7, C8b
	Forearm flexion	Brachioradialis; C5, C6
	Radial hand extension	Extensor carpi radialis
	Forearm supination	Supinator

Muscle Innervation Hip and Lower Extremity

Nerve	Action to Test	Muscle[a]
Femoral	Hip flexion	Iliopsoas, T12, L1,[b] L2, L3
	Leg extension	Quadriceps femoris, L2, L3,[b] L4
Obturator	Thigh adduction	Pectineus
		Adductor longus, brevis, magnus L2, L3, L4
		Gracilis
Superior gluteal	Thigh abduction	Gluteus medius and minimus
	Thigh flexion	Tensor fascia lata
	Lateral thigh rotation	Piriformis
Inferior gluteal	Thigh abduction	Gluteus maximus
Sciatic (trunk)	Leg flexion	Biceps femoris L5, S1,[b] S2
		Semitendinosus
		Semimembranosus
Deep peroneal	Foot dorsiflexion and supination	Tibialis anterior, L4, L5
	Toes 2-5 and foot extension	Extensor digitorum longus/brevis
	Great toe and foot dorsiflexion	Extensor hallucis longus
Superficial peroneal	Plantar flexion foot and eversion	Peroneus longus/brevis; L5, S1
Tibial	Plantar flexion and inversion	Posterior tibialis
	Flex distal phalanx great toe	Flexor hallucis longus
	Flex middle phalanx toes 2-5	Flexor digitorum brevis
	Flex proximal phalanx great toe	Gastrocnemius; L5, S1,[b] S2
	Knee flexion and ankle plantar flexion	Flexor hallucis brevis
	Ankle plantar flexion	Plantaris, soleus
Pudendal	Voluntary pelvic floor contraction	Perineal and sphincters; S3, S4

DIP, distal interphalangeal joint; IP, interphalangeal joint; MCP, metacarpophalangeal joint; PIP, proximal interphalangeal joint.

Reprinted with permission from Tintinalli JE, Stapczynski JS, Cline DM, et al. *Tintinalli's Emergency Medicine: A Comprehensive Study Guide.* 7th ed. New York, NY: McGraw-Hill; 2010.

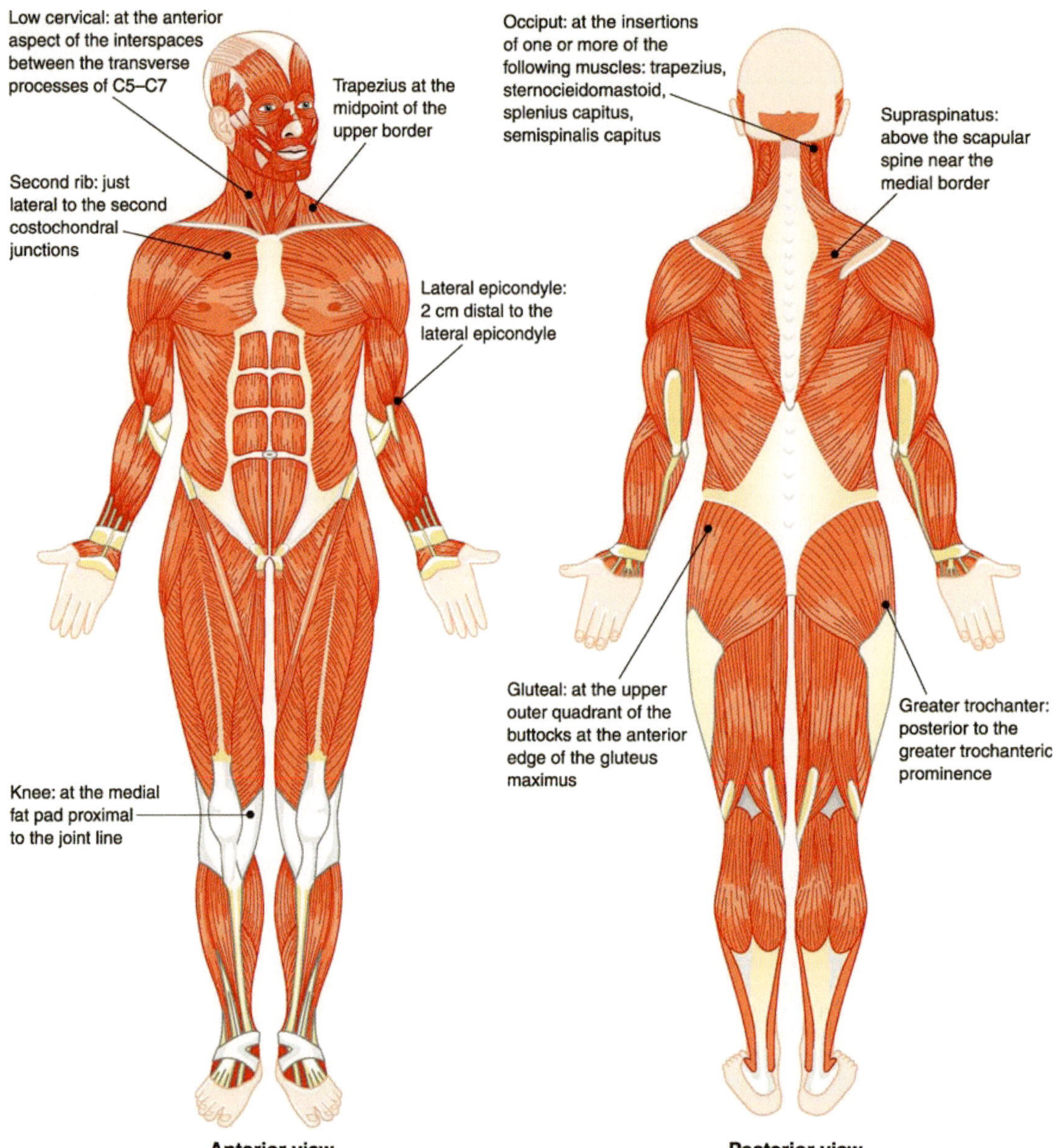

FIGURE 91-5. The 18 primary fibromyalgia tender points. [From The patient with diffuse pain. In: Imboden JB, Hellmann DB, Stone JH, eds. *Current Rheumatology: Diagnosis and Treatment.* 2nd ed. New York, NY: McGraw-Hill; 2004.]

coccyx, (2) entire leg pain, (3) entire leg sensory loss, (4) giveaway weakness of the entire lower extremity, (5) absence of pain-free periods, (6) intolerance to procedural or pharmacologic treatments, and (7) frequent emergency department visits and admissions for intractable pain. These symptoms had little presence in patients who were asymptomatic but had satisfactory test-retest reproducibility in patients with chronic back pain.

The *pain drawing* is another tool commonly used by pain practitioners to evaluate new patients with chronic pain complaints (**Fig. 91-6**).[8] Patients are evaluated by having them draw the areas of their pain and concomitantly having the Minnesota Multiphasic Personality Inventory (MMPI) test scored along with the drawing. The authors found a strong correlation between patients evaluated having a normal MMPI (no evidence of hysteria [Hy] or hypochondriasis [Hs]) and those having fewer than 2 penalty deductions on their pain drawing. The authors reported that the pain drawing might help physicians screen out up to 93% of patients who would have poor psychometrics related to (1) unreal drawings; (2) expansion or magnification of pain (eg, pain outside the bodily limits); (3) areas of excessive annotation of particularly severe pain (stars, circling, lightning bolts, etc); and (4) low back pain radiating pain indicators. Waddell et al[9] described a series of physical examination signs that can be used as an aid in the examination of patients with low back pain.

Increasingly, the pain medicine clinician needs a thorough understanding of contemporary imaging modalities, such as plain radiographs, magnetic resonance imaging, and computed tomography. Imaging complements and reinforces the appraisals and clinical impressions of pain patients.[10] Likewise, correlating imaging study abnormalities with physical examination findings using a thorough understanding of anatomy enables the physician to differentiate significant from confounding findings. For example, it is well known that abnormalities found on imaging studies may not correlate with the patient's pain or examination. Significant changes may be found on spine magnetic resonance studies in 35% of asymptomatic patients.[10,11]

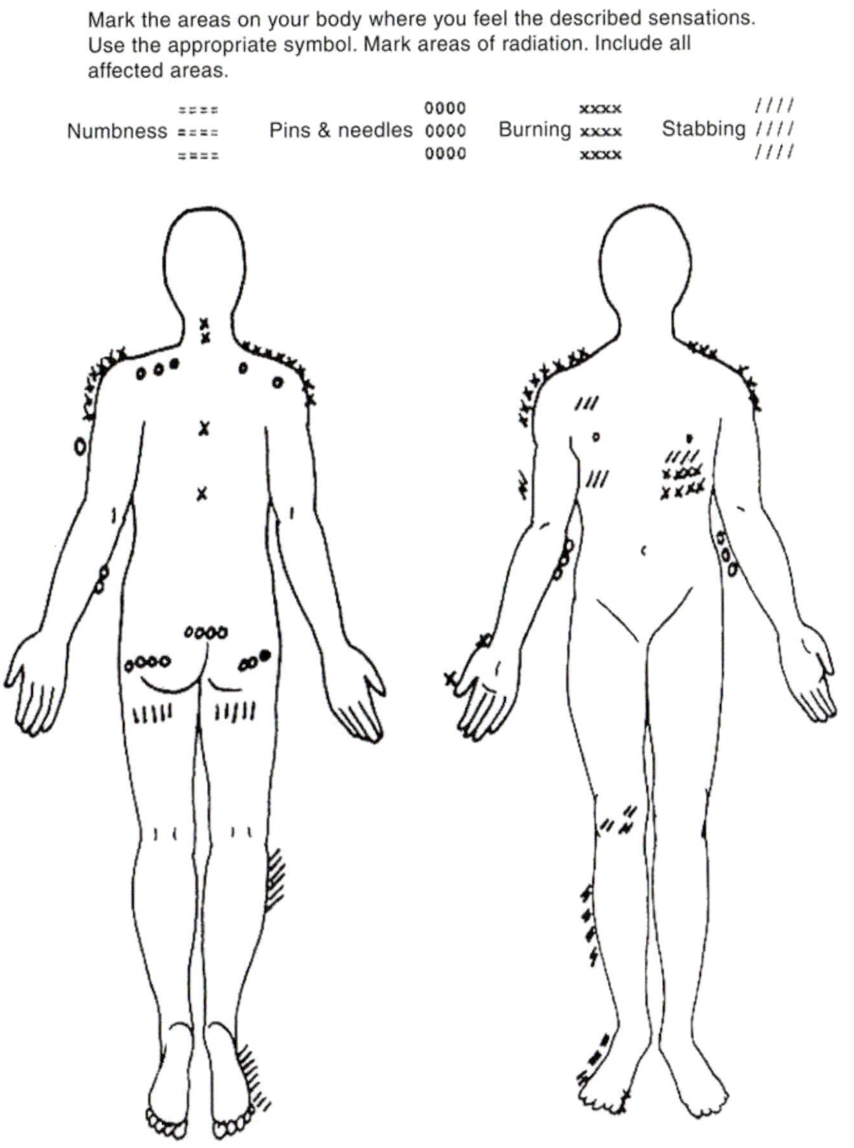

Mark the areas on your body where you feel the described sensations. Use the appropriate symbol. Mark areas of radiation. Include all affected areas.

Numbness ==== Pins & needles 0000 Burning xxxx Stabbing ////

FIGURE 91-6. Example of a pain drawing from a patient with multiple noncontiguous areas of pain with amplification and somatic preoccupation. [From Ransford AO, Cairns D, Mooney V. The pain drawing as an aid to the psychologic evaluation of patients with low back pain. *Spine.* 1976;1:127-134. With permission.]

PHARMACOLOGIC THERAPY

It is quite apparent to physicians who engage in chronic pain therapy that currently available pharmacologic agents often are insufficient as single therapies. Finding treatments through a mechanism-based approach offers the best chance for a rational selection of therapies.[12] It may be difficult to determine what level of clinical improvement actually is significant when performing randomized controlled trials of the various pharmaceutical agents currently available. Farrar et al[13] examined 10 recently completed drug trials using one agent (pregabalin) for treatment of a variety of different pain conditions (diabetic peripheral neuropathies, postherpetic neuralgia, fibromyalgia, chronic low back pain, and osteoarthritis). Essentially, the best correlation of patient global impression of change with the 11-point pain intensity numerical rating scale was determined to be an approximately 30% improvement or a 2-point scale decrease. This approximate relationship persisted regardless of the condition being treated and other patient demographic variables. Thus the authors recommended that application of these standards for all pain studies not only was reasonable but that such standardization of future pain studies would render the studies more readily comparable, valid, and clinically useful. A 30% improvement is seemingly small, but when combination therapies are used, each contributing a small percentage toward clinical improvement, the reason for increased interest by pain clinicians in multimodal therapies is understandable.

SPECIFIC PHARMACOLOGIC ADJUVANTS

Antidepressants Many of the antidepressant agents are useful as either primary or adjuvant therapy for neuropathic pain syndromes as well as other types of pain, such as myofascial pain syndromes. It is generally accepted that the mechanism of action of these drugs in pain is complex and may be related to reuptake inhibition of various neurotransmitters important in descending bulbospinal inhibitory pathways.[14] Additional mechanisms may be important, including effects on *N*-methyl-D-aspartate (NMDA) excitatory amino acid receptors,[15,16] sodium channel blockade,[17] and even other mechanisms. Earlier studies addressed initial speculation that these agents were working as *antidepressants only* in pain patients with concomitant depression.[18] Max et al demonstrated that amitriptyline was effective in patients with diabetic peripheral neuropathy pain both in the presence and the absence of depressed mood. Early comparisons of different types of antidepressants with selective serotonergic or nonselective reuptake inhibition of both noradrenaline and serotonin suggested that

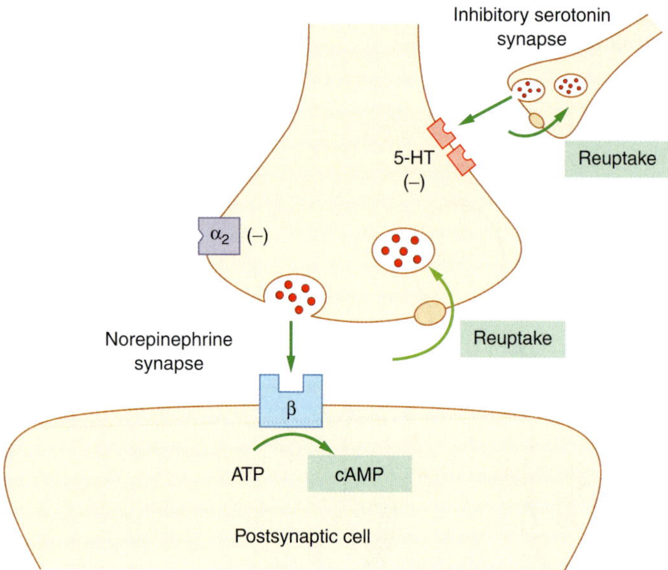

FIGURE 91-7. Mechanism of action of nonspecific reuptake inhibition of neurotransmitters, serotonin (5-HT), and norepinephrine in the descending inhibitory pathway. [From Potter WZ, Hollister LE. Antidepressant agents. In: Katzung BG, ed. *Basic and Clinical Pharmacology.* New York, NY: McGraw-Hill; 2004.]

drugs with nonselective mechanisms were more effective in treating neuropathic pain states (**Fig. 91-7**).[19] The selective serotonin reuptake inhibitors (SSRIs) in particular were generally believed to be devoid of efficacy in pain conditions, but newer studies suggest that these agents have an occasional but less pronounced role.[20-22]

Tricyclic antidepressants (TCAs) have a characteristic 3-ring nuclear structure and are chemically similar to phenothiazines and antihistamines, sharing side effects such as sedative and antimuscarinic actions. These side effects are perhaps the main detractors to the use of these agents in pain treatment, given their limited ability to reach effective doses. Certainly, the sedative properties of tricyclics can be used to advantage in the treatment of concomitant sleep deprivation, which frequently is present in chronic pain syndrome patients. However, many patients feel groggy or cognitively impaired even with introductory doses of these agents. Elderly patients in particular may have cardiac or urinary conditions that are exacerbated by the antimuscarinic actions of tricyclics, and the drugs may be contraindicated in some patients.[23]

Nortriptyline Roose et al[24] studied the specific SSRI paroxetine in comparison with nortriptyline in ischemic heart disease patients with depression. Approximately 60% of patients in both groups experienced improvement in depressive symptoms, but the nortriptyline group had significantly more adverse cardiac events, involving 18% of the study group. The patients in the nortriptyline group were titrated to target plasma levels over the first 3 to 7 days rather than the more typical slow ramping dose used by many physicians treating pain. Nevertheless, the development of adverse events illustrates the precautions that must be considered with the use of tricyclic agents. The prototype TCAs amitriptyline and imipramine are metabolized via mono-demethylation to the active metabolites nortriptyline and desipramine, respectively. Imipramine, similar to amitriptyline, has been successfully used for treatment of painful diabetic neuropathy.[25] However, the second-generation tricyclic agents (nortriptyline and desipramine) tend to be better tolerated because of less intense antimuscarinic and sedative properties and thus are more popular with pain physicians (**Table 91-5**).[26-28]

Amitriptyline Amitriptyline was one of the first agents shown to be effective in the treatment of postherpetic neuralgia[29] and has been a prototypical pain adjuvant drug for more than 2 decades. Although the drug is effective compared with placebo, its individual effects are generally not sufficient to result in complete analgesia. Preemptive use of amitriptyline in elderly patients has been associated with a decreased incidence of pain prevalence 6 months after the diagnosis of herpes zoster. The author recommended early institution of amitriptyline in this group.[30] Dosing of tricyclics for pain treatment generally begins at low evening doses and is increased gradually until limited by side effects or pain improves. Meta-analysis suggests that an average dose of approximately 75 to 100 mg/d of these agents may be required to achieve optimal results.[31]

TABLE 91-5 Pharmacologic Differences Among Several Antidepressants

Drug	Sedative Action	Antimuscarinic Action	Block of Amine Pump for Serotonin	Norepinephrine	Dopamine
Amitriptyline	+++	+++	+++	++	0
Amoxapine	++	++	+	++	+
Bupropion	0	0	+, 0	+, 0	0
Citalopram, escitalopram	0	0	+++	0	0
Clomipramine	+++	++	+++	+++	0
Desipramine	+	+	0	+++	0
Doxepin	+++	+++	++	+	0
Fluoxetine	+	+	+++	0, +	0, +
Fluvoxamine	0	0	+++	0	0
Imipramine	++	++	+++	++	0
Maprotiline	++	++	0	+++	0
Mirtazapine[a]	+++	0	0	0	0
Nefazodone	++	+++	+, 0	0	0
Nortriptyline	++	++	+++	++	0
Paroxetine	+	0	+++	0	0
Protriptyline	0	++	?	+++	?
Sertraline	+	0	+++	0	0
Venlafaxine	0	0	+++	++	0, +
Trazodone	+++	0	++	0	0

0, None; +, slight; ++, moderate; +++, high; ?, uncertain.

[a]Significant α_2-adrenoceptor antagonist.

From Potter WZ, Hollister, LE. Antidepressant agents. In: Katzung BG, ed. *Basic and Clinical Pharmacology.* 9th ed. New York, NY: McGraw-Hill; 2004. With permission.

Studies have demonstrated that amitriptyline and other tricyclic agents have important NMDA-blocking activity[15,16,32,33] as well as significant and long-acting inhibitory action at the neuronal sodium channel. Renewed research interest has focused on the use of these agents for neural blockade.[17,34]

A randomized trial comparing amitriptyline with nortriptyline showed that despite the study's small sample size, there appeared to be no major differences between the 2 drugs with respect to pain scores, patient satisfaction, disability, preference, or mood. Intolerable side effects were more prevalent in the amitriptyline group.[26] Although most studies have been positive, a randomized controlled trial did study the use of amitriptyline for treatment of spinal cord injury pain compared with the pharmacologically active "placebo" benztropine. The study was conducted over only 6 weeks and did not detect any difference between the groups receiving amitriptyline or benztropine.[35] Recently, the role of coadministration of agents acting on different pharmacologic targets has been advocated. Raja et al[27] compared the tricyclic agents nortriptyline and desipramine with the opioid drugs morphine and methadone in a randomized group of 76 patients with postherpetic neuralgia[36] and reported improved analgesia in postherpetic neuralgia and diabetic neuropathy with combination therapy over either agent alone.

Both opioids and tricyclics had statistically significant analgesic effects relative to placebo; however, more patients (54%) preferred the opioids to the tricyclics (30%) despite similar pain reductions. Interestingly, although opioid agents are commonly thought to induce deleterious cognitive effects, the tricyclics were responsible for significant differences in hand-grooved pegboard tests as well as symbol substitution compared with the opioids.

Other Antidepressants Multiple studies have evaluated the potential role of non-TCAs. Previous studies had demonstrated no difference between placebo and fluoxetine.[19] Based on the study by Max et al,[19] it is believed that drugs with properties of nonspecific reuptake inhibition may be superior as analgesics to those with specific serotonin effects. Venlafaxine, a nonspecific reuptake inhibitor of noradrenaline, serotonin, and some actions on dopamine, has been studied in comparison with imipramine. Interestingly, venlafaxine is similar to amitriptyline in terms of reuptake inhibition pattern. In the comparison with imipramine, the authors found that both agents were effective in a painful diabetic neuropathy model.[37] Another double-blind randomized trial of bupropion for treatment of neuropathic pain also was positive (see Table 91-5).[38]

Duloxetine In contrast to fluoxetine, duloxetine—a nonselective serotonin and norepinephrine reuptake inhibitor—has shown promise in the treatment of neuropathic pain and was approved by the US Food and Drug Administration (FDA) for the treatment of diabetic neuropathy. Duloxetine has also been shown to be safe and effective in relieving many symptoms associated with fibromyalgia independent of concurrent depression[39,40] and is also FDA approved for this indication.

The mechanism of action of duloxetine appears to be descending inhibition, with potent inhibition of reuptake of both norepinephrine and serotonin and weak inhibition of dopamine reuptake (see Fig. 91-7).

Duloxetine has no major active metabolites and a long elimination half-life of approximately 12 hours. In studies of duloxetine 60 and 120 mg/d versus placebo for treatment of diabetic neuropathy, both doses were effective in reducing pain and interfering with nighttime pain. Duloxetine appears to be particularly effective for treatment of nighttime pain severity. Significant depression was not present in the study patients with diabetic neuropathy.[41]

Duloxetine therapy had been considered safe, with only the minor risk of elevated serum transaminase levels. Some cases of cholestatic jaundice and hepatitis have been reported postmarketing. Patients particularly at risk seem to be those with preexisting liver disease, with possible increased risk for further liver damage. Deleterious liver effects may be compounded in patients who consumed substantial amounts of alcohol. Gastrointestinal upset, constipation, and other side effects are common findings with use of the drug.[41]

In studies of patients with both painful physical symptoms and depression, duloxetine 60 mg/d was found to be an effective treatment for both.[42]

Evaluating the primary efficacy measure of Brief Pain Inventory average pain scores, improvements in the duloxetine patient groups averaged 25% to 50%. Side effects included nausea, dry mouth, fatigue, and decreased appetite.

Milnacipran Milnacipran is a dual reuptake inhibitor that blocks uptake of norepinephrine 3 times greater than 5-HT (serotonin) reuptake inhibition. It is indicated for the management of fibromyalgia in the United States as well as an antidepressant in Europe. The half-life is 8 to 10 hours, and the therapeutic dose range is 100 to 200 mg daily in a twice-daily dosing schedule. It is eliminated primarily by the kidney, 55% excreted unchanged in the urine. Unlike duloxetine, it has limited hepatic metabolism. During clinical trials by Mease et al[43] and Clauw et al,[44] a larger proportion of patients treated with milnacipran, compared with placebo, have met the 3 criteria of improvement in pain, physical function, and global assessment. Adverse events include, but not limited, to 7 beats per minute increase in heart rate and a 3 mm Hg increase in systolic and diastolic blood pressure. Nausea is the most common side effect when initiating therapy. The practitioner should therefore follow titration recommendations to enhance compliance. Milnacipran is associated with less weight gain than TCAs.

Opioids Opioid use for treatment of chronic pain has increased considerably over the last 2 decades. In 1980, only 2% of patient visits for chronic musculoskeletal pain conditions resulted in opioid prescriptions. In 2000, this number more than quadrupled to 9%,[45] representing a net increase of 4.6 million prescribed opioid visits compared with 20 years earlier. The increase in total musculoskeletal patient visits over the same time period was negligible, indicating that physician-prescribing practices had changed significantly. The authors[45] theorized that the reasons for increased prescribing were related to advocacy by major pain organizations,[46] increased pharmaceutical company direct marketing campaigns to health care consumers, national guidelines published by the Agency for Health Care Policy and Research,[47] and Joint Commission on Hospital Accreditation emphasis on pain assessment and treatment.[45] Chronic pain patients were increasingly referred by noninstitutionally employed ambulatory care providers to pain specialists, 34% in 1980 versus 49% in 2000.[45] Fewer patients were seen for chronic headache complaints, but more were seen for extremity pain. Unfortunately, these increases in opioid prescribing were not without problems.

Prescription opioid mentions in the Drug Abuse Warning Network from 1994 to 2001 were analyzed.[48] During that period, hydrocodone combinations increased form 9320 to 21 567, an increase of 131%. Similarly, oxycodone combinations increased from 4069 to 18 409, an increase of 352% that has not yet plateaued.[49] The authors of a position statement noted that illicit use of opioid prescriptions had risen faster than legal use of these drugs.[49] They also noted that almost no research had determined the abuse liability of different agents. Nonmedical use had increased from 1% to 3% during that period. In 2000, 2 million people used opioids for nonmedical reasons. Another study noted that opioid analgesics accounted for 9.85% of all drug abuse, an increase of 5.75% from 1997.[48] Increases in illicit use may be due in part to unscrupulous physician behavior, the nature of prescribing to chronic pain patients as a group, and illegal substance diversion by some patients. Theft has risen as a new problem for the Drug Enforcement Agency monitoring illicit drug use. A total of nearly 13 000 theft loss events occurred in 22 eastern US states from 2000 to 2003, including 4.4 million dose units of oxycodone alone.[50]

Use of opioids for pain syndromes has been studied, but adverse effects are troublesome. In a study of neuropathic pain patients resistant to treatment, patients received either high-strength or low-strength levorphanol capsules up to a maximum of 21 capsules per day.[51] Pain intensity, quality of life, psychologic and cognitive function, and blood levels were outcome measures. Patients in the high-strength group took

11.9 capsules (89 mg/d), and those in the low-strength group took 18.3 capsules (2.1 mg/d). Pain was reduced by 36% in the high-strength group versus 21% in the low-strength group. Central poststroke neuropathic pain was least likely to improve. Despite obvious analgesic effects, higher doses produced more side effects without significant additional benefits in terms of other outcome measures. More than a fourth of patients withdrew from the study, and episodic anger and irritability were reported more by the daily group.[51] Although the patients had improvement in symptoms, one wonders if the large number of withdrawals and the anger/irritability issues justify this treatment. In contrast to evidence of efficacy in some patients with neuropathic pain taking daily scheduled opioids, other pain states may not be as efficacious. In a population of patients with intractable head pain, 160 sequential patients were monitored, and 70 of these patients qualified for inclusion in the analysis. Of those reviewed, only 26% had more than 50% pain relief. Multiple problems with compliance including requests for early refills of opioids, lost prescriptions, multiple providers of opioids, and other problems occurred in a remarkable 50% of patients. The authors concluded that daily scheduled opioids were associated with low overall efficacy and an unexpectedly high incidence of maladaptive behaviors.[52]

In response to the study by Caudill-Slosberg et al,[45] an editorial discussed the current state of opioid-prescribing practices and the lack of a clear evidence-driven approach to opioid therapies for chronic noncancer pain syndromes.[53] Evidence-based guidelines have been offered to improve patient selection and adherence monitoring.[54]

In an effort to better manage chronic pain patients taking opioids and to avoid legal and regulatory interference, many pain treatment facilities use an opioid agreement or "contract." To determine the key attributes included in the opioid consumption contracts of major academic centers, Fishman et al[55] evaluated the opioid contracts of 39 academic centers and the major care statements/prohibitions for their core meaning. The most common categories included (1) terms of treatment, (2) prohibited behavior, and (3) points of termination. Rank ordering of statements included (1) improper use of medications, (2) disciplining by termination (for missed appointments, medication abuse, etc), (3) limitations on replacement of lost medications or prescription changes, (4) informing physician of relevant information, including side effects and changes in medical condition, and (5) submission to random drug screens. Unfortunately, little evidence indicates that drug contracts improve patient compliance. Monitoring is an intensely time-consuming task that is not possible to accomplish in many clinical settings. Potentially indispensable statements on opioid treatment, including prohibited usage during pregnancy, driving automobiles, prohibition of alcohol use, and many others, are present in less than half of opioid contracts. Long-term opioid studies of chronic pain syndromes generally consist of small numbers and short duration. Short-term data limit the ability to generalize the reproducibility of opioid treatment outcomes to large groups of chronically treated patients.[54,56]

Opioid Side Effects Rajagopal et al[57] noted significant decreases in sex hormone production in male cancer survivors taking opioids for at least 1 year. Evidence of central hypogonadism, including decreased testosterone and reduced sexual desire, was noted in this group. This finding is similar to those in patients taking chronic intrathecal opioids.[58] Immunologic studies have indicated significant impairment immunologic function caused by opioid therapies, particularly natural killer cell cytotoxicity with chronic opioid use.[59,60] In a mouse model,[61] the covalent agent buprenorphine did not significantly suppress immunity in contrast to fentanyl. This finding suggests that differential effects may be associated with different opioids.

Opioid-Induced Hyperalgesia It is well understood that several agents (eg, TCAs) may provide part of their analgesic activity by augmentation of descending inhibitory pathways from the brainstem to the spinal cord.[14] It also appears that just as there are descending inhibitory pathways, there also are descending *facilitatory pathways.* Animal models suggest that the rostral ventromedial medulla (RVM) contains populations of neurons that are characterized as either *on cells* or *off cells,*[62] which may be an important reason for opioid hyperalgesia and apparent opioid-induced pain. The on cells seem to promote nociception, whereas the off cells seem to inhibit nociceptive neural firing. Morphine and other μ-agonists decrease firing of the on cells and increase activity of the off cells. Cholecystokinin (CCK) appears to be a pro-nociceptive peptide neurotransmitter that is important in decreasing morphine antinociception.[63] Researchers have demonstrated that within the RVM, CCK may augment descending pain facilitation in response to ongoing opioid exposure. In an animal model, continuous morphine significantly increased thermal and tactile hypersensitivity after 3 days, and microdialysis of the RVM demonstrated a 5-fold increase in CCK in the RVM.[64] Previous research had demonstrated that either a lesion of the bilateral dorsolateral funiculus (neuronal tracts used for descending modulation) or lidocaine injection into the RVM could abort evidence of opioid-induced hyperalgesia.[65] Evidence indicates that descending facilitation enhances local spinal cord release of dynorphin (a potent algogenic substance), leading to enhancement of spinal afferent nociceptive receptivity. Continuous morphine infusion leads to increasing spinal dynorphin. Dynorphin then evokes release of excitatory peptides such as calcitonin gene-related peptide and substance P at dorsal root ganglia primary afferents.[66] Injection of dynorphin antiserum abolishes the pro-nociceptive opioid pain facilitation.[66] These studies point to a major change in the way we look at concepts such as opioid tolerance. Increased opioid requirements may be a true tolerance, that is, a rightward shift of dose-response curves, or evidence that opioid-induced descending facilitation is occurring (opioid hyperalgesia). Future research to develop compounds that either block CCK activity in the RVM or block the dynorphin-induced excitatory peptides to allow ongoing analgesia from opioid agents may be indicated.[67]

Tolerance Tolerance can be characterized as the state of physiologic adaptation to a certain level of opioid dosing, recognized as declining effects of the opioid over time. This may be related to downregulation of opioid receptors or accumulation of antianalgesic substances. For example, opioid therapy may cause NMDA receptor activation and induce intracellular cascades that result in activated protein kinase C feedback inhibition on available opioid receptors.[68] Tolerance is predominantly a concept relative to analgesia because a right shift in the dose-response curve occurs over time. Some side effects, such as sedation and cognitive slowing, seem to be less of an issue over time, sometimes resolving within the first 1 to 2 weeks of therapy and being less prominent than with other agents.[27] Tolerance is not seen with other side effects such as urinary retention or opioid-induced constipation, which can be an overwhelming problem with higher doses of these agents. Selective opioid receptor antagonists that are unable to cross the blood–brain barrier have been developed to overcome opioid-induced constipation. Methylnaltrexone is administered subcutaneously, and alvimopan is an oral peripheral μ-opioid antagonist. Both have been shown to effectively cause laxation without reversing opioid analgesia.[69] Alvimopan is an oral, peripherally acting, μ-opioid receptor antagonist for the treatment of opioid-induced bowel dysfunction.[70]

Physical Dependence Physical dependence implies a state of requirement for receptor occupancy to prevent a physiologic withdrawal syndrome after abrupt cessation of an opioid agonist. This state of dependence occurs within days to weeks of starting the sustained delivery of a receptor-specific agonist. In contrast to withdrawal of alcohol, benzodiazepines, barbiturates, and other agents, withdrawal of opioids is rarely a life-threatening situation but nonetheless causes symptoms. Symptoms of opioid withdrawal include piloerection, nausea and vomiting, diarrhea, diaphoresis, agitation, dysphoria, nasal congestion, and seizure. Psychologic dependence is more complex and implies that the patient has an expectation of withdrawal or a fear of lack of analgesia and therefore may resist efforts to taper opioid agents.

Addiction Addiction can be defined as a primary chronic neurobiologic disease, with genetic, psychosocial, and environmental factors influencing its development and manifestations. It is characterized by one or more of the following behaviors: impaired control over drug use, compulsive use, continued use despite harm, and craving.[72]

Pseudoaddiction Weissman and Haddox[73] described a state in which patients who had been given drug doses that were inadequate to control their pain or who had abruptly stopped or were tapered too rapidly from a drug manifested what appeared to be drug-seeking behavior (consistent with addiction). However, in reality the patients simply were experiencing a normal reaction in response to pain that previously was well controlled but now had an acute exacerbation caused iatrogenically. These patients may seem to have significant knowledge of opioid agents and dosages that previously worked for them; thus they appear to be drug seekers.

Equianalgesic dosing tables are commonly used to guide therapy with weak or potent opioids based on equivalent doses (**Table 91-6**). In clinical reality, most patients respond well to opioids dosed in this manner. Sometimes a disparity is observed upon switching to another opioid based on equivalency tables, but the results are generally both safe and "close" to the right dose.

The equianalgesic dosing tables are universally used by pain specialists when switching from one drug to another. The referenced doses for these tables are based on single-dose administrations, so use of these tables for chronic dosing of opioid agents is unclear. Pereira et al[74] reviewed the literature from 1966 to 1999 and determined that the literature lacked studies examining long-term dose ratios and that the published studies were not homogeneous, wide ranges existed, methadone in particular was more potent than originally thought and correlated highly with the dose of previous opioid given, the ratios might change depending on the direction of change, and discrepancies existed with respect to fentanyl and oxycodone.

Many researchers have postulated that use of opioid agents in the future may be determined and administered based on pharmacogenomics. An individual's specific genome likely is better suited for specific agents based on the expression of specific receptor characteristics, variations in metabolic processing, and other features. Cloning of opioid μ-type receptors gives credence to this line of reasoning.[75]

Tamper-Resistant Formulation The increased prescribing of opioids for pain has been associated with escalation of diversion and misuse/abuse of the medications. It is a challenge to balance access of these medications for appropriate use while protecting society from the consequences of abuse of the medications. Attempts to combat the abuse and diversion include increased monitoring such as Researched Abuse, Diversion and Addiction-Related Surveillance (RADARS) System. The RADARS system collects data across the United States through surveys and Poison Control Center reports.[76] Additionally, pharmaceutical companies are being asked to submit plans for opioid Risk Evaluation and Mitigation Strategies as part of the FDA drug approval process to ensure that the benefits of the medications outweigh the risks.[77]

Because many medications that are abused are altered to increase the drug delivery, tamper-resistant medications formulations are being developed. In August, 2010 a new formulation of Oxycontin was released. Although not proven to be safer or less likely to be abused the formulation makes it more challenging to crush or dissolve the tablets for nasal inhalation or intravenous injection. Embeda was a sustained-released morphine with a sequestered core of naltrexone. It has been voluntarily withdrawn from the market due to not meeting predetermined product stability benchmarks by the company. If the pellets inside the capsule are tampered with (eg, by crushing), the naltrexone released antagonizing a significant portion of the morphine. The released naltrexone also can precipitate withdrawal if the patient is opioid tolerant. When taken as directed, the naltrexone does not affect the efficacy of the opioid. These two examples highlight some of the challenges related to combating abuse and diversion of opioid medications. It is probably unlikely that all forms of abuse can be deterred (intravenous injection vs intranasal vs swallowing increased dosage of whole pills. Additionally manufacturing complexity may limit pharmaceutical company investment.[78]

Opioids in Neuropathic Pain Opioid use for many pain states is supported by randomized controlled drug studies showing efficacy. Although often characterized as an opioid-resistant type of pain, neuropathic pain syndromes may have the most hearty evidence for efficacy with opioid therapies.[27,79-83] The major neuropathic pain studies generally have examined patients with postherpetic neuralgia, painful diabetic peripheral neuropathy, or central pain syndromes, including postspinal cord injury and postcerebrovascular accident pain. For example, Watson and Babul[79] performed a randomized controlled trial involving 50 patients with postherpetic neuralgia and symptom duration of at least 3 months. In this study, 38 patients completed the study, which compared oxycodone tablets at a dose up to 30-mg controlled-release agent twice daily compared with placebo. Pain scores of patients showed improvement in pain relief of 2.9 points versus 1.8 points for the placebo group and a decrease in allodynia and steady and paroxysmal pain.[79] Raja et al[27] compared the TCA agent amitriptyline to morphine or methadone in a total of 76 patients with postherpetic neuralgia symptoms of long duration. Three treatment periods were studied over 24 weeks, with administration of opioid, TCA, and placebo. Interestingly, although both the TCA and opioid groups had improvements in study end points, 54% of patients favored opioids compared with 30% who favored the TCA. Methadone is commonly thought to be superior to other opioids for treatment of neuropathic pain because of its dual action on μ-opioid receptors as well as NMDA receptors, but this was not demonstrated in the study. In patients with intolerance to morphine, patients switched to methadone achieved doses of only 15 mg versus 91 mg for morphine. Reduction in pain intensity was less for methadone (1.2 points on a visual analogue scale compared with a pain scale reduction of 2.2 points with morphine). Another interesting finding of this study was that although most pain practitioners commonly attribute side effects such as psychomotor and cognitive slowing to opioids, patients taking the TCA actually performed worse on pegboard placement skills and other tests of psychomotor skills.[27]

Tapentadol (Nucynta) A new molecule combines the effect of μ-agonism and norepinephrine reuptake inhibition, and therefore it works on ascending and descending pathways. This new drug embodies the concept of the multimechanistic approach into the treatment of acute pain. Although the long-acting formulation is not available yet, several studies have shown its efficacy in multiple chronic pain entities.[84-87]

The 75-mg dose is equivalent to oxycodone 10 mg in acute pain model. However, it achieves pain control with lesser μ-agonism. Hence the side effects of that stimulation are decreased (eg, less nausea and vomiting). It is metabolized in the liver by conjugation with inactive metabolites. The parent drug and its metabolites are eliminated via renal clearance. Time of maximal concentration is 1.25 hours, and its half-life is 4 hours.

NMDA Antagonists With our enhanced understanding of the development of both peripheral and central sensitization (windup) and the role of excitatory amino acids acting at NMDA receptors, blockade of this central hyperalgesic response has assumed greater therapeutic importance. Likewise, use of NMDA blockers for opioid tolerance and opioid-induced hyperalgesia is a reasonable therapy. Currently available NMDA blockers include ketamine, methadone, dextromethorphan, amantadine, magnesium, and memantine.

Methadone Methadone, an opioid first synthesized in the mid-twentieth century, has become the agent most commonly used for management of long-term opioid addiction. Methadone is highly lipophilic and has high oral bioavailability. Unlike many modern-era formulated long-acting continuous relief opioids, it is inherently long acting. The drug is a racemic mixture[88]; the D-isomer reverses morphine tolerance and blocks development of hyperalgesia thought to be mediated by NMDA receptor activation.[89] Methadone is useful for both the treatment of neuropathic pain and the management of cancer pain, predominantly as a second-line agent when other opioids become ineffective. The

TABLE 91-6 Opioid Analgesics for Adults Aged 15 Years or Older

Drug	IM Dose	IM Duration (h)	Starting Oral Dose	Comments
Agonists Related to Morphine				
Morphine	10 mg	3-6	15-30 mg	Available as 8-12-h sustained-release tablets (MS-Contin, Oramorph-SR), 12-24-h sustained-release capsules (Kadian-Nonformulary), and suppository Oral: Prompt release: 15-30 mg every 4 h as needed; controlled release: 15-30 mg every 8-12 h IV PCA: Usual 1-3 mg (range: 0.1-5 mg); lockout interval: usual 5-20 min; 4-h lockout (usual range: 10-30 mg), maximum 30 mg IV, SC continuous infusion: 0.8-10 mg/h; may increase depending on pain relief/adverse effects
Embeda morphine/naltrexone[a]	N/A		20 mg/0.8 mg	Embeda is morphine sulfate with sequestered naltrexone 100 g/4 mg available as low as 20 mg QD or BID dosing
Hydromorphone dilaudid	1 mg	3-5	4-8 mg	Available as high-potency injectable (Dilaudid-HP) and as suppository
Hydromorphone sustained release (Exalgo)	–	–	8 mg/d	24-h formulation that uses the OROS delivery system. Available in 8, 12, 16 mg. Approved by the FDA for opioid-tolerant patients
Oxymorphone IV (Numorphan)	1 mg	4-6	10 mg PO	PO formulation is 2-3 times compared with MS. Bioavailability is 10/1
Opana IR	–	4-6	10 mg	
Opana ER	–		5-10 mg PO	Dosed every 12 h
Agonists Related to Codeine				
Codeine	15 mg	3-5	30-60 mg	60 mg PO equivalent to 650 mg of aspirin or acetaminophen; usually used orally in combinations with these drugs; some patients resistant to analgesic effect
Hydrocodone (Vicodin, others)	–	–	5 mg	10 mg PO equivalent to codeine 80 mg PO; available in combinations
Oxycodone (Roxicodone, others)	–	–	5 mg	10 mg PO equivalent to codeine 90 mg PO; available in combinations and as 12-h sustained-release tablets (OxyContin)
Synthetic opioid agonists				
Meperidine (Demerol, others)	50-100 mg	2-4	50 mg	Irritating to tissues IM; toxic metabolite with long half-life causes CNS excitation and convulsions
Fentanyl (Sublimaze)	0.1 mg	1-2	–	Transdermal patch (Duragesic) for chronic pain releases fentanyl over 72 h, possibly with less constipation than morphine; Actiq "Transmucosal system" FDA approved for breakthrough pain
Methadone (Dolophine; others)	10 mg	4-6	10-20 mg	Long half-life; risk of CNS depression with repeated use
Propoxyphene HCl (Darvon, others)	–	–	65 mg	65 mg of HCl or 100 mg of napsylate PO equivalent to codeine 32 mg PO; available in combinations with acetaminophen or aspirin; toxic metabolite with long half-life causes convulsions and cardiotoxicity; not better than plain acetaminophen; use discouraged in the elderly
Levorphanol (Levo-Dromoran, others)	2 mg	4-6	2-4 mg	Long half-life; risk of CNS depression with repeated use
Tramadol (Ultram)	–	–	50-100 mg q6h	50 mg equivalent to codeine 60 mg; 100 mg comparable with aspirin 650 mg plus codeine 60 mg
Tapentadol (Nucynta)	–	–	50-100 mg q4-6h	75 mg is equivalent to 10 mg of oxycodone
Partial Agonists and Mixed Agonist/Antagonists				
Buprenorphine (Buprenex, others)	0.3 mg	4-6	–	Partial agonist; virtually no psychotomimetic effects; sublingual preparation effective
Pentazocine (Talwin-NX, Talacen) nonformulary; use discouraged	60 mg	2-4	50 mg	Mixed agonist/antagonist; 60 mg PO equivalent to codeine 60 mg PO, very irritating to tissues; psychotomimetic effects; available in combinations with acetaminophen, aspirin, or naloxone (to discourage IV drug abuse)
Butorphanol (Stadol) nonformulary	1-2 mg	3-6	–	Mixed agonist/antagonist; nasal spray (Stadol NS 1 mg/spray) comparable to IM injection
Nalbuphine (Nubain, others)	10 mg	3-6	–	Mixed agonist/antagonist; less psychotomimetic effect than pentazocine
Dezocine (Dalgan) nonformulary	10 mg	3-6	–	Mixed agonist/antagonist

[a]This drug has been removed from the US market.

CNS, central nervous system; FDA, Food and Drug Administration; N/A, not applicable.

From Inpatient Pain Service Guidelines. MC4398. Mayo Foundation for Medical Education and Research. Mayo Foundation, 2001. With permission.

equianalgesic dosing ratio seems to increase with increasing opioid doses and may exceed 10:1 compared with morphine.[90] Dosing paradigms to change from other opioids[91] have been designed to more effectively load the drug and prevent respiratory depression secondary to methadone's prolonged pharmacologic actions. Possible side effects at high doses include QT-interval prolongation and a propensity to sudden cardiac death.[92] Patients receiving higher doses may be reasonably monitored for QT-interval prolongation.

Ketamine Ketamine, a noncompetitive antagonist at the NMDA receptor, has been found efficacious in the treatment of primary neuropathic pain and hyperalgesic states in both intravenous (IV) and oral applications. When used orally, the drug appears to work primarily through its metabolite norketamine.[93] Psychomimetic effects appear to be most limiting, although the deleterious side effects were minimized at lower doses (40-60 mg/d) and when coupled with oral benzodiazepine therapy. Ketamine therapy has been attempted as intermittent IV infusion for chronic neuropathic pain states such as postherpetic neuralgia[94] and for posttraumatic pain,[95] with some apparent efficacy. In a small study comparing ketamine with magnesium (another NMDA antagonist), ketamine administered IV at 0.3 mg/kg/h resulted in significant improvement in a group of patients with neuropathic pain, but magnesium did not reach significance.[96] Other NMDA agents have been used with inconclusive results. A double-blind placebo-controlled trial of the agent memantine in postherpetic neuralgia patients did not show separation from the placebo group in terms of allodynia, spontaneous pain, or hyperalgesia; both groups improved. The authors concluded that the agent was ineffective in reducing postherpetic pain.[97] Dextromethorphan also has been studied, with inconclusive results. In a randomized double-blind controlled trial of 2 doses of dextromethorphan over a 10-day treatment period, no clinically significant difference between any of the tested outcome measures was observed.[98] Amantadine, better known as an agent for parkinsonism or influenza prophylaxis, is a noncompetitive NMDA antagonist and has been well tolerated from a side-effect profile. IV infusion of amantadine was evaluated for treatment of surgical neuropathic pain (postmastectomy, postthoracotomy, postherniorrhaphy). Amantadine reduced both mean pain intensity and hyperalgesic "windup" pain on a statistically significant basis.[99]

Overall, the NMDA antagonists appear to have therapeutic potential; further well-designed randomized trials with larger numbers of patients are necessary to form conclusions. At this time, methadone and ketamine appear to have better evidence supporting their use.

Clinical Rationale for Antiepileptic Drugs In neuropathic pain, changes in sodium channel expression lead to alterations and accumulation in sensory nerves and nociceptive neural pathways. Voltage-gated sodium channels have critical functions in the neuronal transmission of action potentials. They also play an important role in the genesis of neuropathic pain via an increase in neuronal excitability. For the development of neuropathic pain, complete expression of $Na_V1.8$ seems to be necessary.[100] It appears that injured axons are functionally degraded and do not play a role in neuropathic pain. However, the role of neighboring C-fibers that are not injured appears to expand, with C-fibers playing an important role in the development of aberrant pain transmission (**Fig. 91-8**).

Thus redistribution of the tetrodotoxin-resistant sodium channels $Na_V1.8$ and $Na_V1.9$ to peripheral sites of injury is critical in the development of neuropathic pain. These sodium channel subunits congregate near the site of injury and result in spontaneous neural ectopic firing. Likewise, in addition to the $Na_V1.8$ and $Na_V1.9$ sodium channels, β3 is found in increased concentration at the site of nerve injury. β3 messenger RNA is found in increased concentration within these neurons. Neuropathic pain and epilepsy have functional similarities. In animal models of limbic epilepsy, sodium channel expression and upregulation of $Na_V1.3$ were increased, and changes in β subunits occurred. Thus the ability pharmacologically to block these redistributed, uninjured, unmyelinated C-fiber sodium channels may be the most useful approach to therapy for neuropathic pain caused by partial nerve injuries.

Calcium channels may be altered in neuropathic pain states. A commonly used neural constriction injury animal model shows that, after peripheral ligation injury, the $\alpha_1\delta_1$ segment of the calcium channel is upregulated in dorsal ganglion neuropathy. This change is associated with the production of tactile allodynia (**Table 91-7**).[101]

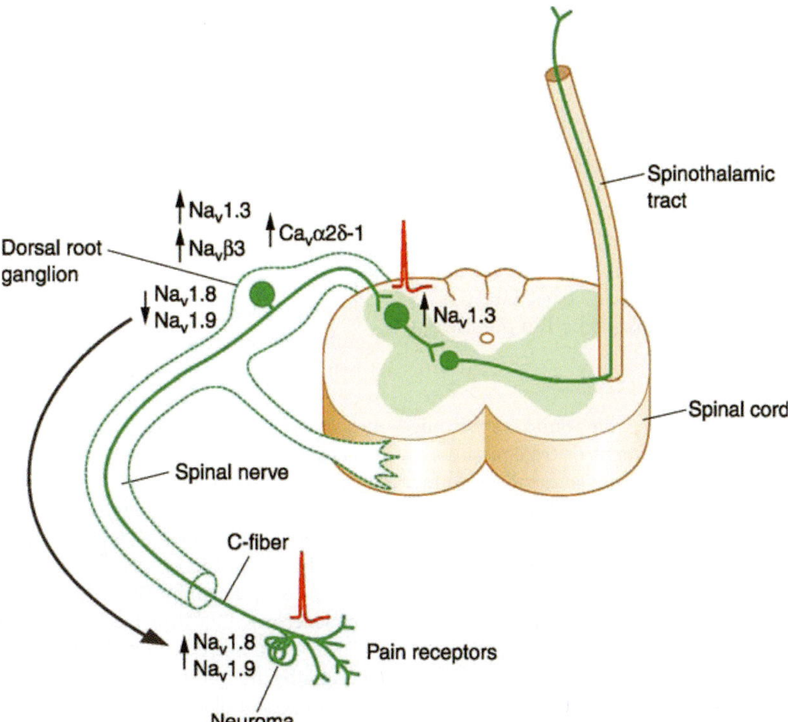

FIGURE 91-8. Injury to peripheral axons results in redistribution of tetrodotoxin-resistant sodium channel subunits ($Na_V1.8$, $Na_V1.9$) from normal areas, leading to spontaneous ectopic firing at sites of injury. Other sodium channel ($Na_V\beta3$) and calcium channel ($Ca_V\alpha2\delta\text{-}1$) alterations also may cause increased neuronal activity. [Reprinted from Rogawski GA, Loscher W. The neurobiology of antiepileptic drugs for the treatment of nonepileptic conditions. *Nat Med.* 2004;10:685-692. With permission.]

TABLE 91-7 Neuropathic Pain States

Vascular	Postischemic myelopathy, central poststroke pain
Infectious	HIV myelopathy, CMV sensory neuropathy; Lyme disease neuropathy, postherpetic neuralgia
Metabolic/nutritional	Thiamine (beriberi) deficiency neuropathy, Niacin (pellagra) deficiency neuropathy, diabetic neuropathy, alcoholic neuropathy
Traumatic/iatrogenic	Postsurgical: postmastectomy syndrome, postnephrectomy syndrome, postthoracotomy syndrome; complex regional pain syndrome, phantom limb pain, brachial plexus avulsion injury; traumatic spinal injury; syringomyelia; postradiation myelopathy
Hereditary	Fabry disease, Guillain-Barré neuropathy
Toxic	Arsenic, thallium, mercury, others
Compressive	Spinal stenosis, foraminal stenosis, entrapment syndromes: carpal tunnel, cubital tunnel, tarsal tunnel, pronator teres, syndrome, others
Inflammatory	Radiculopathy, diabetic lumbosacral radiculoplexopathy, inflammatory demyelinating polyradiculopathy
Drug-induced	Cis-platinum, vincristine, paclitaxel (Taxol), isoniazid, stavudine, zalcitabine
Neoplastic	Nerve infiltration, brachial plexus compression (eg, Pancoast tumor)
Idiopathic	Idiopathic sensory neuropathy, multiple sclerosis, Parkinson disease
Neuropathic pain may be due to a variety of different causes that may have treatment implications	

CMV, cytomegalovirus; HIV, human immunodeficiency virus.

Evidence indicates that neuronal-type voltage-gated calcium channels play a role in neuropathic pain induced by peripheral nerve injury. Agents have been developed for intrathecal use acting via the ω-conopeptide, which is known to inhibit N-type–gated calcium channels.[102] Gabapentin suppresses allodynia. Dorsal root ganglion $\alpha_2\delta$ upregulation likely plays a significant role in the neuroplasticity of pain expression after peripheral nerve injuries and contributes to allodynia development. Peripheral but not central axonal injury significantly upregulates the expression of dorsal root ganglion $\alpha_2\delta$ calcium channel subunits. These precede the onset of allodynia. Evidence also indicates that messenger RNA upregulation occurs after spinal nerve ligation. In a rat model, the L5-L6 dorsal root ganglions ipsilateral to nerve injury showed a 6- to 7-fold increase of $\alpha_2\delta$ expression at 7 days. Likewise, as recovery from tactile allodynia occurs, the upregulation in dorsal root ganglion $\alpha_2\delta$ subunits diminishes.[101]

Specific Anticonvulsant Agents

Carbamazepine Carbamazepine is a tricyclic compound chemically similar to imipramine. It is effective for treatment of trigeminal neuralgia and has long been the drug of choice.[103] It also has been found useful for treatment of bipolar disorder and seizures.[104] No studies have compared imipramine with other recently released anticonvulsants for treatment of trigeminal neuralgia. The drug acts chiefly by blocking sodium channels and is thought to be most useful for treatment of shooting or lancinating types of pain. In experimental neuromas, peripherally located ectopic discharges are suppressed within the typical ranges of serum concentrations.[105] In patients, dosing generally begins at 100-200 mg/d and can be titrated very slowly (4-8 wk) up to 1200 mg/d. Significant side effects can occur, including agranulocytosis, aplastic anemia, hepatic function abnormalities, and Stevens-Johnson syndrome. The chief drawback to use of carbamazepine is poor tolerability in elderly patients, often related to diplopia, sedation, and ataxia.

TABLE 91-8 Anticonvulsant Therapies for Neuropathic/Headache Pain

Drug	Neuropathic Pain	Trigeminal Neuralgia	Migraine Prophylaxis
Phenytoin	+	++	0
Carbamazepine	++	++	0
Oxcarbazepine	++	+	0
Lamotrigine	++	++	+
Zonisamide	+	0	+
Valproate	+	+	++
Topiramate	+	+	++
Gabapentin	++	+	++
Levetiracetam	++	0	+
Benzodiazepines	+	+	0
Tiagabine	+	0	+
Pregabalin	++	?	?

Reprinted and modified from Rogawski MA, Loscher W. The neurobiology of antiepileptic drugs for the treatment of nonepileptic conditions. *Nat Med.* 2004;10:685-692, with permission from Macmillan Publishers Ltd.

In particular, combining carbamazepine with structurally similar agents (such as TCAs) may enhance sedating side effects.[104] Drug interactions may occur due to carbamazepine induction of hepatic microsomal enzymes. Monitoring of carbamazepine should include baseline serum hepatic function tests, complete blood counts, and serum sodium, with particular screening for complications in the first 4 to 6 months of therapy. Carbamazepine is commonly used for treatment of diabetic peripheral neuropathy and other neuropathic pain conditions.[104,107] **Table 91-8** compares various anticonvulsant therapies for neuropathic pain, migraine headache, and trigeminal neuralgia.

Oxcarbazepine Oxcarbazepine is an antiepileptic drug chemically similar to carbamazepine. The drug acts at voltage-gated sodium and calcium channels to block epileptiform or ectopic discharges. The major clinical advantage to carbamazepine may be the requirement for less frequent serum monitoring.

Although carbamazepine may induce agranulocytosis, hyponatremia, and hepatic function abnormalities, it appears that hyponatremia is the only reason for ongoing generalized serum monitoring of this agent. An open-label, 9-week trial of 30 patients with diabetic painful neuropathy demonstrated improvement of patients' visual analogue pain scores of 29 points (48.3%), with side effects of dizziness and drowsiness. Other studies have demonstrated improvements in pain with use of oxcarbazepine.[108-110] Additional randomized controlled studies with oxcarbazepine are needed to predict the effects of this agent reliably in various pain syndromes.

Topiramate Topiramate is a substituted monosaccharide agent that is significantly different from other anticonvulsant drugs. Topiramate has 3 main mechanisms of action. Like other anticonvulsants, the drug is a sodium channel blocker, with some action at voltage-gated calcium channels. It can potentiate γ-aminobutyric acid (GABA)-mediated inhibition at separate sites from the benzodiazepines. Interest also has focused on its action at the kainate and α-amino-3-hydroxy-5-methylisoxazole-4-propionic acid (AMPA) receptors, where it can decrease excitatory amino acid (glutamate) neurotransmission. Topiramate has found its greatest use in headache therapy as a preventive agent for migraine headache. Large trials have demonstrated significant decreases in migraine headache prevalence when the drug has been used as a preventive agent.[111,112]

Three randomized controlled trials of topiramate for painful diabetic neuropathy did not support a statistically significant difference between topiramate and placebo in visual analogue scores or any of the secondary efficacy end points.[113] However, pain reductions were numerically greater in the topiramate study groups in 2 of the studies. Patients were allowed rescue analgesia throughout this study, and it was believed that this may have confounded the results. In another randomized controlled trial, patients with painful diabetic neuropathy were found to have evidence of analgesia with topiramate. In this study, rescue analgesia was only permitted for a 6-week period. The major findings of the study were that pain visual analogue scores decreased from 68 to 46.2 in the topiramate groups versus a decrease from 69 to 54 in the placebo group ($p < 0.003$). Fifty percent of the topiramate patients versus 34% of the placebo patients had more than a 30% response.[114] The other notable finding was that topiramate reduced body weight significantly versus placebo. The weight loss had no adverse effect on serum glycemic control of diabetic patients. Topiramate has been used in diet clinics to aid weight loss and has been used for essential tremor, binge eating disorders, and bipolar disorder.[104] In a study of patients taking topiramate for epilepsy, weight reduction was maintained in 86% of patients despite a return of caloric intake to normal baseline levels. Obese patients appeared to develop reductions in weight of greater magnitude than patients who were not obese.[115] Thus it appears that topiramate is potentially an ideal agent for patients with obesity, diabetes, and painful neuropathy or migraine.

Topiramate is generally started at 25 mg at night and ramped higher every 1 to 2 weeks on a twice-daily schedule to a target dose of 200 to 400 mg/d. Patient side effects are frequent and include cognitive slowing, somnolence, nervousness, fatigue, dizziness, and diarrhea.[104] As with all anticonvulsants, female patients with the potential for pregnancy should be using birth control because of the risks of teratogenicity and altered effectiveness of birth control pills.[104]

Gabapentin Gabapentin is a GABA analogue that binds to the α2-δ1 ligand of voltage-sensitive neuronal calcium channels.[116] There is no evidence that it functions through GABA-mediated actions despite its structural similarity with GABA. Gabapentin is approved by the FDA for adjunctive therapy of tonic-clonic and partial seizures and for postherpetic neuralgia at doses of 1800 mg or more. Early case series showed the drug had some efficacy in other neuropathic pain syndromes, including complex regional pain syndrome.[117] Subsequently, several excellent-quality randomized studies demonstrated the efficacy of gabapentin for a variety of neuropathic pain syndromes (**Tables 91-8 and 91-9**).[118-123]

Backonja et al[117] found that gabapentin was effective for the symptomatic treatment of neuropathic pain in patients with diabetes mellitus. The study compared 70 patients who received gabapentin and 65 who completed the study in the placebo group. Using an intent-to-treat analysis, gabapentin-treated patients had significantly lower mean daily pain scores ($p < 0.001$) compared with placebo patients. Pain scores decreased in the active gabapentin group from 6.4 at baseline to 3.9 compared with baseline scores of 6.5 versus 5.1 at end in the placebo group. Additionally, secondary outcome measures were significantly better in the gabapentin group, including the Short-Form 36 (SF-36) quality-of-life questionnaire and profile of mood states. Similar to other anticonvulsants, gabapentin should be titrated slowly to maximum doses of 3600 mg/d, usually dosed on a 3 to 4 times per day schedule secondary to the short half-life of 5 to 8 hours.[104] Gabapentin is not metabolized, and, unlike carbamazepine, it does not induce hepatic enzymatic function. It is eliminated by the kidneys, and dosage should be reduced according to creatinine clearance in renally impaired patients. Adverse events include somnolence, peripheral edema, memory loss (usually high doses), dry mouth, dizziness, and nausea.

Pregabalin Pregabalin is an agent that causes inhibition at the neuronal calcium ion channel. This mechanism of action and its molecular structure are similar to gabapentin, which has perhaps become the first-line broad-spectrum agent used for many painful neuropathic syndromes. Pregabalin has been found to bind selectively at the $\alpha_2\delta_1$ subunit, an auxiliary protein commonly associated with voltage-gated calcium channels.[116]

Pregabalin binding causes reduction of calcium influx and neurotransmitter release, including substance P, glutamate, and noradrenaline.[124]

In a randomized double-blind, controlled trial, patients received placebo or 150 mg or 300 mg daily of pregabalin, and primary end points

TABLE 91-9 Pharmacologic Therapy for Neuropathic Pain in Peripheral Neuropathy

Medication	Starting Doses	Maintenance Doses and Comments
First Line		
Gabapentin	100-300 mg TID	↑ by 300-400-mg increments every 5-7 d to 3600 mg daily divided in 3-4 doses
Tricyclic antidepressants	10-25 mg qhs	↑ by 10-25-mg increments every 7 d to 100-150 mg qhs; titration can continue following blood levels (stay below 500 ng/mL) and ECG
Tramadol	50 mg QD or BID	↑ by 50-g increments every 5-7 d to a maximum of 100 mg QID
Second Line		
Lamotrigine	25 mg GD or BID	After 2 weeks, ↑ by 25-mg increments weekly to 100-200 mg BID
Carbamazepine	100-200 mg QD or BID	↑ by 100-200 mg every 7 d to 600 mg QD in divided doses; titration can continue following blood levels; extended-release forms can be given on BID schedule
Bupropion SR	150 mg QD	After 1 week, ↑ to 150 mg BID
Venlafaxine XR	75 mg QD	↑ by 75-mg increments every 7 d to 150-225 mg QD
Opiate analgesics	Varying doses; initiate with short-acting agent QID PM	After 1-2 wk, replace with longer-acting agent on QD or BID schedule; careful titration is necessary
Topical Agents		
Capsaicin 0.075%	Apply TID or QID	Continue with starting dose; may be considered

From Sindrup SH, Jensen TS. Review article: Efficacy of pharmacological treatments of neuropathic pain: an update in effect related to mechanism of drug action. *Pain.* 1999;83: 389-400.

included decreased mean pain scores, health-related quality of life, and SF-36 health survey scores. Overall, patients with postherpetic neuralgia had significantly lower pain scores and less sleep interference.[125] In another group of patients with painful diabetic peripheral neuropathy, a placebo-controlled trial demonstrated significant improvements in pain scores and sleep interference.[126] Pregabalin may be better tolerated than gabapentin, and less dose titration is necessary. Pregabalin has been reported to cause symptoms of somnolence, dizziness, and peripheral edema, which are similar to side effects reported with gabapentin.[126] Drug dosage can be started at 50 mg 2 or 3 times daily and increased to 100 mg 3 times daily by 1 week. The drug has been scheduled for both diabetic peripheral neuropathy and postherpetic neuralgia by the FDA. Dosages should be reduced for renal impairment based on creatinine clearance similar to gabapentin.

Levetiracetam Levetiracetam is a novel oral antiepileptic drug with structural features unrelated to those of other antiepileptic drugs. Most antiepileptic drugs are screened for inhibition of epileptiform activity by maximal electroshock or pentylenetetrazol seizure induction. Levetiracetam antiepileptic action seems to occur via inhibition of neuronal hypersynchronization.[127] Levetiracetam appears to have minimal interactions with other agents. It causes occasional increased drowsiness and cognitive dysfunction and may place patients at risk for driving or other activities exacerbated by cognitive dysfunction or altered wakefulness. It has a low protein binding (<10%) and is not hepatically metabolized.[104] Small case series have described 3 patients who achieved partial or complete relief of pain related to sensory motor peripheral neuropathy.[128] At this time, levetiracetam-controlled studies are limited, and no comparison studies exist for other more commonly used antiepileptic drugs.

Lamotrigine Lamotrigine is thought to act similarly to phenytoin in decreasing rapid firing of neurons. It causes use-dependent inhibition of voltage-gated sodium channels.[104] Several studies have demonstrated the efficacy of lamotrigine in a variety of pain syndromes, but because of side effects it is generally relegated to second-line therapy.

In a randomized controlled study of 59 patients with painful diabetic neuropathy, lamotrigine was titrated from 25 mg/d up to 400 mg/d over a 6-week period compared with similar titration of placebo. The lamotrigine group improved compared with the placebo group, and the authors concluded lamotrigine was both safe and effective.[129] Lamotrigine also has been studied in HIV-associated neuropathy, with a small improvement seen compared with the placebo group. In this study, the titration schedule was very slow and similar to that used in other studies, beginning at 25 mg/d up to 300 mg/d over 7 weeks. Despite the gradual titration, the dropout rate was high, with 5 of the 13 dropouts from a sample of 42 patients citing rash.[130] Among a group of 14 patients with refractory trigeminal neuralgia, those given lamotrigine improved significantly better than those on placebo. Although the patients already were taking either phenytoin or carbamazepine, these drugs were continued during the study. The one patient who withdrew from the study did so during the placebo arm of this crossover design.[131]

In a randomized double-blind, placebo-controlled crossover study, lamotrigine was given to 30 patients with spinal cord injury pain syndromes. The drug was titrated from an initial 25 mg/d dosage up to 400 mg/d over a 9-week period, compared with a 9-week placebo titration. There was a 2-week washout period between each arm of the study. Twenty-two patients completed the trial. Daily numerical pain scale in the group treated with lamotrigine was reduced from 6.4 ± 0.1 to 4.2 ± 0.1, and numerical pain scales decreased from 6.5 ± 0.1 to 5.3 ± 0.1 in the control group. The difference between groups was statistically significant ($p < 0.001$ at lamotrigine doses of 200-300 and 400 mg). The primary finding of this study was that, in patients with incomplete spinal cord injuries, lamotrigine significantly reduced the pain at the same level of injury or below the level of injury. Patients who had evidence of central sensitization (windup pain) and brush-evoked allodynia were more likely to have a positive response to lamotrigine. The drug appeared to have no effect in patients with complete spinal cord injuries. The drug was generally well tolerated.[132]

Lamotrigine most notably has been associated with the development of Stevens-Johnson syndrome (a severe exfoliating dermatitis that can be a dermatologic emergency). Pediatric patients may be most prone to these dermatologic complications, which may be seen in up to 1% to 2% of patients in that age group.[104] Significant evidence now indicates that lamotrigine has a role in the treatment of various neuropathic pain syndromes, but side effects (particularly rash) must be closely monitored, and patients must adhere to a slow titration schedule.

Tiagabine Tiagabine has not been studied in a randomized fashion for treatment of pain syndromes. Tiagabine is an inhibitor of the GABA transporter protein GAT-1. It also acts as a GABA reuptake inhibitor, thus increasing available GABA within neuronal synapses and surrounding glia.[104] An open-label study of tiagabine compared with gabapentin in 91 patients with chronic pain suggested that both drugs were efficacious.[133] Notably, the effects of tiagabine on sleep quality in this study suggest that it may be useful for patients who have both pain and sleep disturbances. Further randomized studies will clarify its role in pain management.

Phenytoin Phenytoin has been used for several decades for treatment of epilepsy, cardiac arrhythmias, and various pain syndromes. Phenytoin alters Na^+, Ca^{2+}, and K^+ conductance and inhibits repetitive high-frequency discharges.[104] Phenytoin was used in a study of 40 patients with painful diabetic neuropathy who received either the active drug 100 mg 3 times per day or placebo for 2 weeks, followed by a 1-week washout period before crossing over to the other group. In group 1, 70% of the phenytoin patients versus 25% of the placebo patients had decreased pain. In group 2, similarly 78% of the phenytoin patients had improved scores pain compared with 28% of the placebo patients. Nearly a fourth of the phenytoin patients had complete relief.[134] Although phenytoin is cost effective, it does have significant side effects, including gingival hyperplasia, hirsutism, and rash. Long-term use can result in peripheral neuropathy.[104] One advantage of phenytoin is its availability in IV form. A study of IV infusion of 15 mg/kg phenytoin in patients with neuropathic pain resulted in significant improvement of several features of altered nerve conduction (shooting pain, burning pain, sensitivity, and numbness). The investigator concluded that IV phenytoin could be useful for acute flares of pain (**Table 91-10**).[135]

Topical Agents During a 1-week open-phase segment of a pilot trial studying the analgesic efficacy of a topical formulation of 1% amitriptyline and 0.5% ketamine, 11 patients had a significant analgesic effect for a variety of different neuropathic pain syndromes, including postherpetic neuralgia and painful diabetic peripheral neuropathy. In a follow-up of this initial pilot trial, 92 patients with mixed neuropathic pain syndromes, including postherpetic neuralgia, postsurgical, posttraumatic neuropathic pain, and diabetic neuropathy with evidence of allodynia, hyperalgesia, and pinprick hypesthesia, were randomly assigned to receive placebo, 2% amitriptyline, or 1% ketamine, combined with a primary outcome measure of change in average daily pain intensity.[136] Unfortunately, a reduction in pain score of 1.1 to 1.5 units was observed in all groups, and there were no differences between the groups. Blood concentrations showed no significant systemic absorption. Other studies have shown that higher doses may be required to produce significant analgesia.[137] This abstract detailed a comparison of high-dose amitriptyline-ketamine (4% amitriptyline/2% ketamine) cream for 1 week. Of the 129 subjects who responded, 118 patients were randomized to receive either high dose (4% amitriptyline/2% ketamine) or low dose (2% amitriptyline/1% ketamine) cream, or a placebo cream for 2 additional weeks. After 3 weeks of treatment, results showed the high-dose group had average daily pain intensity that decreased from 6.5 to 3.28 versus the placebo pain intensity score of 4.34. There was no difference between the placebo and the low-dose group. The percentage of subjects with 30% reduction was superior to placebo for patient sleep quality and global satisfaction. Plasma levels were detectable in less than 10% of subjects and were well below therapeutic levels. Topical cream was well tolerated. This finding may imply that, compared with the study by Lynch et al,[136] higher concentrations of amitriptyline-ketamine cream are required to produce analgesia for mixed neuropathic pain syndromes.

Older topical agents for treatment of neuropathic pain include capsaicin. A multicenter double-blind, vehicle control study was conducted by the capsaicin study group.[138] The trial was conducted over 8 weeks, and either capsaicin or vehicle cream was applied to painful areas 4 times per day. Pain intensity and relief were recorded every 2 weeks using the physician's global evaluation as well as visual analogue pain scales. A total of 252 patients were studied. Capsaicin showed 69.5% versus 53.4% improvement according to the physician's global evaluation scale, and 38.1% versus 27.4% decrease in pain intensity (see Tables 91-9 and 91-10). Other studies have also demonstrated efficacy for chronic postherpetic neuralgia.[139] As in previous studies, initial burning at the application site was noted. The mechanism of action of capsaicin is depletion of substance P at peripheral thermal receptors, a process that can take several weeks. Over the past decade, capsaicin has been used less frequently by pain physicians secondary to poor tolerance of the drug when used by patients with postherpetic neuralgia and other peripheral neuropathic conditions.

Intravenous Analgesics

Intravenous Lidocaine Therapy IV lidocaine has been used for the last 2 decades for the control of predominantly neuropathic pain syndromes.

TABLE 91-10 Number Needed to Treat to Obtain One Patient With More Than 50% Pain Relief[a]

	Painful Neuropathy	Postherpetic Neuralgia	Peripheral Nerve Injury	Central Pain	Trigeminal Neuralgia
Antidepressants					
Antidepressants all types	3.0 (2.4-4.0)	2.3 (1.7-3.3)	2.5 (1.4-10.6)	1.7 (1.1-3.0)	ND
TCA all types	2.4 (2.0-3.0)	2.3 (1.7-3.3)	2.5 (1.4-10.6)	1.7 (1.1-3.0)	ND
TCA serotoninergic/noradrenergic	2.0 (1.7-2.5)	2.4 (1.8-3.9)	2.5 (1.4-10.6)	1.7 (1.1-3.0)	ND
TCA noradrenergic	3,4 (2.3-6.6)	1.9 (1.3-3.7)	ND	ND	ND
Optimal dose	1.4 (1.1-1.9)	ND	ND	ND	ND
SSRI	6.7 (3.4-435)	ND	ND	NA	ND
Ion Channel Blockers					
Mexiletine	10.0 (3-∞)	ND	ND	NA	ND
Phenytoin	2.1 (1.5-3.6)	ND	ND	ND	ND
Carbamazepine	3.3 (2-9.4)	ND	ND	3.4 (1.7-105)	2.6 (2.2-3.3)
Lamotrigine	ND	ND	ND	ND	2.1[b] (1.3-6.1)
Gabapentin	3.7 (2.4-8.3)	3.2 (2.4-5.0)	ND	ND	ND
NMDA antagonists					
Dextromethorphan	1.9 (1.1-3.7)	NA	ND	NA[c]	ND
Memantine	ND	NA	ND	ND	ND
$GABA_B$ agonist					
Baclofen	ND	ND	ND	ND	1.4[d] (1.0-2.6)
Opioids					
Oxycodone	ND	2.5[e] (1.6-5.1)	ND	ND	ND
Tramadol	3.5 (2.3-6.4)	ND	ND	ND	ND
Various					
Levodopa	3.4 (1.5-∞)	ND	ND	ND	ND
Capsaicin	5.9 (3.8-13)	5.3 (2.3-∞)	3.5 (1.6-∞)	ND	ND

TCA, tricyclic antidepressants; ND, not done; SSRI, selective serotonin reuptake inhibitors; NA, not active.

[a]In case of more than one study on a drug in the pertinent pain type, number needed to treat is calculated for combined data.

[b]Add-on therapy to carbamazepine.

[c]Low dose of dextromethorphan.

[d]Add-on therapy to carbamazepine or phenytoin in 4 patients.

[e]For 30% of patients, add-on therapy to tricyclic antidepressants.

From Sindrup SH, Jensen TS. Review article: Efficacy of pharmacological treatments of neuropathic pain: an update in effect related to mechanism of drug action. *Pain.* 1999;83:389-400.

IV lidocaine is generally given via a 1-mg/kg bolus and infusion of 4 mg/kg over 30 to 60 minutes. IV lidocaine for phantom and stump pain was compared with morphine infusion, but lidocaine IV infusion was effective only for stump pain.[83] In an animal model, systemic lidocaine suppressed aberrant impulses at the dorsal root ganglia and at sites of experimentally induced nerve injuries. Minimal affect was seen on normal sensory conduction. The median effective dose was lower at dorsal root ganglia sites.[140] Local anesthetics administered systemically also depress evoked unmyelinated C-fiber activity in the dorsal cord.[141] In another study comparing the effects of systemic lidocaine with morphine, both agents relieved the pain of postherpetic neuralgia.[82]

In a study by Finnerup et al,[142] IV lidocaine was found to reduce spontaneous pain significantly in all patients either with or without evoked pain. There was no difference in the number of responders. Both spinal cord injury pain at and below the level of injury as well as brush-evoked dysesthesia were relieved. The authors concluded that agents with systemic sodium channel blocking properties may be treatment options for spinal cord injury pain. IV lidocaine also has been studied for painful chronic diabetic neuropathy pain, with positive results.[143,144] Mexiletine, an oral class IB antiarrhythmic drug, also has been used for pain relief and is thought to have oral lidocaine-like activity. Galer et al[145] studied a small group of patients receiving one of 2 IV lidocaine doses. Although the higher dose of IV lidocaine was more analgesic, both doses were highly correlated with mexiletine responsiveness. The authors concluded that IV lidocaine could be used as a predictor of ultimate response to mexiletine. Previous studies have demonstrated that oral mexiletine is helpful for painful diabetic neuropathy, particularly in reducing symptoms such as burning and stabbing.[146] Mexiletine can often be limited by intolerance to the drug, particularly abdominal symptoms (nausea) and nervousness/tremor in some patients. Dosing should begin with 150 mg twice daily or less, with a goal of at least 10 mg/kg (see Table 91-10).

Combination Therapy Few trials have examined the combination of different antinociceptive agents either from the same class (ie, antiepileptic drugs) or from multiple classes (pairing opioids, antiepileptic drugs, and antidepressant agents). Although most of these medications have numbers needed to treat of 3 or greater,[31] therefore necessitating a multimodal analgesic approach, the rationale for combination therapies has not been adequately studied. A study by Gilron et al[81] evaluated patients with diabetic neuropathy or postherpetic neuralgia, comparing gabapentin, morphine, or the combination of both drugs versus placebo. The study demonstrated a reduction in mean daily pain from 5.72 at baseline to 3.06 with the gabapentin-morphine combination. Both agents were analgesic. At the maximal tolerated doses, the combination was well tolerated but did produce higher frequencies of dry mouth and constipation for gabapentin and morphine, respectively. The authors concluded that there was merit to additional trials of this type comparing combinations of antinociceptive agents as a multimodal approach to pain control. Number-needed-to-treat evaluations can be important in determining the relative effects of different pharmacologic treatments. In a review, Sindrup and Jensen[31] reported numbers needed to treat of various agents in different classes. The comparison is useful in choosing an agent(s) that has high efficacy and is safe, based on numbers-needed-to-harm analysis (see Table 91-10).

Skeletal Muscle Relaxants Skeletal muscle relaxants include a disparate group of medications with multiple modes of action. *Benzodiazepines* include drugs such as diazepam and clonazepam. These agents act to depress the central nervous system via the chloride channel component of the inhibitory neurotransmitter GABA receptor. Benzodiazepines have broad effects on patients, including functioning as anxiolytics, sedatives, and relaxants. Diazepam, as a prototypical benzodiazepine, has rapid onset of action with a prolonged half-life, high lipophilicity, and high protein binding.[147] Although generally not considered potent analgesics in their oral/parenteral forms, research has focused on their use as intrathecal drugs where they are quite analgesic.[148] Clonazepam has perhaps the most robust evidence for conventional oral or topical forms for conditions such as burning mouth pain and other facial neuropathic pain syndromes/trigeminal neuralgia.[149] Clonazepam is perhaps the agent of choice as an inhibitor of myoclonic jerking that can be frequently seen in high-dose opioid patients.[150]

Tizanidine, an α_2-adrenergic agonist chemically, has been used for painful spasm and headache prophylaxis.[151] The drug initially was marketed for control of spasticity in association with brain injury[152] and has been found useful in controlling spastic hypotonia as measured by Ashworth scale improvement.

Baclofen, a $GABA_B$ agonist used for spasticity, has found limited usefulness for the control of neuropathic pain. Three subtypes of the GABA receptor have been described: $GABA_A$, $GABA_B$, and $GABA_C$. $GABA_B$ receptors are primarily located in the lamina I-III area of the dorsal spinal cord.[153] A small trial of oral baclofen given to 15 patients compared the effects of the racemic mixture of baclofen versus the levorotatory form alone and noted greater improvement in patients who received the levorotatory form than in patients treated with the mixed form.[154] A comprehensive review of intrathecal baclofen use indicates several reports of analgesic effects of baclofen in animals and humans.[153]

More conventionally used oral muscle relaxants include agents such as cyclobenzaprine, methocarbamol, orphenadrine, metaxalone, and carisoprodol. Of these agents, cyclobenzaprine has perhaps the best evidence for efficacy in pain control. Chiefly, cyclobenzaprine was compared with ibuprofen as therapy for acute neck and back pain in a randomized trial.[155] In this study, the combination of ibuprofen with cyclobenzaprine provided no advantage over cyclobenzaprine alone. A review of the use of 3 commonly prescribed muscle relaxant agents—carisoprodol, cyclobenzaprine, and metaxalone—demonstrated that these agents represent 45% of all prescriptions for musculoskeletal pain. The review concluded that all were effective, some based on good randomized trial evidence, particularly for cyclobenzaprine. Unfortunately, although carisoprodol represented 13.3% of all prescriptions, its usefulness is significantly limited by its abuse potential.[156] Carisoprodol blocks descending reticular formation interneuronal activity and is metabolized to meprobamate. Meprobamate is a potent anxiolytic and sedative agent with a high propensity for physical and psychologic dependency, which ultimately led to the parent drug's removal from the market. Meprobamate is similar in function to barbiturates.[157] The danger of the effects of carisoprodol on driving have been detailed, with more of the impaired drivers manifesting higher blood carisoprodol levels. Impairment appeared to mimic that seen with benzodiazepine use but with several other manifestations, including horizontal nystagmus, hand tremor, and involuntary movements.[158]

Nonsteroidal Anti-inflammatory Drugs NSAIDs are used on a daily basis by millions of people and on an occasional basis by many more. The proportion of patients using NSAIDs is nearly 4-fold higher in an older age group compared with a younger group.[159] In a study of 3154 elderly patients in Italy, 24.7% were taking NSAIDs, a third chronically.[160] As the percentage of baby-boomer Americans older than 65 years advances in the next 2 decades, the number of patients taking these agents likely will continue to expand. NSAIDs are commonly and appropriately used for many acute pain syndromes, including traumatically induced pain, surgical pain, pain from sprains and strains, temporomandibular joint pain, some headaches, menstrual cramping/dysmenorrhea, and some chronic conditions such as rheumatoid arthritis, seronegative arthritides, osteoarthritis, and other painful states. The ultimate goal of therapy with NSAIDs is to decrease inflammation, harness any ongoing tissue destruction, prevent peripheral sensitization of nociceptors by locally released inflammatory factors (bradykinin, histamine, substance P; **Fig. 91-9**), provide analgesia during restorative healing, and to do so without causing concomitant

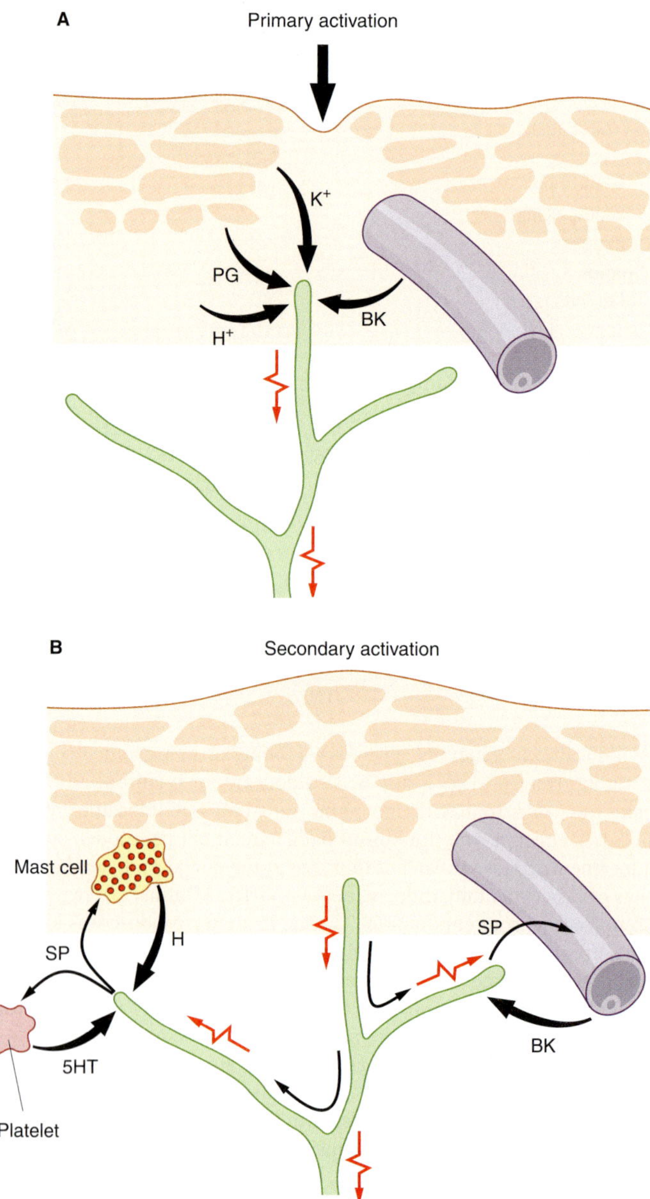

FIGURE 91-9. A. Release of local factors at the site of tissue injury causes primary activation of nociceptors. Release of prostaglandins (PG), bradykinins (BK), hydrogen ion (H^+), and potassium (K^+) contributes to ongoing pain and inflammation. **B.** Release of platelet 5-HT (serotonin) and mast cell histamine, other peptides (substance P), and bradykinin (BK) leads to peripheral sensitization of the nociceptor. [From Pain: pathophysiology and management. In: Kasper DL, Braunwald E, Fauci AD, et al, eds. *Harrison's Principles of Internal Medicine.* 16th ed. Harrison's Online. www.accessmedicine.com. New York, NY: McGraw-Hill; 2004-2005:Figure 11-2. With permission.]

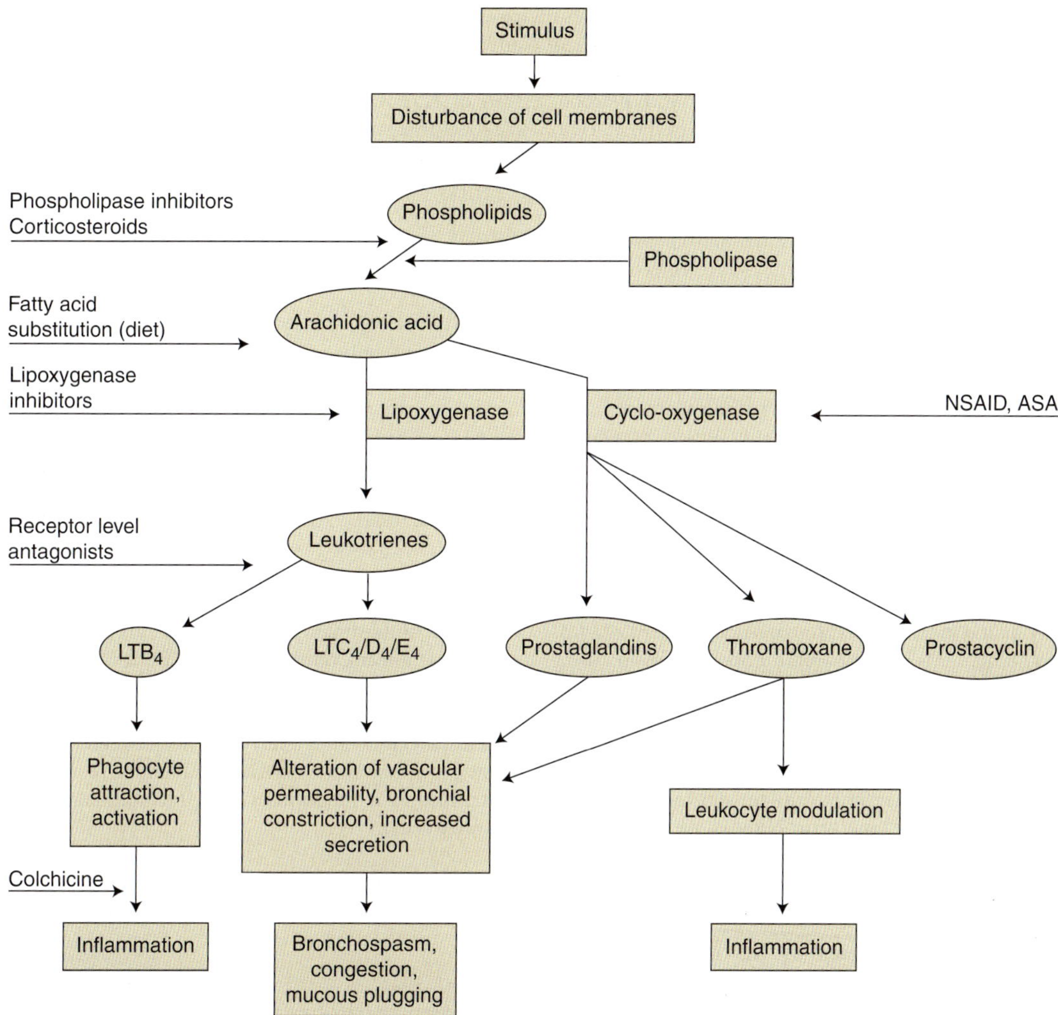

FIGURE 91-10. Cellular disturbance at the membrane level induces production of prostaglandins and leukotrienes active in the inflammatory process. [From Wagner W, Khanna P, Furst DE. Nonsteroidal anti-inflammatory drugs, disease-modifying antirheumatic drugs, nonopioid analgesics, and drugs used in gout. In: Katzung BG, ed. *Basic and Clinical Pharmacology.* 9th ed. New York, NY: McGraw-Hill; 2004:576-577. With permission.]

gastrointestinal injury, renal effects, or cardiovascular thrombotic events. The major mechanism of NSAID action occurs by arresting the action of COX enzyme breakdown of arachidonic acid precursors. The COX enzyme is involved in the synthesis of cyclic endoperoxides from these arachidonic acid precursors to prostaglandins (**Fig. 91-10**). Prostaglandins have varied effects, often as proinflammatory substances, as well as generation of a gastric mucous membrane protective barrier and modulation of renal plasma flow and electrolyte balance. Two isoforms of the cyclo-oxygenase (COX) enzyme exist: COX-1 and COX-2. The COX-1 enzyme normally is present or constitutive and functions in homeostasis, as in the gastric mucosa. One of the main side effects of prolonged NSAID use is gastric ulceration related to inhibition of COX-1 activity. The COX-2 form of the enzyme is constitutive in the central nervous system and renal tissues but is inducible at sites of pain and inflammation. Efforts to block the inducible form of the enzyme at sites of peripheral inflammation (ie, COX-2) led to the introduction of COX-2-selective NSAIDs in the last decade.[161]

The COX-2-specific agents had demonstrated lower risks of gastric ulceration compared with nonspecific COX agents, but all COX inhibitors have a propensity to cause gastrointestinal bleeding depending on dose and duration of therapy. Platelet aggregation is permanently affected with aspirin, which irreversibly acetylates platelet COX. The older nonacetylated salicylates, such as salsalate and magnesium choline salicylate, as well as the selective COX-2 blockers, appear to have less effect on platelet function.[161] Thus some NSAIDs and aspirin, in particular, may react adversely with other anticoagulant agents (eg, warfarin).

Unfortunately, the apparent effects of increased cardiovascular risk have led to the withdrawal from the US market of 2 COX-2 selective drugs (rofecoxib and valdecoxib) and have derailed the ultimate availability of an IV COX-2 form of valdecoxib (parecoxib). Celecoxib, which is much less selective for the COX-2 isoform than rofecoxib and valdecoxib, remains available. It is thought that, to some extent, all NSAIDs as a class may have deleterious effects on the cardiovascular system. Therefore, use of these agents for prolonged periods, particularly by chronic pain patients, should be done with caution and with appropriate balancing of risks versus benefits. An initial study investigated the risks of rofecoxib compared with naproxen was performed (Vioxx Gastrointestinal Outcomes Research [VIGOR]).[162] In the VIGOR study, 8000 patients with rheumatoid arthritis were treated with rofecoxib 50 mg/d or naproxen 1000 mg/d. A statistically significant increase in nonfatal myocardial infarctions was noted in the rofecoxib patients compared with the naproxen patients. In the Celecoxib Long-Term Arthritis Safety Study (CLASS),[163] 20% to 22% of patients were commonly receiving low-dose aspirin in addition to celecoxib. Early recommendations that concomitant low-dose aspirin therapy along with the COX-2 agent might be protective against thrombotic events were discussed with practitioners.

In the Adenomatous Polyp Prevention on Vioxx (APPROVe) trial, 2586 patients with a history of colorectal adenoma were studied because it appeared that NSAIDs might have beneficial effects in primary prevention. Comparing a 25-mg dose of rofecoxib with placebo, 46 patients in the rofecoxib group and only 26 patients in the placebo group had confirmed thrombotic events, which included myocardial coronary syndromes, cerebrovascular events, and cardiac/pulmonary failures. The risks became apparent at 18 months of therapy.[164] Nussmeier et al[165] studied the use of perioperative valdecoxib in coronary bypass patients and found a similar result. As for rofecoxib, valdecoxib appeared to increase the incidence of acute thrombotic events compared with placebo therapy, even though these patients already had diseased vasculature.

NSAIDs as a rule are weak acids and highly protein bound. Particular care is mandatory when prescribing these agents to older debilitated or cachectic patients who are critically ill, are intravascularly volume depleted, or have protein-deficient nutritional states. NSAIDs are metabolized by either the CYP 2C or CYP 3A cytochrome P450 enzymes and are excreted in the urine. It is generally believed that NSAIDs are prescribed according to their specific chemical class. Many of the more popular analgesic agents are propionic acids (eg, ibuprofen, ketoprofen, oxaprozin, naproxen), but multiple classes exist. No evidence indicates that one particular agent or class is superior in specific patients if comparable doses are given. Some clinicians believe that a failed drug trial from one class necessitates a trial with another group, but this has not been demonstrated.[166] Patients with a history of other gastrointestinal problems, who are nicotine or alcohol users, who are taking concomitant oral steroids, or who are taking warfarin or other anticoagulant substances are least likely to do well. The wisdom of long-term NSAID use as a chronic pain treatment appears to be suspect considering the high degree of adverse drug side effects.

An association has been reported between long-term administration of NSAIDs (>180 d) and increased radiographic evidence of osteoarthritis progression. A large group of 1695 patients with either hip or knee osteoarthritis was studied. Radiographs from baseline to a mean of 6.6 years were reviewed. The authors concluded that chronic use of diclofenac, a generally well-tolerated and popular NSAID, was associated with a 2.4-fold (hip) or 3.2-fold (knee) increased risk of osteoarthritis progression compared with short-term use.[167]

Topical NSAIDs may have a therapeutic effect in certain well-localized situations. A systemic review and meta-analysis of topical NSAIDs for musculoskeletal pain concluded that although the number needed to treat was approximately 4.7 to achieve one patient with 50% or more pain relief, the topical agents were well tolerated with few side effects. Interestingly, 3 trials in the meta-analysis demonstrated no difference between oral and topical NSAIDs.[168]

In some cases, acetaminophen may be a safer alternative than NSAIDs. Even though millions of patients take acetaminophen daily, the drug's mechanism of analgesia is not clear. Previously, acetaminophen was considered a weak nonspecific COX inhibitor with little anti-inflammatory action and predominantly central versus peripheral effects, but this may not be correct. An emerging concept of its mechanism of action is that acetaminophen has a COX-3 inhibition profile. COX-3 is expressed in the cerebral cortex and heart in humans and effectively and selectively blocked by acetaminophen as well as some NSAIDs.[169] A more recent proposal is that the acetaminophen functions via supraspinal serotonergic mechanisms (**Table 91-11**).[170]

TABLE 91-11 Available Anti-Inflammatory Drugs and Dosing Strategies

Medication	Daily Dosage Range	Dosage	Frequency
Acetaminophen	2-4 g	325-650 mg	4 h
		650-1000 mg	QID
Salicylic acid derivatives			
Acetylsalicylic acid (aspirin)	2.4-6 g	600-1500 mg	QID
Choline magnesium trisalicylate	1.5-3 g	500-1000 mg	TID
		750-1500 mg	BID
Salsalate	1.5-3 g	750-1500 mg	BID
Propionic acid derivatives (ibuprofen)	1.2-3.2 g for pain	200-400 mg	QID
		400, 600, or 800 mg	TID to QID, to a maximum dose of 3200 mg/d
Naproxen	500 mg-1 g	250, 350, or 500 mg	BID
Naproxen sodium	550-1100 mg	275-550 mg	BID
Flurbiprofen	100-200 mg	50-100 mg	BID
Ketoprofen	75-225 mg	25-75 mg	TID
Acetic acids (diclofenac, etodolac)	150-200 mg	50 mg	TID
		75 mg	BID
	400-1200 mg	200-300 mg	BID, TID, or QID
Indomethacin	<200 mg	25-50 mg	TID or QID
Sulindac	300-400 mg	150 or 200 mg	QD to BID
Tolmetin	800-1800 mg	400, 600, or 800 mg	TID
Enolic acids (meloxicam [Mobic])	7.5-15 mg	7.5 mg for osteoarthritis	QD
		15 mg rheumatoid arthritis	
Piroxicam	10-20 mg	10 or 20 mg	QD
Naphthylalkanones (nabumetone)	1-1.5 g	500 mg	BID up to 1.5 g
Cyclo-oxygenese-2/selective (celecoxib)	200-400 mg	100 or 200 mg	QD to q12 h
Fenamates (meclofenamate)	50-400 mg	50-100 mg	TID to QID
Mefenamic acid (Ponstel)	1-2 g	250 mg	QID

Reprinted from *Guidelines for the Management of Pain in Osteoarthritis, Rheumatoid Arthritis, and Juvenile Chronic Arthritis.* 2nd ed. Table 11, 2002;59-61. With permission of the American Pain Society.

Early studies comparing acetaminophen with NSAIDs have been somewhat surprising, particularly given the fact that acetaminophen's actions are primarily central. Bradley et al[171] compared acetaminophen 4 g/d with ibuprofen up to 2.4 g/d in a randomized double-blind experiment of 182 patients with knee osteoarthritis. The patients had improved rest pain and less disability independent of which agent they given, and the authors concluded that presumptive evidence of synovial inflammation does not necessarily predict which agent will provide a greater response. In another study of 382 patients comparing rofecoxib, celecoxib, and acetaminophen, patient functional end points including measures such as walking pain, rest pain, and morning stiffness improved in all groups, but only significantly for rofecoxib. In terms of average 6-week functional disability score, only the 25-mg rofecoxib group was statistically different than acetaminophen. No cardiac events were noted, and adverse events were generally limited.[172] Given that rofecoxib is no longer clinically available, these results indicate that practitioners should be wary in potentially higher-risk groups and strongly consider acetaminophen.

Acetaminophen-induced hepatic failure has been thought to be a risk for patients with existing hepatic disease as well as those ingesting toxic levels of the drug. Patients ingesting 2 oz or more of alcohol per day should have dose reductions to a maximum of 2.5 g/d acetaminophen.[166] Risk of analgesic nephropathy is possible with acetaminophen but is a rare occurrence. Evidence suggests that even in patients with hepatic disease, although the serum half-life of acetaminophen may be prolonged, glutathione stores are not sufficiently depleted to critical levels at recommended doses.[173] Overall, according to American Pain Society guidelines, the favorable risk-to-benefit ratio of acetaminophen warrants ongoing use if efficacy is present during the first few weeks at doses of at least 2 to 3 g/d.[166]

PAIN REHABILITATION STRATEGIES

Anesthesiologists are extremely well prepared in the application of pharmacologic and interventional principles because of excellent command of the perioperative care of complex patients. However, chronic pain patients often defy treatment in a strictly biomedical model of care. The biomedical model presupposes a definable injury, disease, or process that can be treated.[174] Unfortunately, despite extensive and often expensive evaluations to explain patient pain syndromes, a precise diagnosis cannot always be made. Furthermore, patients presenting to a chronic pain treatment facility have often tried multiple therapies without significant improvement. Thus a biopsychosocial model of care, in which the patient is treated holistically, understanding their reaction, beliefs, and coping mechanisms regarding the physical pain within the broad context of their work and family and social environments, often is an option.

For example, more than half of patients admitted to a pain rehabilitation program had already tried opioids, NSAIDs, physical therapy, antidepressants, injections, anticonvulsants, and other therapies; many also had tried alternative medical treatment and surgery. Many of these trials had temporary effects, but ultimately they all failed for a variety of reasons inherent to many chronic pain patients.

Gallagher[174] recommended multiple approaches to maximizing the results of pharmacologic trials: (1) carefully plan medication trials; (2) consider alternative (nonpharmacologic) treatments for pain fluctuation; (3) select medications based on pain mechanism and consider associated medical and psychologic morbidities; (4) utility of a goal-oriented management plan for each problem with "time-limited" target outcome measures; (5) close scrutiny during initial 2-week medication trials with frequent patient contact; and (6) upon failure of a drug trial, gradual reduction of the dose, keeping other agents at stable levels.

The most common reasons for failed drug trials are improperly low (inadequate dose) or too high (side effects limit trial) doses or inadequate durations of trials.

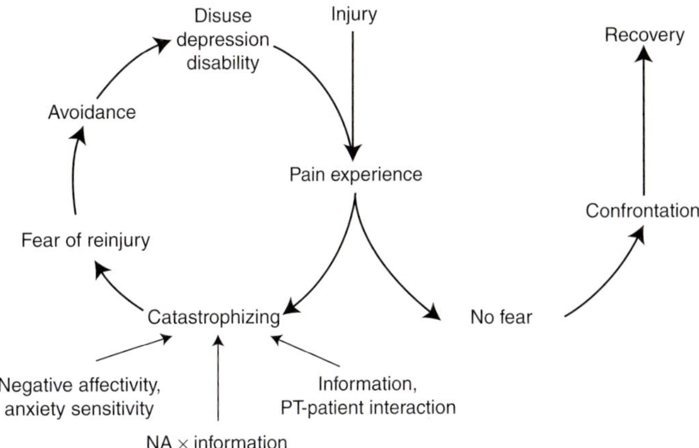

FIGURE 91-11. Injury occurs, and the patient experiences pain. Some patients have a "catastrophizing" coping response to the experience of pain, reinforced by physicians and physical therapists, who may encourage abstinence from the painful activity. Further activity induces fear of (re)injury and gradual social, sexual, and functional disability. This continued cycle of pain is difficult to overcome. [Reprinted from Vlaeyen JWS, Crombez G. Fear of movement/(re)injury, avoidance and pain disability in chronic low back pain patients. *Man Ther.* 1999:4:187-195.]

Modern pain rehabilitation programs aim to treat the whole patient to modify maladaptive behaviors, overcome psychosocial detractors, allow functional restoration, and improve coping skills. These programs generally include physical reconditioning/exercise, aided by physical and occupational therapists, and cognitive-behavioral therapies, including biofeedback, relaxation, stress management, substance use educational interventions, introduction of concepts of pacing and pain-inducing activity moderation, and use of positive reinforcements of appropriate instead of maladaptive behaviors (**Fig. 91-11**). Many of these programs modify or eliminate unnecessary or problematic pharmaceutical agents causing side effects to the patient, particularly opioids and other narcotics or habituating drugs.

Multiple studies have demonstrated that functional improvements are sustained over time, as well as the ability to decrease or eliminate medications (opioids, NSAIDS, muscle relaxants).[175,176] Rome et al[177] studied 356 patients admitted to the pain rehabilitation program for an entire year. Of this group, 274 patients completed both the program and all questionnaires; 99 patients were taking opioids before the program and 175 were not. Only 3 of the opioid patients were still taking opioids at the conclusion of the 3-week program, and significant improvement was noted in all outcome variables in both groups.[177] This is important because it demonstrates that despite a presumed acute increase in pain due to opioid withdrawal, the opioid group was also able to achieve program goals.

Robbins et al[178] evaluated the effect of deleting the behavioral medicine portion of a pain rehabilitation approach and carving out only the physical therapy portion of the care plan. In this study, patients did not fare as well on either short-term or long-term follow-up. Thus insurers and managed care organizations approach to chronic pain care often can be "penny wise and pound foolish."

A number of studies have started to question the role of spinal operations as therapy for chronic lumbar pain due to discogenic disease. Soon many other therapies will be scrutinized for chronic pain care, and evidence, if lacking, will spurn new approaches to care of patients. Spinal fusion for discogenic pain is an example of a quickly growing procedure that seems to be outpacing the growth of other joint replacements for arthritic conditions such as hip or knee replacement.[179] Brox et al[180] studied patients with degenerative disk disease at L4-L5 or L5-LS1 and chronic pain for more than 1 year.

Patients were randomized to spinal instrumented fusion plus postsurgical physical therapy or exercise and cognitive interventions. After 1 year, there was no clear advantage to instrumented fusion over cognitive interventions combined with physical therapy and functional restoration techniques. Surgical patients had improved leg pain, and cognitive interventions/exercise patients had better fingertip to floor distance ability. Oswestry disability scores improved in both groups. Based on a study by Fairbank et al,[181] in which only marginal, not clearly advantageous, improvement was noted in the surgical group versus intensive rehabilitation, a cost study was performed in which the authors determined that surgical stabilization was not a cost-effective use of scarce health care resources in Great Britain.[182] These studies are the first of several that are beginning to clearly demonstrate to patients and payers that the combination of behavioral medicine techniques with physical therapeutics is effective for patients with chronic lower back pain.

PSYCHOLOGIC MANAGEMENT OF PAIN

Psychologic component plays a significant role in managing chronic pain. *Pain catastrophizing*[183] can be summarized as a negative cognitive belief state associated with actual or potential pain experiences. Three major attributes of catastrophizing are (1) magnification, (2) rumination, and (3) helplessness.

Catastrophizing is associated with a heightened pain experience and is one of the most important psychologic factors contributing to perceived pain intensity. Catastrophizing is associated with increased disability, pain-induced health care–seeking behavior, and analgesic use. It is apparent that patients who catastrophize in response to painful experiences have intense emotional distress and increased pain overall. Patients appear more likely to be female than male. Thus the role of gender in pain has been studied. For example, in a large study examining gender differences, women reported greater levels of pain from chronic spinal conditions than men did. Interestingly, the patients taking opioids had poorer function and disability whether they were men or women, but men had more affective distress while taking opioids and women had less.[184]

Psychologic management of chronic pain includes operant-behavioral therapy, cognitive behavioral therapy (CBT), biofeedback, guided imagery, meditation, and relaxation hypnosis. CBT is based on the theory that patients believe they cannot function because of their pain and they are helpless. The treatment in CBT provides patients with techniques to gain a sense of control over the effects of pain on daily living as well as modifying the affective, behavioral, cognitive, and sensory-physical dimensions of experience.[185]

PHYSICAL MODALITIES AND EXERCISE

Physical modalities can be applied within an overall pain treatment plan to aid in functional rehabilitation. Many pain rehabilitation programs provide vigorous inpatient or outpatient programs in which subjects receive both cognitive-behavioral strategies combined with physical therapy and functional restoration techniques. Before beginning any physical training sessions, a functional capacity evaluation can be useful in identifying and quantifying specific limitations of the patient. The practitioner must realize that most chronic pain disorders have evolved over time, so any specific regimens must be applied in a graded and preferably supervised fashion to prevent (re)injury, which would reinforce in the patients' mind once again that they are disabled by the pain. Patients who catastrophize may understand that they need to exercise, but education alone often is insufficient to overcome their fear. Introduction of graded exposure to the feared activity in a sense "teaches" the patient that he or she actually can do the activity (see Fig. 91-11).[186]

Physical modalities include but are not limited to exercise, transcutaneous electrical nerve stimulation (TENS), heat, cold (cryotherapy), iontophoresis, acupuncture, electrical stimulation of the muscles, traction, manipulation, myofascial release techniques, and massage.

VOCATIONAL REHABILITATION

When chronic pain interferes with a patient's ability to return to work, the physician can use programs such as work conditioning and work hardening. Although similar, these 2 programs differ in their content and structure. The work-conditioning program provides structured progressive reconditioning that relies less on passive modalities and more on activities for physical fitness. The program often runs 1 to 2 hours, 3 to 5 times per week for a period of 2 to 6 weeks. In contrast, the work-hardening program provides a more comprehensive approach to the patient who has been off work for prolonged periods. These programs incorporate job-specific work simulation and address psychologic and vocational issues along with physical reconditioning. The programs often are located in environments that appear "worklike" to minimize the patient's perception of illness and to facilitate the return to a work mindset. Education is an important part of both types of programs and includes proper body mechanics, safe lifting techniques, stress management, and promotion of a healthy lifestyle.

Vocational rehabilitation assists the chronic pain patient when return to his or her former occupation is unlikely. Vocational counseling may be provided by individual rehabilitation facilities or accessed through local or state agencies when available. Physical modalities are used in conjunction with therapy to provide temporary pain relief, improve stiffness, and allow the patient to more fully participate in performance of specific tasks that will manifest long-term gains in functionality.

EXERCISE

A review of randomized controlled trials and observational studies of therapeutic exercise in adults with chronic low back pain supports the theory that therapeutic exercise is effective for reducing chronic pain.[187]

Individually tailored programs that emphasize stretching or strengthening may be superior. A typical physical therapy regimen may include low-impact forms of movement education, such as aquatic therapies, walking, and passive and active stretching, with gentle progression to the patient's tolerance. Occupational therapy is used to teach patients energy conservation techniques or to assess for adaptive equipment needs such as gait and grasp aids, braces, and orthotics, which may be useful for promoting independence and protecting against injury. One important goal supported by both the physician and physical therapist is patient autonomy. A home-based therapy routine should be encouraged from the onset of physical/occupational therapy and monitored or modified regularly as needed. The patient should be encouraged to adopt a more active lifestyle, incorporating the skills acquired in physical/occupational therapy into daily life. In aquatherapy, exercises can be performed with decreased weightbearing stress on the joints.

TRANSCUTANEOUS ELECTRICAL NERVE STIMULATION

The gate control theory—activation of specific large fiber afferents carried in A-fibers might compete at the dorsal horn with slower unmyelinated sensory afferent (C-fibers) and functionally "close" the gate to this slower noxious information—may explain the rationale for transcutaneous electrical nerve stimulation (TENS) analgesia. TENS may be one of the most useful therapies based on these concepts. TENS units are multichannel devices in which surface electrical stimulation is applied through gel pads with an external generator over sites of pain. To maximize analgesia, different amplitudes, frequencies, and pulse waveforms are used to decrease pain perception. TENS has been studied for treatment of several types of pain, with some studies demonstrating benefit and others showing equivocal results. Most reports of benefit have derived from studies in which stimulation was below motor threshold strength. High-frequency stimulation may give long-lasting pain relief.[188]

ICE AND HEAT

Cryotherapy and heat are the most commonly used physical modalities available to the patient because of their efficacy, ease of use, and safety profiles. Both heat and cold produce analgesia; heat also produces hyperemia, whereas cold decreases nerve conduction.[189] The decrease in blood flow found with cryotherapy may decrease delivery of inflammatory chemicals to the site of injury. Some patients with chronic low back pain have found ice massage to be as effective as TENS.[190]

Heat applications via superficial heat combined with exercise are commonly used for various arthritic and musculoskeletal injuries.[191,192] Heat can be provided in the form of moist heat (hot packs), heat lamps (incandescent or infrared), hydrotherapy, ultrasound, paraffin baths, and short-wave diathermy. Cryotherapy is provided in more limited forms, such as hydrotherapy, ice packs, ice massage, and iced compression wraps; it also can be applied through vapocoolant sprays, such as ethyl chloride.

IONTOPHORESIS

Iontophoresis involves the application of low-level electrical current directly to skin or indirectly via the dosage form to enhance permeation of the topically applied therapeutic agent.[193] In pain management, iontophoresis is usually used to deliver steroids to the inflamed area noninvasively.

ACUPUNCTURE

The ancient art of acupuncture has been used for several millennia for treatment of a variety of medical conditions including pain. The Chinese typically are credited for developing acupuncture. The premise of acupuncture is that energy flow, called *qi,* is important to good health, which is maintained by a smooth flow of the qi. Thus disease or pain results from disruptions or stagnation of the flow of qi.[194] Qi is thought to reside in specific channels or meridians located along specific anatomic regions of the body. Along these meridians are multiple points considered important for accessing qi, called *acupuncture points.* Over the past several decades, acupuncture has grown in popularity as an option for treatment of multiple pain conditions.

On a neurobiologic basis, the needling that occurs at specific acupuncture points has been shown to cause release of peptides such as endorphins and enkephalins.[195] Functional magnetic resonance imaging studies have shown patterns of activation in distinct regions of the brain such as the auditory/visual cortex when traditional acupuncture points for hearing and vision are used[196] as well as common activation areas between healthy volunteers when identical acupuncture points are selected.[197]

Data regarding the efficacy of acupuncture in chronic pain states are conflicting.[198,199] However, a 1998 National Institutes of Health consensus panel extensively reviewed the available literature and concluded that use of acupuncture was acceptable as "an adjunct treatment or acceptable alternative or may be included in a comprehensive management program" for the treatment of headache, tennis elbow, fibromyalgia, myofascial pain, low back pain, and osteoarthritis.[200]

COMPLEMENTARY AND ALTERNATIVE MODALITIES

Complementary medicine includes the use of alternative modalities like yoga, tai chi, aromatherapy, and herbal remedies. These can be used for maintaining health in a holistic approach.

CONCLUSION

Chronic pain management is an evolving discipline that requires broad knowledge and management skills. Peak physician performance demands well-trained compassionate providers who are familiar with not only pharmacologic and interventional therapies but also with the patient's overall cognitive, emotional, and functional state. Pain mechanisms now are better understood, and therapies can be better targeted, often from a multimodal approach. Comparative studies of different pharmacologic, cognitive-behavioral, and interventional therapeutics are needed to determine which are the most efficacious based on solid evidence.

KEY REFERENCES

- Ballantyne JC, Mao J. Opioid therapy for chronic pain. *N Engl J Med.* 2003;349:1943-1953.
- Fairbank J, Frost H, Wilson-MacDonald J, et al. Randomised controlled trial to compare surgical stabilization of the lumbar spine with an intensive rehabilitation programme for patients with chronic low back pain: the MRC spine stabilization trial. *BMJ.* 2005;330:1233-1239.
- Farrar JT. Young JP, LaMoreaux L, et al. Clinical importance of changes in chronic pain intensity measured on an 11-point numerical pain rating scale. *Pain.* 2001;94:149-158.
- Gilron I, Bailey JM, Tu D, et al. Morphine, gabapentin or their combination for neuropathic pain. *N Engl J Med.* 2005;352:1324-1334.
- Gold MS, Weinrich D, Kim C-S, et al. Redistribution of NA_V 1.8 in injured axons enables neuropathic pain. *J Neurosci.* 2003;23:158-166.
- Raja SN, Haythronthwaite JA, Pappagallo M, et al. Opioids versus antidepressants in postherpetic neuralgia. A randomized, placebo-controlled trial. *Neurology.* 2002;59:1015-1021.
- Sabatowski R, Galvez R, Cherry DA, et al. Pregabalin reduces pain and improves sleep and mood disturbances in patients with postherpetic neuralgia: results of a randomized placebo-controlled clinical trial. *Pain.* 2004;109:26-35.
- Sindrup SH, Jensen TS. Review article: Efficacy of pharmacological treatments of neuropathic pain: an update in effect related to mechanism of drug action. *Pain.* 1999;83:389-400.
- Trescot A, Helm S, Hansen H, et al. Opioids in the management of chronic non-cancer pain: an update of American Society of the Interventional Pain Physicians (ASIPP) guidelines. *Pain Physician.* 2008;11;S5-S62.
- Vanderah TW, Suenaga NM, Ossipov MH, et al. Tonic descending facilitation from the rostral ventromedial medulla mediates opioid-induced abnormal pain and antinociceptive tolerance. *J Neurosci.* 2001;21:279-286.
- Vlaeyen JWS, Crombez G. Fear of movement/(re)injury, avoidance and pain disability in chronic low back pain patients. *Man Ther.* 1999:4:187-195.

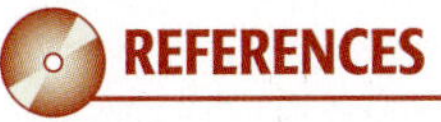

REFERENCES

Complete references available on DVD and online version at www.LongneckerAnesthesiology.com

CHAPTER 92

Interventional Management of Chronic Pain

Carlos A. Pino
James P. Rathmell

KEY POINTS

1. The best pain medicine practitioners strike a reasonable balance between interventional and noninterventional management. This practice pattern is sustainable, and those adopting a balanced style of practice will be able to adapt to evolving scientific evidence that appears to support pain treatment, regardless of the type of treatment.
2. Although the evidence supporting the need for routine radiographic guidance is still evolving, the intuitive appeal of this more precise approach has evolved to the point where most practitioners now perform at least a portion of their injections using fluoroscopic guidance.
3. The key to safety and success of any interventional pain technique is a clear understanding of normal anatomy. The procedures described in this chapter require an understanding of the normal anatomy of the spine, including the epidural and subarachnoid spaces, zygapophyseal joints, intervertebral disks, and, most importantly, the spinal cord with its somatic and sympathetic components.
4. Epidural steroid injections are efficacious in the treatment of acute lumbosacral radicular pain or in radiculopathies secondary to herniated or bulging disks. Epidural steroid injections also have been used to treat back pain secondary to degenerative disk disease, spinal stenosis, trauma, spondylolysis or spondylolisthesis, and in pain following laminectomy. The epidural space can be approached through the interlaminar space (median or paramedian), intervertebral foramen (transforaminal), or sacral hiatus (caudal). The approach selected depends on patient selection, indication for injection, practitioner's experience, and availability of imaging. We are still lacking large-scale studies comparing clinical outcomes with the transforaminal versus the interlaminar approach.
5. Many practitioners continue to use sympathetic blockade as a part of a multidisciplinary approach to treating complex regional pain syndrome. Sympathetic blocks are one tool that can reduce pain and facilitate functional recovery.
6. Intra-articular facet injection has been largely supplanted by radiofrequency treatment techniques for facet-related pain. Clinical experience and a limited number of published observational studies suggest that intra-articular injection of local anesthetic and steroid leads to relief of facet-related pain that is of limited duration. In contrast, radiofrequency treatment is safe and effective in producing longer-term pain relief in the same group of patients.
7. Discography is a diagnostic test in which radiographic contrast is injected into the nucleus pulposus of the intervertebral disk. Although originally developed for the study of disk herniation, discography now is used most commonly to identify symptomatic disk degeneration. The usefulness of this diagnostic test remains controversial.
8. Intrathecal morphine and other opioids are now widely used as adjuncts in the treatment of acute and chronic pain, and a number of agents show promise as analgesic agents with spinal selectivity. Patient selection for intraspinal pain therapy is empiric and remains the subject of debate. In general, intrathecal drug delivery is reserved for patients with severe pain that does not respond to conservative treatment.
9. Direct electrical stimulation of the dorsal columns, known as spinal cord stimulation or dorsal column stimulation, has proven effective, particularly for treatment of chronic radicular pain. Patient selection for spinal cord stimulation is empiric and remains the subject of some debate. In general, spinal cord stimulation is reserved for patients with severe pain that does not respond to conservative treatment. The pain responds best when relatively well localized because success of spinal cord stimulation depends on the ability to cover the entire painful region with electrical stimulation.

The subspecialty of interventional pain medicine involves minimally invasive treatments and minor surgery as part of pain care, including neural blockade and implantable analgesic devices. Despite the paucity of scientific evidence to guide pain practitioners, a number of techniques appear to have efficacy based on limited observational data and have been adopted into widespread use. As practitioners we are left to choose among available treatment modalities, often with only anecdotal evidence and personal experience to guide us in treating a group of desperate patients with intractable pain who are willing to accept almost any treatment, even those that remain unproven. There is no single practice pattern that a pain specialist can point toward as the correct way to treat patients with chronic pain. Training programs vary widely in the scope of what they train practitioners to do. The best pain medicine practitioners strike a balance between interventional and noninterventional management. This practice pattern is sustainable, and those adopting a balanced style of practice will be able to adapt to evolving scientific evidence that appears in support of pain treatment, regardless of the type of treatment. A balance between treatment modalities also allows practitioners to switch from one mode to another or to incorporate multiple treatment approaches simultaneously. Although this chapter focuses on interventional treatments used to treat chronic pain, use of these interventional modalities is just a small part of the armamentarium of the skilled pain practitioner.

USE OF IMAGE-GUIDED TECHNIQUES IN PAIN MEDICINE

A little more than a decade ago, radiographic guidance was used infrequently by pain practitioners; it was reserved for use in major procedures such as neurolytic celiac plexus block. During the last several years, 2 forces have been at work. First, pain practitioners are now being called on to serve as diagnosticians. Patients and referring practitioners expect pain physicians to have familiarity with imaging modalities and their usefulness in diagnosing pain conditions. At the same time, pain practitioners have come to realize the usefulness of radiographic guidance in achieving precise anatomic placement of needles and catheters. Although the evidence supporting the need for routine radiographic guidance is still evolving, the intuitive appeal of this more precise approach has evolved to the point where most practitioners now perform at least a portion of their injections using fluoroscopic guidance.[1] In some cases (eg, patients with intractable pain associated with metastatic cancer), radiographic guidance has proven invaluable in the planning and implementation of therapy directed toward pain relief.

Some years ago, our research group examined the distribution of injectate in a series of patients who received epidural steroid injections for radicular pain associated with new herniated disks.[2] We found that the injectate often spread to the side opposite the disk herniation. This finding is not at all surprising. A disk herniation present on one side might well obstruct the flow of fluid through the relatively confined epidural space. The fluid would follow the path of least resistance, spreading preferentially to the contralateral unaffected side and exiting the contralateral intervertebral foramina. This study and others[3,4] have challenged the conventional wisdom that suspending the steroid in a modest volume is sufficient to consistently produce spread of the injectate to the affected levels, regardless of where the solution is placed within the epidural space. Using this line of reasoning, investigators have concluded that the blind loss-of-resistance technique is not the best way to deliver steroid to the site of inflammation.[3,4] Using radiographic guidance, bony structures can be visualized directly and in real time. The needle can be seen within the radiographic field, and simple geometry can be used to guide the needle directly from the skin's surface to its destination.

More recently, ultrasound-guided nerve blocks have become commonplace for providing regional anesthesia for surgery, and multiple techniques have been described.[5-8] Growing experience with ultrasound among anesthesiologists, as well as improvement in image resolution and processing, have sparked the interest of pain physicians to learn more about the usefulness of ultrasound for pain procedures.[9,10] Proponents of ultrasound-guided pain procedures point to advantages such as reduced radiation exposure for patients and providers and improved visualization of soft tissues, vessels, and nerves. Most of the experimental work published to date consists of cadaver studies and case reports describing various techniques.[11-14] In the only available randomized controlled trial, Galiano et al randomized 40 patients with low back pain to undergo facet joint injections guided by ultrasound versus computed tomography.[15] The duration of the procedure and radiation dose was significantly less in the ultrasound group; however there was no difference in pain relief between the groups in this small study.[15] The data available to date are scant, and although the technology is appealing, clinical trials are needed to investigate the efficacy and safety of ultrasound-guided pain procedures.[16,17] For now, radiographic guidance remains the standard means for conducting most interventions in the pain clinic.

SPECIFIC TECHNIQUES USED IN IMAGE-GUIDED INTERVENTION FOR CHRONIC PAIN

This chapter provides an overview of the most common techniques used in interventional pain medicine. The section begins with a discussion of the anatomy relevant to image-guided interventions for treating chronic pain. Then the clinical usefulness of each technique and the technical aspects of conducting each intervention are described. Illustrations for the most common techniques are provided. We have published detailed technical descriptions of these and other pain treatment techniques elsewhere.[18]

ANATOMY RELEVANT TO IMAGE-GUIDED INTERVENTION FOR CHRONIC PAIN

The key to safety and success of any interventional pain technique is a clear understanding of the normal anatomy. The procedures described in this chapter require understanding of the normal anatomy of the spine, including the epidural and subarachnoid spaces, the zygapophyseal (facet) joints, intervertebral disks, and, most importantly, the spinal cord with its somatic and sympathetic components. The basic anatomy relevant to common interventions used in the treatment of chronic pain is reviewed here.

Anatomy of the Spine The spinal cord is protected within the vertebral canal and extends from the foramen magnum to the first or second lumbar vertebra in human adults. Its is covered by 3 meninges. The most internal pia mater lies in close apposition to the cord. It is separated from the thin arachnoid mater by the free-flowing cerebrospinal fluid (CSF). The dense dura mater lies most external, surrounding the arachnoid and accompanying the segmental nerve roots well into the vertebral foramen. The epidural space lies within the bony vertebral canal surrounding the dura matter and spreads from the base of the skull to the sacrococcygeal membrane.

Normally, the vertebral canal is nearly triangular, surrounded by the bony components of the vertebrae. There are 33 vertebrae: 7 cervical, 12 thoracic, 5 lumbar, 5 fused elements that make up the sacrum, and 4 to 5 fused ossicles that form the coccyx (**Fig. 92-1**).[19] A typical vertebra consists of a vertebral body and 2 pedicles that extend posteriorly surrounding the spinal canal and epidural space to join a pair of arched laminae (**Fig. 92-2**). The laminae fuse in the midline to form a dorsal projection called the *spinous process.* Near the junction of the pedicles and the laminae are found the lateral projecting transverse processes, the superior and the inferior articular processes (zygapophyses or facets). The pedicles and their articulating processes form the superior and inferior vertebral notches. In the articulated spine, these notches form the intervertebral foramina.[19]

The zygapophyseal, or "facet," joints are paired structures that lie posterolaterally on the bony vertebrae at the junction of the lamina and pedicle medially and the base of the transverse process laterally. The facet joints are true joints, with opposing cartilaginous surfaces and a true synovial lining. They are subject to the same inflammatory and degenerative processes that affect other synovial joints throughout the body.[19] Two opposing articular surfaces compose each facet joint. The facet joint articular processes are named for the vertebra to which they belong. Thus each vertebra has a superior articular process and an inferior articular process. This nomenclature can be confusing because the superior articular process of a given vertebra actually forms the inferior portion of each facet joint.

The intervertebral disk is composed of glucosaminoglycans with a relatively fluid inner nucleus pulposus surrounded by a stiff, lamellar outer annulus fibrosus.[19] With aging, hydration of the intervertebral disks declines, leading to loss of disk height and fissure formation in the annulus fibrosus. These fissures begin centrally near the border between the nucleus pulposus and the annulus fibrosus and can extend to the periphery of the disk space. This process of degradation is called *internal disk derangement* and is believed responsible for producing discogenic pain. The annulus contains neural elements from the sinuvertebral nerve, which are believed to be responsible for pain transmission.[20] These same radial fissures within the annulus represent paths through which nuclear material can pass and extrude as a herniated nucleus pulposus. When this extruded material is adjacent to a spinal nerve posterolateral to the intervertebral disk, it can lead to intense inflammation, nerve root compression, and radicular pain with or without radiculopathy. Radicular pain is common; radiculopathy of nerve root dysfunction in the form of numbness, weakness, and/or loss of deep tendon reflexes is less common. The paired facet joints, along with the vertebral bodies and intervertebral disks, form the 3 weight-bearing support columns that distribute the axial load on the vertebral column while allowing for movement. The structure of the vertebrae varies from cephalad to caudad and should be thoroughly familiar to the practitioner, especially when using imaging (see Figs. 92-1 and 92-2). Of importance when performing injections, the spinous processes of the cervical and lumbar regions approach the lamina in a nearly perpendicular fashion, which facilitates a midline approach when performing epidural or subarachnoid injections. The cervical facet joints are oriented nearly parallel to the axial plane where the atlas (C1) articulates with the occiput and become gradually more steeply angulated in a cephalad to caudad direction at lower cervical levels. The orientation of the cervical facet joints in a plane close to the axial plane allows for a great degree of rotation of the neck as well as flexion and extension.

The midthoracic (T5-T9) spinous processes are acutely angled caudad, making the midline approach to the epidural space more difficult than the paramedian approach. The thoracic facet joints are so steeply angulated that they approach the frontal plane, which makes intra-articular injection difficult or impossible. At midthoracic levels, the inferior articular process of the vertebra forming the superior portion of each thoracic facet joint lies directly posterior to the superior articular process forming the inferior portion of each joint. This allows for some degree of flexion and extension but limited rotation of the spinal column in the thorax region.

The spinous processes of the lumbar vertebrae approach the lamina in a nearly perpendicular fashion. The lumbar facet joints are angled with a somewhat oblique orientation, allowing for flexion, extension, and rotation that is greater than that in the thorax but less than in the cervical region. The sacral hiatus is the area where the fifth sacral vertebra lacks both the laminae and the spinous process posteriorly (**Fig. 92-3**). The 2 sacral cornua lie on either side of the sacral hiatus and cephalad to the coccyx and are useful landmarks when performing an epidural from a caudal approach.

The midline distance from the ligamentum flavum to the dural sac varies considerably, depending on the vertebral level, increasing from 2 mm at C3-C6 to 5 to 6 mm in the midlumbar region.[21] The epidural space narrows posterior and laterally toward the intervertebral foramina. The anterior boundary of the epidural space is provided by the posterior longitudinal ligament covering the vertebral

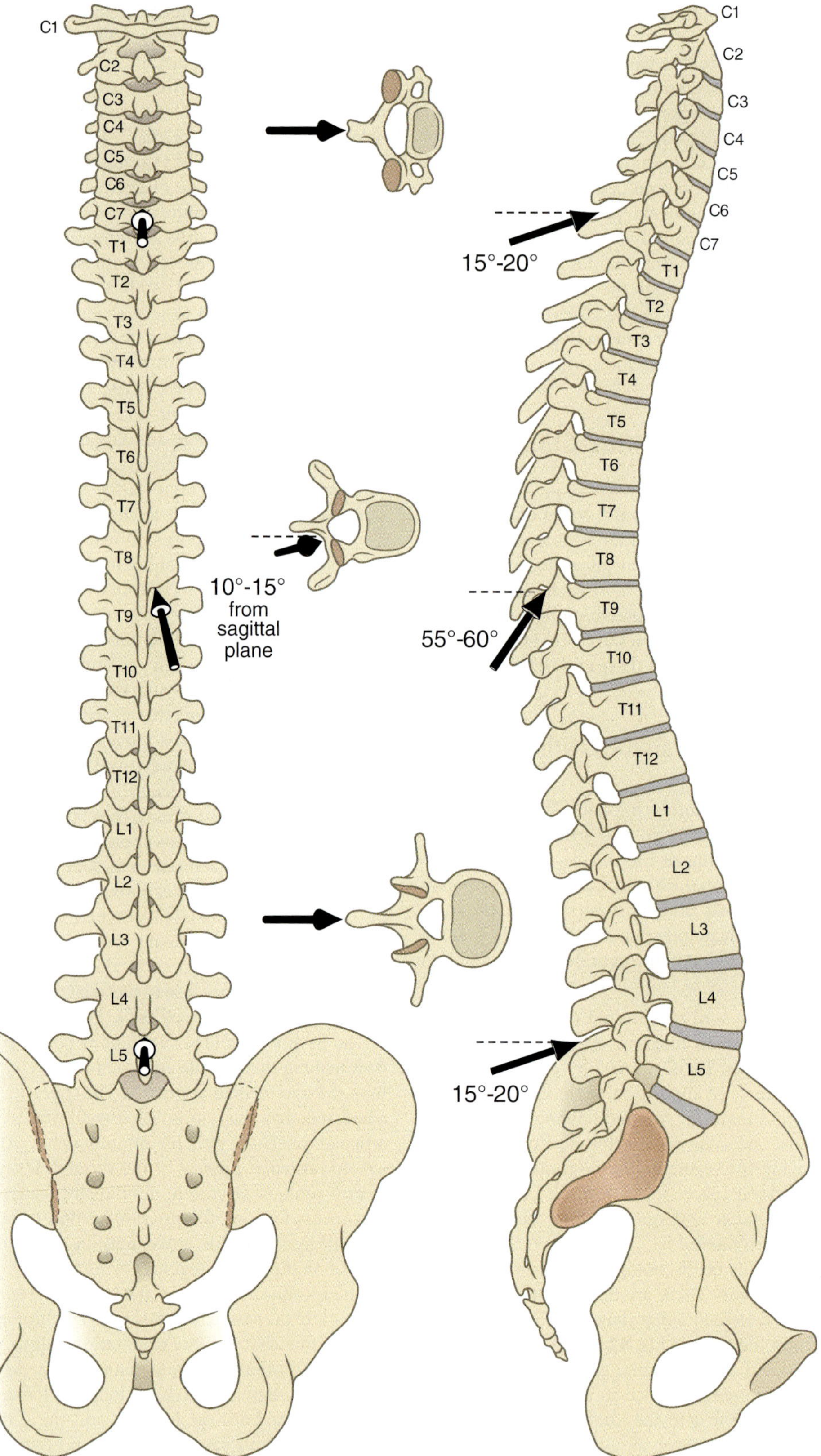

FIGURE 92-1. Anatomy of vertebral column. In most humans, the most prominent spinous process at the base of the neck is C7 (the vertebrae prominens). Note the angle of the spinous processes changes dramatically from cervical to lumbar levels, with the steepest angle in the midthoracic region. The approximate plane of needle entry for interlaminar epidural injection is shown for cervical, thoracic, and lumbar levels. [Adapted from Rathmell JP. *Atlas of Image-Guided Intervention in Regional Anesthesia and Pain Medicine.* Philadelphia, PA: Lippincott Williams & Wilkins, 2006:33 (Figure 5-3). With permission.]

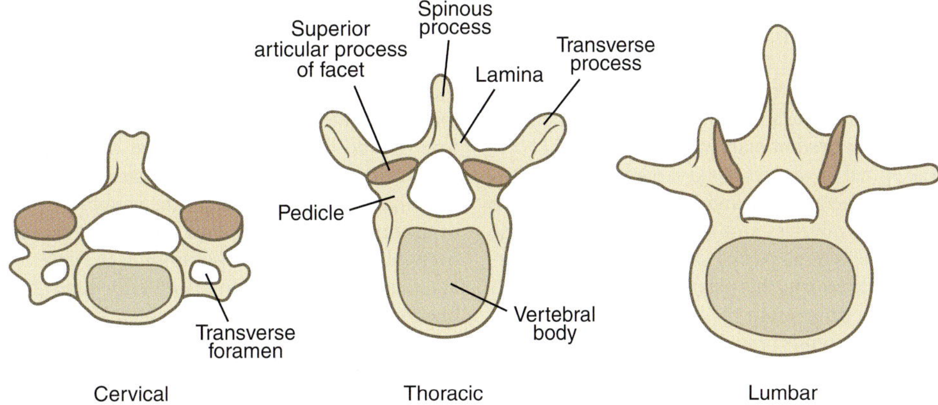

FIGURE 92-2. Anatomy of the cervical, thoracic, and lumbar vertebrae. [Adapted from Rathmell JP. *Atlas of Image-Guided Intervention in Regional Anesthesia and Pain Medicine.* Philadelphia, PA: Lippincott Williams & Wilkins, 2006:32 (Figure 5-1). With permission.]

bodies and the intervertebral disks. Posteriorly, the epidural space is limited by the periosteum of the anterior surfaces of the laminae, the articulating facet processes (zygapophyses), and the ligamentum flavum. Laterally, the pedicles and the intervertebral foramina limit the epidural space.

Knowledge of surface anatomy enhances safety when performing procedures under image guidance and is an absolute necessity when imaging is not available. Important surface landmarks include the spinous process at C7 *(vertebra prominens),* which is the most prominent cervical spinous process palpable when the neck is flexed. The spinous process at T7 lies opposite the inferior angle of the scapula when the arm is at the side. A line joining the superior aspects of the iliac crests passes through the spinous process of the fourth lumbar vertebrae. The spinal cord generally terminates at the L2 level and the dural sac ends at S2, which corresponds to the level of the posterior superior iliac spines. The tip of an equilateral triangle drawn between the posterior superior iliac spines and directed caudally overlies the sacral cornua and sacral hiatus.

Additionally, the articulated spine is supported by the anterior and posterior longitudinal ligaments, the supraspinous and interspinous ligaments, and the ligamentum flavum.[21] Many of the procedures discussed here make reference to the ligamentum flavum. The ligamentum flavum, or "yellow ligament," is a structure of variable thickness and completeness, composed of elastic fibers, that defines the posterolateral soft tissue boundaries of the epidural space. Because its leather-like consistency resists active expulsion of fluid from a syringe, loss of this resistance as a needle passes through the ligamentum flavum is valuable in signaling entry into the epidural space. The ligament's structure is steeply arched and tent-like, so much so that the lateral reflection may be up to 1 cm deeper than at the midline. In the cervical and thoracic epidural space, the ligamentum flavum often does not fuse in the midline, which can become problematic during loss-of-resistance techniques. When the dense ligamentum flavum is absent in the midline, it is possible to enter the epidural space without ever sensing significant resistance to injection. The ligamentum flavum is thickest at the lumbar and thoracic levels and thinnest at the cervical level. Its thickness also diminishes at the cephalad aspect of each interlaminar space and as the ligamentum flavum tapers off laterally. In patients who have undergone spinal surgery, scarring of the posterior epidural space is common, such that the loss of resistance and the flow of injected solutions are less predictable.

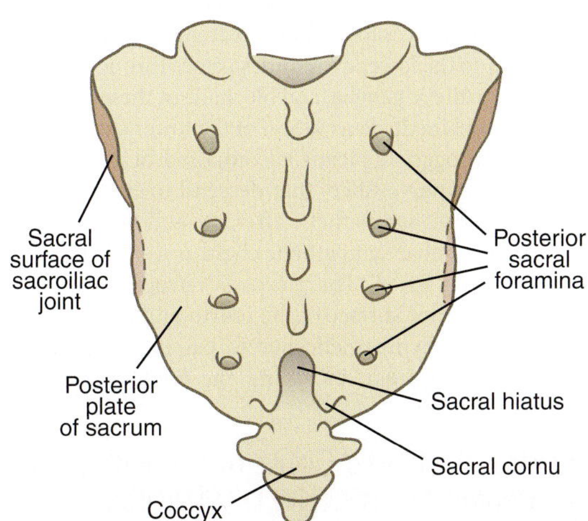

FIGURE 92-3. Anatomy of the posterior sacrum and coccyx. [Adapted from Rathmell JP. *Atlas of Image-Guided Intervention in Regional Anesthesia and Pain Medicine.* Philadelphia, PA: Lippincott Williams & Wilkins, 2006:32 (Figure 5-2). With permission.]

The spinal cord is a cylindrical structure composed of an external white matter and internal gray matter that is protected by the bony vertebral column. White matter represents the myelinated ascending and descending tracts of the spinal cord, which conduct information to and from the brain. The gray matter contains axons, dendrites, and synaptic terminals arranged grossly in the shape of butterfly wings when viewed in cross section. The spinal cord receives its vascular supply from arteries of the brain and from segmental spinal arteries arising from the subclavian artery, aorta, and iliac arteries.[19] The posterior spinal cord receives its blood supply from a paired system of posterior spinal arteries arising from the posterior inferior cerebellar arteries. The anterior spinal artery is a single discontinuous vessel formed by the union of a terminal branch from each vertebral artery that descends along the anterior midline of the spinal cord. In all regions of the cord, the anterior spinal artery provides nutrition to approximately 75% of the cord tissue, including all of the gray matter,[21] which makes this territory most vulnerable to ischemia.

The segmental spinal arteries reach the spinal cord by way of the intervertebral foramina and the epidural space, to reach the spinal nerve roots. Although the main purpose of these segmental arteries is to provide blood supply to the nerve roots (and thus they have been termed *radicular arteries*), some send branches that penetrate the dura to join the anterior and posterior spinal arteries, providing blood supply to the spinal cord. The largest of the segmental arteries is the *artery radicularis magna* (artery of Adamkiewicz), which supplies the anterior spinal artery for the thoracolumbar region of the cord. In 78% of cases, it enters by way of a left intervertebral foramen between T8 and L3; in 15%

of cases, the artery of Adamkiewicz takes off more cephalad, at about the level of T5.[21] Many of our pain procedures are performed in this region, and damage to or embolization caused by particulate steroid injected into the artery of Adamkiewicz or other spinal segmental arteries can result in ischemia and infarction of the anterior two-thirds of the lumbar spinal cord, with its resultant predominantly motor lesion.[22]

Venous drainage of the spinal cord occurs via large epidural veins, which are more prominent in the anterior and lateral portions of the epidural space. These veins are valveless and connect to the systemic circulation via the basivertebral venous plexus (Batson plexus), intracranial veins, and azygos veins. Inferiorly, this plexus communicates with the sacral venous plexus, which drains into the uterine and iliac veins. At each level, the vertebral plexus sends branches through the intervertebral foramina that anastomose with the thoracic and abdominal veins. The extensive communication between the epidural venous plexus and the systemic circulation is responsible for the distension of the epidural veins that occurs with increases in intra-abdominal pressure. Thus significant obstruction of the inferior vena cava results in rerouting of the venous return through the epidural venous plexus to the azygos vein.

The spinal nerve at each level traverses the intervertebral foramen and divides into anterior and posterior primary rami. The anterior ramus contains most of the sensory and motor fibers at each vertebral level. Of importance, a small branch of the anterior ramus, the sinuvertebral nerve, provides neural branches to the posterior outer layers of the annulus of the disk.[20] The posterior primary ramus, in turn, divides into a lateral branch, which provides innervation to the paraspinous musculature, and a small variable sensory distribution to the skin overlying the spinous processes; the medial branch passes over the base of the transverse process where it joins with the superior articular process of the facet joint and courses along the articular process to supply sensation to the joint. Each facet joint receives sensory innervation from the medial branch nerve at the same vertebral level as well as from a descending branch from the vertebral level above; thus 2 medial branch nerves must be blocked to anesthetize each facet joint (eg, medial branch blocks at the base of the L4 and L5 transverse processes are needed to anesthetize the L4-L5 facet joint). The specific course of the medial branch nerves and cannula position for radiofrequency treatment at specific spinal levels is discussed in the following sections.

Anatomy of the Sympathetic Nervous System Because we cover sympathetic nerve block techniques, a brief review of the anatomy is warranted. The sympathetic nervous system is part of the autonomic nervous system that innervates cardiac, smooth muscle, and glandular tissues, mediating a variety of reflexes. In certain pathologic pain states, neuronal activity in the sympathetic nervous system may be involved in the maintenance of chronic pain.[23] Anatomically, the peripheral sympathetic system arises as efferent preganglionic fibers that leave their cell bodies in the intermediolateral column of the spinal cord, which extends from the first thoracic spinal segment to approximately the second lumbar segment. These axons leave the spinal cord within the ventral root and initially proceed as part of the spinal nerve. They separate from the somatic motor neuron, forming the white rami communicantes, and project to the sympathetic chain, located along the anterolateral surface of the vertebral bodies. Within the sympathetic nerve trunk, the preganglionic fibers can transverse variable distances cephalad and caudad, forming synapses with many postganglionic neurons in different ganglia at other levels in the chain. The ratio of preganglionic sympathetic fibers to postganglionic fibers is estimated to be 1:10, permitting coordinated activity at several spinal levels.[23] The axons of the postganglionic neurons are predominantly unmyelinated and exit the ganglia as the gray rami communicantes, which join the spinal nerves en route to their peripheral targets. In addition to the multiple ganglia located in the thoracolumbar chain, there are classically 3 cervical ganglia, 4 to 5 lumbar ganglia, 4 sacral ganglia, and 1 coccygeal ganglion (the ganglion impar).

In the cervical region, the sympathetic chain lies at the anterolateral aspect of the vertebral bodies. Most sympathetic fibers traversing to and from the head, neck, and upper extremities pass through the stellate ganglion. In most individuals, the stellate ganglion is formed by fusion of the inferior cervical and first thoracic sympathetic ganglia; in some individuals the 2 ganglia remain separate. The ganglion is commonly found just lateral to the longus colli muscle, anterior to the neck of the first rib and the transverse process of the seventh cervical vertebra. In this position, the ganglion lies posterior to the first portion of the subclavian artery at the origin of the vertebral artery posterior to the dome of the lung. Although several approaches to stellate ganglion block have been described, the most common is the anterior paratracheal approach at C6 using surface landmarks. Performing the block at C6 reduces the likelihood of pneumothorax, which is more likely when the block is carried out close to the dome of the lung at C7. The anterior tubercle of the transverse process of C6 (Chassaignac tubercle) is palpable in most individuals.

Sympathetic innervation to the abdominal viscera arises from the anterolateral horn of the spinal cord between the T5 and T12 levels. Nociceptive information from the abdominal viscera is carried by afferents that accompany the sympathetic nerves. Pain transmitted via the celiac plexus originates from the upper abdominal structures, including the pancreas, diaphragm, liver, spleen, stomach, small bowel, ascending and proximal transverse colon, adrenal glands, kidney, abdominal aorta, and mesentery. The celiac plexus is composed of a diffuse network of nerve fibers and individual ganglia that lie over the anterolateral surface of the aorta at the T12-L1 vertebral level. Presynaptic sympathetic fibers travel from the thoracic sympathetic chain toward the ganglion, traversing over the anterolateral aspect of the inferior thoracic vertebrae as the greater (T5-T9), lesser (T10-T11), and least (T12) splanchnic nerves. Presynaptic fibers traveling via the splanchnic nerves synapse within the celiac ganglia, over the anterolateral surface of the aorta surrounding the origin of the celiac and superior mesenteric arteries at approximately the L1 vertebral level. Postsynaptic fibers from the celiac ganglia innervate all of the abdominal viscera with the exception of the descending colon, sigmoid colon, rectum, and pelvic viscera.

The lumbar sympathetic chain consists of 4 to 5 paired ganglia that lie over the anterolateral surface of the second through fourth lumbar vertebrae. The cell bodies that send projections to the lumbar sympathetic ganglia lie in the anterolateral region of the spinal cord from T11 to L2, with variable contributions from T10 and L3. As in the thoracic area, the lumbar preganglionic fibers leave the spinal canal with the corresponding spinal nerve, join the sympathetic chain as white communicating rami, and then synapse within the appropriate ganglion. Postganglionic fibers exit the chain to join the diffuse perivascular plexus around the iliac and femoral arteries or via the gray communicating rami to join the nerves that form the lumbar and lumbosacral plexus. Sympathetic fibers accompany all of the major nerves to the lower extremities. Most of the sympathetic innervation to the lower extremities passes through the second and third lumbar sympathetic ganglia, and blockade of these ganglia results in near-complete sympathetic denervation of the lower extremities.

The superior hypogastric plexus is composed of a flattened band of intercommunicating nerve fibers that descend over the aortic bifurcation. The plexus carries sympathetic afferents and postganglionic efferent fibers from the lumbar sympathetic chain as well as parasympathetic fibers that arise from S2-S4. The plexus is retroperitoneal in location and lies over the anterior surface of the fourth and fifth lumbar and the first sacral vertebrae. Sympathetic nerves passing through the plexus innervate the pelvic viscera, including the bladder, uterus, rectum, vagina, and prostate.

INTERLAMINAR EPIDURAL INJECTION STEROIDS AND TRANSFORAMINAL INJECTION OF STEROIDS

Overview The theoretical background supporting the use of epidural steroids is based on the existence of inflammation as the basic pathophysiologic process. Nerve root edema has been demonstrated surgically and with computed tomography (CT) in patients with herniated disks.[24] Inflammation of nerves in the presence of a herniated disk has further been confirmed during surgery,[25] myelography,[26] and histologic examinations.[27,28] More recently, phospholipase A_2 (PLA_2), the rate-limiting enzyme in the conversion of arachidonic acid to prostaglandins and leukotrienes, has been found in high levels in the extruded disk material of patients undergoing discectomy for herniated disk.[29] Other inflammatory mediators such as prostaglandins have also been shown to produce hyperalgesia.[30] Clinically, improvement of pain has been shown to coincide with resolution or decrease in nerve root edema, despite a persistent herniated disk.[20]

In laboratory animals, PLA_2 has been implicated as a primary inflammatory mediator. Its administration adjacent to lumbar spinal nerves produces motor weakness and decreased mechanical withdrawal thresholds.[31] Histologic examination shows reversible demyelination, vacuolar degeneration in the nerve roots, and unclear axonal margins.[27] In another animal model of radiculopathy, Hayashi et al[32] ligated the left L4 and L5 nerve roots while surgically placing an epidural catheter with the tip between the ligated nerve roots. All rats demonstrated reversible motor weakness that resolved completely in 4 weeks, and all of the animals exhibited thermal hyperalgesia. The rats were separated into groups and treated with epidural betamethasone alone, normal saline, or epidural betamethasone plus bupivacaine. All treatment groups demonstrated a transient reduction in thermal hyperalgesia, but both betamethasone groups showed prolonged benefit lasting 3 to 4 weeks.

Steroids decrease inflammation by inducing the biosynthesis of a PLA_2 inhibitor, preventing prostaglandin generation.[33,34] Steroids also suppress ongoing discharge in chronic neuromas and prevent the development of ectopic neural discharges from experimental neuromas, which has been attributed to direct action on the membrane.[35] Steroids may block nociceptive input. Local application of methylprednisolone was found to reversibly block transmission in the unmyelinated C-fibers but not in Aβ-fibers.[36]

Patient Selection Many investigators have attempted to identify which patients are most likely to benefit from epidural steroid injections. In 1960, Goebert et al[37] administered 3 consecutive epidural hydrocortisone and procaine injections in 239 patients with low back pain. Fifty-eight percent of the patients had more than 60% relief for 3 months or longer, and 8% of patients claimed 40% to 60% pain relief.

In a prospective study, White et al[38] followed the response of 304 patients with low back pain to epidural steroid injection. They found longer pain relief in patients with less than weeks of pain and in those patients without "psychologic overlay." Eighty-seven percent of the patients reported good short-term success, without significant differences between the acute and chronic pain groups, whereas 34% of patients in the acute pain group still reported pain relief at 6 months compared with 12% in the chronic pain group. Twenty-four percent of patients without psychologic overlay were still relieved of their pain at 6 months compared with only 1.5% of patients with psychologic overlay.

One prospective randomized study of lumbar epidural steroid injections followed 36 patients younger than 50 years with radicular pain, positive straight-leg raising test, and a prolapsed disk at L4-L5 or L5-S1 confirmed by magnetic resonance imaging (MRI).[39] These patients were randomized to 2 groups; both received identical conservative therapy, and one of the groups also received a series of 3 epidural steroid injections. At 2-week follow-up, patients in the epidural steroid injection group had a significantly greater increase in straight-leg raise measurements compared with the control group. In addition, a trend in pain relief favoring the epidural steroid group was noted but did not reach significance. This study was not blinded, and all injections were given within 14 days of randomization, so the interval from onset to injection was very brief.

The effectiveness of epidural steroids in the relief of radicular pain attributable to herniated disk has been documented by many studies.[40-47] In 2 fairly recent systematic reviews, national organizations have assembled practice guidelines based on the best available scientific evidence; both groups concluded the epidural steroid injections are useful in speeding the resolution of acute radicular pain associated with disk herniations.[48,49] Although their usefulness has not been clearly documented by controlled studies, epidural steroid injections also have been used to treat back pain secondary to degenerative disk disease,[40,44,45] spinal stenosis,[50] trauma,[37] spondylolysis or spondylolisthesis,[38,40,42] and in pain following laminectomy.[37,51]

There has been some recent data suggesting that the transforaminal and interlaminar routes of injection may vary in their effectiveness. In a 2009 study, Lee et al studied a cohort of patients with disk herniations and spinal stenosis.[52] Patients were randomized to receive an interlaminar epidural steroid injection versus bilateral transforaminal epidural steroid injections. There was no difference in pain scores or patient satisfaction in the disk herniation group. However, in patients with spinal stenosis, there was significant improvement in pain scores and satisfaction in those that received bilateral transforaminal epidural when compared with the group receiving interlaminar injections.

In a large observational study on the frequency of epidural steroid injections and patient characteristics, Fanciullo et al[53] collected information on 25 479 patients seen at 23 specialty spine centers in the United States from 1995 to 1998. Epidural steroid injection formed part of the treatment plan for only 2002 patients (7.9%). Lumbar problems were far more likely in patients who had an epidural steroid injection (12.6%) than in patients with cervical (3.7%), thoracic (1.8%), or sacral problems (2.4%). The most frequent diagnoses in patients who were offered epidural steroid injection were spinal stenosis (40.1%) and herniated disk (34.3%), followed by spondylolisthesis (7.8%) and compression fractures (1.6%). Evidence supports the use of epidural steroids in patients with disk herniations and other presumed inflammatory conditions that cause acute radicular pain, such as spinal stenosis or spondylolisthesis, but the efficacy of epidural steroids is undocumented in patients with compression fractures. Thus patient selection for epidural steroid injections is not always consistent with existing data, and concordance between clinical practice and reported evidence of efficacy is variable. Indeed, epidural injection of steroids is one of the most overused treatments for back pain in the United States.

Drug Selection for Epidural Steroid Injection Most studies reported in the literature used a mixture of local anesthetic and steroid, saline with steroid, or steroid alone. The steroids most commonly used are either methylprednisolone acetate (Depo-Medrol) or triamcinolone diacetate (Aristocort). The doses of methylprednisolone most widely used vary from 80 to 120 mg, and the doses of triamcinolone most commonly used vary from 50 to 75 mg.[44,45,54,55]

Methylprednisolone acetate has been approved for intramuscular, intrasynovial, soft tissue, and intralesional injection. It is a glucocorticoid with an elimination half-life of 139 hours and a range from 58 to 866 hours.[56] Triamcinolone diacetate, which has an elimination half-life of 18 to 36 hours, possesses glucocorticoid properties while being essentially devoid of mineralocorticoid activity, thus causing little or no sodium retention. It has been approved for administration by intramuscular, intra-articular, and intrasynovial routes.[57]

Serious injury to the central nervous system has been reported following transforaminal epidural steroid injections.[58-60] The likely etiology is embolization of steroid particles into the vertebral artery or a segmental spinal artery causing end-arteriolar occlusion, resulting in posterior circulation strokes or spinal cord infarction. The resulting injuries are catastrophic: quadriplegia, paraplegia, cortical blindness, or death. The most recent and convincing evidence that embolization of particulate steroid can result in stroke comes from a large animal study. Okubadejo et al[61] administered particulate (methylprednisolone) and nonparticulate (dexamethasone) directly in to the vertebral arteries of anesthetized swine; those animals receiving particulate steroid never regained spontaneous respiratory function, and MRI demonstrated changes consistent with acute stroke, whereas those receiving dexamethasone had no changes on MRI and recovered fully with no apparent harm. In an effort to avoid microembolic complications, practitioners have started using dexamethasone for transforaminal injections, specifically in the cervical spine. Dexamethasone sodium phosphate is a synthetic glucocorticoid that has an elimination half-life of only 1.8 to 3.5 hours in patients with normal renal function but a biologic half-life of 36 to 54 hours. Because dexamethasone is water soluble and has been approved for intravenous administration, it is thought that the risk of vascular microembolization is diminished. Derby et al[62] evaluated particle size of various steroid preparations of dexamethasone, triamcinolone, betamethasone, and methylprednisolone. They found that dexamethasone particles measured about 0.5 μm, smaller in diameter than a red blood cell, and no aggregation was observed when mixed with local anesthetic or contrast medium. There are no randomized studies comparing clinical efficacy with different formulations of corticosteroids; however, observational studies did not find any statistical differences between particulate and nonparticulate steroids in cervical transforaminal epidural injections.[63,64] We have recently changed our practice to use dexamethasone in cervical transforaminal epidural steroid injection as detailed later.

In a review of the literature, Kepes and Duncalf[65] found that methylprednisolone was the least irritating, the most beneficial, and the longest acting, although Delaney et al[66] prefer triamcinolone because of its excellent anti-inflammatory effect and low potential for sodium retention. No study has compared the effectiveness of triamcinolone and methylprednisolone, which likely are equally effective. Both of these preparations contain polyethylene glycol, which has been found to impair nerve transmission in rabbit vagus nerve and cause degenerative lesions in rat sciatic nerves.[67,68] Both preparations also contain benzyl alcohol, which is potentially toxic when administered locally to neural tissue.[44] Neither of these preparations should be used intrathecally.

Most practitioners dilute the steroid with local anesthetic or sterile saline, and the results are apparently comparable with either diluent.[43] Some authors have recommended use of local anesthetics "in the presence of muscle spasms."[39,69] However small the dose, use of local anesthetic carries some risks, including hypotension, arrhythmias, and seizures from intravascular injections. Brown[44] suggests that because the results are comparable, use of saline probably is sufficient. Some investigators have combined epidural methylprednisolone with morphine.[70,71] In an initial study, Cohn et al[70] showed encouraging results in postlaminectomy patients; however, a subsequent study was unable to repeat such beneficial effects. Epidural morphine carries significant risk of respiratory depression and should be used with caution in the outpatient setting.

Traditionally, the volume of diluent has depended on the site of injection: lumbar, caudal, or transforaminal. When using a caudal approach, 20 to 25 mL of a solution has been recommended to ensure epidural spread cephalad to the desired level.[40,43] When using a lumbar interlaminar approach, a volume of 5 to 10 mL has been recommended to reach the areas most commonly involved in the lumbar region.[38] Other practitioners use smaller volumes (2-3 mL), especially when using the transforaminal approach. Some authors have suggested that several nerve roots may be inflamed in addition to those adjacent to the herniated or bulging disk, and they recommend against using a small volume of diluent.[72] Wood et al[68] suggested diluting the steroid after their study showed degenerative lesions in rat sciatic nerves attributable to the polyethylene glycol vehicle in the steroid preparation. The optimal volume of injectate and site of epidural placement remain unresolved.

Epidural steroids have been associated with glucose intolerance and pituitary-adrenal axis suppression for up to 3 weeks after repeated administration.[73-75] Ward et al measured insulin sensitivity and fasting blood glucose, fasting plasma insulin, and fasting serum cortisol levels in 10 healthy individuals 24 hours before and 1 week after epidural administration of triamcinolone 80 mg via a caudal route.[76] They found that 24 hours after epidural steroid injection, insulin sensitivity had decreased to nearly half the baseline, fasting insulin levels increased 1.4-fold, and fasting glucose levels had increased 1.1-fold. All of these values normalized by 1 week after injection, and they demonstrate the marked changes in insulin sensitivity occurring in nondiabetic healthy individuals after epidural steroid injection.

Technique The epidural space can be approached through the interlaminar space (median or paramedian), intervertebral foramen (transforaminal), or sacral hiatus (caudal). The approach selected depends on patient selection, indication for injection, practitioner's experience, and availability of imaging. The patient can be positioned in the lateral decubitus position, sitting or prone, depending on the technique to be used.

Interlaminar Technique for Epidural Steroid Injection The term *interlaminar* has been given to the traditional posterior approach to the epidural space to easily differentiate it from the transforaminal or caudal approach. The interlaminar approach can be either midline or paramedian. Correct epidural placement with this technique is facilitated by the use of image guidance. As reported by Sharrock et al,[77] anesthesiologists have a high success rate of epidural anesthesia using loss of resistance; however, use of image guidance can confirm proper placement in all cases. When using the midline approach, the point of insertion depends on the level of entry and angle of the corresponding spinous processes. For the cervical and lumbar midline approach, the needle should be almost perpendicular to the neuraxis, in line with the corresponding spinous process. This is also true with the low thoracic approach below T9. In the midthoracic region, the spinous processes are sharply angled caudad, such that the tip of the spinous processes lies opposite the lamina of the inferior vertebral body. In this region, the midline approach requires that the needle be inserted with a steep cephalad angle, often approaching 130°. Many practitioners prefer the paramedian approach in the midthoracic region. The choice of needles when using the interlaminar approach is similar to those available for anesthesia; the most common type is the 18- or 20-gauge Tuohy needle.

For cervical interlaminar epidural injections, most practitioners place the patient in a sitting or prone position. When in the sitting position, the patient is asked to sit comfortably and flex the neck anteriorly. The forehead can be leaned against a sturdy, padded horizontal surface to minimize involuntary movement. This position avoids rotation of the spine and widens the lower cervical epidural space. Because of its large interlaminar distance, the most common approach is C6-C7 or C7-T1, especially because the long spinous process of C7 (the vertebra prominens) serves as a reliable surface marker.

When the prone position is used for the cervical interlaminar approach, most practitioners prefer to use image guidance. This allows for good visualization of the interlaminar space and needle advancement between adjacent spinous processes.

Cervical Epidural Steroid Injection Technique Classically, the epidural space has been identified using loss of resistance to saline. Regardless of the approach, sterile technique must be strictly observed. The skin and subcutaneous tissues overlying the interspace where the block is to be performed are anesthetized with local anesthetic. The cervical interspaces with the largest interlaminar distance typically are found at C6-C7 and C7-T1. Because of the ease of entry, many practitioners place the needle via one of these larger interspaces, regardless of the level of pathology, and they rely on the flow of steroid in the epidural space to reach the level of pathology. The same technique can be used in all cervical interspaces below C3-C4. Interlaminar injections above the C2-C3 level have not been described.

An 18- or 20-gauge Tuohy needle is placed through the skin and advanced several centimeters until the needle is firmly seated in the interspinous ligament. An anteroposterior (AP) image is taken, and the needle is redirected toward midline. We use the loss-of-resistance technique with saline to find the epidural space. Repeat images taken after every few millimeters of needle advancement will ensure that the needle direction does not stray from midline. A firm grasp of the adjacent structures and the proximity of the spinal cord is essential during a cervical interlaminar epidural injection. After the needle tip enters the epidural space, the position is confirmed by injecting nonionic radiographic contrast, and adequate spread is verified in the AP and lateral planes. If lateral imaging of the cervicothoracic junction and low cervical spine is hindered by the adjacent structures of the torso and arms, a second lateral image taken just above the shoulders often can be much simpler to interpret when trying to confirm epidural contrast flow. Once epidural needle position has been confirmed, a solution containing steroid diluted in preservative-free saline is injected. In our practice, we routinely use 80 mg of methylprednisolone acetate or the equivalent diluted in 3 to 5 mL of total volume.

Midthoracic Epidural Steroid Injection Because of the steep angulation of the spinous processes at this level, image guidance is often used. The patient lies prone, with the head turned to one side. The C-arm is rotated 40° to 50° caudally from the axial plane without any oblique angulation. This allows for good visualization of the interlaminar space and needle advancement between adjacent spinous processes.

The skin and subcutaneous tissues approximately 1 cm lateral and 2 to 3 cm caudad to the interspace where the block is to be performed are anesthetized. An 18- or 20-gauge Tuohy needle is placed through the skin and advanced several centimeters until the needle is firmly seated in tissue. An AP image is taken, and the needle is directed toward the superior margin of the lamina below the interspace that is to be entered, near the junction of the spinous process and the lamina. Although a midline approach can be used at low thoracic levels, the spinous processes are angled too steeply to allow for true coaxial needle placement at the midthoracic levels. Thus the needle is best directed toward the superior margin of the lamina. While advancing, repeat images are taken and care must be taken to keep the needle tip over the lamina until bone is gently contacted. The periosteum is then anesthetized, and the needle is slowly advanced over the superior margin of the lamina until loss of resistance occurs. Because the needle is unlikely to lie within the interspinous ligament when using a paramedian approach, there will be little resistance to injection until the needle enters the interlaminar space and traverses the ligamentum flavum. A firm understanding of the adjacent structures and the proximity of the spinal cord is essential for thoracic interlaminar epidural injection. After the needle tip enters the epidural space, the position is confirmed by injecting nonionic radiographic contrast, and spread is verified in the AP and lateral planes. Once epidural needle position has been confirmed, a solution containing steroid diluted in preservative-free saline is injected, and the needle is removed.

Lumbar Epidural Steroid Injection Epidural injection at the lumbar level can be administered with the patient in a sitting or prone position. The patient is asked to sit comfortably with his or her back to the practitioner, curving the spine posteriorly and pushing the lumbar region against the examiner's fingers in an attempt to separate the spinous processes. If the procedure is to be performed in the prone position under fluoroscopic imaging, a pillow is placed under the mid and lower abdomen to reduce the lumbar lordosis and increase the separation between adjacent spinous processes. The C-arm is rotated 15° to 20° caudally from the axial plane without any oblique angulation. This allows for good visualization of the interlaminar space and needle advancement between adjacent spinous processes.

The skin and subcutaneous tissues overlying the interspace where the block is to be performed are anesthetized. An 18- or 20-gauge Tuohy needle is placed through the skin and advanced 1 to 2 cm until the needle is firmly seated in the interspinous ligament. If the patient is prone, a lateral image should be taken as the needle is advanced, until loss of resistance occurs. If the patient is sitting, adequate positioning will allow a proper midline approach. A firm knowledge of the adjacent structures and the proximity of the thecal sac and cauda equina are essential for lumbar interlaminar epidural injection (**Fig. 92-4**). After the needle tip enters the epidural space and aspiration is negative for CSF or blood, the position is confirmed by injecting nonionic radiographic contrast, and spread is verified in the AP and lateral planes. Lateral imaging of the lower lumbar spine is hindered by the overlying iliac crests, and visualization can be difficult in the obese patient. Once epidural needle position has been confirmed, a solution containing steroid diluted in preservative-free saline is injected, and the needle is removed. In the lumbar region, we usually use 80 mg of methylprednisolone acetate or the equivalent diluted in 5 to 10 mL of total volume. When larger injectate volumes are used, the solution spreads extensively in both the anterior and posterior aspects of the epidural space. In patients with significant lumbar pathology, the injectate tends to follow the path of least resistance, often flowing toward the side opposite the pathology.[2]

Caudal Epidural Steroid Injection Anesthesiologists will be familiar with caudal injections administered to pediatric patients in the operating room. Because of difficulty identifying the sacral hiatus clinically in adults, these procedures usually are performed under fluoroscopy. The patient lies prone with the head turned to one side. The C-arm is rotated 20° to 30° caudally from the axial plane without any oblique angulation. This allows for good visualization of the sacrum, sacral hiatus, and coccyx.

Once the sacral hiatus is identified radiographically, the overlying skin and subcutaneous tissues are anesthetized. The sacral hiatus can be difficult to visualize radiographically. The approximate location can be identified by palpating the paired sacral cornua in the midline, near the superior extent of the gluteal cleft. An 18- or 20-gauge Tuohy needle can be used, but a smaller 22-gauge, 3.5-in spinal needle is adequate. The needle is placed through the skin and advanced directly through the sacrococcygeal ligament. Once the needle has passed through the sacrococcygeal ligament and is within the caudal spinal canal, the angle of the needle is decreased to lie closer to the plane of the sacrum, and the needle is advanced into the spinal canal an additional 1 to 2 cm. AP and lateral imaging confirm the needle's position within the caudal epidural space. The caudal epidural space is generously supplied with veins, and intravascular needle placement is ruled out by injecting nonionic radiographic contrast under live fluoroscopy. Once caudal epidural needle position has been confirmed, a solution containing steroid diluted in preservative-free saline is injected, and the needle is removed. The caudal epidural space is distant from the usual sites of nerve root inflammation near the lumbosacral junction; thus a significant volume of injectate usually is required to effect spread to the level of the lumbosacral junction. For this approach, we use 80 mg of methylprednisolone acetate or the equivalent diluted in at least 10 mL of total volume.

Complications of the interlaminar approach include dural puncture with subsequent postdural puncture headache, which can occur when this technique is used at any level of the spine. Although in a different patient population, the incidence of dural puncture in parturients undergoing lumbar epidurals ranges between 0% and 2.6%.[78] Postdural puncture headaches occur frequently after unintended dural puncture with large epidural needles. The incidence of headache following cervical dural puncture is lower than that following lumbar puncture, likely because of the diminished column of CSF cephalad to the point of dural puncture.

Although cervical and thoracic epidural blood patches using small volumes of autologous blood have been described, most practitioners manage postdural puncture headaches following cervical or thoracic epidural injection conservatively with fluids and oral analgesics. Dural puncture also can occur during caudal epidural injection but usually only if the needle is advanced several centimeters cephalad within the caudal spinal canal. The thecal sac extends to the level of approximately S2, and the position can be approximated by palpating the adjacent posterior superior iliac spines, which lie at the same level. Epidural blood patch using autologous blood is a safe and effective treatment that relieves headache symptoms promptly in 70% to 98% of patients who fail to improve after 24 to 48 hours of conservative treatment and oral analgesics.[79] The incidence of unintentional dural puncture may be higher in patients with previous lumbar surgery because of scarring within the epidural space and adhesion of the dura to the posterior elements.

Although direct neurologic needle trauma is rare (<0.6%),[80] injury to the spinal cord with catastrophic consequences, including quadriplegia, has been described, particularly in heavily sedated patients.[81-83] The level of sedation during this procedure should allow for direct conversation between the practitioner and the patient to ensure that the patient

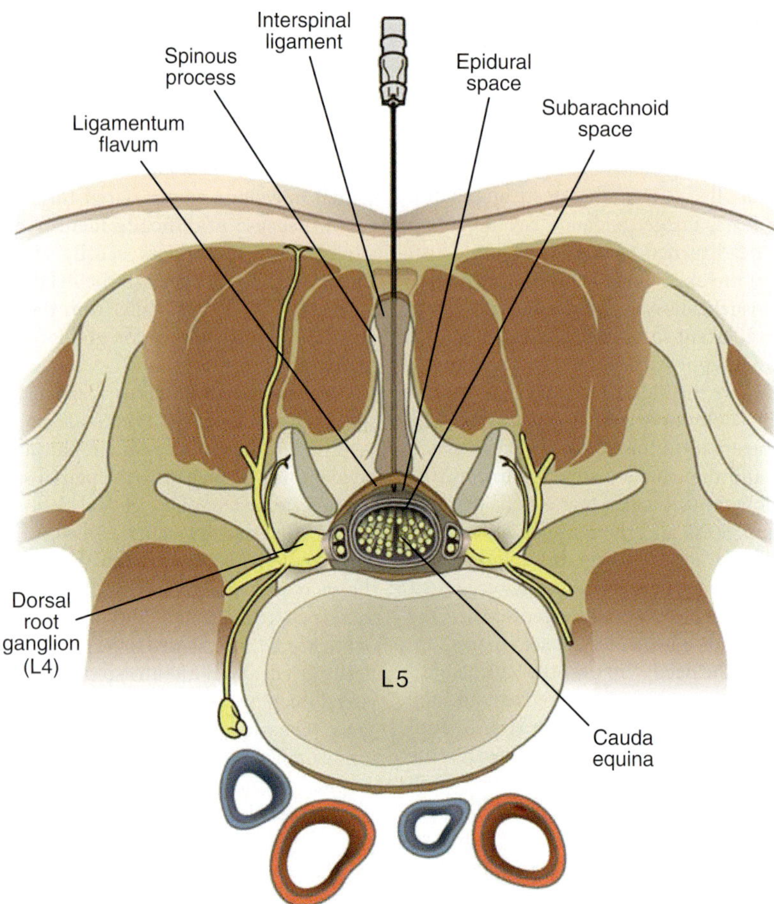

FIGURE 92-4. Axial diagram of interlaminar lumbar epidural injection. The epidural needle is advanced in the midline between adjacent spinous processes to traverse the ligamentum flavum and enter the dorsal epidural space in the midline. The normal epidural space is approximately 4-6 mm wide (from the ligamentum flavum to the dura mater in the axial plane). Note the proximity of the underlying cauda equina during the lumbar epidural injection. [Adapted from Rathmell JP. *Atlas of Image-Guided Intervention in Regional Anesthesia and Pain Medicine.* Philadelphia, PA: Lippincott Williams & Wilkins, 2006:47 (Figure 5-20). With permission.]

can report contact with neural elements before significant traumatic injury occurs. Caution should be taken to avoid interlaminar epidural injection at any level where there is effacement of the epidural space.[84] Complete effacement of the epidural space as well as the CSF column surrounding the spinal cord within the thecal sac occurs in high-grade spinal stenosis, particularly that due to a large central or paramedian disk herniation. Direct trauma to the cauda equina or spinal nerve is unlikely during lumbar epidural injection when disciplined use of radiographic guidance is used to ensure that the needle tip does not stray from the midline. Direct trauma to the cauda equina or the exiting nerve roots is unlikely with the caudal approach.

Regardless of the level of injection, epidural bleeding or infection can occur. Epidural hematoma or abscess can lead to significant compression of the spinal cord or cauda equina. Interlaminar epidural injection should be avoided or postponed in patients receiving anticoagulants.[85]

Transforaminal Technique for Epidural Steroid Injection Transforaminal epidural steroid injection and selective nerve root injection can be performed using similar techniques. The distinction between the 2 techniques is questionable because the fascial sheath surrounding the spinal nerves is contiguous with the dura mater within the epidural space. A solution injected around a spinal nerve may well enter the epidural space, whether or not the needle tip is advanced through the intervertebral foramen before injection. Nonetheless, many practitioners reserve the term *selective nerve root injection* for injections performed with the needle tip adjacent to the spinal nerve, outside of the intervertebral foramen and the term *transforaminal injection* for injections performed with the needle tip within the intervertebral foramen. Unlike the interlaminar technique, the transforaminal approach requires the use of radiographic imaging to proceed with safety.[86]

Several important anatomic aspects are unique to transforaminal epidural and selective nerve root injections. At cervical levels, the ventral and dorsal roots converge in the vertebral canal to form the spinal nerve in the intervertebral foramen. The foramen faces obliquely anterior and laterally. Its roof and floor are formed by the pedicles of the articulated vertebrae. Its posterolateral wall is formed largely by the superior articular process of the lower vertebra and in part by the inferior articular process of the upper vertebra and the capsule of the zygapophysial joint. The anteromedial wall is formed by the lower end of the upper vertebral body, the uncinate process of the lower vertebra, and the posterolateral corner of the intervertebral disk. Immediately lateral to the external opening of the foramen, the vertebral artery ascends within the *foramen transversarium* in close proximity to the spinal nerve and anterior to the articular pillars of the zygapophysial joint. The spinal nerve, in its dural sleeve, lies in the lower half of the foramen, whereas the upper half is occupied by epiradicular veins. Arterial branches arise from the vertebral arteries to supply the nerve roots (radicular arteries) or the spinal cord via the anterior and posterior spinal arteries (spinal segmental or medullary arteries). Medullary and radicular arterial branches also may arise from the deep or ascending cervical arteries and traverse through the entire length of the foramen adjacent to the spinal nerve. It is these spinal segmental arteries that are at risk for penetration during cervical transforaminal injection.

At the lumbar levels, the ventral and dorsal roots of the spinal nerves descend within the vertebral canal to form the spinal nerve in the intervertebral foramen. Its roof and floor are formed by the pedicles of consecutive vertebrae. Its posterior wall is formed largely by the superior articular process of the lower vertebra and in part by the inferior articular process of the superior vertebra and the capsule of the zygapophysial joint. The anterior wall is formed by the vertebral body and the intervertebral disk. The spinal nerve, in its dural sleeve, lies in the anterior and superior portions of the foramen, just inferior to the pedicle.

The most common indication for a transforaminal approach or selective nerve root injection is for placing the corticosteroid immediately adjacent to the inflamed nerve root causing the radicular symptoms. Nerve root inflammation may stem from an acutely herniated intervertebral disk causing nerve root irritation or other causes of nerve root impingement, such as isolated foraminal stenosis due to spondylitic spurring of the bony margins of the foramen. Although some studies[87,88] have shown better ventral dye spread with transforaminal and parasagittal approaches versus interlaminar injection, there is scant evidence that better clinical outcomes result from one or the other approach.[86] Selective nerve root injection with local anesthetic has been used diagnostically to determine which nerve root is causing symptoms when pathology exists at multiple vertebral levels. This information can prove invaluable in planning surgical intervention.

Cervical Transforaminal Steroid Injection The patient lies supine, facing directly forward. The C-arm is rotated 45° to 55° lateral oblique until the neural foramina are clearly visualized. The patient may also be asked to rotate the head away from the side of injection. Although this position facilitates access to the side of the neck, the neural foramina and bony elements of the cervical spine will no longer be aligned, which may prove confusing to the inexperienced practitioner.

A 25-gauge, 1.5- to 2.5-in blunt-tipped needle is sufficient in length for all but the most obese patients. To avoid the vertebral artery and the spinal nerve, the needle is advanced toward the posterior and middle aspect of the intervertebral foramen. Care is taken ensure that the needle tip remains superimposed on the bone of the facet column during advancement. In this way, the superior articular process of the facet just posterior to the foramen is contacted first, preventing needle advancement through the foramen and into the spinal canal. Once the needle contacts the facet, it is walked anteriorly into the foramen and advanced no more than another 2 to 3 mm. The depth is assessed by obtaining an image in the direct AP plane. To avoid direct trauma to the spinal cord and intrathecal injection, the needle should be advanced no further than halfway across the facet column. Many practitioners place a small length of flexible tubing between the needle hub and the syringe, so that once the needle is in final position, small changes in needle position do not occur as the syringe is taken on and off of the needle itself. Nonionic radiographic contrast is injected under "live" or real-time fluoroscopy (or digital subtraction cineradiography) to ensure that the needle tip lies in close proximity to the nerve root without any intravascular or intrathecal spread. The solution containing the steroid can then be injected safely. We have stopped using particulate steroid in cervical transforaminals and currently use four 4 to 12 mg of dexamethasone sodium phosphate (in 1-2 mL).

Lumbar Transforaminal Steroid Injection The patient lies prone on the fluoroscopy table. The C-arm is rotated 20° to 30° lateral oblique to allow direction of the needle toward the superolateral aspect of the intervertebral foramen. A somewhat less oblique approach will result in a final needle position slightly lateral to the intervertebral foramen, which some practitioners advocate as a means of limiting spread of the injectate to a single nerve root. However, even small volumes of injectate are often seen to track along the exiting nerve root to enter the lateral epidural space.

A 22- or 25-gauge, 3.5-in spinal needle is sufficient in length for patients of average build, whereas a 5-in needle may be needed in obese patients. To avoid the spinal nerve, the needle is advanced coaxially toward the superior aspect of the intervertebral foramen, just inferior to the pedicle and inferolateral to the pars interarticularis. This serves as an effective depth marker. Once this bony margin is contacted, the C-arm is rotated to a lateral view and the needle is slowly advanced toward the anterior and superior aspect of the foramen. If the patient reports paresthesia at any time during needle advancement, the needle should be withdrawn slightly and the position confirmed with radiographic contrast. With the needle in final position, nonionic radiographic contrast is injected under real-time fluoroscopy (or digital subtraction cineradiography) in the AP position to ensure that the needle tip lies in close proximity to the nerve root without any intravascular or intrathecal spread. Obtaining a final lateral image will allow assessment of the extent of spread of the injectate.

Complications of the transforaminal technique can be catastrophic. A firm grasp of the anatomy of adjacent vascular and neural structures is essential to avoid complications during cervical and lumbar approaches (**Fig. 92-5**). Direct intravascular injection into the vertebral artery may produce generalized seizures when local anesthetic is used or cerebral ischemia when particulate steroid solutions are used.[86,89] Direct injection of particulate steroid into a spinal segmental artery supplying the spinal cord at the cervical or lumbar level can lead to catastrophic infarction of the spinal cord. Needle positioning toward the posterior aspect of the foramen and advancing the needle in a plane parallel to the nerve root reduces the risk of entering a vascular structure. Again, particular care should be taken when performing transforaminal injection on the left between T8 and L3 because the artery of Adamkiewicz lies between these levels. However, use of radiographic contrast injected during "live" or "real-time" fluoroscopy (or digital subtraction cineradiography) to visualize final needle position and detect any hint of intravascular injection is the only means to verify accurately that injectate is not located within an artery.

Subarachnoid injection may occur if the needle is advanced too far medially and pierces the dural cuff as it extends laterally onto the exiting nerve root. Direct trauma to the spinal nerve or the spinal cord itself also may occur. Intradiscal placement of the needle during attempted transforaminal epidural steroid injection has been reported but usually is without sequelae.[90]

SYMPATHETIC BLOCKS

Overview The sympathetic nervous system is involved in the pathophysiology of a number of different chronic pain conditions, including complex regional pain syndrome (CRPS) and ischemic pain. These chronic pain states often are referred to as sympathetically maintained pain because they share the characteristic of pain relief following blockade of the regional sympathetic ganglia.[91,92] In an extensive review, Cepeda et al[93] questioned the efficacy of sympathetic blockade in the diagnosis and treatment of CRPS. In a review of 29 studies that included 1144 patients, only 29% of patients reported "full positive response," and 41% had a "partial positive response." According to these authors, most of the studies were retrospective and of poor quality. Sympathetic blockade is still widely used despite the scant evidence supporting its diagnostic and therapeutic role.[92,93] Many practitioners continue to use sympathetic blockade as a part of a multidisciplinary approach to treating CRPS; sympathetic blocks are one tool that can reduce pain and facilitate functional recovery. Blockade of the stellate ganglion has been used in the diagnosis and treatment of sympathetically maintained pain of the head, neck, and upper extremity, and a second lumbar sympathetic block is used for diagnosis and treatment of sympathetically maintained pain of the lower extremities. Celiac plexus block has been used for malignant and nonmalignant pain involving the upper abdominal viscera, and several techniques have been described.[95] Celiac plexus neurolysis has been used successfully to treat pain from pancreatic cancer.[96,97] Superior hypogastric block for treatment of chronic pain arising from the bladder, uterus, rectum, vagina, and prostate has been well described.[98]

Stellate Ganglion Block Stellate ganglion block has long been the standard approach to diagnosis and treatment of sympathetically

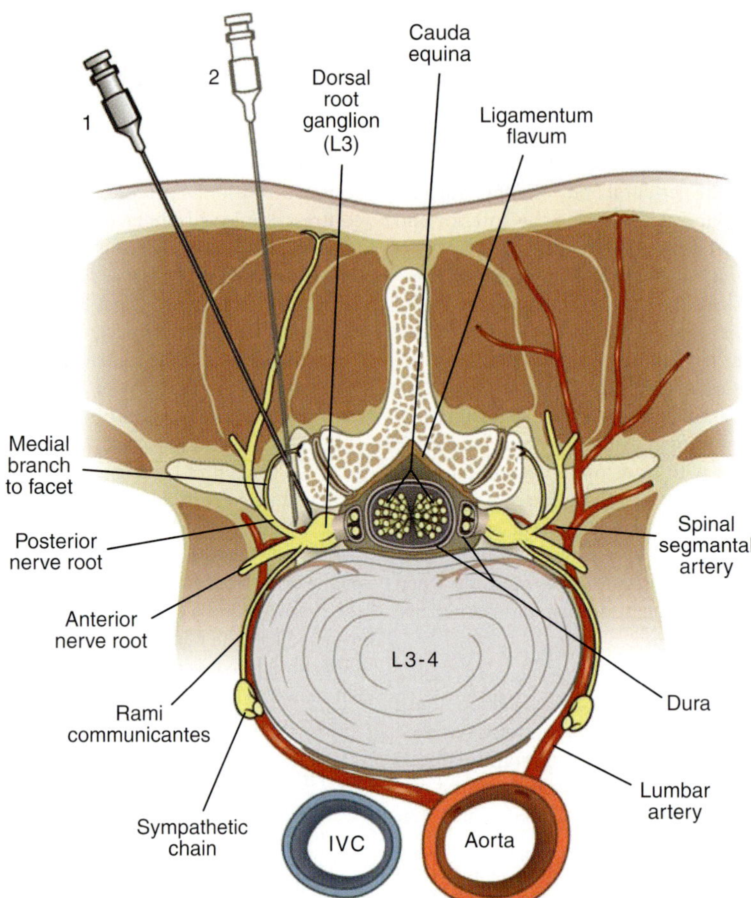

FIGURE 92-5. Axial view of lumbar transforaminal and selective nerve root injection. The anatomy and proper needle position (axial view) for right (1) L3-4 transforaminal injection and (2) L3 selective nerve root injection. [Adapted from Rathmell JP. *Atlas of Image-Guided Intervention in Regional Anesthesia and Pain Medicine.* Philadelphia, PA: Lippincott Williams & Wilkins, 2006:58 (Figure 6-7). With permission.]

maintained pain syndromes involving the upper extremity, such as CRPS. Other neuropathic pain syndromes, including ischemic neuropathies, herpes zoster (shingles), early postherpetic neuralgia, and postradiation neuritis, also may respond to stellate ganglion block. Blockade of the stellate ganglion has proven successful in reducing pain and improving blood flow in vascular insufficiency conditions such as intractable angina pectoris,[100] Raynaud disease,[101] frostbite,[102] vasospasm, and occlusive and embolic vascular disease.[103] The sympathetic fibers control sweating; thus stellate ganglion block can be quite effective in controlling hyperhidrosis.[104]

Patients with signs and symptoms of CRPS of the upper extremities may gain significant pain relief from stellate ganglion block.[99] Unfortunately, the duration and magnitude of the pain relief are unpredictable.[93] This led to the use of repeated sympathetic blocks, sometimes as often as daily or weekly over an extended period of time in attempt to improve the duration of pain relief. No controlled studies have ever verified this practice, and experts currently agree that repeated sympathetic blocks alone rarely eliminate the pain and disability associated with CRPS. Nevertheless, incorporating sympathetic blockade into a coordinated multidisciplinary rehabilitation plan is essential for effective treatment of patients with CRPS. This treatment plan typically includes physical therapy, oral neuropathic pain medications, and supportive psychotherapy. Neuroablation has been used to destroy the sympathetic chain in patients who attain excellent pain relief of temporary duration with local anesthetic blocks. Few data evaluating the success of sympathetic ablation are available, and expert opinion regarding the usefulness of this approach in the long-term treatment of CRPS is varied.

To perform a stellate ganglion block, the patient is placed supine, facing directly forward with a pillow under the upper back and lower neck to hold the neck in a slight extension. To perform the block without radiographic guidance, the operator palpates the cricoid cartilage and then slides a finger laterally into the groove between the trachea and the sternocleidomastoid muscle, retracting the muscle and adjacent carotid and jugular vessels laterally. Chassaignac tubercle typically is palpable in this groove at the C6 level. Once the tubercle has been identified, a needle is advanced through the skin and seated on the tubercle, where local anesthetic is injected. The local anesthetic spreads along the prevertebral fascia, ideally in a caudal direction to anesthetize the stellate ganglion, which lies just inferior to the point of injection in the same plane. In practice, marked variations in the size and shape of the Chassaignac tubercle reduce the rate of successful block. The adjacent vertebral artery and C6 spinal nerve must be avoided to optimize conduct of this block. A simple modification of technique in which the needle is directed medially toward the base of the transverse process using radiographic guidance is a simple means of improving the reliability of stellate ganglion block and is described here.

When using fluoroscopic imaging, the C-arm is centered over the lower cervical spine without angulation. The position of the vertebral bodies and transverse processes of C6 and C7 are identified. The skin and subcutaneous tissues overlying the base of the transverse process of C6 or C7 on the affected side are anesthetized. The transverse processes are often difficult to distinguish from the underlying facet columns, but the transverse process joins the vertebral body just inferior to the uncinate process of the vertebral body, a structure that is easy to identify on the posteroanterior (PA) radiograph. The block can be carried out at either the C6 or C7 level when using radiographic guidance. However, it is important to realize that the vertebral artery passes near the base of the transverse process at C7, and many individuals lack a bony foramen transversarium at this level. Thus, at C7, care must be taken to keep the needle tip in line or medial to a line connecting the uncinate process of C7 and T1. Straying more lateral will risk penetration of the vertebral artery. The overlying carotid artery must be retracted laterally to perform the classic technique for stellate ganglion block over the C6 transverse process, but this is unnecessary when the needle is directed toward the base of the transverse process because the needle passes medial to the great vessels of the neck.

A 25-gauge, 2.5-in needle is placed through the skin and advanced coaxially until it is seated in the tissues. The needle is adjusted to remain coaxial as it is directed toward the base of the transverse process, just inferior to the uncinate process using repeat PA images after every 2 to 4 mm of needle advancement. Once the surface of the vertebral body is contacted, the needle is in its final position. Intravascular placement is ruled out and proper position is assured by injecting radiographic contrast. The contrast should spread along the anterolateral margin of the vertebral bodies in both PA and lateral radiographs. Thereafter, 10 mL of local anesthetic (0.25% bupivacaine) is injected incrementally. Repeat radiographs following local anesthetic injection should show dilution of the contrast and spread of the solution inferiorly to the T1 level where the stellate ganglion lies. Sympathetic block should ensue within 20 minutes following injection and is assured by seeing a 1°C or greater rise in temperature of the ipsilateral hand. **Table 92-1** lists the signs of successful stellate ganglion block.

Many important structures lie within the immediate vicinity of the needle's tip once it is properly positioned for stellate ganglion block. Commonly, diffusion of local anesthetic blocks the adjacent recurrent laryngeal nerve. This often leads to hoarseness, a feeling of having a lump in the throat, and subjective feelings of shortness of breath and difficulty swallowing. Bilateral stellate ganglion block should not be performed because bilateral recurrent laryngeal nerve blocks may lead to loss of laryngeal reflexes and respiratory compromise. The phrenic nerve is also commonly blocked by direct spread of local anesthetic and leads to unilateral diaphragmatic paresis. Diffusion of local anesthetic as well as direct placement of local anesthetic adjacent to the posterior tubercle results in somatic block of the upper extremity. This may take the form of a small area of sensory loss due to diffusion of local anesthetic or a complete brachial plexus block when the local anesthetic is placed within the nerve sheath.

Major complications associated with stellate ganglion block include neuraxial block (spinal or epidural) and seizures. Extreme medial angulation of the needle from a relatively lateral skin entry point may lead to needle placement into the spinal canal through the anterolaterally oriented intervertebral foramen. In this manner, local anesthetic can be deposited in the epidural space, or, if the needle is advanced far enough, it may penetrate the dural cuff surrounding the exiting nerve root and lie within the intrathecal space. Medial angulation will direct the needle toward the trachea and esophagus and risk penetration of these structures. More likely is placement of the needle tip on the posterior tubercle and spread of local anesthetic proximally along the nerve root to enter the epidural space. In this case, partial or profound neuraxial block, including high spinal or epidural block with loss of consciousness and apnea, may ensue. Airway protection, ventilation, and intravenous sedation should be promptly administered and continued until the patient regains airway reflexes and consciousness. Because the maximal effect of epidural local anesthetic may require 15 to 20 minutes to develop when longer-acting local anesthetics are used, it is imperative that patients be monitored for at least 30 minutes after stellate ganglion block.

Intravascular injection during stellate ganglion block likely will result in immediate onset of generalized seizures. The carotid artery lies just anteromedial to the Chassaignac tubercle, whereas the vertebral artery lies within the bony transverse foramen just posteromedial to the tubercle. If injection occurs into either structure, the local anesthetic injected enters the arterial supply traveling directly to the brain, and generalized seizures begin rapidly and after small amounts of local anesthetic. However, because the local anesthetic rapidly redistributes, the seizures typically are brief and do not require treatment. In the event of seizure, halt the injection, remove the needle, and begin supportive care.

TABLE 92-1 Signs of Successful Stellate Ganglion Block

Horner syndrome
Miosis (papillary constriction)
Ptosis (drooping of the upper eyelid)
Enophthalmos (recession of the globe within the orbit)
Anhidrosis (lack of sweating)
Nasal congestion
Venodilation in the hand and forearm
Increase in temperature of the blocked limb by at least 1°C

Celiac Plexus Block Neurolytic celiac plexus block is among the most widely applicable of all neurolytic blocks. Neurolytic celiac plexus block has a long-lasting benefit for 70% to 90% of patients with pancreatic and other intra-abdominal malignancies. A meta-analysis by Eisenberg et al[105] concluded that adequate-to-excellent pain relief can be achieved in 89% of patients in the first few weeks following the block. From 70% to 90% of patients still had complete pain relief during the 3-month interval before their death.[105] Although encouraging, interpretation of these data requires caution because this meta-analysis is based on retrospective studies.

Several techniques for localizing the celiac plexus have been described. In the classic technique, a percutaneous posterior approach uses surface and bony landmarks to position needles in the vicinity of the plexus. Numerous reports have described new approaches for celiac plexus block using guidance from plain radiographs, fluoroscopy, CT, or ultrasound.[106-108] No single methodology has proven clearly superior with regard to safety or success rate. In recent years, it has been generally agreed that radiographic guidance is necessary to perform celiac plexus block. Many practitioners have turned to routine use of CT, taking advantage of the ability to visualize adjacent structures when performing this technique.[109]

The transcrural approach to the celiac plexus (**Fig. 92-6**) places the local anesthetic or neurolytic solution directly on the celiac ganglion, anterolateral to the aorta. The needles pass directly through the crura of the diaphragm en route to the celiac plexus. In contrast, splanchnic nerve block (see Fig. 92-6) avoids the risk of penetrating the aorta and uses smaller volumes of solution, and the success is unlikely to be affected by anatomic distortion caused by extensive tumor or adenopathy near the pancreas. Because the needles remain posterior to the diaphragmatic crura in close apposition to the T12 vertebral body, this has been termed the *retrocrural technique*. Splanchnic nerve block is a minor modification of the classic retrocrural celiac plexus block; the only difference is that, for splanchnic block, the needles are placed more cephalad. In most cases, celiac plexus (transcrural or retrocrural) and splanchnic nerve block can be used interchangeably, with the same results. Although some strongly advocate one approach or the other, there is no evidence that either approach results in superior clinical outcomes.[95]

Celiac plexus and splanchnic nerve block are used to control pain arising from intra-abdominal structures. These structures include the pancreas, liver, gallbladder, omentum, mesentery, and alimentary tract from the stomach to the transverse colon. The most common application of neurolytic celiac plexus block is treatment of pain associated with intra-abdominal malignancy, particularly pain associated with pancreatic cancer.[96,110] Neurolysis of the splanchnic nerves or celiac plexus can produce dramatic pain relief, reduce or eliminate the need for supplemental analgesics, and improve quality of life in patients with pancreatic cancer and other intra-abdominal malignancies.[110] The long-term benefit of neurolytic celiac plexus block in patients with chronic

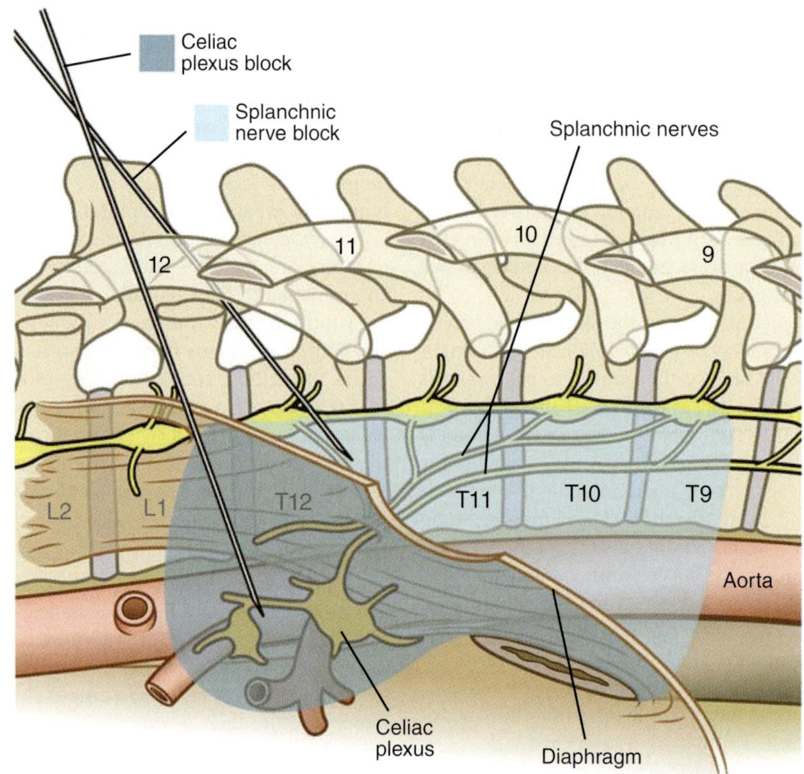

FIGURE 92-6. Anatomy of the celiac plexus and splanchnic nerves. The celiac plexus is composed of a diffuse network of nerve fibers and individual ganglia that lie over the anterolateral surface of the aorta at the T12-L1 vertebral level. Presynaptic sympathetic fibers travel from the thoracic sympathetic chain toward the ganglion, traversing over the anterolateral aspect of the inferior thoracic vertebrae as the greater (T5-T9), lesser (T10-T11), and least (T12) splanchnic nerves. Celiac plexus block using a transcrural approach places the local anesthetic or neurolytic solution directly on the celiac ganglion anterolateral to the aorta. The needles pass directly through the crura of the diaphragm en route to the celiac plexus. In contrast, for splanchnic nerves block, the needles remain posterior to the diaphragmatic crura in close apposition to the T12 vertebral body. Shading indicates the pattern of solution spread for each technique. [Adapted from Rathmell JP. *Atlas of Image-Guided Intervention in Regional Anesthesia and Pain Medicine.* Philadelphia, PA: Lippincott Williams & Wilkins, 2006:124 (Figure 11-1). With permission.]

nonmalignant pain, particularly those with chronic pancreatitis, is debatable.

Transcrural Technique Once the C-arm is aligned over the thoracolumbar junction, the skin and subcutaneous tissues overlying the superior margin of the L1 vertebral body are anesthetized. The aorta lies to the left of midline over the vertebral bodies. By routinely placing the left-sided needle first, a single needle can often be used for the block. If the aorta is penetrated en route, a transaortic technique is used. A 22-gauge, 5-in spinal needle is advanced just caudal to the margin of the 12th rib and cephalad to the transverse process of L1 to contact the anterolateral surface of the L1 vertebral body. The C-arm is then rotated to a lateral projection and the needle advanced to lie 2 to 3 cm anterior to the anterior margin of L1 in the lateral view. Continuous aspiration should be applied as the needle is advanced past the anterior border of L1. If blood appears, the needle has penetrated the aorta and should be advanced through the anterior wall of the aorta until blood can no longer be aspirated. The needle tip should be medial to the lateral border of the L1 vertebral body in the AP view. Final needle position is confirmed by injecting radiographic contrast under live fluoroscopy. The contrast should layer over the anterior surface of the aorta and appear pulsatile. If the contrast spreads to both sides of midline over the anterior surface of the aorta, then only a single needle is necessary for the block. If the contrast remains to the left of midline over the anterolateral surface of the aorta, a second needle is placed from the contralateral side using the same technique described for the left-sided block. Diagnostic celiac plexus block before neurolysis is performed using 10 to 15 mL of 0.25% bupivacaine per side. The dose should be given in increments of 5 mL, aspirating periodically to ensure that the needle has not moved to an intravascular location.

Splanchnic Nerve Block or Retrocrural Technique Once the C-arm is aligned, the skin and subcutaneous tissues overlying the anterolateral margin of the midportion of the T12 vertebral body are anesthetized. For splanchnic nerve block and neurolysis, needles must be placed on both sides. A 22-gauge, 5-in spinal needle is advanced just caudal to the margin of the 12th rib and cephalad to the transverse process of L1 to contact the anterolateral surface of the T12 vertebral body. This requires 20° to 30° of cephalad angulation of the C-arm. The C-arm is then rotated to a lateral projection and the needle advanced 1 to 2 cm to align with the anterior third of the T12 vertebral body in the lateral view. The needle tip should be just medial to the lateral border of the T12 vertebral body in the AP view. Final needle position is confirmed by injecting radiographic contrast under live fluoroscopy. The contrast should layer over the anterolateral surface of the T12 vertebral body. A second needle is placed from the contralateral side using the same technique described for the left-sided block. Diagnostic splanchnic nerve block prior to neurolysis is performed using 5 to 8 mL of 0.25% bupivacaine per side. The dose should be given in increments of 5 mL, aspirating periodically to ensure that the needle has not moved to an intravascular location.

Celiac Plexus and Splanchnic Neurolysis The technique for needle placement is identical for diagnostic local anesthetic block of the celiac plexus or splanchnic nerves and for neurolysis. The 2 commonly used neurolytic solutions are ethyl alcohol and phenol. Phenol is a combination of carbolic acid, phenic acid, phenylic acid, phenyl hydroxide, hydroxybenzene, and oxybenzene. There is no commercially available phenol preparation, but a solution can be prepared by a compounding pharmacist from anhydrous phenol crystals.

Phenol is highly soluble in glycerin and radiographic contrast solutions. Phenol has local anesthetic properties at lower concentrations and is neurolytic at higher concentrations. Concentrations lower than 5% cause protein denaturation, whereas higher concentrations produce protein coagulation and segmental demyelination. Poorly myelinated and unmyelinated nociceptive fibers are destroyed at concentrations of 5% to 6%. Higher concentrations can produce axonal damage, spinal cord infarction, arachnoiditis, and meningitis. Large systemic doses of phenol cause effects similar to those seen with local anesthetic overdose, such as seizures and cardiovascular collapse. A 10% to 12% solution of phenol can be prepared in radiographic contrast. This allows radiographic monitoring of the spread of neurolytic solution as it is injected.

For celiac plexus neurolysis, 10 to 15 mL per side is injected. If the neurolytic solution spreads to both sides of midline over the anterior surface of the aorta, then only a single needle is necessary for the block. If the neurolytic solution begins to spread posteriorly toward the intervertebral foramen, the injection should be halted to avoid nerve root injury. During splanchnic neurolysis, the contrast should layer over the anterolateral surface of the T12 vertebral body. A second needle is placed from the contralateral side using the same technique described for the left-sided block. For splanchnic neurolysis, 5 to 8 mL per side is injected. The needles should be flushed with saline or local anesthetic before they are removed to avoid depositing the neurolytic solution along the needle track.

Neurolysis also can be performed using 50% to 100% ethyl alcohol in similar volumes. Alcohol in excess of 33% results in extraction of cholesterol, phospholipids, and cerebrosides from neural tissues. It produces nonselective destruction of neural tissue. Unlike phenol, the degree of neural blockade increases over the first several days following neurolysis; however, it is intensely inflammatory and has been associated with persistent or worsened pain and neuritis. Phenol has a direct local anesthetic effect and is associated with minimal pain on injection. Because of the intense burning pain on injection, ethyl alcohol is best diluted with local anesthetic prior to injection or injected after placing a small volume of local anesthetic.

Although most cases can be carried out using fluoroscopic guidance alone, CT allows excellent visualization of the anatomic structures that lie in close proximity to the target site during neurolytic celiac plexus block.[111] To directly ablate the celiac plexus, the needles must be advanced through the diaphragm until they lie adjacent to the anterolateral surface of the aorta. This can be accomplished by advancing 2 separate needles adjacent to the anterolateral surface of the aorta or using a single needle advanced through the aorta.

CT-guided celiac plexus block is carried out with the patient positioned prone in the CT scanner gantry. A radiographic marker is placed on the skin surface 1 cm inferior to the inferior margin of the 12th rib and 7 cm from midline, and axial CT images extending from T12 through L1 are taken in 3-mm intervals. In this way, the position of the needle entry site on the skin's surface can be adjusted to form a direct path to the anterolateral surface of the aorta, without passing through adjacent structures. The skin is anesthetized, and a 22-gauge, 5-in spinal needle is seated in a plane that corresponds to the axis seen on CT. With the needle seated in the subcutaneous tissue, but still superficial, a repeat CT image is obtained through the tip of the needle, and the angle of the needle is redirected toward the anterolateral surface of the aorta. The needle is advanced, and repeat CT images are obtained after every 1 to 2 cm of needle advancement. Once the needle is in position, a small volume of radiographic contrast is injected to confirm needle position. A solution of neurolytic drug in radiographic contrast allows radiographic monitoring of the spread of neurolytic solution as it is injected. A repeat CT image is obtained after every 5 mL of injection. If the neurolytic solution spreads to both sides of midline over the anterior surface of the aorta, then only a single needle is necessary for the block.

Following celiac plexus block, several physiologic side effects are expected, including diarrhea and orthostatic hypotension. Blockade of the sympathetic innervation to the abdominal viscera results in unopposed parasympathetic innervation of the alimentary tract and may produce abdominal cramping and diarrhea. Likewise, the vasodilatation that ensues often results in orthostatic hypotension. These effects are invariably transient but may persist for several days after neurolytic block. The hypotension seldom requires treatment other than intravenous hydration.

Complications of celiac plexus and splanchnic nerve block include hematuria, intravascular injection, and pneumothorax. CT allows visualization of the structures that lie adjacent to the celiac ganglion as the block is being performed and may help to avoid these complications.[111] The kidneys extend between T12 and L3, with the left kidney slightly more cephalad than the right. The aorta lies over the left anterolateral border of the vertebral column. The celiac arterial trunk arises from the anterior surface of the aorta at the T12 level and divides into the hepatic, left gastric, and splenic arteries. Using the transaortic technique, caution must be used to avoid needle placement directly through the axis of the celiac trunk as it exits anteriorly. The inferior vena cava lies just to the right of the aorta over the anterolateral surface of the vertebral column.

Neurolytic celiac plexus block carries small but significant additional risks. Intravascular injection of 30 mL of 100% ethanol will result in a blood ethanol level well above the legal limit for intoxication but below the danger limit of severe alcohol toxicity. Intravascular injection of phenol is associated with clinical manifestations similar to those of local anesthetic toxicity: CNS excitation, followed by seizures and, in extreme toxicity, cardiovascular collapse. The most devastating complication associated with neurolytic celiac plexus block is paraplegia. The actual incidence of this complication is unknown but appears to be less than 1:1000. The theoretical mechanism is spread of the neurolytic solution toward the posterior surface of the aorta to surround the spinal segmental arteries, specifically the artery of Adamkiewicz.

Lumbar Sympathetic Block Lumbar sympathetic blockade has been used extensively in the diagnosis and treatment of sympathetically maintained pain syndromes involving the lower extremities.[99] Patients with peripheral vascular insufficiency due to small vessel occlusion also can be treated effectively with lumbar sympathetic blockade. If local anesthetic block improves blood flow and reduces pain, these patients often benefit from surgical or chemical sympathectomy.[112]

Other patients with neuropathic pain involving the lower extremities have shown variable response to lumbar sympathetic block. In those with acute herpes zoster and early postherpetic neuralgia, sympathetic block may reduce pain.[113] However, after 3 to 6 months, once postherpetic neuralgia is well established, sympathetic blockade is rarely helpful. Likewise, deafferentation syndromes such as phantom limb pain and neuropathic lower extremity pain following spinal cord injury have shown variable and largely disappointing responses to sympathetic blockade.[114]

Lumbar sympathetic block typically is carried out using a single-needle technique and a large volume of local anesthetic to spread cephalad and caudad to bathe adjacent ganglia. The patient lies prone with a pillow under the lower abdomen and iliac crest to reduce lumbar lordosis. The C-arm is centered over the midlumbar region. The final needle position for lumbar sympathetic block is over the anterolateral surface of the lumbar vertebral body. The C-arm is rotated obliquely 20° to 30° until the tip of the transverse process of L3 overlies the anterolateral margin of the L3 vertebral body.

The ganglia of the lumbar sympathetic chain vary in number and location among individuals. The ganglia lie between L2 and L4, and in most humans the ganglia lie over the inferior portion of L2 and the superior portion of L3.[115] Thus the optimal location for a single needle is over the anterolateral margin of the inferior portion of L2, the L2-L3 interspace, or the superior margin of L3.

After the skin and subcutaneous tissues are anesthetized, a 22-gauge, 5-in spinal needle is advanced using a coaxial technique toward the anterolateral surface of the L3 vertebral body to gently contact bone. The needle is then walked laterally off the bony margin. The C-arm is rotated to a lateral projection, and the needle is advanced until the tip lies over the anterior third of the vertebral body. Proper needle position is verified in the AP projection where the needle tip should lie medial to the lateral margin of the vertebral body.

Once the needle is in position, aspiration to detect intravascular needle placement is carried out, followed by administration of nonionic radiographic contrast. Contrast spread should be seen anterior to the L3 vertebral body. From 15 to 20 mL of 0.25% bupivacaine is injected incrementally. Signs of successful sympathetic blockade in the lower extremities include venodilation and temperature rise. Skin temperature should be monitored in the contralateral foot to assess for changes unrelated to the block. A rise in temperature of at least 1°C without a rise in temperature of the contralateral limb should occur with successful sympathetic block.

Lumbar Sympathetic Neurolysis Neurolytic lumbar sympathetic block has been used in efforts to provide long-term sympathetic blockade in patients who receive only short-term pain relief with local anesthetic blocks. Lumbar sympathetic neurolysis can be accomplished using either injection of a neurolytic solution or radiofrequency lesioning. Because the locations of the lumbar sympathetic ganglia are variable, injection of neurolytic solution that spreads to encompass an area beyond the needle tip may produce more reliable neurolysis than radiofrequency treatment. Nonetheless, when the needle tips are positioned accurately, the discrete lesions resulting from radiofrequency treatment can produce effective neurolysis.[116] Although the techniques are well described, few data are available to guide the choice among chemical neurolysis, radiofrequency neurolysis, and open surgical sympathectomy.

Chemical Neurolysis Chemical neurolysis of the lumbar sympathetic chain is carried out by placing 3 separate needles at the L2, L3, and L4 levels, as described for local anesthetic block. The needles should be directed to the mid or inferior aspect of L2, the superior aspects of L3, and L4 to correlate with the most frequent anatomic locations of the lumbar sympathetic ganglia. Three needles are placed so that the smallest volume of neurolytic solution can be injected to treat the ganglia at each level. Once proper needle position has been confirmed in the AP and lateral projections, a small volume of radiographic contrast is placed through each needle to ensure that the needles are not located intravascularly and that the injectate will layer in close apposition to the anterolateral margin of the vertebral bodies. Thereafter, 2 to 3 mL of neurolytic solution is placed through each needle.

Radiofrequency Neurolysis Similar to chemical neurolysis, radiofrequency neurolysis of the lumbar sympathetic chain is carried out by placing 3 separate 15-cm radiofrequency cannulas with 10-mm active tips over the anterolateral surface of the L2-L4 vertebral bodies. Once proper needle position has been confirmed, sensory and motor stimulation are conducted. When the cannulas are in proper position over the sympathetic ganglia, the patient typically reports vague back or abdominal discomfort with less than 1.0 V of output and sensory stimulation at 50 Hz. However, the report of any sensation during sensory testing is more variable than during sensory testing before radiofrequency treatment of the facet joints. Motor stimulation is then carried out to ensure that the cannulas do not lie along the course of the anterior primary ramus of one of the spinal nerve roots. There should be no muscle movement in the lower extremities during stimulation at 2 Hz at an output of at least 3 V. Our practice has been to place the lesions if the cannulas appear to be in proper anatomic position even if the patient reports no pain or discomfort during sensory stimulation. Local anesthetic is added and lesions are created at 80°C for 90 seconds.

Significant and potentially toxic levels of local anesthetic can result from direct needle placement into a blood vessel and intravascular injection during lumbar sympathetic block. Hematuria can follow direct needle placement through the kidney but usually is self-limited. Nerve root, epidural, or intrathecal injection can arise when the needle is advanced through the intervertebral foramen and usually is avoided entirely with proper use of radiographic guidance. Following neurolytic lumbar sympathetic block, significant postsympathectomy pain arises in the L1 and L2 nerve root distribution over the anterior thigh in as many as 10% of treated patients. This observation stems from results following open surgical sympathectomy, but such postsympathectomy neuralgia also has been reported after both chemical and radiofrequency sympathectomy. Postsympathectomy neuralgic pain in the anterior thigh has been postulated to result from partial neurolysis of adjacent sensory fibers, most often the genitofemoral nerve.[117]

FACET JOINT INJECTIONS: INTRA-ARTICULAR INJECTIONS, MEDIAL BRANCH BLOCKS, AND RADIOFREQUENCY TREATMENT

Overview Intra-articular facet injection has been largely supplanted by radiofrequency techniques for treatment of facet-related pain. Clinical experience and a limited number of published observational studies suggest that intra-articular injection of local anesthetic and steroid leads to relief of facet-related pain that is limited in duration.[118,119] In contrast, radiofrequency treatment is safe and effective in producing longer-term pain relief in the same group of patients. Nonetheless, an understanding of facet-related pain syndromes and the methods for placing medication directly within the facet joint may still prove useful for those practitioners who are unable to provide radiofrequency treatment.

Osteoarthritis of the spine is ubiquitous and an inevitable part of aging. The degenerative cascade that leads to degeneration of the intervertebral disks causes progressive disk dehydration and loss of disk height. Typically starting in the third decade of life, disk degeneration leads to increased mobility of adjacent vertebrae and increased shear forces on the facet joints themselves. This can lead to a pattern of pain over the axis of the spine that increases with movement, particularly with flexion and extension, but produces little or no pain radiating toward the extremities. In the past, the only treatment available for those with debilitating facet-related pain was segmental fusion of the spine to completely arrest motion within the painful portion of the spine.[120]

Most patients have pain that is gradual in onset and can be localized only to a general region of the spinal axis.[121] However, a subgroup of patients present with sudden onset of pain, often associated with trauma in the form of sudden flexion or hyperextension of the spine in the affected region. Diagnostic studies are invariably unrevealing, showing either no abnormalities or facet arthropathy at multiple levels. In those with pain of sudden onset, it may be possible to isolate one or more facets that are causing the pain. It is in these patients with sudden onset of well-localized pain that intra-articular facet injection with local anesthetic and steroid can prove most beneficial.

Patients with facet-related pain are difficult to distinguish from those with other causes of axial spinal pain. Some patients present with sudden onset of pain following a significant flexion-extension (whiplash) injury, but more commonly the onset is insidious over months to years. Patients with myofascial or discogenic pain as well as those suffering from sacroiliac dysfunction present with similar symptoms. Nonetheless, certain features can be helpful in differentiating facet-related pain from other causes of spinal pain. The pain caused by facet arthropathy is most pronounced over the axis of the spine itself and typically is maximal directly in the region of the most affected joints. The pain tends to be exacerbated by movement, particularly extension of the spine, which forces the inflamed articular surfaces of the facet joints together. However, axial spinal pain at rest or worsening with forward flexion or rotation of the spine is another common feature. The most important historical feature is a predominance of axial spinal pain; patients who report that the predominance of their pain is in the extremities are more likely to have acute or chronic radicular pain than facet-related pain. The quality of the pain typically is deep and aching, with the pain waxing and waning with activity. Burning or stabbing qualities suggest neuropathic pain rather than facet arthropathy.

Diagnostic studies often are unrevealing. Patients with significant facet-related pain may have unremarkable plain x-ray film and/or imaging studies of the spine, or they may show facet arthropathy at multiple levels. Although there is no reported correlation of facetogenic symptoms with plain x-rays or CT, the latter is currently considered to be the optimal imaging modality to visualize facet arthropathy. In recent years, some practitioners have begun using single-photon emission computed tomography (SPECT) to aid in the diagnosis of facet-related pain. Unlike planar views of regular bone scans, SPECT scanning integrates the use of a radioactive isotope and CT by rotating a gamma camera that creates a topographical image to better localize a point of abnormal tracer uptake.[123,124] Radionuclide bone scintigraphy depicts bone areas with increased bone turnover, including synovial changes caused by inflammation and degenerative changes undergoing remodeling. With SPECT, the sensitivity to depict these changes is increased.[125]

Several studies have shown that SPECT results correlate with response to facet joint steroid injections. Dolan et al looked at 58 patients with clinical signs of facet-generated pain. Twenty-two patients had a positive SPECT scan; 36 had negative scans. All patients underwent facet joint injections with steroid and local anesthetic. The group of patients with positive SPECT showed significant improvement in pain relief and the McGill Pain Questionnaire.[123] In a prospective randomized study, Pneumaticos et al identified a group of 47 patients with clinical criteria of facet-generated pain and treated the joints based on SPECT results. In patients with negative SPECT scans, the facets to be injected were determined based on clinical criteria. Patients who underwent facet joint injections based on the results of the SPECT scan had significantly lower pain scores, at 1 and 3 months, than patients whose level had been determined clinically.[126] Although these results suggest that SPECT may prove a useful adjunct in the diagnosis of facet-generated pain, an analysis of cost, risks associated with radiation and use of radioactive isotopes, and potential benefits is needed before this test can be recommended.

The patterns of pain caused by abnormalities in specific facet joints have been established by injecting a mild irritant into a specific facet joints in healthy volunteers and then recording the pattern of pain produced.[127-129] The levels treated are chosen by correlating the patient's report of pain to these pain diagrams. Occasionally a patient presents with evidence of facet arthropathy and a pattern of pain that corresponds to a single level, but this is uncommon. Most patients have more diffuse pain that can only be narrowed to a specific region. Treatment should be directed toward the joint(s) that most closely matches the pattern of referred pain that has been established for each joint and that typically requires treatment at more than one level.

Intra-Articular Facet Joint Injections versus Radiofrequency Treatment Choosing between intra-articular facet injection and diagnostic medial branch blocks followed by radiofrequency treatment is a common clinical scenario. Limited outcome studies of intra-articular injection, particularly at the cervical level, have demonstrated only transient pain relief lasting from days to weeks in most patients.[118,119,130] In a randomized trial, Marks et al[131] showed equal pain relief in patients receiving facet joint injections and medial branch blocks. Patients who obtain significant pain relief from diagnostic blocks of the medial branch nerves may attain significant pain reduction from radiofrequency treatment that is longer lasting. Two randomized controlled trials have shown that radiofrequency ablation provides prolonged pain relief up to 6 months.[132,133] Based on this improved efficacy and a long track record of safety, more practitioners are moving immediately to radiofrequency treatment rather than intra-articular injection. Indeed, a recent study by Cohen et al suggests that omitting diagnostic blocks altogether and proceeding directly to radiofrequency treatment can produce dramatic cost savings.[134] Intra-articular injection remains valuable in patients with recent-onset pain that is discrete in location and suggests involvement of a single facet joint. Intra-articular injection also is a reasonable alternative when the expertise or equipment for radiofrequency treatment is not available, but it will provide only transient symptomatic relief in patients with facet-related pain who have not responded to conservative treatment.

Intra-Articular Facet Injection

Cervical Intra-Articular Facet Injection The patient lies prone, facing directly toward the table with a small headrest under the forehead to allow for air flow between the table and the patient's nose and mouth. The C-arm is rotated 25° to 35° caudally from the axial plane without oblique angulation. This brings the axis of the x-ray path in line with the axis of the facet joints and allows for good visualization of the joints. Although the cervical facet joints also can be entered from a lateral approach with the patient lying on his or her side, advancing a needle using radiographic guidance in the AP plane allows the operator to directly see the position of the spinal canal at all times and avoid medial needle direction that could lead to spinal cord injury.

The skin and subcutaneous tissues overlying the facet joint where the block is to be carried out are anesthetized. The cervical level is easily identified by counting upward from the T1 level, where the T1 vertebra is easily distinguished by the presence of a large transverse process that articulates with the first rib. A 22-gauge, 3.5-in spinal needle is placed through the skin and advanced until it is seated in the tissues in a plane that is coaxial with the axis of the x-ray path. The needle is then advanced in increments of 0.5 to 1 cm using repeat images to redirect the needle toward the facet joint. Once the surface of the joint space is contacted, a lateral radiograph is obtained, and the needle is advanced slightly to penetrate the posterior joint capsule. The needle should not be advanced into the joint between articular surfaces; this serves no purpose and is likely to abrade the articular surfaces and lead to worsened pain once the local anesthetic block subsides. Although intra-articular location of the needle tip can be confirmed with radiographic contrast, this is unnecessary if the needle location is correct in both AP and lateral planes.

Thoracic Intra-Articular Facet Injection Thoracic intra-articular facet injection is not commonly used. The plane of the thoracic facet joints is steeply angled, nearing the frontal plane. Even with steep angulation of the C-arm, the joint space cannot be visualized directly but must be inferred from the position of adjacent structures. The patient is positioned prone with the head turned to one side. The C-arm is angled 50° to 60° in a caudad direction from the axial plane. The plane of the mid and lower thoracic facet joints lies at an angle of 60° to 70° from the axial plane, but further angulation of the C-arm is impractical without the image intensifier resting against the patient's back. This angle allows visualization of structures adjacent to the facet joint from which the position of the joint can be inferred. The inferior articular process (superior aspect of the joint) lies posteriorly, directly over the superior articular process (inferior aspect of the joint). The needle tip is advanced toward the inferior aspect of the joint.

The thoracic level is easily identified by counting upward from the T12 level where the 12th and lowest rib joins the T12 vertebra. A 22-gauge, 3.5-in spinal needle is placed through the skin and advanced until it is seated in the tissues in a plane that is coaxial with the axis of the x-ray path. The needle is adjusted to remain coaxial and advanced toward the inferior margin of the joint space. Because of the joint's steep angle, the needle can be advanced only into the inferior and posterior most extent of the joint. Lateral radiography is difficult to interpret because of the overlying structures of the thorax.

Lumbar Intra-Articular Facet Injection The anatomy of the lumbar facet joint and surrounding structures is illustrated in **Fig. 92-7**. The patient is positioned prone with the head turned to one side. The C-arm is angled obliquely 25° to 35° from the sagittal plane and without caudal angulation. This angle allows direct visualization of the facet joint. The skin and subcutaneous tissues overlying the facet joint where the block is to be carried out are anesthetized. The lumbar level is easily identified by counting upward from the sacrum. A 22-gauge, 3.5-in spinal needle is placed through the skin and advanced until it is seated in the tissues in a plane that is coaxial with the axis of the x-ray path. The needle is adjusted to remain coaxial and advanced toward the joint space.

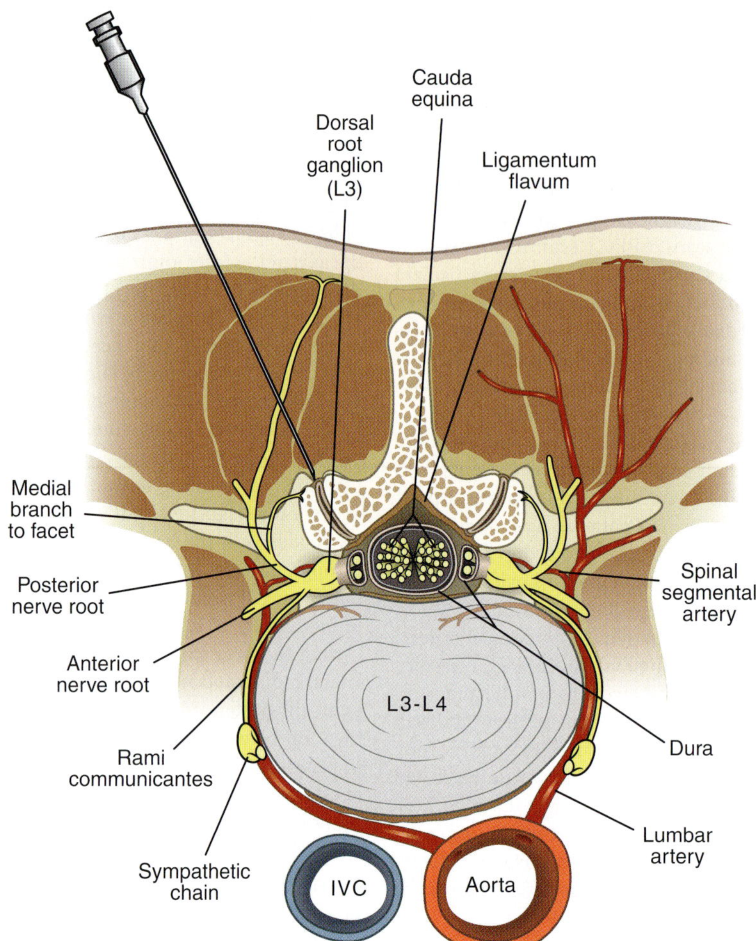

FIGURE 92-7. Axial diagram of intra-articular lumbar facet injection. The axis of the facet joint lies 25-35° from the sagittal plane. Note the innervation to the facet joint. [Adapted from Rathmell JP. *Atlas of Image-Guided Intervention in Regional Anesthesia and Pain Medicine.* Philadelphia, PA: Lippincott Williams & Wilkins, 2006:76 (Figure 7-17). With permission.]

Whether the intra-articular injection is done at the cervical, thoracic, or lumbar level, the facet joint itself holds only limited volume, typically less than 1.5 mL. Placing contrast in the joint limits the ability to place local anesthetic and steroid within the joint. Intra-articular injections are commonly carried out at the lumbar levels. At this level, the articular space is Z-shaped, with the superior recess extending slightly lateral to the axis of the articular surfaces and the inferior recess extending slightly medial to the axis of the articular surfaces. Once needle position has been confirmed, a solution containing steroid and local anesthetic is placed. A total dose of 80 mg of methylprednisolone acetate or the equivalent should be divided over all of the joints to be injected, but more than 40 mg per joint probably is unnecessary. Using concentrated steroid (40 or 80 mg/mL) allows a 1:1 mixture with local anesthetic (0.5% bupivacaine) to provide some immediate pain relief.

Complications associated with intra-articular facet injection are uncommon. The most likely adverse effect is an exacerbation of pain. This is frequent when intra-articular cervical facet injection is carried out and the needle is advanced within the joint space. The joint space is narrow, and advancing the needle within the joint can abrade the articular surfaces, causing increased pain. This exacerbation usually is self-limited. Infection can occur, leading to abscess within the paraspinous musculature, but the incidence is exceedingly low.[135] Bleeding complications have not been associated with intra-articular facet injection.

Facet Medial Branch Blocks and Radiofrequency Treatment In patients who receive only temporary relief from therapeutic intra-articular facet injections or have pain that is more diffuse, requiring treatment at numerous levels, radiofrequency treatment can produce significant, enduring pain relief. Many investigators have pointed to the need for controlled diagnostic injections to determine who will respond to radiofrequency treatment. Despite the value of placebo-controlled injections, they are impractical in most clinical settings. Most practitioners rely on a single set of diagnostic local anesthetic blocks to the medial branch nerves at the levels of suspected pathology to determine who should receive radiofrequency treatment. Patients who report significant pain relief, usually defined as 50% or more pain reduction lasting the average duration of the local anesthetic, go on to radiofrequency treatment. Similar transient pain relief with intra-articular injection of local anesthetic can be used as a reasonable prognostic test before proceeding with radiofrequency treatment.

Conventional radiofrequency treatment produces a small area of tissue coagulation surrounding the active tip of an insulated cannula. When the tip of the radiofrequency cannula is placed in close proximity to a neural structure, the lesion encompasses the nerve, causing denervation. The most commonly used cannulas for facet treatment are 22-gauge SMK (Sluijter-Mehta) cannulas, which come in lengths of 5, 10, and 15 cm. These radiofrequency cannulas have a noninsulated area where coagulation occurs, called the *active tip,* which may be 4, 5, or 10 mm in length. Conventional radiofrequency damages neural tissue by creating an electrical field between the active tip of the needle connected to a voltage generator and an inactive or dispersion electrode at a distance. This induces the movement of a tissue ionic current that follows the alternating current, generating friction and therefore creating heat surrounding the needle tip. Radiofrequency power produces heat by current flow and not through heat transfer from the tip.[136] The lesion, although variable, is well circumscribed and reproducible when the physical parameters are properly controlled. The size mostly depends on needle diameter, length of the active tip, tissue vascularization, tip temperature, and time of exposure. Lesions are characterized by a central core filled with blood related to electrode placement surrounded by an area of coagulation necrosis and separated by a wall of neuroglial proliferation from a zone of liquefaction necrosis. The lesion is surrounded by an area of demyelination.[137,138] For all but the most obese patients, the 10-cm cannulas with 5-mm active tips are used.

In recent years, pulsed radiofrequency treatment has come into frequent use. Studies that investigated the effects of nonheated tissues exposed to the electromagnetic field showed that the so-called *isothermal (42°C-45°C) radiofrequency procedure* induced physiologic changes in tissues.[139] Van Zundert et al[140] showed increase in expression of c-fos in the dorsal horn of experimental animals up to 7 days after pulsed radiofrequency treatment, which suggests sustained activation of a pain-inhibiting process. Although the concept of long-lasting pain reduction without neural destruction is appealing, as yet little clinical evidence supports the efficacy of this new technique.[141]

The key concept when using conventional versus pulsed radiofrequency is understanding where the lesion or pulse radiofrequency energy will occur relative to the active tip. The lesion produced by conventional radiofrequency is along the shaft of the needle surrounding the active tip. There is scant tissue destruction at the tip of the needle; thus the active tip of the cannula must be placed along the course of the nerve. In contrast, the highest density of voltage change during pulsed radiofrequency emanates directly from the tip of the radiofrequency cannula; thus the tip of the needle should be directed perpendicular to the course of the nerve to be treated. Techniques for both conventional and pulsed radiofrequency treatment are discussed here.

Cervical Facet Medial Branch Block and Radiofrequency Treatment The medial branch nerves to the cervical facets course across the articular pillar, midway between the superior and inferior articular processes. The nerves can be anesthetized by placing a needle from a posterior or lateral approach. For the patient, the lateral approach is more comfortable because he or she can lie on one side rather than face down, and the needle must traverse less tissue en route to the target. However, when the needles are inserted from a lateral approach, they are directed toward the spinal cord; even slight rotation of the neck can lead to confusing the left and right articular pillars and result in needle entry into the spinal canal. For performing diagnostic medial branch blocks, either approach is adequate because the local anesthetic will be deposited in the same location in both approaches. For conventional radiofrequency treatment, the cannulas should be placed using a posterior approach, which will allow the entire length of the 5-mm active tip to be placed along the course of the nerve on the articular pillar. For pulsed radiofrequency treatment, the cannulas can be placed from a lateral approach because the voltage fluctuations are maximal at the tip of the cannula.

Posterior Approach The patient lies prone, facing directly toward the table with a small headrest under the forehead to allow for air flow between the table and the patient's nose and mouth. The C-arm is rotated 25° to 35° caudally from the axial plane without any oblique angulation. This brings the axis of the x-ray path in line with the axis of the facet joints and allows for good visualization of the articular pillars.

Lateral Approach The patient lies in the lateral decubitus position with a pillow under the head to keep the neck horizontal and minimizes lateral flexion of the neck to either side. The C-arm is placed directly over the patient's neck without rotation or angulation. Care must be taken to ensure that the left and right articular pillars are aligned directly over one another. This is a point of great confusion among practitioners who are inexperienced with radiographic anatomy of the cervical spine. Even small degrees of rotation can place the left and right facet joints in significantly different locations on lateral radiographs. It is difficult to discern the left side from the right, and if a needle is advanced toward the contralateral facet target in error, the needle can easily penetrate into the spinal canal.

Diagnostic Medial Branch Blocks The cervical level can be identified by counting upward from T1 or downward from C2. Radiographically, T1 is identified in the AP view by its large transverse process that articulates with the head of the first rib, and C2 can be identified by its odontoid process in the AP view and its large spinous process in the lateral view. The skin and subcutaneous tissues overlying the facet target where the block is to be carried out are anesthetized. A 22-gauge, 3.5-in spinal needle is placed through the skin and advanced just until it is seated in the tissues in a plane that is coaxial with the axis of the x-ray path. The needle is adjusted to remain coaxial and advanced toward the facet target in the middle of the articular pillar, midway between superior and inferior articular surfaces of the vertebra. This appears as an invagination, or "waist," on AP radiographs and as a trapezoid on lateral radiographs. From the posterior approach, the needle is gently seated on the lateral margin of the facet column in the middle of the "waist"; from a lateral approach, the needle tip is seated in the middle of the trapezoid. Needle position is confirmed with AP and lateral radiographs. Once needle position has been confirmed, a small volume of local anesthetic is placed at each level and the needles are removed. The patient is instructed to assess the degree of pain relief in the hours immediately after the diagnostic blocks.

Radiofrequency Treatment Radiofrequency cannulas are placed using a technique identical to that described for medial branch blocks. For conventional radiofrequency treatment, 5-cm SMK cannulas with 5-mm active tips are used and placed from a posterior approach. Once the lateral margin of the facet column is contacted, the needle is walked laterally off the facet and advanced 2 to 3 mm to position the active tip along the course of the medial branch nerve. Proper testing for sensorimotor dissociation is conducted. For sensory testing, the patient is asked to report pain or tingling during stimulation at 50 Hz at output less than 0.5 V. Motor testing is carried out at 2 Hz, slowly increasing the output to 3 times the sensory threshold. There should be no motor stimulation to the affected myotome throughout the testing period. We routinely increase the output to 3 V to rule out stimulation of the nerve root before we proceed with the radiofrequency procedure. Thereafter, great care must be taken to prevent any movement of the cannulas. Each level is anesthetized before ablation, and lesions are created at 80°C for 60 to 90 seconds.

For pulsed radiofrequency treatment, 5-cm cannulas with 5-mm active tips are inserted from a lateral approach. The tip is placed in the center of the trapezoid of the target facet, midway between articular surfaces and midway between the anterior and posterior extents of the facet column. Proper testing for sensory thresholds is conducted as for conventional radiofrequency treatment. Each level then is treated with pulsed radiofrequency adequate to maintain voltage fluctuations of 40 to 45 V for 120 seconds, without exceeding a tip temperature of 42°C. Local anesthesia is not needed for pulsed radiofrequency treatment but can be placed before the cannulas are removed.

Thoracic Facet Medial Branch Block and Radiofrequency Treatment The medial branch nerves to the thoracic facets course over the base of the transverse processes where they join with the superior articular processes. The patient lies prone, with the head turned to one side. The C-arm is positioned over the thoracic spine, rotated 25° to 35° caudally from the axial plane without any oblique angulation. The transverse processes of the thoracic vertebrae are best seen from this angle at both high and low thoracic levels.

Diagnostic Medial Branch Blocks The thoracic level can be identified by counting downward from T1 or upward from T12. The skin and subcutaneous tissues overlying the facet target where the block is to be carried out are anesthetized. A 22-gauge, 3.5-in spinal needle is placed through the skin and advanced just until it is seated in the tissues in a plane that is coaxial with the axis of the x-ray path. The needle is adjusted to remain coaxial and advanced toward the base of the transverse process where it joins the superior articular process and seated just on the bony margin. Once the needle is in position, a small volume of local anesthetic is placed at each level and the needles are removed. The patient is instructed to assess the degree of pain relief in the hours immediately after the diagnostic blocks.

Radiofrequency Treatment Radiofrequency cannulas are placed using a technique identical to that described for medial branch blocks. For conventional radiofrequency treatment, 5- or 10-cm SMK cannulas with 5-mm active tips are used. Once the needle is seated against the superior margin of the transverse process where it joins the superior articular process of the facet, the cannula is walked superolaterally off the transverse process and advanced 2 to 3 mm to position the active tip along the course of the medial branch nerve. Proper testing for sensorimotor dissociation is conducted as previously described. Thereafter, great care must be taken to prevent any movement of the cannulas. Each level is anesthetized and lesions are created at 80°C for 60 to 90 seconds. Cannula placement for thoracic pulsed radiofrequency treatment is carried out in the same manner.

Lumbar Facet Medial Branch Blocks and Radiofrequency Treatment The medial branch nerves to the lumbar facets course over the base of the transverse process where they join with the superior articular processes (**Fig. 92-8**). The medial branch nerve lies in the groove between the transverse process and the superior articular process, which slopes inferolaterally. The patient lies prone, with the head turned to one side. A pillow is placed under the lower abdomen in an effort to tilt the pelvis backward and swing the iliac crests posteriorly away from the lumbosacral junction. The C-arm is positioned over the lumbar spine with 25° to 35° of oblique angulation so that the facet joints themselves and the junction between the transverse process and the superior articular process are clearly seen. For medial branch blocks, the needle can be advanced in the axial plane without caudal angulation. However, for radiofrequency treatment, the C-arm should be angled 25° to 30° caudal to the axial plane so that the active tip of the radiofrequency cannulas will be parallel to the medial branch nerve within the groove between the transverse process and the superior articular process as it slopes inferomedially.

Diagnostic Medial Branch Blocks The lumbar level can be identified by counting upward from the sacrum. The skin and subcutaneous tissues overlying the facet target where the block is to be carried out are anesthetized. A 22-gauge, 3.5-in spinal needle is placed through the skin and advanced until it is gently seated in the tissues in a plane that is coaxial with the axis of the x-ray path. The needle is adjusted to remain coaxial and advanced toward the base of the transverse process where it joins the superior articular process and seated just on the bony margin. Once the needle is in position, a small volume of local anesthetic

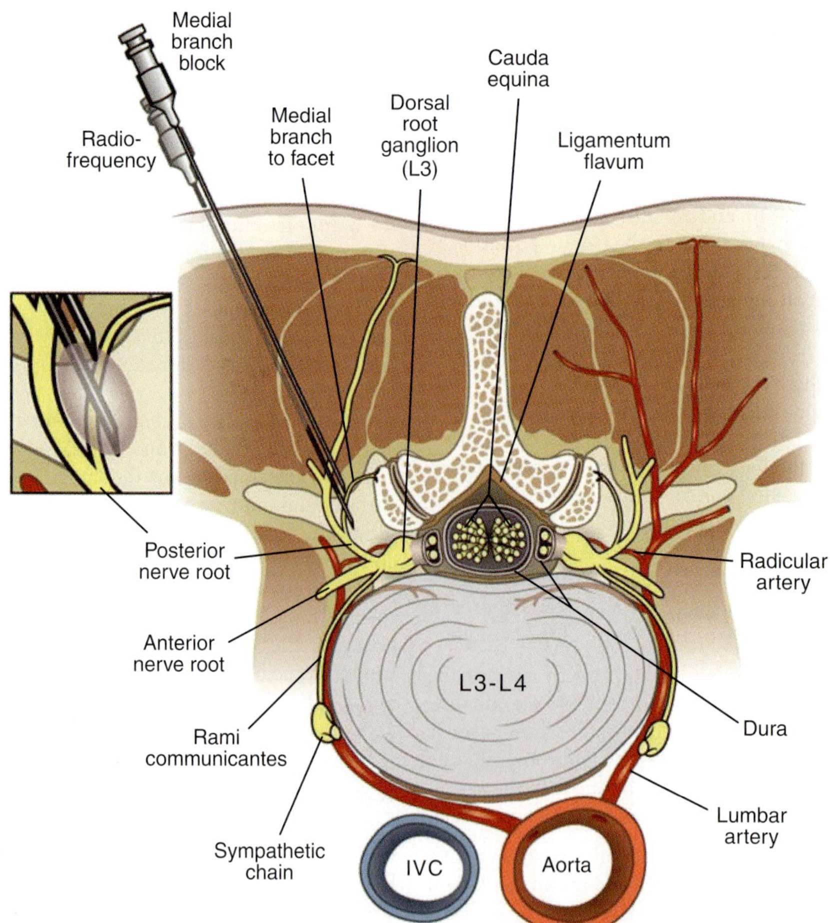

FIGURE 92-8. Axial diagram of lumbar medial branch nerve blocks and radiofrequency treatment. A 22-gauge, 3.5-in spinal needle (or 22-gauge, 10-cm SMK radiofrequency cannula with 5-mm active tip) is advanced toward the base of the transverse process where it joins with the superior articular process. Placement of cannulas for conventional radiofrequency treatment should be carried out with 25°-30° of caudal angulation of the C-arm to bring the axis of the active tip parallel to the course of the medial branch nerve in the groove between the transverse process and the superior articular process. IVC, inferior vena cava. [Adapted from Rathmell JP. *Atlas of Image-Guided Intervention in Regional Anesthesia and Pain Medicine.* Philadelphia, PA: Lippincott Williams & Wilkins, 2006:89 (Figure 7-34). With permission.]

is placed at each level and the needles are removed. The patient is instructed to assess the degree of pain relief in the hours immediately after the diagnostic blocks.

Radiofrequency Treatment Radiofrequency cannulas are placed using a technique identical to that described for medial branch blocks; however, the C-arm is angled 25° to 30° caudal to the axial plane so that the active tip of the radiofrequency cannulas will be parallel to the medial branch. For conventional radiofrequency treatment, 10-cm SMK cannulas with 5-mm active tips are used. Once the needle is seated against the superior margin of the transverse process where it joins the superior articular process of the facet, the cannula is walked off the superior margin of the transverse process and advanced 2 to 3 mm to position the active tip along the course of the medial branch nerve. Proper testing for sensory-motor dissociation is conducted as previously described, assuring there is no stimulation of the motor nerves to the lower extremities. Thereafter, great care must be taken to prevent any movement of the cannulas. Each level is anesthetized and lesions are created at 80°C for 60 to 90 seconds. Cannula placement for lumbar pulsed radiofrequency treatment is carried out in the same manner, except that the active tip need not be parallel to the medial branch nerve.

Complications of Medial Branch Block and Radiofrequency Treatment Complications associated with diagnostic medial branch nerve blocks are uncommon and similar to those following intra-articular facet injections. Unlike intra-articular injection, it is unusual for medial branch blocks to cause an exacerbation of pain. Patients should be warned to expect mild pain at the injection site lasting 1 or 2 days after the procedure. Radiofrequency treatment of the facets also is associated with few complications. Despite the fact that conventional radiofrequency produces actual tissue destruction, injury to the spinal nerve roots is uncommon, perhaps because of sensory and motor testing. Injury to the spinal nerve root has been reported following radiofrequency treatment and could present with new-onset radicular pain with or without radiculopathy. The importance of physiologic testing before each lesion should be emphasized because this will reduce the chance that the active tip of the cannula is close enough to the anterior nerve root to cause injury.

Exacerbation of pain following conventional radiofrequency treatment is common, and patients should be instructed to expect an increase in pain, similar in character to their usual pain, that will last from several days to a week or more. A smaller group of patients report uncomfortable dysesthesia, usually in the form of a sunburn-like feeling of the skin overlying the spinous processes and often accompanied by allodynia. This adverse effect is more common following cervical radiofrequency treatment and usually subsides over several weeks. These dysesthesias likely stem from partial denervation of the lateral branch of the posterior primary ramus, which supplies a variable region of cutaneous innervation overlying the spinous processes. Likewise, some patients report a small patch of complete sensory loss in this same region.

Pulsed radiofrequency treatment does not produce tissue destruction, so it is not surprising that most patients have no worsening of their pain following treatment or have a transient, mild exacerbation that is short lived. Painful dysesthesia and other consequences of nerve injury do not occur with pulsed radiofrequency treatment. It is precisely because of this lack of neural destruction and associated adverse effects that pulsed radiofrequency treatment has become popular among practitioners. If controlled trials emerge to support the efficacy of pulsed radiofrequency treatment, it may rapidly replace conventional radiofrequency.[141]

LUMBAR DISCOGRAPHY AND INTRADISCAL TREATMENTS

Overview Discography is a diagnostic test in which radiographic contrast is injected into the nucleus pulposus of the intervertebral disk. Although originally developed for the study of disk herniation, discography now is used most commonly to identify symptomatic disk degeneration. The 2 components of discography are (1) the anatomic appearance of contrast spread within the disk (using plain radiographs and/or CT) and (2) the presence or absence of typical pain during contrast injection within the disk (pain provocation). The usefulness of discography remains controversial. Some clinicians routinely use discography to identify symptomatic disks before surgical fusion or intradiscal thermal annuloplasty, whereas others believe the test is of unproven benefit in identifying symptomatic disks.[142,143] Discography remains the only test available that attempts to correlate pain response from the patient during provocation with abnormal disks discovered on imaging studies. Improved surgical outcomes following lumbar fusion have been reported when guided by the use of discography.[143-146] Intradiscal electrothermal therapy (IDET) is a minimally invasive procedure that offers an alternative treatment to a subset of those patients with discogenic low back pain. Much like its use prior to fusion, discography is used to identify symptomatic intervertebral disks prior to IDET.[147]

The patient with low back or neck pain originating from the vertebral disk often presents with deep, aching axial midline pain. Pain can be referred to the buttocks and posterior thigh from lumbar disks but does not extend to the distal extremities. Patients with discogenic pain often are young and otherwise healthy. Discogenic pain is common in those with jobs that require repetitive motion of the affected spine segment (eg, package handlers) or expose the spine to excessive vibration (eg, long-distance truck drivers, helicopter pilots, and jackhammer operators). Onset of symptoms usually is gradual. Pain is experienced with prolonged sitting (sitting intolerance), standing, and bending forward. The referred pain usually remains in the proximal part of the extremity. Results of physical examination usually are nonspecific, with limited range of motion at the affected segment or pain with movement, particularly on flexion.

Proponents of discography argue that MRI and CT reveal only nonspecific findings, such as loss of disk height and/or hydration. Jensen et al[148] showed that more than 50% of asymptomatic patients have abnormal findings on MRI scans, in at least one intervertebral disk. The presence of a high-intensity zone on MRI (an area of increased T2 signal intensity at the posterior aspect of the disk) indicates that a radial tear of fissure may be present in the annulus fibrosis, again a nonspecific finding common in individuals without back pain.

Treatment for discogenic pain starts with conservative therapy, including physical therapy and oral nonsteroidal anti-inflammatory drugs. In those with prolonged or disabling pain that is suspected to be of discogenic origin, provocative discography can help to identify the affected level and guide targeted therapy.

Diagnostic Lumbar Discography Lumbar discography is a painful procedure, even when performed by the most skilled practitioners. Intravenous sedation can facilitate the procedure; however, caution must be used to avoid oversedation, which could impede ongoing communication with the patient. The patient must be able to report paresthesias before neural injury occurs. Discography relies on the patient reporting the location and severity of symptoms during provocation, and excessive sedation can make interpretation of the results difficult.[149]

The patient lies prone, with the head turned to one side. A pillow is placed under the lower abdomen, above the iliac crest in an effort to reduce the lumbar lordosis. Having the patient rotate the inferior aspect of the pelvis anteriorly toward the table tips the iliac crest posteriorly and often is key to performing discography successfully at the L5-S1 level. The C-arm is rotated 25° to 35° obliquely centered on the disk space to be studied. The C-arm is then angled in a caudad-cephalad direction; the degree varies among patients, depending on the disk to be studied and each patient's degree of lumbar lordosis. In general, the L3-L4 disk lies close to the axial plane and requires no cephalad angulation to align the vertebral end plates; the L4-L5 disk requires 0° to 15° of cephalad angulation; and the L5-S1 disk requires 25° to 35° of cephalad angulation (**Fig. 92-9**). Proper alignment of the C-arm is critical to the safety and success of discography.

The skin and subcutaneous tissues overlying the disk space where discography is to be carried out are anesthetized, and additional local anesthetic is instilled liberally as the needle is advanced. A 22-gauge,

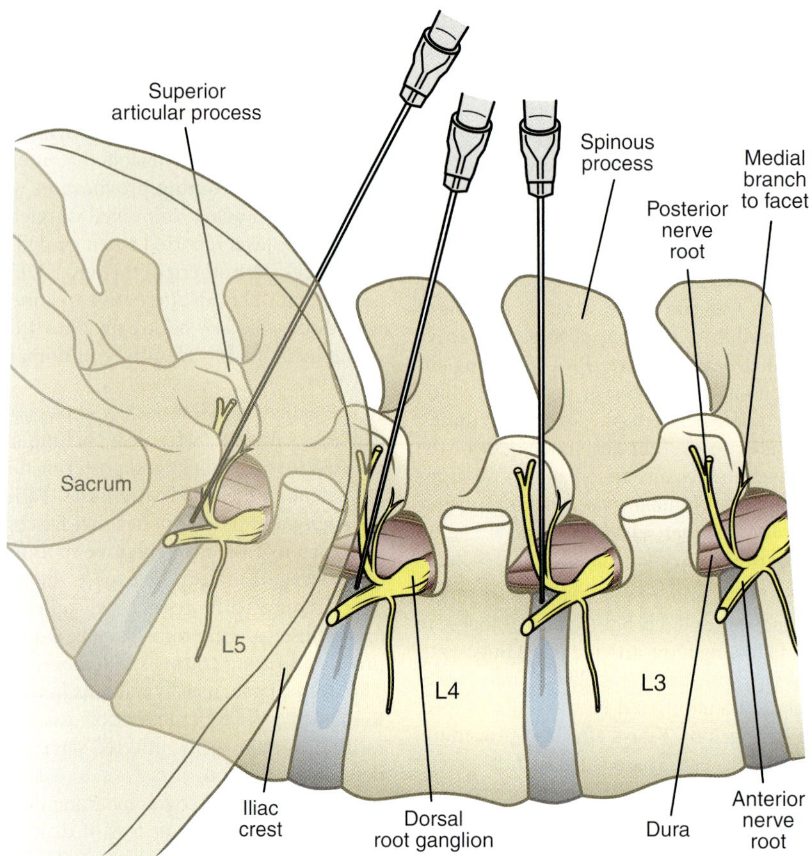

FIGURE 92-9. Anatomy of the lumbar intervertebral disks. In general, the L3-L4 disk lies close to the axial plane, the L4-L5 disk is angled caudally 0°-15°, and the L5-S1 disk is angled caudally 25°-35°. Needles can be safely inserted into each disk through the posterolateral aspect of the annulus fibrosis, just caudal to the exiting nerve root. [Adapted from Rathmell JP. *Atlas of Image-Guided Intervention in Regional Anesthesia and Pain Medicine.* Philadelphia, PA: Lippincott Williams & Wilkins, 2006:102 (Figure 9-1). With permission.]

5-in spinal needle is placed through the skin and advanced just until it is seated in the tissues in a plane that is coaxial with the axis of the x-ray path. A 7- or 8-in spinal needle is often required in obese patients and often needed at the L5-S1 level because of the long and oblique trajectory to the disk space. Without careful use of a coaxial technique throughout the entire course of needle advancement, discography will require multiple repositionings of the needle, if it can be done successfully at all. The direction of the needle should be rechecked after every 1 to 1.5 cm of needle advancement and adjusted to remain coaxial. The position of the exiting nerve root beneath the pedicle should be kept in mind at all times, and efforts to ensure that the needle does not stray cephalad or lateral to the intended point over the middle of the disk will reduce the likelihood of striking the nerve root en route to the disk.

Once the needle is in contact with the surface of the disk, there will be a notable increase in resistance to needle placement. At this point, the C-arm should be rotated to a lateral position and the needles advanced halfway from the anterior to the posterior margin of the disk. Proper final placement is then checked in the AP plane, where again the needle should be in the midportion of the disk space. The nucleus pulposus occupies the central third of the disk space, and placement of the needle tip anywhere within the nucleus should suffice. The final needle path lies just inferior to the exiting nerve root, and in many patients it is difficult or impossible to position the needle exactly in the center of the disk.

Once the needles are in final position at all levels to be tested, provocative testing is carried out. A small volume of radiographic contrast containing antibiotic is placed at each level (<1.5 mL of iohexol 180 mg/mL containing 1 mg/mL of cefazolin). The contrast material is injected under live fluoroscopy to observe the pattern of contrast spread within the disk. As the contrast is injected, the resistance to injection is noted and the patient is questioned about his or her symptoms. Some practitioners use an inline pressure monitoring device to ensure that excess pressure is not delivered during the provocative test. Some evidence indicates that pain reproduction using small volumes without excessive pressure during injection correlates most closely with symptomatic diskogenic pain; injection under high pressure or with large volumes may well produce pain even in normal disks.[150]

A concordant diskogram result occurs when the patient reports his or her typical pattern of severe pain during injection at the level of suspected pathology and the same patient reports no pain on injection of an adjacent disk that is normal in appearance.[149,151] After injection of all levels, final AP and lateral radiographs should be obtained to document the levels tested and the patterns of contrast spread during injection. Some practitioners advocate for subsequent CT to assess the patterns of disk disruption using axial imaging, but the usefulness of CT discography in planning subsequent therapy is unclear.

Complications of Lumbar Discography Most patients experience a marked exacerbation of their typical back pain in the days following discography. They should be warned to expect this pain and given a short course of oral analgesics for treatment of the exacerbation. Less commonly, injury to the exiting nerve roots occurs. The position of the nerve roots is in close proximity to the needle's path. Care must be taken to advance the needle slowly as it passes over the transverse process en route to the posterolateral margin of the disk. If the patient reports a paresthesia to the lower extremity, the needle should be withdrawn and redirected.

Paresthesia occurs in a small proportion of patients, even with good technique. Persistent paresthesias are uncommon and typically ensue only after repeated paresthesias occur during the procedure. In a recent 10-year retrospective case-control study, Caragee et al found that discography resulted in accelerated disk degeneration compared with matched controls, and they call on practitioners to carefully weigh the risks and benefits before recommending disk injection.[152]

Infection can occur, leading to abscess within the presacral musculature, but the incidence is exceedingly low. Infection within the disk space (discitis) is the most feared complication of discography, with an incidence less than 1:1000. Treatment of discitis may require long-term administration of intravenous antibiotics and/or surgical removal of the infection. No cases of discitis occurring in patients who received intradiscal antibiotics during discography have been reported. Bleeding complications have not been associated with intradiscal injection.

Intradiscal Electrothermal Therapy Spinal fusion has been reserved for patients with advanced disk degeneration, with clinical results varying between 46% and 82%.[95,114] Patients who have early degenerative disk disease with preservation of near-normal disk height (>75% of normal disk height remaining) but severe ongoing back pain that does not improve with conservative therapy may be adequate candidates for intradiscal thermal coagulation (intradiscal electrothermal therapy [IDET]).[153] The mechanism of action of IDET is unclear, but thermal energy has been shown to coagulate neural tissue[154] and induce collagen denaturation,[155] thereby addressing both nociceptive and mechanical aspects of discogenic pain.[156] Early prospective studies demonstrated significant pain reduction and improvement in physical function in 30% to 50% of patients treated with IDET.[153,156] However, 2 randomized controlled trials comparing IDET to placebo have reached conflicting conclusions.[157,158] A recent systematic review by Helm et al that examined the 2 randomized controlled trials and 16 observational studies found that IDET produced significant relief in only half of the patients. Currently, strong evidence in support of IDET is lacking, and there has been a dramatic decline in the use of this technique.[159]

Patients with diskogenic pain present with concordant pain on discography at one or 2 spinal levels and no pain during provocation of an adjacent control disk. IDET makes use of a navigable thermal resistance wire that is placed percutaneously and positioned along the posterior aspect of the of the annulus fibrosis. Once in position, the disk is heated using a standardized protocol. Like discography, IDET is a painful procedure, even when performed by the most skilled practitioners. Intravenous sedation can facilitate the procedure, but a level of sedation that allows for ongoing communication with the patient is essential. The patient must be able to report paresthesias or excess discomfort during intradiscal treatment before neural injury occurs. Placement of cannulas for IDET is identical to that for needle placement during discography. The patient lies prone, with the head turned to one side. A pillow is placed under the lower abdomen above the iliac crest in an effort to reduce the lumbar lordosis. The C-arm is rotated 25° to 35° degrees obliquely centered on the disk space to be studies. The C-arm is then angled in a caudad-cephalad direction that varies among patients, depending on the disk to be studied and the degree of lumbar lordosis.

Like discography, the L3-L4 disk lies close to the axial plane and requires no cephalad angulation to align the vertebral end plates; the L4-L5 disk requires 0° to 15° of cephalad angulation; and the L5-S1 disk requires 25° to 35° of cephalad angulation. Proper alignment of the C-arm is critical to the safety and success of IDET. The technique for placing the cannulas through which the IDET catheter is introduced into the disk is similar to that for needle placement for discography. However, the best final position of the introducer is in the anterolateral aspect of the nucleus rather than the central portion of the nucleus. This allows for a more gradual angle as the IDET catheter exits the introducer and curves around the inner aspect of the annulus. The skin and subcutaneous tissues overlying the disk space where IDET is to be carried out are anesthetized, and additional local anesthetic is instilled liberally as the cannulas are advanced. A 17-gauge introducer supplied by the manufacturer is placed through the skin and advanced just until it is seated in the tissues in a plane that is coaxial with the axis of the x-ray path. The IDET introducer is stiff and easy to redirect and advance. The direction of the cannula should be rechecked after every 1 to 1.5 cm of needle advancement and adjusted to remain coaxial. The position of the exiting nerve root beneath the pedicle should be kept in mind at all times, and efforts to ensure that the needle does not stray cephalad or lateral to the intended point over the middle of the disk will reduce the likelihood of striking the nerve root en route to the disk.

Once the needle is in contact with the surface of the disk, there will be a notable increase in resistance to needle placement. At this point, the C-arm should be rotated to a lateral position and the needles advanced halfway from the anterior to the posterior margin of the disk. Proper final placement is then checked in the AP plane, where again the needle should be in the midportion of the disk space.

Once the IDET introducer is in a satisfactory position, the navigable thermal resistance wire (SPINECATH, Smith & Nephew, Andover, MA) is introduced. The tip of the wire slides along the medial circumference of the annulus and can be guided by gently rotating the proximal end of the catheter. The catheter is first advanced beyond the tip of the introducer and into the disk space using lateral radiography. When the tip of the catheter passes to the posterior aspect of the annulus and begins to traverse along the posterior annulus, the C-arm is rotated to the AP view, and the catheter is advanced to final position across the entire posterior annulus. The catheter has 2 radiopaque guides that indicate the active treatment portion of the catheter. These markers should be positioned to either side of the disk to indicate that the entire posterior annulus will be treated.

This brief description is simplistic; guiding the IDET catheter to final position can be quite challenging and requires delicate manipulation of the catheter to keep the tip from advancing into radial tears within the annulus. Overaggressive handling of the catheter causes it to kink, and, once kinked, the catheter is difficult or impossible to steer.

Once the catheter is in final position, heat is introduced using a specific protocol designed to gradually raise the temperature within the disk to 80° to 90°C and maintain that temperature for a minimum treatment period, typically 14 to 16 minutes. It is important that the patient is not overly sedated during the actual heat treatment so that he or she can report discomfort due to excess heat before neural injury occurs.

Complications of IDET Patients should be warned of the typical postprocedural flare-up in pain symptoms that occurs after IDET. This results in an exacerbation of typical axial back pain, often lasting several days to weeks. Less commonly, injury to the exiting nerve roots occurs. The position of the nerve roots is in close proximity to the needle's path. Care must be taken to advance the needle slowly as it passes over the transverse process en route to the posterolateral margin of the disk. If the patient reports a paresthesia to the lower extremity, the needle should be withdrawn and redirected. Paresthesia occurs in a small proportion of patients, even with good technique. Persistent paresthesias are uncommon and typically ensue only after repeated paresthesias occur during the procedure.

Cauda equina syndrome, with severe neuropathic pain in the lower extremities as well as bowel and bladder dysfunction, has been reported to occur from IDET.[160,161] Injury to the cauda equina is more likely to occur when there is an insufficient posterior annulus and the thermal catheter lies in close proximity to the thecal sac. The catheter can exit the disk space to enter the epidural space; however, this should be evident before treatment on lateral radiographs. Assuring that the patient is sufficiently awake to report excessive discomfort during the IDET treatment should reduce the chances of significant neural injury. Finally, overaggressive handling of the IDET catheter leads to kinking of the catheter near the point where it exits the tip of the introducer within the intervertebral disk. Repeated attempts to reposition the catheter once it is kinked can lead to shearing of the catheter tip. Catheter breakage and migration of the tip have been described.[162]

A key to successful outcome following IDET is strict adherence to a structure rehabilitation program that guides the patient through gradual increases in physical activity over a 6-week to 3-month time period. Rehabilitation following IDET is similar to the programs used following lumbar fusion.

Plasma Disk Decompression (Nucleoplasty) Discectomy is one of the most common spine surgeries performed and the standard treatment for persistent radicular pain from disk herniation. With current trends toward less invasive techniques, various percutaneous disk decompression techniques have been introduced into clinical practice.

Plasma-mediated disk decompression, or nucleoplasty, uses a device that is inserted into the nucleus pulposus and creates channels within the nucleus, thereby reducing the intradiscal tissue volume. The device uses radiofrequency energy to excite electrolytes in a conductive medium. The energized particles break down molecular bonds dissolving soft tissue at temperatures ranging from 40°C to 70°C.[163,164] In 2002, Sharps and Isaac[165] prospectively followed 49 consecutive patients after undergoing nucleoplasty. They reported significant improvement in pain scores 1 year after the procedure. In a similar study, Mirzai et al[166] studied 52 consecutive patients and also found decreased pain scores and decrease in analgesic consumption up to 1 year after nucleoplasty. In a recent multicenter prospective trial, Gerszten et al[167] randomized 90 patients with radiculopathy and contained herniations to receive nucleoplasty versus transforaminal epidural steroid injections. At the 2-year follow-up, patients in the nucleoplasty group had significantly better pain scores and quality of life.

Patients who are suitable for nucleoplasty present with persistent radicular pain that has not responded to conservative therapies and a concordant, contained herniation of the nucleus pulposus. Some practitioners have suggested that MRI imaging should reveal a contained disk protrusion less than 6 mm and at least 50% of disk height maintenance.[168] Opinions vary on the use of a discogram before nucleoplasty. Singh and Derby recommend performing discography to recreate the patient symptoms.[169] Other authors have suggested performing discograms to confirm that the herniation is contained within the annular fibers and not as a provocative test[170,171]

Nucleoplasty can be facilitated by intravenous sedation, but a level of sedation that allows for ongoing communication with the patient is essential. The patient must be able to report paresthesias or excess discomfort during intradiscal treatment before neural injury occurs. Placement of the 19-gauge introducer is identical to that for needle placement during discography. The patient lies prone, with the head turned to one side. A pillow is placed under the lower abdomen above the iliac crest in an effort to reduce the lumbar lordosis. As in discography, the C-arm is rotated 25° to 35° degrees obliquely centered on the disk space to be studied. The C-arm is then angled in a caudad-cephalad direction that varies among patients, depending on the disk to be studied and the degree of lumbar lordosis.

Once the introducer needle is placed within the nucleus pulposus under fluoroscopic guidance, the stylet is removed and the nucleoplasty device is introduced in the cannula and advanced slightly into the nucleus. The proximal limit is determined by using a circumferential reference mark on the shaft. The nucleoplasty device is then advanced until it comes into contact with the annulus on the opposite side. Here the depth stop marker on the shaft is advanced to the hub of the cannula to designate the distal limit for advancing the device. The device is then withdrawn to the proximal marker, and the reference line on the device is oriented in the 12 o'clock position. The ablation mode is activated and the device is advanced until the anterior annular border is reached. The coagulation mode is then activated and the device is withdrawn to the proximal marker. The device should be moved at approximately 2 mm/second. The reference line on the device is then rotated clockwise, and the procedure is repeated 6 times at the 2, 4, 6, 8, and 10 o'clock position, creating a total of 6 channels.[172]

Complications of Nucleoplasty Nucleoplasty is a relatively new technique for disk decompression, and complications are thought to be rare. Aside from the well-known potential complications such as bleeding, infection, and nerve damage, 2 complications specific to this procedure have been reported in the literature. Smuck et al[173] reported the case of a patient who developed a radiculopathy several months after nucleoplasty. A repeat MRI revealed epidural fibrosis, and the radicular pain spontaneously resolved. Li et al reported a case of a breakage of the device within the disk. Although the fragment could not be retrieved, the patient had a good clinical outcome.[174]

IMPLANTABLE DRUG DELIVERY SYSTEMS AND SPINAL CORD SIMULATION

Implantable Drug Delivery Systems Intrathecal morphine and other opioids are now widely used as useful adjuncts in the treatment of acute and chronic pain. A number of agents show promise as analgesic agents with spinal selectivity. Continuous delivery of analgesic agents at the spinal level can be carried out using percutaneous epidural or intrathecal catheters, but vulnerability to infection and the cost of external systems typically limit them to short-term use (<6 wk). Reliable implanted drug delivery systems are available that make long-term delivery of medications to the intrathecal space feasible. These systems consist of a drug reservoir/pump implanted within the subcutaneous tissue of the abdominal wall, which is refilled periodically through an access port. The pump may be a fixed-rate, constant-flow device or a variable-rate pump that can be programmed using a wireless radiofrequency transmitter similar to those used for implanted cardiac pacemakers.

The intrathecal catheter is placed directly within the CSF of the lumbar cistern by advancing a needle between vertebral laminae at the L2-L3 level or below. Direct delivery of the opioid at the spinal level corresponding to the dermatome in which the patient is experiencing pain may improve analgesia, particularly when local anesthetics or lipophilic opioids (eg, fentanyl or sufentanil) are used. Thus, in the past, some practitioners advocated threading the catheter cephalad to the appropriate dermatome. Unfortunately, cases of inflammatory mass formation surrounding the catheter tip of some indwelling intrathecal catheters have been reported.[175-179] These inflammatory masses often present with gradual neurologic deterioration caused by spinal cord compression. Currently, many physicians recommend that implanted intrathecal catheters be placed only within the lumbar cistern below the conus medullaris, where the appearance of an inflammatory mass is less likely to directly impinge on the spinal cord.[180]

Patient selection for intraspinal pain therapy is empiric and remains the subject of debate. In general, intrathecal drug delivery is reserved for patients with severe pain that does not respond to conservative treatment.[180,181] Most patients with cancer have ongoing pain despite appropriate oral opioid therapy, or they develop intolerable side effects related to these medications. Randomized controlled trials comparing maximal medical therapy with intrathecal drug delivery for cancer-related pain have demonstrated improved pain control and reduction in opioid-related side effects in patients who received intrathecal pain therapy.[182] Intrathecal drug delivery has been widely used for noncancer pain, particularly for treatment of chronic low back pain.[183] However, use of this therapy in noncancer pain has not been subject to controlled trials and remains controversial.[184]

Once a patient is selected for intrathecal therapy, a trial is performed. Most physicians now conduct trials by placing a temporary percutaneous intrathecal catheter and infusing the analgesic agent over several days to judge the effectiveness of this therapy *before* a permanent system is implanted. Some carry out the trial of intrathecal therapy using a single dose or a continuous epidural infusion. The most common analgesic agent used for spinal delivery is morphine, which remains the only opioid approved by the Food and Drug Administration (FDA) for intrathecal use.

It is important to discuss the benefits and risks involved in the procedure with the patient and his or her family. Before the procedure, discuss with the patient the location of the pocket for the intrathecal pump. Most devices are large, and the only region suitable for placement is the left or right lower quadrant of the abdomen. Once the site is determined, mark the proposed skin incision with a permanent marker while the patient is in the sitting position. The position of the pocket on the abdominal wall is deceptively difficult to determine once the patient is lying on his or her side. If the location is not marked, the pocket is often placed too far lateral within the abdominal wall.

Implantation of an intrathecal drug delivery system is a minor surgical procedure that is performed in the operating room using aseptic precautions, including skin preparation, sterile draping, and use of full surgical attire.[185] The procedure can be conducted under either local anesthesia or general anesthesia using dedicated anesthesia personnel. Performing the initial spinal catheter placement under general anesthesia is controversial, and concerns about neural injury are similar to those associated with any neuraxial technique performed under general anesthesia.[186]

The patient is positioned on a radiolucent table in the lateral decubitus position with the patient's side for the pump pocket nondependent. The arms are extended at the shoulders and secured in position so they are well away from the surgical field. The skin is prepared, and sterile drapes are applied. The radiographic C-arm is positioned across the lumbar region to provide a cross-table AP view of the lumbar spine. Care must be taken to ensure that the x-ray view is not rotated by observing that the spinous processes are indeed in the midline, halfway between the vertebral pedicles.

Surgical Technique The L4-L5 or L5-S1 interspace is identified using fluoroscopy. The spinal needle supplied by the intrathecal device manufacturer must be used to ensure that the catheter will advance through the needle without damage. The needle is advanced using a paramedian approach starting 1 to 1.5 cm lateral to the spinous processes and just inferior to the superior margin of the lamina that forms the inferior border of the interspace you plan to enter. The needle is directed to enter the spinal space in the midline. After dural penetration, the stylette is removed to ensure adequate flow of CSF. Using fluoroscopic guidance, the spinal catheter is advanced through the needle until the tip is well into the spinal space but below L2. Position of the catheter tip is verified using fluoroscopy in the AP and lateral planes. The needle is then withdrawn slightly (~1-2 cm) but left in place around the catheter within the subcutaneous tissues to protect the catheter during the subsequent dissection. The catheter is secured to the surgical field using a small clamp to ensure that it does not fall outside the sterile field.

A 5- to 8-cm incision parallel to the axis of the spine is extended from just cephalad to just caudad to the needle, extending directly through the needle's skin entry point. The subcutaneous tissues are divided using blunt dissection until the lumbar paraspinous fascia is visible surrounding the needle shaft. A purse string suture is created within the fascia surrounding the needle shaft. This suture is used to tighten the fascia around the catheter and prevent backflow of CSF, which may lead to a chronic subcutaneous CSF collection. The needle is removed, taking care not to dislodge the spinal catheter. Free flow of CSF from the catheter should be evident after the needle is removed; if no CSF flows from the catheter, a blunt needle can be inserted within the end of the catheter and gentle aspiration used to ensure that the catheter remains within the thecal sac. If CSF cannot be aspirated from the catheter, it should be removed and replaced. Once the provider is certain that the catheter is adequately placed, it is then secured to the paraspinous fascia using a specific anchoring device supplied by the manufacturer.

Attention is now turned to creating the pocket within the patient's abdominal wall. A 10- to 12-cm transverse incision is made along the previously marked line, and a subcutaneous pocket is created using blunt dissection. The pocket should always be created caudad to the incision. If the pocket is placed cephalad to the incision, the weight of the device on the suture line is likely to cause wound dehiscence. In many patients, the blunt dissection can be accomplished using gentle but firm pressure with the fingers. It is simpler and less traumatic to use a small pair of surgical scissors to perform the blunt dissection. After the pocket is created, the pump is placed in the pocket to ensure that the pocket is large enough. The pump should fit completely within the pocket without any part of the device extending beneath the incision.[185] With the device in place, the wound margins must fall into close apposition. There should be no tension on the sutures during closure of the incision or the wound is likely to dehisce.

After pocket creation is completed, a tunneling device is extended within the subcutaneous tissues between the paraspinous incision and the pocket. The catheter is then advanced through the tunnel (most tunneling devices place a hollow plastic sleeve in the subcutaneous tissue through which the catheter can be advanced from the patient's back to pump pocket). The catheter is trimmed to a length that allows for a small loop of catheter to remain deep to the pump and attached to the pump. The pump is placed in the pocket, with a loop of catheter deep to the device. This loop allows for patient movement without placing tension on the distal catheter and causing it to be pulled from the thecal sac. Two or more sutures should be placed through the suture loops or mesh enclosure surrounding the pump and used to secure the pump to the abdominal fascia. These simple retaining sutures prevent the pump from rotating or flipping within the pocket. The skin incisions are then closed in 2 layers: a series of interrupted subcutaneous sutures to securely close the fascia overlying the pump and the catheter, followed by a skin closure using suture or staples.

Surgical Technique for Permanent Epidural Catheter Placement For placement of a permanent epidural catheter, patient positioning and use of fluoroscopy are similar to those described for intrathecal catheter placement. The interspace of entry varies with the dermatomes that are to be covered, particularly if local anesthetic solution is to be used. A typical loss-of-resistance technique is used to identify the epidural space, and a Silastic catheter is threaded into the epidural space. A paraspinous incision is created, and the catheter is secured to the paraspinous fascia as described for intrathecal catheter placement.

Two types of permanent epidural systems are available: (1) a totally implanted system using a subcutaneous port accessed by a needle placed into the port through the skin and (2) a percutaneous catheter that is tunneled subcutaneously but exits the skin to be connected directly to an external infusion device.

To place a permanent epidural with a subcutaneous port, a 6- to 8-cm transverse incision is made overlying the costal margin halfway between the xiphoid process and the anterior axillary line. A pocket is created overlying the rib cage using blunt dissection. The catheter is then tunneled from the paraspinous region to the pocket as described for intrathecal catheter placement and secured to the port. The port must then be sutured securely to the fascia over the rib cage. Care must be taken to ensure that the port is secured firmly in a region that overlies the rib cage. If the port migrates inferiorly to lie over the abdomen, it becomes difficult to access. The rigid support of the rib cage holds the port firmly from behind, allowing for easier access to the port. The skin incisions are then closed in 2 layers: a series of interrupted subcutaneous sutures to securely close the fascia overlying the catheter, followed by a skin closure using suture or staples.

To place a permanent epidural without a subcutaneous port, a tunneling device is extended from the paraspinous incision to the right upper abdominal quadrant, just inferior to the costal margin. A small incision (~0.5 cm) is made to allow the tunneling device to exit the skin. Percutaneous epidural catheters are supplied in 2 parts: the distal portion of the catheter that is placed within the epidural space, and the proximal portion of the catheter that enters the abdominal wall and connects with the distal portion of the catheter. The proximal portion of the catheter is secured to the tunneling device and pulled through the incision in the abdominal wall subcutaneously to emerge from the paraspinous incision. Many catheters are supplied with an antibiotic-impregnated cuff designed to arrest entry of bacteria along the track of the catheter. This cuff should be placed approximately 1 cm from the catheter's exit site along the subcutaneous catheter track. The proximal and distal portions of the catheter are trimmed, leaving enough catheter length to ensure there is no traction on the catheter with movement. The 2 ends of the catheter are connected using a stainless-steel union supplied by the manufacturer and sutured securely. The paraspinous skin incision is closed in 2 layers with a series of interrupted subcutaneous sutures to securely close the fascia overlying the catheter, followed by a skin closure using suture or staples. The skin incision at the epidural catheter's exit site in the right upper quadrant is closed around the base of the catheter using 1 or 2 simple interrupted sutures.

Complications Bleeding and infection are risks inherent to all open surgical procedures. Bleeding within the pump pocket can lead to a hematoma surrounding the pump that may require surgical drainage. Bleeding along the subcutaneous tunneling track often causes significant bruising in the region but rarely requires treatment. Similar to other neuraxial techniques, bleeding within the epidural space can lead to significant neural compression. Infection of drug delivery devices is infrequent (range: 2.5%-9%), and most infections involve the pump pocket site.[185] Signs of infection within the pump pocket typically occur within 10 to 14 days of implantation but may occur at any time. Some practitioners have reported successful treatment of superficial infections of the area overlying the pocket with oral antibiotics aimed at the offending organism and close observation alone. However, infections within the pocket or along the catheter's subcutaneous course almost universally require removal of all implanted hardware and treatment with parenteral antibiotics to eradicate infection. Catheter and deep tissue infections can extend to involve the neuraxis and result in epidural abscess formation and/or meningitis. Although meningitis is rare, each time a pump is refilled provides an opportunity for the drug to become contaminated during preparation or for the pump reservoir to become contaminated during needle penetration.[185] Permanent epidural catheters without subcutaneous ports have a higher infection rate than those with ports in the first weeks after placement, but both systems have a similar high rate of infection when left in place for more than 6 to 8 weeks.[187]

Spinal cord injury during initial catheter placement has been reported.[188,189] Most practitioners recommend placing the catheter only in the awake patient so that the patient can report paresthesia during needle placement. However, this is a topic of some debate, and placement of the intrathecal catheter under general anesthesia using radiographic guidance below the level of the conus medullaris (~L2) is considered appropriate by some physicians. The catheter can be placed incorrectly within the subdural compartment or the epidural space. In both cases, free flow of CSF will not follow, indicating improper location of the catheter tip.

Wound dehiscence and pump migration are infrequent problems. Assuring that the size of the pocket is sufficient to prevent tension on the suture line at the time of wound closure is essential to minimize the risk of dehiscence. Pump migration usually occurs because retaining sutures were omitted at the time of pump placement. Placing 2 or more sutures through the suture loops or mesh on the pump and securely fastening them to the abdominal fascia will minimize the risk of pump migration.

Subcutaneous collection of fluid surrounding the pump (seroma) can be problematic and typically follows pump replacement. Percutaneous drainage of the sterile fluid collection often is successful in resolving the problem. Subcutaneous collection of spinal fluid, particularly in the paraspinous region, can develop, even many months after pump placement. This complication can be managed with observation alone unless the fluid collection is large or painful; in these instances, neurosurgical exposure of the spinal catheter as it enters the dura and placement of a pursestring suture around the catheter to eliminate the spinal fluid leak may be needed.

Based on a series of deaths reported through the FDA's MedWatch system, the manufacturer of the most widely used intrathecal drug delivery pump conducted a large-scale population study and concluded there is a small increase in unexplained mortality in patients with noncancer pain receiving chronic intrathecal drug delivery.[190]

Spinal Cord Stimulation The idea that direct stimulation of the ascending sensory tracts within the spinal cord might interfere with the perception of chronic pain is founded in everyday observations. We all are familiar with the fact that rubbing an area that has just been injured seemingly reduces the amount of pain coming from that injured region. The advent of transcutaneous electrical stimulation (TENS) whereby a light, pleasant electrical current is passed through surface electrodes in the region of ongoing pain reinforced the observation that stimulation of sensory pathways reduces pain perception in chronic pain states. In 1965, Patrick Wall, a neurophysiologist exploring the basic physiologic mechanisms of pain transmission, and Ronald Melzack, a psychologist working with patients who had chronic pain, together proposed the gate control theory to explain how non-noxious stimulation can reduce pain perception.[191] In their theory, they proposed that second-order neurons at the level of the spinal cord dorsal horn act as a "gate" through which noxious stimuli must pass to reach higher centers in the brain and be perceived as pain. If these same neurons receive input from other sensory fibers entering via the same set of neurons within the spinal cord, the non-noxious input can effectively close the gate, preventing simultaneous transmission of noxious input. Thus the light touch of rubbing an injured region or the pleasant electrical stimulation of TENS closes the gate to the noxious input of chronic pain. From this theory, investigators developed the concept of direct activation of the ascending fibers within the dorsal columns that transmit nonpainful cutaneous stimuli as a means of treating chronic pain.

We have learned much about the anatomy and physiology of pain perception since the gate control theory was first proposed. It is unlikely that the simplistic notion of a gate within the dorsal horn is responsible for our observations, but the theory served as a useful concept in the development of spinal cord stimulation. Both the peripheral nerve fibers and second-order neurons within the dorsal horn transmitting pain signals become sensitized after injury, and anatomic changes, cell death, and altered gene expression all likely have a role leading to chronic pain.[192,193] Direct electrical stimulation of the dorsal columns, known as *spinal cord stimulation* (SCS) or *dorsal column stimulation,* has proved effective, particularly in the treatment of chronic radicular pain.[193] North et al[193] reported a prospective, randomized, crossover trial comparing SCS with reoperation in patients with persistent radicular pain after lumbosacral spine surgery. Patients randomized to SCS were considered more "successful" and less likely to cross over than those randomized to surgery. Although the sample was small, there was no difference in activities of daily living and work status. The mechanisms behind SCS remain unclear, but direct electrical stimulation within the dorsal columns may produce retrograde changes within the ascending sensory fibers that modulate the intensity of incoming noxious stimuli.

The epidural SCS lead is placed directly within the dorsal epidural space just to one side of midline using a paramedian, interlaminar approach. Entry into the epidural space is performed several levels below the final intended level of lead placement. Typically, leads for stimulation of the low back and lower extremities are placed via the L1-L2 interspace and those for upper extremity stimulation are placed via the C7-T1 interspace. Investigators have mapped the patterns of electrical stimulation of the dorsal columns and the corresponding patterns of coverage reported by patients with leads in various locations.[194] In general, the epidural lead must be positioned just 2 to 3 mm to the left or right of midline on the same side as the painful region to be covered.

For lower extremity stimulation, successful coverage usually is achieved by placing the lead between the T8 and T10 vertebral levels, although upper extremity stimulation usually requires lead placement between the occiput and C3 vertebral levels. If the lead ventures too far from midline, uncomfortable stimulation of the exiting nerve roots will result. If the lead is placed too low, overlying the conus medullaris (at or below L1-L2), unpredictable patterns of stimulation may result. In the region of the conus, the fibers of the dorsal columns do not lie parallel to the midline; rather, they arc from the corresponding nerve root entering the spinal cord toward their eventual paramedian location several levels cephalad.

Patient selection for SCS is empiric and remains a subject of debate. In general, SCS is reserved for patients with severe pain who do not respond to conservative treatment. The pain responds best when relatively well localized because success of SCS depends on the ability to cover the entire painful region with electrical stimulation Attaining adequate coverage is more difficult when pain is bilateral, often requiring 2 leads, 1 to each side of midline.[195,196] When the pain is diffuse, it may be impossible to get effective coverage with stimulation using SCS. Among the best established indications for SCS is chronic radicular pain with or without radiculopathy in either the upper or lower extremities. Use of SCS for treatment of chronic axial low back pain has been less satisfactory, but results seem to be improving with the advent of dual-lead systems and electrode arrays that allow for a broad area of stimulation.[197] Randomized controlled trials comparing SCS with repeat surgery for patients with failed back surgery syndrome have demonstrated greater success in attaining satisfactory pain relief in those treated with SCS.[193,198] In a more recent randomized controlled trial, Kumar et al demonstrated sustained improvements over 24 months in pain relief, functional capacity, and health-related quality of life in patients with persistent pain after prior lumbar surgery who received SCS.[199] A small randomized controlled trial by Kemler et al[200] also suggested significant improvement of pain relief in patients with CRPS who were treated with SCS in conjunction with physical therapy compared with physical therapy alone. Functional status did not improve in either group.[200] The usefulness of psychologic screening before SCS remains controversial; some investigators have suggested that screening for patients with personality disorders, somatoform disorder, or hypochondriasis may improve the success rate of SCS.[197,201]

Once a patient is selected for therapy with SCS, a trial is carried out by placing a temporary percutaneous epidural lead. The screening is conducted using an external device as an outpatient procedure to judge the effectiveness of this therapy *before* a permanent system is implanted. Some carry out the trial of SCS using a surgically implanted lead that is tunneled using a lead extension that exits percutaneously. The strictly percutaneous trial lead is simpler to place and does not require a full operating room setup for placement. The surgically implanted trial lead requires placement in the operating room and surgical removal if the trial is unsuccessful. If the trial is successful, the implanted trial lead can remain, and the second procedure to place the impulse generator is brief, not requiring placement of a new epidural lead. In either case, after successful trial stimulation, a permanent system is placed and the lead is positioned to produce the same pattern of stimulation that afforded pain relief during the period of trial stimulation.

Placement of a percutaneous trial spinal cord stimulator lead can be carried out in any location that is suitable for epidural catheter placement. This may be done in the operating room but also can easily and safely be carried out in any location that allows for adequate sterile preparation of the skin and draping of the operative field. Fluoroscopy must be available to guide anatomic placement. Using a strictly percutaneous trial, the trial lead is placed in the same fashion used for permanent lead placement, but the lead is secured to the skin without any incision for the trial period.

Before permanent spinal cord stimulator implantation, discuss with the patient the location of the pocket for the impulse generator. The regions most suitable for placement are the lower quadrant of the abdomen and the lateral aspect of the buttock. Once the site is determined, mark the proposed skin incision with a permanent marker while the patient is in the sitting position. As with the pump reservoir, the position of the pocket is deceptively difficult to determine once the patient is lying on his or her side. If the location is not marked, the pocket is often placed too far lateral within the abdominal wall. Placement of the impulse generator within the buttock allows for the entire procedure to be carried out with the patient in the prone position and simplifies the operation by obviating the need to turn from the prone to lateral position halfway through implantation. If the impulse generator is placed in a pocket overlying the buttock, it must remain well below the superior margins of the iliac crest.

Implantation of a spinal cord stimulator lead and impulse generator is a minor surgical procedure that is carried out in the operating room using aseptic precautions, including skin preparation, sterile draping, and use of full surgical attire. The procedure must be conducted using local anesthesia and light enough sedation that the patient can report where he or she feels the electrical stimulation during lead placement.

The patient is positioned on a radiolucent table in the prone position. Initial lead placement can be carried out with the patient in a lateral decubitus position, but even small degrees of rotation along the spinal axis can make positioning of the lead difficult. The arms are extended upward so they are in a position of comfort well away from the surgical field. The skin is prepared and sterile drapes are applied. For stimulation in the low back and lower extremities, the radiographic C-arm is positioned directly over the thoracolumbar junction to provide an AP view of the spine. Care must be taken to ensure that the x-ray view is not rotated by observing that the spinous processes are in the midline, halfway between the vertebral pedicles.

Surgical Technique The L1-L2 interspace is identified using fluoroscopy. The epidural needle supplied by the device manufacturer must be used to ensure that the lead will advance through the needle without damage. The needle is advanced using a paramedian approach starting 1 to 1.5 cm lateral to the spinous processes and somewhat caudad to the interspace to be entered. The needle is directed to enter the epidural space in the midline with an angle of entry not more than 45° from the plane of the epidural space. If the angle of attack of the needle on initial entry into to the epidural space is too great, the epidural lead will be difficult to thread as it negotiates the steep angle between the needle and the plane of the epidural space. The epidural space is identified using a loss-of-resistance technique. The electrode is then advanced through the needle and directed to remain just to one side of midline in the dorsal epidural space as it is threaded cephalad under fluoroscopic guidance. The electrode contains a wire stylette with a slight angulation at the tip. Gentle rotation of the electrode as it is advanced allows the operator to direct the electrode's path within the epidural space. For stimulation in the low back and lower extremities, the electrode initially is positioned 2 to 3 mm from the midline on the same side as the patient's pain between the T8 and T10 vertebral levels.

Final electrode position is attained by connecting the electrode with an external impulse generator and asking the patient where the pattern of stimulation is felt. In general, cephalad advancement results in stimulation higher in the extremity and caudad movement leads to stimulation lower in the extremity. However, if the lead is angled even slightly from medial to lateral, the pattern of stimulation may change less predictably with movement of the electrode (eg, cephalad advancement can lead to stimulation lower in the extremity under these circumstances). Final electrode position should be recorded using radiography so that a permanent lead can be placed in the same position. For trial stimulation, the needle is then removed, the electrode is secured to the back, and a sterile occlusive dressing is applied. The patient is instructed on the use of the external pulse generator and scheduled to return in 5 to 7 days for assessment of his or her response and for removal of the trial lead.

During permanent implantation, the procedure for initial lead placement is identical to that for trial stimulation. Once final lead position is attained and the optimal pattern of stimulation is confirmed, the lead must be secured, a pocket for the impulse generator created, and the lead tunneled beneath the skin to connect with the impulse generator. Following initial lead placement, the epidural needle is withdrawn slightly (~1-2 cm) but left in place around the lead within the subcutaneous tissues to protect the lead during the subsequent incision and dissection. A 5- to 8-cm incision parallel to the axis of the spine is extended from cephalad to caudad to the needle, extending directly through the needle's skin entry point. The subcutaneous tissues are divided using blunt dissection until the lumbar paraspinous fascia is visible surrounding the needle shaft. The stylette is then removed from the lead and needle is withdrawn, taking care not to dislodge the electrode. The lead is secured to the paraspinous fascia using a specific anchoring device supplied by the manufacturer.

If lead placement has been carried out in the prone position and the impulse generator is to be placed over the buttock, this site is included in the initial skin preparation and draping, ensuring that it is below the superior margins of the iliac crest. If the generator is to be placed in the abdominal wall, the lead must be coiled beneath the skin, the paraspinous incision temporarily closed using staples, and a sterile occlusive dressing applied. The sterile drapes are then removed, and the patient is repositioned in the lateral decubitus position with the side where the abdominal pocket will lie upward. After repeat preparation of the skin and application of sterile drapes, attention is turned to creating the pocket within the patient's abdominal wall or overlying the buttock. An 8- to 10-cm transverse incision is made along the previously marked line, and a subcutaneous pocket is created using blunt dissection. The pocket should always be created caudad to the incision. If the pocket is placed cephalad to the incision, the weight of the impulse generator on the suture line is likely to cause wound dehiscence. Blunt dissection is accomplished using gentle but firm pressure with the fingers or using a small pair of surgical scissors. After the pocket is created, the impulse generator is placed in the pocket to ensure that the pocket is large enough. With the device in place, the wound margins must fall into close apposition. As with the pump reservoir, there should be no tension on the sutures during closure of the incision or the wound is more likely to dehisce.

After the pocket creation is completed, a tunneling device is extended within the subcutaneous tissues between the paraspinous incision and the pocket. The electrode is advanced through the tunnel (tunneling devices vary and are specific to each manufacturer). The means with which the electrode is connected to the impulse generator also varies by manufacturer. Some devices use a lead extension that connects the impulse generator and the lead; others use a one-piece lead that is connected directly to the impulse generator. After tunneling, the lead and/or lead extension are connected with the impulse generator. Any excess lead is coiled and placed behind the impulse generator within the pocket. This loop allows for patient movement without placing tension on the distal electrode and causing it to be pulled from the epidural space.

The skin incisions are closed in 2 layers: a series of interrupted subcutaneous sutures to securely close the fascia overlying the impulse generator within the pocket and the electrode over the paraspinous fascia, followed by a skin closure using suture or staples.

Complications Bleeding and infection are risks inherent to all open surgical procedures. Bleeding within the impulse generator pocket can lead to a hematoma surrounding the device that may require surgical drainage. Bleeding along the subcutaneous tunneling track often causes significant bruising in the region but rarely requires treatment. Similar to other neuraxial techniques, bleeding within the epidural space can lead to significant neural compression. According to Follett et al,[185] the complexity of lead implantation, including the trial period and a second-stage implant operation, may contribute to the higher multiple-site infection rate observed for SCS patients in postmarket surveillance data. Signs of infection within the impulse generator pocket also appear within 10 to 14 days after implantation but may occur at any time. Infections within the pocket or along the lead's subcutaneous course almost universally require removal of all implanted hardware and treatment with parenteral antibiotics to eradicate infection. Lead and deep tissue infections can extend to involve the neuraxis and result in epidural abscess formation and/or meningitis.

There is a significant risk of dural puncture during initial localization of the epidural space using the loss-of-resistance technique. The epidural needle used for electrode placement is a Tuohy needle that has been modified by extending the orifice to allow the electrode to pass easily. This long bevel often results in equivocal loss of resistance; it is not uncommon to have minimal resistance to injection along the entire course of needle placement. To minimize the risk of dural puncture, the needle tip can be advanced under fluoroscopic guidance and first seated on the margin of the vertebral lamina. In this way, the depth of the lamina is certain and the needle need be advanced only a small distance over the lamina, through the ligamentum flavum, and into the epidural space. Loss of resistance is used only during the final few millimeters of needle advancement over the lamina. If dural puncture does occur, there is no clear consensus on how to proceed. Some practitioners abandon the lead placement and allow 1 to 2 weeks before reattempting placement; this approach allows the practitioner to watch and treat postdural puncture headache, which is nearly certain to occur. Other practitioners proceed with lead placement through a more cephalad interspace; if postdural puncture headache ensues and does not respond to conservative treatment, an epidural blood patch is placed at the level of the dural puncture. Spinal cord and nerve root injury during initial lead placement have been reported. Placing the epidural needle and lead in the awake, lightly sedated patient who is able to report paresthesias should minimize the risk of direct neural injury.

The most frequent complication following spinal cord stimulator placement is lead migration. The first line of defense is ensuring that the lead is firmly secured to the paraspinous fascia. Suturing the lead to loose subcutaneous tissue or fat is not adequate. Postoperatively, the patient must be clearly instructed to avoid bending and twisting at the waist (lumbar leads) or bending and twisting the neck (cervical leads) for at least 4 weeks after lead placement. Placing a soft cervical collar on those who had a cervical lead placed provides an easy reminder to avoid movement. Lead fracture may occur, often months or years after placement. Avoiding midline placement or tunneling the lead across the midline will reduce the incidence of fracture caused by compression of the lead on bone. Lead fracture is signaled by a sudden loss of stimulation and is diagnosed by checking lead impedance using the spinal cord stimulator programmer.

TRAINING IN INTERVENTIONAL PAIN MEDICINE

In the rapidly changing world of modern health care, new technologies are appearing at a dizzying rate. Many of these new treatments require physicians to acquire detailed new knowledge and technical skills. Interventional pain medicine is evolving as a distinct discipline that requires detailed new knowledge and expertise. Familiarity with radiographic anatomy for the conduct of image-guided injection and the minor surgical skills needed to place implanted devices such as spinal cord stimulators and implanted drug delivery systems are just a few of the techniques that practitioners must master. As we set out to introduce new interventional techniques to our own pain practices, we must be properly trained to conduct these techniques to ensure safety and success.

FUTURE DIRECTIONS

The field of evidence-based medicine has emerged as a new paradigm to guide practicing physicians.[202] This field endeavors to educate practitioners about how to frame specific questions based on the clinical problems they are faced with every day. They then venture to the published scientific literature with focused questions about prevention, treatment, and diagnosis of specific clinical conditions. Many evidence-based medicine centers offer concise and periodically updated summaries about specific clinical conditions. The idea is to get the best information available to the practicing clinician. It describes the best available evidence, and if there is no good evidence, it says so. In pain medicine, we are faced with an expanding array of treatment options that strike us as logical developments that *should* provide pain relief for our patients. However, there is a dearth of clinical evidence to guide rational choice and application of most of these emerging treatments.

Merrill[203] has presented a detailed analysis of the current state of evidence guiding the use of interventional treatments in the field of pain medicine. He points out the frequent flaws in existing studies including the lack of valid comparators (eg, no treatment) and concludes that "the practice of invasive pain medicine teeters at a particularly critical juncture . . . crippled by a lack of vigorous self-evaluation of its role in the treatment of chronic pain." Merrill goes on to detail the means by which we, as scientists and clinicians, can proceed to build a better body of evidence for the treatments we are using.

The field of pain medicine is young and early in development, and it is perhaps unreasonable to expect an accumulation of randomized clinical trials just yet. The evidence-based medicine movement gives little guidance to practitioners whose tools are still under development. It simply reminds us that no evidence regarding many of our techniques exists. As individual practitioners, we must monitor our own outcomes using valid measures, be more reflective and systematic in studying our own outcomes and patterns of care, and provide this information to our patients as part of the decision-making process. As pain practitioners we have an expanding range of treatment options available to us, few with convincing evidence of efficacy superior to alternate treatments. We must evaluate each patient and use the limited evidence available to us today to guide compassionate and rational, if not evidence-based, use of therapy for our patients.

KEY REFERENCES

- Buchner M, Zeifang F, Brocai DRC, et al. Epidural corticosteroid injection in the conservative management of sciatica. *Clin Orthop.* 2000;375:149-156.
- Cepeda MS, Lau J, Carr DB. Defining the therapeutic role of local anesthetic sympathetic blockade in complex regional pain syndrome: a narrative and systematic review. *Clin J Pain.* 2002;18:216-233.
- Cohen SP, Larkin TM, Barna SA, et al. Lumbar discography: a comprehensive review of outcome studies, diagnostic accuracy and principles. *Reg Anesth Pain Med.* 2005;30:163-183.
- Horlocker TT, Wedel DJ, Benzon H, et al. Regional anesthesia in the anticoagulated patient: defining the risks. (The second ASRA consensus conference on neuraxial anesthesia and anticoagulation). *Reg Anesth Pain Med.* 2003;28:172-197.
- North RB, Wetzel FT. Spinal cord stimulation for chronic pain of spinal origin. *Spine.* 2002;27:2584-2591.
- Pauza KJ, Howell S, Dreyfuss P, Peloza JH, Dawson K, Bogduk N. A randomized, placebo controlled trial of intradiscal electrothermal therapy for the treatment of discogenic low back pain. *Spine J.* 2004;4:27-35.
- Rathmell JP. *Atlas of Image-Guided Intervention in Regional Anesthesia and Pain Medicine.* Philadelphia, PA: Lippincott Williams & Wilkins; 2006.
- Smitt PS, Tsafka A, Teng-van de Zande F, et al. Outcome and complications of epidural analgesia in patients with chronic cancer pain. *Cancer.* 1998;83:2015-2022.
- Tehranzadeh J. Discography 2000. *Radiol Clin North Am.* 1998;36:463-495.
- Van Kleef M, Barendse GAM, Kessels A, et al. Randomized trial of radiofrequency lumbar facet denervation for chronic low back pain. *Spine.* 1999;24:1937-1942.
- Ward A, Watson P, Wood C, et al. Glucocorticoid epidural for sciatica: metabolic and endocrine sequelae. *Rheumatology.* 2002;41:68-71.
- Wong GY, Schroeder DR, Carns PE, et al. Effect of neurolytic celiac plexus block on pain relief, quality of life, and survival in patients with unresectable pancreatic cancer. A randomized controlled trial. *JAMA.* 2004;291:1092-1099.

REFERENCES

Complete references available on DVD and online version at www.LongneckerAnesthesiology.com

CHAPTER 93 Cancer Pain and Palliative Care

Rodolfo Gebhardt
Phillip C. Phan
Allen W. Burton

KEY POINTS

1. Cancer pain remains a significant problem. Studies show approximately 30% of ambulatory cancer patients suffer moderate to severe pain. With progressive disease, the incidence is far higher. Incident pain or episodic severe pain often is problematic for cancer patients.
2. Elucidation of the painful syndrome helps guide effective treatment. In most cases, cancer pain stems from the tumor itself. Tumors cause pain due to invasion of bone, soft tissues, muscle, and nervous structures. A less frequent cause of cancer pain is treatment-related pain, including postchemotherapy neuropathic pain, postsurgical pain syndromes, and postradiation pain syndromes.
3. Neuropathic pain is usually more difficult to treat. Neuropathic pain is seen with chemotherapy-induced painful peripheral neuropathies, postherpetic neuralgias, phantom limb pain, and others. Nociceptive pain syndromes typically are opioid responsive, whereas in neuropathic pain states, adjuvant analgesics may be needed to obtain adequate analgesia.
4. Treat opioid-related side effects aggressively. In some patients, opioid doses are limited by intolerable side effects, including sedation, confusion, constipation, nausea, and pruritus. These side effects are best managed by changing opioids, adding agents to treat the side effect, or using neuraxial, neural blockade, or other interventional pain techniques to lower systemic opioid doses.
5. Stick with the basic tenets of cancer pain management. These include the use of oral opioids whenever possible, often with combinations of long-acting opioids for constant pain with short-acting opioids for incident pain. It also includes the use of adjuvant coanalgesics, including nonsteroidal anti-inflammatory drugs, anticonvulsants, antidepressants, and topicals to minimize opioid doses and concomitant opioid-related side effects.
6. Treat constipation and nausea prophylactically.
7. Advance to interventional therapies when the risk-to-benefit ratio is favorable. Interventional options for pain control include nerve blocks, parenteral infusions, neuraxial infusions, palliative radiotherapy, palliative chemotherapy, and surgery in combination for optimal patient quality of life. The optimal blend of these techniques currently is empirical and based largely on availability of services.
8. Cancer pain management is rewarding. In most cases, adequate pain and symptom control can be obtained through regular assessment and application of the relatively straightforward principles outlined.

EPIDEMIOLOGY

The American Cancer Society reports that the cancer death rate for men and women combined decreased by 1.6% per year during the period 2001 to 2006, in keeping with the steady downward trend that started in the early 1990s. New diagnoses for all types of cancer combined also decreased, approximately 1% per year. Men saw greater declines, but overall death and incidence rates still are much higher among men than women. Rates of the most common cancer types in men (prostate, colorectal, and lung) are falling, but unfortunately others are rising: kidney, liver, esophageal, myeloma, melanoma, and leukemia.

Among women the rates for breast and colorectal cancer has declined, but lung, thyroid, pancreatic, bladder, kidney, myeloma, melanoma, and leukemia have increased.[1]

TABLE 93-1 Barriers to Effective Cancer Pain Control

I. Barriers by health care providers
  A. Inadequate assessment by physicians
  B. Lack of knowledge regarding current treatments by providers
  C. Outdated beliefs by practitioners
    1. Cancer pain expected with disease progression
    2. Opioids prescribed only for dying patients
    3. Patient's pain complaints unreliable
  D. Reluctance to prescribe opioids by physicians
    1. Fear of regulatory controls
    2. Fear of increasing liability for overprescribing
    3. Increased work and effort for opioid management
II. Patient and family-related barriers
  A. Fear of developing addiction to "narcotics"
  B. Reluctance to discuss pain with physician
  C. Fear of acknowledging pain as disease progression
III. Barriers from health care system
  A. Lack of coordination for effective treatment of pain
  B. Inadequate resource for dedicated pain treatment

Approximately 11.1 million Americans live with cancer, and an estimated 1.48 million new cases were diagnosed in 2009. The 5-year survival rate for all cancers has increased to 66% due to earlier detection and better treatment.[2]

Greater survival does not translate to better quality of life. A total of 67% of patients with metastatic disease have pain, and 62% of those suffer from severe pain.[3]

Cancer-related pain is not only due to tumor growth into tissue but can also be the result of some treatment modalities. Thus pain is one of the most feared consequences of cancer.

CANCER PAIN AND RELATED SYMPTOM BURDEN

The diagnosis of cancer is distressing to patients in many ways. First, patients fear that cancer will shorten their life. Second, patients are apprehensive that cancer will bring significant pain and suffering with disease progression. Pain is already experienced by 20% to 50% of cancer patients at the time of diagnosis. With cancer progression, 75% of patients with advanced cancer experience pain.[4] Up to 80% of cancer patients described their pain as having moderate to severe intensity.

According to the World Health Organization (WHO), an estimated 6.6 million people worldwide die of cancer every year.[5] WHO studies point out that cancer-related pain continues to be a significant source of global health concern. With advances in therapeutic modalities, approximately 80% of cancer pain can be readily controlled.[6] Unfortunately, even with these advances, cancer pain remains widely undertreated, even in developed countries.[7] In the United States, the reasons for undertreatment of cancer pain are complex and encompass many barriers (**Table 93-1**).

In recent years, there has been a growing awareness that pain control is an essential part of comprehensive cancer care. Some studies have shown a direct correlation between good pain control and the cancer patient's length of survival as well as responsiveness to timely oncologic treatment.[8,9] In addition to problems stemming from immobility (deep venous thrombosis, pneumonia), uncontrolled pain has proved to be major risk factor in cancer-related suicides.[10,11]

ASSESSMENT

Pain is always subjective and experienced only by the patient. Over the past 20 years, the assessment of pain has been the subject of much research and refinement of techniques and instruments. A brief review is presented in here; see the references for more details on the assessment of cancer pain. In addition to evaluating the pain symptoms, the physician must focus on a myriad of related symptoms. The cancer patient often experiences fatigue, insomnia, depression, anxiety, somnolence, and even cognitive impairment. The psychosocial symptoms, such as anxiety and depression, often can have a large impact on the patient's perception and expression of pain. Furthermore, the patient can develop symptoms from side effects of therapeutic intervention, such as nausea, vomiting, and headaches. Thus the cancer patient commonly presents with a constellation of symptoms that have a profound impact on the patient's psychological well-being, functional status, and quality of life.

SCREENING INSTRUMENTS

Many pain clinics use a questionnaire to aid and standardize the assessment. The Wisconsin Brief Pain Inventory (BPI) and Memorial Pain Assessment Card are well-accepted standard tools for evaluating cancer pain.[12,13] At The University of Texas MD Anderson Cancer Center, an institutionally approved MD Anderson questionnaire (modified BPI) is used for initial and follow-up assessment of patients (**Fig. 93-1**).

Advantages to the Wisconsin BPI include the following:

1. It is a 15-minute questionnaire that can be self-administered.
2. It includes several questions about the characteristics of the pain and associated symptoms, including the origin of the pain and the effects of prior treatments.
3. It incorporates 2 valuable features of the McGill Pain Questionnaire, a graphic representation of the location of pain and groups of qualitative descriptors. Severity of pain is assessed by a series of scales from 0 to 10 (11-point numerical rating scale [NRS]) that score pain at its best, worst, and on average. The perceived level of interference with normal function is also quantified with an NRS.
4. Consistent evidence suggests that the BPI is cross-culturally valid and is useful, particularly when patients are not fit to complete a more through or comprehensive questionnaire.[14,15] Further evidence shows its validity and usefulness in documenting outcomes and health status of patients without cancer pain.[16]

Pediatric cancer pain assessment is a complex topic beyond the scope of this chapter, but pain assessment in the child should be organized in an age-appropriate manner using the proper tool. Examples of pediatric assessment tools include Beyer's The Oucher, Eland's color scale-body outline, Hester's poker chip tool, and McGrath's faces scale.[17]

PAIN HISTORY

Objective observations of grimacing, limping, and vital signs (tachycardia) may be useful in assessing the patient, but these signs often are absent in patients with chronic pain. Pain evaluation should be integrated with a detailed oncologic, medical, and psychological history. The initial evaluation should include determination of the patient's feelings and attitudes about pain and disease, family concerns, and the psychological history. A comprehensive but objective approach to assessment instills confidence in patients and family that will be valuable throughout treatment.

A comprehensive evaluation of the patients with cancer pain includes the following:

- The *chief complaint* is obtained to ensure appropriate triage (ie, may need to send patient who has severe pain with a bowel obstruction to the emergency center for urgent treatment).
- The *oncologic history* is obtained to gain the context of the pain problem. The oncologic history includes diagnosis and stage of disease, therapy and outcome (including side effects), and patient's understanding of the disease process and prognosis.
- The *pain history* should include information on any preexisting chronic pain and the following data for each new pain site: onset and evolution, site and radiation, pattern (constant, intermittent, or unpredictable), intensity (best, worst, average, current) using NRS from 0 to 10,

quality, exacerbating and relieving factors, pain interference with usual activities, neurologic and motor abnormalities (including bowel and bladder continence), vasomotor changes, and current and past analgesics (use, efficacy, side effects). Prior analgesic use, efficacy, and side effects should be cataloged. Prior treatments for pain should be noted (radiotherapy, nerve blocks, physiotherapy, etc).

- *Review of medical record and radiologic studies.* Many treatments of cancer themselves can cause pain (eg, chemotherapy- and radiotherapy-induced neuropathies or postoperative pain syndromes; **Table 93-2**).[18] Many specific cancers can cause well-established pain patterns as a result of known likely sites of metastasis: (1) breast to long bones, spine, chest wall, brachial plexus, and spinal cord; (2) colon to pelvis, hips, lumbar plexus, sacral plexus, and spine; and (3) prostate to long bones, pelvis, hips, lung, and spine.[19]
- *Psychological history* should include marital and residential status, employment history and status, educational background, functional status, activities of daily living, recreational activities, support systems, health and capabilities of spouse or significant other, and history of drug or alcohol use.[20]
- *Medical history* (independent of oncologic history) should include coexisting systemic disease, exercise intolerance, allergies to medications, previous and current medication use, prior illness and surgery, and thorough review of systems including the following:
  - General (including anorexia, weight loss, cachexia, fatigue, weakness, insomnia)
  - Neurologic (including sedation, confusion, hallucination, headache, motor weakness, altered sensation, incontinence)
  - Respiratory (including dyspnea, cough, pneumonia)

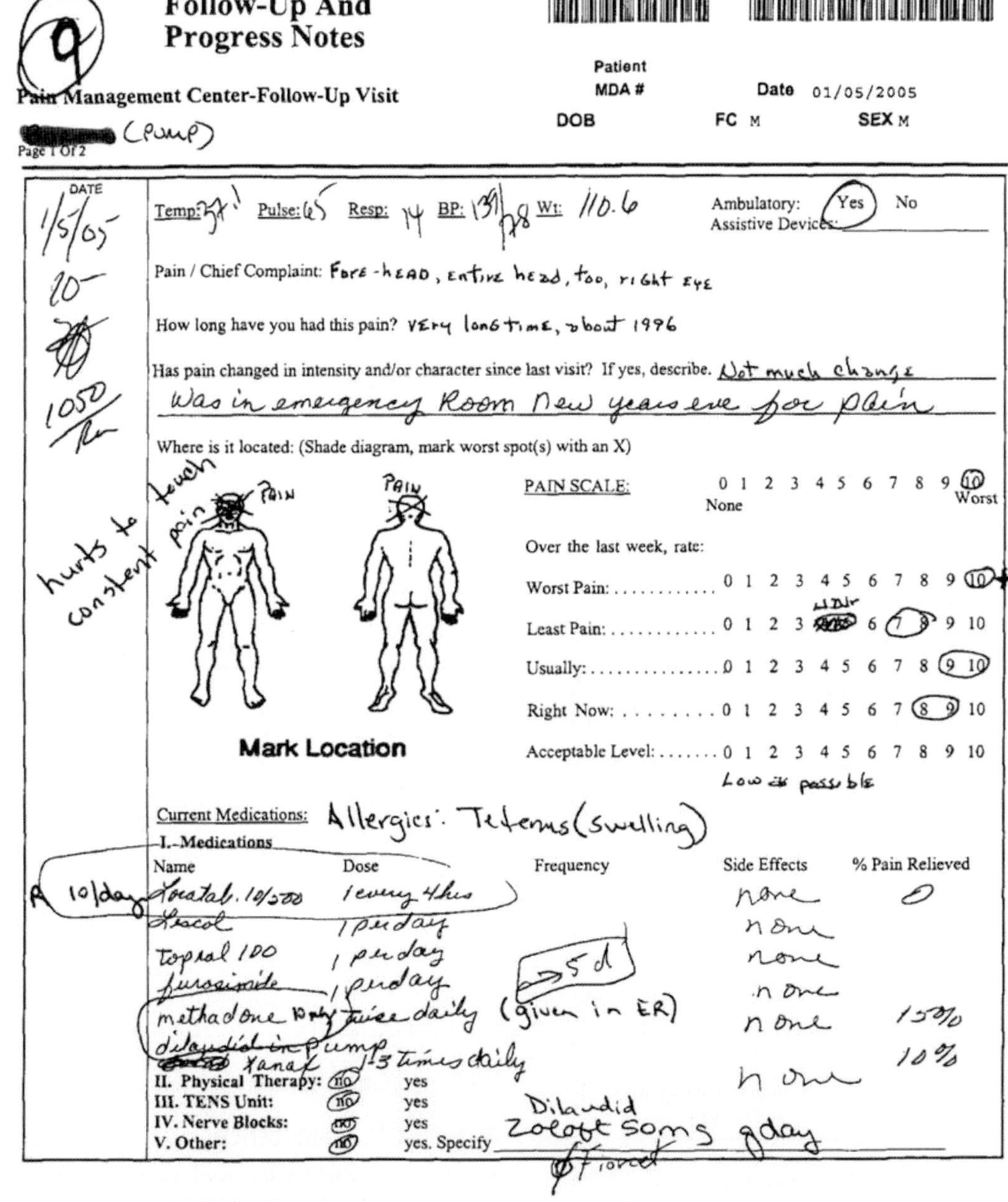

THE UNIVERSITY OF TEXAS MD ANDERSON CANCER CENTER

Follow-Up And Progress Notes

Pain Management Center-Follow-Up Visit

(Pump)

Page 1 Of 2

Patient MDA #

Date 01/05/2005

DOB

FC M

SEX M

DATE 1/5/05

Temp: 97.1 Pulse: 65 Resp: 14 BP: 139/78 Wt: 110.6

Ambulatory: Yes No

Assistive Devices:

Pain / Chief Complaint: Fore-head, entire head, too, right eye

How long have you had this pain? very long time, about 1996

Has pain changed in intensity and/or character since last visit? If yes, describe. Not much change

Was in emergency Room New years eve for pain

Where is it located: (Shade diagram, mark worst spot(s) with an X)

hurts to touch

constant pain

PAIN SCALE: 0 1 2 3 4 5 6 7 8 9 10

None Worst

Over the last week, rate:

Worst Pain: 0 1 2 3 4 5 6 7 8 9 10

Least Pain: 0 1 2 3 4 5 6 7 8 9 10

Usually: 0 1 2 3 4 5 6 7 8 9 10

Right Now: 0 1 2 3 4 5 6 7 8 9 10

Acceptable Level: 0 1 2 3 4 5 6 7 8 9 10

Low as possible

Mark Location

Current Medications: Allergies: Tetems (swelling)

I. Medications

Name	Dose	Frequency	Side Effects	% Pain Relieved
Lortab 10/500	1 every 4 hrs		none	0
Lescol	1 per day		none	
Toprol 100	1 per day		none	
furosemide	1 per day		none	
methadone	twice daily (given in ER)		none	15%
dilaudid in pump				10%
Xanax	3 times daily		none	

II. Physical Therapy: no yes

III. TENS Unit: no yes

IV. Nerve Blocks: no yes

V. Other: no yes. Specify Dilaudid Zoloft 50mg qday

Follow-Up and Progress Notes

File Under: Progress Notes/Dictated Reports

FIGURE 93-1. MD Anderson modified brief pain inventory (BPI) assessment form.

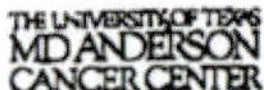

THE UNIVERSITY OF TEXAS MD ANDERSON CANCER CENTER

Follow-Up And Progress Notes

Pain Management Center-Follow-up Visit

Patient MDA # Date 01/05/2005

DOB FC M SEX M

Page 2 Of 2

DATE

Other Symptoms:

Bowel Patterns: Usual Frequency: 2-3 days Consistency: med

Last B M: 2days ago Bowel Regimen: ✓ No ___ Yes

Sexual Disfunction: No ___ Yes ✓

Other Symptoms:

	NONE (Best)										Worst
Fatigue	0	1	2	3	4	5	(6)	7	8	9	10
Nausea	(0)	1	2	3	4	5	6	7	8	9	10
Depression	0	1	2	3	4	5	6	(7)	8	9	10
Anxiety	0	1	2	3	4	5	6	7	(8)	9	10
Drowsiness	0	1	2	3	4	(5)	6	7	8	9	10
Difficulty Thinking Clearly	0	1	2	3	4	(5)	6	7	8	9	10
Shortness of Breathe	0	1	2	3	4	5	6	7	(8)	9	10
Poor Appetite	0	1	2	3	4	(5)	6	7	8	9	10
Insomnia	0	1	2	3	4	5	(6)	7	8	9	10
Feeling of Well-Being	0	1	2	3	4	5	6	7	(8)	9	10

Anything Else We Can Help You With Today?

Needs refill on Zoloft & Lortab

IT pump refill done in clinic

Plan Of Care:

Teaching: see ITPR → see IPOCTR

Treatment Plan of Care: see IPTP

Other: RTC- 1/6/05 for IT pump refill

Signature: [illegible] Meyer RN, R.N.

Follow-Up and Progress Notes

File Under: Progress Notes/Dictated Reports

FIGURE 93-1. *(Continued)*

Type of Surgery	Reported Incidence of Chronic Pain
Limb amputation	30-80%
Thoracotomy	22-70%
Cholecystectomy	3-56%
Inguinal hernia	0-37%

TABLE 93-2 Incidence of Chronic Postoperative Pain by Type of Surgery

Data from Perkins FM, Kehlet H. Chronic pain as an outcome of surgery. *Anesthesiology*. 2000;93:1123-1133.

- Gastrointestinal (including dysphagia, nausea, vomiting, dehydration, constipation, diarrhea)
- Psychological (including irritability, anxiety, depression, dementia, suicidal ideation)
- Genitourinary (including urgency, hesitancy, hematuria)

PHYSICAL EXAMINATION

The physical examination must be thorough, although at times a focused examination may be appropriate. In patients with spinal pain and known or suspected metastatic disease, a complete neurologic examination is mandatory. Gonzales et al[21] found new evidence of metastatic disease in 64% of patients, which resulted in new antitumor therapy for 18% of patients evaluated by their pain service.[21]

CLINICAL PLAN OF CARE

The clinical plan of care should include the following considerations:

- It is important to formulate a clinical impression *(diagnosis)*. Multiple diagnoses usually apply, and it is optimal to use the most specific known diagnosis, for example, (1) T11 compression fracture (pathologic versus osteoporotic) with severe pain, (2) metastatic breast carcinoma (with known bony metastasis), (3) nausea with dehydration, and (4) constipation.
- It also is important to formulate recommendations *(plan)* and alternatives for each problem. For example (related to the preceding problem list): (1) MRI of the T-spine with consideration of vertebroplasty/kyphoplasty if appropriate; (2) oxycodone slow-release 10 mg twice daily, with oral transmucosal fentanyl citrate for breakthrough pain; (3) management including further chemotherapy, radiotherapy, or bisphosphonates as deemed appropriate by the patient's oncologist; (4) Metoclopramide 10 mg orally 30 minutes prior to meals and as needed for nausea; (5) addition of Senokot-S twice daily for constipation.
- A call to the referring oncologist and/or primary care provider helps ensure good communication among all of the patient's physicians. An exit interview with the patient, ideally conducted by the physician, or any trained professional can be designated for this important duty. The exit interview may include the following:
  - Explaining the probable cause of symptoms in terms the patient can understand.
  - Discussing the prognosis for symptom relief, management options, and specific recommendations. In addition to writing prescriptions, oral and written instructions should be provided. Educational material regarding medications, pain management strategies, procedures, or others should be provided. Potential side effects should be discussed.
  - Arranging for follow-up with clinic contact information.
  - A dictated summary (in addition to the phone call) should be sent to referring and consulting physicians to keep them apprised of the patient's present status and treatment offered.

ETIOLOGY AND CLASSIFICATION OF CANCER PAIN SYNDROMES

Pain in cancer patients can have many causes. Most cancer pain syndromes are tumor related, but an increasing array of treatment-related painful syndromes are being seen now with increasing life expectancy. Numerous schemas for classification of cancer pain syndromes have been explored. This chapter discusses time course and pathophysiology as relevant classifications as they relate to treatment strategies.

PAIN SYNDROME TIME COURSE

Acute A vast majority of cancer pain is due to tumor invasion of pain-sensitive structures. The invasion causes a derangement of physiologic processes, including inflammation, edema, acidosis, and necrosis of pain-sensitive tissues. Other pathologic processes may include invasion of bone or soft tissues, obstruction of lymphatic or vascular vessels, distension of hollow organs, distortion of solid organs, and compression of nervous system structures.[22] All of these processes cause typical acute cancer pain syndromes, most of which are diagnosed during the oncologic workup. Many of these same pains improve with successful treatment of the tumor, so reassessment is important given the dynamic nature of tumor-related pain.

Chronic A significant source of pain can be related to cancer treatments. Most times, pain is more chronic with a gradual onset and often delayed diagnosis and treatment. Certain types of chemotherapy often cause painful peripheral neuropathy, including the taxanes, platinum compounds, vincristine and its analogues, and some newer agents such as bortezomib.[23] Neuropathy is often dose related and resolves with lowering of the dose of the offending agent in subsequent courses of chemotherapy. However, in some patients, the painful neuropathy is permanent and very disabling. It can lead to problems with gait or fine motor tasks of the hands in addition to severe pain.

Radiation treatment may cause neural injury in the form of plexopathy, chronic radiation myelopathy, chronic radiation enteritis, and proctitis. Nonspecific postradiation head and neck pain is reported, often involving a myofascial pain syndrome.[24]

Surgical treatment can lead to chronic postoperative pain syndromes. For example, the post radical mastectomy patient often has pain to the posterior upper arm, axilla, and anterior chest wall secondary to damage of the intercostobrachial nerve.[25] Similarly, nerve damage during thoracotomy and radical neck dissection can cause pain in the distribution of the affected nerves.[26]

After amputations, patients can develop different kind of sensations:

1. Phantoms: the patient still feels the amputated limb as being present.
2. Stump pain: pain at the distal part of the limb: most commonly caused by a neuroma.
3. Phantom limb pain: the patient feels the amputated limb is still present and it hurts.[27]

As pain syndromes become chronic, that is, they last beyond the expected healing time course, the treatment algorithms become similar to treatment of noncancer chronic pain. Many confusing issues are developing in this patient population, such as patients with very slowly progressive cancer and associated pain that may last many years. In many cases, the lines between treating cancer pain or so-called malignant versus nonmalignant pain syndromes are blurring.[28]

CANCER PAIN PATHOPHYSIOLOGIC CLASSIFICATION

In the assessment of cancer pain, an understanding of pain classification is helpful in delineating both the mechanism of pain and its responsiveness to therapeutic interventions. Pain can be broadly classified into nociceptive and neuropathic pain.

Nociceptive Pain Nociceptive somatic pain occurs when nonneurologic tissues suffer insult or injury. However, the associated neurologic structures are not injured and remain functional. Consequently, the injuries of the damaged tissues are detected as noxious stimuli that are transmitted along the classic pain pathways. The pain perceived by the central nervous system (CNS) is proportional to the degree of tissue damage caused by the cancer. The pain experienced by the patient often is responsive to nonsteroidal anti-inflammatory drugs (NSAIDs) because tissue damage from cancer inevitably initiates activation of cellular phospholipase A_2 to release arachidonic acid from cell lipid membrane. Cyclo-oxygenase (COX) enzymes then act on arachidonic acid to produce potent inflammatory mediators such as thromboxanes, prostaglandins, and leukotrienes. NSAIDs, including the COX inhibitors, attenuate this initial inflammatory reaction at the site of the tissue damaged by cancer and thus reduce the initial pain signals. The physician must be aware of the growing concerns about the cardiovascular side effects of this group of compounds.[29]

Opioid therapy also is effective in helping to control nociceptive pain. Opioid analgesics act on pain receptors at the level of spinal cord and in the brain to modulate pain pathways in the CNS. Nociceptive pain responds to opioids in a scaled manner, such that pain control is generally proportional to opioid dosage.[30]

Nociceptive somatic pain results from activation of nociceptive receptors in somatic tissues. These nociceptors are sensitive to mechanical, chemical, and thermal stimuli. They are located in skin, bone, muscle, tendon, joint, and connective tissues. The pain signals from these nociceptors are carried along sensory nerve fibers. The patient's perception of nociceptive somatic pain typically is characterized as aching, dull, sharp, throbbing, and well localized to the injured tissue site.

Nociceptive visceral pain, in contrast, is poorly localized. It originates typically from solid organs of the chest, abdomen, and pelvis.

The nociceptive receptors in these solid organs typically do not respond to cutting or burning stimuli. However, they are extremely sensitive to any mechanical stress or torsion of organs as well as tension or traction on mesenteric or vascular attachments to organs. Visceral nociceptive pain signals are carried by autonomic sympathetic fibers. This pain is poorly localized by the patient and often described as vague, dull, aching, or pressure-like.[31] The patient often perceives this nociceptive visceral pain as a referred pain that is falsely localized to a distant site. For example, pancreatic cancer pain often presents as a referred mid-back pain, and cancer involvement of diaphragm causes pain in the right shoulder.

Neuropathic Pain The second major class of cancer pain is neuropathic pain. This pain differs from nociceptive pain in that the cancer causes direct injury to neural tissues. Tumor destruction of peripheral nerves causes abnormal and exaggerated pain signal transmission. Tumor invasion of peripheral or CNS results in abnormal pain signal processing, integration, and perception. Common descriptions include burning, tingling, and shooting pain. The cancer patient often reports extraordinary pain perception, with the pain feeling different from the usual pain sensation. Neuropathic pain often is described as diffuse and excessively sensitive (hyperesthesia), even with nonnoxious stimuli (allodynia). Neuropathic pain is thought to be less responsive to opioid analgesics and instead requires adjuvant medications and interventional therapy for effective control.[32]

TREATMENT MODALITIES

PHARMACOLOGIC THERAPY

WHO Guidelines As intimated, the barriers to effective pain control are multifold. As a result, clinicians have traditionally undertreated cancer pain. A growing recognition of this health issue has led to the development of numerous guidelines for treating cancer pain, including the famous WHO stepladder approach to treating cancer pain (**Fig. 93-2**). Although too simple to serve as a comprehensive treatment algorithm, the principle of treating more resistant cancer-related pain with stronger doses of opioids is generally sound.

Nonopioid Analgesics The nonopioid class of analgesics includes both acetaminophen and NSAIDs. Nonopioids are commonly used for mild cancer pain, as directed by the WHO analgesic ladder. Even in the patient with advanced cancer, nonopioid analgesics combined with opioid analgesics are effective in treating pain at both central and peripheral sites. Nonopioids help to reduce the requirement for opioids, thus decreasing the opioid-associated side effects of nausea, constipation, somnolence, and cognitive impairment. Nonopioid analgesics must be used with caution, if at all, in cancer patients who are immunosuppressed. Both acetaminophen and NSAIDs can suppress a fever response indicative of a mounting infection in the immunocompromised patient.

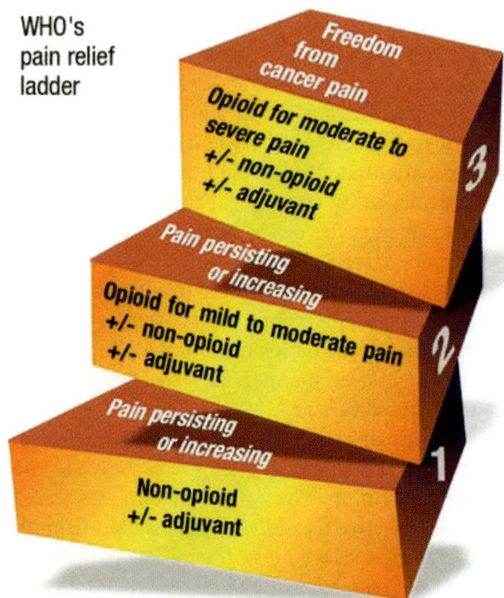

FIGURE 93.2. Pain relief ladder from the World Health Organization (WHO). [Redrawn from http://www.who.int/cancer/palliative/painladder/en].

TABLE 93-3 Adjuvant Drugs for Treatment of Cancer Pain

I. Antidepressants
Amitriptyline
Nortriptyline
Imipramine
Desipramine
Duloxetine
Maprotiline
Paroxetine
Venlafaxine
II. Anticonvulsants
Gabapentin
Carbamazepine
Oxcarbazepine
Pregabalin
Clonazepam
Topiramate
III. Local Anesthetics
Mexiletine
Transdermal lidocaine
IV. Corticosteroids
Dexamethasone
Methylprednisolone
Prednisolone
Cortisone
V. Miscellaneous
Psychostimulants: Dextroamphetamine, Methylphenidate, Modafinil
GABA agonist: Baclofen
A_2 antagonist: Clonidine
NMDA antagonist: Ketamine, dextromethorphan
Antiemetics[a]: Metoclopramide, ondansetron, dronabinol
Laxatives/stool softeners[a]: Senna, docusate

[a]Recommended in all patients receiving opioids.

GABA, γ-Aminobutyric acid; NMDA, *N*-methyl-D-aspartate.

Adjuvant Medications This heterogeneous class of adjuvant medications has a defined role in the WHO 3-step analgesic ladder. They fall into 5 general categories: antidepressants, anticonvulsants, local anesthetics, corticosteroids, and miscellaneous (**Table 93-3**).

These adjuvant medications act to promote certain desirable effects (or prevent opioid-related side effects) in the cancer patient. Tricyclic antidepressants are useful for certain types of neuropathic pain, especially burning dysesthetic pain. They have the significant side effect of sedation at high doses. Consequently, they can be helpful in cancer pain patients with insomnia and depression.

Anticonvulsants and local anesthetics have a membrane-stabilizing effect and are effective for neuropathic pain secondary to nerve injury in both peripheral and CNSs.

Corticosteroids have a potent anti-inflammatory effect and are helpful in cancer patients with spinal cord compression, intracranial tumors, organ capsule distension, and bone infiltration. Steroids also have CNS effect in improvement of mood and sense of well-being in the cancer patient.

Antiemetics and stool softeners should routinely be prescribed along with opioids. The other miscellaneous adjuvant medications have

TABLE 93-4 "Weak" Opioids for Treatment of Moderate Cancer Pain

Generic Name	Examples
Hydrocodone	Lortab, Vicodin, Lorcet, Norco
Codeine	Tylenol 3, 4
Tramadol	Ultracet, Ultram ER

variable effects and are tailored to the patient's individual pain and associated symptoms.

Opioid Analgesics Opioid analgesics are a mainstay for the treatment of cancer pain. In the WHO 3-step analgesic ladder, "weak" opioids are recommended for treatment of moderate cancer pain, whereas "strong" opioids are prescribed for severe cancer pain. The "weak" opioids have less potency and fewer side effects. **Table 93-4** lists some common oral "weak" opioids.

The "weak" opioids are often produced containing acetaminophen or aspirin. They are "weak" because of the limitation of their ceiling dose of acetaminophen or aspirin, above which the patient has a higher risk of renal and hepatotoxicity.

The "strong" opioids are more potent because they are made in pure form, without addition of aspirin or acetaminophen. Thus these opioids do not have a maximum ceiling dose. However, with higher dosages of the "strong" opioids, patients tend to experience more significant side effects like nausea and vomiting, constipation, pruritus, somnolence, and cognitive impairment. Some common "strong" opioids are listed in **Table 93-5**.

Failure of Noninterventional Therapies It has been estimated that up to 70% to 90% of patients with cancer pain have satisfactory pain relief from pharmacologic therapies alone, following the WHO guidelines for cancer pain.[33] However, this means that 10% to 30% of patients have pain that cannot be treated with medications alone. The reasons for this failure of pharmacologic treatment are variable.[34] They vary from physician-related factors to patient-related factors. The physician-related reasons for pharmacologic failure include inaccurate assessment of pain and deficiency in knowledge of current analgesics and adjuvant medications. Patient-related reasons range from fear of addiction to adverse side effects.[35,36] Most commonly, the patient cannot tolerate adverse side effects of the medication regimen, especially opioid use.[36] Failure of pharmacologic control of cancer pain is commonly seen with progression of cancer. Patients with advanced disease can present with intractable pain from multiple metastases and multiple pain sites.

INTERVENTIONAL THERAPIES

Goal of Intervention Patients who fail to respond to conservative pharmacologic treatments may be candidates for interventional therapies. A large armamentarium of invasive procedures is available to achieve better control of cancer pain. However, the role of interventional therapies must be placed in the proper context. They cannot be used as the sole treatment of cancer pain, especially for advanced cancer patients. Rather, they should be used as part of a multimodal approach in the treatment of cancer pain.[37,38] The etiologies of cancer pain are diverse, and the pain symptom is interrelated with the constellation of symptoms experienced by cancer patients. Consequently, a global multimodal approach to the treatment of cancer pain is necessary. It includes appropriate antineoplastic therapy, management of analgesics and adjuvant pain medications, behavioral and psychiatric support, and finally interventional therapies. Interventional pain procedures do not completely eliminate the need for pain medications. The therapeutic goal of such procedures is to help alleviate cancer pain and reduce the overall analgesic need, thereby minimizing associated opioid-related side effects.

TABLE 93-5 "Strong" Opioids for Treatment of Severe Cancer Pain

Generic Name	Examples
Morphine/MS-CR	MSIR, MS Contin, Oramorph, Kadian, Avinza
Oxycodone/oxycodone	CR Roxicodone, OxyContin
Fentanyl	Duragesic (time-released transdermal), Actiq (PO immediate release), Fentora
Hydromorphone	Dilaudid
Methadone	Dolophine
Oxymorphone	Opana , Opana ER

Communication Before proceeding with any invasive pain procedure, communication between the pain physician and the relevant parties is mandatory. The patient must first be educated on the risks and benefits of the interventional procedure. All questions about the procedure should be extensively and satisfactorily answered. At the same time, the patient must be grounded in realistic expectations for outcomes of this procedure. The patient should be made aware of the efficacy of the procedure, duration of effectiveness, and possibility of failure of the procedure to provide complete or even partial pain relief. All potential complications from procedure are explained to the patient. He or she must understand that the interventional procedure is part of a multimodal approach for pain control.

With cancer patients, especially those critically ill or preterminal, family members and caregivers are often involved in the decision-making process. Family support helps the patient cope emotionally with cancer and undergo the procedural intervention. The patient, family members, and caregivers must be educated and have realistic expectations about the procedure.

Effective communication with other professional members of the care team is important. They include the patient's oncologists, primary care providers, and all relevant consultants. Treatment of cancer is a multidisciplinary effort. The interventional procedure should be planned in coordination with the overall cancer treatment. For example, the cancer patient may undergo chemotherapy with resultant thrombocytopenia. In such cases, interventional procedures must be carried out before chemoinduction or afterward when the patient's platelet count has normalized. Typically, other members of the patient's care team are informed about the planned interventional procedure and given a chance to voice their input or concerns.

Detailed Physical Examination A thorough physical examination of the patient before the procedure is critical. This entails a complete neurologic evaluation. Interventional procedures for pain control are invasive and involve neurologically sensitive tissues such as peripheral nerves or CNS structures. The objective of some interventions is to disrupt or modulate pain pathways involved in nociception. Interventional procedures such as neurolysis of peripheral nerves will block not only pain transmission but also sensory and motor innervations. Consequently, it is important to document before and after the procedure a complete and thorough physical examination, with focus especially on pain and neurologic changes. Changes such as sensory and motor blockade are closely monitored after procedures.

Categories of Interventional Techniques Interventional therapies can be categorized into 3 groups: neurolytic techniques, neuromodulation techniques, and surgical techniques.

Neurolytic or *neuroablative techniques* are procedures that target destruction of nerves or neural structures involved in generation or transmission of pain signals. Neurolytic lesions can be created by a variety of agents. Lysis is achieved with chemicals (glycerol, alcohol, or phenol), heat (radiofrequency coagulation), or cold (cryotherapy).

Neuromodulation techniques have as their basis the original Wall and Melzack[39] gate control theory of pain. This theory proposes that all nerve fiber endings except those that innervate hair cells are alike and that supra-threshold stimulation of these nonspecific receptors initiates pain signals. According to Melzack and Wall,[39] substantia gelatinosa functions as a primary gatekeeper in the transmission of pain from the periphery to the CNS. Neuromodulation techniques aim at modulation of pain signals along the transmission pathway. These techniques include local anesthetic blockade; regional infusion of drugs at epidural, intrathecal, intraventricular, or perineural sites; and electrical stimulation of the CNS.

Surgical techniques are the third class of interventional pain procedures. Surgical procedures range from minimally invasive percutaneous vertebroplasty and kyphoplasty to extremely invasive neurosurgical destructive techniques.

Neurosurgical techniques include percutaneous cordotomy, thalamotomy, cingulotomy, hypophysectomy, and trigeminal tractotomy. Most of these procedures are performed stereotactically under monitored anesthesia care and fluoroscopy or computed tomography (CT) guidance.

Neurolytic Procedures Over the past century, many chemical and physical ablative techniques have been developed with the goal of disrupting the transmission of pain signals along neural pathways. An ideal agent would selectively disrupt A-delta and C nerve fibers. Unfortunately, such an agent does not exist, and all commonly used agents cause an indiscriminate neural destruction. Chemical neurolysis is achieved with alcohol (50%-100%), phenol (5%-15%), and glycerol. These agents produce nerve injury resulting in degeneration of nerve fibers distal to the lysis lesion (Wallerian degeneration).[40] The injury disrupts nerve cell transmission of pain and results in a nociceptive block. However, with Wallerian degeneration, the nerve axon can begin to regenerate within 3 months. Thus chemical neurolysis provides a temporary block of nociception for approximately 1 to 3 months.[41]

Alcohol is the chemical classically used for neurolysis.[42] Today many clinicians favor the use of phenol for peripheral neurolysis because it is less neurotoxic than alcohol.[43] Alcohol is used in concentration up to 100%. It causes nonselective destruction of all nerves as well as surrounding soft tissues. Alcohol is rapidly soluble in blood and is hypobaric relative to cerebrospinal fluid (CSF). If injected into the intraspinal space, it rises rapidly, diffusing away from the initial injection site. Specifically, it damages nerves by extracting fatty substances and precipitating proteins in the nerve axon, resulting in Wallerian degeneration.[44] The injury is proportional to both the concentration and volume of alcohol used. A higher risk of neuritis is associated with alcohol injection compared with phenol.[45] Patients often experience intense burning pain initially with alcohol injection.

Phenol is associated with a lower risk for neuritis.[45] Phenol 5% is equivalent to alcohol 40% concentration in neurolytic potency.[46] Phenol is less water soluble than alcohol, so it tends to concentrate more around the injection site. It is diffusible and able to penetrate neural axon and denature proteins, causing Wallerian degeneration.[45]

Phenol is available at a concentration of 6.7% when prepared with water, but it can be concentrated to 15% when mixed with glycerol or radiopaque contrast.

Phenol at higher concentrations can be injurious to vascular structures, and toxicity (usually at doses >5 g) can result in seizures, cardiovascular collapse, nausea, and vomiting.[47]

Many clinicians prefer phenol because the intensity and duration of neural blockade are less with phenol, theoretically providing a wider margin of safety.

Glycerol is less commonly used in peripheral neural blockade. It is used primarily for the treatment of trigeminal neuralgia. It is injected directly into the trigeminal cistern (Meckel cave), with good efficacy in blocking trigeminal neuralgia. Other neurolytic chemicals that have been attempted include ammonium salt compounds and hypertonic and hypotonic saline solutions, with variable results.[45]

Radiofrequency thermocoagulation is also used to produce a physical nociceptive block.[48] A lesion created by radiofrequency heating is discrete, and lesion size is controlled by the temperature of the probe and the duration of application. Some studies have shown that radiofrequency ablation can produce a longer lasting block.[49]

TABLE 93-6 Potential Risks of Neuroablation Techniques

Dysesthetic pain: Painful neuralgia due to deafferentation, neuritis, or neuroma formation
Tissue damage: Accidental injury to nontargeted neurologic and nonneurologic tissues
Motor paralysis: Especially with intrathecal neurolysis
Sensory deficit: Areas of paresthesia or numbness
Failure to relieve pain: Due to incomplete ablation or incorrect nerve target
Short-term pain relief: Due to central nervous system plasticity, axonal regrowth, or tumor progression

Cryotherapy can be used to achieve neurolytic lesioning. Applying extreme cold to the nerve results in long-lasting nerve blockade. Cryoneurolysis of intercostal nerves intraoperatively has good efficacy in controlling postthoracotomy pain.[50] Wide application of cryoablation has been hindered by the large probe size and the relative complexity of the equipment involved.

Patient selection for chemical neurolysis, radiofrequency ablation, and cryoneurolysis techniques is extremely important in achieving the desired outcome. The patient should have an advanced progressive cancer with a limited life expectancy (6-12 months). The pain should be severe, persistent, refractory to conservative treatment, and consistent with a nociceptive somatic or visceral pain. Neuropathic pain usually does not respond well to neuroablation therapy. **Table 93-6** lists the potential risks associated with neuroablation.

Despite the inherent risks of neuroablation, patients with advanced cancer and well-localized nociceptive pain can benefit greatly from neurolytic blockade. Peripheral neurolysis has been proven to alleviate the suffering of cancer patients with intractable pain.[51] Regional blocks are extremely useful in disrupting pain signals transmitted along the sympathetic and parasympathetic nerves.

NEURAL BLOCKADE IN HEAD AND NECK

More than 40 000 patients are diagnosed with head and neck cancer each year in the United States, and more than 500 000 patients are diagnosed worldwide.[52] Cancer of the head and neck constitutes approximately 5% of all malignant diseases in the United States and affects approximately 6.6 million patients worldwide.[53] Because of dense facial and neck innervations, cancer commonly causes not only disfiguring facial lesions but also disabling pain in the face and neck. Blocking relevant trigeminal nerve or cervical nerve branches can control the pain. However, the efficacy of interventional nerve blocks can be affected by tumor distortion of anatomy, radiation-induced fibrosis of local tissues, and possible overlapping sensory innervations of neighboring cranial nerves V, VII, IX, and X and upper cervical nerves. Careful evaluation of facial pain and proper selection of nerve block provide patients with relief.

Trigeminal Nerve Block

Indications Blockade of trigeminal ganglion or specific branches of trigeminal nerves alleviates somatic and neuropathic pain from cancer.

Anatomy The trigeminal or gasserian ganglion is formed from 2 nerve roots that arise from the ventral pons of the brainstem. These roots fuse anteriorly and enter the Meckel cave, a recess in the middle cranial fossa. Three sensory divisions then exit anteriorly as the ophthalmic nerve (V1), maxillary nerve (V2), and the mandibular nerve (V3). Destruction of the gasserian ganglion is useful for intractable pain from invasive tumors of the orbit, maxillary sinus, and mandible.[54] Conversely, each individual sensory nerve can be blocked separately if selective blockade is desired.

Techniques The patient is placed in a supine position, with the cervical spine extended on a foam pad or pillow. The cheek skin is aseptically prepped and then anesthetized with 1% lidocaine, 2.5 cm just lateral to the corner of mouth. Using C-arm fluoroscopic guidance, a 3.5-inch,

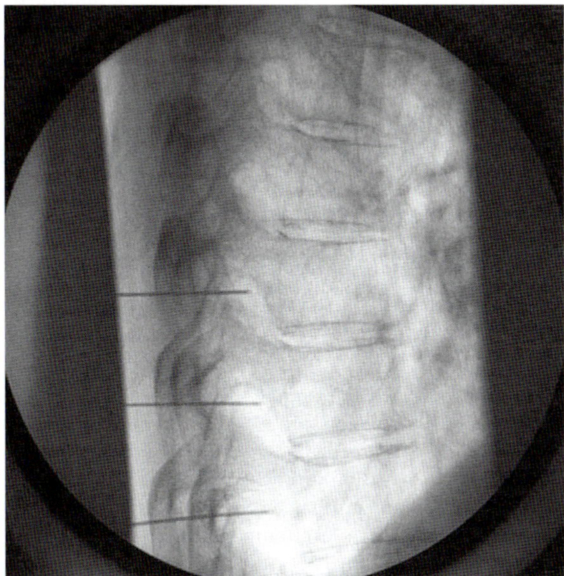

FIGURE 93-3. Lateral view of and intercostal dorsal root ganglion radiofrequency ablation.

20-gauge spinal needle is advanced slowly through the anesthetized skin area, 2.5 cm lateral to the corner of the lips. The direction of the spinal needle should be cranial, dorsal, and medial, with the foramen ovale as the target (**Fig. 93-3**). It may be easier to have the patient gaze straight ahead and then aim the needle in the cephalad direction, perpendicular to the midpupillary line. The needle is directed through the pterygopalatine fossa until the needle reaches the skull base. The needle then is walked posteriorly into the foramen ovale. Once the needle enters the foramen ovale, its tip should be located within the Meckel cave. Careful aspiration is important to ensure that the needle tip is not in a vascular structure. First a local anesthetic is injected (0.5 mL) to obtain a diagnostic block, and if adequate results in analgesia are obtained, this can be followed by injecting 0.5 mL of 100% alcohol.

Neuroablation of the trigeminal nerve can also be achieved using radiofrequency, both conventional and pulsed.

Complications Unintentional dural puncture can lead to neurotoxicity, including seizures and death. When the needle is directed through the pterygopalatine fossa, injury to vessels can result in facial hematoma or ocular subscleral hematoma. Postprocedural neuritis can cause significant dysesthetic pain in trigeminal sensory areas. Masticator weakness is possible with trigeminal block.

Occipital Nerve Block

Indications Occipital nerve block is effective for the treatment of oncologic pain in the posterior scalp and occipital region.

Anatomy Most of the posterior scalp is innervated by the greater occipital nerve, which arises from the dorsal rami of the C2 nerve root. It emerges subcutaneously in the posterior scalp just slightly inferior to the superior nuchal line and 2 to 3 cm lateral to the greater occipital protuberance. At this point of emergence, it is just medial to the occipital artery.[55]

Techniques The patient is placed in a sitting position, with the neck slightly flexed. The greater occipital protuberance and the mastoid process are palpated. In addition, a third of the distance between these 2 structures, the greater occipital artery can be palpated (3-4 cm lateral to the greater occipital protuberance on the superior nuchal line). The greater occipital nerve lies just medial to the greater occipital artery. It can be blocked at this site with local anesthetic or neurolytic injection.

The skin is aseptically prepped, and a short 1-inch, 25-gauge needle is introduced after the skin is infiltrated with local 1% lidocaine. Bony contact is made at a minimal depth of approximately 2 to 3 mm. A diagnostic block with 1 to 2 mL of local anesthetic (1% lidocaine) can be injected. For neurolytic block, a volume of 3 to 5 mL is used.

Complications Because of the superficial location of the greater occipital nerve and the relative ease of this block, complications are minimal. The close proximity of the greater occipital artery may increase the risk of intravascular injection, which can be avoided by frequent aspiration while the neurolytic solution is slowly injected. Neuritis also can occur with neurolytic agents, especially with alcohol.

Current advances in ultrasonography allow for better visualization of vascular nerve structures and dispersion of injectate, thus decreasing the incidence of side effects.

Superficial Cervical Plexus Block

Indications Superficial cervical plexus block is often used to treat cancer pain in the neck in areas innervated by the superficial cervical plexus.

Anatomy The superficial and deep cervical plexus arises from the first 4 cervical nerves. The cervical plexus begins just lateral to the first cervical vertebrae. It is located anterior to the levator scapulae and middle scalene muscles and posterior to the sternocleidomastoid (SCM) muscle. The plexus gives off both superficial sensory branches and deep motor branches. This anatomic division of sensory and motor nerves allows for selective sensory blockade of the superficial sensory branches of the cervical plexus without compromising the motor function of the neck muscles.

These superficial branches arise from the plexus and pierce the deep fascia of the neck at the posterior border of the SCM muscle. It is at this point where the bundle of the superficial cervical plexus emerges that sensory innervation to the plexus can be blocked easily.[56] The superficial cervical plexus gives rise to the sensory nerves that supply sensation to the skin and superficial fascia of the head, neck, and shoulder. These nerves include the lesser occipital, greater auricular, accessory, anterior cervical nerve, and suprascapular nerves.[57]

Techniques The patient is placed in a supine position, with the head turned away from the site to be blocked. The mastoid process is identified with the attached SCM muscle. The patient may have to raise the head slightly to allow for identification of SCM muscle. The neck is aseptically prepped. Just lateral to the SCM midpoint, a 1-inch, 25-gauge needle is inserted subcutaneously. A 5-mL volume of local anesthetic (1% lidocaine) is injected subcutaneously at this point. The needle then is directed superiorly and inferiorly along the posterior border of the SCM. A total volume of 10-20 mL of local anesthetic can be injected to achieve a diagnostic block. This block, if successful, can be followed with neurolytic agents to achieve a longer blockade. As a note of caution, the external jugular vein crosses the midpoint of the lateral border of the SCM. Careful aspiration before infiltration is helpful to avoid intravascular injection.[58]

Complications Few complications are associated with this superficial cervical block. The most common complication is intravascular injection into the external or internal jugular vein, with resulting systemic toxicity. Placement of the needle into jugular vein may result in hematoma or even air embolism.

NEURAL BLOCKADE IN UPPER EXTREMITY

Brachial Plexus Block

Indications Malignancy can involve the upper extremity. Such cancers include sarcomas, both of bone and soft tissue. In the United States, almost 13 000 new cases of bony sarcoma and 7000 new cases of soft tissue sarcomas are diagnosed each year.[59] In most cases, surgical resections of sarcomas with limb-sparing procedures are performed with good results. However, these patients often have severe pain from direct tumor invasion of neurovascular bundle or as a consequence of surgical resection of tumor. Neural blockade of the brachial plexus is effective in controlling somatic nociceptive pain in upper extremity cancer.

For short-term palliation of cancer pain, brachial plexus block can be performed with a catheter left in place for continuous infusion of local anesthetic. In cases of severe intractable pain from invasive tumors of brachial plexus or soft tissues and bone of shoulder and upper extremity, destruction of the brachial plexus is indicated. The patient should be made aware of the full consequences of neurolysis of brachial plexus, including paralysis of the upper extremity.

Anatomy The brachial plexus is formed from fusion of ventral rami of C5-T1 nerve roots. These nerve roots, with possible contribution from C4 and T2, emerge from the lateral aspect of the vertebral bodies and run laterally and inferiorly in the interscalene compartment. These nerves of the brachial plexus run down the interscalene compartment and pass behind the clavicle, cephalad to the first rib and then into the axilla.

Techniques Multiple approaches to brachial plexus blockade include interscalene block, supraclavicular, infraclavicular, and axillary blocks. For cancer pain from tumor involvement of the shoulder, interscalene block is preferred.[60]

The patient is placed in a supine position, with the head turned away from the site to be blocked. The posterior border of the SCM muscle is identified. The patient can cooperate by slightly flexing his or her head. The groove between the posterior border of SCM muscle and the anterior scalene muscle can be palpated by rolling fingers posteriorly off the edge of SCM muscle. The neck is then aseptically prepped. At the level of the cricoid cartilage (C6) in the interscalene groove, a 1.5-inch, 25-gauge needle is inserted in a slightly caudal, medial, and posterior angle. The skin is infiltrated with local anesthetic. The needle is inserted as described until paresthesia of shoulder, arm, or hand is obtained. Such paresthesia is encountered at a needle depth of 1 cm. Once a paresthesia is achieved or a motor response is obtained via verve stimulator, the needle is known to be near the brachial plexus. If aspiration is negative for CSF and blood, 30 to 40 mL of local anesthetic solution is injected incrementally, with frequent aspiration. Throughout injection, the patient is monitored for signs of local anesthetic toxicity and subarachnoid injection.

Once the efficacy of local anesthetic blockade in relieving cancer pain has been proven, the patient may wish to proceed with a longer lasting neurolytic block with phenol. A 20-mL volume of 6% phenol is slowly injected into the intrascalene compartment of the brachial plexus. Motor paralysis of upper extremity can be expected with this neurolysis of brachial plexus.

If a shorter prolonged blockade of brachial plexus is desired, a continuous local anesthetic infusion of the brachial plexus can be performed. The infraclavicular approach for brachial plexus block is preferred because the catheter can remain in the same position for 3 weeks or more.[61] The infraclavicular entry site permits easy catheter threading near the plexus, and the catheter's position is minimally affected with patient movement. For the infraclavicular approach, the patient is placed in a supine position with the head turned away from the site to be blocked. The clavicle is identified by palpation and fluoroscopy. The axillary artery also is palpated and marked. The ipsilateral neck, anterior shoulder, and axillary region are prepped with povidone iodine (Betadine) in a sterile manner. At the inferior border of the clavicle at the midpoint, local anesthetic (1% lidocaine) is generously infiltrated subcutaneously. A 16-gauge spinal needle is introduced at this midclavicular point and directed laterally toward the marked axillary artery location. The needle is directed at a 45° angle to the skin and then connected to a nerve stimulator by an alligator clip. As the needle advances, fluoroscopy allows for visualization of the needle tip. Once the tip nears the brachial plexus, muscles innervated by the plexus are stimulated, with visible flexion and extension of the elbow, wrist, and fingers. At this point, 2-3 mL of contrast dye is injected to confirm under fluoroscopy the spread along axillary sheath. The catheter then is threaded through the spinal needle and 3-5 cm beyond the tip. The needle is withdrawn, and the catheter is sutured in place. Infusion of 0.125% to 0.25% bupivacaine or 0.2% ropivacaine is used to provide continuous brachial plexus analgesia. It is effective in controlling somatic pain for several days and sympathetically mediated pain for up to a few weeks.

Complications Complications of interscalene block are possible because of proximity to many structures in the neck. Intravascular injection, as mentioned earlier, leads to systemic toxicity. Subarachnoid injection can cause sensory, motor, or total spinal anesthesia and even death. Phrenic nerve block is an expected side effect of interscalene block.

Complications of infraclavicular brachial plexus block are similar to those of interscalene block. Proximity to the subclavian artery and vein increases the potential for intravascular injection.

With the advance of imaging devices, the use of a high-definition ultrasound machine is now advocated for all this peripheral blocks. This allows the provider with an image of the nerves, surrounding structures, and spread of the agent injected.

Neural Blockade in Thorax Intercostal Nerve Block

Indications Lung cancer is the number-one cancer killer among both men and women.[59] It accounts for 15% of malignant disease in men and 13% in women. Patients diagnosed with lung cancer often require thoracotomy with surgical biopsy or resection of tumor mass. Many patients experience chest wall pain from either direct tumor involvement of the chest wall or surgical trauma to intercostal nerves. In addition to lung cancer, aggressive breast cancer may invade the ribs and intercostal nerve bundles, causing pain.

Tumor invasion of lung parenchyma and visceral pleura does not cause pain because these structures are nociceptive insensitive. However, cancer involvement of the parietal pleura does elicit a pain response. Pain is transmitted from parietal pleura along the somatic nerve, including the intercostals nerves from T1-12. Intercostal nerve blockade is effective in blocking this somatic pain.[62]

Anatomy The intercostal nerves are formed from ventral rami of thoracic nerves from T1 to T12. Each nerve, joined by intercostal vein and artery, runs in a neurovascular bundle in the subcostal groove. It gives off 4 branches as it runs anteriorly in the intercostals space. The first is the gray rami communicantes, which joins the sympathetic ganglion. The second branch is the posterior cutaneous nerve, which innervates the paravertebral region. The third branch is the lateral cutaneous nerve, which innervates the axilla and lateral chest wall. The fourth branch is the anterior cutaneous nerve, which innervates anterior thorax. There is considerable sensory overlap between those branches as well as between the intercostal nerves themselves. Thus pain from one area may require blockade of multiple adjacent intercostal nerves.[63]

Techniques For neurolytic block, the procedure should be performed under fluoroscopic guidance. The patient is placed in a prone position. The relevant ribs are identified by palpation and under fluoroscopy. The inferior border of each rib is indicated with a marking pen. The intercostal block is classically performed at the angle of the rib, just lateral to the paraspinal muscle groups. The relevant paraspinal area is prepped aseptically. Using a 1-inch, 25-gauge needle, the skin is infiltrated subcutaneously with local anesthetic. The clinician should palpate to obtain a gross estimation of the depth from skin to bone of rib. The needle is slowly advanced perpendicular to the skin, with fluoroscopic guidance. The C-arm should be in the anteroposterior projection with a caudal tilt. The needle tip should hit the body of the rib and then walk inferiorly off the lower border of rib into the subcostal groove. Water-soluble contrast dye injected into this groove should show a spread along the inferior border of rib. A neurolytic solution of 10% phenol can be injected with 3-5 mL for each intercostal block.

Complications Common complications of intercostal nerve blockade include pneumothorax and systemic toxicity. Pneumothorax results from needle puncture through parietal and visceral pleura. This creates an air leak from lung into pleural space. A simple pneumothorax may infrequently progress into a tension pneumothorax with its life-threatening implications. The patient should be closely monitored after the procedure, and a postprocedural chest radiograph is recommended.

Another complication of intercostal nerve blockade is systemic toxicity from absorption of anesthetic or neurolytic solution into the intercostal neurovascular bundle. Because of the close proximity of intercostal artery and vein to the nerve, rapid absorption of injected solution into the circulation is common. However, systemic toxicity is infrequent because of the small volume used for neurolysis. A less likely complication is neuraxial spread of the anesthetic or neurolytic solution.

Instead of chemical neurolysis, cryoanalgesia and radiofrequency ablation have been used for intercostal nerve blockade. Cryoanalgesia or "freezing" of intercostal nerves has been shown to control pain in postthoracotomy patients if performed under direct visualization of intercostal nerve at termination of surgery.[50] After surgery, percutaneous intercostal cryolysis has not been shown to be as effective.[64]

Intercostal nerve radiofrequency ablation can be used for long-lasting blockade. A blunt-tipped 100-mm, 22-gauge radiofrequency electrode with a 5-mm active tip is inserted into the intercostal space. One milliliter of 2% lidocaine is injected into the electrode cannula. Lesioning is accomplished by coagulation at 80°C for 60 seconds. The technique of proximal intercostal nerve radiofrequency lesioning, including ablation of the dorsal root ganglion, is being used with favorable preliminary results (Fig. 93-3).

SYMPATHETIC BLOCKADE FOR CANCER PAIN

Visceral pain arises from cancer involvement of sympathetically mediated organs. Insults to these organs can result from abnormal distension of organ wall or viscus, tension or torsion on mesenteric vessels, and ischemia. Such visceral pain is commonly seen with gastrointestinal malignancies, such as hepatic metastases, intestinal tract tumors, and pancreatic cancers. Sympathetically mediated pain can involve neuropathic pain, as occurs with direct injury to nervous tissue such as brachial plexopathy and lumbosacral plexopathy. Blockade of sympathetic chain has been shown to be effective in controlling sympathetically mediated pain.[65,66]

The sympathetic axis is made up primarily of a pair of ganglionated paravertebral chains that run from base of skull to the tip of coccyx. It also consists of several major vertebral plexuses, including celiac, cardiac, and hypogastric plexuses. **Table 93-7** lists major sympathetic structures and the corresponding tissues innervated.[67]

These sympathetic structures are attractive targets for blockade of sympathetically mediated pain. Interruption of pain pathways at these discrete sites has been demonstrated to have a useful role in controlling oncologic pain.[68,69]

Stellate Ganglion Block

Indications Stellate ganglion block helps control sympathetically mediated pain in the head, neck, and upper extremity. Sympathically mediated pain is commonly seen in tumor invasion of brachial plexopathy as in Pancoast tumors.[70]

TABLE 93-7 Sympathetic Structures

Sympathetic Structures	Innervated Tissues
Stellate ganglia	Brain, ear, tongue, pharynx, larynx, skin of neck, head, and upper extremity
Thoracic ganglia	Mediastinal contents, esophagus, trachea bronchus, pericardium, heart, lung
Celiac plexus	GI tract (from distal esophagus to mid–transverse colon), liver, adrenals, ureters, abdominal vessels
Lumbar ganglia	Skin and vessels of lower extremity, kidneys, ureters, transverse colon, testes
Hypogastric plexus	Descending and sigmoid colon, rectum, vaginal fundus, bladder, prostate, prostatic urethra, testes, seminal vesicles, uterus, and ovaries
Ganglion impar	Perineum, distal rectum and anus, distal urethra, vulva and distal third of vagina

Anatomy Stellate or cervicothoracic ganglion is formed from fusion of the inferior cervical and the first sympathetic ganglia. This ganglion controls sympathetic afferent nociceptive signals to the head, neck, and upper extremity. The ganglion is located at the base of the neck and anterior to the neck of the first rib. It is bounded anteriorly by subclavian artery and the origin of vertebral artery, posteriorly by the vertebral body and longus colli muscle, laterally by the scalene muscles, and inferiorly by the dome of the pleura.

Techniques Because of many important structures in the neck adjacent to stellate ganglion, fluoroscopic imaging is recommended. The patient is placed in a supine position with the neck slightly extended. The classic technique is to identify the Chassaignac tubercle at C6 and insert the needle at this site. However, many clinicians recommend the Racz technique for a possible improved safety margin.[71] The patient's neck is aseptically prepped, and the skin over the body of the C7 vertebral body is anesthetized with 1% lidocaine. The nondominant hand is used to palpate the carotid artery at the level of C7 and retract it laterally. The dominant hand introduces a 1.5-inch, 22-gauge needle just medial to the palpated carotid artery and directs the needle in a medial direction. The target of the needle tip is the ventrolateral aspect of the C7 vertebral body, not the transverse process as seen in the classic approach. Once the needle tip contacts the C7 vertebral body, it is withdrawn slightly, approximately 1 mm. The needle then is aspirated for CSF or blood. From 1-2 mL of contrast dye is injected to confirm the caudocephalad spread anterior to the prevertebral facia. For gangliolysis, a mixture of 3% phenol, local anesthetic, and steroid is used (ie, 5 mL of 6% phenol in saline, 5 mL of 0.5% bupivacaine, and 80 mg of methylprednisone).

The volume of this mixture injected depends on the extent of blockade desired. Ten milliliters of neurolytic mixture is adequate for stellate ganglion blockade of sympathetically mediated pain to the head and upper extremity. If blockade of pain from thoracic viscera is desired, a volume of 15-20 mL of neurolytic mixture is necessary. During injection, the clinician must exercise caution to minimize intravascular injection. Even 1 mL of local anesthetic injected into the carotid or vertebral artery can cause loss of consciousness and seizure. An initial test dose, frequent aspiration, and slow injection are good suggested measures.

Efficacy Evidence of sympathetic blockade in the head can include a myriad of signs of Horner, syndromes such as miosis, ptosis, enophthalmos, facial anhidrosis, and nasal congestion. Sympathetic blockade to upper extremity results in visible engorgement of veins in the hands and forearm.

Complications Because of anatomic proximity to critical structures, serious complications of stellate ganglion block can include pneumothorax, anesthetic-induced seizure from intravascular injection, and total spinal anesthesia from subarachnoid injection. Other less serious problems include localized hematoma, infection, and neck muscle tenderness. Many clinicians fear a permanent Horner syndrome with neurolysis. However, Racz and Holubec[71] did not observe any long-term Horner syndrome with their modified technique.

Celiac Plexus Blockade

Indications Celiac plexus blockade continues to be an effective intervention for pain from pancreatic cancer and malignancies involving the upper and midabdomen.[68,72] Pancreatic cancer carries a poor prognosis, and palliation of pain symptom is a priority in these patients, with survival rates typically less than 6 months. Patients often present initially with upper abdominal pain with referred pain to the back.[73] The pain is described as severe, increasing with disease progression, and poorly relieved by opioids or other medications. Celiac plexus block is the treatment of choice for pain control in pancreatic cancer patients.

Anatomy Sympathetic innervations of abdominal organs arise in the anterolateral horn cells in the spinal cord. Preganglionic fibers from T5 to T12 leave ventral roots of spinal cord to join with white rami communicans.

Passing from the sympathetic ganglia to the celiac plexus, the preganglionic fibers travel along the discrete splanchnic pathways.

Preganglionic fibers from T5 to T9 coalesce to form the greater splanchnic nerve. This greater splanchnic nerve passes through the diaphragm and synapse onto the celiac plexus. Preganglionic nerves from T10 to T11 join to form the lesser splanchnic nerve before synapsing within the celiac plexus. The least splanchnic nerve arises from the T12 sympathetic ganglion and courses through anteriorly to join the celiac plexus. Blockade of sympathetically mediated pain in this region is accomplished by neurolysis of either the celiac plexus or the splanchnic nerves that became the plexus.

The celiac plexus is located anterior to the aorta at the level of the L1 vertebral body and anterior to the crura of the diaphragm. This plexus contains 2 large discrete ganglia on either side of the aorta. The left celiac ganglion is slightly lower than the right ganglion.

Techniques Multiple techniques (up to 13 approaches) have been described for sympathetic blockade at the level of celiac plexus.[74,75,76] Using a posterior approach, clinicians can use the classic retrocrural, transcrural, or transaortic technique.

Anteriorly, percutaneous gangliolysis with CT guidance or direct intraoperative celiac gangliolysis can be used.

Another method is the transgastric approach, using an endoscope with an ultrasound probe to better visualize the aorta, celiac artery, and injectate spread.

Because of the proximity of vascular structures, patients with coagulopathy should have those corrected before needle placement. Skin infections, intra-abdominal infections, or sepsis represent contraindications to the neurolytic celiac plexus block.

Due to the subsequent unopposed parasympathetic activity, the technique should be avoided in patients with bowel obstruction.[8]

An intravenous cannula should be placed and the patient should receive approximately 500 mL of intravenous crystalloid before performing the procedure to minimize hypotension due to vasodilation.

Monitoring electrocardiogram, blood pressure, and pulse oximetry is strongly recommended. Intravenous sedation is not always necessary but may help patients tolerate and sustain the proper position.

For the posterior classic retrocrural approach, the patient is placed in a prone position with a pillow under the lower abdomen to minimize lordosis. The back is prepped aseptically. Using fluoroscopy, the relevant landmarks are identified and marked: the spinous processes of T12 and L1, and the inferior border of the 12th rib. It is very important to correctly identify the T12 spinous process by following the 12th rib medially and by counting cephalad from the L5 spinous process. The skin is infiltrated with local anesthetic at a distance 5 to 8 cm lateral to the L1 spinous process and inferior to the 12th rib.

A bilateral needle technique is used. Under direct fluoroscopic guidance, using both the anteroposterior (AP) and lateral views, two 5- or 7-inch 22-gauge spinal needles are slowly advanced. The anterolateral inferior border of the T12 vertebral body is identified as the final target point. Local anesthetic is infiltrated along this needle path.

In the AP fluoroscopic view, the needle tip should be no further medial than a third of the distance from the lateral vertebral border (**Fig. 93-4**). In the lateral fluoroscopic view, the needle tip should lie just anterior to the vertebral body (Fig. 93-4). After negative aspiration for blood, urine, and CSF, contrast dye is injected. Fluoroscopic images should demonstrate linear spread along the anterior vertebral bodies on the lateral view and vertical spread on the AP view. Caution should be taken to avoid intravascular, intrathecal, intraneural, intradiscal, or intracrural injection. If observed, needle position should be adjusted appropriately. Contrast dye should never spread dorsally toward the exiting thoracolumbar spinal nerve roots. After acceptable contrast dye spread patterns have been confirmed bilaterally, the celiac plexus is anesthetized with 10 mL local anesthetic (a mixture of 2% lidocaine and 0.5% bupivacaine 1:1 can be used) through each needle. After 15 minutes a careful neurologic exam should reveal no neurologic deficits (both sensory and motor). At this point 10 mL of 98% ethyl alcohol is injected into each needle slowly over 1 to 2 minutes. The needles are flushed with local anesthetic as they are removed from the skin.

Efficacy Celiac plexus blockade has been found to provide significant relief of pancreatic cancer pain. Pain relief has been reported between 70% and 94% of patients.[73] Studies have shown a higher success rate, corresponding to better patient selection and technologic advances.

Complications Although not strictly a complication, sympatholysis with its side effects should be considered in celiac blockade. Orthostatic

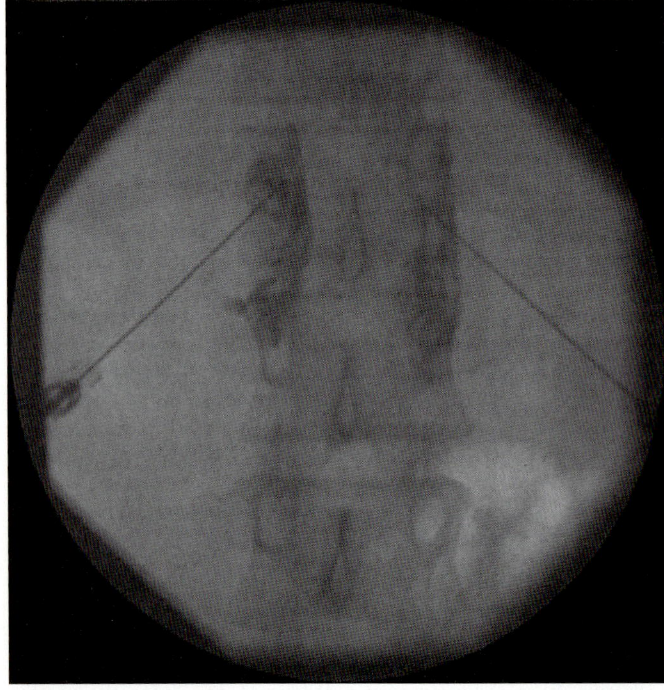

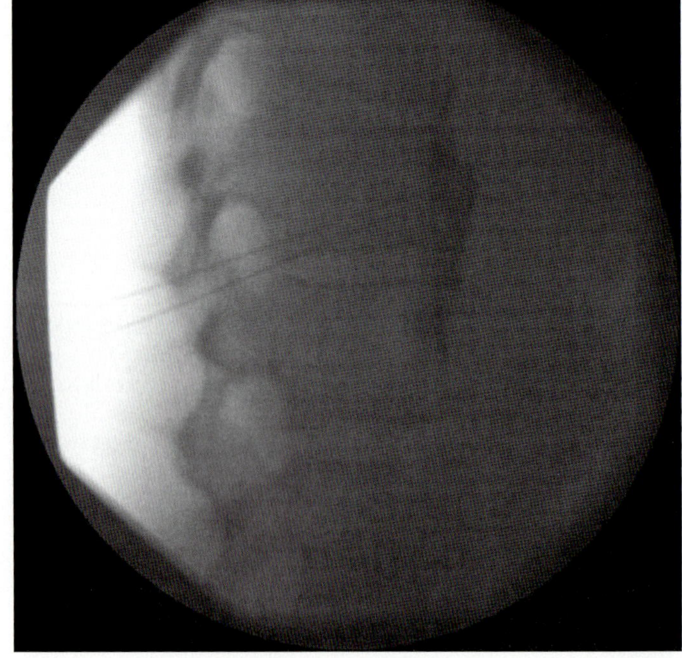

FIGURE 93-4. Anteroposterior and lateral views of retrocrural celiac plexus block.

hypotension may occur and should be anticipated. Unopposed parasympathetic activity leads to gastrointestinal hypermotility. The consequent diarrhea is transient and does not last more than 2 days. Serious complications can include visceral injury, renal trauma with hematoma, and intravascular or subarachnoid injection. Pneumothorax is possible.

Lumbar Sympathetic Block

Indications Lumbar sympathetic blockade has been used to treat sympathetically mediated cancer pain due to tumor invasion or metastases to the lumbosacral region, chemotherapy- or radiation therapy-induced lumbar plexopathy, phantom limb pain, and lower extremity neuropathy secondary to malignancy.[77]

Anatomy Lumbar sympathetic chain is variable in size and location. The sympathetic ganglia usually are located between the L2 and L4 vertebral bodies. Classically, the sympathetic chain lies in the fascial plane anterolateral to lumbar vertebral bodies, just anterior and medial to psoas muscles.

Techniques The patient is placed in a supine position, with a pillow under the lower abdomen to minimize lordosis. The back is prepped aseptically. Using fluoroscopy, surface landmarks of L2, L3, and L4 spinous processes are identified and marked. At a distance 5 to 8 cm lateral to each spinous process, the skin and underlying muscle tissue are generously infiltrated with local anesthetic. A 7-inch, 22-gauge needle is introduced at the selected site and directed at a 45° angle with the midline. The needle is advanced until vertebral body is confirmed. The depth of the needle is noted, and the needle is withdrawn and redirected at a steeper angle (60° with midline) to walk off the vertebral body. Once the needle slides past vertebral body, it is advanced approximately 1 cm further into the prevertebral fascial plane. This sequence is repeated bilaterally for L2, L3, and L4 levels. Contrast dye, 1-3 mL, at each needle site can be used to visualize the spread radiographically. A diagnostic block with 20-30 mL of 2% lidocaine can be performed, with the patient awakened to rule out any neurologic (sensory and motor) deficit. Neurolysis then can be performed with 6% phenol with a volume of 5 mL at each needle site.

Complications Side effects of lumbar sympatholysis include hypotension and diarrhea. Intestinal hypermotility is self-limited.[78] Other complications include psoas muscle necrosis and renal or visceral damage. The most common complication with lumbar sympatholysis is genitofemoral neuralgia. Most cases are transient and resolve in a few weeks.

Superior Hypogastric Plexus Block

Indications Pelvic malignancies can affect multiple organs in the pelvis and include gynecologic and prostate cancers. Each year in the United States, 18 400 new cases of gynecologic cancer of the uterine cervix, vulva, and vagina are diagnosed, resulting in approximately 6300 deaths.[52] Patients with pelvic malignancy often experience initial visceral pelvic pain. The pain often is described as vague, poorly localized in the pelvic region, and colicky in character. Surgical destruction of the hypogastric plexus has been shown to relieve pelvic pain.[79,80] Plancarte et al[81] reported a technique for hypogastric blockade with good results for controlling pelvic pain secondary to cancer. In that study, all 28 cancer patients with intractable pelvic pain reported good pain relief after the procedure.

Anatomy The superior hypogastric plexus arises from the coalescence of nerve branches descending from the celiac plexus and lumbar sympathetic chains. This hypogastric plexus is a bilateral retroperitoneal structure located usually anterolaterally, extending from the level of the L5 vertebral body to upper third of the S1 vertebral body. The plexus is just medial to the bifurcation of iliac arteries and veins on each side.

Techniques The patient is placed in a prone position. A pillow is placed under the lower abdomen to minimize lumbar lordosis. The back is prepped aseptically. Under fluoroscopy, the spinous processes of L4 and L5 are identified and marked. The entry point is 5 to 7 cm off midline at the level of the L4-5 interspace. The skin and underlying tissue at this point are well anesthetized with local anesthetic (1% lidocaine). A 7-inch, 22-gauge needle is introduced at an orientation 30° caudal and 45° mesiad off midline. Under fluoroscopy in AP and lateral views, the needle is slowly advanced, with the target the anterolateral aspect of the L5 vertebral body. The iliac crest and L5 transverse process can be obstacles along the needle trajectory. The needle may have to be reoriented slightly to bypass these anatomic structures. Once bony contact is made with the L5 vertebral body, the needle is reoriented to a more mesiad angle to walk the needle tip off the body of the L5 vertebra. The tip of the needle should be advanced past the anterolateral border of the L5 vertebral body under direct lateral fluoroscopic guidance. A loss of resistance may be felt as the needle tip passes beyond the psoas muscle fascia and into the retroperitoneal space where the hypogastric plexus lies. Because of close proximity to the bifurcation of iliac vessels, careful aspiration is helpful to ensure the needle tip is not intravascular. Contrast dye can be injected to visualize even dye spread to the paramedian space at L5, anterior to the psoas fascia. Each side can be injected with 10 mL of 2% lidocaine for diagnostic block, and neurolysis can be achieved with 10 mL of 10% phenol at each site.

Complications Because of close proximity to the iliac vessels, the clinician should be cautious about intravascular injection. Vascular puncture may lead to hemorrhage. Other less likely complications include subarachnoid injection, sacral nerve injury, and bladder or bowel injury.

Ganglion Impar Block

Indications In the perineum, there is a diffuse network of mixed sympathetic and somatic innervations. Thus perineal pain usually involves both somatic and sympathetic pathways. In cancer patients with perineal pain, cancer can involve the lower colon, rectum, bladder, cervix, and endometrium. Blockage of ganglion impar with the goal of disrupting sympathetically mediated pathways is effective in managing some intractable perineal cancer pain.[82]

Anatomy Ganglion impar is a solitary retroperitoneal structure located at the level of the sacrococcygeal junction. The 2 parallel sympathetic chains fuse together anterior to superior borders of the coccyx, forming the ganglion impar or ganglion of Walther.

Technique The patient is placed in a prone position; sedation is optional. Using fluoroscopy, the patient's sacrococcygeal junction is visualized from an anterior-posterior image. After anesthetizing the overlying tissues with 1% lidocaine, a 2.5-inch, 22 gauge needle is slowly advanced through the midline of the sacrococcygeal junction until the needle tip appears 2-3 mm anterior to the ventral sacrococcygeal ligament from a lateral perspective.

After a negative aspiration through the needle, 1 to 2 mL of contrast dye is injected. A confirmatory dye spread pattern from a lateral view should resemble a "comma" shape staying immediately on the ventral aspect of the sacrum and coccyx (**Fig. 93-5**) in the retroperitoneal space. From an AP view, most of the dye spread should remain in the midline. For diagnostic and accuracy purposes, and before neurolysis, 5 mL of 2% lidocaine is injected. The patient is assessed over the next 15 minutes for improvement of their pain, as well as for the lack of a motor conduction block affecting the lower extremities. If the preliminary results are satisfactory (ie, at least 50% reduction of their pain and no neurologic deficits), neurolysis is accomplished using 5 mL of 98% ethyl alcohol. The needle is gently flushed with local anesthetic before removal from the skin.

Complications This block of ganglion impar may cause rectal perforation because of proximity to the rectum. Because most of this region is dually innervated by both somatic and sympathetic fibers, complete pain relief may be difficult to achieve by this block alone.

Neuromodulation Techniques

Intraspinal Drug Delivery Significant side effects from systemic high-dose opioid administration can be minimized with intraspinal delivery of opioids. Delivery of opioids in close proximity to the spinal cord

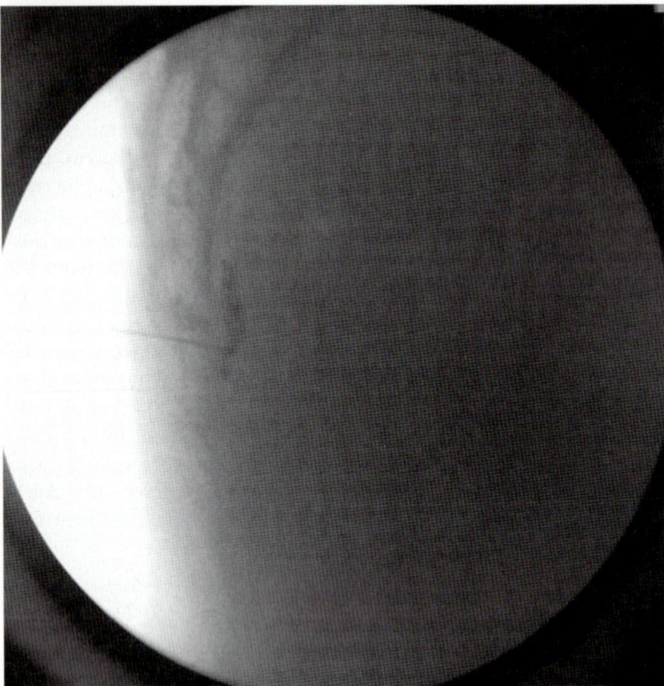

FIGURE 93-5. Lateral view of ganglion impar block.

provides for more potent analgesia and fewer side effects.[9] If the opioid dose is delivered into epidural location, only 20% to 40% of the systemic dose is required to achieve similar analgesia.[83,84] The intrathecal dosage is even lower, requiring only 10% of the systemic dose.

In cancer patients, the intraspinal drugs can be delivered by percutaneously tunneled epidural catheters, tunneled epidural or spinal catheters connected to subcutaneously implanted injection ports, or fully implanted spinal infusion pump systems (**Fig. 93-6**).[85] The SynchroMed pump system (Medtronic Inc, Minneapolis, MN) is an example of a fully implantable system that is sophisticated yet easy to use. The pump can easily be reprogrammed to meet the patient's changing pain condition. Advantages of a fully implantable intrathecal pump include effective pain control, increased independence and mobility of the patient, and a reduced risk of infection with an internalized pump system. However, the initial cost of system hardware and implantation surgery can be prohibitive and hard to justify for patients with a predicted survival less than 3 months.[86,87] With survival time less than 3 months, a simple tunneled epidural catheter or subcutaneous infusion is more economically feasible and beneficial for the patient. The epidural space is further from the spinal cord and thus requires a higher dose or rate of infusion, usually mandating an external pump.

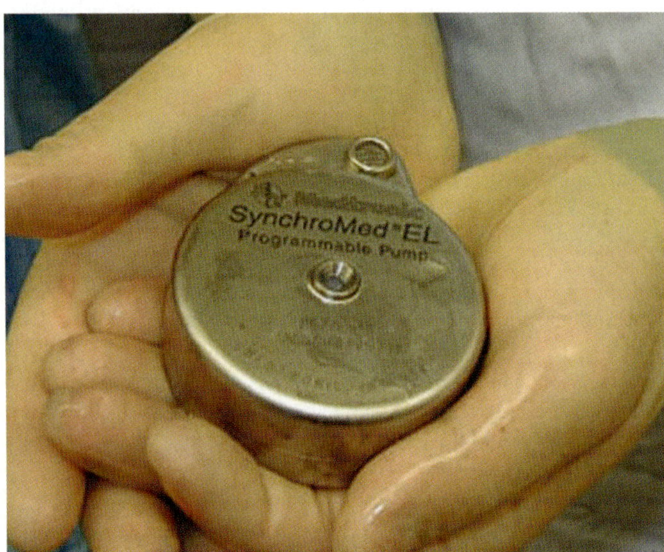

FIGURE 93-6. Implantable programmable pump.

Other Techniques

Vertebroplasty Neurosurgical procedures can be used to treat intractable pain. Vertebroplasty is one procedure that provides significant pain relief in patients with vertebral compression fractures secondary to malignant diseases. Malignant tumors include metastasis, lymphomas, and myeloma. Vertebroplasty involves injection of polymethylmethacrylate (PMMA) cement into the diseased vertebral body (**Fig. 93-7**).[88,89]

Kyphoplasty Percutaneous kyphoplasty is the placement of balloons into the vertebral body with an inflation/deflation sequence to create a cavity before the cement injection. These procedures are most often performed percutaneously on an outpatient (or short stay) basis. The procedure is indicated for painful vertebral compression fractures due to osteoporosis or malignancy, and painful hemangiomas. The procedure may have efficacy in painful vertebral metastasis and traumatic compression fractures. Much evidence favors the use of this procedure for pain associated with these disorders.[90]

Kyphoplasty is a refinement of the vertebroplasty procedure. In addition to the reduction of fracture-related pain, some or all of the height is restored to the compressed vertebral body. Normalizing the height of the fractured vertebra reduces the focally exaggerated curvature of the spine (ie, kyphosis). The restoration of a more normal-appearing configuration of the vertebral body and improvement in the load-bearing physics is accomplished with the intravertebral inflation of 1 or 2 high-pressure balloons (KyphX; KYPHON). As with vertebroplasty, access is via a transpedicular or peripedicular approach. The procedure distracts the fragments and elevates the collapsed vertebral endplate. The inflated balloons create cavities in the vertebral body, the margins of which are

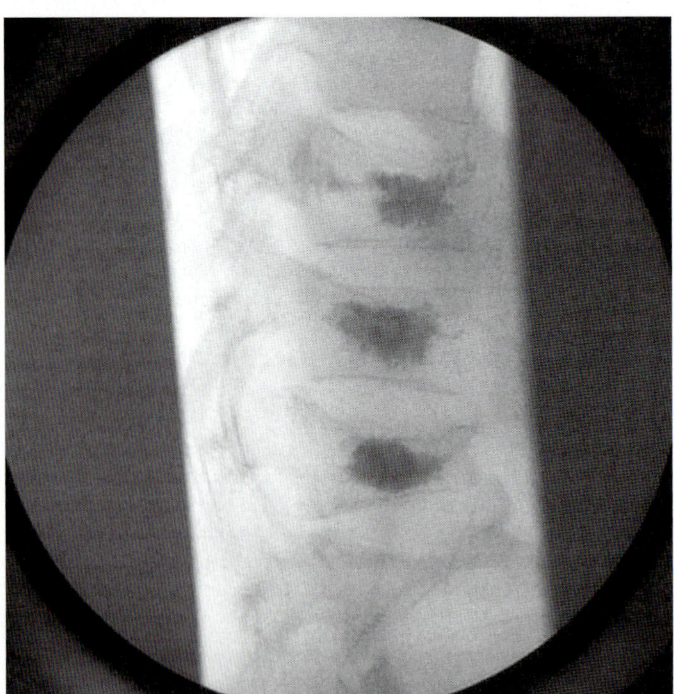

FIGURE 93-7. Lateral view of a vertebroplasty.

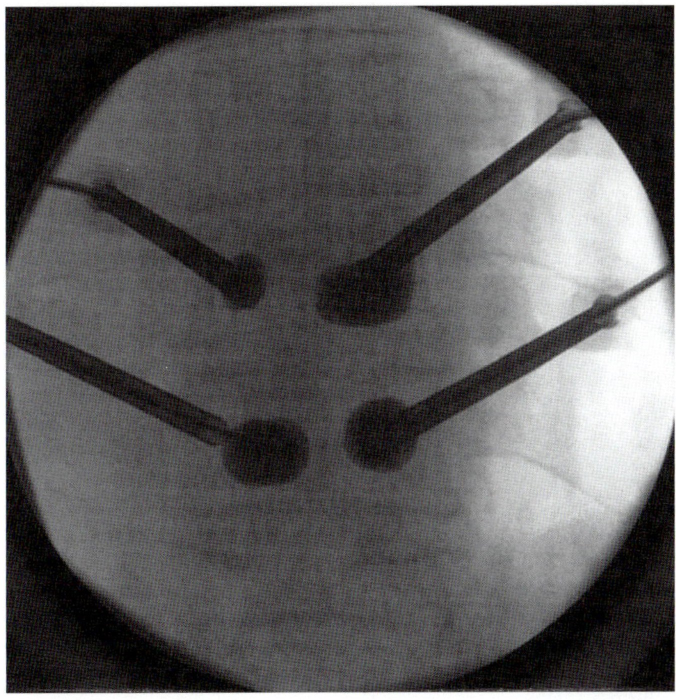

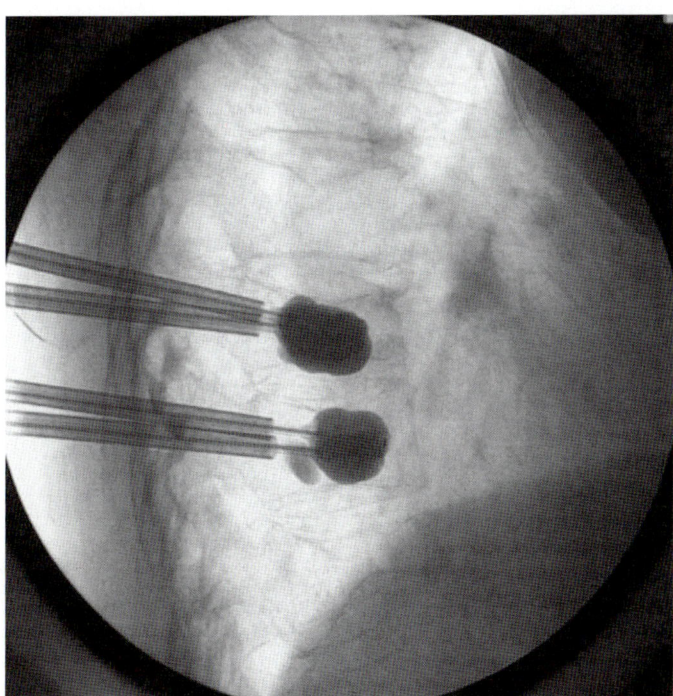

FIGURE 93-8. Two radiographic views of kyphoplasty.

lined by the displaced, fragmented trabeculae. These are later filled with the injection of PMMA (**Fig. 93-8**).

The overall risks of the procedure are low, but serious complications (including spinal cord compression) can occur. With good patient selection and careful technique, these complications are avoidable, making the risk-to-benefit ratio highly favorable.

PALLIATIVE CARE

Palliative care is defined as comprehensive care of the terminally ill patient. In overall oncologic care, much effort and treatment is used in the palliative treatment mode. Many patients have meaningful life-extending and life-enhancing palliative (as distinct from "curative") treatments. Treatments include chemotherapy, radiotherapy, tumor ablative procedures, surgery, and the interventional treatments outlined in this chapter.

Effective palliation in the patient with advanced cancer always starts with complete assessment and appropriate pharmacologic management. In some patients in whom the risk-to-benefit ratio is favorable and more conservative therapies are failing, interventional pain techniques may be helpful. When treating the advanced cancer patient, it is important to keep in mind some tenets of palliative medicine, such as these adopted from Field et al.[91] Symptom control is a paramount concern. It is critical to discuss openly and compassionately the patient's goals of care and to tailor treatments in accordance with the patient's wishes. The patient's overall well-being has a direct impact on the caregiver's quality of life. Clinicians must be honest with patients and family members while being cautious not to extinguish hope.[92]

CONCLUSION

Cancer pain management is a complicated challenge. It requires a thorough understanding of the cancer disease process, pain diagnosis, and treatment modalities available to treat the pain condition. In addition to pain, the patient often presents with a constellation of symptoms arising from cancer and its treatment. Both pharmacologic and interventional modalities of treatment are necessary to help the patient control pain and reach a satisfactory quality of life. In carefully selected cases, diverse interventional techniques help the physician and patient to achieve effective control of cancer pain, thereby optimizing quality of life.

KEY REFERENCES

- Burton AW, Rajagopal A, Shah HN, et al. Epidural and intrathecal analgesia is effective in treating refractory cancer pain. *Pain Med.* 2004;5:239-247.
- Cata JP, Weng HR, Lee BN, et al. Clinical and experimental findings in humans and animals with chemotherapy-induced peripheral neuropathy. *Minerva Anestesiol.* 2006;72:151-169.
- Eisenberg E, Carr DB, Chalmers TC. Neurolytic celiac plexus blockade for treatment of cancer pain: a metaanalysis. *Anesth Analg.* 1995;80:290-307.
- Ferrante FM, Bedder M, Caplan KA, et al. Practice guidelines for cancer pain management. *Anesthesiology.* 1996;94:1243-1257.
- Hassenbusch SJ, Paice JA, Patt RB, et al. Clinical realities and economic considerations: economic of intrathecal therapy. *J Pain Symptom Manage.* 1997;14:536-548.
- Lyss AP, Portenoy RK. Strategies for limiting the side effects of cancer pain therapy. *Semin Oncol.* 1997;24:S128-S133.
- Perkins FM, Kehlet H. Chronic pain as an outcome of surgery. *Anesthesiology.* 2000;93:1123-1133.
- Smith TJ, Coyne PJ, et al. An implantable drug delivery system (IDDS) for refractory cancer pain provides sustained pain control, less drug-related toxicity, and possibly better survival compared with comprehensive medical management (CMM). *Ann Oncol.* 2005;16:825-833.

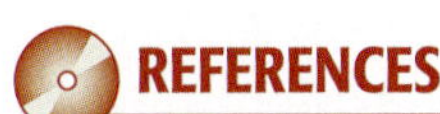

REFERENCES

Complete references available on DVD and online version at www.LongneckerAnesthesiology.com

PART 9

Practice-Related Issues

CHAPTER 94

Legal Issues in Anesthesiology

C. Lee Parmley

KEY POINTS

1. Elements of negligence: To succeed in a medical malpractice action, the plaintiff must prove four elements by preponderance of the evidence. (1) Duty: The defendant owed a duty of care to the plaintiff. (2) Breach of duty: The defendant failed to act consistent with the standards of care. (3) Causation: The injury suffered by the plaintiff is linked to or caused by the defendant's breach of duty. (4) Damages: There is actual compensable loss resulting from the defendant's breach of duty.
2. Exclusive contracts: Exclusive arrangements used by hospitals to contract for anesthesiology service and may be challenged on allegation of antitrust and restraint of trade.
3. National Practitioner Data Bank: Information contained in this databank is protected from unrestricted public inquiry but is queried when medical staff application is made.
4. HIPAA (Health Insurance Portability and Accountability Act): Protects health care information while asking acknowledgment that it may be released for uses related to medical treatment, payment, and/or health care operation, such as auditing performance evaluation and training program.
5. Informed consent: Process by which a patient chooses to accept or refuse treatment offered once there has been exchange of information sufficient to establish an understanding of potential risks and benefits of both treatment and nontreatment options.
6. Do not resuscitate orders: Should be reconsidered when patients with these orders are taken for surgery and anesthesia. A patient-oriented approach requires an individualized look at goal-directed and procedure-directed option.
7. Parents are the natural guardian of their children and are expected to seek care that is in their children's best interest when needed. Courts usually appoint a guardian other than the parent and support decisions for medical care deemed to be clearly in the child's best interest.

LEGAL SYSTEM

The American legal system is composed of federal and state court systems, the latter of which is the usual forum for matters pertaining to anesthesia practice.[1] State courts are established to adjudicate civil and criminal actions. Many consider our legal system to be cumbersome, overburdened, and often ineffective and unfair. Despite this reputation, it is our route to dispute resolution and protection of interests both personal and public. When contracts are formed by private parties, the legal system is called on to interpret language and hold parties to their contractual obligations. When one party is injured by another, the legal system is expected to resolve the matter and make whole the injured party to the extent possible. When criminal actions are taken, punitive action is imposed by the legal system.

CRIMINAL

Criminal courts deal with violation of criminal and other statutes and regulations for which penalties beyond those available in the civil system can be imposed. Penalties include fines and loss of privileges, including liberty. An occasional publication can be found that refers to cases where the practice of anesthesia resulted in criminal penalties.[2] A finding of gross negligence can in some jurisdictions lead to a charge of homicide.[3] These cases though are in fact rare, and anesthesia providers ideally will have little need to interface with the criminal court system. Violation of criminal statutes and some state regulations represent the possibility of being indicted as a criminal defendant. Legal representation in such proceedings is seldom provided through malpractice insurance coverage, and effective representation is necessary and usually quite costly.

Occasionally health care providers, including those in the field of anesthesia, are needed to testify as witnesses in criminal proceedings that involve patients who were the victims of criminal activity. Participating in such proceedings represents a considerable inconvenience, although often the court makes every effort to accommodate scheduling needs. Although in this situation the witness usually is called to provide factual evidence, the attorneys also may rely on the witness's expertise and ask for explanations and opinions, which ordinarily are in the realm of the expert witness.

CIVIL

Civil courts impose financial penalties and at times require or prevent a particular action of an individual. Most frequently the practice of anesthesiology interfaces with the civil court system, which is the forum for resolution of disputes based in contract and tort law, which includes actions in medical malpractice or medical negligence cases.

EVIDENTIARY STANDARDS

For legal proceedings, evidence is offered to establish the factual basis of the case. The finder of fact is ordinarily a jury but in some cases may be a judge. Evidence is presented to the finder of fact, who then weighs the evidence and determines the true factual basis. How convincing the evidence must be to make a determination is thought of as the burden of proof. For criminal cases, the evidence must be sufficient to eliminate reasonable doubt. Civil cases, such as medical malpractice, ordinarily rely on a preponderance of the evidence standard. Language frequently applied is "more likely than not" or "with a reasonable degree of medical probability." Medical practitioners are trained to look at evidence supporting a p value of 0.01 or 0.05 or a confidence interval of 95% to 99%. The preponderance of the evidence standard is much lower, just enough to tip the evidentiary scale at more than 51%.

BURDEN OF PROOF

For civil and criminal cases, the party bringing the case has the burden of proof, which means the responsibility to provide evidence sufficient to meet the evidentiary standard. There is a presumption of innocence until the evidence is sufficient to establish facts that are legally sufficient to prove otherwise. For medical malpractice, the plaintiff brings the case and has the burden of proving with the preponderance of evidence that every element of the tort claim is present.

Occasionally there are cases where the burden of proof shifts to the defendant, who must prove he or she is not negligent. With *res ipsa loquitur* (meaning "the things speaks for itself"), the plaintiff's case is much easier to prove. Surgery on the wrong part of the body would be such a case. For *res ipsa* to apply, (1) the injury must ordinarily not occur in the absence of negligence, (2) the instrumentalities involved in the injury must be under the exclusive control of the defendant, (3) the plaintiff must be free of any contribution to the injury, and (4) the evidence or factual details must be more readily available to the defendant than the plaintiff. When *res ipsa loquitur* applies, there exists a rebuttable presumption that negligence exists, making it the defendants' burden to prove otherwise.[4]

MEDICAL LIABILITY

ELEMENTS OF NEGLIGENCE

Humans owe each other a duty of ordinary care to avoid injury to each other. When one individual is injured due to the failure of another to exercise ordinary care, a case in negligence can arise. For the medical arena, the injury involves the care provided by a health care provider or institution. Four elements must be proven.

The first of the elements is referred to as "Duty." Usually established through the development of a doctor–patient relationship, the duty is the requirement to provide care, although ordinary or standard care is all that the duty requires. The second element of negligence is a "Breach" of the established duty. The breach occurs when the individual with a duty fails to provide ordinary care or act within the standards of care.

"Causation" is the third element and is the causal link between the breach of duty and the injury sustained by the plaintiff. At times a patient may suffer an injury, and there may be one or more breaches of the standards of care. Unless the breach can be shown to have caused the injury sustained, the case will lack causation. Causation can be proven by 2 legal tests, the "but for" test and the "substantial factor" test. The plaintiff may succeed if he or she can show by a preponderance of the evidence that "but for" the defendant(s)' breach of duty the injury would not have occurred. Alternatively, the plaintiff may succeed if it can successfully be shown that the defendants' breach of duty represented a substantial factor in causing the plaintiff's injury, despite the presence of other factors, which may include ones introduced through action or inaction of the plaintiff.

The fourth element of negligence is called "Damages." This is the economic value assigned to the injury sustained by the plaintiff. Although losses may be physical, economic, and emotional, damages will be calculated to compensate the plaintiff such as to make him or her whole. The calculated damages will include medical expenses (current and future), loss of earnings, and earning capacity as well additional amounts added for pain, suffering, and loss of consortium, all of which will be computed in economic terms. Punitive damages intended to punish the defendant may be sought and awarded for gross negligence, that is, willful and wanton disregard for the well-being of the plaintiff.

STANDARDS OF CARE AND EXPERT TESTIMONY

The duty to provide ordinary care is basic tort law and expressed in the terms of doing what would be done by the reasonably prudent person in the same or similar circumstances. Ordinary care requires a slightly different perspective for purposes of establishing standards of care in medical negligence litigation. For that purpose, standards of care are those actions that would be taken by physicians of similar training and experience in the same of similar circumstances. For anesthesia cases, the defendant can expect to face the standards, practice parameters, and guidelines promulgated by the American Society of Anesthesiologists (ASA).[5]

There are clear times when an anesthesia provider, under extenuating circumstances, may waive some requirements, but if this is done it should be documented as to why the requirement is waived.[6] The ASA's introductory language for practice parameters and guidelines expresses their appropriate application, seeming to limit their application as standards of care. Nonetheless, the finder of fact likely will be influenced by the fact that these guidelines have been developed by practitioners of apparently similar training and experience within the national society, which makes it seem a reasonable expectation that practitioners within the specialty would follow them. Certainly an adverse event occurring when the recommendations of the ASA are being ignored will be more difficult to defend than if it occurs when full compliance is well documented.

In addition to published information that can be used to help establish standards of care, expert witnesses[7] will be called by both parties to testify as to the appropriate action that was or should have been taken by the defendant practitioner. Expert testimony will seek to establish the existence of a physician–patient relationship, with associated duty of care, and breach of that duty as a violation of the standards of care. Expert testimony also will be required to establish that, in fact, the breach of duty was a causative factor that resulted in the plaintiff's injury. Interestingly, it seems always possible to find expert opinion sufficiently diverse to support both the plaintiff's and the defendant's position.[8]

Expert testimony should follow ethical principles, and in 2008 the ASA Committee on Professional Liability set forth guidelines for providing such testimony. It would be unethical for an expert to testify that the action of a defendant anesthesia provider were negligent and caused postoperative vision loss (POVL) when the cause of POVL itself is not known.[9,10]

ANESTHESIA MALPRACTICE CLAIMS

Notorious multimillion-dollar verdicts in cases against anesthesiologists such as the $20 million award in an Alabama case where aspiration resulted in death make exciting news clips and captivate public attention.[11] They do not, however, truly reflect the trend of decline in the number of claims against anesthesia providers as well as the amount paid on such claims. The National Practitioner Data Bank shows for 2002 that the mean medical malpractice payment due to anesthesia-related malpractice was $338,190; the median was $150,000. This is consistent with recent information flowing from the ASA Closed Claim Project.[12]

Medical negligence cases involving anesthesia have declined over the past several decades. In fact, in 1999 the Institute of Medicine recognized anesthesia as an area in which very impressive improvements in safety have been made.[13] Historically, adverse outcomes related to respiratory events were the single largest class of injury, and consequences of brain damage and death led to high-damage claims. This is true across adult, pediatric,[14,15] and obstetric[16-18] populations. Review of anesthesia-related claims in England from 1995 to 2007 reported similar findings.[19] Most commonly, respiratory adverse events resulting in significant injury were inadequate ventilation, esophageal intubation, and difficult tracheal intubation. Advances in technology with the development of oximetry and capnography in conjunction with the creation and implementation of practice guidelines appear significant when considering factors that have both improved patient safety and reduced anesthesia malpractice cases.[20]

Perhaps lagging behind this trend is anesthesia practice at remote locations (ie, outside the operating room) where there are higher numbers of adverse events associated with inadequate oxygenation/ventilation and oversedation. These are often deemed preventable by better monitoring.[21,22] This pattern highlights a clear need for similar standards for anesthesia and monitoring in all anesthesia areas. Office-based surgery facilities are accredited by 3 organizations, each setting standards for administration of anesthesia and sedation, which fortunately are readily tied to ASA standards and guidelines.[23]

The next generation of quality improvement in the practice of anesthesiology seems to be through collective efforts across the professional society. The creation of registries for POVL[10] and pediatric perioperative cardiac arrests[24,25] have allowed collection of data for analysis which, without collective effort, would not be sufficient to further guide practice to improve delivery of care. Guidelines for anesthetic and perioperative management can be expected to flow from these efforts.

Despite the reduction in the number and cost of claims against anesthesia providers, medical malpractice cases continue to be filed and likely will continue despite the efforts made to curb them through tort reform. The process is initiated by a notice letter, which establishes the intent of the injured party or plaintiff to take legal action. This must be done within the statue of limitations and begins with filing a complaint or petition in state court and serving notice on the defendants being sued. The defendants thereafter file a responsive pleading, which answers the allegations in the original petition.[26]

DISCOVERY

Once filed, the case enters the discovery phase, where both plaintiff and defendants acquire evidence to be used to prove their case. This involves requests for production of documents such as medical records and other written or recorded information that may reflect facts pertaining to the plaintiff's injury and the economic loss associated with it. Discovery also includes depositions whereby sworn testimony from parties as well as fact and expert witnesses is taken and preserved in preparation for trial. Discovery allows the plaintiff and defendants to develop their cases and possibly enter settlement negotiations and avoid trial.

TRIAL

At trial, the plaintiff is required to prove all elements of the negligence case against each defendant with sufficient evidence to meet the burden of proof. Defense of the medical practice case requires that the defendant defeat only one of the elements of the plaintiff's case. Although attack is made on multiple elements, failure of the plaintiff on only one element results in a verdict for the defendant. The trial concludes with a verdict for the plaintiff or defendant. An award of damages in some dollar amount for the plaintiff will be divided such that costs of litigation and the attorney's contingency fee are paid prior to money going to the injured party. A verdict for the defendant puts an end to the experience, although the memories will remain.

AVOIDING AND SURVIVING LAWSUITS

The most effective protection against a medical malpractice lawsuit is the rapport a health care provider develops with the patient.[27] In obstetrics patients unhappy with their peripartum care or who feel mistreated and/or ignored are more likely to file lawsuits. It may be that malpractice litigation serves both for reparation of injury for substandard care as well as for emotional vindication.[28] In general, if the provider is personable, available, and trustworthy, the injured patient will want to keep him or her out of the defendant pool, even if there is reason to be included. By contrast, poor bedside manner and distrust increases the likelihood of being named in malpractice cases. Angry patients and those who sense they are getting less than the whole truth often resort to the legal system for resolution. Those who have generated the anger and distrust can expect to participate in the legal action.

Although provider apology for medical error does not decrease the number of lawsuits filed, it does tend to expedite settlement of claims for fewer dollars.[29,30] In the past, standard practice was to adopt a policy of total silence,[31] believing that disclosure would increase the incidence of litigation.[32] The older approach now faces one of counterintuition in which disclosure and apology are made when adverse events and medical errors occur. Current information indicates that physician communication skills can decrease claims for medical malpractice.[33] The process of interaction following an adverse event helps fulfill needs of both physician and patient,[34] should be undertaken as close to the time of error as possible when the patient is capable of full comprehension, and after consultation with legal counsel that does not have power of veto. The truth-based apology may eliminate the perception that details are being withheld and is consistent with the recommendations of several professional societies and associations.[35]

When involved in a case with an undesired outcome, it is wise to anticipate the possibility of adverse legal action. Notifying one's insurance carrier and the hospital risk management officer are appropriate early steps, soon after the event and long before legal action is initiated. It is crucial to avoid discussing the matter with others and never to alter medical records. Records kept in the ordinary course of business, with the exception of those generated as part of the peer review and quality improvement processes, are discoverable and will end up in the hands of the plaintiff's attorney.[26] The protection of quality improvement documents is now coming under review.

Protected from discovery are products generated in anticipation of litigation and communications between the attorney and client. Some have recommended that after a mishap a personal record of the events be created that may prove extremely useful in subsequent legal proceedings. But this should be started with a heading reading "this is being composed in anticipation of legal action" to provide protection from discovery.[36] Liability insurance policies ordinarily provide legal counsel for the insured health care provider, and their recommendations should be heeded. If there is reason to believe that the attorney provided by the insurance company is not zealously representing the case filed against one, it is best to ask for alternative representation or to employ individual counsel. Individual counsel is also recommended when the damages sought exceed the coverage afforded by the liability policy.

As a defendant in a medical malpractice lawsuit, a practitioner's competence will be called into question. Extent of training and experience is of interest to both plaintiff and defense counsel. Board certification has also been a point of contention. The American Board of Anesthesiology believes that certification identifies anesthesiologists more likely to recognize or avoid untoward events and more likely to rescue patients from such events should they occur.[37,38] Failure to pass board examinations, however, has been considered not relevant as proof of negligence (*Campbell v Minjamuri,* 19 F.3d 1274 8th Cir 1994) because a person's performance on an examination, oral or written is not determinative of an anesthesia provider's ability to act within the standard of care on any particular occasion.[39]

Hospital credentials committees are increasingly driven to focus on providers' maintaining competence for practice within their specialty and/or subspecialty areas. Deeming someone competent who subsequently is involved in medical mishaps or deeming someone incompetent restricting his or her ability to make a livelihood both represent significant liability issues. Simulation-based programs to provide evidence of continued competence are being developed. These can be used only to determine whether a practitioner acted within standards of care in a particular situation and cannot be considered a guarantee of proper action in other situations.[40]

ECONOMIC RELATIONSHIPS AND CONTRACTS

CORPORATIONS

It is common for groups of anesthesia providers to join forces to provide services for hospitals, outpatient centers, and clinic operations. The legal entity that frequently does this is the professional corporation, which is formed and regulated under state law.[4] A corporation is a separate entity, which in many ways has attributes of a person in that it can enter into contracts, employ workers, earn and lose money, and be a party to litigation. Such corporations may be owned by one or more individuals, often those who form the practice together and thereafter employ others who eventually become shareholders.

Medical practice corporations take on numerous expenses, including billing and other costs of business, malpractice insurance premiums, educational expenses, and at times the costs of travel and transportation. Earnings of the group practice are pooled, overhead expenses paid, and salaries to shareholders and other employees paid. The corporation is also the entity with which a hospital might contract to obtain coverage for anesthesia services needed to maintain business operations. Corporations file returns and pay taxes on profits, so they may pay out bonuses to employees and stockholders at the end of each fiscal year.

Corporations and other practice groups contract with providers, frequently in employee, pre-partnership, and partnership arrangements. Most such contracts include provisions setting forth how monies are to be billed, collected, and distributed and consequences and restrictions in the event a practitioner leaves the practice if the contract is breeched. Litigation within practice groups has proven costly, as demonstrated when a jury in Dallas, Texas, ordered an anesthesia group to pay $6.3 million to an anesthesiologist wrongly terminated after he had challenged the validity of the group's billing practices and was thereafter fired based on false allegations of alcohol and drug abuse.[41]

HOSPITALS

Hospitals, also legal entities, often enter into explicitly exclusive supplier arrangements for the provision of "hospital-based physician" services, which includes anesthesiology.[42] Typically this contract is made between a hospital and a corporation. The contract spells out compensation, billing, minimum services, and management responsibilities; at the same time it excludes other anesthesiologists or groups from providing services at the hospital.[42] For the hospital, this provides an assurance that necessary services will be provided and is an alternative to hiring anesthesia providers as employees salaried by the hospital. For the corporation and anesthesia group, it prevents others from entering the practice area and capturing revenue, which will be theirs and protected by the exclusivity clause of the contract.

The bargaining power of the hospital compared with the practice groups is seldom equal, and at times the group may find itself in the position of being controlled by the hospital's business plan and driven to cut costs and corners. This may prove problematic at times because hospitals are most often responsible for providing adequate supplies and monitoring anesthesia equipment as well as its maintenance. Patient care problems may also arise when qualified practitioners are excluded by the contract, which may also circumvent peer review activities.[43]

At times, exclusive contracts are legally challenged based on allegations of restraint of trade and antitrust.[44] Often the plaintiff to such action is a practitioner who is not a party to the contract or employed by the contracting entity and therefore cannot practice in the defendant hospital. The pleadings will cite violations of procedural due process, not unlike those involving the termination of staff privileges,[45] and also allege that the exclusive contract seeks to monopolize the market and is a restraint of trade. Although the contracts usually are upheld at trial, the courts have not been totally insensitive to the argument.

Courts have concluded that certain types of provisions in exclusive contracts are unreasonable "per se," and if these exist the contract imposes an unreasonable restriction on competition. The per se violations include agreements to fix prices, agreements between competitors to divide markets, and, in some cases, group boycotts and tying arrangements. Short of per se violations, contracts may be found unlawful if they are not supported by the "rule of reason," which states that contracts are lawful if the participants lack market power or the results are significant efficiencies that outweigh the anticompetitive effects.[46]

When patients can easily travel to an alternative hospital to receive care, the institution and contracting group lack market power as considered under the rule of reason. However, exclusive contracts have been found unlawful when a hospital has high market share, and the contract tends to insulate the physician group from competition. At times, courts have upheld exclusive contracts when they allow hospitals and physician groups to control cost or quality of services provided to patients.[46]

SUPERVISION

Anesthesiologists who supervise certified registered nurse anesthetists (CRNAs) and/or residents are held accountable for the actions of those under their supervision. Although there is really not an alternative to direct supervision of residents, CRNA supervision is somewhat different.

A substantial portion of the total number of anesthetics administered in the United States is performed by CRNAs either with or without the supervision of anesthesiologists. This supervisory relationship, when it exists, is known as the anesthesia care team, and is described in the Statement on the Anesthesia Care Team from the ASA House of Delegates.[47] It should be no surprise that malpractice attorneys are familiar with the concepts of medical direction, supervision, and the idea of an anesthesia care team.[6]

The distribution of anesthesia providers in this country is highly skewed toward metropolitan areas, where supervision in the anesthesia care team is more prevalent.[48] CRNAs working in the anesthesia care team model are found to be more limited in their scope of practice when employed by the anesthesiology group rather than the hospital, and many find their practice to be noncollaborative.[49] The scope of practice of CRNAs in rural hospitals[50] is broader than in metropolitan practice.

To date no studies have shown a difference in anesthesia quality of care or outcomes based solely on the distinction of the provider being a CRNA or anesthesiologist. In 2001, the Centers for Medicare and Medicaid Services (CMS)[51] published its ruling allowing state governments exemption from the requirement for CRNA supervision. This required written notification of CMS by the state governor after consultations with the boards of medicine and nursing, determination that opting out was consistent with state law and that, upon decision, was in the best interests of the citizens of the state.

In addition to being seen as favorable to CRNAs, this allowed an option to relieve supervising physicians of liability, which concerned some, especially supervising physicians who were not anesthesiologists.

PRIVATE AND PUBLIC INFORMATION

Health care records are customarily maintained by a health care entity that requires and enforces their timely and accurate completion. The necessity for medical information in the delivery of health care is paired with their necessity for billing and to a lesser degree for research and teaching. The evolution of electronic recordkeeping and communication has driven the development of information technology systems in health care. Commonly hospitals have multiple data management systems that represent challenges to interface on a single electronic medical record.

Anesthesia Information Management Systems (AIMS) have been available for nearly 2 decades, but hospitals often resist requests to invest in them.[52] Arguments favoring the AIMS investment include improvements in efficiency, cost reductions, improved coding throughput, and, for purposes of this chapter, support of risk management. Rather than increasing medicolegal exposure for providers, AIMS seem to be useful in documenting absence of negligence and facilitating agreements to settle cases and even in cases that proceeded to litigation.[53]

HEALTH INSURANCE PORTABILITY AND ACCOUNTABILITY ACT

Whereas the regulations under the Health Insurance Portability and Accountability Act of 1996 (HIPAA) are relatively new, the underlying concept of privacy of medical information is not.[54,55] In fact, some consider the HIPAA regulations to be unduly complex, long, and laden with excess commentary, although the underlying principle is quite simple. The recognized right for a patient's personal medical information to be kept private has been present from the time of Hippocrates.[56,57] Understandably, patients are willing to disclose to their physician the information required for diagnosis and treatment when they understand that the information will remain confidential.

In the era of electronic communications, management of health care information has become more complex and protection of privacy more problematic. Some computer experts believe that, for all practical purposes, privacy is dead, and that personal control of private information is a mere illusion in the computer age. Apparently denying the legitimacy of this perception, HIPAA regulations seek to inform and educate patients about their privacy rights. Patients are to receive a notice of privacy, setting forth who will be able to use their medical information and for what purposes. Patients are asked to acknowledge that they have been informed their information may be disclosed for uses related to medical treatment, payment, and/or health care operations such as auditing, performance evaluations, training programs, and the like. Some providers still obtain authorization to disclose medical information, which is necessary when the disclosure is for reasons other than treatment, payment, or operations, for example, medical research.

Patients have a right to access and copy their entire medical history with limited exception, and parents have rights to access the medical records of their minor children unless precluded through court action. Emergency treatment need not be delayed while HIPAA notice is provided, but once the emergency condition has stabilized, privacy notice is to be provided. HIPAA regulations stipulate that the information to be disclosed is to be the minimum necessary and specifically include the conducting of training programs where health care trainees learn under supervision. Significant penalties can be imposed for violations of HIPAA regulation. Civil monetary penalties up to $25,000 annually[58] may be imposed for violations, and criminal penalties for those who knowingly obtain to disclose identifiable health information can be as high as 10 years of imprisonment and $250,000 if the intent is to use the information for commercial advantage.[58]

Not surprisingly HIPAA regulations pose increasing risk for private lawsuits where plaintiffs allege privacy of their health care information has been violated. The civil or criminal penalties outlined by HIPAA for privacy violations include fines or imprisonment or both, assuming anyone is bothering to enforce the rules.[59]

Courts in Utah (*Sorensen v Barbuto,* 143 P.3d 295 (Utah Ct. App. 2006)) and North Carolina (*Acosta v Byrum,* 638 S.E. 2d 246 [N.C. Ct. App. 2006]) have relied on HIPAA regulations to establish a duty of confidentiality and standards of care. Although these have not yet encroached on the anesthesia world, more of these cases will no doubt be coming in the future, and anesthesia providers must reassess the risk of not having adequate HIPAA compliance programs in place.

NATIONAL PRACTITIONER DATA BANK

The National Practitioner Data Bank (NPDB) was established in 1986 through the Health Care Quality Improvement Act.[60] Seeking to improve the quality of health care, the NPDB was intended to restrict the ability of incompetent physicians to move from state to state without disclosing their incompetence. The NPDB is a flagging system to facilitate a review of health care practitioners credentialing. Hospitals, medical boards, professional societies, and others that take adverse actions against professional licensure, as well as those that make payments as a result of medical malpractice actions, are required to report to the NPDB. Any actions taken to reduce, restrict, suspend, revoke, or deny clinical privileges or membership are to be reported, as are monetary payment and adverse judgments resulting from medical malpractice lawsuits.

When health care practitioners apply for clinical privileges, a hospital must query the NPDB and repeat the query every 2 years thereafter. Information obtained through this query is restricted to use only for the purpose for which it was obtained. Civil penalties can be imposed for violation of the confidentiality of the NPDB information. Although the general public cannot obtain information regarding a particular practitioner from the NPDB, a plaintiff's attorney can request information pertaining to a practitioner against whom he or she has filed suit, if through discovery it is disclosed that the hospital failed to do so. Defense attorneys cannot query the NPDB, but a practitioner may make a query to obtain information concerning himself or herself to see which, if any, incidents have been reported.

In general, those involved in the credentialing of health care practitioners enjoy qualified immunity. They cannot be held liable for providing information regarding the health care practitioner unless the information provided is false and the individual providing the information actually knew it to be false. Courts have held that hospitals are immune for reporting peer review information to the NPDB, as long as the reports are made without knowledge of falsity.

CONSENT

Among the legal documents most frequently seen by anesthesia providers are those associated with the process of informed consent.[61,62] In general, patients come to the health care industry seeking care, and it would be presumed that they would agree to receive the care they are seeking. That presumption is incorrect if there are aspects of the care they would consider sufficient to make them think it over and perhaps choose not to be treated. The process of informed consent in essence represents the foundation of the physician–patient relationship. The patient seeks diagnosis and treatment; the physician makes a diagnosis and offers options for treatment. The patient cannot compel the physician to treat contrary to his or her will, just as the physician cannot compel the patient to accept treatment that he or she does not want. A full disclosure and comprehension of treatment risks and benefits is necessary if the consent is to be truly informed.

Elements of the informed consent process include (1) competency and capacity, (2) discussion with patient, (3) disclosure of information, (4) treatments and alternatives, (5) material risks—common and rare serious, (6) autonomous authorization, and (7) documentation.[63]

Competency pertains to the patient legal decision making authority. Adult patients, 18 years or older, are generally deemed competent to make their own decisions about health care unless a court has determined otherwise. Consent to treat a minor is given by a parent or legal guardian unless emancipated under provisions of state law.

Capacity is determined by the medical professionals as to whether a patient has the ability to make a particular health care decision at a particular time. Capacity includes the ability to understand and reason about a medical condition and appreciate risks, benefits, and proposed alternatives. If capacity is lacking, consent must be obtained from an authorized decision maker.

Discussion with the patient includes *disclosure of information* necessary to make an informed decision about the treatment being offered. Required disclosure includes the potential benefits of the recommended treatment, alternative treatment(s), and nontreatment as well as the risks represented by each option.

Material risks include those that are frequent and likely to occur despite having little if any long-term consequence and those that are rare although serious including permanent disability and death. Special attention must be paid to risks of anesthesia, which are distinct and frequently more serious that those associated with the surgical treatment to be undertaken; at times, separate consent forms are appropriate.[64] The extent of risk disclosure has been a topic of disagreement over the years. The "professional-practice" standard, requiring disclosure of risks deemed appropriate by physicians, has largely been replaced by the "reasonable person" standard.

Autonomous authorization occurs when a patient or authorized agent gives consent for a recommended procedure after discussion and an opportunity to ask questions that are satisfactorily answered. The consent for constitutes *documentation* of the process that included discussion or the treatment, alternatives, risks, and agreement to proceed. Some insurers and some but not all states require a separate consent for anesthesia; others include the anesthesia on the same consent form used for the procedure.

BLOOD PRODUCTS

Although many standard surgical consent forms include provision for blood product administration, it is common practice in some areas to have separate consent documents pertaining to their administration. This is in part due to the inherent risks, although small, of transmitting infectious disease, as well as to allow those who might refuse administration of blood products for religious reasons to engage in meaningful informed consent dialogue. The refusal of blood products, as is frequently encountered when Jehovah's Witnesses undergo anesthesia and surgery, may present an ethical conflict for practitioners. Although uncommon, being asked to stand by and allow a patient to die for lack of a lifesaving blood transfusion generates a conflict of conscience for the health care providers involved.[65] Nonetheless, it is well-recognized that patients do have the right to refuse treatment even when that treatment is necessary to sustain life.

Frequently the issue is made far complex when individual Jehovah's Witness patients allow administration of some blood components, such as albumin and immune globulins, but not red blood cells; each individual is allowed to make decisions regarding these matters.[66] When minor children are involved and the need for administration of blood product arises, courts routinely intervene to require treatment for children whose parents deny consent for lifesaving medical interventions.[4]

EMERGENCY

There are exceptions to the duty to disclose. The legal system recognizes the rights of a physician in a true emergency to act without patient consent, so long as his or her actions are consistent with those customarily done in the particular emergency. In emergency situations, there may be a presumption of consent that patients would want treatment that would be lifesaving. There are rare occasions when the mere discussion of treatment risks may be detrimental to a patient's health. When discussion of risks generates emotional distress, such as to foreclose a rational discussion, a physician may exercise what is known as *therapeutic privilege* and forgo full risk disclosure to the patient. Careful documentation and discussion with family members regarding the situation is appropriate in this case.

SURROGACY AND FAMILY CONSENT

Incompetent patients requiring surgery and anesthesia traditionally have family members in attendance who can be engaged in the consent process. This long-standing practice has gained legal acceptance and is based on the presumption that the family is generally most concerned about the good of the patient and ordinarily is the most knowledgeable about the patient's preferences, goals, and values. Since the 1980s, many states have enacted family consent statutes, which set forth the hierarchy of family members and close friends who are to be looked to for medical decision making. Ordinarily the hierarchy runs in descending order from the spouse, parents, most of the reasonably available adult children, and nearest living relative. Some states have freestanding statutes, although others incorporate this into their statutes addressing living will, advance directive, and health care decision making.[67]

ETHICAL ISSUES

Busy anesthesia practice usually is conducted without undue attention to biomedical ethics for its own sake. Although daily activities are filled with a balancing of risks and benefits and providing care consistent with the patient's wishes, the ethical principles of autonomy, beneficence, and nonmaleficence are not necessarily the terminology commonly applied. These principles are more in focus when dealing with end-of-life decisions, as may be faced when terminally ill patients are brought to the operating room, when life-sustaining treatment is to be withdrawn, and when transplantable organs are retrieved from the cadaveric donor.

END-OF-LIFE CARE

The past several decades have been characterized by tremendous advances in technology, pharmacology, and health care in general. Populations are aging, and medical conditions that once were terminal have found treatments that prolong life considerably. Prior years saw deaths in the hospital occur despite every effort that could be made. More frequently today we see hospital deaths when decisions are made that not everything that can be done really should be done.[68] Decisions to limit care by either withholding or withdrawing treatments are commonly made in the process of caring for patients at the end of life.

DO NOT RESUSCITATE ORDERS

Probably the most basic of decisions regarding end-of-life care is a decision to withhold advanced cardiac life support in the event of a cardiac arrest. In 1974, the American Heart Association and American Medical Association stated that the purpose of cardiopulmonary resuscitation is to prevent sudden, unexpected death; it is not indicated in cases of terminal illness where death is expected.[69-73] The 2005 guidelines for Advance Cardiac Life Support published by the American Heart Association state, "CPR is inappropriate when survival is not expected."[74] Although currently this concept is not difficult to grasp, historically orders to withhold cardiopulmonary resuscitation, or "do not resuscitate (DNR)" orders, were often spoken rather than written.[75] But with time there evolved a more sound recognition that continuation of life-sustaining treatments[76] as well as cardiopulmonary resuscitation may not always be appropriate, and the distinction between sustaining life and prolonging the dying process emerged.

There are really 2 reasons to withhold cardiopulmonary resuscitation: when it is medically inappropriate and when a patient refuses to have such treatment[74,77] even if it might be deemed medically appropriate by the health care team. Ethically speaking, there is no obligation to provide care that is of no benefit to the patient, especially if such treatment could be considered harmful or cause pain. Likewise, treatment offered and considered appropriate can be refused by the patient whose autonomy we must respect.

Conflict has arisen when patients with DNR orders are brought to the operating room to undergo surgical procedures and anesthesia.[78] Cardiac arrest is among the recognized risks of anesthesia, and practitioners would choose to have every opportunity to correct problems caused by their care. For some time, there was a pattern of universal suspension of DNR orders when patients were in the operating room and under the effects of anesthesia. Currently such practices are being reconsidered and replaced by more patient-oriented and individualized policies and practices with goal-directed and procedure-directed options.[79] This reevaluation process regarding DNR orders before surgery is appropriate for the pediatric population as well.[80] The ASA recommends the development of a policy that provides 4 options and requires a reconsideration of the decision for the DNR and the implications of the procedure and anesthetic to be undertaken.[81,82]

WITHDRAWAL OF TREATMENT

Life-sustaining treatment is ordinarily initiated when organ failure is sufficient to risk loss of life. When underlying conditions are corrected and organ function restored, life-sustaining treatment is no longer needed and can be discontinued. This is commonly seen when patients require mechanical ventilation postoperatively while temporary pulmonary insufficiency would put them at risk of death without such support. However, if organ function is not restored or the patient's condition deteriorates further, it may become apparent that survival can no longer be expected. At this time, it will be appropriate to entertain the option of withdrawing life-sustaining treatment that is merely delaying the moment of death or prolonging the dying process.[83] Even when life-sustaining treatment is withdrawn, physicians have a duty to care for the dying patient, administering medications to provide comfort and assuring the continuation of other care for preservation of dignity. Often medications administered for comfort also have depressant effects that could hasten death, a double effect. Such medications are to be administered to provide comfort even if they may also hasten death.[83]

Some patients have executed a directive to physicians, or a living will, which specifies desire regarding the application of life-sustaining treatment in the event they have a terminal or irreversible condition and they are incompetent to express their desire at that point in time. Most frequently the directive asks that treatments be discontinued so that the individual may die naturally, although other instructions may also be given. A directive to withdraw or withhold life-sustaining treatments can be considered a statement of refusal of treatment in the process of informed consent.

Even without a written directive, decisions to limit life-sustaining treatment are frequently made for the incompetent patient. Family members who would otherwise be involved in the consent process can engage in discussions regarding the discontinuation of life-sustaining treatment. At times they may be aware of the specific desire of the patient in this regard, but even if this was never clearly expressed, the decision can be made based on the patient's values and what is in his or her best interest.[67]

FUTILITY

At times patients, or more often families, demand administration or continuation of treatment that is medically inappropriate.[84] When there is no expectation for survival, treatment directed at cure can be considered futile.[85,86] Although there is no obligation to provide futile care, there is reluctance to discontinue such treatment demanded by families, when to do so would soon be followed by the patient's death. Consultation of clinical ethics is appropriate and may help resolve such situations. Some institutions and state laws provide a due process means by which discontinuation of futile life-sustaining treatment, even contrary to the demands of the patient or family, can be accomplished with protection from legal liability.[87,88]

ORGAN DONATION AFTER CARDIAC DEATH

Although historically organs for transplantation were retrieved from patients immediately following cardiac death, this practice was largely abandoned with the evolution of the concept of brain death. Anesthesia practitioners are commonly called on to provide intraoperative management for the brain-dead cadaveric organ donor.[89] The procedure, unlike most cases, is somewhat unique in that administration of anesthetic is not necessary to render the patient insensitive to pain, and once the heart is arrested the intraoperative management of the anesthesia provider is essentially complete despite continuation of the surgical procedure.

With the high demand for transplantable organs and the increased public awareness of organ donation, there is rekindled interest in organ donation after cardiac death. Such an option at times occurs when there is a decision to discontinue life-sustaining treatment for a patient who will die soon and who has preserved function of transplantable organs such as kidney and liver. The end-of-life process usually occurs in the intensive care unit (ICU) and includes administration of medications to provide comfort at the time life-sustaining treatment is removed. Moving this process to the operating room allows control of the circumstances surrounding death and the possibility for retrieval of transplantable organs.[90]

Understandably, some who work in the operating room environment are troubled by this practice. They may need to reconsider what really is taking place and, if necessary, be excluded from the process. Although withdrawal of life-sustaining treatment and administration of medications for comfort predictably will be followed by death, the death is not caused for purposes of obtaining transplantable organs. The "dead donor rule," which applies here as well as for the brain-dead donor, prohibits the practice of causing death to obtain organs.[91]

Anesthesiologists have resisted the opportunity to participate in this practice. Rather than bringing in the anesthesia provider solely for participation in the end-of-life process, this is often done with providers who have cared for the patient in the ICU. Regardless of whether or not anesthesiologists directly participate in these procedures, their involvement in the development of hospital policies and procedures is appropriate, and they should seek to ensure that the protection of patient dignity and comfort is paramount throughout.[92]

PEDIATRIC ISSUES

CONSENT

Generally speaking, the legal system protects individual rights regardless of a person's age. The ability of some individuals to comprehend the nature of medical care and its impact on their person is limited, which is the case in the pediatric population. Cognitive development throughout childhood as well as developments of emotional reactions based on a broadening experiential foundation leads eventually to the competencies associated with adulthood. Ethical arguments that consent of the pediatric patient should not be based on an arbitrary age but rather on the development of personhood place high value on the child's input in the consent process.[93]

The ability to consent for and refuse treatment requires a level of maturity and understanding. Although it is generally accepted that it is important to consider the autonomous capacity of children and involve them in their treatment decision, this involvement will be inconstant, and legal guidelines in this area are lacking.[94] Certainly a child may refuse to be subject to the pain of an injection despite the fact that immunization may have an effect in prolonging life. Clearly the consent for a surgical procedure is even more complex, and with younger children it would be unrealistic to expect an understanding of a procedure and its inherent risks and potential benefits. A progression is recommended for use in obtaining consent from or for children; this allows involvement of the child based on age and developmental maturity. For ages 6 years and younger, in whom decision-making capacity is highly limited, consent is made on the child's behalf and in his or her best interest. With increasing age and development of decision-making capacity, the child's participation and contribution to the process increase through informed permission and assent to informed consent at maturity.[95] Even though the capacity to truly give consent may be present with older children and teenagers, parents still are ordinarily asked to execute consent documents on their children's behalf.

Parents are the natural guardian of their children and are expected always to seek care that is in the best interest of the children. When there is question as to whether or not the consent for treatment or refusal of treatment is truly in the child's best interest, it may be necessary to seek intervention by the legal system. Every state has a statutory framework set up to protect abused or neglected children, and statutes allow any person to petition the court for guardianship for the protection of a person lacking legal capacity.[4,62] Courts traditionally support decisions for medical care deemed to be clearly in the child's best interest and ordinarily will not appoint a guardian other than the parent unless there is good reason.

NEGLECT AND ABUSE

Child protective services are established by state governments to allow the state to take custody of children who are being denied the necessities of life, such as housing, clothing, food, education, and medical care. There is some variation among the states, but most allow the state to take custody of the child on little or nothing more than a verified petition alleging neglect or abuse.[62] Temporary custody may be sufficient to allow provision of medical care, but ultimately unless the state shows by clear and convincing evidence that all statutory requirements are met, there is little chance of terminating parental rights and maintaining custody.

Children are commonly the victims of injury, with trauma and accidents the leading causes of death between the ages of 1 and 14 years.[96] At times, patterns of injury may be of concern, especially with acute injuries seen in conjunction with signs of prior trauma, such as bruises, contusions, and healing fractures, which may be suggestive of the "battered child syndrome."[97] Abuse may be sexual or may take the form of neglect, with failure to meet a child's needs for shelter, clothing, food, and health care.[98] Stories telling the sequence of events leading to the current and prior injuries may seem inadequate to explain the degree of trauma, and details related may change over time.[99]

The immediate matter of consent for treatment when a child requires treatment that a parent declines is directed to the court, where a judge can and almost always will issue a court order that permits the health care provider to care for the child. A more long-term plan is activated when child protective services intervenes in the situation.

KEY REFERENCES

- American Society of Anesthesiologists. Ethical Guidelines for the Anesthesia Care of Patients with Do-Not-Resuscitate Orders or Other Directives That Limit Care. 1999.
- Fallat ME, Deshpande JK. Do-not-resuscitate orders for pediatric patients who require anesthesia and surgery. *Pediatrics.* 2004;114(6):1686-1692.
- Feld AD. The Health Insurance Portability and Accountability Act (HIPAA): its broad effect on practice. *Am J Gastroenterol.* 2005;100(7):1440-1443.
- Gallagher TH, Studdert D, Levinson W. Disclosing harmful medical errors to patients. *N Engl J Med.* 2007;356(26):2713-2719.
- Jones JW, McCullough LB, Richman BW. Informed consent: it's not just signing a form. *Thorac Surg Clin.* 2005;15(4):451-460, v.

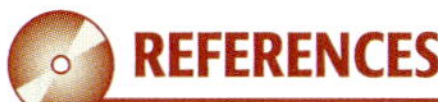

REFERENCES

Complete references available on DVD and online version at www.LongneckerAnesthesiology.com

CHAPTER 95 Substance Dependence and Abuse in Anesthesia Care Providers

Margaret F. Brock
Raymond C. Roy

KEY POINTS

1. The incidence of opioid abuse among anesthesia providers is 1%.
2. Addiction is a treatable chronic, relapsing disease with a genetic predisposition.
3. Seventy-five percent of addicts declare themselves by age 27 years.
4. Drugs change the brain. The brain changes associated with addiction are independent of drug of abuse.
5. Addiction among anesthesia providers is most commonly detected through observed behavioral changes.
6. Interventions should be based on concern over wellness. Substance abuse is only one of several potential diagnoses that threaten wellness.
7. Intervention at an early stage of addiction is associated with greater treatment success than intervention at later stages.
8. Evidence-based treatment of addiction reduces relapse rates.
9. Most addicts have psychiatric comorbidities that must be treated concurrently to prevent relapse.
10. Reentry requires a contract between the abstinent colleague and his employer.

"[T]here is always *soma,* delicious *soma,* half a gramme for a half-holiday, a gramme for a weekend . . . A gramme is better than a damn . . . I wish I had my *soma.*"

—Aldous Huxley,
Brave New World, 1932

The United States manifests a significant ambivalence toward drugs. While the federal government wages war against the illicit drug industry and organized medicine campaigns against the nonmedical use of prescription drugs, the entertainment and advertising industries, in the spirit of Lieutenant Milo Minderbinder in Joseph Heller's *Catch-22*, bombard its citizens daily with prodrug references. Lyrics from Toby Keith's popular country music song "Get Drunk and Be Somebody" reflect a common mantra:

All week long, we're real nobodies,
But we just punched out: it's paycheck Friday.
Weekend's here, good God Almighty:
People, let's get drunk an' be somebody

Comedians receive knowing laughs and applause from their audiences when they reference or parody recreational drug use. Television, Internet, and movie advertisements suggest that life is more enjoyable in social settings involving alcohol and more manageable with medications ("Ask your doctor if this medication is right for you."). Helping people to "pass" drug tests is also a big business. For example, if "urine luck" is entered into an Internet search engine, almost 2 million citations are offered. Physicians and major pharmaceutical companies tout the benefit of medications to relieve pain. Anesthesia providers make their living daily demonstrating that drugs of high abuse potential can be safely administered. Even a brochure for the Wood Library Museum of Anesthesiology proclaims, "Thank Goodness They Inhaled." Drug and alcohol misuse is commonly associated with youthful experimentation. However, misuse also is triggered by internal and external pressures to improve self-confidence and performance on the athletic field, in the classroom, on competitive examinations, in the workplace, and in the bedroom to achieve a better body image, to feel more comfortable socially, to cope with the stresses of highly competitive work and study environments, and to escape from dysfunctional social relationships and unsatisfactory living situations. College students call this "pharming."[1] The economic costs of drug misuse are staggering. If health care, law enforcement, prosecution, incarceration, and loss of productivity are taken into account, the annual cost associated with drug misuse, excluding nicotine and caffeine, is $465 billion, an amount greater than that linked to heart disease ($290 billion), cancer ($187 billion), or obesity ($123 billion).[2] The number of people who misuse drugs is also staggering. According to the 2003 National Survey on Drug Use and Health sponsored by the Substance Abuse and Mental Health Services Administration, 9.1% of the population of the United States older than 12 years, an estimated 21.6 million people, has a substance misuse disorder. Substance misuse disorders run the gamut from smoking marijuana to driving under the influence to chemical dependency. According to the National Institute of Mental Health National Comorbidity Survey Replication, the prevalence of substance misuse disorders in the US English-speaking population is 14.6%.[3]

ANESTHESIA PROVIDER VULNERABILITY

STATISTICS

An argument can be made that the prevalence of substance abuse among physicians is less than for society as a whole. Because 75% of addicts declare themselves by 27 years of age,[3] they may be less likely to complete medical training. Supporting this premise is a 1992 study that determined the lifetime prevalence of substance abuse among all physicians, regardless of specialty, to be 7.9% versus the 14.6% previously mentioned.[4] There are no published data for the incidence or prevalence of substance misuse or abuse specific to the entire population of practicing anesthesia providers. Surveys of anesthesia residency and student registered nurse anesthetists (SRNAs) training programs consistently report an incidence of 1% to 2%.[5] Despite the paucity of data there appears to be a consensus that the incidence (snapshot) and prevalence (professional lifespan) of abuse among anesthesia providers are approximately 1% and 10%, respectively. Thus, if there are 8500 anesthesia residents and SRNAs in training at any given time, then 95 are likely to have a problem severe enough to require suspension from training over any 3-year period or 32 per year. Likewise, if there are 80 000 practicing anesthesiologists and CRNAs, then 8000 will have a problem during their professional life.

VULNERABILITY HYPOTHESES

Anesthesiologists are consistently overrepresented in analyses of data from physician health programs (PHPs). In Florida, anesthesiologists represent 4.7% of the total physician workforce, but 12% of those enrolled in the PHP.[6] It is tempting to accept this data as evidence confirming increased vulnerability of anesthesia providers to substance abuse and propose 5 explanations: (1) Drug abusers seek opportunities. Substance-abusing medical trainees seek to practice anesthesia to gain direct access to opioids and other anesthetic drugs for abuse. (2) Opportunity creates abusers. Unlike most physicians who must write prescriptions or orders for drugs to be administered by persons other than themselves, anesthesiologists personally administer drugs and are daily presented with the opportunity to divert drugs for their own abuse. (3) The stress of administering anesthesia is overwhelming. Susceptible anesthesia providers seek relief from the pressure of administering drugs that can lead to patient death or injury. (4) Personalities of anesthesia providers predispose them to addiction. What makes anesthesia attractive to some are the short-term rewards for effort, the risk of doing something daily with life-or-death consequences, and the adrenaline rush of the occasional need-to-rescue situations. This phenotype is shared by those who view experimenting with illicit drugs attractive. (5) Environment creates abusers. Chronic inhalation of trace amounts of anesthetic drugs in the operating room may increase the susceptibility to abuse. If hypotheses 2 and 5, and possibly 3 and 4, are ever proved, then drug addiction would definitely be considered an occupational hazard. Even though each of these hypotheses has face validity, no studies specifically designed to test any of the first 4 have been performed. Gold et al, exploring the fifth hypothesis, propose that "secondhand" exposure may produce changes in the brain that predispose susceptible anesthesia providers to chemical dependence.[6] They have detected propofol and fentanyl in air sampled from cardiac surgery operating rooms. The highest concentrations were in samples from air around the patient's head.[7]

There are several reasons not to accept *at this time* an increased vulnerability of anesthesiologists to substance abuse based solely on PHP enrollment data. (1) The percentage enrollment in PHPs has not been verified as a valid cross-sectional sample for addicted physicians. The percentage of individuals enrolled in treatment programs is less than those who need such treatment. The cumulative lifetime probability of patients with substance abuse disorders receiving any treatment is 52.7% to 76.9%.[8] (2) The effect of the drug abused on admission to a PHP has not been studied. Anesthesia providers could have the same prevalence of substance misuse disorders as other medical practitioners, but the time span over which they are diagnosed and treated may be compressed into a younger age range because they are more likely to abuse drugs with a higher addictive potential (eg, fentanyl vs alcohol). (3) The effect of the preferred drug of abuse (eg, high with opioids, cocaine, or methamphetamine vs low with alcohol) on peer and legal pressure to enroll in PHPs has not been studied. Alcohol is a legal substance, socially acceptable if consumed without intoxication and legally acceptable if blood alcohol levels while driving are below a certain threshold. "An estimated 8 million adults in the United States are alcoholics. Of this number, only a minority ever receive treatment for the disorder, even when treatment is defined broadly to include participation in Alcoholics Anonymous."[9] (4) The effect of the diagnosis of abuse versus dependence, made according to the *Diagnostic and Statistical Manual of Mental Disorders, Fourth Edition* (*DSM-IV*), is not taken into account in most of these analyses. In the National Epidemiologic Survey on Alcohol and Related Conditions, which included 42 392 respondents, 22% of those who met the *DSM-IV* definition of drug dependence did not meet the definition of drug abuse.[10] An unknown percentage of dependent individuals carefully avoid behaviors at work associated with abuse so as to protect their primary source of drugs and to escape detection and subsequent enrollment in PHPs. (5) The effectiveness of specialty-dependent substance abuse awareness efforts has not been determined. Educational initiatives have not reduced the incidence in anesthesia training programs over the last 4 decades, perhaps because most of the trainees who declare themselves during training were in early stages of addiction before the start of their residency. But awareness programs may have increased the detection and intervention rates for anesthesiologists more than for other physicians.

SUBSTANCE MISUSE TERMINOLOGY

TOLERANCE, DEPENDENCE, WITHDRAWAL

Terms associated with both appropriate and inappropriate drug use are *tolerance, physical dependence,* and *withdrawal.*[11] Each represents an aspect of normal physiologic adaptations seen in all patients after repeated administration of certain drugs. The American Academy of Pain Medicine, the American Pain Society, and the American Society of Addiction Medicine issued a consensus document in 2001 defining physical dependence and tolerance.[12] "Tolerance is a state of adaptation in which exposure to a drug induces changes that result in a diminution of one or more of the drug's effect over time." Either a given dose of a drug yields a decreased effect after repetitive administration or an increasingly larger dose of the drug is required to produce an effect of intensity comparable to the first dose. "Physical dependence is a state of adaptation that is manifested by a drug class specific withdrawal syndrome that can be produced by abrupt cessation, rapid dose reduction, decreasing blood level of the drug, and/or administration of an antagonist." All chronic pain patients who are treated with opioids develop tolerance and physical dependence. All patients initiate the physiologic processes that lead to tolerance and dependence with their first exposure to the drug.

ABUSE, INTOXICATION, ADDICTION

Terms specifically applied to inappropriate drug use are *abuse, intoxication,* and *addiction.*[11] Abuse is the inappropriate use of a drug. Intoxication refers to reversible "clinically significant maladaptive behavioral or psychological changes developing during or shortly after use of" a drug of abuse. Addiction is not used in the first through the fourth editions of the *DSM,* copyright by the American Psychiatric Association, or the *International Classification of Diseases* (*ICD-9* or *ICD-10*), copyright by the World Health Organization. These 2 systems classify all substance misuse disorders with the terms *abuse, intoxication, withdrawal,* and *dependence* (**Table 95-1**). In this setting what the layperson considered addiction was what the psychiatrist called dependent use, typically associated with withdrawal after intoxication and recurrent use either to limit withdrawal symptoms or give into cravings. Recognizing that the term *dependence* is misused for addiction when it is actually a normal physiologic response to both licit and illicit drugs, *DSM* will replace it with addiction in its fifth edition due to be published in 2013. In *DSM-V,* "Substance-Related Disorders" will become "Addiction and Related Disorders"; tolerance and withdrawal will not be counted as symptoms in the diagnosis of substance use disorders when they occur within the context of appropriate medical treatment; and drug craving and compulsive drug seeking will be added to the list of symptoms for addiction.[13] The National Institute on Drug Abuse and the National Institute on Alcohol Abuse and Alcoholism differentiate dependence and addiction as follows: "Physical dependence refers to adaptations that result in withdrawal symptoms when drugs such as alcohol and heroin are discontinued. Those are distinct from the neuroadaptations that result in addiction, which refers to the loss

TABLE 95-1 Outline of Substance-Related Disorders: *DSM-IV* General Criteria

I. Intoxication: Reversible substance-specific syndrome

II. Abuse

A. Recurrent use associated with ≥1 of the following within 12 months:
   1. Failure to fulfill major role obligations at work, school, or home
   2. Use in hazardous situations
   3. Use-related legal problems
   4. Use despite recurrent social or interpersonal problems caused or exacerbated by effects of intoxication

B. Symptoms have never met criteria for substance dependence for this substance class

III. Dependence:[a] Recurrent use with ≥3 of the following manifestations:

A. Tolerance
B. Self-treatment to relieve or avoid withdrawal symptoms
C. Overdoses
D. Persistent unsuccessful efforts to stop
E. High percent of time devoted to drug acquisition, use, recovery
F. Reduction in social, occupational, or recreational activities in order to use
G. Use despite acknowledging threat to physical or mental health
H. Drug craving[b]

[a]Replaced by addiction in *DSM-V*.

[b]To be added in *DSM-V*.

Reprinted with permission from the *Diagnostic and Statistical Manual of Mental Disorders*, Fourth Edition, Text Revision, (Copyright ©2000). American Psychiatric Association.

TABLE 95-2 Important Federal Legislation Regarding Substance Abuse

Year	Legislation
1914	**Harrison Narcotic Tax Act** Felony for doctors to prescribe narcotics to *maintain* addiction but not to treat withdrawal leading to abstinence
1970	**Comprehensive Drug Abuse Prevention and Control Act** Five schedules for controlled substances Drug Enforcement Administration (DEA) DEA number
1973	**Methadone Control Act** Methadone maintenance clinics
1986	**Health Care Quality Improvement Act** National Practitioner Data Bank (NPDB)
1988	**Drug-Free Workplace Act (DFA)** Institutional and medical licensing board substance abuse policies, including counseling, rehabilitation Notification of federal agencies (eg, NPDB) of drug-related offense by employee
1992	**Americans with Disability Act (ADA)** Protects abstinent employees, rehabilitated or in employee assistance programs, or PHPs who maintain reasonable performance standards with no/reasonable accommodations and who relapse (if they do so) away from the workplace.
2000	**Drug Addiction Treatment Act** Qualified physicians may dispense FDA-approved drugs to maintain addiction (eg, buprenorphine) in office setting (substitution therapy)

of control over the intense urges to take the drug even at the expense of adverse consequences."[14]

PSEUDOADDICTION

Pseudoaddiction is a diagnosis made in chronic pain patients who develop drug-seeking behaviors because their pain is inadequately treated.[15] The diagnosis requires 4 conditions: an appropriately diagnosed and documented pain condition, inadequate pain treatment unrecognized by the medical staff, analgesia-seeking behavior misinterpreted by the medical staff as inappropriate non–pain-related drug seeking, and resolution of drug-seeking behavior when sufficient analgesia is provided. If the drug seeking is not pain related, then the diagnosis becomes either substance (opioid) abuse or dependence.

OPIOID VERSUS OPIATE

Although the terms *opiate* and *opioid* are frequently used interchangeably, *opioid* actually refers to any agent that binds to opioid receptors. There are 4 classes of opioids: (1) endogenous peptides, such as endorphins, enkephalins, and dynorphins; (2) opiates, such as morphine and codeine, which are the naturally occurring alkaloids derived from the opium poppy *(Papaver somniferum);* (3) semisynthetic derivates of opiates, such as heroin, hydrocodone, hydromorphone, oxycodone, and oxymorphone; and (4) synthetic drugs, such as meperidine, methadone, fentanyl, sufentanil, alfentanil, remifentanil, butorphanol, nalbuphine, and buprenorphine.

OPIOID VERSUS NARCOTIC

Narcotic is a general term that refers to substances that induce a sleep state or narcosis. Before the twentieth century, opium was used to create a "daydreaming" state of drowsiness rather than the "high" or "rush" now sought from heroin, cocaine, and methamphetamine. Thus this definition of narcotic was more appropriate then than now. *Narcotic* is also a legal term that applies to drugs identified in the Harrison Narcotics Tax Act of 1914, the Controlled Substances Act of 1970, and the United Nations Single Convention on Narcotic Drugs of 1961. In this context, opioids, the stimulants cocaine and methamphetamine, and cannabinoids are referred to as narcotics (**Table 95-2**).

ADDICTION

ADDICTION AS A DISEASE

Addiction has 3 hurdles to overcome before it achieves the ultimate goal of most addictionologists, its recognition as a disease that, once contracted, does not prevent anesthesia providers from returning to work if it is appropriately treated. The first hurdle, disease designation, was cleared in 1956 and 1987, respectively, when the American Medical Association declared that alcoholism and then substance abuse satisfied all 5 criteria for a disease: (1) identified vector: the drug of abuse; (2) an organic lesion: same "core" pathology in the brain regardless of drug of abuse; (3) typical signs and symptoms: acute withdrawal signs may be drug dependent, but abstinence behavior is the same for all drugs of abuse (ie, there is a "core" addiction syndrome); (4) predictable natural course; and (5) evidence-based treatments that alter the natural course. The second hurdle, chronic disease recognition, has almost been cleared. For years addiction was viewed as an acute disease that resolved after the acute withdrawal symptoms subsided rather than a chronic disease with relapses and remissions that must be managed. "Relapse among patients with diabetes, hypertension, and asthma following cessation of treatment has been considered evidence of the effectiveness of those treatments and the need to retain patients in medical monitoring. In contrast, relapse to drug or alcohol use following discharge from addiction treatment has been considered evidence of treatment failure."[16] The third hurdle, reliable treatment consistently provided, has not been cleared sufficiently for all anesthesia providers to return to work in the same capacity as they left. But the discouraging data from decades ago regarding relapse need to be replaced with the more optimistic current data *when addiction is diagnosed at an early enough stage and appropriate treatment is provided and sustained.*[9,17]

DRUGS OF ABUSE

Although longer-acting opioids are the drugs most likely to be abused by anesthesia providers in surveys that commonly exclude alcohol, caffeine, cannabinoids, and nicotine, case reports document abuse of inhaled agents (eg, sevoflurane[18,19]), intravenous inducing agents,[20,21] and the shorter-acting opioid remifentanil.[22] All addictive drugs cause the release of dopamine and glutamate in specific brain regions depending on the stage of addiction. The mechanisms by which concentration of dopamine increases in these regions vary with the drug of abuse in the early stages of addiction, but the mechanism by which most of the dopamine and glutamate increase is independent of the drug of abuse in later stages of addiction. The acute withdrawal symptoms vary with the drug of abuse, but the abstinence behavior of addiction is essentially the same regardless of the drug of abuse.[23,24]

Despite the considerable diversity in their molecular structures, all drugs of abuse either increase dopaminergic transmission from the ventral tegmental area (VTA) or exaggerate the effects of normal dopamine released into the nucleus accumbens (NAc), prefrontal cortex (PFC), and amygdala (AMG). Dopaminergic neurons in the VTA form a synaptic cleft with neurons in the NAc. Cocaine, methamphetamine, amphetamine, and methylphenidate directly increase the concentration of dopamine in the synaptic cleft by blocking the reuptake of dopamine into the presynaptic VTA neuron. They accomplish this by interfering with the ability of the dopamine transporter (DAT), a carrier protein, to move extracellular dopamine intracellularly. To induce a "high," 50% of DAT must be blocked. Above this threshold the intensity of the "high" is increased with the increasing percentage of DAT blocked.[25] Opioids increase dopamine indirectly by acting on γ-aminobutyric (GABA)ergic interneurons in the VTA. By binding to opioid receptors on GABAergic cells, they stop the inhibitory action of GABAergic neurons on dopaminergic cells. The activity of dopaminergic neurons increases, and more dopamine appears in the synaptic cleft in the NAc. Ethanol releases endorphins that block the inhibition of dopaminergic neurons by GABAergic neurons.[23,24]

DRUG HIGHS VERSUS NATURAL REWARDS

Because of their pharmacokinetic profiles, drugs of abuse produce a longer and stronger "dopamine high" than do natural rewards or threats. Dopamine homeostasis limits the high from natural rewards. The sustained high concentrations of dopamine in the synapses of the NAc, PFC, and AMG exaggerate the value or perceived importance of the drug experience and imprint cues more strongly to repeat the drug experience than to pursue natural rewards. Individuals become chemically dependent by "overlearning of the motivational significance of cues that predict the delivery of drugs."[26] Over the same time period, the sustained high concentrations of dopamine with repeated drug intake lead to a downregulation of dopamine receptors, which devalues natural rewards and creates a "reward deficiency syndrome" or "negative emotional state."[24,26] Changes in the PFC and AMG lead to an increase in glutamatergic output to the NAc in response to drug cues (eg, passing a street corner where drug was previously purchased or hearing a pop when vial of medicine is opened), drug reinstatement (eg, social pressure to have a drink or requiring postoperative analgesic therapy), or stress that direct the addict to restrict the focus of his or her activity to drug acquisition and administration. An addict will seek drugs despite intellectually knowing and openly acknowledging that doing so will jeopardize marriage, career, health, or life. There is an actual or relative decrease in descending inhibitory influences due to a direct loss of neural traffic saying "do-not-do-this" behavior, an increase in neural traffic insisting on "got-to-have-it" behavior, or a combination of the two.

DOPAMINE RECEPTORS

Dopamine is no longer viewed solely as the mediator of pleasure but as the primary neurotransmitter for learning from experience what is pleasurable, aversive, novel, and predictable.[23,24] Initially, all experience and all drugs of abuse increase firing of dopaminergic neurons in the VTA. A molecule of dopamine released from VTA neurons into the synapses in the NAc, AMG, and PFC binds to 1 of 5 different dopamine receptor subtypes grouped into 2 families: the D1 family, which includes receptors D1 and D5, and the D2 family, which includes receptors D2, D3, and D4. The dopamine D2 receptor density is important in determining an individual's perception of drug experience as pleasurable or aversive and his or her susceptibility to addiction. The brain lesion associated with substance abuse manifests a greater of number D1 receptors and fewer D2 receptors. The density of dopamine D2 receptors decreases approximately 4% to 6% per decade, but advancing age is not associated with an increase in addiction risk. Within a given age range, there is wide individual variability in the density of dopamine D2 receptors. Those with a high density of dopamine D2 receptors are more likely to view a recreational drug experience as unpleasant and thus not develop behaviors that lead to addiction.[27] With increasing chemical dependence, the number of D2 receptors and the ratio of the number of D2 receptors to D1 receptors decreases in the NAc and PFC. High levels of dopamine D2 receptors protect against alcohol abuse. When an adenoviral vector is used to deliver the dopamine D2 receptor into the NAc of rats previously trained to self-administer alcohol, the rats reduce their alcohol intake.[28] Thus focusing on means to increase the number of dopamine D2 receptors could produce new therapies to treat alcoholism and possibly other addictions.

GLUTAMATE RECEPTORS

Sustained exposure to cocaine or amphetamine causes endocytosis of the AMPA glutamate receptor in the postsynaptic cells of the NAc. A reduced density of postsynaptic AMPA-type subunit GluR2 in the NAc is associated with drug craving in addicts. When a viral protein vector was used to deliver a peptide decoy of the AMPA receptor into the NAc (but not the VTA) of addicted rats, the NAc cells retracted the receptor decoy rather than the receptor itself. Restoring the postsynaptic density of GluR2 in this manner extinguished craving-like behavior in the rats and suggests a new direction for treatment of addiction.[29] Another new direction may focus on the cystine-glutamate transporter mechanism.[30] Cystine is the oxidized dimeric form of cysteine. Administration of prodrugs for cysteine may increase the extracellular glutamate in the NAc, decrease the amount of glutamate released into the NAc with PFC stimulation, and reduce drug-seeking behavior.

BRAIN LESIONS

Addiction is the end result of a pathologic hardwiring of brain circuits that control learned behavior. The addicted brain is a brain reorganized in 3 parallel phases as described in **Table 95-3** that yield

TABLE 95-3 Neurocircuitry and Neurotransmitters of Addiction

Neuroplasticity of addiction is divided into 3 phases that occur in parallel but at different rates and a final common pathway.
Binge/Intoxication Phase (dopamine)
VTA ⟶ NAc (reward)
VTA ⟶ PFC (executive control)
VTA ⟶ AMG (habitual action)
Withdrawal/Negative Affect Phase (CRF)
AMG ⟶ Brainstem, hypothalamus
Preoccupation/Anticipation (Craving) Phase (glutamate)
Drug seeking induced by drug taking or stimuli paired with drug taking
Reinstatement (drug): PFC ⟶ NAc
Reinforcement (cues): (PFC) ⟶ AMG ⟶ NAc
Stress (norepinephrine, CRF as well as glutamate)
(+) stress: Brainstem ⟷ AMG ⟶ NAc
(–) stress [withdrawal, (–) emotional state]: Brainstem ⟷ AMG⟶ NAc
Relapse (final common pathway) [GABA, peptides (eg, dynorphin)]: NAc ⟶ VP

AMG, amygdala; CRF, corticotropin-releasing factor; GABA, γ-aminobutyric acid; NAc, nucleus accumbens; PFC, prefrontal cortex; VP, ventral pallidum; VTA, ventral tegmental area.

Data from Kalivas and O'Brien C[23] and Koob and Volkow.[24]

TABLE 95-4 Brain Lesions Common to Addiction Regardless of Drug of Abuse

Hypofrontality
Decrease is directly proportional to years of abuse
Decreased VTA volume
Increased dopamine in AMG, PFC
Replaces increased dopamine in NAc
Change in neural input to NAc
Dopaminergic from VTA becomes glutaminergic from PFC, AMG
Downregulation of D2 receptors

VTA, ventral tegmental area; AMG, amygdala; PFC, prefrontal cortex; NAc, nucleus accumbens.

the lesions summarized in **Table 95-4**. Three key elements in the reorganization are the development of hypofrontality, the conversion of the NAc from a dopaminergic responsive center to a glutamatergic responsive center, and the shift in VTA dopaminergic activity from the NAc to the PFC and AMG. Frontal lobe volume losses occur in cocaine-, alcohol-, and heroin-dependent subjects, with a negative correlation between normalized prefrontal volumes and years of abuse. The pyramidal neurons in the PFC decrease in size and show diminished baseline glutamatergic activity. But presented with drug cues or the drug itself, the amount of glutamate they release in the NAc is exaggerated. Similarly, the size of dopaminergic neurons in the VTA decrease and their baseline activity diminishes. When stimulated by drug administration or drug cues, the amount of dopamine they release in the PFC and AMG is exaggerated. Finally, the number and density of dendritic spines on the medium spiny cells in the NAc and pyramidal neurons in the PFC increase when the drugs of abuse are cocaine or amphetamine but not opioids. These changes in neuron morphology are long lasting. Synapses and postsynaptic dopamine and glutamate receptors are located on these spines. The increase in dendritic arborization appears to be mediated through induction of the transcription factor ΔFosB and its set of target genes and brain-derived neurotrophic factor.[23]

Three principles appear to govern the reorganization of the brain with addiction.[31] *Principle 1:* An important pathway for drug-seeking behavior involves glutamatergic projections from the PFC to the NAc. Laboratory support for this principle comes from 4 key observations: (1) inactivation of the PFC prevents resumption of drug-seeking behavior in abstinent rats challenged by relapse stimuli; (2) injection of α-amino-3-hydroxy-5-methylisoxazole-4-propionic acid (AMPA) glutamate receptor antagonists into the NAc prevents drug- or cue-induced relapse; (3) increased glutamate release occurs in the NAc following drug- or stress-induced relapse; and (4) treatments that prevent the release of glutamate prevent or reduce drug seeking in both animal and human subjects. *Principle 2:* Relapse may be triggered by cues from past drug abuse activity, stress, or a single dose of the drug of abuse (reinstatement/priming). Each of these relapse stimuli involves a different neural circuit. *Principle 3:* Craving and relapse require dopaminergic transmission from the VTA, not to the NAc, as happens with initial or acute administration of a drug of abuse, but to the PFC and AMG. In humans, the greater the increase in dopamine concentration in the PFC and AMG, the greater the craving or desire for drugs. The more advanced the addiction, the greater the increase in dopamine concentration in the PFC and AMG with a given cue. In human addicts, there is no increase in dopamine concentration in the NAc with drug cues. Laboratory support for this principle comes from the following 4 observations: (1) inactivation of the VTA inhibits relapse from all stimuli in laboratory animals; (2) dopamine release in the PFC precedes glutamate release in the NAc; (3) if dopamine release into the PFC is prevented, glutamate release in the NAc is prevented, and relapse does not occur; and (4) if dopamine release occurs in the PFC after injection of glutamate antagonists in the NAc, relapse does not occur.

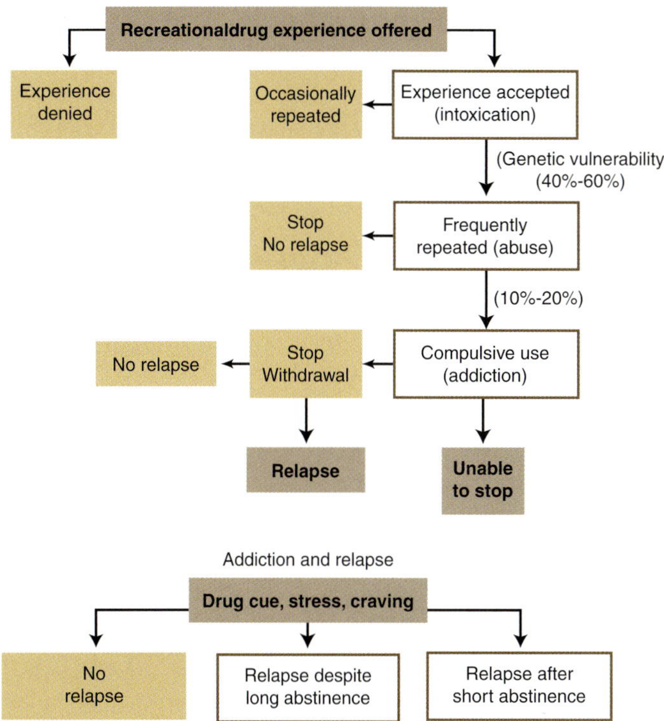

FIGURE 95-1. Natural history of exposure to drugs of abuse.

NATURAL HISTORY

The neuroadaptations that occur in the brain as it responds to abuse and transitions to dependence and addiction can be divided into 4 stages chronologically: (1) initial drug experience (hours to days), (2) repetitive drug exposure (weeks to months), (3) early addiction (months to years), and (4) late addiction (years). In the first 2 "recreational drug" stages, the abuser typically is sharing the drug experience with others. In the last 2 stages, the abuser tends to isolate himself or herself. The rate at which a susceptible individual passes through these stages depends in part on the drug of abuse: slower (years) for alcohol and faster (months to years) for opioids, and even faster for cocaine, and methamphetamine (weeks to months). Not only is the pathophysiology different for each stage, but the success rates for intervention, treatment, and reentry into anesthesia practice are different for each stage. The earlier the intervention, the greater the likelihood of successful treatment and reentry (**Fig. 95-1**).

EVIDENCE-BASED TREATMENT

Over the last decade, 3 major advances have been made in the treatment of addiction caused by any drug.[32,33] First is the recognition that addiction is a chronic relapsing disease. This means that successful treatment requires more than detoxification and graduation from a rehabilitation program. It must include rest-of-life management. Second is the development of anti-craving drugs to combat the changes in the neural circuitry in the brain that create the compulsion to repeat the drug experience. Third is the emergence of addictionologists, physicians who specialize in the treatment management of these complex patients (**Table 95-5**).

Treatment regimens for anesthesia providers seeking reentry are designed to maintain abstinence with opioid antagonists and control cravings with drugs prescribed by addictionologists, active participation in PHP-endorsed behavioral health programs, and active treatment of psychiatric comorbidities, such as depression. If this approach is unsuccessful, as defined by short periods of abstinence, multiple relapses, or failure to remain enrolled in treatment programs, then administration

TABLE 95-5 Treatments of Opioid Addiction

- Prevention
- Surveillance
  - Investigation
  - Recognition
- Intervention on colleague in early stage of addiction (diversion)
  - Detoxification
    - Initiate abstinence
    - Control/reduce/monitor withdrawal signs and symptoms
    - Retain in addiction control program
  - Addiction control
    - Rehabilitation program
    - Comorbidity treatment
    - Antagonist therapy[32]
    - Anti-craving therapy[32]
  - Consider reentry as anesthesia provider
- Intervention of colleague in late stage of addiction
  - Detoxification
    - Transition to maintenance program
    - Control/reduce/monitor withdrawal signs and symptoms
    - Retain in addiction control program
  - Addiction control
    - Rehabilitation program
    - Comorbidity treatment
    - Agonist therapy (replacement or maintenance)
  - Not a candidate for reentry as anesthesia provider.

TABLE 95-6 Recognition of Colleague Misusing Drugs

- Physical symptoms and signs
  - Drug related
    - Intoxication
    - Withdrawal
    - Injection site abscess[36]
    - Puffy-hand syndrome[37]
  - Adulterant related[38]
- Behavior changes
  - Acute drug effects
    - Intoxication
    - Withdrawal
  - Addiction
    - Work habits
    - Personal life
    - Professionalism
    - Drug acquisition
  - Competence
- Comorbidities
  - Psychiatric comorbidity (dual diagnosis)
    - Depression
  - Infectious disease
  - Cardiac complaints at younger age than is typical
    - Chest pain[39,40]
    - Dysrhythmias (torsade de pointes)[41]
  - Monitoring
    - Medical records
    - Pharmacy records
    - Time sheets
    - Fellow worker complaints
    - Patient complaints
  - Drug testing
    - For cause
    - Monitoring for compliance
    - Random

of agonist drugs, such as methadone or buprenorphine, are considered. This substitution may enable a colleague to control his or her addiction but precludes the person from returning to the practice of anesthesia.

RECOGNITION OF COLLEAGUE MISUSING DRUGS

THE DIFFICULT ONES

Inexperienced opioid misusers and end-stage abusers often present intoxicated, comatose, or dead, but experienced users who do not meet the *DSM-IV* criteria for abuse are very difficult to identify. They compose approximately 20% of the dependent drug population.[14] They remain outwardly competent and professional but inwardly miserable as they contrive to sustain their addiction while hiding it from family, friends, and colleagues and protecting their job and source of drugs. Only late in the addictive process, when the amount of opioid these dependent individuals require becomes too great to acquire at work, when their drug-seeking behavior overcomes their ability to sustain their charade, or when they give in to suicidal ideation do they declare themselves.

EXISTING SURVEILLANCE SYSTEMS

Early identification of an errant colleague requires a surveillance system. The Drug-Free Workplace Act (DFA) requires employees to comply with their institution's substance abuse policy and employers to document efforts to maintain a drug-free workplace. However, the DFA does not mandate any specific surveillance system for health care organizations. Some non–health care businesses and institutions have adopted drug testing as their primary surveillance system. In alcohol and drug rehabilitation programs, drug testing alone misses many noncompliant participants. More accurate results in this setting are obtained when behavioral observations are combined with some form of drug testing. How well behavioral assessment and drug testing in a homogeneous population, 100% of whom are known to have a substance abuse problem, translates to the inhomogeneous population in surgical suites, only 1% of whom may have a substance abuse problem, remains to be determined. The primary monitoring activity in health care institutions is for quality of care and compliance and not for drug misuse behavior. Unlike the case for surgeons, few outcome data tend to be collated specific to individual anesthesia providers. Thus surveillance systems that rely on quality assessments are unlikely to detect gradually deteriorating performance or subtle changes in behavior (**Table 95-6**). There is considerable reluctance on the part of health care workers to report colleagues whom they only suspect of drug abuse. Random drug testing has the potential to reveal a problem earlier than quality of care or behavioral assessments. The complexities of the collection process, the relative ease by which addicts can subvert the system, and the high cost-to-benefit ratio in large systems with low anticipated positive findings have deterred most programs from implementing random urine drug testing.[34,35] Most large health care institutions have a drug awareness program and a response system rather than a true surveillance system. They rely on an alert, educated, concerned health care provider reporting suspicious or abnormal behavior to the department head, the professional advisory or wellness committee, or employee assistance program for subsequent investigation. Thus our current systems do not favor early detection of a colleague with a substance misuse problem, especially if he or she meets *DSM-IV* criteria for dependence but not abuse.

IDEAL SURVEILLANCE SYSTEM

The ideal surveillance system should not be created specifically to detect substance misuse. Rather, it should focus on anesthesia provider well-being in general. If behavioral changes are found to be due not to substance abuse but to some other cause, such as sleep deprivation, stress,

TABLE 95-7 Barriers to Recognition of Colleague Misusing Drugs

Continued competent performance until late in the addiction process
Symptoms for abuse and addiction overlap with other common conditions such as stress, sleep deprivation
Limited observations of single provider by same observer
Academic medical center: Multiple attendings and/or multiple trainees
Large practices: Multiple attendings and multiple certified registered nurse anesthetists or anesthesia assistants
Physician-only practice: No other anesthesia provider critiquing anesthetic
Wide variability in acceptable anesthetic management
No system that identifies outliers in opioid administration in the operating room
No system that identifies outliers in pain scores in the postanesthesia care unit
Limited substance abuse education of, or feedback from, nurses in operating room or postanesthesia care unit
Ease of drug diversion with current drug accounting and monitoring systems
Unwillingness to believe it could happen
Fear of being bad guy, ruining career of colleague, or being wrong ("false alarm")
Abuser feeling either he or she can control the addiction or that it is worth the risk
Family fear loss of "face" or security and hope abuser overcomes problem on own

TABLE 95-8 Signs and Symptoms of Withdrawal

Common to Nonstimulant Drugs of Abuse
Central nervous system: agitation, anxiety, dysphoria, irritability, panic
Autonomic nervous system: tachycardia, hypertension
Gastrointestinal system: nausea
Opioid
Influenza-like symptoms: fever, diaphoresis, myalgia, arthralgia, tearing, rhinorrhea, sneezing
Central nervous system: tremors, yawning, insomnia, suicidal ideation
Autonomic nervous system: piloerection, mydriasis
Gastrointestinal system: stomach cramps, vomiting, diarrhea
Alcohol
Central nervous system: insomnia, tremors, delirium tremens, hallucinations, grand mal seizures, status epilepticus
Gastrointestinal system: vomiting, poor appetite
Stimulant Drugs of Abuse (Cocaine and Methamphetamine)
Central nervous system: depression, exhaustion, fatigue, sleepiness, lack of motivation, cravings, psychotic reactions, suicidal ideation
Gastrointestinal system: intense hunger

Data from Kosten and O'Connor.[42]

a medical illness such as diabetes mellitus, or side effects of medications prescribed for a medical illness, they still must be addressed. The ideal system should have observers who can witness the behavior of the same providers frequently enough to recognize a change. The observational standard should be a change in behavior, a more sensitive but less specific finding, rather than a specific behavior that has reached a certain threshold for inappropriateness or diagnosis. The ideal system collects and integrates different kinds of information from different sources: (1) observation of signs and symptoms of acute drug intoxication or withdrawal; (2) behavioral changes related to dress, work habits, professionalism, personal life, competence, and drug acquisition; (3) signs and symptoms of psychiatric comorbidities associated with addiction, especially depression; (4) analyses of information from anesthesia information systems (AIMS) and evaluations; and (5) drug testing. For example, do AIMS queries reveal anesthesiologists whose opioid use is 2 standard deviations greater than the others, especially if they also record high delivered concentrations of potent inhaled agents, or whose patients consistently have higher pain scores in the recovery room than expected? Without an aggressive surveillance system, the barriers to recognition (**Table 95-7**) are formidable.

SIGNS AND SYMPTOMS

Most people have no difficulty recognizing the intoxicated individual. Alcoholics are more likely to come late to work intoxicated, but "experienced" users chemically dependent on intravenous opioids are more like to come early to work, check out drugs for the first case, and immediately divert opioids for acute self-administration to treat withdrawal symptoms. These same "experienced" users also request breaks during the day to sequester themselves to inject opioids to prevent withdrawal symptoms. **Table 95-8** lists the signs and symptoms of withdrawal.[42] When experienced addicts run out of viable veins or when "inexperienced" addicts miss their veins, they frequently resort to subcutaneous or intramuscular injections. Because of poor sterile technique, the sites of this "skin popping" become infected. Abscesses, especially in the lower extremities of anesthesia providers, are red flags suggesting possible substance abuse.[36] Intravenous drug users who inject primarily in the upper extremity may develop the puffy hand syndrome.[37] Other red flags include keeping injection sites away from public eyes by wardrobe changes, such as switching to wearing long pants rather than short pants to and from work, wearing long-sleeved shirts in clinical settings, or wearing operating room scrubs to and from work, or changing clothes in the privacy of their office or in dressing room stalls rather than out in the open.

CHEST PAIN AND COCAINE

The appearance of chest pain, malignant dysrhythmias (ventricular fibrillation, ventricular tachycardia, supraventricular tachycardia), or signs and symptoms of an acute coronary syndrome in a young colleague should include substance abuse in the differential diagnosis. The average age of patients presenting with cocaine-associated chest pain was 37.6 ± 9.3 years, considerably younger than the typical coronary heart disease population.[39,40] Both cocaine and crystal methamphetamine reach peak blood concentrations within seconds to minutes after smoking or intravenous injection, minutes after nasal insufflation or "snorting," and too long after oral ingestion for significant abuse. They increase the catecholamine concentration in the synaptic cleft by interfering with the ability of the catecholamine transporter, a carrier protein, to return extracellular catecholamines intracellularly to presynaptic neurons. The increased catecholamine residence time in the synapse leads to α-adrenergic effects, such as hypertension and coronary spasm, and β-adrenergic effects, such as tachycardia and dysrhythmias. The combined increase in oxygen demand and decrease in oxygen supply leads to anginal symptoms, frequently in the absence of occlusive coronary lesions, myocarditis, and dilated cardiomyopathy. Chronic use accelerates atherosclerosis and produces hypertrophic cardiomyopathy. Although the risk of these myocardial infarctions is greatest within 1 hour of drug administration, they may occur up to 1 to 2 days later.

DETECTING DIVERSION OF ANESTHETIC DRUGS

Two papers evaluated the use of an AIMS to monitor for diversion of controlled substances. In a retrospective study in 2007, Vigoda et al[43] compared the medications secured from the automated medication dispensing system to administration records on an AIMS record. Discrepancies, found in 15% of cases, occurred mostly due to documentation errors in AIMS or amount of drug waste in the dispensing system. The authors recommended a utilization of an electronic interface between the AIMS and dispensing system to alert users of medication entry errors before closing a record. Epstein et al[44] used records from the drug-dispensing machine to identify behavioral patterns associated with abuse of controlled substances. Based on 2 known cases of drug diversion and their onset, the authors used database queries to identify atypical drug transactions. Examples include frequent transactions an hour or more after the end of a procedure or checking out drugs from a machine in a location different than the anesthetizing site. Use of a surveillance system could result in recognition of diversion. In the accompanying editorial, Dexter[45] suggests collaboration by anesthesiologists and data analysts to improve drug surveillance. A survey conducted by Wischmeyer et al[20] reported that 71% of anesthesia training programs had no established system to control or monitor propofol use. Because propofol abuse had been implicated in 7 anesthesia provider deaths (6 of whom were residents), a monitoring system for its use was recommended. As part of their Substance Abuse Prevention Protocol, Tetzlaff et al[46] report the use of an interface between the AIMS and the electronic controlled substance dispensing system to detect "excessive use, excessive wastage, inappropriate transaction site identification, frequent transactions after the close of the case and any regular pattern of failure to correctly reconcile use/wastage/returns." Chisholm and Harrison[47] run chart methodology, plotting standardized units of opioid usage against anesthetists' operating room time, to demonstrate a means to detect abnormal patterns of use.

Observing that the frequency of substance abuse remains unchanged despite improved education efforts, Fitzsimmons et al[48] initiated a program for random urine drug testing of all residents. Brock and Roy[35] commented that their use of a positive urine test as surrogate marker for the reduction in incidence of substance abuse is not dependable. They also questioned the integrity of urine samples brought in any time during a 36-hour response window. Depending on the chain of custody, this allows time for the individual to dilute, contaminate the sample, or supply another person's urine. In response, Fitzsimmons responded that the window had subsequently been reduced to 10 hours.[49] Acknowledging that drug screening will not detect all incidents of misuse, the authors reiterated that their intent was to reduce the incidence of abuse as well as to provide a means of earlier detection of abuse. Recent ingestion of poppy seeds can lead to false-positive results for opioid abuse, diminishing the usefulness of random urine drug screens. Due to short half-lives and diluted concentrations, many of the drugs abused by anesthesia providers can be missed by urine drug screens (UDSs). Hair analysis provides a reliable, although expensive, means to detect chronic exposure to drugs, including fentanyl.[50] Limitations to the use of hair include lack of hair (shaving, trimming scalp hair), in which case alternative areas (pubic area, underarms, chest) can be used; and environmental exposure to particular agents (sample should be taken gloved, after thorough hand cleansing and in a site away from the tested drug's use). According to 2008 information from a New York State laboratory,[51] costs for a UDS including a fentanyl assay were $32.50, including propofol assay were $290, and were over $1000 for hair analysis. Oral fluid testing is also undergoing validation.[52]

Systematic surveillance of the AIMS interface with medication dispensing units (electronic or manual) combined with random analysis of returned waste drugs is a useful means of screening for drug misuse. Diversion detection should also include continued education on the risk factors for as well as the typical signs and symptoms of substance abuse. The authors also recommend "for-cause" testing rather than random screening. The American Society of Anesthesiologists' (ASA) Web site includes a model department policy for drug and alcohol testing[53] that was developed by the Committee on Occupational Health's Task force on Chemical Dependence. A position statement on security of medications in the operating room was approved by the ASA Executive Committee in October 2003.[54]

INTERVENTION

DEFINITION AND GOALS

Intervention is an "advocacy-oriented" confrontation of a colleague whose behavior has suggested that he or she *may* have a problem with chemical dependence.[51,55] Its goal is to convince a colleague with documented detrimental changes in behavior to enter an evaluation program voluntarily. Treating a colleague for apparent signs of intoxication, side effects of the abused drug or its adulterants, or withdrawal and resuscitating a colleague from an overdose are acute emergency medical treatments. These actions are not included in the scope of the term *intervention,* although they should trigger a subsequent intervention. More commonly intervention is required in the absence of these medical issues. It is divided into 3 phases: investigation of suspicious behavior, preparation of a plan for confronting the suspect, and the confrontation itself. Each phase of intervention should be conducted with the assistance of specifically trained personnel who are not members of the Anesthesia Department. Intervention does not include diagnosis or treatment. It is important to remember that most interventions are prompted by documented observations of inappropriate behavior, which could have many causes, and not the witness of actual drug administration.

KEYS TO SUCCESS

The 3 keys to a successful intervention are a thorough investigation, an experienced intervention team, and rehearsed intervention plan. These factors are well discussed in the review by Silverstein et al[51,55] and summarized as follows. The investigation, which may take weeks, is ideally performed confidentially by an experienced team drawn from the human resources, employee assistance, or risk management departments or physician well-being committee of the medical center, with a representative from the Anesthesia Department. The purpose of the investigation is not to make the diagnosis of substance misuse, substance abuse, or chemical dependency but to gather sufficient evidence of behavioral changes, drug diversion, or drug use to mandate an evaluation. No intervention should be attempted based only on suspicion without evidence.

INTERVENTION TEAM

The intervention team should consist of 2 or more members with experience in confronting people who deny their problems. If behavioral changes are the only evidence of suspected drug misuse, the team cannot assume that drug misuse is the problem. Rather, the team should accept that the evidence suggests it is reasonable and necessary for the individual to have an evaluation before he or she is allowed to return to work. It is the purpose of the subsequent medical and psychiatric evaluation to determine the cause of the behavioral changes. There should never be a one-on-one intervention. The gender and cultural makeup of the team is important to avoid charges of harassment or assault. Ideally, one team member should be someone who is either a certified addictionologist, a former impaired professional, or an experienced employee assistance professional. A spouse or family member could be motivated to either facilitate or sabotage the process. Advice from an experienced interventionalist is recommended to determine suitability of the spouse as a member of the intervention team. Interventions take time, sometimes hours, if diversion is to be successfully accomplished. It is important for team members to devote their full attention to the intervention by turning off their beepers and cell phones and canceling all other commitments until the intervention is completed.

INTERVENTION PLAN

The intervention plan should include preparation for immediate drug testing, inpatient admission to a hospital or treatment center, accompanied transfer to testing site and inpatient facility, and contingency plans if the suspect refuses to accept testing and evaluation. The purpose of the intervention is not to accuse the individual of a crime or to make the diagnosis of drug misuse. It is to convince the health professional colleague to submit to drug testing and an evaluation. Drug testing should be required as a routine part of institutional policy and procedure related to risk management of untoward events or inappropriate or unaccountable behavior. Because the suspect may become physically hostile, security personnel should be alerted to be in the vicinity of the intervention, but they should remain out of sight unless needed to avoid the perception of an impending arrest. Finally, an individual once confronted must be regarded as a suicide risk and not be left alone until he or she has been admitted to an evaluation center or accompanied by a responsible individual away from the medical center if he or she refuses evaluation and leaves against medical advice.

DIVERSION

Unfortunately, *diversion* is a term used for 2 opposing activities. *Diversion* is the term used when drugs designated for analgesia, sedation, or anesthesia are diverted by an anesthesia provider for personal use. Intervention with the goal of detoxification, treatment, and monitored reentry into the workforce is also called diversion. Cooperation between the state medical boards and the PHPs is essential to enable the practitioner with a problem to walk the bureaucratic tightrope between confidentiality and ability to return to work versus public safety issues and loss of ability to practice medicine. Unfortunately, the protection afforded by PHPs tends not to extend to CRNAs.

OPIOID DETOXIFICATION

TECHNIQUES

Medically supervised opioid withdrawal, or detoxification, can be divided into 4 general approaches in order of decreasing duration of time required to complete the process: (1) substitution of abused opioid with an approved opioid, methadone, or buprenorphine, and a slow taper (weeks to months) of the approved opioid to minimize withdrawal symptoms; (2) complete discontinuation of any opioids and administration of medications, such as clonidine and benzodiazepines, to attenuate withdrawal symptoms (1-2 wk); (3) precipitation of withdrawal by administration of antagonists, naloxone or naltrexone, and the administration of medications to attenuate the withdrawal symptoms (rapid detoxification in 3-5 d); and (4) precipitation of withdrawal by administration of antagonists during general anesthesia or sedation (ultrarapid opioid detoxification [UROD] in 6-8 h).[56] When clonidine-assisted, buprenorphine-assisted, and anesthesia-assisted detoxifications were compared with naltrexone as preparation for antagonist therapy, no differences in the rate of retention in treatment programs or frequency of opioid-positive urine specimens were observed. There was a significant increase in morbidity with UROD blamed, perhaps somewhat questionably by nonanesthesiologists, on the use of general anesthesia.[57] The accompanying editorial by another nonanesthesiologist stated "anesthesia-assisted detoxification should have no significant role in the treatment of opioid dependence."[58] When UROD was combined with subcutaneous implantation of naltrexone pellets, pulmonary edema, aspiration pneumonia, prolonged debilitating withdrawal, delirium, and death occurred after discharge home.[59] However, there are experienced advocates in Europe for UROD in select patients.[60-62]

UROD POSITION STATEMENT

Currently in the United States, UROD should be considered only if it is part of a clinical study approved by an institutional review board. The American Society of Addiction Medicine (ASAM) has published a public policy statement regarding opioid antagonist agent detoxification under sedation or anesthesia stating: (1) "ASAM does not support the initiation of acute opioid detoxification interventions unless they are part of an integrated continuum of services that promote ongoing recovery from addiction," and (2) "[UROD] is a procedure with uncertain risks and benefits, and its use in clinical settings is not supportable until a clearly positive risk-benefit relationship can be demonstrated. Further research on UROD should be conducted."[63] It is unethical to provide general anesthesia or deep sedation for ultrarapid detoxification to patients who are not enrolled in approved treatment programs under the care of credentialed addictionologists and who just want to "get clean" to go back to work. Doing so facilitates illegal drug use, enables addictive behavior, and puts patients at risk for significant morbidity and mortality if they are discharged directly home from the recovery room.

RELAPSE AND REENTRY

RELAPSE

Addiction now is recognized as a chronic relapsing disease. Unfortunately, most of the data regarding relapse come from abstinence programs that either are too short term or too limited with patients who are far less motivated than most health care providers or have been identified and treated too late in the addiction process. The reported relapse rates are so high that antagonist therapy with its goal of no relapse typically is rejected in favor of agonist therapy with methadone or buprenorphine with a goal of fewer relapses. However, there is a group of patients who do get close to optimum therapy, physicians in PHPs.[9] In this group, the results for abstinence programs are far more optimistic. In their study of relapse in the Washington Physician Health Program, Domino et al[17] observed an overall relapse rate of 25% over 10 years. To express the results more positively, 75% of physicians did not relapse. Three factors predicted relapse: a family history of substance abuse, a coexisting psychiatric illness, and major but not minor opioid use. Major opioids included fentanyl, sufentanil, morphine, meperidine, methadone, heroin, and controlled-release oxycodone. Minor opioids included butorphanol, codeine, hydrocodone, pentazocine, propoxyphene, and tramadol. Relapsed rates decreased with increasing time in treatment. All who avoided relapse in the first 5 years successfully returned to the practice of medicine. With specific regard to anesthesiologists, the study had insufficient power to separate out a contribution of anesthesiology as a profession independent of the abuse of major opioids. However, the authors did refer to data from the New Jersey Physician Health Program and California Physicians Diversion programs that did not reveal a risk for anesthesiologists higher than for other specialists.

REENTRY

Both the Joint Commission on Accreditation of Health Care Organizations (JCAHO) and the American Board of Anesthesiology (ABA) support the intent of the Americans with Disabilities Act: protection of individuals with a history of alcohol or substance abuse who are not currently abusing alcohol or using drugs illegally. The JCAHO now mandates that hospital medical staffs have "a process to identify and manage matters of individual health for licensed independent practitioners. The purpose of this process is to help with rehabilitation, rather than discipline, to aid a practitioner in retaining and regaining optimal professional functioning that is consistent with protection of patients."[64] The ABA's Booklet of Information[65] contains a specific policy admitting qualified applicants with a history of alcohol or illicit drug use into the examination system, if the ABA receives "acceptable documentation" that "they do not pose a direct threat to the health and safety of others" and are "not currently engaged in the illegal use of drugs." After a candidate satisfies the examination requirements, "the ABA will determine whether it should defer awarding its certification to the candidate for a period of time" usually several years after the candidate enters a rehabilitation program, to assure a reasonable period of abstinence, monitored compliance with reentry contracts, and safe care of patients. The ABA receives notifications of actions by state medical boards from The Federation of State Medical Boards and "will initiate proceedings to revoke certification(s) of diplomats with a medical license that is revoked, suspended or surrendered in lieu of revocation or suspension upon notice of such action."

The return of successfully treated anesthesia care providers to the clinical practice of anesthesia (reentry) remains controversial. Currently, the decision to return the practitioner to the operating room is made on an individual basis. Many studies have suggested that upon completion of treatment, anesthesiology trainees should be redirected into another specialty. In 1990 Menk et al published results from a survey of 159 anesthesiology training programs; 34% of the parenteral opioid abusing group successfully reentered training versus 70% of the nonopioid using group.[66] Unfortunately death was the presenting relapse symptom in 16% of the reentering parenteral opioid using group. From a survey of academic chairs and program directors, Booth et al[67] reported occurrence of addictive disorders in 1% of faculty members and 1.6% of residents. Of note, 18% of these cases were detected by death or near death. In the most recent study of treatment outcomes among 199 residents in anesthesiology involved in drug misuse, 167 returned to medicine, 100 continued as anesthesia residents, 9 died, and 91 completed their anesthesia training, for a 79% overall reentry rate in medicine and a 46% reentry rate into anesthesia.[5] Fry provided dismal results from a small 10-year survey of anesthesiologists and anesthesia trainees in Australia and New Zealand.[68] Only 19% of abusing trainees were successful in a return to any specialty of medicine, 15% of those reentering anesthesia were successful in training completion, and there was 31% mortality among all the trainees (5 of 16). Collins and McAllister reanalyzed Fry's data to demonstrate 14% mortality for those residents returning to anesthesia.[69] Wischmeyer et al conducted a survey of academic chairs that included abuse of propofol; 18% of departments reported abuse of propofol, of which 28% presented by death.[20] In 2009, Bryson published another survey of US residency program directors' experience with trainee substance abuse over a 10-year period. He reported 29% relapse rate and 10% incidence of death as the presenting symptom of relapse in residents returning to anesthesia training.[70] All of these studies were retrospective studies that relied heavily on the opinion of the program director of departmental chair, who may not have been in position during the survey time period.

Controversy over the subject of routine reentry after successful treatment has recently become a topic of considerable discussion. A review of indexed literature from 1993 to 2008 by Bryson and Silverstein[51] concluded that there was no guarantee against relapse after successful completion of treatment. Stating that despite educational and program efforts "deaths from opioid abuse continue" and based on the subjective report of "nearly 100% relapse" of 12 nurse anesthetists over the course of 20 years, the ensuing editorial by Berge et al recommended "one strike, you're out" rather than return to the operating room.[71] Six letters to the editor responded to both documents. Cohen described the Physician Health Committee of the Medical Society of the District of Columbia's monitoring program for reentering anesthesiologists. This program includes individual consideration, long-term close surveillance, and aftercare by a specialist in addiction medicine.[72] Skipper and Dupont[73] included reports by Pelton and Ikeda,[74] Paris and Canavan,[75] and Domino et al[17] in support of individual consideration for return to the operating room. Paris and Canavan used data from the New Jersey PHP to demonstrate no difference in relapse rate between 32 anesthesiologists and 36 physician controls, as well as no significant difference between practicing physicians and residents. In addition, Skipper and Dupont cited the outcomes report of McClellan et al[76] after a 5 or more year follow-up of 904 physicians from 16 PHPs, which supported individualized treatment. Earley and Berry[77] cited Angres et al[78] in support of using specific factors in making the decision to return immediately after treatment. Noting that none of the published studies contained specifics of treatment, follow-up care, or previously mentioned factors, they recommended research evaluating the various assessment and management protocols. Katz[79] criticized Berge for not making a distinction between residents and attending physicians, the effect on relapse and death upon redirection to another specialty or not practicing medicine, as well as abuse of different drugs. Citing the "one strike, you're out" default position, Specht was concerned that individuals would be less likely to seek help due to fear of career loss.[80] In the only letter of support of "one strike, you're out," Torri mentioned concerns for patient safety under the care of the relapsing anesthesia care provider before detection.[81] Berge et al responded that reentry criteria that predict success upon return to anesthesia practice, particularly within the framework of a well-functioning PHP, as well as life-long monitoring may provide a platform for reentry. They also supported research with valid study design, outcome metrics, and appropriate data analyses.[82]

Oreskovich and Caldeiro reviewed in 2009 the indexed literature on the subject of reentry of anesthesiologists after successful treatment for chemical dependency and found that most PHPs "did not define the role of monitoring programs, type or duration of treatment, role of hair and nail testing to confirm recent opioid use, or the effect of the use of depot naltrexone."[83] Review of "the subset of PHPs that incorporated trimodal monitoring (chemical, behavioral, and workplace), aggressively tested hair and fingernails for high-potency opioids, required administration of depot naltrexone, and followed up anesthesiologists for five years after residential treatment that averaged three months" supported the individualized return to clinical practice.[83] They note the need to address the inconsistency among the various states' PHP programs and the absence of PHP in several states. When available, they recommend a requirement for participation in a PHP-mandated monitoring and aftercare program. In the previously cited study from the Washington Physician Health Program,[17] only 5 of 22 anesthesiologists who misused fentanyl were able to return to practice (23%), but no information about the 11 anesthesiologists whose drug of choice was not fentanyl was presented. Presumably, they were less likely to relapse and more likely to have successfully reentered practice. The authors concluded that risk of relapse was increased in those who used a major opioid, had a coexisting psychiatric illness, or family history of a substance use disorder.

DuPont et al published results from McClellan's 5-year longitudinal cohort study involving 904 physicians enrolled into 1 of 16 responding PHPs. Over the 5-year period, 78% of the participants had negative drug testing, and posttreatment 72% of all physicians continued to practice medicine.[84] Skipper et al conducted an analysis of a subset of 102 anesthesiologists from this study.[85] Anesthesiologists had a higher rate of opioid and intravenous drug use in comparison with other physicians. There was no statistical difference in completion of contracts (71% anesthesiologists vs 64% nonanesthesiologists) or continuation in other medical practice specialties (76% anesthesiologists vs 73% nonanesthesiologists). There was no report of physician death or significant patient harm due to relapse. Fitzsimmons and Baker's editorial comments that Skipper et al demonstrate that recovery and successful return to practice are very likely for the trained anesthesiologist who receives the support of a PHP.[86] They suggest that residents who are referred to a PHP and successfully complete a course of treatment should be considered for reentry into anesthesiology training. In response to a letter to the editor by Silverstein and Bryson,[87] Skipper noted that 12% of the returning anesthesiologists changed specialties.[88] Citing DuPont's study, he also refuted their suggestion that many addicted anesthesiologists, including the more severe cases, are not referred to PHPs. Thus successful reentry can occur. The question is when and how.

Based on their experience with 5 addicted anesthesia residents, Bryson and Levine recommend a gradual return to the operating room.[89] The accompanying editorial by Tetzlaff and Collins commented that relapse risk stratification could lead to development of case-by-case system for reentry.[90] Criteria used by PHPs for consideration for reentry has been published. Talbot's original return to work classification has not undergone research evaluation but remains a useful template.[78] The literature supports 3 criteria for a negative outcome: positive family history, comorbid psychiatric disorder, and history of relapse. The Earley Consultancy[91] is in the process of developing and implementing a reentry evaluation tool: the Medical Personnel Addiction Recovery Inventory (MPARI). This was initially created for anesthesiologists (APARI). The tool is based on expert consensus only and has not been analyzed for validity or interrater reliability. The ASA Web site contains a model curriculum on drug abuse and addiction for residents in anesthesiology.[92] It was developed by the Committee on Occupational Health and includes a useful section on reentry with a sample reentry agreement. Talbot's criteria for reentry are listed on the site. Successful reentry requires completion of an effective treatment program, motivation, supportive environment, involvement of family/significant others, as well as a reentry agreement, including monitoring. Although not all states have a well-functioning PHP, the Federation of State Physician Health Programs contains an active list of state programs.[93] The North Carolina Physician's Health Program[94] contains a list of available services: training in identification of impairment and intervention procedures, assessment of referrals and treatment recommendations, advocacy for successful treatment participants, monitoring and support, and financial assistant for indigent participants.

REENTRY CONTRACT

Reentry should involve a work reentry contract stipulating what is expected of the reentering individual by the employer and what the reentering individual should expect from the employer if he or she meets the contractual obligations. Becoming increasingly common are *last chance agreements,* which clearly describe how substance abuse has affected the employee's performance in the past, how the employee's performance has put the employer at risk, what is expected of the employee if employment is to continue, and what the employee can expect if his or her performance does not meet expectations.

CALL TO ACTION

Substance abuse has gotten the attention of professional organizations in anesthesia. The Committee on Occupational Health for the ASA has prepared 2 useful documents: "Model Curriculum for Substance Abuse" and "Model Department Policy for Drug and Alcohol Testing as Part of a Comprehensive Intervention for Suspected Substance Abuse in Anesthesia Professionals." The Society of Academic Anesthesia Chairs and Academic Anesthesia Program Directors (SAAC/AAPD) has sponsored 2 instructional videos: the original *Wearing Masks* and *Collateral Damage: Drug Abuse and Anesthesiology.* The American Association of Nurse Anesthetist (AANA) has sponsored the making of several instructional videos that are sequels to *Wearing Masks.* Both the ASA and AANA have established wellness committees. Anesthesiologists who have an interest in addressing the problems of substance abuse should become members of the Association of Medical Education and Research in Substance Abuse (AMERSA).[95] As C. Everett Koop, MD, former US surgeon general remarked in the McGovern Lecture, Hanover, New Hampshire, May 1, 2003,

> I try to remember not to call people with addictions—drug addicts. I propose that you do the same. The word *addict* carries a very negative connotation and suggests that the person is the problem rather than the disease.

KEY REFERENCES

- Bryson EO, Silverstein JH. Addiction and substance abuse in anesthesiology. *Anesthesiology.* 2008;109:905-917.
- Collins GB, McAllister MS, Jensen M, et al. Chemical dependency treatment outcomes of residents in anesthesiology: results of a survey. *Anesth Analg.* 2005;101:1457-1462.
- Kalivas PW, O'Brien C. Drug addiction as a pathology of staged neuroplasticity. *Neuropsychopharmacy.* 2008;33:166-180.
- Koob GF, Volkow ND. Neurocircuitry of addiction. *Neuropsychopharmacy.* 2010;35:217-238.
- Levine MR, Rennie WP. Pre-employment urine drug testing of hospital employees: future questions and review of current literature. *Occup Environ Med.* 2004;61:318-324.
- McLellan AT, Lewis DC, O'Brien CP, et al. Drug dependence, a chronic medical illness: implications for treatment, insurance, and outcomes evaluation. *JAMA.* 2000;284:1689-1695.
- O'Brien CP. Evidence-based treatments of addiction. *Phil Trans R Soc B.* 2008;363:3277-3286.
- O'Connor PG. Methods of detoxification and their role in treating patients with opioid dependence. *JAMA.* 2005;294:961-963.
- Samet JH, Galanter M, Bridden C, et al. Association for Medical Education and Research in Substance Abuse (AMERSA). *Addiction.* 2006;101:10-15.
- Skipper GE, Campbell MD, DuPont, RL. Anesthesiologists with substance use disorders: a 5-year outcome study from 16 state physician health programs. *Anesth Analg.* 2009;109:891-896.

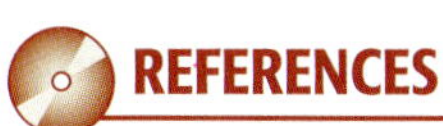

REFERENCES

Complete references available on DVD and online version at www.LongneckerAnesthesiology.com

CHAPTER 96 The Economics of Operating Room Anesthesia Practice

Franklin Dexter
Richard H. Epstein

KEY POINTS

1. Efforts to increase anesthesia group productivity are essentially indistinguishable from efforts to increase the efficiency of use of operating room (OR) time and vice versa.
2. To describe operational reality, the mathematics of service-specific staffing is based on the surgeon and patient having open access to OR time on the workday of their choosing.
3. Scheduling cases and making decisions on the day of surgery to increase OR efficiency are worthwhile interventions to increase anesthesia group productivity. However, the most important step, by far, is the allocation of OR time (ie, the planning of service-specific staffing) appropriately 2 to 3 months before the day of surgery.
4. Reducing surgical, turnover times, or first case of the day start delays generally provides small increases in anesthesia group productivity, but results vary widely because they are highly sensitive to both the OR allocations (ie, staffing) and the appropriateness of those OR allocations.

This chapter focuses on the determinants of anesthesia labor productivity and costs in operating rooms. It is intended to help physicians apply evidence-based management as they plan staffing for their facilities (ie, hospitals, day surgery centers, etc). Although the concepts are the same worldwide, the specific examples and their relevance to daily practice focus on US nonfederal facilities. Both productivity and the cost of providing operating room (OR) anesthesia care are inextricably linked to the choices of how many ORs to open at the start of the day and how to schedule cases into those locations. That is, evaluation of anesthesia care (productivity, costs, efficiency) within an OR is a surrogate for evaluation of OR management (productivity, costs, efficiency) and vice versa. The principles and processes for the evaluation discussed can be used equivalently for anesthesia OR care and OR management.

DEFINITIONS

SCHEDULING AND ASSIGNMENT

Staff scheduling is the process of deciding which anesthesia providers work each shift on each day. Staff scheduling for a future date usually is performed before the surgical cases to be performed on that date have been scheduled.

For example, an anesthesia group creates its work schedule 2 months in advance. Drs Jones and Green are scheduled to work 8 AM to 4 PM on March 8.

Staffed hours are hours that an anesthesia group schedules its providers to cover when not on call (eg, 8 AM-4 PM).

Staff assignment is the process of deciding who will take care of a specific patient on a specific day. Most assignments are typically made on the weekday before the date of surgery.

For example, tomorrow, Dr White will be medically directing 3 certified registered nurse anesthetists in ORs 11, 12, and 13.

ELECTIVE, URGENT, AND EMERGENT CASES

We are not aware of any one best answer as to what constitutes an elective, urgent, or emergent case.[1] Still, differentiating among such cases is necessary to plan staffing. The following is a set of reasonable definitions that provide for different operational decisions.

An *elective case* can be defined as one for which the patients can wait at least 3 days for surgery without sustaining additional morbidity.[2] The choice of 3 days corresponds to patients waiting from Friday to Monday. At a facility with patients scheduled for elective surgery on Saturdays, 2 days would be used as the threshold. For example, tonsillectomy and knee arthroscopy are elective cases.

An *emergent case* can be defined as one for which the patient is likely to sustain additional morbidity and/or mortality unless surgical care is started in less time than needed for a team to be called in from home. In this context, "likely" to have a worse outcome means based on scientific studies, such as published observational studies. By using this evidence-based definition, the appropriateness of the relevant staffing decision can be made by reviewing data on prior emergent cases.[2] For example, cesarean delivery because of a prolapsed umbilical cord and a ruptured aortic aneurysm are emergent cases.

An *urgent case* is defined as one for which the safe waiting time lies between that of an emergency and an elective case.[2] Almost all nonelective cases are urgent cases.

For example, liver transplantation and nailing of a femoral neck fracture are urgent cases. They are not emergency cases because the patient can wait long enough for an OR team to come to the hospital from home.

From a practical viewpoint, sufficient staff need to be present in-house to deal with emergent cases, whereas providing staff who take calls from home to cover urgent cases that cannot be covered by the in-house call team is a viable approach. The cost differential between having sufficient staff in-house to handle urgent cases versus having them taking call from home can be considerable.[2,3]

DEFINITIONS RELATED TO SERVICE-SPECIFIC STAFFING AND OPERATING ROOM ALLOCATION

Surgical service refers to a group of surgeons who share allocated OR time (ie, service-specific staffing). An individual surgeon, a group, a specialty, or a department can function as a surgical service, depending on how OR time is allocated. *Service* simply refers to the unit of OR allocation.

For example, 2 ORs are allocated to the cardiothoracic surgeons practicing at a hospital, any of whom can schedule cases in these rooms. Then, "cardiothoracic surgery" is a service.

For example, 2 gynecologists are partners in 1 of 3 gynecology groups that practice at a hospital. If the 2 gynecologists are together allocated OR time, then they represent a service.

For example, a busy general surgeon is personally allocated 8 hours of OR time every Friday. Then, from the perspective of allocating OR time and scheduling cases on Fridays, that surgeon represents a surgical service, even though there may also be a general surgery service. The service-specific staffing is that one OR for 8 hours every Friday.

Even when a surgical suite does not have a formal organizational plan for allocating ORs (ie, "block schedule"), there can be service-specific staffing (ie, OR allocations). In this regard, "services" need not be specific clinical subspecialties in the medical staff organizational structure. Rather, they reflect the activities of individuals or groups of surgeons who use the OR facilities and thus require organized staffing to support those activities. In some circumstances, several disparate subspecialties may share OR time and thus function as a service.

For example, a 10-OR surgical suite has the official policy that all of its cases are scheduled on a first-scheduled, first-served basis. However, in reality, cases of the same specialty usually are scheduled into the same ORs because this simplifies the distribution of resources (eg, surgical equipment, tables, video towers) and assignment of nursing and anesthesia teams who specialize in the area of surgical practice. Some nurses and anesthesia providers preferentially care for patients undergoing neurosurgery and otolaryngology cases, some mostly gynecology or general surgery, and so forth. In this case, the services correspond to the specialty teams.

Allocated operating room time is the interval of OR time with a specified start and end time on a specified day of the week assigned by the facility to a surgical service for scheduling cases. Some facilities have OR time that is staffed and available for cases but not allocated to a specific service. Such OR time has been allocated to a "pseudo-service," variably named the "Open," "Unblocked," "First-Scheduled, First-Served," or "Other" service.

For example, Urology is allocated OR time in 2 rooms from 8 AM to 5 PM on Monday to Friday. This does not mean that the department's surgeons are limited to scheduling cases only if they can be completed by 5 PM. Instead, it means that staffing has been *planned* for the department's surgeons between 8 AM and 5 PM. The definition applies whether or not at that hospital it happens the department's surgeons actually finish by 5 PM. If the Urology service's cases run past 5 PM, and if nursing and anesthesia teams were to plan its staff scheduling to match the allocated OR time, then they would need to work beyond the end of regularly scheduled hours.

OR time of a case is defined as the time from when a patient enters an OR until he or she leaves the OR (ie, "wheels-in" to "wheels-out"). This definition is used often because these events are unequivocal and thus have good interrater reliability. Future use of anesthesia information management systems (AIMS) to provide such data automatically may make OR management easier.[4]

Turnover time is the time from when one patient exits an OR until the next patient on that day's OR schedule enters the same OR.[5,6] Separating turnover time from the OR time of a case permits the 2 to be studied statistically as separate processes (discussed later in the section on impact of reducing times on productivity). Cleanup times and setup time are characteristically recorded separately from OR times. In part, this is because it is hard to define when cleanup has ceased and setup has begun for the next case, and these activities may overlap. Turnover times include cleanup times and setup times but should exclude planned or unplanned delays between cases (eg, when a to-follow surgeon is given a scheduled 1:30 PM start time and the prior case in the room ended at noon, or if the second of third cases in a room cancels and the third patient is not available). Hospital surgical suites may consider times between cases that are longer than a defined interval (eg, 1 h) to represent delays, not turnovers, when computing turnover times to focus statistics on the latter cleanup and setup times.[5] This is because it is difficult to determine retrospectively the cause of such outliers, and these are usually unrelated to the process of room setup and cleanup.

For example, staffing is planned from 7 AM to 3 PM. A patient arrived at the holding area at 7:45 AM, her IV was placed at 7:50 AM, she entered the OR at 7:59 AM, the trachea was intubated at 8:12 AM, the operative site was prepared at 8:15 AM, and the incision was made at 8:23 AM. The patient left the OR at 10:59 AM. From the perspective of OR scheduling, the case started at 7:59 AM. The OR time of the case was 3 hours.

For example, a surgeon is scheduled to perform a hepatic resection. However, soon after incision, the patient is found unexpectedly to have widespread metastases and the incision is closed without performing the planned procedure. The patient exits from his OR 2.5 hours earlier than planned. Including a planned 0.5-hour turnover, the second case of the day could start 3 hours earlier than planned. However, the second case of the day in that OR will be performed by a different surgeon. He is unavailable, caring for patients in his outpatient office. The result is a delay of 3 hours. That delay should not contribute to the calculation of turnover times.

Operating room workload for a service is its total hours of cases including turnover times. This excludes the urgent cases for that service if separate OR time is allocated for urgent cases performed by all services. Turnover times are applied, by convention, to the service performing the prior case in the OR, and there is no turnover time included for the last case of the day in the room.

Underutilized operating room time = [Allocated OR time] − [OR workload], or zero if this value is negative[7] means that underutilized OR time equals the allocated OR time minus the OR workload, provided the allocated OR time is larger than the OR workload. Otherwise, the underutilized OR time is 0 hour. See **Figure 96-1** for a graphical representation of these definitions.

METRICS RELATED TO SERVICE-SPECIFIC STAFFING AND OPERATING ROOM ALLOCATION

Based on the preceding definitions, the following metrics are derived:

Adjusted utilization = 100% × (1 − [Underutilized OR time] ÷ [Allocated OR time]).[6]

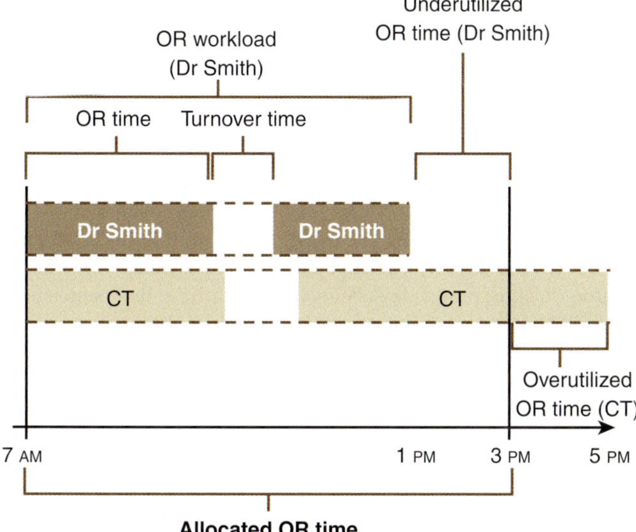

FIGURE 96-1. Graphic representation of OR allocation definitions and metrics. In this figure, Dr Smith and CT are *surgical services*, both of which had been given 8 hours or *allocated OR time* (7 AM to 3 PM). The Dr Smith service finished its last case of the day at 1 PM, resulting in 2 hours of *underutilized time*, an *OR workload* of 6 hours, and a 75% *adjusted utilization*. The CT Service finished its last case at 5 PM, resulting in 2 hours of *overutilized time*, an *OR workload* of 10 hours, and a 100% *adjusted utilization*. Had the CT service finished at 7 PM instead of 5 PM, there it would have generated 4 hours of *overutilized time* but still a 100% *adjusted utilization*. Assuming that overutilized time is 1.5 times more expensive than underutilized time (ie, "time and a half"), the *inefficiency of use of OR time* by the Dr Smith service would have been 2 hours, whereas it would have been 3 hours if the CT service finished at 5 PM and 6 hours if it had finished at 7 PM. This highlights the inadequacy of using *adjusted utilization* to examine the appropriateness of OR allocations for surgical services and shows why *inefficiency of use of OR time* is the appropriate metric.

For example, staffing is planned from 7 AM to 3 PM. An OR's last case of the day ends at 1 PM. The OR workload is 6 hours. There are 2 hours of underutilized OR time. The adjusted utilization is 75%.[6]

Overutilized operating room time = [OR workload] − [Allocated OR time], or zero if this value is negative.[7]

For example, an OR is staffed from 7:30 AM to 5 PM. The last case of the day in the OR ends at 7 PM. There are 2 hours of overutilized OR time.

Inefficiency of use of operating room time
= [(Cost per hour of underutilized OR time)
× (Hours of underutilized OR time)]
+ [(Cost per hour of overutilized OR time)
× (Hours of overutilized OR time)].[7-9]

Operating room efficiency is the value maximized when the inefficiency of use of OR time has been minimized.[7] "Efficiency" is characteristically thought of as the ratio of an output to the necessary input. When surgeons and patients are provided open access to OR time on any future workday, the output (eg, number of cases performed) is a constant (see Tactical Versus Operational Decisions to Increase Productivity section). Thus maximizing "efficiency" is achieved by minimizing the input. That occurs when service-specific staffing and case scheduling are so good there are both 0 hours of underutilized OR time and 0 hours of overutilized OR time. In practice, this is an unachievable goal, due to variance in surgical times for identically scheduled cases.

For example, why would a surgical department be allocated 2 ORs on Mondays? If the department's surgeons were allocated 3 ORs, then much of the OR time would be underutilized. That would reduce OR efficiency. If the department was allocated 1 OR, then the surgeons would be working late to finish their cases, resulting in much overutilized OR time. That would reduce OR efficiency. The choice of 2 ORs provides the best balance.

In our experience, this example provides what most facilities consider the objective of OR allocation: providing the right amount of OR time to get the cases done (ie, not too much or too little). That is the essence of operational OR management decision making. That *must* be differentiated from the longer term tactical stage of OR allocation, wherein an increase or reduction in allocated OR time is expected to result in a change in OR workload.[10]

The example also shows why good operational decisions cannot be made based on OR utilization. True, OR allocation would not be 3 ORs based on either OR efficiency or OR utilization because there would be many hours of underutilized OR time. However, the choice of 1 or 2 ORs would not be clear based on OR utilization because the resulting hours of overutilized OR time are not included in the calculation of utilization (which, by definition, cannot be higher than 100%). In contrast, decision making based on OR efficiency considers both the expected underutilized and overutilized OR time.

For example, Dr Abrams is an orthopedic surgeon in a solo practice. She is allocated OR 1 on Mondays and Wednesdays for 10 hours, from 7 AM to 5 PM. Dr Yue is another orthopedic surgeon in a solo practice. He is allocated OR 1 on Tuesdays and Thursdays for 10 hours, also from 7 AM to 5 PM. Both Drs Abrams and Yue consistently perform slightly less than 10 hours of cases in their allocated OR time, virtually never more. Both perform spinal surgery cases. However, Dr Abrams tends to perform one more case of the same type as Dr Yue within the allocated OR time because Dr Abrams operates much more quickly than Dr Yue. OR efficiency is identical and unaffected by how quickly Dr Abrams operates.

MANAGERIAL COST ACCOUNTING

Labor cost equals the sum of 2 products: staffed hours multiplied by the cost per hour of staffed hours and hours worked late multiplied by the cost per hour of hours worked late. More complicated managerial accounting models generally are not needed for purposes of OR allocation and case scheduling. Labor cost can generally be estimated as the sum of the allocated OR time multiplied by the cost per hour of staffed hours and the hours of overutilized OR time multiplied by the cost per hour of overutilized OR time.

Operating room productivity equals the OR workload divided by the labor costs. *Anesthesia group productivity* equals anesthesia workload divided by labor costs.

For example, the only anesthesia service that a group provides at an outpatient surgery facility is OR anesthesia. Staffing is planned for 5 ORs from 7 AM to 3 PM. There is virtually never any overutilized OR time. Then, each increase in OR workload (ie, the cases performed) results in an increase in OR and anesthesia group productivity.

For example, an anesthesia group practices at a hospital both with substantial underutilized OR time and overutilized OR time. Recent increases in elective OR workload have resulted in cases finishing in the early evenings, resulting in increased overutilized OR time. Then, the increase in OR workload could be reducing anesthesia group productivity. That would be happening if the cost per hour of overutilized OR time is much higher than the cost per hour of regularly staffed hours.

Although it may seem good to make operational OR management decisions based on increasing anesthesia group productivity, we recommend against the approach. Instead, make operational OR management decisions to maximize OR efficiency. Usually the decisions will be the same but not always.

We recommend decision making based on OR efficiency, for 2 reasons.[1,11] First, whereas decisions based on OR efficiency are invariant to the perspective of the cost assessment, decisions based on labor cost are not. There is no one best answer as to whose labor costs should be used to make decisions. Although from the perspective of the anesthesia group, the ideal would be to make the decisions based on its labor costs, other reasonable options include the labor cost of the hospital or society. Second, labor costs vary depending on staff scheduling and staff assignment, whereas OR efficiency does not. If labor costs were used, distributed decision making would no longer be consistent depending on the perspective of who makes the decision. For example, if one anesthesia provider works overtime to cover for another anesthesia provider who has called in sick, that would affect decisions based on labor costs but would not affect decisions based on OR efficiency.

Revenue is the money received from third parties to provide care for a specific patient. *Variable costs* are costs that increase proportionate to the volume of patients receiving care.[12]

For example, the amount of endotracheal tubes and medications used varies with the number of patients who receive anesthesia care. Hence disposable equipment and pharmacy costs are variable costs.

Fixed costs are those costs unrelated to the volume of patients receiving care. For example, an anesthesia machine costs the same regardless of how often it is used. An anesthesia machine is a fixed cost.

For example, a new 8-OR ambulatory surgery center has virtually no overutilized OR time but much underutilized OR time. On a short-term basis, labor costs can be viewed as fixed. Even if OR workload was increased, all the cases would still be completed within allocated OR time. The number of anesthesia providers needed to staff the ORs would be unchanged. However, on a longer term basis, labor costs could be reduced by closing an OR if the OR workload does not increase sufficiently.

Contribution margin equals revenue minus the variable costs for providing care to those patients. These include revenue and variable costs associated both with the current case and those related to subsequent care due to complications.

For example, consider the calculation of contribution margin for a colon resection in which the wound becomes infected. Revenue and variable costs need to be included due to the original surgery as well as the full hospitalization including 3 trips back to the OR to wash out the wound.

Profit equals revenue minus the sum of fixed and variable costs. This is the same as contribution margin minus fixed costs.

For example, let us return to the orthopedic surgeons, Drs Abrams and Yue, who were described previously. Dr Abrams performs one extra spinal surgery case in the same number of hours of OR time as Dr Yue. For the anesthesia group, Dr Abrams is more profitable than Dr Yue because the anesthesia group gets more revenue for the same fixed costs of staffing the OR. However, the implants that Dr Adams chooses cost 80% of the revenue, whereas those that Dr Yue chooses cost 50% of the revenue. Thus, for the hospital, Dr Abrams is less profitable than Dr Yue.[13] Both still have a positive contribution margin but only slightly so for Dr Adams.

OPERATING ROOM EFFICIENCY ON THE DAY OF SURGERY

OR efficiency is maximized by choosing staffing and scheduling cases to minimize the [(Cost per hour of underutilized OR time) × (Hours of underutilized OR time)] + [(Cost per hour of overutilized OR time) × (Hours of overutilized OR time)]. If one considers that cost of 1 hour of overutilized time to 1 hour of underutilized time as a fixed ratio, R,(typically 1.5-2.0), the value to be minimized can be expressed in terms of hours: (Hours of underutilized OR time) + R × (Hours of overutilized OR time). This relationship is further simplified on the day of surgery.

At most surgical facilities, OR nurses are full-time hourly or salaried employees. Thus, on the day of surgery, the increment in nursing labor cost from 1 hour of underutilized OR time is negligible relative to the cost from 1 hour of overutilized OR time. Finishing cases early, but still before the end of staffed hours, reduces labor costs negligibly versus the labor cost that would result from a reduction in overutilized OR time. The same applies to nurse anesthetists and/or anesthesiologists who are employees of the surgical facility or corresponding anesthesia group.

Few anesthesiologists and nurse anesthetists in private practice can earn enough money to cover the cost of their salary plus benefits unless they are scheduled to care for whatever patients may need urgent surgery along with patients having elective scheduled surgery. Thus the incremental revenue lost on the day of surgery by having 1 hour of underutilized OR time is negligible relative to the indirect/intangible costs from working late unexpectedly (ie, the opportunity cost of being idle is effectively zero).[14,15]

Consequently, on the day of surgery, the cost per hour of underutilized OR time is negligible relative to the cost per hour of overutilized OR time.[1,16] Thus, on the day of surgery, minimizing the inefficiency of use of OR time (see Definitions earlier) requires only that management minimize the hours of overutilized OR time because the cost per hour of this time is a constant.[1,16]

Case scheduling to maximize OR efficiency minimizes hours of overutilized OR time, as previously reported for surgical suites.[17] The following 2 scenarios illustrate the implications of the results.

For example, an anesthesiologist is assigned to an OR staffed from 8 AM to 3 PM, but with 1 expected hour of overutilized OR time. The anesthesiologist works quickly. She places every intravenous catheter and arterial cannula on the first attempt and performs a fiberoptic intubation in 10 minutes. Because of her rapid work, the cases finish at 3 PM, preventing 1 hour of overutilized OR time. Thus the anesthesiologist increased OR efficiency.[16]

A different anesthesiologist is assigned to another OR staffed from 8 AM to 3 PM, but with 7 hours of scheduled cases. The anesthesiologist works equally quickly, resulting in cases finishing at 2 PM instead of at 3 PM. Because overutilized OR time was not reduced, the anesthesiologist did *not* increase OR efficiency.[16]

These scenarios show that "working fast" is *not* synonymous with increasing OR efficiency. The last scenario of the preceding section showed that working fast is not synonymous with maximizing profit either.

For example, a different anesthesiologist is supervising resident physicians in 2 ORs. Staffing is planned from 8 AM to 4:30 PM.

The anesthesiologist needs to decide which of the 2 ORs to start first. One OR is scheduled with 2 cases from 8 AM to 6:30 PM, the other with 5 cases from 8 AM to 3:30 PM. To maximize OR efficiency, the anesthesiologist should first start the OR expected to have 2 hours of overutilized OR time.[16]

By following this simple principle, individual and collective decision making can be closely linked to enhancing OR efficiency. Without understanding the principles of OR efficiency, the anesthesiologist is likely to have made the opposite decision because there are more cases in the other OR.

The same principles and use of scenarios can be applied to housekeepers, OR nurses, managers, postanesthesia care unit nurses, and so on.[4,9] In essence, all decision making on the day of surgery that has "improving efficiency" as the goal revolves around this concept of reducing overutilized time. Working faster per se does *not* increase OR efficiency; rather, OR efficiency is increased only when working faster reduces overutilized time.

For example, staffing is planned from 7 AM to 3:30 PM. Recently the hospital hired a new OR nurse. On Monday, she assisted in OR 12, resulting in cases finishing at 2 PM instead of 3 PM. On Tuesday, she assisted in OR 14, resulting in cases finishing at 4:30 PM instead of 5:30 PM. She increased OR efficiency more on Tuesday than Monday because reducing 1 hour of overutilized OR time increases OR efficiency more than does reducing 1 hour of underutilized OR time.

TACTICAL VERSUS OPERATIONAL DECISIONS TO INCREASE PRODUCTIVITY

Consider a common OR management problem: staffing is planned from 7 AM to 3 PM. A surgeon has been allocated 8 hours of OR time every Monday for years, and the hospital has an "official" policy that elective cases may only be scheduled into allocated time. The surgeon has always underestimated the OR times of his cases to bypass this constraint. The surgeon has never finished before 6 PM and usually ends between 7 and 8 PM.

The anesthesiologists and OR nurses may complain about working late every Monday because the surgeon is being allowed to "overbook" his schedule. They may lobby to have a committee meet to rectify the situation. Simultaneously, the administrators may discuss the surgeons' lack of respect for rules and hospital resources. Nevertheless, physicians who refer their patients to the surgeon reward him by continuing to send him work because their patients are pleased with his expeditious service.

The fundamental issue is the surgeon's frequent misrepresentation of the estimated OR times of his cases to get them onto the OR schedule.[18] The merits of the tactical issue (ie, whether this is overall good or bad practice) have little relevance to anesthesia productivity. The relevant operational decision is clear: on a short-term basis, managers should change staffing to match the reality of the existing workload. Doing so neither increases nor reduces OR capacity or convenience for the surgeon and his or her patients. What it does is to reduce labor costs by reducing the hours worked late in lieu of staffed hours. From the surgeon's perspective, the only thing that will change is that he can provide more realistic estimated operating times because there will no longer be a need to fabricate to get the cases running past the end of the regular workday on the schedule. From the perspective of the anesthesiologists and the OR nurses, complaints about working "late" will disappear because the regular hours in the surgeon's room now extend to 12 hours, and staff working in that room can expect to work for this period of time.

For example, when an anesthesiologist was hired, the job description said that work hours were 7 AM to 5 PM. Yet every Monday for the past 5 years, the anesthesiologist has finished working between 7 and 8 PM. Staffing is planned to 8 PM because that is the reality of the existing OR workload. Planning the staffing to 8 PM does not change the workload; however, it results in the work being planned for long in advance.

In the 2 preceding scenarios, the surgeon and patient are choosing the day of surgery. Cases are not being turned away, provided they can be done safely, even if they will likely be performed in overutilized OR time.[19] Subject to that priority, OR time can be allocated based on maximizing OR efficiency. To describe operational reality, mathematics needs to be based on the surgeon and patient having open access to OR time on the workday of their choosing.

For example, all ORs are allocated at a hospital for 8 hours. The adjusted utilizations range from 75% to 85% among the surgical services. Thus there is essentially only underutilized OR time. At this hospital, allocating OR time based on OR efficiency would give precisely the same result as allocating OR time based on adjusted utilization. This is because virtually no OR ever finishes late. A zero has been substituted for the hours of overutilized OR time in the equation for the inefficiency of use of OR time (see earlier, Inefficiency of Use of OR Time). The surgeons can be considered to have open access to OR time on the workday of their choosing, and they have chosen to perform cases only when they can be completed within allocated hours.

The 2 preceding scenarios demonstrate that service-specific staffing can be considered for any facility when decisions are made based on OR efficiency and on surgeon and patient open access to OR time on any future workday. The next scenario shows that the assumption of fixed hours applies only to a minority of surgical suites.[8]

For example, an ambulatory surgical center has a policy that OR time is allocated based on OR utilization. Staffing is planned from 8 AM to 3:30 PM. This policy is enforced strictly. A surgeon asks to book a case to start at 1:30 PM, with an expected (realistic) OR time for the case of 2.5 hours. He is told "No"; that would be unacceptable because the case will likely end at 4 PM.

The preceding scenario will seem unreal to most clinicians in the United States. That is the point. Only scheduling cases if they can reasonably be expected to finish by the end of allocated OR time is not the reality of short-term operational decision making at many facilities. Although considering a facility to have fixed hours of OR time is an accurate and practical model from a tactical perspective, it is not realistic for day-to-day decision making for all surgeons at a surgical suite.[1,19-21]

We return to the first scenario of this section, which describes persistent overutilized OR time. Should the surgeon be encouraged to continue to schedule cases beyond the hours that have been allocated? That is a reasonable tactical question, which includes consideration of the financial impact of the surgeon's cases versus the long-term effects on hiring and retention of OR nurses and anesthesia providers.[10] The tactical decision can, and probably should, be considered from multiple perspectives, including societal. However, the operational decision making focuses on the reality of the existing workload. Operational decisions, specifically service-specific staffing, are what most managers can control.

Truly not having fixed hours of OR time, despite an official policy against overbooking elective cases, is particularly common at hospitals at which surgeons mischaracterize cases as "urgent" to get them onto the OR schedule.

For example, an academic department is allocated 3 ORs from 7 AM to 3 PM on all weekdays. No elective case is scheduled unless it will fit into the 8 hours based on mean historical OR time data from the OR information system. The service schedules 20% of its OR hours as urgent cases. Many of these patients likely could have waited safely for several days for surgery. Thus these were elective cases. The surgeons called the cases "urgent" to achieve open access to OR time and thus bypass the policy against overbooking. OR efficiency would have been greater had more OR time been allocated originally. This would have allowed the cases to be performed in allocated, rather than overutilized, OR time.

Suppose that on a long-term (tactical) basis, the behavior of the academic surgeons was considered so bad that penalties are applied. Then, there would be very little overutilized OR time. The methods described in this chapter would be valid and appropriate but not necessarily a useful improvement. Consequently, there is reason to consider whether the behavior of the surgeons just described is inherently bad.

From the societal, hospital, and surgeons' perspective, likely the behavior is good, or at least not bad enough to penalize the surgeons. They are serving as their patients' advocates, assuring timely surgery. Most patients only have 2 preoperative visits with the surgeon, making surgeon flexibility to schedule initial consultations very important to growth in surgical practices.[22] Further, in some health care systems, including that in the United States, the more cases that the surgeons perform, the higher the hospital and physician contribution margins.

Hospitals receiving fee-for-service reimbursement achieve an overall positive contribution margin for the elective cases of almost all surgeons,[10,20,23] because a large percentage of OR costs are fixed (eg, anesthesia machines, surgical robots, video equipment for minimally invasive surgical suites, operative navigation systems, OR tables and lights, etc). If professional revenues for the anesthesia providers and surgeons were also considered in the calculation of contribution margin, then every surgeon would provide an overall positive contribution margin for their elective cases. The implication, then, is that if a case can be performed safely, it is economically irrational not to perform the case.[10,20,24]

The rationale for providing surgeons with open access to OR time, provided a case can be performed safely, makes particular sense for hospitals with intensive care units (ICUs) that often are full. For patients needing such care, the ICU is a frequent bottleneck that results in delays or cancellations of surgical cases. There are 2 ways to approach this problem, other than simply providing and staffing more ICU beds.

One strategy to reduce the risk of delays or cancellations is to adjust the days that services are scheduled to perform surgery.[25] Although such techniques can be implemented practically,[25] the incremental benefit to hospitals may be small. If most surgeons schedule patients for ICU admission on the same days of the week, usually the cause of case cancellations is visible to the surgeons. The surgeons generally suffer more, financially, from case cancellations and delays than the hospitals and anesthesiologists. In this situation, the hands-on facilitation of a local OR manager or an expert in managing organizational conflict can help. Such interventions are valuable and important.[26] However, they are not commonly decisions made by anesthesia group managers, although they can facilitate such processes.

The second of the 2 strategies is to provide surgeons with flexibility in the days when they have OR time. Cases should get onto the OR schedule to assure that the expensive bottleneck (the ICU) is always full. For example, although 90% of patients may have ICU lengths of stay less than 2 days following coronary artery bypass graft, there can be marked variability in length of stay.[27] Consequently, it can be very difficult to predict when a relatively full ICU will have an open bed as a result of a patient transfer from the unit. When the bottleneck to doing surgery is downstream from ORs and the service time for that downstream process is highly variable, then flexibility in scheduling the OR cases is needed to maximize throughput. This does present some inconvenience to surgeons and patients in that they do not know with certainty the date when the procedure will be performed until very close to the day of surgery, but it is preferable to having the case cancelled on the day of surgery due to inadequate ICU resources.

The same logic applies to expensive capital equipment (eg, surgical robots or minimally invasive surgical suites), that, like the ICUs, is a fixed cost that is best kept as fully utilized as possible. ORs in the future will include more technologically advanced equipment, resulting in even higher capital costs. The percentage of hospital costs for surgery that are attributed to labor likely will decrease as capital costs increase to support these and other expensive technologies. To maximize use of that equipment, surgeons should have open access to OR time to do a case on whatever future workday they are available, provided the case can be performed safely using existing equipment. For example, if 2 surgical services have allocated time on the same day of the week and are vying for the one operative robot, providing the services the ability to book elective cases on days other than on the date of their surgical block will increase the utilization of this expensive resource.

The caveat of allowing open access to OR time "provided the case can be performed safely" is of strikingly large importance. Safety includes access to limited ICU beds, hospital ward beds, postanesthesia care unit beds, fluoroscopy equipment, nonfatigued staff, implants, and so forth. What can be done safely limits how much work can be done in a surgical suite on any given day.[1,9,10,28] Characteristically, tactical decision making limits what can be done safely. Then, operational decision making functions within these boundaries.

Based on these arguments, realistic operational decision making needs to function within a structure that allows the surgeon and patient to choose the day of surgery. The reason why this is so important is that surgeons are not the individuals primarily responsible for OR efficiency through their filling of the OR time allocated to them. Rather, the parties primarily responsible for OR efficiency are the nursing and anesthesia group managers who choose the OR allocations to match staffing to the surgeons' workloads.

For example, for 1 week each year, most of the thoracic surgeons are away at a conference. There is substantial underutilized OR time, resulting in poor OR efficiency. This is an example of poor OR management. The managers should have increased OR efficiency by adjusting staffing to match the surgeons' and patients' hours (eg, by making that time available for the extra staff to use some of their accrued vacation).

ALLOCATING OPERATING ROOM TIME AND SCHEDULING CASES BASED ON OPERATING ROOM EFFICIENCY TO INCREASE PRODUCTIVITY

Allocating OR time (ie, planning service-specific staffing) and scheduling cases based on OR efficiency can increase OR and anesthesia group productivity by reducing labor costs.

PERFORMING CALCULATIONS USING COMPLETE ENUMERATION

In practice, OR allocations that are calculated based on OR efficiency are done by service and day of the week. That is because day of the week is the best predictor of a service's workload.[8,29] Calculating an OR allocation means determining how many ORs should be staffed daily for each service and, for each of these ORs, how many hours of staffing should be planned (eg, 8, 10, or 13 h).[8,29] Calculations of optimal allocations can be done by complete enumeration. Details are reviewed in McIntosh et al. Specifically, all possible staffing solutions are considered, starting with 0 hour and progressively increasing staffed hours until additional increases in the staffed hours cause the efficiency of use of OR time to decrease for that service.[29] If shifts of 8, 10, and 13 hours are considered, then the successive choices are 0, 8, 10, 13, 16, 18 hours, and so on. Increasing the staffed hours causes the efficiency of use of OR time to increase progressively to a maximum, after which it decreases. The complete enumeration can be constructed such that every series of cases performed by the same surgeon on the same day would be performed in its original sequence and take the same amount of OR time. The only change is in the start times.

For example, a surgeon is currently allocated 8 hours of OR time individually on Thursdays (**Fig. 96-2**). The surgeon historically has done 9 hours of cases every Thursday. The hospital calculates that the expense of 1 hour of overutilized time is twice that of 1 hour of underutilized time, and inefficiency is expressed in terms of the number of equivalent underutilized hours. Candidate allocations are 0, 8, 10, and 13 hours. The inefficiency of use of OR time for each potential allocation is determined from the cost of the underutilized and overutilized hours that would have resulted. A 0-hour allocation (A) would have resulted in 9 hours of overutilized time, with an inefficiency of 18. An 8-hour allocation (B) would have resulted in 1 hour of overutilized time, with

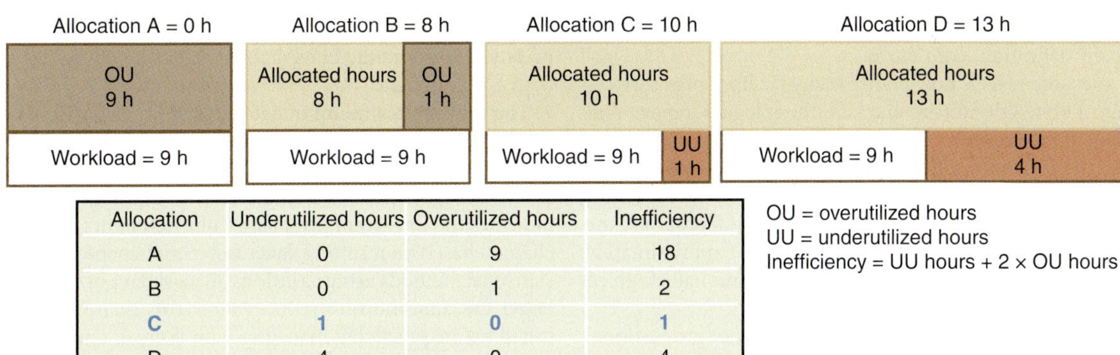

Allocation	Underutilized hours	Overutilized hours	Inefficiency
A	0	9	18
B	0	1	2
C	1	0	1
D	4	0	4

FIGURE 96-2. Simple example of calculating the optimal allocation for a surgical service performing exactly 9 hours of cases every Thursday. The method of determining the optimal allocation for a hypothetical surgical service performing exactly 9 hours of surgery (workload) every Thursday, as determined from the OR information system over the past 12 months, is shown. Currently, the service has an 8-hour allocation, and the question is whether this should be changed. Four candidate allocations, A, B, C, and D of 0, 8, 10, and 13 hours, respectively, are considered, and the inefficiency of use of OR time ("inefficiency") is determined for each potential allocation by determining the number of underutilized (UU) and overutilized (OU) hours that would have resulted had the candidate allocation been in place during the time period of the historical data. The hospital has determined that the cost of 1 hour of OU time is twice as expensive as that of 1 hour of underutilized time. This factor of 2 incorporates the direct cost of overtime ("time-and-a-half pay" or 1.5) and an increment of 0.5 to account for the indirect costs of staff dissatisfaction and recruitment and training to replace staff who resign as a result of having to work late. Thus inefficiency = UU hours + 2.0 × OU hours. For each allocation, the number of UU and OU hours that would result are shown graphically and tabulated below the figure. Allocation C (10 hours) results in the smallest inefficiency and thus is the optimal solution. The surgical service in question should have its allocation increased from 8 hours to 10.

an inefficiency of 2. A 10-hour allocation (C) would have resulted in 1 underutilized hour with an inefficiency of 1. Finally, a 13-hour allocation (D) would have resulted in 4 hours of underutilized time with an inefficiency of 4. Because the most efficient solution (ie, smallest value of inefficiency) is Allocation C, the surgeon should be allocated 10 hours of OR time to maximize the efficiency of use of OR time.

There is a unique solution to the choice of the OR allocation that will maximize OR efficiency if OR allocations can be of any duration (eg, 7.3 h)[8] but not necessarily when fixed choices (eg, 8, 10, 13 h) are considered. When 2 choices provide nearly the same inefficiency of use of OR time, the OR workload can be reviewed to consider which most closely matches how the surgeons in the service have historically been using their OR time.

For example, a gynecology group performs an average of 14 hours of cases each Monday, with a range of 13.0 to 14.5 hours. Forecasted OR efficiency would be nearly identical whether 13 hours of OR time were allocated in 1 OR or 8 hours in each of 2 ORs. The gynecology group has had 2 ORs (ie, reliable first case of the day start times) for the past 6 years. They have consistently scheduled cases into those ORs such that there is only underutilized OR time, not overutilized OR time. Two ORs would be the most reasonable choice. In this example, planning OR allocation based on OR efficiency versus adjusted utilization results in no effective improvement.

Maximizing OR efficiency is the same as minimizing the sum of underutilized hours and overutilized hours multiplied by the relative cost of overutilized to underutilized OR hours.[8] Thus only the relative cost of overutilized to underutilized OR hours needs to be known, not the costs per se.[8] A commonly used[29] value for this ratio of costs is 1.75. This includes the direct costs of overtime at "time and a half" (1.50) and an increment (0.25) for indirect (intangible) costs of employee dissatisfaction, resignation, and recruitment and training.[29] Because of the marked effect of limiting consideration to common staff schedules (eg, 8 or 13 h), the resulting inefficiency in use of OR time is characteristically highly insensitive to local experts' uncertainty in the choice of the value of this parameter.[30]

For example, on 3 Fridays, a service performed 12, 7, and 15 hours of cases, including turnover times. There are 8-hour shifts, with overtime scheduled by rotation using a late list. The relative cost of overutilized to underutilized hours is considered 1.75. If the service were allocated 8 hours of OR time each Friday, then the cost of the Friday of use of OR time would be 20.25 hours (0 underutilized + 1 underutilized + 0 underutilized + 1.75 × [4 overutilized + 0 overutilized + 7 overutilized]). If the allocation were two 8-hour ORs each Friday, the cost would be 14 hours (4 underutilized + 9 underutilized + 1 underutilized). If the allocation were three 8-hour ORs each Friday, the cost would be 38 hours (12 underutilized + 17 underutilized + 9 underutilized). Therefore, the service should be allocated two 8-hour ORs to maximize OR efficiency.

There is only one answer to the question "How close are current OR allocations to those that would maximize OR efficiency?" In contrast, there is no one answer to the question "How close are current OR allocations to those that are optimal based on OR utilization?" because there is then the subsequent question of how to determine the optimal OR utilization. The best OR utilization varies among services because it is sensitive to many parameters, such as staffed hours, turnover times, day-to-day variability in OR workload, statistical distribution of OR times of cases, and so forth.[19,31] Years of data can be required to estimate these parameter values sufficiently accurately to use them to decide on the OR utilization to use as the service's goal.[32] Allocating OR time based on OR efficiency simultaneously takes into account all of these issues. When a manager says, "We allocate OR time based on OR efficiency," that is close to a sufficient statement to describe precisely what happens in practice because the choice of the relative cost of overutilized to underutilized OR time is invariably close to 1.75 and insensitive to any differences. In contrast, when a manager says, "We allocate OR time based on OR utilization," that alone says virtually nothing about what happens in practice at the surgical suite.

CALCULATED OPERATING ROOM ALLOCATIONS DIFFER FROM THOSE IN CURRENT PRACTICE

Managers' efforts to reduce labor costs must focus predominantly on OR allocation and case scheduling because almost all of anesthesia providers' costs are labor costs. For 11 of 12 facilities studied, allocating

OR time based on OR efficiency achieved significantly lower labor costs than the plans that were being used by the local managers.[29,33,34] For 10 of the 11 facilities, the statistical method approach resulted in plans that reduced labor costs by at least 10%.[29,33,34] The percentage increases in OR efficiency were, by definition, even more.

A common anecdote reveals how poorly many facilities plan service-specific staffing. Often OR nurses and anesthesiologists report that every OR finishes at least an hour or two late every day. To consider the irrationality[35] of the situation, suppose that the relative cost of overutilized to underutilized OR time were 2.0. Then, it is twice as expensive to finish late versus early. Thus, with appropriate OR allocations, the odds for each service and OR to finish early should be approximately 2 chances in 3. That is, if staffing decisions were made rationally, a given OR would finish early on 2 of every 3 days.

In practice, percentage reductions in labor costs are not proportional to the number of ORs.[29,33] Even at facilities for which allocations are virtually all for 1 room, either for 8 hours or 10 hours, savings are found.[36] Surgical suites at which many hours of OR time are allocated to services do not have the largest percentage improvements from applying the operations research to OR management.

The explanation for this observation is that the principal challenge faced by managers is not the number of ORs to be allocated to services but how to manage variability in OR workload from week to week. The fact that the OR allocation decision is stochastic is the conceptual problem in the practicing managers' decisions. This is caused by psychological bias that is observed for such decisions in other industries.[35] Implementation is not achieved by education but rather by automating reliance on decision-support software.[35]

For example, consider a service with OR workload averaging 6 hours every Tuesday.[37] Because there are no overutilized hours, allocation based on OR efficiency is identical to allocation based on OR utilization.[36] Once the principle is understood by managers, analysis is unneeded in the future. One analysis is sufficient. In contrast, suppose that the same facility has 3 of its 8 ORs as unblocked, open, first-come, first-served "other" time. The surgical suite staffs in 8-, 10-, and 13-hour shifts. Then, those 3 ORs could be allocated as 8/8/8, 8/8/10, 8/10/10, 10/10/10, 8/8/13, 8/13/13/, 13/13/13, 8/10/13, 10/10/13, and 10/13/13. Intuition will not help with this complex decision. If education has value, and this is unknown, then it is by increasing trust in relying on the statistical results.[36]

URGENT CASES

Some hospitals have one or more ORs allocated for urgent cases during the regular workday. Typically, the appropriate number of ORs is chosen for such urgent cases by considering them to be performed by a pseudo-service, the "Urgent" service. Then, the preceding methods are applied. At facilities not planning an OR for urgent cases, when calculating OR allocations for elective cases, each urgent case should be attributed to its surgical service.

The relative cost of overutilized to underutilized OR time may be appropriately higher for the urgent service than the other elective services because the choice affects not just how often staff work late, but also patient waiting time for urgent surgery. However, urgent cases often cannot start immediately because of a lack of availability of personnel or equipment, such that overutilized OR time would occur regardless of calculations. In practice, the use of the same relative cost for overutilized to underutilized OR time as above (eg, a factor of 1.75) can provide answers that clinicians consider reasonable.

AMOUNT OF DATA REQUIRED FOR EFFECTIVE CALCULATIONS

To assess how much data are required to produce acceptable results, a long series of data from a surgical suite was divided into training and testing data sets, with different training periods.[11] The complete enumeration was applied to the training data, and the expected labor costs that would have occurred during the subsequent testing period were calculated. Each increase in the number of months of data up to 9 months resulted in a statistically significant reduction in expected labor costs. There were large incremental benefits in using at least 7 months of data. For the studied hospital, there was no advantage to using more than 1 year of data.

The minimum amount of data needed for calculating OR allocations based on OR efficiency can be particularly important to managers at facilities purchasing a new OR information system, anesthesia information system, or anesthesia billing system. The minimum period of data indicates the time from installation of the system to when management changes based on resulting data can be implemented. Application of the statistical methods using as little as 30 workdays of system data provided better OR allocations to reduce labor costs than OR allocations established by the practicing managers with years of data.[11]

SOURCES OF DATA

Data for analysis can come from an OR information system, an electronic anesthesia patient record information system, or anesthesia billing data.[38] OR information system data have the advantage of virtually always having necessary data fields completed. Anesthesia billing data have the advantage of accuracy, because billing errors can be costly or even lead to challenges of fraudulent behavior. When using anesthesia billing data, the anesthesia provider is substituted for the room field to calculate turnovers.

Facilities with OR information systems that do not have data review at the time of data entry often have data sets that contain errors or omissions, including lack of knowledge of the actual ORs in which some cases were performed. This can occur if cases are moved during the day without correcting the corresponding information systems or if the times of OR entry or exit are incorrectly entered. This manifests as the false appearance of 2 cases overlapping in the same OR at the same time. The typical fix is to change the recorded OR of each case that overlaps to a unique unknown OR. For example, suppose that one case is listed as being performed in OR 1 from 9 AM to 10 AM and another in OR 1 from 9:30 AM to 11 AM. Among all cases in the data set, the latter case is the 129th for which the true OR is unknown. The second case can be considered to have been completed in the fictitious room "Unknown129." Making such a change affects calculated turnover times because some turnovers between cases will be altered and thus may affect OR allocations. Nonetheless, studies demonstrated that the impact of this adjustment on the labor costs that result from poor OR allocations is of negligible importance, for 3 reasons.[39,40] First, OR allocations are based on each service's total hours of cases, a large number, plus total hours of turnover times, a much smaller number. Second, for cases in an OR that have a preceding case and a following case, 2 turnover times are lost. Yet the turnover time between the remaining cases is increased between the 2 cases surrounding the reassigned case to the default maximum turnover time.[39] Third, the effect of allocating OR time only in fixed increments (eg, 8 or 13 hours) is of larger importance.

ASSESSING TRENDS, SEASONAL VARIATION, AND DATA ERRORS

Use of complete enumeration assumes that there are no systematic differences among weeks in the expected OR workload (ie, there are no trends or seasonal variation).[29] National survey data show that these assumptions hold for most facilities.[41] Raw data were reanalyzed from the 1994 to 1996 National Survey of Ambulatory Surgery. As a positive control, to assure that seasonal variation could be detected if present, the average number of myringotomy tubes inserted each day in ambulatory surgery centers of the United States was examined. As expected, myringotomy tube insertions peaked each winter, corresponding to the peak incidence of middle ear infections. Specifically, the average number of tubes inserted each day varied systematically among months for all 26 of the overlapping 11-month periods in the 36 months of the survey. In contrast, the average number of ambulatory surgery cases performed with an anesthesia provider each day in the United States per 10 000 population was found not to vary systematically month to month on an 11-month basis.

Good routine practice is to test for statistically significant trends[42] or seasonality, to confirm that analysis is reasonable for each surgical suite. For example, the runs test can be applied to the total labor cost over each consecutive 4-week period.[29,43] Calculate the total labor cost for each 4-week period. Subtract the median from each value. Delete zero differences. Assign a "+" to positive differences and a "–" to negative differences. A "run" is defined as a series of one or more consecutive values that are the same. Finally, compare the number of runs of +'s and –'s to a critical value from appropriate statistical tables. For example, if over 10 weeks the values were +-0---+-++ there would be 5 runs (2 +, 1 ++, 1 ----, and 1 -). At $p < 0.05$, the expected number of runs is between 2 and 10, so the null hypothesis that there is a trend would be rejected. This test, the Wald-Wolfowitz one-sample runs test, is available in statistics packages such as SYSTAT (Systat Software, Inc, Chicago, IL) and StatXact (Cytel, Inc, Cambridge, MA).

It is almost never necessary to incorporate methods appropriate for data with trends and seasonality into the analysis. When the runs test detects trends or seasonality, characteristically this reflects a problem with the data or special conditions[42] that need to be modeled separately. For example, if a hospital opens a new 4-room minimally invasive OR suite in the middle of the data collection period, this may result in a positive trend in OR workload. Opening of a new surgery center may result in a rapid decline in workload.[42]

In addition to using the runs test, plot each service's OR workload for the days of the week when the service is allocated OR time. The graphs are helpful to detect unrecognized errors in the data. For example, plotting OR workload for a service against time can show if a service had no cases listed for a day of the week for some part of the data period being used. This usually occurs when the data sent for analysis include one or more surgeons who recently left the facility and operated on the empty days.

Finally, look for the presence of many zero values in the histogram of OR workload for each combination of the day of the week and the service allocated OR time. This usually happens when the service's scheduling is characteristic of an individual surgeon rather than a group of surgeons. These holes often represent time when an individual surgeon is away (eg, on vacation). These can be hard to identify in a graph of OR workload versus time. Such services should have their allocations of OR time combined with another service to achieve reliable staffing predictions.

SERVICES WITH LOW OPERATING ROOM WORKLOADS

Provided cases are scheduled sequentially into ORs (see later, then services with average OR workloads that are consistently less than 8 hours have no overutilized hours. Allocating OR time based on adjusted utilization does not differ from doing so based on OR efficiency. Many facilities appropriately apply a minimum adjusted utilization for OR allocations.[44,45] For example, based on the relative cost ratio of 1.75 described earlier, if services' workloads were always the same each weekday, then the optimal value would be 68%.[44,45]

For example, a service's OR workload averages 6 hours every Monday. The facility bases its decisions on the efficiency of use of OR time. The service's adjusted utilization is 75%. Thus the service is allocated a single OR for 8 hours. There are 2 underutilized hours and 0 overutilized hours. Because there are no overutilized hours, allocation based on OR efficiency is identical to allocation based on OR utilization. There are 0 hours of underutilized time caused by OR allocation and case scheduling.

Each service not receiving an OR allocation on a given day (due to low historical workload) can be combined into an "Other" service (ie, open, unblocked, first-scheduled, first-served time). At facilities without substantial cross-training of staff, there may be different "Other" services for different nursing teams. The calculations of the preceding sections are repeated for the "Other" service(s) on each workday.

Importantly, do not simply measure the average OR workload of a service; observe that it is too low for an allocation of an 8-hour OR for the day, and then automatically pool it into "other" service time. Apply the graphical methods of the preceding section to assure that the reason for a low OR workload reflects an actual low workload, not a service that operates every other week on the studied day of the week.[9] Likewise, assure that incomplete data or a trend in OR workload is not being observed.

USING QUALITATIVE INFORMATION TO IMPROVE FORECASTS

Qualitative information not available from information system data should be used when finalizing OR allocations. For example, a surgeon operates at an outpatient surgery center on Fridays in her 8 hours of allocated OR time. For years, she has consistently performed 7.0 to 7.5 hours of cases at the surgery center in that 8 hours of OR time. The OR allocations are being updated for the next quarter. Based on historical data, she would, of course, be allocated 8 hours of OR time on Fridays. However, she is 8 months pregnant and has requested 3 months of maternity leave. She should not be allocated OR time during the next quarter because it would be underutilized, thereby reducing OR efficiency. Even without personally allocated OR time, the surgeon would continue to have open access to OR time on any future workday, if she were to change her mind and work for a few days during her period of maternity leave. Note that if she were not provided open access to OR time, then there would be an adversarial relationship between the facility not wanting to plan a "block" for her versus her desire to keep some block time to provide herself and her patients some flexibility.[35]

While doing this though, focus on the psychological bias that results in most of the inefficiency of use of anesthesia time, the bias being lack of use of the mathematics. The qualitative information should be used to update the forecasts of workload but not used in an ad hoc manner to convert from workload to OR allocations. We humans can be good at forecasting changes in workload but not in making the mathematical conversions from mean workloads into appropriate OR allocations (staffing).[35]

FORECAST REMAINING UNDERUTILIZED OPERATING ROOM TIME

A concern at some facilities is that underutilized OR time is needed for nonclinical, but nonetheless important activities. For example, equipment for the next day's cases may be set up by nurses whose ORs finish earlier than the end of their shift. The manager of such a facility may express concern that changing OR allocations to increase OR efficiency will impair processes that function well by taking advantage of existing underutilized OR time.

Expected underutilized time can be estimated empirically after future OR allocations have been determined. Applying the allocations, each historical day's resulting total underutilized hours are calculated. The statistical distribution of each day's total hours of underutilized OR time can be described using histograms or percentiles.

CASE SCHEDULING TO MAXIMIZE OPERATING ROOM EFFICIENCY

Allocating OR time to increase OR efficiency is of little value unless cases are also scheduled into the OR time appropriately. A series of thought experiments and computer simulations were performed to evaluate case scheduling based on maximizing OR efficiency.[16] The performances of different case scheduling heuristics were compared. The analyses showed that managers can achieve efficient OR scheduling while leaving case scheduling decisions to the convenience of the surgeons and patients, provided 3 simple scheduling rules are followed.

In other words, there were small differences in resulting OR efficiency among several different scheduling heuristics, with these 3 exceptions.

The first of 3 scheduling rules is that a service should not schedule a case into another service's OR time if the case can be completed within its own allocated OR time.[16] For example, 2 gynecologists are partners in a group that has been allocated 10 hours of OR time on Tuesdays. One of the gynecologists has scheduled 6 hours of cases into the OR time, leaving 4 hours of allocated but unscheduled OR time. An orthopedic surgeon has scheduled 2 hours of cases into his personally allocated 8 hours of OR time. Nine days before the day of surgery, the second gynecologist wants to schedule a new 2-hour case. The available start time would be after her partner who has already scheduled cases. The case would not be scheduled into the orthopedic surgeon's OR time, even if the second gynecologist wants to start earlier. The reason is that the gynecology group has available OR time for the case.

The reason for this result is that OR allocations are calculated based on expected OR workload on the day of surgery. Services fill their allocated OR time at different rates.[46] Almost all facilities with allocated OR time follow the preceding scheduling rule. Thus the importance of this finding was not that it showed a new way to schedule cases but that it showed that most facilities make decisions based on OR efficiency.[16]

The second of the 3 scheduling rules is that a case should not be scheduled into overutilized OR time if it can start earlier in another of the service's ORs.[17] This applies to services allocated 2 or more ORs. Suppose that OR workload is 23 hours. The hours of overutilized OR time would be considered slightly less if 2 ORs were allocated for 13 hours (total: 26 hours) versus 3 ORs for 8 hours (total: 24 hours). This result may not apply unless the case scheduling results in similar packing of the cases into the allocated OR time.[16,47] Simulations show this does occur generally.

For example, a service has been allocated OR 1 and OR 2 from 7 AM to 3 PM. One surgeon in the service has scheduled cases in OR 1 to finish around 2 PM. OR 2 is empty. A second surgeon in the service wants an afternoon start. He asks to start an elective 3-hour case at 2:30 PM in OR 1. Even though OR workload would be the same, scheduling the case into OR 1 would be expected to result in overutilized OR time and thereby reduce OR efficiency. His request should be denied. The surgeon should take the first case of the day, start in OR 2, or schedule the case on a different workday.

The preceding scenario matches what is done at most surgical suites. Cases are generally not scheduled in overutilized OR time when a service has another allocated OR that is empty. Consequently, as the first rule, this rule shows that scheduling cases based on maximizing OR efficiency differs little from what is commonly done in practice.[16] Changes resulting from decision making based on OR efficiency generally do not affect case scheduling. Rather, they affect OR allocations (as above) and in the third rule regarding how OR time is released.

The third of the 3 scheduling rules is that if a service has already filled its allocated OR time, then, to maximize OR efficiency, its new case should be scheduled into another service's OR time instead of into overutilized OR time.[16,47]

For example, a service has filled its allocated OR time but has another elective case that it desires to schedule. If the OR time of another service were not released, the case would be performed in overutilized OR time. OR efficiency is greater by performing that case in the OR time allocated to another service that otherwise would be underutilized on the day of surgery.

For example, a surgeon may be subverting the case scheduling system for the "Other" service, which provides first-scheduled, first-served OR time. The surgeon may be creating fictitious patients to "hold" OR time for his cases (eg, at the desirable 8 AM start time). At a Surgical Services Committee meeting, a manager suggests that there be the policy that, when a case is cancelled, first access to cancelled OR time goes to other surgeons with waiting cases, not the surgeon canceling the case. That recommendation is not sound. When a service has filled its allocated OR time and has another case to schedule, OR efficiency is enhanced by releasing the OR time of the service expected to have the most underutilized OR time. No cases should be waiting to be scheduled.

To evaluate which service should have its OR time released, simulations were performed scheduling new hypothetical cases into actual OR schedules. Services fill their allocated OR time at different rates. Thus, theoretically, the service that should have its OR time released for a new case should be the service that is predicted, at the time the new case is booked, to be the service that will have the most underutilized OR time on the scheduled day of surgery. Yet performance is only slightly better versus scheduling the case into the OR time of the service with the largest difference between allocated and scheduled OR time at the time when the new case is scheduled.[46] The latter is far easier to implement practically.

In contrast, releasing the OR time of the service with the second most, instead of the service with the most, allocated but unscheduled OR time has a large negative effect on OR efficiency.[46] The reason is that usually a particular case can only be scheduled into a few services' OR time without resulting in overutilized OR time. The differences among those few services in their amount of expected open OR time often are large. This occurs because day-to-day variability in the OR workload of services on a day of the week generally exceeds variability due to the timing of how quickly different services filled their allocated OR time.

The timing of when allocated OR time should be released has been studied.[48] Potentially, the scheduling office could wait to release the allocated OR time until closer to the day of surgery when data may be available on subsequently scheduled cases, to improve the quality of the decision. Simulation results were equivocal as to the benefit of such a decision. Under 2 conditions, postponing the decision of which service had its OR time released for the new case until early the day before surgery had a negligible effect on resulting OR efficiency versus releasing the allocated OR time when the new case was scheduled.[48] This finding applies to an ambulatory surgery center with brief cases. At such facilities, typically there is only one good choice for the service to have its OR time released.[46] Thus, there is no good reason to wait in making the decision. This finding often also applies to large surgical suites in which cases are scheduled as if there were many smaller suites. For example, at a 25-OR surgical suite, one nursing and anesthesia team may staff the 6 ORs used for urology and general surgery. From the perspective of releasing OR time for a new urology or general surgery case, only 6 ORs are available, not all 25.

For example, a hospital contains a team cross-trained in neurosurgery and otolaryngology. One week hence, on next Monday, neurosurgery has been allocated one 8-hour OR. Otolaryngology has been allocated one 8-hour OR also. The otolaryngologists have scheduled 9 hours of cases into their OR. A third otolaryngologist wants to schedule another 2-hour case. The neurosurgeons have scheduled a case for 3 hours from 7 AM to 10 AM. The otolaryngologist with the new case can book the case because the surgeons have open access to OR time on whatever workday they choose. Provided the otolaryngologist is available at 10:30 AM, then the neurosurgeons' OR time would be released. There is no advantage to waiting to schedule the case. Yet if the neurosurgeon with the 7 AM to 10 AM case was to schedule another case, ideally the otolaryngologist could be persuaded to start his case later in the day.

Despite this consideration of how best to release allocated OR time, it is important to appreciate that results are highly sensitive to the OR time being allocated appropriately based on OR efficiency. Issues of when to release allocated OR time pale in practical importance versus OR allocation and staffing. Although OR management problems are observed on the day of surgery, often the root cause and only practical way to fix the problem is to plan OR allocations and staffing properly several weeks or months before the day of surgery.[49]

For example, OR information systems data are used to calculate OR allocations, which then are reviewed by an OR committee. An ophthalmologist complains that his allocated OR time on Wednesdays has been "released" for 2 of the past 3 weeks. Each time, the otolaryngology service has filled its allocated 8 hours of OR time and so has booked cases into his OR time. The ophthalmologist is upset that the schedulers are treating him unfairly by repeatedly releasing his allocated OR time. Although he schedules many cases a couple of days before the day of surgery, his OR workload is consistently at least 7 hours each Wednesday. The ophthalmologist's concerns are well founded; this should not be happening. However, the problem is not that the schedulers are releasing his OR time. Rather, they are making the proper decision to maximize OR efficiency. The problem is that the otolaryngology service should be allocated more than 8 hours of OR time.

Finally, although this chapter has focused on decision making before the day of surgery, the same principles apply to decisions made on the day of surgery.[1,50] The principles described can also be used to decide how cases are moved on the day of surgery,[51] how staff are assigned on the day of surgery,[52] and how cases are sequenced in each OR.[53-55]

IMPACT OF REDUCING TIMES ON PRODUCTIVITY

IMPACT OF REDUCING SURGICAL AND TURNOVER TIMES

The impact of interventions on labor costs can be forecast using each facility's own data, along with corresponding confidence intervals.[9-14] For example, turnover times can be reduced between each case.[9-14] Surgical times can be reduced to national average values for each procedure.[15] First case of the day starts can all be on time.[9,45] For all interventions, first the labor cost is calculated assuming that OR time is allocated and cases are scheduled based on OR efficiency. Second, the intervention is performed, thereby reducing OR workload by service. Third, using the revised workload values, OR time is reallocated based on OR efficiency and the new estimates for labor costs projected. Fourth, the differences are calculated. By analyzing the differences in 4-week periods, to prevent effects of variation by day of the week, confidence intervals can be calculated for the differences.[14,15,29]

For example, consider a hospital that allocates OR time to many small services, each having adjusted utilizations of more than 85% with 8-hour allocations.[15] Cases are being scheduled based on OR efficiency (ie, sequentially into ORs[16]). Reducing OR times cannot result in reduced overutilized hours because there are none. Labor costs will not be reduced (ie, they are fixed to achievable reductions in OR times).

For example, a different hospital has few surgical services, most with more than one OR, and many ORs with workloads exceeding 8 hours.[15] Conclusions are different than in the preceding example. Reducing OR times can result in reductions in workload sufficient to reduce allocated OR time (eg, an OR allocated for 10 hours would now be allocated for 8 hours). Thus, at this hospital, there would be financially important reductions in labor costs from reducing OR times.

Equivalent analyses can be performed at teaching facilities to calculate[15] the impact of longer OR times (due to factors such as teaching time and development of skills in trainees)[56,57] on labor costs.

These examples show that, generally, cost reduction from reducing OR or turnover times can only be achieved provided OR allocations are reduced.[9] The initial impact is increased underutilized OR time and reduced overutilized OR time. This initial step is evident to clinicians. The secondary step is revisions of OR allocations based on the new values of decreased OR workload. The latter step provides for the large reductions in labor cost. Whereas the former is often a welcome change, the latter can be less popular politically.

Usually, reductions in labor costs from reducing turnover times tend to be small. At 4 academic tertiary hospitals studied, reductions in average turnover times of 3 to 9 minutes would result in 0.8% to 1.8% reductions in labor cost.[14] Reductions in average turnover times of 10-19 minutes would result in 2.5% to 4.0% reductions in labor costs.[14] These analyses can be fruitful in educating stakeholders that achievable reductions in the times to complete tasks often have less effect on OR efficiency than does good management decision making.

IMPACT OF NOT CHANGING OPERATING ROOM ALLOCATIONS

Some facilities do not make decisions systematically based on increasing OR efficiency and are unlikely to change their practices.[35] Then the methodology outlined here can be used to calculate the higher labor costs that the facility sustains from OR time not being allocated and cases not being scheduled based on OR efficiency.[11,29,33]

For example, anesthesia group expenses exceed revenue at a facility. The calculation is performed using labor costs of anesthesia providers. The estimate of the resulting additional labor costs is used by the head of the anesthesiology group when she negotiates an appropriate administrative support agreement from the hospital.[44]

Calculations of administrative support agreements can also apply to negotiations with medical schools, ambulatory surgical facilities, or a multispecialty group. At 2 academic medical centers, estimated annual excess labor costs were $1.6 million and $1.0 million, respectively.[33]

IMPACT OF NOT REDUCING THE NUMBER OF ALLOCATED OPERATING ROOMS

Some organizations aim to adjust their OR allocations to be as close as possible to those that are expected to maximize OR efficiency while not reducing the number of allocated ORs. This approach does not result in maximal OR efficiency. Instead, it reflects organizational pressure to open as many ORs as are available for first case of the day starts. The mathematics can be weighted to allocate more ORs by repeating the analyses using a higher relative cost of overutilized to underutilized hours. An increase in the relative cost gives an increase in how many ORs are allocated.[9,19] The smallest value is chosen for which the allocated number of staffed ORs matches the desired, usually current, number of ORs. This analysis is run separately for each day of the week.[19]

Increasing the number of allocated ORs results in a slightly smaller percentage increase in OR labor cost than in staffing.[19] The reason is that opening more ORs than are needed to maximize OR efficiency does not change OR workload. Thus the increase in allocated OR hours increases underutilized OR time and reduces overutilized OR time. The cost per hour of overutilized OR time exceeds that of underutilized OR time. Consequently, the percentage reduction in OR efficiency is less than the percentage increase in allocated OR hours. The same argument applies to labor costs.

FORECASTING THE TIME REMAINING IN ONGOING CASES

The preceding sections have focused almost entirely on decision making before the day of surgery because good decision making *cannot* be done on the day of surgery unless the OR allocations chosen months ahead are appropriate. As considered in the section "Operating Room Efficiency on the Day of Surgery," when there is consistent overutilized time on the day of surgery, first and foremost this was a failure months before in statistical forecasting of workload and managerial decision making. However, to use those OR allocations in practice on the day of surgery, another set of data are needed: the forecasted time remaining in cases that are ongoing. In most hospital ORs, the cases running at the end of the day are those that took longer than scheduled.[1] Therefore, good decision making cannot be done in the late afternoon without estimating the time remaining in late running cases. The solution to this problem is not intuitive.

Forecasting the time remaining in cases is one of the most important determinants of decision making on the day of surgery because it affects decisions such as calling for the next patient, moving cases, and staff relief. Even where there is no bias between scheduled times provided by surgeons and the actual durations from the OR information system (ie, the average difference is close to 0 min), there is substantial variance among historical case lengths for the same scheduled procedure or procedures that comprise a case.

Consider a laparoscopic small bowel resection scheduled for 2 hours that has been in the OR for 0.5 hour: The median expected time remaining is around 1.5 hours. In contrast, suppose that the patient has been in the OR 1.8 hours. The median expected time remaining is not 0.2 hour, but longer. The reason is that many of these resections took less than 1.8 hours, so the median duration of the cases that took longer than 1.8 hours is more than 2.0 hours because the shorter duration cases are excluded. For some of these longer cases, the laparoscopic approach may have been abandoned in favor of an open resection due to the presence of adhesions, or a complication ensued requiring additional time.

For any given combination of surgeon and procedure, there is considerable variation between the time when skin closure begins and when the patient leaves the OR (eg, from 15 minutes to 90 minutes).[58] This "extra time" comprises the time to close the incision, for the patient to recover sufficiently from anesthesia to allow removal of the endotracheal tube, for monitors to be removed and intravenous lines secured, and for the patient to be transferred to the stretcher and transported out of the OR.

The time remaining in a case can be forecast[58,59] using Bayesian methods by combining the scheduled OR time, historical case duration data, and elapsed times in the OR determined from real-time AIMS data. Practically, this requires computerization for 2 reasons. First, many cases running late at the end of the day include rare combinations of procedures with little or no historical data.[60-62] These cases have a markedly disproportionate impact on the overall variability in decisions involving case durations on the day of surgery.[62] Second, accurate predictions require data about how long cases have been underway and in which OR they are being performed. That can be inferred automatically based on the identifier of the AIMS workstation transmitting pulse oximetry, electrocardiogram heart rate, and end tidal carbon dioxide partial pressures.[63] The method of automatic forecasting of the remaining time works well even in the absence of any historical data, and it automatically incorporates variance due to changes from the scheduled procedure.[58]

CONCLUSION

OR allocation is a 2-stage process.[10] During the initial tactical stage of allocating OR time, considering OR hours to be fixed is reasonable. For operational decision making on a shorter term basis, such a conceptual model produces results markedly inconsistent with how surgical suites are and should be run. Consider the workload to be fixed on a short-term basis. Provide staff flexibly to match the existing workload, not vice versa. Do so by making operational decisions based on maximizing OR efficiency because this is an important step to maximizing anesthesia group productivity.

KEY REFERENCES

- Dexter F, Epstein RH. Calculating institutional support that benefits both the anesthesia group and hospital. *Anesth Analg.* 2008;106:544-553.
- Dexter F, Epstein RH, Lee JD, Ledolter J. Automatic updating of times remaining in surgical cases using Bayesian analysis of historical case duration data and instant messaging updates from anesthesia providers. *Anesth Analg.* 2009;108:929-940.
- Dexter F, Traub RD. How to schedule elective surgical cases into specific operating rooms to maximize the efficiency of use of operating room time. *Anesth Analg.* 2002;94:933-942.
- Strum DP, Vargas LG, May JH. Surgical subspecialty block utilization and capacity planning. A minimal cost analysis model. *Anesthesiology.* 1999;90:1176-1185.

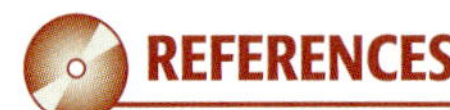

REFERENCES

Complete references available on DVD and online version at www.LongneckerAnesthesiology.com

CHAPTER 97 Practice Management

Philip J. Mesisca
Susan Chapman Moss

KEY POINTS

1. Practice structure considers and clarifies lines of authority, decision making, communication processes, information flow, and levels of authority that define how centralized or decentralized the practice functions.
2. Staffing models require careful consideration of several issues, including the complexity of the case, experience of the provider, physical status of the patient, hospital regulations, surgeon expectations, and provider/resident/student nurse anesthetist teaching rules.
3. Charges and payments for professional anesthesia services generally include base relative value units (accounting for anesthetic complexity), plus time units, plus additional unit modifiers multiplied by a dollar conversion factor.
4. Successful negotiations with third-party payers and hospitals hinge on the clear articulation of needs by both parties and willingness of both parties to accept a reasonable offers as well as an accurate understanding of the value your group brings to the hospital or contracting organization.
5. Billing systems must ensure that every service rendered is captured and that all monies contractually obligated for those services are collected.
6. From a billing compliance perspective, if the service is not appropriately documented, then it did not happen. Compliance with various rules and regulations is both important and essential for the financial health of the practice. Further, the consequences of not knowing, or not following, these regulations can be substantial, both legally and financially.
7. Monthly information that should be tracked for trend purposes includes total cases and units, cases and units per location, payer mix, charge lag, charges, contractual adjustments, cash collections, accounts receivable, net collection rate, days in accounts receivable, aged accounts receivable, total credit balances, and collection agency net collections.

Practice management details are often delegated to nonphysician administrative professionals and their support staff, but it is important that all physicians have a global comprehension of basic practice management topics. Practice management, in its simplest form, focuses on the nonclinical pieces of a medical practice. There are entire textbooks just on practice management, so this chapter provides a brief overview of practice management for anesthesiologists. It broadly covers some global practice management areas that relate to all physicians, and when appropriate, it covers details and issues specific to anesthesia, such as billing and compliance, staffing models, and data analysis and reporting.

To many physicians, worrying about the business side of their practice is something that they may have no interest in or even something they are embarrassed about because that is not why they decided to become a doctor. If, however, more money goes out than comes in, no business or physician will be able to continue to do what matters most to them. So, however confusing or distasteful the practice management side of the business may be, it is a necessary one.

We hope this brief chapter complements the other chapters in this book and helps you become a physician who can face the challenges of the future of medicine by understanding basic business practice processes and relating them to the practice of anesthesiology.

GOVERNANCE AND ORGANIZATIONAL DYNAMICS OF A PRACTICE

What is the practice's mission? Are decisions made to influence the strategic direction of the practice? How does the practice facilitate decision making? How are conflicts resolved? What are the plans for the future? How is the practice going to get there? The answers to these questions help to determine a practice's governance and group dynamics.

PRACTICE MODELS

Most anesthesiologists join either an academic or a private-practice organization. Academic medical groups have always had complex, multiple missions: teaching, advanced clinical practice, and research. Generally most academic anesthesiologists do have some percentage of their time that is nonclinical, often devoted to research and/or academics, whereas this is uncommon in community practice (except perhaps for those with significant administrative responsibilities, either for the practice or for the facility). Whatever the model, efficient, effective management and financial health are essential foundations for personal and group satisfaction.

STRUCTURE AND CONTRACTUAL ISSUES

Practice structure, at the highest level, considers and clarifies lines of authority (chain of command), decision-making process, communication flows and processes, as well as levels of authority that relate to how centralized or decentralized the practice prefers to function.

An example of a private-practice model might consist of a general partnership as the overriding entity. There may then be an executive committee that might be considered the second level of decision making. This group may be empowered to make operational decisions and financial commitments to a maximum threshold established by the general partnership. Depending on the size of the practice, there may be smaller groups or specific individuals who also have authority and operational decision making for smaller units or divisions.

There are other practice models, such as employment by a health system, the US military, Public Health Service, or Department of Veterans Affairs, where the anesthesiologist is fully employed to perform clinical duties and generally does not need to worry about the economics of billing or case volumes. Other anesthesiologists may work as locum tenens, essentially temporary contracted physicians who are hired by groups and hospitals to cover staffing shortfalls. For any of these arrangements, the structure of the practice must be clear and understood in a written format. Buy-in formulas for new partners should be understood and clear. Issues such as who can leave or be asked to leave, why, and with how much notice is required should be clearly described, as well as the financial repercussions of such actions. Noncompete clauses, if included, should be clearly understood and explained. The process of assigning and requesting time off, call coverage, and overall assignments should be clear and in writing as well.

COMPENSATION ARRANGEMENTS

The total amounts of monies available for physician compensation are relatively easy to calculate. Revenue less all other expenses leaves an amount of money. That money can be paid fully to physicians as base salary and bonus, as base salary and incentive, or as base salary with some monies saved for the future. The size of the pie, so to speak, is influenced by numerous factors discussed throughout this chapter. How the pie is divided is the basis for understanding the compensation model for a practice.

In an academic practice, the compensation arrangement often considers the teaching, administration, and research responsibilities, funding, and performance in addition to clinical responsibilities. In a private practice, the focus is on the clinical workload. The best compensation arrangement for a practice is the one that meets the needs of the group and allows the group to fulfill its missions while retaining and recruiting physicians as needed.

There are 2 main compensation formulas. At one end of the spectrum, the group splits the bottom line. This equal-share method takes into account that the anesthesiologist is assigned to cover a specified location (or locations) and does not control volume or the payer mix at those sites. Some consider this model fairer because it does not penalize an anesthesiologist who might work with a slower surgeon or at an inefficient location. At the other end of the compensation spectrum is a more individual model that pays the provider for the amount of work he or she performs. Proponents of this model argue that this rewards the anesthesiologist who improves turnover times, takes extra calls, does a late-day elective case, or uses less vacation time. Many anesthesia groups follow a hybrid of these 2 models to balance the needs and priorities of the members.

HOSPITAL RELATIONSHIPS

NEGOTIATING COVERAGE AND STIPENDS

The relationship between hospital administrators and anesthesia groups has evolved over the past decade as financial pressures on both parties have grown due to third-party reimbursement trends, erosion of hospital operating margins, and rising physician compensation levels.

Successful negotiations hinge on the clear articulation of needs by both parties and willingness to accept a reasonable, mutually beneficial offer. The hospital should set expectations related to daytime and call requirements, number of anesthetizing locations and services, growth and new programs, and administrative activities. To justify financial support, the anesthesia group may need to educate hospital administrators about the local and national physician compensation and recruitment market, efficiency concerns that have an impact on anesthesia productivity (operating room utilization rates, turnover times) and the financial health of the practice (revenue cycle, practice overhead). Stipends typically include those for administrative activities (directorships, participation in hospital committees, etc), call coverage (obstetrics, trauma), income guarantees, and recruitment costs associated with new anesthetizing locations. These costs may be justified based on full-time equivalent (FTE) calculations and market-rate compensation data. Academic groups may receive support for educational expenses, such as residency program director and salary and benefits for residents and fellows.

CREDENTIALING

To meet regulatory requirements and maintain clinical standards, physicians must obtain hospital appointments through a credentialing process involving verification of state medical licensure, board certification status, state and federal Drug Enforcement Administration licenses, employment and training history, and other key documentation.

PROVIDERS

PHYSICIAN ANESTHESIOLOGIST

An anesthesiologist in the United States has completed a 4-year undergraduate degree that includes satisfying premed requirements, 4 years of medical school, and 4 more years of an anesthesia residency. Following successful completion of a residency program, candidates are eligible to sit for the American Board of Anesthesiology certification examination. Almost 90% of anesthesiologists are board certified.

Following residency, many anesthesiologists also complete an additional fellowship year of specialty training in specific areas such as pain management, cardiac anesthesia, pediatric anesthesia, neuroanesthesia, obstetric anesthesia, or critical care medicine.

Anesthesiologists may also seek certification in one of the following subspecialties, which require additional training and examinations: critical care medicine, hospice and palliative medicine, pain medicine.[1]

CERTIFIED REGISTERED NURSE ANESTHETIST

The requirements for becoming a certified registered nurse anesthetist (CRNA) mainly include a bachelor's degree in nursing or other appropriate baccalaureate degree, registered nurse licensure, a minimum of 1 year of acute care experience (eg, intensive care unit [ICU], emergency department), and the successful completion of both an accredited nurse anesthesia educational program and the certification examination.[2]

OTHER TYPES OF PROVIDERS

Anesthesiologist assistants (AAs) have first completed an undergraduate degree that includes a core of required courses in biomedically related sciences, followed by satisfactory completion of a graduate degree (typically 2 years) in an accredited AA education program. Upon completion of a program, a student may become certified by passing the National Commission for Certification of Anesthesiologist Assistants examination (NCCAA). As nonphysician anesthetists, AAs work under the direction of licensed anesthesiologists to implement anesthesia care plans. An AA may not practice outside the field of anesthesia or apart from the supervision of an anesthesiologist.[1]

Physician assistants (PAs) are licensed to practice medicine with physician supervision. Graduation from an accredited PA program and passage of the national certifying examination are required for state licensure. The average PA program curriculum takes approximately 26.5 months to complete.[3]

Nurse practitioner (NPS) first earn a bachelor's degree in nursing (4 years of education), followed by their graduate NP degree (2-4 years of education), which (depending on state regulations) may provide opportunities for independent practice; such programs also permit specialization in career tracks such as oncology, pediatrics, and geriatrics although not specifically in anesthesia practice because this area is covered by the CRNA programs. However, NPs may assist practices in such areas as preoperative evaluation, postoperative care, and so on.

Anesthesia technician/technologists support the work of anesthesia clinical providers and often assist with monitoring lines, patient transport, patient and room preparation, and stocking of equipment at the anesthetizing site.

STAFFING MODELS

Staffing models require careful consideration of several issues, including the complexity of the case, experience of the provider, physical status of the patient, hospital regulations, surgeon expectations, and provider/resident/student nurse anesthetist teaching rules.

PERSONALLY PERFORMED

From a billing perspective, for a Medicare case, personally performed means the following:

- The physician personally performed the entire anesthesia service alone (full payment to physician); or,
- The physician is involved with 1 or 2 anesthesia cases with residents, and the physician is the teaching physician as defined by Medicare rules and regulations (full payment to physician); or,
- The physician is continuously involved in a single case involving a student nurse anesthetist (full payment to physician); or,
- The physician is continuously involved in one anesthesia case involving a CRNA (or AA); both the CRNA (or AA) and the physician may be paid pursuant to the medical direction payment policy (50% payment to physician and 50% payment to CRNA or CRNA's employer such as the hospital or physician group); or,
- The physician and the CRNA (or AA) are involved in one anesthesia case, and the services of each are found to be medically necessary. Upon review of documentation, if it is determined that both were necessary for the case, then full payment may be made for each of the 2 providers (full payment to physician and full payment to CRNA or CRNA's employer, ie, the hospital or physician group).[5]

CARE TEAM

If not performing a case independently, an anesthesiologist generally oversees CRNAs, student registered nurse anesthetists, AAs, interns, residents, or combinations of these individuals. In some care team models, Medicare considers that medical direction has been met, and 50% payment made, if the physician medically directs qualified individuals in 2, 3, or 4 concurrent cases and the physician performs each of the following activities:

1. Performs a preanesthetic examination and evaluation
2. Prescribes the anesthesia plan
3. Personally participates in the most demanding procedures in the anesthesia plan, including, if applicable, induction and emergence
4. Ensures that any procedure in the anesthesia plan that he or she does not perform are performed by a qualified anesthetist
5. Documents his or her presence during some portion of the anesthesia monitoring and monitors the course of anesthesia administration at frequent intervals
6. Remains physically present and available for immediate diagnosis and treatment of emergencies
7. Provides indicated postanesthesia care

These "7 steps," as they are known, must be met to bill Medicare for a medically directed service. Also, the total number of rooms that could be covered at any given time is limited to 4. Exceptions to these medical direction rules allow a physician to perform other specific services and not violate the medical direction rules described. The overall medical direction rules apply to cases involving student nurse anesthetists if the physician directs 2 concurrent cases, each of which involves a student nurse anesthetist or the physician directs one case involving a student nurse anesthetist and another involving a CRNA, AA, or resident.

If anesthesiologists are in a group practice, one physician member may provide the preanesthesia examination and evaluation while another fulfills the other criteria. Similarly, one physician member of the group may provide postanesthesia care while another member of the group furnishes the other component parts of the anesthesia service.

A physician who directs the administration of anesthesia to not more than 4 surgical patients cannot ordinarily be involved in furnishing additional services to other patients. However, addressing an emergency of short duration in the immediate area, administering an epidural or caudal anesthetic to ease labor pain, or periodic rather than continuous monitoring of an obstetric patient does not substantially diminish the scope of control exercised by the physician in directing the administration of anesthesia to surgical patients. It does not constitute a separate service for the purpose of determining whether the medical direction criteria are met. Furthermore, while directing concurrent anesthesia procedures, a physician may receive patients entering the operating room suite for the next surgery, check or discharge patients in the recovery room, or handle scheduling matters without affecting fee schedule payment.[5]

IN- AND OUT-OF-OPERATING-ROOM COVERAGE

Health care advances have led to the significant growth of interventional/procedural medicine, and anesthesia providers are being asked to respond to this trend. Anesthesiologists have expanded their workplace beyond the confines of the operating rooms and are traversing the hospital campus to anesthetize patients undergoing a diverse mix of procedures in locations such as electrophysiology or cardiac catheterization laboratories, radiology suites, in vitro fertilization sites, and endoscopy rooms. In addition to off-site procedural locations, anesthesia providers often cover diverse services, such as preoperative assessment clinics, recovery areas, obstetric services, inpatient pain consultative services, outpatient pain clinics, and critical care units. Each location requires a unique anesthesia staffing pattern influenced by volume, clinical complexity, geographic proximity to other anesthesia locations and providers (an important factor for emergency backup and coverage for personal breaks), efficiency demands (turnover times in the operating rooms, patient visits in preoperative or pain clinics), and service/availability demands (dedicated ICU or obstetrics staff). Meeting these multiple and often competing demands for clinical services can be challenging. Coverage of multiple hospitals and other locations requires either dedicated staff for each location or staff that is highly flexible about assignments.

Staffing patterns vary widely by location, from 1:1 coverage of complex surgical cases to 1:4 coverage of routine surgical cases. Financial performance associated with each location is closely linked to efficiency, case volume, and payer mix and should be closely monitored by the group.

FINANCIAL MANAGEMENT

Viewed from a national perspective, academic anesthesia departments and private practice anesthesia groups both face a myriad of financial challenges due to both revenue and expense concerns. Revenue constraints include contract rates and reimbursement policies dictated by Medicare and other payers, billing office performance, and hospital support for medical administration, CRNA expenses, and trauma or other call coverage. Expenses are heavily influenced by recruitment and retention needs because professional staff salaries and fringe benefits compose most of the anesthesia practice expenses.

Successful financial management requires a thorough understanding of financial statements, effective budgeting, strong financial oversight, and paying great attention to detail. In today's health care environment, thin operating margins require innovative approaches to important business problems. Often the best business solutions may be technology intensive (eg, electronic charge capture and billing systems, electronic staff scheduling/deployment systems).

UNDERSTANDING FINANCIAL STATEMENTS

Although a detailed understanding of financial statements may be daunting to clinicians, a basic understanding of them is necessary for effective practice management oversight. Many business managers use at least 3 basic financial statements to document and assess their practice's financial performance: the income statement (or profit-and-loss statement), the balance sheet, and the cash flow statement.

The income statement summarizes a practice's revenue (primarily from professional services rendered to patients) less expenses (support staff compensation, benefits, malpractice insurance premiums, etc) for a particular month, quarter, or year. The final net figure, usually referred to as the bottom line, is of most concern, but understanding the details that have an impact on that number is also very important.

The balance sheet is used to describe the financial position at a given point in time by detailing practice assets, liabilities, and equity. Assets represent things of value that a practice owns or something that will be received and can be measured objectively. What a practice owes to others are considered liabilities. These include taxes collected from employees but not yet remitted, payments due to an agency for services already provided, and so on. They are obligations that must be paid under certain conditions and time frames. A practice's equity represents funds contributed or retained by the partners or shareholders, who accept the uncertainty that comes with ownership risk in exchange for a potential long-term return on their investment. Assets must always equal liabilities plus equity.

The cash flow statement provides an explanation of uses of cash (ie, cash from patients and insurance companies, investment income, etc). Understanding how much cash a practice has and how much cash a practice needs is essential to ensure that bills can be paid on time, payroll can be processed, and so on.

BUDGETING

A budget is a quantitative financial plan for a defined period of time that serves to articulate financial and operational goals, objectives, and strategic plans. A budget allows you to quantify and prioritize these goals, objectives, and plans and provides you with a way to measure financial and operational performance. Approaches to budgets include the historical (uses historical data updated with new facts, trends, and assumptions), zero-based/bottom-up (assumes all costs must be justified), and flexible budgeting methodologies (updated throughout the budget period according to major cost drivers such as volume). Capital budgets focus on projects or tangible assets (eg, property, plant, or equipment items) that exceed a certain expense threshold. Important operating budget considerations include professional staff salaries and fringe benefits, payer reimbursement assumptions, malpractice costs, operational changes (such as additional anesthetizing locations), and investment income returns. Revenue budget assumptions should address volume growth of anesthetic procedures, contract rates for payment, payer mix, and collection rates, although expense budget assumptions should consider the impact of staffing needs (resignations and hiring), compensation and incentive plans, and inflationary costs. Operating room utilization and efficiency influence both staffing needs and revenue generation, and therefore they should be carefully reviewed as part of the budgetary process.

REVENUES AND EXPENSES

The 3 main sources of anesthesia practice revenues are patient services revenue, contract revenue, and nonoperating revenue (interest and investment income). For the purposes of this discussion, we exclude other income sources such as research grants, philanthropy, royalty income, and endowments.

Clinical volume and type of service, contract rates, payer mix, and billing performance are the main drivers of patient services revenue. Contract revenue may be derived from professional services agreements, hospital stipends, or other management service contracts. Major expense categories include physician and CRNA compensation and benefits, support staff expenses, malpractice fees, billing and overhead fees, depreciation, bad debt (mostly for uninsured or underinsured patients), and other operating expenses such as rent, utilities, and information technology. It is important to understand which expenses are fixed (costs that remain constant despite changes in case volume, eg, anesthesia machines) rather than variable (costs that fluctuate with volume, eg, anesthetic drugs), particularly if volume predictions are uncertain. For example, when hiring additional staff to cover a new anesthetizing location, the practice will incur a fixed and incremental compensation expense, but revenue will depend on the volume and efficiency of the newly added site unless otherwise negotiated in advance with the hospital.

FINANCIAL ANALYSIS

Practice profitability requires an ongoing analysis of performance against expectations, goals, and targets. Essential financial analyses should include periodic budget analyses of the variance between actual and budgeted performance, service-specific margin analyses (percentage by which revenues exceed expenses; may be calculated on a direct, total, or contribution basis), and benchmarking analyses (comparison to published compensation,* productivity, billing, and expenses† data).

CAPITAL

Large capital (tangible asset) items such as anesthesia machines, monitoring equipment, and electronic medical records typically are purchased through the hospital and may require advanced planning via the capital budgeting process. Smaller items, such as computers for administrative use, may be purchased through practice funds.

BILLING AND PAYMENT FOR ANESTHESIA SERVICES

PROFESSIONAL VERSUS TECHNICAL BILLING

The provision of anesthesia services is paid for by 2 separate reimbursement mechanisms: a technical or facility fee and a professional fee. Third-party payers compensate the hospital for the technical or nonprofessional costs of anesthesia services via the facility fee (eg, anesthesia equipment, supplies, and technicians), although professional and practice expenses are reimbursed through professional fees. Facility fees or charges are derived from the duration and type of anesthetic services rendered and reimbursed via payer-specific contract rates (eg, diagnosis-related group (DRG) or case rate, percentage of charges, fee for service).

PROFESSIONAL BILLING FOR ANESTHESIA, OBSTETRIC, CRITICAL CARE, AND PAIN MANAGEMENT SERVICES

Medicare payments for most physician services are made on the basis of a standardized fee schedule (resource-based relative value scale [RBRVS]) that was implemented in 1992, which replaced the traditional customary and prevailing charge system. However, Medicare's method of calculating anesthesia professional reimbursement for anesthesia services differs from that used for other physician services in that the relative value units (RVUs) are based on a schedule developed and maintained by the American Society of Anesthesiologists (ASA). The anesthesia RVUs for any service are described as "base units" and correlate to work effort (ie, estimated anesthetic intensity or complexity). In addition to base units, payment for anesthesia services reflect time units (often 15 minutes per unit), additional modifying units (eg, physical status), on occasion, and an anesthesia-specific conversion factor (or per unit payment rate). Professional fee schedules for most other payers are reflective of Medicare's approach under the RBRVS system. Monitoring catheters and nerve blocks administered during time-based anesthesia services are billed separately.‡

Concurrency modifiers are used to indicate the type of oversight rendered by the attending anesthesiologist in conjunction with a resident and/or CRNA. Personally performed (modifier AA) indicates that an attending anesthesiologist was present for the entire case, whereas medical direction (QK or QY) denotes concomitant involvement in 1, 2, 3, or 4 anesthetics in conjunction with a resident or CRNA. The CRNA portion of a medically directed case is billed with a QX modifier. Medical supervision (AD) indicates physician involvement in more than 4 concurrent cases.

Billing for nonsurgical obstetric anesthesia (ie, labor epidurals) typically follows 1 of 4 methods recommended by the ASA: (1) base units plus patient contact time plus one time unit per hour, (2) base units plus time units subject to a reasonable cap, (3) a flat fee, and (4) an incremental fee schedule.§

Critical care, acute pain, and chronic pain management services are billed as evaluation and management services and procedures and reimbursed under the RBRVS system. Critical care services are billed based on physician time expended (eg, <30 min, 30-74 min). Acute and chronic pain services are billed via a variety of current procedural terminology (CPT) codes,** including inpatient consultations, subsequent hospital day care, new patient visits, follow-up visits, and interventional procedures.

DOCUMENTATION AND CODING

Adequate medical record documentation is required to substantiate billing for all anesthesia services with specific criteria established by local payers based on current Medicare rules or the payer's specific policies. The coding of anesthesia services (assignment of appropriate nationally standardized codes indicating the type of procedure or service rendered) typically is performed by professional coders employed directly by the practice or by the billing office. Documentation and coding are essential for compliance purposes and for negotiating the claims denial and appeals process.

CHARGES VERSUS PAYMENTS

A professional charge for a time-based anesthesia service is generated based on the total number of ASA units (base, time, and additional modifying units) and procedures where the unit and procedure charges are set by the physician practice. The payment or reimbursement usually is based on negotiated contract rates and varies by payer. The key differences between charges and payments are the result of contractual adjustments and write-offs. For example, for a practice with a $100 per ASA unit charge, a 7-hour triple coronary artery bypass would generate a charge of $4800 (for 20 time units plus 28 base units). Medicare reimbursement†† for this case if personally performed, however, would total $1080 based on the $22.50 conversion factor (Philadelphia, 2010)‡‡ with a $3720 contractual adjustment.

Reimbursement for invasive monitors (arterial or pulmonary arterial catheters, etc), regional anesthetic blocks, evaluation and management services, and other procedures are based on a flat fee schedule negotiated with each payer rather than ASA units. Whereas charges are influenced by volume and service mix, payments are affected by payer mix, contract rates, and payer policies, and the speed of payment depends on submission of "clean claims."

BILLING SERVICES

Anesthesia practices may choose to bill and collect for their own professional fees or outsource these activities to a billing company. Given the complexities of anesthesia billing, it is essential to employ a service with expertise in this area. Such expertise often is difficult to recruit and retain in-house for small to midsize anesthesia groups and may be outsourced to a billing company. The accuracy of claims is the responsibility of the physician group independent of billing service arrangements, so it is imperative that billing functions be monitored closely and include a robust compliance plan (see "Billing Compliance" later). Billing performance should be closely monitored by the practice/department to continually ensure accuracy, effectiveness, and efficiency (**Table 97-1**).

*The Association of American Medical Colleges (AAMC), Society of Academic Anesthesiology Chairs (SAAC)/Association of Anesthesiology Program Directors (AAPD), Medical Group Management Association (MGMA) academic and private practice compensation surveys.

†MGMA best performing practices.

‡Assumes that these services were not the primary mode of anesthesia and were not included in the calculation of anesthesia time units unless clinically appropriate.

§Reimbursement for surgical obstetric anesthesia is based on time and base units as described earlier.

**CPT Code Book.

††Sample calculation only; not reflective of Medicare payment reduction for concurrency.

‡‡2010 Medicare anesthesia conversion factor for metropolitan Philadelphia.

TABLE 97-1 Analysis of Billing Performance

1. Monthly review of key statistics (budgeted vs actual, current vs prior year)
   a. Volume, charges, and payments
   b. Payer mix
   c. Days in accounts receivable, aged accounts receivable
   d. Charge or front-end lag (number of days from date of anesthetic service to date of claim submission)
   e. Case reconciliation (verification that all cases performed resulted in sending out a claim to the correct payor)
2. Collection rate variance and volume/service mix variance by payer
3. Per unit reimbursement analysis (actual vs contract rate)
4. Write-offs by type (free care, account settlement, bad debt, payer policy, filing limits, provider enrollment, missing referral/authorization, etc)
5. Matched collection rates at 2-, 6-, and 9-month intervals (gross collection rate, net collection rate, adjudication rate)

MANAGED CARE CONTRACTING

NEGOTIATION STRATEGIES

Before you begin negotiations, be sure you have an accurate and realistic understanding of the value your group brings to the hospital or contracting organization. That is important because if you cannot come to an agreement with the payer, your only option will be not to contract with them. If the hospital has a contract with that payer and many of the surgeons have a contract with that payer, you will be under tremendous pressure to obtain a contract with that payer. If you do not, you must be in a position to present data that can explain why.

It is critical to educate the payer and the hospital about anesthesia salaries in the local market, what others pay, the national shortages, and other issues that are well known to you but may not be known to the payer or the hospital. Make sure what you are asking for is reasonable and your explanation is understandable.

Understand each payer's fee schedule, not just their anesthesia per unit rate. Many practices are provided a fair anesthesia per unit rate; however, their fee schedule for procedures (eg, pulmonary arterial catheter insertion) or for pain or critical care services may be inadequate. Understand where your primary business volumes incur, and be sure you can prioritize what services are most important when negotiating your fee schedule.

Do not allow a payer to dictate policies and fee schedules; however, you also must be realistic regarding a fair-market payment scale in your local community. Like most negotiations, it is best if the final agreement is a win/win. An important but frequently overlooked contract issue is being sure that if the payer does not pay quickly or underpays, there should be clear language regarding the penalties and next steps to resolve the problem.

DATA ANALYSIS AND REPORTING

Physicians and many administrators tend to want too much data that may not be pertinent to understanding their practice and practice operations. Focusing on the key issues leads to more effective analysis with fewer distractions.

TRACKING WHAT YOU NEED TO KNOW

Tracking what you need to know falls into 3 categories:

1. Information needed to ensure that your billing process is collecting all the money that should be collected
2. Information to be comfortable that your billing process is meeting all billing compliance rules and regulations
3. Information that notes trends to which your practice may need to react or form a strategic plan

In general, you want to be sure that every service you rendered is captured and whatever monies that contractually should be collected for those services are collected. You want to be sure that services are reconciled against case logs (eg, operating room final schedules) so you know what services were rendered and you have a charge to submit for that service. You need to know what bills have been paid and whether or not they have been paid correctly. Of all the bills that are not yet fully paid, how old (aged) are they, and what is being done to collect the remainder (payment plan has been set up, etc)?

Following a statistically valid sample of random accounts through the revenue cycle process is a helpful method for fully understanding how the system is working and validate some of the monthly data. If you review randomly selected cases from the operating room schedules and track each through the billing cycle, you will have a very good sense of how your billing process is working. Sometimes reports of average data and group numbers do not always tell the entire story. This sampling process, although somewhat time consuming, is a great way to know what is truly happening and whether or not your monthly reports are accurate.

BILLING METRICS AND TRENDS

Trends are important for strategic purposes. Remember, 1 month does not a crisis make. Some of the monthly information that should be tracked for trend purposes includes the following:

- Total cases and total anesthesia units (is volume increasing or decreasing?)
- Cases and anesthesia units per location and per FTE physician
- Payer mix (especially if better payers are being replaced by poorer payers over time)
- Charge lag (how long it takes from when you render the service until the charge is entered into the billing system)
- Charges, contractual adjustments, and cash collections in total and by division/location/FTE (eg, ambulatory surgery center, multiple hospitals, acute pain, chronic pain, critical care, etc)
- Accounts receivable (is the total accounts open and still due to be paid growing or decreasing over time?)
- Net collection rate (collections divided by gross charges less contractual adjustments plus refunds). This should not be confused with gross collection rate, which is a more common measure that has less value in our opinion. Essentially, the net collection rate is a measure of how much money is being collected as a percentage of what is collectable. For example, if your charge was $1500 and you have a contract that payer X agrees to pay you 60% of your charges, then your expected payment would be $900. If you are paid $850, then your net collection rate is 94%. Generally, depending on factors such as self-pay or charity care, a net collection rate in the high 80s to mid-90s would be expected.
- Days in accounts receivable (how long it takes to collect the money due on your charges)
- Percentage of accounts receivable older than 90 days from date of service (the older past due accounts age, the less likely it is that you will eventually collect them)
- Total credit balances (many times credit balances grow and mask other problems)
- Collection agency net collections (many practices worry about what a collection agency charges, yet what really matters is how much money they collect for you net of their fees). Some larger practices always have 2 collection agencies and split what is turned over to each evenly and then track the net results. When one agency outperforms the other over time, they may drop the lower performer and contract with a new agency.

BILLING COMPLIANCE

Although it may seem at times that all the myriad of rules and regulations are in place just to make the practice of anesthesiology more difficult, there are reasons why compliance with various rules and regulations is both important and pertinent. The consequences of not knowing or not following these regulations can be substantial, both legally and financially.

Note that Medicare rules and regulations change occasionally, and sometimes they are interpreted differently by various carriers and agencies, so always check with your practice leadership and billing compliance experts as well as your local carrier to ensure that your understanding of billing practices rules and regulations are up-to-date and correctly interpreted for the state in which you are located.

COMMON PROBLEMS

What scenarios seem to present the most opportunities for anesthesia billing compliance problems?

- *Physicians not understanding the billing rules and regulations.* Anesthesia time starts when the anesthesia practitioner begins to prepare the patient for anesthesia services in the operating room or an equivalent area and ends when the anesthesia practitioner is no longer furnishing anesthesia services to the patient, that is, when the patient can be placed safely under postoperative care. It rarely correlates with the surgical start and stop times or the in- or out-of-operating-room times. Because the stop time often occurs after the patient leaves the operating room and the begin time often starts before the patient is brought into the operating room, the chance for overlap is obvious. Overlap is not a problem as long as it is properly documented and the impact on medical direction billing is understood and followed. The problem occurs when the billing does not accurately reflect the existence or extent of simultaneous care (ie, "concurrency").
- *Medically directing more than 4 concurrent cases.* When the physician is responsible for more than 4 concurrent cases, he or she is no longer medically directing any of them. Exceeding 4 cases has significant negative ramifications on your overall reimbursement. Even a 1-minute overlap invokes billing concurrency that may have an impact on billing regulations and reimbursement amounts. **Figure 97-1** illustrates a typical workday and the consequences of 1 minute of overlap that affects reimbursement significantly. In this illustration, Case 1 in Room A started at 7:31 and finished at 11:32. Case 2 in Room B started at 7:52 and finished at 8:46. Case 3 in Room C started at 8:00 and finished at 14:12. Case 4 started in Room D at 7:15 and finished at 8:42. Case 5 started in Room B at 8:42 and finished at 13:14. During the 8:42 interval, the anesthesiologist actually was responsible for 5 cases. Even though it was only for that 1 minute, all 5 cases now are considered nonmedically directed.
- *Rounding.* It is a mistake, and wrong, to round your start and/or stop times, even if you are rounding to less time. Many physicians believe that because different clocks may not be synchronized, then they can just round because it really is only a matter of minutes. That rationalization may seem appropriate, but in reality billing compliance requires exact minutes to be reported, not more and not less. It may seem obvious why rounding up would be inappropriate, but why would rounding down? The situation just described is a good example to illustrate the reasoning for this seemingly innocent action. If the physician had rounded down, then Case 5 would have been noted as starting at 8:45 instead of 8:42. Case 4 would have been noted as ending at 8:40 instead of 8:42. The total minutes charged to each case actually would be less than the total minutes the physician was responsible for each case, so it would appear that, if anything, the physician would be shortchanging his or her reimbursement by several minutes. In reality, it would mean that instead of 5 cases being handled concurrently, the maximum concurrent cases now would appear to only be 4, thus greatly improving reimbursement because all the cases now would be considered medically directed, resulting in much greater payment.
- *Not meeting the other noted necessary criteria for medical direction* (eg, relieving a CRNA in a room for a break while still being responsible for the other rooms). Taking over a case by yourself does not allow you to medically direct other concurrent cases. Likewise, not being present for induction or emergence would prevent that particular case from being considered medically directed.
- *Forgetting that if it is not documented, it did not happen.*
- *Having a written policy in place and then not following it.* If you have a policy, you had better make sure you can follow it, do follow it, and have a process in place to monitor compliance and take corrective action if individuals do not comply.

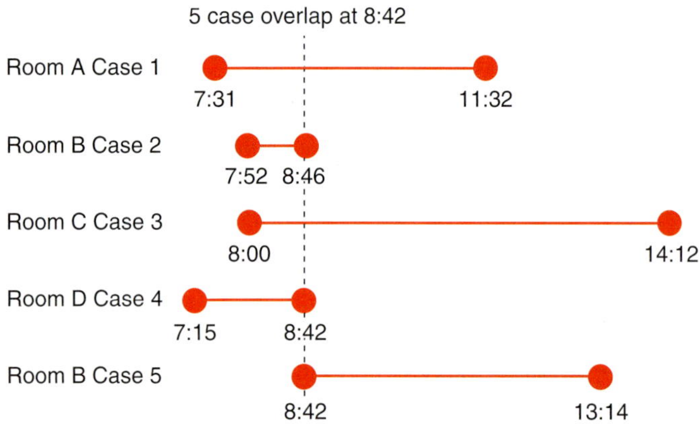

FIGURE 97-1. Example of an overlap of 5 concurrent cases.

SUMMARY

Practice management is the structure that supports the primary function of anesthesia practice, that of delivering anesthesia care to needy patients in operating rooms, obstetric units, radiology suites, intensive care units, and pain management centers. Effective communication, management, and billing functions are essential for individual provider satisfaction and for the vitality of the practice group. As with clinical care, it is often the small details that make the difference between a thriving cohesive practice and one that is failing or fraught with dissension.

KEY REFERENCES

- American Academy of Nurse Practitioners. Position statement on nurse practitioner curriculum. http://www.aanp.org/AANPCMS2/AboutAANP/NPCurriculum.htm. Accessed June 16, 2010.
- American Academy of Physician Assistants. Becoming a physician assistant. http://www.aapa.org/about-pas/becoming-a-physician-assistant. Accessed June 16, 2010.
- American Association of Nurse Anesthetists. Becoming a CRNA. http://www.aana.com/BecomingCRNA.aspx?id=98&linkidentifier=id&itemid=98. Accessed June 16, 2010.
- American Society of Anesthesiologists What is an anesthesiologist? http://www.asahq.org/providers/homepage.htm. Accessed June 16, 2010.
- CMS Centers for Medicare & Medicaid Services—Anesthesiologists Center. Medicare Claims Processing Manual. Chapter 12: Physicians/Nonphysician Practitioners, pp. 111-119. http://www.cms.gov/manuals/downloads/clm104c12.pdf. Accessed June 16, 2010.

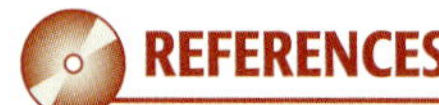

REFERENCES

Complete references available on DVD and online version at www.LongneckerAnesthesiology.com

APPENDIX

Formulary

Mark Dershwitz
Carl Rosow

TABLE A-1 Analgesic Agents

Drug	Route	Usual Dose	How Supplied	Form	Cost*
Oral COX Inhibitors					
Acetaminophen	PO	325-1000 mg	325, 500 mg	Tablet	0.01
Aspirin	PO	325-1000 mg	325, 500 mg	Tablet	0.05
Celecoxib	PO	100-400 mg	100 mg 200 mg 400 mg	Capsule Capsule Capsule	2.03 3.32 4.98
Choline magnesium trisalicylate	PO	500-1000 mg	500 mg 1000 mg	Caplet Caplet	0.35 0.86
Diclofenac	PO	50-75 mg	50 mg 75 mg	Tablet Tablet	0.80 1.10
Diflunisal	PO	500-1000 mg	500 mg	Tablet	0.66
Ibuprofen	PO	200-800 mg	200 mg 400 mg 600 mg 800 mg	Tablet Tablet Tablet Tablet	0.02 0.04 0.05 0.08
Indomethacin	PO	25-50 mg	25 mg	Capsule	0.04
Ketorolac	PO	10 mg	10 mg	Tablet	0.68
Naproxen	PO	250-500 mg	250 mg 375 mg 500 mg	Tablet Tablet Tablet	0.10 0.08 0.08
Piroxicam	PO PO	10-40 mg	10 mg 20 mg	Capsule Capsule	0.09 0.11
Sulindac	PO	150 mg	150 mg	Tablet	0.33
Oral Opioids					
Codeine	PO	30-60 mg	30 mg 60 mg	Tablet Tablet	0.47 0.86
Codeine/acetaminophen	PO	30-60 mg/300 mg	30/300 mg 60/300 mg	Tablet Tablet	0.47 0.75
Hydrocodone/acetaminophen	PO	5-7.5 mg/500-1000 mg	5 mg/500 mg 7.5 mg/750 mg	Tablet Tablet	0.15 0.27
Hydromorphone	PO	2-4 mg¶	2 mg	Tablet	0.36
Levorphanol	PO	2 mg¶	2 mg	Tablet	0.80
Methadone	PO	10-20 mg¶	10 mg	Tablet	0.18
Morphine	PO	30-60 mg	30 mg 2 mg/mL, 5 mL	Tablet Solution	0.23 0.58
Morphine sustained release	PO	30-60 mg¶	30 mg	Caplet	1.20
Oxycodone	PO	5-10 mg	5 mg	Tablet	0.26
Oxycodone/acetaminophen	PO	5-10 mg/500-1000 mg	5 mg/500 mg	Caplet	0.20
Oxycodone sustained release	PO	10-20 mg¶	10 mg 20 mg 40 mg 80 mg	Tablet Tablet Tablet Tablet	1.52 2.93 5.18 9.75
Tramadol	PO	50-100 mg	50 mg	Tablet	0.09
Tramadol/acetaminophen	PO	75 mg/650 mg		Tablet	0.77

(*Continued*)

TABLE A-1 Analgesic Agents (*Continued*)

Drug	Route	Usual Dose	How Supplied	Form	Cost*
Transdermal and Transmucosal Opioids					
Fentanyl	Transdermal	25-100 mcg/h	25 mcg/h 50 mcg/h 75 mcg/h 100 mcg/h	Patch Patch Patch Patch	9.75 17.81 27.17 36.05
Fentanyl	Transbuccal	200-1600 mcg	200 mcg 400 mcg 800 mcg	Lozenge Lozenge Lozenge	17.67 25.68 41.08
Parenteral COX Inhibitors					
Acetaminophen	IV	1000 mg	10 mg/mL, 10 mL	Solution	10.60
Ketorolac	IV IM	30 mg 60 mg	30 mg/mL, 1 mL 30 mg/mL, 2 mL	Solution Solution	1.00 1.07
Parecoxib[§]	IV/IM	20-40 mg	40 mg	Powder	§
Parenteral Opioids					
Alfentanil	IV	0.3-3 mcg/kg/min	500 mcg/mL, 2 mL 500 mcg/mL, 5 mL	Solution Solution	3.87 7.25
Codeine	IV/IM	30-60 mg	30 mg/mL, 2 mL	Solution	2.18
Fentanyl	IV	0.5-5 mcg/kg	50 mcg/mL, 2 mL 50 mcg/mL, 5 mL 50 mcg/mL, 20 mL	Solution Solution Solution	0.53 0.72 2.70
Hydromorphone	IV/IM	0.5-2 mg	2 mg/mL, 1 mL	Solution	0.68
Meperidine	IV/IM/SC	12.5-100 mg	100 mg/mL, 1 mL	Solution	0.63
Methadone	IV	1-10 mg	10 mg/mL, 20 mL	Solution	101.25
Morphine	IV/IM/SC	1-10 mg	10 mg/mL, 1 mL	Solution	0.57
Oxymorphone	IV/IM	1.5 mg	1 mg/mL, 1 mL	Solution	2.35
Remifentanil	IV	0.01-1 mcg/kg/min	1 mg 2 mg 5 mg	Powder Powder Powder	23.58 44.69 92.30
Sufentanil	IV	0.05-0.5 mcg/kg	50 mcg/mL, 1 mL 50 mcg/mL, 5 mL	Solution Solution	3.14 12.64
Epidural Opioids					
Fentanyl[‡]	Epidural Epidural	25-100 mcg 1-4 mcg/mL, 5-10 mL/h	50 mcg/mL, 2 mL	Solution	0.53
Hydromorphone[‡]	Epidural Epidural	0.75-1.5 mg 10-100 mcg/mL, 5-10 mL/h	2 mg/mL, 1 mL	Solution	0.68
Meperidine[‡‡]	Epidural	25-75 mg	100 mg/mL, 1 mL	Solution	0.63
Methadone	Epidural	1-5 mg	10 mg/mL, 20 mL	Solution	101.25
Morphine	Epidural	2-5 mg	0.5 mg/mL, 10 mL	Solution, preservative-free	9.83
Morphine extended-release liposome injection	Epidural	10-20 mg	10 mg/mL, 1 mL 10 mg/mL, 1.5 mL	Solution, liposomal Solution, liposomal	309.09 463.64
Sufentanil	Epidural	20-50 mcg	50 mcg/mL, 1 mL	Solution	3.14
Intrathecal Opioids					
Fentanyl[‡]		10-25 mcg	50 mcg/mL, 2 mL	Solution	0.53
Meperidine[‡‡]		10-20 mg	100 mg/mL, 1 mL	Solution	0.63
Morphine		0.25-0.5 mg	0.5 mg/mL, 10 mL	Solution, preservative free	9.83
Sufentanil[‡]		3-10 mcg	50 mcg/mL, 1 mL	Solution	3.14

(*Continued*)

TABLE A-1 Analgesic Agents (*Continued*)

Drug	Route	Usual Dose	How Supplied	Form	Cost*
Opioid Agonist/Antagonists					
Buprenorphine	IV	0.3 mg	0.3 mg/mL, 1 mL	Solution	2.52
Butorphanol	IV/IM Nasal	0.5-2 mg 1-2 mg (1-2 sprays)	2 mg/mL, 1 mL 10 mg/mL, 2.5 mL	Solution Solution	2.70 59.45
Nalbuphine	IV/IM	5-10 mg	10 mg/mL, 1 mL	Solution	1.50
Opioid Antagonists					
Alvimopan	PO	6-12 mg	12 mg	Tablet	56.25
Methylnaltrexone	SC	8-12 mg	20 mg/mL, 0.6 mL	Solution	36.00
Naloxone	IV/IM	0.04-1 mg	0.4 mg/mL, 1 mL	Solution	3.06
Naltrexone	PO	50 mg	50 mg	Tablet	3.03
Opioid Adjuncts					
Carbamazepine	PO	200-400 mg	200 mg	Tablet	0.08
Gabapentin	PO	300-1800 mg	300 mg	Capsule	0.12
Pregabalin	PO	50-100 mg	50 mg	Capsule	2.02

*Reflects the cost to a hospital that is part of a large buying group for the size and form listed.

†The required preservative-free preparation is generally not available in the United States.

‡Not approved by the Food and Drug Administration for this indication in the United States.

§An investigational agent in the United States.

¶Much higher doses are commonly used in opioid-tolerant patients.

TABLE A-2 Sedative, Hypnotic, and General Anesthetic Agents

Drug	Route	Usual Dose	How Supplied	Form	Cost*
Barbiturates					
Methohexital	IV PR	1-2 mg/kg 25 mg/kg	500 mg	Powder	38.64
Thiopental	IV	3-6 mg/kg	500 mg	Powder	†
Benzodiazepines					
Diazepam	IV PO	2-10 mg 5-10 mg	5 mg/mL, 2 mL 5 mg	Solution Tablet	2.74 0.07
Lorazepam	IV/IM	1-5 mg	2 mg/mL, 1 mL	Solution	0.95
Midazolam	IV/IM PO	1-5 mg 0.5-0.75 mg/kg	1 mg/mL, 2 mL 2 mg/mL, 118 mL	Solution Solution	0.59 60.94
Benzodiazepine Antagonist					
Flumazenil	IV	0.5-1 mg	0.1 mg/mL, 5 mL	Solution	6.30
Antihistamines					
Diphenhydramine	IV/IM	25 mg	50 mg/mL, 1 mL	Solution	0.33
Hydroxyzine	IM	25 mg	50 mg/mL, 1 mL	Solution	0.70
Promethazine	IV/IM	6.25-12.5 mg	25 mg/mL, 1 mL	Solution	0.60
Neuroleptics					
Chlorpromazine	IV/IM	25-100 mg	25 mg/mL, 1 mL	Solution	1.35
Droperidol	IV/IM	2.5-10 mg	2.5 mg/mL, 2 mL	Solution	1.00
Haloperidol	IV/IM	1-5 mg	5 mg/mL, 1 mL	Solution	5.70

(*Continued*)

TABLE A-2 Sedative, Hypnotic, and General Anesthetic Agents (*Continued*)

Drug	Route	Usual Dose	How Supplied	Form	Cost*
Volatile Anesthetics					
Desflurane	Inhalation	MAC = 6.0%	240 mL	Liquid	136.03
Enflurane	Inhalation	MAC = 1.8%	250 mL	Liquid	102.78
Halothane	Inhalation	MAC = 0.75%	250 mL	Liquid	44.76
Isoflurane	Inhalation	MAC = 1.2%	250 mL	Liquid	33.33
Sevoflurane	Inhalation	MAC = 2.0%	250 mL	Liquid	169.20
Others					
Etomidate	IV	0.15-0.3 mg/kg	2 mg/mL, 10 mL	Solution	8.86
Ketamine	IV IV IM	0.2-2 mg/kg 0.2-2 mg/kg 2-5 mg/kg	10 mg/mL, 20 mL 50 mg/mL, 10 mL 100 mg/mL, 5 mL	Solution Solution Solution	14.85 5.63 7.31
Propofol	IV	0.5-2.5 mg/kg 25-150 mcg/kg/min	10 mg/mL, 20 mL 10 mg/mL, 50 mL	Solution Solution	1.98 4.95
Fospropofol	IV	6.5 mg/kg loading dose 1.6 mg/kg supplemental doses	35 mg/mL, 30 mL	Solution	32.40
Dexmedetomidine	IV	0.2-0.7 mcg/kg/h	100 mcg/mL, 2 mL	Solution	61.97

*Reflects the cost to a hospital that is part of a large buying group for the size and form listed.

†Currently not available in the United States.

TABLE A-3 Muscle Relaxants and Reversal Agents

Drug	Route	Usual Dose	How Supplied	Form	Cost*
Depolarizing					
Succinylcholine	IV IM	1-2 mg/kg 4-6 mg/kg	20 mg/mL, 10 mL	Solution	1.68
Nondepolarizing					
Atracurium	IV	0.4 mg/kg	10 mg/mL, 10 mL	Solution	6.30
Cisatracurium	IV	0.2 mg/kg	2 mg/mL, 10 mL	Solution	19.17
Pancuronium	IV	0.1 mg/kg	1 mg/mL, 10 mL	Solution	1.44
Rocuronium	IV	0.6 mg/kg	10 mg/mL, 10 mL	Solution	35.18
Vecuronium	IV	0.1 mg/kg	10 mg	Powder	2.66
Reversal Agents					
Edrophonium	IV	0.5-1 mg/kg	10 mg/mL, 15 mL	Solution	22.50
Neostigmine	IV	0.04-0.08 mg/kg	1 mg/mL, 10 mL	Solution	1.34
Pyridostigmine	IV	0.2-0.4 mg/kg	5 mg/mL, 2 mL	Solution	20.46

*Reflects the cost to a hospital that is part of a large buying group for the size and form listed.

TABLE A-4 Local Anesthetics

Drug	Route	Maximum Dose	Contents	Size	Form	Cost*
Topical						
Cetacaine	Topical	2-s spray	14% benzocaine 2% butamben 2% tetracaine	56 mL	Liquid spray	59.25
Cocaine	Topical	3 mg/kg	4%	10 mL	Solution	46.67
EMLA cream	Topical	20 g	2.5% lidocaine + 2.5% prilocaine	5 g	Cream	8.54
Lidocaine	Topical	5 mg/kg	4% 2% 5%	50 mL 100 mL 35 g	Solution Viscous solution Ointment	6.90 12.40 6.87

(*Continued*)

TABLE A-4 Local Anesthetics (*Continued*)

Drug	Route	Maximum Dose	Contents	Size	Form	Cost*
Spinal						
Bupivacaine	Intrathecal	†	0.75% bupivacaine + 8.25% glucose	2 mL	Solution	1.32
	Intrathecal	†	0.5% bupivacaine[§]	10 mL	Solution	1.73
Lidocaine	Intrathecal	†	1.5% lidocaine + 7.5% glucose	2 mL	Solution	9.00
Tetracaine	Intrathecal	†	1% tetracaine	2 mL	Solution	3.95
Tetracaine	Intrathecal	†	Tetracaine powder	20 mg	Powder	11.25
Epidural/Nerve Block/Local Infiltration[‡]						
Bupivacaine	Injection	3 mg/kg	0.25-0.75% bupivacaine	10 mL	Solution	1.67
				30 mL	Solution	2.41
Chloroprocaine	Injection	12 mg/kg	2% chloroprocaine	30 mL	Solution	5.88
	Injection		3% chloroprocaine	30 mL	Solution	7.46
Lidocaine	Injection	7 mg/kg	0.5% lidocaine	50 mL	Solution	2.84
	Injection		1% lidocaine	2 mL	Solution	1.09
	Injection		1% lidocaine	20 mL	Solution	1.02
	Injection		2% lidocaine	20 mL	Solution	1.45
Mepivacaine	Injection	7 mg/kg	1% mepivacaine	30 mL	Solution	4.11
	Injection		1.5% mepivacaine	30 mL	Solution	4.35
	Injection		2% mepivacaine	20 mL	Solution	6.30
Ropivacaine	Injection	3 mg/kg	0.5% ropivacaine	30 mL	Solution	13.13
	Injection		1% ropivacaine	20 mL	Solution	14.58
IV Regional (Bier Block)						
Lidocaine	Injection	0.75 mL/kg	0.5% lidocaine	50 mL	Solution	2.84

*Reflects the cost to a hospital that is part of a large buying group for the size and form listed.

†Toxic plasma concentrations are unlikely to be achieved via the intrathecal route.

‡This list does not include every concentration and package size available.

§Not approved by the FDA for this indication in the United States.

TABLE A-5 Antiemetics

Drug	Route	Usual Dose	How Supplied	Form	Cost*
Dopamine Antagonists					
Droperidol	IV/IM	0.625-1.25 mg	2.5 mg/mL, 2 mL	Solution	1.00
Haloperidol	IV/IM	1 mg	5 mg/mL, 1 mL	Solution	5.70
Prochlorperazine	IV/IM	10 mg	5 mg/mL, 2 mL	Solution	2.25
Serotonin Antagonists					
Dolasetron	IV	12.5 mg	20 mg/mL, 0.625 mL	Solution	14.06
Granisetron	IV	1 mg	1 mg/mL, 1 mL	Solution	140.54
Ondansetron	IV	4 mg	2 mg/mL, 2 mL	Solution	0.86
Palonosetron	IV	0.075 mg	0.05 mg/mL, 1.5 mL	Solution	39.60
Antihistamines					
Diphenhydramine	IV/IM	25 mg	50 mg/mL, 1 mL	Solution	0.33
Hydroxyzine	IM	25 mg	50 mg/mL, 1 mL	Solution	0.70
Promethazine	IV/IM	6.25-12.5 mg	25 mg/mL, 1 mL	Solution	0.60
Neurokinin Antagonist					
Aprepitant	PO	40 mg	40 mg	Tablet	39.56
Glucocorticoids					
Dexamethasone	IV	4 mg	4 mg/mL, 1 mL	Solution	0.75
Antimuscarinic					
Scopolamine	Transdermal	14 mcg/h	14 mcg/h	Patch	8.19

*Reflects the cost to a hospital that is part of a large buying group for the size and form listed.

TABLE A-6 Cardiovascular Drugs

Drug	Route	Usual Dose	How Supplied	Form	Cost*
Anticholinergic Agents					
Atropine	IV	0.01-0.02 mg/kg	0.4 mg/mL, 1 mL 0.1 mg/mL, 10 mL	Solution Solution	0.61 1.87
Glycopyrrolate	IV	0.005-0.01 mg/kg	0.2 mg/mL, 1 mL	Solution	0.48
Scopolamine	IV	0.2-0.8 mg	0.4 mg/mL, 1 mL	Solution	4.20
Antidysrhythmic Agents					
Adenosine	IV	6-12 mg	3 mg/mL, 2 mL	Solution	8.19
Amiodarone	IV	5-10 mg/kg	50 mg/mL, 3 mL	Solution	1.25
Digoxin	IV	0.125-0.5 mg	0.25 mg/mL, 2 mL	Solution	0.92
Isoproterenol	IV	0.5-4 mcg 0.1-1 mcg/kg/min	0.2 mg/mL, 5 mL	Solution	12.30
Lidocaine	IV	1-2 mg/kg 1-4 mg/min	20 mg/mL, 5 mL	Solution	1.40
Phenytoin	IV	5-15 mg/kg	50 mg/mL, 5 mL	Solution	2.07
Procainamide	IV	5-15 mg/kg	100 mg/mL, 10 mL	Solution	8.06
Inotropes					
Dobutamine	IV	2-20 mcg/kg/min	12.5 mg/mL, 20 mL	Solution	2.94
Dopamine	IV	2-20 mcg/kg/min	80 mg/mL, 10 mL	Solution	1.04
Inamrinone	IV	0.5-1.5 mg/kg 5-10 mcg/kg/min	5 mg/mL, 20 mL	Solution	94.50
Milrinone	IV	50 mcg/kg 0.5 mcg/kg/min	1 mg/mL, 10 mL	Solution	5.63
Vasopressors					
Ephedrine	IV/IM	5-50 mg	50 mg/mL 1 mL	Solution	0.58
Epinephrine	IV	0.01-1 mg	1 mg/mL, 1 mL 0.1 mg/mL, 10 mL	Solution Solution	0.60 1.75
Norepinephrine	IV	1-20 mcg/min	1 mg/mL, 4 mL	Solution	4.14
Phenylephrine	IV	40-80 mcg 10-80 mcg/min	10 mg/mL, 1 mL	Solution	0.61
Vasopressin	IV	0.01-0.04 U/min	20 U/mL, 1 mL	Solution	6.34
Antihypertensive Agents					
Enalaprilat	IV	1.25-2.5 mg	1.25 mg/mL, 2 mL	Solution	2.79
Hydralazine	IV	2-20 mg	20 mg/mL, 1 mL	Solution	11.14
Labetalol	IV	5-40 mg	5 mg/mL, 20 mL	Solution	2.22
Methyldopa	IV	250-500 mg	50 mg/mL, 5 mL	Solution	37.50
Phenoxybenzamine	PO	10-20 mg	10 mg	Tablet	5.80
Phentolamine	IV	1-5 mg	5 mg/mL	Powder	48.60
β-Blockers					
Esmolol	IV	10-40 mg	10 mg/mL, 10 mL	Solution	9.45
Metoprolol	IV	1-10 mg	1 mg/mL, 5 mL	Solution	0.94
Propranolol	IV	1-10 mg	1 mg/mL, 1 mL	Solution	7.39
Calcium Channel Blockers					
Diltiazem	IV	0.25-0.35 mg/kg 5-15 mg/h	5 mg/mL, 10 mL	Solution	2.12
Nicardipine	IV	5-15 mg/h	2.5 mg/mL, 10 mL	Solution	23.10
Nifedipine	SL	10 mg	10 mg	Capsule	0.45
Nimodipine	PO	60 mg	30 mg	Capsule	6.87
Verapamil	IV	2.5-5 mg	2.5 mg/mL, 2 mL	Solution	3.57

(*Continued*)

TABLE A-6 Cardiovascular Drugs (*Continued*)

Drug	Route	Usual Dose	How Supplied	Form	Cost*
Vasodilators					
Alprostadil	IV	0.05-0.4 mcg/kg/min	0.5 mg/ml, 1 mL	Solution	27.90
Fenoldopam	IV	0.1-1 mcg/kg/min	10 mg/mL, 1 mL	Solution	72.00
Nitroglycerin	IV SL	0.5-10 mcg/kg/min 0.4 mg	5 mg/mL, 10 mL 0.4 mg	Solution Tablet	5.25 0.10
Nitroprusside	IV	0.5-10 mcg/kg/min	50 mg	Powder	3.83
Diuretics					
Acetazolamide	IV	250 mg	500 mg	Powder	38.81
Bumetanide	IV	0.5-2 mg	0.25 mg/mL, 2 mL	Solution	1.22
Ethacrynic acid	IV	50-100 mg	50 mg	Powder	89.06
Furosemide	IV	5-40 mg	10 mg/mL, 2 mL	Solution	0.67
Mannitol	IV	0.25-1 g/kg	250 mg/mL, 50 mL 200 mg/mL, 500 mL	Solution Solution	0.98 13.51

*Reflects the cost to a hospital that is part of a large buying group for the size and form listed.

TABLE A-7 Agents Affecting Blood Clotting

Drug	Route	Usual Dose	How Supplied	Form	Cost*
Anticoagulants Affecting the Clotting Cascade					
Antithrombin III	IV	2000-5000 U	1000 U	Powder	2655.00
Antithrombin III, recombinant	IV	2000-5000 U	1750 U	Powder	3071.00
Argatroban	IV	2 mcg/kg/min	100 mg/mL, 2.5 mL	Solution	1115.25
Bivalirudin	IV	750 mcg/kg 30 mcg/kg/min	250 mg	Powder	585.00
Dalteparin	SC	2500-10 000 IU	12 500 IU/mL, 0.2 mL 10 000 IU/mL, 1 mL	Solution Solution	16.97 55.03
Drotrecogin	IV	24 mcg/kg/h	5 mg/mL	Powder	277.82
Enoxaparin	SC	0.5-1.5 mg/kg	100 mg/mL, 0.4 mL 100 mg/mL, 1 mL	Solution Solution	27.06 67.73
Fondaparinux	SC	2.5-10 mg	5 mg/mL, 0.5 mL 12.5 mg/mL, 0.8 mL	Solution Solution	32.63 102.73
Heparin	IV SC	5000-25 000 U 5000 U	1000 U/mL, 10 mL 5000 U/mL, 1 mL	Solution Solution	3.22 1.68
Lepirudin	IV	0.4 mg/kg 0.15 mg/kg/h	50 mg	Powder	204.88
Tinzaparin	SC	50-175 IU/kg	20 000 IU/mL, 2 mL	Solution	136.08
Anticoagulants Affecting Platelets					
Abciximab	IV	0.25 mg/kg 0.125 mcg/kg/min	2 mg/mL, 5 mL	Solution	584.14
Aspirin	PO	81-325 mg	81 mg, 325 mg	Tablet	0.01
Cilostazol	PO	100 mg	100 mg	Tablet	1.37
Clopidogrel	PO	75 mg	75 mg	Tablet	3.16
Dipyridamole	PO	75 mg	75 mg	Tablet	0.62
Eptifibatide	IV	180 mcg/kg 1-2 mcg/kg/min	2 mg/mL, 10 mL 2 mg/mL, 100 mL	Solution Solution	93.09 805.24
Ticlopidine	PO	250 mg	250 mg	Tablet	1.44
Tirofiban	IV	0.4 mcg/kg/min 0.1 mcg/kg/min	50 mcg/mL, 100 mL 50 mcg/mL, 250 mL	Solution Solution	215.66 372.00

(*Continued*)

TABLE A-7 Agents Affecting Blood Clotting (*Continued*)

Drug	Route	Usual Dose	How Supplied	Form	Cost*
Fibrinolytic Activators					
Alteplase (tPA)	IV	100 mg	100 mg	Powder	3584.78
Hemostatic Agents					
Aminocaproic acid	IV	4-5 g	250 mg/mL, 20 mL	Solution	0.84
Desmopressin	IV	0.3 mcg/kg	4 mcg/mL, 1 mL	Solution	5.31
Eptacog alfa (factor VIIa)	IV	90 mcg/kg	4800 mcg	Powder	5904.00
Phytonadione (Vitamin K)	IV	5-25 mg	2 mg/mL, 0.5 mL	Solution	4.00
Protamine	IV	25-250 mg	10 mg/mL, 5 mL	Solution	6.75
Tranexamic acid	IV	10-100 mg/kg	100 mg/mL, 10 mL	Solution	66.00

*Reflects the cost to a hospital that is part of a large buying group for the size and form listed.

TABLE A-8 Anesthetic Adjuncts

Drug	Route	Usual Dose	How Supplied	Form	Cost*
Antacid and Aspiration Prophylaxis					
Cimetidine	PO IV/IM	300 mg 300 mg	300 mg 150 mg/mL, 2 mL	Tablet Solution	0.13 2.51
Citric acid/sodium citrate solution	PO	30 mL	30 mL	Solution	0.46
Famotidine	PO IV/IM	20 mg 20 mg	20 mg 10 mg/mL, 2 mL	Tablet Solution	0.15 0.53
Metoclopramide	PO IV/IM	10 mg 10 mg	10 mg 5 mg/mL, 2 mL	Tablet Solution	0.21 0.47
Omeprazole	PO	20 mg	20 mg	Capsule	2.38
Pantoprazole	PO IV/IM	40 mg 40 mg	40 mg 40 mg	Capsule Powder	2.95 10.80
Ranitidine	PO IV/IM	150 mg 50 mg	150 mg 25 mg/mL, 2 mL	Tablet Solution	1.14 3.02
Sucralfate	PO	1 g	1 g	Tablet	0.37
Bronchodilators and Other Drugs for Asthma					
Albuterol	Inhalation Inhalation	90 mcg 2.5 mg	200-dose 0.83 mg/mL, 3 mL	Inhaler Nebulizer solution	19.46 0.35
Aminophylline	IV	5 mg/kg 0.5-1 mg/kg/h	25 mg/mL, 10 mL	Solution	0.60
Beclomethasone	Inhalation	42 mcg	100-dose	Inhaler	28.60
Budesonide	Inhalation	90 mcg	200-dose	Inhaler	87.97
Flunisolide	Inhalation	25 mcg	100-dose	Inhaler	34.87
Fluticasone	Inhalation	50 mcg	120-dose	Inhaler	56.45
Ipratropium	Inhalation	17 mcg	200-dose	Inhaler	107.04
Levalbuterol	Inhalation	45 mcg	200-dose	Inhaler	39.37
Metaproterenol	Inhalation	650 mcg	200-dose	Inhaler	26.37
Mometasone	Inhalation	220 mcg	30-dose	Inhaler	98.60
Montelukast	PO	10 mg	10 mg	Tablet	3.28
Omalizumab	SC	150-300 mg	150 mg	Solution	520.94
Terbutaline	IV/SC	0.25 mg	1 mg/mL, 1 mL	Solution	3.60
Tiotropium	Inhalation	18 mcg	18 mcg	Powder for inhalation	5.75
Zafirlukast	PO	20 mg	20 mg	Tablet	1.29
Zileuton	PO	600 mg	600 mg	Caplet	4.68

(*Continued*)

TABLE A-8 Anesthetic Adjuncts (*Continued*)

Drug	Route	Usual Dose	How Supplied	Form	Cost*
Intravenous Dyes					
Fluorescein	IV	500 mg	100 mg/mL, 5 mL	Solution	0.49
Indigotindisulfonate	IV	40 mg	8 mg/mL, 5 mL	Solution	6.26
Methylene blue	IV	10 mg	10 mg/mL, 1 mL	Solution	3.56
Glucocorticoids					
Dexamethasone	IV	1-10 mg	4 mg/mL, 5 mL	Solution	0.82
Hydrocortisone	IV	100 mg	100 mg	Powder	2.81
Methylprednisolone	IV	40-1000 mg	40 mg 1000 mg	Powder Powder	2.25 31.20
Other Hormones					
Glucagon	IV	0.5-1 mg	1 mg	Powder	63.00
Insulin, human	IV/SC	1-20 U	100 U/mL, 10 mL	Solution	28.50
Levothyroxine	IV	50-150 mcg	200 mcg	Powder	18.00
Octreotide	IV/SC	50-150 mcg	100 mcg/mL, 1 mL	Solution	7.56
Oxytocin	IV	10 mU/min	10 U/mL, 1 mL	Solution	0.95
Secretin	IV	0.2-0.4 mcg/kg	16 mcg	Powder	311.25
Miscellaneous Agents					
Baclofen	Intrathecal	50 mcg	50 mcg/mL, 1 mL	Solution	63.00
Caffeine sodium benzoate	IV	250-500 mg	125 mg/mL, 2 mL	Solution	6.09
Carboprost tromethamine	IM	250 mcg	250 mcg/mL, 1 mL	Solution	83.53
Dantrolene	IV	1-10 mg/kg	20 mg	Powder	75.94
Doxapram	IV	0.5-1 mg/kg	20 mg/mL, 20 mL	Solution	37.80
Hydroxocobalamin	IM	1 mg	1 mg/mL, 10 mL	Solution	5.63
Methylergonovine	IM	0.2 mg	0.2 mg/mL, 1 mL	Solution	5.86
Physostigmine	IV	1 mg	1 mg/mL, 2 mL	Solution	3.65
Sodium nitrite	IV	300 mg	30 mg/mL, 10 mL	Solution	40.50
Sodium thiosulfate	IV	12.5 g	250 mg/mL, 50 mL	Solution	16.88

*Reflects the cost to a hospital that is part of a large buying group for the size and form listed.

TABLE A-9 Intravenous Antibiotics

Drug	Route	Usual Dose	How Supplied	Form	Cost*
Acyclovir	IV	5-10 mg/kg	50 mg/mL, 20 mL	Solution	31.94
Amikacin	IV	7.5 mg/kg	250 mg/mL, 2 mL	Solution	2.70
Amphotericin B	IV	0.25-1 mg/kg	50 mg	Powder	8.73
Ampicillin	IV	1-2 g	1 g	Powder	6.23
Ampicillin/sulbactam	IV	2 g/1 g	2g/1g	Powder	6.33
Azithromycin	IV	500 mg	500 mg	Powder	6.56
Aztreonam	IV	1-2 g	2 g	Powder	60.23
Caspofungin	IV	70 mg	70 mg	Powder	315.80
Cefazolin	IV	1 g	1 g	Powder	0.95
Cefepime	IV	1-2 g	1 g	Powder	15.25
Cefotaxime	IV	1-2 g	1 g	Powder	3.27
Cefoxitin	IV	1-2 g	1 g	Powder	9.84
Ceftazidime	IV	1-2 g	1 g	Powder	10.67
Ceftriaxone	IV	1-2 g	1 g	Powder	3.47

(*Continued*)

TABLE A-9 Intravenous Antibiotics (*Continued*)

Drug	Route	Usual Dose	How Supplied	Form	Cost*
Cefuroxime	IV	0.75-1.5 g	1.5 g	Powder	4.79
Chloramphenicol	IV	12.5-25 mg/kg	1 g	Powder	22.41
Ciprofloxacin	IV	400 mg	10 mg/mL, 40 mL	Solution	5.40
Clindamycin	IV	600 mg	150 mg/mL, 4 mL	Solution	3.45
Dalfopristin/quinupristin	IV	7.5 mg/kg	350 mg/150 mg	Powder	143.31
Daptomycin	IV	4-6 mg/kg	500 mg	Powder	191.33
Ertapenem	IV	1 g	1 g	Powder	52.04
Erythromycin	IV	1 g	1 g	Powder	16.25
Fluconazole	IV	400 mg	2 mg/mL, 200 mL	Solution	13.50
Ganciclovir	IV	5 mg/kg	500 mg	Powder	60.80
Gentamicin	IV	1-7 mg/kg	40 mg/mL, 2 mL	Solution	0.64
Imipenem/cilastatin	IV	0.5-1 g	500 mg/500 mg	Powder	30.95
Levofloxacin	IV	0.5 g	5 mg/mL, 100 mL	Solution	32.87
Linezolid	IV	600 mg	2 mg/mL, 300 mL	Solution	90.08
Meropenem	IV	0.5-1 g	1 g	Powder	58.64
Metronidazole	IV	0.5-1 g	5 mg/mL, 100 mL	Solution	1.88
Nafcillin	IV	1 g	1 g	Powder	7.77
Oxacillin	IV	1 g	1 g	Powder	7.77
Penicillin G	IV	1 000 000 U	20 000 U/mL, 50 mL	Solution	9.50
Piperacillin/tazobactam	IV	3 g/0.375 g	3 g/0.375 g	Powder	16.10
Rifampin	IV	600 mg	600 mg	Powder	102.23
Telavancin	IV	10 mg/kg	750 mg	Powder	135.00
Ticarcillin/clavulanic acid	IV	3 g/0.1 g	3 g/0.1 g	Powder	12.23
Tobramycin	IV	1-7 mg/kg	40 mg/mL, 2 mL	Solution	1.86
Vancomycin	IV	0.5-1 g	1 g	Powder	5.81
Voriconazole	IV	4-6 mg/kg	200 mg	Powder	107.63

*Reflects the cost to a hospital that is part of a large buying group for the size and form listed.

TABLE A-10 Intravenous Fluid Solutions and Electrolytes

Solution	Contents	How Supplied	Cost*
Albumin	5% albumin 25% albumin	250 mL 50 mL	43.50 43.50
Calcium chloride 10%	13.6 mEq calcium chloride	10 mL	1.70
Calcium gluconate	4.7 mEq calcium gluconate	10 mL	0.67
Dextran 40	10% dextran 40 in 0.9% sodium chloride	500 mL	20.75
Dextran 70	6% dextran 70 in 0.9% sodium chloride	500 mL	10.80
Dextrose (D5)	5% glucose (dextrose) 10% glucose (dextrose)	1000 mL 1000 mL	1.20 1.20
Dextrose + 0.5 normal saline (D5/½ NS)	5% glucose (dextrose) 66 mEq/L sodium chloride	1000 mL	1.48
Dextrose + normal saline (D5/NS)	5% glucose (dextrose) 132 mEq/L sodium chloride	1000 mL	1.61
Hetastarch	6% hetastarch 132 mEq/L sodium chloride	500 mL	11.66

(*Continued*)

TABLE A-10 Intravenous Fluid Solutions and Electrolytes (*Continued*)

Solution	Contents	How Supplied	Cost*
Isolyte H[†]	5% glucose (dextrose) 39 mEq/L sodium 13 mEq/L potassium 3 mEq/L magnesium 44 mEq/L chloride 16 mEq/L acetate	1000 mL	3.45
Isolyte P[†]	5% glucose (dextrose) 23 mEq/L sodium 20 mEq/L potassium 3 mEq/L magnesium 29 mEq/L chloride 23 mEq/L acetate 3 mEq/L phosphate	1000 mL	5.73
Isolyte S[†]	140 mEq/L sodium 5 mEq/L potassium 3 mEq/L magnesium 98 mEq/L chloride 27 mEq/L acetate 23 mEq/L gluconate	1000 mL	2.33
Lactated Ringer solution	130 mEq/L sodium 109 mEq/L chloride 4 mEq/L potassium 3 mEq/L calcium 28 mEq/L lactate	1000 mL	1.23
Magnesium sulfate 50%	40 mEq magnesium sulfate	10 mL	0.70
Normal saline	132 mEq/L sodium chloride	1000 mL	1.22
Potassium chloride	2 mEq/mL	10 mL	0.90
Sodium bicarbonate 8.4%	1 mEq/mL sodium bicarbonate	50 mL	1.71
THAM	3.6% tromethamine	500 mL	180.37

*Reflects the cost to a hospital that is part of a large buying group for the size and form listed.

[†]This represents one brand name. Similar solutions are available under other brand names such as Normosol and Plasma-Lyte.

Index

Note: Page numbers followed by b indicate boxed material; those followed by f indicate figures; those followed by t indicate tables.

E

G

H

J

O

U